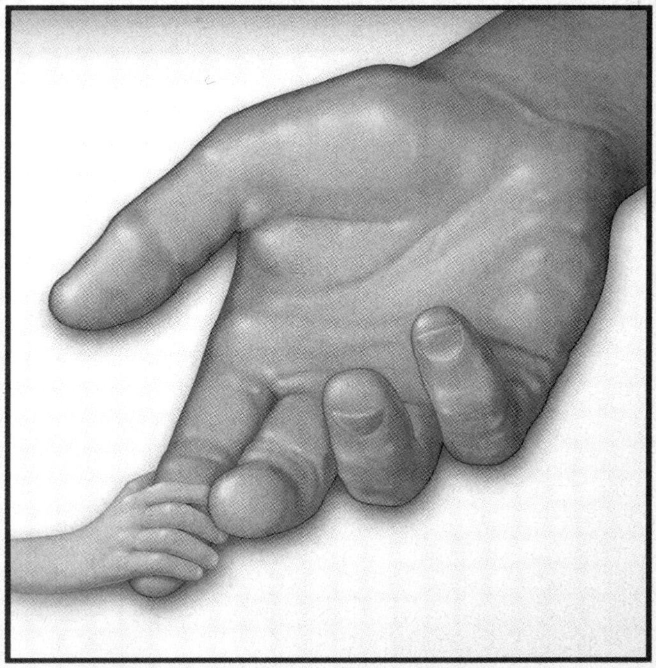

小 儿 外 科 学

Pediatric Surgery

（第 6 版·上卷）

注 意

小儿外科学

Pediatric Surgery

（第6版·上卷）

主　　编　Jay L. Grosfeld
　　　　　James A. O'Neill, Jr.
　　　　　Eric W. Fonkalsrud
　　　　　Arnold G. Coran

主　　译　吴晔明

副主译　施诚仁　蔡　威　刘锦纷
　　　　刘国华　董其刚

主译助理　顾　松

北京大学医学出版社

Peking University Medical Press

图书在版编目(CIP) 数据

小儿外科学：第6版 /（美）格罗斯费尔德（Grosfeld，J. L.）等主编；吴晔明等译. — 北京：北京大学医学出版社，2008

书名原文：Pediatric Surgery: Sixth Edition

ISBN 978-7-81116-311-7

Ⅰ. 小… Ⅱ. ①格… ②吴… Ⅲ. 儿科学：外科学 Ⅳ. R726

中国版本图书馆 CIP 数据核字（2008）第 154800 号

北京市版权局著作权合同登记号：图字：01-2006-5582

Pediatric Surgery, 6th edition
Jay L. Grosfeld, James A. O'Neill, Jr., Eric W. Fonkalsrud and Arnold G. Coran
ISBN-13: 978-0-323-02842-4
ISBN-10: 0-323-02842-X

978-981-259-755-7
981-259-755-7
Elsevier (Singapore) Pte Ltd.
3 Killiney Road, #08-01 Winsland House I, Singapore 239519
Tel: (65) 6349-0200, Fax: (65) 6733-1817
First Published 2009
2009 年初版

小儿外科学

主　　译： 吴晔明
出版发行： 北京大学医学出版社（电话：010-82802230）
地　　址：（100191）北京市海淀区学院路 38 号 北京大学医学部院内
网　　址： http://www.pumpress.com.cn
E－mail： booksale@bjmu.edu.cn
印　　刷： 北京画中画印刷有限公司
经　　销： 新华书店
责任编辑： 马联华　李　娜　董彩萱　　**责任校对：** 杜　悦　　**责任印制：** 郭桂兰
开　　本： 889 mm × 1194 mm　1/16　**印张：** 75　**插页：** 2　**字数：** 2406 千字
版　　次： 2009 年 1 月第 1 版　2009 年 1 月第 1 次印刷
书　　号： ISBN 978-7-81116-311-7
定　　价： 760.00 元（上下卷）

编著者名单

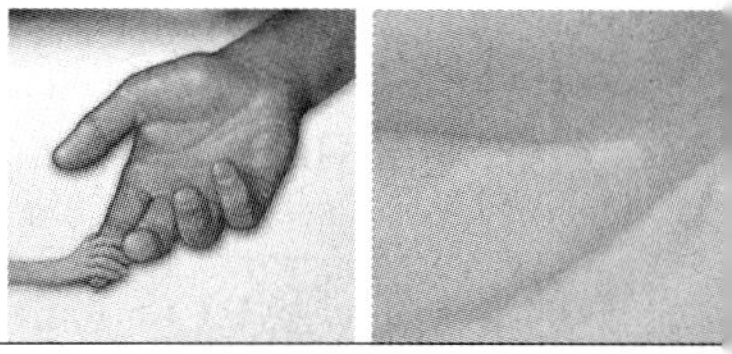

Mark C. Adams, MD, FAAP
Professor of Urology and Pediatrics, Vanderbilt University School of Medicine; Pediatric Urologist, Monroe Carell Jr. Children's Hospital at Vanderbilt, Nashville, Tennessee
Magaureter and Prune-Belly Syndrome

N. Scott Adzick, MD
C. Everett Koop Professor of Pediatric Surgery, University of Pennsylvania School of Medicine; Surgeon-in-Chief, The Children's Hospital of Philadelphia, Philadelphia, Pennsylvania
Cysts of the Lungs and Mediastinum

Craig T. Albanese, MD
Professor of Surgery, Pediatrics, and Obstetrics and Gynecology, and Chief, Division of Pediatric Surgery, Department of Surgery, Stanford Hospital & Clinics, Stanford; John A. and Cynthia Fry Gunn Director of Surgical Services, Lucile Packard Children's Hospital at Stanford, Palo Alto, California
Necrotizing Enterocolitis

Fred Alexander, MD
Associate Professor of Surgery, Cleveland Clinic Lerner School of Medicine of Case Western Reserve University; Staff Surgeon, Cleveland Clinic Foundation, Cleveland, Ohio
Crohn's Disease

R. Peter Altman, MD
Professor of Surgery, Columbia University College of Physicians and Surgeons; Surgeon-in-Chief, Morgan Stanley Children's Hospital of New York Presbyterian, New York, New York
The Jaundiced Infant: Biliary Atresia

Richard J. Andrassy, MD
Denton A. Cooley Professor and Chairman, Department of Surgery, University of Texas Medical School at Houston; Executive Vice President of Clinical Affairs and Associate Dean for Clinical Affairs, University of Texas at Houston, Houston, Texas
Rhabdomyosarcoma

Walter S. Andrews, MD
Professor of Surgery, University of Missouri–Kansas City School of Medicine; Director, Transplantation Program, Children's Mercy Hospital, Kansas City, Missouri
Gallbladder Disease and Hepatic Infections

Harry Applebaum, MD
Clinical Professor of Surgery, David Geffen School of Medicine at UCLA; Head, Division of Pediatric Surgery, Kaiser Permanente Medical Center, Los Angeles, California
Duodenal Atresia and Stenosis—Annular Pancreas

Marjorie J. Arca, MD
Assistant Professor of Surgery, Medical College of Wisconsin; Attending Surgeon, Children's Hospital of Wisconsin, Milwaukee, Wisconsin
Atresia, Stenosis, and Other Obstructions of the Colon

Robert M. Arensman, MD
Professor of Surgery, Louisiana State University School of Medicine; Attending Surgeon, Ochsner Clinic Foundation, New Orleans, Louisiana
Gastrointestinal Bleeding

James B. Atkinson, MD
Professor and Chief, Division of Pediatric Surgery, Department of Surgery, David Geffen School of Medicine at UCLA, Los Angeles, California
Liver Tumors

Richard G. Azizkhan, MD, PhD(Hon)
Professor of Surgery and Pediatrics, Lester Martin Chair of Pediatric Surgery, and Vice Chair, Department of Surgery, University of Cincinnati College of Medicine; Surgeon-in-Chief and Director, Division of Pediatric Surgery, Cincinnati Children's Hospital Medical Center, Cincinnati, Ohio
Teratomas and Other Germ Cell Tumors

Anwar Baban, MD
Laboratory of Molecular Genetics, Gaslini Children's Hospital, Genoa, Italy
Hirschsprung's Disease and Related Neuromuscular Disorders of the Intestine

Douglas C. Barnhart, MD, MSPH
Assistant Professor, Departments of Surgery and Pediatrics, University of Alabama at Birmingham School of Medicine; Attending Surgeon, The Children's Hospital of Alabama, Birmingham, Alabama
Biopsy Techniques for Children with Cancer

Robert H. Bartlett, MD
Professor of Surgery, University of Michigan Medical School, Ann Arbor, Michigan
Extracorporeal Life Support for Cardiopulmonary Failure

Laurence S. Baskin, MD
Professor of Urology, University of California, San Francisco, School of Medicine; Chief, Pediatric Urology, UCSF Children's Hospital at UCSF Medical Center, San Francisco, California
Hypospadias

Spencer W. Beasley, MB, ChB, MS
Clinical Professor of Pediatrics and Surgery, Christchurch School of Medicine and Health Sciences, University of Otago; Chief of Child Health Services, Division of Child Health, and Clinical Director, Paediatric Surgery, Christchurch Hospital, Christchurch, New Zealand
Torticollis

Michael L. Bentz, MD, FAAP, FACS
Professor of Surgery, Pediatrics, and Plastic Surgery, and Chairman, Division of Plastic Surgery, University of Wisconsin School of Medicine and Public Health; Chief of Plastic Surgery, University of Wisconsin Hospital and Clinics, Madison, Wisconsin
Hand, Soft Tissue, and Envenomation Injuries

Victor E. Boston, MD, FRCSI, FRCSEng, FRCSEd
Honorary Senior Lecturer, Department of Surgery, The Queen's University of Belfast Faculty of Medicine; The Royal Belfast Hospital for Sick Children, Belfast, Northern Ireland
Ureteral Duplication and Ureteroceles

Scott C. Boulanger, MD, PhD
Assistant Professor of Surgery, Division of Pediatric Surgery, University of Mississippi Medical Center School of Medicine, Jackson, Mississippi
Inguinal Hernias and Hydroceles

Edward L. Bove, MD
Professor of Surgery, University of Michigan Medical School; Head, Section of Cardiac Surgery, C.S. Mott Children's Hospital, Ann Arbor, Michigan
Congenital Heart Disease and Anomalies of the Great Vessels

Mary L. Brandt, MD
Professor and Vice Chair, Michael E. DeBakey Department of Surgery, Baylor College of Medicine, Texas Children's Hospital, Houston, Texas
Disorders of the Breast

John W. Brock III, MD
Professor of Urologic Surgery, Vanderbilt University School of Medicine; Director, Pediatric Urology, Vanderbilt Medical Center; Surgeon in Chief, Monroe Carell Jr. Children's Hospital at Vanderbilt, Nashville, Tennessee
Bladder Exstrophy

Rebeccah L. Brown, MD
Assistant Professor of Clinical Surgery and Pediatrics, University of Cincinnati College of Medicine; Associate Director of Trauma Services, Cincinnati Children's Hospital Medical Center, Cincinnati, Ohio
Genitourinary Tract Trauma

Marybeth Browne, MD
Surgical Resident, McGaw Medical Center of Northwestern University, Chicago, Illinois
Gastrointestinal Bleeding

Terry L. Buchmiller, MD
Formerly Assistant Professor of Surgery, Weill Medical College of Cornell University of New York, New York; Currently Assistant Professor of Surgery, Harvard Medical School; Assistant in Surgery, Children's Hospital Boston, Boston, Massachusetts
The Jaundiced Infant: Biliary Atresia

Ronald W. Busuttil, MD, PhD
Professor and Executive Chairman, Department of Surgery, David Geffen School of Medicine at UCLA; Chief, Division of Liver and Pancreas Transplantation, Dumont-UCLA Liver Cancer Center; Director, Pfleger Liver Institute, UCLA Medical Center, Los Angeles, California
Liver Transplantation

Michelle S. Caird, MD
Lecturer, Department of Orthopaedic Surgery, Alfred Taubman Health Care Center, University of Michigan, Ann Arbor, Michigan
Musculoskeletal Trauma

Anthony A. Caldamone, MD, FAAP
Professor of Surgery (Urology) and Pediatrics, Brown University School of Medicine; Chief of Pediatric Urology, Hasbro Children's Hospital, Providence, Rhode Island
Renal Infection, Abscess, Vesicoureteral Reflux, Urinary Lithiasis, and Renal Vein Thrombosis

Darrell A. Campbell, Jr., MD
Professor of Surgery, University of Michigan Medical School; Chief of Clinical Affairs, University of Michigan Health System, Ann Arbor, Michigan
Renal Transplantation

Donna A. Caniano, MD
Professor of Surgery and Pediatrics, The Ohio State University College of Medicine and Public Health; Surgeon-in-Chief, Children's Hospital, Columbus, Ohio
Ethical Considerations

Michael G. Caty, MD
Associate Professor of Surgery and Pediatrics, University at Buffalo School of Medicine and Biomedical Science; Surgeon-in-Chief, Women and Children's Hospital of Buffalo, Buffalo, New York
Adrenal Tumors

Dai H. Chung, MD
Associate Professor of Surgery and Pediatrics, The University of Texas Medical Branch School of Medicine at Galveston; Chief, Section of Pediatric Surgery, UTMB Children's Hospital, Galveston, Texas
Burns

Robert E. Cilley, MD
Professor of Surgery and Pediatrics, Penn State College of Medicine; Chief, Division of Pediatric Surgery, Milton S. Hershey Medical Center, Hershey, Pennsylvania
Disorders of the Umbilicus

Paul M. Colombani, MD
Professor of Surgery, Pediatrics, and Oncology, and Robert Garrett Professor of Surgery, Johns Hopkins University School of Medicine; Chief, Division of Pediatric Surgery, Johns Hopkins Medicine; Pediatric Surgeon-in-Charge, Johns Hopkins Hospital, Baltimore, Maryland
Surgical Implications Associated with Bone Marrow Transplantation

Joel D. Cooper, MD
Professor of Surgery, University of Pennsylvania School of Medicine; Chief, Division of Thoracic Surgery, Hospital of the University of Pennsylvania, Philadelphia, Pennsylvania
Lung Transplantation

Arnold G. Coran, MD
Professor of Pediatric Surgery, University of Michigan Medical School, Ann Arbor, Michigan
Nutritional Support; Congenital Anomalies of the Esophagus; Hirschsprung's Disease and Related Neuromuscular Disorders of the Intestine; Abnormalities of the Female Genital Tract

Robin T. Cotton, MD
Professor of Otolaryngology, University of Cincinnati School of Medicine; Director, Pediatric Otolaryngology–HNS, Cincinnati Children's Hospital Medical Center, Cincinnati, Ohio
Lesions of the Larynx, Trachea, and Upper Airway

Michael C. Dalsing, MD
Professor of Surgery and Director, Section of Vascular Surgery, Indiana University School of Medicine, Indianapolis, Indiana
Venous Disorders in Childhood

Alan Daneman, MBBCh, BSc, FRANZCR, FRCPC
Professor of Radiology, University of Toronto Faculty of Medicine; Staff Radiologist, Hospital for Sick Children, Toronto, Ontario, Canada
Intussusception

Andrew M. Davidoff, MD
Associate Professor, Department of Surgery and Pediatrics, University of Tennessee School of Medicine; Chief, Division of General Pediatric Surgery, St. Jude Children's Research Hospital, Memphis, Tennessee
Principles of Pediatric Oncology, Genetics of Cancer, and Radiation Therapy

Richard S. Davidson, MD
Associate Professor, University of Pennsylvania School of Medicine; Attending Surgeon, Children's Hospital of Philadelphia and Shrener's Hospital, Philadelphia
Musculoskeletal Trauma

Romano T. DeMarco, MD
Assistant Professor of Urologic Surgery, Division of Pediatric Urology, Vanderbilt University School of Medicine, Nashville, Tennessee
Bladder Exstrophy

Daniel A. DeUgarte, MD
Pediatric Surgery Fellow, University of Michigan Medical School and C.S. Mott Children's Hospital, Ann Arbor, Michigan
Liver Tumors

Eric Devaney, MD
Assistant Professor of Surgery, University of Michigan Medical School; Attending Surgeon, C.S. Mott Children's Hospital, Ann Arbor, Michigan
Congenital Heart Disease and Anomalies of the Great Vessels

William Didelot, MD
Professor of Pediatric Orthopaedics, Indiana University School of Medicine; Staff Surgeon, Riley Hospital for Children, Indianapolis, Indiana
Major Congenital Orthopedic Deformitites

John W. DiFiore, MD
Clinical Assistant Professor of Surgery, Case School of Medicine; Staff Pediatric Surgeon, Children's Hospital at Cleveland Clinic, Cleveland, Ohio
Respiratory Physiology and Care

Patrick A. Dillon, MD
Assistant Professor of Surgery, Washington University in St. Louis School of Medicine; Attending Surgeon, St. Louis Children's Hospital, St. Louis, Missouri
Gastrointestinal Tumors

Peter W. Dillon, MD
Professor of Surgery and Pediatrics, Penn State College of Medicine; Vice Chair, Department of Surgery, and Chief, Division of Pediatric Surgery, Penn State Children's Hospital, Hershey, Pennsylvania
Congenital Diaphragmatic Hernia and Eventration

Patricia K. Donahoe, MD
Marshall K. Bartlett Professor of Surgery, Harvard Medical School; Director, Pediatric Surgical Research Laboratories and Chief, Pediatric Surgical Services Emerita, Massachusetts General Hospital, Boston
Ambiguous Genitalia

James C. Y. Dunn, MD, PhD
Assistant Professor of Surgery, David Geffen School of Medicine at UCLA; Attending Surgeon, Mattel Children's Hospital at UCLA, Los Angeles, California
Appendicitis

Simon Eaton, BSc, PhD
Senior Lecturer in Pediatric Surgery and Metabolic Biochemistry, Department of Pediatric Surgery, Institute of Child Health, University College London, London, United Kingdom
Neonatal Physiology and Metabolic Considerations

Martin R. Eichelberger, MD
Professor of Surgery and Pediatrics, George Washington University School of Medicine and Health Sciences; Director, Emergency Trauma, Burn Service, and Senior Attending, Pediatric Surgery Service, Children's National Medical Center; President and CEO, Safe Kids Worldwide, Washington, DC
Accident Victims and Their Emergency Management

Sigmund H. Ein, MDCM, FRCSC, FAAP, FACS
Associate Professor of Surgery, Adjunct Clinical Faculty, Department of Surgery, University of Toronto Faculty of Medicine; Honorary Staff Surgeon, Division of General Surgery, The Hospital for Sick Children, Toronto; Courtesy Staff, Department of Surgery, Lakeridge Health Corporation, Oshawa, Ontario, Canada
Intussusception

Carolyn Ells, RTT, PhD
Assistant Professor of Medicine, McGill University Faculty of Medicine; Clinical Ethicist, Sir Mortimer B. Davis Jewish General Hospital, Montreal, Quebec, Canada
Ethical Considerations

Barry L. Eppley, MD, DMD
Professor of Plastic Surgery, Indiana University School of Medicine, Indianapolis, Indiana
Cleft Lip and Palate

Mary E. Fallat, MD
Professor of Surgery, and Director, Division of Pediatric Surgery, University of Louisville; Chief of Surgery, Kosdir Children's Hospital, Louisville, Kentucky
Ovarian Tumors

Diana L. Farmer, MD
Professor of Clinical Surgery, Pediatrics and Obstetrics, Gynecology, and Reproductive Medicine, University of California, San Francisco, School of Medicine; Surgeon-in-Chief, UCSF Children's Hospital, San Francisco, California
Cysts of the Lungs and Mediastinum

Douglas G. Farmer, MD
Associate Professor of Surgery, David Geffen School of Medicine at UCLA; Director, Intestinal Transplantation, Dumont-UCLA Transplant Center, Los Angeles, California
Liver Transplantation; Intestinal Transplantation

Steven J. Fishman, MD
Professor of Surgery, Harvard University Medical School; Senior Associate in Surgery, Children's Hospital Boston, Boston, Massachusetts
Vascular Anomalies: Hemangiomas and Malformations

Alan W. Flake, MD
Professor of Surgery and Obstetrics and Gynecology, University of Pennsylvania School of Medicine; Director, Children's Institute for Surgical Science, The Children's Hospital of Philadelphia, Philadelphia, Pennsylvania
Molecular Clinical Genetics and Gene Therapy

Robert P. Foglia, MD
Associate Professor of Surgery and Division Chief, Pediatric Surgery, Washington University in St. Louis School of Medicine; Surgeon-in-Chief, St. Louis Children's Hospital, St. Louis, Missouri
Gastrointestinal Tumors

Eric W. Fonkalsrud, MD
Professor of Surgery, David Geffen School of Medicine at UCLA; Emeritus Chief of Pediatric Surgery, UCLA Medical Center, Los Angeles, California
Ulcerative Colitis; Lymphatic Disorders

Henri R. Ford, MD
Vice-Chair and Visiting Professor of Surgery, Keck School of Medicine of USC; Surgeon-in-Chief and Vice President, Surgery, and Medical Director, Burtie Green Bettingen Surgery Center, Children's Hospital Los Angeles, Los Angeles, California
Sepsis and Related Considerations

Stephanie M. P. Fuller, MD
Clinical Fellow, Division of Cardiothoracic Surgery, The Children's Hospital of Philadelphia and Thomas Jefferson University Hospital, Philadelphia, Pennsylvania
Heart Transplantation

Victor F. Garcia, MD
Professor of Surgery, University of Cincinnati College of Medicine; Director of Trauma Services, Cincinnati Children's Hospital Medical Center, Cincinnati, Ohio
Genitourinary Tract Trauma; Bariatric Surgery in Adolescents

John M. Gatti, MD
Assistant Professor of Surgery and Urology, University of Missouri–Kansas City School of Medicine; Director of Minimally Invasive Urology, Children's Mercy Hospital of Kansas City, Kansas City, Missouri
Abnormalities of the Urethra, Penis, and Scrotum

Michael W. L. Gauderer, MD
Professor of Surgery and Pediatrics (Greenville), University of South Carolina School of Medicine, Columbia; Adjunct Professor of Bioengineering, Clemson University, Clemson; Chief, Division of Pediatric Surgery, Children's Hospital, Greenville Hospital System, Greenville, South Carolina
Stomas of the Small and Large Intestine

James D. Geiger, MD
Associate Professor of Surgery, University of Michigan Medical School; Staff Surgeon, C.S. Mott Children's Hospital, Ann Arbor, Michigan
Biopsy Techniques for Children with Cancer

Keith E. Georgeson, MD
Professor of Surgery, University of Alabama at Birmingham School of Medicine; Chief of Pediatric Surgery, The Children's Hospital of Alabama, Birmingham, Alabama
Gastroesophageal Reflux Disease

Cynthia A. Gingalewski, MD
Assistant Professor of Surgery and Pediatrics, George Washington University School of Medicine and Health Science; Pediatric Surgeon, Children's National Medical Center, Washington, DC
Other Causes of Intestinal Obstruction

Kenneth I. Glassberg, MD
Professor of Urology, Columbia University College of Physicians and Surgeons; Director, Division of Pediatric Urology, Morgan Stanley Children's Hospital of New York–Presbyterian, New York, New York
Renal Agenesis, Dysplasia, and Cystic Disease

Philip L. Glick, MD, MBA
Professor of Surgery, Pediatrics, and Obstetrics and Gynecology, University of Buffalo School of Medicine and Biomedical Sciences; Executive Director, Miniature Access Surgery Center (MASC), Women and Children's Hospital of Buffalo, Buffalo, New York
Inguinal Hernias and Hydroceles

Sherilyn A. Gordon, MD
Assistant Professor of Surgery, Division of Liver and Pancreas Transplantation, David Geffen School of Medicine at UCLA, Los Angeles, California
Intestinal Transplantation

Tracy C. Grikscheit, MD
Senior Fellow in Pediatric Surgery, Children's Hospital and Regional Medical Center and University of Washington School of Medicine, Seattle, Washington
The Impact of Tissue Engineering in Pediatric Surgery

Jay L. Grosfeld, MD
Lafayette Page Professor of Pediatric Surgery Emeritus, Indiana University School of Medicine; Surgeon-in-Chief Emeritus, Riley Hospital for Children, Indianapolis, Indiana
Neuroblastoma; Jejunoileal Atresia and Stenosis; Abnormalities of the Female Genital Tract

Angelika C. Gruessner, MS, PhD
Associate Professor of Surgical Science, University of Minnesota Medical School, Minneapolis, Minnesota
Pancreas and Islet Cell Transplantation

Rainer W. G. Gruessner
Professor of Surgery, University of Minnesota Medical School, Minneapolis, Minnesota
Pancreas and Islet Cell Transplantation

Philip C. Guzzetta, Jr., MD
Professor of Surgery and Pediatrics, George Washington University School of Medicine and Health Sciences; Interim Chief of Pediatric Surgery, Children's National Medical Center, Washington, DC
Nonmalignant Tumors of the Liver

Carroll M. Harmon, MD, PhD,
Associate Professor of Surgery, University of Alabama at Birmingham School of Medicine; Attending Surgeon, Children's Hospital, Birmingham, Alabama
Congenital Anomalies of the Esophagus

Michael R. Harrison, MD
Professor of Surgery, Pediatrics, and Obstetrics, Gynecology, and Reproductive Sciences, University of California, San Francisco, School of Medicine; Director, Fetal Treatment Center, UCSF Children's Hospital and Medical Center, San Francisco, California
The Fetus as a Patient

Andrea A. Hayes-Jordan, MD
Assistant Professor of Surgery and Pediatrics, University of Texas Medical School at Houston and M.D. Anderson Cancer Center; Pediatric Surgeon, Memorial Hermann Children's Hospital and M.D. Anderson Cancer Center, Houston, Texas
Lymph Node Disorders

Stephen R. Hays, MD, MS, FAAP
Assistant Professor of Anesthesiology and Pediatrics, Vanderbilt University School of Medicine; Director, Pediatric Pain Services, Vanderbilt Children's Hospital, Nashville, Tennessee
Pediatric Anesthesia

John H. Healey, MD
Professor of Orthopaedic Surgery, Weill Medical College of Cornell University; Chief of Orthopaedic Surgery, Memorial Sloan-Kettering Cancer Center, New York, New York
Bone Tumors

W. Hardy Hendren III, MD, FACS, FAAP, FRCS (Irel&Engl), FRCPS(Glasgow), DSc(Drexel), MD(HonCausa) Université Aix Marseilles
Robert E. Gross Distinguished Professor of Surgery, Harvard Medical School; Chief of Surgery Emeritus, Children's Hospital Boston; Honorary Surgeon, Massachusetts General Hospital, Boston, Massachusetts
Megaureter and Prune-Belly Syndrome

Bernhard J. Hering, MD
Assistant Professor of Surgery, University of Minnesota Medical School; Associate Director, Diabetes Institute for Immunology and Transplantation, University of Minnesota Medical Center, Fairview, Minneapolis, Minnesota
Pancreas and Islet Cell Tranplantation

David N. Herndon, MD
Professor of Surgery and Pediatrics and Jesse H. Jones Distinguished Chair in Burn Surgery, University of Texas Medical Branch School of Medicine at Galveston; Chief of Staff and Director of Research, Shriners Burns Hospital, Galveston, Texas
Burns

Ronald B. Hirschl, MD
Professor of Surgery, University of Michigan Medical School; Head, Section of Pediatric Surgery, and Surgeon-in-Chief, C.S. Mott Children's Hospital, Ann Arbor, Michigan
Extracorporeal Life Support for Cardiopulmonary Failure

George W. Holcomb III, MD, MBA
Katharine Berry Richardson Professor of Surgery, University of Missouri–Kansas City School of Medicine; Surgeon-in-Chief, Children's Mercy Hospital, Kansas City, Missouri
Gallbladder Disease amd Hepatic Infections

Charles B. Huddleston, MD
Professor of Surgery, Washington University in St. Louis School of Medicine; Chief, Pediatric Cardiothoracic Surgery, and Surgical Director, Lung Transplant Program, St. Louis Children's Hospital, St. Louis, Missouri
Lung Transplantation

Raymond J. Hutchinson, MS, MD
Professor of Pediatrics, University of Michigan Medical School; Director of Clinical Services, Pediatric Hematology/Oncology, C.S. Mott Children's Hospital, Ann Arbor, Michigan
Surgical Implications of Hematologic Disease

John M. Hutson, MD(Monash), MD(Melb), FRACS, FAAP(Hon)
Professor of Pediatric Surgery, Department of Pediatrics, University of Melbourne Faculty of Medicine, Melbourne; Director of General Surgery, Royal Children's Hospital, Parkville, Victoria, Australia
Undescended Testis, Torsion, and Varicocele

Thomas Inge, MD, PhD
Associate Professor of Surgery and Pediatrics, University of Cincinnati College of Medicine; Surgical Director, Comprehensive Weight Management Program, Cincinnati Children's Hospital Medical Center, Cincinnati
Bariatric Surgery in Adolescents

Vincenzo Jasonni, MD
Professor of Pediatric Surgery, University of Genoa Medical School; Surgeon-in-Chief and Chair of Pediatric Surgery, Gaslini Children's Hospital, Genoa, Italy
Hirschsprung's Disease and Related Neuromuscular Disorders of the Intestine

Nishwan Jibri, MD
Department of Pediatric Surgery, Gaslini Children's Hospital, Genoa, Italy
Hirschsprung's Disease and Related Neuromuscular Disorders of the Intestine

Byron D. Joyner, MD
Associate Professor of Urology, University of Washington School of Medicine; Residency Director, University of Washington Urology Program, and Faculty/Staff, Children's Hospital and Regional Medical Center, Seattle, Washington
Ureteropelvic Junction Obstruction

Martin Kaefer, MD
Associate Professor, Department of Urology, Indiana University School of Medicine; Pediatric Urologist, Riley Children's Hospital, Indianapolis, Indiana
Disorders of Bladder Function

Henry K. Kawamoto, Jr., MD, DDS
Clinical Professor of Surgery, Department of Surgery, Division of Plastic Surgery, David Geffen School of Medicine at UCLA; Director, Craniofacial Surgery, UCLA Medical Center, Los Angeles, California
Craniofacial Anomalies

Robert M. Kay, MD
Associate Professor of Orthopedic Surgery, Keck School of Medicine of USC; Orthopedic Surgeon, Children's Hospital Los Angeles, Los Angeles, California
Bone and Joint Infections

Kosmas Kayes, MD
Staff Surgeon, Riley Hospital for Children and St. Vincent Children's Hospital, Indianapolis, Indiana
Major Congenital Orthopedic Deformities

Mark L. Kayton, MD
Assistant Member, Memorial Sloan-Kettering Cancer Center; Assistant Attending Surgeon, Division of Pediatric Surgery, Memorial Hospital, New York, New York
Surgical Implications Associated with Bone Marrow Transplantation

Robert E. Kelly, Jr., MD, FACS, FAAP
Associate Professor of Clinical Surgery and Pediatrics, Eastern Virginia Medical School, Children's Hospital of the King's Daughters, Norfolk, Virginia
The Nuss Procedure for Pectus Excavatum [Chapter 59]

Stephen S. Kim, MD
Assistant Professor of Surgery, University of Washington School of Medicine; Attending, Division of Pediatric Surgery, Children's Hospital and Regional Medical Center, Seattle, Washington
Necrotizing Enterocolitis

Michael D. Klein, MD
Arvin I. Philippart Chair and Professor of Surgery, Wayne State University School of Medicine; Surgeon-in-Chief, Children's Hospital of Michigan, Detroit, Michigan
Congenital Defects of the Abdominal Wall

Giannoula Klement, MD
Instructor in Pediatrics (Hematology-Oncology), Harvard University Medical School; Assistant in Pediatrics, Children's Hospital Boston, Boston, Massachusetts
Vascular Anomalies: Hemangiomas and Malformations

Matthew J. Krasin, MD
Assistant Member and Radiation Oncologist, St. Jude Children's Research Hospital, Memphis, Tennessee
Principles of Pediatric Oncology, Genetics of Cancer, and Radiation Therapy

Thomas M. Krummel, MD, FACS
Professor in Surgery, Stanford University School of Medicine; Service Chief, Surgery, Stanford Hospital & Clinics, Stanford; Susan B. Ford Surgeon-in-Chief, Lucile Packard Children's Hospital at Stanford, Palo Alto, California
New and Emerging Surgical Technologies and the Process of Innovation

Jean-Martin Laberge, MD, FRCSC, FACS
Professor of Surgery, McGill University Faculty of Medicine; Director, Division of Pediatric General Surgery, The Montreal Children's Hospital, Montreal, Quebec, Canada
Infections and Diseases of the Lungs, Pleura, and Mediastinum

Ira S. Landsman, MD
Associate Professor of Anesthesiology and Pediatrics, Vanderbilt University School of Medicine; Director, Division of Pediatric Anesthesia, Vanderbilt Children's Hospital, Nashville, Tennessee
Pediatric Anesthesia

Michael P. La Quaglia, MD
Professor of Surgery, Weill Medical College of Cornell University; Chief, Pediatric Surgical Service, Memorial Sloan-Kettering Cancer Center, New York, New York
Hodgkin's Disease and Non-Hodgkin's Lymphoma

Stanley T. Lau, MD
Pediatric Surgery Fellow, Women and Children's Hospital of Buffalo, Buffalo, New York
Adrenal Tumors

Steven L. Lee, MD
Regional Pediatric Surgeon, Kaiser Permanente, Los Angeles Medical Center, Los Angeles, California
Duodenal Atresia and Stenosis—Annular Pancreas

Joseph L. Lelli, Jr., MD
Assistant Professor of Surgery, Wayne State Medical School; Pediatric Surgeon, The Children's Hospital of Michigan, Detroit, Michigan
Polypoid Diseases of the Gastrointestinal Tract

Marc A. Levitt, MD
Assistant Professor of Surgery and Pediatrics, University of Cincinnati College of Medicine; Associate Director, Colorectal Center for Children, Cincinnati Children's Hospital Medical Center, Cincinnati, Ohio
Anorectal Malformations

Harry Lindahl, MD, PhD
Lecturer in Pediatrics, University of Helsinki School of Medicine; Chief of Pediatric Surgery, Hospital for Children and Adolescents, Helsinki; University Central Hospital, Helsinki, Finland
Esophagoscopy and Diagnostic Techniques

Thom E. Lobe, MD
Professor of Surgery and Pediatrics, University of Tennessee School of Medicine, Memphis, Tennessee; Pediatric Surgeon, Blank Children's Hospital, Des Moines, Iowa
Other Soft Tissue Tumors

Randall T. Loder, MD
Garceau Professor of Orthopaedic Surgery, Indiana University School of Medicine; Director of Pediatric Orthopaedics, Riley Hospital for Children, Indianapolis, Indiana
Amputations in Children

Thomas G. Luerssen, MD
Professor of Neurological Surgery, Indiana University School of Medicine; Chief, Pediatric Neurosurgery Service, Riley Hospital for Children, Indianapolis, Indiana
Central Nervous System Injuries

Jeffrey R. Lukish, MD
Associate Professor of Surgery and Pediatrics, Uniformed Services University of the Health Sciences F. Edward Hébert School of Medicine, Bethesda, Maryland; Chief, Division of Pediatric Surgery, and Attending Pediatric Surgeon, The National Naval Medical Center and Walter Reed Army Medical Center, Washington, DC
Accident Victims and Their Emergency Management

Dennis P. Lund, MD
Chairman, Division of General Surgery, University of Wisconsin-Madison, and Surgeon-in-Chief, UW Children's Hospital, Madison, Wisconsin
Alimentary Tract Duplications

Mary Beth Madonna, MD
Assistant Professor of Surgery, Northwestern University Feinberg School of Medicine; Attending Surgeon, Children's Memorial Hospital and John H. Stroger, Jr. Hospital of Cook County, Chicago, Illinois
Gastrointestinal Bleeding

John C. Magee, MD
Associate Professor of Surgery, University of Michigan Medical School; Director, Adult and Pediatric Renal Transplantation, and Director, Pediatric Liver Transplantation, University of Michigan Health System, Ann Arbor, Michigan
Renal Transplantation

Giuseppe Martucciello, MD
Associate Professor of Pediatric Surgery, Faculty of Medicine, University of Genoa, Genoa, and University of Pavia, Pavia; Director, and Surgeon-in-Chief, Department of Pediatric Surgery, IRCCS Scientific Institute Policlinico San Matteo, Pavia, Italy
Hirschsprung's Disease and Related Neuromuscular Disorders of the Intestine

Stephen J. Mathes, MD
Professor of Surgery and Head, Division of Plastic and Reconstructive Surgery, University of California, San Francisco, School of Medicine, San Francisco, California
Congenital Defects of the Skin, Connective Tissues, Muscles, Tendons, and Hands

Eugene D. McGahren III, MD
Associate Professor of Surgery and Pediatrics, University of Virginia School of Medicine; Pediatric Surgeon, University of Virginia Health System, Charlottesville, Virginia
Laryngoscopy, Bronchoscopy, and Thoracoscopy; Ascites

Leslie T. McQuiston, MD, FAAP
Staff Pediatric Urologist, Urology Associates of North Texas, Cook Children's Hospital, Fort Worth, Texas
Renal Infection, Abscess, Vesicoureteral Reflux, Urinary Lithiasis, and Renal Vein Thrombosis

Peter Metcalfe, MD, FRCSC
Pediatric Urology Fellow, Indiana University School of Medicine and Riley Hospital for Children, Indianapolis, Indiana
Incontinent and Continent Urinary Diversion

Alastair J. W. Millar, MBChB(Cape Town), FRCS, FRACS, FCS(SA), DCh
Honorary Professor, Paediatric Transplantation and Hepatopancreaticobiliary Surgery, University of Birmingham; Consultant, Paediatric Liver and Intestinal Transplantation and Hepatopancreaticobiliary Surgery, Birmingham Children's Hospital, Birmingham, United Kingdom
Caustic Strictures of the Esophagus

Eugene Minevich, MD, FACS, FAAP
Assistant Professor of Surgery, Cincinnati Children's Hospital Medical Center, Cincinnati, Ohio
Structural Disorders of the Bladder, Augmentation

Edward P. Miranda, MD
Professor of Surgery, Division of Plastic Surgery, University of California, San Francisco, School of Medicine, San Francisco, California
Congenital Defects of the Skin, Connective Tissues, Muscles, Tendons, and Hands

Michael E. Mitchell, MD
Professor of Urology, University of Washington School of Medicine; Chief, Pediatric Urology, Children's Hospital and Regional Medical Center, Seattle, Washington
Ureteropelvic Junction Obstruction

Takeshi Miyano, MD, PhD
Professor, Department of Pediatric Surgery, Juntendo University School of Medicine; Director, Juntendo University Hospital, Tokyo, Japan
The Pancreas

Delora Mount, MD, FACS, FAAP
Assistant Professor of Surgery and Pediatrics, University of Wisconsin School of Medicine and Public Health; Chief of Pediatric Plastic Surgery, University of Wisconsin Hospital and Clinics; Director, Craniofacial Anomalies Clinic, American Family Children's Hospital, Madison, Wisconsin
Hand, Soft Tissue, and Envenomation Injuries

Pierre Mouriquand, MD
Professor of Pediatric Urology, Claude-Bernard University Medical School; Head, Department of Pediatric Urology, Debrousse Hospital, Lyon, France
Renal Fusions and Ectopia

Noriko Murase, MD
Associate Professor of Surgery, University of Pittsburgh School of Medicine, Pittsburgh, Pennsylvania
Principles of Transplantation

J. Patrick Murphy, MD
Professor of Surgery, University of Missouri–Kansas City School of Medicine; Chief, Urology Section, Children's Mercy Hospital of Kansas City, Kansas City, Missouri
Abnormalities of the Urethra, Penis, and Scrotum

Saminathan S. Nathan, MD
Director, Musculoskeletal Oncology Service, Department of Orthopaedics, National University Hospital, Singapore, Singapore
Bone Tumors

Kurt D. Newman, MD
Professor of Surgery and Pediatrics, George Washington University School of Medicine and Health Sciences; Surgeon-in-Chief, Children's National Medical Center; Executive Director, Joseph E. Robert, Jr. Center for Surgical Care, Washington, DC
Lymph Node Disorders

Alp Numanoglu, MD, FCS(SA)
Senior Lecturer in Paediatric Surgery, University of Cape Town School of Child and Adolescent Health; Senior Specialist, Department of Paediatric Surgery, Red Cross Children's Hospital, Institute of Child Health, Cape Town, South Africa
Caustic Strictures of the Esophagus

Donald Nuss, MB, ChB, FRCS(C), FACS, FAAP
Professor of Clinical Surgery and Pediatrics, Eastern Virginia Medical School; Children's Hospital of the King's Daughters, Norfolk, Virginia
The Nuss Procedure for Pectus Excavatum [Chapter 59]

Richard Ohye, MD
Assistant Professor of Surgery, University of Michigan Medical School; Surgical Director, Pediatric Cardiac Transplantation, and Director, Pediatric Cardiovascular Surgery Fellowship Program, C.S. Mott Children's Hospital, Ann Arbor, Michigan
Congenital Heart Disease and Anomalies of the Great Vessels

Keith T. Oldham, MD
Professor of Surgery, Medical College of Wisconsin; Surgeon-in-Chief, Children's Hospital of Wisconsin, Milwaukee, Wisconsin
Atresia, Stenosis, and Other Obstructions of the Colon

James A. O'Neill, Jr., MD, MA(Hon)
J.C. Foshee Professor and Chairman Emeritus, Section of Surgical Sciences, Vanderbilt University School of Medicine; Surgeon-in-Chief Emeritus, Vanderbilt University Medical Center, Nashville, Tennessee
Choledochal Cyst; Bladder and Cloacal Exstrophy; Conjoined Twins; Arterial Disorders

Evelyn Ong, MBBS, BSc, FRCS(Eng)
Joint Royal College of Surgeons of England/British Association of Paediatric Surgeons Research Fellow; Department of Paediatric Surgery, Institute of Child Health, University College London; Clinical Research Fellow, Great Ormond Street Hospital for Children NHS Trust, London, United Kingdom
Neonatal Physiology and Metabolic Considerations

William L. Oppenheim, MD
Professor of Orthopedic Surgery, David Geffen School of Medicine at UCLA; Director of Pediatric Orthopedics, UCLA Medical Center; Consultant, Shriners Hospital of Los Angeles, Los Angeles, California
Bone and Joint Infections

H. Biemann Othersen, Jr., MD
Professor of Surgery and Pediatrics and Emeritus Head, Division of Pediatric Surgery, Medical University of South Carolina College of Medicine; Attending Surgeon, MUSC Children's Hospital, Charleston, South Carolina
Wilms' Tumor

Mikki Pakarinen, MD, PhD
Consultant Pediatric Surgeon, Hospital for Children and Adolescents, University of Helsinki Medical Faculty, Helsinki, Finland
Other Disorders of the Anus and Rectum, Anorectal Function

Keshav Pandurangi, MD
Vascular Surgery Fellow, Indiana University School of Medicine, Indianapolis, Indiana
Venous Disorders in Childhood

Richard H. Pearl, MD, FACS, FAAP, FRCSC
Professor of Surgery and Pediatrics,University of Illinois College of Medicine at Peoria; Surgeon-in-Chief, Children's Hospital of Illinois, Peoria, Illinois
Abdominal Trauma

Alberto Peña, MD
Professor of Surgery and Pediatrics, University of Cincinnati College of Medicine; Director, Colorectal Center for Children, Cincinnati Children's Hospital Medical Center, Cincinnati, Ohio
Anorectal Malformations

Rafael V. Pieretti, MD
Chief, Section of Pediatric Urology, Department of Pediatric Surgery, Massachusetts General Hospital, Boston, Massachusetts
Ambiguous Genitalia

Agostino Pierro, MD, FRCS(Eng), FRCS(Ed), FAAP
Nuffield Professor of Paediatric Surgery and Head of Surgery Unit, Institute of Child Health, University College London; Consultant Paediatric Surgeon, Great Ormand Street Hospital for Children NHS Trust, London, United Kingdom
Neonatal Physiology and Metabolic Considerations

William P. Potsic, MD, MMM
Professor of Otorhinolaryngology–Head and Neck Surgery, University of Pennsylvania School of Medicine; Director, Division of Otolaryngology, and Vice Chair for Clinical Affairs, The Children's Hospital of Philadelphia, Philadelphia, Pennsylvania
Otolaryngologic Disorders

Pramod S. Puligandla, MD, MSc, FRCSC
Assistant Professor of Surgery and Pediatrics, McGill University Faculty of Medicine; Attending Staff, Division of Pediatric Surgery and Pediatric Critical Care Medicine, The Montreal Children's Hospital of the McGill University Health Center, Montreal, Quebec, Canada
Infections and Diseases of the Lungs, Pleura, and Medistinum

Devin P. Puapong, MD
Senior Surgical Resident, Kaiser Permanente Medical Center, Los Angeles,California
Duodenal Atresia and Stenosis—Annular Pancreas

Prem Puri, MS, FRCS, FRCS(Edin), FACS
Professor of Paediatrics, University College Dublin; Consultant Paediatric Surgeon and Director of Research, Children's Research Centre, Our Lady's Hospital for Sick Children, Crumlin, Dublin, Ireland
Intestinal Neuronal Dysplasia

Judson G. Randolph, MD
Professor of Surgery Emeritus, George Washington University School of Medicine and Health Sciences; Former Surgeon-in-Chief, Children's National Medical Center, Washington, DC
A Brief History of Pediatric Surgery

Frederick J. Rescorla, MD
Professor of Surgery, Indiana University School of Medicine; Surgeon-in-Chief, Riley Hospital for Children, Indianapolis, Indiana
The Spleen

Jorge Reyes, MD
Professor of Surgery, University of Washington School of Medicine; Chief, Division of Transplant Surgery, University of Washington Medical Center, Seattle, Washington
Principles of Transplantation

Richard R. Ricketts, MD
Professor of Surgery, Emory University School of Medicine; Chief, Division of Pediatric Surgery, Children's Health Care of Atlanta at Egleston, Atlanta, Georgia
Mesenteric and Omental Cysts

Richard C. Rink, MD
Robert A. Garrett Professor of Pediatric Urologic Research and Professor of Urology, Indiana University School of Medicine; Chief, Pediatric Urology, Riley Hospital for Children, Indianapolis, Indiana
Incontinent and Continent Urinary Diversion

Risto J. Rintala, MD
Professor of Pediatric Surgery, University of Helsinki Medical Faculty; Chief, General Pediatric Surgery, Hospital for Children and Adolescents, Helsinki, Finland
Other Disorders of the Anus and Rectum, Anorectal Function

Albert P. Rocchini, MD
Professor of Pediatrics and Director of Pediatrics Cardiology, University of Michigan Redical School; Director of Pediatric Cardiology, University of Michigan Hospital, Ann Arbor
Neonatal Cardiovascular Physiology and Care

Heinz Rode, M Med(Chir), FCS(SA), FRCS(Edin)
Professor of Paediatric Surgery, University of Cape Town School of Child and Adolescent Health; Head of Pediatric Surgery, Red Cross Children's Hospital, Institute of Child Health, Cape Town, South Africa
Caustic Strictures of the Esophagus

Bradley M. Rodgers, MD
Professor of Surgery and Pediatrics, University of Virginia School of Medicine; Chief, Division of Pediatric Surgery, Department of Surgery, University of Virginia Medical Center; Chief, Children's Surgery, UVA Children's Hospital, Charlottesville, Virginia
Laryngoscopy, Bronchoscopy, and Thoracoscopy

A. Michael Sadove MD, MS
James Harbaugh Professor of Surgery (Plastic), Indiana University School of Medicine; Chief of Plastic Surgery, Riley Hospital for Children, Indianapolis; Chairman of Surgery, Clarian North Medical Center, Carmel, Indiana
Cleft Lip and Palate

Bob H. Saggi, MD
Assistant Professor of Surgery, Department of Surgery, Division of Immunology and Organ Transplantation, University of Texas Medical School at Houston; Staff Surgeon, Memorial Hermann Hospital, Houston, Texas
Liver Transplantation

Arthur P. Sanford, MD
Assistant Professor of Surgery, The University of Texas Medical Branch School of Medicine at Galveston; Staff Physician, Shriners Burns Hospital, Galveston, Texas
Burns

L. R. Scherer III, MD
Associate Professor of Clinical Medicine, Indiana University School of Medicine; Director of Trauma, Riley Hospital for Children, Indianapolis, Indiana
Peptic Ulcer and Other Conditions of the Stomach

Jay J. Schnitzer, MD, PhD
Associate Professor of Surgery, Harvard Medical School; Associate Visiting Surgeon, Massachusetts General Hospital, Boston, Massachusetts
Ambiguous Genitalia

Marshall Z. Schwartz, MD
Professor of Surgery and Pediatrics, Drexel University College of Medicine; Director, Pediatric Surgery Research Laboratory, and Surgical Director, Pediatric Renal Transplantation, St. Christopher's Hospital for Children, Philadelphia, Pennsylvania
Hypertrophic Pyloric Stenosis

Robert C. Shamberger, MD
Robert E. Gross Professor of Surgery, Harvard Medical School; Chief, Department of Surgery, Children's Hospital Boston, Boston, Massachusetts
Congenital Chest Wall Deformities

Nina L. Shapiro, MD
Associate Professor of Surgery/Pediatric Otolaryngology, David Geffen School of Medicine at UCLA; Attending Surgeon, UCLA Medical Center, Los Angeles, California
Salivary Glands

Curtis A. Sheldon, MD
Professor, University of Cincinnati College of Medicine; Professor and Director (Pediatric Urology), Cincinnati Children's Hospital Medical Center, Cincinnati, Ohio
Structural Disorders of the Bladder, Augmentation

Stephen J. Shochat, MD
Professor of Surgery and Pediatrics, University of Tennessee School of Medicine; Surgeon-in-Chief and Chairman, Department of Surgery, St. Jude Children's Research Hospital, Memphis, Tennessee
Tumors of the Lung

Michael A. Skinner, MD
Associate Professor of Surgery and Pediatric Surgery, Duke University School of Medicine, Durham, North Carolina
Surgical Diseases of the Thyroid and Parathyroid Glands

C. D. Smith, MD, MS
Associate Professor of Surgery and Pediatrics, Medical University of South Carolina College of Medicine; Attending, Division of Pediatric Surgery, MUSC Medical Center, Charleston, South Carolina
Cysts and Sinuses of the Neck

Jodi L. Smith, MD, PhD
Assistant Professor of Neurological Surgery, Department of Neurological Surgery, Indiana University School of Medicine; Pediatric Neurosurgeon, Riley Hospital for Children, Indianapolis, Indiana
Management of Neural Tube Defects, Hydrocephalus, Refractory Epilepsy, and Central Nervous System Infections

Samuel D. Smith, MD
Professor of Surgery, University of Arkansas for Medical Sciences College of Medicine; Chief of Pediatric Surgery, Arkansas Children's Hospital, Little Rock, Arkansas
Disorders of Intestinal Rotation and Fixation

Charles L. Snyder, MD
Associate Professor of Surgery, University of Missouri–Kansas City School of Medicine, Kansas City, Missouri; Clinical Assistant Professor of Surgery, University of Kansas School of Medicine, Kansas City, Kansas; Director of Clinical Research, The Children's Mercy Hospital, Kansas City, Missouri
Meckel's Diverticulum

Lewis Spitz, MBChB, MD(Hon), PhD, FRCS, FRCPCH, FAAP(Hon), FCS(SA)(Hon)
Emeritus Nuffield Professor of Pediatric Surgery, Institute of Child Health, University College London; Consultant Paediatric Surgeon, Great Ormond Street Hospital, London, United Kingdom
Esophageal Replacement

Thomas L. Spray, MD
Professor of Surgery, University of Pennsylvania School of Medicine; Chief, Division of Cardiothoracic Surgery, and Alice Langdon Warner Endowed Chair in Pediatric Cardiothoracic Surgery, The Children's Hospital of Philadelphia, Philadelphia, Pennsylvania
Heart Transplantation

Thomas E. Starzl, MD, PhD
Distinguished Service Professor of Surgery, University of Pittsburgh School of Medicine; Director Emeritus, Thomas E. Starzl Transplantation Institute, Pittsburgh, Pennsylvania
Principles of Transplantation

Charles J. H. Stolar, MD
Professor of Surgery and Pediatrics, Columbia University College of Physicians and Surgeons; Chief, Pediatric Surgery, Morgan Stanley Children's Hospital of New York–Presbyterian, New York, New York
Congenital Diaphragmatic Hernia and Eventration

Phillip B. Storm, MD
Assistant Professor of Neurosurgery, University of Pennsylvania School of Medicine; Attending Neurosurgeon, Hospital of the University of Pennsylvania and The Children's Hospital of Philadelphia, Philadelphia, Pennsylvania
Brain Tumors

Steven Stylianos, MD
Professor of Surgery, University of Miami Leonard M. Miller School of Medicine; Chief, Department of Pediatric Surgery, Miami Children's Hospital, Miami, Florida
Abdominal Trauma

Wendy T. Su, MD
Fellow, Pediatric Surgical Service, Memorial Sloan-Kettering Cancer Center, New York, New York
Hodgkin's Disease and Non-Hodgkin's Lymphoma

Riccardo Superina, MD, CM, FRCSC, FACS
Professor of Surgery, Northwestern University, Director, Transplant Surgery, Children's Memoral Hospital, Chicago, Illinois
Portal Hypertension

David E. R. Sutherland, MD, PhD
Professor of Surgery, University of Minnesota Medical School; Head, Transplant Division, and Director, Diabetes Institute for Immunology and Transplantation, University of Minnesota Medical Center, Fairview, Minneapolis, Minnesota
Pancreas and Islet Cell Transplantation

Leslie N. Sutton, MD
Professor of Neurosurgery, University of Pennsylvania School of Medicine; Chairman, Division of Pediatric Neurosurgery, The Children's Hospital of Philadelphia, Philadelphia, Pennsylvania
Brain Tumors

Edward P. Tagge, MD
Professor of Surgery and Pediatrics, Division of Pediatric Surgery, Medical University of South Carolina College of Medicine; Attending Surgeon, MUSC Children's Hospital, Charleston, South Carolina
Wilms' Tumor

Daniel H. Teitelbaum, MD
Professor of Surgery, University of Michigan Medical School; Pediatric Surgeon, C.S. Mott Children's Hospital, Ann Arbor, Michigan
Nutritional Support; Hirschsprung's Disease and Related Neuromuscular Disorders of the Intestine

Claire L. Templeman, MD
Assistant Professor of Clinical Gynecology and Surgery, Keck School of Medicine at USC; Pediatric Surgeon, Children's Hospital Los Angeles, Los Angeles, California
Ovarian Tumors

Gonca Topuzlu Tekant, MD
Associate Professor of Pediatric Surgery,
Istanbul University School of Medicine;
Pediatric Surgeon, Cerrahpasa Medical Faculty,
Istanbul, Turkey
Gastroesophageal Reflux Disease

Joseph J. Tepas III, MD
Professor of Surgery and Pediatrics, University of
Florida College of Medicine;
Staff Physician, Shands Jacksonville,
Jacksonville, Florida
Vascular Injuries

Patrick B. Thomas, MD
Pediatric Surgery Fellow, Texas Children's Hospital,
Baylor College of Medicine, Houston, Texas
Wilms' Tumor

Dana Mara Thompson, MD, MS
Associate Professor of Otorhinolaryngology,
Mayo Graduate School of Medicine;
Attending, Otorhinolaryngology Department,
Mayo Clinic, Rochester, Minnesota
Lesions of the Larynx, Trachea, and Upper Airway

Juan A. Tovar, MD, PhD
Professor of Surgical Pediatrics, Department of
Pediatrics, Universidad Autonoma de Madrid;
Head, Department of Pediatric Surgery,
Hospital Universitario LaPaz, Madrid, Spain
Disorders of Esophageal Function

Jeffrey S. Upperman, MD, MA
Assistant Professor of Surgery, Keck School of
Medicine of USC; Attending Surgeon, Children's
Hospital Los Angeles, Los Angeles, California
Sepsis and Related Considerations

Joseph P. Vacanti, MD
John Homans Professor of Surgery, Harvard Medical
School; Chief, Pediatric Surgery, Massachusetts
General Hospital, Boston, Massachusetts
The Impact of Tissue Engineering in Pediatric Surgery

Dennis W. Vane, MD, MS, MBA
Professor of Surgery, University of Vermont College
of Medicine; Chair, Pediatric Surgery, and Vice-Chair,
Clinical Affairs, Department of Surgery,
Fletcher Allen Health Care, Burlington,
Vermont
Child Abuse and Birth Injuries

Mirjana Vustar, MD
Assistant Professor of Anesthesiology and Pediatrics,
Vanderbilt University School of Medicine; Director,
Pediatric Anesthesia Education, Vanderbilt Children's
Hospital, Nashville, Tennessee
Pediatric Anesthesia

Brad W. Warner, MD
Professor of Surgery and Pediatrics, University of
Cincinnati College of Medicine; Attending Surgeon and
Director of Surgical Research, Division of Pediatric
General and Thoracic Surgery, Cincinnati Children's
Hospital Medical Center, Cincinnati, Ohio
Short-Bowel Syndrome

Thomas R. Weber, MD
Professor of Surgery, Saint Louis University School
of Medicine; Director, Pediatric Surgery, Cardinal
Glennon Children's Hospital, St. Louis, Missouri
Esophageal Rupture and Perforation

David E. Wesson, MD
Professor of Surgery and Chief, Division of Pediatric
Surgery, Baylor College of Medicine; Chief,
Pediatric Surgery Service, Texas Children's
Hospital, Houston, Texas
Thoracic Injuries

Karen W. West, MD
Professor of Surgery, Indiana University School of
Medicine; Director of ECMO, Riley Hospital for
Children, Indianapolis, Indiana
Primary Peritonitis

Ralph F. Wetmore, MD
Professor of Otorhinolaryngology–Head and Neck
Surgery, University of Pennsylvania School of Medicine;
Senior Surgeon, The Children's Hospital of
Philadelphia, Philadelphia, Pennsylvania
Otolaryngologic Disorders

Eugene Wiener, MD
Professor, Department of Surgery (Pediatric), University
of Pittsburgh School of Medicine; Executive
Vice President and Chief Medical Officer, Children's
Hospital of Pittsburgh, Pittsburgh, Pennsylvania
Testicular Tumors

Jay M. Wilson, MD
Associate Professor of Surgery, Harvard
Medical School; Attending, Children's Hospital Boston,
Boston, Massachusetts
Respiratory Physiology and Care

Russell K. Woo, MD
Instructor in Surgery, Department of Surgery,
Stanford University School of Medicine;
Staff Physician, Stanford Hospital and Clinic, Stanford,
and Lucile Packard Children's Hospital at Stanford,
Palo Alto, California
*New and Emerging Surgical Technologies and
the Process of Innovation*

Hsi-Yang Wu, MD
Assistant Professor of Urology, University of Pittsburgh School of Medicine; Director of Pediatric Urology Research, Children's Hospital of Pittsburgh, Pittsburgh, Pennsylvania
Testicular Tumors

Elizabeth Yerkes, MD
Assistant Professor of Urology, Feinberg School of Medicine at Northwestern University; Attending Urologist, Children's Memorial Hospital, Chicago, Illinois
Incontinent and Continent Urinary Diversion

Daniel G. Young, MBChB, FRCS(Edin, Glasg), DTM&H
Honorary Senior Research Fellow, University of Glasgow; Former Head (Retired), Department of Surgical Pediatrics, Royal Hospital for Sick Children, Glasgow, United Kingdom
A Brief History of Pediatric Surgery

Moritz M. Ziegler, MD
Professor of Surgery, Division of Pediatric Surgery, University of Colorado School of Medicine; Surgeon-in-Chief, The Children's Hospital, Denver, Colorado
Meconium Ileus

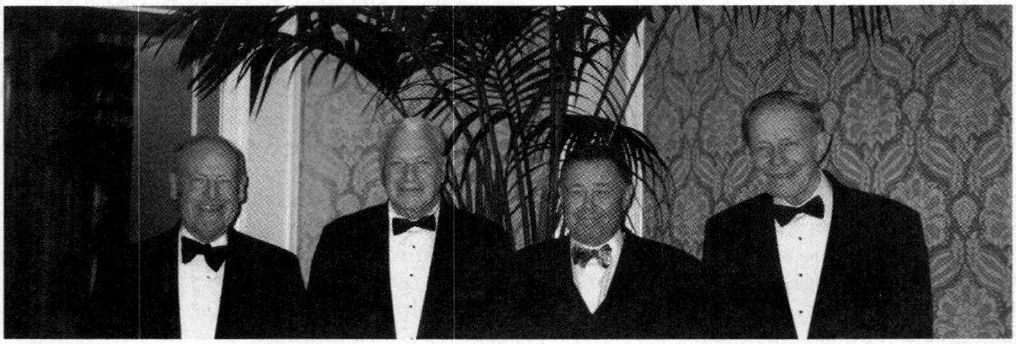

主编（从左到右）：James A. O'Neill, Jr.、Jay L. Grosfeld、Arnold G. Coran 和 Eric W. Fonkalsrud。

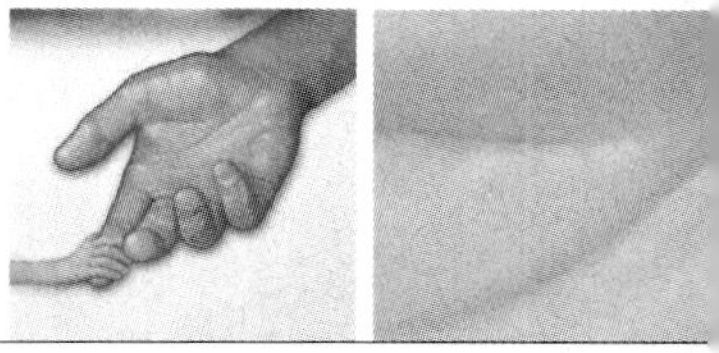

译校者名单

主　译

吴晔明　上海交通大学医学院附属上海儿童医学中心

副主译

施诚仁　上海交通大学医学院附属新华医院
蔡　威　上海交通大学医学院附属新华医院
刘锦纷　上海交通大学医学院附属上海儿童医学中心
刘国华　上海交通大学医学院附属上海第一人民医院
董其刚　上海交通大学医学院附属新华医院

主译助理

顾　松　上海交通大学医学院附属上海儿童医学中心

译校者（按姓氏笔画排序）

重庆医科大学附属儿童医院　王　珊
南京医科大学附属南京市儿童医院　王　浩
郑州大学第一附属医院　文建国
天津市儿童医院　叶祖萍
复旦大学附属儿科医院　吕志葆
苏州大学附属儿童医院　朱锦祥
上海交通大学医学院附属上海第一人民医院　刘国华
上海交通大学医学院附属瑞金医院　许　恩
宁夏医学院附属医院　杜　勇
北京首都儿科研究所　李　龙
浙江大学医学院附属儿童医院　李民驹
安徽省立医院　李巍松
苏州大学附属儿童医院　汪　健

首都医科大学附属北京儿童医院　陈永卫
湖南省儿童医院　周小渔
上海交通大学医学院附属上海第一人民医院　金惠明
广州市儿童医院　夏慧敏

上海交通大学医学院附属新华医院

沈涤华　陈锡民　周　莹　赵　黎　施诚仁　董其刚　蔡　威　潘伟华

上海交通大学医学院附属上海儿童医学中心

王　伟　王　俊　王宇鹏　王耀平　叶启东　刘锦纷　孙　杰　孙彦隽
严志龙　李　菁　吴晔明　何　蓉　张　震　张瑞冬　陈　盛　陈其民
胡　明　赵海腾　洪　莉　顾　松　顾　硕　徐　敏　徐建民　黄　萍
葛翼华　褚　珺　鲍　南

中文版序言

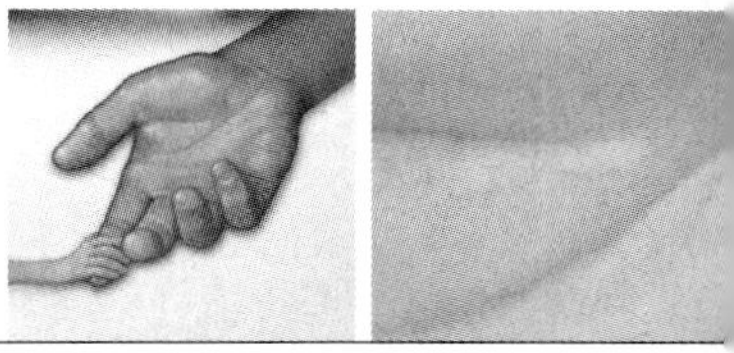

我国对应用科学的发展一向是主张“古为今用、洋为中用”，对医学的发展更是如此。国际上现代小儿外科学基本上是以 Ladd 和 Gross 的观点为主线的体系。小儿外科学在世界各国均有发展，而美国仍然是小儿外科学发展的前沿中心。我国小儿外科起步较晚，受时代背景的影响，创建了具有中国特色的小儿外科，并且在一个有 13 亿人口的发展中大国做出了令人瞩目的成绩。

回顾过去有利于未来。1950 年，我国始建小儿外科。其时正值西方国家对我国实行孤立与封锁。我国小儿外科的四位主要开创者从不同渠道间接引进了 Gross 观点：马安权毕业于圣约翰大学，使用英语渠道；佘亚雄毕业于震旦大学，用法语；童尔昌毕业于同济大学，用德语；我毕业于国立上海医学院，也用英语。四人分别在不同风格的医院通过实践开创了小儿外科。虽然基本观点仍是 Gross 体系，但是思路更宽。1960 年后又有李正等人留苏回国，带来了一些苏联的观点。难得的是，这一代人又都接受过系统的中医学补课教育。这样在多元化学术基础上，结合国情，融入自己的经验，形成了现时的中国小儿外科体系。

改革开放以后，我国小儿外科学书刊的出版空前繁荣，并且都反映了我国的特色。通过各种形式的国际交流，我国的小儿外科学在国际上也取得了一定地位。然而，作为占世界人口 1/4 的、有五千多年文明史的大国，在新的信息时代，随着经济发展，应该有责任也有能力为人类做出更大的贡献。我们小儿外科同道首先需要进一步提高我国小儿外科学水平，与国际先进学术接轨；还应该融入更多的中医精华，创立一个崭新的小儿外科学，作为 21 世纪对全世界儿童的献礼。因此当前需要的是充分、广泛、深入了解国际小儿外科学的体系和动态。

我国小儿外科队伍庞大，分布地域辽阔，水平参差不齐，对国际信息的获取很大程度上仍有语言和经济方面的障碍。上世纪 60 年代初，马安权曾组织翻译了 1953 年版《Gross 小儿外科学》。因为当时经济困难，只摘译出版了前半部。以后因国内十年动乱、盲目排外等等，再无一人出面问津。今天吴晔明教授主译本书正是填补空缺，将为我国小儿外科学界了解美国和国际学术体系提供很大便利。我国小儿外科能在贫困中以惊人的速度发展并壮大，这种精神已经闻名世界，有这本书出版，更将如虎添翼。

本书英文原版在国际上颇具盛名，已是第 6 次更新再版。本书译者校者都是我国当代小儿外科学界的精英，在小儿外科领域都有各自的专长造诣，并且都曾在国外学习，多次参加国际交流。相信本书译本质量必有保障，当为中国小儿外科一项时代硕果。我们国家提出“自主创新”，必先了解世界，了解历史。这部国际经典巨著正是一个理想的参考资料。我为本书的出版干杯。

张金哲

2008 年 2 月 23 日

中国工程院院士

小儿外科学教授

首都医科大学附属北京儿童医院

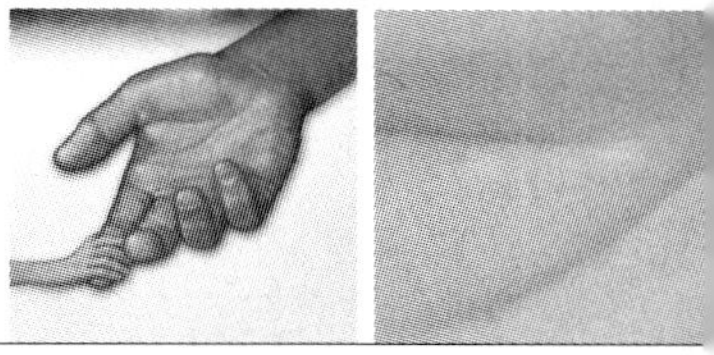

译者前言

《小儿外科学》自1962年第1版出版以来，一直都是国际小儿外科界公认的最权威的经典教科书之一。该书因其为小儿外科领域内容最全面、与临床技术进步同步而深受小儿外科同行的推崇。四十多年来，该书先后出版了6版。在相隔8年后，这本最新的第6版在第5版的基础上，增加了大量的最新理论和临床新技术，极具参考价值。

由于《小儿外科学原则》一书的成功翻译和出版，我受北京大学医学出版社委托，翻译《小儿外科学》第6版。面对如此繁重和艰巨的任务，深感能力不足，一度动摇，后来在上海儿童医学中心全体小儿外科同仁的鼓励和支持下，我鼓起勇气承接了翻译任务。这一工作还得到了施诚仁老师、蔡威学兄的支持，也得到了我的同仁刘锦纷教授的支持，还获得了师长董其刚、刘国华教授的帮助；本书的翻译和校对工作也获得了来自全国各地的、近年来活跃于小儿外科领域的中青年专家的支持和协助，在此对他们表示衷心的感谢，他们是：浙江大学医学院附属儿童医院李民驹教授；天津市儿童医院叶祖萍教授；苏州大学附属儿童医院朱锦祥教授；复旦大学附属儿科医院吕志葆教授；苏州大学附属儿童医院汪健教授；首都医科大学附属北京儿童医院陈永卫教授；首都儿科研究所李龙教授；郑州大学第一附属医院文建国教授；广州市儿童医院夏慧敏教授；湖南省儿童医院周小渔教授；重庆医科大学附属儿童医院王珊教授。没有他们的帮助，本书的翻译和校对工作将更为困难。

我特别要感谢我的同事顾松博士，他为翻译稿的整理、校对、译校者的联系及出版事务做了大量工作。

希望本书的出版有助于我国小儿外科的普及和发展，并成为广大小儿外科专科医生的常用工具书之一。大多数译校者都是利用工作之余完成此项任务，由于时间较为仓促，在翻译和审校中难免存在错误之处，敬请批评指正，以便在再版中得以改正。

吴晔明

2008年1月21日

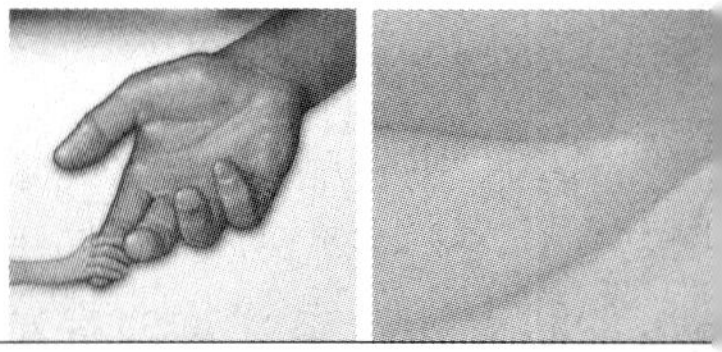

著者前言

《小儿外科学》第 1 版是 1962 年由医学年鉴出版社出版的，编委会由 Kenneth Welch、William Mustard、 Mark Ravitch、Clifford Benson 和 William Snyder 五位医生组成。其目的是为了满足小儿外科的总体工作需要，重点是放在普外、胸外和泌尿外科这些传统领域上。这本内容全面的教科书融入了众多著者的辛勤劳动，自第 1 版出版后，本书又先后出版了 4 版。44 年来各版一直是小儿外科领域中最好的世界闻名的综合性图书。

自 1998 年第 5 版出版以来又过去了 8 年。在这期间，我们经历了一场真正意义上的新的科学信息爆炸，其特征是人类基因组解读、组织工程发展和其他对诊断和如何处理病人已产生明确影响的新技术的引进。

本书第 6 版包含 133 章，拥有国际视角，著者来自美国、加拿大、欧洲、亚洲、澳大利亚、新西兰和非洲。主编者的目的是使本书融入各位专家各自感兴趣领域的重要或独特的经验，以便所有章节都遵循同一个目标：作为当代综合性和权威性教科书，提供可参考使用和实用的信息。本书第 6 版的写作还有很多新作者和共同作者参加。在新加的章节中有一章是小儿外科学简史，描述了英国、美国和亚洲小儿外科专业发展的简要背景。其他新的章节包括：临床分子遗传学和基因治疗、组织工程对小儿外科学的影响、先进而新兴的外科技术和创新历程、儿科肿瘤学 / 遗传学和放射治疗原理、小肠移植以及青春期肥胖治疗。

其他所有章节也都进行了大量修改和更新，并根据大量的最新参考文献进行了扩展。如胎儿作为患者的最新进展；先天性胸壁畸形，包括有关 Nuss 手术的最新信息；小儿麻醉；伦理学和法律问题；先天性巨结肠的遗传学；短肠综合征的新信息（即分期手术）；并且在适当的章节，将微创外科技术（腹腔镜、胸腔镜）融入其中。

第 6 版还包含其他重要修改和更新。第Ⅰ部分：新生儿生理学和代谢问题、呼吸生理学和监护、新生儿心血管生理学和护理、心肺衰竭的体外生命支持、脓毒症及相关问题、血液病和营养。第Ⅱ部分：创伤（包括烧伤护理）。第Ⅲ部分：儿童的主要肿瘤。第Ⅳ部分：器官移植（肝、肺、心脏、胰、肾和骨髓移植的外科含意），这部分也根据最新护理技术和结果的新指南和信息进行了重新组织和更新。第Ⅴ部分：累及头颈部的疾病。第Ⅵ部分：胸部疾病（包括食管闭锁和食管气管瘘以及其他各种食管病变、肺囊肿、先天性膈疝）；第Ⅶ部分：常见的先天性和获得性腹部疾病（包括疝、腹壁缺损、肠闭锁、胎粪性肠梗阻、先天性巨结肠、肛门直肠畸形、肠重复畸形、炎症性肠道疾病、胆道闭锁、胆总管囊肿、胰腺疾病、脾脏、门脉高压和其他）；第Ⅷ部分：泌尿生殖系统疾病；第Ⅸ部分：特殊的小儿外科疾病（联体儿、先天性心脏病、手和软组织、骨科、神经系统和血管疾病）。很多章节有很好的图解，并大量使用了图表、影像学、大体病理照片和组织学照片以及手术操作图示。

第 6 版的编委会由 Jay L. Grosfeld、James A. O'Neill Jr.、Eric W. Fonkalsrud 和 Arnold G. Coran 组成。这四位医生也是第 5 版编委会的成员。最初各章节的编写是由四位主编平均负责的。很高兴，Anthony A. Caldamone 医生作为第Ⅷ部分泌尿生殖系统疾病副主编，Grosfeld 医生作为编委会的主席和总编，成为整部手稿的最终审核者。《小儿外科学》第 6 版承袭的编辑标准承蒙我们之前的本书前 5 版的编辑所设立。

还要感谢我们的行政助理和秘书 Karen Jaeger、Donna Bock、Gale Fielding、Cheryl Peterson 和 Carol Simmons，他们除了完成日常工作外，还自愿帮助我们完成这一著作。没有他们的帮助，这一工作很难完成，非常感谢他们对本书的贡献。我们还要向来自世界各地的、在第 6 版的准备工作中做出重要贡献的众多著者表示我们诚挚的赞赏和感谢，感谢他们主动与我们分享他们的知识和经验，并能按照教科书的特殊格式准时完成写作，使我们能在限定时间内出版本书。

我们还要感谢 Elsevier/Mosby 的出版团队，感谢他们在第 6 版的准备和出版中保持高标准的支持和合作。我们感谢高级发展编辑 Janice Gaillard 女士和文字编辑 Faith Voit 为本书的编辑所做的贡献；感谢出版部主任 Judith Fletcher 和高级项目经理 Linda Grigg 女士为本书的整个出版过程所做的贡献。

本书主编者的照片摄于 2005 年 4 月，是在美国外科学会的一次会议期间。编者们将编写《小儿外科学》第 6 版视作他们钟爱的一项工作，我们希望这本教科书能成为从事小儿外科临床工作的医生、接受培训的医生以及其他对婴幼儿感兴趣的专业人员的专业参考书。我们希望这本教科书可成为有益于全世界遭受外科疾病困扰的儿童的一种知识资源。

主编

（吴晔明译）

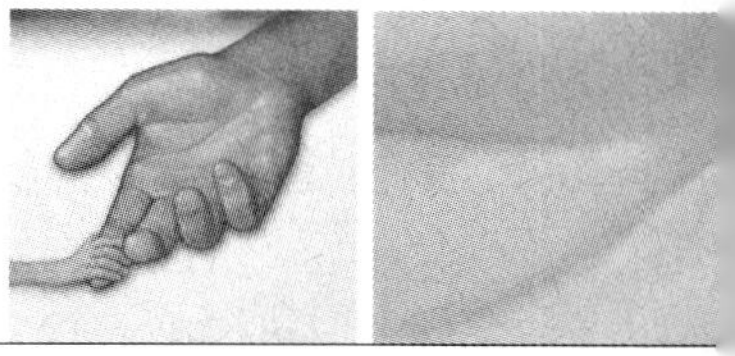

目　录

上　卷

下 卷

彩 图

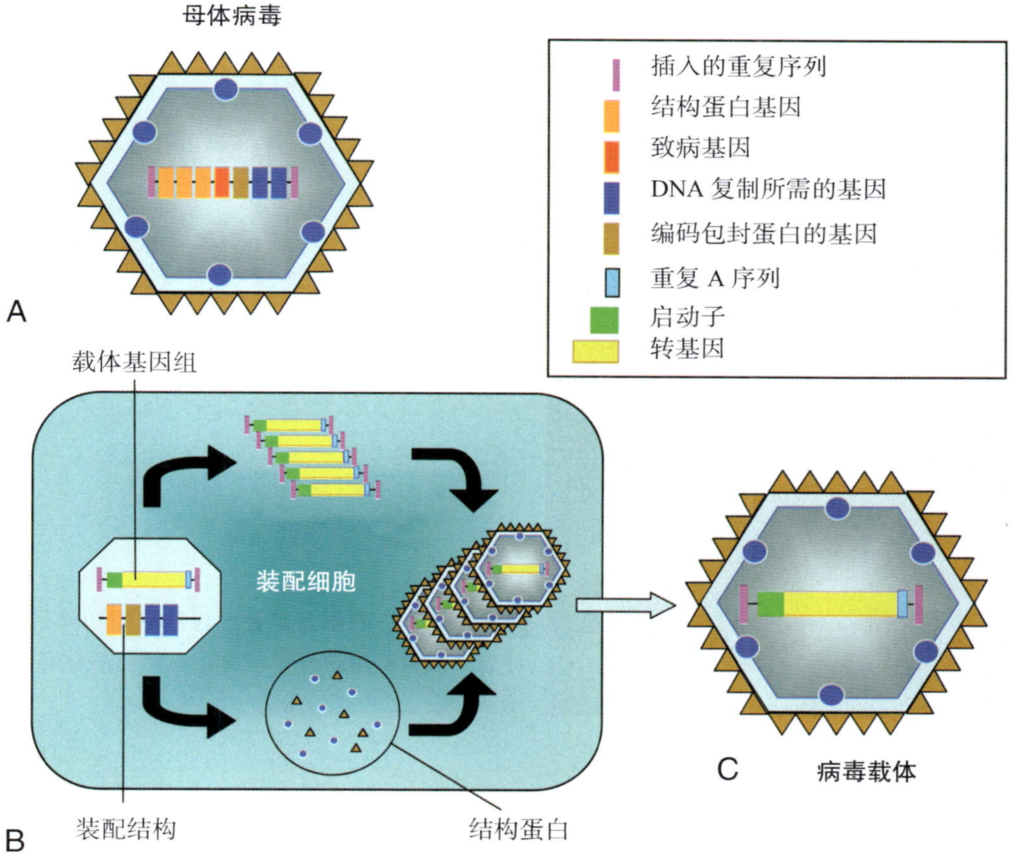

图 2-3 对创建一个遗传学病毒载体的要求。A. 选定的母体病毒所用的基本细胞器包括：编码特异性结构蛋白、包封蛋白和 DNA 复制所需蛋白的基因，但不包括编码致病相关蛋白的基因。B. 病毒载体在装配细胞中进行装配。包装（辅助病毒）结构，包括来源于母体病毒的基因，能够作为一种脂质体或辅助病毒进行转染，或能够稳定地整合进装配细胞的染色质中。致病功能和病毒衣壳化所需的基因序列被剔除出辅助病毒结构，所以不能被装配到病毒颗粒中。相反，病毒载体的基因组包含了转基因表达框，两侧是插入的中止重复序列和 *cis*-作用序列，这些是基因组衣壳化所需的基因序列。病毒结构蛋白和病毒载体 DNA 复制所需的蛋白在装配结构中进行表达，复制的病毒载体基因组被装配到病毒颗粒中。C. 病毒载体颗粒从装配细胞中释放，其中只包含有病毒载体基因组。

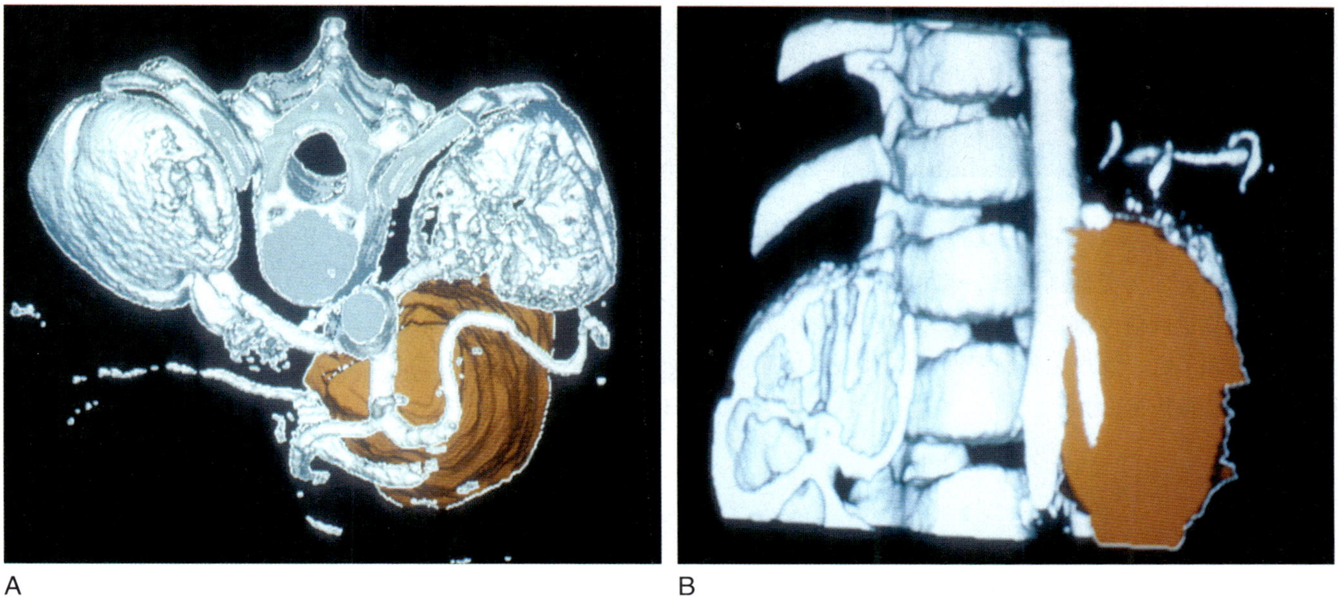

图 28-6 螺旋 CT 扫描三维重建来源于近腹腔干的神经母细胞瘤。A. 前面像提示肿瘤未侵犯腹腔干分支动脉。B. 侧位像证实肠系膜上动脉穿过肿瘤。

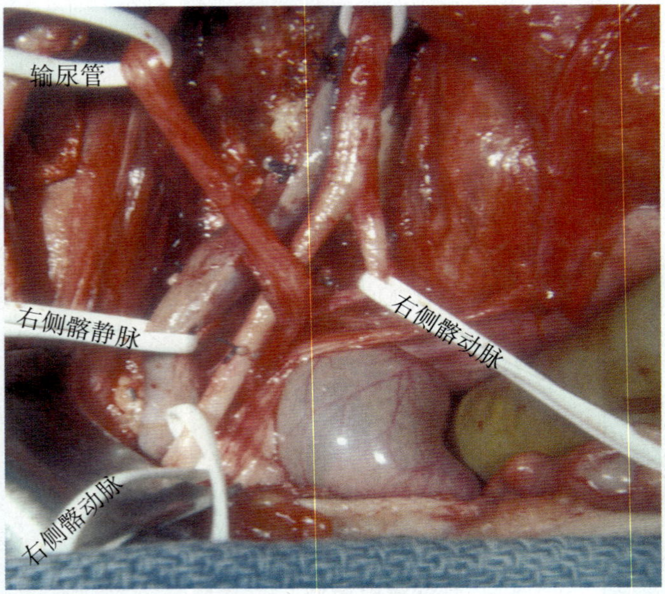

图 28–10 C. 右侧盆腔神经母细胞瘤切除后手术野的照片。注意用血管袢牵拉开髂动脉，右侧髂静脉和输尿管以便于安全切除。

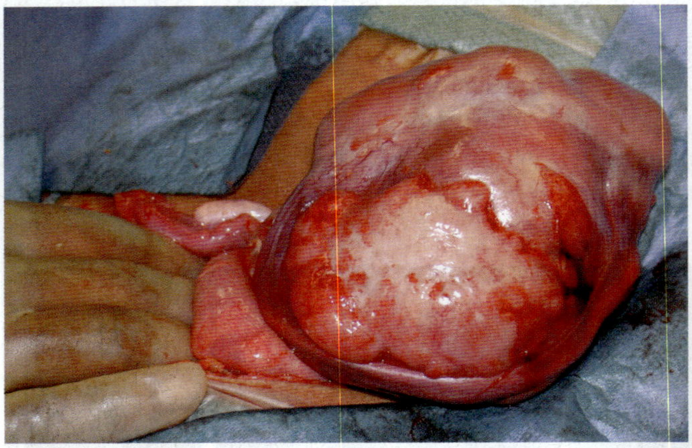

A

图 36–7 A. 从一名 5 岁急性腹痛的女孩体内切除的有完整包膜的肿块，证实为无性细胞瘤。术中发现患儿对侧的输卵管和卵巢靠近肿瘤左侧。术后的标本中包含有小部分同侧的输卵管和子宫，发现无肿瘤浸润。B. 肿瘤的切面可见由薄的纤维中隔分成的小叶。

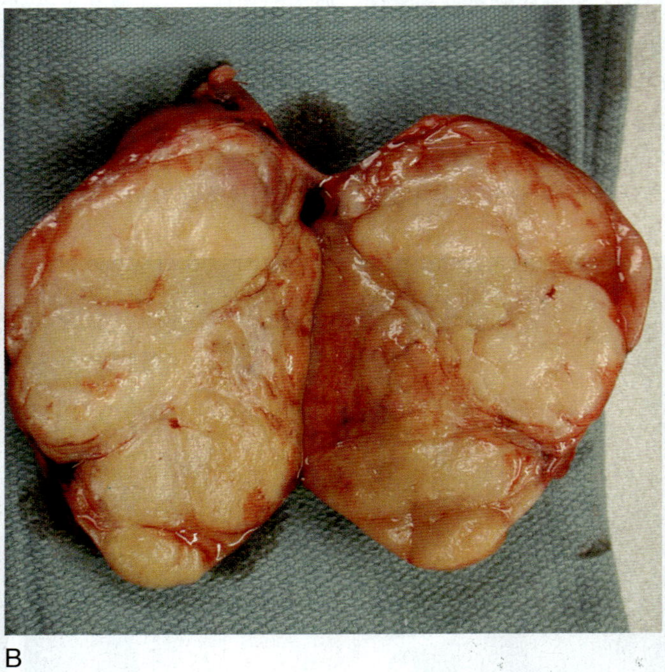

B

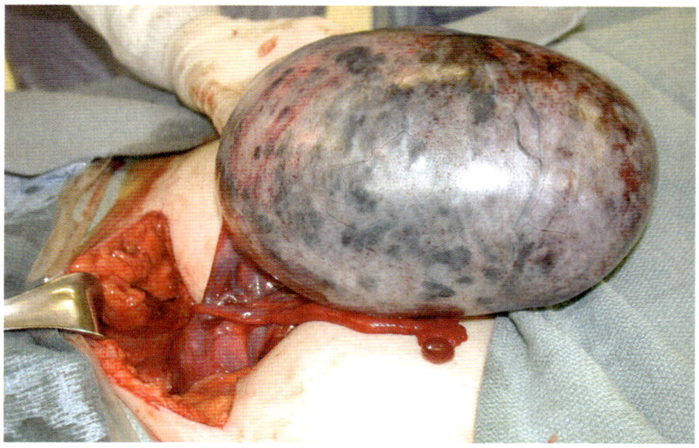

A

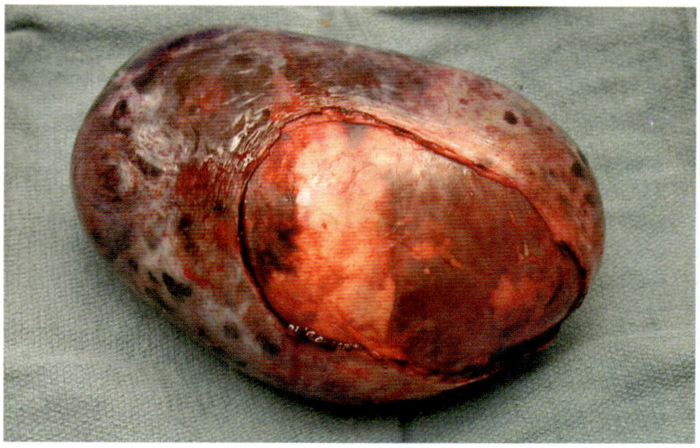

B

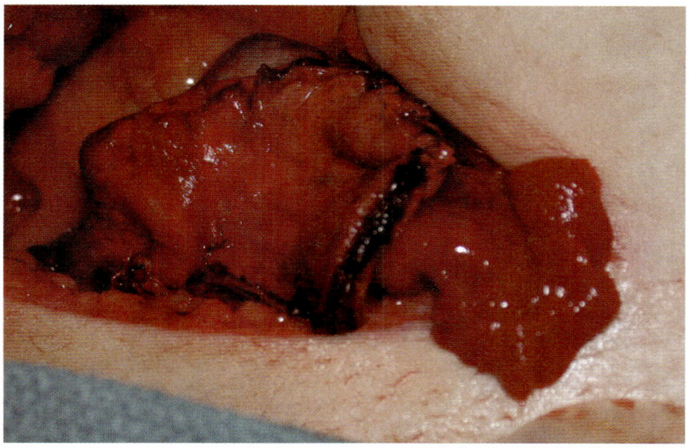

C

图 36–9 A. 一位醒来时突发剧烈腹痛的 14 岁女孩的巨大卵巢畸胎瘤，肿瘤下方可以看到输卵管。B. 肿瘤切除后，可以看到囊肿剥离后的卵巢表面。C. 肿瘤切除后，卵巢组织（左侧）和输卵管（右侧）仍然保留。

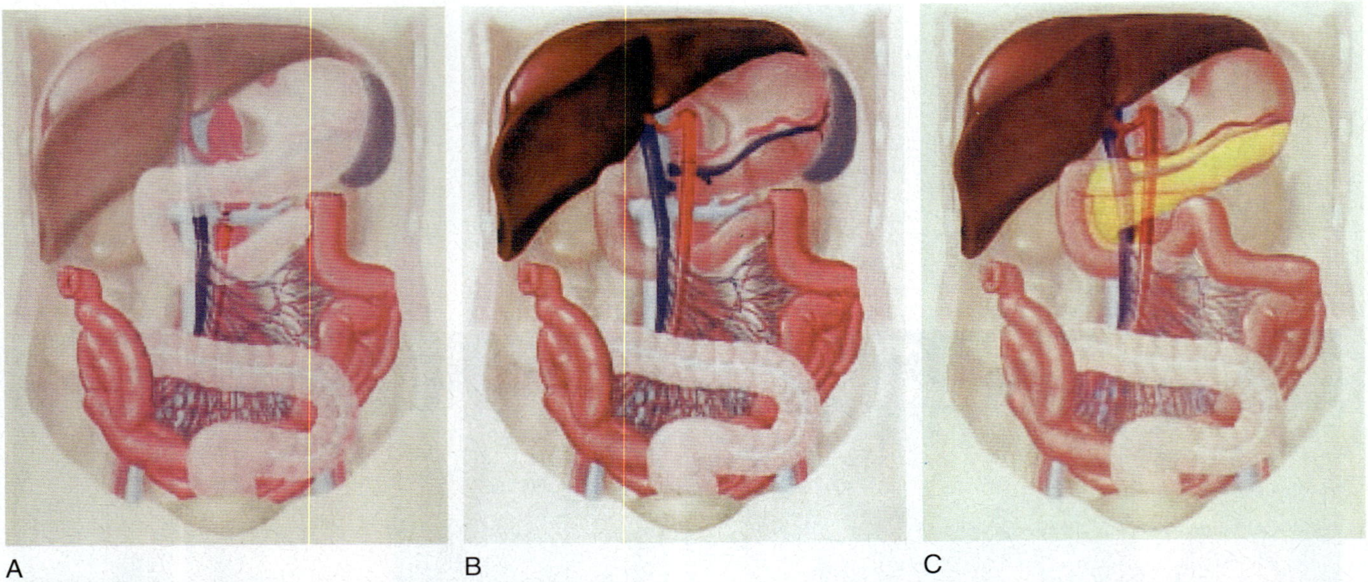

图 46–2 A. 单独的肠移植。B. 肝肠联合移植。C. 多脏器移植。（From Fishbein TM, Gondolesi GE, Kaufman SS: Intestinal transplantation for gut failure. Gastroenterology 2003;126:1615.）

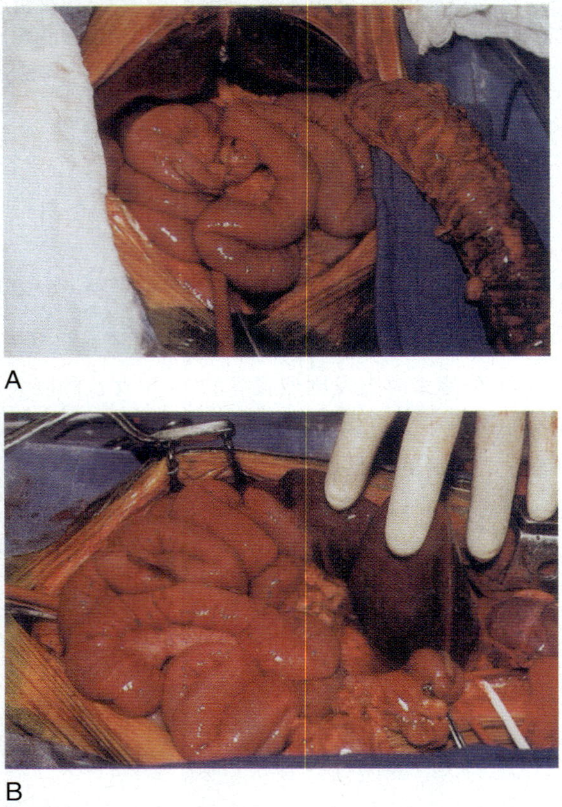

图 46–4 多脏器移植的手术入路。A. 肝圆韧带和镰状韧带已分离，肝完全游离，另外，左侧结肠移到脾曲，末端回肠已缝合（左下角），主动脉插管位置暴露。B. 插管位置在脐带周围的腹主动脉（右下）。供体进行肝素准备，然后钳夹，灌注器官。(From Yersiz H, Renz J, Histaki G, et al: Multivisceral and isolated intestinal procurement techniques. Liver Transpl 2003;9:881.)

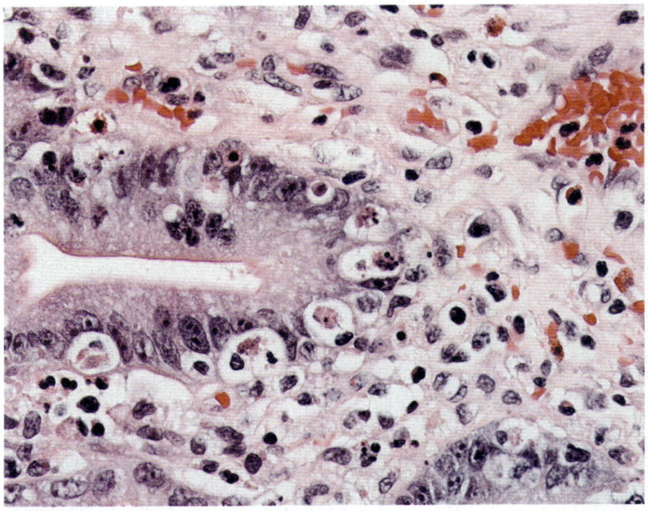

图 46–6 小肠移植物急性细胞排异反应的组织学表现，包括隐窝变形、凋亡，广泛的炎性细胞浸润。

第一部分

概　论

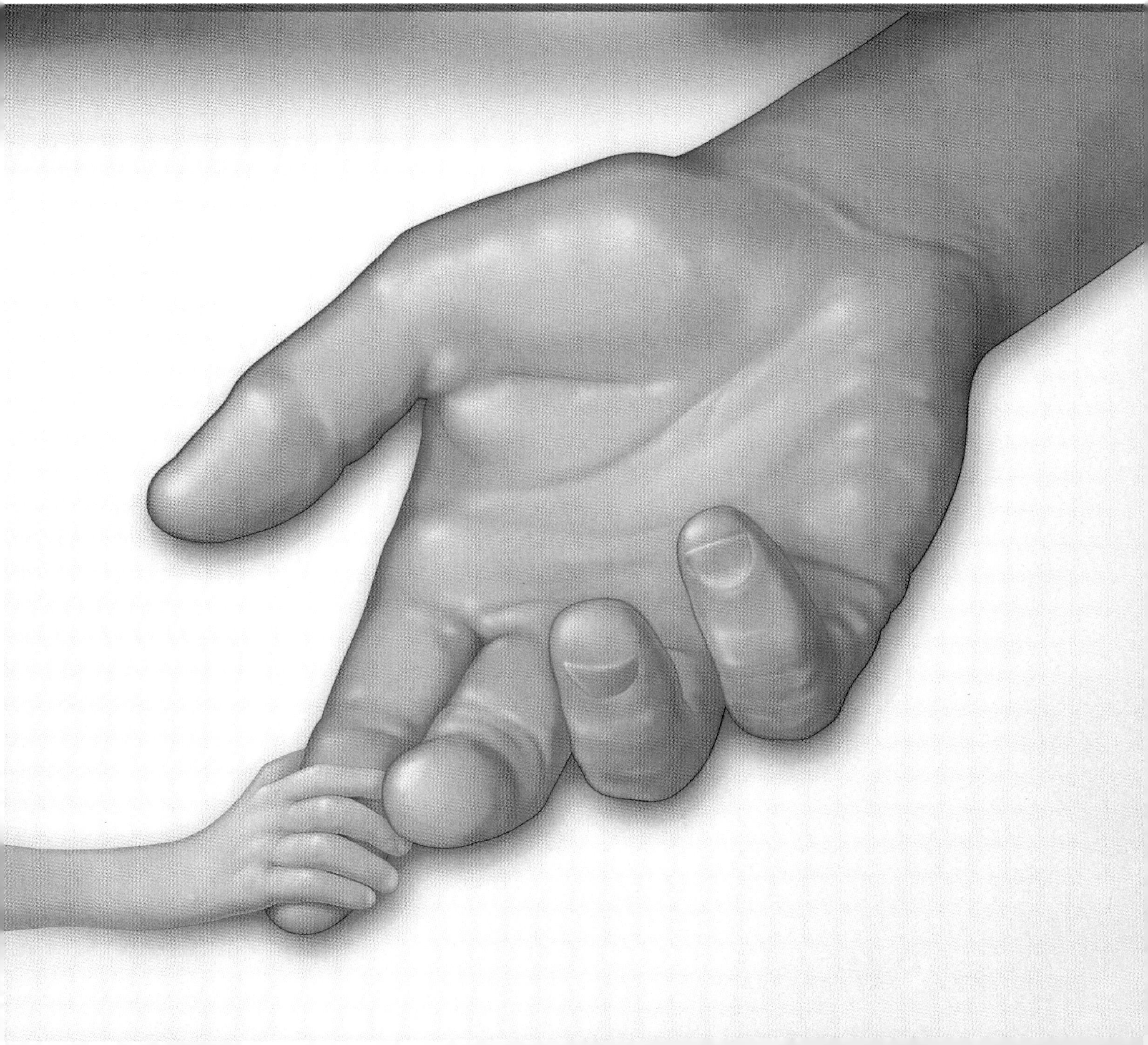

第 1 章

小儿外科学简史

Judson G. Randolph 和 Daniel G. Young

北美

美国

3 小儿外科的临床实践有一相当偶然的开始，但在美国任何关于小儿外科学发展的叙述都必须从 William E. Ladd 开始（图 1-1）。Ladd 出生于 1880 年，1903 年毕业于哈佛大学，并于 1906 年毕业于哈佛医学院。他曾跟当时几位著名的波士顿外科医生学习。第一次世界大战结束后， Ladd 才开始在波士顿儿童医院工作，他将大量时间用在救助需要手术的婴儿和儿童上，无疑他那时仍受到 Halifax 灾难的影响。1927 年，47 岁的 Ladd 被任命为儿童医院的外科主任。

在美国，第一位纯粹的小儿外科开业医生是西雅图的 Herbert Coe 医生。他曾到东部的波士顿儿童医院参观学习，其间 Ladd 偶尔也会出现在那里的手术室。Coe 回到西雅图后于 1919 年建立了美国第一个纯粹的小儿外科专业（直到 1927 年 Ladd 才放弃成人外科学工作）。

如果说 Ladd 是美国小儿外科学的教父，那么他的第一位学生 Robert E. Gross 医生则注定要成为该学科的一代宗师。Gross 生于 1905 年，长于巴尔的摩，是一位钢琴制作师的儿子。他的父亲让年轻的 Bob 跟随一位技师朋友工作，希望他能够掌握细致的技术和工艺。事实上，他做到了。在卡尔顿学院，Gross 最初的专业是化学。然而，在他上大学 3 年级时，当他读了 William Osler 爵士的 Cushing 传记后，他申请进入哈佛医学院并被录取。1931 年他以优异的成绩毕业，但没有得到他期望的外科实习医生资格，所以他参加了 S. Burt Wohlbach 医生负责的哈佛病理学培训项目（图 1-2）。这种病理学背景大大影响了以后他对外科领域问题的研究。

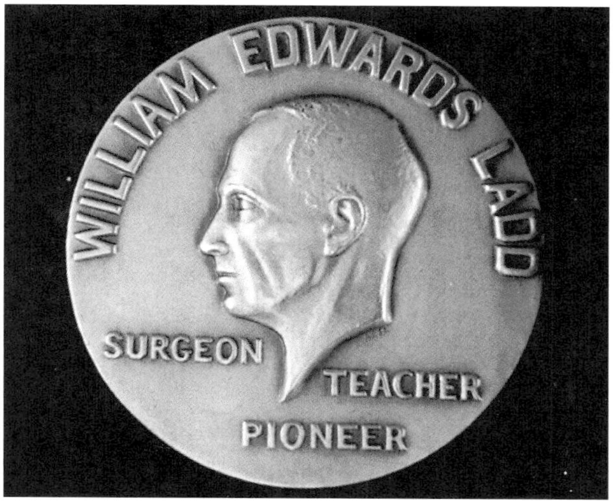

图 1-1 Ladd 奖章，由美国儿科学会外科学分会授予，以表彰在小儿外科领域取得的成就。

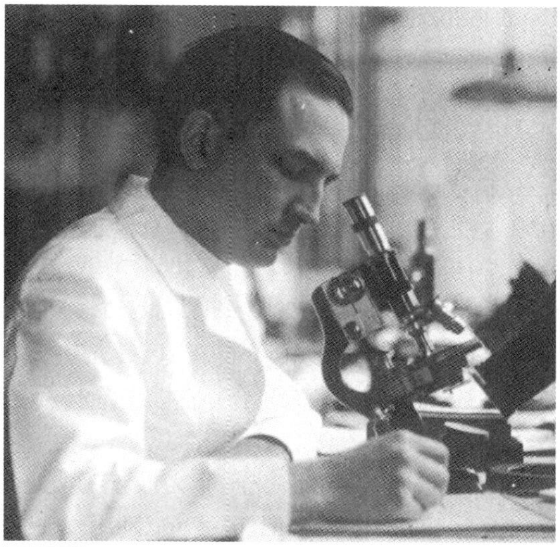

图 1-2 1932 年，Robert E. Gross 在哈佛做病理科住院医师时，在显微镜前。

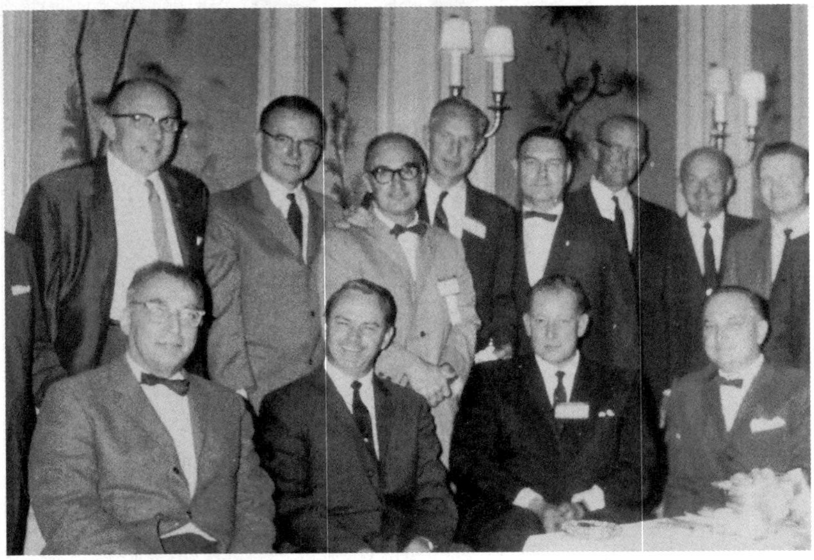

图 1-3　1964 年，一组出席英国小儿外科医生协会会议的北美外科医生。前排（从左到右）：Mark Ravitch、Robert G. Allen、Harvey Beardmore（加拿大人）和Robert E. Gross。后排（从左到右）：Lawrence K. Pickett、H. William Clatworthy、Hugh Lynn、Alexander Bill、C. Everett Koop、Willis Potts、Dan Cloud 和 George Dorman。

在 Peter Bent Brigham 医院和儿童医院的外科联
4 合培训项目中，Gross 开始展露他的才华。在工作中，作为一名生理学家，他更像一名技术精湛的技师。在对死于动脉导管未闭的亚急性细菌性心内膜炎的儿童的尸检研究中，细心的观察促使他去寻找一种外科解决方法。先是用病理标本，然后是进行动物实验，终于 Gross 创造了一套精巧的导管分离技术。最终在 1938 年，他选择了一名因导管未闭而濒临死亡的 8 岁女孩作为他的第一位手术候选人并进行了手术。患儿的恢复和后来的随访都非常令人满意。

Gross 取得这一惊人的临床成就时才 33 岁，只是 Brigham 医院外科的一名助理住院医生。这一广受称道的事件成为先在研究中心研究临床问题、再带回手术室解决问题的一个里程碑。1939 年，在完成外科住院医生的培训后，Gross 接受了 Ladd 的邀请加入了后者在儿童医院的团队。此后，Gross 在整理编辑 Ladd 在婴儿和儿童腹部外科的大量经验方面起了重要作用。1941 年，Gross 和 Ladd 一起出版了一本全新的教科书《小儿腹部外科学》。这本非凡的教科书收录了 Ladd 纠正肠旋转不良的手术方法（1936 年首次描述）和其他一些纠治新生儿畸形的特殊手术方法。

Ladd 退休后，Gross 被任命为波士顿儿童医院外科主任，他也成为 William E. Ladd 在小儿外科领域的继位者，小儿外科是 1941 年在哈佛医学院的支持下建立的。

Ovar Swenson 医生是儿童医院的另一位外科医生，也对小儿外科学做出了杰出的贡献，尤其是在先天性巨结肠病的处理方面，他解决了难点问题并确立了手术方法。1950 年，Swenson 成为波士顿 Tuft 医学院 Floating 医院的外科主任。

在 20 世纪 40 年代，许多先后在儿童医院接受过 Ladd 和 Gorss 培训的医生后来都成为了著名的小儿外科医生（图 1-3）。其中最著名的是 C. Everett Koop 医生和芝加哥的 Willis Potts 医生，他们都曾于 1946 年在波士顿儿童医院学习。Koop 学习了 7 个月后离开波士顿回到了费城，并开始了其在费城儿童医院的长而杰出的小儿外科医生及宾夕法尼亚大学教授的生涯。而 Potts 回到了芝加哥并在 Memorial 儿童医院建立了一个同样强的小儿外科项目，培养了许多杰出的小儿外科医生。

在波士顿儿童医院学习过的 H. William Clatwothy 医生是 Ladd 培训过的最后一位住院医生，也是 Gross 培训过的第一位医生。1950 年，Clatworthy 开始了他在俄亥俄州州立大学哥伦布儿童医院作为外科主任的显赫职业生涯。Tague Chisholm 医生于 1946 年离开波士顿并加入 Oswald Wyatt 医生在明尼阿波利斯（Minneapolis）的团队。Alexander Bill 医生也是在波士顿完成的培训，在波士顿学习期间，他在 Swenson 领导的对巨结肠病手术的实验室研究中起了重要作用，他于 1947 年加入了 Coe 在西雅图的儿童整形医院。Luther Longino 医生是一位来自阿肯色州（Arkansas）的沉默寡言的外科医生，1948 年他在 Gross 指导下完成了住院医生训练并留在波士顿医院，成为 Gross 的第二个病区的助手。在那里他工作了 20 年，指导了大批住院医生的外科技术方面的训练。

怀着梦想并经过不懈的努力，1948 年 Coe 促使美国儿科学会建立了外科分会[17]。这一新建立的分会成为美国小儿外科医生的全国性论坛，并成为美国外科界的一支新力量而获得承认。

到 1950 年，除波士顿儿童医院的培训项目外，在 Potts 领导下的芝加哥 Memorial 儿童医院，Koop领
5 导下的费城儿童医院，Swenson 领导的波士顿 Floating 医院，Thomas Samtulli 医生领导的纽约儿童医院，以及在 William Snyder 医生领导的洛杉矶儿童医院，小儿外科医生都可作为 1 年或 2 年的住院医生接受培训[6]。另外，加拿大的多伦多和蒙特利尔也建立了很好的小儿外科医生训练项目。这些培训项目的内容并不是固定的，有些是心脏外科培训，有些是泌尿外科培训，但所有人均接受过扎实的小儿普通外科培训。

随着 1953 年 Gross 的《小儿外科学》一书的出版，北美的小儿外科专业更加规范。这本著名的教科书详细描述了波士顿儿童医院在小儿普通外科、心脏外科和泌尿外科方面的经验。

20 世纪 50 年代，在美国和加拿大，小儿外科医生的数量通过各种训练项目得到了增加，这些人中许多人进入了私人诊所。随后各儿童医院开始积极寻求训练有素的小儿外科医生去领导他们的外科。医学院也意识到需要在婴幼儿外科疾病方面加强专科训练。

1965 年，发生了一件小儿外科学教育史上的分水岭事件，Clatworthy 非常有远见地要求美国儿科学会外科分会组成一个教育委员会，对美国和加拿大现行的小儿外科医生教育状况进行评估。虽然委员会的最初要求是对已存在的训练项目做评估，但对小儿外科医生教育的基本原则和要求也做出了建议。最初，Clatworthy 报告中由委员会会议通过并列出标准的推荐培训项目在美国有 11 项，在加拿大有 2 项。

一系列重要的事件促使小儿外科学在北美成为一门真正的外科专业[16]。Stephen Gans 医生认为，小儿外科学作为一个专科应有自己的杂志，在 Koop 的帮助下，1966 年创办了《小儿外科杂志》，Koop 任主编。1969 年，Lucian Leape 医生和 Thomas Boles 医生的一次会面导致了建立一个新的外科学会的想法。他们认为这一学会应不受其他任何相关学会如美国儿科学会的限制。这个想法很快就实现了，并有许多知名人物参与。1970 年美国小儿外科学会成立，Gross 为首位主席。Clatworthy 组织的委员会仔细评估了一些培训项目，并将其纳入小儿外科教育的标准课程。

20 世纪 50 年代和 60 年代期间，几次要求美国外科委员会建立一个专门的小儿外科委员会的建议都没有被采纳。尽管有一个新的独立的外科组织的支持，有经过评估的标准化培训项目和一本专业的杂志，以及遍及全国并逐渐列入普通外科的培训项目，但还缺少一位向美国外科委员会再次提出建议的代言人[10]。这个角色后来落到了蒙特利尔的 Harvey Beardmore 医生身上（图 1–4），这是一位亲切、老练、非常机智和有说服力的人物。在其他人失败后，Beardmore 用事实说话并取得了成功。美国外科委员会收到了一份精心准备的申请，并于 1975 年同意授予所有合格的小儿外科专业申请者一份新的证书。

20 世纪 30 年代和 40 年代，对小儿外科专业的研究加强了该专业的发展并首先表现在临床进展上[16]。Ladd 纠正肠旋转不良的手术是一个标志性事件。Gross 的创新技术，包括对心脏周围大血管——动脉导管未闭、主动脉缩窄、血管弓畸形——的治疗都值

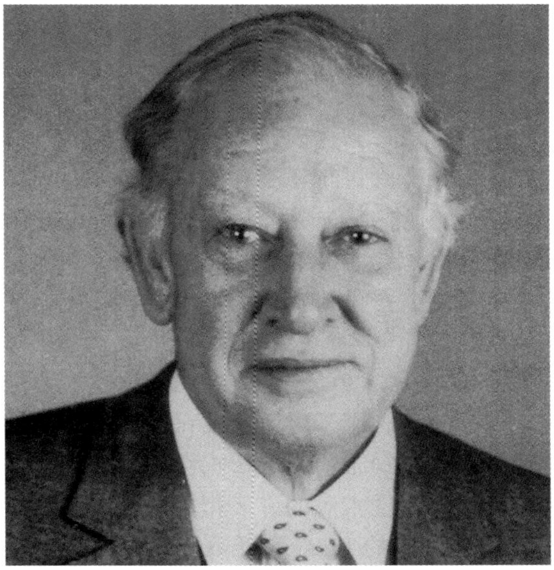

图 1–4　Harvey Beardmore，加拿大著名的小儿外科医生，美国小儿外科学会第 5 任主席，说服美国外科委员会为合格的小儿外科专业人员颁发证书的领导人。

得一提。同时，Blalock 为患 Fallot 四联症的患儿成功进行的“体-肺”短路手术是另一个里程碑。Potts 将主动脉-肺动脉直接短路的手术达到了相同的生理效果，但需要一种特殊的夹子。Potts 和 Smith 研发出一种具有许多精细的齿痕并能安全轻柔地夹住跳动的血管的夹子，他们将这种夹子应用于手术。这一技术至今仍应用于所有血管外科领域。为了治疗狭长的血管挛缩性狭窄，Gross 采用了经过辐射的干冻主动脉做同种异体移植，并证明有长期的临床功能。这一发现是所有周围血管外科发展的基础，得到了国际上的公认。另外，Swenson 对无神经节细胞巨结肠进行了谨慎研究，并采用了 Hochenegg 手术来切除直肠，使数以千计的巨结肠患儿得到了治疗。

针对成年手术患者的生物学影响的研究也开始针对儿童做专门的研究。Francis D. Moore 对机体成分
6 的研究成果已被 Rowe、Moore、Artz、Moncrief 和 Pruitt 纳入对烧伤的处理中，他们早期的学生之一 James O'Neill 又将这些知识应用于处理烧伤儿童。Stanley Dudrick 最先与 Rhoads 和 Wilmore 使用静脉内营养支持手术患者，创立了外科营养学，挽救了各个年龄段的无数患者。Bartlett 应用体外氧合扩展治疗有暂时性肺功能不良的婴儿；这一技术现在已发展成为抢救大龄儿童和成人的重要技术。之后，这一理念已由 Haller、Eichelberger、O'Neill、Tepas 和许多其他医生应用于儿童的治疗中。由 Cowley 最早倡导的对创伤患者要自始至终地进行准确的处理，拯救了许多遭受创伤并有可能失去生命的孩子。

令人畏惧的移植领域是由 Murray、Starzl、Shumway 引导的，后继者们继续在更大范围内、在更多的年龄组患者进行拓展。继 Richmond 的 Jackson 之后，旧金山的 DeLorimier 开始进行胎儿外科的实验研究。DeLorimier 的杰出学生 Harrison 和他的团队现在正从事将这一外科治疗的新形式从临床研究推向临床实践。

Patricia Donohoe 医生正在开展实验室胎儿基础研究，即研究生长因子对胚胎发育的影响。她的工作已明确，Müller 抑制物质可影响性别的形成。在对影响成人和儿童恶性疾病的许多相关研究中，没有人比波士顿儿童医院的 Judah Folkman 的工作更为重要或更有潜力。Folkman 发现了恶性肿瘤的血管形成，这促使他假设并探索使用抗血管生成来抑制癌症作为一种治疗癌症的方法，在肿瘤领域创立了一门全新的学科。

如今，小儿外科临床、教育和研究的重要进步在过去的成就基础上继续深入，并且许多成就也延伸到成人外科。

加拿大

当美国小儿外科在经历各种历程时，加拿大的小儿外科也经历了同步的发展历程，最初主要是在三个大医院。Alexander Forbes，一位整形外科医生，1904—1929年间在蒙特利尔儿童医院发挥了重要作用。Dudley Ross 医生，1937—1954 年间领导蒙特利尔儿童医院外科，主要负责在魁北克省建立现代小儿外科科室。1948 年，Ross 报告了加拿大第 1 例成功治疗的食管闭锁婴儿病例[4]。继 Ross 之后，1954—1974 年，David Murphy 医生作为小儿外科主任和新兴的小儿外科培训项目主任，在 Herbert Owen 医生、Gordon Karn 医生和他的第一个受培训者（1954 年）Harvey Beardmore 医生帮助下，树立起国际声誉。20 世纪 70 年代，Beardmore 就任蒙特利尔儿童医院外科主任，1981—1994 年由 Frank Guttman 接任。

在多伦多，1875 年 Samuel McMaster 夫人建立了儿童医院（the Hospital for Sick Children）。她的丈夫曾创立了 McMaster 大学[5]。在加拿大，19 世纪末和 20 世纪初，同美国一样，治疗成人的外科医生也负责小儿的外科治疗。在多伦多，当时最著名的外科医生也许是 W. Edward Gallie 医生。1921—1929 年，Gallie 担任儿童医院的外科主任，Gallie 还被任命为多伦多大学的外科系主任，在那里他建立了 Gallie 外科培训项目。在加拿大，Gallie 外科学院与美国 Johns Hopkins 的由 William Halsted 医生领导的外科学院齐名。随着职位升迁，Gallie 将小儿外科主任的位置交给了 Donald Robertson 医生。Donald Robertson 医生是一位具有冒险精神的胸外科医生，他担任主任一职直到 1944 年，退休时他几乎与波士顿的 Ladd 齐名。Arthur Lemesurer 医生是一位善于创造的整形外科医生，于 1949 年开始了他的小儿普通外科培训项目。这一项目先后造就了 Clinton Stephens、James Simpson、Robert Salter、Phillip Ashmore、Donald Marshall 和 Stanley Mercer 等杰出的小儿外科医生。所有杰出的毕业生都成为加拿大小儿外科领域的领导人。

1956 年，Alfred Farmer 医生被选为多伦多儿童医院外科主任，他立即组建了几个外科专科，包括小儿普通外科。按照 Clinton Stephens 的说法，这是一个里程碑事件，这使得各个专科都有了各自的领导。1956—1966 年由 Stewart Thomson 任主任，1966—1976 年由 Stephens 本人亲自领导（S. Ein，个人交流）。在这 20 年中，临床工作和临床研究都有巨大的成绩，完成培训项目的人数激增。1977 年，对 Robert Filler 医生的任命更使得小儿外科各方面的优秀传统得到发扬。

第三个对小儿外科做出了很大贡献的儿童医院是蒙特利尔 Sainte-Justine 医院。该医院是由 Justine Lacoste-Beau-Bien 夫人于 1907 年建立的，与蒙特利尔 Francophone 产科医院联合成为北美地区最大的妇女儿童医疗中心之一。1954 年 Pierre-Paul Collin 医生进入 Sainte-Justine 医院，带来了胸外科经验，并开展了针对儿童的治疗。Collin 培训了大批加拿大近代小儿外科界的领军人物，包括 Frank Guttman、Herve Blanchard、Saleem Yazbeck 和 Jean-Martin LaBerge。

这三个主要的小儿外科中心领导并推进了加拿大小儿外科发展，其产生的影响在美国也相当广泛。

英国

18 世纪中叶，瑞士-法国哲学家和伦理学家 Jean-Jacques Rousseau 曾说："出生后有一半人死于 8 岁前，这是自然法则，为什么要试图去抗拒？"。这
7 一看法在 18 世纪很普遍，而小儿外科也直到相当晚的时候才开始发展，尽管当时有资料显示，"外科医生和药剂师比许多著名的内科医生更常出诊治疗儿童"。

随着育婴堂在英国和欧洲各地的发展，儿科开始引起医生和普通大众的注意。在英国，最知名且至今还存在的有 Coram 基金会[13]。Coram 基金会最初创立于伦敦的 Holborn（1739 年），接近现在 Great Ormond 街儿童医院的位置。像其他许多这类机构一样，虽然被称为医院，但与其说是治疗中心，不如说是养育院。按我们今天的理解，儿童医院是 19 世纪发展起来的。

在欧洲，儿童医院和小儿外科发展的重要里程碑是 1802 年巴黎建立的 Hôpital des Enfants Malades。该医院拥有 200 张床位，可为患有内外科疾病的儿童提供治疗。在巴黎，其他医院不允许收入年龄小于 7 岁的儿童。随后，欧洲主要城市也都逐步建立了儿童医院。

1852 年，在 Great Ormond 街的一处经改建的房子里开办了儿童医院[7]。这所医院是 Charles West 医生在 Bence Jones 医生帮助下设计建立的。West 认为，内科性质的患儿应有专门的设施给予处理和特别的关注，而外科性质（当时大多涉及创伤）的患儿应在综合性医院进行治疗。这一观点在一些儿科医生心中持续了很长时间，现在在世界上有些地区仍然存在。

West 反对聘用外科医生作为儿童医院的职员，但董事会的意见却不同，并聘用了 G. D. Pollock。不久 Pollock 辞职，1853 年由 Athol Johnson 接替。Johnson 对小儿外科的认识主要体现在他于 1861 年在《英国医学杂志》上发表的三篇论文[9]。Johnson 之后，T. Holmes 在 1868 年出版了长达 37 章的《新生儿和儿童疾病的外科治疗》一书[8]。虽然当时儿科专业还没有发展，更别提小儿外科，但该书已清楚认识到，小儿外科是一个专门的领域。

19 世纪，儿科被分为两种模式，一种是巴黎建立的模式，患儿在专门治疗儿童疾病的医院进行治疗；另一种是 West 模式，后者在 19 世纪下半叶的英国非常普遍[11]。那时英国的许多儿童医院，如在伯明翰和爱丁堡的儿童医院，只提供药物治疗，没有针对儿童的外科治疗。大约在同一时代，Charles Dickens[12]，一位儿童医院的重要支持者，认为对于所有需要住院的儿童来说，专科医院是非常重要的。一些中心也认识到患有外科疾病的儿童有特殊需要，如在格拉斯哥，在酝酿了 21 年后建立了皇家儿童医院（the Royal Hospital for Sick Children，RHSC）。该院董事会聘用了同等数量的内科和外科医生[19]。非专业人士似乎也理解了对于儿童，内科和外科治疗都很重要。

在 19 世纪后期，由于 19 世纪中叶乙醚麻醉和氯仿麻醉的发展，人们逐渐接受手术，小儿外科有了显著发展。虽然早期已使用苯酚，但英国外科医生 Joseph Lister 为手术消毒的概念做了大量的推动工作。他在伦敦获得资格后，在格拉斯哥（Glasgow）发明了他的手术消毒方法，之后他转到爱丁堡，而后又到伦敦皇家医院。在格拉斯哥，Lister 有一位名叫 William Macewen（即后来的 William 爵士）的年轻助手，后者被誉为神经外科之父，是最早的皇家儿童

医院外科医生之一。

在苏格兰，儿科发展总体上是走在英国其他地区的前面。1860 年，皇家爱丁堡儿童医院（the Royal Edinburgh Hospital for Sick Children，REHSC）成立，但直到 1887 年，其董事会才决定将一个病区用于外科患者，并将缝纫间作为手术室使用[14]。Joseph Bell（爱丁堡皇家外科学院院长）、Harold Styles 爵士（他在 Conrad Ramstedt 之前一年就开始了幽门肌层切开术）、John Fraser 爵士（广泛使用的上下卷《小儿外科学》教科书作者）和 James J. Mason Brown（也是爱丁堡皇家外科学院的一位院长和一本名为《小儿外科学》的作者）都是 1887—1964 年间该院的资深外科医生。有趣的是，1919—1947 年间 Gertrude Hertzfeld 被爱丁堡皇家儿童医院聘为外科医生，她是那个年代很少见的几位女性外科医生之一。

回顾 19 世纪，在格拉斯哥，小儿外科学的培训独立于普通外科。在格拉斯哥，圣蒙哥学院（St. Mungo College）的讲课提纲涉及面很广，表 1–1 列出了 1889—1890 年的一份课程提纲。相似的内科疾病相关的讲座课程共 15 个。

表 1–1 圣蒙哥学院课程提纲：1889—1890 年

小儿外科疾病

讲师：James A. Adams，MD，FFPSG，皇家医院助理外科医生

讲课于夏季的星期二和星期四的上午 11:30 开始，课程包括下列内容：

1. 患病小儿的处理
2. 致病因素——出血、结核、甲状腺肿、佝偻病等
3. 梅毒
4. 骨折
5. 脱臼
6. 关节疾病
7. 骨和骨膜疾病
8. 腺体疾病——颈部、腋窝、腹股沟、Hodgkin 病
9. 先天性畸形——兔唇、腭裂、脊柱裂、脑膨出、畸形足、斜颈、肛门直肠闭锁、手和足畸形
10. 肿瘤——良性、恶性、先天性
11. 白喉——喉炎、假膜性喉炎、气管切开术和其适应证
12. 烧伤——烫伤、并发畸形
13. 脊柱疾病——骨溃疡、成角和侧弯
14. 脓胸——胸腔积液
15. 瘫痪——假性肥大、手足抽搐、痉挛性麻痹、神经元病（neuroninesis）等
16. 泌尿生殖系疾疾病——膀胱反翻、尿道下裂、包茎、轻度包茎、手淫、两性畸形、结石、切开取石、碎石术、尿失禁
17. 疝
18. 腹部疾病——腹膜炎、肠梗阻、消瘦、肿瘤、肛门和直肠
19. 特殊感觉器官
20. 听觉疾病——对颅内脓肿形成的影响
21. 鼻、眼、耳异物等

这些医院开办不久，其董事会就认识到需要开办诊所或门诊部。在曼彻斯特的 Pendelbury，诊所实际上先于医院处理患者，这些诊所处理了许多外科患者，而且大部分的小儿外科手术也在那里做。James Nicoll，那个时代最杰出的外科医生之一，在 1909 年作了一个他的 10 年工作报告[15]，后者是他所发表的 100 多篇文章中的一篇。现在他被称为现代外科之父，但他同样也可以被称为小儿外科医生。虽然，他仅有部分时间致力于小儿外科的工作（表 1–2）。在 19 世纪后期，他成功施行了幽门肌层切开术，其术式与 Styles 和 Ramstedt 术式有所不同。

虽然在 1914 年，Nicoll 曾被邀请担任两个小儿外科部门中的一个的负责人，但他拒绝了，因为如果他出任，他就得放弃成人外科手术。他选择出任了影响较小的诊所的外科医生职位而非客座外科医生职位。当时，皇家儿童医院的董事会要求医院聘任的内
8 科或外科医生必须是全职的，一些特殊的工作可以例外，但任职者在儿童医院的工作必须是优先的。这样，显然在儿童医院外进行的医疗活动是不受欢迎的。

1902 年，Alex MacLennan 首次被皇家儿童医院聘为诊所的外科医生，1914 年又被聘为客座外科医生。1919 年，格拉斯哥大学设立了内科讲师职位和外科讲师职位，这是英国最早的专业分科。1919 年，MacLennan 被聘为格拉斯哥大学小儿外科和骨科疾病的 Barclay 讲师，直到 1938 年他在这个位置上退休。MacLennan 的兴趣主要是骨科。他的继任者，Matthew White 是一位胸腹部外科医生。Matthew White 1924 年在诊所任职，1930 年成为客座外科医生，1938 年成为 Barclay 讲师。还有 Wallace Dennison 和 Dan Young，他们后来也担任了这些职务的外科医

表 1-2　格拉斯哥皇家儿童医院 James Nicholl 开展的门诊手术种类：1899—1908 年 *

结核
畸形足
兔唇和腭裂
乳突积液
脊柱裂
骨折
幽门狭窄

* 在这 10 年中，Nicholl 做了 8988 例手术中的 7392 例。

生。

当时在爱丁堡，小儿外科和成人外科仍紧密相连，直到 Mason Brown 成为主任。有一种说法是，“苏格兰很早就有小儿外科医生，但他们只做小儿外科手术，直到成人外科职位有空缺”[18]。与该说法相反的是，在爱丁堡和格拉斯哥两地的儿童医院，外科医生因致力于儿科工作而拒绝接受具有很高声望的成人外科职位。这些医院的档案记录了这些事实。

第二次世界大战后，小儿外科在很短的时间里得到了很大的发展。促进这一发展的原因有许多，如英国国民健康保险制度的建立，可为各年龄和各社会阶层提供免费治疗。除药物研发以外，20 世纪中叶整形外科业和许多其他技术的创新发展也使小儿外科的这种进步成为可能，尤其是在新生儿外科方面。然而更近的回顾显示，虽然第一个外科性质的儿科“俱乐部”——苏格兰小儿外科“俱乐部”和美国儿科学会外科分会至 1948 年才成立，但小儿外科的发展已经有好几十年[1, 2, 17]。

专业的发展与致力于该专业的人密切相关。Denis Browne，1924 年最早被伦敦儿童医院聘任的澳大利亚人，将他的整个职业生涯献给了小儿外科。当时在伦敦和英国的其他城市，对小儿外科感兴趣的普通外科医生，在从事成人外科手术的同时也进行儿科手术。经济方面的考虑无疑是重要的因素，不管他们的愿望如何，很少人能仅仅依靠小儿外科手术维持生计。Browne 是伦敦第一位将自己定位于小儿外科的外科医生。几年中他便拥有了大量的拥护者和追随者，知名度很高，并且由于他身材高大，很容易被人认出来。所有认识他的人都认为，他有点专横和专制，并且不容易接受别人反驳他的理论和观点。与 Browne 长期共事的 James Crooks 称他是一位“聪明的冒险家，一位叛逆者和一位愤世嫉俗者”。甚至在他去世前几天，Browne“仍极其强调自我”[3]。他的忠实的秘书回忆，当她试图使 Browne 缓和一点他信件中的语气时，一位朋友对她说：“您肯定是疯了！Denis Browne 花了一生的时间建立了他粗鲁的名气，你却要在最后时刻改变他”[20]。我们中的一位 9
（Young）作为他的最后一位助手，发现他富有激情、为人正直。Denis Browne 金质奖章显示了他的风范且清楚地展示了他的观点（图 1-5）。

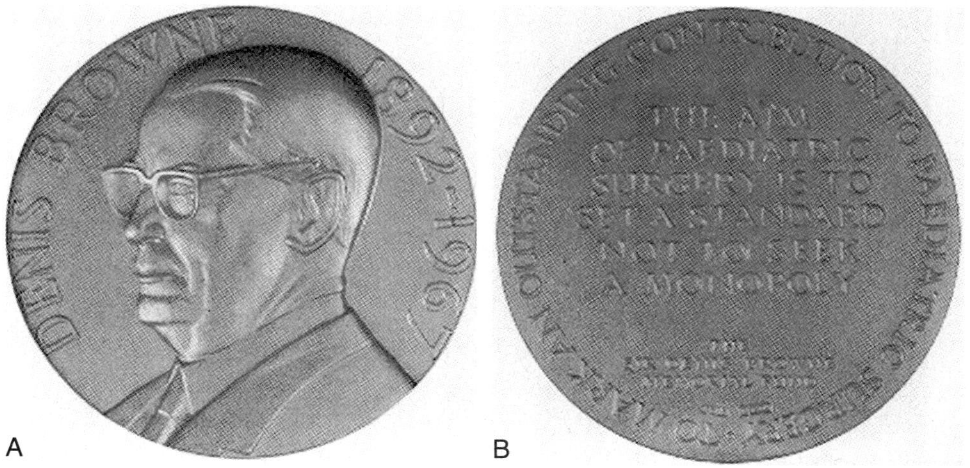

图 1-5　Denis Browne 金质奖牌。A. 奖牌的正面。B. 奖牌的背面，上面写道：“小儿外科的目标是建立一个标准，而不是寻找一个专利”。

第二次世界大战后，许多来自海外的外科医生在英国停留了一段时间，其中大多数人访问了儿童医院。在那里他们受到了 Denis Browne 和其他一些之前提到的外科医生的影响。后来，在许多大陆建立了许多国际知名的中心，Jannie Louw、Douglas Stephens、Durham Smith 和 Christian Barnard 是其中的几个例子。

Browne 主要关注的是解剖结构异常。他提出，宫内压力是导致或引起此类异常的观点得到了广泛的认可。在儿童医院，Browne 有一批与他同时代的资深同事，如 L. Barrington-Ward 和 T. Twistington Higgins，都是相当有地位的外科医生。Browne 在他的晚年成为 Grand Ormond 大街重要的外科医生。在伦敦，Higgins 第一个发起讨论并促使英国小儿外科医生协会成立。那时，Browne 是儿童医院的资深外科医生且是该协会第一任主席和任职时间最长的主席。Browne 晚年在国家健康服务部任过职，他的同事包括 George McNab（用于脑积水的 Holter 瓣的提出者）、David Waterston（早期的小儿心外科医生）和 David Innes Williams 爵士（英国小儿泌尿外科前辈），所有这些杰出人物都为小儿外科的发展作出了重要贡献。

同时也有许多其他方面的发展。Andrew Wilkinson 和其他一些人，如从奥斯陆（Oslo）来的 Ole Knutrud 对新生儿的代谢进行了研究。富有爱心的外科医生 Isabella Forshall（Rickham 后来加入）尽管没有做出什么重大的科学贡献，但她建立了一个卓越的临床服务模式，在她的 1959 年的圣诞卡中，她描绘了许多出席英国小儿外科医生协会会议的杰出人物（图 1-6）。

总之，在大西洋东边，小儿外科学的发展历史揭示，小儿外科的各种分歧多集中在 19 世纪和 20 世纪的主要发展阶段。最近几十年已较少有分歧，但各个社团都提出了各自的方法来稳定地改善对需要手术的新生儿和儿童的护理和照顾，过去 50 年中可看到许多变化。进一步的详细描述见其他各章节。

亚洲

由于篇幅的限制，不能对亚洲小儿外科的发展进行全面的叙述。然而，必须承认，全世界范围的文献

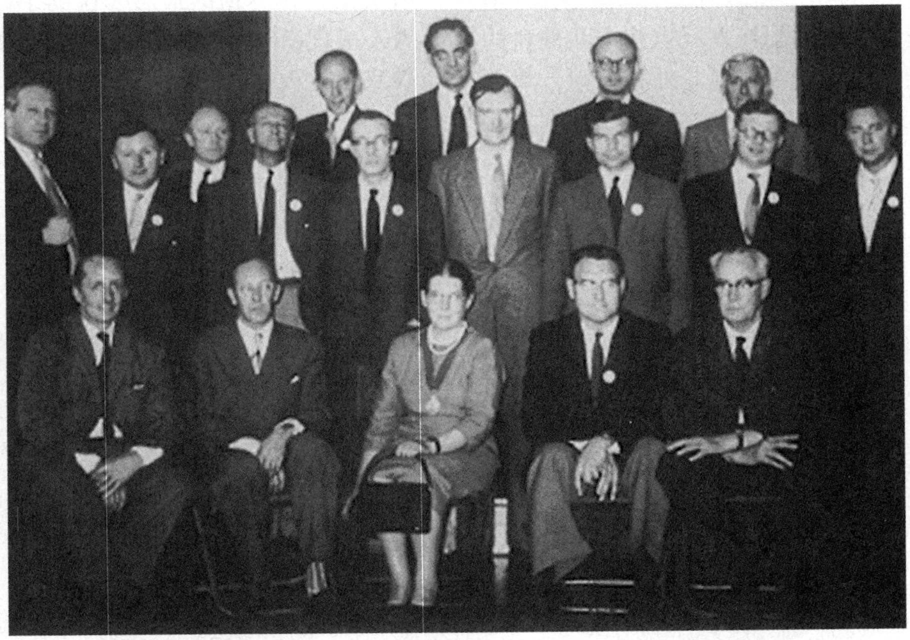

图 1-6 1959 年 Isabella Forshall 的圣诞卡。前排坐者（从左到右）：D. Waterston、M. Grob、I. Forshall、C. Koop 和 D. Browne。后排站立者：H. Beardmore、R. Zachary、I. Kirkland、T. Ehrenpries、W. Dennison、H. Johnson、A. Wilkinsoon、A. Jolleys、J. Bentley、B. Smyth、V. Swain、H. Nixon 和 B. O'Donnell。照片中缺少者是 G. McNab。

中也凝集着来自亚洲国家和地区的专家们的贡献。在中国，张（金哲）被誉为中国的小儿外科之父。目前也已涌现出新一代的小儿外科医生。

日本的小儿外科直到二次世界大战结束后几年才得到发展。20 世纪 50 年代早期出现了第一代小儿外科医生。如大阪的 Ueda、东京 Juntendo 大学的 Suruga、仙台的 Kasai 和福冈的 Ikeda。1952 年，Suruga施行的第一例手术是小肠闭锁。1955 年，Kasai 为胆道闭锁患者施行了第一次肝门肠吻合术。1965 年，日本第一所国家儿童医院在东京建立。1968 年，Suruga 在东京 Juntendo 大学建立了第一个小儿外科学系。而今天在日本，几乎所有的主要大学的医疗中心都有小儿外科培训课程。日本的小儿外科学会及其杂志创立于 1964 年，这些与世界其他国家的发展相平行。日本的第二代小儿外科医生包
10 括大阪的 Okamoto 和 Okada、东京的 Akiyama、Tsuchida 和 Miyano 以及仙台的 Ohi 和福冈的 Suita。这些人分别在营养、胆胰疾病、肿瘤和肠道疾病等领域中作出了重要贡献。

近几十年来，在亚洲，尤其是在日本，众多实验室和临床中心在临床和基础生物学方面都传来了令人振奋的消息，并继续不断丰富着小儿外科领域。在临床发展、教育和研究各方面，小儿外科已真正实现国际化，而其未来似乎也相当有发展前景。

（吴晔明译　董其刚校）

参考文献

1. Bisset W, Carachi R: The forerunner in the north: The Scottish Paediatric Surgical Society. J Pediatr Surg 2003;37(Suppl 7):2-6.
2. Campbell JR: History of the Section of Surgery, the American Academy of Pediatrics: The second 25 years. J Pediatr Surg 1999;34(Suppl 1):19-98.
3. Crooks J: In Nixon HH, Waterston DJ, Wink CSA (eds): Selected Writings of Sir Denis Browne. Farnborough, Inkon Printers, 1983, p 1.
4. Delaure NC: Thoracic Surgery in Canada. Toronto, BC Decker, 1989.
5. Ein S: History of the Division of General Surgery at HSC, Toronto. Unpublished manuscript.
6. Glick PL, Azizkhan RG: A Genealogy of North American Pediatric Surgery. St Louis, Quality Medical Publishing, 1997.
7. Higgins TT: Great Ormond Street, 1852-1952. London, Odhams Press, 1952.
8. Holmes T: Surgical Treatment of the Diseases of Infancy and Childhood. London, Longmans, Green, Reader & Dyer, 1868.
9. Johnson A: Surgery of childhood. BMJ 1861;1:1-4, 41-47, 61-63.
10. Johnson DG: Excellence and search of recognition. J Pediatr Surg 1986;22:1019-1031.
11. Lomax EMR: Small and Special: The Development of Hospitals for Children in Victorian Britain. London, Wellcome Institute for the History of Medicine, 1996.
12. Markel H: Charles Dickens' work to help establish Great Ormond Street Hospital, London. Lancet 1999;354:6357.
13. McLure RK: Coram's Children. New Haven, Conn, Yale University Press, 1981.
14. Minutes of the Board of the Royal Edinburgh Hospital for Sick Children, 1887.
15. Nicoll JH: Surgery of infancy. BMJ 1909;2:753-754.
16. Randolph JG: The first of the best. J Pediatr Surg 1985;20:580-591.
17. Randolph JG: History of the Section of Surgery, the American Academy of Pediatrics: The first 25 years. J Pediatr Surg 1999;34(Suppl 1):3-18.
18. Rickham PP: Jpn J Paediatr Surg 2002;38:210-233.
19. Robertson E: The Yorkhill Story. Glasgow, Robert MacLehose & Co, 1972.
20. Waterman R: In Nixon HH, Waterston DJ, Wink CSA (eds): Selected Writings of Sir Denis Browne. Farnborough, Inkon Printers, 1983, p15.

第2章

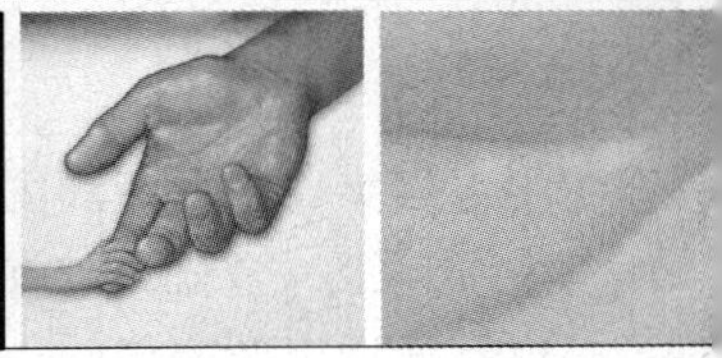

临床分子遗传学和基因治疗

Alan W. Flake

11 本章的主题范围较广，超出了小儿外科学的传统核心教育领域。然而在不久的将来，在包括小儿外科学在内的所有医学专业中，分子遗传学和基因治疗将越来越具有临床重要性。对此一些保守的预期包括：诊断准确性及表型预测的进展、对许多疾病的新的治疗方式以及根据患者的基因型采取最佳的药物疗法，但也可能还有很多其他用途。在此对与小儿外科有关或可能有关的这方面的近期发展做一概述。

临床分子遗传学

虽然人们对遗传性疾病的认识已有几个世纪，但是直到最近遗传才成为许多人类疾病的主导解释。20世纪70年代之前，医生们还曾认为，遗传病相对罕见且与临床治疗无关。然而随着分子遗传学的迅速进步，现在我们已认识到，基因实际上是人类所有疾病的关键因素。McKusick的《人类孟德尔遗传》一书中的条目已从1965年的1500条增加至2000年的10 000条，虽然不是全面的指标，但这确实表明了人类基因学知识的增加[44]。即使是以前曾被认为是纯粹的获得性疾病，如感染，目前也已认识到，其受到内在易损性基因机制和遗传驱动的免疫系统应答的影响。

虽然基因信息及其相关的人类疾病的知识明显增加，但在确认与人类表型相关的基因型异常和治疗的实际应用之间还有很大距离。除了遗传咨询和产前诊断外，目前分子遗传学对日常药物治疗或小儿外科方面的影响很小，然而其前景是不可否认的。明确人类疾病和个体对环境、药理、疾病导致干扰的反应机制是认识下游途径的第一步，后者可能对临床治疗有深刻影响。遗传学的最终应用将是可以纠正受累个体及其后代的种系缺陷。虽然种系纠正仍是具有伦理争议的幻想[56]，但毫无疑问，今后10年内分子遗传学将通过许多方式影响临床实践。有关分子遗传学领域的广泛讨论不在本章讨论的范围，本书另有许多有关小儿外科疾病的临床遗传学方面的信息。

人类分子遗传学和小儿外科疾病

快速确定与人类疾病相关的基因已彻底改变了医学遗传学领域，提供了更准确的诊断、预后及可能的治疗工具。然而，知识的增加常伴随着复杂性的增加。传统模型假设，家族中某种特征的传播与单一分子缺陷的传递有关——个体等位基因分离至家族是根据孟德尔法则。现在的模型发现，只有很少表型可用单一基因位点突变给予满意的解释。现在发现，以前曾被认为是单基因的疾病具有表型多样性，这使遗传病的概念重新建立。虽然孟德尔模型在确定家族性疾病的主要原因方面仍然有用，但它们已不再是疾病的真正生理学和细胞学本质的完整模型[15,66,71]。许多起初 12
认为是单基因引起的疾病现在已被证实是由少数位点引起或调节的。这些疾病被称为寡基因疾病，这是一种发展性概念，包含了一大类既不是单基因也不是多基因的表型。与所知甚少的、由许多基因与环境相互作用引起的多基因或复杂性状不同，寡基因疾病的病因主要是遗传，但需要少数位点等位基因突变的协同作用。现代分子遗传学被视为传统孟德尔性状和复杂性状之间的概念连续体（图2–1）。任何特定疾病在此连续体中的位置取决于三个主要变量：（1）主要位点是否对表型起到主导性作用；（2）影响表型的位点的数目；（3）环境对表型的影响及程度。

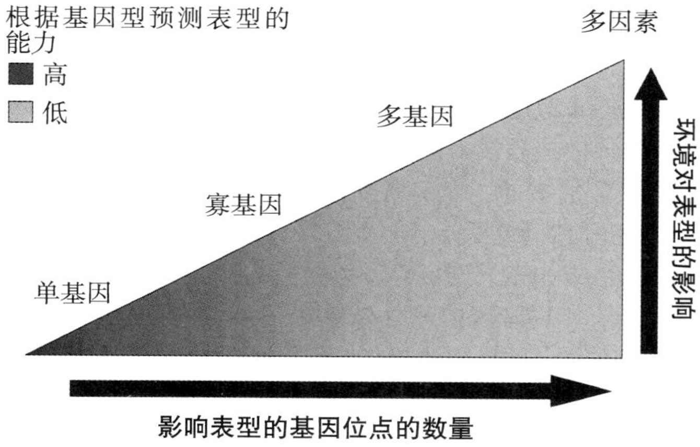

图 2–1　现代分子遗传学的概念连续体。一种疾病的遗传特征取决于：（1）主要位点是否在表型中起到主要作用；（2）影响表型的基因位点数量；（3）环境对表型的影响及程度。疾病越靠近右侧，遗传分析越复杂，表型的基因型越难以预测。

改变分子遗传学概念的疾病特例

单基因疾病

囊性纤维化（CF）是一个接近连续体单基因末端的例子，但它也可说明一些疾病的遗传学复杂性，即使主要位点突变是表型的主要决定因素时。基于观察到的常染色体隐性遗传特征，囊性纤维化跨膜调节蛋白（*CFTR*）基因在人类首先被定位于染色体 7q31.2[68]。一旦 *CFTR* 基因被克隆[62]，可以预期突变分析可能就足以预测患儿的临床结果。然而，对大样本及不同种族人群的 *CFTR* 的突变分析显示，此假设过于简化了此表型的真正遗传本质，特别是在一些囊性纤维化患儿中观察到大量的表型变异。例如，虽然 *CFTR* 突变与胰腺疾病的严重程度有一定关联，但肺表型的严重性（是死亡的主要原因）难以预测[1,16,45]。认识到单纯单基因模型的局限性使人们对更复杂的遗传模型进行评价。这就需要找出人和鼠囊性纤维化肠道的修饰位点[63,73]。进一步的表型分析发现了其他几个与表型有关的位点，包括：（1）低表达甘露糖结合凝集素（*MBL*，也称为 *MBL2*）的等位基因、人白细胞抗原（*HLA*）Ⅱ型多态性以及 α 肿瘤坏死因子（*TNFα*）和 β1 转化生长因子（*TGFβ1*）的变异体与肺疾病的关系[5,6,21,30]；（2）体内一氧化氮合酶 1（*NOS1*）多态性与微生物感染的频率和严重性的关系[22]；（3）黏蛋白 1（*Muc1*）在鼠囊性纤维化表型中对胃肠道的作用（图 2–2）[55]。最近已进一步发现 *CFTR* 及其相关表型的复杂性。第一，杂合性囊性纤维化突变与鼻窦炎易感性有关，这是已确立的多基因特征[69]。第二，更惊奇的是，最近一项研究报道，一些囊性纤维化表型较轻的患者 *CFTR* 无突变。这说明有关 *CFTR* 基因功能障碍是囊性纤维化发生所必需的假说不一定正确[23]。 13

寡基因疾病

在定义先天性巨结肠（HD）的分子遗传学的最新进展上，可举例说明遗传学上一个相对新的概念——寡基因疾病。虽然寡基因的数学分析超出了本章讨论的范围[18,47]，但重要的是要认识到，对传统连锁方式进行的修改是对研究寡基因疾病的有用工具，特别是已知主要位点对表型起很大作用时。可根据神经节细胞缺失的程度来区别先天性巨结肠的两种主要表型组：短段型先天性巨结肠（S–HD）和较为严重的长段型先天性巨结肠（L–HD）。已发现，L–HD 为

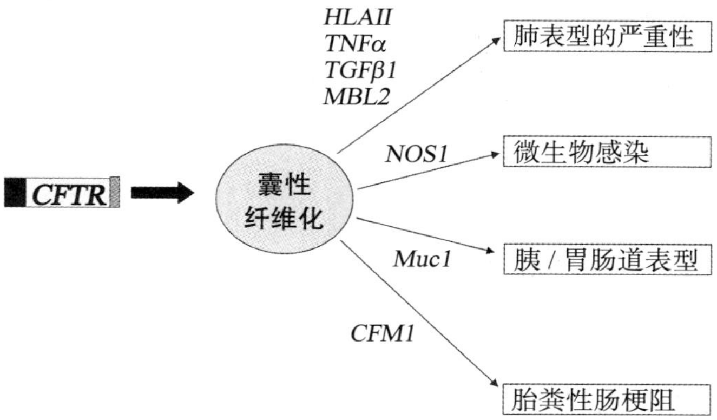

图 2–2　单基因疾病的复杂性。囊性纤维化跨膜调节蛋白（*CFTR*）总能引起囊性纤维化（CF）表型。由于其他遗传因素的修饰效应，*CFTR* 位点突变的出现和本质不能预测该病的表型。因此，虽然 CF 被认为是孟德尔隐性遗传病，每个患者的表型取决于不同位点等位基因的独立数目。*CFM1*：囊性纤维化修饰基因 1；GI：胃肠道；HLA Ⅱ：主要组织相容性复合物Ⅱ类抗原；*MBL2*：甘露醇结合凝集素（C 蛋白）2；*Muc1*：黏蛋白 1；*NOS1*：一氧化氮合酶 1；*TGFβ1*：β1 转化生长因子；*TNFα*：肿瘤坏死因子 α 编码基因。

常染色体显性遗传伴不全外显率；S–HD 的遗传较复杂，为常染色体隐性遗传。凭借一些因素的效力可确立两种先天性巨结肠变异体的寡基因性：复发的风险为 3%～25%，取决于神经节细胞缺失的长度及患儿的性别；遗传率接近 100%，提示有完全遗传基础；明显的临床变异性及降低的外显率；以及非随机地伴有内皮素 B 型受体（*EDNRB*）形态学改变，并有转染中重排（*RET*）多态性和先天性巨结肠[54,57]。迄今为止，连锁、位置克隆研究和功能型候选基因分析相结合的方法已确定了八种先天性巨结肠基因（表 2–1）[2]，其中原癌基因 *RET* 被认为是主要易感位点，特别对于 L–HD 高发的家族[20]。

先天性巨结肠的非孟德尔遗传方式干扰了通过常规连锁方式确定易感修饰位点。当这些方法（参数及非参数连锁研究）用于研究一组 12 个 L–HD 家族时发现，与 9q31 的关联非常微弱。然而基于只有轻度 *RET* 突变的假说，可能与另一位点产生关系，家族按 *RET* 突变资料分类。对具有潜在性微弱 *RET* 突变的家族进行的独立分析发现，其与 9q31 有明显关联[39]，提示轻度 *RET* 等位基因连同 9 号染色体上的未知等位基因可能与发病有关。已证明 S–HD 的遗传模式比 L–HD 的更复杂，需对连锁方法进行进一步调整。近来应用了无模式连锁，不考虑分离因素的数量和遗传模式假设，发现三位点分离对于显示 S–HD 是必需且足够的，*RET* 是主要位点，易感等位基因的传递是附加的[20]。

在诸如先天性巨结肠等疾病中观察到的遗传模式已显示其具有可解释外显率降低和表型变异的两种疾病遗传的扩展模式的能力，及用这些模型去寻找寡基因疾病遗传位点的能力——这是确定它们的潜在基因的第一步。更重要的是，非孟德尔模式的建立改变了人们对人类遗传学的认识，反过来促进了对寡基因性状的发现。

多基因或复杂性疾病

多基因或复杂性疾病被认为是由所知甚少的多基因与环境间相互作用引起的。与小儿外科有关的多基因疾病是肥厚性幽门狭窄（HPS）。肥厚性幽门狭窄的遗传因素很久以前已被识别，其常有家族聚集性，单卵双胎间的同病率为 25%～40%，男性和女性的复 14

表 2–1　与先天性巨结肠有关的基因以及与伴发畸形的关系

基因	基因位点	基因产物	遗传	人口频率（%）	伴发畸形	HD 发生率（%）
RET	10q11.2	GDNF 复合受体	AD	17～38（S–HD）	CCHS	1.8～1.9
				70～80（L–HD）	MEN2A	2.5～5.0
				50（家族性）	MEN2B	未知
				15～35（散发性）		
GDNF	5p12–13.1	RET 和 GFRα–1 配体	AD	<1*	CCHS	1.8～1.9
NTN	19p13.3	RET 和 GFRα–2 配体	AD	<1*	未知	—
GFRα–1	10q26	GDNF 复合受体	未知	†	未知	—
EDNRB	13q22	EDN3 受体	AD/AR	3～7	Waardenburg 综合征	未知
EDN3	20q13.2–13.3	EDNRB 配体	AD/AR	5	CCHS	1.8～1.9
					Waardenburg 综合征	未知
ECE–1	1p36.1	EDN3 处理基因	AD	<1	未知	—
SOX10	22q13.1	转录因子	AD	<1	4 型 Waardenburg 综合征	未知

* 数据有限。

† 迄今未在人类中测到突变，但与鼠发生 HD 相关。

AD：常染色体显性；AR：常染色体隐性；CCHS：先天性中枢性肺换气不足综合征（Ondine 呼吸困扰）；ECE–1：内皮素转化酶 1；EDNRB：内皮素 B 型受体；EDN3：内皮素 3；GDNF：胶质细胞系源性神经营养因子；GFRα–1：GDNF 家族受体 α–1；HD：先天性巨结肠；L–HD：长段型巨结肠；MEN：多发性内分泌瘤病；NTN：neurturin；RET：转染中重排；S–HD：短段型巨结肠；SOX：Sry 样HMG 盒。

发率分别为 10%和 2%。与普通人群相比，一级亲属的危险性高 18 倍[46]。然而，此危险性明显低于根据孟德尔遗传模式的预测[10]。此外据报道，在多次定义的遗传性综合征[9,35,36,59,67]、染色体异常[12,27,29,60,70]以及多种其他缺陷中，肥厚性幽门狭窄是一个相关特征，提示其具有多基因基础。肥厚性幽门狭窄的分子遗传学基础还不清楚，其可能的最终途径通常为幽门肌内神经一氧化氮合酶（nNOS）的表达改变[51]。对这种改变的分子机制的详细分析已经发表，即在肥厚性幽门狭窄患儿中，nNOS 外显子 1c 的信使 RNA（mRNA）表达减少，而 nNOS 外显子 1f 的变异型 mRNA 代偿性上调[51]。已对 16 例肥厚性幽门狭窄患儿和 81 例对照者的 DNA 样本的 nNOS 外显子 1c 启动子突变和单核苷酸多态性（SNP）进行了分析。对外显子 1c 的 5'区进行排序后发现，在 16 例肥厚性幽门狭窄患儿中有 3 例有突变，而在 81 例对照中只有野生型序列。以前未定性的 nNOS 外显子 1c 启动子 SNP（–84G/A SNP）的 A 等位基因携带者发生肥厚性幽门狭窄的风险增加（优势比为 8.0，95%的可信区间为 2.5～25.6），说明–84G/A 启动子 SNP 可改变 nNOS 外显子 1c 的表达，或与 nNOS 转录单位中其他部位的功能性重要序列变异体发生了连锁平衡失调，因此可能可以作为功能性遗传改变的信息标记。观察到的–84G/A SNP 与肥厚性幽门狭窄风险增加之间的关系与报道的 nNOS 基因微卫星多态性与 HPS 家族型间的强相关是一致的[13]。但–84G/A SNP 并不是所有肥厚性幽门狭窄病例的原因，故一氧化氮依赖性信号传导途径或附加机制及基因等成分可能也与肥厚性幽门狭窄的发病有关。这与其他认为肥厚性幽门狭窄是多因素性病因的观察是一致的[46]。总之，nNOS 外显子 1c 调节区域的遗传改变可影响 nNOS 基因的表达，并可能与肥厚性幽门狭窄的发病有关，但肥厚性幽门狭窄的发生可能还与其他许多基因以及环境影响有关。

这些例子说明了目前分子遗传学模式的复杂性，也说明了这些模式在确定疾病（特别是对于多基因疾病）的遗传学原因上尚有不足。目前，大多数小儿外科疾病被归为未定义的多因素遗传，与已经描述的遗传分类相比，对其所知更少。在这些疾病中，尚未确定病原性、易感性或影响性基因位点。孤立的区域畸形可能由环境和多基因间的相互作用引起。多因素遗传以家族中出现大量危险基因为特征。畸形具有遗传基础的假设是基于具有再现风险。虽然多因素遗传疾病的再现风险一般较低，但高于普通人群。如果有一个以上的家族成员受累，或先证者的畸形更严重，或父母是近亲，则再现风险增加。除了这些概括性的东西，遗传学很少能为疾病分类提供特殊信息。

分子遗传学在临床小儿外科中的应用

遗传咨询和产前诊断

正如上文提到的，在认识一种疾病的基因型与其临床治疗的直接应用之间仍有距离。而例外的是遗传咨询和产前诊断。小儿外科医生可能需要一些分子遗传学知识，因为后者在产前咨询中的作用越来越大。分子遗传学可通过提供表型异常的基因型证明、已证实的基因型的表型关联以及在许多情况下随后妊娠的再现风险和对其他家族成员的担心，提供一个受累胎儿的有关信息。再举一个先天性巨结肠的例子可说明分子遗传学在遗传咨询中作用非常大[8,64]。先天性巨结肠患者的同胞患病风险一般为 4%，且随着受累肠段的长度增加而增加。在伴发已知综合征的先天性巨结肠中，与再现风险相比，遗传咨询更关注与综合征有关的预后。对于单纯性先天性巨结肠，可制定更精确的风险表。受累女性亲属比受累男性亲属的再现风险更大，与短段型先天性巨结肠相比，长段型先天性巨结肠患者的亲属再现风险更大。例如，从结肠脾曲近端开始无神经节的女性患者的男性同胞的再现风险为 23%，而女性同胞的再现风险为 18%；同样的男性患者的男性同胞再现风险为 11%，而女性同胞的再现风险为 8%。短段型先天性巨结肠患者的同胞的再现风险降至 6%以下。如果家族内的突变已知，产前诊断是可能的。然而，由于单个基因突变的外显率低（除了 Waardenburg 综合征的 *SOX10* 突变外），产前诊断的临床应用受限。

更常见的是，遗传学的一般知识可为诊断为多因素遗传缺陷胎儿的父母提供复发风险的准确咨询和保证。最常见的情况为涉及小儿外科医生的产前咨询。在发生多发畸形的情况下，小儿外科医生也应该意识到对流产胎儿的组织的遗传学评估价值，经过遗传咨询，父母亲可以选择中止妊娠。不把胎儿送到适当的医学中心进行详细的大体检查，以及在适当的时候不进行最新的分子遗传学评估，对胎儿的家庭来说是一种伤害。

随着分子遗传学不断发现导致某些疾病的基因——其倾向性和修正的基因位点以及其他遗传学相互作用——随之而来的必然是预测特异性基因显性存在及严重程度的能力不断提高。这种情况使产前遗传咨询对特殊的胎儿更适合并可使预后准确性更高，给父母亲一个可在更多信息基础上做出产前选择的机会。

出生后的治疗

在将来，分子遗传学将可为不同父母提供最佳的特异性治疗。这也许包括为不同患者提供基于基因型以及预期对特异性术后并发症起作用的药物的治疗，如感染或术后应激反应。当然，对一位受累个体及其后代的最终治疗是纠正造成一种特殊基因显性的种系遗传学改变。虽然在考虑这些治疗以前有许多科学和伦理学上的障碍需要克服，但是可以想象，分子遗传学与基因转移技术相结合将可以纠正种系的基因突变，即通过整合一个正常基因来替代一个异常基因，最后提供最终的预防性治疗。虽然基因转移技术的现状还远远没有达到这种最终治疗的水平，但是在过去 30 年中取得的进展只能被描述为惊人。本章下一个部分将回顾基因转移现状及其潜在的治疗应用。

基因治疗

在争论中基因治疗仍然是令人困扰的，似乎其最终的潜力在被不断的失望和最近的负面事件所笼罩。2000 年出现了第一例临床上基因治疗成功的病例——治疗 X 连锁的重症联合免疫缺陷（XSCID）[11]——只是没想到这个戏剧性的成功却因为两名患者发生了白血病而被低估。这一事件以及其他负面事件差一点使近年来在基因转移技术领域中取得的坚实进展黯然失色。虽然缓慢，但是基因转移方法确实在不断发展，基因转移比以前变得更加安全、特异和高效。虽然有一些复杂的问题还没有解决，但在未来几年内成功的基因治疗策略很可能会制定出来。基因转移技术可以分为基于病毒载体和非病毒载体的基因转移。这部分内容因为篇幅限制以及基于非病毒载体基因转移的效率限制，下面只回顾一下基于病毒载体基因转移的现状。

用于基因转移的病毒载体

病毒具有高度进化的生物学机制，能够高效地穿透宿主细胞膜，利用宿主的细胞器来促进它们的复制。理想情况下，病毒载体可利用病毒的感染途径，但可避免随着病毒基因复制表达产生的毒性。传统上是从病毒基因组中剔除部分或全部编码区域，留下载体功能所需要的完整基因序列，如将病毒 DNA 包裹到病毒衣壳中或将载体 DNA 整合到宿主染色质中所需要的基因序列。然后将所选择的目的基因表达框克隆到病毒基因骨架中被部分剔除基因的地方。被剔除的编码参与病毒复制或衣壳或包封的蛋白质的蛋白基因，是包含在一个独立的包裹性结构中。然后将载体基因组和包裹性结构共转染到包裹性细胞以产生重组的病毒载体颗粒（图 2-3）。

鉴于涉及基因转移的治疗策略和目标疾病的多样性，已设计出数目如此众多的基因转移载体就不奇怪了。虽然没有一种载体适合所有的基因转移，但是期望所有临床有用的载体都具有某种特性：（1）具有复制和稳定繁殖的能力；（2）能够被纯化和具有较高的滴度；（3）具有介导靶向性基因转移的能力（如避免载体广泛扩散）；（4）可实现基因转移和表达而无毒副作用。目前有五种主要的载体种类至少在一些特殊情况下能够满足这些需要：即致肿瘤 RNA 病毒、慢病毒、腺相关病毒（AVV）、腺病毒和疱疹病毒。表 2-2 对这些载体的总体特性进行了比较。

致肿瘤 RNA 病毒和慢病毒是“整合性”的，也就是说，它们是将其自己的基因组插入到宿主细胞的染色质中。因此，它们具有持续性基因表达的优点。非整合性病毒在未分裂的细胞中可以实现持续性基因表达，但是如果需要维持稳定的遗传性状的改变，在分裂的细胞中，整合性载体是首选的基因转移工具。然而，重要的是要知道，稳定的基因转录不是通过整合来保证的，来自整合的病毒基因组

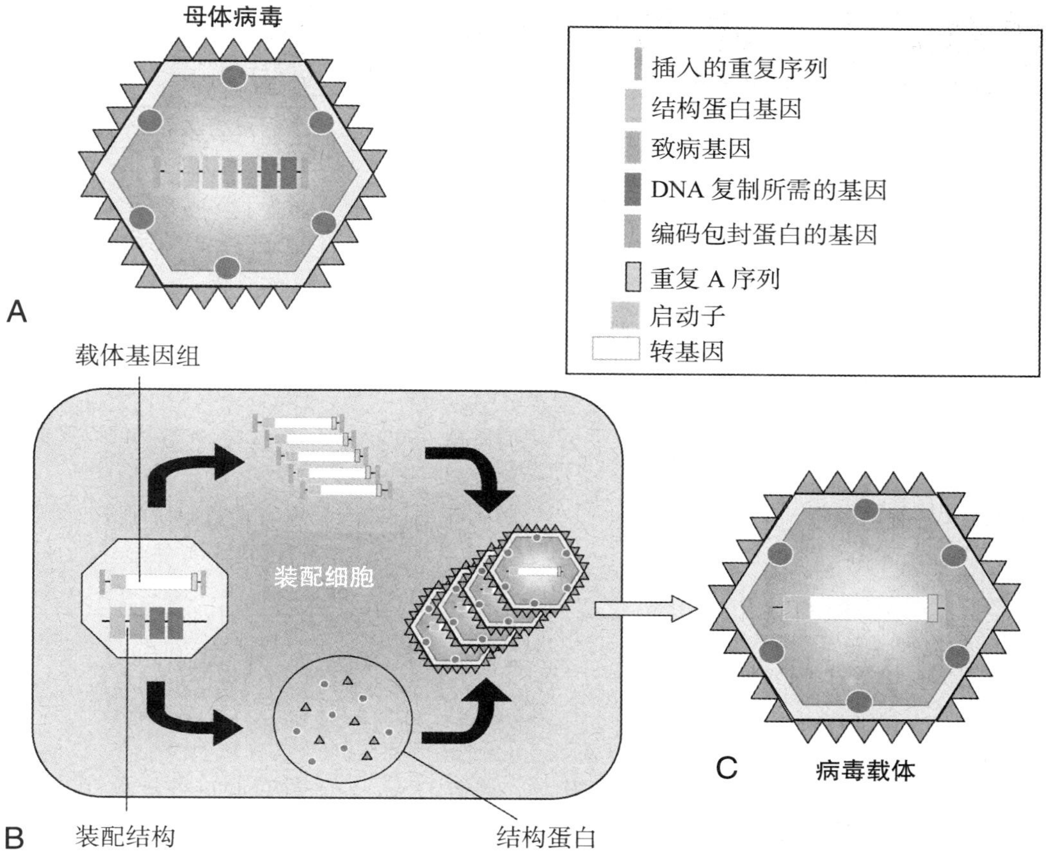

图 2-3　对创建一个遗传学病毒载体的要求。A. 选定的母体病毒所用的基本细胞器包括：编码特异性结构蛋白、包封蛋白和 DNA 复制所需蛋白的基因，但不包括编码致病相关蛋白的基因。B. 病毒载体在装配细胞中进行装配。包装（辅助病毒）结构，包括来源于母体病毒的基因，能够作为一种脂质体或辅助病毒进行转染，或能够稳定地整合进装配细胞的染色质中。致病功能和病毒衣壳化所需的基因序列被剔除出辅助病毒结构，所以不能被装配到病毒颗粒中。相反，病毒载体的基因组包含了转基因表达框，两侧是插入的中止重复序列和 *cis*-作用序列，这些是基因组衣壳化所需的基因序列。病毒结构蛋白和病毒载体 DNA 复制所需的蛋白在装配结构中进行表达，复制的病毒载体基因组被装配到病毒颗粒中。C. 病毒载体颗粒从装配细胞中释放，其中只包含有病毒载体基因组（也见彩图）。

的转基因表达会随着时间的流逝而变得沉默[53]。致肿瘤 RNA 病毒与慢病毒之间的区别在于：穿透完整的细胞核膜的能力。反转录酶病毒只能转导分裂象的细胞，而慢病毒能够自然穿透细胞核膜并转导非分裂象的细胞，使它们在干细胞靶向转基因中显得尤为有用[19,74]。因为有这些差异，在大多数基因转移中，慢病毒载体已取代了反转录酶病毒。因为这两种病毒载体都具有基因组整合能力，所以都有改变
16 宿主细胞基因组的危险。这可能会导致人们不愿意看到的并发症：人类种系改变或插入性基因突变，这些问题在进行儿童或胎儿基因治疗时尤为重要。不过，已经证实这些载体在基因长期转移快速增殖组织的细胞中以及干细胞介导的基因转移中是最为有效的基因转移载体。

非整合性的基因转移载体包括腺病毒载体、腺相关病毒载体（AAV）和疱疹病毒载体。腺病毒载体具有转染谱广泛、病毒包裹能力适中、基因转移高效的优点，但是它们通常也会出现高免疫原性和随之产生的基因表达持续时间较短的缺点。对腺病毒载体的改良是减少免疫原性，进一步增强转染基因的能力，其主要是删除可导致细胞毒性免疫反应的编码免疫原性病毒蛋白的“早期”（E1–E4）病毒基因[3,18]。然而，最重要的进步是发展了辅助病毒依赖型腺病毒载体（HD–Ad），它删除了所有的病毒基因，因此就消除

表 2-2　五种主要的病毒载体组

载体类型	编码物质	装配能力(kb)	组织的取向性	载体基因组	优点	缺点
反转录病毒	RNA	8	只有分裂期细胞	整合型	基因可持久转移到分裂细胞中	需要细胞分裂；可诱导肿瘤生成
慢病毒	RNA	8	广泛，包括干细胞	整合型	可整合进非分裂细胞中；基因可持久转移	潜在的肿瘤生成作用
HSV-1	dsDNA	40	中等	游离型	炎症反应；组织定向性有限	巨大的装配能力；对神经元具有较强的定向性
AAV	ssDNA	<5	广泛	游离型（90%） 整合型（<10%）	无炎症；无致病性	较小的装配能力
腺病毒	dsDNA	8 30*	广泛	游离型	在大多数组织中基因可极有效地转移	衣壳介导的有力的免疫反应；在分裂细胞中短暂表达

* 辅助病毒依赖。

AAV：腺相关病毒；ds：双链；HSV-1：单纯疱疹病毒-1；ss：单链。

了对腺病毒相关蛋白的免疫反应。在基因长期转染极少有细胞分裂的组织时，例如肌肉或脑组织，这些载体可能最终成为最有价值的基因转移载体。

腺相关病毒载体（AAV）是一种辅助病毒依赖型细小病毒，在出现腺病毒或疱疹病毒感染时，AAV就会开始增殖性复制循环。AAV载体是一种单链DNA载体，也是一种在非增殖性组织中实现长期安全基因转移和表达的最有前景的载体系统。AAV是没有已知人类病原性的唯一一种野生型病毒载体系统，因此其基因转染的安全性较高。另外，AAV病毒载体颗粒较小，结构简单，因此全身大剂量应用成为可能。AAV也不会引起急性炎症反应或其他毒性
17 反应。虽然大多数AAV载体基因组经过基因转导以后仍可保持附加型，但是已经发现有接近10%的基因组发生整合[50]。AAV载体的局限性主要有两个。首先是需要将单链DNA基因组转化成双链DNA，而这会限制基因转导的效率。近来这种障碍已经通过研制双链DNA载体得到了克服，即研发了AAV复制循环中的一种发卡状中间体[43]。虽然这些载体在体外和体内实验中能够介导10～100倍的转移基因表达的增加，但是它们只能装载2.4kb的双链DNA，这就限制了其基因治疗的实用性。这与AAV载体的第二个主要局限性有关，这就是有限的装载能力（4.8kb的单链DNA）。一种克服这种局限性的办法是：将基因表达框分开装载到AAV载体中，即利用体内的rAAV基因组的环化连接。在细胞核内这可导致环化连接以后功能性基因框重构[17,49]。最后，一种常用的增强或重新定向AAV载体的组织嗜性的方法是：利用来自另一种血清型AAV病毒的衣壳蛋白来制作转基因载体的假体[58]。虽然大多数的rAAV病毒载体都起源于AAV2病毒，但是迄今为止已经发现了血清型截然不同的8种AAV病毒，这些病毒在特异性细胞类型的基因转导效率上都有所不同。已经证实，AAV病毒载体在肌肉、肝脏和中枢神经系统为靶向的基因转移中尤其有用。

单纯疱疹病毒（HSV-1）载体在目前使用的所有载体系统中是最大最复杂的一种载体。它的主要优势在于它拥有非常大的基因装载能力（40kb）和很强的神经靶向性，在感觉神经元中转移的基因可以实现终身表达。所以HSV-1介导的基因转移的主要目标是神经系统的疾病。

基因转移中临床相关的挑战

近来的不良事件表明，采用病毒载体为基础的基

因转移具有潜在的灾难性后果。必须采取主动的态度去说明采用的特异性病毒载体的基因转移的潜在并发症，以使医生和公众对进一步的临床试验的安全性感到信服。不过，因为病毒载体具有潜在的优点，所以研究人员肯定会不断努力以开发出安全有效的临床基因转移载体。

对成功的基因治疗而言，一个主要的障碍始终是宿主的免疫反应。完整的免疫系统有高度激活能力来对抗病毒载体，使用的是与对抗野生型病毒感染相同的防御系统。病毒产物或新转染基因编码的蛋白可被识别为异物，能够激活不同强度的免疫反应。在所有类型的病毒载体中，腺病毒载体是最具有免疫原性的一种载体，可以诱导多种成分的免疫反应，其中包括细胞毒性 T 淋巴细胞反应，中和病毒的体液免疫反应，以及有效的细胞因子介导的炎症反应[7]。通过开发 HD-Ad 载体来减少拮抗腺病毒抗原的 T 细胞免疫反应已经获得了巨大进展，HD-Ad 载体删去了所有腺病毒的基因。这些载体已显示可降低可矫正小鼠模型的长期表现型的免疫原性，只产生微不足道的毒性[14,34]。然而，即使是 HD-Ad 载体或免疫原性较少的载体系统，如 AAV 或慢病毒载体，也可以针对衣壳蛋白或转基因编码的异常蛋白诱导产生免疫反应，在由无效突变导致的大多数人类蛋白缺陷性疾病中，这是一个潜在的限制性因素。因此，将基因转染技术
18 应用于多种人类疾病时，可能需要开发出有效的无毒性载体系统以避免诱导产生免疫反应。

另一个主要的兴趣点，即有可能促进新的基于病毒载体的基因的转染安全性，是能够特异性靶向治疗受累的组织或器官。野生型病毒感染通常局限于通过传播途径可进入的组织，而重组的病毒载体不会受到同样的生理限制。病毒载体的乱交是一个显著的缺点，因为一种病毒载体的全身或局部应用可导致不希望的病毒载体在多个器官中被多种不同类型的细胞摄取。例如，1999 年发生了 1 例与基因治疗相关的病例死亡，与腺病毒载体缺乏特异性而诱导的全身免疫反应直接相关[7]。因为许多基于病毒载体的基因转染的毒副作用直接与使用的剂量相关，增强病毒载体感染特异性细胞群的效率应该能够减少使用的病毒剂量，从而提高基因治疗的安全性。

现在已经有多种很有前景的方法来实现病毒载体靶向性作用于特异性器官或细胞类型。或许最简单的办法就是病毒载体的假体，其已经被应用于制作反转录病毒、慢病毒和 AAV 病毒载体。通过改变衣壳包裹蛋白来改变病毒的类型或血清型分类，一种具有不同趋化性的病毒载体包皮就能够产生[40]。另一种办法是将衣壳蛋白融合成分子连接器，如具有与特异性受体结合特性的双重特异性抗体[33,61]。第三种办法是通过遗传工程引导衣壳蛋白本身改变它们的受体结合位点（即废除它们的正常受体结合位点），或编码一个小片段的多肽配体来对应另一个受体[28]。这些方法以及其他的办法，当与适当的组织特异性启动子联合使用时，可能会显著降低基于病毒载体的基因治疗产生毒性的可能性。

另一个重要的障碍是：针对人类基因治疗——尤其是胎儿的基因治疗——当使用整合型的病毒载体时，有潜在的产生插入性基因突变的可能。直到最近，这种风险仍被认为非常低，以至于可以忽略不计，这是基于肿瘤产生需要多种遗传病变的假设，以及在许多基因治疗的临床试验中，成百上千例采用反转录病毒载体治疗的病例没有 1 例观察到导致肿瘤发生的事实。然而，近来在另外一个成功的临床试验中[11,25]，11 例因 XSCID 采用反转录病毒载体基因治疗的病例中有 2 例出现了白血病[26]。证据表明，这种情况是由于反转录病毒基因组插入或接近原癌基因 *LMO2* 所致。还有证据表明，反转录病毒的基因并不是随机性插入，如先前所认为的那样，而是选择性地整合到转录活跃的基因中[65]，这些更加重了人们的担心。虽然这些事件更可能是发生在 XSCID 的独特的选择性影响之下，但是很明显插入性突变的风险不能再被忽视。已设计了一些当不良事件发生时可以中和表达转染基因细胞的办法，如诱导自杀基因进入病毒载体就是一种选择，但是这种办法可能也会中和基因治疗的效果。更加令人兴奋的办法是基于位点特异性的整合，例如，吸取噬菌体 ΦX31 的位点整合方法的优点[52]。这种方法毫无疑问只是将来所使用的位点特异性整合的许多办法中的一种，如果获得成功，应该能够忽略插入性基因突变带来的风险。

最后，在处于生殖年龄的人类体内采用整合型病毒载体进行基因转染，其中的一个决定性问题是有可能会使种系产生基因转移而改变人类的基因组。这种事件的风险目前还很难确定，很可能非常低，但是在某些情况下（如胎儿基因转移），这种风险可能会增加[56]。虽然在技术上还没有成为可能，但是目标位点

特异性纠正种系缺陷将会是基因治疗的最终目标。然而，即使技术上成为可能，有目的地去改变人类基因组将会带来深刻的伦理问题和社会问题，在实施这种基因组改变以前需要进行彻底的讨论。这些考虑类似于在插入性基因突变中所面临的问题，对于基因瞄靶和减少潜在性插入性基因突变的风险，先前所提及的许多方法也同样适用。

基因转移目前状况的概述

目前很清楚，病毒载体是将基因有效地转移到绝大多数组织中的最佳转移工具。在早期的临床试验中，数个基因治疗的应用已经显示出很有前景。虽然在 XSCID 试验中提到的不良事件打击了一些研究者的积极性，但是它仍然是通过基因治疗初步成功治愈一种疾病的代表。采用 rAAV 病毒治疗血友病 B 型也非常有前景[32,41]。今后几年，在采用条件复制型溶瘤病毒治疗某种类型的癌症以及采用表达血管生长因子的病毒载体的基因治疗血管和冠状动脉疾病方面将会取得新的进展。将来，通过病毒载体介导的基因转移与其他技术的融合，如 RNA 干扰——一种强有力的实现基因沉默的工具，新的疾病靶向治疗将会变为可能。这些载体将可以用于治疗一大类的疾病，如显性遗传的遗传性疾病、感染性疾病和癌症。随着对病毒载体技术、DNA 进入细胞和细胞核方面的认识的加深，将来有可能出现更加有效的非病毒载体系统，其可能在有效性和较高的安全性方面与病毒载体形成竞争。将来的基因载体系统可能与现在使用的载体有很大的区别，将会最终得到目标特异性、可调节性、转入基因表达持续时间适当且有效的转移基因。

（顾 松 陈 盛译 吴晔明校）

参考文献

1. Acton JD, Wilmott RW: Phenotype of CF and the effects of possible modifier genes. Paediatr Respir Rev 2001;2: 332-339.
2. Amiel J, Lyonnet S: Hirschsprung disease, associated syndromes, and genetics: A review. J Med Genet 2001;38:729-739.
3. Andrews JL, Kadan MJ, Gorziglia MI, et al: Generation and characterization of E1/E2a/E3/E4-deficient adenoviral vectors encoding human factor VIII. Mol Ther 2001;3: 329-336.
4. Angrist M, Kauffman E, Slaugenhaupt SA, et al: A gene for Hirschsprung disease (megacolon) in the pericentromeric region of human chromosome 10. Nat Genet 1993;4: 351-356.
5. Arkwright PD, Laurie S, Super M, et al: TGF-beta(1) genotype and accelerated decline in lung function of patients with cystic fibrosis. Thorax 2000;55:459-462.
6. Aron Y, Polla BS, Bienvenu T, et al: HLA class II polymorphism in cystic fibrosis: A possible modifier of pulmonary phenotype. Am J Respir Crit Care Med 1999;159: 1464-1468.
7. Assessment of adenoviral vector safety and toxicity: Report of the National Institutes of Health Recombinant DNA Advisory Committee. Hum Gene Ther 2002;13:3-13.
8. Badner JA, Sieber WK, Garver KL, Chakravarti A: A genetic study of Hirschsprung disease. Am J Hum Genet 1990;46:568-580.
9. Balci S, Ercal MD, Onol B, et al: Familial short rib syndrome, type Beemer, with pyloric stenosis and short intestine, one case diagnosed prenatally. Clin Genet 1991;39:298-303.
10. Carter CO, Evans KA: Inheritance of congenital pyloric stenosis. J Med Genet 1969;6:233-254.
11. Cavazzana-Calvo M, Hacein-Bey S, de Saint Basile G, et al: Gene therapy of human severe combined immunodeficiency (SCID)-X1 disease. Science 2000;288:669-672.
12. Cekada S, Kilvain S, Brajenovic-Milic B, et al: Partial trisomy 13q22→qter and monosomy 18q21→qter as a result of familial translocation. Acta Paediatr 1999;88:675-678.
13. Chung E, Curtis D, Chen G, et al: Genetic evidence for the neuronal nitric oxide synthase gene (NOS1) as a susceptibility locus for infantile pyloric stenosis. Am J Hum Genet 1996;58:363-370.
14. DelloRusso C, Scott JM, Hartigan-O'Connor D, et al: Functional correction of adult mdx mouse muscle using gutted adenoviral vectors expressing full-length dystrophin. Proc Natl Acad Sci U S A 2002;99:12979-12984.
15. Dipple KM, McCabe ER: Modifier genes convert "simple" mendelian disorders to complex traits. Mol Genet Metab 2000;71:43-50.
16. Drumm ML: Modifier genes and variation in cystic fibrosis. Respir Res 2001;2:125-128.
17. Duan D, Yue Y, Yan Z, Engelhardt JF: A new dual-vector approach to enhance recombinant adeno-associated virus-mediated gene expression through intermolecular cis activation. Nat Med 2000;6:595-598.
18. Feingold E: Regression-based quantitative-trait-locus mapping in the 21st century. Am J Hum Genet 2002;71: 217-222.
19. Follenzi A, Ailles LE, Bakovic S, et al: Gene transfer by lentiviral vectors is limited by nuclear translocation and rescued by HIV-1 pol sequences. Nat Genet 2000;25: 217-222.
20. Gabriel SB, Salomon R, Pelet A, et al: Segregation at three loci explains familial and population risk in Hirschsprung disease. Nat Genet 2002;31:89-93.
21. Garred P, Pressler T, Madsen HO, et al: Association of mannose-binding lectin gene heterogeneity with severity of lung disease and survival in cystic fibrosis. J Clin Invest 1999;104:431-437.

22. Grasemann H, Knauer N, Buscher R, et al: Airway nitric oxide levels in cystic fibrosis patients are related to a polymorphism in the neuronal nitric oxide synthase gene. Am J Respir Crit Care Med 2000;162:2172-2176.
23. Groman JD, Meyer ME, Wilmott RW, et al: Variant cystic fibrosis phenotypes in the absence of CFTR mutations. N Engl J Med 2002;347:401-407.
24. Gupta AK, Berry M: Recessive polycystic kidney disease and congenital hypertrophic pyloric stenosis. Pediatr Radiol 1991;21:160.
25. Hacein-Bey-Abina S, Le Deist F, Carlier F, et al: Sustained correction of X-linked severe combined immunodeficiency by ex vivo gene therapy. N Engl J Med 2002; 346:1185-1193.
26. Hacein-Bey-Abina S, von Kalle C, Schmidt M, et al: A serious adverse event after successful gene therapy for X-linked severe combined immunodeficiency. N Engl J Med 2003;348:255-256.
27. Heller A, Seidel J, Hubler A, et al: Molecular cytogenetic characterisation of partial trisomy 9q in a case with pyloric stenosis and a review. J Med Genet 2000;37: 529-532.
28. Hidaka C, Milano E, Leopold PL, et al: CAR-dependent and CAR-independent pathways of adenovirus vector-mediated gene transfer and expression in human fibroblasts. J Clin Invest 1999;103:579-587.
29. Hodgson SV, Berry AC, Dunbar HM: Two brothers with an unbalanced 8;17 translocation and infantile pyloric stenosis. Clin Genet 1995;48:328-330.
30. Hull J, Thomson AH: Contribution of genetic factors other than CFTR to disease severity in cystic fibrosis. Thorax 1998;53:1018-1021.
31. Kaplan BS, Gordon I, Pincott J, Barratt TM: Familial hypoplastic glomerulocystic kidney disease: A definite entity with dominant inheritance. Am J Med Genet 1989;34:569-573.
32. Kay MA, Manno CS, Ragni MV, et al: Evidence for gene transfer and expression of factor IX in haemophilia B patients treated with an AAV vector. Nat Genet 2000; 24:257-261.
33. Khare PD, Liao S, Hirose Y, et al: Tumor growth suppression by a retroviral vector displaying scFv antibody to CEA and carrying the iNOS gene. Anticancer Res 2002;22: 2443-2446.
34. Kim IH, Jozkowicz A, Piedra PA, et al: Lifetime correction of genetic deficiency in mice with a single injection of helper-dependent adenoviral vector. Proc Natl Acad Sci U S A 2001;98:13282-13287.
35. Konig R, Fuchs S, Kern C, Langenbeck U: Simpson-Golabi-Behmel syndrome with severe cardiac arrhythmias. Am J Med Genet 1991;38:244-247.
36. Krantz ID, McCallum J, DeScipio C, et al: Cornelia de Lange syndrome is caused by mutations in NIPBL, the human homolog of *Drosophila melanogaster* Nipped-B. Nat Genet 2004;36:631-635.
37. Liede A, Pal T, Mitchell M, Narod SA: Delineation of a new syndrome: Clustering of pyloric stenosis, endometriosis, and breast cancer in two families. J Med Genet 2000; 37:794-796.
38. Lusky M, Christ M, Rittner K, et al: In vitro and in vivo biology of recombinant adenovirus vectors with E1, E1/E2A, or E1/E4 deleted. J Virol 1998;72:2022-2032.
39. Lyonnet S, Bolino A, Pelet A, et al: A gene for Hirschsprung disease maps to the proximal long arm of chromosome 10. Nat Genet 1993;4:346-350.
40. MacKenzie TC, Kobinger GP, Kootstra NA, et al: Efficient transduction of liver and muscle after in utero injection of lentiviral vectors with different pseudotypes. Mol Ther 2002;6:349-358.
41. Manno CS, Chew AJ, Hutchison S, et al: AAV-mediated factor IX gene transfer to skeletal muscle in patients with severe hemophilia B. Blood 2003;101:2963-2972.
42. Martucciello G, Torre M, Pini Prato A, et al: Associated anomalies in intestinal neuronal dysplasia. J Pediatr Surg 2002;37:219-223.
43. McCarty DM, Monahan PE, Samulski RJ: Self-complementary recombinant adeno-associated virus (scAAV) vectors promote efficient transduction independently of DNA synthesis. Gene Ther 2001;8:1248-1254.
44. McKusick VA: Mendelian Inheritance in Man: A Catalog of Human Genes and Genetic Disorders, 12th ed. Baltimore, Johns Hopkins University Press, 1998.
45. Mickle JE, Cutting GR: Genotype-phenotype relationships in cystic fibrosis. Med Clin North Am 2000;84:597-607.
46. Mitchell LE, Risch N: The genetics of infantile hypertrophic pyloric stenosis: A reanalysis. Am J Dis Child 1993;147:1203-1211.
47. Moore JH, Williams SM: New strategies for identifying gene-gene interactions in hypertension. Ann Med 2002; 34:88-95.
48. Morsy MA, Caskey CT: Expanded-capacity adenoviral vectors—the helper-dependent vectors. Mol Med Today 1999;5:18-24.
49. Nakai H, Storm TA, Kay MA: Increasing the size of rAAV-mediated expression cassettes in vivo by intermolecular joining of two complementary vectors. Nat Biotechnol 2000;18:527-532.
50. Nakai H, Yant SR, Storm TA, et al: Extrachromosomal recombinant adeno-associated virus vector genomes are primarily responsible for stable liver transduction in vivo. J Virol 2001;75:6969-6976.
51. Ohshiro K, Puri P: Pathogenesis of infantile hypertrophic pyloric stenosis: Recent progress. Pediatr Surg Int 1998;13:243-252.
52. Olivares EC, Hollis RP, Chalberg TW, et al: Site-specific genomic integration produces therapeutic factor IX levels in mice. Nat Biotechnol 2002;20:1124-1128.
53. Pannell D, Osborne CS, Yao S, et al: Retrovirus vector silencing is de novo methylase independent and marked by a repressive histone code. EMBO J 2000;19:5884-5894.
54. Parisi MA, Kapur RP: Genetics of Hirschsprung disease. Curr Opin Pediatr 2000;12:610-617.
55. Parmley RR, Gendler SJ: Cystic fibrosis mice lacking Muc1 have reduced amounts of intestinal mucus. J Clin Invest 1998;102:1798-1806.
56. Prenatal gene transfer: Scientific, medical, and ethical issues: A report of the Recombinant DNA Advisory Committee. Hum Gene Ther 2000;11:1211-1229.
57. Puffenberger EG, Hosoda K, Washington SS, et al: A missense mutation of the endothelin-B receptor gene in multigenic Hirschsprung's disease. Cell 1994;79:1257-1266.
58. Rabinowitz JE, Rolling F, Li C, et al: Cross-packaging of a single adeno-associated virus (AAV) type 2 vector genome into multiple AAV serotypes enables transduction with broad specificity. J Virol 2002;76:791-801.
59. Ramirez-Gomara A, Castejon-Ponce E, Martinez-Martinez M, et al: [Smith-Lemli-Opitz syndrome type II: Neonatal diagnosis and review of the most interesting clinical features]. Rev Neurol 2002;34:946-950.

60. Repetto GM, Wagstaff J, Korf BR, Knoll JH: Complex familial rearrangement of chromosome 9p24.3 detected by FISH. Am J Med Genet 1998;76:306-309.
61. Reynolds PN, Nicklin SA, Kaliberova L, et al: Combined transductional and transcriptional targeting improves the specificity of transgene expression in vivo. Nat Biotechnol 2001;19:838-842.
62. Riordan JR, Rommens JM, Kerem B, et al: Identification of the cystic fibrosis gene: Cloning and characterization of complementary DNA. Science 1989;245:1066-1073.
63. Rozmahel R, Wilschanski M, Matin A, et al: Modulation of disease severity in cystic fibrosis transmembrane conductance regulator deficient mice by a secondary genetic factor. Nat Genet 1996;12:280-287.
64. Russell MB, Russell CA, Niebuhr E: An epidemiological study of Hirschsprung's disease and additional anomalies. Acta Paediatr 1994;83:68-71.
65. Schroder AR, Shinn P, Chen H, et al: HIV-1 integration in the human genome favors active genes and local hotspots. Cell 2002;110:521-529.
66. Scriver CR, Waters PJ: Monogenic traits are not simple: Lessons from phenylketonuria. Trends Genet 1999;15: 267-272.
67. Sponseller PD, Sethi N, Cameron DE, Pyeritz RE: Infantile scoliosis in Marfan syndrome. Spine 1997;22:509-516.
68. Tsui LC, Buchwald M, Barker D, et al: Cystic fibrosis locus defined by a genetically linked polymorphic DNA marker. Science 1985;230:1054-1057.
69. Wang X, Moylan B, Leopold DA, et al: Mutation in the gene responsible for cystic fibrosis and predisposition to chronic rhinosinusitis in the general population. JAMA 2000;284:1814-1819.
70. Webb AL, Sturgiss S, Warwicker P, et al: Maternal uniparental disomy for chromosome 2 in association with confined placental mosaicism for trisomy 2 and severe intrauterine growth retardation. Prenat Diagn 1996;16: 958-962.
71. Weiss KM: Is there a paradigm shift in genetics? Lessons from the study of human diseases. Mol Phylogenet Evol 1996;5:259-265.
72. Yamamoto Y, Oguro N, Nara T, et al: Duplication of part of 9q due to maternal 12;9 inverted insertion associated with pyloric stenosis. Am J Med Genet 1988;31:379-384.
73. Zielenski J, Corey M, Rozmahel R, et al: Detection of a cystic fibrosis modifier locus for meconium ileus on human chromosome 19q13. Nat Genet 1999;22:128-129.
74. Zufferey R, Nagy D, Mandel RJ, et al: Multiply attenuated lentiviral vector achieves efficient gene delivery in vivo. Nat Biotechnol 1997;15:871-875.

第 3 章

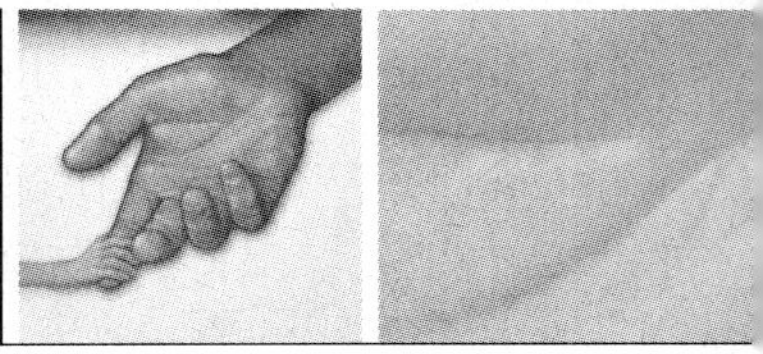

组织工程对小儿外科学的影响

Tracy C. Grikschei　和　Joseph P. Vacanti

21 摘除手术经常需要重建而使切除组织的功能和形态得到替代。在先天性畸形中，组织缺如本身可能就存在。组织工程和器官构建的目的是创建有活力的器官和组织替代物，使之能够更精确地替代并具有更好的与细胞增殖和自体修复相对应的耐用性优点。这些技术已开始从实验室应用向手术室过渡，从而可为患有先天性畸形或器官组织切除的患者提供更好的具有一定外观和功能的替代物。

早期外科医生开始尝试的功能替代术或美容术包括在公元前 6 世纪左右 Sushruta Samhita 中详细记录的内容，其中描述了采用前额皮瓣的鼻成形术，以及在 Talmud 中提到的各种木质和金属假体替代法。这些方法一直延续到现代并已取得很多发展，多种手术要么依赖组织替代，如用足趾替代手指的换位，要么采用人造替代物，如涤纶主动脉移植物。天然替代物的局限在于：很难分清不同组织的优先次序且必须进行替换。在小儿外科领域，供体组织相当有限，且与被替代组织存在差异。人造替代物亦存在已知的问题：材料匮乏、感染率增加和外来材料对免疫系统的破坏。此外，无活力的材料不能与患者一同生长或适应环境变化，所以儿科患者可能需要经历多次越来越复杂的手术。没有一种方法可以解决复合组织的替代问题。

器官移植，作为一种天然组织替代的现代手段，已经证实功能替代可以挽救生命，但是存在供体有限和发生多种相关并发症的障碍。

在小儿外科领域，组织器官替代手术的复兴尤其受到关注，手术结果可以在几十年后进行评价，并且外科重建具有更好的活力和生理变化适应力。另外，在一些先天性畸形中，可提供的供体器官数量不足，且假体材料不能满足与失去器官相近的功能和美容需要，包括生长发育的需要。

短肠综合征、颅面缺损和先天性心脏病患儿的外科治疗问题迫切需要解决。组织工程皮肤和软骨已用于人类。我们盼望在血管、小肠和实体器官的替代方面取得有意义的进展，这些被证实是进行复制的最精致的系统。

组织工程技术与原理

单层细胞培养是一个定义明确的科学，但是使细胞组织连接成复杂的具有功能的三维结构则依赖于细胞结构和会聚在结构上的细胞之间的众多联系。在限定了细胞成分和工程器官的结构之外，足够的血管化和在正常组织中指导细胞信号传导的产生是最大的挑战。

组织工程构建的多种方法可以概括为体内法和体外法。所有方法均尝试采用细胞的支持物或支架——合适的细胞群和细胞外基质替代物。细胞和细胞外基质之间的相互作用需要细胞迁移、增殖、分化和凋亡，所有这些对组织工程结构而言都是关键[60]。

体外模型构建通常依赖一个生物反应器系统或单
层细胞共培养研究中的细胞模式[20,42,58,101]。生物反应器 22
是动态的组织培养装置，其种类从简单的机械设计到更复杂的具有氧气交换、精确的流速和电机械刺激系统。组织工程构建复杂性小的组织，如细胞片，仅需对工程结构进行培养液交换以免生长停滞的简单方法。旋转培养瓶或容器也是一些简单的方法[22]。

更加复杂的生物反应器被设计为可提供一定张力用于骨骼肌培养[94]，一定剪切力用于内皮细胞的培养[96]，以及一定压力用于软骨细胞的培养[12]。有良好的结果显示，在拉伸状态和周围细胞营养液流动的生理条件下，细胞多聚体结构体外生长与体内结果接近，细胞形态生长特点得到改善，代谢活动得到提高[55,68,81]。对生长在聚羟基乙酸结构上的软骨细胞施以流体压力培养的研究显示，细胞增殖率几乎超过 50%，氨基葡聚糖产生增加 60%，细胞外基质中胶原产生增加 125%[4,32]。

其他用于组织工程的体外模型还包括在单层或三维培养中的细胞模式。确定的组织结构可产生更可预测的生长和分化模式。在更复杂的器官构建中，如在肝脏中，组织特异性培养液共培养将成为成功设计的必要条件[5]。影印石刻技术已经用于将 N-（2-氨乙基）-3-氨丙基-三甲氧基硅烷和二甲基二氯硅烷的结构域进行替换，可通过玻璃体结合蛋白介导优先将人类骨源性细胞种植在前者的结构域中[58]。高溶解型聚左旋赖氨酸已应用于微米尺度的微接触印刷术中，通过特异的寡肽微接触印刷技术[101]黏附培养的神经元可使其得到排列[42]。细胞伸展限制和非随机共培养技术可更接近人类组织的三维结构的复制[58]。结构地形信息可能同一些生物信号一样重要。

微加工工程学与对体外组织培养系统的改良的交叉显示具有良好的前景，可产生更小、更智能的生物反应器。在这种反应器中，微流体学、质量转移、营养摄取和细胞生长都可以与已知的细胞结构一起研究，并在微米尺度进行标准化微加工。正像在后面肝组织工程部分中描述的那样，这种方法对复杂器官的构建是至关重要的。

体内研究将动物作为复杂的生物反应器，将复合结构植入血管化的空间，如大网膜、系膜、肩胛间的脂肪垫或背阔肌处，这些地方内源性血供可以参与血管生成[93]。支架以细胞外基质替代物的形式载入细胞后被植入[52]。多聚体海绵在载入细胞前植入数天或数周进行预血管化可以提高细胞的存活率[87]。

在一种较早期的体内模型中，肝、小肠和胰腺实质细胞体外培养 4 天后被种植在可降解的生物聚合体上可产生有活力的细胞，可见有丝分裂象和生长细胞团的血管化[93]。在这个研究中用的一种聚合体是聚羟基乙酸和聚乳酸的一种 90∶10 比例的共聚物，商品名为 Vicryl。随着可供生物材料的最新成果的不断涌现，研究者们成功地使用了不断增加的各类支架，包括小肠黏膜下层，后者可作为小口径静脉移植体与肝细胞移植一起吻合在门静脉和上腔静脉之间[49]。此外藻酸钙胶、市售表面活性剂、琼脂糖、纤维蛋白胶和微加工生物可降解材料的成功应用显示了化学和组织工程学之间的合作的必要性[1,35,36,95]。

体内和体外方法的结合已经使一些简单组织的构建问题得到解决，且将继续在自体组织切除、实验室中扩增并最终在体内替代方面继续起重要作用。

软骨和骨组织工程

小儿外科医生面临着许多以先天性和后天性结构缺损为特征的问题。一些开拓性的治疗已经使原位组织工程得到应用，如采用牵拉骨生成技术之后进行骨移植来治疗 Treacher Collins 综合征[57]。在 20 世纪 60 年代，Tessier 开展了广泛游离大段颅骨和眼睛易位来治疗 Apert 和 Crouzon 综合征[83]。

为了支持这些前沿的方法，已寻求通过组织工程来生产大量的骨和软骨。这开始于观察到：从关节软骨面获取的软骨细胞可在培养中形成软骨，而从骨膜获取的软骨细胞在培养中最初可形成类似的软骨，而随着发展最后可形成新骨[92]。

相对简单的软骨组织在破坏之后有一定限度的自我再生能力[24,26,59]。大多数关节软骨缺损是通过纤维软骨组织形成进行修复，与自体软骨相比，其有不同的生物化学和生物力学特点[39]。修复不全可以产生骨关节疼痛和功能降低[18]。1988 年，Vacanti 等人将牛软骨细胞种植在多聚体支架上产生了新生透明软骨[90]。

在随后的研究中，采用非编织聚羟基乙酸网眼或聚羟基乙酸和聚乳酸共聚物制成了按预先决定的形状进行的构建[90]。利用此方法在人耳[88]和颞下颌关节盘[66]形状的支架上可产生软骨，用同样的方法将软骨塑形成特殊形状可用于替代撕裂的半月板关节软骨[38]。组织工程软骨已经可以作为一个组织结构用于重建猪的乳头[14]和关闭动物的颅骨缺损[53]。软骨管内衬呼吸道上皮结构已经产生，可作为气管替代物植入体内，3 周时一些上皮细胞中可见纤毛形成[69]。

骨组织工程起源于软骨组织工程，是将牛骨膜细
胞种植在聚羟基乙酸支架上植入无胸腺小鼠体内。这 23
些植入物经降钙素染色后进行显微镜下评估可显示局灶样骨形成。然后将这些植入的结构用于修补裸大鼠的顶骨、额骨和颞骨缺损；采用未种植细胞的多聚体作为对照[89]。在采用组织工程构造物修补组中可以观察到骨修复现象，而在对照组中骨缺损没有改变。该技术也已被用于股骨干缺损的修复中，是将股骨干与

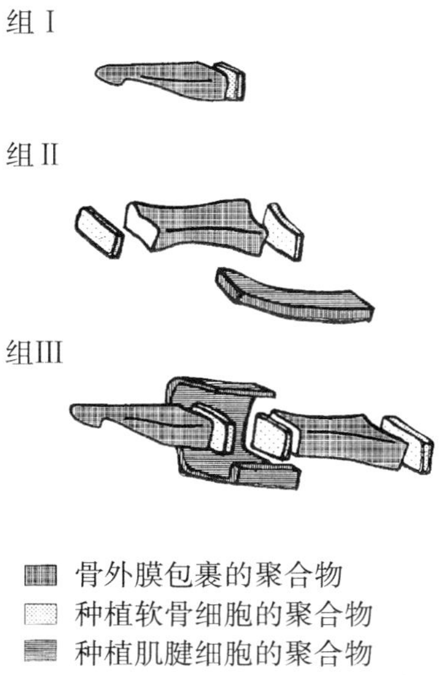

图 3-1 三种不同类型的组织结构成分组成了一个组织工程手指。通过缝合创建有一个末节指骨（组 I）、一个中节指骨（组 II）和一个远端指间关节（组III）的模型，在体外进行结构构建。然后将缝合的组织植入无胸腺小鼠皮下。（From Isogai N, Landis W, Kim TH, et al: Formation of phalanges and small joints by tissue-engineering. J Bone Joint Surg Am 1999;81: 306-316.）

托板一起固定以维持一个关键的间隙。在对照组中可见骨不连接，而在组织工程组中可见大量生长旺盛的骨痂形成。

骨和软骨组织工程相结合已用于构建手指的替代物[41]。牛的三种类型细胞——骨膜细胞、软骨细胞和肌腱细胞——被种植在聚羟基乙酸和左旋聚乳酸共聚体上，形成一个类似关节的合成组织（图 3-1）。各部件以远端指骨、中间指骨和远端指间关节的形式被组装缝合在一起。然后将这个组装体植入无胸腺小鼠皮下。在 20 周时，得到一个带有关节的具有人指外形和组织学的手指，具有成熟的关节软骨、软骨下骨和腱鞘。骨和软骨组织工程在关节重建中具有很好的前景，尤其是儿童矫形外科医生必须纠正的复杂先天性畸形。

心血管组织工程

在美国，每年每 1000 个活产儿中有 5～8 例先天性心脏畸形患儿，包括瓣膜异常[17]。小儿外科治疗先天性心脏病通常需要非自体血管或瓣膜[56,71]。20 世纪 60 年代早期，40%以上的瓣膜替代物是用戊二醛保存的牛或猪的组织[71]。组织瓣膜替代物可避免机械瓣膜的问题，包括全身性血栓栓塞[21]，但由于假体相关问题，包括结构性和非结构性功能丧失、进行性损毁变形（钙化和非钙化）以及感染，仍然有 50%～60%的再手术率[21,33]。另外，大多数常见的用于替代的组织瓣膜由于进行性损毁均有限定的耐用年限[71]。

完美的瓣膜替代物应该是不会引起梗死、血栓形成并可在患者体内生长的可以自我修复的组织，并且可以对体内刺激产生应答而重新塑形[71]。这些标准自从 1962 年 Harken 等人最初概括之后一直没有改变过[34]。一期修复对于儿科患者来说是难能可贵的，目前他们一生中需要进行多次手术。

通过传统的组织工程方法已经制成了组织工程心脏瓣膜。开始是将种子细胞种植在脱细胞的异种来源的瓣膜支架上，后来发展成将种子细胞种植在尺寸合适的单纯多聚体铸模上[2,62,72]。在初期研究中，是将人类大隐静脉的内皮细胞种植在猪的主动脉瓣膜上，采用 Triton 去污剂去除瓣膜上的自体细胞，保留细胞外基质用于对种植细胞的支持[2]。作为肺动脉的替代物植入绵羊体内后，瓣膜具有血流动力学功能，取材时显示没有钙化形成[2]。采用来自不同的瓣叶和导管的生物假体复合物得到了相似的结果，在种植细胞前将它们再脱细胞化[62]。

将一个多聚体支架工程化而不是破坏一个已存在瓣膜的细胞和再注入细胞，是获得一个有生命力的瓣膜的关键，这样后者才可能生长。当自体细胞群种植在多聚体支架时，随着支架降解，细胞也可分泌细胞外基质来维持机械张力[76]。最初的研究采用聚羟基乙酸支架种植绵羊内皮细胞和肌纤维母细胞，在去除绵羊自体肺动脉瓣的右后瓣叶后植入，结果没有狭窄产生，且具有合适的细胞结构和基质形成[72]。当时植入的细胞用细胞标志物标记，结果显示瓣叶胶原含量增加了，弹力蛋白也增加了，最初的细胞持续存活，并且心电图描记证明其具有瓣膜功能[10]。

加入机械生物反应器可增加工程化瓣膜的应力并可促进多聚体支架的改良（聚羟基脂肪酸酯），可使肺动脉瓣反流降低到最低限度，无血栓形成，瓣膜具有分层的纤维组织，以及细胞外基质增加[76]。工程化瓣膜在体内接近收缩期压力的机械应力下生长可超过 5 个月[77]，在基质形成、组织学和生物机械性能方面与天然瓣膜相似。

虽然组织工程瓣膜已经符合部分 Harken 标准，
24 与宿主一同生长的关键能力可能也已符合标准，但瓣膜仍需检测并能在主动脉部位应用成功，因为主动脉部位最常患病，最常被研究和进行瓣膜替代[71]。

血管组织工程

除了瓣膜修复，提供足够的血管管道是治疗儿童先天性心脏病的第二个关键因素，因此自体血管移植或假体材料替代得到了应用。这些替代物由于不能生长，可因钙化和生长停滞而功能退化，需要进行多次手术替代。越小的血管，如直径小于 6mm 的血管，不能通过纺织物或聚四氟乙烯（PTFE）得到满意的构建，必须通过自体动脉或静脉架桥替代，由于血供有限，需要多次手术[86]。

鉴于这些缺点，组织工程被作为一个逻辑策略方法应用于构建大小血管的替代物。2001 年 2 月，Shin'oka 等报道了首例用于一位 4 岁女孩的人类组织工程化血管（图 3–2），之前在 3 岁 3 个月时，她曾因为右心室和肺动脉闭锁经历了 Fontan 手术和肺动脉血管成形术[73]。随后的血管造影显示其右肺动脉中段完全闭塞。一个长 2cm 的自体外周静脉被获取，其分离细胞经 8 周体外培养扩增为 12×10^6 个细胞。聚已酸内酯和聚乳酸的 1∶1 共聚物塑形编织的聚羟基乙酸管作为支架种植细胞，种植后 10 天植入以重建闭塞的肺动脉。7 个月后随访没有发现并发症。

组织工程血管构建始于 1978 年，其时 Herring 成功地从静脉中分离出内皮细胞，并将它们种植到合成支架上[98]。几位科学家通过改变种植方法、支架构成和培养条件，改良了构建组织的功能和结构。1998 年 Shin'oka 等培养了与人类替代物培养条件相似的羊的动脉和静脉内皮细胞，用于替代羊羔 2cm 长的肺动脉[74]。无细胞对照有血栓形成，而组织工程化的组织有内皮层、胶原和弹力蛋白腔，植入后没有血栓形成[74]。同样，将羊静脉细胞种植在不同多聚体（聚羟基丁酸）上并缝合在肺动脉上进行补片扩大，结果蛋白多糖、弹力蛋白和胶原增加，且动脉保持通畅[78]。聚羟基脂肪酸酯和聚羟基乙酸共聚物种植羊主动脉细胞也产生了管腔持续开放的移植物，且机械张力应力曲线开始随时间推移接近自体血管[75]。

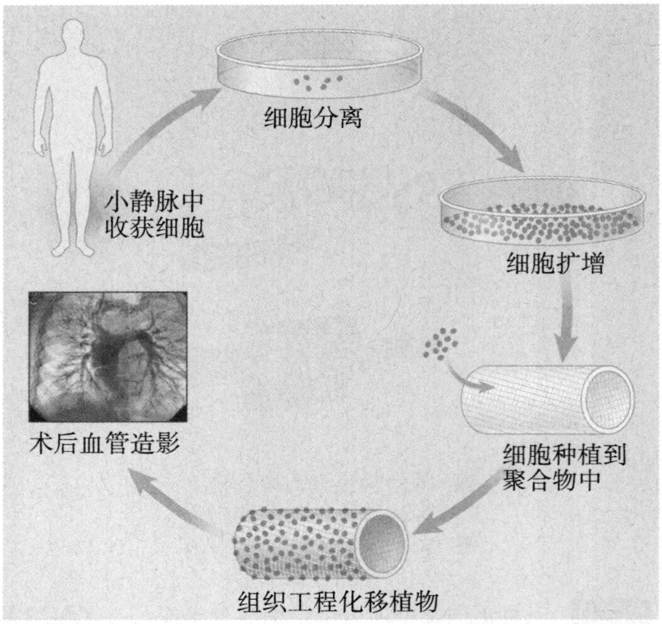

图 3–2　基本的组织工程技术。细胞取自自体静脉，分离后进行体外扩增并种植在生物可降解聚合物支架上，以形成组织工程肺动脉，随后植入一位儿童体内，结果良好。（From Shin'oka T, Imai Y, Ikada Y: Transplantation of a tissue engineered pulmonary artery [letter to the editor]. N Engl J Med 2001;344:532-533.）

提高血管的张力、存活能力和耐久力很可能可以促进细胞之间和细胞与支架间的相互作用，导致包括细胞外基质、腔内表面覆盖平滑的内皮细胞以及胶原和弹力蛋白纤维在内的结构的再生。应用包含有多细胞类型的组织碎片种植在支架上，包括骨髓细胞，据报道可加速移植物的愈合和预防内膜的过度增生[61]。同样，在多聚体材料特性方面的改进已提高了血管发育的速度和质量[75,100]。

肠管组织工程

与疾病相关的肠管切除后，短肠综合征是最严重的后遗症。该综合征的特点为进行性体重下降、营养不良、维生素缺乏和由于经常通过血管途径进行支持而导致的患者感染[99]。典型的短肠综合征发生于由于大量切除或多种肠道疾病予以手术治疗后肠管存留少于三分之一的患者，尽管有一些革新的手术用于治疗该综合征以促进肠黏膜生长[65,97]，包括肠管移植[13]、肠袢反向术[19]、循环肠袢术[84]和裁剪延长术，但仍没有完美的手术治疗方法。肠移植已经取得一些初步的成功，但还没有广泛应用。组织工程小肠构建的最初研究包括自体浆膜层补片或蒂血管化，结果喜忧参半[7,51,54]。组织工程小肠构建还试验了包含聚合物、异体真皮无细胞基质（AlloDerm）和小肠黏膜下层（SIS）（肠黏膜下层胶原肠组织）在内的补片[3,15,40]。
25 在构建与自体肠腔连接之前，在以肠管替代为目标方面，组织工程方法提供了一个具有吸引力的替代物。

组织工程肠管构建始于将胎儿小肠移植到多聚体支架上观察到增殖和小肠形态形成[93]。组织工程构建肠管产品已经从单纯的大鼠小肠模型扩展到胃、胃食管连接、食管和结肠（图 3-3 和 3-4）[27-29,31]。1998 年首次报道了类器官单位的异位移植肠细胞产生了与小肠结构相似的组织[16]。类器官单位是从全层肠壁中获取，在差异离心前通过手术分离、酶消化和研碎而纯化。上述步骤之后的产物——类器官单位——在植入大网膜前被载入 2mm 厚的、其外包被聚乳酸的非编织聚羟基乙酸圆柱状多聚物中。尽管植入的多聚物最初肯定处于低氧状态，但仍有血管生成。工程化的肠管表现为上皮细胞朝向囊腔内面极化生长，包括肌肉和神经。伴随生长有实质性的血管化[16]。

将组织工程化的小肠与切除 75%的小肠的雄性 Lewis 大鼠自体空肠吻合后长期随访显示，其体重增加、肠腔通畅，并且组织工程化小肠的尺寸统计学上明显增加[45,48]。用于救治小肠大量切除时，采用组织工程小肠替代治疗的动物体重增长速度更快，可达到它们术前的体重；没有采用组织工程小肠替代的动物没有得到纠治[30]。吻合后的小肠免疫系统研究显示，新生黏膜免疫细胞群对暴露于肠腔抗原和获取时间具

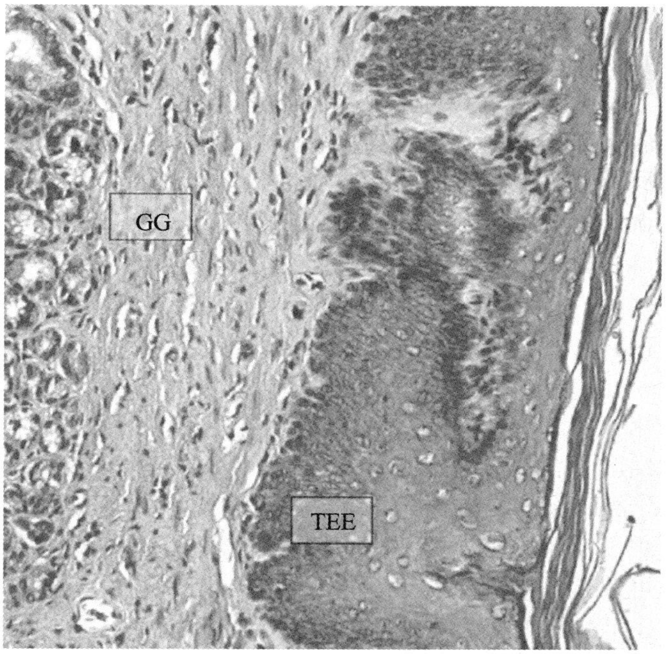

图 3-3 在胃食管连接部的组织工程食管（TEE），工程化的食管（EE）与具有胃腺（GG）的自体胃紧密接触。（From Grikscheit T, Ochoa ER, Srinivasan A, et al: Tissue-engineered esophagus: Experimental substitution by onlay patch or interposition. J Thorac Cardiovasc Surg 2003;126:537-544.）

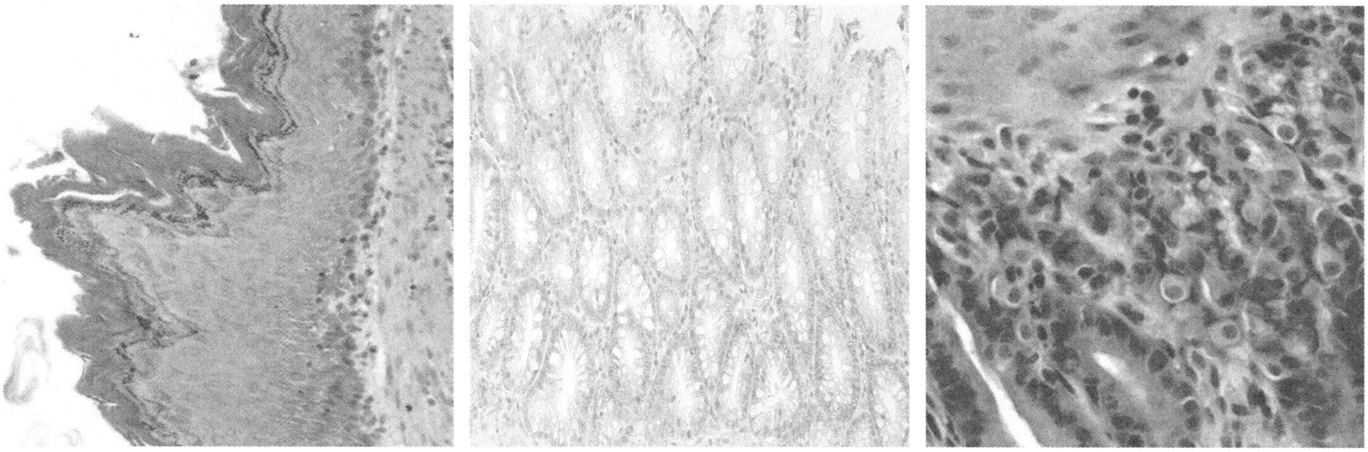

A　B　C

图 3-4 组织工程 Lewis 大鼠模型。A. 组织工程食管(原始放大 20 倍)。B. 组织工程结肠（原始放大 20 倍）。C. 组织工程胃。可见大的半透明壁细胞和腺体结构。（Courtesy of Dr. T. Grikscheit.）

有一定功能[64]。吻合后 20 周获取的组织工程化小肠黏膜其免疫细胞亚群的密度和分布与正常空肠一致。上皮 SGLT1（一种肠钠-葡萄糖协同转运蛋白）的 mRNA 表达在吻合后的组织工程小肠壁内也可探及。同样，一种铁转运蛋白 DCT1 的表达也可探及。但是血管上皮生长因子和碱性纤维母细胞生长因子水平与自体肠管水平相比有差异[25,82]。这些转运体的分布类
26 型显示，工程化的小肠可重复自体空肠的分布类型，提示这种管腔样物对缺乏小肠的患者具有治疗潜力。

随着器官样单位组织工程肠管构建方法的精细化，大量具有更大表面积的肠管被构建，并且工程化结肠、胃及食管已可构建（见图 3-3）[30]。超过 20 倍植入聚合物体积的组织工程肠管已可生成[27,30]。组织工程化结肠作为替代物植入 Lewis 大鼠体内 41天可具有功能，可维持钠平衡、液体吸收、生成粪便中短链脂肪酸及延长肠道通过时间，并且结构上包括神经节细胞和真正的结肠组织学特征[27,29]。在初步研究中，组织工程食管已经应用，或作为补片或作为间置物移植入大鼠体内（参见图 3-3）[28]。在组织工程胃构建中，精确替代的思想得到扩展，一系列研究显示，组织工程化的胃食管连接部可以进行构建，胃窦部也可以进行构建，并且不论年轻的或年老的大鼠，都可以作为自体的供体[31]。对胃泌素进行的适当组织染色显示，壁细胞可具有精确的类似自体胃的结构。组织工程胃可以用病毒蛋白（绿色荧光蛋白）标记以进行随后的鉴定，由此打开了未来对“设计小肠”的转染之门；如组织工程结肠可用于转染 SGLT1 使其可以吸收糖类[31]。

工程化肠管替代物对许多危重儿外科疾病的治疗都很重要，在未来的十年中，随着表面积的增加、转运功能的提高、免疫特点和结构的改进，其对患者的治疗会产生重大影响。随着小量的组织工程小肠和胃合为一体的成功生长，一些实验室已开始大动物的实验研究。

肝替代物和组织工程

肝是一个必不可少的复杂器官，可提供重要功能，包括代谢、分泌、解毒、贮存和吞噬作用。在美国，每年因急性或慢性肝功能障碍导致整体器官衰竭而死亡的人数达到 3 万，急性衰竭的死亡率超过 80% [85]。在美国，慢性肝衰竭是导致死亡的第六大原因，在重大疾病经济花费中列第八位。目前严重肝衰竭的唯一的确定性治疗是原位肝移植，该手术每年开展 3000 例。组织工程构建肝脏作为替代物的尝试包括：细胞直接注射或聚合物支架种植，用或不用肝营养因子刺激；体外生物人工肝（BAL）装置的发展；以及新的用于体内的三维微结构的构建。

肝组织工程构建最初始于细胞移植，即当选择的细胞群替代物可以治疗肝功能不全时观察到，原位肝移植可能是不必要的[68]。独创性的肝脏再生使肝细胞移植的思想更具有吸引力。

在早期研究中，当将肝细胞注入缺乏尿苷二磷酸葡萄糖醛酸转移酶的 Gunn 大鼠的门静脉时，与注射盐水的对照动物相比，这些移植细胞可维持较低的胆红素水平[55]。用二乙基亚硝胺诱导肝衰竭后，肝细胞被注入门静脉或腹腔[81]。与对照组大鼠相比，接受肝细胞注射的大鼠生存期明显延长。在几个将肝细胞注入脾、胰腺和腹腔的研究中也注意到，肝功能可以维持并肝细胞可迁移。将带有乙肝病毒表面抗原的肝细胞异位植入，可观察到表面抗原迁移至胰腺、肺和脾，同时肝功能可维持[32]。这种方法的局限性在于：随着移植时间的推移，注入细胞维持整体肝功能的能力降低。细胞迁移和损耗可导致肝细胞团分离而不能维持肝功能。

组织工程构建肝团块可通过肝营养因子刺激和促进细胞分泌而增加体积。肝营养因子刺激，存在于接受组织工程肝脏治疗的肝功能衰竭患者中，可通过部分肝切除、门腔分流手术以及肝毒素注射再现。众所周知，肝切除后剩余肝可在多种生长因子刺激下迅速增殖，其中包括表皮生长因子、肝细胞生长因子、胰岛素和胰高血糖素[11]。当组织工程构建物被植入肠系膜或大网膜内时，这些因子在门静脉血流中的含量增加可引起移植物宿主动物体内门腔分流的形成，给予移植物丰富的营养因子供应。当将组织工程肝移植入动物体内时行部分肝切除和门腔分流术，可导致移植肝细胞增殖增加，细胞存活时间延长，组织形成更佳，并且在 Gunn 大鼠体内胆红素清除率升高[46,70,87]。

细胞移植，即使有最大限度的肝营养因子刺激，仍不能提供足够的可使暴发性肝衰竭患者的血浆得以解毒的肝细胞团。因此，一种组织工程肝脏提供了一种临时的生物人工肝，就是体外 BAL 设备，或者是

近期的微型预制体内装置。体外生物人工肝的目标是作为向肝移植过渡的桥梁，目的是降低术后发病率和死亡率[79]，并对急性肝功能衰竭患者等待肝脏再生时给予支持，或对合并有肝功能衰竭不适于做肝移植的患者提供支持。

在组织工程化支架-细胞复合体中，大鼠、猪或人来源的肝细胞株实验模型已经用于急性重型肝炎患者血液的解毒[43,80]。在一种已经用于人类肝衰竭患者试验的装置，在透析膜上与胶原覆盖的微载体结合猪肝细胞已于体外被贴附[67]。

虽然已开发了稳定的肝细胞培养系统，包括胶原
27 夹心和双面胶系统，但是在微结构生物反应器中，血浆对培养肝细胞的暴露时间延长可使细胞内三酰甘油小滴明显增加而导致细胞功能严重降低。现在的生物人工肝的寿命是数小时到数天，要用于长期治疗则必须改进。在最近更多的研究中，肝细胞和非实质细胞共培养已可更加耐受血浆环境[6]。

肝细胞共培养的提出源于观察到：宫内脐静脉和卵黄静脉的间充质细胞可诱导外胚层“肝芽”增殖、分支和分化[37]。成年肝脏可为许多复杂的细胞和细胞间相互作用（胆管、Kupffer 细胞、窦内皮细胞和肝细胞）提供支架平台，以使器官功能相协调。这些细胞间的相互作用可能对间充质细胞和实质组织间隔之间的细胞信号传导是必需的。

肝的细胞生理是复杂的，尽管随着培养条件的改进，成熟肝细胞的寿命可延长，但仅为数周。

随着现代显微铸造的进展，对细胞共培养的观察可能会开发出一种可植入组织工程肝脏。血管向移植物内生长对于肝脏这么复杂的器官来讲永远是不够的。因此，我们的实验室已经在寻求构建一个达毛细血管水平的血管系统，然后再添加复杂器官的实质细胞[9]。特殊的血管系统可能可以作为一个模板制成任意厚度和复杂的组织，如心、肝或肾，所有这些都有赖于广泛的血管化，克服单独宿主内生长的限制[9]。

有序排列的肝细胞管道带有局部设计的细胞黏附蛋白，最先是用三维印记方法制造出来的[50,63]，由计算机辅助设计聚合物支架结构，将排放的液体聚合物进行干燥，通过一个类似喷墨打印机的仪器喷出粉末状聚合物。当固化的聚合体被分层构建时，由于高分辨率的缘故可以形成复杂的三维结构。这样，血管供应管道和细胞支持物可以被设计和构建。

未来方向：更好的结构、更好的细胞

随着微电子机械系统（MEMS）的出现及其被用于惯性的向导和导航中[9]，硅片显微加工已经被用于血管网络支架的改良。管道沟渠的类型为仿制血管网络的形式，被蚀刻到硅片和硼硅酸玻璃（Pyrex）模板上，分辨率为 10μm（图 3-5）。内皮细胞和肝细胞在 MEMS 模板上培养可保持生命力和增殖活力而产生白蛋白[9]。然后单层细胞可以被增厚并形成三维结构。将这些层堆积可以合成一个胆管系统，并可以增加各种血管化组织的可供表面积及其加入该系统的实质细胞。进一步的研究已确定，显微构建技术可以被用来形成大的片状活性组织，并且显微加工腔表面内皮细胞可用于有序的共培养（图 3-6）[9]。增厚的分层组织可作为永久移植物植入体内。

伴随着这些先进技术发展的是寻找一个更合适的细胞群，包括在特殊支架上混合培养。麻省理工学院与 Draper 实验室合作已经对显微加工模板进行了改进，对期望的微液流和营养传递建立了数学模型。随着复杂器官血管化问题的解决，许多困难的组织工程 28
构建目标最终将能够达到。

组织工程构建实体的一个显而易见的延伸方向是未来应用干细胞或多能细胞系，必须强调，它涉及伦理和政治问题。值得注意的是，大多数组织工程构建都是围绕类似或同源细胞构建而不是直接采用干细

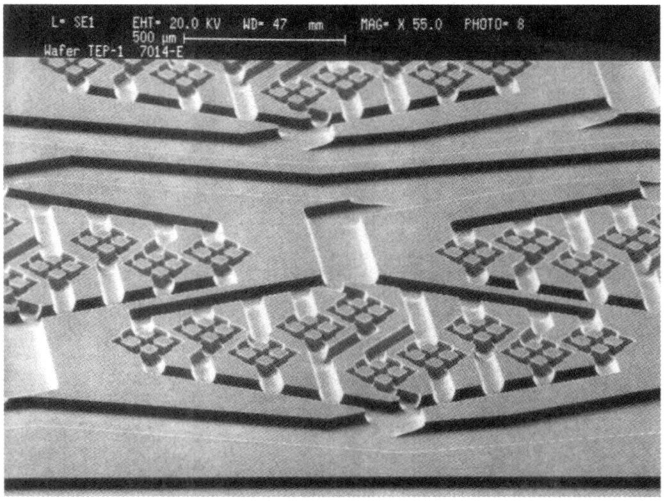

图 3-5　用微电子机械系统蚀刻在硅晶片上的部分毛细血管网络的光学显微照片。（Courtesy of Dr. J. Borenstein.）

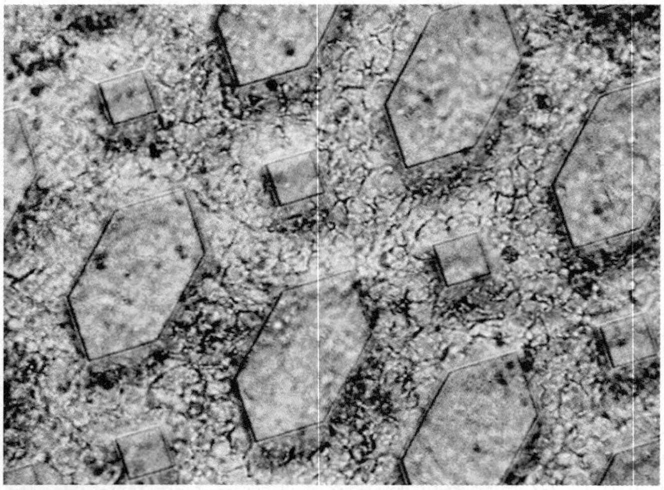

图 3-6　培养 4 天后生长在 Vitrogen 胶包被（30μg/ml）的硼硅酸玻璃晶片上的内皮细胞。（From Kaihara S, Borenstein J, Koka R,et al: Silicon micromachining to tissue engineer branched vascular channels for liver fabrication. Tissue Eng 2000;6:105-117.）

胞。应用间充质干细胞进行构建的课题数量迅速增加，在这一领域一些人已经在寻求将羊水细胞作为间充质干细胞的来源用于胚胎组织工程[47]。此外，对胎儿组织，包括应用软骨细胞进行胸壁构建，已经开展从羊胎中获取细胞后实验室扩增，到动物出生时将构建物植入，植入后观察结构替代物 10 周以上[23]。大多数不基于干细胞方式的组织工程策略可能利用了所用组织内的祖细胞，因此已经被用于组织工程的干细胞没有得到明确的认定。有趣的是注意到，这些细胞已经具有一定程度的分化，可以用于产生足够的许多组织。

通过与工程师、化学家、外科医生、物理学家、生物学家和许多其他领域的科学家的创造性合作，组织工程的迅速蜕变已经发生，随着材料学、细胞生理学和外科应用方面的同步进展，正在取得真正的进步。生物反应器装置的进化，包括给予细胞合适的生理条件刺激，也已经产生了更好的组织。机械工程、组织工程和外科研究的结合代表了组织工程用于解决普通外科和小儿外科问题的未来。

（周　莹译　吴晔明校）

参考文献

1. Atala A, Cima LG, Kim W, et al: Injectable alginate seeded with chondrocytes as a potential treatment for vesicoureteral reflux. J Urol 1993;150:745-747.
2. Bader A, Schilling T, Tebken OE, et al: Tissue engineering of heart valves—human endothelial cell seeding of detergent acellularized porcine valves. Eur J Cardiothorac Surg 1998;14:279-284.
3. Badylak S, Meurling S, Chen M, et al: Resorbable bioscaffold for esophageal repair in a dog model. J Pediatr Surg 2000;35:1097-1103.
4. Balis UJ, Behnia K, Dwarakanath B, et al: Oxygen consumption characteristics of porcine hepatocytes. Metab Eng 1999;1:49-62.
5. Bhatia SN, Balis UJ, Yarmush ML, et al: Probing heterotypic cell interactions: Hepatocyte function in microfabricated co-cultures. J Biomater Sci Polym Ed 1998;9:1137-1160.
6. Bhatia SN, Yarmush ML, Toner M: Controlling cell interactions by micropatterning in co-cultures: Hepatocytes and 3T3 fibroblasts. J Biomed Mater Res 1997;34:189-199.
7. Binnington HB, Tumbleson ME, Ternberg JL: Use of jejunal neomucosa. Surgery 1982;91:293-300.
8. Borenstein JT, Gerrish ND, Currie MT, et al: New ultra-hard etch-stop layer for high precision micromachining. Proceedings of the 12th IEEE International Conference on Micro Electro Mechanical System, MEMS, 1999, Orlando, Fla, pp 205-210.
9. Borenstein JT, Terai H, King KR, et al: Microfabrication technology for vascularized tissue engineering. Biomed Microdevices 2002;4:167-175.
10. Breuer CK, Shin'oka T, Tanel RE, et al: Tissue engineering lamb heart valve leaflets. Biotech Bioeng 1996;50:562-567.
11. Bucher NLR: Liver regeneration: An overview. J Gastroenterol Hepatol 1991;6:615-624.
12. Buckley MJ, Banes AJ, Jordan R: Effects of mechanical strain on osteoblasts in vitro. J Oral Maxillofac Surg 1998; 48:276-282.
13. Bueno J, Ohwada S, Kocoshis S, et al: Factors impacting the survival of children with intestinal failure referred for intestinal transplantation. J Pediatr Surg 1999;34:27-33.
14. Cao YL, Lach E, Kim TH, et al: Tissue engineered nipple reconstruction. Plast Reconstr Surg 1998;102:2293-2298.
15. Chen MK, Badylak SF: Small bowel tissue engineering using small intestinal submucosa as a scaffold. J Surg Res 2001;99:352-358.
16. Choi RS, Pothoulakis C, Kim BS, et al: Studies of brush border enzymes, basement membrane components, and electrophysiology of tissue-engineered neointestine. J Pediatr Surg 1998;33:991-997.
17. Clark EB: Epidemiology of congenital cardiovascular malformations. In Emmanouilides GC, Riemenschneider TA, Allan HD, Gutesell HP (eds): Moss and Adams' Heart Disease in Infants, Children, and Adolescents. Baltimore, Williams & Wilkins, 1995, pp 60-70.
18. Davis MA, Ettinger WH, Neuhaus JM, et al: The association of knee injury and obesity with unilateral and bilateral osteoarthritis of the knee. Am J Epidemiol 1989;130: 278-288.
19. Diego MD, Miguel E, Lucen CM, et al: Short gut syndrome: A new surgical technique and ultrastructural study of the liver and the pancreas. Arch Surg 1982;117:789-795.
20. Folch A, Ayon A, Hurtado O, et al: Molding of deep polydimethylsiloxane microstructures for microfluidics and biological applications. J Biomech Eng 1999;121:28-34.

21. Fowler VG, Durack DT: Infective endocarditis. Curr Opin Cardiol 1994;9:389-400.
22. Freed LE, Vunjak-Novakovic G: Microgravity tissue engineering in vitro. Cell Dev Biol 1997;33:381-385.
23. Fuchs JR, Terada S, Hannouche D, et al: Fetal tissue engineering: Chest wall reconstruction. J Pediatr Surg 2003; 38:1188-1193.
24. Fuller JA, Chadially FN: Ultrastructural observations on surgically produced partial thickness defects in articular cartilage. Clin Orthop 1972;86:193-205.
25. Gardner-Thorpe J, Grikscheit TC, Ito H, et al: Angiogenesis in tissue-engineered small intestine. Tissue Eng 2003;9: 1255-1261.
26. Ghadially FN, Thomas I, Oryschak AF, et al: Long term results of superficial defects in articular cartilage: A scanning electron microscope study. J Pathol 1977;121:213-217.
27. Grikscheit TC, Ochoa ER, Ramsanahie A, et al: Tissue-engineered large intestine resembles native colon with appropriate in vitro physiology and architecture. Ann Surg 2003;238:35-41.
28. Grikscheit T, Ochoa ER, Srinivasan A, et al: Tissue-engineered esophagus: Experimental substitution by onlay patch or interposition. J Thorac Cardiovasc Surg 2003;126:537-544.
29. Grikscheit TC, Ogilvie JB, Ochoa ER, et al: Tissue-engineered colon exhibits function in vivo. Surgery 2002;132:200-204.
30. Grikscheit TC, Siddique A, Ochoa E, et al: Tissue-engineered small intestine improves recovery after massive small bowel resection. Ann Surg (in press).
31. Grikscheit T, Srinivasan A, Vacanti JP: Tissue-engineered stomach: A preliminary report of a versatile in vivo model with therapeutic potential. J Pediatr Surg 2003;38:1305-1309.
32. Gupta S, Aragona E, Vemuru RP, et al: Permanent engraftment and function of hepatocytes delivered to the liver: Implications for gene therapy and liver repopulation. Hepatology 1991;14:144-149.
33. Hammermeister KE, Sethi GK, Henderson WG, et al: A comparison in men 11 years after heart valve replacement with a mechanical valve or bioprosthesis. Veterans Affairs Cooperative Study on Valvular Heart Disease. N Engl J Med 1993;328:1289-1296.
34. Harken DF, Taylor WJ, LeFemine AA, et al: Aortic valve replacement with a caged ball valve. Am J Cardiol 1962;9: 292-299.
35. Hendrickson DA, Nixon AJ, Grande DA, et al: Chondrocyte-fibrin matrix transplants for resurfacing extensive auricular cartilage defects. J Orthop Res 1994;12:485-497.
36. Homminga GN, Buma P, Koot HW, et al: Chondrocyte behavior in fibrin glue in vitro. Acta Orthop Scand 1993;64:441-445.
37. Houssaint E: Differentiation of the mouse hepatic primordium: An analysis of tissue interactions in hepatocyte differentiation. Cell Differ 1990;9:269-279.
38. Ibarra C, Janetta C, Vacanti CA, et al: Tissue engineered meniscus: A potential new alternative to allogeneic meniscus transplantation. Transplant Proc 1997;29:986-988.
39. Ibarra C, Langer R, Vacanti JP: Tissue engineering: Cartilage, bone, and muscle. Yearbook of Cell and Tissue Transplantation 1996/1997. Netherlands, Kluwer Academic Publishers, 1996, pp 235-245.
40. Isch JA, Engum SA, Ruble CA, et al: Patch esophagoplasty using AlloDerm as a tissue scaffold. J Pediatr Surg 2001; 36:266-268.
41. Isogai N, Landis W, Kim TH, et al: Formation of phalanges and small joints by tissue-engineering. J Bone Joint Surg Am 1999;81:306-316.
42. James CD, Davis R, Meyer M, et al: Aligned microcontact printing of micrometer scale poly-L-lysine structures for controlled growth of cultured neurons on planar microelectrode arrays. IEEE Trans Biomed Eng 2000;47:17-21.
43. Jauregui HO, Gann KL: Mammalian hepatocytes as a foundation for treatment in human liver failure. J Cell Biochem 1991;45:359-365.
44. Kaihara S, Borenstein J, Koka R, et al: Silicon micromachining to tissue engineered branched vascular channels for liver fabrication. Tissue Eng 2000;6:105-117.
45. Kaihara S, Kim SS, Kim BS, et al: Long-term follow-up of tissue engineered intestine after anastomosis to native small bowel. Transplantation 2000;69:1927-1932.
46. Kaufmann PM, Sano K, Uyama S, et al: Heterotopic hepatocyte transplantation: Assessing the impact of hepatotrophic stimulation. Transplant Proc 1994;26:2240-2241.
47. Kaviani A, Guleserian K, Perry TE, et al: Fetal tissue engineering from amniotic fluid. J Am Coll Surg 2003;196:592-597.
48. Kim SS, Kaihara S, Benvenuta M, et al: Regenerative signals for tissue engineered small intestine. Transplant Proc 1999;31:657-660.
49. Kim SS, Kaihara S, Benvenuta MS, et al: Small intestinal submucosa as a small-caliber venous graft: A novel model for hepatocyte transplantation on synthetic biodegradable polymer scaffolds with direct access to the portal venous system. J Pediatr Surg 1999;34:124-128.
50. Kim SS, Utsunomiya H, Koski JA, et al: Survival and function of hepatocytes on a novel three-dimensional synthetic biodegradable polymer scaffold with an intrinsic network of channels. Ann Surg 1998;228:8-13.
51. Kobold EE, Thal AP: A simple method for management of experimental wounds of the duodenum. Surg Gynecol Obstet 1963;116:340-344.
52. Lanza RP, Langer R, Vacanti J: Principles of Tissue Engineering. San Diego, Calif, Academic Press, 2000.
53. Lee IW, Vacanti JP, Yoo J, et al: A tissue engineering approach for dural and cranial grafts. Paper presented at Congress of Neurological Surgeons, 1997, New Orleans.
54. Lillemoe KD, Berry WR, Harmon JW, et al: Use of vascularized abdominal wall pedicle flaps to grow small bowel neomucosa. Surgery 1982;91:293-300.
55. Matas AJ, Sutherland DER, Stefes MW, et al: Hepatocellular transplantation for metabolic deficiencies: Decrease in plasma bilirubin in Gunn rats. Science 1976;192:892-894.
56. Mayer J: Uses of homograft conduits for right ventricle to pulmonary artery connections in the neonatal period. Semin Thorac Cardiovasc Surg 1995;7:130-132.
57. McCarthy JG: Lengthening the human mandible by gradual distraction. Plast Reconstr Surg 1992;89:1-8.
58. McFarland CD, Thomas CH, DeFilippis C, et al: Protein adsorption and cell attachment to patterned surfaces. Biomed Mater Res 2000;49:200-210.
59. Meachim G: The effect of scarification on articular cartilage in the rabbit. J Bone Joint Surg Br 1963;45:150-161.
60. Mooney DJ, Langer RS: Engineering biomaterials for tissue engineering: The 10-100 micron size scale. In Bronzino JD (ed): The Biomedical Engineering Handbook. Boca Raton, Fla, CRC Press, 1995.
61. Noishiki Y, Yamane Y, Okoshi T, et al: Choice, isolation, and preparation of cells for bioartificial vascular grafts. Artif Organs 1998;22:50-62.
62. O'Brien MF, Goldstein S, Walsh S, et al: The synergraft valve: A new acellular (nongluteraldehyde-fixed) tissue heart valve for autologous recellularization: First experimental studies before implantation. Semin Thorac

Cardiovasc Surg 1999;11:194-200.
63. Park A, Wu B, Griffith LG: Integration of surface modification and 3D fabrication techniques to prepare patterned poly(L-lactide) substrates allowing regionally selective cell adhesion. J Biomater Sci Polym Ed 1998;9:89-110.
64. Perez A, Grikscheit TC, Ashley SW, et al: Tissue engineered small intestine: Ontogeny of the immune system. Transplantation 2002;74:619-623.
65. Pokorny WJ, Fowler CJ: Isoperistaltic intestinal lengthening for short bowel syndrome. Surg Gynecol Obstet 1991;172:39-43.
66. Puelacher WC, Wisser J, Vacanti CA, et al: Temporomandibular joint disc replacement made by tissue-engineered growth of cartilage. J Oral Maxillofac Surg 1994;52:1172-1177.
67. Rozga J, Williams F, Ro M-S, et al: Development of a bioartificial liver: Properties and function of hollow-fibre module inoculated with liver cells. Hepatology 1993;17:258-265.
68. Russell PS: Selective transplantation. Ann Surg 1985;201:255-262.
69. Sakata J, Vacanti CA, Schloo B, et al: Tracheal composite tissue engineered from chondrocytes, tracheal epithelial cells, and synthetic degradable scaffolding. Transplant Proc 1994;26:3309-3310.
70. Sano K, Cusick RA, Lee H, et al: Regenerative signals for heterotrophic hepatocyte transplantation. Transplant Proc 1996;28:1857-1858.
71. Schoen FJ, Levy RJ: Tissue heart valves: Current challenges and future research perspectives. J Biomed Mater Res 1999;47:439-465.
72. Shin'oka T, Breuer CK, Tanel RE, et al: Tissue engineering heart valves: Valve leaflet replacement study in a lamb model. Ann Thorac Surg 1995;60:S513-S516.
73. Shin'oka T, Imai Y, Ikada Y: Transplantation of a tissue engineered pulmonary artery [letter to the editor]. N Engl J Med 2001;344:532-533.
74. Shin'oka T, Shum-Tim D, Ma PX, et al: Creation of viable pulmonary artery autografts through tissue engineering. J Thorac Cardiovasc Surg 1998;115:536-545.
75. Shum-Tim D, Stock U, Hrkach J, et al: Tissue engineering of autologous aorta using a new biodegradable polymer. Ann Thorac Surg 1999;68:2298-2304.
76. Sodian R, Hoerstrup SP, Sperline JS, et al: Early in vivo experience with tissue-engineered trileaflet heart valves. Circulation 2000;102:III22-III29.
77. Stock UA, Nagashima M, Khalil PN, et al: Tissue engineered valved conduits in the pulmonary circulation. J Thorac Cardiovasc Surg 2000;119:732-740.
78. Stock UA, Sakamoto T, Hatsuoka S, et al: Patch augmentation of the pulmonary artery with bioabsorbable polymers and autologous cell seeding. J Thorac Cardiovasc Surg 2000;120:1158-1167.
79. Sussman N, Kelly J: The artificial liver. Sci Am Sci Med 1995;3:68-77.
80. Sussman N, Kelly J: Temporary liver support: Theory, practice, predictions. Xenop 1995;3:63-67.
81. Sutherland DER, Numata M, Matas AJ, et al: Hepatocellular transplantation in acute liver failure. Surgery 1977;82:124-132.
82. Tavakkolizadeh A, Stephen AE, Kaihara S, et al: Epithelial transporter mRNA expression topography in the tissue-engineered small intestine. Transplantation 2003;75:181-185.
83. Tessier P: Osteotomies totales de la face: Syndrome de Crouzon, Syndrome d'Alpert, Oxycephalies, Scaphocephalies, Turricephalies. Ann Chir Plast Esthet 1967;12:273-286.
84. Thompson JS, Vanderhoot JA, Antonson DL, et al: Comparison of techniques for growing small bowel neomucosa. J Surg Res 1984;36:401-406.
85. Trey C, Burns DG, Saunders SJ: Treatment of hepatic coma by exchange blood transfusion. N Engl J Med 1966;274:473-481.
86. Tu JV, Pashos CL, Naylor CD, et al: Use of cardiac procedures and outcomes in elderly patients with myocardial infarction in the United States and Canada. N Engl J Med 1997;336:1500-1505.
87. Uyama S, Kaufmann PM, Takeda T, et al: Delivery of whole liver-equivalent hepatocyte mass using polymer devices and hepatotrophic stimulation. Transplantation 1993;55:932-935.
88. Vacanti CA, Cima LG, Ratkowski D, et al: Tissue engineered growth of new cartilage in the shape of a human ear using synthetic polymers seeded with chondrocytes. Mat Res Soc Symp Proc 1992;252:367-373.
89. Vacanti CA, Kim WS, Mooney D: Tissue engineered composites of bone and cartilage using synthetic polymers seeded with two cell types. Orthop Trans 1993;18:276.
90. Vacanti CA, Langer R, Schloo B, et al: Synthetic polymers seeded with chondrocytes provide a template for new cartilage formation. Plast Reconstr Surg 1991;87:753-759.
91. Vacanti CA, Paige KT, Kim WS, et al: Experimental tracheal replacement using tissue engineered cartilage. J Pediatr Surg 1994;29:201-204.
92. Vacanti CA, Upton J: Tissue engineered morphogenesis of cartilage and bone by means of cell transplantation using synthetic biodegradable polymer matrices. Clin Plast Surg 1994;21:445-462.
93. Vacanti JP, Morse MA, Saltzmann M, et al: Selective cell transplantation using bioabsorbable artificial polymers as matrices. J Pediatr Surg 1988;23:3-9.
94. Vandenburgh H, Del Tatto M, Shansky J, et al: Tissue engineered skeletal muscle organoids for reversible gene therapy. Hum Gene Ther 1997;7:2195-2200.
95. Wakitani S, Kimura T, Hirooka A, et al: Repair of rabbit articular surfaces with allograft chondrocytes embedded in collagen gel. J Bone Joint Surg Br 1989;71:74-80.
96. Wang DL, Wung BS, Peng YC, et al: Mechanical strain increases endothelin-1 gene expression via protein kinase C pathway in human endothelial cells. J Cell Physiol 1996;163:400-406.
97. Weber TR, Vane DW, Grosfeld JL: Tapering enteroplasty in infants with bowel atresia and short gut. Arch Surg 1982;117:684-688.
98. Williams SK: Endothelial cell transplantation. Cell Transplant 1995;4:401-410.
99. Wilmore DW, Byrne TA, Persinger RL: Short bowel syndrome: New therapeutic approaches. Curr Probl Surg 1997;34:389-444.
100. Yue X, van der Lei B, Schakenraad JM, et al: Smooth muscle seeding in biodegradable grafts in rats: A new method to enhance the process of arterial wall regeneration. Surgery 1988;103:206-212.
101. Zhang S, Yan L, Altman M, et al: Biological surface engineering: A simple system for cell pattern formation. Biomaterials 1999;20:1213-1220.

第 4 章

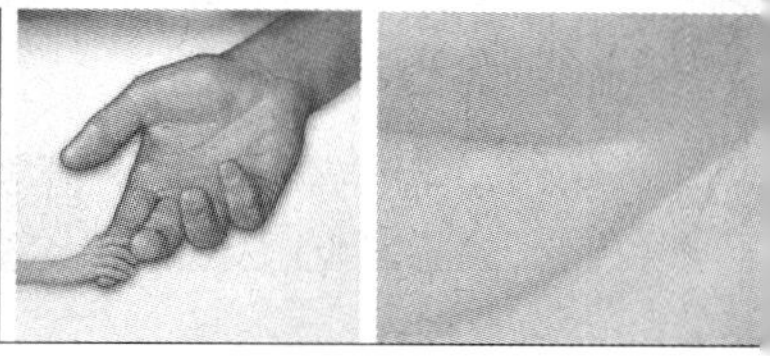

先进而新兴的外科技术和创新历程

Russell K. Woo 和 Thomas M. Krummel

31 “改变是不可避免的。改变是持续不断的”(Benjamin Disraeli)。从经过无数代的进化人类才拥有一个能够对掌的拇指，到每一分钟病情都会发生改变的新生儿手术，改变以及适应改变的反应，决定了是成功还是失败。

工具和技术的使用及其发展仍然是人类的一个显著特征。最初猎人聚居者们是为满足特殊的需要而创造、制造和改良工具。自史前时期应用最初的骨针以来，不断以同样方式进行的创新取得了不断的发展，外科工具和技术的使用决定了我们的技艺和治疗方式。

本章将着重讨论先进而新兴的外科技术，是它们奠定了外科学的现状和今后的变革方向。本章还提出了一个有利于对即将到来的变革进行思考和行动的框架。最后，本章将讨论外科医生在伦理变革过程中所起的重要作用。

由于外科技术取得的进步，我们的事业一直在向前推进，这经常是一种量的飞跃。看一看我们的手术室、治疗小组、重症监护病房，甚至我们的教学机构，都能反映出我们对工具和技术的依赖。血管钳、导管、牵引器、能源以及监护仪器占据着这些空间，目的是加强外科医生在诊断、影像学检查、生命体征监护、分子学上疾病分类以及手术操作过程中的能力。外科医生通常是这些技术的使用者，因此，理解这些技术的基本原理有助于进一步有创造性地使用这些技术。在没有理解药物作用机制和副作用的情况下使用药物，可能会被认为是一种治疗失当。对外科工具和技术的采用也必须制定类似的规范。

新技术源于不断创新的无尽循环。这样的一个循环可能始于一个基本原理的研究发现，也可能始于患者的一个未解决的问题的床边发现。通常，创新需要这两者之间的一个复杂相互影响。外科医生并不是唯一的贡献者，甚至也不是这个循环的决定者。未能解决问题的患者是我们有责任去推进事业的提醒者。Theodore Kocher 在甲状腺外科中的成功是通过他将现有血管钳改良成锯齿状以利于甲状腺手术而取得的。Thomas Fogarty 医生发明的球囊导管是在目睹了动脉切开取栓术的多次失败及灾难性结果以后，才开始作为外科辅助器械出现的。His 角——一个杰出的概念——曾经引发了基于导管操作整个领域的大讨论。John Gibbon 医生成功创建的心肺机，最初也是从肺栓塞患者需要进行手术切除而获得灵感的。虽然他的最初意向因 Lazar Greenfield 的吸引栓子切除导管和腔静脉过滤器而黯然失色，且因在心脏外科中的效用而相形见绌，但是这个故事依旧流传了下来。存在未能解决的问题和外科医生执意寻求解决问题的办法，导致了无数已经永远改变了我们事业的创新。外科医生的作用应该延伸到手术室之外。外科医生应该时刻保持清醒并对诊断、监护和教育的工具和技术保持关注。Mark M. Ravitch——一名非凡的小儿外科医生、发明者和 20 世纪最博学的外科医生之一——把外科学描述为有外科手术操作者特征的知识性学科，但是，更为重要的是，把外科学定义为对患者进行救治的一种态度或责任。Ravitch 医生对缝合器发明的贡献值得无数人的赞颂[203]。

外科手术可以被定义为“用器械或通过外科医生的手进行的一种活动”。这种定义包含着一种影像和
一种操作；而操作意味着一种能动的源泉。历史上我 32
们把“影像”当作是一种直接的视觉图像，把“操作”当作是用两只手或手术工具直接接触进行的操作。腹腔镜技术的革命教会了我们：影像可以是一种视频图像，而操作可以在两只手应用较长的手术工具

表 4-1 外科手术——影像和操作

影像	操作
直接的视觉	两只手直接操作
视频影像	两只手，较长的操作工具
	机器人
超声	冷的，热的
计算机断层扫描（CT）	射频
磁共振成像（MRI）	光力学能量
	聚焦超声能量

下进行。现在这些较长的手术工具偶尔也可以放在手术机器人上进行手术操作。我们关于影像的概念已经包括了超声成像（US）、计算机断层成像（CT）和磁共振成像（MRI），而操作的能源可以包括诸如冷、热、射频（RF）和光力学或化学能。体外震波碎石术是将这种学科应用于肾结石的一种重要的泌尿外科学范例。将来这种“影像”和“操作”将会如何存在（表 4-1）？

诊断学技术

外科疾病的明确诊断已经成为外科实践的一个至关重要的方面，它总是领先于外科学的发展。无论在临床实践、急诊室还是在床边，准确的诊断评估决定了外科判断和治疗。完整的病史和详细的体格检查将永远作为进行诊断评估的根本；然而，附加的影像学检查加上深思熟虑，可以极大地提高对外科患者的诊断评估。受药物、工程和生物学方面技术进步的驱动，诊断评估技术变得更加精细，将来这些检查可以提供更为详尽的解剖学、功能学甚至分子方面的信息。

过去的 30 年间，US、CT 和 MRI 技术的引进和不断改善极大地改变了外科疾病的临床诊断评估。其所提供的精确的解剖学数据促进了多种不同疾病的精确诊断。功能学成像技术，如正电子发射断层成像（PET）和功能性 MRI，已经出现并可提供精确的、经常是实时的生物学或生理学信息。在小儿外科领域，这些影像学检查可以应用于疾病的诊断、术前的手术计划安排和术后的评估。本章将对应用于小儿外科的影像学检查做一个概述，讨论的重点在于新兴的技术和系统。

超声检查

在小儿外科患者的诊断评估中，超声成像已经成为一种真正无法估量的工具。在提供解剖学成像的同时，其还可提供实时功能性方面的信息，超声检查具有的独特品质使其尤其实用，包括费用相对低廉、设备轻便、便于携带以及使用时没有电离辐射而比较安全。正因为如此，这个部分将重点介绍超声成像及其在技术和实践中的进展，包括三维（3-D）超声成像、超声造影成像和超声谐波成像。

超声检查应用发射和反射声波来对身体结构进行成像。超声检查应用与主动声波定位仪（主动声纳）相同的工作原理运行，主动声波定位仪是通过超声检查仪探头发射一束声波进入身体，基于“听到”回声的时间可以计算达到目标结构的距离[123]。在身体内，声波主要在组织界面反射，返回声波的强度主要与组织特性有关。超声成像具有无电离辐射、运动中实时成像和操作时间短的优点[213]。

现代超声检查仪的许多传感器的器件是并排放置在传感器探头中。目前大部分超声检查仪采用线性和扇形的扫描传感器。这些传感器是由单排放置的 64～256 个压电器件组成，传感器可以接受一个层面组织的回声，扫描的厚度与传感器器件的厚度直接有关[123]。这种信息被用于构建实时、动态、二维（2-D）的图像。颜色、能量和脉冲波多普勒成像技术是对这种技术进行改进的成果，可以呈现颜色或运动的可视化的图像[213]。传统的多普勒成像是在一个目标区域内通过追踪散射目标而提供有关血流速度和血流方向的信息[61]。而能量多普勒可显示多普勒信号的能量，在信 / 噪比和低血流探测方面是一种更为敏感的方法[72]。

在小儿外科领域，超声成像已广泛应用于阑尾炎、睾丸扭转、肠套迭、肥厚性幽门狭窄、胆道和胰腺疾病及骨盆病理学方面的评估[54,74]。另外，超声检查还可对先天性畸形进行产前诊断，如对腹壁缺损、膈疝、骶尾部畸胎瘤、囊性腺瘤样畸形、肺隔离症、神经管缺损、梗阻性尿路疾病、面裂和双胎综合征，是一种有力而又相对安全的工具[163]。在实施更多侵袭性的产前诊断技术中，如羊水诊断和胎儿血采样[163]，超声引导也是所必需的。

超声成像和胎儿外科

产前超声检查对正在发育中的胎儿可进行最初观察，有助于确定异常胎儿的自然病史并提示进行产前干预策略[85]。超声评估对诊断和定性可进行胎儿外科
33 治疗的疾病已经成为日益重要的无创性方法[237]。现在胎儿外科技术已经在选定的医疗中心应用于进行各种不同的手术，包括脊髓脊膜膨出的手术修补，非免疫性水肿胎儿的骶尾部畸胎瘤切除手术，对胸腔羊水分流术无效的不断增大的先天性囊性腺瘤样畸形的手术切除，以及采用气管夹塞治疗严重的左侧先天性膈疝[42,45]。目前超声检查仍具有安全、实时的能力，所以仍然是胎儿诊断和治疗的首选检查方法。另外，对于子宫内进行胎儿外科手术患者，超声成像对术后护理和随访也是至关重要的方法。

三维超声检查

尽管 2-D 超声系统在过去的 30 年间得到了显著的改进，但是它的超声成像需要有经验的操作者进行解释。由于这种成像仅显示为目标解剖结构的一个横截面或一个层面，因此需要在大脑中重建的 3-D 图像来解释。由于这些局限性，近来已经出现了可以提供立体图像而不是横截面图像的 3-D 超声系统，并已被越来越多地应用于许多方面。

临床使用 3-D 超声系统的最初报道是在 1986 年，当时 Baba 通过微型计算机处理 2-D 图像后成功地获得了胎儿的 3-D 图像（http://www.ob-ultrasound.net/history-3D.html）。从此以后，发展了多个 3-D 超声系统以提供更详尽的解剖学信息。一般情况下，这些多层面或立体图像是通过两种方法中的一种来获得：（1）利用 2-D 阵列，采用多排器件的传感器来一次捕捉多个层面，从真正的 3-D 数据来呈递一个立体图像；（2）采用一个一维定相的阵列，随着时间的推移获取数个 2-D 层面。然后通过超声检查仪的计算机重建算法融合后得到合成的 3-D 图像。

经由这些技术得到的 3-D 信息可用于进行重建，并可通过信号最大化强度处理、体积补偿或表面补偿来显示 3-D 影像。当这些 3-D 影像以实时方式显示时，它们就能同时提供解剖和功能方面的信息，如采用实时超声检查来评估心脏的功能。实时 3-D 超声有时候是指所谓的四维超声（包括时间维），但本质上还是提供一种 3-D 影像。子宫内胎儿的 3-D 超声影像见图 4-1。

在小儿外科和胎儿外科领域，3-D 超声系统已经可以应用于先天性畸形的详尽的产前诊断评估。Dyson 等人分别前瞻性采用 2-D 和 3-D 超声技术扫描了 63 例患者的 103 种先天性畸形。每一种畸形都进行了回顾以决定：3-D 超声影像是否优于、相当于或不如 2-D 超声影像。在这些畸形中，51%的病例的 3-D 超声影像可以提供额外的信息，45%的病例的 3-D 超声可以提供相等的信息，而 4%的病例的 3-D 超声不如 2-D 超声。尤其是 3-D 超声技术可以为面部畸形、手和足部的畸形、脊柱轴和神经管缺陷的胎儿提供最为有益的评估。总体上在所研究的选择性病例中，约半数的 3-D 超声影像具有诊断学上的优势，

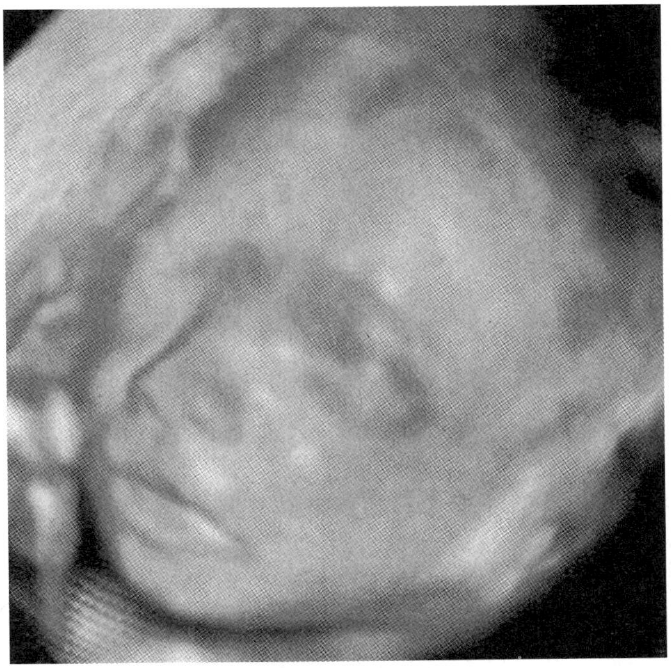

图 4-1　胎儿脸部的三维超声图像。(From Tonni G, Centini G, Rosignoli L: Prenatal screening for fetal face and clefting in a prospective study on low-risk population: Can 3- and 4-dimensional ultrasound enhance visualization and detection rate? Oral Surg, Oral Med Oral Pathol Oral Radiol Endod 2005;100:420.)

在 5%的病例中对患者的处理具有显著性作用。因此，他们得出 3–D 超声在先天性畸形的产前评估中是除了 2–D 超声以外的另一种强有力的工具的结论[52]。

Chang 等人报道了几个采用 3–D 超声技术有效评估胎儿器官体积的研究。他们应用 3–D 超声来精确地估计胎儿肺体积以评估肺发育不全[30]、大脑体积[27,28]、心脏体积[21]、肾上腺体积[29]和肝脏体积[32]。在这些研究中，3–D 超声影像比 2–D 超声图像可提供更为精确的数据[32]。

除了进行产前评估以外，3–D 超声系统已经应用于新生儿和婴幼儿的心室系统成像，以帮助神经内镜治疗术前进行计划安排[104,105]。同样，3–D 超声系统也已经相对广泛应用于评估先天性心脏畸形的经胸超声心动成像领域[122,137]。Cannon 等人研究了在模拟内镜环境下 3–D 超声指导基础手术操作的能力[25]。他们发现与 2–D 超声相比，3–D 超声成像系统指导这些手术操作更加有效和精确[25]。与 2–D 超声相比，3–D 超声系统是以一种更为直觉的方式把复杂的结构变得更形象化。另外，它们似乎能够更加精细地测量体积和相对的结构方位[222]。随着技术的改进，这些技术在小儿外科领域的应用还会不断增加。

34 **超声增强成像和超声谐波成像技术**

除了 3–D 超声以外，超声增强成像和超声谐波成像技术方面也取得了显著进步。超声增强成像技术目前已应用于呈现清楚的心脏内的血流，以评估心脏的结构异常[22]。超声增强造影剂可以分为游离气体泡沫和压缩气体泡沫。这些气体泡沫当被超声波异质化时可呈现出一种独特的回声现象。它们呈现出一种频率依赖的容积震动，可使共振的气体泡沫变成一种声源，而不是原来超声波的反射声波[61]。现在已经出现了一些提高增强成像效果的新方法，包括超声谐波成像、超声谐波能量多普勒成像、脉冲倒置成像、释放脉冲成像和超声亚谐波成像[61]。随着这些方法学的改进，超声增强成像技术可以给临床医生提供更为详细的心脏血流灌注影像，以及肿瘤、动静脉畸形和其他疾病状态下的血流灌注成像。图 4–2 描述了采用微气体泡沫增强的左心室的超声成像。

对超声谐波成像技术进行关注是在 1996 年 Burns 发现超声增强造影剂可产生谐波以后[21]。从此以后，在利用声波谐波特性改进超声成像的质量上得到了显著的发展。声波是各种不同频率成分——基础频率（初始谐波）和谐波频率——的总汇，谐波频率是多种基础频率的整合体。基础频率和其特异性谐波的结合可给予一种信号—种独特的性质。谐波是由组织本身产生的；当应用超声增强造影剂时，谐波是由注入造影剂的反射波来产生，而不是由组织的反射波来产生[221]。

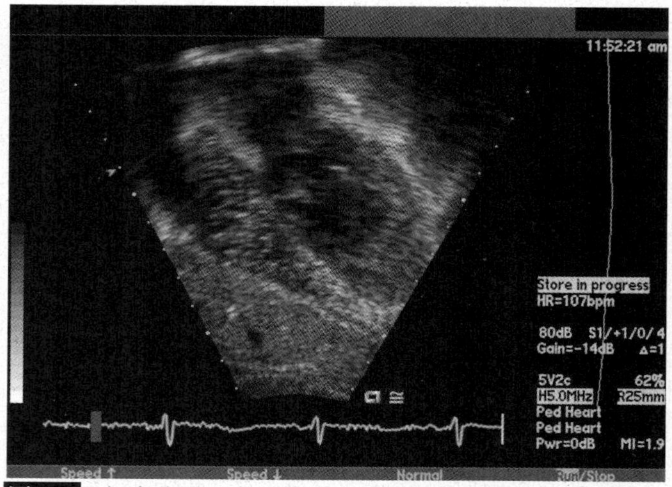

图 4–2 超声造影超声波心动描记图显示在右侧心脏内的微小泡沫。（Courtesy of the Lucille Packard Children's Hospital Echocardiography Laboratory.）

基础频率是由组织分界面产生的回声组成的，组织不同则基础频率不同，而谐波是由组织本身产生的。因此在这种方法中，谐波强度随着到达组织深度的增加而增强，直到自然组织的衰减掩盖了这种效应。相反，基础频率的强度随着深度的增加而出现线性衰减[221]。

组织谐波成像技术是通过利用由组织产生的谐波信号并过滤掉由暂时性声学能量产生的基础频率的回声信号，而利用这些特性的优点[60]。在理论上，这样的过滤可以导致信号–噪音比例和造影剂–噪音比例提高。超声谐波成像技术的其他优点在于：可提高空间定位能力而更好地显示深部的结构，并可减少由超声增强造影剂产生的伪影[29]。图 4–3 比较了由超声谐波成像技术和标准的2–D 超声所得到的图像。

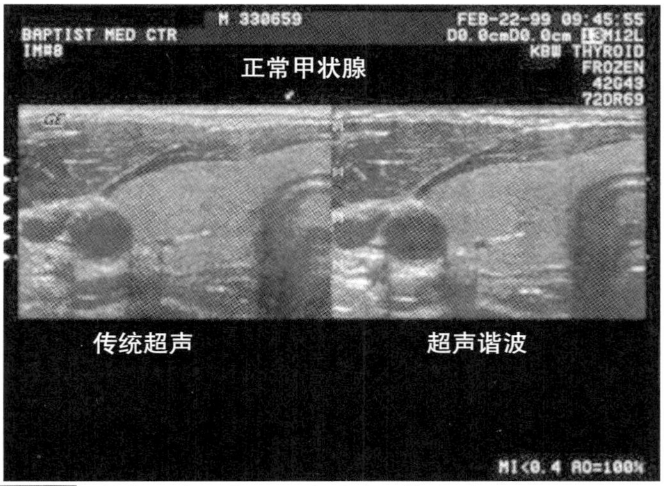

图 4-3 传统超声图像和超声谐波图像的对比。

计算机断层成像（CT）

CT 是 1972 年由英国 EMI 实验室的工程师 Godfrey Hounsfield 发明的，并由马塞诸塞州 Tufts 大学的出生于南非的物理学家 Allan Cormack 研制成了样品。从此以后，CT 被广泛应用于医学实践中。目前，这项技术的发展是改进了成像速度、舒适性和成像质量。近期的发展，如多探头螺旋 CT（MDCT）和立体重建技术或 3-D CT，在儿科手术患者的治疗中可能尤其具有价值。本章这一部分将对 CT 成像技术进行简短的回顾，着重点在多探头螺旋 CT 和立体成像，以及它们在小儿外科中的应用。

多探头螺旋计算机断层成像

CT 是采用一种圆形环绕在患者周围的紧密排列的放射线发射器和探测器带获取 X 射线衰减数值的 2-D 图像。然后用数字衰退技术把这种衰减数值阵列还原成一幅 2-D 的薄层图像。自从 CT 发明以来，CT已经经历了数次重大的发展。

20 世纪 90 年代早期，通过采用滑环得到持续成
35 像，单探头螺旋状或螺旋形 CT 扫描的引入使诊断性 CT 成像取得了彻底改革[127]。在这一技术出现以前，每得到一次薄层扫描图像后，检查平台和患者都得移动以进行下一次扫描，这样扫描过程花的时间就相对较长。螺旋 CT 扫描器是采用滑环技术，使 X 线球管和探测器可以围绕患者进行持续的旋转。当与检查平台持续性移动相结合时，通过旋转的构架可以显著提高扫描的速度。螺旋 CT 扫描器扫描速度的提高使在单次呼吸屏气期内即可获得大量的数据，促进了其在儿科的应用。

螺旋 CT 在过去 8 年里又取得了进步，构架旋转速度更快、X 线球管功率更高以及插补运算法则更完善[183]。然而，最大的进步来自于多探头螺旋 CT 扫描器的引进。相对于单排探测器的 CT，多探头螺旋 CT 采用的是多排平行探测器同时螺旋状围绕在患者的周围。目前可以同时获得四个通道的螺旋状数据，多探头螺旋 CT 扫描器显著快于单探头螺旋 CT 扫描器。这种优势对于 CT 成像的临床应用具有深刻的意义，尤其是在儿科患者中，因为在后者中，组织射线暴露和患者合作问题都被夸大了。与早期型号的 CT相比，多探头螺旋 CT 具有的基本优势包括：充分缩短图像获取时间，从同一未加工数据创建回顾性的更薄或更厚的切面图像，以及减少螺旋 CT 伪影来改进 3-D 重建成像[183]。

在儿童人群中，与标准的螺旋 CT 相比，多探头螺旋 CT 具有许多优势，包括缩短或减少镇静剂的需求，减少患者人为的运动，在更多的解剖部位中有潜在的更为理想的造影增强效果。获取的立体数据也提供了进行多平面重建的能力，这可能是解决问题的一种重要工具。多探头螺旋 CT 在儿童创伤、肿瘤、实性腹部实质器官肿块的评估、可疑的脓肿或炎性疾病[63]以及腹部疼痛[49]的评估中的应用不断增长。Callahan 等人采用多探头螺旋 CT 来评估儿童阑尾炎患者，减少了住院的天数、阴性剖腹手术比例及患者医疗费用[24]。此外，多探头螺旋 CT 可以有效地鉴别儿童腹部疼痛，包括肠道、卵巢以及泌尿系的疾病[49]（图 4-4）。

同样，多探头螺旋 CT 在评估泌尿系结石病和炎性肠病方面可能也具有价值。多探头螺旋 CT 可作为评估儿童腹痛和可疑尿石形成的患儿血尿的一种基本方法[49]。CT 检查可以发现不透 X 线的结石、输尿管或集合系统的扩张、肾脏不对称的增大以及肾周的纤维[49]。另外一种应用不断增长的疾病是儿童炎性肠病[49]。在其评估中，CT 可以显示肠道内炎性改变，同时也可以显示炎性肠病的肠腔外表现，如脓肿，可能比荧光透视法更有优势[49]。

在胸部，多探头螺旋 CT 已经应用于儿童感染性

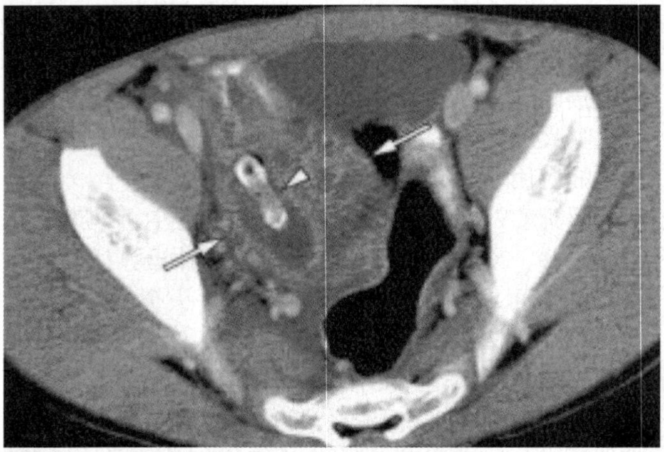

图 4–4 一名患有阑尾炎的 8 岁男孩的多探头 CT 图像。箭头所示为右下腹的一个炎症包块，可能伴有一个阑尾石（小箭头所示）。

疾病，用于探查和监测炎症，以及用于评估肺、纵隔和心脏的先天性畸形。尤其是多探头螺旋 CT 可能还可用于评估支气管肺前肠源性畸形，其中肺隔离症是一种需要考虑的畸形[62]。多探头螺旋 CT 在儿童心血管系统的评估中的应用尤其具有价值[47]。多探头螺旋 CT 在心血管疾病的评估中，如在主动脉动脉瘤、主动脉解剖和血管环的评估中，可能要显著优于超声心动图的效果。最后，多探头螺旋 CT 在定量评估胸壁畸形患儿中具有优势，因为它使用较低剂量的放射线即可完成扫描[49]。

三维计算机断层成像

对 3–D CT 重建的个体研究的处理过程已经可以通过多探头螺旋 CT 来完成。这些 3–D 重建对复杂手术的术前计划安排是有价值的。虽然 3–D CT 已经应用了近 20 年，但是这些技术的质量、速度和能力只是经过近期的改进才进入常规临床实践中[100]。目前，有四种主要的可视化技术应用于 CT 重建以创建 3–D CT 影像：多平面再现、最大强度投射、阴影表面显示和体积呈递（rendering）。多平面再现和最大强度投射局限于外部的可视化，而阴影表面显示和体积呈递可以进行沉浸式或内部可视化，如虚拟的内镜[183]。

3–D CT 可用于儿童颅面、血管和脊髓的手术术前计划安排。特别是 3–D CT 还可用于评估颌面部骨折[58]、颅面部畸形（图 4–5）和血管畸形。3–D CT 已经应用于胸腰部先天性畸形中半椎体切除手术的计划安排[87]。

一个特别有意思的 3–D CT 应用是：创建“虚拟内镜”图像。管腔结构如肠管、气道、血管和泌尿道的内表面被重建[183]。应用 3–D CT 的虚拟内镜可能有助于诊断小肠肿瘤以及用标准检查方法经常难以发现的病变[100]（图 4–6）。 36

磁共振成像（MRI）

1977 年，第一次应用于人类的 MRI 检查是由 Dammadian、Minkoff 和 Goldsmith 医生完成的。这个 MRI 检查用了 5 个小时才得到一幅质量较差的图像。从此以后，技术进步使 MRI 检查的分辨率和速度得到提升。今天，MRI 已经能够提供人体的不平行的无创伤图像。目前最新的 MRI 系统可以在亚秒时间内获取图像，因此促进了快速、近于实时的 MRI 的出现。MRI 技术现在正在发展成为能够提供有关人体生理状态的功能性信息。这部分将对 MRI 做一个简短回顾，重点在于近期技术的进步，如超快速 MRI 和功能 MRI。

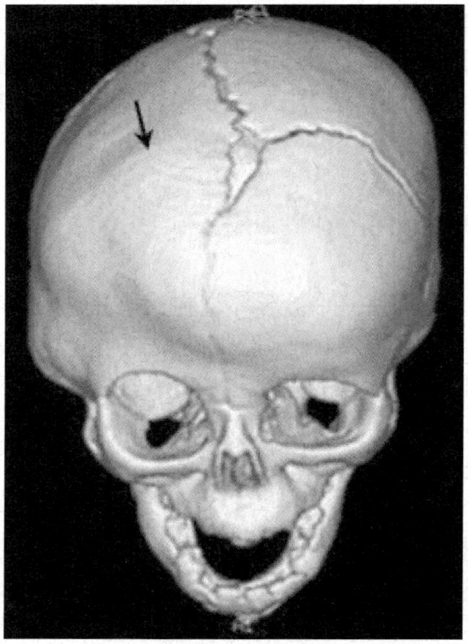

图 4–5 一名婴儿头骨的三维 CT 重建图像，显示右侧冠状颅缝产前早闭（箭头所示）。

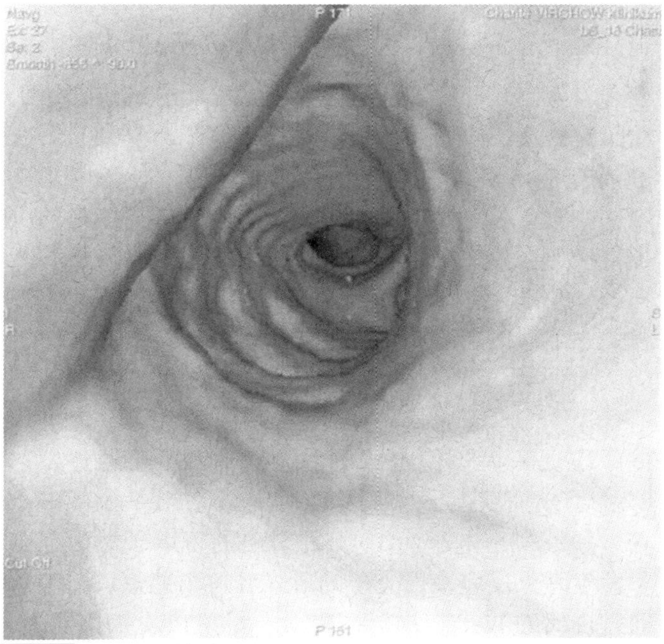

图 4–6　虚拟内镜检查。

MRI 通过强烈而单一的磁场使人体内自旋的氢质子排列而成像。然后应用射频脉冲使一些质子吸收能量并向不同方向旋转。关闭射频脉冲时，质子重新排列并释放贮存的能量。释放能量时发出的信号被检测、定量并输入计算机。不同组织对磁场及射频脉冲的反应不同，因此发出不同的能量信号。经过数学算法，这些信号就可用于 MRI 成像。

超快速 MRI

高速 MRI 中的第一个重大进展发生在 1986 年，当时引进了梯度回声脉冲序列技术（GRE），后者可以减少临床扫描时间，使需要的时间缩短至 10 秒钟。除了可以增加患者进出 MRI 扫描器的次数，更加快速的扫描时间还可以显著增加 MRI 对人体部位的应用（例如腹部），而暂停呼吸能够清除大多数运动相关性的图像扭曲变形[53,226]。自此以后，GRE 技术经历了更新换代和进一步的发展，现在已经达到亚秒级的扫描时间。目前，超快速的 MRI 已经能够在 1/10 秒钟的时间内获得高分辨率的扫描图像。这些超快速 MRI 技术通过减少运动伪影已使 MRI 在临床医学中的应用得到了革命性的发展。它促进了更新的、动态成像方式，包括心脏 MRI、胎儿 MRI 和生理成像技术，如弥漫性灌注扫描（在评估休克期间大脑的生存能力方面具有潜在的价值）和功能 MRI。

超快速 MRI 在儿童的治疗中提供了一种显著优势。大多数传统的 MRI 检查方式需要 30～40 分钟，在此期间患儿必须保持静止不动[199]。因此对儿童经常需要用镇静剂、全身麻醉、甚至是肌肉阻滞剂，以使患儿保持长时间静止不动以便完成 MRI 检查。这些是儿童进行 MRI 检查的主要障碍。超快速 MRI 检查可以显著减少这种需求，因此不仅降低了常规 MRI 检查所使用的镇静剂的潜在副作用，也促进了 MRI 检查在不能进行足够的镇静或麻醉的具有高风险的患儿中的应用[243]。

另外，超快速 MRI 可显著减少发生在腹部和胸部的运动伪影，而这些运动伪影是正常呼吸和肠蠕动的结果。扫描时间足够快速以至 MRI 扫描在一个呼吸暂停期间和相对快于腹部运动时间内就可以完成。
超快速 MRI 尤其有助于降低肠道 MRI 检查期间与使 37
用口服造影剂相关的拖尾效应伪影[81]。此外，通过减少运动伪影和获取快速成像，超快速 MRI 检查促进了心脏 MRI 和胎儿 MRI 的实际应用。胎儿 MRI目前已经应用于更好地鉴别和描述胎儿大脑的特征以及脊柱畸形[73,174]。

功能 MRI（fMRI）

功能 MRI 是一种快速发展的影像学技术，它采用大脑中血流之间的差别来提供神经元活性的体内成像。最初的相关描述仅仅是在 10 年前，目前功能 MRI 已经广泛应用于成年人群的临床和科学研究中。功能 MRI 是建立在有关神经元活性和代谢的两种基本生理假设上的。尤其是，它假定是神经元的活性诱导了与局部脑血流量增加相关的局部葡萄糖代谢的增加。通过检测局部血流量的微小改变，功能 MRI 技术能够提供大脑活性的“功能性”影像。目前，采用的最为常见的技术就是众所周知的“血氧水平依赖（BOLD）”增强造影，即把血液当作一种体内的造影增强介质[48]。BOLD 成像是利用氧合血红蛋白与去氧血红蛋白在磁性方面的微小差异的优点。因为随着局部脑血流量增加和相对过量，神经元激活，更多的氧合血红蛋白会出现在大脑活性区域的静脉毛细血管中。这些差异在功能 MRI 磁场中可呈现为微小的扭曲变形而被检测出来，因而可被用于创建一种大脑活性的功能性影像[236]。

在儿童人群中，功能 MRI 需要大量的患者准备工作，以使患儿在扫描仪器内保持静止不动直到检查完成。已有减少儿童对检查的焦虑和不确定性的各种准备技术的描述，包括播放教育录像，由放射科工作人员陪同的参观，以及进行检查练习。与解剖 MRI 不同，患者进行功能 MRI 检查不能应用镇静剂或麻醉剂，因为这会影响神经元的活性。

直到目前，功能 MRI 在儿科人群中的使用仍然处于早期阶段。然而，功能 MRI 在评估中枢神经系统的组织和发育、大脑可塑性的特征以及在评估和理解神经运动功能性疾病方面仍然有极大的希望[236]。另外，目前功能 MRI 的临床应用包括：描绘近于空间占位性病变的大脑语言皮层和确定大脑语言优势半球。这些临床应用的目的是为了在实施神经外科手术之前提供术前的功能性信息[236]。

正电子发射断层成像（PET）

正电子发射断层摄影术是一项不断被采用的影像学技术，它可提供有关人体的功能状态的信息。PET 最初是在 1973 年由 Hoffman、TerPogossian 和 Phelps 在华盛顿大学开发出来的，现在 PET 已经成为最为常见的一种核医学检查方法[94]。虽然 CT、MRI 和超声技术可提供有关人体解剖学的详细信息，但 PET 可提供患者组织当前的代谢状态信息[107]。以这种方式，PET 经常能够发现预示一种疾病状态的代谢性改变，通常在解剖学改变出现以前就可以发现这些代谢性改变。

PET 成像是基于探测放射性核素发射的正电子和电子发生湮灭反应时释放的光子[209]。这些放射性核素是通过质子轰击靶物质产生的，后者是在回旋加速器中加速的[209]。发射正电子的放射性核素然后被用于合成放射性药物，作为人体生化反应途径中的一部分。最常用的放射性核素是氟化的葡萄糖相似物，2–脱氧–2–[^{18}F] 氟脱氧葡萄糖（FDG）。类似于葡萄糖，FDG 是通过细胞内的己糖激酶来磷酸化[219]。在其磷酸化形式中，FDG 不会穿过细胞膜，因此在代谢活性细胞内发生积聚。在这种方法中，利用 FDG 的 PET 成像可提供有关不同人体组织利用葡萄糖的信息[107,219]。

为了进行探测，FDG 是用 ^{18}F 来进行合成，一种半衰期为 110 分钟的放射性同位元素。合成过程始于在回旋加速器中加速带负电荷的氢离子，直到它们获得接近 8 MeV 的能量。然后通过穿过一种碳箔来祛除这些氢离子上的轨道电子。随后产生的高能量的质子直接通向盛有稳定的富含 ^{18}O 水的靶室。质子和富含 ^{18}O 的水发生核反应形成氢 ^{18}F–氟化物。下面的方程式详细列出了该核反应[107]：

$$H_2(^{18}O) + {}^{1}H + 能量 \rightarrow H_2(^{18}F)$$

^{18}F 是一种不稳定的放射性同位素，可通过发射 β^+ 粒子或捕获电子而发生衰变并放射出一个微中子（υ）和一个正电子（β^+）。发射出的正电子然后与电子发生湮灭反应，以光子的形式释放出能量，后者可通过现代的 PET 扫描器探测出来。在 PET 扫描器中，探测器是闪烁晶体结合光电倍增管。目前，大多数 PET 扫描器采用由锗酸铋、掺铈硅酸镥或掺铈硅酸钆组成的晶体。因为 PET 扫描采用不稳定的放射性同位素，所以 PET 探针必须是在 PET 检查以前即刻进行合成的。这个缺点限制了 PET 成像的直接和广泛的可用性，因此 PET 检查必须要提前预约。FDG 是一种方便的探针，因为其半衰期有 110 分钟，因此它有足够的时间从一个远处的回旋加速器转运到 PET 扫描器中进行典型的全身 PET 成像检查（≥30 分钟）。

在一个典型的 PET 检查中，供诊断或治疗用的放射性药物是经静脉应用的。患者是通过 PET 扫描器成像来探测全身的放射活性（如上文所描述的光子放射），并创建 3–D 图像或组织功能成像。目前，PET 成像广泛已应用于评估和监测肺部、结肠、乳腺、淋巴结和皮肤的肿瘤[193]。PET 成像已用于协助肿瘤的诊断、定位和分期，监测抗肿瘤治疗、肿瘤组织的特征、 38
放射性核素治疗和筛查肿瘤的复发[202,212]。尽管是非特异性检查，FDG 还是经常会用到，因为恶性细胞总体上会显示出葡萄糖利用的增加伴己糖激酶活性上调。

PET 成像也已经应用于评估非肿瘤组织的活性以提供有关其生存能力或代谢活性的信息。在成年人中，PET 扫描经常用于确定心肌组织的存活能力，以确定患者是否能从冠状动脉旁路移植中受益[75,76]。近来，PET 的这种应用已经扩展到儿童人群中，在疑有心肌梗死的患儿行动脉转换手术后评估心脏的功能[177]。同样，PET 扫描可显示大脑组织的存活能力，在休克以后可以进行确诊[173]。最后，PET 成像已经用于鉴别大脑组织中出现异常活动的区域，有助于癫痫灶的定位或诊断功能性疾病，如 Parkinson 病和阿尔茨海默病[157,158]。

虽然 PET 成像提供了重要的有关人类组织代谢活性的功能性信息，但是相对于传统的解剖学成像，它提供的经常是相对模糊不清的图像。在术前计划期间，这种图像可能难以采用，因为它不能精确地将可疑的区域与详细的解剖学信息联系在一起。近来，组合型的 PET/CT 扫描器已经出现，它能够同时进行 PET 扫描和高分辨率的 CT 扫描[192]。这种组合型扫描器的引进只有 5 年的时间，这些扫描器提供了从 PET 扫描得到的功能性信息和从 CT 扫描绘制出的精确的细微的解剖学细节[220]（图 4–7）。

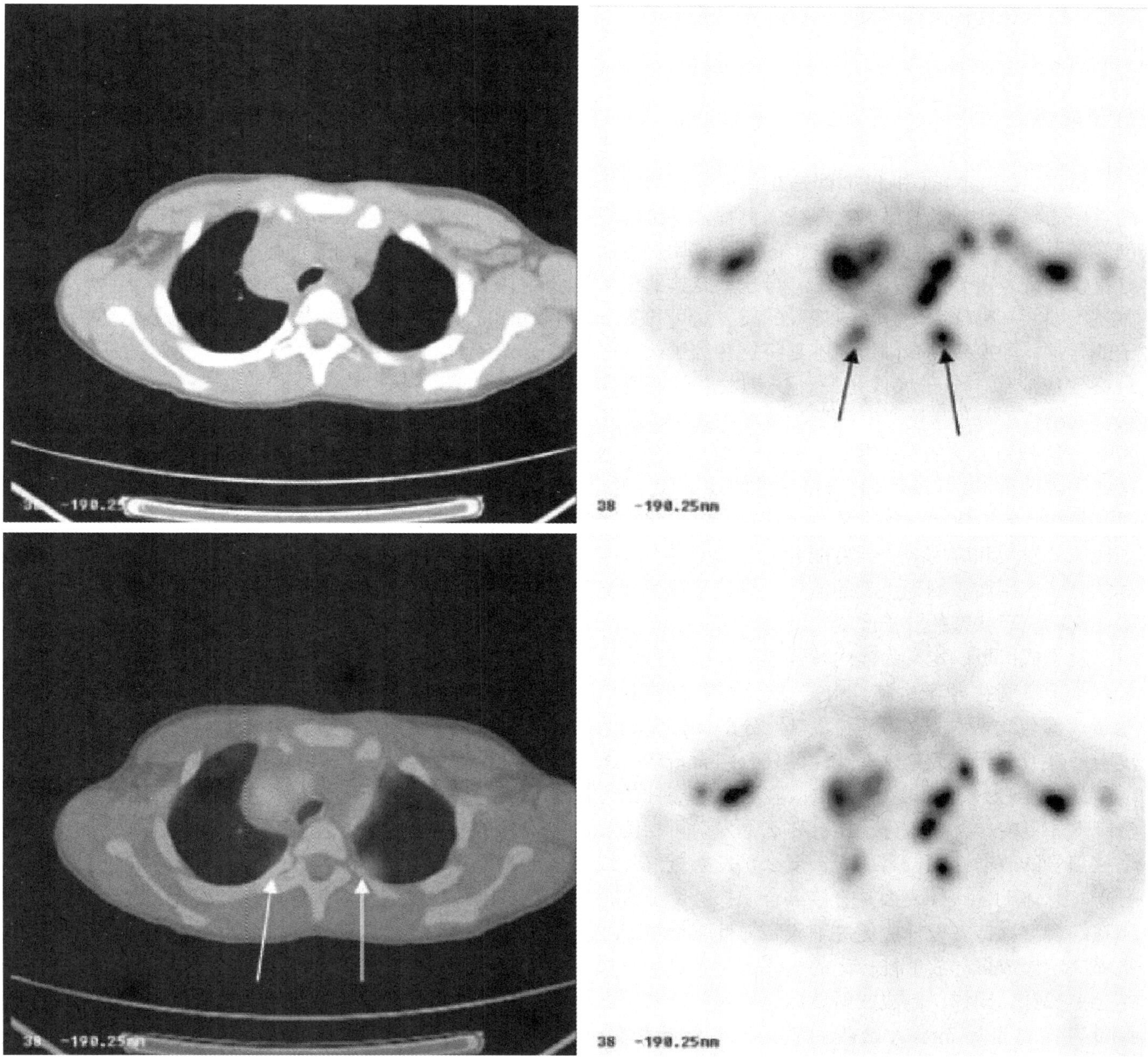

图 4–7　一名患有坏死性肉芽肿的 7 岁女孩的上胸部 PET/CT 组合图像（轴向的）。可以看到 ^{18}F–FDG 在腋窝淋巴结的多个部位和纵隔肿块内部多个病灶中出现浓集。（From Kaste SC: Issues specific to implementing PET–CT for pediatric oncology: What we have learned along the way. Pediatr Radiol 2004;34:205.）

在小儿外科领域，PET/CT 扫描成像代表了一种全新的成像方式，在有关术前计划和术后随访方面具有极大的潜能。然而，儿童人群的一些特异性问题使 PET 成像的应用面临挑战，包括需要禁食、静脉内通路、膀胱内插管、镇静和从泌尿道进行清除[109,180]。目前，组合型 PET/CT 扫描成像在儿童中的临床应用还没有进行广泛的研究。然而，这种有精细解剖学数据的功能性信息组合对于手术计划具有明显优势，将来在外科实践中有可能发挥更大的作用。

分子成像

超声、CT、MRI 和 PET 都是在儿童患者治疗中的常用的确定性技术。虽然这些技术可提供详细的解剖学甚至功能性的信息，但是它们的临床应用仍然没有提供细胞 / 分子水平上的信息。与这些经典的成像方式不同，一种称为“分子成像”的新方法可探查分子的异常，即疾病的基础，而不是将这些分子改变的最终效应成像。分子成像是一种快速发展的研究学科，其结合了分子生物学和细胞生物学的无创成像技术[233]。这种新方法的目标是开发用于在细胞 / 分子水平将生理改变和活体组织的通路成像的技术和方法，尤其是在特异性疾病过程中是关键性目标的通路。分子成像的发展和应用有一天可能会通过阐明潜在性疾病的分子机制而影响到患者的治疗，导致早期发现显示“疾病前”状态的分子改变[91]。

分子成像可以定义为体内特征描记和在细胞和分子水平上测量生理学机制。根据一个简单化的标准，分子成像包含两种基本元素：（1）分子探针，其浓度、活性或发光（或是这些特性的任意组合）随探测的特异性生理过程而改变；（2）监测这些探针的方法[151,145]。目前，大多数分子探针要么是发射可探测放射性信号的放射性同位素或光，要么是发射近红外线分子。总体上，探针要么是直接结合型探针，要么是间接结合型探针。设计成促进细胞特异性表面抗原或抗原决定簇成像的放射性标记的抗体，是常见的直接结合型探针。同样，制成放射性标记的寡核苷酸反义探针直接与目标 mRNA 或蛋白质进行特异性杂交，体内成像是最近出现的方式[38]。放射性标记的寡核苷酸代表小片断的目标 mRNA 或 DNA 的互补序列，因此可以在转录水平对内源性基因表达直接成像。最后，发射正电子的多巴胺类似物被用于大脑多巴胺受体的成像，是其他类型的直接结合型探针。

直接结合型探针有助于进行其目标总量或浓度的成像，而间接结合型探针可反映其目标大分子的活性。也许间接结合型探针应用最为广泛的例子是己糖激酶底物 FDG。临床 PET 成像中最常用的探针，FDG 已经应用于神经系统、心血管疾病和肿瘤的探查。基本上对所有组织应用全身性 FDG 都是可以接受的。

报告转基因技术的应用是采用间接结合型探针进行分子成像的另一个强有力的工具。报告基因是核酸序列，编码容易测定的蛋白质。这样的报告基因已经长期应用于分子生物学和遗传学研究中，以检测细胞内特性和事件，如启动子的功能 / 强度、蛋白质转运和基因转染。通过分子成像技术，报告基因现在已经用于分析基因转染、免疫细胞治疗和在动物模型中检测体内抑制性 mRNA 的效应[191]。采用萤火虫或 Rinella 虫荧光素酶的体内生物发光成像和采用绿色荧光蛋白质或 DsRed 的荧光光学成像，是这种技术的光学成像例子。

在免疫学和免疫治疗研究领域中，Costa 等人应用编码一种含有绿色荧光蛋白和虫荧光素酶的双份通讯蛋白的一种反转录病毒，以及一种 40kDa 单体白 39
介素-12 作为一种治疗性蛋白，转导了对髓磷脂基底蛋白特异的自身抗原反应性 $CD4^+$ T 细胞群[44]。然后将体内生物发光成像技术用于监测一个多发性硬化动物模型中细胞迁移方式。体内生物发光成像显示，在有症状的动物中，导致髓磷脂破坏的免疫细胞转移到了中枢神经系统。而且，他们还发现，白介素-12 免疫调节的 $CD4^+$ T 细胞表达导致了一种疾病严重程度的临床降低[44]。

同样，Vooijs 等人培育了转基因小鼠，其中荧光素酶表达的活化与视网膜母细胞瘤（Rb）抑制基因的剔除被联系起来[230]。在他们的动物模型中，*Rb*抑制基因的丧失触发了垂体肿瘤的发生，使他们可以通过反复的荧光素酶活性成像和电荷耦合器（CCD）监测肿瘤的发生、发展以及动物个体对治疗的反应[230]。虽然光学成像技术比较常用，报告基因也能编码细胞外或细胞内的受体，或结合或转运一种放射性标记或 40
顺磁性探针的转运体，因此可以进行 PET、单光子发射计算机断层显像术（SPECT）或基于 MRI 的分子成像。分子成像的第二种主要要素是成像的方式 / 技术本身。直接和间接结合型探针能够进行放射性标记，可以进行基于核医学的目标细胞 / 分子事件的体内成像，或通过 MRI或 SPECT 进行成像。事实上，已经出现微型 PET 和微型 SPECT 系统，可特异性地针对动物模型中的分子进行成像研究。同样，光学成像技术，如体内生物发光成像，近红外线分光镜检查，采用感光的电荷耦合器进行的可见光成像，以及活体内的成像，可以采用光学活性探针显示目标细胞事件。最后，解剖学成像方式，如 MRI、CT 和超声，都已经被采用，并应用于基于动物的分子成像研究中。

目前，分子成像领域主要还是实验性的，在实验室中具有显著的活性，还没有应用于临床中。然而，分子成像研究已经着眼于探测临床疾病状态的分子学基础及其潜在的治疗方法。目前，分子成像技术正在应用于检测有关细胞凋亡、血管新生、肿瘤生长和发展以及基因治疗的作用机制。

DNA 微阵列（基因芯片）

基因组学这个描述性术语承认了一种转变：一种从理解单个基因的作用和它们各自的功能的渴望到一种理解多个基因的同时作用的更为整体化的渴望，以及随之发生的对细胞行为的影响。DNA 微阵列，或基因芯片，是一种近期的新技术，可以同时检测成千上万条基因[17]。微阵列技术已经应用于重新定义肿瘤的生物学行为，交叉物种间基因组比较，以及在各种疾病中基因表达的大规模分析。本质上，它代表了一种全新的患者和疾病分类方式，即分子分类方式。

治疗技术

外科手术需要两种关键的要素：一个是“影像”，或更广泛地说，是有关目标区域的解剖学信息；另一个是对患者组织的“操作”，以达到一种治疗效果的目标。经典情况下，“影像”是通过外科医生的双眼来获得的，“操作”是用外科医生的双手和简单而传统的手术器械来实施。在过去的数十年间，这个范例已经通过可增强这两种基本要素的技术得到了扩展。

与标准的视线影像不同，现在可以通过手术显微镜、软式内镜或腹腔镜来获得“影像”。内镜可以是单目镜的也可以是双目镜的，可提供 2-D 或 3-D 的影像。这些技术可以给外科医生提供解剖区域的高质量的放大影像，在裸眼下这些影像可能是难以看到的。同样，组织的外科“操作”可以是通过一种导管、软式内镜或更长的腹腔镜来完成。而且，一些器械，如吻合器、电烙器、以超声为能量的手术器械和射频发生器，都已经用于手术操作并可通过目标治疗影响组织。这些技术已经改变了手术操作的方式；它们已经能够创建新的手术域，如腹腔镜外科、干预治疗性的内镜和基于导管的干预治疗。除了这些进展之外，几种涌现的技术平台也有希望进一步拓展手术的定义，包括立体定向的放射外科学和手术机器人工程学。这个部分将回顾这些技术，重点放在目前止血和组织烧蚀器械、立体定向的放射外科学和手术机器人的使用状况。

止血和组织烧蚀器械

设计用来提供止血和组织烧蚀的手持能量设备是广泛使用的外科手术技术。自从在 20 世纪 20 年代有关电外科的最初报道出现以来，已经发展出多种的设备和能量形式来减少血液丧失，包括单极和双极的电烙器、超声解剖器、氩气光束凝固器、冷冻疗法和红外线凝固器。这个部分提供了各种不同的止血和组织烧蚀器械的广泛概述，着眼于它们操作的原理和使用技术。

单极电烙器

虽然早在 16 世纪晚期就已出现了将电流应用到活体组织的概念的报道，但是一直到 20 世纪早期，手术中实际应用电烙器才开始发展。在 1908 年，Lee deForest 发明了一种高频发生器，能够传送一种可控制的电切电流。然而，由于他采用了昂贵的真空管，严重地限制了这种设备的临床应用。在 20 世纪 20 年代，W. T. Bovie 发明了一种价格低廉的电火花裂隙发生器。在 1926 年的一次演示中，Harvey Cushing 认识到将这种设备应用于外科手术的潜力，并且很快第一个实用的电烙器设备就投入到应用中。

能源

电烙器

高频烧蚀电流的应用现在已知道有各种不同的形式，如电烙器、电外科或单纯的“Bovie”。电流可以通过单极或双极机制来传送。在应用单极电烙器时，电流是通过发生器经应用的电极，流经患者人体，
41 再回流到接地的垫板。没有接地垫板的患者会在电流寻找重新进入的地方遭到热烧伤。接触的区域很关键，因为热量与所用电烙器的大小成反比。因此，电烙器的头部通常做得比较小以产生足够而有效的热量，而回流电极做得较大以广泛消散能量。其他三种有关的设置是：电流的频率（电源设置）、电流激活时间和高频发生器产生的波形特征（间歇性或连续性）。

在“电切”模式中，热量可快速产生而很少侧面传播。结果电烙可分离组织而没有显著地凝固下面的血管。在“电凝”模式中，电烙器是以一种较慢的频率产生较少的热量，而且有较多的热量向侧面传播。结果，组织会变干而血管会有血栓形成。

双极电烙器在电烙器的两个电极之间会产生一个短的回路；因此，在电极之间通过被抓握的组织可完成电流的回路。因为热量只在较短回路的组织中间产生，所以侧面热量传播较少，组织浓缩有机械性优势，同时具有热量凝固的特点。

氩气光束凝固器

氩气光束凝固器在凝固器头部与靶组织之间是通过离子化的氩气流动气体来产生一个电流回路。电流是经过氩气传导到组织并产生热量性凝固。氩气的气流可提高能见度并可消散各种表面血管，因此可增强电凝效果。氩气光束凝固器在肝脏手术中的应用具有无可比拟的优势。

手术激光

激光发射器（即光线通过辐射的刺激发射来放大）是可产生一种高强度的和几近非散射的单色辐射光束的设备，其光束通常是在可见光区域内。当光束聚焦在近范围内时，激光能够产生强大的热量而具有凝固组织的功效。激光的散射最小，且激光束能够通过一种纤维光学系统来传播。

基于能量的设置和光子的选择，激光到达的组织深度可以进行控制。在组织内的穿透深度以氩气激光最浅，二氧化碳（CO_2）激光可达到中等深度，钕钇铝石榴红（Nd-YAG）激光可达到的组织深度最深。光敏剂可提供另外一种靶向性优势。光吸收程度以及因此产生的破坏效应依赖于所选择的波长和基于密度、纤维化和血管分布的组织光吸收特性。

光力学的治疗

光能的新应用是在光力学治疗中。光敏剂是靶细胞特异性的，服用后聚集在其被清除的组织中。光敏剂可以用光源进行激活以诱导组织破坏。这种技术已得到了广泛的应用[209]。化生细胞，尤其是在 Barrett 食管炎中，可能也是易感的[185]。

超声

除了诊断性使用的低频超声以外，高频超声输出可以用于分离和凝固组织。现在聚焦的声波已经广泛应用于肾脏结石的治疗中，如体外冲击波碎石术。能量聚焦可产生一种冲击波，导致结石破碎成可以自发排出的大小。

谐波解剖刀

当采用的超声能量到达非常高的频率（55 000Hz）时，组织可被分离而周围组织的损害非常小。这样的高频能量可产生振动、摩擦、热量和最终组织破坏。

高强度聚焦超声

当高强度的超声能量从多个超声波束聚焦到一个点后作用于组织时，结果可导致组织升温和热坏死。没有一个单独的超声波束具有足够的导致损害的能量；只有聚焦到一点后才能产生热量损害效应。结果是可把皮下的小结节作为目标而不损伤皮肤，或可以破坏位于实质性器官的实质内部的小结节而不会穿透器官的表层。然而，迄今为止，聚焦点非常小，这限制了它的临床应用。

汽蚀装置

超声刀（CUSA）——一种具有汽蚀作用的超声吸引器，是应用较低频率的超声能量以及伴随的吸引器。富含水分的组织的破碎可进行实质破坏，而留下血管组织不动，可进行准确的凝固。

射频能量

高频交流电（350～500kHz）可用于组织分离、血管淋巴管封闭或组织消融。应用这种能源可加热靶组织，导致蛋白质变性和坏死。反馈环传感器在一个选择点可中止电流，因此可使周围组织的损伤减少到最低程度。已有将其靶向性应用于调节食管下端括约肌以治疗胃食管反流的报道[223]。

微波能量

微波能量（2450 MHz）可以经过一个探针传送到靶组织。这种快速交替改变的电信号可产生热量，因此可使组织凝固坏死。

冷冻疗法

在温度谱的另外一端，一种冷冻和融解的循
42 环——在冷冻相冰晶形成，在融解相组织解体——可用来进行低温组织破坏。迄今这种治疗方式很少得到临床应用，因为高流量的血流，尤其是在肿瘤组织中，有吸收冷冻能量的倾向。

影像引导系统

计算机技术近来的发展已经深刻地增强了医学影像的作用，从以前的诊断性描述到计算机辅助外科（CAS）。在最近的十年间，医学成像方法已经从早期的基于人类解剖学模型的物理学上的使用，成长为应用计算机视频和绘图技术来计划和分析手术步骤。随着高速计算机的快速发展，汇编和视觉化临床数据的任务已经变得非常便利，为实时、交互式计算机应用在手术操作期间创造了新的机会[40,142,197,212]。这个发展领域，术语称影像引导外科，已经慢慢进展为一个最好称之为信息引导性治疗（IGT）的领域，因为为实现最佳的治疗干预，它要涉及各种数据源的使用。这样的治疗性干预可以想象应该包括从活检、到组织刺激、到直接的医疗植入、到放射治疗可以进行。所有这些高科技干预的共同点是：要在一个特异性位点采用治疗性方式进行精确的干预。

然而，生物医学工程、计算机和信息引导性治疗的影像概念的有效应用都还没有达到其全部的潜力。基础科学和数学框架方面的发展仍然面临着重大挑战，它们是通过应用有关的信息资源来提高治疗性干预方法的基础。

意义

如 1995 年美国国家卫生研究院（NIH）在《支持生物工程的研究报告》（http://grants.nih.gov/grants/becon/externalreport.html）中阐述的那样，科技的适当应用可能会使无创技术替代传统的有创操作。目前对研究计算机辅助外科或信息引导性治疗中的兴趣可能部分归因于充分认识到微创外科（MAS）的好处，尽管也认识到其局限性。

另一方面，基于影像的手术指导有其技术局限性。影像引导性手术导航系统现在已经变成治疗颅脑神经外科手术的标准方法，其中术中的精确定位和穿过大脑的运动是最为重要的。

患者特异性的影像数据组，如 CT 或 MRI，一经与固定的解剖学参照点或基准点发生关联，就能给外科医生提供详细的有关目标区域的空间信息。外科医生就能够利用这些信息精确地瞄准和定位病变位置。术中计算机辅助成像是通过显示位置和最佳方向来提高外科医生依从术前计划的能力。因此，CAS 加计算机辅助外科可为微创外科提供更大的手术精度的额外益处，增加完全和精确切除的可能性。计算机辅助外科和微创外科之间的结合对世界各地的影像学家和外科医生来说是研究机会和挑战。

总体需求

患者特异性模式

与模拟不同，信息引导性治疗（IGT）需要模型数据特异性地与将治疗的患者匹配，因为基于典型解剖学标准制作的模型对一个具体患者进行的实际手术操作是不充分的。患者的特异性成像能够在术前（如通过 CT 或 MRI）或术中（如通过超声或传统的 X 射线照相术）来产生。

高质量成像

信息引导性治疗（IGT）依赖于空间精确的模型。为了描绘逼真而一致的信息，成像需要特别高的分辨率。

实时反馈

目前的系统使外科医生需要等待新的图像被分割和更新。因此，需要快速的动态反馈，与可视化分割和注册有关的反应时间应该缩短。

高度精确和准确

美国神经外科医生协会近期的一项对 250 名神经外科医生进行的调查显示[177]，外科医生很少能够忍受成像系统的错误（总体上为 1～2mm 的精确性，在脊柱和骨科应用中为 2～3mm 的精确度）。可视化、注册和轨迹的所有要素都必须是精确和准确的，并特别关注与术中组织变形有关的错误。

可重复性和耐用性

信息引导性治疗（IGT）必须能够自动合并各种不同的数据，以便于在任何情况下算法都能持续可信任地进行运算。

术前图像与术中信息的相关性

这个要求对生物医学工程师来说是最关键的兴趣点，并且对组织变形的补偿而言尤其重要。是否由显微镜、内镜、荧光镜、电子记录、生理性模拟或其他成像技术来产生，术前和术中成像和信息需要结合起
43 来并由手术引导系统进行相关性分析。

直观的仪器和用户界面

信息引导性治疗（IGT）系统的最为重要的部分是它的可用性。外科医生的注意力必须集中在患者身上，而不是在计算模型的细节上。

立体定向放射外科学

腹腔镜在普通外科中已经成为近来技术发展的主要舞台，而其他外科学科则采用了其他微创方法，这个部分重点讨论由此而来的“影像”和“操作”这个手术主题。例如，血管内的干预治疗，如经皮穿刺冠状动脉血管成形术、药物洗脱冠状动脉支架和主动脉支架移植物，已经使心血管疾病的外科治疗发生了革命性变化[8,22,23]。在耳鼻咽喉学和神经外科学领域，计算机成像引导系统已经用于将术中所遇到的结构与术前影像进行精确关联[112,113]。立体定向放射外科学这一学科将影像引导外科学的概念更加深入了一步。

立体定向放射外科学采用精确的靶向和大量的交叉火力、高度校准的高能量离子射线束来无损伤地切除组织。这种概念是在 20 世纪 50 年代由瑞典的神经外科医生 Lars Leksell 首先提出的，这项技术已用于治疗 / 切除各种良性和恶性颅内病变而不留下手术切口[119]。正常大脑组织的损害，如三叉神经（三叉神经的神经痛）、丘脑（震颤）和癫痫灶（难以处理的癫痫）的损害，都是这项技术的重要临床适应证[34]。其间许多研究显示，对于多种耳鼻喉科疾病，包括颅底和头颈部肿瘤，放射外科学是一项重要的治疗选择[4,9,16,66]。最近，放射外科学技术已经应用于颅脑外疾病的治疗，如脊髓肿瘤和胸腹腔内的病变[215,216]。立体定向放射外科学的许多最新的应用都受到普通外科传统领域的影响，包括肺癌、肝癌和胰腺癌[78,152,154,171,175,206,224,235]。随着对科学技术的认识和放射外科学发展的临床实践，这项技术可能会成为一种价值不断提升的无创手术方式，可以治疗一大类儿童普通外科疾病。这个部分的目的是概述立体定向放射外科学的原则及其目前在儿童中的应用情况。另外，这个部分也将讨论立体定向放射外科学在颅脑外部位的相对较新的应用，重点是不断涌现的科技发展方向。

放射生物学

自 1895 年伦琴发现 X 射线以来，科学家和临床医生们已经研究了电离辐射对生物组织的作用，这个领域称作放射生物学。1906 年，Bergonié 和 Tribondeau 进行了一系列实验研究，实验显示，在更低的放射剂量下，未成熟的分裂期细胞比成熟的非分裂期细胞更易受到损伤[12]。他们的观察导致了 Bergonié-Tribondeau 法则形成，后者阐明了电离辐射可更为有效地杀伤未分化的有丝分裂活跃的细胞[12]。后来的研究证实了这个法则，并进一步优化了我们目前对放射治疗学生物学基础的理解[19,117,119,198]。

所有带电的粒子（β 粒子、质子束，或是电子束）和高能光束（γ 射线和 X 射线）都可以对靶细胞的 DNA 产生直接或间接的损害[83]。密集的粒子辐射的电离特性可导致细胞内 DNA 的直接损害。相反，大多数高能光束（X 射线）的作用机制是从细胞的组成分子（绝大多数情况下是水分子）中喷出电子（辐射分解作用）[82,124]。喷出的电子能够直接损害 DNA，导致细胞损害性自由基形成。这样产生的自由基可以与其他自由基结合形成新的分子，如过氧化氢，其对重要的细胞结构具有毒性作用（细胞膜和溶酶体）。这些自由基也有潜在的继发性损害染色体 DNA 的作用。这些高能辐射造成的损害有许多分子作用机制：一种机制涉及含氮基团的丢失，第二种机制涉及两条 DNA 分子链中间氢键的损害，第三种机制涉及对 DNA 支柱的损害[82,124]。

对 DNA 分子单链的损害是没有什么重要的，因为这种损害通常可以进行修复。然而如果辐射光束的作用足够集中，可使两条邻近的单链 DNA 分子破裂，就会产生一种不可纠正的 DNA 双链破裂[176]。在随后的细胞分裂循环中，一种严重染色体组不稳定性可能会导致细胞的灭活[196]。这种细胞死亡的有丝分裂期后模型是主要的模式，但是如果对 DNA的损害启动了 p53-和 Bcl-2-依赖性机制，也可以发生凋亡性细胞死亡。这些机制能够启动一种瀑布式反应，导致效应物胱门蛋白酶激活，从而瞄准多个重要的细胞死亡底物[228]。另外，辐射损害可能会影响到细胞分裂的比例，因此会导致一种（细胞分裂的）延迟以及伴随的细胞数量下降。最后，如果电离辐射杀死了处于 G1、S 或 G2 期内的细胞，就可能会发生细胞间期死亡。在 G2 和 M 期内，细胞对电离辐射是最为敏感的[228]。

由电离辐射的粒子形式诱导的细胞损害的数量与电离辐射的线性能量迁移（LET）有关。LET 描述的是从电离光束迁移到组织（直接穿过组织）的能量的数量；它可以通过每微米迁移距离上沉积的以千电子伏特计的能量来计算[82,83]。X 射线和 γ 射线归类为具有较低的 LET，因为它们的电子分布在组织中较长的一段距离。电离辐射的线性能量迁移水平是非常重要的，因为相同剂量的电离辐射线性能量迁移水平不同时可产生不同的生物学反应。术语“相对生物学反应”描述的是一种在损害更大的重粒子与 X 射线束之间比较生物学效应的方法[82]。

各种物理、化学和生物学因素都可以影响给定细胞对电离辐射反应的敏感性。影响细胞反应的重要物 44
理学因素包括：线性能量迁移水平和电离辐射的剂量比例[198]。最理想的线性能量迁移大约是 160 keV/μm，其可以产生最高水平的双链 DNA 分子破裂。同时更高的电离辐射剂量比例可防止细胞修复亚致死量的染色体损害。

某种化学因素称为放射敏化剂和辐射防护剂可调节电离辐射的应。最有效的放射敏化剂——氧气——可促进间接损害性自由基的形成[198]。缺氧的细胞，如经常在较大的恶性肿瘤中见到的，对电离辐射具有抵抗力。

在细胞对高能电离辐射反应中，两种重要的生物学因素是：处于细胞周期的时期和细胞修复亚致死性损害的能力。处于 C2 和 M 期的细胞对电离辐射是最为敏感的。暴露于相同电离辐射累积剂量而为多次暴露——分级暴露的细胞，这样的细胞可能比在一段时间或一次暴露整个电离辐射剂量的细胞具有更高的存活率[117]。这种现象是源自于细胞在下一次电离辐射暴露以前修复亚致死性损害的能力，对于放射外科学的作用效力，它形成了一个重要的理论基础[117]。

放射治疗和分级治疗

放射治疗学或放射线疗法指的是利用电离辐射来治疗病理性疾病。利用电离辐射治疗癌症的最初报道是在 1899 年，即在伦琴 1895 年发现 X 射线的不久以后[35]。在 20 世纪 30 年代，Coutard 描述了实用的“分级”，其指的是将全部剂量的电离辐射分成多个较小的剂量，根据每天的基础量来给予[35]。分级是放射治疗学领域的一个基本原则[117,118]。通过以多个每天分级剂量给予电离辐射数周时间，就有可能用一个更高的总剂量来照射肿瘤，同时相对地使周围的正常组织免遭放射治疗的大多数损害。电离辐射对组织的作用取决于多个因素，通常指的是以下四个"R"：再增殖（repopulation）、再分布（redistribu tion）、修复（repair）和再氧化（reoxygenation）[218]。再增殖是指在肿瘤以及邻近正常组织中存活细胞的分裂和随后的增殖。理想情况下，放射治疗以后只有邻近正常组织会发生再增殖。再分布是指处于放射敏感期（G2 期和 M 期）的细胞会发生死亡，处于 S 期的细胞会继续存活。理想情况下，当肿瘤细胞处于放射敏感期而其邻近正常组织细胞处于细胞周期中相对对放射不敏感的 S 期时才给予放射治疗。在分级的电离辐射剂量之间，修复亚致死性损害取决于氧气[218]。肿瘤细胞呈缺氧状态，因此相对缺乏修复其 DNA 的能力。而且，氧气在电离辐射用于杀死肿瘤细胞的自由基机制中是非常重要的。肿瘤细胞获取氧气并在放射治疗中变得更为敏感的方式称为再氧化。虽然确切机制还不清楚，肿瘤中缺氧的区域经常倾向于更好的氧化，因此在一段更长的时期内更加具有放射敏感性。这种现象能够在某些临床情况中使分级治疗比单次剂量治疗更有效[218]。总体上，分级治疗在放射治疗学中是一个非常重要的概念，是作为将正常组织和病理组织暴露于电离辐射下的标准技术。通过分级治疗，正常组织在病理组织被破坏时应该得到恢复。虽然分级治疗方法依据特异性病理学而有所不同，但是目前的方法经常包括有 30 种治疗分级治疗方法[35]。

在 20 世纪 50 年代以前，放射治疗仪只能发出相对较低能量的 X 射线，其特征是快速的能量衰减和浅层的穿透照射[35]。而新的放射治疗仪能够发出百万电子伏特（MeV）的 X 射线，可以穿透更深层的组织，因此更加适用于治疗更深部位的病变。目前，放射治疗主要是采用线性加速器或直线加速器来进行放射治疗。直线加速器采用电磁波来加速带电的粒子穿过直线加速管。这些从直线加速器出来的粒子撞击金属靶，然后产生 X 射线。这个过程称为韧致辐射[35]。较为少见的是采用钴 60 进行放射治疗，即采用放射性同位素作为高能放射源[35]。钴 60 放射源的射线穿透深度相对较浅，最大剂量的深度接近 0.5cm，因此它们较少用于深部病变的放射性治疗。放射治疗已经是一种大家接受的治疗颅内和颅外病变的方法[4,9,34,116,119]。有关放射治疗学应用的医学文献非常广泛，超出了这个概述的范围。

立体定向放射外科学

立体定向放射外科学是指将单次高剂量电离辐射释放到精确定位目标的方法和相应的技术。它具有可以释放大得多的电离辐射剂量到一个病变部位，而周围正常组织不会超出电离辐射的耐受范围这样的潜在优势。这种单次辐射或局限性辐射，可以通过大量的辐射束瞄准组织来达到小范围组织内较大的放射治疗剂量。"立体定向"是指放射外科学采用计算机运算法则将治疗中的患者的实时解剖和术前影像调整一致以便于进行精确的瞄准。为了达到这个目标，患者的解剖位置是通过立体定向框架来固定[34,35]。然后应用术前检查的影像资料将立体定向框架固定到位。这种立体定向框架可严格地固定在患者的头颅上，从而可限制目标解剖区域的运动。另外，框架还可作为外在的基准系统，在术前影像检查和手术计划期间与确定的目标组织关联一致。这项技术是 Leksell 于 1951 年首先报道的，并显示出在剂量和时间之间有一种指数关系，超过时间就会发生坏死。通过在不同角度采用多束电离辐射束，可在目标区域外围产生陡峭的辐射剂量衰减。因为这个原因，定义其在放射外科学的适当的确定目标区域是最为重要的。现在在一个手术中，局限性的分级治疗可以联合立体定向放射外科学一起应用，目前已经将此称为分级或分期放射外 45
科学[35]。分期治疗概念是利用"四个 R"的一个让周围正常组织修复的时间。因为细胞的组成，单次巨大的分级辐射倾向于对缓慢增殖的组织比较有效，如良性肿瘤和动脉静脉畸形（AVM）[35]。相反，分期放射外科学涉及的技术可以使一些正常组织进行修复，当切除体积巨大的肿瘤或邻近重要的正常解剖结构的病变时可能是有优势的。

目前已有几种立体定向放射外科治疗系统在应用中，包括重粒子放射外科治疗系统、伽玛刀放射治疗系统、直线加速器放射治疗系统和无框架的影像引导放射外科治疗系统。

立体定向放射外科治疗系统：目前的技术

重粒子放射外科治疗系统：基于质子的放射外

科治疗系统是最早采用的立体定向放射外科治疗系统[55,56,134,135]。带电的粒子（质子或氦离子）相对于光子对放射外科治疗具有独特的优势[136]。采用光子的放射外科是依赖从多个方向进行辐射的交叉光束来达到高度瞄准组织的电离辐射释放，同时可减少周围正常组织的电离辐射暴露，因为光子衰减能量是沿着光束的整个路径进行的，而带电粒子释放能量的衰减是沿着其辐射束穿透的深度不均匀地进行的。尤其是它们会在入口部位产生一种中间能量剂量的区域，其后是高剂量能量的地带，称为 Bragg 电离峰，然后是能量最小的出口处辐射剂量[35]。Bragg 电离峰可以调节以精确地对目标组织区域释放峰值能量[136]。虽然这种现象是有优势的，但是重粒子放射外科治疗系统有几种缺点，限制了其在临床中的广泛使用。尤其是这种治疗系统的建造和使用非常昂贵，需要回旋加速器参与运转。而且，这样的系统需要辐射束调节设备，必须根据每一个患者的情况进行定制，并且需要患者穿上一种固定的塑料面罩或咬合阻滞器以实现固定。由于这些限制因素，重粒子放射外科治疗系统目前仅限于在美国的两个医疗中心使用，且只用于治疗颅内病变[35]。

伽玛刀放射治疗系统：与重粒子放射外科治疗系统不同，伽玛刀放射治疗系统的价格明显低廉而易于使用。其最初是 1967 年由 Leksell 研制的，Leksell 伽玛刀（Elekta Instruments，Inc.，Norcross，GA）采用钴 60 作为放射源[35]。最初的伽玛刀是用于 Parkinson 病的苍白球切开术治疗，以及治疗颅内肿瘤和血管畸形[34,35,67,90,101]。因为伽玛刀采用一种立体定向框架，采用这种系统的放射外科治疗是不进行分级的，主要是由一次性的治疗性照射组成[113]。图 4–8A 和 B 描绘了伽玛刀。

直线加速器放射治疗系统：直线加速器或线性加速器，很久以来便是标准的分级放射治疗的中流砥柱[5,18,39,116]，并在 1982 年更改为直线加速器放射治 46
疗系统[35]。直线加速器放射治疗随后变成一种性 / 价比卓越的、除了伽玛刀放射外科治疗系统以外被广泛使用的放射治疗系统。当用于放射外科治疗时，直线加速器是通过患者头部周围的多个弓形途径的运动来释放交叉光束。光束交叉的区域就是多个辐射光束交叉以接受高剂量辐射的地方，而周围正常组织很少暴

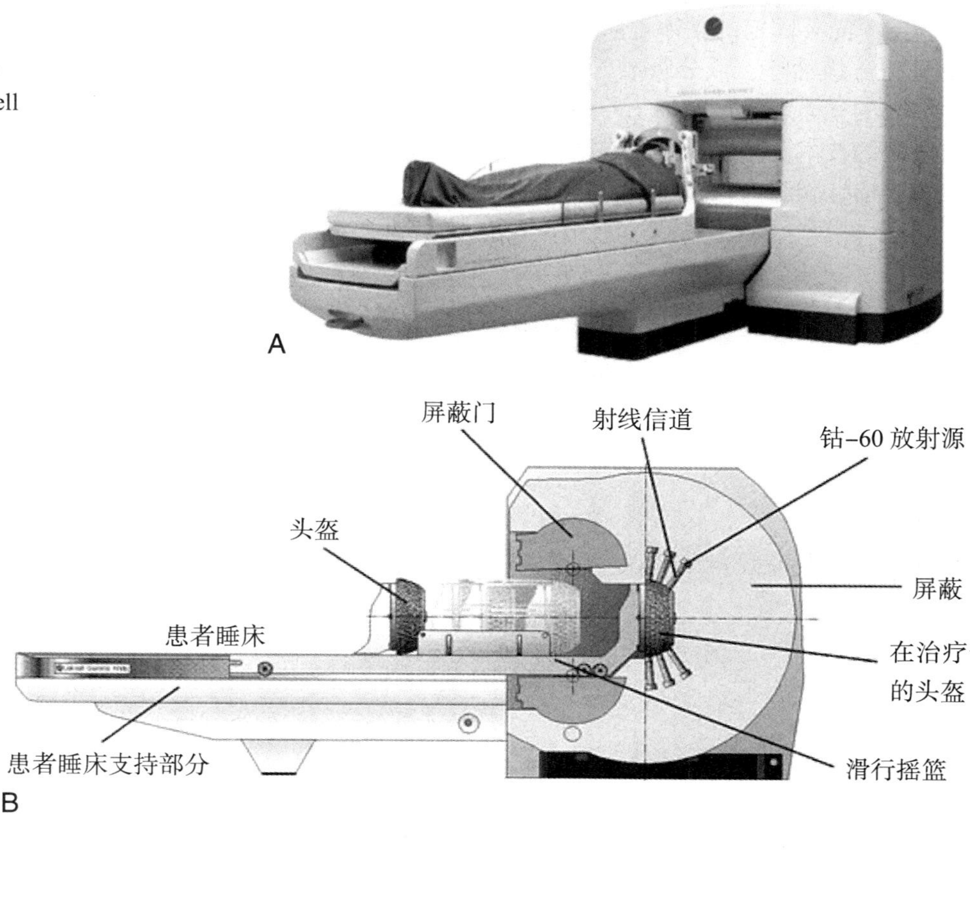

图 4–8　A. Leksell 伽玛刀。（Courtesy of Elekta Instruments，Inc.，Norcross，GA.）B. Leksell 伽玛刀的布局。（http://www.sh.Isuhsc.edu.neurosurgery/gammaknife/gamma-knife/）

露于电离辐射中[35]。采用直线加速器进行放射外科治疗的患者也必须戴上一种固定于头颅的立体定向框架以进行术前的影像学检查和治疗。在美国，目前直线加速器放射外科学治疗是主要的方式，大约比伽玛刀放射外科学系统的应用多 6 倍[35]。

无框架的影像指导放射外科治疗系统：近来出现了一种新奇的直线加速器放射外科治疗系统改良版，可以实现无框架的影像指导放射外科治疗系统。这种系统，商业上已经有现成的产品可用，即 CyberKnife（Accuray，Inc.，Sunnyvale，CA），采用专门为放射外科治疗系统设计的轻量级的直线加速器，装配有一个具有高度机动性的机械臂[33]。机械臂能够定位，有 6 度自由度来瞄准直线加速器，有 0.3mm 的精确度。另外，CyberKnife 系统突出了影像指导性，排除了骨骼固定的需要[34,36]。CyberKnife 需要一系列立体定向射线照片，用于识别术前放置的金基准系统。这种基准系统在术前影像检查和手术计划期间在局麻下进行放置，以便将患者的目标解剖区域与术前用以治疗的影像学检查关联一致。通过在治疗期间主动获取射线照片，系统能够在治疗期间进行导航，以几乎实时的方式追踪目标解剖区域[33,34]。采用影像指导系统以后，CyberKnife 不需要固定的立体定向框架即可运作，因此能够进行分级治疗（低分级放射外科学），同时可用于身体外的立体定位。在小儿外科中，这种系统可能具有显著的技术优势，因为它或许就能够将放射外科学应用于治疗胸腔内和腹腔内的疾病（图 4–9）。

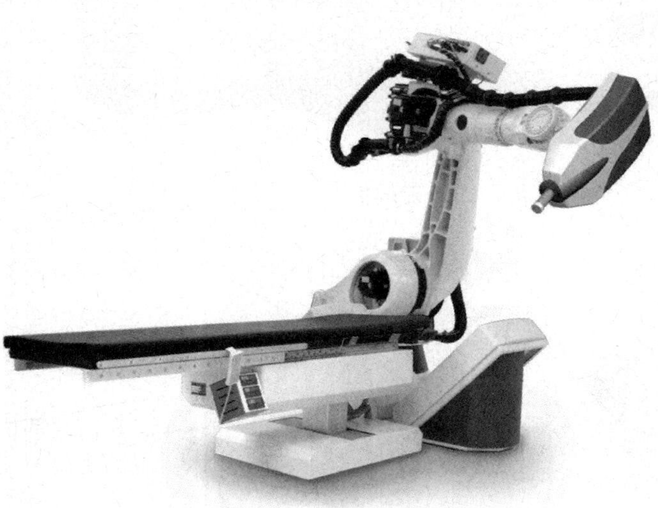

图 4–9　CyberKnife 系统。（http://www.sky.sannet.ne.jp/ybaba/main.html）

立体定向放射外科学在儿童中的应用

颅内病变的立体定向放射外科学治疗许多年以前就已成为一种人们普遍接受的治疗模式。从放射外科学的观点来看，颅内容量是相对静止不变的这个事实导致了本质上静止不动的目标组织，因此高剂量的电离辐射能够在一个或数个治疗分级内传递而对邻近的正常组织很少有损害风险。通过采用将头颅固定于一个给定位置的立体定向头颅框架，可以精确地瞄准目标组织，最大限度地提高治疗的精确度。这种优势使立体定向放射外科技术在成年人中得到了广泛的应用，用于治疗包含在坚硬的颅骨内的良性和恶性耳鼻咽喉部病变[4,39,41,131,132]和神经外科病变[67,68,80,129,168,201]。已有多个研究小组报道了可以安全有效地应用立体定向放射外科学技术来治疗儿童脑部和颈部的恶性病变。除了儿童脑部肿瘤以外，也有立体定向放射外科学用于治疗儿童非恶性颅内病变的报道。采用放射外科学来治疗大脑的动静脉畸形已有很多文献报道[102,133,138,156,200]。在一项有 30 例儿童颅内动静脉畸形病例（平均年龄为 11.2 岁）的研究中，放射外科学治疗以后的完整切除率为 35%。作者的结论是：立体定向放射外科学技术对于有动静脉畸形的患儿是一种有效的治疗选择，并发症的发生率较低，在可接受的水平[200]。

当与成年人群相比时，立体定向放射外科学在儿童中应用的经验仍然是有限的。早期报道突出了放射外科学作为一种治疗模式的安全性和有效性，但是临床随访仍然是早期的，许多研究只限于将放射外科学技术应用于外科不可切除的病变。尽管应用经验相对有限，立体定向放射外科学在儿童中的应用可能有几种对儿童人群的特殊的理论优势。与标准的分级放射治疗相比，立体定向放射外科学技术释放等角的电离辐射治疗，具有毫米对厘米的精确度。在儿童患者，正常组织和病理组织之间的距离可能是非常小的。另外处于发育中的儿童大脑可能比成年人的大脑对电离辐射效应更加敏感。已有报道称在对大脑进行放射治疗以后患儿可能会出现潜在的认知和内分泌障碍[69,70,201]。这些担心大多数局限于应用电离辐射来治疗婴幼儿的颅内肿瘤。因此，立体定向放射外科学治疗精确度的改进在儿童人群中显得尤为重要。

除了精确性，立体定向放射外科学技术与放射治疗学也有所不同，它们只涉及一个到很少几个治疗期间。标准的分级放射治疗学经常需要数十个治疗期间来使治疗效果的收益最大化，而使对正常组织的损害最小化。在儿童，多个治疗期间可能是一种重大
47 的挑战。在年幼的儿童中，可能需要应用镇静剂或麻醉剂来避免患儿运动。这样的干预治疗不是没有风险的，可能会限制治疗期间的数量来减少患儿总体的风险。

虽然立体放射外科学在儿童中的优势显得很有前景，但是也有特殊的劣势和局限性必须给予克服。总体上放射外科学技术需要一种立体定向的框架来将术前影像和实际的电离辐射释放协调一致。然而，这些框架必须采用钉和螺孔可靠地固定在头颅上。在成年人中，这项操作经常可以在局部麻醉下进行，但是在儿童中可能需要足够的镇静剂，甚至可能需要全身麻醉。而且，婴幼儿的头颅比较柔软而不够坚硬，因为颅缝还没有融合，经常不能采用标准的立体定向框架。同样放射外科学治疗期间需要患者保持静止不动，以便系统能够精确地释放电离辐射以进行治疗。成年人能够配合而不需要使用镇静剂，而年幼的儿童和婴幼儿可能需要有意识地使用镇静剂或进行全身麻醉。虽然这种缺点因放射外科学治疗时需要相对很少的治疗期间而是有限的，但与在成年人中的应用相比时，其放射治疗的微创的特性仍然会下降。

近来，已经出现了无框架的影像指导的立体定向放射外科学，即 CyberKnife 系统，采用直线性速器配机器人手臂来释放电离辐射能量。另外，该系统采用实时影像指导以追踪治疗期间内患者解剖部位的运动。因此，这种模式的放射外科学技术不需要采用立体定向的框架。近来，Giller 等人描述了这种系统在儿童中应用的情况[68,70]。他们采用 CyberKnife 系统治疗了 21 例有大脑肿瘤的儿童；后者的年龄从 8 个月到 16 岁不等[69]。没有发生治疗操作相关的死亡或并发症，在过半数的患儿中实现了肿瘤局部控制。71%的患儿只接受了 1 次治疗期间，38%的患儿不需要进行全身麻醉。没有一个患儿需要严格的头颅固定[69]。在另外一个报告中，同一个研究小组强调了，使用 CyberKnife 系统讨论了对 5 例婴幼儿进行的放射外科学治疗[70]。虽然不需要采用标准的立体定向框架，患儿是通过全身麻醉、外形匹配的头部支持、面罩和身体铸型来实现静止不动。没有遇到治疗相关的毒性反应，作者得出的结论是：无毒性的放射外科学学技术能够采用一种不需要严格固定的机器人控制系统来实现对婴幼儿的治疗[69]。

头颅以外的立体定向放射外科治疗学——普通外科中的应用

尽管采用立体定向放射外科学技术治疗颅内病变已经被人们广泛接受，但是它在治疗头颅以外的病变的应用，尤其是在治疗胸腔内和腹腔内疾病的应用，仍处于发展初期。虽然颅内的解剖结构通过立体定向框架能够轻易实现静止不动，但是胸腔和腹腔内的器官经常因为呼吸、蠕动和其他因素而有显著的运动。结果，目前只有一小部分文献是有关将立体定向放射外科治疗应用于头颅以外病变的。近来已有几个研究描述了将立体定向放射外科学技术应用于治疗肝脏[114,216,217,238,244]、胰腺[141,153,154]、肺脏[236,238,240]和肾脏病变[171,175]的效果——解剖区域传统上属于普通外科医生的领域。采用新奇的影像指导技术以及软组织固定设备已使这些治疗变为可能[35,152,216,235]。

目前，大多数临床文献为个案报道和详述研究头颅以外放射外科学技术的安全性和可行性的报道。另外，其中许多报道着重于应用放射外科学技术治疗头颅以外目标组织的技术和工程学方面，有关患者结果的数据很少。所有这些报道都着重于成年患者人群。然而，尽管这个方面经验不足，但是围绕立体定向放射外科学治疗的技术正在快速发展中，显示出对于潜在的不易接近病变的微创治疗具有非常大的前景。最新的系统，如无框架的影像指导 CyberKnife系统，某一天就可能使微创治疗各种儿童恶性肿瘤成为可能。

放射免疫引导的外科学

采用放射性同位素标记抗体，进行全身注射以后，可能会特异性与肿瘤结合，从而可以用伽马探测器进行探测[125,190,204]。对大多数情况，非特异性结合和持续全身分布其信号-噪音比率很低，限制了这种办法的应用。近来，美国食品药品管理局（FDA）已经批准了几种新的有前景的放射性标记的抗体，用于辅助鉴定功能性内分泌肿瘤患者的隐藏的远处转移，以及在乳房癌和黑色素瘤患者中评价受累的淋巴结转移。

外科机器人

内镜技术和装备的创新不断拓展了微创外科（MAS）应用的范围。而许多微创外科操作已替代了传统的开放性手术。在一个有边界限制的操作空间内要达到灵巧和精确的器械控制仍然有困难。这个问题进一步又混合了通过 2-D 视频影像进行手术操作的问题。现在机器人外科手术系统已进步到可能会着手突破这些限制。

自从 20 世纪 90 年代后期引进了机器人外科手术系统以来，计算机增强型机器人外科手术系统的应用得到了快速的发展。最初是设想用于促进战场手术，现在这些系统已经能够用于操作复杂的微创外科手术[7,10,54,57,61,86,105,121,147,148,183,208]。在儿童中，早期的报道表明，手术机器人能够完成普通的和相对简单的小儿外
48 科手术操作。最近，机器人外科手术系统的应用已经写进了多个外科分科中，包括小儿外科学、小儿泌尿外科学和小儿心胸外科学[128,140]。另外，复杂的技术上具有挑战性的手术操作，如机器人辅助的胎儿外科，已经有在动物模型中的应用报道[1,96,97,139,148]。

标准的微创外科技术和方法的限制

虽然微创外科技术已经大事改革了许多手术操作，但是它们具有必然的独特复杂性，不会在传统的开放性手术中出现。有必要强调特殊的外科机器人能够胜任的技术挑战。

运动限制

微创外科器械穿透腹壁来进行工作。进入腹腔的端口作为支点会颠倒器械头部相对于器械手柄活动的运动方向。为了将器械头部运动到在体腔的左边，外科医生的手就必须运动到身体外部的右边。这种运动颠倒需要非倒装的器械控制，是一种精神上费力的工作，尤其是当手术操作的复杂性增加的时候。

微创手术的大多数器械都含有一种末端受动器，装配在较长的刚硬的杆状物头部。内镜套管可使这些器械以体壁内固定点周围为支点，但是运动限定于横向运动。因此开放性手术器械的位置和方向的 6 个自由度（定义为沿 X、Y 和 Z 轴方向运动，以及在这些轴周围进行旋转）在微创外科操作中被缩减为 4个自由度的运动（上下倾斜、左右摇摆、旋转和插入）（图 4-10A）。微创外科器械的另外 2 个自由度可以通过在远端构造的关节来得到恢复，经过套管支点的位置（图 4-10B）。然而，在手术操作期间没有计算机辅助的控制，这些远端关节的精巧的动态控制可能会难以进行协调。

触觉的限制

微创外科器械的长杆迫使外科医生的手远离手术操作的解剖结构，这会显著降低触觉和反作用力。延长的手术器械长度也放大了任何现有的手部的震动。而且，器械头部的偏移高度依赖于它插入体腔内的深度。例如，插入较浅的器械需要相当大的手部运动才能完成体腔内一个给定的器械头部动作，而插入较深的器械仅需要少得多的手部运动就可以扫过器械头部

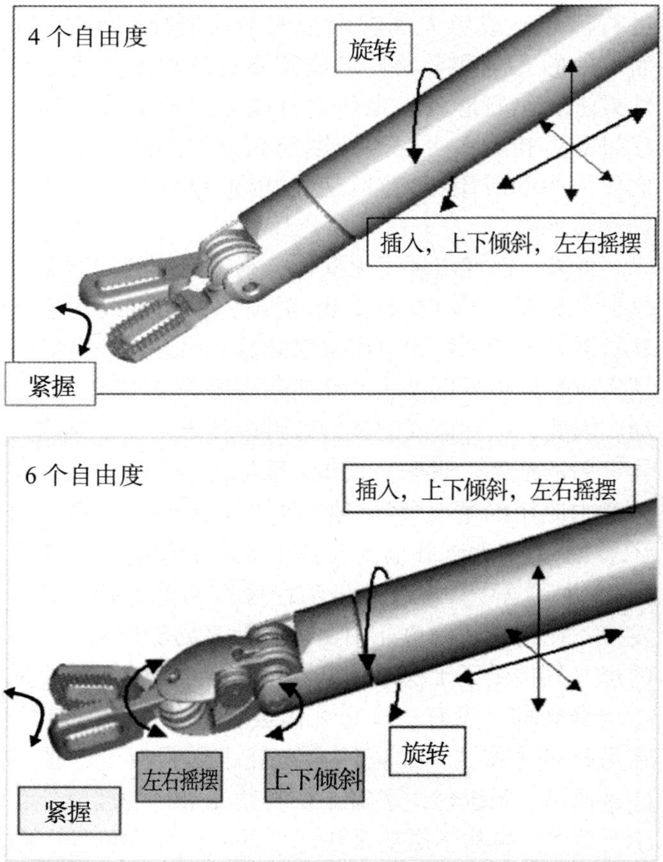

图 4-10 A. 传统的 4 个自由度（DOF）的内镜下手术器械。B. 全部铰接的 6 个自由度的机器人手术器械。（Courtesy of Intuitive Surgical, Sunnyvale, CA）

周围的距离。因此，器械的动力学在整个手术操作中经常发生改变。与标准的开放性手术技术相比，这些因素可能会导致手术的精确度和可预测性运动下降。

视觉的限制

内镜技术的引进需要外科医生接受视频影像的导而不是直接的视觉指导。视频监视器经常位于患者的远侧，内镜、手术器械和监视器之间方向上的不同需要外科医生在视觉和电动调整画面之间进行一种有难度的精神上的转换[214]。当采用有角度的内镜系统时，这个问题将进一步恶化。

传统的内镜是建立在单个镜头行列基础上的，其显示的影像是平面 2–D 形式的。这种形式去除了正常情况下双目并用时视觉的许多深度方面的信息，可使一些操作变得更加复杂，如在组织水平之间进行解剖时。虽然有一些立体定向视频系统存在，但是它们的性能受到内镜本身的分辨率和对比度特性以及显示技术的限制。另外，传统的内镜经常需要一个助手来扶持内镜并进行相关的操作。助手正常的震动和运动经常被放大的影像所夸大。

在外科手术中的机器人技术

在过去的数十年间，机器人已经承担起许多不同的工作，如制造加工、深海探测、弹药引爆、军事监
49 测和娱乐表演。而机器人技术在外科中的应用仍然是一个相对年轻的领域。最初服务于工业机器人的在机械设计、运动学和控制算法方面的改进，都已直接应用到外科手术机器人中了。

最初有记录的外科手术机器人应用是 1987 年用于 CT 引导下立体定向脑组织活检术[242]。从此以后，技术的进步导致了数种不同类型的机器人系统诞生。这些系统在复杂性和功能方面都有显著的不同。

机器人外科手术系统的分类

机器人分类的一种方法是根据它们自动化的水平。目前在外科手术中采用的有三种类型的机器人：自主机器人、外科手术协助设备和远距离遥控机器人（表 4–2）。

表 4–2　机器人外科手术系统的分类

系统的类型	定义	举例
自动化的机器人	系统执行治疗时没有外科医生的即刻指令	CyberKnife 机器人
手术辅助机器人	外科医生和机器人共享控制	伊索机器人
远程遥控机器人	外科医生指令指导手术器械的运动	直觉的外科手术达·芬奇系统 计算机化的运动宙斯系统

自主操作机器人是执行术前的计划而不接受任何来自于外科医生的即刻控制。操作的任务是典型的聚焦或重复性操作，但是需要一定程度的精密度，不是通过人类的双手可以达到的。一个例子就是 Robodoc 系统用于矫形外科中精确地碾磨出股骨槽以便于股骨头植入。另外一个例子是 CyberKnife 系统，其中直线加速器装配在机器人手臂上以便于精确地释放电离辐射到颅内和脊柱内的肿瘤中[2,120]。

第二种类型的机器人是外科手术协助设备，外科医生和机器人共享控制系统。这类机器人中最众所周知的例子是伊索（AESOP）机器人系统（用于理想定位的自动化内镜系统；Computer Motion, Inc.,Goleta,CA）。这种系统允许外科医生将一个内镜配备到机器人手臂上，可提供一种稳定的影像，去除了助手扶持内镜时产生的固有的正常的运动。外科医生可以通过语音命令重新确定内镜的位置。现在，伊索机器人已经应用于许多不同的外科分科中，包括普通外科[6,108]、妇产科外科[149]、心胸外科[160]和泌尿外科[130]。

最后一种类型的机器人是远距离遥控机器人，其每一个功能都明确地由外科医生来控制。在一个控制台上，外科医生手部的运动都会被电子控制器追踪，然后转播给一个受控机器人，以便于器械头部能够完美的反映出外科医生的每一个动作。因为控制台与受控机器人在物理上分离的，这些系统就作为远距离遥控机器人来提及。在机器人辅助外科手术系统中，所有这些近年来的进展都包括了后一种类型的机械。

远距离遥控机器人的历史

远距离遥控机器人外科手术系统的基础可以追溯到 1970 年代，当时美国国家航空和宇宙航行局（NASA）开始发展远距离遥控机器人外科手术系统，用于在太空中向在空间站中生活的宇航员们提供急诊手术。在 1980 年代后期和 1990 年代早期，机器人外科手术系统的目标是发展能够开展战场手术的机器人系统，而外科医生可很好地躲在前线的后方，通过装在轮式装甲车上的机器人为受伤的军队开展手术治疗。这些计划是试图开发一种远距离遥控的机器人，将人类手术者的动作转移到一定距离以外的机器人机械手臂的活动中。虽然将这种“主人-奴隶”式的系统应用到外科手术中是一种革命性的思想，但是这种技术早已应用于其他不同种类的工业中了。最初的机械式主人-奴隶系统是 1948 年由 Raymond Goertz 在 Argonne 国家实验室中开发的。这个机器人，叫做 M1，是采用一系列钢索和机械链连接到主人操作者，通过人类操作者对同一个受控操作者的控制来完成手术，人类操作者在铅玻璃屏障的另外一侧以免受放射线暴露。

斯坦福研究所[72]（现在是斯坦福国际研究所，斯坦福，CA）开发了最初的能够进行手术操作的“主人-奴隶”式远距离遥控机器人外科手术系统。该系统包括有外科医生的工作站和远距离手术系统，这种系统是为进行远距离开放式战场外科手术服务而设计的。它的特征是远距离控制机器人的手臂、立体感的影像、基本的力反馈和一种人类环境改造学的设计。虽然这种系统从来就没有完全的得到发展，但是它形成了今天所使用的商业化机器人系统的基础。

目前在小儿外科领域中使用的机器人技术的状况

目前在小儿外科学文献中已经有两种机器人外科手术系统应用的报道；宙斯（Zeus）系统（原来的 Computer Motion，Goleta, CA；现在由 Intuitive Surgical 掌控，Sunnyvale, CA）和达·芬奇(da Vinci)外科手术系统（Intuitive Surgical）。这两种系统都可以归类为远距离遥控机器人。这两个公司近来进行了合并，这就意味着达·芬奇系统将成为主要的机器人手术平台。然而，目前这两种机器人系统仍然在临床中得到积极应用。

即使这些系统通常被称为外科手术机器人，但是这个词用词不当，因为“机器人”就意味着拥有自主的运动。不管是达·芬奇系统还是宙斯系统其操作都不能离开外科医生的即刻指令来进行。一个比较好的术语可能是“计算机增强的远距离遥控机器人”。然而，出于对已经出版的文献一致性考虑，这个部分仍 50
将继续把这些系统称作机器人。

宙斯系统

宙斯系统包括外科医生控制台和三个机械手臂（图 4-11A 和 B）。外科医生在离开手术台数尺开外的控制台进行操作，采用手持操纵器来控制两条机器人手臂和外科手术器械，脚踩踏板来激活计算机驱动系统，采用语音指令来指挥由伊索机器人手臂控制的照相机[96]。与达·芬奇系统一样，宙斯系统提供了减少震颤和定标运动的功能。

宙斯系统包括三个模块独立式的机器人手臂，这三个手臂都配备在手术台上。这种设计使宙斯系统能够适应许多不同的配置。宙斯系统也是以 5mm 手术器械为特征，能够通过宙斯微小的腕关节来增加关节。这种关节可使手术器械在手腕处具有一种额外的自由度，因此总共有 6 个自由度。最近，已经出现了 3.5mm 的手术器械。这些手术器械的特征是具有较小的直径和头部尺寸，这使它们在小儿外科中显得尤其有用。宙斯系统提供了各种不同的成像选择（3-D 和 2-D）和望远镜尺寸。

宙斯系统在 CE（Conformité Européenne）方针下已经接受了用于外科的普及性审查。在美国，宙斯系统接受了 FDA 用于一般性的腹腔镜外科的审查，现在已经应用于胸腔和心脏的手术。

达·芬奇外科手术系统

达·芬奇外科手术系统包括了两个主要组成部分[140]（图 4-12 A 和 B）。第一个组成部分是外科医生的控制台，其中包含视频显示系统、外科医生控制手柄和使用者的界面面板。第二个组成部分是患者的侧面手推车，其中包含有 2～3 个控制手术器械的手臂以及控制视频内镜的另外一个手臂[50]。

进行操作的外科医生坐在外科医生控制台上，后者可以位于手术台 10m 开外的地方。在控制台内部

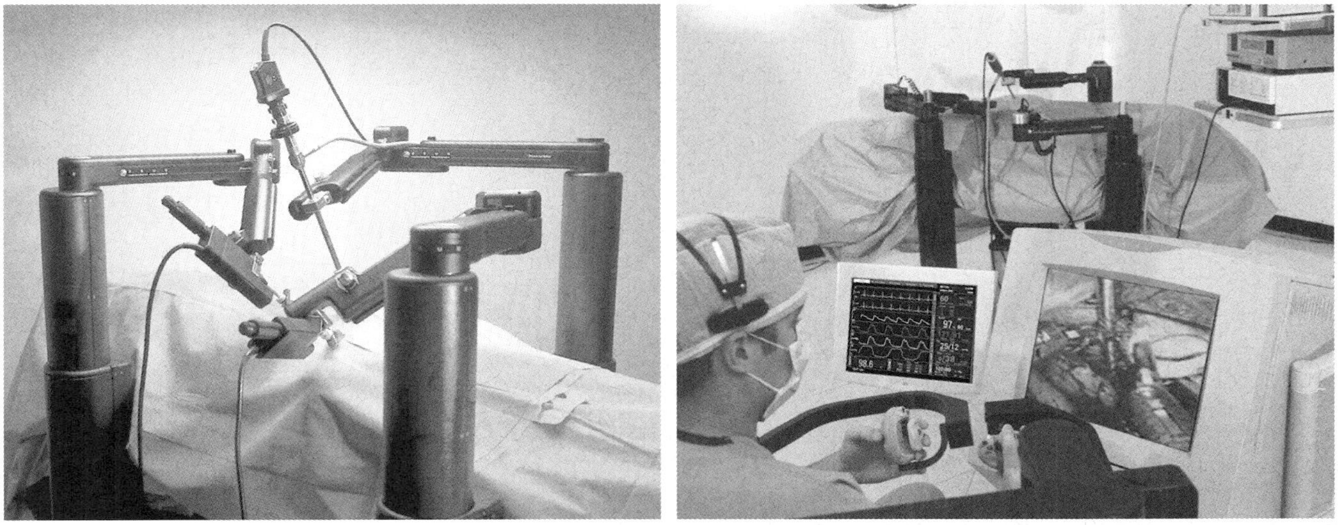

A　　B

图 4-11　A. 计算机化运动的宙斯机器人外科手术系统。B. 宙斯外科医生控制台和它的视频显示器以及熟练的控制。（Courtesy of Intuitive Surgical, Sunnyvale, CA）

装有外科医生控制手柄或母机，后者可担当能够从外科医生的指尖读取位置、方向和控制指令的高分辨率输入设备。这种控制系统也加入了计算机增强功能，如运动成比例缩放和震动衰减。

操作部位的影像可通过高分辨率的立体显示系统放映给外科医生，该系统采用了两个医学等级的阴极射线管监视器来显示单独的影像给外科医生每一只眼睛。然后外科医生的大脑将两幅单独的影像融合成一幅虚拟的 3-D 构造。立体浏览器的影像平面添加上母机的运动范围可恢复视觉协调和手-眼配合。另外，因为内镜下手术器械头部的影像覆盖在外科医生的手感之上，最终的效果就变成外科医生感觉到他们的手事实上就在患者的身体里面。小儿外科方面的应用已经出现了一种新的 2-D 视频 5mm 内镜系统。

标准的达·芬奇手术器械平台包括一组 8.5mm 直径的器械。这些手术器械经过缆索驱动系统可提供 7 个自由度的活动。近来，一套 5mm 的手术器械已经投入使用。这些器械采用一种新的“蛇腕”设计，也能提供 7 个自由度的活动（图 4-12 C）。

自从 1995 年开始应用以来，达·芬奇手术系统在 CE 方针下接受了应用于所有外科手术操作的普及性
51 审查；在美国，它接受了应用于普通外科、胸外科和泌尿外科手术的审查。另外，近来达·芬奇系统接受了应用于涉及心切开术的心脏手术的 FDA 审查。

目前机器人小儿外科手术的优势和局限

不同的机器人手术系统的效用受到儿科患者的体积较小和许多小儿外科手术为重建性手术的高度影响。总体上，机器人系统的优势来自于能够直接突破许多标准的内镜技术和器械受限的技术的特性和能力。与传统的腹腔镜器械需要颠倒操作不同，机器人手术器械的运动可使手术器械直接追踪外科医生的手的活动。在保留了微创外科特性的同时，直观的非颠倒的手术器械控制得到恢复。对于腹腔镜操作初学者来说，手术器械的直观控制是一种特别的优势。

在婴幼儿和新生儿中，经常需要采用经操作器械上的小型放大镜或内镜放大影像来提供微小结构的更加精确的视频[207]。这种增强的视频随着机器人系统的应用得到了进一步的发展，因为它们能够提供一种高倍放大的 3-D 影像。3-D 视频系统加上另外的安全和手术控制措施所能提供的功能超出了传统内镜系统。3-D 显示改善了深度感觉，并且影像通过一个 10 的因数放大，手术器械的敏感性和精确性更高。在控制台上视觉轴与外科医生手部运动的协调一致进一步加强了手-眼配合，这是传统腹腔镜手术很难达到的程度。

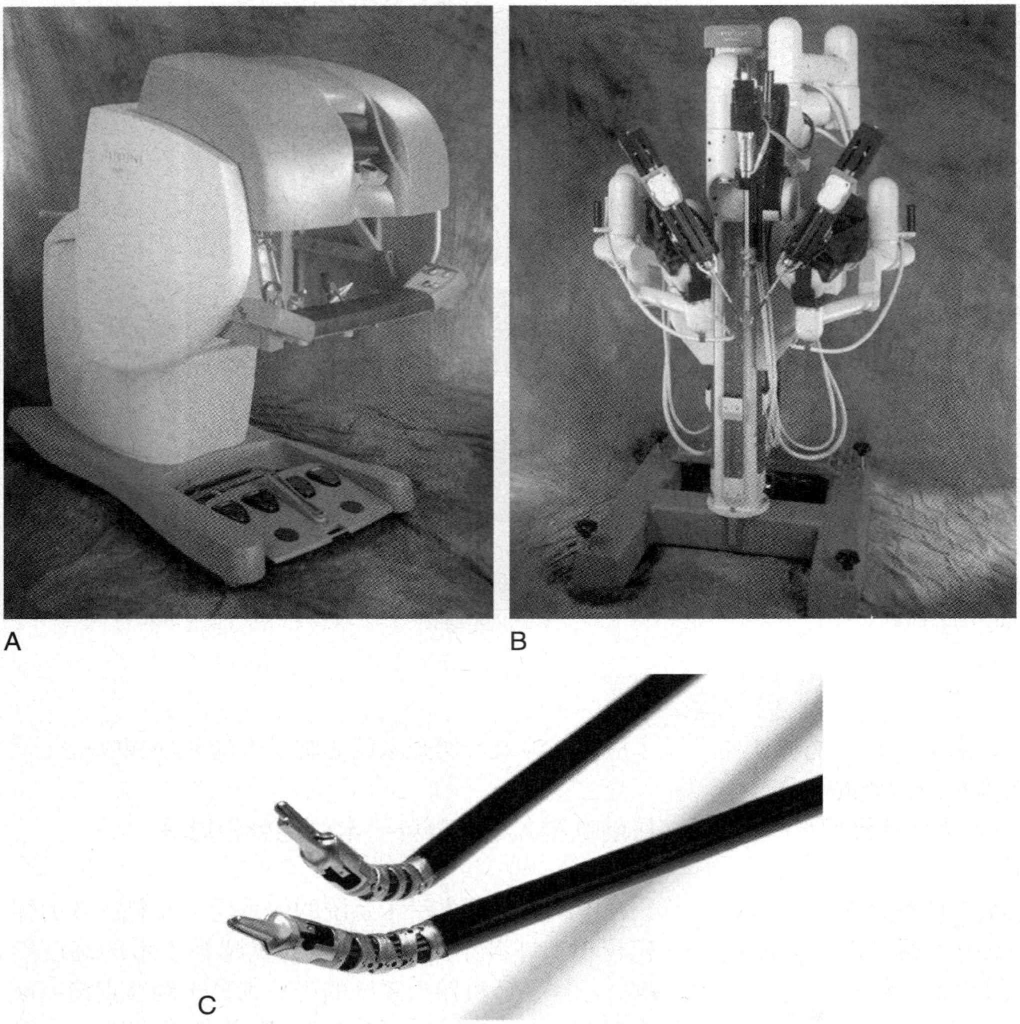

图 4-12　直觉的外科手术达·芬奇机器人外科手术系统是由外科医生控制台（A）和患者床边手推车（B）组成。C. 有关节的 5mm 直径的机器人外科手术器械。（Courtesy of Intuitive Surgical, Sunnyvale, CA）

同样计算机控制系统可以滤过电子震颤，使内镜和手术器械头部的运动比手单独操作更加稳定。另外，该系统可改变从外科医生的手部到器械头部的不同运动的缩放比例。例如，一个 3∶1 的比例可把外科医生手上 3cm 的运动转换成器械头部 1cm 的运动。
52 联合从视频内镜中得到的放大的影像，运动缩放比例可以使较小解剖区域中的精巧动作更加容易完成，动作更加精确[88]。

两种系统在器械远端都采用了工程加固的关节或“手腕”，相对于传统的微创外科器械来说，这些关节或手腕可增加器械的灵活性。这种技术可以使器械进行更大范围的运动和旋转，与人类手腕关节本身的运动范围类似，在有限操作空间内这种技术可能显得尤其有用。特别是达·芬奇手术系统提供的手术器械具有 7 个自由度，其中包括了抓紧动作，而宙斯手术系统手术器械拥有 6 个自由度，也包括抓紧动作。标准的腹腔镜手术器械只拥有 5 个自由度，其中包括抓紧动作。这种增加的灵活性在进行复杂的需要精细的解剖和体内缝合的重建手术时，可能具有特别优势。

最后，通过外科医生和手术患者的分离，远程手术系统的特征是：控制台以工效学原理设计，可以减少经常与长时间进行微创手术有关的劳累。随着小儿肥胖外科领域的发展，这种技术可能成为一种更有意义的技术，因为青少年肥胖患儿的体积更大、腹壁更厚。表 4-3 详细列出了机器人外科手术系统与标准腹腔镜手术技术的技术挑战有关的潜在优势。

虽然机器人外科手术系统与标准的微创外科手术相比可提供多种重要的优势，但是其技术上的许多局限性对小儿外科来说尤其成问题。首先是机器人手术系统的大小问题。当与许多小儿外科手术患者相比

表 4–3　目前远程遥控手术系统的潜在优势

系统	潜在优势	标准的微创外科技术的局限性
达·芬奇	3–D 的视频	2–D 的视频及丧失深度的感觉
	有 6 个自由度的手术器械	刚性的腹腔镜手术器械导致要完成复杂的任务需要一个较高的学习曲线，例如体内缝合
	成比例缩放的运动	因为腹腔镜器械长度较长导致震动被放大
	震动缩减	因为腹腔镜器械长度较长导致震动被放大
	直观的手术器械控制	因为腹腔镜套管的支点作用而会违反直觉的器械头部控制
宙斯	3–D 的视频	2–D 的视频及丧失深度的感觉
	有 5 个自由度的手术器械	刚性的腹腔镜手术器械导致要完成复杂的任务需要一个较高的学习曲线，例如体内缝合
	成比例缩放的运动	因为腹腔镜器械长度较长导致震动被放大
	震动缩减	因为腹腔镜器械长度较长导致震动被放大
	直观的手术器械控制	因为腹腔镜套管的支点作用而会违反直觉的器械头部控制

时，达·芬奇手术系统的手推车或宙斯标准组件机器人手臂可能显得过于庞大了。使用机器人手臂时，这种大小的不协调可能会限制对患者在床边进行的外科手术辅助通道，可能会需要麻醉医生小组进行特殊的术前准备以确保患者气道即刻畅通[207]。

相对于提供标准腹腔镜手术的器械，机器人手术系统可用的手术器械的大小和种类有限。目前，达·芬奇手术系统是唯一的在工业水平正在进一步发展的机器人手术平台。目前达·芬奇手术系统已经引进了一套新的 5mm 直径的拥有 7 个自由度的手术器械。虽然这些器械在最初的 8.5mm 直径基础上显示出显著的改进，但是其提供的手术器械的数量仍然是有限的。而且，这些手术器械采用了一种新的“蛇型手腕”关节，需要稍微大一点的体内操作空间来充分发挥它们增强的灵活性的优势。特别是器械受到的限制比器械头部踞远端连接的关节或手腕 10mm 时更大。同样宙斯外科手术系统提供了数种 5mm 直径的器械，能够拥有 6 个自由度，特征是器械头部和远端连接的关节之间的距离更短，因此它们可以在一个更小的工作空间内发挥其全部的功能。然而它们同时放弃了 1 个自由度。不幸的是，自从两个公司合并以后，再也没有应用新的资源来进一步发展宙斯外科手术系统。

最后，目前可用的机器人外科手术系统中存在很多一般性的限制，在它们广泛应用于小儿外科领域以前必须要克服，包括机器人外科手术系统初期高昂的费用和器械及维护的相对较高的日常费用[140]。另外，没有一个机器人外科手术系统能够提供真正的触觉反馈[207]。相对于开放性手术操作，即使是标准的微创外科手术这样的触觉反馈也减少了，但是在机器人外科手术系统中触觉反馈进一步减少了。这种不利因素部分可以通过机器人外科手术系统提供的改良的视野来补偿，但是当进行精细的外科手术解剖时还是需要一种有效的触觉反馈。

最后，对于整个手术室团队，机器人外科手术系统需要额外的特殊训练。这种操作训练翻译成机器人操作所需时间预计要比传统的腹腔镜手术的训练时间更长，至少要等到外科手术团队熟练掌握新技术的使用。即使是一组有经验的团队，有报道称在每一个机器人辅助手术开始以前，装备的时间也需要额外的 10～35 分钟[207]。毋庸置疑，随着技术的不断发展，53
这些问题中有许多将在下一代机器人外科手术系统中得到解决。

机器人技术在小儿外科中的应用

到目前为止，只有一小部分有关机器人外科手术技术在小儿外科手术中应用的文献显示出机器人辅助外科手术的可行性。这些报道详细描述了在学龄期儿童中完成相对常规的腹腔镜手术操作的情况。最近，有报道称机器人外科手术技术在年轻很多的患者中已经在多个领域中展开，包括小儿普通外科、小儿泌尿外科和小儿心胸外科（表 4–4）。此时大多数文献为

IV类证据，包括病例报告和病例研究，没有I类的证据。然而，最近的报道呼吁对机器人外科手术技术进行更严格的分析。下面一部分详细描述了到目前为止已经出版的文献，重点在于目前和将来机器人外科手术技术在小儿外科领域的应用。

小儿普通外科

描述机器人外科手术系统应用于儿童腹部手术的最初报道是在2002年，是由Gutt等人和Heller等人发表的[79,88]。他们报道了11名儿童（平均年龄12岁，范围在7～16岁）进行了机器人辅助Thal手术或Nissen胃底折叠术治疗胃食管反流性疾病。另外，2名儿童进行了机器人辅助的胆囊切除术治疗有症状的胆石症，1名儿童进行了两侧的卵巢切除术治疗性腺胚细胞瘤。他们采用的是达·芬奇外科手术系统、8.5mm直径的手术器械和12mm直径的内镜。进行胃底折叠术的平均手术时间为146分钟（范围105～180分钟），没有发生显著的术中或术后并发症。

在2003年，多名作者报道了另外的一项病例研究，描述了机器人辅助小儿普通外科手术的安全性和可行性。Luebbe等人描述了一项有20例采用达·芬奇外科手术系统治疗的病例研究[140]，其中包括10例Nissen胃底折叠术（3例同时行胃造口术，1例同时行幽门成形术）、3例胆囊切除术、2例脾切除术、1例脐尿管切除术、1例单侧髂部和腹膜后淋巴结切除术、1例骶骨前肿块活检术、1例肝脏肿块活检术、1例Gore-Tex补片修补Morgagni膈疝手术和1例良性的纵隔肿块活检术[1,140]。患者的平均年龄为8.4岁，但是最年轻的患者只有4个月大，最小的体重只有6.8kg。平均控制台操作时间为93分钟，平均手术室装备时间为45分钟。术中并发症的发生率为15%，包括2例脾脏切除手术中试图控制脾门处出血时中转为剖腹手术，1例在Morgagni膈疝修补手术期间术中经皮抽空气胸。有报道称中转剖腹手术的发生非常迅速。

作者认为，3-D视频、关节化手术器械和运动成比例缩放是机器人外科手术系统的主要优势。其主要的不足是花费昂贵、需要专门训练、丧失触觉感和需要额外的手术室时间进行系统装备和对接。作者详细描述了他们的一些技术，包括患者的体位、通道的放置以及机器人手推车的位置和对接，并描述了他们采用泡沫塑料垫板将体重小于20kg的患者从手术操作台上抬高的技术。这样可使机器人外科手术系统器械通道能够更多地从侧面放置，从而使机器人手臂和辅助外科医生有更大的可动性可以离开而不会碰到手术操作台。我们已经采用了这项技术并发现在较小的患者中这是必需的技术。

Lorincz等人描述了7例采用宙斯外科手术系统进行机器人辅助手术的病例[139]。其中5例儿童行Nissen胃底折叠术（其中3名同时进行了胃造口术），1例行胆囊切除术，1例行Heller肌切开术及部分胃底折叠术。有关患者年龄和体重的特殊性以及并发症没有提及。然而，作者提到随着他们手术团队采用机器人外科手术系统的经验的获得，他们的手术总共时间和装备时间快速下降。第1例Nissen胃底折叠术用了4.5个小时，而他们最近做的1例Nissen胃底折叠术只用了1.5个小时。他们认为组织的解剖和缝线的放置是精确的且打结比较安全。

最近，Knight等人描述了15例采用宙斯外科手术系统进行的胃底折叠术[115]。他们进行了1例Heller肌切开术和Dor胃底折叠术以及14例Nissen胃底折叠术，得到了关于装备时间、手术时间和结果的数据。患者平均年龄为4.3岁（范围为2个月到18岁），平均体重为13kg（范围3.4～37.7kg）。他们的平均手术时间为195分钟，从第1例所用时间为323分钟下降到最后1例为180分钟。没有发生术后并发症。

小儿泌尿外科

机器人外科手术系统在小儿泌尿外科的应用正在不断引起人们的兴趣，近来的报道描述了它们在复杂重建手术中的应用（见表4-4）。Pedraza等人报道了在1名7岁大的男孩身上完成的腹腔镜下阑尾膀胱造口术（Mitrofanoff手术），采用了一个四通道经腹膜入路和达·芬奇外科手术系统[165]。总共的手术时间为6个小时，没有发生术中或术后的并发症。作者发现机器人外科手术系统在进行阑尾膀胱吻合术中具有优势。同样相同的研究小组还在1名4岁大的女孩身上实施机器人辅助的腹腔镜下双侧肾输尿管部分切除术[164]。这个手术所用的总共手术时间为7小时20分钟，没有发生并发症。作者认为机器人界面有利于肾门和血管的解剖，可完成复杂的微创外科手术。

表 4–4　机器人外科手术系统在小儿普通外科中的临床经验

作者	机器人系统	研究类型	患者(N)	手术操作	结果	评注
Gutt 等人[79]和 Heller 等人[88]	达·芬奇	病例研究	14	11 例胃底折叠术，2 例胆囊切除术，1 例双侧的输卵管－卵巢切除术	手术时间：胃底折叠术 146 分钟（平均）；胆囊切除术 105 和 150 分钟；输卵管－卵巢切除术 95 分钟	没有发生并发症或中转为开腹手术
Luebbe 等人[139]	达·芬奇	病例研究	20	10 例胃底折叠术，3 例胆囊切除术，2 例脾切除术，1 例脐尿管切除术，1 例 Morgagni 膈疝修补术，3 例活检术，1 例淋巴结切除术	平均时间：OR 装备 45 分钟；患者准备 17 分钟；控制台操作时间 93 分钟（范围 10～229 分钟）	15% 并发症发生率（2 例因为出血而中转为开腹手术，1 例气胸）
Lorincz 等人[139]	宙斯	病例研究	7	5 例 NISSEN 胃底折叠术，1 例胆囊切除术，1 例 Heller 肌切开术	胃底折叠术的手术时间从 4.5 小时缩减为 1.5 小时	随着团队的进步，沿着学习曲线，病例的手术时间快速缩减
Knight 等人[115]	宙斯	回顾性病例综述	15	14 例 NISSEN 胃底折叠术，1 例 Heller 肌切开术加 Dor 胃底折叠术	手术时间，6 小时，没有发生并发症	学习以后可快速改善，认识到在打结和缝合处放置有更加轻松和自信的好处
Pedraza 等人[164]	达·芬奇	病例报告	1	阑尾膀胱造口术（Mitrofanoff 手术）	平均手术时间 195 分钟，术后最初 30 天内发生 2 例并发症	阑尾膀胱吻合手术期间机器人手术操作是有用的
Pedraza 等人[164]	达·芬奇	病例报告	1	双侧半肾输尿管切除术	手术时间 7 小时 20 分钟，没有发生并发症	机器人手术界面使肾门和肾血管的解剖更容易
Peters 等人[167]	达·芬奇	综述性文章	未提供	肾切除术，肾盂整形术（都是经腹膜和腹膜后），抗反流手术（经腹膜和经膀胱），阑尾膀胱造口术，巨输尿管重建术	未提供	对于目前的机器人外科手术系统，经腹膜手术途径更容易进行
Le Bret 等人[128]	宙斯	回顾性临床试验	56	动脉导管未闭结扎术（28 例胸腔镜，28 例机器人手术）	手术室时间：胸腔镜 83 分钟；机器人手术 162 分钟手术操作时间：胸腔镜 24 分钟；机器人手术 50 分钟	对于机器人手术组具有更长的手术时间，1 例中转为视频胸腔镜手术，在并发症和结果方面没有显著性的差异
Mihaljevic 等人[150]	达·芬奇	病例研究	2	血管环切断术	总共的手术时间：172.5 分钟（平均）机器人手术时间：106.5 分钟（平均）	因为需要装备的时间，所以总共的手术时间要比标准的胸腔镜手术通常所需的时间更长，机器人手术组解剖时间稍微有所缩短。

在一篇机器人外科手术系统在小儿泌尿外科中的应用综述中，Peters 描述了采用机器人辅助（达·芬奇外科手术系统）有利于进行复杂的泌尿外科手术[167]。虽然没有提供详细的病例，但是作者描述了采用
55 机器人辅助进行的各种不同的手术，包括肾切除术、肾盂成形术（经腹膜和腹膜后都有）、膀胱输尿管反流手术（经腹膜和经膀胱）、阑尾膀胱造口术、巨输尿管重建手术、肾盂切开取石术和大的 müller管残留物切除术。作者认为虽然机器人外科手术系统能够用于进行腹膜后的手术，但是因为机器人手术器械的大小和手臂的缘故，经腹膜手术是最为容易进行的操作，并认为应建立一个专业团队来提高使用机器人外科手术系统的效率。

小儿心胸外科

到目前为止，只有两篇机器人外科手术系统在小儿心胸外科中的应用的报道（见表 4-4）。Le Bret 等人报告了一项病例数相对较大的研究，在 56 例动脉导管未闭患儿进行了手术关闭的报道[128]。手术患儿被分为两组，一组进行标准的胸腔镜修补 PDA 手术，另一组采用宙斯外科手术系统进行机器人辅助的修补手术。作者没有详细描述小组分配的办法。虽然患儿的病情特征总体上相似，但是相对于标准的胸腔镜手术组患儿（平均年龄 33 个月；平均体重 13.3kg），机器人辅助组患儿（平均年龄 20 个月；平均体重 10.7kg）倾向于由年龄更小、体重更轻的患儿组成。在两组患儿中都没有发生术中并发症。分配到机器人辅助组的 28 例患儿手术中完成了 27 例，1 例患儿由于不能获得足够的暴露而需要中转为标准的胸腔镜手术。相对于标准的胸腔镜手术组（平均总共手术室时间为 83 分钟；平均外科手术时间为 24 分钟），机器人辅助组的总共手术室和外科手术时间（平均总共手术室时间为 162 分钟；平均外科手术时间为 50 分钟）显著延长，具有统计学显著意义。

在术后并发症、重症监护病房中所需时间或住院所需时间方面，两组之间没有显著性差异。作者总结，虽然机器人辅助行动脉导管未闭修补手术在较小的儿童是安全可行的，但是相对于标准的胸腔镜手术，它没有任何优势。而且作者认为，行机器人辅助手术所需要的额外的操作时间没有随着经验获得而下降，所以这个额外的操作时间应该归咎于机器人系统的复杂性且不呈一种学习型曲线。

在最近的一个报道中，Mihaljevic 等人描述了在 2 例患儿（年龄分别为 10 岁和 8 岁，体重分别为 48kg 和 27kg）采用达·芬奇外科手术系统切断血管环的手术[150]。总共的手术室时间分别为 180 分钟和 165 分钟，外科手术操作时间分别为 115 分钟和 98分钟。作者认为，相对于标准的胸腔镜手术，机器人系统提高的增强视频和增大的灵活性显示了显著的优势，并认为体内手术器械灵活性的改进是一种重要特征，有助于在气管和食管附近进行所有纤维性束带分离。作者认为，虽然相对于标准的胸腔镜手术，机器人辅助手术中的解剖时间稍微缩短一些，但是总共的手术室时间通常更长，因为需要装备的时间。

实验性外科手术

虽然已经出版的人类外科手术的经验大部分着眼于相对常规的微创外科手术，但是多名作者已经报道了在动物模型中进行更多的复杂重建手术的可行性。Hollands 等人[96,98]、Knight 等人[115]和 Lorincz 等人[115]都报道了宙斯外科手术系统在猪动物模型中的应用。技术上具有挑战性的手术，如肠肠吻合术、肝脏空肠吻合术、肝门肠吻合术、食管食管吻合术，都已经证实在技术上是可行的（表 4-5）。机器人辅助的手术和标准的腹腔镜手术都有合情合理的相似的手术时间和并发症发生率。另外，生存研究表明，机器人辅助的手术是可以耐受的，具有合理的长期结果。

同样，Aaronson、Malhotra、Olsen 和他们的同事们已报道了达·芬奇外科手术系统在动物模型中的应用，以实施复杂的小儿心血管外科、神经外科和泌尿外科手术[1,143,161]，包括在年幼羔羊中进行主动脉吻合术[143]、经膀胱外科手术[161]和在胎羊动物模型中进行模拟的脊髓脊膜突出修补术[1]。在最近的研究中，机器人外科手术系统能够完成腹腔镜下通过小的子宫造瘘来进行子宫内修补全层皮肤缺损[1]。

结论

目前机器人外科手术系统已经应用于小儿外科领域，主要是作为一种便于进行微创外科手术的工具。目前发表的应用机器人进行小儿外科手术的临床经验还是有限的，主要由显示手术安全可行的回顾性的病

表 4-5 动物模型中实验性小儿机器人外科手术

作者	手术操作	机器人系统	研究类型	手术时间，腹腔镜手术（平均）	手术时间，机器人手术（平均）	额外的结果
Hollands 等人[96,98]	猪的肠-肠吻合术（5 例腹腔镜，5 例机器人）	宙斯	急性	麻醉 176 分钟，手术时间 143 分钟，吻合时间 109 分钟	麻醉 154 分钟，手术时间 139 分钟，吻合时间 93 分钟	所有的吻合都通畅，没有发生狭窄；每一组都有 1 例发生小的渗漏；统计学上没有显著性差异
	猪的肝管空肠吻合术（5 例腹腔镜，5 例机器人）	宙斯	急性	吻合时间 66 分钟	吻合时间 93 分钟	对照组发生 5 例并发症（3 例渗漏和 2 例中转手术）；机器人手术组发生 1 例并发症（中转手术）
	猪的食管食管吻合术（5 例腹腔镜，5 例机器人）	宙斯	急性	麻醉时间 124 分钟，手术时间 97 分钟，吻合时间 89 分钟	麻醉时间 151 分钟，手术时间 131 分钟，吻合时间 125 分钟	所有的吻合都通畅，没有发生狭窄；1 例吻合术有小的渗漏；统计学上没有显著性差异
	猪的肝门肠吻合术（10 例腹腔镜，10 例机器人）	宙斯	急性	麻醉时间 125 分钟，手术时间 98 分钟，吻合时间 60 分钟	麻醉时间 164 分钟，手术时间 137 分钟，吻合时间 94 分钟	对照组发生 4 例并发症（1 例吻合口狭窄和 3 例吻合口破裂）；机器人手术组发生 4 例并发症（1 例渗漏，1 例吻合口狭窄，2 例吻合口破裂）
Lorincz 等人[139]	猪的肝门肠吻合术（8 例机器人）	宙斯	生存（1 个月）	N/A	总共手术时间 380 分钟，装备时间 20 分钟，端侧吻合 129 分钟，胆道解剖 36 分钟，肝门肠吻合 96 分钟	8 例动物中有 5 例术后存活时间 >1 个月；所有的实验室指标均正常；没有发生吻合口狭窄，吻合口均愈合良好。
	猪的食管食管吻合术（7 例机器人）	宙斯	生存（1 个月）	N/A	平均手术时间 120 分钟	8 例动物中有 5 例术后存活时间达到 1 个月；所有的动物均需要 1～2 次的术后扩张术，尸体检查发生吻合口均愈合良好
Malhotra 等人[143]	幼年绵羊的胸腔大动脉吻合术（5 例机器人手术）	达·芬奇	生存（6～12 小时）	N/A	主动脉夹钳时间 47 分钟，吻合时间 26 分钟	所有的 5 例羔羊经过手术过程均存活；平均吻合口破裂压力为 163± 9mmHg
Aaronson 等人[1]	子宫内胎绵羊的模拟脊髓脊膜突出修补术（6 例机器人手术）	达·芬奇	生存（7～11 天）	N/A	子宫内手术时间，在 6 例手术中沿陡峭的学习曲线，从正好 120 分钟急剧下降为 30 分钟	6 例羔羊中有 4 例存活到观察期取标本时间；子宫内内镜手术是可行的。
Olsen 等人[161]	猪的 Cohen 交叉三角形输尿管再植术（14 例机器人再植术）	达·芬奇	生存	N/A	平均手术时间 68 分钟	术后评估显示膀胱输尿管反流得到解决

例报告和病例研究报道组成。相对于标准的腹腔镜手术，采用机器人辅助手术的病例的平均年龄、手术装备时间和手术时间都要更长一些。然而，发生并发症或中转为开腹手术的比例都比较低。到目前为止，在临床结果的长期随访方面任何有意义的差异还没有报道。因为已经发表的有关机器人辅助人类手术的经验的文献大部分都为相对简单和常规的微创外科手术，所以在表现出有任何显著的临床意义之前，它可能还需要一段时间。

相对人类手术的文献，已经发表的动物实验性手术的报道显示，在动物模型上进行机器人辅助性手术是可行的，偶尔可以有效地进行一些复杂的重建手术。这些应用代表将来机器人小儿外科手术的需求，因为机器人外科手术界面的好处在于可以很容易地进行精细的解剖和体内缝合。一些手术，如食管闭锁修补术、肝门肠吻合术和输尿管再植术，都可以用目前现有的腹腔镜手术器械来完成。然而，在微创外科手术环境中掌握这些复杂的技术是极具挑战性的任务。机器人外科手术系统具有完成这些技术上具有挑战性手术的潜力，它以微创的方式保留促进美观、降低术
57 后疼痛和可能缩短住院时间的好处。

相对标准的微创外科技术而言，目前正在使用的两个机器人外科手术系统可提供许多同样的优势：3-D视频、关节化手术器械、直观的运动、减少震颤和运动的成比例缩放。另外，它们也有许多同样的局限性，这些局限性限制了机器人手术系统在小儿外科领域的广泛应用，如高昂的前期投资和日常费用、相对局限的手术器械的选择、需要致力于专门的训练、较长的装备时间以及缺乏触觉的反馈。尤其是对于小儿外科患者而言，大型机器人外科手术系统的尺寸和手术器械的尺度还是一个主要的问题，必须通过进一步的发展来解决这些问题。然而，研究者们总体上赞同机器人外科手术系统在技术上的特色[50,128,140]。虽然定量的临床价值还没有得到证实，但是大多数作者已经在主观上得出结论，认为机器人外科手术系统似乎能增强手术操作的精细程度，使复杂的微创外科手术更容易进行。因此进一步的研究要完整地评价机器人外科手术系统在小儿外科人群中的应用和潜在利益。

微创外科的出现给患者带来了大量的潜在利益。然而，采用腹腔镜设备进行手术操作时其本身固有的局限性对于外科医生而言具有极大挑战，当手术变得更加复杂时，如在小儿外科中遇到的手术，这种挑战只会变得更大。机器人和计算机技术的结合对于这个领域的发展可有非常显著的潜在性贡献。随着技术的持不断进步，机器人外科手术系统最终要得到人们接受，费用问题、训练问题、手术器械的大小、安全性、效率和临床通用性问题等都要得到解决。

微米技术和纳米技术——尺度问题

新技术将来自材料科学，其应用原理是微米机电系统（MEMS）和纳米机电系统（NEMS）[211]。如电子工业是通过处理硅电子特性的能力而转变一样，现在在一个相似尺度内处理生物材料也已经成为可能。过去40年间，普通材料如不锈钢、聚丙烯、聚酯和聚四氟乙烯一直没有什么变化。最近这种可能性的一个例子是镍钛记忆合金（等原子的镍和钛）的应用，一种具有性状记忆特性的金属合金。

在设备的制造中，一个重要的概念和特征是“top down”与“bottom up”组装。Top down是指从原材料开始到加工成一种设备的概念。在一种典型的MEMS设备中，硅被蚀刻、加热和处理直至成为它的最终形式。在新生的纳米技术领域，概念原理的基础是自组装。这里，成分组件是放置在一起，在最佳条件下自组装成一种材料。这个过程更多是一种生物学组装。

微米机电系统（MEMS）

外科学技术的进步是由大多数企业——应用更小、更有效率和更有力的技术的趋势——来设定的。这种趋势，其在医学和外科学领域中的应用，具体体现在MEMS设备上[179]。

大多数MEMS设备都小于人类头发的尺度，并且虽然它们是在微米水平进行度量的，它们可以进行单独使用或成组投入使用。MEMS设备已在汽车气囊系统和喷墨打印机中应用了多年。

由于医学领域越来越依赖计算机来加强治疗计划，因而也越来越需要具有功能性和诊断性功能的MEMS设备。这种水平的性能涉及MEMS设计技术的中心，后者是以开发出能够驱动、感觉和在微米尺度修饰外周的世界的设备为基础。大多数MEMS设

备的基本设计和制造与标准的集成电路的制造相似，后者包括晶体生长、造模和蚀刻。

设备和举例

MEMS 设备在生物学应用中特别有用，因为它们体积较小、能量低和公称压力[65]。设备效能增强和新的应用领域也出现在 MEMS 在生物医学的应用中。现有两种基本类型的 MEMS 设备：传感器和微马达。传感器能将一种形式的能量（如机械能、光能、热能或其他类型的能量）转换成电能或信号。微马达能接受能量并将它转换成一种动力。

传感器

传感器能够将能量转换或转变成一种电信号。输入的能量可以是机械能、热能、光能或磁能。传感器可以是主动性的系统，也可以是被动性的系统。主动性传感器能从输入的信号中获取它们自身的能量，而被动性传感器需要一个外在的能源来进行工作。几乎所有的这些设备都处于发展阶段，但是可以形成这种概念。

数据刀和 H–探针型手术器械：MEMS 设备尤其适合于外科手术的应用，因为它们较小的尺度可以自然集成到外科手术器械的头部。一个例子就是“数据刀”（Verimetra, Inc., Pittsburgh），其采用显微制造的压力传感器贴覆到手术刀刀口上（图 4–13）。在进行切割时，数据刀压力传感器可与以前收集的体外数据相互参照，以通知外科医生有关正在分离的组织的
58 类型。在内镜下进行手术操作时，由于触觉反馈的感觉下降或完全消失，这种信息就变得尤其有用。

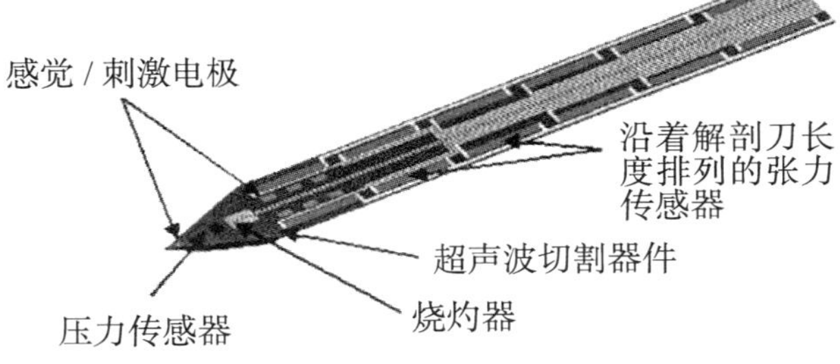

图 4–13　数据刀是基于微机电的解剖刀。（Courtesy of Verimetra, Inc., Pittsburgh.）

Verimetra 公司的 H–探针采用相似的传感器，在进行冠状动脉旁路移植手术期间可透壁“触摸”钙化的斑块。这种技术的目的就是为了在动脉切开术之前，通过更加精确地瞄准一个理想的吻合部位来排除冠状动脉旁路移植管道的定位不良。

动脉血气分析仪：MEMS 技术能够应用于动脉血气分析。这种基于 MEMS 的分析仪是建立在已经确立的红外分光镜检查方法上。它由一个红外光光源、一个红外光传感器和一个光学过滤器组成。红外光穿过过滤器，而过滤器设计用来监测氧气、二氧化碳和其他相关血气的红外光光谱。因为大多数气体都有一种已知的红外光吸收谱，传感器就能设计成具有红外光信号的特殊值。

再一次因为微米尺度的技术和相对较小的采样体积，标本的检测比传统的动脉血气分析需要更少的时间即可完成。一个特殊的例子是用于监测早产儿血液的动脉血气导管，可通过氧气和二氧化碳特异性传感器来收集实时数据。

血压传感器：在医学 MEMS 技术中最大的成功范例就是一次性使用的血压传感器。一次性使用的血压传感器已替代了可重复使用的硅柱或石英电容性压力传感器，后者每个售价可高达 600 美元，而且不得不进行消毒和重新校准以便再次使用。这些昂贵的设备是采用一种生理盐水充填的导管和必须直接接到动脉腔内的振动膜排列来测量血压。在硅 MEMS 血压传感器中，压力符合显微机械加工振动膜的偏转。一个抵抗成分——一个张力表，被离子植布在薄的硅振动膜上。压电晶体管可随着不同的压力变化而改变输出电压。温度补偿和校准能够整合在一个传感器上。

医学中其他的 MEMS 传感器：Wheatstone 桥压阻现象的硅压力传感器是在医学中广泛采用的一种主要 MEMS 设备。它可测量的血压范围为不到 0.1 到超过 10 000 psi（1 psi ＝6894.75729 帕斯卡），这种传感器结合了电阻器和蚀刻的振动膜结构来提供一种随压力而改变的电信号。最初，这种类型的传感器被用于血压监测设备中，但是它们在医学领域中的应用要远远超出这些。这些类型的传感器可见于呼吸监测器、透析机、输液泵和医疗钻孔设备中。它们也用于充气的病床空气垫或用于当一种呼吸暂停监测器探测

到经过一段时间仍然缺乏运动时的信号报警。

微马达

微马达是一种以流体能量的或电能驱动的设备，能提供压力和运动。几种微马达已经应用于 MEMS 设备中，包括静电微马达、压电微马达、热能微马达、磁能微马达和相位恢复微马达。在医学中，微马达应用于阀门、加速计和药物输送系统。预计将来还可用于生产肌肉激活剂或“人工肌肉”。

药物输送系统： MEMS 设备以微泵的形式应用于药物输送系统[126]。一种典型的药物泵由泵室、入口阀、出口阀、可变形的横隔膜和电极组成。当一个电流作用于电极时，横隔膜发生变形可增加泵室的容积。泵室容积改变可引起泵室内压力下降。泵室压力下降即可打开入口阀。当电流终止时，泵室压力回归正常，随着入口阀关闭和出口阀开放，液体得以流出。

其他微泵可通过合并的活塞或加压的气体来开放出口阀。更为吸引人的应用之一是胰岛素输送系统的可植入式泵。

目前的胰岛素微泵有缺点，大多数价格非常高昂。这种药物供给系统必须每隔 3 个月充填一次，每一个微泵的花费在 10 000～12 000 美元之间。而且胰岛素在核心温度下是不稳定的，因此胰岛素类似物必须是合成的、在生理温度下稳定的化合物。进一步的考虑是，一种能够感应葡萄糖和胰岛素水平以及胰岛素滴定量的生物力学胰腺，其可能是一种有趣的组合传感器和微马达的 MEMS 设备。

下一步

目前 MEMS 设备正处于与 20 世纪 60 年代的半导体工业相同的发展状态。就像最初的半导体一样，MEMS 设备现在大部分是由政府部分资助研发的，例如美国国防先进技术研究计划署（DARPA）。相对很少的商业性公司才把 MEMS 设备作为一种主要产品。然而，在 1960 年没有一个人能够预言在 40 年以后，在美国半导体将会处现在每一人的桌面上。那么如此预言 MEMS 设备的潜在的价值，包括在外科手术中的应用，就不会内有道理了。用于激素和多肽生长因子的留置性微型传感器可能会替代插曲式的检查、实验室测定或 CT 扫描以监测肿瘤的复发。随着更多的设备得到组合，设计过程就变得更加容易，下一步的技术就能基于最近学到的知识。在将来某一点上，当更多的承受得起的技术变得实际可用时[179]，我们将会把 MEMS 设备视为普通外科手术方法、精巧的手术器械、在线的实验室、监视设备以及也许是细胞或甚至是 DNA 插入。

纳米机电系统（NEMS）

近来有人综述了纳米技术和 NEMS 在医学和外科手术中的应用[68]。大小至关重要。在医学和生物学中，大小尺度下降的主要优势在于，它可以使材料或微粒进入其他方式不能进入的人体间隔内。在外科 59
手术方面，目前和将来的应用包括包被和表面改性、自组装或是存生物学系统的生物模仿和肿瘤的靶向性治疗。

包被和表面改性

虽然大多数医用装置是由疏松材料组成，但是生物学融入或相互作用只是发生在表面的最薄层。为了优化这种表面的相互作用，已经出现了烧结的整形外科生物学材料。小球表面的一薄层是在疏松材料表面经过加热处理后熔接或“烧结的”[169]。这种小球表层的处理优化了骨骼的向内生长，而疏松材料起到了加强装置机械稳定性的作用。羟基磷灰石包被的植入物具有一种生物学优势，其中植入物采用陶瓷羟基磷灰石包被，因此可以通过模拟（生物学模拟）骨结晶的性质来诱导骨骼的向内生长。进一步的尝试涉及包被 RGD 多肽，在许多细胞结构蛋白中它是主要的细胞连接蛋白。

心脏血管支架和现在的药物释放性支架，是一种类似的表面包被的例子。当代的药物释放性支架具有微米级厚的包被物，由一种植入时就开始释放药物的单体聚合物制成[99]。包被的西罗莫司或紫杉醇药物可以缓慢地弥散到组织微环境中以防发生纤维化反应。将来理想的支架将有可能通过工程设计来优化疏松材料和包被物。实际上，完美的生物相容性材料可能是一种人工合成的疏松材料，其表面接种有患者自身的细胞，如一种内皮细胞化的 Gore-Tex 血管支架。

自组装

NEMS 的材料是采用自导向或自组装的过程来制造，其中材料混合物可以凝结成微粒、材料或复合物[126]。因此，NEMS 的制造过程从纳米固体相开始——一种典型的溶液，并通过控制溶液所处的环境，就可以制造出 NEMS。

近来，生物大分子，包括蛋白质和 DNA，都已经用于稳定纳米微粒晶体并利用独特的性质来制造材料，因此开启了下一代纳米微粒和材料中无限多样性的大门[144,194]。这样的过程模拟了自然界的能力来制造一些材料，如珍珠、珊瑚和胶原。

肿瘤学

与其他领域相比，微米尺度和纳米尺度的技术将给肿瘤学领域提供更多关键性的治疗优势。考虑到恶性肿瘤转化和扩散的反常生物学过程，我们目前的治疗是粗略的和非靶向性的。图 4-14 描绘了一个复杂的纳米微粒[84]，是由一个三氧化二铁核心包被了氧化硅外壳组成。配位体可以连接到包被的氧化硅表面，然后可以通过三氧化二铁核心瞄准到一个特殊部位。这种技术可用于基于肿瘤浸润性的诊断性目的或用于肿瘤的治疗或同时用于肿瘤的诊断和治疗。

Harisinghani 等人[84]在前列腺癌的者中采用三氧化二铁纳米颗粒来鉴别淋巴结中的肿瘤转移。作者正式了在鉴别最后含有肿瘤的淋巴结时，纳米颗粒的敏感性和特异性都有提升。进一步的工作采用含有肿瘤特异性抗体的功能化磁性纳米颗粒将可增强肿瘤的特异性摄取。

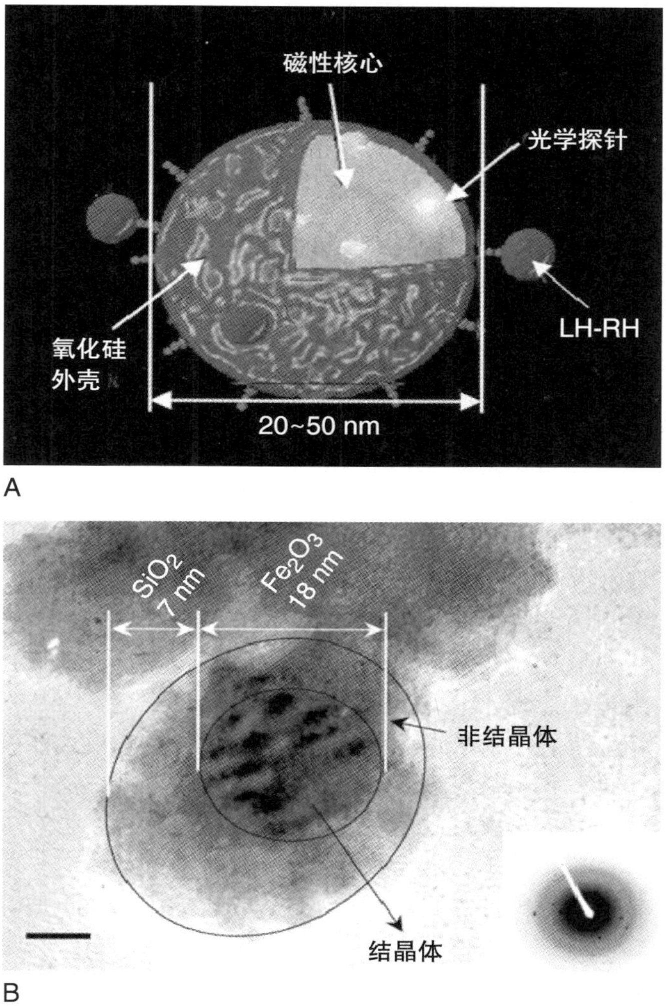

图 4-14　纳米微粒的示意图。一个三氧化二铁核心被氧化硅外壳包裹。连接到氧化硅的配位体能够将三氧化二铁核心瞄准到一个特异性部位或潜在的肿瘤部位。这个三氧化二铁核心可以在磁场中进行加热。另外，这个三氧化二铁核心可以携带毒素、基因或药物。

外科模拟和虚拟现实技术

模拟和虚拟现实技术[71,146]是可能会改变我们思考外科教育、演练和实践方式的两个概念。外科的实践是直观的、认知的和手工操作的艺术和科学，需要医生来处理越来越大量的信息。技术正在变得更加的特异和复杂，并且决定经常要在急诊情况下快速做出，甚至是在处理罕见的问题时。

外科模拟

模拟是一种在试验条件下，能够让参与者进行再现或重试的设备或练习，可能发生的现象与实际操作时发生的类似。必须有足够的现实主义态度来暂停参与者的怀疑。在商业化航空公司的业务中，模拟飞行是作为最具成本效益的训练飞行员的方法而被坚定地广为接受。飞行员必须在模拟器上达到某种水平的熟练程度，才允许去操纵一种特殊的飞行器，而且在模拟器上飞行员必须通过定期的熟练水平测试来保留他们的飞行执照。军事组织采用一种类似的方法来训练基本的飞行技能，他们发现，模拟飞行可用于教授在复杂作战情境中进行格斗的技能。因此外科模拟是植根于其他高绩效、高风险组织机构中得到确认的技术和经验之上的。

学习飞行的费用和风险激发了 Wdward Link 来构建一套称为“飞行员制造者”的机械设备（Link, http://www.link.com/history.html）。混合仪器的累加可以训练飞行员在恶劣天气中进行飞行。在第二次世界大战刚开始时，随着对飞行员训练学员的空前需求，成千上万的训练学员在 Link 飞行模拟器中进行了训练[89]。

医学社团也正在数个领域中开始采用模拟器来训练医护人员，特别是外科医生、麻醉医生、抽血者、护理人员和护士。模拟器可以反复进行临床实践中预演形式的认知练习的能力使外科训练与飞行员训练有相同的感觉。

外科治疗必须承担与潜在疾病和治疗的模式都相关的一种人类风险因素。通过训练可以降低风险。其中一种办法就是通过模拟来实现这些目标。

模拟的不严格定义为假定向外性质的动作或一种既定目标的外观或是一系列过程[181]。通常的设想是模拟器外加一台计算机，但这不是必不可少的设备。模拟是一项技术（不是工艺学），用于替代或详述真实的体验，在现实世界真实性方面的经验指导下，以一种完全交互式的形式[64]。为了进行模拟，在一个任务或充分“沉浸式（immersive）”的环境中，使用者能够暂停现实性来学习或想象一个外科教学点，其只需要影响到使用者。然后将获得的知识用于教学中或类似任务的活体手术操作中。外科医生可通过基于 Linux 的计算机来学会打结，或通过一个代表腹腔的纸板箱来模拟腹腔镜阑尾切除术的动作。

模拟器中的视频显示系统

模拟器技术涉及训练系统的设计，该训练系统必须是安全而有效率的，能够有效地使新受训者适应或可为临床医生提供先进的培训。这种系统涉及教授特殊的技能、产生模拟极限或急诊情况下进行处置的提纲。到目前为止，娱乐行业是主要的使用者和视频显示系统的研发者。在视频技术的进步中，娱乐业取得了如此多的进展，以至模拟器中采用的许多视频设备都是借助于这些基础。考虑到 1990 年价格为 100 000 美元的超级计算机具备的图形计算能力与 1998 年价格为 150 美元的视频游戏系统的图形计算能力基本相当，现在可用的技术更是超出了代表外科手术模拟技术的能力[232]。

小道具是模拟器视频动作的关键性组成部件。虽然腹腔镜外科手术操作能够呈现在一台台式计算机上，但是一个更加沉浸式的体验可以通过包括监视器和在实际手术室采用的手术器械来完成。举一个例子，人体模型模拟器，尽管内部是复杂的，但是可以用作模拟环境的补充。手术操作模拟器，如腹腔镜外科手术，应该采用类似于在实际的手术室出现的显示方式。

另一个方面，开放性手术的模拟，需要的系统目前正处于发展阶段。外科医生和模拟的患者之间交互的水平需要一种沉浸式显示系统，如头戴显示器（HMD）。对于一个开放性手术模拟器的研发者来说，最佳的办法可能是选择一个具有良好光学质量的系统，集中发展一种清晰稳定的影像。这种类型的视频显示系统的设计包括“通过显示系统观察”部分，其中在实际的模型中添加了合成的影像[186]。这些系统在手术台水平采用了一种高分辨率的监视器显示屏，因为显示的影像特征必须具有很高的清晰度。

人 / 模拟器界面和触觉反馈

力反馈是在虚拟世界中模拟重力或阻力[106]。触觉反馈是一种应用于皮肤感觉的感知，皮肤感觉的感知通常是对触觉的反应。发展触觉反馈和力反馈都是必需的，因为使用者在接触虚拟目标时要有触觉感知。这种所谓的触觉环或人–设备界面，最初是为远程外科手术开发出来的，对外科手术模拟的发展提供了许多借鉴。

呈现触觉反馈的技术正在不断成熟，得到了美国、欧洲和日本的触觉设计工业以及许多大学研究中心的快速发展的支持[106]。触觉反馈技术已经应用于模拟腹腔镜外科手术操作中；然而，要想将这 61
种技术应用于开放性手术中，要能像外科医生那样随意地选择各种不同的手术器械，还需要关键性的创新。

影像的产生

外科领域的 3-D 交互式的图形影像是外科手术模拟的下一代水平。在现实世界中观察和操作一个物体，不同于在虚拟世界中操作相同的物体。对于模拟器来说，模型化的大多数物体都是假定为固体。在人类组织中，可能除了骨骼以外，假定的固体都不会存在。许多器官都是可以变形的半固体，具有潜在空间。虚拟的物体必须能够真实反映真实世界中物体的特性。即使采用今天的计算能力，创建一个可以工作的外科手术操作界面的任务（无论是皮肤、器官，还是血管）也是极其困难的。

在创建交互式外科操作物体中，主要的挑战是真实展现外科医生通过解剖来改变术野的结构面。在一个模拟器中，对于切开或切除一处病变所产生的强力改变这种复杂问题，计算机程序支持的模拟经常不能处理。这种模拟还没有包括血流组织，因为在模拟器官的外观中，血流组织会导致另外的改变。而且，模拟的情形必须实时呈现，这就意味着必须要瞬间出现变化。

为了在身体上得以实现，模拟外科手术操作的表面和内部器官必须是可以压缩的，可以响应作用于表面的力量，或钝性接触或切割。计算机图形设计中已有多种可创建可变形的可压缩物体的方法。

通常，模拟器的图形设计是基于体素（voxel）制图学。体素是体积的一种近似值，而像素是面积的一种近似值。想象一个体素作为空间中的一个立方体，具有长度、宽度和深度。就像像素具有固定的长度和宽度，体素具有固定的长度、宽度和深度。然而，应用体积作为唯一的特征来定义一种“可变形的物体”，并没有具体表现出压力、应力或张力的物理学性质。因此，图形影像将不是对外科操作的精确反应。体素方法不能代表器官结构模拟切割以后发生的实时真实改变。

这个问题的解决可采用一种更为独特的限定要素的办法。限定要素允许程序员采用体积、压力、应力、张力和密度作为体积的变量。这种方法创建了一种更为详细的影像，能够通过钝性压力或切割来进行操作。实时的拓扑改变也可以支持。

目前，一种较好的可供选择的解决这个问题的方法是避免计算模型。一些研究小组已经采用中空的人体模型和连接有记录位置的追踪设备的手术器械。任务教练员可直接应用带有通道的纸板箱等效物插入内镜手术器械，来使受训员练习腹腔镜操作技能。这些工具可用于完成某种任务，如打结或目标操作。

在教学、培训和实践中模拟

历史上，外科培训一直是与学徒的年限联系在一起的。住院医生是通过参与并在患者治疗或手术操作中担当更加积极的作用来学习外科学并积累自己的经验。尽管这种模式有潜在的缺点，但是这种模式在全世界已经成功地训练了一代又一代的外科医生。在传统教育模式中，对患者治疗来说，差错和风险是与生俱来的，尽管外科领域一直在做着诚实的努力，但这始终是一种因素，无论怎样进行教学。现在外科培训有了新方法，无论如何它们将有助于减少治疗差错和风险[155,189]。

模拟环境下的训练具有很多优势。第一个优势是可以真实地模拟症结：它提供了一种结果差错无妨或可以失败的环境。基于模拟器的训练不会招致对虚拟的患者的真实伤害、损害或死亡。如果一名学生在一个模拟的胆囊切除术中横断了胆总管，这名学生只需记住这个技术性差错并从中吸取教训。而且，模拟能够自定义和由一个计算机老师来定义，或能够由一个真实的教师来监控和代理，这就意味着学生们能在手术室外利用自己的时间来学习[187]。

模拟器是灵活的工具。通过一种特殊的模拟器目标评价，任务能够进行修订以适应教学目标。例如，自我容纳的“箱式训练器”可用于教授一种特别熟练的技能，可进行修改以更容易、更难，或用来教授抓取及打结技术。在更为复杂的基于计算机的模拟器中，可以由计算机自动修改各种参数，或由教师手动操作修改各种参数，甚至在模拟期间就可以修改参数。这些参数可包含从图形覆盖的改变，到一个未预期的医学紧急事件的引入。在人体内部学习腹腔镜导航技能的方法已经从这类模拟技术中获得很多收益。外科教学的主要目标是在一个 3-D 环境下，学习如何思考和熟练地操作。外科的“飞行直达”计划是可用于学习这种人体内部特殊定位的无价资源[37]。

也许外科模拟的最大好处之一是：使早期学习者能够成为基本任务的技能熟练者，而这些任务以前是不会出现在正规训练中的。医学生的定位，现在经常把患者的治疗任务排除在外，会有助于他们与外科职业的衔接、教育和进入。因此，模拟器最为一致成功是，对于先前对模拟任务很少或没有经验的个人具有最大的好处[170]。

展望

模拟的成功，特别是在航空工业中，强烈提示了其可以有效地应用于内科和外科的实践中。随着各种
62 形式的新技术的出现，其进步将依赖于多种因素。一个只是出于技术兴趣而制造的产品注定是要失败的；因此，模拟器市场必须是由临床和教育需求驱动的。在外科模拟的早期发展阶段，更简单的基于人体模型的训练器已经被证实更加的有用。然而，随着图形设计和人类界面技术的发展，模拟将变得更加逼真，设备价格将下降，更加融入的由计算机产生的模型，将会引领继续医学教育的这种独特形式的发展之路。

虚拟现实技术

虚拟现实技术虽然与模拟密切相关，但是它有许多独特的地方。模拟是用于教育和训练的方法；虚拟现实技术是使模拟看上去更加真实的一种形式。虚拟现实技术，简单地讲，就是创建一种 3-D 的人工环境，模拟使用者在真实世界中可能发生的事物。相对于模拟技术，虚拟现实技术几乎总是依靠计算机和计算机软件来产生一种虚拟的环境。而且，虚拟现实技术还需要一种界面设备来使使用者沉浸于虚拟世界中[195]。这种设备可以像计算机鼠标或键盘一样简单，也可以像基于虚拟现实技术的护目镜或耳机一样复杂。虚拟现实技术的基本目的是：将使用者的注意力从外部世界转移到人工的虚拟世界，并有详细的基于视觉、声音和触觉的交互式内容。当进行优化后，这样的一种体验让参与者感觉到真实的世界变成了这种虚拟的环境。

开始

虽然虚拟现实技术这个术语是 1989 年由 Jaron Lanier 引进的，但是就我们目前所知道的虚拟现实技术的概念，在此之前很早就出现了。1963 年，Ivan Sutherland 发明了画板，一种最初的图形设计工具。目前，Sutherland 正在研发头盔显示器（HMD），后者通告了现代融入式技术的理论和主题（图 4-15A），并导致了为贝尔直升机实验室研发的场景生成器。有了场景生成器（图 4-15B），计算机制图法就可以取代标准的用于飞行模拟器中的视频照相机生成显示系统。Sutherland 和 Evans 设计了数种基于虚拟现实技术的产品，Sutherland 在 1971 年研发了第一代动脉吻合模拟技术。

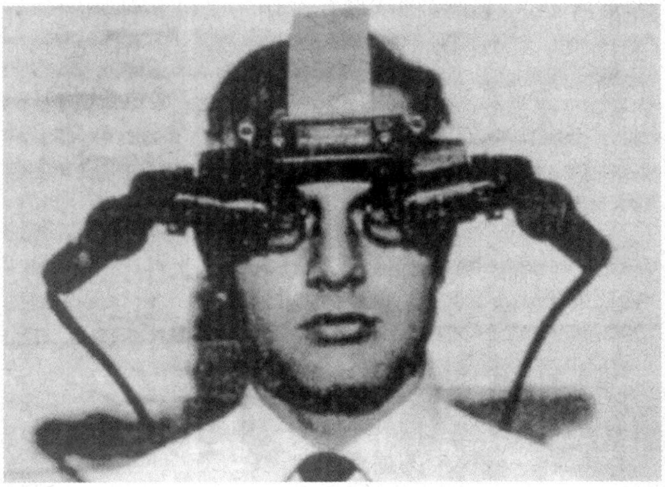

A

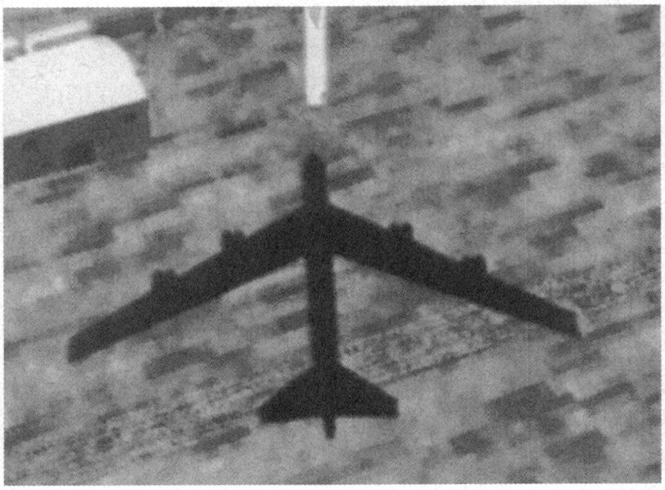

B

图 4-15 A. Sutherland 的头盔式显示器。B. 场景生成器软件，Evans 和 Sutherland。（From National Systems Contractors Association Multimedia Online Expo, “Science for the New Millennium.”）

随着计算机界面工具的同时发展，如鼠标，虚拟现实沉浸变为可能，因为在计算机上普通用户可以用一种比键盘可能更加直觉的方式更轻易地进行互相作用。20 世纪 70 年代，技术上的重大进步意味着计算机正在变得更加强有力、更小和更便宜；个人计算机、鼠标、激光打印机和桌面的结构都得到了发展[92]。

科学，娱乐业甚至更是如此，开始将虚拟现实技术作为增强他们各自的商业性的一种方法。虚拟现实技术在制造令人眼花缭乱的特殊效果（如星球大战、终结者和完美风暴）的一鸣惊人的电影时具有明显的应用价值。在 DNA 搜索中进行基因组的 3-D 制图使虚拟现实技术进入医学应用中。计算机辅助设计模型的实时修改第一次成为可能。Thomas Zimmerman 设计了一种“数据手套”，一种人类界面设备，希望能把手势转换成音乐，即通过把一些手势直接输入计算机，后者就能将这些运动翻译成声音。1982 年，Zimmerman 取得了这种手套的发明专利权。这种手套能够翻译穿戴者的手部运动和手指的弯曲状态，使它们与一种 3-D 环境发生相互作用。

1986 年，Jaron Lanier 第一次将头盔显示器（HMD）与数据手套结合起来，给这个世界一种更加逼真的融入式虚拟现实技术版本。使用者不仅能够看到 3-D 环境，而且能够通过感觉物体与其发生交互作用，并能看到他们自己正在与虚拟现实发生交互作用。从此以后，出现了许多热衷于探索和增加对这个领域的全面认识的研究小组、组织和个人。

虚拟现实技术在外科中的发展开始于 1980 年代。人们很快就认识到，模拟和虚拟现实技术对于外科手
63 术来说不会只依赖于特别详细的图形地形，像复杂的专业飞行模拟器那样。事实上，即使适度详细的外科手术虚拟现实系统即可以完成“训练任务”的目的。这强调了这个事实，即对外科医生来说，训练的基本目标之一是确立技术技能。因此，表现两根中空的管子以及持针器和镊子的简单图像的界面，就足以教授受训者有关肠吻合的原则。在 20 世纪 80 年代晚期，斯坦福大学的 Delp 研发了一种基于虚拟现实技术的用于下肢肌腱转移的最初的外科手术模拟器。1991 年，Satava 和 Lanier 设计了世界上第一台腹腔内交互式模拟器。在外科手术虚拟现实技术中，在这些初期的发明之后接着就出现了改进的版本，新版本是基于类似的计算机辅助数字化和绘制技术。虽然这些早期的重复缺乏计算能力以综合最大限度的细节来表现外科适应性及动态改变，但是它们的确建立了虚拟现实技术的概念。

组成

虚拟环境的构建需要一个计算机系统、一台显示器、一种界面设备和计算机软件。外科手术模拟和人工环境都是基于相同类型的设计方法。计算机速度必须足以驱动制图以传递最低限度的画面帧数，以便用户感觉不到闪烁或感觉不到显示器上画面改变。为了达到这个目的，模拟器应该以不少于 30Hz（或是每秒 30 帧画面）的速度将画面传递给用户的双眼，相当于大多数电视机的设置。5 年以前，这种类型的图形生成器需要高端的图形加速卡（Silicon Graphics, Mountain View, CA）或一个工作站来完成（Sun, Mountain View, CA）。现在，双核处理器或单核处理器的个人电脑就可以以这个速度呈递图像。

产生虚拟世界的软件有特殊要求。首先，程序员必须设计软件来匹配真实世界的物理限制。例如心脏，模拟冠状动脉旁路移植时，不能漂浮在稀薄的空气中。它必须有一些重力、可压缩性、体积和质量表现。这些限制，甚至更多的限制，在构建虚拟世界时必须要考虑以接近逼真。其次，软件必须设计为用户交互性的，可被汇编并有效而精确地处理，并且不会出现用户动态改变模拟时系统变得不稳定的情形。例如，当镊子牵拉组织时必须要恰当地呈现组织改变的图像。软件也必须能传达力反馈，通过外部设备，实时传达到用户。

从患者的数据生成虚拟人体

外科解剖，虽然对外科医生是第二天性，但是编程进入计算机系统却相当困难。成千上万的解剖学交互作用可以轻易超出处理器的计算能力，所以数字化呈递患者的数据必须要尽可能有效地进行。

用于虚拟现实技术的患者的特异性数据来自于多种渠道。核磁共振、磁共振血管成像术、CT 影像、PET 扫描、超声扫描和 SPECT 影像都是常见的形式。传统上，内科医生在头脑中将这些 2-D 数据集组织起来，在大脑中编译成可视化的患者 3-D 表现，而不像看得见的人类数据组合（图 4-16）。有了虚拟现

实技术，这些影像集就可被计算机捕捉，以 3-D 形式自动实现数据呈现；这就是以前手术以前外科医生大脑中需要进行的任务[26]。

应用不同类型的数据源，如 MRI 或 CT 扫描，可使虚拟现实技术程序员吸收不同种类扫描方法具有的独特的优势。如 CT 扫描对扫描骨骼特别管用。MRI 对软组织扫描特别有用。这些特性可以整合起来创建一种逼真的虚拟现实影像。

3-D 影像在系统内部的呈现方式对模拟的总体表现可产生深远的影响。从 CT 扫描、MRI 和其他方法获取的患者数据集合形成体素[3,210]。体素图形学是基于体积的，可形成一种包含无数数据点的影像。计算每一点上的改变对任何一台计算机都会产生极大的压力。然而，其他形式的虚拟现实技术能够减轻这种对系统的压力并加速模拟速度。

表面呈现

呈现是数字化数据的过程，是通过应用对数据的参数将数据呈现为计算机化的影像。为了减少需要计算的数据点的数量，表面呈现把基于体积的影像转换成简单的几何学图形，只有少得多的数据点[26]。这种几何学图形可以是基于影像中不同区域分界线的一种多边形拼凑物。分界线区域可以位于筋膜和脂肪之间或灰色物质和白色物质之间。这样的分界需要了解每一个区域的特性，因为体素影像中会有一些模糊，如 CT 扫描。描影算法可以混合层或区域，所以最终的产物有一种平滑的外观（图 4-17）。几何学元素的数量在虚拟现实技术的表面呈现方法中极其重要。必须记住，在虚拟的空间中由用户模拟的每一个动作需要通过计算机对真实世界中的每一个几何学物体进行重新计算。如果有太多的多边形需要快速重新生成，模拟就会发生“痉挛”，因此就会失真或根本就不可用。与基于体素的肖像比较时，表面呈现的物体能明确地跑得更快。

体积呈现

体积呈现需要特殊设备来处理无限数量必须进行

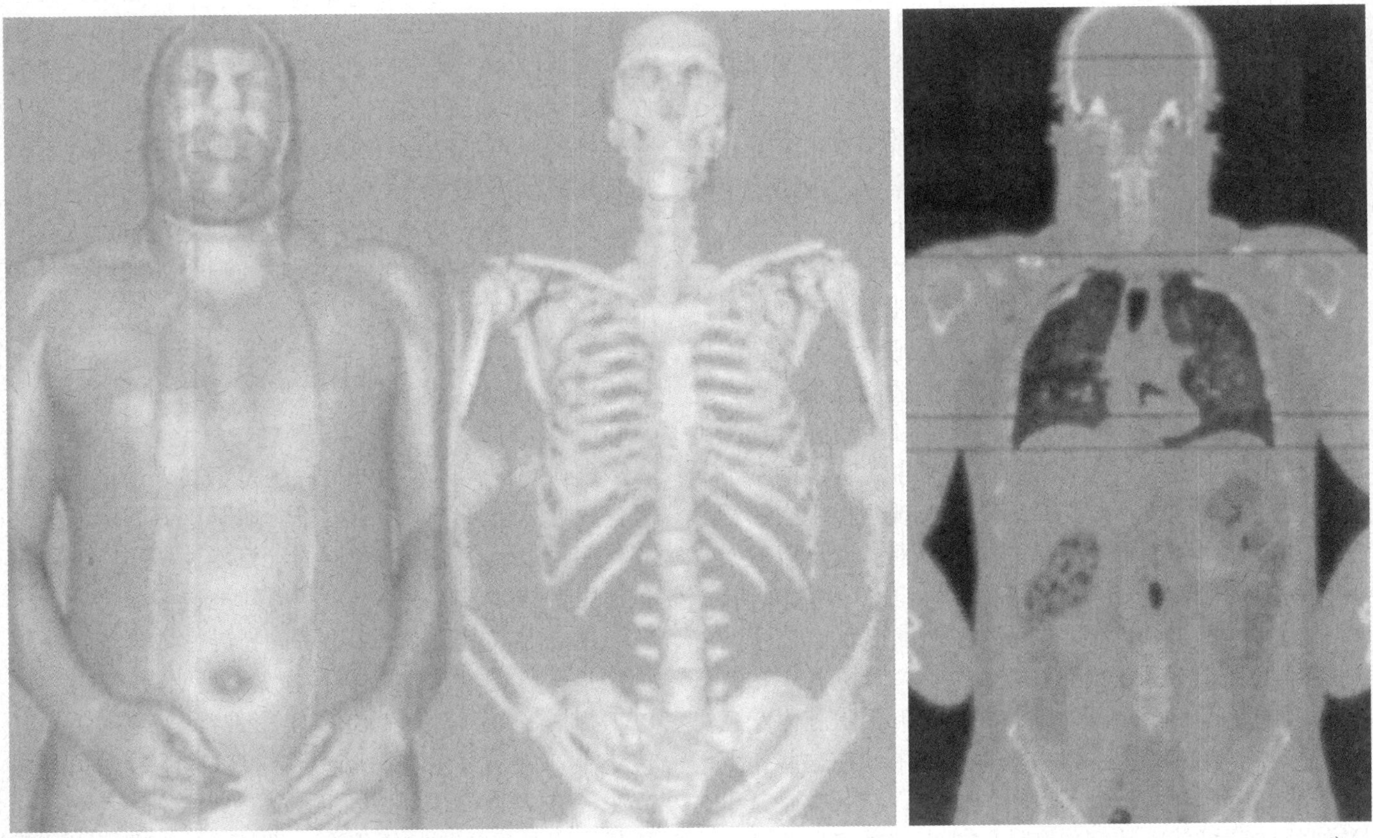

图 4-16　可视化人体计划。基于 MRI 和 CT 数据的人体三维模型的重建。（Courtesy of the National Library of Medicine Dataset.）

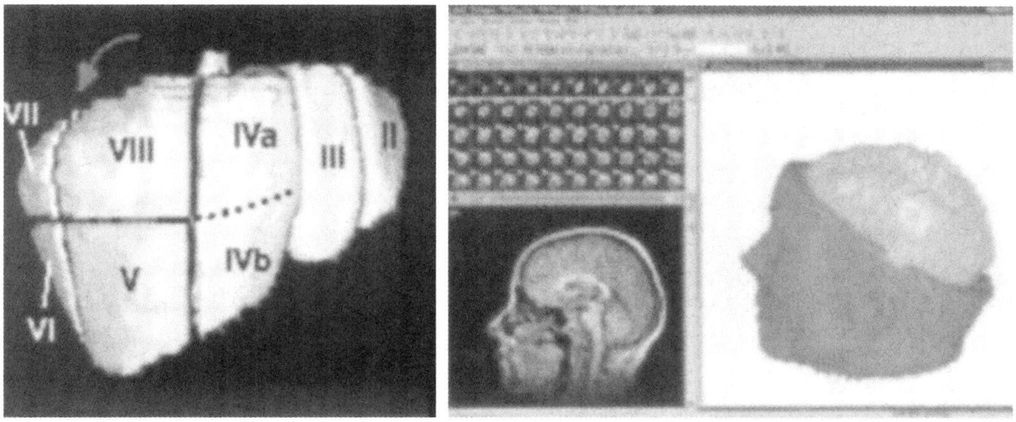

图 4-17 肝脏的表面呈现图像。（Courtesy of 3-D Doctor: 3-D Imaging, Rendering, and Measurement Software for medical Images, Lexington, MA.）

整合的数据。这种方法采用体积数据进行工作，并且每一次呈现它们，数据组都是由用户操作。这种方法与表面呈现不同在于，表面呈现是将体积分离为多组
64 表面的多边形。当外科医生想要局限性地观察物体的表面时，表面呈现的物体是精美的，但是就如它的名字所示，表面呈现只是显示数据组的表面部分。目前，更加高端的计算机设备，如图形工作站，需要用来呈现基于体积的图像。

有限的元素

有限的元素是基于几何学的网络而被放置于物理学约束之下。压力、弹力、应力和张力会影响正在被操作物体的性状和性质。这样的操作不仅影响到模型的表面，也会影响到体积。当与详细的图形叠加进行整合时，有限元素的模型能够提供迄今为止最为精确的模拟[210]。

虚拟显示

在一个完美的世界中，虚拟现实技术能够整合我们五种感觉中的任何一种或全部，但是它通常主要依
65 赖于我们最为重要的视觉。我们视觉系统分类为三组：深度感觉、视野和临界的融合频率。

人类的深度感觉局限于大约 30 米，因为与观察的距离相比，双眼是靠近在一起的。虚拟现实系统必须可使用户能够再现这种机制，或达到真实世界中不能够达到的适当的深度。眼睛只需要有限的视野来感觉，仿佛它就是虚拟环境中的一部分。临界融合频率是指在这个频率上，静止的画面快速连续出现，看起来是无衔接缝的运动数据流。这种情形很像古老的动画方法，其中拖曳的闪光卡给人以活生生的卡通片印象。平滑视频的近似频率大约在 30～40Hz。这种画面必须能够递送一种 3-D 的影像。虚拟现实视频画面最具有动感的形式就是头盔显示器（HMD）。虽然虚拟现实能够呈现并经常呈现在桌面监视器中，但是当参与者并不是处于一个封闭的系统中时，如头盔显示器（HMD），那种沉浸其中的感觉并不完全。在桌面监视器中，一种 3-D 的环境是被投影到一种 2-D 的屏幕中。

现有两种清楚的呈现 3-D 环境的基本方法。第一种方法是采用两个单独的显示器，每一只眼睛配一个显示器，以此达到有立体感的效果。第二种方法是采用装配在头上的跟踪系统，后者可以改变系统的透视来匹配用户正在观看的方向。这种跟踪的方法必须与用户头部和手部的运动协调一致。

许多不同类型的头盔显示器（HMD）已经投入使用。某种眼罩式显示系统的能力取决于它的最终目的。眼罩式显示系统可应用于个人视频游戏、建筑学和导弹的发射指挥等。头盔显示器（HMD）也有许多模式。例如，不透明的显示器，完全闭塞与外部世界的任何视线接触。任何视觉输入都单独来自于装配在头上的视频显示系统。

Fakespace, Inc.（Menlo Park, CA）提供了一种双目全方位监视器（BOOM）。这种与头连接的显示器外形上是由一个平衡架子支持的。因为它不是让用户进行穿戴的，而是由一个外部平台支持的，所以 BOOM 系统可以加入另外的硬件技术到该系统中，

因此可以创造高度高保真的视觉能力。分辨率为1280×1024，高于大多数计算机显示器的分辨率，而在 Fakespace 系统中是标准配置。当然，BOOM 设备对于用户来说是无重量的，依靠一种运动追踪系统来保持面对式视角。这种旋转的架子可使系统具有较高的自由度和视野。

一种更加新奇的沉浸式视频显示系统是洞穴自动虚拟环境（CAVE；Fakespace/ 电子可视化实验室），这是一种房间大小的多用户系统。图像是立体地向墙壁和地面投影并通过百叶窗式眼镜来观看。用户戴着位置追踪器，在洞穴自动虚拟环境中通过一台超级计算机来监视用户的位置。随着用户在这种“狭窄的”空间内运动，视角的改变被持续不断地更新。单目的头盔显示器可使佩带者在数据传递时还可以接触外部的世界（图 4–18A）。外科中的应用包括：在处理有关患者生命体征和影像学检查数据的同时，还有能力
66 进行手术操作。

虚拟视网膜显示器可将扫描光线直接投影到观察者的视网膜上（图 4–18B）。因为具有这种特征，所以观察者会感知到一个特别宽广的视野。虽然仍然处于发展阶段，但是视网膜显示器具有接近人类视觉分辨率的可能，同时可以被装入一个轻量的便携式系统中[229]。虚拟视网膜显示器已经在华盛顿大学的人类界面技术实验室中开发出来了。

输入设备

与虚拟世界交互作用的最佳方法就是用一个人的手。这种办法既自然又直觉。数据手套系统（VPL Research, Redwood City, CA[图 4–19]）就是一种典型的系统。

数据手套系统可将用户的手从键盘上解放出来。命令被简单化，任务可通过基本的指点或在虚拟环境中抓紧来执行。自从数据手套的概念出现以后，许多厂商已开发出了类似的界面产品。数据手套是通过许多不同的方法来处理信息。有一些数据手套采用手关节上面的机械传感器或压力测量来确定位置。另一些数据手套则采用纤维光学电路来测量光强度的改变和纤维光学带子的角度作为手弯曲和伸展的程度。有些数据手套也采用了追踪器来监视它在自由空间中的位

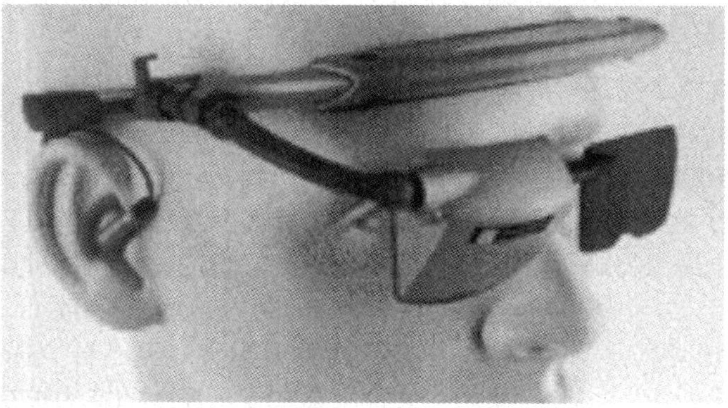
A

图 4–18　A. 电子眼镜Ⅱ，有眼镜阻挡片（虚拟视频，Redmond, WA）。B. 视网膜显示器理论（人类界面技术实验室，华盛顿大学）。驱动电子从电子源聚集成一种影像，如一台计算机。从计算机或其他视频源获得的像素定向成 1 像素，同一时间通过透镜，直接投影到视网膜。“扫描仪”以每秒钟 1800 万像素的速率将一幅图像水平和垂直地“画”到视网膜上。光学系统可将这种图像折射到观察者的眼镜中。

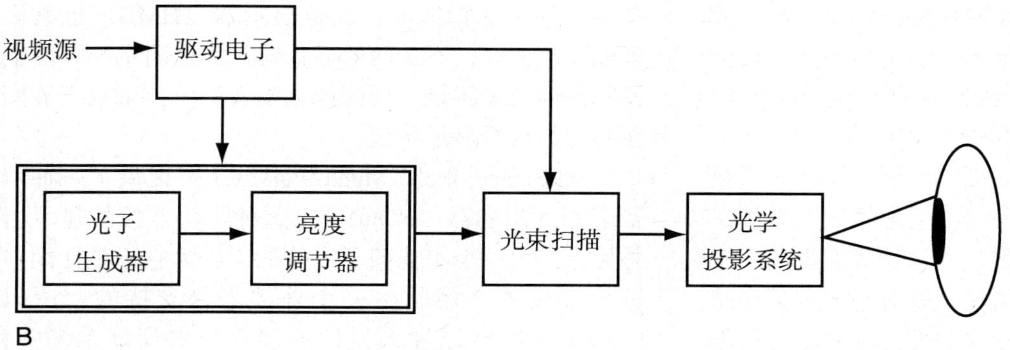

B

置。在各种配置中，数据手套仍然是一种直觉的复杂问题的解决方法。

力反馈和触觉反馈

力量（阻力）和触觉（接触或触摸）反馈可能是两种最为重要的外科手术虚拟现实技术的目标，然而，它们也是最难以实现的目标。外科医生在人类环境中依赖于接触和阻力的敏锐感觉，如果没有这些感觉，逼真度就会受损。腹腔镜检查就是触觉如何从外科医生手上发生转移的一个例子[182]。

触觉非常难以人工产生[178]。人类能够轻易地判断力量的大小，从而举起一杯水并流畅地送入口中。一个计算机如果没有正确编程，可能就会把举起一个杯子误解成举起一块空心砖，而导致将虚拟的水杯扔过整个房间。一直到近期，虚拟现实模拟技术缺少的一个主要的组成部分还是接触的感觉或触觉。

触觉反馈需要两种基本的特征来给用户呈现接触的感觉。首先，系统需要一台计算机，能够计算模拟的 3–D 图像和用户的手之间的交互作用，所有的计算都是实时进行的。其次，触觉反馈环需要某种形式的界面设备（不管是操纵杆、数据手套，还是其他设备），使用户能够与计算机发生交互作用。支持触觉反馈的计算机系统是典型的具有硬件视频加速的 3–D 图像工作站[46,106]。这些系统与界面设备连接，例如流行的 PhanToM 操纵杆（SenseAble Technologies, Woburn, MA [图 4–20]）。这样的基于操纵杆的设备能够提供 6 个自由度的功能。而且，计算机的视频必须能以每秒钟大约 30 次的速率刷新，以便于创建一种流畅的模拟。

与骨骼与肌肉连接一样，因为所有力量的产生必须与固定的点和活动的轴联系在一起，目前力量反馈系统需要一种机械连接的外骨骼。目前力量反馈系统可以采用两种办法来得到这种外骨骼。第一种办法包含装配在手的外部的一种外骨骼，这种外骨骼类似于机电跟踪系统中采用的外骨骼。这种连接包含数个与有长线缆的小马达相连的滑轮。马达配置时远离手部以减轻重量，但是能够通过牵引适当的线缆对不同的手指节点施加作用力。第二种办法包含指尖与手掌上的底盘之间一套小的装满空气的活塞。通过对活塞施加压力可以只对指尖施加作用力。

因为这些系统都可以将它们的作用力反馈给手或手腕上的某些节点，它们可以使你抓紧一个虚拟的物体并感觉它的性状，但是它们不能阻止你将你 67
的手穿过那个物体。为了防止这一点，外骨骼必须伸展到底盘部，后者是沿着手臂和身体或是一个类似于机器人手臂的外部系统，通过更多的连接装配在地板上。

已经开发了多种方法来产生力反馈和触觉反馈[178]。当模拟接触时，压电震动系统可以对用户的指尖产生轻微的震动。电触觉反馈是以相同的指尖感觉原理进行工作，但是没有运动的部分。在虚拟的接触时，一股小电流会流过皮肤表面。微针阵列是由一层纤细的微针组成，可延伸到指尖以产生极度精细的清晰度。微针能够再现边缘的感觉。充气式反馈采用手套内部放置有气袋的手套。这些气袋在期望的时间可发生膨胀以再现接触表面的感觉。温度反馈是采用在手上加

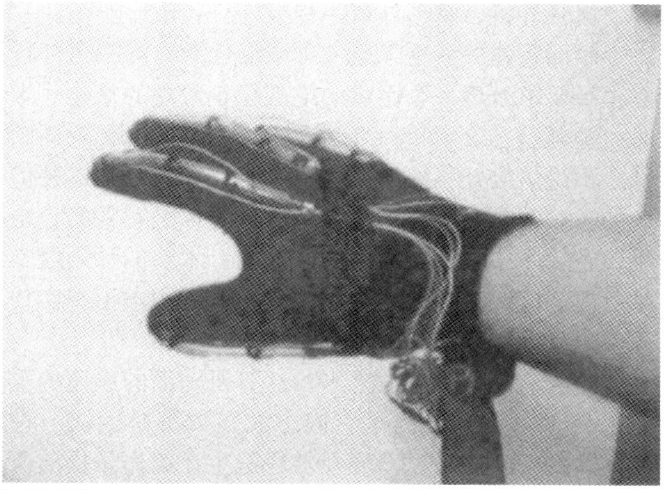

图 4–19　一般的数据手套。

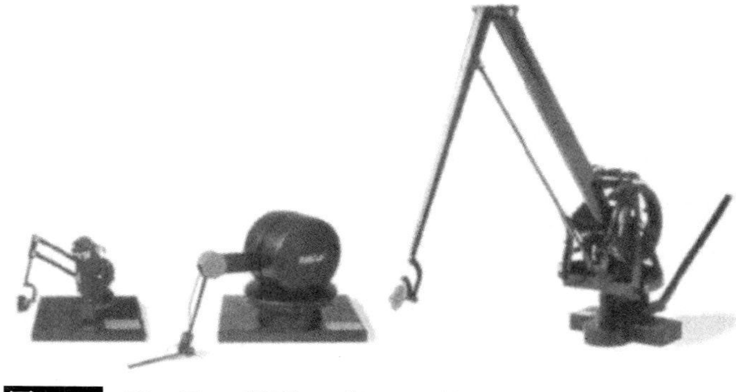

图 4–20　PhanTom 界面。（SenseAble Techologies, Woburn, MA）

热线圈来再现温度的改变。

虚拟现实技术中的跟踪

虚拟现实技术是基于空间的关系。即使呈现给用户的是某种物体的虚拟表象，但是计算机必须要知道相对于这样的物体用户现在处于何处。否则，用户的手将会穿过一个虚拟的杯子而不是去抓紧它。有一些虚拟现实系统通过跟随或追踪来解决这个问题，关键性界面点在用户和计算机之间。追踪系统是放置在头盔和手套上，以便计算机知道何时开始作用。现在已经有数种追踪方法[178]。

机械式追踪系统在物理上是与用户的界面相连接。用户的头盔拴在一端，有计算机的界面在另外一端。这种直接的连接速度较快，但是受试者总是与系统相连限制了活动性。

与小的闪光灯相连的照相机被放置在身体上，能够用作光学追踪的方法。从不同的视角拍摄照片，多个照相机就可以分析身体上发射闪光的二极管的配置。这些 2-D 的数据就可以整合成一种单纯 3-D 影像。这样的处理需要花费时间，这是光学追踪的一个关键性缺点。可以采用磁场信号；磁场源点可放置在手上，采用传感器来追踪。缺点包括受到附近磁场源的干扰和有最大可用的追踪距离。

声学追踪器采用的是高频声音源，在工作区域内对声音源做三角测量。这些系统是依赖声音源与麦克风之间的视线，如果周围有硬的墙面或其他声学反射性表面，就能受到声学反射。如果将多个声学追踪器一起使用，它们必须采用非冲突的频率进行工作，这种策略在磁场追踪中也被采用。

虚拟现实技术的挑战

随着各种新兴技术的出现，有低潮、有骗局，也有希望[46]。虚拟现实技术也不例外。具有最大的改进空间的领域是图像和触觉反馈领域。因为有大规模处理能力以创建完全虚拟现实的产物，目前人们必须在图像的细节与流畅的运行之间进行权衡。这意味着目前虚拟现实技术可以由以下短语来定义：“它可以更好、更快和更便宜；但只能选择其中两个”。这样的权衡导致：模拟只能有动画的质量以便它们能够具有一种合情合理的运行时间。甚至随着图像细节上的被迫删减，在用户界面和虚拟现实技术的反应时间之间还是有一点轻微的延迟或滞后的感觉。手术切开的视觉呈现仍然非常难以精确地实现。

触觉反馈需要相当的计算能力（如果不是更多），可能导致系统不稳定或不精确。许多虚拟现实的力反馈系统可能由于“设法完成”力反馈和毁灭错觉而被迫舍弃。

虚拟现实技术的术前计划

除了简单的任务训练，虚拟现实技术的巨大优势和目标之一是，在同一个患者身上进行实际手术以前，能够根据患者的特异性数据来计划并执行虚拟的手术操作。这个能力远远超出了一个普通任务或人体的早期学习。当计划一个手术时，外科医生通常会将一些数据，如 CT 或 MRI 扫描，以及患者的体格检查和图表，在头脑中整合成一种想象的解决方案。这样的想象需要数年的经验和训练来掌握，特别是当需要将多个 2-D 影像翻译成一种 3-D 影像时。

对于许多外科学专业，虚拟现实技术可以将患者的特异性数据聚集成 “前后” 影像，可在术前由外科医生进行操作，以便病例的结果是可以预测的。这些结果是将基于外科医生在手术期间的决策。而且，随着更多的程序开发出来，虚拟现实的预先计划能够用作一种基于患者实际数据的研究模型，可能可以用于预测一种新的外科手术方案的结果。通过给外科医生提供一份预先设计好的手术操作要点，虚拟现实技术也可加速对复杂病例的决定过程，因此可使医院系统更加有效。虚拟现实技术的术前计划可用于普通外科、血管外科、整形外科、神经外科和矫形外科。

颅面重建外科手术是一项艰巨任务。当一名外科医生被要求处理一个困难的或甚至是常规的重建手术时，他就会从 2-D 的 CT 或 MRI 扫描来重建 3-D 图像。不论这名外科医生如何有经验，如果采用这种传统的方法，其对整形重建结果的预测都是有限的。结果，在手术室内进行手术操作期间，术前的计划经常被更改。因为这些原因，在这个领域利用虚拟现实技术来进行演练和准备的频率正在不断增加[110,111]。

现在有许多种办法来进行计算机辅助的颅面的重建外科手术设计，但是它们中大多数都是生成一种 3-D 的交互式影像，以便在外科医生在工作站提前所做工作的基础上预测手术结果。这种处理是从患者特 68

异性的 CT 或 MRI 扫描显示的横断切面开始，就像面部重建用于创伤和畸形的方法一样[151]。一旦从患者处得到扫描影像，它们就被分割并指定为骨窗和软组织窗。这种处理方式导致了进行 2-D 切面的肿块必须重建为一种 3-D 的环境。患者特异性的 CT 影像通常是在一台图像工作站上进行处理的。

德国的 Erlangen 大学已经演示了一种包括“临界立方体”的用于 2-D 的 CT 扫描到 3-D 重建方法[227]。在这种处理中，Cyberware（Cyberware, Mon terey, CA）扫描仪被用于扫描患者皮肤表面的特征，然后进行压缩以减少数据的体积。皮肤窗和骨窗类似地编译成一种 3-D 影像。这种影像能够在任何平面进行切割以便聚焦于一个感兴趣的特殊区域。Keeve 和其同事们[110]采用这种技术模拟了一种下颌骨的 Dal-Pont 截骨术。经过 3-D 影像呈现以后，可以进行任何数量的切割、移动和操作步骤，其在手术室内将可以预测重建手术的结果（图 4-21）。对真实患者采用这种计算机辅助设计模型进行面部重建手术而形成的“前后”图像已经生产了积极成果。

斯坦福大学的国家生物计算中心采用了一种稍微有所不同的呈现范例，后者是基于 CT 影像基础之上的；它被称作外科手术计划和分析的虚拟环境（）。Montgomery 和其同事们[151]开发了 VESPA 用于颅面部的手术重建，以及乳腺的外科手术、软组织的重建和先天性缺陷的手术修补。一旦获得 CT 扫描影像，体素或基于体积的影像就可被聚焦于感兴趣的区域，就可产生非常特异性的片断性数据。3-D 影像就被播送到一台高清晰的 CRT（阴极射线管）监视器上，戴有履带式 CrystalEyes（一种轻便、无线的用于立体 3D 成像的液晶立体眼镜）（StereoGraphics, San Rafael, CA）快门眼镜和手持一种 FasTrak（三维运动跟踪和数字化系统）（Polhemus, Colchester, VT）记录笔用于输入的用户，就可以看到并操作虚拟的物体。

面部重建外科手术的复杂性要求有这种类型的术前能力，因为按照惯例，常规采用 2-D 的外科医生能够进行的也只有这么多的手术设计和预测。预先计划可使外科医生和患者看到几乎保证的结果；这不仅可使外科医生和患者都安心，而且也可以减少麻醉的时间。

基于虚拟现实技术的三维外科手术模拟器

外科手术的实际施行是高度视觉化的，随后是持续视觉化和触觉反馈以及修改的手工的操作任务[166]。这代表了一种难以克服的挑战。为了创建一种虚拟现实外科手术模拟器用于教育或实践，程序员必须开发一种能充分代表外科手术环境的系统；它必须对外科手术的改变（如切开、解剖、切除）发生反应，其中如果外科医生影响到手术野，就必须给出适当的力反馈。这些先决条件必须以一种对外科医生是透明的方式来完成（即虚拟的手术室应该模拟一个真实的手术室）。依赖于目标听众和应用，已经开发了许多种外科手术模拟器。虚拟外科手术模拟器已经被应用于开放性手术操作、腹腔镜外科手术和远程遥现外科手术。

Karlsruhe 的“VEST”内镜外科训练器（IT VEST Systems AG, Bremen，Germany）可能是最为发达的内镜外科手术模拟器（图 4-22）。这种设备模拟了外科中有窗孔的人类腹部，可以插入多个腹腔镜手

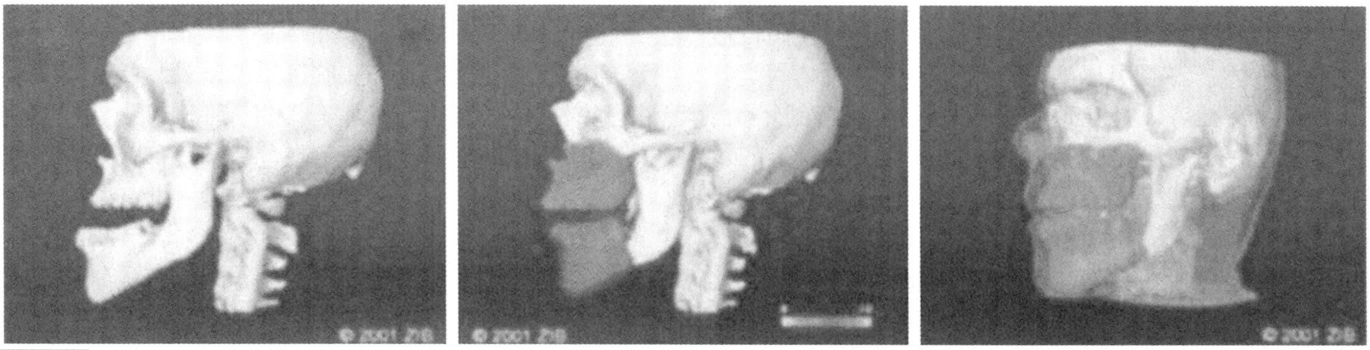

图 4-21　高度 Le Fort I 截骨术的三维手术设计（Konrad-Zue-Zentrum for Informationstechnik, Berlin, Germany）。(Courtesy of SenseAble Techologies, Woburn, MA.)

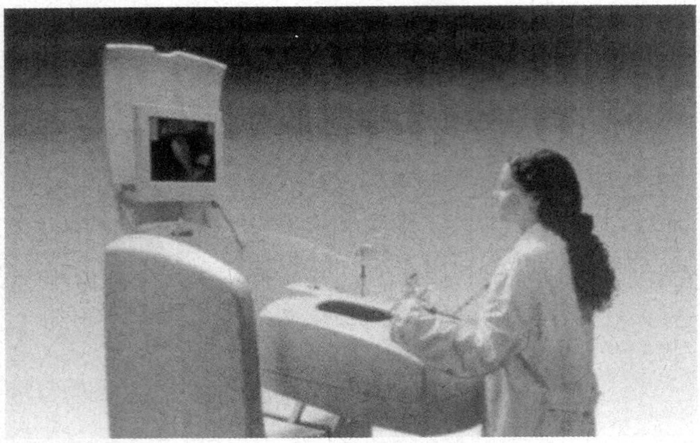

图 4-22 VEST/LapSim 一种内镜外科手术训练器（IT VEST Systems AG, Bremen, Germany）。(Courtesy of IT VEST Systems AG.)

术器械和内镜照相机。力反馈可提供并应用于腹腔镜手术器械。虚拟显示是由专利产品 KISMET（运动学上的模拟、监视和用于遥控机器人的离线程序化环境）3-D 生成外科手术环境来产生的[77]。这种软件可使用户沉浸于高度逼真的虚拟的微创胆囊切除术的腹腔镜情境中，它是采用实时组织动力学和对用户的动作产生动态组织反应来完成虚拟手术。腹腔镜手术器械采用传感器追踪，模拟放置在人类腹腔内的实际的内镜手术器械的自由度。这种系统是由一种图像工作站进行处理，有能力支持全部的沉浸式护目镜和遥控
69 训练。随着计算能力和图像能力的进一步发展，图像的呈现将会变得更加详细，并有望达到实际手术室中的视频监视器的效果。

现在也可有其他外科手术模拟系统。波士顿动力学（剑桥，MA）和宾夕法尼亚州立大学已经开发出一种吻合模拟器，这种模拟器是基于力反馈的外科手术器械和有快门护目镜的 3-D 视频。这种系统使用户可将缝线放置在肠道或血管之上以模拟精巧而自然的吻合手术。一种可以实时分析外科医生成绩的“外科手术报告卡”，是在这个系统的一个独特的用途。有关性能的评论标准包括时间、精确性、针进入的角度和组织损害[162]。

用于支气管镜、导管插入和内镜检查的虚拟现实模拟器是如此的真实，以至住院医生和实习医生可采用这样的模拟器来获得还没有经验的手术暴露。斯坦福大学已经采用 BronchSim 和 CathSim 设备（沉浸式医疗技术，Gaitherburg, MD）以及虚拟现实的上消化道钡餐造影模拟器（第五代的沉浸式技术，Pretori,南非）来评估外科手术操作训练。一项包含 BronchSim 设备的研究由三个部分组成：实践、导航与可视化和诊断与治疗。这个题目被引入到支气管镜和由训练小组叙述的模拟中，由四个视频根据基本的支气管镜进行补充，并由沉浸式医疗技术软件进行支持。其中一个任务涉及从 CT 扫描图像和胸部 X 光平片进行腔内的支气管壁内肿瘤的诊断，以及随后采用活检工具进行安全的肿瘤组织采样和控制出血。

BronchSim 设备能够将专家与新手鉴别开来，从 Likert 调查问卷得到的主观性数据表明，采用支气管镜可提升手术操作能力和熟悉性。类似的教育研究已采用相同的内部机构评估完成了。这些研究得到了同样令人鼓舞人心的结果。

随着计算机辅助医学的出现，对于医学教育规划，虚拟现实技术训练工具从来没有像今天一样变得如此的易于接近。我们的结果以及许多其他研究者的结果都表明，结合虚拟现实系统的外科手术教育可以应用于医学生和住院医生的训练计划中。经验表明，许多虚拟现实模拟器界面具有足够的逼真度，不仅可以作为一种教学工具，而且可以作为一种磨炼目前技能的方法。

在外科教育中的模拟

在外科教育中，目前的训练着重于核心知识、患者保健、团队训练和手术操作技能。外科手术模拟器能够用于加强上面的每一项内容。在初期教育和继续教育中，模拟都可以用于住院医生和开业外科医生的技能训练、患者的治疗和危机训练。

外科手术模拟通过“外科手术模拟中心”的形式已经被数个外科中心和住院医生培养计划接受。人体模型模拟器正在作为一种正式的认证训练方法，被用于外科实习医生和住院医生在危象治疗、高级心脏生命支持（ACLS）和高级创伤生命支持（ATLS）方面的训练。

作为一个基于人体模型核心知识训练的例子，已经开发了一种初始烧伤外科治疗的模拟。急性烧伤的治疗是一种核心的外科技能，其正确治疗与心肌梗死的治疗一起归类于紧急事件中。尽管需要专门的技术

来治疗烧伤，但是只有 20%的外科住院医生有正式的烧伤外科轮转实习。

MedSim 人类患者模拟器（HPS）采用的是一种人体大小的男性人体模型，其与定制的计算机系统相连。人类患者模拟器可以可靠地模拟正常生理状态和病理状态，被证明可用于高级心脏生命支持（ACLS）和高级创伤生命支持（ATLS）的认证训练。模拟的输出是通过标准的床边监护设备、自发性呼吸、睁眼、动脉搏动、声音反应和机器人肢体运动。测试方案演示了一种 40%的三度烧伤。

最初，模拟方案的精确性和关联性是由重症监护和烧伤外科医生验证的。后来，又由高年资外科住院医生进行了 30 分钟的模拟。对每一个项目都提供了 Lichert（等级为 1～5 级）调查问卷和专门的任务报告。每一个住院医生的成绩都被拍成电影以便于由主治医生进行专门的评估。在采用补液、气管插管和焦痂切开术治疗烧伤患者时，人类患者模拟器的计算机驱动的反应是根据住院医生执行高级创伤生命支持（ATLS）的能力。

对于 ATLS 方案和烧伤的治疗，主治医生的反馈是建议的方案可精确地反映关键的治疗点。这些专家也认识到，接受过模拟训练的住院医生能够在类似的情形中担当起作为一名医生的功能。在听取汇报以后，对烧伤治疗、补液计算、气管插管与通气管理以及胸腔与四肢的焦痂切开术每一个项目都更有信心。
70 烧伤治疗模拟能够教会住院医生如何处理没有经历过的情形，能够担当新的才能的一种可信任的平台。这种对应用人类患者模拟器模拟的烧伤治疗训练的第一次确认表明，这是解决重症患者治疗教育两难选择的一种可行方案。

外科手术的“fly-through”基于虚拟现实技术的工具也同样受到欢迎，这些工具是设计用来为医学生或住院医生提供最初的展示外科手术解剖学 3-D 关系的一种工具。包括虚拟人类男性的方案已经吸收了从这种模型获取的数据组的优势，创建了一种模拟的人类解剖学资源，使医学生可以从任何角度和途径来接近各种解剖结构。这种虚拟人类方案数据组可以以一种 3-D 的方式呈现而创建模拟详细的 fly-through 电影。这些 fly-through 能够进行修改以显示许多常见手术操作的前后效果，提供了一种腹腔内的“内镜式”观察视角。随着需要更为详细和特异外科手术关系知识的更多手术操作的开发，并随着外科教育时间的持续下降，虚拟现实技术 fly-through 可能会提供一种教育解决方案。

外科创新

技术持续快速发展，已经变得越来越复杂，并且是跨学科发展；同时临床外科学要求变得越来越多，需要特别的关注。结果，技术的发展和创造性外科医生之间的差距正在不断加大。这个章节就是试图缩小这种差距。

实际上如果变化是不断的，并且不断的循环已经提升了我们的领域，我们有责任去理解、全面地整合以及甚至直接引导外科创新的实用性变化方向。外科医生具有无可否认的独特地位，有义务对这种循环有所贡献，但是这种不断增大的差距已经构成了一个特殊的知识领域，需要一种专门的教育计划。

一种教授年轻外科医生创新步骤的正式教育计划已经确定为一种 2 年期的研究生课程（http://surgery.stanford.edu/innovation）。在第一年中，学员参加听讲课程，讨论实际问题，即进行评估、技术解决方案、智力、所有权、FDA 申请程序和有关经济学。基于团队的课程占第一年的大部分内容。

第二年用于进一步发展一种经确认的计划。在完成这个计划后，学员将拥有必备的技能，以便在下一个外科创新周期成为一个重要的贡献者。取决于学员的背景，生物工程学的硕士学位也是可以完成的。

在 Lucile Packard 儿童医院，外科创新计划重点在于很好制定的生物设计计划，由 Paul Yock 和 Joshua Makower 博士领导（http://innovation.standford.edu/isp/home.isp）。这个网络着重于显示技术转移，可给床边到长椅子周期带来双向的创新。这种独特的学术研究计划在新兴的生物医学工程的前沿通过跨学科研究和教育，着重于新的健康保健技术的发明和实施。

外科创新计划和生物设计是题目为“斯坦福大学生物-X 启蒙”的校园内跨学科研究计划的一部分；它有 500 多名来自生命科学、工程学、化学和物理学的科学家，在生物计算、生物物理学、染色体组学与蛋白质组学、再生医学和化学生物学方面具有广泛的研究主题。

结论

如果小儿外科仍要继续积极参与到无穷的变革中，就应该承认核心技术在促进我们医疗和护理中的作用，并积极从事和推动这种过程以一种符合伦理的方式发展。严肃地讲，我们如果不采取积极的措施，那么我们小儿外科医生、我们所从事的这个事业以及我们的使命都会慢慢地蒙受损失。这部两卷的著作是给我们之前的先驱者的献礼，他们在不到50年的时间内来确定了我们的专业。我们作为这一代的小儿外科医生必须要构建下一个50年的发展。

（顾 松译 陈永卫校）

参考文献

1. Aaronson OS, Tulipan NB, Cywes R, et al: Robot-assisted endoscopic intrauterine myelomeningocele repair: A feasibility study. Pediatr Neurosurg 2002;36:85.
2. Adler JR Jr, Chang SD, Murphy MD, et al: The CyberKnife: A frameless robotic system for radiosurgery. Stereotact Funct Neurosurg 1997;69:124-128.
3. Aharon S, Robb RA: 3-D surface reconstruction of patient-specific anatomic data using a pre-specified number of polygons. Stud Health Technol Inform 1997;39:430.
4. Ahn YC, Lee KC, Kim DY, et al: Fractionated stereotactic radiation therapy for extracranial head and neck tumors. Int J Radiat Oncol Biol Phys 2000;48:501.
5. Alexander E 3rd, Loeffler JS: Radiosurgery using a modified linear accelerator. Neurosurg Clin North Am 1992;3:167.
6. Arezzo A, Testa T, Ulmer F, et al: Positioning systems for endoscopic solo surgery. Minerva Chir 2000;55:635.
7. Argenziano M, Oz MC, Kohmoto T, et al: Totally endoscopic atrial septal defect repair with robotic assistance. Circulation 2003;108(Suppl 1):II191.
8. Arjomand H, Turi ZG, McCormick D, et al: Percutaneous coronary intervention: Historical perspectives, current status, and future directions. Am Heart J 2003;146:787.
9. Bajada C, Selch M, De Salles A, et al: Application of stereotactic radiosurgery to the head and neck region. Acta Neurochir Suppl (Wien) 1994;62:114.
10. Ballantyne GH, Moll F: The da Vinci telerobotic surgical system: The virtual operative field and telepresence surgery. Surg Clin North Am 2003;83:1203.
11. Bargar WL, Bauer A, Borner M: Primary and revision total hip replacement using the Robodoc system. Clin Orthop 1998;354:82.
12. Bergonié J: De quelques resultats de la radiotherapie et essai de fixation d'une technique rationelle. C R Acad Sci (Paris) 1906;143:983.
13. Billotte W: Ceramic biomaterials. In Bronzino JD (ed): Biomedical Engineering Handbook, 2nd ed. Boca Raton, Florida, CRC Press, 1999.
14. Black PM, Tarbell NJ, Alexander E 3rd, et al: Stereotactic techniques in managing pediatric brain tumors. Childs Nerv Syst 1993;9:343.
15. Blasberg RG, Gelovani J: Molecular-genetic imaging: A nuclear medicine–based perspective. Mol Imaging 2002;1:280.
16. Blomgren H, Lax I, Naslund I, et al: Stereotactic high dose fraction radiation therapy of extracranial tumors using an accelerator. Clinical experience of the first thirty-one patients. Acta Oncol 1995;34:861.
17. Brown PO, Botstein D: Exploring the new world of the genome with DNA microarrays. Nat Genet 1999; 21(Suppl 1):S33.
18. Buatti JM, Friedman WA, Bova FJ, et al: Linac radiosurgery for locally recurrent nasopharyngeal carcinoma: Rationale and technique. Head Neck 1995;17:149.
19. Buatti JM, Friedman WA, Meeks SL, et al: The radiobiology of radiosurgery and stereotactic radiotherapy. Med Dosim 1998;23:201.
20. Buatti JM, Meeks SL, Marcus RB Jr, et al: Radiotherapy for pediatric brain tumors. Semin Pediatr Neurol 1997;4:3049.
21. Burns PN: Harmonic imaging with ultrasound contrast agents. Clin Radiol 1996;51(Suppl 1):S50.
22. Bush RL, Lin PH, Lumsden AB: Endovascular treatment of the thoracic aorta. Vasc Endovasc Surg 2003;37:399.
23. Bush RL, Lin PH, Lumsden AB: Endovascular management of abdominal aortic aneurysms. J Cardiovasc Surg (Torino) 2003;44:527.
24. Callahan MJ, Rodriguez DP, Taylor GA: CT of appendicitis in children. Radiology 2002;224:325.
25. Cannon JW, Stoll JA, Salgo IS, et al: Real-time three-dimensional ultrasound for guiding surgical tasks. Comput Aided Surg 2003;8:82.
26. Carmine J, Allen P, Ardrey P, et al: Medical Applications of Virtual Reality. Raleigh, NC, Department of Biological and Agricultural Engineering, North Carolina State University, 1999.
27. Chang CH, Chang FM, Yu CH, et al: Three-dimensional ultrasound in the assessment of fetal cerebellar transverse and antero-posterior diameters. Ultrasound Med Biol 2000;26:175.
28. Chang CH, Chang FM, Yu CH, et al: Assessment of fetal cerebellar volume using three-dimensional ultrasound. Ultrasound Med Biol 2000;26:981.
29. Chang CH, Yu CH, Chang FM, et al: Assessment of fetal adrenal gland volume using three-dimensional ultrasound. Ultrasound Med Biol 2002;28:1383.
30. Chang CH, Yu CH, Chang FM, et al: Volumetric assessment of normal fetal lungs using three-dimensional ultrasound. Ultrasound Med Biol 2003;29:935.
31. Chang FM, Hsu KF, Ko HC, et al: Fetal heart volume assessment by three-dimensional ultrasound. Ultrasound Obstet Gynecol 1997;9:42.
32. Chang FM, Hsu KF, Ko HC, et al: Three-dimensional ultrasound assessment of fetal liver volume in normal pregnancy: A comparison of reproducibility with two-dimensional ultrasound and a search for a volume constant. Ultrasound Med Biol 1997;23:381.
33. Chang SD, Adler JR: Robotics and radiosurgery—the cyberknife. Stereotact Funct Neurosurg 2001;76:204.
34. Chang SD, Adler JR Jr: Current status and optimal use of radiosurgery. Oncology (Huntingt) 2001;15:209.
35. Chang SD, Adler JR, Steinberg GK: General and Historical Considerations of Radiotherapy and Radiosurgery, vol 3. Philadelphia, WB Saunders, 2003.

36. Chang SD, Main W, Martin DP, et al: An analysis of the accuracy of the CyberKnife: A robotic frameless stereotactic radiosurgical system. Neurosurgery 2003;52:140.
37. Chopra V, Gesink BJ, de Jong J, et al: Does training on an anesthesia simulator lead to improvement in performance? Br J Anaesth 1994;73:293.
38. Choy G, Choyke P, Libutti SK: Current advances in molecular imaging: Noninvasive in vivo bioluminescent and fluorescent optical imaging in cancer research. Mol Imaging 2003;2:303.
39. Chua DT, Sham JS, Kwong PW, et al: Linear accelerator–based stereotactic radiosurgery for limited, locally persistent, and recurrent nasopharyngeal carcinoma: Efficacy and complications. Int J Radiat Oncol Biol Phys 2003;56:177.
40. Cleary K, Anderson J, Brazaitis M, et al: Final report of the technical requirements for image guided spine procedures workshop, April 17-20, 1999, Ellicott City, Maryland, USA. Comput Aided Surg 2000;5:180.
41. Cmelak AJ, Cox RS, Adler JR, et al: Radiosurgery for skull base malignancies and nasopharyngeal carcinoma. Int J Radiat Oncol Biol Phys 1997;37:997.
42. Coleman BG, Adzick NS, Crombleholme TM, et al: Fetal therapy: State of the art. J Ultrasound Med 2002;21:1257.
43. Colombo F, Benedetti A, Casentini L, et al: Stereotactic radiosurgery of intracranial tumors in childhood. J Neurosurg Sci 1985;29:233.
44. Costa GL, Sandora MR, Nakajima A, et al: Adoptive immunotherapy of experimental autoimmune encephalomyelitis via T-cell delivery of the IL-12 p40 subunit. J Immunol 2001;167:2379.
45. Crisera CA, Marosky JK, Longaker MT, et al: Organogenesis particularly relevant to fetal surgery. World J Surg 2003; 27:38.
46. Delany B, Abouaf J: The Market for Visual Simulation/Virtual Reality Systems, 4th ed. New York, CyberEdge Information Services, 2001.
47. Denecke T, Frush DP, Li J: Eight-channel multidetector computed tomography: Unique potential for pediatric chest computed tomography angiography. J Thorac Imaging 2002;17:306.
48. Detre JA, Wang J: Technical aspects and utility of fMRI using BOLD and ASL. Clin Neurophysiol 2002;113:621.
49. Donnelly LF, Frush DP: Pediatric multidetector body CT. Radiol Clin North Am 2003;41:637.
50. Drasin T, Gracia C, Atkinson J: Pediatric applications of robotic surgery. Pediatr Endosurg Innovative Tech 2003;7:377.
51. Dunbar SF, Tarbell NJ, Kooy HM, et al: Stereotactic radiotherapy for pediatric and adult brain tumors: Preliminary report. Int J Radiat Oncol Biol Phys 1994;30:531.
52. Dyson RL, Pretorius DH, Budorick NE, et al: Three-dimensional ultrasound in the evaluation of fetal anomalies. Ultrasound Obstet Gynecol 2000;16:321.
53. Edelman RR, Hahn PF, Buxton R, et al: Rapid MR imaging with suspended respiration: Clinical application in the liver. Radiology 1986;161:125.
54. Even-Bendahan G, Lazar I, Erez I, et al: Role of imaging in the diagnosis of acute appendicitis in children. Clin Pediatr (Phila) 2003;42:23.
55. Fabrikant JI, Levy RP, Steinberg GK, et al: Heavy-charged-particle radiosurgery for intracranial arteriovenous malformations. Stereotact Funct Neurosurg 1991;57:50.
56. Fabrikant JI, Lyman JT, Frankel KA: Heavy charged-particle Bragg peak radiosurgery for intracranial vascular disorders. Radiat Res Suppl 1985;8:S244.
57. Falk V, Jacobs S, Gummert J, et al: Robotic coronary artery bypass grafting (CABG)—the Leipzig experience. Surg Clin North Am 2003;83:1391.
58. Fox LA: Images in clinical medicine. Three-dimensional CT diagnosis of maxillofacial trauma. N Engl J Med 1993;329:102.
59. Freeman CR, Souhami L, Caron JL, et al: Stereotactic external beam irradiation in previously untreated brain tumors in children and adolescents. Med Pediatr Oncol 1994;22:173.
60. Freiherr G: Harmonic imaging: What is it, how it works. Diagnostic Imaging Europe 1998;HU6.
61. Frinking PJ, Bouakaz A, Kirkhorn J, et al: Ultrasound contrast imaging: Current and new potential methods. Ultrasound Med Biol 2000;26:965.
62. Frush DP, Donnelly LF: Pulmonary sequestration spectrum: A new spin with helical CT. AJR Am J Roentgenol 1997;169:679.
63. Frush DP, Donnelly LF: Helical CT in children: Technical considerations and body applications. Radiology 1998;209:37.
64. Gaba DM: The future vision of simulation in health care. Qual Saf Health Care 2004;12(Suppl 1):i2.
65. Garcia-Ruiz A, Gagner M, Miller JH, et al: Manual vs robotically assisted laparoscopic surgery in the performance of basic manipulation and suturing tasks. Arch Surg 1998;133:957.
66. Gardner E, Linskey ME, Penagaricano JA, et al: Stereotactic radiosurgery for patients with cancer of the head and neck. Curr Oncol Rep 2003;5:164.
67. Gerosa M, Nicolato A, Foroni R: The role of gamma knife radiosurgery in the treatment of primary and metastatic brain tumors. Curr Opin Oncol 2003;15:188.
68. Gertner ME, Krummel TM: Micro- and nanoelectromechanical systems in medicine and surgery. In Greco R (ed): Nanobiology: Nano Scale Fabrication of New Generation of Biomedical Devices. Boca Raton, FL, CRC Press, 2005, pp 25-38.
69. Giller CA, Berger BD, Gilio JP, et al: Feasibility of radiosurgery for malignant brain tumors in infants by use of image-guided robotic radiosurgery: Preliminary report. Neurosurgery 2004;55:916.
70. Giller CA, Berger BD, Pistenmaa DA, et al: Robotically guided radiosurgery for children. Pediatr Blood Cancer 2005;45:304.
71. Gorman P, Krummel T: Simulation and virtual reality in surgical education: Real or unreal? Arch Surg 1999; 134:1203.
72. Greco R (ed): Nanobiology: Nano Scale Fabrication of New Generation of Biomedical Devices. Boca Raton, FL, CRC Press 2005, pp 1-24.
73. Gressens P, Luton D: Fetal MRI: Obstetrical and neurological perspectives. Pediatr Radiol 2004;34:682.
74. Gritzmann N, Hollerweger A, Macheiner P, et al: Transabdominal sonography of the gastrointestinal tract. Eur Radiol 2002;12:1748.
75. Gropler RJ: Methodology governing the assessment of myocardial glucose metabolism by positron emission tomography and fluorine 18–labeled fluorodeoxyglucose. J Nucl Cardiol 1994;1(2 Pt 2) (Suppl):S4.
76. Gropler RJ, Soto P: Recent advances in cardiac positron emission tomography in the clinical management of the cardiac patient. Curr Cardiol Rep 2004;6:2026.
77. Gruener G: Telementoring using tactile cues. In Mechanical Engineering. Boulder, CO, University of Colorado, 1998.

78. Gunven P, Blomgren H, Lax I: Radiosurgery for recurring liver metastases after hepatectomy. Hepatogastroenterology 2003;50:1201.
79. Gutt CN, Markus B, Kim ZG, et al: Early experiences of robotic surgery in children. Surg Endosc 2002;16:1083.
80. Hadjipanayis CG, Kondziolka D, Gardner P, et al: Stereotactic radiosurgery for pilocytic astrocytomas when multimodal therapy is necessary. J Neurosurg 2002;97:56.
81. Hahn PF, Saini S, Cohen MS, et al: An aqueous gastrointestinal contrast agent for use in echo-planar MR imaging. Magn Reson Med 1992;25:380.
82. Hall E: Radiobiology for the Radiologist, vol 5. Philadelphia, JB Lippincott, 2000.
83. Hall EJ, Brenner DJ: The radiobiology of radiosurgery: Rationale for different treatment regimes for AVMs and malignancies. Int J Radiat Oncol Biol Phys 1993;25:381.
84. Harisinghani M, Barentsz J, Hahn PF, et al: Noninvasive detection of clinically occult lymph-node metastases in prostate cancer. N Engl J Med 2003;348:2491.
85. Harrison MR, Evans MI, Adzick NS, et al (eds): The Unborn Patient: The Art and Science of Fetal Therapy, 3rd ed. Philadelphia, WB Saunders, 2001.
86. Hashizume M, Shimada M, Tomikawa M, et al: Early experiences of endoscopic procedures in general surgery assisted by a computer-enhanced surgical system. Surg Endosc 2002;16:1187.
87. Hedequist DJ, Hall JE, Emans JB: The safety and efficacy of spinal instrumentation in children with congenital spine deformities. Spine 2004;29:2081.
88. Heller K, Gutt C, Schaeff G, et al: Use of the robot system da Vinci for laparoscopic repair of gastro-oesophageal reflux in children. Eur J Pediatr Surg 2002;12:239.
89. Henriksen K, Moss F: From the runway to the airway and beyond. Qual Saf Health Care 2004;13(Suppl 1):S11.
90. Hernandez L, Zamorano L, Sloan A, et al: Gamma knife radiosurgery for renal cell carcinoma brain metastases. J Neurosurg 2002;97(5 Suppl):S489.
91. Herschman HR: Molecular imaging: Looking at problems, seeing solutions. Science 2003;302:605.
92. Hiltzik M (ed): Dealers of Lightning: Xerox PARC and the Dawn of the Computer Age. New York, HarperBusiness, 1999.
93. Hirth A, Pedersen PH, Baardsen R, et al: Gamma-knife radiosurgery in pediatric cerebral and skull base tumors. Med Pediatr Oncol 2003;40:99.
94. History of PET and MRI. Advanced Biomedical Technology Research [website] 11/17/03; accessed 12/9/04.
95. Hodgson DC, Goumnerova LC, Loeffler JS, et al: Radiosurgery in the management of pediatric brain tumors. Int J Radiat Oncol Biol Phys 2001;50:929.
96. Hollands CM, Dixey LN: Applications of robotic surgery in pediatric patients. Surg Laparosc Endosc Percutan Tech 2002;12:71.
97. Hollands CM, Dixey LN: Robotic-assisted esophago-esophagostomy. J Pediatr Surg 2002;37:983.
98. Hollands CM, Dixey LN, Torma MJ: Technical assessment of porcine enteroenterostomy performed with ZEUS robotic technology. J Pediatr Surg 2001;36:1231.
99. Honda Y, Fitzgerald P: Stent thrombosis: An issue revisited in a changing world. Circulation 2003;108:2.
100. Horton KM, Fishman EK: Multidetector-row computed tomography and 3-dimensional computed tomography imaging of small bowel neoplasms: Current concept in diagnosis. J Comput Assist Tomogr 2004;28:106.
101. Hoshi S, Jokura H, Nakamura H, et al: Gamma-knife radiosurgery for brain metastasis of renal cell carcinoma: Results in 42 patients. Int J Urol 2002;9:618.
102. Humphreys RP, Hoffman HJ, Drake JM, et al: Choices in the 1990s for the management of pediatric cerebral arteriovenous malformations. Pediatr Neurosurg 1996;25:2775.
103. Jacob BP, Gagner M: Robotics and general surgery. Surg Clin North Am 2003;83:1405.
104. Jodicke A, Berthold LID, Scharbrodt W, et al: Endoscopic surgical anatomy of the paediatric third ventricle studied using virtual neuroendoscopy based on 3-D ultrasonography. Childs Nerv Syst 2003;19:325.
105. Jodicke A, Daentzer D, Kastner S, et al: Risk factors for outcome and complications of dorsal foraminotomy in cervical disc herniation. Surg Neurol 2003;60:124.
106. John N: Surgical Simulators on the World Wide Web—This Must Be the Way Forward? Manchester, England, Manchester Visualisation Centre, University of Manchester, 1999.
107. Kapoor V, McCook BM, Torok FS: An introduction to PET-CT imaging. Radiographics 2004;24:523.
108. Kasalicky MA, Svah J, Fried M, et al: AESOP 3000—computer-assisted surgery, personal experience. Rozhl Chir 2002;81:346.
109. Kaste SC: Issues specific to implementing PET-CT for pediatric oncology: What we have learned along the way. Pediatr Radiol 2004;34:205.
110. Keeve E, Girod S, Girod B: Computer aided craniofacial surgery. In Computer Assisted Radiology. Paris, Telecommunications Institute, University of Erlangen, 1996.
111. Keeve E, Girod S, Kikinis R, Girod B: Deformable modeling of facial tissue for craniofacial surgery simulation. Comput Aided Surg 1999;3:228.
112. Kelly PJ: State of the art and future directions of minimally invasive stereotactic neurosurgery. Cancer Control 1995;2:287.
113. Kelly PJ: Stereotactic surgery: What is past is prologue. Neurosurgery 2000;46:16.
114. Kitamura K, Shirato H, Seppenwoolde Y, et al: Tumor location, cirrhosis, and surgical history contribute to tumor movement in the liver, as measured during stereotactic irradiation using a real-time tumor-tracking radiotherapy system. Int J Radiat Oncol Biol Phys 2003;56:221.
115. Knight CG, Lorincz A, Gioell KM, et al: Computer-assisted robot-enhanced laparoscopic fundoplication in children. J Pediatr Surg 2004;39:864.
116. Kocher M, Voges J, Staar S, et al: Linear accelerator radiosurgery for recurrent malignant tumors of the skull base. Am J Clin Oncol 1998;21:18.
117. Kondziolka D, Lunsford LID, Flickinger JC: The radiobiology of radiosurgery. Neurosurg Clin North Am 1999;10:157.
118. Kondziolka D, Lunsford LID, Loeffler JS, et al: Radiosurgery and radiotherapy: Observations and clarifications. J Neurosurg 2004;101:585.
119. Kondziolka D, Lunsford LID, Witt TC, et al: The future of radiosurgery: Radiobiology, technology, and applications. Surg Neurol 2000;54:406.
120. Kuo JS, Yu C, Petrovich A, et al: The CyberKnife stereotactic radiosurgery system: Description, installation, and an initial evaluation of use and functionality. Neurosurgery 2003;53:1235.
121. Lanfranco AR, Castellanos AE, Desai JP, et al: Robotic surgery: A current perspective. Ann Surg 2004;239:14.
122. Lange A, Mankad P, Walayat M, et al: Transthoracic three-dimensional echocardiography in the preoperative assessment of atrioventricular septal defect morphology. Am J Cardiol 2000;85:630.

123. Langer SG, Carter SJ, Haynor DR, et al: Image acquisition: Ultrasound, computed tomography, and magnetic resonance imaging. World J Surg 2001;25:1428.
124. Larson DA, Flickinger JC, Loeffler JS: The radiobiology of radiosurgery. Int J Radiat Oncol Biol Phys 1993; 25:557.
125. LaValle GJ, Martinez DA, Sobel D, et al: Assessment of disseminated pancreatic cancer: A comparison of traditional exploratory laparotomy and radioimmunoguided surgery. Surgery 1997;122:867.
126. Lavan D, McQuire T, Langer R: Small-scale systems for in vivo drug delivery. Nat Biotechnol 2003;21:1184.
127. Lawler LP, Fishman EK: Multidetector row computed tomography of the aorta and peripheral arteries. Cardiol Clin 2003;21:607.
128. Le Bret E, Papadatos S, Folliguet T, et al: Interruption of patent arteriosus in children: Robotically assisted versus videothoracoscopic surgery. J Thorac Cardiovasc Surg 2002;123:973.
129. Lederman G, Wronski M, Fine M: Fractionated radiosurgery for brain metastases in 43 patients with breast carcinoma. Breast Cancer Res Treat 2001;65:145.
130. Lee BR, Chow GK, Ratner LE, et al: Laparoscopic live donor nephrectomy: Outcomes equivalent to open surgery. J Endourol 2000;14:811.
131. Lee N, Millender LE, Larson DA, et al: Gamma knife radiosurgery for recurrent salivary gland malignancies involving the base of skull. Head Neck 2003;25:210.
132. Lee N, Xia P, Quivey JM, et al: Intensity-modulated radiotherapy in the treatment of nasopharyngeal carcinoma: An update of the UCSF experience. Int J Radiat Oncol Biol Phys 2002;53:12.
133. Levy EL, Niranjan A, Thompson TP, et al: Radiosurgery for childhood intracranial arteriovenous malformations. Neurosurgery 2000;47:834.
134. Levy RP, Fabrikant JI, Frankel KA, et al: Stereotactic heavy-charged-particle Bragg peak radiosurgery for the treatment of intracranial arteriovenous malformations in childhood and adolescence. Neurosurgery 1989; 24:841.
135. Levy RP, Fabrikant JI, Frankel KA, et al: Heavy-charged-particle radiosurgery of the pituitary gland: Clinical results of 840 patients. Stereotact Funct Neurosurg 1991;57:22.
136. Levy RP, Schulte RW, Slater JD, et al: Stereotactic radiosurgery—the role of charged particles. Acta Oncol 1999;38:165.
137. Light ED, Idriss SF, Wolf PD, et al: Real-time three-dimensional intracardiac echocardiography. Ultrasound Med Biol 2001;27:1177.
138. Loeffler JS, Rossitch E Jr, Siddon R, et al: Role of stereotactic radiosurgery with a linear accelerator in treatment of intracranial arteriovenous malformations and tumors in children. Pediatrics 1990;85:774.
139. Lorincz A, Langenburg S, Klein M: Robotics and the pediatric surgeon. Curr Opin Pediatr 2003;15:262.
140. Luebbe B, Woo R, Wolf S, et al: Robotically assisted minimally invasive surgery in a pediatric population: Initial experience, technical considerations, and description of the da Vinci Surgical System. Pediatr Endosurg Innovative Tech 2003;7:385.
141. Machado LG, Savi MA: Medical applications of shape memory alloys. Braz J Med Biol Res 2003;36:683.
142. Mack M: Minimally invasive and robotics surgery. JAMA 2001;285:568.
143. Malhotra SP, Le D, Thelitz S, et al: Robotic-assisted endoscopic thoracic aortic anastomosis in juvenile lambs. Heart Surg Forum 2002;6:38.
144. Mao C, Flynn CE, Hayhurst A, et al: Viral assembly of oriented quantum dot nanowires. Proc Natl Acad Sci U S A 2003;100:6946.
145. McCaffrey A, Kay MA, Contag CH: Advancing molecular therapies through in vivo bioluminescent imaging. Mol Imaging 2003;2:75.
146. Meier AH, Rawn RI, Krummel TM: Virtual reality: Surgical application, a challenge for the new millennium. J Am Coll Surg 2000;192:372.
147. Menkis AH, Kodera K, Kiaii B, et al: Robotic surgery, the first 100 cases: Where do we go from here? Heart Surg Forum 2004;7:1.
148. Menon M, Srivastava A, Tewari A, et al: Laparoscopic and robot assisted radical prostatectomy: Establishment of a structured program and preliminary analysis of outcomes. J Urol 2002;168:945.
149. Mettler L, Ibrahim M, Ionat W: One year of experience working with the aid of a robotic assistant (the voice-controlled optic holder AESOP) in gynaecological endoscopic surgery. Hum Reprod 1998;13:2748.
150. Mihaljevic T, Cannon JW, del Nido PJ: Robotically assisted division of a vascular ring in children. J Thorac Cardiovasc Surg 2003;125:1163.
151. Montgomery K, Stephanides M, Schendel S: User Interface Paradigms for VR-Surgical Based Planning, Lessons Learned over a Decade of Research. Stanford, CA, Stanford University, 1996-2000.
152. Murphy MJ, Adler JR Jr, Bodduluri M, et al: Image-guided radiosurgery for the spine and pancreas. Comput Aided Surg 2000;5:278.
153. Murphy MJ, Chang SD, Gibbs IC, et al: Patterns of patient movement during frameless image-guided radiosurgery. Int J Radiat Oncol Biol Phys 2003;55:1400.
154. Murphy MJ, Martin D, Whyte R, et al: The effectiveness of breath-holding to stabilize lung and pancreas tumors during radiosurgery. Int J Radiat Oncol Biol Phys 2002;53:4752.
155. Murray W, Schneider A: Using simulators for education and training in anesthesiology. Anesthesia Patient Safety Foundation Newsletter, 1996.
156. Nicolato A, Gerosa M, Ferraresi P, et al: Stereotactic radiosurgery for the treatment of arteriovenous malformations in childhood. J Neurosurg Sci 1997;41:359.
157. Nordberg A: Application of PET in dementia disorders. Acta Neurol Scand Suppl 1996;168:71.
158. Nordberg A: PET imaging of amyloid in Alzheimer's disease. Lancet Neurol 2004;3:519.
159. Nugent H, Edelman E: Tissue engineering therapy for cardiovascular disease. Circ Res 2003;92:1068.
160. Okada S, Tanaba Y, Yaegashi S, et al: Initial use of the newly developed voice-controlled robot system for a solitary pulmonary arterio-venous malformation. Kyobu Geka 2002;55:871.
161. Olsen LH, Deding D, Yeung CK, Jorgensen TM: Computer assisted laparoscopic pneumovesical ureter reimplantation. In Cohen: Initial experience in a pig model. APMIS Suppl 2003;109:23.
162. O'Toole RV, Playter RR, Krummel TM, et al: Measuring and developing suturing technique with a virtual reality surgical simulator. J Am Coll Surg 1999;189:127.
163. Paek B, Goldberg JD, Albanese CT: Prenatal diagnosis. World J Surg 2003;27:27.
164. Pedraza R, Palmer I, Moss V, et al: Bilateral robotic assisted laparoscopic heminephroureterectomy. J Urol 2004;171:2394.

165. Pedraza R, Weiser A, Franco I: Laparoscopic appendicovesicostomy (Mitrofanoff procedure) in a child using the da Vinci robotic system. J Urol 2004;171:1652.
166. Peitgen H, Preim B, Selle D, et al: Risk Analysis for Liver Surgery. Center for Medical Diagnostic Systems and Visualization. Bremen, Germany, 1999.
167. Peters C: Robot assisted surgery in pediatric urology. Pediatr Endosurg Innovative Tech 2003;7:403.
168. Petrovich Z, Jozsef G, Yu C, et al: Radiotherapy and stereotactic radiosurgery for pituitary tumors. Neurosurg Clin North Am 2003;14:147.
169. Pilliar RM: Powder metal-made orthopedic implants with porous surface for fixation by tissue ingrowth. Clin Orthop 1983;176:242.
170. Pimentel K, Teixeira K: Virtual Reality: Through the New Looking Glass. Windcrest, New York, McGraw-Hill, 1993.
171. Ponsky LE, Crownover RL, Rosen MJ, et al: Initial evaluation of Cyberknife technology for extracorporeal renal tissue ablation. Urology 2003;61:498.
172. Powers JE, Burns PN, Souquet J: Imaging instrumentation for ultrasound contrast agents. In Nanda N, Schlief R, Goldberg B (eds): Advances in Echo Imaging Using Contrast Enhancement. Dordrecht, The Netherlands, Kluwer Academic, 1997, p 139.
173. Powers WJ, Zazulia AR: The use of positron emission tomography in cerebrovascular disease. Neuroimaging Clin North Am 2003;13:741.
174. Prayer D, Brugger PC, Prayer L: Fetal MRI: Techniques and protocols. Pediatr Radiol 2004;34:685.
175. Qian G, Lowry J, Silverman P, et al: Stereotactic extracranial radiosurgery for renal cell carcinoma. Int J Radiat Oncol Biol Phys 2003;57(2 Suppl):S283.
176. Radford IR: Evidence for a general relationship between the induced level of DNA double-strand breakage and cell-killing after X-irradiation of mammalian cells. Int J Radiat Biol Relat Stud Phys Chem Med 1986;49:611.
177. Rickers C, Sasse K, Buchert R, et al: Myocardial viability assessed by positron emission tomography in infants and children after the arterial switch operation and suspected infarction. J Am Coll Cardiol 2000;36:1676.
178. Riva G, Bolzoni M, Melis L: Sensing in VR. Milan, Applied Technology for Psychology Laboratory, 1996.
179. Roberts B: Is there money in MEMS? Electronic Business Magazine, May 1999.
180. Roberts EG, Shulkin BL: Technical issues in performing PET studies in pediatric patients. J Nucl Med Technol 2004;32:5.
181. Rosen J, Lasko-Harvill A, Satava R: Virtual reality and surgery. In Taylor R (ed): Computer Integrated Surgery. Cambridge, MA, MIT Press, 1996.
182. Rosenberg LB, Stredney D: A haptic interface for virtual simulation of endoscopic surgery. Stud Health Technol Inform 1996;29:371.
183. Rubin GD: 3-D imaging with MDCT. Eur J Radiol 2003; 45(Suppl 1):S37.
184. Rutten I, Deneufbourg JM: Radiotherapy in pediatric head and neck tumours. Acta Otorhinolaryngol Belg 2000;54:1.
185. Salo JA, Salminen JT, Kiviluoto TA, et al: Treatment of Barrett's esophagus by endoscopic laser ablation and antireflux surgery. Ann Surg 1998;227:40.
186. Salzberg A, Krummel TM (eds): Patient Safety: The Surgeon's Role. Patient Safety Manual. Chicago, American College of Surgeons, 2001.
187. Salzberg A, Krummel TM: Use of a virtual reality flexible bronchoscopy simulator for use in medical and surgical training. Paper presented at a meeting of the Society of Critical Care Medicine, 2001, San Diego, CA.
188. Salzberg D, Bloom M, Krummel TM: Current problems in surgery. Curr Probl Surg Adv Technol 2003;39:733.
189. Satava RM: Virtual endoscopy: Diagnosis using 3-D visualization and virtual representation. Surg Endosc 1996;19:173.
190. Schneebaum S, Papo J, Graif M, et al: Radioimmunoguided surgery benefits for recurrent colorectal cancer. Ann Surg Oncol 1997;4:371.
191. Schnepp R, Hua X: A tumor-suppressing duo: TGFbeta and activin modulate a similar transcriptome. Cancer Biol Ther 2003;2:171.
192. Schoder H, Erdi YE, Larson SM, et al: PET/CT: A new imaging technology in nuclear medicine. Eur J Nucl Med Mol Imaging 2003;30:1419.
193. Schoder H, Larson SM, Yeung HW: PET/CT in oncology: Integration into clinical management of lymphoma, melanoma, and gastrointestinal malignancies. J Nucl Med 2004;45(Suppl 1):72S.
194. Seeman N, Belcher A: Emulating biology: Building nanostructures from the bottom up. Proc Natl Acad Sci U S A 2002;99(Suppl 2):S6451.
195. Semwal SK, Barnhart BK: Ray casting and the enclosing-net algorithm for extracting shapes from volume data. Comput Biol Med 1995;25:261.
196. Seymour CB, Mothersill C, Alper T: High yields of lethal mutations in somatic mammalian cells that survive ionizing radiation. Int J Radiat Biol Relat Stud Phys Chem Med 1986;50:167.
197. Shahidi R, Clarke L, Bucholz RD, et al: White paper: Challenges and opportunities in computer-assisted interventions, January 2001. Comput Aided Surg 2001; 6:176.
198. Shrieve DC, Klish M, Wendland MM, et al: Basic principles of radiobiology, radiotherapy, and radiosurgery. Neurosurg Clin North Am 2004;15:467.
199. Singh RK, Smith JT, Wilkinson ID, et al: Ultrafast MR imaging in pediatric neuroradiology. Acta Radiol 2003;44:550.
200. Smyth MD, Sneed PK, Ciricillo SF, et al: Stereotactic radiosurgery for pediatric intracranial arteriovenous malformations: The University of California at San Francisco experience. J Neurosurg 2002;97:48.
201. Somaza SC, Kondziolka D, Lunsford LD, et al: Early outcomes after stereotactic radiosurgery for growing pilocytic astrocytomas in children. Pediatr Neurosurg 1996;25:109.
202. Stahl A, Wieder H, Wester JH, et al: PET/CT molecular imaging in abdominal oncology. Abdom Imaging 2004;29:388.
203. Steichen FM, Ravitch MM (eds): Stapling in Surgery. Chicago, Year Book, 1984.
204. Stigbrand T, Ullen A, Sandstrom P, et al: Twenty years with monoclonal antibodies: State of the art—where do we go? Acta Oncol 1996;35:259.
205. Suh JH, Barnett GH: Stereotactic radiosurgery for brain tumors in pediatric patients. Technol Cancer Res Treat 2003;2:141.
206. Takacs I, Hamilton AJ: Extracranial stereotactic radiosurgery: Applications for the spine and beyond. Neurosurg Clin North Am 1999;10:257.
207. Talamini MA: Robotic surgery: Is it for you? Adv Surg 2002;36:1.
208. Talamini MA, Chapman S, Horgan S, et al: A prospective analysis of 211 robotic-assisted surgical procedures. Surg Endosc 2003;17:1521.

209. Tanaka H, Hashimoto K, Yamada I, et al: Interstitial photodynamic therapy with rotating and reciprocating optical fibers. Cancer 2001;91:1791.
210. Taylor CA, Hughes TJ, Zarins CK: Finite element modeling of three-dimensional pulsatile flow in the abdominal aorta: Relevance to atherosclerosis. Ann Biomed Eng 1998;26:975.
211. Taylor R, Stulberg D: Excerpts from the final report for the second international workshop on robotics and computer assisted medical interventions, June 23-26, 1996, Bristol, England. Comput Aided Surg 1997;2:78.
212. Tempany C, McNeil B: Advances in biomedical imaging. JAMA 2001;285:5627.
213. Temple MJ, Langer JC: Image-guided surgery for the pediatric patient: Ultrasound, computerized tomography, and magnetic resonance imaging. Curr Opin Pediatr 2003;15:256.
214. Tendick F Jr, Tharp G, Stark L: Sensing and manipulation problems in endoscopic surgery: Experiment, analysis and observation. Presence 1993;2:66.
215. Timmerman R, Papiez L, McGarry R, et al: Extracranial stereotactic radioablation: Results of a phase I study in medically inoperable stage I non–small cell lung cancer. Chest 2003;124:1946.
216. Timmerman R, Papiez L, Suntharalingam M: Extracranial stereotactic radiation delivery: Expansion of technology beyond the brain. Technol Cancer Res Treat 2003; 2:153.
217. Tokuuye K, Sumi M, Ikeda H, et al: Technical considerations for fractionated stereotactic radiotherapy of hepatocellular carcinoma. Jpn J Clin Oncol 1997;27:170.
218. Tome WA, Mehta MP, Meeks SL, et al: Fractionated stereotactic radiotherapy: A short review. Technol Cancer Res Treat 2002;1:153.
219. Townsend DW: Physical principles and technology of clinical PET imaging. Ann Acad Med Singapore 2004;33:133.
220. Townsend DW, Carney JP, Yap JT, et al: PET/CT today and tomorrow. J Nucl Med 2004;45(Suppl 1):4S.
221. Tranquart F, Grenier N, Eder V, et al: Clinical use of ultrasound tissue harmonic imaging. Ultrasound Med Biol 1999;25:889.
222. Treece GM, Prager RW, Gee AH, et al: Correction of probe pressure artifacts in freehand 3D ultrasound. Med Image Anal 2002;6:199.
223. Triadafilopoulos G, DiBaise JK, Nostrant TT, et al: The Stretta procedure for the treatment of GERD: 6 and 12 month follow-up of the U.S. open label trial. Gastrointest Endosc 2002;55:149.
224. Uematsu M: [Stereotactic radiation therapy for non small cell lung cancer.] Nippon Geka Gakkai Zasshi 2002; 103:256.
225. Uhlendorf V: Physics of ultrasound contrast imaging: Scattering in the linear range. IEEE Trans Ultrasonics Ferroelectrics Frequency Control 1994;41:70.
226. Unger EC, Cohen MS, Gatenby RA, et al: Single breath-holding scans of the abdomen using FISP and FLASH at 1.5 T. J Comput Assist Tomogr 1988;12:575.
227. van Leeuwen MS, Obertop H, Hennipman AH, Fernandez MA: 3-D reconstruction of hepatic neoplasms: A preoperative planning procedure. Baillieres Clin Gastroenterol 1995;9:121.
228. Verheij M, Bartelink H: Radiation-induced apoptosis. Cell Tissue Res 2000;301:133.
229. Viirre E, Pryor H, Nagata S, Furness TA 3rd: The virtual retinal display: A new technology for virtual reality and augmented vision in medicine. Stud Health Technol Inform 1998;50:252.
230. Vooijs M, Jonkers J, Lyons S, et al: Noninvasive imaging of spontaneous retinoblastoma pathway–dependent tumors in mice. Cancer Res 2002;62:1892.
231. Wara W, Bauman G, Gutin P, et al: Stereotactic radiosurgery in children. Stereotact Funct Neurosurg 1995; 64(Suppl 1):118.
232. Waterworth JA: Virtual Reality in Medicine: A Survey of the State of the Art. Umea, Sweden, Umea University, 1998, p 1.
233. Weissleder R, Mahmood U: Molecular imaging. Radiology 2001;219:316.
234. Weprin BE, Hall WA, Cho KH, et al: Stereotactic radiosurgery in pediatric patients. Pediatr Neurol 1996;15:193.
235. Whyte RI, Crownover R, Murphy MJ, et al: Stereotactic radiosurgery for lung tumors: Preliminary report of a phase I trial. Ann Thorac Surg 2003;75:1097.
236. Wilke M, Holland SK, Myseros JS, et al: Functional magnetic resonance imaging in pediatrics. Neuropediatrics 2003;34:225.
237. Wilson RD: Prenatal evaluation for fetal surgery. Curr Opin Obstet Gynecol 2002;14:187.
238. Wulf J, Hadinger U, Oppitz U, et al: Stereotactic radiotherapy of extracranial targets: CT-simulation and accuracy of treatment in the stereotactic body frame. Radiother Oncol 2000;57:225.
239. Wulf J, Hadinger U, Oppitz U, et al: Stereotactic radiotherapy of targets in the lung and liver. Strahlenther Onkol 2001;177:645.
240. Wulf J, Hadinger U, Oppitz U, et al: Impact of target reproducibility on tumor dose in stereotactic radiotherapy of targets in the lung and liver. Radiother Oncol 2003;66:141.
241. Yin F, Kim JG, Haughton C, et al: Extracranial radiosurgery: Immobilizing liver motion in dogs using high-frequency jet ventilation and total intravenous anesthesia. Int J Radiat Oncol Biol Phys 2001;49:211.
242. Young RF: Application of robotics to stereotactic neurosurgery. Neurol Res 1987;9:123.
243. Zimmerman RA, Haselgrove JC, Wang Z, et al: Advances in pediatric neuroimaging. Brain Dev 1998;20:275.
244. Zissiadis Y, Dutton S, Kieran M, et al: Stereotactic radiotherapy for pediatric intracranial germ cell tumors. Int J Radiat Oncol Biol Phys 2001;51:108.

第 5 章

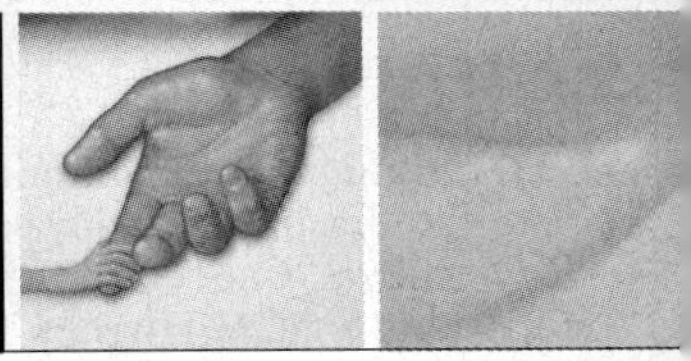

胎儿患者

Michael R. Harrison

77 现在令许多小儿外科医生感兴趣的先天性缺陷在小儿出生前即可被发现。有一些遗传性解剖畸形需要特殊探查，而绝大多数异常情况都是在有产科指征进行超声检查时偶然发现的。导致进行产前诊断的临床情况往往与潜在的胎儿畸形有关，如羊水过少与胎儿尿路梗阻有关，羊水过多与胎儿肠梗阻有关。

产前诊断能促进围生期保健。如能及早发现严重的胎儿损害，即可行孕期咨询以及终止妊娠。对于许多可矫正的缺陷，最好的办法是从产院转运至合适的医疗中心，近足月时分娩后治疗；改变分娩时机或分娩方式对某些先天缺陷有利（表 5-1）。最后，一系列关于受累胎儿的研究将有助于阐述一些可经手术矫正的损害的发育病理生理学机制，从而改进出生前和出生后的治疗方法。非常重要的是，熟悉出生后手术矫正这些先天缺陷的外科医生应该参与制订孕期治疗决策和家庭咨询工作[28]。

胎儿成像技术

近 30 年来，胎儿直接成像技术发展迅速。超声检查能精确描绘胎儿解剖学，包括正常和异常情况。这一非侵入性技术对胎儿和母亲都较为安全，现已常规应用于绝大多数孕期检查。超声诊断还应用于其他方面，但是必须注意，该技术依赖于实际操作者，这是很重要的。所得信息的范围和可靠度与超声检查者的技能和经验直接相关，而这些信息是制订治疗决策的关键。例如，治疗一种胎儿缺陷必须先彻底评估胎儿是否还存在其他畸形，因为各种畸形可能是一种症候群的部分表现。三维超声检查没有提高该技术的精确性和敏感度，但被证实其有利于各种超声引导下的干预方法。

实时超声检查可提供胎动和胎儿重要功能（心率变异性、呼吸运动）的重要信息，以此可反映胎儿的健康状况。连续的超声检查评估对于定义胎儿疾病的自然病史和进展更有用。胎儿颈半透明度增高是一种与染色体和一些结构畸形有关的发现；因而在胎龄 11～14 周时，超声检查可作为一种无创筛查技术使用。最后，在实时超声引导下可以抽取胎儿液体（尿液、腹水、胸水、血液、脑脊液）用于诊断和治疗[28]。以我对 500 例胎儿进行的超声检查经验来看，这一技术既安全又相对简单。

尽管超声检查已取代了很多传统的放射成像检查，但在许多情况下应用快速计算机断层成像和磁共振影像检查获得胎儿影像时无需实施麻醉或使胎儿麻痹。在确定预后方面，可以施行器官的体积测量（如发育不良的肺），但这个方法被证实并不优于早期的超声检查（如肺-头比例）。磁共振影像检查的优势在于发现中枢神经系统的先天畸形和获得性损伤，因此是确定神经系统预后的重要手段[28]。

生化筛查

孕妇血清和羊水的甲胎蛋白（AFP）水平升高是胎儿发育异常的一个可靠指标。以往 AFP 是用于筛查神经管缺陷，但在另一些胎儿缺陷时它也会升高，如脐膨出、腹裂和骶尾部畸胎瘤，此时胎儿血清渗出增加。AFP 是胎儿血清的主要糖蛋白，它的分子量、氨基酸序列和免疫学特性都与白蛋白相仿。在 13～15 孕周时，胎儿血清 AFP 水平达到峰值，为 3mg/ml。羊水 AFP 浓度的变化曲线与血清 AFP 浓度的相似，但具体数值为后者浓度稀释 150 倍。测定其他标志物（如雌三醇和绒毛膜促性腺激素）可以筛查出非整倍体儿。 78

表 5-1 产前诊断的缺陷的处理

以下缺陷的通常治疗方法是终止妊娠
无脑儿、积水性无脑畸形、前脑无叶无裂畸形
与染色体异常有关的严重畸形（如 13 三体综合征）
双侧肾脏发育不全、婴儿多囊肾
严重的、无法治疗的遗传性代谢障碍（如 Tay-Sachs 病）
致命性骨发育异常（如致死性发育不全、隐性成骨不全）
宫内可发现的胎儿缺陷，但最好近足月分娩后纠治
食管、十二指肠、空肠回肠和肛门直肠闭锁
胎粪性肠梗阻（囊性纤维化）
肠囊肿和重复畸形
小的、未受损的脐膨出和腹裂
单侧肾多囊性发育异常、肾积水
颅面、肢体和胸壁畸形
单纯性水囊状淋巴管瘤
小型骶尾部畸胎瘤、中胚叶肾瘤、成神经细胞瘤
良性囊肿（如卵巢、肠系膜、胆总管）
可能需要实施剖宫产娩出的胎儿缺陷
联体双胎
巨型或破裂的脐膨出、腹裂
严重肾积水、大的或破裂的脊髓脊膜膨出
大型骶尾部畸胎瘤或颈部水囊状淋巴管瘤
出现不能耐受产程或胎儿应激，需要提早分娩的所有畸形
可能导致早产的先天缺陷
进行性扩大的脑积水、胸腔积液
腹裂或破裂的脐膨出伴有肠损伤
肠扭转或胎粪性肠梗阻继发肠缺血和坏死
进行性胎儿水肿
宫内生长迟缓
心律失常（如室上性心动过速伴心力衰竭）
可能需要施行产时宫外治疗的先天缺陷
先天性高气道阻塞综合征（CHAO）
大型颈部肿瘤（如畸胎瘤）
阻塞气管或口腔的肿块（如水囊状淋巴管瘤）
需要立即行 ECMO 套管插入术
妨碍肺膨胀的胸部占位

ECMO：体外膜式氧合器；EXIT：产时宫外治疗。

胎儿采样

采集样本获得的细胞可以用于许多遗传缺陷和遗传性代谢异常疾病的染色体核型分析和 DNA 诊断。（经阴道或经腹部）采集绒毛膜绒毛样本可用于孕期第一个 3 个月的宫内诊断，而羊水穿刺术通常在孕期第二个 3 个月时方可进行。最常见的操作指征是高龄妊娠、已知的携带者状态或前一胎为遗传性疾病患者。从胎龄 14 周起，即可在超声引导下，行经皮穿刺脐带血管获得胎儿血样。血细胞培养可获得更快的染色体核型结果（2 天，羊水穿刺获得染色体核型结果需 7 天）。胎儿皮肤和肝活检可在超声检查或胎儿镜下进行。因采样技术导致胎儿流产的风险范围是 1%～5%。

应用新的、强效的采样技术可以从母亲血循环中分离到胎儿细胞，所以一些疾病诊断只需采集母血进行遗传测试即可。分子分析以及人类基因组图谱的快速发展已使通过遗传诊断的疾病种类不断增加[28]。

胎儿评估

尽管大多数通过产前超声检查诊断的解剖畸形可在出生后经内、外科治疗而得到最好的处理，但有一些简单而可预见的会对发育产生破坏性后果的解剖畸形可能需要在产前进行纠治[18,19,29]。在 20 世纪 80年代，应用动物模型研究了严重的、可能可以纠正的宫内损害的发育病理生理学；自然病史是通过对人类胎儿的连续观察确定；干预的入选标准已制定出来；子宫切开术和胎儿手术的麻醉、抗分娩和外科技术得到了提高[2,19,21,23,28,29]。

这些对基础和临床研究的投资已经惠及一些存在相对少见缺陷的胎儿患者，采用新的治疗方法也将有利于更多胎儿患者的治疗，这些技术包括干细胞移植、组织工程学和基因治疗，可用于多种解剖和生化缺陷。表 5-2 列出了胎儿治疗发展史上的里程碑。

图 5-1 是为胎儿手术行子宫切开术的平面图，该技术经 30 多年的实验和临床工作发展而来[28]。由于子宫切开术存在明显的风险（尤其是早产），现已产生可避免切开子宫的电子内镜下进行胎儿手术的技术（FETENDO）（图 5-2）[17]。开多个通道的复杂胎儿镜手术需要给母亲做微小的剖腹术（如放置 FETENDO 夹或 FETENDO 气囊以闭合气管）。经皮胎儿镜介入

表 5-2 胎儿治疗的里程碑

事件	地点	年份
Rh 溶血病的宫内治疗（IUT）	国立妇女医院，奥克兰，新西兰	1961
子宫切开术建立胎儿血管通路——IUT	波多黎各大学	1964
胎儿镜——诊断用	耶鲁大学	1974
实验病理生理学（羊模型）	UCSF	1980
子宫切开术和母体安全（猴子模型）	UCSF	1981
尿路病变的膀胱羊水分流术	UCSF	1982
脑积水的脑室羊水分流术	丹佛大学	1982
国际胎儿内、外科学会成立	圣巴巴拉，加利福尼亚	1982
开放式胎儿手术治疗尿路病变	UCSF	1983
CCAM 切除术	UCSF	1984
《未出生的患者：围生期诊断和治疗》（第 1 版）发行	UCSF	1984
胎儿血管内输液	国王学院，伦敦大学	1985
CDH 开放修补	UCSF	1989
双胎脐带连接异常的 RFA 治疗	国王学院，伦敦大学	1990
NIH 试验：CDH 开放修补	UCSF	1990
主动脉球部瓣膜成形术	国王学院，伦敦大学	1991
SCT 切除术	UCSF	1992
胎盘血管的激光消融术	圣约瑟夫医院，密尔沃基；国王学院，伦敦大学	1995
EXIT 治疗胎儿气道梗阻	UCSF	1995
胎儿镜手术（FETENDO）	UCSF	1996
SCIDS 的干细胞治疗	底特律	1996
CDH——FETENDO 夹、气囊	UCSF	1997
脊髓脊膜突出的开放修补	Vanderbilt	1997
NIH 试验：FETENDO 气囊用于 CDH	UCSF	1998
心包畸胎瘤切除术	UCSF	2000
胎-胎输血综合征的 EuroFetus 试验	大学医院，Gasthuisberg，比利时；巴黎-Ouest 大学，凡尔赛，法国	2001
颈部畸胎瘤切除术	UCSF	2001
NIH 试验：脊髓脊膜突出的开放修补	UCSF，CHOP，Vanderbilt	2002
NIH 试验：双胎输血综合征	CHOP，UCSF，围生期工作网	2002
心脏发育不全的球囊扩张术	哈佛大学	2003

CCAM：先天性囊性腺瘤样畸形；CDH：先天性膈疝；CHOP：费城儿童医院；EXIT：产时宫外治疗；IUT：宫内输液；NIH：国家卫生研究院；RFA：射频消融；SCIDS：严重联合免疫缺陷综合征；SCT：骶尾部畸胎瘤；UCSF：加州旧金山大学。

法已用于临床诊断性活组织检查、胎-胎输血综合征的胎盘血管激光消融术[53]、胎儿膀胱镜检查和尿道减压[40]、脐带绕结或联体双胎分离术[12,45]以及羊膜索切断术。超声引导下的经皮介入法已用于导管分流置管术（膀胱、胸部）[40,47]、建立血管通路（心脏、脐血管）、巨大肿瘤或联体双胎的射频消融术[55]、从胎儿体腔中抽吸液体[50]以及将药物或细胞直接输入胎儿体内[16]。

母亲和胎儿的管理

无论是穿刺还是切开，都是对子宫的破坏，会引起子宫收缩。尽管目前技术先进，但胎膜破裂和早产

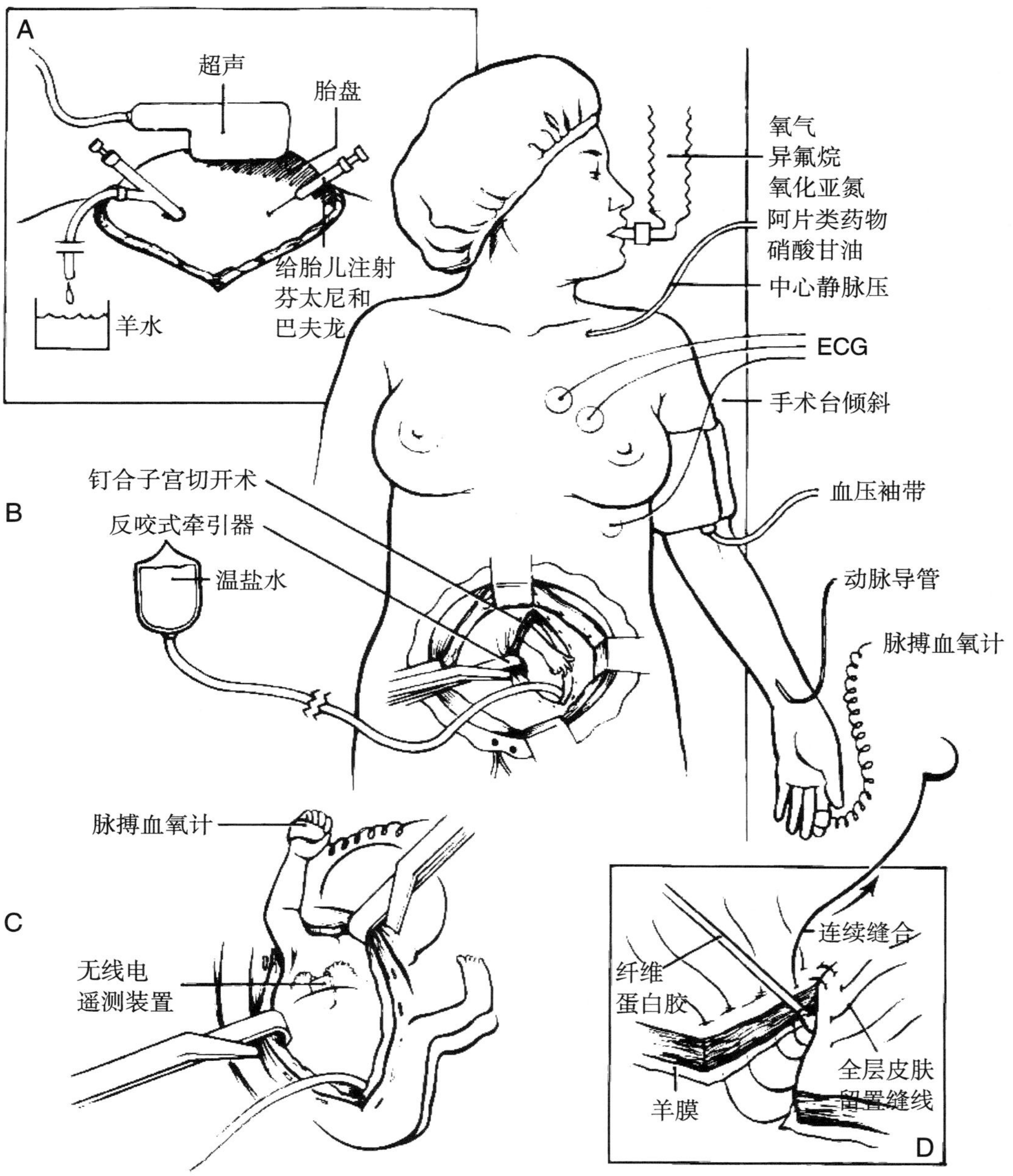

图 5-1 开放式胎儿手术概要。A. 经腹部低位、横切口暴露子宫。超声检查进行胎盘定位、给胎儿注射纳洛酮和肌松剂并吸出羊水。B. 用U形钉开放子宫可以止血和封闭胎膜。在胎儿周围持续灌注加温的盐水溶液。孕妇麻醉、子宫收缩抑制和监护如图所示。可吸收的U形钉和反咬钳有利于子宫切开术时暴露胎儿的相关部位。C. 一个小型的脉搏血氧计记录术中脉搏次数和氧饱和度。一个无线电遥测装置用来监护术中和术后的胎儿心电图（ECG）和羊膜腔压力。D. 胎儿修补术后，用可吸收的缝线和纤维蛋白胶关闭子宫切口。用温和的乳酸林格液恢复羊水量。

分娩是胎儿治疗的致命弱点。虽然，吸入卤化物能为母亲和胎儿提供满意的麻醉，但要达到术中子宫舒张的麻醉深度则会引起胎儿和母亲的心肌抑制并影响胎盘灌注[52]。吲哚美辛能使胎儿的动脉导管收缩，合并使用硫酸镁和拟 β 受体类药物会造成母亲肺水肿。在寻找更有效的和毒性更低的抗分娩药物疗法过程中，发现外源性一氧化氮可以消除猴子子宫切开术诱发的早产[39]。静脉注射硝酸甘油能够延迟分娩，但要求严格控制速度以防严重并发症。

术后的管理在胎儿重症监护室中进行。持续监测母亲的动脉压、中心静脉压、尿量和氧饱和度。用分娩力计在体表记录胎儿安全和子宫活动度。患者自控镇痛术、持续硬膜外麻醉或两种方法并用，可以减轻母亲应激和帮助保胎。当分娩得到控制且胎儿稳定时，即可将患者转送到产科病房。继续进行门诊监测和保胎，胎儿超声检查至少每周一次。子宫切开术后要求此次和今后妊娠都要行剖宫术分娩[11,43]。

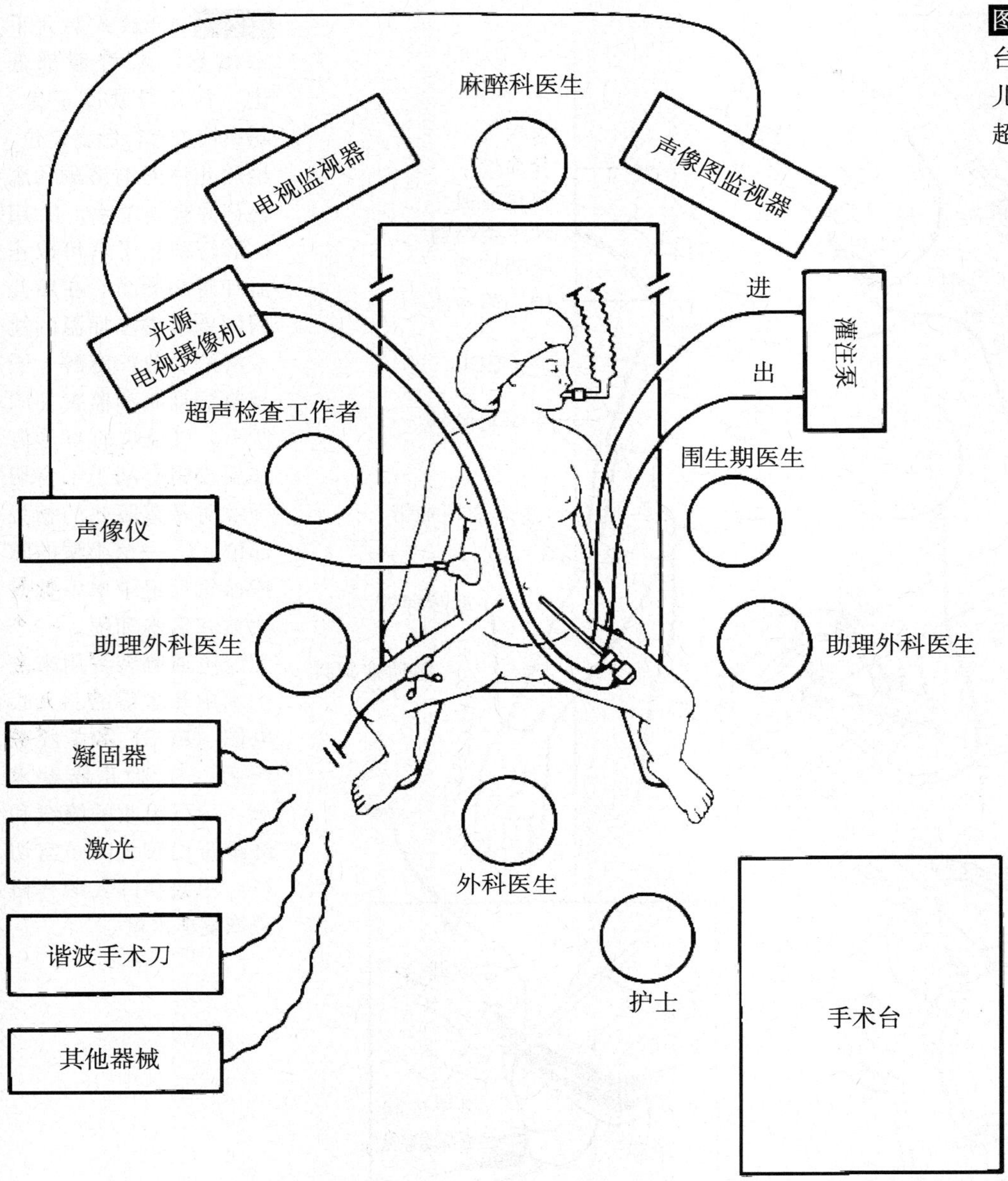

图 5-2 手术室布局。注意手术台头端有两个监视器：一个是胎儿镜图像监视器；另一个是实时超声影像监视器。

孕妇-胎儿手术的危险性

对胎儿来说，手术的风险与手术纠正致命或致病缺陷带来的裨益是要进行权衡的。手术对母亲的风险和益处很难评估。许多胎儿畸形并不直接威胁孕妇的健康，然而孕妇在手术中要经受明显的风险和不适。孕妇可能选择为了未出世的胎儿承担手术风险，这样也可以减轻抚养一个严重畸形儿的负担。

涉及胎儿手术干预对母亲的影响的文献很少[43]。我和我的同事分析了不同类型的胎儿干预方法（子宫切开术、各种内镜操作和经皮技术）中孕妇的发病率和死亡率，并以此对手术中孕妇的危险率进行了量 80
化。我们对 1989 年 7 月至 2003 年 5 月间加州大学旧金山分校胎儿治疗中心的 187 例病例进行了回顾性评估。其中采取开放式子宫切开术的有 87 例，采取内镜技术的有 69 例，经皮技术的有 31 例。没有发生母亲死亡。接受内镜操作者，即使同时进行剖腹术，其发病率也比接受开放式子宫切开术者低，差异有统计学意义：最终分娩方式为剖宫产（94.8%对 58.8%，$P<0.001$）需要重症监护的比例（1.4%对 26.4%，

$P<0.001$）、住院天数（7.9 对 11.9 天，$P=0.001$）和需要输血者（2.9%对 12.6%，$P=0.022$）。组间胎膜早破、肺水肿、胎盘剥离、术后阴道出血、难免早产或胎儿手术至分娩的间期无显著差别。内镜组绒毛膜羊膜分离的发生率较高（64.7%对 20.3%，$P<0.001$）。经皮技术组的发病率最低[11]。该研究证实，胎儿手术可在不导致孕妇死亡的情况下实施。但近期并发症可能比较严重，如影响孕妇健康、孕期长短和胎儿存活率。

孕中期子宫切开术不会在子宫下段进行，因此，胎儿手术后的分娩和之后的分娩都应行剖宫产术。在我们的研究病例中，有 2 例在后来的妊娠中发生了子宫破裂；但子宫关闭和新生儿情况都很好。最后，胎
81 儿手术不会危害母亲以后怀孕和分娩的能力。

产前诊断指导围生期处理

先天缺陷的种类决定其围生期处理（见表 5-1）[28]。对于不能适应出生后生活的严重畸形，如能尽早诊断，家长就可以选择终止妊娠。许多在宫内诊断出的、可被纠正的畸形最好在近足月分娩后行适当的内、外科处理；已产前诊断的可以让孕妇在治疗中心分娩，因为后者有新生儿外科团队并可做好术前准备。如胎儿畸形会引起难产或可在无菌环境立即施行外科修补，则选择性剖宫产分娩优于阴道试产。

如胎儿需在诊断后尽快治疗，可考虑提早分娩，但必须认真权衡早产风险。每一种畸形行提早分娩的基本病变不同，但其原则是相同的：继续妊娠对胎儿会产生进行性不良影响。某些情况下，一个特殊器官系统的功能会因损害而下降（如肾盂积水），而且不纠正其功能损伤会继续恶化。某些畸形对胎儿产生的进行性不良影响的直接原因是胎儿仍处于宫内环境（如腹裂的肠损伤是由于肠暴露在羊水中）。

有些胎儿缺陷状态可经产前治疗得到缓解（见表 5-3）。例如，血液可输入腹膜腔或直接输入脐动脉，经胎盘给予抗心律失常药可逆转胎儿室上性心动过速。当必需物质、药物或营养素不能经胎盘转运
82 时，可将其注入羊水而使胎儿吞咽和吸收。将来，应用恰当的干细胞移植或基因工程可能纠正细胞功能缺陷[14,16]。

表 5-3　可能需要产前治疗的胎儿缺陷

疾病	治疗
胎儿溶血（红细胞缺陷）	红细胞——腹膜内或静脉输注
肺未成熟（表面活性物质缺乏）	糖皮质激素——经胎盘给药
代谢障碍（如甲基丙二酸血症、多种羧化酶缺陷）	B_{12}——经胎盘给药 生物素——经胎盘给药
心律失常（室上性心动过速）	洋地黄——经胎盘给药 普萘洛尔——经胎盘给药 普鲁卡因胺——经胎盘给药
内分泌缺陷（如甲状腺功能减退、肾上腺增生）	甲状腺剂——经羊膜给药 皮质类固醇——经胎盘给药
营养缺乏（如宫内生长迟缓）	蛋白质热卡——经羊膜或静脉输注

需要产前外科纠正的胎儿问题

被批准考虑进行产前治疗的仅有的解剖畸形是那些会干扰胎儿器官发育以及一旦减轻能使胎儿继续正常发育的畸形（表 5-4）。起初，重点研究的是一些致命和可成功纠正的畸形。近十年来，更多的胎儿缺陷被确认，新的治疗方法不断被研发[21,28]。随着侵入性干预技术逐步减少，一些不致命的畸形（如脊髓脊膜膨出）也成为胎儿手术纠正的对象[10,38,58]。最后，干细胞移植、基因治疗和组织工程学可望用于治疗许多遗传疾病[14,16,32,51]。 83

尿路梗阻

胎儿尿路梗阻会造成肺发育不良和肾发育异常，但这些常见致死的后果经尿道减压可改善[1]。未经治疗的胎儿尿路梗阻的自然病程已被确证，根据胎儿尿液电解质和 β_2 微球蛋白以及胎儿肾脏超声图像制定的选择标准也已证明是可靠的[40]。在所有存在尿道扩张的胎儿中，90%是无须干预的。但是，因尿路梗阻引起双侧肾积水的胎儿表现出羊水过多、过少者应给

表 5–4 应产前治疗的胎儿疾病

	对发育的影响（治疗的基本原理）	不进行治疗的结果	推荐的治疗方法
致命缺陷			
尿路梗阻（尿道瓣膜）	肾积水 肺发育不全	肾衰竭 肺衰竭	经皮膀胱羊水分流术 胎儿镜瓣膜消融术 开放式膀胱造口术
先天性囊性腺瘤样畸形	肺发育不全、水肿	水肿、死亡	开放式肺叶切除术 消融术（激光、RFA） 类固醇 开放式彻底修复术
先天性膈疝	肺发育不全	肺衰竭	暂时性气管闭塞术：气管夹（开放式手术或胎儿镜）、胎儿镜球囊（经皮、可逆）
骶尾部畸胎瘤	高排血量衰竭	水肿、死亡	开放式肿瘤切除术 血管闭塞：RFA、酒精、RFA
双胎输血综合征	供体–受体经胎盘的盗血	胎儿水肿、死亡；存活者的神经系统损害	胎儿镜胎盘血管射频消融术（NIH 试验） 羊膜复位术（NIH 试验） 选择性复位术
无心畸胎或异常双胎（TRAP）	血管盗血 栓塞形成	死亡或损害存活双胎	选择性复位术 脐带闭塞或切断术 RFA
中脑导水管硬化	脑水肿	脑损伤	脑室羊水分流术
心瓣膜闭锁	心脏发育不全	心功能衰竭	瓣膜成形术
先天性高气道阻塞综合征（CHAO）	肺液引起过度膨胀	水肿、死亡	胎儿镜气管造口术 EXIT
颈部畸胎瘤	气道梗阻 高排血量衰竭	水肿、死亡	开放式切除术 EXIT 血管闭塞：酒精、RFA RFA
非致命缺陷			
脊髓脊膜膨出	脊髓损伤	麻痹、神经源性膀胱或肠、脑水肿	开放式修复术（NIH 试验） 胎儿镜覆盖术
腹裂	肠损伤	营养不良、短肠	连续的经羊膜置换术
唇腭裂	面容缺陷和畸形	永久性	胎儿镜修复术 * 开放式修补术
代谢或细胞功能缺陷			
干细胞或酶缺陷	血红蛋白病 免疫缺陷 贮积病	贫血、水肿 感染、死亡 发育迟缓、死亡	胎儿干细胞移植 胎儿基因治疗 *
预测的器官缺陷	心、肺、肾功能缺陷或发育不全	新生儿心、肺、肾衰竭	为生后器官移植诱导容受性 * 组织工程学 *

* 还没试用于人类胎儿。

EXIT：产时宫外治疗；NIH：国家卫生研究院；RFA：射频消融；TRAP：双胎可逆动脉灌注。

予治疗。如胎儿肺部成熟，可提早娩出接受生后减压术。如胎儿肺部不成熟，可在超声引导下经皮置管行 Harrison 膀胱羊水分流术、胎儿镜下膀胱切开术或胎儿镜下尿道瓣膜消融术完成宫内膀胱减压[40,47]。许多医疗机构对数百例胎儿的经验性治疗表明，目前的选择标准能够很好地避免不恰当的干预，而且羊水重建术能预防胎儿肺发育不良的发生。迄今，尚不清楚减压术能在多大程度上逆转肾功能的损害。

囊性腺瘤样畸形

尽管先天性囊性腺瘤样畸形常表现为婴儿和儿童的良性肺部肿块，但一些有巨型组织损伤的胎儿会因水肿和肺发育不良在宫内或出生时死亡。已有动物实验研究水肿的病理生理学和胎儿切除术的可行性。200 多例经验性治疗提示，大多数损害在生后可被成功治愈，有些损害可在出生前解决。然而，只有一些存在巨型组织损伤的胎儿在 26 周胎龄前出现水肿，这样的损害可能进展迅速，造成胎死宫内。应该用超声检查密切监测巨型组织损伤，以及时发现水肿征兆，因为对出现这种情况的胎儿可在宫内行急诊囊性肺叶切除术而成功治愈[25]。在两个大型胎儿外科中心，已证实胎儿肺叶切除术是惊人的简单和相当成功[1]。胸腔羊水分流术也已成功用于治疗单个巨型囊肿[59]。经皮消融技术处于研究阶段。孕妇接受类固醇治疗对胎儿超巨型组织损伤缩小和水肿减轻的意义尚在观察中[56]。

先天膈疝

先天膈疝（CDH）已能在孕中期准确诊断出来，而且个体的预后可以通过测量肺 / 头比（LHR）和肝脏是否疝入胸腔来预测。在三级医疗中心足月分娩的无肝脏疝入和 LHR 较好（＞1.4）的胎儿死亡率低。尽管近年来新生儿重症监护技术不断发展，包括应用体外膜肺（ECMO）、一氧化氮吸入、高频通气和膈疝的延迟修复术，但是有肝脏疝入和 LHR 较低的胎儿的死亡率和发病率仍较高[4-6,8,23,41,50]。

CDH 婴儿的基本问题是肺发育不良。近 20 年来，实验动物模型和后来以人类为主体的研究目的是促进胎儿发育不良的肺的生长，改善产时的气体交换。已证实，经开放式子宫切开术行疝的解剖修复虽可行，但死亡率并不降低，已弃之不用[22,26]。胎儿气 84
管闭塞术可防止正常肺液外流而促进胎肺生长，是可供选择的治疗办法。在不同动物模型中，已显示胎儿气管闭塞术能刺激胎肺生长[9,13,46]。可逆的胎儿气管闭塞技术是先在动物模型中研究，然后应用于临床，气管闭塞已从经开放式子宫切开术或胎儿镜下颈部切开术将金属夹外置于气管上，发展到经一个 5mm 子宫开孔在胎儿气管镜下内置可分离的硅树脂气囊完成[3,7,27]。

最初的经验提示，胎儿内镜气管闭塞术能提高严重 CDH 人类胎儿的存活率[27,31,33]。为了评价这一新的治疗方法，我和我的同事进行了一项随机对照研究，比较气管闭塞组和标准监护组的差别[30]。胎儿内镜气管闭塞术的存活率达到期望值（实际值 73%；预测值 75%），优于历史对照组（37%），但不高于同期随机对照组。标准监护组存活率高于期望值的原因可能是因为：该研究设计要求两个治疗组的患者在一个对肺发育不良有经验的重症新生儿医疗单位中分娩、复苏和加强治疗[30]。

无论是产前还是产后，试图改善严重 CDH 预后的治疗都是一把双刃剑。产后重症监护可提高存活率，但也增加了存活者的长期后遗症，而且治疗费用昂贵[5,6,8,25,50]。产前干预可提高肺容量，但干预本身引起的早产是有害的[15,20,22,24,31]。在我们的研究中，产前接受气管闭塞术的严重 CDH胎儿术后平均出生胎龄为 31 周。他们的存活率和呼吸道预后（包括需要用氧的持续时间）与那些未在产前行气管闭塞、在 37 周分娩的婴儿相比结果显示，气管闭塞术可改善肺发育不良，但肺生长的情况受到与提早出生有关的肺不成熟的影响[30]。

这些结果突出了随机研究在评价新的、有前途的治疗方法方面的重要作用。这是国家卫生学会批准资助的第二项评价一个新的产前干预严重胎儿 CDH 方法的项目。第一项研究显示，对解剖缺陷的彻底外科修复（需要子宫切开术）尽管可行，但在提高存活率方面并不优于生后修补，且对治疗肝脏和肠段疝入一样无效[22]。这一研究导致我们单位放弃开放式彻底修复术，以后全世界都放弃了这一方法。来自该研究的有关肺发育不良严重度的测量信息（包括肝脏疝入和 LHR 的发展）引导出一个可供选择的生理学方法，即现代应用气管闭塞扩大发育不全的胎肺的方法[20,24,33]，并引导了发展减少侵入操作的胎儿内镜技术，现在无须子宫切开术就可完成可逆的气管闭塞术[3,17,27]。

我们准确诊断 CDH 和评价其严重度的能力取得了引人注目的提高。CDH 胎儿合并相关畸形者预后不良，而单纯 CDH、不合并肝疝入和 LHR＞1.4 的胎儿预后良好（我们的经验是存活率为 100%）。我们的研究显示，LHR 为 0.9～1.4 者在三级医疗机构娩出的存活率高于 80%。小部分 LHR 低于 0.9 的胎儿在两个治疗组的预后都很差，应在今后进行重点研究[30]。

由于气管闭塞术能有效扩大发育不全的肺，其他气管闭塞的方法也可能有益。虽然本研究的闭塞持续时间（36.2±14.7 天）可与动物模型的研究比拟，但人类闭塞的最佳时机和持续时间仍未知。在动物模型中已研究了妊娠后期的短期闭塞和早期闭塞（可能在宫内逆转）[13,46]，且已应用于人体[7]。采用经皮 2mm 的小型胎儿镜和新型密封胎膜的技术可能会减少由于胎膜早破引起的提早生产和分娩的风险。

脊髓脊膜膨出

脊髓脊膜膨出是一种破坏性的出生缺陷，对中枢和外周神经系统可产生不良影响。脑脊液动力学的变化可造成 Chiari Ⅱ 畸形和脑积水。暴露脊髓的损伤可导致终身下肢神经缺陷、尿失禁、性功能障碍和骨骼异常。这种缺陷会带来许多个人、家庭和社会支出，这是由于受累儿童有接近正常的生命周期，却表现为要住院治疗、进行多次手术、残疾和被送进专门机构。有人推测，有此缺陷的小儿的脊髓本身有畸形，但近期研究提示，生后神经损伤是宫内脊髓暴露和创伤引起的，而且覆盖住暴露的脊索可预防 Chiari 畸形的发展[10,49,58]。

从 1997 年起，接受宫内脊髓脊膜突出关闭术的开放式胎儿手术的胎儿已超过 200 名。初步的临床证据提示此操作可减少由于分流导致的脑水肿的发生率，并重建小脑和脑干，使之更接近正常结构[58]。但脊髓脊膜膨出胎儿手术的临床效果是基于与历史对照组的比较得出的；只探究有效性，没观察安全性；而且缺乏长期随访。

国家卫生学院资助了一项涉及 200 名患者的多中心、随机临床试验（脊髓脊膜膨出治疗的研究，MOMS），在三个胎儿外科中心——加州大学旧金山分校、费城儿童医院和 Vanderbilt 大学医学中心进行；乔治·华盛顿生物统计中心是独立资料和研究合作中心。这项随机试验的首要目的是确定：（1）在 85
胎龄 19～26 周进行的标准多层关闭脊髓脊膜膨出的宫内修补术是否能改善预后，通过计算死亡率或观察 1 岁内是否需要施行脑室减压术的情况，并与标准产后监护组比较来判断预后；（2）脊髓脊膜膨出的宫内修补术是否能提高认知功能，在 30 个修正的月龄时通过 Bayley 婴儿发育量表测量智力发育指数来判断认知功能。在结果公布之前，试验以外的这种手术方法将暂停进行。

气道梗阻

胎儿 CDH 的气管闭塞方法先要发展用于产时安全逆转气道梗阻的技术。产时宫外治疗（EXIT）操作是一项遵循胎儿手术原理的技术（孕妇和胎儿的麻醉、彻底的子宫松弛和维持脐循环以保证胎儿生命支持），在剖宫产术分娩时进行，使胎儿尚在母体旁路中时即开放气道。EXIT 操作已被成功用于逆转气管闭塞、气管修补、行气管切开术开放气道、切除巨大颈部肿瘤、放置血管套管以应用 ECMO 行即刻体外生命支持以及治疗先天性高气道阻塞综合征的喉部梗阻[1,35,36]。

EXIT 操作为外科医生、围生期医生、新生儿科医生和麻醉师提供了一个学会一起工作的绝佳机会，是应该在新建立的胎儿治疗中心首先进行的操作项目之一。

骶尾部畸胎瘤

大多数患有骶尾部畸胎瘤的新生儿都能存活，而且恶性侵入性病变并不常见。但是产前诊断出骶尾部畸胎瘤（超声检查或甲胎蛋白升高）的患者预后很少令人满意。患巨大肿瘤的胎儿中有一亚类（＜20%）可出现水肿，是继发于来自肿瘤的高血流引起的高输出衰竭。由于快速进展的水肿可致死，因此必须进行频繁的超声检查随访。肿瘤切除术如在孕妇镜像综合征（母亲子痫）发生之前进行，就能逆转其病理生理改变[28,34]。通过注射酒精或形成栓塞去除肿瘤的血流供应阻断血管盗血的尝试尚未成功。超声引导下的血管蒂射频消融术已证实有效，但对邻近结构可造成无法接受的损害。

双胎输血综合征

双胎输血综合征（TTTS）是单绒毛膜多胎或一卵双胎妊娠经血管交通引起血流不平衡的并发症，即双胎中的一个血供缺乏，而另一个血供增多。它是单绒毛膜双胎妊娠最常见的严重并发症，此类妊娠的发生率为 4%～35%，在美国每年发病率大约为 0.1‰～0.9‰。虽然 TTTS 发病率相对较低，但可造成双胎妊娠相关的围生期死亡率高达 17%，与其发病率不成比例。标准疗法尚局限于连续羊膜复位术，此方法虽然能改善总体预后，但对于较严重的 TTTS，终末效果不大。此外，连续羊膜复位术后 TTTS 存活者中有 18%～26%合并明显的神经系统和心血管系统后遗症。一卵双胎妊娠时，选择性胎儿镜激光凝固术已可作为一种备选方案，欧洲的一项随机试验显示，其即使不是更好，也与连续羊膜复位术相当[12,53]。

双胎可逆动脉灌注综合征

无心双胎是一种罕见的畸形，即双胎中的一胎能正常“泵”血，负责灌注另一个无心畸胎，形成可逆动脉灌注综合征。在单绒毛膜的无心双胎中，形态学正常的泵血胎儿的生长发育也会受到不良影响。现在有许多可用于完成无心双胎的选择性血流减少或血管闭塞的方法，包括无心胎儿切除术；脐带结扎、分离和烧灼术；以及采用酒精注射、电烙术或射频消融术进行畸形双胎的循环闭塞[12,45]。我和我的同事应用 14–或 17–标准计量厚度的探针在实时超声引导下进行了微创、经皮射频消融术，有效地阻断了无心畸胎的血供，并保护了泵血胎儿[55]。我们已有超过 30例的操作经验，结果极好。

中脑导水管硬化

该病是脑脊液循环受阻使脑室扩大压迫发育中的脑组织并最终损害神经系统功能。对于伴有宫内病情进展的严重病例，脑室减压能缓解压迫对发育脑的不良影响；而经皮置管行脑室羊膜分流术不能改善预后[47]。因此在阐明自然病程、明确入选标准和更好的胎儿分流技术尚未得到之前，需延缓治疗，密切关注[37]。

主动脉闭锁和心发育不全

一些简单的、影响发育的心脏结构畸形可于产前纠正而获益。如果经肺动脉或主动脉瓣膜的血流阻塞影响心室或肺部或全身脉管系统的发育，解除这些解剖梗阻可使发育正常，并改善预后[48]。例如，先天性主动脉瓣狭窄会导致左心发育不全综合征。狭窄的主 86
动脉瓣已可经皮或孕妇接受剖腹手术经子宫置入一个球囊导管进行扩张[42,57]。此法具有应用前景，但操作技术难度高。一些中心正进行纠正胎儿心脏缺陷技术的实验室研究。

腹裂

出生时有腹裂的患儿应在生后立即接受一期或分期腹壁闭合术。尽管腹壁缺损闭合会使许多婴儿面临长时间的营养素吸收和肠道活动障碍。这些患儿出生时常出现肠道增厚，表面覆有一层纤维素“皮”。肠系膜缩短和肠闭锁也可见。肠损伤可能是由于肠系膜收缩（像一个套餐巾用的小环）造成的，后者可造成肠淋巴回流和静脉引流不畅，或是肠浸泡时对羊水中的多种物质产生的炎症反应[54]。

连续羊水置换术已用于稀释假定的炎症介质，以试图预防肠损伤[60]。但是，挑选出有肠损伤胎儿的能力有限，而且置换量可能不足以改变预后。

唇腭裂

由于观察到胎儿创伤修复可无瘢痕形成，这激发了研究者对宫内纠正唇腭裂以避免瘢痕、面中线部位生长迟缓和继发鼻畸形的可能性的兴趣。但是，这类修补术的有效性及干预风险尚未得到证实[44]。

胎儿干细胞移植可纠正的遗传缺陷

有可能经造血干细胞（HSC）移植治愈的多种遗传缺陷（如免疫缺陷、血红蛋白病、贮积病）现已能在妊娠期尽早发现。生后骨髓移植受到供体来源、移植物排异反应、移植物抗宿主病以及移植前病情恶化（常自宫内起）的限制。妊娠早期胎儿 HSC 移植可防止这些难题的发生[14,32,51]。

宫内移植优于生后移植的基本原理是：免疫前的胎儿（<15 周）不应排斥植入的细胞，而且胎儿骨髓主要接受来自胎儿肝脏移行来的 HSC。因而，无需进行骨髓去除和免疫抑制。此外，宫内移植可使胎儿在健康受到潜在疾病损伤之前获得治疗。宫内治疗的缺点是：很难对胎儿做出诊断和治疗评估。运用分子基因技术确诊需要经阴道或经腹部绒毛膜绒毛采样、羊膜穿刺或胎儿血样采样来获得胎儿组织。经腹内或静脉注射递送哪怕少量细胞（<1ml）进入妊娠早期的胎儿体内都是需要技巧的，而且会带来重大危险。宫内 HSC 移植潜在的最大问题是移入物等级或嵌合程度不足以治愈或缓解某些疾病。对于慢性肉芽肿病和严重联合免疫缺陷，较少的正常供体细胞即能提供足够的酶活性以缓解症状。对于改变一些疾病的病程，外周供体细胞移入物等级和表达水平较高是必要的，如对 β-地中海贫血或镰状细胞病。对于需要较高比例供体细胞的疾病，目前有希望的策略是：在宫内诱导耐受性，以便出生后注射来自亲属的移植物。用于宫内移植的供体 HSC 的最佳来源还不太清楚。供体细胞可以从成人骨髓或外周血、新生儿脐带血或流产胎儿的肝脏中获得。

胎儿 HSC 移植的临床经验有限。尽管对严重联合免疫缺陷综合征的移植获得成功，但在其他多数疾病中，注射后的移入物等级较低限制了其临床疗效[14,16,32,51]。

胎儿干预的过去和未来

虽然目前只有一些胎儿缺陷可接受手术治疗，但随着胎儿手术的进展，意外地产生了一些有用的附带物，引发了超越这一狭窄治疗领域的研究兴趣。对于儿科医生、新生儿科医生和畸形学家来说，对宫内疾病发生发展的追踪随访阐明了许多以前认为很神秘的新生儿病情的自然病程和病理生理。对于产科医生、围生期医生和胎儿学家来说，羊和猴的动物实验中的技术发展将被证实可有效地应用于治疗高危妊娠。例如，一个发展用于胎儿手术的可被吸收的 U 形钉装置已在剖宫产中应用，无线电遥测装置也被用于胎儿手术以外的领域，经视频内镜可完成以前需行子宫切开的胎儿操作。这些技术将大大扩展胎儿干预的适应证。最后，在着重解决胎儿手术中子宫切开术后恼人的早产问题的过程中，产生了氧化亚氮对子宫肌层收缩作用的新视点以及氧化亚氮治疗自发早产的研究兴趣。

胎儿外科研究带动了胎儿生物学的发展，其意义超过胎儿治疗学。偶然发现的胎儿切口愈合不留瘢痕引发了新的创伤愈合的生物学研究，并激发了出生后模仿胎儿愈合过程的努力。胎儿组织似乎从生物学和免疫学上都存在移植和基因治疗的优势，而且胎儿的 87
免疫耐受性使许多非外科遗传疾病可经胎儿 HSC 移植获得治愈。

胎儿治疗的最大好处是：对一些疾病，尽可能早地干预（出生前）可能产生最好的结果（一定资源消费下获得最佳生命质量）。但是，由于成本效果的约束，预防性胎儿治疗有可能被失去引导的临床应用所破坏，例如一个仅能部分挽救一个患有致死性疾病的胎儿的复杂宫内操作，其后患儿将在重症监护室（并且是昂贵的）中度生。对胎儿干预的兴趣还应与孕妇及其家庭的意愿相结合，应首先在实验胎儿动物模型中和未经治疗的胎儿中仔细研究疾病，并且在适当的对照研究中未能证明有效和成本效果的治疗方法应当放弃。

（李　菁译　黄　萍校）

参考文献

1. Adzick NS: Management of fetal lung lesions. Clin Perinatol 2003;30:481-492.
2. Adzick NS, Harrison MR, Glick PL, et al: Fetal surgery in the primate. III. Maternal outcome after fetal surgery. J Pediatr Surg 1986;21:477-480.
3. Albanese CT, Jennings RW, Filly RA, et al: Endoscopic fetal tracheal occlusion: Evolution of techniques. Pediatr Endosurg Innov Techn 1998;2:47-53.
4. Albanese CT, Lopoo J, Goldstein RB, et al: Fetal liver position and perinatal outcome for congenital diaphragmatic hernia. Prenat Diagn 1998;18:1138-1142.
5. Boloker J, Bateman DA, Wung JT, Stolar CJ: Congenital diaphragmatic hernia in 120 infants treated consecutively with permissive hypercapnea/spontaneous respiration/elective repair. J Pediatr Surg 2002;37:357-366.
6. Congenital Diaphragmatic Hernia Study Group: Does extracorporeal membrane oxygenation improve survival in neonates with congenital diaphragmatic hernia? J Pediatr Surg 1999;34:720-724.
7. Deprest J, Gratacos E, Nicolaides KH, FETO Task Group: Fetoscopic tracheal occlusion (FETO) for severe congenital diaphragmatic hernia: Evolution of a technique and preliminary results. Ultrasound Obstet Gynecol 2004;24:121-126.
8. Desfrere L, Jarreau PH, Dommergues M, et al: Impact of delayed repair and elective high-frequency oscillatory ventilation on survival of antenatally diagnosed congenital diaphragmatic hernia: First application of these strategies in the more "severe" subgroup of antenatally diagnosed newborns. Intensive Care Med 2000;26:934-941.
9. DiFiore JW, Fauza DO, Slavin R, et al: Experimental fetal tracheal ligation reverses the structural and physiologic effects of pulmonary hypoplasia in congenital diaphragmatic hernia. J Pediatr Surg 1994;29:248-256.
10. Farmer DL, von Koch CS, Peacock WJ, et al: In utero repair of myelomeningocele: Experimental pathophysiology, initial clinical experience, and outcomes. Arch Surg 2003;138:872-878.
11. Farrell JA, Albanese CT, Jennings RW, et al: Maternal fertility is not affected by fetal surgery. Fetal Diagn Ther 1999;14:190-192.
12. Feldstein VA, Machin GA, Albanese CT, et al: Twin-twin transfusion syndrome: The "select" procedure. Fetal Diagn Ther 2000;15:257-261.
13. Flageole H, Evrard VA, Piedboeuf B, et al: The plug-unplug sequence: An important step to achieve type II pneumocyte maturation in the fetal lamb model. J Pediatr Surg 1998;33:299-303.
14. Flake AW: Stem cell and genetic therapies for the fetus. Semin Pediatr Surg 2003;12:202-208.
15. Flake AW, Crombleholme TM, Johnson MP, et al: Treatment of severe congenital diaphragmatic hernia by fetal tracheal occlusion: Clinical experience with fifteen cases. Am J Obstet Gynecol 2000;183:1059-1066.
16. Flake AW, Harrison MR, Adzick NS, Zanjani ED: Transplantation of fetal hematopoietic stem cells in utero: The creation of hematopoietic chimeras. Science 1986;233:776-778.
17. Fowler SF, Sydorak RM, Albanese CT, et al: Fetal endoscopic surgery: Lessons learned and trends reviewed. J Pediatr Surg 2002;37:1700-1702.
18. Harrison MR: Unborn: Historical perspective of the fetus as a patient. Pharos 1982;45:19-24.
19. Harrison MR: Fetal surgery. Am J Obstet Gynecol 1996;174:1255-1264.
20. Harrison MR: Fetal surgery: Trials, tribulations, and turf. J Pediatr Surg 2003;38:275-282.
21. Harrison MR: The University of California at San Francisco Fetal Treatment Center: A personal perspective. Fetal Diagn Ther 2004;19:513-524.
22. Harrison MR, Adzick NS, Bullard KM, et al: Correction of congenital diaphragmatic hernia in utero. VII. A prospective trial. J Pediatr Surg 1997;32:1637-1642.
23. Harrison MR, Adzick NS, Estes JM, Howell LJ: A prospective study of the outcome of fetuses with congenital diaphragmatic hernia. JAMA 1994;271:382-384.
24. Harrison MR, Adzick NS, Flake AW, et al: Correction of congenital diaphragmatic hernia in utero. VIII. Response of the hypoplastic lung to tracheal occlusion. J Pediatr Surg 1996;31:1339-1348.
25. Harrison MR, Adzick NS, Jennings RW, et al: Antenatal intervention for congenital cystic adenomatoid malformation. Lancet 1990;336:965-967.
26. Harrison MR, Adzick NS, Longaker MT, et al: Successful repair in utero of a fetal diaphragmatic hernia after removal of herniated viscera from the left thorax. N Engl J Med 1990;322:1582-1584.
27. Harrison MR, Albanese CT, Hawgood S, et al: Fetoscopic temporary tracheal occlusion by means of detachable balloon for congenital diaphragmatic hernia. Am J Obstet Gynecol 2000;185:730-733.
28. Harrison MR, Evans MI, Adzick NS, Holzgreve W (eds): The Unborn Patient: The Art and Science of Fetal Therapy, 3rd ed. Philadelphia, WB Saunders, 2001, pp 297-314.
29. Harrison MR, Golbus MS, Filly RA: Management of the fetus with a correctable congenital defect. JAMA 1981;246:774-777.
30. Harrison MR, Keller RL, Hawgood SB, et al: A randomized trial of fetal endoscopic tracheal occlusion for severe fetal congenital diaphragmatic hernia. N Engl J Med 2003;349:1916-1924.
31. Harrison MR, Mychaliska GB, Albanese CT, et al: Correction of congenital diaphragmatic hernia in utero. IX. Fetuses with poor prognosis (liver herniation and low lung-to-head ratio) can be saved by fetoscopic temporary tracheal occlusion. J Pediatr Surg 1998;33:1017-1022.
32. Harrison MR, Slotnick RN, Crombleholme TM, et al: In utero transplantation of fetal liver haematopoietic stem cells in monkeys. Lancet 1989;2:1425-1427.
33. Harrison MR, Sydorak RM, Farrell JA, et al: Fetoscopic temporary tracheal occlusion for congenital diaphragmatic hernia: Prelude to a randomized controlled trial. J Pediatr Surg 2003;38:1012-1026.
34. Hedrick HL, Flake AW, Crombleholme TM, et al: Sacrococcygeal teratoma: Prenatal assessment, fetal intervention, and outcome. J Pediatr Surg 2004;39:430-438.
35. Hedrick MH, Ferro MM, Filly RA, et al: Congenital high airway obstruction (CHAOS): A potential for perinatal intervention. J Pediatr Surg 1994;29:271-274.
36. Hirose S, Farmer DL, Lee H, et al: The ex utero intrapartum treatment procedure: Looking back at the EXIT. J Pediatr Surg 2004;39:375-380.
37. Hudgins RJ, Edwards MS, Goldstein R, et al: Natural history of fetal ventriculomegaly. Pediatrics 1988;82:692-697.
38. Jennings RW, MacGillivray TE, Harrison MR: Nitric oxide inhibits preterm labor in the rhesus monkey. J Matern Fetal Med 1993;2:170.
39. Johnson MP, Bukowski TP, Reitleman C, et al: In utero surgical treatment of fetal obstructive uropathy: A new comprehensive approach to identify appropriate candidates for vesicoamniotic shunt therapy. Am J Obstet Gynecol 1994;170:1770-1776.

40. Johnson MP, Sutton LN, Rintoul N, et al: Fetal myelomeningocele repair: Short-term clinical outcomes. Am J Obstet Gynecol 2003;189:482-487.
41. Keller RL, Glidden DV, Paek BW, et al: Lung-to-head ratio and fetoscopic temporary tracheal occlusion: Prediction of survival in severe left congenital diaphragmatic hernia. Am J Obstet Gynecol 2003;21:244-249.
42. Kohl T, Sharland G, Allan LD, et al: World experience of percutaneous ultrasound-guided balloon valvuloplasty in human fetuses with severe aortic valve obstruction. Am J Cardiol 2000;85:1230-1233.
43. Longaker MT, Golbus MS, Filly RA, et al: Maternal outcome after open fetal surgery: A review of the first 17 human cases. JAMA 1991;265:737-741.
44. Longaker MT, Whitby DJ, Adzick NS, et al: Fetal surgery for cleft lip: A plea for caution. Plast Reconstr Surg 1991;88:1087-1092.
45. Lopoo JB, Paek BW, Machin GA, et al: Cord ultrasonic transection procedure for selective termination of a monochorionic twin. Fetal Diagn Ther 2000;15:177-179.
46. Luks FI, Wild YK, Piasecki GJ, De Paepe ME: Short-term tracheal occlusion corrects pulmonary vascular anomalies in the fetal lamb with diaphragmatic hernia. Surgery 2000;128:266-272.
47. Manning FA, Harrison MR, Rodeck C: Catheter shunts for fetal hydronephrosis and hydrocephalus: Report of the International Fetal Surgery Registry. N Engl J Med 1986;315:336-346.
48. Marshall AC, van der Velde ME, Tworetzky W, et al: Creation of an atrial septal defect in utero for fetuses with hypoplastic left heart syndrome and intact or highly restrictive atrial septum. Circulation (online), June 28, 2004.
49. Meuli M, Meuli-Simmen C, Hutchins GM, et al: In utero surgery rescues neurologic function at birth in sheep with spina bifida. Nat Med 1995;1:342-347.
50. Muratore CS, Kharasch V, Lund DP, et al: Pulmonary morbidity in 100 survivors of congenital diaphragmatic hernia monitored in a multidisciplinary clinic. J Pediatr Surg 2001;36:133-140.
51. Peranteau WH, Hayashi S, Kim HB, et al: In utero hematopoietic cell transplantation: What are the important questions? Fetal Diagn Ther 2004;19:9-12.
52. Rychik J, Tian Z, Cohen MS, et al: Acute cardiovascular effects of fetal surgery in the human. Circulation 2004;110:1549-1556.
53. Senat MV, Deprest J, Boulvain M, et al: Endoscopic laser surgery versus serial amnioreduction for severe twin-to-twin transfusion syndrome. N Engl J Med 2004;351:136-144.
54. Sydorak RM, Nijagal A, Sbragia L, et al: Gastroschisis: Small hole, big cost. J Pediatr Surg 2002;37:1669-1672.
55. Tsao K, Feldstein VA, Albanese CT, et al: Selective reduction of acardiac twin by radiofrequency ablation. Am J Obstet Gynecol 2002;187:635-640.
56. Tsao K, Hawgood S, Vu L, et al: Resolution of hydrops fetalis in congenital cystic adenomatoid malformation after prenatal steroid therapy. J Pediatr Surg 2003;38:508-510.
57. Tworetzky W, Marshall AC: Balloon valvuloplasty for congenital heart disease in the fetus. Clin Perinatol 2003;30:541-550.
58. Walsh DS, Adzick NS: Foetal surgery for spina bifida. Semin Neonatol 2003;8:197-205.
59. Wilson RD, Baxter JK, Johnson MP, et al: Thoracoamniotic shunts: Fetal treatment of pleural effusions and congenital cystic adenomatoid malformations. Fetal Diagn Ther 2004;19:4113-4120.
60. Wilson RD, Johnson MP: Congenital abdominal wall defects: An update. Fetal Diagn Ther 2004;19:385-398.

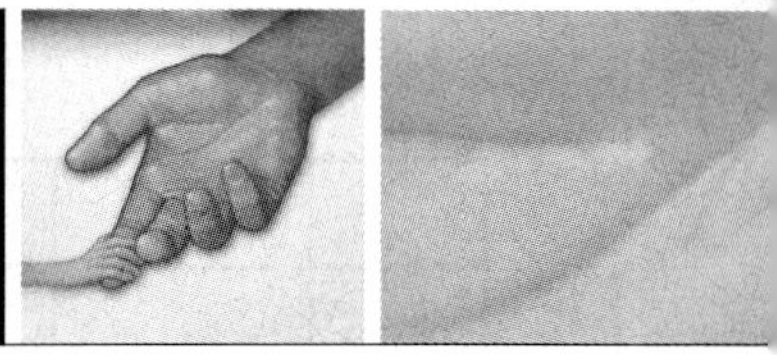

第 6 章

新生儿生理学和代谢问题

Agostino Pierro、Simon Eaton 和 Evelyn Ong

89 新生儿重症监护和外科技术的显著发展提高了患有先天性或获得性畸形新生儿的成活率。与此契合的是，我们在婴儿生理学和他们对饥饿、麻醉、手术应激和全身炎症的代谢反应方面的理解也有进步。新生儿不仅是小型成人，他们的生理学，包括体温调节、液体和热卡需要，可与成人迥异，尤其是早产或发育迟缓的新生儿。本章着重讲述经历手术后新生儿的生理和代谢情况，特别强调早产儿的特征。我们在此讨论液体和电解质平衡、新生儿能量代谢和体温调节以及糖类、脂肪和蛋白质的代谢。此外，我们还讨论当前有关新生儿手术创伤和败血症的反应的认识，这是引起新生儿生理改变的两个主要原因。

早产、小于胎龄和宫内发育迟缓的新生儿

胎儿期的生长速率最快。事实上，从一个受精细胞发育为一个 3.5kg 的新生儿其过程包含身长增加 5000 倍，体表面积增加 61×10^6 和体重增加 6×10^{12}。出生后生长速率最快的时期是在出生后不久。而新生儿病危或手术后一段时期出现生长缓慢或停止并不罕见。

依照胎龄可将新生儿分为早产儿、足月儿或过度成熟儿。孕 37 周之前出生的婴儿为早产儿，37～42 周出生的婴儿为足月儿，42 周之后出生的为过期产儿。以前，出生体重低于 2500g 的婴儿均称为早产儿。现在认为这一定义是不恰当的，因为许多出生体重低于 2500g 的新生儿是足月儿或过度成熟儿，为小于胎龄儿；他们的外表和存在的临床问题与早产儿不同。胎龄评估可在出生前进行，也可在出生后头几天内应用巴拉德评分法（图 6–1）进行。通过绘制体重–胎龄标准曲线图（图 6–2），可将新生婴儿分为小于、适于或大于胎龄儿。对照不同胎龄绘制的头围和身长标准曲线图也用于评估宫内发育（图 6–3）。出生体重低于同胎龄新生儿第 10 百分位者称为小于胎龄儿。出生体重高于同胎龄新生儿第 90 百分位者称为大于胎龄儿（见图 6–2）。大体上，早产儿体重低于 2500g，头顶–足跟长度小于 47 厘米，头围小于 33 厘米，以及胸围小于 30 厘米。由于早产婴儿的诸多器官功能和解剖不成熟，而存在生理障碍：体温难以维持、呼吸困难常见、肾功能不成熟、抗感染能力不足、结合和排泄胆红素功能受损，同时出血倾向较多见。

根据出生体重可将早产婴儿分组如下：

1. 低出生体重（1501～2500g）。该组占所有早产儿的 82%。其死亡率是足月儿的 40 倍。
2. 极低出生体重（1001～1500g）。该组占所有早产儿的 12%。其死亡率是足月儿的 200 倍。
3. 超低出生体重（≤1000g）。该组占所有早产儿的 6%，但新生儿死亡率极高。其死亡率是足月儿的 600 倍。

在医学文献中，宫内发育迟缓（IUGR）的定义常混淆不清。IUGR 通常是指经胎儿超声检查发现宫内生长减慢者。IUGR 可以是一过性的，新生儿出生时仍可为正常大小。IUGR 分为两种类型：匀称型和非匀称型。匀称型 IUGR 是指体型正常（小头和小身
体），但为临床问题较严重的 IUGR 类型[165]。非匀称 90
型 IUGR 是指腹围较小、皮下和腹部脂肪减少、骨骼肌质量缩小以及头围正常者。尽管 10%～30%的 IUGR 婴儿在儿童和成人期仍然生长落后，但非匀称型 IUGR 婴儿的生长追赶比匀称型 IUGR 者常见。早产儿预期在 2 岁时完成生长追赶。胎龄 29 周后出生者

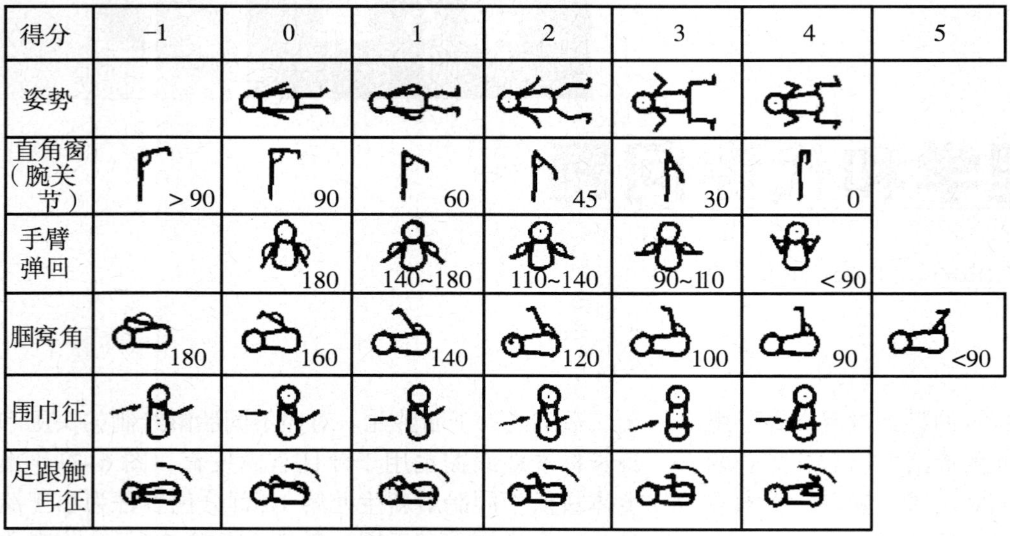

身体成熟度

皮肤	胶胨状易破，透明	凝胶状，红色，半透明	光滑，粉红色，可见静脉	表皮脱屑和(或)见皮疹，少量的静脉影	皮肤裂缝，苍白区域；稀疏静脉影	羊皮纸样，皮肤深裂缝；无血管影	皮革样强韧，有皮肤裂缝，起皱
毳毛	无	稀疏	丰富	细毛状	有无毛区域	大部分区域无毛	
跖纹	足跟至足趾长度40~50mm：-1 <40mm：-2	>50mm，无足纹	模糊的红色足痕	仅见前部横向足纹	前部2/3可见足纹	整个足底可见足纹	
乳腺	难以观察到	几乎看不见	乳晕平坦，没有突起	斑点状乳晕，1~2mm突起	乳晕高起，3~4mm突起	乳晕丰满，5~10mm突起	
眼睛/耳朵	眼睑并合松弛：-1轻易分开：-2	眼睑睁开；耳廓垂下；不能弹回	耳廓微成形；软；慢慢弹回	耳廓成形；软，但能迅速弹回	成形并直立，瞬间弹回	软骨丰富，耳朵坚挺	
生殖器（男性）	阴囊平坦，光滑	阴囊空虚，皱褶模糊	睾丸居上未降，皱褶稀疏	睾丸下降，可见少量皱褶	睾丸已降，较多皱褶	悬垂状睾丸，较深皱褶	
生殖器（女性）	阴蒂明显凸起，阴唇平坦	阴蒂明显凸起，小阴唇较小	阴蒂明显凸起，小阴唇扩大	大阴唇和小阴唇都较明显	大阴唇较大，小阴唇较小	大阴唇遮盖阴蒂和小阴唇	

成熟度等级评定

得分	孕周
-10	20
-5	22
0	24
5	26
10	28
15	30
20	32
25	34
30	36
35	38
40	40
45	42
50	44

图 6-1 Ballard 胎龄评分。(From Ballard JL, Khoury JC, Wedig K, et al: New Ballard score, expanded to include extremely premature infants. J Pediatr 1991;119:417-423.)

通常出现生长追赶，而胎龄 29 周前出生者常在生后头 1 周至 2 年内出现身长和体重增加速度减慢[32,66,68]。

新生儿预期死亡率

引起新生儿死亡的因素很多。最常见的原因见表 6-1。总体而言，过去 10 年来新生儿的死亡率有所下降（图 6-4）[48]。出生体重和胎龄是死亡率的强项指标。胎龄 22 周、出生体重 500g 的新生儿存活率大约为 0%。随着胎龄增长，新生儿存活率逐渐提高，胎龄 23 周者存活率约为 15%，胎龄 24 周者存活率约为 56%，胎龄 25 周者存活率约位 79%。预期死亡率的评分系统对于新生儿外科医生制订治疗计划、家长咨询服务和各医疗中心比较预后非常有用。这些新生儿评分系统虽然可用，但不适用于需要外科手术的解剖异常者。评分系统可基于生理学异常，如低血压或高血压、酸中毒、低氧血症、高碳酸血症、贫血和中性粒细胞减少症（新生儿急性生理学状况评分，SNAP），或基于临床参数，如胎龄、出生体重、畸形、酸中毒和吸入氧浓度（婴儿临床危险指数，

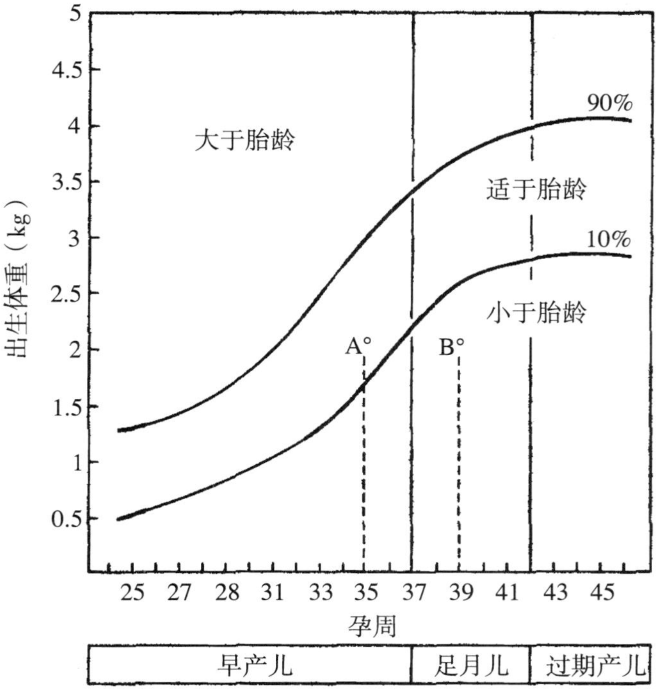

图 6-2 依据活产单胎白种婴儿的出生体重和胎龄评估宫内生长水平。（From Disturbances in newborns and infants. In Beers MF, Berkow R [eds]: The Merck Manual of Diagnosis and Therapy, 17th ed. White House Station, NJ, Merck Research Laboratories, 1999, pp 2127-2145.）

91 CRIB）[4,141]。CRIB 包括 6 个参数，要求在生后 12 小时内采集；SNAP 包括 26 个参数，要求在生后 24 小时内采集；每个评分系统都有不同的修订本[63]。我们最近应用的是修订的器官衰竭评分（见表 6-2），它来源于成人和儿童的脓毒血症相关的器官衰竭评估（SOFA），可用于监测有手术指征的新生儿急腹症患儿的临床情况。将外科医生的判断和目标评分情况结合起来可以对重症新生儿的临床进展做出准确的评估，并估计其死亡危险性。

表 6-1 外科疾病新生儿的主要死因

早产新生儿	足月新生儿
坏死性小肠结肠炎	先天畸形
先天畸形	感染
重度脏器不成熟	持续性肺动脉高压
呼吸窘迫综合征	胎粪吸入
脑室内出血	产时窒息，产伤
感染	
支气管肺发育不良	

电解质和液体平衡

体液成分

体液总量（TBW）分为两部分：细胞内和细胞外。妊娠第一个 3 个月时，胎儿 TBW 约为体重的 90%；细胞外液占体重的 65%，细胞内液占体重的

图 6-3 依据胎龄、出生时的身长（A）和头围（B）评估宫内生长。

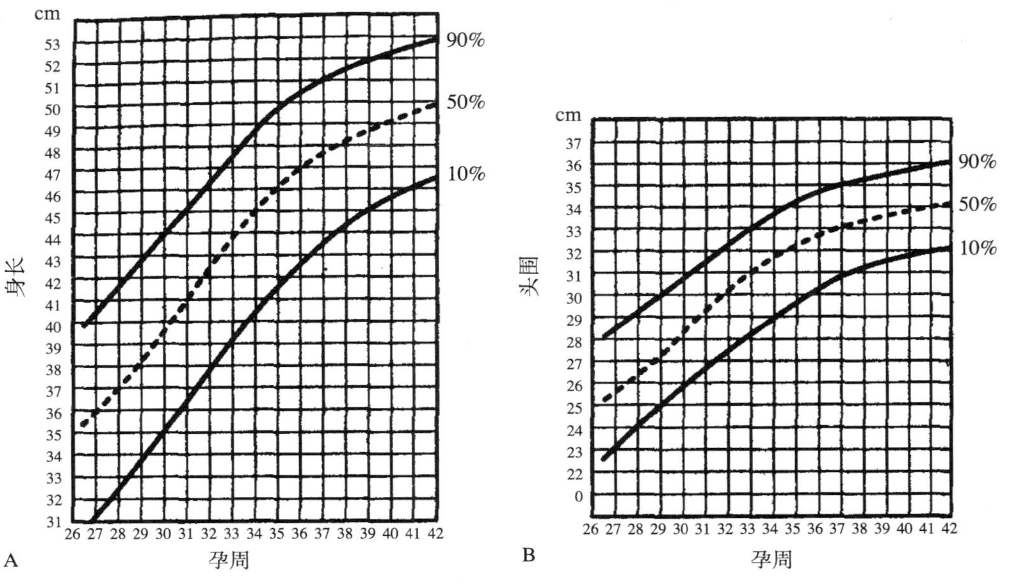

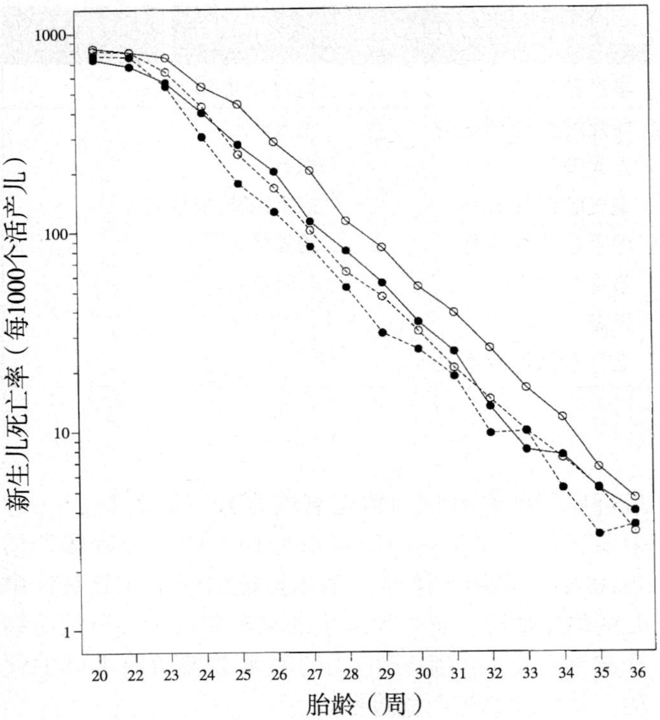

图 6-4 美国不同胎龄新生儿的死亡率，（●）代表黑人，（○）代表白人。实线表示 1989 年的资料，虚线表示1997 年的资料。以上资料只包括 37 周胎龄以下的新生儿。(From Demissie K, Rhoads GG, Ananth CV, et al: Trends in preterm birth and neonatal mortality among blacks and whites in the United States from 1989 to 1997. Am J Epidemiol 2001;154: 307-315.)

25%[61]。脂肪只占体重的 1%。但在整个妊娠期内，随着体内蛋白质和脂肪的增加，体内水分的百分比不断变化。在胎龄 32 周时，TBW 降至 80%，近足月时约为 68%～75% [60]。3 月龄时，TBW 占总体重的 60%，并随着细胞外液（ECF）与细胞内液（ICF）的比值下降。在胎龄 20 周时，ECF 占总体
92 重的 60%，足月时降至 40%，而 ICF 在胎龄 20 周时占总体重的 25%，足月时升至 35%，在 2 月龄时为 43%。此后，ECF 和 ICF 与体重的关系都随时间的推移而减少。早产小于胎龄儿的体液比例（约 90%）比适于胎龄儿的（约 84%）明显增高[78]。

除了在成人中所见的体液分布外，胎儿的肺内也明显含有液体。胎儿的肺部液体是由分泌入肺泡腔的氯化物组成的。肺部液体是积聚在气管中并可从气管中流出，其与羊水液囊是相通的，占羊水总量的 1/3[108]，或可被吞咽。肺部液体一直增加直至胎龄 36周，至足月时达到高峰[67,92,99]。肺泡液和血液循环间的液体交换量尚不明确。胃在胎儿期也可作为一个大型的体液储存池。以前认为每天被吞咽的羊水量约为 200～1500ml；现在认为每天被吞咽的羊水量等于胎儿总体重的 20%～25%[22,155]。这些羊膜囊内的液体通路如图 6-5 所示。

新年儿体液转移

新生儿的液体平衡代表其稳态机制对新生儿围生期的环境和循环的明显改变的适应（图 6-5）。

围生期

产前，肺内液体产生减少，而现存液体被重吸收。产程中，气管中的水分溢出增加并不断加速，因此肺部脱水；动脉压可升高并造成水分从血管腔隙移入血浆中及轻度的血细胞比容升高。如果脐带结扎延迟和新生儿位置等于或低于胎盘位置，则会发生胎盘输血，引起红细胞和血容量增加 50%。红细胞增多症可造成严重后果，如神经系统损害、血栓形成和局部组织缺血[146]。 93

出生后

产后第 1 天时，新生儿出现少尿。度过接下来的 1～2 天后，液体明显从细胞内向细胞外转移可引起多尿和尿钠增多；这是造成约 5%～10%的足月儿和 10% ～20%的早产儿在生后第 1 周出现体重减轻的原因。从 ECF 和 ICF 中丧失的液体比例尚有争议，其机制不明。这一多尿现象与液体入量或不显性失水无关，可能与生后心钠素的波动有关[116]。测量 ECF 和 ICF 的方法有限，因而限制了我们对此过程的理解。已证实，大量增加水和热卡的摄入是减轻体重损失的必需条件。仅高热卡摄取可使减轻体重损失，但 ECF 仍降低。以后的体重增加是组织质量和每公斤体重 ICF 增加的结果，而不是每公斤体重 ECF 增加的结果。生后第 5 天以后，尿排量才开始反映婴儿的体液状态。

表 6–2 修改版器官衰竭评分表

器官系统	得分 * 0	1	2	3	4
呼吸系统（PaO_2/FiO_2 比值）	＞400	≤400	≤300	≤200，并应用呼吸支持	≤100，并应用呼吸支持
肾脏（排尿量）			每小时＜1ml/kg，持续 6 小时	每小时＜0.5 ml/kg，持续 6 小时	无尿
肝脏［血清胆红素 μmol/L（mg/ml）］		20～32（1.17～1.9）	33～101（2.0～5.9）	102～204（6.0～12.0）	＞204（＞12.0）
心血管系统（低血压）	无低血压	MAP（mm Hg）＜胎龄＋年龄（周）	需多巴胺每分钟＜5.0 μg/kg，或任何剂量的多	需多巴胺每分钟＞5.0 μg/kg，肾上腺素每分钟＜0.1μg/kg，或去甲肾上腺素每分钟＜0.1μg/kg	需多巴胺每分钟＞15.0μg/kg，肾上腺素每分钟＞0.1μg/kg，或去甲肾上腺素每分钟＞0.1μg/kg
凝血功能（血小板计数）	＞150	≤150	≤100	≤50	≤20 或需输注血小板

* 计算累计得分，记录每次评分间期的每一项参数的最差得分。

MAP：即平均动脉压。

From reference 12、118、179、180.

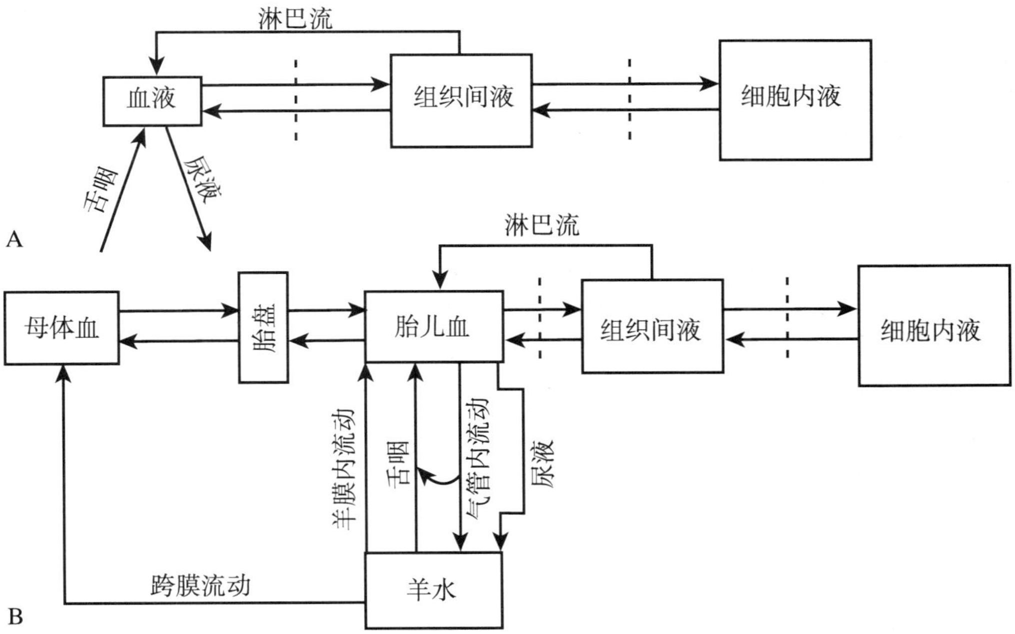

图 6–5 体液移动的主要路线：A. 成人。B. 近足月胎儿。（From Brace RA: Fetal and amniotic fluid balance. In Gluckman PD, Heymann MA (eds): Pediatrics and Perinatology: The Scientific Basis, 2nd ed. London, Arnold, 1996, pp 233-241.）

肾功能

第一个功能肾单位在胎龄第 8 周出现，胎龄 34 周时肾小球数量已达成人水平。肾小球滤过作用始于胎龄第 9～12 周之间。肾动脉是在 T12～L2 水平发自主动脉并分出节段终动脉，且在围生期易受局部缺血的损害。在宫内时，胎儿的肾血流量和肾小球滤过率（GFR）随新的肾单位的发育而渐渐增加。肾血管阻力初时较高；因此，尽管在妊娠期内肾脏所占的心排出量比例逐渐增加，宫内胎儿的肾血流量仍较少。

出生的第 1 天时，肾皮质灌注的分布情况的变化表现在皮质外层灌流增加。虽然肾血流总量未改变，但 GFR 在此时迅速升高。在出生后的头几天里，当皮质外层灌流增加时，皮质内层灌流不变。最终，肾血管的阻力降低，使 GFR 在出生后 3 月中迅速升高，然后缓慢升高，在 12～24 月龄时达成人水平。早产儿和低出生体重儿的 GFR 低于足月儿，无生后早期的迅速上升。但是，GFR 在早产儿出生后为逐渐升高直至达到 40 周胎龄足月儿的水平。由于 GFR 存在这些迅速的变化，生后很难用血浆肌酐来判断肾功能状况。

尿渗透压受两个机制控制。依赖髓质间质的渗透压利用逆流系统在亨氏袢浓缩尿液。新生儿期，肾髓质的低渗透压使逆流系统不太有效；尿液浓缩能力在 500～700 mOsm/kg，与成人肾脏的 1200mOsm/kg 相比，显得对液体过多时的耐受力不够。

如同在成人期，新生儿能应答血清渗透压的变化。抗利尿激素（ADH）从胎龄 12 周起即可由脑垂体合成，它通过增加肾集合管对水的重吸收来调节血清渗透压。围生期时 ADH 分泌增加，早产儿和足月儿在应对适宜刺激时都能合成 ADH。足月儿的 ADH 浓度测得值为 275～280 mOsm/kg，其分泌水平几乎达到成人水平。但与成人比较，新生儿的肾小管对 ADH 相对不敏感，可能是 ADH 受体较少或肾髓质较
94 低的浓度梯度降低了它的作用。

ADH 分泌异常（过多）综合征（SIADH）可继发于肺损害、手术创痛或缺氧引起的脑损害。其表现可为体重增加、低钠血症、少尿伴尿渗透压增高以及与血浆钠呈比例的高尿钠。治疗方法是液量限制和经鼻给予合成的去氨加压素（DDAVP）。

钠

新生儿的正常血清钠浓度为 135～140mmol/L，由弱化的肾脏排泄控制。血清钠是血清渗透压和细胞外液量的主要决定因素。尿钠外排依赖于 GFR，因此，新生儿比成人少。此外，新生儿的肾小管对钠的重吸收能力有限，所以尿钠丢失较多，早产儿较足月儿更明显。在生后第 1 天的少尿期，正常情况下不需要补充钠。在接下来的正常利尿期，正常维持钠的需要量是 2～4 mmol/kg。

低钠血症

血容量减少、正常血容量和血容量过多（表 6–3）时都可发生血清钠浓度低于 135mmol/L。临床常无明显症状，直至血清钠低于 120mmol/L 时可表现出脑水肿症状：淡漠、恶心、呕吐、头痛、抽搐和昏迷。症状的严重程度与低钠血症的起病速度和程度直接相关。

肾脏对血清钠降低的反应表现为排出更多的稀释尿，但由血容量减少引起的 ADH 分泌可影响该表现。因此，尿钠检验可用于帮助确定低钠血症的潜在病因。尿钠浓度低于 10mmol/L 提示为肾脏对等容性低钠血症做出的适当反应。如尿钠浓度高于 20mmol/L，则提示钠从受损的肾小管中漏出或血容量过多。

高钠血症

高钠血症（血清钠＞145mmol/L）可见于不同的水合状态（见表 6-3）。儿童期最常继发于低渗性液体丢失，如腹泻。临床体征包括黏膜干燥、皮肤弹性差、昏睡、烦躁不安、肌张力增高、抽搐和昏迷。脑组织中液体丢失可造成血管撕裂和脑出血。保留在细胞内的牛磺酸可使脑组织中的细胞外水分向细胞内回流增加。低钙血症常伴发于高钠血症。

钾

钾是最多的细胞内阳离子，对维持细胞膜的离子梯度至关重要。其正常的血清浓度为 3.5～5.8mmol/L。生后最初 24～72 小时，大量钾离子从细胞内向细胞外的移动可造成血浆钾升高。这种情况常伴发于多尿期，通过限制有效水分和钠来减少肾小

表 6–3　血钠异常和水化状态

	低容量性	等容性	高容量性
低钠血症	胃肠道丢失：呕吐、腹泻、小肠瘘、回肠造口术 摄入低张溶液 肾脏疾病 脑性失盐综合征 出汗：囊性纤维化、肾上腺皮质功能不全	抗利尿激素分泌异常综合征 利尿剂	充血性心衰 肝硬化 肾病综合征 肾衰竭
高钠血症	尿崩症 出汗过多 不显性丢失增加	抗利尿激素分泌不足	钠摄入过多

管排钾量。此结果直接与早产的提早程度有关，并可明显提高发病率。在多尿期末和钾排出增加时，血清钾最终下降。因此，生后第 1 天无需补充钾，但多尿期后，每天需要摄入维持量 1～3mmol/kg。

低钾血症

低钾血症最常见的原因是医源性原因，可因钾摄入不足或应用利尿剂，但也可因呕吐、腹泻、碱中毒（造成钾内流）或多尿型肾衰竭。胰岛素和交感神经系统兴奋也会引起钾内流而加重已存在的低钾尿症。正常的离子梯度可被破坏并可诱发肌肉电位传导异常，如心
95 律失常、麻痹性肠梗阻、尿潴留和呼吸肌麻痹。

高钾血症

高钾血症的病因包括严重的代谢性酸中毒、细胞坏死引起细胞内钾释放（如严重的坠落伤）、急性肾衰竭、医源性过度摄入、肾上腺功能不全、胰岛素依赖性糖尿病或严重溶血。合并缺氧、代谢性酸中毒、分解代谢状态和少尿时会加重高钾血症。早产儿还会因高的不显性失水而发生高钾血症。如低钾血症一样，高钾血症可改变细胞膜的电梯度，因此患者易发生心律失常，包括心搏暂停。

钙

钙在酶活性、肌肉收缩舒张、凝血级联系统、骨代谢和神经传导方面起重要作用。新生儿总钙的血清浓度维持在 1.8～2.1mmol/L，足月婴儿为 2.0～2.5mmol/L，可分成三个部分。30%～50%的钙与蛋白质结合，5%～15%与柠檬酸、乳酸、重碳酸盐和无机离子形成复合物。剩下的游离钙离子具有代谢活性，其浓度随血清白蛋白水平波动。氢离子可与钙可逆性地竞争白蛋白结合位点；因此，在酸中毒时游离钙浓度升高。

钙代谢受很多激素调控，但主要是受二羟胆钙化醇（钙的胃肠吸收、骨吸收，增加肾脏对钙的重吸收）、甲状旁腺素（骨钙吸收，降低尿钙排除）和降钙素（骨钙沉积和增加尿钙排除）调控。钙可逆浓度梯度从母体主动转运至胎儿循环中，造成围生期的高钙血症。出生后可暂时出现血钙下降至 1.8～2.1 mmol/L，24～48 小时后可逐渐上升到正常婴儿水平。

低钙血症

在新生儿期，除了通常是无症状的生理性低钙血症，其他引起低钙血症的原因有甲状旁腺功能减退，包括 DiGeorge 综合征，以及糖尿病母亲所生婴儿对甲状旁腺素不敏感，后者也可与低镁血症有关。临床表现有震颤、抽搐和心电图上 QT 间期延长。

高钙血症

高钙血症较低钙血症少见，但可由先天性代谢缺

陷引起，如家族性低钙尿和高钙血症或原发性甲状旁腺功能亢进。医源性原因有维生素 A 过量或饮食中磷摄入不足。儿童期较少见的原因有散发性甲状旁腺功能亢进、瘤外综合征和转移性骨病。

镁

镁作为一个重要的酶辅助因子，影响三磷酸腺苷（ATP）代谢和糖酵解。体内镁总量中只有 20%能以生物活性自由离子形式进行交换。剩余的镁是结合于骨组织中或与主要在肌肉和肝脏中的细胞内蛋白质、RNA 或 ATP 结合。镁的胃肠吸收受维生素 D、甲状旁腺素和钠的重吸收调控。如上文所述，低镁血症常与低钙血症有关。

酸碱平衡

酸碱平衡依靠细胞内外的缓冲系统、呼吸作用和肾功能维持。细胞内系统包括平衡的共轭酸碱对，公式如下：

$$HA \rightarrow H^+ + A^-$$

此处 H 为质子，A 是酸。pH 由计算缓冲系统 pH 的公式（Henderson-Hasselbalch 公式）得出：

$$pH = pK + \log [A^-] / [HA]$$

此处 pK 是弱酸的解离常数，$[A^-]$是被解离的酸的浓度，[HA]是酸的浓度。碳酸酐酶系统是最重要的细胞内缓冲系统：

$$CO_2 + H_2O \rightarrow H^+ + HCO_3^-$$

细胞外缓冲系统是相似的，但质子与蛋白质、血红蛋白或磷酸松散缔合，需要数小时才能达到平衡。

呼吸代偿是利用碳酸酐酶系统清除二氧化碳，并因此使反应式向左转移达到平衡和质子数量减少。转移程度受碳酸氢盐入血脑屏障的主动转运影响，因此可兴奋呼吸中枢。

正常细胞外液 pH 维持在 7.35～7.45。正常代谢过程可产生碳酸、乳酸、酮酸、磷酸和硫酸，所有这些物质或排出或受多种缓冲系统的调控。

胎儿的酸碱平衡

碳酸酐酶-碳酸氢盐缓冲系统对于胎儿尤为重要，因为 CO_2 能很容易地经由胎盘循环排出。发育中的胎儿的细胞内缓冲系统比儿童或成人的明显小，但仍比细胞外缓冲系统的能力大。胎儿呼吸代偿受到胎盘功能、母胎循环和母体呼吸代偿作用的限制。肾脏代偿对维持酸碱平衡的意义更大。 96

新生儿的酸碱平衡

出生后失去了母胎循环和母体呼吸及肾脏代偿机制作用的新生儿被迫去适应环境，其系统不断发育成熟。有资料提示，如果新生儿呼吸中枢对 pH 变化的敏感性高，则能更好地调控酸碱平衡。细胞内蛋白质质量增加可使细胞内缓冲系统的作用增强。此时，细胞外缓冲系统已经具有功能。

呼吸代偿在建立有效呼吸后才能起作用。因为此机制有赖于肺功能和肺成熟，患有肺部疾病的新生儿其呼吸代偿受损。CO_2 能自由地通过血脑屏障，使呼吸动力中枢对呼吸性酸中毒产生速发型应答。对代谢性酸中毒的应答是迟发的，因为细胞间质的碳酸氢盐需要几个小时才能与脑中的碳酸氢盐达到平衡。

肾脏代偿是新生儿可用于维持酸碱平衡的最重要的机制。已发现，新生儿生后数小时就能调整尿液酸度，但肾脏代偿功能的全面成熟需 2～3 天。如上文所述，肾功能和灌注的变化可造成新生儿生后头几天调控酸碱平衡的能力受限。近端小管能重吸收 85%～90%被滤过的碳酸氢盐，但早产儿的这一功能不足。新生儿的重吸收功能还会受到一些摄入药物的影响。多巴胺可抑制近端小管钠质子泵的活性，因此能减少碳酸氢盐重吸收的量。其余的碳酸氢盐在远端小管重吸收，但与近端小管不同的是：此处缺乏碳酸酐酶。醛固酮是影响远端小管功能和促进质子从此处排出的最重要激素。但早产婴儿的远侧肾单位对醛固酮不敏感。从尿中排出的质子有磷酸盐、硫酸盐和铵盐。排泌量随年龄和胎龄的增加而增多。而应用含磷酸盐的药物能增加转运至远端小管的磷酸盐的量，因此能提高 H^+ 的排出能力。多巴胺可减少远端小管重吸收质子的量，因此能增加质子排出。

酸碱平衡失调的原因

动脉血气用于帮有助确定酸碱平衡失调的原因（表 6–4）。酸–碱平衡状况可用 pH 表示，而依据碳酸氢盐和 CO_2 分压的高或低可提示为代谢性或呼吸性原因。首要治疗的应是所有潜在的问题，如脱水或脓毒症引起的代谢性酸中毒。缓慢输注缓冲液应作为辅助治疗，如碳酸氢钠或三羟甲氨基甲烷（一种不含钠的缓冲液）。碳酸氢钠用量可参照以下计算公式：

$NaHCO_3$ (mmol) ＝碱剩余 × 体重(kg) / 3

能量代谢

能量是做功的能力，也是所有生活过程必需的。能量的单位是热卡或焦耳。1 卡等于 4.184 焦耳；相当于使 1g 水的温度从 15℃升高到 16℃所需要的能量。应用最广的医用能量单位是千卡（kcal），1 千卡等于 1000 卡。1 焦耳能量相当于将 1kg 物体移动 1 米所需的牛顿力。热力学第一定律说明能量是无法创造或消失的。因此：

摄入的能量＝消耗的能量＋储存的能量

至于新生儿，可表达如下：

能量摄入＝排泄物中的能量损失＋能量储存
　　　　＋组织合成的能量
　　　　＋活动耗费的能量
　　　　＋基础代谢率 97

表 6–4　胎儿和新生儿酸碱失衡的原因

	胎儿	新生儿
代谢性酸中毒	胎盘功能不全继发的缺氧	缺氧
	母亲缺氧	围生期窒息
	母亲患糖尿病	严重肺部疾病
	败血症	低血容量
	肾小管发育异常	早产儿心肌功能障碍
		血管活性调节功能异常
		败血症
		代谢紊乱
		早产儿（肾脏发育不成熟）
代谢性碱中毒	妊娠剧吐	长期使用利尿剂
呼吸性酸中毒	母亲通气不足：哮喘	呼吸窘迫综合征
	气道阻塞	
	麻醉剂过量	
	麻醉	
	硫酸镁毒性作用	
呼吸性碱中毒	母亲通气过度	发热
		医源性过度通气
		尿素循环紊乱

能量摄入

粮食中的主要物质是糖类、脂肪和蛋白质（见下文）。从这些食物中可获得的势能是当这些食物被完全吸收和氧化时释放的能量。可代谢的能量要少于摄入的能量，因为能量可从粪便中丢失，也可以不完全的代谢混合物的形式丢失，如来自氨基酸的尿素或来自脂肪的酮体。因此，可代谢的能量应计算如下：

可代谢的能量＝摄入的能量－从尿和粪中损失的能量

食物代谢可经过多种复杂的代谢途径。食物的完全代谢时其被氧化成 CO_2 和水，至于蛋白质，是经代谢成为尿素和氨。这一代谢反应与预测的化学计算方程式相符[109]。氧化作用释放的能量通常不是直接利用，而是依据某处某时的需要，由释放的能量产生高能中间产物。这些中间产物包括 ATP、三磷酸鸟苷、三磷酸胞苷、尿嘧啶核苷、三磷酸肌苷和磷酸肌酸。这些中间产物的储能形式是高能磷酸键。高能磷酸键水解时释放能量。这些高能中间产物的产生是代谢途径中的一个直接步骤。而更常见的是，它们由氧化磷酸化作用间接产生，这一过程是指一种化合物以其氢离子被连续去除的方式被氧化，然后氢离子经过多种黄素蛋白和细胞色素传递，直至与氧结合产生水。这一过程可释放大量能量用于产生含有高能磷酸键的中间产品。因此，食物中的能量是用于产生高能中间产品，所有的生命进程均以此种能量形式供能。

呼吸商是经耗氧产生的 CO_2 来计算，不同的氧化底物有不同的呼吸商。葡萄糖氧化的呼吸商数值为 1.0，脂肪氧化的呼吸商数值为 0.70～0.72，取决于被氧化的脂肪链长度。因此用间接测热法测得的呼吸商反映的是底物利用的平衡性。然而，这种情况是复杂的，如脂肪经不完全氧化方式转化为酮体或糖类转变为脂质会造成呼吸商大于 1.0。糖类、脂肪和氨基酸的精确呼吸商值如表所列[109]。

出生代表由胎儿状态而来的一个过渡期，此时糖类是主要的能量底物（约占能量消耗的 80%），婴儿期时，糖类和脂肪都能提供能量[69]。这一过渡期的佐证是呼吸商的变化，它从出生时的 0.97 下降到 3 小时龄时的 0.80[74,153]，此时脂肪供能占 60%～70%。这可能是由于新生婴儿出生初期很难获得外源性能量以满足其能量需求这个事实，因此新生婴儿更依赖于内源性能量储存。此后，呼吸商在生后 1 周内缓慢增高[28,29,153]，提示新生婴儿在第一时间内优先代谢脂肪。低出生体重儿的呼吸商大于 0.90[138]。

能量贮存

能量主要以脂肪形式储存。一个正常的体重 70kg 的男子约有 17kg 脂肪，这些脂肪氧化能产生 150 000 kcal 的能量——足够用于禁食 2 月所需的能量。能量还以糖原形式储存在肝脏、肾脏和肌肉组织中。肌糖原只能在原位利用，但肝糖原和肾糖原可用以产生葡萄糖并可在其他部位代谢。糖原储存含有 1000～3000kcal 的糖原代谢值，足够用于禁食 6～24小时所需的能量。除了能量储存，蛋白质还可执行其他功能，一个正常的体重 70kg 的男子含有的 11kg 蛋白质（7kg 在细胞内，4 kg 在细胞外），在严格禁食时约有一半（约等于 22 000 kcal）可被用于供能。蛋白质被代谢的严重后果包括消瘦、创伤愈合减慢、水肿、生长和神经系统发育停滞以及对感染的抵抗力减弱。对成长中的婴儿的研究提示，每增加 1 克体重（即每 1 克能量储存）平均需要 5kcal 的能量。完成组织沉积所需的能量包括：(1) 储存在组织本身中的能量（如 9 kcal/g 脂肪）；(2) 投入在转化食物为可储存和可利用的底物所需的能量。研究显示，这一额外的能量投入占组织能量值的 5%～30%[94]。

生长和组织合成所需的能量

在情况稳定、发育成熟的成人，用于生长的能量很少。但在新生儿，生长所需的能量非常大。在婴儿期，高达 50%以上的能量摄入用于生长[35,143]。生长所需的能量包括组织中储存的能量和投入组织合成的能量。能量储存的测定可通过计算可代谢的摄入能量和能量消耗的差值得到。现认为，组织合成所需的能量与饮食诱导的生热作用一样（即用以代谢、合成和沉积的营养素互变作用的能耗）[13,27,143]。记录进食前后的静态能量消耗（REE）的差值，Reichman 等人[143]估计，每天组织合成消耗的能量为 3～6kcal/kg。对成长中的婴儿的能量消耗进行的数周纵向研究发现，组织合成的能耗为每天 9.3kcal/kg，或占总能量摄入的 7.6% [35]。正常早产儿的生长速度为每天 17～19g/kg[36]，足月儿为每天 4～8g/kg[185]。因此，早产儿 98
的生长能耗要大得多[130]。早产儿相关研究提示其生长的代谢耗能与蛋白质增长的速度有关[33,59,115,130]。这是因为蛋白质每单位重量产生的能量值较脂肪的低，但却需要更多的能量投入。生长迅速的早产儿其生长的代谢消耗主要用于蛋白质合成代谢，其估计值为 1.2kcal/g 体重增长值，约占能量消耗总量的 30%[33,115]。

能量损耗

婴儿能量可从排泄物中丢失。由于其消化道和肾脏发育不成熟，以及其胆汁酸供给可能不足，粪和尿中的能量丢失可能相应地比成人高。

活动的能量

研究显示，能量消耗的变异很大程度上与一个婴儿的活动有关。旺盛活动度，如啼哭时，能量消耗是双倍的[130]，但婴儿大多数时间是在睡觉[130]，花费在活动上的能量不足每日热能消耗总量的 5% 。

研究提示，日耗能量与活动的持续时间和程度有关[29,59]。

基础代谢率和静息能量消耗

出于医学伦理学考虑，绝不可能让一个新生婴儿彻底禁食 14 小时以测定其基础代谢率。因此，静息能量消耗（REE）是更常用于基础代谢研究。REE 受许多因素影响，包括年龄、身体组分、生命器官的大小和能量摄入。

年龄：一个足月适于胎龄儿的 REE 出生时为每日 33 kcal/kg，至生后 1 周末增加到每日 48kal/kg[85,149]。接着维持不变，1 月后开始下降。早产儿和小于胎龄儿的 REE 较高[117]。这些与年龄相关的差异可能反映出身体组分的不同[85]，此外已有研究认为，生后第 1 周基础代谢的增加可能提示功能器官的酶活性提高[93]。

机体组分：生后头几周内，婴儿丢失体液，同时伴有公认的体重减轻[74]。出生前，胎儿体内水分约为 75%，但到 1 个月龄时，水分下降为 45%[56,57]。因此，生后头几周内观察到 REE 的增加可能反映了体内组织的增加和体液的相对减少。

生命器官的大小：在成人，脑、肝、心和肾脏占基础代谢率的 66%，但只占总体重的 7%。婴儿的这些器官（尤其是脑）占体重的比例较大。目前认为，生后第 1 个月单是脑组织就占基础代谢率的 60%～65%。早产儿和小于胎龄儿的生命器官受宫内和宫外营养不良的影响较其他器官小[85,117]。因此，它们占基础代谢的比例更高[36]，单是脑组织就占基础代谢率的 70% [88]。同时，早产儿和小于胎龄儿所含代谢活跃的棕色脂肪组织的比例往往较代谢不活跃的白色脂肪组织的高[130]。足月儿和适于胎龄儿只有 40g 棕色脂肪组织，其白色脂肪组织为 520g[85]。

饮食摄入：婴儿的 REE 与热卡摄入和体重增加有关。已证实，REE 增长值与能量摄入增长水平之间呈显著的线性相关[35]。一项研究提示，餐后 REE 每天增加 8.5kcal/kg，相当于总能量摄入的 5.7%；这与生长耗能相关[35]。Salomon 等人 150 在婴儿测定了每种食物成分的饮食诱导的生热作用。他们发现，氨基酸能将 REE 提高 11%（热卡摄入的 4.4%），脂肪能提高 8%（热卡摄入的 3%），而葡萄糖不能提高 REE。此研究结果与其他一些研究相悖，即认为摄入葡萄糖后 REE 明显提高，尤其是大剂量时[1,134]。

新生儿的能量代谢与成人和儿童不同，反映出其特殊的生理状况。新生婴儿每单位体重的代谢率和能量需求比儿童和成人明显高（图 6–6）[170]。他们每天需要约 40～70kcal/kg 能量维持新陈代谢，50～70kcal/kg 的能量满足生长（组织合成和能量储存），还有 20kcal/kg 为排泄物中的能量丢失（见图 6–6）[59,130]。计 99
算机化和小型化的间接热量计实现了新生儿能量代谢的非侵入性研究[130,132,137,170]。一个经肠道喂养的新生婴儿每天总的能量需求量为 100～120kcal/kg，而一名 10 岁儿童为 60～80kcal/kg，一名 20 岁成人为 30～40kcal/kg。接受全肠外营养的新生婴儿所需热卡较低（每天 80～100 kcal/kg）。这是由于没有排泄物中的能量丧失，有事实证明，当婴儿处于双绝缘保温箱孵育的中性温度护理环境时，没有体温调节的能量需求。

现已公布一些可用于预测成人能量消耗的公式。情况稳定的新生儿，其 REE 可应用一些参数，如体重、心率和年龄，并根据以下公式预测[132]：

$$\text{REE（cal/min）} = -74.436 + (34.661 \times \text{公斤体重}) + (0.496 \times \text{每分钟心率}) + (0.178 \times \text{日龄})$$

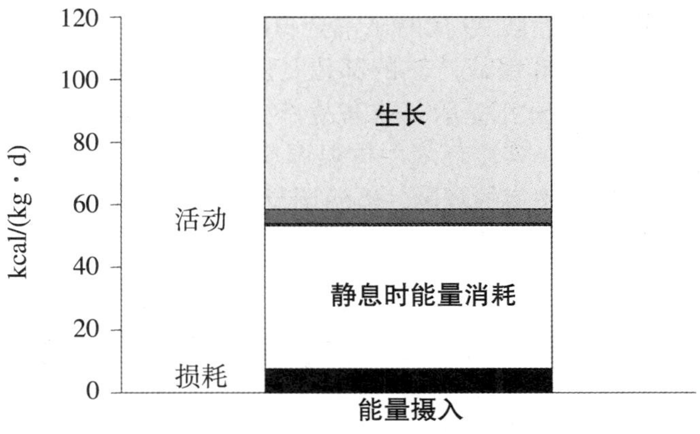

图 6–6　接受手术之新生儿的能量摄入的分配。（Adapted from Pierro A, Carnielli V, Filler RM, et al: Partition of energy metabolism in the surgical newborn. J Pediatr Surg 1991;26: 581-586.）

以上公式中体重对 REE 有重要预测价值，它也是 REE 的最有力的预测指标，并代表生命组织的总质量。心率能间接测量婴儿的血流动力学和代谢状态，而生后年龄在出生后头几个星期内也能影响 REE。

体温调节

分娩后，相对低的环境温度和残留羊水的蒸发可使新生婴儿失热增加。新生儿是恒温的。他们对环境温度的变化远比成人敏感，因为他们的质量较小而体表面积相对较大，他们的绝缘组织如脂肪和毛发较少，他们无法进行明显的行为和衣物修正，如启动体温调节装置或穿上额外的衣服，并且其能量储备有限[28]。热平衡的范围对婴儿很关键[85]，而且比成人的高（足月适于胎龄儿为 32℃～34℃）[86]。已发表许多有关不同体重和年龄的婴儿最佳环境温度的表格[86]。许多研究显示，处在热平衡的范围之外的婴儿的发病率和死亡率均明显上升。

热能可经辐射、传导和对流（70%）以及蒸发（25%）丧失；进食时体温升高（3%）及排泄（2%）时也会丧失[85]。婴儿对冷的反应依赖下丘脑调节中心的成熟和生热作用底物的存在[85]。交感神经系统介导的原始反应是通过寒战和非寒战的生热作用和血管收缩来减少热能丧失。新生婴儿对寒冷暴露没有寒战反应，但有高度特异组织——棕色脂肪组织——能不经过寒战而产热。棕色脂肪组织在胎龄 22 周时已很完善，在胎龄 29 周时已占全身脂肪的 90%[114]。这是最重要的非寒战产热的部位；其他部位包括脑、肝和肾脏。研究提示，非寒战产热的最优燃料是游离脂肪酸[31]。寒冷环境中体温调节的能量消耗相当大。即使在热平衡的范围，体温调节仍占能量消耗总量的 8%[157]。当完全依赖非寒战产热时，REE 升高 1 倍。

在全身麻醉下接受大手术后的新生儿常发生低体温[122,152]。面对寒冷环境的挑战，新生婴儿要维持生理体温所经历的困难比成人的要大。低体温时可能会使手术后并发症的发生率上升，如酸中毒、免疫功能受损和创伤愈合延迟[105]。当环境温度下降时发现，棕色脂肪储备的血流量增加且是由棕色脂肪的线粒体产热。手术中，新生儿不但暴露在寒冷环境中，而且还有多种麻醉剂和肌松剂会对产热（能量消耗）和核心温度产生不利影响[95,97]。实验动物的非寒战产热可被麻醉剂抑制[2,121]。Albanese 等人[2]的研究显示，对寒冷暴露下的兔子施行全身麻醉终点时，可引起迅速和极度的非寒战产热增加。这可用于解释婴幼儿手术结束时能量消耗突然和迅速增加[41,97]。

长久以来已知棕色脂肪组织含有一种蛋白质——解连蛋白[1]，它能在底物氧化过程中消除跨线粒体内膜的质子梯度[31]。但是，最近有假说认为，质子渗漏可促进肝脏的生热作用[141]。质子渗漏强度可能是代谢率的决定因子[135]。营养素的氧化分解能释放能量，氧化磷酸化时能在细胞线粒体中转化出可应用的化学燃料（ATP）。这通常是体内能量消耗过程的推进力。氧化磷酸化时，质子从线粒体基质被泵入到膜间隙。质子泵与氧消耗量（VO_2）的比率和产生与维持跨内膜质子电化学电位的差异直接相称。质子回流入基质的途径有两条：经磷酸化作用途径产生 ATP，或经渗漏途径不产生 ATP 而释放热能。成人静止肝细胞氧消耗量的 20%～30%是用以启动热能产生的质子渗漏[25]。这一渗漏途径在肝脏和其他器官是构成标准 REE 的重要机体反应，可导致静息热产生[26,145]。鼠肝线粒体内膜对质子的渗透性在胎内时较高，生后早期 100
明显降低并维持最低水平直至成年[175]。Valcarce 等人[175]研究发现，这是围生期鼠在棕色脂肪组织生热作用建立之前的一个温度适应的保护性机制。可以认为新生儿也有相似的保护性机制的“预设程序”，使他们能在出生（冷适应）、手术（断脐）和饥饿（暂时性低血糖）的应激状态中存活。

糖类、脂肪和蛋白质的新陈代谢

围生期发生的营养和新陈代谢的极大变化反映了生理学的同样的极大变化。胎儿生存在一个热稳定环境中，且营养不断从静脉途径输入而废物可有效地排出。出生时，这种持续的营养素供给突然终止可造成暂时性饥饿。这一饥饿期结束时，营养素从来自胎盘的葡萄糖供给变成乳汁供给，后者脂肪含量高而糖类含量低。此外，新生儿的肾脏和肺部代谢活性明显增强，而且新生儿必须激活生热作用和热量守恒的代谢和生理学机制以维持自己的体温。新生儿要成功适应宫外环境，需要仔细调节葡萄糖和脂肪代谢的变化并要在建立蛋白质或氨基酸足量供应之前利用蛋白质储备。到新生儿期末，当婴儿开始摄入糖类含量比乳汁的高和脂肪含量低的饮食时，营养再次发生变化。因此，一个健康的新生儿是处于代谢变化状态，对于这些变化必须谨慎调节才能在此关键时期维持生长和脑发育。现在已经知道，新生儿期的营养和生长是以后心血管疾病和神经发育的重要决定因子。由早产、感染、胃肠功能障碍、麻醉和手术导致的额外生理学应激情况是对新生儿维持代谢稳态的重大挑战。内科医生和外科医生应慎重处理营养和代谢问题以避免由营养不良、低血糖和高血糖引起的神经系统后遗症而导致额外的发病率和死亡率[40]。对新生儿期手术、肠外营养或脓毒症的长期代谢、神经系统和心血管系统后遗症尚不清楚，但关注此期手术患者的今后发育和营养管理对其成人期健康意义重大。

新生儿的葡萄糖代谢

胎儿大部分能量供给（约 70%的总热卡来源于糖类，＜10%来源于脂肪）来自母体提供的葡萄糖。出生时从高糖类膳食变为高脂肪和低糖类饮食（约 40%的总热卡来源于糖类，50%来源于脂肪）[69]表示，新生儿不但必须适应糖类供给时间和数量的变化，还要通过胰岛素和胰高血糖素、葡萄糖异生以及其他葡萄糖稳态机制调节自己的血糖。脑组织只能利用葡萄糖和酮体，不能直接氧化脂类。因而，在新生儿期维持血糖正常对良好的神经系统预后尤为重要。尽管脂肪作为燃料来源在新生儿期较成人期供应量大，葡萄糖循环在新生儿期（每分钟 3～5mg/kg）仍较成人（每分钟 2～3mg/kg）多，部分原因是由于脑-体质量比相对增高。早产儿葡萄糖循环速率更大（每分钟 5～6mg/kg）[120]。在早产儿和足月儿中，90%的葡萄糖被脑组织利用；成人期该比例下降到 40%左右[5]。足月儿有两种产生葡萄糖的重要方法以维持血糖正常：糖原分解和葡萄糖异生。足月儿葡萄糖产生于糖原分解（约 40%）和甘油（20%）、丙氨酸和其他氨基酸（10%）以及乳酸（30%）的葡萄糖异生[100]。

围生期的胰高血糖素-胰岛素轴

尽管胎儿能合成和释放胰高血糖素和胰岛素，但孕期的胰岛素功能可能是促进合成代谢和促进生长而不是调节外周血糖[120]。孕期胰高血糖素对诱导葡萄糖异生酶很重要，出生时由于断脐造成的胰高血糖素冲击现象可能是生后葡萄糖异生能力迅速提高的原因[160]。胰岛细胞在新生儿生后头 2 周内相对应答迟钝，以致于对葡萄糖浓度升高引起的胰岛素分泌增加和胰高血糖素分泌减少的反应相对较慢[120]。新生儿对低血糖的反应也同样慢，因此如果新生儿出现低血糖，有可能是在胰岛素分泌减少和胰高血糖素分泌增加以刺激葡萄糖异生之前。此外新生儿终末器官的胰岛素敏感度较成人的低；因此血浆胰岛素与血糖的关系不太密切，而胰高血糖素与血糖的关系较为密切[81,82]。早产儿对葡萄糖应答功能的成熟比足月儿更慢[43]。

围生期的糖原和糖原分解

在妊娠第 3 个 3 月期中，母体葡萄糖以糖原形式储存。许多储存在胎儿肝脏里，有些糖原储存在胎儿骨骼肌、肾和肠中，只有少量储存在脑中。肝和肾糖原在出生时和生后不久可被动用以维持外周的葡萄糖浓度；但是早产儿（妊娠后 3 个 3 月期缩短或缺如）、
小于胎龄儿或经历较大围生期应激者由于产生早期肝 101
糖原的儿茶酚胺兴奋性动员，其肝糖原储备在生后 24 小时或更短时间内就会耗竭。其他组织，如心脏、骨骼肌和肺部，能代谢细胞内储存的糖原，但由于缺乏葡萄糖-6-磷酸酶而不能将其动员至循环中。围生期胰高血糖素或儿茶酚胺冲击能引起糖原储存的动员和利用反应。

新生儿糖原异生

葡萄糖异生的关键酶可在妊娠胎儿早期出现，并在整个妊娠期和新生儿期不断升高。但是胎儿体内的葡萄糖异生尚未被证实，并且不知道细胞溶质中的磷酸丙酮酸羧激酶（氨基酸或乳酸的葡萄糖异生所必需的）或葡萄糖-6-磷酸酶（所有底物的葡萄糖异生和糖原分解后葡萄糖输出所必需的）在胎儿肝脏的表达是否足以支持葡萄糖异生。胎儿葡萄糖-6-磷酸酶表达较低，但足月儿生后数天内该酶表达上调[30]。测定早产儿的甘油葡萄糖异生的研究提示，有一些甘油葡萄糖异生[169]，但由于早产儿的葡萄糖-6-磷酸酶浓度可能有限，故此途径只能部分代偿外源性葡萄糖供应

减少[177]。肠外甘油补充能提高早产儿葡萄糖异生速率[166]，但混合氨基酸制剂[167]或丙氨酸[178]的供给不能使之增高，这一现象符合如下假设，即早产儿氨基酸或乳酸的葡萄糖异生受限与其磷酸丙酮酸羧激酶缺乏有关。早产儿的肠外脂类能刺激葡萄糖异生[167]，可能是其提供了含碳底物（甘油）和脂肪酸。脂肪酸氧化作用在葡萄糖异生过程中是必不可少的，它既可提供能量源（ATP）支持葡萄糖异生，也可提供乙酰辅酶 A 以激活丙酮酸羧化酶。对人类新生儿葡萄糖异生的诱导因素迄今知之甚少，但在动物实验中发现，出生时胰高血糖素–胰岛素比值增高能刺激参与葡萄糖异生的酶的成熟，尤其是磷酸丙酮酸羧激酶。足月新生儿生后 4～6 小时之内可出现明显的葡萄糖异生[58,101]。

新生儿低血糖症

生后血糖水平立刻下降，但既可因糖原分解或葡萄糖异生而自发升高，也可为进食而升高。临床对此期低血糖不太重视，但认为后续的低血糖应该避免。对于多少血糖浓度以下应诊断为低血糖以及低血糖持续多长时间应进行预防或检查，目前仍有相当大的争议[80]，主要因为此期代谢、生理学和营养方面的巨大变化会使葡萄糖浓度波动明显。此外，新生儿低血糖的症状是非特异性的，可能包括表 6–5 所列出的症状，且多为主观性的。近来，外周葡萄糖浓度的干预阈值在足月儿伴异常临床体征者为小于 45mg/dL（2.5mmol/L），足月儿有高危因素而欠缺代谢适应能力者为持续低于 36mg/dL（2.0mmol/L），早产儿（但资料有限）为低于 47mg/dL（2.6mmol/L），同时，经肠外喂养的婴儿其血糖应一直高于 45mg/dL（2.5mmol/L），因为这些婴儿的胰岛素可能增高（且因此抑制了脂解作用和生酮作用）[42]。

新生儿的低血糖病因见表 6–6。在此关键发育期内，葡萄糖代谢对脑组织尤其重要，且血糖低于 2.6mmol/L 的低血糖症与近期神经生理学变化[103]和神经发育预后不良有关[51,111]。但是，这些研究很难从低 102
血糖的并发症和病因（如早产儿、先天性高胰岛素血症[111]、小于胎龄儿[51]或糖尿病母亲[164]之新生儿）中确切描绘出低血糖是一个引起神经系统问题的独立危险因子，还有一些引起神经系统问题的不确定因素，即低血糖的发作频率、程度和持续时间[79]。近期新生儿脑显像方式的进展已可显示出由新生儿低血糖引起的

表 6–5 新生儿低血糖的症状和体征

激惹	哭声异常
震颤	心跳停止
呼吸暂停	低体温
青紫	呼吸急促
疲软、淡漠、嗜睡	惊厥发作

表 6–6 新生儿低血糖的原因

与母亲代谢变化有关
- 产时给予葡萄糖
- 药物治疗
  - 特布他林、利托君、普萘洛尔
  - 口服降糖药
- 妊娠糖尿病；糖尿病母亲的婴儿
- 严重的母婴 Rh 血型不相容性

与新生儿问题有关
- 特发病情或适应不良
- 围生期缺氧缺血
- 感染、败血症
- 低体温
- 高血黏度
- 胎儿成红细胞增多症、胎儿水肿
- 换血疗法
- 其他
  - 医源性原因
  - 先天性心脏畸形

宫内生长发育迟缓

内分泌和代谢紊乱
- 高胰岛素血症（如先天性高胰岛素血症、Beckwith–Wiedemann 综合征）
- 其他内分泌紊乱
  - 全垂体功能减退症
  - 单纯性生长素缺乏症
  - 皮质醇分泌不足
- 先天性代谢缺陷
  - 糖原累积病 1a 和 1b
  - 1,6–二磷酸果糖磷酸酶缺乏
  - 丙酮酸羧化酶缺乏症
  - 脂肪酸氧化异常

特征性征象，但研究的病例数较少，还是很难将这些特征与低血糖的并发症区分开来[178]。

新生儿低血糖的治疗依赖喂养途径以及是否已明确危险因素。应频繁地进行血糖监测，并且治疗性或调查研究性计算法提示，如出现低血糖临床体征，还应在增加肠道喂养的同时给予静脉输注葡萄糖[80]。

新生儿高血糖

新生儿高血糖也可发生，并被认为代表若干特定的临床疾病。尽管较少，糖尿病也可见于新生儿期，发生率约为 1/400 000～1/500 000 活产儿[156,181]。新生儿持久性和短暂性糖尿病均可发生。新生儿短暂性糖尿病约占 50%，常在生后 3～6 个月龄内缓解；但也可能到儿童或青春期时发展为持久性糖尿病。持久性新生儿糖尿病也占 50%左右。短暂性新生儿糖尿病归咎于父系印迹[64,112]，且持久性新生儿糖尿病的一个分子组成因素已被阐明[70]。

大多数新生儿的高血糖是自限性的，可自发缓解，并且只有少数糖尿病的共同特征。此症发生频率随着经肠外喂养和接受皮质类固醇治疗的极低出生体重婴儿存活率的升高而增高。新生儿高血糖的病因学尚不太明了，但可能的原因是：在葡萄糖液输注、过快的葡萄糖液输注速率、终末器官的胰岛素抵抗或低血浆胰岛素伴高儿茶酚胺水平（如由于皮质类固醇给药）时不能抑制葡萄糖异生；感染；或对疼痛或手术（见下文）的反应[80]。新生儿高血糖的处理是病因治疗（如治疗感染或疼痛、减缓过快的葡萄糖液输注速率）。对于胰岛素给药目前仍有争议[168]；一方面，输注胰岛素时可高速度输注葡萄糖；另一方面，有副作用的报道。对新生儿高血糖症的急性或远期后遗症尚不清楚；高血糖不会引起酮症或代谢性酸中毒，但渗透性利尿和糖尿可能会导致脱水。尽管由于新生儿高血糖造成脑部病理改变和神经发育预后不良的证据不足，但渗透性改变会增加脑出血的风险。根据 Van den Berghe 等人[176]的研究结果，近来在成人重症监护室中，医生对严格控制患者血糖产生了很大的研究兴趣。对于新生儿或特殊亚群的新生儿，严格控制其血糖是否能带来裨益尚有待证实，但已证明，血糖峰值和高血糖持续时间与儿童死亡率有关[162]，而且高血糖与新生儿坏死性小肠结肠炎的发病率和死亡率升高有关[76]。

新生儿脂质和脂肪代谢

脂肪是新生儿的主要能量来源，乳汁或配方奶中 40%～50%的热卡是由脂肪提供。如上文所讨论的，生后 3 小时之内脂肪氧化成为主要燃料[74,153]。此外，脂肪是机体的主要储能形式。尽管大多数脂肪酸链的长度有利于供能，而组成磷脂和其他脂肪衍生类脂的脂肪酸是构成细胞膜的极为重要的成分，这些细胞膜的功能有赖于脂肪酸的正确链长和不饱和程度。因此，在整个新生儿生长期间，饮食或机体代谢都可提供不同的脂肪酸组成，这对生长支持很重要，尤其是对富含复合脂类的脑组织。

新生儿脂肪酸氧化作用和生酮作用

脂肪酸 β-氧化是脂肪酸氧化的主要方式。从酰基链连续去除二碳单位的过程是为心脏和骨骼肌提供 ATP 的主要来源。肝脏 β-氧化所起的作用不同，它可使酮体（乙酰乙酸和 β-羟丁酸）进入外周循环，并提供 ATP 和乙酰辅酶 A 激活丙酮酸羧化酶支持肝脏葡萄糖异生。此外，肾脏[172]、小肠[19]、白色脂肪组织[173]和脑星形胶质细胞[45]可能在某些情况下产生酮体。酮体是肝外器官的另一种重要燃料，特别是在血糖降低时的脑组织。由此可知，喂养期间以及对生理学和代谢方面稳态的适应过程中引起葡萄糖浓度波动时，生酮作用是脑部极其重要的供应代用燃料的途径。储存、摄取或输入的三酰甘油的酰基团发生氧化作用时，非酯化脂肪酸必须释出。以上反应可发生在脂肪细胞中远离激素敏感性脂肪酶的作用位点，或位于内皮脂蛋白脂肪酶的作用位点[55,71]。非酯化脂肪酸与白蛋白结合后可提供主要底物，在组织中吸收和氧化。此外，细胞内三酰甘油的储存可为心脏和骨骼肌中的 β-氧化提供重要的酰基部分，而且也需要激素 103
敏感性脂肪酶的作用。激素敏感性脂肪酶和脂蛋白脂肪酶受激素和营养状况的调控，因此组织中非酯化脂肪酸的供应对脂肪酸氧化有部分控制作用（图 6-7）[52]。肝脏脂肪酸氧化作用和生酮作用的途径如图 6-8 所示。在产后期即刻，分娩和断脐可造成胰高血糖素-儿茶酚胺冲击，激发脂解作用和胰岛素的下降，此应激反应的结果是引起血浆非酯化脂肪酸浓度迅速升高[119,127]。这一脂解作用还可释放出甘油，后者可作为葡萄糖异生的前体（见上文）[119,127]。出生后不久即可有

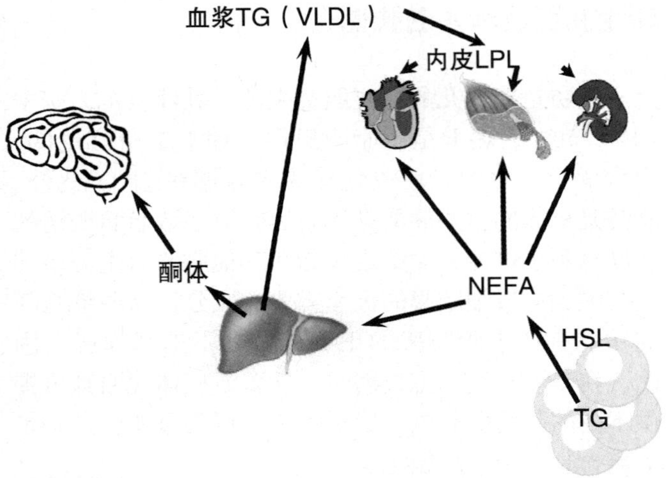

图 6-7 脂肪酸的代谢生理学。在激素敏感性脂肪酶（HSL）的作用下，脂肪组织储存的三酰甘油（TG）释放出脂肪酸（非酯化脂肪酸，NEFA）。NEFA 可在心脏、肌肉和肾脏被吸收，并氧化为二氧化碳，产生三磷酸腺苷（ATP）；它们可在肝脏被氧化为酮体或再酯化为循环 TG 极低密度脂蛋白（VLDL）。酮体在脑组织被氧化，脑中不能直接氧化脂肪酸。在内皮脂蛋白脂肪酶（LPL）作用下，循环 TG可释放 NEFA，继而后者被吸收和氧化。

酮体生成[22,47,69,84,126,183]，出生后头 2 天达到 0.2～0.5mmol/L，5～10 天时为 0.7～1.0mmol/L[183]，但在早产儿或小于胎龄儿，此功能可能受损[47,83,84]。低血糖时，酮体水平可升高至 1.5～5.0mmol/L[183]。实验动物出生后，它们参与脂肪酸氧化作用和生酮作用的酶活性均增高，因而其脂肪酸氧化作用和生酮作用的能力增强[69]，但对人类脂肪酸氧化作用的酶的诱导作用所知甚少。羟甲基戊二酰辅酶 A 合酶对生酮作用具有极其重要的控制作用，此酶可被胰高血糖素短期激活，这可能是出生时生酮作用迅速冲高的原因[39]。

酮体的利用

我们对人体组织中利用酮体的酶的个体发生学知之甚少。心脏、肌肉、肾脏和脑都能利用酮体，所需的酶类已在人体组织中发现[62,123,124]。在小鼠，酮体酶类的活性在新生儿脑组织中很高，断乳时下降，但在新生儿肌肉和肾脏中的水平较成人的低，提示脑组织能优先利用[69]。 104

新生儿的蛋白质和氨基酸代谢

与处于氮平衡中立状态的健康成人相反，婴儿在正氮平衡时才能达成满意的生长和发育。婴儿能有效率地保留氮，并且能保留 80%的经口和静脉摄入的可代谢蛋白质[33,159,190]。蛋白质代谢依赖蛋白质和能量摄

图 6-8 肝脏的脂肪酸氧化。循环非酯化脂肪酸（NEFA），与白蛋白连接，可被肝细胞吸收。脂肪酸在线粒体内可被氧化或酯化为三酰甘油并再排出。来自脂肪酸氧化的乙酰辅酶 A 可经三羧酸循环产生三磷酸腺苷（ATP），或用于产生酮体为外周利用。

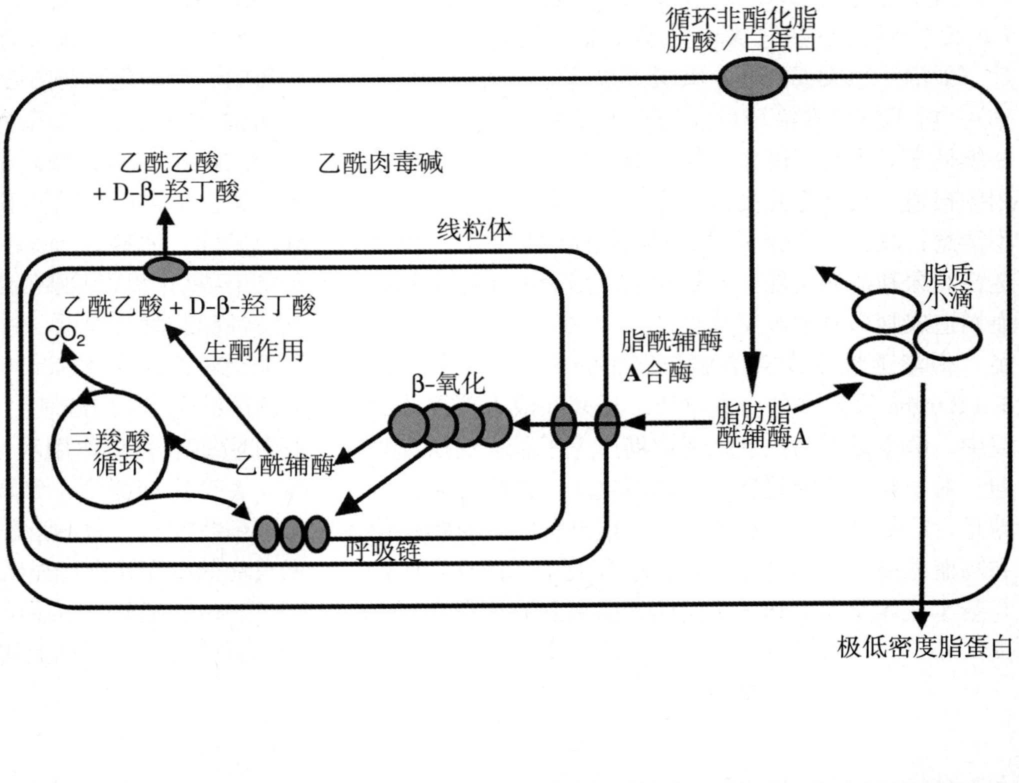

入。饮食蛋白质的影响已经确立。蛋白质摄入增加可增强蛋白质合成[65,72]、减少内源性蛋白质分解[125]，因此增加蛋白质净沉积。非蛋白质能量摄入对蛋白质代谢的影响尚有争议。摄入糖类和脂肪能增强蛋白质沉积[16,34,110,128,147,174]，因而称为蛋白质节约。尽管一些研究提示糖类的蛋白质节约效应比脂肪的强[34,110,174]，但另一些研究结果认为脂肪的蛋白质节约效应与糖类相等或更强[16,128,147]。给新生儿手术患者静脉输注脂肪供能可以减少蛋白质氧化和用于蛋白质的能量消耗而增加蛋白质沉积[128]。为进一步研究这一蛋白质代谢的正效应，我们已利用间接测热法和一种稳定同位素（^{13}C-亮氨酸）示踪剂的技术组合来研究整个蛋白质代谢的各个组分。两组新生儿均接受全肠外营养供给热量和氮源：一组营养配方为高脂肪，另一组营养配方为高糖类[95]。两组间的全身蛋白质代谢组分无显著差异：即蛋白质合成、蛋白质分解、蛋白质氧化和排泄以及蛋白总量无显著差异。这项研究证实了以前的观察，有报道认为，婴儿蛋白质周转率、合成和分解速度高，是成年人的 8 倍。新生儿接受肠外营养者，内源性身体蛋白质的合成和分解远远超过外源性蛋白质的摄入和氧化。婴儿很能保留氮源，而且糖类及脂肪在蛋白质代谢方面具有同等作用。这些研究结果支持在手术新生儿的静脉营养中使用脂肪。

新生儿每天所需的蛋白质量为 2.5～3.0 g/kg。氨基酸，蛋白质的构件成分，可广泛地相互转换，因此有几个氨基酸被认为是可有可无的（或非必需的）：丙氨酸、天冬氨酸、天冬酰胺、谷氨酸和丝氨酸。其他氨基酸则被认为是不可缺少的（或必需的）：组氨酸、异亮氨酸、亮氨酸、赖氨酸、蛋氨酸、苯丙氨酸、苏氨酸、色氨酸和缬氨酸。还有其他一些氨基酸（精氨酸、半胱氨酸、甘氨酸、谷氨酰胺、脯氨酸和酪氨酸）通常情况下不是必需的，但在应激状态（如败血症）的代谢过程中是重要的。含硫氨基酸（半胱氨酸、蛋氨酸）及酪氨酸，在急性期蛋白质中尤为丰富，因此在急性期反应中供给尤为重要。人类母乳以蛋白质和游离氨基酸形式提供氨基酸。奶蛋白质的重要性不仅因为它的营养价值；还因为它们有其他重要特性，如抗感染活性（免疫球蛋白 A、免疫球蛋白 M、免疫球蛋白 G、乳铁蛋白、溶菌酶）[77]。有人认为，人乳中的微量成分——血小板活化因子乙酰水解酶——对母乳的保护作用具有一定作用，可对抗坏死性小肠结肠炎。谷氨酰胺在手术早产儿和新生儿中特别受关注。

全肠外营养的氮源通常是结晶氨基酸的混合物。市面上供应的营养溶液包含八种已知的必需氨基酸加组氨酸，后者是儿童的必需氨基酸[191]。接受静脉高氨基酸的患者会出现一些并发症，如氮质血症、高氨血症和代谢性酸中毒[102]，但氨基酸摄入量为每天 2～3g/kg 者很少出现这些并发症[4]。重症营养不良或额外损失（如空肠、回肠）的患者，其蛋白质需要量更高[191]。对理想的氨基酸溶液的定量组成尚有争议。半胱氨酸、牛磺酸和酪氨酸似乎是新生儿的必需氨基酸。但是，在新生儿肠外营养中添加半胱氨酸其增长率或氮潴留没有差异[190]。这些氨基酸的重要性在于它们与递质、胆盐和激素的合成有关。没有这些氨基酸供给可能导致长期的神经系统或胃肠功能障碍[140]。肠外营养者血浆异常氨基酸谱的发生率低。在新生儿中，还没有令人信服的数据支持哪一种结晶氨基酸溶液优于另外一种。谷氨酰胺是一种具有许多重要生物学功能的氨基酸，如作为免疫系统和肠道的优先燃料。有作者假设，在败血症时，谷氨酰胺有可能成为“有条件的必需”氨基酸，同时给早产儿或手术新生儿的肠外营养中添加谷氨酰胺可能有助于维持黏膜结构、防止细菌定植，因而有可能减少感染发生并缩短建立全肠道内喂养的时间。

应激时的代谢反应

身体已经形成了能够应对各种危及生命的有害刺激的系统。在某些方面，这些反应都是刻板的，可导致所谓的应激反应。应激可被定义为“引起机体出现不平衡状态并因此威胁其稳态的因素”[184]。新生儿应激反应的启动因素包括手术创伤和败血症。本章我们将讨论手术创伤引起的应激反应；败血症引起的生理学变化在第 10 章讨论。

应激反应是由数个信息分子启动和协调的，可影响全身系统。手术创伤的损害可被认为是一种“有控制的”损害，损害结果可改变代谢、炎症、内分泌和免疫反应。这些反应在无医源性干预的情况下演变为损害和感染生存率的提高。它们限制患者损伤范围内的活动性可避免二次损伤，并通过炎症信号的产生开始愈合过程。新陈代谢的变化可使参与组织再生和愈合所需的底物供应增加。为迅速清除任何原因或继发机会性微生物入侵引发的免疫刺激，以及之后的免疫不全麻痹，可削弱这个刺激而使机体随之愈合。

与成人不同，经历大手术的婴儿和儿童其能量需求似乎很少被手术创伤本身改变。成年人外伤或手术后可引起短暂的代谢率降低的“低潮”期，接着是一个“流出”期，特征是耗氧量增加以支持器官之间的大规模物质交换（图 6–9）[87]。新生儿经历重大腹部手术后，其耗氧量和 REE 中度（15%）和即时（高峰期为 4 个小时）升高，并在术后 12～24 小时迅速返回基线水平（见图 6–9）[97]。手术后 5～7 天能量消耗没有进一步增加。据 Anand 等人描述，这些变化出现的时间符合术后儿茶酚胺水平的上升。内分泌及生化的最大变化出现在术后即时，并在之后 24 小时逐步恢复。有趣的是，婴儿在出生后第 2 天接受大手术者其 REE 较之出生头 48 小时内接受手术者有较大幅度的增加。这可能是由于新生儿分泌的内源性阿片。曾有人提出，手术中的疼痛刺激可造成内分泌和代谢方面的应激反应，而阿片可能抑制这些刺激[9,10]。有研究支持以上观点，认为中等剂量的阿片可抑制婴儿手术引起的内分泌和代谢应激反应。新生儿脐带血中的内源性阿片水平高出成年人休息时血浆水平的 5 倍[54]。因此，48 小时龄以内的婴幼儿，血循环中高浓度的内源性阿片有可能减少其代谢应激反应。这可能构成了一种保护机制，可减少围生期的应激反应。

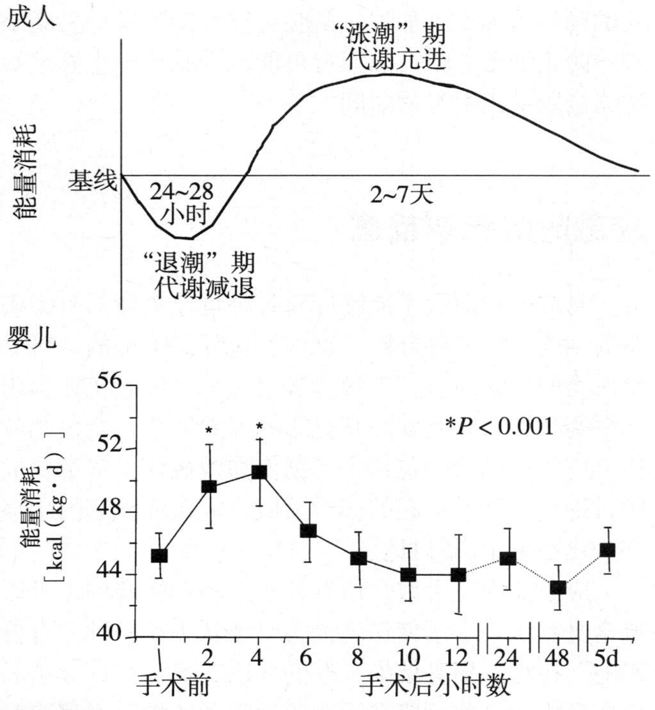

图 6–9 经历大手术后，成人和新生儿的能量消耗变化。婴儿数据用均值 ± SEM 表示。（Adapted from Jones MO, Pierro A, Hammond P, et al: The metabolic response to operative stress in infants. J Pediatr Surg 1993;28:1258-1262; and Pierro A: J Pediatr Surg 2002; 37: 811-822.）

Chwals 等人[38]的研究表明，术后能量消耗增加是由于严重的潜在急性疾病（如败血症、重症炎症）。健康婴儿的 REE 与其生长速度成正比，而急性代谢应激状态下出现生长迟缓。这些作者认为，能量是被用于使婴儿在手术的急性损害反应后恢复生长。他们指出，术后连续测定 REE 可用于损害严重程度分级，并可能是手术后婴儿回归正常生长代谢的有效监测参数。

手术创伤会引发一连串的炎症反应以调节整个机体的手术应激反应，这与损伤后反应类似。化学或激素信号和神经传入信号都可以促发并控制该反应。有些引发这些反应的化学信号可促发与手术创伤有关的细胞损害。

细胞因子

细胞因子是控制和协调对损害的应答的主要的化学传递系统的组成之一。它们是一组低分子量糖肽或糖蛋白，作用是调节局部和全身的免疫功能及调控炎症反应。细胞因子的活性浓度极低，通常在皮克水平，而且它的产生通常是短暂的。细胞因子的作用是改变靶细胞的基因表达。在皮摩尔至纳摩尔浓度范围内，细胞因子的作用方式是旁分泌和自分泌，但如果外溢入循环则可影响全身。 10

细胞因子在体内一般有多种作用。它们通常不储存在细胞内，而必须在适宜的刺激和基因转录下重新合成并被释放到组织中。细胞因子基因调控的一个关键控制因子是核因子 κB[21,89]，它是一种蛋白质转录因子，可提高多种细胞因子基因的执行。淋巴细胞在损伤部位可被激活。首先出现在炎症部位的细胞是单核细胞和中性粒细胞，它们在手术或创伤发生后头几个小时内可产生细胞因子[104]。这些细胞因子是其他白细胞的趋化因子。

根据它们是否刺激免疫系统或抑制免疫反应，细胞因子分为促炎和抗炎两类。虽然大多数细胞因子有明确的促炎或抗炎性，但少数具有双重特性。一些细胞因子在一种特定的细胞中或某些条件下表现出促炎作用，但在不同的细胞中或不同的条件下可能表现出抗炎作用[188]。抗炎因子的产生对抑制免疫反应以防过多组织破坏和死亡有重要意义。天然炎症抑制剂的存在有助于减轻灾难性的正反馈回路，后者可能导致炎症过度引起广泛组织破坏。创伤后释放的细胞因子通常包括促炎的白细胞介素（IL）-1、IL-6 和肿瘤坏死因子（TNF）-α 和抗炎的 IL-1ra 和 IL-10。

手术应激时，促炎和抗炎细胞因子都会产生。实际的细胞因子级联具有异质性，取决于各种因素，包括手术的类型和量级。成年人手术引起的细胞因子级联已有详尽报道，但在新生儿，同类研究有限。细胞因子可与靶器官的特异性膜受体结合。它们在急性应激中的作用包括：（1）改变基因表达和扩增，从而影响伤口愈合和免疫活性；（2）释放反向调节激素；（3）促进细胞之间的信息交通。细胞因子的释放还可影响物质利用。TNF 可使葡萄糖转运增加，IL-1 可刺激肝脏葡萄糖异生，IL-1、IL-6 和 TNF 可刺激肝脏脂肪合成。IL-1 和 TNF 还可促进肌蛋白水解。在新生儿期，大手术后 12 小时，IL-6 增高可达峰值；此增高程度与手术创伤的量级成正比，表明这种细胞因子是新生儿应激反应的标志物。IL-1 和 TNF 可能对损害和感染后产生的代谢反应有协同作用。但是，全身细胞因子释放不能解释损害后产生的所有代谢变化，因为受伤患者的血流中不是始终都有细胞因子存在，而且全身给予细胞因子不能引发所有受伤成人出现的代谢反应。

其他组织损伤反应的介质包括组胺，它是著名的急性炎症化学介质，可引起血管扩张和即时的短暂的血管通透性增加；5-羟色胺（血清素），一种强力血管收缩剂；激活的中性粒细胞、单核细胞和巨噬细胞释放的溶酶体复合物；淋巴因子，炎症级联涉及的具有血管活性作用或趋化特性的化学物质；补体系统；以及激肽系统。这些介质能使血管舒张、增加血管通透性以及白细胞迁移和激活。术后出现的变化也会影响免疫系统。免疫麻痹之后常出现一个免疫激活期。促炎症反应可与抗炎症反应平衡。此平衡往往决定和预示并发症的发展以及发病率和死亡率的结果。

其他反应可由周围和中枢神经系统刺激启动。如来自疼痛受体的周围传出神经可以反馈到中枢神经系统，产生一些临床炎症反应征象以及手术应激后出现的反应。封闭这一传入刺激的确可抑制应激反应。芬太尼和吗啡常用于小儿麻醉止痛。研究表明，早产儿和新生儿应用芬太尼可减轻手术应激产生的代谢反应[9-11]。

内分泌反应

多项研究已描述了婴儿和儿童手术的内分泌反应特点[7,8,73]。这些研究显示，术后反应持续 24～48 小时；成人持续时间较长[20,171]。与一夜禁食所得数值相比，术后早期胰岛素水平有所增加；但是，胰岛素的增高与葡萄糖增加不成比例。术后胰岛素-血糖比值发生了变化，超过 24 小时[8,182]。Anand 等人[8]发现，新生儿术后即时胰岛素-葡萄糖比值先下降，6 小时时恢复。Ward-Platt 等人[182]发现，年长婴儿和儿童术后该比值出现即时和持续的上升。

术后皮质醇明显升高，并持续升高达 24 小时，同时伴有儿茶酚胺升高[75,148]。这两种激素都有抗胰岛素作用。皮质醇和儿茶酚胺上升可局部带动术后高血糖反应，有可能造成术后胰岛素相对不敏感。Anand 等人[8]发现，新生儿腹部手术结束时的葡萄糖与肾上腺素水平明显相关。术后成年人和婴幼儿的乳酸水平都增加[6,9,91]。乳酸水平的提高与葡萄糖代谢变化有关[8]，更与手术引起的低组织灌注相关[91]。乳酸升高的程度可用来判断手术的大小量级。激素水平的变化与手术应激的量级有关，107
并已证实在一些（但不是全部）操作中减弱，如在腹腔镜手术。

新生儿手术对糖代谢的影响

众所周知，成人手术会造成高血糖，新生儿手术后的高血糖反应也有案可查[8-11,23,53,106,133,161]，而高血糖的程度与年龄呈负相关[161]。但是，与成年人术后数天血糖水平持续升高不同，新生儿血糖水平上升短暂，仅持续 12 小时。在一项很好的研究中，Anand 和 Aynsley-Green[7]发现，手术应激程度与血糖升高水平之间存在强相关关系。同一研究显示，应激评分也与血浆肾上腺素、去甲肾上腺素、胰高血糖素和胰岛素水平呈强正相关，而与血皮质醇的相关性稍弱[7]。手术后的高血糖反应可能是多因素的，包括血儿茶酚胺升高以及随后的胰高血糖素升高引起的糖原分解和葡萄糖异生增加。此外，高血糖引发的胰岛素反应可能不适当地较低，尤其是术后的早产儿，且组织对胰岛素的反应相对难以控制。Anand 小组的研究支持这些假设，证明儿茶酚胺释放能促发以上这些结果，他们发现，调整手术麻醉疗程以减少手术引起的儿茶酚胺反应可使术后高血糖和内分泌反应减弱[9-11]。新生儿手术后肾上腺素、去甲肾上腺素和葡萄糖反应时间如图 6-10 所示。

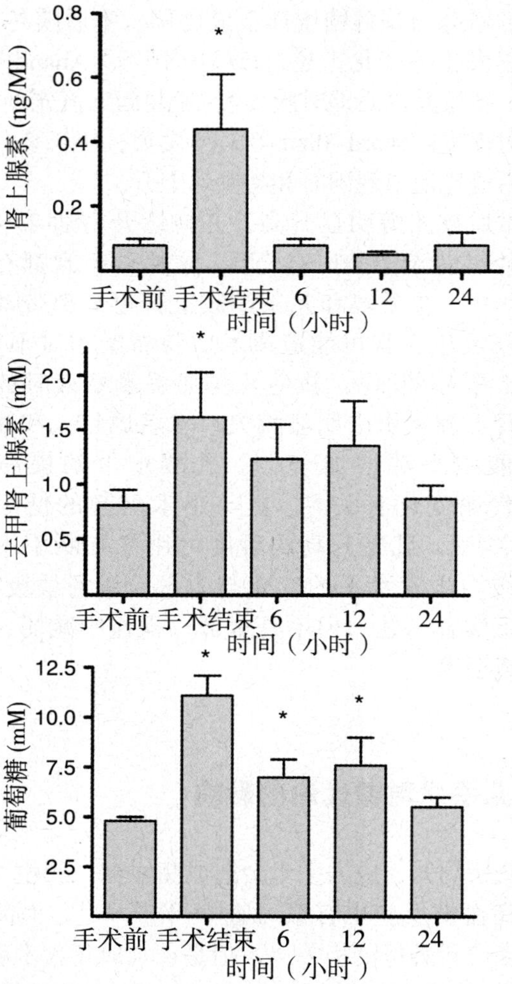

图 6-10　新生儿手术中的肾上腺素、去甲肾上腺素和葡萄糖反应。（Data from Anand KJS, Brown MJ, Causon RC, et al: Can the human neonate mount an endocrine and metabolic response to surgery? J Pediatr Surg 1985;20:41-48.）

葡萄糖摄入量超过代谢所需时，糖类可转化为脂肪（脂肪合成）。与这一过程相关的风险是双重的：新合成的脂肪堆积在肝脏[163]和二氧化碳生成量增加导致呼吸性酸中毒加重，尤其是在肺功能受损的患者[14]。Jones 等人[96]报道，术后接受肠外营养的婴儿，每天以克 / 公斤表示的葡萄糖摄入量与脂肪利用（氧化和转化为脂肪）呈线性负相关（$y = 4.547 - 0.254x$；$r = -0.937$；$P \leq 0.0001$）。据此计算，当葡萄糖摄入量大于每天 18g/kg 时，体内由葡萄糖合成的脂肪超过脂肪氧化。Jones 等人[96]还发现，葡萄糖摄入量与二氧化碳生成量之间明显相关性（$y = 3.849 + 0.183x$；$r = 0.825$；$P \leq 0.0001$）。这一线性相关的斜率在每天葡萄糖摄入量超过 18g/kg（$y = 2.62 + 0.244x$，$r = 0.746$；$P \leq 0.05$）这比在葡萄糖摄入量小于 18g/kg 者（$y = 5.30 + 0.069x$，$r = 0.264$；$P = 0.461$）更陡。因此葡萄糖向脂肪转化造成的二氧化碳生成量增加。葡萄糖摄入量每天超过 18g/kg 还可引起呼吸明显增快和血浆三酰甘油水平显著升高。总之：

1. 葡萄糖摄入是糖类和脂肪利用的主要决定因素。
2. 手术婴儿中，最大的葡萄糖氧化能力是每天 18g/kg，这相当于婴儿的能源消耗。
3. 如果葡萄糖摄入量超出最大氧化能力，则（a）净脂肪氧化停止；（b）净脂肪合成开始；（c）葡萄糖生热效应增加，同时伴有葡萄糖代谢降低；（d）二氧化碳生成量和呼吸速率增加；（e）血浆三酰甘油浓度升高。

因此，建议手术后稳定新生儿的肠外营养的静脉葡萄糖摄入量每天不超过 18g/kg[96,129]。

新生儿手术对脂肪代谢的影响

在新生儿，手术可造成非酯化脂肪酸和酮体浓度
升高[8,9,11,133]，而通过调节儿茶酚胺的释放可以降低它 108
们浓度[9,11]，这提示儿茶酚胺对脂肪分解的刺激作用与其浓度升高有关。Pierro 等人[129]通过静脉输注 4 小时 10% 的脂肪乳剂，之前给予等热量和等容量的葡萄糖和氨基酸混合物，研究了脂肪利用情况。患者的氧耗量和二氧化碳生成以及体内脂肪利用是用间接热量测定法测量气体交换而计算出。研究提示：

（1）手术婴儿可很快（2 小时之内）适应静脉输注脂肪；（2）超过 80%的外源性脂肪能被氧化；（3）输注脂肪时糖类停止向脂肪转化，因而二氧化碳生成减少[129]。这项研究并未测量混合静脉营养（包括糖类、氨基酸和脂肪）的脂肪利用率。最近有关稳定手术新生儿接受固定剂量的糖类和氨基酸以及不同剂量的静脉用长链三酰甘油脂肪乳剂的研究显示，在糖类摄入量达到每天 15g/kg（每天 56.3cal/kg）时，即使脂肪摄入量高达每天 6g/kg，来自脂肪氧化的能量代谢的比例也不超过 20%。在糖类摄取量为每天 10g/kg 时，这一比例可高达 50% [131]。这项研究似乎显示，在术后接受肠外营养的婴儿中，大部分静脉输入的脂肪没有被氧化而被储存起来。新生儿体内的脂肪氧化似乎主要受糖类摄入量和 REE 的影响。当婴儿葡萄糖热卡摄入量超过 REE 时，无论脂肪摄入量为多少，体内脂肪氧化水平最低[131]。因此，要将静脉用脂肪作为能量来源（即氧化为二氧化碳和水），糖类摄入量必须保持在低于基本能量需要水平。

通常用于儿科肠外营养的脂肪乳剂主要是长链三酰甘油（LCT）。理论上，全肠外营养时在静脉营养中加入 L-肉毒碱或中链三酰甘油（MCT）能增快静脉内脂肪氧化的速率。MCT 与 LCT 之间的重要区别在于其生理学和代谢特性。与 LCT 相比，MCT 从血流中清除的速度更快，且氧化产生能量更完全。因此，它们似乎是优先的机体能量来源。我们调查了两组手术后稳定新生儿接受全肠外营养静脉时 MCT 在静脉脂肪利用方面的影响。一组输注以 LCT 为主的脂肪乳剂（100% LCT），另一组输注等热量的以 MCT 为主的脂肪乳剂（50% MCT + 50% LCT）。在接受的糖类热量超过实测的 REE（每天 56 kcal/kg）的婴幼儿，供给以 MCT 为主的脂肪乳剂不会提高其脂肪氧化。相反，摄取的糖类热量低于 REE（每天 41kcal/kg）婴儿，供给以 MCT 为主的脂肪乳剂可增加体内的脂肪氧化，从每天 0.6 ± 0.2g/kg 上升到 1.7 ± 0.2g/kg。给予以 MCT 为主的脂肪乳剂不会增加婴儿代谢率。脂肪不被利用可成为游离脂质过氧化反应和自由基生成的底物。过氧化反应与肠外营养中的脂质有特别关联[18,186]，并已证实依赖于糖类的摄入量：如果因为糖类摄入量高使体内不发生脂肪氧化，则更多脂质会出现过氧化反应。

新生儿手术对蛋白质和氨基酸代谢的影响

在成人中，大部分手术应激可造成肌肉蛋白分解而引起负氮平衡。在新生儿，氮平衡已经处于一种极不稳定的状态，所以如果发生大部分蛋白质分解，其生长和其他重要功能就会受损。新生儿术后氮丢失会增加[39,90,151,189]，而且肌肉蛋白的分解已为 3-甲基组氨酸排泄增加所证实。但是，以上变化比较短暂，并能通过提供额外饮食氮源或热卡而缓解。Powis 等人[136]研究了经历大手术的婴儿和幼儿的蛋白质代谢动力学。患者观察时段设在术前 4 小时和术后头 6 小时。研究发现，术前和术后的全身蛋白质流出、蛋白质合成、氨基酸氧化和蛋白降解无显著差异，显示婴儿和儿童在接受大手术后全身的蛋白质转换没有增加。这可能是婴儿和儿童能够将用于生长的能量转化到用于创伤修复和愈合，从而可避免出现像成人一样的能量消耗和分解代谢的全面增加。迄今，有关新生儿的蛋白质转换的成分知之甚少。唯一一项有价值的研究是对 6 名罹患坏死性小肠结肠炎的新生儿的研究，结果显示，在疾病急性期和恢复期，蛋白质转换是无差别的[137]。

（李　菁译　黄　萍校）

参考文献

1. Acheson KJ, Schutz Y, Bessard T, et al: Nutritional influences on lipogenesis and thermogenesis after a carbohydrate meal. Am J Physiol 1984;246:E62-E70.
2. Albanese CT, Nour BM, Rowe MI: Anesthesia blocks non-shivering thermogenesis in the neonatal rabbit. J Pediatr Surg 1994;29:983-986.
3. Alroomi L, Barclay S, Beattie J, et al: CRIB (Clinical Risk Index for Babies), mortality, and impairment after neonatal intensive-care. Lancet 1995;345:1020-1022.
4. American Academy of Pediatrics Committee on Nutrition: Commentary on parenteral nutrition. Pediatrics 1983;71: 547-552.
5. American Academy of Pediatrics Committee on Nutrition: Hypoglycemia in infants and children. In Kleinman RE (ed): Pediatric Nutrition Handbook, 5th ed. Elk Grove, IL, American Academy of Pediatrics, 2004, pp 515-535.
6. Anand KJS: Neonatal stress responses to anesthesia and surgery. Clin Perinatol 1990;17:207-214.
7. Anand KJS, Aynsley-Green A: Measuring the severity of surgical stress in newborn infants. J Pediatr Surg 1988;23: 297-305.

8. Anand KJS, Brown MJ, Causon RC, et al: Can the human neonate mount an endocrine and metabolic response to surgery? J Pediatr Surg 1985;20:41-48.
9. Anand KJS, Hickey PR: Halothane-morphine compared with high-dose sufentanil for anesthesia and postoperative analgesia in neonatal cardiac surgery. N Engl J Med 1992;326:1-9.
10. Anand KJS, Sippell WG, Aynsley-Green A: Randomised trial of fentanyl anaesthesia in preterm babies undergoing surgery: Effects on the stress response. Lancet 1987;1:62-66.
11. Anand KJS, Sippell WG, Schofield NM, et al: Does halothane anaesthesia decrease the metabolic and endocrine stress responses of newborn infants undergoing operation? BMJ 1988;296:668-672.
12. Antonelli M, Moreno R, Vincent JL, et al: Application of SOFA score to trauma patients: Sequential Organ Failure Assessment. Intensive Care Med 1999;25:389-394.
13. Ashworth A, Bell R, James WP, et al: Calorie requirements of children recovering from protein-calorie malnutrition. Lancet 1968;2:600-603.
14. Askanazi J, Nordenstrom J, Rosenbaum SH, et al: Nutrition for the patient with respiratory failure: Glucose vs fat. Anesthesiology 1981;54:373-377.
15. Ballard JL, Khoury JC, Wedig K, et al: New Ballard score, expanded to include extremely premature infants. J Pediatr 1991;119:417-423.
16. Bark S, Holm I, Hakansson I, et al: Nitrogen-sparing effect of fat emulsion compared with glucose in the postoperative period. Acta Chir Scand 1976;142:423-427.
17. Basu R, Muller DPR, Eaton S, et al: Lipid peroxidation can be reduced in infants on total parenteral nutrition by promoting fat utilisation. J Pediatr Surg 1999;34:255-259.
18. Basu R, Muller DPR, Papp E, et al: Free radical formation in infants: The effect of critical illness, parenteral nutrition, and enteral feeding. J Pediatr Surg 1999;34:1091-1095.
19. Bekesi A , Williamson DH: An explanation for ketogenesis by the intestine of the suckling rat—the presence of an active hydroxymethylglutaryl-coenzyme-A pathway. Biol Neonate 1990;58:160-165.
20. Bellon JM, Manzano L, Larrad A, et al: Endocrine and immune response to injury after open and laparoscopic cholecystectomy. Int Surg 1998;83:24-27.
21. Blackwell TS, Christman JW: The role of nuclear factor-kappa B in cytokine gene regulation. Am J Respir Cell Mol Biol 1997;17:3-9.
22. Bougneres PF, Lemmel C, Ferre P, et al: Ketone-body transport in the human neonate and infant. J Clin Invest 1986;77:42-48.
23. Bouwmeester NJ, Anand KJS, van Dijk M, et al: Hormonal and metabolic stress responses after major surgery in children aged 0-3 years: A double-blind, randomized trial comparing the effects of continuous versus intermittent morphine. Br J Anaesth 2001;87:390-399.
24. Brace RA: Physiology of amniotic fluid volume regulation. Clin Obstet Gynecol 1997;40:280-289.
25. Brand MD: The proton leak across the mitochondrial inner membrane. Biochim Biophys Acta 1990;1018:128-133.
26. Brand MD, Chien LF, Ainscow EK, et al: The causes and functions of mitochondrial proton leak. Biochim Biophys Acta 1994;1187:132-139.
27. Brooke OG, Ashworth A: The influence of malnutrition on the postprandial metabolic rate and respiratory quotient. Br J Nutr 1972;27:407-415.
28. Bruck K: Temperature regulation in the newborn infant. Biol Neonate 1961;3:65-119.
29. Bruck K, Parmlee AH, Bruck M: Neutral temperature range and range of "thermal comfort" in premature infants. Biol Neonate 1962;4:32-51.
30. Burchell A, Gibb L, Waddell ID, et al: The ontogeny of human hepatic microsomal glucose-6-phosphatase proteins. Clin Chem 1990;36:1633-1637.
31. Cannon B, Nedergaard J: Brown adipose tissue: Function and physiological significance. Physiol Rev 2004;84:277-359.
32. Casey PH, Kraemer HC, Bernbaum J, et al: Growth patterns of low birth weight preterm infants: A longitudinal analysis of a large, varied sample. J Pediatr 1990;117: 298-307.
33. Catzeflis C, Schutz Y, Micheli JL, et al: Whole-body protein-synthesis and energy-expenditure in very low birth-weight infants. Pediatr Res 1985;19:679-687.
34. Chessex P, Gagne G, Pineault M, et al: Metabolic and clinical consequences of changing from high-glucose to high-fat regimens in parenterally fed newborn-infants. J Pediatr 1989;115:992-997.
35. Chessex P, Reichman BL, Verellen GJ, et al: Influence of postnatal age, energy intake, and weight gain on energy metabolism in the very low-birth-weight infant. J Pediatr 1981;99:761-766.
36. Chessex P, Reichman B, Verellen G, et al: Metabolic consequences of intrauterine growth retardation in very low birthweight infants. Pediatr Res 1984;18:709-713.
37. Chwals WJ: The newborn as a surgical patient: Metabolic considerations. In O'Neill JA Jr, Rowe MI, Grosfeld JL, et al (eds): Pediatric Surgery, 5th ed. St Louis, Mosby-Year Book, 1998, pp 57-70.
38. Chwals WJ, Letton RW, Jamie A, et al: Stratification of injury severity using energy-expenditure response in surgical infants. J Pediatr Surg 1995;30:1161-1164.
39. Colle E, Paulsen EP: Response of the newborn infant to major surgery. 1. Effects on water, electrolyte, and nitrogen balances. Pediatrics 1959;23:1063-1084.
40. Coran AG: Nutrition of the surgical patient. In Welch KJ, Randolph JG, Reed DJ (eds): Pediatric Surgery. Chicago, Year Book, 1986, pp 96-108.
41. Coran AG, Pierro A, Schmeling DJ: Metabolism of the neonate requiring surgery. In Cowett RM (ed): Principles of Perinatal-Neonatal Metabolism, 2nd ed. New York, Springer, 1998, pp 1131-1151.
42. Cornblath M, Hawdon JM, Williams AF, et al: Controversies regarding definition of neonatal hypoglycemia: Suggested operational thresholds. Pediatrics 2000;105:1141-1145.
43. Cowett RM, Farrag HM: Neonatal glucose metabolism. In Cowett RM (ed): Principles of Perinatal-Neonatal Metabolism, 2nd ed. New York, Springer, 1998, pp 683-722.
44. Cruickshank AM, Fraser WD, Burns HJ, et al: Response of serum interleukin-6 in patients undergoing elective surgery of varying severity. Clin Sci (Colch) 1990;79:161-165.
45. Cullingford TE, Dolphin CT, Bhakoo KK, et al: Molecular cloning of rat mitochondrial 3-hydroxy-3-methylglutaryl-CoA lyase and detection of the corresponding mRNA and of those encoding the remaining enzymes comprising the ketogenic 3-hydroxy-3-methylglutaryl-CoA cycle in central nervous system of suckling rat. Biochem J 1998;329:373-381.
46. Cunningham JJ: Body composition as a determinant of energy expenditure: A synthetic review and a proposed general prediction equation. Am J Clin Nutr 1991;54:963-969.
47. Deboissieu D, Rocchiccioli F, Kalach N, et al: Ketone-body turnover at term and in premature newborns in the first 2 weeks after birth. Biol Neonate 1995;67:84-93.
48. Demissie K, Rhoads GG, Ananth CV, et al: Trends in preterm birth and neonatal mortality among blacks and whites in the United States from 1989 to 1997. Am J Epidemiol 2001;154:307-315.
49. Disturbances in newborns and infants. In Beers MF, Berkow R (eds): The Merck Manual of Diagnosis and Therapy, 17th ed. White House Station, NJ, Merck Research Laboratories, 1999, pp 2127-2145.

50. Donnell SC, Lloyd DA, Eaton S, et al: The metabolic response to intravenous medium-chain triglycerides in infants after surgery. J Pediatr 2002;141:689-694.
51. Duvanel CB, Fawer CL, Cotting J, et al: Long-term effects of neonatal hypoglycemia on brain growth and psychomotor development in small-for-gestational-age preterm infants. J Pediatr 1999;134:492-498.
52. Eaton S: Control of mitochondrial β-oxidation flux. Prog Lipid Res 2002;41:197-239.
53. Elphick MC, Wilkinson AW: The effects of starvation and surgical injury on the plasma levels of glucose, free fatty acids, and neutral lipids in newborn babies suffering from various congenital anomalies. Pediatr Res 1981;15:313-318.
54. Facchinetti F, Bagnoli F, Bracci R, et al: Plasma opioids in the first hours of life. Pediatr Res 1982;16:95-98.
55. Fielding BA, Frayn KN: Lipoprotein lipase and the disposition of dietary fatty acids. Br J Nutr 1998;80:495-502.
56. Fomon SJ: Body composition of male reference infant during first year of life—Borden Award address, October 1966. Pediatrics 1967;40:863-870.
57. Fomon SJ, Nelson SE: Body composition of the male and female reference infants. Annu Rev Nutr 2002;22:1-17.
58. Frazer TE, Karl IE, Hillman LS, et al: Direct measurement of gluconeogenesis from [2,3-C-13(2)]alanine in the human neonate. Am J Physiol 1981;240:E615-E621.
59. Freymond D, Schutz Y, Decombaz J, et al: Energy-balance, physical-activity, and thermogenic effect of feeding in premature-infants. Pediatr Res 1986;20:638-645.
60. Friis-Hansen B: Body water compartments in children: Changes during growth and related changes in body composition. Pediatrics 1961;28:169-181.
61. Friis-Hansen B: Water distribution in the foetus and newborn infant. Acta Paediatr Scand Suppl 1983;305:7-11.
62. Fukao T, Song XQ, Mitchell GA, et al: Enzymes of ketone body utilization in human tissues: Protein and messenger RNA levels of succinyl-coenzyme A (CoA), 3-ketoacid CoA transferase and mitochondrial and cytosolic acetoacetyl-CoA thiolases. Pediatr Res 1997;42:498-502.
63. Gagliardi L, Cavazza A, Brunelli A, et al: Assessing mortality risk in very low birthweight infants: A comparison of CRIB, CRIB-II, and SNAPPE-II. Arch Dis Child 2004;89: F419-F422.
64. Gardner RJ, Mungall AJ, Dunham I, et al: Localisation of a gene for transient neonatal diabetes mellitus to an 18.72 cR(3000) (similar to 5.4 Mb) interval on chromosome 6q. J Med Genet 1999;36:192-196.
65. Garlick PJ, Clugston GA, Swick RW, et al: Diurnal pattern of protein and energy metabolism in man. Am J Clin Nutr 1980;33:1983-1986.
66. Gibson AT, Carney S, Cavazzoni E, et al: Neonatal and postnatal growth. Horm Res 2000;53(Suppl 1):S42-S49.
67. Gilbert WM , Brace RA: Amniotic fluid volume and normal flows to and from the amniotic cavity. Semin Perinatol 1993;17:150-157.
68. Gill A, Yu VY, Bajuk B, et al: Postnatal growth in infants born before 30 weeks' gestation. Arch Dis Child 1986;61: 549-553.
69. Girard J, Ferré P, Pégorier J-P, et al: Adaptations of glucose and fatty-acid metabolism during perinatal-period and suckling-weaning transition. Physiol Rev 1992;72:507-562.
70. Gloyn AL, Pearson ER, Antcliff JF, et al: Activating mutations in the gene encoding the ATP-sensitive potassium-channel subunit Kir6.2 and permanent neonatal diabetes. N Engl J Med 2004;350:1838-1849.
71. Goldberg IJ: Lipoprotein lipase and lipolysis: Central roles in lipoprotein metabolism and atherogenesis. J Lipid Res 1996;37:693-707.
72. Golden M, Waterlow JC, Picou D: The relationship between dietary intake, weight change, nitrogen balance, and protein turnover in man. Am J Clin Nutr 1977;30:1345-1348.
73. Gruber EM, Laussen PC, Casta A, et al: Stress response in infants undergoing cardiac surgery: A randomized study of fentanyl bolus, fentanyl infusion, and fentanyl-midazolam infusion. Anesth Analg 2001;92:882-890.
74. Gudinchet F, Schutz Y, Micheli J-L, et al: Metabolic cost of growth in very-low birthweight infants. Pediatr Res 1992;16:1025-1030.
75. Hakanson E, Rutberg H, Jorfeldt L, et al: Endocrine and metabolic responses after standardized moderate surgical trauma: Influence of age and sex. Clin Physiol 1984;4: 461-473.
76. Hall NJ, Peters M, Eaton S, et al: Hyperglycemia is associated with increased morbidity and mortality rates in neonates with necrotizing enterocolitis. J Pediatr Surg 2004;39:898-901.
77. Hamosh M: Human milk composition and function in the infant. In Polin RA, Fox WW, Abman SH (eds): Fetal and Neonatal Physiology, 3rd ed. Philadelphia, WB Saunders, 2004, pp 275-284.
78. Hartnoll G, Betremieux P, Modi N: Body water content of extremely preterm infants at birth. Arch Dis Child Fetal Neonatal Ed 2000;83:F56-F59.
79. Hawdon JM: Hypoglycaemia and the neonatal brain. Eur J Pediatr 1999;158:S9-S12.
80. Hawdon JM, Aynsley-Green A: Disorders of blood glucose homoeostasis in the neonate. In Rennie JM, Roberton NRC (eds): Textbook of Neonatology. Edinburgh, Churchill Livingstone, 1999, pp 939-956.
81. Hawdon JM, Aynsley-Green A, Alberti K, et al: The role of pancreatic insulin-secretion in neonatal glucoregulation. 1. Healthy term and preterm infants. Arch Dis Child 1993; 68:274-279.
82. Hawdon JM, Aynsley-Green A, Bartlett K, et al: The role of pancreatic insulin-secretion in neonatal glucoregulation. 2. Infants with disordered blood-glucose homeostasis. Arch Dis Child 1993;68:280-285.
83. Hawdon JM, Ward-Platt MP: Metabolic adaptation in small-for-gestational-age infants. Arch Dis Child 1993;68:262-268.
84. Hawdon JM, Ward-Platt MP, Aynsley-Green A: Patterns of metabolic adaptation for preterm and term infants in the 1st neonatal week. Arch Dis Child 1992;67:357-365.
85. Heim T: Homeothermy and its metabolic cost. In Davis JA, Dobbing J (eds): Scientific Foundations of Paediatrics. London, Heinemann, 1981, pp 91-128.
86. Hey EN, Katz G: The optimum thermal environment for naked babies. Arch Dis Child 1970;45:328-334.
87. Hill AG, Hill GL: Metabolic response to severe injury. Br J Surg 1998;85:884-890.
88. Hofman MA: Energy metabolism and relative brain size in human neonates from single and multiple gestations: An allometric study. Biol Neonate 1984;45:157-164.
89. Holmes-McNary M: Nuclear factor kappa B signaling in catabolic disorders. Curr Opin Clin Nutr Metab Care 2002;5:255-263.
90. Hughes EA, Stevens LH, Toms DA, Wilkinson AW: Oesophageal atresia: Metabolic effects of operation. Br J Surg 1965;52:403-410.
91. Ishida H, Murata N, Yamada H, et al: Effect of CO_2 pneumoperitoneum on growth of liver micrometastases in a rabbit model. World J Surg 2000;24:1004-1008.
92. Jain L: Alveolar fluid clearance in developing lungs and its role in neonatal transition. Clin Perinatol 1999;26: 585-599.

93. Jansky L: Non-shivering thermogenesis and its thermoregulatory significance. Biol Rev Camb Philos Soc 1973;48:85-132.
94. Jequier E: The influence of nutrient administration on energy-expenditure in man. Clin Nutr 1986;5:181-186.
95. Jones MO, Pierro A, Garlick PJ, et al: Protein metabolism kinetics in neonates: Effect of intravenous carbohydrate and fat. J Pediatr Surg 1995;30:458-462.
96. Jones MO, Pierro A, Hammond P, et al: Glucose utilization in the surgical newborn infant receiving total parenteral nutrition. J Pediatr Surg 1993;28:1121-1125.
97. Jones MO, Pierro A, Hammond P, et al: The metabolic response to operative stress in infants. J Pediatr Surg 1993;28:1258-1262.
98. Jones MO, Pierro A, Hashim IA, et al: Postoperative changes in resting energy-expenditure and interleukin-6 level in infants. Br J Surg 1994;81:536-538.
99. Kalache KD, Chaoui R, Marks B, et al: Does fetal tracheal fluid flow during fetal breathing movements change before the onset of labour? Br J Obstet Gynaecol 2002;109:514-519.
100. Kalhan SC: Metabolism of glucose and methods of investigation in the fetus and newborn. In Polin RA, Fox WW, Abman SH (eds): Fetal and Neonatal Physiology, 3rd ed. Philadelphia, WB Saunders, 2004, pp 449-464.
101. Kalhan SC, Parimi P, Van Beek R, et al: Estimation of gluconeogenesis in newborn infants. Am J Physiol Endocrinol Metab 2001;281:E991-E997.
102. Kerner JA: Carbohydrate requirements. In Kerner JA (ed): Manual of Pediatric Parenteral Nutrition. New York, Wiley, 1983, pp 79-88.
103. Koh THHG, Aynsley-Green A, Tarbit M, et al: Neural dysfunction during hypoglycaemia. Arch Dis Child 1988; 63:1353-1358.
104. Kondo T, Ohshima T, Mori R, et al: Immunohistochemical detection of chemokines in human skin wounds and its application to wound age determination. Int J Legal Med 2002;116:87-91.
105. Kurz A, Sessler DI, Lenhardt R: Perioperative normothermia to reduce the incidence of surgical-wound infection and shorten hospitalization: Study of Wound Infection and Temperature Group. N Engl J Med 1996;334:1209-1215.
106. Larsson LE, Nilsson K, Niklasson A, et al: Influence of fluid regimens on perioperative blood-glucose concentrations in neonates. Br J Anaesth 1990;64:419-424.
107. Latal-Hajnal B, von Siebenthal K, Kovari H, et al: Postnatal growth in VLBW infants: Significant association with neurodevelopmental outcome. J Pediatr 2003;143:163-170.
108. Laudy JA, Wladimiroff JW: The fetal lung. 1. Developmental aspects. Ultrasound Obstet Gynecol 2000;16:284-290.
109. Livesey G, Elia M: Estimation of energy expenditure, net carbohydrate utilization, and net fat oxidation and synthesis by indirect calorimetry: Evaluation of errors with special reference to the detailed composition of fuels. Am J Clin Nutr 1988;47:608-628.
110. Long JM, Wilmore DW, Mason AD, et al: Effect of carbohydrate and fat intake on nitrogen excretion during total intravenous feeding. Ann Surg 1977;185:417-422.
111. Lucas A, Morley R, Cole TJ: Adverse neurodevelopmental outcome of moderate neonatal hypoglycaemia. BMJ 1988;297:1304-1308.
112. Ma D, Shield JPH, Dean W, et al: Impaired glucose homeostasis in transgenic mice expressing the human transient neonatal diabetes mellitus locus, TNDM. J Clin Invest 2004;114:339-348.
113. Menni F, de Lonlay P, Sevin C, et al: Neurologic outcomes of 90 neonates and infants with persistent hyperinsulinemic hypoglycemia. Pediatrics 2001;107:476-479.
114. Merklin RJ: Growth and distribution of human fetal brown fat. Anat Rec 1974;178:637-645.
115. Micheli JL, Schutz Y: Protein metabolism and postnatal growth in very low birthweight infants. Biol Neonate 1987;52(Suppl 1):S25-S40.
116. Modi N, Betremieux P, Midgley J, et al: Postnatal weight loss and contraction of the extracellular compartment is triggered by atrial natriuretic peptide. Early Hum Dev 2000;59:201-208.
117. Montgomery RD: Changes in the basal metabolic rate of the malnourished infant and their relation to body composition. J Clin Invest 1962;41:1653-1663.
118. Moreno R, Vincent JL, Matos R, et al: The use of maximum SOFA score to quantify organ dysfunction/failure in intensive care: Results of a prospective, multicentre study. Working Group on Sepsis Related Problems of the ESICM. Intensive Care Med 1999;25:686-696.
119. Novak M, Melichar V, Hahn P: Postnatal changes in blood serum content of glycerol and fatty acids in human infants. Biologia Neonatorum 1964;7:179-184.
120. Ogata ES: Carbohydrate homeostasis. In Avery GB, Fletcher MA, MacDonald MG (eds): Neonatology: Pathophysiology and Management of the Newborn, 5th ed. Philadelphia, Lippincott Williams & Wilkins, 1999, pp 699-714.
121. Ohlson KB, Mohell N, Cannon B, et al: Thermogenesis in brown adipocytes is inhibited by volatile anesthetic agents: A factor contributing to hypothermia in infants? Anesthesiology 1994;81:176-183.
122. Okada Y, Powis M, Mcewan A, et al: Fentanyl analgesia increases the incidence of postoperative hypothermia in neonates. Pediatr Surg Int 1998;13:508-511.
123. Page MA, Williams DH: Enzymes of ketone-body utilisation in human brain. Lancet 1971;2:66-68.
124. Patel MS, Johnson CA, Rajan R, et al: Metabolism of ketone-bodies in developing human brain—development of ketone-body-utilizing enzymes and ketone-bodies as precursors for lipid-synthesis. J Neurochem 1975;25:905-908.
125. Pencharz PB, Masson M, Desgranges F, et al: Total-body protein-turnover in human premature neonates—effects of birth-weight, intrauterine nutritional-status and diet. Clin Sci 1981;61:207-215.
126. Persson B: Determination of plasma acetoacetate and D-beta-hydroxybutyrate in new-born infants by an enzymatic fluorometric micro-method. Scand J Clin Lab Invest 1970;25:9-18.
127. Persson B, Gentz J: Pattern of blood lipids, glycerol and ketone bodies during neonatal period, infancy and childhood. Acta Paediatr Scand 1966;55:353-362.
128. Pierro A, Carnielli V, Filler RM, et al: Characteristics of protein sparing effect of total parenteral nutrition in the surgical infant. J Pediatr Surg 1988;23:538-542.
129. Pierro A, Carnielli V, Filler RM, et al: Metabolism of intravenous fat emulsion in the surgical newborn. J Pediatr Surg 1989;24:95-101.
130. Pierro A, Carnielli V, Filler RM, et al: Partition of energy metabolism in the surgical newborn. J Pediatr Surg 1991; 26:581-586.
131. Pierro A, Jones MO, Hammond P, et al: Utilisation of intravenous fat in the surgical newborn infant. Proc Nutr Soc 1993;52:237A.
132. Pierro A, Jones MO, Hammond P, et al: A new equation to predict the resting energy expenditure of surgical infants. J Pediatr Surg 1994;29:1103-1108.

133. Pinter A: Metabolic effects of anesthesia and surgery in newborn infant—changes in blood levels of glucose, plasma free fatty-acids, alpha-amino-nitrogen, plasma amino-acid ratio and lactate in neonate. Z Kinder Grenzgebiete 1973; 12:149-162.
134. Pittet P, Gygax PH, Jequier E: Thermic effect of glucose and amino acids in man studied by direct and indirect calorimetry Br J Nutr 1974;31:343-349.
135. Porter RK, Brand MD: Body-mass dependence of H^+ leak in mitochondria and its relevance to metabolic-rate. Nature 1993;362:628-630.
136. Powis MR, Smith K, Rennie M, et al: Effect of major abdominal operations on energy and protein metabolism in infants and children. J Pediatr Surg 1998;33:49-53.
137. Powis MR, Smith K, Rennie M, et al: Characteristics of protein and energy metabolism in neonates with necrotizing enterocolitis—a pilot study. J Pediatr Surg 1999;34:5-10.
138. Putet G: Lipids as an energy source for the premature and full-term neonate. In Polin RA, Fox WW, Abman SH (eds): Fetal and Neonatal Physiology, 3rd ed. Philadelphia, WB Saunders, 2004, pp 415-418.
139. Quant PA, Robin D, Robin P, et al: Control of hepatic mitochondrial 3-hydroxy-3-methylglutaryl-CoA synthase during the fetal neonatal transition, suckling and weaning in the rat. Eur J Biochem 1991;195:449-454.
140. Rassin DK: Amino acid requirements and profiles in total parenteral nutrition. In Lebenthal E (ed): Total Parenteral Nutrition: Indications, Utilization, Complications, and Pathophysiological Considerations. New York, Raven Press, 1986, pp 5-15.
141. Rautonen J, Makela A, Boyd H, et al: CRIB and SNAP: Assessing the risk of death for preterm neonates. Lancet 1994;343:1272-1273.
142. Reber KM, Nankervis CA: Necrotizing enterocolitis: Preventative strategies. Clin Perinatol 2004;31:157-167.
143. Reichman BL, Chessex P, Putet G, et al: Partition of energy metabolism and energy cost of growth in the very low-birth-weight infant. Pediatrics 1982;69:446-451.
144. Rolfe DF, Brand MD: The physiological significance of mitochondrial proton leak in animal cells and tissues. Biosci Rep 1997;17:9-16.
145. Rolfe DF, Hulbert AJ, Brand MD: Characteristics of mitochondrial proton leak and control of oxidative phosphorylation in the major oxygen-consuming tissues of the rat. Biochim Biophys Acta 1994;1188:405-416.
146. Rosenkrantz TS: Polycythemia and hyperviscosity in the newborn. Semin Thromb Hemost 2003;29:515-527.
147. Rubecz I, Mestyan J, Varga P, et al: Energy metabolism, substrate utilization, and nitrogen balance in parenterally fed postoperative neonates and infants: The effect of glucose, glucose + amino acids, lipid + amino acids infused in isocaloric amounts. J Pediatr 1981;98:42-46.
148. Rutberg H, Hakanson E, Anderberg B, et al: Effects of the extradural administration of morphine, or bupivacaine, on the endocrine response to upper abdominal surgery. Br J Anaesth 1984;56:233-238.
149. Rutter N, Brown SM, Hull D: Variations in the resting oxygen consumption of small babies. Arch Dis Child 1978; 53:850-854.
150. Salomon JW, Swyer PR, Jequier E: Thermic effects of glucose, amino acid and lipid in the term newborn. Biol Neonate 1979;35:8-16.
151. Schmeling DJ, Coran AG: The hormonal and metabolic response to stress in the neonate. Pediatr Surg Int 1990;5:307-321.
152. Sellden E, Brundin T, Wahren J: Augmented thermal effect of amino-acids under general-anesthesia—a mechanism useful for prevention of anesthesia-induced hypothermia. Clin Sci 1994;86:611-618.
153. Senterre J, Karlberg P: Respiratory quotient and metabolic rate in normal full-term and small-for-date newborn infants. Acta Paediatr Scand 1970;59:653-658.
154. Shanbhogue RLK, Lloyd DA: Absence of hypermetabolism after operation in the newborn- infant. JPEN J Parenter Enteral Nutr 1992;16:333-336.
155. Sherer DM: A review of amniotic fluid dynamics and the enigma of isolated oligohydramnios. Am J Perinatol 2002;19:253-266.
156. Shield JP, Gardner RJ, Wadsworth EJ, et al: Aetiopathology and genetic basis of neonatal diabetes. Arch Dis Child Fetal Neonatal Ed 1997;76:F39-F42.
157. Sinclair JC: Heat production and thermoregulation in the small-for-date infant. Pediatr Clin North Am 1970;17: 147-158.
158. Singhal A, Lucas A: Early origins of cardiovascular disease: Is there a unifying hypothesis? Lancet 2004;363:1642-1645.
159. Snyderman SE, Boyer A, Kogut MD, et al: The protein requirement of the premature infant. I. The effect of protein intake on the retention of nitrogen. J Pediatr 1969;74:872-880.
160. Sperling MA, DeLamater PV, Phelps D, et al: Spontaneous and amino acid-stimulated glucagon secretion in the immediate postnatal period: Relation to glucose and insulin. J Clin Invest 1974;53:1159-1166.
161. Srinivasan G, Jain R, Pildes RS, et al: Glucose-homeostasis during anesthesia and surgery in infants. J Pediatr Surg 1986;21:718-721.
162. Srinivasan V, Spinella PC, Drott HR, et al: Association of timing, duration, and intensity of hyperglycemia with intensive care unit mortality in critically ill children. Pediatr Crit Care Med 2004;5:329-336.
163. Stein TP: Why measure the respiratory quotient of patients on total parenteral nutrition? J Am Coll Nutr 1985;4:501-513.
164. Stenninger E, Flink R, Eriksson B, et al: Long term, neurological dysfunction and neonatal hypoglycaemia after diabetic pregnancy. Arch Dis Child 1998;79:F174-F179.
165. Styne DM: Endocrine factors affecting neonatal growth. In Polin RA, Fox WW, Abman SH (eds): Fetal and Neonatal Physiology, 3rd ed. Philadelphia, WB Saunders, 2004, pp 266-275.
166. Sunehag AL: Parenteral glycerol enhances gluconeogenesis in very premature infants. Pediatr Res 2003;53:635-641.
167. Sunehag AL: The role of parenteral lipids in supporting gluconeogenesis in very premature infants. Pediatr Res 2003;54:480-486.
168. Sunehag AL, Haymond MW: Glucose extremes in newborn infants. Clin Perinatol 2002;29:245-260.
169. Sunehag AL, Haymond MW, Schanler RJ, et al: Gluconeogenesis in very low birth weight infants receiving total parenteral nutrition. Diabetes 1999;48:791-800.
170. Teitelbaum DH, Coran AG: Perioperative nutritional support in pediatrics. Nutrition 1998;14:130-142.
171. Thorell A, Efendic S, Gutniak M, et al: Insulin resistance after abdominal surgery. Br J Surg 1994;81:59-63.
172. Thumelin S, Forestier M, Girard J, et al: Developmental-changes in mitochondrial 3-hydroxy-3-methylglutaryl-CoA synthase gene-expression in rat-liver, intestine and kidney. Biochem J 1993;292:493-496.
173. Thumelin S, Kohl C, Girard J, et al: Atypical expression of mitochondrial 3-hydroxy-3-methylglutaryl-CoA synthase in subcutaneous adipose tissue of male rats. J Lipid Res 1999;40:1071-1077.
174. Tulikoura I , Huikuri K: Changes in nitrogen metabolism in catabolic patients given three different parenteral nutrition regimens. Acta Chir Scand 1981;147:519-524.
175. Valcarce C, Vitorica J, Satrustegui J, et al: Rapid postnatal developmental changes in the passive proton permeability

of the inner membrane in rat-liver mitochondria. J Biochem 1990;108:642-645.
176. Van den Berghe G, Wouters P, Weekers F, et al: Intensive insulin therapy in critically ill patients. N Engl J Med 2001;345:1359-1367.
177. van Kempen AA, Romijn JA, Ruiter AF, et al: Adaptation of glucose production and gluconeogenesis to diminishing glucose infusion in preterm infants at varying gestational ages. Pediatr Res 2003;53:628-634.
178. van Kempen AA, Romijn JA, Ruiter AF, et al: Alanine administration does not stimulate gluconeogenesis in preterm infants. Metabolism 2003;52:945-949.
179. Vincent JL, De Mendonca A, Cantraine F, et al: Use of the SOFA score to assess the incidence of organ dysfunction/failure in intensive care units: Results of a multicenter, prospective study. Working Group on Sepsis-Related Problems of the European Society of Intensive Care Medicine. Crit Care Med 1998;26:1793-1800.
180. Vincent JL, Moreno R, Takala J et al: The SOFA (Sepsis-Related Organ Failure Assessment) score to describe organ dysfunction/failure. On behalf of the Working Group on Sepsis-Related Problems of the European Society of Intensive Care Medicine. Intensive Care Med 1996;22:707-710.
181. Vonmuhlendahl E, Herkenhoff H: Long-term course of neonatal diabetes. N Engl J Med 1995;333:704-708.
182. Ward-Platt MP, Tarbit MJ, Aynsley-Green A: The effects of anesthesia and surgery on metabolic homeostasis in infancy and childhood. J Pediatr Surg 1990;25:472-478.
183. Williamson DH, Thornton PS: Ketone body production and metabolism in the fetus and neonate. In Polin RA, Fox WW, Abman SH (eds): Fetal and Neonatal Physiology, 3rd ed. Philadelphia, WB Saunders, 2004, pp 419-428.
184. Wilmore DW: From Cuthbertson to fast-track surgery: 70 years of progress in reducing stress in surgical patients. Ann Surg 2002;236:643-648.
185. Winthrop AL, Jones PJ, Schoeller DA, et al: Changes in the body composition of the surgical infant in the early postoperative period. J Pediatr Surg 1987;22:546-549.
186. Wispe JR, Bell EF, Roberts RJ: Assessment of lipid peroxidation in newborn infants and rabbits by measurements of expired ethane and pentane: Influence of parenteral lipid infusion. Pediatr Res 1985;19:374-379.
187. Yager JY: Hypoglycemic injury to the immature brain. Clin Perinatol 2002;29:651-674.
188. Yasukawa H, Ohishi M, Mori H, et al: IL-6 induces an anti-inflammatory response in the absence of SOCS3 in macrophages. Nat Immunol 2003;4:551-556.
189. Zlotkin SH: Intravenous nitrogen intake requirements in full-term newborns undergoing surgery. Pediatrics 1984;73:493-496.
190. Zlotkin SH, Bryan MH, Anderson GH: Intravenous nitrogen and energy intakes required to duplicate in utero nitrogen accretion in prematurely born human infants. J Pediatr 1981;99:115-120.
191. Zlotkin SH, Stallings VA, Pencharz PB: Total parenteral nutrition in children. Pediatr Clin North Am 1985;32: 381-400.

第 7 章

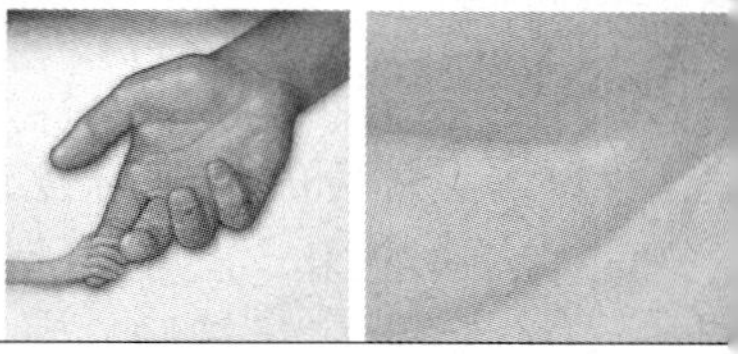

呼吸生理学和监护

Jay M. Wilson 和 John W. DiFiore

“人体只不过是一对钳子固定住一个风箱和一只炖锅以及支撑它们的支柱” [35]。本章将讨论正常的肺发育、肺生理、监护仪器（创伤性及无创性）和支持通气的仪器。最后我们将讨论如何将这些相关的信息应用于现代监护病房处理的呼吸衰竭患者。

肺发育

虽然肺组织结构的发育很复杂，但以下由 Reid 提出的三条“肺发育定律”提供了有用的总结[157,158]。

气道：支气管树在孕 16 周时已完全发育成熟。

肺泡：肺泡在出生以后开始发育，直至 8 岁其数目不断增长。肺泡的直径不断增大直至成年期胸腔停止发育。

血管：腺泡前的血管（动脉和静脉）随着气道的发育而发育，腺泡内的血管随着肺泡的发育而发育。腺泡内血管肌增长速度远不及新生血管的增长速度。

肺发育分为五个阶段：胚胎期、假腺泡期、微管期、囊泡期和肺泡期。各期的分界并不明显，在整个肺中可见到不同的发育阶段混杂在一起。个体之间也有差别[148]。

胚胎期

人类胎儿的肺起源于胚胎 3 周时前肠尾端的喉气管沟的腹侧憩室。这个憩室向尾端生长形成原始气管[28]。在胚胎 4 周时该憩室的尾端分叉，形成两个初始肺芽。这些肺芽发育成叶芽，最终形成最终的肺叶（右边 3 叶，左边 2 叶）。在胚胎 6 周时，叶芽继续分化形成支气管肺段。

原始肺芽由内胚层分化来的上皮细胞分隔形成。该上皮细胞进一步分化成分隔气道的呼吸上皮细胞[30]以及分隔肺泡和执行气体交换的特殊上皮细胞[198]。肺芽长入圆形团块组织，后者将最终形成血管、平滑肌、软骨和其他构成肺分化支架的结缔组织。肺的神经支配来源于外胚层（图 7–1A）。

假腺泡期

胚胎第 7～16 周起，传导气道通过不断的分叉样分化而形成，在胚胎 16～25 周形成原始气道。在这期间，肺已经形成明显的腺体化外观（假腺泡化），由丰富的间叶细胞包围的小的上皮细胞分隔的管道样组织形成（图 7–1B）[107]。在胚胎 16 周时，所有的支气管都已经形成[155,157,158]。在这之后的发育只是现有的气道增长及增宽，而不存在继续分叉的变化。与此同时，呼吸道上皮开始分化，纤毛出现在近端气道，软骨开始形成。

在假腺泡期，间叶细胞的相互作用对于正常肺部气道形态的形成是必需的[116]。在体外实验中，只有当支气管中胚层存在的情况下，内胚层的肺芽才会进行正常的支气管分叉分化。其他的中胚层，包括气管，都不能诱发支气管分叉分化。更有甚者，支气管分叉的速度和程度与存在的间叶细胞的数量成正比[116]。

除了对支气管分叉的影响，间叶细胞的存在对于

支气管的细胞分化也是必需的。随着间叶细胞数量的增加，上皮细胞的分化从支气管（纤毛柱状细
115 胞和杯状细胞）向肺泡（主要是Ⅱ型肺上皮细胞）转移[116]。同样只有在肺上皮细胞和间叶细胞共存的情况下，肺间叶细胞才会分化成平滑肌、血管及软骨[183]。

微管期

微管期发生在胚胎 16～24 周。此时，肺气体交换部分的基本结构已经形成，并且血管化。

在微管期的初期，肺只有很简单的空间结构。潜在的气体交换结构是内壁光滑和盲端的管道，由立方

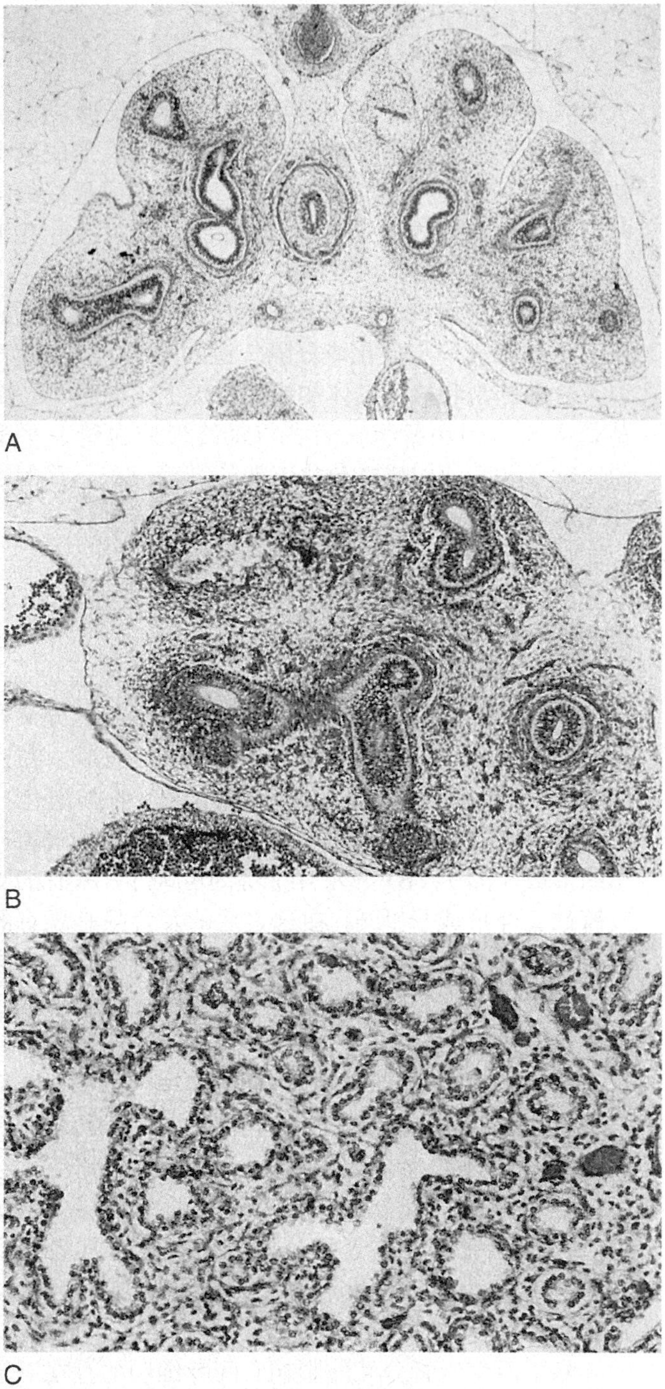

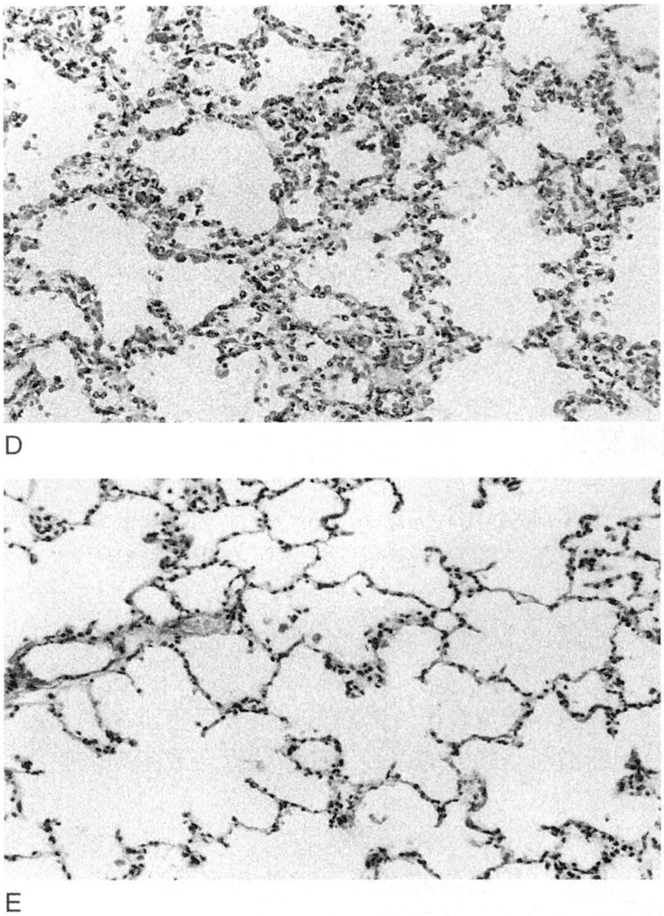

图 7–1 肺发育阶段：A. 胚胎期：0～6 周。B. 假腺泡期：7～16 周。C. 微管期：16～24 周。D. 终极囊泡期：24～40 周。E. 肺泡期：出生以后。

上皮细胞分隔，并由大量疏松间质及散在的血管支持。随着微管期发展，毛细血管的发育增加。这些“管道”将呈现一种更复杂和不规则的样式
116 (图 7–1C)。

在大约孕 20 周时，原始上皮细胞开始分化。原始气体交换通道的上皮细胞下的毛细血管的生长提供了这个分化阶段的形态学证据。在一群上层上皮细胞，毛细血管的生长可导致细胞浆变稀，气–血交换界面变窄，以及分化为 I 型肺泡上皮，后者最终负责气体交换。在其他上层上皮细胞中，开始出现与表面活性物质合成有关的板层体；II 型细胞通过这些结构可确认，后者最终可产生表面活性物质。虽然有些研究人员认为，原始 I 型细胞是未分化的上皮细胞，一个更有说服力的证据说明，I 型细胞是由分化的 II 型上皮细胞发展而来的[3,4,64,173,177]。在微管期末期，肺的结构发育已达到有可能进行气体交换的程度。

终末囊泡期

肺发育的终末囊泡期为孕 24 周至出生时，伴随着肺的形态的显著改变。间质组织将明显减少，气腔壁将明显变薄。凸入远端气腔的组织可将其分隔成囊泡，此处毛细血管一般只暴露于一层呼吸界面（图 7–1D）。此后，在成熟肺泡中，每一根毛细血管同时暴露于至少两个肺泡内[34]。

在此发育阶段，人类胎儿的肺囊泡细胞是可分辨的 I 型及 II 型肺泡上皮。在形态学上，它们和新生儿及成人肺组织的相应细胞并无不同。但是，早期胎儿肺脏产生的表面活性物质的生化特性与孕后期的不同。尽管板层体的形态学无差异，未成熟肺生成的表面活性物质富含磷脂酰肌醇，而孕后期肺生成的表面活性物质富含磷脂酰甘油[80]。

出生后或肺泡期

一个肺泡即一个肺泡管的外翻开放部分，几乎只由薄层的 I 型肺泡上皮细胞排列而成。其间质中的毛细血管同时暴露于两个肺泡内，由于所有细胞的细胞核都远离气体交换界面，气体交换屏障通常只有几个纳米厚度[148]。肺泡内气体和毛细血管中血液的屏障由三层结构组成：薄层排列的 I 型上皮细胞，常见于内皮细胞和肺泡细胞的基底膜，以及内皮细胞的薄层延伸部分（图 7–2A）。I 型上皮细胞负责气体交换，而 II 型上皮细胞合成并分泌表面活性物质。

出生时，肺部没有成熟肺泡，代之以将近 2000 万个原始终末囊泡[26,27,51,60]。这些囊泡由成熟的肺泡上

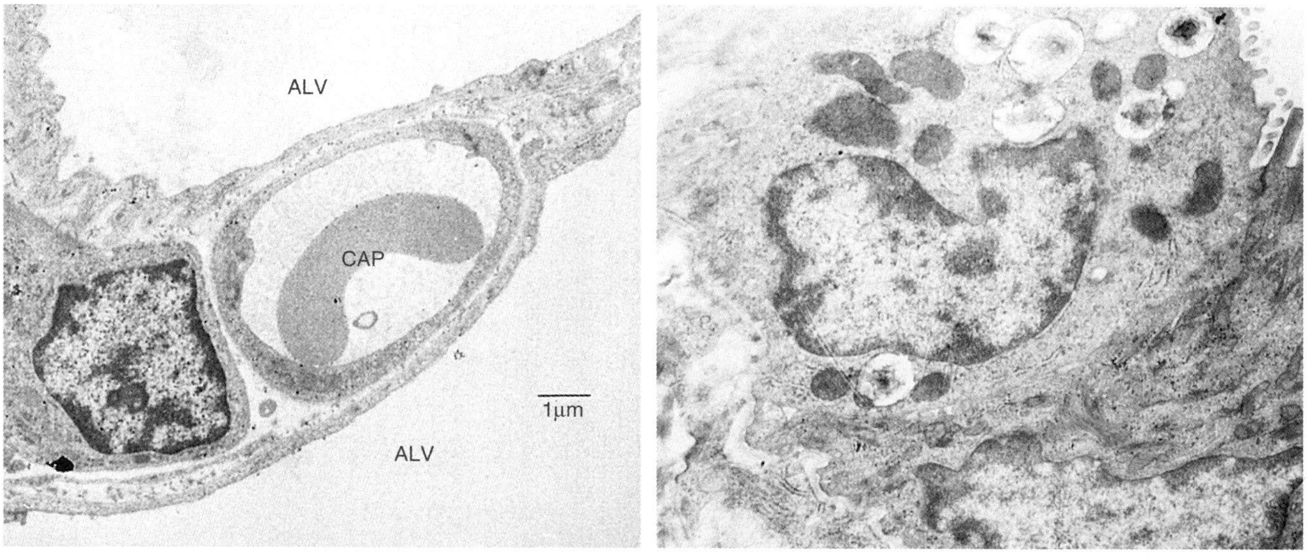

A B

图 7–2 A. I 型肺泡上皮细胞的电镜照片。注意薄的肺泡–动脉界面。B. II 型肺泡上皮细胞的电镜照片。注意富含表面活性物质的板层体。ALV：肺小动脉；CAP：毛细血管。

皮细胞排列组成；它们形似大的空杯子[26,27,51,60,157]。大约出生后5周，这2000万个原始终末囊泡开始分化为肺泡，至8岁时肺泡数量将达到3亿个，期间最快的增殖期在4岁之前（图7-1E）[51,60,199]。8岁以后，肺容量的增加是由于肺泡体积增大而不是由于数量增
117 多[51]。

动脉的生长

肺动脉的生长方式根据对应于腺泡的所在位置而有所不同。腺泡前区是指传导气道，包括气管、主支气管和支气管分叉直至终末细支气管。腺泡是指肺的功能性呼吸单位，包括终末细支气管的远端结构（特别是呼吸性细支气管、肺泡管和肺泡）。在腺泡前区，肺动脉发出的分支伴随每一个气道分支——一条“常规”动脉最终供应终末细支气管至腺泡。常规动脉发出许多额外分支，并穿行进入邻近的呼吸组织供应支气管周围的肺实质；这些分支称为“额外”动脉[89,156]。

腺泡前常规动脉及额外动脉的发育在孕16周时完成，这与支气管气道的分叉同步[88,89]。以后，腺泡前动脉的变化只涉及大小，不涉及数量。在腺泡内区，常规肺动脉的终末分支供应毛细血管床。为与肺泡的发育一致，这些肺部小血管在出生后快速增长以赶上肺泡的增长速度。

在成人，肺动脉的完全肌肉化见于整个腺泡，甚至于紧靠胸膜下的肺泡壁上。但胎儿肺动脉的完全肌肉化出现在终末细支气管或其近端。因此，腺泡内部的动脉只有部分肌肉化或无肌肉化。儿童早期出现的新肺泡与腺泡内动脉同步发生。然而，这些血管的肌肉化进程很缓慢[157]。

胎肺发育的介质

有大量的证据支持肺内液体对正常及实验胎肺生长的作用。人体自然状态下发生的气道闭塞可导致巨大的富含液体的肺，其组织学表现为正常的或轻微扩张的肺泡[2,74,77,110,125]。在其他情况下，子宫内气道闭塞会导致巨肺，也可合并其他解剖结构异常，如Potter综合征或先天性膈疝，此时通常会造成肺发育不良[145,146,202]。

对羊胎肺的研究提供了肺液体动力学可能在肺发育中起关键作用的线索。在孕末期，羊肺内液体的生成速度与气管内-肺内的压力一样显著增加。更明显的是，这些变化发生在肺增长的最快阶段，在肺液体动力学变化后的12～14天，肺容量和肺泡总数量明显增加[6,58]。

对正常胎羊的实验证明，肺内滞留的液体可导致肺增生，而液体引流后会导致肺发育不良。胎的气管闭塞可防止双侧胚胎肾切除和实验性胎的膈疝所导致的肺泡和肺血管部分发育不良[56,57,161,203]。这些初始实验后，许多动物胚胎实验显示，气管闭塞后肺的生长明显增快。但是，持续的闭塞可导致肺的过度生长、表面活性物质生成和Ⅱ型肺泡上皮细胞数量明显减少[32,67,108,138,143]。短时间气管闭塞可以缓解这种影响，同时也不会导致由于长时间闭塞引起的Ⅱ型肺泡上皮细胞明显减少[52,53,140]。出生以后的肺膨胀可促进新生儿的肺发育，但对成人肺脏无此作用，提示未成熟肺的可延展性[135]。

虽然在气管闭塞模型中，肺内压力增高被认为是肺生长的原发刺激，但它可能只是更复杂的下游调节变化的起点。研究涉及气管闭塞模型中肺内液体化学组成的变化[141]。气管闭塞与许多生长因子表达增强与生成增加有关，包括角质化细胞生长因子、血管内皮生长因子、转化生长因子-β2、胰岛素样生长因子Ⅰ、肝细胞瘤产生的生长因子、核糖体蛋白S24和微管不稳定蛋白，所有这些生长因子均参与肺发育的一个复杂调节通道，且气管闭塞可加强其作用[43,119,130,134,150]。

最近通过肺发育和肺发育不良的其他动物模型揭示了调控肺发育的信号和通道的细节[164]。关于激素对肺发育影响的研究很少，但现有的证据提示，激素对肺发育不起主要作用[31,37,62,101,105]，然而激素对表面活性物质系统的发育有较多影响。表皮生长因子、肝细胞瘤产生的生长因子和角质化细胞生长因子都被认为与肺发育有关[38,115,124,139,181]。孕妇接受皮质醇治疗可导致胎儿肺结构变化，这与表面活性物质的分泌无关[18,33,99,179]。

肺的生理学

呼吸是复杂的过程，涉及吸气肌收缩而在气管内

产生负压使新鲜空气进入肺部。在肺内，摄取氧气和排出二氧化碳的过程是经由通过极薄的肺泡毛细血管膜发生扩散的。这个过程的重要性不仅在于为新陈代谢提供氧气而给身体细胞加油，而且在于通过小心地调节二氧化碳来保持适当的酸碱平衡。这个过程中的任何一个部分发生功能障碍都会导致呼吸衰竭和需要机械通气的支持。

要了解呼吸作用的过程，就有必要先了解评估肺
118 功能的相关术语。

肺容量

肺的总容量被分成如下各亚成分，定义如下（图 7–3）。

功能残气量（FRC）：是存在于正常呼气末的肺内气体量，此时肺内气流为零且肺泡内的压力等于外界气压。

补呼气量（ERV）：这段额外气体可被呼出超出 FRC 的部分以达到残气量。

残气量（RV）：尽可能最小的肺容量。这是所有可以呼出的气体都被排出后依然残留在肺内的气体量。

肺总量（TLC）：肺内总的容量。

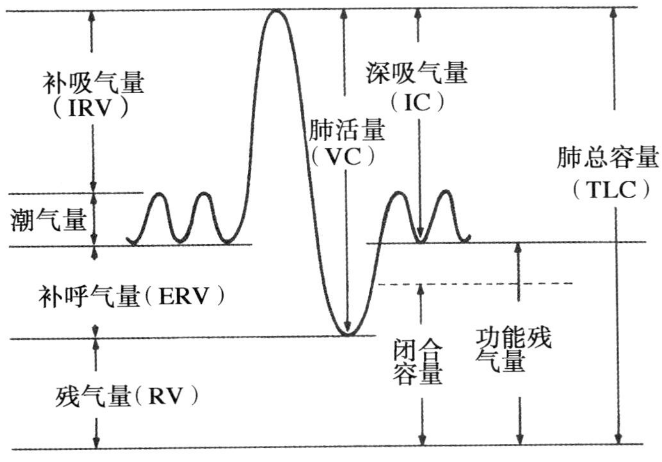

图 7–3 肺容量的功能组成。

深吸气量（IC）：从功能残气量至肺总量被吸入的气体量的差值。

肺活量（VC）：从残气量至肺总量间所吸入的气体。

补吸气量（IRV）：从正常吸气量峰值至肺总量被吸入的气体量。

潮气量（V_T）：正常吸气量。

有关简称和标志参见表 7–1，表 7–2 为相关公式。

潮气量、肺活量、深吸气量、补吸气量和补呼气量都可用肺量计直接测量。相反肺总量、功能残气量和残气量无法用肺量计测量，必须使用以下技术之一来测量：（1）氮清洗试验，即在吸入纯氧时测量从肺内排出的氮；（2）氦稀释试验，测量进入肺内的平衡氦量；或（3）全身体积描记法，应用 Boyle 法则通过测量身体体积和压力的变化来计算
FRC[127]。 119

闭合容量

吸气压力可随着气体传至远端而降低。最终，管腔内压力与周围实质组织的压力相等以支撑气管保持开放；这被称之为等压点[122]。在等压点下游区，管腔内压力下降至低于周围实质组织的压力，气道关闭导致肺泡无通气和生理性分流。在正常肺部，FRC时很少或没有无通气区域。但是，任何引起 FRC 降低的情况（多发生在肺部病变时）都将导致肺部更多区域关闭容量，并形成肺不张和分流增加[120]。相反在 FRC 增加的情况下（正压通气时）也许能打开某些闭合区域，从而减少生理性分流。

肺的顺从性

肺的顺从性的定义是：每单位压力变化可引起的肺容量改变[114]。动态顺从性等于容量变化除以吸气相跨胸腔峰压。静态顺从性等于容量变化除以吸气压力的平台值[71]。在吸气初始，跨胸腔压梯度增加到一个

表 7-1　简称和标志

CaO_2	动脉血氧含量
CCO_2	毛细血管末端血氧含量
$C\bar{v}O_2$	混合静脉血氧含量
D_LCO	肺一氧化碳弥散量
D_LO_2	肺氧弥散量
ERV	补呼气量
FiO_2	吸入气的氧浓度
FRC	功能残气量
IC	深吸气量
IRV	补吸气量
$P\bar{A}CO$	平均肺泡气一氧化碳分压
$PaCO_2$	动脉血二氧化碳分压
P_ACO_2	肺泡气二氧化碳分压
$P\bar{A}CO_2$	平均肺泡气二氧化碳分压
PaO_2	动脉血氧分压
P_AO_2	肺泡气氧分压
$P\bar{A}O_2$	平均肺泡气氧分压
PCO_2	二氧化碳分压
$P\bar{C}O_2$	毛细血管血平均氧分压
$P\bar{E}CO_2$	混合呼出气平均二氧化碳分压
PO_2	氧分压
$\dot{Q}s$	分流量
$\dot{Q}t$	心输出总量
R	呼吸交换比率
RQ	呼吸商
RV	残气量
SaO_2	动脉含氧血红蛋白饱和百分数
SvO_2	混合静脉含氧血红蛋白饱和百分数
TLC	肺总容量
V_A	肺泡气容量
VC	肺活量
V_D	无效腔气容量
V_T	潮气量
$\dot{V}_A/\dot{Q}c$	肺泡通气与肺毛细血管血量的比值
$\dot{V}CO_2$	每分钟二氧化碳排出量
$\dot{V}_E$	每分钟通气呼气量
$\dot{V}_I$	每分钟通气吸气量
$\dot{V}O_2$	每分钟摄取氧气的速率

峰值。这是肺和胸壁的弹性阻力以及气道阻力共同作用的结果。当气体在肺泡内重新分布时，气道内压力

表 7-2　公式

弥散能力	$D_{LCO}=\dot{V}CO/P\bar{A}CO$
无效腔	$V_D=V_T\ (P\bar{A}CO_2-P\bar{E}CO_2/P\bar{A}CO_2)$
分流比率	$\dot{Q}s/\dot{Q}t=CCO_2-CaO_2/CCO_2-CVO_2$
呼吸商	$R=CO_2$ 输出速度 $/O_2$ 输出速度
混合静脉氧饱和度	$S\dot{v}O_2=SaO_2-\dot{V}O_2/13.9\times\dot{Q}\times(Hb)$
肺血流量	$\dfrac{\text{氧摄取量}}{\text{动-静脉氧含量的差值}}$
Henderson–Hasselbalch 公式	$pH=\dfrac{pK+\log[HCO_3^-]}{0.03PCO_2}$

下降至平台值。结果是动态顺从性总是低于静态顺从性。图 7-4 展示的是一个静态顺从性的标准曲线[151]。通气常发生在曲线的陡峭部分，此时较小的压力变化即可引起很大的容积变化。而在低容量和高容量情况下，较大的压力变化可引起最小的容积变化。肺部病变时，肺顺从性降至曲线的平坦部分，机械通气的目标是让它回到陡峭部分。呼吸机所提供的过高压力可导致通气在曲线的顶部进行，使该过程再次无效[91]。

在一个正常呼吸周期内，肺容量和胸膜压的变化反映了肺的弹性和气流阻力特性，可显示在压力-容量环上（图 7-5）。呼气末和吸气末连线的斜率可以用来测量肺的动态顺从性。这条线的下方和曲线之间的区域其右边和左边分别代表在吸气和呼气时因克服气流阻力所做的额外功。

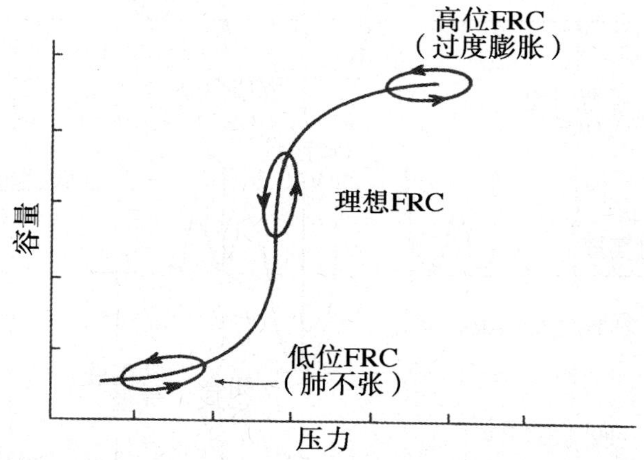

图 7-4　高位、低位和理想功能残气量（FRC）的静态顺应性曲线及动态流量容量环。

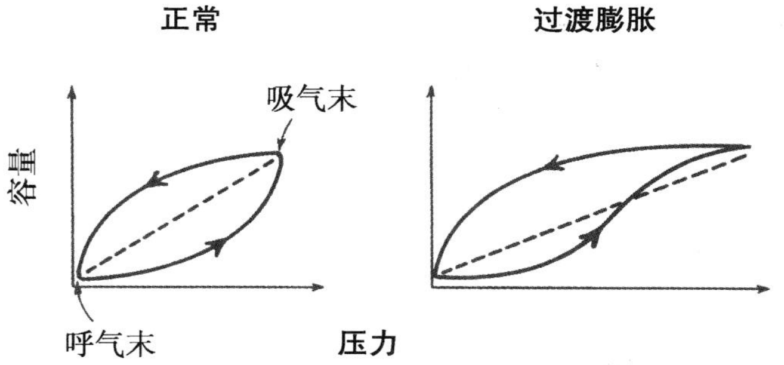

图 7-5 动态压力-容量环显示出一个理想的通气周期和在正压通气时的过度膨胀。

气道阻力

气流阻力是气体（分子间及分子与气管壁间）物理特性的一种作用，也是气体穿行的管道长度。更重要的是，阻力是管道内径的一种作用。由于小儿的气道较窄，继发于气道水肿的内径的轻微变化即可导致阻力的急剧增加。由于肺底部气道较小，所以此处的阻力高于肺尖部的[121]。另外，气流速度也影响阻力，这是因为在临界速度以下，气流为层流。而在临界速度以上，气流是湍流，并且阻力也增加。

时间常数

时间常数是肺顺应性和阻力的乘积，可用来计算呼气有多快。由此，增加单个肺泡单位或肺区的顺应性或阻力可以增加时间常数。一个时间常数被定义为呼出 63%的潮气量所需的时间（二、三和四个时间常数分别为 87%、95%和 99%）[137]。由于各肺泡内的气道阻力各不相同，这取决于肺泡的位置，而且由于各肺泡的顺应性也不同，因此测得的时间常数实际上是
120 整个肺部许多不同时间常数的平均值。当机械辅助通气受到关注时，理解时间常数的重要性就变得明显了。高顺应性或高阻力肺部的时间常数延长。因而，机械通气的设置需调整至达到近似完全的呼气（三个时间常数，或 95%的呼气量）以避免呼吸堆积和过度膨胀。相反低顺应性或低阻力肺部的时间常数缩短；在此情况下，要增加每分通气量，需通过增加呼吸率而不是潮气量来实现。由于低顺应性，潮气量更易导致高压和气压伤。

肺循环

混合静脉血是从体循环汇入右心房，再到达右心室，然后进入肺毛细血管床，并在此进行气体交换。接着血液流入左心房，在此被泵入左心室和最后进入体循环。来自体循环的不饱和血通过支气管和胸膜循环后代表流出左心房血液总量的 1%～3%。在病理情况下，这一解剖右向左分流可接近 10%[65]。此外，在任何情况下右心房压力超过左心房压力时，卵圆孔（所有新生儿和 20%～30%年长儿呈解剖性开放）成为另一个肺外右向左分流的主要部位。

由于血液是液体并受重力影响，因此在直立个体，肺尖部肺毛细血管床的血压和血流最低，而肺底部最高。正常情况下，肺动脉压力足以使部分血液到达肺尖；然而，在病理情况下，如出血或休克，到达肺尖的血流可降至零而形成一个只有通气、没有灌注的区域；这种区域被称为无效腔。肺部可划分为四个区域，命名从肺尖到肺底部向尾部方向进行。在 1 区（肺尖），肺泡压超出肺动脉压，很少或没有血流通过。在 2 区，肺动脉压超出肺泡压，但肺泡压超出静脉压。在这个区域，血流取决于肺动脉压和肺泡压的差值。在 3 区，肺静脉压超出肺泡压，其血流取决于肺动脉压和静脉压的差值。在 4 区（肺底），肺间质压超过肺静脉压和肺泡压，这个区域的血流取决于肺动脉压与间质压的差值[106]。

由于氧气是肺血管舒张剂，缺氧是使肺毛细血管床收缩的有效刺激。此外，酸中毒是肺血管收缩剂，而碱中毒是肺血管舒张剂，因此二氧化碳分压（PCO_2）因其对 pH 的影响而可间接作用于毛细血管床。

肺气体交换

扩散

氧气和二氧化碳通过被动扩散通过肺泡和肺毛细血管床。由于在气体环境里扩散是分子量的作用，氧气在空气中的扩散比二氧化碳迅速。但是，跨毛

细血管肺泡膜的扩散涉及从气相到液相的转变，所以气体在液体中的溶解度会限制扩散速度，二氧化碳（因为它比氧气更易溶解）的扩散速度比氧气快20倍[162]。

扩散驱动力不仅取决于溶解度差异，还取决于跨毛细血管肺泡膜的气体分压差。因而，在毛细血管初始部的气体交换最快，这是因为此处的肺泡和毛细血管间的氧分压（PO_2）和 PCO_2 差最大；实质上，在通过肺毛细血管床 1/3 时，气体交换已完成[194]。其结果是，正常个体在静息状态或在锻炼期间摄入氧气的主要限制因素为肺血流[201]。虽然在健康状态下，扩散率不限制扩散速率，但在毛细血管膜变厚的情况下，扩散可被削弱至足以阻止可利用的血红蛋白的完全饱和。一氧化碳与氧气有相似的扩散特征，可被用以测量扩散能力。

无效腔

每分通气量是指每分钟吸入的空气总量，是潮气量和呼吸率的乘积。但并不是全部吸入气体都参与气体交换；每次潮式呼吸的部分，即只在口咽部、喉、气管和主传导支气管（解剖无效腔）通气的气体，不参与气体交换[196]。除解剖无效腔，在无灌注的肺泡内通气的一定量气体也不参与气体交换。这被称为肺泡无效腔，在没有疾病时最小。解剖和肺泡无效腔统称为生理性无效腔，约等于正常潮气量的 1/3；无效腔超出这个值的应考虑为病理性[152]。

通气 –灌注匹配

为优化气体交换，在给定肺段，通气（V）和灌注（Q）应该匹配[200]。不同肺单位的 V/Q 比是不同的[193]，而肺泡通气与肺血流的平均比率约为 0.8。肺尖的 V/Q 比较高；而肺底的比值较低。正常情况下，V/Q
121 不匹配最小且无关紧要。但在疾病状态下，不匹配可能造成明显的气体交换受损。血液流经肺部无通气区域时，会明显降低动脉氧饱和度的右向左分流会发生。

氧气运输

氧气在血液中的运输有两种方式。或以水溶液的形式在血浆中运输，或以与血红蛋白化学合成的形式在红细胞中运输。以溶液形式运输的氧气量微不足道。因而，大多数氧气是与红细胞中的血红蛋白结合而被运输的。在饱和情况下，1 克血红蛋白能运载 1.34 毫升氧气。但是，由血红蛋白实际运载的氧气量是不同的，是由称为氧离解曲线的 S 形曲线来定义的（图 7-6）。正常情况下，血红蛋白的氧饱和度为 100%；但是，S 形曲线保证了血红蛋白能保持相对高的携氧能力，甚至在 PO_2 低至 60 时。结果是轻度肺功能紊乱并不影响氧的释放。同时，氧离曲线的陡峭区域保证了当 PO_2 下降时有大量氧气被释放入周围组织。当血红蛋白与氧的亲和力发生改变时，氧离曲线可以左移或右移。左移可导致血红蛋白与氧气的高亲和力，可由碱中毒、低温[90]、红细胞 2,3–二磷酸甘油酸（2,3–DPG）[21]降低（常见于旧的库血）[17]或胎儿血红蛋白所致。在此情况下，给定一个 PO_2，血红蛋白氧饱和度比正常时高，因此组织灌注增加以释放同等量的氧气来满足新陈代谢的需要。右移可导致血红蛋白与氧气的低亲和力，由酸中毒[90]、高温和红细胞 2,3–DPG 增加所致[21]。右移导致在给定一个 PO_2 时血红蛋白氧饱和度降低，因此在周围组织中血流速度降低以使更多氧气释放。

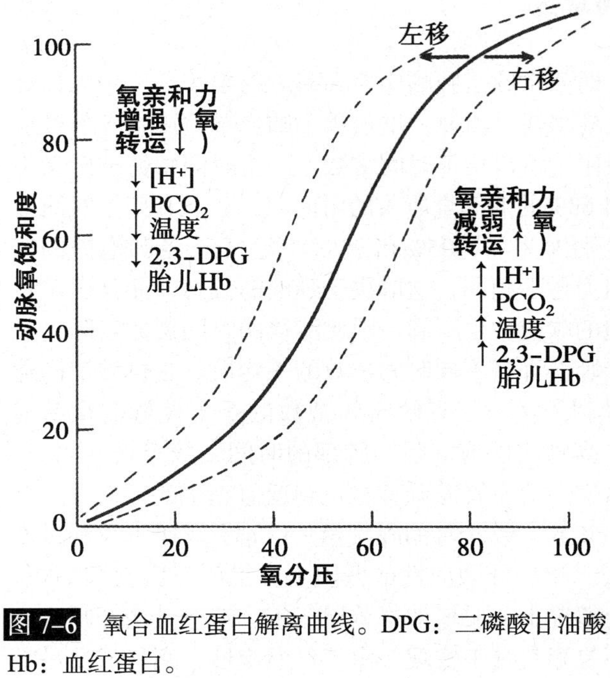

图 7-6 氧合血红蛋白解离曲线。DPG：二磷酸甘油酸；Hb：血红蛋白。

二氧化碳平衡和酸碱调节

由于二氧化碳是新陈代谢的最终产物，它的产生速度是新陈代谢率的作用。在正常情况下产生，二氧化碳量稍少于耗氧量。这是由呼吸商（R）来定义的：

$$R = \frac{CO_2\text{生成率}}{O_2\text{摄取率}}$$

在正常情况下，呼吸商为 0.8，但主要根据营养来源是糖类还是脂肪，它可从 1.0 变为 0.7。肺的主要功能是清除二氧化碳，清除率取决于肺血流和肺泡通气。二氧化碳在血液中可以几种方式运载。在水溶液中，它以溶化的二氧化碳和碳酸形式在平衡状态下存在（$CO_2 + H_2O \rightleftharpoons H_2CO_3$）。通常这个等式方向明显向左。但在红细胞中碳酸酐酶催化的反应下，等式方向向右[102,103]。碳酸的溶解和重结合（$H_2CO_3 \rightleftharpoons H^+ + HCO_3^-$）能力是缓冲血浆以维持生理性 pH的重要因素。Henderson–Hasselbalch 等式可用来说明此关系。还有少量的二氧化碳与血红蛋白结合，以氨基甲酸血红蛋白的形式运输[102]。

监测

由于患急性病的婴儿和儿童的情况可能迅速恶化，故需连续监测他们的生理状况以提供理想管理。在现代监护病房中，临床医生可选择许多生理监测方式；这个部分讨论是最有用的。

无创监测

脉氧仪

脉氧仪可对血红蛋白氧饱和度进行连续的无创监测。脉氧仪的原理是基于分光光度测定法，并依赖于氧合和脱氧血红蛋白以不同的频率发射光线这个事
122 实。氧合血红蛋白选择性吸收红外光（940 nm）并发射红光（660 nm），而脱氧血红蛋白吸收红光并发射红外线。脉氧饱和仪的探头含有两个发光二极管，可将之前测得的通过一个组织灌注区域的特定波长的光发射到另一侧的光敏探测器上。光电二极管可比较探测到的红外线、红光和周围光线来计算动脉血氧饱和度（SaO_2）[7,185]。

脉氧仪的优点是无创性和有一个快速反应时间，可使临床状况的变化显而易见。其缺点是对氧离曲线上部末端的动脉 PO_2 的巨大变化不敏感。另外，当氧饱和度低于 70%时，大多数脉氧仪会明显低估真正的 SaO_2 值。当 SaO_2 常规低于 85%时，有必要通过动脉插管抽取血样来获得实际动脉血氧分压（PaO_2），与其比较相关性。当存在其他形式的血红蛋白时也会发生错误[165]。当出现氨基甲酸血红蛋白和高铁血红蛋白时，SaO_2 读出值会虚假地升高[17]。反之，某些染料，如亚甲蓝，可导致 SaO_2 测得值明显降低[197]。胎儿血红蛋白与成人血红蛋白有相似的吸收光谱，因而对 SaO_2 的测量精度并无影响。生理因素，包括外周灌注差、在传感器放置部位的组织异常增厚或水肿、涂指甲油以及周围光线过强，都可导致读数不准确[36,144,166]。

二氧化碳分压仪

二氧化碳分压仪是一个测量潮气末呼出气体中二氧化碳分压的无创性方法[172]。与脉氧仪一样，二氧化碳分压仪的原理是基于二氧化碳能吸收红外线。呼出气体穿过一个采样腔，其一边为红外线光源，另一边是光敏探测器。根据光敏探测器测得的红外线量，可计算出气体中二氧化碳的量。根据所用设备，报出数据可以是最高二氧化碳浓度（潮气末二氧化碳），也可以显示整个呼出的二氧化碳波形；后者称为二氧化碳描记图[178]。

现有两类二氧化碳监测仪：主流显示器和侧流显示器[83]。主流显示器的采样单元连接在气道和呼吸机及气管内插管之间，能更快地反映二氧化碳的变化，但必须加热以防止水凝结。因此，这些重且热的采样腔必须得到支撑以避触碰到患者。侧流显示器从呼吸循环中抽取连续样本进入监测单元。这个系统轻，因此理论上可用于未插管的患者[25]；但是，由于气流转运到采样单元的时间较长，因而它对二氧化碳的变化反应迟缓。

由于在呼出气体中检测到的二氧化碳是代谢率、肺循环和肺泡通气的产物，因此在解释潮气末二氧化碳测得量的变化时，应将这些变量全部考虑进来。

经皮测量气体压力

用经皮监测的方法可以在皮肤表面测量 PO_2 和 PCO_2[126]。这一装置的原理是基于当血流量超过组织新陈代谢所需血量时，PO_2 和 PCO_2 事实上接近动脉血实际值。为了增加血流量，用于测量经皮 PO_2 和 PCO_2 的仪器具有一个采样电极和一个加热装置来增加局部血流量[186]。经皮监测的好处是：它可以减少（但不排除必要的）患病个体所需的血气分析次数。该装置的一个局限性是：经皮测量的 PO_2 和 PCO_2并不等于动脉血气张力，并且经常比动脉数值高或低5～10mmHg。休克或血管升压药引起的外周灌注变化可造成这些测量值更不准确[187]。另一个缺点是：因为其加热部分可在电极放置部位造成烫伤或水泡。这就需要经常改变监测部位并需重新校准。

肺阻抗描记

肺阻抗描记是测量呼吸频率和呼吸模式的无创性方法[15]。它的原理是基于在吸气和呼气时，由于肺部气流量的差异可使对通过胸腔的电流产生的阻抗（电阻）发生变化[94]。该技术是比较容易执行的。该系统的缺点是：它对身体运动相当敏感而可导致假象。另外，由于该装置只测量阻抗，不能用来评估呼吸做功的质量和潮气量的明显变化[133]。

有创监测

混合静脉血氧监测

测量混合静脉血氧饱和度（Svo_2）在确定氧运输到组织的重大损失中（通常认为当 Svo_2＜60%）时可能是单个最有用的测量方法。因为混合静脉血氧饱和度是动脉饱和度、心排出量和血红蛋白浓度共同作用的结果，因此它们中任何一项发生偏差时都可出现混合静脉血氧饱和度异常。

虽然低 Svo_2 并不能指出受损原因，但它可提供解决问题的几种线索。增加吸入气的氧浓度（FiO_2）
123 来提高 SaO_2，应用升压药或扩容以增加心排出量或经输血来提高血红蛋白浓度，都可用来纠正极低的 SVO_2。SVO_2 可经间歇性从肺动脉插管中抽血测量获得，也可用配备光纤束的肺动脉插管来连续监测[174]。

动脉插管

留置动脉插管可提供连续监测动脉血压和间歇采集血气样本的途径。这种方法适用于需要频繁采集血气样本或血流动力学不稳定的患者。

儿童最常见的放置动脉插管的部位是桡动脉、胫后动脉或足背动脉。当放置桡动脉插管时，一定要确定尺动脉是否通畅，可压迫桡动脉并评估朝向手和手指的血流（Allen 测试）[93]。否则可能发生手的缺血性坏死[20]。新生儿的脐部可提供另外两条动脉通道。一般导管尖端可置于两个位置中的一个。高位（T6～T8）可将导管尖端置于动脉导管之下、腹主动脉分支之上。低位（L3～L4）可将导管尖端置于肾动脉和肠系膜下动脉之间。这些部位的优点是：可使血栓或栓子进入分支血管的并发症的发生率降到最低。

放置直接动脉插管的好处在于：可提供最精确的连续血压测量，并可以最准确地评估 PO_2 和 PCO_2。此技术的缺点是有创的，有感染[149,176]、栓塞[118]和血栓[19]的危险；这些风险可随时间的延长而增加[72]。另一个并发症是可能发生贫血，因为留置动脉插管与过量血液测试有关[128]。因此，必需每日评估直接动脉监测的必要性，一旦对患者的管理无须依赖这些插管时，应尽快拔除它们。

在婴儿，右桡动脉的独特之处在于：它是导管前血液的外周动脉通道（即血液是在与来自开放的动脉导管血在主动脉内混合之前从左心室射出的）。肺动脉高压时（如先天性膈疝），导管前和导管后的动脉氧饱和度有显著差异，监测这两个位点有益于指导治疗。

肺动脉插管

肺动脉插管 PAC 可直接测量右心房压力、右心室舒张末压力、肺动脉压力和 SVO_2[13,44,48,49,169,190]。此外，还可间接计算心排出量和左心充盈压。测量心排出量是基于热稀释技术[69]，即向右房内的肺动脉插管注射一剂冷液。通过测量肺动脉内温度的下降，用 Stuart Hamilton 方程计算心排出量[131]。

左心房压力近似于测得的肺动脉闭合压，即通过给肺动脉插管上的气囊加压直至前向流的血流受阻。

并发症包括：心律失常，可见于多达 50%的危重患者；传导缺陷（6%）；肺梗死（<1%）；肺动脉破裂（0.2%）；导管打结；气囊破裂（5%）；以及感染[16,61,68,142,171,176,184]。最近，肺动脉插管的功效受到质疑，因为几个大型的成人病例研究提示，肺动脉插管不能改善结果，并且与患病率升高和资源耗费增加有关[49]。因为存在这些问题，并且微创性方法有进展，如心动超声图，现在非心脏病的儿科患者已很少使用肺动脉插管。

机械通气

对小儿外科医生而言，具备基本的机械通气知识是重要的，因为呼吸衰竭是最常见的需要收入小儿重症监护病房的诊断[63]。机械通气的目的是：通过保持肺泡通气来充分排泄二氧化碳，维持足够的动脉氧合，增加肺容积来扩张肺不张的区域，以及减少呼吸的机械做功。实现这些目标的同时，还必须避免由气压损伤、氧中毒或两者兼而有之造成的进一步损伤[41]。

1968 年 O'Dwyer 研制了第一代呼吸器由脚踏泵供能，其后无明显改进直至 1970 年，西门子推出 900A。自此，呼吸机从根据循环压力和时间传送大量气体的简单装置进化成：更先进的有间歇指令通气（IMV）、同步 IMV 和呼气末正压（PEEP）的机型。在 80 年代，微处理器的到来给呼吸机提供了新的功能，如压力支持通气（PSV）、指令每分通气、气道压力释放通气及最新的比例辅助通气和容量保证 PSV。

循环机制

机械的呼吸相

所有的机械呼吸周期都经过四个不同的阶段：吸气、切换、呼气和触发。吸气点在于呼气瓣关闭时，新鲜气体在压力引导下进入肺部。切换点在吸气向呼气转换时，其产生与达到耗用时间、传送气体量或压力有关。此时，气体的流入停止，呼气瓣开放使气体
124 从肺部被动释放。触发点是由呼气向吸气转换，其产生与达到耗用时间（控制模式）或由患者初始活动（辅助模式）引发，如气道压力或气流量的改变。最近有关呼吸机的设计改进旨在缩短患者呼吸作用力和呼吸机反应间的机械延迟时间，以提高患者的舒适度和降低患者的呼吸做功。

呼吸机大致分为两类——容量和压力控制的——依据为控制呼吸切换的特定参数。

压力通气

压力通气是用压力作为主要参数来定义吸气；这种方法是目前最常用的婴儿机械通气形式。在这种呼吸机中，当达到预设的吸气峰压（PIP）时，吸气相终止。有些被称为时间切换的呼吸机是使用预定吸气时间来确定吸气相，但因受压力限制，也被归类为压力呼吸机。压力通气的主要优点是：能严格控制 PIP 和平均气道压力从而避免气压伤。其缺点是：潮气量不仅受 PIP 和 PEEP 差值的影响，而且也受吸气时间和顺应性的影响。因此，在疾病过程中当肺顺应性发生改变时，潮气量可能急剧变化。因此，使用压力切换呼吸机需要特别注意设定的潮气量，以避免顺应性恶化时的通气不足或顺应性改善时的过度通气和气压伤（见图 7-5）。

容量切换通气

容量通气是使用预设的潮气量来定义吸气。这种呼吸机的主要优点是：可传送稳定的潮气量。其缺点是：PIP 和平均气道压可随顺应性变化而不同。在病理过程进展中，有必要经常调整潮气量和呼吸频率来保持期望的每分通气量，并防止高气压和气压伤。为了避免危险的高 PIP，大部分容量切换通气呼吸机有一个压力限制阀，在达到预设的压力极限额时可以提早打断吸气。因为高 PIP 会导致明显的肺泡过度通气，这种情况发生时，压力极限警报声会提醒临床医生。容量切换通气常用于年长儿，但也可用于婴儿[41]。

通气模式

通气模式可指示呼吸机如何与患者的自主呼吸作用力共处[25]。大多数呼吸功能提供几种模式，从完全的通气控制到简单的保持 PEEP 而无辅助呼吸。

控制模式

完全控制用于需要完全控制患者通气时[25]。由于不具备患者触发的辅助模式机制，一般要使患者麻痹和镇静以消除其与呼吸机非同步的呼吸。控制模式一般用于需要极端通气时，如需要快速呼吸频率以达到非常高的每分通气量。

辅助控制模式

辅助控制与控制模式的相似之处在于：都可以预设容量压力和吸气时间变量。但在辅助控制模式下，患者可以通过自身触发的呼吸而凌驾于预设的呼吸频率之上，因而患者触发的呼吸完全受呼吸机的支持。在辅助控制模式时，无论是患者还是呼吸机触发的每一次呼气都受到呼吸机的充分支持。如果目标是减少呼吸做功，这个方法可能有利，但如果希望锻炼患者的呼吸肌时，如脱离呼吸机时，这个方法是不利的[9]。其他缺点是：在小婴儿中常出现高呼吸频率、过度换气以及与呼吸机不同步。

间歇指令通气

间歇指令通气（IMV）不同于控制和辅助控制通气之处在于：可预设呼吸机控制完成指令性送气，但也允许自发的、不受呼吸机支持的通气。其优点是：能锻炼呼吸肌。IMV 也是优异的脱离呼吸机的技术，并且可避免高呼吸频率婴幼儿出现过度通气，后者可见于控制模式时。其有一个缺点是：与呼吸机不同步，因为机器触发的吸气可能会叠加在患者的自主呼气相。这会增加呼吸做功，而且可能导致通气不足甚至气胸[75]。

同步间歇指令通气

同步 IMV 时，呼吸机传送的呼吸与患者的自主呼吸同步。这种模式显而易见的优点是：呼吸同步能减少呼吸做功[47]。其缺点则与同步机制的敏感性有关，因为自发的吸气作用力（通常用气道压力的改变来确认）不能立即对同步呼吸做出反应，从而实际上增加了呼吸做功[9]。

压力支持通气

压力支持通气（PSV）是一种自发的通气模式，是一种以恒压送气支持的模式，每次呼吸都是由患者启动。这种方法能增加吸气效率和降低呼吸做功[98,111]。 125
与 IMV 相同，PSV 可用于患者脱离机械通气。IMV 的撤机方式是减少指令呼吸次数并维持吸气压，而 PSV 的撤机方式不同，它是稳步降低压力支持水平，因为呼吸次数由患者控制的。

持续气道正压和呼气末正压

持续气道正压（CRAP）是在患者的整个呼吸周期中预设一个气道正压[10]。而由患者决定潮气量的产生。这种方式能增加 FRC，并常能通过预防肺不张而改善氧合[195]。然而，这一技术会增加呼吸做功。

PEEP 在整个通气周期中提供持续正压，可以防止肺不张、增加 FRC 和改善氧合。尽管大部分呼吸机可提供更高的 PEEP，新生儿 PEEP 的常用范围是 2～10cmH_2O，年长儿为 5～20cmH_2O。

气道压力释放通气

气道压力释放通气可向周围气压短暂地呼气，继而迅速再膨胀以再次生成基线 CRAP。理论上，这样维持压力可在增加二氧化碳排出的同时尽量减少肺不张的发生。动物试验和人体预试验支持这种说法[42,182]。

指令性每分通气

指令性每分通气是一种比较新的模式，呼吸机可调整呼吸频率或压力来维持预设的呼气量。这种模式在撤机时可能有用，因为呼吸机会随着患者的呼吸活动增加而逐渐减少它的支持作用。

成比例的辅助通气

成比例的辅助通气对每次呼吸的支持不同，可视患者的呼吸作用力而定。它是基于来自患者的顺应性和吸气阻力参数的放大[205]。目的是改进患者的呼吸同步性和对呼吸机的舒适度。到目前为止，还没有报道有关的儿童临床试验结果以支持或反驳上述这些益处。

容量辅助压力支持通气

容量辅助压力支持通气旨在确保：接受 PSV 的患者当吸气需求低于预设水平时能保持足够呼气量[8]。成人的人体预试验研究结果已显示这种模式是有前途的[78]。

反比通气

在反比通气时，吸–呼比大于 1，与通常的比例 1∶2 到 1∶5 相反。现已提倡将这种模式应用于重症急性呼吸窘迫综合征（ARDS）或急性肺损伤，以在尽可能减小容量伤或气压伤的同时改善氧合[1]。这是因为反比通气在提高气道平均压时不增加潮气量或 PIP。其应用仍有争议；尽管几个小型研究支持其使用，但其他研究认为，它比更传统的通气方式有较高的并发症发生率[1,123,129,154,163]。但当常规通气模式已用高气道压力也未能扭转低氧血症时，应考虑应用此模式[168]。

高频通气

高频通气（HFV）是指给予超生理呼吸速率（每分钟＞150 次呼吸）传送潮气量小于或等于无效腔的机械通气[22]。高频通气的潜在优点包括：在呼吸周期中容量及压力变化小，在明显低压情况下可进行气体交换，以及对内源性表面活性物质生成的抑制作用较小。大量动物实验数据表明，呼吸机诱导的肺损伤是由肺容量变化造成的而不是压力变化的结果[82]。常规通气中的大的循环容量变化会破坏肺泡毛细血管界面，由此可导致微血管通透性增加和肺间质水肿[117]。这种存在于间质和肺泡腔内的液体和蛋白质混合物可抑制表面活性物质的作用，进而降低肺顺应性。反之，保持肺部高容量及尽可能少的肺泡压或肺泡容量变化不会造成明显的肺损伤[180]。

现已有几种高频通气技术。高频正压通气是常规压力限制呼吸机的改进，可提供的呼吸频率高达每分钟 150 次[23]。高频断流通气可传送高压、短程呼吸和被动呼气[39]。高频喷射通气可在气管内插管的远端发送短喷射呼吸；呼气是被动的[24]。高频振荡通气（HFOV）是使用非常小的潮气量在很高的频率下传送[46,153]。它不同于其他形式的高频通气，其呼气相是主动的。

HFV 的气体交换机制还不清楚。当潮气量低于无效腔量时，肺泡通气应该等于零，且该技术应该是无用的。但可能的机制是大量的轴向气流、区域间的气体混合（摆动呼吸）和分子扩散。

恢复或维持肺容量可以改善氧合。与常规通气需要提高峰压的方法不同，HFV 可在相对固定的肺内压时保持平均肺容量以实现通气[40]。二氧化碳清除对潮气量变化的敏感度比对呼吸频率改变的大[70]。因 126
此，可通过降低呼吸频率来得到期望的较低的二氧化碳分压，因为增加每搏排出量的裨益可超过降低呼吸频率的害处。

目前运用高频通气的策略有两种。高容量策略是设计用于有肺不张倾向的患者。平均气道压是在监测氧合的情况下稳步、小幅提高。此方法的风险包括：压力不足而加剧肺不张，或压力过大导致损伤和气漏[100]。低容量策略是用于气胸或空气陷闭的患者[45]。这个策略常需要较高的 FiO_2，并常可耐受较高的 $PaCO_2$（50～60 mmHg）。

最早使用 HFOV（目前使用最广泛使用的高频通气）的临床经验来自早产儿肺透明膜病[84]。初期研究并未显示 HFV 比常规通气更好，但其方法受到批评，且其结论并未被随后的研究确证。后来对新生儿应用 HFOV 的研究显示，其可明显减少慢性肺病的发生率[46]，改善氧合，并减少气漏综合征的发病率[153]。其他研究显示，在婴儿需行体外膜肺（ECMO）治疗时，HFOV 是其适当的替代方法[50,189]。

年长儿的临床数据很少；但波士顿儿童医院的病例研究显示，对那些符合 ECMO 标准的儿科患者，HFOV 是有些功效的解救治疗[12]。在这项研究中，高容量策略是用于迅速达到并保持最佳肺容量。一项多中心的前瞻性随机试验现已完成，该研究比较了 HFOV 与常规机械通气在弥漫性肺泡疾病和气漏综合征的儿科患者中的应用[11]。资料显示，HFOV 能迅速达成和持续改善氧合，而且尽管使用了较高平均气道压，在 HFOV 中气压伤的发病率仍低于常规机械通气。

气体交换的极端方式

体外生命支持

体外生命支持（ECLS）在气体交换范围的极限

端。它是以一个体外机械装置来支持或暂时代替心脏、肺或两者的功能。使用详情及适应证的讨论见第 8 章。

血管内氧合

血管内氧合包括一个插入下腔静脉的体内气体交换装置，后者与 ECLS 回路的功能相似。下腔静脉的有限空间可限制它的支持性作用。第 8 章将进行更详细的讨论。

体外去除二氧化碳

二氧化碳的体外去除方法类似于 ECLS，但只在清除二氧化碳成为主要问题时使用。第 8 章将会进一步讨论。

液体通气

虽然 30 年前已在实验室内首次证实在液体介质中可以进行气体交换，但直到 1990 年才第一次在患有呼吸窘迫综合征的垂死早产儿中进行临床应用评估[76]。这项研究首次显示，临床可使用液体介质实现气体交换。之后，另外一些临床研究对成人和儿童液体通气的安全性和疗效进行了评估[73,86,87,104]。

现在的液体通气临床试验是采用氟化碳作为液体媒介物。氟化碳是无色、无味的清澈液体，其表面张力低并可携带大量氧气和二氧化碳。目前液体通气的方式有两种：总液体通气（TLV）和部分液体通气（PLV）。在 TLV 中，肺完全充满氟化碳达到 FRC。随后将相当于潮气量的额外氟化碳经类似于 ECMO 的回路装置注入。相当于潮气量的氟化碳在注入肺之前，必须穿过一个外部膜氧合器（在此进行气体交换）。由于这一过程的复杂性，目前 TLV 还只在实验室中进行。相反，PLV 很容易实施，并非常类似于标准机械通气。在 PLV 中，肺被氟化碳液体填充至 FRC。而潮气量是用标准呼吸机使用气体提供[85,167]。在肺的传导气道中，液体和气体的混合使气体可在两种介质中转运。由于 PLV 容易使用，目前在所有液体通气的临床试验中只采用 PLV 方法。

液体通气改善气体交换的机制可能是氟化碳的表面张力低所起的表面活性物质效应和从外周气道中清除渗出物的灌洗效应的共同作用。这两种效应可使肺不张部分的通气恢复，并改善肺部通气灌注匹配。

继初期临床评估氟化碳液体对治疗新生儿的呼吸窘迫综合征之后，其他一些有关成人和儿科患者的临床非对照研究也已完成；这些研究普遍显示，液体通气能改善肺功能[73,86,87,104]。对羊先天性膈疝新生儿应用 PLV 的功效进行评估的实验室研究也提示，液体通气组的气体交换和肺顺应性可得到改善。目前已有 9 个 127
先天性膈疝婴儿在 ECMO 支持的同时接受了 PLV 治疗（J.Wilson，资料尚未发表）[147]。

机械通气的辅助研究

俯卧位

将 ARDS 患者置于俯卧位的目的是通过依赖性体位使重力依赖的血液再分布进入非依赖性肺不张区域而改善氧合。几项小规模研究显示，这样至少可以短暂地改善氧合[132,191]，但最近完成的一项研究显示，儿科患者采用俯卧位不能缩短不用呼吸机的天数，也不能明显改善生存率。此外，这项研究还发现这种技术可有重大的并发症[136]。这个辅助治疗的价值有待继续研究。

一氧化氮吸入

一氧化氮是一种强力短效的肺血管扩张剂，临床试验已应用 10 多年了。对原发性肺动脉高压新生儿，它能改善其氧合并减少使用 ECLS。但尽管能暂时改善氧合，三个大型 ARDS 患者的临床试验显示，它不能使患者尽早脱离呼吸机或不能提高存活率[54,79,109]。

急性呼吸窘迫综合征中的药物辅助治疗

已建议给予 ARDS 患者几种药物辅助治疗，包括前列腺素 E、乙酰半胱氨酸、大剂量皮质类固醇、表面活性物质和多种抗氧化剂。不幸的是，尽管数个小型病例研究的结果令人鼓舞，但最近发表的一项对所有临床试验的荟萃分析表明，这些药物不能改善早期死亡率，而且在前列腺素、表面活性物质和类固醇的有效性治疗试验中出现了较多副作用[5]。因此，目前这些药物中还没有哪一个可以作为呼吸衰竭或ARDS的常规推荐药物辅助措施，需做进一步研究。

呼吸衰竭的处理

呼吸衰竭定义为氧合不足导致缺氧或通气不足导致高碳酸血症。呼吸衰竭的治疗第一步是保持气道通畅。通常用经口或经鼻的气管内插管来完成。2年以上儿童的气管内插管的内径大致可用以下公式来估算：

$$\frac{16+\text{儿童年龄}}{4}$$

8岁以上的儿童常使用无套囊的导管，正压达到20～30cmH_2O时应出现空气泄漏。如果护理得当，这些导管可留置几个星期。

机械通气的目标是恢复正常的肺泡通气和氧合，并且不造成气压伤或氧中毒。一般来说，相当于PaO_2为50～80mmHg，$PaCO_2$为40～60mmHg，pH介于7.35～7.45之间，混合静脉血氧饱和度小于70。

压力切换呼吸机的呼吸机初始设置值应为FiO_2=100%，呼吸频率＝20～30次/分钟，PIP＝20～30cm H_2O，PEEP＝3～5cmH_2O，吸呼比＝1∶2。目标的初始潮气量为6～8ml/kg。如果出现弥漫性肺损伤，应施加PEEP以支持氧合。PEEP支持应从2.0cmH_2O开始，增加幅度为1～2cmH_2O。婴儿PEEP很少需要大于10.0cmH_2O，而年长儿很少超过15.0cmH_2O。镇静作用常可通过患者与机器同步而加强对机械支持的反应。待患者稳定后给予通气管理，且必须根据其基础生理状况给予个性化的通气管理。

呼吸机的设置操作

大部分呼吸机可以预置各种参数，包括呼吸频率、PIP、PEEP、吸气时间和气流速度。调整这些参数时，要考虑到肺部存在的病理疾病。原发性肺动脉高压婴儿的肺顺应性很好，故容易过度膨胀。这些患者可通过低PIP和PEEP、短吸气时间和中等呼吸频率达到充足的每分通气量。反之，ARDS患儿的肺顺应性极差，需要相对较高的PIP和PEEP、短吸气时间和高呼吸频率以达到足够的肺泡通气。阻塞性疾病，如胎粪吸入综合征或哮喘，时间常数较长，并需要低呼吸频率通气。初始设置决定后，必须评估患者的反应，根据肺顺应性和阻力的动态变化随时进行必要的调整。

二氧化碳分压的调整

$PaCO_2$与肺泡通气直接相关，并进而可影响每分通气量（潮气量×呼吸频率）。调节潮气量或增加频率即呼吸频率都可提高每分通气量。然而，高呼吸频率或肺的时间常数延长时，增加呼吸频率可导致呼吸叠加、过度膨胀、肺泡通气减少及随后出现PCO_2上升。 128

氧分压的调整

在大部分需要机械通气的情况下，由于FRC下降至闭合容量引起的片状肺不张会导致明显的肺内分流，而肺对提高FiO_2相对不敏感。此时，增加平均气道压使肺不张区域恢复通气似乎能更有效地提高PaO_2。这可通过增加PIP、PEEP或吸呼比实现。高PIP会造成气压伤，最可能是肺顺应性好的部分（即健康部分）过度膨胀的结果[151]。因此，增加PIP要有节制。一般宁可增加PEEP而不是PIP，因为PEEP可以使塌陷肺泡恢复通气（通过增加FRC），从而减少肺内分流而无明显气压伤的危险。但是，如果使用压力切换呼吸机增加PEEP而不改变PIP，则将导致潮气量降低，故需要调整呼吸频率以保持每分通气量。还有，监测顺应性可确保在通气曲线的最适应部分产生呼吸。

撤机

撤机是机械通气慢慢撤出的过程，以便让患者承担越来越多的呼吸做功。具体的撤机技术取决于所用的通气方式。在合适的呼吸机设置下，只有当患者的血流动力学稳定，而且能够自主维持合适的$PaCO_2$，才可以试着撤机。一般而言，即FiO_2为＜0.4，PIP＜30，PEEP＜5，且呼吸机辅助呼吸每分钟＜15次。小儿还应有足够营养，并且无效腔与潮气量的比值＜0.6（正常为0.3）。

从IMV支持方式撤机包含逐渐减少呼吸机送气频率。撤机速度取决于患者的临床状况和反应。监测患者的自主呼吸作用力和血气参数对这一过程有帮助。在年长患者，拔管前IMV的呼吸频率可减至每分钟2～4次。由于年幼患者的气管内插管较小，其内部气道阻力较高，一般当呼吸频率降至每分钟8～10次时才可尝试拔管。

从PSV方式撤机涉及在监测患者自主呼吸作用力的质量和数量的同时，缓慢下降压力支持水平。一般在这种通气方式下，可每次降低1～2cmH_2O的压力来撤机。

撤机失败

尽管可预测成功撤机的指标很多，10%的患者将会拔管失败。大多数情况下这是由于呼吸负荷过重。临床表现为浅快呼吸、肺力学恶化和呼吸肌负荷增加[96,97]。撤机失败的相关因素包括：伴随浅快呼吸出现的无效腔与潮气量的比值增高；呼吸做功增加导致过量二氧化碳生成；以及有时摄入过多的糖类热卡。由呼吸负荷增加导致的呼吸肌疲劳会造成长时间（＞24小时）的膈肌和呼吸肌功能损害[159]。因此，在尝试再次撤机前必须有充裕的恢复时间。代谢异常，如急性呼吸性酸中毒，会降低膈肌的收缩力和耐力[95]。磷酸盐、钙、钾和镁失衡以及甲状腺功能减退都会损伤呼吸肌功能[103]。纠正这些异常指标可确保能够估算患者的最佳作用力。

机械通气的并发症

气压伤是机械通气的主要并发症。这是由不适当的高PIP或PEEP或过高潮气量引起肺泡过度膨胀造成的。气压伤的后果包括气胸、纵隔积气和肺间质气肿[59]。此外，由于气压伤似乎与容量变化而不是压力变化的关系更密切，要有效地降低气压伤的发生率和严重程度可选择低潮气量（5～7 ml/kg）以及适当低的pH和较高的PCO_2——称为容许性高碳酸血症通气技术[204]。

氧中毒是另一个机械通气并发症。损伤机制大致是氧自由基所致的毛细血管内皮细胞、Ⅰ型和Ⅱ型肺泡上皮细胞损伤[92]。应尽可能通过调节平均气道压以改善肺内分流，并通过适当的PO_2边缘值（50～60 mmHg）来保持FiO_2低于0.6，只要Svo_2保持适当。

支气管肺发育不良是一种进行性慢性疾病，15%的需要机械通气的婴儿可患此症。目前还不清楚造成这种发育不良的原因是否与气压伤、氧中毒或两者有关。因此，避免支气管发育不良的最好方法是尽量注意以最低的可能压力和氧浓度提供足够的通气支持。

这些并发症都是对一个器官正压充气的直接后果，而此器官原是在负压环境下工作的。因此，现在或将来无论正压呼吸机怎么变化都不可能绝对安全。

其他常见的、与通气力学本身不直接相关的并发症包括医源性肺炎，后者是由于重症监护室中普遍存在的自然病原体及气管内插管破坏了上呼吸道防御机制导致的获得性感染。深静脉血栓和肺栓塞在较年长 129
的儿科患者并不少见，对此应该进行预防性治疗。除常见并发症之外，还有插管引起的喉部创伤、错误置管和长时间插管造成的气管狭窄，以及主要由鼻插管导致的鼻窦炎。只要注意细节问题，以上多数并发症可以避免或可以得到治疗。

（李　菁译　黄　萍校）

参考文献

1. Abraham E, Yoshihara G: Cardiorespiratory effects of pressure controlled inverse ratio ventilation in severe respiratory failure. Chest 1989;96:1356.
2. Adams FH, Fujiwara T, Rowshan G: The nature and origin of the fluid in the fetal lamb lung. J Pediatr 1963;63:881.
3. Adamson IY, Bowden DH: The type 2 cell as progenitor of alveolar epithelial regeneration: A cytodynamic study in mice after exposure to oxygen. Lab Invest 1974;30:35.
4. Adamson IY, Bowden DH: Derivation of type 1 epithelium from type 2 cells in the developing rat lung. Lab Invest 1975;32:736.
5. Adhikari N, Burns KE, Meade MO: Pharmacologic treatments for acute respiratory distress syndrome and acute lung injury: Systematic review and meta-analysis. Treat Respir Med 2004;3:307.
6. Alcorn DG, Adamson TM, Maloney JE, et al: A morphologic and morphometric analysis of fetal lung development in the sheep. Anat Rec 1981;201:655.
7. Alexander CM, Teller LE, Gross JB: Principles of pulse oximetry: Theoretical and practical considerations. Anesth Analg 1989;68:368.

8. Amato MB, Barbas CS, Bonassa J, et al: Volume-assured pressure support ventilation (VAPSV): A new approach for reducing muscle workload during acute respiratory failure. Chest 1992;102:1225.
9. American College of Chest Physicians: Consensus conference: Mechanical ventilation. Chest 1993;104:1835.
10. American College of Chest Physicians–American Thoracic Society Joint Committee on Pulmonary Nomenclature: Pulmonary terms and symbols. Chest 1975;67:583.
11. Arnold JH, Hanson JH, Toro-Figuero LO, et al: Prospective, randomized comparison of high-frequency oscillatory ventilation and conventional mechanical ventilation in pediatric respiratory failure. Crit Care Med 1994;22:1530.
12. Arnold JH, Truog RD, Thompson JE, et al: High-frequency oscillatory ventilation in pediatric respiratory failure. Crit Care Med 1993;21:272.
13. Artery Catheter Consensus Conference: Consensus statement. Crit Care Med 1997;25:910.
14. Aubier M, Viires N, Piquet J, et al: Effects of hypocalcemia on diaphragmatic strength generation. J Appl Physiol 1985; 58:2054.
15. Baird TM, Goydos JM, Neuman MR: Optimal electrode location for monitoring the ECG and breathing in neonates. Pediatr Pulmonol 1992;12:247.
16. Barash PG, Nardi D, Hammond G, et al: Catheter-induced pulmonary artery perforation: Mechanisms, management, and modifications. J Thorac Cardiovasc Surg 1981;82:5.
17. Barker SJ, Tremper KK: The effect of carbon monoxide inhalation on pulse oximetry and transcutaneous Po_2. Anesthesiology 1987;66:677.
18. Beck JC, Mitzner W, Johnson JW, et al: Betamethasone and the rhesus fetus: Effect on lung morphometry and connective tissue. Pediatr Res 1981;15:235.
19. Bedford RF: Long-term radial artery cannulation: Effects on subsequent vessel function. Crit Care Med 1978;6:64.
20. Bedford RF, Wollman H: Complications of percutaneous radial-artery cannulation: An objective prospective study in man. Anesthesiology 1973;38:228.
21. Benesch R, Benesch RE, Yu CI: Reciprocal binding of oxygen and diphosphoglycerate by human hemoglobin. Proc Natl Acad Sci U S A 1968;59:526.
22. Bland RD, Kim MH, Light MJ, et al: High frequency mechanical ventilation in severe hyaline membrane disease an alternative treatment? Crit Care Med 1980;8:275.
23. Borg U, Eriksson I, Sjostrand U: High-frequency positive-pressure ventilation (HFPPV): A review based upon its use during bronchoscopy and for laryngoscopy and microlaryngeal surgery under general anesthesia. Anesth Analg 1980;59:594.
24. Boros SJ, Mammel MC, Coleman JM, et al: Neonatal high-frequency jet ventilation: Four years' experience. Pediatrics 1985;75:657.
25. Bowe EA, Boysen PG, Broome JA, et al: Accurate determination of end-tidal carbon dioxide during administration of oxygen by nasal cannulae. J Clin Monit 1989;5:105.
26. Boyden EA: The terminal air sacs and their blood supply in a 37-day infant lung. Am J Anat 1965;116:413.
27. Boyden EA: The pattern of the terminal air spaces in a premature infant of 30-32 weeks that lived nineteen and a quarter hours. Am J Anat 1969;126:31.
28. Boyden EA: Development and growth of the airways. In Hodson WA (ed): Development of the Lung. Philadelphia, Marcel Dekker, 1977, p 121.
29. Branson RD, Campbell RS, Davis K Jr, et al: Comparison of pressure and flow triggering systems during continuous positive airway pressure. Chest 1994;106:540.
30. Breeze RG, Wheeldon EB: The cells of the pulmonary airways. Am Rev Respir Dis 1977;116:705.
31. Brumley GW, Chernick V, Hodson WA, et al: Correlations of mechanical stability, morphology, pulmonary surfactant, and phospholipid content in the developing lamb lung. J Clin Invest 1967;46:863.
32. Bullard KM, Sonne J, Hawgood S, et al: Tracheal ligation increases cell proliferation but decreases surfactant protein in fetal murine lungs in vitro. J Pediatr Surg 1997;32:207.
33. Bunton TE, Plopper CG: Triamcinolone-induced structural alterations in the development of the lung of the fetal rhesus macaque. Am J Obstet Gynecol 1984;148:203.
34. Burri PH: Fetal and postnatal development of the lung. Annu Rev Physiol 1984;46:617.
35. Butler S: In Wilkins R (ed): The Doctor's Quotation Book. New York, Barnes & Noble Books, 1992, p 81.
36. Cahan C, Decker MJ, Hoekje PL, et al: Agreement between noninvasive oximetric values for oxygen saturation. Chest 1990;97:814.
37. Carpenter G, Cohen S: Epidermal growth factor. Annu Rev Biochem 1979;48:193.
38. Catterton WZ, Escobedo MB, Sexson WR, et al: Effect of epidermal growth factor on lung maturation in fetal rabbits. Pediatr Res 1979;13:104.
39. Cavanaugh K, Bloom B: Combined HFV and CMV for neonatal air leak. Respir Manage 1990;20:43.
40. Chang HK: Mechanisms of gas transport during ventilation by high-frequency oscillation. J Appl Physiol 1984;56:553.
41. Chatburn RL: Principles and practice of neonatal and pediatric mechanical ventilation. Respir Care 1991;36:569.
42. Chiang AA, Steinfeld A, Gropper C, et al: Demand-flow airway pressure release ventilation as a partial ventilatory support mode: Comparison with synchronized intermittent mandatory ventilation and pressure support ventilation. Crit Care Med 1994;22:1431.
43. Cilley RE, Zgleszewski SE, Chinoy MR: Fetal lung development: Airway pressure enhances the expression of developmental genes. J Pediatr Surg 2000;35:113.
44. Clark C, Harman E: Hemodynamic monitorying: Pulmonary artery catheters. In Civetta J, Taylor R, Kirby R (eds): Critical Care. Philadelphia, JB Lippincott, 1988, p 319.
45. Clark RH, Gerstmann DR, Null DM, et al: Pulmonary interstitial emphysema treated by high-frequency oscillatory ventilation. Crit Care Med 1986;14:926.
46. Clark RH, Gerstmann DR, Null DM Jr, et al: Prospective randomized comparison of high-frequency oscillatory and conventional ventilation in respiratory distress syndrome. Pediatrics 1992;89:5.
47. Clear J: Improved oxygenation during synchronized vs intermittent mandatory ventilation in VLBW infants with respiratory distress: A randomized crossover design. Pediatr Res 1993;33:1226A.
48. Coleman SS, Anson BJ: Arterial patterns in the hand based upon a study of 650 specimens. Suvr Med (Sofiia) 1961; 113:409.
49. Connors AF Jr, Speroff T, Dawson NV, et al: The effectiveness of right heart catheterization in the initial care of critically ill patients. SUPPORT investigators. JAMA 1996;276:889.
50. Cornish JD, Gerstmann DR, Clark RH, et al: Extracorporeal membrane oxygenation and high-frequency oscillatory ventilation: Potential therapeutic relationships. Crit Care Med 1987;15:831.
51. Davies G, Reid L: Growth of the alveoli and pulmonary arteries in childhood. Thorax 1970;25:669.
52. De Paepe ME, Johnson BD, Papadakis K, et al: Temporal

pattern of accelerated lung growth after tracheal occlusion in the fetal rabbit. Am J Pathol 1998;152:179.
53. De Paepe ME, Papadakis K, Johnson BD, et al: Fate of the type II pneumocyte following tracheal occlusion in utero: A time-course study in fetal sheep. Virchows Arch 1998;432:7.
54. Dellinger RP, Zimmerman JL, Taylor RW, et al: Effects of inhaled nitric oxide in patients with acute respiratory distress syndrome: Results of a randomized phase II trial. Inhaled Nitric Oxide in ARDS Study Group. Crit Care Med 1998;26:15.
55. Dhingra S, Solven F, Wilson A, et al: Hypomagnesemia and respiratory muscle power. Am Rev Respir Dis 1984; 129:497.
56. DiFiore JW, Fauza DO, Slavin R, et al: Experimental fetal tracheal ligation reverses the structural and physiological effects of pulmonary hypoplasia in congenital diaphragmatic hernia. J Pediatr Surg 1994;29:248.
57. DiFiore JW, Fauza DO, Slavin R, et al: Experimental fetal tracheal ligation and congenital diaphragmatic hernia: A pulmonary vascular morphometric analysis. J Pediatr Surg 1995;30:917.
58. Docimo SG, Crone RK, Davies P, et al: Pulmonary development in the fetal lamb: Morphometric study of the alveolar phase. Anat Rec 1991;229:495.
59. Dreyfuss D, Soler P, Basset G, et al: High inflation pressure pulmonary edema: Respective effects of high airway pressure, high tidal volume, and positive end-expiratory pressure. Am Rev Respir Dis 1988;137:1159.
60. Dunnill M: Postnatal growth of the lung. Thorax 1962;17:329.
61. Elliott CG, Zimmerman GA, Clemmer TP: Complications of pulmonary artery catheterization in the care of critically ill patients: A prospective study. Chest 1979;76:647.
62. Erenberg A, Rhodes ML, Weinstein MM, et al: The effect of fetal thyroidectomy on ovine fetal lung maturation. Pediatr Res 1979;13:230.
63. Esteban A, Anzueto A, Alia I, et al: How is mechanical ventilation employed in the intensive care unit? An international utilization review. Am J Respir Crit Care Med 2000; 161:1450.
64. Evans MJ, Cabral LJ, Stephens RJ, et al: Renewal of alveolar epithelium in the rat following exposure to NO_2. Am J Pathol 1973;70:175.
65. Finch CA, Lenfant C: Oxygen transport in man. N Engl J Med 1972;286:407.
66. Fisher J, Magid N, Kallman C, et al: Respiratory illness and hypophosphatemia. Chest 1983;83:504.
67. Flageole H, Evrard VA, Piedboeuf B, et al: The plug-unplug sequence: An important step to achieve type II pneumocyte maturation in the fetal lamb model. J Pediatr Surg 1998;33:299.
68. Foote GA, Schabel SI, Hodges M: Pulmonary complications of the flow-directed balloon-tipped catheter. N Engl J Med 1974;290:927.
69. Forrester JS, Ganz W, Diamond G, et al: Thermodilution cardiac output determination with a single flow-directed catheter. Am Heart J 1972;83:306.
70. Fredberg JJ, Glass GM, Boynton BR, et al: Factors influencing mechanical performance of neonatal high-frequency ventilators. J Appl Physiol 1987;62:2485.
71. Fry DL, Hyatt RE: Pulmonary mechanics: A unified analysis of the relationship between pressure, volume and gas flow in the lungs of normal and diseased human subjects. Am J Med 1960;29:672.
72. Gardner RM, Schwartz R, Wong HC, et al: Percutaneous indwelling radial-artery catheters for monitoring cardiovascular function: Prospective study of the risk of thrombosis and infection. N Engl J Med 1974;290:1227.
73. Gauger P: Initial experience with partial liquid ventilation in pediatric patients with the acute respiratory distress syndrome. Crit Care Med 1996;24:4.
74. Goodlin R, Lloyd D: Fetal tracheal excretion of bilirubin. Biol Neonate 1968;12:1.
75. Greenough A, Morley C, Davis J: Interaction of spontaneous respiration with artificial ventilation in preterm babies. J Pediatr 1983;103:769.
76. Greenspan JS, Wolfson MR, Rubenstein SD, et al: Liquid ventilation of human preterm neonates. J Pediatr 1990; 117:106.
77. Griscom NT, Harris GB, Wohl ME, et al: Fluid-filled lung due to airway obstruction in the newborn. Pediatrics 1969;43:383.
78. Groeger JS, Levinson MR, Carlon GC: Assist control versus synchronized intermittent mandatory ventilation during acute respiratory failure. Crit Care Med 1989;17: 607.
79. Groupe d'Etude sur le NO inhale au cours de lards (GENOA): Inhaled NO in ARDS: Presentation of a double blind randomized multicentric study [abstract]. Am J Respir Crit Care Med 1996;275:383.
80. Hallman M, Kulovich M, Kirkpatrick E, et al: Phosphatidylinositol and phosphatidylglycerol in amniotic fluid: Indices of lung maturity. Am J Obstet Gynecol 1976; 125:613.
81. Hellegers AE, Schruefer JJ: Nomograms and empirical equations relating oxygen tension, percentage saturation, and pH in maternal and fetal blood. Am J Obstet Gynecol 1961;81:377.
82. Hernandez LA, Peevy KJ, Moise AA, et al: Chest wall restriction limits high airway pressure-induced lung injury in young rabbits. J Appl Physiol 1989;66:2364.
83. Hess D: Capnometry and capnography: Technical aspects, physiologic aspects and clinical applications. Respir Care 1990;35:557.
84. High-frequency oscillatory ventilation compared with conventional mechanical ventilation in the treatment of respiratory failure in preterm infants. The HIFI Study Group. N Engl J Med 1989;320:88.
85. Hirschl RB, Merz SI, Montoya JP, et al: Development and application of a simplified liquid ventilator. Crit Care Med 1995;23:157.
86. Hirschl RB, Pranikoff T, Gauger P, et al: Liquid ventilation in adults, children, and full-term neonates. Lancet 1995;346:1201.
87. Hirschl RB, Pranikoff T, Wise C, et al: Initial experience with partial liquid ventilation in adult patients with the acute respiratory distress syndrome. JAMA 1996;275:383.
88. Hislop A, Reid L: Intra-pulmonary arterial development during fetal life: Branching pattern and structure. J Anat 1972;113:35.
89. Hislop A, Reid L: Pulmonary arterial development during childhood: Branching pattern and structure. Thorax 1973;28:129.
90. Hlastala MP, Woodson RD: Saturation dependency of the Bohr effect: Interactions among H^+, CO_2, and DPG. J Appl Physiol 1975;38:1126.
91. Hoppin F, Hildebrandt J: Mechanical properties of the lung. In West J (ed): Lung Biology in Health and Disease: Bioengineering Aspects of the Lung. New York, Dekker, 1978, p 263.
92. Jenkinson S: Oxygen toxicity in acute respiratory monitor-

ing. Respir Care 1983;28:614.
93. Jordan W: Arterial catheters. In Blumer J (ed): A Practical Guide to Pediatric Intensive Care, 3rd ed. St Louis, Mosby-Year Book, 1990, p 263.
94. Jordan W: Electrographic and respiratory monitoring. In Blumer J (ed): A Practical Guide to Pediatric Intensive Care, 3rd ed. St Louis, Mosby-Year Book, 1990, p .
95. Juan G, Calverley P, Talamo C, et al: Effect of carbon dioxide on diaphragmatic function in human beings. N Engl J Med 1984;310:874.
96. Jubran A, Tobin MJ: Pathophysiologic basis of acute respiratory distress in patients who fail a trial of weaning from mechanical ventilation. Am J Respir Crit Care Med 1997;155:906.
97. Jubran A, Tobin MJ: Passive mechanics of lung and chest wall in patients who failed or succeeded in trials of weaning. Am J Respir Crit Care Med 1997;155:916.
98. Kacmarek R: The role of pressure support ventilation in reducing work of breathing. Respir Care 1988;33:99.
99. Kauffman SL: Acceleration of canalicular development in lungs of fetal mice exposed transplacentally to dexamethasone. Lab Invest 1977;36:395.
100. Kinsella JP, Gerstmann DR, Clark RH, et al: High-frequency oscillatory ventilation versus intermittent mandatory ventilation: Early hemodynamic effects in the premature baboon with hyaline membrane disease. Pediatr Res 1991;29:160.
101. Kitterman JA, Liggins GC, Campos GA, et al: Prepartum maturation of the lung in fetal sheep: Relation to cortisol. J Appl Physiol 1981;51:384.
102. Klocke R: Carbon dioxide transport. In Farhi L, Tenney S (eds): Handbook of Physiology. Washington, DC, American Physiological Society, 1987, p 88.
103. Laroche CM, Cairns T, Moxham J, et al: Hypothyroidism presenting with respiratory muscle weakness. Am Rev Respir Dis 1988;138:472.
104. Leach D: Partial liquid ventilation with perflubron (LiquiVent): A pilot safety and efficacy study in premature newborns with severe RDS who have failed conventional therapy and exogenous surfactant. Paper presented at the American Academy of Pediatrics meeting, 1994, Dallas.
105. Liggins GC, Kitterman JA, Campos GA, et al: Pulmonary maturation in the hypophysectomised ovine fetus: Differential responses to adrenocorticotrophin and cortisol. J Dev Physiol 1981;3:1.
106. Lloyd TC Jr, Wright GW: Pulmonary vascular resistance and vascular transmural gradient. J Appl Physiol 1960; 15:241.
107. Loosli CG, Potter EL: Pre- and postnatal development of the respiratory portion of the human lung with special reference to the elastic fibers. Am Rev Respir Dis 1959;80:5.
108. Luks FI, Roggin KK, Wild YK, et al: Effect of lung fluid composition on type II cellular activity after tracheal occlusion in the fetal lamb. J Pediatr Surg 2001;36:196.
109. Lundin S, Mang H, Smithies M, et al: Inhalation of nitric oxide in acute lung injury: Results of a European multicentre study. The European Study Group of Inhaled Nitric Oxide. Intensive Care Med 1999;25:911.
110. MacGregor A: Pathology of Infancy and Childhood. London, Livingston, 1960.
111. MacIntyre N: Weaning from mechanical ventilatory support: Volume-assisting intermittent breaths versus pressure-assisting every breath. Respir Care 1988;33:121.
112. Major D, Cadenas M, Cloutier R, et al: Combined gas ventilation and perfluorochemical tracheal instillation as an alternative treatment for lethal congenital diaphragmatic hernia in lambs. J Pediatr Surg 1995;30:1178.
113. Maren TH: Carbonic anhydrase: Chemistry, physiology, and inhibition. Physiol Rev 1967;47:595.
114. Marshall R: The physical properties of the lungs in relation to the subdivisions of lung volume. Clin Sci (Colch) 1957;16:507.
115. Mason RJ, Leslie CC, McCormick-Shannon K, et al: Hepatocyte growth factor is a growth factor for rat alveolar type II cells. Am J Respir Cell Mol Biol 1994;11:561.
116. Masters JR: Epithelial-mesenchymal interaction during lung development: The effect of mesenchymal mass. Dev Biol 1976;51:98.
117. Mathieu-Costello OA, West JB: Are pulmonary capillaries susceptible to mechanical stress? Chest 1994;105(Suppl): 102S.
118. Matthews JI, Gibbons RB: Embolization complicating radial artery puncture. Ann Intern Med 1971;75:87.
119. McCabe AJ, Carlino U, Holm BA, et al: Upregulation of keratinocyte growth factor in the tracheal ligation lamb model of congenital diaphragmatic hernia. J Pediatr Surg 2001;36:128.
120. McCarthy DS, Spencer R, Greene R, et al: Measurement of "closing volume" as a simple and sensitive test for early detection of small airway disease. Am J Med 1972;52:747.
121. Mead J, Takishima T, Leith D: Stress distribution in lungs: A model of pulmonary elasticity. J Appl Physiol 1970;28:596.
122. Mead J, Turner JM, Macklem PT, et al: Significance of the relationship between lung recoil and maximum expiratory flow. J Appl Physiol 1967;22:95.
123. Mercat A, Graini L, Teboul JL, et al: Cardiorespiratory effects of pressure-controlled ventilation with and without inverse ratio in the adult respiratory distress syndrome. Chest 1993;104:871.
124. Messmer TO, Armour R, Holley RW: Factors influencing the growth of alveolar type II epithelial cells isolated from rat lungs. Exp Cell Res 1982;142:417.
125. Milles G, Dorsey DB: Intra-uterine respiration-like movements in relation to development of the fetal vascular system: A discussion of intra-uterine physiology based upon cases of congenital absence of the trachea, abnormal vascular development, and other anomalies. Am J Pathol 1950;26:411.
126. Monaco F, McQuitty JC: Transcutaneous measurements of carbon dioxide partial pressure in sick neonates. Crit Care Med 1981;9:756.
127. Morris A: Clinical Pulmonary Function Testing: A Manual of Uniform Laboratory Procedures. Salt Lake City, Intermountain Thoracic Society, 1984.
128. Muakkassa FF, Rutledge R, Fakhry SM, et al: ABGs and arterial lines: The relationship to unnecessarily drawn arterial blood gas samples. J Trauma 1900;30:1087.
129. Munoz J, Guerrero JE, Escalante JL, et al: Pressure-controlled ventilation versus controlled mechanical ventilation with decelerating inspiratory flow. Crit Care Med 1993;21:1143.
130. Muratore CS, Nguyen HT, Ziegler MM, et al: Stretch-induced upregulation of VEGF gene expression in murine pulmonary culture: A role for angiogenesis in lung development. J Pediatr Surg 2000;35:906.
131. Nadeau S, Noble WH: Limitations of cardiac output measurements by thermodilution. Can Anaesth Soc J 1986; 33:780.
132. Nakos G, Tsangaris I, Kostanti E, et al: Effect of the prone position on patients with hydrostatic pulmonary edema compared with patients with acute respiratory distress syn-

drome and pulmonary fibrosis. Am J Respir Crit Care Med 2000;161:360.
133. Neuman M: The biophysical and bioengineering bases of perinatal monitoring. Part V. Neonatal cardiac and respiratory monitoring. Perinatal Neonatal 1979;3:17.
134. Nobuhara KK, DiFiore JW, Ibla JC, et al: Insulin-like growth factor-I gene expression in three models of accelerated lung growth. J Pediatr Surg 1998;33:1057.
135. Nobuhara KK, Fauza DO, DiFiore JW, et al: Continuous intrapulmonary distension with perfluorocarbon accelerates neonatal (but not adult) lung growth. J Pediatr Surg 1998;33:292.
136. Offner PJ, Haenel JB, Moore EE, et al: Complications of prone ventilation in patients with multisystem trauma with fulminant acute respiratory distress syndrome. J Trauma 2000;48:224.
137. Otis AB, McKerrow CB, Bartlett RA, et al: Mechanical factors in distribution of pulmonary ventilation. J Appl Physiol 1956;8:427.
138. O'Toole SJ, Sharma A, Karamanoukian HL, et al: Tracheal ligation does not correct the surfactant deficiency associated with congenital diaphragmatic hernia. J Pediatr Surg 1996;31:546.
139. Panos RJ, Rubin JS, Csaky KG, et al: Keratinocyte growth factor and hepatocyte growth factor/scatter factor are heparin-binding growth factors for alveolar type II cells in fibroblast-conditioned medium. J Clin Invest 1993;92:969.
140. Papadakis K, De Paepe ME, Tackett LD, et al: Temporary tracheal occlusion causes catch-up lung maturation in a fetal model of diaphragmatic hernia. J Pediatr Surg 1998;33:1030.
141. Papadakis K, Luks FI, De Paepe ME, et al: Fetal lung growth after tracheal ligation is not solely a pressure phenomenon. J Pediatr Surg 1997;32:347.
142. Patel C, Laboy V, Venus B, et al: Acute complications of pulmonary artery catheter insertion in critically ill patients. Crit Care Med 1986;14:195.
143. Piedboeuf B, Laberge JM, Ghitulescu G, et al: Deleterious effect of tracheal obstruction on type II pneumocytes in fetal sheep. Pediatr Res 1997;41:473.
144. Poets CF, Samuels MP, Noyes JP, et al: Home monitoring of transcutaneous oxygen tension in the early detection of hypoxaemia in infants and young children. Arch Dis Child 1991;66:676.
145. Potter E: Bilateral renal agenesis. J Pediatr 1946;29:68.
146. Potter E, Bohlender G: Intrauterine respiration in relation to development of the fetal lung. Am J Obstet Gynecol 1941;42:14.
147. Pranikoff T, Gauger PG, Hirschl RB: Partial liquid ventilation in newborn patients with congenital diaphragmatic hernia. J Pediatr Surg 1996;31:613.
148. Pringle K: Lung development in congenital diaphragmatic hernia. In Puri P (ed): Congenital Diaphragmatic Hernia. New York, Karger, 1989, p 62.
149. Puri VK, Carlson RW, Bander JJ, et al: Complications of vascular catheterization in the critically ill: A prospective study. Crit Care Med 1980;8:495.
150. Quinn TM, Sylvester KG, Kitano Y, et al: TGF-beta2 is increased after fetal tracheal occlusion. J Pediatr Surg 1999;34:701.
151. Rahn H: The pressure-volume diagram of the thorax and lung. Am J Physiol 1946;146:161.
152. Raine JM, Bishop JM: A-a difference in O_2 tension and physiological dead space in normal man. J Appl Physiol 1963;18:284.
153. Randomized study of high-frequency oscillatory ventila-
153. Randomized study of high-frequency oscillatory ventilation in infants with severe respiratory distress syndrome. HiFO Study Group. J Pediatr 1993;122:609.
154. Rappaport SH, Shpiner R, Yoshihara G, et al: Randomized, prospective trial of pressure-limited versus volume-controlled ventilation in severe respiratory failure. Crit Care Med 1994;22:22.
155. Reid L: The embryology of the lung. In Ciba Foundation Symposium: Development of the Lung. London, Churchill, 1967, p 109.
156. Reid L: Structural and functional reappraisal of the pulmonary artery system. In British Postgraduate Medical Federation: Scientific Basis of Medicine, Annual Reviews. London, Athlone Press, 1968, p 235.
157. Reid L: 1976 Edward B. D. Neuhauser lecture: The lung: growth and remodeling in health and disease. AJR Am J Roentgenol 1977;129:777.
158. Reid LM: Lung growth in health and disease. Br J Dis Chest 1984;78:113.
159. Reid WD, Huang J, Bryson S, et al: Diaphragm injury and myofibrillar structure induced by resistive loading. J Appl Physiol 1994;76:176.
160. Richardson JB: Nerve supply to the lungs. Am Rev Respir Dis 1979;119:785.
161. Roubliova XI, Verbeken EK, Wu J, et al: Effect of tracheal occlusion on peripheric pulmonary vessel muscularization in a fetal rabbit model for congenital diaphragmatic hernia. Am J Obstet Gynecol 2004;191:830.
162. Roughton FJ, Forster RE: Relative importance of diffusion and chemical reaction rates in determining rate of exchange of gases in the human lung, with special reference to true diffusing capacity of pulmonary membrane and volume of blood in the lung capillaries. J Appl Physiol 1957;11:290.
163. Sassoon CS, Mahutte CK, Light RW: Ventilator modes: Old and new. Crit Care Clin 1990;6:605.
164. Schnitzer JJ: Control and regulation of pulmonary hypoplasia associated with congenital diaphragmatic hernia. Semin Pediatr Surg 2004;13:37.
165. Severinghaus JW, Kelleher JF: Recent developments in pulse oximetry. Anesthesiology 1992;76:1018.
166. Severinghaus JW, Spellman MJ Jr: Pulse oximeter failure thresholds in hypotension and vasoconstriction. Anesthesiology 1990;73:532.
167. Shaffer TH, Moskowitz GD: Demand-controlled liquid ventilation of the lungs. J Appl Physiol 1974;36:208.
168. Shanholtz C, Brower R: Should inverse ratio ventilation be used in adult respiratory distress syndrome? Am J Respir Crit Care Med 1994;149:1354.
monitoring of critically ill adults, with and without low flow shock. Crit Care Med 1981;9:706.
188. Tutuncu AS, Cakar N, Camci E, et al: Comparison of pressure- and flow-triggered pressure-support ventilation on weaning parameters in patients recovering from acute respiratory failure. Crit Care Med 1997;25:756.
189. Varnholt V, Lasch P, Suske G, et al: High frequency oscillatory ventilation and extracorporeal membrane oxygenation in severe persistent pulmonary hypertension of the newborn. Eur J Pediatr 1992;151:769.
190. Varon A: Hemodynamic monitoring: Arterial and pulmonary artery catheters. In Civetta J, Taylor R, Kirby R (eds): Critical Care, 2nd ed. Philadelphia, JB Lippincott, 1992, p 321.
191. Voggenreiter G, Neudeck F, Aufmkolk M, et al: Intermittent prone positioning in the treatment of severe and moderate posttraumatic lung injury. Crit Care Med 1999;27:2375.

192. Wagner PD: Diffusion and chemical reaction in pulmonary gas exchange. Physiol Rev 1977;57:257.
193. Wagner PD, Laravuso RB, Uhl RR, et al: Continuous distributions of ventilation-perfusion ratios in normal subjects breathing air and 100 per cent O_2. J Clin Invest 1974;54:54.
194. Wagner PD, West JB: Effects of diffusion impairment on O_2 and CO_2 time courses in pulmonary capillaries. J Appl Physiol 1972;33:62.
195. Waldhorn RE, Herrick TW, Nguyen MC, et al: Long-term compliance with nasal continuous positive airway pressure therapy of obstructive sleep apnea. Chest 1990;97:33.
196. Wasserman K, Whipp BJ: Exercise physiology in health and disease. Am Rev Respir Dis 1975;112:219.
197. Watcha MF, Connor MT, Hing AV: Pulse oximetry in methemoglobinemia. Am J Dis Child 1989;143:845.
198. Weibel ER: Morphological basis of alveolar-capillary gas exchange. Physiol Rev 1973;53:419.
199. Weibel ER, Gomez DM: A principle for counting tissue structures on random sections. J Appl Physiol 1962;17:343.
200. West JB, Wagner PD, Derks CM: Gas exchange in distributions of VA-Q ratios: Partial pressure-solubility diagram. J Appl Physiol 1974;37:533.
201. Whipp BJ, Wasserman K: Alveolar-arterial gas tension differences during graded exercise. J Appl Physiol 1969; 27:361.
202. Wigglesworth JS, Desai R, Hislop AA: Fetal lung growth in congenital laryngeal atresia. Pediatr Pathol 1987;7:515.
203. Wilson JM, DiFiore JW, Peters CA: Experimental fetal tracheal ligation prevents the pulmonary hypoplasia associated with fetal nephrectomy: Possible application for congenital diaphragmatic hernia. J Pediatr Surg 1993; 28:1433.
204. Wung JT, James LS, Kilchevsky E, et al: Management of infants with severe respiratory failure and persistence of the fetal circulation, without hyperventilation. Pediatrics 1985;76:488.
205. Younces M, Roberts D, Light R, et al: Proportional assist ventilation: A new approach to ventilatory support [abstract]. Am Rev Respir Dis 1989;139:A363.

第 8 章

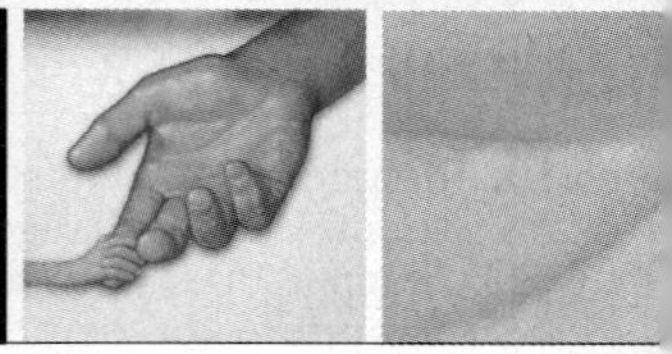

心肺衰竭的体外生命支持

Ronald B. Hirschl 和 Robert H. Bartlett

体外生命支持（ECLS）或体外膜式氧合（ECMO）意味着对那些对常规医疗或药物措施无效的、有急性可逆的心脏或呼吸衰竭患者使用长时间的体外心肺转流，通常要通过胸外插管进行[7,42]。重要的是要认识到，ECLS 不是一种治疗措施；它只是在可逆的病理生理学过程无法自行缓解或通过医疗或手术干预无法缓解的时候提供心肺支持，以便患者可以免受高气道压力、高吸入氧浓度（FiO_2）、血管活性药物和灌注损伤的不利影响。所有运用的 ECLS 都是采取相同的技术，但是对于有呼吸或心力衰竭的成人、儿童和新生儿，其适应证、治疗和结果最好分别考虑。本章只讨论有呼吸或心力衰竭的新生儿和儿童。

1989 年，许多活跃的 ECLS 中心组成了体外生命支持组织（ELSO），对 ECLS 的许多方面进行了标准化。ELSO 对各个成员中心的所有治疗病例进行了登记。在此提供的许多信息是建立在 ELSO 的登记基础上的。

背景

1975 年，ECLS 首次成功应用于一个有呼吸衰竭的新生儿的治疗[9]。到 1982 年，已用 ECLS 治疗了 45 个有呼吸衰竭的新生儿，其中有早产儿，也有足月产儿，结果有 55%的新生儿存活，且 80%的存活者其短期生长和发育都正常[8-10]。三项前瞻性随机试验比较了 ECLS 和传统机械通气对有严重呼吸功能不全的足月产婴儿的效果。1985 年，我们的小组使用了一种称为“乘胜追击法（或胜方策略，play-the-winner）”的适应性设计，对成功和不成功的干预措施进行了随机比较[12]。随机方案的结果为：11 例 ECLS 患者存活，1 例对照组患者死亡。虽然在登记的患者中，预期死亡率为 80%～90%，统计学上是有显著性的，但是这项研究是有高度争议的且不为医学界接受。1989 年，O'Rourke 等人[68]使用相同的适应性设计进行了一项随机试验。对照组 10 例患者中有 6 例存活（60%），ECLS 组 29 例患者中有 28 例存活（97%）。在英国进行的一项传统的随机前瞻性研究证实，在使用 ECLS 治疗的足月新生儿的存活率（72%）和采用传统方法治疗的足月新生儿的存活率（41%）之间存在显著差异[30]。基于这些研究，ECLS 被认为适用于有高死亡率风险的呼吸衰竭的新生儿的。到 2004 年 7 月，ELSO 登记数据库已有 27 407 例心肺衰竭的成人、儿科和新生儿患者进行了 ECLS，整体生存率为 73%[28]。

1991 年，Timmons 等人[94]进行了一次儿科呼吸衰竭的多中心数据汇总研究。唯一与结果改善有关的治疗变量就是 ECLS。Green 等人[39]对这个庞大的数据库进行了进一步的评估。他们对采用 ECLS 治疗（74%存活率）和采用传统治疗（53%存活率）的患者进行了配对研究。到 2004 年 7 月，有 2762 例年龄超过 30 天的呼吸衰竭儿童登记在册，其整体生存率为 56%。

1972 年以来，ECLS 已成功用于儿科心力衰竭患者的治疗。术中或术后心力衰竭是最普遍的适应证。ECLS 是儿童唯一可用的机械支持系统，成人则不同，成人可以使用球囊泵和心室支持装置。到 2004 年 7 月，共登记了 5584 例儿童心力衰竭患者，整体生存率为 41%。

适应证

当预期 2～4 周内可以康复时，ECLS 可用于急

35 性严重呼吸或心力衰竭。严重心力衰竭或呼吸衰竭可定义为死亡风险＞50%的急性衰竭；各类不同的患者的存活率在 50%～90%。在一些病例中，风险很容易判别（例如，在手术室内，停止心肺转流后的心脏停搏或抑制）。在另一些病例中，风险则难以定量（例如，处于中等通气条件设定和一氧化氮治疗下的新生儿，其氧合为 80%，处于临界状态）。一些评分系统已设计出来，用于对这些患者进行分类并尝试定义高死亡风险。

新生儿呼吸衰竭的死亡风险可以在给予所有适当治疗后，用基于动脉氧合（PaO_2）和气道平均压（MAP）的氧指数（OI）来测量。OI 可根据下列公式进行计算：

$$OI = (MPA \times FiO_2 \times 100) / PaO_2$$

在早期的 ECLS 研究中，每隔 30～60 分钟抽取动脉导管后血样进行血气分析，其中 3/5 的 OI＞40时，即预测死亡风险＞80% [11,69]。我们的小组进行了一项随机对照研究，结果提示，在 OI＞25、预期死亡率为59%的基础上，“早期”开始 ECLS 的患者与对照组中 OI＞40 才开始 ECLS 的患者相比，其 1 岁时精神发育评分有升高的趋势，且发病率也较低[79]。我们目前认为，当一系列动脉导管后动脉血气结果证实 OI＞25时，可使用 ECLS，在 OI＞40 时，必须使用 ECLS。

在有呼吸衰竭的年长儿童中，高死亡风险的标准是建立在 OI 或肺泡动脉氧梯度（AaO_2）基础上的。Rivera 等人[75]认为，通气指数（呼吸频率 × $PaCO_2$ × 吸气峰压 /1000）＞40 且 OI＞40 时，死亡率为 77%，合并吸气峰压≥40cmH_2O 和 $AaDO_2$＞580 mmHg 时，死亡率为 81%。我们认为，FiO_2 为 1.0、$AaDO_2$＞600 mmHg——在给予正确治疗后——是儿童高死亡风险的征象。

在有心力衰竭的儿科患者开始 ECLS 的标准是：虽然给予了变力性药物和容量复苏，但患者还存在外周灌注降低临床体征，包括少尿（每小时尿量＜0.5 ml/kg）、代谢性酸中毒和低血压[22,60]。在儿科心脏病患者中，ECLS 是应用于心源性休克（20%）、心搏骤停（20%）和病情急性恶化（10%）；另有 20%的患者是因无法脱离心肺转流而在手术室直接放置了 ECLS。

目前相对的禁忌证为下列情况：

1. 早产儿。新生儿体重下限为 1 kg 和孕 30 周，因为体重更轻和年龄更小的婴儿其颅内出血的发生率更高[18,44]。
2. 使用 ECMO 前颅内出血程度高于 2 级[73]。
3. 长时间机械通气。新生儿和儿科患者使用机械通气超过 7 天被认为是 ECLS 的禁忌证，因为其支气管肺发育不良和不可逆性纤维增生性肺病的发生率高。但对 ELSO 登记数据的回顾提示， 在 ECLS 前已经使用 14 天机械通气的呼吸衰竭新生儿和儿科患者中，存活率约保持在 50%～60%[72]。我们目前对机械通气不超过 14 天的患者使用 ECLS。要牢记，发病率和死亡率会随着机械通气的时间延长而升高。
4. 心搏骤停。在进行 ECLS 前的时间段内，需要进行心肺复苏的心搏骤停被认为是建立体外支持的禁忌证。但是在插管之前或插管过程中发生心搏骤停的新生儿中，观察到的存活率最高有60%[25,99]。至于那些存活者，至少 60%的人有较理想的神经病学预后。在有心力衰竭且在建立 ECLS 之前发生心搏骤停、时间为 65 ± 9 分钟的儿科患者中，也观察到同样的存活率（64%），且无长期后遗症[23]。基于这些数据，许多中心现在也将在 ECLS 之前有心搏骤停的患者作为体外支持的候选人。
5. 先天性膈疝（CDH）合并双侧发育不良。虽然 CDH 最初是一个禁忌证[40]，但随后证实，很多存在这种排除标准的患者能存活下来。因此，大多数中心现在把 CDH 患者都作为 ECLS 的候选人[66,87]。Stolar 等人[90]建议，无法形成动脉导管后，PaO_2＞100 mmHg 和 $PaCO_2$＜50 mmHg 可准确确认无法救治的 CDH 婴儿，这些人应该排除在 ECLS 之外。
6. 严重的神经损害、多发性先天性畸形或其他无法取得长远生命的情况。

年长儿童的其他相对禁忌证是多器官系统衰竭、严重烧伤、免疫缺陷、活动性出血和出现无法治愈的疾病过程。

体外支持的方法

ECLS 的目的是将温暖的动脉化血液灌注到患者

体内[7]。为了达成这一目的，使用静脉–动脉（VA）模式的体外血流来进行心脏支持，使用静脉–静脉（VV）模式的血流来进行呼吸支持。VA 模式提供了完全的支持，但是也有显著的缺点：（1）必须在大动脉上插管，并至少会临时性损害大动脉；（2）实际存在细微颗粒播散或体循环气栓的危险；（3）肺灌注可能明显降低；（4）左心室输出可能降低，因为存在 ECLS 回路流量升高造成的后负荷阻力；（5）冠状动脉主要由相对缺氧的左心室血流进行灌注[80]。
136 VV 通路可以使用两根管道，也可以使用一根双腔管道支持气体交换，这避免了 VA 支持的缺点。VV 或双腔 VV 模式的 ECLS 目前可用于任何年龄组的无需心脏支持的患者（图 8–1）[20]。来自 ELSO 登记的数据和一个非随机化的多中心研究提示，使用双腔 VV 结构的转流可能可提高存活率和降低新生儿颅内出血发生率。但是，根据 ECLS 前心肺功能障碍的严重程度进行校正的配对分析表明，在使用双腔 VV 或 VA 结构转流的患者之间，不存在参数差异[32]。没有可用于体重超过 10 kg 儿童的双腔管。至于年长儿，则使用股静脉和颈静脉插管。

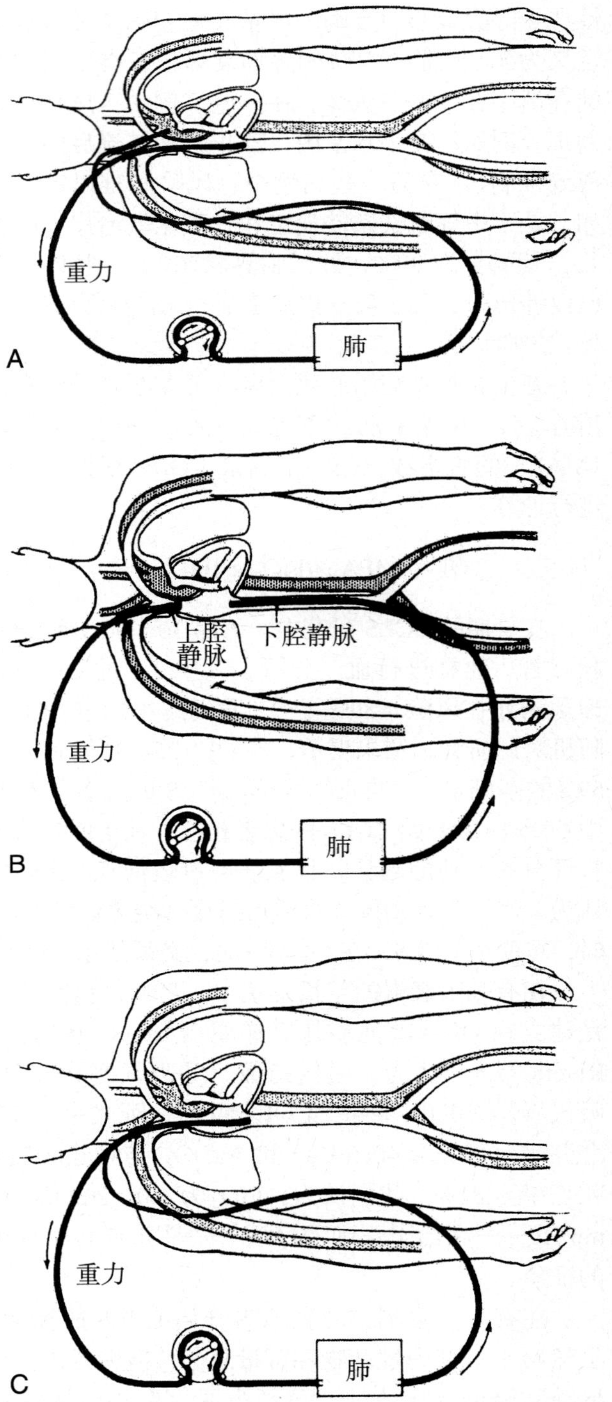

图 8–1 三种最常用的体外转流结构。A. 静脉–动脉模式，通过颈内静脉引流，颈动脉回灌。B. 静脉–静脉模式，通过颈内静脉引流，股静脉回灌。C. 静脉–静脉模式，通过放置在颈内静脉内的双腔管进行转流。

体外生命支持回路

ECLS 回路包括一个泵、一个膜肺和一个热交换器（图 8–2），以及其他用于安全和监测的相关装置。有关功能装置和功能故障的完整技术描述可参阅 ELSO 的教科书[27]。右心房血液借助重力虹吸效应，通过一根经右侧颈内静脉或右侧股静脉置入的管道进行引流。滚动泵是最常用的灌注装置，需要进行持续的伺服调节和监测，以防止引流回路部分负压过大和正压过大。存在回路断开风险时，灌注肢体的回路部分应该能够进行关闭。使用高负压引流回路（例如使
137 用离心泵）会造成溶血，对右心房或腔静脉的内皮细胞造成损害，并且当气体从液体中抽出时形成空泡效应。

最常用的人工肺是 Kolobow 螺线管固体硅胶膜肺。根据表 8–1 所示的患者体重来选择不同尺寸的 ECLS 功能部件。使用多微孔材料制造的中空纤维人工肺在气体交换方面有高功效，其血流阻力低，并且易于使用。多微孔膜肺的缺点是：水在气体相时凝集率升高，并由于发生血浆渗漏而需要频繁更换[62]。磷脂吸附于中空纤维上 5μm 微孔的血液接触界面，是造成血浆渗漏的原因[62]。无空的中空纤维人工肺解决

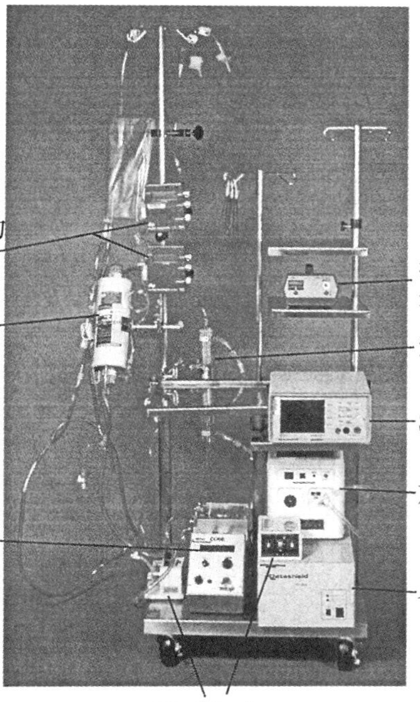

图 8-2 体外生命支持回路。基本部件包括滚动泵、膜肺和热交换器。所示装置的其余部分用来执行监测和安全功能。

了这一问题，可作为 ECLS 的首选。这些装置在欧洲和日本都已经使用，但是在美国没有用过。

新生儿回路的预充容量约为 400～500 毫升，这是新生儿自身血容量的 1～2 倍。因此在转流开始时，必须认真使用回路对新生儿进行灌注，以保持血液的 pH，血细胞比容，钙，凝血因子和电解质在合理的水平，且要保持合适的温度。但是，如表 8–1所示，对于体重超过 35 kg 的患者，使用 ECLS 时可能无需加入额外的血液预充。

患者管理

ELSO 的教科书中详细阐述了对患者的管理。静脉插管的尺寸是决定血流比率的因素，因此也决定了体外支持的水平。应该尽可能放置最大号的静脉管道；其尺寸应该能满足在 100cmH_2O 的重力虹吸压的支持下提供合理的血流（每分钟 100ml/kg）。既定管道的流量–压力特征取决于很多几何因素，包括长度、内径和侧孔位置。采用 M 编号为描述不同的血管通路装置中的流量–压力关系提供了一个标准化的手段[63,83]。

静脉通路的第一选择是颈内静脉，因为其管径大，且使用短插管即可很方便地进入右心房。股静脉是 ECLS 过程中静脉引流通路的第二选择和进行 VV 支持时的第一引流选择。对年龄低于 5 岁的儿童，股静脉太细而不能作为主要引流通路，且对幼儿是使用颈静脉到股静脉方式进行 VV 支持的。近端的静脉引

表 8–1 不同体重的患者进行静脉–静脉支持时的回路组件与使用

	体重（kg）					
	2～4	4～15*	15～20	20～30	30～50	50⁺
引流管（英寸）	1/4	NA	3/8	3/8	1/2	1/2
缆线管道（英寸）	1/4	NA	3/8～1/2	1/2	1/2	1/2
氧合器（m^2）	0.8～1.5	NA	2.5～3.5	3.5～4.5	4.5	4.5 × 2
插管†（F）	12～15	NA	Inf: 16～19	Inf: 17～21	Inf: 21	Inf: 21
	DLVV‡	NA	Dr: 14～19	Dr: 17～21	Dr: 19～23§	Dr: 21～23§
预充	RBC: 1～2 U	NA	RBC: 3 U	RBC: 4 U	RBC: 4 U¶	RBC: 5 U¶
	FFP: 50～100 ml	NA	FFP: 1/2 U	FFP: 1 U	FFP: 1 U	FFP: 1 U

* 静脉–静脉 ECLS 目前不推荐体重在 4～15kg（年龄＜3 岁）的患者使用。

† 特殊尺寸中最短的 Biomedicus 管道是插管时可用的。这些仅是指南，应该考虑不同的患者个体差异。

‡ 12～15F 的 DLVV 插管是由 Jostra 生产的。14F 的 DLVV 插管是由 Kendall 生产的。

¶ 通常使用每 3 升 Normosol 溶液中加入 12.5 g白蛋白和 1g $CaCl_2$。

DLVV：双腔静脉–静脉模式；Dr：引流；ECLS：体外生命支持；FFP：新鲜冰冻血浆；Inf：灌注；NA：不可用；RBC：红细胞；U：单位。1 英寸 = 25.4 毫米。

流管可以放置在近端的颈内静脉内，以促进体外回路中的静脉引流[85]。一个研究证实，与历史上的对照组比较，开始使用这类插管后，颅内出血有所减少[67]。但是，一个 ELSO 登记研究并未能证实常规使用近端静脉引流插管，对颅内出血和生存率有影响[29]。

回输管尺寸的重要性不如静脉插管的尺寸重要，虽然它也必须足够大以耐受在全转流水平时预期的血流率，而不会在膜肺近端产生高于 350 mmHg 的压力。在所有年龄组患者，动脉循环中放置插管的第一选择是颈静脉，因为其容易进入主动脉弓。新生儿和儿童的颈静脉插管和结扎的并发症很少[58,77]。动脉通路的第二选择是股动脉。股动脉插管时，需要对下肢
138 远端动脉循环进行灌注。

通常在局部麻醉下直接切开行插管手术（图 8-3）。动脉和静脉插管的尖端（尺寸参见表 8-1）通常分别置于右侧头臂动脉的开口处和右心房下侧。双腔静脉-静脉插管必须如此放置，以便尖端位于右心房中部，使回灌孔朝向三尖瓣，以减少回灌血流的再次循环。成人和年龄大于 3 岁的儿童在插管之前，优先采取颈内静脉和股静脉的经皮穿刺路径。随后经导引丝放入较大的扩张器，使用 Seldinger 技术取得最终血管通路，将插管放入这些大型静脉。12F 或 15F 的双腔静脉-静脉插管可以比较顺利地经皮置入新生儿的颈内静脉。

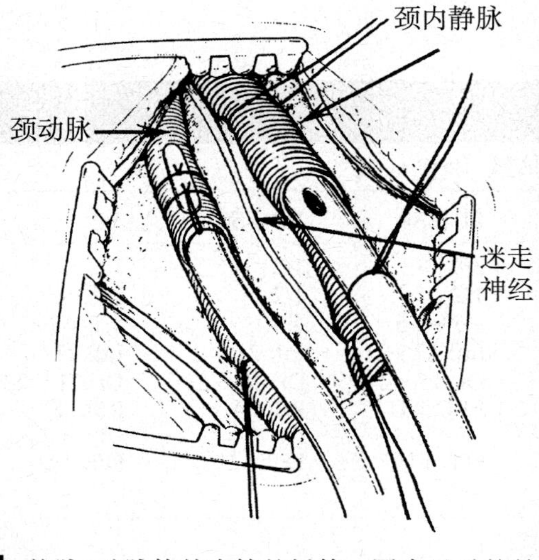

图 8-3 静脉-动脉体外支持的插管。图中显示的是右侧锁骨上切口。在新生儿中，插管置入动脉2.5cm，置入静脉6.0 cm。使用 2-0 丝线环绕结扎固定插管，并在结扎线下发放置一小片塑料管袢，以便在拔管时保护血管不受损伤。标志结扎线的一端系在最远端的环绕线上作为外固定。

插管连上 ECLS 回路，并开始心肺转流。确保 10～15 分钟内流量上升到 100 ml/kg 水平。一旦患者开始了体外支持，心肺状况会迅速获得稳定。在进行静脉-动脉支持过程中，终止使用所有的肌松药物，血管活性药物和其他输液；当使用静脉-静脉转流时、可能还是需要使用一些加压药物或正性肌力药物支持。呼吸机参数调节到最低水平（吸气峰压＜25，且 FiO_2＜0.4），以便让肺休息，并封闭任何由于气压伤引起的空气泄漏。已经证实，在体外支持过程中，使用 12～14cmH_2O 的呼气末正压，可将 ECLS 的持续时间从 132 ± 55 小时降低到 97 ± 36 小时。因为仅使用了部分转流，所以氧合与二氧化碳清除还是取决于自体肺功能和体外血流的作用。放置在回路中静脉肢体内的光纤血氧测定导管可很方便地监测混合静脉血氧饱和（SvO_2），以便能根据氧耗来判定合理的氧输送。调节泵流量来保持氧输送，因此在静脉-动脉支持时，SvO_2 要高于 70%，静脉-静脉支持时，SvO_2 要高于 85%。$PaCO_2$ 和膜肺中的气体通气流量比成反比。

心脏支持插管

能观察到大约 7%的新生儿在开始 ECLS 后心肌功能恶化[26,43,57]。这种“心肌顿抑制（myocardial stun）”通常发生在极度缺氧、较频繁发生心搏骤停以及在 ECLS 之前就需要多次使用肾上腺素加压药物的患者中。在开始 ECLS 的头 24～48 小时内，这种情况通常会缓解。

如果左心室不射血（没有动脉脉搏波形），左心室和心房将扩张并引起肺水肿。如果发生了这种情况，可能需要实施球囊或切开房间隔造口术来进行左心减压，缓解肺水肿和最终改善心功能[51]。

逐步增高肝素剂量以防在 ECLS 过程中血栓形成。通过每小时测定全血活化凝血时间（ACT）来监测抗凝水平[7,42]。ACT 保持在大于正常值（Hemochron 仪测定为 180 秒）的 50%～60%。时常需要输注红细胞保持血细胞比容大于 45%，输注新鲜冰冻血浆保持纤维蛋白原水平大于 200 mg/dL。虽然血小板功能和计数降低与体外支持有关，且给予血小板也仅能一过性纠

正这种情况[76]，但是还是要输注血小板以保持血小板计数大于 100 000/mm³。Stallion 等人[86]提出，血小板计数维持在 200 000/mm³ 以上可能可降低出血并发症。我们持续将血小板计数保持在 100 000/mm³ 以上，除非患者存在出血的高危因素或正在出血，对于后者，我们把血小板计数保持在 150 000/mm³ 以上。

逐步增加利尿药物和血液过滤使体重保持到正常“干”重。在 ECLS 时，肾功能可能会一过性受损；因此对于有些患者，可能需要在回路中安装血液过滤器来增加尿排出量[41]。在 ECLS 前或 ECLS 时发生的肾功能不全也易于处理，可在必要时在体外回路中安装血液过滤器[81]。需要 ECLS 的危重患者对营养存在高度优先的需求。

在 ECLS 期间，实施的大多数手术操作都在重症监护室内进行[6]。可以实施通过 ECLS 回路中的氧合器进行异氟烷气体麻醉或静脉内芬太尼或舒芬太尼和
139 维库溴铵麻醉[65]。Nagaraj 等人[65]阐述了对 37例进行 ECLS 的新生儿进行的 44 次手术操作。这些操作包括再插管或插管重定位（14）、管状胸廓造口术（11）、心脏手术（6）、心导管术（4）、先天性膈疝纠治术（5）和胸廓切开术（4）。46%～55%的患者存在出血并发症，且合并更高的死亡率。因此，必须认真考虑是否有必要进行手术操作，例如，对于少量气胸是否要放置胸腔引流管，或是否将手术推迟到 ECLS 结束以后。在对处于 ECLS 过程中的患者实施手术时，要广泛使用电刀烧灼止血，将 ACT 降低到 160～180 秒，且血小板计数＞150 000/mm³。也应该考虑围术期使用氨基己酸[106]。

先天性膈疝可在 ECLS 之前、之中和之后进行手术修复。当我们认识到肺功能不全是由于发育不良和血管痉挛引起而不是疝引起时，治疗就要改变。Connors 等人[19]最先阐述了对 6 例开始 ECLS 平均 25 小时左右的新生儿进行先天性膈疝修补手术，其中 4 例存活。Lally 等人[54]报道了 42 例在体外支持时进行膈疝修复手术的新生儿的生存率为 43%。Vazquez 和 Cheu[98]报道了高达 48%的需要 ECLS 的先天性膈疝患者在体外支持时进行了手术修复。其他研究提示，可在停止 ECLS 和肺动脉高压持续缓解和脱离呼吸机以后，对先天性膈疝的新生儿实施手术。根据来自 ELSO 登记的数据，Vazquez 和 Cheu[98]证实，在 ECLS 期间进行手术修复的患者，38%因出血需要输血，而在 ECLS 之前或以后进行手术着，则分别为 18%和 6%。Wilson 等人[106]观察了一组 22例在 ECLS 拔管前进行选择性手术修复的患者，发现出血和输血需求有所降低。对这些患者，ACT 维持在 180～200 秒水平，所有患者术后持续使用氨基己酸 72 小时或一直用到拔管。不需要再开胸探查止血。我们目前的实践是脱离 ECLS 后实施疝修补。

当肺功能改善时，ECLS 流量降低，可进行“试脱机”（不进行 ECLS）。在静脉-静脉转流时，膜肺的气相端可单纯封闭，这样患者就仍处于体外血流支持，但并无人工肺参与气体交换。进行静脉-动脉转流的患者可尝试夹闭管线（无血流）。在日常使用合适的加压药物支持下可进行这类试验，并可反复同时进行超声心动图的评估。

一旦决定停止 ECLS，则打开插管部位的切口，结扎右侧颈动脉或颈内静脉或两者都结扎。虽然并未证实存在益处，且存在远端栓塞、远期狭窄和发生动脉粥样硬化的潜在风险，但是还是可以在静脉-动脉体外支持结束后修补颈动脉。经皮放置的插管可以单纯拔出并给予压迫，不用关注患者的抗凝状态。

呼吸衰竭新生儿的 ECLS 持续时间（均数 ± 标准差）为 149 ± 162 小时，呼吸衰竭的儿童为 280 ± 204 小时，先天性心脏病患者为 140 ± 113 小时。在心肺功能改善时可考虑停止心肺支持，其他原因包括出现不可逆的脑损害、其他致命的器官衰竭和无法控制的出血。先天性膈疝或肺炎新生儿和存在心脏或肺衰竭的儿科患者，可能需要在心肺病程缓解之前进行更长时间的 ECLS。

并发症

通常与 ECLS 相关的并发症分为三个主要大类：（1）与肝素化有关的出血；（2）技术上的失败；（3）神经病学后遗症。大部分都是由于开始体外支持前发生的缺氧和血流动力学不稳定引起的。

平均每个 ECLS 病例发生并发症 2.1 次[108]。因为全身进行了肝素化，所以出血并发症是最常见且最具破坏性的[96]。约 13%的新生儿、5%的儿科患者和 4%的心脏病患者发生颅内出血。这是导致接受 ECLS治疗的新生儿死亡的最多见原因[46]。因为存在肝素化，颅内出血的范围和位置异乎寻常[15,16]。处于 ECLS 的

新生儿的发病机制是多因素的。除了使用肝素以外，在停止 ECLS 后 48 小时内，血小板功能和数量也降低，凝血因子水平也降低[2]。Wilson 等人[105]注意到，与历史对照组相比，一组 42 例认为有出血并发症高危因素的新生儿，在插管前或插管后接受了 100 mg/kg 氨基己酸，并持续给予每小时 30mg/kg 剂量直至拔管，其颅内出血发生率降低。早产患儿的颅内出血发生率明显升高，特别是孕龄低于 37周的患儿。虽然对正常动物进行 ECLS 并结扎颈动脉并不会影响颈动脉或脑血流，但在缺氧情况下开始 ECLS 会导致颈动脉和脑血流增高，并丧失脑的自身调节[82]。此外，$PaCO_2$ 降低可导致脑血流显著减少[100]。因此，颈动脉和颈内静脉结扎并迅速启动 ECLS，缺氧或高碳酸血症会引起脑血流和脑自身调节的改变，对抗凝患
140 者存在引起颅内出血的潜在可能。

已观察到 21%的新生儿病例、44%的儿科呼吸病例和 40%的新生儿及儿科心脏病例存在颅外部位的出血：包括胃肠道出血（2%～5%）；插管位置出血（最高为 6%）；其他手术部位出血（新生儿呼吸病例为 6%；儿科呼吸病例为 24%；新生儿和儿科心脏病例为 28%）；其他部位出血组群，包括心包、胸腔内和腹膜后（7%～15%）出血。可以通过将血小板计数维持在 150 000/mm^3 以上和把 ACT 降低到 160～180 秒以内来治疗 ECLS 期间的出血[104]。偶尔中断给予肝素，或如果可以耐受，暂时中断转流使凝血状态恢复正常，这些可能对解决出血问题来说是必须的。如果出血持续存在，则有进行进一步手术干预的适应证。我们发现，腹腔内或胸腔内填塞和计划性每日再探查可控制大部分情况下的出血。仅在极端环境下，应该考虑对一个持续心肺衰竭的患者完全停止转流。

ECLS 开始前后引发的神经损伤受到持续的关注。进行转流前，许多新生儿必须耐受缺氧或缺血性损伤。Streletz 等人[92]注意到，在 145 例新生儿在 ECLS 之中和之前所表现出来的脑电图异常无升高。此外，Walsh-Sukys 等人[102]在一项对 26 例进行传统机械通气治疗的新生儿和 43 例进行 ECLS 治疗的新生儿进行的前瞻性评估中发现，两组患者在 8～20 个月大时出现的神经发育损害的发生率相同，为 25%。英国的新生儿随机研究显示，两组存活者中，1 岁时的任何神经发育损害的发生率为 28%[30]。这提示在ECLS 开始前数分钟时结扎颈动脉，其时低氧血症和血流动力学不稳定程度最大，会导致脑组织氧合的进一步降低，这可能会加重神经损伤[55]。

发现有 10%～13%的患者在 ECLS 过程中出现癫痫发作[17]。新生儿在 ECLS 时出现癫痫发作预示着预后差：50%～65%在 ECLS 过程中有脑电图癫痫的患者死亡，或在 1～2 岁内发展成严重残疾。6%～12%的患者发生溶血（血清血红蛋白＞100 mg/dL）。这个并发症可能是由体外支持过程中红细胞损伤引起的，通常与回路中血块形成、滚压泵极度梗阻或使用离心泵等有关。发现 8%的患者有高胆红素血症，10%的患者有肾功能不全。气胸（发生率为 4%～14%）和心脏压塞是危及生命的胸腔内并发症，表现为 PaO_2 升高和外周灌注与 SvO_2 降低，随后出现 ECLS 流量降低和进行性恶化。先紧急放置胸腔或心包引流管，再开胸对心脏压塞进行决定性治疗，可能可以挽救生命。

ELSO 登记资料显示，有 27%的病例发生技术性并发症[91]。每个 ECLS 病例发生机械类并发症的均数为 0.75。最值得注意的技术性并发症包括：回路中出现血栓（26%）、插管位置不正确（6%～15%）、氧合器失效（5%～17%）、泵功能失灵（1%～4%）和回路中出现气体（6%）。虽然在新生儿患者中，生存率存在显著降低——无技术性并发症者的生存率为 84%，而有技术性并发症者的生存率为 80%，技术性并发症对生存的影响并不重大。

结果和随访

ELSO 登记资料中，自 1975 年以来报道了总计 27 520 个病例[28,91,95]。在这些病例中，新生儿呼吸衰竭 19 296 例，儿科呼吸衰竭 2762 例，儿科心力衰竭 5157 例。表 8-2 中给出了新生儿呼吸衰竭存活者的数量和诊断。总体存活率为 77%，在新生儿患者中，观察到的最佳存活率的诊断是胎粪吸入综合征（94%的存活率）、呼吸窘迫综合征（84%）和新生儿持续性肺动脉高压（78%）。在接受 ECLS 的患者中，先天性膈疝患者的存活率最差，可能是因为在那种状况下同时存在“不可逆的”肺发育不良。实际上，需要 ECLS 治疗的先天性膈疝患者的死亡率从 1987 年高达 71%已降低到现在的 53%。对新生儿呼吸疾病进行的 ECLS 治疗病例总数在 1992 年达到顶峰，为

141 1488 例。1993 年（1306 例）和 1994 年（1151 例）的新生儿病例总数存在下降趋势，因为新生儿呼吸治疗的效果得到了改善，包括使用一氧化氮和高频振荡通气[28]。

表 8-3 显示了密歇根大学采用 ECLS 治疗呼吸衰竭的儿科患者的经验。虽然自 1982 年以来的总体生存率为 75%，但是在最近 2 年的生存率为 88%[93]。此外，证实了患者年龄越小，其存活率越高，包括年龄小于 1 岁的婴儿存活率为 100%。ELSO 登记资料证实，儿科呼吸衰竭病例的累计发病率为每年 150～200 例，总体存活率为 56%（表 8-4）[28]。最常见诊断之一为病毒性肺炎，主要由呼吸道合胞病毒引起，其实际存活率为 49%～58%[61,89]。来自其他个别中心的研究也提示，采用 ECLS 治疗的呼吸衰竭儿科患者的存活率为 41%～53%[64,103]。已注意到，有多器官系统衰竭的儿科患者和进行 ECLS 治疗的极重症败血症休克患者其存活率约为 50%[14]。Green 等人[38]分析了来自 ELSO 登记资料的数据，证实使用 ECLS 时间超过 2 周的呼吸衰竭儿科患者的存活率与接受较短时期支持的患者的存活率相似。但是，必须考虑到呼吸功能障碍的可逆性本质，出现合并的多器官系统衰竭，发生与 ECLS 相关的并发症，这些可以用来判断是否要在长时间 ECLS之后继续使用这一治疗。

表 8-5 显示了 ELSO 登记数据的心脏支持病例的总结[28]。每年报给登记部门的心脏病病例为 200～300 例，大部分为儿科心脏手术病例。总体存活率为 41%。几乎所有患者都采用静脉-动脉转流治疗。单心室类畸形患者的存活率特别差（0～25%）[53]。虽然

表 8-2 体外生命支持组织登记资料：体外生命支持治疗新生儿呼吸衰竭的数据总结（至 2004 年 7 月）

主要诊断	患者总数	存活数	存活百分比
先天性膈疝	4491	2367	53
胎粪吸入综合征	6560	6160	94
新生儿持续性肺动脉高压 / 持续性胎儿循环	2914	2287	78
呼吸窘迫综合征 / 透明膜病变	1380	1161	84
肺炎 / 败血症	2650	1857	70
气体渗漏综合征	96	69	72
其他	1205	777	64
总计	19 296	14 678	76

表 8-3 密歇根大学 1982 年 11 月至 2004 年 7 月间采用体外生命支持治疗的儿科呼吸衰竭病例

主要诊断	患者总数	存活数	存活百分比
病毒性肺炎	53	44	83
细菌性肺炎或败血症	17	10	59
误吸	13	10	77
创伤	7	7	100
急性呼吸窘迫综合征	67	42	63
其他	40	34	85
总计	197	147	75

表 8-4 体外生命支持组织登记资料：采用体外生命支持治疗儿科呼吸衰竭病例的数据总结（至2004 年 7 月）

主要诊断	患者总数	存活数	存活百分比
细菌性肺炎	290	157	54
病毒性肺炎	728	457	63
创伤	70	44	63
误吸	168	110	65
肺炎	22	9	41
急性呼吸窘迫综合征	278	144	52
其他	1206	615	51
总计	2762	1536	56

表 8-5 体外生命支持组织登记资料：采用体外生命支持治疗心力衰竭病例（儿童年龄为 1 天至 16岁）的数据总结（至 2004 年 7 月）

主要诊断	患者总数	存活数	存活百分比
心脏手术	4064	1564	38
心脏停搏	98	30	31
心肌炎	156	89	57
心肌病	333	181	54
其他	933	409	44
总计	5584	2273	41

Ziomek 等人[107]证实了 17 例在手术室内就开始 ECLS 的患者的存活率为 47%，但是其他研究提示，在手术室内开始 ECLS 或在手术后超过 50 小时后开始 ECLS 或进行 ECLS 治疗超过 6～9 天的患者的预后不良[107]。来自许多中心的数据证实，存活率在 46%～53%波动 [47,74]。Klein 等人[50]在 39 例婴儿和儿童中观察到的存活率为 61%。死亡原因为：37%的患者心血管功能缺乏改善，15%的患者存在重大中枢神经系统损害，这提示了更早进行 ECLS 干预能改善预后[74]。在费城儿童医院的大型病例研究中，3.4%的进行心脏手术的儿童使用了 ECLS，总体存活率为 39% [59]。采用 ECLS 作为等待心脏移植的过渡手段的患者存活率为 40%～60% [31]。心脏移植后心力衰竭的儿科患者使
142 用 ECLS 的远期存活率为 35%～41%。

在其他临床情况下，ECLS 也是有用的，如儿童和成人创伤的存活率约为 65% [4,88]。虽然以前将热损伤考虑为禁忌证，但是 ECLS 也用于儿科烧伤患者(平均烧伤面积为总体表面积的 46%)，5 个患者中有 3 个存活[37]。ECLS 也成功用于接受气管修复的患者、需要进行肺灌洗的肺泡蛋白沉积症患者和因宫内肾功能不全引起肺发育不良的患者，以及哮喘、镰状细胞病和肺移植后肺衰竭患者[33-35,45,49,84,101]。其他 ECLS 使用方式为：给存在心源性休克、创伤后低血压、体温过低、心律失常和心脏停搏的成年或儿科患者作为体外心肺支持[24]。

针对新生儿和儿科患者在一段时间的 ECLS 后的长期随访进行了很多研究。大部分证实，70%～80%的患者神经功能正常[1,5,36,78]。这些研究证明，在 ECLS 治疗的新生儿和采用传统机械通气治疗的新生儿中，神经损伤发病率无差异。

已证实进行 ECLS 治疗的先天性膈疝患者的发病率高，包括胃食管反流的发生率高达 81%，需要管饲的高达 69%，发生慢性肺病变的高达 62%，出现神经轴外液体聚集或脑室扩大的有 30%，40%～50%的人有发育迟缓[21,56,97]。这些问题似乎可以随着时间而缓解。先天性膈疝新生儿的神经发育预后与其他 ECLS 治疗的儿童不同。虽然大多数心脏病患者和呼吸衰竭儿科患者证实了随访中出现的后遗症很少，但是对这些组群的长期研究尚不完整。

三项研究比较了采取 ECLS 治疗新生儿患者的费用与更传统治疗方式的费用。全部都证实，住院费用没有显著差异：ECLS 患者为 485 000 美元，采取传统机械通气治疗患者为 537 000 美元[79]。Pearson 和 Short[70]发现，接受 ECLS 的新生儿的平均日花费为接受传统机械通气患者日花费的 2 倍，但是 ECLS 组的平均住院天数降低了 50%。如只考虑存活者的话，ECLS 组的住院费用比传统治疗组的低 43%。

一个持续进行数天或数周的体外支持的患者需要一个有内科医生、呼吸治疗师、护士和 ECLS 技术员组成的、有准备、有组织、训练有素且技术娴熟的专业队伍。这并非是在需要时就可以不作准备和不用组织就随意使用的技术。目前美国儿科学会委员会给予胎儿和新生儿的推荐标准建议，仅能在通过认证的三级地区中心建立新生儿 ECLS 中心，并要具备合理的教学计划、开展研究活动和婴儿随访程序[71]。

体外生命支持的前景

虽然现有的装置可以进行安全而有效的长时间体外支持，但是未来的 ECLS 依赖于部件技术的改善和相关回路的简化和自动调节。可能可以通过潮流量单根插管系统来进行静脉-静脉支持，该系统通过一根经皮放置的静脉插管，以一个非封闭滚压泵和交互夹闭来产生循环性引流和再灌注。一旦发展出可提供体外支持用途且无需抗凝的紧凑型伺服调节装置，ECLS 将从一个复杂而高劳动强度的干预手段转变成一个简单的技术。在那时，体外支持的适应证将拓宽，同时此技术将更多地用于心肺功能不全程度较轻的人群。

ECLS 经验中的一个主要益处在于有益于探索心脏和呼吸衰竭的病理生理学。加深对肺和心脏器官衰竭的理解可催生出新的预防措施并改进治疗模式，并最终消除心脏呼吸衰竭患者对 ECLS 的需求。

（孙彦隽译　刘锦纷校）

参考文献

1. Adolph V, Ekelund C, Smith C, et al: Developmental outcome of neonates treated with extracorporeal membrane oxygenation. J Pediatr Surg 1990;25:43.
2. Anderson H, Cilley RE, Zwischenberger JB, et al: Thrombocytopenia in neonates after extracorporeal membrane oxygenation. ASAIO Trans 1986;32:534.
3. Anderson H, Snedecor SM, Otsu T, et al: Multicenter comparison of conventional venoarterial access versus venovenous double-lumen catheter access in newborn infants undergoing extracorporeal membrane oxygenation. J Pediatr Surg 1983;28:530.
4. Anderson HL, Shapiro MB, Delius RE, et al: Extracorporeal life support for respiratory failure after multiple trauma. J Trauma 1994;37:266.
5. Andrews AF, Nixon CA, Cilley RE, et al: One- to three-year outcome for 14 neonatal survivors of extracorporeal membrane oxygenation. Pediatrics 1986;78:692.
6. Atkinson JB, Kitagawa H, Humphries B: Major surgical intervention during extracorporeal membrane oxygenation. J Pediatr Surg 1992;27:1197.
7. Bartlett R: Extracorporeal life support for cardiopulmonary failure. Curr Probl Surg 1990;27:621.
8. Bartlett RH, Andrews AF, Toomasian JM, et al: Extracorporeal membrane oxygenation for newborn respiratory failure: Forty-five cases. Surgery 1982;92:425.
9. Bartlett RH, Gazzaniga AB, Huxtable RF, et al: Extracorporeal circulation (ECMO) in neonatal respiratory failure. J Thorac Cardiovasc Surg 1977;74:826.
10. Bartlett RH, Gazzaniga AB, Huxtable RH, et al: Extracorporeal membrane oxygenation (ECMO) in newborn respiratory failure: Technical consideration. Trans Am Soc Artif Intern Organs 1979;25:473.
11. Bartlett RH, Gazzaniga AB, Toomasian J, et al: Extracorporeal membrane oxygenation (ECMO) in neonatal respiratory failure: 100 cases. Ann Surg 1986;204:236.
12. Bartlett RH, Roloff DW, Cornell RG, et al: Extracorporeal circulation in neonatal respiratory failure: A prospective randomized study. Pediatrics 1985;76:479.
13. Baumgart S, Streletz LJ, Needleman L, et al: Right common carotid artery reconstruction after extracorporeal membrane oxygenation: Vascular imaging, cerebral circulation, electroencephalographic, and neurodevelopmental correlates to recovery. J Pediatr 1994;125:295.
14. Beca J, Butt W: Extracorporeal membrane oxygenation for refractory septic shock in children. Pediatrics 1994;93:726.
15. Bowerman RA, Zwischenberger JB, Andrews AF, et al: Cranial sonography of the infant treated with extracorporeal membrane oxygenation. AJR Am J Roentgenol 1985; 145:161.
16. Bulas DI, Taylor GA, Fitz CR, et al: Posterior fossa intracranial hemorrhage in infants treated with extracorporeal membrane oxygenation: Sonographic findings. AJR Am J Roentgenol 1991;156:571.
17. Campbell LR, Bunyapen C, Gangarosa ME, et al: Significance of seizures associated with extracorporeal membrane oxygenation. J Pediatr 1991;119:789.
18. Cilley RE, Zwischenberger JB, Andrews AF, et al: Intracranial hemorrhage during extracorporeal membrane oxygenation in neonates. Pediatrics 1986;78:699.
19. Connors RH, Tracy T Jr, Bailey PV, et al: Congenital diaphragmatic hernia repair on ECMO. J Pediatr Surg 1990;25:1043.
20. Cornish JD, Heiss KF, Clark RH, et al: Efficacy of venovenous extracorporeal membrane oxygenation for neonates with respiratory and circulatory compromise. J Pediatr 1993; 122:105.
21. D'Agostino J, Bernbaum J, Gerdes M, et al: Outcome for infants with congenital diaphragmatic hernia requiring extracorporeal membrane oxygenation: The first year. J Pediatr Surg 1995;30:10.
22. Dalton HJ, Siewers RD, Fuhrman BP, et al: Extracorporeal membrane oxygenation for cardiac rescue in children with severe myocardial dysfunction. Crit Care Med 1993;21:1020.
23. del Nido PJ, Dalton HJ, Thompson AE, et al: Extracorporeal membrane oxygenator rescue in children during cardiac arrest after cardiac surgery. Circulation 1992;86 (Suppl II):II-300.
24. Dembitsky WP, Moreno-Cabral RJ, Adamson RM, et al: Emergency resuscitation using portable extracorporeal membrane oxygenation. Ann Thorac Surg 1993;55:304.
25. Dickey LA, Cheu HW: Neonates requiring cardiopulmonary resuscitation before extracorporeal membrane oxygenation: Prognostic factors for survival and neurologic outcome. Paper presented at the 9th Annual Children's National Medical Center ECMO Symposium, Feb 28, 1993, Keystone, Colo.
26. Dickson ME, Hirthler MA, Simoni J, et al: Stunned myocardium during extracorporeal membrane oxygenation. Am J Surg 1990;160:644.
27. ECMO Extracorporeal Cardiopulmonary Support in Critical Care. Ann Arbor, Mich, ELSO, 1995.
28. ELSO: The Registry of the Extracorporeal Life Support Organization. (updated annually). Available at elso@med.umich.edu.
29. Fazzalari FL, Hirschl RB, Delosh T, et al: The routine use of a proximal venous cannula in neonatal ECLS does not reduce the incidence of intracranial hemorrhage. Paper presented at the American Academy of Pediatrics, 1994.
30. Firmin R: United Kingdom neonatal ECMO study. Paper presented at the 7th International ELSO Conference, Sep 30, 1995, Dearborn, Mich.
31. Galantowicz ME, Stolar CJ: Extracorporeal membrane oxygenation for perioperative support in pediatric heart transplantation. J Thorac Cardiovasc Surg 1991;102:148.
32. Gauger PG, Hirschl RB, Delosh TN, et al: A matched pairs analysis of venoarterial and venovenous extracorporeal life support in neonatal respiratory failure. ASAIO J 1995; 41:M573.
33. Geiduschek JM, Inglis A Jr, O'Rourke PP, et al: Repair of a laryngotracheoesophageal cleft in an infant by means of extracorporeal membrane oxygenation. Ann Otol Rhinol Laryngol 1993;102:827.
34. Gibbons MD, Horan JJ, Dejter S Jr, et al: Extracorporeal membrane oxygenation: An adjunct in the management of the neonate with severe respiratory distress and congenital urinary tract anomalies. J Urol 1993;150:434.
35. Gillett DS, Gunning KE, Sawicka EH, et al: Life threatening sickle chest syndrome treated with extracorporeal membrane oxygenation. BMJ 1987;294:81.
36. Glass P, Miller M, Short B: Morbidity for survivors of extracorporeal membrane oxygenation: Neurodevelopmental outcome at 1 year of age. Pediatrics 1989;83:72.
37. Goretsky MJ, Greenhalgh DG, Warden GD, et al: The use of extracorporeal life support in pediatric burn patients with respiratory failure. J Pediatr Surg 1995;30:620.
38. Green TP, Moler FW, Goodman DM: Probability of survival after prolonged extracorporeal membrane oxygenation in pediatric patients with acute respiratory failure: Extracorporeal Life Support Organization. Crit Care Med 1995;23:1132.

39. Green TP, Timmons OD, Fackler JC, et al: The impact of extracorporeal membrane oxygenation on survival in pediatric patients with acute respiratory failure. Paper presented at the Society of Critical Care Medicine, 1994.
40. Heiss K, Manning P, Oldham KT, et al: Reversal of mortality for congenital diaphragmatic hernia with ECMO. Ann Surg 1989;209:225.
41. Heiss KF, Pettit B, Hirschl RB, et al: Renal insufficiency and volume overload in neonatal ECMO managed by continuous ultrafiltration. ASAIO Trans 1987;33:557.
42. Hirschl RB, Bartlett RH: Extracorporeal membrane oxygenation support in cardiorespiratory failure. Adv Surg 1987;21:189.
43. Hirschl RB, Heiss KF, Bartlett RH: Severe myocardial dysfunction during extracorporeal membrane oxygenation. J Pediatr Surg 1992;27:48.
44. Hirschl RB, Schumacher RE, Snedecor SN, et al: The efficacy of extracorporeal life support in premature and low birth weight newborns. J Pediatr Surg 1993;28:1336.
45. Hurrion EM, Pearson GA, Firmin RK: Childhood pulmonary alveolar proteinosis: Extracorporeal membrane oxygenation with total cardiopulmonary support during bronchopulmonary lavage. Chest 1994;106:638.
46. Jarjour IT, Ahdab-Barmada M: Cerebrovascular lesions in infants and children dying after extracorporeal membrane oxygenation. Pediatr Neurol 1994;10:13.
47. Kanter KR, Pennington G, Weber TR, et al: Extracorporeal membrane oxygenation for postoperative cardiac support in children. J Thorac Cardiovasc Surg 1987;93:27.
48. Keszler M, Ryckman FC, McDonald J Jr, et al: A prospective, multicenter, randomized study of high versus low positive end-expiratory pressure during extracorporeal membrane oxygenation. J Pediatr 1992;120:107.
49. King D, Smales C, Arnold AG, et al: Extracorporeal membrane oxygenation as emergency treatment for life-threatening acute severe asthma. Postgrad Med J 1986; 62:855.
50. Klein MD, Shaheen KW, Whittlesey GC, et al: Extracorporeal membrane oxygenation for the circulatory support of children after repair of congenital heart disease. J Thorac Cardiovasc Surg 1990;100:498.
51. Koenig PR, Ralston MA, Kimball TR, et al: Balloon atrial septostomy for left ventricular decompression in patients receiving extracorporeal membrane oxygenation for myocardial failure. J Pediatr 1993;122 (Suppl):S95.
52. Kolobow T, Boman RL: Construction and evaluation of an alveolar membrane artificial heart lung. ASAIO Trans 1963;9:238.
53. Kulick TJ, Moler FW, Palmisano JM, et al: Outcome-associated factors in pediatric patients treated with ECMO following cardiac surgery. Circulation (in press).
54. Lally KP, Paranka MS, Roden J, et al: Congenital diaphragmatic hernia: Stabilization and repair on ECMO. Ann Surg 1992;216:569.
55. Liem KD, Hopman JC, Oeseburg B, et al: Cerebral oxygenation and hemodynamics during induction of extracorporeal membrane oxygenation as investigated by near infrared spectrophotometry. Pediatrics 1995;95:555.
56. Lund DP, Mitchell J, Kharasch V, et al: Congenital diaphragmatic hernia: The hidden morbidity. J Pediatr Surg 1994;29:258.
57. Martin GR, Short BL, Abbott C, et al: Cardiac stun in infants undergoing extracorporeal membrane oxygenation. J Thorac Cardiovasc Surg 1991;101:607.
58. Matsumoto JS, Babcock DS, Brody AS, et al: Right common carotid artery ligation for extracorporeal membrane oxygenation: Cerebral blood flow velocity measurement with Doppler duplex US. Radiology 1990;175:757.
59. Meliones JN, Custer JR, Snedecor S, et al: Extracorporeal life support for cardiac assist in pediatric patients: Review of ELSO Registry data. Circulation 1991;84:168.
60. Moler FW, Custer JR, Bartlett RH, et al: Extracorporeal life support for severe pediatric respiratory failure: An updated experience, 1991-1993. J Pediatr 1994;124:875.
61. Moler FW, Palmisano JM, Green TP, et al: Predictors of outcome of severe respiratory syncytial virus-associated respiratory failure treated with extracorporeal membrane oxygenation. J Pediatr 1993;123:46.
62. Montoya J, Shanley C, Merz S, et al: Plasma leakage through microporous membranes: Role of phospholipids. ASAIO J 1992;38:M399.
63. Montoya JP, Merz SI, Bartlett RH: A standardized system for describing flow/pressure relationships in vascular access devices. ASAIO Trans 1991;37:4.
64. Morton A, Dalton H, Kochanek P, et al: Extracorporeal membrane oxygenation for pediatric respiratory failure: Five-year experience at the University of Pittsburgh. Crit Care Med 1994;22:1659.
65. Nagaraj HS, Mitchell KA, Fallat ME, et al: Surgical complications and procedures in neonates on extracorporeal membrane oxygenation. J Pediatr Surg 1992;27:1106.
66. Newman KD, Anderson KD, Van Meurs K, et al: Extracorporeal membrane oxygenation and congenital diaphragmatic hernia: Should any infant be excluded? J Pediatr Surg 1990;25:1048.
67. O'Connor TA, Haney BM, Grist GE, et al: Decreased incidence of intracranial hemorrhage using cephalic jugular venous drainage during neonatal extracorporeal membrane oxygenation. J Pediatr Surg 1993;28:1332.
68. O'Rourke PP, Crone RK, Vacanti JP, et al: Extracorporeal membrane oxygenation and conventional medical therapy in neonates with persistent pulmonary hypertension of the newborn: A prospective randomized study. Pediatrics 1989;84:957.
69. Ortega M, Ramos AD, Platzker AC, et al: Early prediction of ultimate outcome in newborn infants with severe respiratory failure. J Pediatr 1988;113:744.
70. Pearson GD, Short BL: An economic analysis of extracorporeal membrane oxygenation. J Intensive Care Med 1987;2:116.
71. Poland RL, Cassady G, Erenbery A, et al: Recommendations on extracorporeal membrane oxygenation. Pediatrics 1990;85:618.
72. Pranikoff T, Hirschl RH, Custer JR, et al: Survival is inversely proportional to the duration of mechanical ventilation prior to pediatric extracorporeal life support. Paper presented at the American Academy of Pediatrics Section on Surgery, Oct 22, 1994, Dallas, Tex.
73. Radack DM, Baumgart S, Gross GW: Subependymal (grade 1) intracranial hemorrhage in neonates on extracorporeal membrane oxygenation: Frequency and patterns of evolution. Clin Pediatr 1994;33:583.
74. Raithel SC, Pennington DG, Boegner E, et al: Extracorporeal membrane oxygenation in children after cardiac surgery. Circulation 1992;86:305.
75. Rivera RA, Butt W, Shann F: Predictors of mortality in children with respiratory failure: Possible indications for ECMO. Anesth Intensive Care 1990;18:385.
76. Robinson TM, Kickler TS, Walker LK, et al: Effect of extracorporeal membrane oxygenation on platelets in newborns. Crit Care Med 1993;21:1029.
77. Schumacher RE, Barks JD, Johnston MV, et al: Right-sided

brain lesions in infants following extracorporeal membrane oxygenation. Pediatrics 1988;82:155.
78. Schumacher RE, Palmer TW, Roloff DW, et al: Follow-up of infants treated with extracorporeal membrane oxygenation for newborn respiratory failure. Pediatrics 1991;87:451.
79. Schumacher RE, Roloff DW, Chapman R, et al: Extracorporeal membrane oxygenation in term newborns: A prospective cost-benefit analysis. ASAIO J 1993;39:873.
80. Secker-Walker JS, Edmonds JF, Spratt EH, et al: The source of coronary perfusion during partial bypass for extracorporeal membrane oxygenation (ECMO). Ann Thorac Surg 1976;21:138.
81. Sell LL, Cullen ML, Whittlesey GC, et al: Experience with renal failure during extracorporeal membrane oxygenation: Treatment with continuous hemofiltration. J Pediatr Surg 1987;22:600.
82. Short BL, Walker LK, Traystman RJ: Impaired cerebral autoregulation in the newborn lamb during recovery from severe, prolonged hypoxia, combined with carotid artery and jugular vein ligation. Crit Care Med 1994;22:1262.
83. Sinard JM, Merz SI, Hatcher MD, et al: Evaluation of extracorporeal perfusion catheters using a standardized measurement technique—the M-number. ASAIO Trans 1991;37:60.
84. Slaughter MS, Nielsen K, Bolman RD: Extracorporeal membrane oxygenation after lung or heart-lung transplantation. ASAIO J 1993;39:M453.
85. Spector ML, Wiznitzer M, Walsh-Sukys MC, et al: Carotid reconstruction in the neonate following ECMO. J Pediatr Surg 1991;26:357.
86. Stallion A, Cofer BR, Rafferty JA, et al: The significant relationship between platelet count and hemorrhagic complications on ECMO. Perfusion 1994;9:265.
87. Steimle CN, Meric F, Hirschl RB, et al: Effect of extracorporeal life support on survival when applied to all patients with congenital diaphragmatic hernia. J Pediatr Surg 1994; 29:997.
88. Steiner RB, Adolph VR, Heaton JF, et al: Pediatric extracorporeal membrane oxygenation in posttraumatic respiratory failure. J Pediatr Surg 1991;26:1011.
89. Steinhorn RH, Green TP: Use of extracorporeal membrane oxygenation in the treatment of respiratory syncytial virus bronchiolitis: The national experience, 1983 to 1988. J Pediatr 1990;116:338.
90. Stolar C, Dillon P, Reyes C: Selective use of extracorporeal membrane oxygenation in the management of congenital diaphragmatic hernia. J Pediatr Surg 1988; 23:207.
91. Stolar CJ, Snedecor SM, Bartlett RH: Extracorporeal membrane oxygenation and neonatal respiratory failure: Experience from the extracorporeal life support organization. J Pediatr Surg 1991;26:563.
92. Streletz LJ, Bej MD, Graziani LJ, et al: Utility of serial EEGs in neonates during extracorporeal membrane oxygenation. Pediatr Neurol 1992;8:190.
93. Swaniker F, Kolla S, Moler F, et al: Extracorporeal life support outcome for 128 pediatric patients with respiratory failure. J Pediatr Surg 2000;35:197.
94. Timmons OD, Dean JM, Vernon DD: Mortality rates and prognostic variables in children with ARDS. J Pediatr 1991;119:896.
95. Toomasian JM, Snedecor SM, Cornell RG, et al: National experience with extracorporeal membrane oxygenation for newborn respiratory failure: Data from 715 cases. ASAIO Trans 1988;34:140.
96. Upp J Jr, Bush PE, Zwischenberger JB: Complications of neonatal extracorporeal membrane oxygenation. Perfusion 1994;9:241.
97. Van Meurs KP, Robbins ST, Reed VL, et al: Congenital diaphragmatic hernia: Long-term outcome in neonates treated with extracorporeal membrane oxygenation. J Pediatr 1993;122:893.
98. Vazquez WD, Cheu HW: Hemorrhagic complications and repair of congenital diaphragmatic hernias: Does timing of the repair make a difference? Data from the Extracorporeal Life Support Organization. J Pediatr Surg 1994;29:1002.
99. von Allmen D, Ryckman FC: Cardiac arrest in the ECMO candidate. J Pediatr Surg 1991;26:143.
100. Walker LK, Short BL, Gleason CA, et al: Cerebrovascular response to carbon dioxide in lambs receiving extracorporeal membrane oxygenation. Crit Care Med 1994;22:291.
101. Walker LK, Wetzel RC, Haller J Jr: Extracorporeal membrane oxygenation for perioperative support during congenital tracheal stenosis repair. Anesth Analg 1992; 75:825.
102. Walsh-Sukys MC, Bauer RE, Cornell DJ, et al: Severe respiratory failure in neonates: Mortality and morbidity rates and neurodevelopmental outcomes. J Pediatr 1994; 125:104.
103. Weber TR, Tracy T Jr, Connors R, et al: Prolonged extracorporeal support for non neonatal respiratory failure. J Pediatr Surg 1992;27:1100.
104. Whittlesey GC, Drucker DE, Salley SO, et al: ECMO without heparin: Laboratory and clinical experience. J Pediatr Surg 1991;26:320.
105. Wilson JM, Bower LK, Fackler JC, et al: Aminocaproic acid decreases the incidence of intracranial hemorrhage and other hemorrhagic complications of ECMO. J Pediatr Surg 1993;28:536.
106. Wilson JM, Bower LK, Lund DP: Evolution of the technique of congenital diaphragmatic hernia repair on ECMO. J Pediatr Surg 1994;29:1109.
107. Ziomek S, Harrell J Jr, Fasules JW, et al: Extracorporeal membrane oxygenation for cardiac failure after congenital heart operation. Ann Thorac Surg 1992;54:861.
108. Zwischenberger JB, Nguyen TT, Upp J Jr, et al: Complications of neonatal extracorporeal membrane oxygenation: Collective experience from the Extracorporeal Life Support Organization. J Thorac Cardiovasc Surg 1994; 107:838.

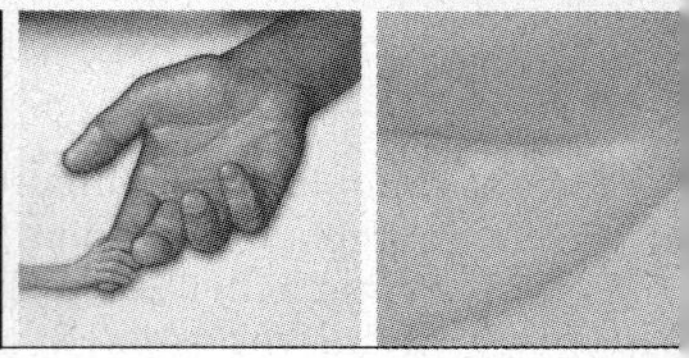

第 9 章

新生儿心血管生理学和护理

Albert P. Rocchini

146 为了适当地满足患者的心血管需求，理解正常的心血管生理学是重要的。本章概述了正常胎儿和新生儿的心血管生理学，并阐述了一些新生儿共有的心血管问题的药物治疗原则。

心血管生理学

不管年龄如何，影响心血管功能的重大变量都是前负荷（舒张末容量）、心率、动脉压（后负荷）和收缩力（心脏的收缩性状态）[5,6,58]。在所有年龄段，心肌肌肉长度、心率和其他改变心脏收缩性状态的因素增加时，会对心功能产生一个正性效应，而增加后负荷则会产生一个负性效应。但是，在未受到损伤的动物或人，几乎不可能去改变这些因素中的任何一个而又同时不影响其他因素。真实的生理学反应是针对干预手段的一个复合性效应。例如，在离体肌肉制备后，提升对肌肉的刺激率可引起收缩力增强。但是，在动物和儿童中，如用更快的速率进行心脏起搏，则会导致每搏排出量降低、心排出量无变化或轻微降低。这些反向效应是由于难以控制静脉回流、舒张末容量、收缩性状态、心率和后负荷之间的交互作用所致。

此外，患者的年龄可影响心血管功能。例如，对于胎儿，增加体循环后负荷对胎儿右心室功能（降低）的影响比对左心室功能的影响更大，而对于婴儿，增加体循环后负荷对左心室功能（降低）的影响比对右心室功能的影响更大[50]。以下各节分别就胎儿和新生儿的心率、前负荷、后负荷和收缩性进行阐述。

心率

对未成熟心脏和成人心脏，心率变化对心室输出的影响是相同的。采用心房起搏来提升心率也可以引起心室效能降低。随着心率升高，相应的舒张末充盈时间缩短且舒张末容量降低，可引起每搏排出量降低；但是，因为每搏排出量的降低通常与心率升高存在比例关系，实际效应是心排出量要么无变化，要么轻微降低。与成人相比，胎儿和新生婴儿的静息心率相对较高。由于基础心率高，提升心率也很少能增加新生儿的心排出量。同样，对于新生儿或胎儿，将其心率降低到接近成人水平，约每分钟 60 次左右，通常会伴有显著的心排出量下降。与起搏不同，自发的心率上升通常伴有心排出量升高。自发性心率变化与因心房起搏引起的类似变化不同，因为导致自发性变化的基础刺激同时也影响收缩、静脉回流或后负荷。例如，尽管心率引起的舒张充盈时间缩短，但是维持舒张末容量的静脉回流增加可引起每搏排出量增加。同样，如果提升心率的刺激也能增加收缩性的话，即便静脉回流可能不增加，心率的上升也将引起心排出量上升。自发性心率上升对心排出量的正性效应也存在例外情况，通常可以通过动脉压升高来解释。后负荷对心室功能的负面效应可导致每搏排出量和心排出量的降低。

前负荷

在所有年龄段的人，心室输出依赖于舒张末容量。当舒张末容量升高（Frank-Starling 关系）时，147
每搏排出量或心排出量上升。这种关系依赖于既定的肌小节长度下的横桥数量，而肌小节长度依赖于肌丝对钙的敏感性。虽然这些关系在新生儿和成人中都存在，但是在新生儿中，这些关系强度时常减弱。广为人知的是，当左心室舒张末压力高时，只有进一步升高充盈压，才会有舒张末容量和每搏排出量的小幅升高。从图 9–1 中可以看出，舒张末压力的进一步升高可引起心排出量的细小变化，这称为前负荷储备。新生儿由于心肌不成熟且僵直度高（顺应性降低），产生前负荷储备的压力比成人低[28]。

后负荷

未成熟和成年心脏的心血管功能会受到后负荷升高的负面影响[32,46,58]。后负荷对心肌功能的影响上存在成熟度差异。未成熟心室无法在成年心脏可耐受的动脉压下射血。这个对后负荷所产生的反应的量化差异是因为：未成熟心肌的收缩性差（根据肌肉横截面积校正），且未成熟心脏的心室壁较薄。后负荷对右心室和左心室的影响也存在量化差异。对于新生儿和成人，动脉压升高对右心室产生的负面效应比对左心室产生的要大得多。在胎儿和存在粗大动脉导管未闭得新生儿，这种差异是右心室每搏排出量、舒张末容量和当左右心室游离壁厚度相同的情况下，右心室游离壁曲率相对较大的结果[46]。因为根据 Laplace 定律，在相同的动脉压下，右心室的收缩期室壁应力高于左心室的。右心室收缩期室壁应力上升，使得动脉压上升对右心室射血产生的负面效应更大。

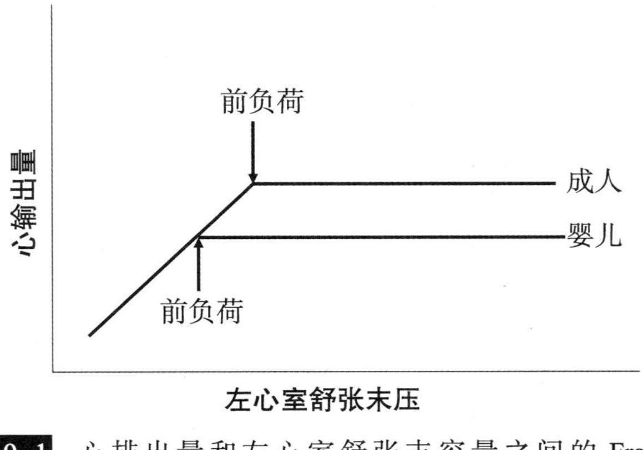

图 9–1　心排出量和左心室舒张末容量之间的 Frank-Starling 关系。进一步增加舒张末容量却无法进一步提升心排出量的点称为前负荷储备（箭头所示）。因为新生儿心肌僵直度高、顺应性低，产生前负荷储备的压力比成熟的成人心脏低。

收缩性

一个不改变前负荷或后负荷、但可以提升收缩力或增加心排出量的干涉措施，称为存在正性变力效应。这种正性效应通常来源于肌丝对钙的敏感性升高或细胞溶质的钙转移增多。未成熟心脏对正性变力药物的反应为左心室输出量升高；但是，与成人相比，这种反应相对较弱。心肌中的钙通过二氢吡啶敏感性钙通道移动，这对钙诱导的肌浆网钙释放是必须的[24,27,35,43,59]。钙诱导的钙释放放大了钙离子流对细胞溶质的钙浓度的影响[54,59]。在缺乏钙诱导的钙释放的情况下，跨膜钙流引起的收缩仅为在有增益系统存在时取得的收缩的数分之一。二氢吡啶敏感性钙通道和肌浆网钙释放通道（斯里兰卡肉桂碱受体）对钙诱导的钙释放是必须的。与成人心脏相比，未成熟心脏更多地依赖于细胞外钙，因为它降低了钙诱导的钙释放。成人心肌对细胞外钙的依赖型降低，这是由于肌浆网已经成熟。绝对和相对肌浆网容量随年龄增长而增长，肌浆网的钙释放也是一样。例如，斯里兰卡肉桂碱对新生儿心肌的收缩力效应很小。肌浆网不成熟和极大地依赖于细胞外钙浓度是对钙通道阻滞剂作用的两个解释，诸如新生儿对维拉帕米的耐受性很差。

胎儿循环

在理解了前负荷、后负荷、心率和收缩性是如何对新生儿心血管功能产生影响之外，还要理解出生对心血管系统的影响。胎儿循环和成人循环在很多方面都有不同。成人循环的特征是血流为串联结构。那就是说，来自静脉系统的血流回到心脏的右心房和右心室，然后再射入肺进行氧合。然后氧合血通过肺静脉回流到左心房和左心室，并摄入动脉系统。右心室在肺循环的低后负荷条件下工作，而左心室在体循环的 148
高后负荷条件下工作。胎儿的氧合与二氧化碳清除在胎盘中进行。氧合的血流通过脐静脉进入胎儿，脐静脉通过静脉导管与下腔静脉连接[16,47,52]。氧合脐带血流与来自胃肠道的低氧合门脉血流混合。因为右心房内有下腔静脉瓣，饱和度较高的脐静脉血优先通过卵圆孔进入左心房[21,36]，而来自下腔静脉远端和上腔静脉的低饱和度血流进入三尖瓣并直接流入右心室。虽然存在优先模式的血流，但是一些来自胎盘的血流也进入三尖瓣，且一些来自远端下腔静脉和上腔静脉的血流也进入卵圆孔。左右心室都向体循环泵血。右心室输出血流直接通过动脉导管进入胸部降主动脉，而左心室输出血流也通过主动脉瓣进入升主动脉。由于脐静脉回流存在优先血流，大部分的氧合血进入左心室并供应分布到心脑循环，而氧合程度较低的血流进入右心室并分布到肺动脉、腹部器官和胎盘动脉[52]。

由于这种独特的胎儿循环，许多种出生后无法存活的先天性心脏病却能在宫内良好地耐受。例如，左右心室发育不良或左右心室流出道闭锁的婴儿，在宫内的发育是正常的，而在出生后，这些病变是致命的，除非进行手术治疗。出生时，胎儿循环会迅速转变为成人循环。这一变化涉及脐带–胎盘循环消失，建立起正确的肺循环，以及通过关闭动脉导管和卵圆孔将心脏左右两侧分开。图 9–2 描绘了胎儿、出生后即刻和出生后数天的血流动力学[51]。出生后持续性胎儿循环通常意味着没有产生正确的肺循环及胎儿通道并未闭合。例如，先天性膈疝婴儿存在的持续性胎儿循环是因为氧合差和卵圆孔与动脉导管持续开放引起的肺阻力高。

常见的新生儿心血管问题的处理

充血性心力衰竭

新生儿心力衰竭的常见原因包括心律失常和先天性心血管畸形。表 9–1 列出了常见的先天性心脏病变和可能发生充血性心力衰竭的年龄。对于有发绀型先天性心脏病的婴儿来说，有大量肺血流或房室瓣反流的疾病通常会发生充血性心力衰竭。对这类心力衰竭的根本治疗方法就是对基础的先天性畸形进行治疗；但是，也必须使用药物治疗使婴儿保持稳定，以促使在低风险下进行手术纠治。标准的药物治疗规则包括：控制心率、控制前负荷、控制后负荷及改善收缩力。由于新生儿的静息心率高，不能采用提升心率的方法来增加心排出量。实际上，慢性室上性心动过速通常都是心房的异位节律点引起的，这是引起充血性心肌病的一个原因。

控制前负荷是处理心力衰竭的主要对症治疗。使用利尿药物来达成目的。治疗心力衰竭的最常用利尿药物是呋塞米（速尿）。表 9–2 列出了一些常用的利尿药物和目前推荐的使用剂量。有一个能很好地进行对症治疗的利尿药物是螺内酯（安体舒通）[13,33]。最近的证据提示，除了引起液体潴留以外，醛固酮还能引起心肌纤维化。现在有很多成人的临床试验提示，慢性阻断盐皮质激素受体可改善心脏重塑[33]。当使用利尿药物时，要考虑避免利尿过度。如果儿童的前负荷降低到前负荷储备以下，心排出量将会降低（见图 9–1）。

后负荷药物是通过降低心室负荷来发挥作用的，主要是通过降低体循环血管阻力。用来改变后负荷的最有效的药理学制剂是血管扩张药（见表 9–2）。这些药物是用来治疗因大型左向右分流、严重房室瓣和半月瓣反流、扩张性心肌病和术后低心排状态引起的心力衰竭婴儿的重要的治疗制剂[7–10,29]。血管紧张素转化酶抑制剂是最常用的降低后负荷药物[38,42,55,61]。除了可以降低心室后负荷，其还表现出能够改善充血性心肌病成人的心血管重塑[33]。其他控制后负荷的方法是阻滞 β 受体。低剂量的 β 受体阻断药可成功用于治疗充血性心肌病。它们通过干扰交感神经活动增强带来的有害作用而起效[3,22]。

最后一类用来治疗婴儿和幼儿充血性心力衰竭的药物是增加心脏收缩的药物（见表 9–2）。这个类别中最老的药物是洋地黄。地高辛仍然是最常用的慢性变力性药物。通过抑制钠–钾–三磷酸腺苷酶泵来提高收缩性，引起细胞内钠增加，转而刺激钙通过钠–钙交换通道进入细胞；细胞内钙增加可使收缩性升高。近来的研究提示，洋地黄也有助于通过抑制交感神经活动量来改善心力衰竭，从而降低心脏代谢需求[25]。除地高辛以外，还有其他静脉内用变力性药物，其中大部分是刺激心脏上的 β 肾上腺素能受体，从而提高腺苷酸环化酶活性并最终提高收缩性。这些药物在治疗严重的急性充血性心力衰竭和心源性休克时特别有用。根据不同的药物，血压可升高或轻微升高。例如，多巴胺可以引起 α 受体刺激和

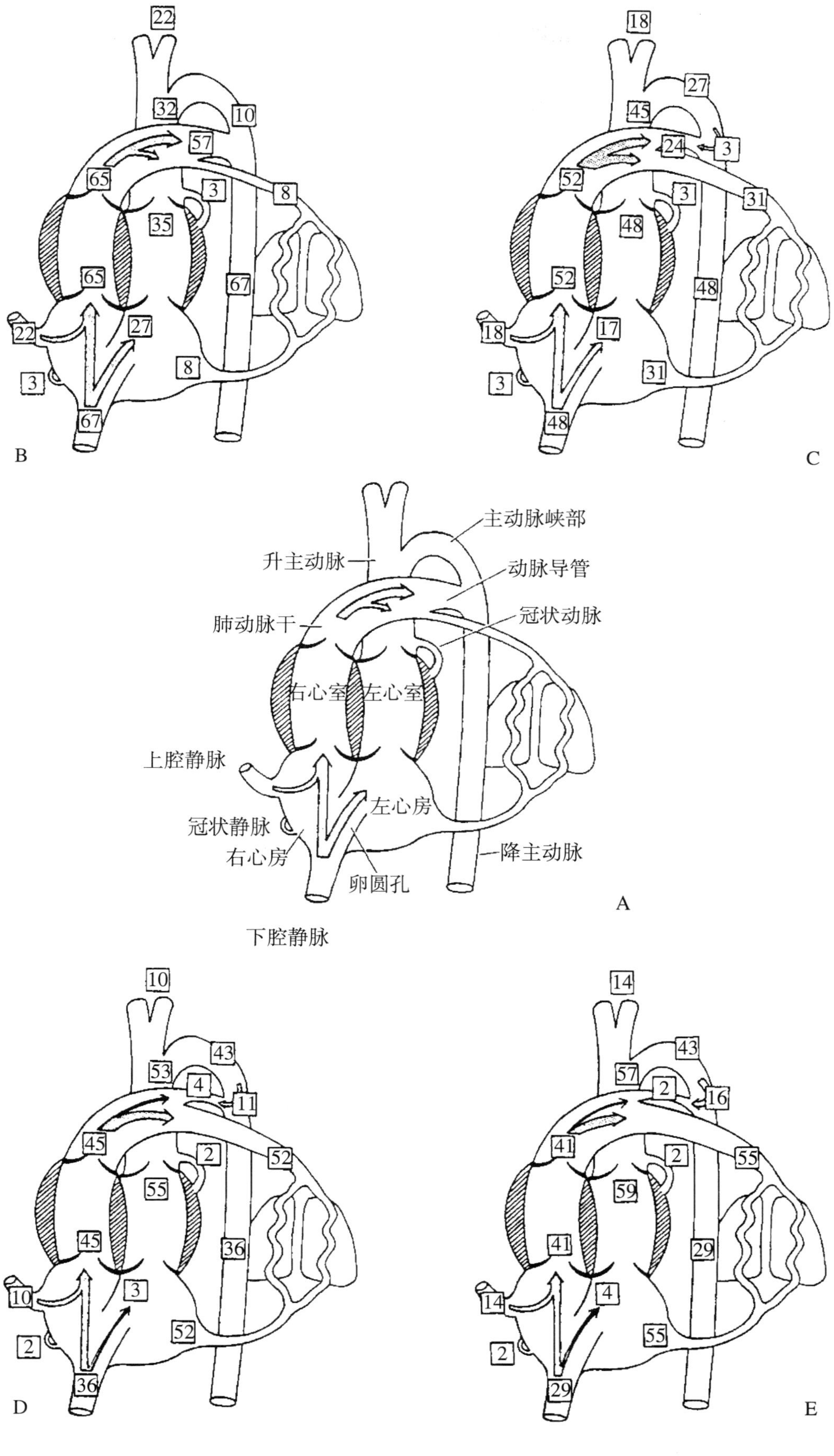

图 9-2 胎羊的循环分布。方框中显示出混合心室输出量的百分比。A. 胎儿循环的解剖。B. 安定状态。C. 给予 3%的氧通气后，胎儿血气未改变。D. 给予氧气通气之后。E. 氧气通气并阻断脐带之后。（From Rudolph AM: The fetal circulation and its adjustments after birth. In Moller JH, Hoffman JIE [eds]: Pediatric Cardiovascular Medicine. Philadelphia, Churchill Livingstone, 2000, p 62.）

表 9-1 不同年龄充血性心力衰竭的原因

胎儿到出生后1天	出生后第 1～6 周	出生后 6 周到 3 月	出生后 6 个月后
快速性心律失常	重症主动脉瓣狭窄	室间隔缺损	心肌心包炎
贫血或溶血性疾病	主动脉缩窄（单纯性或复杂性）	动脉导管未闭	心内膜炎
		房室间隔缺损	原发性肺动脉高压 *
房室瓣反流	左心发育不良综合征	房间隔缺损 *	风湿性心脏病
心脏阻滞	主动脉弓中断	快速性心律失常	川崎病
心脏或心包肿瘤 *	重症肺动脉瓣狭窄	左冠状动脉异常起源于肺动脉	先天性心脏病术后神经肌肉疾病
动静脉畸形（通常为脑或肝）*	共同混合型病变（如永存动脉干、单心室）	心肌炎或心肌病	
出生时窒息	快速性心律失常	非梗阻型完全性肺静脉异位引流	心肌病（限制性、肥厚性、扩张性）
胎儿-母体或胎儿-胎儿输血症	梗阻型或非梗阻型完全性肺静脉异位引流		体循环高压
心肌炎	心肌炎或心肌病		胶原血管病
血黏度高	体循环高压 *		药物：蒽环类抗生素、吐根、可卡因、重金属
卵圆孔早闭或动脉导管未闭	内分泌紊乱：甲状腺疾病、肾上腺功能障碍、甲状旁腺疾病 *		贫血：镰状细胞、地中海贫血、溶血 *
半月瓣关闭不全（如肺动脉瓣缺如、主动脉-左心室通道）*	持续性肺动脉高压		
	动脉导管未闭（特别在早产儿）		
	糖尿病母亲的婴儿		

* 引起心力衰竭的罕见原因。

表 9-2 用于治疗心力衰竭的药物

分类	药物	剂量	用药间隔	备注
利尿药物	氢氯噻嗪	2.0～3.0mg/kg，最高 50mg/d	每日 2 次	升高尿酸水平
	呋塞米	0.5～2.0mg/kg，最高每天 6.0mg/kg	每日 1 次或每日 2 次	
	螺内酯	1.0～3.3mg/kg	每日 2 次	保钾；与转化酶抑剂同时使用时要注意
	甲苯喹唑磺胺	0.2～0.4mg/kg	每日 1 次	
ACE 抑制剂	贝那普利	0.2mg/kg，最高 10mg/kg	每日 1 次	孕妇忌用；查血清钾、肌酐；咳嗽和血管性水肿也是副作用
	卡托普利	0.3～0.5mg/kg，最高 6.0mg/kg	每日 3 次	
	依纳普利	0.08mg/kg，最高 5.0mg/d	每日 1 次到每日 2 次	
	赖诺普利	0.07mg/kg，最高 40mg/d	每日 1 次	
ACE 抑制剂	依贝沙坦	6～12 岁：75～150 mg/d	每日 1 次	孕妇忌用；查血清钾、肌酐
	氯沙坦	每天 0.7mg/kg，最高 50mg/d	每日 1 次	
β 受体阻断药	美托洛尔	1.0～2.0mg/d，最高每天 6.0mg/kg	每日 1 次	
血管扩张药	肼屈嗪	0.75mg/kg，最高 7.5mg/kg	每日 4 次	可能会引起心动过速、液体潴留、狼疮样综合征
	哌唑嗪	0.05～0.1mg/kg，最高 0.5mg/kg	每日 3 次	
变力性药物	地高辛	洋地黄化剂量：20～40μg/kg，根据年龄维持剂量：5～10μg/kg		
	多巴酚丁胺	每分钟 2～20 μg/kg，静脉		
	多巴胺	每分钟 2～20 μg/kg，静脉		
	米力农	负荷剂量 0.05～1.0 mg/kg，然后每分钟 0.5～0.75 μg/kg		
	肾上腺素	每分钟 0.05～2.0 μg/kg，静脉		

ACE：血管紧张素转化酶。

一定程度的血管收缩[11]，而多巴酚丁胺可能会引起更多的体循环血管舒张，并会轻微降低体循环血压或不对其产生影响[20,44]。米力农是另一种静脉内使用的变力性药物，常多用于婴儿。它是一种磷酸二酯酶抑制剂，通过抑制环一磷酸腺苷的分解来提高收缩性。除了是一种正性变力药物，米力农也可以降低后负荷。因此米力农可能会轻微降低血压，也有助于产生一定程度的肺动脉血管扩张，因此这是一种用于严重充血性心力衰竭和肺动脉高压婴儿的理想的药物[19]。

如果药物治疗不足以维持合理的心排出量，可用机械装置来支持循环。最常用的机械支持装置是体外膜式氧合。最近，心室辅助装置也用于终末期的心肌病婴儿，作为等待心脏移植的过渡手段[17,30,56]。

心律异常

心脏阻滞

心率慢和心率快都会严重损害婴儿的心血管循环。完全性心脏阻滞可以是先天性的或后天性的，在每 20 000 例活产婴儿中有 1 人发生[12,41,53]。母亲结缔组织病与先天性心脏阻滞之间存在强烈的关联。例如，一个系统性红斑狼疮的父母，如其抗 Ro 为阳性，则其生下完全性心脏阻滞儿的风险为 1/20[48]。母亲对可溶性核蛋白抗原产生的 IgG 抗体（抗 Ro 和抗 La）在孕第 12～16 周后会通过胎盘。这种抗体的转运可导致胎儿心脏产生炎性应答，特别是传导系统，可破坏房室结[34,37,40,48,49,53,57]。新生儿完全性心脏阻滞可能需要也可能不需要治疗。是否要给一个心脏阻滞的婴儿放置起搏器的决定，取决于是否有宫内心力衰竭（水肿）的表现或出生后是否发生充血性心力衰竭。单心率问题通常不是放置起搏器的适应证；但是，如果婴儿的心率降低到 50 次 /分钟以下，大多数都要放置起搏器。一些类型的先天性心脏病也有很高的心脏阻滞的发生率。这些病变包括三尖瓣的 Ebstein 畸形和纠正性大动脉错位。

心动过速

婴儿和幼儿常发生心动过速，并导致心力衰竭。最常见的心动过速是室上性心动过速。阵发性室上性心动过速的发病率在每 250～1000 儿童中为 1 人[31]。在年龄低于 4 个月的男性婴儿中最常见，通常在胎儿期就有所表现。心动过速的基本病理机制通常是 Wolff-Parkinson-White 综合征（心房和心室之间有附加旁路）或房室结折返（房室结内双传导通路）。如果一直存在室上性心动过速，可能在 24～48 小时内发生心力衰竭。如不考虑病因，室上性心动过速的治疗都是相同的。如果婴儿出现酸中毒或低血压，应该立刻给予同步直流电心脏复律，剂量是 1～2 瓦秒 / 公斤[2]。如果婴儿病情稳定且相对无症状，任何增加房室结不应性的干预措施可能都会奏效。直接在婴儿脸部中央放置冰袋或冰水袋会产生潜水反应并终止心动过速。快速静脉内输注腺苷，对治疗室上性心动过速也是很有效的[15]。常用剂量是 100μg/kg 快速注射，每次增加 100μg，直至最大剂量 400μg/kg。与使用腺苷有关的一些严重副作用包括心房纤颤、室性心动过速、心搏暂停、呼吸暂停和支气管痉挛。因此，必须在有条件进行心脏复律和心肺复苏的条件下使用腺苷。

对存在室上性心动过速和轻到中度充血性心力衰竭的儿童可以先用腺苷进行治疗；如果腺苷未能消除心动过速，其他诸如地高辛、胺碘酮和普鲁卡因胺等药物也有一定的帮助。表 9-3 列出了一些常用的抗心律失常药物和目前的推荐剂量。婴儿使用地高辛时，优先采用静脉内给药。洋地黄化剂量可以每 2～4 小时的频度给予。如果给予三次剂量以后仍持续有心动过速，可再给予一次相当于洋地黄化总量四分之一的剂量。如果心动过速仍然没有消除，在洋地黄化之后，采用迷走刺激或腺苷可能有效。地高辛的维持剂量取决于终止心动过速的洋地黄化的总需求剂量：其是洋地黄化总量的 1/8，每日 2 次。对 QRS 波增宽的心动过速患者和可能是 153
Wolff-Parkinson-White 综合征引起心动过速的患者，应避免给予地高辛。Wolff-Parkinson-White 综合征伴有心房纤颤时，使用地高辛会导致心室应答加速并产生心室纤颤。

艾司洛尔或普萘洛尔可能进一步抑制心功能，在充血性心力衰竭的危重婴儿使用时，应该多加注意。一旦心动过速终止且充血性心力衰竭得以控制，β 阻滞剂可有效地用于有室上性心动过速的婴儿的长期抗心律失常治疗。

表 9-3 用于治疗快速性心律失常的药理学制剂

药物	剂量	起效时间	潜在不良反应	药物相互作用	心血管禁忌证	备注
腺苷	100～150 μg/kg 快速静脉注射；此后给予双倍剂量，最高为 300 μg/kg	<5 秒	呼吸困难、支气管痉挛、头痛、胸痛、房室传导阻滞 / 心搏暂停、室性早搏、心房纤颤、尖端扭转型室性心动过速、低血压	茶碱：腺苷作用减弱 地高辛：室性心动过速风险增加 地西泮：增强腺苷的作用	QT 间期延长 II 度或 III 度房室传导阻滞，使用起搏器患者除外 病窦综合征	心室率增快、尖端扭转型室性心动过速、心室纤颤患者使用时，需有可用的除颤仪备用
胺碘酮	推注：5mg/kg，持续 10 分钟输注：每天 10～15μg/kg	首次推注后 5 分钟内	低血压、窦性停搏或心动过缓、房室传导阻滞	地高辛：增加地高辛浓度 普鲁卡因胺：引起浓度增加 华法林：INR 指标升高	病窦综合征或房室传导阻滞，除非已使用起搏器 心源性休克	密切监测血压、心率和心律 可使用扩容和钙剂治疗低血压
艾司洛尔	负荷量：500μg/kg，1～2 分钟内使用 维持量：每分钟 50～200μg/kg	1～2 分钟内	低血压、头晕、头痛、恶心、支气管痉挛、心排出量降低	地高辛：浓度增加 吗啡：引起艾司洛尔浓度增加	窦性心动过缓，II 或 III度心脏阻滞，心源性休克，明显的心力衰竭	肾功能降低、糖尿病或哮喘患者使用时需注意
普鲁卡因胺	负荷量：婴儿 7～10 mg/kg，45 分钟内使用；年长儿 12 mg/kg 输注：每分钟 40～50μg/kg；偶尔可能需要增加到每分钟 100μg/kg	30 分钟内	低血压、心室对心房扑动的反应增加、心动过缓、心搏暂停、抑制心室功能、发热、肌痛、房室传导阻滞、心烦、头晕、头痛	胺碘酮：导致普鲁卡因胺浓度增加 地高辛：引起地高辛浓度增加	无起搏器者，会引起 II 或III度房室传导阻滞 充血性心力衰竭 QT 间期延长	持续心电图和血压监测监测 钾浓度，如低钾，可能加重心律失常

INR：国际标准化比率。

现在越来越多地使用胺碘酮作为室上性心动过速的紧急治疗药物，特别对术后患者。有报道静脉内使用胺碘酮首次快速注射剂量后 2 小时内，超过 40%的患者心动过速消失[26,45]。胺碘酮的主要副作用包括低血压、心室功能下降和心动过缓。

折返性室上性心动过速患者静脉内使用普鲁卡因胺也非常有效。联合使用普鲁卡因胺和 β 阻滞剂在治疗新生儿折返性心房扑动时特别有效。

维拉帕米虽然是一个治疗成人室上性心动过速的有效药物，但是对充血性心力衰竭婴儿来说是禁忌的。婴儿使用维拉帕米会导致心血管衰竭和死亡[1,23]。

在我们单位，我们多用食管超速起搏来消除婴儿的室上性心动过速。食管起搏的优点在于：不仅可以治疗心律失常，还可以有助于达成心动过速的最终诊断。超速起搏通过食管来起搏心房，其速率比心动过速的心率稍微快一点。终止起搏，则通常恢复窦性心律。食管起搏在大多数类型的室上性心动过速中有效，包括心房扑动[18,39]。

室性心动过速在新生儿中极少见。通常见于有心脏内肿瘤的婴儿，如横纹肌瘤也可见于 QT 间期延长综合征的婴儿。

先天性心脏病

某些特定类型的先天性心脏病很多都合并有其他先天性病变，需要在新生儿期一并实施手术治疗。例如，法洛四联症和室间隔缺损常见于有气管食管瘘、肛门闭锁和其他与十二指肠乳头有关的复杂病变的婴儿。主动脉弓中断、永存动脉干和法洛四联症通常见于 DiGeorge 综合征的婴儿。有报道先天性膈疝的婴儿有左心发育不良综合征。超过 60%的 Down综合征婴儿有先天性心脏病（动脉导管未闭、室间隔缺损、房室间隔缺损和法洛四联症）。因为先天性心脏病和其他需要在新生儿期一并手术的先天畸形之间存在强关联，通常在外科手术前，需要进行一次心脏科会诊和超声心动图检查。确切的治疗取决于先天性心脏病的类型。

对诸如法洛四联症或肺动脉闭锁等存在肺血流受限的婴儿来说，动脉导管对维持适当氧合是必需的。如果在胎儿期存在动脉导管，通常可以通过使用前列腺素 E_1 来保持开放，常用的初始剂量是每分钟 0.1～0.05μg/kg。如果导管开放，可使用低剂量的前列腺素（每分钟 0.02～0.03μg/kg）来维持其开放；如果导管实际上关闭了，可开始使用较高剂量的前列腺素，直到导管开放，然后减量到低剂量治疗。与使用前列腺素有关的副作用包括：呼吸暂停、癫痫发作、发热、低血压和面红。一旦婴儿稳定，则要考虑更多的根本治疗。在我们单位，无论何时，只要有可能，我们都选择对这些病变进行根治治疗，而不是姑息性的体肺动脉分流。

左心发育不良综合征的婴儿，初始治疗是需要建立一个房间隔缺损并保持动脉导管开放。这些婴儿的体循环血流与肺动脉阻力正相关，而氧饱和度和肺动脉阻力呈负相关（即当肺动脉阻力降低、肺血流增多、导致氧饱和度升高和体循环血流减少）。左心发育不良综合征婴儿的理想体循环氧饱和度在80%左右。当氧饱和度高于 80%且低于 90%时，肺循环血流和体循环血流的比值通常高于 4∶1，通常会出现体循环低血压；当氧饱和度高于 70%且低于80%时，肺循环血流和体循环血流接近平衡。理想情况下，可让这些患者保持自主呼吸并撤离氧疗。在一些病例中，可能需要将婴儿放置在一个空气和氮气混合的空间内来造成肺动脉血管收缩。较低的吸入氧浓度可以导致肺动脉血管收缩，引起肺血流降低，并维持合理的体循环灌注。一旦婴儿稳定，原则上应进行 Norwood 手术。在一些选择性病例中，心脏移植可能是婴儿的最佳手术选择。

室间隔缺损或房室间隔缺损的婴儿通常在出生后头一个月内没有症状。室间隔缺损的充血性心力衰竭通常是由于肺血流过多引起。室间隔缺损左向右分流的两大决定性因素是：缺损的位置和肺小动脉与体小动脉阻力的比值。足月婴儿通常要经过 4～6 周才能使肺阻力降低到正常水平；因此，存在大型间隔缺损的婴儿在出生后第 2 月之前，通常不会发生心力衰竭。引起室间隔缺损婴儿发生早期心力衰竭的原因包括早产和其他相关心脏病变。与早期发生充血性心力衰竭关系最大的两个常见病变为主动脉缩窄和房室瓣反流严重的房室间隔缺损。

（孙彦隽译 刘锦纷校）

参考文献

1. Abinader E, Borochowitz Z, Berger A: A hemodynamic complication of verapamil therapy in a neonate. Helv Paediatr Acta 1981;36:451.
2. Adkins DL, Kerger RE: Pediatric defibrillation: Current flow is improved by using "adult" electrode paddles. Pediatrics 1994;94:90.
3. Anderson JL, Bilbert EM, O'Connell JB, et al: Long term (2 year) beneficial effects of beta receptor blockade with bucindolol in patients with dilated cardiomyopathy. J Am Coll Cardiol 1991;17:1373.
4. Anderson PAW, Glick KL, Killman AP, et al: The effect of heart rate on in utero left ventricular output in the fetal sheep. J Physiol (Lond) 1986;372:557.
5. Anderson PAW, Glick K, Manring A, et al: Developmental changes in cardiac contractility in fetal and postnatal sheep: In vitro and in vivo. Am J Physiol 1984;247:H371.
6. Anderson PAW, Manring A, Glick K, et al: Biophysics of the developing heart. III. A comparison of the left ventricular dynamics of the fetal and neonatal lamb heart. Am J Obstet Gynecol 1982;143:195.
7. Artman M, Graham TP: Guidelines for vasodilator therapy of congestive heart failure in infants and children. Am Heart J 1987;113:994.
8. Beekman RH, Rocchini AP, Dick M, et al: Vasodilator therapy in children: Acute and chronic effects in children with left ventricular dysfunction or mitral regurgitation. Pediatrics 1983;52:112.
9. Beekman RH, Rocchini AP, Rosenthal A: Hemodynamic effects of hydralazine in infants with a large ventricular septal defect. Circulation 1982;65:523.
10. Bengur AR, Beekman RH, Rocchini AP, et al: Acute hemodynamic effects of captopril in children with a congestive or restrictive cardiomyopathy. Circulation 1991;83:523.
11. Bhatt-Mehta V, Nahata MC: Dopamine and dobutamine in pediatric therapy. Pharmacology 1989;9:303.
12. Chameides LM, Truex RC, Vetter VL, et al: Association of maternal systemic lupus erythematosus with congential complete heart block. N Engl J Med 1977;297:1204.
13. Chatterje K: Congestive heart failure: What should be the initial therapy and why? Am J Cardiovasc Drugs 2002;2:1.
14. Clyman RI, Teitel D, Padbury C, et al: The role of β-adrenergic receptor stimulation and contractile state in the preterm lamb's response to altered ductus arteriosus patency. Pediatr Res 1988;23:316.
15. Crosson JE, Etheridge SP, Milstein S, et al: Therapeutic and diagnostic utility of adenosine during tachycardia evaluation in children. Am J Cardiol 1994;74:155.
16. Dawes GS, Mott JC, Widdicombe JG: The foetal circulation in the lamb. J Physiol 1952;126:563.
17. delNido PJ, Armitage JM, Fricker FJ, et al: Extracorporeal membrane oxygenation support as a bridge to pediatric heart transplantation. Circulation 1994;90:66.
18. Dick M II, Scott WA, Serwer GS, et al: Acute termination of supraventricular tachyarrhythmias in children by transesophageal pacing. Am J Cardiol 1988;61:925.
19. DiDomenico RJ, Park HY, Southworth MR, et al: Guidelines for acute decompensated heart failure treatment. Ann Pharmacother 2004;38:649.
20. Driscoll DJ, Gillete PC, Duff DF, et al: Hemodynamic effects of dobutamine in children. Am J Cardiol 1979;43:581.
21. Edlelstone DI, Rudolph AM, Heymann MA: Liver and ductus venosus blood flows in fetal lambs in utero. Cir Res 1978; 42:426.
22. Eichhorn EJ: Paradox of beta-adrenergic blockade for the management of congestive heart failure. Am J Med 1992; 92:527.
23. Epstein MC, Kiel EA, Victoria BE: Cardiac decompensation following verapamil therapy in infants with supraventricular tachycardia. Pediatrics 1985;75:737.
24. Fabiato A: Appraisal of the physiological relevance of two hypotheses for the mechanisms of calcium release from the mammalian cardiac sarcoplasmic reticulum: Calcium-induced release versus charge-coupled release. Mol Cell Biochem 1989;89:135.
25. Ferguson DW, Berg WJ, Sanders SJ, et al: Somatoinhibitory responses in digitalis glycosides in heart failure patients: Direct evidence from sympathetic neural recordings. Circulation 1989;80:65.
26. Figa FH, Bow RM, Hamilton BF, et al: Clinical efficacy and safety of intravenous amiodarone in infants and children. Am J Cardiol 1994;74:573.
27. Fisher DJ, Tate CA, Phillips S: Development regulation of the sarcoplasmic reticulum calcium pump in the rabbit heart. Pediatr Res 1992;31:474.
28. Friedman WF: The intrinsic physiologic properties of the developing heart. Prog Cardiovasc Dis 1972;15:87.
29. Friedman WF, George BL: Medical progress—treatment of congestive heart failure by altering loading conditions of the heart. J Pediatr 1985;106:697.
30. Gajarski RJ, Mosca RS, Ohye RG, et al: Use of extracorporeal life support as a bridge to pediatric cardiac transplantation. J Heart Lung Transplant 2003;22:28.
31. Garson A Jr, Ludomirsky A: Supraventricular tachycardia. In Garson A Jr, Bricker JT, McNamara DG (eds): The Science and Practice of Pediatric Cardiology. Philadelphia, Lea & Febiger, 1990, p 1809.
32. Gilbert RD: Control of fetal cardiac output during changes in blood volume. Am J Physiol 1980;238:H80.
33. Gonzalez A, Lopez B, Diez J: Fibrosis in hypertensive heart disease: Role of the renin-angiotensin-aldosterone system. Med Clin North Am 2004;88:83.
34. Hartley JB, Kaine JL, Fox OF, et al: Ro(SS-A) antibody antigen in a patient with congenital complete heart block. Arthritis Rheum 1985;28:1321.
35. Hille B: Calcium channels. In Ionic Channels of Excitable Membranes, 2nd ed. Sunderland, Mass, Sinauer Associates, 1991, p 83.
36. Kiserud T, Eik-Nes SH, Blaas HG, et al: Foramen ovale: An ultrasonographic study of its relation to the inferior vena cava, ductus venosus and hepatic veins. Ultrasound Obstet Gynecol 1992;2:389.
37. Lee LA, Coutler S, Erner S, et al: Cardiac immunoglobulin deposition and congenital heart block associated with maternal anti-Ro autoantibodies. Am J Med 1987; 83:793.
38. Lewis AB, Chabot M: The effect of treatment with angiotensin converting enzyme inhibitors on survival of pediatric patients with dilated cardiomyopathy. Pediatr Cardiol 1993;14:9.
39. Lister JW, Cohen LS, Bernstein WH, et al: Treatment of supraventricular tachycardia by rapid atrial stimulation. Circulation 1968;38:1044.
40. Litsey SE, Noonan JA, O'Connor WN, et al: Maternal connective tissue disease and congenital heart block: Demonstration of immunoglobulin in cardiac tissue. N Engl J Med 1985;312:98.
41. McCue CM, Mantakas ME, Tingelstad JB, et al: Congenital heart block in newborns of mothers with connective tissue disease. Circulation 1977;56:82.
42. Montigny M, Davignon A, Fouron JC, et al: Captopril in infants in congestive heart failure secondary to a large ventricular left-to-right shunt. Am J Cardiol 1989; 63:631.
43. Ogawa Y: Role of ryanodine receptors. Crit Rev Biochem Mol Biol 1994;29:229.

44. Opie LH: Drugs for the Heart, 3rd ed. Philadelphia, WB Saunders, 1991, p 142.
45. Perry JC, Fenrich AL, Hulse JE, et al: Pediatric use of intravenous amiodarone: Efficacy and safety in critically ill patients from multicenter protocol. J Am Coll Cardiol 1996;27:1246.
46. Pinson CW, Morton MJ, Thornburg KL, et al: An anatomic basis for fetal right ventricular dominance and arterial pressure sensitivity. J Dev Physiol 1987;9:253.
47. Pohlman AG: The fetal circulation through the heart. Bull Johns Hopkins Hosp 1907;18:409.
48. Ramsey-Goldman R, Hom D, Deng J, et al: Anti-SS-A antibodies and fetal outcome in maternal systemic lupus erythematosus. Arthritis Rheum 1986;28:1321.
49. Reed BR, Lee LA, Harmon C, et al: Autoantibodies to SS-A/Ro in infants with congenital heart block. J Pediatr 1983;6:889.
50. Reller MD, Morton MJ, Reid DL, et al: Fetal lamb ventricles respond differently to filling and arterial pressures and to in utero ventilation. Pediatr Res 1987;22:621.
51. Rudolph AM: The fetal circulation and its adjustments after birth. In Moller JH, Hoffman JIE (eds): Pediatric Cardiovascular Medicine. Philadelphia, Churchill Livingstone, 2000, p 62.
52. Rudolph AM, Heymann MA: The circulation of the fetus in utero: Methods for studying distribution of blood flow, cardiac output and organ blood flow. Circ Res 1966; 21:163.
53. Scott JS, Maddison PJ, Taylor PV, et al: Connective-tissue disease, antibodies to ribonucleoprotein, and congenital heart block. N Engl J Med 1983;309:209.
54. Sham JSK, Cleemann L, Morad M: Gating of the cardiac Ca^{2+} release channel: The role of Na^+ current and Na^+-Ca^{2+} exchange. Science 1992;255:850.
55. Stern H, Weil J, Genz T, et al: Captopril in children with dilated cardiomyopathy: Acute and long-term effects in a prospective study of hemodynamic and hormonal effects. Pediatr Cardiol 1990;11:22.
56. Takano H, Nakatani T, Tanaka Y, et al: Clinical experience with ventricular assist systems in Japan. Ann Thorac Surg 1993;55:250.
57. Taylor PV, Scott JS, Gerlis LM, et al: Maternal antibodies against fetal cardiac antigens in congenital complete heart block. N Engl J Med 1986;315:667.
58. Thornburg KL, Morton MJ: Filling and arterial pressures as determinants of left ventricular stroke volume in fetal lambs. Am J Physiol 1986;251:H961.
59. Valdivia HH, Kaplan JH, Ellis-Davies GC, et al: Rapid adaptation of cardiac ryanodine receptors: Modulation by Mg^{2+} and phosphorylation. Science 1997;267:1997.
60. Wang Y-P, Fuchs F: Osmotic compression of skinned cardiac and skeletal muscle bundles: Effects on force generation, Ca^{2+} sensitivity and Ca^{2+} binding. J Mol Cell Cardiol 1995;27:1235.
61. Webster MW, Neutze JM, Calder AL: Acute hemodynamic effects of converting enzyme inhibition in children with intracardiac shunts. Pediatr Cardiol 1992;13:129.

第 10 章

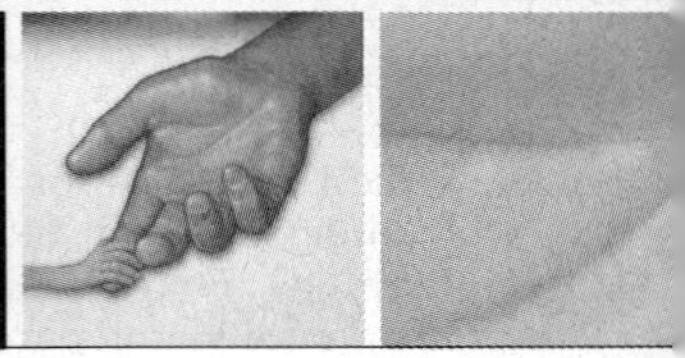

脓毒症及其相关问题

Jeffrey S. Upperman 和 Henri R. Ford

156 近年来，尽管新生儿学和儿科重症监护的研究取得了不少进展，广谱抗微生物药物得到了广泛使用，但感染仍然是导致婴儿和儿童患病和死亡的首要原因。微生物感染常常是由于宿主内源性防御机制无法对抗入侵的微生物毒力所致。免疫受损的婴儿和儿童，以及宿主防御系统功能受损的早产儿和足月新生儿，尤其容易罹患细菌感染。这种感染开始时只在局部引起炎症反应以杀死细菌。若感染本身或针对感染的炎症反应无法得到控制，则可能产生临床症候群，曾被定义的脓毒综合征。

脓毒症这个术语传统上是指受感染个体对血液中存在的革兰阴性或阳性微生物病原体做出的生命体征、内环境及代谢反应的临床改变。然而，越来越多的证据显示，发展为脓毒综合征并不依赖于菌血症及活动性感染。在很多严重受伤且死于脓毒症危象的患者，并没有找到明确的感染源[54]。在这些患者中，大量的坏死或受损组织足以激活炎症级联反应，最终导致严重的血流动力学紊乱，其特征表现是发热、休克或心血管虚脱、低灌注，伴有器官功能异常以及全身水肿。这一连串的事件现被定义为全身炎症性反应综合征（SIRS）。因此，SIRS 也可以在没有明确的全身感染时发生。SIRS 代表了严重感染导致宿主最终死亡的共同途径。

脓毒症是在 SIRS 病因被认为是感染的时候定义的，目前脓毒症在美国仍是引起患病和死亡的主要原因。事实上，Martin 等人[90]回顾了 1979—2000 年间大约 750 000 000 例住院患者的出院资料，发现其中有 10 319 418 例是脓毒症患者。在研究期间，脓毒症的发病率每年增长 8.7%，从大约 164 000 例增长到接近 660 000 例。Watson 等人报道[141]，一项全国性调查结果显示，在约 1 600 000 例年龄在 19 岁及以下的住院患者中，每年发生严重脓毒症的患者有 42 364例。婴儿脓毒症的发生率最高（5.16/1000），年长儿的发生率显著下降（10～14 岁儿童中约为 0.20/1000），男孩的发病率较女孩高。报道还称，符合严重脓毒症诊断标准的患者的住院死亡率约为 10%，或全国死亡 4383 例（6.2/10 万人口）。在患者的宿主防御机制发生改变的患者，如糖尿病、肝功能衰竭、烧伤、创伤、恶性肿瘤及药物诱导的免疫抑制患者，脓毒症是其最常见的死因。大约 30%的脓毒症患者血液中可以查到革兰阴性菌。成人和年长儿体内最常见的微生物包括大肠杆菌、绿脓杆菌、克雷白杆菌以及类细菌等[28,156]。在新生儿中，最常见的病原微生物是 B 族链球菌和革兰阴性肠杆菌（主要是大肠杆菌）。虽然这些微生物引起的特异性临床症状随着宿主的发育成熟度而有所改变，但是此类感染（如果得不到控制的话）其最终结果仍可能是 SIRS 或死亡。

外科遇到的新生儿和儿童的特殊感染如何进行详细检查不属于本章的讨论范围。本章将阐述新生儿和儿童感染后发生 SIRS 的机制。为了更好地理解 SIRS 的发病机制，我们首先应该了解病原微生物进入组织或体循环而引起感染和诱发炎症级联反应的机制。同样我们还应该了解宿主内源性防御系统如何被细菌侵入或有害的可溶性炎症反应介质如何被放大而诱发 SIRS 的过程。

本章的第一部分主要讨论感染的决定因素，如细菌的毒力和宿主防御机制。细胞和体液（包括抗体、补体和细胞因子）对感染和组织损伤的反应将进行详细讨论，因为它们是发生 SIRS 的最终共同途径。新生儿宿主防御机制的改变分开讨论。第二部分讨论年
长儿和新生儿中 SIRS 的发病机制及血流动力学和代 157
谢结果。本章第三部分讨论新生儿脓毒症的诊断方法，最后一部分讨论一些新的治疗方法，特别是生物反应的调控治疗。

感染的决定因素

感染的屏障

正常人体内寄生着众多的微生物。细菌普遍地存在于皮肤、口咽部、呼吸道、胃肠道和泌尿生殖道。然而，除非细菌丛与宿主的局部防御机制之间的内在平衡发生改变，一般不会发生临床感染。体内原有的菌丛可通过阻断病原微生物黏附于上皮屏障或通过与其竞争营养物阻止病原微生物生长。其他器官系统所具有的特殊防御机制也可减少病原微生物的生长机会。例如，皮肤不仅能维持相对的酸性环境以限制细菌繁殖，而且还会定期脱皮，从而有效地阻碍细菌黏附。肠黏液及肠蠕动可以防止细菌附着于肠上皮细胞，而呼吸道上皮的纤毛可以防止细菌黏附于呼吸道。胃酸能阻止细菌的生长繁殖。口咽、鼻咽和气管支气管分泌物中富含免疫球蛋白 A（IgA），IgA 可以降低细菌对黏膜细胞的黏附能力。因此，一旦发生感染，一定是原本完整的防御屏障出现了缺口，以致细菌得以黏附并随后穿透进入（图 10-1）。此外，病原微生物的毒力必须足够强大才能穿透防御屏障。最后，入侵的细菌还要能逃避宿主的局部细胞和体液防御机制，才能在宿主体内生存和繁殖。

在局部或全身感染的过程中，保护屏障的破坏起到了重要的作用。多种损害可以导致保护屏障的破坏，包括创伤或组织的直接损伤、手术、营养不良、烧伤、免疫抑制、休克及缺血再灌注损伤[142]。例如，缺血期间动用三磷酸腺苷可导致二磷酸腺苷、腺苷酸、肌苷及次黄嘌呤等产物蓄积。黄嘌呤氧化酶活性 158
会增强，但由于次黄嘌呤氧化为黄嘌呤时需要氧参与，黄嘌呤氧化酶活性增强的效应在初期并不明显。然而，在再灌注期间，氧得到补充后次黄嘌呤会被氧

图 10-1 肠道屏障被想象成一系列跨栏，细菌必须穿透上皮层，才能波及全身。第一道跨栏：胃酸可降低胃内 pH，对细菌生长来说提供了一个恶劣环境；第二道跨栏：协调的肠蠕动持续地顺流扫除细菌，因此可限制其与黏膜表面相连；第三道跨栏：原有的微生物菌丛（需氧菌和厌氧菌）可防止致病性革兰阴性需氧菌过度生长；第四道跨栏：IgA 是非杀菌性免疫球蛋白，能包被和聚集细菌，防止其附着到黏膜表面；第五道跨栏：肠黏液形成网状屏障，防止细菌附着到肠上皮细胞。

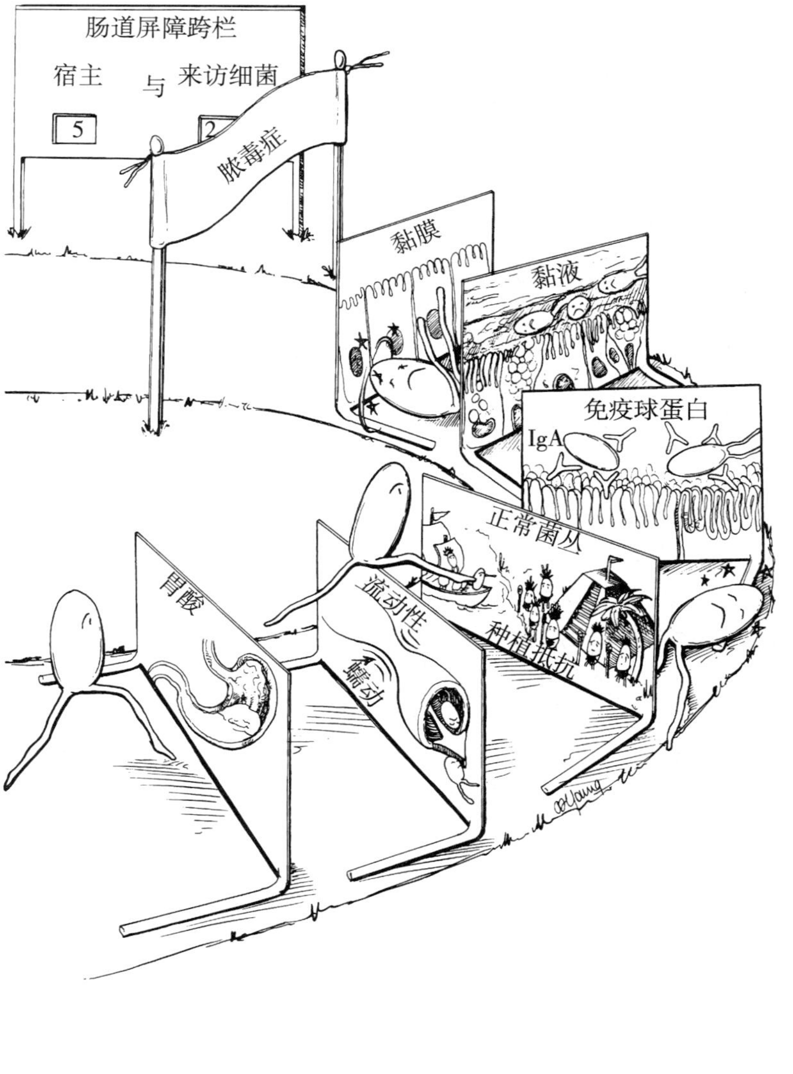

化，形成过氧化物（O_2^-）和过氧化氢（H_2O_2）等毒性活性氧中间体（ROI）。这些 ROI 可直接介导组织损伤而使肠保护屏障遭到破坏[7,32,33,143]。因此，细菌能够黏附于受损上皮表面并侵入，或者细菌也可经受损的黏膜直接进入血流。如上文所述，微生物一旦入侵成功，是否会发生临床感染主要取决于微生物的毒力与宿主局部防御机制之间的相互作用。

细菌毒力

病原微生物具有独特的生物化学属性，即毒力因子，使其能在宿主体内引起感染。如果病原微生物的毒力因子能成功地躲避宿主的免疫系统，就能在宿主体内大量繁殖并持续存在，而引起局部组织破坏或将病原体传递给其他易感者。

微生物感染过程的第一步可能也是最关键的一步是：病原微生物黏附于细胞表面。有些病原体就在黏附部位进行繁殖，而另一些则将黏附作为入侵的前提。因此消除微生物感染过程的第一步就可以彻底地防止病原微生物的生长和入侵。

微生物的黏附过程是细菌表面的特殊分子（即黏附因子）与宿主细胞特殊受体之间复杂的相互作用的结果。有研究表明，细菌菌毛可能是最有研究价值的黏附因子，能促进细菌黏附于黏膜表面。肠杆菌家族的成员具有明显的、形态学相似的菌毛——I 型菌毛，使之能够与上皮细胞上的 D-甘露糖受体相连[26,28]。进而，某些细菌，如大肠杆菌，能同时表达不同类型的黏附因子-I 型、X 型和 P 型菌毛，其特点是明显增强了微生物黏附于宿主表面的能力[48]。其他黏附因子包括透明质酸酶（是一种不仅能够介导细菌黏附还能加速细菌进入宿主的蛋白质）和血细胞凝集素（可表达的病原体有百日咳杆菌、鼠伤寒沙门杆菌及流感病毒）[45]。宿主也可以分泌一些蛋白质而间接促进细菌黏附，包括细胞外基质中的蛋白质，即纤连蛋白、层粘蛋白、胶原及玻连蛋白。这些蛋白质拥有共同的精氨酸-甘氨酸-天冬氨酸（RGD）肽序列，这在许多与哺乳纲动物细胞结合的病原微生物中也能找到[48]。例如，已知金黄色葡萄球菌和化脓性链球菌能与上皮表面的纤连蛋白结合[48]。幸运的是，细菌与细胞外基质蛋白相连的亲和力通常较低，很少引起微生物的入侵。

细菌黏附为微生物穿过宿主的完整上皮细胞屏障并进行繁殖创造了条件。然而，细菌只有黏附力还不足以使其进入宿主细胞。细菌入侵需要黏附因子与细胞表面受体之间的高度亲和作用。因整合因子受体能结合细菌的黏附因子和细胞外基质蛋白，如纤连蛋白、层粘蛋白、胶原及玻连蛋白，因此，整合素受体是细胞表面两者相互作用的主要目标。事实上，据报道多种病原微生物能与宿主细胞整合素受体结合。微生物是否侵入或只是附着在宿主细胞表面取决于相互作用的亲和力[69]。

其他的细菌毒力因子可能也可以促进细菌入侵。例如，发现耶尔森菌属的细胞表面蛋白透明质酸酶具有双重作用，既可充当黏附因子，又可作为细菌入侵的增强剂。耶尔森菌可与细胞表面的 β_1 整合子结合，从而侵入细胞内部。将透明质酸酶基因转移至非治病性大肠杆菌后，其也会具有入侵和浸润宿主组织的能力[69,97]。另外一种透明质酸酶基因变体，即所谓的黏附侵入位点，被认定只存在于致病性耶尔森菌属而不存在于非致病性菌属中。这种分子可作为细菌毒力的潜在的标记。

一旦细菌侵入，微生物会处于细胞内吞噬体中，且必须逃避细胞内宿主的防御机制（详见下文）才能进行繁殖。侵入的细菌为了生存：（1）必须避免宿主细胞溶酶体和吞噬体融合形成吞噬溶酶体；（2）必须防止吞噬溶酶体酸化；（3）必须中和吞噬溶酶体的抗菌活性。成功逃避了宿主防御机制的微生物能在宿主体内生存和繁殖。在此过程中，细菌毒素可以直接损伤宿主细胞或干扰宿主防御机制而起重要的作用。例如，白喉毒素可以生成死细胞层充当细菌生长的介质。艰难梭菌能分泌可以破坏上皮黏膜的肠毒素（毒素 A）和细胞毒素（毒素 B）。产气荚膜梭菌可以分泌大量的外毒素，也具有毒力作用。这些毒素都是具有不同靶目标的酶，包括有透明质酸酶、胶原酶、蛋白酶、脱氧核糖核酸酶和卵磷脂酶。如流感嗜血杆菌、肺炎链球菌、脑膜炎奈瑟菌及其他可导致口腔感染的细菌能产生蛋白酶，后者能使局部宿主防御机制失去作用[47]。金黄色葡萄球菌能通过产生过氧化氢酶灭活过氧化氢等 ROI。同样，细菌内毒素也具有强效的生物学特点。脂多糖（LPS）由三个部分组成：O-特异性侧链、核心多糖及内部脂质 A 区域。LPS（又称内毒素）的大多数生物学特点归因于脂质 A 区域。事实上，脂质 A 被认为是脓毒性休克主要介质。LPS 159

（脂质 A）能触发炎症级联反应而释放各种炎症介质，包括花生四烯酸衍生物、白细胞三烯、前炎症细胞因子，同时可激活补体。内毒素通过与炎症细胞结合成可溶性的膜结合受体复合物而与炎症细胞相互作用。于是引起了信号级联反应，增加了前炎症细胞因子的表达。这些炎症介质与 SIRS 的特征性血流动力学和代谢改变相关。LPS 的结合机制将在后面做详细介绍。

细菌逃避宿主防御机制的另一种方法是躲避吞噬作用或避免被特异性的吞噬细胞吞食，如中性粒细胞和巨噬细胞。链球菌分泌的链球菌溶血素能抑制中性粒细胞移行或趋化，并能损伤吞噬细胞的细胞毒性。除非存在受调理素作用的特异性抗体，与细菌表面结合并促进细菌黏附于中性粒细胞的 Fc 受体，否则包裹微生物无法被清除。这些微生物能使脾切除患者致病，尤其是 4 岁以下的患者。最后，IgG 的 Fc 受体与细菌细胞壁蛋白 A 结合可使某些病原微生物逃避吞噬作用，如葡萄球菌毒株。这种相互作用防止了 IgG 抗体的 Fc 受体与中性粒细胞的 Fc 受体结合。

宿主防御

当细菌黏附、入侵并有能力逃避细胞内和细胞外宿主防御机制时，才会发生感染。吞噬细胞（包括中性粒细胞、单核-巨噬细胞、淋巴细胞和体液成分）构成宿主抵抗病原微生物入侵的主要防线。免疫系统为了消灭入侵病原微生物，常会发动一系列反应。然而，这种反应过分剧烈时会使宿主自身组织遭受破坏。

中性粒细胞

中性粒细胞是最终分化的效应器细胞，构成针对感染、组织损伤或其他刺激释放炎症介质或细胞因子事件的第一线防御反应。正常情况下，中性粒细胞在血流中循环 6～7 小时。从骨髓释放后，将近 50%的血液循环中的中性粒细胞黏附于血管内皮。从功能上说，中性粒细胞是免疫系统中居于底层的“步兵”。正因为这样，中性粒细胞必须通过细胞渗出过程离开血液循环，定居于组织中并在那里继续存活 48 小时，从而发挥吞噬和杀死微生物的作用。中性粒细胞的渗入组织的过程受到精确的调节，涉及吞噬细胞与与血管内皮细胞上受体之间的相互作用。这种相互作用至少部分受细胞因子或其他炎症介质的调控，会产生三种结果：（1）中性粒细胞黏附于内皮；（2）中性粒细胞通过内皮移行至受伤和炎症部位（细胞渗出）；（3）继而刺激或引发中性粒细胞的杀伤作用。中性粒细胞的黏附受到中性粒细胞和内皮细胞上黏附分子的调控。中性粒细胞与内皮细胞之间的相互作用涉及三种重要的黏附分子：选择素、整合素和免疫球蛋白超级家族。黏附级联反应的第一步是中性粒细胞沿血管内皮滚动，此过程受到选择素的调控——总体来讲即白细胞（L）–选择素。白细胞（L）选择素与内皮（E）选择素和血小板（P）–选择素相结合，后两者均存在于活化的内皮细胞上[13]。损伤、感染或炎症可在几分钟内刺激 P 选择因子在内皮细胞表达上调。此过程使中性粒细胞上的 L 选择素与内皮上的 P 选择素可以低度亲和性黏附，这也有利于白细胞的滚动。中性粒细胞移行至炎症部位需要中性粒细胞和内皮细胞间形成稳固的黏附。此过程受到中性粒细胞上的 β_2 整合因子 CD11b/CD18 和细胞间黏附分子 1（I-CAM–1）的操控，后者是免疫球蛋白超级家族的成员，存在于内皮细胞上。

细菌释放的 LPS 通过刺激释放炎症介质，如肿瘤坏死因子–α（TNF–α）、白细胞介素–1（IL–1）及干扰素–γ（IFN–γ），可使 ICAM–1 和 E 选择素在内皮细胞上表达上调，从而对中性粒细胞的黏附和移行起到重要作用[13,135]。E 选择素上调可增强中性粒细胞的滚动，而 ICAM–1 上调可促进中性粒细胞和内皮细胞间的高度亲和，促进中性粒细胞移行至炎症部位。此外，LPS 与脂多糖结合蛋白（LBP）结合形成复合物，然后与中性粒细胞（和单核细胞）上的 CD14 分子和 Toll 样受体 4（TLR–4）结合，导致 β_2 整合素 CD11b/CD18 上调。因此，细菌 LPS 能直接或间接增强中性粒细胞和内皮细胞间的相互作用[68,118]。

中性粒细胞与内皮细胞相互作用的结果是使中性粒细胞产生牢固的黏附。中性粒细胞通过内皮细胞移出或移行受到血小板–内皮细胞黏附分子 1（PECAM–1）的调控[98–100,106]。PECAM–1 在血管内高度表达，特别是在内皮细胞表面和中性粒细胞内。这会对维持血管屏障的通透性、调节细胞移行及单核细胞和中性粒细胞透过内皮细胞的移行产生影响。PECAM–1 抗体会导致屏障渗漏并抑制中性粒细胞移

160 行[71]。除了 PECAM-1 之外，中性粒细胞移出需要细胞外基质中存在趋化梯度。已有大量的趋化因子被发现，包括小细菌肽、单核细胞趋化蛋白 1（MCP-1）、血小板活化因子（PAF）及白三烯 B_4。炎症部位布满了趋化因子。对于中性粒细胞移行最重要的两种趋化因子可能是 IL-8 和 C5a，后者是补体激活经典途径和替补途径的产物（详见下文）。中性粒细胞对趋化因子的反应性和敏感性极高，即使趋化因子的浓度低至 0.1%也能觉察出来[87,126,127]。中性粒细胞上的受体与趋化因子相互作用后会引起一系列细胞内信使事件，导致蛋白激酶 C 从细胞浆转移至细胞膜、蛋白激酶 C 依赖的磷酸化作用及细胞液内游离钙增加。上述反应可使中性粒细胞的细胞骨架发生改变，而中性粒细胞能经内皮移出并随着趋化梯度快速移动[37]。

中性粒细胞与内皮细胞的黏附作用使炎症部位的中性粒细胞可以移行。中性粒细胞是第一种在损伤部位聚集的炎症细胞，并可通过强大的吞噬作用和细胞毒作用限制感染。有证据表明，损伤或感染后早期释放的某种炎症介质或趋化因子可以增强中性粒细胞和内皮细胞间的相互作用，并使中性粒细胞发动更强大的细胞毒反应[3]。利用特异性单克隆抗体抗黏附分子而阻断中性粒细胞和内皮细胞间的相互作用，可以抑制受损部位中性粒细胞的趋化性，因此也可能会削弱机体抵抗细菌感染的能力[95]。事实上，患者缺乏 β_2 整合素受体 CD11b/CD18，会使白细胞黏附功能下降，从而容易反复发生细菌感染。其结果是中性粒细胞不能黏附于内皮细胞，从而不能外渗至组织。不能合成选择素配体（白细胞黏附功能缺陷Ⅱ）的患者不具备招募中性粒细胞至炎症区域的能力，患者同样会发生反复的细菌感染[43,63]。

在组织中，中性粒细胞要有效地处理微生物需要能够吞噬微生物及其后将其在细胞内杀死（图 10-2）。经免疫球蛋白预先调理的微生物可以明显增强中性粒细胞的吞噬功能。这个过程激活了补体，导致其他配体或受体沉积在细菌表面。这有利于中性粒细胞黏附于微生物上。中性粒细胞和细菌间相互作用其结果产生了信号传导，引起继发性膜流动性改变，形成伪足，并将细菌完全包裹在细胞内形成吞噬体。预先采用炎症细胞因子或趋化因子刺激中性粒细胞可以激活中性粒细胞，使其具有更为强大的杀伤功能。溶酶体内含有强大的杀微生物成分，通过溶酶体与吞噬体融合可以影响其对细菌的杀伤功能。在吞噬溶酶体中，

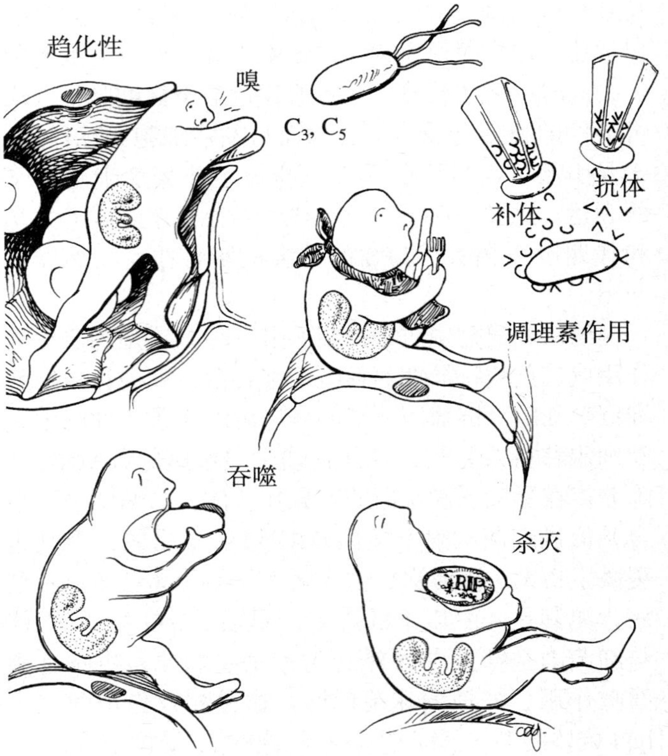

图 10-2 中性粒细胞杀伤细菌的步骤总结。A. 中性粒细胞的趋化性受到中性粒细胞和内皮细胞上的黏附分子、炎症细胞因子、趋化因子的控制，如受到C5a、白细胞介素-8的控制。B. 细菌在被吞食（吞噬作用）前"做"准备或被调理。C. 调理后的细菌被中性粒细胞吞食入胞浆即形成了吞噬体。D. 中性粒细胞通过溶酶体与吞噬体的融合破坏摄入的细菌，其中溶酶体中含有强效的杀菌物质。在吞噬溶酶体中存在需氧和无氧两种杀伤方式。

杀伤细菌可以通过需氧和无氧两条途径。

主要的需氧机制涉及在 NADPH 氧化酶催化下形成 ROI。激活的酶聚集在细胞膜处，并催化分子氧（O_2）还原为过氧化物（O_2^-），即所谓的呼吸暴发。过氧化物再在过氧化物歧化酶的催化下转变为过氧化氢（H_2O_2）。H_2O_2 再与铁或其他金属的过氧化物发生反应，从而提供强效的 ROI 羟基（^oOH）。或者 H_2O_2 在髓过氧化物酶作用下也可以与氯化物（Cl^-）反应，生成高活性的次氯酸（HOCL），髓过氧化物酶存在于细胞浆的颗粒中。继而 HOCL 与内源性含氮化合物发生反应形成强效的氧化剂氯胺，氯胺是中性粒细胞细胞毒性的主要成分[110,114]。

中性粒细胞的无氧性杀菌途径主要受特异性的细

161 胞浆颗粒中大量多肽的影响。分别是溶菌酶、弹性蛋白酶、乳铁蛋白、组织蛋白酶及防御素。这些肽中很多能协同提高中性粒细胞的杀伤微生物能力。例如，防御素和弹性蛋白酶可增加细菌细胞膜的通透性，允许其他具有杀伤功能的多肽及 ROI 穿透细菌。然而在某些情况下，如通过细胞因子中性粒细胞前启动或存在强烈的刺激，中性粒细胞的细胞毒储备可以通过强效的脱颗粒及特殊颗粒（溶酶体）与细胞膜融合（不仅是吞噬体）不加选择地融合，导致向周边的微环境中释放 ROI 及其他杀伤微生物成分。

单核-巨噬细胞

单核-巨噬细胞代表了一类表现型相关的异质细胞群，起源于与粒细胞相同的干细胞。正因为这样，在宿主防御微生物方面，单核-巨噬细胞的很多表现与中性粒细胞相似。原单核细胞起源于原始干细胞，前单核细胞获得骨髓中的某些特殊颗粒后分化成为原单核细胞。原单核细胞进一步成熟形成单核细胞，其吞噬细胞的能力也得到增强。单核细胞释放进入血后会移行到各种组织和器官中，并在那里分化为成熟的巨噬细胞，其特点是获得了某些特殊的颗粒（酶）以及生长因子和补体的受体[70,80,136]。尽管巨噬细胞的功能和代谢特点中存在区域性差异，但总体来说，组织巨噬细胞能够识别各种炎症性和免疫性刺激，包括细菌及其副产物、补体片段和细胞因子。然后这些刺激经过处理传递至特异性免疫反应中，导致各种细胞因子的释放，以加强组织修复能力或对抗微生物的细胞毒性作用。

巨噬细胞是机体抵御侵入细胞内病原体的主要效应器，这些病原体包括一些细菌、分枝杆菌及疟原虫。虽然，巨噬细胞的效率不如中性粒细胞，但巨噬细胞能够吞噬和杀伤很多常见的细菌。同中性粒细胞一样，巨噬细胞也能产生黏附分子，如 L 选择素、β_2 和 β_1 整合素。后者是巨噬细胞与中性粒细胞的重要区别，因为 β_1 整合素能使 β_2 整合素缺乏症患者（白细胞黏附功能缺陷）体内的巨噬细胞移行到损伤或炎症部位。巨噬细胞移行到炎症或组织损伤部位是对各种趋化因子的反应，包括补体（C5a）、细菌多肽、异体抗原及细胞因子，如 IL-1、TNF-α和 MCP-1。这些细胞因子能以自分泌（起源细胞）或旁分泌（远处细胞）的方式补充额外的巨噬细胞或其他炎症细胞至损伤或感染部位。配体与受体间的相互作用会产生吞噬细菌作用，并继而在细胞内进行杀伤。由这些细菌产生的抗原碎片被巨噬细胞处理，然后被呈递给具有主要组织相容性复合体（MHC）Ⅱ型分子背景的 T 淋巴细胞。巨噬细胞和 T 细胞间的同族作用可引起特异性免疫应答，从而放大细胞因子（和细胞）对进一步增强杀菌活性的反应。这种高度特异性的功能是巨噬细胞在宿主防御微生物中的一个主要特征。

巨噬细胞杀伤微生物的机制与中性粒细胞杀伤微生物的机制十分相似。吞噬体包裹细菌，然后吞噬体与溶酶体融合释放细胞毒物质（颗粒），对细菌产生杀伤作用。巨噬细胞既可采用需氧机制，也可采用无氧机制。与中性粒细胞相似的是，巨噬细胞可以生成 ROI，此外，巨噬细胞还可以产生大量强效的一氧化氮分子（NO）。NO 被证明具有多种生物学特点，包括抗菌活性。LPS 和 IFN-γ 可以引起巨噬细胞前启动，如导致 ROI 和 NO 的产量增加。这种现象有利于消灭微生物，但如果失去控制或以宿主组织为目标则可造成伤害。

NO 是精氨酸在一氧化氮合酶（NOS）的作用下转化为瓜氨酸的产物。NOS 有三种异构体：NOS-1（神经元 NOS）和 NOS-3（内皮的 NOS）是钙依赖性的且基本上都处于低水平表达状态；它们可生成皮摩尔数量的 NO。NOS-2（也称为诱导性 NOS 或 iNOS），除了在炎症介质（如 LPS、细胞因子）作用下受到诱导时，通常情况下都不存在；NOS-2 也是在巨噬细胞中发现的主要异构体[4,121]。研究表明，无论在体外还是在体内，NO 对很多种微生物都具有细胞毒性作用和抑制细胞生长作用；这些微生物包括寄生虫、分枝杆菌、真菌、病毒、细菌及衣原体[30]。然而，还没有明显的证据表明，人类吞噬细胞能产生足量的 NO 发挥抗微生物作用[121]。事实上，有证据提示，NO 必须与 ROI 相互作用才能发挥其细胞毒性作用[84]。但是，迄今尚未完全了解此反应的精确本质；在某种情况下，NO 可能抑制细胞生长或具有细胞毒性，然而在其他情况下，NO 可能具有细胞保护作用[31,75,121]。

目前已鉴定出多种 NO 的靶分子。NO 可直接抑制血红素蛋白，如肌红蛋白、血红蛋白、过氧化氢酶、过氧化物酶、细胞色素 *c* 以及非血红素铁蛋白，如铁蛋白、核糖核苷酸还原酶、合成 DNA 过程中的限速酶[103]。另外 NO 也可以诱导参与线粒体的电子传输链的酶催化域中的铁硫键构象改变，如 NADH-辅酶 Q 氧化还原酶、NADH-琥珀酸氧化还原酶以及 Krebs 循环中的乌头酸酶[103]。此外，NO 可以通过脱氨基反应，去除抗氧化剂如巯基来增加氧化应激，或与 ROI 反应生成毒性更强的代谢物，如过氧亚硝基阴离子，直接破坏 DNA[31]。NO 可诱导 DNA 链断裂，结果可能会激活 DNA 修复酶多（ADP）核糖转移酶，引起无效的修复循环，导致还原当量（NAD^+）耗竭
162 以及生物能的剥夺[137]。受刺激后，激活的巨噬细胞中的 NO 产量会增加，同时也能诱导 ROI 生成[67]。NO 具有未配对电子，会优先与其他具有未配对电子的物质反应，如血红素铁、非血红素铁蛋白及过氧化物。更多有关 NO 的生物学反应如表 10-1 所示[67]。

NO 的生物学效应可分为直接和间接两种。直接效应即 NO 与生物学目标发生特异性反应，如与金属或其他基团；间接效应为 NO 首先与氧或过氧化物反应形成氧化还原性物质，再介导大分子的转变。与 NO 相关的生物学反应中最迅速最普遍的是 NO 与 O_2^-反应，后者可生成强效的氧化剂过氧亚硝基阴离子（$ONOO^-$）（表 10-1，方程 1）。在生理性 pH下，$ONOO^-$发生质子化形成高反应性的过氧亚硝酸（ONOOH，未显示），过氧亚硝酸（理论上）可发生均裂反应形成 OH 和 NO_2。然而，在后一种反应中，这两个自由基团的反应迅速，以至于平衡几乎完全趋向方程的左侧，因此，该反应在热力学上是不利的[27]。有证据提示，过氧亚硝基阴离子是一种关键的活性氮中间物，常在活体内发生炎症损害时生成，也与 NO 病理性或细胞性的病变效应有关[27]。NO 也可以与血红蛋白反应形成高铁血红蛋白和硝酸盐，产物基本上没有毒性。NO 或 $ONOO^-$也可以与金属蛋白反应生成亚硝阳离子（NO^+），亚硝阳离子再被氧化为硫醇（R—SH），形成 S-亚硝基硫醇（R—SN=O）（方程 2）。S-亚硝基硫醇是一种具有生物活性的化合物，已被证明能抑制鼠伤寒沙门杆菌生长[31]，并能作为 NO（方程 3a 和 3b）或作为 NO^+ 的供体[27,130]。NO 或 $ONOO^-$与金属蛋白或 Fe^{3+}反应（方程 2）释放出结合态的铁，在 Haber-Weiss反应（方程 4）中，通过 °OH 的形成提供必要的催化剂而导致进一步的氧化性损伤。

NO 在体外的化学性质相当复杂。在某种情况下，NO 可与 O_2^-反应生成 ONOO，使过氧亚硝基阴离子分解为硝酸盐（方程 1），能减少氧化剂介导的损伤。事实上，NO 与 O_2^-相互作用后可在早期降低 O_2^-介导的葡萄球菌的杀伤力，但是在持续的潜伏期内 NO 的杀伤力会增强[75]。Pacelli 等人[108]报道在大肠杆菌中也有相似的发现。然而，其他的机制可以增强 NO 的细胞毒效应。例如，NO 正常代谢后的终末产物亚硝酸盐（NO_2^-）是无害的，但在 pH为 5.0 时能转化生成亚硝酸，吞噬溶酶体通常为这种条件[21]。然后亚硝酸还可生成 NO。事实上，这种反应与自然抵抗相关的巨噬细胞蛋白 1 有关[104]。这种基因可通过将附近细胞产生的 NO_2^-运输到自身酸性溶酶体或吞噬溶酶体中，而使不产生 NO 的细胞得到该分子，在那里 NO_2^-进行质子化后生成亚硝酸。亚硝酸再经歧化作用生成 NO。因此，微生物可在不制造 NO 的细胞内的吞噬体被杀伤。

从前面的讨论中可以看出，NO 的抗微生物作用主要由 $ONOO^-$、NO^+、OH 及 R—SN=O 介导。然

表 10-1 一氧化氮反应

1. $°NO + °O_2^-$（过氧化物）$\longrightarrow$ $ONOO^-$（过亚硝酸盐）$\underset{H^4}{\rightleftarrows}$ $°OH$（羟基）$+ °NO_2$（二氧化氮）

   $ONOO^- \downarrow$ NO_3^-（硝酸盐）

2. $°NO$ 或 $ONNO^-$ $+ Fe^{+3} \longrightarrow Fe^{+2}$ $NO^+ \xrightarrow{R—SN}$ RS—N=O

3. a. RS—N=O $+ °O_2^-$ $H^+ \longrightarrow$ R—SH $+ °O_2 + °NO$

   b. $°NO + °O_2^- \longrightarrow ONNO^-$

4. $°O_2^- + H_2O_2 \xrightarrow{Fc} O_2 + OH^- + OH$

而，巨噬细胞激活后持续产生过量的此类化合物也可能会导致细胞损伤、多系统器官功能衰竭或 SIRS。

淋巴细胞

尽管中性粒细胞和单核-巨噬细胞是宿主防御微生物的主要效应器，但某些微生物，特别是在细胞内的病原体却能逃避其细胞毒作用。因此，必须通过不同的方法消灭这些微生物。淋巴细胞及自然杀伤细胞（NK）构成了防御这些微生物的第二道防线。

淋巴细胞起源于骨髓中的造血干细胞。在分化早期，淋巴样远祖细胞在骨髓的一个腔室内发育成熟，并在那里获得表型和功能特征。某些细胞离开骨髓
63 后，在胸腺处接受“教育”或成熟化处理。这些成熟的 T 细胞从胸腺移行到外周淋巴器官定居，如在脾脏、淋巴结和肠 Peyer 淋巴集结。其他淋巴远祖细胞可在骨髓中或在胎儿肝脏中发育成熟，成为合成免疫球蛋白的淋巴细胞（B 细胞）。

B 细胞和 T 细胞在消灭微生物中都具有重要的作用。尤其是 B 细胞能够产生调理性抗体，后者有助于吞噬被包围的微生物。B 细胞还可以分泌其他的免疫球蛋白，如 IgA，通过预防细菌黏附和入侵而在黏膜免疫反应中起重要作用。此外，B 细胞还参与抗体依赖性的由细胞介导的细胞毒作用。与之相反，T 淋巴细胞在细胞介导的抵御细胞内病原体的免疫反应中起重要作用。T 细胞介导的杀伤过程包括：（1）抗原或微生物的识别；（2）细胞激活；（3）复制增殖；（4）杀伤靶目标。抗原呈递和识别部分受到正常存在于细胞表面的蛋白的控制[7]，即受 MHC 蛋白质家族的控制。MHC 蛋白分为两种类型：Ⅰ型于所有的有核细胞中表达，而Ⅱ型主要于抗原呈递细胞中表达，如在巨噬细胞、树突状细胞及 B 淋巴细胞中。这些细胞吞噬细菌并将其加工或分解成小碎片或多肽，再捆绑于 MHC Ⅱ型蛋白并被插入到呈递抗原细胞的细胞膜中。具有相同 MHC 分子的 T 细胞能识别出这种抗原呈递细胞上的 MHC-多肽复合物。这种复合物与 T 辅助（TH）细胞（CD_4^+）上的特异性配体相互作用产生细胞因子、招募其他吞噬（炎症）细胞，并使各种淋巴细胞增生，即 B 细胞、CD_8^+细胞毒性 T 淋巴细胞（CTL）及 TH 细胞增生。最后在杀灭微生物的过程中，CTL 起主要作用。具有 MHC Ⅱ型蛋白但无法处置抗原的细胞被感染后，细胞内的 MHC Ⅰ型分子与入侵病原体的抗原肽结合生成复合物。这种复合物容易被识别并被当作 CTL 破坏的目标。因此，尽管只有抗原呈递细胞能处理具有 MHC Ⅱ型分子的抗原并引发 TH 反应，但所有被细胞内病原体感染的细胞都能通过 MHC Ⅰ型分子与外来抗原结合生成复合物的方式，为 CTL 提供攻击的靶目标。

T 细胞的激活需要两个重要条件：通过 T 细胞受体信号传导蛋白复合物 CD3 给予刺激，以及在抗原呈递细胞或受感染细胞上同时发生 CD4 或 CD8 配体与合适的 MHC-多肽复合物之间发生交联。信号传导可启动级联反应，导致钙动员、蛋白激酶激活、转录和翻译某些特殊基因编码的蛋白质，以帮助消灭病原体。这些蛋白质包括 CTL 中的穿孔素和丝氨酸蛋白酶以及 TH 细胞中的各种细胞因子。TH 细胞根据其细胞因子分成两种：TH1 细胞产生 IL-2 和 IFN-γ，TH2 细胞产生 IL-4、IL-5、IL-10 及 IL-13。其他细胞因子，如 IL-3 和粒细胞-巨噬细胞克隆刺激因子，则由 TH1 和 TH2 细胞共同产生。分泌的细胞因子与靶细胞上的特异性受体结合并激活信号传导途径，导致新的蛋白质生成及细胞增生或分化，同时根据所释放的细胞因子的种类获得相应的效应器表现型。例如，TH1 细胞因子主要引起 T 细胞介导的反应，其部分特点是招募巨噬细胞至炎症部位，然后由 IFN-γ 激活巨噬细胞[22,101]。与之相比，TH2 细胞因子将平衡移向体液（B 细胞）反应。激活的 CTL 与表达 MHC-多肽复合物的细胞结合并释放细胞毒性颗粒，如穿孔素，后者能在细胞膜上打“洞”，导致细胞渗透性分解。另为这些 CTL 也可释放丝氨酸蛋白酶诱导受感染细胞发生凋亡（程序性细胞死亡）而不影响效应器细胞（CTL）[65,91,113]。

与 CTL 相似，代表了淋巴细胞家族变体的 NK细胞同样也能利用颗粒胞吐作用杀死受感染的靶细胞。此外，这些细胞具有免疫球蛋白的 Fc 受体，因此 NK 细胞能参与抗体依赖性的细胞介导的细胞毒作用。

体液因子

上文讨论了细胞介导的免疫应答在宿主防御微生物中的重要性。然而，应当明确细胞反应是一种非常复杂的现象，通常在不同体液因子的作用下启动和完善，其中包括免疫球蛋白、补体激活及细胞因子。

免疫球蛋白

免疫球蛋白或抗体代表的是由成熟B淋巴细胞或浆细胞合成的一类蛋白质，主要是由TH细胞与具有MHC-多肽复合物的抗原传递细胞之间的相互作用产生的。这种相互作用可以导致细胞因子合成和B细胞增生及成熟，并产生特殊类的免疫球蛋白。在宿主防御微生物的过程中，抗体的主要作用是防止细菌黏附和入侵易感的宿主细胞。其机制包括调理微生物使其易于被吞噬，激活补体并将其碎片沉积于细菌细胞膜上，以进一步增强吞噬作用及细菌杀伤力，中和内源性微生物毒素或毒力因素，以阻止细菌黏附于细胞表面。免疫球蛋白主要分成五种：IgA、IgG、IgM、IgD和IgE。其中IgG、IgM和IgA是介导宿主防御微生物的主要抗体。

IgM是分子量最大的免疫球蛋白，也是启动感染
164 或抗原刺激反应的主要成分。正因为这样，IgM的半衰期只有5～6天，且随着IgG水平升高其水平会稳步下降。由于IgM的分子较大，其只存在于血管内，充当有效的细菌凝集素及补体系统的强效激活剂作用。

IgG也许是数量最多的抗体，约占血清免疫球蛋白的85%左右。IgG在血管内和血管外（组织）均存在。IgG是唯一一种能穿过母体胎盘进入胎儿的免疫球蛋白。IgG是直接抵御细菌和病毒的主要抗体。其分子的生物学强度在于其能通过分子上的Fab成分结合抗原，同时利用其Fc成分结合中性粒细胞、单核细胞或巨噬细胞上的Fc受体，从而调理细菌。进而，IgG复合物可激活补体系统。

IgA同型抗体在局部黏膜免疫中起关键作用。IgA由浆细胞在位于上皮组织下方的淋巴组织中合成及分泌。IgA以二聚体的形式释放，并在穿过上皮细胞时获得分泌形成分，以分泌性IgA的形式存在于黏膜表面。分泌性IgA可作为捆绑病原微生物的抗菌涂料，因此能防止病原微生物黏附、定植及其后侵入组织。但要注意的是，除了IgG和IgM之外，IgE在局部黏膜的免疫反应中也发挥作用，特别是在先天性IgA缺乏的患者。

补体系统

虽然抗体能有效地识别病原微生物上的抗原决定簇，但是抗体不能独立地杀伤微生物。经过调理后，抗体必须依靠吞噬细胞摄入微生物，并依靠补体激活进一步增强其调理作用以中和并最终杀伤摄入的病原体。补体激活途径有两条：经典途径和替代途径（图10-3）。抗原抗体复合物是经典途径的主要起始物。而细菌细胞壁碎片、内毒素（LPS）、细胞表面、烧伤和受伤的组织以及多糖复合物可激活替代（备解
素）途径。刺激任何一条途径都能启动级联反应，作 16
为复杂的放大处理的结果，可导致明显的补体激活。级联反应中最关键一步是C3，两条途径会聚集于此形成C3a和C3b。C3a既是血管舒张剂，又是吞噬细胞趋化因子。而C3b分子是补体级联反应中最关键的成分，因为此酶可通过进一步促进C3分解为C3a和C3b使系统得到明显放大，并且可通过替代途径增加C3b的产量。进而，C3b是最强效的生物调理素，大多数吞噬细胞上存在C3b的细胞表面受体。C3b沉积可以在细菌表面激活补体级联反应的远端部分（C8和C9）而插入和破坏细胞膜，导致细菌渗透性溶解。在此过程中，另一种更为强效的趋化因子C5a也被释放，其同样可以在吞噬细胞中诱导呼吸暴发，因此有助于杀伤细菌。

细胞因子

在抵抗微生物过程中，起细胞毒性作用的协调或调控各种细胞效应器之间的复杂的相互作用的介质统称为细胞因子。细胞因子代表异种糖蛋白，可由不同的细胞分泌，包括中性粒细胞、单核-巨噬细胞、B和T淋巴细胞、NK细胞、内皮细胞及成纤维细胞。这些细胞在遇到炎症和抗原刺激（如LPS）时可合成和释放新的细胞因子。由于细胞因子的生物学活性强大，其生产、分泌及活性周期受到严格的调节，特别是在信使RNA（mRNA）水平。细胞因子分别通过与邻近的、起始的或远端靶细胞表面的特殊受体结合，可以旁分泌、自分泌或内分泌方式发挥作用。细胞因子与其受体间的相互作用可产生信号传导并导致新基因转录、mRNA翻译和蛋白质合成。例如，蛋白质的合成能使靶细胞的表型发生改变，使之具有细胞毒性效应器功能，也可下调或上调其他细胞因子的生成。一般来说，细胞因子的功能广泛而重复。某些细胞因子可以放大炎症反应，但其他因子可限制其程度。前炎症因子，如TNF-α、IL-1、IL-6、IL-8、

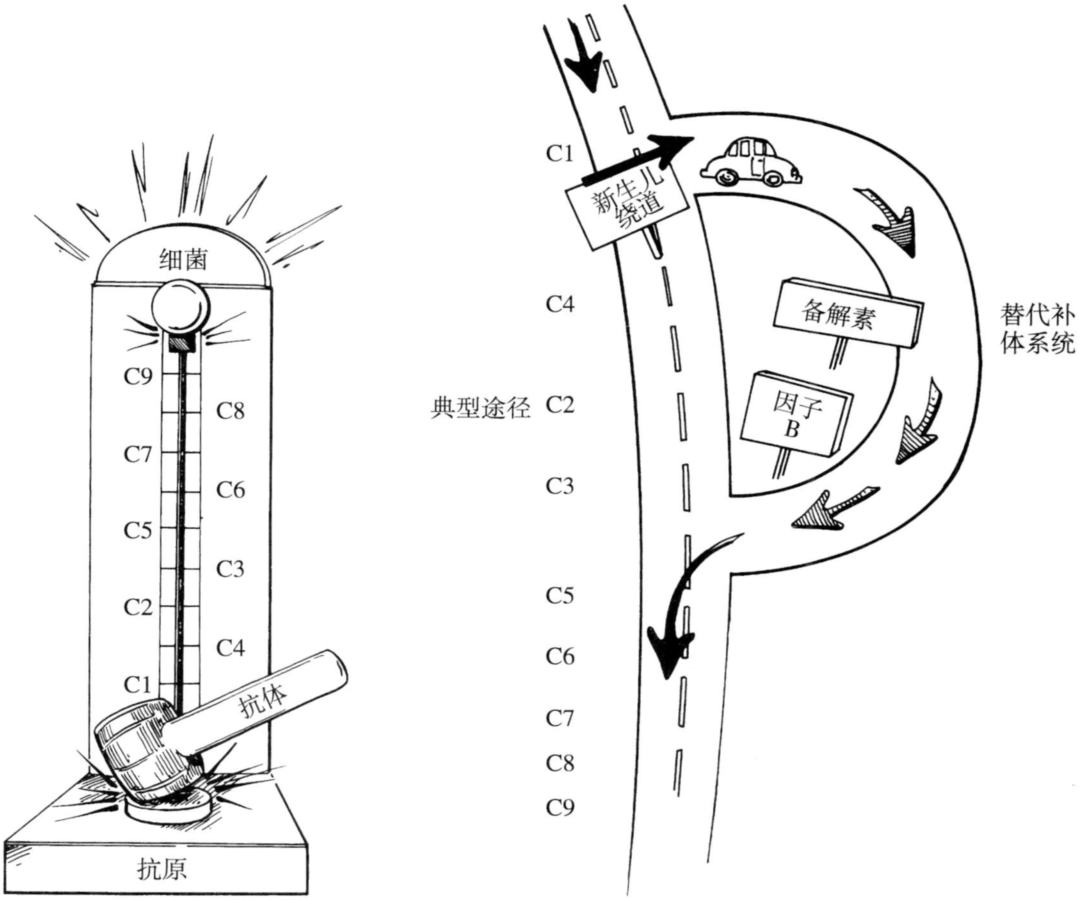

图 10-3　补体激活的经典和替代途径。经典途径通过抗原抗体复合物激活。替代途径（备解素）途径可被很多因素激活，包括细菌细胞壁碎片和脂多糖。补体级联反应的关键点在 C3，两条途径在此汇聚形成 C3a 和 C3b。C3b 能导致补体系统明显放大。C3b是一种强效的调理素，能激活远处的级联成分。

IL-11 和 IL-18，具有很多相似的特征；其他对某种病原体具有更强免疫力的细胞因子，如 IL-2、IL-4、IL-12 和 IL-13，也表现出很多的相似性。抗炎细胞因子，如 IL-10 及改变生长因子-β，可中和邻近炎症介质的生物学活性——单核-巨噬细胞及其分泌产物。

TNF-α 是感染后最早释放出来的炎症介质之一。TNF-α 主要来源于单核-巨噬细胞，尽管 NK 细胞、柱状细胞及部分激活后的 T 细胞也能生成 TNF-α，但都不如前者。TNF-α 在炎症反应中能发挥很多重要的功能。TNF-α 水平低时会：（1）增强内皮细胞与白细胞的黏附性；（2）提高炎症部位中性粒细胞的趋化性或补充中性粒细胞；（3）刺激生成其他与 TNF-α 功能相似的前炎症细胞因子，如 IL-1、IL-6 和 IL-8；（4）促使中性粒细胞和单核-巨噬细胞杀伤微生物；（5）为提高杀伤了，上调 MHC Ⅰ 型分子在靶细胞上的表达。然而，若 TNF 生产过度或失去控制，如严重脓毒症时的状况，则可因心血管功能衰竭、心肌收缩力抑制及引起弥散性血管内凝血而导致复杂的血流动力学紊乱。应当指出的是，TNF-α 水平明显升高的创伤患者的血清中很容易检测到可溶性 TNF-α，因此持续监测有助于限制 TNF-α 过多产生的有害效应[64]。

IL-1 是炎症反应期间相对较早释放出来的细胞因子。IL-1 可以由单核-巨噬细胞产生，上皮细胞、内皮细胞及树突状细胞受到内毒素或 TNF 刺激时也能产生 IL-1。IL-1 分子存在两种生物活性形式：IL-1α 可能与膜有关，而 IL-1β 溶解后产生活性。两者的作用与 TNF 相似，包括诱导其他细胞因子，如 IL-2、IL-6 及 IL-8。而与 TNF 不同的是，IL-1 对 MHC

Ⅰ型分子的表达影响很小或几乎没有。可能是因为IL-1受体拮抗剂同时释放了，后者在结构上与IL-1α、IL-1β具有同源性，因此，IL-1不会引起血流动力学紊乱。

IL-6是肝脏产生急性期蛋白质最重要的调节剂。在组织损伤、感染、TNF及IL-1发生反应时，多种细胞产生IL-6，包括单核巨噬细胞、TH2细胞及成纤维细胞。IL-6可刺激B细胞分化，促进CTL成熟。IL-6通过膜结合受体发挥作用，而膜结合受体能在远离生成部位调节IL-6的活性[72]。

IL-8是单核-巨噬细胞、T细胞、内皮细胞及血小板受到炎症、IL-1和TNF刺激时分泌的。IL-8是最强效的中性粒细胞趋化因子和活化因子之一。IL-8属于化学吸引剂家族，化学吸引剂家族还包括MCP-1、-2和-3，巨噬细胞炎性蛋白（MIP-1a、MIP-1b），以及RANTES（调节活化，正常T细胞表达和分泌）等趋化因子。这些介质在炎症早期主要由单核-巨噬细胞生成，也可由中性粒细胞和血小板产生。MIP-1a和MIP-1b可以通过自分泌方式招募其他单核吞噬细胞至炎症部位，因此可潜在放大炎症反应。其他前炎症巨噬细胞产物，即移行抑制因子，可能是由TNF在炎症部位诱导的，可在该部位“押获”巨噬细胞，进一步增加TNF-α的产量。RANTES是一种起源于淋巴细胞的化学吸引剂，能提高巨噬细胞的趋化性，上调黏附分子，增加炎症介质的释放[64]。其他化学吸引剂包括PAF和白三烯B_4，PAF是由内皮细胞和巨噬细胞分泌产生的。PAF除了可作为中性粒细胞的化
166
学吸引剂外，还可上调中性粒细胞上的CD11b/CD18（$β_2$整合因子）。一般来说，化学吸引剂不仅可将吞噬细胞招募至炎症部位，似乎还可以促使这些细胞发挥细胞毒效应器的功能[77,117,153]。

其他细胞因子在消灭入侵病原微生物的过程中也发挥了重要作用，包括TH1细胞产物（如IL-2、IFN-γ）与TH2细胞产物（如IL-4、IL-3）。一般说来，TH1细胞因子主要针对细菌、病毒或原虫感染，TH2细胞因子主要针对多细胞生物或过敏原[122,123]。IL-2是原始T细胞生长因子，通过诱导细胞增生可直接放大免疫反应，通过激活NK细胞也可增加杀伤力。IFN-γ可能是一种最重要的巨噬细胞激活因子。IFN-γ可刺激巨噬细胞表达MHC Ⅱ型分子，这对于抗原处理及放大免疫反应是必需的。此外，IFN-γ还可诱发NOS活性（NOS-2），这对于在细胞内杀伤入侵病原体是至关重要的[30,36]。IFN-γ可以通过诱导TNF-α生成、巨噬细胞表达TNF-α受体及NK细胞激活，增强对微生物的杀伤力。CTL受到IL-2及表达MHC Ⅰ型分子的抗原刺激后、NK细胞受到IL-12刺激后均能生成IFN-γ。

巨噬细胞的主要产物IL-12是诱导NK细胞产生IFN-γ的最强效物质。此外，IL-12可影响未定型的TH细胞分化成TH1表型，分泌IL-2和IFN-γ[51]。IL-12能支持IL-2的大多数功能，但其增生效应除外。因此，IL-12对消灭细胞内微生物可起到重要的作用。

TH2细胞因子如IL-4、IL-13的作用尚不清楚。虽然，TH2细胞因子可部分促进单核细胞分化及诱导黏附分子在内皮上表达，但TH2主要负责B细胞中免疫球蛋白的同型转换，主要导致IgG4和IgE的生成。

通常血浆细胞因子水平与局部组织状况之间没有直接联系。这可能是由于出现了针对炎症级联反应起始物的抗炎或调节细胞因子。例如，IL-1受体拮抗物及TNF-α的可溶性受体可分别中和IL-1β及TNF-α的生物学活性[25,42,64]。TH2细胞因子IL-10能通过抑制TNF-α及IL-1受体拮抗剂的生成下调巨噬细胞的功能[25,137]。IL-10能通过下调MHC Ⅱ型分子的表达阻止巨噬细胞作为抗原递呈细胞放大免疫反应的能力[64]。转化生长因子-β由脱颗粒的血小板和激活的巨噬细胞释放，可通过自分泌方式下调巨噬细胞的功能。同样，前列腺素E_2、儿茶酚胺及糖皮质激素在损伤和炎症时大量释放，并已证明能抑制巨噬细胞的功能[64]。虽然儿茶酚胺能增加IL-10产量，糖皮质激素能减少IFN-γ、TNF-α及IL-1β生成，但确切机制尚不清楚[60,76,140]。

除了前面提到的调节性细胞因子之外，近来的研究表明还存在其他种类的蛋白质抑制细胞因子信号传导[79]。这类蛋白是被称为细胞因子信号抑制物（SOCS），属于负性调节细胞因子信号传导的蛋白质家族。这些蛋白质通过Janus酪氨酸激酶、信号转导物及转录激活物发出信号。其生物学结果为减弱细胞因子的反应。目前尚不清楚SOCS的下游靶目标，但可以肯定的是，如果能阐明此条途径，则可能提供治疗目标。

脓毒症反应的核心是生成细胞因子和发出信号。但在临床和人种相似的情况下，不同个体可对完全相

同的刺激可表现出其独特的反应。虽然所有个体均存在内在差异的说法过分简单，但事实上，不同个体之间基因结构的唯一性可以解释两个相似患者存在细胞因子反应独特性的原因。一种可能的解释是两个患者之间蛋白质的表达存在差别。例如，某些患者受到创伤可能导致严重的脓毒症，需要入住重症监护病房接受治疗，而另一些创伤患者可能仅出现以发热、心动过速为特点的程度较轻的炎症，并且只持续症状数小时便消退。蛋白质表达存在差异可有很多原因，但一个重要的因素可能是个体的基因结构。基因多态性或单个核苷酸的多态性差异在于核酸碱基对，每 100 个碱基发生 1 次。发生在基因启动子区域的碱基对改变可以导致基因产物过剩或不足。例如，镰状细胞病患者与基因多态性有关，此类患者还可发生恶性血液病，但当同样的个体接触疟疾抗原（恶性疟原虫）时，基因程序的偏差可保护患者防止发生疟疾。近来有证据提示，一种基因多态性的存在可作为其他保护性基因多态性的标志[134]。细胞因子的基因多态性可以解释不同个体之间为何有炎症反应差异[151]。该领域中多项研究正在进行，尽管复杂情况不断涌现，但有望借助超级计算机简化数据量繁多的问题，并提供一个解读个体的细胞因子变异性的简明方法。这类进展可能可以提供有助于临床医生做出合理的治疗决策提供数据，如同现在手术前需要测定凝血参数那样。

新生儿的宿主防御

一般来说，新生儿特别是早产儿更容易发生细菌
67 感染和脓毒症。这种易感性与新生儿的宿主防御系统存在内源性不足密切相关。此处我们将讨论一些导致新生儿易患感染的原因。

新生儿时，人体中性粒细胞的产量接近最高水平。中性粒细胞数量约占循环中中粒细胞数量的 60%，其中 15%的中性粒细胞是未成熟的。在早产儿中这些百分率数值更低。新生儿易患细菌感染的一个最重要原因是：对应于应激或感染，相对来说他们无法使循环中中性粒细胞的数量显著增加，这主要是由于中性粒细胞的贮备量有限，此外较次要的是，中性粒细胞没到达目标的却增多了[24,139]。事实上，从新生小鼠获得的实验数据表明，新生小鼠的中性粒细胞贮备量只有成年水平的 20%～30%[24]。感染时中性粒细胞的增加依赖于骨髓原始干细胞的形成增加，此过程至少需要 5～7 天，才能形成新的中性粒细胞。由于新生儿循环中中性粒细胞的数量无法充足地增加，结果新生儿全身感染常导致其严重的中性粒细胞减少症。事实上，中性粒细胞贮备排空的相对程度是预测新生儿脓毒症的致命性后果的指标。

除了贮备消失之外，有证据表明，新生儿的中性粒细胞与活化内皮的黏附力也下降了[6,125]。这可能是由于 L–选择素在新生儿中性粒细胞表面的表达减少以及细胞表面 β_2 整合素无法上调所致[6,125]。结果中性粒细胞不能与内皮形成高度亲和性黏附，而这对趋化梯度做出有效反应并移行至炎症组织处是必需的。事实上，一些研究表明，新生儿中性粒细胞的趋化性较成人中性粒细胞的趋化性显著低下[66,114]。进而，累积的证据提示，新生儿中性粒细胞的膜受体与趋化性受体结合可导致信号传导异常，这也可以损伤趋化性。

在正常情况下，新生儿中性粒细胞结合、摄入和杀伤细菌的能力并不逊于成人的中性粒细胞。然而，在调理素浓度低于最适浓度的情况下，新生儿的中性粒细胞的吞噬作用效率下降[96]——一个重要的因素，因为新生儿血清中的调理素不足。

新生儿的中性粒细胞的过氧化物产量正常，但是羟自由基和特殊颗粒（防御素）的数量相对减少[5]。因此，它们可能显示出依赖氧的和不依赖氧的微生物杀伤力下降[5]。然而，除了可能存在大量细菌负荷——杀菌能力变得至关重要时之外，与微生物杀伤活性不足相比，新生儿的中性粒细胞贮备大量减少及中性粒细胞趋化性受损更为重要。

虽然新生儿的中性粒细胞贮备可能消失，但是足月新生儿的单位血容量中单核细胞的数量与成人的似乎相等甚至超出[23]。然而，婴儿的单核细胞移行至炎症处的时间较成人明显延迟。其原因可能包括单核细胞的化学吸引因素生成减少、单核细胞的趋化性受损（在中性粒细胞中已做介绍）、无法上调新生儿单核细胞表面的黏附分子。很多研究显示新生儿单核细胞具有正常的趋化性；还有一些研究显示新生儿的单核细胞可能具有正常的移行能力，但不能根据趋化梯度适当定位。同样关于新生儿的单核细胞表面黏附分子的表达也有一些相矛盾的研究报道。一些研究显示 β_2 整合素可表达增加，但另一些研究显示在新生儿的活化态及静息态的单核细胞上，这些分子下调[3]。然而，

一旦新生儿的单核细胞到达活性炎症部位，其吞噬和杀伤细菌的能力与成人单核细胞相比同样有效。新生儿的单核细胞也可生成与成人水平相当的 ROI，因此其杀伤微生物的机制与成人的相似。但相对于成人单核细胞来说，有关新生儿单核细胞 NO 产量的研究资料仍然缺乏。活化的新生儿单核细胞及巨噬细胞生成 IL-6 和 TNF-α 的量大大低于成人水平。相反，新生儿和成人的 IL-1 量是相当的。

足月新生儿的循环中 T 淋巴细胞的含量远高于成人。同样，其 $CD4^+$ 与 $CD8^+$ T 细胞的比值也高于成人。由于相对缺乏异体抗原暴露，这些 T 细胞主要呈现原始表型。然而在促有丝分裂刺激下，T 细胞也能有效地增殖。新生儿 T 细胞受到刺激后产生大量的 IL-2。相反，其他细胞因子如 TNF-α、IFN-γ、IL-3、IL-4、IL-5 和 IL-10 的量则为中等或明显受到抑制[40,41,83]。新生儿表现出 T 细胞介导（CTL）的细胞毒性下降；这种现象部分是由于原先抗原暴露相对缺乏及细胞因子的合成不足所致。单核-巨噬细胞的趋化性受损可能也会造成 T 细胞功能相对下降，导致抗原呈递细胞和 TH 细胞之间的 MHC 限制性同族相互作用消失。因此，细胞因子产量显著下降，且炎症反应无法得到放大。

足月新生儿同样也表现出 B 细胞功能及发育的相对不成熟。尽管新生儿 B 细胞能分化成为分泌 IgM的浆细胞，但其直到后期也不会分化成分泌 IgG 或 IgA 的浆细胞。新生儿 IgM 的分泌量大于成人。而新生儿的血清 IgG 均来源于母体胎盘转移。事实上，直到出生后第 3 个或第 4 个月，新生儿的 IgG 在循环中的比例才开始增加。因此若母体循环中 IgG 水平正常，则其胎儿可免遭大多数感染介质的危害，但无法防御引起不同免疫球蛋白同型的微生物，如大肠杆菌和沙门杆菌。由于早产儿不能接受大量来自母体
168 的 IgG，其特别容易罹患感染。在新生儿出生 1 周后，IgM 和分泌性 IgA 在分泌物中就可检测出，它们在母乳中大量存在，通过母乳喂养可补偿性地防御细菌感染。

NK 细胞可以通过非 MHC 限制性方式促进靶细胞分解，在防御细胞内病原体方面发挥重要的作用。对于足月新生儿来说，其所含 NK 细胞的百分比与成人相仿。然而，新生儿的 NK 细胞功能和表型不成熟（$CD56^-$）[74,91]。出生时其溶解能力只能达到成人的 50%，直到婴儿期末才能达到成熟水平。这种现象可能部分是由于新生儿的细胞因子量（特别是 IFN-γ）较低造成，如上文已讨论的那样。

一般来说，因为新生儿的免疫球蛋白水平低下，其主要依靠补体激活替代（不依赖抗体的）途径（图 10-3）。然而绝大多数足月儿和早产儿的资料显示，补体激活经典途径和替代途径中的成分均显著下降。C9 是补体系统的终末成分，对于杀伤革兰阴性微生物起着关键作用，新生儿的 C9 水平下降，特别是早产儿。无论是足月新生儿还是早产儿其调理能力也受到伤害。这可能是调理素 C3b 沉积在微生物上导致交联无效的结果。另外也可表现为纤连蛋白消失，而纤连蛋白对于细胞黏附具有重要的作用，同时也有利于某些细菌与吞噬细胞结合。新生儿还表现出强效趋化因子 C5a 的生成减少。足月儿和早产儿除中性粒细胞贮藏池的存量下降外，免疫球蛋白水平也下降了，因而不能有效地使用最强效的生物学调理素 C3b，而 C3b 能够放大补体途径。此外，C5a 和 C9的减少造成炎症部位的吞噬细胞内流减少及炎症处杀伤功能受损，这些缺陷可使足月儿和早产儿进一步易患细菌感染。

全身炎症反应综合征的发病机制

宿主内在的防御机制与微生物病原体的毒力因素之间的复杂作用从较大程度上控制了临床感染的发生。若免疫系统防御细菌入侵失败，将导致微生物在侵入门户或感染病灶处增生。这些感染最初会在局部引起炎症反应，其目的是破坏微生物。巨噬细胞受到细菌及其副产物如内毒素（LPS）激活后，会在局部释放出炎症细胞因子，如 TNF-α 和 IL-1β。LPS 的脂质 A 部分会与 LBP 结合，后者是正常人血清中存在的一种 60-kD 蛋白质。这种 LPS-LBP 复合物继而与 CD14 分子（存在于巨噬细胞、中性粒细胞和内皮细胞上的一种受体）结合，然后再与细胞上的 TLR 相互作用，诱导释放出细胞因子，如 TNF-α、IL-6 及 PAF（图 10-4）。LPS-LBP 与 TLR 结合，并通过有丝分裂原激活的激酶发出信号[14]。有趣的是，巨噬细胞在 LPS 诱导下生成细胞因子是随着年龄增长而逐步递减的，提示年龄越小的个体其前炎症反应越复杂[14]。这些分子可上调内皮细胞和中性粒细胞上黏附分子的表达。随后释放的 IL-8 有助于在感染部位招募和激活其他炎症细胞，特别是中性粒细胞。中性粒

图 10-4 全身炎症反应综合征（SIRS）的发病机制。屏障破坏后细菌侵入，导致局部释放脂多糖（LPS），继而在中性粒细胞、巨噬细胞及内皮细胞上形成 LPS-脂多糖结合蛋白（LBP）-CD14-Toll 样受体 4（TLR-4）复合物，从而激活细胞。释放炎症细胞因子后，上调黏附分子，提高中性粒细胞和巨噬细胞的趋化性。（补体系统、凝血级联及淋巴细胞群同样被激活，未在图表中表示）。激活的细胞释放杀伤微生物物质，特别是杀伤细菌的物质，但如果炎症过程未得到控制，则其可能有害并造成远处器官损伤，引起 SIRS。ICAM：细胞间黏附分子；IL：白细胞介素；MCP：单核细胞趋化蛋白；MIP：巨噬细胞炎症蛋白；NO：一氧化氮；PAF：血小板活化因子；PECAM：血小板-内皮细胞黏附分子；ROI：活性氧中间物（或类）；TNF：肿瘤坏死因子。

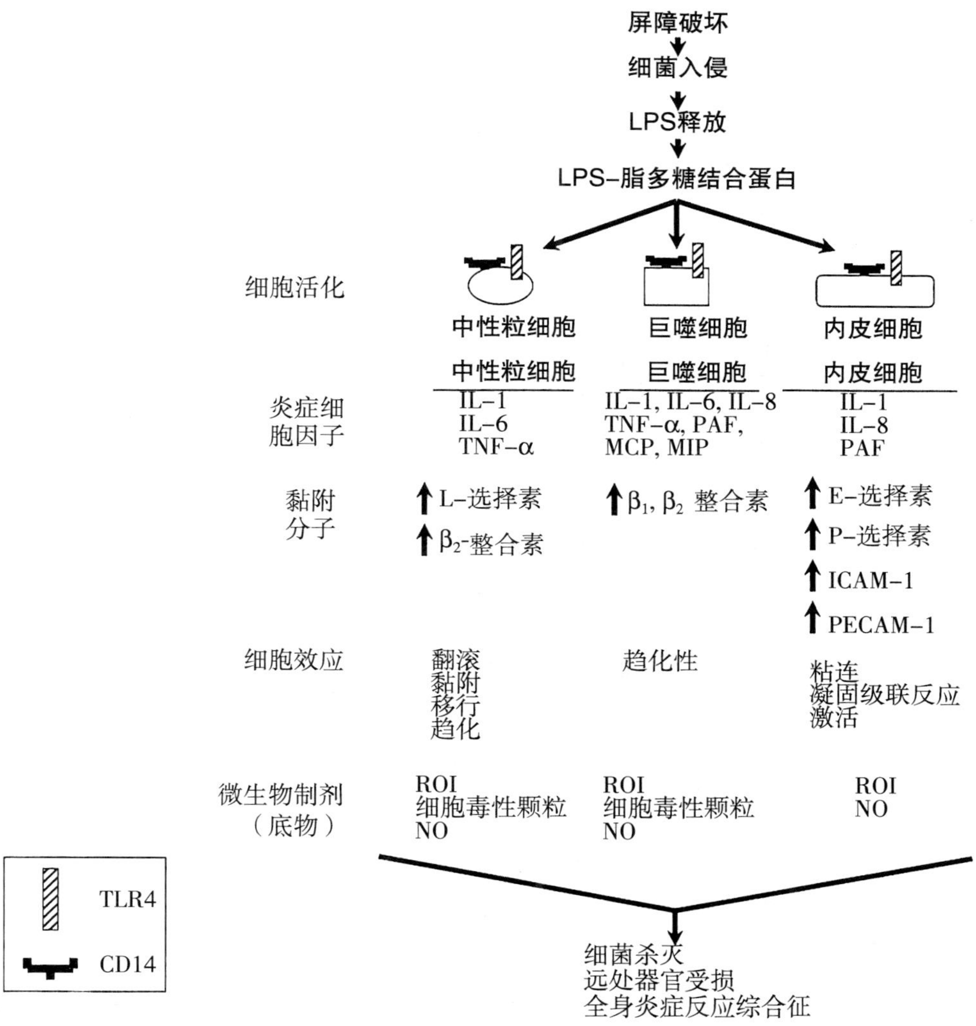

细胞通过滚动、粘连并随趋化梯度渗出内皮而发生移行。激活的中性粒细胞在感染处吞噬病原体并在吞噬溶酶体中杀伤微生物。其他外源性因素如抗生素有助于控制和消除感染。然而，若感染控制失败或治疗明显拖延，则可能引起细菌增生，并侵入全身（血流），进一步激活和放大炎症级联反应。个别情况下，即使感染得到了成功治疗，也会发生后一种现象。炎症级联反应的刺激未得到控制的标志是 SIRS，其特点是生命体征、体内平衡及代谢均发生临床改变，并伴有器官功能异常。

诊断年长儿及成人 SIRS 至少需要存在下列标准的两项：(1) 体温＞38℃或＜36℃；(2) 心率＞90次 / 分；(3) 呼吸频率＞20 次 / 分或 $PaCO_2$＜32mmHg；(4) 白细胞计数＞12 000/mm^3 或＜4000/mm^3，或带宽超过 10%。很多非感染性疾病，如创伤、烧伤及急性胰腺炎，均能诱发 SIRS。因此，“脓毒症”这个术语只用于感染导致的 SIRS。SIRS患者发展成进行性器官功能异常的危险因素包括感染或炎症病灶持续存在，如未经引流的脓肿、持续低灌注及持续的炎症反应本身。

未经控制的炎症反应可以导致激活的巨噬细胞持续释放细胞因子（TNF-α 和 IL-1β）。全身性释放细胞因子可上调远处器官内皮细胞上的黏附分子，如肺，因此可强化中性粒细胞介导的急性肺损伤。IL-8 招募和激活中性粒细胞；后者可以通过未成熟的脱颗粒及细胞毒性颗粒或 ROI 释放直接引起内皮细胞的细胞毒性损伤。这种现象会导致肺间质损伤、毛细管渗漏及呼吸衰竭。此外，通过增加 L-选择素的释放[94]，以及减少自然凋亡率（这可能与释放 IL-6 或 PAF 有关）[15]，SIRS 患者循环系统中可持续存在中性粒细胞。其结果造成中性粒细胞的半衰期延长，因此这些激活的中性粒细胞能介导多种器官的损伤，从而导致
169 毛细管渗漏综合征、灌注减少以及终末器官损伤。

组织低氧可通过刺激巨噬细胞额外释放 TNF-α、IL-1 和 IL-8 以及上调中性粒细胞和内皮细胞上的黏附分子，从而进一步放大炎症级联反应[9,119,145]。

还有不少其他机制有助于延长炎症反应。例如，TNF-α 和 IL-1β 均能激活转录调节因子——核因子 κB，核因子 κB 可以与每个基因的启动子区结合。激活后基因转录可增加，并额外生成前炎症细胞因子[1,78,86,152]。进而，TNF-α 和 IL-1β以自分泌方式激活巨噬细胞生成其他前炎症细胞因子。巨噬细胞与 $CD4^+$ TH 淋巴细胞相互作用后会生成 IFN-γ，后者是一种最强的巨噬细胞激活剂之一。经过上述多种相互作用后，巨噬细胞有能力维持自身的炎症表型，延长炎症级联反应。事实上，一向对 97 例脓毒症患者的细胞因子的回顾性分析研究表明，全身炎症反应的程度（定义为血浆中炎症介质的浓度）可明显影响死亡率[15,20]。最后，TNF 位点上基因的多态性可能影响在染期间血浆中 TNF-α 的水平，因此也可能影响患者的预后。与 *TNFB2* 等位基因纯合子或 *TNFB1* 及 *TNFB2* 杂合子的患者相比，*TNFB1* 等位基因纯合子患者的血浆中 TNF-α 水平较低，感染后死亡率也较低[131]。

生理和代谢结果

SIRS 或脓毒症患者最突出的临床和血流动力学改变是全身血管阻力下降和外周氧摄取量减少[109]。因此，必须持续增加氧运输或氧供以维持适当的组织氧合。全身血管阻力下降可能部分缘于 NO 以及前列环素或补体激活。然而，还没有任何报道能阐明患者发生出血性休克后，诱导性 NOS 在血流动力学代偿失调时的作用[76]。通过增加心排出量和每分通气量可
170 以增加氧的运输。因心肌功能抑制、肺衰竭或因器官功能异常导致的细胞代谢减少，患者无法满足氧需求的增加与氧传递之间的平衡，死亡的危险性增加。这些患者可表现出无氧代谢明显增加，乳酸产量过剩[12]。

去脂肪体重的大量丢失是 SIRS 或脓毒症患者的典型特征。前炎症细胞因子激活神经体液轴后会释放出促肾上腺皮质激素、皮质醇、儿茶酚胺及其他糖异生激素，如胰高血糖素，以增加能量底物。当为了产生能量，机体尝试肝糖原异生及合成蛋白质而形成底物时，可发生骨骼肌断裂。TNF-α、IL-1 和 IL-6 介导的发热反应可进一步提高分解代谢率。虽然提供外源性氨基酸可在肝脏中合成蛋白质，但是增加的分解代谢率不会对外源性氨基酸产生反应。TNF-α 和 IL-1 也可以降低脂蛋白脂肪酶活性（脂蛋白脂肪酶引起总体脂肪生成）[85,133]，减少外周三酰甘油的清除率。

新生儿脓毒症

新生儿由于宿主防御系统存在内源性不足，在出生后 4 周内特别容易发生细菌感染。这些“脆弱的”宿主无法有效地将细菌感染限制在局部，因而有可能发生菌血症或脑膜炎，还有可能发生新生儿脓毒症。经过修订的 Bone 标准更加精确地定义了小儿群体的脓毒症，包括：（1）脓毒症的临床证据，伴有发热（直肠温度＞38.0℃）或体温过低（＜35.6℃）；（2）心动过速（心率＞同年龄组的第 95 位百分位数）；（3）呼吸急促（呼吸频率＞同年龄组的第 95 位百分位数）；（4）低血压（平均动脉压＜同年龄组的第 5位百分位数）；（5）精神状态改变，代谢性酸中毒（动脉血 pH＜ 7.35 或碱缺乏＞-5），少尿（每小时尿量＜1ml/kg），或出现外周灌注不良的征象，如毛细管再灌注延迟[38]。尽管临床证明活产儿发生新生儿脓毒症的比率只有 1/1000～5/1000，但其死亡率很高，约为 30%～50% [129]。进而幸存下来的患者都经历了严重的病情。新生儿脓毒症的危险因素可以归纳为两个方面：即母体因素和新生儿因素。

母体因素

早产、破膜时间过长（＞24 小时）、临床证明存在绒膜羊膜炎、生殖道中致病菌繁殖（如 B 组链球菌或大肠杆菌）、尿路感染及邻近预产期进行性交，这些都是导致新生儿感染的危险因素。这些因素增加

了新生儿在子宫内及在经阴道分娩期间暴露于病原体而发生感染的危险。事实上，这些危险因素可使全身感染的发生率上升 10 倍以上[129]。

新生儿因素

如上文所述，新生儿的宿主防御机制显著受损。其主要原因有中性粒细胞贮藏量减少、中性粒细胞和单核细胞趋化性异常、细胞因子和补体产量下降以及特异性 IgG、分泌性 IgA、IgM 水平下降等，这些连同血管内留置导管可导致解剖屏障受损。这些不足会使早产儿的病情更加恶化。出生体重低也是一个独立的危险因素，体重低于 2500g 的新生儿比体重高于 2500g 的新生儿感染的几率增加将近 8 倍。

新生儿脓毒症最常见的致病微生物是 B 组链球菌和大肠杆菌 K–1。这些细菌通常聚集在母体的胃肠道中，在直肠或阴道培养物中也能检测到。导致新生儿脓毒症的其他病菌包括表皮葡萄球菌及细胞内病原体单核细胞增多性李斯特菌。除了新生儿宿主防御机制存在内源性缺陷之外，这些细菌的毒力因素也影响全身感染的发生率。B 组链球菌具有夹膜多糖，可在缺乏适当调理素的情况下防止链球菌被中性粒细胞吞噬，如上文所述新生儿体内缺乏足够的调理素[45,147]。同样大肠杆菌 K–1 的夹膜多糖也是其最重要的结构性毒力因素之一。其他潜在的毒力因素包括菌毛、特殊的 O 抗原以及大肠杆菌 K–1 的 α–溶血素、B 组链球菌的神经氨酸酶和毒素[45,147]。表皮葡萄球菌的内在致病性源于其生成黏附素的能了，后者可提高细菌与上皮的黏附力，同时其表面的黏质物可保护细菌，防止细菌被吞噬并抵御抗生素的毒性效应[55,111]。与细菌感染不同，单核细胞增多性李斯特菌及某些病毒（如单纯疱疹病毒）所致的新生儿感染反映了 T 细胞介导的免疫反应存在缺陷。

新生儿脓毒症的典型特征是体温失调、呼吸暂停、呼吸窘迫、心血管功能衰竭、嗜睡、喂养困难及其他胃肠道功能紊乱。足月儿及早产儿可能会在出生后 96 小时内暴发性发生 B 组链球菌感染。患儿可在 24 小时内出现呼吸窘迫、低血压及弥散性血管内凝血，如不及早进行支持治疗和给予抗生素，可导致死亡。低血糖也是新生儿脓毒症的常见症状。这主要是由于糖原分解、糖异生减少（尽管促进糖异生作用的激素产量增加，如胰高血糖素）及组织利用葡萄糖增加所致。

有证据表明，在成人和年长儿中，前炎症细胞因子，如 TNF–α、IL–1、IL–6、IL–8 和 PAF，在血流动力学紊乱中起着重要的作用，而这也是新生儿脓毒 171
症的特点。Sullivan 等人[132]报道，革兰阳性和革兰阴性细菌感染患儿的体内 IL–1、IL–6 和 TNF–α 水平均升高。同样发现 IL–6（特别是与 C–反应蛋白联合）是诊断新生儿细菌感染的敏感指标[18]。给予 B 组链球菌感染脓毒症的新生小猪己酮可可碱（一种 TNF–α 的抑制剂）后，TNF 的产量可以减少，并可改善小猪肺部的血流动力学[52]。Wong 等人[49]发现，早罹患脓毒症的婴儿和儿童血浆中，NO 的稳定的终末代谢产物亚硝酸盐和硝酸盐水平升高，提示 NO 也可能是造成脓毒症新生儿血流动力学紊乱的重要介质。

诊断

SIRS 和脓毒症的各种临床征象已被回顾，但这些征象都是非特异性的。例如，有研究报道，在发热的足月新生儿中，只有 10%有细菌感染的记录；在早产儿中，这个数字下降至 3% [129]。迅速而准确的诊断一直是临床医生的基本目标，特别是对足月儿和早产儿，这样才能给予适当的抗生素治疗，从而减少新生儿脓毒症的发病率和死亡率。虽然从血液、脑脊液、尿液、体液或组织中分离出微生物仍然是诊断细菌感染的金标准，但这些培养物的结果可能是阴性的。即使只有 0.5ml 血液标本也能增强血培养物的敏感性。应从外周血或留置导管中获取培养基。尿培养物应从耻骨弓上穿刺抽吸或直接通过膀胱置管获取，尿液应浓缩 25～50 倍。出生后 7 天（特别是出生后 72 小时）内如尿液培养物结果呈阳性，则可推测新生儿原先患有菌血症。高达 1/3 的脓毒症新生儿可同时患有脑膜炎，因此，还应给这些患儿进行腰穿。如果出现下列表现，应怀疑有脑脊膜感染：（1）脑脊液中白细胞计数＞32 $/mm^3$，同时中性粒细胞＞60%；（2）脑脊液中葡萄糖浓度低于同时抽取的血清葡萄糖浓度的 50%；（3）脑脊液中蛋白质含量＞150mg/dL；（4）通过革兰染色或对流免疫电泳发现细菌。

已有不少实验室检测方法能为诊断细菌感染提供直接或间接证据。但遗憾的是，还没有一种单一的方法能有效地确定或排除细菌性脓毒症的诊断。

总白细胞计数：总白细胞计数本身在新生儿脓毒症的诊断中价值有限。在最终确诊为感染的新生儿中，白细胞计数＜5000/mm^3 或＞20 000/mm^3 者不到 50%[112,128]。由于总白细胞计数预测的准确性不高，很多研究者开始寻找其他诊断新生儿感染的中性粒细胞指标。总中性粒细胞计数（考虑到成熟和未成熟两种形式）也不可靠，因为只有 2/3 的脓毒症患儿存在中性粒细胞计数异常。同样未成熟中性粒细胞计数的诊断价值不大，因为感染时释放入血的晚幼粒细胞数目与感染病程并不一致，不具有预测性，这也反映了新生儿中性粒细胞贮备不足这一事实。一项最有用但不够可靠的指标是中性粒细胞总数中未成熟中性粒细胞所占的比率；正常情况下，该比率约为 0.2。比率正常可提示感染的可能性很低。在没有围生期窒息或妊娠诱发高血压的情况下，比率超过 0.2 是诊断感染的一个敏感指标。严重的中性粒细胞减少症（比率＞0.8）通常意味着骨髓重度衰竭，预后不佳。

血小板计数：血小板减少症已证明是新生儿脓毒症的非特异性、晚期预测指标。在病毒、真菌及细菌感染中均可见。另外血流动力学发生改变后才能发现血小板减少症。

急性期反应物：发生感染时，肝脏会合成大量的蛋白质，即急性期反应物。这些蛋白质绝大多数是在受到 IL-6、C-反应蛋白、白蛋白、纤维蛋白原和结合珠蛋白刺激后产生的。C-反应蛋白是研究最广泛的蛋白质。其主要作用是作为载体蛋白于具有潜在毒性的微生物副产品结合并提高其清除率。然而，如 C-反应蛋白水平达到正常值的 10 倍，则有可能是由其他非感染性病因引起的，包括围生期窒息、胎粪误吸及呼吸窘迫综合征。测定 C-反应蛋白水平有助于监测治疗反应。C-反应蛋白浓度在感染后的最初 8 小时内升高，并在 2～3 天内达到峰值；当炎症过程消退时，其水平迅速下降。结合珠蛋白、纤维蛋白原及红细胞沉降率对于诊断细菌感染没有任何价值或价值有限。

研究者们一直在尝试将各种筛查试验的数据组合起来从而提高预测的准确性。与单个试验相比，这些组合的筛查试验在诊断感染方面并没有显示出优越性。然而，如果这些试验的预测结果呈阴性，则意味着经过正常试验排除细菌性脓毒症的可能性接近 100%。至今，也没有证明测定血浆中各种细胞因子的水平有助于诊断细菌性感染。

PIRO 系统是在脓毒症研究中新出现的概念。这是一种以患者的易患情况（P）、感染的性质和程度（I）、宿主反应的性质和程度（R）和伴发器官功能异常的程度（O）为基础对患者进行评估的方法[81,82]。PIRO 模型可区分感染直接导致的疾病与宿主对感染反应导致的继发疾病。此外，PIRO 系统还可说明感染发生前的疾病状况，即可能有加重病情的危险性而 172
与感染过程本身无关。

治疗

只有迅速识别脓毒症和 SIRS 的症状和体征并及早进行积极干预，才能成功治疗脓毒症和 SIRS。需要特别指出的是，必须给予患者适当的心血管和肺功能的支持，特别是在 SIRS 的早期阶段，当毛细管渗漏综合征和全身血管阻力下降可能影响血压及组织氧合时，因为外周氧利用减少而氧需求增加。因此，首要目标是恢复向组织输送氧。这个目标可通过确保患者复苏来达到。有证据提示，脓毒症患儿基本上无法得到足够的复苏[19,61]。SIRS 患者容量补充不足会导致低血压、组织灌注减少和氧债加重。为了改善这些患者的预后，应主动尽早进行复苏[19,61]。首先应纠正容量不足，然后才能给予血管加压药。患者出现明显的肺功能失调或衰竭时，机械通气是一种重要的辅助手段。应当密切监测尿量和血流动力学参数，并适当地加以调整。应尽早开始给予营养支持（尤其是肠道营养）以减轻分解代谢状态并为肠道提供营养物。对足月儿和早产儿更是如此，因为他们的糖原贮备较少并常出现严重的低血糖。

除了液体复苏和呼吸支持之外，抗生素治疗是脓毒症治疗的基础。应毫不迟疑地开始经验性广谱抗生素治疗。脓毒症或 SIRS 通常是全身性革兰阴性感染的结果，虽然 SIRS 患者血培养呈阳性者不足 50%。最常见的致病微生物包括大肠杆菌、绿脓杆菌、克雷白杆菌及拟杆菌。在足月儿和早产儿中，B 组链球菌、大肠杆菌及单核细胞增生性李斯特菌占分离后细菌的大部分。在这些人群中，氨苄西林和庆大霉素在早期治疗中可覆盖足够多的菌种，因为表皮葡萄球菌及其他微生物（如念珠菌）的感染较晚才会发生。在抗生素治疗开始后 24～48 小时内应进行血培养，以判断患者对治疗是否有反应。积极治疗后如患者培养物结果仍连续呈现阳性，提示患者对抗生素耐药、存在未引流的感染灶或留置导管处细菌感染。

抗生素治疗脓毒症初期，患者的病情可发生急性或亚急性恶化。这种现象缘于被杀死的细菌释放的大量内毒素进入血流。事实上，静脉给予抗生素可使人体内游离的内毒素水平升高 50 倍[124]。LPS 与 LBP结合形成复合物后作用强度是 LPS 的 1000 倍以上。LPS–LBP 复合物可与巨噬细胞、中性粒细胞或内皮细胞上的 CD14 分子及 TLR–4 相连，诱导合成和释放大量的前炎症细胞因子，进一步激活或放大炎症级联反应，这正是 SIRS 的特征。因此，近年来有大量研究尝试采用 LPS 的脂质 A 部分的单克隆抗体阻断脓毒症患者的炎症反应。

首先在 SIRS 患者中采用人单克隆（IgM）抗脂质 A 抗体（HA–1A）的试验研究表明，血培养有阳性发现的革兰阴性菌菌血症患者最有可能从这项治疗中受益[156]。然而，随后在革兰阴性菌菌血症及脓毒性休克的患者中进行的临床试验其结果不支持这一理论，与接受安慰剂的患者相比，接受 HA–1A 的患者的死亡率没有显著差异[92]。Rogy 等人[116]对接受大肠杆菌注射的狒狒进行了 HA–1A 和杀菌性通透性增加蛋白质（BPI，人类产生的内源性 LPS 中和蛋白）比较，得到了相似的观察结果。另一项临床研究采用了另一种不同的抗 LPS 单克隆抗体——E5，结果发现革兰阴性菌脓毒症非休克患者的死亡率并没有获得任何改善；然而，E5 治疗大大缓解了器官衰竭并防止了向成人型呼吸窘迫综合征的发展。抗 LPS 治疗不能改善脓毒症死亡率可能与持续内毒素血症、感染无法控制、抗体中和 LPS 不足等因素有关[28]。还有另一种可能，即一旦 LPS 启动了炎症级联反应， HA–1A 或其他抗 LPS 抗体中和都会无效。此外，由于其他因素也可能导致 SIRS，包括革兰阳性菌感染、严重创伤或烧伤，因此尝试阻断邻近的炎症反应中的可溶性介质要比以 LPS 为阻断目标更实际一些。其他研究者在使用 CDP57 时也采取了相同的策略，CDP57 是一种完全人类化的抗 TNF–α 抗体。快速进展为脓毒性休克的患者在给予 CDP57 后，循环中的 TNF–α 水平迅速下降（30 分钟内），而且循环中的 IL–1β 和 IL–6 水平会相对缓慢地下降；然而患者的生存率却不受影响[34]。一项Ⅲ期试验评估了 SIRS 患者接受 IL–1 受体拮抗剂后的状况，除了终末期器官功能异常或采用急性生理学和慢性健康评估（APACHE）Ⅲ评分预测死亡风险大于 242 分的患者，在生存率方面并没有显示出任何优势[49,50]。

激活细胞因子级联可触发各种反应，包括激活凝血级联反应及抑制纤维蛋白溶解途径[29]。激活凝血会导致凝血酶产生，使纤维蛋白沉积在微脉管系统，从而导致微血管和大血管内血栓形成。此过程具有进化意义，因为其目的在于限制微生物在宿主体内弥散，但若不加以控制，结果反而可能使患者发生器官功能异常并最终导致死亡。激活后的蛋白 C 是一种凝血[58,88]和炎症的内源性调节剂[11,29,135]。一旦蛋白
C 被凝血酶–血栓调节素复合物激活，会产生抗血栓 173
和纤维蛋白原溶解效应。激活的蛋白 C可以通过抑制核因子 κB 易位[73]、细胞因子形成[56,62]及选择素活性[57]直接产生抗炎效应。因为很多重症脓毒症患者存在获得性蛋白 C 激活不足及死亡率危险性增加，因此激活的蛋白 C 有希望成为治疗的靶位[46]。近来，在成人和小儿的有关重组人类活化蛋白 C（活化的 drotrecogin alfa）的研究结果显示，这种药是安全和有益的。PROWESS 研究[120]是在重症脓毒症成人患者中开展的多中心大规模随机、双盲对照研究。结果表明，与接受安慰剂的患者相比，各种原因导致的脓毒症成人患者接受 drotrecogin alfa（活化的）后 28 天内的死亡率显著下降。在对成人的试验进行评估分析期间开始了儿科患者的研究，这是一项在美国和英国开展的国际性多中心的开放性、非随机性序列研究。研究者发现，在整个研究期间，蛋白 C 和抗凝血酶[70]基线水平明显升高[3]；另外还发现约 5%的患者发生了严重出血。这些结果与成人的试验结果类似，为开展大规模的Ⅲ期随机对照研究提供了依据。

在抗细胞因子治疗药物中，给予可溶性 TNF 受体或 BPI 可被证明是相当有效的。特别是 BPI（正常情况下由中性粒细胞产生）与 LPS 具有高度的亲和力，对内毒素激发的脓毒症模型具有保护性[50,89]。其

他不少潜在的免疫调节剂已开始应用，包括牛磺罗定（一种抗内毒素药物[146]）及单磷酰脂质 A（来源于沙门杆菌明尼苏达 R595 的内毒素水解衍生物）。然而，至今未发现其有任何益处[10]。其他关于脓毒症的生物学治疗方法是以内皮细胞及其产物为靶物的。抗氧化剂治疗和 PAF 受体拮抗剂能减轻 ROI 及 PAF 损害效应造成的损伤。然而，至今还没有开展相关的临床试验。针对 P-选择素、E-选择素、ICAM-1、CD11/CD18 整合素及 PECAM-1 的抗体在再灌注损伤实验模型中的结果已显现出希望[87]。

磷酸二酯酶抑制剂代表了另一类重要的免疫调节剂。这些药物可增加细胞内环磷酸腺苷（cAMP）的水平，使 LPS 刺激后 TNF-α 的 mRNA 累积下降。己酮可可碱是这一类药物中最为有名的，它可以减少内毒素性休克实验模型及志愿者 TNF-α 的产量[115,120,154]。β 和 α 激动剂对于稳定脓毒症患者的心血管功能具有重要的作用，且被证明能减少 TNF-α 的产量，推测是由于增加了细胞内 cAMP 水平[76]。皮质类固醇在各种脓毒性休克模型中具有保护作用。其机制可能与 TNF-α 的翻译激活被抑制有关[53]。给予小儿脑膜炎患者小剂量的地塞米松可降低脑脊液中细胞因子的水平，改善炎症及神经病的总体预后。相反，大剂量的皮质类固醇对于脓毒症休克患者是有害的，因为阻断 TNF-α 的 mRNA 翻译只需要小剂量，大剂量应用可能引起不必要的长时间免疫抑制，反而不利于 TNF 阻断的有益效应[17,39]。在开始抗生素治疗前给予类固醇可发挥出最大的抗炎效应，这是由于类固醇可阻断 TNF-α 增加，正常情况下，TNF-α 水平升高主要缘于抗生素诱导细菌分解后产生的内毒素血症。有关给药最佳时机的争论同样也存在于其他生物学反应修饰因子中。

静脉给予 γ 球蛋白和新鲜冷冻血浆已成为脓毒症新生儿的辅助治疗手段，特别是在缺乏 IgG、IgM、IgA 和补体的早产儿。还没有一项临床对照研究能够说明给极低体重出生儿经静脉预防性使用 γ 球蛋白对于治疗能带来任何好处[44]。同样给疑似感染的婴儿预防性地使用新鲜冷冻血浆也没有发现具有任何益处[2]。重症革兰阴性脓毒症的早产儿常由于坏死性小肠结肠炎继发肠穿孔，有数据显示，这些早产儿静脉给予 γ 球蛋白（700mg/kg）可能有用。

（张瑞冬译　陈锡明校）

参考文献

1. Abraham E: Alterations in transcriptional regulation of proinflammatory and immunoregulatory cytokine expression by hemorrhage, injury, and critical illness. New Horiz 1996;4:184-193.
2. Acunas BA, Peakman M, Liossis G, et al: Effect of fresh frozen plasma and gammaglobulin on humoral immunity in neonatal sepsis. Arch Dis Child Fetal Neonatal Ed 1994;70: F182-F187.
3. Albelda SM, Smith CW, Ward PA: Adhesion molecules and inflammatory injury. FASEB J 1994;8:504-512.
4. Albina JE, Cui S, Mateo RB, Reichner JS: Nitric oxide-mediated apoptosis in murine peritoneal macrophages. J Immunol 1993;150:5080-5085.
5. Ambruso DR, Altenburger KM, Johnston RB Jr: Defective oxidative metabolism in newborn neutrophils: Discrepancy between superoxide anion and hydroxyl radical generation. Pediatrics 1979;64(Suppl):722-725.
6. Anderson DC, Abbassi O, Kishimoto TK, et al: Diminished lectin-, epidermal growth factor-, complement binding domain-cell adhesion molecule-1 on neonatal neutrophils underlies their impaired CD18-independent adhesion to endothelial cells in vitro. J Immunol 1991;146:3372-3379.
7. Ar'Rajab A, Dawidson I, Fabia R: Reperfusion injury. New Horiz 1996;4:224-234.
8. Arnaout MA: Leukocyte adhesion molecules deficiency: Its structural basis, pathophysiology and implications for modulating the inflammatory response. Immunol Rev 1990;114:145-180.
9. Arnould T, Michiels C, Remacle J: Increased PMN adherence on endothelial cells after hypoxia: Involvement of PAF, CD18/CD11b, and ICAM-1. Am J Physiol 1993;264:C1102-C1110.
10. Astiz ME, Rackow EC, Still JG, et al: Pretreatment of normal humans with monophosphoryl lipid A induces tolerance to endotoxin: A prospective, double-blind, randomized, controlled trial. Crit Care Med 1995;23:9-17.
11. Bajzar L, Kalafatis M, Simioni P, Tracy PB: An antifibrinolytic mechanism describing the prothrombotic effect associated with factor V Leiden. J Biol Chem 1996;271: 22949-22952.
12. Beal AL, Cerra FB: Multiple organ failure syndrome in the 1990s: Systemic inflammatory response and organ dysfunction. JAMA 1994;271:226-233.
12a. Bernard GR, Vincent JL, Laterre PF, et al: Recombinant human protein C Worldwide Evaluation in Severe Sepsis (PROWESS) Study group. Efficacy and safety of recombinant human activated protein C for severe sepsis. N Engl J Med 2001;344:699-709.
13. Bevilacqua MP, Nelson RM: Selectins. J Clin Invest 1993; 91:379-387.
14. Boehmer ED, Goral J, Faunce DE, Kovacs EJ: Age-dependent decrease in Toll-like receptor 4-mediated proinflammatory cytokine production and mitogen-activated protein kinase expression. J Leukoc Biol 2004;75:342-349.
15. Bone RC: Sepsis and its complications: The clinical problem. Crit Care Med 1994;22(Suppl):S8-S11.
16. Bone RC, Balk RA, Fein AM, et al: A second large controlled clinical study of E5, a monoclonal antibody to endotoxin: Results of a prospective, multicenter, randomized, controlled trial. The E5 Sepsis Study Group. Crit Care Med 1995;23:994-1006.
17. Bone RC, Fisher CJ Jr, Clemmer TP, et al: A controlled clinical trial of high-dose methylprednisolone in the treatment of severe sepsis and septic shock. N Engl J Med

1987;317: 653-658.
18. Buck C, Bundschu J, Gallati H, et al: Interleukin-6: A sensitive parameter for the early diagnosis of neonatal bacterial infection. Pediatrics 1994;93:54-58.
19. Carcillo JA, Davis AL, Zaritsky A: Role of early fluid resuscitation in pediatric septic shock. JAMA 1991;266:1242-1245.
20. Casey LC, Balk RA, Bone RC: Plasma cytokine and endotoxin levels correlate with survival in patients with the sepsis syndrome. Ann Intern Med 1993;119:771-778.
21. Chan J, Xing Y, Magliozzo RS, Bloom BR: Killing of virulent *Mycobacterium tuberculosis* by reactive nitrogen intermediates produced by activated murine macrophages. J Exp Med 1992;175:1111-1122.
22. Cher DJ, Mosmann TR: Two types of murine helper T cell clone. II. Delayed-type hypersensitivity is mediated by TH1 clones. J Immunol 1987;138:3688-3694.
23. Christensen RD: Hematopoiesis in the fetus and neonate. Pediatr Res 1989;26:531-535.
24. Christensen RD, Rothstein G: Exhaustion of mature marrow neutrophils in neonates with sepsis. J Pediatr 1980;96: 316-318.
25. Cinat M, Waxman K, Vaziri ND, et al: Soluble cytokine receptors and receptor antagonists are sequentially released after trauma. J Trauma 1995;39:112-118.
26. Clegg S, Gerlach GF: Enterobacterial fimbriae. J Bacteriol 1987;169:934-938.
27. Crow JP, Beckman JS: Reactions between nitric oxide, superoxide, and peroxynitrite: Footprints of peroxynitrite in vivo. Adv Pharmacol 1995;34:17-43.
28. Danner RL, Elin RJ, Hosseini JM, et al: Endotoxemia in human septic shock. Chest 1991;99:169-175.
29. de Fouw NJ, van Tilburg NH, Haverkate F, Bertina RM: Activated protein C accelerates clot lysis by virtue of its anticoagulant activity. Blood Coagul Fibrinolysis 1993; 4:201-210.
30. De Groote MA, Fang FC: NO inhibitions: Antimicrobial properties of nitric oxide. Clin Infect Dis 1995;21(Suppl 2): S162-S165.
31. De Groote MA, Granger D, Xu Y, et al: Genetic and redox determinants of nitric oxide cytotoxicity in a *Salmonella typhimurium* model. Proc Natl Acad Sci U S A 1995;92: 6399-6403.
32. Deitch EA, Rutan R, Waymack JP: Trauma, shock, and gut translocation. New Horiz 1996;4:289-299.
33. Deitch EA, Specian RD, Berg RD: Endotoxin-induced bacterial translocation and mucosal permeability: Role of xanthine oxidase, complement activation, and macrophage products. Crit Care Med 1991;19:785-791.
34. Dhainaut JF, Vincent JL, Richard C, et al: CDP571, a humanized antibody to human tumor necrosis factor-alpha: Safety, pharmacokinetics, immune response, and influence of the antibody on cytokine concentrations in patients with septic shock. CPD571 Sepsis Study Group. Crit Care Med 1995;23:1461-1469.
35. Dillon HC Jr, Khare S, Gray BM: Group B streptococcal carriage and disease: A 6-year prospective study. J Pediatr 1987;110:31-36.
36. Ding A, Nathan C, Stuehr D: Release of reactive nitrogen intermediates and reactive oxygen intermediates from mouse peritoneal macrophages: Comparison of activating cytokines and evidence for independent production. J Immunol 1988;141:2407.
37. Ding J, Badwey JA: Neutrophils stimulated with a chemotactic peptide or a phorbol ester exhibit different alterations in the activities of a battery of protein kinases. J Biol Chem 1993;268:5234-5240.
38. Duke T, South M, Stewart A: Activation of the L-arginine nitric oxide pathway in severe sepsis. Arch Dis Child 1997; 76:203-209.
39. Effect of high-dose glucocorticoid therapy on mortality in patients with clinical signs of systemic sepsis. The Veterans Administration Systemic Sepsis Cooperative Study Group. N Engl J Med 1987;317:659-665.
40. Ehlers S, Smith KA: Differentiation of T cell lymphokine gene expression: The in vitro acquisition of T cell memory. J Exp Med 1991;173:25-36.
41. English BK, Burchett SK, English JD, et al: Production of lymphotoxin and tumor necrosis factor by human neonatal mononuclear cells. Pediatr Res 1988;24:717-722.
42. Ertel W, Keel M, Bonaccio M, et al: Release of anti-inflammatory mediators after mechanical trauma correlates with severity of injury and clinical outcome. J Trauma 1995;39: 879-885.
43. Etzioni A, Doerschuk CM, Harlan JM: Of man and mouse: Leukocyte and endothelial adhesion molecule deficiencies. Blood 1999;94:3281-3288.
44. Fanaroff AA, Korones SB, Wright LL, et al: A controlled trial of intravenous immune globulin to reduce nosocomial infections in very-low-birth-weight infants. National Institute of Child Health and Human Development Neonatal Research Network. N Engl J Med 1994;330:1107-1113.
45. Ferrieri P: Neonatal susceptibility and immunity to major bacterial pathogens. Rev Infect Dis 1990;12(Suppl 4): S394-S400.
46. Fijnvandraat K, Derkx B, Peters M, et al: Coagulation activation and tissue necrosis in meningococcal septic shock: Severely reduced protein C levels predict a high mortality. Thromb Haemost 1995;73:15-20.
47. Finlay BB, Falkow S: Common themes in microbial pathogenicity. Microbiol Rev 1989;53:210-230.
48. Finlay BB, Falkow S: Salmonella interactions with polarized human intestinal Caco-2 epithelial cells. J Infect Dis 1990; 162:1096-1106.
49. Fisher CJ Jr, Dhainaut JF, Opal SM, et al: Recombinant human interleukin 1 receptor antagonist in the treatment of patients with sepsis syndrome: Results from a randomized, double-blind, placebo-controlled trial. Phase III rhIL-1ra Sepsis Syndrome Study Group. JAMA 1994;271:1836-1843.
50. Fisher CJ Jr, Marra MN, Palardy JE, et al: Human neutrophil bactericidal/permeability-increasing protein reduces mortality rate from endotoxin challenge: A placebo-controlled study. Crit Care Med 1994;22:553-558.
51. Gazzinelli RT, Hieny S, Wynn TA, et al: Interleukin 12 is required for the T-lymphocyte-independent induction of interferon gamma by an intracellular parasite and induces resistance in T-cell-deficient hosts. Proc Natl Acad Sci U S A 1993;90:6115-6119.
52. Gibson RL, Redding GJ, Henderson WR, Truog WE: Group B streptococcus induces tumor necrosis factor in neonatal piglets: Effect of the tumor necrosis factor inhibitor pentoxifylline on hemodynamics and gas exchange. Am Rev Respir Dis 1991;143:598-604.
53. Giroir BP: Mediators of septic shock: New approaches for interrupting the endogenous inflammatory cascade. Crit Care Med 1993;21:780-789.
54. Goris RJ, te Boekhorst TP, Nuytinck JK, Gimbrere JS: Multiple-organ failure: Generalized autodestructive inflammation? Arch Surg 1985;120:1109-1115.
55. Gray ED, Peters G, Verstegen M, Regelmann WE: Effect of extracellular slime substance from *Staphylococcus epidermidis* on the human cellular immune response. Lancet 1984;1: 365-367.

56. Grey ST, Tsuchida A, Hau H, et al: Selective inhibitory effects of the anticoagulant activated protein C on the responses of human mononuclear phagocytes to LPS, IFN-gamma, or phorbol ester. J Immunol 1994;153: 3664-3672.
57. Grinnell BW, Hermann RB, Yan SB: Human protein C inhibits selectin-mediated cell adhesion: Role of unique fucosylated oligosaccharide. Glycobiology 1994;4:221-225.
58. Gruber A, Hanson SR, Kelly AB, et al: Inhibition of thrombus formation by activated recombinant protein C in a primate model of arterial thrombosis. Circulation 1990;82: 578-585.
59. Hack CE, Zeerleder S: The endothelium in sepsis: Source of and a target for inflammation. Crit Care Med 2001; 29(Suppl):S21-S27.
60. Han J, Thompson P, Beutler B: Dexamethasone and pentoxifylline inhibit endotoxin-induced cachectin/tumor necrosis factor synthesis at separate points in the signaling pathway. J Exp Med 1990;172:391-394.
61. Han YY, Carcillo JA, Dragotta MA, et al: Early reversal of pediatric-neonatal septic shock by community physicians is associated with improved outcome. Pediatrics 2003;112: 793-799.
62. Hancock WW, Grey ST, Hau L, et al: Binding of activated protein C to a specific receptor on human mononuclear phagocytes inhibits intracellular calcium signaling and monocyte-dependent proliferative responses. Transplantation 1995;60:1525-1532.
63. Harlan JM: Leukocyte adhesion deficiency syndrome: Insights into the molecular basis of leukocyte emigration. Clin Immunol Immunopathol 1993;67(Suppl):S16-S24.
64. Hauser CJ: Regional macrophage activation after injury and the compartmentalization of inflammation in trauma. New Horiz 1996;4:235-251.
65. Hayes MP, Berrebi GA, Henkart PA: Induction of target cell DNA release by the cytotoxic T lymphocyte granule protease granzyme A. J Exp Med 1989;170:933-946.
66. Hill HR: Biochemical, structural, and functional abnormalities of polymorphonuclear leukocytes in the neonate. Pediatr Res 1987;22:375-382.
67. Hogg N, Darley-Usmar VM, Wilson MT, Moncada S: Production of hydroxyl radicals from the simultaneous generation of superoxide and nitric oxide. Biochem J 1992;281:419-424.
68. Huber AR, Kunkel SL, Todd RF 3rd, Weiss SJ: Regulation of transendothelial neutrophil migration by endogenous interleukin-8. Science 1991;254:99-102.
69. Isberg RR, Tran Van Nhieu G: Binding and internalization of microorganisms by integrin receptors. Trends Microbiol 1994;2:10-14.
70. Iwama A, Wang MH, Yamaguchi N, et al: Terminal differentiation of murine resident peritoneal macrophages is characterized by expression of the STK protein tyrosine kinase, a receptor for macrophage-stimulating protein. Blood 1995;86:3394-3403.
71. Jackson DE: The unfolding tale of PECAM-1. FEBS Lett 2003;540:7-14.
72. Jones SA, Horiuchi S, Topley N, et al: The soluble interleukin 6 receptor: Mechanisms of production and implications in disease. FASEB J 2001;15:43-58.
73. Joyce DE, Gelbert L, Ciaccia A, et al: Gene expression profile of antithrombotic protein C defines new mechanisms modulating inflammation and apoptosis. J Biol Chem 2001;276:11199-11203.
74. Kaplan J, Shope TC, Bollinger RO, Smith J: Human newborns are deficient in natural killer activity. J Clin Immunol 1982;2:350-355.
75. Kaplan SS, Lancaster JR Jr, Basford RE, Simmons RL: Effect of nitric oxide on staphylococcal killing and interactive effect with superoxide. Infect Immun 1996;64:69-76.
76. Kern J, Lamb R, Reed J, et al: Dexamethasone inhibition of interleukin-1 beta production by human monocytes: Posttranscriptional mechanisms. J Clin Invest 1988;81:237.
77. Koefoed-Johnsen V, Ussing HH: The nature of the frog skin potential. Acta Physiol Scand 1958;42:298-308.
78. Kolesnick R, Golde DW: The sphingomyelin pathway in tumor necrosis factor and interleukin-1 signaling. Cell 1994;77:325-328.
79. Krebs DL, Hilton DJ: SOCS: Physiological suppressors of cytokine signaling. J Cell Sci 2000;113:2813-2819.
80. Leonard EJ, Skeel A: A serum protein that stimulates macrophage movement, chemotaxis and spreading. Exp Cell Res 1976;102:434-438.
81. Levy MM, Fink MP, Marshall JC, et al: 2001 SCCM/ESICM/ACCP/ATS/SIS International Sepsis Definitions Conference. Crit Care Med 2003;31:1250-1256.
82. Levy MM, Fink MP, Marshall JC, et al: 2001 SCCM/ESICM/ACCP/ATS/SIS International Sepsis Definitions Conference. Intensive Care Med 2003;29:530-538.
83. Lewis DB, Yu CC, Meyer J, et al: Cellular and molecular mechanisms for reduced interleukin 4 and interferon-gamma production by neonatal T cells. J Clin Invest 1991;87:194-202.
84. Lipton SA, Choi YB, Pan ZH, et al: A redox-based mechanism for the neuroprotective and neurodestructive effects of nitric oxide and related nitroso-compounds. Nature 1993;364:626-632.
85. Lowry SF: Anticytokine therapies in sepsis. New Horiz 1993;1:120-126.
86. Machleidt T, Wiegmann K, Henkel T, et al: Sphingomyelinase activates proteolytic I kappa B-alpha degradation in a cell-free system. J Biol Chem 1994;269: 13760-13765.
87. Maier RV, Bulger EM: Endothelial changes after shock and injury. New Horiz 1996;4:211-223.
88. Marlar RA, Kleiss AJ, Griffin JH: Human protein C: Inactivation of factors V and VIII in plasma by the activated molecule. Ann N Y Acad Sci 1981;370:303-310.
89. Marra MN, Thornton MB, Snable JL, et al: Endotoxin-binding and -neutralizing properties of recombinant bactericidal/permeability-increasing protein and monoclonal antibodies HA-1A and E5. Crit Care Med 1994;22: 559-565.
90. Martin GS, Mannino DM, Eaton S, Moss M: The epidemiology of sepsis in the United States from 1979 through 2000. N Engl J Med 2003;348:1546-1554.
91. Masson D, Tschopp J: A family of serine esterases in lytic granules of cytolytic T lymphocytes. Cell 1987;49:679-685.
92. McCloskey RV, Straube RC, Sanders C, et al: Treatment of septic shock with human monoclonal antibody HA-1A: A randomized, double-blind, placebo-controlled trial. CHESS Trial Study Group. Ann Intern Med 1994;121:1-5.
93. McDonald T, Sneed J, Valenski WR, et al: Natural killer cell activity in very low birth weight infants. Pediatr Res 1992;31:376-380.
94. McGill SN, Ahmed NA, Hu F, et al: Shedding of L-selectin as a mechanism for reduced polymorphonuclear neutrophil exudation in patients with the systemic inflammatory response syndrome. Arch Surg 1996;131:1141-1146.
95. Mileski W, Borgstrom D, Lightfoot E, et al: Inhibition of leukocyte-endothelial adherence following thermal injury. J Surg Res 1992;52:334-339.

96. Miller ME: Phagocyte function in the neonate: Selected aspects. Pediatrics 1979;64(Suppl):S709-S712.
97. Miller VL, Falkow S: Evidence for two genetic loci in *Yersinia enterocolitica* that can promote invasion of epithelial cells. Infect Immun 1988;56:1242-1248.
98. Muller W, Weigl S, Deng X, Phillips DM: PECAM-1 is required for transendothelial migration of leukocytes. J Exp Med 1993;178:449-460.
99. Muller WA: The role of PECAM-1 (CD31) in leukocyte emigration: Studies in vitro and in vivo. J Leukoc Biol 1995;57:523-528.
100. Muller WA: Migration of leukocytes across endothelial junctions: Some concepts and controversies. Microcirculation 2001;8:181-193.
101. Murray HW, Spitalny GL, Nathan CF: Activation of mouse peritoneal macrophages in vitro and in vivo by interferon-gamma. J Immunol 1985;134:1619-1622.
102. Mustafa MM, Ramilo O, Saez-Llorens X, et al: Cerebrospinal fluid prostaglandins, interleukin 1 beta, and tumor necrosis factor in bacterial meningitis: Clinical and laboratory correlations in placebo-treated and dexamethasone-treated patients. Am J Dis Child 1990;144: 883-887.
103. Nathan C: Nitric oxide as secretory product of mammalian cells. FASEB J 1992;6:3051-3064.
104. Nathan C: Natural resistance and nitric oxide. Cell 1995;82:873-876.
105. Nguyen T, Brunson D, Crespi CL, et al: DNA damage and mutation in human cells exposed to nitric oxide in vitro. Proc Natl Acad Sci U S A 1992;89:3030-3034.
106. O'Brien CD, Lim P, Sun J, Albelda SM: PECAM-1-dependent neutrophil transmigration is independent of monolayer PECAM-1 signaling or localization. Blood 2003;101:2816-2825.
107. Odio CM, Faingezicht I, Paris M, et al: The beneficial effects of early dexamethasone administration in infants and children with bacterial meningitis. N Engl J Med 1991;324:1525-1531.
108. Pacelli R, Wink DA, Cook JA, et al: Nitric oxide potentiates hydrogen peroxide-induced killing of *Escherichia coli*. J Exp Med 1995;182:1469-1479.
109. Parrillo JE, Parker MM, Natanson C, et al: Septic shock in humans: Advances in the understanding of pathogenesis, cardiovascular dysfunction, and therapy. Ann Intern Med 1990;113:227-242.
110. Partrick DA, Moore FA, Moore EE, et al: Neutrophil priming and activation in the pathogenesis of postinjury multiple organ failure. New Horiz 1996;4:194-210.
111. Peters G, Locci R, Pulverer G: Adherence and growth of coagulase-negative staphylococci on surfaces of intravenous catheters. J Infect Dis 1982;146:479-482.
112. Philip AG, Hewitt JR: Early diagnosis of neonatal sepsis. Pediatrics 1980;65:1036-1041.
113. Podack ER, Young JD, Cohn ZA: Isolation and biochemical and functional characterization of perforin 1 from cytolytic T-cell granules. Proc Natl Acad Sci U S A 1985;82: 8629-8633.
114. Raghunathan R, Miller ME, Everett S, Leake RD: Phagocyte chemotaxis in the perinatal period. J Clin Immunol 1982;2:242-245.
115. Refsum SE, Halliday MI, Campbell G, et al: Modulation of TNF alpha and IL-6 in a peritonitis model using pentoxifylline. J Pediatr Surg 1996;31:928-930.
116. Rogy MA, Moldawer LL, Oldenburg HS, et al: Anti-endotoxin therapy in primate bacteremia with HA-1A and BPI. Ann Surg 1994;220:77-85.
117. Rollins BJ, Sunday ME: Suppression of tumor formation in vivo by expression of the JE gene in malignant cells. Mol Cell Biol 1991;11:3125-3131.
118. Rosengren S, Olofsson AM, von Andrian UH, et al: Leukotriene B4-induced neutrophil-mediated endothelial leakage in vitro and in vivo. J Appl Physiol 1991;71: 1322-1330.
119. Scannell G: Leukocyte responses to hypoxic/ischemic conditions. New Horiz 1996;4:179-183.
120. Schade UF: Pentoxifylline increases survival in murine endotoxin shock and decreases formation of tumor necrosis factor. Circ Shock 1990;31:171-181.
121. Schoedon G, Schneemann M, Walter R, et al: Nitric oxide and infection: Another view. Clin Infect Dis 1995; 21(Suppl 2):S152-S157.
122. Scott P: IL-12: Initiation cytokine for cell-mediated immunity. Science 1993;260:496-497.
123. Scott P, Kaufmann SH: The role of T-cell subsets and cytokines in the regulation of infection. Immunol Today 1991;12:346-348.
124. Shenep JL, Flynn PM, Barrett FF, et al: Serial quantitation of endotoxemia and bacteremia during therapy for gram-negative bacterial sepsis. J Infect Dis 1988;157:565-568.
125. Smith JB, Kunjummen RD, Kishimoto TK, Anderson DC: Expression and regulation of L-selectin on eosinophils from human adults and neonates. Pediatr Res 1992;32: 465-471.
126. Snyderman R, Goetzl EJ: Molecular and cellular mechanisms of leukocyte chemotaxis. Science 1981;213:830-837.
127. Snyderman R, Pike MC: Chemoattractant receptors on phagocytic cells. Annu Rev Immunol 1984;2:257-281.
128. Squire E, Favara B, Todd J: Diagnosis of neonatal bacterial infection: Hematologic and pathologic findings in fatal and nonfatal cases. Pediatrics 1979;64:60-64.
129. St Gene J, Polin R: Neonatal sepsis: Progress in diagnosis and management. Drugs 1988;36:784-800.
130. Stamler JS: Redox signaling: Nitrosylation and related target interactions of nitric oxide. Cell 1994;78:931-936.
131. Stuber F, Petersen M, Bokelmann F, Schade U: A genomic polymorphism within the tumor necrosis factor locus influences plasma tumor necrosis factor-alpha concentrations and outcome of patients with severe sepsis. Crit Care Med 1996;24:381-384.
132. Sullivan JS, Kilpatrick L, Costarino AT Jr, et al: Correlation of plasma cytokine elevations with mortality rate in children with sepsis. J Pediatr 1992;120:510-515.
133. Tracy K: Tumor necrosis factor (cachectin) in the biology of septic shock syndrome. Circ Shock 1991;35:123.
134. Upperman JS, Pillage G, Siddiqi MQ, et al: Dominance of high-producing IL-6 and low-producing IL-10 and IFN-γ alleles in glucose-6-phosphate dehydrogenase deficient trauma patients. Shock (in press).
135. van Hinsbergh VW, Bertina RM, van Wijngaarden A, et al: Activated protein C decreases plasminogen activator-inhibitor activity in endothelial cell-conditioned medium. Blood 1985;65:444-451.
136. VanFurth R, Hirsh J, Fedurko M: Morphology and peroxidase cytochemistry of mouse promonocytes, monocytes, and macrophages. J Exp Med 1970;132:794.
137. Vannier E, Miller L, Dinarello C: Coordinated anti-inflammatory effects of interleukin 4: Interleukin 4 suppresses interleukin1 but up-regulates gene expression and synthesis of interleukin1 receptor antagonist. Proc Natl Acad Sci U S A 1992;89:4076-4080.
138. VonAndrian U, Hansell P, Chambers J, et al: L-selectin function is required for β_2-integrin-mediated neutrophil

adhesion at physiologic shear rates in vivo. Am J Physiol 1992;263:H1034-H1044.
139. Walker RI, Willemze R: Neutrophil kinetics and the regulation of granulopoiesis. Rev Infect Dis 1980;2: 282-292.
140. Warren MK, Vogel SN: Opposing effects of glucocorticoids on interferon-gamma-induced murine macrophage Fc receptor and Ia antigen expression. J Immunol 1985; 134:2462-2469.
141. Watson RS, Carcillo JA, Linde-Zwirble WT, et al: The epidemiology of severe sepsis in children in the United States. Am J Respir Crit Care Med 2003;167:695-701.
142. Waxman K: Shock: Ischemia, reperfusion, and inflammation. New Horiz 1996;4:153-160.
143. Waxman K: What mediates tissue injury after shock? N Horiz 1996;4:151-152.
144. Weiss SJ: Tissue destruction by neutrophils. N Engl J Med 1989;320:365-376.
145. West MA, Wilson C: Hypoxic alterations in cellular signal transduction in shock and sepsis. New Horiz 1996;4: 168-178.
146. Willatts SM, Radford S, Leitermann M: Effect of the antiendotoxic agent, taurolidine, in the treatment of sepsis syndrome: A placebo-controlled, double-blind trial. Crit Care Med 1995;23:1033-1039.
147. Wilson CB: Immunologic basis for increased susceptibility of the neonate to infection. J Pediatr 1986;108:1-12.
148. Wilson RF: Special problems in the diagnosis and treatment of surgical sepsis. Surg Clin North Am 1985;65: 965-989.
149. Wong HR, Carcillo JA, Burckart G, et al: Increased serum nitrite and nitrate concentrations in children with the sepsis syndrome. Crit Care Med 1995;23:835-842.
150. Wright SD, Ramos RA, Tobias PS, et al: CD14, a receptor for complexes of lipopolysaccharide (LPS) and LPS binding protein. Science 1990;249:1431-1433.
151. Wunderink RG, Waterer GW: Genetics of sepsis and pneumonia. Curr Opin Crit Care 2003;9:384-389.
152. Yang Z, Costanzo M, Golde DW, Kolesnick RN: Tumor necrosis factor activation of the sphingomyelin pathway signals nuclear factor kappa B translocation in intact HL-60 cells. J Biol Chem 1993;268:20520-20523.
153. Yoshimura T, Yuhki N, Moore SK, et al: Human monocyte chemoattractant protein-1 (MCP-1): Full-length cDNA cloning, expression in mitogen-stimulated blood mononuclear leukocytes, and sequence similarity to mouse competence gene JE. FEBS Lett 1989;244:487-493.
154. Zabel P, Wolter DT, Schonharting MM, Schade UF: Oxpentifylline in endotoxaemia. Lancet 1989;2:1474-1477.
155. Zhong W, Chavali S, Utsunomiya T, et al: Cytokine regulation by a β-adrenergic agonist improves mortality in mice with severe endotoxemia. Surg Forum 1995;46:99-101.
156. Ziegler EJ, Fisher CJ Jr, Sprung CL, et al: Treatment of gram-negative bacteremia and septic shock with HA-1A human monoclonal antibody against endotoxin: A randomized, double-blind, placebo-controlled trial. The HA-1A Sepsis Study Group. N Engl J Med 1991;324:429-436.
157. Zingarelli B, O'Connor M, Wong H, et al: Peroxynitrite-mediated DNA strand breakage activates poly-adenosine diphosphate ribosyl synthetase and causes cellular energy depletion in macrophages stimulated with bacterial lipopolysaccharide. J Immunol 1996;156:350-358.

第 11 章

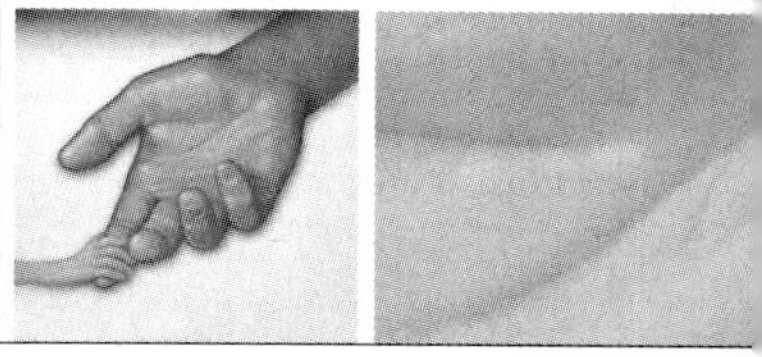

与外科有关的血液疾病

Raymond J. Hutchinson

78 就如何全面处理小儿外科患者，血液科医生和小儿外科医生经常进行交流。贫血、血小板减少症、血小板功能异常、凝血因子缺乏和血栓形成的评估和处理则是他们经常谈论的话题；另外，如何合理地进行输血治疗也是他们关注的话题。这里将讨论这些领域中的一些最重要的问题。

贫血

红细胞数量不足可导致向组织输氧不足，其病理生理学原因主要有三种：（1）骨髓中红细胞产生或成熟异常（例如，Diamond–Blackfan 贫血、儿童短暂性成红细胞减少）；（2）出血造成红细胞丢失（例如，Meckel 憩室引起的胃肠道出血）或脾隔离造成的红细胞丢失（如同在镰状细胞病中所见；（3）红细胞破坏（溶血性疾病）[75]。很明显，当给一位面色苍白的孩子制定治疗计划或对全血细胞计数报告中血细胞比容低下或血红蛋白浓度低下进行评价时，一份完整的病史和体格检查报告可提供宝贵的信息。在小儿内科和外科患者中，先天性贫血和遗传性贫血的发生率与个人史和家族史明显相关。当然，小儿诊断时的年龄至少是部分决定了新生期相关因素或遗传因素的重要性。

在病史方面，要注意下列情况：母亲子宫内出血或新生儿溶血（例如，可分别缘于胎盘分离或胎儿成红细胞增多症）、新生儿黄疸或新生儿出血、面色苍白的进展程度、巩膜黄疸的表现以及直肠出血史等。确定家族其他成员是否有贫血或治疗贫血、进行脾切除术或胆囊切除术等有关的家族史。全面的体格检查包括评价黄疸和苍白的程度、脾和淋巴结的大小、出血体征（包括化验便血）及心血管的稳定性。

全血细胞计数能提供很多关于贫血病因的信息。除了红细胞谱系之外，全血细胞计数还能提供白细胞和血小板两个谱系的信息。当一个以上的造血谱系异常时通常提示问题发生在骨髓。因此，在处理由多发性血细胞减少症的儿童时要及早进行骨髓抽吸检查和组织活检。按平均细胞容积（MCV）可将贫血分为小红细胞性、正常红细胞性和大红细胞性贫血三类，这种有助于提供诊断线索和制定处理方案。同样当平均细胞血红蛋白浓度值超过 36 时，强烈提示存在大量的球形红细胞，如在遗传性球形红细胞症所见的那样[66]。红细胞分布宽度指数提供了循环中红细胞分布状况的信息，有利于内科医生将红细胞群按同类的大小或不同类的双相或多相特征进行分类。红细胞宽度指数与 MCV 结合起来考虑将使治疗有更好的成本效益。图 11–1 为一名贫血患者的诊断流程。

非溶血性贫血

由于骨髓衰竭或缺乏必需营养素（如缺铁），红细胞产量低下，这是引起严重贫血的常见机制。这种贫血会妨碍外科急症的处理。

骨髓衰竭

骨髓衰竭存在的一条主要线索是患者出现多谱系血细胞减少症。若贫血伴发中性白细胞减少症或血小板减少症，则提示存在：（1）由体质性（Fanconi） 179
贫血或获得性再生障碍性贫血引起的骨髓衰竭；（2）由浸润性疾病造成的骨髓衰竭，发生于急性白血病或转移性神经母细胞瘤患者。骨髓抽吸检查以及

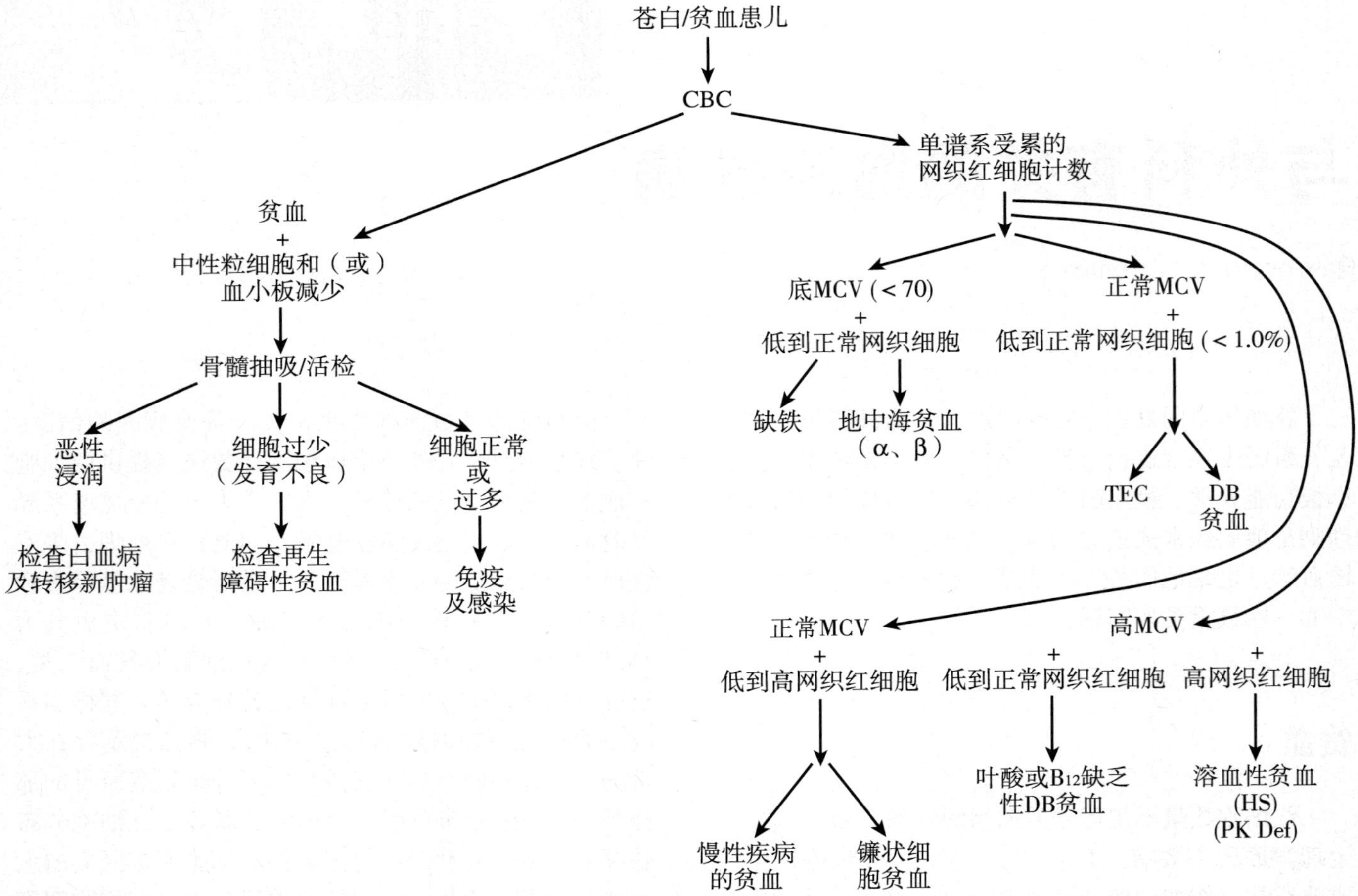

图 11-1 贫血的诊断流程图。Asp/Bx：抽吸 / 活检；CBC：全血细胞计数；DB：Diamond-Blackfan；Def：缺乏；HS：遗传性球形红细胞症；MCV：平均细胞容积；Nl：正常；PK Def：丙酮酸激酶缺乏；TEC：小儿暂时性成红细胞减少症。

活检常有助于迅速做出明确诊断。

Fanconi 贫血是常染色体隐性遗传，但男性的发病率略高于女性（1.3∶1）[8]。血液病学表现各异，最初多表现为单谱系细胞受到影响，进而发展到多谱系再生障碍性贫血。发病年龄从出生至 35 岁不等（平均年龄为 8 岁，中位数年龄为 7 岁）[8]。Fanconi贫血患者经常伴有先天性畸形（例如，皮肤色素沉着过多、拇指和前臂桡侧异常、身材矮小和精神发育迟缓）[40]。患者可因相关的染色体断裂易患白血病和肝脏肿瘤等恶性肿瘤[20,86]。

获得性再生障碍性贫血患者中至少有 50%表现为特发性贫血，患者发病前常有乙型肝炎或服用了诸如氯霉素、磺胺、酚噻嗪以及抗惊厥药等药物[7]。Fanconi 贫血患者使用类固醇药物后血细胞计数会暂时性升高[88]；但该类药物对获得性再生障碍的患者无效[61]。Fanconi 贫血患者和获得性再生障碍性贫血患者可以使用合适配型的同种异体骨髓移植进行治疗，来自同胞兄弟姊妹者更合适[38,79]。目前，重组人类造血生长因子，如红细胞生成素、粒细胞集落刺激因子、粒细胞–巨噬细胞集落刺激因子和白细胞介素–3，由于疗效短暂或反应不佳而较少使用[33,58,100]。

单谱系红细胞再生障碍的特征是白细胞和血小板计数正常、网织红细胞计数低下（<1.0%）以及骨髓涂片中缺乏红细胞系前体。当遇到这种情况时，应当想起两种疾病：Diamond–Blackfan 贫血（先天性再生障碍性贫血）和小儿暂时性成红细胞减少症（TEC）。前者的特征是持续生成胎儿性红细胞，例如血红蛋白电泳中胎儿血红蛋白百分比很高、胎儿红细胞抗原 i 持续表达以及红细胞 MCV 高[5]。TEC 患者通常没有这些特征[105]。TEC 常在 2～8 周内消失，可能与病毒

引起的细胞生成抑制有关[34]。皮质类固醇是治疗 Diamond-Blackfan 贫血的主要方法；开始时每天使用泼尼松 2mg/kg，只要患者的情况允许，可以逐渐减量至隔天服用或更少[6]。Diamond-Blackfan 贫血患者偶尔会依靠输血维持生命，极少的病例需要进行同种异体骨髓移植[57]。虽然 TEC 患者偶尔需要输注红细胞，但多数患者因痊愈很快而不需要治疗。

失血

贫血是急性和慢性出血的一种重要表现。严重的急性出血通常伴有心血管应激体征，包括外周血管收缩、低血压、心动过速和少尿[69]。如果患者的失血量超过总血容量的 30%，经常会发生低血容量性休克。急性出血后，可能需要数个小时才能测出血红蛋白和血细胞比容水平的改变；如出血后 1～2 小时内这些值即急剧下降，通常表示失血量已超过总血容量的 20%[54]。

相反，缓慢或间歇性出血引起的慢性失血通常不会产生心血管应激症状。慢性贫血患者经常有代偿性表现，不需要进行输血干预。当输血不可避免时，应当采取审慎态度，因为反复输血具有明显的危险性，包括传播病毒感染[55]以及输血性含铁血黄素沉着症[21]。

血液在脾内隔离是造成明显失血的另一种机制，也能导致贫血[87]。溶血性贫血、门静脉血管畸形或肝脏原发性疾病引起的脾大会使血液在扩张的脾窦状隙内隔离。

失血性贫血的治疗根据贫血发展程度而有所不同。为了恢复大量失血患者的血容量和携氧能力，可能需要快速输血。快速输血通常都能在 15～30 分钟以内安全完成，即使是在幼儿，只要输血量和速度根据患儿的体型和失血估计量调整。通过监测心率、动脉血压、静脉压以及中心和外周温度可防止血容量过度扩张[69]。慢性贫血患者的心肺功能已经逐渐受损，因此输注红细胞时只要将心肺功能恢复至代偿水平即可。应该避免过度输血，特别是当慢性贫血患儿需要反复输血时。对于这种患儿，经常输血会导致输血性含铁血黄素沉着症；输注红细胞的量越多，输注的铁负荷也就越多。血清铁蛋白超过 1000 μg/L 后，转铁蛋白饱和，患者有心脏和肝脏内铁沉积的危险[21]，对这些患者可采用去铁胺进行螯合治疗。因失血或进行性溶血而导致贫血的患者要缓慢地输血至基线水平，可将输血量按 5～10ml/kg 分成若干份，每次输血 2 小时以上，每次输血之间要有一定的时间以保证血液的再平衡和患者循环状况的重新评估。

营养性贫血

缺铁性贫血的病因有食物中铁摄取不足、吸收不良、转运缺陷造成不能合理利用铁、出血丢失铁以及铁在异常部位分离（如在含铁血黄素沉着症患者，铁沉着在肺部）。不论性别，患者的年龄都可影响铁缺乏。婴儿在生长发育期间，血容量迅速扩增，30% 的铁用于血红蛋白生成且需从饮食中获取。在成人，只有 5%的铁来自饮食[25]，其余部分通过红细胞降解获得。

美国儿科学会[9-11]推荐，足月儿每天需从饮食中摄入 1.0mg/kg 铁，最高 15mg/d，开始时间不迟于 4 个月龄，持续至 3 岁。体重 1500～2500g 的早产儿每天需摄入 2mg/kg 铁，最高 15mg/d，开始时间不迟于 2 个月龄。推荐给予极低出生体重儿的量更大：出生体重在 1500g 以下的婴儿每天需摄入 4mg/kg 铁。年长儿和成人食物中铁需要量各异，取决于生长发育水平和性别：

4～10 岁	10mg/d
11～16 岁	18 mg/d
成年男性	10mg/d
成年女性	18 mg/d

发生营养性铁缺乏的高峰年龄段为 6 月至 2 岁。在此期间，小儿从依赖母乳或富铁乳品过渡为以来混合性奶制品（通常为牛奶）以及固体食物。食物中的铁含量取决于小儿的饮食构成。对牛奶依赖严重的小儿摄入固体食物量较少，特别容易罹患缺铁性贫血。这些小儿的典型表现为渐进性苍白，血红蛋白浓度为 3.0～6.0g/dL，MCV 为 45～60fL。年龄较大者罹患缺铁性贫血的可能性较少，特别是因饮食摄入不足而致者很少，除非存在偏食习惯。

喂养未经加工的牛乳、肠道寄生虫感染以及原先存在铁缺乏都可能导致婴儿肠道失血。使用阿司匹林或含有阿司匹林的药物可能引起肠道失血，量大时可能导致贫血。其他造成失血和铁缺乏的原因包括：围生期——胎儿-母体出血、分娩时胎盘损伤以及双胞胎通过胎盘交通输血；年长儿——罹患 Meckel 憩室、肠重复畸形、出血性毛细血管扩张以及罕见的出血性溃疡或胃食管反流。

若发现有小细胞低色素性贫血及临床致病原因，则可确诊为铁缺乏。MCV 低下和平均血红蛋白小体应通过细致的血涂片检查才能确认。测定血清铁水平、总铁结合力以及血清铁蛋白水平的血清铁检测可最终做出诊断。典型病例可表现为血清铁水平低下、总铁结合力升高、血清铁蛋白水平低下以及总铁储存下降。最后进行铁试验性治疗，网织红细胞应在 1 周内增加，血红蛋白和血细胞比容应快速升高。

治疗包括给予口服铁（硫酸亚铁），按每天 6mg/kg 的剂量补充铁元素。由于硫酸亚铁中的铁元素只占 20%，计算剂量时必须加以考虑（如 1 片 325mg 的硫酸亚铁中只含有 65mg 铁元素）。补充铁剂必须持续 3～4 月。在此期间，通常贫血、小红细胞症可以纠治，并可提高游离红细胞原卟啉水平。

溶血性贫血

小儿外科医生都有可能接触到镰状细胞病、β-地中海贫血、遗传性球形红细胞症以及丙酮酸激酶缺乏症患儿。

镰状细胞病

镰状血红蛋白病发病于出生后早期，可以有疼痛危象、急性胸部综合征、菌血症以及脾隔离等一系列表现[36]。一项镰状细胞病的合作研究报告报道，纯合子镰状细胞病患者和镰状细胞-血红蛋白 C 病患者的疼痛危象、急性胸部综合征和菌血症的发生率明显升高。但在一项针对 694 例婴儿的跟踪随访 10 年的队列研究中，20 例死亡患儿均为镰状细胞病纯合子患者[36]。该研究还发现，手足综合征患者多为镰状细胞性贫血患者，且多发生于出生后的 3 年内。

小儿外科医生十分关注镰状细胞病的一些后遗症。疼痛性血管闭塞危象偶尔会被误诊为急腹症（如阑尾炎）而进行手术治疗。因为疼痛危象常伴有白细胞计数升高，因此后者无助于鉴别阑尾炎和疼痛危象。疼痛危象发生时，进行一系列检查并与对镰状细胞病评估富有经验的血液学专家合作，可以降低外科误诊的发生率。

急性胸部综合征可以表现为病危状态。治疗可以通过快速输血提高血液的携氧能力和降低血红蛋白 S 的百分比，以逆转细胞镰状化过程。

对于反复发生脾隔离的患者，可以进行脾切除术，以减少再次发生脾隔离的危险。脾隔离的特征是血红蛋白、血细胞比容和血小板计数急剧下降。有时，进行性脾隔离可导致低血容量性休克，有可能是致命的。通常在有两次脾隔离发作后才可进行脾切除术，即使是年幼的患者（年龄小于 4 岁）也不例外。相似地，胆石病出现症状常提示需要进行胆囊切除术[81]。

镰状细胞贫血患者的围术期发病率很高[29]。镰状细胞病患者手术时，主要的并发症有疼痛危象、急性胸部综合征以及输注同种异体红细胞产生的输血反应。

小儿外科医生在处理镰状细胞病患儿时还需考虑镰状血红蛋白的百分比以及全身麻醉的安全性。过去常采用输注红细胞使镰状血红蛋白百分比降到 30%以下。但资料显示，如果对患者采用更保守的方法使其术前血红蛋白水平达到 10g/dL 左右，而不是将其血红蛋白 S 的水平下降到任意临界值，患者术后的状况会同样良好[103]。手术期间，应加强监护以确保血液的适当氧合，但应避免输血过度。

此外，减少术前输血可以降低产生同种异体免疫和输血反应的风险。8%～50%镰状细胞病患者可产生非 ABO 红细胞抗体，且抗体量随着输注红细胞次数而改变[27]。很明显，这些抗体的生成会增加外科手术的复杂性，也会增加后续输血反应的风险[27]。推荐输注表现型与 E、C 和 Kell 群抗原相匹配的红细胞，以减少发生同种异体免疫的风险[19,104]。几项已发表的研究质疑了术前积极输血的益处，建议对年幼的患儿实施低风险手术时不需要输血[44,103]。相对于积极输血以降低血红蛋白 S 的做法来说，增加血浆血红蛋白浓度使其达到 10g/dL 的保守输血治疗可提供更多的益处，即发生并发症的风险下降[103]。

术后并发症各异，取决于手术操作的类型、患者的年龄、疾病状态和受累器官的功能状况、是否存在感染、是否患有慢性肺部疾病、女性患者是否妊娠以及镰状细胞病的遗传类型[29]。术前通过胸片、血氧饱和度以及肺功能监测评估肺功能，并通过测定血清尿素氮和肌酐、血压以及筛检尿路感染和蛋白尿评估肾 182

功能，是降低围术期风险的有效策略。

β-地中海贫血

β-地中海贫血的特点是无法合成正常数量的 β 链血红蛋白多肽[101]，导致不能有效地生成红细胞。纯合子 β-地中海贫血患者在生命早期就需依靠输注红细胞维持生命。作为髓外造血的结果，脾大常发生。红细胞脾隔离会常常增加输血需要。当每年输注红细胞超过 250ml/kg 时，应考虑实施脾切除术，这样可减少输血。

遗传性球形红细胞症和红细胞酶缺陷

遗传性球形红细胞症和红细胞酶缺陷，如丙酮酸激酶缺陷，可导致溶血性贫血，并常与胆石的形成有关。当胆石病出现症状时，需行胆囊切除术。若遗传性球形红细胞症患者存在中至重度贫血却维持相对较高的网织红细胞计数（≥10%）时，患者 5～6 岁时应考虑实施脾切除术。脾切除术可降低发生胆石的危险性；当遗传性球形红细胞症患者发生病毒感染时，脾切除术可以减少血红蛋白急剧下降的可能性。对于其他类型的溶血性贫血患者，如丙酮酸激酶缺陷和难治性自身免疫性溶血性贫血，同样要考虑脾切除术的治疗价值。

血小板减少症和血小板功能性疾病

血小板减少症

通常认为 150 000/μL 为血小板计数正常值范围的下限，血小板计数下降低于此值时就认为存在血小板减少症。血小板减少症的病因可以是遗传性的也可以是获得性的。

遗传性血小板减少症

在出生后早期诊断血小板减少症时应考虑几种遗传方式。出生时伴有桡骨缺如的血小板减少症为常染色体隐性遗传，常在 1 岁以后自行改善。但是，这些患儿在 1 岁内可能发生中枢神经系统和胃肠道出血，死亡率高达 35%[46]。单纯无巨核细胞性血小板减少症可在出生时或出生后不久出现症状，不伴有躯体异常，但进展为再生障碍性贫血的发生率很高[28,45]。如其名称所示，单纯无巨核细胞性血小板减少症是一种骨髓衰竭状态，为常染色体隐性遗传。如前文所述，Fanconi 贫血在完全表现为再生障碍性状态之前，可仅表现为血小板减少症；但可通过躯体特征和 Fanconi 贫血伴有染色体断裂与单纯无巨核细胞性血小板减少症区别。此外，家族性血小板减少症可为常染色体显性遗传、常染色体隐性遗传以及性连锁遗传等。Wiskott-Aldrich 综合征是性连锁遗传的例子，发生血小板减少症的同时伴有湿疹或经常罹患感染。这种综合征主要见于男性，如遗传学所预期的那样。患者常有 T 淋巴细胞功能异常的背景[76]。

获得性血小板减少症

暴露于母体内抗血小板表面抗原的抗体（由于服用某种药物或罹患病毒感染或由于自身免疫状况）会导致获得性血小板减少症。某些种类的药物更易诱发血小板减少症，包括抗菌药（如甲氧苄啶-磺胺甲噁唑）、抗惊厥药（如苯妥英和卡马西平）以及酚噻嗪类（如氯丙嗪）。需要特别指出的有两种疾病：新生儿同种免疫性血小板减少症和特发性血小板减少性紫癜。

当母体被胎儿的来自父方的并在妊娠期表达的血小板抗原致敏后，有可能发生新生儿同种免疫性血小板减少症。当胎儿母体血屏障遭到破坏，胎儿的血小板进入母体循环后，母体会产生抗血小板抗体 IgG。常引起致敏反应的血小板抗原是 PL[A1]，此抗原在人群中的阳性为 98% [32]。盲目输注血小板通常不会提高婴儿的血小板计数，特别是当普通抗原（如 PL[A1]）引起致敏后，输入的血小板会迅速遭到破坏。相反，采用来自母体的血小板（PL[A1]阴性）通常可持续提高婴儿的血小板计数；孕妇产后条件允许时可采集血小板，这有可能成为一种有效的治疗方法[4]。

特发性血小板减少性紫癜可发生于任何年龄段的儿童和青少年，但最常见于 2～5 岁小儿[64]。该病常发生于病毒感染之后，一般认为是由于抗病毒免疫反应出错，形成与血小板产生交叉反应的抗体导致脾内破坏所致。治疗包括静脉注射免疫球蛋白（IgG）、静脉注射抗 D 免疫球蛋白以及口服泼尼松[31]。尽管这三种治疗方法均能提高血小板计数，但是静脉注射 IgG 和服用泼尼松起效更快，1～2 天即可测出血小板计数有所提高。在使用泼尼松前，应进行骨髓检查以排除白血病，因泼尼松可能会对白血病产生部分效果，但其并不适用于治疗白血病。这些治疗的作用期短暂，但即使时间不长，仍可有 55%～75%的患者在确诊后的第 1 个月完全恢复，80%～90%的患者在确诊后的 6 个月内恢复[65,68]。对于罹患新生儿同种免疫性血小板减少症的患儿，血小板会被网状内皮系统迅速消耗，因此，输注供体的血小板没有任何治疗效果。若患儿对其他治疗无反应，有时可以实施脾切除术治疗血小板减少症；约有 70%的患儿在脾切除术后症状可获得完全缓解[80]。

血小板的功能性疾病

即使血小板计数正常，皮肤或黏膜出血仍提示存在血小板功能异常。很多年前就已认识到阿司匹林对血小板的功能有副作用。阿司匹林可抑制血小板环氧化酶，导致血栓烷 A_2 缺乏，抑制血小板聚集[47]。由于服用阿司匹林或存在其他缺陷，出血时间延长成为血小板功能异常的特征。

Von Willebrand 病的特征是血小板粘连和聚集功能异常。该病与Ⅷ因子前体活性和 von Willebrand 因子水平低于正常有关[53,72]。已知该病存在多个变型，尽管多数病例是由于遗传因素，为常染色体显性遗传。输注冷沉淀物常可纠正血小板功能缺陷，每单位冷沉淀物含有 60～80 单位的Ⅷ因子前体活性。只要冷沉淀物能提供每公斤体重 10 单位的Ⅷ因子活性，就能充分地满足手术中的止血要求。若对 von Willebrand 病患者的术前纠治失败，患者术中黏膜、体表或两者出血的风险会增加。

另外两种疾病可能也与小儿外科医生相关，即 Glanzmann 血小板功能不全和 Bernard-Soulier 综合征[37]。这两种疾病均可遗传，伴有血小板功能严重缺陷。筛检可发现，这两种疾病患者的出血时间大于 20 分钟。输注 0.2U/kg 或 4 U/m² 的浓缩血小板可以有效地纠治严重出血。但是由于患儿发生同种异体免疫的风险很大，患儿可迅速对血小板输注产生抵抗作用。

凝血疾病

评估小儿出血倾向时，内科医生应从回顾与出血史相关的项目开始。包括术后出血（如包皮环切术或拔牙术）、脐带残端迟发性出血、肌内注射形成血肿、轻微创伤出现青肿、关节内出血、撕裂伤后出血不止、月经过多、血尿以及胃肠道出血。应查明有无使用阿司匹林、含有阿司匹林成分的药物或抗凝药的病史。同时应注意是否有易导致出血的全身性疾病（如红斑狼疮、肾病、甲状腺功能减退、脓毒症）。最后，必须考虑是否有出血倾向家族史，这样可以增加或减少诊断出血性疾病的可能性（图 11-2）。

体检可以为诊断出血性疾病提供进一步的资料。应注意皮肤或黏膜出血（瘀点、瘀斑）、软组织出血（血肿）、关节出血以及检眼镜检查中的出血情况。

实验室筛查包括：血小板计数、出血时间、凝血酶原时间（PT）以及活化部分促凝血酶原激酶时间（APTT）（表 11-1）。出血时间反映了血小板数量和功能。由于标准化程度提高，模板方法比以往的方法更优越。然而，出血时间的变异性很大，与实验操作者的经验、患者的皮肤温度、切口的长度和深度有关。出血时间的正常值范围为 3.5～11.5 分钟。出血时间为 12～15 分钟时要慎重对待，数值超过 15 分钟时为延长和异常。当想要获得出血时间或出血时间延长的检测结果时，由于阿司匹林会明显延长出血时间，内科医生应当询问患者是否使用过阿司匹林或含有阿司匹林成分的药物。

有几种试验可用于筛查凝血因子缺乏或凝血因子缺陷。筛检时全血凝血时间不够敏感，而活化凝血时间较敏感，但并不适用。在常规筛检试验中，APTT 最为敏感。在该试验中，血浆与无活性物质一起保温（如白陶土），采用部分促凝血酶原激酶替代血小板，随后添加钙。APTT 可检测内源性和共同途径中缺乏的凝血因子。然而，APTT 无法检出Ⅷ因子和Ⅸ因子轻度缺乏，对检测是否缺少Ⅶ因子和ⅩⅢ因子则根本无效。APTT 的正常值范围为 25～35 秒；精确的上限值取决于试剂和采用的方法[63]。其他主要筛查检测，如 PT，在血浆中添加了组织因子（一种完整的促凝血酶原激酶），并同时或先后进行再钙化来完成。PT 正常值范围为 11～12 秒[63]；其可用于检测Ⅶ因子和共同途径中凝血因子的缺乏。

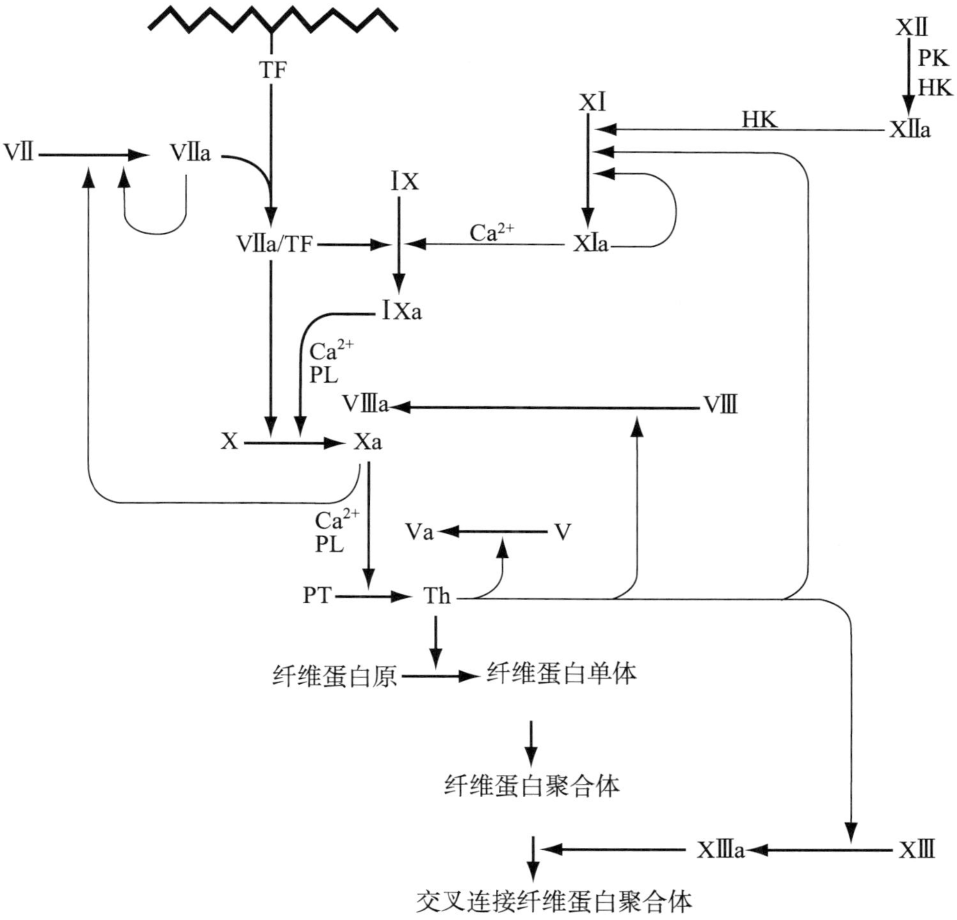

图 11-2 凝血级联反应过程简图。HK：高分子量激肽原；PK：前激肽释放酶；PL：磷脂；PT：凝血酶原；TF：组织因子；Th：凝血酶。(From Schafer AI: Coagulation cascade: An overview. In Loscalzo J, Schafer AI [eds]: Thrombosis and Hemorrhage. Boston, Blackwell Scientific, 1994.)

表 11-1　出血性疾病的检测试验

试验	测量参数
血小板计数	血小板数量
出血时间	全身主要的止血 血小板数量缺乏或功能缺陷 血小板-血管壁相互作用的缺陷 原发性血管疾病
凝血酶原时间（PT）	外源性及共同途径：因子Ⅶ、X、V；凝血酶原；纤维蛋白原
活化部分促凝血酶原激酶时间（APTT）	内源性及共同途径：因子Ⅻ、Ⅸ、Ⅺ、Ⅷ、X、V；凝血酶原；纤维蛋白原；前激肽释放酶；高分子量激肽原
凝血酶时间	纤维蛋白原
纤维蛋白原定量	血浆中纤维蛋白原的水平（mg/dL）
纤维蛋白降解产物	纤维蛋白原或纤维蛋白的裂解产物——纤维蛋白溶解增加时或弥散性血管内凝血时升高
D-二聚体测定	纤维蛋白降解产物；凝血酶和纤维蛋白溶酶生成的指示物
优球蛋白溶解时间	纤维蛋白溶解活性的筛查试验
混合检测（利用 PT 或 APTT）	血液循环中出现抗凝物质
抗凝血酶III（AT III）活性	抗血栓形成的 AT III的水平
蛋白 C，蛋白 S 抗原活性	抗血栓形成的蛋白 C 和蛋白 S 的水平
活化蛋白 C 抵抗力测定	出现突变的、功能缺陷的 Leiden V因子（容易导致血栓形成）

From Schafer AI: Approach to bleeding. In Loscalzo J, Schafer AI (eds): Thrombosis and Hemorrhage. Boston, Blackwell Scientific, 1994; Comp PC: Approach to thrombosis. In Loscalzo J, Schafer AI (eds): Thrombosis and Hemorrhage. Boston, Blackwell Scientific, 1994; and Santoro SA: Laboratory evaluation of hemostatic disorders. In Hoffman R, et al (eds): Hematology: Basic Principles and Practice. New York, Churchill Livingstone, 1991.

可采用特异的方法测定单一因子的缺乏。若无法鉴别一种或多种因子缺乏，应考虑检测血浆中的抗凝物质。可以综合考虑通过 APTT 或 PT 来完成，但要取决于何者更为异常。在这些研究中，按照不同比例（1∶3、1∶1、3∶1）将正常人的血浆与患者的异常血浆混合。在检测中，若 3∶1 混合（正常人∶患者）无法完全纠正，则说明存在抑制物。而 1∶3 及 1∶1 混合时缺乏的因子应可完全纠正。

凝血因子缺乏

最常见的遗传性凝血因子缺乏包括血友病 A（Ⅷ因子缺乏）和血友病 B（Ⅸ因子缺乏）。这两种疾病均为 X 染色体连锁隐性遗传，受累的几乎均为男性。血友病 A 患者的Ⅷ因子前体的活性不足或存在缺陷，其出血严重程度与Ⅷ因子水平密切相关；Ⅷ因子水平低于 3%时常伴有关节和软组织自发性出血。血友病 B 的特征是Ⅸ因子缺乏或存在缺陷。Ⅸ因子水平极度低下（低于正常值的 3%）时可以导致关节和软组织自发性出血。不同凝血分子的缺陷构成了血友病 A和血友病 B 的不同亚型。血友病 A 比血友病 B 更多见。在美国，前者在男性中的发病率为 1/10 000，而后者在男性中的发病率为 1/40 000。

一般来说，Ⅷ因子或Ⅸ因子水平高于正常值的 30%就能正常止血。凝血因子水平处于 8%～20%的个体生活基本接近于正常，患者只有在手术后或受到严重创伤后才会发生大量出血[63]。

Ⅷ因子缺乏在出生时就可以做出诊断。最终确诊为血友病 A 的患儿的特征是 APTT 延长。进一步的研究表明，功能性Ⅷ因子缺乏的程度可以通过特异方法检测。在评估是否存在Ⅸ因子缺乏时，内科医生必须考虑到婴儿中维生素 K 依赖的凝血因子在达到正常水平前可以产生生理性延迟。虽然这种生理性延迟使对婴儿Ⅸ因子水平的解释更复杂，但若出现像血友病 B 那样Ⅸ因子水平接近于零的情况，这种延迟现象不会导致错误的解释。APTT 延长伴有Ⅸ因子水平低于 10%符合血友病 B 的诊断。若婴儿的检测水平处于 10%～50%，应待其长大到 3～6 个月龄时复查；若患儿发生大量出血，应尽快进行复查。

其他因子缺乏

先天性纤维蛋白原缺乏血症患者常在出生后早期发生异常出血（如黑便、呕血、黏膜出血、血肿、脐带出血）。年长儿可能在发生轻微创伤后出血、月经过多、关节积血以及脑出血。通过定量地测定纤维蛋白原可以进行诊断。在其他方法（如沉淀和凝结的方法）无效时，免疫学方法仍可检测出少量的纤维蛋白原。纤维蛋白原水平在 50mg/dL 以上时患者通常能够正常止血[3]。使用全血、血浆以及冷沉淀物能够纠正纤维蛋白原水平。

异常纤维蛋白原血症是纤维蛋白原功能性疾病，是由蛋白质结构缺陷造成的。现已发现 300 多种异常的纤维蛋白原[15,63]。很多异常纤维蛋白原血症患者并没有临床出血病史，是通过常规筛查诊断出来的。有出血倾向的患者可有月经过多、容易发生青肿及轻微创伤后或手术后出血时间延长病史。纤维蛋白原缺乏血症为常染色体隐性遗传，而异常纤维蛋白原血症为常染色体显性遗传。对于异常纤维蛋白原血症，免疫定量或沉淀反应技术得到的结果常为正常，但在测定评价纤维蛋白原对凝血的贡献时会出现异常。多数异常纤维蛋白原血症患者不需要治疗，但患者严重出血时可以输注血浆或冷沉淀物。

表 11–2 列举了已知的凝血因子及其与临床出血相关的特征。凝血酶原（Ⅱ因子）、Ⅴ因子和Ⅺ因子缺乏患者可能有轻度出血倾向，然而，Ⅶ因子和Ⅹ因子缺乏患者的出血倾向各不相同，有些患者可发生严重的出血事件。值得注意的是，接触活化因子——Ⅻ因子（Hageman 因子）、前激肽释放酶（Fletcher 因子）以及高分子量激肽原缺乏均与出血无关，缺乏这些因子也不应成为推迟手术的理由。 18

获得性缺陷

严重的肝脏疾病常伴有大量的凝血因子缺乏。健康的肝脏是合成大部分凝血因子（纤维蛋白原、凝血酶原、Ⅴ因子、Ⅶ因子、Ⅸ因子、Ⅹ因子、Ⅺ因子、Ⅻ因子和ⅩⅢ因子；前激肽释放酶；以及高分子量激肽原）的器官[63]。肝脏也能合成某些天然抗凝物质[如抗凝血酶Ⅲ（AT Ⅲ）、蛋白 C 和蛋白 S］及纤维蛋白溶解抑制物（抗纤维蛋白溶酶和 α_1 抗胰蛋白

表 11-2　凝血因子缺乏

缺乏因子	临床关联
Ⅰ	水平低于 50mg/dL 有出血的风险
Ⅱ	受伤、拔牙、手术后轻度出血倾向
Ⅴ	轻度出血倾向（月经过多、受伤或手术后明显出血）
Ⅶ	出血倾向各异（新生儿颅内出血、月经过多）
Ⅷ	水平低于 5%时导致中度至重度出血倾向
Ⅸ	水平低于 5%时导致中度至重度出血倾向
Ⅹ	出血倾向各异（新生儿出血、创伤后出血、月经过多）
Ⅺ	轻度出血倾向（月经过多、鼻出血、术后出血）
Ⅻ	常没有症状
前激肽释放酶	无症状
高分子量激肽原	无症状

酶）。肝脏还是清除活化凝血因子的器官，因此，当肝功能衰竭无法清除活化凝血因子且不能合成 AT Ⅲ时，会出现弥散性血管内凝血（DIC）。然而，肝脏严重损伤和肝功能衰竭更常导致与凝血因子生成减少相关的出血倾向。肝脏合成的抑制物减少导致的纤维蛋白溶解增加也可能会导致出血倾向。

婴儿维生素 K 缺乏会产生严重的出血倾向。引起维生素 K 缺乏的原因包括：饮食中维生素 K 摄入不足、吸收不良或特殊药物的拮抗作用[63]。维生素 K 缺乏可妨碍在维生素 K 依赖的凝血因子[78]（包括凝血酶原、Ⅶ因子、Ⅸ因子和Ⅹ因子）上形成必要的钙结合位点。新生儿依靠摄入外源性维生素 K，较大的婴儿从结肠吸收维生素 K，且主要并通过细菌合成。在年长儿和成人，维生素 K 则通过回肠吸收。每日维生素 K 的大约需要量 1μg/kg，可从食用的绿叶蔬菜中得到补充[74]。维生素 K 吸收后储存在肝脏中。

大多数正常婴儿体内维生素 K 储存量不足，但很少会发展成现出血体质。如果早期未得到补充，婴儿可能出现青肿、头部血肿、胃肠道和脐部出血以及穿刺部位的渗血。这些婴儿的血小板和纤维蛋白原水平基本正常，但由于缺乏Ⅱ因子、Ⅶ因子、Ⅸ因子和Ⅹ因子，其 PT 和 APTT 显著延长。通过胃肠外途径给予维生素 K 后，可以快速纠正凝血试验异常和出血。母乳喂养会加重维生素 K 缺乏，因为母乳中维生素 K 的含量（2～15μg/L）远低于牛奶中的含量（60μg/L）[48]。在新生儿出生后短期内给予肌内注射维生素 K，可以预防出血性疾病。推荐 0.5～1.0mg 维生素 K_1的氧化物，这个剂量远大于 25μg的需要量[49]。

除了新生儿期，吸收不良也可以引起维生素 K 缺乏并导致出血倾向。囊性纤维化、胆道闭锁、慢性溶血性贫血伴继发性胆石病和阻塞性黄疸以及疾病导致近端小肠功能异常均能引起维生素 K 吸收不良。使用香豆素类化合物可引起维生素 K 缺乏，造成出血。维生素 K 缺乏引起的出血可从包括大块瘀斑和明显的黏膜出血，也包括中枢神经系统出血。PT 和 APTT 测定结果通常延长，但给予维生素 K 治疗后能恢复正常。维生素 K 静脉注射 5～10mg 可在数小时内改善临床症状，并可在 24 小时之内纠正凝血试验异常[63]。

DIC 发生于机体内凝血机制激活时、纤维蛋白原转变成纤维蛋白之后。大量病理生理状况可引起 DIC，包括宫内感染、母体毒血症、胎盘早剥、严重的呼吸窘迫综合征、坏死性小肠结肠炎、播散性细菌感染、病毒和立克次体感染、白血病和其他恶性肿瘤、巨大海绵状血管瘤、严重创伤、急性过敏反应以及蛇咬伤[63]。广泛的内皮破坏或组织损伤伴前凝血物质释放可激活Ⅻ因子和血小板黏附于受损内皮之上，随后发生血小板聚集并释放磷脂。

通过外周血涂片检测找到红细胞碎片及证实血小板数目少，有助于诊断 DIC。应当进行凝血参数检测，包括血小板计数、PT、APTT、凝血酶时间以及纤维蛋白原定量。因凝血酶活性以及继发于纤维蛋白溶解形成的纤维蛋白降解产物会形成纤维蛋白单体，进行相关检测以及 D 二聚体水平检测有助于确诊 DIC。

DIC 的治疗包括纠治基础疾病、去除诱发因素并给予支持治疗。进一步的治疗则取决于患者的全身情况以及出血或血栓形成表现。暴发性紫癜以及伴有血栓形成的患儿可采用肝素治疗；然而，DIC 不严重时，是否采用肝素治疗尚有疑问。AT Ⅲ水平下降时，肝素可能不再有效。可通过输注新鲜冷冻血浆或 AT Ⅲ浓缩物补充 AT Ⅲ。患者的血小板计数和纤维蛋白原水平可作为治疗反应的监测指标。对于原先已有出血且不伴有血栓形成的患者，在出现中重度出血并伴有血小板计数下降和 PT、APTT 延长时，可以输注血小板和新鲜冷冻血浆。

血栓形成性疾病

天然生成的抗凝物 AT Ⅲ、蛋白 C 和蛋白 S 能防止体内凝血过度。这些抗凝物活性缺乏时常会引起血栓形成。此外，遗传性Ⅴ因子（G1691A）和凝血酶
187 原（G20210A）异常以及同型半胱氨酸和脂蛋白（a）水平异常也与小儿血栓形成有关[67]。而抗磷脂抗体（如狼疮抗凝物、抗心肌磷脂抗体）则与静脉血栓形成的风险增加相关。

AT Ⅲ是肝素治疗所必需的肝素辅因子，也是一种主要的凝血抑制物。AT Ⅲ是凝血酶和活化的Ⅹ因子的生理抑制物。AT Ⅲ在肝脏中合成，生理半衰期为 2～5 天。先天性 AT Ⅲ缺乏的发病率为 1/2000～1/5000[89,73]。血栓性疾病常在 20～30 岁时首先被发现。手术、创伤、感染以及妊娠容易导致血栓性疾病。AT Ⅲ是肝素保持全部活性所必需的，因此有效地给患者抗凝治疗时需要大量的肝素。可以采用免疫学、酶学以及凝血方法测定 AT Ⅲ，以获得诊断。虽然很多患者表现为 AT Ⅲ数量上的缺乏，但也有部分患者存在 AT Ⅲ质量上的缺陷，而后者在免疫学测定中可能被忽略。口服抗凝药是主要治疗方法。但现已有纯化的 AT Ⅲ浓缩物，可以使用 50 IU/kg 的剂量用于短期预防高危状态下的血栓形成，如预防急性血栓形成、手术期间或妊娠 6 个月后的血栓形成[59,98]。应可以获得 80%及以上的水平。长期预防可采用华法林。

蛋白 C 和蛋白 S 是维生素 K 依赖的血浆蛋白，均可灭活凝血物质前体，因此可降低血栓形成的风险。蛋白 C 的功能是灭活Ⅴ因子和Ⅷ因子，其激活后，也可间接地促进血块溶解[63]。蛋白 C 缺乏是常染色体显性遗传。纯合子婴儿的特征是暴发性紫癜、视网膜血栓形成，伴有视网膜脱离和视力丧失以及其他部位血栓形成[43]。杂合子婴儿在儿童期常不出现任何症状，但在青春期和青年期会发生静脉血栓形成。杂合子患儿通常约占 50%，但这些个体仍具有血栓形成的危险性。蛋白 C 可通过功能性和免疫学方法测定。对于纯合子个体，蛋白 C 虽然能起到预防血栓形成的作用，但对这些患者使用华法林应谨慎，因为华法林有可能进一步减少维生素 K 依赖的蛋白 C 而增加血栓形成的风险。事实上，杂合子个体在服用华法林期间常会发生紫癜性、血栓性皮肤损伤，因此杂合子个体也是华法林使用的禁忌证。这些副作用可能是蛋白 C 水平进一步降低所致。急性静脉血栓形成时应采用肝素治疗，蛋白 C 缺乏患者在急性血栓形成时可采用蛋白 C 浓缩物治疗。

蛋白 S 是蛋白 C 的辅因子。缺乏蛋白 S 与反复静脉血栓形成相关。只有该蛋白正常水平的 35%～50%的杂合子在青春期和青年期可反复形成血栓[85]。对于蛋白 S 缺乏（以及 AT Ⅲ和蛋白 C 缺乏）患者的静脉血栓治疗，肝素使用原则同样适用，对使用华法林应保持谨慎。

近年来已证明Ⅴ因子突变（如 Leiden Ⅴ因子）与活化的蛋白 C 无法灭活Ⅴ因子相关[14,24]。蛋白 C 常通过灭活Ⅴ因子和Ⅷ因子预防血栓形成，因此，蛋白 C 对Ⅴ因子的作用失效时，理论上会导致血栓形成的危险性增加。事实上，对于血栓栓塞发病率很高的家族的研究表明，活化蛋白 C 抵抗、Ⅴ因子突变和血栓形成存在相关性[106]。Ⅴ因子突变可能是静脉血栓栓塞最常见的原因。

输血治疗

合理使用血制品可通过增加患者的氧输送、扩张血管内容量及改善凝血功能从而提高危重患者的生存率。婴儿和体重 10～30kg 的幼儿其血容量估计约为 75.4ml/kg[84]。输注红细胞可用于纠正病理生理情况下的不恰当的氧输送及组织缺氧。输注红细胞应基于以下几个因素：组织缺氧的体征（心动过速和呼吸急促）、失血程度、贫血发展速度、患者年龄以及患者可能经历的伴随性或继发性生理应激（如感染、肺功能衰竭和手术）。输注的红细胞可以相对存活较长时间；每天被破坏的红细胞少于输注量的 1% [69]。一般来说，输入患者体内的红细胞的存活时间通常超过 110～120 天[106]。

过去，急性重度失血的患者更多的是输注全血。然而，随着血液分离更多应用于血制品的生产，如果需要的话，现在更强调使用浓缩红细胞和血浆代用

品。对于中度出血的患者，浓缩红细胞与含有枸橼酸盐的全血同样有效[84]。对于严重出血的患者，为了防止输注浓缩红细胞后引起无法接受的血细胞比容增加，需要输注适量的血浆代用品[69]。

为了使大量失血的患者的血容量和携氧能力尽快恢复，必须快速输血。这种做法通常与前面讨论过的对贫血引起的失血的处理基本相同。非紧急情况时，可以在 1～2 小时内按 10～15ml/kg 输血。大量输血使患者 24 小时内的输血量与患者的血容量相等时，
88 会有引起枸橼酸中毒、电解质失衡、红细胞 2,3-二磷酸甘油酸分解导致组织氧释放量减少、肺微栓塞、中心体温下降（如大量输入未经加温的血液）、血小板减少症以及 DIC 的风险。若要预防和成功治疗大量输血带来的副作用，需要在输血期间和输血后对患者进行仔细的评估。

已有多种血浆代用品，如右旋糖酐、改良的液体明胶以及羟乙基淀粉，已被用于扩张低容量患者的血浆容量。然而，因有可能引起过敏反应并导致异常出血，对这些血浆代用品的使用热情有所下降。全氟化碳具有高度氧可溶性，在动物实验中被证明能有效地替代血液来输送氧[70]。但是，包括血小板计数下降[80]、巨噬细胞功能抑制[35]以及激活补体造成肺部改变[23]的副作用大打阻碍了全氟化碳的应用。目前全氟化碳正处于临床试验评估阶段[95]。

癌症或免疫缺陷患者的输血

免疫缺陷患者和癌症患者的输血原则是纠正异常的血流动力学并改善氧输送不足。不存在外周血红蛋白或血细胞比容低于某个最低值就必须输血的绝对值。事实上，考虑到输血的风险、输血治疗的高成本，以及目前越来越多的人认为患者能够耐受比以前所知更低的血红蛋白值而不发生不良后果，很多医疗中心正在放弃输血的绝对阈值标准。很明显，患者的年龄、血红蛋白或血细胞比容下降的速率以及伴随疾病均影响是否输血的决定。10 岁以下儿童的血红蛋白可以低至 6～7g/dL 而不产生不良反应。但是，当血红蛋白快速下降至此水平时通常需要输注红细胞。同样伴有感染、肺部占位性疾病、胸膜渗出、心肌病、中枢神经系统受损或其他主要脏器受伤时也需要早期输血。要根据患者的免疫状态考虑选择红细胞制品的种类及进行相关处理。对原发性免疫缺陷及继发性免疫缺陷患者，为了防止输注血制品后发生移植物抗宿主病，血制品应用之前应对至少按照 1500cGy 水平进行辐射。此外，对接受骨髓移植的患者及其他重度免疫抑制患者，若巨细胞病毒（CMV）血清学检测为阴性，则输血时应给予巨细胞病毒阴性或不含巨细胞病毒（减白细胞）的血制品。事实上，很多血库现只向受血者提供减白细胞的细胞制品。

红细胞制品的选择

当对患者进行换血治疗及当患者由于急性出血而大量失血时，新鲜全血是合适的选择。对由于过分扩容而导致问题的患者，使用其他红细胞制品可能更为适合。

对急性中度失血及红细胞生成低下或溶血导致慢性贫血的患者，可以选择应用浓缩红细胞。浓缩红细胞的优点包括去除了抗凝物质枸橼酸及 60%～70%的血浆[17]。对于容量超负荷、心功能差或两者兼有的患者来说，这种考虑尤其重要。

洗涤红细胞的优点之一是去除了 85%～90%的白细胞以及 95%以上的血浆[17]。然而，这种红细胞制品的生产会使医疗费用增加。洗涤红细胞可用于有非溶血性输血反应病史的患者。

冷冻去甘油化红细胞已去除 90%以上的白细胞，并保留了少量的血浆（<0.5%的原始血浆）[17]。这种制品常用于需要长期输血的患者。

减白细胞红细胞比较地没有白细胞（>70%被去除）[107]，因此传播 CMV 以及其他病毒的可能性减少。这种血制品适合于有输血反应病史及存在感染 CMV 疾病风险的患免疫缺陷患者。

上述每一种血制品在输血治疗中各有其用途。内科医生应记住每种血制品的适应证及红细胞经额外处理后（如洗涤、冷冻和解冻）相关费用会增加。

输血反应和中毒

输血时，血浆抗凝物枸橼酸与钙离子结合可导致枸橼酸中毒，出现低钙血症的症状。发生这种中毒是使用全血快速补充红细胞和容量时的主要障碍。

输血反应由多种形式，通常是由于患者接触来自血浆、红细胞、白细胞以及血小板中的具有天然或获得性敏感性蛋白质而发生。输血反应的发生率约为2%～3%。发生输血反应的患者中，41%出现发热而没有溶血，58%发生荨麻疹，而发生延迟性溶血的患
189 者为 1% [12]。对于反复发生荨麻疹的患者，输注洗涤红细胞或冷冻红细胞，联合对受血者进行抗组胺或皮质类固醇药物预处理，可以降低复发率。非溶血性发热反应常常由于血浆蛋白或白细胞同种抗原产生抗体而引起，主要发生于以往有输血史或妊娠史的患者。经退热药、抗组胺药或皮质类固醇药物预处理后，患者症状可以减轻。目前由于现代化血库实施精密的质控措施，溶血反应已经很少见。主要的血型不相容可以导致溶血反应，出现发热、寒战、腹部和腰部疼痛、心动过速、低血压、肾衰竭以及休克的症状。当怀疑这些症状与输血有关时，应立即停止输血，并采集患者的血样与残余的血制品一起送至血库检验。延迟性输血反应发生于输血后 3～10 天，是由于以前的输血使得次要血型致敏所致，通常没有因主要血型不相容引起的反应严重。

由于获得性免疫缺陷综合征（AIDS）的流行，通过血制品传播疾病的风险再次受到关注。虽然，不足 5% AIDS 病例是由输血导致，但由于人类感染人免疫缺陷病毒（HIV）后死亡率很高，人们对于输注血制品仍然十分恐惧。优先从无偿献血者中采集血制品以及 HIV 筛检已将 HIV 传播几率降至 1/ 153 000。输血时还应考虑肝炎病毒、CMV 和 EB 病毒的传播风险。事先筛查 B 型肝炎和 C 型肝炎可大大降低通过输血传播这些病毒的风险；A 型肝炎传播与输血无关。采集无偿供血者的血液及筛检 B 型肝炎病毒抗原可使由输血获得 B 型肝炎的几率降至 1/1000[12]。有可能需要反复输血的患者推荐注射 B 型肝炎疫苗。现已能对 C 型肝炎病毒做出鉴定，并在献血者中开展 C 型肝炎病毒的筛查。希望通过这项检测使输血导致感染的概率下降 6% [52]。CMV 是以淋巴细胞作为载体，免疫缺陷患者输注携带 CMV 的淋巴细胞后可以引起严重感染。免疫缺陷患者输注冷冻或洗涤红细胞以及来自 CMV 阴性供血者的减白细胞红细胞制品可以减少感染 CMV 相关疾病的风险[30,96]。

对免疫缺陷个体，移植物抗宿主病是与输血相关的潜在问题之一。该病以往报道常发生于同种异体骨髓移植后，而现在报道与免疫缺陷患者输血相关的发病一直在增加。输血相关的移植物抗宿主病已报道 131 例[3]。输血相关的移植物抗宿主病其特征是高热、鳞状斑丘疹样红疹、腹泻、肝细胞损害引起病理性肝酶升高以及全血细胞减少。该病通常在输血后 8～12 天发病。该病的总体死亡率为 90%，并且绝大多数在发病后的 1 个月内死亡。类固醇、抗胸腺细胞球蛋白、环磷酰胺及抗 T 细胞单克隆抗体对治疗该病均无效。将所有的细胞制品进行辐射后再行输注可避免免疫缺陷患者罹患输血相关的移植物抗宿主病。按照 1500～5000cGy 剂量辐射的血制品可杀死淋巴细胞，而不会对红细胞、血小板及中性粒细胞造成不利影响。处理后的血制品不带有放射性，可按常规在医院中使用。目前尚无输注新鲜冷冻血浆或冷沉淀物后发生输血相关的移植物抗宿主病报道。

输注血小板

正常儿童和成年人的血小板计数为 150 000～450 000/μL[51]，新生婴儿的血小板水平偶尔可低至 80 000/μL。血小板一旦释放进入血流，生存期约为 8～10 天。血小板计数低于 10 000/μL 的个体明显有出血风险[116]，而血小板计数低于 50 000/μL 的个体在手术中有出血风险[1]。血小板计数低于 10 000/μL 的患者输注血小板浓缩物可降低自发性出血风险，而血小板计数低于 50 000/μL 的患者输注血小板浓缩物后可以降低围术期和术后出血的风险。

随机供体血小板浓缩物可通过全血两步离心后获得[39]。通过初步低速旋转处理可以去除红细胞，而血小板悬浮于上层的血浆中。然后将血小板富集的血浆进行高速离心，结果血小板沉积在底部而非悬浮在血浆中。之后将血小板浓缩物放在 20～24℃温度下储存，最多可以保存 5 天。储存时其 pH应维持在 6.0 或 6.0 以上。

单个献血者的血小板可经血液成分单采技术收集。200～400ml 血浆中血小板的含量约为 3×10^{14}，相当于 6～8 名献血者所献血液中可得到的量[39]。这些血小板最多能存放 5 天。对随机供血者的浓缩物产生同种异体免疫的患者，可以输注单个供血者的浓缩物。对血小板产生同种抗体的患者，通过反复试验或 HLA 配型鉴定单个供血者的相容性，输血后血小板的计数常常会大量增加。对来自随机供血者的血小板

190 浓缩物产生同种异体免疫的患者，在输血后 1 小时测定血小板计数，对于判断是否需要单个供血者的血小板或 HLA 相配的血小板具有很高价值[90]。若患者无脓毒症或血小板未在脾脏内隔离，输注来自随机供血者的浓缩物 1 小时后循环中血小板计数未增加，则通常表明存在血小板同种抗体。

血小板浓缩物常用于治疗血小板减少症伴出血或血小板明显减少以致给手术和其他侵袭性操作带来严重威胁的患者。当血小板计数低于 50 000/μL 的血小板减少症患者必须进行手术和侵袭性操作时，预防性输注血小板是合理的[39]。该阈值同样适用于伴有血小板减少症的头外伤患者。很多肿瘤医学中心给予癌症患者预防性输注血小板，血小板输注阈值为 10 000～30 000/μL[2,26,77]。有研究认为，血小板计数在 10 000/μL 以上时出血的危险性很小，即使患者有发热和感染[16]。最后，很重要的一点是要知道，输注浓缩血小板可以治疗由血小板功能受损（如 Glanzmann 血小板功能不全、Bernard–Soulier 综合征）或获得性血小板功能缺陷（如服用阿司匹林）导致的出血。

要止住血小板减少症患者的出血，血小板计数需要增加 40 000/μL[50]。对于小儿，每公斤体重给予 0.1U 的血小板浓缩物通常能产生血小板 40 000/μL的增加。同样，4U /m^2 体表面积也能达到相同的结果[56]。在临床上，即使是婴儿，也必须至少给予 2U 血小板浓缩物。这种算法同样适用于实施外科手术的血小板减少症患者。输注血小板后 1 小时测定血小板计数常可精确地评估血小板增量。对于出血患者，出血停止是最终指标。输入血小板的半衰期平均约为 4 天。伴有发热、感染及血小板消耗性疾病时，血小板生存期缩短[91]。ABO 相容的血小板的生存期可以延长，但对此尚有争议[18,92]。对同种致敏的受体给予单个供血者的血小板或 HLA 相配的血小板常可延长血小板生存期。对于连续 2～3 次输入随机供血者的血小板后血小板增量低于 10 000/μL 的患者，应考虑更换单个供血者或 HLA 相配的血小板。然而，若血小板减少症患者准备移植亲属供体骨髓，要避免使用来自家庭成员的相配的血小板，以防止对少量抗原致敏，因为这有可能增加潜在的移植物排斥反应。

血小板浓缩物可通过血液过滤器输注。标准的 170μm 筛滤器可去除血凝块，常被用于输注血小板浓缩物[39]。当前的微聚物血液过滤器可去除淋巴细胞，同时允许血小板通过。这种过滤器可以减少发生输血性发热反应的危险，并通过去除淋巴细胞可以预防 HLA 抗原的致敏。而用于输注减白细胞红细胞的输血器由于同时可以去除大多数血小板，不能用于输注血小板浓缩物[60]。以 1500cGy 剂量辐射血小板后再行输注，可以降低移植物抗宿主病高危患者的风险。按照这种剂量辐射后，血小板功能体外测定没有发生改变[62,71,83,94]。

血小板浓缩物中含有少量 Rh 阳性红细胞可能足以使 Rh 阴性个体产生抗 D 抗体[41]。Rh 阴性女性受血者输注血小板浓缩物时，给予 Rh 免疫球蛋白可以预防发生这种致敏反应。白细胞凝集素联合白细胞、血小板输注引起的输血反应可以发生在输注血小板期间或输注后的短期内[39]。发热和寒战通常与血小板输注反应相关。减慢输注速率可以降低发热反应的风险。给予对乙酰氨基酚、静脉注射皮质类固醇以及经胃肠外途径给予哌替啶可以改善这种反应。过敏性输血反应的特征是荨麻疹及偶尔发生低血压或支气管痉挛[39]。抗组胺药物，以及偶尔应用肾上腺素可治疗过敏性反应。

输注血小板浓缩物后感染病毒的风险很小。此外，由于血小板储存于室温下，患者输注血小板后发生发热、寒战、低血压或 DIC 时，应该考虑到血小板可能被细菌污染。

（张瑞冬译　陈锡明校）

参考文献

1. Aballi AJ, Puapondh Y, Desposito F: Platelet counts in thriving premature infants. Pediatrics 1968;42:685.
2. Aderka D, et al: Bleeding due to thrombocytopenia in acute leukemias and reevaluation of the prophylactic platelet transfusion policy. Am J Med Sci 1986;291:147.
3. Adler SP: Transfusion associated cytomegalovirus infections. Rev Infect Dis 1983;5:977.
4. Adner MM, et al: Use of "compatible" platelet transfusions in treatment of congenital isoimmune thrombocytopenic purpura. N Engl J Med 1969;280:244.
5. Alter BP: Fetal erythropoiesis in stress hematopoiesis. Exp Hematol 1979;7:200.
6. Alter BP: The bone marrow failure syndromes. In Nathan DG, Oski FA (eds): Hematology of Infancy and Childhood, 3rd ed. Philadelphia, WB Saunders, 1987.
7. Alter BP, Potter NU: Long-term outcome in Fanconi's anemia: Description of 26 cases and review of the literature. In German J (ed): Chromosome Mutation and Neoplasia. New York, AR Liss, 1983.
8. Alter BP, et al: Classification and aetiology of the aplastic anemias. Clin Haematol 1978;7:431.
9. American Academy of Pediatrics, Committee on Nutrition: Iron balance and requirements in infancy. Pediatrics 1969; 43:134.

10. American Academy of Pediatrics, Committee on Nutrition: Iron supplementation for infants. Pediatrics 1976;58:765.
11. American Academy of Pediatrics, Committee on Nutrition: Iron fortification of infant formulas. Pediatrics 1999; 104:119.
12. American Medical Association: General Principles of Blood Transfusion, 3rd ed. Chicago, AMA, 1985.
13. Bernard J, Soulier J: Sur une nouvelle variété de dystrophie thrombocytaire hemorragipore congenitale. Sem Hop Paris 1948;24:3217.
14. Bertina RM, et al: Mutation in blood coagulation factor V associated with resistance to activated protein C. Nature 1994;369:64.
15. Bolton PHB, et al. The rare coagulation disorders—review with guidelines for management from the United Kingdom Haemophilia Centre Doctors' Organisation. Haemophilia 2004;10:593.
16. Brecher G, Schneiderman M, Cronkite EP: The reproducibility and constancy of the platelet count. Am J Clin Pathol 1953;23:15.
17. Bucala R, Kawakami M, Cerani A: Cytotoxicity of a perfluorocarbon blood substitute to macrophages in vitro. Science 1983;220:965.
18. Cable R: Platelet transfusion. In Nathan DG, Oski FA (eds): Hematology of Infancy and Childhood. Philadelphia, WB Saunders, 1987.
19. Castro O, et al: Predicting the effects of transfusing only phenotyped-matched RBCs to patients with sickle cell disease: Theoretical and practical implications. Transfusion 2002;42:684.
20. Cattan D, et al: Maladie de Fanconi et cancer du foie. Arch Fr Mal App Dig 1974;63:41.
21. Cohen A: Management of iron overload in the pediatric patient. Hematol Oncol Clin North Am 1987;1:521.
22. Cohen A, Markenson AL, Schwartz E: Transfusion requirements and splenectomy in thalassemia major. J Pediatr 1980;97:100.
23. Colman RW, et al: Effects of a perfluoro erythrocyte substitute on platelets in vitro and in vivo. J Lab Clin Med 1980;95:553.
24. Dahlbäck B, Hildebrand B: Inherited resistance to activated protein C is corrected by anticoagulant cofactor activity found to be a property of factor V. Proc Natl Acad Sci U S A 1994;91:1396.
25. Dallman PR: Iron deficiency and related nutritional anemias. In Nathan DG, Oski FA (eds): Hematology of Infancy and Childhood, 3rd ed. Philadelphia, WB Saunders, 1987.
26. Daly PA, et al: Platelet transfusion therapy: One-hour posttransfusion increments are valuable in predicting the need for HLA-matched preparations. JAMA 1980;243:435.
27. Davies SC: Blood transfusion in sickle cell disease. Curr Opin Hematol 1996;3:485.
28. Eisenstein EM: Congenital amegakaryocytic thrombocytopenic purpura. Clin Pediatr 1966;5:143.
29. Firth PG, Head CA: Sickle cell disease and anesthesia. Anesthesiology 2004;101:766.
30. Fosburg MT, Kevy SV: Red cell transfusion. In Nathan DG, Oski FA (eds): Hematology of Infancy and Childhood, 3rd ed. Philadelphia, WB Saunders, 1987.
31. Gadner H: Management of immune thrombocytopenic purpura in children. Rev Clin Exp Hematol 2001;5:201.
32. Galea P, et al: Isoimmune neonatal thrombocytopenic purpura. Arch Dis Child 1981;56:112.
33. Ganser A, et al: Effects of recombinant human interleukin-3 in aplastic anemia. Blood 1990;76:1287.
34. Gasser C: Akute erythroblastopenie. Schweiz Med Wochenschr 1949;79:838.
35. Geyer RP: "Bloodless" rats through use of artificial blood substitutes. Fed Proc 1975;34:1499.
36. Gill FM, et al: Clinical events in the first decade in a cohort of infants with sickle cell disease. Blood 1995; 86:776.
37. Glanzmann E: Hereditaire haemorrhagische thromboasthenie E in beitrag zur pathologie der blut plattchen. Jahrb Kinderheilk 1918;88:1.
38. Gluckman E, et al: Bone marrow transplantation in Fanconi anaemia. Br J Haematol 1980;45:557.
39. Gmur J, et al: Safety of stringent prophylactic platelet transfusion policy for patients with acute leukemia. Lancet 1991; 338:1223.
40. Gmyrek D, Syllm-Rapoport I: Zur Fanconi-Anämie FA: Analyse von 129 beschriedenen Fällen. Z Kinderheilk 1964; 91:297, 1964.
41. Goldfinger D, McGinniss MH: Rh-incompatible platelet transfusions: Risks and consequences of sensitizing immunosuppressed patients. N Engl J Med 1971; 284:942.
42. Greenbaum BH: Transfusion-associated graft-versus-host disease: Historical perspectives, incidence, and current use of irradiated blood products. J Clin Oncol 1991; 9:1889.
43. Griffin JH: Clinical studies of protein C. Semin Thromb Hemost 1984;10:162.
44. Griffin TC, Buchanan GR: Elective surgery in children with sickle cell disease without preoperative blood transfusion. J Pediatr Surg 1993;28:681.
45. Gross S, Kiwanuka J: Chronic ITP terminating in aplastic anemia. Am J Pediatr Hematol Oncol 1981;3:446.
46. Hall JG, et al: Thrombocytopenia with absent radius (TAR). Medicine 1969;48:411.
47. Hamberg M, et al: Isolation and structure of two prostaglandin endoperoxides that cause platelet aggregation. Proc Natl Acad Sci U S A 1974;71:345.
48. Haroon Y, et al: The content of phylloquinone (vitamin K_1) in human milk, cows' milk and infant formula foods determined by high-performance liquid chromatography. J Nutr 1982;112:1105.
49. Hathaway WE: New insights on vitamin K. Hematol Oncol Clin North Am 1987;1:367.
50. Higby DJ, et al: The prophylactic treatment of thrombocytopenic leukaemic patients with platelets: A double blind study. Transfusion 1974;14:440.
51. Hillyer CD, et al: Methods for the reduction of transfusion-transmitted cytomegalovirus infection: Filtration versus the use of seronegative donor units. Transfusion 1994;34:929.
52. Holland PV, Schmidt PJ (eds): Committee on Standards, American Association of Blood Banks: Standards for Blood Banks and Transfusion Services, 12th ed. Arlington, Va, American Association of Blood Banks, 1987.
53. Howard MA, Firkin B: Ristocetin—a new tool in the investigation of platelet aggregation. Thromb Diath Haemorrhag 1971;26:362.
54. Howarth S, Sharpey-Schafer EP: Low blood pressure phases following hemorrhage. Lancet 1947;1:19.
55. Hutchinson RJ: Blood products. Semin Pediatr Surg 1992;1:231.
56. Ilett SJ, Lilleyman JS: Platelet transfusion requirements of children with newly diagnosed lymphoblastic leukemia. Acta Haematol 1979;62:86.
57. Iriondo A, et al: Complete recovery of hemopoiesis following bone marrow transplant in a patient with

unresponsive congenital hypoplastic anemia (Blackfan-Diamond syndrome). Blood 1984;64:348.
58. Kojima S, et al: Treatment of aplastic anemia in children with recombinant human granulocyte colony-stimulating factor. Blood 1991;77:937.
59. Laharrague P, et al: Antithrombin III: Substitutive treatment of the hereditary deficiency. Thromb Haemost 1980;1:72.
60. Lee EJ, Schiffer CA: ABO compatibility can influence the results of platelet transfusion: Results of a randomized trial. Transfusion 1989;29:384.
61. Li FP, et al: The mortality of acquired aplastic anemia in children. Blood 1972;40:153.
62. Lohrmann HP, et al: Platelet transfusions from HL-a compatible unrelated donors to alloimmunized patients. Ann Intern Med 1974;80:9.
63. Lusher JM: Diseases of coagulation: The fluid phase. In Nathan DG, Oski FA (eds): Hematology of Infancy and Childhood, 3rd ed. Philadelphia, WB Saunders, 1987.
64. Lusher JM, Iyer R: Idiopathic thrombocytopenic purpura in children. Semin Thromb Hemost 1977;3:175.
65. Lusher JM, et al: Idiopathic thrombocytopenic purpura in children. Am J Pediatr Hematol Oncol 1984;6:149.
66. MacKinney AA, et al: Ascertaining genetic carriers of hereditary spherocytosis by statistical analysis of multiple laboratory tests. J Clin Invest 1962;41:554.
67. Manco-Johnson MJ, et al: Recommendations for tPA thrombolysis in children. On behalf of the Scientific Subcommittee on Perinatal and Pediatric Thrombosis of the Scientific and Standardization Committee of the International Society of Thrombosis and Haemostasis. Thromb Haemost 2002;88:157.
68. McClure PD: Idiopathic thrombocytopenic purpura in children: Diagnosis and management. Pediatrics 1975; 55:68.
69. Mollison PL, Engelfriet CP, Contreras M: Blood Transfusion in Clinical Medicine, 8th ed. Oxford, Blackwell Scientific, 1987.
70. Mollison PL, Young IM: In vivo survival in the human subject of transfused erythrocytes after storage in various preservative solutions. Q J Exp Physiol 1942;31:359.
71. Moroff G, et al: The influence of irradiation on stored platelets. Transfusion 1986;26:453.
72. Nilsson IM, Blombäck M, Von Francken I: On an inherited autosomal hemorrhagic diathesis with antihaemophilic globulin (AHG) deficiency and prolonged bleeding time. Acta Med Scand 1957;159:35.
73. Odegard OR, Abildgaard U: Antifactor X a activity in thrombophilia: Studies in a family with AT III deficiency. Scand J Haematol 1977;18:86.
74. Olson RE: Vitamin K. In Colman PW, et al (eds): Hemostasis and Thrombosis: Basic Principles and Clinical Practice. Philadelphia, JB Lippincott, 1982.
75. Oski FA: The erythrocyte and its disorders. In Nathan DG, Oski FA (eds): Hematology of Infancy and Childhood, 3rd ed. Philadelphia, WB Saunders, 1987.
76. Perry GS III, et al: The Wiskott-Aldrich syndrome in the United States and Canada (1892-1979). J Pediatr 1980; 97:72.
77. Pisciotto PT, Snyder EL: Platelet defects and their therapy. In Luban NLC (ed): Transfusion Therapy in Infants and Children. Baltimore, Johns Hopkins University Press, 1991.
78. Prydz H: Vitamin K-dependent clotting factors. Semin Thromb Hemost 1977;4:1.
79. Ramsay NKC, et al: Total lymphoid irradiation and cyclophosphamide as preparation for bone marrow transplantation in severe aplastic anemia. Blood 1980; 55:344.
80. Reid NM: Chronic idiopathic thrombocytopenic purpura: Incidence, treatment, and outcome. Arch Dis Child 1995; 72:125.
81. Rennels MB, et al: Cholelithiasis in patients with major sickle hemoglobinopathies. Am J Dis Child 1983; 138:66.
82. Robertson HD, Polk HC: Blood transfusions in elective operations: Comparison of whole blood versus packed red cells. Ann Surg 1975;181:778.
83. Rock G, Adams GA, Labow RS: The effects of irradiation on platelet function. Transfusion 1988;28:451.
84. Russell SJM: Blood volume studies in healthy children. Arch Dis Child 1949;24:88.
85. Schafer AI: The hypercoagulable states. Ann Intern Med 1985;102:814.
86. Schaison G, et al: L' anémie de fanconi. fréquence de l' évolution vers la leucémie. Presse Med 1983;12:1269.
87. Seeler RA, Shwiaki MZ: Acute splenic sequestration crises (ASSC) in young children with sickle cell anemia. Clin Pediatr 1972;11:701.
88. Shahidi NT, Diamond LK: Testosterone-induced remission in aplastic anemia of both acquired and congenital types: Further observations in 24 cases. N Engl J Med 1961;264:953.
89. Shapiro SS, Anderson DB: Thrombin inhibition in normal plasma. In Lundblad R, Fenton J, Mann K (eds): Chemistry and Biology of Thrombin. Ann Arbor, Mich, Science Publishers, 1977.
90. Simpson MB: Platelet function and transfusion therapy in the surgical patient. In Schiffer CA (ed): Platelet Physiology and Transfusion. Washington DC, American Association of Blood Banks, 1978.
91. Slichter SJ: Controversies in platelet transfusion therapy. Annu Rev Med 1980;31:509.
92. Slichter SJ, Harker LA: Preparation and storage of platelet concentrates. II. Storage variables influencing platelet viability and function. Br J Haematol 1976; 34:403.
93. Smedley JC, Bellingham AJ: Current problems in haematology. 2. Hereditary spherocytosis. J Clin Pathol 1991; 44:441.
94. Snyder EL, DePalma L, Napychank P: Use of polyester filters for preparation of leukocyte-poor platelet concentrates. Vox Sang 1988;54:21.
95. Squires JE: Artificial blood. Science 2002;295:1002.
96. Stevens CE, et al: Hepatitis B virus antibody in blood donors and the occurrence of non-A, non-B hepatitis in transfusion recipients: An analysis of the transfusion-transmitted viruses study. Ann Intern Med 1984; 101:733.
97. Stuart MJ, Kelton JG: The platelet: Quantitative and qualitative abnormalities. In Nathan DG, Oski FA (eds): Hematology of Infancy and Childhood, 3rd ed. Philadelphia, WB Saunders, 1987.
98. Thaler E, et al: Antithrombin III replacement therapy in patients with congenital and acquired antithrombin III deficiency. Thromb Haemost 1979;42:327.
99. Thomas WJ, et al: Free erythrocyte protoporphyrin: Hemoglobin ratios, serum ferritin and transferrin saturation levels during treatment of infants with iron deficiency anemia. Blood 1977;49:455.
100. Vadhan-Raj S, et al: Stimulation of myelopoiesis in patients with aplastic anemia by recombinant human granulocyte-macrophage colony-stimulating factor. N Engl J Med 1988;319:1268.
101. Valentine WN, Neel JV: Hematologic and genetic study of transmission of thalassemia (Cooley's anemia: Mediterranean anemia). Arch Intern Med 1944;74:185.

102. Vercellotti GM, et al: Activation of plasma complement by perfluorocarbon artificial blood: Probable mechanism of adverse pulmonary reactions in treated patients and rationale for corticosteroid prophylaxis. Blood 1982; 59:1299.
103. Vichinsky EP, et al: A comparison of conservative and aggressive transfusion regimens in the perioperative management of sickle cell disease. N Engl J Med 1995; 333:206.
104. Vichinsky EP, et al: Prospective RBC phenotype matching in a stroke-prevention trial in sickle cell anemia: A multicenter transfusion trial. Transfusion 2001;41:1086.
105. Wang WC, Mentzer WC: Differentiation of transient erythroblastopenia of childhood from congenital hypoplastic anemia. J Pediatr 1976;88:784.
106. Zöller B, Dahlbäck B: Linkage between inherited resistance to activated protein C and factor V gene mutation in venous thrombosis. Lancet 1994;343:1536.

第 12 章

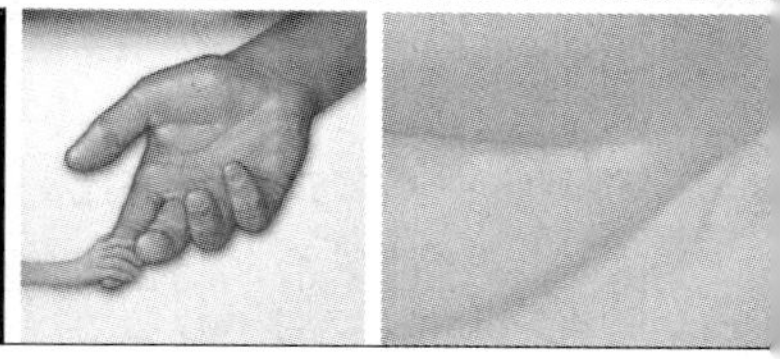

营养支持

Daniel H. Teitelbaum 和 Arnold G. Coran

现代营养支持的发展是近 350 年来许多研究学者努力的结果。1658 年，第一位在促进静脉营养方面有名的人物是伦敦圣保罗大教堂的建筑师 Christopher Wren 先生。他应用中空的鹅毛管为狗灌注葡萄酒。在 19 世纪，第一位生理学家 Claude Bernard 为动物灌注了大量物质。他发现糖在事先被胃液消化后再静脉给予能有效地代谢。这一发现促进了对糖类消化吸收过程的最初的了解[172]。在 20 世纪 30 年代，Elman[62]第一次成功地给患者输注了蛋白质，即酪蛋白的水解产物。1949 年，Rhoads 等人[171]发明了持续为狗输注静脉物质的装置，并证明了通过静脉营养方式能绝对增加幼犬的体重。严格应用消毒技术的中心静脉插管，使 Dudrick 以及他的同事们可以为患者输注高渗糖和蛋白质营养液[59,60,228]。这一技术允许对成人和儿科患者应用全胃肠外营养（Total parenteral nutrition，TPN）。TPN 应用最引人注目的一个病例是一位十二指肠闭锁的新生儿，维持了超过 22 个月的 TPN，并获得了体重和头围的增长[228]。应用这一技术使一些原先可能死亡的先天畸形的新生儿手术后存活率戏剧性地升高。过去的 50 年婴儿及儿童的肠内和肠外营养产品有了迅速的发展。应用静脉输注装置及中心静脉插管允许对大量外科患者进行胃肠外营养（parenteral nutrition，PN），否则这些患者会因为长期的饥饿而导致营养不良。

正常儿童生长

儿科患者最重要的是生长和发育。足月新生儿在生命最初的 6 个月以 25～30g/d 的速率生长，使 5 个月时体重达到出生体重的 2 倍[125]，在 12 个月时平均达到出生体重的 3 倍。3 岁时，体重是出生体重的 4 倍。在 10 岁时，体重增加 20 倍。身长在 1 岁时增加 50%，到 10 岁时增加到 3 倍。早产儿的生长方式与足月儿是不同的。许多营养素在怀孕的第三期在胎儿体内积聚。所以，1kg 的早产婴儿脂肪仅占体重的 1%～2%，而 3.5kg 的足月儿占到 16%。在生命的最初 7～10 天，早产儿预期的体重丧失是 15%，而足月儿常常仅丧失 7%～10%。在这最初的体重丧失期之后，小于 27 周的早产儿体重以较慢的大约 10～20g/d 的速度增长，因为他或她还没进入体重快速增长的第三孕期阶段[176]。

营养评价

营养评价是对外科患者最初评估中重要的一个方面[13]。外科患者中营养不良的发生率在许多文献中报道[25]。Cooper 等人[46]经典的研究显示小儿外科患者中 18%～40%面临营养不良；这一比例在其他一些儿科患者中也有报道[84]。其他存在营养不良危险的患者包括：有大的开放性的伤口、伴有蛋白质丧失以及代谢增长需要；如大面积的烧伤、钝性损伤、败血症等。一个重要的问题是：大手术以后多长时间胃肠道处于功能低下状态。这一信息应被整合到围术期的营养支持中。营养评价分为主观和客观的部分。

主观的整体评价是在病史询问和体检中进行。包括体重减轻（5%说明轻度营养不良；10%，中度到重度营养不良）、厌食、呕吐以及体检示肌肉萎缩（显示重度营养不良）的评估；这些评估对儿科患者需要校正，但不像对成人评价那样确定[184]。客观的整体的评价是应用准确的方法对住院患者和门诊患者营养不良进行评估。

客观评价的部分从基本人体测量的身长、体重、头围开始。将测量值放在国家健康统计中心的标准生长曲线中。从这些量表中可以计算出期望的体重别身长指数。因为身长和头围较少受到额外脂肪或手术后液体变动的影响，身长是一个很好的长期身体生长的指标。营养状态的急性改变更多地影响到体重而非身长，并减少儿童的体重别身长指数。相反慢性营养不良会导致身长和体重的落后。

营养状态的生化检测

血清白蛋白水平是作为慢性营养状态的指标。然而，白蛋白转化慢（半衰期 18 天）。所以，其他一些蛋白指标，如前白蛋白（半衰期 2 天）和维生素 A结合蛋白（半衰期 12 小时），可作为更接近现状的指标。目前没有建立婴儿和儿童前白蛋白和维生素 A结合蛋白的标准范围。理想的是，先测得基本水平值，然后可以用测定水平来判定疾病或营养供给的影响效果。其他有用的检测营养状态的指标包括骨龄和牙齿状况。营养不良常常导致骨骼成熟的延迟[58]。

身体组分的直接测量

过去 25 年来，发明了许多方法能更直接地测量儿童和成人的身体组分。这些方法大多不容易被临床医生接受。然而，有一些方法在儿科中心变得普及。同位素稀释技术测量人体水分已应用好几年。这一方法的原理是脂肪是无水的，绝大部分同位素能直接进入人体含水的部分[48]。尽管这一假设并不是始终是真的，但这个方法能得出最接近人体的很好的脂肪和水的数值[47,90]。生物电阻抗分析方法通过测量人体对电流的阻抗从而测定人体总含水量。利用这些方法可以推断人体其他组分，包括人体总脂肪含量。近来，双光子分光光度法和双能量 X 线分光测量法被用来测量骨矿物含量以及脂肪和人体水总量[28,173]。由于设备精确度非常好，而且放射暴露很低，双能量 X 线分光测量法可能最终成为测量儿童身体组分的方法之一。

营养需要

能量需要

婴儿和儿童的能量需要是独特的。据估计早产儿每 kg 体重仅有 4 天营养储备，而足月儿能无营养存活 1 月[83,154]。在儿童，能量需要用来维持身体代谢和生长。根据儿童的年龄和理想体重得出推荐膳食需要量（RDA）的能量需要，能大致估计出卡路里消耗。能量需要根据儿童年龄和生理的状态是不同的（表 12–1）。活跃的生长时期和剧烈的生理活动增加能量的需要。在一份良好平衡的膳食中热量的平均分布是：蛋白质 15%；脂肪 35%；糖类 50%。

尽管仔细的临床体检对判定儿童的营养状态是重要的，Baker 等人认为，检测体重身高比值、肱三头肌皮褶厚度、中上臂围、手力量、白蛋白浓度、总蛋白水平、或肌酐身高比值这些数值不能可信地测定衰竭状态。对代谢率实际的测量或估计是最好的追踪营养状态的方法。常用的列线图可能高估或低估能量的消耗[97,130,138]。一种最准确地测量能量消耗的方法是间接热量测定[42]。这种方法测定了二氧化碳产物和氧的消耗。样本最好检测暖箱内婴儿的静息能量消耗（REE）。能量消耗或代谢率可以检测每分钟氧耗的立方厘米，如果底物已知可转换成每小时或每天的卡路里。所有的检测只是接近实际热卡需要；医生必须根据患儿的临床表现来调节。这是一个很好的监测患儿的途径，尤其当患儿处于重症监护时[225]。与成人比较，儿童术后 REE 的升高很少。Mitchell 等人[138]发现心脏患儿术后 REE 值低于正常、健康、未手术的儿童。这一发现被 Letton 等人[115]证实，他检测了小婴儿术后能量消耗。这些研究建议依赖 RDA值可能导致术后患儿过度喂养（后面讨论）。然而间接热量测定在气管插管的小婴儿中可能较困难，因为漏气可能

表 12–1 热卡和蛋白质需要

年龄（岁）	千卡（每公斤体重）	蛋白质（克 / 公斤体重）
0～1	90～120	2.0～3.5
1～7	75～90	2.0～2.5
7～12	60～75	2.0
12～18	30～60	1.5
＞18	25～30	1.0

导致结果不准确。

水

婴儿体内水含量高于成人（体重的 75%比 65%）。液体提供了水的主要来源；但有部分由食物氧化和人体组织提供。水的需求与热卡消耗有关，所以婴儿单位体重需要的水高于成人。总的来说，热卡的需要量（每天 kcal/kg）与水的需要量匹配（每天 ml/kg）。健康婴儿日常液体的消耗量等于体重的 10%～15%，而成人仅占 2%～4%。另外，婴儿和儿童食物水含量大大高于成人；婴儿和儿童消耗的水果和蔬菜含大约 90%水。仅有 0.5%～3%的液体摄入被婴儿和儿童保留。大约 50%由肾脏排泄，3%～10%通过消化道丢失，40%～50%不显性丧失。

蛋白质

婴儿蛋白质的需要根据生长和维持日常的需求（表 12-1）。平均蛋白质摄取大约占总热卡需要的 15%。婴儿体重的 2%由氮组成（成人为 3%）。身体氮生成的主要增长在生命的第一年。蛋白质营养价值不仅在提供氮源的数量上，而且在蛋白质的氨基酸组成上[103]。蛋白质提供 4kcal/g 的能量，应该包括在能量产生估计中。

20 种氨基酸可分类，其中 9 种是婴儿必需的（表 12-2）。新生组织不能形成除非这 9 种氨基酸在饮食中同时存在。缺乏任何一种氨基酸都会导致负氮或蛋白质平衡。所以蛋白质的需要在足月儿和婴儿中明显升高（与大儿童相比），范围在每天 2～3g/kg 。这一估计根据几种来源。根据胎儿从胎盘吸收数据外推证明在胚胎第三期蛋白质需要是每天 2.2g/kg[113,238]。新生儿大量蛋白质的需求与升高的血尿素氮水平相关。早产儿蛋白质需求较足月儿高，范围是每天 3.0～3.5g/kg[238]。在极低出生体重儿，可达到每天 3.85g/kg[237]。如此高的蛋白质负荷要由不成熟的肾脏来平衡，所以需要监测尿素氮的变化。三种氨基酸对新生儿是条件必需氨基酸：组氨酸、半胱氨酸、酪氨酸[82,137]。有建议认为，脯氨酸也是早产儿必需氨基酸，尽管还需要进一步证实[179]。另外，牛磺酸对正常神经元和视网膜发育是必需的[236]，并且牛磺酸补充显示可降低胃肠外营养（PN）相关胆汁淤积[194]。早产儿存在一定风险，由此小儿专用氨基酸溶液应该应用 PN 使用患儿（PN＞2 周）。

表 12-2　必需氨基酸

苏氨酸	色氨酸
白氨酸	组氨酸 *
异亮氨酸	酪氨酸 †
缬氨酸	半胱氨酸 †
赖氨酸	脯氨酸 ‡
蛋氨酸	谷氨酰胺 ‡
苯丙氨酸	精氨酸 †

* 仅婴儿必需。
† 可能在未成熟儿必需。
‡ 可能在额外应激和能量要求时必需。

2 种氨基酸对消化道黏膜的完整性和机体免疫状态是有益的：谷氨酰胺和精氨酸。尽管这些氨基酸不是真正必需的，机体在应激状态下需要更多量。谷氨酰胺已被证明在动物或可能在人体中可阻止 TPN 相关的肠道萎缩[191,235]。最近，谷氨酰胺在肠道耐受性的效应受到质疑[34,73,233]。精氨酸显示能提高氮潴留、伤口愈合及免疫状态[12,180]。然而，至少在动物模型中显示，早期给予精氨酸会由于激活消化道的一氧化氮而使预后恶化[109]。

糖类

糖类通过肠外和肠内的途径提供了一种主要的营养来源。糖类可由三种形式供给：单糖（葡萄糖和果糖）、双糖（乳糖、蔗糖、麦芽糖）和复合糖类（淀粉）。由于人体可以由氨基酸形成糖，所以没有必需糖类的量。然而，少量额外的糖类能阻止自身蛋白质来源的消耗，所以可作为少量蛋白质的底物[104]。这种效应导致内源性葡萄糖产物的抑制和内源性葡萄糖的氧化，所以阻止骨骼肌产生的氨基酸的氧化。机体储 197
备葡萄糖的能力有限，尽管作为底物是必需的，而且中枢神经系统需要连续的葡萄糖供给。葡萄糖是糖类最主要的来源，它提供每克 3.4kcal 的能量。葡萄糖代谢通过需氧的三羧酸循环，每摩尔葡萄糖产生 38

摩尔三磷酸腺苷（ATP）；或通过厌氧的糖酵解循环，每摩尔葡萄糖产生 2 摩尔 ATP 和乳酸作为最终产物。葡萄糖在肝脏通过糖原异生的方式形成，使用骨骼肌来源的氨基酸和通过科里循环（葡萄糖乳酸盐循环）（一次转化为丙酮酸盐）由骨骼肌的糖原破坏产生的乳酸。餐后葡萄糖立即吸收，促使循环葡萄糖容量增加。餐后 4 小时，这些来源迅速消失，肝脏糖原作为接下来 8～12 小时能量的主要来源。新生儿糖原储备受限（34 克），大部分存于肝脏。因此，禁食相当短的时间也会导致低血糖状态。

新生儿和小婴儿最早给予的肠内糖类是乳糖[2]。乳糖由双糖酶（例如乳糖酶）分解为葡萄糖和半乳糖，位于肠上皮边界。因为乳糖是小儿童占优势的糖类，乳糖酶在大部分儿童维持很丰富水平直到至少 2～3 岁。无乳糖配方奶以大豆为基础，包含蔗糖或玉米糖浆能提供适合的糖类数量（常见肠内营养章节）。早产儿可能不能消化这类糖类，特别是乳糖，因为乳糖酶在肠道（通过柠檬酸循环）活性是不够的。因此，对早产儿而言，具有 50∶50 混合乳糖和葡萄糖聚合体的配方奶是理想的。

摄入不适合的葡萄糖可能导致酮症状态，这时脂肪和肌肉会由于糖原异生而破坏。稳定的婴儿接受大约占总热卡 40%～45%的糖类。葡萄糖不耐受确实会产生，不仅会表现为高葡萄糖血症，而且更常见的是高甘油三酸酯血症（见后）。摄入高于机体能使用的糖类会产生高血糖症或脂肪形成（在并发症章节讨论）。

脂肪

脂肪在三种营养素中具有最高的产热密度(9kcal/g)。通常，静脉内输注脂肪占所有非氮原热卡的 30%～50%。脂肪的优点是一种很好的能量来源而且提供必需脂肪酸。亚麻酸对新生儿，大儿童及成人都是必需的。亚麻酸缺乏在新生儿可能迅速产生。新生儿 PN 中不提供脂肪 3 天就可能导致脂肪酸缺乏[72,116]。在婴儿，当亚麻酸摄入少于 1%热卡是就会产生脂肪酸缺乏；通常，2%～4%食物热卡应该来自必需脂肪酸。脂肪酸缺乏表现包括鳞状皮肤、头发脱落、腹泻和伤口愈合不良[66]。缺乏微量亚麻酸也可能是视觉或行为疾病的原因。脂肪酸是机体所有组织最好的能量来源，除了红细胞和脑组织。然而，当它们转化为酮体时，脑也能利用脂肪酸作为能量来源。脂肪酸能进入线粒体通过肉毒碱转化酶系统进行 β 氧化（见下文）。

脂肪酸有两种类型的存在形式：即饱和与不饱和脂肪酸。饱和脂肪酸缺乏双碳键，常来源于动物。不饱和脂肪酸至少有一个双键，它的位置由 Ω 前缀来标示。有两种主要的多聚不饱和脂肪酸是亚麻酸，是一种 Ω–6 脂肪酸和 α 亚麻酸，后者是 Ω–3 脂肪酸。Ω–6 脂肪酸主要来源于植物，Ω–3 脂肪酸主要来源于鱼油。这两种多聚不饱和脂肪酸对细胞膜和中枢神经系统的发育以及花生四烯酸和前列腺素的合成都是必需的。来源于 Ω–6 脂肪酸的血栓素是潜在的血小板聚合的调节剂，而来源于 Ω–3 脂肪酸的血栓素是抗凝血的。Ω6 脂肪酸可形成花生四烯酸，可促进前列腺素 E2 的合成，是一种已知的免疫抑制剂，而 Ω–3 脂肪酸可促进前列腺素 E1（PGE_1）和前列腺素 E3（PGE_3）形成，没有免疫抑制的效应（图 12–1）。50/50 比例的 Ω–6 脂肪酸对 Ω–3 脂肪酸看起来是理想的，仅基于从烫伤后存活的动物实验数据[3]。但没有新生儿和儿童理想病例的可靠数据。

可通过计算三烯对四烯比例＞0.4（正常≤0.2）来监测是否缺乏；三烯包括 5, 8, 11–二十碳三烯酸，四烯包括亚麻酸和花生四烯酸和二十碳三烯酸–花生四烯酸。

19

矿物质、微量元素和维生素

最近美国食品和药品管理局修改了每日正常需要

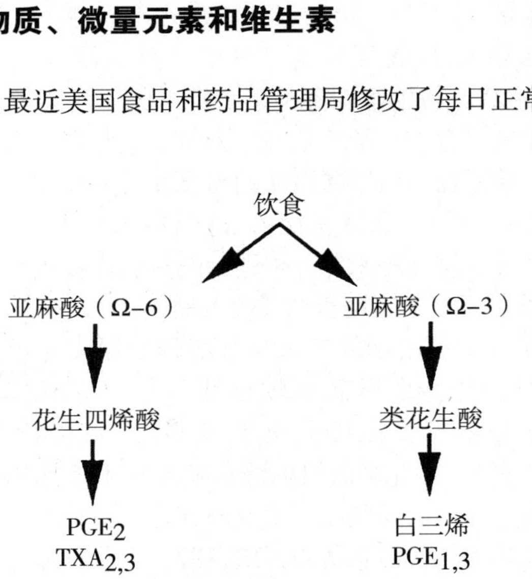

图 12–1 由 Ω–3 和 Ω–6 脂肪酸衍生的前列腺素（PG）和血栓素（TX）的形成。

的维生素[101]。维生素是不同代谢反应必需的组分或辅助因子。许多商品化的婴儿配方奶包含了适当数量的维生素以满足已知的日常需要。这种需求在 1970年代由美国医学协会建立[7]。婴儿如果接受其他种类的配方或母乳可能需要额外的维生素供给。

脂溶性维生素

维生素 A

维生素 A 主要储存在肝脏，与形成视觉与协调细胞循环的维甲酸有关。缺乏维生素 A 可导致夜盲、干眼症、生长不良以及对感染耐受削弱。维生素 A 是否能提高支气管肺发育不良仍然不清楚[102]。然而，有一点是清楚的，就是低水平的维生素 A 使婴儿易罹患长期的肺部疾病[193]。过多的维生素 A 对婴儿是有害的。少于 6000mg 的每日维生素 A 会导致厌食、皮肤脱屑、增加颅内压[122]。

维生素 D

维生素 D 对骨的形成和矿物质的稳态是必需的；缺乏可能导致脂肪吸收不良；然而，维生素 D 过度应用可能导致高钙血症[143]。大多配方奶包含合适的维生素 D（大约 60IU/100kcal）。现在没有证据表明超过标准配方的维生素 D 供给会促进更好的骨的生长。

维生素 E

维生素 E 看来具有明显的抗氧化效应。维生素 E 可能阻止胆道闭锁婴儿的神经病变，以及囊性纤维化儿童的肌肉无力[190]。维生素 E 足月新生儿大约需要 0.7IU/100kcal 能量摄入。因为它的抗氧化作用，维生素 E 用在减轻支气管肺发育不良的新生儿的肺损伤，关于这一点维生素 E 看来是有效的[64]。还不太清楚维生素 E 是否对防止早产儿的视网膜病有效；它也可能减少颅内出血的发生率[156]。

维生素 K

维生素 K 出生时即需要防止凝血疾病，应在生后立即给予[202]。维生素 K 包括在很多配方中，但在婴儿长期的发作性腹泻时需要更大。是否缺乏的评估根据凝血时间很容易做到。

水溶性维生素

水溶性维生素缺乏在人工喂养与母乳喂养婴孩中很少见到。维生素 B 在糖类、蛋白质、脂肪代谢中以及氧化和还原反应中是需要的。缺乏可能在短肠综合征和嗜睡症候群中见到。维生素 B 缺乏首发的症状通常为维生素 B_1（维生素 B_1）水平异常，可用红细胞酮醇基转移酶测定来检测。维生素 C 在几种最优化的酶反应中需要，有直接的抗氧化效应。过多的维生素 C 可能导致肾结石，干扰维生素 B_{12} 的吸收。孕期过量的抗坏血酸可能导致正常喂养婴儿的坏血症。

微量元素

微量元素占人体体重构成不到 0.01% [133]。它们常作为金属酶起作用，这是最大的酶反应，但它们也可作为可吸收离子的辅助因子或非蛋白器官分子。如果没有供给，这些因子特殊的缺乏可能在临床上表现症候群，例如在长期 TPN 时，以及短肠综合征或吸收不良状态。表 12–3 列出了推荐的微量元素剂量。

锌

锌具有多种生物化学功能，包括形成金属酶、

表 12–3　儿科和青春期患者接受全胃肠外营养时推荐的每天微量元素补充量

元素	婴儿 * [μg/(kg·d)]	青春期 [μg/(kg·d)]	缺乏的结果
锌（磷酸盐）	250†	50	皮炎
铜（磷酸盐）	20	20	贫血、中性粒细胞减少
镁（磷酸盐）	1.0	1.0	没有区别
铬（氯化物）	0.20	0.05～0.20	高血糖
硒（作为硒酸）	2.0	2.0	肌炎、心肌病

* 数量超过正常推荐量，推论有明显比例的肠内微量元素未被吸收。

† 每天 400μg/kg 应该给予未成熟儿。

RNA 构成以及膜的稳定[22]。而且，锌看来在维持正
199 常免疫系统功能中扮演重要角色。缺锌可能有多种原因，在儿科手术患者中常见，包括短肠综合征、烧伤、腹膜透析、炎症性肠病以及其他原因的腹泻。锌缺乏的临床表现包括生长迟缓、脱发、皮肤病变（肠病性肢端皮炎）、削弱的淋巴细胞功能以及伤口愈合不良[206]。早产儿最少每日供给 400μg/kg。由于在发作性腹泻和败血症时经肠道丢失较多，这时需要提供较多剂量。另外，锌缺乏可能使肠道大范围切除术后恢复减弱[204]。

铜

铜是一种对金属酶功能很重要的微量元素。主要的铜储存、分布、分泌的部位在肝脏。铜缺乏常见在接受 PN 配方中未添加铜的患者中[99]。铜缺乏的表现包括小红细胞、低色素性贫血，粒细胞缺乏，在儿童包括生长迟缓、骨骼脱钙。婴儿或儿童缺铜可导致再生障碍性贫血而致死[195]。

硒

在过去 20 年，硒被认为是必需的微量元素。它可组成含硒酶，帮助催化谷胱甘肽抗氧化物酶，一种去除氧自由基的必需的酶。一种测量硒水平的可行的方法是测定红细胞内谷胱甘肽抗氧化物酶活性。硒水平在 TPN 6 周后戏剧性地下降[79]。不添加硒，缺乏的征候表现为心肌病变和外周肌炎伴有肌肉压痛。

锰、铬和钼

尽管没有明确的锰缺乏病例的文献记录，锰仍然被认为是多个器官和人体必需的元素。动物缺乏锰会导致生长迟缓、新生儿期共济失调[9]。铬主要的作用是胰岛素作用的调节因子，铬缺乏会导致糖耐受不良。钼对含嘌呤和硫磺复合物的氧化代谢很重要[167]。钼缺乏与血清尿酸水平升高有关。

肠内营养

肠内营养（EN）包括口服营养供给和管饲。如果胃肠道是有功能的，EN 是首选的营养供给方式。即使在完全喂养不能耐受时，小剂量的经口喂养可能防止消化道功能进一步恶化。

适应证

婴儿在术前或创伤前健康良好，能耐受 5～7 天没有充足的能量摄入而不会产生严重的后果，之后开始提供适当的营养支持。小于 32 孕周的早产儿常常没有成熟协调的咀嚼吞咽反射。所以肠内喂养必须采用每 2～3 小时推注一次或持续喂养的方式。在术后肠梗阻解决后即可开始肠内喂养。有很多配方可供不同需要（表 12-4 和 12-5）。有特殊疾病伴有吸收不良的儿童可以从特别配方中得到益处。

营养给予方式

口服摄入以外，有许多可靠的肠内给予方式。这些包括鼻胃和鼻空肠喂养。儿童接受胃的喂养较经小肠喂养能耐受更高的渗透压。而且，胃酸对消化有益，有杀菌作用，更少产生胃肠道并发症[124]。听诊空气吹入管道来判断管的位置是不适合的，确证必须吸到胃内容物或造影证实[136]。对需要超过 4～8 周喂养的患者，更持久的喂养装置（如胃造瘘管）应该考虑。术前的评估包括在 24 小时 pH 测定结果显示上消化道异常后的上消化道系列检查。如果其中一个检查显示有反流，在胃造瘘手术时要考虑行胃底折叠术。术前胃排空也要评估[70,150]。更常用的胃造瘘方法是经皮胃镜胃造瘘（PEG）置管[76]。一种改进的胃造瘘管是胃造瘘"纽扣"，用无反应的硅胶成分制成。它在低侧面的装置内有一个瓣膜，几乎与腹壁平面，能在使用时盖上[75]。这些纽扣在 PEG 同时能够放置[200]。据报道应用 PEG 方法并发症较其他方法少；然而，有几种并发症被描述，包括不合适的位置（即接近幽门），疏忽放置通过邻近的肠道环，胃造瘘管途径的坏死，以及技术上失败要求剖腹手术[17]。

运用空肠管是有麻烦的，问题包括经幽门放置管
随意地移动，因为喂养物浓缩导致管腔堵塞。外科手 20
术放置 J 管近期的并发症包括腹腔内脓肿和肠扭转梗死。长期的并发症包括肠梗阻和腹膜炎。当应用远端

表 12–4 婴儿配方

配方	kcal/ml	蛋白质 (g/L)	蛋白质 (% kcal)	蛋白质来源	糖类来源	糖类 (% kcal)	脂肪来源	脂肪 (% kcal)	指征
Similac Special Care (Ross)	0.81	22	11	脱脂牛奶，乳清	乳糖，玉米糖浆固体	42	中链脂肪酸油，大豆油，椰子油	47	早产
Neosure (Ross)	0.73	19	10	脱脂牛奶，乳清	乳糖，玉米糖浆固体	42	中链脂肪酸油，大豆油	48	早产，出院配方
Enfamil (Mead Johnson)	0.67	14	9	乳清，脱脂牛奶		43	棕榈油精，大豆油，椰子油，葵花子油	48	标准
Similac (Ross)	0.67	14	8	脱脂牛奶，乳清	乳糖	43	大豆油	49	标准
	0.81	22	11	脱脂牛奶，乳清	乳糖	42	椰子油	47	
Prosobee (Mead Johnson)	0.67	20	12	大豆分离，蛋氨酸	玉米糖浆固体	42	棕榈油精，大豆油，椰子油，葵花子油	48	乳糖不耐受，半乳糖血症
Isomil (Ross)	0.67	17	10	大豆分离，蛋氨酸	玉米糖浆，蔗糖	41	大豆油，椰子油，	49	乳糖吸收不良，半乳糖血症
Nutramigen (Mead Johnson)	0.67	19	11	水解酪蛋白，胱氨酸，酪氨酸，色氨酸	玉米糖浆固体，改良玉蜀黍淀粉	44	棕榈油精，大豆油，椰子油，葵花子油	45	蛋白质不耐受
Pregestimil (Mead Johnson)	0.67	19	11	水解酪蛋白，胱氨酸，酪氨酸，色氨酸	玉米糖浆固体，改良玉蜀黍淀粉，葡萄糖	41	中链脂肪酸油，玉米油，大豆油，红花油	48	蛋白质不耐受，囊性纤维病，新生儿胆汁淤积，短肠综合征
Alimentum (Ross)	0.67	19	11	水解酪蛋白，胱氨酸，酪氨酸，色氨酸	蔗糖，改良木薯淀粉	41	中链脂肪酸油，红花油，大豆油	48	蛋白质不耐受，新生儿胆汁淤积
Neocate (Scientific Hospital Supplies)	0.69	20	12	游离氨基酸	玉米糖浆固体	47	红花油，玉米油，大豆油	41	食物过敏，蛋白质不耐受，短肠综合征

MCT：中链三酰甘油。

Enfamil 和 Similac 都是以牛奶为基本蛋白质，包含乳糖作为糖类的来源。仅有受限的原因应用大豆配方，例如 Prosobee 和 Isomil。两者都包含玉米糖浆固体作为糖类来源；Isomil 也包含蔗糖。大豆配方有指征应用于半乳糖血症和原发性或继发性乳糖缺乏，但它们不应用于有过敏记录或对牛奶蛋白不耐受的患者，因为这些患者中 1/3 也对大豆不耐受。水解蛋白或要素配方推荐应用于对牛奶蛋白不耐受的婴儿。水解蛋白包括 Nutramigen、Alimentum 和 Pregestimil。Alimentum 和 Pregestimil 也提供 50%～55%中链脂肪酸的脂肪。当婴儿消化水解蛋白持续出现蛋白不耐受症状时，可提供一种氨基酸基础的配方。对婴儿总体来说，Neocate 是仅有的一种可靠的氨基酸基础配方。大于 12 月的儿童如果对牛奶蛋白持续不耐受，可能对 Peptamen Jr（Clintec）反应良好，这是一种乳清蛋白水解物；如果大于 12 月儿童需要氨基酸基础配方，选择包括 Neocate 1＋（scientific Hospital supplies）、L–emental（GalaGen/Nutrition Medical）和Elecare（Ross）(见表 12–5)。Neocate 1+ 和 Elecare 都有长链三酰甘油。L–emental 的 68%的脂肪来源于中链脂肪酸。

表 12–5 儿科配方

配方	kcal/ml	蛋白质 (g/L)	蛋白质 (% kcal)	蛋白质来源	糖类来源	糖类 (% kcal)	脂肪来源	脂肪 (% kcal)	指征
PediaSure (Ross)	1.0	30	12	酪蛋白酸钠，乳清蛋白	水解玉蜀黍淀粉，蔗糖	44	红花油，大豆油，中链脂肪酸油	44	标准，口服喂养，管饲喂养
Kindercal (Mead Johnson)	1.06	34	13	酪蛋白酸钠	糊精–麦芽糖复合剂，蔗糖	50	椰子油，中链脂肪酸油，玉米油，红花油	37	标准，口服喂养，管饲喂养
Boost (Mead Johnson)	1.06	43	17	牛奶	玉米糖浆，蔗糖	53	椰子油，玉米油，红花油	30	标准，口服喂养，管饲喂养
Peptamen Jr. (Clintec)	1.0	30	12	水解玉蜀黍淀粉	糊精–麦芽糖复合剂	55	中链脂肪酸油	33	短肠综合征，胆汁淤积，胰腺炎
L-emental (GalaGen/Nutrition Medical)	0.8	24	12	L–氨基酸	糊精–麦芽糖复合剂，改良玉蜀黍淀粉	63	中链脂肪酸油，黄豆油	25	短肠综合征，IBD，胰腺炎
Elecare (Ross)	1.0	30	15	L–氨基酸	玉蜀黍淀粉固体	44	红花油，椰子油，大豆油	42	吸收不良，食物过敏
Suplena (Ross)	2.5	30	6	酪蛋白酸钠，酪蛋白酸钙	水解玉蜀黍淀粉，蔗糖	51	红花油，大豆油	43	肾衰竭

IBD：炎性肠病。

进入幽门的管道时，开始推荐应用滴注管饲以预防腹泻和倾倒综合征的发生。在肠内喂养之前要确认管道位置可调，这需要吸引肠道内容物或造影来确定。

肠内配方

配方选择依据患者的年龄和胃肠道的状况。总体来说，足月儿应该维持母乳喂养（见后）或标准 20 千卡 / 盎司的配方（1 盎司 = 28.4 毫升）（见表 12–4 和 12–5）。乳糖基本配方是首选的，因为生理上更接近母乳和更经济。大豆配方是治疗半乳糖血症和原发或继发乳糖酶缺乏的指征。大豆配方不能用于有过敏记录或对乳蛋白不耐受的患者，因为有 1/3 的婴儿对牛乳和大豆不耐受。所以，含蛋白水解酶或要素配方推荐应用于乳蛋白不耐受的婴儿。通过提高给予的量、增加配方的浓度或补充喂养来增加热卡。配方浓度可增加到 30kcal/ounce，但如此高浓度的配方对有些婴儿消化困难，增加肾脏负荷；对婴儿来说可能需要时间来建立对高浓度配方的耐受。高浓度配方也偶尔可能与坏死性小肠结肠炎过程有关[31]。配方补充可通过加入葡萄糖聚合物或脂肪来达到，例如中链三酰甘油或植物油。每 0.5g 葡萄糖聚合物加入一盎司标准配方可增加能量约 0.06kcal/ml，所以产生总热卡为 0.73kcal/ml。加入 0.5g 油入配方增加热卡 0.13kcal/ml，总热卡为 0.8kcal/ml。通过这种方式增加热卡一定要注意，因为如果配方中蛋白和矿物质数量受限的话将影响婴儿充分消耗蛋白质和矿物质的能力。然而，每盎司配方最高加入 2.0g 葡萄糖聚合物或 1.0g 油是安全的。

早产儿标准配方是母乳基础的配方，提供 22～24 卡 / 盎司以及维生素、矿物质、微量元素使之完善。脂肪的部分由中链三酰甘油提供可补充小婴儿受限的胆盐池。中链三酰甘油可直接由内皮细胞基底外侧表面吸收而不需要胆盐。然而，中链三酰甘油不能用于防止必需脂肪酸的缺乏（这要求长链三酰甘油）。糖类由葡萄糖聚合物以及乳糖构成，当乳糖酶活性受限发生时使糖类吸收更完善。早产儿患坏死性小肠结肠炎的风险增加。这风险并不是由于胃肠道启动喂养而增加；然而，喂养增加速率太快显示将新生儿置于高风险。一般来说，喂养增加不应超过每天 20ml/kg[116]。喂养是否通过推注或持续方式给予显示不影响住院结果或达到完全喂养的时间[21,189]。最后，早产儿直到 32 孕周吸吮及吞咽功能才发育充分。

如果一个孩子体重增加不良，热卡密度增加可通过增加配方浓度或粉末而不增加液体的方式。增加配方浓度必须注意，迅速增加浓度可能导致不耐受，以及很少的小肠结肠炎的病例[31]。

母乳

母乳较商业配方有很多优点。美国儿科学会建议母乳喂养到 1 岁，但多数美国母亲在婴儿第二个月停止母乳喂养。母乳对新生儿提供营养和被动免疫保护[6]。母乳包括 87%的水，提供 0.64～0.67kcal/ml。母乳中脂肪含量相当高为 3.4g/dL。母乳蛋白含量（0.9%）较牛乳和商业配方低，但更容易吸收因为其含较高的乳清蛋白。酪蛋白，在牛乳中占优势，是蛋白和钙的混合物。乳清部分包括原始乳清蛋白和乳铁蛋白，一种铁结合蛋白，提供限制铁活性成为金黄色葡萄球菌和大肠杆菌的抑菌剂[120]。母乳含较多的半胱氨酸，对新生儿是必需的，还含有牛磺酸，对胆盐分泌和神经、视网膜发育是必需的。除了微量元素数量适合，母乳较商业配方更有效的吸收微量元素。另外，摄入母乳通过从母体转运免疫球蛋白和淋巴细胞采集被动免疫[162]。尽管母乳有很多优点，更高的对钙、磷、电解质、维生素和微量元素的需要不能仅由母乳提供。因此，母乳增强剂（每盎司一包）应该加入到母乳喂养的早产儿。补充支持应该延续到孩子达到足月儿的体重。

并发症

一旦术后的肠梗阻缓解胃肠道能很好地耐受喂养。重症患儿常丧失一部分吸收功能，由于这些患者常存在乳糖酶缺乏，开始无乳糖饮食症状常常表现为痉挛性腹痛、腹泻和呕吐。给予其他饮食的改变能提高喂养耐受。首先，已明显证明的，胃肠道较渗透压的增加更能耐受稳定的量的增加。所以，通过从 1/8 或 1/4 强度的配方开始，缓慢增加浓度能避免这些副反应。第二，给予配方通过持续滴注的方式可能较推注喂养更能耐受。胃食管反流和倾倒综合征由此而减

203

少。吸入是肠内喂养最大的风险。从鼻胃管快速推注可能导致更高的反流发生率。应用慢的，持续的方式或更好的空肠喂养将减少并发症[140]。然而，后一种方法是有争论的。尽管患者有延迟的胃排空（例如，婴儿有败血症，最近的创伤，电解质不平衡，或接受阿片类药物）或昏迷的有吸入的风险，在情况稳定的患者，通过鼻胃管持续灌注比鼻十二指肠管灌注吸入更少发生[198]。第三，应该注意确定肠内配方不被污染，无论在准备时或在床边，到期时间应该观察。最后，胶质、地芬诺酯、鸦片樟脑酊、盐酸洛哌丁胺等用于失去显著长度的肠道的患者（见后短肠综合征讨论）。对适当的糖类吸收的评估通过测量粪 pH和还原底物可以稳定测定。粪 pH小于 5.5 或还原底物大于 0.5%证明未吸收的包裹的糖类进入粪便。一旦测出，配方中糖类浓度应该减少。

肠外营养（PN）

PN 是通过静脉给予平衡和完全的营养来支持合成代谢，防止体重丧失，或促进体重增加。因为疾病急性期促进能量动员和蛋白储存，应该提供合适和及时的营养来防止营养不良促进逐步的恢复[146]。PN 的指征是当口服或肠内喂养不可能或当肠内营养不能满足营养需要时作为营养的补充。PN 应当应用尽可能短的时间，口服或肠内营养在临床可能的情况下尽快开始。尽管肠内营养能防止肠道萎缩和减少 PN 相关肝胆并发症的风险[226,227,229]，最近的荟萃分析显示肠内和肠外营养的并发症概率几乎相等[30]。

适应证

TPN 对不能耐受肠内营养的婴儿和儿童来说是理想的。临床需要 PN 的状况包括胃肠道疾病（短肠综合征、吸收不良、难治性腹泻、肠梗阻、迁延性呕吐、炎性肠病、肠皮肤瘘）、先天性异常（腹裂、巨结肠、肠闭锁、肠扭转、胎粪性肠梗阻）、胃肠道放疗化疗导致胃肠道功能低下和早产儿严重的呼吸窘迫综合征。极低出生体重（VLBW）婴儿常常对肠内营养不耐受，在生后 24～48 小时需要 PN。在营养不良的早产儿中禁食 1～2 天即可见到表现。大儿童和成人一般不需要 TPN，除非饥饿时间超过 7～10 天。然而，小婴儿如果禁食时间超过 4～5 天就需要 TPN。

静脉通路

根据患者营养需要静脉通路方式是不同的。对婴儿维持短期的 TPN（＜10～14 天），外周 TPN 是理想的。然而，外周 TPN 最大的风险是液体外渗、促使炎症反应和潜在的皮肤坏死。从 1990 年代中期以来，经皮的静脉内管道开始应用。这种管道直径相对较小（2F 或 22G），从孩子的外周静脉放入，在上肢或下肢，进入中央静脉系统。这种管道对儿童和成人都完全适用；常常能维持数周，感染率很低[119,182]。与 Broviac 型管放置要求局部或全身麻醉不同，PICC 常在 NICU 放置，仅需稍微镇静。另外的优点是避免气胸，因为静脉通路经过四肢而不是胸部。外周通路装置费用较 Broviac 型管少，感染率和并发症相当[69]。

如果婴儿和儿童需要更长时间的静脉灌注，中央静脉 PN 应用通过埋置的硅胶管（例如 Broviac2.7 或 4.0F），常常有波形的涤纶套囊。尽管埋置管道和套囊没有显示减少管道的败血症，应用套囊能防止突发的移动[222]。管道可能放入上腔或下腔静脉。最理想的位置是管道头端位于上腔静脉和右心房交界处。孩子的面静脉、颈外静脉、锁骨下静脉、和隐静脉是理想的通路部位。如果儿童体重小于 750g，颈内静脉或股静脉可能需要，因为其他静脉的口径太小。一种聚乙烯氯化物中心静脉管道可以应用于短期的中央静脉营养（如 14 天）。

给药

新生儿一般维持在葡萄糖和电解质溶液（例如，D-10-W，0.2%的生理盐水，20mEq KCl/L）维持速率（第一天 80ml/kg，第二天 100 ml/kg）并在生后 24～48 小时开始 PN。在生后的 2～3 天新生儿倾向 20
于不能耐受高的葡萄糖和氨基酸。葡萄糖溶液浓度一般从 10%～12.5%开始，然后浓度逐日缓慢增加到 20%～25%。检测患者的血糖水平和电解质平衡和检查尿糖来证实患者是否耐受给予的葡萄糖水平。PN

可能从外周或中央静脉系统给予。外周静脉发生静脉炎的风险在 PN 溶液渗透性超过 600～900mOsm/L 时很高[89]。溶液渗透压很高必须通过中央静脉给予。外周静脉给予的儿童最大葡萄糖浓度是 12.5%。因为脂肪乳剂是等渗的，所以外周 PN 是同时给予脂肪能保护静脉延长外周静脉插管[127]。因为 PN 溶液内的钙磷沉淀可能是致命的，所以美国食品药品管理局推荐 PN溶液灌注时通过管道内滤器。0.22μm 的过滤器用于无脂肪内容物的 PN 溶液，而 1.2μm 的过滤器用于完全的营养混合物，允许脂肪颗粒（直径 0.5μm）通过过滤器。PN 应该开始连续灌注超过 24 小时。对接受长期 PN 的患者，给予时间可以稍短（如 16 小时）。重要的是为避免高或低血糖症，在每天开始后或结束灌注前 1～2 小时将速度减慢一半。另外，新生儿，尤其是早产儿，糖原储存受限，常常不能耐受 PN 循环。新生儿 PN 的指导方针见图 12-2。

维护管道防止感染需要精心护理，因为管道常是新生儿败血症的来源[111]。皮肤部位必需隔日用消毒药水清洗并用干燥敷料覆盖[169]。管道和灌注袋每72小时更换一次，给予脂肪的管道必需每 24 小时更换。

肠外配方组成

PN 包括大营养素（氨基酸、葡萄糖、脂肪乳剂）、微量营养素（复合维生素、微量矿物质）、液体和电解质。

氨基酸

儿科肠外晶状氨基酸提供了必需和非必需的特殊平衡来配合儿童发育的需要。新生儿特殊氨基酸配方（Aminosyn-PF，TrophAmine）设计参照母乳喂养婴儿的血浆氨基酸谱。这种配方与标准氨基酸配方比较能促进婴儿更好的体重获得和提高氮平衡[19]。有的氨基酸，如半胱氨酸、酪氨酸、甘氨酸和牛磺酸，被认为是条件必需氨基酸（见表 12-2）。给予早产儿补充牛磺酸是必需的，可以促进胆汁酸结合和提高胆汁流[149]以及降低 PN 相关胆汁淤积的程度。早产儿牛磺酸缺乏的另一个风险是：作为肾脏牛磺酸丢失增加的结果，由于胱硫醚酶活性降低，使牛磺酸合成能力低下[40,236]。氨基酸作为一种能量来源（4kcal/g）和蛋白质合成的氮源。肠外氨基酸大概提供总热卡的 10%～15%。氨基酸开始给予每天 1.0g/kg，2～3 天达到目标数量。为了刺激宫内蛋白质增长速率，低出生体重婴儿需要直到每天 3.85g/kg 的氨基酸[212,237]。足月儿每天氨基酸需要量是 2.5～3.0g/kg，大儿童 1.5g～2.0g/kg，青春期 1.0～1.5g/kg。氨基酸剂量要根据患者的临床情况和营养状态来调整。例如，伤口愈合和透析治疗或持续肾脏替代治疗的患者需要高氨基酸剂量来补充通过透析膜和过滤丢失的氨基酸[53,128]。有肝功能衰竭和高氨血症的患者需要低氨基酸剂量。

葡萄糖

含葡萄糖液是能量的主要来源和提供组织生长的碳骨架。葡萄糖也作为蛋白质不足的底物通过抑制糖异生来防止躯体蛋白质储存的破坏[185]。在大多儿童和青春期接受 PN 时，肠外葡萄糖提供总热卡的 50%～60%。含葡萄糖液的热卡值是 3.4kcal/g。在婴儿，PN 开始葡萄糖灌注速率是每分钟 4.0～8.0mg/kg，来维持适当的血清葡萄糖浓度。新生儿低的葡萄糖数量可由于肝脏产生葡萄糖不适合导致低葡萄糖血症。以后葡萄糖灌注每日提高每分钟 2.0mg/kg，直到达到营养目标。最大葡萄糖灌注率不能超过每分 10～14mg/kg，当 PN 通过中央静脉系统给予时能容易达到[65,197]。

脂肪乳剂

脂肪乳剂是能量和必需脂肪酸的浓缩的来源，提供 9kcal/g 的能量。热卡值根据脂肪乳剂的浓度而不同；脂肪乳剂浓度为 10%、20%和 30%浓度时分别提供 1.1kcal/ml、2.0kcal/ml 和 3.0kcal/ml。美国市场上静脉内脂肪乳剂由长链三酰甘油制成。脂肪常常提供 30%～50%非氮原热卡需要，或总热卡的 20%～
30%。典型的，婴儿和儿童的脂肪乳剂开始剂量是 205
1.0g/kg/d，逐日增加 1.0g/kg，最大达到每天 3.0g/kg。逐渐增加每日脂肪摄取（每天 0.5 或 1.0g/kg）看起来不会增加脂肪清除。然而，当脂肪 24 小时持续灌注而不是间歇或一天中部分给予时脂肪乳剂，能很好

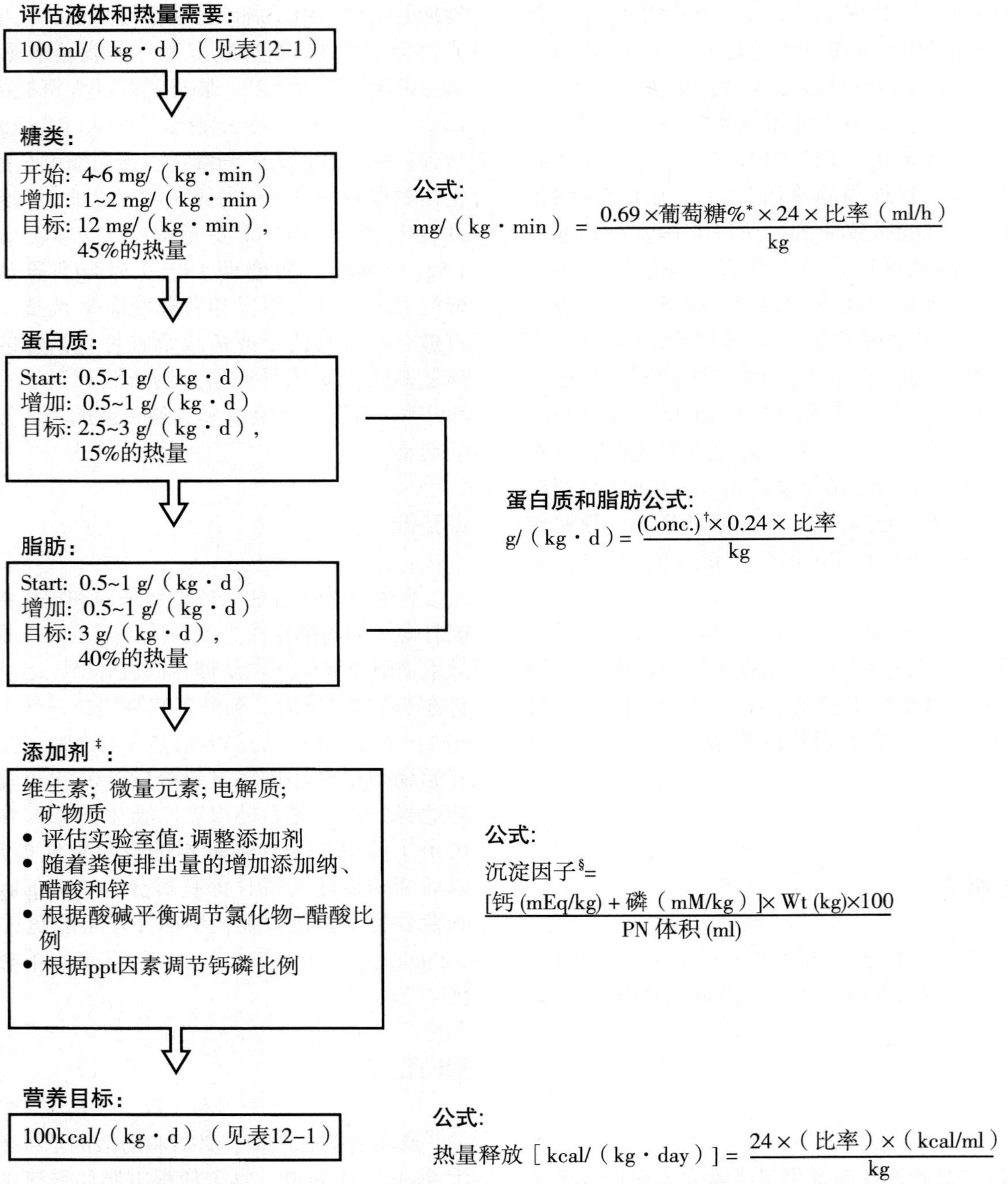

图 12-2 图示如何写新生儿和小婴儿的肠外营养顺序。液体需要应该根据婴儿孕周和体重来调节。* 葡萄糖浓度应该用百分数表示（如 20 指 20%）。† 这种配方浓度应该写成百分数（如 4.25 是指 4.25%）。‡ 见每一种添加剂的相关表格。§ 如果氨基酸浓度大于 1.5%，沉淀因素应该小于 3；如果最后氨基酸浓度大于 1%和小于 1.5%，沉淀因素应该小于 2；如果氨基酸浓度小于 1%，不应该添加钙和磷。如果添加剂（例如胱氨酸）加入肠外营养这些配方必须调整。

清除[29,96]而且脂肪利用增加[77]。脂肪乳剂也存在清除率不同。20%脂肪乳剂比 10%脂肪乳剂好，因为它的低磷脂含量而能更好清除[80,205]。由于脂肪乳剂衍生于植物油，它们也是不同数量的维生素 K 和维生素 E 异构体的自然来源。假设，由于脂肪部分代谢为脂肪酸和单酸甘油酯，游离脂肪酸可能与胆红素竞争白蛋白结合位点，潜在替换游离胆红素进入血清。尽管在过去高胆红素血症患者脂肪限制应用，最近许多动态研究没有显示核黄疸的高风险，除非这个孩子有换血的风险。

复合维生素

儿科肠外复合维生素包括水溶性和脂溶性的。加入每日 PN 中。美国有几种可靠的复合维生素配方，但没有特别设计针对未成熟婴儿的需要。儿科肠外复合维生素提供低剂量的维生素 A 和高剂量的水溶性维生素给未成熟婴儿。高的维生素 A 摄入对低出生体重婴儿是必需的，它们有增加的肺部疾病的风险[102]。在应激状态下水溶性维生素快速丢失。维生素 B_1 是正常葡萄糖代谢的辅助因子。葡萄糖通常代谢为丙酮酸盐，然后转化为乙酰辅酶 A，它通过柠檬酸循环氧化。如果维生素 B_1 缺乏产生，丙酮酸盐替换转化为乳酸，可能导致乳酸酸中毒[175]。乳酸酸中毒曾报道在接受没有维生素 B_1 补充的葡萄糖输注的患者中产生[16,106]，而且在循环复合维生素短缺时致使维生素 B_1 缺乏而导致乳酸酸中毒的死亡率在美国也有报道。

微量元素

标准儿科微量矿物质配方包括锌、铜、锰和铬；有的配方加入硒。微量元素配方是根据美国医生协会营养咨询组和临床营养协会的在缺乏时每日静脉内补充微量矿物质的推荐来设计的[7]。

微量元素状态在患者处于不同临床情况下是不同的。例如，患者在慢性腹泻、营养吸收不良、短肠综合征、烧伤时，锌丢失增加[20,21,129]。锌缺乏典型表现是头发脱落、口鼻周围脂溢性皮炎，偶尔功能性肠梗阻。锌缺乏也与最佳水平以下生长有关，部分由于它在生长激素–胰岛素样生长因子轴中的作用[38,144]。在这样的情况下，额外的锌是需要的，这在标准日常微量元素添加剂中不常遇到。

患者严重胆汁淤积时，铜和锰分泌降低，因为两个微量元素都主要通过胆汁分泌。在长期 PN 有胆汁淤积的患者由于高浓度锰导致神经毒性曾有报道[67,207]。无论给予微量元素的剂量是受限或补充，血的微量元素浓度必须定期检测避免缺乏或中毒。微量元素缺乏并不常见。铜缺乏表现为低色素性贫血、正常红细胞贫血，中性粒细胞减少，皮肤和头发色素缺失，张力减退，意识运动迟缓，以及骨质疏松症。曾有由于铜缺乏导致各类血细胞减少症的报道，一个 PN 依赖的患者伴有胆汁淤积在 PN 溶液中铜受限[195]。

铬缺乏也很少见，可导致糖尿病样症状。硒缺乏长期 PN 潜在的并发症表现为肌肉疼痛和心肌病。这些缺乏在常规接受微量元素添加剂的患者中很少见到，仍然至少每年进行水平监测。

液体和电解质

PN 溶液不能作为急性水和电解质丢失的治疗。替换是，患者需要接受独立的静脉液体来补充水和电解质（表 12–6）。在家庭应用时，液体和电解质常常为了方便加入 PN 混合剂中给予。PN 电解质调整基于血清电解质浓度。调整时应该计算所有电解质来源和丢失，酸碱状态、临床情况和给药影响电解质平衡。

钠

钠通过 PN 溶液提供，可以是氯化物、醋酸盐或磷酸盐形式。新生儿和特别未成熟儿在最初 1～2 周由于肾功能不成熟产生尿钠增多。因为适当的钠摄取对蛋白质合成和组织发育是必需的，必需根据血清和尿钠水平来补充[41]。早产儿可能需要最多每天

表 12–6　患儿每日电解质需要

电解质	日常维持需要
对体重小于 10 公斤的患者	
钠	2.0～4.0 mEq/kg
钾	2.0～4.0 mEq/kg
钙	0.5～3.0 mEq/kg
磷	0.5～1.5 mM/kg
镁	0.25～1.0 mEq/kg
对体重为 10 ~ 30 公斤的患者	
钠	20～150 mEq
钾	20～240 mEq
氯	20～150 mEq
醋酸盐	20～120 mEq
钙	5～20 mEq
磷	4～24 mM
镁	4～24 mEq

207 8.0mEq/kg 的钠。PN 溶液中最大钠浓度不能超过生理盐水水平（154mEq/L）。

钾

钾通过 PN 溶液提供，可以是氯化物、醋酸盐或磷酸盐形式。高钾需要在合成代谢[32]和改善任何胃肠道或肾脏钾丢失的情况下是必需的。PN 溶液中钾浓度不能超过 80mEq/L，钾输注速率在婴儿和儿童不能超过每小时 0.5mEq/kg[203]。患者接受高钾输注必须在 ICU 密切监测心功能。

氯化物和醋酸盐

PN 溶液中氯化物和醋酸盐比例根据患者的酸碱状态调节。醋酸盐在体内以 1∶1 摩尔比例转化为碳酸氢盐。高醋酸盐-低氯化物比例证明有助于改善由于低的胃肠道液体和电解质丢失导致的代谢性酸中毒。高醋酸盐也用于帮助儿童呼吸性酸中毒。早产儿特别有酸碱变化的风险因为肾脏亲水离子的分泌和碳酸氢盐的重吸收功能不全[41,95]。低醋酸盐-高氯化物比例减少由于过多的胃肠道液体和电解质丢失导致的代谢性碱中毒患者的碳酸氢盐负荷。当调整氯化物-醋酸盐比例时必须警惕，因为 2～3 天可能产生戏剧性酸碱变化。

钙和磷

钙和磷在婴儿和儿童由于生长增加的需求大于成人的需要。皮质内固醇和环状利尿剂，常常用于新生儿和儿科重症监护患者，由于钙丢失增加而大大增加钙需求。出生后，早产儿由于尿高磷酸分泌科观察到低磷酸血症。由于磷酸分解为单碱和双碱的形式，根据溶液的 pH，它们应该用毫摩尔而不是毫当量计算来避免剂量错误。钙磷应该以适当的比例和数量提供来优化骨矿化和防止代谢性骨病[165]。骨矿化最优化摄入比例是 2.6 毫当量钙比 1 毫摩尔磷（1.7 毫克钙对 1 毫克磷）[153]。不适当的钙磷比例给予是有问题的，因为其溶解可受限；这样肠内钙磷给予是要求的。盐酸化半胱氨酸，一种可以加入 PN 溶液的酸性化合物，可以用来降低溶液的 pH，允许更高地给予钙磷数量。一种酸性的媒介物，更喜欢单价的磷酸盐而不是两价的磷酸盐，可以另外与钙结合。盐酸半胱氨酸以 40mg/g 氨基酸的剂量加入新生儿 PN 溶液[68]。钙磷能安全地加入 TPN 当用下面的公式来计算浓度：

钙（mEq）＋磷（mM）≥30（每 1000ml TPN 溶液）

对组织和骨生长最佳的需要不能满足除非通过肠内提供钙磷。

添加剂

肝素

在 PN 溶液中加入肝素到浓度 0.5～1.0U/ml[139]能维持静脉管道的通畅[214]和减少静脉刺激[231]。而且，肝素是脂蛋白酯酶的辅助因子，这是血管内皮细胞分泌的一种酶，可以增强脂肪的清除[234]。肝素不能用于有出血或有出血风险或有血小板减少的患者。

组胺$_2$受体拮抗剂

组胺$_2$受体拮抗剂,如雷尼替丁、法默替丁和西咪替丁，与 PN 溶液是可配伍的，可加入 PN 溶液用于应激性溃疡的预防。

常规胰岛素

尽管常规胰岛素与 PN 溶液可配伍，在婴儿胰岛素治疗调节困难。所以静脉内胰岛素应该用单独的输注允许胰岛素剂量的安全滴定。

右旋糖酐铁

铁并不常规加入 PN，缺铁性贫血可能在 PN 依赖的患者中产生。当口服吸收不可靠或胃肠道不耐受时，右旋糖酐铁是外周最常见应用的可靠的铁剂。因为铁能作为细菌增殖的底物， 右旋糖酐铁应该避免用于感染的患者。因为严重的过敏性副反应可能产生，在全剂量使用前应该静脉内试验剂量应用。尽管没有制造商推荐，许多有质量组在生后 4 月内患者中安全应用右旋糖酐铁。每日右旋糖酐铁剂量为

1.0mg/kg 加入新生儿 PN 溶液中以避免缺铁性贫血。铁替代计算见于表 12-7。估计的总右旋糖酐铁剂量能平均的分为增加剂量和加入每日提供的不含脂肪 PN 溶液中直到给予总的替代剂量。治疗剂量右旋糖酐铁不能与脂肪乳剂配伍[220]。一种潜在的安全的静脉内应用铁剂是葡萄糖酸铁（Ferrlecit，R&D 实验室，Marina Del Rey, Calif）。它能优先应用于肾衰竭的患
208 者，也能有效地应用于儿童[145]。

卡尼丁

卡尼丁是一种季胺，在转运长链脂肪酸进入线粒体时需要，在线粒体内进行氧化[26]。早产儿有卡尼丁缺乏的风险，由于他们卡尼丁储存受限和卡尼丁合成减少[181]。脂肪酸氧化减少和血清卡尼丁浓度升高与血浆低的卡尼丁浓度有关。尽管许多肠内配方包括卡尼丁，PN 溶液没有卡尼丁。PN 补充左旋卡尼丁能使血浆卡尼丁浓度正常[27]和提高脂肪酸氧化。早产儿在脂肪输注时不能解释的高三酰甘油血症每天补充 10mg/kg 的卡尼丁可能有益[213]。

并发症

经过 40 年 PN 应用的经验，并发症仍然是儿科患者应用的障碍。PN 主要的并发症分为代谢性、肝胆系统的和感染性。

表 12–7 静脉内铁补充治疗

总铁补充剂量计算
右旋糖酐铁 ml ＝ 0.0476 × 体重（kg）×（Hb_n–Hb_o）＋每 5kg 体重 1ml（最大为 14ml）
1ml 右旋糖酐铁 ＝ 50mg 元素铁
Hb_n ＝要求的血红蛋白（g/dL）。如果患者体重＜15kg，则血红蛋白是 12。如果患者体重＞15kg，则为 14.8。
Hb_o ＝ 测量血红蛋白（g/dL）
最大每日铁补充剂量
婴儿体重＜5 kg：25mg
儿童体重 5～10kg：50mg
儿童体重＜10kg：100mg

代谢性并发症

高血糖症

接受 PN 的患者产生高血糖原发于过多的葡萄糖输注的结果。加剧葡萄糖不耐受的因素包括败血症、手术、糖尿病、胰腺炎、早产儿、和皮质内固醇治疗。血糖在 PN 开始时一致性升高，但内源性胰岛素分泌常常在 48～72 小时调整。未经治疗的高糖血症可促使渗透性利尿电解质紊乱[197]、吞噬作用减弱[4]以及肝脂肪变[71]。在重症监护室严格控制葡萄糖水平显示能明显提高成人抗感染的作用，这一策略可能也适用于儿科人群[216]。

处理高糖血症第一步是降低葡萄糖负荷或减慢输注速率。然而，这可能与营养摄入相矛盾，因为葡萄糖是 PN 热卡的主要来源。如果减少葡萄糖剂量不能改善高糖血症，是胰岛素治疗的指征。因为婴儿对胰岛素治疗有不同反应，PN 溶液中加入胰岛素应该避免。相反，规则的胰岛素滴注应该根据系列的葡萄糖检查。

低血糖症

PN 时低血糖症常常是 PN 输注速率突然减缓的结果。在一天中的一段时间接受 PN 的患者中（循环的），在结束前 1～2 小时逐渐减少输注速率可避免低血糖症。未成熟儿由于代谢反应低下有增加发生低血糖症的风险，这组患者循环应用 PN 是不安全的。如果非持续性的 PN 是不可避免的，静脉给予 10%的葡萄糖水可防止症状性低血糖症[13]。

高三酰甘油血症

PN 患者中高葡萄糖输注是高三酰甘油血症的原发原因。过多的糖类摄入增强了肝脏和脂肪组织的脂肪合成[1]。其他在儿科患者易造成高三酰甘油血症的因素包括未成熟[180]、脂肪过度喂养[10,11]、重症疾病和败血症[152]。尽管逻辑上应该减少脂肪输注，但减少葡萄糖更为有效。如果减少葡萄糖摄入高三酰甘油血症仍持续，脂肪乳剂剂量和速率应该下调，维持三酰甘油水平在 275mg/dL 以下。在儿童脂肪剂量每天 0.5～1.0g/kg 可防止必需脂肪酸缺乏。如果使用 10%

脂肪乳剂，推荐转换为20%脂肪乳剂，因为其更好被清除。卡尼丁缺乏可能也是高三酰甘油血症的常见原因，尤其在早产儿（见上文）。

代谢性酸中毒

代谢性酸中毒可能由于PN中过多的氯化物或氨基酸负荷的结果。为提高钙磷的溶解性而增加到PN中的盐酸半胱氨酸是另一个酸中毒的原因[82]，它能导致钙从婴儿骨中析出。早产儿和肝肾疾病的患者有高的代谢性酸中毒的风险，应该紧密地监测酸碱变化。

电解质紊乱

低钾，低镁，低磷血症在合成代谢和蛋白质合成（重复综合征）中需要增加所致。这在严重营养不良的患者中特别常见，在喂养增加缓慢时应该监测[32]。细胞内常常需要磷来产生高能量磷结合物和骨
209 形成，当糖类输注时可产生细胞内磷转移[168]；缺乏可能导致低通气和昏迷。高钾、高镁和高磷血症可能由于摄入增加伴肾功能降低和高代谢。营养不良患者表现低钙血症常常继发于血清白蛋白浓度减少，伴有成比例的低的总血清钙。

代谢性骨病

代谢性骨病，包括骨减少、骨软化和佝偻病，是一种PN依赖患者的并发症。诊断常常是困难的，没有证据直到观察到病理性骨折。生化标记可能显示为升高的血清碱性磷酸酶浓度、高尿钙、低或正常的甲状旁腺激素和低的1,25二羟维生素D[55,187]。几种易导致PN相关代谢性骨病的因素包括：钙磷缺乏，由于利尿导致钙丢失过多，过多维生素D摄取[188]，以及铝中毒[151]。加大钙磷摄入对提高骨矿化是很重要的。钙缺乏是钙补充受限和继发性代谢性酸中毒[51]氨基酸高尿钙的结果[118]。铝，PN溶液组分，是另外可能导致代谢性骨病的原因。铝通过削弱钙的骨沉积促使骨重塑[219]，减少甲状旁腺激素分泌，减少活性维生素D的形成[107]。早产儿和肾衰竭患者有铝中毒的高风险由于铝排除的减弱。增加的维生素D服用可能事实上是危险的，因为维生素D可能在代谢性骨病病理生成中起作用；然而，确切的机制还不知道。从这些患者中撤除维生素D可导致骨的去矿化增加，解决骨痛，正钙平衡[188]，使血清活性维生素D浓度和甲状旁腺激素正常[221]。

肝胆并发症

PN相关肝胆并发症包括胆汁淤积、脂肪变性和胆石病。多种因素可能导致PN相关肝胆并发症，包括未成熟、过度喂养、PN依赖、缺少肠内刺激使胆囊收缩、短肠综合征和反复败血症[18,210]。胆汁淤积是接受PN儿童最常见肝胆并发症。黄疸可能在PN开始后2～3周产生。血清结合胆红素浓度在2mg/dL或以上常作为胆汁淤积生化指标[210]。预防或减轻PN相关胆汁淤积的策略包括开始肠内喂养、停用PN、避免过度喂养[135]、平衡热卡[35]、循环PN、避免或彻底治疗败血症[35]。药物干预可能包括胆汁酸或胆囊收缩素应用提高胆汁流；然而，两者的前瞻性对照研究证明没有防止作用[85,211]。口服抗生素，例如口服庆大霉素和甲硝唑，用来降低肠道细菌过度生长和减少细菌移位[218]。迅速的直接胆红素的增加是一个强烈的预示即将来临的肝脏衰竭。使用补充牛磺酸的PN溶液显示减少早产儿和坏死性小肠结肠炎的胆汁淤积的程度[194]。在短肠综合征的婴儿中，血清直接胆红素水平大于2.5mg/dL超过4月有80%死亡率[209]，建议一个潜在的移植评估的参考标准[33]。

感染性并发症

败血症是婴儿和儿童经中心输注PN最常见和严重的并发症[56]。发热和突然的葡萄糖不耐受显示败血症发生。持续的高血糖证明增加感染的发生率，推荐进行密切控制[217]。尽管应用严格的消毒技术后很少见，当怀疑微生物污染时应该进行PN溶液的微生物培养。导管相关的感染仍然是接受PN患者最主要的败血症原因。微生物能进入血流：（1）沿着管道路径，开始于皮肤穿刺点；（2）通过污染的静脉内溶液；（3）在抽血或清洗静脉内管道时管道针孔处无菌破坏；或（4）通过远处的感染灶或胃肠道。在这些病例管道作为外来物细菌生长的焦点。减少败血症并发症发生率最重要的因素是管道替换在严格无菌条件下和对管道部位精确的照顾。与管道相关并发症有关的因素包括长期插管、多种目的使用管道、管道针

孔的人工操作和长期 PN 治疗。大多数研究报告，在无免疫抑制患者应用中央静脉插管时，每 1000 插管-天感染发生率 0.5～2.0[105,232]。对免疫抑制患者（例如血液病或肿瘤患者），通常报道每 1000 插管-天感染率 2～3[54,91]。一个高的感染发生率在短肠综合征儿童中发现——每 1000 插管-天感染率 7～9[37,111,140,157]。

几种方法被证明有效预防管道相关感染，包括应用无菌屏障和在管道穿刺处应用表面抗菌剂、抗微生物外套的管道以及规则的管道冲洗。防止和管理管道相关感染的指南已有发表[131,148]。一般非永久性聚氯乙烯管在导管败血症时应该去除；然而，在超过 80%应用硅胶管（如 Broviac 或 Hickman）的患者中，静脉内抗生素应用能清除感染。另一种治疗这些感染的方法是抗生素锁定技术；这允许明显高剂量的抗生素通过导管给予，当它未使用时抗生素保留在管腔内[50,134]。这种技术允许抗生素的应用在正常情况下有如此高的小抑制浓度全身应用时可能导致肾衰竭（例如乙氧萘胺青霉素对金黄色葡萄球菌感染）。抗生素锁定技术在几个中心作为常规使用，但常常在患者不能耐受氨基糖苷和万古霉素时更有效。尽管有高的抗生素失败率，大部分皮下导管感染的患者应该移去管道。大多有真菌感染的患者也应该移走管道。当用抗真菌治疗补救管道时有报道死亡率和高的失败率[43]。念珠菌感染时，保留管道有高达 25%的致死率，很少有机会（13%）清除导管部位的感染[63]。在移除导管后仅需短期（7～14 天）的抗真菌药物治疗；然而，血培养结果必须阴性[37]。在不常见的病例因为先前放置了几种管道，中央静脉通路丢失了，一系列导管部位的抗真菌治疗可以尝试。一种不常见的与 TPN 相关的真菌微生物是糠皮马拉色霉菌。这种微生物在脂肪丰富的环境生长，但是只要离开脂肪，在未移走导管的情况下它对抗真菌治疗有反应。

过度喂养导致并发症

过度喂养能导致许多副反应。过度的葡萄糖摄入由于血清葡萄糖水平超过肾小管重吸收阈值可能导致渗透性利尿和脱水。免疫抑制也与过度喂养有关，并被认为与补体系统失活及抑制自然杀伤细胞的活性有关。过度喂养也可能导致肝脏损害，因为过多葡萄糖不能氧化转化为脂肪（脂肪生成）。这种变化可能导致血清三酰甘油水平升高和肝脏脂肪变性。另外，糖类过度喂养相关的脂肪生成导致高的二氧化碳产生，以升高的呼吸商反映[230]。任何呼吸商值超过 1.0 表示过度喂养；这种高水平可能使重症患儿呼吸削弱加剧，因为它产生过多的二氧化碳。强调在重症监护室评估营养需要的重要性，避免过度喂养可能是困难的。热卡需要最好用间接能量测定评估。对重症患儿过度喂养可能导致液体潴留，这可能使呼吸功能进一步损害。

技术并发症

近年来由于技术不断改进以及用放射技术确认导管位置，在婴儿和儿童中，由于中心静脉导管放置导致的技术性并发症大大减少了。由于导管激惹导致的心律失常已大大减少，因为管道的尖端放于上腔静脉与右心房结合部。另外一个重要点是要保证导管位置不要太中间，因为这可能导致导管在第一肋和锁骨之间捏挤，潜在剪切远端管道进入心脏[87]。甚至适当地放置硅酮导管，在管道处也可能产生静脉内栓子，特别在有败血症和循环减少的重症患者中。大血管内栓子要求抗凝治疗和移除管道。这些栓子导致的肺栓塞和感染在婴儿和小儿童中有报道[208]。溶栓治疗被证明能有效清除导管凝血块避免管道重新放置[92]。这种步骤必须重复至少两次以确保栓子去除。长期体内置管的患者可能由于脂肪或钙沉积导致管道梗阻。这些患者需要接受一系列酒精和稀释盐酸冲洗。PN给予通过外周进入中央导管（PICC）在过去 10 年中大大增加，从 1996 年起，这成为美国 PN 的主要方式[93]。这种方法有避免很多中央静脉置管并发症的优点，而且管道可以在小剂量或无镇静剂的基础上置入[5,39]。然而，栓塞事件比中央置管发生频率更多。

实验室检查监测

监测实验室值是必需的，因为这些值在儿科患者中偏差常见，尤其在 TPN 开始时。表 12－8 给予了监测的指南。全血计数，葡萄糖，血尿素氮，肌酐，和电解质（钠、钾、氯、二氧化碳）水平在开始时和应用期间测定。肝功能（谷丙转氨酶、谷草转氨酶、乳酸脱氢酶、碱性磷酸酶、总直接胆红素）检测应该进行，镁、白蛋白、钙和磷水平应该在开始时和逐渐

表 12–8 全胃肠外营养患儿血液实验室监测指南

	开始	每日	每周 2～3 次	每周	作为指征
葡萄糖	X	X	X		
血尿素氮，肌酐	X	X	X		
钠、钾、氯、二氧化碳	X	X	X		
AST、ALT、LDH、碱性磷酸（酯）酶、总直接胆红素、GGTP	X			X	
镁、钙、磷	X		X		
白蛋白、总蛋白	X			X	
三酰甘油	X*			X	
血红蛋白、血细胞比容、全血计数、血小板、凝血酶原时间	X				X
铜、锌、硒、铬、锰、铁					X
总铁结合力、铁蛋白					X
维生素浓度					X
糖、蛋白质、pH、酮体和白细胞测试片＜诊断用药＞					X
氨					X
血培养					X

* 一旦达到脂肪输注目标，就测量。

ALT：丙氨酸转氨酶；AST：天冬氨酸转氨酶；GGTP：γ–谷氨酰转肽酶；LDH：乳酸脱氢酶。

增加的间期检查。三酰甘油水平应该维持直到达到需要的脂肪摄入水平。

手术患儿中的特殊问题

手术患儿对手术应激与大儿童和成人十分不同。
211 儿童代谢明显受到手术应激影响。然而，能量消耗增加时期明显比成人短[94]。麻醉明显影响机体代谢，例如芬太尼对减少代谢反应有益处[8]。而且在新生儿，蛋白转化和代谢不受大手术影响。然而，PN与增加氧自由基产生有关，可能促使抑制免疫状态。因此，使用 PN 必须考虑潜在的伤害和潜在的利益。

术前营养支持

在营养不良成人，术前给予肠内营养 2～3 周可能减少术后伤口感染、吻合口瘘、肝肾衰竭和住院时间。PN 支持时间不太清楚。一个荟萃分析证明，在轻到中度营养不良患者中术前 PN 仅有最低限度的益处可能增加并发症[108]。最明显的效应在重度营养不良患者中有记录，如果接受术前 PN 发展最少的非感染性并发症（术前 7～15 天，术后 3 天）[36]。然而，PN 患者观察到有感染率增加不能完全由中央静脉置管来解释。这显示应用 PN 可能确实容易引起感染并发症增加。因此，除非有清楚的严重营养不良的指征（见前面的主观总体评估讨论），一种延迟的手术治疗提供术前的 PN 不被推荐[13]。这些发现外推到新生儿是困难的，因为他们的营养储备受限。然而，因为对手术的代谢反应相似，对儿科患者提供相似的结论是合理的。

术后营养支持

术后应用营养支持更加有争议。在成人，供应肠内营养假设能减少败血症发生率和花费更少。然而，营养素不耐受是需要考虑的限制。数据表明当术后营养支持提供时，应该早期应用 PN 和 EN 结合的方式直到胃肠道完全恢复。一项对照研究检查了儿童术后 PN 效应证明对氮平衡和胰岛素样生长因子–1 水平有正性作用；然而没有临床效应观察到[126]。术后 PN效应处理被忽略了[108]。术后时期，PN 患者有高的感染率。荟萃分析研究显示有确实的术后 PN 副反应。当然，术后长期的禁食置患者处于风险[178]。通常，术后 PN 应该限制应用，不可能开始 EN 至少 5～7天的大儿童（在青春期 10 天）可考虑应用[13]。

重症外科患者

对重症患者或败血症术后患者营养管理显示有很大的挑战。临床上，重症儿童表现为肠内喂养不足，厌食，常常有麻痹性肠梗阻。胰岛素抵抗结果是高血糖和高三酰甘油。控制高血糖显示有明显的效应来预防败血症[217]。脏器蛋白质储存随着时间逐渐减少。尽管白蛋白测量由于它的长的半衰期（>8 天）可能变化缓慢，其他脏器蛋白质状态的检测例如前白蛋白水平（半衰期 2 天）更好地反映代谢紊乱。在这时评估能量需要是重要的，而且这些需要在术后或败血症，重症婴儿中常常过高估计。几乎 1/3 的婴儿能量需求倾向于支持生长（每天 30～35kcal/kg）。因为在败血症和重症疾病时生长有停止，明显的能量需求减少可能跟着发生。在一个重症疾病的研究中，术后婴儿，平均测到的基础能量消耗仅有每天 43kcal/kg[115]。然而，结果格外的不同，更加强调间接能量测定的应用，这方法也能提供呼吸商的信息（见前面）。目的是防止过度喂养。尽管没有新生儿的研究，成人荟萃分析数据建议 PN 在大多重症疾病手术患者中没有益处，应该在最初几天有限应用，直到证明禁食时间超过 5～7 天[86]。

胆道闭锁

伴有胆道闭锁的婴儿，甚至在临床成功进行肝门肠吻合以后，通常有低于正常数量的胆汁流进入小肠，这导致在脂肪消化和吸收方面的严重缺陷。这种缺陷可能导致婴儿必需脂肪酸的缺乏和不适合的脂溶性维生素的吸收[100]。这能导致骨矿化的缺少和生长发育迟缓。对这种婴儿必需的目标是用一种配方最大化脂肪摄入来提供适当的热卡。这种患者常常应用的配方是 Pregestimil（Mead Johnson）。这种配方有大数量的中链脂肪酸（MCT）和丰富的亚油酸，当面对吸收降低时来防止脂肪酸缺乏。在这些患者中应用这种配方显示能增加生长。Portagen（Mead Johnson）不能用于淤胆的婴儿因为它不能提供充足的必需脂肪酸来预防缺乏。当 PN 需要时，标准晶状氨基酸溶液应该使用；没有证明对肝脏有益的配方。母乳，对婴儿通常是理想的，可能对胆道闭锁的婴儿是有害的，因为母乳比商业化可靠配方含有更高浓度的脂肪，这些孩子不能很好耐受。

胆道闭锁患者维生素补充是严格的（表 12–9）。不幸的是，补充维生素很少有保险的策略覆盖，除非医学上必要的。经常对维生素水平进行监测是必要的以保证达到充足的补充。给那些提供给婴儿的标准配方补充水溶性维生素应该准备复合维生素。铁、锌和钙缺乏也应该仔细监测。从实践来看，给一个小婴儿服用这许多维生素是困难和昂贵的。许多使用结合形式的脂溶性维生素（ADEK 0.5ml/kg）；然而，维生素 k 可能不适合用这种形式，而应该给予另外的补充（2.5mg/d）。维生素水平应该随访，用个体化维生素纠治缺乏。

胆道闭锁儿童蛋白质代谢削弱；在健康婴儿需要 4%～9% 的能量消耗，但在胆道闭锁患儿需要 17%[160]。Pierro 等人[159]显示，胆道闭锁婴儿 REE（静息能量消耗）比预期的高 29%，仅占代谢能量摄入的 35% 被这些儿童生长应用。

短肠综合征

对短肠综合征儿童的营养支持是复杂的和需要

表 12–9　胆汁淤积症的维生素治疗

维生素（商品名，制造商）	剂量	给药
维生素 A (Aquasol A; Centeon, LLC)	10 000～15 000 IU/d	3.0-mg 片剂 3.0-、7.5- 或 15-mg 胶囊 50 000 IU/ml 滴剂 *
维生素 D: 25(OH)D_3 (Calderol; Organon Teknika Corp)	2.0～4.0 μg/(kg·d)	20- 和 50-mg 片剂
维生素 D: 1,25$(OH)_2D_3$ (Rocaltrol; Roche Labs)	0.01～0.05 μg/(kg·d)	0.25- 和 0.5-μg 胶囊 0.1μg/ml 液体
维生素 E: TPGS (Liqui-E;Twin Labs)	25 IU/(kg·d)	26.7 IU/ml 液体
维生素 K	2.5～5.0 mg/d	5-mg 片剂

* 50 000 IU = 15mg。

TPGS：水溶性维生素 E。

多种方法，需要儿外科医生、儿科消化医生、药剂师和营养医生一起工作。尽管开始的基础或主要的能量来源是 PN，肠内喂养应该尽可能在短肠综合征产生以后就开始。肠内喂养能刺激小肠的适应和防止 PN 相关胆汁淤积的发展。理想的肠内溶液是等渗的，蛋白质来源应该主要是要素。双肽和三肽常常推荐使用因为这种蛋白质来源更容易和更有效地吸收[215]。尽管数据有限，其他人发现更多要素（纯
213 氨基酸）肠内配方喂养能更好地耐受[23]。这种溶液应该有相当数量的 MCT，因为这种来源的脂肪能更好地通过小肠内皮细胞基底层吸收并进入门静脉系统。然而，MCT 没有包含必需脂肪酸；由此，这种脂肪不能作为这类患者的基本脂质来源。表 12–4 和 12–5 列出了为婴儿和儿童分别推荐的配方。除了在早期喂养应用要素配方，更复杂的饮食对达到小肠适应有更大的益处，最后改良的常规饮食应该用来替代[24]。

大量大便排出与锌、镁、钠、碳酸氢盐和钾的过多丢失相关[201]。这些丢失必须被监测。总的机体钠的丧失与生长发育迟缓有关，除非摄入适当数量的热卡[183]。一种简单的检测这种缺失的方法是尿钠测定。尿钠水平低于 10mEg/L 可能说明机体总钠缺失，口服补充（氯化钠或碳酸氢钠）应该作为日常基础给予[177]。大量粪便排出可能是提高肠内喂养主要的障碍。导致大量粪便排出的原因可能包括感染、吸收不良、肠蠕动加快和胆汁酸对结肠上皮的激惹[164]。儿童大便应该间歇性评估有无感染。另外，粪便 pH、还原底物和定性粪便脂肪应该检查。粪便 pH 小于 5.5 和升高的还原底物水平（＞0.5%）说明糖类吸收不良。大便体积应该少于每天 45ml/kg。糖类蔗糖配方不能产生阳性还原底物测验，除非糖类吸收不良。粪便脂肪升高提示脂肪吸收不良，这可能要求修改儿童肠内饮食（如增加 MCT 百分比）。粪便 α_1–抗胰蛋白酶增加说明蛋白质吸收不良，尽管这种情况很少碰到。应用树脂结合物（如考来烯胺）明显减少胆汁酸激惹在许多患者中证明相当有效。然而，过多应用胆汁酸结合物可能导致循环胆汁酸池丧失，更加限制脂肪酸吸收。因为许多短肠综合征患儿肠道运动降低，只有在其他因素去除后（如感染、细菌过度生长、胆汁酸激惹，潜在可纠正的吸收不良）才考虑用药物来减少肠道活动。

肥胖

肥胖成为一个世界性问题，在北美、欧洲和亚洲有报道令人震惊的肥胖增加率[15,45]。在美国，证明肥胖发生率较过去 30 年有 3 倍的增加。肥胖这种增加是令人担忧的。首先，超过 50%诊断为肥胖的儿童会带着这些额外的体重进入成人。第二，许多继发性并发症在这些儿童中证实，包括 X 综合征的前糖尿病状况、2 型糖尿病、冠状动脉疾病和梗阻性睡眠呼吸暂停[142,161]。其他问题包括骨和关节疾病和胆结石。许多这类儿童确定肥胖困难妨碍鉴别和治疗。尽管国家健康研究所一致建立了体重指数（BMI）大于 40 为病理性肥胖[74]，BMI 在青春期有戏剧性的变化，不能跟随线性曲线[166]。更符合的定义是根据疾病控制和预防中心的标准生长曲线的均数和标准差数值。用这种标准，“处于超重风险”定义为：处于 85 百分位数，“超重”定义为在 95 百分位数[15]。影响肥胖发展因素是环境和遗传[121]。肥胖危险在父母之一肥胖时增加到 80% [224]。

治疗这种状况是复杂的，没有先进理想的方法。然而必须有一组方法提供[88]；这包括儿科医生、护士、营养师和精神病学家的支持。关键的问题是当考虑外科干预青春期肥胖患者时需要仔细评估和基于充分成熟到理解这个关系到一生的决定来选择，以及愿意参与到一生的随访。维生素和营养素缺乏在这类患者中常见需要每 6 个月监测 1 次[112]。常见缺乏包括蛋白质、维生素 B_{12}、叶酸、铁、钙、维生素 D、和维生素 B_1。

发育迟滞

营养不良在儿童与生长和发育不良相关。生长发育迟滞的诊断是根据体重低于平均体重百分位数超过 2 个标准差（Z 值为 2.0），结果是儿童落于 2.3 百分位数[170]。生长发育迟滞可能是全身性的，包括身高、体长和其他身体器官发育低于第 5 百分位数，也可能是非全身性的，体重低于第 5 百分位数，但身长和头围在正常范围。通常全身性生长发育迟滞的患者比非全身性生长发育迟滞有更严重的营养不良和患有更大可能的神经系统发育低下；后一种患者有相关的正常认知发育。近来研究显示异常认知发育在生长发

育迟滞的患者可能存在不良的社会环境，常可以逆转[117,199]。

喂养生长发育迟滞患者的方法应该包括多学科参与包括医学 / 社会学和心理学因素。一个系统性评估包括神经病学、吞咽疾病、喂养厌恶、吸收不良和代谢性疾病是需要的。对婴儿营养支持应该从大约每天 50kcal/kg 开始，增加每天 20～25kcal/kg，直到胃肠道耐受适当的喂养。粪便重量在小婴儿应该少于 150g/d。喂养可能每天增加 150～40kcal/kg 到达到适
14 当的追赶生长[155]。也可能要求在营养恢复的第一周配方中补充额外的钾（最大到每天 5.0mEq/kg）。钾、镁和磷水平需要密切监测，因为它们常常在喂养开始时迅速跌落。一个简单的计算热卡需要的方法是每天获得每一克体重增长应该额外提供 5 个卡路里。

残疾儿童

美国 10%～20%儿童因为慢性疾病和发育问题有特殊健康照顾需求[174]。为几个这类疾病，儿外科医生积极参与到患者的营养照顾中；这类疾病包括神经系统发育不良、发育延迟、脑瘫和遗传性疾病如 13、18、21 三体和 Cornelia de Lange 和 Rett 综合征。儿外科医生常常负责为许多这类患者提供营养通路，以及在术前和术后维持营养照顾。潜在的促进这些患儿营养不良的因素包括喂养问题、不协调的舌运动、并列的吞咽反射不良、胃食管反流伴有营养素丧失和由于肌肉痉挛或手足徐动症（肌紧张太多或太少的混合类型）而增加的能量消耗。因为测定这类患者的能量消耗可能不实际，估计的能量需要可以基于先前的 REE 研究。患有痉挛性（高肌张力）脑瘫的儿童可能较正常有低的能量需要；青春期要求总的热卡大约 1200～1300kcal/d。患有手足徐动症的儿童需要可能高于正常热卡摄入－有时甚至高于 RDA 两倍。患有脊髓脊膜膨出的儿童远远少于同龄人的活动；由于这个原因，他们的能量需要只有正常儿童的 50%～60%（表 12-10）。

如果儿童机体体质明显异常，更适合的能量需要的估计根据体表面积而不是体重。在营养补充期间重复评估儿童生长是必需的，因为这些儿童中肥胖常见。因为增加移动超重儿童的困难，肥胖可能增加对家庭和给予照顾者的负担。

表 12-10 发育障碍儿童根据身高估计热量需要指南

状态	推荐热卡
能走动的，年龄 5～12 岁	13.9kcal/cm身高
不能走动的，年龄 5～12 岁	11.1 kcal/cm 身高
脑瘫伴有严重活动受限	10 kcal/cm 身高
脑瘫伴有轻到中度活动	15 kcal/cm 身高
手足徐动症样大脑麻痹，青春期	最多至 6000 kcal/d
Dowm 综合征，男孩，年龄 1～14 岁	16.1 kcal/cm 身高
Dowm 综合征，女孩，年龄 1～14 岁	14.3 kcal/cm 身高
脊髓脊膜膨出	大约 50%的婴儿期后年龄推荐的膳食供给量 可能需要少到 7kcal/cm 身高来维持正常体重
Prader-Willi 综合征	10～11 kcal/cm 身高(维持） 9 kcal/cm 身高（促进体重减轻）

RDA：允许的推荐饮食。

From Nelson JK, et al: Mayo Clinic Diet Manual, 7th ed. St Louis, Mosby-Year Book, 1994.

（洪 莉译 蔡 威校）

参考文献

1. Aarsland A, Chinkes D, Wolfe RR: Hepatic and whole-body fat synthesis in humans during carbohydrate overfeeding. Am J Clin Nutr 1997;65:1774-1782.
2. Akintorin SM, Kamat M, Pildes RS, et al: A prospective randomized trial of feeding methods in very low birth weight infants. Pediatrics 1997;100:E4.
3. Alexander J, Saito H, Trocki O: The importantce of lipid type in the diet after burn injury. Ann Surg 1986;204:1-8.
4. Alexiewicz JM, Kumar D, Smogorzewski M, et al: Polymorphonuclear leukocytes in non-insulin-dependent diabetes mellitus: Abnormalities in metabolism and function. Ann Intern Med 1995;123:919-924.
5. Alhimyary A, Fernandez C, Picard M, et al: Safety and efficacy of total parenteral nutrition delivered via a peripherally inserted central venous catheter. Nutr Clin Pract 1996;11:199.
6. American Academy of Pediatrics: Pediatric Nutrition Handbook, 4th ed. Elk Grove Village, Ill, AAP, 1998.
7. American Medical Association Nutrition Advisory Group: Department of Food and Nutrition: Multivitamin preparations for parenteral use. JPEN J Parenter Enteral Nutr 1979;3:258.

8. Anand K, Sippell M, Aynsley-Green A: Randomised trial of fentanyl anaesthsia in preterm babies undergoing surgery: Effects on the stress response. Lancet 1987;1:243-248.
9. Anderson RA: Selenium, chromium and manganese. In Shils M, Young V (eds): Modern Nutrition in Health and Disease, 7th ed. Philadelphia, Lea & Febiger, 1988, pp 274-277.
10. Andrew F, Chan G, Schiff D: Lipid metabolism in the neonate. I. The effects of Intralipid infusion on plasma triglyceride and free fatty acid concentrations in the neonate. J Pediatr 1976;88:273-278.
11. Andrew F, Chan G, Schiff D: Lipid metabolism in the neonate. II. The effects of Intralipid on bilirubin binding in vitro and in vivo. J Pediatr 1976;88:279-284.
12. Angele M, Smail N, Ayala A, et al: L-Arginine: A unique amino acid for restoring the depressed immune functions following trauma-hemorrhage. J Trauma Injury Infect Crit Care 1999;46:34-41.
13. August D, Teitelbaum DH: Guidelines for the use of parenteral and enteral nutrition in adult and pediatric patients. JPEN J Parenter Enteral Nutr 2002;26:1SA-137SA.
14. Baker J, Detsky A, Wesson D: Nutritional assessment: A comparison of clinical judgement and objective measurements. N Engl J Med 1982;306:969-972.
15. Ball G, Willows N: Definitions of pediatric obesity. CMAJ 2005;172:309-310.
16. Barrett TG, Forsyth JM, Nathavitharana KA, et al: Potentially lethal thiamine deficiency complicating parenteral nutrition in children. Lancet 1993;341:901-902.
17. Beasley SW, Catto-Smith AG, Davidson PM: How to avoid complications during percutaneous endoscopic gastrostomy. J Pediatr Surg 1995;30:671-673.
18. Beath SV, Davies P, Papadopoulou A, et al: Parenteral nutrition-related cholestasis in postsurgical neonates: Multivariate analysis of risk factors. J Pediatr Surg 1996; 31:604-606.
19. Beck R: Use of a pediatric parenteral amino acid mixture in a population of extremely low birth weight neonates: Frequency and spectrum of direct bilirubinemia. Am J Perinatol 1990;7:84-86.
20. Berger MM, Cavadini C, Bart A, et al: Cutaneous copper and zinc losses in burns. Burns 1992;18:373-380.
21. Berger MM, Cavadini C, Chiolero R, Dirren H: Copper, selenium, and zinc status and balances after major trauma. J Trauma Injury Infect Crit Care 1996;40:103-109.
22. Bettger WJ, O'Dell BL: A critical physiological role of zinc in the structure and function of biomembranes. Life Sci 1981;28:1425-1438.
23. Bines J, Francis D, Hill D: Reducing parenteral requirements in children with short bowel syndrome: Impact of an amino acid-based complete infant formula. J Pediatr Gastroenterol Nutr 1998;26:123-128.
24. Bines J, Taylor R, Justice F, et al: Influence of diet complexity on intestinal adaptation following massive small bowel resection in a preclinical model. J Gastroenterol Hepatol 2002;11:1170-1179.
25. Bistrian BR: Nutritional assessment and therapy of protein-calorie malnutrition in the hospital. J Am Diet Assoc 1977;71:393-397.
26. Boehm KA, Helms RA, Christensen ML, et al: Carnitine: A review for the pharmacy clinician. Hosp Pharm 1993; 28:843-850.
27. Bonner CM, DeBrie KL, Hug G, et al: Effects of parenteral L-carnitine supplementation on fat metabolism and nutrition in premature infants. J Pediatr 1995;126:287-292.
28. Braillon PM, Salle BL, Brunet J, et al: Dual energy x-ray absorptiometry measurement of bone mineral content in newborns: Validation of the technique. Pediatr Res 1992; 12:77-80.
29. Brans YW, Andrew DS, Carrillo DW, et al: Tolerance of fat emulsions in very-low-birth-weight neonates. Am J Dis Child 1988;142:145-152.
30. Braunschweig C, Levy P, Sheean P, Wang X: Enteral compared with parenteral nutrition: A meta-analysis. Am J Clin Nutr 2001;74:534-542.
31. Braunschweig CL, Wesley JR, Clark SF, Mercer N: Rationale and guidelines for parenteral and enteral transition feeding of the 3- to 30-kg child. J Am Diet Assoc 1988;88:479-482.
32. Brooks MJ, Melnik G: The refeeding syndrome: An approach to understanding its complications and preventing its occurrence. Pharmacotherapy 1995;15:713-726.
33. Btaiche IF, Khalidi N: Parenteral nutrition-associated liver complications in children. Pharmacotherapy 2002;22: 188-211.
34. Buchman AL: The role of glutamine: Counterpoint. Nutr Clin Pract 2003;18:391-396.
35. Buchmiller CE, Kleiman-Wexler RL, Ephgrave KS, et al: Liver dysfunction and energy source: Results of a randomized clinical trial. JPEN J Parenter Enteral Nutr 1993;17:301-306.
36. Buzby GP, Williford WO, Peterson OL, et al: A randomized clinical trial of total parenteral nutrition in malnourished surgical patients: The rationale and impact of previous clinical trials and pilot study on protocol design. Am J Clin Nutr 1988;47:357-365.
37. Caniano DA, Starr J, Ginn-Pease ME: Extensive short-bowel syndrome in neonates: Outcome in the 1980s. Surgery 1989; 105:119-124.
38. Castillo-Duran C, Rodriguez A, Vengas G, et al: Zinc supplementation and growth of infants born small for gestational age. J Pediatr 1995;127:206-211.
39. Chait PG, Ingram J, Phillips-Gordon C, et al: Peripherally inserted central catheters in children. Radiology 1995; 197:775-778.
40. Chesney RW: Taurine: Is it required for infant nutrition? Am J Nutr 1988;118:6-10.
41. Chevalier RL: Developmental renal physiology of the low birth weight pre-term newborn. J Urol 1996;156:714-719.
42. Chwals WJ, Lally KP, Woolley MM: Indirect calorimetry in mechanically ventilated infants and children: Measurement accuracy with absence of audible airleak. Crit Care Med 1992;20:768-770.
43. Clarke DE, Raffin TA: Infectious complications of indwelling long-term central venous catheters. Chest 1990;97:966-972.
44. Cohen M, Gartner L: The use of medium chain triglycerides in the management of biliary atresia. J Pediatr 1971; 79:379-381.
45. Cole T, Bellizzi M, Flegal K, Dietz W: Establishing a standard definition for child overweight and obesity worldwide: International survey. BMJ 2000;320:1240-1243.
46. Cooper A, Jakobowski D, Spiker J, et al: Nutrition assessment: An integral part of the preoperative pediatric surgical evaluation. J Pediatr Surg 1982;16:554.
47. Coran AG, Drongowski RA: Body fluid compartment changes following neonatal surgery. J Pediatr Surg 1989; 24:829-832.
48. Coran AG, Drongowski RA, Wesley JR: Changes in total body water and extracellular fluid volume in infants receiving total parenteral nutrition. J Pediatr Surg 1984;19:771-776.
49. Cornblath M, Hawdon JM, Williams AF, et al: Controversies regarding the definition of neonatal hypoglycemia: Suggested operational thresholds. Pediatrics 2000;105:

1141-1145.
50. Cowan CE: Antibiotic lock technique. J Intraven Nurs 1992;15:283-287.
51. Cunningham J, Fraher LJ, Clemens TL, et al: Chronic acidosis with metabolic bone disease. Am J Med 1982;73:199-204.
52. Dahlstrom KA, Ament ME, Moukarzel AA, et al: Low blood and plasma carnitine levels in children receiving long-term parenteral nutrition. J Pediatr Gastroenterol Nutr 1990; 11:375-379.
53. Davies SP, Reaveley DA, Brown EA, et al: Amino acid clearances and daily losses in patients with acute renal failure treated by continuous arteriovenous hemodialysis. Crit Care Med 1991;19:1510-1515.
54. Dawson S, Pai MKR, Smith S, et al: Right atrial catheters in children with cancer: A decade of experience in the use of tunnelled, exteriorized devices at a single institution. Am J Pediatr Hematol Oncol 1991;13:126-129.
55. de Vernejoul MC, Messing B, Modrowski D, et al: Multifactorial low remodeling bone disease during cyclic total parenteral nutrition. J Clin Endocrinol Metab 1985;60:109.
56. Donnell S, Taylor N, van Saene H, et al: Infection rates in surgical neonates and infants receiving parenteral nutrition: A five-year prospective study. J Hosp Infect 2002;52:273-280.
57. Donowitz LG, Hendley JO: Short-course amphotericin B therapy for candidemia in pediatric patients. Pediatrics 1995;95:888-891.
58. Dreizen S, Spirakis CN, Stone RE: A comparison of skeletal growth in maturation in under nourished and well nourished girls before and after menarche. J Pediatr 1967;70:256.
59. Dudrick S, Groff D, Wilmore D: Long term venous catheterization in infants. Surg Gynecol Obstet 1969;129:805-808.
60. Dudrick S, Wilmore D, Vars H, Rhoads J: Can intravenous feeding as the sole means of nutrition support growth in the child and restore weight loss in an adult? An affirmative answer. Ann Surg 1969;169:974-984.
61. Eddy T, Nicholson A, Wheeler E: Energy expenditures and dietary intakes in cerebral palsy. Dev Med Child Neurol 1965;7:377-380.
62. Elman R: Amino acid content of blood following intravenous injection of hydrolyzed casein. Proc Soc Exp Biol Med 1937;37:437.
63. Eppes SC, Troutman JL, Gutman LT: Outcome of treatment of candidemia in children whose central catheters were removed or retained. Pediatr Infect Dis J 1989;8:99-104.
64. Falciglia H, Johnson J, Sullivan J, et al: Role of antioxidant nutrients and lipid peroxidation in premature infants with respiratory distress syndrome and bronchopulmonary dysplasia. Am J Perinatol 2003;20:97-107.
65. Farrag HM, Nawrath LM, Healey JE, et al: Persistent glucose production and greater peripheral sensitivity to insulin in the neonate vs the adult. Am J Physiol 1997;272:E86-E93.
66. Feuerstein G, Hallenbeck JM: Leukotrienes in health and disease. FASEB J 1987;1:186-192.
67. Fitzgerald K, Mikalunas V, Rubin H, et al: Hypermanganesemia in patients receiving total parenteral nutrition. JPEN J Parenter Enteral Nutr 1999;23:333-336.
68. Fitzgerald KA, MacKay MW: Calcium and phosphate solubility in neonatal parenteral nutrient solutions containing TrophAmine. Am J Hosp Pharm 1986;43:88-93.
69. Foley MJ: Radiologic placement of long-term central venous peripheral access system ports (PAS Port): Results in 150 patients. J Vasc Interv Radiol 1995;6:255-262.
70. Fonkalsrud EW, Ellis DG, Shaw A, et al: A combined hospital experience with fundoplication and gastric emptying procedure for gastroesophageal reflux in children. J Am Coll Surg 1995;180:449-455.
71. Forsyth JS, Crighton A: Low birthweight infants and total parenteral nutrition immediately after birth. I. Energy expenditure and respiratory quotient of ventilated and non-ventilated infants. Arch Dis Child Fetal Neonatal Ed 1995;73:F4-F7.
72. Friedman Z, Danon A, Stahlman MT, Oates JA: Rapid onset of essential fatty acid deficiency in the newborn. Pediatrics 1976;58:640-649.
73. Fukatsu K, Ueno C, Hashiguchi Y, et al: Glutamine infusion during ischemia is detrimental in a murine gut ischemia/reperfusion model. JPEN J Parenter Enteral Nutr 2003;27:187-192.
74. Gastrointestinal surgery for severe obesity: Proceedings of a National Institutes of Health Consensus Development Conference. Am J Clin Nutr 1992;55:487S-619S.
75. Gauderer ML, Picha GJ, Izant RJ Jr: The gastrostomy "button"—a simple skin-level, non-refluxing device for long-term enteral feedings. J. Pediatr Surg 1984;19:803-805.
76. Gauderer ML, Ponsky JL, Izant RJ Jr: Gastrostomy without laparotomy: A percutaneous endoscopic technique. J Pediatr Surg 1980;15:872-875.
77. Ghisolfi J, Garcia J, Thouvenot JP, et al: Plasma phospholipid fatty acids and urinary excretion of prostaglandins PGE_1 and PGE_2 in infants during total parenteral nutrition, with continuous or sequential administration of fat emulsion. JPEN J Parenter Enteral Nutr 1986;10:631-634.
78. Gutcher GR, Lax AA, Farrell PM: Tocopherol isomers in intravenous lipid emulsions and resultant plasma concentrations. JPEN J Parenter Enteral Nutr 1984;8:269-273.
79. Hankins DA, Riella MC, Scribner BH, Babb AL: Whole blood trace element concentrations during total parenteral nutrition. Surgery 1976;79:674-677.
80. Haumont D, Deckelbaum RJ, Richelle M, et al: Plasma lipid and plasma lipoprotein concentration in low birht weight infants given parenteral nutrition with 20 or 10 percent lipid emulsions. J Pediatr 1989;115:787-793.
81. Haumont D, Richelle M, Deckelbaum RJ, et al: Effect of liposomal content of lipid emulsions on plasma lipid concentrations in low birth weight infants receiving parenteral nutrition. J Pediatr 1992;121:759-763.
82. Heird WC, Gomez MR: Parenteral nutrition in low-birth-weight infants. Annu Rev Nutr 1996;16:471-499.
83. Heird WC, Kashyap S, Gomez MR: Protein intake and energy requirements of the infant. Semin Perinatol 1991; 15:438-448.
84. Hendricks K, Duggan C, Gallagher I: Malnutrition in hospitalized pediatric patients: Current prevalence. Arch Pediatr Asolesc Med 1995;149:1118-1120.
85. Heubi JE, Wiechmann DA, Creutzinger V, et al: Tauroursodeoxycholic acid (TUDCA) in the prevention of total parenteral nutrition-associated liver disease. J Pediatr 2002;141:237-242.
86. Heyland DK, MacDonald S, Keefe L, Drover JW: Total parenteral nutrition in the critically ill patient: A meta-analysis. JAMA 1998;280:2013-2019.
87. Hinke DH, Zandt-Stastny DA, Goodman LR, et al: Pinch-off syndrome: A complication of implantable subclavian venous access devices. Radiology 1990;177: 353-356.
88. Inge T, Zeller M, Garcia V, Daniels S: Surgical approach to adolescent obesity. Adolesc Med Clin 2004;15: 429-453.
89. Isaacs JW, Millikan WJ, Stackhouse J, et al: Parenteral nutrition of adults with 900-milliosmolar solution via peripheral veins. Am J Clin Nutr 1977;30:552-559.

90. Jensen MD: Research techniques for body composition assessment. J Am Diet Assoc 1992;92:454-460.
91. Johnson PR, Decker MD, Edwards KM, et al: Frequency of Broviac catheter infections in pediatric oncology patients. J Infect Dis 1986;154:570-578.
92. Jones GR, Konsler GK, Dunaway RP, et al: Prospective analysis of urokinase in the treatment of catheter sepsis in pediatric hematology-oncology patients. J Pediatr Surg 1993; 28:350-355.
93. Jones K, Kovacevich D, Teitelbaum D: Establishing a comprehensive database for home parenteral nutrition: Six years of data. Nutr Clin Pract 2000;15:279-286.
94. Jones M, Pierro A, Hammond P, Lloyd D: The metabolic response to operative stress in infants. J Pediatr Surg 1993; 28:1258-1263.
95. Kalhoff H, Wiese B, Kunz C, et al: Increased renal net acid excretion in prematures below 1600 g body weight compared with prematures and small-for-date newborns above 2100 g on alimentation with commercial preterm formula. Biol Neonate 1994;66:10-15.
96. Kao LC, Cheng MH, Warburton D: Triglycerides, free fatty acids, free fatty acids/albumin molar ratio, and cholesterol levels in serum of neonates receiving long-term lipid infusions: Controlled trial of continuous vs intermittent regimens. J Pediatr 1984;104:429-435.
97. Kaplan AS, Zemel BS, Neiswender KM, Stallings VA: Resting energy expenditure in clinical pediatrics: Measured versus prediction equations. J Pediatr 1995;127:200-205.
98. Karlen J, Aperia A, Zetterstorm R: Renal excretion of calcium and phosphate in preterm and term infants. J Pediatr 1985;106:814-819.
99. Karpel JT, Peden VH: Copper deficiency in long-term parenteral nutrition. J Pediatr 1972;80:32-34.
100. Kaufman S, Murray N, Wood R: Nutritional support for the infant with extrahepatic biliary atresia. J Pediatr 1987; 110:679-685.
101. Kelly D: Guidelines and available products for parenteral vitamins and trace elements. JPEN J Parenter Enteral Nutr 2002;26:S34-S36.
102. Kennedy KA, Stoll BJ, Ehrenkranz RA, et al: Vitamin A to prevent bronchopulmonary dysplasia in very-low-birth-weight infants: Has the dose been too low? Early Hum Dev 1997;49:19-31.
103. Keshan TH, Miller RG, Jahoor F, Jaksic T: Stable isotopic quantitation of protein metabolism and energy expenditure in neonates on- and post-extracorporeal life support. J Pediatr Surg 1997;32:958-963.
104. Kien L: Carbohydrates. In Tsang RC, Lucas A, Vauy R (eds): Nutritional Needs of the Preterm Infant: Scientific Basis and Practical Guidelines. Baltimore, Williams & Wilkins, 1993, pp 47-63.
105. King DR, Komer M, Hoffman J, et al: Broviac catheter sepsis: The natural history of an iatrogenic infection. J Pediatr Surg 1985;20:728-733.
106. Kitamura K, Takahashi T, Tanaka H, et al: Two cases of thiamine deficiency-induced lactic acidosis during total parenteral nutrition. Tohoku J Exp Med 1993;171:129-133.
107. Klein GL, Berquist WE, Ament ME, et al: Hepatic aluminum accumulation in children on total parenteral nutrition. J Pediatr Gastroenterol Nutr 1984;3:740-743.
108. Klein S, Kinney J, Jeejeebhoy K, et al: Nutrition support in clinical practice: Review of published data and recommendations for future research directions. JPEN J Parenter Enteral Nutr 1997;21:133-156.
109. Kozar R, Verner-Cole E, Schultz S, et al: The immune-enhancing enteral agents arginine and glutamine differentially modulate gut barrier function following mesenteric ischemia/reperfusion. J Trauma 2004;57: 1150-1156.
110. Krick J, Murphy P, Markham J, Shapiro B: A proposed formula for calculating energy needs of children with cerebral palsy. Dev Med Child Neurol 1992;34:481-487.
111. Kurkchubasche AG, Smith SD, Rowe MI: Catheter sepsis in short-bowel syndrome. Arch Surg 1992;127:21-25.
112. Kushner R: Managing the obese patient after bariatric surgery: A case report of severe malnutrition and review of the literature. JPEN J Parenter Enteral Nutr 2000;24:126-132.
113. Lemons J: Fetal-placental nitrogen metabolism. Semin Perinatol 1979;3:177-190.
114. Lennon C, Davidson KW, Sadowski JA, et al: The vitamin K content of intravenous lipid emulsions. JPEN J Parenter Enteral Nutr 1993;17:142-144.
115. Letton RW, Chwals WJ, Jamie A, Charles B: Early postoperative alterations in infant energy use increase the risk of overfeeding. J Pediatr Surg 1995;30:988-993.
116. Leung FY: Nutrient needs and feeding of premature infants: Nutrition Committee, Canadian Paediatric Society. Trace elements in parenteral micronutrition. Can Med Assoc J 1995;152:1765-1785.
117. Levitsky DA, Strupp BJ: Malnutrition and the brain: Changing concepts, changing concerns. J Nutr 1995;125: 2212S-2220S.
118. Lipkin EW, Ott SM, Chesnut CHI: Mineral loss in the parenteral nutrition patient. Am J Clin Nutr 1988;47: 515-523.
119. Lundberg G, Wahlberg E, Rickberg A, Olofsson P: PAS-Port: A new implantable vascular access device for arm placement: Experiences from the first two years. Eur J Surg 1995;161:323-326.
120. Mackie R, Sghir A, Gaskins HR: Developmental microbial ecology of the neonatal gastrointestinal tract. Am J Clin Nutr 1999;69:1035S-1045S.
121. Maffeis C: Childhood obesity: The genetic-environmental interface. Best Pract Res Clin Endocrinol Metab 1999;13: 31-46.
122. Mahoney C, Margolis M, Knauss TA, Labbe R: Chronic vitamin A intoxication in infants fed chicken liver. Pediatrics 1980;65:893-896.
123. Maini B, Blackburn GL, Bistrian BR, et al: Cyclic hyperalimentation: An optimal technique for preservation of visceral proteins. J Surg Res 1976;20:515-525.
124. Marian M: Pediatric nutrition support. Nutr Clin Pract 1993;8:199-209.
125. Marian M, Rappaport W, Cunningham D, et al: The failure of conventional methods to promote spontaneous transpyloric feeding tube passage and the safety of intragastric feeding in the critically ill ventilated patient. Surg Gynecol Obstet 1993;176:475-479.
126. Marvin V, Rebollo M, Castillo-Duran C, et al: Controlled study of early postoperative parenteral nutrition in children. J Pediatr Surg 1999;34:1330-1335.
127. Matsusue S, Nishimura S, Koizumi S, et al: Preventive effect of simultaneously infused lipid emulsion against thrombophlebitis during postoperative peripheral parenteral nutrition. Surg Today 1995;25:667-671.
128. Maxvold N, Smoyer W, Custer J, et al: Amino acid loss and nitrogen balance in critically ill children with acute renal failure: A prospective comparison between classic hemofiltration vs hemofiltration with dialysis. Crit Care Med 2000; 28:1161-1165.
129. McClain CJ: Zinc metabolism in malabsorption syndromes. J Am Coll Nutr 1985;4:49-64.

130. Mendeloff E, Wesley J, Deckert R: Comparison of measured resting energy expenditure (REE) versus estimated energy expenditure (EEE) in infants. JPEN J Parenter Enteral Nutr 1986;10(Suppl):65.
131. Mermel LA: Prevention of catheter-related infections. Ann Intern Med 2000;132:391-402.
132. Merritt RJ, Kalsch M, Roux LD: Significance of hypoalbuminemia in pediatric oncology patients—malnutrition or infection? JPEN J Parenter Enteral Nutr 1985;9:303-306.
133. Mertz W: The essential trace elements. Science 1981;18: 1332-1338.
134. Messing B, Peitra-Cohen S, Debure A, et al: Antibiotic-lock technique: A new approach to optimal therapy for catheter-related sepsis in home-parenteral nutrition patients. JPEN J Parenter Enteral Nutr 1988;12:185-189.
135. Messing B, Zarka Y, Lemann M, et al: Chronic cholestasis associated with long-term parenteral nutrition. Transplant Proc 1994;26:1438-1439.
136. Metheny N, Dettenmeier P, Hampton K, et al: Detection of inadvertent respiratory placement of small-bore feeding tubes: A report of 10 cases. Heart Lung 1990;19:631-638.
137. Miller RG, Jahoor F, Jaksic T: Decreased cysteine and proline synthesis in parenterally fed, premature infants. J Pediatr Surg 1995;30:953-957.
138. Mitchell IM, Davies PSW, Day JME, et al: Energy expenditure in children with congenital heart disease, before and after cardiac surgery. J Thorac Cardiovasc Surg 1994;107: 374-380.
139. Moclair A, Bates I: The efficacy of heparin in maintaining peripheral infusions in neonates. Eur J Pediatr 1995;154: 567-570.
140. Montecalvo M, Steger K, Farber H, et al: Nutritional outcome and pneumonia in critical care patients randomized to gastric versus jejunal tube feedings. Crit Care Med 1992;20:1377-1387.
141. Moukarzel AA, Haddad I, Ament ME, et al: 230 Patient years of experience with home long-term parenteral nutrition in childhood: Natural history and life of central venous catheters. J Pediatr Surg 1994;29:1323-1327.
142. Must A, Jacques P, Dallal G, et al: Long-term morbidity and mortality of overweight adolescents: A follow-up of the Harvard Growth Study of 1922 to 1935. N Engl J Med 1992;327:1350-1355.
143. National Academy of Sciences: Hazards of overuse of vitamin D. Am J Clin Nutr 1975;28:512-516.
144. Ninh N, Maiter D, Veniers J, et al: Failure of exogenous insulin-like growth factor-I to restore normal growth in rats submitted to dietary zinc deprivation. J Endocrinol 1998;159:211-217.
145. Nissenson A, Lindsay R, Swan S, et al: Sodium ferric gluconate complex in sucrose is safe and effective in hemodialysis patients: North American clinical trial. Am J Kidney Dis 1999;35:360-361.
146. Nordenstrom J, Pesson E: Energy supply during total parenteral nutrition—how much and what source? Acta Anaesthesiol Scand 1985;29:95-99.
147. Offenbacher EG, Pi-Sunyer FX: Chromium in human nutrition. Annu Rev Nutr 1988;8:543-563.
148. O'Grady NP, Alexander M, Dellinger EP, et al: Guidelines for the prevention of intravascular catheter-related infections: Centers for Disease Control and Prevention. MMWR Morb Mortal Wkly Rep 2002;51:1-29.
149. Okamoto E, Rassin DK, Zucker CL, et al: Role of taurine in feeding the low-birth-weight infant. J Pediatr 1984;104: 936-940.
150. Okuyama H, Urao M, Starr G, et al: A comparison of the efficacy of pyloromyotomy and pyloroplasty in patients with gastroesophageal reflux and delayed gastric empyting. J Pediatr Surg 1997;32:316-320.
151. Ott SM, Maloney NA, Klein GL, et al: Aluminum is associated with low bone formation in patients receiving chronic parenteral nutrition. Ann Intern Med 1983;98:910-914.
152. Park W, Paust H, Schroder H: Lipid infusion in premature infants suffering from sepsis. JPEN J Parenter Enteral Nutr 1984;8:290-292.
153. Pelegano JF, Rowe JC, Carey DE, et al: Effect of calcium/phosphorus ratio on mineral retention in parenterally fed premature infants. J Pediatr Gastroenterol Nutr 1991;12:351-355.
154. Pereira GR, Zeigler MM: Nutritional care of the surgical neonate. Clin Perinatol 1989;16:233.
155. Peterson KE, Washington J, Rathbun JM: Team management of failure to thrive. J Am Diet Assoc 1984;84:810-815.
156. Phelps DL: The role of vitamin E therapy in high-risk neonates. Clin Perinatol 1988;15:955-963.
157. Piedra P, Dryja D, LaScolea L Jr: Incidence of catheter-associated gram-negative bacteremia in children with short bowel syndrome. J Clin Microbiol 1989;6:1317-1319.
158. Pierro A: Metabolism and nutritional support in the surgical neonate. J Pediatr Surg 2002;37:811-822.
159. Pierro A, Jones MO, Hammond P, et al: A new equation to predict the resting energy expenditure of surgical infants. J Pediatr Surg 1994;29:1103-1108.
160. Pierro A, Koletzko B, Carnielli V: Resting energy expenditure is increased in infants and children with extrahepatic biliary atresia. J Pediatr Surg 1989;24:534-539.
161. Pinhas-Hamiel O, Dolan LM, Daniels SR, et al: Increased incidence of non-insulin-dependent diabetes mellitus among adolescents. J Pediatr 1996;128:608-615.
162. Pittard WBI: Breast milk immunology: A frontier in infant nutrition. Am J Dis Child 1987;133:83-87.
163. Pollack A, Cowett RM, Schwartz R, Oh W: Glucose disposal in low-birth-weight infants during steady-state hyperglycemia: Effects of exogenous insulin administration. Pediatrics 1978;61:546-549.
164. Potter G: Bile acid diarrhea. Dig Dis 1998;16:118-124.
165. Prestridge LL, Schanler RJ, Shulman R, et al: Effect of parenteral calcium and phosphorus on mineral retention and bone mineral content in very low birth weight infants. J Pediatr 1993;122:761-768.
166. Prevention CfDCa: CDC growth charts. In Report no. 314. Atlanta, Department of Health and Human Services, National Center for Health Statistics, 2000.
167. Rajagopalan KV: Molybdenum—an essential trace element. Nutr Rev 1987;45:321-328.
168. Rasmussen A: Carbohydrate induced hypophosphatemia. Acta Anaesthesiol Scand 1985;29:68-70.
169. Reed CR, Sessler CN, Glauser FL, Phelan BA: Central venous catheter infections: Concepts and controversies. Intensive Care Med 1995;21:177-183.
170. Report of the Dietary Guidelines Advisory Committee for the 2000 Dietary Guidelines for Americans, Washington, U.S. Dept. of Health, 2005.
171. Rhoads CM, Parkins W, Tourtelotte D, Vars HM: Method for continuous intravenous administration of nutritive solutions suitable for prolonged metabolic studies in dogs. Am J Physiol 1949;159:409.
172. Rhoads JE, Dudrick SJ: History of intravenous nutrition. In Rombeau JL, Caldwell MD (eds): Clinical Nutrition: Parenteral Nutrition. Philadelphia, WB Saunders, 1986, pp 1-10.
173. Rico H, Revilla M, Villa LF, et al: Body composition in

children and Tanner's stages: A study with dual-energy x-ray absorptiometry. Metabolism 1993;42:967-970.
174. Roche A: Growth and assessment of handicapped children. Diet Curr 1970;6:25.
175. Romanski SA, McMahon M, Molly M: Metabolic acidosis and thiamine deficiency. Mayo Clin Proc 1999;74: 259-263.
176. Rose J, Gibbons K, Carlson SE, Koo WWK: Nutrient needs of the preterm infant. Nutr Clin Pract 1993;8:226-232.
177. Sacher P, Hirsig J, Gresser J, Spitz L: The importance of oral sodium replacement in ileostomy patients. Prog Pediatr Surg 1989;24:226-231.
178. Sandstrom R, Drott C, Hyltander A, et al: The effect of postoperative intravenous feeding (TPN) on outcome following major surgery evaluated in a randomized study. Ann Surg 1993;217:185-195.
179. Sangild P, Petersen Y, Schmidt M, et al: Preterm birth affects the intestinal response to parenteral and enteral nutrition in newborn pigs. J Nutr 2002;132:3786-3794.
180. Schilling J, Vranjes N, Fierz W, et al: Clinical outcome and immunology of postoperative arginine, omega-3 fatty acids, and nucleotide-enriched enteral feeding: A randomized prospective comparison with standard enteral and low calorie/low fat IV solutions. Nutrition 1996;12:423-429.
181. Schmidt-Sommerfeld E, Penn D: Carnitine and parenteral nutrition of the neonate. Biol Neonate 1990;58:81-88.
182. Schuman E, Ragsdale J: Peripheral ports are a new option for central venous access. J Am Coll Surg 1995;180: 456-460.
183. Schwarz K, Ternberg J, Bell M, Keating J: Sodium needs of infants and children with ileostomy. J Pediatr 1983;102: 509-513.
184. Sermet-Gaudelus I, Poisson-Salomon A, Colomb V: Simple pediatric nutritional risk score to identify children at risk of malnutrition. Am J Clin Nutr 2000;72:64-70.
185. Shaw JH, Holdaway CM: Protein-sparing effect of substrate infusion in surgical patients is governed by the clinical state, and not by the individual substrate infused. JPEN J Parenter Enteral Nutr 1988;12:433-440.
186. Shennan AT, Bryan MH, Angel A: The effect of gestational age on Intralipid tolerance in newborn infants. J Pediatr 1977;91:134-137.
187. Shike M, Shils ME, Heller A, et al: Bone disease in prolonged parenteral nutrition: Osteopenia without mineralization defect. Am J Clin Nutr 1986;44:89-98.
188. Shike M, Sturtridge WC, Tam CS, et al: A possible role of vitamin D in the genesis of parenteral nutrition-induced metabolic bone disease. Ann Intern Med 1981;95:560-568.
189. Silvestre MAA, Morbach CA, Brans YW, et al: A prospective randomized trial comparing continuous versus intermittent feeding methods in very low birth weight neonates. J Pediatr 1996;128:748-752.
190. Sokol RJ: Vitamin E and neurological deficits. Adv Pediatr 1990;37:119-148.
191. Souba WW, Herskowitz K, Austgen TR, et al: Glutamine nutrition: Theoretical considerations and therapeutic impact. JPEN J Parenter Enteral Nutr 1990;14:237S-243S.
192. Spear ML, Stahl GE, Hamosh M, et al: Effect of heparin dose and infusion rate on lipid clearance and bilirubin binding in premature infants receiving intravenous fat emulsions. J Pediatr 1988;112:94-98.
193. Spears K, Cheney C, Zerzan J: Low plasma retinol concentrations increase the risk of developing bronchopulmonary dysplasia and long-term respiratory disability in very-low-birth-weight infants. Am J Clin Nutr 2004;80:1589-1594.
194. Spencer A, Yu S, Tracy T, et al: Parenteral nutrition-associated cholestasis in neonates: multivariate analysis of the potential protective effect of taurine. JPEN J Parenter Enteral Nutr 2005;29:337-344.
195. Spiegel JE, Willenbucher RF: Rapid development of severe copper deficiency in a patient with Crohn's disease receiving parenteral nutrition. JPEN J Parenter Enteral Nutr 1999;23:169-172.
196. Steephen AC, Traber MG, Ito Y, et al: Vitamin E status of patients receiving long-term parenteral nutrition: Is vitamin E supplementation adequate? JPEN J Parenter Enteral Nutr 1991;15:647-652.
197. Stonestreet BS, Rubin L, Pollak A, et al: Renal functions of low birth weight infants with hyperglycemia and glucosuria produced by glucose infusions. Pediatrics 1980;66: 561-567.
198. Strong R, Condon S, Soling M, et al: Equal aspiration rates from postpylorus and intragastric-placed small bore nasoenteric feeding tubes: A randomized prospective study. JPEN J Parenter Enteral Nutr 1992;16:59-63.
199. Strupp BJ, Levitsky DA: Enduring cognitive effects of early malnutrition: A theoretical reappraisal. J Nutr 1995;125: 2221S-2232S.
200. Stylianos S, Flanigan LM: Primary button gastrostomy: A simplified percutaneous, open, laparoscopy-guided technique. J Pediatr Surg 1995;30:219-220.
201. Sundaram A, Koutkia P, Apovian C: Nutritional management of short bowel syndrome in adults. J Clin Gastroenterol 2002;34:207-220.
202. Suttie J: Vitamin K responsive hemorrhagic disease of infancy. J Pediatr Gastroenterol Nutr 1990;11:4-6.
203. Taketomo CK, Hodding JH, Kraus DM: In Inc L-C, Hudson OH (eds): Pediatric Dosage Handbook, 8th ed. Hudson, OH, Lexi-Comp, 2001, pp 816-818.
204. Tamada H, Matsuo Y, Nezu R, et al: Zinc deficient diet impairs adaptive changes in the remaining intestine after massive small bowel resection in rats. Br J Surg 1992;79: 959-963.
205. Tashiro T, Mashima Y, Yamamori H, et al: Intravenous Intralipid 10% vs 20%, hyperlipidemia, and increase in lipoprotein X in humans. Nutrition 1992;8:155-160.
206. Tasman-Jones C, Kay RG, Lee SP: Zinc and copper deficiency, with particular reference to parenteral nutrition. Surg Annu 1978;10:23-52.
207. Taylor S, Manara AR: Manganese toxicity in a patient with cholestasis receiving total parenteral nutrition [letter]. Anaesthesia 1994;49:1013.
208. Teitelbaum D, Caniano D, Wheller J: Resolution of an infected intracardiac thrombus. J Pediatr Surg 1989;24:1118-1120.
209. Teitelbaum D, Drongowski R, Spivak D: Rapid development of hyperbilirubinemia in infants with the short bowel syndrome as a correlate to mortality: Possible indication for early small bowel transplantation. Transplant Proc 1996;28:2677-2678.
210. Teitelbaum DH: Parenteral nutrition-associated cholestasis. Curr Opin Pediatr 1997;9:270-275.
211. Teitelbaum DH, Tracy TJ, Aouthmany M, et al: Use of cholecystokinin-octapeptide for the prevention of parenteral nutrition-associated cholestasis. Pediatrics 2005;115: 1332-1340.
212. Thuren P, Hay WJ: Intravenous nutrition and postnatal growth of the micropremie. Clin Perinatol 2000;27:197-234.
213. Tibboel D, Delemarre FMC, Przyrembel H, et al: Carnitine deficiency in surgical neonates receiving total parenteral nutrition. J Pediatr Surg 1990;25:418-421.
214. Treas LS, Iatinis-Bridges B: Efficacy of heparin in peripheral venous infusion in neonates. J Obstet Gynecol Neonatal

Nurs 1992;21:214-219.
215. Tremel H, Kienle B, Weilemann LS, et al: Glutamine dipeptide-supplemented parenteral nutrition maintains intestinal function in the critically ill. Gastroenterology 1994;107:1595-1601.
216. van den Berghe G, Wouters PJ, Bouillon R, et al: Outcome benefit of intensive insulin therapy in the critically ill: Insulin dose versus glycemic control. Crit Care Med 2003;31:359-366.
217. van den Berghe G, Wouters PJ, Weekers F, et al: Intensive insulin therapy in the critically ill patient. N Engl J Med 2001;345:1359-1367.
218. Vanderhoof JA, Langnas AN, Pinch LW, et al: Short bowel syndrome. J Pediatr Gastroenterol Nutr 1992;14:359-370.
219. Vargas JH, Klein GL, Ament ME, et al: Metabolic bone disease of total parenteral nutrition: Course after changing from casein to amino acids in parenteral solutions with reduced aluminum content. Am J Clin Nutr 1988;48: 1070-1078.
220. Vaughan LM, Small C, Plunkett V: Incompatibility of iron dextran and a total nutrient admixture. Am J Hosp Pharm 1990;47:1745-1746.
221. Verhage AH, Cheong WK, Allard JP, et al: Increase in lumbar spine bone mineral content in patients on long-term parenteral nutrition without vitamin D supplementation. JPEN J Parenter Enteral Nutr 1995;19:431-436.
222. von Meyenfeldt MM, Stapert J, de Jong PC, et al: TPN catheter sepsis: Lack of effect of subcutaneous tunnelling of PVC catheters on sepsis rate. JPEN J Parenter Enteral Nutr 1980;4:514-517.
223. Werlin SL, Lausten T, Jessen S, et al: Treatment of central venous catheter occlusions with ethanol and hydrochloric acid. JPEN J Parenter Enteral Nutr 1995;19:416-418.
224. Whitaker R, Wright J, Pepe M, et al: Predicting obesity in young adulthood from childhood and parental obesity. N Engl J Med 1997;337:869-873.
225. White MS, Shepherd RW, McEniery JA: Energy expenditure measurements in ventilated critically ill children: Within- and between-day variability. JPEN J Parenter Enteral Nutr 1999;23:300-304.
226. Williamson RC: Intestinal adaptation (first of two parts): Structural, functional and cytokinetic changes. N Engl J Med 1978;298:1393-1402.
227. Williamson RC: Intestinal adaptation (second of two parts): Mechanisms of control. N Engl J Med 1978; 298:1444-1450.
228. Wilmore DW, Dudrick SJ: Growth and development of an infant receiving all nutrients exclusively by vein. JAMA 1968;203:860.
229. Wilmore DW, Smith RJ, O'Dwyer ST, et al: The gut: A central organ after surgical stress. Surgery 1988;104:917-923.
230. Wolfe RR, O'Donnell TF, Stone MD, et al: Investigation of factors determining the optimal glucose infusion rate in total parenteral nutrition. Metabolism 1980;29: 892-900.
231. Wright A, Hecker J, McDonald G: Effects of low dose heparin on failure of intravenous infusions in children. Heart Lung 1995;24:79-82.
232. Wurzel CL, Halom K, Feldman JG, Rubin LG: Infection rates of Broviac-Hickman catheters and implantable venous devices. Am J Dis Child 1988;142:536-540.
233. Yang H, Larsson J, Permert J, et al: No effect of bolus glutamine supplementation on the postresectional adaptation of small bowel mucosa in rats receiving chow ad libitum. Dig Surg 2000;17:256-260.
234. Zaidan H, Dhanireddy R, Hamosh M, et al: Lipid clearing in premature infants during continuous heparin infusion: Role of circulating lipase. Pediatr Res 1985;19:23-25.
235. Zeigler T, Young L, Benfell K: Clinical and metabolic efficacy of glutamine-supplemented PN after bone marrow transplantation. Ann Intern Med 1992;116: 821-828.
236. Zelikovic I, Chesney RW, Friedman AL, et al: Taurine depletion in very low birth weight infants receiving total parenteral nutrition: Role of renal immaturity. J Pediatr 1990;116:301-306.
237. Ziegler EE: Protein in premature feeding. Nutrition 1994; 10:69-71.
238. Zlotkin SH, Bryan MH, Anderson GH: Intravenous nitrogen and energy intakes required to duplicate in utero nitrogen accretion in prematurely born human infants. J Pediatr 1981;99:115-120.

第 13 章

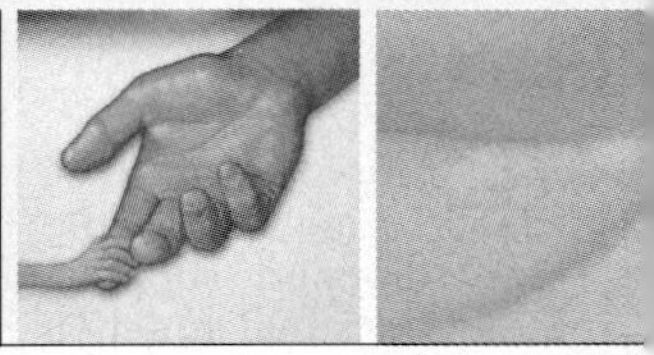

小儿麻醉

Ira S. Landsman、Mirjana Vustar 和 Stephen R. Hays

221 小儿外科学前辈 Marc Rowe 医生曾说过：“无论小儿外科医生多么有技术和经验，要想让新生儿安全度过围术期，都需要与能力相当的小儿麻醉医生合作”[242]。在给新生儿和年长儿麻醉时都要考虑其快速生长发育过程。小儿的解剖学、生理学、药理学和心理特点以及外科问题的多样性，均影响麻醉护理。本章将对小儿麻醉和疼痛处理中与临床相关的重要问题进行讨论。

生理学问题

出生后最初的 3 个月中，婴儿的循环系统和呼吸系统的适应过程逐渐完成，其温度调节过程发生改变，体液分布向成人方向转变，骨骼肌增多，肝脏酶系统和肾功能渐趋成熟。2 岁后，小儿的生理功能趋向于成人，但是心理还不成熟。在 6 个月至 1 岁间，婴儿对周围环境充满警觉，应注意心理保护。在此年龄段，术前准备可以使用镇静药。对于麻醉医生来说，健康学龄前儿童（2～6 岁）出现麻醉技术性问题相对较少，但是需要注意患儿的恐惧心理及其对手术缺乏理解与合作的情况。术前对学龄儿童（6～18 岁）的恐惧心理也需加以适当处理。

新生婴儿能够感受急性疼痛和术后疼痛。出生时，外周伤害性感受器的功能已趋于成熟[99]。然而，将即时的化学性、温度性和机械性疼痛刺激传递至中枢神经系统的神经传导通路尚未完全发育成熟，中枢神经系统的抑制性传出通路也未成熟[100]。过去，由于人们对新生儿的疼痛反应认识不足，在对新生儿实施能引起成人疼痛的手术操作时，没有给予适当的镇痛措施[230,279,319]。一系列可测定的生理、代谢和临床改变已表明，不同孕龄的新生儿都会对疼痛刺激产生明显的反应，而镇痛和麻醉能够减轻这些反应[8,9]。

新生儿对麻醉剂非常敏感且对药物的代谢和清除机制尚不完善[39]。1 个月大的婴儿在容量分布、中枢神经系统的敏感性和转运蛋白（如白蛋白、α1–酸糖蛋白）的质量和数量方面仍存在着明显的个体差异，导致新生儿对麻醉剂的反应差异极大，常常难以预测。

出生几周之后，婴儿的药物代谢功能逐渐成熟，许多鸦片类药物，如芬太尼和吗啡，在婴儿和幼儿的半衰期要短于年长儿和成人。对出生后 6 月内的婴儿，静脉给予麻醉剂的单位体重剂量，如硫喷妥钠和异丙酚，要大于其他年龄段的（图 13–1）[145,316]。对于维持适当的麻醉深度，吸入麻醉剂的浓度在 1 岁以内的婴儿要明显高于其他年龄段的儿童（表 13–1，图 13–2）。然而婴儿心脏对这些高浓度的麻醉剂却更加敏感。

麻醉风险

在给患者麻醉前评价患者的疾病严重程度是麻醉医生日常工作的一部分。为此，美国麻醉医生协会（ASA）早在 1941 年就创立了生理状况分级系统。因为 ASA 分级系统没有将手术操作类型考虑在内，故不能预测风险[215]。ASA 分级允许麻醉医生根据患者的疾病选择麻醉方式。ASA 的五个级别如下所示：

ASA 1：患者为正常健康人
ASA 2：患者有轻度全身性疾病
ASA 3： 患者有重度全身性疾病
ASA 4： 患者有重度持续威胁生命的全身性疾病 22
ASA 5： 濒死的患者，如果不手术可能就无法存活。

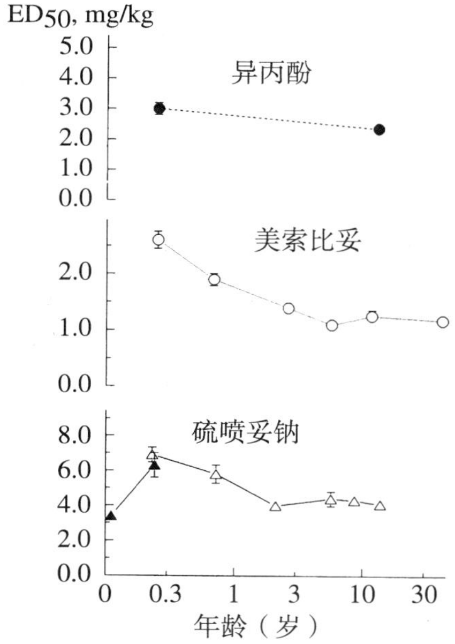

图 13–1 不同年龄组患者的 ED_{50}（50%的患者产生麻醉作用的药物剂量）的估计值 ± 标准差。美索比妥以空心圆圈表示，硫喷妥钠以空心或实心三角表示，异丙酚以实心圆圈表示。为便于比较，所引图的纵坐标已作相应的调整，对于年龄 7～16 岁的儿童，可在相同高度得到 ED_{50} 值。(From University and University Hospital of Lund: Intravenous Induction of Anesthesia in Infants and Children. Lund, Sweden, Studentlitteratur, 1991.)

表 13–1 小儿年龄与吸入麻醉剂平均最低肺泡气有效浓度

年龄（月）	氟烷 *	异氟烷 †	地氟烷 ‡	七氟烷§
1	0.87	1.6	9.16	3.2～3.3
2	1.08	1.9	9.4	3.2～3.3
14	0.97	1.8	8.72	2.5
44	0.91	1.6	8.54	2.5
480	0.76	1.2	7.5	2.5

* From Cook DR, Marcy JH: Pediatric anesthetic pharmacology. In Cook DR, Marcy JH (eds): Neonatal Anesthesia. Pasadena, Calif, Appleton Davies, 1988.

† From Cameron CB, Robinson S, Gregory GA: The minimum anesthetic concentration of isoflurane in children. Anesth Analg 1984;63:418.

‡ From Taylor RH, Lerman J: Minimum alveolar concentration of desflurane and hemodynamic responses in neonates, infants, and children. Anesthesiology 1991;75:975.

§ From Lerman J, et al: The pharmacology of sevoflurane in infants and children. Anesthesiology 1994;80:814.

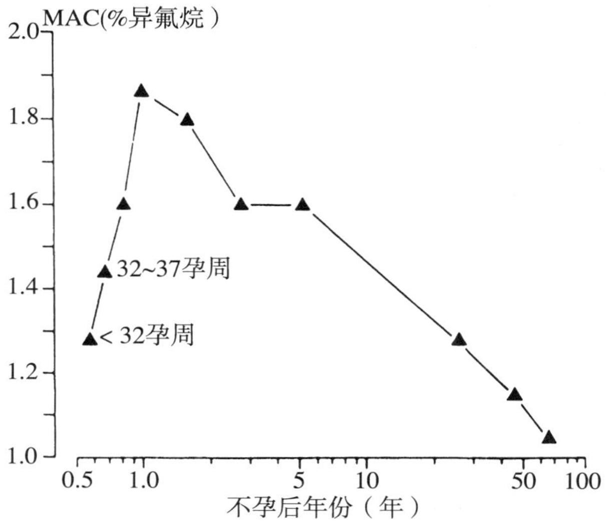

图 13–2 根据妊娠龄计算的异氟烷的最低肺泡气有效浓度（MAC）。(From LeDez KM, Lerman J: The minimum alveolar concentration [MAC] of isoflurane in premature neonates. Anesthesiology 1987;67:301.)

鉴于小儿疾病的复杂性，ASA 3 和 4 级患者术前需由麻醉医生进行会诊。

单纯由麻醉导致的死亡并不常见。在英国，总体麻醉死亡率约为 1/185 000[48]。小儿麻醉相关的死亡危险性高于成人。巴尔的摩麻醉研究委员会发现，麻醉死亡率在成人为 3.3/10 000，而在儿科患者则要增加 5 倍。其中 20% 发生在出生 7 天以内的新生儿。Keenan 和 Boyan 报道[151]，小于 12 岁的小儿发生心搏骤停的风险要高 3 倍（4.7/10,000）。在 Morray 等人[202]的综述中提到，小儿由于呼吸问题引起的麻醉并发症和死亡率明显要高于成人。

小儿围术期心搏骤停登记制度建立于 1994 年，目的是为了研究小儿麻醉后发生心搏骤停的相关临床因素和后果[203]。结果发现，与麻醉相关的心跳骤停最常见于 1 岁以内的婴儿和患有严重基础疾病的小儿。急症手术，特别是对有严重基础疾病的患儿实施的手术，如果在麻醉期间发生了心搏骤停，则死亡率明显上升。在这项研究中，37%的发生心搏骤停的患儿与用药有关，而在 ASA 1 和 2 级患者，64%的心跳骤停与用药有关。美国减少使用氟烷（一种强效的心脏抑制药）后，今后的统计结果将大为改观。

一般来说，大型儿科医疗中心的麻醉死亡率较低。例如，在 1966—1978 年期间，波士顿儿童医院

0～10 岁年龄组的麻醉死亡率是 0.8/10, 000，10～20 岁年龄组的麻醉死亡率是 0.6/10 000。多数麻醉死亡发生在实施急症手术的患儿。此外，Keenan 等人[152]认为，如果所有小于 1 岁的婴儿都由小儿麻醉专科医生实施麻醉，该组患儿的麻醉死亡率可能会降低。
223 Auroy 等人[18]发现，要降低并发症的发生率及提高小儿麻醉的安全性，每位小儿麻醉医生每年至少要完成 200 例小儿麻醉工作。

喉痉挛

喉痉挛是对小儿实施吸入麻醉期间常见的并发症。虽然多数喉痉挛是自限性的或对保守疗法有效，但麻醉医生必须时刻准备好肌松药来处理喉痉挛并恢复正常通气，因为喉痉挛可能导致呼吸衰竭和心搏骤停。小儿喉痉挛的发生率高于成人。Olsson 和 Hallen[212]研究了1967—1978 年的 11 年间 136 929例各年龄段患者喉痉挛的发生率，发现其发生率为 8.7‰。据报道，全身麻醉期间喉痉挛的发生率与年龄呈负相关，其中新生儿至 9 岁小儿的发生率较高（17.4‰），而新生儿至 3 个月大的婴儿最高（28.2‰）。在青少年患者中，男性发生率比女性发生率明显升高（12.1‰：7.2‰）[212]。研究还显示，患有上呼吸道感染或支气管哮喘的患儿麻醉期间发生喉痉挛的概率非常高（95.8‰）。

治疗喉痉挛引起的不完全性呼吸道梗阻的措施包括去除手术刺激，清除喉头部位的分泌物和异物，以及增加麻醉深度。可选用与患儿匹配的面罩，用纯氧进行正压通气。如果这些措施还不能改善通气，就需要使用肌松药。肌肉或静脉注射琥珀胆碱可以放松声带，得到适当的正压通气。

术后呼吸暂停

早产儿术后发生呼吸暂停危险性尚有争议。已有的研究结果因样本量太小而不可靠[67]。早产儿和少于 44 周的足月新生儿，不论其是否有呼吸暂停史，术后都有可能发生呼吸暂停[168,274,312]。术后呼吸暂停定义为呼吸停止在 15 秒及以上，或呼吸停止少于 15 秒但伴有心动过缓。发生术后呼吸暂停的原因尚不清楚。全麻后的苏醒时间可能暴露中枢性呼吸调节功能未成熟或上呼吸道紧张性降低；这些因素都被认为与术后呼吸暂停有关[67]。

尽管术后呼吸暂停通常发生在术后最初 2 小时内，但也可能发生在麻醉后 12 小时。一些研究者试图确定一个妊娠周数，使在其后出生的无新生儿呼吸暂停史的健康早产儿可在手术当天出院。结果发现，妊娠周数为 44[186]～60 周[107,169,312]，存在显著差异。部分原因是监护程度不同。监护越多，发现呼吸暂停的概率越高。由于争议颇多，每个医院必须制定自己的对策。一般认为，如果早产儿的妊娠周龄在 50周或以下，术后需要监护 24 小时。很明显，对患有严重疾病或有神经病学问题或有反复的新生儿呼吸暂停史的小儿应制订更为有效的监护措施。

迄今为止，贫血是唯一确认的在此类危险人群可增加术后呼吸暂停危险的独立危险因素[67,309]。对伴有贫血且血细胞比容低于 30%的早产儿，建议推迟选择性手术，并且补充铁剂直到血细胞比容大于 30%。如果贫血小儿的手术不能延期，则必须加强监护，以防发生术后呼吸暂停。

麻醉前评估和准备

术前访视的基本目的是获取患者外科疾病和病史等方面的信息，以估计其对麻醉的反应。术前评估可了解应在麻醉前给以纠治的患者的异常，包括重度贫血、镰状细胞异常、急性全身感染及下呼吸道疾病活动期（如哮喘、支气管肺发育不良和囊性纤维化）。

除此之外，术前访视需向孩子和家长解释择期手术和麻醉的简要过程以消除他们的焦虑。术前行为评估在大型儿科医院很常见。这些准备活动包括信息介绍、医院参观、角色预演和小儿生活指导[147]。门诊手术可以减轻幼儿与家长分离后的焦虑情绪。通常在麻醉诱导前给予患者简单解释以减轻其恐惧心理并强化术前宣教效果。在年长儿中，术前访视可使麻醉医生和患者之间建立起融洽的关系，培养信任感并加强合作。在一些医院，家长可参与麻醉诱导过程。对家长和学龄前儿童来说，这种经历可缓解恐惧和焦虑。但对个别家长来说，参与是一种情感创伤。

术前禁饮

为了确保麻醉安全，患者必须排空胃，但又需防
224 止患者发生脱水。这两个目标是一致的，不难达到。如果手术安排在第二天早晨，那么患者术前一天可按常规进食和睡眠，不存在特殊的问题。

尚无研究证明放松禁示指南会增加肺误吸的风险[137,272]。围术期禁示指南由 ASA 制定的，如表 13-2 所示[303]。这些指南允许小儿在择期手术前 2 小时摄入清饮料。婴儿在术前 4 小时可以哺食母乳，婴幼儿在术前 6 小时可以按常规进食。

如果不详细交代这些细节，就有可能造成小儿禁饮时间过长，特别是婴儿。手术应该按照孩子的年龄来排序，最小的孩子应该第一个做手术。手术时间若被推迟，外科医生和麻醉医生应注意对婴儿的禁饮限制做相应的修改。

麻醉前用药

术前用药包括不同药物以及不同的给药途径。过去很多医院的麻醉科都将镇静催眠药、麻醉剂和止涎药制成自己独特的混合剂，而且通常采用肌内注射途径给药。术前用药的目的在于减轻焦虑、镇痛、减少自主（迷走）反射、减少气道分泌物和胃液容量以及降低胃液酸度。目前趋向于采用口服和经鼻途径给药。

表 13-2 为了降低发生肺误吸的风险推荐的禁食方案 *

摄入原料	最短禁食时间（小时）†
清饮料 ‡	2
母乳	4
婴儿配方奶	6
非母乳§	6
清淡饮食¶	6

* 适用于择期手术的健康小儿。不适用于产妇。遵守这些原则不能保证胃排空完全。

† 禁食期限适用于所有年龄段。

‡ 清饮料包括水、不含果肉的果汁、碳酸饮料、清茶和清咖啡。

§ 非母乳的胃排空时间与固体相似，在决定禁食时间时还需考虑摄入量。

¶ 典型的清淡饮食由吐司和清饮料组成。油煎、脂肪类食物或肉类可以延长胃排空时间。决定禁食时间时还需考虑摄入食物的量和种类。

术前用药应为快速的短期水平的镇静，以使小儿与家长分离并使麻醉诱导更加平稳。小儿在选择性手术前一般没有疼痛，所以不需将阿片类药物作为标准术前用药的一部分。过去吸入麻醉剂用乙醚和环丙烷时常使用止涎药。新一代的吸入麻醉剂不会明显增加口腔分泌物，因此，不必再将止涎药作为术前用药。

咪达唑仑是一种常用的短效的苯二氮䓬类药物，目前常用于术前镇静。它是一种催眠、抗焦虑、抗惊厥药物，具有顺行性而非逆行性遗忘特性[233,292]。在生理 pH 情况下，咪达唑仑具有亲脂性，能快速通过胃肠道吸收，并能迅速进入中枢神经系统[233]。静脉注射镇静剂量的咪达唑仑能够抑制低氧性通气驱动，减弱心血管和呼吸对低氧血症的反应[4]。静注咪达唑仑合用阿片类药物时，未给予监护的患者容易发生呼吸暂停和低氧血症[20]。

对小儿可以通过鼻内、口服、直肠、静脉或肌肉途径给予咪达唑仑以产生镇静作用。Walbergh[300]研究表明，经鼻滴注咪达唑仑生物利用度只有静脉给药的 51%，起效速度比直肠途径快 45%。Wilton 等人报道[320]，18 个月至 5 岁的小儿经鼻滴注咪达唑仑 0.2mg/k g，给药后 5～10 分钟可产生镇静作用。Tome[288]发现，对实施门诊短小外科手术的婴幼儿经鼻给予咪达唑仑 0.2～0.3mg/kg，能产生良好的镇静作用且不会延长麻醉恢复时间或出院时间。还没有健康小儿术前镇静时采用鼻内滴注（0.2～0.3mg/kg）或口服（0.5～0.75mg/kg）咪达唑仑后发生心血管呼吸抑制的报道[83,194,320]。口服商品剂型的咪达唑仑能在给药后 10～20 分钟后产生令人满意的镇静和抗焦虑作用[65]。口服静脉剂型的咪达唑仑后起效时间为 20～30 分钟。

鼻内滴注咪达唑仑能引起轻微的短暂性鼻黏膜刺激，如果 0.5%的药液（5mg/ml）用量大于 1ml，还可能发生窒息和呛咳。因此 0.5%的咪达唑仑如用量大于 1ml，则采取口服途径更容易让患者接受。将咪达唑仑静脉剂型调配成口服液时，为了掩盖其苦味，应添加糖水或糖浆。已经证明，咪达唑仑口服剂型具有更为一致的生物利用度和 pH特性。这种稳定性使其剂量低至 0.25mg/kg 时也能够产生足够的镇静作用[65]。

225 小儿发生肺内误吸极其罕见，故对健康儿童术前不必使用增加胃液 pH或加速胃排空的药物[63,284]。婴儿、儿童和成人术前 2 小时饮用清饮料不会增加胃残余容量[70]。事实上，部分小儿术前 2小时饮用清饮料反而能减少胃残余容量，提高胃液 pH。

输液

液体维持

足月儿和儿童的液体治疗有不同的计算方法，涉及体重、体表面积和热卡消耗等[22,136,243]。体重和热卡消耗，以及非显性失水量、肾需水量、粪便失水量和生长需水量决定了液体维持量。热卡消耗与体重有关：1～10kg 的婴儿为 100cal/kg；10～20kg 为 1000cal/d，另加超过 10kg 的部分每天 50cal/kg；大于 20kg 的年长儿为 1500cal/d，另加超过 20kg 的部分每天 25cal/kg。患者每消耗 100cal 热量，需要 67ml 水来排泄溶质；另外每消耗 100cal 热量还需 50ml 水，与非显性失水有关，而每 100cal 物质氧化后可产生水分 17ml。因此，婴儿和儿童每消耗 100cal 热量需要消耗 100ml 水。假设一天以 25 个小时进行计算，那么有个简单的公式可以计算健康足月婴儿和儿童每小时的液体维持量。1～10kg 的小儿每小时的液体维持量为 4ml/kg。10～20kg 小儿的每小时的液体维持量分为：第一个 10kg 为 4ml/kg，10～20kg 之间为 2ml/kg。20kg 以上的患者的每小时液体维持量分为第一个 10kg 为 4ml/kg，第二个 10kg 的 2ml/kgh，超过 20kg 的部分为 1ml/kg。例如，一个体重为 28kg 的小儿的每小时液体维持量为 68ml。

每当给予婴儿和儿童 100ml 水分时，还需要补充 3mEqNa^+、2mEqK^+、2mEqCl^-和 5g 葡萄糖以防酮症发生。更方便的做法是将钠和氯的补充量均以 3mEq 计算。作为常规静脉液体治疗，将 5%的葡萄糖添加到 0.25%的正常盐水中常能够满足这些需求。但是，这并不是术中补液的理想选择。

早产儿或危重病婴儿

对早产儿或危重病婴儿患者来说，很多因素会影响水和电解质的平衡。婴儿的妊娠周龄、产后龄、体重、肾脏溶质负荷和肾脏最大浓缩能力各不相同。疾病、应激、感染、肠道活动减弱、光线疗法以及胃或肠道引流引起的组织破坏和分解代谢均可对液体疗法产生显著影响。Rowe、Hammarlund 等人[123]、Bell和 Oh[22]已经对这些问题做过系统回顾。

术中补液

术中补液包括初始补液和维持补液。补液可以单纯补充术前禁食导致的体液不足并给予液体维持量，也可以在给予液体维持量的同时纠正术前缺失、液体异位分布和血液中不同成分的丢失。

估计液体缺失量

禁食引起的液体缺失应该在麻醉期间得到补充。一个健康儿童禁食后，液体缺失量是通过每小时液体维持量 MFR 乘以禁食的小时数来估计。在麻醉后第 1 个小时内可补充估计液体缺失量（EFD）的一半，在随后的 2 个小时内补足剩余量[105]。液体维持量应联合液体缺失量同时给予。因此，对一位正在进行体表手术的婴儿来说，手术进行 3 小时且只伴有极少或不伴有第三间隙缺失时，手术期间需补充液体量的计算如下：

EFD = 禁食时间 × MFR（每小时 ml/kg）
第 1 小时补液量 = MFR + 1/2 的 EFD
第 2 小时补液量 = MFR + 1/4 的 EFD
第 3 小时补液量 = MFR + 1/4 的 EFD

葡萄糖的作用

由于手术可引起应激激素释放而降低胰岛素的敏感性，术中血糖水平通常升高。血糖浓度过高会产生糖尿和渗透性利尿。高血糖可加重局部组织的缺血、缺氧而导致神经系统损害[113,143,172,208,226,311]。几项研究显示，健康婴儿和儿童在禁食开始至 17 小时后仍能保持正常血糖水平。这些研究显示，健康婴儿和儿童在手术期间不需要补充糖溶液[19,311]。对存在发生低血糖高危风险的患者（如早产儿和对妊娠周数而言太小的婴儿以及行完全胃肠外营养的小儿、糖尿病患儿）来说，在液体治疗和补糖的同时需加强血糖监测。

术中补液的选择

对大多数患者来说，术中液体维持和补充术中液体缺失可以选择乳酸林格液。乳酸林格液的电解质组分与血清相似。如果采用低张液体作为液体维持和补充第三间隙液体丢失的液体，可能发生低钠血症以及
26 相关的神经系统并发症。

大多数外科疾病都会发生等张液体从细胞外腔室转移至更小的间隙和从细胞内移至非功能性间隙的情况[241]。液体转移至非功能性间隙的急性分离过程叫做第三间隙丢失。血浆容量可同时被累及。第三间隙丢失量因外科操作不同而有所不同，对婴儿来说丢失量最大的是腹腔内手术。此外，暴露肠管和使用灯照加温会增加蒸发量。对婴儿来说，每小时第三间隙丢失量腹腔手术估计为 6～10ml/kg，胸腔手术为 4～7 ml/kg，体表手术或神经外科手术为 1～2 ml/kg。液体移位可能意味着大量的额外的功能性液体丢失。因此，脱水程度的临床征象可用来估计所需补液量。通常使用乳酸林格液补充第三间隙液体丢失。如果丢失量过大，一些学者认为丢失量的 1/4～1/3 应用 5%的白蛋白来补充。补充第三间隙液体的目的是维持合适的血压、组织灌注和尿量。

输血

输血取决于患者的需要，外科医生和麻醉医生之间的交流起决定性作用。准确测量婴儿的失血量和评价失血量的安全限度是输血治疗的重要组成部分。失血量通过称重纱布、使用校准的小型吸引瓶和视觉估计判断。允许失血量通过患者的初始血容量和血红蛋白或血细胞比容来计算[38,105]。需考虑的其他因素包括患者的年龄、心肺功能状态和患者的一般状况。这些因素也决定了输血的利弊。输注晶体液进行等容量血液稀释可达到预定的血细胞比容。

允许失血量的估计

通过患者的血容量、体重和血细胞比容来计算允许失血量（ABL）的方法有数种。公式由简单至复杂，但是都包括估计血容量。允许失血量可以通过下列方程计算：

$$ABL = 体重(kg) \times EBV \times [Ho - Hl] / H$$

EBV 为估计血容量，Ho 为初始血细胞比容，Hl 为血细胞比容可接受的最低值，H 为平均血细胞比容 [(Ho − Hl) ÷ 2]。

该方程假定血液丢失和补充的过程是呈指数形式的渐变过程。估计的血容量新生儿为 90ml/kg，婴儿和儿童为 80ml/kg，青少年为 65～78ml/kg。这个方程适用于所有年龄组的患者。

是否在血细胞比容达到最低允许值才给予输液补充血容量尚存争议。通常按照估计失血量的 2～3 倍给予乳酸林格液。

血液制品

血液成分治疗取决于临床状况和不同血液制品的供应情况。新鲜全血（采血时间为 4 个小时以内）来源有限。患有脓毒症的婴儿可从中获得凝血因子和免疫因子、血小板以及白细胞。当失血量预计达到 40%或以上时，新鲜全血有助于补充血小板和凝血因子。然而，通常给予的是血液成分而不是新鲜全血[47]。浓缩红细胞（RBC）的血细胞比容在 55%～75%之间，含钾相对较高（K ± 15～20mEq/L），呈酸性（pH＜7.0），而钙离子水平较低。快速给予浓缩红细胞后，患者血液成分会发生明显变化。每输入 10ml/kg 的浓缩红细胞（血细胞比容约为 70%）后估计的患者血细胞比容增加值取决于患者的年龄、体型和估计血容量（表 13–3）。

当患者的失血量接近于其血容量时，凝血因子明显减少；正常凝血需要 5%～20%的Ⅴ因子和 30%的Ⅷ因子。新鲜冷冻血浆（FFP）中含有正常数量的所有凝血因子（除血小板外）。当患者大量失血时（血细胞比容在 35%～40%），可输入接近等量的 FFP 和浓缩红细胞。

手术期间是否需要输注血小板可以通过术前血小板计数进行预测。出血时，机体可释放出脾和骨髓中储

表 13-3 随着输血后血容量的增加，血细胞比容升高的估计值

年龄	血容量 (ml/kg)	血细胞比容升高的估计值 *
早产儿	100	6.30
足月儿	90	7.00
学龄前儿童	80	7.7
学龄儿童	75	8.2
成人	65	9.3

* 每次输注 10ml/kg 浓缩红细胞（血细胞比容约为 70%）后，血细胞比容升高的估计值取决于患者的年龄、体型和估计的血容量。

存的血小板。对术前血小板计数较高（>250 000/mm³）的婴儿可以到失血达到血容量 2～3 倍时再考虑输注血
227 小板，但是对术前血小板计数较低（<150 000/mm³）的婴儿在失血量达到血容量后就需输注血小板。每 10kg 体重输注两袋血小板后，血小板约克升高 10 000～15 000/mm³。

快速输注冷的含有枸橼酸盐的血液制品十分危险，因此这种血液制品在输注前应当加温。所有血液制品均含有枸橼酸盐，以 FFP 含量最高。因此，快速输注 FFP 会导致患者的血浆游离钙浓度明显改变。在大多数情况下，机体钙动员和肝脏代谢枸橼酸盐的速度足以防止血浆游离钙浓度的下降。但是，由于婴儿的钙储备十分有限，快速输注 FFP 会急剧降低游离钙并引起动脉血压的明显下降[63,64]。静脉输注氯化钙（10～20mg/kg）或葡萄糖酸钙（30～60mg/kg）可以治疗急性低钙血症，能有效补充游离钙并改善血流动力学改变。枸橼酸盐代谢后，经血液的缓冲作用可能产生严重的代谢性碱中毒。

吸入麻醉剂

有几种吸入麻醉剂可用于麻醉诱导和维持。药物的选择取决于小儿的年龄和疾病进程。每一种吸入麻醉剂都有其优点和缺点（表 13-4）。没有一种药物能够完全保证血流动力学稳定。对心肌明显抑制的患者或血流动力学紊乱的患者，应避免使用吸入性药物或应降低吸入麻醉剂的浓度。对健康小儿，不论其年龄，很多吸入麻醉剂都能安全和成功地使用。

为了避免静脉注射对小儿造成伤害，常采取吸入麻醉诱导。但是，小儿吸入麻醉也存在风险，可增加发生心动过缓、低血压甚至心搏骤停的发生率[151,228]。强效吸入麻醉剂的不良反应的高发生率同与年龄相关的药物摄取、麻醉剂物需要量和心血管系统敏感性有关。由于血-气溶解系数、血-组织溶解系数、身体构成、肺泡通气与功能性余气量之比以及心排出量分布均存在明显的不同，婴儿和幼儿比成人能更快地摄取吸入麻醉剂[40,174,177,271,275]。因而，在麻醉诱导初期，婴儿脑部、心脏和肌肉组织中的药物浓度要高于成人的[59]。

麻醉剂物的摄取受到心脏分流的影响。右向左分流可减慢难溶性（氧化亚氮）和中等溶解性（氟烷）
麻醉性气体的吸入诱导时间。心内分流对易溶性药物 22
的影响很小[276,281]。溶解度较小的药物在肺泡内的浓度要比在血液中高。由于右向左分流，部分血液不流经肺而直接进入体循环，故进入体循环到达血管丰富器官的吸入麻醉剂较少。溶解度高的药物在血液中的浓度远高于肺泡内的浓度。因为大多数药物留在血液中，肺灌注虽然减少，但仍然携带着大量的药物。诱导的速率减慢。多数情况下左向右分流不影响麻醉诱导的速[281]度。

最低肺泡气有效浓度

最低肺泡气有效浓度（MAC）是指在 1 个大气压下，能防止 50%的患者对外科切口产生体动反应的吸入麻醉剂浓度，是测量吸入麻醉剂强度的标准方法。吸入麻醉剂的 MAC 随患者年龄而改变（见表 13-1）。Lerman 等人[178]发现，1 个月月龄以内的新生儿中氟烷的 MAC 值约比 1 个月～1 岁婴儿的低 25%。LeDez 和 Lerman 的研究表明[174]，妊娠龄小于 32 周的早产儿中异氟烷的 MAC 值低于妊娠龄较长的新生儿。对于所有麻醉剂来说，6～12 个月的婴儿的 MAC 值最大。MAC 需要量的增加以及麻醉剂的快速摄取可使婴儿和儿童容易发生麻醉剂过量[151,228]。

氧化亚氮

氧化亚氮是一种弱效的吸入麻醉剂，MAC 值

表 13-4 吸入麻醉剂

药物	优点	缺点和注意事项
氧化亚氮	价廉 无味 迅速起效，恢复快 与其他强效吸入麻醉剂联合使用时，可以减少强效吸入麻醉剂的副作用 可兴奋交感神经系统，减轻心脏抑制或强效吸入麻醉剂引起的血管扩张	用于扶助其他吸入麻醉剂或静脉麻醉剂以提供完全的全身麻醉 在危重病患者中可以产生强效的血管扩张作用 可扩张空腔，如肠或中耳；可加重气胸和颅腔积气 手术室空气污染可引起神经病变
氟烷	无刺激性气味 有效的吸入麻醉诱导药物 可使支气管扩张（与其他强效吸入药物类似）	可抑制心脏，表现为心动过缓和心肌收缩力下降 可引起氟烷相关性肝炎（儿童中罕见） 可增加心肌对肾上腺素引起心律失常的敏感性；但与青少年和成人相比，更大剂量的肾上腺素才会诱发婴儿和儿童的室性心律失常
异氟烷	可维持心肌收缩力和心率 可降低心肌对肾上腺素引起心律失常的敏感性	有刺激性气味 不是一种有效的吸入麻醉诱导药物 可使新生儿和小婴儿发生心动过缓 可通过降低全身血管阻力导致低血压
七氟烷	无刺激性气味 有效的吸入麻醉诱导药物 血气系数低 可维持心肌收缩力和心率 可降低心肌对肾上腺素引起心律失常的敏感性	比氟烷昂贵 通过肝脏代谢，释放出游离的氟离子；理论上有导致肾性尿崩症的危险 可在氢氧化钡石灰和碱石灰中降解，形成有潜在毒性的代谢物 麻醉后谵妄的发生率增加
地氟烷	血气系数低 可维持心肌收缩力和心率 可降低心肌对肾上腺素引起心律失常的敏感性	有刺激性气味 不适于作为吸入诱导药物 喉痉挛发生率高 价格昂贵 麻醉后谵妄的发生率增加

为 105%，通常被当作强效吸入性药物的辅助药物。氧化亚氮通过减少强效吸入性药物镇痛时所需的剂量来减少其副作用。在麻醉诱导阶段，氧化亚氮能促进强效吸入麻醉剂的摄取。Eger 和 Saidman[88]指出，氧化亚氮比氮气更易溶于血液中，因此，可以扩张空腔，如肠腔。因此，氧化亚氮通常禁止用于存在闭合式气胸、肠梗阻或气脑的患者。已经证明，氧化亚氮能抑制淋巴细胞、破坏睾丸和导致出生缺陷。长期接触可引起流产，因此，确保手术室的排气系统能有效清除麻醉废气十分重要。

氟烷

氟烷因对气道的刺激性低于异氟烷和地氟烷，曾经是小儿麻醉中最常用的吸入麻醉剂。但是，氟烷可引起心动过缓、低血压和室性心律失常，故不是一种理想的麻醉诱导剂。在很多医学中心，七氟烷（因其心血管安全性较高）已经替代了氟烷作为麻醉诱导剂的地位[253]。氟烷相关性肝炎尽管在成人中备受关注，但是在青春期前的儿童中却很少见，即使反复暴露后[49,301]。Warner 等人[302]报道，60 例至少接受了 10 次氟烷麻醉的小儿没有发生肝功能障碍。

氟烷在动物和人类均可抑制心脏功能[28,44,60,61,89]。除了对心功能的直接作用之外，氟烷还与儿茶酚胺产生相互影响。氟烷能使心肌对肾上腺素致心律失常作用敏感化，尽管心律失常在成人中要比在儿童中更常见[144,148,150]。Johnston 等人[144]报道了在恩氟烷、异氟烷和氟烷麻醉的患者中，使患者产生 3 次或 3 次以上室性早搏的肾上腺素静脉注射剂量的反应曲线（图 13-3）。Karl 等人[148]发现，对儿童静脉注射肾上腺素剂量超过 1.7μg/kg 时并没有发生室性心律失常。研究同样表明，对进行腭裂修补的小儿实施氟烷麻醉时，其能耐受 7.8μg/kg 的肾上腺素和 1%的利多卡因而不出现室性心律失常。心动过速和高血压是最常见的副作用。Cote[63]将 10μg/kg 的肾上腺素添加到局麻药给药，时间超过 20 分钟时并没有发生明显的心律失常。

229 异氟烷

异氟烷的溶解系数低于氟烷，所以从理论上来说，异氟烷诱导和恢复要比氟烷迅速。但是，异氟烷麻醉诱导时常引起中重程度的气道刺激反应。

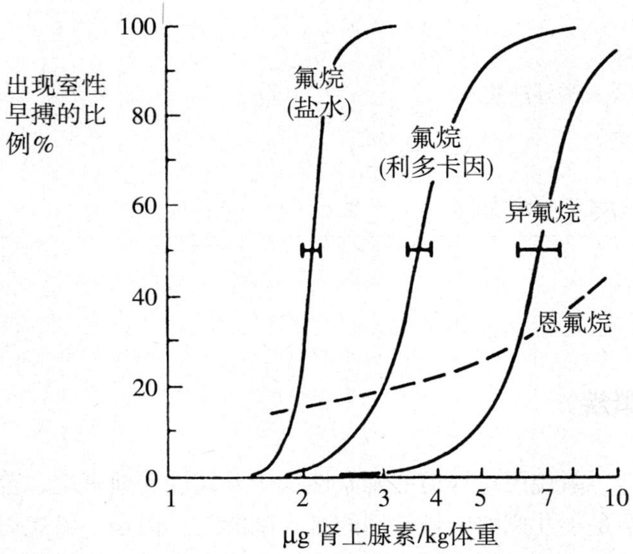

图 13-3 在这个统计分析中，横条线表示 ED50（使 50%的患者产生麻醉诱导的药物剂量）的标准差。肾上腺素（μg/kg）的 ED50 与氟烷和异氟烷的明显不同（$P<0.01$）。在氟烷组，肾上腺素加 0.5%的利多卡因注射后对室性早搏具有显著的保护作用。(From Johnson RR, Eger EI, Wilson C: A comparative interaction of epinephrine with enflurane, isoflurane, and halothane in man. Anesth Analg 1976;55:709.)

异氟烷对小儿心血管的作用已经有不少资料。与成人不同，对术前未用药的 5～26 周龄婴儿实施异氟烷麻醉时，常出现与氟烷麻醉时相似的心率减慢以及氟烷麻醉时一半的血压下降[105]。对大于 2 岁的术前不用阿托品的小儿，异氟烷与氟烷相比可更好地保持心率和心功能[323]。氟烷和异氟烷都会使血压下降。异氟烷可降低外周血管阻力，但不影响心排出量。Gallagher 等人[109]在 15 位年长儿中应用脉搏多普勒超声心动图比较了氟烷和异氟烷对心功能的作用[109]。异氟烷可使心排出量、心率和心肌收缩性保持不变，但氟烷会使心肌收缩性下降。Kotrly 等人[163]发现，在成人中异氟烷保持压力感受器的反应优于氟烷。

地氟烷

地氟烷是一种强效的吸入麻醉剂。地氟烷的血气溶解度低，与氧化亚氮相似[87]。因其具有刺激性气味，地氟烷作为小儿麻醉诱导药物时，喉痉挛、咳嗽和低氧血症的发生率非常高[282,283,334]。地氟烷麻醉苏醒较快。但在小儿中，地氟烷麻醉后谵妄或兴奋的发生率较高[30]。Cohen 等人[57]认为，补充芬太尼可减少与地氟烷相关的小儿兴奋的发生率而不延迟麻醉苏醒。

地氟烷对心血管功能的影响与年龄相关[282]。吸入地氟烷 1MAC 时，在切口前，与清醒时相比，动脉血压约下降 30%，且心率明显下降或保持不变。因此，当吸入 1MAC 时，地氟烷与异氟烷和氟烷相同，可减轻小儿压力感受器的反应。Weiskopf 等人[308]也证明，在成人中，将吸入地氟烷的 MAC 值从 0.55 快速增加到 1.66 时，会出现短暂的血压升高和心率增快现象。这种兴奋现象与交感神经和肾素-血管紧张素系统活性增强有关。

七氟烷

七氟烷是一种强效的吸入麻醉剂，血-气溶解系数低，无刺激性气味，现正逐步取代氟烷成为婴儿和儿童的吸入麻醉剂[176,270]。临床研究发现，小儿使用七氟烷麻醉后恢复时间早于氟烷[81,253]，这可能与其血气溶解度较低有关。与氟烷相比，七氟烷对心血管的副作用较少。Wodey 等人[321]在婴儿中比较了等效浓度的七氟烷和氟烷对心血管的影响。结果发现，七氟烷降低心排出量的程度低于氟烷。心肌收缩力的轻度下降可被体循环阻力（SVR）的明显下降所代偿，故心率没有改变[321]。与氟烷不同，七氟烷不增加心肌对肾上腺素诱发心律失常的敏感性[209]。七氟烷可使呼吸道阻力明显下降，是一种有效的支气管扩张药物[115]。研究显示，与氟烷相比，七氟烷导致的麻醉恢复后兴奋的发生率升高[293,299]。Weldon等人[314]发现，复合咪达唑仑术前用药和术后用骶管阻滞提供可有效镇痛，能够减少小儿七氟烷麻醉后的激动和兴奋现象。其他研究证实，使用酮咯酸[82]、芬太尼[69,106]或可乐定进行适当的镇痛，能够显著地减少麻醉恢复后兴奋的发生率。

使用七氟烷主要要关注其在肝脏通过细胞色素系统代谢之后释放的氟化物以及可能引起的肾性尿崩症。但是，研究表明，成人志愿者持续暴露于七氟烷后其肾脏浓缩能力和肌酐清除率均正常。除了在活体内代谢之外，七氟烷经钠石灰和氢氧化钡石灰降解时可产生两种具有潜在毒性的烯烃，化合物 A 和化合物 B。尽管患者经呼吸环路吸入七氟烷证明不存在毒性作用，但动物研究发现其具有化学诱导毒性的组织学证据[34,109,116]。Frink 等人[104]报道，小儿经呼吸环路吸入 2L/min 流量的七氟烷，麻醉后 24 小时，其化合物 A 的浓度仍很低，且没有肾或肝功能异常。

神经肌肉阻滞药

神经肌肉阻滞药（即肌松药）可阻断神经肌肉连接处的乙酰胆碱受体，常用于气管内插管、手术时需要肌松以及控制机械通气时。神经肌肉阻滞药可减少强效吸入麻醉剂或静脉镇静催眠药的用量，因此，可降低低血压、心动过缓和心搏骤停的发生率。在婴儿期，由于在生理上和生物化学上神经肌肉连接逐渐成熟，骨骼肌的收缩特点发生改变，肌肉量与体重按比例增加，神经肌肉连接部位对肌松药的敏感性发生改
30 变[187]。此外，肌松药的分布容量、再分布、清除以及代谢率均随着年龄变化而有所变化。这些因素都影响肌松药的剂量反应关系和肌松时效[59,71,117]。

除分布容量、麻醉方法和麻醉剂剂量这些因素之外，婴儿对琥珀胆碱相对抗药，而对非去极化肌松药较为敏感（表 13-5）。琥珀胆碱作为去极化肌松药存在很多副作用，在选择性手术病例中已不再使用。

手术期间，应采用神经刺激器监测神经肌肉的阻 231
滞程度，并给予患者足够剂量的药物以达到理想的阻滞程度。除非术后打算进行机械通气，否则在手术结束时需拮抗非去极化肌松药产生的肌肉麻痹。常应用抗胆碱酯酶药（如新斯的明或依酚氯铵）联合抗胆碱能药防止毒蕈碱样副作用。肌松拮抗效果可以通过肌张力、通气幅度和对神经刺激的反应来判断。撤离辅助通气的最低标准应当包括肌张力良好、屈曲手臂和腿以及通气效果满意。很多麻醉医生认为，对 50～100Hz 的强直刺激不出现衰退是拮抗完善的最佳标准。在重症监护病房也经常使用肌松药以控制机械通气。神经肌肉阻滞药物无镇静、催眠或镇痛作用，但可以间接降低代谢需求，防止寒战，减少机械通气不同步，降低颅内压，以及增加胸壁顺应性。重要器官功能衰竭、乙酰胆碱受体上调、营养不良、电解质紊乱和酸碱失衡、药物相互作用以及肌肉萎缩等因素会对肌松药的动力学产生明显的影响。此外，在未监测神经肌肉传导的情况下，长时间反复使用肌松药可能导致肌肉持续无力。了解有关神经肌肉药理学与年龄、联合用药和疾病进程的相互影响有助于在重症监护患者中更加合理地使用神经肌肉阻滞药。

并发症

肌性神经病

在给予重症监护患者肌松药之后出现长时间的意外麻痹是常见的[258,286]。罹患“重症监护病房神经肌肉综合征”的患者都接受过不同时间的多种肌松药治疗，表现为不同程度的肌无力，并伴有各种严重的疾病。这种综合征与失用性萎缩、严重疾患的多神经病以及类固醇性肌病之间存在着相当多的重叠。某些病例可仅表现为肌松药过量，也可表现为具体的神经肌肉病理变化[175,305]。病理学改变包括Ⅰ型和Ⅱ型肌纤维明显萎缩以及肌肉结构破坏，基本没有炎症，运动和感觉神经基本正常。这种综合征可能与严重疾病和使用肌松药导致的乙酰胆碱受体协同性功能不良性上调有关[175]。有研究表明，通过监测神经肌肉传导和减少

表 13–5 肌松药

药物	类型	剂量	代谢和排泄	优点	缺点和注意事项
琥珀胆碱	短效；去极化	静脉注射：1.0～2.0mg/kg 肌内注射：小于 6 个月者，4.0～5.0mg/kg；大于 6 个月者，3.0～4.0mg/kg	拟胆碱酯酶	起效迅速，恢复快，可以通过血管内或肌肉途径给药	咬肌痉挛，触发恶性高热，心动过缓，高钾血症可引起致命的心律失常，肌红蛋白血症（肌肉损伤），肌肉自发性收缩，眼内压增加，拟胆碱酯酶缺乏延长神经肌肉阻滞时间 下列患者应避免使用：肌营养不良，多发性创伤＞24 小时，烧伤＞24 小时，脊柱损伤＞24 小时，恶性高热易感
米库氯铵	短效；非去极化	气管插管：0.2mg/kg 维持：0.1mg/kg	血浆胆碱酯酶	恢复时间 10 分钟；输注可能	组胺释放；气管插管条件不可预料
阿曲库铵	中效；非去极化	气管插管：0.5mg/kg 维持：0.15mg/kg	酯水解；Hoffman 降解	不论年龄，恢复时间均为 30 分钟；可用于肾脏疾病患者；输注可能	组胺释放；（Hoffman 降解的代谢物）；大剂量致癫痫
顺阿曲库铵	中效；非去极化	气管插管：0.1mg/kg 维持：0.3mg/kg	酯水解；Hoffman 降解	恢复时间 30 分钟；无心血管效应；输注可能	
罗库溴铵	中效；非去极化	气管插管：0.6mg/kg（起效 50～80 秒）或 1.2mg/kg（起效 30 秒）维持：0.1mg/kg	肝脏和肾脏	恢复时间 15～40 分钟（剂量依赖）；可用于快速顺序插管；输注可能	轻度迷走神经松弛
维库溴铵	中效；非去极化	气管插管：0.1mg/kg 维持：0.02mg/kg	肾脏和肝脏	小儿的恢复时间约为 30 分钟；剂量高达 0.4mg/kg 是无组胺释放；无心血管系统效应	对于婴儿肌松作用持久，恢复时间大约为 70 分钟
泮库溴铵	长效；非去极化	气管插管：0.1mg/kg 肌松：0.02mg/kg	肾脏和肝脏	恢复时间大约为 50 分钟；价格便宜	迷走神经松弛，心动过速，高血压，组胺释放

单位时间肌松药用量可降低长时间麻痹的危险性。Lele[75]建议，定期停用肌松药，进行药效学、神经病学以及电生理学方面的检查有助于早期发现该综合征。婴儿和幼儿长时间使用神经肌肉阻滞药有可能干扰其肌肉的正常生长和发育，导致持续数月的中重度肌无力。肌肉发育不能逆转因制动引起的肌萎缩。因此，年长的婴儿和儿童更可能恢复肌肉功能，因为他们的神经肌肉发育已达到一定水平，而出生后不久即被制动的新生儿（特别是早产儿）则较难恢复[264]。

恶性高热

恶性高热（MH）是一种威胁生命的疾病，其特点是接触某些药物后产生高热、高代谢和肌肉损伤。

强效的吸入麻醉剂（不包括氧化亚氮）和去极化肌松药琥珀胆碱是最有可能触发儿童恶性高热的药物。恶性高热的触发物能引起骨骼肌肌浆网内 Ca^{2+} 过量释放入肌浆，导致一系列代谢性改变，最终造成热量产生、细胞损伤、高钾血症和肌红蛋白血症[183]。恶性高热引起的人肌细胞内钙水平升高可被丹曲林所对抗[183]。恶性高热若不予处理，其死亡率可超过 60%。若迅速给予丹曲林治疗，死亡率可下降接近于零。

在使用琥珀胆碱的全麻患者中，恶性高热的发生率大约是 1/60 000；若不使用琥珀胆碱，则为 1/220 000[213]。多数恶性高热患者平素基本健康。恶性高热是一种多基因遗传的家族性疾病。一级亲属处于高危状态；二级亲属的危险性较低，但遇到触发药物后诱发恶性高热的危险性很高。Duchenne 肌营养不良患者发生恶性高热的危险性很高。其他与发生恶性高热相关的疾病还有中心核病和 King-Denborough 综合征。

恶性高热的典型体征包括心动过速、室性心律失常、呼吸急促、体温迅速升高超过 39.5℃、下颌僵硬或全身性僵硬、代谢性和呼吸性酸中毒以及混合静脉血氧饱和度下降。相关的实验室检查结果包括高钾血症、高碳酸血症、呼吸和代谢性酸中毒、肌酸磷酸激酶和乳酸增加、凝血因子异常以及出现肌红蛋白尿。

应当在出现高代谢体征和体温达到极端之前考虑恶性高热的诊断。疾病的早期征象包括呼吸急促、心动过速、呼气末二氧化碳（$ETCO_2$）升高和室性心律失常。这些征象应当给予迅速评估以排除以下各种原因，如医源性高热、脓毒症、嗜铬细胞瘤、甲状腺功能亢进、呼吸机瓣膜功能异常导致二氧化碳重复吸
32 入、麻醉深度不够以及体温和 $ETCO_2$ 监测发生错误。

急性恶性高热的处理如表 13-6 所示。治疗重点是静脉使用丹曲林，该药需用不含防腐剂的无菌蒸馏水稀释。尽管可能需要更大的剂量，静脉用丹曲林的初始剂量是 2.5mg/kg。需要的话，剂量可以超过常规的极限（10mg/kg）[238]。丹曲林的应用应当根据临床征象和实验室检查给予指导，每 5 分钟重复一次直至代谢性酸中毒纠正为止。丹曲林可通过减少钙离子移动或骨骼肌特有的钙转运蛋白穿透细胞膜，减少肌浆网释放钙[199,227]。丹曲林可降低肌肉的高代谢，减轻肌肉僵硬并恢复肌肉的正常功能。随着骨骼肌功能恢复正常，血清钾减少，乳酸产生减慢[247]。患者会在 20 分钟内对丹曲洛林产生反应。$ETCO_2$ 在 6 分钟内开始下降，而动脉血气分析证明，20分钟内代谢性和呼吸性酸中毒可得到明显改善[247]。45 分钟后，代谢性和呼吸性酸中毒应当被消除。如果代谢异常持续存在，则有必要采用更大剂量的丹曲洛林进行治疗[238]。

表 13-6 急性恶性高热的处理

表 13-6 急性恶性高热的处理
立刻停止吸入麻醉剂。
尽可能快地取消或终止手术。
高流量 100%纯氧强力呼吸。
静脉注射丹曲林（2mg/kg），并根据需要重复注射。
如果体征再次出现，则加大丹曲林的剂量。
开始时予以降温毯降温，静脉注射冷生理盐水（15ml/kg，持续 10 分钟），在腋窝和腹股沟部位放置冰袋，如果中心体温＞38℃，则用冷生理盐水灌洗体腔。当中心体温回落到 38℃时，停止降温。
纠正代谢性酸中毒，给予碳酸氢钠，初始剂量为1.0～2.0mEq/kg。
给予钙（氯化钙 10mg/kg）或在 50%的葡萄糖（1mg/kg）中添加胰岛素（0.2U/kg）治疗高钾血症。
给予利多卡因（1mg/kg）治疗室性心律失常。
给予呋塞米（1mg/kg）以使尿量维持在每小时2ml/kg 水平，如果需要的话，再添加甘露醇。
动脉和中心静脉置管。
每 15 分钟 1 次重复进行静脉血气和电解质分析，直到疾病征象消失和生命体征正常。

受累儿童的父母可能希望进行肌肉活检和挛缩试验，因为结果若为阴性则意味着其他亲属罹患恶性高热的危险性不增加。理想情况下，应告知受累儿童的同胞兄弟姊妹并进行肌肉活检。

在有恶性高热个人史和强烈家族史的患者，实施区域或局部麻醉后可安全地进行手术。若不应用触发药物，也可进行全身麻醉。所有非去极化肌松药和静脉麻醉剂都可安全地用于恶性高热易感者。用丹曲林预防恶性高热的做法尚存争议[102,214]。对这些患者最重要的是要监测恶性高热的早期征象既迅速开始治疗。

乳胶过敏

自 1979 年首例乳胶过敏病例确诊以来，乳胶过

敏的发生率一直在上升。乳胶过敏可引起患者严重反应，甚至可导致患者死亡。有必要鉴别小儿是否处于乳胶过敏的危险之中，并采取适当的措施防止术中发生乳胶过敏。有特异反应性病史和有脊柱裂或泌尿生殖系统异常的小儿在实施多次手术时发生乳胶过敏的危险性增加。即使没有经过多次手术，脊柱裂患者也是发生乳胶过敏的独立的危险因素。

患者经非胃肠途径接触乳胶或经黏膜接触乳胶后不久就可能发生严重的反应，包括面部潮红、血管舒张、严重支气管痉挛和血管通透性增加伴水肿和心血管虚脱。轻微的过敏反应（如荨麻疹和血管神经性水肿）可能会因患者覆盖手术单而被掩盖。治疗措施包括持续纯氧通气、静脉补液和给予肾上腺素来维持血压。肾上腺素是一线治疗药物，其作用机制是维持血压和舒张支气管平滑肌。其他有效药物包括抗组胺药（静脉注射苯海拉明 0.5～1.0mg/kg）、吸入支气管扩张药、H_2 受体阻断剂和皮质类固醇（甲泼尼龙 0.5mg/kg）。皮质类固醇虽不是一线治疗药物，但其对迟发反应和后期反应有益。在手术室里创造一个没有乳胶的环境是预防乳胶过敏的最佳方法。

静脉麻醉剂

硫喷妥钠

硫喷妥钠是巴比妥类麻醉诱导剂，可经静脉或直肠途径给药。静脉麻醉诱导的剂量随年龄不同而异。Westrin 等人[317]认为，硫喷妥钠的 ED50（可使 50%的患者麻醉的药物剂量）在新生儿为 3.4 ± 0.2mg/kg，1～6 月婴儿为 6.3 ± 0.7mg/kg。Jonmarker等人[145]发现，硫喷妥钠诱导剂量的 ED50 在婴儿为 7～8mg/kg，1 岁以上的小儿为 4～5mg/kg（图 13-4）。这些研究证实了之前 Cote 等人[66]以及 Brett 和 Fisher[41]的发现，即小儿使用硫喷妥钠的剂量较大。巴比妥类药物能减少脑血流，降低颅内压。健康小儿能够很好耐受硫喷妥钠导致的心肌抑制和静脉舒张作用[317]。对血流动力学不稳定的患者，这种心血管效应可导致明显的低血
233 压。脱水、心力衰竭以及明显失血的患儿应该尽量避免使用硫喷妥钠。硫喷妥钠诱导的副作用包括呃逆、呛咳和喉痉挛。Valtonen 等人[296]报道，在 1～6 岁的小儿中这些副作用的发生率约为 20%。硫喷妥钠外渗会引起组织损伤，这可能与硫喷妥钠的强碱性有关。巴比妥类药物也可引起组胺释放。静脉注射硫喷妥钠可引起过敏反应，需要给予积极的处理，给予肾上腺素、抗组胺药物和类固醇。

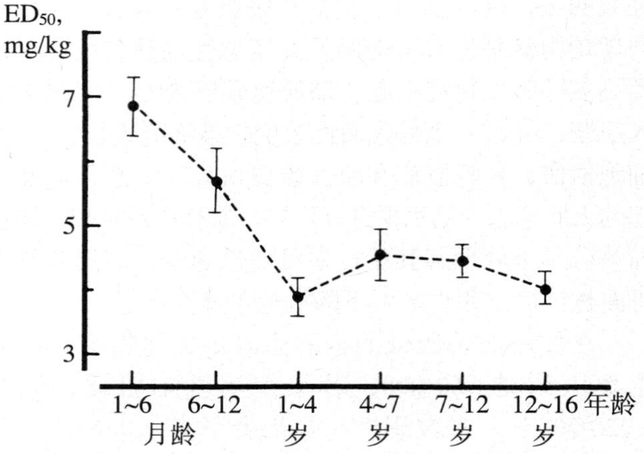

图 13-4 不同年龄组硫喷妥钠的 ED_{50}（使 50%患者产生麻醉诱导的药物剂量）估计值 ± 标准差。(From Jonmarker C, et al: Thiopental requirements for induction of anesthesia in children. Anesthesiology 1987;67:104.)

异丙酚

异丙酚是一种具有镇静、催眠作用的亲脂性静脉麻醉剂，常用于麻醉诱导和维持。异丙酚的药物动力学特点是分布、代谢和清除都很迅速。注射结束后，异丙酚再次分布于外周组织可使血浆浓度迅速下降。异丙酚是通过肝脏结合转换成无活性的代谢物并经肾脏排泄[333]。

Westrin[316]发现，1～6 个月大的术前未用药的婴儿所需异丙酚的诱导剂量（3.0 ± 0.2mg/kg）大于 10～16 岁儿童的剂量（2.4 ± 0.1mg/kg）。Aun 等人[16]的报道与之相似。Hannallah 等人[126]发现，3～12岁术前未用药的儿童的异丙酚有效麻醉诱导剂量是 2.5～3.0mg/kg[124]。虽然年幼儿和年长儿需要不同剂量的异丙酚的机制尚不清楚，但是 Westrin[316]提出，可能是因为婴儿与体重相关的心排出量较高，血管分布的腔室较大，而到达脑内动脉的药物峰值浓度比成人低有关。

异丙酚联合阿片类药物麻醉时减慢了充分麻醉所

需的注射速度。McClune 等人[191]、Short 和 Chui[266]发现，给予成人异丙酚联合咪达唑仑镇静时，两种药物剂量各减少了 44%。添加咪达唑仑 0.13mg/kg 能减少全身麻醉时异丙酚所需的输注速率的 52%。异丙酚具有止吐作用，亚催眠剂量同样有此功效[37]。

异丙酚可引起低血压，但作用机制尚未完全清楚[17,124,257]。Aun 等人[17]比较了在 41 例 8 个月～12 岁健康儿童对硫喷妥钠（5mg/kg）和异丙酚（2.5mg/kg）诱导剂量的血流动力学反应。该研究测量了心率、血压和血流速度。静注异丙酚后平均动脉压下降了 28%～31%，比硫喷妥钠（14%～21%）明显。心指数下降了 10%～15%，两种药物相似。在研究中，这些儿童能耐受低血压，不需要药物干预。Hannallah 等人[124]指出，像成人一样，小儿异丙酚麻醉后心率减慢比吸入麻醉性气体明显。采用异丙酚和阿片类药物维持麻醉时，阿托品可减轻幼儿的心动过缓。Keyl 等人[154]认为，在异丙酚麻醉期间，迷走神经介导的外周压力感受反射刺激的心率反应明显受到抑制，同时循环压力感受器刺激的血压反应受到损害。

经手背静脉注射异丙酚引起的疼痛的发生率可以高达 50%[295]。通过肘前静脉注射异丙酚或在注射器中按每 2～3mg/kg 异丙酚添加 0.1mg/kg 利多卡因可减轻或消除疼痛。

监测

无创监测

对麻醉患者，麻醉医生应注意无创监测的三个方面。第一个方面是直接观察患者而不使用机械或电子设备。第二个方面包括定期或连续测量和记录生命体征、尿量、失血量、补液和输血量，以及调整心血管和呼吸参数。这方面可以再细分为必要监测（即麻醉后为了保障安全而必须进行的测量）和针对某些病例进行的特殊监测。第三个方面是监测与患者相连的机器的表现（例如，加温器的温度、通气报警以及分光计对吸入和呼出气体的分析）。

34 ASA 已经建立了麻醉监测基本标准，包括使用麻醉剂期间连续评估患者的氧合、通气、循环和体温。在麻醉机上安置氧浓度分析仪，通过测量患者的呼吸回路中吸入气的氧浓度确保输送合适的氧浓度，通过脉率氧饱和度仪测量血氧状况。通过定性观察临床体征确保通气，例如胸廓起伏、观察呼吸囊和听诊呼吸音。通过定量方法，例如二氧化碳描记法、二氧化碳测量法或质谱法，连续监测二氧化碳。当机械通气时，使用连续监测装置以防管道意外脱落。使用连续显示心电图、动脉血压和心率的监测仪检测循环，至少每 5 分钟评价一次。此外，可以通过听诊心音、触诊脉搏、监测动脉内压力波形、超声脉搏监测或脉搏体积描记法或血氧定量法确保循环稳定。麻醉期间，温度监测有助于维持患者的体温正常[12]。

体温监测

在婴儿中，体温测定最常用的部位是直肠，但是存在下列缺点：（1）僵硬的热敏电阻探头导线有可能造成肠壁穿孔；（2）探头有可能移位；（3）使用水温毯时，肛周和尾骨区域的组织受热，影响测定结果。更重要的是，总体来说直肠温度不能迅速随着全身温度变化而变化，如在控制性降温和复温期间。食管中段温度或鼻咽温度更能反映患者的中心温度。理论上，鼓室温度最接近脑部温度，因此可提供更为理想的信息。目前使用的鼓室探头对于婴儿的外听道来说可能太大，而且使用时存在发生鼓室创伤的可能。

麻醉和手术期间，应监测其他部位的温度，如吸入气、加温毯和手术室内的温度。考虑到经常需要监测患者的多个部位的温度，因此，多通道热敏电阻温度监测仪最为有用。

脉率氧饱和度监测

通过脉率氧饱和度监测仪可以连续无创地监测动脉血氧饱和度（SaO_2）。通常将探头置于手指或足趾上，但是只要有搏动性血管床，任何部位都可进行监测。采用对氧合血红蛋白和去氧血红蛋白吸收系数不同的两种波长的光线分别照射探头下的组织。探测光的透射量随着搏动血管的收缩和舒张改变光线经过的距离而改变，表现为特征性的体积描记波形，且消除了来自血液、皮肤、结缔组织或骨骼的影响。这种技术在氧饱和度 70%～100%的范围内能精确地工作。血管搏动减弱会降低仪器测量氧饱和度的性能，如在低温、低血压或使用血管收缩药物时。除了连续显示 SaO_2 之外，脉率氧饱和度仪还连续提供脉率读数以及振幅。

二氧化碳描记法

二氧化碳描记法是一种方便的通气监测方法。此外，二氧化碳描记法可确定待测样品的气体成分和浓度。常用于氧气、二氧化碳、氮气、氧化亚氮和常用吸入性麻醉剂的测定。

显示的吸入和潮气末数值的精确性取决于二氧化碳描记曲线的可靠性。实时二氧化碳描记图中，图 13-5A 表示平静呼吸且没有再呼吸时的二氧化碳曲线。平滑的、水平肺泡平台最大值（4）代表肺泡气
235 体，与动脉二氧化碳张力保持平衡或接近。在这种情况下，当通气肺部血流分布良好时，两值差在 2～4 torr 之内。若通气和灌注不匹配，就会发生明显的偏离（肺泡-动脉二氧化碳梯度），特别是存在大量死腔通气并伴有肺栓塞时。

在实际操作中并不总能获得理想的二氧化碳描记曲线，但是异常的曲线可用于诊断或高度提示患者、麻醉回路或通气技术发生了某些问题。图 13-5B（1）中的切迹表明，神经肌肉阻滞不全时可产生自主呼吸。图 13-5B（2）中缓慢、陡峭的呼气波形表明气道阻塞，图 13-5B（3）中的圆形曲线反映了持续压力缺乏，如呼吸回路出现明显漏气时。婴儿麻醉期间常用浅快的控制呼吸。此时，如图 13-5B（4）所示，发生了呼气不全和部分重呼吸。实时二氧化碳描记图的缺陷是不能精确地知道吸气和呼气的开始时间，因为吸气期重复吸入二氧化碳在监测时肺泡平台延长。Bhavani-Shankar 和 Philip[33]建议，同时监测气流波形可以精确地定位吸气和呼气的时程，有利于监测重复呼吸。该项技术的临床意义尚有待于进一步研究证实。

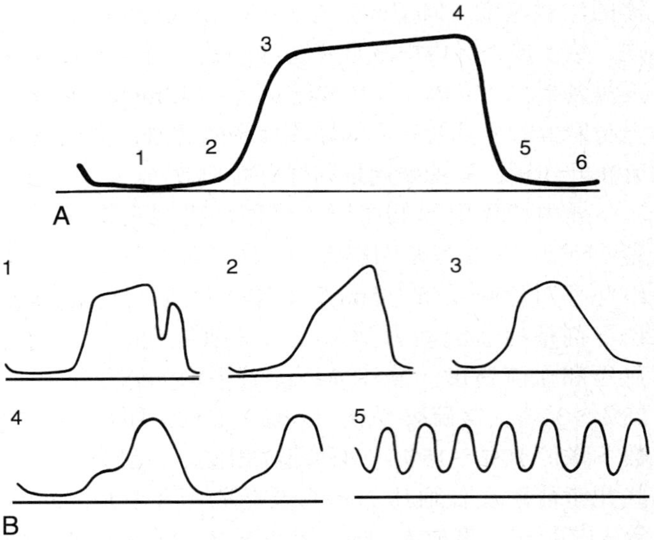

图 13-5 A. 理想的二氧化碳描记曲线：（1）呼气开始。（1～2）解剖死腔气排空。（2～3）死腔气与肺泡气混合。（3～4）肺泡平台。（4）潮气末最大值；吸气开始。（4～5）死腔气排空。（5～6）吸入气中没有二氧化碳。B. 二氧化碳描记曲线的类型：（1）神经肌肉阻滞不全时的自主呼吸。（2）呼吸道梗阻。（3）呼吸回路存在大量漏气，不能持续正压。（4）在 Mapleson D 回路中，新鲜气流很大量而潮气量很小时，呼出的二氧化碳被稀释，不能达到稳定的肺泡平台。（5）当新鲜气流量很小时，从 Mapleson D 回路的呼出端部分重呼吸二氧化碳，表现为呼吸过快而潮气量很小。

神经肌肉功能监测

唯一让人满意的监测神经肌肉功能的方法是：刺激外周运动神经，然后观察或测量受此神经支配的骨骼肌的反应。市场上现已有能提供理想的矩形或正方形脉冲且作用时程不长于 0.2 毫秒的各种神经刺激器。通常通过肘部或腕部表面的电极刺激尺神经，观察拇内收肌的反应。应使用较小表面积的电极或针型电极以减少对肌肉的直接刺激。应确保整个神经兴奋采用超强电刺激。0.1Hz 单次重复刺激或低频率(2Hz 持续 2 秒)的 4 个成串刺激，可用于使用肌松药后的神经肌肉传导的连续监测。强直刺激（50 Hz）、4 个成串刺激、双重暴发刺激可用于药物拮抗后神经肌肉功能的评估。

在成人，神经肌肉传导功能良好的临床征象包括维持抬头 5 秒，肺活量至少达到 15～20ml/kg，或吸气负压达到 30cmH$_2$O。因为对婴儿不能持续抬头 5 秒钟，因此，具备屈臂或屈腿能力是神经肌肉传导适度的可靠征象。由于婴儿的肺活量不容易获取，因而以测量吸气压代替。强直刺激（30～50Hz）下 5 秒无衰减，或 4 个成串反应接近正常（>0.7）也是神经肌肉传导功能恢复良好的可靠征象。

有创监测

各种高级的无创监测设备已经减少了有创监测的需求。有创监测更多是由患者疾病驱动的而非手术操作[13]。重症患者常需应用动脉内、中心静脉和肺动脉导管在术中和术后对脉搏、血管内压力和一系列动脉血气分析、血液化学以及凝血功能检查进行短期的连续测量。

右侧桡动脉的氧浓度与颈动脉最接近，是最理想的动脉采血部位。当存在右向左分流时，动脉导管后的血氧张力较低，且可能在主动脉缩窄修补术等操作时被箝闭。当不能在桡动脉置管时，可选择股动脉、足背动脉或胫后动脉。在婴儿中，通常避免在肱动脉和腋动脉置管，因为存在截肢的风险。股动脉置管有可能引起关节损伤，颞浅动脉置管进行冲洗时可引起逆行血液灌注，有引发脑颞叶梗死的危险。尽管脐动脉在出生后 10 天内可用于置管，但感染发生率高，故较少使用。另外，因为存在血栓形成和栓塞的风险，股动脉导管末端应仔细定位于膈肌之上或第三或第四腰椎之下，以便远离腹腔动脉、肠系膜动脉和肾动脉的起始部。此外，对右向左分流的患者在未闭的动脉导管以下部位采血时，脐动脉血氧饱和度可能低于颈动脉或右侧桡动脉，因此有可能错误判断低氧血症而使用过高浓度氧进行治疗。

中心静脉置管，特别是血流导向的肺动脉导管（Swan-Ganz）在婴儿和小儿中应用有限。而且相对于手术室患者，中心静脉置管可能更常适用于在重症监护病房中的患者。手术患者需行中心静脉置管的指征包括大量失血、休克和低流量状态。虽然可选择锁骨下静脉或股静脉置管，但更推荐颈内静脉作为置管通路。置管和监测大静脉回心血流的压力可用于指导维持或调控患者的循环血容量[13]。可能的并发症有房性或室性心律失常、血栓栓塞、血胸、气胸和感染。

6 疼痛管理

各个年龄段的小儿都能感受疼痛。虽然小儿疼痛管理有待于完善，但是近来由于对小儿疼痛的兴趣和意识增长，以及哲学观点的转变和技术的进步，小儿疼痛管理已经明显改善了[7,14]。

给予小儿手术患者合适的互利，需要给患儿进行相应的疼痛处理，而疼痛处理应与其让年龄、情感和身体发育的成熟度以及手术过程相匹配。小儿感受疼痛的能力经常被忽视，其耐受强效镇痛的能力也常被质疑[92,255]，这使很多患儿在手术时没有得到充分的疼痛处理。历史上，高达 40%的小儿在手术后第一天主诉有中度到重度的疼痛[188]。尽管很多小儿持续遭受着术后疼痛的折磨，但随着多学科的共同努力，小儿围术期疼痛处理已明显改善了[233]。主要是通过手术计划、术后疼痛的预期程度、麻醉技术和预期恢复过程制定术前、术中和术后的镇痛策略[216]。患儿的疼痛状况需定期评估，必要时应调整镇痛方案。

除外科手术之外，小儿还经常遭受其他的疼痛刺激。静脉穿刺、静脉插管的疼痛以及其他类似的操作都能带来短暂但剧烈的疼痛，这经常被小儿及其家长描述为患病和住院期间最痛苦的事情[92]。在这种情况下，适当的疼痛处理既可为患儿镇痛，又可增强患儿的合作，有利于成功地完成操作[259]。给予适当的干预可以使大多数患儿能够在无痛、无焦虑和应激的情况下接受诊断性和治疗性操作。

急性疼痛是对已发生的或即将发生的组织损伤的一种生理性反应，可提供损伤或疾病的部位以及性质等有用信息。因此，在基础外科疾病确诊之前，常不给予患者有效的镇痛。这些患者不予治疗的疼痛，特别是在儿童，已逐渐被人们所认识[210]。适当的镇痛不仅能缓解患者的疼痛和减轻痛苦，还有助于进行更加全面和精确的评估，特别是对恐惧或不合作的小儿患者。例如，急性腹痛患儿静脉注射吗啡能提供有效的镇痛，且不会掩盖病灶处的触痛，也不影响阑尾炎的临床诊断[155]。传统上认为不应对未确诊的患者（包括儿童）进行强效镇痛，这种做法站不住脚，应予以摒弃。

围术期计划和常用方法

围术期的疼痛处理应使患者尽可能舒适，但要避免过度镇静或呼吸抑制。可以采用多种方法，应根据小儿的不同情况进行选择和调整。镇痛计划在术前麻醉评估时就应开始实施，并应贯穿于整个手术操作和术后阶段。

很多非药技术可增强镇痛效果，增加患者的配合，并可减少药物用量 *。常用的非阿片类镇痛药包括对乙酰氨基酚和非甾体类抗炎药，而氯胺酮在特定病例中的应用日益增多。口服阿片类药物适用于治疗轻度至中度的疼痛，而静脉注射阿片类药物仍是治疗中度至重度疼痛的主要方法。对长时间需要静脉阿片类药物的患者可以采用连续输注或患者控制镇痛等方式。很多局麻技术也可应用。

世界卫生组织提出的镇痛三阶梯方案是一个有用的镇痛范例（图 13-6）[327]。早在 1986 年，该方案首先作为科研报告提出，建议用于癌痛处理，如今镇痛阶梯方案已经成为普遍有效处理各种病例的疼痛模型，且可用于儿科手术患者。该方案提供了各种水平的辅助用药和非药物技术，强调疼痛是一种主观感受，每个患者的反应各不相同。并且在该方案中镇痛药分层次使用，轻度疼痛使用非阿片类药镇痛药，中度疼痛使用低强度的阿片类药物，严重疼痛使用高效阿片类药物。该方案最重要的可能是，将患者的疼痛完全缓解作为最终的目标。

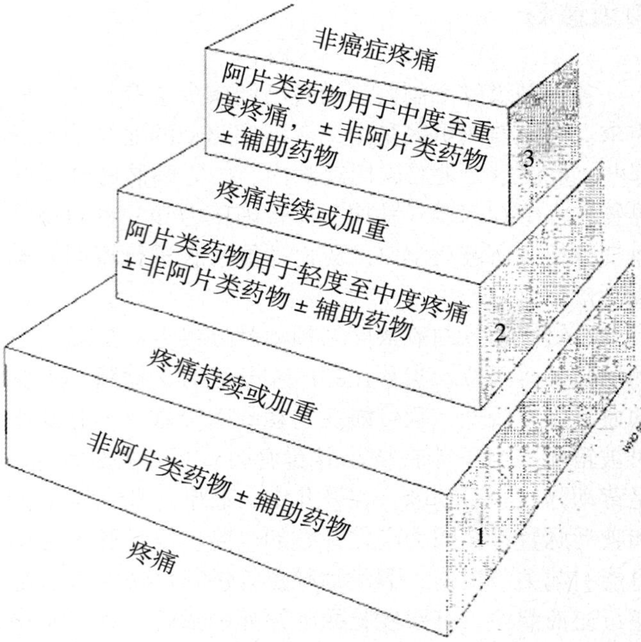

图 13-6 三阶梯镇痛于 1986 年首次被推荐作为癌症疼痛处理方案，现已普遍及有效地用作各种情况的疼痛处理模型，并且适用于儿科手术患者。(From World Health Organization: Cancer Pain Relief: With a Guide to Opioid Availability, 2nd ed. Geneva, WHO, 1996, p 15.)

发育和生理学

各年龄段的小儿都能感受疼痛，但是疼痛的类型和强度可能存在显著差异。尽管外周伤害感受器的功能在出生时已经发育完善[99]，但是对小儿的中枢调节和痛觉感受尚未研究清楚。此外，在新生儿和婴儿中，很多表达痛觉的反射通路在结构上和功能上尚不成熟[10]。因此，尽管小儿外周伤害感受器能接受到疼痛刺激，但是神经中枢对疼痛的处理差异较大，感知疼痛的能力也较为有限。故婴幼儿对疼痛的反应较难预测，特别是早产儿[101]，这也构成小儿不能得到恰当的镇痛治疗的常见原因。

痛觉敏感和超前镇痛

急性疼痛是对组织损伤的一种生理性反应。持续或严重的疼痛未得到适当治疗时可引发严重的病理生理反应[101,325]。组织损伤和炎症可使外周伤害感受器的活性增强，导致对机械性和化学性刺激高度敏感。在动物模型中，背角神经元可对传入刺激产生神经生理学和形态学改变，同时兴奋性增加。外周和中枢的高敏反应可能改变正常的感觉（感觉迟钝），加重伤害性刺激引起的疼痛（痛觉过敏），或对正常的无害性操作也产生疼痛（异常性疼痛），这表明高敏反应在细胞和神经生理学上与临床上疼痛敏感有关。

在组织损伤发生前进行超前镇痛可以抑制疼痛通路上传的刺激，减弱神经内分泌性应激反应，并防止发生外周和中枢高敏反应[325]。单纯全身麻醉不能有效地达到这些目的；在动物模型中已对非甾体类抗炎药(NSAID)、阿片类药物以及一系列局部麻醉技术进行过研究，结果各不相同[55,56,326]。通常动物模型显示，在伤害性刺激之前进行超前镇痛，可降低背角神经元高度兴奋性，减轻疼痛反应，并可减少临床上镇痛药的用量。然而，在人体研究中出现了矛盾的结果，且常为负面结果，特别是在儿童的研究[6,15,96,135,138,166,278]。

* 见参考文献 1, 3, 45, 53, 58, 91, 130, 133, 153, 170, 181, 192, 196, 205, 206, 224, 246, 250, 265。

在术前不同时间或术后开始进行镇痛的研究表明，大多数患者的主观性疼痛评分、客观性评估和镇痛药用量常无明显影响。因此，对超前镇痛作为防止痛觉敏感和减少围术期疼痛的确切效果仍然存在着争论，需要进一步研究[73,157,197]。

疼痛评估

对儿科患者的疼痛评估具有挑战性。学语前或发育迟缓的儿童无法向监护人表达有无疼痛及其严重程度。在各个年龄段的患者中，都可能存在区分疼痛和烦躁的困难。尽管如此，小儿疼痛仍应得到迅速地识别、评估和处理。

已经发明了不少工具，并已得到验证，可用于不同年龄段和发育程度的小儿的定量疼痛评估[23,86]。这些工具通常依靠主观自述或客观评估。对于能够理解和合作的年长患儿，常采用模拟评分等方法对疼痛强度进行主观性自述。对于学语前、年幼的或发育延迟的小儿，采用疼痛相关的行为客观性评估。模拟评分采用脸部图画或照片描述不同程度的疼痛，通常为患者提供颜色、箭头、线条或数字（通常 0～10）以表达疼痛水平。学龄儿童和年长儿童通常有能力进行模拟评分。对学语前、年幼的或发育延迟的患者可使用数字性工具客观评价各种与疼痛相关的行为来得到疼痛评分，从而定量地评价疼痛强度。此法类似于评价新生儿活力的 Apgar 评分。主观性自述模拟疼痛评分和客观性行为评估疼痛评分的结果在小儿中经常不一致[30]，这可能反映了在区分疼痛、烦躁和其他原因引起的痛苦之间存在着困难。选择合适的人群持续使用一种疼痛评估方法并进行趋势分析，要比选择某种特定的方法更重要。

非阿片类镇痛药

非阿片类镇痛药是小儿疼痛处理中重要的辅助药物但常被忽视。非阿片类镇痛药足以治疗轻度至中度疼痛，且可以减少中度至重度疼痛患者的阿片类药物的需要量[159]。与阿片类药物不同，非阿片类镇痛药通常存在封顶效应，即超过推荐剂量是不能明显改善镇痛效果，反而会增加副作用和中毒的危险[190]。小儿常用的非阿片类镇痛药包括对乙酰氨基酚、各种非甾体类抗炎药以及氯胺酮（表 13-7）。其他镇静催眠药和诱导药物包括水合氯醛、苯二氮䓬类、巴比妥类、依托咪酯以及异丙酚，但都缺少镇痛作用。

对乙酰氨基酚

对乙酰氨基酚常用于治疗小儿轻度至中度疼痛， 238
还可以用作退热药。对乙酰氨基酚是强效的环加氧酶抑制剂，没有抗炎活性，因此很少引起胃肠道、肾脏或血液方面的并发症。对乙酰氨基酚的主要毒性是肝脏损伤，可见于急性和慢性过量使用的患者。对乙酰氨基酚对轻度至中度疼痛可提供完全的镇痛，并可减少中度至重度疼痛治疗中阿片类药物的需要量，特别是当按计划给予时。非甾体类抗炎药可以增强围术期使用对乙酰氨基酚的镇痛效果[236]。

在美国，对乙酰氨基酚有口服和直肠两种剂型；其他国家还有静脉用剂型。对乙酰氨基酚常用的口服剂量是每 4 小时 15mg/kg（最大量为 1000mg），口服负荷剂量为 20mg/kg（最大量为 1000mg），特别适用于操作期镇痛和围术期镇痛。总量不宜超过 4g/d。

与口服相比，直肠吸收对乙酰氨基酚较缓慢，生物利用度变异较多，且需要更大的剂量才能达到等价的镇痛效果[245]。已经证明，经直肠使用对乙酰氨基酚能够在某些手术后减少疼痛评分，减少阿片类药物的用量，包括鼓膜切开置管术和腹股沟疝修补术[162]，使用剂量不小于 40mg/kg[236]。直肠用对乙酰氨基酚的维持剂量为每 4 小时 20mg/kg（最大量 1300mg），常用于不合作或不能耐受口服的患者。总量不超过 4 g/d。

非甾体类抗炎药

同对乙酰氨基酚一样，对于轻度至中度疼痛，非甾体类抗炎药可以提供足够的镇痛效果；处理中度至重度疼痛时，非甾体类抗炎药常与阿片类药物合用[160,304]。对于肌肉骨骼痛，非甾体类抗炎药特别有效。与对乙酰氨基酚不同的事，非甾体类抗炎药具有明显的抗炎活性，因此可引起胃肠道、肾脏以及血液等方面的副作用。非甾体类抗炎药可减少肠系膜和肾脏灌注，损害血小板功能，可能引起胃肠道局部缺血、肾功能不全和出血。大剂量或长期使用时风险增加。

三柳胆镁是非甾体类抗炎药中唯一不会引起血小

表 13-7 小儿常用的非阿片类镇痛药

药物	剂量	评价
对乙酰氨基酚	20mg/kg 口服负荷量（最大 1000mg），然后 15mg/kg 口服（最大 1000mg），每 4 小时 1 次 40mg/kg 经直肠负荷量（最大 1300mg），然后 20mg/kg 经直肠（最大 1300mg），每 4 小时 1 次 最大 4g/24h 口服或经直肠	有良好的退热作用 过量会产生肝脏毒性
选择性非甾体类抗炎药（NSAID）		
三柳胆镁	10mg/kg 口服或经直肠（最大 1000mg）每 6 小时 1 次 最大 4g/24h	有良好的退热作用 只有非甾体类抗炎作用而不会导致血小板功能异常 与 Reye 综合征无关
布洛芬	10mg/kg 口服或经直肠（最大 800mg），每 6 小时 1 次 最大 4g/24h	有良好的退热作用
酮咯酸	0.5mg/kg 肌内注射或静脉注射（最大 30mg），每 6 小时 1 次 总疗程＜5 天	退热作用差 有可能导致明显的血小板功能异常
氯胺酮（需要专业人员和监护）	4.0～10.0mg/kg 口服（成人剂量为 300～500mg） 3.0～5.0mg/kg 肌内注射（成人剂量为 150～300mg） 0.5～1.0mg/kg 静脉注射（成人剂量为 50～100mg）	抗胆碱能药物，可减少流涎 苯二氮䓬类药物，可以防止躁动 可增加颅内压，可能诱发癫痫发作

板功能异常的药物，因此被用于罹患凝血方面疾病或存在手术出血危险的患者。因有罹患原发性水痘的小儿服用阿司匹林后发生 Reye 综合征的报道，阿司匹林在小儿中的使用已明显减少[190]。尽管三柳胆镁是阿司匹林的一种衍生物，但目前无与 Reye 综合征相关的报道。然而，对于以前曾患原发性水痘或接受过水痘免疫的小儿来说，仍需限制三柳胆镁的使用。三柳胆镁有液体和片剂两种剂型，常用剂量为每 6 小时 10mg/kg（最大量 1000mg）。对于不愿意或无法口服片剂的患者，可以通过直肠给予相同剂量的液体剂型。总量不超过 4 g/d。

在美国，小儿最常用的口服非甾体类抗炎药是布洛芬，后者有液体、片剂和胶囊等剂型。布洛芬为中效镇痛药，退热效果明显，小儿使用安全。但布洛芬在小儿操作性和围术期镇痛的应用较少[160]。布洛芬的口服剂量为每 6 小时 10mg/kg（最大量 800mg）。可以经直肠使用相同剂量的液体剂型。总量不超过 4 g/d。

酮咯酸是非甾体类抗炎药中唯一可经静脉使用的镇痛药。吲哚美辛可经静脉使用，但只允许针对罹患动脉导管未闭的婴儿促进动脉导管关闭之用。酮咯酸是一种高效非甾体类抗炎药，其镇痛效果与很多阿片类药物相似；与其他非甾体类抗炎药或对乙酰氨基酚相比，酮咯酸能提供良好的围术期镇痛作用[204]。酮咯酸特别适用于不能耐受阿片类药物或存在围术期恶心和呕吐的高度风险的患者。该药上市初期，只能经肌肉途径给药，现已证实酮咯酸经静脉给药也是安全有效的[232]。口服酮咯酸给药只用于成人，尚不能用于小儿。

肌注或静注酮咯酸的常用剂量是每 6 小时 0.5mg/kg（最大量 30mg）。小儿酮咯酸分布容积和血浆清除率约为成人的 2 倍，但是总体清除半衰期与成人相似[211]。作为最强的非甾体类抗炎药，酮咯酸的副作用的发生率也是最高的，其总疗程不得超过 5天，以免发生严重的胃肠道和肾脏的并发症。酮咯酸可影响肠系膜灌注，因此禁止用于罹患坏死性小肠结肠炎的婴儿。

单次使用酮咯酸可引起严重的血小板功能异常，对于有高度出血危险性的患者来说，酮咯酸的应用存在着争议。初期的经验表明，在小儿扁桃体切除术的围术期应用酮咯酸可能会增加术中失血量[245]，回顾性研究也报道术后出血率增加[108,146]。然而，其他的回顾性研究和前瞻性随机研究数据并不能证实酮咯酸有出血增加的倾向[21]。产品说明书警告具有高危出血风险的患者：使用酮咯酸需慎重。在得到更多明确的信息之前，这类患者慎重起见应避免使用酮咯酸。

氯胺酮

氯胺酮是一种与苯环己哌啶相似的镇静催眠药。与其他镇静催眠药物不同，氯胺酮是一种有效的分离麻醉剂。氯胺酮为 N–甲基–D–天冬氨酸受体拮抗剂，尽管其作用机制尚未完全清楚，但其对阿片类和许多其他受体具有轻度激活作用。氯胺酮的镇痛和镇静作用与剂量相关，全身麻醉诱导作用需要较大的剂量，而其遗忘作用变化较大。与其他苯环己哌啶衍生物相似，幻觉和谵妄并不少见，但在年幼患者中的发生率较低、程度较轻[119]。氯胺酮具有支气管扩张作用，但也可导致严重的流涎。氯胺酮可促进内源性儿茶酚胺释放，因而可保持血流动力学参数相对稳定。氯胺酮可增加颅内压，有致惊厥作用，所以罹患颅内病变或有癫痫发作的患者使用时要谨慎。

对于年幼儿或有潜在血流动力学不稳定的婴儿和儿童来说，氯胺酮是最常用的静脉诱导药物。氯胺酮肌注适用于不合作或缺乏静脉通路的患者。氯胺酮也可在围术期和重症监护病房内用作辅助镇痛药。近来，氯胺酮被推荐用于罹患各种疾病的小儿的操作性镇痛和镇静[119,287]。在得到氯胺酮有利的安全性资料后，其在小儿急诊科特别受到欢迎[219,221]。氯胺酮通常静脉用剂量为 0.5～1.0mg/kg（成人为 50～100mg），肌肉用剂量 3.0～5.0mg/kg（成人为 150～300mg），口服用剂量为 4.0～10.0mg/kg（成人为 300～500mg）；其镇痛和镇静效果好，严重并发症发生率低。口服给药后，可能导致恢复期延长，特别是大剂量时，恢复时烦躁并不少见。为了预防流涎，推荐同时给予抗胆碱能药物，如阿托品或格隆溴铵。同时给予苯二氮䓬类药物可以减少幻觉和谵妄的发生。儿童给予氯胺酮后，必须进行充分监护，而且要配备相应的复苏设备和人员[85]。

阿片类镇痛药

不愿给小儿使用阿片类药物是小儿未得到充分镇痛治疗的一个常见原因。阿片类药物是处理中重度疼痛的主要药物，已在小儿操作性和围术期镇痛中发挥了重要作用[329]。通过作用于中枢神经系统中各种阿片受体的亚型，阿片类药物可产生与剂量相关的镇痛作用和呼吸抑制；其他副作用包括嗜睡、瞳孔缩小、胃肠道动力下降、恶心和尿潴留。很多阿片类药物会引起组胺释放，引起荨麻疹、瘙痒、恶心、支气管痉挛，偶尔发生低血压。经椎管内给药时，瘙痒更加多见，且通常程度更加剧烈，可能是由中枢神经系统的阿片效应而不是组胺释放引起的。阿片类药物的副作用可通过其他药物给予治疗（表 13–8）。

阿片受体的拮抗剂纳洛酮能快速地逆转阿片类药物的作用。轻度呼吸抑制或嗜睡时，可以静脉注射纳洛酮 1.0μg/kg，必要时可每 1～2 分钟重复和调整用量；10～100μg/kg 的纳洛酮可以逆转阿片类药物过量时引起的呼吸暂停或昏迷。必要时可以加大剂量或重复使用。纳洛酮可能会促使阿片依赖的患者出现戒断症状，有报道大剂量时可以引起肺水肿。

阿片类镇痛药通常不存在最大有效剂量。首次使用阿片类药物的患者开始给药时建议使用推荐剂量；逐渐增量至产生临床效应，必要时加大剂量。长期用药或持续疼痛的患者常需增大剂量（耐受，快速减敏）。阿片类药物治疗超过 7～10 天时可能产生药物依赖性，在中断治疗前需逐渐减量以免发生戒断症状[262]。药物耐受和药物依赖可以分别发生。药物成瘾是一种执意搜寻药物的精神病理性状态，但在接受正规剂量镇痛的小儿中极少发生，故不应成为妨碍治疗的理由[329]。

阿片类药物经常与镇静催眠药物联合应用，特别 240
是与苯二氮䓬类药物，这可增加呼吸抑制和缺氧的危险[20,267,331]。药物剂量必须仔细滴定，给予适当监护，并应有能力处理包括呼吸抑制和呼吸暂停的并发症[20,267,331]。必须准备好适当的拮抗药物。

新生儿和小婴儿使用阿片类药物已成为很多研究的题目和争论的话题。以往在小鼠和人体的研究中表明，新生儿的血脑屏障对阿片类药物的通透性增加，特别是吗啡，可能引起较严重的呼吸抑制[167,306]。目前，已经越来越清楚地认识到，在新生儿中，吗啡[31,32,52,131,185]、芬太尼[134]以及事实上所有阿片类药物的药理学特点和临床效果都存在着明显的个体差异。一般而言，与年长儿相比，新生儿对阿片类药物的清除率较低，排除时间较长，且出生几个月后才可接近成人水平。没有理由阻止给予任何年龄段的小儿阿片类药物治疗，应给每一位患者提供个体化剂量，并调

表 13-8 阿片类药物副作用的药物治疗

副作用	药物	剂量	评价
呼吸暂停，昏迷	纳洛酮	10~100μg/kg 静脉注射或肌内注射，必要时每 1~2 分钟 1 次 通常初始最大量：400μg 可能需要加大剂量或重复注射	可再次发生镇静作用 阿片类药物依赖患者可产生撤退症状 大剂量可能会引起肺水肿
轻度呼吸抑制，轻度镇静	纳洛酮	1.0μg/kg 静脉注射或肌内注射，必要时每 1~2 分钟 1 次 通常初始最大量：400μg 可能需要加大剂量或重复注射	可再次发生镇静作用
便秘	多库酯	5.0mg/kg 口服（最大 100mg），每日 2 次	可软化粪便
恶心	甲氧氯普胺	0.1mg/kg 静脉注射（最大 10mg），必要时每 6 小时 1 次	有锥体外系副作用
	恩丹西酮	0.1mg/kg 静脉注射（最大 4.0mg），必要时每 6 小时 1 次	价格昂贵
	异丙嗪	0.25~0.5mg/kg 口服、经直肠或静脉注射（最大 25mg），必要时每 6 小时 1 次	可能引起嗜睡
瘙痒	苯海拉明	0.5~1.0mg/kg 口服或静脉注射（最大 50mg），必要时每 6 小时 1 次	可能会引起嗜睡
	羟嗪	0.5~1.0mg/kg 口服或静脉注射（最大 50mg）每 6 小时 1 次 必要时	可能会引起嗜睡
	纳布啡	0.05μg/kg 静脉注射（最大 5.0mg），必要时每 4 小时 1 次	针对椎管内用阿片类药物产生的瘙痒
	纳洛酮	每小时 1.0μg/kg 静脉输注	针对椎管内用阿片类药物产生的瘙痒

整剂量至产生临床效果。

口服阿片类药物

因疼痛所需且胃肠道功能许可时，口服阿片类药物提供了经胃肠道的治疗。口服阿片类药物起效相对较慢，不适合紧急重度疼痛的处理。几种低效口服阿片类药物常用于儿童（表 13-9），对轻度至中度疼痛的镇痛效果良好。

可待因有液体和片剂剂型，常与对乙酰氨基酚联

表 13-9 小儿口服弱效阿片类药物

药物	剂量	评价
可待因	1.0mg/kg 口服，每 4 小时 1 次（成人剂量，30～60mg）	有片剂和液体剂型 常与对乙酰氨基酚制成复方使用 胃肠道副作用的发生率高
氢可酮	0.2mg/kg 口服，每 4 小时 1 次（成人剂量为 10～15mg）	有片剂和液体剂型 常与对乙酰氨基酚或 NSAID 制成复方使用 胃肠道副作用的发生率中等
羟考酮	0.1mg/kg 口服，每 4 小时 1 次（成人剂量为 5～10mg）	有羟考酮片剂和与对乙酰氨基酚或 NSAID 制成复方剂 有羟考酮口服液 胃肠道副作用的发生率低 缓释剂用于慢性治疗

合使用，常用剂量为 1.0mg/kg（成人剂量为 30～60mg），每 4 小时 1 次。可待因引起胃肠道不适的发生率很高。氢可酮有液体和片剂剂型，常与对乙酰氨基酚联合使用或给予一种非甾体类抗炎药联合使用，常用剂量为 0.2mg/kg（成人剂量为 10～15mg），每 4 小时 1 次。氢可酮引起胃肠道不适的
241 发生率低于可待因。羟考酮片剂有两种，分别为单纯羟考酮配方和含有对乙酰氨基酚或含有一种非甾体类抗炎药的复合配方；液体剂型只含有羟考酮。羟考酮常用剂量为 0.1mg/kg（成人剂量为 5～10mg），每 4 小时 1 次。羟考酮很少引起胃肠道不适，患者常能很好地耐受。缓释羟考酮剂型可用于慢性疼痛的治疗。

高效阿片类药物常经静脉途径给药，但也可经口服给药（表 13–10）。吗啡口服的起始剂量为 0.3mg/kg（成人为 15～30mg），每 3 小时 1 次。但吗啡可以引起组胺释放，产生荨麻疹、瘙痒、支气管痉挛等副作用，大剂量时甚至发生低血压，虽然这些副作用在口服给药时比较少见。口服缓释吗啡可用于治疗慢性疼痛。氢吗啡酮口服起始剂量为 20～40μg/kg（成人为 2～4mg），每 3 小时 1 次，其引起组胺释放的程度较吗啡轻。哌替啶口服起始剂量为 1.0mg/kg（成人为 50～100mg），每 3 小时 1 次。哌替啶不应长期使用，因为积聚的代谢产物去甲哌替啶具有神经毒性，有可能导致癫痫发作[114,201]。去甲哌替啶通过肾脏排泄，因此肾脏疾病患者发生癫痫的危险性增加。美沙酮口服起始剂量为 0.1mg/kg（成人为 5.0～10.0mg），每 6～12 小时 1 次，特别适用于对阿片类药物依赖的患者的慢性治疗[285]。在美国只有获得国家专项证书的机构才有资格采用美沙酮治疗阿片类药物成瘾的患者。

经口腔黏膜吸收的枸橼酸芬太尼（OTFC）制成了棒棒糖的剂型。虽然 OTFC 常可引起恶心和呕吐，但 OTFC 可为小儿提供有效的麻醉前镇静[103,227]，并可给疼痛性操作提供镇痛和镇静[254]。通常的剂量为 5～15μg/kg（成人剂量为 400μg）；儿童需要的单位剂量可能比成人大。使用 OTFC 的患者需要适当的监护[328]。

表 13–10　小儿用的强效阿片类药物

药物	剂量 *	评价
芬太尼	5～15μg/kg 口服（成人剂量为 400μg）	有单次剂量的口服剂型
	0.5～1.0μg/kg 静脉注射（成人剂量为 50～100μg），每 1 小时 1 次	婴儿快速注射可能会引起胸壁僵直
	静脉输注：每小时 0.5～1.0μg/kg（成人剂量为 50~100μg/h）	经皮贴剂不用于急性疼痛的治疗
	贴剂：25μg = 1mg/h 静脉注射吗啡	
氢吗啡酮	20～40μg/kg 口服（成人剂量为 2.0～4.0mg），每 3 小时 1 次	组胺释放作用轻于吗啡
	10～20μg/kg 肌内注射、静脉注射或皮下注射（成人剂量为 1.0～2.0mg），每 3 小时 1 次	
	静脉输注：每小时 4μg/kg（成人剂量为 0.2～0.3mg/h）	
哌替啶	1.0mg/kg 口服、肌内注射、静脉注射或皮下注射（成人剂量为 50～100mg），每 3 小时 1 次	神经毒性代谢物可引起癫痫发作，肾脏疾病患者的风险较高
	静脉输注：不推荐	无肝胆方面的优点
美沙酮	0.1mg/kg 口服（成人剂量为 5～10mg），每 6～12 小时 1 次	可用于长期治疗，包括姑息治疗
	0.05mg/kg 静脉注射（成人剂量为 2.5～5.0mg），每 6～12 小时 1 次	阿片类药物成瘾治疗应在联邦专业机构中进行
	静脉注射：通常不用	
吗啡	0.3mg/kg 口服（成人剂量为 15~30mg），每 3 小时 1 次	组胺释放可引起荨麻疹、瘙痒、支气管痉挛、低血压
	0.1mg/kg 肌内注射、静脉注射或皮下注射（成人剂量为 5～10mg），每 3 小时 1 次	大剂量和快速给药可增加组胺释放
	静脉输注：每小时 0.02mg/kg（成人剂量为 1.0～1.5mg/h）	口服缓释剂型可用于慢性疼痛的治疗

* 在可使用阿片类药物的患者中推荐使用的初始剂量；调整到所需要的临床效果，可能需要更高的剂量；在新生儿及幼儿中剂量减少 25%～50%。

静脉用阿片类药物

静脉用阿片类药物是治疗中度至重度疼痛的主要药物（表 13-10）。尽管从药理学上来说，皮下或肌肉途径给药都是有效的，但会引起额外的疼痛和不是，特别是对儿童，应避免使用[25,26,248]。静脉用阿片类药物的副作用更为常见和严重，因此需适当的监护并对并发症进行迅速处理。新生儿和小婴儿静脉给予阿片类药物之后，必须特别仔细地予以监护，而且剂量也需减少 25%～50%。等效剂量的阿片类药物产生副作用的风险基本相似[329]。

吗啡是传统的静脉用阿片类镇痛药，初始剂量为 0.1mg/kg（成人为 5～10mg），每 3 小时 1 次。静脉用氢吗啡酮的初始剂量为 10～20μg/kg（成人为 1～2mg），每 3 小时 1 次，其引起组胺释放的程度较吗啡轻。哌替啶的初始剂量为 1.0mg/kg（成人为 50～100mg），每 3 小时 1 次，但不能用于长期治疗，静脉用药发生癫痫并发症明显早于口服给药[114,201]。尽管曾经很受欢迎，哌替啶并不优于其他阿片类药物，等效剂量时诱发肝胆管痉挛也不少见[262,329]。但目前哌替啶已不再推荐作为一线镇痛药，尽管小剂量的哌替啶可有效治疗寒战。美沙酮的初始剂量为 0.05mg/kg（成人为 2.5～5mg），每 6～12 小时 1 次。术中给予美沙酮的小儿外科患者随后镇痛的需要量要低于术中
242 给予吗啡的患者[26]。呼吸抑制的危险和其他阿片类药物的副作用在应用美沙酮的患者组较迟发生。

芬太尼起效快、作用时间短，常用于小儿操作性和围术期镇痛。静脉用芬太尼的初始剂量通常为 0.5～1.0μg/kg（成人为 50～100μg），每小时 1 次，多在操作中或操作后立即开始使用。芬太尼具有高亲脂性，大剂量、反复或持续给药会导致明显的组织蓄积作用，作用时程明显延长[207]。芬太尼经皮贴剂可提供连续性经皮吸收，作用与静脉注射相似。一块 25μg 的芬太尼贴片相当于静脉注射吗啡 1.0mg/h。贴剂起效缓慢，吸收存在个体差异。虽然芬太尼贴剂对处理某些慢性疼痛有效，但不适用于处理急性疼痛患者[110,329]。

对于需要多次静脉注射阿片类药物的婴儿和儿童来说，连续输注镇痛的有效方法。对于健康的患者按照推荐剂量给药时，很少发生呼吸抑制，不会影响自主呼吸，也不会延迟机械通气支持的撤离[184]。每小时静脉注射剂量：吗啡为每小时 10～20μg/kg（成人为 1.0～1.5mg/h），氢吗啡酮为每小时 2.0～4.0μg/kg（成人为 0.2～0.3mg/h），芬太尼为每小时 0.5～1.0μg/h（成人为 50～100μg）。哌替啶具有潜在的神经毒性，因此不推荐用于连续输注。美沙酮半衰期较长，因此，小儿连续输注美沙酮既无必要，也无帮助。药量应从小剂量开始，逐渐加量使用，并需严密观察镇痛效果、镇静水平以及呼吸抑制的程度。所有接受连续阿片类药物输注的患者应当尽可能进行连续脉搏血氧饱和度监测，新生儿和小婴儿还需监测心肺功能指标。新生儿和小婴儿第一次使用阿片类药物时药物剂量通常要减少 25%～50%[95,161]。

患者自控镇痛

传统上，通常是在患者感到疼痛后才给予阿片类药物。出现疼痛症状后再用药常会耽误用药时机，导致疼痛恶性循环，有形成持续疼痛或过度镇静的危险（图 13-7）[118]。这种模式只能使患者得到短暂镇痛，而且有发生阿片类药物的严重副作用的风险。较为理想的是，将阿片类药物的水平维持在镇痛阈值之上而低于引起功能紊乱或呼吸暂停的阈值，在有效水平和中毒水平之间保持一个平衡（图 13-8）[25]。在患者感到疼痛之前，按照适当的间隔间断性静脉注射阿片类药物，可以维持阿片类药物的浓度在镇痛窗内，但是这种方法颇为费时，且存在药物蓄积的危险。持续输注阿片类药物可以建立药理学稳态，但不易进行短期调节。患者自控镇痛（PCA）为小儿静脉输注阿片类药物提供了一种安全、有效和容易调整用药的方法[118,235,318]。

PCA 是利用微处理器来控制输注阿片类药物，这使患者能根据需要按压按钮，随时输注小剂量的药
物。为防止药物输注过量，需设置一个适当的锁定间 243
隔。PCA 镇痛效果优越，剂量合适，很少发生严重的并发症[26]。通过适当的指导，大多数学龄儿童能够安全有效地使用 PCA 输注阿片类药物[26,111]。护士或家长控制的镇痛可用于没有能力或不愿意自己控制的小儿[5,182,313]，如果时间间隔调节不合理，特别是联合背景输注时，发生呼吸抑制的危险性增加[198]。

吗啡是 PCA 最常用的药物，也可用氢吗啡酮或芬太尼（表 13-11）。哌替啶不推荐用于 PCA，因为持续用药会增加中毒的危险。对于阿片类药物需要量

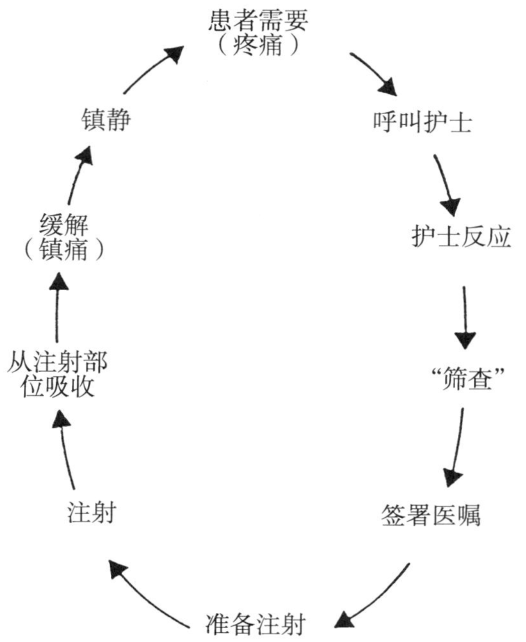

图 13-7 传统阿片类药物治疗的恶性循环示意图。(From Graves DA, Foster TS, Batenhorst RL, et al: Patient-controlled analgesia. Ann Intern Med 1983;99:360-366.)

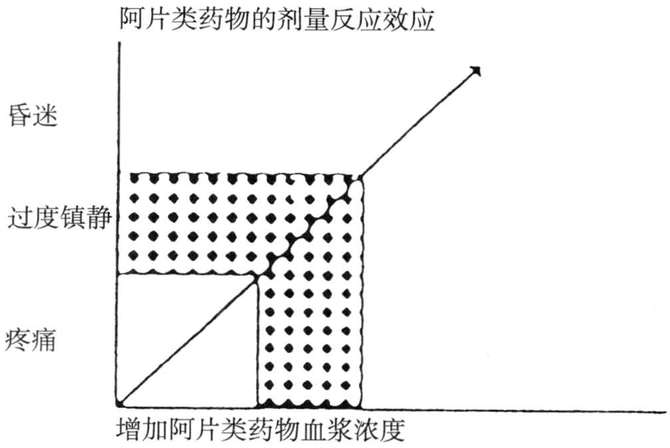

图 13-8 阿片类药物治疗的镇痛窗。理想的剂量反应曲线显示了随着血浆中阿片类药物浓度的升高，从疼痛至镇痛再至昏迷的连续性过程。阴影区域描绘了镇痛不当与过度镇静之间的镇痛窗。(From Berde CB: Pediatric postoperative pain management. Pediatr Clin North Am 1989; 36:921-940.)

很大且对其他药物耐受的小儿癌症患者，PCA 可以采用美沙酮[249]，但是对于大多数小儿来说，使用美沙酮既不需要也没有帮助，因为该药半衰期太长。PCA 常用的方案有吗啡 0.02mg/kg（成人为 1.0～1.5mg），氢吗啡酮 4μg/kg（成人为 0.2～0.3mg）或芬太尼 1.0μg/kg（成人为 50～100μg）。患者自控时锁定间隔时间为 8～10 分钟，护士或家长控制时锁定时间为 15～60 分钟。对年幼的或病重的患者，延长给药的间隔可能更加安全。开启背景输注以确保持续镇痛和维持睡眠期间的药物浓度，这种做法得到了提倡[128]，但是还没有证明这样做能够显著增加镇痛效果[195,315]。研究表明，成人 PCA 采用背景输注会增加发生呼吸并发症的危险[94,217]，但在小儿中还没有观察到这种现象。小儿 PCA 采用背景输注尽管安全，但对镇痛效果的帮助有限。

接受 PCA 的患者应定时进行疼痛评估，以及时调整剂量和给药间隔。对使用任一阿片类药物治疗的小儿都推荐进行连续性脉率氧饱和度监测。年幼和危重的小儿应进行心肺功能监测。向患者、家长和护理

表 13-11 小儿患者自控镇痛的用药方案

药物	需要剂量 *	背景输注（如果使用）
芬太尼	0.5~1.0μg/kg 静脉注射（成人剂量为 50~100μg）	每小时 0.5~1.0μg/kg 静脉注射（成人剂量为 50~100μg/h）
氢吗啡酮	4μg/kg 静脉注射（成人剂量为 0.2~0.3mg）	每小时 4μg/kg 静脉注射（成人剂量为 0.2~0.3mg/h）
哌替啶	不推荐使用	
美沙酮	通常不用	
吗啡	0.02mg/kg 静脉注射（成人剂量为 1.0~1.5mg）	每小时 0.02mg/kg 静脉注射（成人剂量为 1.0~1.5mg/h）

* 通常患者自控镇痛的锁定时间为 8~10 分钟；护士或家长控制镇痛的锁定时间为 15~60 分钟。推荐剂量是针对以前从未使用过阿片类药物的患者的初始用药。剂量需要逐步调整至产生临床效果，可能需要较大剂量。新生儿和小婴儿的剂量减少 25%~50%。

人员介绍有关 PCA 的用法是必要的。

局部麻醉

利多卡因能有效镇痛，但作用时程相对较短，且常可导致运动神经阻滞。在局麻药配方中，利多卡因常与丙胺卡因配伍使用，丙胺卡因可引起高铁血红蛋白血症，特别是当大剂量使用或用于小儿时。布比卡因广泛用于小儿，因为其作用时程较长，且阻滞感觉神经强于运动神经。布比卡因有高度的心脏毒性，且对心脏和神经的毒性阈值相似；在感觉麻木或抽搐发作之前可出现心律失常。两种较新的药物，左旋布比卡因[121]和罗哌卡因[290]的毒性作用较小。左旋布比卡因是布比卡因的左旋同分异构体，神经传导阻滞的作用与布比卡因相似，但对心脏的毒性阈值较高。与布比卡因相比，罗哌卡因可以高度选择性地阻滞感觉神经，而对心脏的毒性阈值相对较高。但由于价格昂贵，这些新药的应用受到了限制。按照最大推荐剂量应用（表 13–12）可以降低中毒的危险。

局部麻醉可以通过表面应用局麻药，局部直接浸润，以及外周神经、神经丛或椎管内阻滞来进行。局部麻醉的一个优点是镇痛不需要依靠阿片类药物或其他全身麻醉剂，尽管部分小儿局部麻醉时仍常需使用这些药物[261]。小儿较多使用辅助镇痛药物与其理解能力和情感与身体发育差异较大有关。与全身使用阿片类药物相比，小儿局部麻醉发生副作用的风险较低，
244 副作用包括恶心、镇静以及呼吸抑制[25,78,261,289,291]。对阿片类药物敏感性增加的患者，如新生儿和罹患慢性呼吸系统疾病的小儿，采用局部麻醉特别有利。在一些病例中已经证明，小儿局部麻醉能够改善手术效果[195]。

表 13–12 局麻药的最大推荐剂量

局麻药	最大推荐剂量（mg/kg）*
布比卡因	3.0
左旋布比卡因	3.0
利多卡因	5.0
丙胺卡因	7.0
罗哌卡因	4.0

* 在局麻药药液中添加血管收缩药，如肾上腺素或去氧肾上腺素，可能会延长局麻药的吸收时间，并可适度地加最大推荐剂量，但这并不可靠。

小儿可在不用镇静或全身麻醉下使用表面麻醉。浸润麻醉可用于愿意合作或年长的儿童，或在手术操作期间进行。与成人操作不同，小儿的外周神经、神经丛以及椎管内阻滞多在全身麻醉诱导以后进行[75,239]。理论上，这种做法可妨碍对并发症的观察，后者包括感觉异常、阻滞失败、注射到其他部位或组织。幸运的是，在全身麻醉情况下，小儿使用局麻技术而发生严重并发症的现象非常罕见[25,220,324]。在麻醉诱导后至外科手术前实施局部麻醉可以降低术中全身麻醉的深度，加速术后苏醒和恢复[330]。

表面麻醉

很多局麻药配方都可经皮肤镇痛而不再需要注射（表 13–13），潜在地减少或消除了全身使用镇痛药及镇静药的需要。

EMLA 乳膏是由 2.5%的利多卡因和 2.5%的丙胺卡因混合组成的。使用时可在皮肤上涂一厚层，用密闭的敷料覆盖至少 60 分钟。EMLA 可为小手术提供有效的经皮镇痛，如包皮环切术和胸引管拔除[23,51,122,237,280]。其镇痛作用可长达 4 小时。EMLA 乳膏使用方法简

表 13–13 表面麻醉剂配方

产品	成分	评价
ELA–Max	4%～5%的利多卡因脂质体	30 分钟前使用 不需要敷料 为非处方药
EMLA	2.5%的利多卡因 + 2.5%的丙胺卡因	1～4 小时前使用 需要密闭的敷料 丙胺卡因可引起高铁血红蛋白血症
Numby Stuff	Iontocaine（2%的利多卡因 +1/100 000 的肾上腺素）	10 分钟前使用 需要特殊的电极和仪器 麻刺感可使小儿感到不适
TAC	4% ～11.8% 的可卡因 + 0.5%～1%的丁卡因 + 1/2000 ～1/4000 的肾上腺素	20 分钟前使用 避免接触黏膜 避免在末端灌注区域使用 有潜在的可卡因毒性

单，患者及其家长可以在家里使用。其副作用有红斑、皮肤苍白和皮疹。EMLA 中的丙胺卡因成分有引起高铁血红蛋白血症的危险，特别是在大剂量使用或用于婴儿时。在合理使用的情况下，副作用很少发生。

还有其他一些表面麻醉药剂型。ELA–Max 是一种含 4%或 5%的利多卡因的脂质体剂型，属于非处方药[90]。Numby Stuff 是一种独特的表面麻醉装置，是利用弱电流将含有 2%的利多卡因和 1∶100 000 的肾上腺素的药液以离子化方式快速透入皮内起作用[14,273]。TAC（丁卡因、肾上腺素、可卡因）已有多种制剂，可以为表皮撕裂伤的小儿修补伤口提供有效的镇痛[36,93,132,268]。

浸润麻醉

局麻药浸润能为短小手术提供有效的镇痛，合作的或较年长的患者使用时不需应用镇静或镇痛药物。可以采用任何一种适用药物。很多局麻药液的酸性pH可增加其溶解度而延长作用时间，但这也是注射时产生疼痛的主要原因。缓冲 pH有助于减轻清醒患者的疼痛，而且可以增强局麻效果。在 10ml 局麻药液内加入 1.0mEq 碳酸氢钠可以明显减轻注射痛，且不会使药液发生沉淀[54]。碳酸氢钠应在使用前才加入。

浸润麻醉还能为小手术提供有效的术后镇痛，但对大手术无效[34]。如果不超过最大推荐剂量，浸润麻醉发生局麻药中毒的危险性很小。小儿腹股沟疝修补术时在伤口处实施浸润麻醉，作用时间可达 2～4小时，与髂腹股沟–髂腹下神经阻滞[50,231]或骶管阻滞[256]的镇痛效果相似。但是，浸润麻醉不能提供长时间的镇痛[260]。

外周神经和神经丛阻滞

只要设备合适、操作医生本人有兴趣，成功阻滞任何外周神经或神经丛都是有可能的[76,260]，神经阻滞可以优化镇痛效果，减少阿片类药物的需要量并改善肺功能[189]。外周神经阻滞容易在小儿中实施，其中有几种方法特别适用于小儿外科患者。与成人相比，小儿较少实施神经丛阻滞，主要是由于医生缺乏经验，但也有可能是在将应用于成人的操作技术应用于小儿时要战胜各种挑战。肢体局部静脉麻醉或称 Bier 阻滞，已有在小儿中应用的报道[80]，但其应用因局麻药的毒性反应而受限。理论上，在手术切口前进行外周神经和神经丛阻滞可提供超前镇痛并减轻整体的疼痛经历，但是在临床实践中尚未得到可靠的论证[6,15,278]，特别是在小儿中。因此，何时进行阻滞并不如实施阻滞本身重要。

腹直肌阻滞 245

近来由于对小儿脐部手术的兴趣，特别是在腹腔镜技术的应用，促进了在这些手术中应用局部麻醉的研究。胸部下方肋间神经的终末皮支支配着腹部前方中线处的皮肤。尽管这个区域很容易实施浸润麻醉，但进行具体的神经阻滞可延长镇痛的时间。已有对进行脐疝和脐旁疝修补的小儿实施腹直肌鞘阻滞的报道[97]，而且稍作改良后已被称为脐旁阻滞[68]。

在脐部和一侧白线的中点处进行注射（图 13–9）[68]。将针尖磨钝的针头按照中等角度刺入皮肤，直到感觉到明显的弹性或“噗”的一声，即直到感觉到针尖穿过腹直肌外鞘的突破感为止。为了减少发生注入血管的情况，在回抽和试验剂量结果均为阴性之后，注入 0.25～0.5ml/kg 的局麻药。注药时阻力感轻微或无阻力。可以把针后退一点，然后在皮下朝脐部进针，这样可以增加覆盖到远端皮支的效果。在对侧重复注射一次。腹直肌阻滞可用于脐上或脐下其他皮区的中线腹疝修补术的麻醉[76]。

髂腹股沟–髂腹下神经阻滞

髂腹股沟神经和髂腹下神经是腰丛的终末皮支。髂腹股沟神经起源于第一腰段脊神经根，支配外生殖器的大部分以及大腿近端部分。髂腹下神经起源于第十二胸段和第一腰段脊神经根，支配腹股沟韧带以上部分的腹壁前部皮肤。通常是联合阻滞这两根神经可为同侧腹股沟部位的手术提供镇痛[127]，如腹股沟疝修补术和睾丸固定术。

注射穿刺点在髂前上棘向内后上各旁开 1～2cm 处（图 13–10）[330]。将针尖磨钝的针头垂直刺入皮肤，直到感觉有明显的弹性或“噗”的一声，即直到感觉到针头刺破了 Scarpa 筋膜的突破感觉并触及外斜肌腱膜为止。为了减少发生注入血管内的情况，在回抽和试验剂量结果均为阴性之后，注入 0.5～1.0ml/kg 的局麻药。注药时阻力感轻微或无阻力。可以把针后退一点，然后在皮下向脐部进针，以改善阻滞髂腹下神经远端皮支的效果。髂腹股沟-髂腹下神经阻滞只能提供皮肤镇痛，涉及内脏操作时还需辅助其他麻醉
246 技术。因为没有阻滞内脏神经，所以在行睾丸固定术时，对于减弱神经内分泌应激反应方面，髂腹股沟-髂腹下神经阻滞的效果不如骶管阻滞[269]。可以进行双侧阻滞，但是由于受到局麻药用量的限制，其在幼儿中的应用受到限制。

髂筋膜阻滞

股骨和大腿前部受股神经支配。大腿中部和近端外侧则分别受闭孔神经和股外侧皮神经支配。各种技术可同时用于阻滞这三根神经，如髂筋膜阻滞，可在大腿近端产生镇痛作用，但对大腿后部无作用。这种阻滞方法适用于涉及大腿近端的股骨或软组织的手术；而对于为了确诊肌病而进行四头肌活检的小儿则特别有用，因为这类患者最好避免使用挥发性吸入麻醉剂。髂筋膜阻滞在儿科中的应用已逐渐增加[76,142]，与传统的三合一进路相比，其操作更容易，成功率更高[79]。

髂前上棘向内向下各旁开 1～2cm 处为穿刺注射点，相当于在腹股沟韧带中外三分之一交界处的下方进针（图 13-11）[260]。将针尖磨钝的针头以下外侧角度垂直于髂前上棘方向进针，直到感觉到两次明显的弹性感突破或两次“噗”声音，即直到感觉到针尖先后穿透阔筋膜和髂筋膜的突破感为止，其中阔筋膜的突破感较为明显。也可采取直接进针方式直到遇到骨性障碍再后退少许。为了减少发生注入血管的情况，在回抽和试验剂量结果均为阴性之后，注射 0.5～

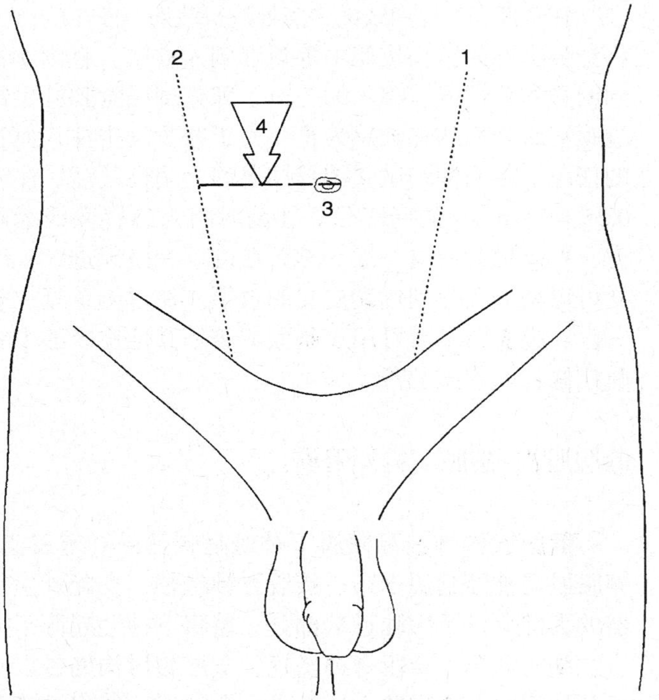

图 13-9 脐部进行腹直肌阻滞的体表标志。在脐部和一侧白线的中点处进行注射。（1 和 2）左侧和右侧白线。（3）脐部。（4）右侧注射点。左侧注射点的定位与之对称。(From Courreges P, Poddevin F, Lecoutre D: Para-umbilical block: A new concept for regional anaesthesia in children. Paediatr Anaesth 1997;7:211-214.)

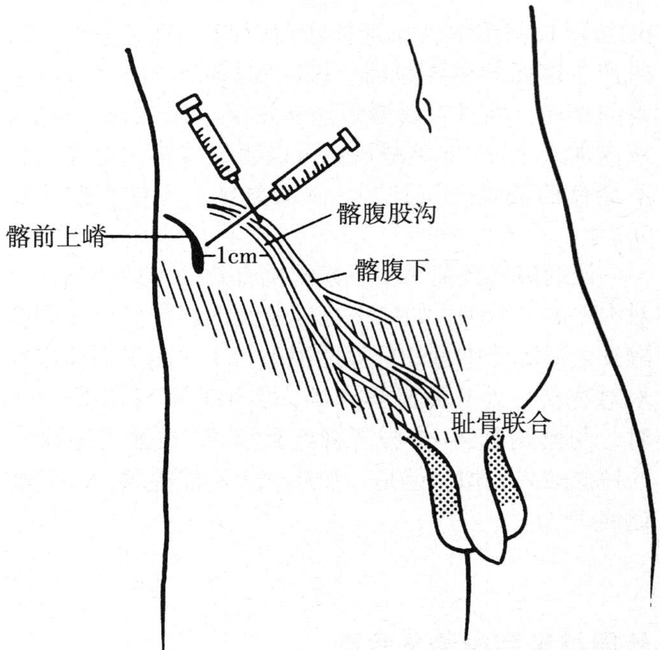

图 13-10 髂腹股沟-髂腹下神经阻滞的标志。在髂前上棘的中、上方 1～2cm 处分别进针。受髂腹股沟神经支配的皮区包括大部分外生殖器和部分大腿近端。受髂腹下神经支配的皮区包括腹股沟韧带上方的腹壁前部皮肤。(From Yaster M, Maxwell LG: Pediatric regional anesthesia. Anesthesiology 1989;70:324-338.)

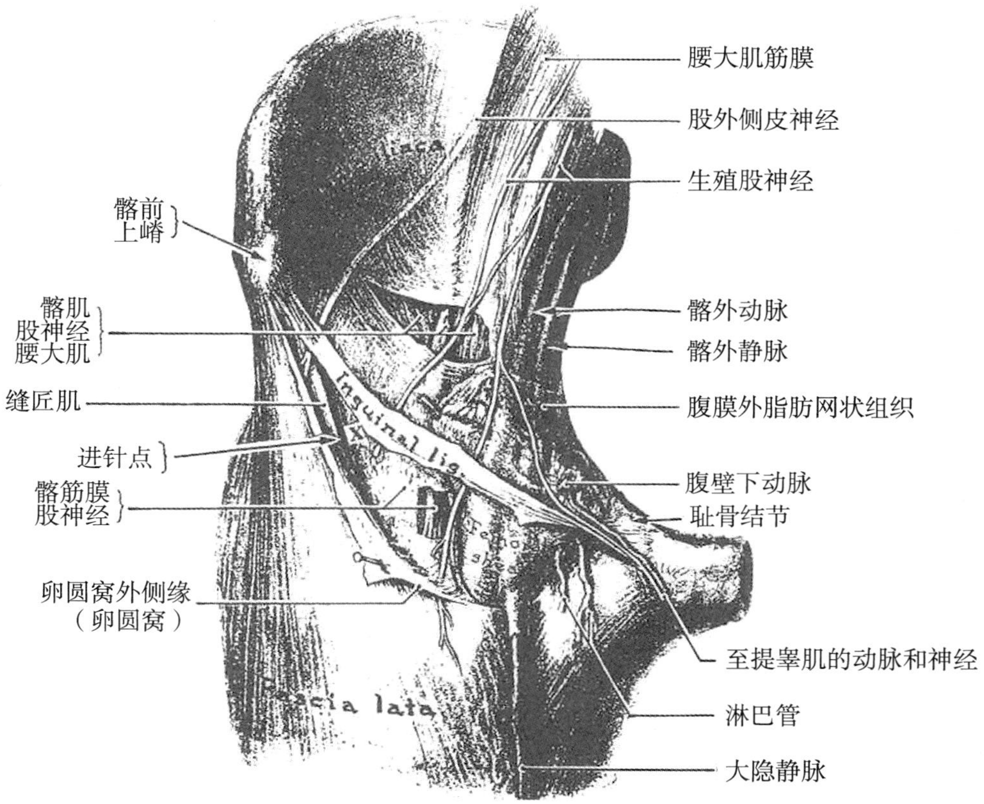

图 13-11 髂筋膜阻滞的体表标志。在髂前上棘往中、下方 1～2cm 处分别进针，即在腹股沟韧带的中、外三分之一交界处的下方分别进针。(From Sethna NF, Berde CB: Pediatric regional anesthesia. In Gregory GA [ed]: Pediatric Anesthesia, 3rd ed. New York, Churchill Livingstone, 1994, pp 281-318.)

1.0ml/kg的局麻药。注药时阻力感轻微或无阻力。已有在小儿中采用连续性髂筋膜阻滞的报道[218]。可以进行双侧阻滞，但是由于受到局麻药用量的限制，在幼儿中的应用受到限制。

阴茎阻滞

阴茎阻滞可为包皮环切术和其他一些阴茎远端的手术提供镇痛，如简单的尿道下裂修补术；而阴茎近端的手术则多采用骶管阻滞，如复杂的尿道下裂修补术[35,141,297,332]。一般来说，与骶管阻滞相比，阴茎阻滞的并发症较少，特别是运动神经阻滞的发生率较低。但是，骶管阻滞的成功率更高并能提供更加持久的镇痛作用。阴茎阻滞也存在一定的风险，刺破阴茎背血
47 管可能引起血肿[43]，而且还有阴茎头坏疽的报道[252]。阴茎阻滞中的局麻药液不可含有肾上腺素或其他血管收缩药。

在阴茎根部中线外侧大约是 10 点钟和 2 点钟的位置进行注射（图 13-12）[234,330]。也可以在中线处注射。将针尖磨钝的针头垂直刺入皮肤，直到感觉到明显弹性或“噗”的一声，即感觉到针尖穿透 Buck 筋膜的突破感为止。为了减少发生血管内注射的情况，在回抽和试验剂量结果均为阴性之后，注入 0.5～1.0ml/kg 的局麻药，药量最多为 10ml。注药时阻力感轻微或无阻力。然后在对侧进行同样操作。在阴茎根部 Buck 筋膜的浅层中进行环形阻滞可提供相同的镇痛作用，而且发生血肿的危险减少[43]。

椎管内阻滞

椎管内阻滞包括蛛网膜下腔阻滞和硬膜外阻滞。蛛网膜下腔阻滞是将局麻药直接注入脊髓蛛网膜下腔的脑脊液中，几乎只应用于全身麻醉后有发生呼吸暂停较大风险的婴儿。但连续蛛网膜下腔阻滞技术偶尔也用于姑息性镇痛。硬膜外阻滞是将局麻药注入黄韧带和硬膜之间潜在的腔隙，是小儿手术和围术期镇痛

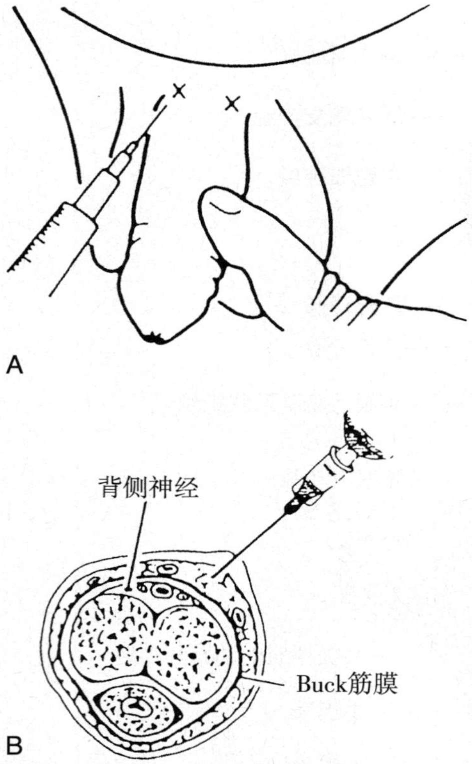

图 13-12 阴茎阻滞的标志。A.在阴茎根部中线外侧大约10点和2点的位置进针。B.一根背静脉、两根背动脉、两根背神经以及三个海绵体位于 Buck 筋膜下方。(A, From Yaster M, Maxwell LG: Pediatric regional anesthesia. Anesthesiology 1989;70:324-338. B, From Rice LJ, Hannallah RS: Local and regional anesthesia. In Motoyama EK, Davis PJ [eds]: Smith's Anesthesia for Infants and Children, 5th ed. St Louis, CV Mosby, 1990, pp 393-426.)

的常用技术。可以单次注入局麻药，可重复给药，也可以通过留置导管进行连续给药。

椎管内阻滞的禁忌证包括患者或家属拒绝、凝血病（可能发生椎管内血肿）、局部或全身感染（有引起椎管内脓肿或脑膜炎的危险）、颅内压增加以及解剖畸形。很多禁忌证都是相对的，对每个患者需权衡利弊。

骶管阻滞

小儿中最常用的椎管内阻滞是骶管阻滞[330]。骶管阻滞是通过第5骶椎未融合而形成的骶裂孔穿刺进入硬膜外腔。这种技术相对简单，成功率高，而并发症的发生率低[42,77]。

在骶角之间及稍下方出进针（图 13–13）[330]。将针尖磨钝的针头按照向头侧约 45° 进针，直到感觉到明显弹性或“噗”的一声，即直到感觉到针头刺破了骶尾韧带为止。骶尾韧带是黄韧带的最下方。如果遇到骨质，通常意味着是骶骨后壁，可退回针头少许，改为以与皮肤更加平行的角度再次进针。注药时无阻力意味着针尖在硬膜外腔中。为了减少发生血管内注射的情况，在回抽未见血或脑脊液且试验剂量结果阴性之后，才能注入全量的麻醉药。与骶管阻滞相关的严重并发症包括血管内或骨内注射、硬脊膜意外刺破造成全脊麻、盆腔脏器损伤和血肿形成，但这些并发症很少见[225]。

骶管阻滞最常采用单次注射，给予 1.0ml/kg 的麻 248
醉药可为 30kg 以下的患者提供脐部以下的有效镇痛。也许因为婴儿和儿童整体的交感张力较低，因此在行椎管内阻滞之后，通常不会显示出血流动力学紊乱。儿科患者骶管阻滞后会发生局部血流的明显改变，但心率和血压不发生变化[173]。

骶管阻滞的镇痛时程与所用的麻醉药有关。常规剂量的麻醉药可以提供数小时的镇痛，且不会引起尿潴留[98]。0.0625%～0.25%的布比卡因最为常用。添加阿片类药物可以延长镇痛作用，但会增加副作用，特别是呼吸抑制。随着阿片类药物的亲水性增加，脑脊液吸收药物的速度加快且作用范围扩大，因此镇痛时程和副作用均会增加。芬太尼属于高亲脂性阿片类药物，可在骶管内应用，对于门诊患者和门诊外科手术，小儿的剂量为 0.5～1.0μg/kg。吗啡属于高亲水性阿片类药物，骶管内用药剂量为 30～70μg/kg 时能提供 12 小时以上的镇痛作用，但是会发生明显的副作用，包括瘙痒和呼吸抑制，最长可达 24 小时[164,294]。

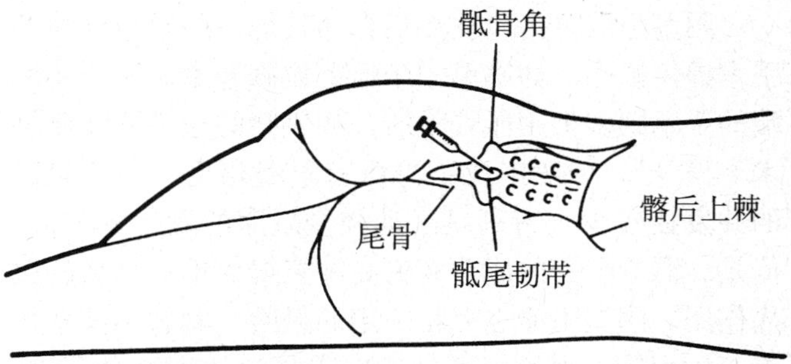

图 13–13 骶管阻滞的体表标志。在骶角之间及稍下方进针注射。(From Yaster M, Maxwell LG: Pediatric regional anesthesia. Anesthesiology 1989;70:324-338.)

门诊患者不能在椎管内使用吗啡镇痛。与骶管内用芬太尼相比，骶管内应用氢吗啡酮时，5.0～10.0μg/kg 的剂量能提供更加持久的镇痛作用，而发生呼吸抑制的危险要比骶管内用吗啡明显减少。现已有报告在骶管内使用可乐定[129,263]和氯胺酮[307]的报道。对于对阿片类药物敏感性增加的患者，这两种药物特别有利，如对新生儿和罹患慢性呼吸系统疾病的小儿。

连续性技术

单次骶管阻滞的镇痛作用一般少于 24 小时，骶管内使用吗啡的镇痛作用也不会超过这个时间长度。需长时间镇痛的患者可采用连续性技术。通过硬膜外置管反复注射或连续性注射麻醉药可提供良好的镇痛作用，对于小儿，可以通过骶管、腰段或胸段进路放置硬膜外导管[24,84,120]。已有在颈段硬膜外置管为小儿提供临终关怀的报道[222,298]，此外，也有隧道型导管用于长期镇痛的报道[11]。

硬膜外导管也可经骶管置入，并可放置到腰段或胸段脊椎水平，特别是对新生儿和幼儿，其硬膜外脂肪多呈凝胶状，且其硬膜外腔中基本没有纤维隔膜[77]。可以利用带管芯的导管通过骶管在远端留置硬膜外导管。也可以直接在腰段或胸段放置硬膜外导管，这种方法常用于体重超过 5～10kg 的患者。经腰段或胸段放置硬膜外导管不能可靠地到达预定的远端椎骨水平。导管的行走方向常常难以预料，当导管超出针头 3cm 后，常会在穿刺点水平发生导管卷曲[180]。以往对于小儿在全身麻醉下放置硬膜外导管的安全性的关注多限于理论上的讨论，虽然已有神经系统并发症的报道[149]。与含碘消毒液相比，皮肤准备时采用氯己定可使导管拔除后导管细菌培养的阳性率明显下降[156]。选择硬膜外注射的药物取决于与疼痛部位相对的导管尖端的皮区位置，以及镇痛的分布区域和强度。在美国，经常联合使用局麻药和阿片类药物（表 13-14）；其他国家还使用其他药物[200,251]。局麻药和阿片类药物联合使用可产生协同作用而减少两种药物的剂量，并可减轻运动神经的阻滞程度，从而减少阿片类药物的副作用[27,193]。如果硬膜外导管尖端的定位接近疼痛部位所在的皮肤区域，可使用含有亲脂性阿片类药物（如芬太尼）的低浓度局麻药，这样镇痛效果较好。如果硬膜外导管的尖端远离疼痛部位所在的皮肤区域水平，或这个区域覆盖有多重皮肤区域，那么可能需要在局麻药内添加亲水性阿片类药物（如氢吗啡酮或吗啡）。硬膜外使用阿片类药物可提供良好的镇痛作用，但是也可产生相关的副作用，包括瘙痒、恶心、尿潴留以及呼吸抑制。随着阿片类药物的亲水性增加，发生副作用的危险性也增加[282]。阿片类药物的副作用可采用其他药物进行处理（表 13-8）。可乐定可替代阿片类药物用于硬膜外镇痛，提供的镇痛效果相似而避免了阿片类药物的副作用[72,158]。这对于对阿片类药物敏感性增加的患者特别有利，包括新生儿和罹患慢性呼吸系统疾病的小儿。

必须密切观察接受硬膜外注射的患者。对于接受硬 249
膜外阿片类药物的所有小儿来说，推荐进行连续性脉率氧饱和度和呼吸与心电监测[193]。或者对全部接受硬膜外镇痛的患者给予连续脉率氧饱和度监测，而对有呼吸抑

表 13-14　小儿硬膜外注射的药物 *

局麻药†	阿片类药物 †, ‡
0.0625% ~0.1% 的布比卡因（最大剂量为每小时 0.4mg/kg）	芬太尼为每小时 0.5~1.0μg/kg（成人为 50~100μg/h）
或	或
0.0625% ~0.1% 的左旋布比卡因（最大剂量为每小时 0.4mg/kg）	氢吗啡酮为每小时 2.0~4.0μg/kg（成人为 150~300μg/h）
或	或
0.1%~0.5%的利多卡因（最大剂量为每小时 3mg/kg）	吗啡为每小时 3.0~6.0μg/kg（成人为 250~500μg/h）
或	和（或）
0.1%~0.2%的罗哌卡因（最大剂量为每小时 0.5mg/kg）	可乐定为每小时 0.25~0.5μg/kg（成人为 25~50μg/h）

* 胸段导管给药通常为每小时 0.2～0.3ml/kg（最大为 5～10ml/h），腰段导管给药为每小时 0.3～0.4ml/kg（最大为 10～15ml/h），骶管导管给药为每小时 0.4～0.5ml/kg（最大为 15～20ml/h）。

† 在新生儿和小婴儿中，推荐的局麻药和阿片类药物的剂量要减少 25%～50%。

‡ 推荐的阿片类药物的剂量是针对以前从未使用过阿片类药物的患者的初始用量，剂量需要逐步调整至产生临床效果，可能需要更大的剂量。

制危险的患者再加上呼吸和心电监测。对新生儿和小婴儿、罹患神经系统疾病或肺部疾病的小儿以及接受亲水性阿片类药物的患者，如吗啡，均应加强监护[25]。对所有接受硬膜外注射的患者应该经常并定期评价其意识水平、镇痛强度、运动和感觉神经被阻滞的程度以及副作用。连续椎管内镇痛技术需要监护人付出更多辛劳和专业知识，但可为重度疼痛的小儿提供了良好的镇痛。

评价

合理地处理小儿疼痛需要认识儿科患者所特有的生长发育和生理学问题。应当制定完整的围术期计划，提供相应的镇痛并尽可能地进行超前疼痛处理。有不少工具可用于定量评估各年龄段小儿的疼痛状况。

一些非药物性措施可以减少药物的使用量，非阿片类镇痛药可以减少阿片类药物的用量。但阿片类药物仍然是治疗中度至重度疼痛的主要药物，只要剂量合理，可用于各年龄段的患者。局部麻醉可优化镇痛效果，而且可减少全身用药的需求。可以进行表面麻醉和浸润麻醉，或进行外周神经、神经丛以及椎管内阻滞。疼痛处理应该个性化，应定期评估疼痛的程度，及时调整用药方案以优化镇痛效果，减少副作用，促进患者恢复。

（张瑞冬译　陈锡明校）

参考文献

1. Adams ML, Brase DA, Welch SP, et al: The role of endogenous peptides in the action of opioid analgesics. Ann Emerg Med 1986;15:1030-1035.
2. Agrawal A, Gerson CR, Seligman I, et al: Postoperative hemorrhage after tonsillectomy: Use of ketorolac tromethamine. Otolaryngol Head Neck Surg 1999;120:335-339.
3. Akman I, Ozek E, Bilgen H, et al: Sweet solutions and pacifiers for pain relief in newborn infants. J Pain 2002;3:199-202.
4. Alexander CM, Gross JB: Sedative doses of midazolam depress hypoxic ventilatory responses in humans. Anesth Analg 1988;67:377-382.
5. Algren J, Deegear C, Skjonsby B, et al: Efficacy and safety of patient-parent, or nurse-controlled analgesia in children. Anesthesiology 1998;89:3.
6. Altintas F, Bozkurt P, Ipek N, et al: The efficacy of preversus postsurgical axillary block on postoperative pain in paediatric patients. Paediatr Anaesth 2000;10:23-28.
7. American Academy of Pediatrics Task Force on Pain in Infants, Children, and Adolescents: The assessment and management of acute pain in infants, children, and adolescents. Pediatrics 2001;108:793-797.
8. Anand KJ, Hickey PR: Pain and its effects in the human neonate and fetus. N Engl J Med 1987;317:1321-1329.
9. Anand KJ, Sippell WG, Aynsley-Green A: Randomised trial of fentanyl anaesthesia in preterm babies undergoing surgery: Effects on the stress response. Lancet 1987;1:62-66.
10. Andrews K: The human developmental neurophysiology of pain. In Schechter N, Berde C, Yaster M (eds): Pain in Infants, Children, and Adolescents. Philadelphia, Lippincott Williams & Wilkins, 2003, pp 19-42.
11. Aram L, Krane EJ, Kozloski LJ, et al: Tunneled epidural catheters for prolonged analgesia in pediatric patients. Anesth Analg 2001;92:1432-1438.
12. ASA: ASA House of Delegates standards for basic anesthetic monitoring. 1986.
13. ASA: ASA House of Delegates statement on intravascular catheterizaion procedure. 2000.
14. Ashburn MA, Gauthier M, Love G, et al: Iontophoretic administration of 2% lidocaine HCl and 1:100,000 epinephrine in humans. Clin J Pain 1997;13:22-26.
15. Ates Y, Unal N, Cuhruk H, et al: Postoperative analgesia in children using preemptive retrobulbar block and local anesthetic infiltration in strabismus surgery. Reg Anesth Pain Med 1998;23:569-574.
16. Aun CS, Short SM, Leung DH, et al: Induction dose-response of propofol in unpremedicated children. Br J Anaesth 1992;68:64-67.
17. Aun CS, Sung RY, O'Meara ME, et al: Cardiovascular effects of IV induction in children: Comparison between propofol and thiopentone. Br J Anaesth 1993;70:647-653.
18. Auroy Y, Ecoffey C, Messiah A, et al: Relationship between complications of pediatric anesthesia and volume of pediatric anesthetics. Anesth Analg 1997;84:234-235.
19. Ayers J, Graves SA: Perioperative management of total parenteral nutrition, glucose containing solutions, and intraoperative glucose monitoring in paediatric patients: A survey of clinical practice. Paediatr Anaesth 2001;11:41-44.
20. Bailey PL, Pace NL, Ashburn MA, et al: Frequent hypoxemia and apnea after sedation with midazolam and fentanyl. Anesthesiology 1990;73:826-830.
21. Bailey R, Sinha C, Burgess LP: Ketorolac tromethamine and hemorrhage in tonsillectomy: A prospective, randomized, double-blind study. Laryngoscope 1997;107:166-169.
22. Bell EF, Oh W: Fluid and electrolyte balance in very low birth weight infants. Clin Perinatol 1979;6:139-150.
23. Benini F, Johnston CC, Faucher D, et al: Topical anesthesia during circumcision in newborn infants. JAMA 1993;270:850-853.
24. Berde C, Sethna N, Yemen T, et al: Continuous epidural bupivacaine-fentanyl infusions in children following ureteral reimplantation. Anesthesiology 1990;73(3A):A1128.
25. Berde CB: Pediatric postoperative pain management. Pediatr Clin North Am 1989;36:921-940.
26. Berde CB, Beyer JE, Bournaki MC, et al: Comparison of morphine and methadone for prevention of postoperative pain in 3- to 7-year-old children. J Pediatr 1991;119:136-141.
27. Berde CB, Sethna NF, Levin L, et al: Regional analgesia on pediatric medical and surgical wards. Intensive Care Med 1989;15(Suppl 1):S40-S43.
28. Berry FA: Preoperative assessment and general management of outpatients. Int Anesthesiol Clin 1982;20:3-15.
29. Bevan JC, Johnston C, Haig MJ, et al: Preoperative parental anxiety predicts behavioural and emotional responses to induction of anaesthesia in children. Can J Anaesth 1990;37:177-182.

30. Beyer JE, McGrath PJ, Berde CB: Discordance between self-report and behavioral pain measures in children aged 3-7 years after surgery. J Pain Symptom Manage 1990;5:350-356.
31. Bhat R, Abu-Harb M, Chari G, et al: Morphine metabolism in acutely ill preterm newborn infants. J Pediatr 1992;120: 795-799.
32. Bhat R, Chari G, Gulati A, et al: Pharmacokinetics of a single dose of morphine in preterm infants during the first week of life. J Pediatr 1990;117:477-481.
33. Bhavani-Shankar K, Philip JH: Defining segments and phases of a time capnogram. Anesth Analg 2000;91:973-977.
34. Bito H, Ikeda K: Closed-circuit anesthesia with sevoflurane in humans: Effects on renal and hepatic function and concentrations of breakdown products with soda lime in the circuit. Anesthesiology 1994;80:71-76.
35. Blaise G, Roy WL: Postoperative pain relief after hypospadias repair in pediatric patients: Regional analgesia versus systemic analgesics. Anesthesiology 1986;65:84-86.
36. Bonadio WA, Wagner V: Efficacy of TAC topical anesthetic for repair of pediatric lacerations. Am J Dis Child 1988;142:203-205.
37. Borgeat A, Wilder-Smith OH, Saiah M, et al: Subhypnotic doses of propofol possess direct antiemetic properties. Anesth Analg 1992;74:539-541.
38. Bourke DL, Smith TC: Estimating allowable hemodilution. Anesthesiology 1974;41:609-612.
39. Bouwmeester NJ, Hop WC, van Dijk M, et al: Postoperative pain in the neonate: Age-related differences in morphine requirements and metabolism. Intensive Care Med 2003;29:2009-2015.
40. Brandom BW, Brandom RB, Cook DR: Uptake and distribution of halothane in infants: In vivo measurements and computer simulations. Anesth Analg 1983;62:404-410.
41. Brett CM, Fisher DM: Thiopental dose-response relations in unpremedicated infants, children, and adults. Anesth Analg 1987;66:1024-1027.
42. Broadman L, Hanallah R, Norden J, et al: "Kiddie caudals": Experience with 1154 consecutive cases without complications. Anesth Analg 1987;66:S18.
43. Broadman LM, Hannallah RS, Belman AB, et al: Post-circumcision analgesia—a prospective evaluation of subcutaneous ring block of the penis. Anesthesiology 1987;67:399-402.
44. Brower RW, Merin RG: Left ventricular function and compliance in swine during halothane anesthesia. Anesthesiology 1979;50:409-415.
45. Brown JL: Imagination training: A tool with many uses. Contemp Pediatr 1995;12:22-26, 29-30, 32.
46. Browne BL, Prys-Roberts C, Wolf AR: Propofol and alfentanil in children: Infusion technique and dose requirement for total IV anaesthesia. Br J Anaesth 1992;69:570-576.
47. Buchholz DH: Blood transfusion: Merits of component therapy. I. The clinical use of red cells, platelets, and granulocytes. J Pediatr 1974;84:1-15.
48. Buck N, Devlin H, Lunn J: Report on the confidential inquiry into perioperative deaths. Nuffield Provincial Hospitals Trust, London, the King's Fund Publishing House, 1987.
49. Carney FM, Van Dyke RA: Halothane hepatitis: A critical review. Anesth Analg 1972;51:135-160.
50. Casey W, Rice L, Hannallah R, et al: A comparison between bupivacaine instillation versus ilioinguinal/iliohypogastric nerve block for postoperative analgesia following inguinal herniorrhaphy in children. Anesthesiology 1990;72: 637-639.
51. Cassidy KL, Reid GJ, McGrath PJ, et al: A randomized double-blind, placebo-controlled trial of the EMLA patch for the reduction of pain associated with intramuscular injection in four- to six-year-old children. Acta Paediatr 2001;90:1329-1336.
52. Chay P, Duffy B, Walker J: Pharmacokinetic-pharmacodynamic relationship of morphine in neonates. Clin Pharmacol Ther 1992;51:334-342.
53. Christensen J, Fatchett D: Promoting parental use of distraction and relaxation in pediatric oncology patients during invasive procedures. J Pediatr Oncol Nurs 2002;19: 127-132.
54. Christoph RA, Buchanan L, Begalla K, et al: Pain reduction in local anesthetic administration through pH buffering. Ann Emerg Med 1988;17:117-120.
55. Coderre TJ, Melzack R: Cutaneous hyperalgesia: Contributions of the peripheral and central nervous systems to the increase in pain sensitivity after injury. Brain Res 1987;404:95-106.
56. Coderre TJ, Vaccarino AL, Melzack R: Central nervous system plasticity in the tonic pain response to subcutaneous formalin injection. Brain Res 1990;535:155-158.
57. Cohen IT, Hannallah RS, Hummer KA: The incidence of emergence agitation associated with desflurane anesthesia in children is reduced by fentanyl. Anesth Analg 2001;93: 88-91.
58. Collins SK, Kuck K: Music therapy in the neonatal intensive care unit. Neonatal Netw 1991;9:23-26.
59. Cook D: Clinical use of muscle relaxants in infants and children. Anesth Analg 1981;60:335.
60. Cook D, Davis P: Pediatric anesthesia pharmacology. In Lake C (ed): Pediatric Cardiac Anesthesiology. Norwalk, Conn, Appleton & Lange, 1993.
61. Cook DR, Brandom BW, Shiu G, et al: The inspired median effective dose, brain concentration at anesthesia, and cardiovascular index for halothane in young rats. Anesth Analg 1981;60:182-185.
62. Cooper CM, Gerrish SP, Hardwick M, et al: EMLA cream reduces the pain of venipuncture in children. Eur J Anaesthesiol 1987;4:441-448.
63. Cote C (ed): A Practice of Anesthesia for Infants and Children, 2nd ed. Philadelphia, WB Saunders, 1982.
64. Cote C: Calcium chloride versus calcium gluconate: Comparison of ionization and cardiovascular effects in children and dogs. Anesthesiology 1987;66:465.
65. Cote CJ, Cohen IT, Suresh S, et al: A comparison of three doses of a commercially prepared oral midazolam syrup in children. Anesth Analg 2002;94:37-43.
66. Cote CJ, Goudsouzian NG, Liu LM, et al: The dose response of intravenous thiopental for the induction of general anesthesia in unpremedicated children. Anesthesiology 1981;55:703-705.
67. Cote CJ, Zaslavsky A, Downes JJ, et al: Postoperative apnea in former preterm infants after inguinal herniorrhaphy: A combined analysis. Anesthesiology 1995;82:809-822.
68. Courreges P, Poddevin F, Lecoutre D: Para-umbilical block: A new concept for regional anaesthesia in children. Paediatr Anaesth 1997;7:211-214.
69. Cravero JP, Beach M, Thyr B, et al: The effect of small dose fentanyl on the emergence characteristics of pediatric patients after sevoflurane anesthesia without surgery. Anesth Analg 2003;97:364-367.
70. Crawford M, Lerman J, Christensen S, et al: Effects of duration of fasting on gastric fluid pH and volume in healthy children. Anesth Analg 1990;71:400-403.
71. Crumrine RS, Yodlowski EH: Assessment of neuromuscular function in infants. Anesthesiology 1981;54:29-32.
72. Cucchiaro G, Dagher C, Baujard C, et al: Side-effects of postoperative epidural analgesia in children: A randomized study comparing morphine and clonidine. Paediatr Anaesth 2003;13:318-323.
73. Dahl JB, Kehlet H: The value of pre-emptive analgesia in the treatment of postoperative pain. Br J Anaesth 1993;70:434-439.

74. Dahl JB, Moiniche S, Kehlet H: Wound infiltration with local anaesthetics for postoperative pain relief. Acta Anaesthesiol Scand 1994;38:7-14.
75. Dalens B: Regional anesthesia in children. Anesth Analg 1989;68:654-672.
76. Dalens B: "Small blocks" in paediatric patients. Baillieres Clin Anaesthesiol 2000;14:745-758.
77. Dalens B, Hasnaoui A: Caudal anesthesia in pediatric surgery: Success rate and adverse effects in 750 consecutive patients. Anesth Analg 1989;68:83-89.
78. Dalens B, Tanguy A, Haberer JP: Lumbar epidural anesthesia for operative and postoperative pain relief in infants and young children. Anesth Analg 1986;65:1069-1073.
79. Dalens B, Vanneuville G, Tanguy A: Comparison of the fascia iliaca compartment block with the 3-in-1 block in children. Anesth Analg 1989;69:705-713.
80. Davidson AJ, Eyres RL, Cole WG: A comparison of prilocaine and lidocaine for intravenous regional anaesthesia for forearm fracture reduction in children. Paediatr Anaesth 2002;12:146-150.
81. Davis P, et al: Emergency and recovery from sevoflurane in pediatric ambulatory patients: A multicenter study. Anesthesiology 1993;79:A1166.
82. Davis PJ, Greenberg JA, Gendelman M, et al: Recovery characteristics of sevoflurane and halothane in preschool-aged children undergoing bilateral myringotomy and pressure equalization tube insertion. Anesth Analg 1999;88:34-38.
83. DeJong P: Comparison of rectal to intramuscular administration of midazolam and atropine for premedication of children. Acta Anaesthesiol Scand 1988;32:485.
84. Desparmet J, Meistelman C, Barre J, et al: Continuous epidural infusion of bupivacaine for postoperative pain relief in children. Anesthesiology 1987;67:108-110.
85. Drugs AAoPCo: Guidelines for monitoring and management of pediatric patients during and after sedation for diagnostic and therapeutic procedures: Addendum. Pediatrics 2002;110:836-838.
86. Duhn L, Medves J: A systemic integrative review of infant pain assessment tools. Adv Neonatal Care 2004;4:126-140.
87. Eger E, et al: Partition coefficients of I-653 in human blood, saline, and olive oil. Anesth Analg 1987;66:971.
88. Eger EI 2nd, Saidman LJ: Hazards of nitrous oxide anesthesia in bowel obstruction and pneumothorax. Anesthesiology 1965;26:61-66.
89. Eger EI 2nd, Smith NT, Stoelting RK, et al: Cardiovascular effects of halothane in man. Anesthesiology 1970;32:396-409.
90. Eichenfield LF, Funk A, Fallon-Friedlander S, et al: A clinical study to evaluate the efficacy of ELA-Max (4% liposomal lidocaine) as compared with eutectic mixture of local anesthetics cream for pain reduction of venipuncture in children. Pediatrics 2002;109:1093-1099.
91. Eland J: The use of TENS with children. In Schechter N, Berde C, Yaster M (eds): Pain in Infants, Children and Adolescents. Baltimore, Williams & Wilkins, 1993, pp 331-340.
92. Eland J, Anderson J: The experience of pain in children. In Jacox S (ed): Pain: A Sourcebook for Nurses and Other Health Professionals. Boston, Little, Brown, 1977, pp 453-473.
93. Ernst AA, Marvez E, Nick TG, et al: Lidocaine adrenaline tetracaine gel versus tetracaine adrenaline cocaine gel for topical anesthesia in linear scalp and facial lacerations in children aged 5 to 17 years. Pediatrics 1995;95:255-258.
94. Etches RC: Respiratory depression associated with patient-controlled analgesia: A review of eight cases. Can J Anaesth 1994;41:125-132.
95. Farrington EA, McGuinness GA, Johnson GF, et al: Continuous intravenous morphine infusion in postoperative newborn infants. Am J Perinatol 1993;10:84-87.
96. Fassoulaki A, Sarantopoulos C, Zotou M, et al: Preemptive opioid analgesia does not influence pain after abdominal hysterectomy. Can J Anaesth 1995;42:109-113.
97. Ferguson S, Thomas V, Lewis I: The rectus sheath block in paediatric anaesthesia: New indications for an old technique? Paediatr Anaesth 1996;6:463-466.
98. Fisher QA, McComiskey CM, Hill JL, et al: Postoperative voiding interval and duration of analgesia following peripheral or caudal nerve blocks in children. Anesth Analg 1993;76:173-177.
99. Fitzgerald M: Pain and analgesia in neonates. Trends Neurosci 1987;9:254.
100. Fitzgerald M, Anand K: Developmental neuroanatomy and neurophysiology of pain. In Schechter N, Berde C, Yaster M (eds): Pain in Infants, Children, and Adolescents. Baltimore, Williams & Wilkins, 1993.
101. Fitzgerald M, Howard R: The neurobiologic basis of pediatirc pain. In Schechter N, Berde C, Yaster M (eds): Pain in Infants, Children, and Adolescents. Philadelphia, Lippincott Williams & Wilkins, 2003, pp 19-42.
102. Flewellen EH, Nelson TE, Jones WP, et al: Dantrolene dose response in awake man: Implications for management of malignant hyperthermia. Anesthesiology 1983;59:275-280.
103. Friesen RH, Carpenter E, Madigan CK, et al: Oral transmucosal fentanyl citrate for preanaesthetic medication of paediatric cardiac surgery patients. Paediatr Anaesth 1995;5:29-33.
104. Frink EJ Jr, Green WB Jr, Brown EA, et al: Compound A concentrations during sevoflurane anesthesia in children. Anesthesiology 1996;84:566-571.
105. Furman EB, Roman DG, Lemmer LA, et al: Specific therapy in water, electrolyte and blood-volume replacement during pediatric surgery. Anesthesiology 1975;42:187-193.
106. Galinkin J, Fazi L, Cuy R, et al: Use of fentanyl in children undergoing myringotomy and tube placement during halothane and sevoflurane anesthesia. Anesthesiology 2000;93:1378-1383.
107. Galinkin J, Kurth D: Neonatal and pediatric apnea syndromes. Problems in Anesthesia 1988;10:444-454.
108. Gallagher JE, Blauth J, Fornadley JA: Perioperative ketorolac tromethamine and postoperative hemorrhage in cases of tonsillectomy and adenoidectomy. Laryngoscope 1995;105:606-609.
109. Gallagher T, Black S, Black G: Isoflurane does not reduce aortic peak flow velocity in children. Br J Anaesth 1986;58:1116.
110. Gaukroger P: Novel techniques of analgesic delivery. In Schechter N, Berde C, Yaster M (eds): Pain in Infants, Children, and Adolescents. Baltimore, Williams & Wilkins, 1993, pp 195-202.
111. Gaukroger PB, Tomkins DP, van der Walt JH: Patient-controlled analgesia in children. Anaesth Intensive Care 1989;17:264-268.
112. Gehan G, Karoubi P, Quinet F, et al: Optimal dose of lignocaine for preventing pain on injection of propofol. Br J Anaesth 1991;66:324-326.
113. Glauser TA, Rorke LB, Weinberg PM, et al: Acquired neuropathologic lesions associated with the hypoplastic left heart syndrome. Pediatrics 1990;85:991-1000.
114. Goetting MG, Thirman MJ: Neurotoxicity of meperidine. Ann Emerg Med 1985;14:1007-1009.
115. Goff MJ, Arain SR, Ficke DJ, et al: Absence of bronchodilation during desflurane anesthesia: A comparison to sevoflurane and thiopental. Anesthesiology 2000;93:404-408.
116. Gonsowski CT, Laster MJ, Eger EI 2nd, et al: Toxicity of compound A in rats: Effect of increasing duration of administration. Anesthesiology 1994;80:566-573.

117. Goudsouzian NG: Maturation of neuromuscular transmission in the infant. Br J Anaesth 1980;52:205-214.
118. Graves DA, Foster TS, Batenhorst RL, et al: Patient-controlled analgesia. Ann Intern Med 1983;99:360-366.
119. Green SM, Nakamura R, Johnson NE: Ketamine sedation for pediatric procedures. Part 1. A prospective series. Ann Emerg Med 1990;19:1024-1032.
120. Gunter JB, Eng C: Thoracic epidural anesthesia via the caudal approach in children. Anesthesiology 1992;76:935-938.
121. Gunter JB, Gregg T, Varughese AM, et al: Levobupivacaine for ilioinguinal/iliohypogastric nerve block in children. Anesth Analg 1999;89:647-649.
122. Hallen B, Olsson G, Uppfeldt A: Pain-free venipuncture: Effect of timing of application of local anaesthetic cream. Anaesthesia 1984;39:969-972.
123. Hammarlund K, Sedin G, Stromberg B: Transepidermal water loss in newborn infants. VIII. Relation to gestational age and post-natal age in appropriate and small for gestational age infants. Acta Paediatr Scand 1983;72:721-728.
124. Hannallah R, et al: Propofol anesthesia in paediatric ambulatory patients: A comparison with thiopentone and halothane. Can J Anaesth 1983;41:12.
125. Hannallah R, Rosales J: Experience with parent's presence during anesthesia induction in children. Can Anaesthesiol Soc J 1983;30:286.
126. Hannallah RS, Baker SB, Casey W, et al: Propofol: Effective dose and induction characteristics in unpremedicated children. Anesthesiology 1991;74:217-219.
127. Hannallah RS, Broadman LM, Belman AB, et al: Comparison of caudal and ilioinguinal/iliohypogastric nerve blocks for control of post-orchiopexy pain in pediatric ambulatory surgery. Anesthesiology 1987;66:832-834.
128. Hansen LA, Noyes MA, Lehman ME: Evaluation of patient-controlled analgesia (PCA) versus PCA plus continuous infusion in postoperative cancer patients. J Pain Symptom Manage 1991;6:4-14.
129. Hansen T, Henneberg S, Walther-Larsen S, et al: Caudal bupivacaine supplemented with caudal or intravenous clonidine in children undergoing hypospadias repair: A double-blind study. Br J Anaesth 2004;92:223-227.
130. Harrison D, Johnston L, Loughnan P: Oral sucrose for procedural pain in sick hospitalized infants: A randomized-controlled trial. J Paediatr Child Health 2003;39:591-597.
131. Hartley R, Green M, Quinn MW, et al: Development of morphine glucuronidation in premature neonates. Biol Neonate 1994;66:1-9.
132. Hegenbarth MA, Altieri MF, Hawk WH, et al: Comparison of topical tetracaine, adrenaline, and cocaine anesthesia with lidocaine infiltration for repair of lacerations in children. Ann Emerg Med 1990;19:63-67.
133. Hernandez-Reif M, Field T, Largie S, et al: Children's distress during burn treatment is reduced by massage therapy. J Burn Care Rehabil 2001;22:191-195.
134. Hertzka RE, Gauntlett IS, Fisher DM, et al: Fentanyl-induced ventilatory depression: Effects of age. Anesthesiology 1989;70:213-218.
135. Ho JW, Khambatta HJ, Pang LM, et al: Preemptive analgesia in children. Does it exist? Reg Anesth 1997;22:125-130.
136. Holliday M, Segar W: The maintenance need for water in parenteral fluid therapy. Pediatrics 1957;19:823.
137. Hollinger I: Current trends in pediatric anesthesia. Mt Sinai J Med 2002;69:51-54.
138. Holthusen H, Eichwede F, Stevens M, et al: Pre-emptive analgesia: Comparison of preoperative with postoperative caudal block on postoperative pain in children. Br J Anaesth 1994;73:440-442.
139. Holzman RS, van der Velde ME, Kaus SJ, et al: Sevoflurane depresses myocardial contractility less than halothane during induction of anesthesia in children. Anesthesiology 1996;85:1260-1267.
140. Howard RF: Current status of pain management in children. JAMA 2003;290:2464-2469.
141. Irwin MG, Cheng W: Comparison of subcutaneous ring block of the penis with caudal epidural block for post-circumcision analgesia in children. Anaesth Intensive Care 1996;24:365-367.
142. Ivani G, Tonetti F: Postoperative analgesia in infants and children: New developments. Minerva Anestesiol 2004;70:399-403.
143. Jensen BH, Wernberg M, Andersen M: Preoperative starvation and blood glucose concentrations in children undergoing inpatient and outpatient anaesthesia. Br J Anaesth 1982;54:1071-1074.
144. Johnston RR, Eger EI II, Wilson C: A comparative interaction of epinephrine with enflurane, isoflurane, and halothane in man. Anesth Analg 1976;55:709-712.
145. Jonmarker C, Westrin P, Larsson S, et al: Thiopental requirements for induction of anesthesia in children. Anesthesiology 1987;67:104-107.
146. Judkins JH, Dray TG, Hubbell RN: Intraoperative ketorolac and posttonsillectomy bleeding. Arch Otolaryngol Head Neck Surg 1996;122:937-940.
147. Kain ZN, Caldwell-Andrews A, Wang SM: Psychological preparation of the parent and pediatric surgical patient. Anesthesiol Clin North Am 2002;20:29-44.
148. Karl H, et al: Epinephrine-halothane interactions in children. Anesthesiology 1983;58:142.
149. Kasai T, Yaegashi K, Hirose M, et al: Spinal cord injury in a child caused by an accidental dural puncture with a single-shot thoracic epidural needle. Anesth Analg 2003;96:65-67.
150. Katz R, Epstein R: The interaction of anesthetic agents and adrenergic drugs to produce cardiac arrhythmias. Anesthesiology 1968;29:763-784.
151. Keenan R, Boyan C: Cardiac arrest due to anesthesia: A study of incidence and causes. JAMA 1985;253:2373.
152. Keenan R, Shapiro J, Dawson K: Frequency of anesthetic cardiac arrests in infants: Effect of pediatric anesthesiologists. J Clin Anesthesiol 1991;3:433.
153. Kemper KJ, Sarah R, Silver-Highfield E, et al: On pins and needles? Pediatric pain patients' experience with acupuncture. Pediatrics 2000;105:941-947.
154. Keyl C, Schneider A, Dambacher M, et al: Dynamic cardiocirculatory control during propofol anesthesia in mechanically ventilated patients. Anesth Analg 2000;91:1188-1195.
155. Kim M, Strait R, Sato T, et al: A randomized clinical trial of analgesia in children with acute abdominal pain. Acad Emerg Med 2002;9:281-287.
156. Kinirons B, Mimoz O, Lafendi L, et al: Chlorhexidine versus povidone iodine in preventing colonization of continuous epidural catheters in children: A randomized, controlled trial. Anesthesiology 2001;94:239-244.
157. Kissin I: Preemptive analgesia. Anesthesiology 2000;93:1138-1143.
158. Klamt JG, Garcia LV, Stocche RM, et al: Epidural infusion of clonidine or clonidine plus ropivacaine for postoperative analgesia in children undergoing major abdominal surgery. J Clin Anesth 2003;15:510-514.
159. Kokinsky E, Thornberg E: Postoperative pain control in children: A guide to drug choice. Paediatr Drugs 2003;5:751-762.
160. Kokki H: Nonsteroidal anti-inflammatory drugs for postoperative pain: A focus on children. Paediatr Drugs 2003;5:103-123.
161. Koren G, Butt W, Chinyanga H, et al: Postoperative morphine infusion in newborn infants: Assessment of disposition characteristics and safety. J Pediatr 1985;107:963-967.

162. Korpela R, Korvenoja P, Meretoja OA: Morphine-sparing effect of acetaminophen in pediatric day-case surgery. Anesthesiology 1999;91:442-447.
163. Kotrly KJ, Ebert TJ, Vucins E, et al: Baroreceptor reflex control of heart rate during isoflurane anesthesia in humans. Anesthesiology 1984;60:173-179.
164. Krane EJ, Tyler DC, Jacobson LE: The dose response of caudal morphine in children. Anesthesiology 1989;71: 48-52.
165. Kulka PJ, Bressem M, Tryba M: Clonidine prevents sevoflurane-induced agitation in children. Anesth Analg 2001;93:335-338.
166. Kundra P, Deepalakshmi K, Ravishankar M: Preemptive caudal bupivacaine and morphine for postoperative analgesia in children. Anesth Analg 1998;87:52-56.
167. Kupferberg HJ, Way EL: Pharmacologic basis for the increased sensitivity of the newborn rat to morphine. J Pharmacol Exp Ther 1963;141:105-112.
168. Kurth C: Posoperative apnea in premature infants. Anesthesiology 1987;66:488.
169. Kurth CD, LeBard SE: Association of postoperative apnea, airway obstruction, and hypoxemia in former premature infants. Anesthesiology 1991;75:22-26.
170. Kuttner L, Solomon R: Hypnotherapy and imagery for managing children's pain. In Schechter N, Berde C, Yaster M (eds): Pain in Infants, Children, and Adolescents. Philadelphia, Lippincott Williams & Wilkins, 2003, pp 317-328.
171. Lambert SA: The effects of hypnosis/guided imagery on the postoperative course of children. J Dev Behav Pediatr 1996;17:307-310.
172. Lanier WL, Stangland KJ, Scheithauer BW, et al: The effects of dextrose infusion and head position on neurologic outcome after complete cerebral ischemia in primates: Examination of a model. Anesthesiology 1987;66:39-48.
173. Larousse E, Asehnoune K, Dartayet B, et al: The hemodynamic effects of pediatric caudal anesthesia assessed by esophageal Doppler. Anesth Analg 2002;94:1165-1168.
174. LeDez KM, Lerman J: The minimum alveolar concentration (MAC) of isoflurane in preterm neonates, Anesthesiology. 1987;67:301-307.
175. Lee C: Intensive care unit neuromuscular syndrome? Anesthesiology 1995;83:237-240.
176. Lerman J, Davis PJ, Welborn LG, et al: Induction, recovery, and safety characteristics of sevoflurane in children undergoing ambulatory surgery: A comparison with halothane. Anesthesiology 1996;84:1332-1340.
177. Lerman J, Gregory GA, Willis MM, et al: Age and solubility of volatile anesthetics in blood. Anesthesiology 1984;61: 139-143.
178. Lerman J, Robinson S, Willis MM, et al: Anesthetic requirements for halothane in young children 0-1 month and 1-6 months of age. Anesthesiology 1983;59:421-424.
179. Lerman J, Sikich N, Kleinman S, et al: The pharmacology of sevoflurane in infants and children. Anesthesiology 1994;80:814-824.
180. Lim YJ, Bahk JH, Ahn WS, et al: Coiling of lumbar epidural catheters. Acta Anaesthesiol Scand 2002;46: 603-606.
181. Lin Y: Acupuncture. In Schechter N, Berde C, Yaster M (eds): Pain in Infants, Children, and Adolescents. Philadelphia, Lippincott Williams & Wilkins, 2003, pp 426-470.
182. Lloyd-Thomas A, Howard R: A pain service for children. Paediatr Anaesth 1994;4:3-15.
183. Lopez J: Myoplastic free Ca^{++} during malignant hyperthermia episode in swine. Muscle Nerve 1985;11:82.
184. Lynn AM, Opheim KE, Tyler DC: Morphine infusion after pediatric cardiac surgery. Crit Care Med 1984;12: 863-866.
185. Lynn AM, Slattery JT: Morphine pharmacokinetics in early infancy. Anesthesiology 1987;66:136-139.
186. Malviya S, Swartz J, Lerman J: Are all preterm infants younger that 60 weeks postconceptual age at risk for postanesthetic apnea? Anesthesiology 1993;78:1076.
187. Martin LD, Bratton SL, O'Rourke PP: Clinical uses and controversies of neuromuscular blocking agents in infants and children. Crit Care Med 1999;27:1358-1368.
188. Mather L, Mackie J: The incidence of postoperative pain in children. Pain 1983;15:271-282.
189. Matsota P, Livanios S, Marinopoulou E: Intercostal nerve block with bupivacaine for post-thoracotomy pain relief in children. Eur J Pediatr Surg 2001;11:219-222.
190. Maunuksela E, Olkkola K: Nonsteroidal anti-inflammatory drugs in pediatric pain management. In Schechter N, Berde C, Yaster M (eds): Pain in Infants, Children, and Adolescents. Philadelphia, Lippincott Williams & Wilkins, 2003, pp 171-180.
191. McClune S, McKay A, Wright P: Synergistic interaction between midazolam and propofol. Br J Anaesth 1992; 69:240.
192. McDonnell L, Bowden ML: Breathing management: A simple stress and pain reduction strategy for use on a pediatric service. Issues Compr Pediatr Nurs 1989;12:339-344.
193. McIlvaine WB: Spinal opioids for the pediatric patient. J Pain Symptom Manage 1990;5:183-190.
194. McMillan CO, Spahr-Schopfer IA, Sikich N, et al: Premedication of children with oral midazolam. Can J Anaesth 1992;39:545-550.
195. McNeely JK, Farber NE, Rusy LM, et al: Epidural analgesia improves outcome following pediatric fundoplication: A retrospective analysis. Reg Anesth 1997;22:16-23.
196. Merkel S, Gutstein H, Malviya S: Use of transcutaneous electrical nerve stimulation in a young child with pain from open perineal lesions. J Pain Symptom Manage 1999;18:376-381.
197. Moiniche S, Kehlet H, Dahl JB: A qualitative and quantitative systematic review of preemptive analgesia for postoperative pain relief: The role of timing of analgesia. Anesthesiology 2002;96:725-741.
198. Monitto CL, Greenberg RS, Kost-Byerly S, et al: The safety and efficacy of parent-/nurse-controlled analgesia in patients less than six years of age. Anesth Analg 2000;91:573-579.
199. Morgan KG, Bryant SH: The mechanism of action of dantrolene sodium. J Pharmacol Exp Ther 1977;201:138-147.
200. Moriarty A: Postoperative extradural infusions in children: Preliminary data from a comparison of bupivacaine/diamorphine with plain ropivacaine. Paediatr Anaesth 1999;9:423-427.
201. Morisy L, Platt D: Hazards of high-dose meperidine. JAMA 1986;255:467-468.
202. Morray JP, Geiduschek JM, Caplan RA, et al: A comparison of pediatric and adult anesthesia closed malpractice claims. Anesthesiology 1993;78:461-467.
203. Morray JP, Geiduschek JM, Ramamoorthy C, et al: Anesthesia-related cardiac arrest in children: Initial findings of the Pediatric Perioperative Cardiac Arrest (POCA) Registry. Anesthesiology 2000;93:6-14.
204. Morrison NA, Repka MX: Ketorolac versus acetaminophen or ibuprofen in controlling postoperative pain in patients with strabismus. Ophthalmology 1994;101:915-918.
205. Moss VA: Music and the surgical patient: The effect of music on anxiety. AORN J 1988;48:64-69.
206. Mullooly VM, Levin RF, Feldman HR: Music for postoperative pain and anxiety. J N Y State Nurses Assoc 1988;19:4-7.

207. Murphy MR, Olson WA, Hug CC Jr: Pharmacokinetics of 3H-fentanyl in the dog anesthetized with enflurane. Anesthesiology 1979;50:13-19.
208. Nakakimura K: Glucose administration before cardiac arrest worsens neurologic outcome in cats. Anesthesiology 1990;72:1005.
209. Navarro R, et al: Humans anesthetized with sevoflurane or isoflurane have similar arrhythmic response to epinephrine. Anesthesiology 1994;80:545.
210. O'Donnell J, Ferguson L, Beattie T: Use of analgesia in a paediatric accident and emergency department following limb trauma. Eur J Emerg Med 2002;9:5-8.
211. Olkkola KT, Maunuksela EL: The pharmacokinetics of postoperative intravenous ketorolac tromethamine in children. Br J Clin Pharmacol 1991;31:182-184.
212. Olsson GL, Hallen B: Laryngospasm during anaesthesia: A computer-aided incidence study in 136,929 patients. Acta Anaesthesiol Scand 1984;28:567-575.
213. Ording H: Incidence of malignant hyperthermia in Denmark. Anesth Analg 1985;64:700-704.
214. Ording H, Hedengran AM, Skovgaard LT: Evaluation of 119 anaesthetics received after investigation for susceptibility to malignant hyperthermia. Acta Anaesthesiol Scand 1991;35:711-716.
215. Owens WD: American Society of Anesthesiologists physical status classification system is not a risk classification system. Anesthesiology 2001;94:378.
216. Panel of the Agency for Health Care Policy & Research: Acute Pain Management: Operative or Medical Procedures and Trauma. Clincial Practice Guideline. Rockville, Md, Agency for Health Care Policy & Research, Public Health Service, US Department of Health & Human Services, 1992.
217. Parker RK, Holtmann B, White PF: Effects of a nighttime opioid infusion with PCA therapy on patient comfort and analgesic requirements after abdominal hysterectomy. Anesthesiology. 1992;76:362-367.
218. Paut O, Sallabery M, Schreiber-Deturmeny E, et al: Continuous fascia iliaca compartment block in children: A prospective evaluation of plasma bupivacaine concentrations, pain scores, and side effects. Anesth Analg 2001;92:1159-1163.
219. Petrack E, Marx C, Wright M: Intamuscular ketamine is superior to meperidine, promethazine, and chlorpromazine for pediatric emergency department sedation. Arch Pediatr Adolesc Med 1996;150:676-681.
220. Pietropaoli JA Jr, Keller MS, Smail DF, et al: Regional anesthesia in pediatric surgery: Complications and postoperative comfort level in 174 children. J Pediatr Surg 1993;28:560-564.
221. Pitetti R, Singh S, Pierce M: Safe and efficacious use of procedural sedation and analgesia by nonanesthesiologist in a pediatric emergency department. Arch Pediatr Adolesc Med 2003;157:1090-1096.
222. Plancarte R, Patt R: Intractable upper body pain in a pediatric patient relieved with cervical epidural opioid administration. J Pain Symptom Manage 1991;6:98-99.
223. Polkki T, Pietila A, Vehvilainen-Julkunen K: Hospitalized children's descriptions of their experiences with postsurgical pain relieving methods. Int J Nurs Stud 2003;40:33-44.
224. Pomeranz B: Scientific research into acupuncture for the relief of pain. J Altern Complement Med 1996;2:53-60.
225. Pullerits J, Holzman RS: Pediatric neuraxial blockade. J Clin Anesth 1993;5:342-354.
226. Pulsinelli WA, Waldman S, Rawlinson D, et al: Moderate hyperglycemia augments ischemic brain damage: A neuropathologic study in the rat. Neurology 1982;32:1239-1246.
227. Putney JW, Biancri CP: Site of action of dantrolene in frog sartorius muscle. J Pharmacol Exp Ther 1974;189:202-212.
228. Rackow H, Salanitre E, Green LT: Frequency of cardiac arrest associated with anesthesia in infants and children. Pediatrics 1961;28:697-704.
229. Rauck R, et al: Comparison of the efficacy of epidural morphine given by intermittent injection or continuous infusion for the management of postoperative pain. Reg Anesth 1994;19:316.
230. Rawlings DJ, Miller PA, Engel RR: The effect of circumcision on transcutaneous Po_2 in term infants. Am J Dis Child 1980;134:676-678.
231. Reid MF, Harris R, Phillips PD, et al: Day-case herniotomy in children: A comparison of ilio-inguinal nerve block and wound infiltration for postoperative analgesia. Anaesthesia 1987;42:658-661.
232. Reinhart D, Palladinetti T, Patel M, et al: IV ketorolac vs sufentanil for outpatient ENT surgery, a double-blind, randomized, placebo-controlled study. Anesthesiology 1992;77:3.
233. Reves JG, Fragen RJ, Vinik HR, et al: Midazolam: Pharmacology and uses. Anesthesiology 1985;62:310-324.
234. Rice L, Hannallah R: Local and regional anesthesia. In Motoyama E, Davis P (eds): Smiths' Anesthesia for Infants and Children. St Louis, CV Mosby, 1990, pp 393-426.
235. Rodgers BM, Webb CJ, Stergios D, et al: Patient-controlled analgesia in pediatric surgery. J Pediatr Surg 1988;23:259-262.
236. Romsing J, Moiniche S, Dahl JB: Rectal and parenteral paracetamol, and paracetamol in combination with NSAIDs, for postoperative analgesia. Br J Anaesth 2002;88:215-226.
237. Rosen DA, Morris JL, Rosen KR, et al: Analgesia for pediatric thoracostomy tube removal. Anesth Analg 2000;90:1025-1028.
238. Rosenberg H: International workshop on malignant hyperpyrexia. Anesthesiology 1981;54:530.
239. Ross AK, Eck JB, Tobias JD: Pediatric regional anesthesia: Beyond the caudal. Anesth Analg 2000;91:16-26.
240. Rowe M: Fluid and electrolyte management in pediatric surgery. In Welch K (ed): Pediatric Surgery, vol 2. Chicago, Year Book Medical Publishers, 1986.
241. Rowe MI, Arango A: Colloid versus crystalloid resuscitation in experimental bowel obstruction. J Pediatr Surg 1976;11:635-643.
242. Rowe MI, Rowe SA: The last fifty years of neonatal surgical management. Am J Surg 2000;180:345-352.
243. Roy RN, Sinclair JC: Hydration of the low birth-weight infant. Clin Perinatol 1975;2:393-417.
244. Russell IA, Miller Hance WC, Gregory G, et al: The safety and efficacy of sevoflurane anesthesia in infants and children with congenital heart disease. Anesth Analg 2001;92:1152-1158.
245. Rusy L, Houck C, Sullivan L, et al: A double-blind evaluation of ketorolac tromethamine versus acetaminophine in pediatric tonsillectomy: Analgesia and bleeding, Anesth Analg 1995;80:226-229.
246. Rusy LM, Weisman SJ: Complementary therapies for acute pediatric pain management. Pediatr Clin North Am 2000;47:589-599.
247. Ryan J: Malignant hyperthermia. In Cole C (ed): A Practice of Anesthesia for Infants and Children. Philadelphia, WB Saunders, 1993.
248. Rylance G: Clinical pharmacology: Drugs in children. BMJ (Clin Res Ed) 1981;282:50-51.
249. Sabatowski R, Kasper SM, Radbruch L: Patient-controlled analgesia with intravenous L-methadone in a child with cancer pain refractory to high-dose morphine. J Pain Symptom Manage 2002;23:3-5.
250. Sahler OJ, Hunter BC, Liesveld JL: The effect of using music therapy with relaxation imagery in the management of

patients undergoing bone marrow transplantation: A pilot feasibility study. Altern Ther Health Med 2003;9:70-74.
251. Sanders JC: Paediatric regional anaesthesia: A survey of practice in the United Kingdom. Br J Anaesth 2002;89: 707-710.
252. Sara CA, Lowry CJ: A complication of circumcision and dorsal nerve block of the penis. Anaesth Intensive Care 1985;13:79-82.
253. Sarner JB, Levine M, Davis PJ, et al: Clinical characteristics of sevoflurane in children: A comparison with halothane. Anesthesiology 1995;82:38-46.
254. Schechter N, Weisman S, Rosenblum M, et al: The use of oral transmucosal fentanyl citrate for painful procedures in children. Pediatrics 1995;95:335-339.
255. Schechter NL: The undertreatment of pain in children: An overview. Pediatr Clin North Am 1989;36:781-794.
256. Schindler M, Swann M, Crawford M: A comparison of postoperative analgesia provided by wound infiltration or caudal analgesia. Anaesth Intensive Care 1991;19:46-49.
257. Sebel PS, Lowdon JD: Propofol: A new intravenous anesthetic. Anesthesiology 1989;71:260-277.
258. Segredo V, Caldwell JE, Matthay MA, et al: Persistent paralysis in critically ill patients after long-term administration of vecuronium. N Engl J Med 1992;327:524-528.
259. Selbst S, Zempsky W: Sedation and analgesia in the emergency department. In Schechter N, Berde C, Yaster M (eds): Pain in Infants, Children, and Adolescents. Philadelphia, Lippincott Williams & Wilkins, 2003, pp 651-668.
260. Sethna N, Berde C: Pediatric regional anesthesia. In Gregory G (ed): Pediatric Anesthesia. New York, Churchill Livingstone, 1994, pp 281-318.
261. Shandling B, Steward DJ: Regional analgesia for postoperative pain in pediatric outpatient surgery. J Pediatr Surg 1980;15:477-480.
262. Shannon M, Berde CB: Pharmacologic management of pain in children and adolescents. Pediatr Clin North Am 1989;36:855-871.
263. Sharpe P, Klein JR, Thompson JP, et al: Analgesia for circumcision in a paediatric population: Comparison of caudal bupivacaine alone with bupivacaine plus two doses of clonidine. Paediatr Anaesth 2001;11:695-700.
264. Shear CR: Effects of disuse on growing and adult chick skeletal muscle. J Cell Sci 1981;48:35-54.
265. Shenkman Z, Holzman RS, Kim C, et al: Acupressure-acupuncture antiemetic prophylaxis in children undergoing tonsillectomy. Anesthesiology 1999;90:1311-1316.
266. Short TG, Chui PT: Propofol and midazolam act synergistically in combination. Br J Anaesth 1991;67:539-545.
267. Sievers TD, Yee JD, Foley ME, et al: Midazolam for conscious sedation during pediatric oncology procedures: Safety and recovery parameters. Pediatrics 1991;88:1172-1179.
268. Smith SM, Barry RC: A comparison of three formulations of TAC (tetracaine, adrenalin, cocaine) for anesthesia of minor lacerations in children. Pediatr Emerg Care 1990;6:266-270.
269. Somri M, Gaitini LA, Vaida SJ, et al: Effect of ilioinguinal nerve block on the catecholamine plasma levels in orchidopexy: Comparison with caudal epidural block. Paediatr Anaesth 2002;12:791-797.
270. Splinter W: Halothane: The end of an era? Anesth Analg 2002;95:1471.
271. Splinter WM, Schaefer JD, Zunder IH: Clear fluids three hours before surgery do not affect the gastric fluid contents of children. Can J Anaesth 1990;37:498-501.
272. Splinter WM, Schreiner MS: Preoperative fasting in children. Anesth Analg 1999;89:80-89.
273. Squire S, Kirchhoff K, Hissong K: Comparing two methods of topical anesthesia used before intravenous cannulation in pediatric patients. J Pediatr Health Care 2000;14:68-72.
274. Steward D: Premature infants are more prone to complications following minor surgery than are term infants. Anesthesiology 1982;56:304.
275. Steward DJ, Creighton RE: The uptake and excretion of nitrous oxide in the newborn. Can Anaesth Soc J 1978;25:215-217.
276. Stoelting RK, Longnecker DE: The effect of right-to-left shunt on the rate of increase of arterial anesthetic concentration. Anesthesiology 1972;36:352-356.
277. Streisand JB, Stanley TH, Hague B, et al: Oral transmucosal fentanyl citrate premedication in children. Anesth Analg 1989;69:28-34.
278. Suresh S, Barcelona S, Young N, et al: Does a preemptive block of the great auricular nerve improve postoperative analgesia in children undergoing tympanomastoid surgery? Anesth Analg 2004;98:330-333.
279. Taddio A, Katz J, Ilersich AL, et al: Effect of neonatal circumcision on pain response during subsequent routine vaccination. Lancet 1997;349:599-603.
280. Taddio A, Nulman I, Goldbach M, et al: Use of lidocaine-prilocaine cream for vaccination pain in infants. J Pediatr 1994;124:643-648.
281. Tanner G: Effects of left-to-right mixed left-to-right, and right-to-left shunts on inhalation anesethetic induction in children: A computer model. Anesth Analg 1985;64:101.
282. Taylor RH, Lerman J: Minimum alveolar concentration of desflurane and hemodynamic responses in neonates, infants, and children. Anesthesiology 1991;75:975-979.
283. Taylor RH, Lerman J: Induction, maintenance and recovery characteristics of desflurane in infants and children. Can J Anaesth 1992;39:6-13.
284. Tiret L, Nivoche Y, Hatton F, et al: Complications related to anaesthesia in infants and children: A prospective survey of 40240 anaesthetics. Br J Anaesth 1988;61:263-269.
285. Tobias J, Schleien C, Haun S: Methadone as treatment for iatrogenic narcotic dependency in pediatric intensive care unit patients. Crit Care Med 1990;18:1292-1293.
286. Tobias JD, Lynch A, McDuffee A, et al: Pancuronium infusion for neuromuscular block in children in the pediatric intensive care unit. Anesth Analg 1995;81:13-16.
287. Tobias JD, Phipps S, Smith B, et al: Oral ketamine premedication to alleviate the distress of invasive procedures in pediatric oncology patients. Pediatrics 1992;90:537-541.
288. Tome J: Intranasal midazolam does not delay discharge in patients having ultrashort surgical procedures. Anesth Analg 1993;40:A66.
289. Tree-Trakarn T, Pirayavaraporn S: Postoperative pain relief for circumcision in children: Comparison among morphine, nerve block, and topical analgesia. Anesthesiology 1985;62:519-522.
290. Tsuchiya N, Ichizawa M, Yoshikawa Y, et al: Comparison of ropivacaine with bupivacaine and lidocaine for ilioinguinal block after ambulatory inguinal hernia repair in children. Paediatr Anaesth 2004;14:468-470.
291. Tverskoy M, Cozacov C, Ayache M, et al: Postoperative pain after inguinal herniorrhaphy with different types of anesthesia. Anesth Analg 1990;70:29-35.
292. Twersky R: Midazolam enhances anterograde but not retrograde amnesia in pediatric patients. Anesthesiology 1993;78:51.
293. Uezono S, Goto T, Terui K, et al: Emergence agitation after sevoflurane versus propofol in pediatric patients. Anesth Analg 2000;91:563-566.
294. Valley RD, Bailey AG: Caudal morphine for postoperative analgesia in infants and children: A report of 138 cases. Anesth Analg 1991;72:120-124.
295. Valtonen M, Iisalo E, Kanto J, Rosenberg P: Propofol as an induction agent in children: Pain on injection and pharmacokinetics. Acta Anaesthesiol Scand 1989;33:152-155.

296. Valtonen M, Iisalo E, Kanto J, Tikkanen J: Comparison between propofol and thiopentone for induction of anaesthesia in children. Anaesthesia 1988;43:696-699.
297. Vator M, Wandless J: Caudal or dorsal nerve block? A comparison of two local anaesthetic techniques for postoperative analgesia following day case circumcision. Acta Anaesthesiol Scand 1985;29:175-179.
298. Veyckemans F, Scholtes JL, Ninane J: Cervical epidural analgesia for a cancer child at home. Med Pediatr Oncol 1994;22:58-60.
299. Voepel-Lewis T, Malviya S, Tait AR: A prospective cohort study of emergence agitation in the pediatric postanesthesia care unit. Anesth Analg 2003;96:1625-1630.
300. Walbergh E: Pharmacokinetics of intravenous and intranasal midazolam in children. Anesthesiology 1989;71:A1066.
301. Wark H, O'Halloran M, Overton J: Prospective study of liver function in children following multiple halothane anaesthetics at short intervals. Br J Anaesth 1986;58:1224-1228.
302. Warner LO, Beach TP, Garvin JP, et al: Halothane and children: The first quarter century. Anesth Analg 1984;63: 838-840.
303. Warner M, et al: Practice guidelines for preoperative fasting and the use of pharmacologic agents to reduce the risk of pulmonary aspiration: Application to healthy patients undergoing elective procedures. A report by the American Society of Anesthesiologists Task Force on Preoperative Fasting. Anesthesiology 1999;90:896-905.
304. Watcha MF, Jones MB, Lagueruela RG, et al: Comparison of ketorolac and morphine as adjuvants during pediatric surgery. Anesthesiology 1992;76:368-372.
305. Watling S, Dasta J: Prolonged paralysis in intensive care unit patients after the use of neuromuscular blocking agents: A review of the literature. Crit Care Med 1994;22:884.
306. Way WL, Costley EC, Leongway E: Respiratory sensitivity of the newborn infant to meperidine and morphine. Clin Pharmacol Ther 1965;11:454-461.
307. Weber F, Wulf H: Caudal bupivacaine and s(+)-ketamine for postoperative analgesia in children. Paediatr Anaesth 2003;13:244-248.
308. Weiskopf RB, Moore MA, Eger EI 2nd, et al: Rapid increase in desflurane concentration is associated with greater transient cardiovascular stimulation than with rapid increase in isoflurane concentration in humans. Anesthesiology 1994;80:1035-1045.
309. Welborn L, Hannallah R: Anemia and postoperative apnea in former preterm infants. Anesthesiology 1991;74: 1003-1006.
310. Welborn LG, Hannallah RS, Norden JM, et al: Comparison of emergence and recovery characteristics of sevoflurane, desflurane, and halothane in pediatric ambulatory patients. Anesth Analg 1996;83:917-920.
311. Welborn LG, McGill WA, Hannallah RS, et al: Perioperative blood glucose concentrations in pediatric outpatients. Anesthesiology 1986;65:543-547.
312. Welborne L: Postoperative apnea in former premature infants: Prospective comparison of spinal and general anesthesia. Anesthesiology 1990;72:838.
313. Weldon B, Connor M, White P: Nurse-controlled versus patient-controlled analgesia following pediatric scoliosis surgery. Anesthesiology 1991;75:3.
314. Weldon BC, Bell M, Craddock T: The effect of caudal analgesia on emergence agitation in children after sevoflurane versus halothane anesthesia. Anesth Analg 2004;98:321-326.
315. Weldon BC, Connor M, White PF: Pediatric PCA: The role of concurrent opioid infusions and nurse-controlled analgesia. Clin J Pain 1993;9:26-33.
316. Westrin P: The induction dose of propofol in infants 1-6 months of age and in children 10-16 years of age. Anesthesiology 1991;74:455-458.
317. Westrin P, Jonmarker C, Werner O: Thiopental requirements for induction of anesthesia in neonates and in infants one to six months of age. Anesthesiology 1989;71: 344-346.
318. Wilder R, Berde C, Troshynski T, et al: Patient-controlled analgesia in children and adolescents: Safety and outcome among 1589 patients. Anesthesiology 1992;77:1187.
319. Williamson PS, Williamson ML: Physiologic stress reduction by a local anesthetic during newborn circumcision. Pediatrics 1983;71:36-40.
320. Wilton NC, Leigh J, Rosen DR, et al: Preanesthetic sedation of preschool children using intranasal midazolam. Anesthesiology 1988;69:972-975.
321. Wodey E, Pladys P, Copin C, et al: Comparative hemodynamic depression of sevoflurane versus halothane in infants: An echocardiographic study. Anesthesiology 1997;87:795-800.
322. Wodey E, Senhadji L, Pladys P, et al: The relationship between expired concentration of sevoflurane and sympathovagal tone in children. Anesth Analg 2003;97: 377-382.
323. Wolf W, Neal M, Pertson M: The hemodynamic and cardiovascular effects of isoflurane and halothane anesthesia in children. Anesthesiology 1986;64:328.
324. Wood CE, Goresky GV, Klassen KA, et al: Complications of continuous epidural infusions for postoperative analgesia in children. Can J Anaesth 1994;41:613-620.
325. Woolf CJ, Chong MS: Preemptive analgesia—treating postoperative pain by preventing the establishment of central sensitization. Anesth Analg 1993;77:362-379.
326. Woolf CJ, Wall PD: Relative effectiveness of C primary afferent fibers of different origins in evoking a prolonged facilitation of the flexor reflex in the rat. J Neurosci 1986;6:1433-1442.
327. World Health Organization: Cancer Pain Relief: With a Guide to Opioid Availability, 2nd ed. Geneva, WHO, 1996.
328. Yaster M: Pain relief. Pediatrics 1995;95:427-428.
329. Yaster M, Kost-Byerly S, Maxwell L: Opioid agonists and antagonists. In Schechter N, Berde C, Yaster M (eds): Pain in Infants, Children, and Adolescents. Philadelphia, Lippincott Williams & Wilkins, 2003, pp 181-224.
330. Yaster M, Maxwell LG: Pediatric regional anesthesia. Anesthesiology 1989;70:324-338.
331. Yaster M, Nichols DG, Deshpande JK, et al: Midazolam-fentanyl intravenous sedation in children: Case report of respiratory arrest. Pediatrics 1990;86:463-467.
332. Yeoman PM, Cooke R, Hain WR: Penile block for circumcision? A comparison with caudal blockade. Anaesthesia 1983;38:862-866.
333. Zuppa AF, Helfaer MA, Adamson PC: Propofol pharmacokinetics. Pediatr Crit Care Med 2003;4:124-125.
334. Zwass MS, Fisher DM, Welborn LG, et al: Induction and maintenance characteristics of anesthesia with desflurane and nitrous oxide in infants and children. Anesthesiology 1992;76:373-378.

第 14 章

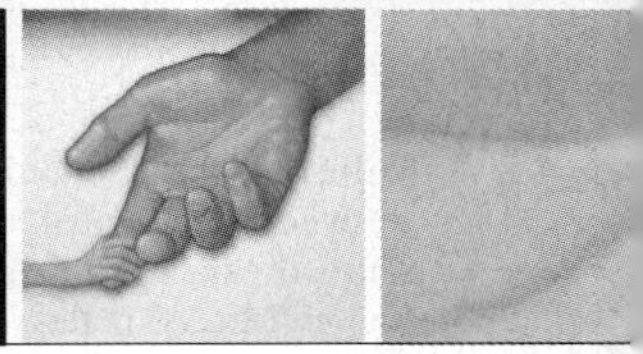

伦理学问题

Donna A. Caniano 和 Carolyn Ells

257 Potts 在其经典著作《外科医生与孩子》中曾写道，“给一个有先天畸形的新生婴儿进行的满意的手术有赖于：这个孩子的完整生活是否由此展现在其面前这个事实。家长们期望奇迹出现，但更感激的是这个孩子能得到仅仅作为一个人可以得到的最好的对待”[19]。这句意味深长的表述揭示了小儿外科手术的要点，即是否纠正了一个严重的先天性异常，是否治疗了一个严重的毁损性损害，或是否切除了一个恶性肿瘤。对小儿外科医生来说，每一项为患儿缓解病痛及为其将来获得完整而活力的生活的努力都会给自己带来喜悦。小儿外科医生面对的伦理学挑战包括：医学实践的基本道德原则、外科专业的特殊问题和婴儿与儿童医疗护理中特有的其他问题。本章回顾了一些有关小儿外科伦理学的基本伦理学概念和责任，也探讨了一些伦理学的新领域和有关外科手术的争议，包括对病态肥胖患儿的手术处理和对两性畸形患儿的性别确定手术。

小儿外科伦理学

外科伦理学的特性首先是源于外科医生与其患者之间关系的特性。Little[11]曾提出外科医生与患者关系的道德范畴的五根支柱：拯救、亲近、考验、后果及在场。这些因素在其他治疗关系中也可能存在，但在手术中表现得尤为突出。

拯救是指当患者面对严重威胁生命的疾病时，为了得到手术救治，患者及其家属将处于无助和完全依赖的情况。此时患者不得不接受侵袭性和创伤性的手术治疗，对此患者及其家属无法掌控，此时，外科医生将起主导作用，外科医生和患者及其家属（小儿外科多数是孩子的家长）需要相互配合，共同面对和协商患者的治疗。

亲近是指外科医生与患者之间密切相互作用的情况。很显然，外科医生做手术与做其他治疗是有区别的。外科医生探查和接触、切除和缝合患者的部分身体是患者自身无法想象的。这种亲近可使外科医生了解及明白患者的病痛，这种作用是无法互换的。患者是无法知道给他们做手术的外科医生是采用如此密切的工作方式，也无法得知外科医生是如何了解他们的情况的。

外科医生必须认识到手术对患者来说是一种严峻的考验，是一种患者必须忍受的极端经历。Little 认为[11]，手术会使患者放弃自主权、依靠他人、给予信任、面对风险、面对身体切口和死亡、丧失对时间和空间的控制以及要经历隔离、疼痛、恐惧、不适、病痛和厌倦。在手术过程中，患者的身份认知感会不可避免地遭受挑战或改变。

对于手术的后果，外科医生必须认识到，有些患者虽然术后能迅速康复，但手术可能有远期问题。生理和情感上的创伤、不适、危险和其他类型的病痛可能常使患者处于经历过的疾病或伤痛的阴影之中，使患者日后易受疾病或伤痛的困扰。了解手术的后果有助于外科医生理解其对患者现存状况以及他们自身的威胁。在小儿外科中，手术后果呈现出独特的双重性，既影响到患儿，又影响到患儿的家长。

对外科医生来说，在场既是美德，也是职责。在整个手术过程中他们必须始终在场并投身其中。在小儿外科中，这种专业职责还要延伸到患儿的长期随访，经常要延伸到青春期。例如，对于一个在新生儿期做过胃肠和肝胆系统重大重建手术的患儿来说，小儿外科医生可能是唯一一个了解其潜在的远期并发症和功能障碍的专家。履行这样的职责要有以患者为中心的思想，外科医生要根据患者的特殊情况和经历培育医患关系并促进患者的收益。

258 外科医生应将其专业价值和伦理学原则溶于医患关系中，把患者的利益放在首位。McCullough 等人[12]在《外科伦理学》一书中将患者的权利与外科手术联系在一起，认为他们的每一种权利都意味着一种重要的专业价值。作者提醒我们，患者有权利“不成为外科医生故意或无意的牺牲品，不被外科医生有意或粗心大意地伤害……不被外科医生欺骗……能被充分地告知手术的利弊，能由有水平的有能力医生给予治疗，能使自己的健康和利益高于外科医生的经济利益，并能在疾病被告知的情况下决定是否接受治疗”[12]。

在小儿外科中，使患者完全知情的专业责任，使其能够决定选择与不选择治疗以及不被欺骗，通常需要借助于第三方（多数情况下是患儿的父母）——作为婴儿、儿童和青少年的监护人来完成，包括要充分告知病情，获取理解和认同。虽然孩子的决策代理人常为家长，但根据相关法律，指定的监护人及其他代理人也能充当这一角色。在某些地区和某些特殊情况下，青少年患者有权对自己接受的治疗做出决定。这种情况特别适用于罹患慢性疾病的青少年，如镰状细胞病、囊性纤维化和恶性肿瘤进展期。但是，当青少年患者违背父母意愿做出同意或拒绝手术治疗时，可能需要社会机构的帮助或法律援助。

家庭或决策代理人并不一定有权代表患者接受（或拒绝）手术。以患者为中心的治疗需要懂得患者是生活在一个家庭中，他或她是家庭中的一员。同样要懂得，年龄很小的患者有着明显的弱势——在做出治疗决定的过程中很少或不能表达意愿，并且很少或根本无法理解手术过程。这些患儿应得到能够优化他们所需要治疗方式的支持和对其所处弱势地位给予保护的支持。医患关系扩展有助于外科医生了解患者并给予患者于他们最有益的建议，这也有助于其他人提供这些患者所需要的支持。

一个经常摆在小儿外科医生（及决策代理人）面前的伦理学挑战是：当患者在价值观尚未完全形成时如何判断其意愿。小患者治疗计划应综合考虑其性格、目标、价值观及喜好等因素并与予以权衡后做出。

小儿外科医生在做出伦理学决策及解决问题时需要调动一切手段。Baylis 和 Caniano[1]提倡以团队的方式解决在婴幼儿手术治疗时遇到的伦理学难题。他们认为，在三级儿童医院中，当代卫生服务离不开多个团队：即患儿和家长、护理和相关卫生服务成员以及外科专业人员。对于任何一个既定的患者而言，卫生服务团队必须遵循一个共同的道德规范及与患者特殊情况相关的伦理学问题的理解。例如，对于罹患多发性先天畸形的早产儿来说，服务提供者和决策代理人必须有伦理学问题的实践和认知。团队或团队的领导人必须有能力向患儿家长及其他相关家庭成员阐明其重要价值观和目标。当患儿家长及其家庭的文化或宗教背景与卫生团队的价值观和目标存在明显分歧时，需要特别关注。例如，在某些文化中，为患儿的治疗做出最后决定的可能不是其父母，而是祖父母或社区的长者。最后，团队必须按照特定的决策方式做出决定。

适用于小儿外科中存在的伦理学棘手问题的几句格言是：（1）好的伦理始于好的事实；（2）理性的人可以持有不同的或反对的观点；（3）一般地说，最佳的决定来自大家的一致认识；（4）大多数决定不需要匆忙做出；（5）对于罹患严重疾病的新生儿和儿童，大多数决定都是痛苦的，很多都没有乐观的解决办法。

当外科专业人员与患者及其家长之间的观点存在分歧时，大多就会处于伦理窘境。分歧通常集中在如何使患者获取最大利益（如继续存活而伴有严重的疾病负担）以及能够使人接受的患者生活质量是什么。Glover 和 Caniano[7]概括了一个包含几种成分的伦理决策过程，包括确认决策者的身份、搜集所有提示最佳预后的手术资料、弄清“关系人”（对婴儿来说通常是其家长和关系密切的家庭成员）的相关价值观、详细说明现有的治疗和非治疗选择、评估所有的选择并提出建议（通常是小儿外科医生的责任）并获得一致意见（万一存在明显的分歧，需要伦理学顾问或中间人参与）。下文讨论小儿外科医生面对的新的伦理学挑战，一些方法还将继续讨论。

创新和研究

发达国家的居民都非常看重各个领域的创新，包括医学领域的创新。在小儿外科领域，要获得进步和技术更新，个人和集体的作用都很重要。社会期望外科医生能取得创新并发明出新的治疗方法和技术。患者则倾向于能够提供更有益的新的手术方法，如胆囊 259

切除术在 20 年间已从开腹手术快速地转变为腹腔镜手术。同时患者给予外科医生很大的空间，允许甚至是期盼他们改良必须实施的传统手术。McKneally[13]观察到，外科医生通常是将自己原创的手术方法和技术成就冠以个人的名字。小儿外科中大量的手术都是以首次报道的医生名字来命名的，如用于肠旋转不良的 Ladd 手术和用于治疗 Hirschsprung 病的 Duhamel 根治术。

在其他医学领域，引进新药和新的治疗手段之前要进行随机临床试验。与之相比，外科领域可以比较宽松地开展新手术而较少受到严厉的法律和专业条例的限制[6]。虽然有些经典的手术，如治疗肠套迭的空气灌肠术和治疗 Hirschsprung 病的 Swenson 根治术，最初是在动物模型上试验成功的，但多数小儿外科手术是在患者身上直接试验并完善起来的。新的手术方法通常是在小儿外科专业会议上进行交流并随后发表在专业杂志上。创立新手术的小儿外科医生通常会报告他或她的经验、说明相关并发症和结果以及在同一家医院中患者的跟踪随访结果。

未经严格的审查即在人体上行改良手术方法的理由包括以下几方面：（1）缺乏适当的动物模型以满足特殊解剖条件的需要；（2）新手术意味着标准的延伸，即以一种创新的方式使用可接受的技术；（3）开展新手术可使患者获益而不是以学习为目的；（4）缺少有关新手术的专业标准；（5）手术应何时开展临床试验尚无明确规定；（6）对患者的安全和利益保障而言，当前的体系运行良好。事实上，大量术式已被放弃，或因术后没有获得理想效果（如用于治疗 Hirschsprung 病的交感神经切除术），或因术后的发病率和死亡率高得使人难以接受（如用于治疗病态肥胖的空肠回肠分流术）。

研究应该是一种系统性研究，其设计是为了得到知识或对知识进行概括总结。在小儿外科中，会有对某个患儿以新的方式进行手术的情况；因此从严格意义上说，这种手术并不是研究。但随着这种手术量增加及其资料增多，最后这种手术方式往往会形成并写成文章发表。从为一个患者进行的治疗开始到进入临床研究，这本身就是人体研究的伦理学对象。

1966 年 Beecher 在《新英格兰医学杂志》上发表了一篇有关生殖医学方面的文章，详细地阐述了若干刊登在权威杂志上的违背知情同意伦理学规范和安全性的手术案例[2]。虽然第二次世界大战后纽伦堡审判揭露了二战期间一些令人发指的非人道的人体试验，但是在美国，主流医学研究仍不规范，仍有一些不符合伦理学的悬而未决的研究案例。Beecher 的报告激起了公众的关注，并促使联邦政府要求所有与人体试验有关的研究（医学、行为学和手术）必须进行机构审查，以使其符合伦理学规范。

通过 1974 年的国家研究法，国家人体生物医学和行为学研究保护委员会召集了一批权威临床科学家、医生以及伦理学、宗教和法律方面的专家，审议并制定了开展人体试验研究的基本原则和确保伦理学研究的方针。1979 年该委员会发表了总结性报告，即 Belmont 报告[17]。该报告确认了尊重试验对象（又分为尊重自主权和保护弱者）、仁慈和公正的原则，尤其是与研究伦理学相关时。虽然具体应用不同，但这些原则在随后的临床实践中发挥了重要作用。Belmont 的报告提到了对小儿外科医生来说至关重要的两个特点：受试者知情同意的作用，以及对弱势受试者如儿童的保护。

家长和社会希望小儿外科医生在手术创新中采取相对保守的态度。通常手术的安全性有赖于长期考验和纠治先天性畸形效果的改进。Levine[10]将一些新的手术方式归类为效果未知的手术，即认为其存在伦理学和医学风险且有可能被创新的命名掩盖。对小儿外科医生和家长来说，效果未知的手术这个概念更加透明和诚实。它意味着推荐的新手术尚未经过严格的临床研究这个事实。事实上假定一种新式手术的效果优于传统术式的假设，是一种假定其只缺乏经验数据的假设。某种效果未知的手术其临床试验也许可以说明其效果优于、等同或劣于传统手术。例如，近期国家卫生研究所资助的一项在胎儿期通过内镜在气管内封堵治疗先天性膈疝的临床研究被叫停，原因是 24 例受试患儿的生存率低于接受标准治疗（按计划分娩并在出生后接受三级医疗中心治疗）的患儿。

现有的手术创新体制还没有严格的监管，因此对于一种既定的疾病，这可能会妨碍最佳外科治疗方式的选择。治疗方式存在争议会促使小儿外科医生在参加设计良好的前瞻性、多中心合作的临床试验以确定最佳手术或治疗方式中承担伦理学义务[3]。患儿及其家长有权期望小儿外科医生实施好的外科治疗，包括效果已得到证明的外科治疗和手术方案。当小儿外科医生对其患者实施效果未知的手术时，无论是出于多好的意愿，这种手术都可能不是最佳的，因为手术疗效尚未经过严格的试验研究。

减肥手术

在许多发达国家，儿童和青少年肥胖被认为是一个公众关注的重大健康问题。在美国，约 6%的儿童有肥胖问题，其中 1/3 为病态性肥胖。虽然这种情况的原因尚未完全明了，但美国儿童的体育活动减少及进食高热量的食物可能是主要原因。

儿童和青少年肥胖对个人健康和公众健康都是重要问题。因为肥胖常与严重的疾病相关，如高脂血症、高血压和 2 型糖尿病，并且经济和社会负担沉重。与儿童和青少年肥胖相关的负面心理因素还没有得到很好的研究。由于儿童和青少年肥胖会带来一系列严重的生理、精神卫生和长期的健康问题，卫生服务专业人员和各种社会团体对此给予了普遍关注。

治疗病态肥胖有药物和手术等方法。这些方法的成功率各不相同，需要进一步进行研究和评估，特别是在儿童中。在成人患者中，包括完善的锻炼和饮食计划在内的药物治疗长期以来并未获得成功。儿童医院很少有全面的肥胖治疗方案；因此，有关这些方案的治疗效果的文献很少。

在成人病态肥胖患者中，手术治疗非常普遍，因为其可成功地减轻患者的体重，并且并发症和死亡率均在可接受的范围之内。有鉴于对成人肥胖患者的疗效良好，小儿外科医生常被公众请求——特别被求医心切的患儿及其家长请求——为有病态肥胖的儿童和青少年实施减肥手术治疗（见第 78 章）。

在北美和欧洲一些国家，成人肥胖患者最常在腹腔镜下进行 Roux-en-Y 胃改道术和胃捆扎减容术。尽管两者均可获得减轻体重的疗效，但胃捆扎减容术不改变患者解剖结构，是可逆性的，胃改道术则不可逆地改变患者解剖结构。胃改道术不仅会缩小胃容积，还会引起患者吸收不良，因此胃改道术后体重减轻的效果更明显。在成人的长期研究结果表明，胃捆扎减容术后患者体重减轻效果不理想，但其合并的高血压和糖尿病病情会减轻。

小儿外科医生应注意减肥手术中存在的若干伦理学问题[9]。目前两种减肥手术对儿科患者均属效果未知的手术，且在这类人群中进行的多中心临床试验证明，其既没有安全性也没有有效性。患儿及其决策代理人在决定做减肥手术之前，应该了解这些手术疗效的未知性质。此外，如果可能的话，实施这些手术的小儿外科医生应参加精心设计的临床试验，以便确定这些手术对病态肥胖患儿的安全性、有效性并获得术后长期随访结果。同其他效果未知的治疗一样，在设计评价减肥手术的安全性和有效性试验时，应注意不能影响患者的治疗目标。

由于没有足够的有关儿科患者减肥手术的研究资料，其开展时间也不长（只有零星的青少年病例报道），这些手术的风险及潜在的益处很难评价。虽然早期的研究结果表明其对青少年患者是安全的，但长期的随访结果尚不明了。胃改道术已引起人们对慢性营养问题的关注，如维生素缺乏及可能伴随终身的长期副作用。另一个问题是患者必须严格执行饮食方案，并应不定期地接受身体检查。已经得到的一致看法是，患者大多无法长期坚持规律的身体检查，尤其是当其不存在身体不适时。由于这种减肥手术对青少年患者的远期风险尚不知晓，最好对患者进行密切的监测以发现隐匿的生理改变，因为后者可能被忽视而导致严重的后果。

手术风险并不单由不符合伦理学的治疗带来。手术风险的伦理学评估要考虑风险的严重性、风险发生的概率以及患者可能获得的潜在益处。患者的潜在利益应以现有的证据及患者的特殊情况来评价。若研究存在空白点，小儿外科医生应采用成人的数据并依据自身的经验外推至青少年患者。在告知手术方案环节，小儿外科医生应对患儿及其决策代理人诚实，说明什么是已知的，什么是未知的，以及他们向特定的患者推荐的减肥手术的理由。

对于罹患病态肥胖儿童和青少年来说，手术的减肥效果可能比非手术效果来的要快，且容易“稳固”。快速和简单的解决办法当然是人们希望的，但是如果非手术方法或损伤小的手术是（或证明是）更安全或更有效的，或如果它们对儿童和青少年的意愿（如对自身的健康、身体和将来的生活做出重要决定的能力）是一种保护，小儿外科医生应该考虑同意进行。
小儿外科医生，作为儿童健康的维护者，对病态肥胖 261
患儿的治疗选择负有权衡多方反馈意见并进行评估的专业责任。总之，如果延迟手术是安全的，那么对于缺乏决策能力的患儿，外科医生应延迟为其手术直至其具备了相应的能力。当手术的效果是不可逆转的以及手术的安全性和有效性未知时，这种做法尤其重要。小儿外科医生不仅应当考虑减肥手术是否是这类特殊患者的治疗选择，还应考虑手术是否是这类患者的最佳选择。虽然是否选择手术最终取决于患者及其决策代理人，但外科医生的意见通常是重要因素。对于一些患者来说，这可能意味着推荐一种有效性略差但可逆的外科技术，或延迟手术直至患儿长大一些且在此期间寻求治疗时再做决定。

性别确定手术

婴儿罹患下列疾病时可能应进行性别确定手术，包括性器官不明、泄殖腔外翻及阴茎发育不良。在过去 10 年中，治疗新生儿性器官不明的传统医疗和外科处理已引发了争议，一些曾在婴儿期接受"重建"治疗的人士对这些治疗的正确性及结果是否成功给予了质疑。尽管有若干组织支持，如北美两性畸形协会和雄激素不敏感支持组织，但是这些有两性畸形的成年人（大多数在婴儿期和儿童期接受了性别确定手术）还是对他们过去接受的医疗和手术的一些方面公开表示了极度不满。

如今两性畸形这个术语在医学专业领域和公众两方面都是指导致男性或女性生殖器解剖学异常的先天性畸形。性别确定手术依据的主要假设是：两性畸形可以导致心理伤害，这种伤害可以通过实施手术使患儿生殖器官外观正常化来避免或减轻，并且患儿能够按照他或她的相应的生殖器外观确定养育性别。通常性器官不明的婴儿出生时都会考虑有急病，需要迅速做出诊断，排除威胁生命的先天性肾上腺增生，并主要根据解剖学因素决定适合的养育性别。新生儿学家、小儿内分泌学家和小儿外科医生的处理都是基于 Money[16] ——John Hopkins 大学著名的心理学家——的性心理发育学理论。该理论认为，个体的性别取决于性器官，而个体的性身份取决于个体采纳的性角色。Money 的性心理分化理论认为，出生前的因素影响个性特征，包括挑衅行为和母性意识，但是性身份的主要决定因素是出生后的环境。从本质上说，Money 的理论认为：男性或女性的行为内涵主要取决于社会文化而并非完全由生物学因素决定。

对于两性畸形婴儿，Money 的理论在按照何种性别予以养育的决定方面起重要作用。首先，由于后天环境是决定婴儿性身份的重要因素，成功的治疗将为其提供明确的性身份认证。其次，由于性身份并不取决于性器官不明的原因，性别和性转换应依据解剖学条件（及重建手术潜力）、生育潜力和性交能力赋予。因此，在个体的性别已定的情况下，医学决定的性身份在大多数情况下可以通过在婴儿期进行外科重建手术赋予。

来自两性畸形组织的支持者、社会学家和其他一些人士引用了一些有关早期进行性别确定手术的资料。他们找到了一些有关性功能、性快感及性心理结果的客观的、长期的、多中心研究数据[14]。一项包含婴儿期接受女性化手术的小样本单中心的研究报告，患者的解剖、功能及性心理结果均可接受[18]。近期更多的报告（评价者最初并不是小儿外科医生）表明，女性化手术的远期效果并不理想，存在功能障碍和外观不佳[4,15]。最近的一项对罹患泄殖腔外翻的遗传学男性患儿的研究发现，14 例在新生儿阶段接受女性性别确定手术的病例有 8 例发生了与性别身份不一致情况，后者仍将自己识为男性[20]。由于有关各种两性畸形的预后报告很少，因此还不清楚反对在早期进行性别确定手术的人士其不满是少数患者的声音，还是多数患者预后欠佳的反映。

对传统方法的主要伦理学担心是医学和外科专业人士的家长式决策方式。家长通常没有被完整地告知诊断真相，即使被告知，外科医生也会对孩子的某些情况加以保留以减轻性别身份冲突。大多数两性畸形患者的家长和医生不会向他们透露诊断结果。因此，当他们长大至成年或青少年时，如果他们遇到性身份问题或性别难题并最终发现真相时，他们会对自己在婴儿和儿童期接受的治疗表示巨大的怨恨。对患者隐瞒两性畸形病史除了会引起他们对家长和医生的无礼和不信任外，还会剥夺他们逐步认知他们是谁和发生了什么、接受心理咨询以及向与他们有相同或相似经历的人寻求帮助的机会。知情同意的伦理学责任要 26
求：两性畸形患儿的家长应得到所有有关诊断、治疗选择（包括不在早期进行性别确定手术）、预期结果（包括有关长期预后的全面数据）及拥护者组织和获得咨询的相关信息。

大多数情况下，早期性别确定手术对婴儿身体健康并不是必需的。事实上，来自两性畸形组织的拥护者认为：早期手术对孩子的心理健康是不必要的，有时甚至可以引起伤害。Daaboul 和 Frader 认为，对罹患严重两性畸形及性别完全不相符的患儿应采取"折中”的方法[5]。他们认为，在这些患儿中延迟外科重建手术会导致他们在学龄期和青少年阶段发生相当严重的心理障碍。此外，发达国家尚无两性畸形儿童长期随访的可靠数据。这些患儿的家长应可以对是否早期进行性别确定手术做出决定，只要他们了解有关功能和性别结果相关知识。

与给予两性畸形患儿家长完整和诚实告知相关的伦理学义务应包括：小儿内分泌学家和小儿外科医生尊重家长的选择，包括拒绝早期施行性别确定手术。只要延期手术对患儿身体不会带来危险（感染、发育不全的性腺发生恶性肿瘤），这些患儿的家长就应该得到与其他家长相同的自主决定权。

（张瑞冬译　陈锡明校）

参考文献

1. Baylis F, CanianoDA: Medical ethics and the pediatric surgeon. In Oldham KT, Colombani PM, Foglia RP (eds): Surgery of Infants and Children: Scientific Principles and Practice. Philadelphia, Lippincott-Raven, 1997, p 382.
2. Beecher H: Ethics and clinical research. N Engl J Med 1966;274:1354.
3. Caniano DA: Ethical issues in the management of neonatal surgical anomalies. Semin Perinatol 2004;28:240.
4. Creighton SM, Minto CL, Steele SJ: Objective cosmetic and anatomical outcomes at adolescence of feminizing surgery for ambiguous genitalia done in childhood. Lancet 2001; 358:124.
5. Daaboul J, Frader J: Ethics and the management of the patient with intersex: A middle way. J Pediatr Endocrinol Metab 2001;14:1575.
6. Frader J, Caniano DA: Research and innovation in surgery. In McCullough LB, Jones JW, Brody BA (eds): Surgical Ethics. New York, Oxford University Press, 1998.
7. Glover JJ, Caniano DA: Ethical considerations in newborn surgery. In Puri P (ed): Newborn Surgery. Oxford, Butterworth-Heinemann, 2003.
8. Harrison MR, Keller Rl, Hawgood SB, et al: A randomized trial of fetal endoscopic occlusion for severe fetal congenital diaphragmatic hernia. N Engl J Med 2003;349:1916.
9. Inge TH, Krebs NF, Garcia VF, et al: Bariatric surgery for severely overweight adolescents: Concerns and recommendations. Pediatrics 2003;114:217.
10. Levine RJ: Ethics and Regulation of Clinical Research, 2nd ed. New Haven, Conn, Yale University Press, 1988.
11. Little M: Invited commentary: Is there a distinctively surgical ethics? Surgery 2001;129:668.
12. McCullough LB, Jones JW, Brody BA: Principles and practice of surgical ethics. In McCullough LB, Jones JW, Brody BA (eds): Surgical Ethics. New York, Oxford University Press, 1998.
13. McKneally MF: Ethical problems in surgery: Innovation leading to unforeseen complications. World J Surg 1999;23:786.
14. Meyer-Bahlburg HF: Gender assignment and reassignment in 46,XY pseudohermaphroditism and related conditions. J Clin Endocrinol Metab 1999;84:3455.
15. Minto CL, Liao LM, Woodhouse CRJ, et al: The effect of clitoral surgery on sexual outcome in individuals who have intersex conditions with ambiguous genitalia: A cross-sectional study. Lancet 2003;361:1252.
16. Money J: Gender: History, theory and usage of the term in sexology and its relationship to nature/nurture. J Sex Marital Ther 1985;11:71.
17. National Commission for the Protection of Human Subjects of Biomedical and Behavioral Research: The Belmont Report. OPPR Reports. Washington, DC, US Government Printing Office, 1979.
18. Newman K, Randolph J, Parson S: Functional results in young women having clitoral reconstruction as infants. J Pediatr Surg 1992;27:180.
19. Potts WJ: The Surgeon and the Child. Philadelphia, WB Saunders, 1959, p 3.
20. Reiner WG, Gearhart JP: Discordant sexual identity in some genetic males with cloacal exstrophy assigned to female sex at birth. N Engl J Med 2004;350:333.

第二部分

创　伤

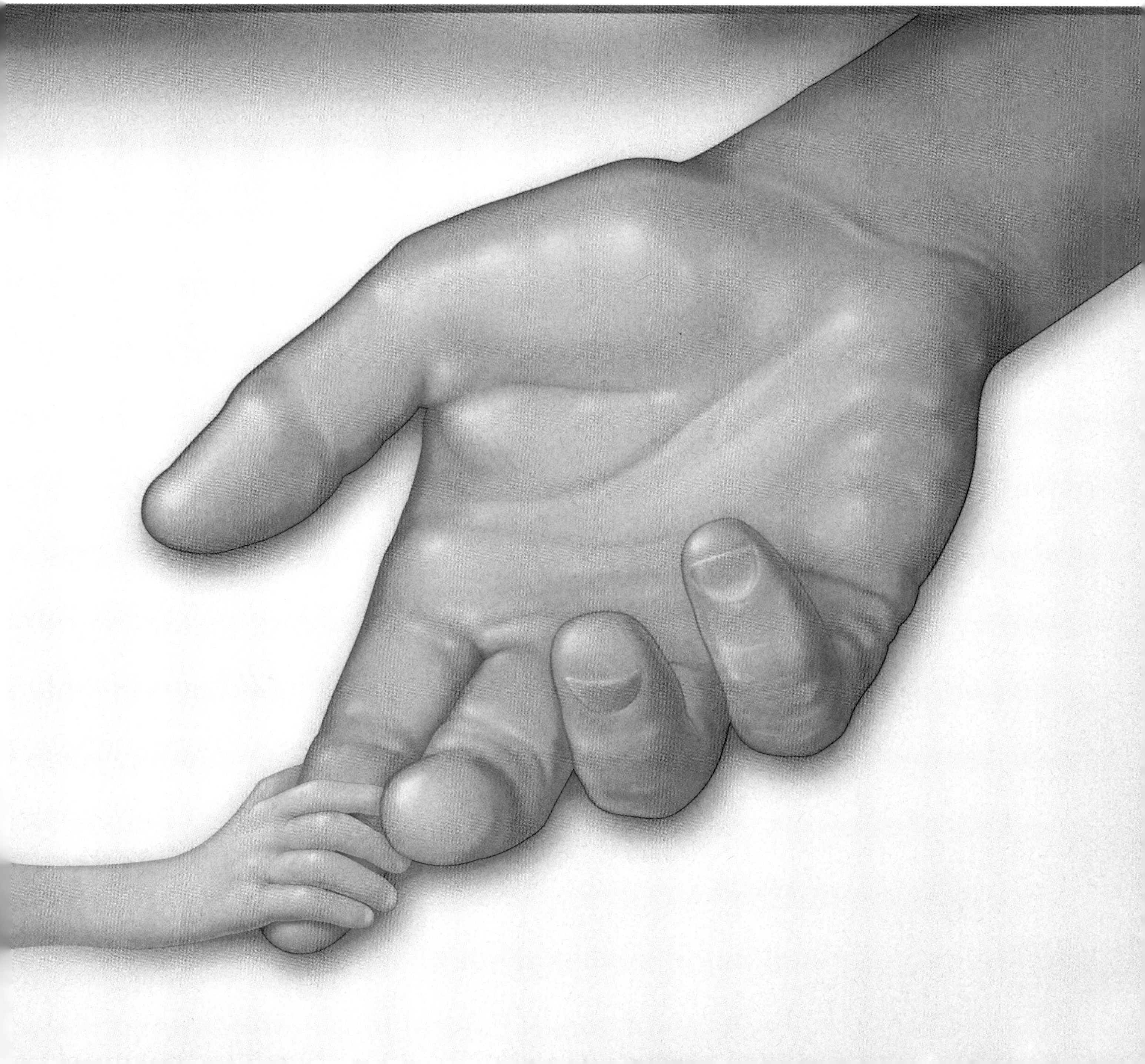

第 15 章

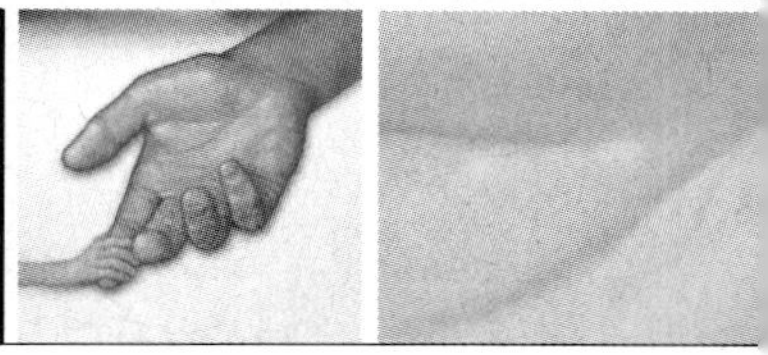

意外伤害及其急救处理

Jeffrey R. Lukish 和 Martin R. Eichelberger

儿童期意外伤害的流行病学

65 可预防的意外伤害对受伤害儿童及其家庭可带来巨大的经济和感情负担，对整个社会也是如此。在美国，意外伤害是 14 岁及以下儿童死亡的首要原因，据称每年至少夺去 5600 个生命或平均每天 15 个儿童死亡[2]。另外，在美国，2000 年大约有 1180 万人次 14 岁及以下儿童因意外伤害就诊，或者说每 5 个就诊儿童中就有 1 个是因为意外伤害。在所有因意外伤害住院的儿童中，16%会发生永久性残疾[4]。

1987—2000 年，14 岁及以下儿童的意外伤害死亡率下降了 39%；1～14 岁儿童的意外伤害死亡率下降了 42%。然而在美国，意外伤害导致的死亡仍是该年龄组儿童死亡的首要原因。2000 年，儿童致命性意外伤害的首要原因是车祸（28%），其次是溺死（16%）和气道梗阻（14%）。2001 年，跌倒是医院急诊室见到的非致命性伤害的首要原因（36%）[20]。

意外伤害相关的死亡的主要原因随儿童年龄而不同，取决于儿童的发育能力和潜在危害的接触，另外也与父母对儿童能力和损伤危险的认识有关。1 岁以下婴儿的伤害死亡率下降最少，只有 10%，比较而言，1～4 岁年龄组儿童伤害死亡率下降 42%，5～9 岁年龄组下降 42%，10～14 岁年龄组下降 40%。1 岁以下婴儿意外伤害相关的死亡率最高，是所有儿童的 2 倍以上。气道梗阻是这个年龄组的首要致死原因。在 1～4 岁年龄组，溺死占意外伤害死亡的 27%，是意外伤害致死的首要因素。5～9 岁年龄组的意外伤害死亡率最低；在这组和 10～14 岁年龄组中，最常见伤害原因是车祸（图 15-1）[20]。

在所有年龄组，男孩的意外伤害风险均比女孩的高。这可能是由于男孩进行的可导致伤害的活动、危险和粗暴的游戏更多。人种和种族也是儿童意外伤害的重要危险因素。美国印第安纳州和阿拉斯加州的儿童意外伤害死亡率最高，非洲裔美国儿童意外伤害死亡率排在第二位。这种人种和种族上的不同说明，我们更应该对贫穷社区的人们采取更多措施，这种因素比生物学差异更有意义[17,20]。

故意伤害和死亡可能是因为谋杀、儿童虐待或自杀。然而确定这些原因需要儿童保护组织进行评估。这些儿童的恢复具有挑战性，因为虐待往往是慢性的，最终可导致儿童只剩下有限的生理储备（参见第 24 章儿童虐待）。

复苏和预后效果

对受伤儿童的复苏包括给予有效措施以逆转和控制由受伤引起的生理平衡方面的变化。儿童恢复能力较好，但年龄越小初期的稳定时间明显变短[19]。因此，在确定损伤已得到治疗及不再进行干预的患儿的生理已稳定之前，不能结束复苏。

在伤害模式、生理表现和处理方面，儿童和成人之间是有区别的，尤其是在 2 岁以下儿童。治疗受伤害儿童的医生必须认识和理解这些重要区别，才能使复苏措施符合儿童的特殊需要。

有关成人意外伤害的死亡和发病三峰模型的原则应用于儿童时必须进行修改。在三峰模型中，儿童受 266
伤害的第一个死亡高峰发生在受伤害后数秒至数分钟，是由于损伤了中枢或周围神经系统和中央脉管系统。这组儿童的存活率只有通过努力预防来提高。儿童受伤害的第二个死亡高峰发生于受伤害后数分钟到数小时内，是因为中枢神经系统的占位病灶所致，通常是硬膜下和硬膜外血肿、实质脏器损伤或胸膜和心包间隙积液。这些损伤需要快速识别和治疗，因为儿

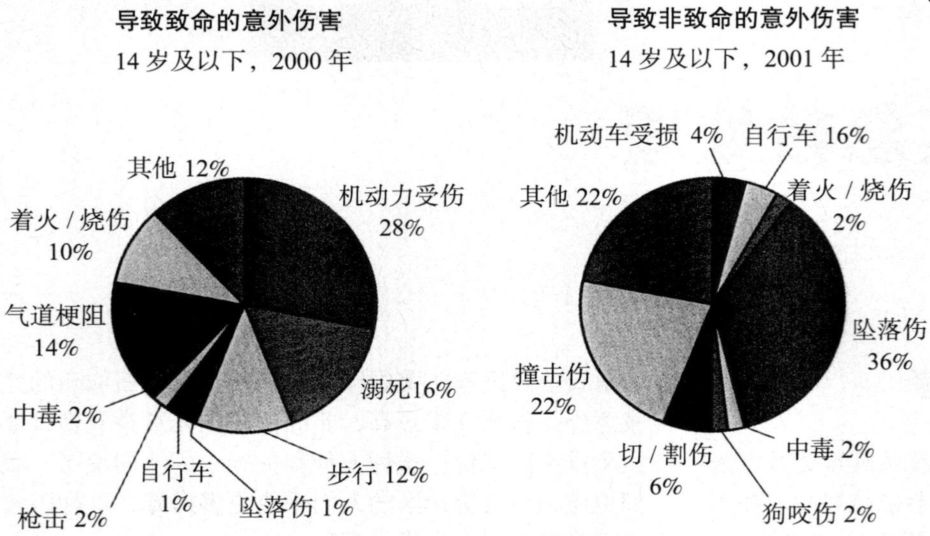

图 15-1 美国 2000—2001 年 14 岁及以下儿童致命和非致命意外伤害的百分比。(From National Center for Health Statistics, Centers for Disease Control and Prevention: National Electronic Injury Surveillance System All Injury Program, 2003.)

童的有效复苏时间范围比成人的短 50%；高级创伤生命支持方案尤其关注了这类损伤。尽管初始生理代偿可能足以产生一些临时调节作用，但进展性功能障碍和能量储备耗尽将导致氧输送不足和儿童的最后死亡。儿童急救医疗服务和转运系统的完善已经对防止儿童死亡起了有益的作用。儿童受伤害死亡的第三个高峰出现在最初受伤害发生后的几天到几周，是由于损伤导致的并发症，如败血症和全身炎症反应综合征，这些并发症可导致多脏器功能衰竭[18]。最后一个高峰在幼年儿童中导致的死亡通常比较少。

复苏原则

入院前急救

系统性处治对受伤害儿童的存活是首要的。急救人员在野外发现儿童受伤时，应立刻开始处治。儿童的命运取决于这第一个至关紧要的决定和措施。儿童意外伤害相关的死亡率在院外复苏期间是成人的 2 倍。而儿童在院外心脏停搏中的存活率只有成人的一半[15]。尽管儿童和成人心脏停搏的不同原因会引起部分这种差异，但没有儿童处治经验和不恰当的培训同样可造成不良后果。在野外，儿童复苏干预的失败率是成人的 2 倍；入院前气管插管的失败率接近 50% [11]。缺乏有关儿童复苏技巧是可以理解的；尽管这类创伤是儿童急救转运的最常见类型，但在大多数都市里其只占所有急救患者的 10%以下。

在野外，急救人员的最重要目标是：

1. 识别和处理紧急致命的功能障碍。
2. 评估创伤机制和损伤程度。
3. 提供有关医疗资料。
4. 转至水平合适的儿童创伤治疗机构。

除了上述情况外，还要努力安慰受到惊吓的受伤儿童及其焦虑的父母。因此，急救人员的任务是很艰难的。所以要想把入院前急救工作做好，就要通过采取严格的程序治疗受伤儿童。儿童野外复苏相关程序和技巧与稍后描述的在急诊部门的处理方法相似。

对致命性伤害的初步检查和处理

当医护人员碰到一个受伤儿童时，无论是在野外还是在急救室，都应该按照设计好的快速流程来识别和治疗急性损伤。这种系统途径考虑了诊断标准和治疗决策，所以损伤的个体差异不会妨碍治疗人员去识别和处置对预后有深远影响的损伤。这种系统性程序包括初期检查、复苏阶段和确定性再次检查。初步检查是确定即刻致命伤害的最初程序，是按 ABCDE 顺序进行检查，即气道、呼吸、循环、意识丧失和暴露。这个系统依靠简单观察来评估生理紊乱和即刻干预以防止死亡。

气道和颈椎的处理

进行气道控制可能是儿童创伤处理的所有优先措施中最没有争议的。无法建立和维持儿童气道会导致组织缺氧和通气不当，这仍然是心搏和呼吸骤停的常见原因。当氧饱和度低于 95%时可以发现明显的临床缺氧。

评估气道包括：口腔检查，清除碎片、松脱牙齿和软组织碎片，用吸引器吸除血液和分泌物。如果患儿神经反应完整、发声正常、通气无喘鸣和窘迫，无需采用有创性气道处理。有自主呼吸的儿童可以通过上推下颌来明显改善通气。

由昏迷、烦躁不安、休克或直接气道损伤导致气道不安全时需要气管插管。在球囊面罩通气中，鼻咽和口咽气道能同期改善，但这只是建立确切控制前的临时措施。在大多数患者，经口气管插管同时行轴向颈椎固定是气道控制的常用方法。尽管在颈椎可能损伤而无呼吸暂停的成人患者推荐经鼻气管插管，但这不是儿童的指征，儿童也难以耐受。

儿童的气道解剖独特，会影响治疗技术的运用。儿童喉部解剖位置比成人高且靠前，需要有向上成角的喉镜才能恰当置入气管导管。去除前半部分颈托可以使气管导管进入颈部而轻压环状软骨。儿童会厌比较短，不易变形，自后面翘起盖在声门入口上。因此，必须用直的叶片直接控制会厌来获得良好的声门暴露。声门脆弱易损。儿童气道最狭窄处位于声门下环状软骨环，而成人则在声门。所以，气管导管通过声门并不能确保进一步安全地进入气道，也不能避免声门下方的损伤。在儿童复苏中选择合适的气管导管是非常重要的。新生儿气管导管内径范围为 3.0～3.5mm，1～2 岁为 4.5mm。2 岁以后内径选择可以通过以下公式估算：内径 = 年龄 / 4 + 4。用患者的小指直径估算同样有效。因为有声门下气管狭窄，所以 8 岁及以下儿童用无气囊的气管导管（图 15-2）[11,13]。

运用什么气管插管取决于建立气道的紧迫程度。对于有低血压、低血氧和昏睡的儿童，复苏首要步骤是立即经口气管插管。在有其他选择时，应该更多使用合适的 100%的球囊面罩通气给氧和给药。胸部损伤会影响插管或不能达到合适的氧饱和度。通过高频通气引起低碳酸血症 [二氧化碳分压（$PaCO_2$）为 30～35mmHg] 是有益的。

当用面罩给氧后，需注射硫酸阿托品（0.01～0.02mg/kg）以确保插管时的高心率。维持适当的心率是重要的，这与心排出量直接相关，每搏排出量在儿童没有大的变化。还应该静脉注射止痛剂和肌松剂。循环容量正常时，短效巴比妥酸盐，如戊硫代巴比妥钠（5.0mg/kg），是合适的止痛剂。血容量减少时应用苯二氮䓬类，如咪达唑仑（0.1mg/kg）。肌松剂和短效非去极性剂（维库溴铵 0.1mg/kg）或短效去极性剂（氯化琥珀胆碱 1.0mg/kg）可以联合使用。烧伤和有失活组织时使用琥珀胆碱，因为有血钾过高的危险。必须持续监测插管儿童的潮气末 CO_2 和动脉血氧饱和度。

在一些病例，当有口或上颌外伤或先天性畸形不能行气管插管时，有指征建立外科性气道。环甲膜切开术是 10 岁以上儿童的常用方法。通过横行皮肤切口容易暴露环甲膜以放置小的无气囊气管导管。因为环甲膜位置表浅，其并发症发生率低于紧急气管切开术。当儿童情况稳定后，为避免声门下狭窄，环甲膜切开应转换成正式的气管切开术。

在年幼儿童，环状软骨是脆弱的结构，但可提供对气管的主要支撑。紧急环甲膜切开会损伤这层膜而导致明显的病态，产生终身喉气管软化。为避免这个并发症，10 岁以下儿童应进行环甲膜针刺切开和气管内喷气法。用 16～18 号静脉穿刺针经环甲膜进入气道内腔，再连接浓度 100%的 10～12 升 / 分钟的氧气即可。在儿童，针式喷气受限制，因为 30 分钟后会发生高碳酸血症；所以这种方法只能短时有效。随着儿童病情稳定，必须行气管内插管或
正规气管切开[13]。 268

呼吸

儿童头部受伤（自发通气动力障碍）或胸部受伤（肺膨胀障碍）时，常出现危害呼吸和通气的结果。识别头部外伤通常很容易，但识别肺膨胀障碍的胸部外伤需要仔细地观察。应强调这些伤害的潜在危害，
因为儿童胸部外伤死亡率接近 25%[14]。 269

胸部损伤后，气体、液体或内脏就会危害胸膜腔。压迫肺实质能引起气体交换不足而产生呼吸窘迫。在创伤性膈肌破裂病例，失去肌肉的完整性同样

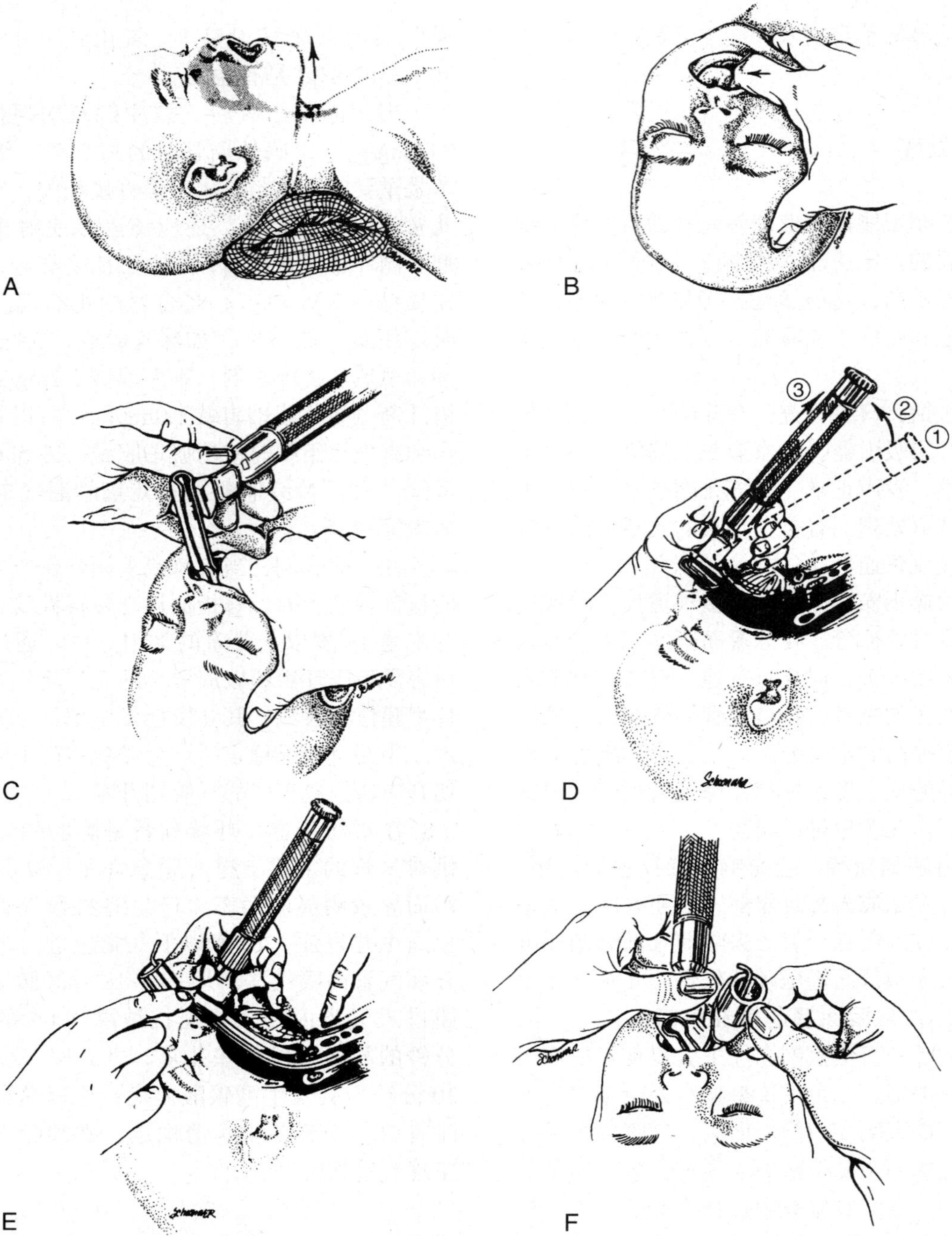

图 15-2 气管插管。A．儿童的喉和声门上间隙与成人相比要靠前，且与头部成角，抬起后颈能理想暴露儿童的声门。B．相对于口腔来说，儿童的舌较大。舌应该被推到口腔一侧以便于暴露咽后部和声门上区域。C．喉镜的镜片从口腔右侧插入，沿着沟向后滑。D．镜片到位后将儿童颈部在吸气位置轻度拉伸，抬起手柄（位置 1、2、3）提起会厌，使声门处于直视下。E．除了新生儿外，直的镜片应放在会厌上并连着舌根抬起以暴露喉。前端稍弯的导芯置于气管导管内能成功帮助插管。F．喉镜取出时固定气管导管，然后在确认双侧呼吸音后固定好气管导管。(From Eichelberger MR: Pediatric Trauma, Prevention, Acute Care, Rehabilitation. St. Louis, Mosby, 1993.)

直接影响肺膨胀。儿童纵隔极易移动，当胸膜腔压力增高时，纵隔移向对侧，导致对侧肺被压缩。纵隔血管结构扭曲和胸内压力升高可引起静脉回流减少危象。

连枷胸可造成胸壁完整性丢失，从而可削弱通气和氧合。因此，吸气时会发生反常胸壁运动，阻止肺的完全膨胀。正压辅助呼吸是最好的办法。因为儿童胸部易变形，引起肋骨多发性骨折的力量是巨大的且能传递到下方的肺实质，可导致肺挫伤。肺实质出血和水肿会削弱通气-灌注比，并且肺顺应性降低会显著增加呼吸做功；以上都会促使呼吸衰竭。

识别通气损害通常不难，尤其是在高度怀疑时。评估口鼻通气的声音以及频率、深度和呼吸费力通常有效。望诊时，胸壁不对称运动提示通气异常。叩诊浊音或回音过强，则是因为胸膜间隙存在液体或气体使呼吸音降低所致。张力性血气胸、纵隔移位可通过气管偏离、心脏搏动点移位以及由于静脉回流减少所致的颈部静脉扩张来发现。

在初级复苏期间，机械通气失败是致命的，需要立即处理。所有儿童需要通过鼻导管、面罩或气管内导管来供氧。气管内插管和辅助通气足以治疗由于头部损伤、肋骨骨折疼痛、连枷胸和肺挫伤所致的肺通气不足。单纯的血气胸通过供氧可以坚持到初期复苏后行胸腔引流术（图 15-3）。在血气胸引起危及通气和血压过低的病例中，需要行胸腔引流术，并经常联合气管插管和建立静脉通路以快速输注液体。如果有张力性气胸和血流动力学紊乱，可通过锁骨中线第二肋间隙胸腔穿刺排气来减轻，随后可留置胸腔引流管。

应该选用适当口径的胸腔引流管插入胸膜腔以排出血和气体。年幼儿童肋间隙狭窄，限制了引流管的大小，应该选择可使用的最大口径引流管。引流管放在乳头水平（第四或第五肋间隙）的腋前线上以避免通过抬高的横膈进入腹腔。将引流管指向后部和头部以便排出血和气体，并连接到密封的硅胶 Pleurovac 引流系统，压力设置在-15 cmH_2O（见图 15-3）。胸腔引流管的长期引流在儿童中不常见。然而，引流量达到每小时 1～2 ml/kg 体重是一个重要的信号，提示血管或纵隔损伤的持续出血，可能需要开胸手术以确定和控制出血。

进行气管插管时，儿童吸入的氧分数应该是 100%，潮气量是 10～12 ml/kg，频率是 15～20 次 / 分。给氧和通气应该维持动脉的氧分压（PO_2）在大于 80mmHg 和 PCO_2 在 30～35mmHg，呼气末正压不超过 5cmH_2O，目的是通过最优化给氧和降低颅内压（ICP）增加脑灌注来防止继发性脑损伤。头外伤的儿童可以通过适当的过度通气造成低碳酸浓度（PCO_2 为 30～35 mmHg）来减少 ICP 以得到最佳的治疗[6,13,18]。

血液循环和血管通路

初期复苏的第三步是迅速评估循环系统和建立静脉通路。严重受伤的儿童时常有正常的生命体征，即使是在血容量明显减少时也是如此。因为他们的心血管储备推迟了低血容量的早期血流动力学变化，直到复苏过程的相对晚期才出现异常。对受伤机制的了解，持续仔细检查生理学参数和临床的体征，对于降低死亡率是必需的。

是否有效灌注的一个可靠参数是正常的神志状态。如果儿童处于正在复苏过程中，复苏有效的临床征象应该得到监测。下列参数的改善代表复苏成功和血流动力学稳定：

1. 心率减慢（＜100 次 / 分钟)）。
2. 脉压增高（＞20 mmHg）。
3. 恢复正常皮肤颜色和周围灌注。
4. 肢体末端温暖。
5. 感觉神态清晰（Glasgow 昏迷评分改善）。
6. 心脏收缩压升高（＞80 mmHg）。
7. 婴儿每小时尿量 1～2 ml/kg，青少年每小时尿量 1 ml/kg。

在建立有效通气之后，为一个低血容量儿童准备静脉通路常是一种挑战。对受严重伤害的病例最好建立两条通路。最好是在横膈上方和下方各建立一条静脉通路，以防复苏液体从隐藏的腹部损伤静脉中溢出这种潜在的风险。儿童的任何周围静脉通路都是有用的。

上肢放置大口径的周围血管导管有两种方法。如果静脉穿刺不成功，骨髓穿刺导管适用于年龄小于 6 岁的儿童（见下文）。年龄大于 6 岁的儿童，最好在脚踝静脉处切开皮肤。在内踝向上向前 0.5～1cm 处的短横切口很容易暴露大隐静脉。暴露的血管用一根 270
丝线牵引，在直视下把最大的合适的静脉导管插入血管腔内。不必横断或结扎血管（图 15-4）　。

中央静脉置管能引起严重的并发症，如锁骨下或股动脉的破裂，因此成为不太实用的技术。由于易于进入，常选择股静脉入路。如果一定要选择锁骨下静脉通路，儿童应该置于 Trendelenburg 体位，使头部

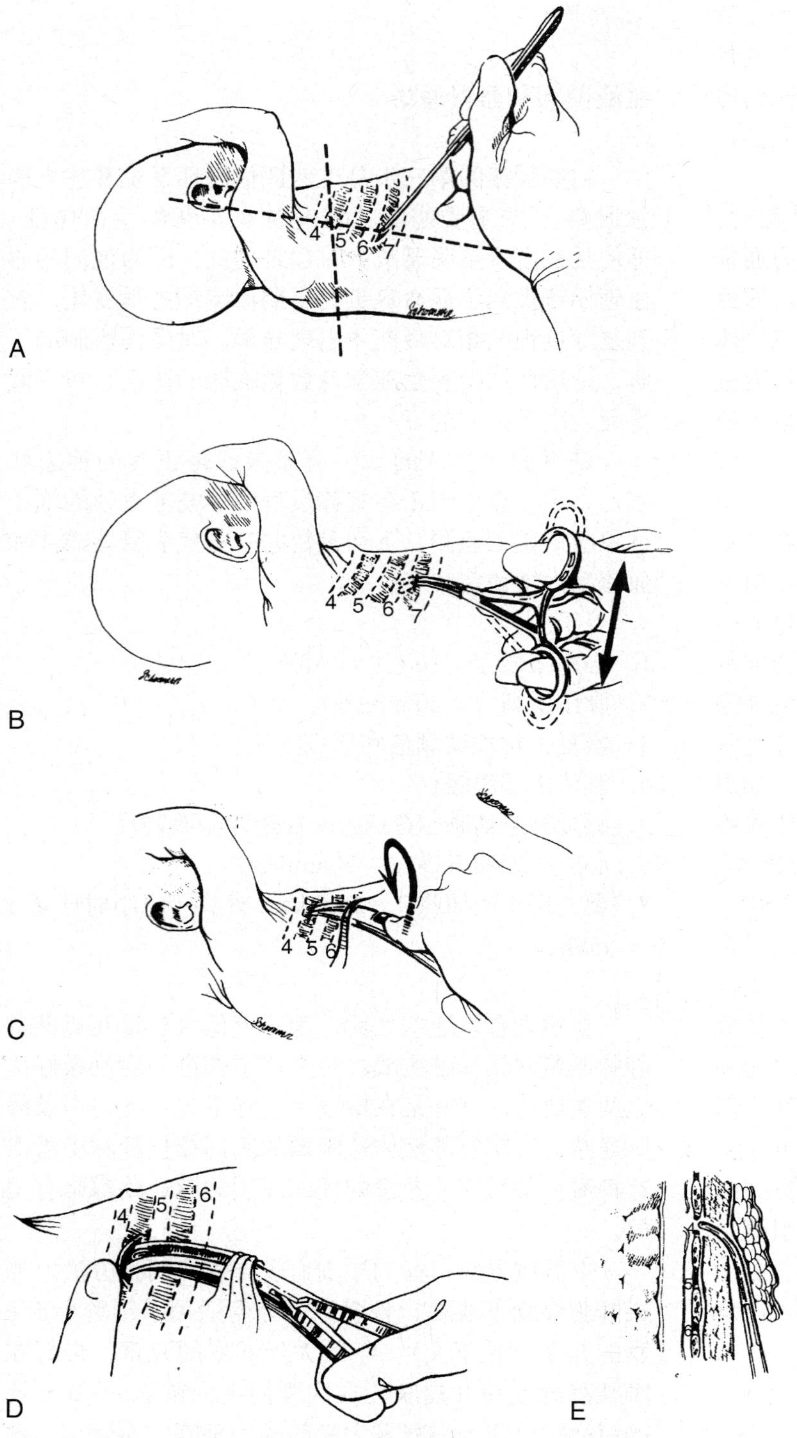

图 15-3 放置胸腔引流管。A. 在腋中线做一切口，在男性刚好低于乳头，在女性在乳房下（第 4 肋间隙）。B. 在皮下向头端分离至两根肋骨上。在儿童应采用长的皮下通道以减少导管周围气体泄露。C. 第 4 肋间隙是放置胸腔引流管的理想位置。D. 进入胸膜腔的位置应做在刚好肋骨上方以避免损伤肋间血管。E. 操作侧面视图。(From Eichelberger MR: Pediatric Trauma, Prevention, Acute Care, Rehabilitation. St. Louis, Mosby, 1993.)

在中间的位置，不需在肩后垫物体。这一位置是建立儿童和成人锁骨下静脉通路的最理想进入部位[12]。

骨髓内通路是一条给予液体、血制品和药物的简单、可靠和安全的路径。因为骨髓在儿童早期能很好地灌注，所以该技术适用于 6 岁以下的儿童。较好的骨髓穿刺位置为经过胫骨前中的平坦表面，大约在胫骨粗隆下方的 2～3 cm 处。穿刺针指向脚与水平成 60°角。穿透骨皮质，然后可通过骨髓腔抽出血液和骨髓来检测发现。可选的部位包括远端股骨中线，在儿童膝关节上方向头端 3cm 和内踝上远端胫骨，或

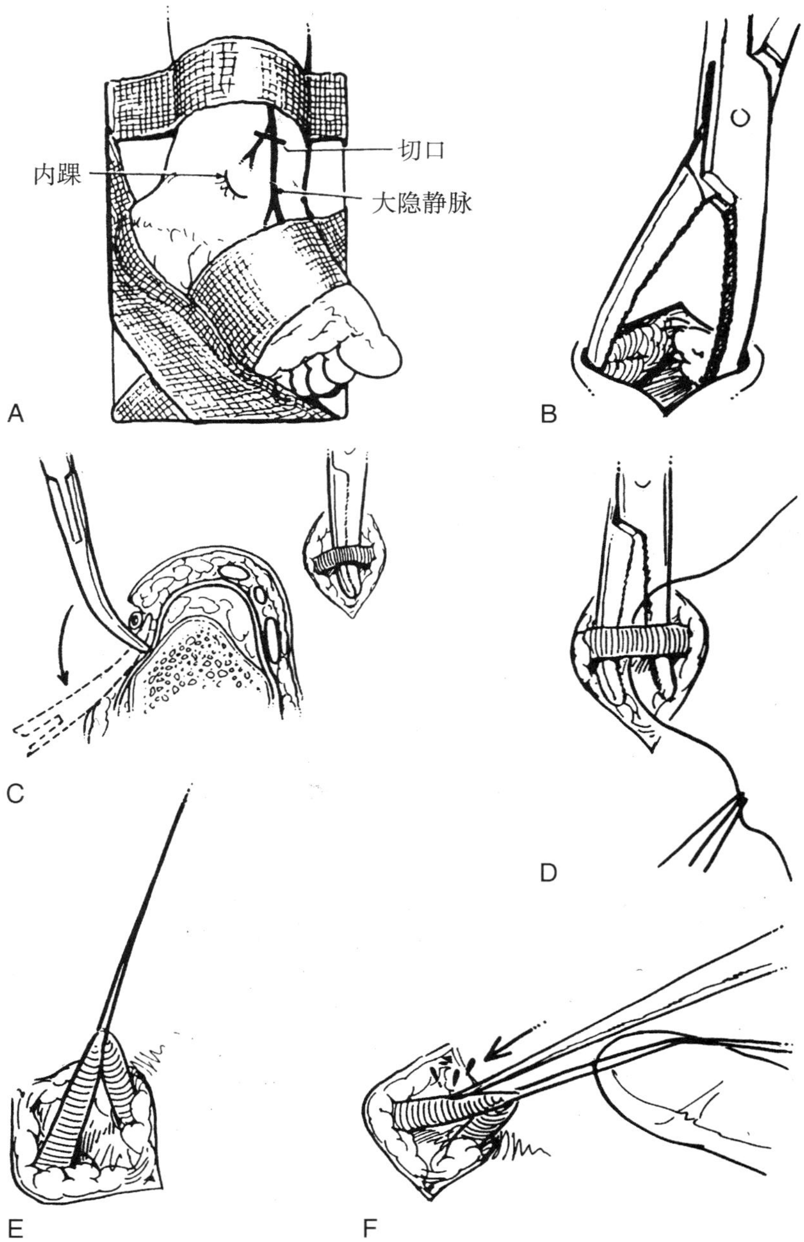

图 15-4 大隐静脉置管术。A. 始终可获得的紧急静脉通路位于踝部，大隐静脉位于内踝前方。B. 在内踝前方做横切口（向前 1cm，头侧 1cm），切口内垂直解剖暴露大隐静脉。C. 解剖血管周围。D. 将缝线在血管下方穿过留置。E 和 F. 轻轻牵引缝线便于静脉置管。(From Eichelberger MR: Pediatric Trauma, Prevention, Acute Care, Rehabilitation. St. Louis,Mosby, 1993.)

在青少年中近端肱骨，尽管骨髓通路在青少年组很少用。应该在儿科的复苏房间中放置特别设计的骨髓穿刺针，以使这一操作易于进行；14～16 号的针都可使用。该技术并发症发生率低，潜在并发症包括骨髓炎、蜂窝织炎、骨折、生长板损伤、脂肪栓塞和间隔综合征。

一旦建立了血管的通路，就可开始进行一定量的液体复苏。通常用等张晶体液，如乳酸林格液，以 20 ml/kg 的增量给予。如果在给予 40 ml/kg 之后仍然持续停留在低血容量，则开始输注 10ml/kg 的 ABO 血型-匹配的浓缩红细胞。浓缩红细胞能提升胶体渗透压，而且能比晶体液产生更迅速持久的血管扩张作用。除此之外，红细胞可提供血红蛋白来增加氧的携带能力。所有的液体（晶体、胶体和血）应该在注入前加温。这可以由微波加热晶体液或使用一个加热装置来完成。

不断地反复评估患儿对复苏的反应、确定受伤害的性质和程度、避免过度液体复苏的并发症都非常重

要。当灌注恢复之时，逐渐地减少液体注入的速率以
272 避免不必要的输液。健康肺很少出现肺水肿，但是肺或脑挫伤区域的液体积聚却可使肺水肿有相当高的发生率。如果给予晶体液和血液复苏后血流动力学仍不稳定，可能有腹部或骨盆部位的出血。心脏功能障碍可能是由于填塞、张力性血气胸、脑脊髓受伤、寰枕移位或极深的低体温导致[7,13]。

意识丧失

快速神经系统评估包括在主要检查之中，以识别可能需要立即处治的严重损伤。描述脑功能的一个快速的方法是 AVPU 记忆法：灵敏、语言回答、疼痛反应或无反应。对瞳孔反射和对称的评估同样有用。小脑幕裂孔疝继发于扩张的颅内血肿，可引起同侧的瞳孔扩大和光反射消失。对眼睛的直接伤害常使一侧瞳孔大小不等，通常很明显。去皮质或去大脑时的极端姿势特征为丧失皮质和大脑功能。对于一个一侧瞳孔固定和扩大的昏睡患儿，需采取紧急措施降低 ICP。这些措施包括早期控制气管插管保持合适的 PCO_2（30～35mmHg），可伴适度的过度通气，CO_2 能引起脑血管收缩和减少脑血流。这些方法可降低脑体积和 ICP，并增加脑的灌注压（CPP）。采用反 Trendelenburg 体位，即把头抬高 30°，也能降低颅内高压，但是只能在心脏功能正常的患儿中应用。

暴露

完全暴露患儿对于全面的检查和确认伤势十分重要。一个意识清醒的儿童不理解这样做的需要，因此，暴露必须小心行事。对于 Glasgow 昏迷评分正常的稳定儿童，全面的初期检查不必同时除去所有衣物。暴露先前包扎的伤口时，孩子会特别关注疼痛，这种特别关注经常能保证更有效的评估。

对儿童而言，体温降低会影响生理学参数，如认知功能、心脏和凝血功能。核心温度维持在 35～36℃非常重要。温暖的复苏房间有利于保持身体核心温度，可将热损失降低到最小。同样复苏液体和吸入气体应该加温加湿。头顶上和床上加热设施很有必要，对于一个受伤的婴儿来说，最好使用加温器。

复苏期

持续反复评估儿童对治疗的反应是复苏的基础。任何时候出现恶化都需要重复进行初步检查。在完成 ABCDE 检查和致命性伤害稳定之后，应该放置一根胃管和一根导尿管，随后抽血做血气分析以及安置心脏监视器。

儿童的急性胃扩张能引起呼吸窘迫和迷走神经反应性心搏缓慢。胃减压可以排空胃，减少呕吐和吸入的危险，这对所有受伤害儿童都很重要，尤其是对意识水平低的儿童。在放置胃管减压之前评估面中部和脑脊液鼻漏的出现很重要。如果检查结果不正常，应该经口放置胃管。

彻底的会阴部检查包括进行直肠指检之后放置导尿管。有高位骑跨伤时，前列腺、会阴出血或阴囊淤斑或不稳定的前部骨盆骨折，在导尿管插入之前要做逆行尿道造影。

虽然很少有不正常发现，但用心电图来监测心脏的节律是必需的。偶尔会遇到继发性的异常，如由于后期休克导致的窦性心动过缓，血容量过少引起的电机械分离，张力性气胸或心脏压塞，体温降低或酸中毒所致的室颤。心室异位、低电压和缺血表现常伴有心肌挫伤。除了评估实际节律，弥散的低电压可能是心包膜积血的第一表现。

建立血管通路之后，应取血样和尿样做实验室检查，包括血常规和代谢检查、尿液分析和动脉血气分析。血酒精含量和毒物学荧屏检查在儿童中不是常规检查，但在青少年中常见。同时应做血型和交叉配对试验[5,7]。

神经系统复苏

儿童时期导致获得性残疾和死亡的最常见原因是脑外伤。据估计，美国每年每 500 个儿童中就有 1 个遭受脑外伤，每年有 7000 个儿童因为脑外伤死亡，28 000 个儿童永久残疾[1,10]。由于预防策略和地区创伤系统的建立，严重创伤性脑外伤的总死亡率从 1970 年代的大约 50%下降至现在的 36%。目前儿童意外伤害的总死亡率是 3%。这些病例死亡的主要原因 70%是中枢神经系统损伤。总的来说，3 岁以上儿童的预后比受同样损伤的成人要好；而 3 岁以下的患

儿的预后常比较差[3,13,18]。

创伤性脑外伤可以分为原发性和继发性。原发性脑损伤是大脑的结构性紊乱，是由于直接机械性撞击，引起细胞和血管的破裂、侵害或组织丢失。儿童大脑易于出现深部白质的损伤，如剪切伤、点状出
273 血、脑肿胀和线性非凹陷性骨折，而不是成人常见的硬膜下和脑内血肿和压迫性骨折。然而，儿童硬膜外血肿的发生率较高，可能因为薄而柔软的颅骨更易于破裂及切割硬膜血管。儿童相对较大的头颅、较少的肌肉以及松弛的颈椎韧带可能导致儿童弥漫性轴索损伤的发生率较高。

原发性脑损伤只有积极预防一种办法，而继发性脑损伤则是临床神经复苏的目标。继发性脑损伤的发生是因为创伤后脑灌注降低。弥漫性和局限性脑肿胀影响氧气和基础物质的运输，这是 ICP 升高及其影响 CPP 的结果。CPP、ICP 和平均动脉压（MAP）的相关性为：CPP = MAP – ICP。复苏应该通过控制 ICP 和维持 MAP 而使 CPP 最佳化。当 ICP 超过静脉的流出压力（脑肿胀的结果）时，就像是一个 Starling 电阻，决定脑血流的压力梯度。在患有严重脑损伤的儿童，正常的 CPP 值和 ICP 的理想范围并不清楚[8]。在儿童中，良好的预后可能是通过维持所有年龄儿童的 ICP 低于 20mmHg、8 岁以下儿童的 CPP 维持在 45mmHg 以上、8 岁以上儿童的 CPP 维持在 70～80mmHg 实现的[3]。

减少继发性脑损伤的重点在维持 ICP 和 CPP 在治疗水平，并使 MAP 处于正常。最迅速的方法是插管和控制性正压通气，最初可使 PCO_2 降到 30～35mmHg，PO_2 高于 100mmHg，pH 到 7.40 ± 0.05。低碳酸血症和碱中毒可促进脑血管收缩，限制脑血容量和降低 ICP。这个效果很快，但是会在脑脊液 pH 重新平衡期间受到限制。发生效果的最长时间尚不清楚，可能从几小时到几天。现在的治疗是使 PCO_2 维持在 30～35mmHg。这样可以避免因过度正压通气，对严重的脑损伤患者后者有可能加重脑缺血转变成脑梗死[8]。通常进行脑室造瘘术，使脑脊液排出以进一步优化 CPP。伤后 24～48 小时需要重复行头颅 CT 扫描，以评估脑水肿的程度、识别新的梗死或发现新发展的血肿和可能需要处理的严重挫伤。通气状态和液体输注在最初 48 个小时内需再评估从而保持最佳状态。

如果经过上述措施仍不能控制 ICP，应进行渗透压治疗，每 4～6 小时快速输注 20%的甘露醇，剂量为 0.25 ～0.5g/kg。甘露醇在血浆钠浓度大于 145mEq/L、血浆渗透压摩尔浓度大于 310mOsm、尿量少于每小时 0.5 ml/kg 或血压低时停止使用。甘露醇通过在脑的微环境中创造高渗状态来发挥治疗效果；还可通过利尿排除来自脑的间隙的自由水以改善脑的氧运输及血流[8]。

轻度或中度高血压可通过改善脑干微血管灌注来逆转异常 ICP 和升高 CPP[16]。治疗方法是静脉内注入多巴胺，剂量为每分钟 5～20μg/kg。

创伤性脑损伤后常见高热和惊厥，这可以影响 ICP 和 CPP 的治疗。高热和惊厥通过增加已经受伤的大脑的代谢需求可进一步加重继发性脑损伤。因此，应该每 4～6 小时用对乙酰氨基酚 10mg/kg，以使核心温度维持在一个正常范围（35～36℃）。冷却毯在顽固发热时是必须的。头部受伤儿童单次惊厥而神经系统评估正常，则不需要治疗。受伤后 1 周之内发生的惊厥在 1 岁以下儿童用苯巴比妥治疗，1 岁以上儿童用苯妥英治疗。剂量是一次静脉注射 10～20mg/kg，随后每天 5mg/kg 的剂量，7 天后停止。迟发惊厥的患儿需要长期抗惊厥药物治疗。对昏迷的患儿在没有证实惊厥活动时是否需要在复苏期间进行抗惊厥药物预防尚有争论。

凝血功能障碍

凝血障碍发生在以下一些情况：极低体温、大量输血和严重的脑损伤。低体温通过减少促进凝固的酶的活性而引起过度出血。大量输血，指急性给予血制品≥一个血容量（65～80 ml/kg），同样可引起凝血障碍。另外一个机制是由于抗凝的库存血中含乙二胺四乙酸或柠檬酸盐（柠檬酸盐-磷酸盐-葡萄糖）的抗凝剂，两者都可以螯合钙而限制凝血反应中的钙-依赖步骤。急性低血钙是大量输血的另一个结果。

大量输血引起凝血障碍的最常见机制是：稀释性血小板减少。因为其他凝血因子有非常好的功能储备，所以这些凝血因子的稀释引起的凝血障碍非常少。当持续的出血耗尽循环中的血小板，而血液被红细胞代替，就会发生血小板计数的进一步减少。在急性损伤，血小板的计数减少到 50 000 会产生外科出

血。血小板水平在 100 000 以下有明显的凝血障碍，在 50 000 水平或以下需要输注血小板。给予 ABO 匹配的血小板，初始剂量为每公斤体重 0.1U 浓缩血小板或每平方米体表面积 4U，可以使体内血小板水平提升大约 40 000。

严重的头部损伤也与凝血障碍有关，而与血小板稀释无关。据推测是大量的促凝血的组织凝血酶原激
274 酶从脑损伤区域释放出来，导致播散性血管内凝血和消耗性凝血病，这样所有凝血因子、纤维蛋白原和血小板就被消耗。头部损伤后凝血障碍是预后不良的表现。需要给予相匹配的新鲜冰冻血浆，剂量为 15～30 ml/kg。冷沉淀物包含大量纤维蛋白原、VIII 因子、XIII 因子和 von Willebrand 因子，除了新鲜冰冻血浆，可以给予 0.1U/kg。给予新鲜冰冻血浆、冷沉淀物或两者同时给予可能在先前有凝血障碍疾病情况下需要，如有血友病、von Willebrand 病和严重的肝脏疾病时[13]。

疼痛管理

急性疼痛管理的主要目标是降低受伤儿童的应激反应和改善预后。急性疼痛是一种有害的刺激，会导致生理性应激反应的激活。结果使神经内分泌反应激活，这对新陈代谢、温度调节、创伤愈合和免疫方面有极大的副作用。以下是受伤儿童疼痛处理的要点：

1. 有一个由全身心投入疼痛管理的临床医生领导的富有经验的多学科团队。
2. 有一个确保最少疼痛的承诺。
3. 有效的疼痛管理需要持续的可调整的认识过程。
4. 重视对焦虑的认识和处理的必要性，因为它可能改变疼痛治疗的效果。
5. 具有与其他儿童支持性护理和治疗计划相融合的、有效进行所有疼痛治疗的能力和知识。

一个团队性的、基于规程来控制疼痛的方法会提高儿童急救处理的总的成功率[9]。

结论

系统地处理受伤害儿童能解救生命。然而，对伤害的预防是必要的。

在过去 16 年间，儿童意外伤害死亡率下降了将近 40% [20]。预防所取得的最瞩目的进步是：儿童意外火器伤害的死亡率下降了 72%，自行车相关的伤害死亡率下降了 60%。火灾和烧伤死亡率下降了 56%，步行伤害死亡率降低了 51%。不幸的是，机动车伤害死亡率下降缓慢，特别是在 5～9 岁的孩子中，为主要死亡原因。气道梗阻伤害的死亡率在婴儿中仍保持不变。

许多因素可使儿童期意外伤害的总体死亡率下降。很清楚，首要的是伤害的预防，重点是使较小的孩子和机动车伤害危险降低到最少。然而，一旦发生伤害，正确的复苏仍能解救生命。

（顾　硕译　吕志葆校）

参考文献

1. Centers for Disease Control: Childhood injuries in the United States. Am J Dis Child 1990;144:627-646.
2. Centers for Disease Control and Prevention: Web-based Injury Statistics Query and Reporting System (WISQARS). Fatal Injury Reports 1999-2000. National Center for Injury Prevention and Control, Centers for Disease Control and Prevention. Available at www.cdc.gov/ncipc/wisqars.
3. Chambers IR, Treadwell L, Mendelow AD: Determination of threshold levels of cerebral perfusion pressure and intracranial pressure in severe head injury by using receiver-operating characteristic curves: An observational study in 291 patients. J Neurosurg 2001;94:412-416.
4. Children's Safety Network, Economics and Insurance Resource Center: Special run: Hospitalized unintentional injury among children 15 and under. Feb 2003.
5. Chu UB, Clevenger FW, Imani ER, et al: The impact of selective laboratory evaluation on utilization of laboratory resources and patient call in a level I trauma center. Am J Surg 1996;172:558-562.
6. Committee on Quality Improvement, American Academy of Pediatrics, and Commission on Clinical Policies and Research, American Academy of Family Physicians: The management of minor closed head injury in children. Pediatrics 1999;104:1407-1415.

7. Committee on Trauma of the American College of Surgeons: Advanced Trauma Life Support Instructor Manual. Chicago, American College of Surgeons, 1997.
8. Faillace WJ: Management of childhood neurotrauma. Surg Clin North Am 2002;82:349-363.
9. Golianu B, Krane EJ, Galloway KS, Yaster M: Acute pain in children: Pediatric acute pain management. Pediatr Clin North Am 2000;47:1-24.
10. Kraus JF, Rouk A, Hemyaris P: Brain injury among infants, children, adolescents, and young adults. Am J Dis Child 1990;144:684-691.
11. Losek JD, Bonadio WA, Walsh-Kelly C, et al: Prehospital pediatric endotracheal intubation performance review. Pediatr Emerg Care 1989;5:1.
12. Lukish J, Valladares E, Bulas D, et al: Classical positioning decreases subclavian vein cross sectional area in children. J Trauma 2002;53:272-275.
13. Magnuson DK, Eichelberger MR: Approach to the pediatric trauma patient. In Surgery of Infants and Children. Philadelphia, Lippincott-Raven, 1997, pp 391-414.
14. Peclet MH, Newman KD, Eichelberger MR, et al: Thoracic trauma in children: An indicator of increased mortality. J Pediatr Surg 1990;25:961.
15. Ramenofsky ML, Luterman A, Quindlen E, et al: Maximum survival in pediatric trauma: The ideal system. J Trauma 1984;24:818.
16. Rosner MJ: Pathophysiology and management of increased intracranial pressure. In Andrews BT (ed): Neurosurgical Intensive Care. New York, McGraw-Hill, 1993, pp 57-112.
17. Scheidt PC, et al: The epidemiology of nonfatal injuries among US children and youth. Am J Public Health 1995; 85:932-938.
18. Stafford PW, Blineman TA, Nance ML: Practical points in evaluation and resuscitation of the injured child. Surg Clin North Am 2002;82:273-302.
19. Taylor GA, Eichelberger MR: Abdominal CT in children with neurological impairment following blunt trauma. Ann Surg 1989;210:229-233.
20. Wallace AL, Cody BE, Mickalide AD: Report to the Nation: Trends in Unintentional Childhood Injury Mortality, 1987-2000. Washington, DC, National Safe Kids Campaign, May 2003.

第 16 章

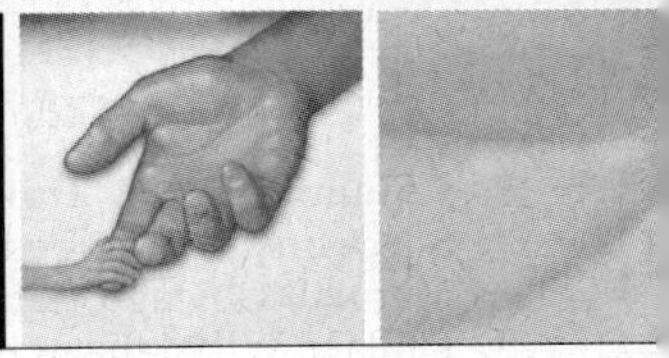

胸部损伤

David E. Wesson

流行病学和预防

275 胸壁、膈肌、肺和纵隔的结构损伤占一级儿童创伤中心处理病例的 25%，通常发生在高能钝性损伤或锐性创伤后。低能量的损伤，如从游戏场设备上跌下，很少导致胸部损伤。胸部损伤程度可以轻微也可以迅速致死，但如果能够及时诊断，所有胸部损伤都能成功治疗。尽管胸部损伤没有腹部、软组织和外轴骨骼损伤常见，但却是更加致命的。因为这种损伤要撞击才会出现，患者有较大的死亡危险。胸部损伤在非中枢神经系统损伤导致的创伤死亡中占很高比例。

与儿科其他外伤的大多数类型相似，胸外伤男女之比在 2∶1 和 3∶1 之间。胸部受伤可以按照解剖部位分类（如肋骨骨折、肺的挫伤、支气管的裂伤），也可以按照机制分类（钝性或穿透性）或按对生命的威胁程度分类（即刻的或潜在的）。尽管大部分胸部的严重钝性损伤在所有年龄组中都是与机动车相关的，儿童作为行人受伤的比例却明显高于成人[22]。青少年中锐性胸部损伤和成人相似，大多是刀伤和枪伤。从气枪中出来的小圆子弹，虽然被认为是相对无害的，但也可能引起致命的损伤。导致青春期前的儿童的穿透性损伤包括一些不常见的其他机制，例如被玻璃碎片或金属竿刺伤[64]。

临床常见的胸部损伤如表 16–1 所示[12]。尸体解剖研究发现，在院前和急诊部死亡病例中，由主要血管和心脏损伤所致的快速死亡占较高的比例[3]。在成人中，肋骨骨折是胸部钝性损伤的最常见类型[12,58]。在儿童中，肺挫伤最常发生。在儿童中，气管、支气管的裂伤比成人更多见，而主动脉的创伤性破裂则相对少见[82]。

最常见的胸部损伤是肺挫伤、气胸、血胸、肋骨的骨折、胸骨骨折或肩胛骨骨折。心脏、主动脉、气管、支气管和横膈的损伤非常少见，但更具有潜在危险。最常见的即刻威胁生命的胸部损伤是气道梗阻、张力性气胸、大量血胸和心脏压塞。开放性气胸和大片的连枷胸罕见。最常见的可能潜在威胁生命的胸部损伤是心肌挫伤、主动脉的破裂、膈肌撕裂、气管、支气管的破裂和食管破裂。

钝性和锐性胸部损伤的相对发生率差异很大，与社区暴力有关。Peterson 等人[64]报告了一项大型成人

表 16–1 来自国家儿科创伤登记的儿科胸部损伤的流行病学

	钝性伤	穿通伤	总计（%）*
气胸 / 血胸	38	64	41
气胸	24	23	23
血气胸	9	24	11
血胸	5	18	7
肺	53	19	48
挫伤	49	14	43
裂伤	1	10	3
心脏	5	13	6
挫伤	4	<1	3
裂伤	<1	8	2
膈肌	2	15	4
肋骨骨折	35	7	30
主动脉	1	1	<1
支气管	<1	0	<1
食管	<1	1	<1

* 每种损伤类型患者的总百分比。总的来说，83%的损伤是钝性的，15%的损伤是穿透性的，2%是其他机制所致。（From Cooper A, Barlow B, DiScala C, String D: Mortality and truncal injury: The pediatric perspective. J Pediatr Surg 1994;29:33.）

276 和儿童胸部损伤病例研究。在 12 岁及以下儿童的胸部损伤中，钝性损伤占 81%，锐性损伤在青少年胸部损伤中占 58%。在 Nakayama 和 Ramenofsky 的研究中[58]，17 岁以下儿童的胸部损伤 97%是钝性损伤。在 Meller 等人研究中[53]，几乎所有受伤青少年是锐性损伤。国家儿科创伤登记（NPTR）反映了整个北美众多儿科创伤中心的经验。1985—1991 年，有 25 000 多个病例报告到 NPTR 处，其中有 1553 个胸部损伤的病例[12]。86%的损伤是钝性损伤（大多数与和机动车有关），其 14% 是锐性损伤（大多数是刺伤或射击创伤）。

钝性损伤和锐性损伤病例的总的死亡率大致相同，分别为 15% 和 14%[12]。死亡率随着复合损伤数量的增加而增加。钝性损伤的大多数死亡原因是由于合并头部损伤，而锐性损伤的大部分死亡是由于胸部本身受伤所致。总的来说，胸部损伤在 NPTR 的致死原因中仅次于中枢神经系统损伤，排在第二位。胸部损伤死亡大多数发生在意外事故现场或在转运到医院的过程中，都是由重要器官的致命损伤所致。能活着到达医院的胸部损伤患者都有可能救活。

虽然在成人和儿童中钝性损伤和锐性损伤的比例不同，但损伤的类型和诊断治疗的基本原则都是相同的。最常见的损伤——肺的挫伤、肋骨骨折、气胸和血胸——能通过简单的治疗来处理，如胸廓造口术、给氧和止痛。大约 20%的患者还需要气管插管和机械通气，这常是为了处理合并的头部损伤。

事实上一些胸部损伤常需要手术处理：如主气道裂伤、主动脉损伤、结构性心脏和心包损伤以及食管穿孔。胸部损伤最大的挑战之一是要尽快识别需要手术的罕见病例。在 Nakayama 的研究中[58]，3 位锐性损伤患者中有 2 位，83 位钝性损伤病人中仅 3 位接受了胸部手术。在 Peterson 的报告中[64]，15%的钝性损伤儿童需要胸廓切开术（与成人的有关报告相同），而 40%的锐性损伤儿童中需要手术（比成人的有关报告高很多）。

虽然临床医生更关心患者的治疗，但关于儿童胸部损伤的讨论总会提及预防。机动车意外伤害和射击创伤引起了相当多的严重的儿科胸部伤。这些损伤都是可预防的。增加安全带和儿童限制器的使用会大量减少机动车伤害的危险。减少武器的违法使用同样会有很大帮助，尤其是对于青少年。胸部保护器在减少胸部损伤发生上可能有效，这些胸部损伤包括年轻运动员中的心脏休克震荡[51,86]。总体来说，这些措施实质上降低了儿童胸部损伤的严重性和这种损伤导致的死亡和残疾。

临床表现

胸部外伤的病理生理学和治疗策略基于儿童和成人之间的解剖和生理学的不同而明显不同。在儿童中，最重要的解剖因素是相对狭窄的气道容易发生梗阻；声门位置靠前上，使经鼻气管插管很困难，因此在紧急情况下不适宜应用；气道较短会增加支气管内插管的危险。儿童增加的耗氧量和低的功能残气量使组织易于缺氧。由于儿童主要依赖横膈呼吸，任何情况引起的腹腔压力增加都会限制膈肌移动而使问题更加复杂。

有严重胸部损伤的儿童可能只表现轻微的症状和体征。一项由马里兰急救医疗服务系统协会（MIEMSS）进行的大型成人研究发现，2/3 的胸部损伤患者到达医院时生命体征平稳[79]，在儿童中也有相似的发现[53]。在 MIEMSS 的研究中，大约 25%的严重胸内损伤患者没有肋骨骨折。这些“不可思议的”损伤包括气胸、血胸、心肌挫伤、心脏破裂、气管支气管损伤、肺的裂伤、横膈破裂和主动脉破裂。

儿童的肋骨比成人柔软。因此在儿童中很少有肋骨骨折。然而值得注意的是，因为儿童胸壁的弹性，可能发生严重的胸部损伤而没有外部表现。在 Nakayama 的研究中[58]，只有不到一半的严重胸部损伤患儿有肋骨骨折。胸壁的柔韧性和可压缩性为儿童所特有，这可能可以解释为什么外伤性窒息几乎只在患儿中发生，以及为什么主气道损伤在患儿中远远超过成人。

纵隔在儿童比在成人更易移动。因此张力性气胸更易于使纵隔移动而危及对侧肺的通气并减少静脉血回流到心脏。

诊断及初期复苏

创伤性胸部损伤患者的诊断和初期治疗必须同时开始。虽然胸部损伤的表现可能立即出现或延迟数小时或数天才出现，但最初的目标是排除即刻致命的损伤，如气道梗阻、张力性气胸、大量血胸和急性心脏压塞。

所有的受伤患者应按照美国外科医生协会的高级创伤生命支持纲要的原则（ATLS）来治疗[1]。总的原
277 则如下：

1．初期评估。
2．生命功能复苏。
3．再次仔细评估。
4．确定治疗。

所有胸部损伤的患儿必须给予供氧，开放两条大静脉，放置鼻胃管以避免胃的扩张。鼻胃管可显示食管和胃的位置异常，提示主动脉损伤或膈肌破裂。应该仔细观察胸部受伤的儿童。应该持续监测生命体征和动脉血氧饱和度（SaO_2）。如果儿童是气管插管，应该持续监测或经常检查潮气末二氧化碳浓度。应准备好血液以备输血。必须具备处理呼吸问题的设备和专业人员以处理气道，如口腔气道、气管导管和喉镜，必须将球囊面罩放在可取之处，尤其在转运和诊断操作时。

在 ATLS 原则的初期复苏阶段，应该立即识别致命的损伤并进行处理。首先是清理和保护气道。可能需要气管内插管。在插管后，气管内导管的位置要通过观察胸部偏移、听两侧气体进入的声音、监测潮气末二氧化碳浓度和胸部 X 光片来检验。一个比色法的二氧化碳探测器可用来查证气管导管的位置，尤其是在入院前的过程中[5]。

第二重要的是要确保适当的通气。如果有张力性气胸，应该在做放射影像前处理。有时对开放性气胸或大块的连枷胸在初始复苏时需要插管和辅助通气。如果输注足够的液体后，休克仍难纠正，通常提示持续性失血（最有可能的是腹腔）。然而如果没有发现明显的低血容量的原因，应当考虑急性心脏压塞的可能性。这种情况通过心包穿刺放液术可以暂时缓解。

紧急开胸的指征可以在任何阶段变得明显（表 16–2）。最常见的指征是大量的出血、大量气体泄漏和心脏压塞。在急诊室或因复苏行胸廓切开术是有争论的，似乎没有明确的指征或反指征[79]。在 MIEMSS 的报告中，39 位在急诊室中无生命体征的成年患者没有一位在紧急胸廓切开术后存活。然而在儿童中，

表 16–2 紧急开胸术的指征
心脏和大血管穿透伤
大量或持续的胸腔内出血
大块胸壁缺损的开放性气胸
主动脉造影照片损伤主动脉或主支气管
大量或持续的气体漏出，显示损伤主气道
心脏压塞
食管穿孔
膈肌破裂
心脏按压仍不能触及脉搏

紧急胸廓切开术可能挽救儿童的生命，尤其是对穿透性心脏损伤的儿童。Powell 等人[66]报告了一组在急诊室行胸廓切开术后的儿童和青少年有 26%的生存率。这些作者建议对创伤后心搏停止或接近心搏停止的患者在急诊室行胸廓切开术有以下三种情形：

1．所有穿透性胸部损伤的病例。
2．钝性损伤在 ER 中出现急性恶化的生命征象。
3．在损伤现场接近医院时，钝性损伤在现场出现危及生命症状时。

紧急开胸手术的切口选在左前外侧胸壁第五肋间隙。使用肋骨撑开器。如果有心脏压塞的证据，在膈神经的前面应该纵向打开心包。心脏创伤采用直接压迫和简单缝合来控制，除非发生冠状动脉的损害，否则不需要修补冠状动脉。如果没有心脏压塞，应该横跨钳闭主动脉。如果患者有严重的肺部损伤，应该夹闭或扭曲关闭肺门（见治疗）。患者如果对这些治疗有反应，应在手术室进行修补。

大多数情况的胸部损伤患儿的生理状态稳定。初期复苏之后，应行下一个步骤的详细再评估。为了避免遗漏重要的器官损伤，必须进行彻底和仔细的评估。对所有的病例均需明确重要的胸部撞击病史。因此尽可能多地获得详细的关于意外事故的细节是非常重要的。与乘员和行人一样，儿童在机动车意外中受伤都需要仔细评估。有呼吸困难的病史也提示重要的胸部损伤。

通过视、触、叩、听系统地检查胸部是再评估的下一个步骤。呼吸急促、触痛和胸壁摩擦音提示胸内损伤[7,26]。应该寻找有无发绀、呼吸困难、呼吸杂音、

气管偏斜、声嘶或喘鸣、皮下气肿、开放的或抽吸的胸部创伤、呼吸音减低或缺失、静脉充血、奇脉和奇脉低血压。呼吸困难和发绀意味着氧合作用不充分。呼吸杂音可能起因于对气道的损害或存在如血、黏液和呕吐物这样的杂质。气管偏斜提示张力性气胸或巨大的血胸。声嘶或喘鸣或合并其他发音困难意味着直接的喉或气管损伤。外科性气肿提示气管或支气管裂伤，但很少有食管穿孔。颈静脉充血、低血压和奇脉超过 10mmHg 提示急性心脏压塞。应该寻找患者急
278 性主动脉缩窄的征象，这可能是由胸腔内主动脉损伤引起。严重的心脏损伤的最敏感的征象是低血压或不能由出血解释的大量液体需求。心脏的损伤也可能出现高调的心脏收缩期杂音。急性充血性心力衰竭可能是由心脏瓣膜损伤或创伤性心室间隔缺损引起。

Holmes 等人[32]在一组 16 岁以下钝性躯干损伤的儿童中确定了一套预示胸部损伤的临床表现，最强的提示表现包括低血压、呼吸频率加快、胸部变形、合并大腿骨折和 Glasgow 昏迷评分小于 15 分。98%的确诊病例至少有上述表现中的一项。视诊和触诊是最敏感的，但是听诊发现异常具有最高的阳性预示价值。这肯定了临床评估对儿童钝性损伤诊断的重要性。最常见的损伤按顺序为肺挫伤、气胸和肋骨骨折。

近几年来，外科医生运用床边超声波检查评估腹部外伤很有帮助，超声检查现在是所有主要创伤病例临床常规评估的一部分[49]。在胸部外伤中超声检查同样也有作用。其对临床诊断气胸、血胸和心包渗液足够准确[41,49,62]。最近有文章报告说，外科医生在急诊室运用超声检查气胸是重要操作[41]。

由于缺乏敏感性和特异性，临床评估通常需要影像诊断来补充，后者通常是确定儿童是否需要手术的关键步骤[27]。虽然一些作者建议：当钝性损伤胸部检查完全正常时，胸部 X 线平片可以不用，但 X 线平片仍是常规检查[7,47]。最好采用标准的后前位和侧位检查，也可采用脊柱后前位照片。即使患者是从另外一所医院转来的，胸部放射学检查在到达创伤中心后仍应重复检查。胸部受伤在 X 光片上的重要表现包括皮下气肿、肋骨或其他骨结构骨折、血胸、挫伤或其他实质损伤（如吸入性肺炎）、纵隔移位或增宽膈肌破裂。

计算机断层扫描（CT）提供了比放射平片更详细的图像，在诊断气胸、肋骨骨折和肺挫伤上敏感性更强。CT 也同样可以帮助诊断膈肌破裂。因为胸片不能 100%诊断，所以一些小组推荐对所有怀疑有胸部损伤的患者进行 CT 扫描。CT 能确认的最常见的损伤是肺挫伤和裂伤[50]，许多 CT 上可以显示出来的气胸在 X 线片上要么不明显要么被低估了[50]。Manson 等人[50]因此得出结论，X 线平片诊断的只是胸部损伤的“大体影像检查”，尤其是在创伤复苏室获得的胸部平片，并建议对临床或 X 线平片诊断为严重胸部损伤的病例均应进行增强 CT 扫描。对这些病例，CT 能够更好地确认已经识别的损伤并可能发现平片不能显示的损伤。Exadaktylos 等人[20]支持这个观点。他们的经验是：即使胸部平片是正常的，CT 也可能显示致命的主动脉损伤。他们认为，胸部损伤患应常规进行 CT 检查。Renton 等人[70]研究了 CT 是否应该取代常规胸部平片检查而成为初始影像检查这个问题，结果给否定了，主要的原因是：增加的费用不能通过因为使用 CT 而改变了相关治疗来确认其合理。他们估计，200 个 CT 检查才改变 1 个患者的临床治疗。因此 CT 应该在怀疑胸部损伤的病例中使用。

有时候其他诊断性检查，包括超声波、经胸廓或经食管心脏超声检查、支气管镜检查、放射性核素骨扫描、血管造影术和甚至胸腔镜检查，都是有帮助的。超声检查比前后（位）的胸部放射检查更敏感且具有 CT 在诊断创伤性气胸上的敏感性[72]。最近的病例报告证明了使用胸腔镜手术诊断心包破裂和心脏疝[65]。在怀疑儿童虐待病例，放射性核素骨扫描有助于发现近期和陈旧的肋骨骨折。虽然在大多数急诊情况下不能使用核磁共振成像（MRI），但 MRI 对确定胸部脊柱损伤很有帮助，特别怀疑有脊髓损伤时。MRI 可能同样有助于在可疑病例识别膈肌损伤[55]。

多年来，血管造影术是诊断主动脉及其主要分支损伤的金标准。然而，一个明显的趋势是使用螺旋 CT 作为对疑似主动脉损伤的初始检查，用血管造影术指导对确诊病例的修补，或一些病例完全不需要主动脉造影检查。

经胸壁超声心脏检查是诊断由挫伤引起的所有类型的结构性心脏损伤和功能障碍的有效方法。它可显示心内损伤或心脏压塞。经食管超声心脏检查（TEE）是诊断创伤性主动脉破裂的有效检查。它能识别在 X 光平片或 CT 上见到的纵隔血肿的病因[46]。

心包穿刺放液术可能在疑为心脏压塞时使用。所有胸部损伤患者应在急诊室评估期间进行连续的心电

监护。在疑为心脏挫伤病例，应进行 12 导联心电图检查以排除心律失常。在疑为主气道损伤的病例，支气管镜检查应该在全身麻醉下在手术室进行。

治疗

胸部损伤的治疗是不同的，依据不同的结构性损伤和受伤严重程度，从支持供氧到简单的干预（气管
279 插管、机械通气、胸廓造口置管），再到手术（微创，开胸手术伴有或不伴有心肺分流术）。大多数患者不需要手术，仅仅通过支持治疗就能愈合，可伴有或不伴有胸廓造口置管术[42]。

当有手术指征时,依据术前的诊断，理想的切口位置是不同的。在第五肋间隙的前外侧做切口，可延长过中线，是急诊手术的最佳位置。一个活盖式切口可能适合于上纵隔的血管损伤。对于食管的损伤，相对的后外侧开胸术可以得到合适的暴露；而对最远端的胸段食管，最好是从侧面探查。正中胸骨切开术对心脏损伤是最佳术式。心肺分流在创伤急诊中很少需要，只在如冠状动脉破裂和胸主动脉破裂时需要。心内损伤到房室瓣或房间隔或室间隔时，需要旁路手术，部分可以选择修补。

目前已经订出控制腹腔内创伤损害的原则，这对选择性胸内损伤病例也同样适用。肺部的非解剖性切除以控制出血和大量气体泄露，用 GIA 吻合器行肺段切除术来处理肺贯穿伤，全肺切除术和肺门扭转[88]可能是有效的。最新的病例报告是已经无法控制出血或肺气体泄漏的病例。分开肺下的韧带、将下叶扭转到上叶前上，这样可以控制病情以便可以将患者送回重症监护室（ICU），以稳定病情并在确定病情控制后再送回手术室行肺切除术。

钝性损伤

胸壁

软组织

尽管临床上认为胸壁软组织损伤并不重要，但仍提示可能有严重的胸内损伤。胸壁软组织损伤应该按照公认的伤口处理原则来处理。

肋骨骨折

儿童时期肋骨强壮且柔软。因此肋骨骨折在儿童中比在成人中少见，而且连枷胸罕见。因为肋骨骨折需要很大的力量，因而是严重受伤的标志。第一肋骨骨折意味着有主要血管损伤的可能性，尤其是锁骨下动脉。第一根肋骨骨折也可能并发 Horner 综合征和胸廓出口综合征。

治疗目标是保持患者舒适同时避免肺膨胀不全和肺炎。治疗肋骨骨折包括休息和止痛。口服或静脉内注射止痛药通常足以控制疼痛，对肋间神经阻滞也可能有帮助。儿童很少有由于胸壁夹板固定而引起的肺膨胀不全。肋骨骨折通常可在 6 周内自然痊愈。全部肋骨骨折的儿童在 NPTR 中的死亡率为 10% [12]。

肋骨骨折在小于 3 岁的幼儿和婴儿常是由于儿童受虐待所致[24,87]。在无意外受伤情况下，儿童有一根或多根肋骨骨折的可能性随年龄增长而减小[87]。在儿童受虐待病例，典型的骨折位置是在肋骨颈部靠近肋（椎骨）横突关节处。Kleinman 等人[40]描述了受虐待婴儿的肋骨头破碎；因为肋骨头是软骨组织，这些损伤通常无法在 X 光片上发现。位于后面的肋骨囊性病灶是儿童受虐待的另一个标志[48]，通常认为是多发肋骨骨折在不同时期的愈合。

连枷胸

连枷胸在儿童中相对少见。它发生在胸壁的某个部分，因毗连的肋骨骨折而变得不稳定时。受伤胸壁可出现反常运动——在吸气时凹陷，在呼气时凸出。因反常运动可使通气无效。连枷胸通常伴有肺挫伤。胸壁肌僵直和无效咳嗽常常合成原发损伤。这可导致受影响的肺被压紧和塌陷，依次造成通气-弥散功能失调和组织缺氧。

连枷胸的初期治疗包括给氧、缓解疼痛（肋间神经阻滞、口服或静脉用止痛药或连续硬膜外阻滞）和物理疗法。液体治疗必须小心监测以避免肺水肿，建议进 ICU 进行监护。只有连枷胸而没有其他重要损伤的儿童很少需要机械通气。如果发展到呼吸衰竭，需要进行数天的气管内插管和呼气末正压通气。气管切开术很少使用。在 NPTR，连枷胸总死亡率是 40%[12]。

胸骨骨折

胸骨骨折在青少年中比在成人中少见，因为胸骨是软骨组织。

胸膜间隙

气胸

气胸可能是因为胸壁、肺实质、气管、支气管树或食管损伤所致。产生气胸需要很高能量，因此被视为其他隐蔽损伤的标记。

80 **单纯的气胸：**单纯气胸可能引起胸痛、呼吸窘迫、呼吸急促、受影响侧的气体进入减少和氧饱和度降低。仔细的体检能显示胸壁摩擦感、捻发音或气管移位。然而，许多患者没有临床体征或症状，由此要强调对所有外伤病例常规行胸部 X 光片检查。X 光片显示的征象包括单侧的或不对称的透亮影、纵隔的一个锐利轮廓和看得见的远离胸壁脏层胸膜的边缘。简单气胸的诊断应该在治疗前由胸部 X 光片确认。

单纯的气胸应该在肋间隙置管引流（图 16–1）。胸部引流最好的插入位置是在腋窝前线的第四或第五肋间隙（乳头水平）。对胸腔引流管的大小建议如下：新生儿为 12～16F，婴儿为 16～18F，学龄儿童为 18～24F，青少年为 28～32F。胸腔引流管应该连接到水下，密封并轻微吸引，当气体停止溢出时可以拔除。对大部分病例来说，这是唯一且必需的治疗。持续的或大量的空气溢出意味着气管支气管树的损伤。

小的无症状的气胸可以选择性进行仔细观察。如果患者要转运到另一所医院或因为任何原因需插管通气，或气胸超过 15%，就应该进行引流。当有怀疑时，就应该插入胸腔引流管。

开放性气胸：开放性气胸在儿童中罕见。在开放性气胸患者，胸膜腔内压力和大气压相等，因而肺被压缩，肺泡通气量减少。对吸气性创伤应该进行临床识别。可以通过放入 Heimlich 活瓣或应用封闭敷裹伤口——只在三面覆盖和粘贴，这样就能形成活瓣功能——或在常规位置插入胸腔引流管来治疗。

张力性气胸：张力性气胸可以在形成单向活瓣时发生，气体只能进入胸膜腔而不能漏出（图 16–2）。潜在原因通常是肺裂伤或损伤到气管或大的支气管。胸膜腔内气压超过了大气压而压迫同侧肺，把纵隔推向对侧，压平横膈，可损害对侧肺的通气，减少静脉血回流到心脏。脉搏和呼吸频率可加快，患者出现严重的窘迫。气管通常偏离受损一侧，颈部静脉充血。同侧胸部叩诊过清音且呼吸音减低。出现发绀是后期表现。最重要的鉴别诊断是心脏压塞，然而，这种异常因为气管不移位和胸部叩诊正常可以与张力性气胸区分。张力性气胸应该在受伤患者中考虑，尤其是机械通气患者突然出现没有明显原因的恶化。患儿有低血压和呼吸窘迫，因为腔静脉的扭转，在开胸引流置 281
管后好转。急性胃扩张和右侧主干插管可能引起左侧呼吸音减低，应该与张力性气胸鉴别。

张力性气胸的治疗是应立即行针式导管引流（不必等待胸部 X 线片），经锁骨中线第二肋间隙或在腋下第四或五肋间隙，随后放置胸腔引流管。

血胸

当大量血液丢失进入胸腔导致休克时，就可以使用大量血胸这个词。大量血胸在锐性损伤比钝性损伤中更常见。

血胸可能来源于肋间动脉或胸廓内动脉、肺或纵隔血管的破裂。从大血管直接出血到胸膜腔，如主动脉或肺门血管，通常是致命的。由于肺循环的压力低，大多数肺出血会自然停止。从体循环血管的出血，如肋间动脉，很容易造成大量血胸，产生低血容量、纵隔移位、呼吸音降低和受累侧叩诊浊音的表现。血胸常合并气胸（见图 16–1）。治疗是在肋间隙放置引流管以防止血胸凝块，并监测血液丢失的比例和总量。应在两条大的静脉内放置导管。一旦有休克表现，就开始休克治疗。因为引流操作会进一步增加出血，在引流大量血胸前就应开始输血。然而，引流和再扩张肺通常能使出血停止。

在大多数病例，肋间隙胸膜腔引流是唯一需要的治疗措施。然而，有以下情况时需要行开胸手术：

1. 初始出血超过全身估计血容量的 20%～25%。
2. 持续出血超过每小时 2～4ml/kg。
3. 出血不断增加。

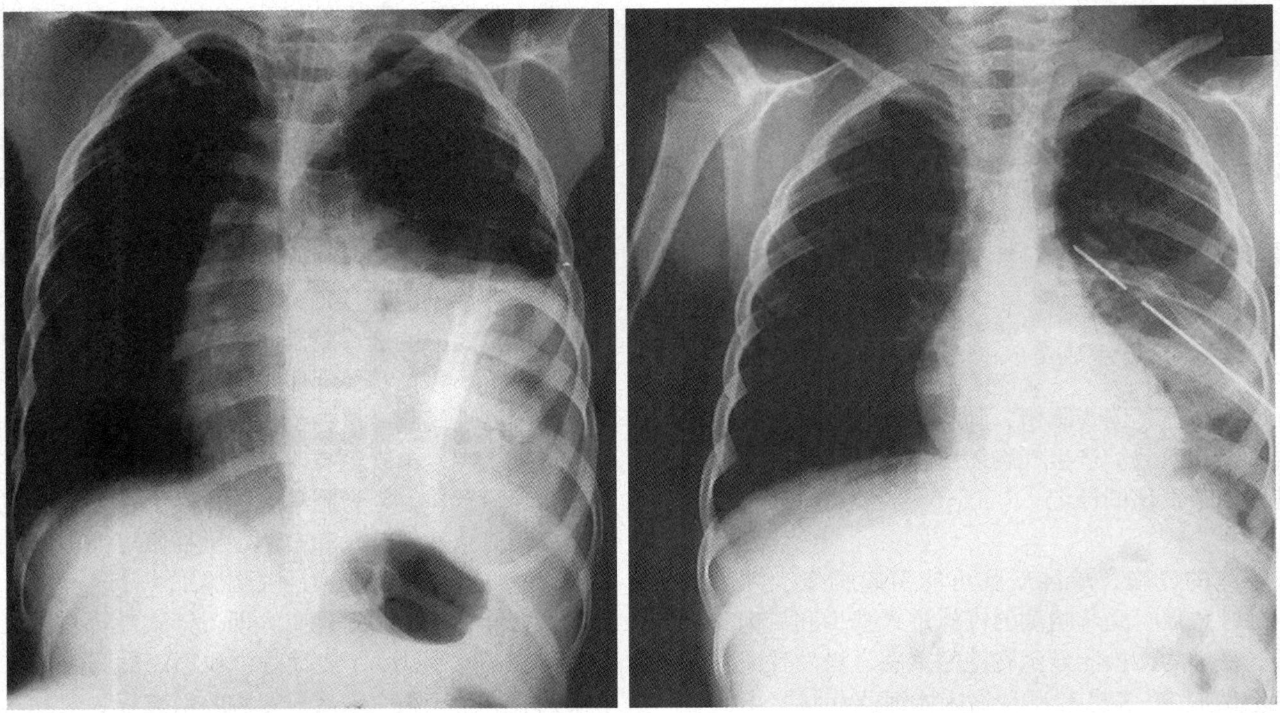

A B

图 16–1 A. 左侧血气胸；注意鼻胃管的位置。B. 同一患者插入肋间引流后；不需要其他治疗。(From Wesson DE: Trauma of the chest in children. Chest Clin North Am 1994;3:423.)

4．胸膜间隙不能有效引流出血和血块。

Hoth 等人[35]报道了对钝性损伤胸腔引流量增加的病例进行开胸时，非治疗性探查的可能性增加。自体输血在大量血胸手术时有帮助。

肺

血肿和挫伤

肺挫伤是儿童胸部钝性损伤的最常见类型。对肺的直接外力可导致肺实质的破裂、出血和非解剖性分布的水肿，而胸壁通常没有明显损伤。尽管可能出现肋骨骨折和胸壁擦伤，但在目前还很少有明显的特异性的症状和体征。

因为缺乏体格检查的特异性，诊断血肿和挫伤的关键是常规胸部放射学检查。肺挫伤通常在就诊时的放射学平片上表现明显（图 16–3），在 CT 上更加显著，通常位于后部和中后部。然而，当挫伤在平片上明显时，不需要进行 CT 检查。肺挫伤可能进展，尤

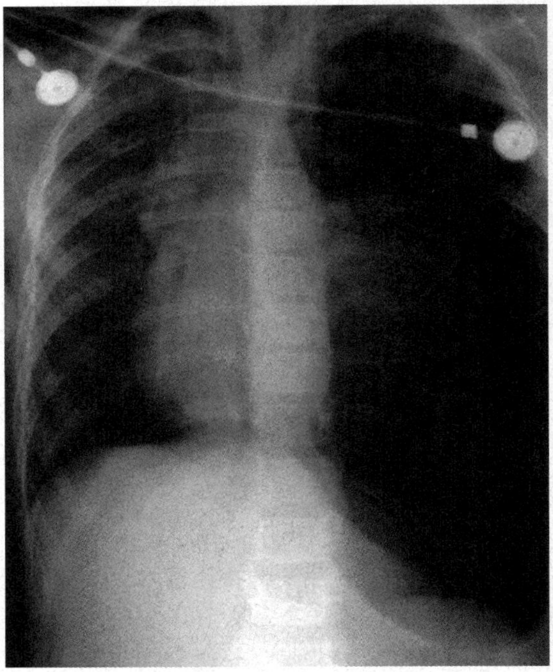

图 16–2 左侧张力性气胸。这张照片显示张力性气胸的典型表现，包括纵隔移位、压平和倒置横膈，受累侧空间增大。此患儿除有因腔静脉扭转引起的呼吸压迫——胸腔穿刺术引流可减轻，还有低血压。

其是当合并水肿和肺膨胀不全时。儿童肺挫伤很少需要机械通气，几乎不会发展到呼吸窘迫综合征。鉴别诊断包括吸入性肺炎，后者是由于在现场、转运途中、插管时或入院后呕吐所导致。其最常累及右下叶。

对有广泛肺血肿和挫伤的患者应该持续检测监护 SaO_2，最好是在 ICU 进行。治疗措施是支持、止痛、物理治疗、给氧和限制液体。与成人相比，气管内插管和机械通气治疗在儿童很少需要。入院后病情恶化少见[8]。重要的是防止水中毒和胃内容物吸入。最常见并发症是肺部感染。如果没有感染大多数肺血肿和
82 挫伤在 10 天内消失。

肺挫伤可以合并气胸、血胸或胸膜渗出，所有这些都可能需要肋间隙引流。这些继发性现象可能在有胸壁骨折表现时更加常见，并且甚至可能延迟到 48 小时之后。因此，肺挫伤患者应该进行系列的胸部放射学检查（见图 16–3）。

偶尔在创伤愈合过程中，肺出现空洞形成创伤后肺气囊。因为肺气囊通常在数月后自然愈合，所以很少需要治疗。

裂伤

肺的裂伤在锐性损伤中很常见，常引起气胸或血胸。它们也可以由肋骨骨折引起。

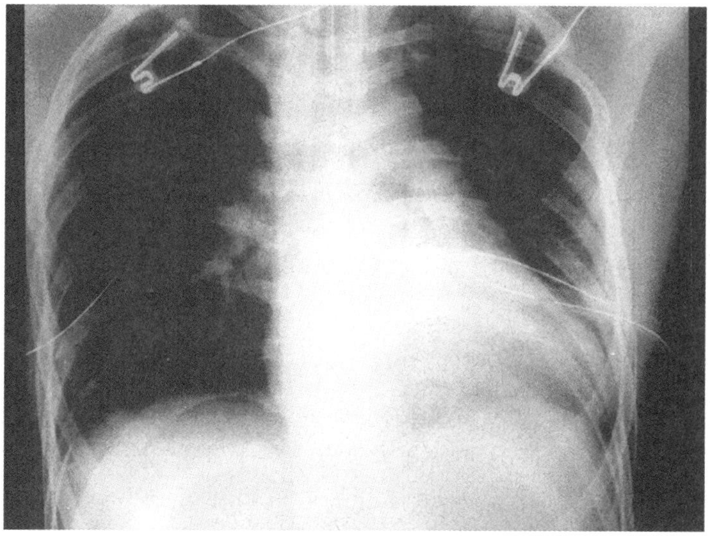

A

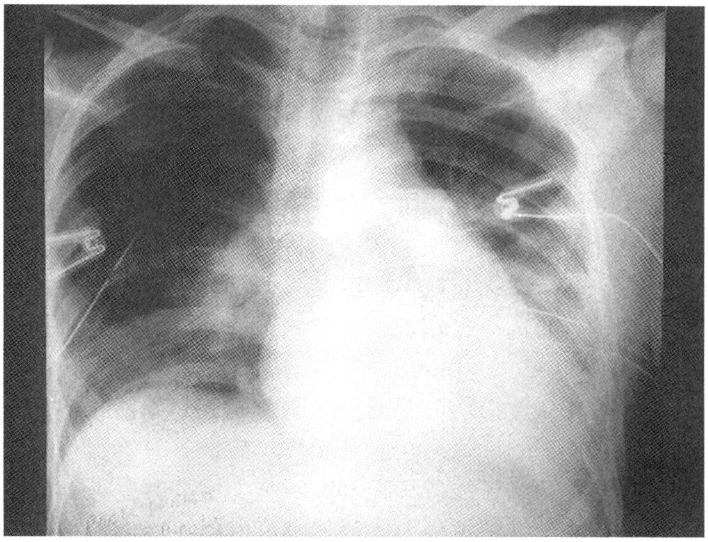

B

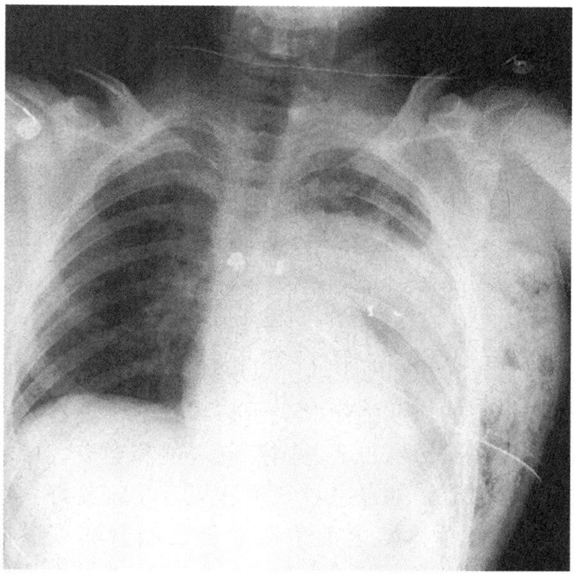

C

图 16–3　肺挫伤。A. 挤压伤伴肺挫伤；注意肋骨多发骨折。B. 同一患者 2 天后；注意病灶的进展。C. 枪击伤有肺挫伤和皮下气肿。(From Wesson DE: Trauma of the chest in children. Chest Clin North Am 1993;3:423.)

气栓是肺裂伤最严重的并发症。儿童胸部损伤病情突然恶化，尤其是在接受正压通气而没有气胸时应该怀疑气栓。气栓可能导致局部神经功能缺失。发现有泡沫的血从动脉插管抽出是气栓形成的证据。急诊开胸，夹紧肺门，从心脏或右心室流出道抽出气体可能挽救生命[36]。

气管和支气管

在儿童，损伤主气道并不常见。几乎所有主气道损伤都是钝性损伤所致[12]。最常见的特殊病变是其中一个主支气管部分或完全横断和气管黏膜撕裂。气管损伤通常发生在隆凸内 2～3cm，如果不能识别和正确治疗可能很快危及生命。损伤远端肺叶支气管比较常见。

283 一些有主气道损伤的患者在到达医院前或到达后短期内因为呼吸衰竭死亡。大多数表现为常因张力性气胸引起的呼吸困难。其他有主气道损伤的患者特征性地表现为嗓音失调、青紫、咯血、大的皮下和纵隔气肿，以及肺不能膨胀或尽管进行了适当的引流，仍持续有大量气体漏出（图 16–4）。虽然不常见，“肺下垂”即肺实际下落到胸膜腔下半部分，在低于损伤支气管水平，实际上有助于主气道损伤的诊断。最后，一些患者因为支气管梗阻随后出现肺慢性塌陷和感染。

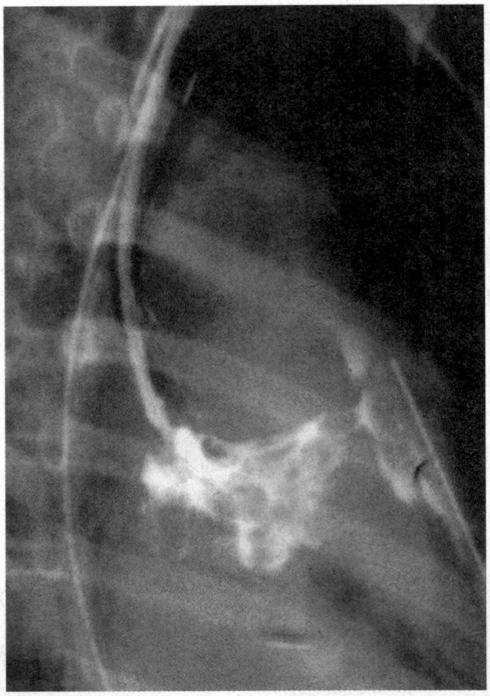

图 16–4 尽管有合适的胸部引流，胸部损伤患者仍有气体持续漏出。右上叶支气管可以看到血，注射造影剂后显示漏出的部位和程度，可以通过注射纤维蛋白胶和胸腔引流控制。有时需要手术关闭或切除术。

在创伤室的初期治疗取决于临床状况。气道损伤的初期治疗是按照 ATLS 原则控制气道和通气。可能需要插管和引流。如果患者气道和氧合状态良好，在把患者转运到手术室之前应避免尝试插管的气道操作。柔软的气管镜有助于在损伤位置外或选择未受损伤的支气管进行插管。低于平均气道压力的高频通气在大量气体泄漏时可能比常规方法有效，并能为手术修补争取时间[69]。

螺旋式 CT 对疑为主气道损伤的稳定患者是最好的初期检查方法，但支气管镜更理想。无论是肺不张还是引流后大量气体持续泄漏，都是支气管镜检查的指征。应该在手术室全身麻醉下用硬的通气支气管镜进行。如果可能，患者在麻醉诱导和支气管镜检查期间允许自主呼吸。进行开胸的医护人员和设备应该准备。对不稳定的或可能或确定有颈椎损伤的患者，用软支气管镜或通过气管插管插入导管同样可能发现病灶。在支气管镜下，可以看见气管壁的缺损。其他支气管镜中的损伤表现有黏膜破裂和软骨暴露。对远端支气管损伤，可能需要支气管造影检查。

小的膜状气管裂伤和一些部分支气管撕裂不超过 1/3 圈的情况可以自然愈合。对于气管或支气管的大的裂伤，经过侧后位开胸进行修补可能是最好的方法，能确保长期良好的结果。肺叶或肺段的远端支气管损伤可能通过纤维蛋白胶封堵或进行肺切除，而不是直接修补。右侧进胸能很好地暴露气管、隆凸和右侧主支气管；左侧进胸能暴露左主支气管远端的损伤。在表现有大量气体泄漏时，在尝试修补气管前应该夹闭肺门。推进气管导管或插入一个消毒管经过手术区域到远端气管可能在修补时有帮助。清创后单纯间断缝合效果很好。尽管可能必须行肺叶或肺段切除，但肺切除只在不稳定的和严重肺损伤的患者才作为最后的选择。肺切除或支气管修补的远期效果通常很好[59]。

支气管损伤可能因自然闭合而一开始被忽略，有气管狭窄的危险。在数月和数年后，支气管损伤自然愈合的儿童可能持续肺膨胀不全，常合并受累部位的肺炎或支气管扩张。这种狭窄可以在一些病例进行扩张治疗，但通常必须开放修补或切除受累肺。有人报道，完全横断主支气管后期修补有可能保留肺[78]。

食管

最常见的导致食管损伤的原因是吞咽了腐蚀性液体和锐性损伤，包括医源性损伤。强烈呕吐和干呕在儿童期很少导致食管撕裂。外部的钝性损伤很少导致
284 食管损伤。钝性损伤导致食管损伤通常认为是胃内排出的气体通过胃食管联合处导致食管内压力的突然增高所致。

食管穿孔可引起发热、胸痛和呼吸急促。偶尔颈部出现皮下气肿。纵隔或胸膜内气体可能在常规胸片或 CT 上见到。如果怀疑食管损伤，可以进行造影剂检查、食管镜检查或两者同时进行。

当食管损伤的诊断是在最初的 12 小时做出时，最好的治疗方法是早期关闭和引流。当诊断较晚时，可能需要唾液分流，即指颈部食管造瘘和胃造瘘，再加上胸部引流。

横膈

尽管横膈损伤在儿童中罕见，但这是由于对腹部的强力冲击或穿透性损伤所致。识别这些损伤很重要，因为胃和肠可能由于这些缺损形成疝和绞窄。90%的横膈损伤出现在左侧。钝性损伤时，撕裂通常靠近中心腱并呈放射状。

横膈损伤的最初表现容易被忽略，因为它们通常都合并其他严重损伤。它们可能没有症状，或可能导致腹部、胸部或同侧肩部顶端疼痛。在诊断横膈损伤中体格检查很少有帮助。诊断通常基于胸部平片，这是最重要的诊断方法（图 16–5）。表 16–3 总结了横膈损伤的放射学表现。常规的胸部平片上任何横膈或靠近横膈的异常都应怀疑横膈损伤。在初期胸部平片

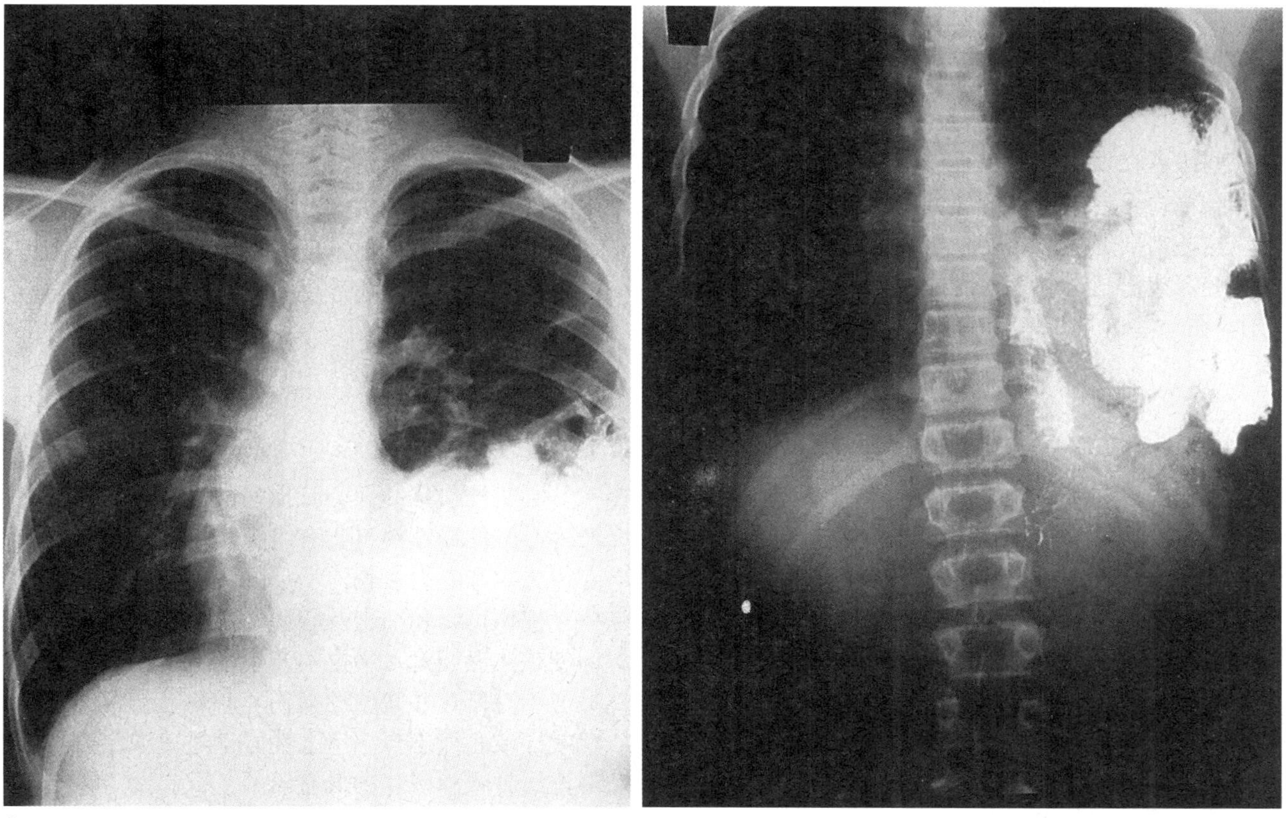

A　　B

图 16–5　横膈破裂。A. 胸部平片。B. 胃肠道造影检查见到疝出的肠道。

表 16-3 横膈损伤的影像学表现
半边横膈影模糊
半边横膈抬高
疝入的内脏引起横膈上的气体形态异常
鼻胃管头端进入到胸腔
不典型的气胸
靠近横膈的肺呈盘状膨胀不全

上，30%～50%的病例表现正常[9]。因此，对疑为横膈损伤病例应该重复行放射学检查。

因为其他损伤的表现经常成为主要表现，所以横膈损伤的诊断经常延误。开始时，腹部脏器疝进入胸腔可能没有发生，尤其是在接受机械通气的患者。然而，正常呼吸的较低的胸内压力可能逐渐使胃和肠道疝入胸腔。这在平片上可以发现，尤其是疝入的胃里有胃管时。如果没有鼻胃管，疝出的胃可能发生急性扩张，导致严重的呼吸窘迫。

如果需要，可以通过上、下消化道放射造影检查来确诊。然而，这些检查不容易对多发急性损伤的患者实施。多维 CT 重建可能有效。横膈损伤在 CT 上
285 的表现包括横膈不连续、腹腔脏器疝入胸腔和胃通过缺损处被压缩[89]。在稳定的患者，MRI 可能对建立诊断有帮助。

一些患者在发生紊乱过程的晚期表现为疝出内脏梗阻和绞窄，可导致严重的腹部和胸部疼痛、恶心和呕吐。这些需要通过腹部切口进行修补。修补通过开放的腹腔探查进行，但近来有一些腹腔镜下修补的报道[52,67]。在一些晚期患者因为有胸腔粘连应进行开胸手术。

心脏和心包

对心脏的钝性损伤能产生不同的损伤类型：休克震荡、挫伤或心肌、瓣膜或分隔的直接破裂[57]。冠状动脉破裂或血栓形成尽管很少，但同样可能发生。心包撕裂可能使心脏疝出到胸膜间隙，从而影响心脏功能并导致心排出量降低。胸部钝性损伤偶尔产生隐蔽性的结构性心脏损害，而没有大的心功能影响和出血或心脏压塞[18]。这些损伤包括动脉或室间隔缺损、二尖瓣或三尖瓣关闭不全以及心室壁瘤形成。常表现为新的杂音或心电图改变。诊断需要心电图和或心导管检查来确定。一旦患者病情稳定就可以进行选择性修补。对所有已知或怀疑心脏损伤的患者应该安排心电图检查。

一些病例显示儿童在受到胸部直接击打后可出现突然心跳停止。心源性休克更适合描述这种情况[51,86]。心源性休克最常出现于有组织的运动比赛如篮球。没有挫伤或损伤的其他表现在尸检时发现，死亡通常归因于心室纤维颤动。

当为心脏创伤进行急诊手术时，外科医生应该牢记几个原则：

1. 准备和包裹整个胸腔。
2. 切口选在左侧第 4 或第 5 肋间隙侧前方向（除了已知心脏损伤的稳定患者进行选择性心脏修补，应该通过胸骨正中切口来修补）。
3. 当打开心包时避开膈神经。
4. 直接压迫控制出血。
5. 必要时利用纱布缝合心脏。
6. 切开心包。

一些作者已经报道使用皮肤代产品来控制心脏伤口，但最好直接缝合。在缝合时可以置入球囊导管来控制出血。

尽管大多数心脏损伤不需要心肺分流就可以修补，但这个方法仍然可以选择。在手术中，外科医生应该经常检查有无震颤，因其可能提示瓣膜破裂或创伤性室间隔缺损。在术后通过听诊新的杂音和进行心电图检查发现心内病灶也很重要。出院后同样应该随访心脏超声检查。

心肌挫伤

心肌挫伤是钝性心脏损伤的最常见形式。它可以产生心脏的局部损害，有组织学改变。能导致致命的心律失常和心力衰竭。治疗的目标是处理并发症。

挫伤可以和冲击及心源性休克相区别，因为后者即使是在显微镜水平也不产生任何结构改变。挫伤常见但不总是合并胸壁的损伤。心肌挫伤可能完全无症状或导致心律不齐（室上性心动过速或室颤）或继发心排出量减少引起的低血压。

不幸的是，尽管许多检查已经可以进行，包括心电图检查、心脏超声检查、心肌酶谱（CKMB、心肌

肌钙蛋白 I、心肌肌钙蛋白 T）检查和放射性核素扫描，但没有一个可以确诊心脏挫伤[30,80,81]。这使应该做多少检查才可以获得诊断难以确定，治疗更加难以确定。Tellez 等人[84]总结说："对所有多发钝性损伤儿童的心脏进行全面评估很难证明什么"。最简单的检查是 12 导联心电图，可能显示 ST 段和 T 波倒置。心脏超声检查可能显示射血分数减少、局限的收缩期室壁运动异常、舒张期室壁厚度增加和回声区域增加。Swaanenburg 等人[80]发现，在 ICU 监护的选择性患者中，心肌肌钙蛋白 I 和 T 水平比其他任何诊断性检查更加正确和可靠。因此，他们建议对入院时怀疑有心肌挫伤而瓣膜正常的患者在入院后应该重复检查。

一项对 41 名钝性胸部损伤的儿童使用综合检查的回顾性研究——这些检查包括血清酶水平、心电图、心脏超声和焦磷酸盐心肌扫描——结果显示，异常结果的发生率高。然而，所有检查结果与临床过程之间
36 几乎没有相关性[45]。作者的结论是：心肌挫伤在儿童胸部创伤中罕有临床意义。因此，当 12 导联心电图和心脏超声显示正常时，可以排除重大心肌挫伤。

治疗心肌挫伤包括肌收缩力的支持，同时进行 12～24 小时的心电图监护并经常测定血压。在受伤早期并发症很少发生[23]。Tellez 等人[84]建议在急诊室和 ICU 心脏监护以确定心律不齐，在心率不齐和明显胸部损伤的患者，需做系列心电图和心肌酶检查。

心肌破裂

心脏的破裂通常会迅速致命。实际上，胸部创伤死亡的最常见原因是心肌破裂。在系列尸检中，Bergman 等人[3]发现，2/3 的患者死在事故现场，1/3 死在急诊室。大多数心脏破裂患者是源于高能撞击，如交通意外或从高处坠落。当在心脏收缩晚期发生撞击时，主动脉易于破裂，心室破裂发生在舒张晚期。右心室是最常破裂的部位。

心肌破裂儿童常表现心脏压塞（见下文），也可发生心肌坏死、动脉瘤形成和延迟破裂[74]。有创伤性动脉隔缺损或室间隔缺损的患者可能表现新的杂音而没有心力衰竭。所有胸部损伤患者都应该在出院前仔细检查有关新的杂音表现。任何新的杂音都是做心脏超声检查的指征。早期诊断和修补可使患者存活。

瓣膜损伤

瓣膜损伤少见，但钝性损伤后容易出现[4,75]。房室瓣最常受累，由于损伤环状部、腱索或乳头肌破裂而导致关闭不全（图 16-6）。这是钝性心脏损伤的一种类型，可以进行半选择性修补。

心脏压塞

心脏压塞由钝性损伤后心包腔内血液积聚引起。心脏压塞的全部表现——奇脉和 Beck 三征（颈静脉压力升高、系统性低血压和心音遥远）——很少在急性损伤患者中发生。心脏压塞通常伴有心动过速、外周血管收缩、颈部静脉扩张，以及尽管积极进行液体复苏，但仍有持续低血压。实际上，存在不能解释的低血压时应该怀疑心脏压塞，尤其当伴有颈部静脉压力升高时。确定诊断的最好方法是通过经胸心脏超声检查，这可由外科医生在床边进行，腹部创伤急诊超声检查[10,62]。

对怀疑心脏压塞的治疗首先是控制气道和呼吸及扩张血容量。诊断应该通过心脏超声检查来确定，后

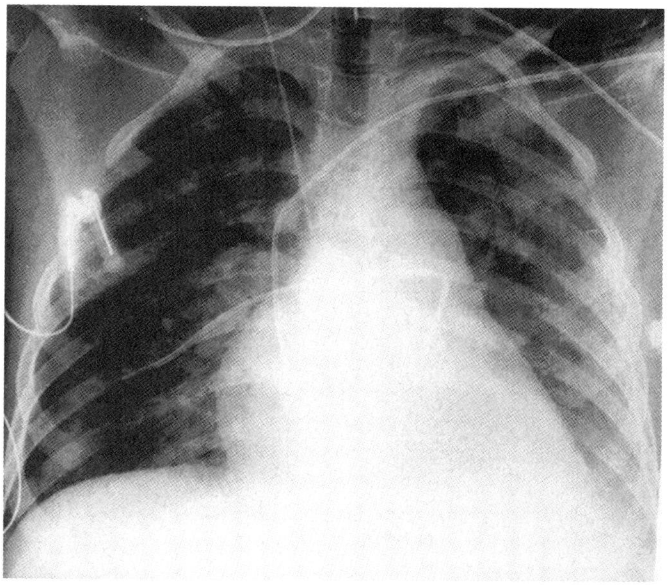

图 16-6 钝性胸部损伤 2 天后，心脏扩大和肺水肿；注意 Swan-Ganz 导管。二尖瓣环和腱索撕裂被成功修补。(From Wesson DE: Trauma of the chest in children. Chest Clin North Am 1993;3:423.)

者是最好的简单的诊断工具。如果患者严重休克，通过心包间隙针式导管引流也许能挽救生命（图 16–7）。因此，在急诊或不能进行心脏超声检查时，应选择心包穿刺放液。针头应该在剑突下呈 45°角向上和向左肩方向进针。成功的标志是抽出不凝的血液。如果需要，应该在确诊后，在治疗期间放置导管以重复抽吸。心包穿刺放液可能并发出血或损伤到左前冠状动脉降支。如果心包穿刺放液时患者情况不能稳定，应该立即开胸以缓解填塞和控制出血。

心包裂伤

心包可能因为钝性损伤撕裂。最常见部位是在左
287 侧膈神经前方。心脏可能通过缺损疝出和扭转而削弱其功能并降低心排出量。这种类型的损伤可以通过 CT 或电视胸腔镜手术确诊[37,85,89]。

主动脉

主动脉和其主要分支的创伤性破裂在儿童不常见[2]。Eddy 等人[17]报道，在华盛顿 King 县的所有儿童的创伤性死因中，2.1%是主动脉损伤。主动脉的创伤性破裂在成人创伤性死亡原因中的比例（约 10%）比儿童高。可能因为成人动脉更易破碎和撕裂。主动脉损伤的预兆有低血压、头部损伤、高速机动车的乘员、骨盆骨折、肢体骨折和其他胸部损伤。然而，这些预兆是否可靠还不清楚。Dyer 等人[16]认为，这些预兆是“有缺点的”和“主观的”。Horton 等人[34]发现，速度超过每小时 20 英里（1 英里 = 1.609 千米）和靠边超过 15 英寸（1 英寸 = 2.54 厘米）的乘客与主动脉损伤强相关。

主动脉的创伤性破裂发生在急剧减速时，这是因为对主动脉壁产生了剪切力。损伤的最常见部位靠近动脉韧带、主动脉根部或其他主要分支点，如无名动脉、椎动脉或颈动脉的开始部位。远侧弓撕裂通常位于主动脉前内侧面和水平方向。Marfan 综合征的儿童在躯干钝性损伤后处于主动脉壁夹层形成的危险中。

尽管主动脉损伤通常迅速致死，但在一些病例，动脉外膜和胸膜可以包住血液和防止出血。没有立即出血的患者其自然进程还不清楚，但突然破裂在这些患者中不太可能发生。因此，没有必要在患者处于稳定状态、彻底诊断和治疗其他损伤之前把他们紧急送入手术室。在修补主动脉前可能需要开腹探查、开颅或两者同时进行。

在儿童，主动脉损伤的治疗与成人一样重要[33,38]。

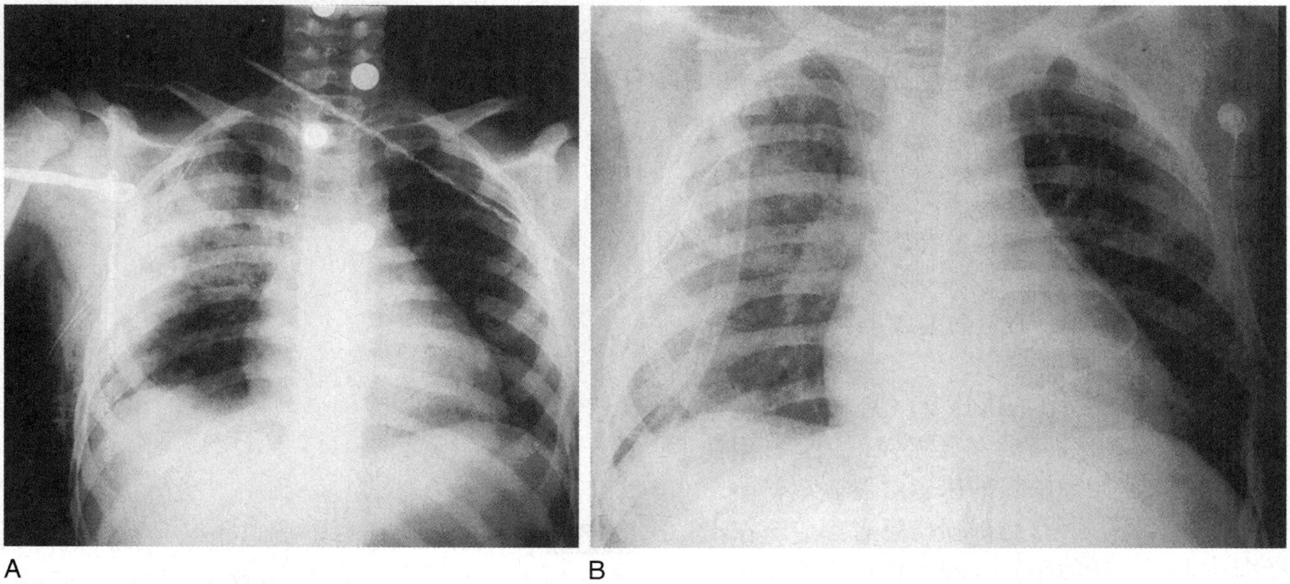

图 16–7 钝性胸部损伤后心脏压塞。患者是后座乘客，前额高速撞击。胸骨下部有保险带痕迹。休克对液体复苏没有反应，心包渗出在胸部心脏超声中证实。A. 胸部平片正常心脏，有肺挫伤表现。B.血性心包渗出导管引流后的胸片。不需要进一步治疗。(From Wesson DE: Trauma of the chest in children. Chest Clin North Am 1993;3:423.)

但诊断不易做出，因为可能没有胸部损伤的临床证据。急性缩窄综合征——上肢高血压、上下肢血压不同、心前区或背部大杂音——尤其罕见的。在 DelRossi 等人[13]报道的 27 例主动脉损伤患者中没有发现 1 例有缩窄综合征。

通常通过胸部平片做出诊断，这方法很敏感（假阴性 2%～7%），但却是非特异性的（假阳性 80%）。主动脉破裂的放射学表现与成人的一样（表 16–4，图 16–8）。几乎所有的病例都显示纵隔增宽（纵隔–胸比例＞0.25）和主动脉轮廓异常。

至今，大多数作者认为主动脉造影是诊断主动脉损伤的金标准。现在许多作者认为，对比增强多阶段的螺旋 CT 是诊断主动脉损伤的确定性检查，它和主动脉造影有相等的敏感性（图 16–9）[16,25,54,61]。如果螺旋 CT 正常，不需要做主动脉造影。这降低了放射线平片对怀疑有钝性胸部损伤的患者做主动脉造影的阴性率。Melton 等人[54]和 Rubin[73]已对螺旋 CT 和 CT 血管成像技术做过综述。造影剂注射的时间、注射量及注射速率都必须仔细控制以获得理想的结果。螺旋 CT 的花费只有主动脉造影的一半[61]。

主动脉造影对可疑病例或为确诊病例进行修补前获得更加详细的解剖情况仍然有帮助[11]。然而，许多权威人士对主动脉损伤的处置单独应用螺旋 CT 是否足够仍有争议[54]。

经食管心脏超声检查在诊断胸主动脉降部的损伤同样有作用，尤其是对于 ICU 内不能去放射科检查的不稳定患者。经食管心脏超声检查对升主动脉及其分支损伤的诊断没有作用。不幸的是，经食管心脏超声检查对操作的依赖性高。Le Bret 等人[46]发现，经食管心脏超声上的三个表现足以确诊主动脉损伤患者：表现为探头和主动脉之间的距离增大（＞3mm）、主动脉壁双重轮廓和主动脉与脏层胸膜之间的超声信号。在这个报道中，经食管心脏超声检查诊断主动脉创伤性破裂的敏感性是 100%；特异性是 75%。作者提议对所有严重胸部创伤的病例进行经食管心脏超声检查。经食管心脏超声检查在 CT 或主动脉造影可疑的病例同样有用，可以避免不必要的开胸手术[63]。

表 16–4 主动脉损伤的影像学表现

纵隔增宽（纵隔–胸比例＞0.25）
主动脉结消失或轮廓异常
左主支气管压低（在水平下＞40°）
气管偏斜（左边缘在 T4 棘突右侧）
食管偏斜（鼻胃管在 T4 棘突右侧）
左侧胸膜帽
左侧血胸

一旦诊断成立，对主动脉损伤治疗选择包括开放修补、血管内支架移植或对一些病例采取非手术观察。主动脉手术有重大并发症的危险，包括颅内高压——可以加剧出血、左心室劳损、肾衰竭和脊髓缺血。肝素可能增加远离损伤部位出血的可能性。

小的内膜活瓣可能自然愈合，但是在患者稳定后通过左后外侧开胸修补是一种治疗选择（其他部位的出血应该首先修补）。安全的推迟手术，在决定手术期间或控制合并的神经系统严重损伤、严重烧伤、脓毒性的或污染伤口、肝素化时易于出血的实质脏器损伤和呼吸衰竭[83]。在这些病例，必须用 β 受体阻断药控制平均动脉压并在 ICU 监护，直到修补能安全完成。艾司洛尔是常用的 β 受体阻断药。

心肺旁路（通常左心旁路）在修补损伤延伸到主动脉根部的病例时经常应用。左肺应该塌陷和收缩。当分离主动脉以横跨钳闭时应仔细，防止损伤其供应脊髓的分支和迷走神经及其返支。一些部分撕裂的病例可以进行一期修补，尤其当撕裂呈环状时，修补通常需要放入圆形涤纶移植片，可以通过三个途径进行这个手术：

1．夹闭和缝合。
2．术中分流。
3．体外循环支持。

最简单的方法是夹闭和缝合而不进行分流或建立心肺旁路。这是最快的方法且横跨钳闭时间最短，在损伤不是非常严重时是适用的。Razzouk 等人[68]报道，夹闭缝合技术在大多数患者是可行的，没有增加死亡率和脊髓损伤。Kwon 等人[43]也同意，夹闭技术不增加死亡率和发病率。然而其他人强烈反对。Hochheiser 等人[31]报道，体外循环修补有较低的截瘫发生率。

另一种观点是可以用肝素保护术中分流。这可能可以降低脊髓的缺血损伤而没有全身肝素化的风险。然而，还没有对照研究来证实这点。

第三种方法是在修补时使用体外循环支持。最常见的选择是心肺旁路，从左上肺静脉或左房到股

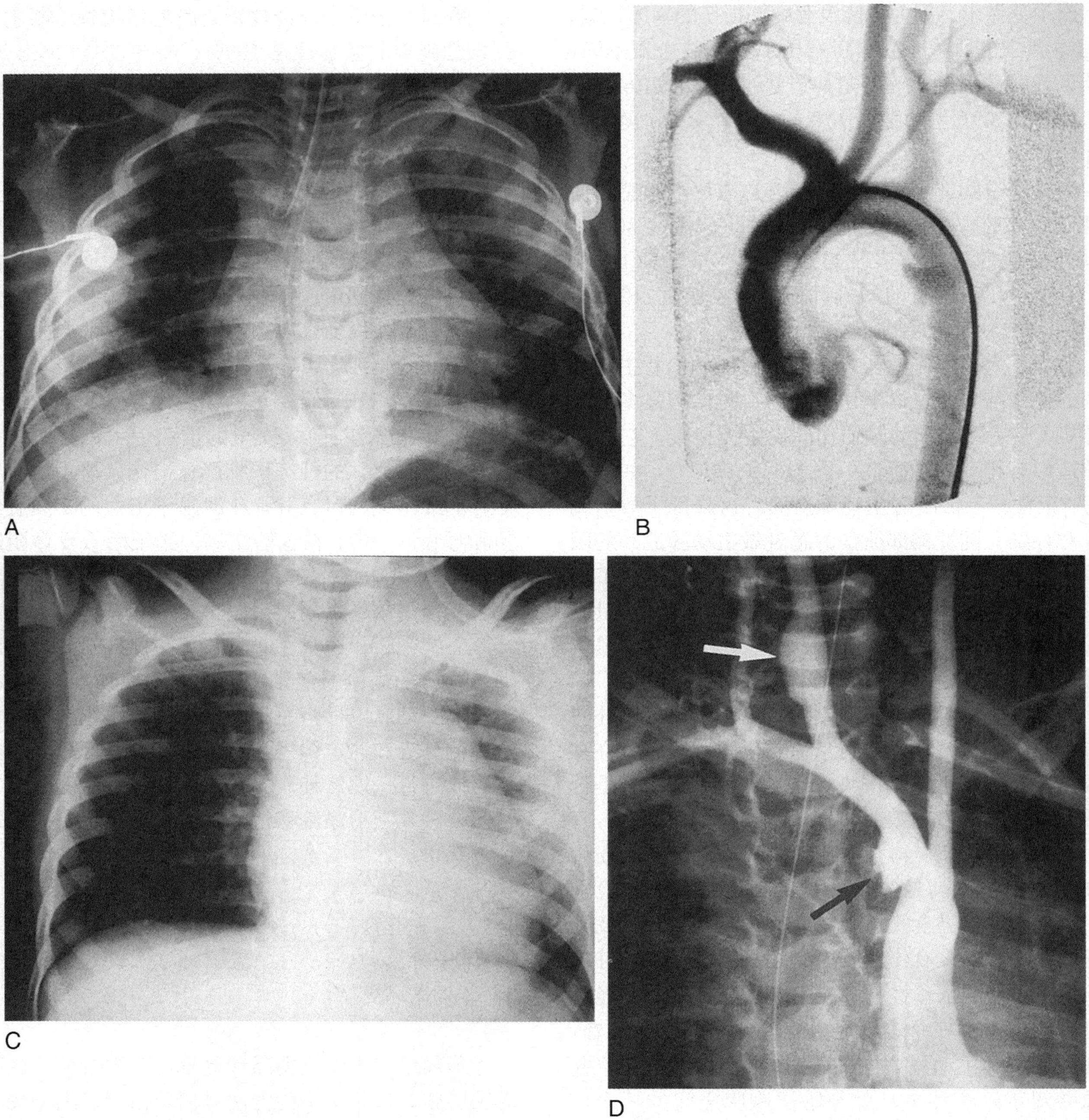

图 16-8 主动脉及其分支的创伤性破裂。A. 纵隔增宽，气管导管和鼻胃管都偏向右侧。B. 与 A 为同一个患者，主动脉损伤经主动脉造影照片证实。C. 在一个不同的胸部钝性损伤患者，纵隔增宽。D. 与 C 为同一个的患者，无名动脉在起始处裂伤（箭头所示）。(From Wesson DE: Trauma of the chest in children. Chest Clin North Am 1993;3:423.)

动脉[56]。股–股旁路和降主动脉远端直接灌注也有使用。一些作者认为，心肺旁路可降低截瘫的危险，但需要全身肝素化，这会增加颅内出血的发生率[44]。主动脉创伤性破裂修补后截瘫的比例大约是 5%～10%。脊髓血供的个体差异、夹闭时间和术中低血压是脊髓损伤的重要决定因素。

近来有些经股动脉插入支架（血管内支架移植）来治疗成人胸主动脉损伤的报道。早期结果显示可能比标准开放修补要好。3 个病例显示截瘫的发生率明显降低[15,39,60]。血管内支架已经在儿童有少量报道，但

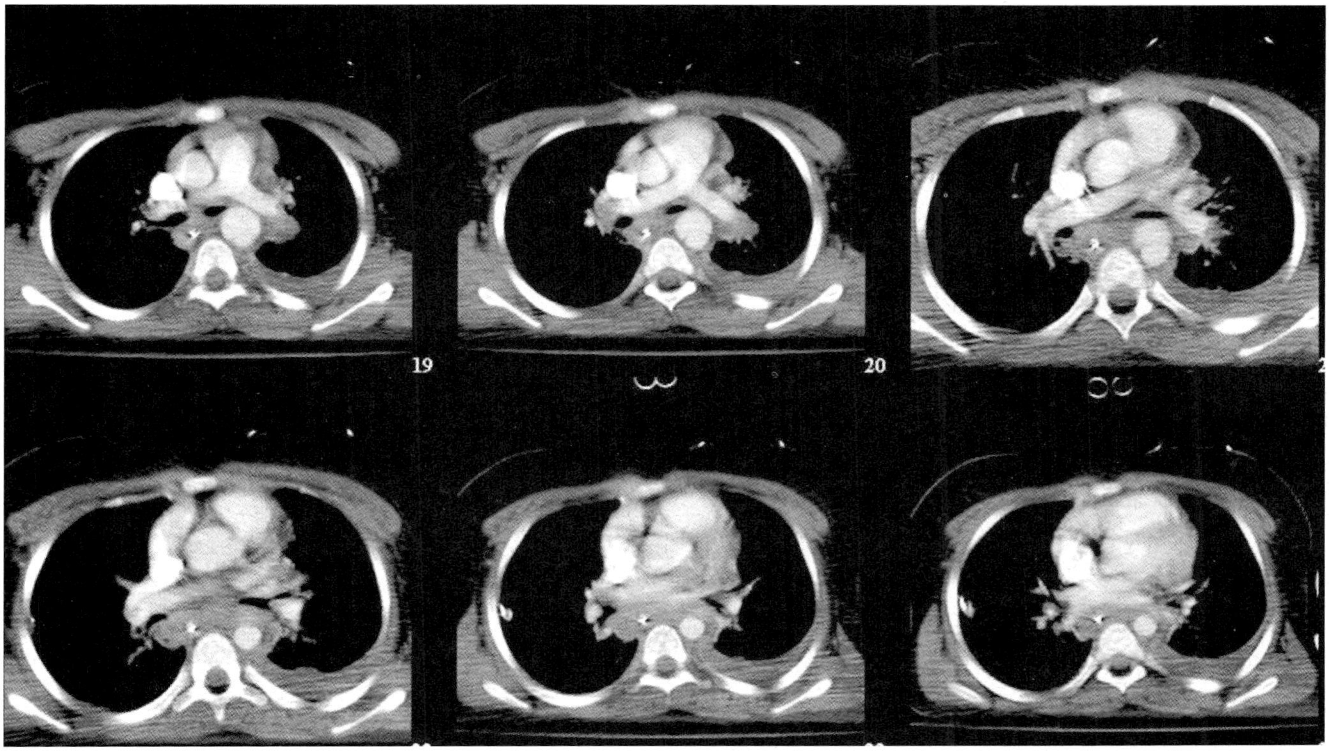

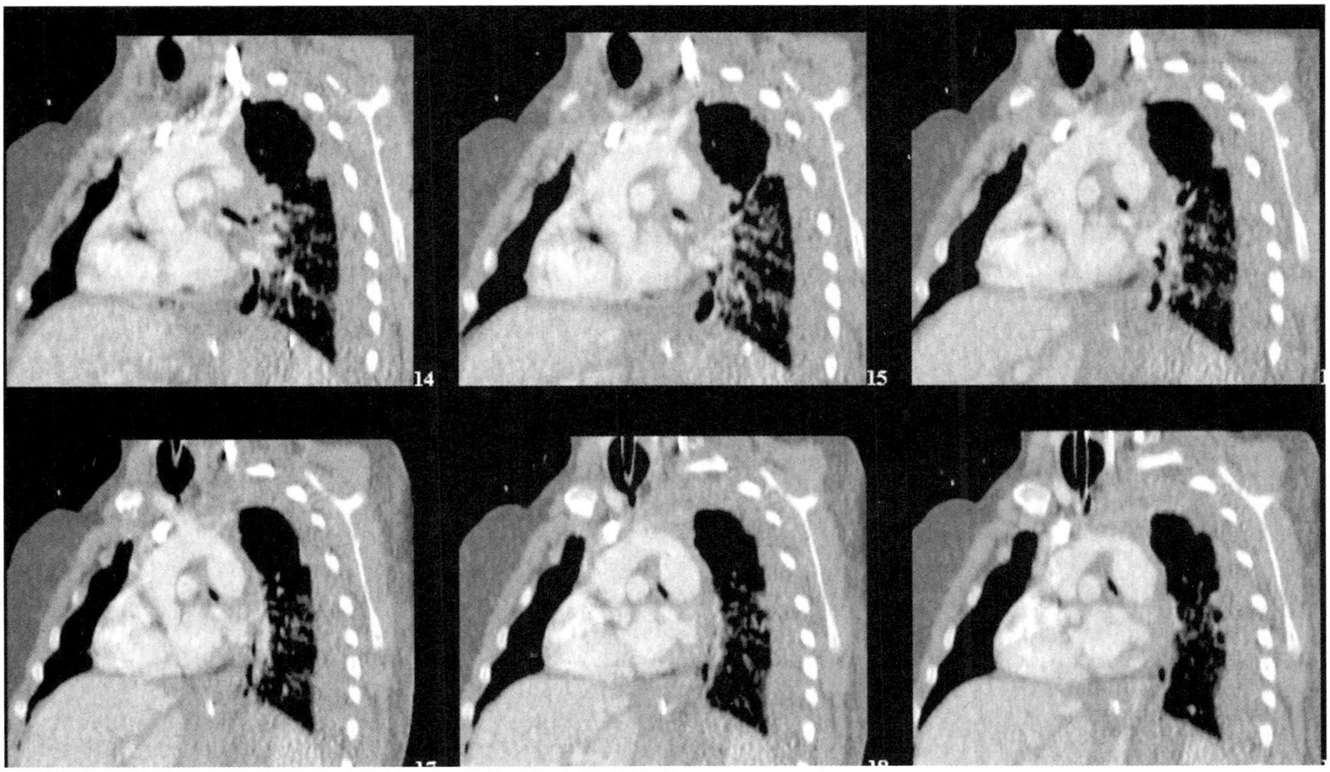

图 16-9　多排 CT 扫描重建显示了一个 14 岁男孩的主动脉创伤性破裂。A. 轴面图。注意峡部的主动脉周围血肿。B. 三维重建。注意峡部血流阻断。

没有长期随访结果[38]。

在 Eddy 的报道中[17]，13 例创伤性主动脉破裂患者中只有 1 例存活。与此相比，DelRossi 等人[13]报道一个临床研究有 75%的存活率。在 DelRossi 的研究中，21 例存活者中有 3 例在修补后发生截瘫，其中 2 例后来康复了。还没有证据表明哪种技术更好。然而，Fabian 等人[21]报道，夹闭-缝合技术比旁路修补更易产生截瘫，尤其在夹闭时间大于 30 分钟的病例。

与许多类型损伤一样，预后同样取决于是否合并有其他损伤[44]。Hormuth 等人[33]报道了总体结果很好的 11 例胸部主动脉损伤儿童患者。他们修补了峡部损伤，同时建立了左心旁路并直接灌注远端胸主动脉，并且主动脉弓损伤是在低温下修补的。

乳糜胸

尽管乳糜胸相对罕见，但损伤到胸导管会产生乳糜胸。大多数病例在营养支持下自然恢复（全胃肠外营养或中链三酰甘油要素饮食）。偶尔可以通过结扎胸导管进行治疗。

291 创伤性窒息

创伤性窒息是只在儿童出现的临床综合征，发生在关闭声门时突然压迫腹部或胸部（或同时都有）[76]。这种情况可导致胸内压力快速升高，并传递到引流到没有静脉瓣的上腔静脉的静脉中。可导致上半身的皮肤、巩膜及脑部血液渗出。脑可能在受伤时或稍后由于组织缺氧而受到伤害。这种损伤的临床表现包括抽筋、定向力障碍、上半身瘀点和呼吸衰竭(图 16-10)。支持治疗是主要方法，大多数患者可完全恢复。

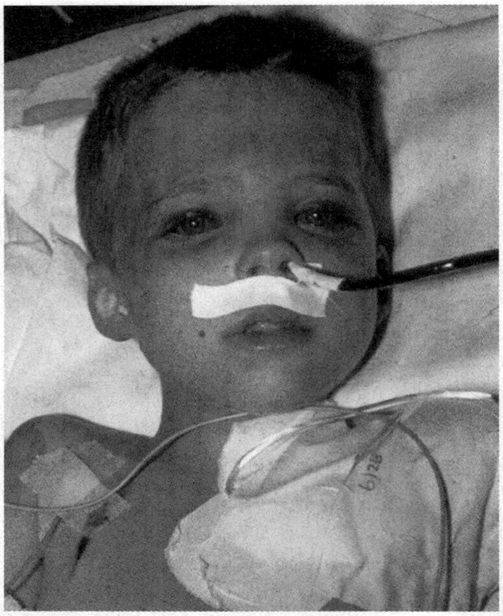

图 16-10 创伤性窒息。这个儿童在机动车意外中受伤，但是仍遭受了胸部的严重压迫损伤。除了上半身躯干皮肤点状出血，还有 48 小时精神错乱，脑部也显示有出血。

锐性损伤

锐性损伤的初期治疗同钝性损伤相似：清理气道、给氧和静脉补液，仔细评估患者，拍摄胸片。通过在平片上标记伤口的进出位置来了解损伤的路径。复苏初期如果需要，行气管插管和置入胸腔引流管。对任何伤口在乳头线水平下的患者应该意识到可能合并腹部损伤，这点非常重要。对怀疑损伤到主气道的患者，可以做支气管镜。如怀疑食管损伤，则有必要进行食管镜和水溶性造影检查。在稳定患者，行心脏超声检查以诊断可能的心脏损伤。

治疗同钝性损伤的相似。大多数患者不需要开胸手术。最常见的手术指征是大量出血、大量气体泄漏和心脏压塞。

锐性损伤最常累及心脏，尤其锁骨中线上的前部伤口。这些损伤可能导致心脏压塞，如果心包有缺损，出血会渗出到胸腔。休克在胸部锐性损伤患者中是紧急开胸的指征。然而，对于生理学参数正常的靠近心脏伤口的患者的处理却存在问题。最保守和安全的做法是把所有这类患者送入手术室进行剑突下心包开窗，如果需要，随后经过胸骨正中切口开胸。近来报道认为，早期心脏超声检查对隐蔽的心脏损伤是敏感的检查，这个技术可以用在需要心包开窗的选择性患者身上，能使不必要的创伤性操作降低到最低[10,57,62]。在一份报告中，只有心脏超声显示心包渗出的患者需要进行剑突下心包开窗。如果发现血液，随后胸骨正中切口开胸。对心脏超声显示正常的患者进行临床观察。Harris 等人[28]报告了一项有关锐性心脏损伤的大型经验性研究，建议在稳定的患者进行心脏超声检查诊断这些疾病。

当锐性心脏损伤需要手术时，经过缺损置入一个 Foley 导管能临时控制出血，有助于缝合缺损。对已控制的心脏损伤，最好行胸骨正中切口开胸。

并发症

在儿童，有关胸部损伤的死亡率和外科处理的并发症的文献资料几乎没有。两个最常见的术后并发症是肺不张和肺炎。最严重的是截瘫，在胸主动脉损伤病例中的发生率是 5%～10%。

结果

胸部损伤死亡的危险基于损伤的类型和合并损伤的数量及严重程度而不同，尤其是是否有中枢神经系统损伤。Roux 和 Fisher[71]报道了南非的 100 个连贯的机动车相关的胸部创伤儿童案例。91 例步行者成为最大的亚组。8 例患者死亡，平均创伤严重程度评分是 34，而存活者的平均评分是 25。8 例死亡儿童中有 7 例死于致命性头部损伤。因此儿童的钝性胸部损
92 伤、损伤的严重性和伴随的头部损伤是决定存活的主要因素。在儿童，由于胸部损伤造成的死亡多在损伤后的最初几天内发生，常是因为其他损伤，而不是成人病例中的呼吸衰竭和败血症。

胸部损伤的总的死亡率在 NPTR 中是 15%，实际上和大多数成人报道一样[12]。死亡率随胸部损伤不同而不同，膈肌破裂 30%，心脏损伤 40%，大血管损伤 50%。

幸存者致病率明显降低。DiScala[14]报道，在 NPTR 中，90%的幸存者在出院时没有功能缺损。

总结

下面几点总结了儿童胸部损伤的治疗：

1. 大多数胸部损伤能通过临床评估并结合胸部平片来诊断。
2. 大多数胸部损伤患者通过支持治疗和胸腔引流可以痊愈。
3. 致命性胸部损伤不常见。
4. 少数胸部损伤需要手术，但如果能确诊和及时治疗，即使是最严重的胸部损伤也可以成功治疗。

（顾　硕译　吕志葆校）

参考文献

1. American College of Surgeons: Advanced Trauma Life Support Program for Physicians. Chicago, American College of Surgeons, 1993.
2. Banks E, Chun J, Weaver F: Chronic innominate artery dissection after blunt thoracic trauma: Case report. J Trauma 1995;38:975.
3. Bergman K, Spence L, Wesson D, et al: Thoracic vascular injuries: A post mortem study. J Trauma 1990;30:604.
4. Bertrand S, Laquay N, El Rassi I, et al: Tricuspid insufficiency after blunt chest trauma in a nine-year-old child. Eur J Cardiothorac Surg 1999;16:587.
5. Bhende MS, Thompson AE: Evaluation of an end-tidal CO_2 detector during pediatric cardiopulmonary resuscitation. Pediatrics 1995;95:395.
6. Blackmore CC, Zweibel A, Mann FA: Determining risk of traumatic aortic injury: How to optimize imaging strategy. AJR Am J Roentgenol 2000;174:343.
7. Bokhari F, Brakenridge S, Nagy K, et al: Prospective evaluation of the sensitivity of physical examination in chest trauma. J Trauma 2003;54:1255.
8. Bonadio WA, Hellmich T, Wisconsin M: Post-traumatic pulmonary contusion in children. Ann Emerg Med 1989;8:1050.
9. Brandt M, Luks FI, Spigland NA, et al: Diaphragmatic injury in children. J Trauma 1992;32:298.
10. Carillo EH, Guin BJ, Ali AT, et al: Transthoracic ultrasonography is an alternative to subxiphoid ultrasonography for the diagnosis of hemopericardium in penetrating precordial trauma. Am J Surg 2000;179:34.
11. Chen MY, Miller PR, McLaughlin CA, et al: The trend of using computed tomography in the detection of acute thoracic aortic and branch vessel injury after blunt thoracic trauma: A single-center experience over 13 years. J Trauma 2004;56:783.
12. Cooper A, Barlow B, DiScala C, String D: Mortality and truncal injury: The pediatric perspective. J Pediatr Surg 1994;29:33.
13. DelRossi AJ, Cernaianu AC, Madden LD, et al: Traumatic disruptions of the thoracic aorta: Treatment and outcome. Surgery 1990;108:864.
14. DiScala C: Biannual Report. National Pediatric Trauma Registry, 1995.
15. Dunham MB, Zygun D, Petrasek P, et al: Endovascular stent grafts for acute blunt aortic injury. J Trauma 2004;56:1173.
16. Dyer DS, Moore EE, Ilke DN, et al: Thoracic aortic injury: How predictive is mechanism and is chest computed tomography a reliable screening tool? A prospective study of 1561 patients. J Trauma 2000;48:682.

17. Eddy AC, Rusch VW, Fligner CL, et al: The epidemiology of traumatic rupture of the thoracic aorta in children: A 13-year review. J Trauma 1990;30:989.
18. End A, Rodler S, Oturanlar D, et al: Elective surgery for blunt cardiac trauma. J Trauma 1994;37:798.
19. Eren S, Balci AE, Ulku R, et al: Thoracic firearm injuries in children: Management and analysis of prognostic factors. Eur J Cardiothorac Surg 2003;23:888.
20. Exadaktylos AK, Sclabas G, Schmid SW, et al: Do we really need routine computed tomography scanning in the primary evaluation of blunt chest trauma in patients with "normal" chest radiograph? J Trauma 2001;51:1173.
21. Fabian TC, Richardson JD, Croce MA, et al: Prospective study of blunt aortic injury: Multi-center trial of the American Association for the Surgery of Trauma. J Trauma 1997;42:374.
22. Fernandez L, Radhakrishna J, Gordon RT, et al: Thoracic BB injuries in pediatric patients. J Trauma 1995;38:384.
23. Frame SB, Thompson TC: Blunt cardiac injuries. Adv Trauma Crit Care 1995;10:15.
24. Garcia V, Gottschall CS, Eichelberger MR, et al: Rib fractures in children: A marker of severe trauma. J Trauma 1990;30:695.
25. Gavant ML, Menke PG, Fabian T, et al: Blunt traumatic aortic rupture: Detection with helical CT of the chest. Radiology 1995;197:125.
26. Gittleman MA, Gonzalea-del-Rey J, Brody AS, et al: Clinical predictors for the selective use of chest radiographs in pediatric blunt trauma evaluations. J Trauma 2003;55:670.
27. Hall A, Johnson K: The imaging of paediatric thoracic trauma. Paediatr Respir Rev 2002;3:241.
28. Harris DG, Bleeker CP, Pretorius J, et al: Penetrating cardiac injuries—current evaluation and management of the stable patient. S Afr J Surg 2001;39:90.
29. Harris GJ, Soper RT: Pediatric first rib fractures. J Trauma 1990;30:343.
30. Hirsch R, Landt Y, Porter S, et al: Cardiac troponin I in pediatrics: Normal values and potential use in the assessment of cardiac injury. J Pediatr 1997;130:853.
31. Hochheiser GM, Clark DE, Morton JR: Operative technique, paraplegia, and mortality after blunt traumatic aortic injury. Arch Surg 2002;137:434.
32. Holmes JF, Sokolove PE, Brant WE, et al: A clinical decision rule for identifying children with thoracic injuries after blunt torso trauma. Ann Emerg Med 2002;39:492.
33. Hormuth D, Cefali D, Rouse T, et al: Traumatic disruption of the thoracic aorta in children. Arch Surg 1999; 134:759.
34. Horton TG, Cohn SM, Heid MP, et al: Identification of trauma patients at risk of thoracic aortic tear by mechanism of injury. J Trauma 2000;48:1008.
35. Hoth JJ, Scott MJ, Bullock TK, et al: Thoracotomy for blunt trauma: Traditional indications may not apply. Am Surg 2003;69:1108.
36. Hu J, Wall MJ Jr, Estrera AL, et al: Surgical management of traumatic pulmonary injury. Am J Surg 2003; 186:620.
37. Janson JT, Harris DG, Pretorius J, et al: Pericardial rupture and cardiac herniation after blunt chest trauma. Ann Thorac Surg 2003;75:754.
38. Karmay-Jones R, Hoffer E, Meissner M, et al: Management of traumatic rupture of the thoracic aorta in pediatric patients. Ann Thorac Surg 2003;75:1513.
39. Kasirajan K, Heffernan D, Langsfield M: Acute thoracic aortic trauma: A comparison of endoluminal stent grafts with open repair and nonoperative management. Ann Vasc Surg 2003;17:589.
40. Kleinman P, Mark SE, Spevak MR, et al: Fractures of the rib head in abused infants. Radiology 1992;185:119.
41. Knudtson JL, Dort JM, Helmer SD, et al: Surgeon-performed ultrasound for pneumothorax in the trauma suite. J Trauma 2004;56:527.
42. Kulshrestha P, Munshi I, Wait R: Profile of chest trauma in a level I trauma center. J Trauma 2004;57:576.
43. Kwon CC, Gill IS, Fallon WF, et al: Delayed operative intervention in the management of traumatic descending thoracic aortic rupture. Ann Thorac Surg 2002;74:1888.
44. Langanay T, Verhoye JP, Corbineau H, et al: Surgical treatment of acute traumatic rupture of the thoracic aorta—timing reappraisal? Eur J Cardiothorac Surg 2002;21:282.
45. Langer JC, Winthrop AL, Wesson DE, et al: Diagnosis and incidence of cardiac injury in children with blunt thoracic trauma. J Pediatr Surg 1989;24:1091.
46. Le Bret F, Ruel P, Rosier H, et al: Diagnosis of traumatic mediastinal hematoma with transesophageal echocardiography. Chest 1994;105:373.
47. Lomoschitz FM, Eisenhuber E, Linnau KF, et al: Imaging of chest trauma: Radiological patterns of injury and diagnostic algorithms. Eur J Radiol 2003;48:61.
48. Magid N, Glass T: A "hole in a rib" as a sign of child abuse. Pediatr Radiol 1990;20:334.
49. Mandavia DP, Joseph A: Bedside echocardiography in chest trauma. Emerg Med Clin North Am 2004;22:601.
50. Manson D, Babyn PS, Palder S, et al: CT of blunt chest trauma in children. Pediatr Radiol 1995;23:1.
51. Maron BJ, Gohman TE, Kyle SB, et al: Clinical profile and spectrum of commotio cordis. JAMA 2002;287:1142.
52. Matthews BD, Bui H, Harold KL, et al: Laparoscopic repair of traumatic diaphragmatic injuries. Surg Endosc 2003; 17:254.
53. Meller JL, Little AG, Shermeta DW: Thoracic trauma in children. Pediatrics 1984;74:813.
54. Melton SM, Kerby JD, McGiffin D, et al: The evolution of chest computed tomography for the definitive diagnosis of blunt aortic injury: A single-center experience. J Trauma 2004;56:243.
55. Mirvis SE, Shanmuganathan K: MR imaging of thoracic trauma. Magn Reson Imaging Clin N Am 2000;8:91.
56. Moore EE, Burch JM, Moore JB: Repair of the torn descending thoracic aorta using the centrifugal pump for partial left heart by-pass. Ann Surg 2004;240:38.
57. Nagy K, Lohmann C, Kim DO, et al: Role of echocardiography in the diagnosis of occult penetrating cardiac injury. J Trauma 1995;38:859.
58. Nakayama DK, Ramenofsky ML: Chest injuries in childhood. Ann Surg 1989;210:770.
59. Nakayama DK, Rowe MI: Intrathoracic tracheobronchial injuries in childhood. Int Anesthesiol Clin 1988;26:42.
60. Ott MC, Stewart TC, Lawlor DK, et al: Management of blunt thoracic aortic injuries: Endovascular stent versus open repair. J Trauma 2004;56:565.
61. Parker MS, Matheson TL, Rao AV, et al: Making the transition: The role of helical CT in the evaluation of potentially acute thoracic injuries. AJR Am J Roentgenol 2001;176:1267.
62. Patel AN, Brennig C, Cotner J, et al: Successful diagnosis of penetrating cardiac injury using surgeon performed ultrasonography. Ann Thorac Surg 2003;76:2046.
63. Patel HN, Hahn D, Comess KA: Blunt chest trauma: Role of intravascular and transesophageal echocardiography in cases of abnormal thoracic aortogram. J Trauma 2003;55:330.
64. Peterson RJ, Tepas JJ 3rd, Edwards FH, et al: Pediatric and

adult thoracic trauma: Age-related impact on presentation and outcome. Ann Thorac Surg 1994;58:14.
65. Place RJ, Cavanaugh DG: Computed tomography to diagnose pericardial rupture. J Trauma 1995;38:882.
66. Powell RW, Gill EA, Jurkovich GJ, et al: Resuscitative thoracotomy in children and adolescents. Am Surg 1988;54:188.
67. Pross M, Manger T, Mirow L, et al: Laparoscopic management of late-diagnosed major diaphragmatic rupture. J Laparoendosc Adv Surg Tech A 2003;10:111.
68. Razzouk AJ, Gundry SR, Wang N, et al: Repair of traumatic aortic rupture: A 25-year experience. Arch Surg 2000; 135:913.
69. Reinoso-Barbero F, Sanabria P, Bueno J, et al: High-frequency ventilation for a child with traumatic bronchial rupture. Anesth Analg 1995;81:183.
70. Renton J, Kincaid S, Ehrlich PF: Should helical CT scanning of the thoracic cavity replace the conventional chest x-ray as a primary assessment tool in pediatric trauma? An efficacy and cost analysis. J Pediatr Surg 2003;38:793.
71. Roux P, Fisher RM: Chest injuries in children: An analysis of 100 cases of blunt chest trauma from motor vehicle accidents. J Pediatr Surg 1992;27:551.
72. Rowan KR, Kirkpatrick AW, Liu D, et al: Traumatic pneumothorax detection with thoracic US: Correlation with chest radiography and CT—initial experience. Radiology 2002;227:305.
73. Rubin GD: CT angiography of the thoracic aorta. Semin Roentgenol 2003;38:115.
74. RuDusky BM: Myocardial contusion culminating in a ruptured pseudoaneurysm of the left ventricle—a case report. Angiology 2003;54:359.
75. Salehian O, Mulji A: Tricuspid valve disruption and ventricular septal defect secondary to blunt chest trauma. Can J Cardiol 2004;20:231.
76. Sarihan H, Abes M, Akyazici R, et al: Traumatic asphyxia in children. J Cardiovasc Surg (Torino) 1997;38:93.
77. Scorpio RS, Wesson DE, Smith CR, et al: Blunt cardiac injuries in children: A postmortem study. J Trauma 1996; 41:306.
78. Shabb BR, Taha M, Nabbout G, et al: Successful delayed repair of a complete transection of the right mainstem bronchus in a five-year-old girl: Case report. J Trauma Injury Infect Crit Care 1995;38:964.
79. Shorr R, Crittenden M, Indeck M, et al: Blunt thoracic trauma: analysis of 515 patients. Ann Surg 1987;206:200.
80. Swaanenburg JC, Klaase JM, DeJongste MJ, et al: Troponin I, troponin T, CKMB-activity and CKMB-mass as markers for the detection of myocardial contusion in patients who experienced blunt trauma. Clin Chim Acta 1998; 272:171.
81. Sybrandy KC, Cramer MJ, Burgersdijk C: Diagnosing cardiac contusion: Old wisdom and new insights. Heart 2002;89:485.
82. Taskinen SO, Salo, JA, Halttunen PE, et al: Tracheobronchial rupture due to blunt chest trauma: A follow-up study. Ann Thorac Surg 1989;48:846.
83. Tatou E, Steinmetz E, Jazayeri S, et al: Surgical outcome of traumatic rupture of the thoracic aorta. Ann Thorac Surg 2000;69:70.
84. Tellez DW, Hardin WD Jr, Takahashi M, et al: Blunt cardiac injury in children. J Pediatr Surg 1987;22:1123.
85. Thomas P, Saux P, Lonjon T, et al: Diagnosis by video-assisted thoracoscopy of traumatic pericardial rupture with delayed luxation of the heart: Case report. J Trauma 1995;38:967.
86. Wang JN, Tsai YC, Chen SL, et al: Dangerous impact—commotio cordis. Cardiology 2000;93:124.
87. Williams RL, Connolloy PT: In children undergoing chest radiography what is the specificity of rib fractures for non-accidental injury? Arch Dis Child 2004;89:490.
88. Wilson A, Wall MJ Jr, Maxson R, et al: The pulmonary hilum twist as a thoracic damage control procedure. Am J Surg 2003;186:49.
89. Worthy S, Kang EY, Hartman TE, et al: Diaphragmatic rupture: CT findings in 11 patients. Radiology 1995; 194:885.

第 17 章

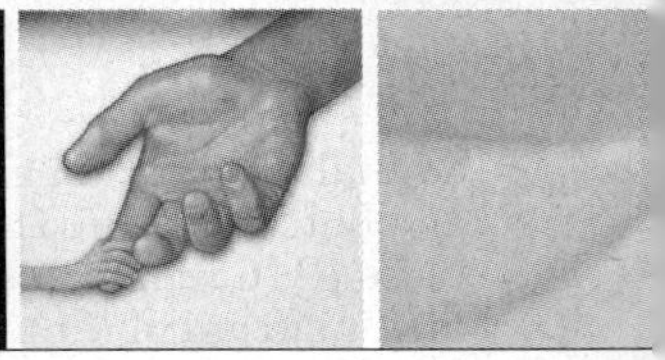

腹部创伤

Steven Stylianos 和 Richard H. Pearl

谁能想象 1968 年 Simpson 发表的关于对可能有
295 脾脏损伤的儿童行选择性非手术治疗取得成功的论文的影响呢[142]？20 世纪 50 年代初期，Toronto 儿童医院的外科主任 Warnsborough 最先提出这种建议。随着 1956—1965 年间 12 例脾脏损伤保守治疗的成功，脾脏损伤的非手术治疗时代由此开始。这组患者的脾脏损伤是通过临床表现、常规实验室检查以及放射线平片做出诊断的。要知道这个报道早于超声、计算机断层扫描（CT）或同位素影像检查。后来，有一个儿童脾脏损伤的诊断是在数年后因为不相关疾病而行剖腹探查术时才确定的，此时，其破裂的脾脏已经愈合成两个独立的部分。40 多年后的今天，对于血流动力学稳定的儿童脾脏损伤，非手术治疗是标准的治疗方法，这个原则现已成功应用于治疗肝脏、肾脏和胰腺等许多脏器的钝性损伤。随着对受伤儿童的解剖模式和生理反应的认识逐渐增加，手术控制变成现在的准则。我们在成人创伤中心的同事已逐渐认识到这个方法的成功，并将许多从儿童创伤中学来的处理原则应用到他们的患者身上[79]。

最近一项国家儿科创伤登记（NPTR）的回顾性研究指出，儿童钝性损伤中 8%～12%有腹部损伤[28]。幸运的是他们中 90%以上可以存活。尽管腹部损伤比胸部损伤多 30%，但腹部损伤可能致命的却比胸部损伤的少 40%。儿童腹部损伤很少需要开腹，这使外科医生在治疗儿童创伤治疗中的作用成为一个辩论的问题。近来对 NPTR 和国家创伤数据库的分析强调，在所有属于外科性质的儿童创伤患者中，超过 25%的受伤儿童需要手术干预[1,141]。很显然，合格的儿童创伤外科医生将是这个治疗的理想人选。

外科医生很少具有手术治疗严重腹腔实质脏器损伤的丰富经验。因此外科医生急需熟悉致命性腹部损伤的当前的治疗流程。对儿童腹部损伤的诊断和治疗的重要贡献要归功于放射科医生和内镜医生。CT 的分辨率和速度、腹部创伤急诊超声检查（FAST）的显示能力和经皮、血管造影以及内镜介入等，这些儿童创伤组的非手术成员的工作可加强患者的治疗并改善预后。本章集中讨论儿童比较常见的损伤和特有的治疗方法。肾脏和泌尿生殖器的损伤将在第 18 章讨论。

诊断方法

儿童急性创伤的初期评估与成人的相似。在初期检查和 ABC 评价（气道、呼吸、循环）后，进行颈椎、胸部和骨盆的 X 线平片检查。其他腹部平片很少用于儿童创伤患者的急性评估。随着影像学诊断技术的发展，在怀疑腹部损伤的儿童中，治疗方法有了重大改变。在大多数儿童中迅速发现潜在的致命性损伤已经成为可能。

计算机断层扫描

基于 CT 有许多优点，CT 现已经成为评估儿童创伤的首选影像学检查。CT 检查在大多数医疗机构都能进行，是鉴别和确定腹部损伤程度的无创和准确方法，可降低非治疗性剖腹探查手术的发生率。

静脉使用造影剂动态扫描可以使血管和实质性组织获得理想的增强效果。在钝性脾脏和肝脏损伤的儿童，对比显影的重要性还有争议，稍后将讨论（图 17-1）[35]。如果有指征，首先行头颅 CT 平扫，以避
免漏诊出血性脑损伤。因为会导致误吸，胃肠道 29
（GI）增强造影一般在急性创伤处理中不需要。

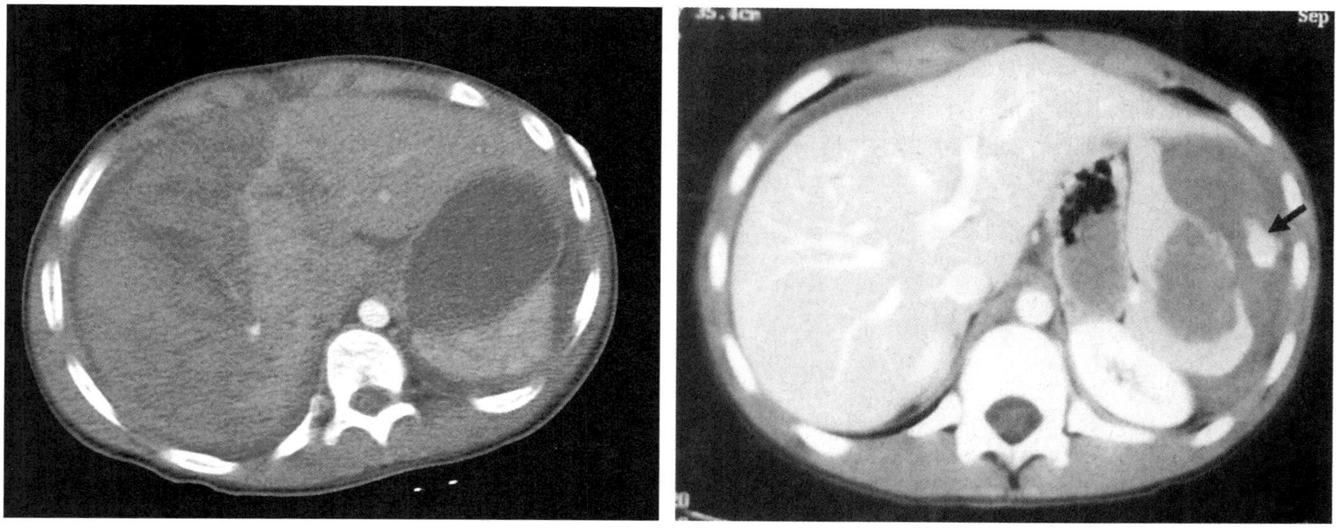

A　　B

图 17-1 A. 腹部 CT 静脉增强扫描显示右肝叶明显损伤。该患者成功应用血管造影栓塞治疗，避免了手术。B. 腹部 CT 静脉增强扫描显示脾脏明显损伤（箭头所示）。该患者保持血流动力学稳定而避免了手术。

不是所有腹部损伤儿童都要做 CT。明显锐性损伤经常需要立即手术干预。血流动力学不稳定的儿童不应该从复苏室带出去做 CT。这些儿童可以选择其他诊断性检查并从中获益，如腹腔灌洗或 FAST，或紧急手术干预。创伤时腹部 CT 的最大限制是不能识别小肠破裂[11,15]。提示但不能诊断小肠穿孔的 CT 表现有：气腹、肠壁增厚、腹腔内游离液体、肠壁增强和肠管扩张[59]。儿童肠损伤高度怀疑的表现是：腹腔内有液体而 CT 检查没有确定的实质脏器损伤[127]。小肠损伤的诊断和治疗将在后面详细讨论。

腹部创伤急诊超声检查

早期由临床医生进行超声检查来评估受伤儿童是最理想的。检查 Morrison 窝、Douglas 窝，检查左侧季肋部，包括脾周解剖。腋下观察心包，采用标准的 FAST 四点检查法（图 17-2）。尤其是当患者非常不稳定而不能去做腹部 CT 扫描时，这种床边检查可能是最好的快速影像学诊断。早期研究已发现，FAST 在儿童中是有效的影像学检查方法，对识别小肠损伤
7 的特异性高（95%），但敏感性较低（33%）[103]，没有发现明显的游离液体不能排除重要损伤。FAST 能降低“可能性”损伤的 CT 扫描次数。根据临床情况

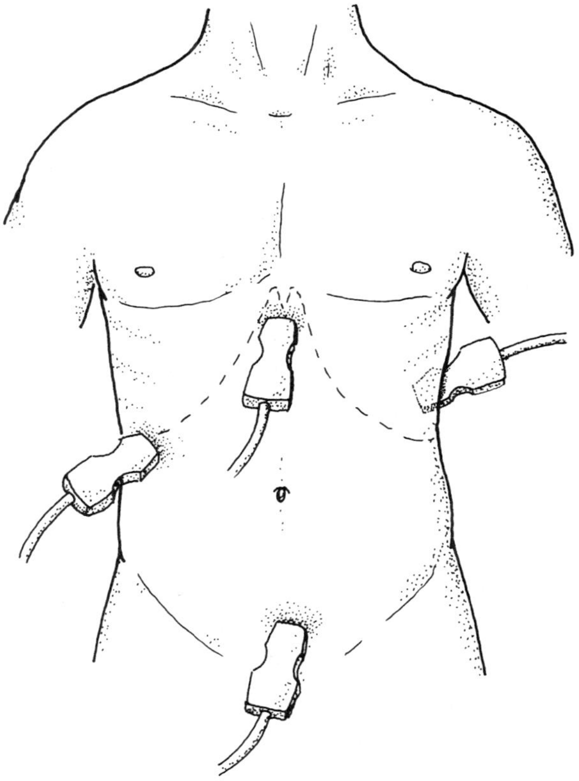

图 17-2 腹部创伤急诊超声检查（FAST），强调观察腋下，右上象限和 Morrison 窝，左上象限和左结肠旁区，和盆腔区域和 Douglas 窝。(Original illustration by Mark Mazziotti, MD.)

重复检查是必要的，发现游离液体并不是手术干预的指征。近来在一项儿童钝性腹部损伤的小样本研究中，是用估计腹腔出血量的一个简单评分系统来预测是否需要开腹手术[101]。对这种 FAST 评分需要进行前瞻性验证。

诊断性腹腔灌洗和腹腔镜检查

诊断性腹腔灌洗（DPL）成为创伤评估的主要手段已经超过 30 年。然而，该方法在儿童创伤中的作用有限。因为超过 90%的实质脏器损伤不需要手术干预，所以通过 DPL 发现腹腔游离血液的临床意义不大。对于腹腔实质脏器损伤而腹腔无血液的患者，血流动力学不稳定和需要持续输血是决定手术的因素。另外，CT 检查的速度和准确性进一步降低了 DPL 在儿童创伤中的应用指征。CT 诊断实质脏器损伤、十二指肠、胰腺和小肠的隐匿损伤的敏感性在不断提高，从而削弱了 DPL 在评估临床怀疑小肠损伤而 CT 没有确定诊断的患者中的作用。在这些患者中，DPL 出现胆汁、食物残渣或其他胃肠道穿孔的证据具有诊断性价值。近来文献建议，腹腔镜不仅能用于诊断还能用于外科治疗，进一步限制了 DPL 的使用。来自 Dundee 和 Scotland 的一组研究显示，DPL 和腹腔镜的敏感性都很高（100%），但腹腔镜有更高的特异性（94%对 83%）[29]。

在成人的前瞻性大样本试验表明，腹腔镜检查可提高诊断的准确性，降低非治疗性剖腹探查的比例，明显缩短住院时间，减少费用。例如，在 Tennessee 大学的一份报告中，55%的腹部创伤患者在腹腔镜评估后避免了剖腹探查[37]。纽约 Jacobi 医疗中心的类似研究也显示了阴性探查的减少及增加腹腔镜诊断与治疗之间的直接关联[126]。多项成人的研究已经显示，腹腔镜不仅可应用在创伤评估方面，而且也可应用于相关损伤的治疗。腹腔镜下修补胃肠穿孔、膀胱破裂、肝脏裂伤、膈肌损伤和脾脏损伤均有报道[21,128,140]。可行性手术的扩展直接与外科医生的技巧及患者的整体稳定性相关。在 Illinois 儿童医院，最近我们应用腹腔镜成功治疗了 2 例因车把导致肠穿孔的患者。同选择性腹部手术一样，随着创伤中心直接用该方法培训住院医生，更多的儿童中心也报道了腹腔镜处理儿童创伤的结果[20,44,52]。

实质脏器损伤

脾脏和肝脏

脾脏和肝脏是钝性腹部损伤最常见的受累器官，各占损伤的 1/3。在单独的脾脏或肝脏损伤且血流动力学稳定的儿童，采取非手术治疗普遍取得成功，现在已成为标准方法。然而，不同小儿外科医生的治疗方法有很大差异。NPTR 的回顾和美国小儿外科医生协会的成员调查显示，在临床实践中存在较大差异[38,133]。争论同样存在于 CT 分级的实用性及增强显影的发现是否可作为肝脾损伤预后的指征[49,82,89,106]。近来一些研究报告：在钝性脾脏损伤儿童中，CT 增强显影达 7%～12%（图 17-1）[25,76,99]。显影组手术的比例接近或超过 20%。作者强调，CT 增强显影比较麻烦，但大多数患者通过保守治疗可取得成功。儿童脾脏损伤中血管造影栓塞的作用还没有确定。

近来 APSA 创伤学会分析了 1995—1997 年北美 32 个中心的 832 名非手术治疗儿童的同期资料（表 17-1）[135]。对单独脾脏或肝脏损伤且血流动力学稳定的儿童（CT I～IV 级）在重症监护室、住院时间、影

表 17-1 832 名有单独脾脏或肝脏损伤的儿童通过 CT 分级的资源利用和活动限制

	I 级 (n=116)	II 级 (n=341)	III 级 (n=275)	IV 级 (n=100)
入住 ICU（%）	55.0	54.3	72.3	85.4
住院天数（平均）	4.3	5.3	7.1	7.6
住院天数（范围）	1～7	2～9	3～9	4～10
输血（%）	1.8	5.2	10.1*	26.6*
剖腹探查（%）	0	1.0	2.7†	12.6†
影像随访（%）	34.4	46.3	54.1	51.8
活动限制（平均周数）	5.1	6.2	7.5	9.2
活动限制（周数范围）	2～6	2～8	4～12	6～12

* III 级与 IV 级比较，$P<0.014$。

† III 级与 IV 级比较，$P<0.0001$。

CT：计算机断层扫描；ICU：重症监护室。

From Stylianos S, APSA Trauma Committee: Evidence-based guidelines for resource utilization in children with isolated spleen or liver injury. J Pediatr Surg 2000;35:164-169.

表 17-2 对 CT 分级的单独脾脏或肝脏损伤儿童的资源利用的建议指南

	I 级	II 级	III 级	IV 级
ICU 天数	0	0	0	1
住院天数（天）	2	3	4	5
出院前影像	无	无	无	无
出院后影像	无	无	无	无
活动限制（周）*	3	4	5	6

CT：计算机断层扫描；ICU：重症监护室。

* 回到全接触，竞争性运动（如足球、摔跤、曲棍球、长曲棍球、登山）应该有专业儿童创伤外科医生来判定。建议指南是指回到无限制的活动，包括与正常年龄相适应的活动。

From Stylianos S, APSA Trauma Committee: Evidence-based guidelines for resource utilization in children with isolated spleen or liver injury. J Pediatr Surg 2000;35:164-169.

像随访和活动限制方面达成意见一致的指南。随后在1998—2000 年，这个指南在 16 个中心用于 312 名脾脏或肝脏损伤未行手术的儿童[136]。有其他轻微损伤（如没有移位的非粉碎性骨折或软组织损伤）但不影响研究结果的患者也包括进来。患者按照 CT 分级判定的损伤程度分组。指南提出，按年龄、器官损伤和损伤分级等参数来分析，所有患者随访至损伤后 4 个月。必须强调，这个指南提出的假设是基于血流动力学稳定。极低的输血和手术比例证明了患者的稳定性。

特别指南的依从程度是：入住 ICU 81%，住院时间 82%，影像随访 87%，活动限制 78%。从第一年到第二年依从性有明显的进步，比如住 ICU 的时间（77%对 88%，$P<0.02$）和活动限制（73%对 87%，$P<0.01$）。而在年龄、性别或损伤器官上的依从性没有差别。指南的偏差中，外科医生选择的占病例的 90%，患者相关的仅占 10%。6 例患者（1.9%）再次入院，但是不需要手术。对比原先研究的 832 名患者，按照推荐指南进行前瞻性处理的 312 名患者明显减少了每组患者入住 ICU 的时间（$P<0.0001$）、住院时间（$P<0.0006$）、影像随访（$P<0.0001$）和体力活动限制的时间（$P<0.04$）。

从这些资料中可以得出的结论是：基于创伤严重程度的特殊治疗指南前瞻性应用在患者处理、改善资源利用和指南安全性确认方面其结果一致。与回顾性资料比较，明显减少了住 ICU 的时间、住院时间、影像随访和活动限制，且没有相关的并发症。

主治医生对脾脏或肝脏损伤决定是否手术最好基于持续血液丧失的证据，如低血压、心动过速、尿量减少和血细胞比容下降以及对晶体液和输血没有反应。目前在大多数儿童创伤中心和拥有强大的儿科团队的成人创伤中心，单纯钝性脾脏和肝脏损伤非手术治疗的比例已经超过 90%（H. N. Lovvorn，个人交流）[87,135,136]。NPTR 的一项超过 100 例患者的研究显示，肝脏、脾脏损伤同时合并头部损伤，即使血流动力学稳定，也是非手术治疗指征[63]。钝性脾脏和肝脏损伤的手术干预比例在是否合并闭合性头颅损伤的患者中无明显差异。

一点也不奇怪，成人创伤机构治疗儿童创伤患者有极高的存活率；然而，治疗脾脏或肝脏损伤的一项分析显示，手术治疗比例之高令人担忧[42,64,87,113]。因为大部分严重儿童创伤不是在专门的儿童创伤中心治疗的，所以手术比例的差异强调了宣传指南的重要性。Mooney 和 Forbes[88]回顾了 1990 年代新英格兰儿童创伤资料，有明确脾脏损伤的儿童为 2500 例，其中 2/3 是由非儿童创伤外科医生治疗的，2/3 是在非创伤中心治疗的。在考虑到多患者相关和医院相关的变量后，作者发现，曾接受过儿科训练的外科医生治疗儿童脾脏损伤时手术风险将降低一半。Rothstein 等人[114]使用 KIDS 2000 管理数据库做了相似的回顾，发现尽管调整了患者和医院相关变量，与儿童专科医院相比，成人综合性医院治疗的儿童进行脾脏切除手术的几率要高 2.8 倍 ($P<0.003$)，有儿科部门的综合性医院则高 2.6 倍 ($P<0.013$)。

成人创伤外科医生治疗受伤儿童时必须考虑儿童和成人创伤患者在解剖、免疫和生理方面的差别，并在治疗原则中有所显示。主要关心的问题是输血增加的潜在危险、遗漏合并损伤和住院时间的延长。通过比较已经显示这些问题都不能得到更好处理[78,86,90,95,104,118,133]。

合并的腹部损伤

对脾脏损伤提倡外科干预的学者认为，如果不做手术会遗漏合并的腹部损伤。Morse 和 Garcia[90]报道了 120 名脾脏损伤的儿童，其中 110 名（91%）非手术治疗成功，且其中 22 名（18%）有合并的腹部损伤。这 120 名患者中只有 3 名（2.5%）有胃肠道损伤，都是因为在早期具备特殊指征行剖腹手术时发现 299

的。没有因为遗漏合并损伤或延迟手术而死亡。同样，NPTR 的一项 1988—1998 年的回顾研究显示，在 2977 个腹腔实质脏器损伤的患者中，只有 96 人（3.2%）合并有空腔脏器损伤[95]。在受暴力打击的患者中，多发性实质脏器损伤和胰腺损伤的患者合并空腔脏器损伤的发生率更高。因为损伤机制的不同可能可以解释脾脏损伤儿童合并腹部损伤发生率的差异。在儿童，单纯进行剖腹探查术以避免遗漏潜在的合并损伤是不正确的。

非手术治疗的并发症

非手术治疗方案在过去 20 年里已经成为大多数儿童钝性肝脏和脾脏损伤的治疗标准。该经验使我们可以评价非手术方法的优缺点。非手术治疗策略成功的根本在于出血能够在早期自发的停止。儿童单纯脾脏或肝脏损伤的输血比例已经降到 10%以下，确定大多数患者没有持续的血液丢失[73,82,87,135,136]。尽管有许多正面报道，但关于延迟性出血严重的副作用也有个别报道[13,40,46,123]。Shilyansky 等人[123]报道了 2 例钝性肝脏损伤后 10 天延迟出血的病例。这两个儿童尽管生命体征和血细胞比容正常，但都有持续的右上象限腹痛和右肩痛。作者推荐持续的院外观察直到症状缓解。其他报道已有描述 II 级脾脏损伤后 38 天和 IV 级肝脏损伤后 24 天的明显出血患者[13,40]。这些罕有的现象提示在恢复无限制活动前要警惕一个最短的安全期。

常规影像随访常常可以发现在脾脏损伤后的假性囊肿和假性动脉瘤（H. N. Lovvorn，个人交流）[41,98]。脾脏假性动脉瘤常没有症状并随时间而消失。自限性的创伤后脾脏假性动脉瘤的确切的发生率还不清楚，因为成功的非手术治疗后，大多数不能坚持常规影像随访。血管造影栓塞技术能成功地治疗这些病灶，避免手术和损失脾脏实质（图 17–3）。脾脏假性囊肿体积可以很大，导致疼痛和胃肠道功能失调（图 17–4）。单纯经皮抽吸有很高的复发率。腹腔镜下切除和袋形缝合术有很好的效果（图 17–5）。

紧急控制策略的结局

如果能对复苏迅速做出反应，即使是最严重的实质脏器损伤也能在不需要手术的情况下获得治疗[108]。而在输液和输红细胞后血流动力学还不稳定的患者，需要紧急剖腹探查、栓塞或二者同时进行。大多数需要手术的脾脏和肝脏损伤对简单的止血方法有较好反应，这些止血方法有手法压迫、直接缝合、局部止血药和网眼包扎[14,72]。在有严重肝脏损伤的患儿，迅速打开胸骨暴露肝上或心包内的下腔静脉，以完全游离肝血管（图 17–6）[150]。只要血容量充足，儿

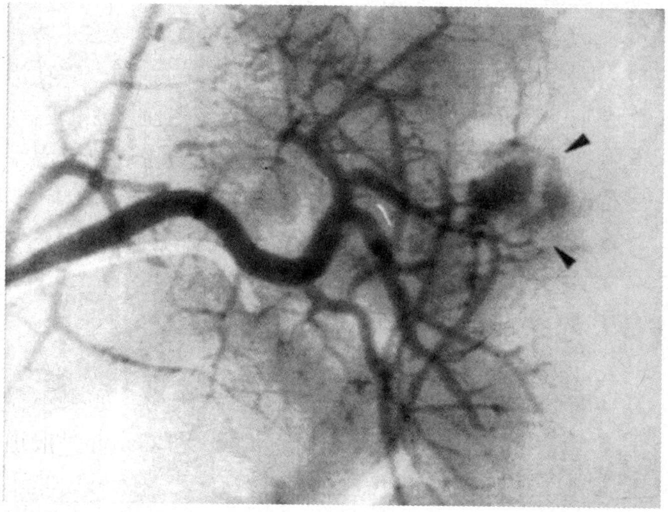

A

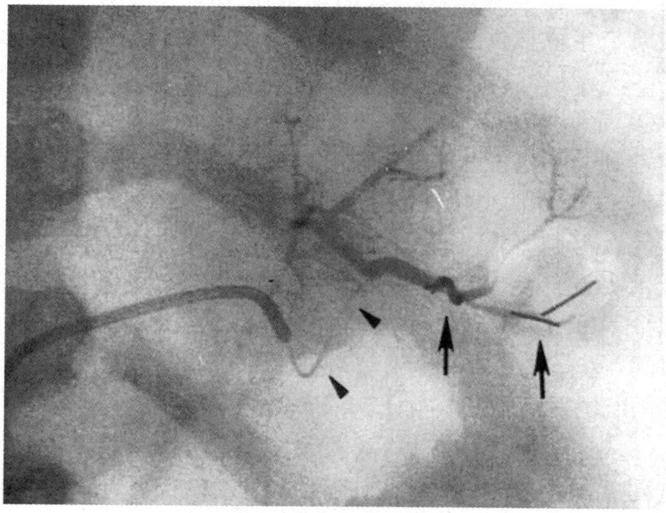

B

图 17–3 A. 钝性脾脏损伤非手术治疗后脾脏假性动脉瘤（箭头所示）。B. 成功的血管造影栓塞（箭头显示破裂血管闭合）。

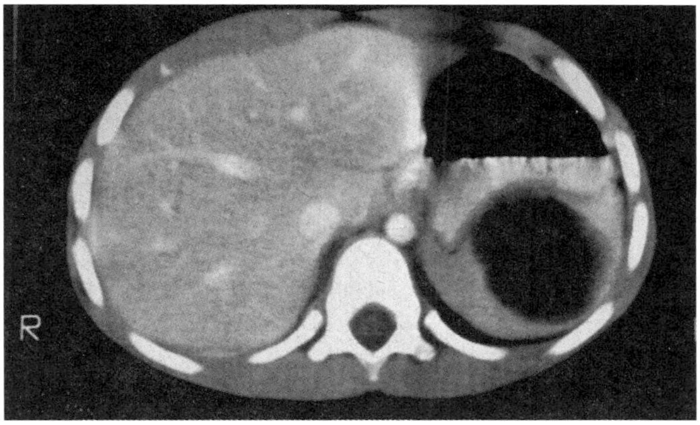

图 17–4 创伤后脾脏假性囊肿的计算机断层扫描成像。

童可以耐受 30 分钟或更长时间的血管阻断。通过这些暴露，肝和主要肝周静脉能得到游离并控制出血，允许直接缝合修补或结扎受损的血管。复杂和危险的心房和腔静脉转流技术已经不再使用，新的血管内球囊导管法可以临时闭塞血管以暴露近肝下腔静脉[4]。

早期的严重肝损伤的致病率和死亡率与大量失血及大量输注冷的血制品有关。手术时间太长和大量输血会导致体温过低、凝血功能障碍和酸中毒。尽管外科手术组尽力抢救，致命性的生理性和代谢性改变仍然不可避免，一旦生理储备耗尽，这些患严重疾病的患者将会死亡。对 8 个学院创伤中心的 537 名患者的研究显示，失血占手术中患者死亡原因的 82% [57]。死亡前，平均 pH 是 7.18，而平均核心体温是 32℃。在 Moulton 等人[93]报道的 12 名肝后血管或严重肝实质损伤的接受手术的儿童患者中，只有 5 例存活（42%）。

在外科控制严重出血期间保持生理状态稳定，即使对最有经验的外科手术组来说也是困难的挑战，尤其当发生体温过低、凝血功能障碍和酸中毒时。这
个三联征建立了一个恶性循环，彼此相互影响，这 301
些生理和代谢的紊乱经常妨碍手术的完成。由稀释、体温过低和酸中毒所致的致命性凝血功能障碍可很快发生[145]。实验性研究已经确定了在不同程度的低体温时，凝血酶原和抗凝血酶、血小板激活和血小板黏附缺陷的变化[147]。

在急诊腹部手术中强调生理和代谢的稳定已经引起阶段性的、多学科治疗计划的发展，包括简短的剖腹手术、肝周填塞、临时腹部关闭、血管造影栓塞和内镜胆管支架置入术[5,32,45,69,149]。Asensio 等人[6]报道了 1991—1999年治疗的 103 例大多数肝脏损伤在 IV 到 V 级的患者，平均失血约 9.4 升，在手术室平均输液量是 15 升。在第一次手术中有 50%的患者使用肝脏的包裹技术，其中有 40%的患者在初次手术控制出血后接受血管造影栓塞（图 17–7）。存活率在 IV 级损伤患者是 63%，在 V 级患者是 24%，提示尽管有较好的手术设计，考虑到分期并采用多学科联合的方法，这类损伤仍然具有较强的致命性。治疗儿童严重损伤的创伤外科医生必须熟悉这些救命的技术。

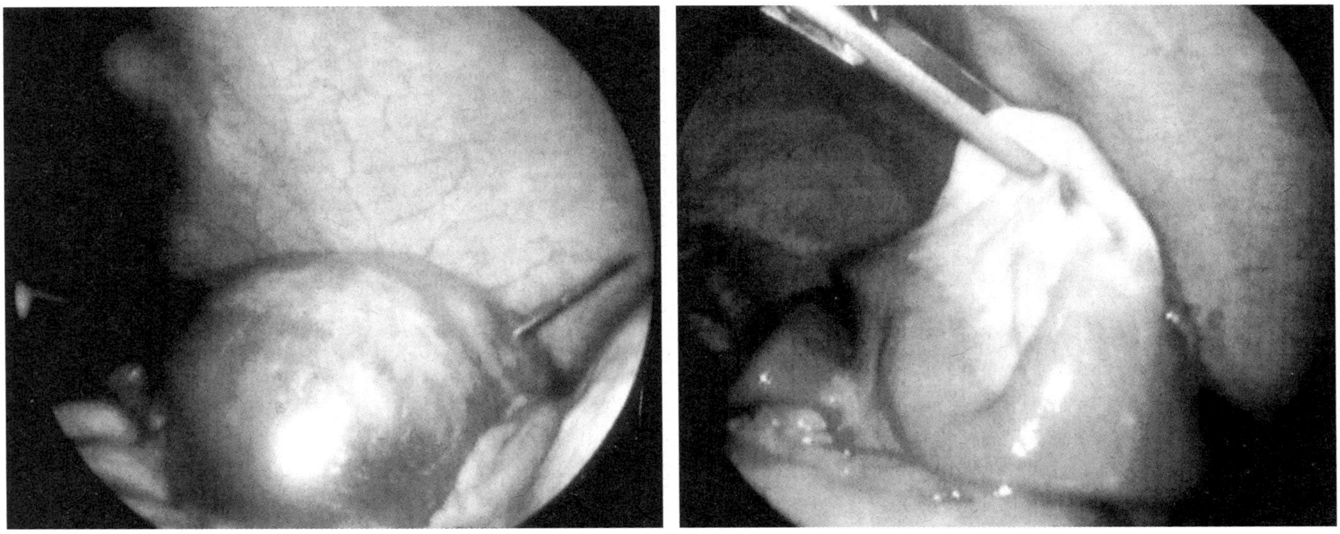

A B

图 17–5 A. 脾脏假性囊肿包膜在腹腔镜下的图像。B. 袋形缝合术前和腹腔镜抽吸后显示的囊肿壁。

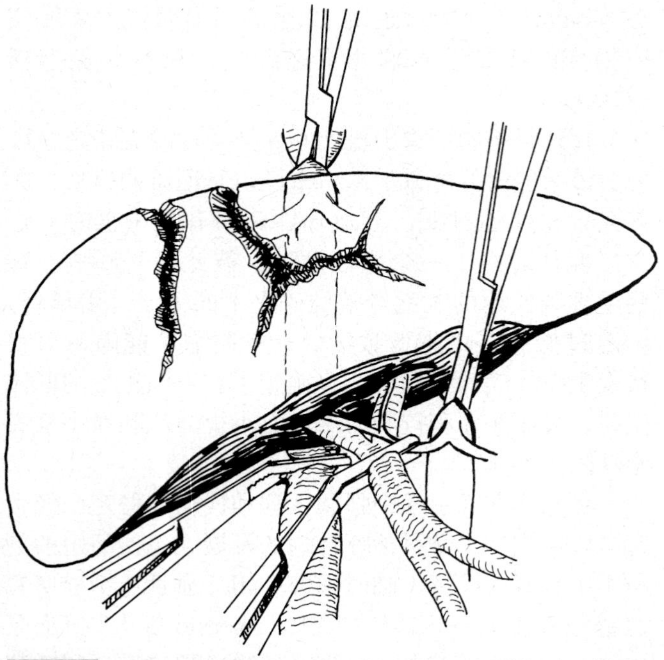

图 17-6 通过阻断门静脉、肝上和肝下下腔静脉和上腹部动脉(可选)，完全游离肝血管。(Original illustration by Mark Mazziotti, MD.)

简短剖腹探查填塞止血，给再次手术争取了复苏时间，对不能控制出血的患儿是另一种可选的治疗方案。这种“损害控制”原理是系统、分期治疗创伤失血的患者[8,119,143]。损害控制的三个阶段详见表 17–3。尽管有争论，复苏终点不仅包括传统的生命体征和尿量，

表 17–3 创伤失血患者的“损害–控制”策略

1 期	简短手术探查
	控制出血和污染
	填塞和临时关闭腹壁
2 期	积极 ICU 复苏
	恢复身体核心温度
	使血容量和氧的传输达到理想状态
	纠正凝血功能障碍
3 期	再次手术取出填塞物
	确定损伤的修补
	关闭腹壁

ICU：重症监护室

还包括血清乳酸盐、碱缺失、混合静脉血氧饱和度和胃黏膜 pH。一旦患者复温，输注凝血因子和给氧，患者回到手术室取出填塞物并确定损伤修补。一项研究回顾了一些机构用腹部填塞包裹治疗的近 700 例患者，发现止血成功率为 80%，存活 32%～73%，腹腔脓肿比例 10%～40%[26,53]。尽管在过去 20 年里先填塞、再手术的方法在成人中的使用增加，但在儿童中应用的报道很少[30,36,56,80,115,132,134,138]。虽然如此，我们仍然相信这个技术可以应用到钝性损伤后大量腹腔出血的儿童中。

我们曾经报道 1 例 3 岁的儿童，有严重肝脏损伤不能关闭腹腔而需要腹腔填塞[138]。我们构造了一个硅胶的“silo”袋来容纳肠管，直到可以取出填塞物， 30

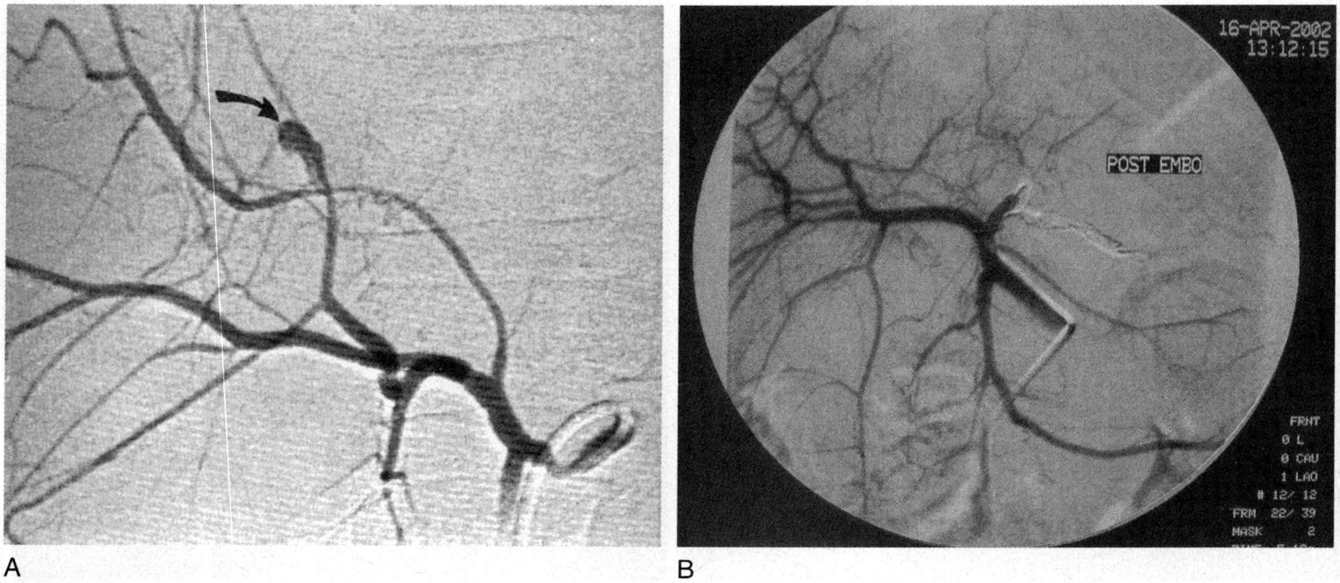

A B

图 17–7 A. 在初期损害–控制剖腹探查手术后持续出血患者的肝动脉血管造影。出血的血管被确定（弯箭头）。B. 实施了成功栓塞。

最后患者彻底康复。填塞和 silo 的结合技术为纠正低体温、酸中毒和凝血功能障碍争取了时间，而没有呼吸方面的危害。一项回顾性研究报道 22 例婴儿和儿童（6 天到 20 岁），由于难以控制出血而需要腹腔填塞[134]。出血的解剖位置在肝脏或肝静脉的有 14 例，腹膜后腔和骨盆的 7 例，胰腺床 1 例。其中 12 例患者完成一期关闭（55%），其他 10 例临时皮肤闭合或使用假体材料。在 22 例患者中 21 例（95%）通过填塞控制出血，18 例（82%）患者在 72 小时内取出填塞物，取出填塞物后患者没有再出血，2 例填塞物尚未取出的患者死亡。7 例患者发生腹部或盆腔脓肿，但都通过剖腹探查（6 例）或经皮穿刺（1 例）而成功引流。7 例腹腔败血症的患者中 6 例存活。总体上，18 例（82%）患者存活。2 例患者因为多器官功能衰竭死亡，一个是因为复杂心脏畸形导致的心力衰竭，另一个是因为钝性肝脏损伤后的失血。存活组和非存活组在手术中血制品输注、开始填塞时间、生理状态或腹部关闭类型上没有差异。

尽管腹腔填塞的效果令人鼓舞，但这可导致严重的疾病发生，如腹腔内败血症、器官衰竭和腹腔内压力增加。腹腔内填塞物被皮肤和肠道菌丛污染，但这些生物体和后来引起患者败血症相关的细菌不同[48]。Adams 等人[2]评估了 28 个腹部填塞患者的液体样本，发现即使是在培养无菌的情况下，腹腔内仍有内毒素和中间产物的蓄积。作者认为剖腹探查术后填塞物液体积聚受损的原因主要是中性粒细胞功能障碍，由于中性粒细胞突发性呼吸增强和中性粒细胞对抗感染所需的趋化性受到抑制。因此，已知的这些患者腹腔内和全身感染倾向可能与中性粒细胞受体状态和与腹腔炎症介质积聚有关的效应器的功能有关。可考虑采用早期清除、重复填塞和其他减少介质积聚的方法。

必须强调在出现不可逆的休克前实施简短手术和再手术是成功的关键。如果不采用腹部填塞作为长时间止血失败后的最后的方法，那么往往会导致失败。腹腔填塞的指征有生理和解剖标准。在大量出血需要大量输注血制品的患者中，大多数指征是手术中的参数，包括 pH（～7.2）、核心体温（＜35℃）和凝血值（凝血酶原时间＞16 秒）。

再次探查的理想时间仍然有争议，因为复苏的生理性终点和延长填塞增加的感染风险都没有明确。填塞提供止血带来的明显好处的同时，增加的腹内压对通气、心排出量、肾脏功能、肠系膜循环和颅内压有潜在损害作用。及时的缓解继发的腹腔间隔综合征可能是拯救患者的关键。填塞时临时关闭腹壁能防止腹腔间隔综合征。我们建议临时关闭腹壁应扩展到所有需要填塞的患者，直到出血停止和内脏水肿消退。

对不稳定创伤患者分期手术策略显示了外科治疗的进步，还需要合理的评估和一定的技术水平。控制大量出血的腹腔内填塞用于有凝血功能障碍、低体温和酸中毒的患者，对这种患儿过多的手术操作会带来生命危险。

腹腔间隔综合征

腹腔间隔综合征一词是描述增加的腹腔内压所产生的有害作用[116]。腹腔间隔综合征包括由于严重的通气–弥散比例失调而致的呼吸不足、由于下腔静脉压迫导致前负荷减小引起的血流动力学的变化、肾脏血管压迫导致的肾脏功能破坏、心排出量减少、通气压增高引起的颅内高压、血流灌注不足和过度腹壁膨胀。创伤患者，导致腹腔内高压的因素包括血腹、腹腔后间隙或肠水肿和腹腔及盆腔填塞物的使用。组织和血流动力学休克可以诱发一系列事件，包括毛细血管漏、缺血–再灌注及血管活性介质和自由基的释放，这些组合增加了细胞外容量和组织水肿。实验显示持续腹腔内压力升高可以导致细胞因子明显改变[100,112]。一旦组织水肿和腹腔内液体的影响很大时，必须考虑腹部减压。

腹腔间隔综合征的不良作用已经逐渐发现，然而，腹腔间隔综合征只在最近才被发现其致命性以及潜在的可治疗性[122,149]。因为大容量复苏规则的应用，近年来该综合征的发生率明显升高。腹腔内压力的测量有益于确定腹腔间隔综合征对生理和代谢参数的影响，腹腔内压力可以由测定膀胱压力来决定[19,31,52]。这包括向 Foley 导管慢慢注入 1ml/kg 盐水并连接到一个
压力转换器或通过一个三通连接到测压计。耻骨联合 303
通常是零点，压力用厘米水柱或毫米汞柱来测量。腹内压力在 20～35cm H_2O 或 15～25mm Hg范围是腹部减压的指征。有些人提出根据其他生理或代谢参数的改变而不是特定的压力测量值来进行干预。Chang 等人[19]报道了 11 例有腹腔间隔综合征的成人创伤患者，他们使用肺动脉导管和胃张力测量法改善了前负荷、肺功能和内脏灌注。对于只有脑外伤而没有腹部腹腔

间隔综合征表现的患者的难治性颅内高压，采用无对照的减压剖腹探查手术进行降压治疗已经获得成功[85]。

在儿童中腹腔间隔综合征的腹部减压经验有限[31,34,97,122,134,138]。在腹腔间隔综合征的儿童，非特异性腹部 CT 发现包括下腔静脉变窄、直接肾脏压迫和移位、增强时肠壁增厚和腹部圆形形态[34]。Neville 等人[97]报道了对 23 例婴儿和儿童使用补片腹壁成形术，其中只有 3 例是创伤患者。这些作者发现，对腹腔间隔综合征使用腹壁成形术有效降低了气道压力和对氧的需求。对气道压力或吸入氧气分数下降无反应，对这些患者来说是不利的症状。有些作者已经发现，对腹腔间隔综合征的儿童进行腹部减压会导致气道压力下降、氧张力升高和尿量增加[31,97,122]。

许多材料在临时补片腹壁成形术中得到使用，包括硅橡胶薄膜、Gore-Tex 膜片、静脉注射袋、膀胱镜检查袋、造口术装置和不同的网眼物质（图 17-8）。在成人成功使用的真空包装技术很有前景[8,80,139]。

胆道损伤

儿童钝性肝脏损伤的非手术治疗有较高的成功率，但有 4%并发持续胆漏[10,117]。在怀疑胆道损伤时推荐应用放射核素扫描[120]。即使早期显影正常，延迟显影也可能发现胆漏。有些报道说明了在钝性肝脏损伤后行内镜逆行胰胆管造影术（ERCP）并经壶腹放置胆管支架的优点。尽管 ERCP 是有创性的，也需要患者镇静，但能精确地找到损伤位置，而且可以不用开放手术就能治疗胆管损伤（图 17-9）。内镜下经壶腹放置胆管支架引流是近来治疗持续胆漏的主要方法。对钝性肝脏损伤后持续胆漏患者在 ERCP 时同时切开括约肌的方法用来减低胆管内压和促进内部减压[22,92,121]。需要注意是内镜下胆管支架可能移位或发生梗阻，需要特殊处理。

十二指肠和胰腺损伤

与肝脏、脾脏相比，十二指肠和胰腺的损伤相当少见，在钝性损伤所致的腹腔损伤的儿童中，不到 10%。其中单独十二指肠和胰腺损伤的发生大约占 2/3 病例，其余的则合并有其他器官损伤。十二指肠和胰腺损伤的程度及其合并损伤决定了是否进行手术治疗。“起保护作用”的后腹膜减少损伤机会，但也增加了早期诊断的难度。另外，合并的腹腔内损伤或多系统损伤，都会增加诊断难度。这些损伤能掩盖十二指肠和胰腺损伤的细微的临床和放射诊断表现。

十二指肠

在一个钝性十二指肠损伤的报道中，Ballard 等 304
人[7]回顾了 6 年宾夕法尼亚州的经验。在 28 个创伤中心的 103 864 个登记患者中，十二指肠钝性损伤发生有 206 例（0.2%），其中只有 30 例（14%）有全层破

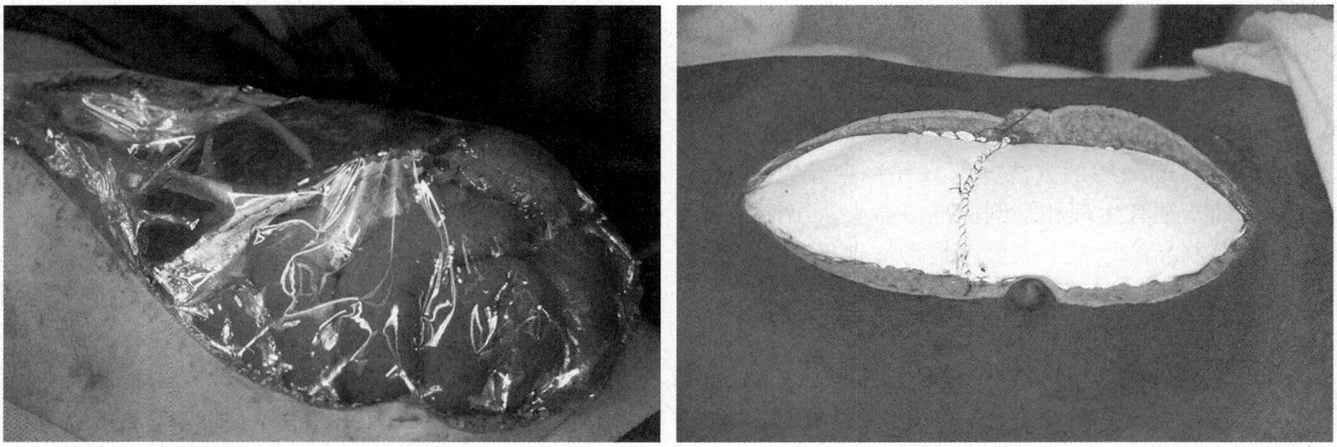

A B

图 17-8 A. 用硅橡胶薄膜进行的腹壁扩张术。B. 用 Gore-Tex 补片进行的腹壁扩张术。

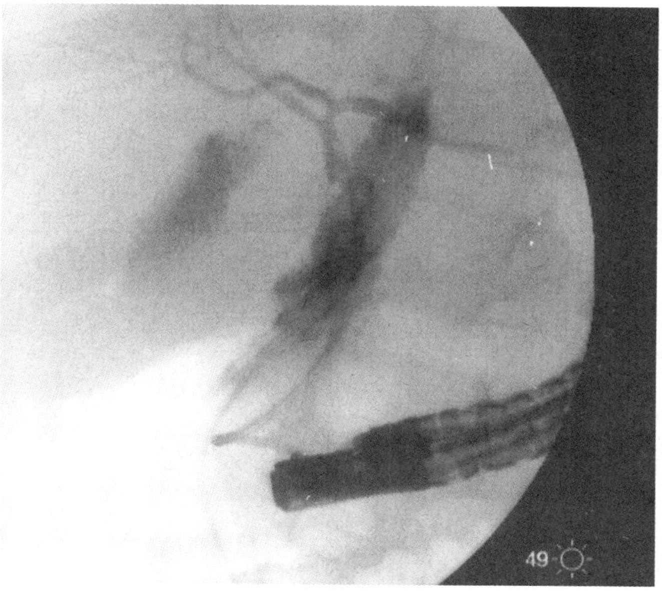

A

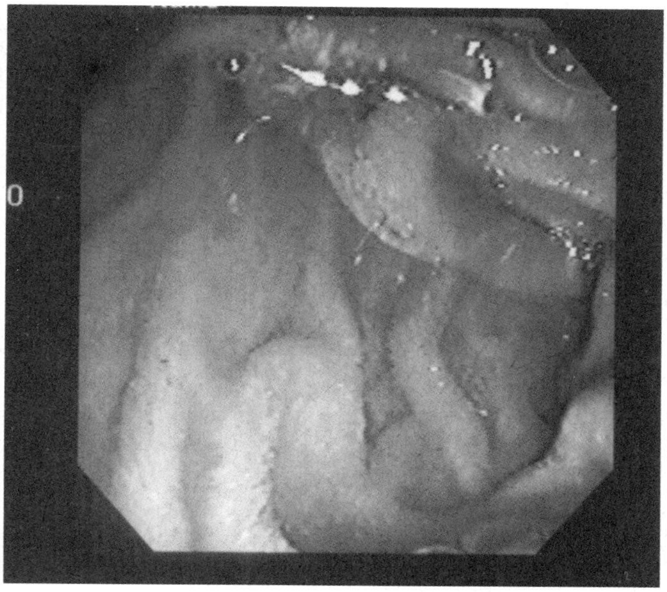

B

图 17-9 A. 内镜逆行胰胆管造影发现钝性肝脏损伤后严重胆漏。B. 经壶腹胆管支架的内镜显示。

裂。损伤的机制中车祸占 70%，包括成人和儿童。这些患者没有明显头部损伤（30 例中的 26 例），92%报道有腹痛或压痛或体检时反跳痛。18 例患者进行了 CT 检查，有后腹膜气体或造影剂外溢表现的占 26%。相同数量的表现是正常的。死亡率是 13%，且不受诊断和治疗延迟的影响。这项研究着重分析了这种损伤的难度，因为只有个别中心（或外科医生）的少量报道。另外，研究者回顾了修补进行的程度——从十二指肠缝合到 Whipple 手术——但是评论不能得出确定的结论，因为患者和许多中心的报道数量很少。

相反，多伦多的一组单中心 10 年（1986—1996 年）的经验研究报告了 27 个遭受钝性十二指肠损伤并接受治疗的儿童（平均年龄 7 岁）[124]。其中 13 个儿童有十二指肠穿孔（平均年龄 9 岁），14 个儿童有十二指肠血肿（平均年龄 5 岁）。19 个患者有合并损伤（10 个胰腺，5 个脾脏，4 个肝脏，2 个长骨骨折，1 个中枢神经系统，1 个肾脏挫伤，1 个空肠穿孔和 1 个胃破裂）。17 个患者是从其他机构转入，平均转运时间 4 小时。穿孔的患者从受伤到手术的平均时间间隔是 6 小时。表 17-4 显示的是十二指肠血肿和穿孔在临床表现、实验室评估和放射学表现上的比较。大多数进行腹部 CT 扫描同时行口服或静脉造影（图 17-10 和 17-11）。这些患者的 CT 结果比较显示在表 17-5。这些资料说明在各组间临床表现十分相似，只

表 17-4 儿童十二指肠血肿和穿孔的体征和症状

患者特征	十二指肠血肿	十二指肠穿孔
数量	14	13
年龄（岁）	5	9*
ISS 得分	10	25*
座椅安全带损伤（%）	6（100）	5（71）
表现		
疼痛或压痛：数量（%）	10（71）	12（92）
擦伤：数量（%）	6（43）	11（85）
GCS 评分	15	15
合并损伤		
胰腺：数量（%）	7（50）	3（23）
腰椎：数量（%）	1（7）	4（31）
总数：数量（%）	11（79）	8（62）
实验室评估		
Hgb：mg%/Hct	12.3/0.36	12.1/0.37
淀粉酶：单位（%）	678（64）	332（46）

* 统计学上有显著差异。

GCS：Glasgow 昏迷评分；Hct：血细胞比容；Hgb：血红蛋白；ISS：损伤程度等级。

From Shilyansky J, Pearl RH, Kroutouro M, et al: Diagnosis and management of duodenal injuries in children. J Pediatr Surg 1997:32: 880-886.

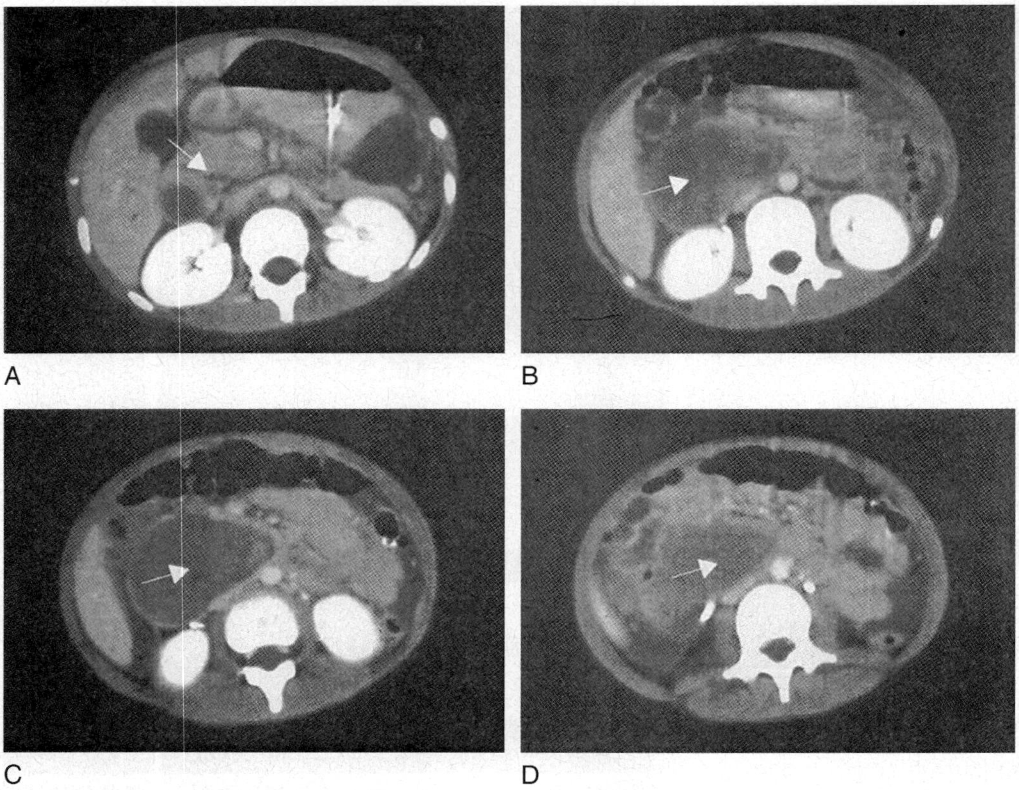

图 17-10 一个 8 岁女孩摔倒在操场上后腹部 CT 发现十二指肠血肿。A. 箭头显示狭窄的十二指肠腔。B 到 D. 箭头指示大的壁内血肿。这个孩子的治疗是鼻胃管吸引和静脉营养。她在损伤后 24 天正常进食。

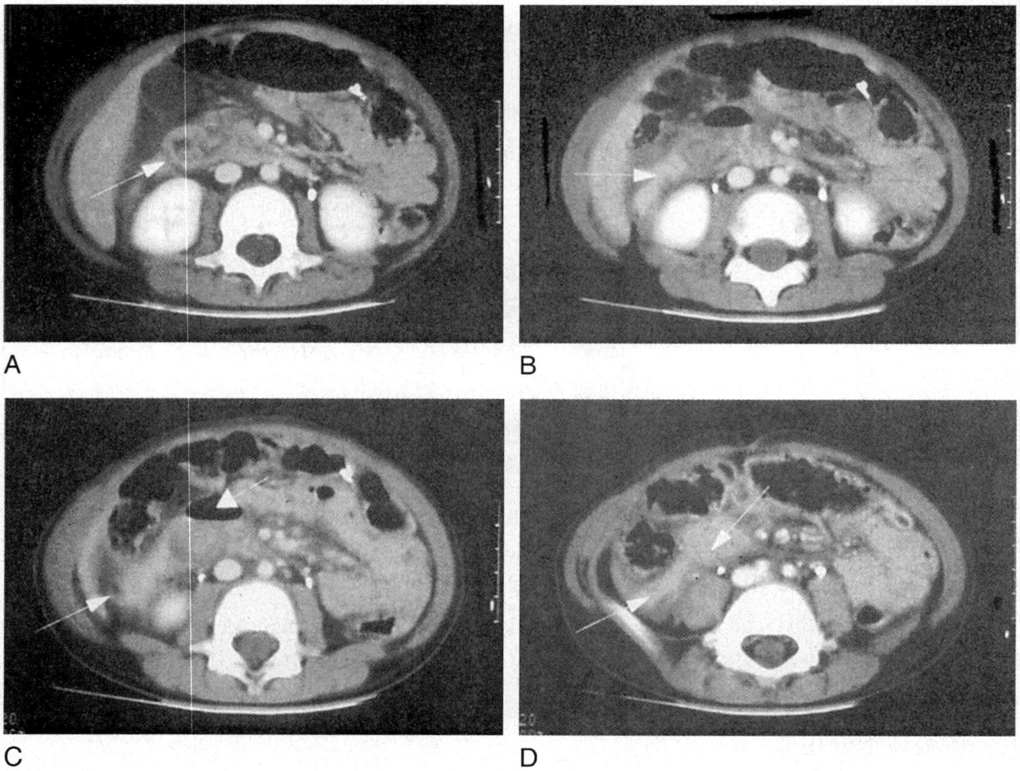

图 17-11 一个 4 岁男孩在机动车意外中腹部 CT 发现的十二指肠穿孔。A. 箭头显示破裂的十二指肠壁。B 到 D. 小箭头指示后腹膜肠道造影剂渗出。C. 大箭头指示后腹膜腔外气体。发现十二指肠第二和第三段的大的缺损。进行了管状十二指肠造瘘和胃空肠吻合。这个儿童在受伤后 5 天开始进食，再过 4 天后回家。

306 有年龄和损伤程度评分有统计学差异（但在个别患者很少有临床相关性）。然而，空气或肠造影剂渗出到后腹膜、十二指肠周围或肾周间隙在每个十二指肠穿孔的儿童中都有发现（9 个患者中发现 9 个），但在十二指肠血肿的 10 个儿童中却没有发现。作者注意到文献中一些先前的报道，描述了这些十二指肠损伤患者的特殊 CT 表现，但无论是综合期刊还是专业期刊，先前的研究都没有关于儿童患者的报道。来自同一中心的一个 1986 年的报道总结了 24 例十二指肠血肿患者，都采取非手术治疗[146]。该报道和前面的报道结果一样。CT 扫描（或可疑患者行 GI 造影检查）显示十二指肠狭窄、螺旋状或没有渗出的梗阻对所有患者都具有诊断意义。最近的 14 例非手术患者，鼻胃管减压的时间是 12 天（平均），给予静脉营养的时间是 18 天（平均）。14 个患者中 13 个症状在伤后平均 16 天时缓解。另外一个儿童发生慢性纤维性狭窄而在伤后 49 天行十二指肠成形术。该儿童还伴有胰腺挫伤。

St. Louis 儿童医院的 Desai 等人[33]回顾了对 24 例腹部十二指肠钝性损伤患者的处理经验[33]。有 19 个十二指肠血肿（15 个通过 CT 诊断，4 个通过 GI 检查诊断），其中 17 个采取非手术治疗。对于 5 个穿孔患者，其中 4 个接受了简单缝合修补。来自盐湖城和匹兹堡的经验发现，十二指肠损伤的常见原因是儿童虐待，尤其是很小的患者[24,43]。因此，如果描述的损伤病史或机制和急性损伤矛盾，单独十二指肠损伤应该高度怀疑儿童虐待。

在所有这些研究中，对十二指肠穿孔患者都采取了不同方法的手术治疗，这些方法的采用是根据损伤的程度和外科医生的喜好。我们建议一期缝合十二指肠穿孔（只要有可能）。一期缝合可以结合十二指肠引流和要么胃空肠吻合术（图 17–12）加幽门缝合，要么胃引流及空肠造口术营养支持。这些外科方法降低了十二指肠瘘的发生率，缩短了胃肠道营养的时间和住院时间。当面对有并发症的十二指肠创伤时，有效的组合是三管技术：十二指肠缝合（一期修补，浆膜补片，或吻合），同时行十二指肠引流减压（管1），经胃造口用可吸收的缝线进行幽门旷置（管 2）和空

表 17–5　儿童十二指肠血肿和穿孔的 CT 表现比较

CT 表现	十二指肠血肿 (n = 10) 数量（%）	十二指肠穿孔 (n = 9) 数量（%）
游离气体	1（10）*	2（22）
游离液体	8（80）	9（100）
后腹膜液体	9（90）	9（100）
肠壁和腹膜增强	2（20）	4（44）
十二指肠口径改变	4（40）	3（33）
增厚的十二指肠	10（100）	8（89）
壁上的血肿	10（100）	0
后腹膜气体	0	8（89）
后腹膜造影剂 †	0	4（57）
后腹膜气体或造影剂	0	9（100）

* 儿童合并空肠穿孔。

† 2 个儿童没有进行肠造影。

From Shilyansky J, Pearl RH, Kroutouro M, et al: Diagnosis and management of duodenal injuries in children. J Pediatr Surg 1997:32: 880-886.

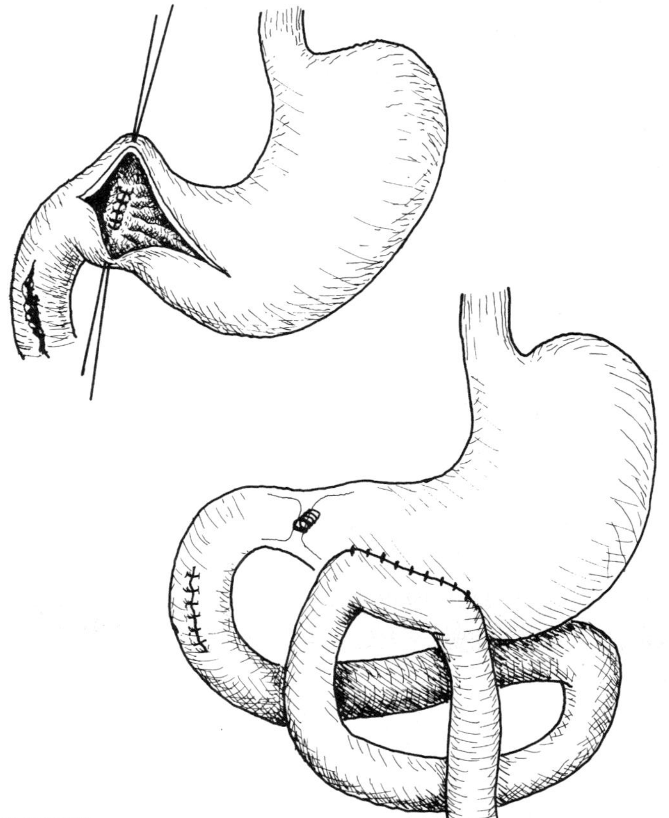

图 7–12　十二指肠侧面损伤行一期修补和包括用可吸收的缝线缝合幽门和胃空肠吻合术。没有描述修补术后的闭式吸引引流。(Original illustration by Mark Mazziotti, MD.)

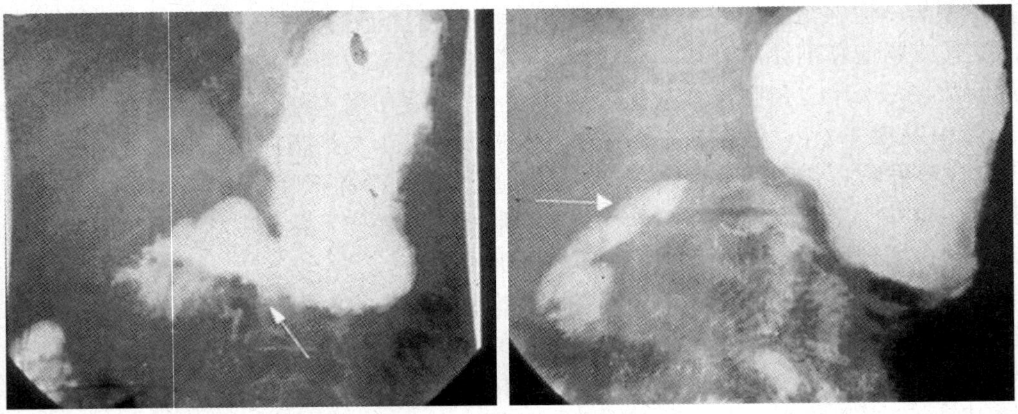

图 17–13 7岁因机动车意外导致的十二指肠穿孔女孩的上消化道检查。患儿接受一期修补、幽门旷置、逆行管状十二指肠造口术、胃空肠吻合术。这个儿童伤后6天接受空肠喂养，伤后12天经口喂养。A. 伤后6周，上消化道检查显示胃空肠吻合自发闭合（箭头所示）。B. 明显开放的幽门（箭头所示）。

肠造口（管3）。当十二指肠缝合后（用可吸收缝线临时关闭幽门），损伤的彻底愈合通常发生在幽门管
307 自发再开放前（图 17–13）。然而，不论外科医生选择哪种修补，文献总结发现，保护十二指肠缝合（引流和排除）和常规肠喂养（胃空肠吻合术或喂养用空肠造口）降低了致病率并缩短了住院时间[39,70]。

外科选择列在表 17–6，举例说明在图 17–12 和 17–14。很少需要采用胰管十二指肠切除术（Whipple 手术）。尽管在文献中偶然有报道，但胰管十二指肠切除术只在主要血液供应已经破坏，而且不能重建的非常严重的十二指肠和胰腺损伤中保留使用[39,70]。

胰腺

胰腺损伤比十二指肠损伤稍微多一些，在儿童钝性腹部损伤中约占 3%～12%[71]。和十二指肠损伤一样，只有个别中心的少量报道，因此不能严格评估其结果。近来，2 个中心（多伦多和圣地亚哥）分别报道了各自在处理钝性胰腺损伤时的不同经验[16,17,61,75,125,144]。这里，我们通过比较这些论文，并结合其他作者的经验来形成整体的治疗建议。

Canty 和 Weinman（圣地亚哥）[17]报道了超过 14

表 17–6 十二指肠创伤的手术选择

修补十二指肠
胃肠道改道（幽门旷置或十二指肠的憩室化）
胃肠减压（置入胃管或胃空肠吻合术）
建立胃肠道的喂养通路（空肠造口管或胃空肠的吻合）
十二指肠减压（十二指肠造口管）
胆管引流
修补区域广泛引流（十二指肠外侧引流）

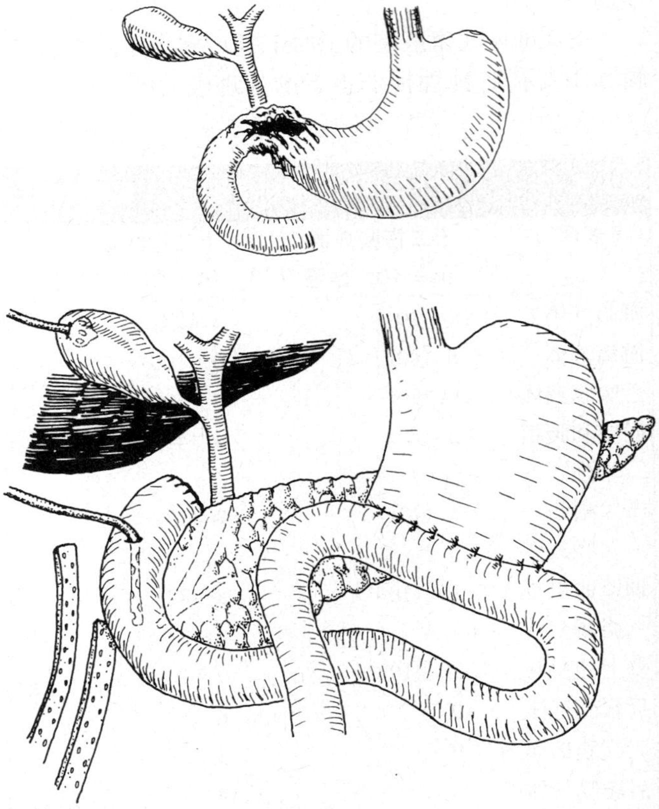

图 17–14 近端十二指肠和胰腺复合伤中十二指肠憩室形成。切除和闭合十二指肠残端，管式十二指肠造口、管式胆囊造口术、胃空肠吻合术和多根闭式吸引引流如图所示。应该强烈推荐建立喂养性空肠造口术（这里没有描述）。(Original illustration by Mark Mazziotti, MD.)

年时间的 18 个严重胰腺损伤的患者。损伤原因是汽车或自行车碾压。18 个患者中 16 入院时做 CT 扫描，其中，11 个提示胰腺损伤，5 个漏诊损伤。对 8 个患者行远端胰腺切除术（44%）。在 6 个近端胰管损伤
308 或初期 CT 漏掉的患者中有 5 个发生假性囊肿，另外 2 个开始症状轻微和入院没有做 CT 扫描的儿童也发生假性囊肿。在这 7 个假性囊肿患者中，2 个自动消退，5 个采取囊肿胃吻合手术治疗。2 个最近治疗的患者接受了 ERCP 并放置导管支架，症状缓解，完全治愈。作者提议远端损伤应该采取胰腺切除术治疗，近端损伤予以观察，假性囊肿进行观察或行囊肿胃吻合术。作者认为急性 ERCP 治疗并放置支架安全有效，CT 具有建议性但不总是对胰腺损伤的类型和部位具有诊断意义[16,17,61]。

来自多伦多的三个报道的经验总结有明显区别[75,125,144]。提示胰腺损伤的 CT 结果详见表 17-7。第一个报道主要是 2 个证实胰腺导管破裂的患者（ERCP 或导管造影）出现导管完全愈合，没有手术干预[75]。随后是 10 年（1987—1996 年）多的连续治疗的 35 例儿童的总结报告[125]。其中 23 个患者早期诊断（＜24 小时），12 个患者延迟诊断（2～14 天）。

表 17-7　儿童胰腺损伤相关的 CT 表现的总结

相关表现	儿童数量
腹腔内液体	21
小囊液体	20
胰腺周围局部液体	20
后腹膜液体	20
右前肾旁液体	16
左前肾旁液体	15
增厚的 Gerota 筋膜（右侧和左侧）	16
肠系膜液体或血肿	13
左后肾旁液体	9
液体分隔脾静脉和胰腺	7
液体围绕肠系膜上静脉和门静脉	7
液体分隔胰腺和十二指肠	6

Data from references 75, 125, 144.

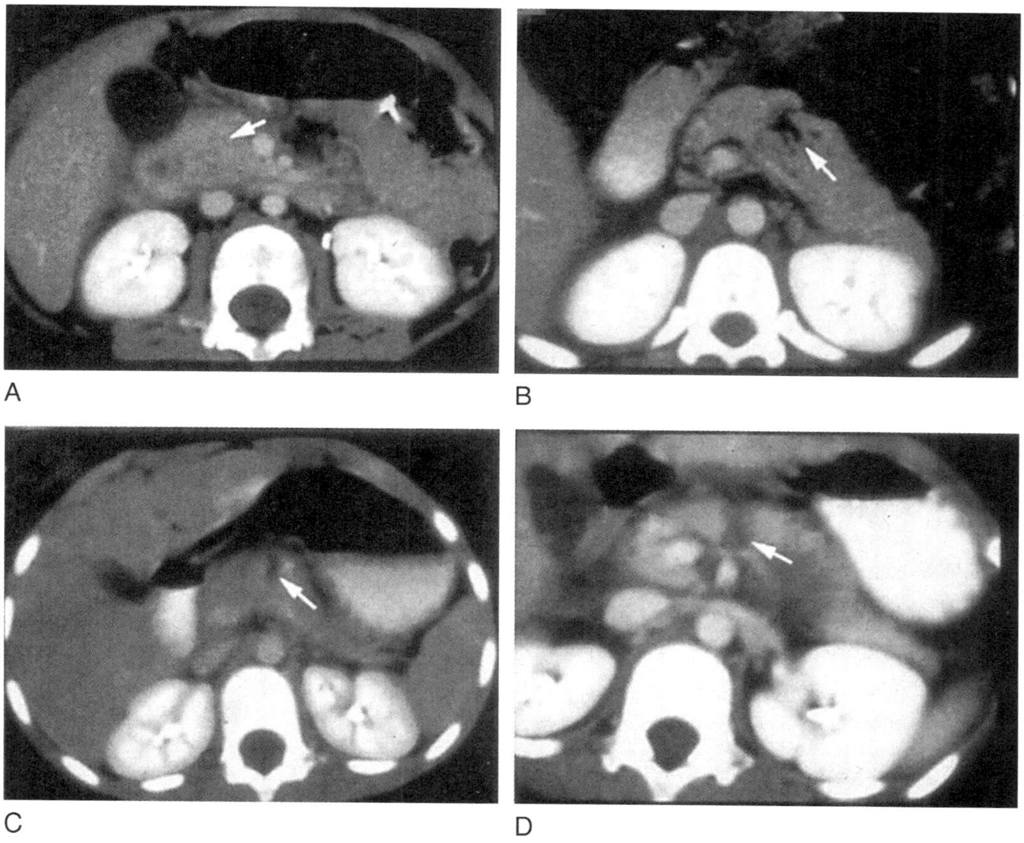

图 17-15　儿童胰腺损伤的 CT 图像。A. 挫伤。B. 星形碎片。C. 部分破裂。D. 横断。

表 17-8 儿童胰腺损伤 CT 表现的建议分级

组（临床）	级别（CT）	胰腺损伤	描述	儿童数量
1	I	挫伤	胰腺弥漫性或局部肿胀	14
2	II	星形碎片	胰腺实质内液体或血液分隔	2
	III	部分破裂	胰腺的两个部分不完全分离	1
3	IV	完全横断	胰腺的两个部分完全分离	8
	V	假性囊肿	持续的胰腺周围液体积聚	3

Data from references 75, 125, 144.

28 个儿童采取非手术治疗，另外 7 个因其他损伤采取手术治疗。28 个非手术治疗的病例，CT 具有诊断意义，显示损伤的五种模式：挫伤、星状碎裂、部分折裂、完全横断和假性囊肿（图 17-15）。患者基于CT分级分到三个临床组（表 17-8）。在这 28 个患者中，发生假性囊肿的有 10 例（第一组 14 个患者中有2个，第二组 11 个患者中有 5 个，第三组 3 个患者有3 个）。第一组没有患者需要引流，而第二组有 4个，第三组全部需要干预处理。这些引流操作发生在受伤后 10～14 天。开始经口喂养的平均时间是 15 天（第
309 一组 11 天，第二组 15 天，第三组 23 天）。所有非手术治疗患者的平均住院时间是 21 天。

圣地亚哥和多伦多的研究的比较情况见表 17-16。这两项研究显著的不同点在于在多伦多研究中 CT 诊断的敏感性为 100%，而在圣地亚哥的研究中是69%，在圣地亚哥病例中手术比例是 44%而在多伦多是 0%。多伦多的一项回顾研究随访了 10 名导管横断的患者[144]。这些儿童中 4 个（40%）发生假性囊肿，其中 3 个经皮引流（图 17-17），平均住院时间是 24 天，所有患者都康复。随访 9 个患者，8 个做了 CT 扫描：其中 6 个远端胰腺萎缩，2 个胰腺完全正常。在平均 47 个月的随访中没有发现外分泌腺的或内分泌腺的功能异常。作者总结在钝性胰腺损伤的非手术治疗后，萎缩（远端）或再通可以发生在所有患者，没有长期致病性。

Dallas 和 Seattle 的报道认为早期对横断于左侧脊柱的病例进行远端胰腺切除术可以缩短住院时间[81,83]。然而，粘连性肠梗阻和内、外分泌腺功能异常的长期后遗症没有得到评价。其他报道证实核磁共振胰腺造影作为诊断工具、早期行 ERCP 干预并行导管支架来诊断和治疗及使用生长抑素来减少胰腺分泌和促进愈合的有效性[12,51,65,111,130]。著名的日本的单中心大系列报

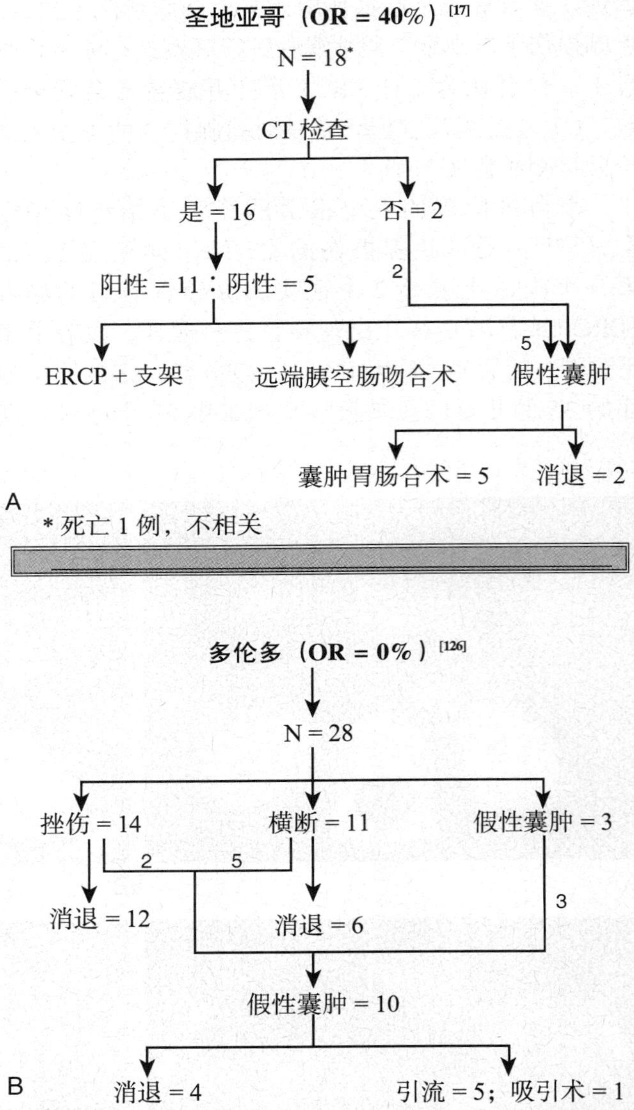

图 17-16 儿童钝性胰腺损伤的治疗方案的比较。A. 圣地亚哥。B. 多伦多。CT：计算机断层扫描；ERCP：内镜逆行胰胆管造影术；OR：手术室。(A, from Canty TG Sr, Weinman D: Management of major pancreatic duct injuries in children. J Trauma 2001;50:1001-1007. B, from Shilyansky J, Sen M, Kreller M, et al: Nonoperative management of pancreatic injuries in children. J Pediatr Surg 1998;33:343-345.)

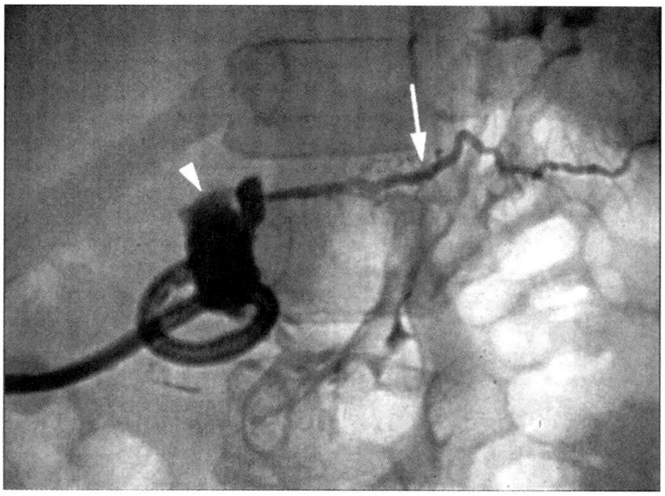

图 17-17 儿童钝性损伤后对胰腺假性囊肿经皮置管引流的造影检查（箭头所示）。主胰腺导管（箭头所示）通畅。假性囊肿消失，没有形成瘘管，未行手术干预。

道了 20 例证实胰腺损伤的儿童，其中 19 例接受非手术治疗（9 例挫伤，6 例撕裂伤，5 例主胰管破裂）[67]。所有病例，都未通过手术而完全康复。该中心关于假性囊肿的形成和治疗及总的结果的经验实质上与多伦多的报道相似。

这些来自大的儿童创伤中心的报告明显有矛盾。一些报道证明了对所有的胰腺损伤实施非手术治疗，包括导管破裂的观察处置的有效性和安全性。其他则倡导积极手术治疗进行清创或切除。因为支持者为这些治疗的每一种方法都提供了资料，因此医院的治疗策略或外科医生的选择将有可能决定选择哪种治疗方案。然而，在脊柱或脊柱左侧行单纯切除胰腺、保留脾脏的远端胰腺切除术疗效确定，并且住院时间短和可接受的致病性（图 17-18）。

由于存在争议，我们认为尽可能实行保守治疗，包括以下方面：

1. 对所有病史、体格检查或损伤机制均提示可能有钝性胰腺损伤的患者早期做螺旋 CT，并经口或静脉对比造影。
2. 损伤证实，并在选择性患者中早期行 ERCP 提供导管支架。
3. 全胃肠外营养的非手术治疗。
4. 对形成的假性囊肿的预期处理。
5. 对有症状的、感染的或增大的假性囊肿行经皮引流。

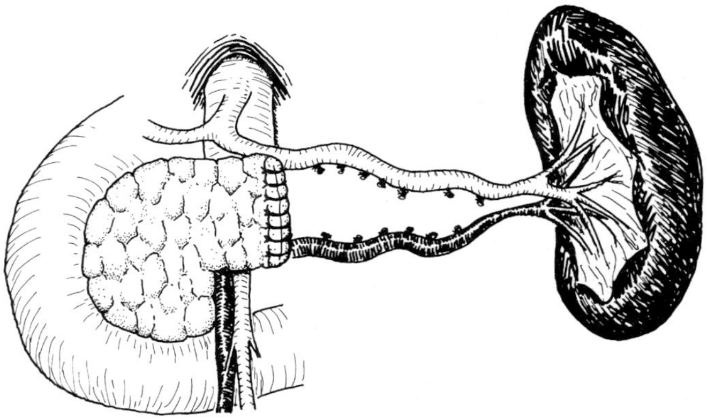

图 17-18 保留脾脏的远端胰腺切除术。(Original illustration by Mark Mazziotti, MD.)

胃、小肠和结肠的损伤

和前面讨论的损伤相比，胃、小肠和结肠的损伤容易诊断和治疗。钝性损伤通过三种不同的机制导致这些器官损伤的特殊模式。第一是发生在胃、空肠、横结肠猛烈压迫在脊柱上的压榨性损伤。可以发生血肿、裂伤、部分或完全横断，伴有即时或延迟发生的穿孔或梗阻。第二，在快速压力传导到一个充满和扩张的空腔脏器时发生爆破性损伤，没有直接的压迫机制。肩带或座位保险带损伤到消化道可以是这种形式。第三是剪切损伤，是由于一端固定的脏器快速加速或减速所致，这些脏器固定于 Treitz 韧带、回结肠区域或直肠乙状结肠连接。减速时，损伤是由固定点组织的撕裂所致。

不管损伤机制如何，穿孔的内脏导致腹腔的快速污染。在初始进行创伤评估时，所有神经系统未受影响的患者都有一些症状（疼痛）和体征（压痛、肌卫、反跳痛）。实际上，许多报道已经证明初期和全面的体格检查对这些损伤比超声和 CT 有更高的诊断意义[23,60,91]。在新墨西哥报道的 48 例小肠损伤患者的研究中，所有清醒患者在就诊时或在系列体格检查后都有异常的生理表现[91]。其他诊断性检查（US、CT、DPL、实验室检查）意义相对较小。这些发现已由 North Carolina 的相似性研究所证实，该研究包括 32 名在剖腹探查时确认的小肠损伤的儿童，其中 94%在入院时的生理表现提示有小肠损伤，84%有弥漫性腹部压痛（腹膜炎症状）[60]。在最初损伤时出现腹腔游离气体和 GI 造影剂渗出到腹腔时，这些损伤可能迅速

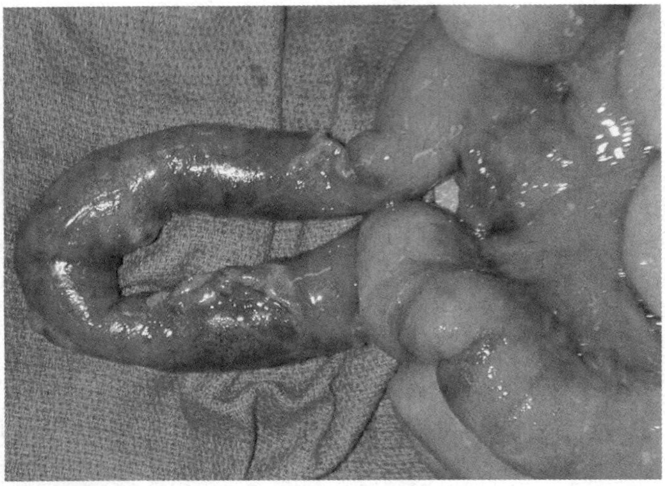

图 17-19 小肠系膜撕裂伴小肠缺血。

得到诊断。然而，当发生部分肠壁裂伤、血肿或肠系膜血管撕开时，发展到全层缺损可以延迟到几小时或几天（图 17-19）。当高度怀疑时，应进行系列的体格检查。

胃和小肠的损伤可以直接修补。饱胃时破裂通常在胃大弯，并呈爆破或星形结构。可以通过直接清创和修补进行处理。小肠损伤的类型包括单纯裂伤、横断及累及小肠的长段撕脱。然而，除非大量污染（或其他损伤需要扩大修补），清创切除和吻合通常足够处理损伤。结肠损伤时，尤其是延迟诊断和粪便污染时，依次进行结肠造口、清除远端黏液瘘管或 Hartmann 储袋术。如果发生单独结肠损伤，

311 进行早期修补，术中肠冲洗，肠吻合和围术期抗生素预防安全有效，能预防吻合口导发的并发症和再次手术。腹腔内消化道损伤需要尽早识别，快速复苏，迅速手术，完全清除污染和失活组织。如果有临床指征，则重建或转移消化道。治疗期间根据污染程度和手术后临床表现（比如，白细胞计数是否正常、有无发热、胃肠道功能是否恢复）应用广谱抗生素。

座椅 - 安全带损伤的体征

对高速碰撞中儿童因腰部安全带造成的损伤亚型需要经常进行体格检查[23]。这些儿童表现为腹部体格检查中可以看到的安全带体征（图 17-20）。多项研究证明该体征常伴有腹部实质和空腔脏器损伤[18,131,148]。

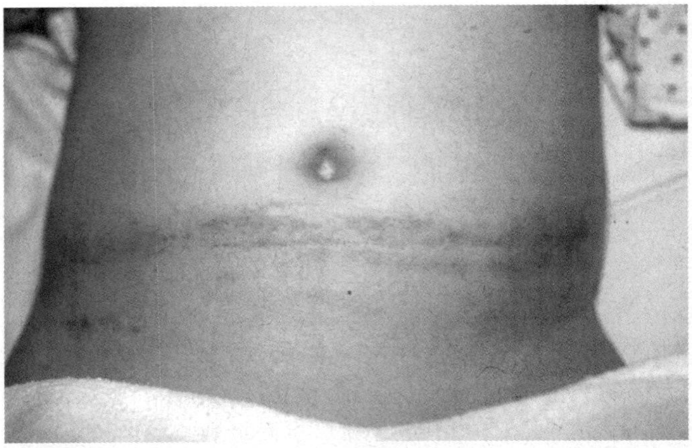

图 17-20 下腹部横行的安全带体征。

损伤的三联征是：腹壁挫伤或腹壁疝，腰椎骨折和单独空肠或回肠穿孔。一项报道回顾了 95 名腹部创伤入院的患者，所有患者损伤时都系了座位安全带，其中 60 个有保险带体征[148]。这 60 个患者中 9 个伴有小肠损伤，相比较而言，35 个没有安全带体征的患者没有小肠损伤。先前描述的更常见的损伤可能分散患者和创伤治疗组的注意，导致大血管如主动脉和髂血管损伤的诊断延迟[94,107]。

在近来来自费城的报告中，一项由州农业保险公司制作的数据被用来分析[147]985 名在机动车碰撞中的儿童乘客[77,96]。在该研究中，1967 名儿童（1.33%）有安全带导致的腹部擦伤。尽管腹壁擦伤不常见，有阳性表现的儿童发生明显腹腔内损伤的几率是没有擦伤的儿童的 232 倍。这些资料进一步显示，9 个有腹部安全带体征的儿童中有 1 个有明显腹内损伤。因此，尽管腹部安全带体征少见，但当其发生时，要求做 CT 扫描（入院和系列）。经常可以见到正确使用（n = 881）和不甚正确使用（n = 1086）座椅安全带的现象。在按年龄和座椅位置调校后，正确使用组儿童比不正确使用组儿童出现腹部损伤的几率低 3 倍（危险因子为 3.51）。

胃肠道损伤的影像学检查

胃肠道损伤的影像学已经发展了十年，螺旋 CT 和外科医生在急诊室进行的 FAST 直接影响了诊断的准确性和治疗方法的选择。CT 诊断的优势和劣势已经讨论。然而，通过这种方式，儿童钝性腹部损伤的

诊断和治疗能力已经明显增强。多伦多的两项研究证实了这些问题。第一项研究在 1992 年，回顾了 12 例 CT 诊断的腹部钝性损伤患者[50]。发现肠壁增强是消化道缺血合并致命性中枢神经系统损伤的表现，或可见于肠壁增厚、游离腹腔液体及肠穿孔。1996 年的一项随访研究回顾了 10 年来 43 名外科手术确定的消化道穿孔的患者[59]。其中 47%发现有腔外气体，一个为假阳性。五项 CT 表现可能有消化道穿孔：腔外气体、腹腔内游离液体、肠壁增厚、肠壁增强和肠管扩张。具备所有五项表现的患者可确诊为肠穿孔。但这只发生在 18%的学龄组儿童。所有患者至少有这五项特征性 CT 表现中的一个。没有假阴性研究。尽管
312 CT 扫描是评估消化道穿孔的可靠方法，但并不能代替系统的临床评估。Calgary 的相似研究回顾了 145 名钝性腹部损伤的儿童[47]。其中 20 名患者的 CT 扫描提示消化道损伤，而 152 名阴性（有些儿童不只做了一次检查）。腹部 CT 在需要手术的肠系膜和小肠损伤的评估中敏感性为 0.93，在这个研究组中，阴性预示值是 0.99。因此，CT 很少遗漏明显的肠系膜或小肠损伤。

在没有实质脏器损伤时出现腹腔游离液体提示有小肠损伤。Hulka 等人[58]报道一组 259 名进行 CT 扫描（所有都经口或静脉内增强）的患者，发现只有 24 名（9%）有单独腹腔内液体，其中 16 名患者有少量腹腔液体，只有 2 名需要剖腹探查手术。其余 8 名腹腔内液体超过一个部位，其中 4 名出现小肠损伤需要手术。作者发现肠道造影对小肠损伤的诊断意义较小。Holmes 等人[55]也曾报道过类似发现，小量腹腔液体临床意义不大。报道称，只有 8%腹部 CT 扫描可发现单独腹腔内液体，其中 17%有可识别的损伤。这些表现是通过对 542名儿童中的 7 名（1.3%）研究得出的。

FAST 是有效的影像工具，在评价儿童损伤中有很高的特异性（95%），但敏感性低（33%）[103]。在对 89个 FAST 阴性儿童的研究中，只有 20 例在外科医生的建议下继续进行了 CT 检查。没有这些发现，他们可能都会进行腹部 CT 扫描。FAST 能减少不必要的 CT 扫描，但不能检测到特殊腹腔脏器的损伤。因此，FAST 在评估这些损伤中的价值有限。最后，匹兹堡的一项大规模的研究中，回顾了 350 名腹部损伤的儿童，30 例（8.5%）需要剖腹探查[3]。19 例进行延迟剖腹探查手术（损伤后 3.5 小时或更长的）的患者中有 5 例 CT 扫描为假阴性（26%）。以上作者总结得出，系统体格检查而不是 CT，是诊断儿童消化道穿孔的金标准。我们的意见一致。

会阴、肛门和外生殖器的损伤

儿童损伤累及到会阴、肛门和外生殖器主要有两种机制：意外坠落和性虐待。意外伤害是由于以两腿叉开的姿势坠落到钝性或锐性物体上造成的。这些损伤的性质有擦伤、挫伤、裂伤或穿透伤，根据物体的击打和坠落高度而不同。意外损伤经常损伤外生殖器、尿道、会阴体和肛门，但很少累及直肠。而性虐待导致的损伤通常是由于剧烈、强迫的动作或故意在这些部位插入物体所造成的直肠或阴道的穿透。因此，当检查儿童会阴损伤时，单独直肠或阴道损伤应怀疑是否是儿童虐待。而会阴部包括生殖器、会阴和肛门的复合损伤是典型的意外损伤[62,110]。

对会阴部损伤程度的诊断需要在麻醉下进行，通过直肠镜检查、乙状结肠镜检查和逆行尿道造影。损伤程度评估以后，外科策略包括尿道修补（直接或通过支架）、在耻骨弓上膀胱造口进行尿流改道、修补直肠损伤、直肠冲洗以及在需要时放置引流。对于更加复杂的损伤，行结肠造口术以粪便改道。恢复后，在准备重建连续性排便、取出尿道支架或尿流改道复原术前必须详细进行放射学检查，以确认是否完全愈合（比如通过静脉肾盂造影图、膀胱 X 线片、尿道造影照片和钡剂灌肠）。

尽管少见，有报道儿童由于被虐待而致直肠穿孔死亡[102]。创伤性分娩导致的新生儿直肠阴道损伤少见，却是致命性的并发症[74]。更常见的是，在新生儿直肠插入温度计、子宫颈扩张器、灌肠管时可以导致明显直肠损伤。需要外科修补。我们最近治疗了一个 3 天大的婴儿，在治疗囊性纤维化顽固性便秘反复灌肠后出现直肠乙状结肠连接部穿孔，需要剖腹探查和结肠造口手术。因此，在新生儿，表面上无害的直肠操作能导致严重的需要外科评估和干预的损伤。

膈肌损伤

膈肌损伤很少见到，即使是在最大的儿童创伤中

心也是这样。在伊利诺伊儿童医院，从1998年到2002年的超过800个入院需要Ⅰ级儿科创伤评估的患者中，只有2个创伤性膈肌损伤。在多伦多的治疗儿童疾病的医院，从1977年到1998年只见到15个这种损伤的儿童[66,109]。在丹佛儿童医院也有相似的报道，从1992年到2002年，1397个钝性腹部损伤儿童入院观察，387个有腹腔内损伤，但只有6个诊断有膈肌破裂（0.5%）[9]。这种损伤是由于巨大压力作用于腹腔，造成腹腔内容物向头部加速运动，撕裂了横膈肌肉。偶尔，锐性创伤也可导致这种损伤。但是，这种损伤经常是由于探查其他损伤时意外发现。在多伦多的系列报道中，15个膈肌破裂的患者中有13个是钝性损伤，平均年龄7.5岁，左右侧膈肌同时累及[109]。在超过一半的患者中只靠胸片做出
313 诊断。在初期评估中有3个患者遗漏。由于导致这种损伤需要较大压力，所以要注意合并多发损伤的可能性。该报道中，81%的患者有多发损伤，包括肝脏裂伤（47%）、骨盆骨折（47%）、大血管损伤（40%）、肠穿孔（33%）、长骨骨折（20%）、肾脏裂伤（20%）、脾脏裂伤（13%）和闭合性头部损伤（13%）。和预期的一样，并发症很多，5例死亡，平均住院时间20天。在有这种合并损伤的儿童，急诊手术应该包括探查两侧膈肌，并把此作为常规腹腔探查中的一部分。在清除失活组织后通常可以直接缝合修补。Pledgeted缝合可以用来加固修补和防止肌肉撕裂，使得缝合更加安全。如果大量膈肌组织被破坏，可以使用2mm的Gore-Tex补片进行无张力缝合，类似于在新生儿修补先天性膈疝。膈肌损伤的腹腔镜和胸腔镜修补的报道是指对没有合并损伤的稳定患者进行延迟修补[84,105]。已有报道在婴儿中这种损伤的诊断延误，该患者肾脏撕裂通过创伤破裂的膈肌进入胸腔[27,129,137]。由于这种损伤很少出现，当损伤机制和其他损伤的程度与位置支持膈肌损伤时，我们必须高度警惕。

总结

近来儿童创伤治疗的进步和重症监护水平的提高已使严重损伤患儿的预后大为改观。小儿外科医生必须清楚致命性腹部创伤的当前治疗规程。放射科医生和内镜医生为腹部创伤儿童的诊断和治疗做出了重大贡献。临床经验和出版物对儿童实质脏器损伤的非手术治疗的特殊关注，以及最近影像学和内镜的应用使得儿童创伤非手术治疗逐渐增加。尽管如此，对危重的儿童，小儿外科医生应该协同内科医生进行多学科治疗。非手术治疗通常由外科决定。

（顾 硕译 吕志葆校）

参考文献

1. Acierno SP, Jurkovich GJ, Nathens AB: Is pediatric trauma still a surgical disease? Patterns of emergent operative intervention in the injured child. J Trauma 2004;56:960-966.
2. Adams JM, Hauser CJ, Livingston DH, et al: The immunomodulatory effects of damage control abdominal packing on local and systemic neutrophil activity. J Trauma 2001;50:792-800.
3. Albanese CT, Meza MP, Gardner MJ, et al: Is computed tomography a useful adjunct to the clinical examination for the diagnosis of pediatric gastrointestinal perforation from blunt abdominal trauma in children? J Trauma 1996;40:417-421.
4. Angeles AP, Agarwal N, Lynd C: Repair of a juxtahepatic inferior vena cava injury using a simple endovascular technique. J Trauma 2004;56:918-921.
5. Asensio JA, Demetriades D, Chahwan S: Approach to the management of complex hepatic injuries. J Trauma 2000;48:66-69.
6. Asensio JA, Roldan G, Petrone P, et al: Operative management and outcomes in 103 AAST-OIS grades IV and V complex hepatic injuries: Trauma surgeons still need to operate, but angioembolization helps. J Trauma 2003;54:647-654.
7. Ballard RB, Badellino MM, Enyon CA, et al: Blunt duodenal rupture: A 6 year statewide review. J Trauma 1997;43:729-733.
8. Barker DE, Kaufman HJ, Smith LA, et al: Vacuum pack technique of temporary abdominal closure: A 7-year experience with 112 patients. J Trauma 2000;48:201-207.
9. Barsness KA, Bensard DD, Ciesla D, et al: Blunt diaphragmatic rupture in children. J Trauma 2004;56:80-82.
10. Bass BL, Eichelberger MR, Schisgall R: Hazards of non-operative therapy of hepatic trauma in children. J Trauma 1984;24:978-982.
11. Bensard DD, Beaver BL, Besner GE, et al: Small bowel injury in children after blunt abdominal trauma: Is diagnostic delay important? J Trauma 1996;41:476-483.
12. Boman-Vermeeren JM, Vermeeren-Walters G, Broos P, et al: Somatostatin in the treatment of a pancreatic pseudocyst in a child. J Pediatr Gastroenterol Nutr 1996;23:422-425.
13. Brown RL, Irish MS, McCabe AJ, et al: Observation of splenic trauma: When is a little too much? J Pediatr Surg 1999;34:1124-1126.
14. Brunet C, Sielezneff I, Thomas P, et al: Treatment of hepatic trauma with perihepatic mesh. J Trauma 1994;37:200-204.
15. Bulas DI, Taylor GA, Eichelberger MR: The value of CT in detecting bowel perforation in children after blunt abdominal trauma. AJR Am J Roentgenol 1989;153:561-564.

16. Canty TG Sr, Weinman D: Treatment of pancreatic duct disruption in children by an endoscopically placed stent. J Pediatr Surg 2001;36:345-348.
17. Canty TG Sr, Weinman D: Management of major pancreatic duct injuries in children. J Trauma 2001;50:1001-1007.
18. Chandler CF, Lane JS, Waxman KS: Seatbelt sign following blunt trauma is associated with increased incidence of abdominal injury. Am Surg 1997;63:885-888.
19. Chang MC, Miller PR, D'Agostino R, et al: Effects of abdominal decompression on cardiopulmonary function and visceral perfusion in patients with intra-abdominal hypertension. J Trauma 1998;44:440-445.
20. Chen MK, Schropp KP, Lobe TE: The use of minimal access surgery in pediatric trauma: A preliminary report. J Laparoendosc Surg 1995;5:295-301.
21. Chen RJ, Fang JF, Lin BC, et al: Selective application of laparoscopy and fibrin glue in the failure of nonoperative management of blunt hepatic trauma. J Trauma 1998;44:691-695.
22. Church NG, May G, Sigalet DL: A minimally invasive approach to bile duct injury after blunt liver trauma in pediatric patients. J Pediatr Surg 2002;37:773-775.
23. Ciftci AO, Tanyel FC, Salman AB, et al: Gastrointestinal tract perforation due to blunt abdominal trauma. Pediatr Surg Int 1998;13:259-264.
24. Clendenon JN, Meyers RL, Nance ML, et al: Management of duodenal injuries in children. J Pediatr Surg 2004; 39:964-968.
25. Cloutier DR, Baird TB, Gormley P, et al: Pediatric splenic injuries with a contrast blush: Successful nonoperative management without angiography and embolization. J Pediatr Surg 2004;39:969-971.
26. Cogbill TH, Moore EE, Jurkovich GJ: Severe hepatic trauma: A multicenter experience with 1335 liver injuries. J Trauma 1988;28:1433-1438.
27. Cohen Z, Gabriel A, Izrachi S, et al: Traumatic avulsion of kidney into the chest through a ruptured diaphragm in a boy. Pediatr Emerg Care 2000;3:180-181.
28. Cooper A, Barlow B, DiScala C, et al: Mortality and truncal injury: The pediatric perspective. J Pediatr Surg 1994; 29:33-38.
29. Cuschieri A, Hennessy TP, Stephens RB, et al: Diagnosis of significant abdominal trauma after road traffic accidents: Preliminary results of a multicentre clinical trial comparing mini-laparoscopy with peritoneal lavage. Ann R Coll Surg Engl 1988;70:153-155.
30. Davies MRQ: Iatrogenic hepatic rupture in the newborn and its management by pack tamponade. J Pediatr Surg 1997;32:1414-1419.
31. DeCou JM, Abrams RS, Miller RS, et al: Abdominal compartment syndrome in children: Experience with three cases. J Pediatr Surg 2000;35:840-842.
32. Denton JR, Moore EE, Codwell DM: Multimodality treatment for grade V hepatic injuries: Perihepatic packing, arterial embolization, and venous stenting. J Trauma 1997;42:964-968.
33. Desai KM, Dorward IG, Minkes RK, et al: Blunt duodenal injuries in children. J Trauma 2003;54:640-646.
34. Epelman M, Soudack M, Engel A, et al: Abdominal compartment syndrome in children: CT findings. Pediatr Radiol 2002;32:319-322.
35. Eubanks JW, Meier DE, Hicks BA, et al: Significance of "blush" on computed tomography scan in children with liver injury. J Pediatr Surg 2003;38:363-366.
36. Evans S, Jackson RJ, Smith SD: Successful repair of major retrohepatic vascular injuries without the use of shunt or
37. Fabian TC, Croce MA, Stewart RM, et al: A prospective analysis of diagnostic laparoscopy in trauma. Ann Surg 1993;217:557-565.
38. Fallat ME, Casale AJ: Practice patterns of pediatric surgeons caring for stable patients with traumatic solid organ injury. J Trauma 1997;43:820-824.
39. Fang JF, Chen RJ, Ling BC: Controlled reopen suture technique for pyloric exclusion. J Trauma 1998;45:593-596.
40. Fisher JC, Moulton SL: Nonoperative management and delayed hemorrhage following pediatric liver injury. J Pediatr Surg 2004;39:619-622.
41. Frumiento C, Sartorelli K, Vane DW: Complications of splenic injuries: Expansion of the nonoperative theorem. J Pediatr Surg 2000;35:788-791.
42. Frumiento C, Vane DW: Changing patterns of treatment for blunt splenic injuries: An 11-year experience in a rural state. J Pediatr Surg 2000;35:985-989.
43. Gaines BA, Shultz BS, Morrison K, et al: Duodenal injuries in children: Beware of child abuse. J Pediatr Surg 2004;39:600-602.
44. Gandhi RR, Stringel G: Laparoscopy in pediatric abdominal trauma. JSLS 1997;1:349-351.
45. Ginzburg E, Klein Y, Sutherland M, et al: Prolonged clamping of the liver parenchyma: A salvage maneuver in exsanguinating liver injury. J Trauma 2004;56: 922-923.
46. Goettler CE, Stallion A, Grisoni ER, et al: Delayed hemorrhage after blunt hepatic trauma. J Trauma 2002;52: 556-559.
47. Graham JS, Wong AL: A review of computed tomography in the diagnosis of intestinal and mesenteric injury in pediatric blunt abdominal trauma. J. Pediatr Surg 1996;31:754-756.
48. Granchi TS, Abikhaled JA, Hirshberg A, et al: Patterns of microbiology in intra-abdominal packing for trauma. J Trauma 2004;56:45-51.
49. Hackam DJ, Potoka D, Meza M, et al: Utility of radiographic hepatic injury grade in predicting outcome for children after blunt abdominal trauma. J Pediatr Surg 2002;237:386-389.
50. Hara H, Babyn PS, Bourgeois D: Significance of bowel wall enhancement on CT following blunt abdominal trauma in childhood. J Comput Assist Tomogr 1992;16:94-98.
51. Harrell DJ, Vitale GC, Larson GM: Selective role for endoscopic retrograde cholangiopancreatography in abdominal trauma. Surg Endosc 1998;12:400-404.
52. Hawegawa T, Miki Y, Yoshioka Y, et al: Laparoscopic diagnosis of blunt abdominal trauma in children. Pediatr Surg Int 1997;12:132-136.
53. Hirshberg A, Mattox KL: Planned re-operation for severe trauma. Ann Surg 1995;222:3-8.
54. Hobson KG, Young KM, Ciraulo A, et al: Release of abdominal compartment syndrome improves survival in patients with burn injury. J Trauma 2002;53:1129-1134.
55. Holmes JF, London KL, Brant WE, et al: Isolated intraperitoneal fluid on abdominal computed tomography in children with blunt trauma. Acad Emerg Med 2000;7: 335-341.
56. Horwitz JR, Black T, Lally KP: Venovenous bypass as an adjunct for the management of a retrohepatic venous injury in a child. J Trauma 1995;39:584-585.
57. Hoyt DB, Bulger EM, Knudson MM: Death in the operating room: An analysis of a multi-center experience. J Trauma 1994;37:426-432.
58. Hulka F, Mullins RJ, Leonardo V, et al: Significance of peritoneal fluid as an isolated finding on abdominal computed tomographic scans in pediatric trauma patients. J Trauma

1998;44:1069-1072.
59. Jamieson DH, Babyn PS, Pearl R: Imaging gastrointestinal perforation in pediatric blunt abdominal trauma. Pediatr Radiol 1996;26:188-194.
60. Jerby BL, Attorri RJ, Morton D Jr: Blunt intestinal injury in children: The role of the physical examination. J Pediatr Surg 1997;32:580-584.
61. Jobst MA, Canty TG Sr, Lynch FP: Management of pancreatic injury in pediatric blunt abdominal trauma. J Pediatr Surg 1999;34:818-824.
62. Kadish HA, Schunk JE, Britton H: Pediatric male rectal and genital trauma: Accidental and nonaccidental injuries. Pediatr Emerg Care 1998;14:95-98.
63. Keller MS, Sartorelli KH, Vane DW: Associated head injury should not prevent nonoperative management of spleen or liver injury in children. J Trauma 1996;41:471-475.
64. Keller MS, Vane DW: Management of pediatric blunt splenic injury: Comparison of pediatric and adult trauma surgeons. J Pediatr Surg 1995;30:221-225.
65. Kim HS, Lee DK, Kim IW, et al: The role of retrograde pancreatography in the treatment of traumatic pancreatic duct injury. Gastrointest Endosc 2001;54:45-55.
66. Koplewitz BZ, Ramos C, Manson DE, et al: Traumatic diaphragmatic injuries in infants and children: Imaging findings. Pediatr Radiol 2000;30:471-479.
67. Kouchi K, Tanabe M, Yoshida H, et al: Nonoperative management of blunt pancreatic injury in children. J Pediatr Surg 1999;34:1736-1738.
68. Kularni R, Daneshmand A, Guertin S, et al: Successful use of activated recombinant factor VII in traumatic liver injuries in children. J Trauma 2004;56:1348-1352.
69. Kushimoto S, Arai M, Aiboshi J, et al: The role of interventional radiology in patients requiring damage control laparotomy. J Trauma 2003;54:171-176.
70. Ladd AP, West KW, Rouse TM, et al: Surgical management of duodenal injuries in children. Surgery 2002;132:748-753.
71. Lane MJ, Mindelzun RE, Jeffery RB: Diagnosis of pancreatic injury after blunt abdominal trauma. Semin Ultrasound CT MR 1996;17:177-182.
72. Lange DA, Zaret P, Merlotti GJ, et al: The use of absorbable mesh in splenic trauma. J Trauma 1988;28:269-275.
73. Lenwand MJ, Atkinson CC, Mooney DP: Application of the APSA evidence-based guidelines for isolated liver or spleen injuries: A single institution experience. J Pediatr Surg 2004;39:487-490.
74. Lickstein DA, Moriary KP, Feins NR: Neonatal rectovaginal tear during cesarean section. J Pediatr Surg 1998;33:1315-1316.
75. Lucaya J, Vasques E, Caballerro F, et al: Nonoperative management of traumatic pancreatic pseudocysts associated with pancreatic duct laceration in children. Pediatr Radiol 1998;28:5-8.
76. Lutz N, Mahboubi S, Nance ML, et al: The significance of contrast blush on computed tomography in children with splenic injuries. J Pediatr Surg 2004;39:491-494.
77. Lutz N, Nance ML, Kallan MJ, et al: Incidence and clinical significance of abdominal wall bruising in restrained children involved in motor vehicle crashes. J Pediatr Surg 2004;39:972-975.
78. Lynch JM, Ford H, Gardner MJ: Is early discharge following isolated splenic injury in the hemodynamically stable child possible? J Pediatr Surg 1993;28:1403-1407.
79. Malhotra AK, Fabian TC, Croce MA, et al: Blunt hepatic injury: A paradigm shift from operative to nonoperative management in the 1990s. Ann Surg 2000;231:804-813.
80. Markley MA, Mantor PC, Letton RW, et al: Pediatric vacuum packing wound closure for damage-control laparotomy. J Pediatr Surg 2002;37:512-514.
81. McGahren ED, Magnuson D, Schauer RT, et al: Management of transection of the pancreas in children. Aust N Z J Surg 1995;65:242-246.
82. Mehall JR, Ennis JS, Saltzman DA, et al: Prospective results of a standardized algorithm based on hemodynamic status for managing pediatric solid organ injury. J Am Coll Surg 2001;193:347-353.
83. Meier DR, Coln CD, Hicks BA, et al: Early operation in patients with pancreas transection. J Pediatr Surg 2001;36:341-344.
84. Meyer G, Huttl TP, Hatz RA, et al: Laparoscopic repair of traumatic diaphragmatic hernias. Surg Endosc 2000;14:1010-1014.
85. Miglietta MA, Salzano LJ, Chiu WC, et al: Decompressive laparotomy: A novel approach in the management of severe intracranial hypertension. J Trauma 2003;55:551-555.
86. Miller K, Kou D, Stallion A, et al: Pediatric hepatic trauma: Does clinical course support intensive care unit stay? J Pediatr Surg 1998;33:1459-1462.
87. Mooney DP, Birkmeyer NJO, Udell JV: Variation in the management of pediatric splenic injuries in New Hampshire. J Pediatr Surg 1998;33:1076-1080.
88. Mooney DP, Forbes PW: Variation in the management of pediatric splenic injuries in New England. J Trauma 2004;56:328-333.
89. Moore EE, Cogbill TH, Jurkovich GJ: Organ injury scaling: Spleen and liver (1994 revision). J Trauma 1995;38:323-324.
90. Morse MA, Garcia VF: Selective nonoperative management of pediatric blunt splenic trauma: Risk for missed associated injuries. J Pediatr Surg 1994;29:23-27.
91. Moss RL, Musemeche CA: Clinical judgment is superior to diagnostic tests in the management of pediatric small bowel injury. J Pediatr Surg 1996;8:1178-1181.
92. Moulton SL, Downey EC, Anderson DS: Blunt bile duct injuries in children. J Pediatr Surg 1993;28:795-797.
93. Moulton SL, Lynch FP, Canty TG: Hepatic vein and retrohepatic vena caval injuries in children: Sternotomy first? Arch Surg 1991;126:1262-1266.
94. Muniz AE, Haynes JH: Delayed abdominal aortic rupture in a child with a seat-belt sign. J Trauma 2004;56:194-197.
95. Nance ML, Keller MS, Stafford PW: Predicting hollow visceral injury in the pediatric blunt trauma patient with solid visceral injury. J Pediatr Surg 2000;35:1300-1303.
96. Nance ML, Lutz N, Arbogast KB, et al: Optimal restraint reduces the risk of abdominal injury in children involved in motor vehicle crashes. Ann Surg 2004;239:127-131.
97. Neville HL, Lally KP, Cox CS: Emergent abdominal decompression with patch abdominoplasty in the pediatric patient. J Pediatr Surg 2000;35:705-708.
98. Norotsky MC, Rogers FB, Shackford SR: Delayed presentation of splenic artery pseudoaneurysms following blunt abdominal trauma: Case reports. J Trauma 1995;38:444-447.
99. Nwomeh BC, Nadler EP, Meza MP, et al: Contrast extravasation predicts the need for operative intervention in children with blunt splenic trauma. J Trauma 2004;56:537-541.
100. Oda J, Ivatury RR, Blocher CR, et al: Amplified cytokine response and lung injury by sequential hemorrhagic shock and abdominal compartment syndrome in a laboratory model of ischemia-reperfusion. J Trauma 2002;52:625-632.

101. Ong AW, McKenney MG, McKenney KA, et al: Predicting the need for laparotomy in pediatric trauma patients on the basis of the ultrasound score. J Trauma 2003;54: 503-508.
102. Orr CJ, Clark MA, Hawley DA, et al: Fatal anorectal injuries: A series of four cases. J Forensic Sci 1995; 40:219-221.
103. Patel JC, Tepas JJ: The efficacy of focused abdominal sonography for trauma (FAST) as a screening tool in the assessment of injured children. J Pediatr Surg 1999; 34:44-47, 52-54.
104. Pearl RH, Wesson DE, Spence LJ: Splenic injury: A five year update with improved results and changing criteria for conservative management. J Pediatr Surg 1989;24:428-431.
105. Pitcher G: Fiber-endoscopic thoracoscopy for diaphragmatic injury in children. Semin Pediatr Surg 2001;10:17-19.
106. Potoka DA, Schall LC, Ford HR: Risk factors for splenectomy in children with blunt splenic trauma. J Pediatr Surg 2002;37:294-299.
107. Prince JS, LoSasso BE, Senac MO: Unusual seat-belt injuries in children. J Trauma 2004;56:420-427.
108. Pryor JP, Stafford PW, Nance ML: Severe blunt hepatic trauma in children. J Pediatr Surg 2001;36:974-979.
109. Ramos CT, Koplewitz BZ, Babyn PS, et al: What have we learned about traumatic diaphragmatic hernias in children? J Pediatr Surg 2000;35:601-604.
110. Reinberg O, Yazbeck S: Major perineal trauma in children. J Pediatr Surg 1989;24:982-984.
111. Rescorla FJ, Plumley DA, Sherman S, et al: The efficacy of early ERCP in pediatric pancreatic trauma. J Pediatr Surg 1995;30:336-340.
112. Rezende-Neto JB, Moore EE, de Andrade MVM, et al: Systemic inflammatory response syndrome secondary to abdominal compartment syndrome: Stage for multiple organ failure. J Trauma 2002;53:1121-1128.
113. Rhodes M, Smith S, Boorse D: Pediatric trauma patients in an "adult" trauma center. J Trauma 1993;35:384-393.
114. Mooney DP, Rothstein DH, Forbes PW: Variation in the management of pediatric splenic injuries in the United States. J Trauma Surg (in press).
115. Rotondo MF, Schwab CW, McGonigal MD: Damage control: An approach for improved survival in exsanguinating penetrating abdominal injury. J Trauma 1993;35:375-383.
116. Saggi BH, Sugerman HJ, Ivatury RR, et al: Abdominal compartment syndrome. J Trauma 1998;45:597-609.
117. Scioscia PJ, Dillon PW, Cilley RE: Endoscopic sphincterotomy in the management of posttraumatic biliary fistula. J Pediatr Surg 1994;29:3-6.
118. Shafi S, Gilbert JC, Carden S: Risk of hemorrhage and appropriate use of blood transfusions in pediatric blunt splenic injuries. J Trauma 1997;42:1029-1032.
119. Shapiro MB, Jenkins DH, Schwab CW, et al: Damage control: Collective review. J Trauma 2000;49:969-978.
120. Sharif K, Pimpalwar AP, John P, et al: Benefits of early diagnosis and preemptive treatment of biliary tract complications after major blunt liver trauma in children. J Pediatr Surg 2002;37:1287-1292.
121. Sharpe RP, Nance ML, Stafford PW: Nonoperative management of blunt extrahepatic biliary duct transection in the pediatric patient. J Pediatr Surg 2002;37:1612-1616.
122. Sharpe RP, Pryor JP, Gandhi RR, et al: Abdominal compartment syndrome in the pediatric blunt trauma patient treated with paracentesis: Report of two cases. J Trauma 2002;53:380-382.
123. Shilyansky J, Navarro O, Superina RA, et al: Delayed hemorrhage after nonoperative management of blunt hepatic trauma in children: A rare but significant event. J Pediatr Surg 1999;34:60-64.
124. Shilyansky J, Pearl RH, Kroutouro M, et al: Diagnosis and management of duodenal injuries in children. J Pediatr Surg 1997;32:880-886.
125. Shilyansky J, Sen LM, Kreller M, et al: Nonoperative management of pancreatic injuries in children. J Pediatr Surg 1998;33:343-345.
126. Simon RJ, Rabin J, Kuhls D: Impact of increased use of laparoscopy on negative laparotomy rates after penetrating trauma. J Trauma 2002;53:297-302.
127. Sivit CJ, Taylor GA, Bulas DI, et al: Blunt trauma in children: Significance of peritoneal fluid. Radiology 1991; 178:185-188.
128. Smith RS, Fry WR, Morabito DJ, et al: Therapeutic laparoscopy in trauma. Am J Surg 1995;170:632-637.
129. Sola JE, Mattei P, Pegoli W Jr, et al: Rupture of the right diaphragm following blunt trauma in an infant: Case report. J Trauma 1994;36:417-420.
130. Soto JA, Alvarez O, Munera F, et al: Traumatic disruption of the pancreatic duct: Diagnosis with MR pancreatography. AJR Am J Roentgenol 2001;176:175-178.
131. Stassen NA, Lukan JK, Carrillo EH, et al: Abdominal seat belt marks in the era of focused abdominal sonography for trauma. Arch Surg 2002;137:718-723.
132. Strear CM, Graf JL, Albanese CT, et al: Successful treatment of liver hemorrhage in the premature infant. J Pediatr Surg 1998;33:849-851.
133. Stylianos S: Controversies in abdominal trauma. Semin Pediatr Surg 1995;4:116-119.
134. Stylianos S: Abdominal packing for severe hemorrhage. J Pediatr Surg 1998;33:339-342.
135. Stylianos S, APSA Trauma Committee: Evidence-based guidelines for resource utilization in children with isolated spleen or liver injury. J Pediatr Surg 2000;35:164-169.
136. Stylianos S, APSA Trauma Study Group: Prospective validation of evidence-based guidelines for resource utilization in children with isolated spleen or liver injury. J Pediatr Surg 2002;37:453-456.
137. Stylianos S, Bergman KS, Harris BH: Traumatic renal avulsion into the chest: Case report. J Trauma 1991; 31:301-302.
138. Stylianos S, Jacir NN, Hoffman MA, et al: Pediatric blunt liver injury and coagulopathy managed with packs and silo. J Trauma 1990;30:1409-1410.
139. Suliburk JW, Ware DN, Balogh Z, et al: Vacuum-assisted wound closure achieves early fascial closure of open abdomens after severe trauma. J Trauma 2003;55: 1155-1160.
140. Taner AS, Topgul K, Kucukel F, et al: Diagnostic laparoscopy decreases the rate of unnecessary laparotomies and reduces hospital costs in trauma patients. J Laparoendosc Adv Surg Tech A 2001;11:207-211.
141. Tepas JJ, Frykberg ER, Schinco MA, et al: Pediatric trauma is very much a surgical disease. Ann Surg 2003;237:775-781.
142. Upadhyaya P, Simpson JS: Splenic trauma in children. Surg Gynecol Obstet 1968;126:781-790.
143. Vargo D, Sorenson J, Barton R: Repair of grade VI hepatic injury: Case report and literature review. J Trauma 2002;53:823-824.
144. Wales PW, Shuckett B, Kim PC: Long term outcome of non-operative management of complete traumatic pancreatic transection in children. J Pediatr Surg 2001;36:823-827.

145. Watts DD, Trask A, Soeken K, et al: Hypothermic coagulopathy in trauma: Effect of varying levels of hypothermia on enzyme speed, platelet function, and fibrinolytic activity. J Trauma 1998;44:846-854.
146. Winthrop AL, Wesson DE, Filler RM: Traumatic duodenal hematoma in the pediatric patient. J Pediatr Surg 1986;21:757-760.
147. Wolberg AS, Meng ZH, Monroe DM, et al: A systematic evaluation of the effect of temperature on coagulation enzyme activity and platelet function. J Trauma 2004;56:1221-1228.
148. Wotherspoon S, Chu K, Brown AF: Abdominal surgery and the seat-belt sign. Emerg Med 2001;13:61-65.
149. Yang EY, Marder SR, Hastings G, et al: The abdominal compartment syndrome complicating nonoperative management of major blunt liver injuries: Recognition and treatment using multimodality therapy. J Trauma 2002;52:982-986.
150. Yellin AE, Chaffee CB, Donovan AJ: Vascular isolation in treatment of juxtahepatic venous injuries. Arch Surg 1971;102:566-573.

第 18 章

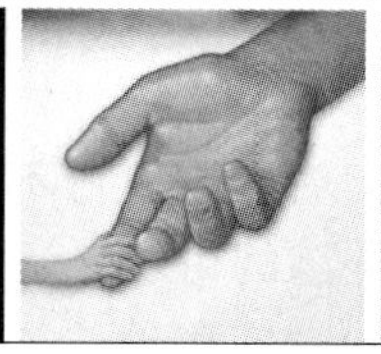

泌尿生殖道外伤

Rebeccah L. Brown 和 Victor F. Garcia

17 ## 流行病学

在美国，外伤是引起儿童和青少年死亡的最主要的原因。钝性外伤或锐性外伤造成的肾脏损伤是最为常见的泌尿生殖道损伤[21,122]，大约有 50%的泌尿系统损伤累及肾脏[121]，腹部的钝伤占泌尿生殖系统外伤原因的 90%[21]。在所有的钝伤中，有 10%～20%会出现肾脏损伤[121,122]。肾脏是最容易出现损伤的实质脏器，比肝脏、脾脏或者胰腺损伤的可能性更大[21,43,130]。严重的肾脏损伤往往伴有其他器官的损伤，在 80%的锐性损伤和 75%的钝性外伤的患者会出现这种情况[172]。最主要的相关外伤是头颅闭合性外伤和肢体骨折[7,43,145]，伴随出现腹部损伤的大约占到患者的 42%～74%，一般是脾脏或者肝脏的钝伤以及结肠的穿透伤[102,104,122,179,182]。一般情况下，大多数单纯的肾脏外伤损伤等级不会很高[40]，单纯肾脏外伤引起死亡的很少见，多发性脏器损伤是患者的死亡原因。

外伤机制

大多数肾脏钝伤是由于突然的减速暴力造成。由于肾脏是限制在 Gerota 筋膜内，所以可能会被挤压到肋骨或脊柱上，导致破裂或挫伤。附近肋骨的尖锐骨折碎片也可能会穿破集合系统和肾盂造成直接损伤。快速的减速可造成动脉或静脉的损伤，这是由固定的肾蒂血管受牵拉所致[21]。因为肾动脉的内膜弹性相对于其他层以及外膜较低，所以在外伤中更容易裂伤，这会导致血管内膜下撕裂和动脉血栓形成[69]。肾脏钝伤的机制包括：行人 / 机动车车祸伤（60%）、高处坠落伤（22.5%）、运动中受到的损伤（10%）、暴力侵犯损伤（3.5%）以及其他原因的损伤（4%）[175]。绝大多数在机动车祸中肾脏受到损伤的儿童是没有系好安全带[122]，然而在使用座位安全带时迅猛减速伴随严重的屈伸，会导致肾蒂的撕裂以及肾盂输尿管连接部（UPJ）损伤的风险增高，这种致伤机制已经得到确认。令人感兴趣的是，在运动损伤中自行车事故是最常见的原因，而且通常出现高等级的肾脏损伤[75]。尽管小儿外科和泌尿科医生一般都会认为参加对抗性的体育活动，如足球、曲棍球以及武术，发生儿童肾脏外伤的风险更大[175]，但是 McAleer 及其同事[123]的回顾性调查显示，24%的外伤是由于自行车事故，而只有 5%的外伤是由对抗性的体育活动造成。这些情况必须让有过严重肾脏外伤和只有单侧肾脏的孩子了解。锐性泌尿生殖道损伤逐渐增多，当患儿胸部、腹部、侧腹部以及腰部区域有锐性外伤时要怀疑有无泌尿生殖道穿通伤[28,65]。医源性损伤比较少见，一般能够迅速得到诊断。行肾脏细针穿刺活检或者内镜进入尿道、膀胱以及输尿管时可以明显增加外伤的风险。还有对邻近脏器的操作也会有引起泌尿生殖道外伤的风险，最常见的导致输尿管损伤的操作发生在妇科和肿瘤手术中。

解剖学因素

儿童泌尿生殖道外伤的风险增大是由于儿童相对于成人的不同的解剖特点造成的[21,109,139]。在儿童肾脏相对身体比例要大，而且在腹部位置相对较低，这使其肾脏暴露更明显，更容易损伤，而且保护也相对较少，如皮下脂肪较少、腹壁肌肉薄弱、胸廓肋骨的骨化程度较低。由于许多儿童的肾脏含有胚胎性的小叶，所以肾脏实质性破裂以及需要行肾下极切除的风险增大。进一步来说，儿童由于肾脂肪囊和 Gerota

筋膜相对成人发育不全，增加了裂伤、非局限性出血
318 和尿外渗的可能性。儿童由于肾脏游离度更大，所以快速的减速可能会造成其肾蒂的损伤以及 UPJ 破裂。在一个关于儿童和成人肾脏钝性外伤的比较性病例研究中，Brown 及其同事[21]的结论表明，儿童相对成人发生较大的肾脏损伤的可能性明显增加，但严重损伤的可能明显降低。

因为类似的原因，存在肾脏病变或者先天性肾脏疾病都会增加钝伤后泌尿生殖道损伤的风险。研究表明，儿童肾脏外伤中合并有肾脏疾病或者先天性泌尿生殖道异常的占 1%～23% [19,38,45,67,121,122,135,146]。尤其是先天性肾脏异常时，例如肾积水（UPJ 梗阻）、肾脏位置异常（马蹄肾、交叉融合异位肾）或者是肾脏的结构异常（如多囊肾、输尿管反流）时，肾脏即使受到的外伤相对轻微，也可能严重受损[45]。大量的血尿伴随外表轻微的外伤，提醒医生要小心泌尿系统存在着病理学变化，这时候需要进一步行影像学检查。尽管先天性泌尿生殖道畸形增加了儿童外伤后的风险，但看上去并不增加外伤后的死亡率和病残率[123]。

临床特征

对严重外伤的患者进行系统而迅速的全身检查，包括对泌尿生殖系统损伤的评价。受伤机制非常重要，对评价外伤的风险有重要作用。在机动车车祸和坠落伤时，出现直接的对腹部或侧腹部的撞击以及明显的减速暴力损伤时，要警惕肾脏损伤。在腹部、侧腹部、背部、胸部及骨盆的锐性外伤时要怀疑有无肾脏损伤的可能。尽管腹部和侧腹部的触痛以及侧腹部的皮下淤血或者包块提示肾脏外伤，但是超过 25%的严重肾脏损伤的患者腹部体检没有明显的体征。在实际当中，55%的肾脏严重损伤儿童表现为肾周的压痛，反过来说，在肾周压痛的患儿中有一半存在比较严重的肾脏外伤[167]。

会阴部皮下淤血、水肿、裂伤和出血都高度提示有泌尿生殖道损伤，尿道口出血或者潮湿的肿块以及男孩直肠指检发现前列腺位置上移均需要进一步行影像学检查，在进行导尿之前应排除尿路损伤。

肉眼血尿高度提示存在泌尿生殖道的外伤，需要进一步的影像学检查。反过来说，没有血尿，包括肉眼血尿甚至镜下血尿，并不能排除泌尿生殖道外伤的可能性。有报道称完全的肾蒂撕裂和 UPJ 的破裂都有可能不出现血尿[14,35-38,43,131,158,166,179]。

然而低位肋骨的骨折以及腰椎的骨折可能会合并有肾脏的外伤，骨盆的骨折可能会合并有膀胱和尿道的损伤，大约 8%的骨盆骨折合并有下尿路损伤。下尿路损伤的发生率在各种骨盆骨折合并耻骨联合骨折的患者是 27%，在骨盆骨折中是 17%，耻骨骨折中是 2% [196]。Aihara 和他的同事[3]的研究表明，一些特定类型的骨盆骨折容易合并出现直肠、膀胱、尿道的损伤。直肠损伤往往伴随着较宽的耻骨分离，膀胱损伤往往伴有骶髂关节增宽和耻骨联合分离以及骶骨的骨折。尿道损伤最常见的是伴有耻骨联合分离和耻骨前支的骨折。这些部位骨折的时候要高度怀疑有无直肠和下尿道损伤，应迅速进行相关的诊断检查。

在骨盆骨折的时候出现大量的血尿提示有膀胱穿孔。骨盆骨折时，任何程度的血尿都是进行膀胱造影的指征，95%的膀胱损伤患者会出现肉眼血尿，其余的存在有镜下血尿。

诊断性评估

对所有的外伤患者都应该取尿样进行检查，以评价有无泌尿生殖道损伤的可能性。肉眼血尿提示可能存在泌尿生殖道损伤，但并不表示损伤严重程度。在没有肉眼血尿的时候，尿样的试纸片检测有无血尿的发生是很可靠的和安全的监测，其假阳性率为 4.3%[58]，试纸片检查血尿阴性的不需要进行显微镜检测[44,58]。如果试纸检查血尿存在，就需要进行显微镜下检查进一步精确的给血尿定量。需要注意的是，有些情况下血尿是由于非外伤因素造成的，例如放置导尿管导致的，这时候血尿一般是微量的，如果每高倍视野超过 5 个红细胞，那么就考虑不是正常的情况了[44,178]。

在怀疑有泌尿生殖道损伤治疗时，一个关键问题就是进行进一步影像学检查的必要和检查的程度，大多数人都会同意给肉眼血尿的患儿进行影像学检查，但是单独在尿液分析中发现的镜下血尿，进行进一步影像学检查的合理性存在着很多争议 *。

* 见参考文献 7,8,22,30,71,90,102,112,114,121,131,140,145,167,170,174,182 和 183。

目前仍不清楚什么程度的儿童镜下血尿需要影像学的检查。有些研究尝试着去了解在成人肾脏外伤时进行进一步的肾脏影像学检查的标准能否适用于儿童，包括肉眼血尿、休克、主要的相关损伤以及明显的减速损伤。虽然在文献报道中不同程度的镜下血尿[112,183]，从 20 个红细胞每高倍视野[91]到 50 个红细胞每高倍视野[145]，都有显著性的差异。在一个对 382 个肾脏外伤儿童的详细研究分析中表明，使用成人进行影像学检查的标准可以使儿童 98%～100%的肾脏外伤得到明确诊断[174]。

通常认为腹部的外伤合并有休克有理由进行泌尿生殖道的影像学检查。有些学者发现，在腹部钝伤病史合并有镜下血尿但没有休克的年轻患者，同时合并有腹部主要脏器损伤以及有明显减速损伤病史的可以在没有肾脏影像学资料的情况下安全治疗[29,128,138,152]。但是超过 25%的各种程度的血尿合并休克的患者有明显的肾脏损伤[89,131,152]。在把成人的标准应用于儿童时要注意一个陷阱，特别是把有无休克作为判断标准的时候，因为儿童在有明显的低血容量的时候仍可保持正常的血压，实际上只有 5%的较重的肾脏外伤儿童会有休克[101,167]，所以有无低血压存在并非是儿童肾脏外伤的可靠指标[167,183]。心动过速通常出现在低血容量之前，是儿童休克的指标之一，是有麻烦的征兆。从以上情况来看，是否给患儿进行影像学检查和成人一样要根据全部的临床表现来决定，而不是根据某一个方面，包括如何受伤（直接的打击、明显的减速损伤、弯曲伸展损伤），生命体征的变化（心动过速、低血压）、体检发现的异常（腹部和侧腹部的压痛、挫伤）、尿液分析（镜下血尿、肉眼血尿）及相关部位的损伤。在大多数情况下，镜下血尿不会单独出现，儿童镜下血尿大多合并有其他的指标，如受伤的机制、体检发现，还有相关的损伤，这些均提示需要进一步的影像学检查以避免误诊的发生。

在儿童腹部外伤处理中，腹部的 CT 检查是标准的评价手段，它可以提供精确的图像以及对肾脏外伤进行分级[18,102,121,201]。它对于分辨实质的挫伤和裂伤、肾周以及腹膜后血肿以及尿外渗、节段性的损伤和大部的损伤有较高的敏感性和特异性，还能显示没有生机、没有血流的组织和节段性的坏死，以及其他的相关损伤。使用先进的快速螺旋 CT 检查的要点就是获得延迟期的肾显像（80 秒后），可以发现实质和静脉的损伤。排泄期（2～10 分钟）的显像可以发现有无尿液和血液的外渗。尿外渗集聚的特点就是动脉期大量的造影剂停留伴稀释[133,176]。

在血流动力学平稳的患者 CT 已经取代了静脉肾盂造影检查，在血流动力学不平稳时，快速的静脉肾盂造影目的是在外科探查之前明确双侧肾脏的功能，这是非常有用的。在儿童快速静脉注射 2～3ml/kg 体重的非碘性造影剂，10 分钟后迅速拍片[133]，需要明确的是静脉肾盂造影只能提供最基本的信息，无法对肾脏外伤进行分级，有些研究表明，大约 20%的有明显肾脏外伤的患者其静脉肾盂造影是正常的。同样在静脉肾盂造影中肾脏无显影并不表示有动脉闭塞和损伤，其他如肾挫伤合并有血管痉挛、水中毒、低血压或者低血液灌注等情况下有一半的患者会出现类似的现象[48]。

在肾脏损伤的诊断和分级中，动脉造影已经几乎被 CT 和 CT 动脉成像所代替，动脉造影比 CT 的侵入性更大，需要有经验的介入放射医生的技巧，而且可能在低龄的儿童有出现血管损伤的危险，因为他们的血管更加细小、脆弱，难以插管以及建立管道。目前动脉造影的目的是应用于延迟性或者进行性的肾脏出血、肾血管损伤、外伤性肾动静脉瘘以及动脉假瘤形成，这些情况下介入技术除了诊断之外还可以通过选择性栓塞[61,64,93,116,137,184]以及血管内支架[23,111,134]同时进行治疗。

超声检查在欧洲作为评价肾脏外伤的手段应用非常广泛，而在美国并非如此。在美国，外伤患者超声检查仅限于腹部外伤急诊超声检查（FAST），该项检查中主要是检查腹腔有无游离液体。对于儿童外伤，FAST 作用不大，除了在合并有闭合性颅脑损伤且有血流动力学不稳定的患儿，可用来排除腹腔内内出血的可能。在血流动力学稳定的患儿 CT 能提供更有用的信息。除了经验丰富的医生，超声对于肾实质损伤并不特别敏感，而且只有多普勒彩色超声检查才能诊断血管损伤，因此它在急诊处理中的作用是相当有限的。

需要特别注意的是，CT 和 IVP 对于膀胱的破裂都不敏感。Hass 和其同事[86]在 15 例怀疑有膀胱损伤的患者中对比了螺旋 CT 和逆行性膀胱造影的准确性，他们发现，膀胱造影可以对 15 例膀胱损伤的患者进行正确的诊断和分级，而 CT 只有 60%的准确性。所以当怀疑有膀胱损伤的时候进行膀胱造影是标准的选择。在常规的造影中，摄片之后，注入少量的

造影剂，然后再次摄片观察有无较多的外溢。如果看
320 到造影剂大量外溢，需要插入气囊导尿管引流，如果没有外溢再将剩下的造影剂注入，然后进行正位、斜位、侧位的摄片，这时需要保持膀胱充盈以避免遗漏小到中等的膀胱壁撕裂伤。青少年的膀胱必须充入300～400ml的造影剂，年幼的儿童必须在重力下滴注，直到患儿有不适的感觉或者可达到膀胱的容积。在2岁以下的儿童，膀胱的容积是7ml × 体重（kg），2～11岁是[年龄（岁）＋2] × 30ml。

作为膀胱造影的一部分，当造影剂从膀胱引流之后需拍摄一张排空片，超过15%的腹膜外膀胱破裂的患者只有通过排空后摄片才能发现，当存在腹膜外膀胱破裂时可以看见造影剂外渗限制在盆腔区域或者非常明显的延伸到盆腔血肿之中，还可能沿着盆腔侧壁分布。当存在腹膜内膀胱破裂时，外渗的造影剂进入腹腔，可以见到造影剂衬托出肠道的外形。

最近发现，CT下的膀胱造影更快，而且对诊断和分级有着同样的精确性，基本需求和普通造影一样，包括膀胱完全扩张、排空前后的摄片等。简单地在CT检查时注入静脉造影剂后夹住气囊导尿管是不够的，会导致更高的损伤遗漏率[113,156]。

当考虑有UPJ损伤时，逆行肾盂造影术在评估输尿管和肾骨盆的完整性中具有重要的作用。在CT中远端输尿管显影不良时，应高度怀疑有输尿管损伤；如果CT不能提供足够的细节，则提示行逆行肾盂造影。

逆行尿路造影术在怀疑有输尿管损伤时应用，在膀胱镜下将小气囊的Foley导尿管插入输尿管开口的凹陷，将大约30ml的造影剂滴注入输尿管下段，正常情况下应该显示整个输尿管径路直到膀胱充满造影剂，当出现缺损和外溢的时候提示有输尿管的破裂。当存在血尿时，在逆行尿路造影之后再进行膀胱造影，即使逆行性尿路造影是正常的也需要进行膀胱造影，因为10%～15%的骨盆骨折伴输尿管损伤的患者合并有膀胱损伤[48]。

泌尿生殖道外伤的分级和评分系统

1989年美国创伤外科学会（AAST）器官损伤评分委员会设计和发表了一个泌尿生殖道外伤的分类或者分级系统（表18-1），用来把外伤的描述标准化以利于研究和资料的收集。表18-1显示和描述了这个分级系统，外伤分为五个级别，从最轻的I级到最复杂的V级，对于肾脏外伤分级是非常有用的。Santucci和其同事[173]研究了2467例肾脏外伤的患者，证实它可以用来评估外伤的严重性，对外科治疗有指导意义，例如I级只需要观察，而V级损伤一般都需要肾脏切除，在这之间的患者（II～IV级）需要根据具体情况处理。随着等级的升高，侵入性治疗有增加的趋势。需要注意的是该项研究是建立在成人的基础上，所以把这个结果推广到儿童时，不能完全照搬。此外在复杂的实质损伤合并有较重的肾血管损伤的IV级和V级患者中，该分级系统受到批评，因为这些患者即使在同一外伤等级中，其治疗也是完全不同的。将来会有改良的系统提出来替代目前的评分系统。AAST对于尿道、膀胱、输尿管的评分系统（见表18-1）没有被广泛的认同，也没有得到大家共同采用。

特定外伤的治疗

肾脏

钝伤

同脾脏、肝脏外伤一样，大多数肾脏钝性的外伤可以通过保守治疗而安全的治愈*。几乎85%的儿童肾脏外伤是相对轻微的，一般是I级和II级，以挫伤和小的实质裂伤为主。这些低等级的肾脏外伤都会完全愈合不留后遗症。较重的肾实质外伤发生率是10%～15%，其余的5%的儿童会发生肾蒂的破裂[48,179]。

CT诊断轻微的肾脏外伤合并有镜下血尿的患儿需要短暂的住院观察，出院时要清楚地交代随访安排。肉眼血尿或（和）CT诊断高等级的肾脏外伤需
要住院卧床休息，严密的检测生命体征的变化，进行 32
一系列的体检和血细胞计数。按照惯例，当患儿完全康复、生命体征平稳、血细胞计数平稳、肉眼血尿消失的时候才能下床活动。当存在有肉眼血尿的时候，可能会因为血凝块导致膀胱出口或Foley导尿管的堵塞，但当患儿出现排尿量减少、膀胱扩张或者膀胱痉

* 见参考文献2,7,8,43,88,109,112,118,120,168,171,179和197。

表 18-1　美国创伤外科学会泌尿系统外伤评分

分级 *	外伤的描述
肾损伤的分级	
I 级挫伤	镜下血尿或者肉眼血尿；泌尿系统检查阴性
血肿	包膜下出血，非扩展性的不伴有实质裂伤
II 级血肿	非扩展性的肾周围血肿局限于肾周后腹膜
裂伤	肾皮质裂伤深度＜1cm 没有尿外渗
III 级裂伤	肾皮质裂伤深度＞1cm 没有尿外渗或集合系统破裂
IV 级裂伤	实质的裂伤穿过皮质、髓质以及集合系统
血管损伤	主要动脉或者静脉的损伤伴有出血
V 级裂伤	肾脏完全破碎
血管损伤	肾蒂撕裂肾脏无血供
输尿管损伤评分	
I 血肿	挫伤性血肿不伴有去血管化
II 裂伤	≤50%横断
III 裂伤	＞50%横断
IV 裂伤	完全离断伴有 2cm 的无血管化
V 裂伤	肾蒂的撕裂伴有肾脏去血管化
膀胱损伤评分	
I 血肿	淤血，黏膜下血肿
裂伤	部分变厚
II 裂伤	腹膜外膀胱裂伤≤2cm
III 裂伤	腹膜外膀胱裂伤＞2cm 或腹膜内膀胱壁裂伤≤2cm
IV 裂伤	腹膜内膀胱壁裂伤＞2cm
V 裂伤	腹膜外或者腹膜内膀胱壁裂伤延伸至膀胱颈或者输尿管开口（膀胱三角）
尿道损伤评分	
I 淤血	出血局限在黏膜下；尿路造影正常
II 伸长性的拉伤	尿道造影有尿道拉长不伴有外渗
III 部分破裂	尿道造影见造影剂在损伤的原位外渗，膀胱有造影剂显影
IV 完全破裂	尿道造影见造影剂在损伤的原位外渗，膀胱无造影剂显影；＜2cm 的尿道断裂
V 完全破裂	完全离断＞2cm，或者造影剂外溢到前列腺或者阴道

* 同一器官的多发性损伤分级增加一级。

† 基于尸检、剖腹探查或影像学检查的精确评估。

From Moore EE, Shackford SR, Pachter HL, et al: Organ injury scaling: Spleen, liver, and kidney. J Trauma 1989;29:1664.

挛性疼痛时，要考虑这种可能性。通过放置 Foly 导尿管或者冲洗甚至更换导尿管可解决问题。虽然通常建议在患者镜下血尿或者肉眼血尿问题解决之前要减少活动，但是在文献中没有循证医学的准则规定限制活动的程度和时间。外伤后需要休息多少时间才能无风险的进行日常活动并不明确，合理时间确定需要前瞻性的研究。

尽管对低等级肾脏外伤的治疗很少有争议，但对血流动力学稳定的稍复杂肾脏外伤以及高级别肾脏外伤合并血流动力学不稳定的患者的治疗尚不明确。尽管 AAST 评分对于外科手术有一定的指导价值，但手术指征更取决于血流动力学的稳定性而不是影像学检

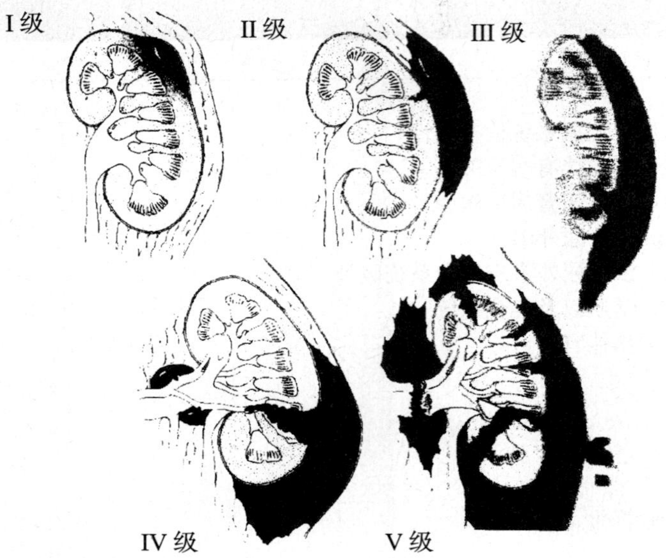

图 18-1 美国创伤外科学会泌尿系统外伤评分图示。(Reproduced with permission from Coburn M: Genitourinary trauma.In Moore E, Feliciano DV, Mattox KL [eds]: Trauma, 5th ed.New York, McGraw-Hill, 2004.)

查上的肾脏损伤的分级，唯一的绝对手术适应证是血流动力学不稳定伴有持续性出血以及需要持续的输血。在影像学上持续的肾脏出血包括 CT 或者动脉造影后腹膜血肿的扩大和非限定性增长、肾主要动脉或者静脉的完全性撕脱伴有尿外渗[94]。

在过去，明确的肾脏外伤伴有尿外渗尽管不是绝
322 对的手术探查指征，至少也是相对的指征。近期的研究表明，在这种情况下，血流动力学稳定的患者大多数都可以通过非手术治疗成功治愈[120,148,161,171]。Matthews 和其同事[120]报道了 27/31（87%）尿外渗的患者自行愈合，其他 4 例因为持续性的尿外渗放置了输尿管支架。同样，Russell 和同事[171]报告了 15 例 IV 级肾脏外伤伴尿外渗的儿童患者，其中 9 例（60%）只需要观察，有 1 例因低血压和持续性出血急诊手术行部分肾脏切除，5 例形成尿性囊肿，2 例行经皮引流，3 例需要输尿管支架。尽管非手术治疗会出现一些并发症，大多数并发症和尿外渗有关，可以通过经皮引流[171]或经输尿管镜放置支架[120,161,171]治疗，这样可以获得很高的肾保留比例。

较重的肾脏外伤合并有肠道或者胰腺的损伤会增加严重感染的风险，例如肾周脓肿或者感染性的尿囊肿。Husmann 和其同事[98]在一个对腹部钝伤后较重的肾裂伤合并有无生机的肾脏碎片的手术治疗和非手术治疗进行对比研究，发现外科手术只是对那些合并有腹腔内损伤的患者的预后有帮助。所以，在儿童较重的肾脏钝伤伴有无生机的碎片合并有消化道穿孔或者合并有较复杂的胰腺损伤时，才是进行肾脏探查的指征以减少严重感染的发生。

在大多数中心，对于血流动力学稳定的高等级肾脏钝性外伤患儿进行保守治疗已经成为一个标准，肾脏外伤病例研究显示，大多数儿童和成人即使是最复杂的肾脏外伤，包括肾脏的破碎、肾完全的离断伴有扩大的肾周血肿和尿外渗，非手术治疗仍可成功[6,171]。对这些患者进行非手术治疗的倡议者提出，虽然缺少前瞻性的研究对比立即手术治疗和保守治疗，没有可靠的资料表明早期手术治疗可以减少近期和远期的并发症。保守治疗避免了由于即刻进行手术探查造成的
肾脏切除的危险，只有 0～13%的患者需要后期的手 32
术治疗[7,8,112,171,179,197]。近期在介入影像学上技术和设备的进步明显减少了后期手术[78]。儿童肾脏外伤的处理流程图见图 18-2。

过去 13 年（1991－2004 年）* 发表的 10 篇儿童肾脏钝性外伤的回顾性病例研究总共包括 668 例患者，损伤等级如下：I 级（342）、II 级（46），、、II 级（64）、IV 级（85）、V 级（24）、IV 级和 V 级（16），I 级和 II 级（50），I 级到 III 级（18），II 级和 III 级（23）。有 45 例（6.7%）需要外科手术治疗，包括 30 例（4.6%）肾脏切除（13 例 IV 级，15 例 V 级，2 例 IV 级和 V 级），10 例（1.6%）半肾切除（其中 8 例 IV 级，1 例 V 级，1 例 IV 级和 V 级），1 例肾网套式压迫止血（IV 级和 V 级），还有 2 例行肾造瘘术（IV 级和 V 级）。所有 I 和 II 级肾脏损伤保守治疗均成功。2 例 III 级肾脏损伤需手术干预，1 例行肾造瘘，1 例行部分肾脏切除术。在 125 例 IV 级和 V 级肾脏损伤中，41 例（33%）需手术干预，其中 30 例肾脏切除，10 例部分肾脏切除，1 例肾修补，2 例肾造瘘。几乎所有的手术指征均是血流动力学不稳定以及持续性的出血，绝大多数需要在 24 小时内急诊手术。广泛且较重的高等级（IV 级和 V 级）的损伤手术率从 1.7%[112]～12.7%[118]不等。非手术治疗的成功率在所有的肾钝性外伤中为 93%，在 III 级外伤中为 97%，IV 级外伤中是 75%，V 级中为 33%。

* 见参考文献 7,8,21,43,112,118,158,171,174 和 179。

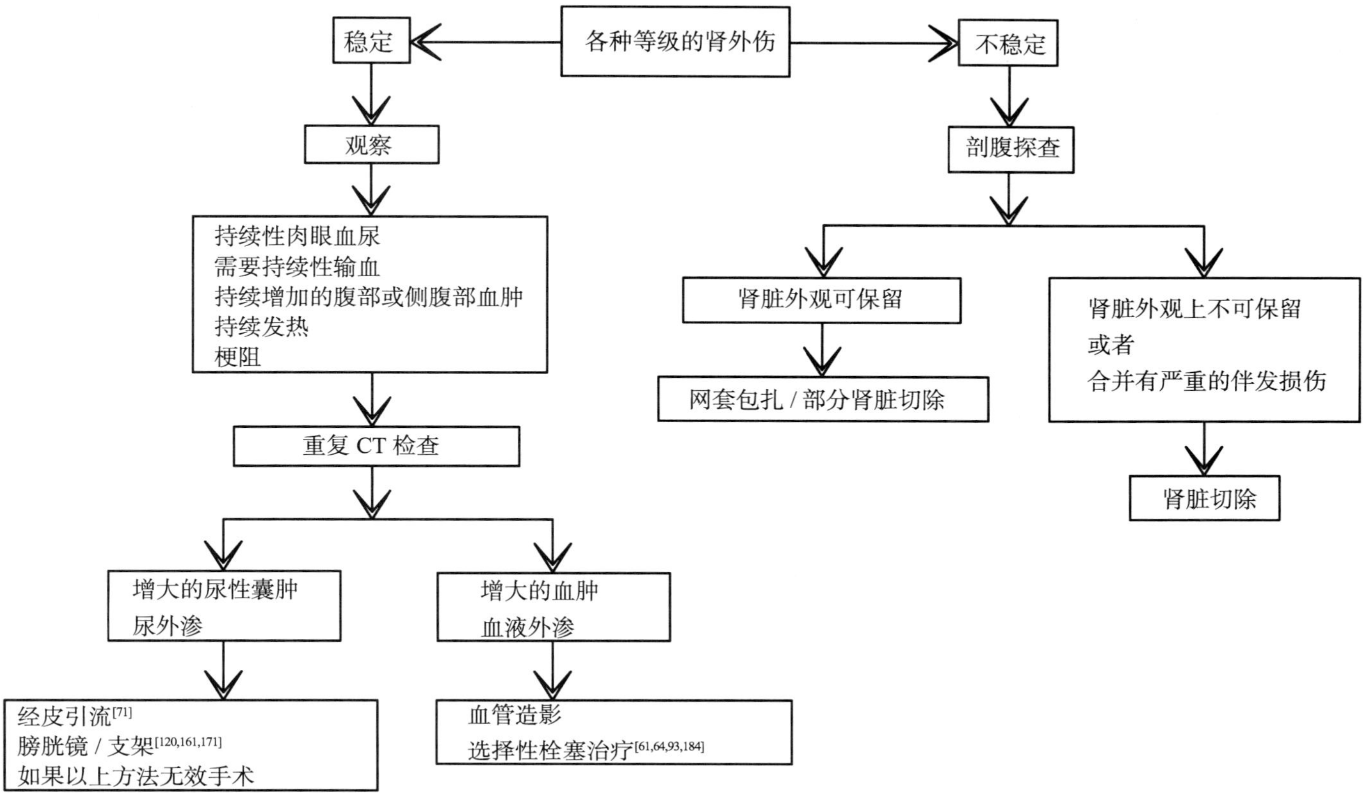

图 18–2 儿童肾脏外伤处理的流程图。

锐性外伤

儿童锐性外伤比较少见。尽管腹部的枪伤均需要进行剖腹探查，但是只有在术前或者术中发现较重的肾脏外伤伴有 Gerota 囊外渗、有明显的泌尿道外的后腹膜脏器的损伤（大血管、十二指肠、胰腺、结肠）以及探查发现有进行性扩大的伴有搏动的后腹膜血肿时，需要切开后腹膜进行探查[191]。McAninch 和其同事[128]将累及到肾脏的枪伤分成五个类别，（1）挫伤 18.4%；（2）轻微的裂伤 13.8%；（3）大的裂伤 50.5%；（4）血管损伤 6.9%；（5）裂伤合并有血管损伤 10.3%。大多数患者存在有多发伤，其中 95%需要相应的处理。即便许多切除的肾脏有潜在的保留可能性，大多数因为危险的血流动力学不稳定而进行了肾脏切除。

对于肾周围的锐性外伤，如果血流动力学稳定且通过 CT 造影扫描三维重建分级同时不伴有其他的损伤，非手术治疗是合适的[68,198]。然而如果采用非手术治疗，那么对有无遗漏的输尿管以及其他相关损伤的怀疑还应该保持。

在一篇回顾性的调查中，McAninch 和其同事[127]发现 55%的肾脏锐伤和 24%的肾脏枪伤可以通过非手术成功治疗，且并发症在可接受的范围。在血流动力学不稳定的锐性外伤或者术中发现后腹膜血肿的患者，给予单次快速的静脉肾盂造影是非常有用的，这可以确定肾脏外伤，同时评价双侧的肾功能，以指导下一步的治疗。

肾血管损伤

严重的肾血管损伤在儿童是比较少见的。Carroll 和其同事[31]以及 Turner 和其同事[190]报告表明，锐性外伤中肾血管损伤占 64%和 68%。而 Cass 和其同事[39]证实 76%的肾血管损伤是由于钝性外伤造成。然而无论是什么受伤机制，这些患者的外伤都比较严重，等级较高，需要大量的输血。在合并有威胁生命的多系统损伤时[31,39,179]，相应的治疗在肾脏外伤治疗前进行。Knudson 和其同事[105]报道，在肾血管损伤后预后不良的因素包括钝伤、V 级的损伤以及试图进行动脉修补。V 级的损伤往往伴有严重的实质损伤，这往往导致重新建立血管的肾脏功能不良。V 级的肾外伤伴有严重的实质损伤，在对侧肾功能完好的情况下立即进行肾脏切除是更好的处理方式。Bruce 和其同事[23]比较了 12 例肾血管钝性外伤的手术患者（9 例肾脏切除。3 例血管重建）和 16 例非手术治疗患者（其中 1 例进行了血管内支架放置），他们得出的结论是非手术治疗单侧钝性肾动脉损伤通常是安全的和成功的，发生外伤后肾血管性高血压的风险是 6%。

肾血管钝性损伤的病理机制是由于迅速的减速导致肾血管结构的牵拉、动脉内膜的破裂以及血栓的形成[31]。肾钝性外伤发生在左侧比发生在右侧更为常见[31,33,34,190]。因为右肾的动脉比左侧要长，所以对减速造成的牵拉损伤更有抵抗力[31]。

13%～56%的肾血管损伤的患者也许没有血尿或者只是镜下血尿[31,39,65,128,179]，大多数患者是由于有其他的症状和体征引起怀疑有肾脏较重的外伤时，才进行进一步的影像学检查[31,179]。

肾血管损伤在 CT 中的表现是：（1）缺乏肾脏增强显影或者是无分泌，但通常有正常的肾轮廓影；（2）静脉增强；（3）中央血肿；（4）增强的肾动脉出现突然中断；（5）肾盂肾盏无造影剂充盈[31,179]。
324 这种损伤的处理决定于确立诊断的时间、血管损伤的程度和种类，还有合并外伤的严重程度[31,105,179]。对于右肾静脉的修补比较困难，这是因为长度短而且更靠近下腔静脉。虽然如此，主肾静脉损伤在大多数的患者中还是可以修补的[31]。左肾静脉起始部的撕裂伤可以通过结扎血管治疗，因为血液完全可以通过肾上腺和性腺的静脉回流[31,83]。

分支的血管难以修补，最好的处理是结扎。如果肾脏坏死的区域超过 15%，可以进行部分肾脏切除术[90]。然而其他的人提出对肾主动脉分支闭塞的患者，如果不合并有不能控制的后腹膜出血、严重的尿外渗或者不合并有其他腹腔内需要手术治疗的病变，可以行保守治疗，这种治疗策略并发症发生率很低[11,31]。

肾动脉修补最适合锐性外伤，也最容易获得成功。尽管有在外伤后 19 小时重建血管的报道[82]，但是对于肾脏，缺血 8 小时后血管重建成功率明显降低[31,69,82,147,177]。Ivatury 和其同事[99]回顾了 40 例穿刺性肾血管外伤的患者，结论是肾血管外伤是否保留肾脏决定于合并外伤的状态和程度，他们还报道试图对肾动脉的修补往往是无意义的。肾静脉的损伤相对容易修补预后较佳。对血流动力学不稳定的多发伤患者施行肾脏切除是首选。

钝伤导致的肾动脉主干损伤很少能获得全部肾脏功能的保留[31,179,190]。Hass 和其同事[85]回顾了 12 例因钝性外伤肾动脉完全闭塞的患者，其中 5 例试图进行肾动脉重建，平均热缺血时间是 5 小时（范围从 4.5～36 小时）。4/5 例患者在血管重建手术当时从技术上看是成功的，但术后肾功能扫描中 3 例患者肾脏无功能，1 例术后只有很少的肾功能。2 例患者因为并发症进行延迟的肾脏切除。其余 7 例患者保守治疗，其中 3 例患者发生明显的高血压进行了肾脏切除。基于这些情况，作者们认为不能提倡对单侧的肾动脉闭塞而对侧肾功能良好的患者进行急诊血管重建，除非患者血流动力学稳定且热缺血时间低于 5 小时。当患者是单侧肾脏损伤、完全的动脉栓塞形成、严重的合并伤以及相当长的热缺血时间，此时应该进行肾脏切除术或者保守治疗，这取决于血流动力学的稳定性。有些报道成功使用血管内支架治疗儿童[134]或者成人[23,111]外伤性肾动脉撕裂和血栓形成。在孤立肾或者双侧肾脏同时出现肾动脉损伤时需要尝试进行肾动脉重建[31,46,160]。肾血管损伤的流程图见图 18–3。

并发症

尽管大多数的儿童肾脏外伤可以保守治疗，但非手术治疗并非没有并发症。选择了非手术治疗患者需要严密的监测。出现血色素下降、需要持续性输血以及持续出现肉眼血尿均提示有进行性的出血。可以重复进行 CT 检查或者动脉造影。动脉造影是非常有用的，因为它可以通过选择性血管栓塞达到止血的目的。实际上在有些选择性的患者动脉造影栓塞可以提高保守治疗的成功性[64]。然而，大量的出血通过栓塞无法缓解需要急诊手术。

长期的肠梗阻、发热、进行性增大的腹部和侧腹部包块或者不适感均提示有持续性的尿外渗或者尿性囊肿，这是肾脏外伤后最常见的并发症。Russell 和其同事[171]报道三分之二的尿性囊肿患儿将会自行缓解，所以小的、非感染性的稳定积液无需手术探查而只需观察，而巨大的扩张的积液可以通过经皮引流[171]或者经皮放置输尿管支架[120,161,171]治疗，同时静脉使用广谱抗生素。

延迟性肾出血并不常见，最常发生在外伤后的两

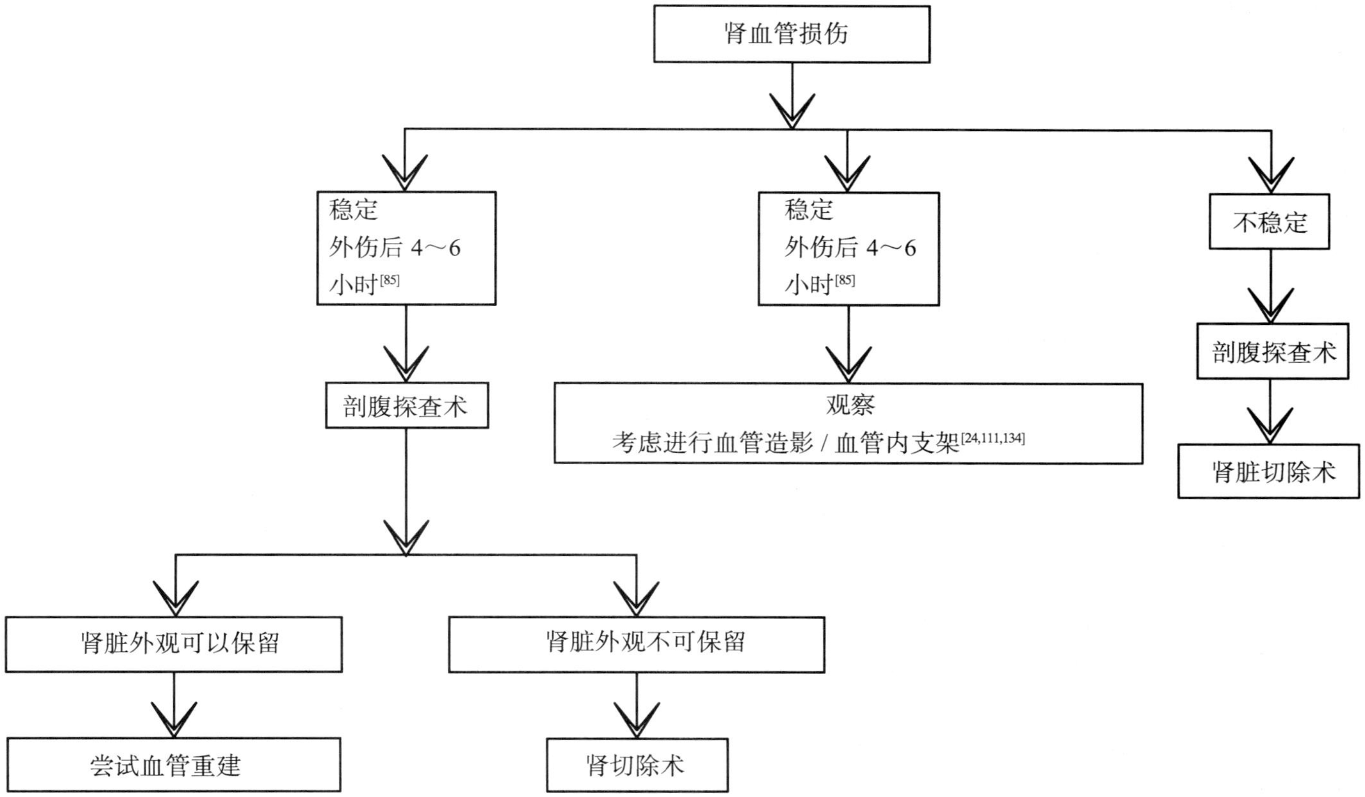

图 18–3 儿童肾血管损伤处理的流程图。

325

周。Teigen 和其同事[184]报道 2 例儿童在最初的肾脏外伤通过动脉造影确诊后，经皮经管道栓塞治疗成功，几周后发生大量的威胁生命的出血。

肾周的脓肿可能伴有肠梗阻、高热和败血症，可以通过 CT 诊断。大多数的患者可以通过静脉广谱抗生素和经皮引流而治愈。多发性脓肿经皮引流效果不佳，一般需要手术引流。

迟发性的并发症可能包括肾积水、动静脉瘘、假性动脉瘤、肾盂肾炎、结石形成以及延迟性肾性高血压。外伤后的动静脉瘘以及假性动脉瘤均可以通过经皮血管栓塞成功治疗[116,137]。创伤后肾性高血压的发病率很低，只有 5%以下的患者发生[85,141,142,194]。尽管肾性高血压通常在外伤后 2 周到几个月出现[85,142,194]，但是有时候延迟到外伤后 10～15 年，所以长时间的随访是非常重要的[160]。

随访和预后

在目前的文献中缺乏以循证医学为基础的儿童肾脏外伤后的随访指南。在回顾性的研究中，Abdalati 和其同事[1]研究了 35 例患者肾脏外伤后分级、并发症的频率以及与康复时间的关系。从该研究中他们推断，I 级和 II 级损伤可以完全康复需要临床随访，不必行影像学的随访。III 级的随访通常伴随很高的并发症（30%），通常需要 4 个月才能完全康复。然而需要强调的是，III 级损伤即使证明完全恢复，还要进行 3～4 次的系列 CT、闪烁扫描、B 超等影像学检查随访，IV 级的损伤通常会伴随有不同程度肾脏的丢失，需要进行影像学上的随访以评价并发症和残余肾脏的功能。虽然 CT 可以提供关于愈合程度、有无并发症的重要信息，但定量 99Tcm 二巯基琥珀酸闪烁扫描（DMSA）对于评价外伤后肾脏功能更有价值[143]。Keller 和其同事[103]对 17 例非手术治疗的儿童肾脏外伤进行了随访研究，在影像学完全愈合之后通过测量血尿素氮（BUN）、肌酐、血压、DMSA 肾脏扫描。Abdalati 和其同事[1]得出同样的结论，在外伤后 3 个月影像学上来看是完全愈合了，肾功能的恢复和肾脏外伤的等级相关，II～IV 级的外伤可以恢复到接近正常的肾功能，而V级外伤往往有明显的肾功能损伤，其原因主要是由于瘢痕形成和肾实质体积的丢失。尽管在DMSA肾脏扫描中有明显的肾功能下降，但所有的儿童均没有症状、血压正常以及血BUN和肌酐正常。需要更大规模的前瞻性的临床和影像学随访研究来进一步评价愈合的时间、并发症的比例、残留的功能以及长期的预后，从而为医生提供一个更符合循证医学的方式来随访和指导外伤儿童的康复。目前通常推荐严重肾脏外伤的儿童外伤后进行血压检测以及CT或者DMSA随访3～6个月，患儿出现泌尿系统症状或者血压上升是进一步的影像学检查的指征。

肾脏外伤的手术治疗

尽管大多数儿童肾脏外伤患者可以通过非手术治疗获得康复，但外科医生必须熟悉肾脏外伤的手术处理技术。前面讨论的对于血流动力学不稳定或者合并有其他严重损伤患者通常采用的手术治疗，往往采取一个正中的剖腹探查切口，虽然传统上认为外科医生首先应该控制肾动静脉进入Gerota筋膜或者血肿的近心端，因为这样可以减少出血以及肾切除的比例
326 [125]，但是近期这个方式受到了挑战。在所有的回顾性研究[4,56]和一个随机性前瞻性研究中[81]，得出的结论表明，在打开Gerota筋膜之前进行肾蒂的控制对肾切除比例、输血量和血液丢失没有作用，却明显的延长了手术时间，增加了1个小时甚至更久。肾切除比例取决于肾脏外伤的程度，而不是肾血管控制的方式[4]。

不管哪一种方式，肾脏需要暴露、肾蒂需要被控制，当有持续性出血的时候，需要迅速的分离出肾脏、用手指控制肾蒂。左肾静脉可以结扎，因为血液可以通过同侧的肾上腺和生殖腺静脉回流，而右肾静脉的外伤需要修补，肾段的动脉可以结扎。如果坏死区域跨度超过肾脏的15%行部分肾脏切除[90]。如果患者的血流动力学是稳定的、肾脏本身是可以保留的、外伤后热缺血时间可以接受，则可以进行肾动脉修补和血管重建，否则要行肾切除术。

如果肾脏外观是可保留的，对肾脏清创保留有活力的组织、清除血肿然后使用可吸收缝线8字缝合止血。如果集合系统破裂需要用细的可吸收单股缝线缝合，因为编织线会割裂肾脏组织[126]，在输尿管和肾盂损伤的时候需要放置内支架。

关闭肾脏包膜以拉近肾脏边缘。如果包膜损毁，那么破裂的边缘覆盖带蒂的大网膜、后腹膜脂肪或聚乙醇酸网[90,126]。接近正常的肾脏外形以及覆盖组织有利于止血和伤口愈合，防治延迟性出血和尿外渗[126]。

输尿管

输尿管损伤并不常见，在儿童威胁生命的外伤中是次要的。虽然如此，诊断和治疗上的延迟仍会造成严重并发症，还会明显增加迟发的致命尿路感染的风险[14,26,76,96]。Boone和其同事[14]报道，钝伤后UPJ损伤在外伤后24小时内诊断其并发症的比例为13%，而如果诊断延误其比例为54%，早期诊断肾脏丢失率为4.5%～9%，比较而言，延误诊断肾脏丢失率为32%～33%[14,96]。

输尿管外伤的分级是依据解剖位置和黏膜损伤的程度（见表18-1）[144]。腹部钝伤后输尿管损伤比较少见，在钝伤中发病率为1%，直接的损伤可能是挤压伤或者是严重的伸直和屈曲伤造成的。直接挤压到脊椎椎体或横突造成的损伤就像前面描述[199]，通常合并有外伤性截瘫[100]。先天性输尿管梗阻的患儿更容易出现集合系统的损伤[89]，而且如果不能认识到病变，没有解除梗阻往往会造成修补失败。

输尿管间接损伤的原因包括坠落伤和减速损伤，就像Boone和其同事[14]注意到的那样，这两种外伤方式特别容易造成UPJ部损伤。Howerton和其同事[96]回顾了54例输尿管撕裂伤在UPJ 4cm以内的患者，发现这种损伤的形式在儿童更常见，发病率是成人的3倍，同样右肾的发病是左肾的3倍。

大约4%的穿刺性外伤会累及到输尿管，往往是刀刺伤和枪伤。尽管这种外伤常见于成人，但同样在儿童中也有一定的发病率[181]。Petrez-Brayfield和其同事[157]回顾了118例输尿管枪伤的患者，根据外伤的部位和严重程度接受相应的外科手术治疗，该报道称并发症比例为20%，所以在此类外伤中要高度怀疑存在输尿管损伤。

儿童输尿管医源性损伤常见于输尿管镜检查和经皮尿路内镜检查，在开放性手术中，当切除腹腔或盆腔肿瘤或者结肠的时候也会导致输尿管损伤，在儿童中有时还会有放射性损伤发生。

由于早期输尿管损伤缺乏症状和体征，造成了非

手术方法诊断的困难，Boone 和其同事[14]在 27%的 UPJ 裂伤的患者中遇到肉眼血尿，26%的患者为镜下血尿同时伴有休克，大约有 1/3 的患者没有血尿。就像 Brandes 和其同事[16]回顾性的报道那样，23%～37%的输尿管损伤的患者没有明显的血尿，侧腹部的肌卫、皮下淤血以及肿块大约只在 7%的输尿管近端损伤的患者中出现[14]。当双侧损伤或孤立肾的患者发生输尿管损伤时候偶尔会出现无尿。

影像学在输尿管外伤中的诊断方法包括 CT 和 IVP，超过 75%的输尿管损伤在 IVP 中会被漏诊[16,165]，同样 CT 诊断输尿管损伤也是比较困难的。目前通常使用快速螺旋 CT 进行诊断，其关键是获得延迟性分泌期的影像（2～10 分钟之内），这样尿外渗就不会被错过。当输尿管没有造影剂的时候，应怀疑有无输尿管损伤的可能性[187]，逆行性肾盂造影术是相当敏感的检查，对血流动力学稳定怀疑有输尿管损伤的患者应该施行该项检查。

大约有一半的输尿管损伤患者会出现延误诊断，其主要原因为临床表现不典型，常无血尿，影像学检查不敏感，以及大多合并有多系统损伤同时伴有循环
27 的不稳定[16,165]。输尿管损伤会继发败血症、血管塌陷或者伤口内尿外渗。输尿管周围纤维化、蜂窝组织炎以及脓肿也较常见，其他的一些并发症例如狭窄引起输尿管梗阻和肾衰竭。

相对于肾脏外伤的处理，在输尿管外伤中保守治疗受到限制。轻微的损伤伴有外渗可以通过逆行性置放支架非手术治疗方式，然而大多数患者可以通过早期手术修补恢复良好。如果诊断明显的延误，则在手术重建之后给予临时性的支架放置或者经皮肾造瘘。因为在外伤 3～5 天之后组织的炎性、脆性增加，这时行修补术，并发症的比例明显增加。

输尿管损伤的处理取决于损伤的位置、受伤的机制、组织丢失的多少以及局部组织的条件。如果输尿管损伤伴有严重的肾脏外伤或者肾脏粉碎，那么最好行肾脏切除；不合并有肾脏外伤应该尝试进行修补；如果 UPJ 破裂可以行肾盂成形修补术；如果肾盂损伤非常严重，行局部清创术缝合肾盂，通过肾盏输尿管吻合恢复输尿管的完整性；如果是输尿管中段的损伤，可以在清创保留有活性的组织后使用可吸收的细线行斜形端端吻合；骨盆部位的输尿管损伤往往通过简单的输尿管再植治疗，有时会将输尿管缝合至腰大肌或者采用膀胱肌管法进行无张力的吻合[84]，通常都会使用输尿管支架。

输尿管枪伤时要进行清创直到边缘血运正常。静脉使用荧光素和 Wood 灯判断活力是有效的方法，有无蠕动并非是有活力的可靠指标。斜形的端端吻合必须使用支架。对于血流动力学不稳定的患者，同时合并有多系统损伤时，最好采取输尿管外置，或者简单的结扎，在术中或术后采用经皮肾造瘘。对于血流动力学不稳定的患者，当有较长的缺损不能一期直接吻合时，简单进行结扎也是一个很好的方法。对长段缺损而平稳的患者可以择期进行重建[12,165,181]。方法包括肾脏游离可以获得 3～5cm 长度[181]，psoas hitch 法或者膀胱肌管法吻合[15]，自体移植[12,193]。另外也可以进行对侧输尿管输尿管吻合和回肠间置[181]。

伴有明显的邻近脏器损伤（即十二指肠或胰腺损伤）的延误性诊断是非常麻烦的，这些损伤很难直接修复。经皮顺行性输尿管支架，后期再进行外科手术处理瘘和狭窄[186]，这也许是在合并有感染性尿性囊肿、脓肿、诊断延误或者是输尿管重建后出现尿外渗并发症等情况下最好的处理方式。

膀胱

解剖学

儿童膀胱位于腹膜外 Retzius 间隙，但仍认为是腹腔内器官[53]。当骨性骨盆生长膀胱进入盆腔，增加了对外伤的抵抗力。在有些外伤的情况下，膀胱的附着部位决定了外伤的形式。膀胱侧方固定于闭孔内肌和脐韧带[53]，在基底部膀胱和泌尿生殖隔相连，Denonvillier 筋膜或直肠膀胱筋膜固定住膀胱后面。和其他部位不一样，膀胱的顶部是可移动和扩张的[154]。

病因

膀胱的外伤一般为钝伤和锐伤。虽然任何一种下腹部的外伤都可能会引起膀胱的损伤，但最常见的是医源性损伤[52,62,80]。引流管的移位和腐蚀、脑室腹腔分流管、子宫内的器械以及 Foley 导管是导致膀胱意外损伤的罕见原因[25,50,53,202]。最常见的故意的锐性伤是枪伤，常常伴有其他腹腔内的损伤。

膀胱损伤中钝性外伤占到 80%，其外伤的程度往往取决于当时膀胱的充盈程度[154]。机动车车祸是最常见的膀胱钝性外伤的病因，骨盆骨折伴有尖锐的骨片可能会划伤膀胱（通常会接近膀胱颈部），剪切力可以将膀胱在其附着处撕裂[53,151]，下腹部的直接的暴力会导致膀胱顶部的破裂而没有周围骨盆骨折[53,180]。

因为膀胱在骨盆的保护之下，只有相当大的暴力才会导致损伤，所以，几乎一半的膀胱损伤合并有其他腹腔脏器的损伤也就并不奇怪了[70]。75%～95%的膀胱损伤合并有骨盆骨折[27,70,151,180]，但是骨盆骨折中只有 4%～20%会有膀胱损伤[13,24,72,163]。

分类和定义

膀胱的钝伤可以分为挫伤、腹膜外破裂和腹膜内破裂，60%～65%的病例会发生腹膜外膀胱破裂，腹膜内破裂的比例为 25%，联合损伤出现的几率为 10%～15%[95]。膀胱的 AAST 分级见表 18–1。

挫伤为膀胱肌肉层损伤而膀胱壁的连续性没有破坏，而破裂为膀胱壁的全层完全破坏[53]。典型挫伤情况可以不做任何处理自动愈合。

328 腹膜外的膀胱损伤通常伴有骨盆骨折[42,52,54]。19%的患者（大多数为男性）合并有尿道损伤，8%会合并有腹膜内脏器损伤[53,54]。

相对腹膜外的膀胱外伤，腹膜内外伤通常不合并有骨盆骨折（表 18–4）。这些损伤通常是由于压榨伤造成（突然发作型）从耻骨弓上直接压向扩张的膀胱或者是迅速的减速暴力损伤[42,52,188]。腹膜内的膀胱破裂一般发生在膀胱的顶部，而腹膜外的损伤通常是骨折穿通或者是撕裂伤[41,55]。在儿童和婴儿，膀胱为腹腔内器官，破裂时通常会造成腹腔内的尿外渗[122]。有些情况下，新生儿会因为严重的膀胱壁血肿造成破裂，或者由于脐动脉置管造成的[20,60]。

处理

膀胱挫伤

膀胱挫伤通常不需要特殊处理而自行愈合。如果骶神经有正常功能，那么膀胱挫伤愈后非常好。骨盆巨大血肿的患者膀胱变形通过放置 Foly 导尿管引流可获得好转。

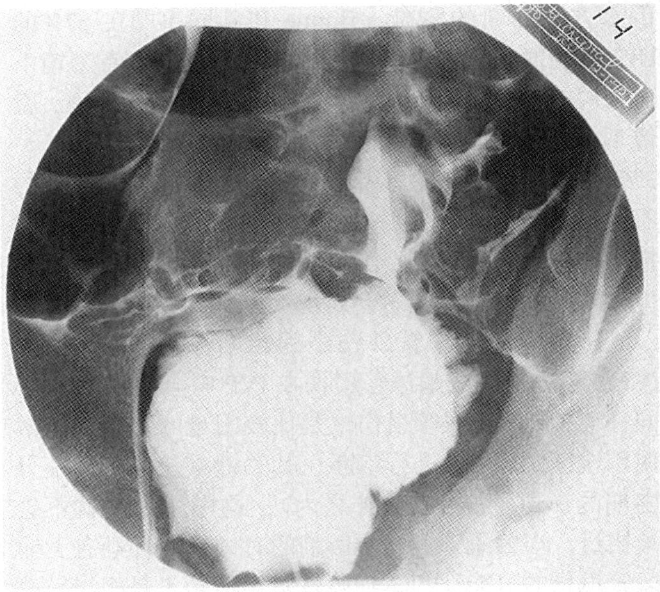

图 18–4 排泄性膀胱造影显示膀胱腹膜内破裂，患者同时合并有双侧坐骨上支和耻骨下支的断裂。

腹膜内破裂

腹膜内膀胱破裂往往合并有其他明显的外伤，需要全面细致的评价患者的状况。最薄弱和移动性最大的顶部是最常见的腹腔内破裂部位，这种情况通常发生在儿童[53,122]。

腹腔内的破裂最好通过手术早期修补。如果腹腔内的尿外渗被延误，会导致患者代谢的异常、败血症以及机械性的紊乱[27,60,92]。病情延误超过 24 小时会出现 BUN、肌酐和血钾上升，血钠下降，实验室检查类似肾衰竭的表现[92]。

手术入路应该从下腹部中线切口，避开侧方的血肿。如果有必要，需要扩大膀胱顶部的裂口探查膀胱内部，同时伴有腹膜外裂伤可以通过膀胱内采用单根可吸收缝线修补。但是外科医生要注意保护输尿管开口，术中可以通过静脉注射靛蓝胭脂红帮助确定输尿管开口的位置和完整性，静脉注射后 10 分钟染料就会在输尿管开口出现。如果裂伤延伸到膀胱颈部要仔细的修补，重建括约肌的完整，避免后期尿失禁的可能性。腹膜内的膀胱破裂需要用可吸收的缝线缝合两层。

修补完成后，放置闭合性负压引流管引流出体外。过去大多数外科医生在腹腔内膀胱破裂修补后，会放置耻骨上膀胱造瘘管代替使用经尿道引流管。近期的文献报道，经尿道放置导尿管不但可行，而且更好。对任何程度的膀胱损伤，通过经尿道放置导尿管同样有效，并发症更少，相对膀胱造瘘管更早拔出[95,185,192]。

尿液的引流通常保留 5～10 天。大多数外科医生在拔管前要进行膀胱造影，明确膀胱恢复的完整性。如果没有尿外渗的表现，那么尿路的引流和闭合性的负压引流就可以去除。

腹膜外破裂

腹膜外膀胱破裂的处理推荐单独使用导尿管引流，这个方法既有效又安全，而且可以免除进行膀胱探查、处理盆腔血肿以及把闭合性的骨盆骨折转变成开放性的必要。这时使用造影检查要注意，有时造影剂外溢量相当惊人，因为能否发现造影剂的外溢取决于裂口的大小和滴入造影剂的量，而造影剂外渗的程度[53,55]和膀胱撕裂损伤的程度可能不相关[27,35-37,54]。在
329 大多数情况下，裂伤通过使用经尿道的导尿管即可以完全愈合，甚至在严重的尿外渗的患者[41,42,55]，大约 90%的腹膜外膀胱破裂会在 10 天内愈合，其余的在 3 周之内康复[55]。几乎不需要手术干预。

锐性损伤

膀胱锐性损伤往往合并有其他损伤，通常都需要首先处理。一般情况下，膀胱锐性外伤的患者均需要剖腹探查，从正中线打开腹腔，首先探查脏器和主要血管结构。

然后探查膀胱，明确膀胱损伤的程度，失活的膀胱和衣物碎屑或者骨片均要清除[27]。输尿管的完整性需要通过静脉注射靛蓝胭脂红来明确。当有尿外渗的时候需要尽可能仔细的探查，必要时放置输尿管导管。

应该避免游离膀胱，否则会导致严重的出血。大而非扩张性的血肿不要去处理。膀胱一般在顶部打开。腹膜外的膀胱缺损应该在膀胱内通过可吸收的单股线连续缝合，无渗漏的关闭是理想的但不是必须的，当有足够的膀胱内引流时稀疏的缝合也能安全愈合，腹腔内的缺损需要进行双层可吸收缝线吻合来缝合。闭合性的引流就像前面谈过那样，经尿道引流，放置 5～10 天。

尿道

尽管在威胁儿童生命的外伤中，尿道损伤是次要的，但是此类外伤会导致相当高比例的长期并发症。目前还不能确定早期修补和后期修补哪一种方式更好，没有前瞻性、随机性的研究报道，能获得的资料主要是来源于成人的回顾性研究，可获得的儿童的资料病例数量比较少。由于解剖上的差异从成人获得的资料，不一定能适用于儿童。例如在儿童后尿道损伤中，没有前列腺的保护，损伤可以发生在任何部位。

钝伤合并有骨盆破裂是导致大多数儿童后尿道损伤的原因，大约有 5%的男性骨盆骨折会同时有后尿道损伤[153]。在这些患者中，大约有 10%～20%会合并有膀胱破裂[55]。90%的尿道损伤的原因是机动车车祸，还有 10%是因为坠落伤和挤压伤以及运动损伤。膀胱侧方的外力没有骨盆骨折也很少引起尿道损伤，后尿道的锐性外伤包括刀刺伤、枪伤以及医源性外伤是非常少见的。

前尿道损伤常常见于骑跨伤，例如高处落下正好跨在围墙或者篱笆上，踢伤或者自行车造成的损伤。锐性的尿道损伤少见，但有时在枪伤和刀刺伤中可以见到。尿道的器械、阴茎外科、性生活中以及手淫也会造成前尿道外伤。

尿道外伤的诊断比较直接明了，其症状主要是不能排空膀胱或者是感觉要排尿但没有小便，外伤后尿道口有血或者肉眼血尿出现均强烈提示有尿道损伤。体检中要注意阴茎、阴囊以及会阴部有可能出现水肿、淤血。Buck、Colle 和 Scarpa 筋膜完整性一旦破坏，根据肿胀的部位可以提示损伤的部位。直肠指检可以发现有无前列腺的上移或者或囊性的肿块，然而这在低龄儿童可能比较困难，所以在诊断时往往需要影像学检查证实。

如果怀疑有尿道损伤，不要盲目试图去插导尿管，因为这会形成错误的假道，有时还会使部分断裂变成全部断裂。逆行性造影在尿道损伤中是标准的处理方法，发现有扩张、充盈缺损、外渗均提示有尿道损伤。如果逆行造影中尿道是完整的，那么可以放置导尿管，然后进行膀胱造影排除膀胱破裂的可能性。

表 18-1 说明了尿道损伤的分级，包括挫伤、拉伤、部分断裂和全部断裂。挫伤和血肿造成的充盈缺损，或者逆行性尿道造影显示尿道拉长，但没有外渗，提示 I 级和 II 级的外伤。尿外渗同时膀胱完整提

示部分断裂（III 级损伤），尿外渗造影剂无法进入近端导尿管提示完全断裂（IV 级损伤），有时尿道周围肌肉痉挛类似全部断裂。图 18–5 提供了一个尿道球
330 部损伤的例子。

尿道外伤长期的后遗症可能是毁坏性的，包括性无能、逆行射精、尿失禁以及尿道狭窄。有些是外伤直接造成的，有些与外科修补有关。

当诊断为前尿道损伤，逆行性造影提示有轻微的尿外渗且尿道完整性较好，同时膀胱能自行排空，这种 I 级和 II 级的损伤可以自行愈合。如果患者一直能自主排空小便，无需进行任何导尿操作。中间程度的前尿道损伤可以通过置放经尿道的 Foley 导尿管来治疗，而更复杂的损伤最好首先放置耻骨上导尿管。延迟性的狭窄是常见的，大多数可以通过尿道成形术来纠正。

前尿道的锐性外伤可以通过探查和 I 期修补术或者耻骨上尿液分流来处理。Husmann 和其同事[97]回顾了 17 例因低速枪伤导致前尿道部分断裂的治疗，结论得出最好的处理方式是大范围的清创、海绵体和尿道的修补以及放置耻骨上导管，这种情况下狭窄的发生率较低（1/8），而单纯耻骨上分流和经导尿管置放支架发生率相对较高（7/9）。

儿童大多数后尿道损伤可以通过非手术治疗。I 级和 II 级损伤，如果膀胱可以自行排空，通过非手术且无需放置尿管即可治愈；如果膀胱不能自行排空，那么可以放置细的 Foley 导尿管治疗。III 级损伤合并有微量的尿外渗，可以在逆行性造影之后，迅速

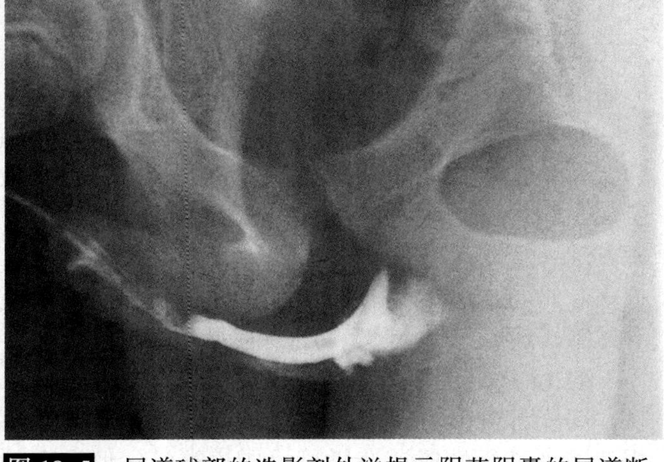

图 18–5 尿道球部的造影剂外溢提示阴茎阴囊的尿道断裂。膜后部和前列腺部尿道是完整的。

在透视下放置细的 Foley 导尿管。如果导管不能轻易通过，那么应该放置耻骨上造瘘管。

复杂的后尿道损伤的修补方法包括：I 期尿道吻合、延期的 I 期尿道吻合、I 期尿道会师、I 期内镜下尿道会师以及耻骨上膀胱造瘘延期手术。

I 期外科修补包括清除骨盆血肿、游离前列腺和尿道、直接进行端端吻合膜部和前列腺部的尿道。这种处理方式会增加损伤部位无法控制性出血的可能性，因为清除血肿后损伤部位血肿压迫止血的作用消失。另外切除了前列腺和尿道周围的组织，增加了性无能的可能性。还有需要分离、游离前列腺和尿道，同时还要清除撕裂的尿道，损伤了尿道内括约肌，增加了尿失禁的可能性[51,53,56,57,108,195]。为了减少这些情况的发生，Mundy[150]提倡延迟性的一期外科修补，在外伤后 7～10 天进行。因为这时候患者病情更加稳定，手术视野因为出血造成的模糊也会减轻，而且纤维化还没有形成。

I 期尿道会师术最早由 Ormond 和 Cothran 在 1934 年介绍，其后许多年来该技术有很多的变化[59,66,73,107]。尽管不需要直接缝合断裂的尿道断端，这项技术还是要求开放性的进入，清除盆腔血肿，伴随有所有的并发症。近期联合使用经尿道和经膀胱内镜的技术，可以获得尿道的会师而且没有探查断裂尿道的风险[47,49,74,77,115,132,164,169]。进一步来说，这种方法没有处理前列腺周围组织而且没有增加海绵体神经的外伤，也不会增加勃起障碍的危险。这些微创技术已经能够获得很好的疗效，但是临床经验仅仅限于小范围的系列患者，这些患者中术后 88%～100%没有尿失禁，14%～39%有不同程度的勃起障碍，大约有一半的患者需要进行尿道内切开。

考虑到 I 期开放性手术修补或者会师术对性功能和尿控功能的影响，所以可选用另一种方式，称为耻骨上膀胱造瘘延期尿道成型。最早由瑞典的 Johanson 在 1953 年提出，不要去探查尿道，仅仅通过耻骨上导尿管分流尿液，狭窄是不可避免的，可以在几个月之后修补。这种方法已经获得广泛的认可，而且被认为是复杂的后尿道断裂的标准处理方式。它的优点包括避免进入新鲜的骨盆血肿从而增加失血和感染的机会，放置耻骨上导管迅速方便，这样因为避免了分离前列腺和尿道而减少了性无能和尿失禁的可能性[73]。缺点是需要长时间的耻骨上造瘘管，感染和结石形成的风险增加，几乎 100%可能发生尿道狭窄，而且在

后期手术中需要复杂和困难的修补[107]。Tunc 和其同事[189]回顾了 77 例后尿道损伤接受延迟性手术的患者，95%的患者显示了尿道的完整性，术后 9%出现尿失禁，16%出现勃起障碍。他们推断延迟性尿道成形是个成功的治疗方法，后期的并发症是可以让人接受的。

在回顾了大量的不同处理方式下复杂后尿道损伤的结果，Holevar 和其同事[95]的结论是这些外伤可以通过经内镜下尿道会师术或者耻骨上膀胱造瘘延期尿道成形治疗，最终的结果是相似的。

331 女性的尿道外伤是比较少见的[31,162]。最常见的致伤机制是机动车后的骨盆骨折，有时是骑跨伤。女性的尿道外伤可以是远端会阴部的撕裂、根部的破裂或者是撕裂伤，后者特点是通常合并有其他的骨盆损伤，包括阴道和膀胱颈部裂伤。

Perry 和其同事[159]回顾性评价了女性尿道外伤合并有骨盆骨折。阴道口有血提示要进行仔细的阴道探查，尿道口也需要仔细的探查，可以通过一个导尿管来明确。然而值得注意的是，即使有明显的尿道损伤导尿管也能置入膀胱，移除导尿管后出现外阴肿胀需要进行进一步探查。由于尿道造影在女孩实施困难，很难实现，尿道镜是个更好的诊断方法。女孩尿道损伤的延误是常见的，而且具有毁损性的后果[159]。此类损伤大约有 50%的误诊率会导致威胁生命的败血症和坏死性筋膜炎，所以在怀疑女孩有尿道损伤时，进行尿道镜检查的门槛应该降低。

治疗方式取决于外伤的程度和部位。尿道损伤至膀胱颈部需要精细的修补，行膀胱出口和尿道端端的吻合，这种情况占三分之二[121,122,126,129]；合并阴道损伤可以进行一期修补；尿道挤压伤如果没有膀胱颈损伤，可以通过延长的经尿道放置导尿管治疗（6～8 周）。如果有必要可以在耻骨上膀胱造瘘管。女性尿道损伤长期明显的并发症包括尿道狭窄、尿道阴道瘘、尿失禁和阴道狭窄[63]。

很明显，应尽力发现这一不常见的损伤，并尽早进行彻底治疗。

外生殖器

女孩

女孩外生殖器外伤相当常见，主要症状是外伤后迅速出现内裤和会阴部血迹[117]。钝性的外伤常见是由于骑跨伤造成。最常见的损伤类型发病率按照降序排列如下：会阴体裂伤和挫伤、阴道、大阴唇、尿道以及直肠。由于对一个清醒的、不舒服、焦虑和害羞的女孩进行完整的泌尿生殖道检查是非常困难的，所以检查最好在全麻下进行。有 76%的患者实际损伤比在急诊室评价更为严重[117]。

女性外生殖器的外伤处理方式取决于外伤的种类和程度。坏死、挫伤组织应该清除，裂伤可以在止血后一期修补。使用可吸收线可以避免拆线，有时需要进行尿道镜和直肠镜做全面的评价。

男孩

最常见的阴茎损伤是行包皮环切过程中的医源性损伤[80]。包皮环切的并发症有阴茎切断、尿道瘘、龟头裂伤、不准确的去除包皮会造成阴茎发生脱套伤。这些损伤可以通过采用合适的技术来避免。

由于钝伤和锐伤造成阴茎的外伤在儿童中是非常少见的。尿道的撕裂伤处理应该和前面叙述的那样。如果发现进行性扩大的血肿、可触摸到的阴茎缺损以及严重的出血提示海绵体损伤，当发生这些情况时需要进行一期修补术[17]，有时候也需要行耻骨上造瘘[79]。外生殖器枪伤局限时，推荐的治疗方法是表面的清创、修复海绵体的缺损以及一期修复尿道损伤[87]。

阴茎的勃起障碍（阳痿）可发生于骨盆和会阴部的钝伤[149]。阳痿可能是由于阴茎血管在骨盆内撕裂造成的，进行阴茎的血管重建可能会有效果[119]。有时候会出现持续性的勃起，这时候进行选择性的阴茎动脉造影对诊断很有帮助，而且可以对动静脉瘘进行栓塞，多普勒彩超对于病变的定性和定位也很有帮助[138]。

由于拉链造成的阴茎绞伤很多在急诊室即可处理，有时需要在全麻下进行[200]。对于束带造成的阴茎钳制伤，可以迅速解除束缚物以解决问题。在儿童，毛发的束缚是个常见的原因，相当难以去除，严重的情况下会造成阴茎前部的皮肤、龟头、阴茎海绵体、尿道的坏死，需要保守的清创和尿路分流[48]。

阴囊的外伤可以是钝性外伤、锐性外伤或者是两者同时造成。高清晰的超声检查对评价此类外伤非常有用[10]。超声可以了解锐性外伤有无睾丸的破裂，睾丸周围组织的异常，还可以了解有无异物和其位置[110]。这项检查对于区分较轻的外伤也很有价值，例如可以将阴囊血肿、睾丸鞘膜积液和鞘膜积血同需要外科急诊处理的情况如睾丸破裂和坏死区分开来。需要注意的是超声不易鉴别附睾的破裂[155]。有鞘膜积血的患者应该考虑进行手术探查，因为手术探查可以清除鞘膜内的积血，减少并发症而且加速恢复。睾丸的破裂可以通过清创和一期缝合治疗[5]。

（李巍松译　吕志葆校）

参考文献

1. Abdalati H, Bulas K, Sivit C, et al: Blunt renal trauma in children: Healing of renal injuries and recommendations for imaging follow-up. Pediatr Radiol 1994;24:573.
2. Ahmed S, Morris LL: Renal parenchymal injuries secondary to blunt abdominal trauma in childhood: A 10-year review. Br J Urol 1982;54:470.
3. Aihara R, Blansfield JS, Milham FH, et al: Fracture locations influence the likelihood of rectal and lower urinary tract injuries in patients sustaining pelvic fractures. J Trauma 2002;52:205.
4. Altala A, Miller FB, Richardson JD, et al: Preliminary vascular control for renal trauma. Surg Gynecol Obstet 1991; 173:386.
5. Altarac S: Management of 53 cases of testicular trauma. Eur Urol 1994;25:119.
6. Altman AL, Haas C, Dinchman KH, et al: Selective nonoperative management of blunt grade 5 renal injury. J Urol 2000;164:27-30.
7. Bass DH, Semple PL, Cywes S: Investigation and management of blunt renal injuries in children: A review of 11 years' experience. J Pediatr Surg 1991;26:196.
8. Baumann L, Greenfield, Aker J, et al: Nonoperative management of major blunt renal trauma in children: In-hospital morbidity and long-term followup. J Urol 1992;148:691.
9. Beaver BL, Colombani PM, Fal A, et al: The efficacy of computed tomography in evaluating abdominal injuries in children with major head trauma. J Pediatr Surg 1987; 22:1117.
10. Berman JM, Beidle TR, Kunberger LE, Letourneau JG: Sonographic evaluation of acute intrascrotal pathology. AJR Am J Roentgenol 1996;166:857.
11. Bertini JE Jr, Flechner SM, Miller P, et al: The natural history of trauma branch renal artery injury. J Urol 1986; 135:228.
12. Bodie B, Novick AC, Rose M, Strafton RA: Long-term results with renal autotransplantation for ureteral replacement. J Urol 1986;136:1187.
13. Bond SJ, Gotschall CS, Eichelberger MR: Predictors of abdominal injury in children with pelvic fracture. J Trauma 1991;31:1169.
14. Boone TB; Gilling PJ, Husmann DA: Ureteropelvic junction disruption following blunt abdominal trauma. J Urol 1993; 150:33.
15. Bracken RB, Sheldon CA: Psoas hitch, Boari flap and transureteroureterostomy. In Fowler JE Jr (ed): Mastery of Surgery: Urologic. Boston, Little, Brown, 1992.
16. Brandes SB, Chelsky MJ, Buckman RF, Hanno PM: Ureteral injuries from penetrating trauma. J Trauma 1994;36:766.
17. Brandes SB, Buckman RF, Chelsky MJ, Hanno PM: External genitalia gunshot wounds: A ten-year experience with 56 cases. J Trauma 1995;39:266.
18. Bretan APN Jr, McAninch JW, Federle MP, et al: Computerized tomographic staging of renal trauma: 85 consecutive cases. J Urol 1986;136:561.
19. Brower P, Paul J, Brosman SA: Urinary tract abnormalities presenting as a result of blunt abdominal trauma. J Trauma 1978;18:719.
20. Brown D, Maghill HL, Block DL: Delayed presentation of traumatic intraperitoneal bladder rupture. Pediatr Radiol 1986;16:253.
21. Brown SL, Elder JS, Spirnak JP: Are pediatric patients more susceptible to major renal injury from blunt trauma? A comparative study. J Urol 1998;160:138.
22. Brown SL, Haas C, Dinchman KH, et al: Radiologic evaluation of pediatric blunt renal trauma in patients with microscopic hematuria. World J Surg 2001;25:1557.
23. Bruce LM, Croce MA, Santaniello JM, et al: Blunt renal artery injury: Incidence, diagnosis, and management. Am Surg 2001;67:550.
24. Burgess AR, Eastridge BJ, Young JW, et al: Pelvic ring disruption: Effective classification systems and treatment protocols. J Trauma 1990;30:848.
25. Burnett DG: Near bladder perforation in urethra-catheter extrusion: An unusual complication of cerebrospinal fluid-peritoneal shunting. J Urol 1982;127:543.
26. Campbell EW, Filderman PS, Jacobs SC: Ureteral injury due to blunt and penetrating trauma. Urology 1992;40:216.
27. Carroll PR, McAninch JW: Major bladder trauma: Mechanism of injury and a unified method of diagnosis and repair. J Urol 1984;132:254, 1984.
28. Carroll PR, McAninch JW: Operative indications in penetrating renal trauma. J Trauma 1985;25:587, 1985.
29. Carroll PR, McAninch JW: Current management of blunt renal trauma. Urol Ann 1987;1:171.
30. Carroll PR, McAninch JW: Staging renal trauma. Urol Clin North Am 1989;16:193.
31. Carroll PR, et al: Renovascular trauma: Risk assessment, surgical management, and outcome. J Trauma 1990;20:547.
32. Carter CT, Schafer N: Incidence of urethral disruption in females with traumatic pelvic fractures. Am J Emerg Med 1993;11:218.
33. Cass AS, Susset J, Khan A, et al: Renal pedicle injury in the multiple injured patient. J Urol 1979;122:728.
34. Cass AS: Immediate radiological evaluation and early surgical management of genitourinary injuries from external trauma. J Urol 1979;122:772.
35. Cass AS: Immediate surgical management of severe renal injuries in multiple injured patients. Urology 1983;21:140.
36. Cass AS: Renal trauma in the multiple-injured child. Urology 1983;21:487.
37. Cass AS: Blunt renal pelvic and ureteral injury in multiple-injured patients. Urology 1983;22:268.
38. Cass AS: Blunt renal trauma in children. J Trauma 1983; 23:123.
39. Cass AS, Bubrick M, Luxenberg M, et al: Renal pedicle injury in patients with multiple injuries. J Trauma 1985; 23:892.
40. Cass AS, Luxenberg M, Gleich P, et al: Clinical indications

for radiographic evaluation of blunt renal trauma. J Urol 1986;136:370.
41. Cass AS, Luxenberg M: Features of 164 bladder ruptures. J Urol 1987;138:743.
42. Cass AS: Diagnostic studies and bladder rupture: Indications and techniques. Urol Clin North Am 1989;16:267.
43. Ceylan H, Gunsar C, Etensel B, et al: Blunt renal injuries in Turkish children: A review of 205 cases. Pediatr Surg Int 2003;19:710.
44. Chandhoke PJ, McAninch JW: Detection and significance of microscopic hematuria in patients with blunt renal trauma. J Urol 1988;140:16.
45. Chopra P, St-Vil D, Yazbeck S: Blunt renal trauma—blessing in disguise? J Pediatr Surg 2002;37:779.
46. Clark DE, Georgitis JW, Ray RS: Renal arterial injuries caused by blunt trauma. Surgery 1981;90:87.
47. Clark WR, Patterson DE, Williams HJ Jr: Primary radiologic realignment following posterior urethral disruption. Urology 1992;39:182.
48. Coburn M: Genitourinary trauma. In Moore E, Feliciano DV, Mattox KL (eds): Trauma, 5th ed. New York, McGraw-Hill, 2004.
49. Cohen JK, Berg G, Carl GH, et al: Primary endoscopic realignment following posterior urethral disruption. J Urol 1991;146:1548.
50. Cohen MS, et al: Bladder perforation after orthopedic hip surgery. Urology 1977;9:291.
51. Coffield KS, Weems WL: Experience with management of posterior urethral injury associated with pelvic fracture. J Urol 1977;117:722.
52. Corriere JN Jr, Sandler CM: Management of the ruptured bladder: Seven years experience with 111 cases. J Trauma 1986;26:830.
53. Corriere JN Jr: Trauma to the lower urinary tract. In Gillenwater JY, et al (eds): Adult and Pediatric Urology. Chicago, Year Book Medical, 1987.
54. Corriere JN Jr, Sandler CM: Mechanisms of injury patterns of extravasation and management of extraperitoneal bladder rupture due to blunt trauma. J Urol 1988;139:43.
55. Corriere JN Jr, Sandler CM: Management of extraperitoneal bladder rupture. Urol Clin North Am 1989;16:275.
56. Corriere JN Jr, McAndrew JD, Benson GS: Intraoperative decision making in renal trauma surgery. J Trauma 1991;31:1390.
57. Crassweller PO, Farrow GA, Robson CJ, et al: Traumatic rupture of the supramembranous urethra. J Urol 1977;118:770.
58. Daum GS, Krolikowski FJ, Reuter KL, et al: Dipstick evaluation of hematuria in abdominal trauma. Am J Clin Pathol 1988;89:538.
59. DeWeerd JH: Immediate realignment of posterior urethral injury. Urol Clin North Am 1977;4:75.
60. Diamond DA, Ford C: Neonatal bladder rupture: A complication of umbilical artery catheterization. J Urol 1989;142:1543.
61. Dinkel HP, Danuser H, Triller J: Blunt renal trauma: Minimally invasive management with microcatheter embolization experience in nine patients. Radiology 2002;223:723.
62. Dmochowski R, Crondell SS, Corriere JN Jr: Bladder injury in uroascites from umbilical artery catheterization. Pediatrics 1986;77:421.
63. Dorai CDRT, Boucaut HAP, Dewan PA: Urethral injuries in girls with pelvic trauma. Eur Urol 1993;24:371.
64. Eastham JA, Wilson TG, Larsen DW, et al: Angiographic embolization of renal stab wounds. J Urol 1992;148:268.
65. Eastham JA, Wilson TG, Ahlering TE: Urological evaluation and management of renal-proximity stab wounds. J Urol 1993;150:1771.
66. Elliott DS, Barrett DM: Long-term follow-up and evaluation of primary realignment of posterior urethral disruptions. J Urol 1997;157:814.
67. Esho JO, Ireland GW, Cass AS: Renal trauma and preexisting lesions of kidney. Urology 1973;1:134.
68. Fairhurst JJ, Rubin CM, Hyde I, et al: Bladder capacity in infants. J Pediatr Surg 1991;26:55.
69. Fay R, Brosman S, Lindstrom R, Cohen A: Renal artery thrombosis: A successful revascularization by autotransplantation. J Urol 1974;111:572.
70. Flancbaum L, Morgan AS, Fleisher M, et al: Blunt bladder trauma: Manifestation of severe injury. Urology 1988;31:220.
71. Fleisher G: Prospective evaluation of selective criteria for imaging among children with suspected blunt renal trauma. Pediatr Emerg Care 1989;5:8.
72. Flint L, Babikan G, Anders M, et al: Definitive control of mortality from severe pelvic fracture. Ann Surg 1990;211:703.
73. Follis HW, Koch MO, McDougal WS: Immediate management of prostatomembranous urethral disruptions. J Urol 1992;147:1259.
74. Gelbard MK, Heyman AM, Weintraub P: A technique for immediate realignment and catheterization of the disrupted prostatomembranous urethra. J Urol 1989;142:52.
75. Gerstenbluth RE, Spirnak JP, Elder JS: Sports participation and high grade renal injuries in children. J Urol 2002;168:2575.
76. Ghali AM, El Malik EM, Ibrahim AI, et al: Ureteric injuries: Diagnosis, management, and outcome. J Trauma 1999;46:150.
77. Gheiler EL, Frontera JR: Immediate primary realignment of prostatomembranous urethral disruptions using endourologic techniques. Urology 1997;49:596.
78. Gill B, Palmer L, Reda E, et al: Optimal renal preservation with timely percutaneous intervention: A changing concept in the management of blunt renal trauma in children in the 1990s. Br J Urol 1994;74:370.
79. Gomez RG, Castanheira AC, McAninch JW: Gunshot wounds to the male external genitalia. J Urol 1993;150:1147.
80. Gonzales ET Jr, Guerriero WG: Genitourinary trauma in children. In Kelalis PP, King LR, Bellman AB (eds): Clinical Pediatric Urology. Philadelphia, WB Saunders, 1985.
81. Gonzales RP, Falimirski M, Holevar MR, et al: Surgical management of renal trauma: Is vascular control necessary? J Trauma 1999;47:1039.
82. Guerriero WG, Carlton SE Jr, Scott R Jr, et al: Renal pedicle injuries. J Trauma 1971;1:53.
83. Guerriero WG: Penetrating renal injuries in the management of renal pedicle injury. Urol Clin North Am 1977;4:3.
84. Guerriero WG: Ureteral injury. Urol Clin North Am 1989;16:237.
85. Haas CA, Dinchman KH, Nasrallah PF, et al: Traumatic renal artery occlusion: A 15 year review. J Trauma 1998;45:557.
86. Haas CA, Brown SL, Spirnak JP: Limitations of routine spiral computerized tomography in the evaluation of bladder trauma. J Urol 1999;162:51.
87. Hall SJ, Wagner JR, Edelstein RA, et al: Management of gunshot wounds to the penis and anterior urethra. J Trauma 1995;38:439.
88. Haller JA Jr, Papa P, Drugas G, Colombani P: Nonoperative management of solid organ injuries in children. Is it safe? Ann Surg 1994;219:625.

89. Hardeman S, Husmann DA, Chinn HK, et al: Blunt urinary tract trauma: Identifying those patients who require radiological studies. J Urol 1989;141:1095.
90. Herschorn S, Kodona RT, Abara EO: Genitourinary trauma. In McMurtry R, McMillan GA (eds): Management of Blunt Trauma. Baltimore, Williams & Wilkins, 1990.
91. Herschorn S, Raadomski SB, Shoskes DA, et al: Evaluation and treatment of blunt renal trauma. J Urol 1991;146:274.
92. Heyns CF, Rimington PD: Intraperitoneal rupture of the bladder causing the biochemical features of renal failure. Br J Urol 1987;60:217.
93. Heyns CF, Van Vollenhoven P: Increasing role of angiography and segmental artery embolization in the management of renal stab wounds. J Urol 1992;147:1231.
94. Holcroft HW, Trunkey DD, Minagi H, et al: Renal trauma and retroperitoneal hematomas: Indications for exploration. J Trauma 1975;15:1045.
95. Holevar M, Ebert J, Luchette F, et al: Practice management guidelines for the management of genitourinary trauma. On Internet site for Eastern Association for the Surgery of Trauma, Copyright 2004.
96. Howerton RA: Proximal ureteral avulsion from blunt abdominal trauma. Milit Med 1991;156:311.
97. Husmann DA, Boone TB, Wilson WT: Management of low velocity gunshot wounds to the anterior urethra: The role of primary repair versus urinary diversion alone. J Urol 1993;150:70.
98. Husmann DA, Gilling PJ, Perry MO, et al: Major renal lacerations with a devitalized fragment following blunt abdominal trauma: A comparison between nonoperative (expectant) versus surgical management. J Urol 1993; 150:1774.
99. Ivatury RR, Zubowski R, Stahl WM: Penetrating renovascular trauma. J Trauma 1989;29:1620.
100. Javadpour N, Guinan P, Bush IM: Renal trauma in children. Surg Gynecol Obstet 1973;136:237.
101. Jetvich MJ, Montero GG: Injuries to renal vessels by blunt trauma in children. J Urol 1969;102:493.
102. Karp MP, Jewett TC Jr, Kuhn JP, et al: The impact of computed tomography scanning on the child with renal trauma. J Pediatr Surg 1986;21:617.
103. Keller MS, Eric Coln C, Garza JJ, et al: Functional outcome of nonoperatively managed renal injuries in children. J Trauma 2004;57:108-110.
104. Knudson MM, McAninch JW, Gomez R, et al: Hematuria as a predictor of abdominal injury after blunt trauma. Am J Surg 1992;164:482.
105. Knudson MM, Harrison PB, Hoyt DB, et al: Outcome after major renovascular injuries: A Western Trauma Association multicenter report. J Trauma 2000;49:1116.
106. Koff SA: Estimating bladder capacity in children. Urology 1983;21:248.
107. Koraitim MM: Pelvic fracture urethral injuries: Evaluation of various methods of management. J Urol 1996;156:1288.
108. Koraitim MM: Pelvic fracture urethral injuries: The unresolved controversy. J Urol 1999;161:1433.
109. Kuszmarov IW, Morehouse DD, Gibson S: Blunt renal trauma in the pediatric population: A retrospective study. J Urol 1981;126:648.
110. Learch TJ, Hansch LP, Ralls PW: Sonography in patients with gunshot wounds of the scrotum: Imaging findings and their value. AJR Am J Roentgenol 1995;165:879.
111. Lee JT, White RA: Endovascular management of blunt traumatic renal artery dissection. J Endovasc Ther 2002; 9:354.
112. Levy JB, Baskin LS, Ewalt DH, et al: Nonoperative management of blunt pediatric major renal trauma. Urology 1993;42:418.
113. Lis LE, Cohen AJ: CT cystography in the evaluation of bladder trauma. J Comput Assist Tomogr 1990;14:386.
114. Livene PM, Gonzales ET: Genitourinary trauma in children. Urol Clin North Am 1985;12:53.
115. Londergan TA, Gundersen LH, Van Every MJ: Early fluoroscopic realignment for traumatic urethral injuries. Urology 1997;49:101.
116. Lupattelli T, Garaci FG, Manenti G, et al: Giant high-flow renal arteriovenous fistula treated by percutaneous embolization. Urology 2003;61:837.
117. Lynch JM, Gardner MJ, Albanese CT: Blunt urogenital trauma in prepubescent female patients: More than meets the eye. Pediatr Emerg Care 1995;11:372.
118. Margenthaler JA, Weber TR, Keller MS: Blunt renal trauma in children: Experience with conservative management at a pediatric trauma center. J Trauma 2002; 52:928.
119. Matthews LA, Herbener TE, Seftel AD: Impotence associated with blunt pelvic and perineal trauma: Penile revascularization as a treatment option. Semin Urol 1995; 13:66.
120. Matthews LA, Smith EM, Spirnak JP: Nonoperative treatment of major blunt renal lacerations with urinary extravasation. J Urol 1997;157:2056.
121. McAleer IM, Kaplan G, Sherz HC, et al: Genitourinary trauma in the pediatric patient. Urology 1993;42:563.
122. McAleer IM, Kaplan GW: Pediatric genitourinary trauma. Urol Clin North Am 1995;22:177.
123. McAleer IM, Kaplan GW, LoSasso BE: Congenital urinary tract anomalies in pediatric renal trauma patients. J Urol 2002;168:1808.
124. McAleer IM, Kaplan GW, LoSasso BE: Renal and testis injuries in team sports. J Urol 2002;168:1805.
125. McAninch JW, Carroll PR: Renal trauma: Kidney preservation through improved vascular control—A refined approach. J Trauma 1984;22:285.
126. McAninch JW: Genitourinary trauma. In Moore EE, Mattox KL, Feliciano DV (eds): Trauma. East Norwalk, CT, Appleton & Lange, 1991.
127. McAninch JW, Carroll P, Klosterman P, et al: Renal reconstruction after injury. J Urol 1991;145:932.
128. McAninch JW, Carroll PR, Armenkas NA, et al: Renal gunshot wounds: Methods of salvage and reconstruction. J Trauma 1993;35:279.
129. McAninch JW, Morey AF, Bruce JE: Efficacy of radiographic imaging in pediatric blunt renal trauma. Proc Am Urol Assoc Suppl 1996;155:526A.
130. Medica J, Caldamone A: Pediatric renal trauma: Special considerations. Semin Urol 1995;13:73.
131. Mee SL, McAninch JW, Rovinson AL, et al: Radiographic assessment of renal trauma: A 10-year prospective study of patient selection. J Urol 1989;141:1095.
132. Melekos MD, Pantazakos A, Daouaher H, et al: Primary endourologic re-establishment of urethral continuity after disruption of the prostatomembranous urethra. Urology 1992;39:135.
133. Mercader VP, Gatenby RA, Curtis BR: Radiographic assessment of genitourinary trauma. Trauma 1996;13:129.
134. Merrott T, Portier F, Galinier P, et al: Trauma of the renal pedicle in children: Report of 2 cases of late revascularization with endovascular prosthesis. Prog Urol 2000; 10:277.
135. Mertz JHO, Wishard WN JR, Nourse MH, et al: Injury to the kidney in children. JAMA 1963;183:830.
136. Miller SF, Chait PG, Burrows PE, et al: Post-traumatic arte-

rial priapism in children: Management with embolization. Radiology 1995;196:59.
137. Miller DC, Forauer A, Faerber GJ: Successful angioembolization of renal artery pseudoaneurysms after blunt abdominal trauma. Urology 2002;59:444.
138. Miller KS, McAninch JW: Radiographic assessment of renal trauma: Our 15-year experience. J Urol 1995;154:352.
139. Monstrey SJ, vander Staak FH, vander Werken C, et al: Urinary tract injuries in children: Are they different from adults? Z Kinderchir 1988;43:31.
140. Monstrey SJ, vanderWerken C, Debruyne FM, et al: Rational guidelines in renal trauma assessment. Urology 1988;31:469.
141. Monstrey SJ, Beerthuizen GI, vander Werken C, et al: Renal trauma and hypertension. J Trauma 1989;29:65.
142. Montgomery RC, Richardson JD, Harty JI: Post-traumatic renovascular hypertension after occult renal injury. J Trauma 1998;45:106.
143. Moog R, Becmeur F, Dutson E: Functional evaluation by quantitative dimercaptosuccinic acid scintigraphy after kidney trauma in children. J Urol 2003;169:641.
144. Moore EE, Shackford SR, Pachter HL, et al: Organ injury scaling: Spleen, liver, and kidney. J Trauma 1989; 29:1664.
145. Morey AF, Bruce JE, McAninch JW: Efficacy of radiographic imaging in pediatric blunt renal trauma. J Urol 1996;156:2014.
146. Morse TS, Smith JP, Howard WHR, et al: Kidney injuries in children. J Urol 1967;98:539.
147. Morton JR, Crawford ES: Bilateral traumatic renal artery thrombosis. Ann Surg 1972;176:62.
148. Moudounie SM, Patard JJ, Manunta P, et al: A conservative approach to blunt renal lacerations with urinary extravasation and devitalized renal segments. Br J Urol 2001;87:290.
149. Munarriz RM, Yan OR, Znehra A, et al: Blunt trauma: The pathophysiology of the hemodynamic injury. J Urol 1995;153:1831.
150. Mundy AR: The role of delayed primary repair in the acute management of pelvic fracture injuries of the urethra. Br J Urol 1991;68:273.
151. Murphy JP: Genitourinary trauma. In Ashcraft KW (ed): Pediatric Urology. Philadelphia, WB Saunders, 1990.
152. Nicolaisen GS, McAninch JW, Marshall GA, et al: Renal trauma: Re-evaluation of the indications for radiographic assessment. J Urol 1985;133:183.
153. Noe HN, Jerkins GR: Genitourinary trauma. In Kelalis PP, Kemp LR, Belman AB (eds): Clinical Pediatric Urology. Philadelphia, WB Saunders, 1992.
154. Oliver JA, Taguchi Y: Rupture of the full bladder. Br J Urol 1964;36:524.
155. Patil MG, Onuora VC: The value of ultrasound in the evaluation of patients with blunt scrotal trauma. Injury 1994;25:177.
156. Peng MY, Parisky YR, Cornwell EE, et al: CT cystography versus conventional cystography in evaluation of bladder injury. AJR Am J Roentgenol 1999;173:1269.
157. Perez-Brayfield MR: Gunshot wounds to the ureter: A 40 year experience at Grady Memorial Hospital. J Urol 2001;166:119.
158. Perez-Brayfield MR, Gatti JM, Smith EA, et al: Blunt traumatic hematuria in children: Is a simplified algorithm justified? J Urol 2002;167:2543.
159. Perry MO, Husmann DA: Urethral injuries in female subjects following pelvic fractures. J Urol 1992;147:139.
160. Peterson NE: Review article: Traumatic bilateral renal infarction. J Trauma 1989;29:158.
161. Philpott JM, Nance ML, Carr MC, et al: Ureteral stenting in the management of urinoma after severe blunt renal trauma in children. J Pediatr Surg 2003;38:1096.
162. Pode D, Shapiro A: Traumatic avulsion of the female urethra: Case report. J Trauma 1990;30:235.
163. Poole GV, Ward EF, Griswold JA, et al: Complications of pelvic fractures from blunt trauma. Ann Surg 1992;58:225.
164. Porter JR, Takayama TK, Defalco AJ: Traumatic posterior urethral injury and early realignment using magnetic urethral catheters. J Urol 1997;158:425.
165. Presti JC, Carroll PR, McAninch JW: Ureteral and pelvic injuries from external trauma: Diagnosis and management. J Trauma 1989;29:370.
166. Pumberger W, Stoll E, Metz S: Ureteropelvic junction disruption following blunt abdominal trauma. Pediatr Emerg Care 2002;18:364.
167. Quinlan DM, Gearhart JP: Blunt renal trauma in childhood. Features indicating severe injury. Br J Urol 1990; 66:526.
168. Radmayr C, Oswald J, Muller E, et al: Blunt renal trauma in children: 26 years clinical experience in an alpine region. Eur Urol 2002;42:297.
169. Rehman J, Samadi D, Ricciardi R Jr, et al: Early endoscopic realignment as primary therapy for complete posterior urethral disruptions. J Endourol 1998;12:283.
170. Rober PE, Smith JB, Pierce JM: Gunshot injuries of the ureter. J Trauma 1990;30:83.
171. Russell TS, Gomelsky A, McMahon DR, et al: Management of grade IV renal injury in children. J Urol 2001;66:1049.
172. Sagalowsky AI, McConnell JD, Peters PC: Renal trauma requiring surgery: An analysis of 185 cases. J Trauma 23:128, 1983.
173. Santucci RA, McAninch JW, Safir M, et al: Validation of the American Association for the Surgery of Trauma organ injury severity scale for the kidney. J Trauma 2001; 50:195.
174. Santucci RA, Langenburg SE, Zachareas MJ: Traumatic hematuria in children can be evaluated as in adults. J Urol 2004;171:822.
175. Sharp DS, Ross JH, Kay R: Attitudes of pediatric urologists regarding sports participation in children with a solitary kidney. J Urol 2002;168:1811.
176. Shuman WP: CT of blunt abdominal trauma in adults. Radiology 1997;205:297.
177. Skinner D: Traumatic renal artery thrombosis: A successful thrombectomy and revascularization. Ann Surg 1973; 172:264.
178. Sklar DP, Diven B, Jones J: Incidence and magnitude of catheter-induced hematuria. Am J Emerg Med 1986; 4:14.
179. Smith EM, Elder JS, Spirnak JP: Major blunt renal trauma in the pediatric population: Is a nonoperative approach indicated? J Urol 1993;149:546.
180. Snyder H, Caldamone AA: Genitourinary injuries. In Welch KJ, Randolph JG, Ravitch MM (eds): Pediatric Surgery, 4th ed. Chicago, Mosby Year Book, 1986.
181. Spirnak JP, Persky L, Resnick MI: The management of civilian ureteral gunshot wounds: A review of 18 patients. J Urol 1985;134:733.
182. Stalker HP, Kaufman RA, Stedje K: The significance of hematuria in children after blunt abdominal trauma. AJR Am J Roentgenol 1990;154:569.
183. Stein JP, Kaji DM, Eastham J, et al: Blunt renal trauma in the pediatric population: Indications for radiographic

evaluation. Urology 1994;44:406.
184. Teigen CL, Venbrux AC, Quinlan DM, Jeffs RD: Late massive hematuria as a complication of conservative management of blunt renal trauma in children. J Urol 1992;147:1333.
185. Thomae KR, Kilambi NK, Poole GV: Method of urinary diversion in nonurethral traumatic bladder injuries. Retrospective analysis of 70 cases. Am Surg 1998;64:77-80.
186. Toporoff B, Sclafani S, Scalea T, et al: Percutaneous antegrade ureteral stenting as an adjunct for treatment of complicated ureteral injuries. J Trauma 1992;32:534.
187. Townsend M, DeFalco AJ: Absence of ureteral opacification below ureteral disruption: A sentinel CT finding. AJR Am J Roentgenol 1995;164:253.
188. Tso EL, Beaver BL, Haller JJ Jr: Abdominal injuries in the restrained pediatric passenger. J Pediatr Surg 1993; 28:915.
189. Tunc HM, Tefekli AH, Kaplancan T, et al: Delayed repair of post-traumatic posterior urethral distraction injuries: Long-term results. Urology 2000;55:837.
190. Turner WW Jr, Snyder WH III, Fry WJ: Mortality and renal salvage after renovascular trauma: A review of 94 patients treated in a 20 year period. Am J Surg 1983;146:848.
191. Velmahos GC, Degiannis E: The management of urinary tract injuries after gunshot wounds of the anterior and posterior abdomen. Injury 1997;28:535.
192. Volpe MA, Pachter EM, Scalea TM, et al: Is there a difference in outcome when treating traumatic intraperitoneal bladder rupture with or without a suprapubic tube? J Urol 1999;161:1103.
193. Wazzan W, Azoury B, Heinady K, et al: Missile injuries of the upper ureter treated by delayed renal autotransplantation and ureteropyelostomy. Urology 1993;42:725.
194. Weaver FA, Kuehne JP, Papanicolau G: A recent institutional experience with renovascular hypertension. Am Surg 1996;62:241.
195. Weems WL: Management of genitourinary injuries in patients with pelvic fractures. Ann Surg 1979;189:717.
196. Werkman HA, Jansen C, Klein JP, et al: Urinary tract injuries in multiply-injured patients: A rational guideline for the initial assessment. Injury 22:471, 1991.
197. Wessel LM, Scholz S, Jester I, et al: Management of kidney injuries in children with blunt abdominal trauma. J Pediatr Surg 2000;35:1326.
198. Wessells H, McAninch JW, Meyer A, et al: Criteria for nonoperative treatment of significant penetrating renal lacerations. J Urol 157:24, 1997.
199. Whitesides E, Kozlowdki DL: Ureteral injury from blunt abdominal trauma: Case report. J Trauma 1994;36:745.
200. Wyatt JB, Scobie WG: The management of penile zipper entrapment in children. Injury 1994;25:59.
201. Yale-Loehr AJ, Kramer SS, Quinlan DM, et al: CT of severe renal trauma in children: Evaluation and course of healing with conservative therapy. AJR Am J Roentgenol 1989; 152:109.
202. Zakin D: Perforation of the bladder by the intrauterine device. Obstet Gynecol Surv 1984;39:59.

第 19 章

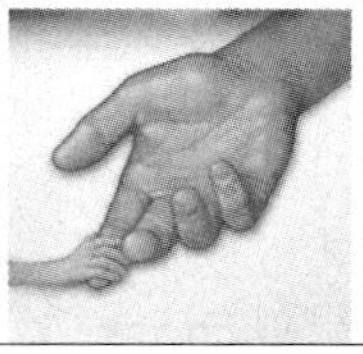

骨骼肌肉系统创伤

Richard S. Davidson 和 Michelle S. Caird

37 骨骼肌肉系统的创伤是最常见的儿童急诊。随着汽车、越野车以及电动割草机的普及，这类创伤的病例数还在继续升高。对于一个多发性创伤的患儿，最佳的治疗需要一个包括各个医疗专业专家组成的团队的合作，这个团队中的成员必须了解各自专业在抢救中的先后次序，分清轻重缓急。对于所有儿科专业的医生来说，最重要的一点是要记住，儿童不是“小大人”。优先考虑的治疗措施不能影响到患儿整体的治疗。

本章回顾了儿童与成人骨骼肌肉系统创伤的重要不同之处，并且强调了对儿童骨骼肌肉系统创伤的评估和处理原则。对于一些高度优先的骨骼肌肉系统创伤做了专门的讨论，包括开放性骨折、骨筋膜室综合征、股骨颈骨折、肢体撕脱伤、脊柱创伤以及可疑的儿童虐待伤。对于儿童骨折创伤治疗的细节问题，读者可以参阅儿童骨折方面的教科书[16,25,27]。

儿童和成人的骨骼肌肉系统

儿童与成人骨骼肌肉系统解剖和生物力学方面的不同决定了儿童期骨骼肌肉系统损伤表现出一些独特的方面。损伤发生在生长中的骨骼时是一把双刃剑：它们可以有巨大的修复和塑性能力，但也会发生过度生长和生长紊乱的问题，其造成的后遗症将是终身的。

解剖学

未成熟的骨在解剖方面主要的特点是骨骺板和骨膜。儿童期长骨包括骨骺、骨骺板、干骺端以及骨干（图 19–1）。骨骺是骨骺板或主要生长板远端的部分区域，包括关节软骨。次级骨化中心在骨骺中出现，并且随着骨成熟过程中软骨的逐渐骨化，次级骨化中心逐渐增大。骨骺板纵向生长并且在干骺端将新生成的软骨转化为骨。骨干或主干被骨膜所包裹，骨膜能产生新骨并提供周缘的骨的生长。到了成年期，生长板闭合，骨重建塑性的潜力极其有限。

生物力学

未成熟的骨多孔，水分含量高，不易碎，较之成熟骨更耐受形变。在压力的作用下，大量的小孔阻止了骨折线的进展，但削弱了骨的强度。因此，儿童骨折较之成人有着更多的变化类型。儿童的骨可以仅仅弯曲但并不骨折（图 19–2）；可以在压力作用下呈现出竹节样的改变；可以像青枝一样骨折，即在张力侧有一条不完全的裂缝，在压力侧弯曲畸形；当然也可以是完全性骨折。

包裹在骨干周围的很厚的骨膜能够防止和最大限度的缩小骨干骨折的移位。骨折时，张力侧的骨膜撕裂，但压力侧的骨膜经常是连续的。这种连续的骨膜起到了铰链和弹性回复的功能，缩小了移位变形。根据损伤机制的不同，骨膜可以使骨折的复位变得简单，也可以使其复杂化（图 19–3）。

在儿童，骨、韧带和软骨的联合体中，骨骺板是最薄弱的部分，因此也是最容易损伤的部分。对于一个青少年，在关节附近施加一个成角的作用力往往导致沿生长板的骨折，然而同样的力施加于成人或青少年往往产生韧带损伤或关节脱位。Frankel 和 Nordin [15] 提供了骨的生物力学方面广泛的信息。当手掌过度牵伸撑地摔倒时，青少年很少发生腕关节扭伤，通

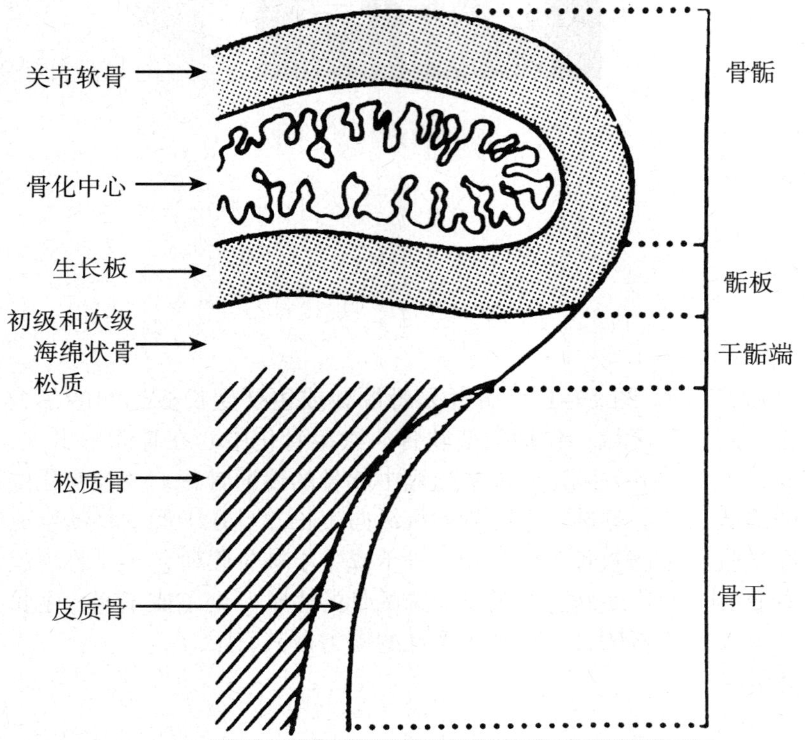

图 19-1 儿童的骨的解剖学。

常，患儿会产生一个移位的桡骨远端骨骺骨折。同样的，取代踝关节扭伤，患儿往往出现腓骨远端骨骺骨折。在低能量的作用力下，这些损伤一般不会

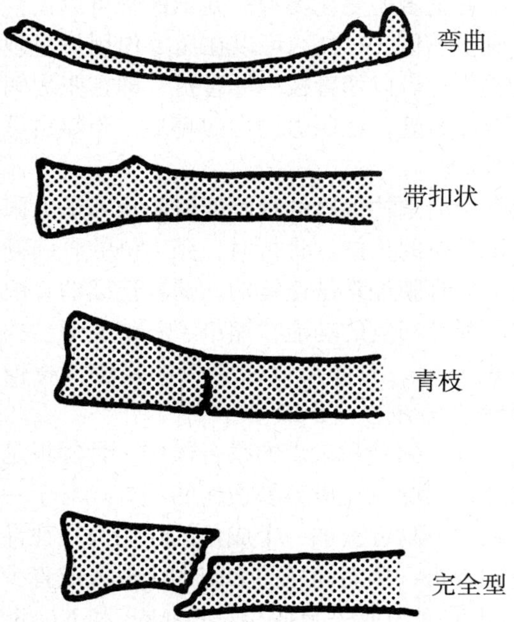

图 19-2 儿童的骨折类型。(From Rang M: Children's Fractures. Philadelphia, JB Lippincott, 1974.)

引起生长紊乱。

骨骺骨折的 Salter-Harris 分型对治疗有指导意义（图 19-4）[28]。1 型骨骺骨折的骨折线延伸至整个骨骺板。2 型骨骺骨折的骨折线包括部分生长板以及部分干骺端。当股骨远端或胫骨近端发生这类骨折时，这些骨折很少引起生长抑制。3 型骨骺骨折的骨折线包括部分骨骺板及穿过骨骺直至关节。由于可能引起关节面不平整，3 型骨骺骨折通常需要切开复位和内固定。4 型骨骺骨折的骨折线是纵向的，从干骺端一直延伸至骨骺内，穿过骨骺板。这类骨折经常导致穿过骨骺板的骨桥形成，从而导致部分骨骺生长抑制，最终产生成角畸形。由于骨折后引起关节不平整以及骨骺早闭的可能性很大，所以 4 型骨骺骨折通常都需要切开复位和内固定。5 型骨骺骨折的诊断是回顾性的，当全部或部分骨骺板停止生长时，可以得出诊断。这种骨骺损伤的假设原因是直接挤压损失或局部血供的破坏。生长紊乱可以是由于纵向生长减少导致，也可以是成角畸形导致。对于任何类型的骨骺骨折，高能量损伤骨骺板都会导致生长不平衡。

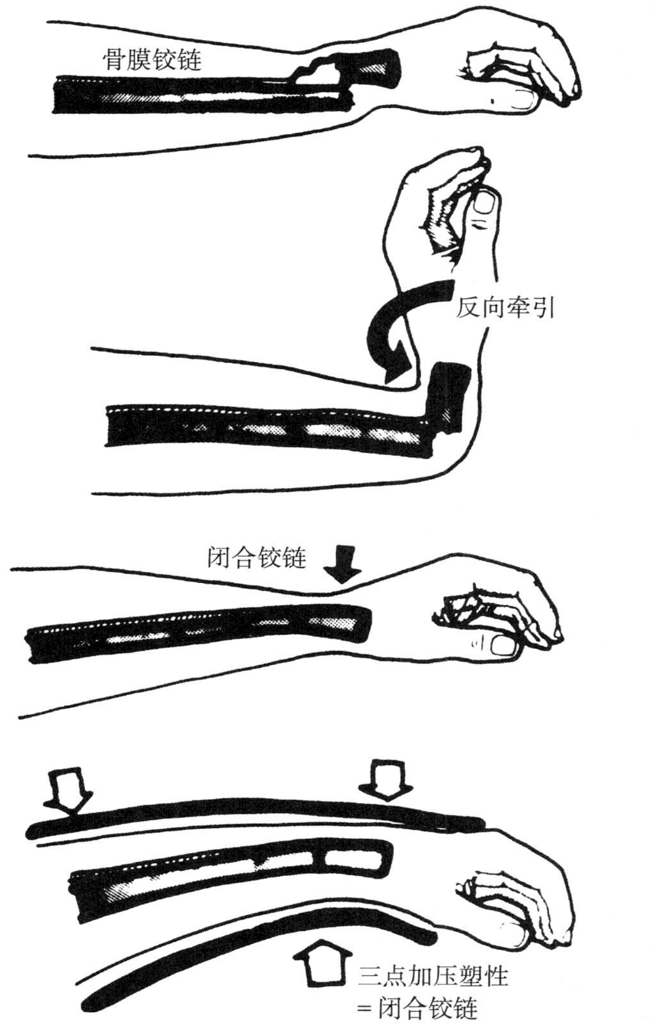

图 19-3 A. 在儿童中，骨折后仍然连接的骨膜牵扯着断端阻止了复位。B. 通过与损伤方向相反方向的牵引可以使骨折复位。C. 合拢骨膜铰链。D. 通过三点加压塑性的石膏可以保证铰链的闭合以及维持骨折的复位。(From Rang M: Children's Fractures. Philadelphia, JB Lippincott, 1974.)

生理学

成人骨骼肌肉系统和儿童骨骼肌肉系统在病理学方面的不同主要表现在骨折的愈合以及塑性重建方面。生长期的骨同样存在发生过度生长以及生长紊乱的风险。

儿童骨折愈合迅速且与年龄有很大相关性。一个新生儿的骨折能够在 1 周内达到临床上的稳定愈合，而同样的骨折发生在青少年身上则需要 6 周的时间愈合。对于儿童，骨折的迅速愈合过程很大程度上依赖
于较厚的骨膜，因为其可以产生自身的骨桥。除了移 339
位的关节内骨折以及软组织嵌入骨折端，儿童中很少发生骨不连。

儿童的骨虽然有很大的塑性重建潜力，但也必须认识到这种潜力的局限性。塑性的潜力与以下因素有关：患儿越小，潜力越大；成角畸形越靠近骨骺板，且与邻近关节的运动方向一致，潜力越大。塑性不能有效纠正与关节运动方向垂直的成角畸形以及旋转畸形，这些畸形应该在骨折愈合开始之前纠正（图 19–5）。

长骨骨折后会出现生长刺激，这一点在下肢表现的更为明显。对于 2 岁以下以及青春期的孩子这种刺激引起腿部不等长的影响相对较小。对于其他年龄段的孩子来说，股骨骨折后平均会造成 1cm 的生长过长[11,29,32]。尽管这种腿部不等长有时是不可预料的，但可以通过在解剖力线的方向允许骨折端重叠 1cm 来降低不等长的可能性。绝大多数的生长刺激发生在损伤后 1 年内，所以推荐 1 年时的随访检查，即使是在毫无症状的完全愈合以后。

骨骺板的损伤会造成严重的短缩畸形、成角畸形或者两者兼而有之。这种损伤可以由于最初的创伤造成，也可以由于骨骺骨折没有达到解剖复位或者反复过度的尝试复位造成（图 19–6）。当较大的（＞2cm）肢体不等长存在时，治疗由骨骼剩余的生长年限以及

图 19–4 骨骺骨折的 Salter–Harris 分型。1 型包括整个骨骺板。2 型包括部分生长板部干骺端。3 型包括部分骨骺，骨折线穿过骨骺进入关节。4 型是纵向的骨折，骨折线从干骺端穿过骺板直至骨骺中。5 型的诊断要等到骨骺生长阻滞时回顾性诊断。各种骨折类型的临床意义见正文。

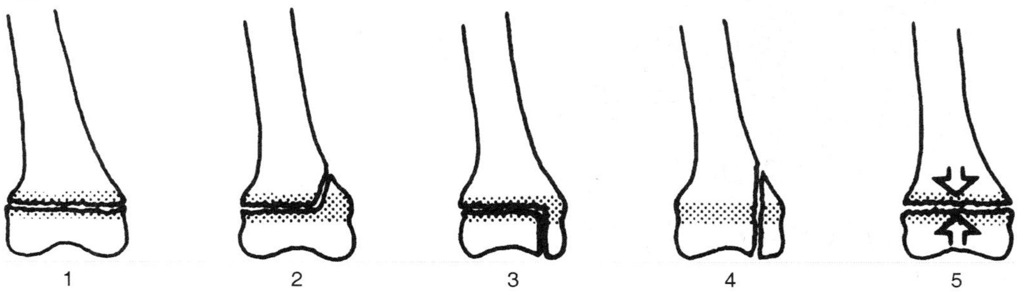

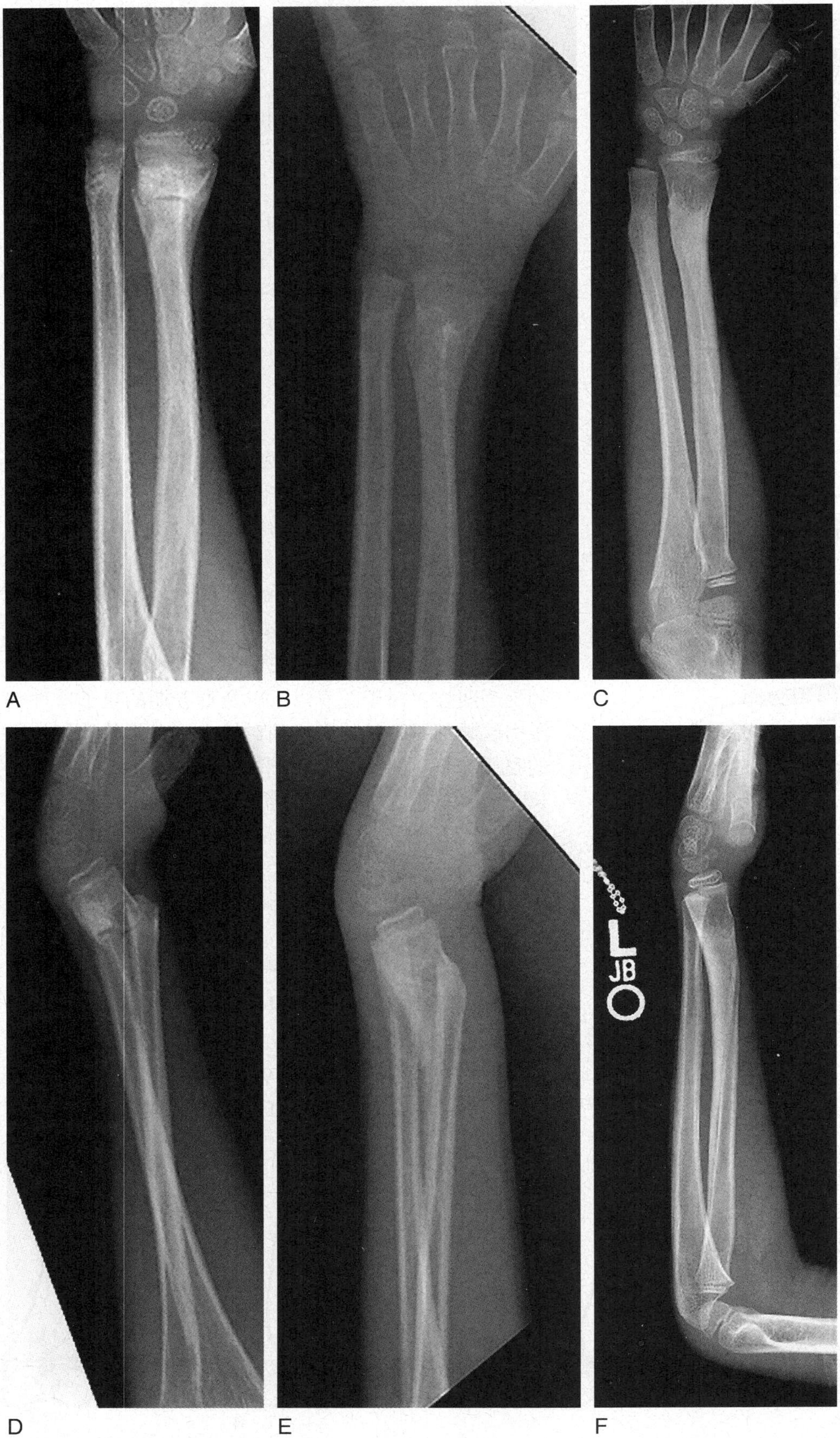

图 19-5 1例7岁男孩的前臂骨折，在9个月的时间里，自身塑性纠正了8°畸形。A至C.前后位平片。D至F.侧位平片。

图 19-6 1 例 13 岁男孩的膝关节前后位片，显示骨折后左股骨远端骨骺生长紊乱（在图右侧）。

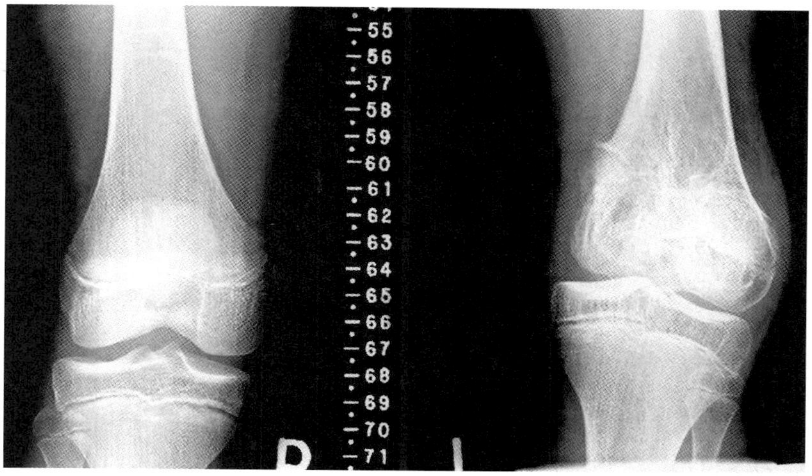

估计的肢体长度差异决定。治疗包括有计划的阻滞正常肢体的生长板、正常肢体的短缩截骨或短缩肢体的骨延长。根据患儿的骨龄和畸形的严重程度，可以考虑矫正成角畸形。

骨骼肌肉系统损伤的评估

临床评估

对多发伤的患儿的最初评估是非常困难的。创伤发生时的细节往往被忽略，患儿的病史往往是不完整的。高级创伤生命支持系统（ATLS）的评估包
1 括首先快速判断危及生命的损伤，随后第二步的评估是寻找和治疗其他重要的损伤。在第二阶段确定的损伤也应得到及时的治疗以免造成终生的后遗症。延迟治疗严重的骨骼肌肉损伤可能会造成不良的预后，难以恢复正常的功能。

骨骼肌肉系统检查从观察患者的情况开始，包括观察畸形、肿胀、擦伤、异常颜色以及开放性骨折的部位。如果怀疑有骨折，明确诊断需要结合全面的体格检查。如果这种检查不能进行，那么必须假定骨折是存在的，被怀疑的部位必须固定，直到骨折诊断明确或排除。固定可以减轻疼痛不适以及进一步的软组织损伤。对于所有被怀疑有损伤的肢体和脊柱进行完整的神经血管检查是非常重要的。如果遇到不合作的患儿不能完成足够的体格检查，或者遇到昏迷的或者未学会说话的患儿，不能提供完整的病史，依靠专项的辅助检查明确诊断是非常重要的。

影像学评估

X 线平片是判断儿童骨骼损伤最早也是最常用的检查手段，但也是在这个年龄段导致误诊的主要原因。因为占了儿童骨骼系统中很大比例的软骨如果骨折了在平片上是不显影的。骨化中心在不同年龄不同的部位出现，其出现的时间和部位存在很大的变化，因此可能被认为是骨折。容易造成混淆的部位主要在肘关节、膝关节和颈椎。对比患侧和健侧肢体的情况非常实用。平片上的软组织特征，例如肘关节损伤时肘后脂肪垫充血反应征，通常表明存在潜在骨折的可
能性很大（图 19-7）[30]。 342

一系列的影像学检查可以作为儿童骨骼肌肉系统损伤的评估手段，并且根据损伤和年龄的不同，可以利用不同的专项检查。超声检查是方便、无创的检查手段，可以用来评估没有骨化的骨骺，尤其是在肘关节损伤中[8]。核磁共振（MRI）也是非常有用的，尤其是评估脊柱损伤，但对于小年龄和不合作的患儿需要应用全身麻醉。CT 扫描对于骨骼接近成熟的患儿发生的关节附近的骨折非常有用。例如，部分骨骺板闭合了的患儿发生踝关节骨骺骨折时，CT 扫描可以最好的显示骨折情况[22]。血管造影成像可以评估骨折造成的血管损伤。极少情况下，胫骨近端骨骺骨折以及肱骨远端髁上骨折可以影响到远端肢体的血液供应。这些损伤需要紧急处理，术中需要动脉造影检查。关节穿刺可以明确关节内有无血液和脂肪，这可以提示 X片上没能显影的关节内骨折。最后，关节造影和关节镜检查可以详细显示关节内的软骨和韧带损伤。

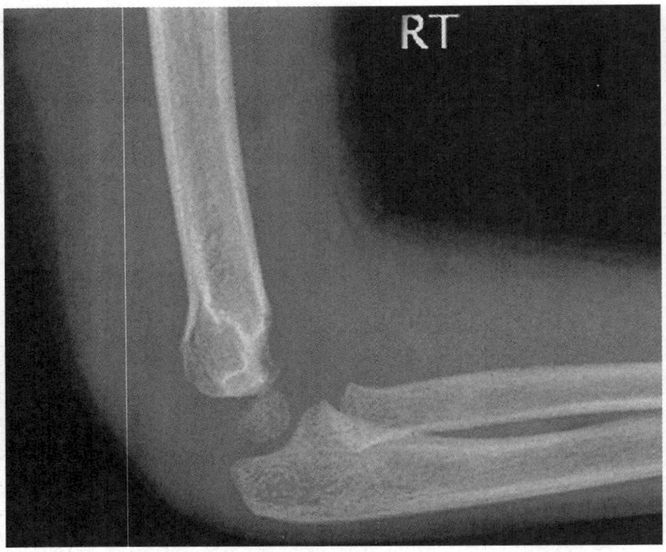

A

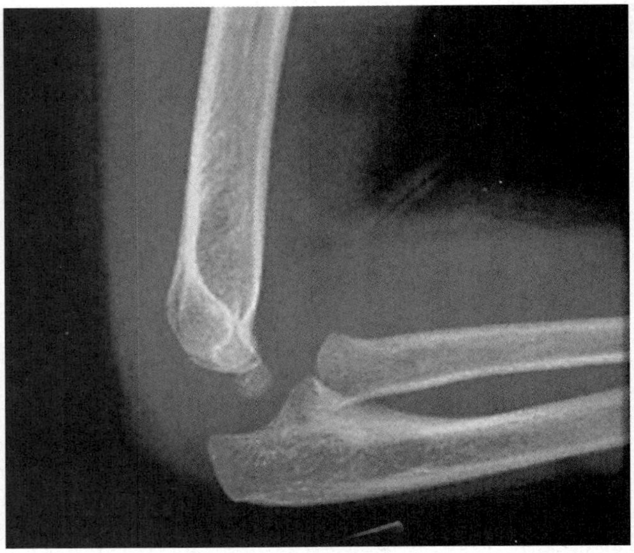

B

图 19-7 1 例 2 岁男孩的肘关节侧位片，显示轻度移位的肱骨髁上骨折和后方脂肪垫征（A）以及一个正常的同年龄对照男孩的肘关节片（B）。

骨骼肌肉系统损伤的治疗

初期治疗

早期的治疗不能影响到患儿的整体治疗。合适的干预时机和与其他专业学科治疗上的合作都是必须的。在其他的检查和治疗完成以前，牵引和支具固定通常能够给骨骼肌肉系统损伤提供足够的固定。制动同时也可以减轻疼痛及止痛药的应用，后者往往会掩盖其他部位损伤的症状，例如腹腔内损伤，从而延误诊断。

尽管支具有许多形式，从石膏到牵引弓，但骨折处理的基本原则是相同的。损伤的部位应予以原位固定，在不影响软组织血供的情况下，固定损伤部位上下两个关节。便携式牵引固定器、传统的石膏或者玻璃纤维支具都可以应用于骨折的初期治疗。没有很好的制动会导致骨折锋利的断端造成进一步的软组织损伤，被牵拉的血管神经束进一步被破坏以及已凝结的小血管再次出血。

最后的骨折处理

适当固定可以防止软组织进一步损伤，通常还能减轻疼痛，同时有利于伤口的处理和患者的转运。儿童骨折固定的技术包括支具、石膏、骨牵引、外固定支架、钢针、弹性髓内钉以及钢板。对于固定方法的选择决定于孩子的年龄、骨折的位置、软组织损伤的存在与否以及程度，还有是否有多发伤存在。

干骺端的无移位的骨折或压缩骨折通常比骨干骨折或移位的骨折要愈合得快。伴有死骨和坏死软组织的骨折需要更长的时间愈合。当确定儿童骨折的愈合时间时，需要结合临床判断和经验进行影像学的评价。

在骨折固定之前，必须在保证不损伤相关软组织的前提下，获得满意的复位，骨折断端必须固定在一起，直到愈合足够好，骨骼强壮到足以抵抗外力。新生儿和小婴儿的骨折的愈合在骨折后的几天内就开始了，而青春期患儿的骨折在 10～14 天内仍可以自由移动。过多的骨折内衬垫、肿胀以及不到位的石膏固定技术都可以导致石膏内骨折的进一步错位。为了防止移位，应该定期复查骨折的 X 片，直到骨折达到完全可靠的愈合。对于不稳定的骨折，更应该在骨痂硬化之前摄片检查，评价对合情况，以便再次进行复位。

在儿童骨折中，很厚的骨膜通常在骨折的张力侧是撕裂的，而在压力侧是完整连续的。完整的骨膜在功能上相当于一个铰链，增加了通过三点成形技术对移位骨折进行闭合复位的成功率（见图 19–3）。复位必须轻柔地进行。对于骨骺骨折进行暴力、反复的复位可能导致医源性损伤和生长紊乱。嵌入骨折端的软组织有时会阻碍一个相对稳定骨折的复位（图 19–8），这种情况通常需要切开复位石膏固定。

在一些病例中，使用交叉钢针、钢板螺钉、髓内钉或由金属钢针和棒或支架组成的外固定支架的内固定是有效的（图 19–9）。这些器械中每种器械的优点必须根据日后是否需要手术取出和是否对生长板有影响来衡量。应用内固定和外固定支架的特定指征包括
44 合并明显软组织损伤的骨折、有闭合性头颅外伤的骨折、存在神经血管损伤的骨折以及非手术治疗失败的病例。粉碎性骨折、斜行骨折以及骨膜完全破裂的骨折如果单纯用石膏固定，可能非常不稳定。对于关节内骨折，如 Salter–Harris 3 型和 4 型骨折，通常需要切开复位和内固定，以避免关节面的不平整和生长紊乱。合并需要修复的血管神经损伤的骨折病例，必须先固定骨折。

需高度优先处理的骨骼肌肉损伤

尽管儿童的许多骨骼肌肉系统损伤可以作为亚急诊而非急诊处理，但一些需要高度优先考虑的骨骼肌肉系统损伤仍需确保足够的重视。即使是对那些非急诊的病例，需要牢记的是，对生长期骨骼的损伤可能会造成终身的后遗症。

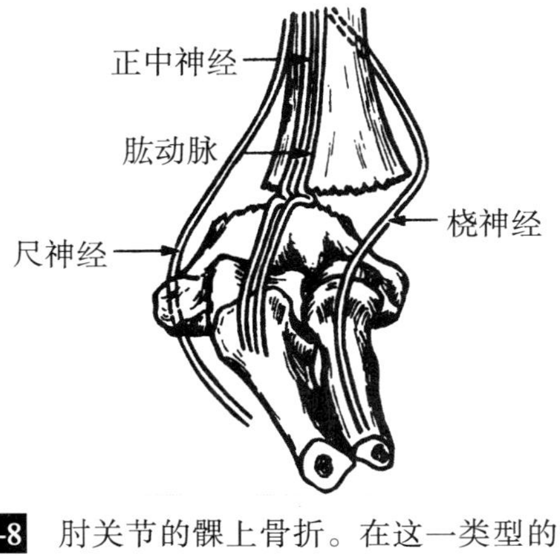

图 19–8　肘关节的髁上骨折。在这一类型的骨折中，软组织可能会嵌插在骨折端之间。

开放性骨折和创伤性关节破裂

开放性骨折是真正的骨科急诊，因为延误了治疗会大大降低挽救肢体的概率。这类损伤通常由高能量的创伤导致。骨折端与外界环境相通，感染的危险大大增加。基础治疗包括合适的抗生素应用、固定骨折以及对伤口迅速及时的冲洗清创。开放性骨折往往需要多次外科手术处理来达到软组织的覆盖和骨折的愈合。

当在骨折部位发现有皮肤破损或磨损时，要考虑是否有开放性骨折。X 线片可以通过反映骨折附近的空气阴影来证实开放性骨折的诊断。尖锐的骨片可以刺破皮肤，当外力消失时，儿童骨骼的柔韧特性很容易使骨折处恢复笔直。此时戳出皮肤的骨折端会回到皮肤以内，同时带入外界的碎片和细菌至深部组织。微小的损伤征象并不代表微小的感染概率。尽量不要在急诊室内探查伤口，那会增加医源性污染的危险，而且很难做到足够的清创。应该在手术室内进行这些操作。

开放性骨折根据伤口的尺寸和软组织损伤的程度进行 Gustilo 分类[17]。1 型指伤口小于 1cm 并且清洁的开放性骨折。2 型指大于 1cm 破口的开放性骨折但不包括严重的软组织损伤、皮瓣损伤和撕脱伤。3 型指的是开放性骨折伴随严重的软组织损伤，又可以分为三个亚型：3A 指尽管软组织有严重的撕脱伤但仍有足够的软组织覆盖骨折端；3B 指包括严重的软组织损伤和骨膜的撕脱，需要植皮或皮瓣来覆盖创面；3C 指开放性骨折伴有需要修补的血管损伤。感染的概率与损伤的严重程度有关：1 型开放性骨折感染概率为 2%，2 型为 2%～10%，3 型可达到 50%[17]。

伤口应该用浸润抗生素的消毒纱布覆盖，用压迫来控制出血。患者应该在第一时间注射破伤风疫苗，以及应用抗生素预防感染。第一代的先锋类抗生素的抗菌谱可以对抗 1 型和 2 型开放性骨折中发现的革兰阳性菌。在 3 型的开放性骨折中加一种氨基糖甙类抗生素，对一些农场中造成的损伤加氨苄西林或青霉素预防厌氧菌感染。

对于所有的伤口必须在基础麻醉下给予足够的清创以及广泛彻底的冲洗。在 2 天或之后的几天内对伤口进行再次评估，必要时再次清创。对于一部分开放性骨折的伤口可以采取一期缝合或者延迟缝合，而对于存在大范围软组织缺损的病例来说，必须采取植皮

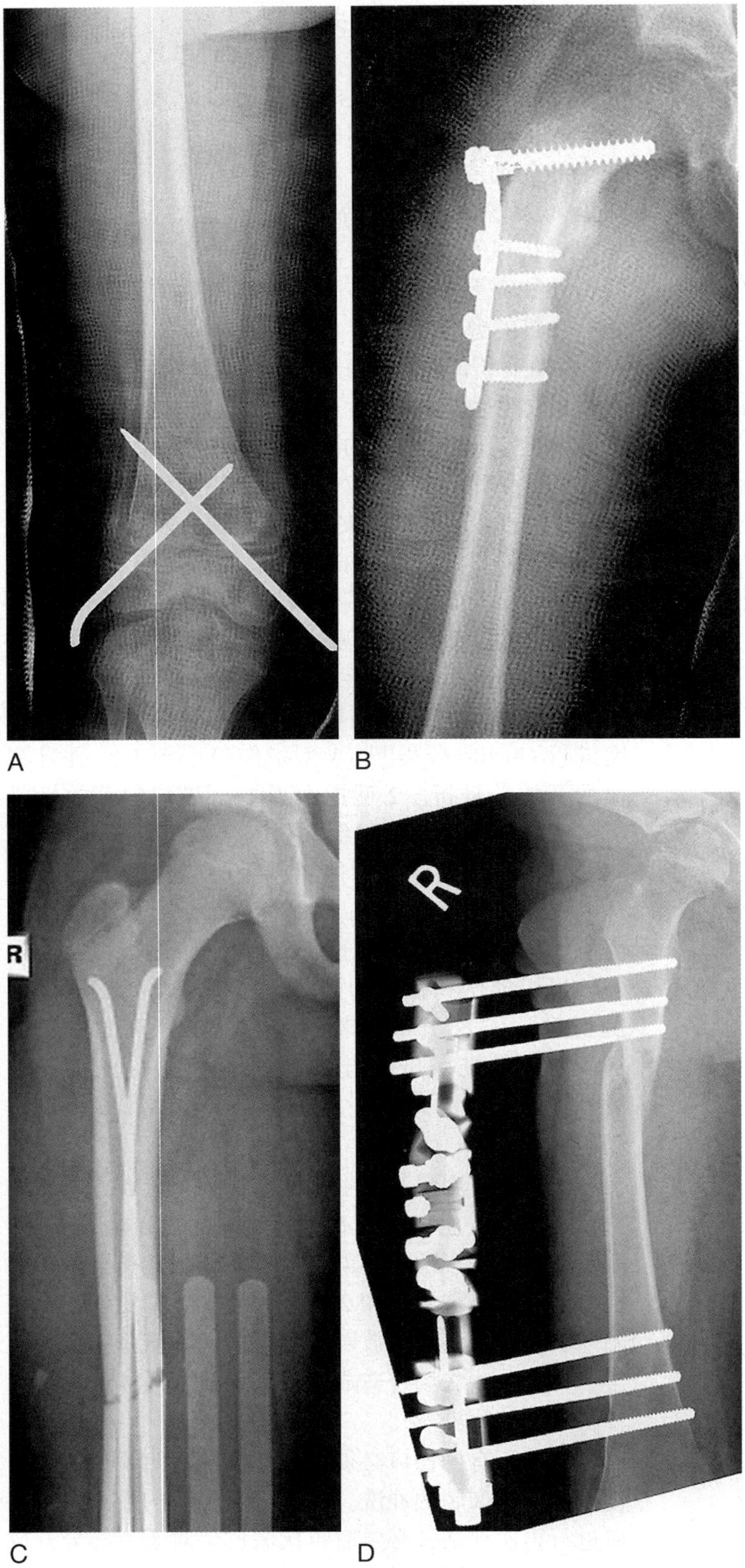

图 19-9 股骨骨折应用不同固定方式的前后位片。A. 一位 9 岁女孩，Salter-Harris 2 型骨骺骨折，应用交叉钢针固定。B. 一位 7 岁男孩，股骨粗隆间骨折，应用螺钉和侧方钢板固定。C. 一位 13 岁男孩的股骨中段横行骨折，应用弹性髓内钉固定。D. 一位 8 岁男孩的股骨粗隆下骨折，应用单臂外固定支架固定。

或皮瓣技术来覆盖创面。清创的目的是去除坏死组织，以防止由于感染而导致的严重的结果，包括肢体坏死以及慢性骨髓炎。充分的固定对于软组织损伤的愈合也是必需的。对于一些小的伤口，石膏固定后开窗观察伤口的情况就足够了。对于大的伤口，通常需要外固定支架，在能接触到伤口的同时又可以提供稳定的固定。

异物外伤导致的关节穿透破裂伤，在诊断方面有时比较困难。如果 X 片上反映出“空气造影样”的变化，往往具有诊断意义。另外还可以诊断性的向关节内注入一些生理盐水，如果从伤口或破口中流出生理盐水，那么说明关节已经穿透，需要进手术室冲洗清创。

骨筋膜室综合征

骨筋膜室综合征发生在限定的石膏绷带空间内压力不断升高时。这不仅会导致循环障碍，并且会进一步发展为组织坏死。闭合性骨折和挤压损伤形成的血肿都会导致骨筋膜室综合征。前臂和腿部的肌间隔是最易发生的部位。当组织压低于平均动脉压 30mmHg 时，缺血损伤开始发生[20]。当怀疑有骨筋膜室综合征发生时，要测定骨折周围肌间隔的压力，可以用市面上可以买到的组织压测定器，或其他的测试装置，例如电子动脉压测定仪。

对于儿童的骨筋膜室综合征的诊断是非常困难的。当成人发生骨筋膜室综合征时，会描述剧烈的疼痛，并且当被动伸展相关肌肉时会出现剧烈疼痛，然而儿童通常很难描述其不适。经典的骨筋膜室综合征的表现是 5P 征：疼痛（Pain）、苍白（Pallor）、感觉异常（Paresthesia）、瘫痪（Paralysis）和无脉（Pulselessness）。这些征象在儿童中常常不明显，并且往往很晚才表现出来。不断增加的镇痛要求往往是儿童骨
筋膜室综合征的一个重要征象[2]。 345

通过早期发现和及时处理，骨筋膜室综合征可以完全恢复。处理时，肢体所有的外固定压力需要去除，测量肌间隔的压力，如果升高，需要手术松解肌间隔。在前臂，需要做掌侧和背侧筋膜松解术，在腿部所有 4 个肌间隔（前，外侧，后侧深部，后侧表浅）都必须松解。这可以通过两个切口来完成。如果没有得到合适的处理，其结果将会使软组织产生不可逆的损伤，包括功能的丧失、残留挛缩和畸形[34]。

股骨颈骨折

尽管儿童中股骨颈骨折和转子间的骨折发生率很低，但还是需要引起注意（图 19-10）。这类骨折通常由高能量损伤引起，包括交通意外和高空坠落[6]，同时这类骨折并发症的发生率很高，包括股骨头缺血坏死、髋内翻、骨不连、骨延长连接以及骨骺早

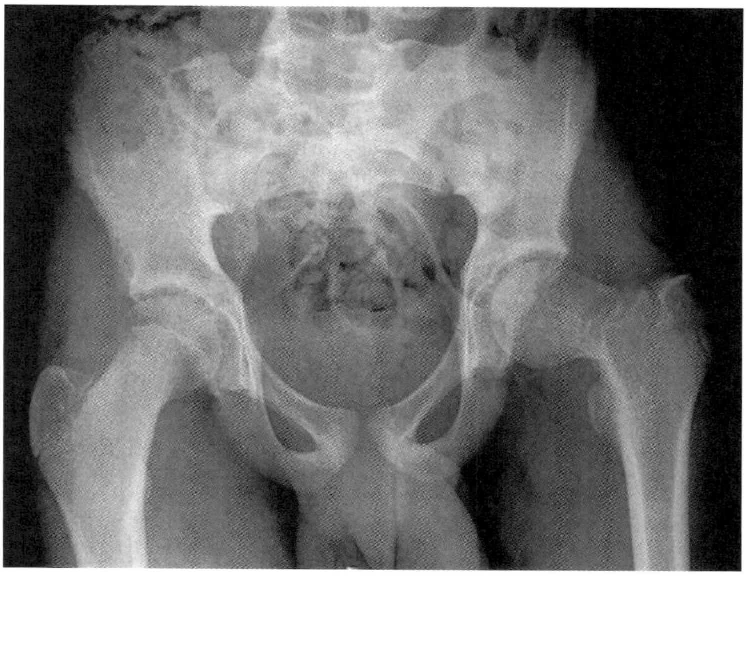

图 19-10 1 例 14 岁男孩的前后位骨盆平片，显示左股骨颈骨折，需要进行内固定治疗。

闭[4,9]。股骨上端处于关节囊的包裹之中，大约在 4 岁之后，股骨头的血供主要来自从股骨颈到股骨头的韧带血管。如果延误了股骨颈骨折的治疗，会导致股骨头缺血坏死的发生率增加，关节破损还会导致终身残疾。早期给髋关节减压、将骨折复位、内固定可以减少并发症发生的概率[6]。

肢体撕脱伤

对儿童的严重创伤性肢体撕脱伤，必须用多学科方法具体问题具体分析地进行评估和治疗。这类创伤包括严重的组织损伤或部分皮肤、肌肉、骨及血管神经的缺损。由于严重的破坏一些肢体可能无法保全，有些可以通过重建手术获得一个没有功能的肢体，有些可以完好的保全下来。撕脱肢体损伤的严重程度评分通过最初表现出来的客观标准来评价。这些标准包括骨和软组织损伤、肢体缺血、休克和患儿的年龄。尽管这一标准最初是应用于成人的[18]，但同样可以应用于儿童下肢的创伤[12]。

节段性的骨缺损在儿童中少见，并且并非一定会导致截肢。如果骨膜能够保留，其成骨的潜力是巨大的。适当的清创和固定，再加上足够长的时间，儿童可能会有良好的预后。外固定技术可以保证骨转运和骨生成，从而修复骨缺损以及纠正轴向的畸形。

电动割草机损伤是一种并不常见、可以预防的损伤，一旦发生会导致儿童严重的残疾[10,13,23]。直接与刀刃接触会导致组织切割伤、截断伤以及肢体碎裂伤。如此的损伤会导致脉管系统和骨骺生长板的严重破坏、关节僵硬、感染以及截肢。如果要保全肢体，治疗方面与开放性骨折类似。

对于截肢的病例，尽可能地保留骨的长度以及所有有活力的软组织对于最终的功能预后是非常重要的。在儿童中，通过骨干中段的截肢手术常会导致骨残端过度生长从皮肤中穿出，这种情况尤其在腓骨、胫骨及肱骨容易发生，可以通过每隔几年切除多余的骨残端来加以解决。

脊柱创伤

儿童脊柱的损伤可以分为伤及颈椎的损伤和伤及胸腰椎的损伤（参见第 21 章）。同身体其他部位的损伤一样，儿童脊柱的损伤与成人的也有许多不同之处。放射影像学有许多不同之处，固定的原则也有所不同。

儿童的颈椎损伤与成人有很大不同[7]。儿童的韧带比较松弛，颈部的肌肉相对较弱，另外相对身体而言，头部较大，这一点在小年龄儿童中尤其明显。在儿童中颈椎损伤，尤其多发于颈部，并且主要发生在韧带和骨突部分而非骨折[19]。当固定一个儿童在担架上时，相对较大的头部应该考虑在内，儿童的担架需要有一个枕部的陷窝或者躯干部的床垫以保持颈椎部的弧度防止颈椎屈曲（图 19–11）[21]。

儿童颈椎的放射学影像评估可能会很困难。假性的半脱位表面上的 C2 相对 C3 向前移位和少见的 C3 相对 C4 向前移位，在正常的 8 岁以下儿童的平片上经常可以看到[5]。另外一些导致读片困难的因素包括未完全骨化、骨骺变异以及椎间盘椎体相对神经结构的移位灵活性。这些因素导致在过度伸展损伤时没有平片上异常的证据，称为无影像异常的脊髓损伤。MRI 对评价软组织损伤非常有帮助，尤其对可能有颈椎韧带损伤的儿童[14]。

在儿童中胸椎和腰椎的损伤非常罕见。椎体的生长发生在每一个椎体头端和尾端的骨突部位或生长中心。当有压力损伤时，青少年儿童常有发生创伤性骨突移位和相应的椎间盘移位至椎管的危险，尤其在腰段[33]。症状与那些中央性椎间盘突出的患者相似，包括肌肉力量减退和生理反射消失。这种损伤需要及早发现和急诊手术减压。

儿童的安全带损伤发生在当儿童坐在安全带保护下剧烈的屈曲时，后方的脊柱收到牵拉[31]。骨折线从椎体后方至椎间盘或者至椎体中部（图 19–12）。除了椎体的损伤，儿童还会有腹部损伤和主动脉的损伤。当患儿的腹部有擦伤或者安全带的勒痕时，要怀疑存在这类损伤。这类损伤需要固定，如果损伤在韧带部分可能需要内固定。

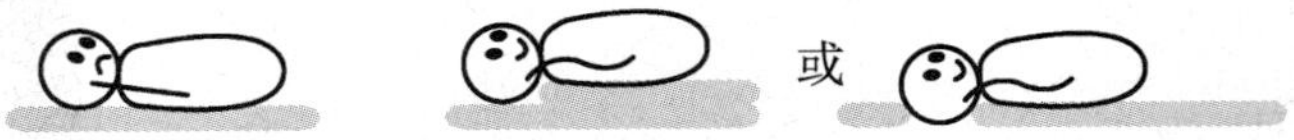

图 19–11 儿童的担架需要在枕部有一个陷窝或者在躯干部后方有床垫来容纳儿童相对较大的头部，防止潜在的颈椎屈曲危险。

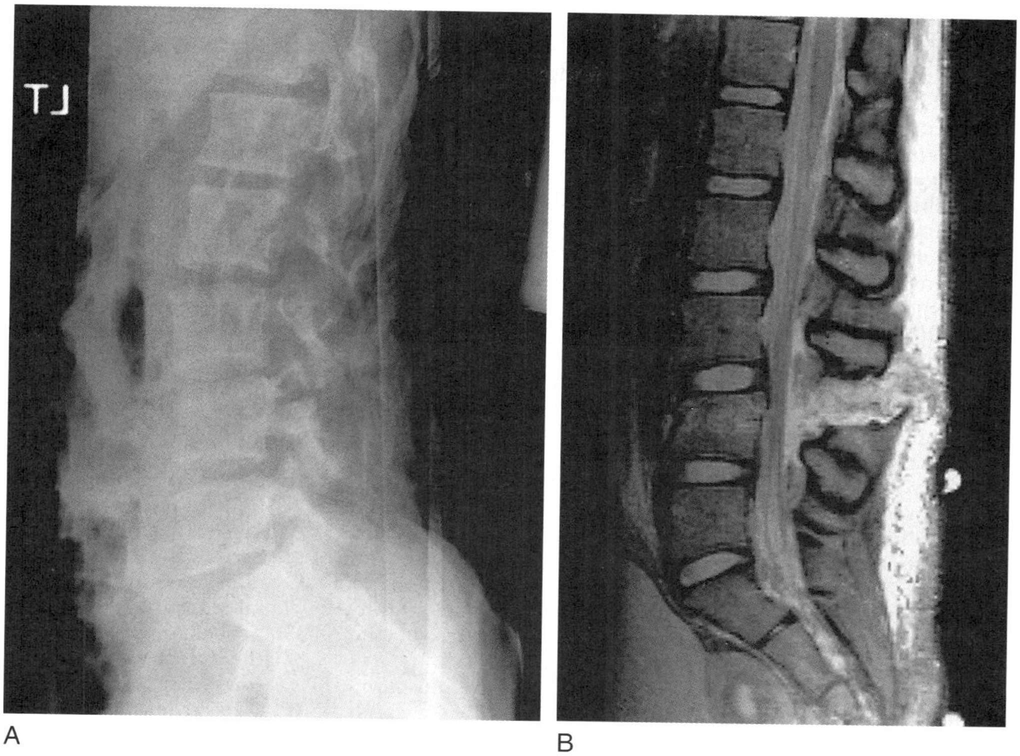

图 19-12 1 例 15 岁女孩在 L4 部位有安全带损伤，但不伴有神经损伤。A. 侧位的腰椎X 片显示 L4 椎体和后方脊柱骨折。B. 矢状位的核磁共振腰椎片显示有严重的骨和软组织损伤。

儿童虐待伤

儿童的虐待伤是一个复杂的医学和社会学问题，识别是处理的关键（参见第 24 章）。如果不存在代谢性疾病或儿童虐待伤，在行走期前的儿童骨折非常少见，骨折是除了皮肤创伤以外第二大判断儿童虐待伤的表现[24]。以下这些情况要怀疑儿童虐待伤：缺乏损伤的病史，存在不同愈合阶段的多处骨折，存在擦伤、干骺段骨折或者 1 岁内的儿童出现长骨骨折[3,26]。所有的社会阶层都有可能出现儿童虐待伤这一问题。

（葛翼华译 赵 黎校）

参考文献

1. Akbarnia B, Torg JS, Kirkpatrick J: Manifestations of the battered child syndrome. J Bone Joint Surg Am 1974; 56:1159.
2. Bae DS, Kadiyala RK, Waters PM: Acute compartment syndrome in children: Contemporary diagnosis, treatment, and outcome. J Pediatr Orthop 2001;21:680.
3. Blakemore LC, Loder RT, Hensinger RN: Role of intentional abuse in children 1 to 5 years old with isolated femoral shaft fractures. J Pediatr Orthop 1996;16:585.
4. Canale ST, Bourland WL: Fracture of the neck and intertrochanteric region of the femur in children. J Bone Joint Surg Am 1977;59:431.
5. Cattell HS, Filtzer DL: Pseudosubluxation and other normal variations in the cervical spine in children. J Bone Joint Surg Am 1965;47:1295.
6. Cheng JCY, Tang N: Decompression and stable internal fixation of femoral neck fractures in children can affect the outcome. J Pediatr Orthop 1999;19:338.
7. Copley LA, Dormans JP: Cervical spine disorders in infants and children. J Am Acad Orthop Surg 1998;6:204.
8. Davidson RS, Markowitz RI, Dormans JP, et al: Ultrasonographic evaluation of the elbow in infants and young children after suspected trauma. J Bone Joint Surg Am 1994;76:1804.
9. Davison BL, Weinstein SL: Hip fractures in children: A long-term follow-up study. J Pediatr Orthop 1992;12:355.
10. Dormans JP, Azzoni M, Davidson RS, et al: Major lower extremity lawn mower injuries in children. J Pediatr Orthop 1995;15:78.
11. Edvardsen P, Syversen SM: Overgrowth of the femur after fracture of the shaft in childhood. J Bone Joint Surg Br 1976;58:339.
12. Fagelman MF, Epps HR, Rang M: Mangled extremity severity score in children. J Pediatr Orthop 2002;22:182.
13. Farley FA, Senunas L, Freenfield ML, et al: Lower extremity lawn-mower injuries in children. J Pediatr Orthop 1996;19:669.
14. Flynn JM, Closkey RF, Mahboubi S, et al: Role of magnetic resonance imaging in the assessment of pediatric cervical spine injuries. J Pediatr Orthop 2002;22:573.

15. Frankel VH, Nordin M: Basic Biomechanics of the Skeletal System. Philadelphia, Lea & Febiger, 1980.
16. Green NE, Swiontkowski MF: Skeletal Trauma in Children, 3rd ed. Philadelphia, WB Saunders, 2003.
17. Gustilo RB, Anderson JT: Prevention of infection in the treatment of one thousand and twenty-five open fractures of long bones. J Bone Joint Surg Am 1976;58:453.
18. Helfet DL, Howey T, Sanders R, et al: Limb salvage versus amputation: Preliminary results of the mangled extremity severity score. Clin Orthop 1990;256:80.
19. Henrys P, Lyne ED, Lifton C, et al: Clinical review of cervical spine injuries in children. Clin Orthop 1977; 129:172.
20. Heppenstall RB, Sapega AA, Scott R, et al: The compartment syndrome: An experimental and clinical study of muscular energy metabolism using phosphorus nuclear magnetic resonance spectroscopy. Clin Orthop 1988; 226:138.
21. Herzenberg JE, Hensinger RN, Dedrick DK, et al: Emergency transport and positioning of young children who have an injury of the cervical spine: The standard backboard may be hazardous. J Bone Joint Surg Am 1989;71:15.
22. Karrholm J, Jansson LI, Laurin S: Computed tomography of intraarticular supination—eversion fractures of the ankle in adolescents. J Pediatr Orthop 1981;1:181.
23. Loder RT, Brown KL, Zaleske DJ, et al: Extremity lawnmower injuries in children: Report by the Research Committee of the Pediatric Orthopaedic Society of North America. J Pediatr Orthop 1997;17:360.
24. McMahon P, Grossman W, Gaffney M, et al: Soft tissue injury as an indication of child abuse. J Bone Joint Surg Am 1995;77:1179.
25. Ogden JA: Skeletal Injury in the Child, 3rd ed. New York, Springer, 2000.
26. Rex C, Kay PR: Features of femoral fractures in nonaccidental injury. J Pediatr Orthop 2000;20:411.
27. Rockwood CA Jr, Wilkins KD, Beaty JH, et al: Fractures in Children, 5th ed. Philadelphia, Lippincott Williams & Wilkins, 2001.
28. Salter RB, Harris WR: Injuries involving the epiphyseal plate. J Bone Joint Surg Am 1963;45:587.
29. Shapiro F: Fractures of the femoral shaft in children: The overgrowth phenomenon. Acta Orthop Scand 1981; 52:649.
30. Skaggs DL, Mirzayan R: The posterior fat pad sign in association with occult fracture of the elbow in children. J Bone Joint Surg Am 1999;81:1429.
31. Smith WS, Kauffer H: Patterns and mechanisms of lumbar injuries associated with lap seat belts. J Bone Joint Surg Am 1969;51:239.
32. Stephens MM, Hsu LC, Leong JC: Leg length discrepancy after femoral shaft fractures in children: Review after skeletal maturity. J Bone Joint Surg Br 1989;71:615.
33. Techakapuch S: Rupture of the lumbar cartilage plate into the spinal canal in an adolescent: A case report. J Bone Joint Surg Am 1981;45:481.
34. Whitesides TE, Heckman MM: Acute compartment syndrome: Update on diagnosis and treatment. J Am Acad Orthop Surg 1996;4:209.

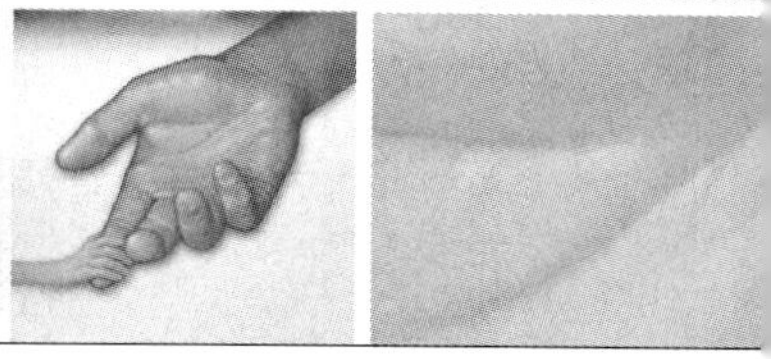

第 20 章

手、软组织损伤及动物咬伤

Michael L. Bentz 和 Delora Mount

8 对儿童手、软组织损伤的评估需要一个对包括创伤部位所有器官系统的全面检查[1]。高度怀疑对于建立准确的诊断和排除其他细小问题是必需的，尤其是对那些不能配合精确检查的婴幼儿。损伤依照其对生活的影响程度而分类。在这样的分类完成后，那些次要的损伤，创伤程度更大的、令人棘手的损伤都能很好地界定出来[6]。病史对于界定损伤前基础功能、以往的损伤、左右利手等情况以及损伤机制和时间是非常重要的。最初的体格检查必须包括血管的检查和灌注情况的检查，因为肢体的缺血和低灌注往往需要紧急的手术干预。其他发现的损伤可以等预约的检查完成后再进行非急诊干预。检查患儿时应该在一个明亮的地方，父母需要陪同在旁边以使患儿保持平静，这样可以提高检查发现的可信度。本章重点是对手、软组织以及动物咬伤的急性期进行评估处理，以便为最初的损伤分类提供一个基础[5,14]。

手、软组织的损伤

评估

血管

早期检查的目的是判断血管损伤、灌注不足和缺血的存在与否及程度。缺血的症状包括苍白、感觉异常、麻木、疼痛和无脉。如果患儿没有在低温下暴露或者肢体近端没有应用止血带，患儿的手指应该是粉红的、温暖的，正常的毛细血管再充盈的时间是 3 秒钟，这可以通过按压远节手指靠近指甲的侧面来准确的测定。充盈时间的延长表明动脉灌注的不足，而快速的充盈则提示静脉压增高或静脉血流不足。脉搏的检查需要检查双侧的桡动脉、尺动脉和肱动脉。如果脉搏测不出或不对称，经皮的多普勒超声可以用来定性和定量血流的流入，Allen 试验对于明确桡动脉和尺动脉对手掌动脉弓的供血相对比例很重要。在 85% 没有损伤的手中，尺动脉及其延续的手掌动脉弓是主要的供血来源[7]。如果在最初的检查中发现有明显的出血，可以予以压迫止血，如果估计到决定性治疗开始的时间比较长，那么可以用近端的止血带止血。不要用止血钳等盲目的在伤口中止血，因为缺血可能导致相应的神经组织损伤。外来的异位应保留在原位，直到最终治疗实施时，因为异物可能正好挡住了血管损伤的部位，去除异物会造成大量出血。

周围神经

周围神经的评估应该在血管检查后进行。单纯的神经损伤，依照损伤部位，会表现出相应的感觉或运动障碍[18]。血管损伤一样可以造成神经功能异常，尤其是在一些亚急性的伤口中，因此，在检查时应该将血管神经检查一并进行。对于肢体断面解剖的清楚的认识有助于明确处于危险中的组织。通过检查远端手部的功能可以有助于明确近端的神经损伤。

正中神经支配桡侧掌侧 3 个半手指的感觉。检查其功能可以通过针尖或两点触觉分辨器来进行。检查正中神经的运动功能可以通过令患儿的示指和拇指做 O 形姿势，感觉拇短展肌和拇对掌肌的收缩来进行（图 20-1）。尺神经支配尺侧 1 个半手指的感觉。运动功能的检查可以通过患儿分指运动时感觉第一背侧 349
骨间肌的收缩来进行（图 20-2）。没有手部固有肌是由桡神经支配的，所以检查桡神经的运动功能可以通过检查患儿伸腕和伸指功能来快速完成（图 20-3）。桡神经支配桡侧背侧 3 个半手指到远节指节水平的感

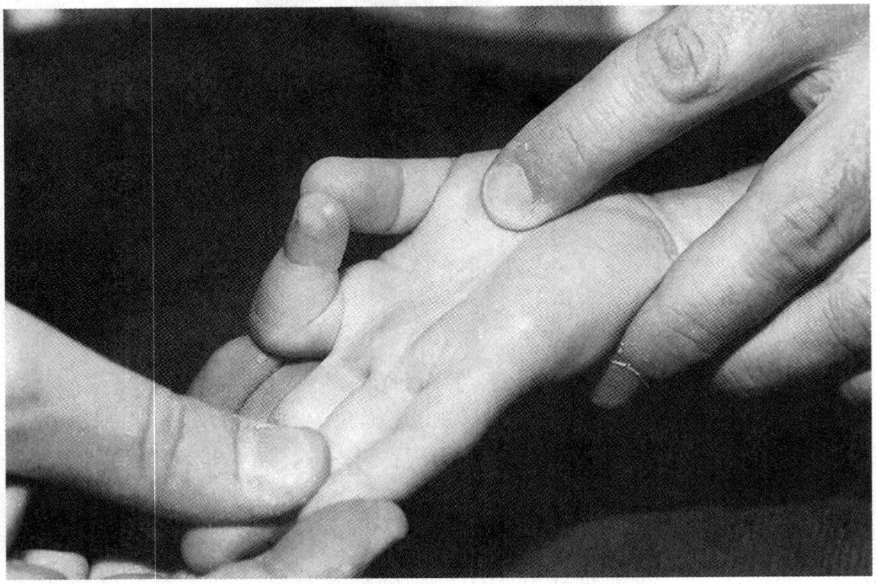

图 20-1 能够用示指和拇指做 O 形姿势，可以感觉到鱼际肌的收缩，提示正中神经连续性完整。

觉功能，交叉支配是很多见的。一系列的检查非常有帮助，孩子合作和集中精神对于取得可靠的评估结果非常重要。另外，肌间隔综合征引起的神经损伤表现不会在最初检查时发现，而是会随着时间的推移逐渐发展变化[13]。

骨骼、肌腱和韧带

尽管有些骨骼损伤在常规体检时表现就非常明显，但大多数还是需要影像学检查。体检可以发现的骨折表现包括：畸形、骨擦音、瘀斑、疼痛、不稳定以及肿胀。除了极小的损伤，对所有的骨折脱位以及异位都要摄正位、侧位和斜位片检查。熟悉儿童骨骺骨折 Salter-Harris 的分型非常重要，因为特殊类型的骨骺骨折通常可以提示预后生长情况（见第 19 章）[16,23]。骨折的表现已经有了详细的描述[12,19]。体检和 X 片表现应该联合起来从而能够准确的描述骨折。开放性骨折包括全层的软组织损伤，而闭合性骨折则没有。单纯骨折导致产生两个骨折端，而粉碎骨折包括多个骨片。青枝骨折包括一侧的连续的皮

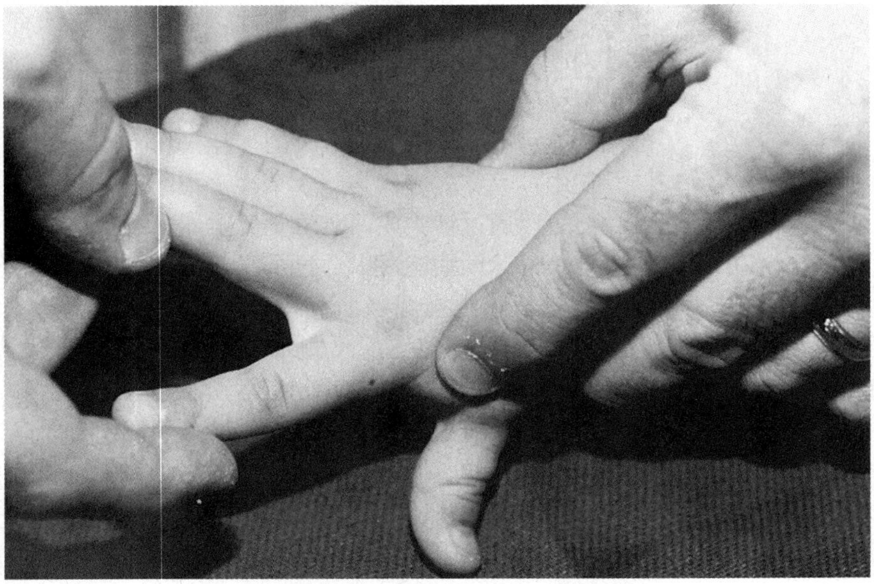

图 20-2 在分指的同时感觉第一骨间背侧肌的收缩可以检查尺神经的完整性。

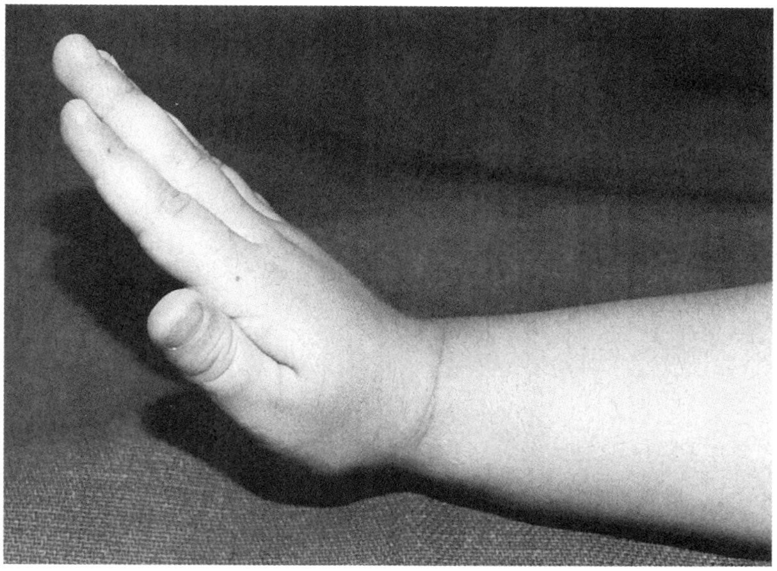

图 20-3　伸指和伸腕功能提示桡神经的功能，因为手部没有肌肉是由桡神经支配的。

质，在儿童中尤其常见，因为儿童的骨骼较有弹性。对骨折的描述还应该包括长度（短缩、延长或正常）、成角（掌侧、背侧、尺侧、桡侧）、旋转（存在或不存在）以及移位相对正常对线的百分比。

肌腱损伤很难诊断，尤其是对不配合检查的幼儿。在这种情况下，必须手术探查以明确损伤。手部在休息时的体位可以提示肌腱的连续性。手部休息时应该是自然屈曲状态，这一体位是由于肌腱被动张力造成的。如果按压前臂远端，由于固定的肌腱被按压，导致所有的手指随之屈曲活动。如果有一个手指保持伸指状态，则提示屈曲机制受到了断裂损伤（图20-4）。检查四个手指中某一指浅屈肌腱可以将相邻指固定，令掌指关节屈曲（图 20-5）。检查指深屈肌腱和拇长屈肌可以持中节指骨观察远节指间关节的屈曲活动。

韧带损伤有时也很难诊断，尤其是当有软组织损伤或骨骼损伤时[24]。异常的关节不稳定提示韧带撕裂损伤[12]。如果对侧没有受伤，那么关节稳定性可以与对侧对比，明确伤前的状态。对于韧带止点的撕脱骨折，平片和应力位摄片可以确定临床检查的发现。

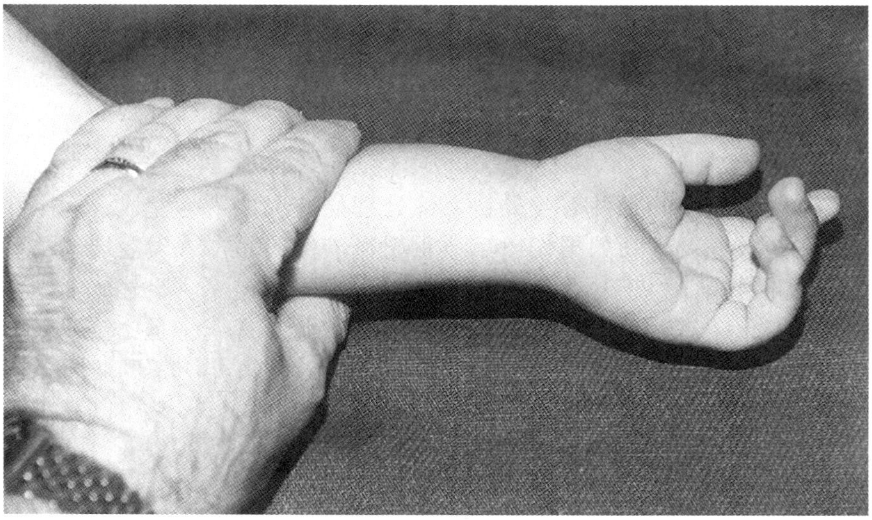

图 20-4　在这个患儿身上，按压其前臂不能使其示指屈曲，提示示指的屈曲机制存在问题。

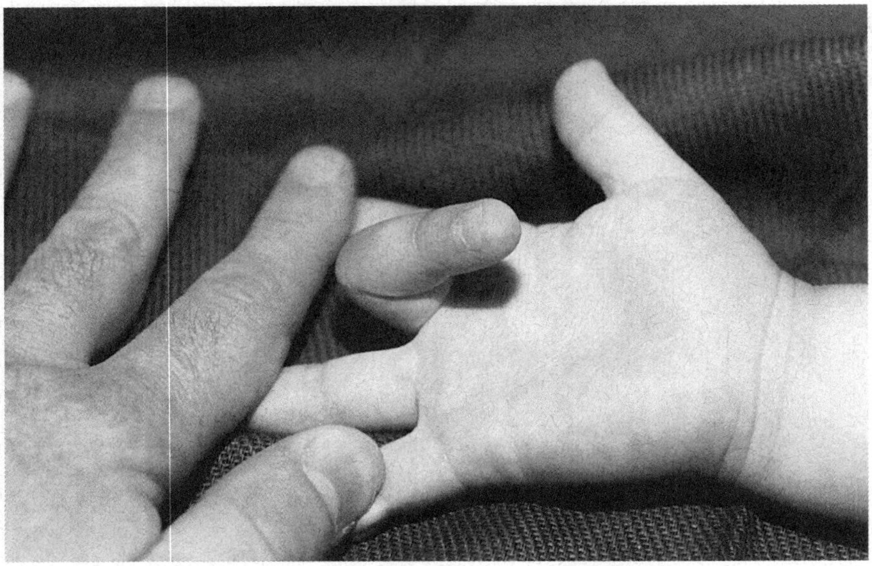

图 20-5 可以通过单独检查掌指关节和近节指间关节的屈曲功能来检查指浅屈肌的功能。指深屈肌的功能可以通过固定中间指节来观察远节指间关节的屈曲来检查。

软组织

详细的检查软组织损伤对于了解伤口愈合的情
351 况非常重要[25]，对长期功能和一期或二期矫形手术的预后结果的评估更为重要。伤口部位的软组织的多少决定了血管、神经和骨骼韧带修复的难易程度，一定量的软组织对于伤口愈合是必须的。需要记录伤口的长度（客观测量）、形状、部位和整体情况，并明确损伤的机制和患儿伤前的状态。明显的异物可以去除，但戳入肢体的异物要留在原位直到进行决定性治疗时。需要注意暴露和骨骼韧带损伤相关的重要组织。

早期治疗

血管

缺血是极少的几种需要外科急诊处理的情况之一。在挽救危及生命的损伤以后，重建血液供应是最首要的目标。由于缺血后 4 小时开始出现不可逆的损伤变化，有时手术暴露介入是必须的，尤其是当缺血累及到肌肉时。早期血管修复是最有效的方法，最好是早期的血管吻合、清创和固定一起完成。如果由于张力或组织缺损导致断端之间很难靠近时，通常使用足背静脉、前臂静脉、大隐静脉或头部静脉的逆行静脉移植，可以广泛的使用。总的来说，所有的接近肘关节的动脉和静脉损伤都应该修复。肘关节以下的动脉损伤也应该修复，以防止对寒冷不耐受，然而，在这些修复手术后仅有一半的血管能够保持通畅[10]。如果有必要，桡动脉可以早期结扎。如果缺血时间较长，软组织损伤严重，或者没有完善的术后监测，那么所有血管修复后都应该做相应的筋膜切开术[13]。随后要进行一系列检查，以早期诊断复发的缺血、术后血栓形成或出血。在这种情况下是否进行溶栓治疗目前存在争议，取决于医生的喜好和经验。

周围神经

周围神经的损伤不是一个需要紧急处理的损伤，可以在血管损伤修复后进行处理。如果伤口清洁、没有感染且血供正常，那么可以考虑做一期的神经损伤端端吻合术。这种修复可以通过固定近远端来方便地完成，这样可以降低张力和增加血供。如果固定近远端后端端之间不能吻合，可以通过移植入神经来完成重建修复。在这些病例中，伤后 10 天内的二期修复是比较理想的选择。为了确保损伤部位的连续性，受累的肢体必须用支具固定，以使断端近端保持最小的移位以及减小吻合口张力。

骨骼、肌腱和韧带

当骨骼、肌腱和韧带损伤的诊断建立后，需要做的是力求达到正常或可接受的解剖对位，然后选用合适的内固定。在儿童中，怀疑有损伤但没有明确的定性的情况很普遍。手部骨折可以在伤后几周内 X 片表现正常，在这种情况下，对于可疑的体检发现和 X 片发现，预防性的治疗可以实施，包括受伤部位的固定。在儿童中，固定很少受到限制，因为固定可以防止进一步的损伤，有助于止痛，并且保持局部的解剖
352 位置。应用支具（代替石膏）是一种理想的选择，因为可以在急性创伤期和复位后阶段使肿胀向非固定区域扩散，防止肌间隔综合征的发生。

对于骨折和脱位的解剖复位可以在损伤当时或伤后一周内进行，都能达到很好的效果[29]。在急诊时，可以通过血肿内阻滞麻醉取得很好的麻醉效果。可以通过在骨折部位注入 2～3ml 不加肾上腺素的 1%的利多卡因来完成麻醉。如果是亚急性的治疗，最常用的是远端的神经阻滞。尤其是在年纪较小的儿童中，必须了解利多卡因的上限剂量是 4mg/kg。对于各种特定骨折的复位方法的详细描述已经超出了本章的范围，但总的来说，轻柔的使用手法牵引或指套牵引，同时旋转和反向旋转在许多骨折和脱位的复位中都很有帮助[8]。复位后的 X 片在大多数的患儿中需要拍摄，分别在外固定前后进行。对于骨折固定的特定位置在儿童中没有成人那么严格，因为儿童韧带僵硬、紧张的倾向较小。在支具固定的最初阶段需要固定在“安全体位”：腕关节伸 30～45°，掌指关节屈 70°，指间关节伸直。对于一些特殊的损伤和临床情况还需要进行一系列体检和放射学检查。

软组织

当确定软组织及其相关的重要组织损伤后，所有的伤口必须用生理盐水进行冲洗，然后去除异物，切除明显坏死的组织。做这些操作需要局部麻醉，在完成彻底的神经学检查后可以进行麻醉。单纯的擦伤和小面积的撕脱伤可以用类似缝合有张力的深部裂伤相同的逐层缝合法进行缝合。线的选择根据伤口的部位、大小、损伤原因以及患儿的年龄来确定。缝合伤口时小患儿需要镇静，同样在拆除缝线时他们也会感觉高度敏感，对于这类患儿，可吸收缝线加无菌免缝创可贴和胶水是最佳的选择。不可吸收缝线可以在年龄较大的儿童和（或）合作的患儿中应用，以减少炎症反应，防止早期瘢痕产生。瘢痕产生的可能性取决于伤口的部位以及损伤的机制。谨慎的伤口缝合可以使瘢痕产生缩小到最低程度。

不能一期缝合的开放性伤口需要更精心的处理。为了在损伤和伤口关闭之间求得平衡，伤口必须在治疗的同时保护起来。生理盐水湿敷是一种简单而有效的方法，可以将需要清创的部位局限下来，允许早期肉芽的生长以及防止干燥。聚维酮碘敷料可以在一些感染伤口中短期使用。乙酸溶液（0.25%）也可以用于已培养证明为假单胞菌类的感染。定量的伤口活检应针对那些非热烧伤的病例。

如果皮肤损伤是表层损伤，没有重要的组织暴露，那么可以用断层皮移植或者用皮肤牵拉法缝合。断层皮移植可以用在大的伤口、对外观要求不高的伤口以及创面由于感染、炎症或者缺血等原因而情况不佳的伤口。全层皮移植在完成血供重建之后，挛缩较少，因此要用于那些有外观需要的伤口，以及那些不希望发生局部瘢痕挛缩的伤口。在这种情况下，局部的皮瓣转移也可以使用，可以提供一个外观较为理想的和周围组织相近的替代组织。如果皮瓣没有特殊的血供，那么可以在任意方向上做转移皮瓣，如果皮瓣的血供是由一特定血管供应的，那么转移必须沿血管轴向进行[17]。局部的带肌肉皮瓣可以在全身各个部位应用，尤其是当需要大块的带血供的组织来覆盖重要结构或填补无效腔时。与轴向皮瓣相似，这些带肌肉的皮瓣也需要以已知的血供方向为基础，这样皮瓣才是可靠的和安全的。最后，如果局部的软组织不够提供伤口关闭的材料，那么需要显微血管外科进行游离带血管蒂的组织皮瓣转移。

断肢损伤

儿童的断肢损伤需要由优秀的显微外科团队进行再植手术，和成人相比效果要好很多[15]。为了提高断肢再植成功的几率，在运送过程中，残肢必须用湿的盐水纱布包好，放置在密封的塑料袋中，再置于一袋冰和生理盐水之中。残肢不能直接接触冰块。

毒液损伤

蛇咬伤

在美国存在 2700 多种蛇，其中有 115 种是本土的种类，只有 19 种是有毒蛇[9]。其中以响尾蛇科的咬伤最为普遍。响尾蛇科毒蛇包括响尾蛇、铜斑蛇以及棉口蛇[28]。银环蛇是另一种类的毒蛇家族。大部分的毒蛇咬伤发生在夏日的清晨、下午的晚些时候以及傍晚。不是所有的蛇咬伤都会出现毒液损伤作用。毒液损伤的表现包括疼痛、水肿、瘀斑、恶心、呕吐、血压降低、DIC、溶血、精神状态改变、癫痫发作，以至于死亡[21]。这些症状的严重程度与毒液的毒性程度呈正比。早期干预包括安慰和支持、固定患肢、抬高患肢、静脉止血带应用，以及迅速转运至最近的医疗
353 单位。冷冻疗法和切开伤口吸引等方法目前已经不再推荐使用。轻度的响尾蛇咬伤（表现为轻度的疼痛，局部水肿，没有全身症状，实验室检查正常）需要最多 5 个单位的抗蛇毒血清；中等程度的毒液损伤（严重的疼痛，扩大的水肿，恶心，呕吐，神经学症状，以及有异常的实验室指标）需要 10～15 单位的抗蛇毒血清，可能还需要再次治疗；严重的毒液损伤（迅速经历从局部症状到全身症状的过程，实验室指标异常）需要早期应用 15～20 个单位的抗蛇毒血清[21]。在皮试后才能静脉应用抗蛇毒血清，以防止发生过敏反应。儿童的抗蛇毒血清用量是成人的 1.5～2 倍，因为儿童的循环血容量小相对蛇毒的浓度大[2,19]。在早期应用抗蛇毒血清后，要积极地进行补液水化处理。可以考虑筋膜切开术，但很少需要这样做[26]。在其他的地区对于蛇咬伤的早期治疗是相似的，根据蛇的类型不同，抗蛇毒血清要做相应的调整[27]。用于对抗北美洲响尾蛇的抗蛇毒血清，对中美洲和南美洲发现的枪头洞蛇、丛林蛇以及双线纹蝮蛇都有效。澳洲能够引起毒液损伤的毒蛇包括普通的褐蛇、本土虎蛇、低地铜头蛇以及红腹黑蛇。

其他动物咬伤

在美国西南发现的毒蜥是墨西哥毒蜥的近亲，在晚春比较活跃。这些毒蜥一旦咬住猎物就会向其体内注射毒液。伤口会出现水肿，但组织损伤没有响尾蛇咬伤严重，然而最终的全身反应是相似的。处理这类损伤首先去除毒蜥，然后应用全身和局部的支持疗法，抗毒血清目前还没有。需要摄片检查，以明确是否有残留毒牙[11]。

黑寡妇毒蜘蛛是一种毒性非常强的新大陆毒蜘蛛。雌性毒蜘蛛呈沙漏形，腹部有红色的标记[3]。咬伤后的局部症状局限，但随后会出现神经系统弥漫性强直和痉挛，1 小时以后可能出现呼吸抑制。黑寡妇毒蜘蛛的毒液损伤可以通过局部伤口处理、补液、心血管系统支持、补充葡萄糖酸钙、肌肉解痉和抗毒血清来治疗[2,5,11,22]。

蝎子蜇伤在儿童中会出现严重的后遗症。树皮蝎是美国唯一的一种毒蝎子，然而在墨西哥和其他中美洲国家还有其他的一些品种。毒液的局部反应很小，然而存在有交感和副交感神经症状。儿童极易在中毒后出现严重的心肺功能不全和神经肌肉系统功能不全。对于蝎子蛰伤的治疗包括局部伤口处理、局部冰敷、特定的抗毒血清以及全身支持，包括保障通气、控制快速性心律失常和镇静。尽管蝎子蜇伤相对较轻，但治疗方面与蜘蛛咬伤相似[20]。

最后，在所有的咬伤中，对于人的咬伤的最终治疗是非常具有挑战性的[4]。根据咬痕来判断咬伤的性质和程度，考虑到可能发生的啮蚀艾肯氏菌感染，进行积极的处理可以达到满意的效果。必须对伤口进行彻底的冲洗，同时应用广谱的抗生素，还要经常检查伤口情况。

（葛翼华译　赵　黎校）

参考文献

1. Ablove RH, Moy OJ, Peimer CA: Pediatric hand disease: Diagnosis and treatment. Pediatr Clin North Am 1998;45:1507-1524.
2. Allen C: Arachnid envenomations. Emerg Clin North Am 1992;10:269-298.
3. Banner W: Bites and stings in the pediatric patient. Curr Probl Pediatr 1988;18:1-69.
4. Bhende MS, Dandrea LA, Davis, HW: Hand injuries in children presenting to a pediatric emergency department. Ann Emerg Med 1993;22:1519-1523.
5. Binder LS: Acute arthropod envenomation: Incidence, clinical features and management. Med Toxicol Adverse Drug Exp 1989;4:163-173.
6. Buncke GM, Buntic RF, Romeo O: Pediatric mutilating hand injuries. Hand Clin 2003;19:121-131.

7. Coleman SS, Anson BJ: Arterial patterns in the hand based on a study of 650 specimens, Surg Gynecol Obstet 1961; 113:409-424.
8. Eaton RG, Littler JW: Joint injuries and their sequelae. Clin Plast Surg 1976;3:85-98.
9. Forks TP: Evaluation and treatment of poisonous snakebites. Am Fam Physician 1994;50:123-130.
10. Gelberman RH, et al: The results of radial and ulnar arterial repair in the forearm: Experience in three medical centers. J Bone Joint Surg Am 1982;64:383-387.
11. Hassen LB: Reptile and arthropod envenomations. Occup Med 1991;6:447-461.
12. Hastings H, Simmons BP: Hand fractures in children: A statistical analysis. Clin Orthop 1984;188:120-130.
13. Holden CEA: Compartmental syndromes following trauma. Clin Orthop 1975;113:95-102.
14. Innis PC: Office evaluation and treatment of finger and wrist injuries in children. Curr Opin Pediatr 1995; 7:83-87.
15. Jaeger SH, Tsai TM, Kleinert HE: Upper extremity replantation in children. Orthop Clin North Am 1981;12: 897-907.
16. Leclercq C, Korn W: Articular fractures of the finger in children. Hand Clin 2000;16:523-534.
17. McGregor IA, Morgan G: Axial and random pattern flaps. Br J Plast Surg 1973;16:202-213.
18. Moberg E: Evaluation of sensibility in the hand. Surg Clin North Am 1960;40:357-362.
19. Nofsinger CC, Wolfe SW: Common pediatric hand fractures. Curr Opin Pediatr 2002;14:42-45.
20. Rimsza ME, Zimmerman DR, Bergeson PS: Scorpion envenomation. Pediatrics 1980;66:298-302.
21. Rudolph R, et al: Snakebite treatment at a southeastern regional referral center. Am Surg 1995;61:767-772.
22. Russell FE: Venomous arthropods. In Schacter LA, Hansen R (eds): Pediatric Dermatology. New York, Churchill Livingstone, 1988.
23. Salter RB, Harris WR: Injuries involving the epiphyseal plate. J Bone Joint Surg Am 1963;45:587-622.
24. Simmons BP, Lovallo JL: Hand and wrist injuries in children. Clin Sports Med 1988;7:495-512.
25. Stewart GM, Quan L, Horton MA: Laceration management. Pediatr Emerg Care 1993;9:247-250.
26. Stewart RM, et al: Antivenin and fasciotomy/debridement in the treatment of the severe rattlesnake bite. Am J Surg 1989;158:543-547.
27. Tibballs J: Diagnosis and treatment of confirmed and suspected snake bite: Implications from an analysis of 46 paediatric cases. Med J Aust 1992;156:270-274.
28. Weber RA, White RR: Crotalidae envenomation in children. Ann Plast Surg 1993;31:141-145.
29. Wood VE: Fractures of the hand in children. Orthop Clin North Am 1976;7:527-542.

第 21 章

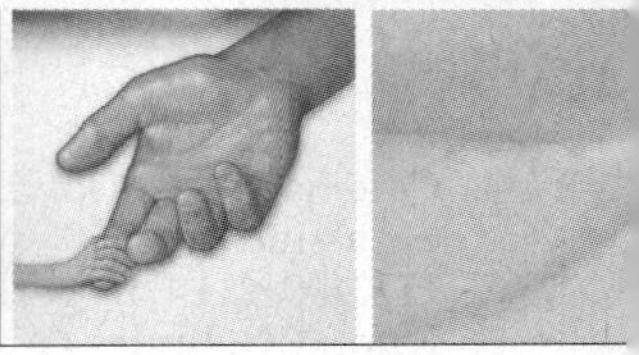

中枢神经系统损伤

Thomas G. Luerssen

355 在儿童创伤中，脑和脊髓的损伤一直是常见情况和主要致死原因。尽管经过 25 年的细致临床研究，目前仍然没有确定的创伤性神经损伤的特效治疗。然而，我们在对于脑和脊髓损伤的自然进程的认识上取得了稳定和实质性地进展；而且，一些改进的治疗方法可以明显改善预后。

我们现在进入了“循证医学”时代，借此对疾病和损伤的处理建议也来自于现有科学研究的严格分析。在过去的 10 年里，中枢神经系统损伤的治疗策略已经来自于这种类型的分析，出版了常规治疗指南[2,21,63,87]。对临床证据的分析和这些建议的产生代表了在这一领域众多顶尖专家的大量工作。不幸的是，这些回顾也能揭示出能用于提出建议的有力科学证据太缺乏了，尤其是在儿童年龄组，因此大多数可获得的推荐认为，神经损伤的诊断和治疗只能由最低程度的医学证据支持。然而，这些发表的实践经验是脑和脊髓损伤的各种治疗的最新方法的有用总结。在本章中这些出版物经常被引用，有兴趣的读者，参阅这些经验和分析文献引文。

治疗中枢神经系统损伤的基本策略

脑和脊髓损伤的管理的最持久的根本原则之一是原发损伤和继发性损伤[124]。原发神经损伤包括神经元、轴突、支持结构和血管组织的即刻破裂。原发损伤的强度和部位，紧跟着发生的一系列不可逆的细胞进程，一些被认为是“延迟的原发损伤”，都直接与损伤的机制相关。这些立即的组织破坏同样被认为是自限性的和基本上不能治疗的。综上情况，我们容易看出，原发性脑损伤是损伤预后的主要决定性因素。

很明显，如果原发损伤是毁坏性的，在许多高能损伤机制中会立即致死。在没有立即致死的患者中，原发损伤引发的一连串细胞内外生物化学改变，无论在受伤区域还是在全身都是有害的，会导致损伤加速和恶化。这些反应性进程表现为所谓的继发性损伤开始。这些继发反应性进程可以在受伤后任何时候开始并持续一段时间。继发性损伤不仅是原来损伤区域和原来未受损伤脑和脊髓的新的损伤，而且对其他器官和全身都产生了有害的影响。

脑和脊髓损伤后的常见全身反应包括低血压和缺氧。很明显即使是轻微和短暂的低血压和缺氧，也会对脑和脊髓损伤的预后造成深远的不良影响[28,123,141]。多发损伤、隐蔽脏器损伤或引起休克的失血的其他因素不是发生这种低血压反应的必需因素。在早期全身并发症中，低血压要比缺氧对急性脑损伤更有害。在急性脊髓损伤中可能也是这样。最后，这些并发症常常可以很早发生，并且在许多病例中很短暂，以至于甚至在现代化监护室里也没有能够发现和报告[12,88]。 35

还有一些其他全身反应，许多在伤后短期发生，但却能在治疗后数天引起进一步损伤。高热，无论是发热还是过度保暖所致，对受伤大脑都是有害的[168]。高血糖常见于应激反应并会因为补液和临时营养而加重，同样对急性神经系统损伤有害[18,27,149]。

组织破裂常指脑和脊髓挫伤，导致损伤区域周围组织迅速发生反应性改变。各种组织因子被释放出来，比如激肽释放酶-激肽系统因子，这些因子能导致微循环障碍和血脑或血脊髓屏障失调，最终引起复杂的结果，一般多为创伤后水肿[113]。神经组织损伤后相关的高代谢反应可能耗尽局部或区域的能量供应。兴奋性氨基酸如谷氨酸和天冬氨酸是从损伤神经中释放出来[56]。创伤后的抽筋发作，尤其是长期亚临床发作，可能就是由于脑损伤的这种反应[172]。同反应性生物化学改变一起，直接血管损伤引起的增大的局部出血能引起相邻血管的进一步压迫，并导致损伤周围区域局部急性缺血。

尽管继发性损伤的全身和生物化学进程是复杂的，但它们的所有病理生理结果是缺血性损伤。缺血性神经损伤在创伤性脑和脊髓损伤患者的神经病理性检查中常可以看到[70,164]。

虽然很多生化进程已经被识别和生理定性，有些已经成为药物干预的目标，但是仍然没有治疗中枢神经系统损伤的特效药物。在对大剂量激素，钙通道阻滞剂，自由基清除剂和谷氨酸拮抗剂的试用中，尽管有少量特殊小组的患者在后期 HOC 分析中被确定从这些治疗中的一种或另一种中受益，但大多数都被否定。更值得关注的是一些组的患者由于给予这些药物后而明显受到伤害[32]。尽管特效治疗没有进展，20 年的临床试验，包括对这些药物的评估，已经显示损伤神经的预后有稳步改善，这种改善在脑损伤要比脊髓损伤更显著。这种预后改善的趋势应当归结于许多缺血性进程可以被受伤复苏开始时和急性治疗期内持续进行的积极的系统的治疗预防。

脑和脊髓损伤基本的治疗策略是：基于通过始终积极维持血容量和血压来预防缺血性损伤。传统认为脑损伤患者要限制补液的观点不再被接受。推荐早期使用血管升压药物。可以通过去除占位来解除局部血管压迫和积极预防治疗脑和脊髓肿胀来保护灌注，减少局部和广泛缺血损伤。支持全身血压、降低颅内压确保脑灌注、去除占位和预防有害并发症是目前治疗脑和脊髓损伤的主要依据。

即刻问题：复苏和转运受伤儿童

有效的支持和预防性治疗应该在伤后尽早开始。初始复苏的目标有两个：防止组织继发性损伤和在进行神经诊断检查之前防止发生任何新的原发损伤。通过尽早补充和维持相应年龄合适的正常血压和血容量可以确保脑和脊髓的氧灌注，这样就能实现第一个目标。这一步再配合补充维持正常通气，至少在这时比给予任何药物都更重要。正确理解实现这个目标的关键：使用何种复苏液体或何种保证通气的方法可能没有实现这个目标本身来得重要。尽管对于使用胶体和更高浓度高渗液体仍在研究，但大多数现在的研究指出等渗和轻微高渗盐溶液对复苏和维持神经系统损伤患者的血压是合适的[21,29,181]。

组织供氧是重要的，在这一点上合适的气道和通气支持是必须的。早期插管和合适麻醉和镇静就能达到这个目标。然而，现场插管在受伤儿童（和成人）中的作用仍然存在争议[77]。因为这个操作伴有相对高的并发症发生率，且在许多情况下不能进行[2,65,127,174]。

对可能有脊柱损伤的患者，防止进一步损伤首先要稳定脊柱。除应用颈托和将患儿固定于硬板上之外，这个操作包含更多内容。维持正常线性解剖位置是重要的。很小的儿童头颅相对大，因此脊柱躺着时相对颈部更易于屈曲[33]。在儿童，单独颈托不能完全固定受伤脊柱[83]。特别注意要固定脊柱于解剖位置，包括头和身体的相对正常位置。小的儿童需要额外抬高身体，这样头部后坠才能保持正常神经位置。一旦获得这些参数，稳定脊柱于解剖位置和建立系统血压和呼吸支持，受伤儿童就可以被转运以确定受伤的诊断和治疗。 357

创伤性脑损伤

流行病学

尽管儿童经常发生头外伤，但这方面的流行病学资料相对有限。英国的一项研究显示，40%在急诊室治疗头外伤的患者是儿童[17]。然而，在讨论预后和治疗上区分“头外伤”和“脑外伤”是重要的，而在讨论机制和预防中分组这些本质则可能是同等重要的。相应的基于人口的研究指出，儿童有临床意义的头外伤的平均发病率大约为 185/10 万，发病率随年龄增长逐渐下降[19,96]。男孩受伤比例大概是女孩的 2 倍。

总体来说，儿童时期所遭受的脑损伤 85% 是轻微的，不会危及生命[97,111]。虽然很少有严重的脑损伤，但是它们仍然是儿科创伤处理的主要关注点。来自儿科创伤中心的报告指出，在所有因钝性创伤导致死亡的孩子中，一半是由脑损伤所引起的[121,171]。

脑损伤的机制和严重程度似乎与预后相关。损伤的原因还和年龄有关。造成儿童头部损伤的最通常的原因是跌落伤，但是儿童跌落通常不引起严重的损伤。造成小年龄孩子严重脑损伤的主要因素应该是虐待。在较年长的儿童中，严重的脑损伤普遍最常被见到和机动车意外事故有关。

在孩子中发生的许多意外脑损伤是可避免的。正确使用乘员安全系统能避免 90% 的对小年龄儿童的严重伤害[147]。在密歇根州的强制性儿童汽车安全法律的落实使儿童在机动车相关的损伤中的数字减少了 25% [116]。虽然关于头盔使用的教育计划迄今只有取得有限的成功[129,148,167]，但与其他娱乐活动一样，如滑板滑行、溜冰、滑雪、骑马，为骑自行车的儿童穿戴头盔就会降低脑损伤的危险[64]。许多跌落伤是可避免的。对于开着的窗户和楼梯保持警觉，包括对门或栏杆的使用，显著地减少了这些损伤的发生。

创伤性脑损伤的范围

现在有许多方法对外伤性脑损伤的主要类型进行概述。作者偏好其中一个包括损伤类型、机制和自然进程之间关系的方法。这样做的最简单的方法是将主要的损伤类型分类为局部的或者弥散的。尽管要注意许多外伤的损伤是局部和弥散损伤的混合，我们仍然可以以脑损伤类型的最初表现作为个体治疗策略的基础。

是局部的还是弥散的脑损伤？

局部损伤包括挫伤、裂伤、外伤性血肿和扩张性肿块引起的局部损伤以及脑的移位和变形。弥散的损伤包括弥漫性轴索损伤（DM）的范畴，它包含常说的脑震荡，以及其他弥漫性损伤，如大脑的局部缺血、全身性缺氧、弥漫性脑肿胀和弥漫性血管损伤。局部损伤通常可在入院时计算机断层（CT）扫描上立刻发现。然而，它们可能临床没有症状。相反，即使是在患者出现意识和神经功能的显著改变时，弥漫性脑损伤也可能很少在早期的神经影像上有显著改变。局部的损伤更可能需要治疗性的外科措施，而弥漫性损伤可能需要广泛的诊断研究来决定损伤的类型和程度。弥漫性损伤也更可能需要长期的颅内压力的监测来指导治疗。分别讨论这些损伤类型的特性是有用的，但是重要的是要记住，在许多病例，尤其是在有比较严重的损伤时，两种损伤类型可能是同时存在的。

局部脑损伤

大多数局部脑损伤与头部冲击相关的机制有关。因为位置不高的跌倒是儿童时期的头部意外损伤的最常见因素，所以头颅打击和它们所产生的局部损伤同样常见。此外，冲击机制与颅骨骨折有关，颅骨骨折在儿科的年龄群体中也是常见的。事实上，住医院治疗的头部伤害的孩子中大约 20%有颅骨骨折[105]。尽管儿童时期的颅骨骨折发生频率高，多数这种损伤的儿童不需要任何的干预或者不会留下直接与骨折相关的任何并发症。因此大多数颅骨骨折的临床重要性是骨折可以作为头部损伤机制的提示和严重性的指标。对颅骨骨折的重要性的大多数研究已经显示在头部损伤的患者发现有颅骨骨折在统计上和张力性颅内血肿或显著脑损伤高度相关[25,82,101,105,166]。此外，复杂颅骨骨折或多发骨折的发生通常与比较剧烈的损伤机制有关，因此会有更严重的脑损害。

如前面所指出的那样，大多数局部脑损伤可立刻在早期的神经影像检查中明显显示出来，根据大小和位置可造成局部的神经功能障碍。源于非锐性损伤机制的最常见的局部损伤是脑的挫伤（图 21–1）。它

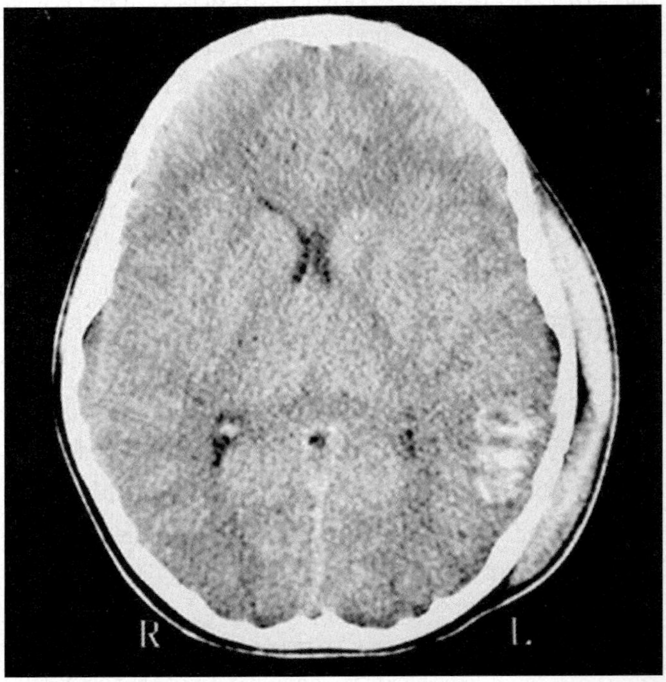

图 21–1 这个线性骨折（未指示）下的脑挫伤是头颅被撞击的结果，这可以被表面的软组织肿胀和出血所证明。患者没有神经缺失症状。

58 通常是脑的表面损害，与头颅冲击部位相对应或与在不规则的头颅内表面上的脑运动相关，抑或是沿着硬脑膜的边缘。脑挫伤的临床表现大都取决于初始损伤的范围、出血量相应引起的占位效应和脑挫伤的部位，即使脑的挫伤可能造成局部脑肿胀，孤立的病灶通常不会对生命构成威胁。许多脑挫伤的神经学症状不明显，只是在初始的 CT 扫描上发现位于颅骨骨折之下或是在前颅底部的损伤。当这些损伤有症状的时候，它们通常引起一个局部的神经缺陷或抽筋发作。后者被认为常发生于急性脑挫伤的成人[38]。但是抽筋发作在脑挫伤的儿童中的发生率并不比那些 CT 扫描正常或有硬膜外血肿的儿童发生率高[73]。

外伤性脑内血肿在儿科年龄组中不是常见的病变形式。出血的致病机制不明确，但是可能与重要动脉血管的破裂有关。因此，这些病变与比较严重的损伤机制有关，而且伴有比较严重的神经功能障碍。在许多情况下，这些病变的表现是稍后会被讨论的脑弥漫性轴索损伤的总的影像表现的一部分。外伤性脑内血肿和出血性挫伤的区别在于前者缺乏与脑表面的接触[67]。外伤性脑内血肿可能相当大，而且因为位置关系，会给儿童留下严重的神经功能缺失。如果颅内压高，应考虑外科清除血肿，但据作者的经验，对这些血肿的清除并没能改善神经方面的预后。

孩子似乎特别易于发生颅骨和脑的非子弹相关的锐性损伤。这些损伤通常是跌落在锐利物体如钉子、铅笔、尖的棍棒或草坪玩具上或被这些物品击伤的结果（图 21–2）。这些损伤的主要危险之一是，除非这个可恶的物体仍旧插在体内，否则损伤入口可能被隐藏或者表现轻微[22,44,126]。从前面刺入颅底可能经眼眶、眶顶或经过鼻或嘴进入。因此，头颅刺入的直接证据可能是看不见的或者可能被局部肿胀所掩盖。

锐性损伤能造成局部挫伤、脑内的出血和脑的裂

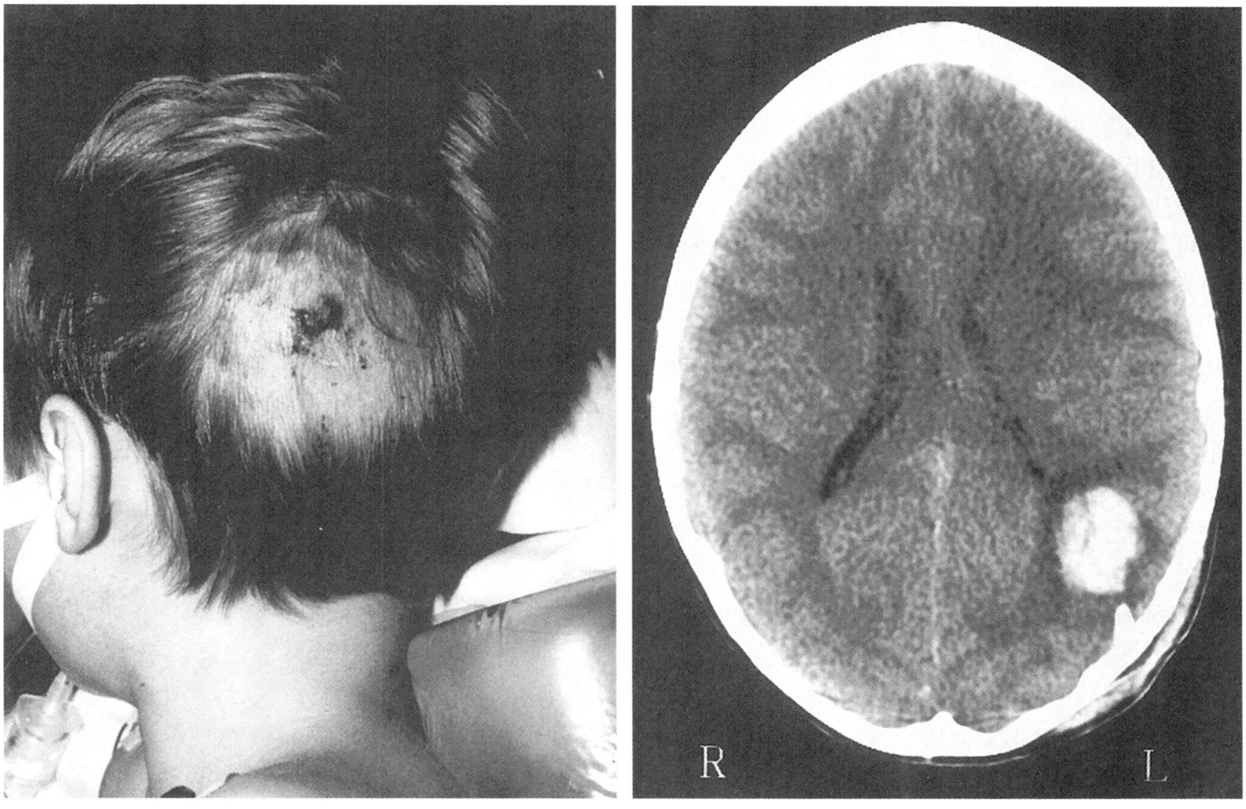

A　　B

图 21–2　显示在小的儿童中、以低速刺入头颅时出现的隐蔽外伤。患者左顶部被草坪飞镖打中，没有发生意识丧失。飞镖立刻掉落。这个损伤被误认是一个较小的头皮撕裂而用蝴蝶绷带包扎。3 天之后，出现发热和头痛。A. 外科探查之前的伤口表现。B. 计算机断层扫描显示一个开放性骨折和大脑内的血肿。在手术中，使头发、污垢和碎骨片从大脑皮层取出。

伤，但是这些病变因为部位置关系和范围小而通常临床症状不明显。较深的刺伤相对来说更可能是具有症状的，不仅是因为组织损伤更广泛，而且因为会伤害主要血管。因为大脑内出血范围逐渐扩张，许多锐性损伤表现延迟的症状出现形式，这是因为脑内出血的扩大、脑脊液漏的出现或显示感染的症状进展。因此无论何时只要有极小的头颅刺伤可能，都要高度怀疑并仔细进行影像检查。木材、玻璃和岩石碎片可能难以在包括 CT 在内的常规影像检查上发现[76]。

头颅的锐性刺伤与直接的脑血管损伤高度相关[51]。每当有深的头颅刺伤的证据或出现重要部位蛛网膜下出血或局部脑内出血时，应该考虑做附加的磁共振血管成影（MRA）、磁共振图像（MRI）或逐渐变得有价值的 CT 血管成像 （CTA）。

弥漫性脑损伤

在儿童期发生的脑损伤主要是弥漫性损伤。弥漫性脑损伤具有在损伤时立刻出现神经功能广泛障碍的特点。尽管如此，脑的结构通常在入院 CT 扫描上维持原样。弥漫性脑损伤的发生是创伤能量在脑的实质里面分散的直接结果或是系统性损伤的结果。所有这些损伤的发生可以是很轻微的，也可以是连续的，可以是完全可逆的，也可以是致命的。通常弥漫性脑损伤的不同类型可以一起发生或者顺序发生，能产生协同作用影响神经状态和预后。

通常弥漫性原发性脑损伤是有角度的或平移的加速（或减速）作用的结果，组织分裂的数量大致与作用于脑组织的能量分散的数量相称[68]。随着神经元分裂数量的增加，神经功能障碍的深度增加和持续时间延长，神经功能预后更差。这些与 CT 扫描出血的表
359 现高度相关，尤其是蛛网膜下腔出血、小的但是广泛的脑内出血和脑室内的出血（图 21–3）[1]。最后，虽然发生外伤，外科上可遇见的占位发生不是弥漫性脑损伤的特性；硬脑膜下血肿常在弥漫性轴索损伤时一同出现，而且一些硬脑膜下血肿很大，以至于一开始必须进行外科手术清除。然而，这些硬脑膜下出血被更多地看成是弥漫性脑损伤的另一个标记，而不是一个像硬膜外血肿或出血性挫伤那样的需要单独治疗的占位病灶。

同所有的脑损伤一样，弥散性原发的脑损伤也有各种不同的表现。在严重范围的一端是很轻微的，出现短暂的神经功能障碍，包括通常的“脑震荡”的症状，而在另一端是进展性进一步损伤和最终出现目前被称为“弥漫性轴索损伤”的致命损伤。

对脑震荡的现代观点是以 Ommaya 和 Gennarelli 的初期工作[130,131]为基础的，这个对脑震荡损伤的定义是按临床症状来分级，显示逐渐增加的意识内容和水平的紊乱。这一个定义允许包括特殊的创伤后损伤，这种损伤在儿童的所谓轻微的头部损伤之后常见，包括没有记忆缺失的意识错乱、有不同程度和持续时间的记忆缺失的意识错乱以及经典的意识丧失，伴有或没有短暂感觉与运动瘫痪和呼吸或循环的紊乱。

随着损伤机制中能量的增加，组织分裂发生且造成弥漫性轴索损伤。现在已经很清楚的是：机械性脑损伤后的长期昏迷的最常见因素是弥漫性轴索损伤。遭受弥漫性轴索损伤的患者从损伤起就是无意识的且保持一个很长的时期[66]。发现瞳孔改变、斜视和去大脑是正常的。这种症状群在磁共振成像前的时期曾经被称为“脑干挫伤”，虽然孤立的脑干挫伤也会发生，但这是极其少有的。相反，大多数的闭合性头部外伤后出现有脑干功能障碍的昏迷患者都是因为遭受了弥漫性轴索损伤。

早期的 CT 扫描上发现取决于受伤的严重度和相关出血的程度。在一些病例，早期的 CT 扫描可能是正常的。随后，特征性的病变可能在磁共振成像上被
发现，并能从广泛的出血性和非出血性的剪力损伤中 36
区别深部白色结构的一些短暂的信号变化。弥漫性轴索损伤的特性 CT 扫描表现是：在深部白质和中央结构中的多个瘀点状出血。然而，特别是桥池部位脑室内出血或局部蛛网膜下腔出血的 CT 表现强烈提示弥漫性轴索损伤。

火器伤

火器伤在儿童中是一个主要的公共卫生问题。因为这些损伤被报道的方式，我们难以确定在儿童中这种损伤的全部发生率。然而最近的报道指出，童年期伤害死亡的 10%与火器有关，这个数字只比车辆意外事故、溺水和房子火灾致死的少一点[62,176]。从治疗和预后的角度看，儿童和成人火器伤的区别很小。与预后差相关的有：昏迷的深度、脑室旁或经脑室的损伤，增高的颅内压和巨大的大脑内出血[138]。尽管会留下重大的神经缺陷和认知障碍[55,125]，大多数

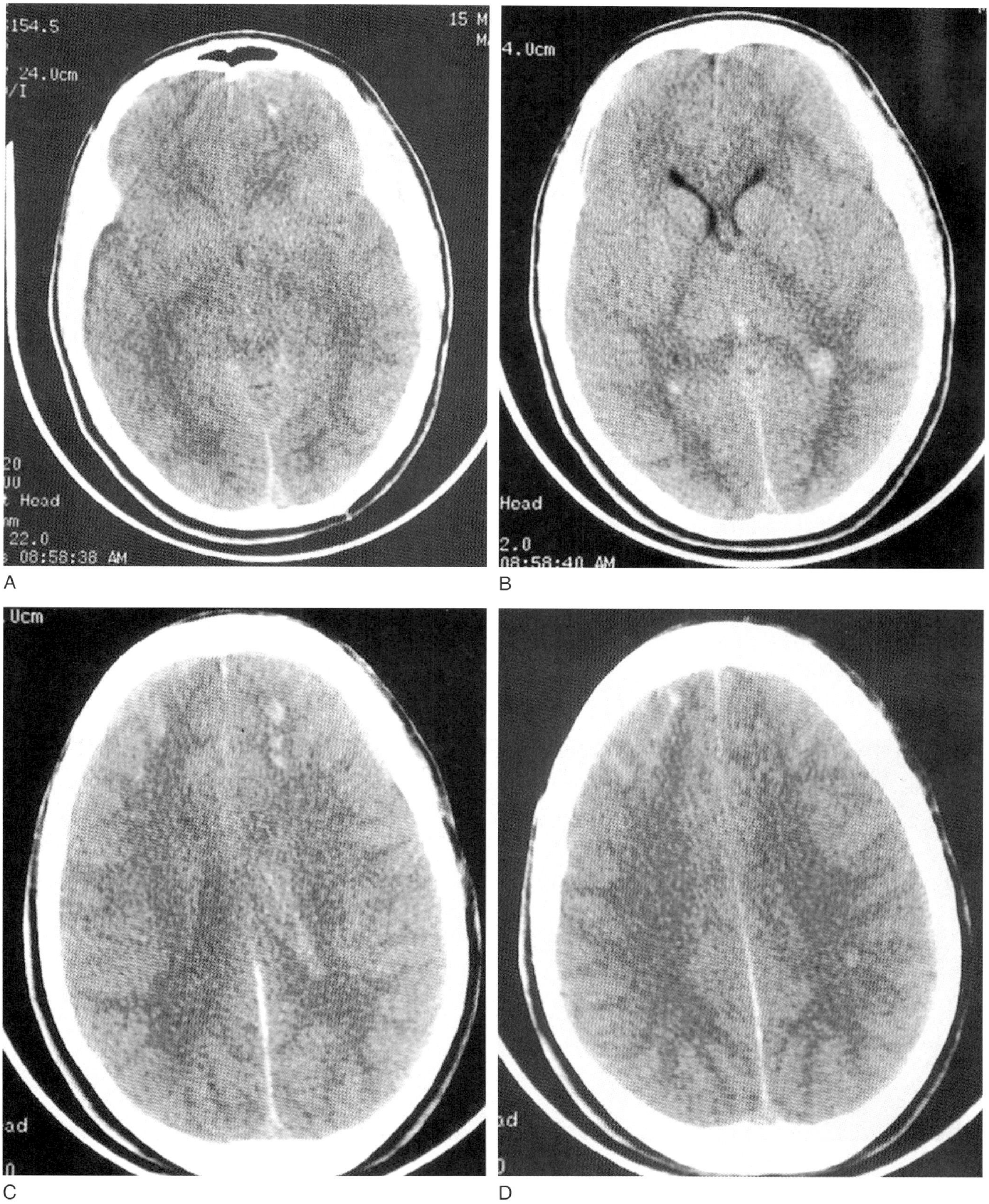

图 21-3　住院 CT 的弥漫性轴索损伤的经典表现包括：蛛网膜下出血和脑室内出血、脑肿胀和脑内遍及的出血瘀点。

的作者建议，对除了明显不能幸存的损伤外的所有患者积极治疗[90]。

由非粉末喷枪如BB枪和铅弹枪所引起的损伤在孩子中的发生率3倍于真正的火器伤[176]，青年期的男性发生损伤的危险度最高[122]。这些损伤一般不太严重，因此死亡率低。BB枪引起的损伤一般不需要外科的治疗。因为球状来福枪弹属速度快口径大的弹道损伤,所以这种损伤更严重而且最好当做真的火器伤来治疗。

压碎性损伤

小的儿童易于发生不寻常的静止负荷类型的颅骨压碎性损伤。这些损伤的发生是由于重物掉落在儿童身上或被车辆碾过。压碎性损伤在临床和放射影像上的发现是引人注目的（图21-4），但是神经预后可能相当好[48]。多发颅骨骨折是典型的表现，包括复杂的颅底颅骨骨折和颜面的骨折。常可见到脑脊液漏和颅神经麻痹。损伤的机制和临床的发现预示严重的损伤和预后不良。但是，尽管有初始的损伤表现，许多主要的皮层结构大多被保留。因此，如果儿童已经平安渡过开始的损伤，积极的多学科治疗能取得满意的长期的功能效果。

加害性损伤

显然，在婴儿中严重的和威胁生命的脑损伤的最常见因素是被施以加害性的损伤（又见第24章）。参与照料受伤孩子的所有医生应该熟悉加害性损伤的临床表现和特征性的放射影像学发现。这个问题最近已经被详细地回顾。婴儿出现意识改变，伴有或没有抽筋发作、视网膜出血和CT显示急性颅内出血，可能已经受到非意外的损伤，尤其是如果是受伤的病史是未知的或报告轻微的时候。另外的发现是：新的或已经痊愈的骨折或其他实质器官损伤是这种损伤的特征性表现。对所有怀疑遭受虐待的儿童，有专业知识的医生应该进行广泛多学科的评价。

儿童脑损伤的初期评估

脑损伤患者的初期评估的目的是双重的。除了其他诊断性检查的计划和协调以及对各种伴随损伤的治疗之外，首先和最重要的是要确定损伤的类型和严重程度，以指导开始治疗的选择。其次，建立一个基线来评估治疗效果，包括治疗的或干预的，积极的，不好的。

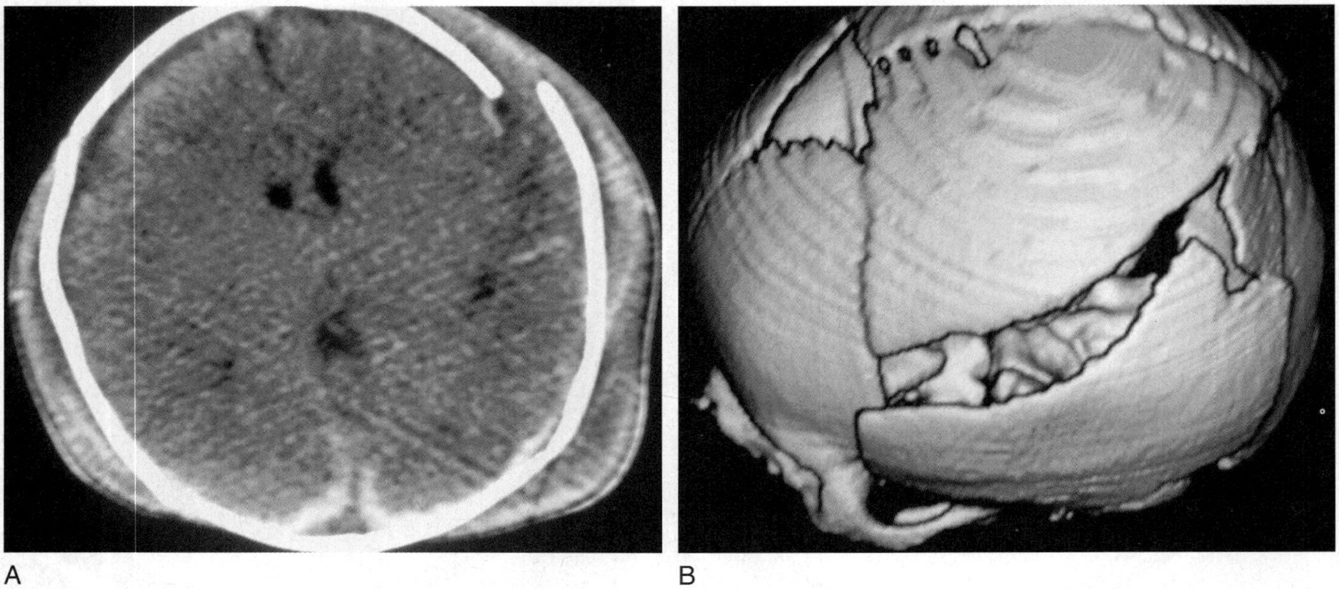

图21-4 一个婴儿的压碎性损伤。计算机断层扫描（A）和3D重建（B）显示头颅“破裂”损伤。尽管颅内出血和硬脑膜撕裂，但脑的结构完整，颅内压降低。这个儿童需要进行脑膜和颅骨重建，但恢复后只会有轻微的后遗症。

在历史上，对脑损伤患者的初始评估主要集中在以评估意识水平以决定损伤的严重程度。对于这个目的，最广泛的评价工具是 Glowgas 昏迷评分[165]。这个评分正如它所设计的那样与预后高度相关[21]。然而，由于对严重受伤患者的转运手段和现场复苏的进步，通常需要院前给予镇痛剂和镇静剂，其对脑损伤的严重程度和类型的神经评估变得不再那么有效[161]。此外，有一小组患者只有轻微的意识改变或没有意识改变，但后来却因为占位病灶或脑肿胀而导致病情恶化[86,95,114]。

最近逐渐清楚的是，在 CT 上的特定发现也和脑损伤的预后显著相关。这种放射学评估能快速地获得，而且不受任何正在进行的治疗影响。不管意识表现的水平怎样，损伤类型的早期影像学识别和适当治疗实质上已经改善了外伤性脑损伤的总的预后。此外现在明确的是，CT 扫描完全正常的头部损伤患者极少出现恶化或不良的预后。根据作者的经验，CT 扫描已经逐渐成为脑外伤的早期诊断的最重要依据，尤其是在年龄小的儿童中。

重要的 CT 扫描发现不只包括有可能采取外科方式处理的占位病灶，还包括弥漫性脑损伤、蛛网膜下出血、脑室内出血或脑实质出血的典型表现和那些可能是早期脑肿胀的非常细微前兆表现，包括中脑周围池被压缩或脑室系统的移位或压缩。CT 扫描上对弥漫性脑损伤表现的早期识别比临床对损伤严重度的印象更重要。这些发现将影响对预后的期待和决定监护和治疗。弥漫性脑损伤的严重程度能通过入院 CT 扫描的表现来分级。如图 21-5 所示，这个特定发现和预后有强相关性[21]，因而能立即做出治疗决策。

目前关于头部损伤的大部分有经验的评估参数都包括了建议进行早期的诊断性 CT 扫描[2,5,21,29,77]。基本 363
上所有可能有严重损伤的患者，有意识改变的患者，应该在生命体征稳定并能安全地转运并度过扫描这段时间时都立刻进行 CT 扫描。对于表面上轻微创伤的头部外伤儿童，如有一个清楚的低强度损伤机制的病史和最多只有一个暂时意识丧失时，现在的建议是可以进行临床评估并观察一段时间而不做神经影像学检查。一个必要条件是，这些孩子应该完全无症状和神经学检查正常并没有合并的病变。另一方面，任何有以下情况的儿童应尽快进行 CT 扫描，包括持续数秒的无意识、抽筋、头颅冲击的临床症状、颅骨骨折、

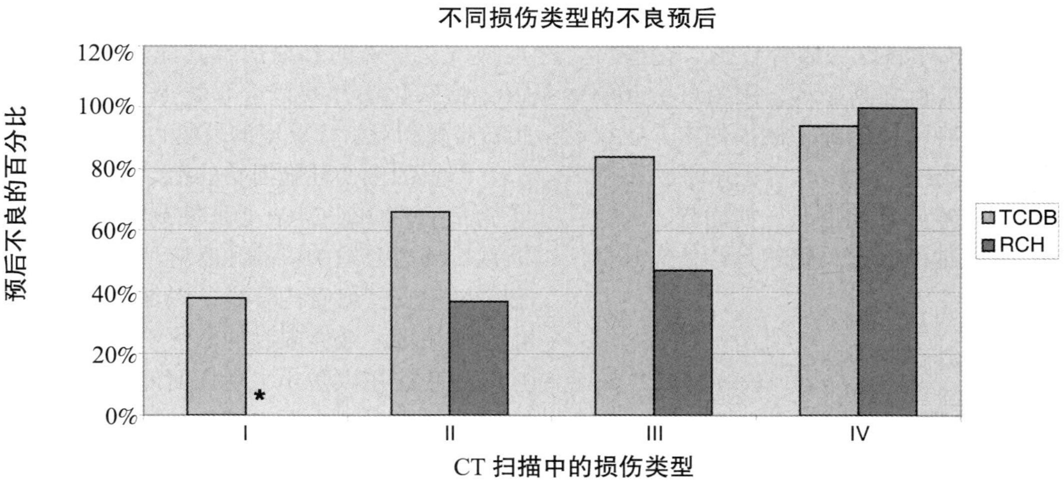

图 21-5 显示入院计算机断层扫描表现对损伤预后的影响。这个图的数据来自创伤昏迷数据库（TCDB）[117]报道的信息和未发表的印第安纳 James Whitcomb Riley 儿童医院的 1000 个连续的儿科脑外伤病例资料。不良预后依照 Glasgow 评分被定义为严重残废的、植物人或死亡[139]。

定义：

弥散性损伤 I：没有在计算机断层扫描上看到的颅内病理改变。

弥散性损伤 II：脑池中线移位 0～5mm 或病变密度表现（或两者都有）；高密度或混合密度病灶小于 25 ml。

弥散性损伤 III：脑池被压缩或消失，中线移位 0～5mm；高密度或混合密度病灶小于 25 ml。

弥散性损伤 IV：中线移位大于 5mm；高密度或混合密度病灶小于 25 ml。

头颅刺伤或脑脊液漏、头痛、持续呕吐、嗜睡或激惹[78,134]。最后如果孩子是经由高能量机制伤害造成的表面上孤立的胸部、腹部或骨骼损伤，那么应该在给予麻醉药、镇痛药或镇静药之前进行头颅的 CT 扫描，因为这些药物会妨碍准确的神经系统检查。

从先前的讨论中清楚的是，头颅平片放射检查在头外伤初始评估中只有有限和次要的作用。CT 扫描将会发现大多数临床重要的颅骨骨折。相反，颅骨放射检查只能提供一些脑损伤的类型和部位的有限信息。磁共振成像在检测大多数脑病变中比 CT 更敏感并在许多神经病变的检查选择上取代了 CT。然而，对于急性的外伤性脑损伤，决定治疗的所有必需信息仍然是由 CT 扫描提供的。在大多数情况下，CT 扫描比磁共振成像更快、更容易获得且花费更少。

最后，尽管神经影像在诊断和治疗创伤性脑损伤中具有重要作用，仔细的体格检查和神经系统检查仍然非常重要。应该检查整个头部以发现撞击的体征：头皮损伤、头颅变形和头颅或眼眶的刺入。颅神经功能的证据，尤其是瞳孔的大小、形状和反应，是必需的，而且应前后比较。前颅底的颅骨骨折的证据表现为眶周瘀肿、鼻出血或 CSF 鼻漏，这是鼻饲管安置的禁忌证，直到能证实前颅底的完整性。耳后擦伤、血鼓室、耳出血和 CSF 耳漏提示颞骨骨折，这些可能不能在标准的筛检 CT 上立刻显示，因为可引起颅神经病变的延迟表现。在可能的加害性损伤中，建议眼科医生进行扩大的检眼镜检查[6]。意识水平状态和运动感觉缺失的表现，连同其他情况，如插管、药物治疗、肿胀、夹板和其他的因素，仍然是评估头外伤患者的必需元素。

严重脑损伤的早期处理

如前所述，脑损害患者复苏的主要目的是在转运和评估期间保持脑的灌注。严重脑损伤治疗的进一步目的是使受损伤的和未受损伤的大脑的灌注最佳化，而且要创造一个环境，使其他继发性损伤机会最小而神经功能恢复程度最大。我们必须这样做来避免或者逆转会造成进一步神经元损伤或者血肿增大的有害过程，后者包括直接影响受损伤脑部的全身并发症，如败血症、急性肺损伤、高血糖和凝血障碍。

已经提出多种治疗策略来治疗创伤性脑损伤。这些治疗大部分包括系统治疗以获得既有治疗作用又有保护作用的反应。所有的“新”的治疗有理论上的吸引力，它的推荐者报道的结果比历史对照要好。然而，至少到现在为止，当这些治疗和已经被定义为“标准治疗”的治疗直接对比测试时，没有被证明有更好的效果。因此，现在的治疗建议仍沿用历史的标准治疗，包括机械通气、液体治疗、镇静、血压和 ICP 的控制。

为了做到这些，我们必须尽可能理解患者的颅内的血流动力学和通过外科清除可及占位获得理想的脑灌注，并且尽可能通过安全的处理来控制 ICP，包括控制脑血容量（动脉和静脉）、脑脊液容量和脑容量[112]。对严重的损伤和部分不太严重的患者，治疗规则和操作要根据 ICP 的监测来进行。ICP 监测为脑损伤患者的许多重要治疗决定提供了基础[107,120]。

个体化治疗的应用超出了本章节的讨论范围。然而，重要的是要认识到，现在对于提高 ICP 的每一种治疗都有一般和特殊效果，且使用每个疗法时都会合并有并发症。历史上常对脑损伤患者给予大剂量类固醇的方法不再被认为是有益的，而且事实上可能是有害的。因此，现在的指导方针不推荐任何的特殊化治疗，举例来说，对脑损害患者预防性或普遍应用过度换气、渗透的利尿剂或其他药物治疗。同时还建议，特殊化治疗要以合乎逻辑的顺序应用，并且由 ICP 监测和对治疗反应的反复再评价来指导。

严重的创伤性脑损伤的治疗的基本要求包括维持正常氧合和 $PaCO_2$ 浓度来控制通气。插管患者任何 36
时候都要有合适的镇静和麻醉。任何时候都要用输血和输液来支持血管内容量，以保持正常的血球容积和电解质浓度。液体限制的做法不予推荐。低渗的液体应该避免应用以防止出现任何低血钠症的倾向。床头可能要抬高以减少颅内的静脉压，只要正常的中央静脉压通过适当的补液来加以维持。对于许多严重的弥漫性脑损伤，这些治疗要求是必需的。

进一步的治疗包括 CSF 引流术的使用。通常方法有放置脑室引流、甘露醇渗透利尿和轻度的过度通气。每当考虑进一步的治疗时，也要为监测治疗效果和并发症加强生理监测。表 21-1 总结了作者基于现在的治疗指导方针的脑损伤加强治疗的方式。少数患者需要更强化的治疗来提高 ICP，包括大剂量巴比妥酸盐、强烈的渗透治疗或强烈的过度通气。这些治疗有较高的并发症发生率，因此应该只有当完全必需的

表 21-1　创伤性脑损伤的医学治疗

治疗	监测
评估和复苏	
恢复正常血压	全身血压和氧合
插管和机械通气	神经系统检查
	潮气末 CO_2
基础治疗	
床头抬高	全身血压和氧合
保持头部在正中位置	颅内压
镇静和肌肉麻痹	动脉 PO_2、PCO_2 和 pH
机械通气维持 $PaCO_2$ 在 35~40mmHg	体重、尿量出量、脉搏和脉压
维持血管内容量正常或稍增加	血色素、电解质、血糖和血尿素氮
正常液体和电解质状态（无液体滞留）；避免贫血、高血糖	对发热和败血症的监测和积极治疗
体温正常或适度的降低	CT
中级治疗	
脑室内脑脊液引流	脑室内导管
甘露醇	中央静脉压
适度过度通气维持 $PaCO_2$ 在 30~35mmHg	血渗透压和电解质
难治性颅内压的重症治疗	
大剂量巴比妥类药物治疗	持续或扁平的光谱脑电图
如有指征则行腰椎脑脊液引流	巴比妥类药物浓度
深度的过度通气	颈静脉氧合监测脑血流

时候由有经验的神经监护医生使用。

为严重受伤的患者做出外科治疗的决策通常是明确的。很明显，头颅的刺伤，包括复杂的颅骨骨折，需要紧急的外科处理。清除大的外科可及的占位病灶可能是严重脑损伤的全部治疗措施的第一个步骤。除此之外，初始的外科步骤可能限于放置 ICP 监视器、脑室引流管或两者都有。这些步骤如有需要可在床边进行。在许多情况下，如闭合性凹陷性骨折、碎片骨折或粉碎性头颅的和颅面的骨折，患者病情稳定或神经损伤改善后就能进行外科矫治。

对脑损伤的典型的主要外科治疗包括清除外伤性颅内的血肿。在儿童中外科可处理的血肿的总的发生率大体上比成人低，而且血肿类型的比例不同。硬脑膜下血肿在婴儿中最常见，但是很少达到需要外科清除的大小。正如在这一个章的开始所讨论的，在比较年长的儿童中，急性硬脑膜下血肿通常更加提示严 365
重的弥漫性损伤（图 21-6）。硬膜外血肿在儿童中是比较常见的外科处理的占位，尤其是在比较年长的儿童头部撞伤时（图 21-7）。在脑的凸面上的，小的硬膜外血肿可能不需外科的清除就能消退。应该更加关注那些发生在比较有限的“腔隙”的血肿，如在颞窝或后颅窝，在这些位置的即使是很小的硬膜外血肿，可能也必须予以清除。大的出血性挫伤或创伤性脑内的血肿在儿童年龄组中非常少见[111]。

基于以上观点，决定清除外伤性颅内的血肿应该是全部的脑损伤治疗策略的一部分。很明显，对于大的硬膜外血肿，手术清除可能是唯一的治疗需要。另一方面，在弥漫性脑损伤的情况下，清除那些在其他方面被认为非手术清除的占位能在颅内容量 / 压力比上取得实质性改善。颅内容量 / 压力比对维持适当的脑灌流是很重要的。在这一个概念上延

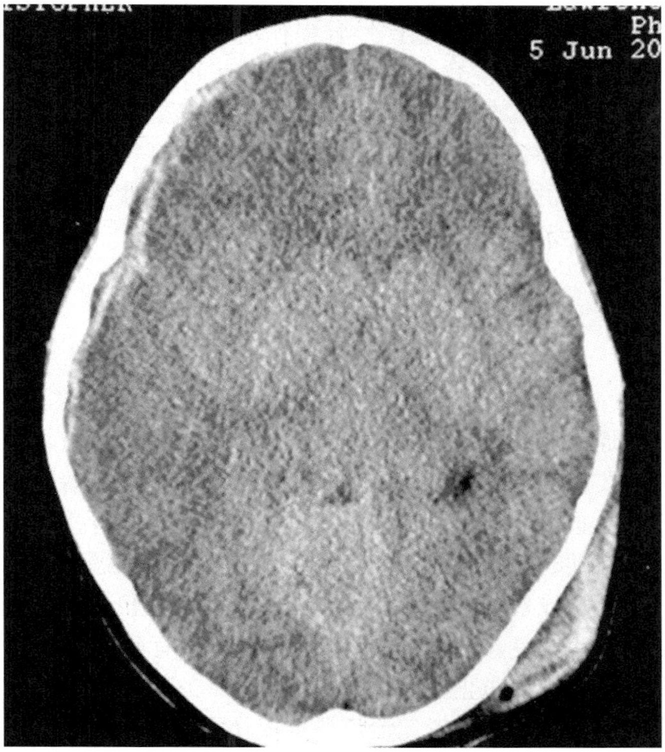

图 21-6　急性的硬脑膜下血肿。出血位于半球表面（图像左侧），似乎很少。然而要注意，脑的广泛移位和半球的肿胀，这能提示严重的弥漫性损伤。

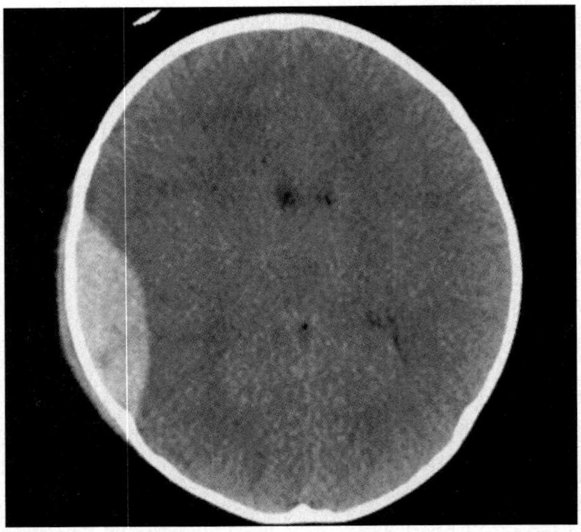

图 21-7 急性硬膜外血肿，注意出血部位的厚度，但也要注意与图 21-6 所示硬膜下血肿的不同：没有中线移位。这种没有肿胀和移位是非损伤性脑膨胀肿块的不常见反应，只要这个肿块在开始昏迷前去除，患儿发病率和死亡率几乎为零。

伸出最近的“治疗性的颅骨切除减压术”的再研究。现在出现有很多关于“治疗性的颅骨切除减压术”在所有严重创伤性脑损伤治疗中的作用的论文数量见涨[2,59]。这个治疗明显增加了可扩展的容积并降低 ICP。然而，现在不明确颅骨切除减压术是否颅骨切除术提供了在标准的治疗之上的一种附加的或独有的效果。同样在损伤治疗期间何时应该进行外科手术也不明确。

“轻微”脑损伤的处理

相当多的头部损伤儿童有轻微的、较小的或很小的原发脑损伤。这些儿童肯定会完全恢复，通常不需要任何治疗。然而在这个大的群体里面隐蔽着一小部分血肿扩大或处在脑肿胀早期的患者。这些患者处在随时间延迟风险增加的状态，且会迅速恶化将造成死亡或残疾。对显然较小的脑损伤的评价重点是识别患者是否处于神经恶化的处境或会有延迟的并发症，且应该防止前面情况的发生[134]。在许多方面，诊断和治疗这些患者比治疗严重损伤更有挑战性且更重要，因为成功的治疗通常产生好的预后[95,114]。

有关这个观点的文章已经发表[5,156]。关于脑损伤的其他类型，早期 CT 扫描是正确诊断和识别处于恶化风险中的脑损伤患者的关键[42,82,106,128]。不管意识的水平如何，有脑池受压、出血性的剪切伤和挫伤或小的创伤性血肿证据则表明患者是处于不断恶化的风险之中。这些患者可以通过反复评估来发现，这包括重复神经影像学检查、ICP 监测和甚至早期使用控制颅内动力学的治疗[110,118]。灌注静脉液体治疗显得更为重要，因为许多表面上轻微脑损伤的儿童似乎在面对即使是轻度低钠血症时也会病情恶化[84,159]。所以关于大多数的脑损伤患者，给他们的维护液体应该是生理盐水或者它的等价物[181]。也应该关注维持正常的血管内的容积和血清的电解质状态。

虽然识别患者处于恶化险境包括 CT 扫描上的明确异常表现，但是关于 CT 扫描和头部外伤近来文献中更重要的发现正在显现出来。特别指出，轻微受伤的患者的完全正常的 CT 扫描基本上和致命性的恶化风险没有关联[36,160]。如作为 CT 正常的意外轻微受伤的儿童，没有颅骨骨折，没有抽筋的病史，而且是无症状的，则可以托付给能胜任的看护者，不用住院观察。

对于因为运动而遭受脑震荡的青少年，现在有出版的指南描述这些个体的评价和治疗，连同关于运动员何时在脑震荡之后能回到运动场的建议[4,23,92,175]。

头部损伤的早期并发症

头部损伤的早期并发症包括损伤相关的颅骨骨折，与头颅的刺入和 CSF 瘘管有关的感染和急性的神经并发症，如创伤后癫痫。关于头部损伤治疗的主要方面是识别由于这些并发症而使受伤患者处于危险之中，而后给以合适的诊断学检查、监护和必要时干预，是达到最佳预后的关键。 36

颅骨骨折的并发症

单纯的非凹陷或轻微凹陷的颅骨骨折会自然愈合。在年龄小的儿童中广泛地颅骨脱离或破裂提示硬脑膜损伤[45]，如果没有外科治疗将难以痊愈。由于有现代的神经影像检查，这些损伤的早期识别使得早期有效修复成为可能，从而避免发生通常在文献中提及的生长性颅骨骨折[140,177]。扩大的颅骨缺损的典型征候和进展的神经系统恶化，两者都相关于颅脑的侵犯和增大的蛛网膜囊肿，可以在受伤后数月到数年内出现[177]，而这完全可以在早期通过修补硬脑膜和颅骨来避免。然而，局部的脑损伤常见于严重的颅骨凹陷，脱离和破裂性骨折，这些患者将会有增高的抽筋和局部神经缺陷发生率。

颅底骨折

对于怀疑颅底骨折的患者，具有紧急临床重要性的主要问题是这些骨折可能是复合伤，因此患者处于发生感染的危险中。鼻或耳 CSF 漏的明显症状只存在于 10%～20%的病例[31,89]。因此，一定要寻找颅底骨折的其他征兆，因为这些骨折在常规神经影像检查容易被遗漏。这些征兆包括双侧的眼眶瘀斑或肿胀、面中部或眼眶骨折的征象、鼓室积血、耳出血和 Battle 征象。在损伤之后的数个星期，这些患者处在增加的脑膜炎危险中。基于这些和对损伤情况的回顾，合并颅底骨折可能比出现 CSF 漏的迹象更多发生，那些被认为可能遭受颅底骨折儿童的家长和看护者必须接受的忠告不仅是识别可能发生在家里的 CSF 耳漏和鼻漏的重要性，而且是对受伤后数周有细微提示细菌性脑膜炎的症状和体征的儿童立即寻求医治的极端重要性。尽管细菌性脑膜炎危险性增高，预防性给予抗生素并没有取得效果。尽管并不清楚疫苗是否降低肺炎球菌性脑膜炎的发生率[53,94,146]。一些医疗中心正在给认为有颅底骨折的患者注射肺炎球菌疫苗。颅底骨折常伴有神经病损。在所有颅神经中，嗅神经最常受伤，尤其是在患者前颅底损伤时。

发生在颅底靠后点的骨折和包括眼眶和面中部的骨折易于损伤视神经。视力丧失可以急性发生也可以延迟发生，应保证有眼科的评估和随访。包含岩部的骨折可能引起听力，前庭或面神经的损伤，或这些损伤合并发生。这些患者需要耳科评估和听力测试[108]。

直接脑血管损伤

尽管闭合性脑外伤后极少发生创伤性颅内动脉瘤，但超过 20%的所有创伤后动脉瘤是发生在儿童年龄组[20]。穿透伤，尤其是刺伤伤口和深的穿透，有合并血管损伤的高的发生率。当大量蛛网膜下出血和局部颅内出血出现在 CT 上时，应该高度怀疑血管损伤，但在一些病例，应进行诊断性血管造影。如果这个造影没有结论，应早期重复影像检查。

创伤后癫痫

癫痫是脑损伤最常见的并发症之一，即使是轻微脑外伤。大多数研究指出儿童创伤后抽搐实质上比成人要高[9,115]。创伤后癫痫的相关危险因子包括较小的年龄和严重创伤[30,73]。然而，并不清楚的是哪些可能具有很高早期癫痫发生的受伤婴儿被排除在这些研究之外[109]。如果分析中去除了这个特殊的组，儿童创伤后癫痫的发生率则会显得相对低。

必须区分早期和晚期创伤后抽搐的差别。早期抽搐一般定义为那些伤后一周内发生的抽搐。对儿科患者，这个定义将包括所谓的撞击相关抽搐，这在轻度头外伤儿童中有达到 10%的发生率[50,73,104]。这些抽搐通常是自限性的而且 CT 显示正常。不必进行治疗，其长期预后好[41,81]。这个特殊综合征在头外伤的成人中几乎见不到，这些成人的早期癫痫与结构性脑损伤或硬膜下血肿显著相关。

严重脑外伤儿童是指昏迷或入院 CT 有结构性损伤的儿童。对他（她）们只有有限和矛盾的信息来评价临床严重程度和处理早期或晚期创伤后癫痫[30,170,179]。现在的建议指出所有有过重复抽搐的严重受伤患者应进行抗惊厥的药物治疗。苯妥英是针对这一目的最广泛的推荐用药[2,26]。已经有一些证据说明在严重头外伤患者预防性应用苯妥英能降低早期创伤后抽搐的发生，尽管还不清楚这个治疗能否改善受伤后的预 367
后[21]。另一方面，强烈的证据显示对严重头外伤患者常规给予抗惊厥治疗既不能降低晚期癫痫的发生也不能改善受伤的预后。因此，超过伤后第一周给予预防癫痫的抗惊厥药物不被推荐[2,21,26]。

脑震荡后综合征

对年幼儿童来说似乎独特的一个神经功能异常的综合征曾被称为“儿童震荡综合征”。轻微头部撞击后短时间内儿童表现出急性发作苍白、发汗和反应淡漠。CT 扫描正常且综合征在发生后很快缓解。根本的机制尚不清楚，尽管已经有研究指出这可能是创伤后癫痫的一种变异[152]。

在儿童中其他更加少见的轻微创伤后的短暂神经功能紊乱也已经被报道，包括短暂皮质性盲、发音障碍、共济失调、接受性言语障碍和长期定向障碍[91,178]。CT 扫描还是正常，症状自行缓解。病因不明。

创伤后脑损伤的预后

儿童期头外伤的预后报道有相当的差异。除去婴儿遭受外加的头部损伤外，儿童总的死亡率大约是成人相当程度头部损伤报道的一半。在大宗病例研究中，儿童头外伤死亡率相对于所有程度的损伤一般低于 5%，对基于 Glasgow 昏迷评分或其他损伤评分系统而定义为严重脑损伤的儿童则低于 20%[102,111,170]。预后不良的相关因素有高能损伤、结构性损伤、入院 CT 脑肿胀和移位、持续和难治的 ICP 升高、合并胸腹部损伤和症状性并发症。

创伤性脑损伤是儿童期获得性丧失功能的首要原因[99]。对于创伤性脑损伤存活的儿童，神经和认知的预后和儿童年龄、损伤严重性、脑的持续性结构损伤的程度相关[8,14,60,102,119]。严重脑损伤儿童易于对智力、记忆、注意力、语言及行为有持续不良作用。这些缺陷似乎不断发展且可能混合作用于学习和社会能力[103]。所以，重大的儿童期头部损伤的总的神经行为预后相对于同样的成人损伤预后来说比较差。

外加性脑损伤的预后另外讨论。这种特殊的损伤有儿童期最高的死亡率和发生率。据报道的死亡率接近 40% [46,49]。发病率同样高，尤其是在婴儿显示出脑梗死和低氧局部缺血性损伤的证据时。

轻微脑损伤的预后

轻微脑损伤是指只对意识产生有限影响和保留脑结构的损伤，也是儿童年龄组最常见的中枢神经系统损伤。所有儿童时期头部损伤的 3/4 以上属于轻微脑损伤[100,111]。直到最近才关注儿童脑震荡的远期预后[154]。尽管定义轻微脑损伤和严重性的分类划分仍有不同[150,157,169]，在可得的文献出现两个一般原则。首先，躯体不适如头痛、视力影响、畏光和噪音、头晕和情感紊乱如抑郁、兴奋或易激和认知减退包括学习困难，在轻微脑损伤儿童伤后数天和数周常见[57]。其次，只要儿童脑受伤前没有任何认知和行为障碍，所有震荡后早期症状被描述在不超过几个月的时间里完全愈合[169]。

脊髓损伤

儿童期脊髓损伤少见，但这些损伤的结果可以是灾难性的。同创伤性脑损伤一样，现代神经影像学为创伤性脊髓病变的诊断和治疗认识作出了贡献。正如本章开始所讨论的，对脊髓损伤的主要治疗努力和脑外伤的一样，目标是阻止新的原发损伤和改善继发性损伤。主要目标在复苏和评估阶段通过保持脊柱正常解剖排列完成。达到第二目标非常困难[3]，由支持血压和氧开始。

一般来说，儿童脊柱和脊髓损伤的诊断和治疗方法和成人相似。最近出版了脊髓损伤治疗指南，总结了最新相关知识[87]。然而，在脊柱损伤儿童，尤其是很小的儿童，临床表现、解剖学、放射影像发现和治疗上仍存在重要的不同点。

流行病学

在儿童每年有少于 10%的脊髓损伤或大约 1000
例新发脊髓损伤[93]。脊柱损伤不累及脊髓非常常见。
在 122 例儿童，只有一半脊椎损伤儿童有神经功能缺 365
失[72]。

受伤的机制和模式和年龄及性别相关。在很小的儿童，男女比例大致相等。在大点的儿童，更成人化的分布出现，男女比例大约 4∶1。大约一半儿童脊柱损伤是因为车祸。1/4 的损伤是因为跳水意外。很明显，直接单独对这两种机制进行预防努力可以显著的降低儿童脊柱损伤的比例。另一个损伤的主要机制是坠落和运动损伤，分别占报道损伤的 10%。年幼儿童更易于坠落损伤所致，而年长儿童更易于源自跳水意外和运动[7,133]。

年幼儿童易于出现颈部区域的脊柱损伤，而年长儿童脊柱损伤的分布和成人相似。儿童更常出现没有合并椎体骨折或错位的脊髓损伤。这些特性被认为和青少年脊椎的解剖性质相关，而和损伤机制无关。儿童脊椎有些重要特性使得椎体能明显的自我回复移位。这些特性包括关节囊和韧带增高的弹性、浅和水平方向上的连接、前方契入的椎体和发育差的钩状突[11,58]。而且，年幼儿童有不相称的较大的头和较弱的颈部肌肉。所有这些因素允许了较广的屈伸范围和头尾牵引。青少年脊柱的运动支点较高，这点解释了儿童头端损伤的高发生率。随年龄增长，这种倾向减少，更特征性的椎体骨折和错位发生增多[10]。最后重点要记住，儿童 10%～15%的脊椎损伤包括在椎体和脊髓不同水平的“跳跃”损伤[72,74]。因此，基于损伤机制，当认定儿童有脊髓损伤或椎体断裂时，需要彻底对脊柱检查以发现另外的损伤。

在儿童，胸腰段脊髓损伤不常见。儿童所有脊髓损伤中少于 20%发生于颈椎以下[143]。主要机制有从高处坠落和高速机动车意外事故，包括由于座椅安全带所致的特征性的牵引性损伤[71]。

脊椎和脊髓损伤的临床分类

因为脊髓损伤在儿童少见，所以可能被忽略，尤其在年龄很小的和那些有多发损伤的儿童更易忽略。正如下一段要讨论的，表现正常的放射平片检查不能完全排除椎体不稳定和脊髓损伤。因此，我们需要根据损伤机制和神经系统发现来提高对此的怀疑。高能机制如机动车意外和高处坠落更易于导致脊椎和脊髓损伤。任何年龄的昏迷患者应怀疑脊髓损伤，直到彻底的评估完成。

清醒患者脊椎损伤的临床表现是疼痛和肌肉痉挛或运动强直。任何儿童在伤后诉说颈部和背部疼痛或强直需要全面评估脊椎的完整性和稳定性。儿童可能因为寰枢（椎）的旋转半脱位而出现斜颈。旋转性半脱位可以是明显轻微的损伤或甚至是一阵咳嗽所导致。这些儿童通常神经学正常。X 线平片可能为阴性，而轴位脊椎 CT 扫描则具有诊断性[162]。

脊髓损伤的主要表现是脊髓运动和感觉水平以下的神经功能异常。在清醒患者容易查出伴有运动功能障碍的完全和严重不完全的脊髓损伤。脊髓损伤一般症状如对称的松弛性麻痹，伴有同一解剖水平的感觉缺失。在昏迷患者或伴多发损伤的患者，有相当比例伴发脊髓损伤。颈部脊髓损伤能导致严重的全身性低血压，这就是所知的“神经性休克”综合征，是由于损伤水平以下交感通路的破坏所致。不像较多见的低血压性休克，神经性休克是由低血压时心动过缓的表现而提示。尽管低体温，这些患者同样血管扩张。低血容量性休克导致低血压、心动过速和血管收缩。其他提示脊髓损伤的全身发现包括反常呼吸，阴茎异常勃起，Horner 综合征和无汗。

严重程度稍轻的损伤可能引起暂时的神经功能障碍、感觉迟钝、局部无力、感觉缺失或感觉和运动功能分离如 Brown-Sequard 或其他中央脊髓综合征。任何暂时神经功能障碍包括四肢、膀胱，不管持续时间和明显彻底康复，都是脊髓损伤的强烈证据。

没有放射影像异常的脊髓损伤

没有放射影像异常的脊髓损伤（SCIWORA）由 Pang 和 Willberger 在 1982 年确立，他们描述了表现有创伤性脊髓病变客观发现的患者，在放射平片和 CT 上没有骨折或连接不稳定的证据[137]。SCIWORA 对儿童也是重要的，尤其在年幼儿童，可能直接与早期幼年脊椎外形的生理特性有关。对于椎体损伤，在小的年龄儿童更易于有喙的损伤。有 SCIWORA 的年 369
幼儿童比年长儿童更易于出现严重或完全的脊髓损伤。在严重脊髓损伤的年长儿童，椎体损伤要比 SCIWORA 更典型[72,132,136]。

诊断这个综合征是复杂的，因为经常发生迟发的神经功能缺陷。许多这种损伤儿童在报道受伤数小时到数天后被证实神经缺陷，而没有进一步的其他损伤[136]。这种延迟恶化的机制不明，但 Pang 推测可能为在已经有轻微损伤的脊髓处重复损伤，这是因为内在的脊椎正常弹性或是因为细微的韧带的损伤伴有增加的损伤位置节段活动[135]。这些论点通过观察到 20%没有颈椎固定的儿童可能发生重复的 SCIWORA 而得到支持，那些固定颈椎的儿童则明显减少了这个现象的发生率[142]。

最后，这个综合征是在 MRI 广泛应用于脊椎疾病的诊断之前被提出的。尽管事实是这些儿童在脊椎平片和 CT 上没有骨的损伤或明显不稳定的证据，大多数（不是全部）患者将在 MRI 上有脊髓或韧带或其他软组织损伤的证据[34,43,69]。因此，对受伤儿童注意到这个异常时，所有医生应给予早期评估，并持续认识到脊椎或脊髓损伤的可能性，即使在最初放射影像检查报告正常时也是这样。

脊椎和脊髓损伤的初期评估

发现儿童脊椎损伤是富有挑战性的。同脑外伤一样，最初的临床发现将决定如何选择诊断性影像。和脑外伤不一样的是脊椎平片仍然是脊椎损伤患者初始评估的重要工具。任何儿童有颈部疼痛、脊椎移动时肌肉抵抗或神经功能缺失，或有高能机制的多发损伤，尤其是包括机动车碰撞时系安全带的乘客发生的脊椎分离，都存在脊椎损伤，直到被证实有其他方面问题。

年长的清醒儿童能表达显示脊椎和神经损伤的临床症状和迹象。目前的建议是，年长儿童如果清醒和熟悉，没有神经功能缺失或其中一样病史，或没有后脊柱中线疼痛或压痛，则不需要进一步放射评估或其他诊断学检查[87]。这不适用于小的儿童，他们有潜在脊椎和脊髓损伤的高风险，因为他们不能表述疼痛[98]。因此，对于小的儿童应放宽放射检查的指征。

在成人，现在有非常好的“决定规则”来进行放射学检查，特别地可以进行前后位、侧位和张口位观察[79,80]。这些检查显示如果患者表现遵循以下五个原则，就会有很低的受伤可能和很少的放射影像发现：没有颈部中线压痛、没有局部神经功能缺失、神志正常、没有沉醉状态和疼痛性分离损伤。对儿科患者的这些决定规则的应用提示了相似的发现，尽管非常小年龄的儿童在这组研究中数量有限[173]。从而，年幼儿童的应用也应遵循这个建议。

儿童患者脊椎的放射学检查由于前面文章描述的幼儿脊椎的正常解剖变异而变得复杂。生长中心和软骨结合会混淆创伤性损伤。脊柱增高的活动度常表现为“假性半脱位”[24,158]。大多数假性半脱位发生在第二和第三椎体，在 8 岁以下儿童允许移位超过 4mm。这种移动与正常的寰椎和齿突之间的前移[163]，能误认为韧带的损伤。因此，儿童脊椎放射学检查必须谨慎解释而且医生应彻底熟悉脊椎的发育解剖。

屈伸位放射检查可用在清醒和配合患者排除脊椎的韧带损伤。然而，对大多数动态影像检查有效性的调查显示，如果在中间位置的常规静态检查显示正常排列，那么在这些动检查究也不容易检测到脊椎不稳定[52,145]。

脊椎 CT 扫描对检测隐蔽的骨折、软组织肿胀和旋转性脱位非常有帮助，同样也能确定先天性异常和在平片上易误认骨折的正常发育变化。而且，CT 是检测创伤后椎管和神经根孔的快速准确的方法。然而，许多脊椎损伤是韧带性的，如果只做 CT 可能会被漏诊。因此，CT 应该被认为是放射平片检查的辅助，而不是替代。

MRI 现在是显示脊髓损伤和隐蔽的韧带及软组织损伤的最好的影像检查方法。如早先所讨论的，许多但非全部的 SCIMORA 患者在 MRI 上显示异常，这证实了临床诊断。MRI 上的发现和脊髓损伤的预后相关[35,69,155]。然而，不清楚的是 MRI 上的发现是否改变了儿童脊髓损伤的治疗决策[87]。

脊髓损伤的早期处理

同创伤性脑损伤一样，积极全身灌注和氧的支持是至关重要的。因为儿童易于发生喙的颈髓损伤，应该关注呼吸功能的减弱。而且，胃扩张常伴随急性脊髓损伤出现，这会加重对有效呼吸的障碍。因此，应该考虑早期置鼻胃管减压。对于中高位颈椎损伤，可能需要选择气管插管来支持呼吸直到损伤的综合评估完成。对脊椎损伤儿童的气管插管有技术上的挑战，应该有专家在不改变头和颈部的相对位置的情况下来操作。

对脊髓损伤患者恢复和维持全身血压将维持其有效灌注。严重脊髓损伤患者，尤其在颈部，最易发生系统性低血压。尽管初始复苏时可以进行血管内容量补充，但神经性低血压应该给予血管加压药物。在脊髓损伤患者复苏和维持正常血压是复杂的，且可能需有创中央静脉压监护的帮助。

脊髓损伤的药物治疗已经成为研究的焦点和科学争论的主题。在第二届国际脊髓损伤研讨会(NASCIS-II)[15]结束和发布后，得到的建议是所有急性脊髓损伤患者接受大剂量甲泼尼龙。这个建议没有正式延伸到儿科患者，但许多中心在所有年龄组中都遵循这个建议。尽管随后的研究显示确认了先前的发现，但这些研究的方法和结论已经有许多质疑[85,87]。现在，脊椎损伤患者应用大剂量激素，包括儿童，只是治疗的一个选择，应该在只有有证据显示有害的副作用比其他临床受益的建议更加一致时才采用[87]。

很少需要早期的外科治疗。大多数儿科骨折和错位可以用不同骨科器械复位和保持解剖排列，包括环状支托。早期外科复位和融合手术只在有明显症状恶化的患者中考虑，这些恶化多发生于不能复位的半脱位或骨折碎片压迫，椎间盘突出或增大的血肿。这些情况在儿童中并不常见。青少年受伤类型和成人相似，可以按照已有的对成人的治疗建议来处理[87]。尽管近来报道显示外科使用器械越来越常见，但对于儿童脊髓损伤患者只有有限的关于手术治疗预后和可取之处的科学信息[54,61]。对畸形的解剖复位，明显不稳定损伤的固定，和神经结构的减压是儿童脊椎损伤手术治疗的指征。大多数这些目标可以通过非手术治疗来完成。现在的研究指出小儿童的椎体损伤大多数应该最初采用非手术治疗，出现持续或进展性畸形或排列不稳定则需手术治疗[87]。

并发症

儿童可以出现脊椎损伤相关的所有并发症，包括皮肤损害、感染、深静脉血栓形成、自主反射障碍、挛缩、痉挛状态、神经性膀胱与肠道和进展性脊椎畸形[180]。然而，儿童主要的急性脊髓损伤并发症是呼吸损害。损伤急性期最常见致命原因是呼吸衰竭[40]。必须积极肺部护理，通气支持可能是必须的，一直到呼吸肌有力才停止。许多其他并发症可能通过物理治疗医生或其他康复专家的早期干预而避免或最小化。

已有报道在脊椎损伤儿童发生静脉血栓形成的发生率，大概同成人相似[180]，这可能不太准确。然而，对儿童患者的研究显示这个并发症很少见[144]。因此，对这个可能并发症预防的特殊治疗的选择差别很大。大概对于成人和年长儿童和青少年来说，血栓预防包括低分子或低剂量肝素结合转动的床，空气压缩长袜，或电刺激仪，推荐应用至伤后 12 周以上[87,180]。

预后

儿童脊髓损伤相关死亡率据报道是 28%，这明显高于成人的报道[75,135]。这些死亡主要发生在现场，不受现代治疗策略的影响。对脊椎损伤的幸存者，预后和受伤水平及严重程度相关。完全损伤依旧是彻底的，尽管长期有有限的功能好转，但不要期望完全康复[72,74,132,136]。儿童不完全损伤有明显功能好转的好机会，甚至完全康复[72,74]。

这些损伤的长期治疗费用是惊人的。儿童脊髓损伤一生的治疗费用在百万美元[39,133,153]。这个花费还要加上伴随这些破坏性损伤的丧失生殖能力。在儿童时期脊髓损伤的成人就业率是 50%[180]。成功就业相关的因素有受伤时年龄小，神经损伤严重度轻，较好的教育，长期和伤后后遗症生活的经验，独立开车的能力。

（顾　硕译　金惠明校）

参考文献

1. Adams JH: Brain damage in fatal non-missile head injury in man. In Braakman R (ed): The Handbook of Clinical Neurology, vol 13, Head Injury. New York, Elsevier, 1990, p 43.
2. Adelson PD, Bratton SL, Carney NA, et al: Guidelines for the acute medical management of severe traumatic brain injury in infants, children and adolescents. Crit Care Med 2003;31:S417.
3. Amar AP, Levy ML: Pathogenesis and pharmacological strategies for mitigating secondary damage in acute spinal cord injury. Neurosurgery 1999;44:1027.
4. American Academy of Neurology: Practice parameter: The management of concussion in sports (summary statement). Neurology 1997;48:581.
5. American Academy of Pediatrics: The management of minor closed head injury in children. Pediatrics 1999;104:1407.
6. American Academy of Pediatrics: Shaken baby syndrome: Rotational cranial injuries—technical report. Pediatrics 2001;108:206.
7. Anderson JM, Schutt AH: Spinal injury in children: A review of 156 cases seen from 1950 through 1978. Mayo Clin Proc 1980;55:499.
8. Anderson V, Catroppa C, Morse S, et al: Recovery of intellectual ability following traumatic brain injury in childhood: Impact of injury severity and age at injury. Pediatr Neurosurg 2000;32:282.
9. Annegers JF, Hauser WA, Coan SP, Rocca WA: A population-based study of seizures after traumatic brain injuries. N Engl J Med 1998;338:20.
10. Apple JS, Kirks DR, Merten DF, Martinez S: Cervical spine fractures and dislocations in children. Pediatr Radiol 1987;17:45.
11. Bailey DK: The normal cervical spine in infants and children. Radiology 1952;59:712.
12. Bekar, A, Ipekoglu Z, Tureyen K, et al: Secondary insults during intrahospital transport of neurosurgical intensive care patients. Neurosurg Rev 1998;21:98.
13. Bergsneider M, Hovda DA, Shalmon E, et al: Cerebral hyperglycolysis following severe traumatic brain injury in humans: A positron emission tomography study. J Neurosurg 1997;86:241.
14. Berryhill P, Lilly MA, Levin HS, et al: Frontal lobe changes after severe diffuse closed head injury in children: A volumetric study of magnetic resonance imaging. Neurosurgery 1995;37:392.
15. Bracken MB, Shepard MJ, Collins WF, et al: A randomized, controlled trial of methylprednisolone or naloxone in the treatment of acute spinal cord injury: Results of the second

National Acute Spinal Cord Injury Study. N Engl J Med 1990;322:1405.
16. Bracken MB, Shepard MJ, Holford TR, et al: Administration of methylprednisolone for 24 or 48 hours or tirilizad mesylate for 48 hours in the treatment of acute spinal cord injury. Results of the third National Acute Spinal Cord Injury randomized controlled trial. National Acute Spinal Cord Injury Study. JAMA 1997;277:1597.
17. Brookes M, MacMillan R, Cully S, et al: Head injuries in accident and emergency departments. How different are children from adults? J Epidemiol Commun Health 1990;44:747.
18. Bruno A, Biller J, Adams HP, et al: Acute blood glucose levels and outcome from ischemic stroke: Trial of ORG 10172 in Acute Stroke Treatment (TOAST) investigators. Neurology 1999;59:280.
19. Bruns J, Hauser WA: The epidemiology of traumatic brain injury: A review. Epilepsia 2003;44:2.
20. Buckingham MJ, Crone KR, Ball WS, et al: Traumatic intracranial aneurysms in childhood: Two cases and a review of the literature. Neurosurgery 1988;22:398.
21. Bullock RM, Chesnut RM, Clifton GL, et al: Guidelines for the management of severe traumatic brain injury. J Neurotrauma 2000;17:451.
22. Caldicott DG, Pearce A, Price R, et al: Not just another 'head lac' ... low-velocity, penetrating intra-cranial injuries: A case report and review of the literature. Injury 2004;35:1044.
23. Cantu RC: Return to play guidelines after a head injury. Clin Sports Med 1998;17:45.
24. Cattell HS, Filtzer DL: Pseudosubluxation and other normal variations in the cervical spine in children. A study of one hundred and sixty children. J Bone Joint Surg Am 1965;47:1295.
25. Chan KH, Mann KS, Yue CP, et al: The significance of skull fracture in acute traumatic intracranial hematomas in adolescents: A prospective study. J Neurosurg 1990;72:189.
26. Chang BS, Lowenstein DH: Practice parameter: Antiepileptic drug prophylaxis in severe traumatic brain injury. Neurology 2003;60:10.
27. Cherian L, Goodman JC, Robertson CS: Hyperglycemia increases brain injury caused by secondary injury after cortical impact in rats. Crit Care Med 1997;25:1378.
28. Chesnut RM: Avoidance of hypotension: Conditio sine qua non of successful severe head injury management. J Trauma (Suppl) 1997;42:S4.
29. Chesnut RM: Management of brain and spine injuries. Crit Care Clin 2004;20:25.
30. Chiaretti A, De Benedictus R, Polidori G, et al: Early post-traumatic seizures in children with head injury. Childs Nerv Syst 2000;16:862.
31. Cooper PR: Cerebrospinal fluid fistulas and pneumocephalus. In Barrow DL (ed): Complications and Sequelae of Head Injury. Park Ridge, IL, American Association of Neurological Surgeons, 1992, p 1.
32. CRASH Trial Collaborators: Effect of intravenous corticosteroids on death within 14 days in 10008 adults with clinically significant head injury (MRC CRASH trial): Randomized placebo-controlled trial. Lancet 2004;364:1321.
33. Curran C, Dietrich AM, Bowman MJ, et al: Pediatric cervical spine immobilization: Achieving neutral position? J Trauma 1995;39:729.
34. Dare AO, Dias MS, Li V: Magnetic resonance imaging correlation in pediatric spinal cord injury without radiographic abnormality. J Neurosurg 2002;97(Suppl):33.
35. Davis PC, Reisner A, Hudgins PA, et al: Spinal injuries in children: Role of MR. AJNR Am J Neuroradiol 1993;14:607.
36. Davis RL, Mullen N, Makela M, et al: Cranial computed tomography scans in children after minimal head injury with loss of consciousness. Ann Emerg Med 1994;24:640.
37. Deputy S: Shaking-impact syndrome of infancy. Semin Pediatr Neurol 2003;10:112.
38. De Santis A, Cappricci E, Granata G: Early post traumatic seizures in adults: Study of 84 cases. J Neurosurg Sci 1979;23:207.
39. De Vivo MJ: Causes and cost of spinal cord injury in the United States. Spinal Cord 1997;35;809.
40. De Vivo MJ, Black KJ, Stover SL: Causes of death during the first 12 years after spinal cord injury. Arch Phys Med Rehabil 1993;74:248.
41. Dias MS, Carnevale F, Li V: Immediate posttraumatic seizures: Is routine hospitalization necessary? Pediatr Neurosurg 1999;30:232.
42. Dias MS, Lillis KA, Calvo C, et al: Management of accidental minor head injuries in children: A prospective outcomes study. J Neurosurg (Pediatrics) 2004;101:38.
43. Dickman CA, Zabramski JM, Hadley MN, et al: Pediatric spinal cord injury without radiographic abnormalities: Report of 26 cases and review of the literature. J Spinal Disord 1991;4:296.
44. DiRoio C, Jourdan C, Mottolese C, et al: Craniocerebral injury resulting from transorbital stick penetration in children. Childs Nerv Syst 2000;16:503.
45. Donahue DJ, Sanford RA, Muhlbauer MS, et al: Cranial burst fracture in infants: Acute recognition and management. Childs Nerv Syst 1995;11:692.
46. Duhaime AC, Christian C, Moss E, et al: Long-term outcome in infants with shaking-impact syndrome. Pediatr Neurosurg 1996;24:292.
47. Duhaime AC, Christian CW, Roarke LB, Zimmerman RA: Nonaccidental head injury in infants—the "shaken-baby syndrome." N Engl J Med 1998;338:1822.
48. Duhaime AC, Eppley M, Margulies S, et al: Crush injuries to the head in children. Neurosurgery 1995;37:401.
49. Duhaime AC, Gennarelli TA, Thibault LT, et al: The shaken baby syndrome: A clinical, pathological, and biomechanical study. J Neurosurg 1987;66:409.
50. Duhaime AC, Sutton LN: Delayed sequelae of pediatric head injury. In Barrow DL (ed): Complications and Sequelae of Head Injury. Park Ridge, IL, American Association of Neurological Surgeons, 1992, p 169.
51. du Trevou MD, van Dellen JR: Penetrating stab wounds to the brain: The timing of angiography in patients presenting with the weapon already removed. Neurosurgery 1992;31:905.
52. Dwek JR, Chung CB: Radiography of cervical spine injury in children: Are flexion-extension radiographs useful for acute trauma? AJR Am J Roentgenol 2000;174:1617.
53. Einhorn A, Mizrahi EM: Basilar skull fractures in children. The incidence of CNS infection and the use of antibiotics. Am J Dis Child 1978;132:1121.
54. Eleraky MA, Theodore N, Adams M, et al: Pediatric cervical spine injuries: Report of 102 cases and review of the literature. J Neurosurg 2000;92(Suppl):12.
55. Ewing-Cobbs L, Thompson NM, Miner ME, et al: Gunshot wounds to the brain in children and adolescents: Age and neurobehavioral development. Neurosurgery 1994;35:225.
56. Faden AI, Demediuk P, Panter SS, et al: The role of excitatory amino acids and NMDA receptors in traumatic brain injury. Science 1989;244:798.
57. Farmer MY, Singer HS, Mellitus ED, et al: Neurobehavioral sequelae of minor head injuries in children. Pediatr Neurosci

1987;13:304.
58. Fesmire FM, Luten RC: The pediatric cervical spine: Developmental anatomy and clinical aspects. J Emerg Med 1989;7:133.
59. Figaji AA, Fieggen AG, Peter JC: Early decompressive craniotomy in children with severe traumatic brain injury. Childs Nerv Syst 2003;19:666.
60. Filley CM, Cranberg LD, Alexander MP, Hart EJ: Neurobehavioral outcome after closed head injury in childhood and adolescence. Arch Neurol 1987;44:194.
61. Finch GD, Barnes MJ: Major cervical spine injuries in children and adolescents. J Pediatr Orthop 1998;18:811.
62. Fingerhut LA, Kleinman JC, Godfrey E, et al: Firearm mortality among children, youth, and young adults 1-34 years of age, trends and current status: United States, 1979-88. Monthly Vital Stat Rep 1991;39(Suppl):1.
63. Gabriel EJ, Ghajar J, Jagoda A, et al: Guidelines for prehospital management of traumatic brain injury. J Neurotrauma 2002;19:113.
64. Garton HJL, Luerssen TG: Head injuries. In Biller J, Bogousslavsky J (eds): Clinical Trials in Neurologic Practice. Boston, Butterworth Heinemann, 2001, p 77.
65. Gausche M, Lewis RJ, Stratton SJ, et al: Effect of out-of-hospital pediatric endotracheal intubation on survival and neurological outcome: A controlled clinical trial. JAMA 2000;283:783.
66. Gennarelli TA, Adams JH, Graham DI: Diffuse axonal injury—a new conceptual approach to an old problem. In Baethmann A, Go KG, Unterberg A (eds): Mechanisms of Secondary Brain Damage. New York, Plenum Press, 1986, p 15.
67. Gennarelli TA, Segawa H, Wald V, et al: Physiological response to angular acceleration of the head. In Grossman RG, Gildenberg, PL (eds): Head Injury: Basic and Clinical Aspects. New York, Raven Press, 1982, p 129.
68. Gennarelli TA, Thibault LE: Biological models of head injury. In Becker DP, Povlishok JT (eds): Central Nervous System Trauma Status Report 1985. Bethesda, MD, NINCDS/NIH, 1985, p 391.
69. Grabb PA, Pang D: Magnetic resonance imaging in the evaluation of spinal cord injury without radiographic abnormality in children. Neurosurgery 1994;35:406.
70. Graham DI: The pathology of brain ischemia and possibilities for therapeutical intervention. Br J Anaesth 1985;57:3.
71. Greenwald TA, Mann DC: Pediatric seatbelt injuries: Diagnosis and treatment of lumbar flexion-distraction injuries. Paraplegia 1994;32:743.
72. Hadley MN, Zabramski JN, Browner CM, et al: Pediatric spinal trauma: Review of 122 cases of spinal cord and vertebral column injuries. J Neurosurg 1988;68:18.
73. Hahn YS, Fuchs S, Flannery AM, et al: Factors influencing posttraumatic seizures in children. Neurosurgery 1988;22:864.
74. Hamilton MG, Myles ST: Pediatric spinal injury: Review of 174 hospital admissions. J Neurosurg 1992;77:700.
75. Hamilton MG, Myles ST: Pediatric spinal injury: Review of 61 deaths. J Neurosurg 1992;77:705.
76. Hansen JE, Gudeman SK, Holgate RC, Saunders RA: Penetrating intracranial wood wounds: Clinical limitations of computed tomography. J Neurosurg 1988;68:752.
77. Haydel MJ, Preston CA, Mills TJ, et al: Indications for computed tomography in patients with minor head injury. N Engl J Med 2000;343:100.
78. Haydel MJ, Shembekar AD: Prediction of intracranial injury in children aged five years and older with loss of consciousness after minor head injury due to nontrivial mechanisms. Ann Emerg Med 2003;42:507.
79. Hoffman JR, Mower WR, Wolfson AB, et al: Validity of a set of clinical criteria to rule out injury to the cervical spine in patients with blunt trauma. N Engl J Med 2000;343:94.
80. Hoffman JR, Wolfson AB, Todd K, et al: Selective cervical spine radiography in blunt trauma: Methodology of the National Emergency X-Radiography Utilization Study (NEXUS). Ann Emerg Med 1998;32:461.
81. Holmes JF, Palchak MJ, Conklin MJ, Kuppermann N: Do children require hospitalization after immediate posttraumatic seizures? Ann Emerg Med 2004;43:706.
82. Hsiang JNK, Yeung T, Yu ALM, et al: High risk mild head injury. J Neurosurg 1997;87:234.
83. Huerta C, Griffith R, Joyce SM: Cervical spine stabilization in pediatric patients: Evaluation of current techniques. Ann Emerg Med 1987;16:1121.
84. Humphreys R, Hendrick EB, Hoffman H: The head-injured child "who talks and dies." A preventable problem? In Marlin A (ed): Concepts in Pediatric Neurosurgery X. Basel, Karger, 1990, p 196.
85. Hurlbert RJ: Methylprednisolone for acute spinal cord injury: An inappropriate standard of care. J. Neurosurg 2000;93(Suppl):1.
86. Iverson GL, Lovell MR, Smith S, Franzen MD: Prevalence of abnormal CT-scans following mild head injury. Brain Inj 2000;14:1057.
87. Joint Section on Disorders of the Spine and Peripheral Nerves of the American Association of Neurological Surgeons and the Congress of Neurological Surgeons: Guidelines for the management of acute cervical spine and spinal cord injuries. Neurosurgery 2002;50(Suppl):S166.
88. Jones PA, Andrews PJD, Midgley S, et al: Measuring the burden of secondary insults in head-injured patients during intensive care. J Neurosurg Anesthesiol 1994;6:4.
89. Kadish HA, Schunk JE: Pediatric basilar skull fracture: Do children with normal neurologic findings and no intracranial injury require hospitalization? Ann Emerg Med 1995;26:37.
90. Kaufman HH: Treatment of civilian gunshot wound to the head. Neurosurg Clin N Am 1991;2:387.
91. Kaye EM, Herskowitz J: Transient post-traumatic cortical blindness: Brief v prolonged syndromes in childhood. J Child Neurol 1986;1:206.
92. Kelly JP, Nichols JS, Filley KO, et al: Concussion in sports: Guidelines for the prevention of catastrophic outcome. JAMA 1991;266:2867.
93. Kewalramani LS, Kraus JF, Sterling HM: Acute spinal cord lesions in a pediatric population: Epidemiological and clinical features. Paraplegia 1980;18:206.
94. Klastersky J, Sadeghi M, Brihaye J: Antimicrobial prophylaxis in patients with rhinorrhea or otorrhea. A double-blind study. Surg Neurol 1976;6:111.
95. Klauber MR, Marshall LF, Luerssen TG, et al: Determinants of head injury mortality: Importance of the low risk patient. Neurosurgery 1989;24:31.
96. Kraus JF: Epidemiological features of brain injury in children: Occurrence, children at risk, causes and manner of injury, severity and outcomes. In Broman SH, Michel ME (eds): Traumatic Head Injury in Children. New York, Oxford University Press, 1995, p 22.
97. Kraus JF, Rock A, Hemyari P: Brain injuries among infants, children, adolescents and young adults. Am J Dis Child 1990;144:684.
98. Laham JL, Cotcamp DH, Gibbons PA, et al: Isolated head injury versus multiple trauma in pediatric patients: Do the

same indications apply? Pediatr Neurosurg 1994;122:431.
99. Lazar MF, Menaldino S: Cognitive outcome and behavioral adjustment in children following traumatic brain injury: A developmental perspective. J Head Trauma Rehabil 1995;10:55.
100. Lescohier I, DiScala C: Blunt trauma in children: Causes and outcomes of head versus intracranial injury. Pediatrics 1993;91:721.
101. Levi L, Guilburd JN, Linn S, Feinsod M: The association between skull fracture, intracranial pathology and outcome in pediatric head injury. Br J Neurosurg 1991;5:617.
102. Levin HS, Aldrich EF, Saydjari C, et al: Severe head injury in children: Experience of the Traumatic Coma Data Bank. Neurosurgery 1992;31:435.
103. Levin HS, Ewing-Cobbs L, Eisenberg HM: Neurobehavioral outcome of pediatric closed head injury. In Michel ME, Broman SH (eds): Traumatic Head Injury in Children. New York, Oxford University Press, 1995, p 70.
104. Lewis RJ, Lee L, Inkelis SH, Gilmore D: Clinical predictors of post traumatic seizures in children with head trauma. Ann Emerg Med 1993;22:1114.
105. Lloyd DA, Carty H, Patterson M, et al: Predictive value of skull radiography for intracranial injury in children with blunt head injury. Lancet 1997;349:821.
106. Lobato R, Rivas J, Gomez P, et al: Head-injured patients who talk and deteriorate into coma: Analysis of 211 cases studied with computerized tomography. J Neurosurg 1991;75:256.
107. Luerssen TG: Intracranial pressure: Current status in monitoring and management. Semin Pediatr Neurol 1997;4:146.
108. Luerssen TG: Skull fractures after closed head injury. In Albright LA, Pollack IF, Adelson PD (eds): Principles and Practice of Pediatric Neurosurgery. New York, Thieme, 1999, p 813.
109. Luerssen TG, Huang JC, McLone DG, et al: Retinal hemorrhages, seizures and intracranial hemorrhages: Relationships and outcomes in children suffering traumatic brain injury. In Marlin AE (ed): Concepts in Pediatric Neurosurgery XI. Basel, Karger, 1991, p 87.
110. Luerssen T, Hults K, Klauber M, et al: Improved outcome as a result of recognition of absent and compressed cisterns on initial CT scans. In Hoff J, Betz A (eds): Intracranial Pressure VII. Berlin, Springer-Verlag, 1989, p 598.
111. Luerssen TG, Klauber MR, Marshall LF: Outcome from head injury related to patient's age: A longitudinal prospective study of adult and pediatric head injury. J Neurosurg 1988;68:409.
112. Luerssen TG, Wolfla CE: Pathophysiology and management of increased intracranial pressure in children. In Andrews BT, Hammer GB (eds): Pediatric Neurosurgical Intensive Care. Park Ridge, IL, American Association of Neurological Surgeons, 1997, p 37.
113. Maier-Hauff K, Baethmann AJ, Lange M, et al: The kallikrein-kinin system as mediator in vasogenic brain edema. Part 2—studies on kinin formation in focal and perifocal brain tissue. J Neurosurg 1984;61:97.
114. Mandera M, Wencel T, Bazowski P, Krauze J: How should we manage children after mild head injury? Childs Nerv Syst 2000;16:156.
115. Mansfield RT: Head injury in children and in adults. Crit Care Clin 1997;13:611.
116. Margolis LH, Wagenaar AC, Liu W: The effects of a mandatory child restraint law on injuries requiring hospitalization. Am J Dis Child 1988;142:1099.
117. Marshall LF, Marshall SB, Klauber LF, et al: A new classification of head injury based on computerized tomography. J Neurosurg 1991;75(Suppl):S14.
118. Marshall LF, Toole BA, Bowers SB: The National Traumatic Coma Data Bank Part 2: Patients who talk and deteriorate: Implications for treatment. J Neurosurg 1983;59:285.
119. Mataro M, Poco MA, Sahuquillo J, et al: Neuropsychological outcome in relation to the Traumatic Coma Data Bank classification of computed tomography imaging. J Neurotrauma 2001;18:869.
120. Mayer SA, Chong JY: Critical care management of increased intracranial pressure. J Intensive Care Med 2002;17:55.
121. Mayer T, Walker ML, Johnson D, et al: Causes of morbidity and mortality in severe pediatric trauma. JAMA 1981;245:719.
122. McNeill AM, Annest JL: The ongoing hazard of BB and pellet gun–related injuries in the United States. Ann Emerg Med 1995;26:187.
123. Megur K, Tator CH: Effect of multiple trauma on mortality and neurological recovery after spinal cord or cauda equina injury. Neurol Med Chir 1988;28:34.
124. Miller JD, Sweet RC, Narayan R, Becker DP: Early insults to the injured brain. JAMA 1978;240:439.
125. Miner ME, Ewing-Cobbs L, Kopaniky DR, et al: The results of treatment of gunshot wounds to the brain in children. Neurosurgery 1990;26:20.
126. Mono J, Hollenberg RD, Harvey JT: Occult transorbital intracranial penetrating injuries. Ann Emerg Med 1986;15:589.
127. Murray JA, Demetirades D, Berne TV, et al: Prehospital intubation in patients with severe head injury. J Trauma 2000;49:1065.
128. Nagy K, Joseph K, Krosner S, et al: The utility of head computed tomography after minimal head injury. J Trauma 1999;46:268.
129. Nelson DE, Bixby-Hammett D: Equestrian injuries in children and young adults. Am J Dis Child 1992;146:611.
130. Ommaya AK: Biomechanics of head injury: Experimental aspects. In Nahum AM, Melvin J (eds): The Biomechanics of Trauma. Norwalk, CN, Appleton-Century-Crofts, 1985, p 245.
131. Ommaya AK, Gennarelli TA: Cerebral concussion and traumatic unconsciousness: Correlation of experimental and clinical observations of blunt head injuries. Brain 1974;97:633.
132. Osenbach RK, Menezes AH: Spinal cord injury without radiographic abnormality in children. Pediatr Neurosci 1989;15:168.
133. Osenbach RK, Menezes AH: Pediatric spinal cord and vertebral column injury. Neurosurgery 1992;30:385.
134. Palchak MJ, Holmes JF, Vance CW, et al: A decision rule for identifying children at low risk for brain injuries after blunt head trauma. Ann Emerg Med 2003;42:492.
135. Pang D: Spinal cord injuries. In McLone DG (ed): Pediatric Neurosurgery, 4th ed. Philadelphia, WB Saunders, 2001, p 660.
136. Pang D, Pollack IF: Spinal cord injury without radiographic abnormality in children—the SCIWORA syndrome. J Trauma 1989;29:654.
137. Pang D, Wilberger JE: Spinal cord injury without radiographic abnormalities in children. J Neurosurg 1982;57:114.
138. Paret G, Barzilai A, Lahat E, et al: Gunshot wounds in brains of children: Prognostic variables in mortality, course, and outcome. J Neurotrauma 1998;15:967.
139. Pettigrew LEL, Wilson JTL, Teasdale G: Assessing disability

after head injury: Improved use of the Glasgow Outcome Scale. J Neurosurg 1998;89:939.
140. Pezzotta S, Silvani V, Gaetani P, et al: Growing skull fractures in childhood. J Neurosurg Sci 1985;29:129.
141. Pigula FA, Wald SL, Shackford SR, Vane DW: The effect of hypotension and hypoxia on children with severe head injuries. J Pediatr Surg 1993;28:310.
142. Pollack IF, Pang D, Sclabassi R: Recurrent spinal cord injury without radiographic abnormalities in children. J Neurosurg 1988;69:177.
143. Proctor MR: Spinal cord injury. Crit Care Med 2002;30(Suppl):S489.
144. Radecki RT, Gaebler-Spira D: Deep vein thrombosis in the disabled pediatric population. Arch Phys Med Rehabil 1994;75:248.
145. Ralston ME, Chung K, Barnes PD, et al: Role of flexion-extension radiographs in blunt pediatric cervical spine injury. Acad Emerg Med 2001;8:237.
146. Rathore MH: Do prophylactic antibiotics prevent meningitis after basilar skull fracture? Pediatr Infect Dis J 1991;10:87.
147. Rivara FP: Epidemiology and prevention of pediatric traumatic brain injury. Pediatr Ann 1994;23:12.
148. Rivara FP, Thompson DC, Thompson RS, et al: The Seattle Children's bicycle helmet campaign: Changes in helmet use and head injury admissions. Pediatrics 1994;93:567.
149. Rovlias A, Kotsou S: The influence of hyperglycemia on neurological outcome in patients with severe head injury. Neurosurgery 2000;46:335.
150. Ruff RM, Jurica P: In search of a unified definition for mild traumatic brain injury. Brain Inj 1999;13:943.
151. Ruge JR, Sinson GP, McLone DG: Pediatric spinal injury: The very young. J Neurosurg 1988;68:25.
152. Ryan CA, Edmonds J: Seizure activity mimicking brain stem herniation in children following head injuries. Crit Care Med 1988;16:812.
153. Sadowsky CL, Margherita A: The cost of spinal cord injury care. Spine 1999;13:593.
154. Satz P, Zaucha K, McCleary C, et al: Mild head injury in children and adolescents: A review of studies (1970-1995). Psychol Bull 1997;122:107.
155. Schaefer DM, Flanders AE, Olsterholm JL, et al: Prognostic significance of MRI in acute phase of spinal injury. J Neurosurg 1992;76:218.
156. Schutzman SA, Barnes P, Duhaime AC, et al: Evaluation and management of children younger than two years old with apparently minor head trauma: Proposed guidelines. Pediatrics 2001;107:983-993.
157. Servadei F, Teasdale G, Merry G, et al: Defining acute mild head injury in adults: A proposal based on prognostic factors, diagnosis, and management. J Neurotrauma 2001;18:657.
158. Shaw M, Burnett H, Wilson A, Chan O: Pseudosubluxation of C2 on C3 in polytraumatized children: Prevalence and significance. Clin Radiol 1999;54:377.
159. Snoek J, Minderhoud J, Wilmink J: Delayed deterioration following mild head injury in children. Brain 1984;107:15.
160. Stein SC, Ross SE: The value of computed tomographic scans in patients with low-risk head injuries. Neurosurgery 1990;26:638.
161. Stocchetti N, Pagan F, Calappi E, et al: Inaccurate early assessment of neurological severity in head injury. J Neurotrauma 2004;21:1131.
162. Suback BR, McLaughlin MR, Albright AL, Pollack IF: Current management of pediatric atlantoaxial rotatory subluxation. Spine 1998;23:2174.
163. Sullivan CR, Bruwer AJ, Harris LE: Hypermobility of the cervical spine in children. A pitfall in the diagnosis of cervical dislocation. Am J Surg 1958;95:636.
164. Tator CH, Koyanagi I: Vascular mechanisms in the pathophysiology of human spinal cord injury. J Neurosurg 1997;86:483.
165. Teasdale G, Jennett B: Assessment of coma and impaired consciousness: A practical scale. Lancet 1974;2:81.
166. Teasdale GM, Murray G, Anderson E, et al: Risks of acute traumatic intracranial hematoma in children and adults: Implications for managing head injuries. BMJ 1990;300:363.
167. Thompson DC, Rivara FP, Thompson R: Helmets for preventing head and facial injuries in bicyclists (Cochrane Review). In The Cochrane Library, Issue 2, 2002. Oxford, Update Software.
168. Thompson HJ, Tkacs NS, Saatman KE, et al: Hyperthermia following traumatic brain injury: A critical evaluation. Neurobiol Dis 2003;12:163.
169. Thompson MD, Irby JW: Recovery from mild head injury in pediatric populations. Semin Pediatr Neurol 2003;10:130.
170. Tilford JM, Simpson PM, Yeh TS, et al: Variations in therapy and outcome for pediatric head trauma patients. Crit Care Med 2001;29:1056.
171. Vane DW, Keller MS, Sartorelli KH, Miceli AP: Pediatric trauma: Current concepts and treatments. J Intensive Care Med 2002;17:230.
172. Vespa PM, Nuwer MR, Nenov V, et al: Increased incidence and impact of nonconvulsive and convulsive seizures after traumatic brain injury as detected by continuous electroencephalographic monitoring. J Neurosurg 1999;91:750.
173. Viccellio P, Simon H, Pressman BD, et al: A prospective multicenter study of cervical spine injury in children. Pediatrics 2001;108:E20.
174. Wang HE, Peitzman AB, Cassidy LD, et al: Out-of-hospital endotracheal intubation and outcome after traumatic brain injury. Ann Emerg Med 2004;44:439.
175. Warren WL, Bailes JE: On the field evaluation of athletic head injuries. Clin Sports Med 1998;17:13.
176. Wilson MH, Baker SP, Teret SP, et al: Saving Children: A Guide to Injury Prevention. New York, Oxford University Press, 1991, p 149.
177. Winston K, Beatty RM, Fischer EG: Consequences of dural defects acquired in infancy. J Neurosurg 1983;59:839.
178. Yamamoto LG, Bart RD: Transient blindness following mild head trauma. Clin Pediatr (Phila) 1988;27:479.
179. Young KD, Okada PJ, Sokolove PE, et al: A randomized, double-blinded, placebo controlled trial of phenytoin for the prevention of early posttraumatic seizures in children with moderate to severe blunt head injury. Ann Emerg Med 2004;43:435.
180. Zidek K, Srinivasan R: Rehabilitation of a child with a spinal cord injury. Semin Pediatr Neurol 2003;10:140.
181. Zornow MH, Prough DS: Fluid management in patients with traumatic brain injury. New Horizons 1995;3:488.

第 22 章

血管外伤

Joseph J. Tepas III

在过去的 10 年间，多系统外伤的处理原则已经发生了显著的改变。损伤控制性手术的发展，对创伤性应激的深入理解，尤其是与全身炎症反应综合征有关的处理，越来越多复杂的影像学技术，都有助于建立重症创伤的更加精确和有效的治疗系统。在这些发展中，包括了不断改进的血管外伤的评价和处理的原则[15]。临床检查预测的精确性得到确认，可以更好地确定动脉造影的指征，就可以更加及时进行手术治疗干预，干预的效果依赖于有效的复苏、精确评估合并的损伤、预计再灌注损伤[13,17]。应用血管内治疗技术，紧急处理一些血管外伤完全可以从手术室移到血管造影室。然而，急诊血管外伤处理的中心，是受损血管的技术性修补和外周灌注的恢复。虽然血管修补需要的基本手术技巧在各个年龄阶段的患者中都是类似的，但是在婴幼儿和儿童中具有独特的特点，可能会存在重大的挑战[9,12,31,32,39]。

流行病学

在成年人群中，大多数的血管外伤是由穿透性创伤所导致的。对于婴幼儿和儿童则不是由穿透性创伤所导致。在儿童人群中主要是由钝性创伤所致，在儿童所有的血管外伤中几乎有一半是由这种类型的损伤机制所导致的。表 22–1 列出了由国家儿童创伤登记（NPTR）所记载的在 1989—2001 年期间 1368 名至少有一处血管外伤儿童的发生机制和死亡率。虽然这只是呈现出了 1.3%的登记病例，但是血管外伤 13%的自然死亡率（相应的整个登记病例为 2.9%的死亡率）显示出这些血管损伤的致命性，以及基于身体不同受累部位的不同结果（表 22–2）。

在成年人群中，血管外伤可以分为涉及主干血管的外伤、破坏外周血液灌注的四肢损伤。在儿童中，后者通常与骨折有关，而不是与穿透性创伤有关。事实上，发生在儿童中的穿透性四肢创伤导致的血管外伤发生率非常的低。Victoroff 等人[46]回顾了国家儿童医学中心 1985—1989 年期间他们治疗的 75 名儿童中 76 例穿透性四肢创伤（枪伤）的经验。没有记载有血管外伤，只有 2 例由子弹或子弹碎片导致的神经损伤。更为大量的损伤是轻微的肌肉骨骼的断裂，可以快速痊愈。根据疾病国际分类第 9 版临床修订版 [ICD–9–CM] 操作码 35～39），来自国家儿童创伤登记的数据在表 22–2 中列出，表明四肢外伤的死亡率同样比较低，但是血管手术治疗的死亡比例显著升高。

表 22–1　国家儿科创伤登记 II 和 III 登记的 1368 例儿童外伤的机制

外伤机制	比例（%）	死亡率（%）
穿透性外伤	52	10
钝性外伤	47	17
碾压性外伤	1	8

表 22–2　国家儿童创伤登记 II 和 III 登记的 1368 例儿童外伤中 1628 个血管外伤的分布

区域	ICD–9–CM	总数	存活数	死亡数（%）	手术数
颈部	900–901	249	196	53（21）	41
胸部	901–902	161	98	63（39）	70
腹部盆腔	902–903	374	248	126（34）	50
上肢	903–904	497	494	3（1）	21
下肢	904–905	326	318	8（3）	36

ICD–9–CM：国际疾病分类，第 9 版，临床修订。

儿童时期的血管外伤有两种截然不同的成分。除由外部的机械作用力所导致的损伤外，使用复杂的血管内诊断和治疗技术的不断增加，伴随而来的是血管结构医源性损伤的虽然低，但是确有发生[24,34,39]。然而，随着技术的不断完善和科技的不断进步，这种血管医源性损伤的发生率似乎在不断的下降[39]。

评价

评价急性血管外伤一般性的原则是根据临床情况作出评价。不考虑血管外伤的原因，怀疑有血管外伤时就必须首先根据患者的病史作出一个合理的临床评价系统。在初始的临床评价期间，必须要回答两个急切的问题：（1）是否有循环系统的完整性受到破坏的证据？（2）血液灌注是否足够？尽管这两个问题之间存在隐含的因果关系，但是每一个问题都可以是紊乱的，而没有即刻影响到另外一个问题。长时间的血管损伤后发生的血管痉挛，是儿童时期血管外伤后的一种常见的特征，可能导致解剖学上完整血管树的外周缺血。反过来，对于非闭塞性血管疾病所导致的损伤，由于存在有效的侧支循环，尽管近端的血流受到损害，但是仍可能会维持远端的血液循环。因此，并不是每一个血流受到损害的患者都会即刻出现外周循环的缺血，出现急性缺血的迹象可能并不预示着是必须要进行手术治疗的血管外伤。不考虑循环的状态，评价任何血管外伤的儿童时，证实或恢复细胞灌注是即刻优先要进行的步骤[32]。

许多研究者证实了彻底的临床体格检查的预测准确性，明确了在检查过程中进行动脉造影术的指征[13,16]。在儿童患者中，后者的问题显得尤其重要，因为它会潜在性的增加额外的医源性损伤。Frykberg 等人[16]显示了血管损伤“硬”体征的预测准确性，对于任何有活动性出血、扩大的血肿、脉搏减弱或出现血管杂音或震颤的患者，建议即刻进行手术治疗。没有扩大的血肿、低血压、外周神经感觉缺乏或存在外伤引起的出血史，这些都考虑为血管损伤的“软”体征，仅仅需要临床观察。这些人群的长期随访已经证实了这种评价办法的预测准确性，验证了作者最初的建议：对于近端血管外伤的处理并不需要常规进行动脉造影术。对于血管外伤的儿童，因为存在医源性损伤微小血管、造影剂毒性，增加作为缺血的主要原因的持续性血管痉挛的频率，所以谨慎进行血管造影术的问题甚至变得更为中肯。Reichard 等人[38]回顾了在 Cook 乡村医院经儿童创伤服务所治疗的 75 例有血管外伤的儿童，分析了他们临床体征的预测准确性。他们报道的一部分包括了对 12 名经动脉造影术“成年人”治疗方案治疗的儿童的比较。所完成的研究中没有一个是单纯性的近端血管外伤。所有 10 名血管外伤儿童都有“硬”体征。77 名没有血管外伤的儿童中有 4 名也表现出至少有一个“硬”体征，因此体格检查出现了 100% 的敏感性和 95% 的特异性。值得注意的是，这些数据证实了 Meagher 等人[30]在 1979 年发表的相似的建议，强调了只有在不能通过病史和临床特征来确定缺血的风险超过动脉造影操作的风险时，急性血管外伤才应该考虑进行动脉造影术[6,29,40]。当考虑到“只有一次”的急诊科动脉造影术，尽管近来出现了动脉造影术安全有效的报道，还是特别注意要进行这种风险的权衡[23]。然而，对于慢性的血管损伤，因为要精确的计划血管重建手术，所以动脉造影术是必须要进行考虑的。

双工多普勒、B 型超声波成像、多探头的计算机 X 射线断层血管造影术和磁共振血管成像技术是最近出现的临床影像学技术。前两种具适当的便携性，能够确定血流和血流速度。然而，它们在诊断急性血管外伤中的作用，还没有得到很好的确定。后两种技术是计算机增强成像技术不断发展的结果。这些技术使得不需要直接侵入动脉血管树就可以看到血管的解剖和血流[44]。近来的报道已经显示这些形式的检查在诊断儿童可疑性血管外伤中的价值。三维重建技术可以完美的确定血管外伤的水平和侧支循环的有效性（图 22-1）。虽然无创技术避免了对动脉血管树进行插管，但是可能会需要更高剂量的造影剂。因此选择患者必须要考虑对比动脉损伤的风险造影剂的潜在毒性。

儿童通常不会患有动脉粥样硬化的血管疾病。因为他们的血管具有弹性，他们通常会伸长并短暂变形，而不是破裂，以此适应所受到的外力。这种变形的即刻效应就是增加了继发于血管内膜撕裂的潜在性血流障碍。这种血流下降的效应可能成为急性缺血或边缘性血供不足，其刺激了侧支循环的增加。然而急性缺血应该容易在临床检查中进行辨别，边缘性血供不足可能会非常的轻微，不会出现临床症状。因此，血液循环在功能和解剖上的完整性必须在临床上得到证实，在每一个血管外伤的儿童中都要进行详细的记

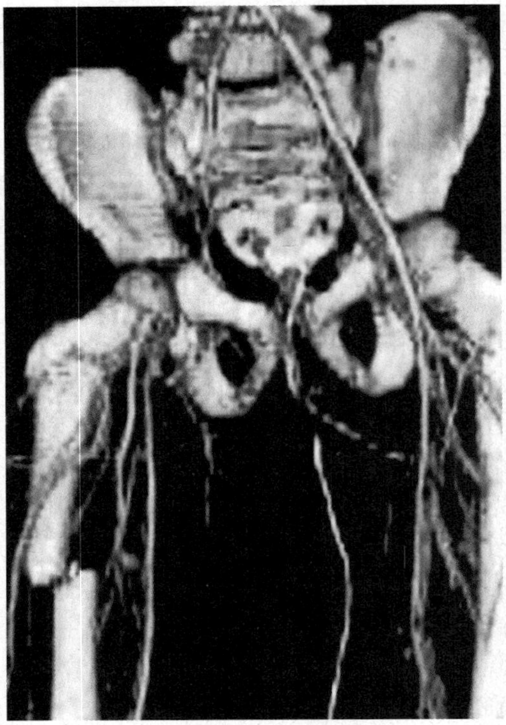

图 22-1 一名 5 岁大的男孩被汽车撞击以后进行的 CT 血管成像图像。他在婴儿时进行了大血管错位血管修补手术，并注意到其右足没有动脉搏动。评估显示了临床上无症状的股动脉破裂。

载。同样重要的是要理解不明原因的可触及动脉搏动的消失，尤其是在下肢，可能是先前就存在而不是急性损伤所导致的。如果灌注压因为其他急性的外伤而突然的下降，侧支循环可能变得不足，就可能会出现进行性缺血的症状。在他们对儿童血管外伤临床发现的预测准确性分析中，Reichard 等人[38]称赞了踝-肱指数（ABI）作为预示外周血流灌注不足的准确性。他们的数据显示了 ABI 小于 0.99 就提示临床上临界
378 性的血管外伤，增强了重症监护病房的出院数据，其提示了血管外伤真正的发病率要高于以前所认为的数字。事实上，由 Seibert 等人[43]报道发现显示了任何采用脐动脉插管治疗的婴儿，外周动脉搏动的评估和 ABI 的测量都应该是出院后常规评估的一部分。

创伤性损伤

创伤性的损伤可以分为涉及躯干的损伤（头颈和躯干）和涉及四肢的损伤（上肢和下肢）。对各个范围进行精确的诊断和及时的治疗都有其独特的挑战性。

躯干部损伤

颈部血管的外伤似乎在儿童时期比较罕见。为了检验他们提出的诊断颈部血管钝性外伤，Rozycki 等人[41]回顾了 797 例机动车祸受害者经过 Grady 纪念医院创伤服务所 17 个月期间治疗，与颈胸部座位安全带体征有关的颈部血管外伤。占到 3%的有颈动脉外伤的患者全部都是成年人。没有遗漏外伤，没有在儿童中出现这种外伤。随着遵守限制儿童法律的逐渐增多，座位安全带体征与显著的血管外伤之间的潜在关系将需要持续进行密切的随访。Cox[2]回顾了 36 名有血管外伤儿童的手术处理，包括 9 名儿童有 11 处颈动脉或颈静脉外伤。其中 8 例是穿透性的颈部外伤。在 3 名血流动力学不稳定的儿童中只有 2 例死亡。

躯干部血管外伤在儿童时期相对比较罕见。这种情况可能是年轻、健康的血管具有更大的弹性所致。虽然儿童对胸部血管的破坏并不具有免疫性，但是大多数的包括儿童外伤患者的文献都显示其发生率比成年人要低。临床报道表明儿童主动脉外伤的自然病史与成年人之间并无差别。死亡率非常的高，尤其是那些出现收缩血压低于 90mmHg 的儿童。Eddy 等人[8]回顾了 King 县验尸官长达 12 年（1975—1987年）的记录，发现有 13 例主动脉破裂的儿童患者。这些儿童中只有 3 名能够成功地活着抵达医院，只有 1 名儿童得以存活。国家儿童创伤登记的资料分析有些更加令人振奋，54 名主动脉破裂的儿童中有 26 名（48%）能够活着出院。这种来自北美的多个有贡献的医院具有代表性，类似于由 Cox 等人[2]做出的单中心的报道，表明这种灾难性外伤的结果可能比一贯报道的成年人的结果要好。较大的胸部静脉外伤甚至更为少见，通常伴有大型的肺破裂。

因为在儿童人群中钝性外伤占优势，尤其是机动车相关的车祸所导致的外伤，就可能会发生腹部血管外伤[7]。动脉破裂比静脉破裂远为罕见。低血压进展到明显的休克是最为常见的发现，当实质性的内脏损伤是最可能的原因时，决定进行剖腹探查相对比较简单。Fayiga 等人[11]回顾了 18 年的手术治疗儿童钝性

血管外伤的经验。17 名患者中出现了 21 处腹部主要静脉的外伤，11 例是致命性的（65%）。在进行剖腹探查手术以前，没有 1 例认识到有腹部主要静脉的外伤。由于在许多其他的病例中，存活率直接跟当时的血流动力学的稳定性有关。大多数的并发症是与非血管性外伤有关。大多数的血管外伤需要直接进行修补手术，类似的经验也可见于 Cox 等人[2]报道的一组相似的 16 例腹部血管外伤的病例中，其中只有 1 例主动脉破裂和 1 例肠系膜上动脉横断的病例需要进行间置移植以修补血管。

四肢外伤

绝大多数的下肢血管外伤都是钝性机械性外伤所导致的结果，是动脉性的外伤，通常合并骨折[9,14,22]。尤其是在腘窝处的外伤，通常是由运动和自行车车祸所导致的。最初的评价必须要证实是否存在可触及的
79 远端动脉搏动和足够的毛细血管灌注。即刻复位错位的骨折片段或是半脱位的关节，经常可使远端动脉搏动恢复。如果缺血的时间持续超过 6 个小时，就有发生骨筋膜室综合征的可能性，应该即刻考虑行筋膜切开术[45]。间置倒转的对侧大隐静脉仍然是治疗所有血管片段性破裂的首选。当不能够收获自体血管以制作成血管补片或是移植血管导管时，就应该考虑合成材料只能作为最后的一种治疗手段[31]。采用单股的单纯缝合线进行血管的吻合[32]。当血管修补完成时，首先释放远端的血管夹以证实有足够的回血。然后在缝合线最后打结以前释放近端的血管夹以冲走任何残留的空气或是血凝块。如果有显著的血管痉挛，通常可以通过采用冠状动脉扩张器进行轻轻的机械扩张来缓解血管痉挛。静脉破裂应该在动脉修补术以前进行修补。进行静脉修补的儿童应该术后持续 48 小时的抗凝治疗。一些作者采用肝素治疗；其他的作者术后单纯应用右旋糖酐溶液持续 2～3 天。Reed 等人[37]报道了他们治疗 7 例儿童因腘动脉外伤即刻进行手术修补的经验。其中 4 例有钝性外伤，3 例是穿透性外伤。相关的合并症包括 3 例骨折、4 例重度的软组织损伤和 1 例神经损伤。所有的患者都进行了血管造影术。3 例在术中进行了血管造影术，因此推测起来 4 例在术前进行的血管造影术是为了证实血管外伤诊断的需要。治疗措施包括 2 例行一期血管修补术和 4 例行静脉旁路移植手术。吻合口是铲形的，以间断缝合的方式进行血管吻合。有 1 名儿童需要进行筋膜切开术。没有死亡、截肢或再手术的病例。在他们报道的时候（1990 年）随访范围在 10～42 个月。所有的患儿都有正常的多普勒压力波或是远端动脉搏动。这些数据表明了即刻积极进行治疗与成功结果之间的关系。其他的研究者报道了类似的建议，强调了长时间血管痉挛的高度倾向性使得儿童时期动脉吻合成为一项特别的挑战[11]。

绝大多数的儿童四肢血管外伤都与中轴线的骨骼破裂有关。在这种最为严重的类型中，骨骼和软组织破坏的复合伤可以导致所谓的“肢体损伤综合征”。它通常的特征是大块的软组织撕裂，可能伴有显著的组织丧失。最初的评估必须要考虑到组织的生存能力、预期的肢体功能、可能因大块组织坏死和败血症而需要进行截肢。已经提出了一种肢体损伤严重程度评分（MESS）作为进行肢体救治的评价和预测的精确系统（表 22-3）。虽然这个系统最初是应用于成年人，但是 Fagelmen 等人[10]证明了当回顾应用于 36 例外伤儿童后，肢体损伤严重程度评分（MESS）的预

表 22-3　肢体损伤严重程度评分（MESS）

因素	得分
骨骼 / 软组织外伤	
低能量（刺伤，单纯骨折，手枪的枪伤）	1
中等能量（开放性或多发性骨折，脱位）	2
高能量（高速碰撞，步枪的枪伤）	3
极高能量（高速外伤，大面积污染）	4
肢体缺血	
搏动减弱 / 消失，正常的血液灌注	1*
没有搏动，感觉异常，毛细血管再充盈不良	2*
冰冷，没有感觉，麻痹，失去知觉	3*
休克	
收缩血压总是大于 90mmHg	1
短暂性低血压	2
持续性低血压	3
年龄（岁）	
＜30 岁	1
30～50	2
＜50	3

* 对于缺血时间＞6 小时的评分加倍。

MESS＞7：预测 100%要进行截肢。

测准确率为93%。与骨折相伴的血管破裂必须要即刻寻找破裂位置，以至于随后进行的中轴骨骼修补产生一个能存活的肢体。可通过暂时的血管旁路以实现血流供应的恢复，直到完成骨折的固定。只要有可能，静脉修补都应该在动脉修补以前进行。丧失活力的组织必须要给予清除，应该要考虑进行筋膜切开术。必须要评价神经功能，并在讨论进行截肢以前进行记录。儿童可能从最初似乎是毁损性的外伤中恢复得好得令人惊讶，虽然这是真实的，但是可能因为没有感觉的、不能移动的四肢而变成永久性的残废，这是一种可怜的选择，在活跃的生命中应用了一个功能性的安装适当的假肢。因此，决定截肢是根据肢体存活能力和预期肢体功能的评估。肢体损伤严重程度评分（MESS）只是作为一种合理的指导原则，但是最终的决定取决于手术医生、患儿的父母亲，可能的时候，还取决于儿童本身。

上肢血管的外伤通常是与髁上骨折有关。腋窝的牵拉伤，尤其是伴有高能量的外力时，例如车辆的弹射，可能会破坏动脉或静脉的结构，产生血肿，其并没有远端外伤中看到的那么精确的描述。除征象明显的血液丢失、腋窝或肩膀区域出现弥漫性的水肿和外周动脉搏动的减弱，都应该即刻行血管造影术以证实血管外伤的存在和损伤的解剖结构。

髁上骨折可能会因直接损伤或因压迫而破坏肱动脉的血流，可伴有或不伴有长时间的血管痉挛。就像在下肢的血管外伤中一样，最终的治疗从评估足够的血液灌注和证实血管的完整性开始。有趣的是近来有一个报道称在发生节段性血管丧失的血管重建手术中，可采用同侧的重要静脉来作为理想的间置移植物[27]。上肢外伤的损伤救治总体上效果良好，功能的恢复与伴发的骨骼肌和神经破坏的性质有关。
380 骨筋膜室综合征作为上肢损伤长期缺血的结果，其发生率要显著低于在下肢外伤中的发生率；然而，仔细的随访保证足够的血流灌注和避免缺血后肌肉挛缩，必须是长期治疗的一部分内容。

医源性损伤

虽然对于婴幼儿和儿童更为尖端的影像学方法不断发展，但是血管造影或血管穿刺对幼年儿童或是较小的婴幼儿血管完整性的潜在性危害仍然存在。在过去的十年间已经有许多的报道来描述这个特别的问题[1,12,34,36]。许多为并发症的个案报道，来自于常规治疗措施的一些通常是无害的操作。例如，Demircin 等人[3]报道了1名婴儿其肱动脉假性动脉瘤是在肘前的静脉穿刺期间无意的穿刺所导致的。这种病变在近端压迫下采用直接缝合修补。Gamba 等人[19]回顾了他们在治疗低出生体重新生儿医源性血管损伤中的经验。在1987年到1994年期间治疗的335例婴儿中，有9例（2.6%）被诊断为血管外伤。平均出生体重为880g（范围为590～1450g），但是在作出诊断时的平均体重为1825g（范围为1230～2730g）。在9例血管外伤中有7例外伤是与静脉穿刺有关，包括6例股动脉静脉瘘，其中2例为双侧的股动脉静脉瘘。1例颈动脉损伤和5例股动脉静脉瘘采用微血管技术进行修补。通过随访临床体格检查和多普勒血流检查来作出的结果非常的好，因而作者强调了积极内科治疗和显微外科处理这些血管外伤的重要性。在1981年 O'Neill 等人[35]回顾了他们手术治疗的41例婴儿与脐动脉插管有关的巨大血栓栓塞性疾病的经验。虽然大多数的并发症是与栓子远端达到股动脉有关，但是有8例婴儿是因为急性主动脉梗阻而需要进行急诊手术治疗。4例婴儿进行了主动脉横断血栓切除术，其中有3例完全恢复。由于脐动脉插管治疗的原则已经建立得更加完善，所以这些问题似乎已经较少发生了。

由于使用体外膜肺氧合器的增加，已经出现了可能需要进行颈部血管重建的问题，尤其是当氧合器支持的过程中涉及同时使用颈动脉和颈静脉的时候。LaQuaglia 等人[26]描述了他们采用显微外科修补术治疗9例医源性动脉损伤儿童的经验。常规使用手术显微镜，采用9-0到11-0的尼龙缝合线进行血管修补。采用局部注射2%利多卡因或罂粟碱来控制血管痉挛。由于显微外科技术的持续发展，更好的缝合线材料可采用，这种手术将变成处理大型外伤到微小血管损伤中一种价值不断提升的辅助技术。

股动脉仍然是最为常见的发生医源性损伤的部位。就如前面在创伤性损伤中所讨论的那样，骨盆和臀部存在有效的侧支循环，可以使这些病变在整个儿童时期的大部分时间内都不会出现临床症状。Lin 等人[28]分析了1986—2001年期间在1431名婴儿中进行的1674例诊断性插管或治疗性的插管手术。在34名儿童中需要进行36例手术。作者将并发症分为非缺血性、急性股动脉缺血性和慢性股动脉缺血性。非缺血性病变包括了假性动脉瘤（n＝4）、动脉静脉瘘（n＝5）和腹股沟血肿（n＝5）。所有的血管损伤都进行了直接修补手术，采用聚二氧六环酮（PDS）或是聚丙烯（Prolene）缝合线进行间断吻合。急性股动脉缺血性病变最为常见，需要进行从血栓切除术到补片修补术等不同的手术。慢性股动脉缺血性病变定义为术后 30 天以后出现血流中断的证据。7 名儿童在标准手术以后平均 193 天时（范围是 31～842 天）出现了临床体征。所有的 7 名儿童症状为跛行、双腿长度的不一致或是步态失调。手术修补 5 例儿童采用倒转的大隐静脉，做髂股动脉旁路手术的重建血管，1 例儿童做股动脉旁路手术的重建血管。只有 1 例儿童需要补片血管成形术。作者对潜在性影响因素的分析表明，统计学上有显著性的预测关系有年龄小于 3 岁，患儿多于三次早先进行过脐动脉插管，治疗性的操作而不是单纯的诊断性操作，采用的导引导管直径大于 6F。这个研究的价值在于鉴别潜在性的预测因素和记录慢性缺血出现症状时需要的相对较短的时间。有任何异常临床发现的儿童都处于血管外伤的风险中，必需随访至少 5 年，最好随访到青春期的早期。肢体长度的差异作为主要血管结构中断的结果，可能不会变得很明显，可能会一直到血管外伤后数年才出现[48]。近来的研究报告表明，医源性血管外伤在青春期以前进行血管重建手术，可纠正一些肢体长度上的差异；然而，这些只是相对较少一组病例，没有代表一致的意见。

如在创伤性血管外伤病例的处理中所示，有高度发生血管痉挛的倾向，需要鉴别长时间的血管痉挛和动脉断裂，这是最初评估中的一项具有挑战性的任务。长时间的血管痉挛被认为是内膜损伤的结果，其可导致一氧化氮产物的紊乱，破坏了动脉壁张力的控制[18,33]。当丧失内皮介导的接触时，如导管尺寸过大或是过于积极的放置导管所引起的剪切力导致的血管外伤一般，在内膜下面的血管平滑肌不能够进行松弛[25]。采用血管造影来证实血管痉挛，需要冒额外的机械性可能会产生问题的风险。CT 血管造影术或是磁共振动脉造影术可能是解决这种临床难题的办法，但是在比较风险和得益时，造影剂的剂量和浓度必须要进行仔细的考虑。在导致坏疽的机制中血管痉挛的作用是有争论的，尽管个案报道提示了其病因和作用[42]。从临床展望中看出，一旦得到证实血管痉挛是外周血液灌注减少的唯一原因，就必须将治疗重点放在证实组织的生存能力，进展成骨筋膜室综合征或是外周缺血的体征上面。假定急性血管痉挛的基本原因至少没有是部分的与血管内膜损伤有关时，发生血栓的风险必须是首先需要考虑的。在过去的数年间，补充溶解血栓剂进行常规的抗凝治疗，特别是尿激酶[20]。尿激酶的推荐剂量各不相同，倾向于完全根据经验进行治疗。在婴幼儿中一直用到每小时 6000U/kg，成功率较高，没有出现并发症。最近，Zenz 等人[49]报道了有关组织型纤溶酶原激活剂的使用，表明使用这种药物可以更快的恢复血流。

手指缺血综合征

静脉内置管相关的同侧手指缺血，可能会在有急性感染性疾病的婴幼儿或幼年儿童中突然发生，通常伴发脱水和血容量减少。在对 104 例病例的回顾分析中，Villavicencio 等人[47]报告，在 68.2%的患者中主要累及到手部，在余下的病例中则累及到足部。患儿的年龄从 29 天到 36 个月不等（平均年龄为 14 个月）。27.8%病例是呼吸道起源的感染，60.5%的病例是来自于胃肠道的感染，来自其他区域的感染病例占到 11.5%。培养出的最为常见的微生物是大肠埃希菌、沙门杆菌、志贺杆菌、链球菌、葡萄球菌、克雷白杆菌和假单胞菌。手指发绀通常发生在静脉置管后不久，可能是留置导管所引发的静脉痉挛导致的结果。如前所述，损伤的内皮细胞可以刺激血管收缩。血流的停滞不动可导致肢体的收缩，减少了肌肉的活动，而肌肉活动可以协助静脉回流。这些情况的持续出现就增加了血管外的压力，可以逐渐产生微循环的衰竭，导致组织坏死，其开始于在手指最远端的区域。

治疗时要立即认识持续性的手指发绀，纠正潜在的全身性疾病，立即取出静脉留置导管。应该立即开始抗凝治疗。应该每天用温水轻轻清洗病变处，累及的肢体通过全部范围的运动进行主动和被动的训练。应该避免进行直接的加热，因为缺血的组织在比正常组织在一个更低的温度时就发生了烧伤。应该将一小片棉花放置于手指或脚趾之间，所有的病变处都应该覆盖无菌的干敷料。发生干性坏疽的区域不需要手术去除。如果在焦痂下面存在发生感染的某些问题时，可以轻轻地从它的一角提起这个区域，以便进行足够的引流。就如动脉病变的病例中，直到已经出现清晰的分界线前，不应该考虑进行截肢。

总结

在儿童人群中，血管外伤显著不同于成年人遇到的血管外伤。创伤性外伤所表现出的一些特征反映出儿童创伤的流行病学特点，如果进行仔细的处理，就可以发现儿童血管系统固有的健康状态。医源性损伤是小型化的代价。它被认为是使许多挽救生命的手术变成可能的技术进步的代价。注意到那些最有风险的细节，可能不会消除问题，但是至少将会减少其发生率，提高知情率。精确的诊断、及时的再血管化治疗和积极处理再灌注损伤是完全康复和正常的长期生长发育所必需的。成功的关键是血管外伤时的高指标，认识到其先前讨论的特征，并采用高精准的技术积极手术治疗血管外伤，这是在儿童血管手术治疗中取得成功的基础。

（顾 松译 陈永卫校）

参考文献

1. Chaikof EL, Dodson TF, Salam AA, et al: Acute arterial thrombosis in the very young. J Vasc Surg 1992;16:428-435.
2. Cox CS Jr, Black CT, Duke JH, et al: Operative treatment of truncal vascular injuries in children and adolescents. J Pediatr Surg 1998;33:462-467.
3. Demircin M, Peker O, Tok M, et al: False aneurysm of the brachial artery in an infant following attempted venipuncture. Turk J Pediatr 1996;38:389-391.
4. Dennis JW, Frykberg ER, Crump JM, et al: New perspectives on the management of penetrating trauma in proximity to major limb arteries. J Vasc Surg 1990;11:84-92.
5. Dennis JW, Frykberg ER, Veldenz HC, et al: Validation of nonoperative management of occult vascular injuries and accuracy of physical examination alone in penetrating extremity trauma: 5- to 10-year follow-up. J Trauma 1998;44:242 (discussion).
6. Dennis JW, Jagger C, Butcher JL, et al: Reassessing the role of arteriogram in the management of posterior knee dislocations. J Trauma 1993;35:692-695.
7. de Virgilio C, Mercado PD, Arnell T, et al: Noniatrogenic pediatric vascular trauma: A ten-year experience at a level I trauma center. Am Surg 1997;63:781-784.
8. Eddy AC, Rusch VW, Marchioro T, et al: Treatment of traumatic rupture of the thoracic aorta: A 15-year experience. Arch Surg 1990;125:1351 (discussion 1355).
9. Eren N, Ozgen G, Ener BK, et al: Peripheral vascular injuries in children. J Pediatr Surg 1991;26:1164-1168.
10. Fagelman MF, Epps HR, Rang M: Mangled extremity severity score in children. J Pediatr Orthop 2002;22:182-184.
11. Fayiga YJ, Valentine RJ, Myers SI, et al: Blunt pediatric vascular trauma: Analysis of forty-one consecutive patients undergoing operative intervention. J Vasc Surg 1994;20:419 (discussion 424).
12. Flanigan DP, Keifer TJ, Schuler JJ, et al: Experience with iatrogenic pediatric vascular injuries: Incidence, etiology, management, results. Ann Surg 1983;198:430-442.
13. Francis H, Thal ER, Weigelt JA, et al: Vascular proximity: Is it a valid indication for arteriography in asymptomatic patients? J Trauma 1991;31:512-514.
14. Friedman RJ, Jupiter JB: Vascular injuries and closed extremity fractures in children. Clin Orthop 1984;188:112-119.
15. Frykberg ER: Advances in diagnosis and treatment of extremity vascular trauma. Surg Clin North Am 1995;75:207-223.
16. Frykberg ER, Crump JM, Dennis JW, et al: Nonoperative observation of clinically occult arterial injuries: A prospective evaluation. Surgery 1991;109:85-96.
17. Frykberg ER, Dennis JW, Bishop K, et al: The reliability of physical examination in the evaluation of penetrating extremity trauma for vascular injury: Results at one year. J Trauma 1991;31:502-511.
18. Furchgott RF, Zawadzki JV: The obligatory role of endothelial cells in the relaxation of arterial smooth muscle by acetylcholine. Nature 1980;288:373-376.
19. Gamba P, Tchaprassian Z, Verlato F, et al: Iatrogenic vascular lesions in extremely low birth weight and low birth weight neonates. Vasc Surg 1997;26:643-646.
20. Giacoia GP: High-dose urokinase therapy in newborn infants with major vessel thrombosis. Clin Pediatr 1993;32:231-237.
21. Harris LM, Hordines J: Major vascular injuries in the pediatric population. Ann Vasc Surg 2003;17:266-269.
22. Hoover JD, Almond PS: Isolated pediatric peripheral vascular injury caused by blunt trauma: A new occurrence. J Trauma 2004;56:198-200.
23. Itani KM, Rothenberg SS, Brandt ML, et al: Emergency center arteriography in the evaluation of suspected peripheral vascular injuries in children. J Pediatr Surg 1993;28:677-680.
24. Klein MD, Coran AG, Whitehouse WM Jr, et al: Management of iatrogenic arterial injuries in infants and children. J Pediatr Surg 1982;17:933-939.
25. Kuo PC, Schroeder RA: The emerging multifaceted roles of nitric oxide. Ann Surg 1995;221:220-235.
26. LaQuaglia MP, Upton J, May JW Jr: Microvascular reconstruction of major arteries in neonates and small children. J Pediatr Surg 1991;26:1136-1140.
27. Lewis HG, Morrison CM, Kennedy PT, et al: Arterial reconstruction using the basilic vein from the zone of injury in pediatric supracondylar humeral fractures: A clinical and radiological series. Plast Reconstr Surg 2003;111:1159 (discussion 1164).
28. Lin Ph, Dodson TF, Bush RL, et al: Surgical intervention for complications caused by femoral artery catheterization in pediatric patients. J Vasc Surg 2001;34:1071-1078.
29. McCorkell SJ, Harley JD, Morishima MS, et al: Indications for angiography in extremity trauma. AJR Am J Roentgenol 1985;145:1245-1247.

30. Meagher DP Jr, Defore WW, Mattox KL, et al: Vascular trauma in infants and children. J Trauma 1979;19:532-536.
31. Milas ZL, Dodson TF, Ricketts RR: Pediatric blunt trauma resulting in major arterial injuries. Am Surg 2004;70:443-447.
32. Mills RP, Robbs JV: Paediatric arterial injury: Management options at the time of injury. J R Coll Surg Edinb 1991; 36:13-17.
33. Moncada S, Higgs A: The L-arginine:nitric oxide pathway. N Engl J Med 1993;329:2002-2012.
34. Nehler MR, Taylor LM Jr, Porter JM: Iatrogenic vascular trauma. Semin Vasc Surg 1998;11:283-293.
35. O'Neill JA, Neblett WW, Born ML: Management of major thromboembolic complications of umbilical artery catheters. J Pediatr Surg 1981;16:972-978.
36. Pigula FA, Buenaventura P, Ettedgui JA, et al: Management of retroperitoneal arterial injury after heart catheterization in children. Ann Thorac Surg 2000;69:1582-1584.
37. Reed MK, Lowry PA, Myers SI: Successful repair of pediatric politeal artery trauma. Am J Surg 1990;160:287-290.
38. Reichard KW, Hall JR, Meller JL, et al: Arteriography in the evaluation of penetrating pediatric extremity injuries. J Pediatr Surg 1994;29:19-22.
39. Reichard KW, Reyes HM: Vascular trauma and reconstructive approaches. Semin Pediatr Surg 1994;3:124-132.
40. Reid JD, Weigelt JA, Thal ER, et al: Assessment of proximity of a wound to major vascular structures as an indication for arteriography. Arch Surg 1998;123:942-946.
41. Rozycki GS, Tremblay L, Feliciano DV, et al: A prospective study for the detection of vascular injury in adult and pediatric patients with cervicothoracic seat belt signs. J Trauma 2002;52:618 (discussion 623).
42. Russo VJ: Traumatic arterial spasm resulting in gangrene. J Pediatr Orthop 1985;5:486-488.
43. Seibert JJ, Northington FJ, Miers JF, et al: Aortic thrombosis after umbilical artery catheterization in neonates: Prevalence of complications of long-term follow-up. AJR Am J Roentgenol 1991;156:567-569.
44. Soares G, Ibarra R, Ferral H: Abnominal aortic injury in a child: intravenous digital substraction angiogram (IVDSA) for the diagnosis of pediatric vascular trauma. Pediatr Radiol 2003;33:563-566.
45. Uslu MM, Altun NS, Cila E, at al: Relevance of mangled extremity severity score to compartment syndromes. Arch Orthop Trauma Surg 1995;114:229-232.
46. Victoroff BN, Robertson WW Jr, Eichelberger MR, et al: Extremity gunshot injuries treated in an urban children's hospital. Pediatr Emerg Care 1994;10:1-5.
47. Villavicencio JL, Gonzalez-Carna JL: Acute vascular problems of children. Curr Probl Surg 1985;22:1-85.
48. Whitehouse WM, Coran AG, Stanley JC, et al: Pediatric vascular trauma: Manifestations, management, and sequelae of extremity arterial injury in patients undergoing surgical treatment. Arch Surg 1976;111:1269-1275.
49. Zenz W, Muntean W, Beitzke A, et al: Tissue plasminogen activator (Alteplase) treatment for femoral artery thrombosis after cardiac catheterisation in infants and children. Br Heart J 1993;70:382-385.

第 23 章

烧　伤

Dai H. Chung、Arthur P. Sanford 和 David N. Herndon

1944 年 Lund 和 Browder[69]开创了用烧伤面积占
383 全身体表面积（total body surface area，TBSA）的百分数的方法来定量评估烧伤的程度。1946 年 Cope 和 Moore[18]在治疗波士顿 Coconut Grove 火灾伤员中计算出了要保持“烧伤性休克”伤员水电解质平衡所需的补液量。20 世纪 60 年代，局部有效的抗菌药物的发现，如 0.5%硝酸银[75]，磺胺咪隆[68]和磺胺嘧啶银[30]，很大程度上降低了烧伤脓毒症的发生。以上这些以及在过去几十年中在烧伤领域取得的其他进展使得严重烧伤患者的总的存活率有了很大提高。最近几年里，在烧伤的一些领域也取得了一系列成果。早期外科切痂和植皮技术的运用使得烧伤脓毒症的发生率大大降低，也缩短了烧伤患者总的住院天数。代谢性药物的应用保证了患者在烧伤后相当长的一段高代谢期保持正氮平衡。对吸入性烧伤的迅速诊断和有效处理也使烧伤患者的预后大大改善。这些还只是使得烧伤死亡率明显降低的重大进展[8]。今天，最明显的进步体现在儿童中严重烧伤患儿总体生存率的提高，目前 14 岁及小于 14 岁的儿童中，98%全身体表面积烧伤的患儿死亡率已经下降到 50%，相对于其他年龄组，相同的死亡率只出现在 75%全身体表面积烧伤的患者[42]。

虽然随着预防性措施和法规的完善，烧伤的总体发生率已经明显下降，但目前在美国每年仍有超过 100 万的烧伤事件发生。幸运的是，大多数烧伤程度都比较轻微，大约有 45 000 名中度到重度烧伤患者需要住院治疗，其中青年男性占 67%，40%是 15 岁以下儿童[3]。烧伤是 5 岁以下儿童中意外事故所致死亡的第二大原因，据统计，2001 年全美国因烧伤而死亡的儿童有 523 名，2002 年大约有 92 500 名 14 岁以下儿童因为烧伤相关创伤被送入医院急诊室抢救（58 100 名因为热灼伤，22 600 名因为烫伤）[12]。因烧伤相关创伤而住院治疗的 4 岁及 4 岁以下儿童中，65%是烫伤，20%是接触性烧伤，剩下的是火焰灼伤。在婴幼儿中，烫伤的最大原因是由热的食物和热的液体所致，其中，热油造成的深度烫伤最为常见。热水龙头也经常造成儿童大面积烫伤，其实如果安装一个温控水龙头，保证流出的水必须低于 48.8℃，这种烫伤就可以避免[2]。儿童也常常由于接触卷发熨斗、烤炉、蒸汽熨斗和烟火而烫伤，接触墙壁插座中的电流以及电线也引起相当一部分儿童的灼伤。虐儿也是儿童烫伤的一个重要原因（图 23-1），两侧对称烫伤、手套或袜子形状的烫伤，特别是手背的烫伤并拖延就诊时间，都要高度怀疑虐儿因素。青少年中，火焰灼伤更为常见，经常发生在玩火或者易燃易爆物品
时。 38

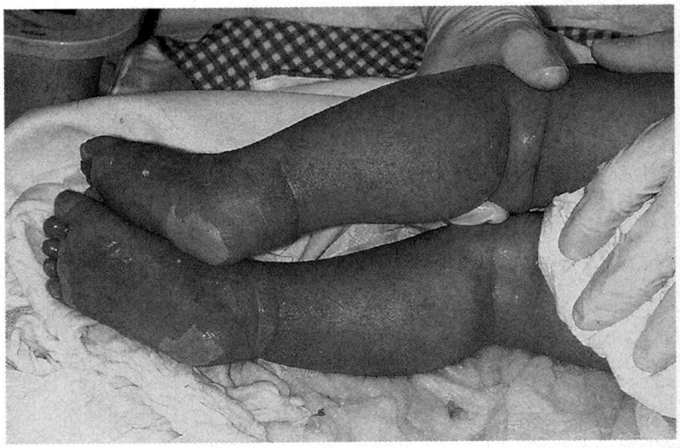

图 23-1 婴儿双下肢烫伤。伤口呈双侧袜子形状分布，边界清晰，符合儿童虐待所致的烫伤表现。

病理生理学

作为人体最大的器官，皮肤保持了体内水分和电解质的平衡，阻断了来自外界的有害侵犯，保护机体免于微生物感染，同时，皮肤也是参与体温调节、进行维生素 D 的合成代谢以及产生神经感觉的重要器官。全身皮肤的总面积在新生儿大约为 0.2～0.3m²，成人大约为 1.5～2.0m²，约占全身体重的 15%。解剖学上，表皮主要是由上皮细胞组成，特别是角质形成细胞，角质形成细胞从基底层逐渐成熟并最终角化脱皮的过程大约需要 2～4 周。真皮主要由分泌胶原蛋白和弹力蛋白的成纤维细胞组成。真皮可以分为表浅的乳头层和深部的网状层，两者之间为一些神经血管丛。网状层和脂肪层中含有皮肤附属器，如毛囊、汗腺和皮脂腺等。所以，真皮深部的烧伤常导致伤处触觉丧失而触痛不明显。

热烧伤可以导致表皮的凝固坏死以及皮下组织不同程度的损伤，损伤的程度取决于温度、暴露时间、皮肤厚度、皮肤传导热的能力以及不同热源特定的热效应。比如，脂肪的热效应要高于水，所以，相同温度相同暴露时间条件下，油脂烫伤的程度往往更为严重。在接触中，通过热传递，热量很容易从温度高的部位传递给温度低的部位，但是，皮肤对热量传递到深层组织起到了屏障的作用，大多数烧伤只局限在皮肤层。当然，局部组织随后对烧伤区域的反应也会导致周围组织的进行性损伤。

烧伤部位的皮肤可以分为三个区域：凝固区、淤血区和充血区（图 23-2）。凝固区由烧伤后的焦痂组成，该区域的细胞在烧伤时已经发生了不可逆的损伤和坏死。凝固区周围的坏死区域是淤血区，该区域的细胞尚未完全死亡，而组织灌注由于局部炎性介质如血栓素 A_2、花生四烯酸、氧化剂和细胞因子的释放而明显增强[95]，在局部微循环中形成血小板血栓、中性粒细胞粘连、纤维素沉积和血管收缩，最终导致细胞死亡。然而适当的伤口处理和复苏能够逆转这一过程并阻断细胞进一步死亡[19]。血栓素 A_2 抑制剂能够显著增加真皮层血流量而缩小淤血层范围，抗氧化剂和缓激肽抑制剂也能改善局部血供[20,79]。用抗 CD18 或抗细胞间粘连分子单克隆抗体阻断白细胞黏附于内皮细胞层而改善组织灌注已经在动物模型上取得了成功[11,72]。淤血区周围的区域是充血区，该区域因为炎症反应而血管扩张，血流增加。

当烧伤面积超过 40%全身体表面积时，烧伤所致的炎症反应往往不能局限在局部伤口，血栓素 A_2 以及其他炎性介质（缓激肽、白三烯、儿茶酚胺、活化的补体、血管活性胺）的大量释放给呼吸循环系统、泌尿系统和消化系统造成了严重的生理负担[97]。毛细血管渗透性增加，血浆大量渗入组织间隙造成血容量急剧下降导致心功能不全。由于心脏搏出量降低、肾血流量减少而造成肾小球滤过率下降，一些其他的升压激素和介质如血管紧张素、醛固酮和血管加压素的活化又进一步影响了肾脏血流，最终导致少尿[78]。如果不及时处理，最终将发展成为急性肾小管坏死和肾衰，这种烧伤患者预后很差[61]。小肠黏膜上皮细胞凋亡的增加和再生的降低导致小肠黏膜萎缩[16,17,100]，那些在正常条件下被完整的小肠黏膜屏障阻断的大分子渗透性增加，其原因主要是短暂的肠系膜缺血，最终可以导致肠内细菌移位和内毒素血症。烧伤也会引起免
疫功能的下降。巨噬细胞会减少；中性粒细胞因为渗 385
出、趋化作用、吞噬作用而损伤，细胞毒性 T 淋巴细胞活性降低，而中性粒细胞、巨噬细胞、T 淋巴细胞功能的损害将导致烧伤后感染的危险性增高[5,6,32,57,64,101]。

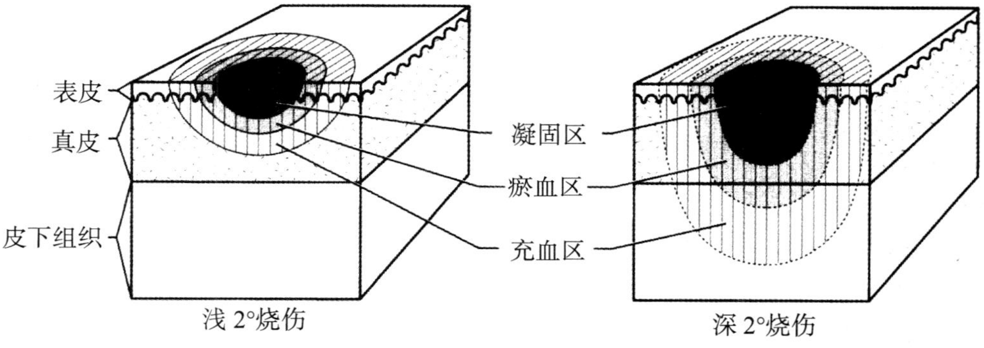

图 23-2 三个烧伤区域：凝固区、瘀血区和充血区。

处理

急救

烧伤的伤员必须迅速脱离热源，对于多发性创伤的伤员还应迅速评估和寻找除了皮肤烧伤以外其他潜在性威胁生命的创伤。脱去烧焦的衣服，取下金属饰物，迅速用凉水冲洗烧伤的伤口，但要防止产生体温过低。脱去衣服后，应将伤员裹在毯子中保暖。对于化学药品灼伤者，必须用大量清水冲洗伤口，并防止残留药品继续损伤周围皮肤。试图中和化学药品被列为禁忌，因为这样只会增加热量并且加重烧伤程度。

和任何创伤患者一样，需要通过两次检查来评估烧伤伤员的伤情。首先要检查的项目是呼吸道、呼吸和循环情况，必须及时发现任何潜在性的威胁生命的情况并迅速处理。喘鸣、气促和声音嘶哑等症状都预示着呼吸道存在问题。气管插管开放呼吸道，并给予纯氧吸入，用脉搏氧饱和度仪检测血氧饱和度，观察胸廓扩张情况确保足够的通气量。然而，氧饱和度正常并不意味着呼吸道已经通畅，因为儿童有相当强大的代偿能力，当氧饱和度下降时就已经接近严重性的气道狭窄了。整个胸背部的全层皮肤烧伤使得躯干收缩，胸廓不能扩张，而导致严重的呼吸功能障碍，必要时需要行切痂术促进胸廓扩张，增加通气量。肢体烧焦的伤员测血压相当困难，脉率可以作为检测血容量的间接指标，如果出现心动过速就提示需要积极地持续给予液体复苏。

烧伤深度的分类要根据累及的皮层而定，包括表皮层、乳头层、网状层、皮下脂肪层及其下方的结构（图 23–3）。I 度烧伤局限于表皮层，皮肤完整，局部红斑并有触痛，治疗上只要在烧伤处外用含有芦荟的软膏，口服非类固醇类抗炎药即可。I 度烧伤（如日晒伤）能在 7～10 天自发愈合，不留瘢痕。II 度烧伤根据累及的真皮深度可以分为浅 II 度烧伤和深 II 度烧伤。浅 II 度烧伤局限在乳头层，具有典型的红斑和水泡，并有疼痛，浅 II 度烧伤能在 10～14 天通过残余的上皮结构进行上皮重建，只留下轻微的色素沉着。深 II 度烧伤累及网状层，由于累及到皮肤附属器，这种烧伤的愈合需要几周时间，并常常会留下明显的瘢痕。III 度烧伤是皮肤全层包括表皮层、真皮层和皮肤附属器的完全性破坏，形成干的、皮革样的焦痂，对触痛不敏感。由于没有残余的上皮或皮肤附属器，这种烧伤从伤口的边缘开始上皮重建。IV 度烧伤常见于长时间的热灼伤或者触电灼伤，累及到皮下的器官，如肌肉和骨胳。

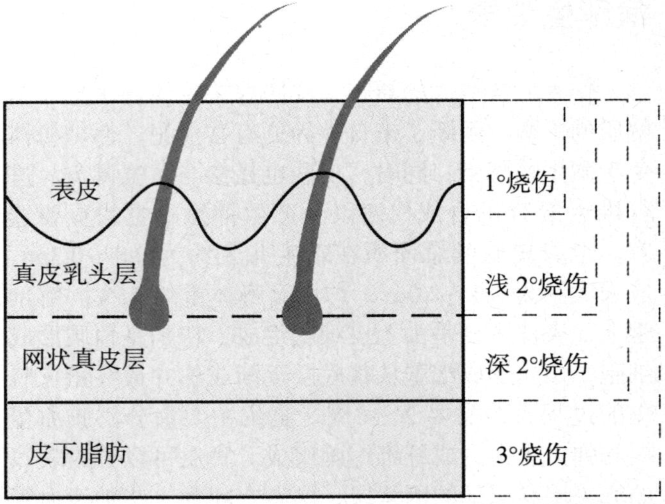

图 23–3 烧伤深度。I 度烧伤局限于表皮层，浅 II 度烧伤累及乳头层，深 II 度烧伤累及网状层，III 度烧伤累及全层皮肤，包括表皮层和真皮层。(Adapted from Wolf S, Herndon DN: Burns. In Townsend CM Jr [ed]:Textbook of Surgery, 17th ed. Philadelphia, WB Saunders, 2004, p 571.)

准确而迅速地评估烧伤深度对于提出合适的烧伤处理方案很重要，特别是区分是表皮层还是真皮层的烧伤，因为这决定着是否需要采用外科手段治疗。不幸的是，就算是一个经验丰富的外科医生，判断明显的深度烧伤是否会在 3 周之内愈合也只有 50%的准确度。对于这种不确定的烧伤，早期切痂并植皮比采用非外科治疗疗效会更好。对烧伤深度更精确的客观检查包括激光多普勒血流仪和荧光素测定血流、超声检测变性的胶原以及伤口的光反射率检测[9,60,80,81]。烧伤伤口活检最终是最精确的诊断手段，但临床价值不大，因为这是一种侵入性检查，并且只能提供静态的伤口情况，而且还需要一个经验丰富的病理学家提供组织学上的检查结果。即使有上述这些现代的检查手段，诊断烧伤深度最可靠的方法仍然是临床观察。

四肢环状的全层烧伤形成收缩性焦痂会影响肢体远端的血管和神经，无弹性的焦痂下方水肿组织的积聚会阻碍静脉回流，造成间隔综合征，并最终影响动脉血供。如果脉搏触诊或多普勒检测不能测出远端肢体的脉搏，在排除全身循环障碍后，对烧伤肢体及时行焦痂切开减张术可以避免烧伤对远端肢体血供的影响。切痂减张可以在床边进行，用解剖刀或者电刀在烧伤肢体的外侧和内侧各做两条纵行切口（图 23-4）。对于手部烧伤，切口应沿着鱼际和小鱼际的隆起部位以及手指的背外侧，并且要避免损伤到血管神经束。因为焦痂切开减张术切开了烧伤的全层皮肤，所以出血较少，但是如果血管受影响的时间较长，切痂减张后的再灌注损伤可能会引起活动性出血和肌肉间隙的进一步水肿。缺血再灌注损伤释放的氧自由基还会造成短暂的低血压。如果注意到隔室压力增加，就必须立即行筋膜切开术以避免神经和软组织的持续性缺血损伤。

根据复苏原则，必须迅速建立静脉通路并输注乳酸林格氏液。首先选择外周静脉，对于大面积烧伤选择股静脉更为理想。如果唯一可用静脉的表面组织也被烧伤，仍然需要立即通过这一静脉建立通路，稍后再改用其他无菌的部位。如果在幼儿烧伤的肢体上建立血管通路有困难，在 6 岁以下的幼儿中可以选择骨内通路。每个严重烧伤的患者都要放置鼻胃管来预防胃肠梗阻。通过经幽门的导管可以直接给予肠内营养。同时还要留置 Foley 导尿管并准确的检测尿量，以作为终端器官灌注的指标。实验室检查包括全血细胞计数、分型以及浓缩人红细胞的交叉配血、生化检查、尿液化验、凝血情况检查以及胸部 X 线检查。

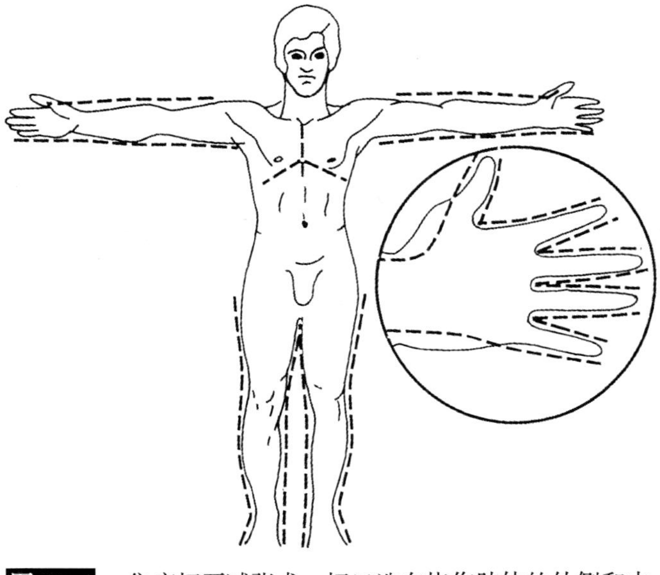

图 23-4 焦痂切开减张术。切口选在烧伤肢体的外侧和内侧。手部焦痂切开减张术切口选在手背部手指的内侧和外侧。(From Eichelberger MR [ed]: Pediatric Trauma: Prevention, Acute Care, Rehabilitation. St Louis, Mosby, 1993, p 569.)

如果怀疑吸入性烧伤，还要测定动脉血气分析和碳氧血红蛋白来指导呼吸系统治疗。

在青少年和成人，烧伤面积通常通过“九分法”来计算，每一侧上肢和头部各占 9%全身体表面积，每一侧下肢和前、后躯干各占 18%全身体表面积，会阴部、外生殖器和颈部共占剩下的 1%。也可以根据患者的手掌面积占 1%全身体表面积来迅速估计烧伤伤口的面积。然而，儿童由于身体比例不同，使用“九分法”会导致估计错误。儿童的头部和颈部占全身体表面积相对较大，而下肢则相对较小，比如婴儿的头部占到 19%全身体表面积，在成人只有 9%。所以，基于婴儿和儿童的相似性和差异性，经过修正的九分法已经用来评估儿童烧伤的面积（图 23-5）。表 23-1 通过患者的年龄和烧伤的部位估计烧伤面积占全身体表面积的百分数。

液体复苏

开放静脉通路后就要进行迅速有效的液体复苏。对于大多数轻到中度烧伤的患者，外周静脉通路补液就已经足够，建立外周通路比较困难时可行大隐静脉切开。而在儿童，经由皮肤的股静脉穿刺置管更为简单和可靠。输注不同比例的胶体和晶体的液体复苏方法很多，Parkland 公式（每公斤体重每 1%烧伤面积输注 4ml 乳酸林格液）最为常用。但是儿童液体复苏需求必须基于体表面积而不是体重，基于体重的公式会使得轻度烧伤的患儿补液不足，而使重度烧伤的患儿总补液量过多[36]。全身体表面积可以通过标准的划线图表根据身高和体重快速估计（图 23-6）。Galveston 公式（Shriners 儿童医院）要求在烧伤后的第一个 24 小时根据每平方米烧伤面积输乳酸林格液 5000ml 加上每平方米全身体表面积输 2000ml 乳酸林格液，而且在前 8 小时内输完一半的量，剩下的一半在后 16 小时内输完（表 23-2）。 387

不管采用哪种方法，液体复苏的首要目的是恢复足够的组织器官灌注。补液需要逐渐增加以保证尿量大于 1ml/（kg·h）。对于 50%全身体表面积烧伤的患者，因为毛细血管渗透性的增加，大约有 50%的补液进入未损伤组织中，特别是在烧伤后的前 6～8 个小时[21]。在这一时期，大分子渗透进入组织间隙使得血管外胶体渗透压增高，所以在烧伤后 12 小时补液中

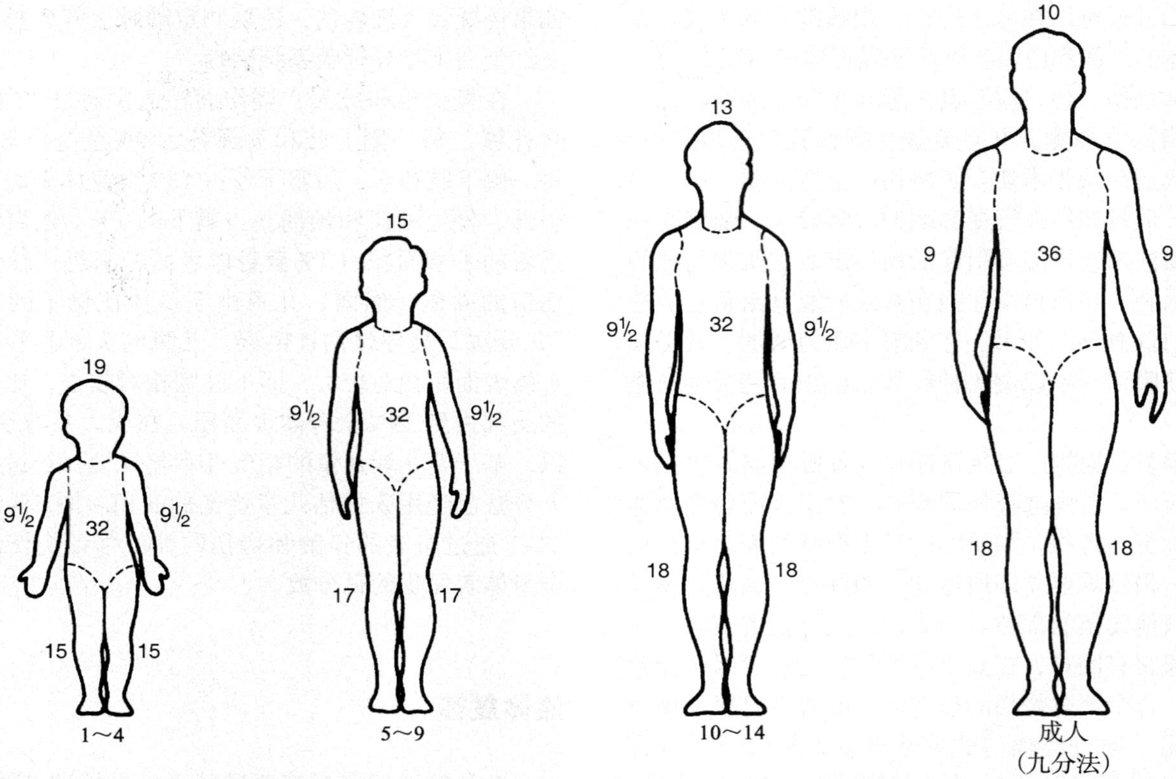

图 23-5 供儿童使用的修订的“九分法”。(From Herndon DN [ed]: Total Burn Care, 2nd ed. Philadelphia, WB Saunders, 2002, p 429.)

需要加入胶体蛋白以维持血管内渗透压。第一个 24 小时之后，每平方米烧伤面积输注 3750ml 乳酸林格液以补充由于蒸发造成的液体丢失，加上每平方米全身体表面积输注 1500ml 乳酸林格液的维持量。含有葡萄糖的液体，比如 5%的葡萄糖加上 1/4～1/2 的生理盐水可以作为补液首选。2 岁以下儿童由于糖原储备有限，对低血糖相当敏感，所以在烧伤后第一个 24 小时给予乳酸林格液的同时需要给予 5%的葡萄糖。

儿童只有在丢失了 25%以上的血容量之后临床上

表 23-1　基于年龄和烧伤部位估计的烧伤面积占全身体表面积的百分数

部位	<1 岁	1～4 岁	5～9 岁	10～14 岁	15 岁	成人
头部	19	17	13	11	9	7
颈部	2	2	2	2	2	2
腹侧躯干	13	13	13	13	13	13
背侧躯干	13	13	13	13	13	13
臀部	2.5	2.5	2.5	2.5	2.5	2.5
外生殖器	1	1	1	1	1	1
上臂	4	4	4	4	4	4
前臂	3	3	3	3	3	3
手	2.5	2.5	2.5	2.5	2.5	2.5
大腿	5.5	6.5	8	8.5	9	9.5
小腿	5	5	5.5	6	6.5	7
足	3.5	3.5	3.5	3.5	3.5	3.5

根据烧伤部位估计儿童烧伤的面积比用“九分法”更精确。

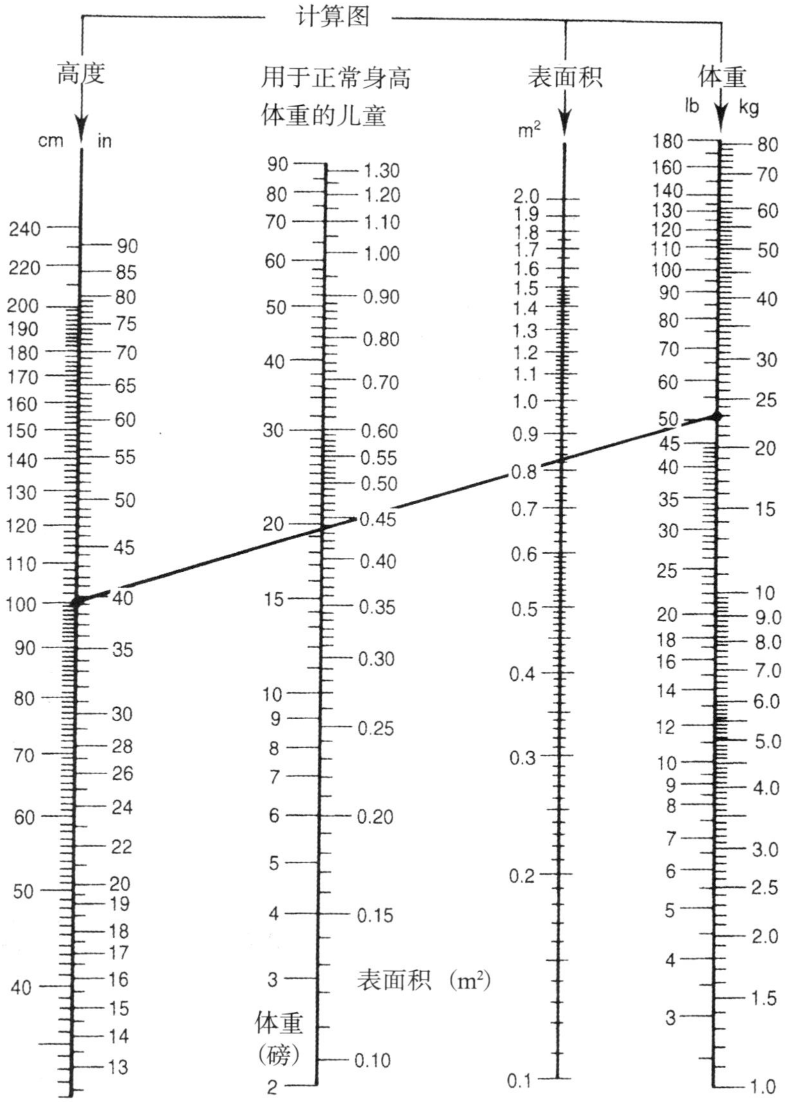

图 23-6　根据身高和体重快速估计全身体表面积的标准的划线图表。在身高和体重间连一条直线就可以获得全身体表面积，单位是 m²。

表 23-2　烧伤快速液体复苏原则

公式	第一个 24 小时	之后
Parkland	每公斤体重每 1%烧伤面积输注 4ml 乳酸林格液，一半的量在前 8 小时内输完，剩下的一半在后 16 小时内输完	5%葡萄糖和 Na^+、K^+ 以及胶体蛋白维持正常的血浆电解质和胶体渗透压
Brooke	每公斤体重每 1%烧伤面积输注 2ml 乳酸林格液（另需胶体液每公斤体重每 1%烧伤面积输注 0.5ml），一半的量在前 8 小时内输完，剩下的一半在后 16 小时内输完	持续静滴以保持每公斤体重每小时 0.5～1.0ml 的尿量
Galveston	每平方米烧伤面积输 5000ml 乳酸格林液加上每平方米全身体表面积输 2000ml 输注乳酸林格液（12 小时后每升加入胶体蛋白 12.5g），一半的量在前 8 小时内输完，剩下的一半在后 16 小时内输完	每平方米烧伤面积输 3750ml乳酸格林液加上每平方米全身体表面积输 1500ml 输注乳酸林格液；可用肠内营养配方代替静脉补液量

才会表现出低血容量的症状，但这时候已经意味着将要发生全身循环衰竭。心动过速是创伤后儿茶酚胺反应的常见表现，但也是血容量不足的代偿性反应，临床上必须警惕且绝不能忽视这一症状。儿童嗜睡、毛细血管再灌注降低、肢端湿冷时必须引起高度重视。动脉血 pH和碱缺失值也能反映液体复苏的程度。烧伤患儿经过积极的液体复苏后常常会并发低钠血症，
389 所以需要随时检测血浆电解质并给予适当的处理，不当地、过快地纠正高钠血症会引起严重的并发症，如脑桥中央髓鞘溶解[1]。

烧伤休克用高渗盐水复苏相当有效[74,96]，它能够通过渗透压差使水分从组织间隙重新吸收到血管中补充血容量，同时明显减轻组织水肿，但是这种方法并不常用，因为高渗盐水有可能导致高钠血症、血浆渗透压过高、肾衰和碱中毒[55,97]。有人建议使用复方高渗盐水——每升乳酸林格液中加入 1 安瓿小苏打——作为第一个 24 小时的液体复苏[26]。

初级急救完成并开始液体复苏后就要考虑将伤员转送到三级烧伤中心作进一步救治，那里拥有处理严重烧伤患者的有经验的多学科专家组。对于一个急性烧伤患者的治疗，除了医生和护士外，呼吸和康复治疗专家也是不能缺少的。任何可以按照美国烧伤协会的标准（表 23–3）定义为“严重烧伤”的患者都应该送往附近的烧伤中心作进一步治疗。

表 23–3 美国烧伤协会对严重烧伤的定义

- Ⅱ度和Ⅲ度烧伤总面积大于 10%全身体表面积，年龄小于 10 岁或大于 50 岁
- Ⅱ度和Ⅲ度烧伤总面积大于 20%全身体表面积，其他年龄组
- Ⅲ度面积大于 5%全身体表面积，在任何年龄组
- 脸部、手、足、外生殖器、会阴以及大关节部位的烧伤
- 严重的化学烧伤
- 严重的电灼伤，包括闪电伤
- 吸入性烧伤
- 烧伤并伴随其他严重创伤
- 烧伤并患有其他严重疾病
- 烧伤并需要特殊的社会、情感、康复上的帮助（包括怀疑儿童虐待和忽视）

局部抗菌剂

烧伤伤口的处理必须根据对伤口深度和面积准确的评估。Ⅰ度烧伤不需包扎，只需避免阳光直晒，并且局部使用止痛的膏药即可。浅Ⅱ度烧伤需要每天换药并局部应用抗菌剂，也可以简单地用油纱布或合成敷料包扎伤口，使伤口迅速地、自发地进行上皮重建。而深Ⅱ度烧伤和Ⅲ度烧伤则需要切痂和植皮。

表 23–4 列出了应用于烧伤伤口的局部抗菌剂。没有一种局部抗菌剂能够阻止藏匿在焦痂中的微生物繁殖，但能够将每克组织中的菌落总数控制在 10^2～10^5。常规伤口活检能够提示即将发生的伤口化脓以及因感染所致的植皮失败。

磺胺嘧啶银是最常用的局部抗菌剂，虽然不能穿透焦痂，但是抗菌谱广，并能减轻Ⅱ度烧伤的疼痛。可以将磺胺嘧啶银单独或与其他抗菌剂如制霉菌素一起涂在细网眼纱布上覆盖伤口，后者可以增加抗真菌的效应，明显减少烧伤患者念珠菌感染的发生[22,24]。最常见的副作用是白细胞减少症，它是由于白细胞靠边引起的，作用时间短暂[59]，当白细胞下降至 3000/mm^3 时，改用另一种局部抗菌剂可以迅速缓解

表 23–4 局部抗菌剂

局部抗菌剂	特性
磺胺嘧啶银	抗菌谱广，无痛，加强上皮生长；不能穿透焦痂，引起白细胞减少
磺胺米隆（10%乳剂或5%浸泡液）	抗菌谱广，包括假单胞菌，能穿透焦痂；对Ⅱ度伤口引起疼痛，引起代谢性酸中毒（碳酸酐酶抑制剂），影响上皮生长
0.5%硝酸银	抗菌谱广，不能穿透焦痂，接触区域色素沉着，引起低钠血症、高铁血红蛋白血症
杆菌肽 / 多链丝霉素	无痛，但抗菌谱窄
制霉菌素	抑制真菌生长；常和磺胺嘧啶银合用
莫匹罗星（百多邦）	对葡萄球菌有效
聚维酮碘	抗菌谱广，但会引起全身吸收
0.025%Dakin 溶液	几乎对所有微生物有效

这一症状。

磺胺米隆可以穿透焦痂，所以经常用于III度烧伤患者。可以将磺胺米隆（10%水溶性乳剂）涂在细网眼纱布上直接覆盖于伤口上。与磺胺嘧啶银相比，磺胺咪隆抗菌谱更广，包括假单胞菌和肠球菌。用5%的磺胺米隆溶液浸泡伤口同样有效，可以减少经常换药的麻烦。磺胺米隆是一种强有力的碳酸酐酶抑制剂，可能会引起代谢性酸中毒，要避免这一副作用，必须限制磺胺米隆的使用面积，不能超过20%全身体表面积，并且每隔几小时和另一种局部抗菌剂，如磺胺嘧啶银，交换作用部位。另外，磺胺米隆会使伤口产生刺激性疼痛，不适于门诊患者使用，特别是儿童。

除了5%的磺胺米隆溶液之外，0.5%的硝酸银和0.025%的次氯酸钠溶液（Darkin 溶液）也很有效。可以将这些溶液直接洒在覆盖伤口的纱布上，而不用频繁地换纱布而造成移植的皮肤或愈合细胞潜在性的丢失。硝酸银无痛，抗菌谱广，但是副作用包括电解质失衡（低钠血症、低氯血症）和褐色或黑色的色素沉着。一种商业上的包含有生物活性银离子（Acticoat）新的敷料既具有硝酸银的活性又可以避免其副作用。Dakin 溶液对所有微生物都有效，包括假单胞菌，但是由于次氯酸遇到蛋白质会失活，使用次数较频繁，而且还能延缓伤口的愈合[38]。

经石油提炼而得的抗菌油膏是无痛、透明的，如多粘菌素 B、杆菌肽和多链丝霉素，便于监测伤口情况。这些药物只对革兰阳性菌有效，并且不能用于脸部、小范围部分全层烧伤以及植皮时的取皮部位。和磺胺嘧啶银一样，这些药物可以和制霉菌素联合使用防止皮肤念珠菌感染。

伤口包扎

浅II度烧伤伤口的处理有很多方法。磺胺嘧啶银局部抗菌包扎最为常用，但使用人工敷料如 Biobrane（临时性皮肤替代品）和 Opsite 能够减少频繁、痛苦伤口换药以及组织、体液的丢失。这些人工产品的原理是对浅II度烧伤伤口进行无菌包扎以使伤口迅速、自发的上皮再生。

Biobrane 是一种薄的人工合成材料，内层是猪胶原蛋白包裹的尼龙，外层是橡胶处理过的硅树脂。它透气而不透水，可以呈片状或者事先做成手套状（图 23-7）[66]。将 Biobrane 铺在无菌的创可贴或敷料上，覆盖在清创后的浅II度伤口上，在 24～48 小时内，Biobrane 会与伤口紧贴。一旦 Biobrane 与伤口紧贴，伤口就直接与空气相通，开始几天要密切观察有无任何感染的征象，直到 Biobrane 下方上皮形成，Biobrane 可以直接从伤口上取下。如果 Biobrane 下方有大量液体积聚，可以用无菌的吸引针吸引积液，而如果有恶臭的液体渗出，就需要取下 Biobrane，用局部抗菌药物包扎伤口。Opsite 或 Tegaderm 也是可用来包扎浅II度伤口的人工敷料。两者由于相对便宜、使用方便以及与外界不相通，常用于外科患者术后伤口的包扎，它们透明的材质也便于对II度伤口监测。虽然没有任何生物材料（如胶原蛋白和生长因子）能加速伤口愈合，但是它们能够促进自发的上皮再生。对于小的浅II度伤口，Biobrane 和 Opsite 要优于一般局部抗菌药物包扎，特别对于门诊患者，可以减轻换药的痛苦。Transcyte 是将人类成纤维细胞培养在 Biobrane 的尼龙网上的人工敷料，也是一种选择。

人工和生物的敷料也可用于全层烧伤伤口的包扎。Integra 是一种用来处理全层烧伤伤口的人工皮肤替代品，它由胶原蛋白基质构成，外覆一层硅树脂。大约 2 周左右，胶原蛋白基质被伤口吸收后，用自体移植的表皮取代外层的硅树脂。自体取皮部位愈合较快并很少感染，而 Integra 覆盖的伤口瘢痕又较少，但是对感染较敏感，需要严密地监测。Alloderm 是另一种皮肤替代品，由脱细胞保存的尸体皮肤制成。这

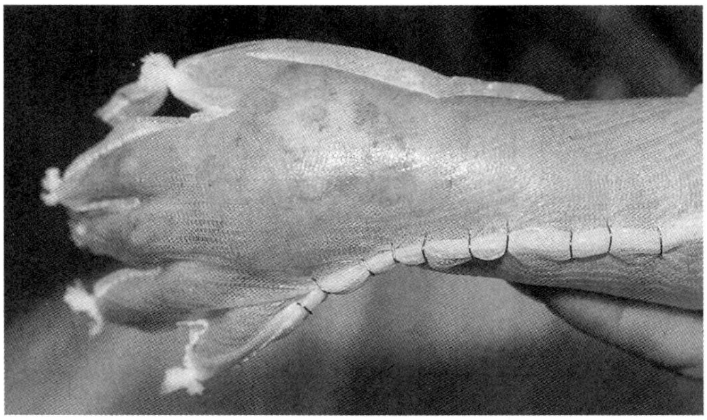

图 23-7 Biobrane 手套。Biobrane 是一种理想的浅II度烧伤伤口人工包扎材料，可以促进上皮再生，并且避免了频繁换药。

些人工皮肤替代品能够最大限度地减少瘢痕收缩，改善外观和功能预后。暂时性的伤口包扎也可以用生物敷料，如来自猪皮肤的异种移植和来自于尸体的同种异体移植。生物敷料具有正常皮肤的免疫性和屏障性功能，特别适用于大面积烧伤。异种移植或同种异体移植的区域最终会因自身免疫系统排斥而脱落，剩下的健康的移植床可供自身移植。虽然很少有报道，但同种异体移植造成的病毒传播也是个应该考虑的问题。

切痂和植皮

早期切痂和植皮能够减少术中出血、缩短住院天
391 数并最终提高烧伤患者的总体存活率[42,46]。在烧伤后的 3 天内，当患者的血流动力学稳定后，就可以对烧伤伤口焦痂进行全层切开。对烧伤深度的准确判断决定了治疗方案的实施，特别是对浅层还是深层真皮烧伤的判断，决定了烧伤伤口只需要换药处理还是需要外科切痂。切痂时，用取皮机（Watson，Weck）或刀片（Zimmer）切去焦痂，显露正常组织。早期切痂（通常烧伤后 24 小时之内）由于血管收缩因子如血栓素、儿茶酚胺的作用，可以减少失血。而如果超过 48 小时切痂，出血就相对较多，因为这时伤口已经充血。应用止血带或是皮下注射肾上腺素溶液能减少出血，但是会干扰外科医生区别有活力组织和无活力组织[70]。局部应用止血药物如凝血酶也有一定疗效，但是价格比较昂贵而且对开放性伤口的大量出血效果有限。对于深度全层烧伤，电灼术能迅速切痂而且失血较少。要再强调一点，对烧伤超过 30%全身体表面积，越早切痂失血越少[23]。然而，对于烫伤患者很难立即判断烫伤深度，就需要采用相对保守的方法而延缓切痂。

烧伤伤口切痂后，理想的方法是进行自体皮肤移植。烧伤面积小于全身体表面积 20%～30%的伤口可以通过一次分层厚皮自体移植而愈合。自体移植的分层厚皮可以通过取皮机而获得，取皮部位可以用油膏如三溴酚铋、猩红处理后包扎，也可以用 Opsite 包扎。大片自体皮肤移植可以获得长期较好的美观效果，但小片网状自体皮肤移植（1∶1 或 2∶1）能够减少取皮量，并能更好地引流植皮部位的渗出液。对于大面积烧伤患者，可以用大块自体皮肤（4∶1 或 6∶1）间隔小块同种异体皮肤（2∶1）的方法进行皮肤移植（图 23-8）。大面积烧伤患者往往需要多次植皮，等到取皮部位完全愈合后再从该部位取分层厚皮。等到自体皮肤逐渐融合时，同种异体皮肤由于排斥作用逐渐脱落，但是这一技术的缺陷是会留下明显的瘢痕。所以，这种方法不适宜应用于颜面部和有重要功能的手部。全层厚皮自体移植包括真皮和表皮结构，对伤口的愈合效果最好，既能减少瘢痕收缩，又没有明显的色素沉着。但是由于全层自体厚皮有限，目前只能用于小面积的伤口。

大面积烧伤患者全身应用重组人生长激素可以解决取皮部位少的问题。生长激素的应用能加速取皮部位愈合，增加反复取皮次数[39,44]。研究表明，生长激素能平均缩短取皮部位愈合时间 2 天左右，最终能使每 1%烧伤面积的住院时间从 0.8 天缩短到 0.54 天[39]。生长激素的这一作用可能是刺激了胰岛素样生长因子-1（IGF-1）的释放，同时诱导了烧伤伤口 IGF-1 受体的表达[44]。单独应用胰岛素也能使取皮部位愈合时间从 6.5 天缩短到 4.7 天[82]。对于那些需要多次植皮的大面积烧伤患者来说，每两次取皮之间缩短 1 天就能明显缩短住院时间。生长激素应用于烧伤儿童也能使烧伤面积占 80%全身体表面积的儿童总住院费用节省 23%[39]。

最近，用培养自身皮肤角质细胞的方法来解决大面积烧伤患者取皮部位少的问题引人关注[31,86,91]。将培养的皮肤移植到烧伤伤口的方法尚存在争议，在广泛应用之前，还有一些问题有待解决。角质细胞的生长相当缓慢，而且即使移植成功，也非常容易受到机械性创伤，只有约 50%～70%可以存活。最近一项报告指出，烧伤面积大于 80%全身体表面积时用常规治疗

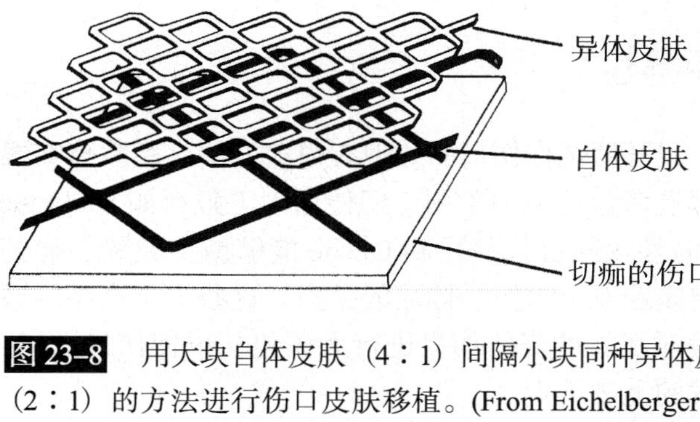

图 23-8 用大块自体皮肤（4∶1）间隔小块同种异体皮肤（2∶1）的方法进行伤口皮肤移植。(From Eichelberger MR [ed]: Pediatric Trauma: Prevention, Acute Care, Rehabilitation. St Louis, Mosby,1993, p 581.)

方法要比用移植培养皮肤的方法住院时间更短[4]，但是这种新技术仍是处理大面积烧伤患者有潜力并值得期待的方法。

高代谢反应

烧伤患者代谢率明显增高。对烧伤患者高代谢反应的认识是过去 30 年中大面积烧伤患者死亡率下降的重要原因之一。高代谢反应包括能量消耗、氧耗、蛋白水解、脂肪水解和氮丢失的增加，代谢率随着烧伤面积的增加而增加，但在 40%全身体表面积的烧伤患者中有一个瓶颈期[43]。高代谢反应是由于促分解代谢的因子如可的松、儿茶酚胺和胰高血糖素的上调而引起的，它们协同增加血糖含量，作为急性炎症期的主要能量来源[89]。可的松刺激糖原异生和蛋白水解，并增加脂肪细胞对脂肪水解激素的敏感性；儿茶酚胺促进肝糖原异生和糖原分解，也促使脂肪水解和外周胰岛素抵抗，后者可以使细胞对血清胰岛素水平的增高产生抵抗作用[58]；胰高血糖素的增加刺激了儿茶酚胺的分泌，进一步促进了糖原异生。

严重烧伤患者中常会有明显的蛋白分解现象。可的松的分解作用可以导致组织蛋白的丢失和负氮平衡。同时，烧伤使得促合成代谢激素如生长激素和 IGF-1 的水平下降，使蛋白合成减少。参与免疫反应的蛋白（也是伤口愈合时胶原形成的必需原料）、抗体和白细胞的生成需要保持正氮平衡。患者烧伤后分泌过多的儿茶酚胺也会造成心动过速和脂肪分解，这可能会导致心衰和肝脏脂肪浸润。

烧伤后生长激素和 IGF-1 水平降低，而烧伤后的药物介入能够减轻分解作用并刺激生长[77]。生长激素、胰岛素、IGF-1、IGF 相关蛋白-3、睾酮和氧雄龙可改善氮平衡并促进伤口愈合[28,37,47,82,99]。使用外源性重组人生长激素可以增加蛋白质合成，改善氮平衡，保持肌肉量并促进伤口愈合[44,98]。生长激素的促合成代谢作用主要是增加蛋白质合成，而 IGF-1 的作用主要是减少蛋白质降解。生长激素也可以通过刺激肝脏和局部组织分泌 IGF-1 增加全身和局部的血液循环来促进伤口的愈合[39]。严重烧伤后血浆生长激素往往会降低，给予严重烧伤患儿重组人生长激素 [0.2mg/(kg·d)]后可以提高血浆生长激素水平，加速取皮部位的伤口愈合，而且住院时间也缩短 25%以上（图 23-9）[34]。对严重烧伤患儿注射重组人生长激素是安全有效的，给予生长激素后严重烧伤患儿在住院期间仍能保持生长[83]，与对照组相比，给予生长激素组的患儿在烧伤后的头 2 年生长速度有所提高。重组人生长激素通过上调 IGF-1 也能刺激骨质形成和肌肉蛋白合成，有效减少肌肉分解和骨质丢失[63]。

对严重烧伤患者给予次于最大剂量的胰岛素可以刺激肌肉蛋白合成，促进肌肉合成代谢。胰岛素同样也能加强取皮部位的愈合和伤口基质的形成[27]。严重烧伤患者睾酮的合成量明显降低，这在成年人中会持续几个月的时间。给患者注射睾酮后可以加强机体对裂解到细胞间隙氨基酸的重新利用，促进氨基酸向细胞内转移，从而增加蛋白合成。维持严重烧伤成人的睾酮水平在正常生理范围可以使净蛋白合成增加[28]。氧雄龙是一种雄化作用较弱的睾酮类似物，已经应用于急性期和恢复期的成年烧伤患者，以期获得正常体重增加。单独应用氧雄龙可以有效加强蛋白合成，增

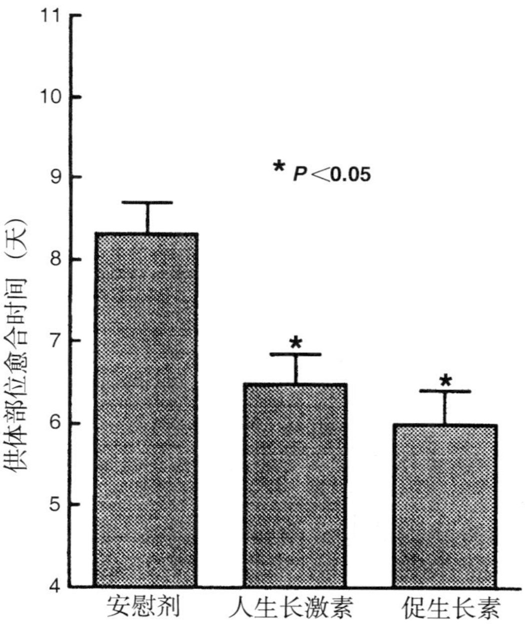

图 23-9 在给予安慰剂（生理盐水，n=26）和重组人生长激素组（人生长激素，0.2mg/(kg·d)，n = 20；促生长素，0.2mg/(kg·d)，n = 20）之间比较取皮部位愈合时间。与对照组相比，任一形式的重组人生长激素都能使平均愈合时间明显缩短（平均值 ± SEM，*$P<0.05$）。(From Gilpin DA, Barrow RE, Rutan RL, et al: Recombinant human growth hormone accelerates wound healing in children with large cutaneous burns. Ann Surg 1994;220:19.)

加严重烧伤患儿肌肉蛋白代谢[90]。

β-受体阻断药普萘洛尔能够在不影响心排出量和机体对冷应激反应的同时减缓心率[14,25,54]、减轻左心室工作负荷、减少外周脂肪代谢并维持去脂体重[7]。最近，对住院治疗的烧伤儿童的研究表明使用β-受体阻断药普萘洛尔可以减弱高代谢反应并可逆转肌肉蛋白的分解代谢（图 23-10）[43]。普萘洛尔起始给予标准剂量[1.98mg/（kg·d）]，维持期要使心率从基础心率大约降低 20%。两周的治疗后，对照组患者在静息状态下的能量消耗和氧耗已经明显上升，而普萘洛尔组这些指标却有显著下降。同时随着能量消耗的降低，β 受体阻断药也能改善骨骼肌蛋白的动力学情
393 况。肌肉蛋白的净平衡与治疗前的基本水平相比增加了 82%，而在对照组这一水平下降了 27%[43]。另外，普萘洛尔和生长激素均有利于改善心血管功能，减少

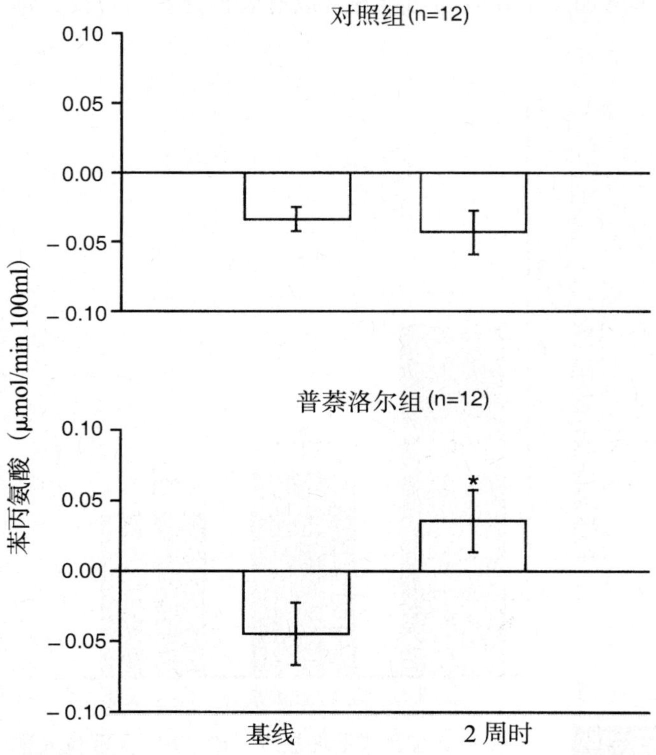

图 23-10 普萘洛尔治疗 2 周后肌肉蛋白合成和分解代谢平衡的平均基线改变。数值通过对同位素标记的苯丙氨酸的 5 小时动力学研究获得。星号（*）表示两组间存在显著性差异（t 检验 $P = 0.001$）以及治疗前后存在显著性差异（配对 t 检验 $P = 0.002$）。(From Herndon DN, Hart DW, Wolf SE, et al: Reversal of catabolism by beta-blockade after severe burns. N Engl J Med 2001;345:1223.)

脂肪组织游离脂肪酸的释放，增加肝脏处理游离脂肪酸和极低密度脂蛋白的能力。普萘洛尔同时也能减少烧伤患儿的外周脂肪分解和肝脏的脂肪沉积[43]。

酮康唑是激素类环状化合物合成阻滞剂，能阻断可的松的合成，具有调节高代谢反应的作用。但是在为了预防溃疡而使胃内 pH 接近中性的患者中，酮康唑很难被吸收。而且我们发现，即使克服了这一问题，口服酮康唑也不能对代谢率或蛋白合成产生很大影响（尚未公布数据）。胰岛素、普萘洛尔和氧雄龙是处理创伤后高代谢反应性价比最高的药物，同时营养支持虽然经常被忽视，但是对创伤后高代谢反应也有明确的作用。

营养

烧伤面积占 25%全身体表面积的患者代谢率增加约 1.5 倍，烧伤面积占 40%全身体表面积的患者代谢率增加约 2 倍[35]，儿童由于脂肪比例小，肌肉量少，当代谢率增加时更易造成蛋白质-热量缺乏性营养不良，从而导致多系统的功能障碍，包括免疫系统功能障碍和伤口愈合延迟。所以，必须给予患者最佳的营养支持以保持并改善患者重要器官的功能。在最初的烧伤评估后就应立即在荧光透视引导下给患者放置胃管，创伤后几小时内就应开始肠内营养。早期的肠内营养能够减少分解代谢激素的水平，改善氮平衡，保持消化道黏膜完整，减少总住院天数[15,73,88]。虽然超高营养能够提供更多的热量，但是对烧伤患者使用超高营养会损害免疫系统，而且使小肠黏膜萎缩，增加细菌移位的机会，最终导致生存率下降[41,48]。肠内营养通常优于肠外营养，能降低烧伤患者的代谢率，减少脓毒症的发生。

计算烧伤患者热量需求有很多公式。Curreri 公式（25kcal/kg + 40kcal/1%烧伤面积）和修正的 Harris-Benedict 公式（静息代谢率 × 损伤因素）遵循基本热卡需求加上与烧伤面积相关的额外热量需求的原则。与液体复苏原则相似，对烧伤儿童的热量计算应该基于患儿的全身以及烧伤部位的面积而不是基于患儿的体重（表 23-5）[50-52]。烧伤患者确切的营养需求尚不明确，但是获得足够的能量需求以及补充蛋白丢失无疑是重要的。推荐的肠内营养热量构成比是 20%～40%来自于蛋白质，10%～20%来自于脂肪，40%～

表 23-5 烧伤患儿的热量需求（Shriners 烧伤医院，Galveston）

年龄组	每日所需热卡
婴幼儿	2100kcal/m^2（全身体表面积）+ 1000kcal/m^2（烧伤面积）
儿童	1800kcal/m^2（全身体表面积）+ 1300kcal/m^2（烧伤面积）
青春期	1500kcal/m^2（全身体表面积）+ 1500kcal/m^2（烧伤面积）

70%来自于糖类。牛奶是最经济也最易耐受的营养来源，但是同时必须增加 Na^+的供给以防止稀释性低钠血症。还有各种商业性的肠内营养公式，如 Vivonex
394 公式和 PediaSure 公式。

药物治疗

镇痛治疗

烧伤伤口的处理和康复治疗都可能给几乎所有的患者带来生理上的疼痛。婴儿和儿童不会像成人一样表达疼痛，而往往表现为恐惧、焦虑、激动、发怒、情绪低落和退缩。允许年长儿童参与自己的伤口治疗能够使他们有一种可控制感，减轻恐惧和痛苦。多种镇痛药和抗焦虑药的组合已经在烧伤治疗和伤口换药的过程中使用（表 23-6）。要成功处理烧伤患儿的疼痛，首先要使患儿知道疼痛与烧伤的深度有关，并且是伤口愈合的征象。制定镇痛治疗计划时必须包括治疗持续性疼痛和治疗过程中相关的刺激性疼痛。物理治疗对获得最佳的预后和功能的恢复相当重要，在镇痛治疗的同时应给予患者有效的物理治疗。但是，需要注意的是运动治疗中必须避免过度运动导致的潜在性并发症的发生。对于大约 5 岁左右的儿童，最好的止痛方法是控制患者止痛法，给予持续性静脉滴注镇静剂，并口服镇痛药物[71]。烧伤对于患儿和他的家庭来说都是一个很大的打击，烧伤治疗专家在帮助烧伤患者走向康复的时候必须竭尽所能地使这一个过程更容易承受。

表 23-6 药物疗法使用的剂量

药物	剂量	适应证
硫酸吗啡	0.05～0.1mg/kg iv.或 0.3mg/kg po.	急性疼痛、处理及换药痛
哌替啶（度冷丁）	1.0～2.0mg/kg po. 或 iv.	急性疼痛、处理及换药痛
氯胺酮	1.0～2.0mg/kg iv. 或 5.0～7.0mg/kg im.	手术、处理及换药痛
安定	1.0～2.0mg/kg po. 或 iv.	术前、焦虑
水合氯醛	250～500mg po.	术前、失眠
咪达唑仑	0.25～0.5mg/kg po. 或 iv.	焦虑、与镇静药物合用
劳拉西泮	0.03mg/kg po. 或 iv.	焦虑

镇静剂和抗焦虑剂

氯胺酮是烧伤患者常用的镇静性麻醉药物，是苯环己哌啶的衍生物，具有分离麻醉的特点，并有很好的镇痛效果。给药方式可以是 1.0～2.0mg/kg 静脉给药或 5.0～7.0mg/kg 肌内注射，氯胺酮起效快，但是作用持续时间相对较短。另外，氯胺酮经常用于手术麻醉，没有呼吸道反射影响。氯胺酮严禁使用于颅内压增高的患者。

苯二氮䓬类药物经常用于控制烧伤后焦虑和增加镇痛药物的镇痛效果。劳拉西泮（Ativan）是一种有效的抗焦虑药，一般 0.03mg/kg 口服或静脉给药，同时它也是一种有效的安眠药，能改善急性期患者的睡眠。安定（Valium）持续时间较劳拉西泮长，更适用于慢性期患者，同时能够增加肌肉放松程度，有利于康复治疗。咪达唑仑（Versed）起效快，30 分钟达到血浆峰值，半衰期在 2～5 小时，经常用来作为一般处理及伤口换药时的镇静剂，同时由于它会导致顺行性遗忘，经常在手术当天使用。

抗生素

在手术期间静脉使用四代抗生素在过去 20 年中大大提高了严重烧伤患者的生存率。寄居在焦痂中的细菌在切痂过程中有可能会发生全身性的转移，导致脓毒症或是其他器官的感染。对于烧伤面积超过 40%全身体表面积的患者手术期间经验性地静脉给予第四代广谱抗生素（如万古霉素、三代头孢菌素和青霉素）能够有效抵抗链球菌、金黄色葡萄球菌和假单胞菌的感染，在这之后通过对切除的焦痂上细菌的药物敏感性检查来调整抗生素的用药。在急性期，一般主要的感染细菌为革兰阳性球菌，革兰阴性菌感染甚至是真菌感染一般见于慢性期伤口，这些伤口在切痂和植皮时必须同时静脉给予四代抗生素。除了烧伤伤口脓毒症，植皮时伤口存在感染以及术后短期移植床的细菌污染还会导致移植失败。最常见的导致移植失败的细菌是乙型溶血性链球菌（化脓性链球菌、无乳链球菌或草绿色链球菌），它们对三代头孢和喹诺酮类敏感。多重耐药细菌的出现，如耐甲氧西林金葡菌，已经成为令烧伤中心头痛的问题。所以，必须重视静脉使用四代抗生素，但只用于手术期间并且首先得明确有感染源存在。

吸入性损伤

吸入性损伤是烧伤患者的主要死因之一。儿童皮肤烧伤的死亡率在1%～2%，但如果同时并发有吸入
395 性损伤，这一比例就立刻上升到40%左右[49,92]。吸入性损伤主要是由吸入性毒素如毒烟、毒气和毒雾引起的。虽然声门上区可同时被热和化学物质烧伤，但是由于热量过了喉部之后就迅速减少，气管支气管以及肺实质很少有直接热源烧伤。损伤上皮释放的一些作用于血管的物质（血栓素 A_2，C_{3a} 和 C_{5a}）可以导致缺氧、呼吸道梗阻增加、肺顺应性降低、肺泡上皮通透性增加和肺血管阻力增加[93]。在这一过程中，中性粒细胞起了相当关键的作用，如果使用配体结合内皮细胞选择素（阻滞中性粒细胞黏附）和抗白介素-8（阻滞中性粒细胞趋化）就可以使呼吸功能得到改善。呼吸道的另一个重要病理改变是纤毛上皮细胞从基底层脱落，导致渗出物形成。这些常由淋巴蛋白组成的渗出物可以融合形成纤维假膜，造成呼吸道阻力增加，并对损伤区域下方的肺组织产生一种“活瓣”作用，最终导致气压性损伤。

对吸入性损伤的诊断是在最初评估时根据病史和体检得出的。屋内着火时患者困在充满浓烟和毒气的屋子里就有可能存在严重的吸入性损伤；脸部烧伤、头发烧焦以及吐出焦炭色的痰均提示有吸入性损伤的存在；声嘶和喘鸣提示明显的呼吸道梗阻，需要立即行气管内插管；患者如果出现定向力障碍和反应迟钝则有可能是一氧化碳水平增高所致（碳氧血红蛋白＞10%）。常见家具燃烧引起的氰化物中毒也能导致不明原因的代谢衰竭。支气管镜检查和氙-133扫描在诊断吸入性损伤中可以达到90%的准确率。床边导光纤维支气管镜呼吸道检查（避免将严重烧伤患者搬动到核医学检查室）可以诊断呼吸道水肿和气管黏膜的炎症改变，如充血、黏膜溃疡和黏膜脱落，仍然是诊断吸入性损伤的金标准[56]。氙-133通气扫描通过评估气体交换情况和肺对氙的排泄情况也能显示吸入性损伤的区域[76]。

烧伤发生后就应该立即对吸入性损伤进行处理。迅速给予100%纯氧能够缩短一氧化碳的半衰期。如果患者出现危急的呼吸衰竭征象就必须迅速通过气管插管开放气道，进行积极的呼吸系统物理治疗以及反复吸痰对防止严重的呼吸系统并发症至关重要。用高流量的湿化气体、支气管扩张药和外消旋肾上腺素解除支气管痉挛，用肝素静脉滴注减少气管支气管假膜形成，改善分钟通气量，降低烟吸入后的最大吸气压力。给予20%乙酰半胱氨酸雾化剂（每4小时3ml）和肝素雾化剂（5000～10 000U溶于3ml生理盐水，每4小时1次）吸入治疗可以有效清除气管支气管分泌物，缓解支气管痉挛，并显著降低再插管率和死亡率[10,62]。

有吸入性损伤存在时，患者的液体复苏一般需要增加液体量，大约在相同程度烧伤的基本补液量上每1%TBSA烧伤每公斤体重再增加2ml。事实上，吸入性损伤导致肺水肿后并不限制补液量，相反，液体补充不足会引起多核细胞的螯合从而加重肺损伤。类固醇被认为对吸入性损伤无效。一般不建议预防性静脉给予抗生素，除非怀疑有肺炎存在。早期肺炎一般是由革兰阳性菌如耐甲氧西林金葡菌引起的，而后期的感染一般是由革兰阴性菌如假单胞菌引起。痰培养和支气管冲洗检查可以指导抗生素的使用。

非热源性烧伤

化学烧伤

儿童经常意外地接触到各种家庭的清洁用品引起化学性烧伤。处理化学性烧伤包括迅速移除化学药

剂，用大量清水冲洗伤口，防止低体温和确保未烧伤区域不再接触污染的液体，同时液体复苏也应相应进行。冲洗伤口不能在木桶内进行，而应该像淋浴一样用水管来冲洗。大量清水冲洗伤口后，伤口敷上局部抗菌剂并包扎，同时制定出适当的外科处理计划。鉴别出致伤的化学药剂对烧伤的治疗相当重要[29]，不能确定致伤药剂时，就需要当地的毒物控制中心参与鉴别药剂的化学组成。

常见的化学药剂可以分为碱类和酸类。碱类，如石灰、氢氧化钾、氢氧化钠和漂白剂，是最容易引起化学烧伤的化学药剂。碱性化学药剂烧伤的主要机制是脂肪的皂化作用，产生的热量进一步损伤细胞，使细胞内水分丢失，并使蛋白和 OH^-结合形成碱性蛋白盐。OH^-还能引起深部组织的进一步化学反应。试图中和碱性是不可取的，因为中和反应会产生更多的热量加重组织损伤。酸性化学药剂烧伤比较少见一些，酸类主要是通过水解作用降解蛋白质，并形成焦痂，所以穿透力不如碱性化学药剂强。甲酸烧伤比较罕见
396 但可以引起多系统的损伤，如代谢性酸中毒、肾衰、血管内溶血和急性呼吸衰竭综合征。氢氟酸烧伤的处理和其他酸性化学药剂烧伤的处理不同[94]。除了用大量清水冲洗伤口外，还需要用 2.5%的葡萄糖酸钙凝胶中和 F^-，否则游离的 F^-能引起组织污染，包括骨骼的液化性坏死。由于可能有低钙血症的危险，伤员需要心电监测有无 QT 间期延长。

电灼伤

儿童电灼伤比较少见，大约占所有收治的烧伤患者的 3%～5%。电灼伤可以分为高压电伤和低压电伤[50]。高压电伤的特点是局部烧伤的程度不同，同时有深部组织的破坏[65,84]。电流从身体一端进入后几乎没有阻力地穿透一些组织，如神经、血管和肌肉，当经过一些阻力相对较高的深部组织，如骨骼，就会产生热量并破坏附近的组织，然而这种损伤并不能从外表看到。皮肤由于对电流的高阻力，往往最容易被灼伤。对电灼伤也应该完成包括心电图在内的两次检查。如果即刻心电图正常，就不需要进一步的心电监护，而如果出现异常情况就需要持续心电监护 48 小时，并及时处理心律失常[85]。

处理电灼伤的关键是对损伤的早期诊断和对深部损伤组织的处理。四肢的水肿和血管反应比较常见，为了避免截肢经常需要做筋膜切开减压。如果尿液中出现肌红蛋白，就需要大量水化并用碳酸氢钠碱化尿液，同时用甘露醇利尿并可作为自由基清除剂。在伤口最终愈合前，需要反复进行伤口探查和清创，因为伤口内会有延迟死亡的细胞和血栓形成。电灼伤损伤细胞的过程可以在毫伏或毫安的水平，所以在即刻创伤中存活下来的细胞也会在接下来的一周时间内由于离子的梯度变性和微血管内血栓形成而逐渐死亡。电灼伤也可能仅仅为热烧伤，而没有传导性烧伤，如电火花灼伤，这种灼伤可以像一般的热烧伤一样处理。低压电伤与一般的热烧伤相似，没有电流向深部组织的传导，一般只需要局部伤口的护理。

门诊烧伤患者

大多数儿童烧伤比较轻微，经常是小于全身体表面积 10%的烫伤或者是接触热的物体后引起的小面积烫伤。这种烧伤一般是浅层的皮肤伤，可以在门诊处理。经过最初的伤情评估，烧伤伤口用水和软肥皂清洗，尽量减少疼痛。水泡，特别是手掌的水泡，如果比较小而且不容易自发破裂的话，尽量保持水泡的完整，因为这对外界环境形成一个天然的屏障，并可避免每天换药，大约 1 周之后随着上皮的再生液体会自发地被重吸收。大面积的水泡需要清创，并敷上局部抗菌剂包扎。磺胺嘧啶银由于广谱抗菌作用和对浅 II 度烧伤伤口的刺激性小，应用最为广泛。但是因为磺胺嘧啶银能够阻碍上皮再生，所以当浅层伤口中已经没有坏死组织并且有上皮再生迹象的时候就要停止磺胺嘧啶银的使用。另外，局部抗菌剂还可以选择三重抗菌软膏（新霉素、杆菌肽和多粘菌素 B 硫酸盐）或者多链丝霉素，后者对上皮再生没有影响。对于小的、浅表性烧伤，用非药物作用的白色凡士林浸渍细网或者多孔纱布（Adaptic）或者浸渍有 3%三溴铋的凡士林细网吸收纱布（Xeroform）包扎就能起到很好的效果，而不需要局部抗菌剂。脸部的浅表性烧伤可以涂以三重抗菌软膏，而不需要包扎。

换药的频率从 2 次 / 天到 1 次 / 周不等，主要看伤口的大小、深度，以及渗出的多少。那些应用了局部抗菌剂，且局部抗菌剂的半衰期在 8～12 小时的伤口换药需要 2 次 / 天，另一些用凡士林或者铋剂浸渍

的纱布包扎的伤口可以减少换药频率——一般 3～5 天一次。人工合成敷料应用于门诊浅表性烧伤的患者是非常理想的[33]，用 Biobrane 包扎干净的浅层伤口后能迅速与伤口黏附，并在 1～2 周内促进伤口的上皮再生（见图 23-7）。Biobrane 包扎的伤口虽然减少了换药的次数，但是仍然要密切监视伤口的感染情况。

康复

急性期治疗

康复治疗是烧伤治疗的基本内容之一。在烧伤的急性期，要用夹板保护患者关节，防止关节变形和挛缩。这种夹板由热塑性材料制成，对热处理具有可塑性，适用于任何一个患者。大面积烧伤的患者整个急性期都要用夹板固定关节，防止关节挛缩，只有到了活动期才可以脱离夹板。患者在植皮后就应该下床活
397 动，并作进一步的物理治疗。

急性期之后，巨大瘢痕的形成是主要的问题。伤口深度、患者年龄以及遗传因素对巨大的瘢痕形成都有很大影响。一般来说，深Ⅱ度烧伤伤口需要 3 周或更长的时间才能愈合，且留下巨大的瘢痕。大概是由于随着生长发育进行的细胞高频有丝分裂，儿童往往比成人更容易形成巨大瘢痕。对伤口 24 小时持续加压是减小巨大瘢痕形成的最有效的方法，在瘢痕成熟之前，可以给患者穿上加压的外衣对伤口加压。瘢痕成熟一般在烧伤后 6～18 个月，在儿童中，瘢痕成熟的速度会更慢。除了夹板和加压外衣，运动治疗也是康复治疗重要的一部分，医生必须建议患者家属制定一项整个活动范围的运动和肌肉训练计划。

长期治疗

烧伤幸存者及其家属都需要长期进行机体上和心理上的康复治疗，必须应对情感从愧疚到创伤后应激的变化。在一项研究中，一组外科医生随访了 12 例全身体表面积 80%以上烧伤和 70%Ⅲ度烧伤的幸存儿童，并对他们对烧伤瘢痕的态度和对未来就业的期望进行了预测。结果表明，所有患者肯定心理上难以适应，很多患者会要求反复的整形手术[45]。事实上，虽然这些患者中很多进行了两次或以上的手术，但是有 3/4 表现出正常的心理适应和情感发育，这项纵向研究进行了 10 年以后，这些儿童的心理评分与未烧伤儿童的心理评分相同。这些幸存者并没有严重的心理问题和社会障碍，体现出了人类惊人的恢复力。

（张　震译　吴晔明校）

参考文献

1. Ayus JC, Arieff AI: Hyponatremia and myelinolysis. Ann Intern Med 1997;127:163.
2. Baptiste MS, Feck G: Preventing tap water burns. Am J Public Health 1980;70:727.
3. Barillo DJ, Goode R: Fire fatality study: Demographics of fire victims. Burns 1996;22:85.
4. Barret JP, Wolf SE, Desai MH, et al: Cost-efficacy of cultured epidermal autografts in massive pediatric burns. Ann Surg 2000;231:869.
5. Bjerknes R, Vindenes H, Laerum OD: Altered neutrophil functions in patients with large burns. Blood Cells 1990; 16:127.
6. Bjerknes R, Vindenes H, Pitkanen J, et al: Altered polymorphonuclear neutrophilic granulocyte functions in patients with large burns. J Trauma 1989;29:847.
7. Breitenstein E, Chiolero RL, Jequier E, et al: Effects of beta-blockade on energy metabolism following burns. Burns 1990;16:259.
8. Brigham PA, McLoughlin E: Burn incidence and medical care use in the United States: Estimates, trends, and data sources. J Burn Care Rehabil 1996;17:95.
9. Brink JA, Sheets PW, Dines KA, et al: Quantitative assessment of burn injury in porcine skin with high-frequency ultrasonic imaging. Invest Radiol 1986;21:645.
10. Brown M, Desai M, Traber LD, et al: Dimethylsulfoxide with heparin in the treatment of smoke inhalation injury. J Burn Care Rehabil 1988;9:22.
11. Bucky LP, Vedder NB, Hong HZ, et al: Reduction of burn injury by inhibiting CD18-mediated leukocyte adherence in rabbits. Plast Reconstr Surg 1994;93:1473.
12. Burn Injury Fact Sheet. Washington, DC, National Safe Kids Campaign; 2004.
13. Carter EA, Gonnella A, Tompkins RG: Increased transcellular permeability of rat small intestine after thermal injury. Burns 1992;18:117.
14. Chance WT, Nelson JL, Foley-Nelson T, et al: The relationship of burn-induced hypermetabolism to central and peripheral catecholamines. J Trauma 1989;29:306.
15. Chiarelli A, Enzi G, Casadei A, et al: Very early nutrition supplementation in burned patients. Am J Clin Nutr 1990; 51:1035.
16. Chung DH, Evers BM, Townsend CM Jr, et al: Burn-induced transcriptional regulation of small intestinal ornithine decarboxylase. Am J Surg 1992;163:157.
17. Chung DH, Evers BM, Townsend CM Jr, et al: Role of polyamine biosynthesis during gut mucosal adaptation after burn injury. Am J Surg 1993;165:144.
18. Cope O, Moore FD: The redistribution of body water. Ann

Surg 1947;126:1016.
19. DelBeccaro EJ, Robson MC, Heggers JP, et al: The use of specific thromboxane inhibitors to preserve the dermal microcirculation after burning. Surgery 1980;87:137.
20. Demling RH, LaLonde C: Early postburn lipid peroxidation: Effect of ibuprofen and allopurinol. Surgery 1990; 107:85.
21. Demling RH, Mazess RB, Witt RM, et al: The study of burn wound edema using dichromatic absorptiometry. J Trauma 1978;18:124.
22. Desai MH, Herndon DN: Eradication of *Candida* burn wound septicemia in massively burned patients. J Trauma 1988;28:140.
23. Desai MH, Herndon DN, Broemeling L, et al: Early burn wound excision significantly reduces blood loss. Ann Surg 1990;211:753.
24. Desai MH, Rutan RL, Heggers JP, et al: *Candida* infection with and without nystatin prophylaxis: An 11-year experience with patients with burn injury. Arch Surg 1992; 127:159.
25. Drost AC, Burleson DG, Cioffi WG Jr, et al: Plasma cytokines following thermal injury and their relationship with patient mortality, burn size, and time postburn. J Trauma 1993;35:335.
26. Du GB, Slater H, Goldfarb IW: Influences of different resuscitation regimens on acute early weight gain in extensively burned patients. Burns 1991;17:147.
27. Ferrando AA, Chinkes DL, Wolf SE, et al: A submaximal dose of insulin promotes net skeletal muscle protein synthesis in patients with severe burns. Ann Surg 1999;229:11.
28. Ferrando AA, Sheffield-Moore M, Wolf SE, et al: Testosterone administration in severe burns ameliorates muscle catabolism. Crit Care Med 2001;29:1936.
29. Fitzpatrick KT, Moylan JA: Emergency care of chemical burns. Postgrad Med 1985;78:189.
30. Fox CL Jr, Rappole BW, Stanford W: Control of *Pseudomonas* infection in burns by silver sulfadiazine. Surg Gynecol Obstet 1969;128:1021.
31. Gallico GG 3rd, O'Connor NE, Compton CC, et al: Permanent coverage of large burn wounds with autologous cultured human epithelium. N Engl J Med 1984;311:448.
32. Gamelli RL, He LK, Liu H: Macrophage suppression of granulocyte and macrophage growth following burn wound infection. J Trauma 1994;37:888.
33. Gerding RL, Emerman CL, Effron D, et al: Outpatient management of partial-thickness burns: Biobrane versus 1% silver sulfadiazine. Ann Emerg Med 1990;19:121.
34. Gilpin DA, Barrow RE, Rutan RL, et al: Recombinant human growth hormone accelerates wound healing in children with large cutaneous burns. Ann Surg 1994; 220:19.
35. Goran MI, Peters EJ, Herndon DN, et al: Total energy expenditure in burned children using the doubly labeled water technique. Am J Physiol 1990;259(4 Pt 1):E576.
36. Graves TA, Cioffi WG, McManus WF, et al: Fluid resuscitation of infants and children with massive thermal injury. J Trauma 1988;28:1656.
37. Hart DW, Wolf SE, Ramzy PI, et al: Anabolic effects of oxandrolone after severe burn. Ann Surg 2001;233:556.
38. Heggers JP, Sazy JA, Stenberg BD, et al: Bactericidal and wound-healing properties of sodium hypochlorite solutions: The 1991 Lindberg Award. J Burn Care Rehabil 1991; 12:420.
39. Herndon DN, Barrow RE, Kunkel KR, et al: Effects of recombinant human growth hormone on donor-site healing in severely burned children. Ann Surg 1990;212:424.
40. Herndon DN, Barrow RE, Linares HA, et al: Inhalation injury in burned patients: Effects and treatment. Burns Incl Therm Inj 1988;14:349.
41. Herndon DN, Barrow RE, Stein M, et al: Increased mortality with intravenous supplemental feeding in severely burned patients. J Burn Care Rehabil 1989;10:309.
42. Herndon DN, Gore D, Cole M, et al: Determinants of mortality in pediatric patients with greater than 70% full-thickness total body surface area thermal injury treated by early total excision and grafting. J Trauma 1987;27:208.
43. Herndon DN, Hart DW, Wolf SE, et al: Reversal of catabolism by beta-blockade after severe burns. N Engl J Med 2001;345:1223.
44. Herndon DN, Hawkins HK, Nguyen TT, et al: Characterization of growth hormone enhanced donor site healing in patients with large cutaneous burns. Ann Surg 1995;221:649.
45. Herndon DN, LeMaster J, Beard S, et al: The quality of life after major thermal injury in children: An analysis of 12 survivors with greater than or equal to 80% total body, 70% third-degree burns. J Trauma 1986;26:609.
46. Herndon DN, Parks DH: Comparison of serial debridement and autografting and early massive excision with cadaver skin overlay in the treatment of large burns in children. J Trauma 1986;26:149.
47. Herndon DN, Ramzy PI, DebRoy MA, et al: Muscle protein catabolism after severe burn: Effects of IGF-1/IGFBP-3 treatment. Ann Surg 1999;229:713.
48. Herndon DN, Stein MD, Rutan TC, et al: Failure of TPN supplementation to improve liver function, immunity, and mortality in thermally injured patients. J Trauma 1987;27:195.
49. Herndon DN, Thompson PB, Traber DL: Pulmonary injury in burned patients. Crit Care Clin 1985;1:79.
50. Hildreth MA, Herndon DN, Desai MH, et al: Caloric needs of adolescent patients with burns. J Burn Care Rehabil 1989;10:523.
51. Hildreth MA, Herndon DN, Desai MH, et al: Current treatment reduces calories required to maintain weight in pediatric patients with burns. J Burn Care Rehabil 1990;11:405.
52. Hildreth MA, Herndon DN, Desai MH, et al: Caloric requirements of patients with burns under one year of age. J Burn Care Rehabil 1993;14:108.
53. Ho-Asjoe M, Chronnell CM, Frame JD, et al: Immunohistochemical analysis of burn depth. J Burn Care Rehabil 1999;20:207.
54. Honeycutt D, Barrow R, Herndon D: Cold stress response in patients with severe burns after beta-blockade. J Burn Care Rehabil 1992;13(2 Pt 1):181.
55. Huang PP, Stucky FS, Dimick AR, et al: Hypertonic sodium resuscitation is associated with renal failure and death. Ann Surg 1995;221:543.
56. Hunt JL, Agee RN, Pruitt BA Jr: Fiberoptic bronchoscopy in acute inhalation injury. J Trauma 1975;15:641.
57. Hunt JP, Hunter CT, Brownstein MR, et al: The effector component of the cytotoxic T-lymphocyte response has a biphasic pattern after burn injury. J Surg Res 1998;80:243.
58. Jahoor F, Herndon DN, Wolfe RR: Role of insulin and glucagon in the response of glucose and alanine kinetics in burn-injured patients. J Clin Invest 1986;78:807.
59. Jarrett F, Ellerbe S, Demling R: Acute leukopenia during topical burn therapy with silver sulfadiazine. Am J Surg 1978;135:818.
60. Jerath MR, Schomacker KT, Sheridan RL, et al: Burn wound assessment in porcine skin using indocyanine green fluorescence. J Trauma 1999;46:1085.

61. Jeschke MG, Barrow RE, Wolf SE, et al: Mortality in burned children with acute renal failure. Arch Surg 1998;133:752.
62. Kimura R, Traber LD, Herndon DN, et al: Treatment of smoke-induced pulmonary injury with nebulized dimethylsulfoxide. Circ Shock 1988;25:333.
63. Klein GL, Wolf SE, Goodman WG, et al: The management of acute bone loss in severe catabolism due to burn injury. Horm Res 1997;48(Suppl 5):83.
64. Klimpel GR, Herndon DH, Stein MD: Peripheral blood lymphocytes from thermal injury patients are defective in their ability to generate lymphokine-activated killer (LAK) cell activity. J Clin Immunol 1988;8:14.
65. Laberge LC, Ballard PA, Daniel RK: Experimental electrical burns: Low voltage. Ann Plast Surg 1984;13:185.
66. Lal S, Barrow RE, Wolf SE, et al: Biobrane improves wound healing in burned children without increased risk of infection. Shock 2000;14:314.
67. LeVoyer T, Cioffi WG Jr, Pratt L, et al: Alterations in intestinal permeability after thermal injury. Arch Surg 1992;127:26.
68. Lindberg RB, Moncrief JA, Switzer WE, et al: The successful control of burn wound sepsis. J Trauma 1965;5:601.
69. Lund CC, Browder NC: The estimation of areas of burns. Surg Gynecol Obstet 1944;79:352.
70. Marano MA, O'Sullivan G, Madden M, et al: Tourniquet technique for reduced blood loss and wound assessment during excisions of burn wounds of the extremity. Surg Gynecol Obstet 1990;171:249.
71. McDonald AJ, Cooper MG: Patient-controlled analgesia: An appropriate method of pain control in children. Paediatr Drugs 2001;3:273.
72. Mileski W, Borgstrom D, Lightfoot E, et al: Inhibition of leukocyte-endothelial adherence following thermal injury. J Surg Res 1992;52:334.
73. Mochizuki H, Trocki O, Dominioni L, et al: Mechanism of prevention of postburn hypermetabolism and catabolism by early enteral feeding. Ann Surg 1984;200:297.
74. Monafo WW: The treatment of burn shock by the intravenous and oral administration of hypertonic lactated saline solution. J Trauma 1970;10:575.
75. Moyer CA, Brentano L, Gravens DL, et al: Treatment of large human burns with 0.5 per cent silver nitrate solution. Arch Surg 1965;90:812.
76. Moylan JA Jr, Wilmore DW, Mouton DE, et al: Early diagnosis of inhalation injury using 133 xenon lung scan. Ann Surg 1972;176:477.
77. Murphy KD, Lee JO, Herndon DN: Current pharmacotherapy for the treatment of severe burns. Expert Opin Pharmacother 2003;4:369.
78. Myers SI, Minei JP, Casteneda A, et al: Differential effects of acute thermal injury on rat splanchnic and renal blood flow and prostanoid release. Prostaglandins Leukot Essent Fatty Acids 1995;53:439.
79. Nwariaku FE, Sikes PJ, Lightfoot E, et al: Effect of a bradykinin antagonist on the local inflammatory response following thermal injury. Burns 1996;22:324.
80. O'Reilly TJ, Spence RJ, Taylor RM, et al: Laser Doppler flowmetry evaluation of burn wound depth. J Burn Care Rehabil 1989;10:1.
81. Park DH, Hwang JW, Jang KS, et al: Use of laser Doppler flowmetry for estimation of the depth of burns. Plast Reconstr Surg 1998;101:1516.
82. Pierre EJ, Barrow RE, Hawkins HK, et al: Effects of insulin on wound healing. J Trauma 1998;44:342.
83. Ramirez RJ, Wolf SE, Barrow RE, et al: Growth hormone treatment in pediatric burns: A safe therapeutic approach. Ann Surg 1998;228:439.
84. Robson MC, Murphy RC, Heggers JP: A new explanation for the progressive tissue loss in electrical injuries. Plast Reconstr Surg 1984;73:431.
85. Robson MC, Smith DJ: Care of the thermal injured victim. In Jurkiewicz MJ, Krizek TJ, Mathes SJ, et al (eds): Plastic Surgery: Principles and Practice. St Louis, CV Mosby, 1990.
86. Rue LW 3rd, Cioffi WG, McManus WF, et al: Wound closure and outcome in extensively burned patients treated with cultured autologous keratinocytes. J Trauma 1993;34:662.
87. Ryan CM, Yarmush ML, Burke JF, et al: Increased gut permeability early after burns correlates with the extent of burn injury. Crit Care Med 1992;20:1508.
88. Saito H, Trocki O, Alexander JW, et al: The effect of route of nutrient administration on the nutritional state, catabolic hormone secretion, and gut mucosal integrity after burn injury. JPEN J Parenter Enteral Nutr 1987;11:1.
89. Shamoon H, Hendler R, Sherwin RS: Synergistic interactions among antiinsulin hormones in the pathogenesis of stress hyperglycemia in humans. J Clin Endocrinol Metab 1981;52:1235.
90. Sheffield-Moore M, Urban RJ, Wolf SE, et al: Short-term oxandrolone administration stimulates net muscle protein synthesis in young men. J Clin Endocrinol Metab 1999;84:2705.
91. Sheridan RL, Tompkins RG: Cultured autologous epithelium in patients with burns of ninety percent or more of the body surface. J Trauma 1995;38:48.
92. Thompson PB, Herndon DN, Traber DL, et al: Effect on mortality of inhalation injury. J Trauma 1986;26:163.
93. Traber DL, Herndon DN, Stein MD, et al: The pulmonary lesion of smoke inhalation in an ovine model. Circ Shock 1986;18:311.
94. Trevino MA, Herrmann GH, Sprout WL: Treatment of severe hydrofluoric acid exposures. J Occup Med 1983;25:861.
95. Vo LT, Papworth GD, Delaney PM, et al: A study of vascular response to thermal injury on hairless mice by fibre optic confocal imaging, laser Doppler flowmetry and conventional histology. Burns 1998;24:319.
96. Warden GD: Burn shock resuscitation. World J Surg 1992;16:16.
97. Warden GD: Fluid resuscitation and early management. In Herndon DN (ed): Total Burn Care. Philadelphia, WB Saunders, 1996, p 53.
98. Wilmore DW, Moylan JA Jr, Bristow BF, et al: Anabolic effects of human growth hormone and high caloric feedings following thermal injury. Surg Gynecol Obstet 1974;138:875.
99. Wolf SE, Barrow RE, Herndon DN: Growth hormone and IGF-I therapy in the hypercatabolic patient. Baillieres Clin Endocrinol Metab 1996;10:447.
100. Wolf SE, Ikeda H, Matin S, et al: Cutaneous burn increases apoptosis in the gut epithelium of mice. J Am Coll Surg 1999;188:10.
101. Zedler S, Faist E, Ostermeier B, et al: Postburn constitutional changes in T-cell reactivity occur in CD8+ rather than in CD4+ cells. J Trauma 1997;42:872.

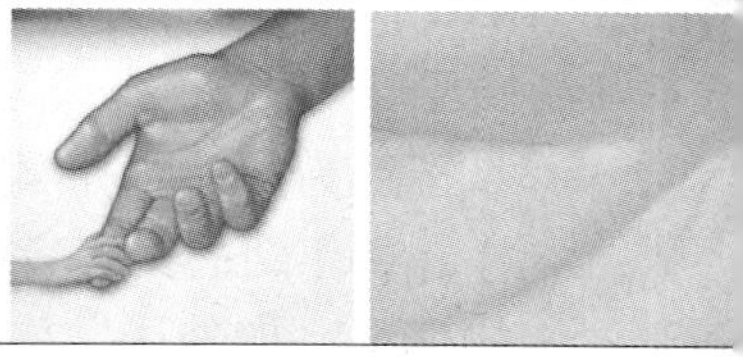

第 24 章

儿童虐待和产伤

Dennis W. Vane

400 ## 儿童虐待

儿童虐待包括肉体虐待、性虐待、心理虐待和忽视。儿童虐待已经成为当今社会的重要焦点问题之一，一些媒体经常对发生在社会各个阶层，包括平民和知名人士中可以鉴定为创伤或者是致命伤害的儿童虐待事件进行暴光，否定了儿童虐待和家庭暴力只有在穷人和文化水平低人群中发生的说法。儿童虐待这一世界性的问题困扰着整个社会，如何避免和采取有效措施来解决这一问题就需要对儿童虐待的流行病学状况进行及时的研究。

不幸的是，只有少数儿童虐待事件有足够的理由来追究家长和看护人的相关责任，在很多国家中，一些宗教或社会的“规则”阻碍了对受害者的鉴定。全世界基本上没有一个国家对这一问题作过完整的陈述[3]。在美国和加拿大，相关法律的制定开始于上世纪 60 年代[71]，从那时起，投诉于当局的相关案件都被移交给处理儿童事务的专业人员。一些法律使原告逃脱责任（比如使用“疑似”和“创伤相关”等词语），限制了委托人的特权，有时甚至对败诉者强加惩罚[47]。

流行病学

据估计，在美国每年大约有 140 万未成年人遭受各种形式的虐待[54]，占全国人口的 2%～3%，其中大约有 16 万儿童遭受了严重的甚至是致命的虐待。全美每年大约因虐待而死亡的儿童 1000～2000，其中 80%小于 5 岁，40%小于 1 岁[48]。虽然大部分死亡案例发生在婴幼儿，但虐待事件在年长儿童中发生率更高。青少年虐待事件发生率是学龄前儿童的 2 倍[54]。

儿童虐待的形式在不同的社会阶层发生率有所不同，性虐待和心理虐待无明显社会阶层相关性，而肉体虐待和忽视在贫困人群中更容易发生[54]。在同一个儿童或者同一个家庭中经常重叠出现几种不同的虐待形式，而且发生儿童虐待的家庭经常同时存在有其他类型的家庭暴力，比如夫妻间或者同胞间的暴力事件[49]。

儿童虐待不断的衍生出了很多社会、经济的问题。在受害儿童中，挥霍和抑郁的发生率要高于普通人群 2～3 倍，而且比一般儿童更具有暴力倾向[22,32]。据估计，大约有 30%的受害儿童将来会虐待自己的孩子[20]。一些学者认为，这种遗传性的暴力倾向部分是由于神经内分泌系统的改变引起的，它能影响个体的觉醒、学习、生长和痛阈[20]。

可以确定上述儿童虐待的发生率是明显少报的，因为专业性的接触和确认必须要求第一时间对虐待事件进行鉴定。如果要预防这一世界性难题，相关医生不但要认识到虐待本身，还必须对发生虐待的高危因素具有很好的认识。

表现

医生必须认识到，受虐待的儿童经常是畏缩的，并且避免和谈话者有目光接触。询问者必须知道，儿童回答提问时经常会迎合询问者的意思，所以要尽量避免干扰儿童的回答。幼儿回答时还常常会加入自己的联想，出现与事实不符甚至相反的情况。对即使这些仍不能对儿童虐待给出精确的诊断，对儿童虐待事件的询问也必须包括家庭成员的详细情况、非亲属的 401
看护者情况、家庭的物质消费以及过去曾经发生的虐待情况。

因为虐待的形式不一，所以表现也随之多种多样。在年幼的受害者中，对虐待的诊断往往依靠客观的表现，如外伤、烫伤、视网膜出血、长骨骨折等。在儿童中，如果出现下列情况就要高度怀疑有儿童虐待：有不同愈合程度的多发伤；伤害程度和看护者提供的受伤病程不符；要求重复病史时与第一次所述不符，特别是“没看到”发生情况的；会阴部的损伤。Wisslow[71]对儿童虐待和忽视的表现作了很好的总结（表 24–1）。在儿童中，任何创伤都有可能是虐待引起的，其中一些创伤和创伤类型与虐待高度相关。

外伤性脑损伤

头部损伤在儿童虐待中可能最为常见，也最具破坏性。贯穿性头部损伤相对少见，大多数头部损伤发生在幼儿中[36]。钝性损伤经常被称为“婴儿摇晃综合征”或者更精确的说是“摇晃冲撞综合征”，它是由于在外力摇晃作用下，大脑在颅室内做加速

表 24–1 提示儿童虐待或忽视的症状和体征

发育不良
体重、身高或两者低于同龄人 5%
体重低于相同身高儿童 5%
生长速度下降
头部损伤
上唇或下唇系带撕裂
不能解释的牙齿损伤
拳击或者坠落引起的双侧黑眼圈
外伤性脱发
视网膜出血
轻到中度跌落伤（<3m）引起的弥漫性或严重的中枢神经损伤
皮肤损伤
擦伤或烫伤，伤口具有一定形状
咬痕
烫伤，呈手套或者袜子外形，以及其他类似浸渍伤
伤口颜色不同（愈合程度不同）
正常不易损伤部位的软组织损伤（大腿，胃部，上臂）
胃肠道或泌尿生殖系统损伤
胆汁性呕吐
只有家长发现的反复呕吐或者腹泻
不明原因的慢性腹部或者会阴疼痛
生殖器或直肠疼痛史
生殖器或直肠损伤
性传播疾病
骨折
排除大的创伤（如摩托车引起的交通事故）后的肋骨骨折
低处坠落（<1.2m）后的复杂头颅骨折
婴儿干骺端长骨骨折
1 岁以下儿童的股骨骨折（任何类型）
愈合程度不同的多发骨折
实验室检查
难以置信或者与生理不符的实验室结果（多种微生物污染的体液，不常见微生物感染，与临床状态或者疾病不符的电解质紊乱，检查结果多变和不稳定）
排除已知饮食和药物因素的中毒试验阳性
婴儿血性脑脊液（表层黄色），意识不稳定，并且无外伤史

From Wissow LS: Child abuse and neglect. N Engl J Med 1995;332:1425-1431.

或者减速运动引起的损伤（图 24–1）。最近研究提出，要引起一般脑损伤必须要接触一定的外物，而引起钝性损伤的外物相对质软，接触外表不会引起创伤[21]。在摇晃中产生的角加速度和导致的冲击力可以引起脑部在颅腔内发生旋转，造成弥漫性轴突损伤和硬膜下桥静脉撕裂，并导致硬膜下出血。儿童自发性或者意外创伤引起的硬膜下出血比较少见，所以如果出现硬膜下出血则要高度怀疑儿童虐待的可能。锐器损伤往往引起特征性的头颅多发性骨折和多发伤。儿童虐待也经常导致继发性脑损伤，常引起脑室内出血、呼吸暂停后的脑部缺氧、心脏停
402 搏以及潜在性的脑干疝出等[35]。据报道，儿童虐待引起的继发性脑损伤死亡率在 15%～38%，明显高于意外创伤引起继发性脑损伤的死亡率[21]，非致命性脑损伤的损伤程度和预后也明显差于意外创伤引起的继发性脑损伤[24]。用 CT 平扫鉴定人为因素引起的头部损伤最为恰当，因为颅内损伤经常伴随颅骨骨折，所以很容易发现[58]。

虽然头部损伤大多数发生在幼儿，但在年长儿中因受虐待而造成头部损伤的也不少见。不同的是，幼儿头部损伤通常看不到外部伤口，而年长儿中则常常可以看到由暴力性外伤引起的外部伤口。这种头部损伤一般相当严重，预后不良[43]。

视网膜出血通常是儿童虐待的特异性病理体征[13]，然而，最近的研究表明意外创伤也会造成视网膜出血，比如阴道分娩，压迫新生儿头颅后造成视网膜出血[18,25]。但是这种情况相当少见，所以，如果出现视网膜出血，就要高度怀疑儿童虐待，一旦出

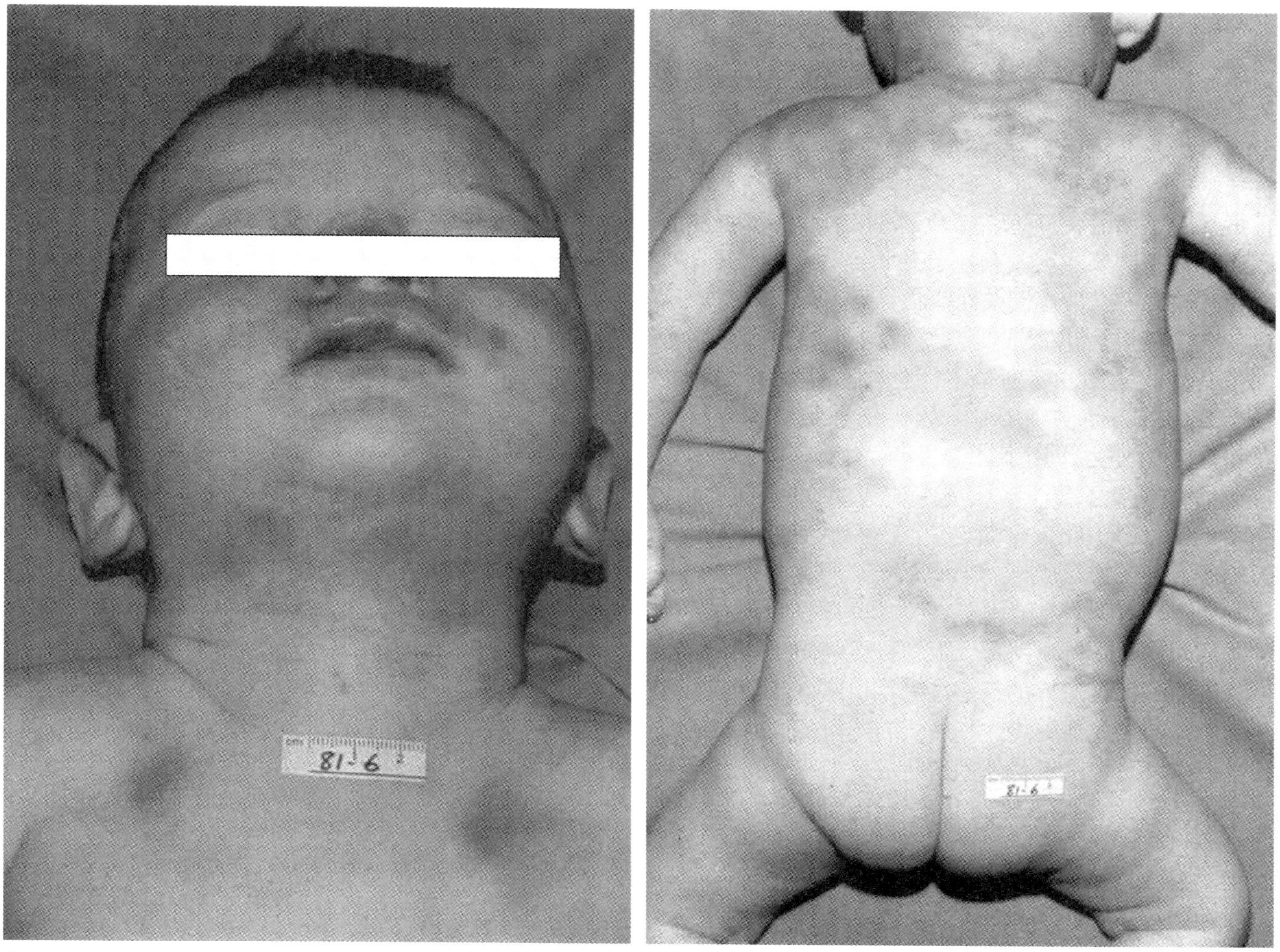

A　B

图 24–1　A 和 B. 婴儿摇晃综合征患儿经常可以在体表看到由手指、手掌引起的胸、肩、颈等部位的伤痕。

现，医生就要开始进行相关的检查。

骨折

据估计，美国大约80%的儿童虐待案件是通过X线证实的[12]。虽然大多数年长儿骨折是由于意外创伤碰撞后造成的，儿童虐待造成的继发性骨折仍可以在各个年龄组中出现[10]。2岁以下的幼儿出现长骨骨折与人为创伤高度相关[14,16]。有关人员曾经对某些骨折类型与虐待的关系做过相关性研究，但是确切地说，
403 所有骨折类型都可以是由多种因素造成的[46]。螺旋形骨折曾被认为是虐待引起的最常见的骨折类型，但是最近的研究已经将单纯性横断骨折放在第一位。螺旋断骨折是由身体某一部分过度扭转引起的扭转力造成的，而横断骨折则是由于对骨的直接创伤造成的。医生在评估时必须将这一点和患儿的创伤史结合起来判断创伤是否和病史相吻合。

长骨骨干骨折，特别是胫骨、股骨和肱骨，是虐待造成的骨折中最常见的类型，卧床患儿发生这些类型的骨折与儿童虐待相关性更高[46]。骨端-干骺端骨折虽然较骨干骨折少见，但是对诊断人为因素造成的骨折具有更高的特异性，造成骨端-干骺端骨折的原因远不只是跌落或者其他小创伤。骨端-干骺端骨折通常又被称为成角骨折或桶柄状骨折。

出生4周后出现股骨或肱骨的1型骨折与儿童虐待高度相关[26]，特别是不能提供受伤史而且有遭受严重的外力创伤经历时，因为这种骨折一般只有在特定人为外力作用下才会发生，如果是意外创伤造成的，一般还会伴随软组织或者其他损伤。其他类型的Salter-Harris骨折与儿童虐待的相关性则相对较小。

锁骨骨折也与儿童虐待有关，但特异性较小。锁骨的任何一端骨折比锁骨骨干骨折更倾向于是由牵拉或者剧烈的摇晃造成的[50]。与锁骨相比，肋骨骨折与儿童虐待的相关性更高。一般认为儿童的肋骨相对有弹性，可以防止由于意外创伤造成的肋骨骨折，如果儿童的肋骨发生骨折，与儿童虐待的相关性上升至82%[8]。

脊椎骨折在儿童比较少见，脊髓损伤同样如此。由于诊断锥体和相对被保护的脊髓的损伤比较困难，导致寻找与儿童虐待相关性的线索难度加大。但是能够肯定的是，要造成脊椎和脊髓的损伤必须是严重的外力创伤，诊断时要仔细调查创伤史。

医生对每一种骨折的发生进行调查很重要，特别是在幼儿年龄组。如果没有其他疾病，小的创伤一般不会引起骨折，所以询问详细的病史很重要。一个有小的创伤病史的患儿出现多发性骨折则需要对潜在的儿童虐待进行调查，因为多发性骨折，特别是骨折的愈合程度不同，是儿童虐待的特异性表现。如果怀疑儿童虐待，一般需要进行骨骼测量，美国放射学会已经发表了相关测量的标准[6]。

烫伤

烫伤和儿童虐待也有一定相关，约20%的儿童烫伤是由虐待引起的。医生必须意识到儿童虐待造成的烫伤伤口通常有一定的特征性外观[45]，比如圆形伤口，特别是不止一个肢体的烫伤；“图案”伤口或者烙印；臀部、外生殖器、会阴的烫伤；斑点伤口或者烟头伤（图24-2）。儿童虐待所致烫伤的患儿一般比意外烫伤的患儿年纪小，提供的烫伤地点经常在盥洗室中[33]。据统计，人为因素烫伤的儿童数目相当惊人，这些儿童常常是由单身母亲扶养或者被他人收养，家庭中的其他孩子往往已经由于遭虐待被其他人带走，如果仔细询问，大约有40%的患儿可以询问到过去发生的虐待史[33]。

烫伤史相当重要，而且经常和烫伤的外形不符。烫伤的表现经常不具有根据病史所应有的特征，比如

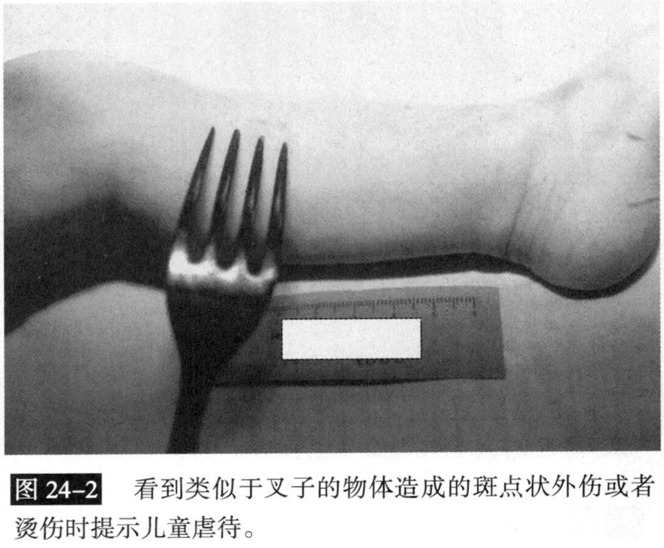

图24-2 看到类似于叉子的物体造成的斑点状外伤或者烫伤时提示儿童虐待。

缺少液体打翻溅出的痕迹，整个伤口深度一致，均超过一般“浅表伤”的深度，以及伤口面积要大于根据病史所应有的伤口大小。一些边界清楚的烫伤伤口常常是由于浸入热水后造成的，暗示事故发生时患儿无法逃脱或者被制服着。臀部和会阴部的烫伤经常发生在幼儿学习自己上厕所的阶段，管理者容易被一些“意外事件”而激怒。烫伤的深度也很重要，一个成年人浸在 65℃的热水中造成Ⅱ度烫伤需要 1.5 秒，这明显长于一般人可以将手浸在 65℃水中的时间。

对烫伤儿童或者怀疑受虐儿童有必要询问完整的病史和做系统的体格检查，受虐儿童其他的体征经常是可见的，比如已愈合和还没完全愈合的骨折以及会阴部的创伤。另外，近来的研究指出有些烫伤的临床表现和慢性皮肤疾病很相似[31]，所以对于发生在非典型部位或对常规治疗无效的皮肤病要高度怀疑虐待的因素。如果烫伤反复发生，医生必须首先确保患儿处
404 在一个安全的生长环境。

胸腹部损伤

幸运的是，儿童虐待引起的胸腹部损伤相对少见，在受虐儿童中发生率在 5%左右[61]，但是，胸腹部损伤是受虐儿童仅次于头部损伤的第二大死因[55]。各种类型的闭合性或开放性腹部损伤都可以由人为因素造成[15,19,38,56,61]，通常由对腹部或者胸腔的重击引起，如前所述，肋骨骨折要高度怀疑儿童虐待因素[8]。最重要的一点是临床医生必须清楚患儿的受伤史，并以此判断患儿的损伤程度是否与病史提供的受伤过程相符，就像最近的一些报告指出的简单地从楼梯或是从椅子上跌落并不能产生足够的破坏力引起内脏穿孔[34]，同样，简单地从床上滚落并不能产生足够的破坏力引起严重的头部损伤。

会阴部损伤必须考虑儿童虐待，除了已经讨论过的会阴部烫伤外，虐待造成的会阴部损伤往往是开放性的。对直肠、阴道以及阴茎和阴囊的撕裂伤需要这方面的常规调查。由于虐待者可能会借助其他外来工具，医生必须对扩张的肛门和阴道口引起重视，特别是引起大便失禁的病例。虐待造成的会阴部创伤常常是慢性的，经常可以看到瘢痕和旧的撕裂伤口。

虐待所致的胸腹部损伤的影像学和诊断性检查与意外创伤引起的胸腹部创伤相同，最新的检测及诊断标准意见已经由美国儿科学会提出[5]。处理方案也与意外创伤引起的胸腹部创伤相同[37,64]。

产伤

在美国，产伤的发生率大约每 1000 个新生儿中有 6～8 个，占新生儿死亡的 2%[65]。产伤最常见于巨大儿，也可继发于胎儿器官巨大症、巨大占位、早产、产程延长、急产、臀位分娩和头盆不称。产前超声以及围生期其他技术的广泛运用使得早期诊断这些高危因素和完善对分娩这些高危婴儿的辅助措施成为可能[28]。

软组织损伤

软组织损伤是最常见的产伤形式，一般表现为血肿（常常是头颅血肿）、单纯的皮肤擦伤或者脂肪坏死形成的皮下肿块。这些损伤一般会在几个月内自发好转，除了安抚家长外不需要治疗。由于器械的使用而造成的撕裂伤很少见，通常可以用免缝胶布或是皮肤胶水闭合伤口而无需缝合，不能达到愈合标准时则需要手术缝合，一般使用精细的缝线，也能达到很好的愈合。撕裂伤一般不深，对于深的撕裂伤必须进行标准的预防性伤口探查。

斜颈可以由产伤或者胎位不正造成，但仍存在争议[63]，因为剖宫产的新生儿也会出现斜颈。斜颈的一般表现为在胸锁乳突肌上出现一个质硬的小肿块，患儿头部朝肿块方向倾斜，脸部转向对侧。大多数斜颈病例只需要家长配合给予物理治疗即可治愈，很少需要手术，但如果不治疗可能会引起脸部不对称。

骨折

产伤造成的最常见的骨折部位在锁骨，发生率大约为每 1000 个新生儿中有 2.7 个[57]。一般，当发现新生儿上臂不会活动或在锁骨部位有肿块才注意到。骨折大多发生在锁骨中段，一般不需要特殊处理，但也有学者建议使用“8”字形夹板或者将患侧的衬衫袖子固定在胸口[41]。偶尔也有当肩位难产时人为将锁骨骨折助产的[9]。

肱骨骨折常常发生在肱骨干或是近端骨骺。因为缺少骨化点，诊断新生儿的骨骺骨折相当困难。肱骨骨折常同时造成神经损伤，形成包括 Erb 麻痹和桡神经麻痹[9,44]。产伤造成肩关节脱位较少，大多是由于宫内因素或者是处理 Erb 麻痹引起的。产伤也会造成肱骨远端骨折和肱骨头脱位，一般常出现在臀位分娩的新生儿[1,66]。对于肱骨近端骨骺骨折的处理一般是将上臂绑在胸前正中，而对于肱骨干骨折一般将上臂固定在外展位或者使用背侧固定板[52]。

产伤可以引起股骨各个部位的骨折，臀位分娩和巨大儿是引发因素[67]。一般表现为下肢的异常扭转、疼痛或触及肿块[68]。治疗可以用牵引、人字形石膏或两者配合，一般要求达到解剖复位，因为股骨的增长和重塑能力并不是很强[51]。

神经损伤

臂丛神经损伤是最常见的神经系统产伤[30]，大约
405 有 21%是由肩位难产造成的。臂丛神经损伤中，Erb 麻痹（C3～C5）最为常见，通常会自发缓解而几乎不留任何后遗症。一般表现为患侧肩部运动障碍[29]，上肢内收和内旋，远端肢体的感觉和手的功能不受影响。经过积极的物理治疗后，大约有 2%的病例会留下永久的功能障碍[29]。低位的颈神经根（C6～T1）损伤（Klumpke 麻痹）表现为手部和腕部的功能障碍，体检发现这种损伤往往伴随 Horner 综合征。微创外科修复已经应用于顽固性臂丛神经损伤的治疗，并取得了不错的疗效，但是这一技术一般只用于对积极的物理治疗效果不佳的患儿[60]。臂丛神经损伤常常并发膈神经损伤，所以一旦发现臂丛神经损伤就要对膈神经功能进行检查。单独的臂丛神经损伤可以引起明显的肩部异常，需要及时的处理[4]。

膈神经损伤也可能单独发生[65]。对膈神经损伤的治疗方案视患儿呼吸系统功能障碍的严重程度而定。无症状的膈神经损伤可以不予处理，如果影响到呼吸功能，可以采用横膈折叠术或者其他能够减少横膈随呼吸产生矛盾运动的手术[42]。

当然，最严重的神经系统产伤是中枢神经系统损伤。颈部脊髓的损伤很少见，但是一旦发生就极具破坏性。颈部脊髓损伤常发生在臀位或者横位阴道分娩的新生儿中[2]，高位的损伤需要机械通气，低位的损伤会留下严重的后遗症。完全脊髓横断的新生儿即使存活也十分危重。另外，有些局部损伤的表现类似于脑性麻痹[40]。

硬膜下、蛛网膜下、脑室内和脑实质内出血也是婴儿产伤的并发症，预后随损伤程度和表现各异而不同。这些损伤常常由胎儿头部吸引术造成[23,70]，胎儿头部吸引同样是头颅帽状腱膜下血肿形成的原因。尽管大多数血肿能够自行吸收且不留后遗症，但还是有大约 25%的患儿最终死亡[69]。也有报道在难产中造成颈内动脉牵拉伤的，预后和血管损伤的程度以及旁路血管代偿的程度有关[62]。也有对视神经直接损伤的相关报道[39]。

新生儿期最常见的中枢神经系统损伤是缺氧性脑损伤以及由此产生的“大脑麻痹”，产生原因尚有争议，但是难产无疑是一个公认的因素。

对神经系统产伤的治疗主要为保守治疗，同时进行积极地物理治疗，对于难治的周围神经损伤可以通过外科手术修复。

胸腹部损伤

胸部的损伤是胸腔压力过大所致，常见损伤有气胸、纵隔积气和乳糜胸[53,69]，食管或者环咽肌穿孔也有发生。大多数胸部的产伤可采用保守治疗，部分需要外科介入。高位食管和环咽肌的穿孔只需要观察或者间断引流[65]，低位的穿孔需要引流或者手术修补，如果早期发现，预后均良好。食管穿孔也会因新生儿期放置胃管不当引起。

产伤引起的腹部损伤中最常见的是肝脏血肿（图 24-3），常表现为贫血，甚至是休克[27]。通常需要靠超声诊断，但是还必须进行彻底地检查以排除新生儿其他肝脏占位的可能。治疗方案一般包括观察、补充血容量以及纠正体温过低和凝血障碍。如果患儿生命体征不稳定或者有持续性出血，就有必要外科介入[11]，然而新生儿肝脏缝合止血往往不及止血剂的运用来的有效。但总的说来，控制新生儿期肝脏出血是相当困难的。

脾破裂比较罕见，表现类似于肝脏破裂，腹腔积血可能是唯一的体征。与肝破裂一样，必须排除其他病理原因[59]。治疗方案包括观察以及纠正体温过低和凝血障碍，外科介入比较困难，常常需要行脾切除。

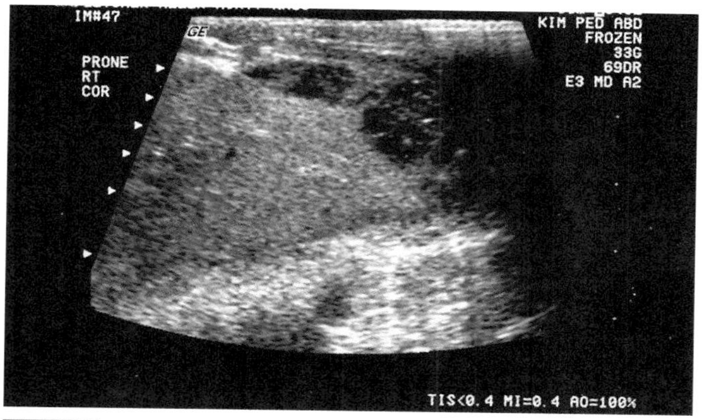

图 24-3 腹部超声明确显示了产伤引起的肝脏血肿，一般可以自行吸收，可以通过腹部超声随访。如果病变持续存在，必须考虑其他原因，如肿瘤等。

止血剂有一定疗效。

因为肾上腺受到肋骨的相对保护，与脾破裂一样，肾上腺损伤也比较少见。一般表现为出血，严重时会引起肾上腺功能障碍，部分病例因在后来的腹部平片中发现钙化点才被证实。对于所有腹腔内实质脏器，要诊断血肿必须完善检查排除其他病理原因，如未知的肿瘤等。

（张 震译 吴晔明校）

参考文献

1. Akbarnia BA, Silberstein MJ, Rend RJ, et al: Arthrography in the diagnosis of fractures in the distal end of the humerus in infants. J Bone Joint Surg Am 1986;68:599-601.
2. Allen JP: Birth injury to the spinal cord. Northwest Med 1986;69:323-326.
3. Al-Moosa A, Al-Shaiji J, Al-Fadhli A, et al: Pediatricians' knowledge, attitudes and experience regarding child maltreatment in Kuwait. Child Abuse Negl 2003;27:1161-1178.
4. Al-Qattan MM: Classification of secondary shoulder deformities in obstetric brachial plexus palsy. J Hand Surg [Br] 2003;28:483-486.
5. American Academy of Pediatrics: Diagnostic imaging of child abuse. Pediatrics 2000;105:1345-1348.
6. American College of Radiology: Standards for Skeletal Surveys in Children. American College of Radiology, 1997.
7. Babbitt DP, Cassidy RH: Obstetrical paralysis and dislocation of the shoulder in infants. J Bone Joint Surg Am 1968;50:1447-1452.
8. Barsness KA, Cha E, Bensard DD, et al: The positive predictive value of rib fractures as an indicator of nonaccidental trauma in children. J Trauma 2003;54:1107-1110.
9. Bianco AJ, Schlein AP, Kruse RI, et al: Birth fractures. Minn Med 1972;55:471-474.
10. Blakemore LC, Loder RT, Hensinger RN: Role of intentional abuse in children 1 to 5 years old with isolated femoral shaft fractures. J Pediatr Orthop 1996;16:585-588.
11. Blocker SH, Ternberg JL: Traumatic liver laceration in the newborn: Repair with fibrin glue. J Pediatr Surg 1986;21:369-371.
12. Brown T: Radiography's role in detecting child abuse. Radiol Technol 1995;66:389-390.
13. Budenz DL, Farber MG, Mirchandani HG, et al: Ocular and optic nerve hemorrhages in abused infants with intracranial injuries. Ophthalmology 1994;101:559-565.
14. Caffey J: Multiple fractures in the long bones of infants suffering from chronic subdural hematoma. AJR Am J Roentgenol 1946;56:163-173.
15. Cameron CM, Lazoritz S, Calhoun AD: Blunt abdominal injury: Simultaneously occurring liver and pancreatic injury in child abuse. Pediatr Emerg Care 1997;13:334-336.
16. Cameron JM, Rae LJ: Atlas of the Battered Child Syndrome. Edinburgh, Churchill Livingstone, 1975.
17. Chapman S: Radiological aspects of non-accidental injury. J R Soc Med 1990;83:67-71.
18. Choi HJ, Lee SY, Yang H, et al: Retinal haemorrhage in vivax malaria. Trans R Soc Trop Med Hyg 2004;98:387-389.
19. Coant PN, Kornberg AE, Brody AS, et al: Markers for occult liver injury in cases of physical abuse in children. Pediatrics 1992;89:274-278.
20. De Bellis MD, Putnam FW: The psychobiology of child maltreatment. Child Adolesc Psychiatr Clin N Am 1994;3:663-678.
21. Deputy S: Shaking-impact syndrome of infancy. Semin Pediatr Neurol 2003;10:112-119.
22. Dodge KA, Bates JE, Petit GS: Mechanisms in the cycle of violence. Science 1990;250:1678-1683.
23. Dwyer D: Problems after vacuum-assisted childbirth. Nursing 2002;32:74.
24. Ewing-Cobbs L, Kramer L, Prasad M, et al: Neuroimaging: Physical and developmental findings after inflicted and noninflicted traumatic brain injury in young children. Pediatrics 1998;102:300-307.
25. Forbes BJ, Christian CW, Judkins AR, et al: Inflicted childhood neurotrauma (shaken baby syndrome): Ophthalmic findings. J Pediatr Ophthalmol Strabismus 2004;41:80-88.
26. Forlin E, Guille J, Kumar S, et al: Transepiphyseal fractures on the neck of the femur in very young children. J Pediatr Orthop 1992;12:164-168.
27. French CE, Waldstein G: Subcapsular hemorrhage of the liver in the newborn. Pediatrics 1982;69:204-208.
28. Friesen CD, Miller AM, Rayburn WF: Influence of spontaneous or induced labor on delivering the macrosomic fetus. Am J Perinatol 1995;12:63-66.
29. Gherman RB, Ouzounian JG, Goodwin TM: Brachial plexus palsy: An in utero injury? Am J Obstet Gynecol 1999;180:1303-1307.
30. Gherman RB, Ouzounian JG, Satin AJ, et al: A comparison of shoulder dystocia-associated transient and permanent brachial plexus palsies. Obstet Gynecol 2003;102:544-548.
31. Heider TR, Priolo D, Hultman CS, et al: Eczema mimicking child abuse: A case of mistaken identity. J Burn Care Rehabil 2002;23:357-359.
32. Holmes SJ, Robins LN: The role of parental disciplinary practices in the development of depression and alcoholism. Psychiatry 1988;51:24-36.
33. Hultman CS, Priolo D, Cairns BA, et al: Return to jeopardy: The fate of pediatric burn patients who are victims of abuse

and neglect. J Burn Care Rehabil 1998;19:367-376.
34. Huntimer CM, Muret-Wagstaff S, Leland NL: Can falls on stairs result in small intestine perforations? Pediatrics 2000; 106:301-305.
35. Johnson DL, Boal D, Baule R: The role of apnea in non-accidental head injury. Pediatr Neurosurg 1995;23: 305-310.
36. Keenan HT, Runyan DK, Marshall SW: A population-based study of inflicted traumatic brain injury in young children. JAMA 2003;290:621-626.
37. Keller MS: Blunt injury to solid abdominal organs. Semin Pediatr Surg 2004;13:106-111.
38. Keller MS, Stafford PW, Vane DW: Conservative management of pancreatic trauma in children. J Trauma 1997;42: 1097-1100.
39. Khalil SK, Urso RG, Mintz-Hittner HA: Traumatic optic nerve injury occurring after forceps delivery of a term newborn. J Pediatr Ophthalmol Strabismus 2003;7:146-147.
40. Koch BM: Neonatal spinal cord injury. Arch Phys Med Rehabil 1979;60:378-381.
41. Kogutt MS, Swischuk LE, Fagan CJ: Patterns of injury and significance of uncommon fractures in the battered child syndrome. Radiology 1974;121:143-149.
42. Langer JC, et al: Plication of the diaphragm for infants and young children with phrenic nerve palsy. J Pediatr Surg 1988;23:749-751.
43. Lee ACW, Ou Y, Fong D: Depressed skull fractures: A pattern of abusive head injury in three older children. Child Abuse Negl 2003;27:1323-1329.
44. Lemperg R, Liliequist B: Dislocation of the proximal epiphysis of the humerus in newborns. Acta Paediatr Scand 1970;59:377-380.
45. Lenoski EF, Hunter KA: Specific patterns of inflicted burn injuries. J Trauma 1977;17:842-846.
46. Loder RT, Bookout C: Fracture patterns in battered children. J Orthop Trauma 1991;5:428-433.
47. Ludwig S, Kornberg AE (eds): Child Abuse: A Medical Reference, 2nd ed. New York, Churchill Livingstone, 1992.
48. McClain PW, Sacks JJ, Froehlke RG, et al: Estimates of fatal child abuse and neglect, United States, 1979 through 1988. Pediatrics 1993;91:338-343.
49. McKibben L, De Vos E, Newberger EH: Victimization of mothers of abused children: A controlled study. Pediatrics 1989;84:531-535.
50. Merten DF, Radkowski MA, Leonidas JC: The abused child: A radiological appraisal. Radiology 1983;146:377-381.
51. Mitchell WC, Coventry MB: Osseous injuries in the newborn. Minn Med 1959;42:1-4.
52. Moucha CS, Mason DE: Distal humeral epiphyseal separation. Am J Orthop 2003;32:497-500.
53. Nakagawa H, Yamauchi M, Kusuyama T, et al: Cervical emphysema secondary to pneumomediastinum as a complication of childbirth. Ear Nose Throat J 2003;82: 948-951.
54. National Center on Child Abuse and Neglect: Study Findings: Study of National Incidence and Prevalence of Child Abuse and Neglect: 1988. Washington, DC, Department of Health and Human Services, 1988.
55. National Pediatric Trauma Registry. Boston, Tufts University.
56. Ng CS, Hall CM, Shaw DG: The range of visceral manifestations of non-accidental injury. Arch Dis Child 1997;77: 167-174.
57. Oppenheim WL, Davis A, Growdon WA, et al: Clavicle fractures in the newborn. Clin Orthop 1990;250:176-180.
58. Pärtan G, Pamberger P, Blab E, et al: Common tasks and problems in paediatric trauma radiology. Eur J Radiol 2003;48:103-124.
59. Perdomo Y, Fiore N, Reyna T: Splenic injury presenting with isolated scrotal findings in a stable newborn. J Pediatr Surg 2003;38:1673-1675.
60. Piatt JH: Birth injuries of the brachial plexus. Pediatr Clin North Am 2004;51:421-440.
61. Purdue GF, Hunt JL: Burn injuries. In Ludwig S, Kornberg AE (eds): Child Abuse: A Medical Reference, 2nd ed. New York, Churchill Livingstone, 1992, pp 105-116.
62. Robertson WC, Pettigrew LC: "Congenital" Horner's syndrome and carotid dissection. J Neuroimaging 2003;13: 367-370.
63. Sanerkin BG, Edwards P: Birth injury to the sternocleidomastoid muscle. J Bone Joint Surg Br 1066;48:441.
64. Sartorelli KH, Vane DW: The diagnosis and management of children with blunt injury of the chest. Semin Pediatr Surg 2004;13:98-105.
65. Schullinger JN: Birth trauma. Pediatr Clin North Am 1993;40:1351-1358.
66. Siffert RS: Displacement of the distal humeral epiphysis in the newborn infant. J Bone Joint Surg Am 1963;45:165-169.
67. Theodorou SD, Ierodiaconou MN, Mitsou A: Obstetrical fracture-separation of the upper femoral epiphysis. Acta Orthop Scand 1982;53:239-243.
68. Towbin R, Crawford AH: Neonatal traumatic proximal femoral epiphysiolysis. Pediatrics 1979;63:456-459.
69. Uchil D, Arulkumaran S: Neonatal subgaleal hemorrhage and its relationship to delivery by vacuum extraction. Obstet Gynecol Surv 2003;58:687-693.
70. Whitby EH, Griffiths PD, Rutter S, et al: Frequency and natural history of subdural haemorrhages in babies and relation to obstetric factors. Lancet 2003;362:846-851.
71. Wissow LS: Child abuse and neglect. N Engl J Med 1995;332:1425-1431.

第三部分

儿童的主要肿瘤

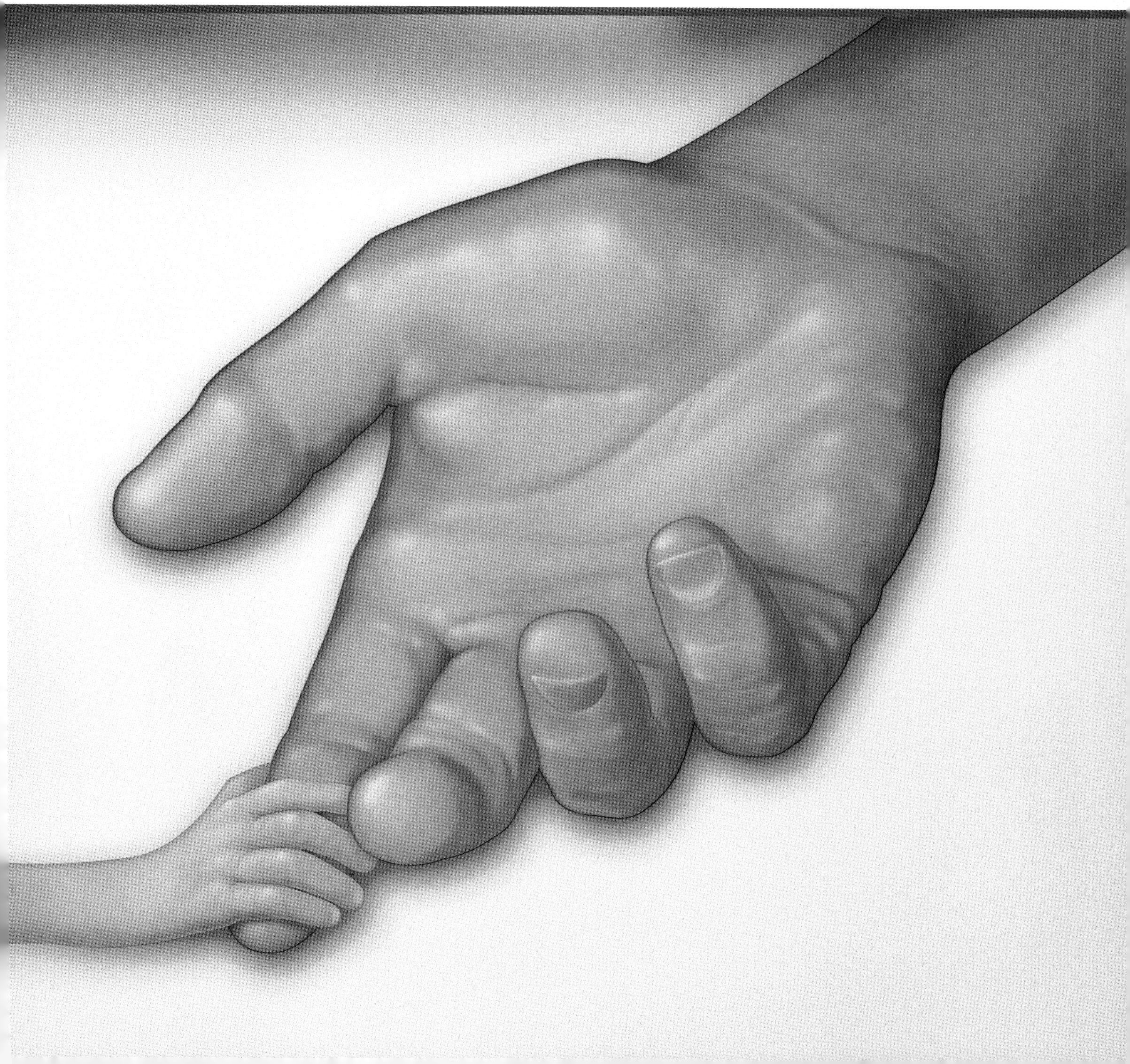

第 25 章

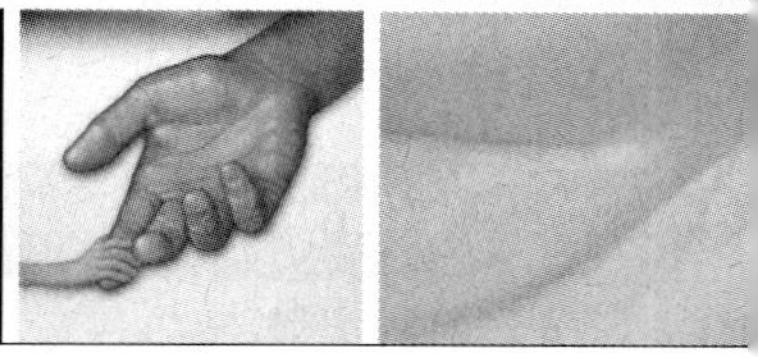

儿科肿瘤学、肿瘤遗传学和放射治疗原理

Matthew J. Krasin 和 Andrew M. Davidoff

11 很久以来，肿瘤治疗发展过程中的许多里程碑来源于儿童肿瘤学领域。最早发现化疗能够有效治疗儿童恶性肿瘤是在 1950 年，当时 Farber[41]报道用叶酸拮抗剂甲氨蝶呤治疗急性淋巴母细胞性白血病（ALL）可获得暂时的缓解[41]。最早成功的通过多学科协作方法治疗肿瘤出现在 20 世纪 50 和 60 年代，通过儿外科、放疗科和儿童肿瘤科专家的合作来提高儿童肾母细胞瘤的疗效[60]。这样的多学科协作方法目前在肿瘤学领域已广泛应用。在 20 世纪 60 年代，由于联合化疗治疗 Hodgkin 病和 ALL 的成功，使得联合化疗在治疗所有类型的儿童肿瘤中广泛应用。从 20 世纪 80 年代后期，神经母细胞瘤成为肿瘤治疗中按不同危险度分级进行不同强度化疗的范例，分级是根据临床和多种生物学指标，包括分子标记而做出的危险度分级。其他在儿童肿瘤学领域的进展包括跨学科、国际合作的临床研究协作组来严格评价新的治疗方法、通过剂量强化化疗来提高晚期实体瘤的疗效，以及通过支持治疗使剂量强化治疗方法能够实现。这些原理和新发展以及应用明显提高了肿瘤患儿的生存率并显著改善了他们的生活质量。

此外，过去 20 年中分子遗传学研究的进展，提高了人们对遗传因素在人类（包括儿童）恶性肿瘤发病机制和病程进展的认识。许多儿童恶性肿瘤已经成为分子遗传学研究的模型。染色体结构改变、相关基因或调控元件的激活或失活性突变、基因扩增和基因印迹在不同类型的肿瘤中各自发挥着作用。有时，这些遗传事件在肿瘤发生的早期出现，并对某一类型肿瘤是特异的，例如 t(11;22)(q24;q12)染色体易位出现于 Ewing 肉瘤；而发生于一系列不同类型的其他的异常几乎总是和遗传学改变有关，例如神经母细胞瘤和 Wilms 肉瘤出现染色体 1p 缺失。某一些改变涉及致癌基因——这些基因激活后直接导致肿瘤发生——而其他则涉及抑癌基因，这些基因的失活将导致肿瘤的发生。这些遗传因素改变的结果，不管其发生的机制如何，导致细胞中个体细胞的增殖和死亡的平衡被破坏。这些发现使分子分析法应用于各种目的，包括诊断、危险度分级和治疗计划制定；对肿瘤相关综合征的理解；遗传病筛查和遗传咨询；预防性治疗，包括手术干预。不久，治疗方案将可能根据每一个患者肿瘤的分子生物学特点来进行。此外，还可能根据肿瘤的分子生物学特点，开发旨在诱导肿瘤细胞的分化、阻止异常的细胞生长途径或重新激活已失活的凋亡途径的新药。

流行病学和生存统计

肿瘤在儿童并不常见；在所有肿瘤病例中约占 2%。然而，在大于 1 岁儿童中，它是位列于外伤后、排位第二的致死因素。每年，在每 1 百万 15 岁以下儿童中，大约有 130 例新发肿瘤病例（约 1∶7000）。这意味着在美国 15 岁以下儿童中，每年有大约 9000 例新发的肿瘤患儿，此外，在 15～19 岁儿童中，还 412
有 4000 例新发的肿瘤患儿[152]。白血病是儿童最常见的肿瘤，而脑瘤是儿童最常见的实体肿瘤（表 25–1）。其次是淋巴瘤，随后分别是神经母细胞瘤、软组织肉瘤、Wilms 肉瘤、生殖细胞肿瘤、骨肉瘤和视网膜母细胞瘤。15～19 岁的儿童中肿瘤分布存在轻微的不同，其中 Hodgkin 病和生殖细胞肿瘤是最常见的恶性肿瘤；非 Hodgkin 淋巴瘤、非横纹肌肉瘤的软组织肉瘤、骨肉瘤、Ewing 肉瘤、甲状腺癌和黑素瘤的发生率也在上升。

总的来说，儿童肿瘤的发生率在出生后第一年中最高，高峰在 2～3 岁幼儿仍存在，然后缓慢下降直

表 25-1 儿童肿瘤的分布频率

肿瘤类型	总百分比
白血病	30
脑瘤	22
淋巴瘤	15
神经母细胞瘤	8
肉瘤	7
肾母细胞瘤	6
生殖细胞肿瘤	5
骨肉瘤	4
视网膜母细胞瘤	2
肝脏肿瘤	1

到 9 岁。随后肿瘤发生率在青少年中又逐渐稳定上升。然而，每一种肿瘤有不同的年龄分布模式。同时有性别的差异性。例如，Hodgkin 病、ALL、脑瘤、神经母细胞瘤、肝母细胞瘤、Ewing 肉瘤和横纹肌肉瘤在 15 岁以下的儿童中男孩多于女孩；而在 15 岁以上的青少年中，骨肉瘤和 Ewing 肉瘤男孩要比女孩多见。尽管如此，在 15 岁以上青少年中，Hodgkin 病和甲状腺癌女孩比男孩多见。肿瘤的分布也与种族有关：白人儿童一般比黑人儿童的肿瘤发生率高 30%。这种差别对于 ALL、Ewing 肉瘤和睾丸生殖细胞肿瘤特别明显。

自从 Farber 在 ALL 患者中首先获得诱导缓解后，儿童肿瘤生存的可能性已经得到明显提高。在 20 世纪 60 年代早期，约 30%患有肿瘤的儿童存活。到 80 年代中期，约 65%患有肿瘤的儿童被治愈，而到 90 年代中期，治愈率上升到接近 75%[122]。这些巨大的进步源于三个重要因素：（1）儿童肿瘤对于化疗药物的敏感性高，至少在初期是这样的；（2）儿童肿瘤接受多学科治疗模式；（3）在大多数儿科治疗中心接受治疗的儿童均使用最新和最有前途的临床研究方案。虽然某些肿瘤类型，如 ALL 和肾母细胞瘤的治疗效果已经比较突出，但其他肿瘤的治疗效果，如转移性神经母细胞瘤和横纹肌肉瘤的治疗效果，仍然不佳。因此，儿童肿瘤的疗效仍然需要进一步提高。

肿瘤分子生物学

在正常细胞的发育和更新过程中，为满足机体的生理需要，细胞进一步进化以执行高度特异的功能。发育和更新涉及严格的调控过程，包括持续的细胞增殖、分化成特定的细胞类型和程序性的细胞死亡（凋亡）。一套复杂的监控和平衡系统确保对这些生理过程的适当的调控。细胞的遗传学特性（基因型）决定了将遵循哪种通路方式或哪些通路来实现这种调控。此外，环境在影响细胞的命运中中起着关键的作用：细胞通过复杂的信号转导途径来对周边的细胞和细胞外微环境产生感受和效应。

肿瘤是遗传性疾病，各种遗传因素和躯体环境影响所致的一系列不断累积的遗传学改变驱动疾病的进展。这些遗传学改变使每个细胞获得一种表型，以使它的生长比周边的正常细胞更好。我们对恶性肿瘤细胞转化过程的理解在不断增长；通过一些儿童肿瘤作为模型，在肿瘤细胞生物学领域已经有许多新的发现。而对肿瘤分子生物学更多的了解对我们去理解正常细胞的生理有显著的帮助。

正常细胞生理学

细胞周期

遗传信息储存在细胞中，并通过染色体上的核酸，以基因形式传给下一代细胞。基因是遗传的功能单位，它存在于染色体的特定部位，能够在每次细胞分裂时准确的自身复制，并能够指导一种酶或其他蛋白的合成。遗传物质以互补的双螺旋链的 DNA 形式存在。每条链的骨架是由连接在一起的糖和磷酸基团组成，互补的碱基——一个嘌呤（腺嘌呤或鸟嘌呤）和一个嘧啶（胞嘧啶或胸腺嘧啶）以氢键连接。正常情况下，细胞核内的组蛋白与 DNA 以一种紧密缠绕的复合物存在。只有激活时，缠绕的 DNA 才能打开。DNA 双链互补的特性保证了它在细胞分裂期间的准确复制：每一条链作为合成的子链的模板。细胞必须确保合成的 DNA（30 亿个碱基对）得到准确地

复制。DNA 错误的复制可改变正常细胞中调控蛋白
13 的功能。

蛋白合成从一条以 DNA 为模板合成的单链信使 RNA（mRNA）的转录开始。RNA 链中的尿嘧啶取代了 DNA 的胸腺嘧啶，戊糖核糖取代了 DNA 链的脱氧核糖。转录后，mRNA 经过修饰，改变了序列、长度、物理性状和稳定性。随后，mRNA 作为模板翻译成氨基酸序列，并形成多肽。然后，这些新合成的蛋白进行翻译后修饰。这些由 DNA 指导合成的蛋白质序列决定着细胞内一系列的活动，特别是调控细胞的分裂周期而影响细胞增殖。

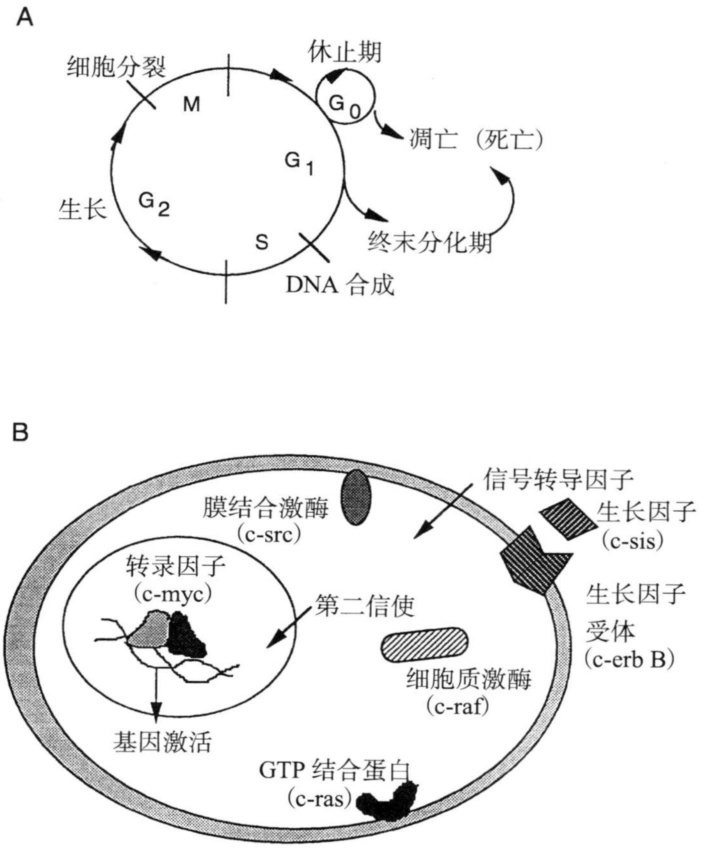

图 25-1 A. 细胞周期。正常细胞按一个有序的模式生长，经历 DNA 复制（S）和核有丝分裂（M 期）。这两个周期被两个细胞生长阶段（G_1 和 G_2）分开。细胞在生长信号作用下离开细胞周期进入静止状态、分化或死亡。B. 细胞信号传导。原癌基因产物（见括号内）作用于信号传导（推动细胞经历各周期）的各个方面。该过程从细胞外生长因子与一个跨膜生长因子受体结合后开始，因此诱导该受体的蛋白激酶活化。其他蛋白与磷酸化受体结合，并通过与膜结合的细胞浆信使将信号传导给细胞核。这激活了与 DNA 结合并影响生长相关的基因转录的细胞核转录因子。GTP：三磷酸鸟嘌呤。

调控细胞周期的分子元件是高度组织和紧密调控的（图 25-1）[134]。正常细胞生长通过 DNA 复制期（S 期）和细胞分裂或有丝分裂期（M 期）完成。这两个细胞周期阶段被两个细胞生长期分隔（G_1 和 G_2）。细胞也能暂时离开细胞周期而进入一个称为 G_0 的休眠期。刺激和抑制细胞生长的信号集中作用于一套驱动细胞周期演变的保守的酶。两种蛋白，即细胞周期调节蛋白和细胞周期调节蛋白依赖的激酶，形成复合体以通过有序的磷酸化靶蛋白来调控细胞周期的进展。细胞周期调节蛋白依赖激酶抑制剂调控细胞周期调节蛋白依赖激酶的活性，并作为细胞周期的“刹车”系统。此外，当出现特定的环境条件或由于合成不正确或损伤而致基因错误时，存在的各种“检查点”能终止细胞周期的进展。研究最多的两个参与细胞周期检查点系统的是 p53 和视网膜母细胞瘤（RB）蛋白[135]。在正常情况下，细胞分裂和最终分化而离开细胞周期，或进入休止期。细胞周期调控效应器的失活或绕过细胞周期检查点能够导致细胞周期的失调——这是恶性肿瘤的一个标志。

信号转导

信号转导途径调控着细胞功能的所有方面，包括代谢、细胞分裂、死亡、分化和运动。多种细胞外和细胞内的增殖或静默信号途径必须被细胞整合，正是这种多种途径的信号整合决定了细胞对各种竞争和互补信号作出应答。细胞外信号包括生长因子、细胞因子和激素；足够的营养物质和氧的提供或缺乏；与其他细胞或细胞外基质的接触。信号介质一般与细胞膜上的受体结合，但他们也可能弥散到细胞与细胞浆或细胞核膜上的受体结合。配体与受体的结合激活蛋白小分子第二信使——信号继续传导所必需的蛋白。信号途径最终影响细胞核转录因子的活性，而核转录因子调控着编码细胞生理过程中所有蛋白的基因的表达和静默。

具有酪氨酸激酶活性的受体是最重要的跨膜受体。它们包括细胞外的配体结合域、跨膜域和细胞内、细胞质的酪氨酸激酶域。配体和受体的结合可导致受体构象的改变，或导致受体和其他一个或多个受体连接。两者均可导致受体的激活。最终，酪氨酸激酶域通过直接对细胞内底物的磷酸化，或通过激活相

关的酪氨酸激酶来传导细胞内信号。

已发现数个重要的有蛋白激酶活性的跨膜受体，
414 并按照相似的结构来分成几个家族[148]。这些家族包括表皮生长因子受体（EGFR）、纤维母细胞生长因子受体、胰岛素样生长因子（IGF）受体、血小板衍生生长因子（PDGF）受体、转化生长因子受体和神经营养蛋白受体（Trks）。在儿童恶性肿瘤中经常发现这些家族成员的异常，因此认为它们在儿童肿瘤发病过程中起作用。这些受体的特异性异常经常用于某些肿瘤类型的鉴别诊断，而且最近，还形成了针对具有这些特异性异常的肿瘤进行靶向治疗的方案。

细胞程序性死亡

多细胞生物已经有一套高度完善和精密调控的细胞自杀机制以维持细胞内环境稳定。正常发育和形态形成过程常伴随有细胞的过多产生，这些细胞将被称为凋亡的遗传程序性过程所清除。凋亡的细胞有明显的形态学特征（质膜上起小泡、体积缩小和核固缩），其 DNA 在核内发生裂解。

“死亡配体”和他们各自的受体之间的相互作用启动凋亡过程，死亡配体包括肿瘤坏死因子-α（TNF-α）、Fas 和 TNF 相关的凋亡诱导配体（TRAIL），以及各自相关的受体。这种相互作用随后发生受体聚集和补充衔接蛋白到质膜上，继而激活半胱氨酸蛋白水解酶（caspase）[105]。Caspase 是一个蛋白水解酶大家族，其功能在于应答凋亡前信号而启动凋亡及随后发生的使细胞拆卸的效应通路。这样，凋亡限制了细胞的扩张和制止细胞的增殖。由于细胞的生存信号可以通过核因子 κB 介导的途径来激活，因此细胞的命运由死亡信号和生存信号间的平衡来决定[85]。由细胞应激过程产生的其他信号（如 DNA 破坏、缺氧和肿瘤基因激活）也可能影响细胞周期的阻滞和凋亡。

除受体和配体结合介导的细胞死亡外，另一条细胞死亡途径是细胞衰老，当染色体达到一个特定长度时被触发。真核细胞染色体有不等长的 DNA 链，其末端称为端粒，为种属特异性的核苷酸重复序列。端粒使染色体末端稳定，否则染色体末端将是极不稳定的[133]。随时间的增加和每一次成功的复制，由于端粒不能完全复制，染色体将缩短。这样，端粒的缩短就像生物时钟限制了细胞的生命全程。然而生殖细胞通过端粒酶能够把端粒序列加到染色体的末端而避免了端粒的缩短。正常情况下，该酶在生物生长和发育早期是失活的。在体细胞内，端粒酶的持续激活或再次激活有助于转化细胞的无限传代。

恶性肿瘤转化

正常细胞调控途径的任何组成部分的改变和失活可能导致生长的失控，这是肿瘤细胞的特征。恶性肿瘤转化的特征是细胞的去分化或分化失败、细胞侵袭和转移能力或药物敏感性下降。肿瘤发生反映在细胞增殖增加和凋亡或衰老下降导致过多细胞的积聚。肿瘤细胞并不比正常细胞的复制要快，但它们对调控信号的反应下降。正性生长信号由原癌基因产生，如此命名是因为它们失控的表达或活化能够促进恶性肿瘤转化。这些原癌基因能够编码生长因子或它们的受体、细胞内信号传导分子和细胞核转录因子（表 25-2）。相反，肿瘤抑制基因，像它们的命名所暗示的那样，控制或限制细胞的生长和增殖。通过各种机制使它们失活可使肿瘤细胞的生长失控。调控细胞死亡的基因也很重要。它们的失活导致抗凋亡和遗传学变异的累积。

肿瘤细胞携带的 DNA 有点突变、病毒基因插入或染色体 / 基因的扩增、缺失或重排。其中的每一个变异都将改变正常细胞生长和分化的背景和过程。虽然基因组的不稳定性是进化过程和正常发育的一种固有的特性，但细胞通过基因组的不稳定性可能出现恶性肿瘤转化。这种固有的不稳定性可能通过遗传或暴露于环境中的去稳定因子而被改变。点突变可以终止蛋白翻译、改变蛋白功能或改变可控制基因表达的调控靶向序列。染色体的改变在基因组内创造了新的遗传背景，导致新的蛋白形成或出现基因失控所致的各种异常事件。

肿瘤相关的遗传学异常可能在体内每个细胞，或只有于肿瘤细胞内检测到。先天性或胚系异常可以是遗传性的，或者是在生殖细胞（精子或卵子）内新发生的。有趣的是，尽管一种可能影响生长调控途径的遗传学异常在所有细胞中出现，但人们一般倾向于只出现某些特定类型的肿瘤。这种选择性充分证明了这样一种现象，即基因功能只在一些特别的微环境或生理条件下才能对生长或发育起作用。当肿瘤来源于胚胎细胞突变时，这种肿瘤发生时间比散发或体细胞改

表 25-2 儿科恶性肿瘤中的原癌基因和抑癌基因

癌基因家族	原癌基因	染色体定位	肿瘤
生长因子和受体	Erb B2	17q21	恶性胶质瘤
	Trk	9q22	神经母细胞瘤
蛋白激酶	Src	7p11	横纹肌肉瘤、骨肉瘤、Ewing 肉瘤
信号传导因子	H-ras	11p15.1	神经母细胞瘤
转录因子	c-myc	18q24	Burkitt 淋巴瘤
	N-myc	2p24	神经母细胞瘤
综合征	**抑癌基因**	**染色体定位**	**肿瘤**
家族性结肠息肉病	*APC*	5q21	小肠息肉、结肠直肠癌
家族性视网膜母细胞瘤	*RB*	13q24	视网膜母细胞瘤、骨肉瘤
WAGR*	*WT1*	11p13	肾母细胞瘤
Denys-Drash†	*WT1*	11p13	肾母细胞瘤
Beckwith-Wiedemann‡	*WT2*（?）	11p15	肾母细胞瘤、肝母细胞瘤、肾上腺
Li-Fraumeni	*p53*	17q13	多种（见正文）
1 型多发性神经纤维瘤	*NF1*	17q11.2	肉瘤、乳腺癌
2 型多发性神经纤维瘤	*NF2*	22q12	神经纤维瘤、神经纤维肉瘤、脑瘤
Von Hippel-Lindau	*VHL*	3p25-26	肾细胞癌、嗜铬细胞瘤、视网膜血管瘤、血管母细胞瘤

* 肾母细胞瘤、虹膜缺失、生殖泌尿道畸形、智力低下。

† 肾母细胞瘤、假两性畸形、肾小球系膜硬化症、肾衰竭。

‡ 多发肿瘤、半侧肢体肥大、巨舌症、高胰岛素血症。

变形成的肿瘤发生早且常是双侧发生。这种情况经常发生在儿童常见的两种肿瘤上：肾母细胞瘤和视网膜母细胞瘤。这些现象促使 Knudson[81]提出肿瘤发病的“二次打击”机制，该理论认为已经出现于胚胎细胞的首发的遗传学缺陷，必须为另一种在肿瘤出现前其他自发的突变所补充。在散发性肿瘤，只
15 有当两个（或更多）自发性突变出现于同一个细胞时才可能发生。

尽管如此，更多见的是，体细胞获得性染色体异常只出现于恶性肿瘤细胞。这些异常影响会生长因子和它们的受体、信号传导和转录因子。常见的与恶性转化相关的染色体变异类型见图 25-2。虽然低水平的染色体不稳定在正常细胞内也存在，但只有当这些变异影响了生长调控途径和促进细胞生长时才会发生肿瘤转化。

DNA 含量

正常细胞包含 23 条染色体的两个拷贝。因此，一个正常的二倍体细胞有 46 条染色体。虽然细胞的 DNA 含量或倍体可以通过染色体核型分析来准确测定，但可以通过较简单的流式细胞仪方法来估计。二倍体细胞的 DNA 指数是 1.0，而亚三倍体的细胞的 DNA 指数范围是 1.26～1.76。大多数（55%）原发神经母细胞瘤细胞是三倍体或亚三倍体（例如 58～80 条染色体），其余的是亚二倍体（35～57 条染色体）或亚四倍体（81～103 条染色体）[76]。亚二倍体或亚四倍体的神经母细胞瘤通常有结构性基因异常（如染色体 1p 缺失和 *MYCN* 肿瘤基因的扩增），而亚三倍体细胞的特征是几乎由完整的三套单倍体染色体构成，几乎没有结构上的异常[16]。重要的是，与亚二倍体或亚四倍体肿瘤比较，亚三倍体肿瘤患者一般有较好的临床和生物学预后因素和极好的生存率[92]。

染色体易位

许多儿童肿瘤，特别是血液恶性肿瘤和软组织肉瘤，存在重复出现的、非随机的染色体结构异常，典

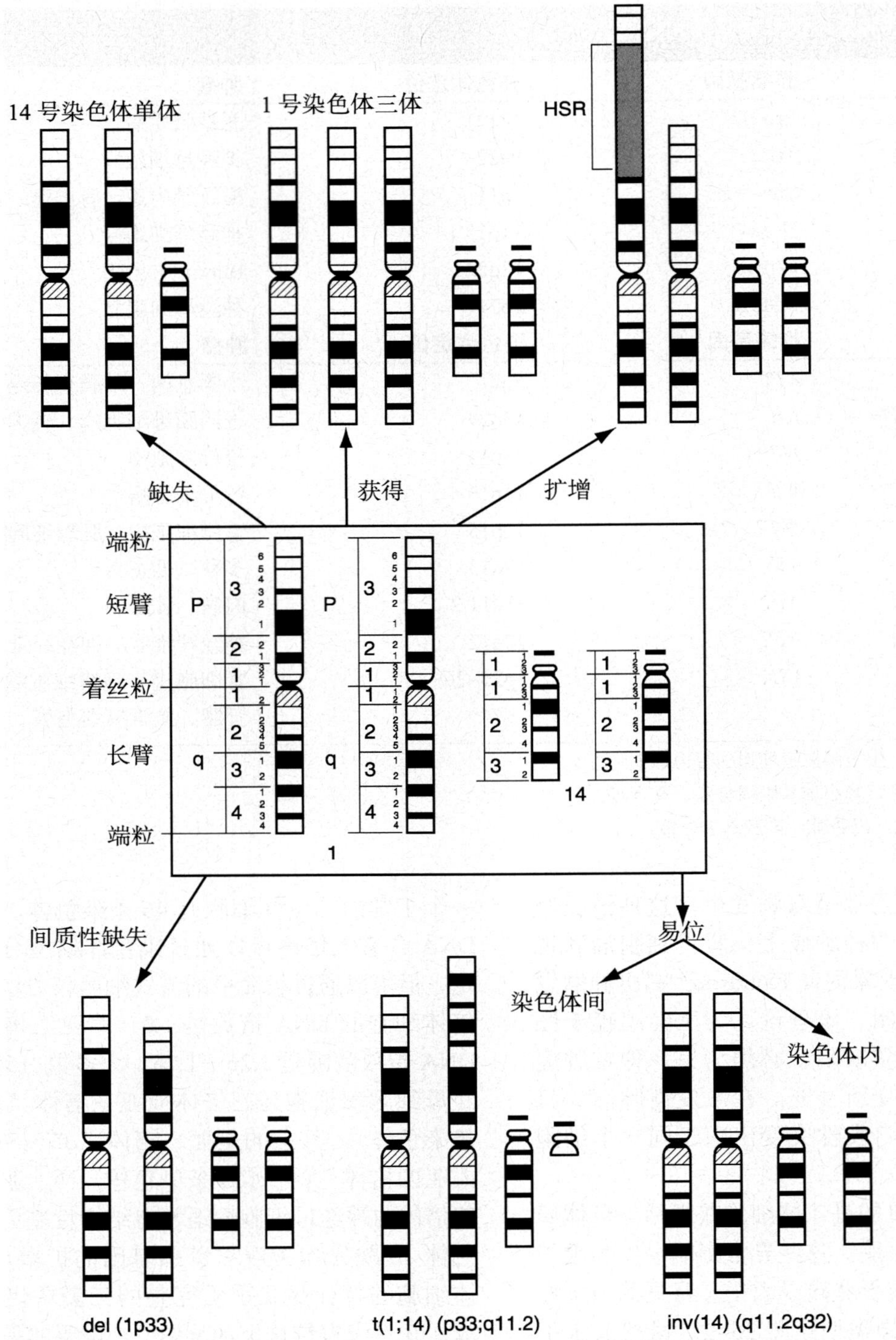

图 25-2 主要的染色体异常图谱，以 1 和 14 号染色体为例。HSR：同源标记区域。

(From Look AT, Kirsch IR: Molecular basis of childhood cancer. In Pizzo PA, Poplack DG [eds]: Principles and Practices of Pediatric Oncology. Philadelphia: Lippincott-Raven, 1997, p 38.)

型的是染色体易位（表 25-3）。非随机易位最常见的结果是来源于不同染色体的两个不同基因发生融合。这些基因的特征是在阅读框架内融合，表达有功能的嵌合性的、有转录因子或蛋白激酶活性的蛋白产物。这些融合蛋白通过激活细胞增殖相关的基因或蛋白而在肿瘤发生中起作用。例如，在 Ewing 肉瘤

表 25-3　软组织肿瘤常见的反复的染色体易位

肿瘤	遗传学异常	融合转录本
Ewing 肉瘤、原发性神经外胚层瘤	t(11;22) (q24;q12)	*FLI1–EWS*
	t(21;22) (q22;q12)	*ERG–EWS*
	t(7;22) (p22;q12)	*ETV1–EWS*
	t(17;22) (q12;q12)	*E1AF–EWS*
	t(2;22) (q33;q12)	*FEV–EWS*
促结缔组织增生小圆细胞瘤	t(11;22) (p13;q12)	*WT1–EWS*
	t(11;22) (q24;q12)	*FLI1–EWS*
滑膜肉瘤	t(X;18) (q11.23;q11)	*SSX1–SYT*
	t(X;18) (q11.21;q11)	*SSX2–SYT*
腺泡型横纹肌肉瘤	t(2;13) (q35;q14)	*PAX3–FKHR*
	t(1;13) (q36;q14)	*PAX7–FKHR*
恶性软组织黑素瘤（透明细胞肉瘤）	t(12;22) (q13;q12)	*ATF1–EWS*
黏液样脂肪肉瘤	t(12;16) (q13;q11)	*CHOP–TLS*（*FUS*）
	t(12;22) (q13;q12)	*CHOP–EWS*
骨骼外黏液样软骨肉瘤	t(9;22) (q22;q12)	*CHN–EWS*
隆突性皮肤纤维肉瘤和巨细胞性纤维母细胞瘤	t(17;22) (q22;q13)	*COL1A1–PDGFB*
先天性纤维肉瘤和中胚层肾瘤	t(12;15) (p13;q25)	*ETV6–NTRK3*
成脂细胞瘤	t(3;8) (p12;q11.2)	?
	t（7;8）（q31;q13）	?

From Davidoff AM, Hill DA: Molecular genetic aspects of solid tumors in childhood. Semin Pediatr Surg 2001; 10: 106-118.

中，t(11;22) (q24;q12)易位的结果是产生由 22 号染色体的一个转录因子基因 *EWS* 和编码 11 号染色体上 ETS 家族转录因子成员之一的基因 *FLI–1* 所形成的融合基因[97]。所产生的嵌合蛋白包含 *FLI–1* 的 DNA 结合域和 *EWS* 的转录激活域，比单纯的 EWS 有更强的转录活性[98]。*EWS–FLI–1* 融合转录体在大约 90% 的 Ewing 肉瘤中能检测到。在 Ewing 肉瘤中，还至少能检测到其他四种 *EWS* 融合基因；存在 *EWS* 和 *ERG*（另一个 ETS 家族成员）融合基因的患者占
16 5%[137]。腺泡型横纹肌肉瘤有特征性的易位，发生在 2 号染色体长臂（75%病例）或 1 号染色体短臂（10%病例）和 13 号染色体长臂之间。这些易位导致 *PAX3*（位于 2q35）或 *PAX7*（位于 1p36）和 *FKHR* 发生融合，*FKHR* 基因是编码转录因子 forkhead 家族的一个成员[53]。存在 *EWS–FLI–1* 和 *PAX7–FKHR* 融合基因的 Ewing 肉瘤和腺泡型横纹肌肉瘤的患者各自预后均较好[8,33]。具有产生增加转录活性的嵌合蛋白的易位特征的肿瘤还有促结缔组织增生的小圆细胞肿瘤[88]、黏液型脂肪肉瘤[120]、骨外黏液软骨肉瘤[27]、软组织恶性黑素瘤[154]、滑膜肉瘤、先天性纤维肉
瘤[149]、中胚层细胞肾瘤[127]和隆突性皮肤纤维肉瘤[109]。 417

原癌基因激活

通常转化细胞内的原癌基因通过点突变或基因扩增而活化。原癌基因通过点突变激活的经典例子是细胞原癌基因 *RAS*。RAS 家族蛋白与细胞质膜的内表面结合，在调控细胞增殖的信号传导途径中起中间体作用。*RAS* 点突变导致 RAS 蛋白的结构激活，因此可使 RAS 信号传导途径持续激活。RAS 途径的激活与一小部分儿童恶性肿瘤的发病机制有关，包括白血病和一些实体瘤。

基因扩增（即选择性的 DNA 序列复制）使肿瘤细胞关键基因的表达增加，而通常这些基因表达的产物是被严格调控的。扩增的 DNA 序列，或称扩增子，可能呈游离（即染色体外形式）的双倍体小片——缺乏着丝粒的成对的染色质小体——或呈染色体内均匀着色区。例如，三分之一神经母细胞瘤的转

录因子和原癌基因 *MYCN* 被扩增。*MYCN* 编码一个 64kDa 的核磷酸蛋白（MycN），它与神经系统和其他组织发育时表达的核蛋白结合形成转录复合物[82]。MycN 表达的增加使 DNA 合成和细胞增殖的效率提高，缩短了细胞周期的 G_1 期[94]。神经母细胞瘤细胞的 *MYCN* 拷贝数能扩增 5～500 倍，而且在原发和转移病灶以及肿瘤进展和治疗的不同时期均保持一致[15]。这种一致性表明 *MYCN* 扩增在神经母细胞瘤的发病早期就已经存在。由于基因扩增通常和疾病进展期、肿瘤快速发展和预后差等有关，而成为一个重要的预后因素[17,132]。细胞表面受体基因 *ERBB2* 是另一个因为基因扩增而过度表达的原癌基因，发生于乳腺癌、骨肉瘤和 Wilm 瘤[114]。

比较基因杂交研究显示，在神经母细胞瘤 17 号染色体长臂（17q）的遗传物质的扩增可能是最常见的遗传异常：这种扩增发生于约 75%的原发肿瘤[146]。这种染色体 17q 扩增与其他已知的一些预后因素有很强的相关性，且可能是一个重要、独立的提示预后差的因素[13]。17q 的扩增最常见的原因是该区域与其他染色体位点发生不平衡的易位，最常见于 1p 或 11q。术语“不平衡”意味着在正常的 17 号染色体外，有额外的 17q 拷贝的出现。虽然尚不明 17q 上有哪些关键基因，以及额外的 17q 拷贝与神经母细胞瘤的恶性肿瘤表型有何相关性，但神经母细胞瘤中存在的 17q 扩增表明 17q 上存在原癌基因。

肿瘤抑制基因的失活

肿瘤抑制基因，或称抗癌基因，对细胞增殖起负调控作用。基因缺失或突变失活使这些基因编码的蛋白功能丧失，将使细胞从生长受约束状态中解放出来，而有助于细胞的恶性转化。使原癌基因激活或肿
418 瘤抑制基因失活的遗传损害的累积效应，使细胞增殖和由于分化或凋亡导致的细胞损失之间平衡被破坏。这种失衡导致一个特异细胞系克隆的过度生长。第一个被认识的肿瘤抑制基因是视网膜母细胞瘤易感基因 *RB*。该基因编码一个作用为细胞周期“守门员”的核磷酸蛋白。当其被磷酸化后，*RB* 允许细胞周期通过 G_1 期，但当其去磷酸化时将阻止细胞分裂。*RB* 基因失活性缺失或点突变导致其蛋白失去调控能力。核磷酸蛋白 *p53* 也被确认是一个重要的肿瘤抑制基因，可能是所有人类肿瘤中最常见的发生改变的基因。*p53* 基因的失活突变导致 *p53* 蛋白调控细胞周期的能力丧失。*p53* 基因失活在儿童实体瘤中常见，包括骨肉瘤、横纹肌肉瘤、脑瘤、间变型肾母细胞瘤和神经母细胞瘤耐药亚型[7,78,86]。此外，遗传性的肿瘤相关 *p53* 肿瘤抑制基因改变发生于 Li-Franumeni 综合征家族，这是一种常染色体显性基因遗传缺陷，易发横纹肌肉瘤、其他软组织和骨肉瘤、绝经前乳腺癌、脑瘤和肾上腺皮质瘤[95]。其他肿瘤抑制基因包括肾母细胞瘤 1（*WT1*）、多发性神经纤维瘤 1（*NF1*）和脑视网膜血管瘤 von Hippel–Lindau（*VHL*）。

我们推测尚存在其他肿瘤抑制基因，但还未得到明确识别。例如，神经母细胞瘤细胞株早期核型分析发现频繁的 1 号染色体短臂缺失[18]。肿瘤遗传物质的缺失表明存在（后来发生丢失）肿瘤抑制基因，但在染色体 1p 上尚未鉴别出特定的肿瘤抑制基因。功能上确认 1p 肿瘤抑制基因的存在的证据是将染色体 1p 转染到神经母细胞瘤细胞株可致发生形态学分化改变，最终细胞出现衰老[5]。通过原位荧光杂交技术（FISH）检测发现大约 20%～35%的原发神经母细胞瘤存在 1p 缺失，缺失最少见的区域在 1p36 内[51]。1p 缺失在肾母细胞瘤中也常见[62]。

转移

肿瘤转移是肿瘤细胞从原发部位播散到远处，是恶性肿瘤的一个标志。肿瘤转移是治疗失败的主要原因，是肿瘤致残和致死的主要因素。虽然肿瘤细胞通过循环播散可能较为常见，但肿瘤转移过程的建立是很低效的。它需要几个因素，包括肿瘤细胞进入血液或淋巴系统、这些细胞在循环中的存活、细胞逃避免疫监测、细胞侵犯异种（异位的）组织和建立血供以允许肿瘤在远隔部位的生长。单纯失控性细胞生长并不足以引起肿瘤的侵袭和转移。许多肿瘤的发展经历了不同的阶段，这可以通过组织病理检查得到证实，包括过度增生、增生异常、原位癌、浸润癌和播散性肿瘤。对这些肿瘤发展的不同阶段进行遗传学分析表明，细胞失控生长源于细胞的癌基因渐进性的改变和抑癌基因的失活，但这些致肿瘤性的遗传学改变与决定肿瘤转移表型的遗传学表现存在明显区别。

组织学上，浸润癌的特征是在扩增的肿瘤周围缺

少基底膜。基质蛋白水解作用看来是肿瘤细胞浸润的关键机制，这种机制使肿瘤细胞能穿透结缔组织屏障，如基底膜，从而从原发部位发生播散。在这个过程中所涉及的蛋白酶包括基质金属蛋白酶和它们的组织抑制因子。靶器官的局部环境可能将明显影响外渗肿瘤细胞的生长能力[44]。介导肿瘤细胞间，以及肿瘤细胞和细胞外基质间相互作用的各种细胞表面受体，包括钙粘蛋白、整联蛋白（α 和 β 亚体通过非共价键结合的跨膜蛋白）和 CD44，细胞和透明质烷黏附相关的一种跨膜糖蛋白[144]。肿瘤细胞必须降低它们的黏附性从而能够从原发部位脱离，但在转移晚期，同一细胞在滞留和经血管到远端部分时需要增加黏附性。

血管生成

血管生成是新生血管生成的生物学过程。这个复杂的侵袭过程包括多个步骤，蛋白水解以降解包绕已形成血管壁的细胞外基质、内皮细胞的趋化性迁徙和增殖、这些内皮细胞形成细管、建立内腔以作为血循环和肿瘤肿块间的导管以及新生血管的功能成熟[50,123]。血管生成需要大量分子的协调活化，包括生长因子、细胞外基质蛋白、黏附性受体和蛋白水解酶。在生理条件下，血管内皮是静止的，细胞分裂比例很低，只有 0.01%的内皮细胞处在细胞分裂期[50,70,123]。然而，在有激素信号、缺氧或缺血等情况时，内皮细胞能被激活而发生迁徙、迅速增殖和产生内腔。

血管生成作为正常生理活动的一部分，如在伤口愈合、炎症、女性的生殖周期和胚胎发育中。在这些过程中，血管生成是通过紧密的、有序的调控实现的。然而，血管生成也出现于一些病理过程，这时正
19 常的调控丧失，导致新生血管的持续生长。这种不衰退的新生血管生成发生于类风湿性关节炎、炎症性肠病、儿童肝血管瘤、眼球新生血管生成和肿瘤的生长和播散[49]。

令人信服的资料显示肿瘤相关的新生血管生成对肿瘤生长、侵袭和转移是必需的[9,47,48,116]。血管生成前阶段（即在新生血管生成前）的肿瘤只能生长至有限的大小，约 2～3mm^3。这时，细胞的快速增殖与相等的细胞快速凋亡所致死亡维持平衡，导致肿瘤大小不变。当肿瘤新生血管的血管源性表型开启后，将导致细胞凋亡率下降，因此，动态平衡偏向了细胞的增殖和肿瘤的生长[71,91]。凋亡下降的发生部分是因为新生血管使灌注增加从而允许有更多的营养和代谢物交换。此外，内皮组织的增生可以旁分泌方式提供许多促进肿瘤生长的因子，如 IGF–I 和 IGF–II[64]。

在实验模型中，肿瘤的血管生成增加和肿瘤的生长增快有相关性，而限制新生血管的形成也抑制了肿瘤的生长。临床上，许多人类肿瘤新生血管的出现与肿瘤生长的增快有一定关系[138]，在晚期恶性肿瘤患者的血和尿中经常检测到高水平的血管生成因子[107]。此外，原发肿瘤内微小血管的数量和密度与肿瘤转移的可能性有相关性，与许多类型的肿瘤患者，包括儿童肿瘤，例如神经母细胞瘤和肾母细胞瘤的总的预后也相关[1,101]。

越来越多的证据表明，肿瘤新生血管生成的调控是很复杂的：新的血管生成是源于多个组织的促进和抑制血管生成信号竞争的结果[23]。特定肿瘤的特异性遗传学变化，例如，*p53* 肿瘤抑制基因[32,153]或人类 *EGFR* 基因[89,113,151]表达的改变，不但影响了细胞周期，而且通过改变关键信号[如上调血管内皮生长因子（VEGF）的表达或下调内源性的血管生成抑制剂血小板反应蛋白 1]而在血管生成中起作用。

显然，肿瘤的转移也有赖于新生血管生成[45,91]。这种依赖性可能与几个因素有关。首先，原发肿瘤内的新生血管为脱落肿瘤细胞进入血液循环提供了更多的机会。此外，增殖中的内皮细胞释放的蛋白酶能破坏基底膜，这对肿瘤的转移能力可能有帮助[19,128]。最后，肿瘤转移细胞在靶器官的成功生长有赖于新生血管的刺激和形成，甚至转移至骨髓也需要如此。

分子诊断学

关于人类基因组信息认知的爆炸性增长促使人们不但增加了对肿瘤形成的分子遗传学基础的认识，也促使一个新学科的形成：把这些分子事件运用到诊断中。分子诊断领域之所以发展是因为需要一种方法来支持常规的组织病理学检查和免疫组化检查相应的基因或染色体结构的异常。在大多数病例中，遗传学检测的结果用于证实光学显微镜和免疫组化的诊断结果。然而，在部分病例中（如原始恶性小圆细胞瘤、未分化滑膜肉瘤和脂肪肉瘤），需要分子分析方法来

做明确的诊断。

最常用于分析肿瘤患者的分子遗传学方法包括直接有丝分裂中期细胞遗传学或核型分析、FISH 和反转录聚合酶链反应（RT–PCR）。其他的方法，如比较基因组杂交、杂合性丢失分析和互补 DNA（cDNA）芯片分析等，可能最终将成为常规诊断技术的一部分，但目前只作为诊断中心和学术机构的研究手段。表 25–4 归纳了每一种方法的标准做法。与任何方法一样，分子遗传学检测有其优点和缺点，理解并认识它们的局限性是很重要的。还有必要了解每一种分子方法对检测材料的特定要求。外科医生最好能在尽可能减少活检相关组织损伤和破坏的同时，又能够获得足够的组织用于诊断、分子遗传学研究和用于将来研究的组织建库。

患者病理组织的分子遗传学分析的价值在不只是有助于佐证组织病理学诊断。许多重要的标记也提供了预后信息。例如，神经母细胞瘤的 *MYCN* 的扩增[16]与生物学上的侵袭性表现明显相关。该基因的扩增可以通过常规的有丝分裂中期细胞遗传学或 FISH 方法来检测，而且目前的神经母细胞瘤治疗方案的分级中包括了是否存在 *MYCN* 的扩增。一些基因融合变异也被认为会影响到预后。在最初的研究中，两个被认为相对预后较好的类型是 Ewing 肉瘤或原始神经外胚层肿瘤的 *EWS–FLI1* 的 1 型变异融合基因[33]和腺泡型横纹肌肉瘤的 *PAX7–FKHR* 基因融合[8]。互补 DNA 芯片分析技术可能会发现许多与预后更有相关性的基因。

可以准确高效分析或描述肿瘤组织谱的新技术正在不断涌现：通过使用 RNA 芯片分析基因表达和通过蛋白质组学分析蛋白表达。这些方法可以用于鉴定特定肿瘤的唯一“指纹”，从而提供诊断或预后的信息。蛋白质组学分析也能发现患者血清或尿液中的特

表 25–4 软组织肿瘤的诊断中应用细胞遗传学和分子学方法的比较

方法	目的	优点	缺点
细胞遗传学	低分辨率分析培养细胞的分裂中期染色体	不需要预先知道遗传学异常 在大多数诊断中心都可采用	需要新鲜、无菌的肿瘤组织用于培养生长 敏感性低；只能检测大的结构异常 无组织学相关性缓慢且技术要求高（可能要数周时间）
原位杂交	通过核酸探针与特异的 DNA 或 RNA 序列杂交检测染色体易位、扩增、和基因缺失	能应用于染色体标本以及细胞学、印片和石蜡切片 有形态学相关性可以同时进行 多个探针检测 快速（通常只要 2 天）	不能检测小的缺失或点突变 解释困难，特别是甲醛固定、石蜡包埋的标本 只有部分特异的核酸探针可以买到
PCR 和 RT–PCR	非常敏感的检测 DNA 序列和 mRNA 转录，用于证明融合基因、点突变和多态性，	是敏感性和特异性最高的分子诊断技术 作为 PCR 产物的 DNA 序列能确认结果和提供额外信息 需要的标本量很少 通用性，能被应用于新鲜组织以及甲醛固定、石蜡包埋的组织 有形态学相关性 正常组织的存在通常不影响检测 结果快速（通常 3～5 天）	甲醛固定降低敏感性 融合基因配对组合的差异性需要合理设计足够的引物以避免假阴性结果 高敏感性要求正确的实验技术以避免假阳性结果

mRNA：信使 RNA；PCR：聚合酶链反应；RT-PCR：反转录酶聚合酶链反应。

From Davidoff AM, Hill DA: Molecular genetic aspects of solid tumors in childhood. Semin Pediatr Surg 2001; 10: 106-118.

异蛋白，这种特征能被用于肿瘤的早期发现、危险度分级和监测复发。

基因芯片分析也能通过分析一个肿瘤细胞 RNA 的整个互补性来检测肿瘤细胞对各种刺激物的效应，如应激、低氧和治疗等。各种商业化的预涂布的试剂盒和简便的使用方法使这种技术已经被广泛使用。这种操作技术涉及将肿瘤中标记的 DNA 或 RNA 互补链与已知的基因或从基因组来的寡核苷酸杂交。而已知的基因或寡核苷酸固定于固体载体，即基因芯片。通过荧光来检测杂交。一旦样品的质量和稳定性能保证，数据处理和统计分析能被确认和标化，基因描记芯片可能被常规用于分析儿童恶性肿瘤。

儿童肿瘤和遗传

分子遗传学技术的进步也提高了我们对肿瘤易感综合征的认识。遗传的（即从父母传给孩子）或非遗传的（即受精前在精子或卵子内发生突变）组成性基因突变估计与 10%～15%儿童肿瘤发生有关[119]。组成性染色体异常是正常的 46 条染色体发生数量异常或结构重排，可能与肿瘤易发相关。如 21 三体（Down 综合征）易发白血病和 Klinefelter 综合征（47XXY）易发生殖细胞肿瘤。染色体结构异常包括间质性基因的缺失导致一个或多个基因的组成性丢失。

肾母细胞瘤可以是散发的、家族性的、或和特定的遗传性疾病或已知的综合征相关。我们通过对该肿瘤后两种类型的研究，已对肾母细胞瘤的分子学基础有了更深入的了解。WAGR 综合征（肾母细胞瘤、虹膜缺失、泌尿生殖系统异常和智力发育迟缓）为可能有共同遗传学异常的患儿群体提供了一个易于识别的遗传学表型。染色体 11p13 的组成性缺失出现于 WAGR 综合征患儿中[121]，也发生于 35%的散发的肾母细胞瘤患者中[31]。一项大样本患者的研究发现染色体 11p13 丢失的基因为 WT1[22]。该基因编码一个对于正常肾脏和生殖腺发育必不可少的核转录因子[118]，同时也是肿瘤抑制因子，但它确切的作用目前尚不清楚。WAGR 综合征患者的虹膜缺失被认为是继发于位于 11 号染色体邻近 WT1 基因的一个 PAX6 基因拷贝发生缺失所致[143]。Denys-Drash 综合征，特征是有极高的肾母细胞瘤、假两性畸形和导致早期肾衰竭的肾小球系膜硬化症发生危险性，与 WT1 的 DNA 结合域的胚系突变相关[112]。发生突变的 WT1 蛋白主要起负面作用。只有 6%～18%的散发肾母细胞瘤有 WT1 突变[112,147]。

在另一个肾母细胞瘤亚型中，在远离 11 号染色体端粒的 *WT1* 位点末端（11p15）存在遗传物质的丢失[30]。因此提示在 11p15 存在第二个肾母细胞瘤的易感基因，暂时命名为 *WT2*。在 Beckwith-Wiedemann 综合征患者中也有报道有该位点的杂合性缺失，该综合征是一个先天性过度生长的综合征，其特征是许多生长的异常以及易于发生各种恶性肿瘤，包括肾母细胞瘤[83]（见第 27 章）。

1 型神经纤维瘤（NF1）是最常见的遗传学异常之一。正常的 NF1 蛋白抑制原癌基因 *RAS*，但在 NF1 患者中，基因的一个拷贝的突变再伴以另一个基因的缺失将使 *RAS* 信号途径被无限制的激活。这些患者将易于发生骨髓疾病、良性肿瘤、脑神经胶质瘤和恶性外周神经鞘瘤。遗传性的儿童肿瘤易发也与 Li-Fraumeni 综合征（源于 *p53* 基因的失活突变性，患者易发生骨肉瘤、横纹肌肉瘤、肾上腺皮质癌和脑瘤的风险）、家族性视网膜母细胞瘤（源于 *RB* 基因的失活突变性，患者易于发生骨肉瘤和视网膜母细胞瘤）、家族性腺瘤性息肉病、和多发性内分泌瘤综合征等相关。另一套遗传性的危险因素以 DNA 修复基因（所谓的看守者基因）突变为代表，见于着色性干皮病和共济失调性毛细血管扩张症[80]。了解这些复杂的综合征和它们的发病机制对于早期发现和可能的预防性治疗是很重要的。

遗传学筛查

随着对遗传性儿童肿瘤分子基础了解的增加，人们有机会来发现易患恶性肿瘤的高危儿童，并且能够对于部分患儿在肿瘤发生前或在仍然可以治疗阶段就能进行干预。两个例子分别是家族性腺瘤性息肉病和家族性甲状腺癌。

家族性腺瘤性息肉病是一个常染色体显性遗传性疾病，患者在 10～30 岁时肠道出现成百上千的腺瘤样息肉。染色体 5q21 上的大肠腺瘤样息肉基因（APC）突变发生于 80%患有该病的家族成员中[108,117]。这些突变允许单个细胞克隆性扩张而导致腺瘤样息肉生长，随着时间的推移再获得其他的遗传学异常，从而导致侵袭性结肠、直肠癌的发生[55]。对于有这种胚系突变的患者推荐作预防性的结肠切除术，但目前对于家族性腺瘤样息肉病儿童的最佳干预时间尚存在争议。这些患者也有更大的患肝母细胞瘤的风险[79]。

髓样甲状腺癌（MTC）是一种少见的恶性肿瘤，它可以是散发的或见于两种综合征：多发性内分泌腺瘤综合征（2A 或 2B 型）或家族性 MTC 综合征。在儿童，MTC 的发生更可能与家族性综合征相关。由于胚系 *RET* 基因突变[104]和 MTC 间存在 100%的相关性，因此建议受累的患者作预防性的甲状腺切除。对于 MTC，除了手术没有其他有效的辅助治疗方法，同时需要强调的是早期干预的必要性。有胚系 *RET* 突变的患者还必须筛查嗜铬细胞瘤，在 2A 型多发性内分泌瘤患者中有 50%将出现此病，以及甲状旁腺功能亢进，在此类患者中发生率为 35%[72]。此外，有 MTC 发病风险的患者或新发的 MTC 患者，以及他们的亲属，必须做胚系 *RET* 突变筛查，以确定合适的手术治疗和给予遗传学咨询。

化疗的一般原则

在发现烷化剂可引起骨髓增生低下后，如第二次世界大战中使用的芥子气，于 20 世纪 60 年代首次注意到细胞毒药物对癌症治疗有效。化疗目前已成为几乎所有癌症治疗方案的一部分。肿瘤化疗的总目标是最大可能的杀灭肿瘤（有效性）而同时尽可能减少毒副作用（毒性）。然而，这个目标的实现可能比较困难，因为化疗药物使肿瘤细胞受影响的剂量常和正常增生的细胞受影响的剂量相似，如骨髓和胃肠道。尽管化疗早期的效果很好，以及大多数肿瘤类型在最初对化疗敏感（通常是很敏感），但化疗的成功常受限于两个因素：耐药的出现并逐步加重和药物对正常组织的毒性。尽管如此，化疗仍然是肿瘤整体治疗所必需的一部分，在局限性肿瘤治疗中作为辅助方法，在播散性或晚期肿瘤治疗中作为主要方法。

许多原则和术语对于理解化疗为抗肿瘤的治疗的一个模式是必不可少的。辅助化疗指对于临床上局限性的原发肿瘤在局部控制（通常是手术切除或放疗）后使用化疗进行全身治疗的方式。该治疗的目标是消灭用常规检查方法不能在原发部位或原发部位外发现的肿瘤。新辅助化疗指在局限性病灶治疗模式前进行的化疗，主要是为了提高治疗的有效性；及当远处肿瘤很小时尽早的治疗微转移肿瘤；或者是为了同时达到以上两个目标。诱导化疗指使用化疗药物作为进展期肿瘤的首选治疗。总体来说，儿童实体肿瘤和诊断时已出现转移的肿瘤化疗的长期无病存活率低于 40%。除了组织学类型预后较好的肾母细胞瘤、生殖细胞瘤和睾丸旁横纹肌肉瘤外，大多数儿童转移性肿瘤有很高的复发和进展风险。联合化疗指使用多个有不同作用机制和无重叠毒性的药物，以提供有效的、协同的抗肿瘤活性并尽可能减少副作用。联合化疗的有效性可用 Goldie-Coldman 假说[56]来解释，该假说认为肿瘤对单个化疗药物的效应反应了单个肿瘤细胞对该药的敏感性。一个肿瘤产生耐药表型的机会取决于突变率和肿瘤细胞数或肿瘤体积。一旦单个肿瘤细胞对某一药物耐药，该肿瘤无法再被该药物治愈。联合应用不同作用机制的药物减少了一个肿瘤细胞对一个或所有药物产生耐药的可能性，因此更可能获得好的治疗效果。

药代动力学指一个药物的作用时间和药物血浆浓度间的关系，药物暴露的定量通过计算药物浓度-时间曲线下面积来表示。一个药物的药代动力学受它的吸收、分布、代谢、清除、半衰期和排泄，及活性代谢产物的存在所影响。药代动力学资料的解释需要理解药物的血浆浓度和它的抗肿瘤效果。一个已知药物的剂量效应曲线通常是 S 形的，有阈值、延滞期、线性效应和平台期。线性期的斜坡常很陡，这个斜度意味着剂量的轻微减少将导致药效的明显下降。因此，给予能承受的最大剂量的药物以确保超过线性期的剂量范围已经成为化疗的一个基本原则。剂量强度的最大化可以通过增加药物的总剂量或缩短给药间期来实现。不合适的减少药物剂量可能将导致不能清除残留的肿瘤细胞。治疗指数是有益的和有害的效应的比值。

正在出现一个关于最佳化疗剂量的理论与长期广泛应用的最大耐受剂量在某种程度上有所冲突，这就是节奏性给药法。这个新的方法是保持小剂量化疗药物的持续给药，其有效性可能是因为两个原因。首先，由于大多数药物是细胞周期特异性的（即它们只能杀灭在特定细胞周期时间点的细胞），任何时候只有一部分肿瘤细胞是易感性的。因此，较长时间的接触一个药物可以导致较多肿瘤细胞被杀灭。其次，节奏性给药可以使药物靶向作用于构成扩张肿瘤脉管系统的内皮细胞，以及肿瘤细胞本身。传统细胞毒性药物治疗的方案——先给予最大耐受剂量，随后给予受影响的正常组织恢复的时间（主要是骨髓和胃肠道）——可能也允许肿瘤内分裂较慢的内皮细胞的恢复和增殖，因此使得肿瘤重新生长[20]。节奏性给药时细胞毒性药物持续给药或至少较为频繁给药，没有休疗间隙，用较低的总剂量可能会更有效控制肿瘤的进展，甚至在肿瘤细胞本身对药物耐药的时候也有效[20]。对于细胞毒性药物和抗血管生成药物，该给药方法显然是正确的。

化疗方案的合理设计和临床试验包含对这些药物作用机制、它们的代谢和它们的毒性特征的了解。大多数用于治疗儿童肿瘤的药物影响恶性肿瘤细胞和正常细胞核酸（DNA 或 RNA）的合成或功能。因此，这些药物能够杀灭肿瘤细胞，但也能影响正常组织。常用化疗药物的作用机制和不良反应见表 25–5。烷化剂通过共价结合 DNA 而干预细胞生长，是非细胞周期特异性药物。抗肿瘤抗生素嵌入 DNA 的双螺旋而破坏 DNA 链。抗代谢药物是真正的细胞周期特异性药物，因为它们干扰了 DNA 和 RNA 合成时所需的正常底物，如嘌呤和胸腺嘧啶。植物碱能够抑制微管功能（长春新碱和紫杉醇）或 DNA 拓扑异构酶（喜树碱抑制拓扑异构酶Ⅰ；鬼臼乙叉甙抑制拓扑异构酶Ⅱ），并且这些作用也导致 DNA 链的破坏。拓扑异构酶是一类能改变 DNA 双链超螺旋结构的酶。它们的作用是暂时性切断 DNA 链的一条（拓扑异构酶Ⅰ）或两条（拓扑异构酶Ⅱ）链，使 DNA 螺旋解开而伸展。DNA 的超螺旋的调控对于 DNA 的转录和复制是必不可少的，DNA 螺旋必须解开从而使这些过程中相关的酶的功能能够正常发挥。因此，拓扑异构酶决定着 DNA 的转录和复制。

这些药物的常见毒副作用也列在表 25–5 中。大多数化疗相关的毒性是可逆的，治疗停止后即可缓解。其他副作用可以通过特异的拮抗剂来缓解，如四氢叶酸用于 MTX 相关毒性的治疗。四氢叶酸与叶酸在体内作用的途径相似，但它不会抵消 MTX 的治疗作用。然而，一些化疗药物可能有长期副作用。值得关注的是那些能够导致第二肿瘤的药物。最值得注意的是应用鬼臼乙叉甙和环磷酰胺后继发的白血病[145]。

最后，了解化疗药物的代谢是重要的。某些药物需要在特定部位或器官代谢以产生活性或在特定的器官消除（见表 25–5）。活化和消除的过程需要器官功能保持正常（如肝脏对于环磷酰胺）；因此，有肝脏或肾脏功能不全的儿童不能给予这些药物。

危险度分级

过去的 30 年中，在治疗儿童肿瘤的众多化疗药物和给药方法的主要进展反映在患儿存活率的改善。化疗方案的毒性（包括化疗后期副作用，这在儿童中特别重要）和治疗的耐药是阻止化疗进一步提高的两个主要障碍。随着更多关于诊断和预后的遗传学标记信息的获得，治疗的策略也将相应发生改变。患者可以根据分子特征分类，这样不但基于肿瘤的组织病理学和分期特征，而且可以根据它的遗传特征接受相应的治疗。一些患者的肿瘤表现出更具侵袭性的生物学特征将需要增加药物剂量以提高他们的存活机会。而肿瘤没有表现出侵袭性生物学特征的患者则将可能从低强度低毒性治疗中获益。这种方法将使这些患者在保持高存活率的同时尽可能减少治疗的长期并发症。

基于危险度分级以使用不同治疗强度的范例是儿童神经母细胞瘤的治疗。越来越多的事实表明，神经母细胞瘤的分子特征对于该肿瘤的临床行为有高度的预测性。当前关于神经母细胞瘤研究的危险度分组是基于临床和生物学两方面的考虑。最重要的临床因素是年龄和诊断时的分期，而最重要的生物学因素看来是 MYCN 状态、染色体倍性（对于小于 1 岁的患儿）和组织病理分类。这些因素目前确定了儿童肿瘤协作组的危险度分级和治疗方法。在这种危险分级的一端，低危患儿只需要手术治疗；而在另一端，有高度复发风险的患者接受强化的多学科协作治疗，包括多药联合大剂量化疗、放疗和干细胞移植。其他因素，如 17q 获得、1p 缺失、caspase 8 失活和 TrKA/B 表达目前正在被评价中，并且可能在将来有助于进一步完善危险度的评估。其他的儿童实体肿瘤的治疗也正向根据危险度分级来治疗的方向发展。例如，肾母细胞瘤患者的下一个治疗方案可能将根据原发肿瘤的 16q 和 1p 缺失的分子分析来进行危险度分级和治疗方法的调整。

表 25-5 常见化疗药物

药物类别	药物	异名	商品名	作用机制	常见毒性作用	活化部位	清除途径	敏感的实体瘤
烷化剂类	卡铂	CBCDCA	伯尔定	铂化、DNA 链内和链间交联	A、H、M（特别是血小板减少症）N/V		肾脏	BT、GCT、NBL、STS
	顺铂	CDDC	顺铂	铂化、DNA 链内和链间交联	A、N/V、R（显著）、耳毒性、神经病变		肾脏	BT、GCT、NBL、OS
	环磷酰胺	CTX	环磷酰胺	烷化、DNA 链内和链间交联	A、N/V、SIADH、M、R、心脏、膀胱炎	肝脏	肝脏、肾脏（少部分）	广谱，BMT
	异环磷酰胺	IFOS	异环磷酰胺	烷化、DNA 链内和链间交联	A、CNS、N/V、M、R、心脏、膀胱炎	肝脏	肝脏、肾脏（少部分）	广谱
	达卡巴嗪		甲嗪咪唑胺	甲基化	H、N/V、M、肝静脉栓塞	肝脏	肾脏	NBL、STS
	替莫唑胺	TMZ	Temodar	甲基化	CNS、N/V、M	自发	肾脏	BT
	氮芥	双氯乙基甲胺	恩比兴	烷化、DNA 链内和链间交联	A、M（显著）、N/V、黏膜炎、起疱、静脉炎、腹泻		自然水解	BT
	美法仑	$_L$-PAM	爱克兰	烷化、DNA 链内和链间交联	M、N/V、黏膜炎、腹泻		自发水解	NBL、RMS、BMT
	白消安		马利兰	烷化、DNA 链内和链间交联	A、H、M、N/V、P、黏膜炎		肾脏	BMT
抗代谢类	阿糖胞苷	Ara-C	赛得萨	抑制 DNA 聚合酶，掺入 DNA/RNA	M、N/V、腹泻、CNS	靶细胞	生物转化	有限
	5-氟尿嘧啶	5-FU	癌肤治	抑制胸腺嘧啶合成，掺入 DNA/RNA	CNS、N/V、M、心脏、腹泻、黏膜炎、皮肤、眼睛	靶细胞	生物转化、肾脏（少数）	胃肠道肿瘤、肝脏肿瘤
	6-巯基嘌呤	6-MP	乐疾宁	抑制胸腺嘧啶合成，掺入 DNA/RNA	H、M、黏膜炎	靶细胞	生物转化、肾脏（少数）	有限
	甲氨喋呤	MTX	氨克生	阻断叶酸代谢、抑制嘌呤合成	CNS、H、M、R、黏膜炎、皮肤		肾脏、肝脏（少数）	OS
抗生素类	放线菌素 D	更生霉素	更生霉素	DNA 插入，链破坏	A、H、M、N/V、黏膜炎、皮肤、起疱		肝脏	RMS、W
	博来霉素	BLEO	博来霉素	DNA 插入，链破坏	P、皮肤、黏膜炎		肝脏、肾脏	GCT
	柔红霉素	Daunorubicin	正定霉素	DNA 插入，链破坏，自由基形成	A、M、N/V、心脏、腹泻、起水疱、增强放疗效应		肝脏	有限

（待续）

表 25-5　常见化疗药物（续表）

药物类别	药物	异名	商品名	作用机制	常见毒性作用	活化部位	清除途径	敏感的实体瘤
	阿霉素	Doxorubicin	多柔比星	DNA 插入，链破坏，自由基形成	A、M、N/V、心脏、腹泻、黏膜炎、起疱、加强、XRT 反应		肝脏	广谱
植物生物碱	表鬼臼毒素	VP-16	依托泊苷	拓扑异构酶 II 抑制剂，破坏 DNA 链	A、M、N/V、黏膜炎、神经病变、腹泻、		肾脏	广谱
	替尼泊苷	VM-26	威猛	拓扑异构酶 II 抑制剂，破坏 DNA 链	A、M、N/V、黏膜炎、神经病变、腹泻		降解	广谱
	长春新碱	VCR	安可平	抑制微管蛋白聚合，阻断有丝分裂	A、SIADH、神经病变、起疱		肝脏	广谱
	长春碱	VLB	硫酸长春碱制剂	抑制微管蛋白聚合，阻断有丝分裂	A、M、黏膜炎、起疱		肝脏	GCT
	紫杉醇		泰素	干扰微管形成	A、M、心脏、黏膜炎、CNS、神经病变			
	多西紫杉醇		泰索帝	干扰微管形成	A、中性粒细胞减少症、心脏、黏膜炎、CNS、神经病变			
	托泊替康	TPT	和美新	拓扑异构酶 I 抑制剂，破坏 DNA 链	A、H、M、N/V、黏膜炎、腹泻、皮肤		肾脏	NBL、RMS
	伊立替康	CPT-11	盐酸伊立替康和山梨醇注射剂	拓扑异构酶 I 抑制剂，破坏 DNA 链	A、H、M、N/V、腹泻	肝脏、胃肠道	肝脏、肾脏（少数）	NBL、RMS
其他	门冬酰胺酶	Erwinia	Elspar	耗尽左旋门冬酰胺，抑制蛋白合成	CNS、H、凝血病、胰腺炎、过敏反应		降解	有限
	皮质类固醇			核受体介导的凋亡	无血管坏死、高血糖、高血压、肌病、胰腺炎、消化性溃疡、精神病、电解质紊乱、体重增加	肝脏	肝脏、肾脏（少数）	BT

毒性反应。A：脱毛症；CNS：中枢神经系统毒性；H：肝脏毒性；M：骨髓抑制；N/V：恶心呕吐；P：肺毒性；R：肾脏毒性；SIADH：抗利尿激素分泌过多综合征；XRT：放疗。实体瘤：BMT：骨髓移植条件；BT：脑肿瘤；EWS：Ewing 肉瘤；GCT：生殖细胞肿瘤；NBL：神经母细胞瘤；OS：骨肉瘤；RMS：横纹肌肉瘤；STS：软组织肉瘤；W：肾母细胞瘤。

靶向治疗

肿瘤治疗方法中另一个主要的变化是靶向治疗的概念。直到最近，抗肿瘤药物的发展仍是基于对大量细胞毒性化合物的经验性筛选，并没有特别考虑到疾病特异性或作用机制。现在，对于改善抗肿瘤药物的治疗指数和克服药物耐药的问题方面，最令人振奋的进展之一是靶向治疗。随着一些恶性肿瘤特异性表型的分子基础被阐明，对于治疗来说重要的新靶点正变得越来越清晰。那些决定肿瘤转化和发展的特征性信号途径促使新药的研发关注于一些关键途径，包括细胞周期调控、受体信号传递、分化、凋亡、侵袭、转移和血管生成，这些在恶性肿瘤组织中可能发生紊乱。某一类型肿瘤分子特征信息的收集可以通过大量现有方法来实现，包括免疫组化、FISH、RT-PCR、cDNA 芯片分析和蛋白质组学。该信息然后能被用于开发新药以对抗肿瘤细胞的分子异常。例如，阻断致癌基因功能或恢复抑癌基因活性可以提供对肿瘤的特异性治疗。此外，分子特征可以用来开发旨在诱导肿瘤细胞分化、阻断生长通路的异常调控，或激活静默的凋亡途径的新药。

一些药物靶向作用于细胞增殖调控。赫赛汀（曲妥单抗）是一个与细胞表面生长因子受体 ERBB2 结合的单克隆抗体，有高度的亲和力，对于 ERBB2 过度表达的肿瘤细胞可以抑制其增殖[99]。目前，它被实验性用于抗 ERBB2 阳性肿瘤，如骨肉瘤和肾母细胞瘤。过度表达 EGFR 的儿童高分化脑神经胶质瘤可能也可以用相似的治疗药物，如 gefitinib（Iressa），这是一个 EGFR（ERBB1）的小分子抑制剂[14]。此外，小分子酪氨酸激酶抑制剂，如伊马替尼（格列卫）被设计用来阻断异常表达的促生长酪氨酸激酶——慢性粒细胞性白血病中的 ABL [142]和胃肠道基质性肿瘤的 c-Kit[21]，这些均处于临床试验阶段。伊马替尼也能被用于治疗那些 PDGF 信号途径在肿瘤细胞存活和生长中起作用的儿童肿瘤。其他激酶抑制剂，如 Flavopiridol 靶向作用于调控细胞周期的细胞周期依赖激酶[77]，而雷帕霉素（西罗莫司）抑制哺乳动物的雷帕霉素靶点（mTOR）[129]，该蛋白的活化导致细胞增殖所必需的蛋白翻译增加。Farnesyl 转移酶（负责激活 RAS 的酶）抑制剂，如 R115777，也正在临床试验中。虽然在成人肿瘤中激活突变是非常多见的，但在儿童肿瘤中很少见。然而，在儿童疾病如幼年型粒单细胞性白血病、某些脑部肿瘤和 NF1 中，RAS 42
信号途径经常被上游生长因子或致癌基因蛋白激活，因此 R115777 等也正被实验应用于这些疾病。还有一些重要的治疗药物是小分子抑制剂，它们能识别独特的融合多肽或具有染色体易位肿瘤（如各种肉瘤）的单一融合多肽的抗原决定簇。那些生长依赖自分泌途径（如横纹肌肉瘤过度产生的 IGF-Ⅱ或隆突性皮肤纤维肉瘤产生的 PDGF）的肿瘤可能对受体阻断剂（如 IGF-Ⅱ或 PDGF 受体抗体）敏感。

其他药物靶向作用于细胞死亡和分化途径的改变。Caspase 8 是调控细胞程序性死亡的半胱氨酸蛋白水解酶，但在肿瘤，如神经母细胞瘤中，DNA 甲基化和基因缺失联合介导 caspase 8 的完全失活，这几乎始终和 MYCN 扩增相关[140]。基因组 DNA 的胞嘧啶残基的甲基化是很常见的，且通常发生在邻近鸟嘌呤的胞嘧啶残基。DNA 甲基化在转录阻抑或某些基因（特别是发育调控基因）的静默中非常重要。Caspase 8 缺乏的肿瘤细胞对死亡受体介导的凋亡和阿霉素耐受；这种耐受表明 caspase 8 可能是一种肿瘤抑制因子。然而，把 caspase 8 缺乏细胞短暂暴露于脱甲基药物（如吉西他滨），或低浓度的 γ-干扰素，能够导致 caspase 8 的再表达，并使细胞对化疗药物诱导的凋亡再次敏感。组蛋白脱乙酰基酶似乎在凋亡耐受相关的基因静默中也有作用[69]；因此，组蛋白脱乙酰基酶抑制剂（如缩酚酸肽）也正在实验用于治疗某些儿童恶性肿瘤。最后，在程序性细胞死亡中由于端粒酶活性持续或再激活发生改变的细胞（这些体细胞一般在出生后端粒酶即丧失），亦可以用各种端粒酶抑制剂进行靶向治疗。

关于靶向细胞分化的一个例子是神经母细胞瘤，其中的不同神经营养因子受体信号途径介导细胞分化和交感神经母细胞恶性转化成神经母细胞瘤细胞的信号传导。神经营养因子在许多类型的神经组织和其他需要神经支配的组织中表达。它们能刺激神经元的存活、成熟和分化，显示出发育调控的表达模式[6,90]。神经营养因子和它们的 TrK 酪氨酸激酶受体在交感神经系统的发育中特别重要，并被认为在神经母细胞瘤的发病机制中起作用。已发现有三种受体-配体配对：TrKA、TrKB 和 TrKC，分别是神经生长因子、脑衍生神经营养因子（BDNF）和神经营养因子 3（NF-3）的主要受体[6]。TrKA 似乎在神经生长因子配体存在时，介导发育中的神经元或神经母细胞瘤发生分化，而在神经生长因子缺乏时介导凋亡[90]。与此相反的是，TrKB-BDNF 途径似乎通过自分泌或旁分泌信号传递促进神经母细胞瘤细胞存活，特别是 *MYCN*-扩增的肿瘤的存活[106]。TrKC 在大约 25%的神经母细胞瘤中表达，与 TrKA 表达明显相关[139]。目前正在进行 TrKA 的激动剂的研究，以试图诱导细胞的分化。相反，用 TrK 特异的酪氨酸激酶抑制剂（如 CEP-751）阻断 TrKB-BDNF 信号途径，以通过阻断重要的生存信号途径而诱导凋亡[40,106]。这种靶向治疗方法与常规细胞毒性化疗比较，在增加特异性和降低毒性方面很具潜力。

抑制血管生成

由于肿瘤生长和扩散依赖于血管生成，抑制血管生成是在理论上可行的抗肿瘤对策。该方法在以下方面特别有吸引力。首先，尽管人类肿瘤在分子和表型上存在很大的异质性，可是大多数（如果不是全部）类型的肿瘤（包括血液肿瘤）需要新生血管来达到所有恶性肿瘤的表型。因此，抗血管生成治疗可能广泛的应用于肿瘤治疗。其次，肿瘤新生血管的内皮细胞虽然增殖很快，但本身是正常的，且变异很慢。因此它们不大可能发展成对血管生成抑制剂耐药的表型，这与增殖很快的肿瘤细胞不同，后者经过高度的自发突变能稳定的产生耐药克隆。最后，肿瘤诱导的新生血管与正常的血管有明显的区别，这允许进行高度特异的靶向治疗[3,131]，这种血管生成抑制剂有高度的治疗指数和很小的毒性。常规化疗药物和血管生成抑制剂的联合应用证实特别有效。

第一个临床证实血管生成抑制剂能使肿瘤退化的报导来自一个患有致命的肺血管瘤患者使用 α-干扰素[150]的时候。此后发现越来越多的自然和合成的血管生成抑制剂，它们抑制不同的血管生成效应器，并且其中许多药物已在临床试用。已发现这些药物的毒性很小。具体的例子有直接抑制内皮细胞的药物，如反应停和考布他汀；阻断血管生成活化剂的药物，如贝伐单抗（Avastin），这是一个重组人抗 VEGF 抗体，或“VEGF 捕捉机”；抑制内皮特异存活信号的药物，如 Vitaxin（一种抗整合蛋白抗体）；非特异作用机制的药物，如塞来昔布（celecoxib）和白介素-12（IL-12）。NCI（美国国立癌症研究所）已经建立了一个网站，列出了所有正在进行临床试验的血管生成抑制剂（http://www.cancer.gov/clinical-trials/developments/anti-angio-table）。

由于抗血管生成治疗可能只有抑制肿瘤进展作用，当抑制血管生成的生长抑制作用中断后，肿瘤可
能恢复进展。因此，可能需要进行抗血管生成药物的 427
长期用药。基因治疗由于其具有持续表达的能力，可以为提供一种较长期应用血管生成抑制剂更为实用的方法[43]。

免疫治疗

免疫系统拥有特效的方法来发现和清除那些被识别为“外来的”分子和病原体。然而，因为肿瘤来源于宿主细胞，它们的免疫源性一般相对较弱。此外，恶性肿瘤细胞有数种机制来逃避免疫系统。这些机制包括下调对于激活许多免疫效应细胞必需的细胞表面主要组织相容性复合分子，产生免疫抑制因子和差异性表达可能作为在抗原漂移过程中免疫系统靶目标的各种不同蛋白。虽然由于癌细胞发生大量的突变和染色体异常，这导致异常、新的或静默蛋白的表达，但大多数（即使不是全部）肿瘤可能具有单一的、肿瘤相关的抗原，这些抗原能被免疫系统识别。例如常见于儿童肉瘤的融合蛋白和神经母细胞瘤持续产生的胚胎性神经外胚层抗原。

动员免疫系统以助清除肿瘤细胞是一个吸引人的方法，原因有以下几条。首先，血循环中的免疫系统细胞能够迅速接近处在隐蔽部位的肿瘤细胞。其次，免疫系统有强大的效应细胞来迅速有效的破坏和清除靶目标，包括肿瘤细胞。最初通过 T 细胞依赖或非依赖的细胞毒性效应来动员免疫系统，使其有效识别和破坏肿瘤细胞，相关研究主要集中于重组细胞因子。细胞因子通过直接刺激免疫系统[66]或通过使肿瘤细胞有更多的免疫源性来起作用。然而，自从最近发现基因转染能显著增加肿瘤免疫源性后，肿瘤细胞为基础的疫苗已开始被使用。例如，转染编码细胞因子基因的肿瘤细胞显示出的免疫源性明显增强，这使它们在被注射入宿主后能起抗肿瘤疫苗作用[4,10,42,57,141]。接受转导基因后的肿瘤细胞似乎比直接注射低剂量细胞因子到病灶的方法有更强的免疫源性。由于细胞因子由转导的肿瘤细胞在局部产生，因此没有为诱导抗肿瘤

效应而全身性高剂量应用细胞因子相关的副作用。这种转基因方法对没有特异相关抗原的肿瘤也有用。

因为考虑到肿瘤细胞可能不表达宿主免疫效应细胞能识别的抗原，因此也使用了另外的疫苗制作方法，即通过把肿瘤的裂解物或抗原性多肽呈递于自身的树突状细胞——免疫系统的抗原递呈细胞。这种方法能使特异性 T 细胞数量增加而介导肿瘤的退化[54]。作为该方法的延伸，一项以应用基因修饰而产生表达细胞因子的树突状细胞的方法正在进行临床前研究[136]。其他的临床前研究表明，通过表达细胞因子的肿瘤细胞形成免疫后，给予免疫激活 CpG 寡聚脱氧核苷酸，肿瘤的特异抗原免疫应答能被进一步提高[130]。

在儿童中，神经母细胞瘤是免疫治疗最常用的对象。通过将细胞因子基因转染进入自体或同种异体肿瘤细胞来治疗神经母细胞瘤的临床研究表明，基因修饰形成的表达细胞因子肿瘤细胞构成的疫苗毒性很低且能诱导抗肿瘤免疫应答[11,12,126]。神经母细胞瘤细胞对抗体依赖的、细胞介导的细胞毒效应敏感，也对补体依赖的细胞毒效应敏感[25]。虽然还没有发现神经母细胞瘤的特异抗原，但已得到鼠的抗神经节苷脂 GD2 单抗，由于 GD2 是一个神经母细胞瘤细胞表面的主要抗原。故这些抗体能起到治疗的作用[26,65]，但有明显毒性，特别是神经性疼痛[111]。由于抗 GD2 抗体诱导的抗体依赖的、细胞介导的细胞毒效应能被细胞因子（如粒单集落刺激因子[111]和 IL-2[67]）强化，目前关于抗神经母细胞瘤抗体的试验正在评价具有这些细胞因子的人源嵌合抗 GD2 抗体（ch14.18）和一个将人源 14.18 抗体通过遗传方法连锁到人重组 IL-2 的融合蛋白（hu14.18:IL2）的使用情况。

放疗的一般原则

放疗是目前治疗儿童肿瘤的三个基本模式之一。它的使用（单用或同手术及全身化疗联合）已成为许多儿童恶性肿瘤的基本治疗。每年，估计有 2000 或更多的儿童初始选择放疗用于治疗多种肿瘤，如白血病、脑瘤、肉瘤、Hodgkin 病、神经母细胞瘤和肾母细胞瘤[36]。考虑到肿瘤治愈性放疗和预期的长期存活（期间可能出现放疗所致的死亡率）之间的均衡性，放疗在儿童的应用方案与成人有所不同。

临床应用

放疗在儿童肿瘤的治疗中常作为多学科治疗计划的一部分，与手术治疗和化疗联合应用。虽然放疗在成人可单独应用，但儿童肿瘤的敏感性要求使用联合治疗来最大限度的控制肿瘤，同时尽可能减少治疗的长期副作用。放疗的应用可以在术前、术后（相对明确的手术切除），或单纯放疗无手术治疗。全身治疗也可以整合入该治疗方法。

根治性放疗

根治性放疗是原发实体肿瘤手术切除的替代治疗方法。它经常是儿童和青少年白血病或淋巴瘤的唯一局部治疗方法[37,52]。虽然它是无法切除肿瘤的唯一治疗选择，根治性放疗也可以用作手术切除的替代治疗，以保留一个器官或一种功能而同时保持最好的局部肿瘤的控制。横纹肌肉瘤的根治性放疗已经作为手术治疗的替代治疗，因后者的可能导致较高的死亡率；放疗已经可以取得较好的局部肿瘤控制而同时保留了正常功能[38]。Ewing 肉瘤家族肿瘤也可以考虑用根治性放疗作为手术的替代治疗。随着病例的仔细筛选，根治性放疗在取得良好的肿瘤局部控制率的同时，可以减少或避免高难度手术切除相关的死亡率[84,125]。

术前放疗

术前放疗可以在几种情况下使用。术前方案中，当肿瘤有不受手术影响的明显边界时，针对局部肿瘤的放疗是简单的。因为能更好地确定受肿瘤侵犯的面积，正常健康组织接受大剂量放疗的面积将减少。术前放疗已经在肾母细胞瘤的治疗中应用，以减少肿瘤的破裂[75]，以及在非横纹肌软组织肉瘤和 Ewing 肉瘤中应用，使手术切除更为容易[34,110]。然而术前放疗应用的限制，特别是在肉瘤患者，可能是术后伤口并发症的发生率轻度升高[110]。

术后放疗

在美国，术后放疗联合手术切除是辅助放疗最常用的方式。除了照射野选择上存在一些难度，术后放疗允许对完整的肿瘤标本进行病理分析，包括分析肿瘤的边界和肿瘤对以前治疗的效应。这种方法的伤口愈合并发症将减少，而且放疗剂量可以按照原发肿瘤切除后的病理学结果进行更为准确的调整。

化疗和放疗的相互作用

大多数的儿童肿瘤通过全身化疗来治疗。和化疗一样，在接受放疗的儿童，必须考虑提高局部治疗的效果及局部或区域性毒性的增强。经常通过联合化疗和放疗来治疗的实体瘤包括肾母细胞瘤、神经母细胞瘤和肉瘤。这些肿瘤可再分成几类，一类是化疗和放疗同时进行[38, 61]，另一类是化疗在放疗前面或后面进行[59,75,96]。当放、化疗同时进行或放疗与化疗的一个疗程很接近时，必须考虑几个问题。

化疗增强局部放疗效应

当即中抗儿童肿瘤的化疗药物同时使用时，可能会提高放疗的效果。例如顺铂、5-FU、丝裂霉素和吉西他滨等是众所周知的放疗增敏剂[2,46,124]。在放疗同时给予任何以上一个药物时需要与单独应用药物时使用不同的剂量和方案。尽管潜在的药物毒性明显增加，但在同时给予化疗和放疗的随机性研究中，肿瘤的局部控制作用明显提高[2,46]。

药物与放疗合用无增敏或只有有限的增敏作用

在儿童恶性肿瘤的治疗中，放疗通常和全身治疗联合应用，并不是为了增强局部效果，而是保证持续给予全身治疗以控制微小转移灶或转移性疾病。在这种情况下，与放疗联用的药物一般用于治疗儿童肉瘤，包括异环磷酰胺和足叶乙甙（它们与放疗联合治疗 Ewing 肉瘤）及长春新碱和环磷酰胺（与放疗联治疗横纹肌肉瘤）[38,61]。虽然这种方法将使局部毒性增加，但持续全身治疗带来的益处却远远超过这种危险性，特别是对微小转移灶高发生率的肿瘤。

增强放疗毒性的药物

一些药物明显增加放疗的局部毒性。因为这个原因，这些药物不与放疗同时使用，而且常在放疗结束后再停止一段时间。两个最明显的药物是阿霉素和放线菌素，当与放疗合用时，两者均能诱发明显的皮肤 429
和黏膜毒性[24,29]。喜树碱类（包括伊立替康和托泊替康）与放疗合用也可能出现黏膜毒性[58,100]。虽然这种毒性增强意味着局部效果的增加，但这种益处在目前的治疗方法和化疗给药剂量指南中并未被提及。因此，这些药物在放疗期间是不可应用的，且在放疗结束 2～6 周后才可再次应用。

随着许多作用于分子通路的新药的应用，目前全身治疗应用的范围日益增宽。很重要的一点是在新药和已知治疗（如放疗）方案联用时需考虑到可能出现的新毒性。

分次放疗

习惯上，外照射束放疗以分次方式进行。分次意味着每天给予放疗，每周 5 天，直到总剂量达到该肿瘤类型的放疗剂量。每天一次（每次剂量在 1.5～2.0Gy），每周 5 天的放疗被认为是“常规的”分次放疗。临近肿瘤的正常组织能够很好耐受这种每日放疗，而且显然许多类型肿瘤都能达到有效的局部控制。

有研究者进行了超分次放疗来治疗儿童恶性肿瘤（主要是脑瘤和实体瘤），以试图克服恶性肿瘤的生物学耐受[38,87]。虽然改良后的分次放疗效果在儿童肿瘤治疗中未得到证实，以下几个原因使人们考虑采用已证实效果与常规分次放疗相等的另一种放疗方案。超分次放疗的每次剂量少于 1.5Gy，能保证给予标准的放疗总剂量时副作用极少。加速的超分次放疗可压缩总的治疗时间，使在其他治疗（包括全身治疗或骨髓移植）之间可应用短程放疗。这种方法已经在儿童神经母细胞瘤的治疗中应用[87]，并且目前正在对接受骨髓移植的 Hodgkin 病患者进行该方法的治疗观察。儿童方案中放疗次数的改变一直在研究中，但它的益处必须与每天多次治疗带来的困难进行均衡，特别是治疗时需要接受全身麻醉的幼儿。

放疗技术

传统放疗

传统或常规放疗的计划及实施是基于非容积的影

像学研究（例如常规的 X 线片）。患者被置于特定的体位使得放射线束由常规的方向射入：即前位、后位和侧位。这种方法的缺陷与常规 X 线精确显示肿瘤组织部位的能力有关。虽然治疗射线束是围绕肿瘤定位的，但邻近的正常组织也受到大剂量的放疗。根据邻近正常组织在 X 线片上轮廓的精确性，这些组织的剂量可能是不能确定的。放疗是通过一个直线加速器产生的光子束来进行。

影像引导的放疗

影像引导的放疗包含用一组将射线照射到通常通过 CT 或 MRI 精确定位描述的治疗部位的技术。邻近的正常组织受到的照射剂量相对较低。当符合以下四个标准时，放疗可以称为影像引导的放疗：（1）获得患者治疗部位的三维影像资料（CT 或 MRI）；（2）影像资料被用于描绘和重建肿瘤三维容积和周边正常组织；（3）放疗束在设计和应用过程中能够在三维上自由定向，放疗束经过的组织可以被发射孔看到；（4）肿瘤和任何正常组织接受的放疗剂量可以基于三维空间的逐点方式进行计算。我们就目前使用的几个应用影像引导的光子放疗方法在这里进行讨论。

适形放疗

三维适形放疗的可以应用于患者在治疗体位进行影像学分析得出的特定的肿瘤容积。这种方法使用多个照射野和入口，将每一个放射束按肿瘤的容积形态而给予，并需每天进行。放射束调节器就像楔子，被用来调节放射束和肿瘤的相对位置，并确保肿瘤得到均一的放射剂量。适形放疗在成人头颈部肿瘤、肺癌和前列腺癌治疗中已经得到广泛研究，其优势在于肿瘤结构呈凸面和重要组织结构没有内陷于目标容积内的情况。目前的资料证实尽管对靶点使用了高放射剂量，但它的毒性仍较低[103]。

强度调控放疗

强度调控放疗是另一个应用外照射束放疗的方法，它需要对患者治疗部位进行影像学分析并描绘肿瘤和正常组织的轮廓。放疗以多个小照射野的方式进行，不围绕整个肿瘤进行，但准确地给予所需的每日
放射剂量。强度调控放疗与适形放疗的不同在于： 430
（1）增加了治疗所需的设计和实施的复杂性和时间；（2）增加了治疗前所需的质控工作量；（3）增加了肿瘤容积的放射剂量不均一性，由此一些肿瘤内部病变区域获得的放射剂量相对较高；（4）能用于凹面的肿瘤，同时重要组织结构内陷于目标容积内部的情况。最后一点意味着该方法能更好地保护正常组织和减少毒副作用。对给予强度调控放疗的成人患者的初步资料显示，它在儿童脑瘤和其他成人肿瘤的应用中有减轻治疗毒性的作用[73]。

近距离放射疗法

近距离放射疗法是通过把放射源置于肿瘤内或邻近部位来实施放疗的方法，通常在手术切除和直视条件下进行。对于肿瘤放疗剂量在切除后设定，并且可能要应用 CT 或 MRI 分析；放射源的合适强度则需预先决定。在儿童通常应用的放射源包括铱 192 和碘 125。近距离放射疗法可以是低剂量强度（大约 40～80cGy/h）或高剂量强度（60～100cGy/min）。低剂量率强度在数天内给予，患者常需要住院，而高剂量率强度分次进行，每次数天，1～2 周内完成。近距离放射疗法的主要好处在于放射源被置于肿瘤内或邻近部位（通常在手术切除时置入）。外科医生和放疗医生有必要进行术前设计和合作以确保合适和准确的进行近距离放射疗法。非横纹肌肉瘤的软组织肉瘤和部分横纹肌肉瘤是儿童肿瘤中最常用到近距离放射疗法的肿瘤类型[102,115]。然而大多数其他儿童实体瘤对近距离放射疗法依从性差，因为受肿瘤的生物学特性（如放疗耐受）或其解剖学定位（如后腹膜）等因素影响。

其他放疗方法

其他几个针对原发肿瘤病灶的放疗方法也在成人和儿童肿瘤患者中应用。术中放疗已经在局部肿瘤切除后开始间歇性应用[63]。虽然在美国这种治疗受到限制，但术中放疗有明显的优点，能在放疗时看到肿瘤病灶，因此提高了放疗的准确性，并提供临时将可移动的关键器官（如肠道和膀胱）搬到照射野以外的机会。限制术中放疗的主要因素是它只能进行单次放

疗，通常在 10～20Gy 的剂量范围。必须考虑到不能从放射野移除的正常组织对放疗的耐受性，这也将限制有效放疗的剂量。

质子放疗和其他应用大带电粒子方法也已经在有限的几个医疗中心进行研究。这些方法的主要优点是具有将放射束终止在特定和可控制深度的属性。这将保护邻近肿瘤的健康正常组织。然而质子放疗的应用受到限制，因为建造合适的治疗设备费用昂贵；只有一小部分机构可以装备。虽然在 20 世纪 90 年代后期对质子放疗的兴趣在下降，但现在已经恢复，在美国有几个新的设备目前正在建设中。通过合理设计，与目前最新的影像引导光子束放疗技术比较，将可以发现这种治疗模式的潜在优势。

姑息性放疗

对于许多患者，肿瘤的治疗，特别是儿童肿瘤，主要集中于可治愈性的将手术、放疗和化疗综合在一起的多学科治疗。尽管儿童肿瘤治疗已取得重大的成功，仍有许多儿童出现复发，并最终死于恶性肿瘤。虽然并没有过多关于姑息性放疗的讨论，它仍然是一个有效的干预性治疗[68]。姑息性放疗的概念提示它的目的是对症治疗。姑息性放疗的最终目的是维持那些不能在疾病中存活患者的生活质量，同时尽可能减少他们必须接受的破坏性治疗。肿瘤放疗专家经常被要求使患者疾病的疼痛部位的症状缓解，特别是那些骨骼浸润和重要脏器（包括脊髓、外周神经和呼吸道）压迫导致的症状。这种情况下的放疗与治疗性放疗相同，都是每日进行。最关注的主要是症状的缓解，同时治疗相关的副作用达到最小。姑息性放疗是高度个体化的，它的成功和失败有赖于组织学诊断、先前的治疗、症状的持续时间和所需治疗的症状如何。

放疗的急性和远期毒性

放疗相关的副作用，包括急性和慢性，在儿童和成人都有完善的描述，但不幸的是，它们的发生率以及和放疗剂量及肿瘤容积的相关性没有特征性[39]。历史上，治疗相关副作用被分成急性或远期作用；一个任意指定的治疗结束后 90 天是这两类作用的分界点。目前评估治疗相关副作用的指南不再用这个任意指定的分界点，但在讨论放疗相关副作用时早期和远期分界点是有意义的。实际上，所有这些副作用源于治疗放射束的范围，通常是大剂量放疗区域。最常见的放疗早期和远期相关副作用见表 25-6。尽管分为早期和远期副作用有任意性，但这种分类将患者中可能完全恢复的副作用和可能永久性存在的副作用区别开来。早期治疗相关副作用，如果正确治疗，将可以恢复正常，邻近肿瘤的健康组织逐渐从放疗副作用中恢复。恢复的时间范围从数天到数月，但患者一般很少有后遗症。放疗结束后，在远期仍可见的治疗相关副作用更可能变成慢性或永久性的。它们显然与被放疗健康组织的正常康复反应相关，导致出现不必要的副作用，如纤维化。许多远期放疗副作用可以被治疗，但是不可逆的。对于接受治愈性放疗的患儿，长期副作用是一个主要的关注点，最好能用可预防远期副作用的方法来治疗。儿童的一些长期副作用可以通过限制接受大剂量放疗的正常组织容积和尽可能减少邻近肿瘤的健康组织的放疗剂量的方法来改善。

干细胞移植的一般原则

输注或移植能够重建造血系统的造血干细胞在两种情况下使用。首先，造血干细胞移植（HSCT）能被用于替代一个有缺陷的造血系统中有缺失或异常的成分。其次，HSCT 能被用于重建实体瘤治疗中被强烈化疗或放疗破坏的造血系统或本身出现异常的造血系统的某一部分。移植的细胞可以是患者本身（即自体移植，其中的细胞在骨髓抑制治疗前采集），也可以来自供体（即同种异体移植，供体一般是 HLA 相合的同胞、不相合的家族成员或部分相合的无关供体）。后两种情况下进行移植需要免疫抑制和移植物预处理来达到移植物成功的植入和避免移植物抗宿主病（GVHD）。造血祖细胞一般从骨髓或外周血获得。它们是移植的主要成分，因为它们能够自我更新，因此，可长期产生造血系统各系细胞。有些情况下，当可获取时，库存的脐带血也可以作为造血干细胞（HSC）的来源。总的来说，虽然自体细胞用于 HSCT 是最安全的，但它们可能被肿瘤细胞污染。GVHD 在同种异体 HSCT时可发生，能危

表 25–6 接受放疗患儿出现的治疗相关副作用

器官 / 部位	急性	慢性
皮肤	红斑	萎缩
	脱皮	色素沉着
皮下组织	水肿	纤维化
黏膜	黏膜炎	溃疡
中枢神经系统	水肿	坏死
	头痛	脊髓炎
		认知下降
眼	结膜炎	白内障
		视网膜病
		干眼
甲状腺	—	甲状腺功能减退
心脏	—	心包炎
		心肌炎
肺	肺炎	肺纤维化
肠道	恶心	坏死
	腹泻	
肾脏	—	肾炎
		肾功能不全
膀胱	排尿困难	出血性膀胱炎
	尿急	
	尿频	
肌肉	水肿	纤维化
		发育不全
骨骼	—	长骨骨骺提前闭合
		发育不全

及生命，但适度的移植物抗宿主反应如果能对抗宿主肿瘤细胞，则可能有益处。

骨髓一般从髂后上棘采集，总量为每公斤受体体重的 10～20ml。外周血干细胞在重组粒细胞集落刺激因子动员后采集，在采集前每日给药至一周。虽然尚不知细胞主要组分对于造血系统重建的应答的确切机制，但表面标记 CD34 的细胞数量与移植物成功植入率相关[35]。在 HSCT 前，受体需要接受预处理（或“净化”）化疗方案的治疗。该治疗有几个目的，包括杀灭残留肿瘤细胞、为异体造血干细胞移植提供免疫抑制、并为移植的造血干细胞提供移植“空间”。在输注前，HSC 采集物可能需体外处理以使假定的祖细胞（例如 $CD34^{+}$或 $CD133^{+}$细胞）浓集，一般用阳性或阴性选择性方法，以利于造血系统重建；除去供体的 T 淋巴细胞，从而减少异体 HSCT 的 GVHD发生危险；或使污染的肿瘤细胞从自体 HSCT 的采集物中清除。

HSCT 可以出现明显的并发症。最常见的早期并发症是感染，这是由于患者短暂但严重的免疫抑制，及同时出现黏膜屏障的破坏所导致的。另一个常见并发症是静脉闭塞病，其临床特征是肝脏肿痛、黄 43
疸和液体潴留。超声检查显示门静脉反流。肝活检显示典型的肝小静脉闭塞和小叶中心肝细胞坏死的组织学表现。这种情况没有特异的治疗方法；只能给予支持治疗，而轻或中度静脉闭塞病是自限性的。其他 HSCT 急性并发症包括 GVHD（是供体 T 细胞介导的过程，因宿主细胞带有抗原差异而被供体 T 细胞攻击）和移植物失活。远期并发症包括慢性 GVHD、内分泌缺乏、继发肿瘤、生长迟缓和其他与作为预处理方案一部分的全身放疗相关的后遗症。然而，尽管其存在这样那样的毒性，HSCT 仍是目前许多儿童高危恶性肿瘤成功的多学科综合治疗的一部分。

临床试验

就像前面提及的，过去的 40 年中儿童恶性肿瘤的整体存活率已经取得显著的提高。取得这种提高是得益于新药的开发和治疗方法的改进、支持治疗的改善和更好的诊断模式使恶行肿瘤能够被更早发现。这些进步的益处已经通过仔细设计和分析的临床试验进行了证实。由于儿童肿瘤相对少见，这些试验的严密的组织和计划是必需的。在美国和其他参与国家中，临床试验主要由儿童肿瘤协作组实施，由各个大的机构或小财团参与小的前导性研究。

临床试验一般分为三个阶段。第 I 阶段研究用来评价一个新的诊断或治疗用药的可能毒性。第 I 阶段常需要一小部分患者，典型的是使用剂量递增方案，在使用更高剂量前观察几组患者的毒性表现。该类研究的终点通常是确定药物的安全剂量或人体最大耐受剂量（或两者均有）。然而，不断增加的生物学试剂的出现和检测将要求研究者转而评估最佳生物学剂量。进入第 I 阶段毒性研究的对象通常限于那些对于常规或“标准”治疗无效的患者。第 II 阶段研究用来检测一个新药或治疗方法是否足够有效以确保值得进一步研究。第 II 阶段研究的药物通常给予初次发病患者，在他们的标准治疗开始前或刚完成后进行。新药在“预测窗口”（即标准治疗前）的测试已经显示对延期的标准治疗有效时不会出副作用。最后，第 III 阶段研究用来比较实验性治疗和标准治疗的有效性。一般第 III 阶段研究最好作前瞻性和随机对照研究，但由于患者数量较少，一般第 III 阶段研究通过比较一个实验性治疗组和过去给予标准治疗对照组的效果来进行。通过这种系统评估来评价新治疗方法的危险性和优点，从而决定拒绝或接受该方法作为新的标准治疗，儿童肿瘤学领域研究也因此不断得到提高。

结论

在过去 20 年，分子遗传学研究的进展已经使我们对人类恶性肿瘤（包括那些儿童恶性肿瘤）病源学和疾病进展过程中遗传因素的了解不断增加。许多儿童恶性肿瘤成为肿瘤分子遗传的模型。儿科学的经验阐明了在许多方面分子分析的使用价值。通过细胞遗传学、FISH 和 RT-PCR 证明肿瘤特异的染色体易位可做出组织病理诊断。染色体异常、基因过度表达和基因扩增的检测可用于危险度分组和选择治疗计划。阐明涉及抑癌基因的信号途径增加了我们对肿瘤相关综合征的了解，并为遗传筛查和咨询及预防性的手术干预指明了道路。在不久的将来，某个肿瘤分子特征的解读将为新治疗方法的形成奠定基础。治疗将实现个体化，那些生物学高危肿瘤患者将接受更强的治疗方案以达到治愈，而生物学低危肿瘤患者将通过低强度治疗而治愈，并因低毒性而获益。阐明肿瘤发病过程中涉及的复杂分子途径，也将促进高效、高特异和高治疗指数的靶向抗肿瘤药物的产生。

（叶启东译 王耀平校）

参考文献

1. Abramson LP, Grundy PE, Rademaker AW, et al: Increased microvascular density predicts relapse in Wilms' tumor. J Pediatr Surg 2003;38:325-330.
2. Al Sarraf M, LeBlanc M, Giri PG, et al: Chemoradiotherapy versus radiotherapy in patients with advanced nasopharyngeal cancer: Phase III randomized intergroup study 0099. J Clin Oncol 1998;16:1310-1317.
3. Arap W, Pasqualini R, Ruoslahti E: Cancer treatment by targeted drug delivery to tumor vasculature in a mouse model. Science 1998;279:377-380.
4. Asher AL, Mule JJ, Kasid A, et al: Murine tumor cells transduced with the gene for tumor necrosis factor-alpha: Evidence for paracrine immune effects of tumor necrosis factor against tumors. J Immunol 1991;146:3227-3234.
5. Bader SA, Fasching C, Brodeur GM, et al: Dissociation of suppression of tumorigenicity and differentiation in vitro effected by transfer of single human chromosomes into human neuroblastoma cells. Cell Growth Differ 1991;2:245-255.
6. Barbacid M: Neurotrophic factors and their receptors. Curr Opin Cell Biol 1995;7:148-155.
7. Bardeesy N, Falkoff D, Petruzzi MJ, et al: Anaplastic Wilms' tumour, a subtype displaying poor prognosis, harbours p53 gene mutations. Nat Genet 1994;7:91-97.
8. Barr FG: The role of chimeric paired box transcription factors in the pathogenesis of pediatric rhabdomyosarcoma. Cancer Res 1999;59:1711s-1715s.
9. Bicknell R, Harris AL: Mechanisms and therapeutic implications of angiogenesis. Curr Opin Oncol 1996;8:60-65.
10. Blankenstein T, Qin ZH, Uberla K, et al: Tumor suppression after tumor cell-targeted tumor necrosis factor alpha gene transfer. J Exp Med 1991;173:1047-1052.
11. Bowman L, Grossmann M, Rill D, et al: IL-2 adenovector-transduced autologous tumor cells induce antitumor immune responses in patients with neuroblastoma. Blood 1998;92:1941-1949.
12. Bowman LC, Grossmann M, Rill D, et al: Interleukin-2 gene-modified allogeneic tumor cells for treatment of relapsed neuroblastoma. Hum Gene Ther 1998;9:1303-1311.
13. Bown N, Cotterill S, Lastowska M, et al: Gain of chromosome arm 17q and adverse outcome in patients with neuroblastoma. N Engl J Med 1999;340:1954-1961.
14. Bredel M, Pollack IF, Hamilton RL, et al: Epidermal growth factor receptor expression and gene amplification in high-grade non-brainstem gliomas of childhood. Clin Cancer Res 1999;5:1786-1792.
15. Brodeur GM, Hayes FA, Green AA, et al: Consistent N-myc copy number in simultaneous or consecutive neuroblastoma samples from sixty individual patients. Cancer Res 1987;47:4248-4253.
16. Brodeur GM, Maris JM, Yamashiro DJ, et al: Biology and genetics of human neuroblastomas. J Pediatr Hematol Oncol 1997;19:93-101.
17. Brodeur GM, Seeger RC, Schwab M, et al: Amplification of N-myc in untreated human neuroblastomas correlates with advanced disease stage. Science 1984;224:1121-1124.
18. Brodeur GM, Sekhon G, Goldstein MN: Chromosomal aberrations in human neuroblastomas. Cancer 1977;40:2256-2263.
19. Brooks PC, Silletti S, von Schalscha TL, et al: Disruption of angiogenesis by PEX, a noncatalytic metalloproteinase fragment with integrin binding activity. Cell 1998;92:391-400.

20. Browder T, Butterfield CE, Kraling BM, et al: Antiangiogenic scheduling of chemotherapy improves efficacy against experimental drug-resistant cancer. Cancer Res 2000;60:1878-1886.
21. Buchdunger E, Cioffi CL, Law N, et al: Abl protein-tyrosine kinase inhibitor STI571 inhibits in vitro signal transduction mediated by c-kit and platelet-derived growth factor receptors. J Pharmacol Exp Ther 2000;295:139-145.
22. Call KM, Glaser T, Ito CY, et al: Isolation and characterization of a zinc finger polypeptide gene at the human chromosome 11 Wilms' tumor locus. Cell 1990;60:509-520.
23. Carmeliet P, Jain RK: Angiogenesis in cancer and other diseases. Nature 2000;407:249-257.
24. Cassady JR, Richter MP, Piro AJ, et al: Radiation-Adriamycin interactions: preliminary clinical observations. Cancer 1975; 36:946-949.
25. Cheung NK: Immunotherapy: Neuroblastoma as a model. Pediatr Clin North Am 1991;38:425-441.
26. Cheung NK, Burch L, Kushner BH: Monoclonal antibody 3F8 can effect durable remissions in neuroblastoma patients refractory to chemotherapy: A phase II trail. In Evans AE, D'Angio GJ, Kundson AG (eds): Advances in Neuroblastoma Research, 3rd ed. Hoboken, NJ: Wiley-Liss, 1991, p 395.
27. Clark J, Benjamin H, Gill S, et al: Fusion of the EWS gene to CHN, a member of the steroid/thyroid receptor gene superfamily, in a human myxoid chondrosarcoma. Oncogene 1996;12:229-235.
28. Clark J, Rocques PJ, Crew AJ, et al: Identification of novel genes, SYT and SSX, involved in the t(X;18)(p11.2;q11.2) translocation found in human synovial sarcoma. Nat Genet 1994;7:502-508.
29. Cohen IJ, Loven D, Schoenfeld T, et al: Dactinomycin potentiation of radiation pneumonitis: A forgotten interaction. Pediatr Hematol Oncol 1991;8:187-192.
30. Coppes MJ, Bonetta L, Huang A, et al: Loss of heterozygosity mapping in Wilms' tumor indicates the involvement of three distinct regions and a limited role for nondisjunction or mitotic recombination. Genes Chromosomes Cancer 1992;5:326-334.
31. Coppes MJ, Haber DA, Grundy PE: Genetic events in the development of Wilms' tumor. N Engl J Med 1994;331: 586-590.
32. Dameron KM, Volpert OV, Tainsky MA, et al: Control of angiogenesis in fibroblasts by p53 regulation of thrombospondin-1. Science 1994;265:1582-1584.
33. de Alava E, Kawai A, Healey JH, et al: *EWS-FLI1* fusion transcript structure is an independent determinant of prognosis in Ewing's sarcoma. J Clin Oncol 1998;16:1248-1255.
34. Delaney TF, Spiro IJ, Suit HD, et al: Neoadjuvant chemotherapy and radiotherapy for large extremity soft-tissue sarcomas. Int J Radiat Oncol Biol Phys 2003;56: 1117-1127.
35. Diaz MA, Vicent MG, Garcia-Sanchez F, et al: Long-term hematopoietic engraftment after autologous peripheral blood progenitor cell transplantation in pediatric patients: Effect of the CD34+ cell dose. Vox Sang 2000;79:145-150.
36. Donaldson SS, Halperin EC: Subspecialty training and certification for radiation oncology. J Am Coll Radiol 2004;1:488-492.
37. Donaldson SS, Hudson MM, Lamborn KR, et al: VAMP and low-dose, involved-field radiation for children and adolescents with favorable, early-stage Hodgkin's disease: Results of a prospective clinical trial. J Clin Oncol 2002; 20:3081-3087.
38. Donaldson SS, Meza J, Breneman JC, et al: Results from the IRS-IV randomized trial of hyperfractionated radiotherapy in children with rhabdomyosarcoma—a report from the IRSG. Int J Radiat Oncol Biol Phys 2001;51:718-728.
39. Emami B, Lyman J, Brown A, et al: Tolerance of normal tissue to therapeutic irradiation. Int J Radiat Oncol Biol Phys 1991;21:109-122.
40. Evans AE, Kisselbach KD, Yamashiro DJ, et al: Antitumor activity of CEP-751 (KT-6587) on human neuroblastoma and medulloblastoma xenografts. Clin Cancer Res 1999; 5:3594-3602.
41. Farber S: Chemotherapeutic studies of tumors, including leukemia, in children. Am J Dis Child 1950;79:961-962.
42. Fearon ER, Pardoll DM, Itaya T, et al: Interleukin-2 production by tumor cells bypasses T helper function in the generation of an antitumor response. Cell 1990;60:397-403.
43. Feldman AL, Libutti SK: Progress in antiangiogenic gene therapy of cancer. Cancer 2000;89:1181-1194.
44. Fidler IJ: The organ microenvironment and cancer metastasis. Differentiation 2002;70:498-505.
45. Fidler IJ, Ellis LM: The implications of angiogenesis for the biology and therapy of cancer metastasis. Cell 1994; 79:185-188.
46. Flam M, John M, Pajak TF, et al: Role of mitomycin in combination with fluorouracil and radiotherapy, and of salvage chemoradiation in the definitive nonsurgical treatment of epidermoid carcinoma of the anal canal: Results of a phase III randomized intergroup study. J Clin Oncol 1996;14:2527-2539.
47. Folkman J: What is the evidence that tumors are angiogenesis dependent? J Natl Cancer Inst 1990;82:4-6.
48. Folkman J: The role of angiogenesis in tumor growth. Semin Cancer Biol 1992;3:65-71.
49. Folkman J: Clinical appli cations of research on angiogenesis. N Engl J Med 1995;333:1757-1763.
50. Folkman J, D'Amore PA: Blood vessel formation: What is its molecular basis? Cell 1996;87:1153-1155.
51. Fong CT, Dracopoli NC, White PS, et al: Loss of heterozygosity for the short arm of chromosome 1 in human neuroblastomas: Correlation with N-myc amplification. Proc Natl Acad Sci U S A 1989;86:3753-3757.
52. Friedmann AM, Hudson MM, Weinstein HJ, et al: Treatment of unfavorable childhood Hodgkin's disease with VEPA and low-dose, involved-field radiation. J Clin Oncol 2002; 20:3088-3094.
53. Galili N, Davis RJ, Fredericks WJ, et al: Fusion of a fork head domain gene to PAX3 in the solid tumour alveolar rhabdomyosarcoma. Nat Genet 1993;5:230-235.
54. Geiger JD, Hutchinson RJ, Hohenkirk LF, et al: Vaccination of pediatric solid tumor patients with tumor lysate-pulsed dendritic cells can expand specific T cells and mediate tumor regression. Cancer Res 2001;61:8513-8519.
55. Giardiello FM: Gastrointestinal polyposis syndromes and hereditary nonpolyposis colorectal cancer. In Rustgi AD (ed): Gastrointestinal Cancers: Biology, Diagnosis, and Therapy. Philadelphia: Lippincott-Raven, 1995, pp 367-377.
56. Goldie JH, Coldman AJ: A mathematic model for relating the drug sensitivity of tumors to their spontaneous mutation rate. Cancer Treat Rep 1979;63:1727-1733.
57. Golumbek PT, Lazenby AJ, Levitsky HI, et al: Treatment of established renal cancer by tumor cells engineered to secrete interleukin-4. Science 1991;254:713-716.
58. Graham MV, Jahanzeb M, Dresler CM, et al: Results of a trial with topotecan dose escalation and concurrent thoracic radiation therapy for locally advanced, inoperable nonsmall cell lung cancer. Int J Radiat Oncol Biol Phys 1996;36:1215-1220.
59. Green DM: The treatment of stages I-IV favorable histology Wilms' tumor. J Clin Oncol 2004;22:1366-1372.

60. Green DM, Jaffe N: Wilms' tumor—model of a curable pediatric malignant solid tumor. Cancer Treat Rev 1978; 5:143-172.
61. Grier HE, Krailo MD, Tarbell NJ, et al: Addition of ifosfamide and etoposide to standard chemotherapy for Ewing's sarcoma and primitive neuroectodermal tumor of bone. N Engl J Med 2003;348:694-701.
62. Grundy P, Coppes MJ, Haber D: Molecular genetics of Wilms' tumor. Hematol Oncol Clin North Am 1995;9: 1201-1215.
63. Haas-Kogan DA, Fisch BM, Wara WM, et al: Intraoperative radiation therapy for high-risk pediatric neuroblastoma. Int J Radiat Oncol Biol Phys 2000;47:985-992.
64. Hamada J, Cavanaugh PG, Lotan O, et al: Separable growth and migration factors for large-cell lymphoma cells secreted by microvascular endothelial cells derived from target organs for metastasis. Br J Cancer 1992;66:349-354.
65. Handgretinger R, Baader P, Dopfer R, et al: A phase I study of neuroblastoma with the anti-ganglioside GD2 antibody 14.G2a. Cancer Immunol Immunother 1992;35: 199-204.
66. Hank JA, Robinson RR, Surfus J, et al: Augmentation of antibody dependent cell mediated cytotoxicity following in vivo therapy with recombinant interleukin 2. Cancer Res 1990;50:5234-5239.
67. Hank JA, Surfus J, Gan J, et al: Treatment of neuroblastoma patients with antiganglioside GD2 antibody plus interleukin-2 induces antibody-dependent cellular cytotoxicity against neuroblastoma detected in vitro. J Immunother 1994;15:29-37.
68. Harris MB: Palliative care in children with cancer: Which child and when? J Natl Cancer Inst Monogr 2004;144-149.
69. Henderson C, Brancolini C: Apoptotic pathways activated by histone deacetylase inhibitors: Implications for the drug-resistant phenotype. Drug Resist Update 2003;6:247-256.
70. Hobson B, Denekamp J: Endothelial proliferation in tumours and normal tissues: Continuous labelling studies. Br J Cancer 1984;49:405-413.
71. Holmgren L, O'Reilly MS, Folkman J: Dormancy of micrometastases: Balanced proliferation and apoptosis in the presence of angiogenesis suppression. Nat Med 1995; 1:149-153.
72. Howe JR, Norton JA, Wells SA Jr: Prevalence of pheochromocytoma and hyperparathyroidism in multiple endocrine neoplasia type 2A: Results of long-term follow-up. Surgery 1993;114:1070-1077.
73. Huang E, Teh BS, Strother DR, et al: Intensity-modulated radiation therapy for pediatric medulloblastoma: Early report on the reduction of ototoxicity. Int J Radiat Oncol Biol Phys 2002;52:599-605.
74. Hug EB, Sweeney RA, Nurre PM, et al: Proton radiotherapy in management of pediatric base of skull tumors. Int J Radiat Oncol Biol Phys 2002;52:1017-1024.
75. Jereb B, Burgers JM, Tournade MF, et al: Radiotherapy in the SIOP (International Society of Pediatric Oncology) nephroblastoma studies: A review. Med Pediatr Oncol 1994;22:221-227.
76. Kaneko Y, Kanda N, Maseki N, et al: Different karyotypic patterns in early and advanced stage neuroblastomas. Cancer Res 1987;47:311-318.
77. Kaur G, Stetler-Stevenson M, Sebers S, et al: Growth inhibition with reversible cell cycle arrest of carcinoma cells by flavone L86-8275. J Natl Cancer Inst 1992;84:1736-1740.
78. Keshelava N, Zuo JJ, Waidyaratne NS, et al: p53 mutations and loss of p53 function confer multidrug resistance in neuroblastoma. Med Pediatr Oncol 2000;35:563-568.
79. Kingston JE, Herbert A, Draper GJ, et al: Association between hepatoblastoma and polyposis coli. Arch Dis Child 1983;58:959-962.
80. Kinzler KW, Vogelstein B: Familial cancer syndromes: The role of caretakers and gatekeepers. In Vogelstein B, Kinzler KW (eds): The Genetic Basis of Human Cancer. New York: McGraw-Hill, 1998, pp 241-599.
81. Knudson AG Jr: Mutation and cancer: Statistical study of retinoblastoma. Proc Natl Acad Sci U S A 1971;68: 820-823.
82. Kohl NE, Kanda N, Schreck RR, et al: Transposition and amplification of oncogene-related sequences in human neuroblastomas. Cell 1983;35:359-367.
83. Koufos A, Grundy P, Morgan K, et al: Familial Wiedemann-Beckwith syndrome and a second Wilms' tumor locus both map to 11p15.5. Am J Hum Genet 1989;44:711-719.
84. Krasin MJ, Rodriguez-Galindo C, Davidoff AM, et al: Efficacy of definitive irradiation and multi-agent systemic therapy for localized Ewing's sarcoma family of tumors (ESFT). Int J Radiat Oncol Biol Phys 2003;57:S197.
85. Kucharczak J, Simmons MJ, Fan Y, et al: To be, or not to be: NF-kappaB is the answer—role of Rel/NF-kappaB in the regulation of apoptosis. Oncogene 2003;22:8961-8982.
86. Kusafuka T, Fukuzawa M, Oue T, et al: Mutation analysis of p53 gene in childhood malignant solid tumors. J Pediatr Surg 1997;32:1175-1180.
87. Kushner BH, Wolden S, LaQuaglia MP, et al: Hyperfractionated low-dose radiotherapy for high-risk neuroblastoma after intensive chemotherapy and surgery. J Clin Oncol 2001;19:2821-2828.
88. Ladanyi M, Gerald W: Fusion of the *EWS* and *WT1* genes in the desmoplastic small round cell tumor. Cancer Res 1994;54:2837-2840.
89. Laughner E, Taghavi P, Chiles K, et al: HER2 (neu) signaling increases the rate of hypoxia-inducible factor 1alpha (HIF-1alpha) synthesis: Novel mechanism for HIF-1-mediated vascular endothelial growth factor expression. Mol Cell Biol 2001;21:3995-4004.
90. Levi-Montalcini R: The nerve growth factor 35 years later. Science 1987;237:1154-1162.
91. Liotta LA, Steeg PS, Stetler-Stevenson WG: Cancer metastasis and angiogenesis: An imbalance of positive and negative regulation. Cell 1991;64:327-336.
92. Look AT, Hayes FA, Nitschke R, et al: Cellular DNA content as a predictor of response to chemotherapy in infants with unresectable neuroblastoma. N Engl J Med 1984;311: 231-235.
93. Look AT, Kirsch IR: Molecular basis of childhood cancer. In Pizzo PA, Poplack DG (eds): Principles and Practices of Pediatric Oncology. Philadelphia: Lippincott-Raven, 1997, p 38.
94. Lutz W, Stohr M, Schurmann J, et al: Conditional expression of N-myc in human neuroblastoma cells increases expression of alpha-prothymosin and ornithine decarboxylase and accelerates progression into S-phase early after mitogenic stimulation of quiescent cells. Oncogene 1996;13: 803-812.
95. Malkin D, Li FP, Strong LC, et al: Germ line p53 mutations in a familial syndrome of breast cancer, sarcomas, and other neoplasms. Science 1990;250:1233-1238.
96. Matthay KK, Villablanca JG, Seeger RC, et al: Treatment of high-risk neuroblastoma with intensive chemotherapy, radiotherapy, autologous bone marrow transplantation, and 13-cis-retinoic acid: Children's Cancer Group. N Engl J Med 1999;341:1165-1173.
97. May WA, Gishizky ML, Lessnick SL, et al: Ewing sarcoma

11;22 translocation produces a chimeric transcription factor that requires the DNA-binding domain encoded by FLI1 for transformation. Proc Natl Acad Sci U S A 1993; 90:5752-5756.
98. May WA, Lessnick SL, Braun BS, et al: The Ewing's sarcoma *EWS/FLI-1* fusion gene encodes a more potent transcriptional activator and is a more powerful transforming gene than FLI-1. Mol Cell Biol 1993;13:7393-7398.
99. McNeil C: Herceptin raises its sights beyond advanced breast cancer. J Natl Cancer Inst 1998;90:882-883.
100. Mehta VK, Cho C, Ford JM, et al: Phase II trial of preoperative 3D conformal radiotherapy, protracted venous infusion 5-fluorouracil, and weekly CPT-11, followed by surgery for ultrasound-staged T3 rectal cancer. Int J Radiat Oncol Biol Phys 2003;55:132-137.
101. Meitar D, Crawford SE, Rademaker AW, et al: Tumor angiogenesis correlates with metastatic disease, N-myc amplification, and poor outcome in human neuroblastoma. J Clin Oncol 1996;14:405-414.
102. Merchant TE, Parsh N, del Valle PL, et al: Brachytherapy for pediatric soft-tissue sarcoma. Int J Radiat Oncol Biol Phys 2000;46:427-432.
103. Merchant TE, Zhu Y, Thompson SJ, et al: Preliminary results from a phase II trial of conformal radiation therapy for pediatric patients with localised low-grade astrocytoma and ependymoma. Int J Radiat Oncol Biol Phys 2002;52:325-332.
104. Mulligan LM, Kwok JB, Healey CS, et al: Germ-line mutations of the RET proto-oncogene in multiple endocrine neoplasia type 2A. Nature 1993;363:458-460.
105. Nagata S: Apoptosis by death factor. Cell 1997;88:355-365.
106. Nakagawara A, Azar CG, Scavarda NJ, et al: Expression and function of Trk-B and BDNF in human neuroblastomas. Mol Cell Biol 1994;14:759-767.
107. Nguyen M, Watanabe H, Budson AE, et al: Elevated levels of the angiogenic peptide basic fibroblast growth factor in urine of bladder cancer patients. J Natl Cancer Inst 1993;85:241-242.
108. Nishisho I, Nakamura Y, Miyoshi Y, et al: Mutations of chromosome 5q21 genes in FAP and colorectal cancer patients. Science 1991;253:665-669.
109. O'Brien KP, Seroussi E, Dal Cin P, et al: Various regions within the alpha-helical domain of the *COL1A1* gene are fused to the second exon of the *PDGFB* gene in dermatofibrosarcomas and giant-cell fibroblastomas. Genes Chromosomes Cancer 1998;23:187-193.
110. O'Sullivan B, Davis AM, Turcotte R, et al: Preoperative versus postoperative radiotherapy in soft-tissue sarcoma of the limbs: A randomised trial. Lancet 2002;359:2235-2241.
111. Ozkaynak MF, Sondel PM, Krailo MD, et al: Phase I study of chimeric human/murine anti-ganglioside G(D2) monoclonal antibody (ch14.18) with granulocyte-macrophage colony-stimulating factor in children with neuroblastoma immediately after hematopoietic stem-cell transplantation: A Children's Cancer Group Study. J Clin Oncol 2000;18: 4077-4085.
112. Pelletier J, Bruening W, Kashtan CE, et al: Germline mutations in the Wilms' tumor suppressor gene are associated with abnormal urogenital development in Denys-Drash syndrome. Cell 1991;67:437-447.
113. Petit AM, Rak J, Hung MC, et al: Neutralizing antibodies against epidermal growth factor and ErbB-2/neu receptor tyrosine kinases down-regulate vascular endothelial growth factor production by tumor cells in vitro and in vivo: Angiogenic implications for signal transduction therapy of solid tumors. Am J Pathol 1997;151:1523-1530.
114. Pinthus JH, Fridman E, Dekel B, et al: ErbB2 is a tumor associated antigen and a suitable therapeutic target in Wilms' tumor. J Urol 2004;172:1644-1648.
115. Pisters PW, Harrison LB, Leung DH, et al: Long-term results of a prospective randomized trial of adjuvant brachytherapy in soft tissue sarcoma. J Clin Oncol 1996; 14:859-868.
116. Pluda JM: Tumor-associated angiogenesis: Mechanisms, clinical implications, and therapeutic strategies. Semin Oncol 1997;24:203-218.
117. Powell SM, Petersen GM, Krush AJ, et al: Molecular diagnosis of familial adenomatous polyposis. N Engl J Med 1993;329:1982-1987.
118. Pritchard-Jones K, Fleming S, Davidson D, et al: The candidate Wilms' tumour gene is involved in genitourinary development. Nature 1990;346:194-197.
119. Quesnel S, Malkin D: Genetic predisposition to cancer and familial cancer syndromes. Pediatr Clin North Am 1997;44:791-808.
120. Rabbitts TH, Forster A, Larson R, et al: Fusion of the dominant negative transcription regulator CHOP with a novel gene FUS by translocation t(12;16) in malignant liposarcoma. Nat Genet 1993;4:175-180.
121. Riccardi VM, Sujansky E, Smith AC, et al: Chromosomal imbalance in the aniridia-Wilms' tumor association: 11p interstitial deletion. Pediatrics 1978;61:604-610.
122. Ries LG: Childhood cancer mortality. In Ries LG, Smith MA, Gurney JG, et al (eds): Cancer Incidence and Survival among Children and Adolescents: United States SEER Program 1975-1995. National Cancer Institute, 1999, pp 165-169.
123. Risau W: Mechanisms of angiogenesis. Nature 1997;386: 671-674.
124. Robinson BW, Ostruszka L, Im MM, et al: Promising combination therapies with gemcitabine. Semin Oncol 2004; 31:2-12.
125. Rodriguez-Galindo C, Spunt SL, Pappo AS: Treatment of Ewing sarcoma family of tumors: Current status and outlook for the future. Med Pediatr Oncol 2003;40: 276-287.
126. Rousseau RF, Haight AE, Hirschmann-Jax C, et al: Local and systemic effects of an allogeneic tumor cell vaccine combining transgenic human lymphotactin with interleukin-2 in patients with advanced or refractory neuroblastoma. Blood 2003;101:1718-1726.
127. Rubin BP, Chen CJ, Morgan TW, et al: Congenital mesoblastic nephroma t(12;15) is associated with *ETV6-NTRK3* gene fusion: Cytogenetic and molecular relationship to congenital (infantile) fibrosarcoma. Am J Pathol 1998; 153:1451-1458.
128. Ruegg C, Yilmaz A, Bieler G, et al: Evidence for the involvement of endothelial cell integrin alphaVbeta3 in the disruption of the tumor vasculature induced by TNF and IFN-gamma. Nat Med 1998;4:408-414.
129. Sabers CJ, Martin MM, Brunn GJ, et al: Isolation of a protein target of the FKBP12-rapamycin complex in mammalian cells. J Biol Chem 1995;270:815-822.
130. Sandler AD, Chihara H, Kobayashi G, et al: CpG oligonucleotides enhance the tumor antigen-specific immune response of a granulocyte macrophage colony-stimulating factor-based vaccine strategy in neuroblastoma. Cancer Res 2003;63:394-399.
131. Schnitzer JE: Vascular targeting as a strategy for cancer therapy. N Engl J Med 1998;339:472-474.
132. Seeger RC, Brodeur GM, Sather H, et al: Association of multiple copies of the N-myc oncogene with rapid progression of neuroblastomas. N Engl J Med 1985;313:

1111-1116.
133. Sharpless NE, DePinho RA: Telomeres, stem cells, senescence, and cancer. J Clin Invest 2004;113:160-168.
134. Sherr CJ: The Pezcoller lecture: Cancer cell cycles revisited. Cancer Res 2000;60:3689-3695.
135. Sherr CJ, McCormick F: The RB and p53 pathways in cancer. Cancer Cell 2002;2:103-112.
136. Shimizu T, Berhanu A, Redlinger RE Jr, et al: Interleukin-12 transduced dendritic cells induce regression of established murine neuroblastoma. J Pediatr Surg 2001;36: 1285-1292.
137. Sorensen PH, Lessnick SL, Lopez-Terrada D, et al: A second Ewing's sarcoma translocation, t(21;22), fuses the EWS gene to another ETS-family transcription factor, ERG. Nat Genet 1994;6:146-151.
138. Srivastava A, Laidler P, Davies RP, et al: The prognostic significance of tumor vascularity in intermediate-thickness (0.76-4.0 mm thick) skin melanoma: A quantitative histologic study. Am J Pathol 1988;133:419-423.
139. Svensson T, Ryden M, Schilling FH, et al: Coexpression of mRNA for the full-length neurotrophin receptor Trk-C and Trk-A in favourable neuroblastoma. Eur J Cancer 1997;33: 2058-2063.
140. Teitz T, Wei T, Valentine MB, et al: Caspase 8 is deleted or silenced preferentially in childhood neuroblastomas with amplification of MYCN. Nat Med 2000;6:529-535.
141. Tepper RI, Mule JJ: Experimental and clinical studies of cytokine gene-modified tumor cells. Hum Gene Ther 1994;5:153-164.
142. Thiesing JT, Ohno-Jones S, Kolibaba KS, et al: Efficacy of STI571, an abl tyrosine kinase inhibitor, in conjunction with other antileukemic agents against bcr-abl-positive cells. Blood 2000;96:3195-3199.
143. Ton CC, Hirvonen H, Miwa H, et al: Positional cloning and characterization of a paired box- and homeobox-containing gene from the aniridia region. Cell 1991;67: 1059-1074.
144. Toole BP: Hyaluronan and its binding proteins, the hyaladherins. Curr Opin Cell Biol 1990;2:839-844.
145. van Leeuwen FE: Risk of acute myelogenous leukaemia and myelodysplasia following cancer treatment. Baillieres Clin Haematol 1996;9:57-85.
146. Vandesompele J, Van Roy N, Van Gele M, et al: Genetic heterogeneity of neuroblastoma studied by comparative genomic hybridization. Genes Chromosomes Cancer 1998;23:141-152.
147. Varanasi R, Bardeesy N, Ghahremani M, et al: Fine structure analysis of the WT1 gene in sporadic Wilms' tumors. Proc Natl Acad Sci U S A 1994;91:3554-3558.
148. Vogelstein B, Kinzler KW: Cancer genes and the pathways they control. Nat Med 2004;10:789-799.
149. Wai DH, Knezevich SR, Lucas T, et al: The *ETV6-NTRK3* gene fusion encodes a chimeric protein tyrosine kinase that transforms NIH3T3 cells. Oncogene 2000;19: 906-915.
150. White CW, Sondheimer HM, Crouch EC, et al: Treatment of pulmonary hemangiomatosis with recombinant interferon alfa-2a. N Engl J Med 1989;320:1197-1200.
151. Xiong S, Grijalva R, Zhang L, et al: Up-regulation of vascular endothelial growth factor in breast cancer cells by the heregulin-beta1-activated p38 signaling pathway enhances endothelial cell migration. Cancer Res 2001;61:1727-1732.
152. Young JL Jr, Ries LG, Silverberg E, et al: Cancer incidence, survival, and mortality for children younger than age 15 years. Cancer 1986;58:598-602.
153. Zhang L, Yu D, Hu M, et al: Wild-type p53 suppresses angiogenesis in human leiomyosarcoma and synovial sarcoma by transcriptional suppression of vascular endothelial growth factor expression. Cancer Res 2000;60: 3655-3661.
154. Zucman J, Delattre O, Desmaze C, et al: EWS and ATF-1 gene fusion induced by t(12;22) translocation in malignant melanoma of soft parts. Nat Genet 1993;4:341-345.

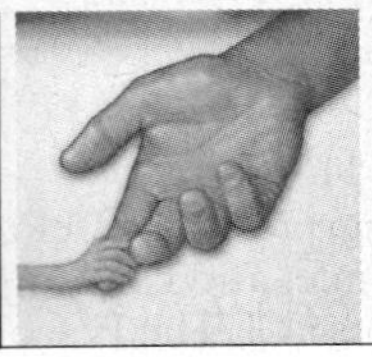

第 26 章

儿童癌症活检原则

James D. Geiger 和 Douglas C. Barnhart

437 随着术前化疗在儿童癌症中的运用越来越多见，活检技术的重要性也在不断提高。过去，最终诊断要在原发肿瘤手术切除时才能实现。目前儿童更多进行经皮或开放活检而不是首次切除。而且随着对恶性肿瘤分子学认识的变化，通过小的标本就能对癌症进行诊断和精确地分期。这就减少了与儿童恶性实体肿瘤诊断相关的并发症。

微创技术诊断的发展有个过程，从完全手术摘除到开放活检再到经皮穿刺活检和微创径路手术。这些实践中的变化不仅源于手术技术的进步，而且源于分子标记物对儿童恶性实体肿瘤的诊断和危险分型认识的提高。这个进步比在个体病例中简化活组织检查的选择要复杂，因为有许多综合因素要考虑。经皮穿刺活检[19,34]、微创径路手术活检[24]和开放手术活检都是安全有效获得诊断以及检验复发或转移的方法。然而，这些技术的成功明显依赖于医疗机构的经验，这在选择活检方法时必须考虑。另外，必须认识到儿童恶性肿瘤治疗的进步和危险分型的进展得益于肿瘤银行的发展及相关生物学的发展。如果没有大量的活检标本，肿瘤银行和细胞系生物研究的发展是不可能的。对于许多肿瘤包括神经母细胞瘤肿瘤，标本的收集对于我们进一步加深对该疾病的认识非常重要。

针对风险分型进行的治疗有显著的进展[18]。当这种分型变得更加复杂时，从活检标本中获得的信息类型也会变得更加个体化。为了选择并发症发生最低且又能获得分型所必需的信息的活检方式，外科医生必须知道有关联合治疗中所采用的分型方案。这个观念可以通过 2 例腹部肿块均疑似神经母细胞瘤的病例来进行说明，2 例都有骨髓转移病灶，他们的治疗均在当前儿童肿瘤组（COG）方案[57]下进行。第一个患者年龄小于 1 岁，其治疗组可分成低危、中危或高危组。分组决定需要通过 N-myc 基因扩增的状态、国际神经母细胞瘤病理学分型状况以及 DNA 的倍体来确定，这些都需要获取原发病变的标本并进行检测才能确定。而一个年龄稍大的有相似临床表现的儿童将被分类到高危组。因此单独的骨髓活检认定可以明确诊断和分组。很显然对多种治疗方式的掌握是选择活检技术的基础。

标本的提取

传统诊断依赖于肿瘤组织伊红染色永久切片的组织学表现。免疫组化可以作为补充的诊断手段，同样运用甲醛溶液固定的标本进行检测。儿童恶性肿瘤分子学诊断有了很大的进展，包括基因变型的认识，它对于诊断和预后都有着重要意义[9,39,41]。检测这些变化的方法包括反转录酶聚合酶链反应[11]、原位荧光杂交[39]、微阵列分析和流式细胞分析。不合适的标本提取可能妨碍这些分析的完成。举例来说，通过甲醛溶液固定淋巴结的流式细胞分析不能完成淋巴瘤的分子形态分型。鉴于分子诊断领域的飞速发展，外科医生在进行 4
活检之前，活检取何处标本需要同病理科医生商讨。

经皮针刺活检

1904 年 Grieg 和 Gray 首次运用细针吸引活检技术为细胞病理学提取标本[17]。Jereb 等 1978 年成功报道运用针刺活检诊断儿童实体肿瘤[29]。随后，多个研究机构的广泛经验证实了针刺吸引和针刺切割活检技术的准确性和安全性。这些技术的吸引力在于诊断不会在联合治疗机构中被延误，在某些情况下，活检可以作为门诊程序进行。

针刺活检通常在普通麻醉或镇静下进行。在特定的大年龄儿童，某些部位的活检可以在局部麻醉下进行[54]。

可触及的肢体肿块和其他体表肿块如淋巴结可以进行经皮针刺活检。深部活检需要超声或 CT 的引导。超声多普勒探头可以清晰地显示大血管和其他结构以及当针头前进时提供最及时的影像[51]。有些切割针头设备放置了一个小的气泡，可以确定活检的部位。CT 可以清晰地显像充气的肺而不会因肠道气体而模糊不清[10]。可以测定和计划活检的深度[19]。同放射科医生合作他们会提供关于影像学监测的情况，最佳方式应该是二者共同参与活检。

细针吸引活检

细针吸引活检因为是微创的活检技术从而明显受到推崇。如果需要对多个病变部位穿刺，标准的操作是运用 22～25G 细针。运用细针吸引活检成功诊断需要有经验的细胞病理医生的合作。为了提高诊断效率，标本取得后应立即进行检查。如果首次标本不够，需要再次穿刺吸引[52]。大量的儿童和成人的细针吸引活检证实该技术的安全性[16,31]。

传统运用细针吸引活检进行诊断是以细胞常规染色以及光镜下细胞的形态为基础。在癌症发生率高的成人患者中，细针吸引活检是一种常见的方法用来确诊可疑病变是否存在癌变。在成人，癌症的诊断以及原发部位的确定足以做出开始治疗的决定。然而患儿的联合治疗方案依赖于组织形态的特异性，因此细针吸引活检在儿童中不是很常用。近来分子技术和电镜对于光镜的补充提高了细针吸引活检的组织形态特异性，增加了细针吸引活检在儿童恶性实体肿瘤中的运用[20,30]。

细针吸引活检最直接的运用是验证转移病灶或原发肿瘤的复发[26]。在这种情况下，证实恶性癌细胞的存在足以指导进一步临床决策。这种微创活检方法特别适合于已经做过免疫学或其他生理学检查的患者。

支持运用细针吸引活检诊断癌症的文献有所增加。细针吸引活检对骨肉瘤的确诊可达到 65%[12]～92%[32]；这项技术在儿童和成人中一样准确。在软组织肿瘤中运用细针吸引活检依赖于对分子基因异常及肿瘤特异性蛋白的认识[30,31]。然而需要注意的是，这一病例研究的报道来源有限数量的细胞学权威机构，所以在这种情况下使用 FNAB 需要非常小心。

细针吸引活检没有广泛用于儿童小圆蓝细胞肿瘤的诊断。然而，随着辅助研究的增加，诸如电子显微镜、细胞免疫组化、DNA 倍体、细胞基因学和荧光原位杂交，细针吸引活检的运用可能会变得普遍[3]。据报道细针吸引活检在儿童头颈部肿块的评估中有很好的敏感性和特异性[35,37]。但解读这些结果仍需要注意，因为大部分吸引活检都是诊断活性的淋巴结病，用来诊断新发恶性肿瘤的病例数量少。此外，通过其他一些诊断技术最终诊断为淋巴瘤的病例假阴性结果经常发生（不是特异性地局限于头颈部）[52]。

芯针活检

与细针吸引活检比较，芯针活检的优势在于能够提供足够的标本进行组织学检查而不只是细胞学检查。另外，它能够提供足够的组织进行分子学评估。尽管该技术在成人中广泛应用，但在儿童中的运用不是很常见。有几个关于该技术在 280 多个儿童病例中运用有效性和安全性的报道[19,34,51,54]。

目前有不同型号的芯针，常用的是 14G[34] 至 18G[19]。针被设计成在中心有一个切割鞘，当针头退出时保证获得组织。这个切割鞘的推进可以是由人工控制的或由螺旋发射装置控制的（图 26–1）。目前没

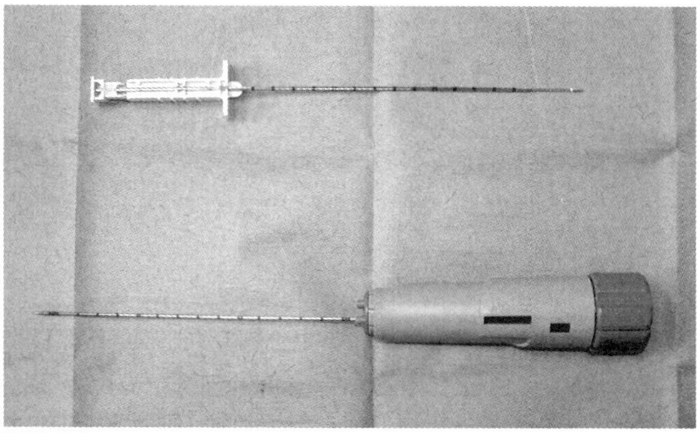

图 26–1　两种常用的切割针刺活检装置。上面一种是直径 14G 的切割针（Allegiance）。它进入需要穿刺的部位，里面的针向前，外鞘手动操作向前覆盖内针得到组织。下面一种是直径 16G 单腔活检设计装置（Bard）。当顶点到达穿刺部位时它是弹射负载被激发。弹射负载机制推动活塞环和套管连续自动前进。

有资料直接比较两种方法从儿童恶性肿瘤所获标本的质量。螺旋发射装置的快速发展使人为挤碎较轻，这
439 在儿童肾脏活检中获得证实[54]。不管用哪种方法，穿刺后都要仔细检查保证获得足够的标本。大多数患者只需要一次穿刺获得足够的组织，如果首次穿刺不能获得足够的标本，那么需要多次穿刺。

芯针活检在不同的解剖部位都已得到成功，包括颈部、纵隔、肺、腹膜腔、肝脏、后腹膜、肾脏、肾上腺、盆腔和肢体[19,34,51,54]。表 26–1 概括了四个病例研究报道的有关芯针活检在恶性肿瘤诊断的准确性。这项技术的敏感性是可以接受的，但也存在明显的误诊病例。这些错误可以通过参考临床病史以及其他标本加以避免[19]。在一些不相符的病例，不明确的诊断需要立刻重新认识，重复经皮穿刺或开放活检。芯针活检检测转移或复发的病变比诊断初发疾病得到的结果准确性高。

在这个报道中没有患者死于与操作有关的死亡以及因操作并发症而需要手术介入。有一文献报道 3% 的芯针活检患者因血细胞容积显著降低需要输血，10%的患者需经胸穿刺放置胸腔引流管[51]。

因存在气胸的风险以及呼吸系统病变部位的变化，肺病变的芯针活检需要特别注意。Connolly 等于 1999 年报道了儿童肺部小病变芯针活检的经验[10]。活检在儿童常规麻醉下 CT 引导下进行。所有的影像检查以及活检都在完全呼气时完成。83%的病例因取到合适的标本而获得诊断，病变平均大小为 9mm。当没有获得合适的标本时，进行吸引细胞学检查，最终诊断率达到 94%。27%的病例出现小的气胸，没有一例有症状或需要引流。

芯针穿刺道肿瘤的复发是这项活检技术的特殊并发症。在成人中这项并发症统计差异很大，从肝细胞癌的 3.4%到颈部肿瘤的 0.01%[33]。有 2 例儿童肾母细胞瘤穿刺道肿瘤复发的报道。此并发症的发生受诸多因素的影响。免疫疗法、化疗、放疗的作用能够减少芯针穿刺道肿瘤的复发。芯针活检使用的大针比吸引活检的小针风险性大[21]。

微创手术

在过去的 15 年里，微创手术包括腹腔镜和胸腔镜的广泛运用对儿童普通外科影响巨大。目前这两项技术被用于癌症的诊断治疗。Gans 和 Beric 在 1971 年报道了在儿童中运用腔镜技术的最初经验。有趣的是，他们提倡的胸腔镜最主要的适应证之一是引导转移植入物的活检。腹腔镜和胸腔镜的适应证变得广泛起来，包括儿童癌症的最初诊断和对转移癌或难治性疾病的评估。

腹腔镜

腹腔镜对于儿童癌症患者腹腔的评价具有以下几个优势。第一它提供了一个检查整个腹腔的机会以及对整个腹膜表面的系统探查。可以检查整个肠管包括肠系膜和淋巴结，可以容易地进行多个活检。第二腹腔镜能够减少手术带给患儿的生理创伤，因为他们病情可能原本已经很重了。第三与所有的微创手术一样术后疼痛减少恢复加快[28]。腹腔镜最主要的缺点是评价后腹膜病变能力有限以及缺少对深部病变的触觉评价。

诊断性腹腔镜和活检在儿童实体肿瘤管理的几种情况下得以运用[24,48]。腹腔镜活检有很高的诊断成功率[24,47]。腹腔镜活检与芯针活检相比能够使外

表 26–1 芯针活检诊断的准确性

作者 / 年份	患者数（总数 / 恶性肿瘤）	敏感性（%）	评论
Klose 等[34]/1991	39/16	100	所有肿瘤组织分型正确
Somers 等[54]/1993	25/23	88	4 例诊断不符，包括神经母细胞被诊断为节细胞瘤
Skoldenberg 等[51]/2002	110/84	82	因为标本不足 16 例得不到诊断
Guimaraes 等[19]/2003	54/54	82	4 例诊断更改，包括肾母细胞瘤被诊断为神经母细胞瘤

科医生获得更大的组织标本。生物学检查特别需要大的标本。在早期诊断中，腹腔镜能够辅助确定腹部巨大肿块的原发来源。在评价腹膜内肿瘤和腹水方面腹腔镜优于 CT[7]。例如，腹腔镜能直接确定盆腔肿块来源于卵巢还是膀胱颈部，放射学检查很难区分这点。腹腔镜的直视作用被用来评价肝母细胞瘤的可切除性[24]。在治疗过程中，腹腔镜用来评价转移性疾病或再次手术时原发肿瘤治疗后的反应。

在肿瘤患者中运用腹腔镜需要注意的一个问题是创口部位的复发。这个并发症在成人各类恶性肿瘤中均有发生，最显著的是直肠和胆囊腺癌[40]。这个并发症最常发生在没有预计的胆囊癌切除术后[49]。创口复发在成人脂肪肉瘤和宫颈癌切除术后也有发生[25,2]。成人上消化道和肾脏恶性肿瘤术后创口复发率非常低[50,15]。在儿童中这方面的相关数据非常有限。COG 回顾研究了 85 例儿童病例均无创口复发[24]。日本儿童腹腔镜外科医生调查随访了 85 例腹腔镜和 44 例胸腔镜病例均无创口肿瘤复发[27]。必须指出这 104 例病例都是神经母细胞瘤，许多是筛查出来的，因此这些资料的广泛适用性可能会受到限制。由于在成人癌症和儿童肿瘤之间存在肿瘤生物学差异，儿童肿瘤通常对新辅助化疗反应明显，因此也很难从成人文献中概括出来。所以，需要对儿童肿瘤创口部位肿瘤复发情况进行进一步监测。

儿童腹腔镜通常在全麻下进行，有助于耐受气腹。腹腔镜检查的绝对禁忌证是心肺功能不稳定，心肺功能不稳定可以阻止腹腔气腹。仰卧位体位最为常用，它能提供腹腔的完整视野。为了获得良好的视野，采用 30 度的腹腔镜，另外至少在两个部位操作和撤出。需要收集腹水进行细胞学检查，并探查整个腹膜表面。可以运用腔镜剪刀进行切割活检。运用电凝和止血药进行止血（在开放活检章节进行讨论），或缝合活检周围组织止血。活检组织通常用标本袋回收。这样做可以减少标本回收时的破坏以及降低创口肿瘤的复发风险。也可以用杯口状活检钳获取标本组织。在腹腔镜引导下进行的切割穿刺活检可以在后腹膜、腹腔内或肝脏肿块上取样进行活检。对于深部肿瘤如肝脏病变，腹腔镜下超声能够用来引导活检，弥补不能触摸组织的缺陷[8,38]。

腹腔镜诊断和治疗儿童实体肿瘤产生的并发症不常见。术中需要转为开放活检的频率很低[24,28,48]。

胸腔镜

胸腔镜最早作为一项分离结核导致的胸膜粘连的技术于 1910 年被 Jacobus 所报告。1976 年 Rodgers 和 Talbert 报道在儿童中运用胸腔镜的最初经验[45]。他们描述了 9 例病例，其中 2 例是肿瘤患者（Ewing 肉瘤和复发的 Hodgkin 淋巴瘤）。随后，胸腔镜在儿童胸部病变的评估中运用得越来越普遍了。有以下几个原因。首先与常规开胸手术相比胸腔镜活检或切除

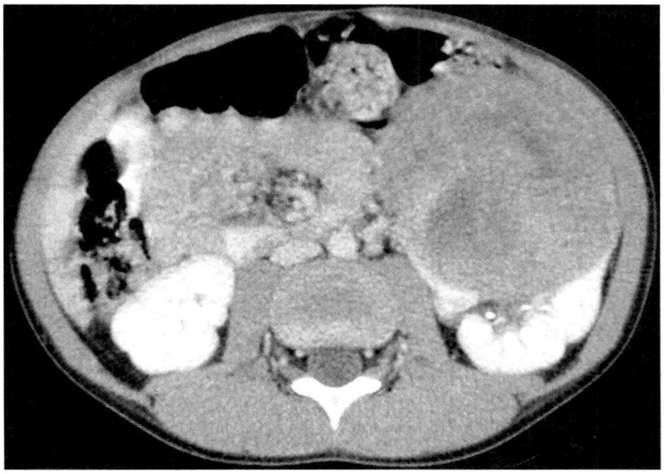

A

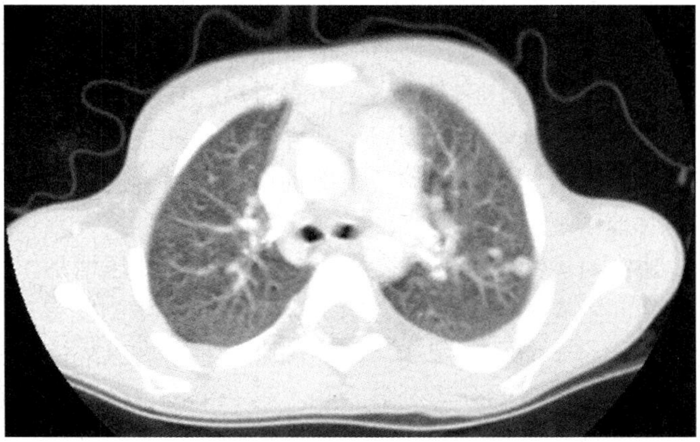

B

图 26–2 一名 5 岁男孩新诊断为腹部肿块时的 CT 扫描图像。A. 腹部盆腔 CT 扫描显示一巨大左侧肾脏肿块。B. 胸部 CT 扫描显示左上叶肺部有单个的 8mm 结节。无其他肺部病灶。肾切除时，同时进行胸腔镜肺部病灶切除活检。肾脏最终病理诊断为 II 期肾母细胞瘤，肺部病理为玻璃样肉芽肿。

术后疼痛显著减轻。其次胸腔镜几乎能够完全显示胸壁和胸膜，这是开胸手术做不到的。另外，绝大多数儿童的纵隔没有大量的脂肪组织，因此能够被胸腔镜探查到。

尽管儿童原发性肺部肿瘤很少发生，但在儿童癌症治疗过程中肺部病变很容易被混淆[56]。最常见的早期肺部转移的肿瘤是肾母细胞瘤。骨软组织肉瘤、肝脏肿瘤、畸胎癌和黑色素瘤的肺部转移也很常见。胸腔镜通常用来评估初诊时或随访阶段的转移病灶，在
441 临床治疗过程中很难鉴别机会致病感染和新转移病变。在地方流行性肉芽肿病中，胸腔镜对诊断非常有帮助（图 26–2），在这种情况下胸腔镜活检的诊断准确性非常高[44,47,48,56]。

纵隔病变也可以用胸腔镜进行活检或者切除[42,44]。胸腔镜能够提供前纵隔和后纵隔良好的视野，甚至在年幼的儿童中。与纵隔镜相比我们更喜欢用胸腔镜来评估儿童纵隔病变。

胸腔镜的绝对禁忌证是胸膜间隙完全阻塞和当需要肺完全塌陷时不能承受单肺通气。

在儿童中胸腔镜手术通常需要在气管插管机械通气下进行。单肺通气以及辅助吹气有利于取得良好的手术视野。在年龄较大的儿童中，双腔的气管插管可以完成上述要求。在年龄较小的儿童中，左肺可以通过右主支气管插管来阻断。左主支气管插管非常困难，插管经常移位到右侧部位。右肺塌陷通过气管插管和右支气管阻断来完成的运用气管阻断器或支气管镜放置 Fogarty 导管可造成右支气管阻塞。Fogarty 导管的尺寸依据年龄而变化，4 岁或小于 4 岁者可用 3 号，5～12 岁者可用 5 号[55]。在插管时可以根据需要充气或放气。如果选择性通气很难做到或患者难以承受，二氧化碳低压气腹（5～10cmH_2O）有助于暴露视野。麻醉医生必须监测因控制性张力气胸带来的副作用。如有需要气体能够被快速抽空，但患者通常能够很好地耐受。

通常对患儿取一侧开胸手术位置。胸腔高压增加了肋间间隙有利于胸腔镜打洞。纵隔病变时体位要有所调整。对于前纵隔病变，需要仰卧一些；后纵隔病变，患者位置需俯卧得更多一些。第一个创口位于腋中线用钝性分离开刀。其余的创口在胸腔镜的引导下根据病变需要进行选择。30 度的胸腔镜有助于完全显示整个胸膜表面的情况。多个创口还有助于彻底探查。

细致地了解每个横断面的影像学是胸腔镜活检成功的基础，尤其是微小病变。当肺塌陷时胸膜或胸膜下的肺部病变通常显而易见，因此可以运用内镜切割钳切割，用标本袋取出。对深部病变的鉴定更具挑战性。当肺完全塌陷后，触摸肺实质可以确诊大的病变，如果 CT 定位准确的话小的病变活检可以按照解剖部位进行如顶部、舌部或基底部病变。CT 引导的定位是通过术前置细金属丝或注射亚甲蓝溶液或自身染色的血液实现的[23,43,36]。这些定位技术在儿童准确诊断中非常有效[36,43]。胸腔内超声有助于定位实质深部病灶。然而，这些技术没有广泛运用，在儿童中的有效性评估也非常有限。在将来，影像学引导的活检将
在术中 MRI 或 CT 引导下完成。 4

组织取样结束以后，气胸排气可通过将小的导管置于有水的密闭容器中完成。除非扩大的肺活检或者肺的其他疾病，否则不需要胸腔引流管。绝大多数儿童术后第二天可以出院，化疗可以马上进行[36]。

胸腔镜技术的诊断效率很高。根据大多数儿科系列报道，几乎所有的病例都取得了准确的诊断组织[24,44,48,56]。胸腔镜诊断的并发症非常少见。气胸以及持续性漏气可能发生在有潜在肺实质疾病或者需要高压呼吸机支持的患者中。在第一个 Trcar 放置过程中因为单肺通气引起的膈肌上升可能损伤膈下脏器。

开放活检术

如果手术不能完全切除，开放活检仍然是取得合适标本的金标准。在直视下腹腔镜和胸腔镜可以获得大的标本，与针刺活检相比提高了诊断性。例如，开放活检在 NWTS–4 中诊断退行发育的成功率高于切割针刺活检的。如果存在可能引起活检错误的肿瘤不均质，同术前影像学检查结合可以在多处取活检标本。

大的标本组织的取得不仅有利于分子标记诊断及预后评估，而且能够为肿瘤银行提供组织及创建细胞系。这些活检提供的临床材料能够完善分子学诊断及早期预后评估。进一步高危分型，获得更为准确的危险分型的治疗方案，目前仍然是儿科肿瘤学研究的焦点。最后，肿瘤银行储存的标本能够用于研究性治疗，如针对个体患者的疫苗。

在进行开放活检的时候有几个重点。最初的活检要考虑到最后的手术治疗。举个例子，肢体的肿块活检应该与肢体的轴线平行，要仔细考虑避免损害皮下及筋膜组织。这样有利于随后的局部扩大切除手术，同时做到最小切除活检的组织。同样，睾丸肿瘤活检只有通过腹股沟进行，如果经阴囊活检，随后睾丸切除时需要附加半侧阴囊切除。腹腔镜活检需要进行计划，允许下次手术可通过延长以前的切口完成。

后腹膜巨大肿瘤可导致解剖关系的显著变异，必须注意避免结构的损伤诸如输尿管、胆道或因肿块发生变化的主要血管结构。儿童腹腔内最常见的肿瘤是血管瘤，活检部位出血是最常见严重的并发症。减少术中出血的方法包括术前纠正出凝血指标和术中充分暴露。电灼肿瘤包膜有助于止血，但我们发现在覆盖着含凝血药物的氧化纤维素的活检部位上直接加压比电灼止血更有效。有可能的话，关闭肿瘤包膜更有助于止血。

其他辅助止血手段包括局部止血药物、纤维蛋白封闭剂和Ⅶa 因子重组体。商品化的有效局部止血产品包括明胶泡沫袋、微纤维胶原蛋白和氧化纤维素，氧化纤维素有纤维和棉花样作用。纤维蛋白封闭剂成分包括纤维蛋白原、凝血酶原和钙。当遇到组织后这些成分的混合物可导致纤维样栓迅速形成。Ⅶa 因子重组体最初用来治疗有阻断子的血友病患者，现在广泛用来治疗严重出血而以往没有凝血异常的患者。有许多报告报道Ⅶa 因子重组体用于治疗创伤患者以及它在前列腺扩大切除术中有效的随机试验。也有报道其在肝母细胞瘤活检后有效地控制出血。我们成功地将其用于控制肾母细胞瘤肝转移引起的出血。这是一个昂贵的治疗方案，尽管风险性总结得不够，但初步经验表明，凝血并发症发生率很低。

外科医生的重要作用在于为诊断和高危分型提供合适的组织。从传统上来说，开放活检能够很好地为此目的服务，且并发症发生率低。但将来由于分子学诊断发展，只需要很少的肿瘤标本或根本不需要原发肿瘤活检，开放活检就会减少。对诊断及治疗的深刻认识以及外科医生和肿瘤科医生的良好合作对于为每个个体患者选择合适活检方式是最为重要的。

(徐　敏译　王　珊校)

参考文献

1. Abramowicz, M: Novoseven for nonhemophilia hemostasis. Med Lett 2004;46:1181.
2. Agostini A, et al: Port site metastasis after laparoscopy for uterine cervical carcinoma. Surg Endosc 2003;17: 1663-1665.
3. Akhtar M, et al: Fine-needle aspiration biopsy diagnosis of small round cell tumors of childhood: A comprehensive approach. Diagn Cytopathol 1999;21:81-91.
4. Aslam A, Spicer RD: Needle track recurrence after biopsy of non-metastatic Wilms' tumor. Pediatr Surg Int 1996;11: 416-417.
5. Ayar D, et al: Needle-track metastasis after transthoracic needle biopsy. J Thorac Imaging 1998;13:2-6.
6. Barro C, et al: Successful use of recombinant factor VIIa for severe surgical liver bleeding in a 5-month-old baby. Haemophilia 2004;10:183-185.
7. Barth RA, et al: A comparison study of computed tomography and laparoscopy in the staging of abdominal neoplasms. Dig Dis Sci 1981;26:253-256.
8. Berber E, Siperstein AE: Laparoscopic ultrasound. Surg Clin North Am 2004;84:1061-1084.
9. Bown N: Neuroblastoma tumour genetics: Clinical and biological aspects. J Clin Pathol 2001;54:897-910.
10. Connolly BL, et al: CT-guided percutaneous needle biopsy of small lung nodules in children. Pediatr Radiol 1999;29: 342-346.
11. Dagher R, et al: Molecular confirmation of Ewing sarcoma. J Pediatr Hematol Oncol 2001;23:221-224.
12. Dodd LG, et al: Utility of fine-needle aspiration in the diagnosis of primary osteosarcoma. Diagn Cytopathol 2002;27:350-353.
13. Friederich PW, et al: Effect of recombinant activated factor VII on perioperative blood loss in patients undergoing retropubic prostatectomy: A double-blind placebo-controlled randomised trial. Lancet 2003;361:201-205.
14. Gans SL, Berci G: Advances in endoscopy of infants and children. J Pediatr Surg 1971;6:199-233.
15. Gill IS, et al: Laparoscopic radical nephrectomy in 100 patients: A single center experience from the United States. Cancer 2001;92:1843-1855.
16. Gonzalez-Campora R: Fine needle aspiration cytology of soft tissue tumors. Acta Cytol 2000;44:337-343.
17. Grieg ED, Gray AC: Lymphatic glands in sleeping sickness. BMJ 1904;1:1252.
18. Grosfeld JL: Risk-based management of solid tumors in children. Am J Surg 2000;180:322-327.
19. Guimaraes AC, et al: Computed tomography-guided needle biopsies in pediatric oncology. J Pediatr Surg 2003; 38:1066-1068.
20. Gurley AM, et al: The utility of ancillary studies in pediatric FNA cytology. Diagn Cytopathol 1992;8:137-146.
21. Haddad FS, Somsin AA: Seeding and perineal implantation of prostatic cancer in the track of the biopsy needle: Three case reports and a review of the literature. J Surg Oncol 1987;35:184-191.
22. Hamilton TE, et al: Open biopsy is superior to needle for detection of anaplasia in patients with Wilms' tumor. Paper presented at the American Pediatric Surgical Association meeting, 2004.
23. Hanninen EL, et al: Computed tomography-guided pulmonary nodule localization before thoracoscopic resection. Acta Radiol 2004;45:284-288.

24. Holcomb GW 3rd, et al: Minimally invasive surgery in children with cancer. Cancer 1995;76:121-128.
25. Horiguchi A, et al: Port site recurrence after laparoscopic resection of retroperitoneal liposarcoma. J Urol 1998; 159:1296-1297.
26. Howell LP: Changing role of fine-needle aspiration in the evaluation of pediatric masses. Diagn Cytopathol 2001;24:65-70.
27. Iwanaka T, et al: No incidence of port-site recurrence after endosurgical procedure for pediatric malignancies. Pediatr Surg Int 2003;19:200-203.
28. Iwanaka T, et al: Endosurgical procedures for pediatric solid tumors. Pediatr Surg Int 2004;20:39-42.
29. Jereb B, Us-Krasovec M, Jereb M: Thin needle biopsy of solid tumors in children. Med Pediatr Oncol 1978;4:213-220.
30. Kilpatrick SE, Garvin AJ: Recent advances in the diagnosis of pediatric soft-tissue tumors. Med Pediatr Oncol 1999;32: 373-376.
31. Kilpatrick SE, et al: Is fine-needle aspiration biopsy a practical alternative to open biopsy for the primary diagnosis of sarcoma? Experience with 140 patients. Am J Clin Pathol 2001;115:59-68.
32. Kilpatrick SE, et al: The role of fine needle aspiration biopsy in the diagnosis and management of osteosarcoma. Pediatr Pathol Mol Med 2001;20:175-187.
33. Kim SH, et al: Needle-tract implantation in hepatocellular carcinoma: Frequency and CT findings after biopsy with a 19.5-gauge automated biopsy gun. Abdom Imaging 2000; 25:246-250.
34. Klose KC, et al: CT-guided percutaneous large-bore biopsies in benign and malignant pediatric lesions. Cardiovasc Intervent Radiol 1991;14:78-83.
35. Liu ES, et al: Fine needle aspiration biopsy of pediatric head and neck masses. Int J Pediatr Otorhinolaryngol 2001;60:135-140.
36. McConnell PI, Feola GP, Meyers RL: Methylene blue-stained autologous blood for needle localization and thoracoscopic resection of deep pulmonary nodules. J Pediatr Surg 2002; 37:1729-1731.
37. Mobley DL, Wakely PE Jr, Frable MA: Fine-needle aspiration biopsy: Application to pediatric head and neck masses. Laryngoscope 1991;101:469-472.
38. Montorsi M, et al: Laparoscopy with laparoscopic ultrasound for pretreatment staging of hepatocellular carcinoma: A prospective study. J Gastrointest Surg 2001;5:312-315.
39. Mora J, Gerald WL, Cheung NK: Evolving significance of prognostic markers associated with new treatment strategies in neuroblastoma. Cancer Lett 2003;197:119-124.
40. Paolucci V, et al: Tumor seeding following laparoscopy: International survey. World J Surg 1999;23:989-995, discussion 996-997.
41. Pappo AS, et al: Biology and therapy of pediatric rhabdomyosarcoma. J Clin Oncol 1995;13:2123-2139.
42. Partrick DA, Rothenberg SS: Thoracoscopic resection of mediastinal masses in infants and children: An evaluation of technique and results. J Pediatr Surg 2001;36:1165-1167.
43. Partrick DA, et al: Successful thoracoscopic lung biopsy in children utilizing preoperative CT-guided localization. J Pediatr Surg 2002;37:970-973, discussion 970-973.
44. Rao BN: Present day concepts of thoracoscopy as a modality in pediatric cancer management. Int Surg 1997;82:123-126.
45. Rodgers BM, Talbert JL: Thoracoscopy for diagnosis of intrathoracic lesions in children. J Pediatr Surg 1976;11: 703-708.
46. Rousou J, et al: Randomized clinical trial of fibrin sealant in patients undergoing resternotomy or reoperation after cardiac operations: A multicenter study. J Thorac Cardiovasc Surg 1989;97:194-203.
47. Saenz NC, et al: The application of minimal access procedures in infants, children, and young adults with pediatric malignancies. J Laparoendosc Adv Surg Tech A 1997;7: 289-294.
48. Sailhamer E, et al: Minimally invasive surgery for pediatric solid neoplasms. Am Surg 2003;69:566-568.
49. Schaeff B, Paolucci V, Thomopoulos J: Port site recurrences after laparoscopic surgery: A review. Dig Surg 1998;15:124-134.
50. Shoup M, et al: Port site metastasis after diagnostic laparoscopy for upper gastrointestinal tract malignancies: An uncommon entity. Ann Surg Oncol 2002;9:632-636.
51. Skoldenberg EG, et al: Diagnosing childhood tumors: A review of 147 cutting needle biopsies in 110 children. J Pediatr Surg 2002;37:50-56.
52. Smith MB, et al: A rational approach to the use of fine-needle aspiration biopsy in the evaluation of primary and recurrent neoplasms in children. J Pediatr Surg 1993;28:1245-1247.
53. Smith MB, et al: A prospective evaluation of an endoscopic ultrasonic probe to detect intraparenchymal malignancy at pediatric thoracoscopy. J Laparoendosc Surg 1996;6: 233-237.
54. Somers JM, et al: Radiologically-guided cutting needle biopsy for suspected malignancy in childhood. Clin Radiol 1993;48:236-240.
55. Tan GM, Tan-Kendrick AP: Bronchial diameters in children—use of the Fogarty catheter for lung isolation in children. Anaesth Intensive Care 2002;30:615-618.
56. Waldhausen JH, Tapper D, Sawin RS: Minimally invasive surgery and clinical decision-making for pediatric malignancy. Surg Endosc 2000;14:250-253.
57. Weinstein JL, Katzenstein HM, Cohn SL: Advances in the diagnosis and treatment of neuroblastoma. Oncologist 2003;8:278-292.

第 27 章

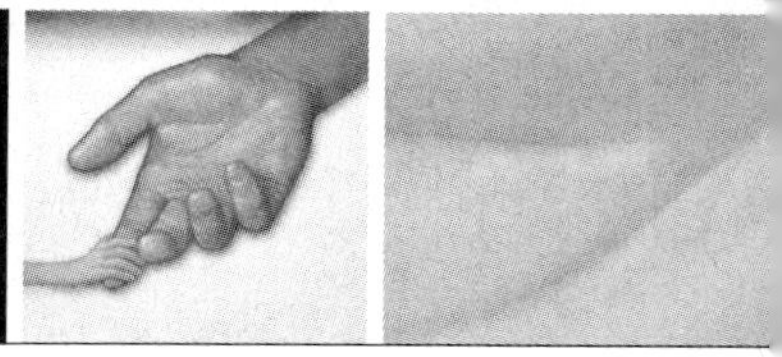

肾母细胞瘤

Edward P. Tagge、Patrick B. Thomas 和 H. Biemann Othersen, Jr.

45 肾母细胞瘤始终是研究的热点，包括临床和基础科学的研究。国家肾母细胞瘤研究组（NWTSG）通过五个合作方案的实施改善了其生存率。在 NWTS-4 中，儿童低危组肾母细胞瘤 2 年无复发存活率超过 91%[60]。尽管如此，还存在一些尚未解决的问题。间变样肿瘤、肾透明细胞肉瘤和肾横纹肌肉瘤对治疗不敏感。10%的患者预后不良，其中包括组织不良病理类型、1p 和 16p 缺失和二倍体。肺和肝脏转移、切除过程中肿瘤破裂、远处淋巴结累及和双侧肾母细胞瘤预后更差。再者，人们对儿童癌症成功治疗方案的远期发病率越来越关注。最后，肾母细胞瘤的基础分子学机制很复杂尚未明确。

本章节简要概括了最新的信息，主要集中在 NWTSG-4 的结论、NWTSG-5 的初步结果讨论和肾母细胞瘤将来治疗的方向。

历史

肾母细胞瘤的病理学描述最早出现在 1872 年[44]。1897 年，Osler 认识到内科医生报道的命名不同的儿童肾脏肿瘤其实是同一类型的实体肿瘤[104]。1899 年，外科医生 Wilms 回顾文献并附加了 7 例自己的病例发表了经典文章，详细描述了临床表现，现在这种肿瘤用他的名字命名[139]。最初手术切除是唯一的治疗选择，预后极差。随后，1916 年 Friedlander 提出放疗，Ladd 改进了手术技术，存活率提高到 20%[50,83]。最终运用放线菌素 D 和长春新碱进行化疗的方法被采用，手术切除、术后放化疗的联合治疗迎来了现代时期，这时的 2 年存活率为 81%。

由于肾母细胞瘤在美国的发生率不高，人们意识到只有合作研究才能保证获得有统计意义的病例数。随后 1969 年建立了 NWTSG。最初合作成员包括来自儿童癌症研究组、西南肿瘤组小儿分组、肿瘤小儿分组和白血病 B 组的机构。NWTSG 最初目标在于改善肾母细胞瘤和其他肾肿瘤患儿的存活率，通过确定副作用研究成功治疗病例的长期结果，肾母细胞瘤的流行病学和生物学，制定为全球内科医生所用的肾母细胞瘤治疗方案。NWTSG 进行的治疗研究涉及来自美国、加拿大和其他一些国家 250 多个儿童肿瘤治疗中心。最后几年里，每年新增 450～500 例肾母细胞瘤病例，其中 70%～80%的病例来自美国。

2001 年，NWTSG 和儿童癌症组、小儿肿瘤组（POG）和横纹肌肉瘤协作组合并成一个新的国家组织——儿童肿瘤组织（COG）。患者进入 NWTSG 临床试验方案于 2002 年完成，远期临床试验将由 COG 肾脏疾病协会制定。NWTS 的命名在晚期疗效的研究中将继续使用。

流行病学

全球统计，肾母细胞瘤在小于 15 岁儿童的发生率为 1/10000[16,19]。肾母细胞瘤占美国儿童癌症的 6%，每年有 450～500 例病例[34]。肾母细胞瘤的发生率在美国和美洲黑人比白人略高，但也只是亚洲人的一半。许多对照研究提示父亲的职业、怀孕期间母亲的 446
激素暴露以及基因易感性可能提高肾母细胞瘤发生的风险。

在 NWTS 资料中平均发病年龄为 38 个月，女孩发病平均比男孩晚 6 个月。患双侧肾母细胞瘤、虹膜缺如、隐睾或尿道下裂、Beckwith-Wiedemann 综合征或叶内肾小体的儿童诊断时年龄小于平均年龄（平均年龄 17～27 个月）。有家族性疾病或多结节肿瘤发病呈中间年龄分布，然而那些叶周肾小体诊断时多年龄较大。

肾母细胞瘤和某些先天性疾病相关：WAGR 综合征（肾母细胞瘤、虹膜缺如、生殖泌尿道畸形和智力障碍）、Beckwith-Wiedemann 综合征（过度生长综合征表现为：脐膨出、巨舌、内脏肥大、高胰岛素型低血糖症）和半侧肢体肥大症[98]。泌尿系统畸形如肾小管疾病、尿道下裂、隐睾在肾母细胞瘤较为多见。

WAGR 综合征是极为少见的基因异常，和 11 号染色体短臂 13 区的缺失有关。因为出生时虹膜缺如很明显所以大多数 WAGR 综合征患儿出生后就得到诊断。尽管如此，不到 1%的肾母细胞瘤患儿伴有 WAGR 综合征。

虹膜缺如是一种严重的眼部疾病，表现为虹膜发育不良。不管是散发病例还是家族性病例多为常染色体显性遗传。有些散发病例与肾母细胞瘤相关染色体缺失有关（WAGR 综合征），结果导致发生肾母细胞瘤的危险性增高。最近对肿瘤和虹膜缺如病例回顾分析发现散发性虹膜缺如的患儿发展为肾母细胞瘤的危险系数为 67（置信区间为 8.1～241）[66]。

Denys-Drash 综合征特征表现为假两性畸形、进行性肾小球病和肾母细胞瘤。基因学上它与 *WT1* 基因突变有关。超过 90% *WT1* 基因突变的 Denys-Drash 综合征患儿存在出现肾母细胞瘤的高危风险。事实上，最近有两例 *WT1* 基因错义突变的患儿预防性双侧肾切除的报道[75]。

有一小部分肾母细胞瘤有家族性。它的遗传方式可能为常染色体显性遗传，含有不完全性或变化的外显率[18,112]。虽然一些家族性病例与 *WT1* 突变有关，但更多与家族肾母细胞瘤基因 *FWT1* 的 17 长臂和 *FWT2*的 19 长臂相关，这些基因图研究正在进行中。

分子生物学和基因组学

肾母细胞瘤的发生与部分功能性控制肾脏正常生长发育的基因的变化有关[32]。大约 2%诊断为肾母细胞瘤的儿童有一个被诊断为肾母细胞瘤的亲戚。这些少见的肾母细胞瘤家庭的出现提示一个变异的基因在肾脏肿瘤发生中起着重要作用。另外一些因素为潜在易感基因。双侧肾母细胞瘤的发生率为 5%～10%[29]。另外，30%～40%肾母细胞瘤患者存在肾小体和潜在的癌前病变。

肾母细胞瘤是研究肿瘤发生机制的一个重要模型。1972 年，Knudson 和 Strong 首次提供了肿瘤抑癌基因在肾母细胞瘤发病中的作用的有关的统计学证据[82]。按照 Knudson 的肿瘤抑癌基因假说，患有家族性癌症综合征的患者遗传了一个含有因胚胎性突变而形成的失活的抑癌基因位点的染色体，一对染色体的另一个抑癌基因随后因体细胞突变失活，最终导致肿瘤发生。Knudson 将他的著名的癌症发生的二次打击模型进一步扩展，最初在视网膜母细胞瘤中运用，而后延伸到肾母细胞瘤。在这个模型中，易发视网膜母细胞瘤或肾母细胞瘤的儿童出生时 DNA 组成中含有一个假设肿瘤抑癌等位基因突变——称为杂合子缺失（LOH）。因此肿瘤发生机制中只需一个新的基因事件，配位基因的缺失或抑制。这些情况增加了双侧肿瘤形成及发病年龄较散发性病例的可能性。随后的染色体 LOH 回顾分析显示，53 例肿瘤中 52 例有母系等位基因缺失[30]。这些震惊事实提示肿瘤染色体缺失不是一个随机事件，肾母细胞瘤抑癌等位基因的位点不是相等的。父系和母系等位基因功能的不同被命名为基因组印痕。

然而，肾母细胞瘤基因学远比最初设想的要复杂。最近更多研究表明，与胚芽性突变相比，双侧和多灶性肾母细胞瘤的发生与体细胞的镶嵌性更相关，这与二次打击模型的宗旨相违背[6]。导致肾母细胞瘤发生的生物途径与几个基因位点相关，包括 11 号染色体短臂上的两个基因，一个位于 11 号染色体短臂 13 区（肾母细胞瘤抑制基因 *WT1*），另一个位于 11 号染色体短臂 15 区（假定的肾母细胞瘤抑制基因 *WT2*）。另外，1 号染色体短臂、7 号染色体短臂、16 号染色体长臂和 17 号染色体短臂（*p53* 肿瘤抑制基因）被认为是与肾母细胞瘤相关的隐匿基因。最近的研究定位了两个位于 19 和 17 号染色体的家族易感基因，不过它们的最终确定正在进行中。众所周知，某些家族易感性不仅与 *WT1* 无关，而且也与 19、17 号染色体基因无关，这提示有其他肾母细胞瘤易感基因存在。

WT1

结合临床观察、核型分析及分子基因学研究得到和肾母细胞瘤相关的基因位点图。1964 年 Miller 等报道虹膜缺如和肾母细胞瘤相关性[98]。随后，有报道少见的复合发育畸形 WAGR 综合征，其中超过 30%的患儿发展为肾母细胞瘤[101]。这些病例的核型分析证实在 11 号染色体短臂 13区存在基因缺失。WAGR 综合征在 11 号染色体短臂 13 区存在间隙性基因缺失，而肿瘤组织在同一位点表现为杂合子缺失，最终导致克隆出第一个肾母细胞瘤基因 *WT1*[20,52]。*WT1* 是一个复合基因由 10 个外显子编码。表达 *WT1* 的细胞产生四种独特的 *WT1* 信使 RNA，这反映出 *WT1* 基因不同拼接形式的转录产物。WT1 分子量在 45～49kD 之间，取决于那种拼接形式的 mRNA 翻译成的蛋白质。WT1 蛋白羧基末端包含 4 个锌指区域，是一个有助于 DNA 在特异性序列模式中捆绑的蛋白质特征。这提示 *WT1* 是一个调节未知靶基因的转译因子。*WT1* 在生殖泌尿道的发育过程中起重要作用，通过它在肾小管前体中高度限制的暂时间隙性表达以及无 *WT1* 基因小鼠肾发育障碍得到证实。除了在生殖泌尿道发育中的作用之外，一些急性成人白血病出现 *WT1* 混乱表达提示其可能在血细胞生成中起作用。*WT1* 同样在间皮细胞中表达，融合 Ewing 肉瘤基因 *EWS* 的 N 末端区域的一个特殊癌基因染色体移位到 *WT1* 的 3 个 c 末端锌指区域导致小圆细胞肿瘤[86]。

90%少见 Denys-Drash 综合征的患者 *WT1* 内有胚芽性突变。大多数是单个氨基酸替代导致的误译突变。WAGR 和 Denys-Drash 综合征患者肾脏显微镜检查通常存在叶内肾性小体[8]。在 Denys-Drash 综合征儿童中观察到的 *WT1* 特异组成突变证实了 *WT1* 显性负性突变的存在[31,109]。和 WAGR 综合征患者不同，WAGR 综合征患者 11 号染色体短臂 13 区存在大的缺失，Denys-Drash 综合征患者只有在 *WT1* 基因存在点突变[108,109]。有趣的是，*WT1* 的结构突变的表型作用远比 *WT1* 完全缺失大，这提示 Denys-Drash 综合征患者突变的 WT1 蛋白是无功能性的，并在显性负性融合中起作用[4,89]。

大约 20%的肾母细胞瘤患者存在 *WT1* 突变。双侧肾母细胞瘤患者胚芽性 *WT1* 突变的频率和肾母细胞瘤标本中可监测到的 *WT1* 突变频率是低的。在绝大多数家族性病例中排除了 *WT1* 位点连锁的存在[77]。在一小部分家族性肾母细胞瘤中观察到遗传性的 *WT1* 改变，但大多数病例研究表明肾母细胞瘤遗传易感性不是由变化的 *WT1* 基因所致。在丹麦对癌症和虹膜缺如进行的回顾发现散发性虹膜缺如患者发生肾母细胞瘤的相对危险指数为 67（置信区间为 8.1～241）[66]。然而，WAGR 和 Denys-Drash 综合征患者在肾母细胞瘤中各自低于 1%。在单侧肾母细胞瘤无先天性综合征的患者中 *WT1* 突变的作用是有限的，因为小于 15%的患者发生 *WT1* 突变[51]。

WT2

在有些肾母细胞瘤中，在 11 号染色体短臂 15 区存在杂合子丢失，在 11 号染色体短臂 13 区保留杂合子[72,114]。肾母细胞瘤核型证实在 11 号染色体短臂 15 区存在 DNA 丢失。在这里，几个调节体细胞生长的基因（*IGF2*、*p57KIP2*、*H19*、*KVLQT1*）受到不良调节影响，包括 BWS 综合征基因。这是推定的肾母细胞瘤基因 *WT2* 的位置，且该基因已被克隆[85]。

BWS 可能是 11 号染色体短臂 15 区一个基因过度表达所致，这个基因正常情况下只有父源性拷贝基因的表达（这个过程叫基因印痕）。事实上，核型分析显示在一些 BWS 儿童中存在父源性 11 号染色体短臂 15 区染色体片断的结构性复制。另外一些该综合征患儿具有 2 条总体正常 11 号染色体拷贝，都遗传自父亲（无母体来源拷贝）——这种现象称单亲同种双染色体[68,71]。可以相信 BWS 遗传获得二个父源性的基因拷贝将加倍表达这个基因，结果导致过度生长的特征。

更多人关注胰岛素样生长因子 2（IGF2），其位于 11 号染色体短臂 15 区，属于 *WT2* 候选基因因为其受基因印痕的影响。然而，到目前，没有直接证据表明它在肾母细胞瘤和 BWS 发病机制中的作用。日本学者证实在这位点上存在一个父源性表达的印痕基因 *PEG8/IGF2AS*。它是 *IGF2* 转录的反相转录，某些基因区域与 *IGF2* 基因共享。有趣的是，在肾母细胞瘤标本中发现 *PEG8/IGF2AS* 和 *IGF2* 过度表达，是肿瘤旁正常肾组织的 10～100 倍。这些发现提示 *PEG8/IGF2AS* 可能是肾母细胞瘤的一个标记，同时也可能是肾母细胞瘤的一个候选基因。

其他肾母细胞瘤位点

因为在大约 20%肾母细胞瘤标本中 16 号染色体长臂上存在杂合子丢失（与 5%的背景发生率相比），

448 所以提出假设 16 号染色体长臂存在其他肾母细胞瘤位点。Grundy 等最初分析了 232 例肾母细胞瘤提出 16 号染色体长臂杂合子丢失是统计学上重要的有害预后因子[69]。与无杂合子丢失的病例相比，存在杂合子丢失的患儿复发率高出 3.3 倍（$P = 0.01$），死亡率高出 12 倍（$P < 0.01$）。相同的研究报道 12%的肾母细胞瘤患儿存在 1 号染色体短臂杂合子丢失，复发率和死亡率比无杂合子丢失病例高出 3 倍（无统计学意义）。鉴于上述资料，NWTS–5 研究了 16 号长臂和 1 号染色体短臂杂合子丢失对肾母细胞瘤预后的意义。

对 4 个遗传性肾母细胞瘤易感性大家族的相关分析提示可能存在其他的肾母细胞瘤基因[66,67]。在这些家族性肾母细胞瘤中 11 号染色体短臂 13 区、11 号染色体短臂 15 区和 16 号染色体长臂不是起同一作用，需要进一步进行详细的相关分析来确定家族性肾母细胞瘤的染色体基因位点。

GPC3 是一种硫酸类肝素蛋白多糖，能交联生长因子如 IGF2。有篇文章报道在肾母细胞瘤和肝母细胞瘤中 GPC3 表达增高，这提示 CPC3 是一个促进生长或神经活性的基因[132]。另一研究确定在从 41 例男性肾母细胞瘤取得的肿瘤和正常组织中存在 GPC3 序列的变异[138]。2个不保守的单个碱基变化仅在于肿瘤组织中，这提示 GPC3 在肾母细胞瘤发生过程中可能起作用。

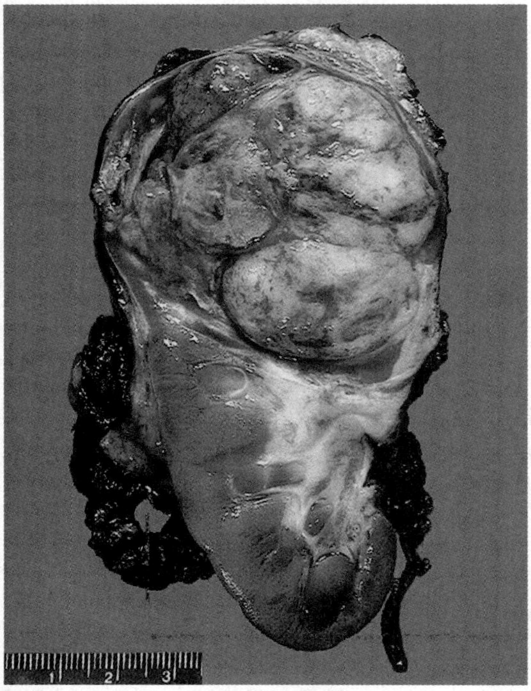

图 27–1 肾上极的巨大肿瘤，由孩子的祖母发现的膨胀肿瘤。

哥伦比亚大学研究员运用寡聚核苷酸微排列调查肾母细胞瘤的基因表达，证实在肾母细胞瘤和正常胎肾有 357 处基因不同表达[87]。肾母细胞瘤系统性基因过度表达相当于后肾发育早期，表达抑制相当于后期。这些标记不仅可以被基因编码转录因子 PAX2[131] 和 HOXA11 也可以被转移相关转录因子 E1AF 加强。

临床表现

在过去，绝大多数儿童表现为无症状的腹部肿块，通常被家属发现（图 27–1）。现代影像学技术的发展，诸如超声和 CT 可以早期评估腹痛从而发现触及不到肿块的肾脏肿瘤。早期症状包括镜下血尿（1/3 的患儿）和其他泌尿道异常、不适、体重下降和贫血。肿瘤膨胀压迫左肾静脉引起左侧精索血管梗阻造成继发性精索静脉曲张。另外，肿瘤瘤栓从下腔静脉生长至右心房导致心功能不全。偶尔，因为腹部一个小的创伤引起肿瘤破裂导致急腹症。

体格检查包括腹部仔细触诊和测量血压。肾母细胞瘤通常表现为圆形光滑可触及的胁腹部肿块。肾母细胞瘤患儿常因肿块压迫肾血管或肿瘤分泌血管紧张肽原酶出现继发性高血压。最后，确定生殖泌尿道畸形和有无虹膜缺如、半侧肢体肥大是非常重要的。

诊断

尽管人们开始关注运用血管内皮生长因子（VEGF）、透明质酸盐和碱性纤维生长因子（bFGF）对肾母细胞瘤进行诊断，但仍没有明确的血、尿诊断指标[81,92,2]。先进的影像学技术提高了检测肾母细胞瘤和它的前体肾胚胎瘤病以及肿瘤侵犯其他脏器的能力[55]。然而，和 NWTSG 推荐的指导原则相比，临床运用影像学检查还需有所变化。儿童疑似肾母细胞瘤的首选影像学方法是 CT（图 27–2），B 超特别适用于血管累及情况的监测。核磁共振（MRI）确定血管浸润情况，尽管这不是 NWTSG 推荐的术前评估方法（图 27–3）。腹部 CT 可以确定对侧肾脏和肝脏的病变。胸部平片用来评估肺部转移状况。胸部 CT 检

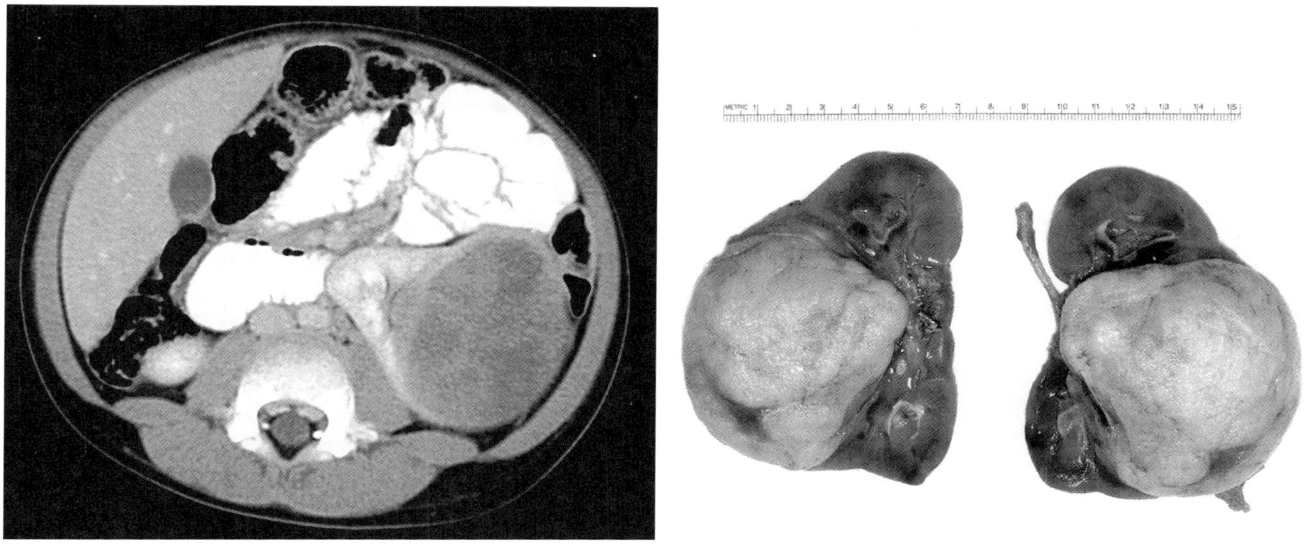

A　B

图 27–2　A. 腹部 CT 显示左肾巨大肿瘤。B. 有两瓣的左肾肿瘤。

查存在争议是因为：在平片不能发现而 CT 可以发现的病变很难解释。最近的研究肾母细胞瘤患儿胸部 CT 发现微转移病灶而胸部平片正常能否预测肺复发危险性的增高[105]。英国儿童肿瘤研究组肾母细胞瘤分组回顾分析了自 1986 年 7 月～1991 年 9 月加入了 UKCCSG 的 449 例病例，当只分析Ⅰ期病例时，CT 阳性组肺复发率为 43%（3/7），CT 阴性组为 10%（5/48），两者存在统计学差异（P ＝0.02）。重要的是，在Ⅰ期病例中，8 例肺部复发中 4 例死亡。

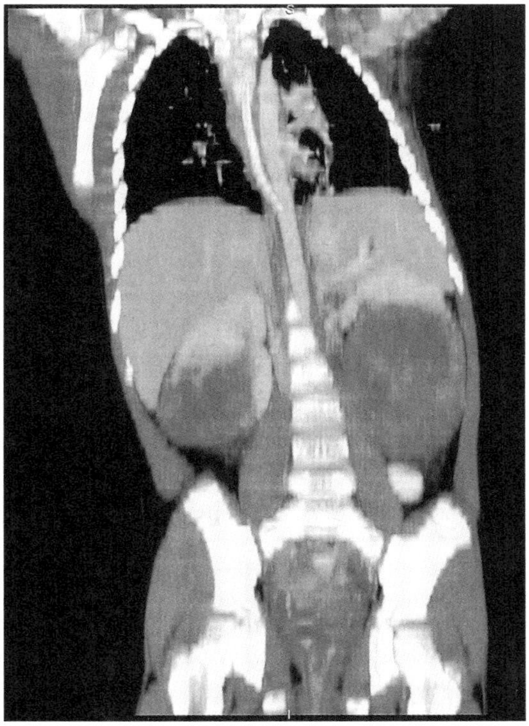

图 27–3　核磁共振冠状面显示双侧肾母细胞瘤几乎替代整个正常肾组织。在该检查中没有累及血管。

筛查

BWS 综合征和半侧肢体肥大患儿发生肾母细胞瘤的风险增高。近来评估登记的 BWS 病例的报告以及以往发表的文章指出 BWS 综合征和半侧肢体肥大患儿在 4 个月或更小的间期内进行 B 超筛查是有益的，尽管假阳性可能导致不必要的手术[24]。国际卫生组织进行了 BWS 综合征患儿的肾母细胞瘤和肝母细胞瘤筛查预算分析[96]。预测从出生到 7 岁，每年 3 次 B 超检查，BWS 患儿从出生到 4 岁每年花费 9642 美元，持续到 7 岁每年需花费 14 740 美元。

病理学

典型的肾母细胞瘤包含正常肾分化中可见到的三种成分：胚基、小管和基质（图 27–4）。这三种成分被认为是正常肾单位分化的重演。典型的肾母细胞瘤是异质的，各种成分比例不同而且出现畸变的脂肪组

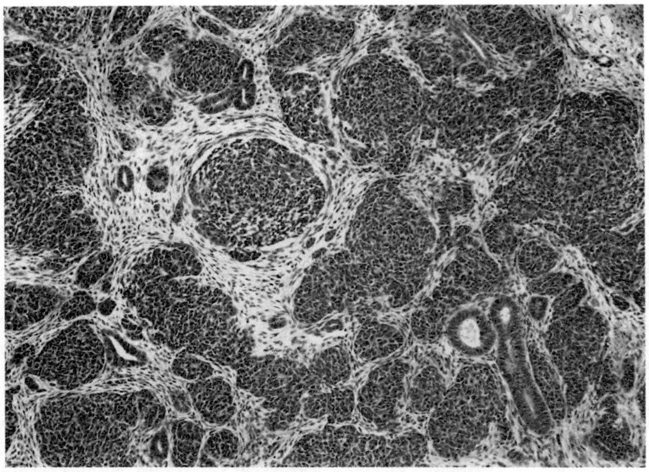

图 27-4 肾母细胞瘤三种成分在中倍光镜下的组织学表现（100 倍；H&E 染色）。上皮样成分包括小管（图右下方所示）和发育不全的小管结构。这张切片主要包含胞浆少的小圆原始细胞组成的细胞胚基。间质成分有疏松的梭状细胞形状。

450 织、骨骼肌、软骨和骨。肾母细胞瘤也可只包含这几种成分中的一种成分（单相的肾母细胞瘤），这类肿瘤难以和其他儿童肿瘤区别。

其他一些临床上易与肾母细胞瘤相混淆的肾脏肿瘤是先天性肾胚胎瘤、肾透明细胞瘤和肾脏横纹肌瘤。先天性肾胚胎瘤是低分化梭型细胞肿瘤的局部复发很少转移。肾透明细胞瘤和肾脏横纹肌瘤最初被认为是变化的肾母细胞瘤，在 NWTS-1 中被包括在组织不良型中。然而，当组织病理、免疫组化和对这两类肿瘤分子特性进行了解后，发现它们与肾母细胞瘤没有关联，这两类肿瘤都有各自特有的组织病理特征，侵袭性并且对治疗反应差。

尽管肾母细胞瘤预后良好，但三种成分的任何一种都可表现为局部或弥漫性的退行发育，这是预后不良的一个主要指标。现在退行发育是肾母细胞瘤组织不良型病理的唯一指标。肿瘤样本的退行发育表明存在巨大的息肉状细胞核。辨识这种变化要求：（1）细胞核直径至少是临近细胞的 3 倍，染色质增多；（2）存在多极或者可辨认的息肉分裂形状。区别局部和弥漫性退行发育的标准目前有所改变。鉴别局部型退行发育和弥漫性退行发育的诊断标准最近有所改变，局部性退行发育的最初定义是根据出现的退行发育的数量制定的。光镜下任何肿瘤间变样核变化小于 10%被明确为局部性退行变化。这个标准允许包括退行发育存在于全部肿瘤内，尽管密度很低，退行发育可在肾外部位或在转移灶内。新的定义强调，退行发育的分布并要求间变样核变化严格控制在原发肿瘤病灶内。退行发育的发生率在 3.2%～7.3%之间[14,141]。退行发育在年龄小于 2 岁的患者很少见。年龄大于 5 岁儿童的退行发育发生率提高至约 13%[57]。有报道在女性和非白种人患者中发生率高。间变型肾母细胞瘤通常显示非整倍体和 *p53* 肿瘤抑制基因突变[113]。

肾脏的透明细胞瘤

作为儿童骨转移性肾肿瘤[94]，肾透明细胞肉瘤是比肾母细胞瘤更具有转移特性的儿童肿瘤，转移包括骨、大脑和软组织。这个肿瘤有高的复发率和死亡率，所以及早确认这种肿瘤并给予比肾母细胞瘤更早更有效的化疗是非常重要的。肾透明细胞肉瘤具有几种类型，包括经典型、玻璃样型和上皮样型。

肾脏的横纹肌样肿瘤

肾脏的横纹肌样肿瘤是一种特殊的肾肿瘤，常发生在年龄小于 1 岁的婴儿中，大于 5 岁的患儿很少见[6,137]。肿瘤侵袭性很强，是预后极差的儿童肾肿瘤。肾脏横纹肌样肿瘤最典型的特征是具有大的囊样细胞核的大细胞（图 27-5）；突出的单个核仁；存在由中等细丝形成的螺纹块构成的细胞浆内容物。另一个典型特性是侵袭性的病变（图 27-6）。肾横纹肌样肿瘤具有不同的免疫组化形态，同一个细胞对许多想象中不相容的表面抗原决定簇包括上皮样、肌源性、神经性和间叶细胞型呈阳性。有助于明确肾横纹肌样肿瘤诊断的特征包括血钙过高以及婴儿广泛的血源性和淋巴源性转移。

肾性小体

在有肾母细胞瘤的肾脏中，通常存在与肾异常发育有关的肾性小体（肾胚胎瘤病）（图 27-7）。这些小体是含有持续原始胚基细胞的小病灶，这些细胞通常在正常新生儿肾脏中存在。实际上所有肾母细胞瘤

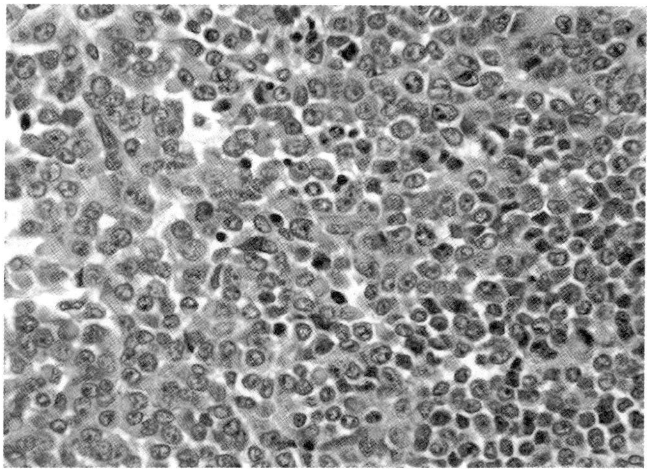

图 27–5　高倍镜下肿瘤细胞含偏心的细胞核和大量玻璃状包涵体嗜酸性细胞浆。这些形态特点描述为“杆状”（肌肉样）。

遗传易感性儿童的肾脏中都包含肾性小体，从而提供
51 了肾脏发育结构缺陷的依据。此外，25%～40%患有散发性肾母细胞瘤的患儿在瘤旁正常肾组织旁中也存在肾性小体[9]。

一份来自我们组的报告注意到在肾母细胞瘤和附近肾性小体中同时存在 *WT1* 的体细胞突变，这提供了肾性小体可能是癌前病变的分子学依据[107]。肾性小体和指示肾母细胞瘤遗传位点之间的联系也在癌前病变的解剖部位反映出来[7,9]。在肾叶周围发生的肾性小体（叶周肾性小体）常在 BWS 儿童中被发现。可发生在肾叶任何部位的叶内肾性小体通常在有虹膜缺如

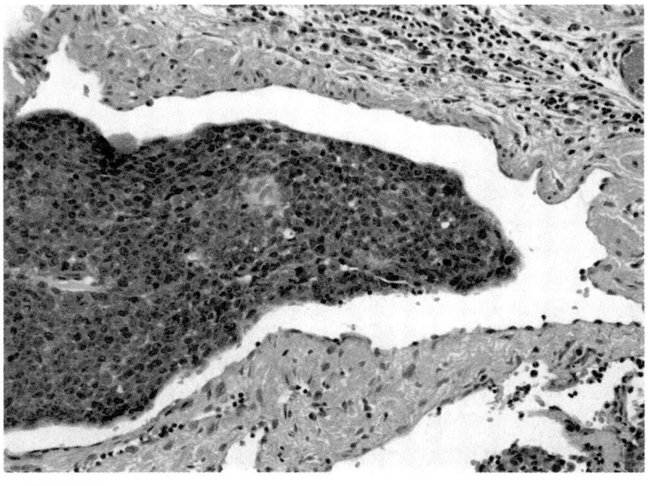

图 27–6　中倍光镜下（X100）显示肿瘤舌形血管通道，提示广泛的血管淋巴浸润。

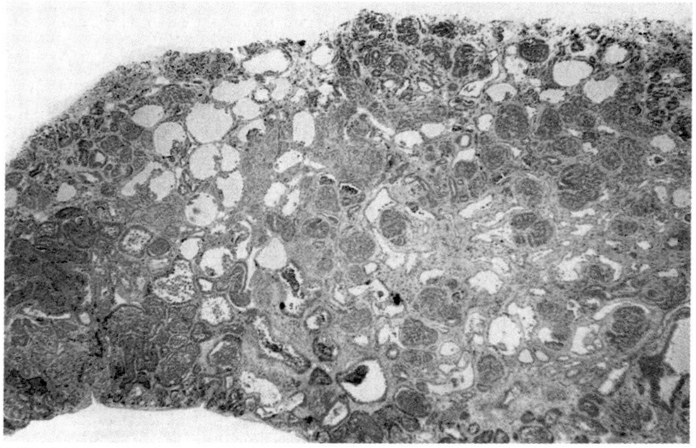

图 27–7　低倍镜下（20 倍）显示肾小体，原始后肾组织聚合体，含有深染胚基和原始小管形状。图片左下部分为正常小管。

或其他与 *WT1* 相关病变的儿童中被发现[9]。这些发现提示不同的肾母细胞瘤基因影响到特定的肾发育旁路，他们的失活能中断特定时期的正常肾发育。

分期

下面是 NWTS–5 分期系统，是以往 NWTSG 的改进。

Ⅰ期：肿瘤局限在肾脏且完整切除。没有破裂，切除前未做活检。肾包膜完整，肾窦血管未被浸润，切除边缘无肿瘤存在。

Ⅱ期：肿瘤超出肾脏但完整切除。局部有肿瘤扩散（穿透肿瘤包膜或肾窦血管有广泛的浸润）。肾实质外血管包括肾窦血管含有肿瘤。肿瘤切除前做过活检（针吸活检除外），或者术前或术中肿瘤破裂但局限于侧腹壁，未累及腹膜。切除边缘无肿瘤。

Ⅲ期：存在非血源性肿瘤残余，局限于腹部。可能发生以下任何一种情况：

1. 肿瘤侵犯腹腔、盆腔淋巴结（肾门、腹主动脉旁或超过）。
2. 肿瘤浸润腹膜表面。
3. 腹膜表面发现肿瘤种植。 452

4. 术后大片或镜下残留（镜下检查肿瘤切除边缘发现肿瘤细胞）。
5. 因肿瘤局部侵犯重要结构而无法完整切除。
6. 术前或术中肿瘤播散，且不仅局限于侧腹壁。

Ⅳ期：存在血源性转移（肺、肝、骨、脑）或腹腔盆腔以外的淋巴结转移。肺部结节在胸部平片未发现而在胸部 CT 中发现，但不需要全肺放疗，这类患者的治疗按照肾肿瘤分期进行。

Ⅴ期：诊断时发现累及双侧肾脏。基于活检前疾病的程度，试图将每侧按照前面的标准分期。

治疗

所有肾母细胞瘤患儿都应受益于肿瘤小组的治疗方案，这个小组包括放射科医生、病理医生、肿瘤科医生、外科医生、麻醉科医生以及放疗科医生。Cosention 等报道[33]芝加哥儿童纪念医院 25 年治疗肾母细胞瘤的经验。他们指出，在他们儿童医院首次接受治疗的肾母细胞瘤患儿存活率比那些肾母细胞瘤由普通外科医生切除、普通泌尿科医生随访治疗的患儿要高。

手术治疗

尽管存在肾母细胞瘤多种治疗模式的进步，但手术分期及肿瘤切除仍是治疗方案的核心组成(图 27–8)。外科医生必须切除肿瘤，通过淋巴结切片检查明确腹腔内分期，仔细检查肝脏和对侧肾脏。即使考虑无法切除肿瘤，开放活检也能够提供足够的肿瘤标本并进行腹腔内分期。

对可能是肾母细胞瘤的手术指南已经清楚列出。为暴露清楚推荐经腹部大的横切口。偶然情况下必须将切口延长至胸部。剖腹切口必须足够大以避免术中过多地挤压肿瘤，否则会增加术中肿瘤播散的机会。要求对腹腔进行完全探查。在一侧肾切除之前必须仔细触摸对侧肾脏以排除双侧肾母细胞瘤。Gerotas 筋膜必须切开，翻转肾脏显示其后面，任何可疑的区域都需做活检。而后，打开肿瘤侧侧腹膜，把结肠翻到中间。必须仔细触摸肾静脉和下腔静脉排除肿瘤侵犯至静脉。最好是在术前用 B 超明确。如果肿瘤浸润存在，需要与肾脏一起切除。如果肿瘤瘤栓侵犯超过肝静脉水平，最好的处理是术前化疗以缩小血管内的瘤栓。

首先尝试暴露和结扎肾血管以减少血源性肿瘤细胞转移的机会，如果操作非常困难或危险，应放弃首

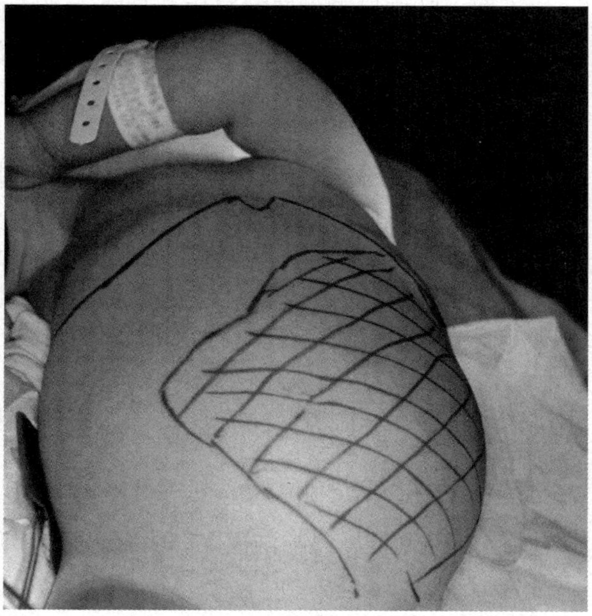
A

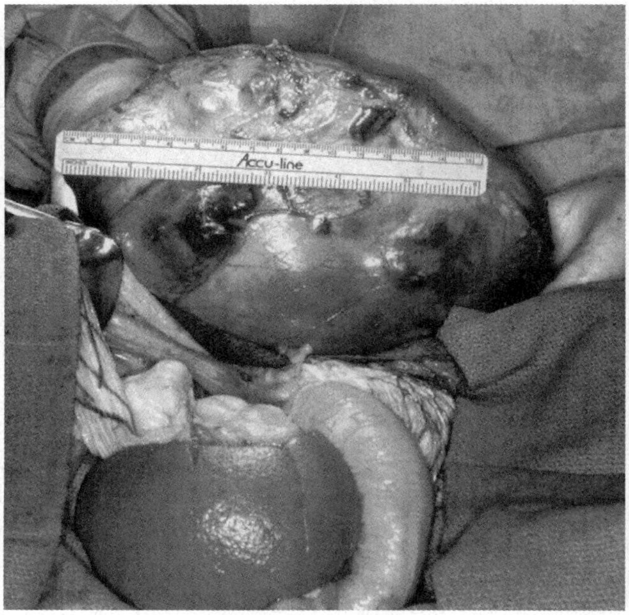

B

图 27–8 A. 巨大肾母细胞瘤范围图示。B. 切除的巨大肿瘤和左肾。

453 先结扎。NWTS-1 和 NWTS-2 对手术因素的分析显示延迟结扎肾静脉未产生任何不良后果[84]。然而，有报道术中发生肺栓塞，早期肾静脉结扎可以防止此并发症[127]。要小心避免肿瘤包膜破裂和肿瘤播散。如果肾上腺与肿瘤没有相连应保留下来。如果相连（上极病变）应同肿瘤一起切除。输尿管被结扎分离到尽可能低的位置，因为输尿管有肿瘤浸润的危险。集合肿瘤和未累及部分的肾脏并一起完整切除。侵犯邻近器官的肿瘤需进行活检和分期。可以对这些患儿进行化疗以缩小肿瘤，然后进行肾切除保护临近器官。只有在外科医生确信肿瘤可以完全切除的情况下能彻底切除肿瘤侵犯的非必须的结构（胰腺尾部、部分膈肌）。如果肯定有肿瘤残留，需做活检，在残留位置留置金属夹标志。推荐使用钛夹，因为含铁的金属夹可以影响 CT 检查。放置的金属夹最好用不吸收的缝合固定标记在结构上。

单侧肾母细胞瘤通常不提倡部分肾切除。除非同时或异时发生的双侧肾母细胞瘤或孤立肾。推荐的疗法是在最终手术切除之前首先对这些患儿进行活检和化疗。

外科医生应该根据术中发现对肿瘤进行局部区域分期。肾门及局部淋巴结是否存在肿瘤对准确分期和选择合适的治疗方案非常重要。为了准确分期，常规髂部、腹主动脉旁及腹腔淋巴结活检必须要做。浸润或可疑的淋巴结应该切除，但不推荐正规淋巴结清扫。为了准确分期，确定腹膜污染情况也非常重要。如果进行过肿瘤活检、肿瘤扩散或肿瘤破裂均认为腹膜受到“污染”。术前切开活检或经前路或后路针刺活检也被认为是局部播散。肾切除前的开放活检被认为是局部播散，除非外科医生确认在手术过程中整个腹膜受到污染（弥漫性播散）。肿瘤有时与邻近结构相粘连（结肠、脾脏、横膈膜）。肿瘤和相粘连的组织一起切除保证无肿瘤播散。这些分离出来的组织（肿瘤组织已被切除）被认为肿瘤播散（局部或弥漫）。当术前肿瘤破裂以及肿瘤细胞播散至整个腹腔，患儿的肿瘤被定为Ⅲ期，整个腹腔表面（腹腔和盆腔）需接受放疗。

可能因为肿瘤体积、肿瘤侵犯下腔静脉肝上部分以及其他一些原因而不能对肿瘤进行手术。NWTSG 过去的经验和国际小儿肿瘤协会 SIOP 的研究表明术前化疗可以缩小肿瘤体积，使得肿瘤能够切除[22,54,56,117,133]。推荐所有患儿首次探查评定可手术性，取肿瘤标本活检，因为在未进行活检的肾脏肿瘤中其错误分期率为 5%～10%。单独通过影像学检查分期的患儿存在过低分期和过高分期的风险，由此导致不恰当的治疗。一旦当肿瘤体积缩小到能够切除的范围，则进行手术切除。通常来说，在第 5 周时重新进行影像学评估。因为存在较多骨骼肌肉或良性成分，肿瘤体积不缩小，影像学检查可能误认为疾病未见缓解。如果肿瘤仍不能手术，需要对原发肿瘤和可见的转移病灶进行活检。肿瘤进展快预示预后差，需要使用不同的加强的化疗方案[121]。

化疗

因为在美国患儿的治疗是按照 NWTSG 方案进行的，所以笔者在本部分提供了最近完成的 NWTS-5 化疗方案。作为一个原则，肾切除和淋巴结检查后要进行化疗，除非在双侧肾母细胞瘤和不能手术病例中。特殊治疗方案按照分期、患儿年龄、肿瘤重量和组织学各异而有所不同。

符合以下方案的患儿给予肾切除和 EE-4A 化疗 454
（表 27-1），药物为长春新碱和更生霉素（放射菌素 D）：

Ⅰ期　组织良好型、年龄小于 24 个月、肿瘤重量小于 550 克。

Ⅰ期　组织良好型、年龄大于 24 个月、肿瘤重量大于 550 克。

Ⅰ期　局部或弥漫间变型。

表 27-1　国家肾母细胞瘤研究-5：Ⅰ期组织良好型或间变型或Ⅱ期组织良好型：化疗 EE-4A

周	0	1	2	3	4	5	6	7	8	9	10	11	12	13	14	15	16	17	18
	A			A			A			A			A			A			A
		V	V	V	V	V	V	V	V	V	V		V*			V*			V*

A：更生霉素（45μg/kg）；V：长春新碱（0.05mg/kg）；V*：长春新碱（0.067mg/kg）。

表 27-2 国家肾母细胞瘤研究-5 Ⅲ期和Ⅳ期组织良好型或Ⅱ至Ⅳ期局部间变型：化疗 DD-4A

周	0	1	2	3	4	5	6	7	8	9	10	11	12	13	14	15	16	17	18	19	20	21	22	23	24
	A			D+			A			D+			A			D*			A			D*			A
			V	V	V	V	V	V	V	V	V		V*			V*			V*			V*			V*
	XRT																								

A：更生霉素（45μg/kg iv）；D*：阿霉素（1.0mg/kg iv）；D+：阿霉素（1.5mg/kg iv）；V：长春新碱（0.05mg/kg iv）；V*：长春新碱（0.067mg/kg iv）；XRT：放疗。

Ⅱ期 组织良好型。

符合下列方案的患儿给予肾切除、腹部放疗和三种药物化疗 DD-4A 方案（表 27-2）：

Ⅲ期 组织良好型。

Ⅱ期或Ⅲ期 局部间变型。

Ⅳ期 组织良好型或局部间变型（不要求对胸部平片无肺部结节而胸部 CT 发现结节的患儿进行整个肺野放疗。是否对整个肺野进行放疗由主治者自行决定。）

符合下列方案的患儿给予肾切除、腹部 1080 cGy 的放疗和四种药物的化疗方案Ⅰ（表 27-3）：

Ⅱ期至Ⅳ期 弥漫间变型。

Ⅰ期至Ⅳ期 肾透明细胞肉瘤。

对于可切除的单侧肾母细胞瘤化疗和手术的时机没有统一规定[54]。30 多年来，SIOP 提倡肾母细胞瘤的诊断依靠影像学、代谢产物的检测排除神经母细胞瘤或术前经皮穿刺活检，治疗从术前化疗开始以改善疾病分期和降低并发症。SIOP 最先进行的研究揭示了术前化疗和放疗可降低术中肿瘤播散的发生率[40]。随后有作者继续强调这种方式的优点，指出术前化疗使得手术提前，同时肿瘤的破裂显著减少，分期分布得到改善，为患儿免除了不断增加的术前发病和生存率降低的风险[22,56]。最近 SIOP 回顾研究比较了在大于 6 个月的患儿中单侧肾母细胞瘤 4 周和 8 周的术前化疗情况[133]。对于以下各种因素延长化疗时间没有任何优势：Ⅰ期分布、术中肿瘤破裂率（1%对 3%），2 年无病存活率（84%），以及 5 年最终存活率（92%对 87%）。

NWTSG 不提倡对单侧肾母细胞瘤进行术前针刺活检，因为标本很小，不能进行腹腔内分期，而且针刺活检可造成局部扩散、肿瘤内出血或者，很少见的破裂。另外，NWTSG 研究没有发现术中肿瘤破裂是主要问题以及没有病理证实的治疗可能导致诊断的错误。Zoeller 等人[40]强调了这一点，他们报道进行急症手术，主要是因为肿瘤破裂或此前错误诊断为肾细胞癌按照 SIOP 方案治疗。

在美国儿童肾母细胞瘤术前化疗的经验不断积累。然而术前化疗被认为对要求实施肾实质分离术的双侧肾母细胞瘤[117]、无法手术的和血管内广泛浸润的

表 27-3 国家肾母细胞瘤研究-5：Ⅱ至Ⅳ期弥漫间变型或Ⅰ至Ⅳ期肾脏透明细胞肉瘤：化疗Ⅰ

周	0	1	2	3	4	5	6	7	8	9	10	11	12	13	14	15	16	17	18	19	20	21	22	23	24
	D						D						D						D						D
		V	V		V	V	V	V	V		V	V	V*	V*					V*						V*
				C			C*			C			C*			C			C*			C			C*
				E						E						E						E			
	XRT																								

C：环磷酰胺[14.7mg/（kg·d）×5 iv.]；C*：环磷酰胺[14.7mg/（kg·d）×3 iv.]；D：阿霉素（1.5mg/kg iv.）；E：鬼臼乙苷（3.3mg/(kg·d）×5 iv.）；V：长春新碱（0.05mg/kg iv.）；V*：长春新碱（0.067mg/kg iv.）；XRT 放疗。

病例最为合适。NWTSG 认为单独依靠影像学分期存在分期过高和过低的风险。如果选择单独依靠影像学诊断（有或无针刺活检）进行术前治疗，局部肿瘤应被认为是III期病变，治疗应该包括针对组织良好型或局部间变型或未知病理型的 DD–4A 方案和针对弥漫间变型的治疗方案 I 。

英国 CCSG 肾母细胞瘤研究–3 对肾母细胞瘤进行术前化疗，但要求化疗前活检明确组织学诊断。最近对化疗前活检的有用性和安全性进行了回顾，指出4%患儿的活检组织未能作出诊断，12%诊断为非肾母细胞瘤性肿瘤[135]。182 名儿童进行了经皮切割针刺活检，血色素下降（20%的病例）和局部疼痛（19%）是最常见的并发症。一例因肿瘤内出血急诊行肾切除术，另一例肿瘤破裂以后死亡。第三例活检后 8 个月出现穿刺径路肿瘤复发。

放疗

自 20 世纪早期，放疗就在肾母细胞瘤的治疗中起着重要作用。在过去，高剂量的放疗和偏心放射野对后期的毒性作用负主要责任；然而，对长期存活者的检查和从 NWTSG、SIOP 获得的研究信息使得我们能够对放射野和剂量进行调整，从而以最小的后期副作用获得高水平的局部肿瘤控制率[39]。

I 期 II 期组织良好型患儿不需要腹部放疗。I 期间变型肾母细胞瘤不需要腹部放疗，但 II 至IV期需要放疗。所有肾透明细胞肉瘤需要术后放疗。

所有III期患者术后放疗总剂量 1080cGy，分 6 次进行。只有存在肾门淋巴结肿大或局限于腹部的肿瘤残余才进行肿瘤床放疗。放射野跨过中线包括所有该水平段的椎体，但不要太远以致与对侧肾脏的任何部分重叠。肾门淋巴结浸润，照射野扩大（整个腹主动脉旁淋巴链）。当有弥散性腹膜种植、术中腹腔大块肿瘤破裂或术前肿瘤破裂需要进行全腹放疗。IV期患者，如果原发性肿瘤像III期一样给予膈下放疗，否则，不需要腹腔放疗。如IV期患者有肺部转移，不管可见病灶的数量和部位双侧肺都需要治疗，包括双侧肺门，尤其是肺尖和后下部位，总剂量 1200cGy，分 8 次进行。

治疗的挑战

腔静脉内和心房浸润

肿瘤侵犯肾静脉和腔静脉是存在的特殊问题[25]。术前 B 超检查可明确存在的问题。肺部肿瘤栓子很危险，提议进行心下静脉阻断和探查。当近端肿瘤瘤栓水平能明确，在该水平之上阻断近端腔静脉，打开取出瘤栓。有人主张不阻断近端，打开静脉置入一个大的有开口和闭口的吸引器，吸除瘤栓。如果肿瘤与腔静脉壁粘连，需要使用球囊导管取出瘤栓。最近有报道少见的病例，腔内肿瘤与血管壁严重粘连，完整切除腔静脉及左肾静脉和部分髂静脉系统[115]。游离和粘连的肿瘤被视为 II 期，但如果肿瘤侵犯血管壁应定为III期[49]。

大多数学者同意肿瘤侵犯肝上腔静脉和心房，手术时需要体外循环[23]。然而，肿瘤定位并控制在心房水平以下，手术切除时不使用体外循环可限制发病率。Lodge等人[90]报道了一项切除瘤栓而不用体外循环的新技术。在切除肝下腔静脉瘤栓之前，他们通过食管超声确定瘤栓的位置、腹部横切口向上中线延伸达到心包内控制下腔静脉的位置（图 27–9A）。

以往资料表明切除血管内瘤栓与手术并发症发生增多相关[119]，尤其是肝静脉水平以上甚至进入右心房的病例中。可通过术前化疗缩小这些血管内肿瘤瘤栓[120]。术前治疗可使血管内肿瘤缩小甚至完全消
失，从而避免通过体外循环手术切除肿瘤瘤栓。最近 456
的一个回顾性研究详述了儿童肿瘤侵入下腔静脉或心房后的预后。NWTS–4 共有 2731例病例，其中 165 例（6%）肾母细胞瘤侵入血管内。侵入水平位于下腔静脉的 134 例（4.9%），心房的 31 例（1.1%）。69 例（55 例累及下腔静脉，14 例侵入心房）接受了术前治疗。5 例出现术前化疗并发症。通过治疗前后影像学检查比较发现，49 例中 39 例血管内肿瘤缩小，包括 12 例中 7 例肿瘤从心房消失，这样避免了体外循环。在心房组手术并发症率为 36.7%,下腔静脉组为 17.2%。一期手术组并发症发生率为 26%，与之相对术前治疗组为 13.2%。当所有的并发症都被考虑进去，术前治疗组的并发症发生率与一期手术组的无统计学差异。3 年无复发存活率（有血管内侵犯的 165

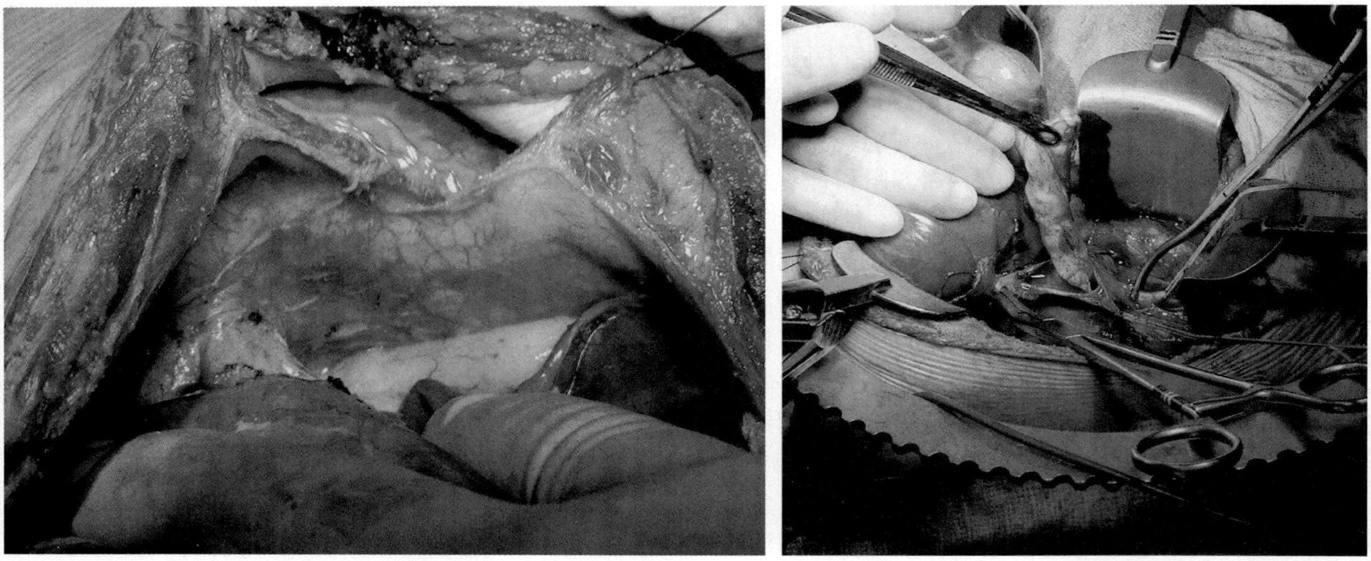

A B

图 27–9 A. 手术过程中的近景。术者的手使肝脏下移，暴露膈下肝上下腔静脉。为心包内控制下腔静脉，沿心包切开膈肌。B. 术中照片为从肝下下腔静脉内切除肿瘤瘤栓。

例为 76.9%，无血管内侵犯的 1622 例为 80.3%）无显著差异。虽然，术前治疗通过减小肿瘤瘤栓的侵犯程度协助手术进行，但手术并发症总发生率两组是相似的。

双侧肾母细胞瘤

双侧肾母细胞瘤（V 期）大约占总病例的 5%（图 27–10）。这些病例的手术治疗存在争议。有些主张双侧肾脏切除然后进行肾移植。另一些采用肿瘤切除然后进行自体移植以保护残留肾组织的功能[41]。然而，对这些按照 NWTS 化疗方案术前化疗的病例的回顾研究表明他们的预后良好；2 年时组织良好型病例[11,13]的存活率超过 80%，诊断后 10 年多达 70%[100]。然而这些患者肾衰竭的风险增高。关注那些肿瘤切除后保留肾实质小于 50%、受高渗透损伤的病例，双侧
457 肾母细胞瘤长期存活者肾衰竭率为 5.4%，结果导致对这些患者进行更保守的手术治疗。初诊时就明确诊断保肾手术非常重要。Coppes 等研究证实诊断时年龄在 1 岁内，叶周肾小体和叶内肾小体同时存在或存在叶周肾小体是重要的危险因素，但这些特征并不能预测所有的将来情况，需要进一步的研究来保证。

术前化疗的患者和进行一期手术的患者的存活率一样，但术前化疗能够保存更多的肾单位。在首次手术时不要进行彻底的切除，只有当肿瘤能够完整切除，双侧绝大多数肾实质能够保留才进行部分肾切除或楔形切除。双侧活检可以确诊双肾肾母细胞瘤及组织类型。4%的病例出现不相符的病理诊断。可疑的淋巴结需做活检，每侧进行手术分期。

病例符合以下情况，首次活检分期后予以 EE–4A

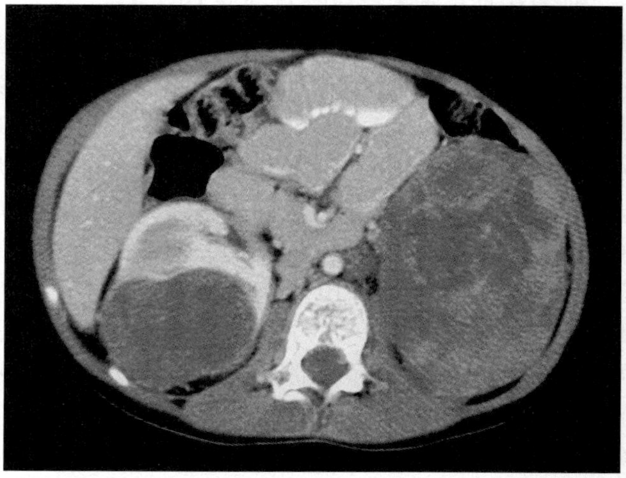

图 27–10 腹部 CT 显示双侧肾母细胞瘤。深色肿瘤组织整个替代左侧肾脏和右侧肾脏的后下部分。

化疗（见表 27–1）：

双侧Ⅰ期，组织良好型或局部或弥漫间变型。
双侧肿瘤，一侧或两侧评估为Ⅱ期，组织良好型。

病理符合以下情况，给予 DD–4A 化疗（见表 27–2）：

双侧Ⅱ期局部间变型。
双侧Ⅲ期或Ⅳ期组织良好型或局部间变型。
双侧Ⅱ期、Ⅲ期或Ⅳ期弥漫间变型，给予化疗方案Ⅰ（见表 27–3）。

治疗 5 周后 CT 检查评估疗效，了解肿瘤体积的缩小情况及部分切除的可行性。在第二次手术时，只有当不影响肿瘤的切除和切除边缘无肿瘤细胞存在的情况下行部分肾切除。如一侧肾脏肿瘤广泛浸润排除了部分肾切除的可能，进行最小浸润侧肾脏肿瘤完整切除。如果术后留有功能的肾脏，则对侧可以积极行彻底肾切除。如果保留的肾有挽救的可能性，需要活检，钛夹标记出病变的范围。追加化疗，12 周前再进行评估，如还有病变，需要进行放疗。

大约 1%的单侧肾母细胞瘤患儿发展成对侧病变。Coppes[27]等评估了所有前 4 次 NWTS 登记的与异时性双侧肾母细胞瘤相关的人口统计学和组织学特点[27]。4669 例中 58 例发展为异时性双侧肾母细胞瘤。初诊 6 年后发生对侧病变的累积发生率由在 NWTS–1 中的大于 3%下降到后续三次研究的 1.5%左右（P＝0.08）。存在肾性小体的患儿发生异时性病变的危险性明显增高，尤其在小年龄儿童中（206 例年龄小于 12 个月的中有 20 例，相比 304例年龄大于 12 个月的中有 0 例）。

一份来自美国费城儿童医院的报告回顾了在双侧肾母细胞瘤患者中进行保肾治疗的经验[26]。从 1982 年至 1997 年，23 例双侧肾母细胞瘤病例行部分肾切除，包括 7 例行内放疗。间变是和预后差相关的最重要的因素（P=0.003）。作者总结后认为：（1）术前化疗辅以保肾手术是双侧肾母细胞瘤的指证，除非弥漫间变型；（2）局部病变包括化疗耐药的可以进行内放疗。

马蹄肾肿瘤

马蹄肾中的肾母细胞瘤面临着诊断和治疗的挑战（图 27–11A）。通常人群中马蹄肾的发生率为 1/400[76]。Neville 等[102]描述，自 1969 年至 1998 年 NWTSG 登记的马蹄肾发生肾母细胞瘤的情况为 8617 例中有 41 例（0.48%），这提示马蹄肾肾母细胞瘤的发生率比通常人群高出 1.96 倍。在他们的研究中，13 例在术前未能诊断出马蹄肾，他们中的 10 例通过 CT 检查作出了诊断。26 例一期手术治疗，15 例活检后术前化疗。手术并发症发生率为 14.6%，包括 2 例尿瘘，2 例尿道梗阻，1 例尿道损伤。尽管 37%马蹄肾来源的肾母细胞瘤在首次探查手术中明确，所有马蹄肾来源的肾母细胞瘤经过化疗后都能手术切除。

目前 NWTSG 推荐的治疗方案如下：在首次探查中，如肿瘤能够切除且只累及马蹄肾的一侧，建议手术切除。如果双侧病例，对所有肿瘤及怀疑转移的淋巴结进行活检，明确手术分期、随后接受按照分期制定的化疗，大约 6 周后进行二次探查手术评估肿瘤对治疗的反应并进行准确切除，如果可能的话（图 27–11B）。尽管在这些复杂病例中大多数肿瘤侵犯肾盂，但马蹄肾最终的手术并发症发生率和 NWTS 报道的其他病例相似[119,122]。

部分肾切除 458

单侧肿瘤进行部分肾切除仍存在争议。一份 SIOP 的报告报道了儿童肾脏肿瘤部分肾切除的经验[21]。部分切除的手术标准包括肿瘤局限于肾脏一极以及侵犯部分小于肾脏的 1/3，未浸润肾脏血管和肾盂，肿瘤边界清楚。运用这些标准，90 例病例中 13 例符合部分肾切除的标准。在这 13 例中，5 例进行了部分肾切除。5 例中无 1 例边缘阳性和复发，同侧的肾功能均得到保留。

疾病复发

Shamberger 等回顾了 100 例 NWTS–4 局部复发的病例的数据（从 2482 例中）。在Ⅲ期患者身上观察到与局部复发最相关的危险因子：组织不良型和术中

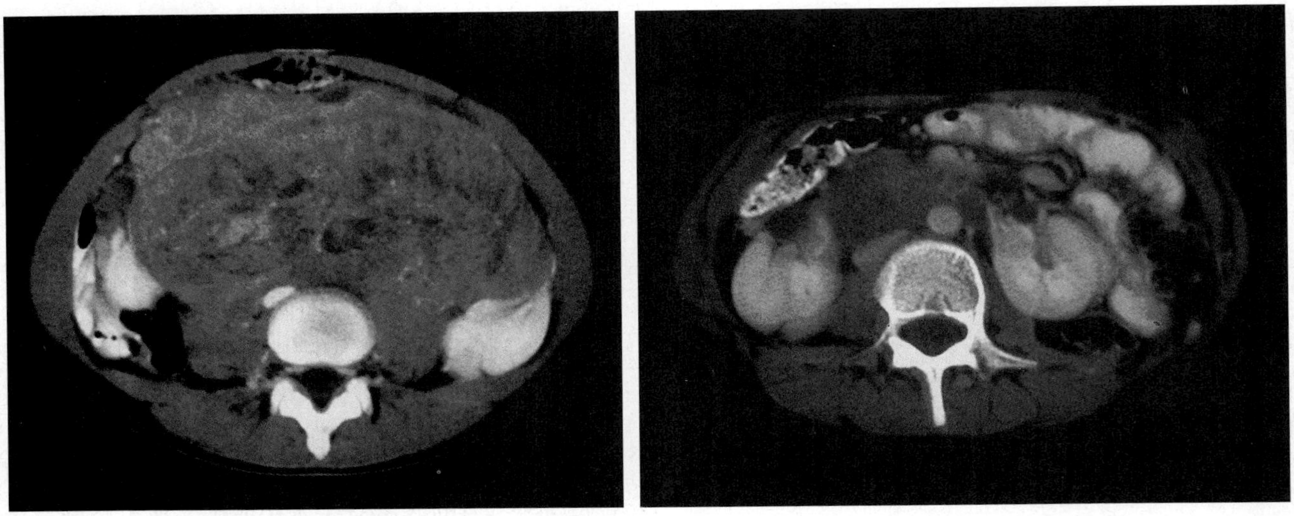

A B

图 27-11 A. 马蹄肾巨大跨中线肾母细胞瘤。B. 术前化疗后的同一肿瘤。肿瘤明显缩小，可以手术切除。脊柱双侧保留了有功能的肾单位。

肿瘤播散。多重回归分析提示肿瘤播散和缺少淋巴结活检与肿瘤复发危险性增高相关。肿瘤复发后存活率差，2 年存活率为 43%。存活率也依赖于最初发病分期，复发前已接受多次治疗的预后差。文章指出肿瘤破裂导致复发风险增高同时强调淋巴结活检的重要性，淋巴结活检可以确保肿瘤分期不会降低，治疗也不会不足。

最近一个追溯性的回顾研究观察了 54 例肾母细胞瘤局部复发的病例后发现 1984 年后接受治疗的患儿 5 年存活率为 63.3%，与之相比 1984 年以前为 20.6%。没有一例间变型病例复发后存活。只有 3 位患儿接受了大剂量化疗结合自体骨髓干细胞移植的治疗，这显示了使用传统化疗方案治疗组织良好型复发肾母细胞瘤的巨大进展。

早期诊断复发可以改善预后。最近英国研究者研究了 13 例肾母细胞瘤患儿的血清 VEGF 水平。在手术前，平均 VEGF 水平为 20ng/ml，手术 1 周后，水平下降到 1.9ng/ml（$P<0.001$，ANOVA）。肿瘤切除后 6 个月，3 例死亡，在这 3 例死亡病例中，术后 3 个月 VEGF 水平大于 10ng/ml 提示肿瘤复发。

预后因素

组织学

在早期，肾母细胞瘤组织学对预后的重要性就已得到了认可，肾母细胞瘤中 12%的组织不良型病理是造成大于半数死亡病例的原因。70 年代后半期，注意到 II 期至Ⅳ期弥漫间变型常规治疗预后差[10,14,141]。NWTSG-3 最初分析结果提示在标准的三种药物长春新碱、更生霉素、阿霉素外增加环磷酰胺可改善无复发存活率[35]。在对局限型和弥漫型定义进行修改后，Faria 等[48]报道了增加环磷酰胺后对弥漫型病例 4 年无复发存活率有显著作用。在局限型病例中未见此作用[58]，他们的预后和组织良好型相似分期的病例相似。尽管运用四种药物治疗，但Ⅳ期弥漫间变型病例 4 年无复发存活率为 16.7%，这提示需要进一步加强治疗。

最近，对 140 例肾母细胞瘤的突变分析显示肾母细胞瘤间变型与 *p53* 突变相关。然而，因为在组织良好型肾母细胞瘤中也发现有 *p53* 突变，所以 *p53* 变化能否作为间变型肾母细胞瘤的生物学标志或预后不良的标志有待进一步确定。鉴于以上问题，研究者研究了 97例肾母细胞瘤 *p53* 基因的表达和相关的表达与预后的关系，他们在 97 例肿瘤中的 13 例中检测到 *p53*，且和疾病复发有关（39%对 17%，$P=0.06$），但不是间变型。在 *p53* 阴性病例中，只有 5%存在转移病变，与之相比，*p53* 阳性病例中为 31%（$P=0.039$）。1 年最终存活率 *p53* 阴性病例为 94%,阳性病例为 85%（$P=0.34$）。

在 2002 年，SIOP 指出某些组织形态在术前化疗后仍然存在，如胚基，对预后有意义，其余没有意义。因此，在 SIOP 以后的试验和研究中，以治疗为目的的肾脏肿瘤分类将被修改：完全坏死（低危肿瘤）、胚基（高危肿瘤）和其他（中危肿瘤）。

DNA 含量

在不同的儿童肿瘤中，肿瘤细胞 DNA 含量的增高与较好的预后有关，包括胚胎型横纹肌肉瘤、神经母细胞瘤[91]和急性淋巴母细胞白血病。然而对于肾母细胞瘤而言，资料比较混乱。在有的文章中，组织良好型病例中的非整倍体与预后差相关[70]，但有的文章结论又不尽相同[5]。最近，Grundy 等[69]通过评估几个染色体片断 DNA 的得失确定了可能的染色体预后因素。对 NWTS-3 和 NWTS-4 登记的 232 例病例研究的结果发现，17.2%肿瘤组织中存在 16 号染色体短臂杂合子丢失，这导致了统计学上显著较差的 2 年无复发和最终存活率。11%肾母细胞瘤患儿的肿瘤组织中存在 1 号染色体长臂杂合子丢失，与较差的无复发存活率和最终存活率相关，为统计学有意义的临界（$P=0.08$ 和 0.12）。与之相对，11 号染色体短臂杂合子丢失或 1 号染色体重复分别出现在 33%和 25%的病例中，但预后无任何差别。NWTS-5 对肿瘤细胞 DNA 含量的预后意义的研究还在继续，希望能够找到新的确定的 DNA 变量来协助治疗方案的修改和判断预后情况。

英国肿瘤基因组 13 个成员组成的实验室提供了互相矛盾的资料[15]。他们回顾了 127 个异常的核型，统一变量存活分析显示核型复合体 1p 或 11p 丢失无显著副作用。存在 16q 丢失的预后差的病例在显著意义的临界，复发风险与 1q 获得之间的相关性不显著。只有 22 号染色体单体性是预后差的重要标志（13 例病例 5 年时无复发存活率为 50%，其余 114 例存活率 79%，$P=0.02$）。

Hing 等[73]对 58 例初诊或复发时组织良好型肾母细胞瘤的标本进行比较基因杂交分析，1q 获得在复发组出现频率显著增高[46 例中 27 例（59%）对 21 例中 5 例（24%），$P=0.019$]这些结果提示诊断时监测 1q 获得可以筛选出复发风险高、早期强化治疗对其有益的患儿。Lu 等[93]证实了上述研究，指出在 18 例组织良好型的病例中，1 号染色体长臂基因相对过度表达在所有复发肿瘤中都有发现，在缓解病例中无一例存在。

基因表达

Eggert 等[46]监测了 39 例肾母细胞瘤酪氨酸激酶受体的表达，指出高水平全长 TrkBmRNA（TrkBfull）表达的患儿，死亡风险明显高于低或无 TrkBfull 表达的患儿（$P=0.02$）。低肿瘤 TrkBfull 表达的患儿 5 年无复发存活率为 100%，与之相比，高肿瘤 TrkBfull 表达的患儿为 65%（$P<0.003$）。相反，肿瘤 TrkBtrunc mRNA 高水平表达的 5 年无复发存活率比低水平表达的要高（95%对 68%，$P=0.005$）。

Ghamen 等[53]在 61 例肾母细胞瘤病例中评估了不同的与凋亡相关的调节蛋白的预后价值，如 Bcl-2、Bax 和 Bcl-X。在病理分期增高的胚基内容物中观察到 Bcl-2 的表达增高，而 Bax 的表达逐步下降。统一变量分析显示胚基 Bcl-2 表达和 Bcl-2/Bax 比值提示临床进展，胚基 Bcl-2 表达是独立于分期的临床进展的预后标记。

生长因子

以往的报告注意到儿童肾母细胞瘤患儿的血清和尿中透明质酸浓度通常增高。通过运用小鼠异体移植模型，Lovvorn 等[92]注意到支持肿瘤生长的小鼠血透明质酸平均浓度为 9379μg/l，与之相对，不支持肿瘤生 460
长的平均浓度为 416μg/l[92]。在患有存有胚基的组织不良型肿瘤的小鼠中血清透明质酸浓度最高。完全切除肿瘤导致血清透明质酸水平回落到异体移植前的浓度。

Lin 等[88]监测了 97 例肾母细胞瘤患儿术前和术后尿 bFGF 的水平，42%术前尿 bFGF 水平升高，肿瘤分期越高术前水平越高，肿瘤复发和顽固性病变术后 bFGF 水平显著升高。

Kayton 等[91]在肾母细胞瘤小鼠模型中检测 VEGF 的升高频率和升高的量。10 例 VEGF 阳性的动物模型中 8 例出现肺转移，但在 11 例 VEGF 阴性中只有 3 例出现肺转移，相关存在统计学意义。在 12 例临床病例标本中的 10 例检测到 VEGF。

Davidoff 等[38]建立了一个腺体相关病毒载体，包含一个可溶性截短的 VEGF 受体-2（FIK-1），这是一个已知的内皮细胞活性抑制剂。在 2 例儿童肾脏肿瘤裸鼠模型中观测到显著的肿瘤抑制效应。在 15 例裸鼠中 10 例（67%）防止了肿瘤生长，其他病例中肿瘤生长也显著受限。

结果

NWTSG 结果

五个方案的研究已经完成：NWTS-1（1969—1974）、NWTS-2（1975—1979）、NWTS-3（1980—1985）、NWTS-4（1986—1995）和 NWTS-5（1995—2002）。NWTS 登记的患儿 5 年存活率 1969—1974 年为 79.7%，1975—1979 年为 81.6%，1980—1984 年为 86.3%，1985—1989年为 88.6%，1990—1995 年为 90.4%。这些在所有儿童癌症中是最高的。

以下是 NWTS-1、NWTS-2 和 NWTS-3 的主要结论：

1. Ⅰ期肿瘤或Ⅱ期组织良好型肿瘤术后肾周不需要放疗。
2. Ⅲ期组织良好型肿瘤治疗方案包括更生霉素、长春新碱、阿霉素结合腹部 1000cGy 放疗，或者更生霉素、长春新碱结合 2000cGy 放疗，这种治疗存活率最佳。
3. 在Ⅳ期组织良好型肿瘤的治疗中增加环磷酰胺不能改善预后。

由于这些研究，确诊的儿童肾母细胞瘤 2 年存活率由 20%上升到 90%[35-37]。

NWTS-4 研究发现放线菌素 D 和阿霉素强化冲击疗法和传统剂量用法相比一样有效且毒性作用更小，且费用减少，每年大约能节约 790 000 美元[60,61]。NWTS-4 同时指出Ⅱ期到Ⅳ期组织良好型肿瘤 6 个月治疗和 15 个月治疗结果相同。Ritchey 等[122]统计了 NWTS-4 登记病例中手术并发症的发生率，在 534 例随机样本中，68 例（12.7%）发生了 76 种并发症，肠梗阻是最常见的并发症（5.1%），以后依次为严重出血（1.9%），伤口感染（1.9%），血管损伤（1.5%）。血管内浸润至下腔静脉、腹部横切口或中线旁切口行肾切除术、肿瘤直径 10cm 或超过 10cm 发生手术并发症的风险增高。NWTS-4 同时强调必须防止术中肿瘤破裂，因为肿瘤播散会导致局部复发风险增高[124]。

NWTS-5 从 1995 年开始，2002 年结束。它有多重的目的：包括（1）评估不同生物预后因子的重要性；（2）通过规范首次治疗减少治疗并发症；（3）改善组织不良型患儿的存活率，包括弥漫间变型肾母细胞瘤、肾透明细胞肉瘤和肾恶性横纹肌样肿瘤；（4）研究双侧肾母细胞瘤患儿的生物和病理特性。关于基因对临床预后的预测，NWTS-5 的结果仍在分析中，未作发表。

NWTS-5 研究中最有意义的是小的Ⅰ期肿瘤的处理。Green 和 Jaffe[63]在 1979 年提出对于年龄小于 24 个月肿瘤小于 550 克的病例单纯肾切除治疗已经足够了。随后一系列 NWTS-1、NWTS-2 和 NWTS-3 治疗结果支持这种假说，认为在这组患儿中 NWTS 治疗方案没有改善原本良好的预后[59]。NWTS-5 建立了对单纯手术做进一步研究的分支，到 1998 年 3 月 31 日，69 例病例进入了单纯手术治疗分支，9 例复发：3 例在肿瘤床和腹部，1 例在胸腔，4 例在双侧肺部，1 例在对侧肾脏。2 年无复发存活率为 82.1%，远低于原有的 95%，因而单纯手术治疗遭到质疑。

欧洲结果

来自欧洲的结果与 NWTS 相似。例如，2000 年来自 UKCCSG 第二肾母细胞瘤研究组报告的结果[99]。4 年无病存活率如下：Ⅰ期组织良好型为 94%，Ⅱ期组织良好型为 91%，Ⅲ期组织良好型为 84%。间变型和横纹肌样型预后差。最近意大利对 98 例连接本次接受 SIOP 方案治疗的肾母细胞瘤患者进行的回顾研究表明其 5 年治愈率结果为 90%[79]。影响临床治疗的主要因素为弥漫间变型和淋巴结浸润。最近包括
461 16 个欧洲国家的 EUROCARE 报告了在 34 个基于人口的癌症登记站登记的 2535 例病例[110]治疗结果，从 1985 年到 1989 年诊断的所有儿童的 5 年存活率为 83%，在以往的社会主义国家爱沙尼亚、波兰和斯洛伐克登记的儿童的存活率显著低下。与来自美国和澳大利亚的结果欧洲的存活率相对稍低。

特殊的肿瘤

回顾 NWTS-3 和 NWTS-4 方案治疗的 4669 例儿童其中 53 例合并 BSW[111]。BWS 患儿倾向于表现为低分期的肿瘤（P=0.0001）。BSW 患儿的 4 年最终存活率与无 BSW 的患儿相似（89%对 90%），21% 的 BSW 患儿为双侧疾病，在 NWTS-4 登记的 BWS 患儿的肿瘤比在 NWTS-3 中的要小（P = 0.02），这提示 B 超筛查是有效的。

Argani 等[1]回顾了 351 例肾脏透明细胞肉瘤病例，包括从 NTWSG-1 到 NTWSG-4 登记的 182 例病例，最终存活率为 69%，多变量分析揭示了 4 个独立的存活预后因子：阿霉素的治疗、分期、诊断时的年龄和肿瘤坏死。

Breslow 等[17]分析并报告了 WAGR 综合征患儿的治疗结果。NWTSG 在 1969 年至 2002 年登记的 8533 例病例中，64 例（0.75%）有 WAGR 综合征。比较合并 WAGR 和无合并的患儿，其平均出生体重（2.94 对 3.45 千克）、诊断时的平均年龄（22 对 39 个月）、双侧病变的百分率（17%对 6%）、转移病变（2%对 13%）、组织良好型与否（100%对 92%）、叶内肾小体存在率（77%对 22%）均不同。4 年存活率两者相似（95%对 92%），但 27 年存活率存在显著差异（48%对 86%）。WAGR 患儿中 5 例晚期死亡死于晚期肾脏疾病。

治疗死亡率和并发症发生率

儿童肾脏癌症治疗无可置疑的进展说明越来越多的肾母细胞瘤患儿预期得到治愈。然而，人们对癌症治疗的远期副作用越来越关注[45]。儿童癌症监测研究观测到肾母细胞瘤标准死亡率为 9.6%，5 年死亡率为 12.1%。10 年、15 年和 20 年时的累计死亡率分别为 1.8%、3.1%和 5.0%[97]。有些副作用在治疗后马上出现（如运用某些化疗药物后），通常为暂时性的，一些可能变为永久性的。尽管儿童耐受治疗的急性毒性作用看似比成人要好，但生长的儿童更易受到延迟的癌症治疗的后遗症的伤害，诸如停止生长、不育症和神经精神功能障碍。

肾母细胞瘤有心脏、肾脏、肺的毒性作用。NWTS-1 证实运用烷化剂治疗后充血性心力衰竭的风险会持续存在 8～12 年或更长时间。对接受 NWTS-1 到 NWTS-4 治疗的患儿进行回顾以确定用阿霉素治疗肾母细胞瘤的充血性心力衰竭发生的频率和危险因素[62]。接受最初治疗 20 年后充血性心力衰竭累计发生率为 4.4%，复发肾母细胞瘤治疗 20 年后的发生率为 17.4%。充血性心力衰竭在女性发生率增高，与累计阿霉素剂量、肺野放疗和左侧腹部放疗相关。一份最近的报告注意到影响心脏功能的最主要的因素是烷化剂运用的总剂量，接受小于 240mg/m^2 剂量的治疗治疗结束 10 余年后无心功能损伤出现[129]。

肾母细胞瘤患儿存在因各种因素造成肾衰竭的风险，包括放疗、运用有肾毒性的化疗药物，高滤过而致的理论性危险[43]，以及可能的基因成分的参与（患儿合并 Denys-Drash 综合征）。1996 年，Ritchey 等报道了 NWTS-1 至 NWTS-4 期间 5823 例病例中 55 例肾衰竭的病例，指出所有单侧疾病 16 年后肾衰竭风险为 0.6%，双侧为 13%。

儿童癌症存活者发生继发性恶性肿瘤的风险也在增加，无论是白血病还是实体肿瘤。几个研究显示，20 年后累计风险在 3%～10%之间，是平常人群发生率的 5～20 倍[65,128]。NWTS 肾母细胞瘤患儿的继发性恶性肿瘤的发生率最先在 1988 年被报道，2438 例病例中 15 例发生继发恶性肿瘤，观察与预期的比率或标准发生率是 8.5%[18]。1996 年结果更新，观察到相似的标准发生率 8.4%，发生了 43 例继发性恶性肿瘤。发现 3 例乳腺癌，多变量分析的相关风险为 12。为了找寻 NWTSG 方案中继发急性髓性白血病的特征，Shearer 等回顾了 43 例继发性恶性肿瘤中的 7 例急性髓性白血病病例、所有病例都接受了化疗包括阿霉素或鬼臼乙叉苷（依托泊苷）[10]，6 例接受膈下放疗。从最初诊断肾脏肿瘤到发展成继发性急性髓性白

血病平均潜伏期为 3 年（1.2～4 年）。

放疗有各种副作用。一个设计评价儿童肾母细胞瘤脊柱放疗导致成年后身高减低情况的研究，指出身高的减低程度依赖于剂量、放射野大小和治疗时的年
462 龄[74]。年龄越小越易受到影响，观察到 57 例平均年龄 55 个月接受 15～24Gy 放疗，身高降低 4.1cm。16 例平均年龄 83 个月接受少于 15Gy 放疗未见身高降低。另一项回顾性研究对放疗、化疗或两者一起对肾母细胞瘤存活者下一代出生、出生体重和先天性畸形发生率的影响。427 位 NWTS-1 至 NWTS-4 治疗存活怀孕者的问题表现如下：接受过腹部放疗的妇女胎位不正或早产的风险增高，她们的婴儿低出生体重、早产、发生先天性畸形的风险高。重要的是，肾母细胞瘤儿童接受上腹部放疗（10～20Gy）不要包括整个盆腔以防止不育症[80]。

展望未来

从 1969 年开始的一段时间，NWTS 没有制定一个临床治疗方案。目前和将来的工作重点会集中在运用以往大量的肾母细胞瘤存活病例研究诊断治疗的长期副作用以及进一步明确肿瘤的发病机制和病因。NWTS 在 1995 年 10 月建立了一个远期作用研究项目（LATE，也被称为 POG9442，CCG4941L），目的在于研究接受了五个方案中任意一个治疗的患儿可能产生的与治疗相关的情况。LATE 是一个联邦基金，研究随访参与者及其子女长期生活的治疗结果及可能的远期作用。其特殊的研究目的包括：

1．确定肾母细胞瘤存活者危及生命的医疗情况的发生率。
2．以往肾母细胞瘤患儿的死亡率。
3．确定肾母细胞瘤存活者严重怀孕并发症风险及其他生育副作用事件。
4．确定儿童肾母细胞瘤和其他癌症发生率及家庭其他成员肾母细胞瘤的发生率。
5．分子生物学家和流行病学家确定最具有信息的肾母细胞瘤亚群。

鉴于对治疗及与高死亡率相关的危险因素的确认，干预治疗应以高风险患儿为目标。目前 90%的肾母细胞瘤患儿可以被治愈，重点应转移到存活者的生存时间生活质量上。通过 COG 将产生新的肾母细胞瘤治疗方案，这些方案在编写本书期间还在酝酿中。

（徐　敏译　王　珊校）

参考文献

1. Argani P, Perlman EJ, Breslow NE, et al: Clear cell sarcoma of the kidney: A review of 351 cases from the National Wilms' Tumor Study Group Pathology Center. Am J Surg Pathol 2000;24:4-18.
2. Argenta PA, Lin RY, Sullivan KM: Basic fibroblast growth factor is a Wilms' tumor marker. Surg Forum 1994; 45:789.
3. Bardeesy N, Falkoff D, Petruzzi MJ, et al: Anaplastic Wilms' tumour, a subtype displaying poor prognosis, harbours p53 mutations. Nat Genet 1994;7:91-97.
4. Bardeesy N, Zabel B, Schmitt K, et al: WT1 mutations associated with incomplete Denys-Drash syndrome define a domain predicted to behave in a dominant-negative fashion. Genomics 1994;21:663-664.
5. Barrantes JC, Muir KR, Toyn CE, et al: Thirty-year population-based review of childhood renal tumours with an assessment of prognostic features including tumour DNA characteristics. Med Pediatr Oncol 1993;21: 24-30.
6. Beckwith JB: Wilms' tumor and other renal tumors of childhood: A selective review from the National Wilms' Tumor Study Pathology Center. Hum Pathol 1983;14: 481-492.
7. Beckwith JB: Precursor lesions of Wilms' tumor: Clinical and biological implications. Med Pediatr Oncol 1993; 21:158-168.
8. Beckwith JB: Nephrogenic rests and the pathogenesis of Wilms' tumor: Developmental and clinical considerations. Am J Med Genet 1998;79:268-273.
9. Beckwith JB, Kiviat NB, Bonadio JF: Nephrogenic rests, nephroblastomatosis, and the pathogenesis of Wilms' tumor. Pediatr Pathol 1990;10:1-36.
10. Beckwith JB, Palmer NF: Histopathology and prognosis of Wilms' tumors: Results from the First National Wilms' Tumor Study. Cancer 1978;41:1937-1948.
11. Bishop HC, Tefft M, Evans AE, et al: Survival in bilateral Wilms' tumor—review of 30 National Wilms' Tumor Study cases. J Pediatr Surg 1977;12:631-638.
12. Blann AD, Li JL, Li C, et al: Increased serum VEGF in 13 children with Wilms' tumour falls after surgery but rising levels predict poor prognosis. Cancer Lett 2001;173: 183-186.
13. Blute ML, Kelalis PP, Offord KP, et al: Bilateral Wilms' tumor. J Urol 1987;138:968-973.
14. Bonadio JF, Storer B, Norkool P, et al: Anaplastic Wilms' tumor: Clinical and pathologic studies. J Clin Oncol 1985; 3:513-520.
15. Bown N, Cotterill SJ, Roberts P, et al: Cytogenetic abnormalities and clinical outcome in Wilms' tumor: A study by the UK Cancer Cytogenetics Group and the UK Children's Cancer Study Group. Med Pediatr Oncol 2002; 38:11-21.

16. Breslow N, Olshan A, Beckwith JB, et al: Epidemiology of Wilms' tumor. Med Pediatr Oncol 1993;21:172-181.
17. Breslow NE, Norris R, Norkool PA, et al: Characteristics and outcomes of children with the Wilms' tumor-aniridia syndrome: A report from the National Wilms' Tumor Study Group. J Clin Oncol 2003;21:4579-4585.
18. Breslow NE, Olson J, Moksness J, et al: Familial Wilms' tumor: A descriptive study. Med Pediatr Oncol 1996; 27:398-403.
19. Bunin GR, Meadows AT: Epidemiology and Wilms' tumor: Approaches and methods. Med Pediatr Oncol 1993;21: 169-171.
20. Call KM, Glaser T, Ito CY, et al: Isolation and characterization of a zinc finger polypeptide gene at the human chromosome 11 Wilms' tumor locus. Cell 1990;60: 509-520.
21. Canning DA: Is partial nephrectomy appropriate treatment for unilateral Wilms' tumor? J Urol 1999;161:367.
22. Capra ML, Walker DA, Mohammed WM, et al: Wilms' tumor: A 25-year review of the role of preoperative chemotherapy. J Pediatr Surg 1999;34:579-582.
23. Chiappini B, Savini C, Marinelli G, et al: Cavoatrial tumor thrombus: Single-stage surgical approach with profound hypothermia and circulatory arrest, including a review of the literature. J Thorac Cardiovasc Surg 2002; 124:684-688.
24. Choyke PL, Siegel MJ, Craft AW, et al: Screening for Wilms' tumor in children with Beckwith-Wiedemann syndrome or idiopathic hemihypertrophy. Med Pediatr Oncol 1999;32: 196-200.
25. Clayman RV, Sheldon CA, Gonzales R: Wilms' tumor: An approach to vena caval intrusion. Prog Pediatr Surg 1983;15:285-290.
26. Cooper CS, Jaffe WI, Huff DS, et al: The role of renal salvage procedures for bilateral Wilms' tumor: A 15-year review. J Urol 2000;163:265-268.
27. Coppes MJ, Arnold M, Beckwith JB, et al: Factors affecting the risk of contralateral Wilms' tumor development: A report from the National Wilms' Tumor Study Group. Cancer 1999;85:1616-1625.
28. Coppes MJ, Bonetta L, Huang A, et al: Loss of heterozygosity mapping in Wilms' tumor indicates the involvement of three distinct regions and a limited role for nondisjunction or mitotic recombination. Genes Chromosomes Cancer 1992;5:326-334.
29. Coppes MJ, de Kraker J, van Dijken PJ, et al: Bilateral Wilms' tumor: Long-term survival and some epidemiological features. J Clin Oncol 1989;7:310-315.
30. Coppes MJ, Haber DA, Grundy PE: Genetic events in the development of Wilms' tumor. N Engl J Med 1994;331: 586-590.
31. Coppes MJ, Huff V, Pelletier J: Denys-Drash syndrome: Relating a clinical disorder to genetic alterations in the tumor suppressor gene WT1.J Pediatr 1993;123:673-678.
32. Coppes MJ, Pritchard-Jones K: Principles of Wilms' tumor biology. Urol Clin North Am 2000;27:423-433.
33. Cosentino CM, Raffensperger JG, Luck SR, et al: A 25-year experience with renal tumors of childhood. J Pediatr Surg 1993;28:1350-1355.
34. Crist WM, Kun LE: Common solid tumors of childhood. N Engl J Med 1991;324:461-471.
35. D'Angio GJ, Breslow N, Beckwith JB, et al: Treatment of Wilms' tumor: Results of the Third National Wilms' Tumor Study. Cancer 1989;64:349-360.
36. D'Angio GJ, Evans AE, Breslow N, et al: The treatment of Wilms' tumor: Results of the National Wilms' Tumor Study. Cancer 1976;38:633-646.
37. D'Angio GJ, Evans A, Breslow N, et al: The treatment of Wilms' tumor: Results of the Second National Wilms' Tumor Study. Cancer 1981;47:2302-2311.
38. Davidoff AM, Nathwani AC, Spurbeck WW, et al: rAAV-mediated long-term liver-generated expression of an angiogenesis inhibitor can restrict renal tumor growth in mice. Cancer Res 2002;62:3077-3083.
39. Davies-Johns T, Chidel M, Macklis RM: The role of radiation therapy in the management of Wilms' tumor. Semin Urol Oncol 1999;17:46-54.
40. de Kraker J, Voute PA, Lemerle J, et al: Preoperative chemotherapy in Wilms' tumour: Results of clinical trials and studies on nephroblastomas conducted by the International Society of Paediatric Oncology (SIOP). Prog Clin Biol Res 1982;100:131-144.
41. Desai D, Nicholls G, Duffy PG: Bench surgery with autotransplantation for bilateral synchronous Wilms' tumor: A report of three cases. J Pediatr Surg 1999;34:632-634.
42. Dome JS, Liu T, Krasin M, et al: Improved survival for patients with recurrent Wilms' tumor: The experience at St. Jude Children's Research Hospital. J Pediatr Hematol Oncol 2002;24:192-198.
43. Donckerwolcke RM, Coppes MJ: Adaptation of renal function after unilateral nephrectomy in children with renal tumors. Pediatr Nephrol 2001;16:568-574.
44. Eberth DJ: Myoma sarcomatodes renum. Virchows Arch Pathol Anat Physiol 1872;10:518-521.
45. Egeler RM, Wolff JE, Anderson RA, et al: Long-term complications and post-treatment follow-up of patients with Wilms' tumor. Semin Urol Oncol 1999;17:55-61.
46. Eggert A, Grotzer MA, Ikegaki N, et al: Expression of the neurotrophin receptor TrkB is associated with unfavorable outcome in Wilms' tumor. J Clin Oncol 2001;19: 689-696.
47. Farber S: Chemotherapy in the treatment of leukemia and Wilms' tumor. JAMA 1966;198:826-836.
48. Faria P, Beckwith JB, Mishra K, et al: Focal versus diffuse anaplasia in Wilms' tumor—new definitions with prognostic significance: A report from the National Wilms' Tumor Study Group. Am J Surg Pathol 1996;20:909-920.
49. Federici S, Galli G, Ceccarelli PL, et al: Wilms' tumor involving the inferior vena cava: Preoperative evaluation and management. Med Pediatr Oncol 1994;22:39-44.
50. Friedlander A: Sarcoma of the kidney treated by roentgen ray. Am J Dis Child 1916;12:328-331.
51. Gessler M, Konig A, Arden K, et al: Infrequent mutation of the WT1 gene in 77 Wilms' tumors. Hum Mutat 1994; 3:212-222.
52. Gessler M, Poustka A, Cavenee W, et al: Homozygous deletion in Wilms' tumours of a zinc-finger gene identified by chromosome jumping. Nature 1990;343:774-778.
53. Ghanem MA, Van der Kwast TH, Den Hollander JC, et al: The prognostic significance of apoptosis-associated proteins BCL-2, BAX and BCL-X in clinical nephroblastoma. Br J Cancer 2001;85:1557-1563.
54. Godzinski J, Tournade MF, de Kraker J, et al: The role of preoperative chemotherapy in the treatment of nephroblastoma: The SIOP experience. Societe Internationale d'Oncologie Pediatrique. Semin Urol Oncol 1999;17: 28-32.
55. Goske MJ, Mitchell C, Reslan WA: Imaging of patients with Wilms' tumor. Semin Urol Oncol 1999;17:11-20.
56. Graf N, Tournade MF, de Kraker J: The role of preoperative chemotherapy in the management of Wilms' tumor: The SIOP studies. International Society of Pediatric

Oncology. Urol Clin North Am 2000;27:443-454.
57. Green DM, D'Angio G J, Beckwith B, et al: Wilms' tumor (nephroblastoma, renal embryoma). In Pizzo PA, Poplack DG (eds): Principles and Practices of Pediatric Oncology, 2nd ed. Philadelphia, JB Lippincott, 1993 pp 713-738.
58. Green DM, Beckwith JB, Breslow NE, et al: Treatment of children with stages II to IV anaplastic Wilms' tumor: A report from the National Wilms' Tumor Study Group. J Clin Oncol 1994;12:2126-2131.
59. Green DM, Breslow NE, Beckwith JB, et al: Treatment outcomes in patients less than 2 years of age with small, stage I, favorable-histology Wilms' tumors: A report from the National Wilms' Tumor Study. J Clin Oncol 1993;11: 91-95.
60. Green DM, Breslow NE, Beckwith JB, et al: Comparison between single-dose and divided-dose administration of dactinomycin and doxorubicin for patients with Wilms' tumor: A report from the National Wilms' Tumor Study Group. J Clin Oncol 1998;16:237-245.
61. Green DM, Breslow NE, Beckwith JB, et al: Effect of duration of treatment on treatment outcome and cost of treatment for Wilms' tumor: A report from the National Wilms' Tumor Study Group. J Clin Oncol 1998;16:3744-3751.
62. Green DM, Grigoriev YA, Nan B, et al: Congestive heart failure after treatment for Wilms' tumor: A report from the National Wilms' Tumor Study Group. J Clin Oncol 2001;19:1926-1934.
63. Green DM, Jaffe N: The role of chemotherapy in the treatment of Wilms' tumor. Cancer 1979;44:52-57.
64. Green DM, Peabody EM, Nan B, et al: Pregnancy outcome after treatment for Wilms' tumor: A report from the National Wilms' Tumor Study Group. J Clin Oncol 2002;20: 2506-2513.
65. Green DM, Zevon MA, Reese PA, et al: Second malignant tumors following treatment during childhood and adolescence for cancer. Med Pediatr Oncol 1994;22:1-10.
66. Gronskov K, Olsen JH, Sand A, et al: Population-based risk estimates of Wilms' tumor in sporadic aniridia: A comprehensive mutation screening procedure of PAX6 identifies 80% of mutations in aniridia. Hum Genet 2001;109:11-18.
67. Grundy P, Koufos A, Morgan K, et al: Familial predisposition to Wilms' tumour does not map to the short arm of chromosome 11. Nature 1988;336:374-376.
68. Grundy P, Telzerow PE, Paterson MC, et al: Chromosome 11 uniparental isodisomy predisposing to embryonal neoplasms. Lancet 1991;338:1079-1080.
69. Grundy PE, Telzerow PE, Breslow N, et al: Loss of heterozygosity for chromosomes 16q and 1p in Wilms' tumors predicts an adverse outcome. Cancer Res 1994;54:2331-2333.
70. Gururangan S, Dorman A, Ball R, et al: DNA quantitation of Wilms' tumour (nephroblastoma) using flow cytometry and image analysis. J Clin Pathol 1992;45:498-501.
71. Henry I, Bonaiti-Pellie C, Chehensse V, et al: Uniparental paternal disomy in a genetic cancer-predisposing syndrome. Nature 1991;351:665-667.
72. Henry I, Grandjouan S, Couillin P, et al: Tumor-specific loss of 11p15.5 alleles in del 11p13 Wilms' tumor and in familial adrenocortical carcinoma. Proc Natl Acad Sci U S A 1989;86:3247-3251.
73. Hing S, Lu YJ, Summersgill B, et al: Gain of 1q is associated with adverse outcome in favorable histology Wilms' tumors. Am J Pathol 2001;158:393-398.
74. Hogeboom CJ, Grosser SC, Guthrie KA, et al: Stature loss following treatment for Wilms' tumor. Med Pediatr Oncol 2001;36:295-304.
75. Hu M, Zhang GY, Arbuckle S, et al: Prophylactic bilateral nephrectomies in two paediatric patients with missense mutations in the WT1 gene. Nephrol Dial Transplant 2004;19:223-226.
76. Huang EY, Mascarenhas L, Mahour GH: Wilms' tumor and horseshoe kidneys: A case report and review of the literature. J Pediatr Surg 2004;39:207-212.
77. Huff V, Compton DA, Chao LY, et al: Lack of linkage of familial Wilms' tumour to chromosomal band 11p13. Nature 1988;336:377-378.
78. Huff V, Reeve AE, Leppert M, et al: Nonlinkage of 16q markers to familial predisposition to Wilms' tumor. Cancer Res 1992;52:6117-6120.
79. Jenkner A, Camassei FD, Boldrini R, et al: 111 Renal neoplasms of childhood: A clinicopathologic study. J Pediatr Surg 2001;36:1522-1527.
80. Kalapurakal JA, Peterson S, Peabody EM, et al: Pregnancy outcomes after abdominal irradiation that included or excluded the pelvis in childhood Wilms' tumor survivors: A report from the National Wilms' Tumor Study. Int J Radiat Oncol Biol Phys 2004;58:1364-1368.
81. Kayton ML, Rowe DH, O'Toole KM, et al: Metastasis correlates with production of vascular endothelial growth factor in a murine model of human Wilms' tumor. J Pediatr Surg 1999;34:743-747.
82. Knudson AG, Strong LC: Mutation and cancer: A model for Wilms' tumor of the kidney. J Natl Cancer Inst. 1972;48:313-324.
83. Ladd WE, White RR: Embryoma of the kidney (Wilms' tumor). JAMA 1941;117:1859-1863.
84. Leape LL, Breslow NE: The surgical treatment of Wilms' tumor: Results of the National Wilms' Tumor Study. Ann Surg 1978;187:351-356.
85. Lee MP, DeBaun MR, Mitsuya K, et al: Loss of imprinting of a paternally expressed transcript, with antisense orientation to KVLZT1, occurs frequently in Beckwith-Wiedemann syndrome and is independent of insulin-like growth factor II imprinting. Proc Natl Acad Sci U S A 1999;96: 5203-5208.
86. Lee SB, Haber DA: Wilms' tumor and the WT1 gene. Exp Cell Res 2001;264:74-99.
87. Li CM, Guo M, Borczuk A, et al: Gene expression in Wilms' tumor mimics the earliest committed stage in the metanephric mesenchymal-epithelial transition. Am J Pathol 2002;160:2181-2190.
88. Lin RY, Argenta PA, Sullivan KM, et al: Diagnostic and prognostic role of basic fibroblast growth factor in Wilms' tumor patients. Clin Cancer Res 1995;1:327-331.
89. Little MH, Williamson KA, Mannens M, et al: Evidence that WT1 mutations in Denys-Drash syndrome patients may act in a dominant-negative fashion. Hum Mol Genet 1993; 2:259-264.
90. Lodge AJ, Jaggers J, Adams D, et al: Vascular control for resection of suprahepatic intracaval Wilms' tumor: Technical considerations. J Pediatr Surg 2000;35: 1836-1837.
91. Look AT, Hayes FA, Shuster JJ, et al: Clinical relevance of tumor cell ploidy and N-myc gene amplification in childhood neuroblastoma. A Pediatric Oncology Group Study. J Clin Oncol 1991;9:581-591.
92. Lovvorn HN 3rd, Savani RC, Ruchelli E, et al: Serum hyaluronan and its association with unfavorable histology and aggressiveness of heterotransplanted Wilms' tumor. J Pediatr Surg 2000;35:1070-1078.
93. Lu YJ, Hing S, Williams R, et al: Chromosome 1q expression profiling and relapse in Wilms' tumour. Lancet 2002;360:385-386.

94. Marsden HB, Lawler W: Bone-metastasizing renal tumor of childhood. Br J Cancer 1978;38:437-441.
95. Maw MA, Grundy P, Millow LJ, et al: A third Wilms' tumor locus on chromosome 16q. Cancer Res 1992;52: 3094-3098.
96. McNeil DE, Brown M, Ching A, et al: Screening for Wilms' tumor and hepatoblastoma in children with Beckwith-Wiedemann syndrome: A cost-effective model. Med Pediatr Oncol 2001;37:349-356.
97. Mertens A, Neglia J, Yasui Y, et al: Mortality rates and causes of death among 5-year survivors of childhood and adolescent cancer. Proc Am Soc Clin Oncol 1999;19:569a.
98. Miller RW, Fraumeni JG, Manning MD: Association of Wilms' tumor with aniridia, hemihypertrophy and other congenital abnormalities. N Engl J Med 1964;270: 922-930.
99. Mitchell C, Jones PM, Kelsey A, et al: The treatment of Wilms' tumour: Results of the United Kingdom Children's Cancer Study Group (UKCCSG) second Wilms' tumour study. Br J Cancer 2000;83:602-608.
100. Montgomery BT, Kelalis PP, BLute ML, et al: Extended followup of bilateral Wilms' tumor: Results of the National Wilms' Tumor Study. J Urol 1991;146:514-518.
101. Narahara K, Kikkawa K, Kimira S, et al: Regional mapping of catalase and Wilms' tumor-aniridia, genitourinary abnormalities, and mental retardation triad loci to the chromosome segment 11p1305-p1306. Hum Genet 1984;66:181-185.
102. Neville H, Ritchey ML, Shamberger RC, et al: The occurrence of Wilms' tumor in horseshoe kidneys: A report from the National Wilms' Tumor Study Group (NWTSG). J Pediatr Surg 2002;37:1134-1137.
103. Okutsu T, Kuroiwa Y, Kagitani F, et al: Expression and imprinting status of human PEG8/IGF2AS, a paternally expressed antisense transcript from the IGF2 locus, in Wilms' tumors. J Biochem 2000;127:475-483.
104. Osler W: Two cases of striated myo-sarcoma of the kidney. J Anat Physiol 1879;14.
105. Owens CM, Veys PA, Pritchard J, et al: Role of chest computed tomography at diagnosis in the management of Wilms' tumor: A study by the United Kingdom Children's Cancer Study Group. J Clin Oncol 2002;20: 2768-2773.
106. Pappo AS, Crist WM, Kuttesch J, et al: Tumor-cell DNA content predicts outcome in children and adolescents with clinical group III embryonal rhabdomyosarcoma. J Clin Oncol 1993;11:1901-1905.
107. Park S, Bernard A, Bove KE, et al: Inactivation of WT1 in nephrogenic rests, genetic precursors to Wilms' tumour. Nat Genet 1993;5:363-367.
108. Pelletier J, Bruening W, Kashtan CE, et al: Germline mutations in the Wilms' tumor suppressor gene are associated with abnormal urogenital development in Denys-Drash syndrome. Cell 1991;67:437-447.
109. Pelletier J, Bruening W, Li FP, et al: WT1 mutations contribute to abnormal genital system development and hereditary Wilms' tumour. Nature 1991;353:431-434.
110. Plesko I, Kramarova E, Stiller CA, et al: Survival of children with Wilms' tumour in Europe. Eur J Cancer 2001; 37:736-743.
111. Porteus MH, Narkool P, Neuberg D, et al: Characteristics and outcome of children with Beckwith-Wiedemann syndrome and Wilms' tumor: A report from the National Wilms' Tumor Study Group. J Clin Oncol 2000;18:2026-2031.
112. Rahman N, Arbour L, Houlston R, et al: Penetrance of mutations in familial Wilms' tumor gene FW1. J Natl Cancer Inst 2000;96:650-652.
113. Re GG, Hazen-Martin DJ, Sens DA, et al: Nephroblastoma (Wilms' tumor): A model system of aberrant renal development. Semin Diagn Pathol1994;11:126-135.
114. Reeve AE, Sih SA, Raizis AM, et al: Loss of allelic heterozygosity at a second locus on chromosome 11 in sporadic Wilms' tumor cells. Mol Cell Biol 1989;9:1799-1803.
115. Renaud EJ, Liu D, Pipe SW, et al: Inferior vena cavectomy for nonexcisable Wilms' tumor thrombus. J Pediatr Surg 2001;36:526-529.
116. Riccardi VM, Sujansky E, Smith AC, et al: Chromosomal imbalance in the aniridia-Wilms' tumor association: 11p interstitial deletion. Pediatrics 1978;61:604-610.
117. Ritchey ML: The role of preoperative chemotherapy for Wilms' tumor: The NWTSG perspective. National Wilms' Tumor Study Group. Semin Urol Oncol 1999;17: 21-27.
118. Ritchey ML, Green DM, Thomas PR, et al: Renal failure in Wilms' tumor patients: A report from the National Wilms' Tumor Study Group. Med Pediatr Oncol 1996;26:75-80.
119. Ritchey ML, Kelalis PP, Breslow N, et al: Surgical complications after nephrectomy for Wilms' tumor. Surg Gynecol Obstet 1992;1992:507-514.
120. Ritchey ML, Kelalis PP, Haase GM, et al: Preoperative therapy for intracaval and atrial extension of Wilms' tumor. Cancer 1993;71:4104-4110.
121. Ritchey ML, Pringle K, Breslow N, et al: Management and outcome of inoperable Wilms' tumor: A report of National Wilms' Tumor Study-3. Ann Surg 1994;220:683-690.
122. Ritchey ML, Shamberger RC, Haase G, et al: Surgical complications after primary nephrectomy for Wilms' tumor: Report from the National Wilms' Tumor Study Group. J Am Coll Surg 2001;192:63-68.
123. Ross JH, Kay R: Surgical considerations for patients with Wilms' tumor. Semin Urol Oncol 1999;17:33-39.
124. Shamberger RC, Guthrie KA, Ritchey ML, et al: Surgery-related factors and local recurrence of Wilms' tumor in National Wilms' Tumor Study 4. Ann Surg 1999;229: 292-297.
125. Shamberger RC, Ritchey ML, Haase GM, et al: Intravascular extension of Wilms' tumor. Ann Surg 2001;234:116-121.
126. Shearer P, Kapoor G, Beckwith JB, et al: Secondary acute myelogenous leukemia in patients previously treated for childhood renal tumors: A report from the National Wilms' Tumor Study Group. J Pediatr Hematol Oncol 2001;23:109-111.
127. Shurin SB, Gauderer MW, Dahms BB, et al: Fatal intraoperative pulmonary embolization of Wilms' tumor. J Pediatr 1982;101:559-562.
128. Smith MB, Xue H, Strong LC, et al: Forty-year experience with second malignancies after treatment of childhood cancer: Analysis of outcome following the development of the second malignancy. J Pediatr Surg 1993;28:1342-1348.
129. Sorensen K, Levitt GA, Bull C, et al: Late anthracycline cardiotoxicity after childhood cancer: A prospective longitudinal study. Cancer 2003;97:1991-1998.
130. Sredni ST, de Camargo B, Lopes LF, et al: Immunohistochemical detection of p53 protein expression as a prognostic indicator in Wilms' tumor. Med Pediatr Oncol 2001;37:455-458.
131. Tagge EP, Hanson P, Re GG, et al: Paired box gene expression in Wilms' tumor. J Pediatr Surg 1994;29:134-141.
132. Toretsky JA, Zitomersky NL, Eskenazi AE, et al: Glypican-3 expression in Wilms' tumor and hepatoblastoma. J Pediatr Hematol Oncol 2001;23:496-499.
133. Tournade MF, Com-Nougue C, de Kraker J, et al: Optimal

duration of preoperative therapy in unilateral and nonmetastatic Wilms' tumor in children older than 6 months: Results of the Ninth International Society of Pediatric Oncology Wilms' Tumor Trial and Study. J Clin Oncol 2001;19:488-500.
134. Trueworthy R, Shuster JJ, Look T, et al: Ploidy of lymphoblasts is the strongest predictor of treatment outcome in B-progenitor cell acute lymphoblastic leukemia of childhood: A Pediatric Oncology Group Study. J Clin Oncol 1992;10:606-613.
135. Vujanic GM, Kelsey A, Mitchell C, et al: The role of biopsy in the diagnosis of renal tumors of childhood: Results of the UKCCSG Wilms' tumor study 3. Med Pediatr Oncol 2003;40:18-22.
136. Vujanic GM, Sandstedt B, Harms D, et al: Revised International Society of Paediatric Oncology (SIOP) working classification of renal tumors of childhood. Med Pediatr Oncol 2002;38:79-82.
137. Weeks DA, Beckwith JB, Mierau GW, et al: Rhabdoid tumor of kidney: A report of 111 cases from the National Wilms' Tumor Study Pathology Center. Am J Surg Pathol 1989;13:439-458.
138. White GR, Kelsey AM, Varley JM, et al: Somatic glypican 3 (GPC3) mutations in Wilms' tumour. Br J Cancer 2002; 86:1920-1922.
139. Wilms M: Die Mischgeschwuelste der Niere. In Leipzig, 1899, Arthur Georgi.
140. Zoeller G, Pekrun A, Lakomek M, et al: Wilms' tumor: The problem of diagnostic accuracy in children undergoing preoperative chemotherapy without histological tumor verification. J Urol 1994;151:169-171.
141. Zuppan CW, Beckwith JB, Luckey DW: Anaplasia in unilateral Wilms' tumor: A report from the National Wilms' Tumor Study Pathology Center. Hum Pathol 1988;19: 1199-1209.

第 28 章

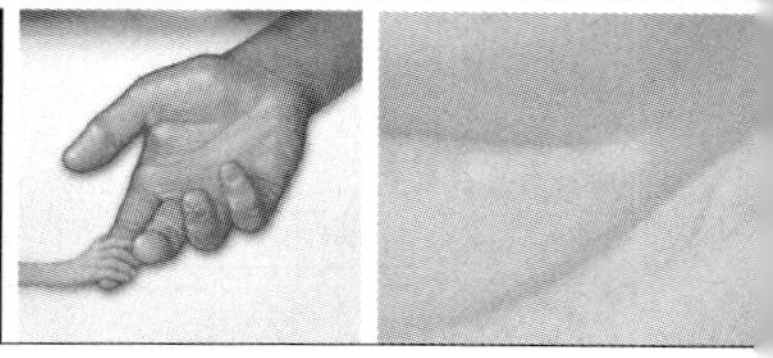

神经母细胞瘤

Jay L. Grosfeld

67 神经母细胞瘤是婴幼儿和儿童最常见的实体肿瘤之一。其来源于神经嵴，可发生在肾上腺髓质以及沿颈部至盆腔的交感神经节链上。因为这个高度恶性的肿瘤特征性地表现出不同寻常的行为，其临床表现也各有不同。虽然观察到肿瘤存在自行消退和恶性向良性的转化[27,43,63,76,83,144,147]，但大多数病例是进展性的。其他恶性肿瘤诸如肾母细胞瘤、横纹肌肉瘤、急性淋巴性白血病、生殖细胞肿瘤、Hodgkin 病和非 Hodgkin 淋巴瘤的存活率通过积极综合治疗已得到了显著提高，但是进展期神经母细胞瘤的预后仍然很差[25,27,67,74,77,83,116]。其肿瘤生物特性表现出很大差异，因此治疗神经母细胞瘤患儿对医生是一个挑战。

原始成神经细胞在宫内第 10 至 12 周胎儿肾上腺中可以发现。在孕 20 周结节数量增长，但在孕周末期数量逐渐减少。每 260 个死于先天性心脏病的新生儿以及每 39 个出生 3 个月内死于其他各种疾病的婴儿中就有 1 个在肾上腺部位发现神经母细胞瘤。临床肿瘤发生率约为 7500 至 10 000 名儿童中 1 例[13,27,73,74]。神经母细胞瘤占儿童所有肿瘤的 10%，占所有癌症死亡的 15%。肿瘤发生的原因还不清楚。在美国每年有 700 例神经母细胞瘤被诊断出来，大约 40%的诊断年龄是 1 岁，7 岁在 75%，10 岁时在 98%[27]。大于 50%的病例诊断时年龄小于 2 岁。神经母细胞瘤在男孩中发病略高于女孩，比例为 1.2∶1.0[27,74]。它是新生儿最常见的腹腔内恶性肿瘤。尽管成人发生率和死亡率有所下降，但 1980 年间到 1990 年间美国婴儿的发病率从 189 例 / 百万上升 220 例 / 百万[115]。男性婴儿中枢神经系统肿瘤、神经母细胞瘤和视网膜母细胞瘤的发病率升高，而女性婴儿畸胎瘤和肝母细胞瘤的发病率升高。神经母细胞瘤的胚胎样性质可以通过产前超声诊断，胎儿期肿瘤很少侵犯胎盘[3,12,56,101,109,146,171,226]。自从 1983 年 Fenart 等最先报道产前诊断神经母细胞瘤后在其他文献中有多于 55 例的病例被报道的。肿块通常在孕 32 周通过超声检查发现，有报道最早在孕 18 周发现[103]。

怀有先天性神经母细胞瘤胎儿的孕妇偶尔因为宫内肿瘤释放儿茶酚胺而经历高血压和潮红。常有肿瘤发生在双胞胎的报道，家庭中父亲和儿子或者母亲和孩子发生肿瘤的情况也有报道[37,70,171]。婴儿期双胞胎同时发生神经母细胞瘤提示遗传性因素可能占主导地位，大龄双胞胎不同时期发病提示随机突变可能更为重要。家族性神经母细胞瘤发病的平均年龄为 9 个月，而普通人群为 18 个月。Maris 等人[145]观察到 20%的家族性神经母细胞瘤有双侧或多灶性肿瘤，并报道遗传性神经母细胞瘤的染色体易感位点为 16 号染色体短臂的 12～13 区。神经母细胞瘤可发生在患有 Beckwith-Wiedemann 综合征、神经纤维瘤病（von Recklinghausen 病）、Hirschsprung 病、中枢性肺换气不足综合征（Ondine's curse）、婴儿酒精综合征以及母亲因癫痫服用苯妥英（婴儿乙内酰脲综合征）的婴儿中[7,59,119,161,206]。虽然环境因素未必在肿瘤的形成中起重要作用，但注意到有神经母细胞瘤患儿的母亲在怀孕期间因阴道感染接受过药物治疗并且父母因职业接触过电磁场[27]。

神经母细胞瘤可以发生在胎内存在神经嵴组织的任何部位。成神经细胞来源于从发育中的脊髓外层迁移而来的原始神经嵴细胞。肿瘤可发生于颈部、后纵隔、腹膜后神经节（脊柱旁）、肾上腺髓质和盆腔主 468
动脉旁体[73,74,79,83]。在 75%的病例中，肿瘤位于后腹膜，在肾上腺髓质（50%）或脊柱旁神经节（25%），在 20%的病例中，原发肿瘤在后纵隔，小于 5%的肿瘤发生在颈部和盆腔（图 28-1）[27,73,74,83]。原发性颅内大脑神经母细胞瘤也可发生[46,246]。此外，婴儿畸胎瘤偶然也可包含神经母细胞瘤病灶。神经母细胞瘤发生

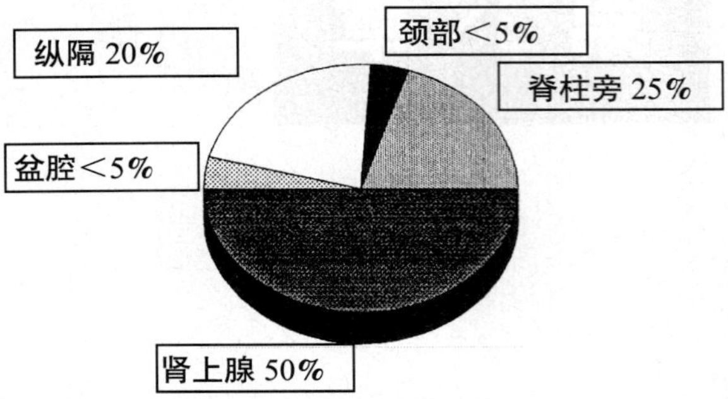

图 28-1　神经母细胞瘤病例在每个原发肿瘤部位的分布。原发肿瘤最常发生于肾上腺。

在膀胱的罕见病例也有报道[60]。成神经细胞临床有三个转归：（1）自行消退；（2）神经母细胞瘤分化成熟为良性神经节细胞瘤；（3）迅速进化成高度恶性的对抗治疗的肿瘤。

肿瘤筛查

为了早期诊断治愈，日本于 1985 开始开展筛选项目，评价 6 个月婴儿尿香草扁桃酸（VMA）及高香草酸（HVA）的水平。这些研究确诊了大量的婴儿神经母细胞瘤，这些病例的存活率比常规检测出来的病例要高。日本筛查出来年龄小于 1 岁的神经母细胞瘤的数量是实际发生率的两倍，但是既没有减少大年龄儿童的发病数，也未提高大于 1 岁患儿的存活率[19,27,199,200]。Sawada 等人[199,200]报道 170 例筛查出来的病例的存活率为 96%。这些观察提示筛查出来的神经母细胞瘤大多是良性的且可以自动消退[199]。然而，一少部分筛查出的患儿为不良生物学特性者且预后差，一部分 6 个月时筛查为阴性的患儿 12～18 个月后会发展成为进行性神经母细胞瘤[106]。

通常来说，筛查可以提供关于这个变化多端的肿瘤的自然组织学信息，确诊出一些与大年龄儿童相反的可以消退的生物学特性良好的肿瘤。在魁北克，通过前瞻性的大样本的对照筛查试验减少了假阳性病例的发生率，但是最终敏感性只有 45%。最终结果与日本的相似[237]。德国一项研究要筛查 260 万个年龄 9～18 个月的婴儿，结果在 1800 例筛查的婴儿中确诊了 149 例神经母细胞瘤，证实了预测价值为 8%[202]。德国研究者统计筛查出来的肿瘤 2/3 将会自行消退。3 例筛查出来的局部病变肿瘤死于治疗的并发症，这个事实说明潜在风险的上升。北美洲和欧洲的研究说明，筛查可能导致过度诊断和治疗[201]。但是对筛查结果的研究是有意义的，它有助于对诊断为早期阶段有成熟或自行消退机会的的神经母细胞瘤患儿减轻治疗[239]。一个数量有限的试验观察了 11 例筛查出来的局部肿瘤，所有的肿瘤在观察期体积都有所缩小[239]。Oue 等人[169]观察了 22 例筛查出来的肿瘤，13 例（59%）自行消退，9 例因体积增大而接受手术治疗。尽管没有 1 例有 N-*myc* 基因扩增，但在 8 例婴儿中发现了其他一些不良的生物学指标，包括二倍体、不良组织分型、染色体缺失（1p），但所有的婴儿均存活[169]。有人认为有令人注目的医疗和心理学理由（尤其是在假阳性病例的父母中）需要停止神经母细胞瘤的筛查[54,238]。鉴于全世界各地已停止筛查工作，日本卫生厅于 2004 年 4 月也停止了筛查工作[169]。

临床表现

神经母细胞瘤临床表现具有多样性，其表现与原发部位、是否存在转移以及与某些肿瘤代谢相关的产物有关。50%～75%已报告的病例存在腹部肿块。肿块质地硬、节结状、活动度差、触诊时疼痛。一般症状包括体重减轻、生长异常、腹部疼痛腹胀、发热和贫血[27,73,74,83]。25%的病例出现高血压，与肿瘤分泌产生儿茶酚胺的代谢产物有关。与神经母细胞瘤相关高钙血症被观察到，因为肿瘤自发破裂导致血腹的病例也有报道[8,24]。

起源于上纵隔或颈部的肿块可侵犯星状神经节并产生 Horner 综合征，表现为患侧上睑下垂、瞳孔缩小、眼球内陷、无汗症和虹膜异色症[73,74,83]。眼眶骨转移可导致眼突出或双侧眼眶淤斑，通常为熊猫眼或棕熊眼（图 28-2）。儿童出现后两种表现而无外伤病史提示可能存在恶性病变。纵隔肿瘤可与呼吸窘迫有关，因为肿瘤影响肺扩张。食管受压可导致吞咽困难（图 28-3）[5,66,74,243]。纵隔和腹膜后脊柱旁病变可以表现为偏瘫，偏瘫与肿瘤从椎间孔侵入成哑铃状或沙漏状病变导致脊髓硬膜外压迫相关[73,118,174,198,242]。有一小部分患儿可存在马尾综合征。盆腔肿瘤可伴有膀胱和肠管功能障碍。贫血通常与骨髓浸润有关。肿瘤过度分泌儿茶酚胺可以导致潮红、出汗和易激惹。也可观

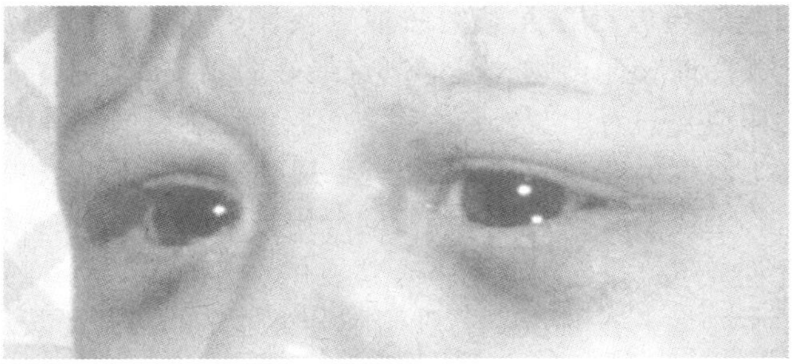

图 28-2 因神经母细胞瘤眼眶转移导致的双侧眼眶淤斑（“熊猫眼”或“浣熊眼”）。

察到表现为眼球震颤和斜视眼阵挛（眼球跳舞综合征）的急性小脑共济失调[9,121,195,196,207]。2/3 病例发生在婴儿纵隔神经母细胞瘤患儿。不自主的肌收缩和随意眼球运动与转移无关。引起神经母细胞瘤这些异常表现的原因还不清楚。可能是由抗原抗体复合物相关的自主免疫现象引起的[9,195,209]。有趣的现象是这些神经系统症状在肿瘤切除后仍然存在。这些儿童在学校通常表现差且有学习困难[195,196]。

婴儿神经母细胞瘤、节细胞神经母细胞瘤及偶尔良性节细胞瘤可出现顽固性腹泻，典型表现为水样、爆破样大便和低钾血症[42,58,127]。腹泻与肿瘤分泌活性肠源性多肽有关[42,58,74,127]。这些肿瘤通常具有生长激素抑制素受体。

神经母细胞瘤可以通过直接侵入周围组织、淋巴浸润或血源性转移播散。局部和远端淋巴结、肝脏、骨髓、骨皮质经常受累[72,74,77,83,91,165]。骨皮质转移的患儿预后差。骨转移经常发生部位包括红髓、长骨干骺端，另外还有颅骨、脊柱、盆骨、肋骨和胸骨体[27,74,77,83]。骨骼病变导致剧烈疼痛，有些病例临床表现为儿童因肿瘤骨转移引起的疼痛而拒绝走路。偶然情况下，进展期患儿表现为出血倾向，与骨髓大量转移引起的血小板减少以及肝脏转移导致的凝血因子生成障碍有关。婴儿Ⅳ-S 期神经母细胞瘤可出现肝脏肿大和皮下多发性结节。血源性转移至大脑、脊柱和心脏不常见。脑部转移在大年龄儿童中表现为头痛和癫痫[25,110]。胸部平片发现只有 4%的病例发生肺部转移[222]。这可能是纵隔淋巴结直接侵入肺部或弥漫性血源性扩散的结果，放射学表现容易与肺水肿或间质性肺炎混淆[222]。偶然情况下，活检时发现肺部淋巴结转移。 470

诊断

通过各种影像学和同位素检查、血清和尿样检查、标本的组织学和基因学评估对神经母细胞瘤做出诊断。在腹部平片中 50%的病例显示点状肿瘤钙化点[73,74,77]。同时也可见因肿块推移造成的肠管气体移位。脊柱旁增宽通常发现腹腔轴旁肿瘤。胸部平片可发现后纵隔肿瘤或腹部肿瘤延伸至横膈上导致的脊柱旁增宽。CT 可以确诊约 80%的肿瘤病例的钙化（图 28-4）[1,73]。通过对此增强 CT，可以从肾上腺和脊柱旁病变区分出肝脏和肾脏以及评估颅骨转移的颅内情况[1,22,74]。核磁共振对于检测脊柱内肿瘤扩张情况以及某些情况下肿瘤与相邻主要血管的关系非常有用。螺

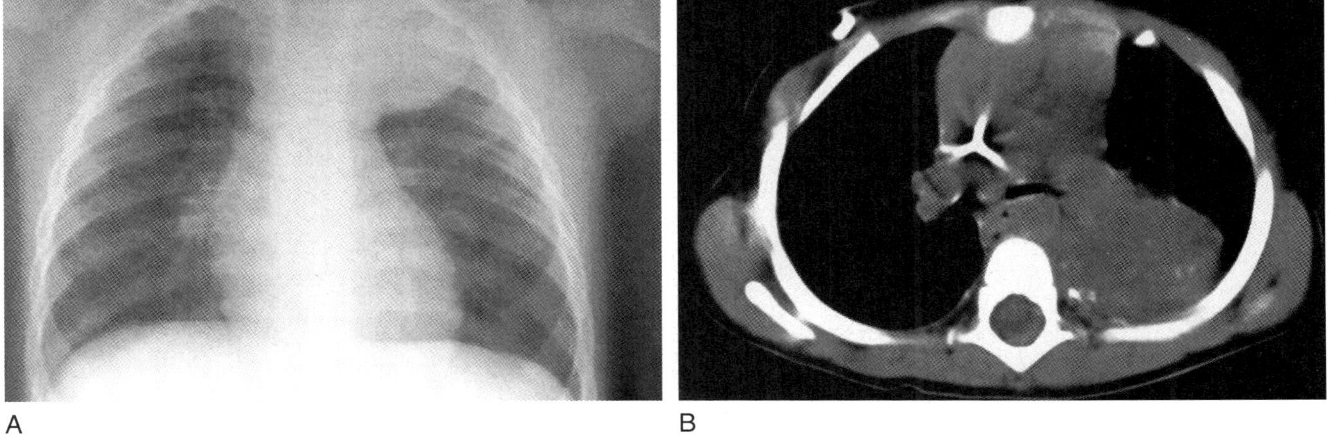

A B

图 28-3 A. 胸部平片显示左上胸腔肿瘤。B. CT 扫描证实后纵隔含有钙化肿块，提示神经母细胞瘤。

旋 CT 三维成像也是一种评估肿瘤与相邻血管的关系的有效方法。后腹膜肿瘤患儿的检查包括初步的腹部平片检查，区分囊性还是实质性病变的超声检查以及下腔静脉推移或梗阻情况的评估。原则上说神经母细胞瘤下腔静脉梗阻提示有不可切除病变的存在[74,75]。腹部 CT 辅助静脉注射造影剂能够一次检查获得腔静脉成像。大多数情况下，脊柱旁和肾上腺神经母细胞瘤引起一侧的肾脏或输尿管（或两者同时）向侧面或向下移位。不需要再做静脉肾盂造影。长骨的检查包括同位素骨扫描（运用骨示踪剂锝和间碘苄胍 MIBG）和多处骨髓穿刺[74,75,77,93]。MIBG 也可作为肾上腺髓质原发肿瘤的检查。骨同位素扫描和放射学骨检查密切相关，偶然会更敏感[93]。骨扫描假阳性发生在近期骨外伤和炎症的病例中。骨示踪同位素被骨骼转移病灶吸收，在原发肿瘤标记为钙化（图 28-5）[73,74]。腹膜后或后纵隔肿块显现骨示踪同位素提示病变为神经母细胞瘤。虽然血管造影曾用来评估儿童肿瘤，但如今这项技术很少使用，因为有许多影像学检查诸如螺旋 CT 或核磁共振血管造影可以很好地识别血管结构（图 28-6）。

盆腔神经母细胞瘤表现为尿路症状或便秘。肿瘤通常通过肛查可以触及，但必须同骶尾部畸胎瘤、卵黄囊瘤、Ewing 肉瘤以及盆腔横纹肌肉瘤鉴别[74,83]。

因为神经母细胞瘤是一种来源于神经嵴细胞的肿瘤，它可以分泌激素产物，是胺前体摄取和脱羧肿瘤（APUD）家族的一员。大于 90%的儿童神经母细胞瘤患者存在儿茶酚胺或其代谢产物水平升高。儿茶酚胺代谢产物分泌的测定最好用收集的 24 小时的尿液[136]。肾上腺素、去甲肾上腺素、多巴胺、异丙肾上腺素、HVA、VMA 和香草扁桃酸水平可以被测定。未成熟低分化的肿瘤倾向分泌特定的高水平的旁代谢产物（HVA）[75]。越成熟的肿瘤分泌越多的 VMA。在极少情况下，肿瘤不分泌过多的儿茶酚胺，Prasad 等人[177]提出副交感神经母细胞瘤分泌高水平的乙酰胆碱但不能将酪氨酸代谢成为多巴胺。进展的恶性肿瘤患者胱硫醚和高丝氨酸的尿浓度升高，血清神经特异性烯醇化酶、血清铁蛋白和乳酸脱氢酶水平升高。25%的病例癌胚抗原阳性[87,167,216,228,244]。尽管人们 471
历来很关注这些检查，但是这些血清水平既不是独立的判断预后的因素，现在也不能用来决定治疗方案。虽然组织病理学检查是神经母细胞瘤诊断的决定性因素，但在有些进展期病例中，骨髓穿刺存在玫瑰样肿瘤细胞和尿 VMA 或其他儿茶酚胺旁代谢产物水平增高提示神经母细胞瘤的诊断。检测肿瘤细胞骨髓穿刺的免疫学检查比常规分析更敏感[156]。对外周血样本进行连续的免疫分子学检测也可以确定循环中的神经母细胞，明确肿瘤的播散程度。

分期

过去神经母细胞瘤有许多不同的分期方法，包括

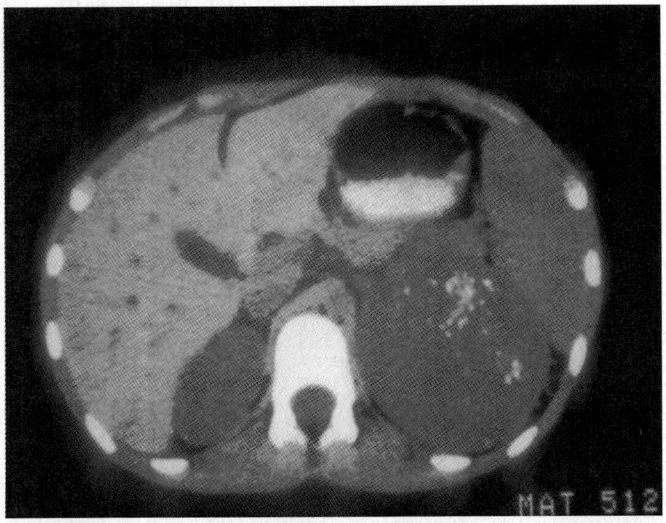

图 28-4　腹部 CT 扫描显示后腹膜肿块具有小点状钙化，同神经母细胞瘤相符。

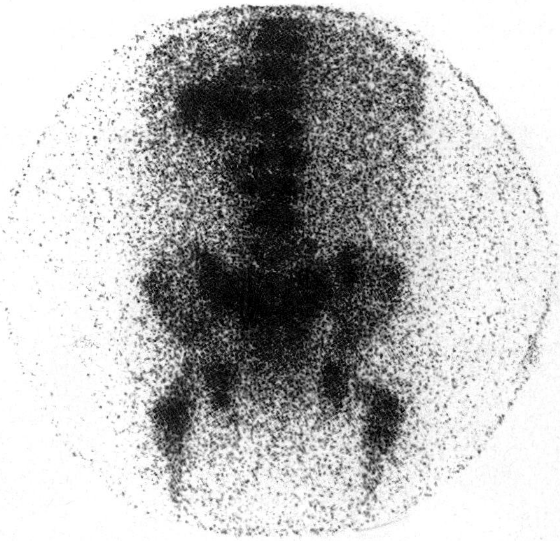

图 28-5　I^{123}-MIBG 同位素扫描显示存在骨转移和肾上腺部位原发肿瘤摄取同位素。

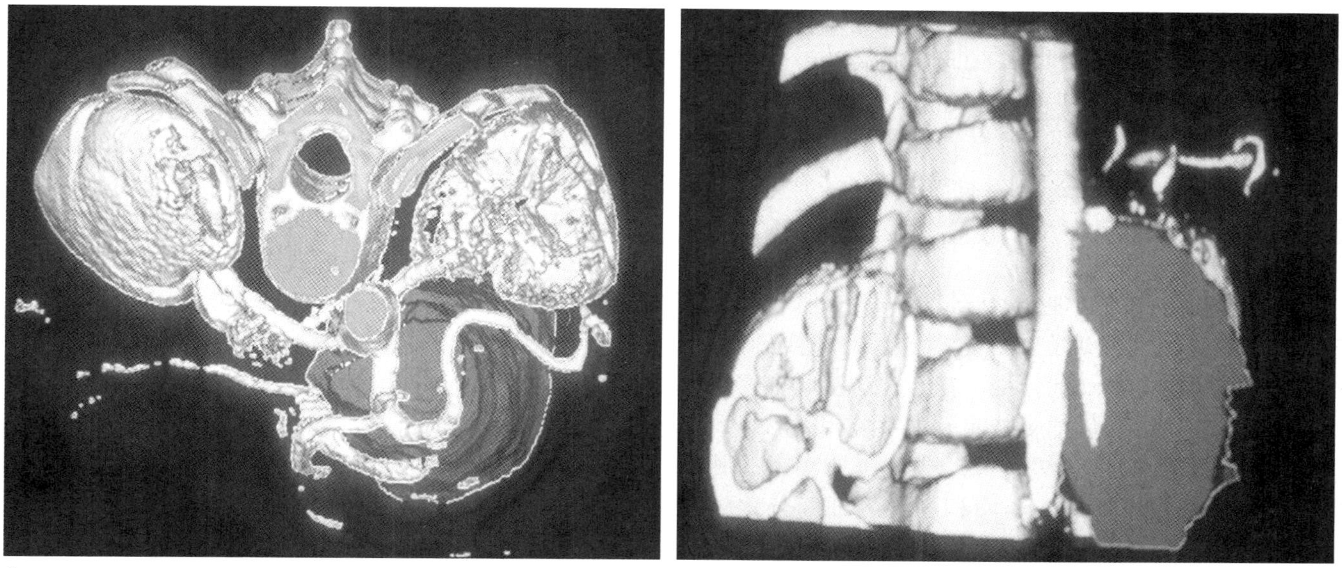

A　　B

图 28-6　螺旋 CT 扫描三维重建来源于近腹腔干的神经母细胞瘤。A. 前面像提示肿瘤未侵犯腹腔干分支动脉。B. 侧位像证实肠系膜上动脉穿过肿瘤（见彩色底片）。

儿童癌症组（CCG）[62]的 Evens 分期法[91]，儿童肿瘤组（POG）运用的 St. Jude 分期系统，欧洲国际抗癌联盟的 TNM 分期系统（肿瘤、淋巴结、转移），以及日本神经母细胞瘤研究组的分期系统。有关部位、病变完全切除、骨皮质存在转移以及婴儿 Evans 分期的Ⅳ-S 期肿瘤的标准基本相同。分期中其他一些方面存在分歧，包括 Evens 分期的Ⅲ期病例和淋巴结浸润的重要性。1988 年国际分期系统（INSS）产生了，建立了一套能够在全球广泛运用的常见标准，有益于大量样本的产生和数据的有效比较（表 28-1）[29]。国际神经母细胞瘤分期系统采用了 POG 和 CCG 系统的一些特点并明确了特有的预后分组。Brodeur 等人
于 1993 年修改了这些标准[28]。2001 年 CCG 和 POG 472
与国家肾母细胞瘤研究组和横纹肌肉瘤研究组合并形成了儿童肿瘤小组 COG，COG 现在采用了 INSS 对所有神经母细胞瘤病例进行分期。在我们机构中，

表 28-1　国际神经母细胞瘤分期系统

分期	描述
Ⅰ期	肿瘤局限于原发部位；完整切除肿瘤，有或无镜下残余；检侧或对侧淋巴结镜检阴性（与原发肿瘤相连的或切除的淋巴结可能是阳性的）
ⅡA	一侧肿瘤部分不完整切除，同侧和对侧淋巴结阴性
ⅡB	肿瘤完整或不完全切除，同侧区域内不相连的淋巴结阳性
Ⅲ期	肿瘤超越中线，有或无淋巴结浸润；或肿瘤未超越中线，对侧淋巴结镜检阳性；或中线部位肿瘤，双侧淋巴结镜检阳性或双侧浸润（不可切除）
Ⅳ期	远处淋巴结、骨、骨髓、肝或其他脏器转移
Ⅳ-S 期	局部原发肿瘤为Ⅰ或Ⅱ期，仅有肝、皮肤或骨髓转移（婴儿年龄小于 1 岁）

From Brodeur GM, Pritchard J, Berthold F, et al: Revision of the international criteria for neuroblastoma diagnosis, staging and response to treatment. J Clin Oncol 1993;11:1466-1477;Brodeur GM, Seeger RC, Barrett A, et al: International criteria for diagnosis, staging, and response to treatment in patients with neuroblastoma. J Clin Oncol 1988;6:1874-1881.

266 例神经母细胞瘤的分期如下：14 例（5.2%）Ⅰ期，52 例（19.6%）Ⅱ期，62 例（23.4%）Ⅲ期，117 例（44%）Ⅳ期，21 例（7.8%）Ⅳ-S 期。

病理学和组织学

神经母细胞瘤的病理分型已经被修改过了，肿瘤的组织学特点也已经确立了，这对预后有重要价值。最有用的系统是 Shimada 分型，基于肿瘤基质丰富还是基质稀少它将神经母细胞肿瘤分为年龄相关的组织良好型和组织不良型（表 28-2）[211]。基质丰富的肿瘤特点是丰富的 Schwann 基质和神经母细胞分化的征兆（成熟的细胞核和节细胞的细胞浆特征）。基质稀少的肿瘤包含不成熟分化差的神经嵴细胞和高的核分裂指数（MKI）。MKI 是指核破裂，它由坏死肿瘤细胞的数量、细胞分裂的数目以及 5000 个细胞中畸形的细胞、分成小叶的细胞、固缩核细胞的数目决定的。MKI 随年龄变化而变化，小于 18 个月的婴幼儿高 MKI 值是大于 200/5000 个细胞，大于 18 个月的是大于 100/5000 个细胞。所有大于 5 岁的儿童为组织不良型。基质稀少的肿瘤通常具有 N-*myc* 扩增，高 MKI 并且预后差。Shimada 等[212]报道组织学和 N-*myc* 扩增二者都可以提供预后信息且独立于分期。有 N-*myc* 扩增的神经母细胞瘤有独特的组织病理学表现型，临床进展很快。

表 28-2 改良的神经母细胞瘤 Shimada 病理学分类

表现	组织良好型	组织不良型
基质丰富	分化良好（节神经细胞瘤） 节细胞神经母细胞瘤，混合	节细胞神经母细胞瘤，结节
基质少（即神经母细胞瘤）		
年龄＜18 月	MKI＜4%	MKI＞4%或未分化
年龄 18～60 月	MKI＜2%和分化	MKI＞2%或未分化/分化差
年龄＞5 岁	无	上述所有表现

MKI：有丝分裂核破裂指数。

From Shimada H, Chatten J, Newton WA Jr, et al: Histopathologic prognostic factors in neuroblastoma: Definition of subtypes of ganglioneuroblastoma and an age-linked classification of neuroblastoma. J Natl Cancer Inst 1984;73:405-416; Shimada H, Stram DO, Chatten J, et al: Identification of subsets of neuroblastomas by combined histopathologic and N-myc analysis. J Natl Cancer Inst 1995;87:1470-1476.

国际神经母细胞瘤病理分型（INPC）采纳了 Shimada 的分型并做了小的改动[208-212,213]。年龄相关的分型既具有预后意义又与生物学相关。目前的系统将未分化亚型分成未分化肿瘤和分化差肿瘤。把基质丰富分化良好的肿瘤改名为成熟型神经节细胞瘤，另外增加 Schwann 基质占优为神经节细胞瘤的特征[208]。年龄仍是一个重要的预后因子，但分化程度和 MKI 也有不同的预后作用，这取决于患儿诊断时的年龄。尽管认为钙化的存在有益于存活，但进一步研究证明，钙化不是一个独立的影响预后的因素[111,208]。Shimada 组织良好型存活率为 85%，与之相比组织不良型为 41%。所有的节细胞神经母细胞瘤结节（GNBn）病例最初都被划分为不良型肿瘤。Umehara 等人[230]最先将表现为不同生物特性的这类特殊肿瘤分类。Peuchmaur 等人[173]最近更改了 INPC 将 GNBn 病例分成两类预后亚型-良好型和不良型。良好型无病存活率为 86%，然而不良型（2/3 的病例）只有 32%。儿童良好型 GNBn 的最终存活率大于 90%，与之相比不良型仅为 33.2%（表 28-7）[172]。大细胞神经母细胞瘤被认为是一类具有明显侵略的临床行为的表现型[229]。这些肿瘤具有不良型的组织学特性，包括多形性未分化的成神经细胞、钙化发生率低和高 MKI。免疫组化检查表现为大的神经母细胞瘤细胞特异性神经烯醇化酶、药物前体基因产物和酪氨酸羟化酶染色阳性；CD99 染色阴性[229]。

在肉眼检查时，神经母细胞瘤表现为血管丰富的紫灰色肿块，通常为实体偶尔为囊性的。肿瘤容易破裂、脆弱的假包膜使得手术操作中易出现大量出血，肿瘤经常坏死尤其是未分化型的。成熟的肿瘤（节细胞神经瘤）质地硬经常为肉白色。组织类型各不相同，原始基质少的神经母细胞瘤可以和其他小的蓝色圆形细胞肿瘤区分开来，诸如 Ewing 肉瘤、横纹肌肉瘤或原始神经外胚层肿瘤。成神经细胞是小的圆形细胞，内含大量细胞核而无许多细胞浆。不成熟的未分化肿瘤的特点是：紧密排列的小的梭形细胞特殊没有任何排列和分化的[142]。细胞核为圆锥状且深染玫瑰状可以观察到，且可以认为是肿瘤早期分化的征象（图

图 28–7 国际神经母细胞瘤病理学分类。FH：组织良好型；GNBn：节细胞神经母细胞瘤结节；MKI：有丝分裂核破裂指数；%MKC：有丝分裂和核破裂细胞；UH：组织不良型；* 标准的 GNBn（单个，肉眼可见，通常在丰富的基质中含出血结节，组织背景基质占优）；**MKC 2%：有丝分裂和核破裂细胞 2%，5000 个细胞中有 100 个；MKC 4%：有丝分裂和核破裂细胞 4%，5000 个细胞中有 200 个。（From Peuchmaur M, d'Amore ES, Joshi VV, et al: Revision of the International Neuroblastoma Pathology Classification: Confirmation of favorable and unfavorable prognostic subsets in ganglioneuroblas toma, nodular. Cancer 2003;98: 2274–2281.）

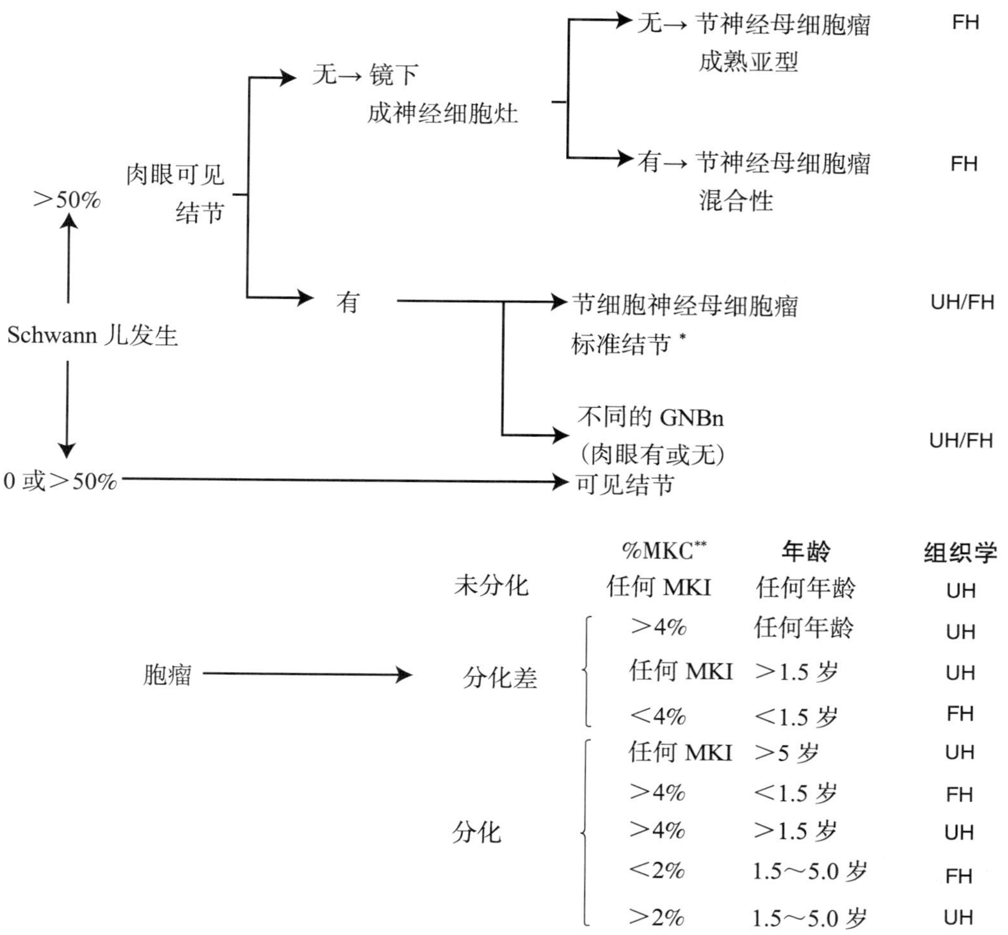

28–8）。每个玫瑰的中心是一团缠绕的细神经纤维。更为成熟基质丰富的肿瘤包含类似正常节细胞的细胞，混合有丰富的神经纤维丝，玫瑰状成神经细胞和节细胞这些组织学成分，所有单个显微镜视野可以见到所有这些成分[70,137]。在电镜下可以观察到神经原纤维和电镜强化细胞膜周围的神经分泌颗粒。神经分泌颗粒可能在多巴胺转化为去甲肾上腺素的部位。这些超微结构的发现以及肿瘤组织的基因认证通常可以将神经母细胞瘤和其他小圆细胞肿瘤区分开来。从高度恶性未分化的神经母细胞瘤发生自发性分化，分化为节细胞神经母细胞瘤最终变为良性节细胞瘤的病例已经被观察发现了。Ambros 等人[11]报道成熟的神经母细胞瘤包含 Schwann 细胞和神经元细胞，包括节细胞。同其他神经元细胞包括节细胞相比较 Schwann 细胞具有正常的染色体数目和三倍体流式细胞[11]。这些观察到的现象提示 Schwann 细胞是正常细胞群的反应，是侵犯神经母细胞瘤的补充或吸收营养因子，与肿瘤的成熟有关，也可作为一个抗神经母细胞瘤的因素[10,11,26]。Schwann 细胞也可产生血管生成抑制剂，诱导内皮细胞凋亡和限制血管生成抑制肿瘤生长[27,40]。

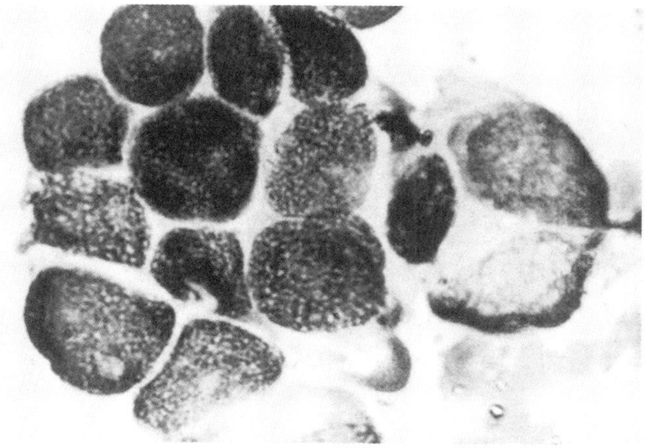

图 28–8 来自骨髓吸引活检的玫瑰样神经母细胞瘤细胞的组织表现，是肿瘤分化的早期特征。

474 ## 生物学和基因改变

肿瘤中观察到独特的癌基因诸如N–*myc*和*ras*癌基因[25,27]。N–*myc*癌基因的扩增（大于10个拷贝）与进展期疾病、肿瘤恶化、预后差相关，尤其是在年龄大于1岁的儿童中。N–*myc*癌基因的过度表达损害细胞的分化，促进了未成熟的神经嵴来源细胞的增殖[25,26]。N–*myc*原癌基因位于2号染色体短臂24区。在这个位点观察到存在长的双微体且未捆绑的染色区域，且可能代表扩增的细胞基因。大约30%的神经母细胞瘤存在N–*myc*扩增。90%N–*myc*扩增的病例疾病进展迅速，对治疗不敏感。肿瘤的DNA流式细胞倍体研究分析提示二倍体肿瘤预后比非整倍体（多倍体或三倍体）肿瘤的差[27,74]。N–*myc*扩增通常与1号染色体缺失和二倍体相关[30,89]。二倍体的肿瘤通常与17号染色体长臂不平衡的获得，甚至N–*myc*缺失相关[11,27,30,144]。11号染色体长臂和14号染色体长臂等位基因的缺失和4、6、11、18号染色体长臂的获得也已经被发现了[27]。

神经素Trk–A（一种高度亲和的神经生长因子的受体）的高度表达与良好的预后相关，与N–*myc*反向相关[157,158]。观察到Trk–A在小婴儿和Ⅰ期和Ⅳ–S期肿瘤中出现，预后非常好。Trk–A和神经细胞分化、肿瘤的消退相关，在血管生长抑制中起重要作用。低亲和性神经生长因子受体基因是另一个原癌基因，具有和Trk–A相似的预后，可能影响细胞的成熟[25,27,120]。相反，Trk–B和其配体BDNF的高表达为不良型肿瘤提供了一种自分泌的生存途径，尤其是在这些N–*myc*扩增的肿瘤中[27,100,159]。这些患儿多患有进展性疾病，年龄通常大于1岁，预后差[27,100,159]。Trk–C的表达被证实在神经母细胞瘤中出现，通常在较低分期，无N–*myc*扩增的肿瘤中可见[27,240]。

另一个克隆的基因，多药耐药相关的蛋白基因（MDR）和化疗耐受、N–*myc*过度表达和预后差相关[166]。相似地，P–糖蛋白水平升高与进展性的疾病及预后差相关[35,235]。肿瘤细胞中端粒酶水平升高，通过保护端粒保护染色体末端结构从而保持细胞的活力[27,191]。在端粒酶水平和神经母细胞瘤预后之间存在

表28–3 神经母细胞瘤的遗传变化

遗传特征	相关因子	危险分组
N–*myc*扩增（2p24位点）	二倍体或四倍体1p等位基因丢失高Trk–B，晚期疾病（Ⅲ、Ⅳ期）	高危
等位基因获得		
17q获得	晚期肿瘤N–*myc*扩增	高危
观察到4q、6p、7q、11q、18q获得	通常发生N–*myc*扩增	危险情况与N–*myc*相关
等位基因丢失		
1p36	与N–*myc*相关，70%～80%为近二倍体与疾病进展相关	高危
11q	很少与N–*myc*扩增相关 与14q杂合子丢失相连	中危，患儿无N–*myc*扩增存活率下降
14q	与11q杂合子丢失相连，与1p和N–*myc*相反关系	中危
易感性		
16p12–13	家族性神经母细胞瘤 多灶性和双侧神经母细胞瘤	低危
相关		
10号染色体（Ret癌基因）	先天性巨结肠	可变的
11p15.5	Beckwith–Wiedemann综合征	低危

LOH：杂合子丢失。

注意：这个表格没有包括Trk–A、–B、和–c以及多药耐药蛋白基因、端粒酶和本章提到的其他一些蛋白的基因表达变化。

反向关系，但在端粒酶水平和 N-*myc* 扩增之间存在正向关系[27]。在部分肿瘤细胞膜表面发现 CD44 糖蛋白，包括神经母细胞瘤。CD44 的高表达和良好的预后相关。相反，在进展性和侵袭性的神经母细胞瘤中发现 nm23 过度表达[140]。发现神经节苷脂 GD2 存在于人类神经母细胞瘤的细胞膜上，其水平升高与疾病活动性和肿瘤进展相关。神经节苷脂抑制肿瘤特异性免疫反应[152]。

475 婴幼儿神经母细胞瘤肿瘤血管生成和预后相关联系的研究显示以微血管密度为特性的肿瘤血管化增强和进展的播散的疾病及易转移性相关[47,49,57,153]。血管化的控制通过激素刺激因子、抑制剂和信号转导途径的平衡来达到[40]。血管化与 N-*myc* 扩增、不良组织类型和预后差相关。神经母细胞瘤产生血管形成因子诱导血管的生长，包括血管内皮生长因子（VEGF）、血小板源性生长因子（PDGF-A）、干细胞因子和它们分别的受体 FIK-1、PDGFR、C-kit[15]。Komuro 等人[122]证实，VEGF-A 的高表达与Ⅳ期病变相关，提出这可能是抗血管治疗的一个靶位。Kaicker 等人[112]提出，在无胸腺小鼠异体移植神经母细胞瘤细胞株 NGP 的神经母细胞瘤动物模型试验中，VEGF 拮抗剂抑制新生血管和肿瘤的生长。他们同时发现反应停抑制血管的生成和降低微血管密度但不能抑制肿瘤的生长。Kim 等人[117]和 Rowe 等人[193]也提出，在神经母细胞瘤模型试验中运用抗血管生成疗法抑制肿瘤的生长。甲磺酸伊马替尼，一种用来治疗消化道基质肿瘤的化合物，在严重联合免疫缺陷小鼠模型中显示其在体内体外能够减少神经母细胞瘤的生长、降低细胞的活性和增加细胞凋亡[15]。Davidaff 等人[49]证实，运用原位肿瘤细胞逆病毒载体转导的基因疗法可以为 FIK-1 受体传递血管生成抑制因子，限制肿瘤诱导的血管生成和肿瘤的生长。

蛋白质 Bcl-2 家族主要负责释放影响肿瘤细胞的消退凋亡信号，其在绝大多数神经母细胞瘤中都表达。Bcl-2 基因产生一种蛋白能够阻止神经元细胞死亡。在进展性疾病中 Bcl-2 表达水平高预后差，表达水平低的病例证实肿瘤凋亡（消退）和分化。Bcl-2 高水平表达在获得性耐药中起重要作用[55]。Bcl 家族亚型一族包括 Bcl-xL，其抑制凋亡，Bcl-xS，诱导自然细胞死亡。VEGF 上调 Bcl-2 表达，通过改变凋亡和它的调节蛋白提高神经母细胞瘤细胞的存活[14]。半胱天冬酶水平升高（负责凋亡信号的酶）和神经母细胞瘤预后改善相关，被证实是一个良好的生物学特性[27]。

基于风险的管理

许多年以来，神经母细胞瘤的治疗因诊断时肿瘤的范围、患儿的年龄和分期不同而有所不同[23,27,41,62]。肿瘤完整切除和局部病变的尽可能多地切除肿瘤可以获得最佳的预后[61,73]。Ⅰ期病变中进行手术治疗[74,83]。Ⅱ期病变进行手术切除，但在许多患儿中镜下有残余病灶或肿瘤侵入椎间孔因而无法进行完整切除，部分这样的患儿接受局部放疗。另一些患儿尽管存在残留肿瘤但只接受手术治疗，这些患儿只有 75%～80%的治愈率[74,124,164]。

因为有残余病灶的Ⅱ期肿瘤患儿的肿瘤特性变化多端以及那些进一步发展的肿瘤（Ⅲ、Ⅳ期）存活率差，所以为了制定合适的治疗方案有必要增加一些信息。在过去的 20 年里，一些生物学和遗传学因素被证实是重要的预后评估标志，可以影响治疗。在新 INSS 的影响、INPC 的使用以及一些生物学和遗传学特性被确认为危险因素和预后因素的基础上建立了危险管理系统来制订治疗方案[27,74,208-210,213]。以危险因素评估预后的新的个体化的治疗方案力争提高生存率、减少长期发病率、改善生活质量。现在的治疗方案以低、中、高危分组为基础（表 28-4）。预后良好包括Ⅰ期、Ⅱ期、Ⅳ-S 期的患儿，他们的年龄小于 1 岁，DNA 流动计数为超二倍体、组织良好型、N-*myc* 扩增少于 1 个、高 Trk-A 表达、1 号染色体短臂无异常。相反，预后差包括进展性肿瘤（Ⅲ、Ⅳ期），年龄大于 1 岁、N-*myc* 扩增大于 10 个、低 Trk-A 表达、双倍的 DNA 倍数、1 号染色体短臂 36 区等位基因丢失和组织不良型。

对于低危组患儿，肿瘤手术切除通常可以治愈，并可以减少化疗相关的危险。通常对中危组患儿进行手术治疗和标准的化疗。预后差的高危组患儿适合高强度的治疗包括联合化疗后彻底手术切除（可能的话），放疗以达到局部控制，骨髓清除治疗和骨髓移植。

手术治疗

在绝大多数病例中完全手术切除原发肿瘤仍然是治疗的最基本要素。手术采用气管插管麻醉，需要严密监测。在上肢留置合适的大口径静脉插管。足够的

表 28-4 神经母细胞瘤风险分组

INSS 分期	年龄	N-*myc* 状态	INPC 组织学	DNA 倍数[†]	风险分组
Ⅰ期	0～21 岁	任何	任何	任何	低
ⅡA/ⅡB	＞365 天	任何	任何	任何	低
	365 天至 21 岁	非扩增	任何	—	低
	365 天至 21 岁	扩增	良好型	—	低
	365 天至 21 岁	扩增	不良型	—	高
Ⅲ期	＜365 天	非扩增	任何	任何	中
	＜365 天	扩增	任何	任何	高
	365 天至 21 岁	非扩增	良好型	—	中
	365 天至 21 岁	非扩增	不良型	—	高
	365 天至 21 岁	扩增	任何	—	高
Ⅳ期	＜365 天	非扩增	任何	任何	中
	＜365 天	扩增	任何	任何	高
	365 天至 21 岁	任何	任何	—	高
Ⅳ-S 期	＜365 天	非扩增	良好型	＞1	低
	＜365 天	非扩增	任何	＝1	中
	＜365 天	非扩增	不良型	任何	中
	＜365 天	扩增	任何	任何	高

*N-*myc* 无扩增＝1 拷贝，扩增大于 1 拷贝。

[†]DNA 指数＞1（非整倍体）或＝1（二倍体）。

INPC：国际神经母细胞瘤病理分型；INSS：国际神经母细胞瘤分期系统。

Modified from Children's Oncology Group protocols by LaBerge JM: Neuroblastoma. In O'Neill JA Jr, Grosfeld JL, Fonkalsrud EW, Coran AG (eds): Principles of Pediatric Surgery, 2nd ed. St Louis, Mosby, 2003.

静脉通路非常重要因为肿瘤血供丰富可能会造成大量失血。体温、氧饱和度、心电图和脉搏需要被监测。手术中需要严密监测血压以发现因肿瘤释放过量儿茶酚胺造成的突发性高血压。

如原发肿瘤来源于后腹膜，手术采用长的、脐上
476 经腹膜横切口。在有些病例中需要双侧肋缘下人字形切口或胸腹切口。进入腹腔，任何一侧，切割侧腹壁的附着使结肠向中前移位。脾脏和胰腺是游离的可向上中移位暴露左侧的肿瘤。对于右侧的肿瘤，十二指肠和胰腺头部可以被移动并向中间牵拉，分离肝脏附着韧带可以改善暴露（图 28-9）。在大多数患有局部病变的儿童中，全部或大部分肿瘤可以被成功切除。不应该由于首次手术中过度追求切除而对患儿的状况造成危害。几乎可以避免切除相邻周围正常结构包括脾脏、胃、胰腺和结肠。在有些病例中，不能将肾上腺或脊柱旁神经母细胞瘤从同侧肾脏中分离出来，因而肾脏必须切除。为分期术中切除可疑的腹主动脉旁淋巴结及肾周淋巴结是非常重要的。后腹膜常规淋巴结清扫通常不必进行。如果需要放疗可以在肿瘤边缘放置钛夹作为标记，同时 CT 随访复查时可以降低放置其他金属夹引起的辐射作用。

因为神经母细胞瘤的假包膜易碎，手术过程中仔细处理以防止肿瘤溃破和出血非常重要。神经母细胞瘤经常粘连或包绕大血管，应仔细检查和保护提供重要脏器血供的血管，诸如腹腔干分支动脉和肠系膜上动脉。原发肾上腺肿瘤由数个小动脉滋养。主要静脉引流通常不变的，右侧直接进入下腔静脉，左侧进入左肾静脉和膈下静脉。尽管没有很好的依据表明对于这些儿童高度恶性肿瘤部分切除或肿瘤减小体积手术有助于改善预后，但是已经观察到肿瘤切除

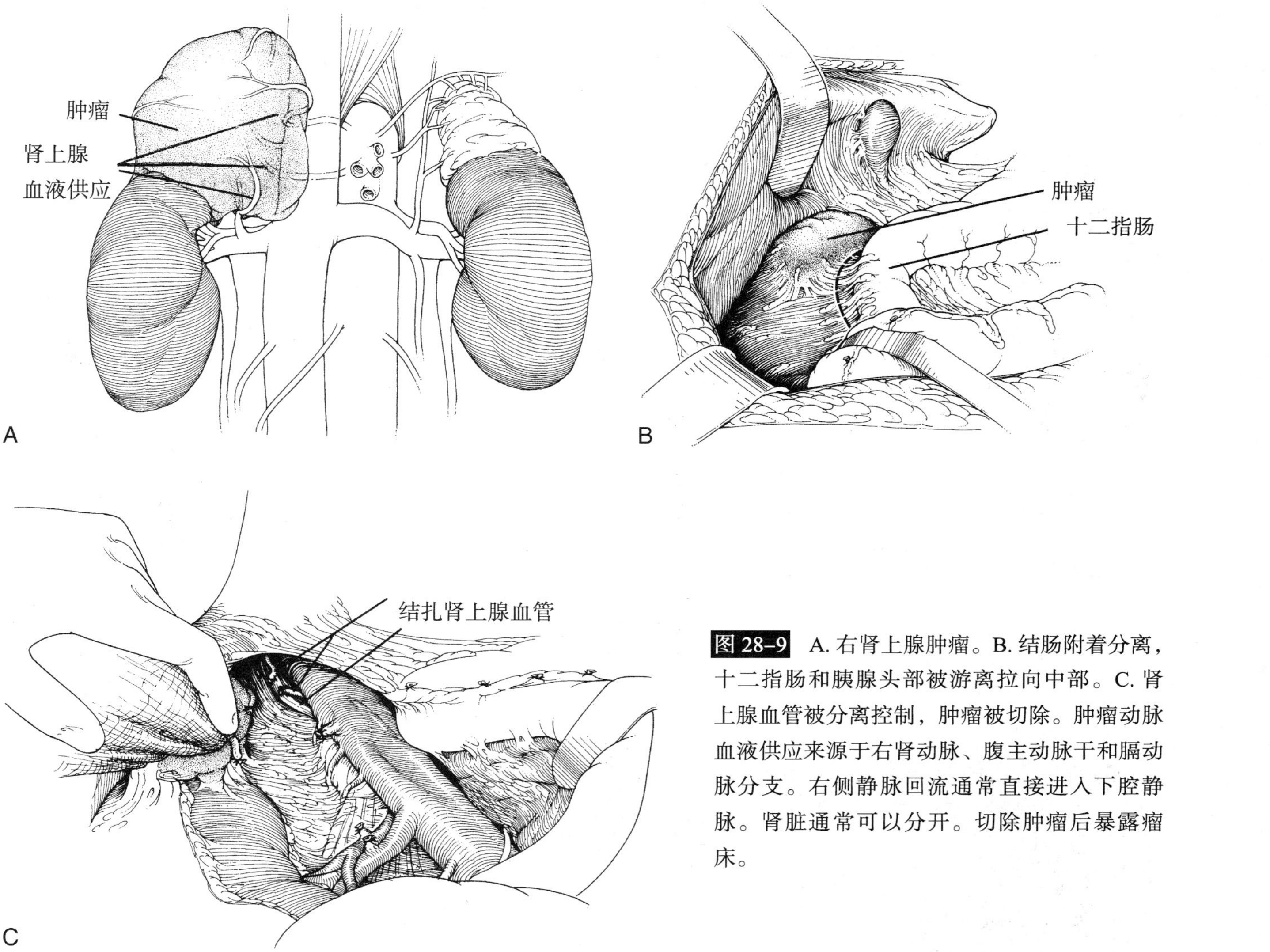

图 28–9　A. 右肾上腺肿瘤。B. 结肠附着分离，十二指肠和胰腺头部被游离拉向中部。C. 肾上腺血管被分离控制，肿瘤被切除。肿瘤动脉血液供应来源于右肾动脉、腹主动脉干和膈动脉分支。右侧静脉回流通常直接进入下腔静脉。肾脏通常可以分开。切除肿瘤后暴露瘤床。

后患儿对辅助治疗的反应有所改善[73,84,134]。过度积极手术切除肿瘤而使儿童出血造成生命危险的做法不提倡。鉴于对初次化疗的敏感反应，肿瘤通常可以在化疗后缩小，可以延迟手术切除或在二次探查手术时被切除[95,78,83,85,194]。位于脊柱旁下段的肿瘤和原发盆腔肿瘤需要仔细解剖分离，将肿瘤与腹主动脉分叉和下腔静脉分离开来。肿瘤经常侵入椎间孔（图 28–10）。

微创手术在一些选出的神经母细胞瘤病例中已经开展[102]。筛查发现的肾上腺肿瘤已经尝试通过腹腔镜切除[123,160]。Yamamoto 等人[239]报道了 3 例直径小于 20mm 的肾上腺神经母细胞瘤病例。他们运用 5 孔技术，腹内压力保持比气腹压力少 4mmHg。包膜完整的肿瘤被完整切除，将肿瘤放入塑料袋从 10mm 的孔拖出。所有病例都为组织良好型，均没有 N–*myc* 扩增。无肿瘤复发。Kouch 等人[125]报道了 6 例运用腹腔镜切除小于 4cm 的肾上腺肿瘤的病例。腹部和开孔 477
部位没有转化和肿瘤复发。Iwanaka 等人[107]运用腹腔镜对进展性神经母细胞瘤进行活检，并通过腹腔镜将微创手术和开腹手术比较，手术时间和失血量两者无显著差异，然而运用腹腔镜切除肿瘤术后开始化疗的时间、术后开始进食的时间和住院的时间要短一些[107,108]。De Lagausie 等人[52]报道了 9 例肾上腺神经母细胞瘤的腹腔镜手术治疗。2例产前发现，7 例产后发现，包括 3 例Ⅳ期。平均年龄 38 个月（2 个月至 9 岁）。8 例完整切除，1 例转为开腹手术。3 例病例中 1 个或更多淋巴结被切除。无死亡和一孔切口感染。这些和其他一些报道提示对选中的患儿进行腹腔镜活检或肿瘤切除是安全有效的[52]。

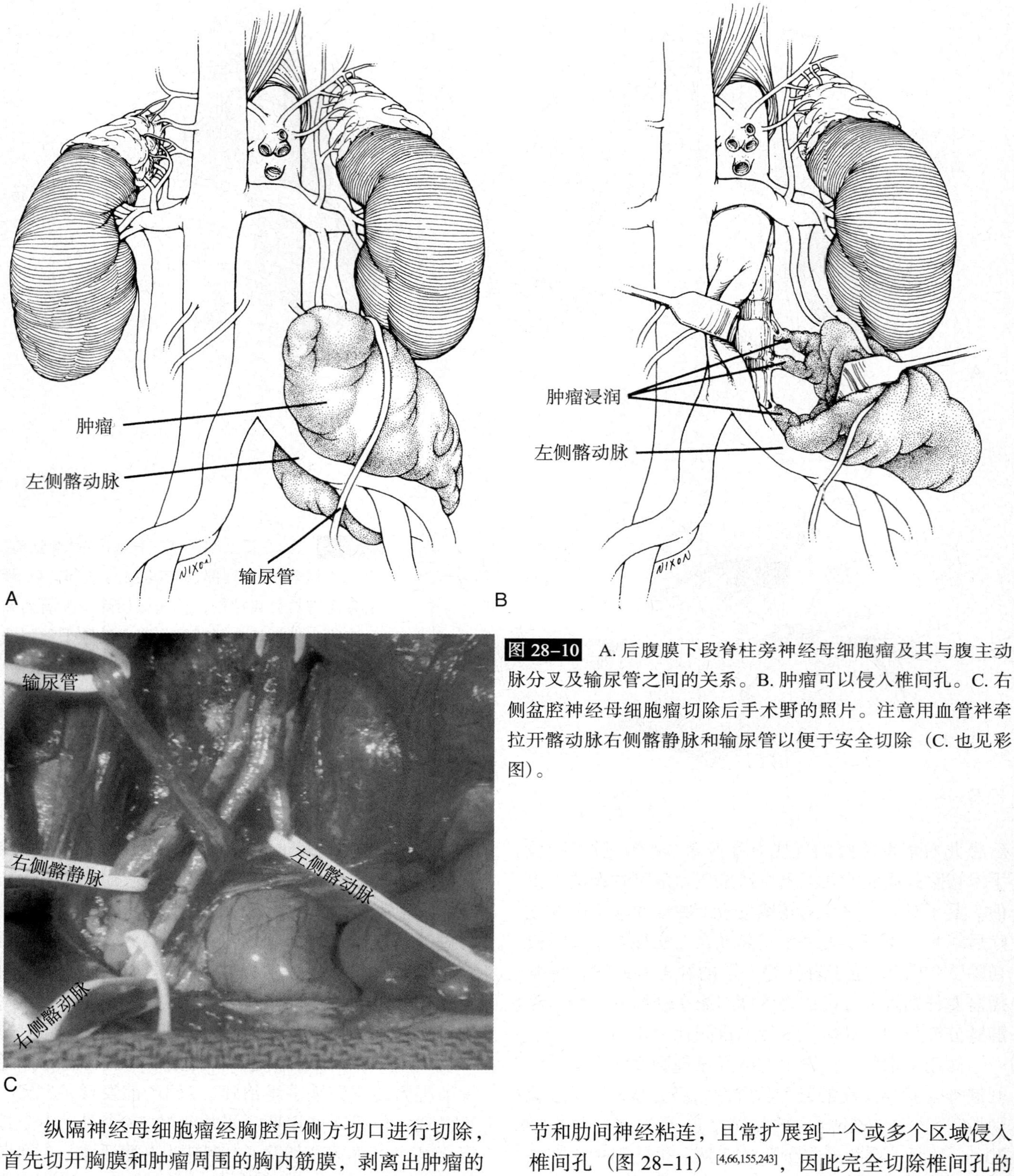

图 28-10　A. 后腹膜下段脊柱旁神经母细胞瘤及其与腹主动脉分叉及输尿管之间的关系。B. 肿瘤可以侵入椎间孔。C. 右侧盆腔神经母细胞瘤切除后手术野的照片。注意用血管袢牵拉开髂动脉右侧髂静脉和输尿管以便于安全切除（C. 也见彩图）。

纵隔神经母细胞瘤经胸腔后侧方切口进行切除，首先切开胸膜和肿瘤周围的胸内筋膜，剥离出肿瘤的一个面，再用锐性或钝性分离出肿瘤与肋骨间的粘连面。术后仔细辨认和结扎或钳夹专供肿瘤的肋间供血血管和引流血管非常重要。肿瘤可能和周围交感神经节和肋间神经粘连，且常扩展到一个或多个区域侵入椎间孔（图 28-11）[4,66,155,243]，因此完全切除椎间孔的肿瘤是不大可能的。小的原发纵隔肿瘤可以通过胸腔镜切除，胸腔镜也可做肿瘤组织活检。

哑铃状肿瘤患者具有神经系统症状（包括偏瘫），

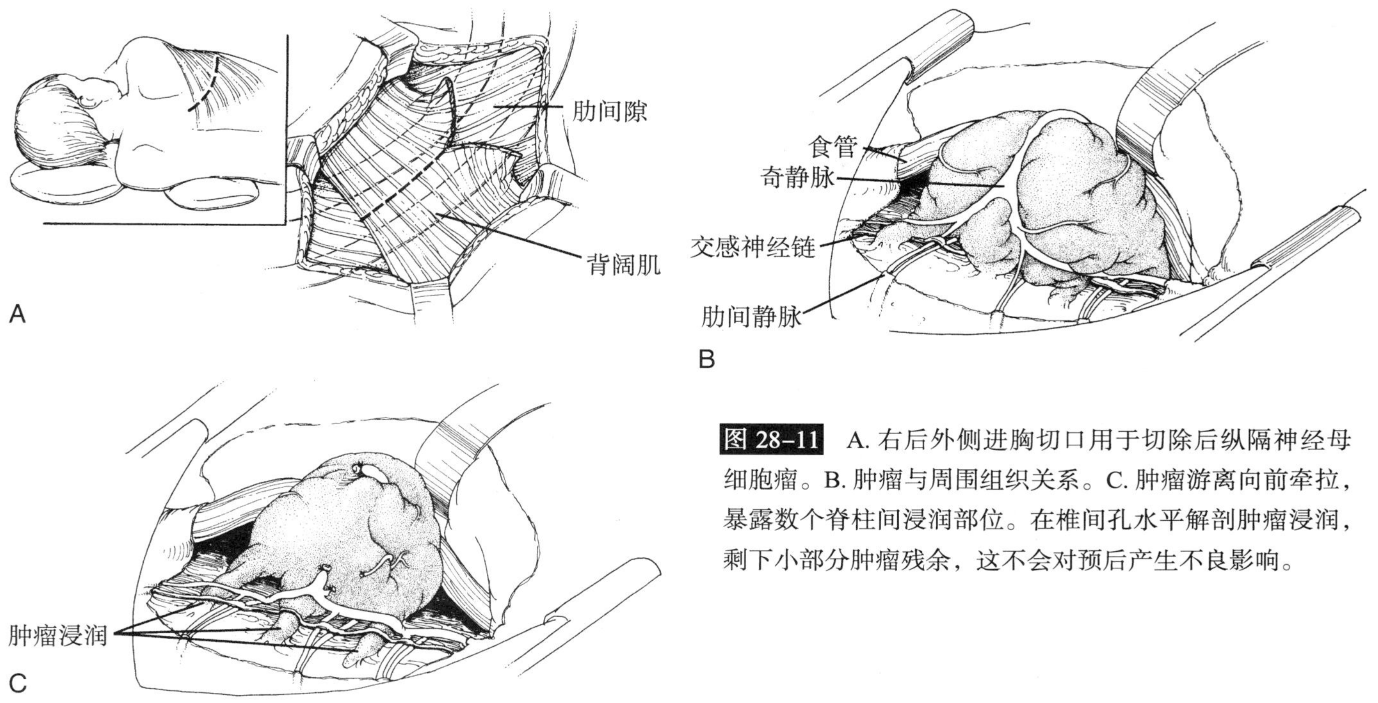

图 28-11 A. 右后外侧进胸切口用于切除后纵隔神经母细胞瘤。B. 肿瘤与周围组织关系。C. 肿瘤游离向前牵拉，暴露数个脊柱间浸润部位。在椎间孔水平解剖肿瘤浸润，剩下小部分肿瘤残余，这不会对预后产生不良影响。

迅速 MRI 检查，在进行胸腔内肿瘤切除前建议急诊行椎板切开术，切除硬膜外肿瘤解除脊髓压迫。纵隔肿瘤的切除可以延期至患者神经系统症状有所缓解。如果影像学检查到硬膜外肿瘤存在而无症状，先进行化疗肿瘤可能缩小，这样可以避免椎板切开术或椎板
8 切除术。肿瘤侵入脊柱的治疗选择某些地方存在争议。Plantaz 等人[174]回顾了法国 42 例病例建议先化疗随后切除残余肿瘤。Yiin 等人[242]报道了 13 例有脊髓压迫症状和神经功能缺失的神经母细胞瘤，所有的患儿首先进行化疗，3 例恢复，4 例改善，6 例进展出现偏瘫。6 例中的 2 例椎板切开后恢复。这些作者建设对化疗过程中神经症状加重的患儿行脊髓减压术。
9 Sandberg 等人[198]报道了 46 例硬膜外或神经椎间孔肿瘤浸润的病例，9 例神经系统检查正常的低危组患儿有完整的手术或化疗的神经系统随访，4 例低危组患儿脊髓压迫症状严重术后有所改善或保持稳定，但是 2 例化疗治疗的患儿神经功能缺陷恶化。12 例高危组中的 11 例神经系统检查正常以及放射检查没有发现严重脊髓压迫表现的给予化疗治疗，神经系统无恶化表现。16 例高危组病例有严重的脊髓压迫症状，10 例中的 7 例首先进行化疗和所有 6 例先进行手术治疗的病例症状改善或保持稳定。未进行手术治疗的患儿中脊髓异常发生率为 12.5%（2/6），进行手术治疗的为 30%（9/30）。这些作者总结出应对高危肿瘤和脊髓浸润但神经系统检查正常的患儿进行化疗，要知道有少部分患儿会因为进行性神经系统异常而需要手术。低危肿瘤患儿可能被治愈的需避免化疗。患儿和他们的家人应该意识到在多达 30%的病例中手术可能产生继发性脊髓异常。

颈部神经母细胞瘤通常是局限性的而且预后良好[82]。Haddad 等人[86]研究了 43 例颈部神经母细胞瘤，确定了与手术并发症增加有关的四种因素；与血管结构粘连、肿瘤大小、肿瘤易碎和哑铃状肿瘤。影像学检查显示血管移位和狭窄的实质肿块[2]。来源于颈部和上纵隔的肿瘤经常浸润星状神经节链。如果术前无症状，手术切除可导致术后 Horner 综合征[2,73]。相对于肿瘤完整切除和存活来说这是个小后遗症，但是应让患儿家属意识到这个可能的并发症。手术中应特别注意保护臂丛、膈神经、迷走神经和喉返神经。II 期肿瘤是否需要辅助治疗取决于基于患儿年龄、肿瘤组织类型和不良生物及遗传因素（例如，N-*myc* 扩增大于 10 个拷贝、1 号染色体短臂缺失、二倍体细胞流动计数、组织不良型病理）的危险评估[74]。13%的 II 期病例具有高危预后因素，需要积极化疗。

进展性疾病（III期）通常需要积极治疗，包括手术切除（能够的话）、多种药物化疗和首次局部放疗。盆腔或接近腹主动脉的III期肿瘤通常最初不能切除，化疗后肿瘤通常会缩小到二次探查手术能够切除的程

度[74,83]。III期肿瘤完整切除后预后得到改善[74,85]。辅助治疗的方案取决于肿瘤的可切除性、组织类型和影响这个特殊肿瘤风险的生物学和遗传学特性。应给予肿瘤完整切除且预后因素满意的患儿温和的化疗。相反，应对肿瘤不能完整切除的患儿进行肿瘤床局部放疗和高强度的化疗。患者高危无反应肿瘤的患儿可能从强化的细胞消除化疗中受益，化疗后会进行自体骨髓移植[31,84,148,149]。III期高危组病例有无不良生物学特
480 性可以预测预后，诸如年龄大于 1 岁、组织不良型和大于 10 个拷贝的 N-*myc*[148,109]。在自体骨髓移植前采用多个单克隆抗体去除肿瘤细胞纯化骨髓[151]。早期采用自体骨髓移植治疗具有高危生物学特性的无反应肿瘤的预后比疾病进展到最后采用该方法作为最后的治疗要好[149,151,178]。最近几年来，在许多儿童癌症中心自体干细胞移植已代替了传统的自体骨髓移植。

对于不能手术的IV期肿瘤 CCG 将诊断时首次手术与延迟的首次手术和二次探查手术的情况进行了比较。完全切除率可能为 62%，延迟首次手术的为 77%，二次探查手术的为 66%[84]。在延迟手术组中儿童肾切除及术后并发症的发生率低[84]。因为三组之间存活率没有差异（3 年时完整切除的为 40%），化疗后延期手术被认为是IV期肿瘤治疗的最佳选择。IV期肿瘤原发灶切除的作用地位尚未明确。患儿对化疗全部或部分敏感，在我们医院进行延期或二次探查手术尽可能切除所有的残余肿瘤。关于IV期肿瘤完全切除的疗效的报道存在争议。向 CCG 报告的 Haase 等人[84]描述，IV期肿瘤化疗后延期手术完整切除肿瘤对存活有益。相反，Kiely[116]和 Shorter 等人[215]报道指出，IV期肿瘤完整切除对延长存活没有帮助。然而，LaQuaglia 等人[134]在一份研究了 70 例IV期肿瘤患儿的报告中指出，肿瘤大部分切除加以高强度的化疗方案能够提高最终存活率。尽管一些研究的报告中显示IV期患儿化疗敏感再加肿瘤手术切除存活率有所提高[78,84,218]，但缺乏有关存活患儿生物学特性的资料，肿瘤大部分切除的独立疗效也未得到证实[134]。最近，LaQuaglia 等人[135]回顾了 141 例 INSS IV期的病例，再次证实强化化疗提高肿瘤的大部分切除率。未切除患儿中 50%局部肿瘤进展，与此相比在肿瘤大部分切除病例中仅为 10%。肿瘤切除者的最终存活率为 50%，未切除者的为 11%[135]。积极手术治疗的存活者偶然发生远期并发症，包括一侧肾上腺切除后肾脏萎缩以及盆腔肿瘤切除后的射精问题[126]。有意思的是来源于盆腔的III、VI期肿瘤完整切除后患儿预后良好[74,84]。

婴儿神经母细胞瘤

诊断时年龄小于 1 岁的婴儿预后明显良好。Riley 儿童医院年龄小于 1 岁的婴儿存活率为 76%，而大年龄儿童仅为 32%（图 28-12）[76]。年龄小于 1 岁的患儿预后良好覆盖所有分期状态，包括婴儿VI期转移病例。在年龄小于 1 岁的患儿中VI期病变的发生率为

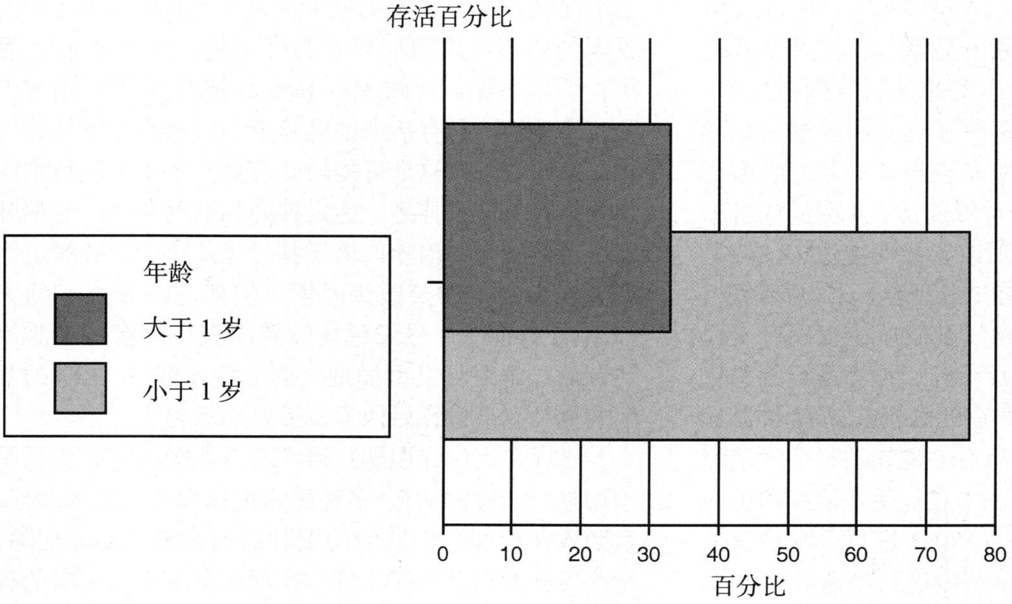

图 28-12 条图提示年龄小于 1 岁的神经母细胞瘤患儿存活率得到改善。

30%，与其相比大年龄组为 60%～70%[76]。

尽管关于Ⅵ期病变原发肿瘤切除存在争议，以我个人的经验，仅有的婴儿存活者进行了原发肿瘤切除[76]。与之相似，CCG 报道 11 例婴儿Ⅵ期病例中的 7 例延期手术肿瘤完整切除后无病存活超过 5 年[84,85]。
1 Ⅵ期婴儿对化疗比大年龄儿童对化疗敏感，50%的婴儿对治疗完全敏感，与之相比大年龄儿童只有 22%。这些现象提示转移病灶的解决对于存活期的影响比手术作用要大。进一步来说在一些婴儿中手术切除是有益的，但应该在转移病灶经化疗得到控制以后进行手术。

Paul 等人[170]报道了 24 例年龄小于 1 岁的Ⅵ期肿瘤病例的 5 年存活率为 75%，与之相比，大年龄儿童的为 10%。患儿化疗治疗药物包括氮芥、长春新碱、达卡巴嗪、阿霉素、环磷酰胺和顺铂，未做骨髓移植。Schmidt 等[204]观察到年龄小于 1 岁、Ⅵ期、无 N-*myc* 基因扩增的婴儿存活率为 93%，然而，N-*myc* 基因扩增大于 10 个拷贝的婴儿疾病进展迅速，尽管接受化疗通常还是失败[204]。因而，为了获得痊愈需要强化化疗和骨髓移植尤其对于存在不良生物标志的高度选择的婴儿来说。

Ⅳ-S 期

神经母细胞瘤患儿中最不寻常的一类是那些年龄小于 1 岁的Ⅳ-S 期患儿，临床表现为肝脏肿大、皮下节结和骨髓侵润，在其他方面表现为Ⅰ期或Ⅱ期原发肿瘤。Ⅳ-S 期病例占 1 岁以内神经母细胞瘤发病的 30%左右[76]。对这些病例的治疗存在一些争议。有些婴儿可能死于Ⅳ-S 期疾病的并发症而不是肿瘤的发展。

严重肝脏肿大并发症包括因为肿瘤浸润的巨大肝脏引起横膈显著上升而造成的呼吸窘迫，凝血功能异常以及肿瘤压迫造成的肾损伤（图 28-13）[21,45,50,76,236]。横膈上升导致胃食管角改变引起呕吐，引起胃食管反流、蛋白质卡路里不足性营养不良和吸入性肺炎。全肠道外营养是一种有效的辅助治疗方法[188,189,231]。Ⅳ-S 期的婴儿死亡大多发生在有肝大相关的严重症状的年龄小于 2 个月的婴儿中，他们不能像大年龄儿童那样承受治疗[76,166]。对肿瘤浸润引起有症状的肝大进行 600～1200Gy 的低剂量放疗是有效的，每天剂量控制在 100～150Gy 之间[21,76,83]。尽管肝脏体积缩小早期可以出现，外周水肿几周内可以缓解，但完全消退需

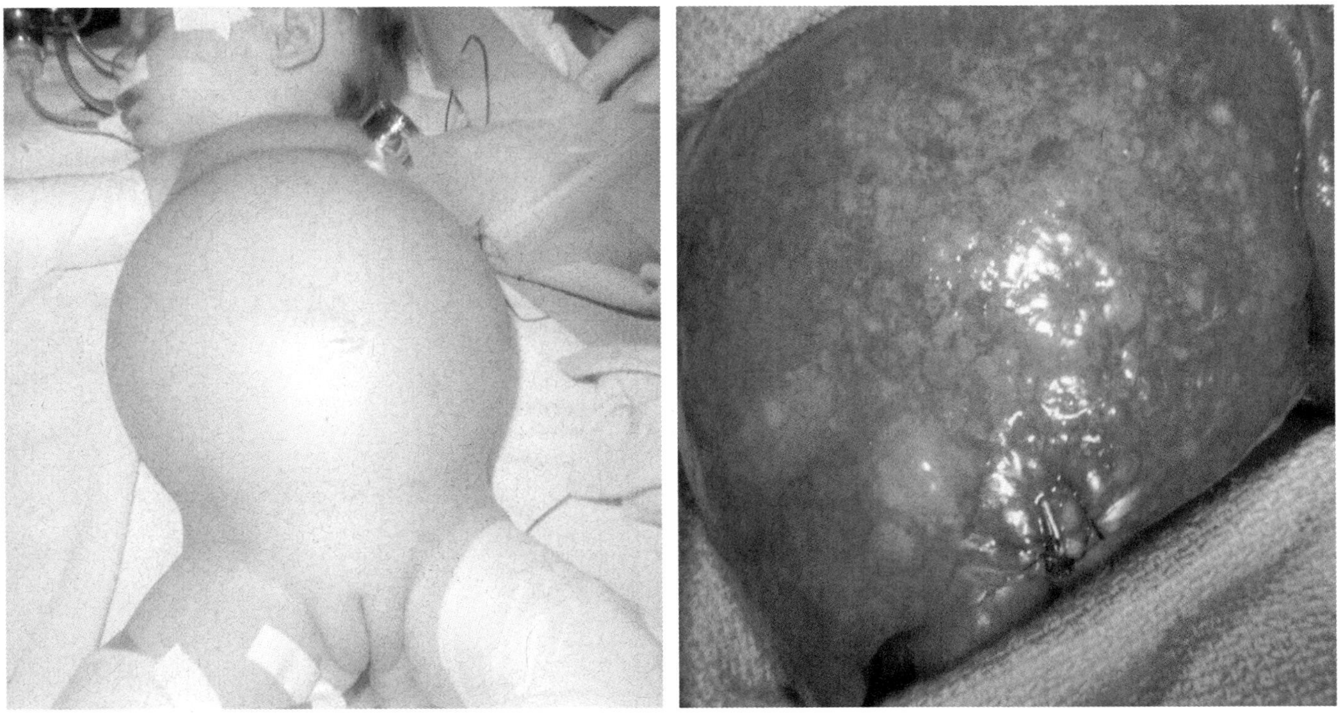

A　　B

图 28-13　A. 一名 6 周大的婴儿表现为腹胀和肝脏肿大。B. 剖腹探查肝脏的发现。有多个转移结节，活检明确诊断为Ⅳ-S 期神经母细胞瘤。

要 6～15 个月[76]。与放疗相比，肝脏肿块的缓解与Ⅳ-S 期病变本身的过程更相关。每天低剂量环磷酰胺 5mg/kg 是合理的替代治疗方法。尽管有些学者提出用合成材料袋制成一个临时腹侧腹壁疝容纳肿大的肝脏以降低腹腔内压力，我没有发现这个技术是有效的[205]。因为可以观察到放置外源性合成袋导致
482 败血症引起的死亡病例[21,76]。为了降低感染的风险，Lee 和 Applebaum 提议运用聚四氟乙烯袋建立暂时腹侧疝，当肝脏肿块一段时间大片缩小后去除。

有远处转移的不寻常患儿的存活率大于 80%，通常不需要特殊治疗。表 82-5 总结了 12 个研究报告的治疗 Ⅳ-S 期神经母细胞瘤的结果，最终存活率为 86%。大多数 Ⅳ-S 期病例（大于 90%）具有良好的遗传和生物因素包括 T-rk 高度表达、没有 N-*myc* 的扩增、组织良好型和无 1 号染色体短臂等位基因的缺失。这提示大多数 Ⅳ-S 期肿瘤能够自行退化。尽管大多数 Ⅳ-S 期疾病预后良好，Wilson 等人报道 18 例有异质性肿瘤表现的病例，存活率只有 50%，其中 3 例有 N-*myc* 的扩增。存在不良遗传和生物预后因子的这部分病例（小于 10%）需要更为积极的治疗。有趣的是有多发皮肤结节的婴儿预后看起来最好。可能是肿瘤存在于多个部位引起增强的免疫反应的结果。神经母细胞瘤肿瘤细胞在体内或体外对组织相容复合性抗原Ⅰ摄入的增加可能改善预后[220]。Ⅳ-S 期疾病的婴儿组织相容复合性表面抗原Ⅰ的表达为正常水平，而那些Ⅰ至Ⅳ期的婴儿为低水平[220]。Sugio 等人[224]报道，组织相容复合性抗原Ⅰ表达的下调和疾病进展期患儿 N-*myc* 癌基因扩增增加相关。

2002 年 Nickerson 等人[162]报道了 80 例 CCG Ⅳ-S 期婴幼儿。58 例未做特殊治疗。所有 44 例无症状患儿都未做治疗但都存活。给予有症状患儿环磷酰胺 5mg/kg 连续 5 天，肝脏放疗 4.5Gy 超过 3 天。6 名小于 2 个月的有症状的婴儿中 5 名死亡。5 年无病存活率为 86%，总的存活率为 92%。有危及生命的并发症（肝脾肿大、凝血异常、肾衰竭）[76,162]的 Ⅳ-S 期患儿需要早期干预。手术切除不改变预后情况。需要对 N-*myc* 拷贝大于 10 个、1 号染色体短臂有缺失或显示其他不良生物标志的肿瘤进行积极的化疗[76,162,203]。12 例 Ⅳ-S 期患儿中的 1 例观察到 N-*myc* 扩增，尽管为预后良好的分期，疾病还是恶化最后治疗失败。在 2003 年 Schleiermacher 等人[203]报道了 94 例法国 Ⅳ-S 期神经母细胞瘤的病例，总的存活率为 88%，建议给予那些需要治疗的病例更为强烈的化疗药物顺铂和依托泊苷。有些存活的 Ⅳ-S 期婴儿未进行原发肿瘤切除（有些原发肿瘤未确诊）。鉴于原发肿瘤的切除对于Ⅵ期肿瘤是有一定益处的，可行的话应

表 28-5　Ⅳ-S 期神经母细胞瘤的存活率

作者（年）	病例数	存活病例数（%）
D'Angio 等人（1971）[45]	16	14（88）
Breslow 等人（1971）[23]	19	18（95）
Nitschke 等人（1980）[165]	11	11（100）
Nickerson 等人（1985）[163]	35	31（89）
Blatt 等人（1987）[21]	11	8（73）
Wilson 等人（1991）[236]	18	9（50）
Suarez 等人（1991）[223]	34	28（75）
DeBernardi 等人（1992）[50]	76	63（83）
Grosfeld 等人（1993）[76]	21	17（81）
Hatchitanda 等人（1996）[88]	45	36（80）
Nickerson 等人（2000）[162]	80	74（92）
Schleiermacher 等人（2003）[203]	94	83（88）
总数	460	392（85）

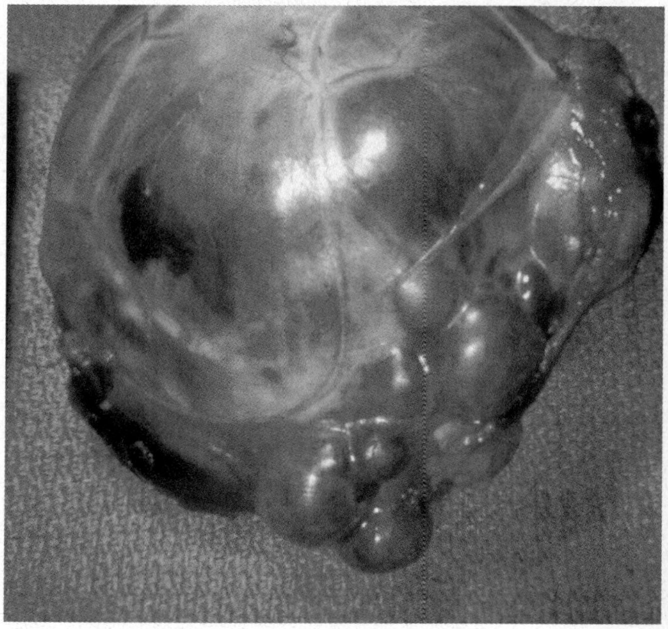

图 28-14　一位 5 个月大的患儿的肾上腺囊性神经母细胞瘤手术被完整切除的图片。患儿只进行了单独手术治疗，长期存活。

切除原发肿瘤，尤其是那些具有不良特性的高危组Ⅳ-S 期病例[76]。

囊性神经母细胞瘤

囊性神经母细胞瘤相对少见，通常在产前超声检查时被发现[227]。其特点是发生在肾上腺，几乎所有病例都在小婴儿期得到诊断（图 28-14）。极少有钙化，
3 只有 10%的病例尿 VMA 和 HVA 水平升高[187]。其有良好的特性和预后[103]。有证据表明这些病变有退化和自动复原的趋势。一些学者建议只进行观察，在出生后前几个月进行严密的超声监测以确定肿块的缩小，肿瘤块小预示肿瘤的退化。那些肿瘤未见退化或体积增大的需要手术切除，如果有手术指征，手术为唯一推荐的方案。CCG 制定了一个前瞻性研究只对这些囊性神经母细胞瘤进行观察。这个研究使用了严格的肿瘤的体积标准（实体的小于 16ml 或囊性的小于 65ml），把新生儿囊性神经母细胞瘤可能是大的肿瘤但有极好的预后这个因素也考虑进去了。

多病灶和双侧神经母细胞瘤

双侧神经母细胞瘤相对不常见，多发生在有家族病例的小婴儿中，他们 16 号染色体短臂 12～13 区的易感位点有改变[145]。在过去，治疗包括单独观察；单侧切除并观察或摘除第二个（小的）病变；双侧肾上腺切除和激素支持。我治疗过 3 例儿童双侧神经母细胞瘤的病例（1 例不是同一时间发生的）。行双侧肾上腺切除术，对所有患儿进行激素支持患儿长期存活。有些双侧肿瘤会自行消退，当一侧持续存在或增大时需要手术干预。预后良好，绝大多数儿童存活。偶然情况下这些婴儿存在其他部位多灶性病变。对这些良好生物标志的病例行肿瘤摘除术以保存肾上腺功能。Hiyama 等人[98]报道了 106 例中的 8 例多病灶神经母细胞瘤（7.5%）。8 例中 7 例为组织良好型，所有病例都表达 Trk-A1 mRNA 和 Ha-ras p21 蛋白。无一例出现 N-*myc* 扩增和端粒酶水平升高。4 例为近三倍体 DNA 流动细胞计数，所有 8 例增殖指数都小于 25%（S 期细胞的百分比）。对 4 例实施了分阶段进行的手术切除。5 例为双侧神经母细胞瘤对其进行了肿瘤摘除术。所有存活病例都无肿瘤复发，且无一需要类固醇替代。作者回顾了 53 例多发病灶的病例指出 18 例有家族性神经母细胞瘤的病史，25 例为偶然发现的病例。因为患儿具有良好的生物特性所以预后极佳，Hiyama 小组建议运用微创技术进行手术切除[98]。

化疗

尽管多药化疗显著提高了许多肿瘤的生存率（如肾母细胞瘤），但化疗对婴儿和儿童生物学和遗传学特性良好的可切除的局限性神经母细胞瘤的疗效并没有这样显著。对Ⅰ期和大多数Ⅱ期患儿，单纯手术切除是必须的[61,74,83]。具有较差生物学和遗传学特性预后因素的Ⅱ期患儿危险性高，需要多药物强化疗，包括顺铂、阿霉素、环磷酰胺和依托泊苷。对于晚期疾病（Ⅲ期和Ⅳ期），从 1970 年到 1980 年早期主要的治疗药物包括环磷酰胺、长春新碱和达卡巴嗪[61,64,67]。如治疗失败加阿霉素和 VM-26。

尽管这些化疗方案不能有效提高Ⅳ期患儿的治愈率，但这些治疗减小了原发肿瘤的体积，清除了骨髓中的肿瘤细胞，偶尔和恶性神经母细胞瘤转化为良性节细胞瘤的组织学成熟有关[67,77]。不幸的是，Ⅳ期患儿中仅 40%对化疗敏感，30%部分敏感，30%不敏感[67]。当剖腹探查评估对患儿对化疗的反应情况时，许多被认为对化疗敏感的实际并未如术前判断的那样，肿瘤持续生长[75,78,218]。

许多研究证实化疗对转移疾病作用有限[67,165]。运用细胞动力学数据，Hayes 等人[98]证实，神经母细胞瘤中肿瘤细胞的增殖分数是非常小的。大部分非增殖的静息细胞对化疗耐药。随后进行了试验在一定的时间相继加入细胞周期特异性药物和非细胞周期特异性药物（环磷酰胺和阿霉素或顺铂加 VM-26 或阿霉素），结果提高了反应率[72,90]。由于这个结果产生了运用多药物更强烈更积极的治疗方案，包括环磷酰胺、阿霉素、顺铂、依托泊苷和 VM-26[165]。运用接近致命计量的苯丙氨酸芥子（美法仑）的骨髓清除法辅助于自体骨髓移植同样可以提高肿瘤的化疗反应[178]。联合运用美法仑、阿霉素、VM-26 以及低计量的全身放疗加上自体骨髓移植进行治疗，无病复发率为 40%排除因毒性而死亡的Ⅳ期 2 年存活率为 34%[44]。

综合上述发现，对Ⅳ期和晚期的Ⅲ期疾病的治疗变得更为积极。联合运用环磷酰胺、阿霉素、顺铂、VM-26或依托泊苷和长春新碱的更大剂量的强化化疗被采用[62,132,149]。附加手术和肿瘤床局部和全身照射残余肿瘤[84,151]。另一个可供选择的治疗方法是接受药物剂量逐渐上升持续输注的骨髓清除化疗，然后进行自体（纯化）骨髓移植，不需要全身放疗[151]。新的化疗药物，包括异环磷酰胺、卡铂和表柔比星已投入使用[233]。添加13顺式维甲酸，一种可引起肿瘤细胞分化和减少骨髓肿瘤细胞浸润的，生物反应调节剂显示
484 有效[151,184,233]。Reynolds等人[183,185]在高危患儿中进行的第三阶段随机试验发现，完成强放化疗（有或无自体骨髓移植）以后使用13顺式维甲酸进行高剂量脉搏治疗，可以显著提高无病存活率。在第一阶段研究中，细胞毒性的合成维甲酸4-HPR（fenretinide）能够对反式和顺式维甲酸耐药的神经母细胞瘤细胞株产生杀伤作用，当酰基鞘氨醇被用来降低毒性作用后能够更好的耐受。Fenretinide还显示出抗血管生成的特性[186]。

其他高强度的压缩的化疗方案包括运用大剂量的环磷酰胺、卡铂和依托泊苷，加上粒细胞集落刺激因子动员外周造血干细胞，增加中性粒细胞和血小板的再生。干细胞通过白细胞去除法采集以后重新回输。美斯纳用于避免大剂量环磷酰胺导致的出血性膀胱炎。大剂量化疗后，手术介入切除原发肿瘤和任何大的转移病灶。外周血干细胞回输用于骨髓清除术后骨髓功能的恢复。监测免疫球蛋白IgG水平并用γ球蛋白替代。预防性地运用磺胺甲异唑和氟康唑防止卡氏肺囊虫和真菌感染。

就骨髓移植而言，接受纯化的自体细胞的患儿比接受同种异体细胞的反应好，因为在后一组中毒性死亡率高且移植抗宿主疾病发生率也有所增加[148]。高危Ⅳ期患儿接受骨髓移植预后较好，尤其是具有N-*myc*癌基因扩增的[148,150,151]。这些新的探索性的化疗项目将年龄大于2岁的Ⅲ期患儿的存活率从36%提高到86%，Ⅳ期患儿（大于1岁）3岁时的存活率由11%提高到37%，6岁时提高到23%[148,149]。运用高强度免疫抑制疗法后EB病毒相关的淋巴增生性疾病发病风险高[176]。同种异体骨髓移植，尤其是运用清除T细胞的干细胞产物时，是一个风险因素。尽管自体骨髓移植后发生的风险低（3.5%），但在大剂量化疗后辅助使用选择性$CD34^+$外周干细胞支持时风险升高。淋巴增生性疾病平均发生在移植后3个月。所有淋巴增生性疾病患儿都在选出的$CD34^+$组。运用利妥昔单抗和更昔洛韦治疗。在许多中心，外周血干细胞移植替代自体骨髓移植成为主要选择。取血可以在门诊完成，痛苦不安可以更少，干细胞移植的并发症发生率低且毒性作用小。肿瘤细胞可以从样本中纯化出来。Kanold等人[114]报道，自体外周血$CD34^+$细胞体外扩增可为神经母细胞瘤患儿提供纯化作用，通过筛查酪氨酸羟化酶mRNA转录数目确诊。

放疗

总的来说，近年来放疗在神经母细胞瘤治疗中的作用变得越来越有限。当作为主要治疗手段时，通常：（1）当肿瘤不能完全切除或局部复发时用来控制局部疾病；（2）骨髓移植前减少肿瘤负荷；（3）用来缓解难治的晚期疾病或减轻转移灶的疼痛[53,81,113,143]。

外部射线放疗与生长期儿童的毒性作用相关，导致生长异常、骨畸形、内分泌缺陷、软组织发育不良改变、皮肤萎缩和最重要的照射野继发性恶性病变。降低放疗诱发的毒性作用的技术包括高分割照射剂量，它通常不降低预期的抗肿瘤疗效，还可以避免同时运用的化疗药物产生的辐射作用[133]。近距放射疗法和术中放疗可以更好的控制放射作用在靶组织上而与周围正常组织分开[80,138]。尽管可以取得早期局部控制，但Ⅳ期患儿术中放疗后3年存活率只有38%。一些患儿仍需要附加的外部射线放疗，放疗后有术后输尿管狭窄、肾动脉狭窄和神经系统疾病的报道出现[83]。Hass-Kogan等人[80]报道了使用术中放疗治疗23例高危神经母细胞瘤患儿的经验，指出该技术的疗效只限于原发肿瘤大部分切除的患儿[80]。所有肿瘤部分切除的患儿尽管接受放疗仍发生复发，最终死亡。支持该治疗有效的资料很少。术中放疗有时难以实施，尤其在有些机构中放射科没有相关的手术配套设施或手术室中没有放疗设备（包括直线加速器）。鉴于这些情况，手术切除后需在麻醉状况下转送治疗。

难治的晚期神经母细胞瘤患儿因广泛转移引起剧烈疼痛。Kang等人[113]运用低于骨髓清除剂量的I^{131}-MIBG靶向放疗缓解疾病症状。这种治疗可以稳定疾病，减轻疼痛或改善生活状态。31%的患儿对治疗有

反应。他们总结认为这种治疗对末期神经母细胞瘤有效。MIBG 靶向放疗也用来同骨髓清除化疗和质子放疗结合治疗复发的和难治的神经母细胞瘤。质子放疗
485 比常规放疗的射线定位更为准确。当质子放疗变得更为广泛应用时，它在需要放疗的神经母细胞瘤的患儿的治疗中会发挥更为重要的作用。

Deutsch 和 Tersak[53] 报道了运用放疗（300～1000cGy）姑息治疗有症状的骨转移的情况。最常见的治疗部位是颅骨、脊柱、髂骨和股骨。29%的患儿存活 1 年或更长（平均 1～52 个月）。只有 8%的患儿存活超过 3 年。

免疫疗法

20 世纪 70～80 年代，观察到的神经母细胞瘤的肿瘤消退提示这可能是一种不寻常的肿瘤宿主关系引起的免疫机制的作用[6,17,20,70]。可以观察到从神经母细胞瘤分离出的淋巴细胞抑制培养中成神经细胞的群落，而其他肿瘤细胞不存在这种现象[20]。进展期患儿血清中包含一种阻断抗体，它可以阻止淋巴细胞介导的细胞毒性反应和抑制淋巴细胞胚细胞样转变为植物血细胞凝集素[94,95]。神经母细胞瘤患儿的淋巴细胞也有降低的全身及原位自然杀伤活性[71]。在试验性研究中，术中电凝[245]和高频超声聚焦引起的高温诱导神经母细胞瘤小鼠的免疫反应。晚期神经母细胞瘤细胞的主要问题是组织相容性抗原 I 缺乏和逃避免疫识别。

尽管免疫治疗进展缓慢，当一种能够介导免疫活性和肿瘤消退的细胞因子重组白细胞介素-2 产生后改变了这种状况[192]。白细胞介素-2 由辅助性 T 淋巴细胞产生。T 淋巴细胞与抗原的相互作用激活淋巴样细胞表达白细胞介素-2 受体。白细胞介素-2 释放的刺激导致免疫细胞扩增和有效的免疫作用。新的分子生物技术发展到能够识别编码癌症抗原和它们的免疫性多肽的基因。可以产生针对癌症细胞表面抗原可能是一种潜在免疫治疗靶点的免疫细胞[192]。

Vertuani 等人[232]报道，类维生素 A 和 T 细胞免疫治疗是治疗神经母细胞瘤的有效组合。类维生素 A 作为组织相容性抗原 I 存在旁路的多步骤调节器并使神经母细胞瘤对细胞毒淋巴细胞敏感[183,185,232]。尝试单独运用被照射细胞转导的白细胞介素-2 或干扰素的肿瘤疫苗、I^{131}-MIBG 靶向疗法和 I^{131} 标记的抗神经节苷脂 GD-2 抗体疗法，或结合骨髓移植，然而，没有有效的数据证实这些治疗的有效性[148]。Raffaghello 等人[180]在神经母细胞瘤裸鼠中运用了抗 GD-2 抗体并指出，与对照组相比，依赖剂量的治疗提高长期生存率同时减少肿瘤的转移。Cheung 等人[39]提出，抗 GD-2 单克隆抗体的免疫治疗应用于轻度疾病，必须和大剂量化疗结合运用才有效。Kushner 等人[130]报道了对 7 例局部神经母细胞瘤单独手术治疗后广泛复发转移的治疗。如果疾病可以被评估的话，他们接受大剂量化疗、抗 GD-2 3F8 抗体和 I^{131} 标记的 3F8 靶向放疗，如有缓解，给予患儿 3F8、粒-巨噬细胞集落刺激因子和 13 反式维甲酸。7 例中 5 例保持缓解 4～8 年[130]。同一组研究人员报道，大剂量的环磷酰胺、伊立替康和拓扑替康化疗可以有效地缓解疾病并诱发一种免疫状态，有益于在顽固性神经母细胞瘤中运用抗体基础上的被动免疫法（运用 3F8 抗体）[131]。

树突状细胞是免疫疗法的潜在靶点。它们可以提高 CD40 激活的 B 淋巴细胞的生长和分化，直接影响自然杀伤细胞的功能，发挥抗原提呈者的作用[181]。Redlinger 等人[182]指出，在采用的免疫治疗中晚期神经母细胞瘤影响树突状细胞的分化和功能。在神经母细胞瘤中可以看到，神经节苷脂抑制树突状细胞的功能。白细胞介素-12 是一个炎性前细胞因子，可以提高 T 淋巴细胞和静息的自然杀伤细胞的细胞毒活性[182]。在神经母细胞瘤的鼠模型中，Shimizu 等人[214]证实，白细胞介素-12转导的树突状细胞疫苗（腺病毒载体表达的白细胞介素-12）导致完全和可持续的抗肿瘤反应。肿瘤退化与树突状细胞和有活力的 T 细胞的高浸润相关。

预后

许多年来，患儿的年龄和疾病诊断时的分期是决定儿童神经母细胞瘤预后的两个重要的独立因素。Evans 等人[62,63]和其他一些学者发现年龄小于 1 岁的患儿和 I 期、II 期、Ⅳ-S 期疾病的患儿预后明显比其他患儿好。年龄大于 1 岁的和那些晚期（III期、Ⅳ期）的患儿预后差[45,77,83,124,206]。Ⅳ期年龄大于 1 岁的和骨皮质转移的患儿预后最差[23,27,73,77,83]。

有些学者提出肿瘤的原发部位也可预测生存情况。与后腹膜肿瘤（脊柱旁或肾上腺）相比发生在颈

部、盆腔和纵隔的预后较好。然而，Breslow 和 McCann[23]和 Koop 和 Schnaufer[24]表示，这些病例预后的改善可以用年龄和分期来解释。尽管有争议，Filler[66]、Young[243]和 Adams 等人[4]报道，对于纵隔病变而言，部位是一个有益的预后因子。Haase 等人[83]指出，不管其他一些因素盆腔肿瘤也同样如此。

有些早期关于神经母细胞瘤的报告提出越成熟越
486 分化的肿瘤预后越好[142]。其他学者指出成熟的组织表现但为未分化的成神经细胞预后同样不佳[124]。在存在转移病灶的患儿中，更多的成熟成分的存在改善预后并与存活率提高相关[66,77,218]。Shimada 等人[211]随后将神经母细胞瘤的组织病理学分为良好型和不良型，前者以基质丰富为特征，后者以基质少为特征。Shimada 分型同样是年龄相关的。Shimada 的组织分型对预后的影响被证实非常重要，特别是当与其他一些预后生物因素相关时，尤其是 N-*myc* 癌基因的扩增和 1 号染色体短臂（1p36）杂合子的丢失[212]。目前 INPC（接受和修改了 Shimada 分型）进一步将良好型和不良型病理分成亚型，是更为有效的独立的预后预测因子[104,173,208,212,213]。约 30%的神经母细胞瘤病例中出现 N-*myc* 基因的扩增，它在调节神经母细胞瘤恶性表型中起重要作用[27,148,157]。N-*myc* 的预后价值独立于年龄和分期。N-*myc* 与治疗不敏感、疾病迅速进展和预后差相关。虽然在实验室研究中成功运用神经生长因子、肾上腺素能增效剂、罂粟碱、前列腺素、外源性环单磷酸腺苷和高温刺激了肿瘤的成熟，但证明其有效的临床证据极少[36,73,97,137,234]。运用类维生素 A 促进分化重新引起关注，在临床试验已经成功地延长了晚期疾病的存活时间[151]。在高危神经母细胞瘤病例治疗中骨髓移植或外周干细胞移植后添加维甲酸已成为一个金标准[27]。

Nakagawara 等人[157,158]报道，婴儿神经母细胞瘤中亲神经的神经生长因子受体原癌基因 Trk-A 高水平表达预后良好。Trk-A 受体由神经生长因子激活，在肿瘤的自发消退和分化中起重要作用。Trk-A 与小年龄患儿、分期低疾病和无 N-*myc* 的表达相关[157,158]。Trk-A 同样可以下调神经母细胞瘤肿瘤细胞株中血管生成因子的表达和微血管的数目。多变量分析显示 N-*myc* 是一个更重要的独立预后因子。相反，Trk-B 另一个亲神经受体通常和 N-*myc* 扩增相关，由于它的配体 BDNF 为肿瘤细胞提供存活或生长的优势[159]。Trk-B-BDNF旁路可以增加血管的生成、致瘤作用、细胞存活和耐药[27,100]。Trk-C（与 Trk-A 相似）存在于分期低无 N-*myc* 扩增的肿瘤[27]。Bcl-2 癌蛋白负责转播凋亡信号，在大多数神经母细胞瘤中表达。神经母细胞瘤中 Bcl-2 表达增高和抑制化疗引导的凋亡以及预后差相关[14,27,32,53]。天冬氨酸特异性半胱氨酸蛋白酶表达下降（负责实施凋亡信号的酶）也同预后差相关。相反，良好生物特性的神经母细胞瘤天冬氨酸特异性半胱氨酸蛋白酶表达的升高改善预后。CD44 高表达的肿瘤通常分化好，导致存活率提高。

婴儿不能切除的神经母细胞瘤中细胞 DNA 含量是对化疗敏感程度的预测因子。流式细胞学分析显示高倍体或三倍体预后好，然而二倍体肿瘤预后差。和 N-*myc* 相似，DNA 倍体具有独立于分期和年龄的预后价值，这两个因子（倍体和 N-*myc*）结合起来能够为婴儿肿瘤提供重要的补充预后信息[11,27]。DNA 流式细胞分析与化疗反应及预后密切相关。

出现眼球震颤和斜视眼阵挛（眼球跳舞综合征）的患儿的存活率约为 90%。这个综合征在原发纵隔肿瘤（大于 60%）、Ⅰ期、Ⅱ期病变和年龄小于 1 岁的婴儿中多见[9,207]。另外，这些肿瘤组织学表现成熟。然而，眼球跳舞综合征患儿如出现疾病进展和 N-*myc* 过度表达则预后差[99]。尽管运用肿瘤切除以及肾上腺皮质激素进行治疗，存活者的神经症状（包括学习和注意力的缺陷）可以持续多年[121,195,196]。

患儿出现因神经性肿瘤分泌血管活性多肽造成的低钾水样腹泻症状预后也较好[42,58,127]。在这些病例中血清血管活性多肽可作为肿瘤标志，肿瘤通常不分泌儿茶酚胺。这些患儿的肿瘤通常更为成熟分化良好（如节细胞神经母细胞瘤）。在某些良性节细胞瘤病变中也可发现血管活性多肽，这再次提示这些病变具有良性特性。在分期低的病变和组织良好型无 N-*myc* 扩增的患儿，肿瘤组织中生长抑素受体的表达多见。这些结果提示生长抑素受体表达是一个好的预后因子[154,179]。

晚期神经母细胞瘤的儿童通常表现出蛋白质热量不足的营养不良，这与对不同皮肤抗原测试无反应性的免疫失活相关[188,189]。Rickard 等人[189]证实，Ⅳ期神经母细胞瘤诊断时存在营养不良的患儿与疾病程度相同营养状况好的患儿比较治疗延长而且预后明显要差。这些观察表明诊断时营养状况的评估是分期的重要组成部分[188]。另外，Van Eys[231]和 Rickard等人[188,189]发现，联合癌症治疗后出现明显的营养耗竭，全肠道

外静脉营养可以恢复和保持患儿在强化肿瘤治疗时的
487 营养状况。在最近研究中，Sala 等人[197]报道了晚期神经母细胞瘤儿童中 50%出现营养不良。他们强调了保持营养的重要性以及营养状态可影响疾病的过程和存活。加拿大多伦多的一项研究发现，原先为了降低神经管缺损发生率强制性地在面粉中补充叶酸，结果在安大略省神经母细胞瘤发生率降低了 60%[69]。

先前，Laug 等人[136]证实，Ⅳ期患儿尿HVA/VMA比值升高预后明显差。大量 HVA 的产生预示原始的不成熟的肿瘤具有更多的潜在恶性。Hann 等人[87]报道，63%的Ⅳ期患儿血清铁蛋白水平升高，预示预后差，尤其是在大于 2 岁的女孩中。有些研究显示神经性肿瘤血清神经特异性烯醇化酶水平升高[167,228]。Zeltzer 等[244]证实，转移病灶患儿中 96%血清神经特异性烯醇化酶升高且高血清水平与预后差相关，尤其是婴儿。局部神经母细胞瘤血清乳酸脱氢酶水平升高与预后不良相关[216]。多耐药基因（*MDR*-1）对神经母细胞瘤的预后作用存在争议[16,166]。然而高水平的 MDR 相关的蛋白基因（位于 16 号染色体）与不良预后相关。这个作用独立于分期、N-*myc* 和 Trk-A 状态[166]。尽管这些早期观察非常有趣且显示了这个神秘的肿瘤的生物特性，但目前年龄、INSS 分期、N-*myc* 状态、1 号染色体短臂 36 区杂合子丢失、不平衡的 17 号染色体长臂获得和 INPC 被认为是神经母细胞瘤最关键的预后因子。目前低危病例存活率大于 90%，中危病例 70%到 75%，高危病例 25%到 30%。3 年时总的存活率为 50%[27]。

总结及未来展望

这个儿童常见的恶性肿瘤因其多变的肿瘤特性至今仍然深不可测。原始神经母性肿瘤按三种可能途径中的一种发展：自发消退（凋亡）、分化成熟为良性的节神经瘤或更常见的肿瘤增殖并快速恶化。胎儿超声和婴儿筛查清楚地证实有些肿瘤自动消退。年龄相关的组织病理学研究阐明有些肿瘤（组织良好型）分化并成熟，其他（不良型）为未分化的肿瘤，对化疗反应差、疾病进展快且预后差。

对重要生物（和遗传）特性的认识可将肿瘤分成危险组（低、中间和高）以确定治疗方案。以危险分组为基准的治疗可以根据年龄、INSS 分期、INPC 组织学以及影响每个肿瘤行为的生物、遗传特性进行个体化治疗[27,94,213]。这样在只需要单独手术治疗的低危组肿瘤患儿中（偶尔在高度选择的患儿中只进行观察）避免了不必要的和潜在危害的治疗。可以让内科医生为最高危组的儿童制定最积极的治疗方案并监测预后。目前，低危患儿预后最好：婴儿年龄小于 1 岁、局部肿瘤为良好 INPC 组织学且能够完整切除（Ⅰ期和Ⅱ期）以及低危的生物和遗传因子、婴儿的Ⅳ-S期。产前超声发现的囊性神经母细胞瘤具有良好的预后。对于Ⅳ-S 期病变，那些囊性、多灶性或双侧肿瘤和具有良好的生物特性的病变而言，进行单独观察是合理的，生后第 1 年严密的超声监测非常重要以确保肿瘤在缩小和退化。肿瘤体积增大是手术介入的指征。中危病例包括无不良生物危险因素的Ⅲ期病例（按照 INSS）和年龄小于 1 岁无生物危险因素的Ⅳ期病例。需要特别关注问题包括：（1）婴儿年龄大于 1 岁；（2）高危患儿包括Ⅱ期年龄大于 1 岁具有 N-*myc* 高度表达，组织不良型的Ⅱ期患儿以及那些有生物及遗传不良预后因素的晚期病变（Ⅲ期、Ⅳ期）；（3）预防和治疗多种积极治疗的并发症。并发症包括常规和全身放疗损伤、免疫抑制、心脏和肾脏毒性、脊柱侧弯、生长和发育的副作用、性成熟延迟、学习障碍和继发性肿瘤的发生，包括肾肿瘤[27,84,194]。

需要更好地了解影响肿瘤消退分化和肿瘤宿主免疫相互作用的因素。在高危儿童中，检测其他肿瘤标志物并把有效对抗肿瘤的单克隆抗体作为目标，发展改进清除骨髓中肿瘤细胞的技术，采用更新更有效化疗方案（有或无全身放疗），回输自体纯化外周血干细胞，运用生长因子（粒细胞集落刺激因子）和其他生物肿瘤调节剂（反式维甲酸）防止感染以及促进消退和分化，可能会控制疾病的进展和改善高度恶性肿瘤的预后。尽管运用高强度治疗改善部分患儿的预
后，但晚期疾病的预后仍然很差，存活小于 50%。今 488
后将毫无疑问改进治疗方案运用毒性作用更小的生物学疗法（凋亡前靶向、抗血管生成和免疫疗法）以改善晚期神经母细胞瘤的预后以及消除目前高强度但相对无效的治疗相关的毒性作用。发生在神经母细胞瘤的遗传变化的明了能够更精确分期系统预测预后和进一步制定选择特异性的治疗方案，这可能包括靶向的基因蛋白质和负责肿瘤恶性进化的信号旁路[27]。

（徐　敏译　王　珊校）

参考文献

1. Abrams HL, Siegelman SS, Adams DF, et al: Computed tomography versus ultrasound of the adrenal gland: A prospective study. Radiology 1982;143:121-128.
2. Abramson SJ, Berdon WE, Ruzal-Shapiro C, et al: Cervical neuroblastoma in eleven infants—a tumor with favorable prognosis: Clinical and radiologic (US, CTR, MRI) findings. Pediatr Radiol 1993;23:253-257.
3. Acharya S, Jayabose S, Kogan S, et al: Prenatally diagnosed neuroblastoma. Cancer 1997;80:304-310.
4. Adams GA, Shochat SJ, Smith EI et al: Thoracic neuroblastoma: A pediatric oncology group study. J Pediatr Surg 1993;28:372-377.
5. Adkins ES, Sawin R, Gerbing RB, et al: Efficacy of complete resection for high risk neuroblastoma: A Children's Cancer Group study. J Pediatr Surg 2004;39:931-936.
6. Akeson R, Seeger RC: Interspecies neural membrane antigens on cultured human and murine neuroblastoma cells. J Immunol 1977;118:1995-2003.
7. Allen RW Jr, Ogden B, Bentley FL, Jung AL: Fetal hydantoin syndrome: Neuroblastoma and hemorrhagic disease in a neonate. JAMA 1980;44:1464-1465.
8. Al-Rashid RA, Cress C: Hypercalcemia associated with neuroblastoma. Am J Dis Child 1979;133:838-841.
9. Altman A, Baehner RL: Favorable prognosis for survival in children with coincident opsomyoclonus and neuroblastoma. Cancer 1976;37:846-852.
10. Ambros IM, Attarbashi A, Rumpler S, et al: Neuroblastoma cells provoke Schwann cell proliferation in vitro. Med Pediatr Oncol 2001;36:163-168.
11. Ambros IM, Zellner A, Roald B, et al: Role of ploidy, chromosome 1p, and Schwann cells in the maturation of neuroblastoma. N Engl J Med 1996;334:1505-1511.
12. Anders D, Kindermann G, Pfeifer U: Metastasizing fetal neuroblastoma with involvement of the placenta simulating fetal erythroblastosis. J Pediatr 1973;82:50-53.
13. Beckwith JB, Perrin EV: In-situ neuroblastoma: A contribution to the natural history of neural crest tumors. Am J Pathol 1963;43:1089-1104.
14. Beirle EA, Strande LK, Chen MK: VEGF upregulates bcl-2 expression and is associated with decreased apoptosis in neuroblastoma cells. J Pediatr Surg 2002;7:467-471.
15. Beppu K, Jaboine J, Merchant MS, et al: Effect of imatinib mesylate on neuroblastoma tumorigenesis and VEGF expression. J Natl Cancer Inst 2004;96:46-55.
16. Bernardi J, et al: Prognostic value of MDR1 gene expression in neuroblastoma: Results of a multivariate analysis. Prog Clin Biol Res 1994;385:111.
17. Bernstein I , Hellstrom KE, Wright PW, et al: Immunity to tumor antigens: Potential implications in human neuroblastoma. J Natl Cancer Inst 1976;57:711-715.
18. Berthold F, Kassenböhmer R, Zieschang J: Multivariate evaluation of prognostic factors in localized neuroblastoma. Am J Hematol Oncol 1994;16:107-115.
19. Bessho F, Hashizume K, Nakajo T, et al: Mass screening in Japan increased the detection of infants with neuroblastoma without a decrease in cases in older children. J Pediatr 1991;119:237-241.
20. Bill AH: Immune aspects of neuroblastoma: Current information. Am J Surg 1971;122:142-147.
21. Blatt JB, Deutsch M, Wollman MR: Results of therapy in stage IV-S neuroblastoma with massive hepatomegaly. Int J Radiat Oncol Biol Phys 1987;13:1467-1471.
22. Blatt JB, Fitz G, Mirro J: Recognition of central nervous system metastases in children with metastatic primary extracranial neuroblastoma. Pediatr Hematol Oncol 1997;14:233-241.
23. Breslow N, McCann B: Statistical estimation of prognosis for children with neuroblastoma. Cancer Res 1971; 31:1098-1103.
24. Brock CE, Ricketts RR: Hemoperitoneum from spontaneous rupture of neonatal neuroblastoma. Am J Dis Child 1982;136:370-371.
25. Brodeur GM: Molecular basis for heterogeneity in human neuroblastoma. Eur J Cancer 1995;31A:505-510.
26. Brodeur GM: Schwann cells as antineuroblastoma agents. N Engl J Med 1996;334:1537-1539.
27. Brodeur GM: Neuroblastoma: Biological insights into a clinical enigma. Nat Rev Cancer 2003;3:203-216.
28. Brodeur GM, Pritchard J, Berthold F, et al: Revision of the international criteria for neuroblastoma diagnosis staging and response to treatment. J Clin Oncol 1993;11:1466-1477.
29. Brodeur GM, Seeger RC, Barrett A, et al: International criteria for diagnosis of staging and response to treatment in patients with neuroblastoma. J Clin Oncol 1988;6: 1874-1881.
30. Caron H, van Sluis B, de Kraker J, et al: Allelic loss of chromosome 1p as a predictor of unfavorable outcome in patients with neuroblastoma. N Engl J Med 1996;334: 225-230.
31. Castel V, Bedal MD, Bezanilla JL, et al: Treatment of stage III neuroblastoma with emphasis on intensive induction chemotherapy: A report from the Neuroblastoma Group of the Spanish Society of Pediatric Oncology. Med Pediatr Oncol 1995;34:29-35.
32. Castel VP, Heidelberger KP, Bromberg J, et al: Expression of the apoptosis-suppressing protein bcl-2 in neuroblastoma is associated with unfavorable histology and N-myc amplification. Am J Pathol 1993;143:1543-1550.
33. Castleberry RP, Pritchard J, Ambros P, et al: The International Neuroblastoma Risk Groups (INRG): A preliminary report. Eur J Cancer 1997;33:2113-2116.
34. Castleberry RP, Shuster JJ, Smith EI: Pediatric Oncology Group experience with the International Staging System criteria for neuroblastoma. J Clin Oncol 1994;12: 2378-2381.
35. Chan HS, Haddad G, Thorner PS, et al: P-glycoprotein expression as a predictor of the outcome of therapy for neuroblastoma. N Engl J Med 1991;325:1608-1614.
36. Chang THT, Prasad KN: Differentiation of mouse neuroblastoma cells in-vitro and in-vivo, induced by cyclic adenosine monophosphate (cAMP). J Pediatr Surg 1976; 11:847-858.
37. Chatten J, Voorhees ML: Familial neuroblastoma: Report of a kindred with multiple disorders including neuroblastoma in four siblings. N Engl J Med 1967;277: 1230-1236.
38. Cheung NK: Monclonal antibody-based therapy for neuroblastoma. Curr Oncol Rep 2000;2:547-551.
39. Cheung NK, Kushner BH, Yeh SD, et al: 3F8 Monoclonal antibody treatment of patients with stage 4 neuroblastoma: A phase II study. Int J Oncol 1998;12:1299-1306.
40. Chlenski A, Liu S, Cohn SL: The regulation of angiogenesis in a neuroblastoma. Cancer Lett 2003;197:47-52.
41. Coldman AJ, Fryer CJ, Elwood JM, Sonley MJ: Neuroblastoma: Influence of age at diagnosis, stage, site and sex on prognosis. Cancer 1980;46:1896-1901.
42. Cooney DR, Voorhees ML, Fisher JE, et al: Vasoactive intes-

tinal polypeptide producing neuroblastoma. J Pediatr Surg 1982;17:821-825.
43. Cushing H, Wolbach SB: Transformation of malignant paravertebral sympathicoblastoma into benign ganglioneuroma. Am J Pathol 1927;3:203.
44. D'Angio GJ, Evans AE: Experience with cyclic low-dose total body irradiation for metastatic neuroblastoma [abstract]. Proc Am Soc Clin Oncol 1982;23:52.
45. D'Angio GJ, Evans AE, Koop CE: Special pattern of widespread neuroblastoma with a favorable prognosis. Lancet 1971;1:1046-1049.
46. Dastur DK: Cerebral ganglioglioneuroblastoma: An unusual brain tumor of the neuron series. J Neurol Neurosurg Psychiatry 1982;45:139-142.
47. Davidoff AM, Kandel JJ: Antiangiogenic therapy for the treatment of pediatric solid malignancies. Semin Pediatr Surg 2004;13:53-60.
48. Davidoff AM, Leary MA, Ng CT, et al: Retroviral vector producer cell mediated angiogenesis inhibition restricts neuroblastoma growth in-vivo. Med Pediatr Oncol 2000;35:638-640.
49. Davidoff AM, Leary MA, Ng CY, et al: Gene therapy mediated expression by tumor cells of the angiogenesis inhibitor Flk-1 results in inhibition of neuroblastoma growth in-vivo. J Pediatr Surg 2001;36:30-36.
50. DeBernardi B, Pianca C, Boni L, et al: Disseminated neuroblastoma (stage IV and IV-S) in the first year of life: Outcome related to age and stage. Italian Cooperative Group on Neuroblastoma. Cancer 1992;70:1625-1633.
51. DeBernardi B, Conte M, Mancini A, et al: Localized resectable neuroblastoma: Results of the 2nd study of the Italian Cooperative Group for Neuroblastoma. J Clin Oncol 1995;13:884-893.
52. de Lagausie P, Berribi D, Michon J, et al: Laparoscopic adrenal surgery for neuroblastoma in children. J Urol 2003;170:932-935.
53. Deutsch M, Tersak JM: Radiotherapy for symptomatic metastases to bone in children. Am J Clin Oncol 2004;27:128-131.
54. Dobrovoljski G, Kerbl R, Strobl C, et al: False-positive results in neuroblastoma screening: The parents' view. J Pediatr Hematol Oncol 2003;25:14-18.
55. Dole M, Nunez G, Merchant AK, et al: Bcl-2 inhibits chemotherapy induced apoptosis in neuroblastoma. Cancer Res 1994;54:3253-3259.
56. Dreyfus M, Neuhart D, Baldauf JJ, et al: Prenatal diagnosis of cystic neuroblastoma. Fetal Diagn Ther 1994;9:269-272.
57. Eggert A, Ikegaki N, Kwiatkowski J, et al: High-level expression of angiogenic factors is associated with advanced tumor stage in human neuroblastomas. Clin Cancer Res 2000;6:1900-1908.
58. El-Shafie M, Samuel D, Klippel CH, et al: Intractable diarrhea in children with VIP-secreting ganglioneuroblastoma. J Pediatr Surg 1983;18:34-36.
59. Emery LG, Shields M, Shah MR, et al: Neuroblastoma associated with Beckwith-Wiedemann syndrome. Cancer 1983;52:176-179.
60. Entz-Werle N, Marcellin L, Becmeur F, et al: The urinary bladder: An extremely rare location of pediatric neuroblastoma. J Pediatr Surg 2003;38:E10-E12.
61. Evans AE, Albo V, D'Angio GJ, et al: Cyclophosphamide treatment of patients with localized and regional neuroblastoma: A randomized study. Cancer 1976;38:655-660.
62. Evans AE, D'Angio GJ, Randolph JG: A proposed staging for children with neuroblastoma. Cancer 1971;27:374-378.
63. Evans AE, Gerson J, Schnaufer L: Spontaneous regression of neuroblastoma. Natl Cancer Inst Monogr 1976;44:49-54.
64. Evans AE, Heyn RN, Newton WA Jr, Leikin SL: Viscristine sulfate and cyclophosphamide for children with metastatic neuroblastoma. JAMA 1969;207:1325-1327.
65. Fenart D, Deville A, Donzeau M, Bruneton JN: Neuroblastome retroperitoneal diagnostique in utero. J Radiol 1983;64:359-361.
66. Filler RM, Traggis DG, Jaffe N, Vawter GF: Favorable outlook for children with mediastinal neuroblastoma. J Pediatr Surg 1972;7:136-143.
67. Finklestein JZ, Klemperer, MA, Evans AE, et al: Multiagent chemotherapy for children with metastatic neuroblastoma: A report from the Children's Cancer Study Group. Med Pediatr Oncol 1979;6:179-188.
68. Fleitz JM, Wooten-Gorges SC, Wyatt-Ashmead J, et al: Renal cell carcinoma in long-term survivors of advanced stage neuroblastoma early in childhood. Pediatr Radiol 2003;33:540-545.
69. French AE, Grant R, Weitzman S, et al: Folic acid food fortification is associated with a decline in neuroblastoma. Clin Pharmacol 2003;74:288-294.
70. Gerson JM, Chatten J, Eisman S: Familial neuroblastoma—a follow-up. N Engl J Med 1974;190:487.
71. Gerson JM, Herberman RB: Systemic and in-situ natural killer activity in patients with neuroblastoma. In Evans AE (ed): Advances in Neuroblastoma Research. New York, Raven Press, 1980.
72. Green AA, Hayes FA, Hustu HO: Sequential cyclophosphamide and doxorubicin for induction and complete remission in children with disseminated neuroblastoma. Cancer 1981;48:2310-2317.
73. Grosfeld JL: Neuroblastoma: A 1990 overview. Pediatr Surg Int 1991;6:9-13.
74. Grosfeld JL: Risk based management of childhood solid tumors. J Am Coll Surg 1999;189:407-425.
75. Grosfeld JL, Ballantine TVN, Baehner RL: Experience with "second-look" operations in pediatric solid tumors. J Pediatr Surg 1978;13:275-280.
76. Grosfeld JL, Rescorla FJ, West KW, Goldman J: Neuroblastoma in the first year of life: Clinical and biologic factors influencing outcome. Semin Pediatr Surg 1993;2:37-46.
77. Grosfeld JL, Schatzlein M, Ballantine TVN, et al: Metastatic neuroblastoma: Factors influencing survival. J Pediatr Surg 1978;13:59-65.
78. Grosfeld JL, West KW, Weber TR: The role of second-look procedures in the management of retroperitoneal tumors in children. J Pediatr Hematol Oncol 1984;6:441-447.
79. Haas D, Ablin AR, Miller C, et al: Complete pathologic maturation and regression of stage IV-S neuroblastoma without treatment. Cancer 1988;62:818-825.
80. Haas-Kogan DA, Fisch BM, Wara WB, et al: Introperative radiation therapy for high risk neuroblastoma. Int J Radiat Oncol Biol Phys 2000;47:985-992.
81. Haas-Kogan DA, Swift PS, Eslch M, et al: Impact of radiotherapy for high risk neuroblastoma: A Children's Cancer Group study. Int J Radiat Oncol Biol Phys 2003;56:28-39.
82. Haase GM: Head and neck neuroblastomas. Semin Pediatr Surg 1994;3:194-202.
83. Haase GM, LaQuaglia MP: Neuroblastoma. In Ziegler M, Azizkhan RG, Weber TR (eds): Operative Pediatric Surgery. New York, McGraw-Hill, 2003, pp 1181-1191.
84. Haase GM, O'Leary MC, Ramsay NK, et al: Aggressive surgery combined with intensive chemotherapy improves

survival in poor risk neuroblastoma. J Pediatr Surg 1991; 26:1119-1123.
85. Haase GM, Wong KY, deLorimier AA, et al: Improvement in survival after excision of the primary tumor in stage III neuroblastoma. J Pediatr Surg 1989;24:194-200.
86. Haddad M, Triglia JM, Helardot P, et al: Localized cervical neuroblastoma: Prevention of surgical complications. Int J Pediatr Otorhinolaryngol 2003;67:1361-1367.
87. Hann JL, et al: Serum ferritin levels as a guide to prognosis in stage IV neuroblastoma [abstract]. Proc Am Soc Clin Oncol 1983;24:72.
88. Hatchitanda Y, Hata J: Stage IV-S neuroblastoma: A clinical, histological and biological analysis. Hum Pathol 1996;27:1135-1138.
89. Hayashi Y, Kanmda N, Inaba T, et al: Cytogenetic findings and prognosis in neuroblastoma with emphasis on marker chromosome 1. Cancer 1989;63:125-132.
90. Hayes FA, Green AA, Casper J, et al: Clinical evaluation of sequentially scheduled cisplatin and VM-26 in neuroblastoma: Response and toxicity. Cancer 1981;48:1715-1718.
91. Hayes FA, Green AA, Hustu HO, Kumar ML: Surgicopathologic staging of neuroblastoma: Prognostic significance of regional lymph node metastases. J Pediatr 1983;102:59-62.
92. Hayes F, Green AA, Mauer AM, et al: Correlation of cell kinetics and clinical response to chemotherapy in disseminated neuroblastoma. Cancer Res 1977;37:3766-3770.
93. Heisel MA, Miller JH, Reid BS, Siegel SE: Radionuclide bone scan in neuroblastoma. Pediatrics 1983;71:206-209.
94. Hellstrom I, Hellstrom KE, Pierce GE, Bill AH: Demonstration of cell bound humoral immunity against neuroblastoma cells. Proc Natl Acad Sci U S A 1968;60: 1231-1238.
95. Hellstrom KE, Hellstrom I: Lymphocyte mediated cytotoxicity and blocking serum activity to tumor antigens. Adv Immunol 1974;18:209-217.
96. Helson L, Ghavimi F, Wu CJ, et al: Carcinoembryonic antigen in children with neuroblastoma. J Natl Cancer Inst 1976;57:725-726.
97. Helson L, Helson C, Peterson RF, Das SK: A rationale for the treatment of metastatic neuroblastoma. J Natl Cancer Inst 1976;57:727-729.
98. Hiyama E, Yokoyama T, Hiyama K et al: Multifocal neuroblastoma: Biologic behavior and surgical aspects. Cancer 2000;88:1955-1963.
99. Hiyama E, Yokoyama T, Ichikawa T, et al: Poor outcome in patients with advanced stage neuroblastoma and coincident opsomyoclonus syndrome. Cancer 1994;74: 1821-1826.
100. Ho R, Eggert A, Hishiki T, et al: Resistance to chemotherapy mediated by TrkB in neuroblastoma. Cancer Res 2002;62:6462-6466.
101. Ho TC, Estroff JA, Kozakewich H, et al: Prenatal detection of neuroblastoma: A ten year experience from the Dana-Farber Cancer Institute and Children's Hospital. Pediatrics 1993;92:358-364.
102. Holcomb GW: Minimally invasive surgery for solid tumors. Semin Surg Oncol 1999;7:184-192.
103. Holgersen LO, Subramanian S, Kirpekar M, et al: Spontaneous resolution of antenatally diagnosed adrenal masses. J Pediatr Surg 1996;31:153-155.
104. Ikeda H, Iehara T, Tsuchida Y, et al: Experience with the International Neuroblastoma Staging System and pathology classification. Br J Cancer 2002;86:1110-1116.
105. Ikeda H, Suzuki N, Takahashi A, et al: Surgical treatment of neuroblastomas in infants under 12 months of age. J Pediatr Surg 1998;33:1246-1250.
106. Ishimoto K, Kiyokawa H, Fujita H, et al: Problems of mass screening for neuroblastoma: Analysis of false negative cases. J Pediatr Surg 1990;25:398-401.
107. Iwanaka T, Arai M, Ito M, et al: Surgical treatment for abdominal neuroblastoma in the laparoscopic era. Surg Endosc 2001;15:751-754.
108. Iwanaka T, Arai M, Kawashima H, et al: Endosurgical procedures for pediatric solid tumors. Pediatr Surg Int 2004;20:39-42.
109. Jennings RW, LaQuaglia MP, Leong K, et al: Fetal neuroblastoma: Prenatal diagnosis and natural history. J Pediatr Surg 1993;28:1168-1174.
110. Jiang TH, Yang CP, Hung IJ, et al: Brain metastases in children with neuroblastoma—a single institution experience. Med Pediatr Oncol 2003;41:570-571.
111. Joshi VV, Cantor AB, Altschuler G, et al: Age-linked prognostic categorization based on a new histologic grading system of neuroblastoma. Cancer 1992;69:2183-2196.
112. Kaicker S, McCRudden KW, Beck L, et al: Thalidomide is anti-angiogenic in a xenograft model of neuroblastoma. Int J Oncol 2003;23:1651-1655.
113. Kang TI, Brophy P, Hickeson M, et al: Targeted radiotherapy with submyeloablative doses of I^{131}-MIBG is effective for disease palliation in highly refractory neuroblastoma. J Pediatr Hematol Oncol 2003;25:769-763.
114. Kanold J, Halle P, Tchirkov A, et al: Ex-vivo expansion of autologous PB CD34+ cells provide a purge effect in children with neuroblastoma. Bone Marrow Transplant 2003;32:485-488.
115. Kenney LB, Miller BA, Gloeker-Reis LA, et al: Increased incidence of cancer in infants in the United States 1980-1990. Cancer 1998;82:1396-1400.
116. Kiely EM: The surgical challenge of neuroblastoma. J Pediatr Surg 1994;29:128-133.
117. Kim ES, Soffer SZ, Huang J, et al: Distinct response of experimental neuroblastoma to combination antiangiogenic strategies. J Pediatr Surg 2002;37:518-522.
118. King D, Goodman J, Hawk T, et al: Dumbbell neuroblastoma in children. Arch Surg 1975;110:888-891.
119. Kinney H, Faix R, Brazy J: The fetal alcohol syndrome and neuroblastoma. J Pediatr 1980;66:130-132.
120. Kogner P, Barbani G, Dominici C, et al: Co-expression of messenger RNA for Trk protooncogene and low affinity nerve growth factor receptors in neuroblastoma with favorable prognosis. Cancer Res 1993;53:2044-2050.
121. Koh PS, Raffensperger J, Berry S, et al: Long-term outcome in children with opsoclonus myoclonus and ataxia and coincident neuroblastoma. J Pediatr 1994;125: 712-716.
122. Komuro H, Kaneko S, Kaneko M, et al: Expression of angiogenic factors and tumor progression in human neuroblastoma. J Cancer Res Clin Oncol 2001;127:739-743.
123. Komuro H, Makino S, Tahara K: Laparoscopic resection of an adrenal neuroblastoma detected by mass screening that grew in size during the observation period. Surg Endosc 2000;14:297.
124. Koop CE, Schnaufer L: The management of abdominal neuroblastoma. Cancer 1975;35:905-909.
125. Kouch K, Yoshida H, Matsunaga T, et al: Extirpation of mass screened adrenal neuroblastoma by retroperitoneoscopy. Surg Endosc 2003;17:1769-1772.
126. Kubota M, Yagi M, Kanada S, et al: Long-term follow up and status of patients with neuroblastoma after undergoing either aggressive surgery or chemotherapy: A single institutional study. J Pediatr Surg 2004;39:

1328-1332.

127. Kudo K, Kitajima S, Munakata H, Yagihashi S: WDHA syndrome caused by VIP-producing ganglioneuroblastoma. J Pediatr Surg 1982;17:426-428.
128. Kumar AM, Wrenn EL Jr, Fleming ID, et al: Preoperative therapy for unresectable malignant tumors in children. J Pediatr Surg 1975;10:657-670.
129. Kushner BH, Cheung NK, LaQuaglia MP, et al: Survival from locally invasive or widespread neuroblastoma without cytotoxic therapy. J Clin Oncol 1996;14:373-381.
130. Kushner BH, Kramer K, LaQuaglia MP, Cheung NK: Curability of recurrent disseminated disease after surgery alone for loco-regional neuroblastoma using intensive chemotherapy and anti-GD-2 immunotherapy. J Pediatr Hematol Oncol 2003;25:512-514.
131. Kushner BH, Kramer K, Modak S, Cheung NK: Campothecin analogs (irinotecan or topotecan) plus high dose cyclophosphamide as preparative regimens for antibody based immunotherapy in resistant neuroblastoma. Clin Cancer Res 2004;10:84-87.
132. Kushner BH, LaQuaglia MP, Bonilla MA, et al: Highly effective induction therapy for stage IV neuroblastomas in children over 1 year of age. J Clin Oncol 1994;12: 2607-2613.
133. Kushner BH, Wolden S, LaQuaglia MP, et al: Hyperfractionated low dose radiotherapy for high-risk neuroblastoma after intensive chemotherapy and surgery. J Clin Oncol 2001;19:2821-2828.
134. LaQuaglia MP, Kushner BH, Heller G, et al: Stage 4 neuroblastoma diagnosed at more than 1 year of age: Gross total resection and clinical outcome. J Pediatr Surg 1994;29:1162-1165.
135. LaQuaglia MP, Kushner BH, Su W, et al: The impact of gross total resection on local control and survival in high-risk neuroblastoma. J Pediatr Surg 2004;39: 412-417.
136. Laug WE, Siegel SE, Shaw KN, et al: Initial urinary catecholamine metabolite concentrations and prognosis in neuroblastoma. Pediatrics 1978;62:77-83.
137. Lazo J, Ruddon RW: Neurite extension and malignancy of neuroblastoma cells after treatment with PGE_1 and papaverine. J Natl Cancer Inst 1977;59:137-143.
138. Leavey PJ, Odom LF, Poole M, et al: Intraoperative radiation therapy in pediatric neuroblastoma. Med Pediatr Oncol 1997;28:424-428.
139. Lee EW, Applebaum H: Abdominal expansion as a bridging technique in stage IV-S neuroblastoma with massive hepatomegaly. J Pediatr Surg 1994;29:1470-1471.
140. Leone A, Seeger RC, Hong CM, et al: Evidence for nm23 RNA overexpression, DNA amplification and mutation in aggressive neuroblastoma. Oncogene 1993;8:855-865.
141. Luttikhuis ME, Powell JE, Rees SA, et al: Neuroblastoma with chromosome 11q loss and single copy MYCN comprise a biologically distinct group of tumours with adverse prognosis. Br J Cancer 2001;85:531-537.
142. Mäkinen J: Microscopic patterns as a guide to prognosis of neuroblastoma in childhood. Cancer 1972;29: 1637-1646.
143. Marcus KJ, Shamberger R, Litman H, et al: Primary tumor control in patients with stage 3/4 unfavorable neuroblastoma treated in tandem double stem cell transplants. Pediatr Hematol Oncol 2003;25:934-940.
144. Maris JM, Matthay KK: The molecular biology of neuroblastoma. J Clin Oncol 1999;17:2264-2279.
145. Maris JM, Weiss MJ, Mosse Y, et al: Evidence for a hereditary neuroblastoma predisposition locus at 16p12-13. Cancer Res 2002;62:6651-6658.
146. Martinez-Mora J, Castellvi A, Coroleu W, et al: Cystic adrenal neuroblastoma: Prenatal diagnosis by ultrasonography. Med Pediatr Oncol 1995;24:109-115.
147. Matsumura M, Tsunoda A, Nishi T, et al: Spontaneous regression of neuroblastoma detected by mass screening. Lancet 1991;338:447-448.
148. Matthay KK: Progress in the treatment of advanced stage neuroblastoma. Pediatric Neoplasms, Postgraduate Course, 82nd Clinical Congress, American College of Surgeons, San Francisco, Oct 1996.
149. Matthay KK, Perez C, Seegar RC, et al: Treatment and outcome for stage III neuroblastoma based on prospective biology staging: A Children's Cancer Group study. J Clin Oncol 1998;16:1256-1264.
150. Matthay KK, Seeger RC, Reynolds CP, et al: Allogeneic vs autologous purged bone marrow transplantation for neuroblastoma: A report from the Children's Cancer Group study. J Clin Oncol 1994;12:2382-2389.
151. Matthay KK, Villlablanca JG, Seegar RC, et al: Treatment of high risk neuroblastoma with intensive chemotherapy, radiotherapy, autologous bone marrow transplantation, and 13-cis-retinoic acid: A Children's Cancer Group study. N. Engl J Med 1999;341:1165-1173.
152. McKallip R, Li R, Ladisch S: Tumor gangliosides inhibit the tumor specific immune response. J Immunol 1999; 163:3718-3726.
153. Meitar D, Crawford SE, Rademaker AW, et al: Tumor angiogenesis correlates with metastatic disease, N-myc amplification and poor outcome in human neuroblastoma. J Clin Oncol 1996;14:405-414.
154. Moertel CL, Reubi JC, Scheithauer BS, et al: Expression of somatostatin receptors in childhood neuroblastoma. Am J Clin Pathol 1994;102:752-756.
155. Molofsky WJ, Chutorian AM: Non-surgical treatment of intraspinal neuroblastoma. Neurology 1981;31:1170-1173.
156. Moss TJ, Reynolds CP, Sather HN, et al: Prognostic value of immunocytologic detection of bone marrow metastases in neuroblastoma. N Engl J Med 1991;324: 219-226.
157. Nakagawara A, Arima M, Azar CG, et al: Inverse relationship between Trk expression and N-myc amplification in human neuroblastoma. Cancer Res 1992;52:1364-1368.
158. Nakagawara A, Arima-Nakagawara M, Scavarda MG, et al: Association between high levels of expression of the Trk gene and favorable outcome in human neuroblastoma. N Engl J Med 1993;328:847-854.
159. Nakagawara A, Azar CG, Scavardo NJ, et al: Expression and function of Trk-B and BDNF in human neuroblastomas. Mol Cell Biol 1994;14:759-767.
160. Nakajima K, Fukuzawa M, Fukui Y, et al: Laparoscopic resection of mass screened adrenal neuroblastoma in an 8 month old infant. Surg Laparosc Endosc 1997;7: 498-500.
161. Nemecek ER, Sawin RW, Park J: Treatment of neuroblastoma in patients with neurocristopathy syndromes. J Pediatr Hematol Oncol 2003;25:159-162.
162. Nickerson HJ, Matthay KK, Seegar RC, et al: Favorable biology and outcome of stage IV-S neuroblastoma with supportive care or minimal therapy: A Children's Cancer Group study. J Clin Oncol 2000;18:477-486.
163. Nickerson HJ, Nesbit ME, Grosfeld JL, et al: Comparison of stage IV and IV-S neuroblastoma in the first year of life. Med Pediatr Oncol 1985;13:261-268.
164. Ninane J, Pritchard J, Morris Jones PH, et al: Stage II neuroblastoma: Adverse prognostic significance of lymph

node involvement. Arch Dis Child 1982;57:438-442.
165. Nitschke R, Cangir A, Crist W, Berry DH: Intensive chemotherapy for metastatic neuroblastoma: A Southwest Oncology Group study. Med Pediatr Oncol 1980;8: 281-288.
166. Norris MD, Bordow SD, Marshall GM, et al: Expression of the gene for multidrug resistance associated protein and outcome in patients with neuroblastoma. N Engl J Med 1996;334:231-238.
167. Odelstad L, Pahlman S, Lackgren G, et al: Neuron specific enolase: A marker for differential diagnosis of neuroblastoma and Wilms' tumor. J Pediatr Surg 1982;17: 381-385.
168. Oue T, Fukuzawa M, Kusafuka T, et al: In situ detection of DNA fragmentation and expression of bcl-2 in human neuroblastoma: Relation to apoptosis and spontaneous regression. J Pediatr Surg 1996;31:251-257.
169. Oue T, Inoue M, Yoneda A, et al: Profile of neuroblastoma detected by mass screening, resected after observation without treatment: Results of the Wait and See pilot study. J Pediatr Surg 2005;40:359-363.
170. Paul SR, Tarbell NJ, Korf B, et al: Stage IV neuroblastoma in infants: Long-term survival. Cancer 1991;67:1493-1497.
171. Pegelow CH, Ebbin AJ, Powars D, Towner JW: Familial neuroblastoma. J Pediatr 1975;87:763-765.
172. Perkins DG, Kopp CM, Haust MD: Placental infiltration in congenital neuroblastoma. Histopathology 1980;4: 383-389.
173. Peuchmaur M, d'Amore ES, Joshi VV, et al: Revision of the International Neuroblastoma Pathology Classification: Confirmation of favorable and unfavorable prognostic subsets in ganglioneuroblastoma, nodular. Cancer 2003; 98:2274-2281.
174. Plantaz D, Rubie H, Michon J, et al: The treatment of neuroblastoma with intraspinal extension with chemotherapy followed by surgical removal of residual disease: A prospective study of 42 patients—results of the NBL 90 study of the French Society of Pediatric Oncology. Cancer 1996;3:521-525.
175. Ponzoni M, Bocca P, Chiesa V, et al: Differential effects of N-4-hydroxyphenylretinamide and retinoic acid on neuroblastoma cells: Apoptosis and differentiation. Cancer Res 1995;55:853-861.
176. Powell JL, Buniz NJ, Callahan C, et al: An unexpectedly high incidence of Epstein-Barr virus lymphoproliferative disease after CD34+ selected autologous peripheral blood stem cell transplant in neuroblastoma. Bone Marrow Transplant 2004;33:651-657.
177. Prasad KN, Mandal B, Kumar S: Demonstration of cholinergic cells in human neuroblastoma and ganglioneuroma. J Pediatr 1973;82:677-679.
178. Pritchard J, McElwain TJ, Graham-Pole J: High dose melphalan with autologous bone marrow for treatment of advanced neuroblastoma. Br J Cancer 1982;45:86-94.
179. Qualman SJ, O'Diorisio MS, Fleshman DJ, et al: Neuroblastoma: Correlation of neuropeptide expression in tumor tissue with other prognostic factors. Cancer 1992; 70:2005-2012.
180. Raffaghello L, Marimpietri D, Pagnan G, et al: Anti-GD2 monoclonal antibody immunotherapy: A promising strategy in the prevention of neuroblastoma relapse. Cancer Lett 2003;197:205-209.
181. Redlinger RE, Shimizu T, Remy T, et al: Cellular mechanisms of interleukin-12 mediated neuroblastoma regression. J Pediatr Surg 2003;38:199-204.
182. Redlinger RE Jr, Mailliard RB, Barksdale EM: Neuroblastoma and dendritic cell function. Semin Pediatr Surg 2004;13:61-71.
183. Reynolds CP: Differentiating agents in pediatric malignancies: Retinoids in neuroblastoma. Curr Oncol Rep 2000;2:511-518.
184. Reynolds CP, Kane DJ, Einhorn PA, et al: Response of neuroblastoma to retinoic acid in vitro and in vivo. Prog Clin Biol Res 1996;366:203-211.
185. Reynolds CP, Matthay KK, Villablanca JG, et al: Retinoid therapy of high risk neuroblastoma. Cancer Lett 2003;197:185-192.
186. Ribatti D, Raffaghello L, Marimpietri D, et al: Fenretinide as an anti-angiogenic agent in neuroblastoma. Cancer Lett 2003;197:181-184.
187. Richards ML, Gundersen AE, Williams MS: Cystic neuroblastoma of infancy. J Pediatr Surg 1995;30:1354-1357.
188. Rickard KA, Detamore CM, Coates TD, et al: Effect of nutrition staging on treatment delays and outcome in stage IV neuroblastoma. Cancer 1983;52:587-598.
189. Rickard KA, Grosfeld JL, Kirksey A, et al: Reversal of protein-energy malnutrition in children during treatment of advanced neoplastic disease. Ann Surg 1979;190:771-781.
190. Rill DR, Santana VM, Roberts WM, et al: Direct demonstration that autologous bone marrow transplantation for solid tumors can return a multiplicity of tumorigenic cells. Blood 1994;84:380-383.
191. Riley RD, Heney D, Jones DR, et al: A systematic review of molecular and biological tumor markers in neuroblastoma. Clin Cancer Res 2004;10:4-12.
192. Rosenberg SA: Development of effective immunotherapy for the treatment of patients with cancer. J Am Coll Surg 2004;198:685-696.
193. Rowe DH, Huang J, Li J, et al: Suppression of primary tumor growth in a mouse model of human neuroblastoma. J Pediatr Surg 2000;35:977-981.
194. Rubino C, Adjadj E, Guerin S, et al: Long-term risk of second malignant neoplasms after neuroblastoma in childhood: Role of treatment. Int J Cancer 2003;107:791-796.
195. Rudnick C, Khakoo Y, Antunes NL: Opsoclonus-myoclonus-ataxia syndrome in neuroblastoma: Clinical outcome and antineural antibodies—a report from the Children's Cancer Group study. Med Pediatr Oncol 2001;36:612-622.
196. Russo C, Cohn SL, Petruzzi MJ, et al: Long term neurologic outcome in children with opsoclonus-myoclonus associated with neuroblastoma: A report from the Pediatric Oncology Group. Med Pediatr Oncol 1997;28: 284-288.
197. Sala A, Pencharz P, Barr RD: Children, cancer and nutrition—a dynamic triangle in review. Cancer 2004;100: 677-687.
198. Sandberg DI, Bilsky MH, Kushner BH, et al: Treatment of spinal involvement in neuroblastoma patients. Pediatr Neurosurg 2003;39:291-298.
199. Sawada T, Sugimoto T, Kawakatsu H, et al: Mass screening for neuroblastoma in Japan. Pediatr Hematol Oncol 1991;8:93-109.
200. Sawada T, Todo S, Fujita K, et al: Mass screening of neuroblastoma in infancy. Am J Dis Child 1982;136:710-712.
201. Schilling FH, Parker C: Mass screening in neuroblastoma: The European experience. In Brodeur GM, Sawada T, Tsuchida Y, Vote PA (eds): Neuroblastoma. Amsterdam, Elsevier, 2000, pp 281-292.
202. Schilling FH, Spix C, Berthold F, et al: German neuroblastoma mass screening study at 12 months of age: Statistical aspects and preliminary results. Med Pediatr Oncol 1998;

31:435-441.
203. Schleiermacher G, Rubie H, Hartmann O, et al: Treatment of stage 4s neuroblastoma—report of 10 years experience of the French Society of Paediatric Oncology (SFOP). Br J Cancer 2003;89:470-476.
204. Schmidt ML, Lukens JN, Seeger RC, et al: Biologic factors determine prognosis in infants with stage IV neuroblastoma: A prospective Children's Cancer Group study. J Clin Oncol 2000;18:1260-1268.
205. Schnaufer L, Koop CE: Silastic abdominal pouch for temporary hepatomegaly in stage IV-S neuroblastoma. J Pediatr Surg 1975;10:73-75.
206. Seeler RA, Israel JN, Royal JE, et al: Ganglioneuroblastoma and fetal hydantoin-alcohol syndrome. Pediatrics 1979; 63:524-527.
207. Senelick RC, Bray PF, Lahey ME, et al: Neuroblastoma and myoclonic encephalopathy: Two cases and a review of the literature. J Pediatr Surg 1973;8:623-632.
208. Shimada H: The International Neuroblastoma Pathology Classification. Pathologica 2003;95:240-241.
209. Shimada H, Ambros IM, Dehner LP, et al: Terminology and morphologic criteria of neuroblastic tumors: Recommendations by the International Neuroblastoma Pathology Committee. Cancer 1999;86:349-363.
210. Shimada H, Ambros IM, Dehner LP, et al: The International Neuroblastoma Pathology Classification (the Shimada system). Cancer 1999;86:364-372.
211. Shimada H, Chatten J, Newton WA Jr, et al: Histopathologic prognostic factors in neuroblastoma: Definition of subtypes of ganglioneuroblastoma and an age-linked classification of neuroblastoma. J Natl Cancer Inst 1984;73:405-416.
212. Shimada H, Stram DO, Chatten J, et al: Identification of subsets of neuroblastomas by combined histopathologic and N-myc analysis. J Natl Cancer Inst 1995;87:1470-1476.
213. Shimada H, Umehara S, Monobe Y, et al: International Neuroblastoma Pathology Classification for prognostic evaluation of patients with peripheral neuroblastic tumors: A report from the Children's Cancer Group. Cancer 2001;92:2451-2461.
214. Shimizu T, Berhanu A, Redlinger RE Jr, et al: Interleukin-12 transduced dendritic cells induce regression of established murine neuroblastoma. J Pediatr Surg 2001;36:1285-1292.
215. Shorter NA, Davidoff AM, Evans AE, et al: The role of surgery in the management of stage IV neuroblastoma: A single institution study. Med Pediatr Oncol 1995;24:287-291.
216. Shuster JJ, McWilliams, MB, Castleberry R, et al: Serum lactate dehydrogenase in childhood neuroblastoma: A POG recursive partitioning study. Am J Clin Oncol 1992; 15:295-303.
217. Shusterman S, Grupp SA, Maris JM: Inhibition of tumor growth in a human neuroblastoma xenograft model with TNP-470. Med Pediatr Oncol 2000;35:673-676.
218. Sitarz A, Finkelstein J, Grosfeld JL, et al: An evaluation of the role of surgery in disseminated neuroblastoma: A report from the Children's Cancer Study Group. J Pediatr Surg 1983;18:147-151.
219. Spurbeck WW, Davidoff AM, Lobe TE, et al: Minimally invasive surgery in pediatric cancer patients. Ann Surg Oncol 2004;11:340-343.
220. Squire R, Fowler CL, Brooks SP, et al: The relationship of class I MHC antigen expression to stage IV-S disease and survival in neuroblastoma. J Pediatr Surg 1990;25: 381-386.
221. Stevens MM: Stage IV-S neuroblastoma: Disseminated malignancy with a favorable prognosis—three case reports. Aust Paediatr J 1979;15:39-43.
222. Stigall R, Smith WL, Francken EA, et al: Intrapulmonic metastatic neuroblastoma. Ann Radiol 1979;22:223-227.
223. Suarez A, Hartmann O, Vassal G, et al: Treatment of stage IV-S neuroblastoma: A study of 34 cases treated from 1982-1987. Med Pediatr Oncol 1991;19:473-477.
224. Sugio K, Nakagawara A, Sasazuki T: Association of expression between N-myc gene and major histocompatibility complex class I gene in surgically resected neuroblastoma. Cancer 1991;67:1384-1388.
225. Suzuki T, Bogenmann, Shimada H, et al: Lack of high affinity nerve growth factor receptors in aggressive neuroblastoma. J Natl Cancer Inst 1993;5:377-384.
226. Suzuki T, Yokota J, Mugishima H, et al: Frequent loss of heterozygosity on chromosome 14q in neuroblastoma. Cancer Res 1989;49:1095-1098.
227. Tanaka S, Tajiri T, Noguchi S, et al: Prenatally diagnosed cystic neuroblastoma: A report of 2 cases. Asian J Surg 2003;26:225-227.
228. Tapia F, Polak JM, Barbosa AJ, et al: Neuron specific enolase is produced by neuroendocrine tumors. Lancet 1981;1:808-811.
229. Tornoczky T, Kalman E, Kajtar PG, et al: Large cell neuroblastoma: A distinct phenotype of neuroblastoma with aggressive clinical behavior. Cancer 2004;100:390-397.
230. Umehara S, Nakagawara A, Matthay KK, et al: Histopathology defines prognostic subsets of ganglioneuroblastoma nodular. Cancer 2000;89:1150-1161.
231. Van Eys J, Copeland EM, Cangir A, et al: A clinical trial of hyperalimentation in children with metastatic malignancies. Med Pediatr Oncol 1980;8:63-73.
232. Vertuani S, De Geer A, Levitsky V, et al: Retinoids act as multistep modulators of the major histocompatibility class I presentation pathway and sensitize neuroblastomas to cytotoxic lymphocytes. Cancer Res 2003;63:8006-8013.
233. Villablanca JG, Khan AA, Avramis VI, et al: Phase I trial of 13 cis-retinoic acid in children with neuroblastoma following bone marrow transplantation. J Clin Oncol 1995;13:894-901.
234. West KW, Weber TR, Grosfeld JL: Synergistic effect of hyperthermia, papaverine and chemotherapy in murine neuroblastoma. J Pediatr Surg 1980;15:913-917.
235. White L: P-glycoprotein expression and progression of neuroblastoma. N Engl J Med 1992;326:1162-1163.
236. Wilson PC, Coppes MJ, Solh H, et al: Neuroblastoma stage IV-S a heterogenous disease. Med Pediatr Oncol 1991;19:467-472.
237. Woods W, Gaor N, Shuster JT, et al: Screening of infants and mortality due to neuroblastoma. N Engl J Med 2002; 346:1041-1046.
238. Woods WG: Screening for neuroblastoma: The final chapter. J Pediatr Hematol Oncol 2003;25:3-4.
239. Yamamoto K, Hanada R, Kikuchi A, et al: Spontaneous regression of localized neuroblastoma detected by mass screening. J Clin Oncol 1998;16:1265-1269.
240. Yamashiro DJ, Nakagawara A, Ikegaki N, et al: Expression of TrkC in favorable human neuroblastoma. Oncogene 1996;12:37-41.

241. Yanik GA, Levine JE, Mattay KK, et al: Pilot study of metiodobenzylguanidine in combination with myeloablative chemotherapy and autologous stem cell support for the treatment of neuroblastoma. J Clin Oncol 2002; 20:2142-2149.
242. Yiin J, Chang CS, Jan YJ, Wang YC: Treatment of neuroblastoma with intraspinal extension. J Clin Neurosci 2003; 10:579-583.
243. Young DG: Thoracic neuroblastoma/ganglioneuroma. J Pediatr Surg 1983;18:37-41.
244. Zeltzer PM, Marangos PJ, Parama AM, et al: Raised neuron specific enolase in the serum of children with metastatic neuroblastoma: A report from the Children's Cancer Study Group. Lancet 1983;2:361-363.
245. Ziegler MM, Vega A, Koop CE: Electrocoagulation induced immunity—an explanation for regression of neuroblastoma. J Pediatr Surg 1980;15:34-37.
246. Zimmerman RA, Bilaniuk CT: CT of primary and secondary craniocerebral neuroblastoma. AJR Am J Roentgenol 1980;135:1239-1242.

第 29 章

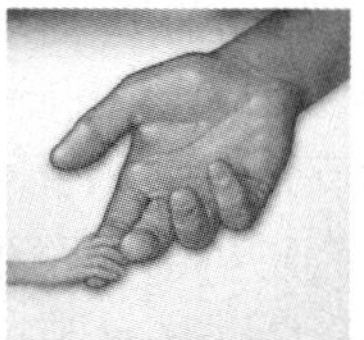

肝脏的非恶性肿瘤

Philip C. Guzzetta, Jr.

95 原发性肝脏肿瘤在儿童肿瘤中所占的比例不到3%，其中只有1/3为良性肿瘤[2,17,30,69]。尽管肝脏良性肿瘤很少，但在从病例数相对较大的各个中心汇合而来的经验基础上，可以制定诊断评估和治疗的推荐方案。良性肿瘤可以是上皮性的（局灶性结节增生、肝细胞腺瘤）、间叶性的（婴儿肝脏血管内皮瘤、海绵样血管瘤、间叶错构瘤），也可以是其他（畸胎瘤、炎性假瘤）。非寄生性囊肿虽然不是真正的肿瘤，但也将在此章讨论。

一个有趣的现象是，儿童肝脏良性肿瘤好发于其父母有某些异常者。很早就发现肝细胞腺瘤与成人口服避孕药有关。当再生障碍贫血儿童接受雄激素治疗，β-型地中海贫血输血造成长期铁超负荷或肾移植后接受糖皮质激素治疗时，儿童发生肝细胞性腺瘤的风险增高[8]。Ⅰ型糖原累积病发生肝细胞性腺瘤[5]和局灶性结节增生的[48]风险增高。患结节性硬化的儿童易发生肝错构瘤[33]。

临床表现

大多数儿童肝脏良性肿瘤表现为右上腹无痛性肿块或肝脏肿大。可出现消化道压迫症状，如便秘、厌食、呕吐。如果为疼痛性肿块，疼痛为钝性疼痛，是因肝脏包膜膨胀或正常周围结构受压引起的。黄疸和体重下降不常见，除非为婴儿肝脏血管内皮瘤(IHH)，这些症状应该引起警惕可能是恶性病变。急性腹部疼痛可能是肿块出血或腹腔内出血，特别是在肝细胞性腺瘤中，但这种情况在儿童中非常少见。当有血管病变时，如IHH，患儿可表现为充血性心力衰竭以及血小板减少症，被称为Kasabach-Merritt综合征。大约半数IHH[35]患儿可见表皮血管瘤[25,55,59]，IHH患儿肝脏迅速肿大可以引起腹腔间隔综合征和呼吸窘迫[52]。在肝脏动静脉畸形或间叶错构瘤[60]中可表现出无显著血小板减少的心力衰竭。某些IHH[21]或间叶性错构瘤产前超声检查可发现胎儿水肿[34]。

诊断

实验室检查

血清甲胎蛋白（AFP）在出生时浓度很高(48 000 ± 35 000ng/ml)，但在8个月时迅速下降至成人水平，即小于10ng/ml（表29-1）[73]。在小于8个月的婴儿中，AFP水平必须通过这种显著变化的递减关系来解释。尽管某些良性病变如间叶错构瘤或畸胎 496

表 29-1 正常婴儿不同年龄血清甲胎蛋白水平

年龄	病例数	AFP 水平 ± 标准差（ng/ml）
早产	11	138 734 ± 41 444
新生儿	55	48 406 ± 34 718
出生2周	16	33 ± 113 ± 32 503
2周至1月	43	9452 ± 12 610
1个月	12	2645 ± 3080
2个月	40	323 ± 278
3个月	5	88 ± 87
4个月	31	74 ± 56
5个月	6	46.5 ± 19
6个月	9	12.5 ± 9.8
7个月	5	9.7 ± 7.1
8个月	3	8.5 ± 5.5

From Wu JT, Book L, Sudar K: Serum alpha fetoprotein (AFP) levels in normal infants.Pediatr Res 1981; 5:50.

瘤[66]也可发生 AFP 中度升高，但儿童肝脏肿瘤 AFP 水平明显升高几乎预示着肿瘤为恶性的。如前面提到的肝脏肿块伴显著的血小板减少通常是 IHH 引起的 Kasabach–Merritt 综合征。甲状腺功能低下也可以出现在 IHH 中[27]，这些儿童需要常规进行甲状腺功能测定，因为甲状腺功能低下显著影响治疗[42]。

影像学检查

儿童出现腹部肿块首选的影像学检查应该是仰卧位的腹部平片，寻找肿块中有无钙化。下一步影像学检查是腹部多普勒超声，以及随后的增强 CT 检查（图 29–1）[6]。是否做核磁共振（MRI）取决于超声和 CT 检查结果，尤其是当准备手术切除以及需要了解更多的和肿瘤相关的血管解剖的详细情况时。动脉血管造影可用于 IHH，或偶尔可用于有充血性心力衰竭的间叶性错构瘤，在后者，治疗需要对肿瘤的血供进行栓塞。肝脾放射性核素扫描对鉴别肝脏肿块很少有诊断价值[45]，在有 CT 和 MRI 的情况下没有必要进行。在超声或 CT 引导下穿刺活检儿童肝脏良性肿瘤通常不予提倡（除非肿瘤切除对患儿有巨大风险），因为对于病理医生来说依靠一小块标本明确诊断存在困难，而且对大多数肿瘤而言手术切除是最佳方案。每个肿瘤的影像学表现将在每节进行讨论。

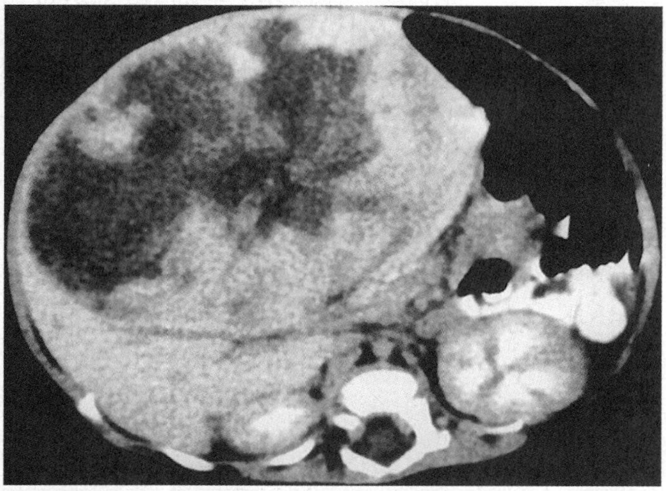

图 29–1　6 个月大的女婴肝左叶的巨大的血管内皮瘤腹部 CT 增强扫描。注意中央区域坏死。

血管性肿瘤

婴儿肝脏血管内皮瘤

IHH 在儿童肝脏良性肿瘤最为常见。IHH 在产前可以诊断，与受影响的新生儿相似，胎儿可以表现为无症状或严重病变[21,55]。有症状的患儿 80%在 6 个月前表现出来，有许多在新生儿期表现出来[25,55,59]。最常见的体格检查表现是肝脏肿大。这个疾病的程度表现不一，有些没有症状，有的有威胁生命的心力衰竭、腹腔间隔综合征和严重的血小板减少症。在多数统计中，男女比例为 2∶1，半数儿童有表皮血管瘤以及 IHH[11,25,59]。在婴儿中，IHH 可以通过腹部超声和动态增强对比 CT 明确诊断。病变通常遍及肝脏但可局限于一些肝段[68]。超声检查中多叶回声增强的结节通常有高流量的血管，而单个病变则具有多异质样回声表现[6]。注射增强造影剂前，这些病变在 CT 上表现为低衰减，增强后弥漫性或向心性增强[6]。IHH 的 MRI 检查可显示疾病的范围，流量的特征和流量结构[6]。尽管影像学技术诊断 IHH 准确率高，但仍需要检查 AFP 和儿茶酚胺水平，因为偶然情况下肝母细胞瘤和Ⅳ–S 期神经母细胞瘤会被误诊为 IHH[29]。

Dehner 和 Ishak[12]确定了 IHH 的两种镜下形态。1 型是一种更为常见的组织类型，特征为血管空间由扩大的和受压的内皮细胞有序地排列而成，由良性细胞学特性的网状纤维支撑。在他们的回顾中，23 例中的 17 例为 1 型。2 型病变为急进型的组织表现，血管管腔是一种更为复杂无规律的分支结构。虽然有丝分裂不常见，但内皮细胞比 1 型染色更深，形态更为多样。在 Dehner 和 Ishak 的文章中，2 型的死亡率比 1 型的要高，但近来发现不管何种类型预后都良好，肿瘤的组织病理类型与预后无关。

肿瘤的治疗取决于症状的严重性以及病变的部位。如果无临床症状仅有轻微的肝脏肿大，通过无损伤的影像学检查诊断明确后，观察是最佳的方案。除非高度怀疑病变可能为恶性病变，否则不提倡经皮或开放活检，因为有大出血的风险。

有症状患儿的治疗首先是药物治疗，包括皮质类固醇[25,55,59]、干扰素[9,18]、长春新碱[47]或环磷酰胺[28]。尽管开始干扰素治疗很热门，但其严重的副作用引起关注，不管是干扰素–α2a[3]还是干扰素 –α2b[6]。另外，该方法需要数周至数月才可以起效，这对临床危重的

49

新生儿来说时间太长。因为疾病的严重程度分布很广以及通常单个中心治疗的病例都小于 20 例；所以任何一种药物治疗的成功率都很难评估。根据我们的经验，弥漫性或多叶病变导致的心功能衰竭和血小板减少的患儿很少通过单独药物治疗得到改善。栓塞运用非常有效但局限于 8 个肝段中少数肝段的病变[68]，但也有一些报告报道弥漫性 IHH 的成功治疗[6]。IHH 病变经常有来源于肠系膜上、横膈、肋间和乳房内动脉的肝外动脉侧枝，以及来源于门静脉系统的血供[6,20]。这些使得通过栓塞完全消除血流最终不能实现。

过去虽然推荐应用肝动脉结扎治疗 IHH，但它妨碍有效的栓塞，应该停止使用。如果已经栓塞但疾病继续恶化，为了存活可以考虑肝切除[11,55]或肝移植[11,36]。虽然放疗用来治疗过这些病变[52,53]，但婴儿肝脏放疗的远期作用还不知道。但有报道说 3 例曾经接受过放疗的 IHH 患儿出现血管肉瘤[19]。因为疾病的多变性和治疗方案的多样性，IHH 存活率的统计不可信，但在小于 6 个月伴有心功能衰竭中的儿童，这种“良性”肿瘤的存活率在 45%～90%之间[11,25,55]。

血管瘤

血管瘤是成人最常见的肝脏血管性肿瘤。在儿童中，血管瘤通常在无症状患儿中偶然被发现[12]。血管瘤镜下检查表现为：大量的扩张无吻合的血管，内膜为扁平的上皮细胞和纤维组织[12]。回顾分析儿童肝脏血管瘤的文献有困难，因为有作者把患儿年龄临床表现相似的血管内皮瘤称之为血管瘤。此外，这些病变的首选治疗不是手术，通常没有标本进行准确组织病理诊断。在儿童，血管瘤出血的风险很低，除非患儿疼痛或肝脏肿大无力，否则一般不需要治疗。相反，成人大的血管瘤（直径大于 4cm）通常需要手术切除[1,57]。

动静脉畸形

动静脉畸形可以在肝实质内或肝动脉和门静脉系统之间。和患儿血管内皮瘤相似，肝门静脉动静脉畸形通常出现在 6 个月之前，也可以出现在新生儿期间，表现为肝脏肿大、心力衰竭和肝区杂音[14]。在年龄较大的儿童和成人中，肝脏动静脉畸形可以以遗传性出血性毛细血管扩张症出现，也称之 Osler-Weber-Rendu 病[6,7]。血管造影可以诊断 AVM，栓塞是治疗有些患儿的方法，但成功关闭动静脉畸形需要根除侧支[6,14]。有报道肝动静脉畸形栓塞导致致命性并发症[71]。对于这些病变而言类固醇治疗没有意义，肝脏动静脉畸形栓塞治疗失败后可以结扎肝动脉进行控制[23,24]。

间叶错构瘤

间叶错构瘤在年龄小于 2 岁的儿童中通常表现为无痛性的右上腹部肿块[13,37,64]。有的患儿可以出现心功能衰竭[45,60]，错构瘤与 IHH 相似可以在产前进行诊断[34]。Edmondson[17]提出，肝脏间叶错构瘤起源于实质小体，它孤立于正常的肝门三联结构独立分化。肿瘤沿胆管生长，可以混合于正常肝组织。因为血管和胆管是实质小体的组成部位，所以肿瘤的生物学特性表现为上述成分为主伴有疏松结缔组织基质包绕。肿瘤可表现为囊性结构为主（图 29-2），因囊液积聚增大迅速[61]；或以血管为主出现心力衰竭[60]。Von 498
Schweinitz 等人[67]提出，未成熟肝脏的脂肪储存细胞可能参与间叶错构瘤的形成和发展。

儿童间叶错构瘤的血清甲胎蛋白水平通常正常，也可以轻度升高[31,40]。这些肿瘤的影像学表现一致且

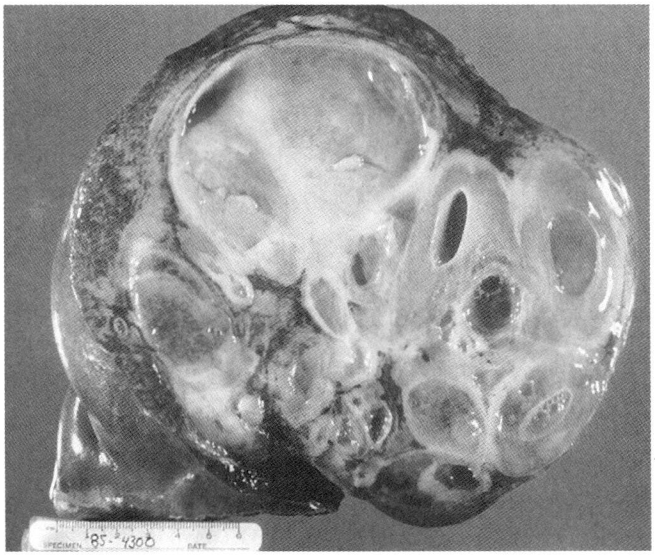

图 29-2 一名 10 个月大的男婴的间叶错构瘤肝左叶切除的病理切面大体标本。

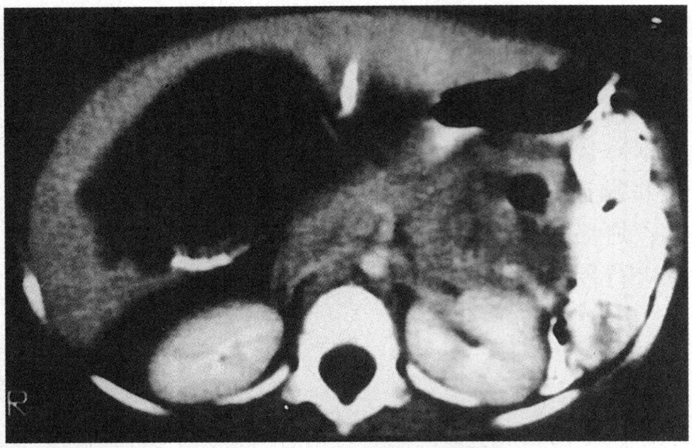

图 29-3 肝脏右叶复发的间叶错构瘤的腹部 CT 增强扫描，先前做过去顶手术。以后成功进行了肝脏右叶部分切除。

为可区分的，腹部超声和 CT 通常表现为单个巨大含有液体的肿块，有囊内分隔，无钙化[62]。

尽管有报道恶性转化，但是间叶错构瘤通常是一个良性的过程[4]，治疗通常是温和的[46,50]。常规来说，如果手术安全，完整手术切除是首选方法。如果病变巨大或累积所有肝叶，采用将囊肿去顶和造袋术的治疗方法，不完全切除病变可能复发（图 29-3）。

间叶错构瘤是一种有别于与结节硬化相关的肝脏错构瘤的病变。后者病变小，多叶病变，可以与其他部位的血管肌脂瘤相关，如肾脏。一般很少有症状，通常发生在年龄大于 2 到 3 岁儿童中。这些错构瘤临床意义小，但它们的存在有助于诊断结节硬化[33]。

肝细胞腺瘤

尽管孤立性病变在儿童中偶然碰到，但在成人中肝细胞腺瘤 HCA 最为常见，与口服合成皮质激素及雌激素有关。HCA 发生在类固醇激素治疗以及慢性贫血长期输血[8]，Ⅰ型糖原累积病的患儿中。Bianchi[5]提出，在Ⅰ型糖原累积病中发生 HCA 的几个机制包括：（1）胰岛素和糖原代谢局部不平衡，因为这些激素对于肝细胞增殖和再生的调节非常重要；（2）糖原过载的反应；（3）癌基因的激活。

这些腺瘤显微镜下检查显示肝细胞沿肝窦呈片状和条索状排列没有管状结构。细胞具有糖原堆积的细胞浆，小的无分裂的细胞核。临近肝脏和血管有压迫但无侵入。儿童通常没有肝硬化[8]。组织学类型和分化良好的肝细胞癌相似，有未切除的 HCA 发展成为肝细胞癌的报道[32,65]。

在儿童，HCA 一般表现为无症状的肝脏肿块。超声和 CT 检查表现为孤立的肿块。肝酶和 AFP 水平正常。这个病变的唯一特性是有因自发破裂而引起的腹腔内出血的倾向。在成人，接受雌激素治疗时几乎都可见腹腔内出血。在激素治疗停止后肿瘤可出现退化。糖原累积病和 HCA 患者，在代谢紊乱纠正后肿瘤可退化[5]。因为知道肝细胞癌和 HCA 之间的联系，所以提倡对未接受激素治疗以及无糖原累积病的患儿进行手术切除治疗。如果肿瘤不能切除且无潜在危险，观察病变监测 AFP 水平是适合的方法。如果 AFP 水平开始上升或病变症状明显，并且手术切除存在无法接受的高风险，那么肝移植是最佳的选择。

局灶性结节增生

局部结节增生 FNH 在儿童表现为形态不规则无张力的肝脏肿块。经常在其他原因剖腹探查时偶然发现或放射检查时发现。FNH 发生的男女之比大约为 4∶1[63]。FNH 偶然同时发现肝脏血管畸形[70]和血管瘤，推测病变是对损伤和缺血不同的反应[17]。腹部超声检查病变为同等回声、低回声或相对于正常肝实质的高回声，10%～15%患儿为多发性。超声可能看不到典型的中央瘢痕。CT 典型表现为密集星状中央瘢痕的高度血管化病变。常规动脉造影或核磁共振血管造影术显示为血管增生的肿块，滋养动脉进入外周在肿瘤的中央部分集中。有些纤维板状肝细胞癌在影像检查中不能和局部结节增生相鉴别，这就是在没有活检就做诊断时要考虑的问题[43]。有些报告报道局部结节增生成人患者同时伴有肝细胞癌[44]。

在标本大体检查时病灶没有胞膜、偶有蒂、较硬（图 29-4）。显微镜检查显示增生的肝细胞、胆道和特定的中央纤维化。这些病变很少恶性，出血也很少见。如果肿瘤切除并发症发生率高，且儿童临床没有症状，应用影像检查、甲胎蛋白水平和活检已作出明确诊断，那么观察是最合适的治疗方案[51]。

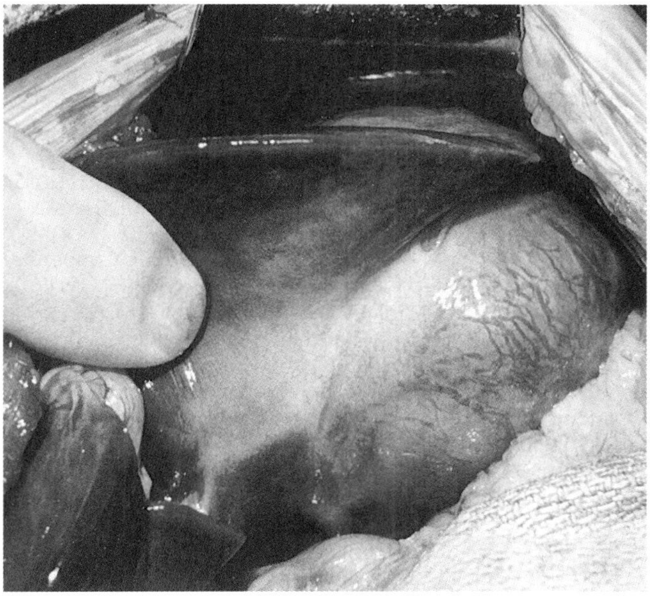

图 29-4 在一位 2 岁大的患儿肝脏左外叶切除手术中见到的局部结节增生。

其他肿瘤

畸胎瘤

有少于 25 例儿童肝脏畸胎瘤的报道[66,72]。这些儿童年龄都小于 1 岁，病灶通常存在钙化，这有助于与其他肿瘤鉴别。有些病变符合肝内胎中胎的标准[41]。畸胎瘤血清甲胎蛋白水平可以升高，但和肝母细胞瘤相比只是轻微升高。肿瘤不成熟的成分有恶化的风险所以切除是畸胎瘤的治疗首选。

炎性假瘤

肝脏炎性假性肿瘤罕见。病变通常发生在年龄大于 3 岁的儿童中，但在小年龄儿童中也有报道。因为病变为实质性的，通过影像检查很难与肝脏其他良性和恶性肿瘤辨别。甲胎蛋白水平正常。儿童肝脏实体肿瘤有发热、白细胞计数升高和高水平反应蛋白，但 AFP 水平正常提示肝脏炎性假性肿瘤的可能。尽管发病的诱因不明，但可能是肝脏对某些侵犯的炎性反应。因为此病变没有大块组织活检或病变切除很难诊断，所以大多数儿童进行肿瘤切除，此病是可以治愈的[22,54]。

非寄生性囊肿

肝脏寄生性囊肿很少见，在成人中比儿童多见。尽管在出生时可能已经存在或有症状，但大多数囊肿没有症状，在探查和尸解时偶尔发现。症状主要和腹胀及相邻结构推移相关。男女发病率相似[15]。非寄生性囊肿通常是单房的，表面覆盖立方或柱状上皮，为胆道样特征。典型囊液为清亮或咖啡色的，胆汁样的很少存在。病理研究提示非寄生性囊肿起源于先天性或继发性胆管周围腺体梗阻。这些腺体正常来源于孕 7 周肝门管状板块，继续增殖一直到成人[15]。有症状的囊肿可通过单纯去顶、造袋术[38]或硬化剂[49]注射而有效地治疗。如果怀疑和胆道相通，胆道造影可以显示起源，完全缝合相通管道。

肝内胆管囊性扩张也可表现为肿块，黄疸和胆囊炎与此相关，切除累及肝叶是治疗的方法[39]。如果肝脏肿块影像检查表现为完全囊性，可以误诊为非寄生性囊肿。外伤后胆道囊肿是因为胆管断裂肝内胆汁淤积所致。这些病变可以通过经皮穿刺引流治疗，有些病例通过胆道括约肌切开降低胆道压力减少胆汁瘘。外伤后囊肿很少需要切除。多发实质囊肿与遗传性多囊肾相关，通常是无症状的，囊肿小的不需要治疗。

表皮样囊肿与非寄生性囊肿不同，表面覆盖上皮细胞为鳞状细胞，多于立方样细胞。组织学特点引导出这样一个理论：这些病变是在肝脏表面发生的前肠芽异常。尽管该病变少见，但报道有恶变倾向，所以切除是最佳的治疗方法[56]。

（徐 敏译 王 珊校）

致谢

The author thanks W. Raleigh Thompson, MD, for his contribution to this chapter in the fifth edition of this book.

参考文献

1. Baer HU, Dennison AR, Moulton W, et al: Enucleation of giant hemangiomas of the liver. Ann Surg 1992;216:673.
2. Baggenstoss AH: Pathology of tumors of liver in infancy and childhood. In Pack G, Islami A (eds): Tumors of the Liver. New York: Springer-Verlag, 1970, p 240.
3. Barlow CF, Priebe CJ, Mulliken JB, et al: Spastic diplegia as a complication of interferon alpha-2a treatment of hemangiomas of infancy. J Pediatr 1998;132:527.
4. Barnhart DC, Hirschl RB, Garver KA, et al: Conservative management of mesenchymal hamartoma of the liver. J Pediatr Surg 1997;32:1495.
5. Bianchi L: Glycogen storage disease I and hepatocellular tumors. Eur J Pediatr 1993;152:S63.
6. Burrows PE, Dubois J, Kassarjian: Pediatric hepatic vascular anomalies. Pediatr Radiol 2001;31:533.
7. Buscarini E, Buscarini L, Danesino C, et al: Hepatic vascular malformations in hereditary hemorrhagic telangiectasia: Doppler sonographic screening in a large family. J Hepatol 1997;26:111.
8. Chandra RS, Kapur SP, Kelleher J, et al: Benign hepatocellular tumors in the young: A clinicopathologic spectrum. Arch Pathol Lab Med 1984;108:168.
9. Chang E, Boyd A, Nelson CC, et al: Successful treatment of infantile hemangiomas with interferon-alpha-2b. J Pediatr Hematol Oncol 1997;19:237.
10. Cohen RC, Myers NA: Diagnosis and management of massive hepatic hemangiomas in childhood. J Pediatr Surg 1986;21:6.
11. Daller JA, Bueno J, Gutierrez J, et al: Hepatic hemangioendothelioma: Clinical experience and management strategy. J Pediatr Surg 1999;34:98.
12. Dehner LP, Ishak KG: Vascular tumors of the liver in infants and children. Arch Pathol 1971;92:101.
13. DeMaioribus CA, Lally KP, Sim K, et al: Mesenchymal hamartoma of the liver. Arch Surg 1990;125:598.
14. Dickman PS, Meza MP, Newman B: Hepatic vascular malformations. Pediatr Pathol Lab Med 1995;15:155.
15. Donovan MJ, Kozakewich H, Perez-Atayde A: Solitary nonparasitic cysts of the liver: The Boston Children's Hospital experience. Pediatr Pathol Lab Med 1995;15:419.
16. Dubois J, Hershon L, Carmant L, et al: Toxicity profile of interferon alfa-2b in children: A prospective evaluation. J Pediatr 1999;135:782.
17. Edmondson HA: Differential diagnosis of tumors and tumor like lesions of liver in infancy and childhood. Am J Dis Child 1956;91:168.
18. Ezekowitz RAB, Mulliken JB, Folkman J: Interferon alfa-2a therapy for life-threatening hemangiomas of infancy. N Engl J Med 1992;326:1456.
19. Falk H, Herbert JT, Edmonds L, et al: Review of four cases of childhood hepatic angiosarcoma—elevated environmental arsenic exposure in one case. Cancer 1981;47:382.
20. Fellows KE, Hoffer FA, Markowitz RI, et al: Multiple collaterals to hepatic infantile hemangioendotheliomas and arteriovenous malformations: Effect on embolization. Radiology 1991;181:813.
21. Gembruch U, Baschat AA, Gloeckner-Hoffmann K, et al: Prenatal diagnosis and management of fetuses with liver hemangiomata. Ultrasound Obstet Gynecol 2002; 19:454.
22. Hata Y, Sasaki F, Matuoka S, et al: Inflammatory pseudotumor of the liver in children: Report of cases and review of the literature. J Pediatr Surg 1992;27:1549.
23. Hazebroek FWJ, Tibboel D, Robben SGF, et al: Hepatic artery ligation for hepatic vascular tumors with arteriovenous and arterioportal venous shunts in the newborn: Successful management of two cases and review of the literature. J Pediatr Surg 1995;30:1127.
24. Heaton ND, Davenport M, Karani J, et al: Congenital hepatoportal arteriovenous fistula. Surgery 1995;117:170.
25. Holcomb GW, O'Neill JA, Mahboudi S, et al: Experience with hepatic hemangioendothelioma in infancy and childhood. J Pediatr Surg 1988;23:661.
26. Howell RR, Stevenson RE, Ben-Menachem Y, et al: Hepatic adenomata with type 1 glycogen storage disease. JAMA 1976;236:1481.
27. Huang SA, Tu HM, Harney JW, et al: Severe hypothyroidism caused by type 3 iodothyronine deiodinase in infantile hemangiomas. N Engl J Med 2000;343:185.
28. Hurvitz SA, Hurvitz CH, Sloninsky L, et al: Successful treatment with cyclophosphamide of life threatening diffuse hemangiomatosis involving the liver. J Pediatr Hematol Oncol 2000;22:527.
29. Ingram JD, Yerushalmi B, Connell J, et al: Hepatoblastoma in a neonate: A hypervascular presentation mimicking hemangioendothelioma. Pediatr Radiol 2000;30:794.
30. Ishak KG: Primary hepatic tumors in childhood. In Popper H, Schaffner F (eds): Progress in Liver Diseases, vol 5. New York, Grune & Stratton, 1976, p 636.
31. Ito H, Kishikawa T, Toda T, et al: Hepatic mesenchymal hamartoma of an infant. J Pediatr Surg 1984;19:315.
32. Janes CH, McGill DB, Ludwig J, et al: Liver cell adenoma at the age of 3 years and transplantation 19 years later after development of carcinoma: A case report. Hepatology 1993;17:583.
33. Jozwiak S, Pedich M, Rajszys P, et al: Incidence of hepatic hamartomas in tuberous sclerosis. Arch Dis Child 1992; 67:1363.
34. Kamata S, Nose K, Sawai T, et al: Fetal mesenchymal hamartoma of the liver: Report of a case. J Pediatr Surg 2003;38:639.
35. Kasabach HH, Merritt KK: Capillary hemangioma with extensive purpura: Report of a case. Am J Dis Child 1940;59:1063.
36. Kasahara M, Kiuchi T, Haga H, et al: Monosegmental living-donor liver transplantation for infantile hepatic hemangioendothelioma. J Pediatr Surg 2003;38:1108.
37. Lack EE: Mesenchymal hamartoma of the liver: A clinical and pathologic study of nine cases. Am J Pediatr Hematol Oncol 1986;8:91.
38. Litwin DEM, Taylor BR, Greig P, et al: Nonparasitic cysts of the liver: The case for conservative surgical management. Ann Surg 1987;205:45.
39. Longmire WP, Mandiola SA, Gordon HE: Congenital cystic disease of the liver and biliary system. Ann Surg 1971;174:711.
40. Luks FI, Yazbeck S, Brandt ML, et al: Benign liver tumors in children: A 25 year experience. J Pediatr Surg 1991; 26:1326.
41. Magnus KG, Millar AJW, Sinclair-Smith CC, et al: Intrahepatic fetus-in-fetu: A case report and review of the literature. J Pediatr Surg 1999;34:1861.

42. Mason KP, Koka BV, Eldredge EA, et al: Perioperative considerations in a hypothyroid infant with hepatic haemangioma. Paediatr Anaesth 2001;11:228.
43. Meyers RL, Scaife ER: Benign liver and biliary tract masses in infants and toddlers. Semin Pediatr Surg 2000;9:146.
44. Muguti G, Tait N, Richardson A, et al: Hepatic focal nodular hyperplasia: A benign incidentaloma or a marker of serious hepatic disease? HPB Surg 1992;5:171.
45. Mulrooney DA, Carpenter B, Georgieff M, et al: Hepatic mesenchymal hamartoma in a neonate: A case report and review of the literature. J Pediatr Hematol Oncol 2001; 23:316.
46. O'Sullivan MJ, Swanson PE, Knoll J, et al: Undifferentiated embryonal sarcoma with unusual features arising within mesenchymal hamartoma of the liver: Report of a case and review of the literature. Pediatr Dev Pathol 2001;4:482.
47. Perez J, Pardo J, Gomez C: Vincristine—an effective treatment of corticoid-resistant life- threatening infantile hemangiomas. Acta Oncol 2002;41:197.
48. Pizzo CJ: Type I glycogen storage disease with focal nodular hyperplasia of the liver and vasoconstrictive pulmonary hypertension. Pediatrics 1980;65:341.
49. Raboei E, Luoma R: Definitive treatment of congenital liver cyst with alcohol. J Pediatr Surg 2000;35:1138.
50. Ramanujam TM, Ramesh JC, Goh DW, et al: Malignant transformation of mesenchymal hamartoma of the liver: Case report and review of the literature. J Pediatr Surg 1999;34:1684.
51. Reymond D, Plaschkes J, Ridolfi Luthy A, et al: Focal nodular hyperplasia of the liver in children: Review of follow-up and outcome. J Pediatr Surg 1995;30:1590.
52. Ricketts RR, Stryker S, Raffensperger JG: Ventral fasciotomy in the management of hepatic hemangioendothelioma. J Pediatr Surg 1982;17:187.
53. Rotman M, John M, Stowe S, et al: Radiation treatment of pediatric hepatic hemangiomatosis and coexisting cardiac failure. N Engl J Med 1980;302:852.
54. Sakai M, Ikeda H, Suzuki N, et al: Inflammatory pseudotumor of the liver: Case report and review of the literature. J Pediatr Surg 2001;36:663.
55. Samuel M, Spitz L: Infantile hepatic hemangioendothelioma: The role of surgery. J Pediatr Surg 1995;30:1425.
56. Schullinger JN, Wigger HJ, Price JB, et al: Epidermoid cysts of the liver. J Pediatr Surg 1983;18:240.
57. Schwartz SI, Husser WC: Cavernous hemangioma of the liver: A single institution report of 16 resections. Ann Surg 1987;205:456.
58. Scioscia PJ, Dillion PW, Cilley RE, et al: Endoscopic sphincterotomy in the management of posttraumatic biliary fistula. J Pediatr Surg 1994;29:3.
59. Selby DM, Stocker JT, Waclawiw MA, et al: Infantile hemangioendothelioma of the liver. Hepatology 1994;20:39.
60. Smith WL, Ballantine TVN, Gonzalez-Crussi F: Hepatic mesenchymal hamartoma causing heart failure in the neonate. J Pediatr Surg 1978;13:183.
61. Srouji MN, Chatten J, Schulman WM, et al: Mesenchymal hamartoma of the liver in infants. Cancer 1978;42:2483.
62. Stanley P, Hall TR, Woolley MM, et al: Mesenchymal hamartomas of the liver in childhood: Sonographic and CT findings. AJR Am J Roentgenol 1986;147:1035.
63. Stocker JT, Ishak KG: Focal nodular hyperplasia of the liver: A study of 21 pediatric cases. Cancer 1981;48:336.
64. Stocker JT, Ishak KG: Mesenchymal hamartoma of the liver: Report of 30 cases and review of the literature. Pediatr Pathol 1983;1:245.
65. Tesluk H, Lawrie J: Hepatocellular ademona: Its transformation to carcinoma in a user of oral contraceptives. Arch Pathol Lab Med 1981;105:296.
66. Todani T, Tabuchi K, Watanabe Y, et al: True hepatic teratoma with high alpha fetoprotein in serum. J Pediatr Surg 1977;12:591.
67. von Schweinitz D, Gomez Dammeier B, Gluer S: Mesenchymal hamartoma of the liver—new insight into histogenesis. J Pediatr Surg 1999;34:1269.
68. Warmann S, Bertram H, Kardorff R, et al: Interventional treatment of infantile hepatic hemangioendothelioma. J Pediatr Surg 2003;38:1177.
69. Weinberg AG, Finegold MJ: Primary hepatic tumors of childhood. Hum Pathol 1983;14:512.
70. Whelan TJ, Baugh J, Chandor S: Focal nodular hyperplasia of the liver. Ann Surg 1973;177:150.
71. Whiting JH, Korzenik JR, Miller FJ, et al: Fatal outcome after embolotherapy for hepatic arteriovenous malformations of the liver in two patients with hereditary hemorrhagic telangiectasia. J Vasc Interv Radiol 2000; 11:855.
72. Witte DP, Kissane JM, Askin FB: Hepatic teratomas in children. Pediatr Pathol 1983;1:81.
73. Wu JT, Book L, Sudar K: Serum alpha fetoprotein (AFP) levels in normal infants. Pediatr Res 1981;15:50.

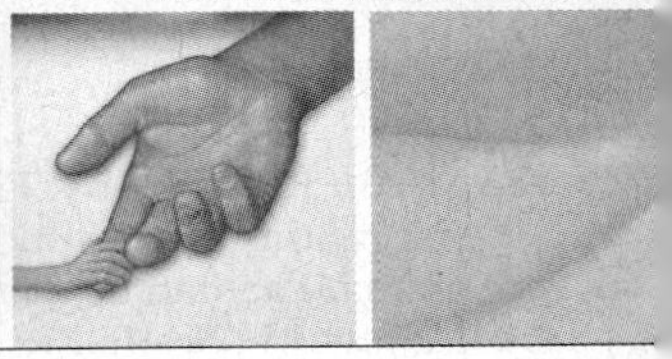

第 30 章

肝脏肿瘤

James B. Atkinson 和 Daniel A. DeUgarte

肝脏恶性肿瘤占所有儿童恶性肿瘤的 1%，是继神经母细胞瘤和肾母细胞瘤之后第三大最常见的腹腔内肿瘤。两大类原发性肝脏恶性肿瘤是肝母细胞瘤和肝细胞癌。随着新化疗方案和肝脏手术技术的进步，肝母细胞瘤患者的存活率显著提高。但肝细胞癌的预后仍然很差，治愈需要完整切除肿瘤。

流行病学

肝母细胞瘤和肝细胞癌有着不同的发生率、年龄分布、基因基础和相关危险因素（表 30-1）。从 1979—1996 年，在美国，小于 20 岁的居民中，肝母细胞瘤的发生率由 0.6/ 百万上升到 1.2/ 百万，而肝细胞癌的发生率由 0.45/ 百万下降到 0.29/ 百万[14]。肝母细胞瘤和肝细胞癌在男性多发[14,50]。肝母细胞瘤通常发生在 6 个月至 3 岁的儿童，而肝细胞癌发生在较大年龄的儿童和成人。

肝母细胞瘤和 Beckwith-Wiedemann 综合征、家族多发性腺瘤样息肉病、半侧肢体肥大症和低出生体重相关[16,23,44,60,62]。最常见基因发生改变的染色体有 1p、1q、2q、4q、7q、8q、12p、17q、20、22q、Xp、Xq[68,71,75]。肝母细胞瘤和 β-连锁蛋白的稳定突变以及 Wnt/β-连锁蛋白信号的激活有关[6]。在肝母细胞瘤中观察到胰岛素样生长因子 II 的上调，可能受到 PLGA1 癌基因过度表达的调控，后者是 8q 染色体上的转录激活剂[78]。细胞遗传学的异常并不能明确致病原因及显示影响预后。肝母细胞瘤的病因还不清楚，但最近的学说提出，肝母细胞瘤可能来源于能够分化为肝细胞和胆道上皮细胞的多潜能肝干细胞或卵圆干细胞。肝母细胞瘤细胞和卵圆干细胞表达这两个细胞系的标记。进一步来说，肝母细胞瘤的结构特性类似于肝细胞生成不同时期的特征[61,79]。

表 30-1　肝母细胞瘤和肝细胞癌的比较

	肝母细胞瘤	肝细胞癌
发病率	1.2/ 百万[12]	0.29/ 百万[12]
年龄分布	6 月至 3 岁	大于 5 岁
高危因素	Beckwith-Weidemann 综合征	乙型肝炎病毒
	家族多发性腺样息肉	肝硬化
	半侧肢体肥大	肝脏疾病
	低出生体重[26,54]	
5 年存活率	52%～75%[12,40,47,55]	18%～28%[11,26]

肝母细胞瘤和极低出生体重之间的联系可以这样解释：遗传畸变的高风险或未成熟肝脏对围生期强化治疗（例如氧疗、利尿剂、放射）作用的易感性。在一个研究中发现，与出生体重控制对照组相比，肝母细胞瘤患者有长时间以及积极的围生期治疗[54]。极低出生体重婴儿发展为进展期肝母细胞瘤的风险较高[26]。有些报道提出，极低出生体重或其他与肝母细胞瘤相关的异常可通过系列超声筛查和甲胎蛋白监测提高早期检测率[11]。然而在进行筛查前必须对高危肝母细胞瘤患者筛查进行常规花费分析评估。

肝细胞癌主要发生于有肝脏疾病和肝硬化的患者。在儿童，肝细胞癌和高酪氨酸血症及其他遗传代谢异常有关[76]。在美国，肝细胞癌的发生率在亚裔及外来儿童中较高[10,14]。在台湾，肝细胞癌多发生于乙型肝炎病毒携带者。乙型肝炎病毒疫苗显著降低了肝细胞癌的发生率[8,36,46]。台湾的一项比较发生在儿童和成人肝细胞癌的研究证实，乙型肝炎病毒感染主要发生在儿童（100%对 80%），肝硬化相近（70%），切除率在儿童较低（18%对 56%）[10]。

临床特征和实验室资料

大多数患者肝脏肿瘤表现为腹部肿块，多于 2/3 的肝脏肿瘤为恶性[11]。尽管大多数患者没有症状，但有些表现为腹胀、厌食、体重下降、疼痛、恶心和乏力。腹部 CT 和超声检查通常显示肝脏实体肿块。实验室检查包括全血细胞计数、全套检查生化、肝功能、凝血状况和血清甲胎蛋白水平。60%的病例出现血小板减少症[73]。有时发现血清氨基转移酶升高和贫血[57]。诊断最终取决于活检。图 30-1 是肝脏恶性肿瘤诊断和治疗的流程图。

肝母细胞瘤和肝细胞癌最敏感的实验室检查是血清甲胎蛋白水平。甲胎蛋白由胎儿肝脏和卵黄囊产生，出生后 6 个月下降至成人水平。尽管甲胎蛋白可以作为肿瘤有效标志物，但不是特异性的。超过 90%的肝母细胞瘤甲胎蛋白水平升高，肝细胞癌大约为 70%[13,31]。甲胎蛋白水平假阳性升高可以发生在肝炎、肝硬化、血管内皮瘤、生殖细胞瘤、睾丸肿瘤和胆囊癌。甲胎蛋白水平正常可以发生在分化良好的和未成熟的肝母细胞瘤以及纤维板块型肝细胞癌[12,13,72]。血清甲胎蛋白可以用来监测化疗反应以及肿瘤复发。偶尔可见肝母细胞瘤分泌与性早熟相关的 β 促绒毛膜性腺激素。 504

影像学检查

影像学检查对于诊断和手术切除可行性评估都是有帮助的。腹部超声或 CT 是肿瘤检查的首选[23]。胸部平片或者 CT 扫描用来排除转移病灶。最终影像学

图 30-1 肝脏肿块的诊断治疗流程图。AFP：甲胎蛋白；CBC：全血计数；CT：计算机断层扫描；CXR：胸片；LFT：肝功能测定；MRI：磁共振扫描；PT/PTT：凝血酶原时间 / 部分促凝血酶原激活时间；US：超声检查。

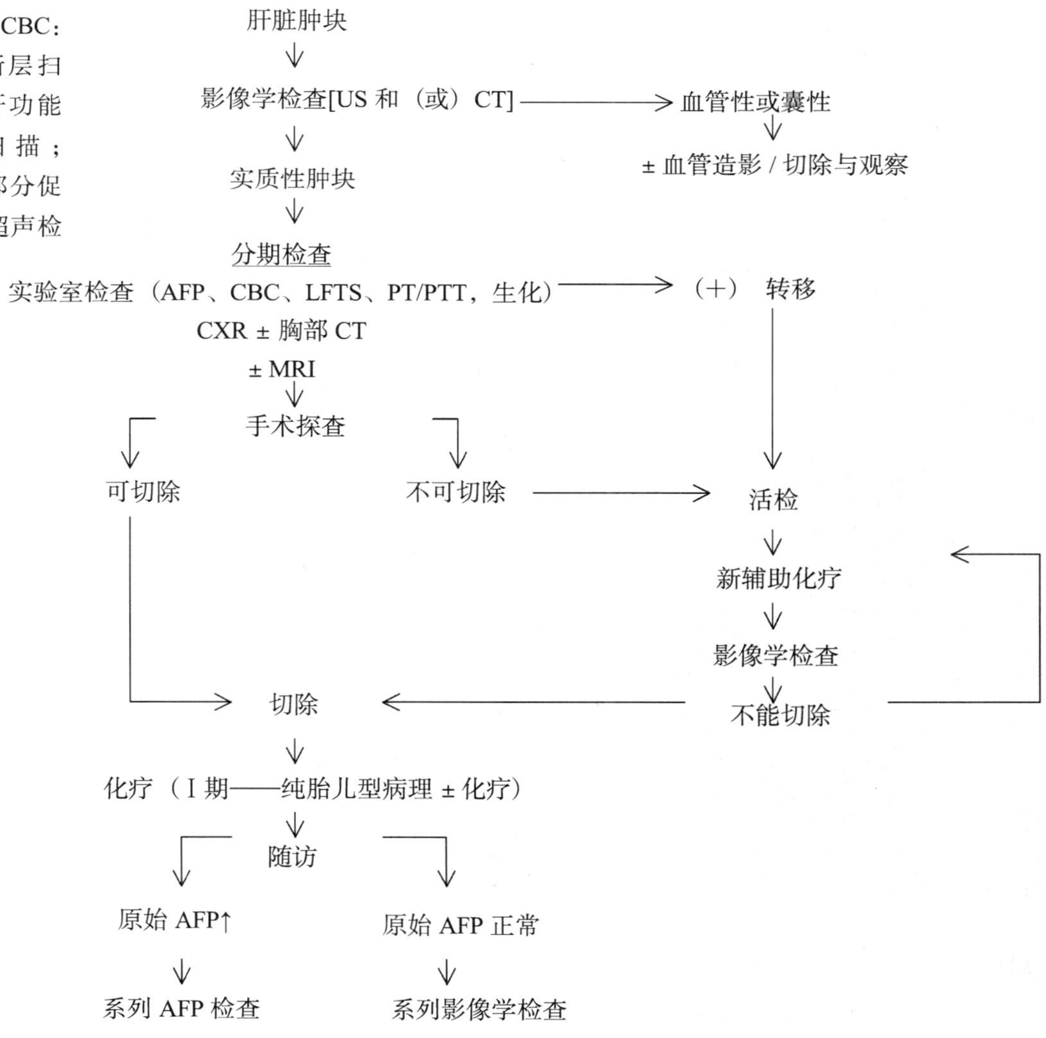

检查应明确肿瘤的大小、部位，评估转移病灶，决定是否存在门静脉、肝静脉或下腔静脉血管浸润。虽然先进的影像学检查提高了预测手术可切除性的能力，但是最终由外科医生在手术中决定。

超声有助于最初评估血管浸润情况。肝脏病变在超声中分成实性的、囊性的和血管性的。肝脏恶性肿瘤超声检查通常表现为边界清的高回声（实性）病变[15]。彩色多普勒超声有助于诊断血管瘤栓和肿瘤内的血管分流[68]。术中超声用来辅助诊断血管浸润和肿瘤可切除性。

血管和胃肠道对照增强 CT 扫描有益于描述肿瘤的类型、大小、部位和检测局部淋巴结肿大。腹部 CT 显示低衰减的肿块。在复杂病例需要非标准手术切除，可以进行螺旋 CT 和三维重建。

核磁共振和磁共振血管成像术特别有助于判断肿瘤和肝脏血管以及胆道解剖之间的联系。肝脏肿瘤在 T1 加权像为同质的低密度，在 T2 加权像为高密度[5]。三维重建可明显提高手术医生预测肿瘤可切除性的能力（图 30–2）。

在过去，用血管造影来检查肝脏血管的解剖结构，随着磁共振和增强 CT 的运用，血管造影已很少用来诊断评估肝脏恶性肿瘤。血管造影作为介入疗法在有些病例需要选择性化疗栓塞时运用。

鉴别诊断和组织学

诊断最后通过经皮穿刺、腹腔镜或开放活检获得。细针抽吸活检可以获得诊断。有些治疗小组根据临床表现高度提示肝母细胞瘤或肝细胞癌首先给予新辅助化疗[13]。然而，鉴于临床上有太多的误诊，我们强调所有病例均行活检[19]。

儿童原发肝脏良性和恶性肿瘤的分布见表 30–2。肝母细胞瘤和肝细胞癌均为上皮来源，占肝脏恶性肿 50
瘤的 90%以上[76]。原发肝脏肿瘤也可间质来源，肉瘤多见。未分化的胚胎肉瘤和横纹肌肉瘤通常发生在 5～10 岁的儿童。他们的甲胎蛋白水平正常，波形纤维蛋白染色阳性[74]。其他恶性肿瘤包括恶性转化的间质错构瘤[58]、血管肉瘤、胆管癌、横纹样瘤[59]、未成熟畸胎瘤和绒毛膜癌[69]。肝脏转移性病变在儿童相对

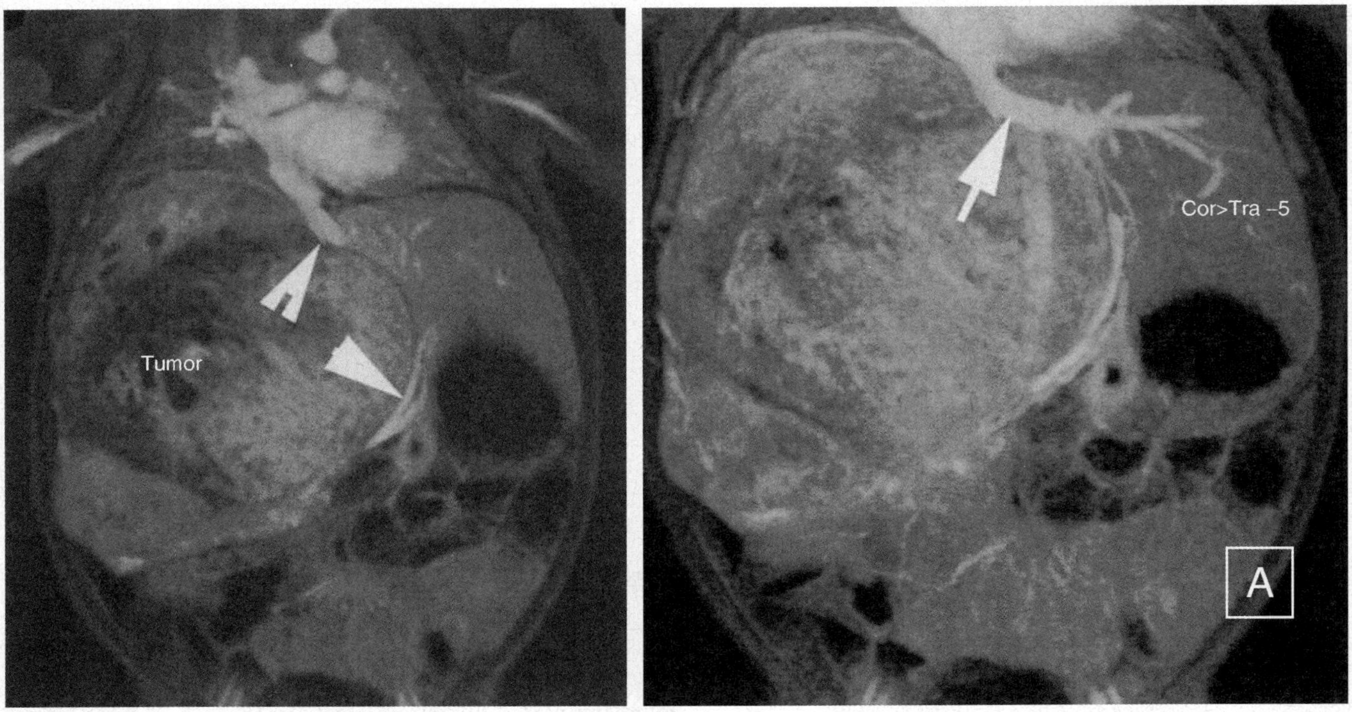

A　　B

图 30–2 A. 核磁共振证实的一位 6 个月大的婴儿的右侧肝脏的 10cm 肿块。B. 核磁共振血管造影三维重建可以旋转并显示血管解剖。推移压迫肝内腔静脉腔证实，肿块不能切除。

表 30-2 儿童原发性肝脏肿瘤的发生率

肿瘤	病人的%
恶性	
肝母细胞瘤	43
肝细胞癌	23
肉瘤	6
良性	
良性血管肿瘤	13
间质错构瘤	6
腺瘤	2
局部结节增生	2
其他	5

Adapted from Weinberg AG, Finegold MJ: Primary hepatic tumors of Childhood. Hum Pathol 1983;14:512-537.

少见。

肝母细胞瘤组织分型在预后评估中作用较小。统一的标准还未制定，但大多数儿童病理医生简化分型为上皮型和混合型（上皮和间质）。上皮型分为婴儿型、胚胎型、巨梁型和小细胞未分化型[60]。小细胞未分化组织类型预后不良[22]。相反，纯婴儿型（PFH）分裂活性低（400 倍镜下小于 2 个有丝分裂 /10 个镜下视野），其无病存活率显著提高（图 30-3）[49,76]。事实上，对于儿童纯婴儿型肝母细胞瘤，完整切除后，COG 不再提倡常规进行辅助化疗。

对于肝细胞癌，有些研究者提出，纤维板层类型患者手术切除率高，预后比其他类型好[12,33]。然而，Katzenstein 等人[30]观察到，尽管中位存活时间延长，但纤维板层类型和其他细胞类型之间进行分期对分期比较时没有差异。

分期

已提出许多有关肝母细胞瘤和肝细胞癌分期系统。目前美国 POG 和德国儿童肝脏肿瘤研究协作组采用的分期系统见表 30-3[21,49]。这个分期系统的核心是建立在术后疾病进展情况基础上的。大约 5%的肝母细胞瘤可完整切除（Ⅰ期），为低有丝分裂活性的 PFH[49]。残余肿瘤定义为肿瘤镜下残余（Ⅱ期）、肉眼残留（Ⅲ期）或肝外病灶或转移（Ⅳ期）。大约

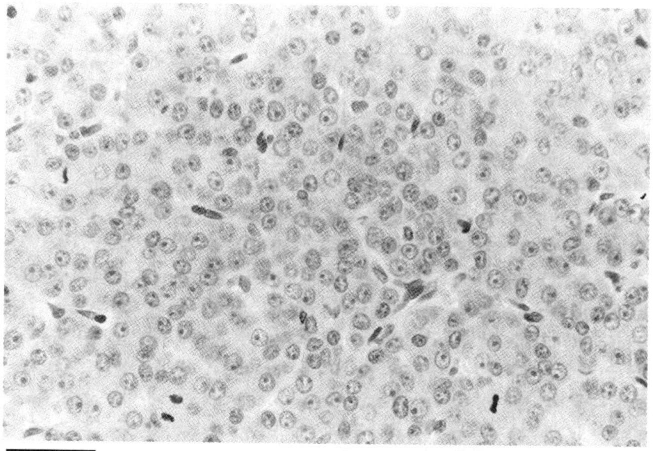

图 30-3 显微镜下照片证实、纯胎儿样组织学（PFH）伴低的有丝分裂活性（400 倍镜下小于 2 个有丝分裂 /10 个镜下视野）。在Ⅰ期肝母细胞瘤中，PFH 明显与良好的无事件存活率相关。

20%的肝母细胞瘤在诊断时已有远处转移[21,49,56,65]。肝细胞癌通常比肝母细胞瘤表现为更快的分期进展[13,29]。尽管 POG 分期系统对术后预后评估有意义，但不能提供术前疾病程度的信息。

为了评估新辅助化疗前后的肿瘤反应及可切除性，国际儿童肿瘤协会 SIOP 发展了 PRETEXT（治疗前疾病进展情况）分期系统[13,57]。PRETEXT 分期系统采用放射检查发现和描述肿瘤侵犯的肝段数目及位置，考虑到肝静脉和门静脉的浸润以及肝外浸润及远处转移情况（图 30-4）。例如，Ⅲ组、p、m 肿瘤为 4
段中 3 段被肿瘤浸润，向门静脉内生长和转移。这个 506
分期系统使得肿瘤科医生能够比较肿瘤对各种不同新辅助化疗方案的反应。其他肝母细胞瘤的分期系统包括日本小儿外科医生协会和 TNM 分期系统[62]。

在儿童，肝细胞癌同样运用 POG 和 PRETEXT 分期系统[13,29]。在成人，Okuda 和 Barcelona 临床分期

表 30-3 母细胞瘤和肝细胞癌的分期

分期	定义
Ⅰ*	完全切除
Ⅱ	镜下残余肿瘤
Ⅲ	肉眼残余肿瘤
Ⅳ	远处转移

* Ⅰ期肝母细胞瘤可以分为：（1）低的有丝分裂活性的纯胎儿型；（2）其他组织类型。

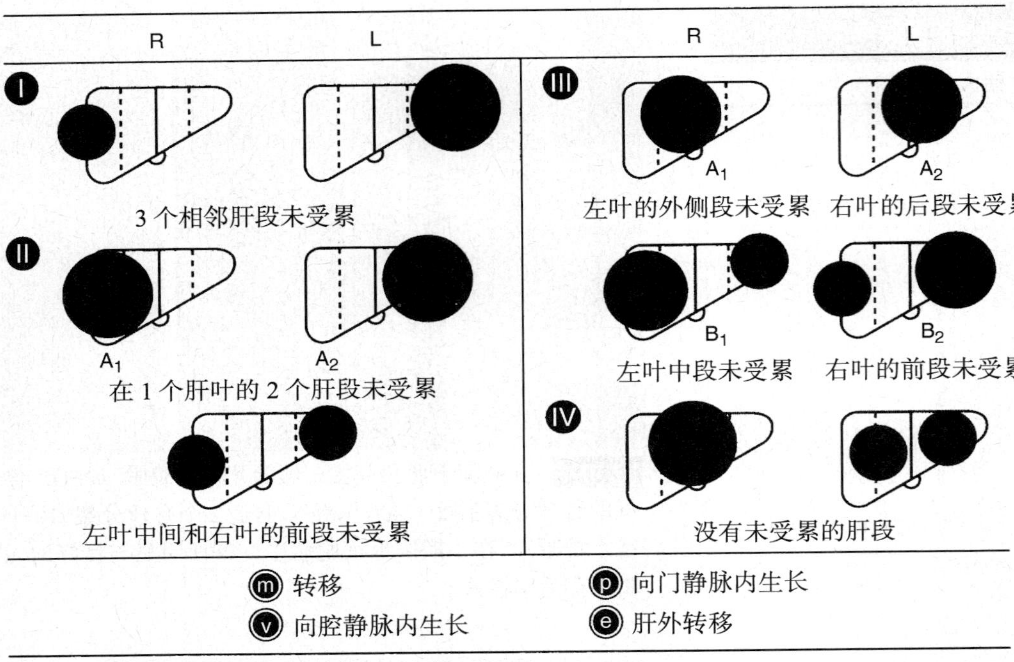

图 30-4 SIOP 治疗前分期系统（PRETEXT）：描述以侵犯肝段数目为基础的肝脏累及程度，并考虑转移（m）、腔静脉（v）和门静脉（p）瘤栓生长和肝外浸润（e）。

系统[38,48]被运用，该系统考虑了肿瘤浸润的程度和肝脏疾病的严重程度。

手术

手术的最初目的是完全解剖切除。肿瘤切除可因为各种缘故而放弃，如多个病灶、两叶浸润、门静脉或下腔静脉瘤栓、血管浸润、腹主动脉旁淋巴结肿大、肝门浸润和远处转移。中央型肿瘤肝静脉累及妨碍了肿瘤安全切除。通常来说，应该避免非解剖学上的肝切除，因为这样做肿瘤不完全切除率高且易局部复发[20]。当病理证实术后镜下肿瘤残存时，如果能够解剖学上切除，那么再次手术切除浸润边缘是有指征的。

成功的肝切除需要仔细的规划和支持护理。有一个具有经验的儿科麻醉医生是基本的。手术的第一步是放置可靠的大口径的静脉插管、动脉监测和辅助的外周静脉插管。病人的体位应该使手术医生能够术中达到颈部、胸部、腹部和腹股沟。如果需要另外的路径或更大的暴露，这些部位的消毒很容易做到。Trendlenburg 体位（头低仰卧位）能够降低腔静脉和肝静脉压力并减少空气栓塞的风险。

最初肋缘下切口能用来评估肿瘤部位和范围。腹部仔细探查有无术前检查可能没有发现的转移病灶。一旦决定进行手术切除，切口延长至整个腹部。在较大年龄儿童，切口中线延伸到剑突有利于更好地暴露肿瘤和肝脏。

肝脏和肿瘤通过解剖韧带完全游离，三角韧带分离从左肝静脉到终点左侧横膈。肝脏右叶从右侧横膈托出，电灼处理裸露的附着韧带。当肝脏从切口托出后，与右侧肾上腺附着组织韧带及膈下下腔静脉的几支分支处理后完全游离肝脏。

接下来游离肝下下腔静脉，使肾静脉以上的腔静脉到与肝实质连接处血管环形游离，并用血管环进行控制。肝脏完全游离后，确定最后的肝脏切除计划。通过 Winslow 孔用双手触摸肝门组织了解肿瘤浸润的情况以及经常碰到的血管异常。肝后下腔静脉需要评估其在肝实质中的部位及肿瘤有无浸润情况。最后仔细评估肿瘤和肝静脉之间的关系。术前影像学增强检查和术中超声可以精确地进行这些评估。未预见的保留肝静脉的浸润会造成切除缘残留、严重的术中出血和术后肝静脉损伤引起急性门脉高压所致的肝功能衰竭（Budd-Chiari 综合征）。当这些评估完成后，游离的肿瘤和肝脏可以进行所要求的切除。手术方式包括标准的左或右肝叶切除术，扩大的左、右肝叶切除术或极少数病例所需的根据解剖进行中央或节段切除。

在所有病例中解剖顺序相似。当肿瘤和肝脏游离以后，手术医生决定肿瘤的可切除性，重点放在肝门血管结构的解剖。在接近十二指肠和胰腺十二指肠动脉分支的末端明确肝动脉、胆总管和门静脉。胆囊从肝脏解剖出来，结扎胆囊管。随后解剖胆总管、肝动脉和门静脉，确定和结扎需切除段或肝叶和肿瘤的血供。当肝动脉和门静脉分支结扎后，会出现明显的分界引导肝实质切除。

肝门解剖完成后，重点放在肝后下腔静脉。肝脏和肿瘤转向左侧，暴露腔静脉走向。从末端开始仔细地解剖腔静脉至肝静脉上方。腔静脉从肝实质游离以后，许多小的成对的分支血管能被确认解剖和结扎。在有些困难的病例，运用 Pringle 手法，阻断保留的肝门脉管结构和膈上或膈下腔静脉有利于解剖。肝门结构的阻断时间限制在 15 分钟，总共阻断时间不超过 60 分钟。这部分手术的最终目的是：需要完全游离除了主要的肝静脉以外的腔静脉。

血管解剖的最后部分是确认和分离适当的肝静脉。左、中、右肝静脉起源非常靠近肝脏表面。直到汇合至心房，静脉的路径非常短。在手术切除之前，肝静脉浸润情况的准确评估非常重要。术中超声对于这些重要结构手术路径的设计非常有帮助。因为肝静脉分支进入肝组织后走行陡直，如果肿瘤边缘允许，可以采用肝实质内分离血管这种较为安全的技术。在肝静脉远端在肝脏表面用电灼标记指导分离肝实质，这比试图在肝外结扎静脉安全。

当肿瘤或解剖原因不允许肝实质内解剖肝静脉时，需要更大范围地暴露和细致解剖分离肝静脉。通常这可以延迟一直到大部分实质解剖完成及标本接近切下准备送至病理医生时。当手术医生很难控制肝静脉时，要毫不犹豫控制膈上腔静脉。

完成血管的解剖后，可以看到线状分界线引导肝实质的解剖。通常用电灼做 3～5mm 深的环状线形标记。在先前解剖的肝门结构和通过先前确定的控制肝静脉路径时，肝实质的解剖要尤为小心。麻醉医生在这时要准备好因肝实质解剖造成的大量失血的处理。标准肝实质手术采用钝性手指剥离或结扎术中的肝实质束，结扎缝合，以及切断实质暴露出血管和胆管。按照手术医生的个人爱好，超声刀（Ethicon 内镜手术，Cincinnati，俄亥俄），Integra 超音波手术吸引器或 Tissuelink 刀都有利于解剖。尽管这些设备可用作精确解剖，但是成功且相对出血少的分离肝实质关键是：在分离肝实质前的完整的血管解剖。

认识 Couinard 描述的肝脏三维节段解剖（图30–5）是肝切除计划的基本（图 30–6）。节段切除包括单个段的切除。肝右叶切除包括：切除Ⅴ、Ⅵ、Ⅶ、Ⅷ段和结扎肝右动脉、门静脉右支、右肝管和右肝静脉。通过胆囊窝和腔静脉连线间的肝中裂分离肝脏实质。508
大的末梢分支和供应这些节段的肝中静脉小的分支都要分离出来。扩大的肝右叶切除（右三肝切除）包括Ⅰ、Ⅳ、Ⅴ至Ⅷ段。肝右和肝中静脉要分离。肝脏实质的分离沿着镰状韧带和左叶间裂。另外，左肝动脉分支、门静脉和通向Ⅰ和Ⅳ段的肝胆管都要结扎。

左叶切除包括切除Ⅱ、Ⅲ、Ⅳ段和结扎左肝动脉、左门静脉、左肝胆管和左肝静脉。肝实质由肝中裂分离。通向Ⅳ段的肝中静脉的分支也要分离。左外侧肝叶切除包括Ⅱ、Ⅲ段。左肝动脉分支、门静脉和通向这些肝段的肝胆管要结扎。扩大的左肝叶切除（左三肝切除）包括Ⅰ至Ⅳ段、Ⅴ和Ⅷ段。肝实质沿着肝右裂分离。结扎左肝动脉、左门静脉、左肝胆管和左、中肝静脉。通向Ⅴ、Ⅷ段的右肝动脉、右门静脉和右肝胆管的分支需要结扎。

如果肿瘤仅浸润Ⅳ、Ⅴ和Ⅷ段，可进行中肝叶切除[34]。在脐部裂隙分离左门静脉进入Ⅳ段的分支。肝中静脉和右前扇形蒂带结扎。中肝叶切除具有保护正常肝实质的优点（不管Ⅰ–Ⅱ段还是Ⅵ–Ⅶ段），这些在标准解剖手术时都需切除（例如扩大右或左肝切除术）。

当肿瘤采用标准手术不能切除，新的技术正在运用。当肿瘤浸润肝静脉或下腔静脉时，肝静脉的重建采用门静脉或人工合成移植物[9]。当所有肝静脉都被浸润时，有一个方法是通过肝下静脉流出通路，切除除了Ⅴ和Ⅵ节段的所有节段（我们没有这项技

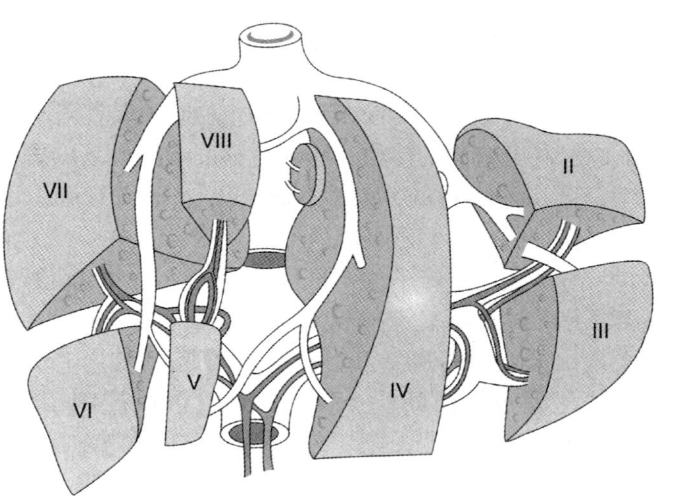

图 30–5　Couinard 描述的肝脏分段的解剖。

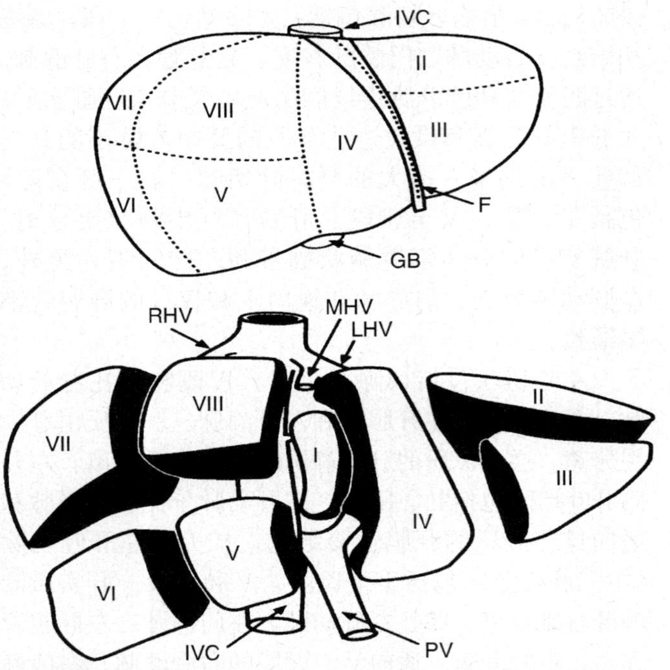

图 30-6 按肝脏节段解剖为基础的肝脏标准解剖切除。左叶切除（以往的左侧节段切除）切除Ⅱ和Ⅲ段。左肝切除Ⅱ、Ⅲ和Ⅳ节段。扩大的左肝切除Ⅱ、Ⅲ、Ⅳ、Ⅴ和Ⅷ（偶尔Ⅰ）。右肝切除Ⅴ、Ⅵ、Ⅶ和Ⅷ节段。扩大的右肝切除（以前右三肝切除）Ⅳ、Ⅴ、Ⅵ、Ⅶ和Ⅷ（偶然Ⅰ）。GB：胆囊；IVC：下腔静脉；LHV：左肝静脉；MHV：肝中静脉；PV：门静脉；RHV：右肝静脉。

术的亲身经验）[67]。

在大多数具有挑战性的病例，运用成为肝移植方法的体外切除法。回心血量通过静脉分流得到保护。肝切除后，肝脏用 Wisconsin 大学保护液灌注，放置在冰盒中，在再移植前，进行肿瘤切除和肝静脉-腔静脉重建[24]。

完全切除后，可以充分进行止血。尤其注意保留下的肝脏毛糙面的渗血和胆漏。在肝上和肝下放置引流。肝切除术后的并发症包括出血、肝下脓肿、胆瘘、伤口感染和胆道梗阻。

麻醉和手术技术的明显进步提高了手术切除率并可将围术期的死亡率降低至小于 5%。如果手术并发大量出血，阻断肝上和肝下下腔静脉，结合 Pringle 手法达到全血阻断[37]。手术切除前可以控制出血。血管夹可以处理肝血管，减少手术时间和出血量[77]。血管夹、超声刀、激光、振荡刀、手指分离、锐性解剖、Kelly 钳都可以分离肝实质。氩气刀和纤维胶可以控制残留肝脏断面出血。成人腹腔镜肝切除已有报道[45]，在儿童有潜在运用的可能。

标准解剖的手术切除导致大部分肝实质丢失：右叶扩大切除 85%，右叶切除 65%，左叶切除 35%，节段或楔形切除 3%～15%。大多数儿童残留的正常肝实质通过代偿性增生易适应手术切除。然而，新生儿肝脏未成熟，特别容易发展成为术后肝功能不全，表现为低血糖、低蛋白血症和低凝血酶原血症。这需要保持静脉输液含 10%的葡萄糖。术后第一周添加白蛋白和维生素 K。2～3 天后可口服。化疗在扩大肝切除术后或损伤的肝功能出现适当的再生前的患者通常暂停 3 周。

肝移植

最终达 6%的肝母细胞瘤患者需要原位肝移植（图 30-7）[23,54]。表现为肝脏所有四个部分浸润或三个部分浸润但不能通过部分肝切除手术来完全切除肿瘤的儿童，都是肝移植的对象。肝移植的禁忌证是化疗后存在肝外病变。

有些报道描述了儿童肝移植后预后良好[1,3,32,51,52,54,61]。肝母细胞瘤新辅助化疗后进行肝移植的儿童患者，10 年存活率达到 85%[51]。在以往尝试肝切除的儿童，肿瘤复发较常见。患儿部分肝切除后进行挽救性肝移植的 5 年最终存活率为 30%～50%。最初手术后切缘阳性与极其不良预后相关。这些资料说明应该避免过激性的部分肝切除，当完全切除存在问题时，应考虑肝移植[51]。

对肝细胞癌来说，肝移植不仅具有完全切除肿瘤的优点，而且还能切除整个瘤体周围的病变肝脏这一理论性优点。许多中心对单个肿瘤为 5cm 或小于 5cm 或三个节结为 3cm 或小于 3cm 的肝细胞癌患者严格限制肝移植[39]。在成人肝细胞癌肝移植后，5 年最终存活率为 60%～70%[48]。

尸体供肝的缺乏，尤其在儿童组，导致进行活体供肝节段移植或劈裂式尸肝移植。活体亲缘关系供体的肿瘤患者肝移植与提高的移植存活率及预后相关[76]。这些病人全肝切除包括切除肝后下腔静脉。这些病例不鼓励进行劈肝移植。在节段移植的病例，腔静脉的重建可以用保存的同种异体的髂静脉或来源于活体供体的颈内静脉[8,41]。移植的缺点在于：相应

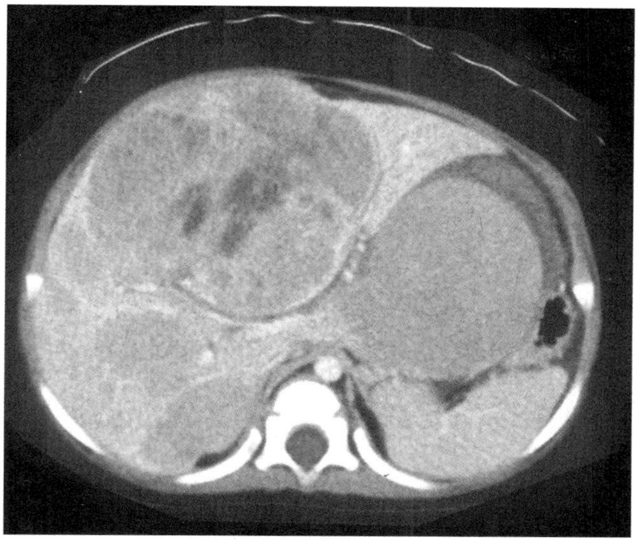

A

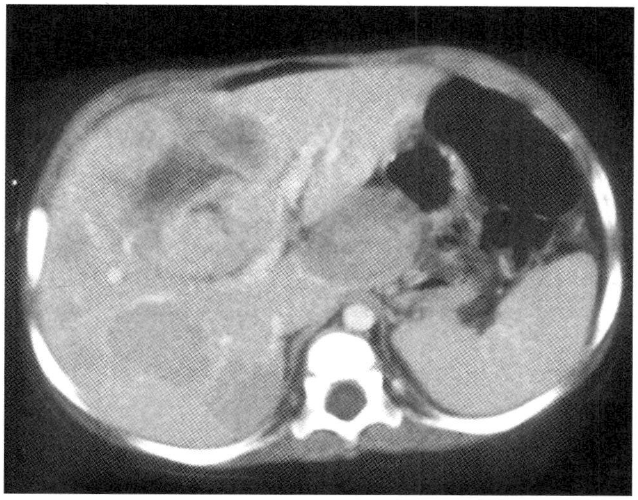

B

图 30–7　CT 扫描证实多病灶的肝母细胞瘤。尽管对化疗很敏感，但是肝移植是治愈的唯一希望。

的费用和一生免疫抑制的风险，可增加肿瘤复发和继发恶性肿瘤。

辅助化疗

尽管最终治愈需要完全手术切除，但肝母细胞瘤和肝细胞癌的辅助化疗仍是主要手段。新辅助化疗用于降低疾病分期、提高完全切除率和最终提高长期存活率[16]。新辅助化疗的缺点在于：治疗不敏感时造成疾病进展，最终肿瘤分期上升或变成无法切除。因而，运用新辅助化疗时需要常规进行影像学和血清甲胎蛋白监测来评估肿瘤的反应性。

化疗有许多方案。治疗结果同顺铂、阿霉素相比，采用顺铂、长春新碱和 5–FU 的治疗结果的相应副作用小[29,49]。SIOP 采用顺铂和阿霉素，且减低阿霉素的剂量后能有较好的顺应性[13]。德国研究组采用顺铂、异环磷酰胺和阿霉素作为化疗方案[21]。治疗结果同 SIOP 相似，但毒性作用较大。VP–16 和卡铂治疗复发和无反应病变。早期报道提出，伊立替康有望成为治疗复发以及难治性肝母细胞瘤的化疗药物[31,35]。应用抗血管生成药物，包括抗血管内皮生长因子抗体和拓扑替康，在肝脏肿瘤实验中能够降低肿瘤的体积[42,43]。

新辅助化疗可显著提高肝母细胞瘤的切除率，但对于儿童肝细胞癌预后影响不明显。50%～70%的III期肝母细胞瘤新辅助化疗后能够切除[49]。但是在III期肝细胞癌中只有 10%～36%经过化疗后能够切除（图 30–8）[13,29]。

放疗在肝母细胞瘤和肝细胞癌治疗中的作用有限。目前综合治疗方案中儿童残余肿瘤给予放疗。然而，最终目的是完整切除，因为后者才是唯一有效的治愈方法。

为了减少标准辅助化疗的全身副作用，新的毒性低的治疗方案仍在探索中。一种选择性作用于肿瘤靶细胞的策略是自杀基因疗法[27]。这个方法涉及一个基因的表达，后者能够只有在肿瘤细胞内把一种膜通透无毒性前药物转变成毒性药物（自杀药物）。举个例子，肝母细胞瘤体内模型运用复制缺陷的腺病毒运载自杀基因，如大肠埃杆菌胞嘧啶[7,28,47]。转录控制因素如甲胎蛋白被用来在肿瘤细胞内选择性表达自杀基因。 511

消融治疗

对病灶不能解剖切除和不能进行肝移植的患者可以采用局部消融治疗，包括化疗栓塞、射频消融法、经病情皮注射乙醇和冷冻疗法[2,35,64]。消融治疗能够减轻和延长存活时间但不能达到治愈。消融治疗可以作为移植的桥梁直到有合适的供体。

射频消融法运用电极针头插入肿瘤内释放变化的不同波长的射频微波引起局部高温损伤。大的病灶需要多次重叠运用，每次持续 10～20 分钟。

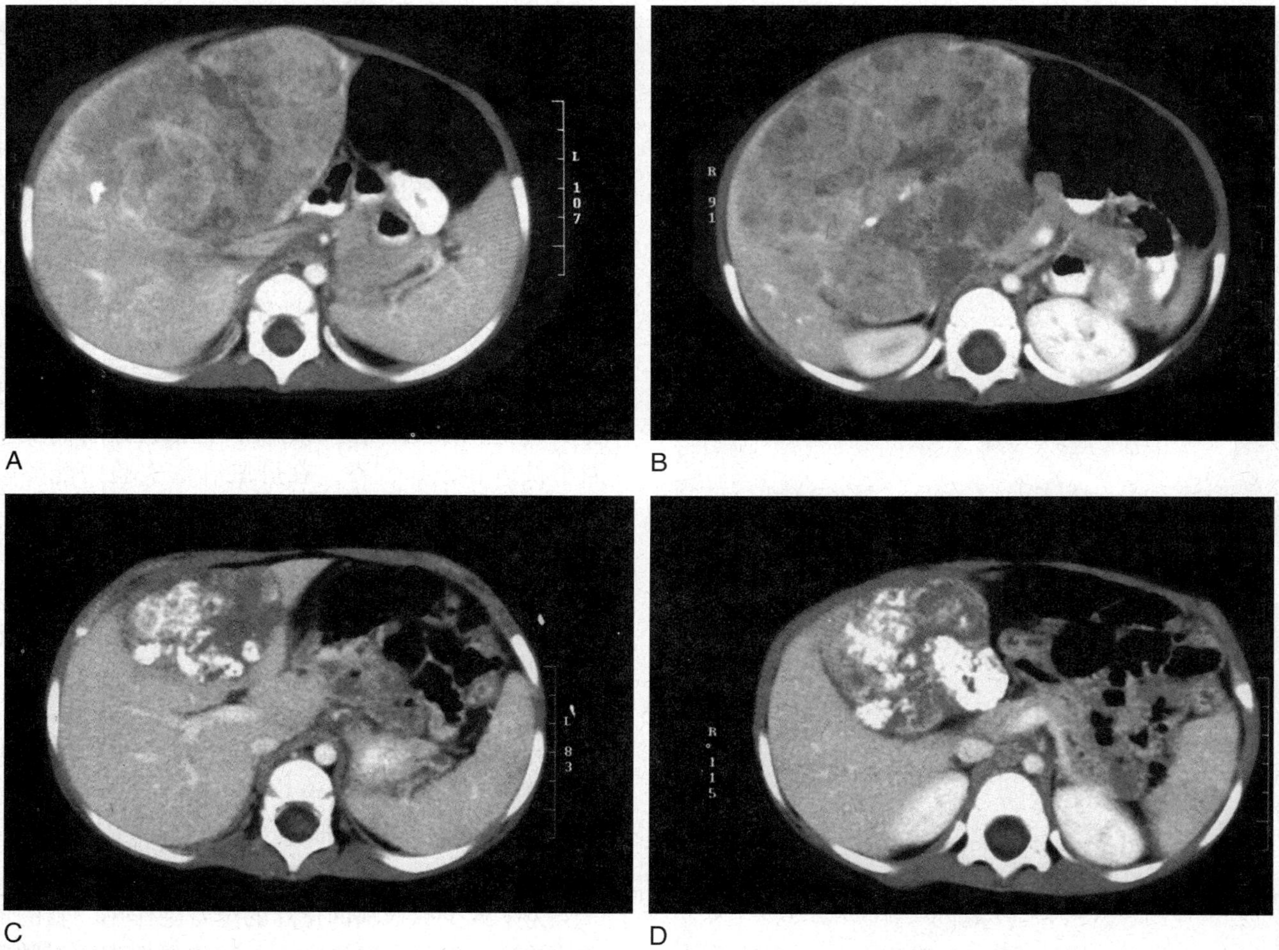

图 30–8　新辅助化疗可以显著减小肿瘤体积，并最后可致安全顺利地进行肝叶切除。化疗后可以看到明显的钙化，门静脉右支清晰可见。

冷冻疗法运用直接冻融引起细胞蛋白质变质、细胞膜破裂和低氧至细胞死亡。在手术中，Pringle 手法可以降低大血管通过或靠近消融部位的热效应。通常两次冷冻循环持续 15～20 分钟伴自行解冻。消融治疗的目标包含正常组织边缘 1cm，这可以通过超声确诊，射频消融存在微小泡回声，冷冻疗法为回声扩大的圆形缘。

肝内动脉化疗栓塞可以潜在提高化疗的反应和使对侧肝脏增生。操作过程包括血管造影并在肿瘤主要滋养动脉放置插管。阿霉素稀释在碘化剂中，顺铂灌注，然后用明胶海绵栓塞[53]。肿瘤内药物浓度可以达到常规化疗的 50～400 倍而不提高药物全身毒性作用。关于儿童化疗栓塞的报道有限，但在有些病例可以达到手术切除[4,40,53]。化疗栓塞的并发症包括肝动脉栓子和胃溃疡。当移植前全身新辅助化疗失败时可以运用化疗栓塞[4]。

预后及随访

一些机构报道，肝母细胞瘤 5 年存活率从 30 年前的 35%显著提高到 75%[14,17,50,57,65]。肝细胞癌的预后极其差，5 年最终存活率小于 18%～28%[13,29]。病灶成功切除者预后良好，肝母细胞瘤 5 年存活率达 91%～100%，肝细胞癌达 30%～54%[10,13,49,57,73]。国际肝肿瘤研究组 5 年无病存活率总结结果见表 30–4。德国儿童肝脏肿瘤协作组报道的肝母细胞瘤无病存活率相似（平均随访时间 58 个月），Ⅰ期（27 例）为 89%，Ⅱ期（3 例）为 100%，Ⅲ期（25 例）为 68%，Ⅵ期（14 例）为 21%[21]。

肝母细胞瘤和肝细胞癌如存在转移疾病，则预后差[10,13,21]。肝细胞癌中多叶、肿瘤大、对化疗反应差都是预后差的因素[13]。尽管转移病灶显示预后差，但有些转移病灶对化疗敏感。有些病人肺部病灶

表 30-4 估计的肝母细胞瘤和肝细胞癌 5 年无事件存活率

分期	肝母细胞瘤	肝细胞癌
Ⅰ（纯胎儿型）	100%（n=9）	
Ⅰ（其他组织类型）	91%（n=43）	
Ⅰ（肝细胞癌）		88%（n=8）
Ⅱ	100%（n=7）	—（n=0）
Ⅲ	64%（n=83）	8%（n=25）
Ⅳ	25%（n=40）	0%（n=13）

Data adapted from Ortega JA, Dougless EC, Feusner JH, et al: Randomized comparison of cisplatin/vincristine/Auorouracil and cisplatin/continuous infusion doxorubicin for treatment of pediatric hepatoblastoma: A report from the Children' s Cancer Group and the Pediatric Oncology Group. J Clin Oncol 2000;18: 2665-2675; and Katzenstein HM, Krailo MD, Malogolowkin MH, et al: Hepatocellular carcinoma in children and adolescents: Results from the Pediatric Oncology Group and the Children' s Cancer Group Intergroup Study. J Clin Oncol 2002;20: 2789-2797.

化疗后持续存在可考虑肺切除。

肝切除术后，大多数病人接受术后化疗。患者需要密切随访以确保甲胎蛋白水平恢复至正常水平，以及肿瘤没有复发。甲胎蛋白水平正常的患者，可用超声和 CT 系列检查筛查肿瘤的复发。

结论

麻醉、手术技术和化疗的进步使儿童肝母细胞瘤的预后得到显著提高。肝细胞癌预后仍很差。肝移植对于肿瘤不能切除者的患者是有用的。为了取得肝脏恶性肿瘤治疗的进步，需要多机构儿童肿瘤研究组的继续合作。

（徐　敏译　王　珊校）

致谢

We are grateful to Marcio Malogolowkin, MD, chair of the Liver Tumor Subcommittee of the Children's Oncology Group and director of the Bone and Soft Tissue Tumor Program at Children's Hospital, Los Angeles, for his review of the manuscript.

参考文献

1. Achilleos OA, Buist LJ, Kelly DA, et al: Unresectable hepatic tumors in childhood and the role of liver transplantation. J Pediatr Surg 1996;31:1563-1567.
2. Ahrar K, Gupta S: Hepatic artery embolization for hepatocellular carcinoma: Technique, patient selection, and outcomes. Surg Oncol Clin N Am 2003;12:105-126.
3. Al-Qabandi W, Jenkinson H, Buckels JA, et al: Orthotopic liver transplantation for unresectable hepatoblastoma: A single center's experience. J Pediatr Surg 1999;34:1261-1264.
4. Arcement CM, Towbin RB, Meza MP, et al: Intrahepatic chemoembolization in unresectable pediatric liver malignancies. Pediatr Radiol 2000;30:779-785.
5. Boechat MI, Kangarloo H, Ortega J, et al: Primary liver tumors in children: Comparison of CT and MR imaging. Radiology 1988;169:727-732.
6. Buendia MA: Genetic alterations in hepatoblastoma and hepatocellular carcinoma: Common and distinctive aspects. Med Pediatr Oncol 2002;39:530-535.
7. Cao G, Kuiryama S, Gao J, et al: Gene therapy for hepatocellular carcinoma based on tumour-selective suicide gene expression using the alpha-fetoprotein (AFP) enhancer and a housekeeping gene promoter. Eur J Cancer 2001; 37:140-147.
8. Chang MH, Chen CJ, Lai MS, et al: Universal hepatitis B vaccination in Taiwan and the incidence of hepatocellular carcinoma in children. N Engl J Med 1997;336: 1855-1859.
9. Chardot C, Saint-Martin C, Gilles A, et al: Living related liver transplantation and vena cava reconstruction after total hepatectomy including vena cava for hepatoblastoma. Transplantation 2002;73:90-92.
10. Chen JC, Chen CC, Chen WJ, et al: Hepatocellular carcinoma in children: Clinical review and comparison with adult cases. J Pediatr Surg 1998;33:1350-1354.
11. Clericuzio CL, Chen E, McNeil DE, et al: Serum alphafetoprotein screening for hepatoblastoma in children with Beckwith-Wiedemann syndrome or isolate hemihyperplasia. J Pediatr 2003; 143:270-272.
12. Craig JR, Peters RL, Edmondson HA, et al: Fibrolamellar carcinoma of the liver; a tumor of adolescents and young adults with distinctive clinico-pathologic features. Cancer 1980;46:372-379.
13. Czauderna P, Mackinlay G, Perilongo G, et al: Hepatocellular carcinoma in children: Results of the first prospective study of the International Society of Pediatric Oncology group. J Clin Oncol 2002;20:2798-2804.
14. Darbari A, Sabin KM, Shapiro CN, et al: Epidemiology of primary hepatic malignancies in US children. Hepatology 2003;38:560-566.
15. de Campo M, de Campo JF: Ultrasound of primary hepatic tumours in children. Pediatr Radiol 1988;19:19-24.
16. Evans AE, Land VJ, Newton WA, et al: Combination chemotherapy (vincristine, Adriamycin, cyclophosphamide, and 5-fluorouracil) in the treatment of children with malignant hepatoma. Cancer 1982;50:821-826.
17. Exelby PR, Filler RM, Grosfeld JL: Liver tumors in children with particular reference to hepatoblastoma and hepatocellular carcinoma: American Academy of Pediatrics Surgical Section Survey—1974. J Pediatr Surg 1975;10: 329-337.

18. Feusner J, Plaschkes J: Hepatoblastoma and low birth weight: A trend or chance observation? Med Pediatr Oncol 2002;39:508-509.
19. Finegold MJ: Chemotherapy for suspected hepatoblastoma without efforts at surgical resection is a bad practice. Med Pediatr Oncol 2002;39:484-486.
20. Fuchs J, Rydzynski J, Hecker H, et al: The influence of preoperative chemotherapy and surgical technique in the treatment of hepatoblastoma—a report from the German Cooperative Liver Tumour Studies HB 89 and 94. Eur J Pediatr Surg 2002;12:255-261.
21. Fuchs J, Rydzynski J, Von Schweinitz D, et al: Pretreatment prognostic factors and treatment results in children with hepatoblastoma: A report from the German Cooperative Pediatric Liver Tumor Study HB 94. Cancer 2002;95:172-182.
22. Haas JE, Feusner JH, Finegold MJ: Small cell undifferentiated histology in hepatoblastoma may be unfavorable. Cancer 2001;92:3130-3134.
23. Helmberger TK, Ros PR, Mergo PJ, et al: Pediatric liver neoplasms: A radiologic-pathologic correlation. Eur Radiol 1999;9:1339-1347.
24. Hemming AW, Reed AI, Langhan MR, et al: Hepatic vein reconstruction for resection of hepatic tumors. Am Surg 2002;235:850-858.
25. Hughes LJ, Michels VV: Risk of hepatoblastoma in familial adenomatous polyposis. Am J Med Genet 1992;43:1023-1025.
26. Ikeda H, Hachitanda Y, Tanimura M, et al: Development of unfavorable hepatoblastoma in children of very low birth weight: Results of a surgical and pathologic review. Cancer 1998;82:1789-1796.
27. Kanai F: Transcriptional targeted gene therapy for hepatocellular carcinoma by adenovirus vector. Mol Biotechnol 2001;18:243-250.
28. Kanai F, Lan KH, Shiratori Y, et al: In vivo gene therapy for alpha-fetoprotein-producing hepatocellular carcinoma by adenovirus-mediated transfer of cytosine deaminase gene. Cancer Res 1997;47:561-565.
29. Katzenstein HM, Krailo MD, Malogolowkin MH, et al: Hepatocellular carcinoma in children and adolescents: Results from the Pediatric Oncology Group and the Children's Cancer Group Intergroup Study. J Clin Oncol 2002;20:2789-2797.
30. Katzenstein HM, Krailo MD, Malogolowkin MH, et al: Fibrolamellar hepatocellular carcinoma in children and adolescents. Cancer 2003;97:2006-2012.
31. Katzenstein HM, Rigsby C, Shaw PH, et al: Novel therapeutic approaches in the treatment of children with hepatoblastoma. J Pediatr Hematol Oncol 2002;24:751-755.
32. Koneru B, Flye MW, Bussutil RW, et al: Liver transplantation for hepatoblastoma: The American experience. Ann Surg 1991;213:118-121.
33. Lack EE, Neave C, Vawter GF: Hepatocellular carcinoma: Review of 32 cases in childhood and adolescence. Cancer 1983;52:1510-1515.
34. LaQuaglia MP, Shorter NA, Blumgart LH: Central hepatic resection for pediatric tumors. J Pediatr Surg 2002;37: 986-989.
35. Lau WY, Leung TW, Yu SC, et al: Percutaneous local ablative therapy for hepatocellular carcinoma: A review and look into the future. Ann Surg 2003;237:171-179.
36. Lee CL, Ko YC: Hepatitis B vaccination and hepatocellular carcinoma in Taiwan. Pediatrics 1997;99:351-353.
37. Liu DC, Vogel AM, Gulec S, et al: Hepatectomy in children under total hepatic occlusion. Am Surg 2003;69:539-541.
38. Llovet JM, Bru C, Bruix J: Prognosis of hepatocellular carcinoma: The BCLC staging classification. Semin Liver Dis 1999;19:329-338.
39. Llovet JM, Burroughs A, Bruix J: Hepatocellular carcinoma. Lancet 2003;362:1907-1917.
40. Malogolowkin MH, Stanley P, Steele DA, et al: Feasibility and toxicity of chemoembolization for children with liver tumors. J Clin Oncol 2000; 18:1279-1284.
41. Martinez JA, Rigamonti W, Rahier J, et al: Preserved vascular homograft for revascularization of pediatric liver transplant: A clinical, histological, and bacteriological study. Transplantation 1999;68:672-677.
42. McCrudden KW, Hopkins B, Frischer J, et al: Anti-VEGF antibody in experimental hepatoblastoma: Suppression of tumor growth and altered angiogenesis. J Pediatr Surg 2003;38:308-314.
43. McCrudden KW, Yokoi A, Thosani A, et al: Topotecan is anti-angiogenic in experimental hepatoblastoma. J Pediatr Surg 2002;37:857-861.
44. Molmenti EP, Wilkinson K, Molmenti H, et al: Treatment of unresectable hepatoblastoma with liver transplantation in the pediatric population. Am J Transplant 2002;2:535-538.
45. Morino M, Morra I, Rosso E, et al: Laparoscopic vs open hepatic resection: A comparative study. Surg Endosc 2003; 17:1914-1918.
46. Ni Y-H, Change M-H, Huang L-M, et al: Hepatitis B virus infection in children and adolescents in a hyperendemic area: 15 years after mass hepatitis B vaccination. Ann Intern Med 2001;135:796.
47. Ohashi M, Kanai F, Tateishi K, et al: Target gene therapy for alpha-fetoprotein-producing hepatocellular carcinoma by E1B55k-attenuated adenovirus. Biochem Biophys Res Commun 2001;282:529-535.
48. Okuda K, Ohtsuki T, Obata H, et al: Natural history of hepatocellular carcinoma and prognosis in relation to treatment: Study of 850 patients. Cancer 1985;56:918-928.
49. Ortega JA, Douglass EC, Feusner JH, et al: Randomized comparison of cisplatin/vincristine/fluorouracil and cisplatin/continuous infusion doxorubicin for treatment of pediatric hepatoblastoma: A report from the Children's Cancer Group and the Pediatric Oncology Group. J Clin Oncol 2000;18:2665-2675.
50. Ortega JA, Krailo MD, Hans JE, et al: Effective treatment of unresectable or metastatic hepatoblastoma with cisplatin and continuous infusion doxorubicin chemotherapy: A report from the Children's Cancer Study Group. J Clin Oncol 1991;9:2167.
51. Otte JB, Aronson DC, Brown J, et al: Liver transplantation for hepatoblastoma: Results from the International Society of Pediatric Oncology (SIOP) study SIOPEL-1 and review of the world experience. Pediatr Blood Cancer 2004; 42:74-83.
52. Otte JB, Aronson D, Vraux H, et al: Preoperative chemotherapy, major liver resection, and transplantation for primary malignancies in children. Transplant Proc 2001; 28:2393.
53. Oue T, Fukuzawa M, Kusafuka T, et al: Transcather arterial chemoembolization in the treatment of hepatoblastoma. J Pediatr Surg 1998;33:1771-1775.
54. Oue T, Kubota A, Okuyama H, et al: Hepatoblastoma in children of extremely low birth weight: A report from a single perinatal center. J Pediatr Surg 2003;38:134-137.
55. Palmer RD, Williams DM: Dramatic response of multiply relapsed hepatoblastoma to irinotecan (CPT-11). Med Pediatr Oncol 2003;41:78-80.
56. Perilongo G, Brown J, Shafford E, et al: Hepatoblastoma presenting with lung metastases: Treatment results of the first cooperative, prospective study of the International Society of Pediatric Oncology on childhood liver tumors. Cancer 2000;89:1845-1853.

57. Pritchard J, Brown J, Shafford E, et al: Cisplatin, doxorubicin, and delayed surgery for childhood hepatoblastoma: A successful approach—results of the first prospective study of the International Society of Pediatric Oncology. J Clin Oncol 2000;18:3819-3828.
58. Ramanujam TM, Ramesh JC, Goh DW, et al: Malignant transformation of mesenchymal hamartoma of the liver: Case report and review of the literature. J Pediatr Surg 1999:34:1684-1686.
59. Ravindra KV, Cullinane C, Lewis IJ, et al: Long-term survival after spontaneous rupture of a malignant rhabdoid tumor of the liver. J Pediatr Surg 2002;10:1488-1490.
60. Rowland JM: Hepatoblastoma: Assessment of criteria for histologic classification. Med Pediatr Oncol 2002:39: 478-483.
61. Ruck P, Xiao JC: Stem-like cells in hepatoblastoma. Med Pediatr Oncol 2002;39:504-507.
62. Sasaki F, Matsunaga T, Iwafuchi M, et al: Outcome of hepatoblastoma treated with the JPLT- 1 (Japanese Study Group for Pediatric Liver Tumor) Protocol-1: A report from the Japanese Study Group for Pediatric Liver Tumor. J Pediatr Surg 2002;37:851-856.
63. Sato M, Ishida H, Konno K, et al: Liver tumors in children and young patients: Sonographic and color Doppler findings. Abdom Imaging 2000;25:596-601.
64. Scaife CL, Curley SA: Complication, local recurrence, and survival rates after radiofrequency ablation for hepatic malignancies. Surg Oncol Clin N Am 2003;12:243-255.
65. Schnater JM, Aronson DC, Plaschkes J, et al: Surgical view of the treatment of patients with hepatoblastoma: Results from the first prospective trial of the International Society of Pediatric Oncology Liver Tumor Study Group. Cancer 2002;94:1111-1120.
66. Sindhi R, Rosendale J, Mundy D, et al: Impact of segmental grafts on pediatric liver transplantation: A review of the United Network for Organ Sharing Scientific Registry Data (1990-1996). J Pediatr Surg 1999;34:107-111.
67. Superina RA, Bambini D, Filler RM, et al: A new technique for resecting “unresectable” liver tumors. J Pediatr Surg 2000;35:1294-1299.
68. Surace C, Leszl A, Perilongo G, et al: Fluorescent in situ hybridization (FISH) reveals frequent and recurrent numerical and structural abnormalities in hepatoblastoma with no informative karyotype. Med Pediatr Oncol 2002; 39:536-539.
69. Szavay PO, Wermes C, Fuchs J, et al: Effective treatment of infantile choriocarcinoma in the liver with chemotherapy and surgical resection: A case report. J Pediatr Surg 2000; 35:1134-1135.
70. Tanimura M, Matsui I, Abe J, et al: Increased risk of hepatoblastoma among immature children with a lower birth weight. Cancer Res 1998;58:3032-3035.
71. Terracciano LM, Bernasconi B, Ruck P, et al: Comparative genomic hybridization analysis of hepatoblastoma reveals high frequency of X-chromosome gains and similarities between epithelial and stromal components. Hum Pathol 2003;34:864-871.
72. Tsuchida Y, Ikeda H, Suzuki N, et al: A case of well-differentiated, fetal-type hepatoblastoma with very low serum-alpha-fetoprotein. J Pediatr Surg 1999;12:1762-1764.
73. von Schweinitz D, Hadam MR, Welte K, et al: Production of interleukin-1β and interleukin-6 in hepatoblastoma. Int J Cancer 1993;53:728.
74. Webber EM, Morrison KB, Pritchard SL, et al: Undifferentiated embryonal sarcoma of the liver: Results of clinical management in one center. J Pediatr Surg 1999;34:1641-1644.
75. Weber RG, Pietsch T, von Schweinitz D, et al: Characterization of genomic alterations in hepatoblastomas: A role for gains on chromosomes 8q and 20 as predictors of poor outcome. Am J Pathol 2000;157:571-578.
76. Weinberg AG, Finegold MJ: Primary hepatic tumors of childhood. Hum Pathol 1983;14:512-537.
77. Yanaga K, Nishizaki T, Yamamoto K, et al: Simplified inflow control using stapling devices for major hepatic resection. Arch Surg 1996;131:104-106.
78. Zatkova A, Rouillard JM, Hartmann W, et al: Amplification and overexpression of the IGF2 regulator PLAG1 in hepatoblastoma. Genes Chromosomes Cancer 2004;39: 126-137.
79. Zimmerman A: Pediatric liver tumors and hepatic ontogenesis: Common and distinctive pathways. Med Pediatr Oncol 2002;39:492-503.

第 31 章

胃肠道肿瘤

Patrick A. Dillon 和 Robert P. Foglia

515 原发性胃肠道（GI）肿瘤在婴儿和儿童中相对少见。GI 恶性肿瘤大约占所有儿童肿瘤的 1.2%[4]。儿童 GI 肿瘤的临床表现和组织病理改变与成人明显不同。此外，虽然遗传学标志物的发现和免疫组化的应用使这些肿瘤能被更明确地鉴别，但同样的进展也使评价它们的真正发病率非常困难。

最常见的症状是非特异性的，包括腹痛、呕吐和便血。症状常在诊断前几个星期出现，出现肠道梗阻时可能需要急诊手术来解决[4,50]。虽然不是常见的诊断，但任何出现肠道梗阻、难治性腹痛和排便习惯改变或 GI 出血表现和症状的患儿必须考虑到 GI 恶性肿瘤的可能性。此外，肠道异常儿童必须接受详细的各种诊断性检查，包括肠道造影检查、超声检查、CT 和内镜检查，以明确诊断和疾病进展程度[31]。

胃肠道间质瘤

流行病学

胃肠间质肿瘤（GIST）是少见的 GI 肿瘤。由于命名、细胞来源和诊断标准不同，其发生率难以确定。已发表文献的病例数很少，良恶性肿瘤混杂，且没有区别原发和复发 GIST，故尚未进行分类[12]。此外，GIST 不管其解剖部位均被归为一类，因此很难预测它们的临床表现[57]。

发病的中位年龄在 50～60 岁；这些肿瘤在小于 40 岁的患者中少见。性别分布相等。最常见的原发部位是胃（50%～70%），其次是小肠（20%～30%）、结肠或直肠（10%）和食管（5%）。肠系膜和大网膜有时也可成为原发 GIST 的部位[39,43]。

GIST 目前分类为胃肠道的间充质肿瘤，被认为起源于肠道的 Cajal 细胞，后者是一种肠道的节律细胞[34]。过去，平滑肌肿瘤（例如平滑肌瘤和平滑肌肉瘤）和神经肿瘤（例如神经鞘膜瘤和恶性外周神经鞘瘤）亦被归类为 GIST。然而，根据组织学和免疫组化特征，现在将 GIST 与平滑肌源性肿瘤区别开来。

与其他疾病的相关性

在 1977，Carney 等人[7]报道了在无关系的年轻女性中，胃平滑肌肉瘤、功能性肾上腺外副神经节细胞瘤和肺软骨瘤的罕见相关性。患者的年龄较小、部位多发和多器官侵犯提示遗传性疾病的可能性，但迄今没有发现遗传学上的连锁性[6]。Carney 三联征的基本特征是胃间质瘤。这些肿瘤通常沿小弯或贲门分布，很少出现局部症状；进一步生长可以导致黏膜溃疡和胃肠道出血，浆膜受侵犯很常见。肿瘤的多发特征可出现局部复发以及广泛播散但进展缓慢的转移病灶。传统的辅助治疗用在转移性肿瘤的治疗是不成功的[6]。尽管在残留胃中有出现胃肿瘤的可能性，但如果可行，胃次全切除术可能是最好的手术方式，可以避免全胃切除术的并发症，特别是十几岁的患儿。做这种手术的患者必须被告知可能出现新的胃部肿瘤，建议每隔 3 年必须复查一次。对患有胃间质肉瘤或肺软骨瘤（或两者均有）的患者应考虑评估有无肾上腺肿 51
瘤，且应该询问 Carney 三联征患者的家族史。然而，目前尚不建议做家族性筛查和遗传咨询[6]。

已发现了 GIST 的一个亚型，通常称作胃肠道自主神经瘤（GANT）。在儿童人群中很少有 GANT 病例的报道。然而在少量该病患儿中以女性为主，症状可包括腹痛、腹胀、呕吐和可触及的腹部肿块[33]。

GANT 可出现于胃肠道的任何部位。在成人，小肠是最常见的发病部位。与 GIST 病例一样，当儿童出现 GANT 时，胃常为肿瘤的原发部位[33]。大多数患儿在诊断时病灶局限，治疗可选择手术切除。目前，化疗和放疗似乎尚无确切的作用。与成人比较，在儿童，病灶局限及诊断时肿块体积小可能是长期预后的有利因素。这些肿瘤与 GIST 鉴别需要免疫细胞化学和超微结构检查，且目前尚无针对儿童的恶性肿瘤的确诊标准[33]。

临床表现

在就诊时，大多数患者已出现一些症状，最常见的有全腹痛、消化不良和隐匿性胃肠道出血。在儿童中出现缺铁性贫血必须做进一步检查，以排除胃肠道源性的贫血[33]。患者较为少见的症状有腹部触及肿块或肠道梗阻[46]。标准的影像学检查有助于诊断，包括腹部平片和 CT；做全身氟脱氧葡萄糖正电子放射断层扫描检查（PET）也有重要的作用[13]。内镜能用来识别肿块，特别是如果肿瘤位于胃或近端的小肠时。

病理学

当免疫组化检查发现表达 KIT（CD117，干细胞因子受体）蛋白的胃肠道出现纺锤形、上皮样或偶尔呈多形性间充质肿瘤时，即可确诊为 GIST。其他细胞标记，如 CD34、平滑肌肌动蛋白、结合蛋白和 S-100 蛋白，用来作为 GIST 的诊断[39]。GIST 疗效的预测有赖于传统的病理学标准，如大小、分期、肿瘤侵犯黏膜或周围器官的程度、有丝分裂指数和核多形性。虽然这些标准对预测 GIST 预后有用，但没有任何单一指标能可靠的与临床预后相一致[27]。与恶性胃间质肿瘤相关的形态学特征包括肿瘤体积大于 7cm、细胞高度密集、黏膜侵犯和分裂象细胞计数在 50 个高倍视野中大于 5 个核分裂象。当区分良恶性胃间质肿瘤时，必须考虑所有这些因素[57]。最近，在 GIST 的 11 外显子的 *c-kit* 基因中发现一个突变。存在这种突变的患者与无突变的 GIST 患者比较，其复发危险性增大，死亡率更高[43]。

治疗

推荐的治疗方法是沿着任何可能存在的假包膜完全切除 GIST。虽然不必考虑扩大切缘，但完整切除可能要求切除整个或部分器官以获得干净的切缘[18]。达到病理切缘阴性一般不难，GIST 倾向于从原发器官悬挂生长，不会广泛浸润。因此，胃的楔形切除和肠道的节段切除已能提供足够的治疗；而广泛切除无明显益处[49]。此外，因为显微镜下切缘的状态对存活并不重要，所以如果能够完全切除肿瘤，则无必要切除重要的器官[12]。GIST 很少转移至淋巴结，因此很少做淋巴结切除术[46]。

局部和远处复发率高说明有必要作辅助治疗。GIST 一般对放疗和预先的所有全身治疗耐受。然而，伊马替尼有明显缩小肿瘤体积的作用，这改变了对 GIST 的治疗策略。伊马替尼是一个信号转导抑制剂，它在 GIST 中通过阻断跨膜受体蛋白酪氨酸激酶 KIT 的三磷酸腺苷结合位点发挥它的活性。伊马替尼已经成功地用于慢性粒细胞白血病和 Ph 染色体阳性白血病的治疗。伊马替尼在 GIST 患者中的应用是基于这样一个假设，即伊马替尼能阻断 GIST 细胞内 KIT 受体酪氨酸激酶的活性[13]。通过使用伊马替尼，对于原来无法做手术的广泛转移的 GIST 患者来说，手术切除成为可能。该治疗也能降低术后 GIST 复发和播散的发生率，从而延长生命。虽然伊马替尼的辅助和新辅助疗法的试验正在进行之中，但看来对于可手术切除的 GIST 患者，推荐首先做手术切除，然后进入伊马替尼的临床试验作为术后辅助治疗，以避免切除不完全、肿瘤泄漏或其他高危因素。对于复发或转移性 GIST 患者，可以考虑伊马替尼试验性治疗，然后做手术切除。

存活

GIST 手术切除后所获得的长期生存在发表的文献中报道各不相同，特别在儿童中评价起来非常困难，因为大多数文章包含的病例数少，或者主要病例是成人患者（表 31–1）。此外，依据最近对本病的认 517
识和病理学分类的改变，许多过去的文章所提及的肿瘤并不是真正的 GIST。尽管存在这些困难，有一些因素看来在预测外科手术后长期生存率方面还是有用

表 31-1 胃肠道间质瘤患者手术切除后的 5 年生存率

单位	统计年份	病例数	完全切除病灶的病例数（%）	5 年生存率（%）
Mayo Clinic	1950—1974	108	52（48）	50
MSKCC	1949—1973	38	20（53）	65
MCV	1951—1984	51	30（59）	63
MDACC	1957—1997	191	99（52）	48
MGH	1962—1986	55	40（73）	35
MSKCC	1982—1998	200	80（40）	54

MCV：Medical College of Viginia；MDACC：MD Anderson Cancer Center；MGH：Massachusetts General Hospital；MSKCC：Memorial Sloan-Kettering Cancer Center。

的：肿瘤的大小、分裂指数和发病部位（表 31-2）。已经注意到肿瘤小于 5cm 的患者生存优于 5～10cm 的肿瘤患者比较；依此类推，后者比那些肿瘤大于 10cm 的患者预后要好。每 50 个高倍视野中，低危肿瘤的分裂指数少于 10 个，而高危肿瘤大于 10 个。已经发现肿瘤发病部位也能预测预后，胃 GIST 比其他部位的预后要好[46]。

食管和胃癌

儿童的食管或胃癌是非常少见的。根据国家癌症统计部的监测、流行病学和最终结果（SEER），在 1988—1996 年间，诊断食管癌的例数为 10 441，只有 3 例（0.03%）是在 10～19 岁，未发现少于 10 岁的患者[20]。

表 31-2 胃肠道间质瘤的预后因素

因素	良性 *	恶性
大小	＜5cm	＞5cm
细胞数量	低	高
核多态性	无或少见	可以很明显
坏死	无	可见
分裂象	＜0～1，每 30～50HPF	1～5 或更多，每 10HPF
浸润生长	无	可以侵犯邻近组织
转移	无	可见
c-kit 突变	无	常见

* 单个因素不能确定是良性。肿瘤大小、有丝分裂指数和有无坏死是预示肿瘤为良性的最重要因素。

HPF：高倍视野，400 倍。

尽管食管癌稀少，但有一些已知的危险因素与肿瘤发展倾向有关。对于食管腺癌，继发于慢性胃食管反流（GERD）的 Barrett 食管是主要的危险因素。儿童中有较高风险出现继发于慢性 GERD 的 Barrett 食管的人群包括严重神经系统缺陷的儿童（如脑瘫）和那些累及食管的先天性缺陷的儿童（如食管闭锁和气管食管瘘）[19]。Hassall 估计[28]在有严重 GERD 和相关危险因素的患儿中，Barrett 食管的发生率为 0.02%；对于那些没有危险因素的人来说，巴雷特食管的发生率更低。尽管如此，长期 GERD 的青少年已证实易患食管腺癌，故通过上消化道内镜和分段活检进行监测，这对那些发生 Barrett 食管黏膜改变的儿童是有益的[29]。

Barrett 食管改变也能见于那些食管替代手术后保留的颈部食管。有这种手术史的患者需要控制胃 pH 和通过内镜对保留的食管上段做活检进行长期监测。由于技术和方法不同，对于食管闭锁患者施行食管替代手术可能导致远端食管残留。这种残留可能导致严重的需要手术切除的慢性食管炎和 Barrett 食管。因为 Barrett 食管是一种癌前病变，能导致食管腺癌，所以在做食管替代手术时，食管的远端必须切除[48]。已经有关于儿童食管化学性损伤后出现食管癌的病例报道。对于那些有 Barrett 食管和食管化学性损伤的患者，必须考虑作内镜下活检来监测恶变的可能[47]。

在 1997—2001 年间，在 SEER 资料报道的总例数为 15 274 例的胃癌患者中，小于 20 岁的患者占 0.1%[55]。尽管儿童胃部腺癌少见，有数个病例报道在小至 2.5 岁的儿童中发现胃部腺癌[17]。肿瘤可以出现于胃的任何解剖部位[38]；症状可能非常不明确，但可出现包括上腹部痛、体重减轻、呕吐和贫血。此外，在胃部腺癌中已经有并发食管失弛缓症相关症状的报道[1,17]。

类癌

流行病学

类癌源于沿原始胃肠道分布的神经内分泌细胞。这些肿瘤与其他胃肠道细胞一样，源于相同的子代细胞，是胺的前体摄取和脱羧（APUD）系统的一部分[59]。儿童类癌能出现于胃肠道——胃、小肠、阑尾（最常见）和直肠——以及肠道外部位，如肺。虽然阑尾类癌在儿童和青少年少见，但它是该年龄组最常见的胃肠道肿瘤[10,40]。该病儿童的发生率很难估计，因为大多数资料的回顾性数据中剔除了某些类型的类癌，但报道的发生率范围看来在 0.08%～0.169%[16, 52]，或约为每年每百万儿童中有 1.14 例[42]，女性比例稍稍占多[23,40]。

诊断

儿童类癌常常在原定为阑尾炎的手术中发现，偶尔也在与类癌无关的手术时发现。虽然临床表现与急性阑尾炎类似或怀疑为妇科病而进行剖腹探查，但常常不能发现阑尾的真正的炎症性改变[10]。缺乏炎症表现可

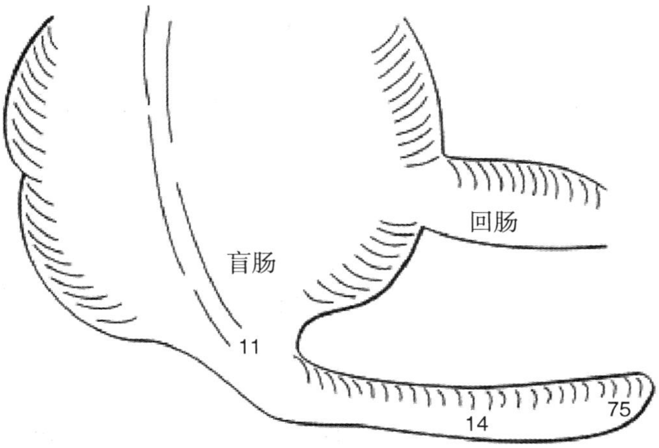

图 31–1 阑尾类癌的发病部位（%）。

能是典型的一般位于阑尾的末端部分的阑尾类癌所致；这样，就没有阑尾腔近端的梗阻（图 31–1）[16,23]。虽然症状不典型，类癌的大小也不同，但没有局限于阑尾的类癌相关的类癌综合征的报道[16,52]。

与阑尾类癌或偶然发现的类癌患者相反，阑尾外类癌（如肺和肝脏）的患儿常常在诊断时有相应症状和扩散表现。Broaddus 等[5]报道，46%的阑尾外类癌患者在初次诊断后出现复发或转移，或者在诊断时即发现肿瘤播散。

治疗

对于局限于阑尾的儿童类癌，手术切除阑尾是治疗的首选，并常可治愈。长期随访结果显示该病很少或没有复发，出现转移的可能性极低[10,40,60]。判断阑尾类癌是否做手术切除的最重要因素是肿瘤大小。对于直径小于 2cm 的类癌，单独做阑尾切除就已足够。不管肿瘤直径大小，组织学上出现浸润阑尾系膜和侵犯阑尾基底的肿瘤是做右半结肠切除术的指征。类癌直径大于 2cm、有高度恶性表现和杯状细胞类腺癌也是做右半结肠切除术的指征[23]。

病理学

肿瘤的重要病理学特征包括大小、组织学亚型、阑尾系膜浸润和淋巴结浸润情况。类癌也能被分成良性、交界性、低度恶性或高度恶性，当然更精确和统一的分类系统可以使那些需要接受更大侵袭性手术的患者得到受益[58]。Van Eden 等人[58]试图通过要求 WHO 将目前肺神经内分泌瘤的分类系统应用于所有胃肠道神经内分泌瘤来解决该问题。

结肠直肠腺癌

结肠和直肠腺癌是最常见的胃肠道肿瘤，美国每年的发病将近 148 300 例，死亡 56 600 例。总人口中发生结肠直肠癌的终身风险是 5%～6%[30]。结肠直肠癌是儿童消化道中仅次于肝脏肿瘤的第二常见肿瘤。虽然结肠直肠癌在儿童中少见，但每百万人中发病率

表 31–3 结肠直肠癌患儿的易感因素
家族性息肉病综合征
炎症性肠病，特别是溃疡性结肠炎
遗传性非息肉病综合征
输尿管乙状结肠吻合术后
慢性寄生虫感染
放疗后
高脂肪和低纤维素饮食
可能暴露于有化学和放射性的环境中

也有 1.3～2[41,56]。虽然曾在一个 9 个月大的患儿中发现结肠癌，但大多数患儿发病时大于 10 岁；诊断时
519 的中位年龄为 15～19 岁[35,45,53]。结肠癌的发病与几个易发因素有关（表 31–3）。这些因素包括高脂和高胆固醇及低纤维饮食、暴露于化学和放射性环境、息肉综合征、炎性肠病、遗传性非息肉病综合征、输尿管乙状结肠吻合术后的尿分流、慢性寄生虫感染和放射治疗后。

肿瘤的发病原因可以分类为散发性（约占 75%患儿）、家族性（约占 10%～20%患儿，这些患儿至少有两个直系亲属患结肠癌，但无明确的遗传学模式）、遗传性（即息肉综合征，约占 1%）、炎症性肠病（约 1%）和遗传性非息肉综合征（约 5%～6%）。

虽然人们公认饮食在成人的结肠癌发病中起作用，但尚无类似关于儿童的研究来支持该说法。各种环境因素与肿瘤的形成有关。在一项研究中发现，在 13 例结肠癌患儿中有 10 例有除草剂接触史[44]。

结肠直肠癌在成人和儿童中存在明显不同。这些区别包括临床表现和症状、肿瘤原发部位、病理学表现、分期和预后。

相关的其他疾病

因为散发性儿童结肠直肠癌约占其中的 75%，这表明 25%的患儿存在一些相关的易感条件。儿童散发性结肠癌显示出侵袭性疾病的特征，其形态学和自然病史与那些家族性腺瘤样息肉、遗传性非息肉结肠直肠癌和成人的结肠癌不同。肿瘤的发生最可能继发于肿瘤抑制基因受累、杂合性缺失或发生突变[11]。

一些遗传性疾病与随后发生的结肠癌明显有关，其特征是息肉综合征。包括 Gardner 综合征（腺瘤样多发息肉、软组织和骨肿瘤）、Tucot 综合征（家族性腺瘤样多发息肉和中枢神经系统肿瘤）、和家族性结肠息肉。加德纳综合征和家族性结肠息肉均为常染色体显性遗传病，与结肠和小肠的腺瘤样息肉有关。

Bassey[3]认为，家族性息肉患者的结肠癌发病率到 28 岁时是 50%，其最终出现结肠癌的可能性接近 100%。那些有 APC 突变或一个以上直系亲属有家族性腺瘤样息肉的患者风险更高，而且纤维乙状结肠镜筛查应该在 10～12 岁间开始。具有结肠息肉、证实 APC 突变、或两者均存在时，需要每年做内镜检查。当患儿到十几和二十几岁时，息肉的增加可能妨碍原本适合的、安全的结肠镜息肉切除术。当发生这种情况时，必须做预防性手术来切除受累的结肠。手术方式包括次全结肠切除术加末端回肠造口术或回肠直肠吻合术，随后每年对保留的直肠进行内镜检查。目前，许多患者可考虑做全腹直肠结肠切除术加恢复性小肠直肠吻合术。

Peutz–Jeghers 综合征与错构性息肉有关。Peutz–Jeghers 综合征的结肠癌发生率为 2%～3%。同样的，幼年型息肉看来发生结肠癌的可能性更高[9,24,54]。

建议做结肠切除是基于发生恶性肿瘤的可能性。这些患者的整个结肠表面可以被覆上千个的息肉。事实上，进行可疑病变的监测和识别的能力还很低。毫无疑问，对于家族性息肉病、Gardner 综合征和 Turcot 特综合征做结肠切除是非常合适的治疗方法。由于 Peutz–Jeghers 综合征和幼年型息肉的恶性变发生率相对较低，合理的治疗策略是进行严密监测。

溃疡性结肠炎患者发生结肠癌的可能性日益增加是肯定的。这种危险性约是一般人群的 20 倍，并与患者的溃疡性结肠炎的患病总时间有关。在患溃疡性结肠炎第一个 10 年后，结肠癌的可能性每年增加 1%～2%[15]。在发生结肠癌的溃疡性结肠炎患者中有一些重要特征，包括发病年龄小、易见多个恶变部位、及全结肠受累的患者其恶性变可能性比只有左侧结肠炎患者要高[25]。

Crohn 病是另一个类型的炎症性肠道疾病，其发生结肠癌的危险性比一般人群高 20 倍[61]。恶性变的可能性与受累肠道的数量有关。然而，肿瘤可能在看来完全正常的部位出现[36]，这在某些方面使 Crohn病
患者的恶性变诊断比溃疡性结肠炎患者的诊断更为困 52
难。因此，常规的监测方案和随机活检特别重要。在

炎症性肠道疾病患者中，作对照性钡灌肠和结肠镜检查是监测的主要方法。在结肠镜检查时，必须对任何可疑部位和随机选择的部位进行活检。

遗传性非息肉性结直肠癌或 Lynch 综合征具有常染色体显性的遗传特性，是遗传性结肠直肠癌的最常见类型[8,37]。它约占所有结肠直肠癌患者的 1%～3%，比家族性息肉相关性结肠癌高 5 倍[8,22]。该类型的结肠直肠癌通常表现为近端结肠病变（约 70%邻近脾曲），患者癌变的年龄（平均约为 45 岁）比一般结肠直肠癌患者更年轻[22,37]。也注意到遗传性非息肉性结肠直肠癌患者发生同时或异时性结肠外肿瘤（如子宫内膜、卵巢、胃、小肠、胰腺、肝胆管、脑和上尿道肿瘤）的倾向[37]。

用于膀胱外翻患者和其他泌尿生殖器异常的尿路分流所做的输尿管乙状结肠吻合术与结肠癌有关。Eraklis 和 Folkman[21]报道，5%做输尿管乙状结肠吻合术的患者出现结肠癌，每一例均发生在输尿管植入部位。实验资料显示在植入部位粪便和尿液的混合导致的慢性炎症是癌变的原因，尤其是当尿液被感染的时候。做该类型尿路分流的患者需保证密切随访，每年行乙状结肠镜检查。

原发肿瘤接受放疗的患儿在照射野有出现结肠直肠癌的风险。LaQuaglia 等人[35]报告了 1 例做肾母细胞瘤切除并做了后腹膜放疗的患者，随后出现左半结肠癌。其他研究者报道了 2 例结肠直肠癌分别继发于后腹膜横纹肌肉瘤和肾母细胞瘤，2 例均接受了切除和放疗[14]。前者是一个 1 岁的男孩，他的后腹膜横纹肌肉瘤接受了术前放疗、手术和化疗。2 岁时他出现放射性结肠炎，随后出现腺瘤样息肉。11 岁时出现直肠腺癌（图 31–2）。后者是肾母细胞瘤，在其 9 个月时进行了手术和放疗。他也出现放射性结肠炎，随后在 42 年后出现多发性结肠腺癌。两例肿瘤的 p53 抗原的免疫组化结果显示，后者的两个肿瘤和前者的腺瘤均为阳性。据此推测放疗导致 p53 突变，进而导致肿瘤发生。

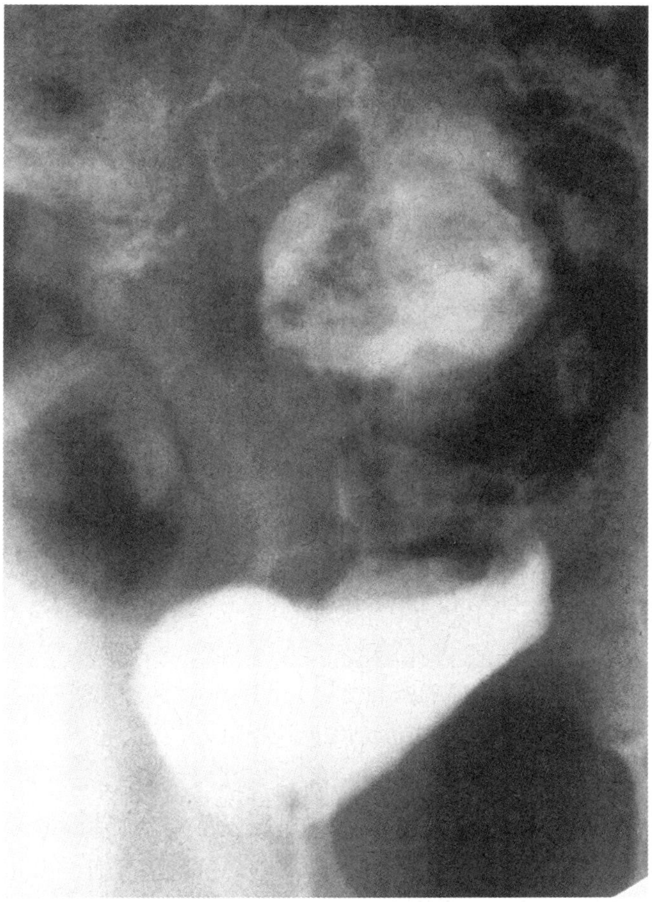

图 31–2　一位以前因后腹膜横纹肌肉瘤接受放疗的 11 岁男孩的气钡造影灌肠。X 线照片显示直肠几乎完全梗阻。

诊断

结肠直肠癌患儿经常出现的症状包括腹痛（几乎所有患者都有）；40%～70%出现恶心和呕吐；排便习惯改变和便秘（特别是左侧结肠病变）。这些患者的体格检查发现经常包括腹胀、触痛和腹部肿块。半数以上患儿的粪便潜血阳性。约 1/3 患儿有直肠出血史，在左半结肠和直肠肿瘤的患者中更为多见。20%～30%的患者出现体重明显减轻。

从症状出现到就诊的中位时间常为数月；至少有一个报道提到在出现症状到诊断之间隔了一年[53]。如果患者的症状被归因于更常见的儿科疾病如阑尾炎、肠套迭或胃肠炎，则可能延误诊断[31]。另一个延误诊断的可能原因是青少年由于害羞而隐瞒症状[51]。直肠出血也可能是良性病变（如息肉或痔）的表现，但需注意结肠直肠癌的可能；早期诊断有赖于是否怀疑到该病[32]。Steinberg 等人[53]认为，如果患者的症状出现大于 3 个月，则已经发生了诊断延误；他们发现，9 例结肠癌患者中有 5 例在诊断肿瘤前已经出现症状 3～36 个月（平均 11 个月）。这种诊断的延误可能是许多患儿处于疾病晚期的一个重要因素。基于就诊时 521

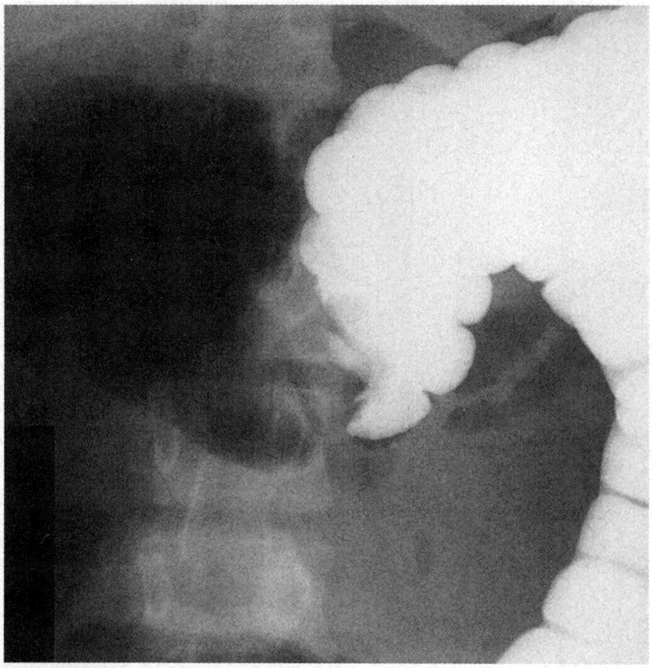

图 31-3 一位出现腹痛和便秘 1 个月的 14 岁患儿的气钡造影灌肠。图中出现横结肠的完全性梗阻。

的表现和症状，可以出现两种情况。首先，临床诊断是一个阑尾炎或腹膜炎所致的急腹症。这种情况时，患儿常直接进入手术室。在第二种情况中，当诊断肠梗阻时，可发生更多可能性。放射科常在诊断结肠中发现肿块，气钡对照灌肠检查发现梗阻部位（图 31-3）。根据病变部位，乙状结肠镜或结肠镜检查进行活检和诊断。在成人，大多数病变位于直肠乙状结肠，可以通过乙状结肠镜诊断。相反，儿童结肠直肠癌相对均匀分布于整个结肠；1/3 肿瘤位于右半结肠[35,45]。结肠镜常用于采集活检组织进行诊断。

病理特征

结肠直肠肿瘤的两个特征在儿童和成人中存在明显不同：分期和腺癌的组织类型。约 40%的成人结肠癌患者的区域淋巴结被侵犯或有远处转移（Duke 分期 C 或 D 期）。在儿童中，80%以上的肿瘤是 Duke 分期的 C 或 D 期[35,45,53]。此外，半数以上结肠直肠癌患儿组织学上显示为黏蛋白型腺癌。黏蛋白亚型的病程具侵袭性，且转移较早[56]。在成人结肠癌中，黏蛋白型腺癌的发生率约大于 5%。没有明确的原因显示为什么该黏蛋白类型在儿童结肠癌中如此多见。诊断时疾病越是晚期，预后差的黏蛋白亚型发生率越高，这两者的协同作用使儿童结肠癌的预后差。

淋巴结的微卫星状态被认为能识别儿童结肠癌中遗传学发生的不同信号途径。结直肠癌患者出现高频微卫星不稳定时更可能有多发性同时或异时结肠直肠癌、且诊断时年龄比微卫星稳定的患者更小[26]。然而，微卫星不稳定不是结肠直肠癌家族史预测性或唯一的表型特征[11]。

在成人，结肠癌和癌胚抗原（CEA）相关性已经得到证实，但在患儿中很少有类似的报告。Rao 等人[45]发现，20 例 Dukes 分期为 C 或 D 期的患儿中有 4 例抗原水平在诊断时正常。在这些患儿的长期评估中，CEA 水平在 60%患儿中与肿瘤负荷的增减相关；不幸的是，其余 40%尽管疾病进展，但抗原水平仍正常。到现在，儿童中的 CEA 水平并未显示出与治疗效应有良好相关性。

治疗

结肠癌患儿的基本治疗手段是手术切除，包括受累结肠、肠系膜和淋巴引流区域的广泛切除。不幸的是，治愈性切除在患儿中的可能性只有 40%～69%；该比例比成人结肠癌患者要低得多[35,45]。卵巢和大网膜是转移的常见部位。如果做根治性手术，应该选择大网膜切除和女性患者中卵巢切除术。

对于这些患儿来说，没有特异的化疗方案可用。大多数研究中，曾给予某些类型的化疗，而对部分患者做过选择性的放疗。虽然无对照的病例报道显示这些方法单用或合用可以获得成功，但没有资料证明化疗或放疗对治愈或姑息治疗有好处。

结肠癌患儿的生存率和生存期是很差的；研究资料常显示患儿 5 年生存率低于 5%[2]。最近，LaQuaglis 等人[35]报道，在中位随访期为 4.7 年时，29 例中的 8 例（28%）存活。生存与肿瘤完全切除直接相关。在做根治性手术的患者中，与预测生存有关的信息包括淋巴结受累或高组织学分级。儿童结肠癌的主要治疗目标是在首次手术时完全切除。即使作了完全切除患者的生存率仍不佳时，可以考虑做辅助性化疗。化疗的使用（部分患者需再做二次探查手术），可能提高生存率。

总结

儿童结肠癌的生物学特性在许多方面与成人不同。临床表现、组织学类型、分期和预后存在显著差别。大多数儿童结肠直肠癌源于先前的腺瘤。出现腺瘤可能性大的家族出现结肠直肠癌的风险较大。该信息表明遗传学比以前想象的可能发挥更重要的作用，仅有极少数病例是真正的散发性。把注意力集中于结肠癌患儿的分子遗传学能有助于更好的了解该疾病。由此，这将有助于发现高危患者，可以早期诊断和早期干预，从而使疾病的分期更低，这些将最终提高患者的生存率。

(叶启东译　王耀平校)

参考文献

1. Aichbichler BW, Eherer AJ, Petritsch W, et al: Gastric adenocarcinoma mimicking achalasia in a 15-year-old patient: A case report and review of the literature. J Pediatr Gastroenterol Nutr 2001;32:103-106.
2. Andersson A, Bergdahl L: Carcinoma of the colon in children: A report of six new cases and a review of the literature. J Pediatr Surg 1976;11:967-971.
3. Bassey HJR: Familial Polyposis Coli. Baltimore, Johns Hopkins University Press, 1975.
4. Bethel CA, Bhattacharyya N, Hutchinson C, et al: Alimentary tract malignancies in children. J Pediatr Surg 1997;32:1004-1008.
5. Broaddus RR, Herzog CE, Hicks MJ: Neuroendocrine tumors (carcinoid and neuroendocrine carcinoma) presenting at extra-appendiceal sites in childhood and adolescence. Arch Pathol Lab Med 2003;127:1200-1203.
6. Carney JA: Gastric stromal sarcoma, pulmonary chondroma, and extra-adrenal paraganglioma (Carney triad): Natural history, adrenocortical component, and possible familial occurrence. Mayo Clin Proc 1999;74:543-552.
7. Carney JA, Sheps SG, Go VL, Gordon H: The triad of gastric leiomyosarcoma, functioning extra-adrenal paraganglioma and pulmonary chondroma. N Engl J Med 1977;296:1517-1518.
8. Chung DC, Rustgi AK: The hereditary nonpolyposis colorectal cancer syndrome: Genetics and clinical implications. Ann Intern Med 2003;138:560-570.
9. Coburn MC, Pricolo VE, DeLuca FG, Bland KI: Malignant potential in intestinal juvenile polyposis syndromes. Ann Surg Oncol 1995;2:386-391.
10. Corpron CA, Black CT, Herzog CE, et al: A half century of experience with carcinoid tumors in children. Am J Surg 1995;170:606-608.
11. Datta RV, LaQuaglia MP, Paty PB: Genetic and phenotypic correlates of colorectal cancer in young patients. N Engl J Med 2000;342:137-138.
12. DeMatteo RP, Lewis JJ, Leung D, et al: Two hundred gastrointestinal stromal tumors: Recurrence patterns and prognostic factors for survival. Ann Surg 2000;231:51-58.
13. Demetri GD, von Mehren M, Blanke CD, et al: Efficacy and safety of imatinib mesylate in advanced gastrointestinal stromal tumors. N Engl J Med 2002;347:472-480.
14. Densmore TL, Langer JC, Molleston JP, et al: Colorectal adenocarcinoma as a second malignant neoplasm following Wilms' tumor and rhabdomyosarcoma. Med Pediatr Oncol 1996;27:556-560.
15. Devroede GJ, Taylor WF, Sauer WG, et al: Cancer risk and life expectancy of children with ulcerative colitis. N Engl J Med 1971;285:17-21.
16. Doede T, Foss HD, Waldschmidt J: Carcinoid tumors of the appendix in children: Epidemiology, clinical aspects and procedure. Eur J Pediatr Surg 2000;10:372-377.
17. Dokucu AI, Ozturk H, Kilinc N, et al: Primary gastric adenocarcinoma in a 2.5-year-old girl. Gastric Cancer 2002;5:237-239.
18. Eisenberg BL, Judson I: Surgery and imatinib in the management of GIST: Emerging approaches to adjuvant and neoadjuvant therapy. Ann Surg Oncol 2004;11:465-475.
19. El Serag HB, Bailey NR, Gilger M, Rabeneck L: Endoscopic manifestations of gastroesophageal reflux disease in patients between 18 months and 25 years without neurological deficits. Am J Gastroenterol 2002;97:1635-1639.
20. Eloubeidi MA, Desmond R, Arguedas MR, et al: Prognostic factors for the survival of patients with esophageal carcinoma in the US: The importance of tumor length and lymph node status. Cancer 2002;95:1434-1443.
21. Eraklis AJ, Folkman MJ: Adenocarcinoma at the site of ureterosigmoidostomies for exstrophy of the bladder. J Pediatr Surg 1978;13:730-734.
22. Fitzgibbons RJ Jr, Lynch HT, Stanislav GV, et al: Recognition and treatment of patients with hereditary nonpolyposis colon cancer (Lynch syndromes I and II). Ann Surg 1987;206:289-295.
23. Goede AC, Caplin ME, Winslet MC: Carcinoid tumour of the appendix. Br J Surg 2003;90:1317-1322.
24. Greenstein AJ, Sachar DB, Smith H, et al: Cancer in universal and left-sided ulcerative colitis: Factors determining risk. Gastroenterology 1979;77:290-294.
25. Greenstein AJ, Slater G, Heimann TM, et al: A comparison of multiple synchronous colorectal cancer in ulcerative colitis, familial polyposis coli, and de novo cancer. Ann Surg 1986;203:123-128.
26. Gryfe R, Kim H, Hsieh ETK, et al: Tumor microsatellite instability and clinical outcome in young patients with colorectal cancer. N Engl J Med 2000;342:69-77.
27. Haider N, Kader M, McDermott M, et al: Gastric stromal tumors in children. Pediatr Blood Cancer 2004;42:186-189.
28. Hassall E: Co-morbidities in childhood Barrett's esophagus. J Pediatr Gastroenterol Nutr 1997;25:255-260.
29. Hassall E, Dimmick JE, Magee JF: Adenocarcinoma in childhood Barrett's esophagus: Case documentation and the need for surveillance in children. Am J Gastroenterol 1993;88:282-288.
30. Jemal A, Thomas A, Murray T, Thun M: Cancer statistics, 2002. CA Cancer J Clin 2002;52:23-47.
31. Karnak I, Ciftci AO, Senocak ME, Buyukpamukcu N: Colorectal carcinoma in children. J Pediatr Surg 1999; 34:1499-1504.
32. Karnak I, Kale G, Tanyel FC, Buyukpamukcu N: Malignant stromal tumor of the colon in an infant: Diagnostic difficulties and differential diagnosis. J Pediatr Surg 2003;38:245-247.

33. Kerr JZ, Hicks MJ, Nuchtern JG, et al: Gastrointestinal autonomic nerve tumors in the pediatric population: A report of four cases and a review of the literature. Cancer 1999;85:220-230.
34. Kindblom LG, Remotti HE, Aldenborg F, Meis-Kindblom JM: Gastrointestinal pacemaker cell tumor (GIPACT): Gastrointestinal stromal tumors show phenotypic characteristics of the interstitial cells of Cajal. Am J Pathol 1998; 152:1259-1269.
35. LaQuaglia MP, Heller G, Filippa DA, et al: Prognostic factors and outcome in patients 21 years and under with colorectal carcinoma. J Pediatr Surg 1992;27:1085-1089.
36. Leichtner AM: Intestinal neoplasms. In Walker WA, et al (eds): Pediatric Gastrointestinal Disease. Philadelphia, BC Decker, 1991.
37. Lynch HT, de la Chapelle A: Hereditary colorectal cancer. N Engl J Med 2003;348:919-932.
38. McGill TW, Downey EC, Westbrook J, et al: Gastric carcinoma in children. J Pediatr Surg 1993;28:1620-1621.
39. Miettinen M, Lasota J: Gastrointestinal stromal tumors—definition, clinical, histological, immunohistochemical, and molecular genetic features and differential diagnosis. Virchows Arch 2001;438:1-12.
40. Moertel CL, Weiland LH, Telander RL: Carcinoid tumor of the appendix in the first two decades of life. J Pediatr Surg 1990;25:1073-1075.
41. Odone V, Chang L, Caces J, et al: The natural history of colorectal carcinoma in adolescents. Cancer 1982;49:1716-1720.
42. Parkes SE, Muir KR, al Sheyyab M, et al: Carcinoid tumours of the appendix in children 1957-1986: Incidence, treatment and outcome. Br J Surg 1993;80:502-504.
43. Pidhorecky I, Cheney RT, Kraybill WG, Gibbs JF: Gastrointestinal stromal tumors: Current diagnosis, biologic behavior, and management. Ann Surg Oncol 2000; 7:705-712.
44. Pratt CB, Rivera G, Shanks E, et al: Colorectal carcinoma in adolescents: Implications regarding etiology. Cancer 1977;40(5 Suppl):2464-2472.
45. Rao BN, Pratt CB, Fleming ID, et al: Colon carcinoma in children and adolescents: A review of 30 cases. Cancer 1985;55:1322-1326.
46. Roberts PJ, Eisenberg B: Clinical presentation of gastrointestinal stromal tumors and treatment of operable disease. Eur J Cancer 2002;38(Suppl 5):S37-S38.
47. Schettini ST, Ganc A, Saba L: Esophageal carcinoma secondary to a chemical injury in a child. Pediatr Surg Int 1998;13:519-520.
48. Shamberger RC, Eraklis AJ, Kozakewich HP, Hendren WH: Fate of the distal esophageal remnant following esophageal replacement. J Pediatr Surg 1988;23:1210-1214.
49. Shiu MH, Farr GH, Papachristou DN, Hajdu SI: Myosarcomas of the stomach: Natural history, prognostic factors and management. Cancer 1982;49:177-187.
50. Skinner MA, Plumley DA, Grosfeld JL, et al: Gastrointestinal tumors in children: An analysis of 39 cases. Ann Surg Oncol 1994;1:283-289.
51. Soper RT: Gastrointestinal neoplasms. In: Ashcraft KW, Holder TM (eds): Pediatric Surgery. Philadelphia, W.B. Saunders, 1993, pp 464-469.
52. Spunt SL, Pratt CB, Rao BN, et al: Childhood carcinoid tumors: The St Jude Children's Research Hospital experience. J Pediatr Surg 2000;35:1282-1286.
53. Steinberg JB, Tuggle DW, Postier RG: Adenocarcinoma of the colon in adolescents. Am J Surg 1988;156:460-462.
54. Stemper TJ, Kent TH, Summers RW: Juvenile polyposis and gastrointestinal carcinoma: A study of a kindred. Ann Intern Med 1975;83:639-646.
55. Surveillance, Epidemiology, and End Results (SEER) Program. SEER 1975-2001. SEER Stat Database. Bethesda, Md, National Cancer Institute, DCCPS, Surveillance Research Program, Cancer Statistics Branch, 2004.
56. Symonds DA, Vickery AL: Mucinous carcinoma of the colon and rectum. Cancer 1976;37:1891-1900.
57. Trupiano JK, Stewart RE, Misick C, et al: Gastric stromal tumors: A clinicopathologic study of 77 cases with correlation of features with nonaggressive and aggressive clinical behaviors. Am J Surg Pathol 2002;26:705-714.
58. Van Eeden S, Quaedvlieg PF, Taal BG, et al: Classification of low-grade neuroendocrine tumors of midgut and unknown origin. Hum Pathol 2002;33:1126-1132.
59. Van Gompel JJ, Sippel RS, Warner TF, Chen H: Gastrointestinal carcinoid tumors: Factors that predict outcome. World J Surg 2004;28:387-392.
60. Volpe A, Willert J, Ihnken K, et al: Metastatic appendiceal carcinoid tumor in a child. Med Pediatr Oncol 2000; 34:218-220.
61. Weedon DD, Shorter RG, Ilstrup DM, et al: Crohn's disease and cancer. N Engl J Med 1973;289:1099-1103.

第 32 章

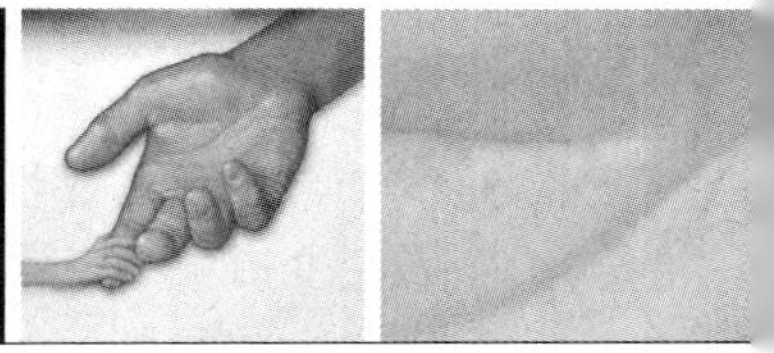

横纹肌肉瘤

Richard J. Andrassy

524 横纹肌肉瘤（rhabdomyosarcoma，RMS，源于希腊词，rhabdos，意为杆状；mys 意为肌；sarkos 意为肉）是见于儿童和青少年的一种原发性恶性肿瘤，源于能分化为骨骼肌的胚胎间充质。RMS 占儿童所有软组织肉瘤的 50%多，因此是最常见的软组织肉瘤。成人肉瘤主要见于四肢，而儿童 RMS 可以见于任何有骨骼肌的部位以及没有骨骼肌的部位（如膀胱、胆道）。RMS 可以出现于除了骨骼外的任何部位和任何组织。最常见的部位是头颈部和泌尿生殖道，只有 20%见于四肢。

最早区分软组织肉瘤和骨肉瘤与上皮和造血系统肿瘤的是 Virchow，他在 19 世纪 50 年代中期提出一个“细胞病理学”理论，把肿瘤起源归因于细胞的特定类型[99]。第一例 RMS 是 Webner 在 1854 年报道，这是一个 21 岁的舌肿瘤患者[97]。在 1946 年，Stout[106] 报道了一系列躯干和四肢出现恶性肿瘤的成人患者。在 1954 年，Pack 等人[79]描述了一群骨骼肌 RMS 患儿。在 1958 年，Horn 等人[50]建议将该肿瘤分成四个亚型：胚胎型、腺泡型、葡萄状和多形型。在这些早期年代，手术切除是唯一的治疗方法，根治性切除是标准治疗。除了一些通过根治性切除能完全切除肿块的选择性部位外（如截肢术和盆腔廓清术），患者生存率很低。根据发病部位不同，其生存率从 7%～70%不等[78]。

1950 年，Stobbe 等人[105]证明，在头颈部不完全切除 RMS 后加用放疗可以提高疗效。在 1961 年，Pinkel 等人[83]建议在完全切除和术后放疗后进行辅助性化疗，这是实体瘤多学科协作治疗的开始。

认识到多学科协作模式的价值，以及这些肿瘤相对少见，美国三个儿童肿瘤研究协作组（儿童肿瘤研究协作组、肿瘤和白血病协作组 B 儿科组和西南肿瘤协作组）在国立癌症研究所的协调下于 1972 年形成了国际横纹肌肉瘤研究（IRS）协作组来研究先前未接受治疗的 21 岁以下患者的 RMS 及未分化肉瘤的治疗及生物学特点。至此，完成了五个包含几乎 5000 例患者的成功临床治疗方案：IRS–I（197—1978）、IRS–II（1978—1984）、IRS–III（1984—1991）、IRS–IV 试验方案（只针对晚期患者；1987—1991）和 IRS–IV（1991—997）[1,2,6-8,11,18]。基于这些研究所获取的经验教训，IRS–V 在 1997 年开始用于低危患者（即预后良好的患者），并于 1999 年开始扩展到其他患者。

虽然趋势是倾向于更少采用截肢手术，外科医生在最初的活检和分期、原发肿瘤再切除、适度局部扩大切除和二次探查手术中发挥重要的作用。在多学科治疗方法中，外科医生应该是一个早期参与者。

流行病学

RMS 在婴儿和儿童中是位于神经母细胞瘤和肾母细胞瘤之后第三位最常见的实体瘤。在美国，RMS 每年约有 250～300 例新发病例。男性的发病率稍高于女性（3∶2），白人和非白人的比例为 12∶5。发病高峰年龄呈双峰型，第一个高峰在 2～5 岁，第二个高峰在 15～19 岁。

RMS 患者的其他先天性异常发生率似乎也较高[98]。RMS 和肾母细胞瘤均与生殖泌尿系统异常高发有关。RMS 也与中枢神经系统异常有关[98]。多发性神经纤维瘤的患者其 RMS 发病危险增加[42,101]。

Li–Fraumeni 家族性癌症综合征首先报道于 1969 年，包括发生于同胞和表亲父母及其他亲戚成员的软组织肉瘤；包括多种恶性肿瘤，包括 RMS、肾上腺 525
皮质癌、恶性胶质瘤、乳腺癌和肺癌[61,62]。该综合征是一个常染色体显性遗传性疾病，并与胚系细胞 p53 基因突变有关[66]。软组织恶性肿瘤患儿家族中相关的主要恶性肿瘤是患儿母亲患乳腺癌[107]。13 例 RMS 患儿母亲的回顾性研究发现她们乳腺癌的发病风险是对照组的 3～13.5 倍[13]。

其他相关性稍差的因素有胎儿酒精综合征、母体吸食大麻或可卡因、X 射线暴露和卫生保健工作者[39,40,95]。

已经观察到，RMS 与 Beckwith-Wiedemann 综合征相关，这是胎儿过度生长综合征，与染色体 11p15 异常有关，因该部位有类胰岛素样生长因子Ⅱ（IGF-Ⅱ）的基因[28]。

RMS 的两个组织学亚型——胚胎型和腺泡型——有不同的遗传学改变（这在这些肿瘤的发病机制上有重要作用）。在腺泡型 RMS 中存在特征性的 2 号染色体长臂和 13 号染色体长臂之间的易位，即 t(2;13)(q35;q14)。该易位使 PAX3 基因（该基因在早期神经肌肉发育过程中有调控转录作用）和 FKHR 基因（转录因子 fox 家族的成员之一）发生融合。目前认为该融合转录因子可能不适当的激活与表型转化有关的基因转录。变异型t(1;13)(p36;q14) 1 号染色体的 PAX7 基因与 FKHR 发生融合。表达 PAX-FKHR 融合基因的肿瘤患者往往年龄较小，且较可能表现出四肢癌变，提示其为不同的临床表型。现在根据这些融合基因的存在，用聚合酶链反应可以证实腺泡型 RMS 的诊断[28,63,72,110]。

已知胚胎型 RMS 有 11p15 位点的杂合性缺失，导致母本遗传学特征的缺失和父本遗传学信息的复制。这是 IGF-Ⅱ基因的位点。已证实 IGF-Ⅱ能刺激 RMS 细胞的生长，而用单克隆抗体阻断该因子能在体内和体外抑制肿瘤生长[113]。其他几种实体瘤与 11 号染色体短臂的缺失相关，包括肾母细胞瘤、肝母细胞瘤和神经母细胞瘤。

MyoD 基因家族编码 DNA 结合蛋白，它能调控编码肌原性蛋白（如结合蛋白、肌酸激酶和肌球蛋白）DNA 序列的转录[59,112]。在 RMS 中，没有发生该基因的下调，因此肿瘤细胞中的 MyoD1 表达保持在高水平[108]。这种过度表达的生物学作用尚未明确；但检测 MyoD1 基因产物的高度表达能用于诊断 RMS[102]。

在许多肿瘤中已报道细胞 DNA 含量的改变，并可能有一些判断预后的作用。胚胎型 RMS 肿瘤的 DNA 含量处于二倍体和超二倍体间（是正常 DNA 数量的 1.1～1.8 倍）。已有报道二倍体胚胎型 RMS 肿瘤比超二倍体肿瘤的预后差。近四倍体与组织学上的腺泡型相关[28,53]。

在 RMS 细胞株和肿瘤标本中已有 RAS 肿瘤基因突变的报道。尚未明确这些改变与 RMS 肿瘤发病机制是否有关、或反映了在肿瘤进展过程中发生的继发性异常[28]。

MET 癌基因在胚胎型和腺泡型 RMS 肿瘤标本及已建立细胞株中的异常表达已有报道。MET 编码 HGF/scatter 因子受体，后者可以调控上皮细胞的运动和侵袭性。据推测，MET 过度表达可以使 RMS 细胞出现类似胚胎成肌细胞的特征，从而使它们可以进入周围的结缔组织[31]。

病理学

RMS 细胞起源于未分化的中胚层组织，分类属于儿童小圆蓝色细胞性肿瘤。光学显微镜、免疫组化、电子显微镜和分子遗传学技术的联合应用可以区分特定的肿瘤类型。识别肌原性谱系的特征可以用来鉴别 RMS。RMS 典型表现是光学显微镜下有骨骼肌或横纹肌母细胞的交叉条纹特征[4,113]。通过免疫组化染色来识别骨骼肌或肌肉特异蛋白。

组织学上，RMS 属于儿童小圆蓝色细胞性肿瘤，该类别也包括神经母细胞瘤、Ewing 肉瘤、小细胞性成骨肉瘤、非 Hodgkin 淋巴瘤和白血病。RMS 的两个亚型中每个均有特征性的组织表现。胚胎型 RMS 是最常见的组织亚型，在所有新诊断 RMS 中占超过 30%的比例。胚胎型亚型，特别是葡萄状和梭形细胞型，目前认为预后较好，但现在关于组织学亚型和肿瘤发病部位二者谁是预后最主要的因素还存在争议。

葡萄状 RMS，被描述为“一串葡萄”，见于成腔结构，预后较好。梭形细胞型不均衡的出现于睾丸旁区域，但也可以见于头颈部，特别是眼眶和四肢[19,60]。这些亚型与经典的胚胎型 RMS 比较几乎都较局限，且较少侵袭，预后非常好；然而，两种亚型在所有 RMS 中只占了 5%～6%[60]。

Horn 等人[50]在 1958 年首先在病理上将 RMS描述为肌原性肿瘤。这些研究者推荐的第一个分型方案把 RMS 分成四个不同的病理学类型（胚胎型、葡萄型、

表 32–1　儿童横纹肌肉瘤的组织学类型：国际横纹肌肉瘤病理学分类

I. 预后良好型
  a. 葡萄状
  b. 梭形细胞
II. 预后中等型
  a. 胚胎型
  b. 多形性（少见）
III. 预后不良型
  a. 腺泡型（包括实质性亚型）
  b. 未分化型

From Asmar L, et al: Agreement among and within groups of pathologists in the classification of rhabdomyosarcoma and related childhood sarcoma: Report of an international study of four pathology classifications. Cancer 1994; 74: 2579.

腺泡型和多形型）。该分类法已经使用了数十年，后被国际儿科病理学专家组于 1994 年修改为一个“通用”系统。该系统根据每一个组织学亚型的预后差别，分为预后良好型、中间型和不良型（表 32–1）[11]。

腺泡型约占肿瘤的 20%，常出现于四肢、躯干和会阴；这些肿瘤预后不良[11]。腺泡型的特征是间质和密集小圆肿瘤细胞呈腺泡状排列，类似于肺组织的结构。其中一个亚型是“实体性”腺泡型 RMS，其特征是缺乏任何细胞间质的致密细胞片结构，但细胞学特征与经典的腺泡型肿瘤类似。未分化肉瘤是一类分类尚不明确的肉瘤，其细胞无肌原性或其他分化的表现[75,76]。组织学亚型的分布见表 32–2。

许多单克隆抗体与 RMS 的成分可发生反应，故已用于诊断。这些包括结合蛋白、肌肉特异的肌动蛋白、肌原纤维节性肌动蛋白、和肌红蛋白的抗体。这些均已用来确定细胞的肌原性，在联合应用时有非常好的特异性和敏感性[121]。MyoD1 早已在应用；其他能用于鉴别这些肿瘤的非肌原性蛋白产物还包括细胞角蛋白、神经元特异的烯醇酶、S–100 蛋白和 Leu–7。

表 32–2　横纹肌肉瘤患者协作组研究–III 的组织学分布

组织类型	百分比（%）
胚胎型	53
腺泡型	19
类型不明确	18
未分化型	7
葡萄状	5
骨外 Ewing 肉瘤	3

临床表现

RMS 的临床表现与原发肿瘤的起源部位、患者的年龄、和有无转移性病灶有关。大多数症状与局部组织结构受压迫相关；偶尔会出现轻度疼痛。没有与 RMS 肿瘤相关的典型的副肿瘤性综合征。

头颈部区域是临床中最常见的部位，在 IRS 研究的患者中约占 35%[25]。头颈部被分成眼眶（10%）、脑膜旁组织（中耳、鼻腔、鼻旁窦、鼻咽部和颞下窝；15%）和非脑膜旁组织（头皮、脸部、口腔、口咽部、喉部和颈部；10%）。这些肿瘤以胚胎型最多见，很少播散到区域淋巴结[56,85,89]。眼眶肿瘤产生突眼，偶尔产生眼肌麻痹。发自脑膜旁部位的肿瘤常产生鼻、耳或窦的阻塞，可伴有或不伴有黏液脓性的或血性的分泌物。起自眼眶或脑膜旁以外部位的头颈部 RMS 常表现为无痛性不断增大的肿块，多为局部生长[114]。脑膜旁肿瘤可侵犯颅内导致出现颅神经瘫痪和脑膜刺激症状。

在 IRS–III 资料中，泌尿生殖系 RMS 肿瘤占所有原发 RMS 肿瘤的 26%[25]。这些肿瘤被分成两个不同的类别：膀胱和前列腺肿瘤（10%）和非膀胱和前列腺肿瘤（16%）。后者发生于睾丸旁、会阴、阴道、和子宫。睾丸旁 RMS 可表现为阴囊或腹股沟管无痛性肿块，最初可被认为是疝气、鞘膜积液或精索静脉曲张。膀胱肿瘤产生血尿和尿道梗阻。前列腺肿瘤能形成盆腔巨大肿块，如果膀胱或肠道发生明显的压迫将导致尿频或便秘。RMS 也可以出现于男性或女性的生殖道中。阴道肿瘤倾向于出现于很年幼的儿童，表现为肿块或阴道出血和分泌物增加。子宫肿瘤一般出现于年长女孩，在诊断时分布已经非常广泛。睾丸旁 RMS 非常易于从淋巴结扩散至后腹膜，特别是年龄大于 10 岁的男孩[121]。阴道肿瘤很少扩散到周围淋巴结。

发生四肢 RMS 的患者约占 20%[7,74]。这些肿瘤表现为肿块，且局部淋巴结扩散发生率高（50%）[7,74]。这些肿瘤大多数为腺泡型，由于部位和可能的组织学类型关系，更具有侵袭性。

大约 15%的 RMS 患儿出现转移性病变，尽管治疗方法已改变，它的预后在过去的 15 年中没有获得显著的改善[25,96]。单独的肺转移看来很少见，做活检可以确诊。

新生儿出现 RMS 是非常少见的，报道的病例只有 14 例（从 IRS-I 到 IRS-IV 中共占 0.4%）[64]。他
527 们在组织学上一般是葡萄状胚胎型或未分化型。

诊断

RMS 通常通过直接的活检做出诊断。没有可用的肿瘤标志物或特异的影像学检查方法。病理学家希望能鉴别 RMS 的组织学亚型来进行充分的分期并指导治疗。为了达到该目的，需要数克的组织。泌尿生殖系的 RMS 活检常通过内镜来进行。用于前列腺 RMS 诊断的针刺活检结果常难于诊断，因此必须获得多条穿刺组织。躯干和四肢 RMS 必须作切除或切开活检，标记切口是为了不干扰随后扩大的局部切除所需要的切口。这通常意味着四肢需要做轴向的切口。扩大的局部切除最终目的要保证切缘清洁。根据原发肿瘤的部位进行区域淋巴结的评估。躯干和四肢病变淋巴结受累的发生率较高，建议做前哨淋巴结活检[73,74]。

RMS 患者在进行根治性手术前需要完整的计划。术前评估包括影像学、外周血和骨髓检查。完整的术前或治疗前评估的概括见表 32-3。

诊断过程中最重要的步骤是获得足够的组织用于组织学和细胞学诊断和分型。该过程一般在全麻下做切开活检来完成。

分期和临床分组

RMS 做治疗前分期以对疾病的程度进行分层，其目的是确定合适的治疗方案，及比较治疗预后。这种分组是 TNM 分期系统的改进，以原发肿瘤部位、原发肿瘤大小、临床区域淋巴结情况和远处转移情况为基础（表 32-4）[58,74]。

表 32-3 术前、治疗前评估
病史和体格检查（身高、体重）
病灶测量（体检或影像学）
全血细胞计数、分类、血小板计数
尿液分析
电解质、肌酐、钙、磷
碱性磷酸酶、乳酸脱氢酶、胆红素、血清谷丙转氨酶
骨髓活检或骨穿
胸片
原发肿瘤的 MRI 或 CT 检查
胸部 CT
头部 MRI 或 CT（对于头部肿瘤）
骨扫描
脑脊液细胞学分析（对于脑膜旁肿瘤）
心电图或心彩超（选择性）

治疗前肿瘤大小根据解剖部位，通过体外测量、MRI 或 CT 检查来进行。该分期是“临床的”，必须由有经验的外科医生根据术前影像学和体格检查结果来进行。术中或病理学结果不影响分期，但将影响临床分组。

IRS 临床分组系统以治疗前和手术结果为基础（表 32-5）。它的前提是原发部位肿瘤完全切除是分层最好的情况，然后根据肿瘤的可切除程度进行分
层。在过去，这种分层导致了大强度的治疗，常进行 52
截肢。该系统并不考虑肿瘤的生物学特性或肿瘤的自然病史，也没考虑到外科医生的经验和手术侵袭性。

随着活检更频繁的使用和新辅助性化疗，已经出现分组Ⅰ或Ⅱ向分组Ⅲ的“转变”，即在活检后进行新辅助性治疗。分组以术中探查和术后病理学表现（包括最终的切缘病理学结果、肿瘤残留、淋巴结浸润、及胸水和腹水细胞学检查）为基础。临床分组和治疗前分期与预后均有相关性[4,27,74]。

根据 IRS-I 至 IRS-V 的结果，在 IRS-V 治疗中建立了危险度分组，这综合了分组、分期和组织学亚型，将患者根据复发风险归类至三个不同的治疗方案（表 32-6）。低危组患者的 3 年无病生存率估计为 88%；中危组患者 3 年无病生存率估计为 55%～76%，高危患者 3 年无病生存率估计低于 30%。故推荐根据组织学亚型、原发部位、诊断时疾病的程度、

表 32-4 治疗前分期

分期	部位	肿瘤	大小	淋巴结	转移性
I	眼眶 头颈部（除脑膜旁） 膀胱-非前列腺	T_1 或 T_2	a 或 b	N_0 或 N_x	M_0
II	膀胱-前列腺 四肢 脑膜旁 其他（包括躯干、后腹膜、会阴、胆道、胸腔）	T_1 或 T_2	a	N_0 或 N_x	M_0
III	膀胱-前列腺 四肢 脑膜旁 其他（与 II 期相同）	T_1 或 T_2	a b	N_1 N_0、N_1、N_x	M_0
IV	所有部位	T_1 或 T_2	a 或 b	N_0、N_1、N_x	M_1

肿瘤：T_1，局限于原发解剖部位：（a）直径 5cm；（b）直径＞5cm；T_2，延伸和（或）固定于肿瘤周围组织：（a）直径 5cm；（b）直径＞5cm。

区域淋巴结：N_0，临床上区域淋巴结无受累；N_1，临床上区域淋巴结受肿瘤浸润；N_x，临床上区域淋巴结的状况不明（特别是不便做淋巴结检查的部位）。

转移：M_0，无远处转移；M_1，出现转移。

表 32-5 国际横纹肌肉瘤协作组研究的临床分组系统

组 I：病灶局限，完全切除。

（区域淋巴结未受侵犯——除了头颈部病变，高度推荐 [9602] 或必须 [9803、9802] 淋巴结活检或取样检查）

（a）局限于原发部位的肌肉或器官

（b）邻近浸润——浸润到原发部位的肌肉或器官外，如穿过筋膜

注：这包括大体检查和镜下确认的完全切除。任何可能无意中与标本一起切除的淋巴结均必须为阴性。如果出现镜下浸润，患者被归类于组 IIb 或 IIc。

组 II：肉眼完全切除，有区域播散的证据。

（a）肿瘤大体切除，有镜下残留（手术医师相信肿瘤被完全切除，但病理医师在边缘发现肿瘤，且再次切除以获得清洁边界是不可行 [9602] 或不合理的 [9803、9802]）。没有肿瘤肉眼残留的表现。没有区域淋巴结浸润的表现。一旦放疗和化疗开始，再次手术探查和切除镜下残留区域不会改变患者的分组。

（b）肿瘤有区域淋巴结浸润、完全切除但有镜下残留。

注：完全切除镜下确认没有肿瘤残留使该组与组 IIa 和 IIc 不同。此外，与 IIa 不同，区域淋巴结受浸润，但最远处淋巴结在组织学上呈阴性。

（c）肿瘤伴有区域性淋巴结浸润、大体切除，但在切除的最远处淋巴结（远离原发部位）有镜下残留或组织学浸润。

注 [只对 9602]：镜下残留的出现使该组与 IIb 不同，而淋巴结浸润使该组与 IIa 不同。

组 III：不完全切除，有肉眼肿瘤残留。

（a）只进行活检术后。

（b）原发肿瘤大体或大部分切除（＞50%）后。

组 IV：病初出现远处转移肿瘤（肺、肝脏、骨骼、骨髓、脑、远处肌肉和淋巴结）。

注 [只对 9602]：上述不包括区域淋巴结和邻近器官浸润，这些患者将属于预后较良好的临床分组（见组 II）。

脑脊液、胸水、腹水、或胸膜、腹膜或网膜的种植物在细胞学检查呈阳性被认为应该属于组 IV。

括号内的数字是 IRS 方案中的具体研究代号。

表 32-6 国际横纹肌肉瘤协作组研究-V 危险度分组

危险度	分期	临床分组、淋巴结状况、部位
低	I	I、II；N_0；所有预后较好部位（眼眶、头颈部、非脑膜旁、生殖泌尿道、膀胱-非前列腺）
	I	III；N_0、Nx；限于眼眶
	II	I；N_0、Nx；所有其他（预后不良）部位；肿瘤最大直径＝5cm
中	I	II；N_1；所有预后较好部位（同上）
	I	III；N_0、Nx、N_1；除眼眶外所有的预后较好部位
	II	II、III；N_0、Nx、N_1；所有其他部位
	III	II、III；N_0、Nx、N_1；所有其他部位
高	IV	IV；N0、Nx、N1；有转移灶的任何发病部位，包括脑脊液、胸水、腹水或网膜种植物

N_0：临床上区域淋巴结无浸润；N_1：临床上区域淋巴结受肿瘤浸润；Nx：临床上区域淋巴结的状况不明（特别是不便做淋巴结检查的部位）。

和治疗效应进行多学科协作。目的是在保留形态和功能情况下，获得局部控制[92]。

治疗

在 30 多年中，RMS 的治疗方法是多样的。对该病生物学和治疗了解的进展主要归功于 IRS（I～V）。
529 RMS 的手术治疗方法采取截肢的越来越少，或手术治疗强度也越来越低，而同时能保持很好的生存率。

RMS 的手术治疗具有部位特异性，后面将按不同部位进行讨论。总的原则是广泛切除原发肿瘤灶和周边未受侵犯的边缘组织，同时保持美观和功能。

除可能切除的小病灶外，早期活检一般进行切开性活检。假包膜能使病灶被剥离，这给了外科医生一个错觉，以为病灶已经被完全切除。许多病灶有视觉或显微镜下残留肿瘤，如果不是截肢则可以再次行切除术[43]。

任何病灶的活检均可能涉及再次手术和扩大切除。在类似四肢等部位，纵向切开通常比水平切开要好。活检确定为恶性时要保证再次手术时切除活检区域；如果活检部位处置不当，则在切除时可能需要比一般切除范围更大。

实体瘤活检传统上被分为切除性活检（标本包含整个肿瘤）和切开性活检（标本只包含肿瘤的一部分）。在切除性活检时，必须仔细标记切缘，以备在检测阳性时能对阳性切缘进行再次切除。理想的切除性活检是能够进行再次切除，以致只留下阴性切缘。如果这种切除性活检将导致再次切除时面积过大，则采用切开性活检更为适合。

如果活检边缘在标本和手术野均未被仔细标记（通常用缝线或夹子），则外科医生随后获得阴性切缘的能力将大打折扣。例如，在睾丸肿块患者中，不合适的活检方法可导致治疗难度增加。任何睾丸肿块手术必须通过腹股沟途径，而不是阴囊切开，以获得精索的近端控制及进行广泛局部切除时肿瘤不会种植在阴囊中。精索近端必须作清洁切缘的检查。如果仍有肿瘤存在则需进一步行高位切除。通过阴囊做肿瘤活检将导致进一步的阴囊切除，并增加了局部复发的风险。

初次活检和新辅助治疗后的第二次切除比部分或不完全切除有更好的治疗效果。已经转入临床分组III的患者，化疗后进行延期或二次探查手术可以使预后更佳，截肢手术更少。在一些选择性的部位，如四肢，应该进行区域淋巴结或前哨淋巴结的活检。

在一些四肢或躯干 RMS 患者，首次肿瘤切除术被认为是完全的，但组织病理发现手术切缘有镜下残留，相当于临床分组 IIa。这些患者中许多可以进行原发灶再次切除（PRE），从而获得更广泛的无病切缘。Hays 等人[43]证明了 PRE 的好处。在 IRS-I 和 IRS-II，154 例四肢或躯干 RMS 患者最初是临床分组 IIa；然后 41 例患者通过成功的 PRE在辅助治疗开始前转入临床分组 I。这些患者与 113 例有镜下残留但未做 PRE 的患者和 73 例首次切除术后无病生存（临床分组 I）的患者进行了比较。在 41例 PRE 患者中，3 年的 Kaplan-Meier 生存分析大约是 91%，相比之下未做 PRE 的分组 IIa 和分组 I 患者均为 74%。该方法也可以应用到其他部位的肿瘤。如果首次切除术不是“肿瘤”（即在首次切除术时未怀疑是恶性肿瘤），即使切缘明显正常，也应该考虑进行 PRE[21,43]。

二次探查手术已经用于数种儿童肿瘤，以评估治疗效果和切除任何手术后的残留肿瘤。二次探查手术在 IRS-III 中进行评估，并在临床分组 II 的 RMS 患者中显出益处[115,117-119]。进行二次探查手术在相当多的患者有良好的反应；12%认为初次手术完全有效的患者被发现有隐匿肿瘤残留，74%部分有效和无效的患者在二次术后被重新归类为完全有效。这些重新分类的患者生存率与那些再次探查时确认为完全有效的患者生存率相似[117,118]。

从 IRS-I 至 IRS-IV 总结的一般手术原则，并由此考虑在 IRS-V 中分为以下几种情况：（1）局部病灶，并完全切除的患者（临床分组 I）5 年 FFS 和总的生存率预后最佳。诊断时即有转移性病灶的患者（分组 IV）预后最差，而那些组 II 和组 III 患者预后中等。这样，如果手术可行且无大的致残率，应尽可能切除所有肉眼可见的肿瘤病灶。（2）病灶被切除后，如果首次手术不是恶性肿瘤，意味着应进行原发灶的再次切除。切缘状况有任何问题均意味着要再次切除。胚胎型的临床分组 I（完全切除）患者不接受术后放疗[123]。（3）理想的状况是保留器官功能，由此使眼、阴道和膀胱等结构得以保留。肿瘤位于或邻近这些部位的患者预后较好。首次化疗后进行放疗是推荐的方法。在首次化疗（加或不加放疗）使肿瘤缩小后，最初未切除的肿瘤进行延期切除能使肿瘤从部分有效改变为完全有效而改善预后。（4）在无转移病灶的睾丸旁 RMS 患儿中，诊断时年龄和区域淋巴结侵犯受累有一定关系。年龄小于 10 岁的 IRS-IV 男孩其无病生存率更好，因为淋巴结复发率比那些 10 岁及以上的患儿更低。我们现在建议对于没有区域淋巴结受累的大男孩进行改良的同侧后腹膜淋巴结剖视。如果这些淋巴结未受侵犯，则不用环磷酰胺和放疗；如果淋巴结内存在肿瘤，则除了长春新碱和放线菌素 D 外，还应给予环磷酰胺和放疗[120,121]。

IRS-V 需考虑的其他事项包括侵袭性更大的淋巴结检查。更早些的研究[56,57]认为，在大多数部位淋巴结受累罕见，因为很少进行淋巴结检查。而最近的研究表明，在四肢原发性肿瘤中，累及淋巴结的发生率比最初估计的要高[68]。前哨淋巴结活检是用活性染料，如异硫蓝，以及同位素标记的锝硫胶体，能对最可能包含肿瘤细胞的区域淋巴结进行定位。外科医生切除被标记的淋巴结，而病理科医生能彻底检查该淋巴结是否有肿瘤存在。前哨淋巴结活检反映了淋巴结区的状况。如果淋巴结阳性，则对淋巴结区进行放疗。前哨淋巴结活检正在应用于 IRS-V 的评估。

对于最初认为肿瘤无法切除的患者，必须在首次化疗后考虑进行二次探查手术。影像学检查在评价疗效时不是始终都有效的。在 IRS-III 中，75%的组 III 患儿和影像学上部分有效或没有效的患儿，但可能在病理学上完全有效、或者通过切除残留的肿瘤转化为完全有效。大多数（但不是全部）影像学上表现为完全有效的患者，可以通过二次手术来确认是否有效。这些转化为完全有效的患者生存状况更好。处于 IV 期的患儿其二次手术益处不大。二次探查手术对于头颈部肿瘤几无用处，但对于躯干和四肢的肿瘤是适合的。在通过二次探查手术转化为完全有效的患者，生存改善的趋势是持久的[117,118]。

化疗

在多学科治疗前，RMS 单纯手术治疗的生存率低于 20%。局部微卫星灶、淋巴结转移或未识别 / 未治疗的远处肿瘤常导致早期复发，随后的死亡主要是由于晚期转移性病变。

辅助性和后来的新辅助性化疗的发展已经使得生存率的明显提高。IRS 研究组资料显示，生存率不断改善、截肢手术不断减少和化疗毒性不断降低[24,25,69,70,83]。

在 RMS 治疗中已知有效的药物包括：长春新碱（vincristine，V）、放线菌素 D（actinomycin D， A）、柔红霉素（doxorubicin）、环磷酰胺（cyclophosphamide，C）、异环磷酰胺（ifosfamide，I）和表鬼臼乙叉甙（etoposide，E）。在局部扩散或转移性肿瘤患者中对美法仑和顺铂的作用进行了评估，结果在临床组 III 或组 IV 患者中进行随机对照研究，该药物与其他药物对照组比较预后没有改善[25,100]。

VAC 在大多数 RMS 患者治疗中已经成为联合化疗的金标准。随后的大样本随机对照研究已经对该方案进行改良，以适应基于临床分组和发病部位的不同亚型的治疗。在临床分组 Ⅰ 的胚胎型 RMS 中，IRS-Ⅲ结果显示，分别给予 VA 和 VAC 治疗，生存率相似[25]。在 IRS-Ⅳ中，临床分组 I 睾丸旁或眼眶肿瘤只接受 VA 治疗 2 年。在 IRS-V 前期研究中，给予“低危”患者单独 VA 化疗，包括 Ⅰ 期、临床分组 Ⅰ 或 Ⅱ（N_0）的眼眶、头颈（nonparameningeal）或生殖泌尿道（非膀胱-前列腺）肿瘤；Ⅱ 期、临床分组 Ⅰ 肿瘤；以及 Ⅰ 期、临床分组Ⅲ（眼眶只是 N_0）肿瘤[28,92]。

当认识到依托泊苷和异环磷酰胺对 RMS的功效后[71]，它们就被整合入 IRS-Ⅳ的治疗方案中。VAC、VAI 与 VIE 治疗的随机对照研究在无转移的 RMS 患者中展开。IRS-Ⅳ的资料显示目前标准的VAC（每次环磷酰胺2.2g/m^2和粒细胞集落刺激因子），在无治疗失败生存率（FFS）和总的存活率方面与VAI和VIE相同[26]。

中危患者的治疗可能因为新药的应用而改善。进行已知活性化疗药物的剂量强化治疗也应该考虑。IRS-Ⅳ的初步研究结果已经显示，中危胚胎型RMS的FFS结果得到改善极可能与环磷酰胺剂量增加有关[2]。环磷酰胺从IRS-Ⅲ的0.9g/m^2增加到IRS-Ⅳ的2.2g/m^2改善了胚胎型RMS患者的FFS，但对腺泡型或未分化型RMS没有影响[2]。

总例数1431的IRS-Ⅰ、IRS-Ⅱ和IRS-Ⅲ的资料显示，不管合并分析还是组Ⅲ和组Ⅳ单独分析，在组Ⅲ和组Ⅳ患者的VAC方案加用柔红霉素没有益处[25,69,70,92]。不管有无依托泊苷，加用柔红霉素和顺铂至VAC方案不会改善IRS-Ⅲ晚期患者的预后[25,69,70]。

尽管进行强化治疗，有转移性病灶的患者预后仍较差。强化的多药联合化疗已经应用以改善生存。国际儿科肿瘤协会（SIOP）报道，在先前未接受治疗的转移性RMS患者联合应用卡铂、表柔比星和长春新碱有效率为53%[33]。

治疗方案中的氨甲蝶呤作为一线用药因骨髓抑制作用相对较轻和其不同的作用机制而具有相对较好的疗效。在Ⅱ期试验中，Pappo等[81]报道在先前未接受治疗的进展期RMS患者，大剂量氨甲喋呤的有效率为33%。

托泊替康是喜树碱（CPT）类似物，是一种拓扑异构酶Ⅰ抑制剂，正在检测其对RMS的潜在作用（拓扑异构酶Ⅰ的抑制剂，可抑制DNA复制）。IRS协作组报道，在初诊的非脑膜旁转移性RMS患者中
531 进行托泊替康的治疗有45%的有效率[82,111]。IRS-V前期研究正在评估转移性RMS在VAC和放疗前的治疗中托泊替康与环磷酰胺联用的效果。似乎托泊替康在新诊断的转移性RMS患者有效，可与VAC联用[82]。

自体骨髓移植已经应用于几种儿童实体瘤中。到目前为止，尚无关于对转移性RMS患者治疗价值相关评估[51,54]。

概括来说，对于目前正在执行的IRS-V的推荐意见如下：

低危患者是那些常见发病部位、局限的胚胎型RMS（Ⅰ期）或不常见发病部位（Ⅱ和Ⅲ期）但已经被完全切除的患者。那些预后最好的患者归类于A组，进行VA方案治疗（加或不加放疗）。其他患者属于B组，进行VAC方案治疗（加或不加放疗）。

中危患者是那些发病部位局限的腺泡型RMS或未分化型肉瘤（Ⅰ～Ⅲ期）或有肉眼残留的（临床Ⅲ组）胚胎型RMS（Ⅱ和Ⅲ期）或诊断时年龄小于10岁有转移的（临床Ⅳ组）胚胎型RMS。他们随机接受VAC或VAC与长春新碱、环磷酰胺加托泊替康交替治疗，同时加用放疗。

高危患者是诊断时年龄大于或等于10岁的胚胎型RMS或年龄小于21岁、诊断时有转移病灶（临床Ⅳ组）的腺泡型RMS及未分化肉瘤。他们接受6周以上的伊立替康试验性治疗，随后给予VAC。最初对伊立替康有效的患者在化疗间歇继续给药，但对无效的患者不再用伊立替康。颅骨脑膜旁肿瘤和诊断时有脑膜侵犯的高危患者接受VAC化疗，不用伊立替康。

放疗

放疗按特定部位和肿瘤的程度进行调整。在某些部位，如头颈部或骨盆，肿瘤通常手术不能完全切除。放疗可以和化疗联合应用以消除残留的肿瘤细胞。放疗剂量的指导原则在IRS协作组相继的研究后已经发生改变。目前剂量已按照残留肿瘤的数量（肉眼或显微镜下）和肿瘤的治疗效应进行调整。

在IRS-Ⅳ，放疗按临床分组来决定。完全切除的临床分组Ⅰ、TNM的Ⅰ和Ⅱ期肿瘤患者不接受放疗。那些完全切除的组Ⅰ、Ⅱ期肿瘤和那些组Ⅱ肿瘤患者接受总剂量4140cGy的常规外照射放疗。临床分组Ⅲ患者随机接受5040cGy外照射放疗或5940cGy的超分割放疗。根据IRS-IV研究，没有迹象表明临床分组Ⅲ肿瘤患儿中，给予总剂量59.4Gy的两个1.1Gy的每日分数（间隔6小时）超分割放疗，与接受总剂量50.4Gy的1.8每日分数放疗的患儿比较，局部控制率更好[29,30]。

组织学亚型为胚胎型的RMS，完全切除的局部肿瘤（组Ⅰ）给予放疗没有显示有何益处[123]。根据患者在进入治疗时的分组，分级的放疗剂量对于所有其他患者是有益的。放疗的区域包括治疗前原发肿瘤部位和受累的区域淋巴结。组Ⅳ患者的原发部位和转移

灶在骨髓能承受的范围内均须接受放疗。

分析 IRS-Ⅰ至 IRS-Ⅳ的组Ⅱ患者资料显示，IRS-Ⅲ和 IRS-Ⅳ的疗效有所改善，可能是由于治疗的强化[103]。

IRS-Ⅲ和 IRS-Ⅳ的组Ⅲ患者的局部复发率在 2000 年由 IRS 的统计室进行了回顾分析。该复发率或保持稳定或已得到改善。在 IRS-Ⅳ，原发眼眶的肿瘤局部复发率是 2%、头颅脑膜旁是 16%，头颈其他部位是 12%，四肢是 7%，泌尿生殖道是 19%，其他部位是 14%。

目前 IRS 协作组的结果表明大多数头颅脑膜旁肉瘤（包括诊断时有邻近局部颅内扩散的）能通过全身化疗和放疗得到成功治疗。放疗针对原发部位，包括任何扩散部位，并需有 2cm 的空白边缘，包括邻近的脑膜。在没有弥漫性脑膜受累（如多发颅内转移）时，全颅放疗和鞘内注射抗肿瘤药物是没有必要的[89,91]。

总的来说，在 IRS-V 中推荐的放疗方案如下：完全切除的（组Ⅰ）胚胎型 RMS 患者不接受放疗。然而，完全切除的（组Ⅰ）腺泡型 RMS 和未分化型肉瘤的原发部位应接受放疗[123]。其他患者根据分组、组织学亚型、和区域淋巴结状态或远处转移来判断接受何等级放疗。有转移的患者应对原发部位和转移灶在骨髓能承受的前提内接受放疗[92]。

不同部位的治疗

头颈部

头颈部肿瘤包括表浅的头颈部、眼眶、腮腺、颊部、喉部、和口咽部。多学科治疗方法使手术侵袭性降低，而同时保持很好的预后。当可行时做广泛切除是合适的，但获得较大边缘的可能性仅限于小的表浅
2 性病变[47]。

眼眶肿瘤对治疗的反应很好，因为肿瘤通常局限于眼眶骨质，且该部位缺少淋巴管。Abramson 等人[1]证明，放疗加化疗是眼眶 RMS 最有效的治疗；该治疗使得摘除眼球的手术不再是必须的。VA 化疗和放疗的患者生存率高于 90%[25,32,114]。区域淋巴结的转移播散发生率低于 3%[56]。颈部淋巴结活检或前哨淋巴结活检似并无必要，除非临床上发现淋巴结受累。有淋巴结受累的患者必须用 IRS 中危方案治疗。这样，除了眼睑部位的小肿瘤，手术对于眼眶原发肿瘤的作用仅限于活检[32,52,114,116]。眶内容物摘除术只选择性应用于复发病例。

非眼眶、非脑膜旁部位包括不会侵犯脑膜的表浅性和深部肿瘤。对于一些肿瘤，如腮腺、喉部、咽部和其他深部肿瘤，手术限于活检，随后进行化疗和放疗来清除肿瘤[116]。该治疗方案生存率可达 83%[3,38]。

烷化剂在眼眶和非眼眶头颈部 RMS 的使用已经遭到质疑[7,52,114,116]。在 IRS-Ⅲ中，眼眶和非脑膜旁头颈部肿瘤的患者在接受强化的 VA 化疗和放疗后与 IRS-Ⅱ中接受类似方案加烷化剂治疗的生存率相同（90%）[24,25]。目前对该低危组的推荐治疗是给予 VA，加或不加放疗[27]。

脑膜旁肿瘤因为有扩散倾向以及有丰富的淋巴管系统而预后较差[3,20,56,116]。此外，脑膜旁 RMS 常发生于隐匿部位，这也常导致诊断延误[32,114,116]。15%的脑膜旁 RMS 患者有转移性病灶[25]。骨骼侵蚀是局部复发的征兆[67]。脑膜旁 RMS 采取的更强化的治疗包括 VAC 化疗、鞘内化疗和全颅脑脊髓放疗，使存活率得到提高[86]。在接受该强化治疗的患者中，无病生存率从 33%提高到 57%，局部肿瘤控制失败率从 28%降至 6%[86]。中枢神经系统的预防性放疗的价值已经受到质疑[35]。在 IRS-III 中，放疗和鞘内化疗根据脑膜受累的程度来定，大多数患者比 IRS-II 中接受的放疗剂量要小。IRS-III 和 IRS-II 比较，患者的无进展生存率没有下降[24,25]。

对于鼻区、鼻旁窦、颞窝和其他前颅底部位的肿瘤，做颅面部切除必须由外科医生中有经验的专家来操作，还应作为最初的化疗和放疗后肿瘤持续存在时的二次治疗的方式。在一些报道中，尽管影像学上有残留肿块，但在切除的标本中未发现活的肿瘤细胞[109,117,118]。其他研究表明，在 CT 上明确存在的残留病灶与随后的局部复发和死亡之间有很好的相关性[36]。这方面内容正在进行进一步研究。

泌尿生殖道

泌尿生殖道包括膀胱、前列腺、睾丸旁区、阴道、子宫、会阴部和偶尔包括的肾脏或输尿管。RMS

是儿童盆腔结构中最常见的恶性肿瘤。该部位的肿瘤根据不同的预后被认为有两种类型：膀胱－前列腺和会阴－阴道、子宫和睾丸旁区。在IRS－Ⅲ，病灶在这些部位的病例约占25%的[25]。在IRS－Ⅰ和IRS－Ⅱ中，6%的盆腔RMS无法明确其盆腔内确切的原发部位。阴道和睾丸肿瘤的预后较好，胚胎型更为多见，常有葡萄状（阴道）或纺锤状细胞（睾丸旁区）亚型。

膀胱RMS和前列腺RMS相互间很难鉴别，因为它们的解剖位置邻近，且肿瘤在诊断前可能长得很大。当可能确诊时，膀胱肿瘤患者的预后比起源于前列腺的肿瘤患者预后明显要好[115]。这些部位的肿瘤大部分是胚胎型（71%）或葡萄状型（20%）；2%在组织学上是腺泡型[75]。

在IRS-Ⅲ中发现膀胱或前列腺RMS患儿接受更强化的化疗和较早放疗后的生存率只比头颈部RMS患儿略低。该发现与IRS－Ⅱ的结果相反[24,25,69,70,87]。

膀胱或前列腺肿瘤一般出现于三角区附近，产生膀胱出口梗阻或血尿症状。诊断常通过膀胱镜检查和活检，以及CT或MRI检查。以前，这些肿瘤患儿的初期治疗方法通常是前部或整个盆腔脏器切除术，随后进行化疗或放疗；这种治疗方法有非常好的长期生存率，在某些研究中接近85%，但它也需要永久性放置导尿管，且部分病例需要结肠造口术[87,90]。目前，保留膀胱是一个重要的目标，所以常用侵袭较小的手术方法[44-46,49]。新辅助化疗和放疗已经使膀胱切除术的比例从50%以上降低到约30%[44-46]。在IRS－Ⅲ中50%的膀胱RMS患者除了长春新碱－阿霉素－环磷酰胺或VAC和放疗外，还接受顺铂的化疗。在IRS－Ⅰ至IRS－Ⅲ中，171例原发性膀胱RMS患儿中，40例在接受新辅助化疗和放疗后做了部分膀胱切除术。9例发生复发（7例为局部复发）。在IRS－Ⅲ中，所有膀胱或前列腺RMS患儿保留膀胱功能的Kaplan－Meier统计生存率为60%。长期生存率超过80%[44-46]。

盆腔脏器切除术不再是前列腺RMS的主要治疗方法。在IRS－Ⅲ诊断的新发病例中，发生于该部位约占5%。诊断时的平均年龄为5.3岁。大多数肿瘤相对较大，组织学上是胚胎型，临床上病灶局限但若想不丧失器官功能则无法切除。44例临床分组Ⅲ肿瘤（有肉眼残留）根据IRS－Ⅲ方案治疗。其中43例只做了活检，1例在首次手术时做了次全切除术。每个患者的平均手术次数是2次（范围为1～5次）。44例中的6例没有做二次手术。其余38例患者中做了二次探查术，包括盆腔脏器切除术[14]、前列腺切除术[4]、膀胱镜或会阴针刺活检[9]、剖腹探查和活检[6]、和保留膀胱的次全切除术[3]。4例患者需要多次手术来探查残留肿块、术后瘘管处理、输尿管狭窄、或小肠梗阻。6例复发或有残留肿物患者经过再次的化疗和后期的脏器切除术[3]、前列腺切除术[1]、或活检[2]。其中4例被治愈，1例接受继发恶性肿瘤的治疗、1例患者在脏器切除术后仍有残留。这样，44例组Ⅲ肿瘤患者中的36例被治愈（至少随访6年；范围为6～11年），而IRS－Ⅱ中则为47例中有23例治愈。那些治愈患者的膀胱保留率也更好（64%比57%）。临床分组Ⅲ前列腺RMS患儿在强化化疗（加或不加放疗）后进行的保守、延期手术能有更高的治愈率，同时有较高的膀胱保留率[65]。

睾丸旁区域

睾丸旁RMS占所有儿童RMS的7%及儿童阴囊肿瘤的12%[120]。大多数睾丸旁RMS是胚胎型、无转移病灶、用多学科综合治疗方式（包括手术、多药联合化疗、对后腹膜淋巴结受累或切除不彻底的患者进行放疗）有较高的治愈率[80]。

大多数肿瘤表现为无痛性阴囊肿块，常容易切除（组Ⅰ）。组Ⅰ和组Ⅱ患者的生存率超过90%[60,96]。邻近睾丸或精索的病灶必须通过睾丸切除术和经腹股沟切开近端暴露精索的方法来切除整个精索。当需要阴囊放疗时，对侧睾丸可以临时移置于邻近的大腿。必须避免打开阴囊活检或肿瘤的播散，否则可以导致腹股沟的复发；肿瘤的溢出或开放式活检者需要行阴囊切除术（加或不加放疗）。如果在睾丸切除术前需要做活检，必须遵循以下步骤：（1）对精索采取高度的无创伤暴露；（2）移动睾丸和精索，仔细从手术野分离；（3）在等待冰冻切片报告时保持活检部位封闭并覆盖睾丸；（4）更换活检时用过的手术衣、手套和器械；（5）如果活检报告呈阳性，切除睾丸和整个精索包括无创夹子；（6）彻底冲洗手术野。有肿瘤播散的患者不管切除是否完全均应归为临床分组Ⅱa[41]。

睾丸旁RMS的淋巴结转移发生率的报道为26%～43%[37,77,86,120]。在IRS－Ⅲ期间，所有患者被要求接受同侧后腹膜淋巴结清扫。在IRS－Ⅳ，后腹膜淋巴结通过 CT 来评估，在该研究中，只有那些 CT 显示有淋巴结受累的患者需要做手术来切除淋巴结。这使约 15%的组 II（淋巴结阳性）患者“降级”至组 I（完全切除，没有淋巴结浸润）。在青少年中有效率更高（＞30%）。这种变化使接受腹膜后腔放疗的患者更少，但也使 IRS–Ⅳ的 FFS 更差和复发率增高。对于小于 10 岁的患儿，IRS–Ⅲ和 IRS–Ⅲ之间的长期生存率没有差别，均很好（IRS–Ⅲ为 100%，IRS–Ⅳ为 98%）。然而，在 IRS–Ⅳ中约 30%归类为组 I 肿瘤的青少年治疗是失败的；这些患者需要重新治疗，补救的效果很差。在 IRS–Ⅳ，给予后腹膜淋巴结放疗和强化的三药联合化疗（包括烷化剂）的患者中，3 年生存率是 100%。基于这些资料，IRS 协作组重新推荐对所有年龄大于 10 岁的患者应进行后腹膜淋巴结清扫。

但这仍存在争议，因为 SIOP 不再推荐对任何患者进行后腹膜淋巴结清扫。Olive 等人[77]发现化疗对于清除隐匿性微小转移是有效的；由此，他们认为，淋巴结清扫在完全切除加化疗的睾丸旁 RMS 患者是不必要的。

后腹膜淋巴结清扫伴有明显的长期并发症。Heyn 等人[48]发现，这些并发症包括与肠梗阻、射精功能丧失、和下肢淋巴水肿。

用强化化疗也有相关的危险性。环磷酰胺是一个 N–磷酸化的环状氮芥的衍生物。环磷酰胺的副作用包括免疫抑制、肺纤维化、不育和男性睾丸萎缩[122]。

目前的推荐是所有睾丸旁 RMS 患者必须做薄层的腹部和盆腔 CT 增强扫描来检查有无淋巴结浸润的表现。大于等于 10 岁的患儿接受同侧后腹膜保留神经束的淋巴结清扫。组 II 患者接受强化治疗（例如 VAC 和后腹膜淋巴结放疗）[16]。小于 10 岁的患儿可以通过腹部薄层 CT 检查（每层 5mm）来分期，对那些检查呈阳性的进行同侧淋巴结清扫。组 I 肿瘤患儿必须接受 VA 化疗，不用放疗。腹股沟淋巴结很少受累，只有临床上呈阳性或阴囊受肿瘤侵犯时需作活检。腹股沟淋巴结被认为不是区域性的淋巴结，当它们呈阳性时，患儿将归为Ⅳ期（临床分组Ⅳ）。

外阴、阴道和子宫

外阴、阴道和子宫 RMS 是最常见的儿科女性生殖系统恶性肿瘤。该肿瘤一般出现于生后最初几年，表现为阴道流血、分泌物、和阴道肿块。如果肿瘤出现于外阴，表现为在阴唇褶内的硬结，或在阴蒂周围。诊断可通过切开或切除活检。阴道病变组织学通常呈胚胎型或葡萄状胚胎型，预后很好[4,6,9]。会阴部病变组织学呈腺泡型，但由于大多数较为局限，预后也较好。阴道病变常出现于胚胎阴道前壁的膀胱阴道隔膜区域（泌尿生殖窦）。膀胱、前列腺囊、前列腺、和阴道下段均起源于泌尿生殖窦。在两性中，这些部位均为 RMS 的好发部位。

在 1972 年前，阴道 RMS 的治疗方式是盆腔脏器切除术。从 1972 年开始，IRS 协作组开始对患者进行前瞻性临床研究。最早的 8 例没有转移病灶的阴道 RMS 患者首先经过手术治疗，随后进行术后 VAC 化疗。3 例患者还接受了放疗。因为阴道 RMS 对化疗有效，IRS–II 先进行化疗，随后进行延期的手术治疗（加或不加放疗）。20 例中的 14 例患者（70%）最终进行手术切除[9]。

在 IRS–Ⅲ，这些患者在活检后（临床分组Ⅲ）先进行包括 VAC 加阿霉素和顺铂的化疗。23 例中只有 7 例患者（30%）在化疗后进行手术切除。其中的 6 例在切除标本中没有活的肿瘤细胞，1 例有成熟的横纹肌母细胞。横纹肌母细胞的出现并不表明肿瘤有持久的活性[49]。在 M. D. Anderson 肿瘤中心，当发现横纹肌母细胞时，我们继续化疗而不进行切除。这些患者在进一步化疗后或随后的活检中没有发现活的肿瘤细胞或横纹肌母细胞。在 IRS-Ⅲ只有 6 例患者进行放疗[6]。

在 IRS–Ⅳ，23 例中只有 3 例（14%）在化疗后进行手术切除。3 例患者只有横纹肌母细胞，1 例进行早期二次探查手术的患者有横纹肌母细胞和少量活的肿瘤细胞。在 IRS-Ⅳ中没有患者进行膀胱切除术，除了 1 例患者外其余患者均仍存活，没有发病的迹象。

早期 IRS 协作组研究表明，原发子宫的肿瘤是一个特别的类型，与那些年长的阴道肿瘤患者不同，通常易于局部复发，且预后很差。早期手术治疗是关键。从 1984 年开始（IRS–Ⅲ），这些患者接受由阿霉素、顺铂、长春新碱、放线菌素 D 和环磷酰胺组成的新辅助化疗。这些治疗使切除范围可以更小，更少的接受放疗，同时可以很好的控制局部和远隔肿瘤。存活率不断提高而更少应用根治性手术治疗[22]。

对于阴道、会阴和子宫 RMS 肿瘤，在 IRS-V 中总的原则包括活检和分期、随后根据分期和分组（即危险度分类）进行化疗。常做二次和三次探查活检手术和膀胱镜检查。阴道远端病变可以是息肉状或局限性的，可以进行早期切除或延期切除。除非复发或持续见到活的肿瘤细胞，否则很少做阴道切除术或子宫切除术。淋巴结受累非常少见。除了晚期或复发肿瘤直接累及卵巢外，不做卵巢切除术。

首先用金标准 VAC 方案进行化疗，随后局部切除，偶尔根据需要使用放疗，这种综合治疗已经取得很好的疗效[10]。1～9 岁的患儿疗效最佳（5 年生存率 98%）；该年龄段以外的患儿在 IRS-Ⅲ或 IRS-Ⅳ中用强化治疗而获益（5 年生存率在 IRS-Ⅰ和 IRS-Ⅱ是 67%，在 IRS-Ⅲ和 IRS-Ⅳ是 90%）[10]。

躯干

原发躯干的 RMS 可以出现于脊柱旁、胸壁、腹壁、腹腔、或骨盆及后腹膜。这些肿瘤腺泡型发生率较高，一些部位的预后极差[8,88]。这些肿瘤的表现根据发病部位而不同，故分别进行讨论。

脊柱旁

脊柱旁 RMS 表现为椎旁肌肉不断增大的肿块。诊断通常需切开性活检，并需与骨外 Ewing 肉瘤鉴别，因为经验告诉我们尤文氏肉瘤在此部位也较常见。对于所有躯干肿瘤，必须沿肿瘤的长轴进行活检（即与肋骨平行），以备以后做扩大的局部切除和必要时切除肋骨的准备。

大多数脊柱旁肿瘤患者在切除前需要化疗，许多在术后还要进行放疗。扩大的局部切除常与整形手术结合，以减少脊柱的不稳定性。在幼儿，如果可行，尽量不进行脊柱旁放疗。

腹壁

该部位相对少见（在所有患者中＜1%），需要切除或切开性活检，随后进行广泛局部完全切除或新辅助化疗，再进行二次探查手术。回顾分析 IRS 患者，5 年的 FFS 是 65%[12]。腺泡型和肿瘤巨大的年长患者预后较差。

胸壁

胸壁和胸廓内的 RMS 在儿童中少见。在 IRS-Ⅰ、-Ⅱ和-Ⅲ登记的 2747 例患者中，只有 105 例是原发于胸壁、胸膜、肺或心脏的肿瘤。已经发现这些部位的肿瘤由于组织类型、疾病有表现时即处于晚期、和难于局部切除而预后较差。早期研究表明局部和远处复发率高[88]。IRS-Ⅱ和 IRS-Ⅲ的回顾性研究[8]包含 84 例胸廓肉瘤：76 例胸壁肿瘤、3 例肺部肿瘤、4 例胸膜肿瘤和 1 例原发于心脏的肿瘤。60 例患者（71%）完成全部治疗。39 例患者有局部复发，22 例患者有远隔复发。42%的患者存活。无进展存活率与组织学类型、发病部位、临床分组或不同 IRS 没有明显相关性。根据单变量分析，总的存活率与临床分组、肿瘤大小和局部或远处复发有显著的相关性，但与组织学类型或不同的 IRS 无关。在多变量分析中，只有临床分组和局部或远处复发有统计学意义。由此，如果存活率要得到改善，必须达到局部肿瘤控制并取得切缘阴性。临床分组Ⅱ的患者接受放疗，其生存率比那些临床分组Ⅰ（完全切除，因此未接受放疗）的要好，这表明手术切除可能有显微镜下或甚至肉眼的肿瘤残留。对于可能有残留的临床分组 I 患者进行二次探查手术或考虑局部放疗可能改善生存[8]。

胸壁 RMS 的特殊手术治疗包括最初的活检（沿肋骨的长轴）和分期。在新辅助化疗后，肿瘤被切除并保留无瘤边缘，附着的胸膜或肺在必要时也可切除。如果需要，扩大的局部切除后可以进行胸壁重建，通常用合成的材料覆盖以肌肉皮瓣。往往肿瘤体积的缩小允许切除时采用一期缝合。

后腹膜和骨盆

后腹膜和骨盆的 RMS 通常表现为大的、成团的肿瘤，其确切的边缘难于界定[23]。这些肿瘤往往侵犯或累及重要的器官或血管；因此，在最初的探查中只能进行活检。早期 IRS 协作组研究显示这些部位的肿瘤预后较差[23]。Blakely 等人[14]报道，在 IRS-Ⅲ和 IRS-Ⅳ实验组的 94 例组Ⅲ患者中，4 年的 FFS 为 57%。他们发现预后良好的因素有：（1）患儿时年龄小于 10 岁；（2）胚胎型组织学类型；（3）在进行化疗和放疗前进行肿瘤减灭术。最近 Raney 等人[93]报道了 56 例局限性的后腹膜和骨盆 RMS 患者。这些患者中有 54 例在最初的诊断性手术后有肉眼肿瘤残留（临床分组Ⅲ）。2 例显微镜下有浸润边缘的患者进行完全切除，没有（组Ⅱa）或有（组Ⅱc）肿瘤累及的区域淋巴结（在开始化疗前被切除）。只有 15 例患者（27%）在化疗前有 50%或更多的肿瘤被切除，这些被认为是肿瘤减灭术；其余 41 例患者被认为只进行了活检。在 15 例化疗或放疗前进行肿瘤减灭术的患者中，迄今没有治疗失败的。相反的是，41 例中的 15 例只进行活检的出现肉瘤复发。这样，看来肿瘤减灭术若在能安全且致残率最少的情况下进行则有一定价值。否则，应该在化疗使肿瘤皱缩后再进行延期切除。

胆囊

胆囊 RMS 患者进行化疗和放疗而不做手术切除，预后也相对较良好[84,104]。大多数患者属于葡萄状胚胎型 RMS，这种类型对化疗反应较好。虽然这些肿瘤表现出明显的梗阻性黄疸，但活检后进行新辅助性化疗常减轻黄疸，而无需做切除或内置、外置胆道引流。手术切除或引流可能会出现明显的并发症。Spunt 等人[104]报道，在 IRS-Ⅰ至 IRS-Ⅳ的 25 例患者中发现做完全切除基本上是不可能的，胆道外置引流常产生感染，肿瘤对联合化疗反应良好，无需做大的手术干预。

会阴和肛周部位

会阴或肛周 RMS 是儿童中少见的肉瘤，其预后相对较差。Blakely 等人[15]报道，在 IRS-Ⅰ至 IRS-Ⅳ中有 71 例患者接受治疗。大多数患者（64%）在出现临床症状时已处于进展期阶段（临床分组Ⅲ和Ⅳ），50%有区域淋巴结受累。所有患者的 5 年 FFS 是 45%，总的生存率是 49%。具备原发肿块小于 5cm、临床分组和分期较低（不属于晚期）、淋巴结阴性、和年龄小于 10 岁这些特征时，患者预后明显较好。当对疾病的程度进行控制做多变量分析时，只有年龄小于 10 岁预示疗效较好。年龄小于 10 岁的 5 年总生存率是 71%，而年长儿童是 20%（$P<0.001$）。因为区域淋巴结受累的发生率高，临床上可疑淋巴结必须接受活检，临床上无可疑淋巴结者必须作前哨淋巴结监测。

四肢

原发于四肢的 RMS 在 IRS-Ⅲ中占 19%[7]，在 IRS-Ⅳ中占 20%[74]。尽管 IRS 协作组在不懈的努力，四肢 RMS 的疗效与其他部位的 RMS 比较仍然不容
乐观。虽然生存率在随后的研究中显示有所改善，但 536
对于没有远处转移灶的患者其 5 年的生存率估计是 74%[7]。这些研究资料的分析表明治疗的改善归因于对预后差患者治疗的强化，而对预后好的患者降低了治疗强度。专家们已提出许多儿童四肢 RMS 相关的预后因素。在 IRS-Ⅳ中应用的 Lawrence-Gehan 分期系统[58]的预后因素有：局部组织侵袭程度、肿瘤大小、淋巴结状况、远处转移和发病部位。因为四肢是相对预后较差的部位，所以在该系统中没有四肢肿瘤被分为 I 期。在 IRS-IV 中共有 139 例四肢 RMS 患者，按照术前分期和临床分组如下：Ⅱ期（n=34），III 期（n=73），Ⅳ期（n=32）；组Ⅰ（n=31），组Ⅱ（n=21），组Ⅲ（n=54），组Ⅳ（n=33）。3 年 FFS 是 55%，总的生存率是 70%。进展期肿瘤患者的 FFS 明显要差。完全切除患者（组 I）的 3 年 FFS 是 91%[74]。

最初的治疗包括进行切开或切除性活检。这必须纵向或轴向进行以便于随后广泛局部切除。如果不用致残就能进行扩大的局部切除，则尽量不致残。标准的 2cm 切缘是任意设定的，在儿童中没有实用性。没有证据表明只有几毫米的清洁边界与更大的切缘比较有更高的复发风险。除非较大的复发或肿瘤持续存在，否则截肢是很少有必要进行的。过去推荐的从起点到插入点切除整个肌肉的方法是不必要的。完全切除的重要性要强调，因为完全切除或只有镜下残留，其生存率明显改善。仔细检查切缘的状态是极为重要的，应保证在首次或再次手术时能够再切除。Hays 等人[43]证实，在淋巴结阴性的四肢和躯干肉瘤患者，因镜下肿瘤残留进行再次切除的生存率，与那些没有进行再次切除或最初切除后没有发现肿瘤残留的患者比较，明显更高。我们的原则是推荐对所有来我们医院的患者在以前手术的基础上再次切除，不管以前的

报告如何。因我们已经在以前报告肿瘤完全切除（可能因为外科医生不知道肿瘤的存在）的患者中发现肿瘤残留，甚至大的肿瘤。

在 IRS-Ⅰ和 IRS-Ⅱ中，四肢 RMS 的淋巴结受累仅占 12%[5,7,56,57]，因为实际上很少有患者进行淋巴结活检。Laquaglia 等人[55]报道淋巴结阳性率为 40%。在 IRS-Ⅳ的回顾性研究中，Andrassy 等人证明，进行淋巴结检查的患者中有 39%在组织学上确定有肿瘤。Neville 等人[74]在 IRS-Ⅳ的回顾性资料中发现，50%淋巴结活检含有肿瘤。在那些临床上淋巴结阴性但因各种原因进行活检的患者中，17%患者被发现有镜下肿瘤。组织学上淋巴结阳性的结果在统计学上是 FFS 的重要预测因素。虽然淋巴结清扫不能改善生存率，但阳性的区域淋巴结必须接受放疗以防止局部的复发。我们已经使用并推荐前哨淋巴结活检来评估区域淋巴结[73,74]。如果不能行前哨淋巴结定位，可考虑侵袭性的取样检查。

并发症

RMS 治疗的并发症是多样、广泛的。这些包括化疗毒性和死亡、放疗相关性急性和长期并发症、和常见的活检和切除手术并发症。具体的并发症及其治疗的讨论不属于本章的范畴。应该对所有患者进行长期随访以观察晚发并发症和继发肿瘤的出现[94]。

转移灶的治疗

转移灶最常见于：肺（58%）、骨骼（33%）、区域淋巴结（33%）、肝脏（22%）和脑（20%）[21]。在 IRS-Ⅲ[25]的患者中，14%在诊断时是临床分组Ⅳ。易发生转移的原发灶包括四肢（23%）、脑膜旁（13%）、和后腹膜、躯干、胃肠道及胸廓内等部位。转移发生率低的原发灶包括眼眶（1.8%）、非脑膜旁或非眼眶的头颈部（4.5%）、和生殖泌尿道等部位[97]。在 RMS 患者中，有无转移是最重要的独立的临床预后预测因素。有转移灶的患者其 3 年 FFS 只有 25%[25,70]。就像前面提及的，发生区域淋巴结转移的可能性随肿瘤原发部位不同而变化（四肢最高），且影响生存率。

肺是转移灶最常见的部位。只有肺部转移的患者与那些有多个部位转移或转移至骨骼或肝脏的患者比较，有较好的预后[96]。只有肺部转移的患者也更可能是预后良好组织类型，且原发四肢的可能较小[96]。因为 RMS 对化疗高度敏感，所以不建议切除多个转移灶。在我们的经验中，肺的单个孤立性转移灶预后比多个转移灶预后更好。因为这个原因，对于单个转移灶值得做活检以确定组织类型。较好的预后可能与除 RMS 外的非转移性肺部病变的治疗有关。化疗后持续存在或复发的肿瘤可能需要做切除以用于诊断，并可能降低肿瘤的负荷。总的来说，有转移患者的生存率几乎未得到改善。它们目前被归类为Ⅳ期、组Ⅳ，并被认为是高危组。

目前正在研究用强化的化疗和放疗以试图改善生存率。在 IRS-Ⅳ中，127 例入选的患者接受两个方案之一来治疗转移灶，这些方案用异环磷酰胺和表鬼臼乙叉甙与长春新碱、放线菌 D 和环磷酰胺或长春新碱、美法仑和 VAC 联合治疗。估计 3 年总生存率和 FFS 分别是 39%和 25%。3 年总的生存率受组织学类型（胚胎型是 47%，其他类型是 34%）和转移灶数量影响。通过多因素分析，两个或两个以下的转移灶是唯一有意义的预测因素[17]。

结果

在每个 IRS 协作组研究中，生存率的总趋势是升高的。生存率有赖于临床分组、分期和原发部位。IRS-Ⅲ的 5 年总生存率是 71%，临床分组Ⅰ的是 90%，组Ⅱ是 80%，组Ⅲ的是 70%，组Ⅳ的是 30%。按照治疗前分期，Ⅰ期生存率是 80%，Ⅱ期是 68%，Ⅲ期是 49%，Ⅳ期是 21%[124]。

总的来说，接受 IRS-Ⅳ治疗的患者 FFS 率与 IRS-Ⅲ中病情相同的患者无差别；估计的 3 年 FFS 率在 IRS-Ⅲ和 IRS-Ⅳ分别是 76%和 77%。IRS-Ⅳ与 IRS-Ⅲ比较，胚胎型 RMS 患者的 3 年 FFS 率得到改善（83%对 74%）。这种改善看来只限于Ⅱ期或Ⅱ～Ⅲ期、组Ⅰ～Ⅱ的胚胎型 RMS 患者。治疗失败的部位中局部性的有 93 例（51%）、区域性的 30 例（17%）、远处的 58 例（32%）。复发后补救性治疗因不同的组而不同。组Ⅰ～Ⅱ的患者在复发 3 年后 41%患者仍存活，而组Ⅲ的患者为 22%存活。

（叶启东译　王耀平校）

参考文献

1. Abramson DH, et al: The treatment of orbital rhabdomyosarcoma with irradiation and chemotherapy. Ophthalmology 1979;86:1330.
2. Anderson GJ, et al: Rhabdomyosarcoma of the head and neck in children. Arch Otolaryngol Head Neck Surg 1990; 116:428.
3. Anderson JR, et al: Improved outcome for patients with embryonal histology but not alveolar histology rhabdomyosarcoma: Results from Intergroup Rhabdomyosarcoma Study IV (IRS-IV). Proc Soc Clin Oncol 1998;17:526a.
4. Andrassy RJ: Rhabdomyosarcoma. Semin Pediatr Surg 1997;6:17.
5. Andrassy RJ: Advances in the surgical management of sarcomas in children. Am J Surg 2002;184:484.
6. Andrassy RJ, et al: Conservative surgical management of vaginal and vulvar pediatric rhabdomyosarcoma: A report from the Intergroup Rhabdomyosarcoma Study-III. J Pediatr Surg 1995;30:1034.
7. Andrassy RJ, et al: Extremity sarcomas: An analysis of prognostic factors from the Intergroup Rhabdomyosarcoma Study (IRS) III. J Pediatr Surg 1996;31:191.
8. Andrassy RJ, et al: Thoracic sarcomas in children. Ann Surg 1998;227:170.
9. Andrassy RJ, et al: Progress in the surgical management of vaginal rhabdomyosarcoma: A 25-year review from the Intergroup Rhabdomyosarcoma Study Group. J Pediatr Surg 1999;34:731.
10. Arndt CA, et al: What constitutes optimal therapy for patients with rhabdomyosarcoma of the female genital tract? Cancer 2001;91:2454.
11. Asmar L, et al: Agreement among and within groups of pathologists in the classification of rhabdomyosarcoma and related childhood sarcomas: Report of an international study of four pathology classifications. Cancer 1994;74:2579.
12. Beech TR, et al: What comprises appropriate therapy for children/adolescents with rhabdomyosarcoma arising in the abdominal wall? A report from the Intergroup Rhabdomyosarcoma Study Group. J Pediatr Surg 1999;34:668.
13. Birch JM, et al: Excess risk of breast cancer in the mothers of children with soft tissue sarcomas. Br J Cancer 1984; 49:325.
14. Blakely ML, et al: Does debulking improve survival rate in advanced-stage retroperitoneal embryonal rhabdomyosarcoma? J Pediatr Surg 1999;5:736.
15. Blakely ML, et al: Prognostic factors and surgical treatment guidelines for children with rhabdomyosarcoma of the perineum or anus: A report of Intergroup Rhabdomyosarcoma Studies I through IV, 1972 through 1997. J Pediatr Surg 2003;38:347.
16. Breneman JC, et al: The management of pediatric genitourinary rhabdomyosarcoma. In Vogelzang NJ, et al (eds): The Comprehensive Textbook of Genitourinary Oncology. Baltimore, Williams & Wilkins, 1996.
17. Breneman JC, et al: Prognostic factors and clinical outcomes in children and adolescents with metastatic rhabdomyosarcoma: A report from the Intergroup Rhabdomyosarcoma Study IV. J Clin Oncol 2003;21:78.
18. Burger RA, et al: Extent of surgery in rhabdomyosarcoma of urogenital structures. Eur Urol 1989;16:114.
19. Cavazzana AO, et al: Spindle cell rhabdomyosarcoma. Am J Surg Pathol 1992;16:229.
20. Coene IMJH, et al: Rhabdomyosarcoma of the head and neck in children. Clin Otolaryngol 1992;17:291.
21. Cofer BR, et al: Rhabdomyosarcoma. In Andrassy RJ (ed): Pediatric Surgical Oncology. Philadelphia, WB Saunders, 1998.
22. Corpron CA, et al: Conservative management of uterine pediatric rhabdomyosarcoma: A report from the Intergroup Rhabdomyosarcoma Study III and IV Pilot. J Pediatr Surg 1995;30:942.
23. Crist WM, et al: Soft tissue sarcomas arising in the retroperitoneal space in children: A report from the Intergroup Rhabdomyosarcoma Study. Cancer 1985;56:2125.
24. Crist WM, et al (for the IRS Committee): Prognosis in children with rhabdomyosarcoma: A report of IRS-I and IRS-II. J Clin Oncol 1990;8:443.
25. Crist WM, et al: Intergroup Rhabdomyosarcoma Study (IRS) III. J Clin Oncol 1995;13:610.
26. Crist WM, et al: Preliminary results for patients with local/regional tumors treated on the Intergroup Rhabdomyosarcoma Study-IV (1991-1997). Proc Am Soc Clin Oncol 1999; 18:18.
27. Crist WM, et al: Intergroup Rhabdomyosarcoma Study-IV: Results for patients with nonmetastatic disease. J Clin Oncol 2001;19:3091.
28. Dagher R, et al: Rhabdomyosarcoma: An overview. Oncologist 1999;4:34.
29. Donaldson S, et al: Hyperfractionated radiation in children with rhabdomyosarcoma: Results of an Intergroup Rhabdomyosarcoma Pilot Study. Int J Radiat Oncol Biol Phys 1995;32:903.
30. Donaldson SS, et al: Results from the Intergroup Rhabdomyosarcoma Study-IV randomized trial of hyperfractionated radiation in children with rhabdomyosarcoma. Int J Radiat Oncol Biol Phys 2000;48:178.
31. Ferracini R, et al: Retrogenic expression of the MET protooncogene correlates with the invasive phenotype of human rhabdomyosarcomas. Oncogene 1996;12:1697.
32. Fiorillo A, et al: Multidisciplinary treatment of primary orbital rhabdomyosarcoma: A single institution experience. Cancer 1991;67:560.
33. Frascella E, et al: Response of previously untreated metastatic rhabdomyosarcoma to combination chemotherapy with carboplatin, epirubicin, and vincristine. Eur J Cancer 1996;32A:821.
34. Furman W, et al: A phase I study of irinotecan (CPT-11) in children with relapsed solid tumors. Proc Am Soc Clin Oncol 1998;17:187a.
35. Gasparini M, et al: Questionable role of CNS radioprophylaxis in the therapeutic management of childhood rhabdomyosarcoma with meningeal extension. J Clin Oncol 1990;8:1854.
36. Gilles R, et al: Head and neck rhabdomyosarcomas in children: Value of clinical and CT findings in the detection of local regional relapses. Clin Radiol 1994;49:412.
37. Goldfarb B, et al: The role of retroperitoneal lymphadenectomy in localized paratesticular rhabdomyosarcoma. J Urol 1994;152:785.
38. Gross M, et al: Therapy of rhabdomyosarcoma of the larynx. Int J Pediatr Otorhinolaryngol 1988;15:93.
39. Grufferman A, et al: In utero x-ray exposure and risk of childhood rhabdomyosarcoma. Paper presented at the Fourth Annual Meeting of the Society for Epidemiologic Research, June 11, 1991, Buffalo, NY.
40. Grufferman S, et al: Parents' use of recreational drugs and risk of rhabdomyosarcoma in their children. Cancer Causes Control 1993;4:217.
41. Hamilton CR, et al: The management of paratesticular rhabdomyosarcoma. Clin Radiol 1989;40:314.

42. Hartley AN, et al: Patterns of cancer in the families of children with soft tissue sarcoma. Cancer 1993;72:923.
43. Hays DM, et al: Primary re-excision for patients with "microscopic residual" following initial excision of sarcomas of trunk and extremity sites. J Pediatr Surg 1989;24:5.
44. Hays DM, et al: Partial cystectomy in the management of rhabdomyosarcoma of the bladder: A report from the Intergroup Rhabdomyosarcoma Study. J Pediatr Surg 1990;25:719.
45. Hays DM, et al: Retention of functional bladders among patients with vesicle/prostatic sarcomas in the Intergroup Rhabdomyosarcoma Studies (IRS) (1978-1990) [abstract]. Med Pediatr Oncol 1991;19:423.
46. Hays DM, et al: Children with vesical rhabdomyosarcoma (RMS) treated by partial cystectomy, with neoadjuvant or adjuvant chemotherapy with or without radiotherapy. J Pediatr Hematol Oncol 1995;17:46.
47. Healy GB, et al: The role of surgery in rhabdomyosarcoma of the head and neck in children. Arch Otolaryngol Head Neck Surg 1991;117:1185.
48. Heyn R, et al (for the IRS Committee): Late effects of therapy in patients with paratesticular rhabdomyosarcoma. J Clin Oncol 1992;10:614.
49. Heyn R, et al: Preservation of the bladder in patients with rhabdomyosarcoma. J Clin Oncol 1997;15:69.
50. Horn RC, et al: Rhabdomyosarcoma: A clinicopathological study and classification of 39 cases. Cancer 1958;11:181.
51. Horowitz ME, et al: Total-body irradiation and autologous bone marrow transplant in the treatment of high-risk Ewing's sarcoma and rhabdomyosarcoma. J Clin Oncol 1993;11:1911.
52. Kao GD, et al: The sequelae of chemoradiation therapy for head and neck cancer in children: Managing impaired growth, development and other side effects. Med Pediatr Oncol 1993;21:60.
53. Kilpatrick SE, et al: Relationship of DNA ploidy to histology and prognosis in rhabdomyosarcoma. Cancer 1994; 74:3227.
54. Koscielniak E, et al: Do patients with metastatic and recurrent rhabdomyosarcoma benefit from high-dose therapy with hematopoietic rescue? Report of the German/Austrian Pediatric Bone Marrow Transplantation Group. Bone Marrow Transplant 1997;19:227.
55. LaQuaglia MP, et al: Factors predictive of mortality in pediatric extremity rhabdomysarcoma. J Pediatr Surg 1990; 25:238.
56. Lawrence W Jr, et al: Lymphatic metastasis with childhood rhabdomyosarcoma. Cancer 1987;60:910.
57. Lawrence W Jr, et al: Surgical lessons from the Intergroup Rhabdomyosarcoma Study (IRS) pertaining to extremity tumors. World J Surg 1988;12:676.
58. Lawrence W Jr, et al: Pretreatment TNM staging of childhood rhabdomyosarcoma: A report of the Intergroup Rhabdomyosarcoma Study Group, Children's Cancer Study Group, Pediatric Oncology Group. Cancer 1997;80:1165.
59. Leader M, et al: Myoglobin: An evaluation of its role as a marker of rhabdomyosarcomas. Br J Cancer 1989;59:106.
60. Leuschner I, et al: Spindle cell variants of embryonal rhabdomyosarcoma in the paratesticular region: A report of the Inergroup Rhabdomyosarcoma Study. Am J Sur Pathol 1993;17:221.
61. Li FP, et al: Soft tissue sarcomas, breast cancer and other neoplasms: A familial syndrome? Ann Intern Med 1969; 71:747.
62. Li FP, et al: A cancer family syndrome in twenty-four kindreds. Cancer Res 1988;48:5358.
63. Li M, et al: Molecular genetics of Beckwith-Wiedemann syndrome. Curr Opin Pediatr 1997;9:623.
64. Lobe TE, et al: Neonatal rhabdomyosarcoma: The IRS experience. J Pediatr Surg 1994;29:1167.
65. Lobe TE, et al: The argument for conservative, delayed surgery in the management of prostatic rhabdomyosarcoma. J Pediatr Surg 1996;31:1084.
66. Malkin D, et al: Germ line p53 mutations in a familial syndrome of breast cancer, sarcomas, and other neoplasms. Science 1990;250:1233.
67. Mandell LR, et al: The influence of extensive bone erosion on local control in non-orbital rhabdomyosarcoma of the head and neck. Int J Radiat Oncol Biol Phys 1989;17:649.
68. Mandell LR, et al: Prognostic significance of regional lymph node involvement in childhood extremity rhabdomyosarcoma. Med Pediatr Oncol 1990;18:466.
69. Maurer HM, et al: The Intergroup Rhabdomyosarcoma Study-I: A final report. Cancer 1988;61:209.
70. Maurer HM, et al: The Intergroup Rhabdomyosarcoma Study-II. Cancer 1993;71:1904.
71. Miser JS, et al: Ifosfamide with mesna uroprotection and etoposide: An effective regimen in the treatment of recurrent sarcomas and other tumors of children and young adults. J Clin Oncol 1987;5:1191.
72. Morison IM, et al: Insulin-like growth factor 2 and overgrowth: Molecular biology and clinical implications. Mol Med Today 1998;4:110.
73. Neville HL, et al: Lymphatic mapping with sentinel node biopsy in pediatric patients. J Pediatr Surg 2000;35:961.
74. Neville HL, et al: Preoperative staging, prognostic factors, and outcome for extremity rhabdomyosarcoma: A preliminary report from the Intergroup Rhabdomyosarcoma Study IV (1991-1997). J Pediatr Surg 2000;35:317.
75. Newton WA, et al: Pathology of rhabdomyosarcoma and related tumors. In Maurer HM, Ruyman FB, Pochedly C (eds): Rhabdomyosarcoma and Related Tumors in Children and Adolescents. Boca Raton, Fla, CRC Press, 1991.
76. Newton WA, et al: Classification of rhabdomyosarcomas and related sarcomas: Pathologic aspects and proposal for a new classification. An Intergroup Rhabdomyosarcoma Study. Cancer 1995;76:1073.
77. Olive D, et al: Paraaortic lymphadenectomy is not necessary in the treatment of localized paratesticular rhabdomyosarcoma. Cancer 1984;54:1283.
78. Ortega JA: A therapeutic approach to childhood pelvic rhabdomyosarcoma without pelvic exenteration. J Pediatr Surg 1979;94:205.
79. Pack GT, et al: Rhabdomyosarcoma of the skeletal muscle: Report of 100 cases. Surgery 1952;32:1023.
80. Pappo AS, et al: Biology and therapy of pediatric rhabdomyosarcoma. J Clin Oncol 1995;13:2123.
81. Pappo AS, et al: A phase II trial of high-dose methotrexate in previously untreated children and adolescents with high-risk unresectable or metastatic rhabdomyosarcoma. J Pediatr Hematol Oncol 1997;19:438.
82. Pappo AS, et al: Up-front window trial of topotecan in previously untreated children and adolescents with metastatic rhabdomyosarcoma: An Intergroup Rhabdomyosarcoma Study (IRSG). J Clin Oncol 2001;19:213.
83. Pinkel D, et al: Rhabdomyosarcoma in children. JAMA 1961;175:293.
84. Pollono DG, et al: Rhabdomyosarcoma of extrahepatic biliary tree: Initial treatment with chemotherapy and conservative surgery. Med Pediatr Oncol 1998;30:290.
85. Raney RB Jr: Rhabdomyosarcoma and related tumors of the head and neck in childhood. In Maurer HM, Ruymann FB, Pochedly C (eds): Rhabdomyosarcoma and Related Tumors in Children and Adolescents. Boca Raton, Fla, CRC Press, 1991.

86. Raney RB Jr, et al: Paratesticular rhabdomyosarcoma in children. Cancer 1978;42:729.
87. Raney RB Jr, et al (for the IRS Committee): Primary chemotherapy with or without radiation therapy and/or surgery for children with localized sarcoma of the bladder, prostate, vagina, uterus and cervix: A comparison of the results in Intergroup Rhabdomyosarcoma Studies I and II. Cancer 1980;66:2072.
88. Raney RB Jr, et al (for the IRS Committee): Soft-tissue sarcoma of the trunk in childhood: Results of the Intergroup Rhabdomyosarcoma Study (IRS), 1972-1976. Cancer 1982;49:2612.
89. Raney RB Jr, et al: Improved prognosis with intensive treatment of children with cranial soft tissue sarcomas arising in nonorbital parameningeal sites: A report from the Intergroup Rhabdomyosarcoma Study. Cancer 1987;59:147.
90. Raney RB Jr, et al: Sequelae of treatment in 109 patients followed from five to fifteen years after diagnosis of sarcoma of the bladder and prostate: A report from the Intergroup Rhabdomyosarcoma Study (IRS) Committee. Cancer 1993; 71:2387.
91. Raney RB Jr, et al: Results of treating localized cranial parameningeal sarcoma on Intergroup Rhabdomyosarcoma (RMS) Studies (IRS)-II through IV. Med Pediatric Oncol 2000;35:178.
92. Raney RB Jr, et al: The Intergroup Rhabdomyosarcoma Study Group (IRSG): Major lessons from the IRS-I through IRS-IV studies as background for the current IRS-IV treatment protocols. Sarcoma 2001;5:9.
93. Raney RB Jr, et al: Results of treatment of 56 patients with localized retroperitoneal and pelvic rhabdomyosarcoma: A report from the Intergroup Rhabdomyosarcoma Study-IV, 1991-1997. Pediatr Blood Cancer 2004;42:618.
94. Rich DC, et al: Second malignant neoplasms in children after treatment of soft tissue sarcoma. J Pediatr Surg 1997; 32:369.
95. Rodeberg DA, et al: Surgical principles for children/adolescents with newly diagnosed rhabdomyosarcoma: A report from the Soft Tissue Sarcoma Committee of the Children's Oncology Group. Sarcoma 2002;6:111.
96. Rodeberg DA, et al: Characteristics and outcomes of rhabdomyosarcoma patients with isolated lung metastases from IRS-IV. J Pediatr Surg 2005;40:256.
97. Ruymann FB: Rhabdomyosarcoma in children and adolescents: A review. Hematol Oncol Clin North Am 1987;1:621.
98. Ruymann FB, et al: Congenital anomalies associated with rhabdomyosarcoma: A report from the Intergroup Rhabdomyosarcoam Study. Med Pediatr Oncol 1988;16:13.
99. Ruymann FB, et al: Epidemiology of soft tissue sarcomas. In Maurer HM, Ruymann FB, Pochedly C (eds): Rhabdomyosarcoma and Related Tumors in Children and Adolescents. Boca Raton, Fla, CRC Press, 1991.
100. Ruymann FB, et al: Comparison of two double chemotherapy regimens and conventional radiotherapy in metastatic rhabdomyosarcoma: Improved overall survival using ifosfamide/etoposide compared to vincristine/melphalan in IRSG-IV. Proc Am Soc Clin Oncol 1997; 16:521a.
101. Seymour-Dempsey K, et al: Neurofibromatosis: Implications for the general surgeon. J Am Coll Surg 2002;195:553.
102. Shapiro DN, et al: Relationship of tumor-cell ploidy to histologic subtype and treatment of outcome in children and adolescents with unresectable rhabdomyosarcoma. J Clin Oncol 1991;9:159.
103. Smith LM, et al: Which patients with rhabdomyosarcoma (RMS) and microscopic residual tumor (group II) fail therapy? A report from the Intergroup Rhabdomyosarcoma Study Group (IRSG). Proc Am Soc Clin Oncol 2000; 19:577a.
104. Spunt SL, et al: Aggressive surgery is unwarranted for biliary tract rhabdomyosarcoma. J Pediatr Surg 2000;35:309.
105. Stobbe GC, et al: Embryonal rhabdomyosarcoma of the head and neck in children and adolescents. Cancer 1950; 3:826.
106. Stout AP: Rhabdomyosarcoma of the skeletal muscle. Ann Surg 1946;123:447.
107. Strong LC, et al: The Li-Fraumeni syndrome: From clinical epidemiology to molecular genetics. Am J Epidemiol 1992;135:190.
108. Tapscott SJ, et al: Deficiency in rhabdomyosarcomas of a factor required for MyoD activity and myogenesis. Science 1993;259:1450.
109. Tefft M, et al: Radiation therapy combined with systemic chemotherapy of rhabdomyosarcoma in children: Local control in patients enrolled into the Intergroup Rhabdomyosarcoma Study. Natl Cancer Inst Monogr 1981;56:75.
110. Turc C: Consistent chromosomal translocation in alveolar rhabdomyosarcoma. Cancer Genet Cytogenet 1986;19:361.
111. Vietti T, et al: Topotecan window in patients with rhabdomyosarcoma (RMS): An IRSG study. Proc Am Soc Clin Oncol 1997;16:510a.
112. Weintraub H, et al: The MyoD gene family: Nodal point during specification of the muscle cell lineage. Science 1991;251:761.
113. Wexler LH, et al: Pediatric soft tissue sarcomas. CA Cancer J Clin 44:211,1994.
114. Wharam M, et al: Management of orbital rhabdomyosarcoma. In Jacob C (ed): Cancers of the Head and Neck, Boston, Martinus Niijhoff, 1987.
115. Wiener ES: Rhabdomyosarcoma: New dimensions in management. Semin Pediatr Surg 1993;2:47.
116. Wiener ES: Head and neck rhabdomyosarcoma. Semin Pediatr Surg 1994;3:203.
117. Wiener ES, et al (for the IRS Committee of CCSG, POG, UKCCSG): Second look operations in children in group III and IV rhabdomyosarcoma (RMS). SIOP XXII Meeting, October, 1990, Rome. Med Pediatr Oncol 1990;18:408.
118. Wiener ES, et al (for the IRS Committee of CCSG and POG): Complete response or not complete response? Second look operations are the answer in children with rhabdomyosarcoma. ASCO Annual Meeting, May 19-21, 1991, Houston, Texas. Proc Am Soc Clin Oncol 1991;10:316.
119. Wiener ES, et al: Rhabdomyosarcoma in extremity and trunk sites. In Maurer HM, Ruymann FB, Pochedly C (eds): Rhabdomyosarcoma and Related Tumors in Children and Adolescents. Boca Raton, Fla, CRC Press, 1991.
120. Wiener ES, et al: Retroperitoneal node biopsy in paratesticular rhabdomyosarcoma. J Pediatr Surg 1994;29:171.
121. Wiener ES, et al: Controversies in the management of paratesticular rhabdomyosarcoma: Is staging retroperitoneal lymph node dissection necessary for adolescents with resected paratesticular rhabdomyosarcoma? Semin Pediatr Surg 2001;10:146.
122. Wiener ES, et al: What is optimal management for children or adolescents with localized paratesticular rhabdomyosarcoma? Results in IRS-III and IRS-IV. J Pediatr Surg (in press).
123. Wolden SL, et al: Indications for radiotherapy and chemotherapy after complete resection in rhabdomyosarcoma: A report from the Intergroup Rhabdomyosarcoma Studies (IRS) I to III. J Clin Oncol 1999;17:3468.
124. Young JL, et al: Cancer incidence, survival, and mortality for children younger than 15 years. Cancer 1986;58:598.

第 33 章

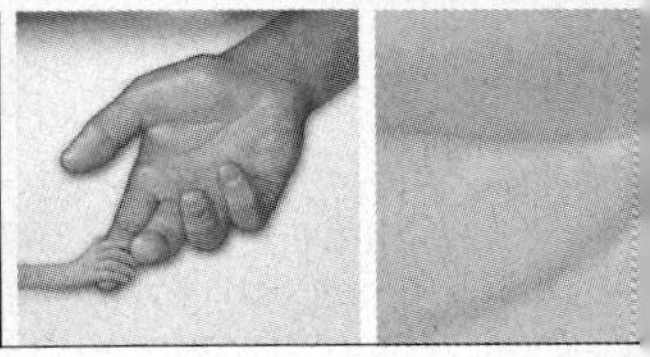

其他软组织肿瘤

Thom E. Lobe

541 软组织肿瘤主要是肉瘤，是一组复杂的不同组织学亚型的儿童恶性肿瘤。预后有赖于组织学类型、年龄、发病部位、浸润程度和许多其他因素。本章集中讨论儿童非横纹肌肉瘤的软组织肉瘤和其他软组织肿瘤。讨论集中于三个方面：（1）分类和命名；（2）目前的多学科协作治疗；（3）不同疑难肿瘤类型和发病部位的手术方法。

儿童的软组织肿瘤构成一组不同的病理学实体，它们表型的变化与间充质组织的多潜能特性相平行。就像表 33–1 所示[86]，良性和恶性肿瘤不同的细胞类型表达出不同的表型。然而，专业名词“良性”和“恶性”肿瘤并不一定与这些肿瘤潜在的临床侵袭性相吻合。一些良性的肿瘤可以通过简单的切除而很容易治愈，如血管瘤；其他一些良性肿瘤能复发，并需要广泛切除，如纤维样纤维瘤。类似的是，恶性肿瘤包括低度恶性的肉瘤，如婴儿纤维肉瘤，几乎无转移倾向；而高度恶性肉瘤常表现出播散性的骨髓病变。这些肿瘤部分在性质上与其认为是肿瘤性增生，不如认为是反应性增生；例子包括结节性筋膜炎和炎性肌纤维母细胞肿瘤。

儿童肉瘤与成人类似肉瘤相比，发生率上存在惊人的区别。最基本的例子是恶性纤维组织细胞瘤，这

表 33–1　儿童软组织肿瘤

组织类型	良性	肉瘤
脂肪	脂肪细胞瘤（相对多见）	脂肪肉瘤（少见）
血管和淋巴管	血管瘤、淋巴管瘤和各种变异型（很常见）	血管肉瘤（少见）、血管外皮细胞瘤、婴儿和成人变异型（较少见）
纤维	损伤后瘢痕（常见）；纤维瘤病和变异型（常见）；结节性筋膜炎（较常见）	纤维肉瘤，婴儿和成人型（较少见）
纤维组织细胞	纤维组织细胞瘤和变异型（常见）	恶性纤维组织细胞瘤（少见）
骨骼肌	横纹肌瘤（少见）	横纹肌肉瘤（常见）
平滑肌	平滑肌瘤（少见）	平滑肌肉瘤（少见）
外周神经组织	神经纤维瘤（较常见）；神经鞘膜瘤（相对不常见）	恶性外周神经鞘膜瘤和变异型；外周原始神经外胚层瘤（较常见）
滑膜	色素沉着绒毛结节性滑膜炎和相关病变（较少见）	滑膜肉瘤（较常见）
骨	骨化性肌炎（较常见）	骨外骨肉瘤（非常少见?）
软骨	软组织软骨瘤（少见）	骨骼外软骨肉瘤，黏液样与间质细胞（较少见）
上皮组织	?	上皮样肉瘤（较少见）
黑色素细胞	?	腱和腱膜透明细胞肉瘤
成肌纤维细胞	炎性肌纤维母细胞瘤（较少见）	肌纤维肉瘤（少见）

是成人最常见的肉瘤，但在儿童中很少见。大多数儿童病理学家发现最常见的只有血管瘤样亚型（表现为低度恶性的交界性恶性行为）。类似的发病率区别亦存在于脂肪肉瘤和平滑肌肉瘤中。相反，横纹肌肉瘤在儿童中是最为常见的软组织恶性肿瘤，但在成人中很少见。在成人，典型的横纹肌肉瘤是多形性亚型，但在儿童，该细胞类型是否存在还存在疑问[80]。滑膜肉瘤和神经肿瘤在儿童中的发生率在增加。

外科医生也必须意识到许多儿科软组织肿瘤的交界“恶性”属性，这与卵巢上皮性肿瘤情况类似。一个例子是前面提及的血管瘤样恶性纤维组织细胞瘤；由于不常见到转移，导致一些研究者将其“恶性”这个名称都略去了[35]。其他交界性病变包括上皮样血管内皮瘤、梭形细胞血管内皮瘤、和隆突性皮肤纤维肉瘤。然而，偶尔这些病变表现出转移性，但组织学表现常不能预测这种能力。

儿科软组织肿瘤的一些类型出现于婴儿和 5 岁以下的儿童时是相对良性的，但在年长儿中则表现出更典型的侵袭性生长方式。婴儿型纤维肉瘤在组织学检查中表现出高度恶性，临床上出现大的、广泛的四肢病变，但众所周知这种肿瘤很少发生转移，并推荐做保守治疗[67]。类似的病变还有婴儿型血管外皮细胞瘤，其表现与婴儿良性血管病类似，但在年长儿和青少年中具有较高的恶性度。

因为肿瘤生物学行为预测的不一致性，儿科软组织肉瘤的分级不但要考虑到成人的细胞组织学特征，还加了一些儿童肿瘤病变的限定（表 33–2）[86,88]。例如，当发生于 5 岁以下的儿童时，不管分裂指数、坏死、或细胞学等特征，纤维肉瘤是低度恶性的（1 级）。然而在年长儿，根据分裂指数是低（<5/10 个高倍视野）是高（>4/10 个高倍视野）或坏死是少（<15%）是多（>15%），来决定它是 2 或 3 级。可根据细胞学特征如多形性和细胞构成来鉴别不明确的病例。该系统不能用于横纹肌肉瘤或外周原始神经外胚层瘤（PNET），因为这些肿瘤始终被认为是高度恶性的，最好接受手术切除、联合化疗和放疗等系统性多学科综合治疗。

纤维瘤病是一组异源性病变，其中部分是可能致命的肿瘤，需要广泛切除和仔细随访。这些肿瘤的主要组分是良性外观的成纤维细胞，但它们随患者的年龄范围、组织学类型、发病部位、多发或软骨样分化倾向和手术切除不完全所致复发可能而变化。一种实体肿瘤——婴儿纤维性错构瘤——包含脂肪、成熟纤维组织和不成熟纤维组织的混合体，典型的位于背部和肩部皮下组织；通常不会复发。相反，婴儿纤维样纤维瘤是一种更具均一性、成熟的成纤维细胞和脂肪广泛浸润的肿块，可以出现于不易进行手术切除的部位；它通过侵犯邻近的解剖结构而导致较高的致残率或死亡率。婴儿纤维样纤维瘤与婴儿纤维肉瘤的区别在于前者缺乏细胞的多形性或分裂活性，且不会转移。年长儿和青少年也可能出现纤维样肌腱膜纤维瘤，其组织学和临床表现与婴儿纤维样纤维瘤类似。已经发现一些能用于治疗的药物[8,31]，但没有大样本的前瞻性、随机性的临床试验证实。另一种类型是婴儿肌性纤维瘤，它可以以单个或多中心病灶出现；后者侵犯内脏时可能是致命的。

表 33–2 儿童肿瘤协作组对非横纹肌肉瘤的儿童肉瘤的分级

1 级
黏液样和分化良好的脂肪肉瘤
深层隆突性皮肤纤维肉瘤
分化良好或婴儿型（<5 岁）纤维肉瘤
分化良好或婴儿型（<5 岁）血管外皮瘤
分化良好的恶性外周神经鞘膜瘤
血管瘤样恶性纤维组织细胞瘤
2 级
没有包含在 1 级或 3 级的肉瘤；<15%肿瘤细胞出现坏死或分裂指数<5/10 个高倍显微镜视野（HPF）
3 级
多形性或圆形细胞脂肪肉瘤
间叶细胞性软骨肉瘤
骨骼外骨肉瘤
恶性蝾螈瘤
腺泡型软组织肉瘤
没有包含在 1 级或 2 级的其他肉瘤，其中>15%的肿瘤出现坏死或分裂指数>4/10 个高倍视野

儿科软组织肿瘤的诊断可以通过常规的组织学检查或甚至细针穿刺活检等来获得[116]，但它经常需要一套专门的技术，可能包括组织化学、免疫组化、电子显微镜、细胞遗传学、流式细胞仪、原位杂交或反转录酶聚合酶链反应（RT–PCR）。总的来说，由于它们的原始、未分化特征，圆细胞肿瘤需要更广泛的检

查，而如果可以得到足够的组织，梭形细胞肿瘤更可能通过常规组织学诊断来诊断。矛盾的是，圆细胞肿瘤在细针吸出做细胞学检查时通常能得到较好的标本，而黏合更强的梭形细胞病变在做此项检查时常不能得到足够的或理想的标本。肿瘤专家、外科医生和病理学家之间需要紧密的合作以得到最好的理想的诊断。偶尔在危及生命的情形下，可能需要在很少的标本中更快的获得诊断。然而，当时间
543 允许时，详细准确的诊断对于临床治疗是非常重要的。辅助检查所需的时间范围从免疫组化和 RT–PCR 的 1 天或更短、电子显微镜的数天、到细胞遗传学的 2 周。这些技术的适用性和可靠性有赖于所获标本的性质和数量；细胞遗传学和 RT–PCR 需要新鲜标本，电子显微镜和免疫组化需要特殊的固定方法。RT–PCR 的好处是非常的敏感，因此只需要很少的标本。如果标本被机体正常组织污染，则细胞遗传学可能会得出错误的结果，而如果标本活力差则不能得到结果。

较为常见的圆形和梭形细胞肉瘤的诊断学特征见表 33–3[86]。最初的病理学检查一般是为了首先确定病变是良性还是恶性，然后检查是圆形还是梭形细胞肿瘤。随后进行鉴别诊断，需要进行特殊的检查以排除或明确可能的诊断。完全未分化圆形肿瘤的鉴别诊断包括许多种病变，最可能的病变有横纹肌肉瘤、淋巴瘤、神经母细胞瘤、PNET 或软组织 Ewing 肉瘤。免疫组化染色用于检查结合蛋白和肌肉特异的肌动蛋白（肌肉的标记）、CD45 和其他淋巴系标记、神经元特异的烯醇化酶和突触素（神经标记）及波形蛋白和 CD99（Ewing 肉瘤的标志）。综合的检查结果通常在进行鉴别时有重要的作用，但仍存在许多局限性。例如，神经元特异的烯醇化酶是一个敏感性的神经标志，但常在横纹肌肉瘤中呈阳性，因此它的表达在没有肌肉的标记表达时会更有用。同样，CD99 是一个非常敏感、相对特异的 PNET 标记，但在 T 细胞淋巴瘤中也较常出现。神经源性的标记可以在 PNET 和神经母细胞瘤中均有出现，但后者是 CD99 阴性的。最后，一些肿瘤（如原始外胚层间质瘤）常表现出多潜能分化模式，用于诊断的不同标志物均可呈阳性。在这些易混淆的情况下，明智的办法是考虑不同方法检查的结果，如电子显微镜和细胞遗传学。

非横纹肌肉瘤的软组织肉瘤

恶性软组织肉瘤来源于间充质细胞，在所有儿童肿瘤中占 7%[74,121]。这些肿瘤包括两个主要的组织学亚型：横纹肌肉瘤和非横纹肌肉瘤的软组织肉瘤。横纹肌肉瘤（见第 32 章）是儿童中最常见的软组织肉瘤，在所有儿童软组织肉瘤中的比例超过半数，在美国每年有 250 例新发患者[87,121]。非横纹肌肉瘤的软组织肉瘤（NRSTS）是一组异源性的恶性肿瘤；在所有儿童软组织肉瘤中占 47%，在所有儿童肿瘤中占 3%[74,75]。这些肿瘤的临床表现仍不是很明确[75,99,121]。它们数量的罕见和组织学异质性阻碍了对它们自然病程和对治疗敏感性的详细研究。因此，许多关于该类肿瘤患儿的治疗资料来源于对成人的研究。此外，尽管它们有侵袭性病理学表现，一些 NRSTS 亚型（如婴儿纤维肉瘤）在单纯接受手术治疗后有相对较好的临床预后[23,75]。

NRSTS 与横纹肌肉瘤类似，可以起自身体的任何部位。两组共计总数 322 例患儿的系列研究显示，最常见的部位是四肢、躯干、及腹腔和骨盆[79,99]。一些部位，如眼和眼眶[18]、乳房[28]等是非常少见的。在这些系列研究中，滑膜肉瘤、神经纤维肉瘤、恶性纤维组织细胞瘤、和纤维肉瘤是最常见的组织类型[97,99]。NRSTS 与 Li–Fraumeni 综合征有相关性，一些肿瘤（如恶性纤维组织细胞瘤）能在以前放疗的部位出现[75]。约 4%的 I 型多发性神经纤维瘤（NF–1）发展成恶性外周神经鞘膜瘤；这些少见恶性肿瘤 40%见于 NF-1 患者[27]。平滑肌肉瘤能发生于感染 HIV 和 EB 病毒的儿童中[70]。

在组织学表现和染色体异常被用于确定肿瘤生物学表现之后，儿童软组织肉瘤正在不断被发现。大多数该类型肉瘤有特异的产生单一融合基因的染色体易位。这些融合基因对患者有诊断、判断预后、和监测作用[5]。

NRSTS 患儿的预后因素包括肿瘤是否能被切除、肿瘤大小、组织学分级、肿瘤侵袭性、和是否有转移灶[84,98]。在 37 例滑膜肉瘤患儿的回顾研究中，完全切除病灶患儿的 5 年生存率是 80 ± 9%，那些未切除或有转移的患儿则为 17 ± 15%[84]。在同一医院接受治疗的 154 例 NRSTS 患儿中，1 或 2 级病灶的患儿 31% 治疗失败，而 3 级病灶的患儿 73%出现复发。同样，那些病灶大、有浸润和 3 级的患儿 88%治疗失败，而

表 33-3 相对常见的儿童软组织肉瘤的鉴别诊断

肿瘤	免疫组化	电镜	细胞遗传学	RT-PCR 或其他分子技术	其他
圆形细胞					
横纹肌肉瘤	结蛋白、肌动蛋白、MyoD	粗和细的细丝、Z带糖原储备、原始胞浆、	t(1;13)；t(2;13)（只限于腺泡型）	PAX7；FHKHR PAX3；FHKHR	糖原 PAS 染色
PNET、Ewing 肉瘤	CD99、突触素、波形蛋白、NSE	神经分泌颗粒、原始胞浆、缺乏细胞间连接	t(11;22)；t(21;22)	Fli-1；EWS ERG；EWS	糖原 PAS 染色 缺乏网硬蛋白
淋巴瘤	CD45、CD45RO、CD20、CD3、CD43、CD30		Burkit 淋巴瘤：t(2;8)；t(8;14)；t(8;22)间变性大细胞性：t(2;5)	Burkit 淋巴瘤：c-myc；IgH：c-myc；Igk：c-myc；Igλ ALK；ALM	流式细胞仪；结外淋巴瘤
促纤维增生性小圆细胞瘤	波形蛋白、细胞角蛋白、结蛋白、突触素、NSE、CD57	无诊断意义	t(11;22) (p13;q12)	WT1；EWS	特征性的促纤维增生性基质
Langerhans 细胞组织细胞增生症	S100、CD1a、花生促凝素	Birbeck 颗粒	无诊断意义	无诊断意义	嗜酸性红细胞常见
神经母细胞瘤	NSE、突触素、嗜铬粒蛋白（弱）	微管形成、神经分泌颗粒、突触连接	1p 缺失、双微染色体、同源染色区	N-myc 扩增（可以在腺泡型横纹肌肉瘤中看到）	神经节分化；尿儿茶酚胺；CD99 阴性
梭形细胞					
滑膜肉瘤	细胞角蛋白、EMA	上皮分化过程、Luse 小体、基膜、假轴突系膜	t(X;18)	SSX1； SYT SSX2；SYT	注意由于神经侵犯而致混淆
恶性外周神经鞘瘤	S100、CD57、GFAP		无	NF-1 缺失？	有过神经纤维瘤病；起源于大的神经；与神经纤维瘤共存
纤维肉瘤、肌纤维肉瘤	波形蛋白、平滑肌肌动蛋白	RER 环孔板、终末网、肌动蛋白微丝、胶原微粒纤维连接、胞饮小泡	无	无	有炎症变异型；认为是炎性肌纤维母细胞肿瘤

PNET：原始神经外胚层瘤；RT-PCR：反转录聚合酶链反应；NF-1：I 型多发性神经纤维瘤；NSE：神经特异性烯醇酶。

病灶小、分级低和没有侵袭的患儿只有 2%治疗失败[99]。

与横纹肌肉瘤对化疗高度敏感不同，NRSTS 的治疗主要是完全手术切除，可加或不加辅助性放疗以防止局部复发。数个前瞻性的成人 NRSTS 研究没有发现辅助化疗对生存有益处[72,127]。唯一针对儿童关于辅助化疗作用的前瞻性研究是由儿童肿瘤协作组（POG）进行的。在该研究中，75 例病灶完全切除的患儿被分配或接受辅助化疗（长春新碱、放线菌素、环磷酰胺和阿霉素），或只进行简单随访。该两组患儿的 3 年无病生存率没有差别（分别是 74%和 76%）。对不同亚型分析发现，3 级病灶患儿明显比那些 1 级或 2 级病灶患儿的预后差（3 年无病生存率分
545 别为 75%和 91%，$P=0.018$）[8]。在 3 级病灶患儿中，远处转移导致超过 80%的患儿治疗失败。这些资料表明，如果针对无法切除或有转移的 NRSTS 患儿的前瞻性研究能够发现有活性的化疗药物，则可以对 3 级病灶、完全切除的 NRSTS 患儿进行辅助化疗的前瞻性研究。

转移的 NRSTS 患儿的疗效仍然很差，3 年无病生存率低于 20%[84,95]。对于大多数 NRSTS，治疗的方法是手术切除。化疗和放疗的作用很不确定。化疗作用的评估由于缺乏随机、对照研究，所以应用很有限。POG 试图对 NRSTS（临床分期Ⅰ和Ⅱ患儿）手术切除后随机分为化疗组（长春新碱、放线菌素 D、环磷酰胺、和阿霉素）和观察组[96]。在 81 例入选的患儿中，只有 30 例接受随机化分组。接受化疗的患儿（随机或非随机）预后更差；然而，这有可能是因为在治疗组中临床分级高的患儿数量更多。治疗 NRSTS 的最有活性的药物包括异环磷酰胺和阿霉素[29]。在 POG 对于未切除或转移性 NRSTS 患儿的前瞻性研究中，比较了 VADRAC（长春新碱、环磷酰胺和阿霉素）和 VADRAC 加达卡巴嗪（DTIC）。结果发现增加 DTIC 没有益处：4 年总生存率和无病生存率分别是 30.6 ± 8.5%和 18.4 ± 6.8%[95]。在Ⅰ期和Ⅱ期试验中发现，新药、已知活性药物强化治疗和同时进行生长因子支持及术前化疗是可能改善 NRSTS 患儿预后的对策。

有转移灶的患儿，特别是大于 10 岁、骨骼或骨髓受累的患儿往往预后较差，需要选择新的治疗方法。对于绝大部分患儿，大剂量单药、多药或放-化疗与干细胞移植联合治疗均没有改善预后，但这仍然是当今临床研究的基础[5]。

放疗一般用于显微镜下有残留病灶或组织学上发现肿瘤延伸非常接近切除边缘的患儿，也可以用于肿瘤大于 5cm 的Ⅰ期患儿。放疗的效果尚未被证明，然而儿童暴露于放疗的副作用（包括对身体生长影响和继发性肿瘤）使其在体积小、完全切除的肿瘤中的应用存在疑问。Spunt 等[114]分析了 121 例在 St. Jude 儿童医院接受治疗的临床Ⅰ和Ⅱ期 NRSTS 患儿。放疗降低了临床Ⅱ期患儿的局部复发风险，但对无病生存率没有影响。放疗对临床Ⅰ期患儿的局部复发没有影响。

作为第二恶性肿瘤的儿童软组织肉瘤可以使用与原发儿童肉瘤一样的对策来治疗[11]。

滑膜肉瘤

滑膜肉瘤是最常见的儿童 NRSTS 之一；大约 30%的滑膜肉瘤见于 20 岁以下患者。只有很少关于滑膜肉瘤患儿的报道[38,63,82,84,107]。至于在成人，大多数该类肉瘤出现于四肢，最常见于下肢。其他常见的部位有躯干和头颈部。对于所有患儿，5 年无病生存率约为 70%；然而，对于临床Ⅰ期和Ⅱ期的肿瘤患儿生存率约为 80%，而Ⅲ和Ⅳ期肿瘤患儿为 0～58%。预后看来与成人的结果类似。因为大多数报道不是只关于成人就是只关于儿童，且使用了不同的分期体系，所以难于进行直接的比较。常见局部复发，转移部位主要是肺，也可以转移至淋巴结[38]。晚期复发常见，且生存曲线在 10 和 15 年时仍在下降。

滑膜肉瘤的主要治疗方法是手术切除。有许多关于对化疗敏感的报道，但没有研究确定显示化疗能改善生存。CW-81 研究对患者的治疗最初用长春新碱、更生霉素、环磷酰胺或异环磷酰胺和阿霉素的联合化疗。在 5 例临床Ⅲ和Ⅳ期的肿瘤患者中，2 例完全有效，3 例是部分有效；所有 5 例患者均做了完全切除并获得长期生存[63]。在 13 例有转移的成人患者中，大剂量异环磷酰胺（14～18g/m^2）的使用在所有患者中取得疗效。大多数是部分或暂时有效，但当结合手术切除残留灶后，4 例患者分别在 3、14、21 和 42 个月仍处于无病状态[103]。这些资料表明，化疗能使肿瘤缩小从而进行随后的手术切除，但作为辅助方案使用的化疗对于滑膜肉瘤的作用未得到证明。因此，对

于滑膜肉瘤治疗方法的选择尚存在争议，有不同的方法用于治疗儿童和成人患者。一个回顾性研究分析了一个医院中 30 年间的各个年龄段的大量病例。该研究包含 271 例患者，年龄 5～87 岁；255 例表现为局部病灶，其中 215 例被大体切除，而 40 例在诊断时已无法切除。41%的患者接受化疗，其中 76%为 16 岁以下的患者和低于 20%的年长患者。28%的病灶大体切除患者接受辅助性化疗。该研究对象总的 5 年无病生存率是 37%，然而，该生存率会随年龄变化（16 岁以下患者为 66%、17～30 岁为 40%、30 岁以上为 31%）。在能够手术切除肿瘤的患者中，接受化疗的 5 年无转移生存率是 60%，而未接受化疗的是 48%。化疗带来的益处对肿瘤大于 5cm 的 17 岁或 17 岁以上的患者中最大（化疗与无化疗组的无转移生存率分别是 47%和 27%）。在可以测量肿瘤大小的患者中，
546 对化疗敏感的比例约为 48%。虽然作者仍在寻求辅助化疗在治疗成人软组织肉瘤中作用的更令人信服的证据，但他们推荐高危滑膜肉瘤患者（肿瘤大小＞5cm）是考虑接受此类治疗的首选对象[40]。

针对滑膜肉瘤的放疗常用于镜下残留或组织学上发现肿瘤接近切缘的患者。同其他 NRSTS 一样，放疗的有效性仍未得到证明，而它对于儿童生长、第二肿瘤的风险和其他远期效应的副作用使其在体积小、完全切除的肿瘤中的应用仍存在疑问[89]。

滑膜肉瘤肿瘤组织的遗传学检查显示 SYT-SSX1 融合型的肿瘤预后更差[62]。在有转移的患者中，该融合型比 SYT-SSX2 类型更多见；在病灶局限的患者中，SYT-SSX1 的患者总的生存时间较短。

某些原发部位，如手滑膜肉瘤，是很少见的。关于它们的治疗尚没有明确的指导原则。必须对每一个病例进行个体化治疗，可以采用功能性的肢体保留方法，又不削弱肿瘤治疗的原则[51]。

原发肾脏的滑膜肉瘤现在是一个大家接受的实体肿瘤，可能是一个以前被认为是肾母细胞瘤成人变异的亚型[3]。

婴儿纤维肉瘤

婴儿纤维肉瘤是婴儿最常见的软组织肉瘤，约占儿童纤维肉瘤的半数。这些肿瘤通常表现为缓慢增大的肿块，可以为数月到数年。大多数出现于四肢，但头颈部肿瘤也常见。名词“婴儿”纤维肉瘤是一个误称，因为其预后已改善、且该肿瘤相关的染色体改变也见于约 5 岁的儿童。幼儿纤维肉瘤也有较好的预后，长期生存率高于 90%。虽然儿童纤维肉瘤的复发率约为 50%，但转移的可能性小于 10%[24,113]。

婴儿纤维肉瘤生长迅速，局部浸润，但很少发生转移。虽然完全切除能够治愈，但通常是不可能达到的。新辅助化疗能使许多肿瘤缩小至可以切除。在完全切除后进行辅助化疗或放疗似乎没有作用。虽然复发较常见，大多数病例能通过再次手术切除。总的生存率大于 90%[37]。

因为 5 岁以下婴儿纤维肉瘤表现出典型的良性病程，推荐进行保守的手术治疗来保留器官功能。婴儿纤维肉瘤一般对化疗还是敏感的，某些病例可成功的作为首选治疗方法[60,110]。也有婴儿纤维肉瘤自发性消退的报道[67]。肺部纤维肉瘤在儿童是一种罕见的恶性肿瘤。由于少有转移，完全切除能治愈[91]。气管纤维肉瘤也是类似的[93]。

血管外皮细胞瘤

只有 5%～10%的血管外皮细胞瘤出现于儿童和青少年[34,57]，其中许多是婴儿血管外皮细胞瘤，与见于年长儿的病程相比，这是一种病程更具良性表现的疾病。婴儿中多出现于头颈部，转移可能性低。

婴儿血管外皮细胞瘤不完全切除者常不必进一步治疗也能治愈[6]。已经有对化疗敏感的报道[4,6]。虽然先天性血管外皮细胞瘤一般不会转移，预后较好，但也有一些转移和死亡的报道[6]。也有单纯活检后肿瘤自愈的报道[21]。

该病可以出现于一些特别的部位，例如偶尔出现于甲状舌导管残基上[50]。该肿瘤与良性动静脉畸形类似，而有时被诊断为“血管瘤”[76]。也有报道肿瘤的出现伴有 15 染色体三体[117]。

神经源性肉瘤

神经源性肉瘤（恶性外周神经鞘膜瘤、神经纤维肉瘤、神经肉瘤和恶性神经鞘膜瘤）常表现出疼痛或神经系统症状，这些症状在诊断前常已出现较长时

间。神经源性肉瘤可以新发或起源于以前存在的纤维瘤。在儿科中，21%～62%患者表达 NF-1 基因[17,32,71]。然而，只有 5%以下表达 NF-1 的患者出现肉瘤[112]。

中枢神经系统原发肉瘤在儿童中罕见。它们起源的细胞是有争议的，但最被广泛接受的理论认为是硬脑膜、小脑膜或它们延伸入脑的部分和沿外膜周围的脊髓、脉络膜和脉络丛间质的有多能造血功能的原始间充质干细胞。由于不同研究的定义不同，报道的该部位肉瘤的发生率为 0.1%～4.3%。这些肿瘤常出现于儿童的天幕上间隙的部位。常可见到硬脑膜结合部和中枢神经系统的播散。虽然侵袭性切除加术后放疗可以提供一个长期生存的机会，但中枢神经系统外的转移往往预后很差。对于局部复发肿瘤应该行重复的开颅术。更新的化疗方案在将来可能有成功的希望[1]。

这些是侵袭性非常强的肿瘤，根治性手术是主要的治疗手段。在有 NF-1 的患者中，肿瘤出现的年龄更早，复发和转移更快更常见[33,71,126]。恶性外周神经鞘膜瘤很罕见，通常是致命的，局部复发和远处转移
547 的风险高[115]。

完全切除是最重要的预后因素，5 年无病生存率为 67%。有镜下残留的 5 年无病生存率为 43%；当肿瘤没有完全切除时，复发是不可避免的，5 年无病生存率降为 22%，大多数肿瘤转移部位是肺[126]。体外放疗似乎对生存无影响，但近距离放射疗法（BRT）和术中放疗是有益处的[126]。

脂肪肉瘤

虽然脂肪肉瘤是成人中较为常见的软组织肉瘤之一，但在儿童中则罕见[19,39,64,111]。大体完全切除是治疗的方法。已经有通过放疗[19]和化疗[39]使肿瘤缩小以获得完全切除的报道。辅助化疗或放疗已经用于有镜下肿瘤残留的患儿，但它的有效性尚未证实[39,64]。成人四肢脂肪肉瘤的 5 年生存率有赖于组织学亚型，分别如下：分化良好肿瘤是 100%；黏液性肿瘤是 88%；成纤维细胞肿瘤是 58%；多形性肿瘤是 56%；脂肪母细胞肿瘤是 40%[20]。儿童脂肪肉瘤与成人比较预后更好，可能与黏液性肿瘤和分化良好型肿瘤比例更高有关（占 70～85%的儿童脂肪肉瘤）。

促结缔组织增生性小圆细胞肿瘤

使结缔组织增生性小圆细胞肿瘤主要见于年青男性，表现为疼痛、腹水、腹胀或肿块、恶心和呕吐、或肠道 / 膀胱梗阻。肝脏、肺和淋巴结的广泛播散转移也常见[45]。虽然确切的肿瘤类型难于确定，但用 RT-PCR 方法检测甲醛溶液固定的标本来确定肿瘤类型的特异性达 94%～100%[43]。

由于就诊时已有广泛的播散，完全手术切除基本上是不可能的。对化疗敏感性（包括大剂量化疗和自体干细胞移植）已有报道[10,36,46,61,104]。长期生存仍有赖于新辅助化疗后切除所有病灶的可能性。放疗对于镜下残留肿瘤的治疗可能有用。用射频清除无法切除的结缔组织增生性小圆细胞肿瘤的肝脏转移灶可能有效[30]。

软组织恶性黑素瘤

约 25%该类肿瘤出现于 20 岁以下患者。大多数患者表现为四肢已存在较长时间的肿物进行性增大[25,106]。常见局部复发。远隔转移常在肺（59%）、淋巴结（53%）和骨骼（22%）。

治疗方法是手术切除。总生存时间的中位数是 49 个月[106]，但诊断时出现转移的患者一般生存时间少于 1 年。局部复发和转移可能在诊断和治疗后数年出现。辅助化疗或放疗的作用对于这些肿瘤尚不确定[44]。

腺泡状软组织肉瘤

大约 25%的腺泡状软组织肉瘤见于 20 岁以下患者。该肿瘤主要见于女性（61%），特别是年轻患者中[66]。临床表现包括四肢无痛性增大的肿块，在儿童也常见到头颈部[16,85]。该肿瘤在儿童中的比例为 0.8%～1.8%。诊断时年龄 0～9 岁的患儿平均生存时间是 20 年，而诊断时年龄 10～19 岁的平均生存时间为 14 年。肿瘤直径大于 5cm 时，转移的风险增加，常在疾病的早期发生。转移灶的切除能影响生存率[83]。约 20%患者在诊断时有转移。肿瘤转移有时在诊断后许多年发生，累及肺、骨骼、和脑。

治疗方法主要是手术，完全切除是最好的治疗。如果切缘足够，则局部复发的风险较低。诊断时有转移灶的患者，中位生存时间是 3 年[66]。年轻患者生存时间更长，但这主要与诊断时转移发生率较低有关[66,85]。根据软组织肉瘤意大利协作组资料，儿童腺泡状软组织肉瘤与成人比较，其预后更好[16]。

特异的诊断和手术选择

新的影像学模式

磁共振波谱学看来在儿童肿瘤中评估肿瘤是有效的，可被用于根据儿童的个体化调整化疗剂量的评估[118]。磁共振波谱学判断预后的作用已经被用于四肢肉瘤，目的是确定是否治疗前波谱可以预测“好”和“坏”的肿瘤，及是否治疗早期出现的变化在预测治疗敏感性中有用[59]。

已经通过系统回顾相关的文献和荟萃分析，评估了氟脱氧葡萄糖正离子发射成像扫描在儿童肉瘤中的诊断和治疗作用。虽然它能被用于检测、分级、治疗和评价局部进展期肉瘤[7]，目前没有认为此模式是标
48 准治疗的方法[7]。

活检和手术

细针抽吸的价值主要在于鉴别实体肿块和含液体肿块或可能需要引流的脓肿。在所有其他情况下，至少应该用 Tru-Cut 针活检[12,52,65,94,99,100]。虽然已经有针刺管道复发的报道，但这些是极为罕见的事件，在癌性患者中更为多见[108]。当获得的组织不足以用于特异的诊断时，或者存在偏差时，应该进行开放式活检。对于四肢病变，切口必须是纵向的或与神经血管束平行。横向活检切口将污染多个组织层次，并因此妨碍了肢体保留手术[73,99,101]。只有在肿瘤较小（<2.5cm）或位于一个能够在最终扩大的局部切除时不影响功能或可避开出现畸形危险的部位时，才考虑采用病灶的切除性活检[119]。在所有其他情况下，切开获得活检组织必须仔细计划和操作，以使切口在根治手术时能够被完全切除。

已经反复表明当计划切除良性肿瘤或当恶性肿瘤的切除没有仔细计划时，肿瘤切除的质量和数量往往是不够的。在这些情况下，在 30%～49%患者中，残留的肿瘤能在随后的再次切除中被发现[12,14,47,99,102,122,124]。如果没有进行根治性切除，会有 50%～90%的局部复发率[13,14,47,55,99,102,128]。因此，不管什么时候，当诊断性影像学检查、手术记录、或病理学检查表明存在肿瘤残留或肿瘤接近切缘，推荐患者只要可能就应进行手术部位的再次切除[12,14,58,99,101,119,125]。

四肢肿瘤

两个主要的因素导致软组织肉瘤患儿截肢术的减少。首先，虽然截肢术的局部控制率较高，但它没有改善总的生存率[14,55,99,102,122,124,125]。其次，肢体保留手术（加或不加辅助放疗）已经将局部复发率减少至 10%以下[22,41,42,77,99,122,124]。虽然截肢术在老年患者中可能是合理的，但对于成长中的儿童来说不是一个最好的选择。成人患者的截肢术避免了肌肉骨骼的畸形或继发恶性肿瘤的风险[14,94,99,101,102]。

手术原则是获得扩大的局部切除，保证有足够的切缘，一般认为是约 2cm[101,119]。根据肿瘤的大小和部位，扩大的局部切除可以通过根治性区域切除、从插入点到肌起点切除肌肉或根治性扩大局部切除来获得[12,14,53,55,92,99,102,119,122,124]。虽然在大多数情况下可获得广泛切缘，在某些情况下，特别是邻近大的神经或血管时，切缘可能只有几毫米。在这种情况下，建议沿着肿瘤切除外膜[55,102]。虽然切除是主要关心的事，但常根据不同患者术前诊断的影像学资料调整切除范围。

以前活检部位的皮肤呈椭圆形，皮瓣被掀起来。切开通常是从肿瘤一侧的 2～3cm 开始。肿瘤深部的切缘常位于血管或神经的上面。在这种情况下，邻近肿瘤的外膜或外周神经鞘必须被切除以获得更多一点的切缘。如果血管大体受到累及，可以考虑切除血管，并做血管重建修复术。如果肿瘤侵犯骨骼，可以考虑剥除骨膜、切除骨骼边缘、或切除部分骨骼。在这些情况下，骨骼的缺陷可以通过带血管腓骨移植或自体移植加髓内钉来弥补。

在腘窝和肘部，因为复杂的神经血管解剖结构、疏松结缔组织和邻近结构的紧密联结，要局部切除肿

瘤且获得满意的切缘基本上是不可能的[90,105,109]。这些肿瘤不受筋膜边界的限制，被认为是区划外型。我的原则是在切除这些肿瘤时，只要可行，不管什么时候都要保留肢体功能，而不管切缘的大小。以间质近距离放射疗法、外照射疗法、或两者联合的方式加用放疗进行局部控制。在有神经血管浸润、局部复发、和骨骼未发育成熟的患儿，应该考虑进行大范围损伤性的手术，如截肢术。

在手和脚的肿瘤中存在类似的情形，这些部位出现原发性肿瘤相对少见。以上部位层次紧密，密布着肌腱和神经血管束，切除时要获得足够的切缘是很困难的。手术方法可以放射状切除一个或多个指 / 趾、扩大局部切除的区域、和补充进行放疗或使用无神经血管转移技术（特别是在切除拇指的病例中）[15,48,49,54]。在下肢，在治疗大的、高危型浸润性肿瘤或当联合治疗将导致肢体功能很差时，截肢术仍有作用。截肢术对控制疼痛也是适宜的，特别是在承重肢体和局部复发的患者。

多学科联合治疗已经使 NRSTS 的肢体保留率达到 90%～95%，而局部复发率缩小到 10%左右[12,99,101,22,124]。近年，对肿瘤生物学有了更好的理解，进行放疗的技术也得到改善。放疗可以在术前、术中、或术后进行[22,26,42,81,122,123]。

肢体淋巴结引流的治疗

在近年，区域淋巴结清扫在软组织肉瘤的作用更为明确。在对 2500 多例 NRSTS 患者的回顾性研究 549
中，淋巴结受累的发生率在 3.9%左右。在同一研究中，作者发现随着肿瘤分期的升高，淋巴结转移的发生率也轻度增加，范围从 1 期的 0%到 3 期的 12%[69]。在 St. Jude 儿童医院关于 NRSTS 的回顾研究中观察到类似的变化范围[114]。在另一个回顾性研究中，204 例患者中有 76 例进行淋巴结清扫或活检；其中 9 例是肿瘤阳性，9 例中的 7 例患儿的肿瘤是分期较高[48,99,101,102]。我的经验是只活检高危肿瘤类型（大于 5cm）的可疑淋巴结，或如果淋巴结出现于原发肿瘤

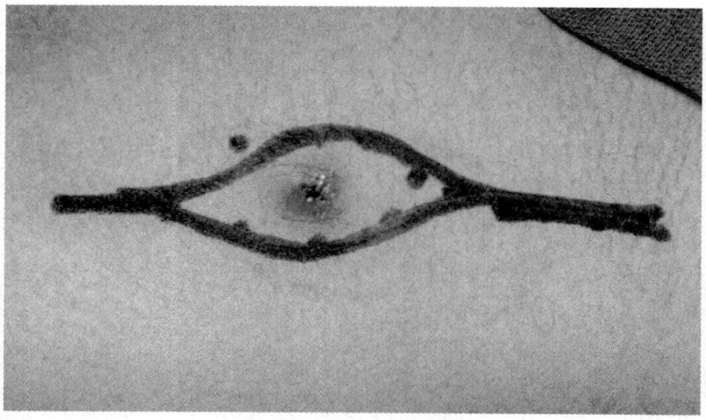
A

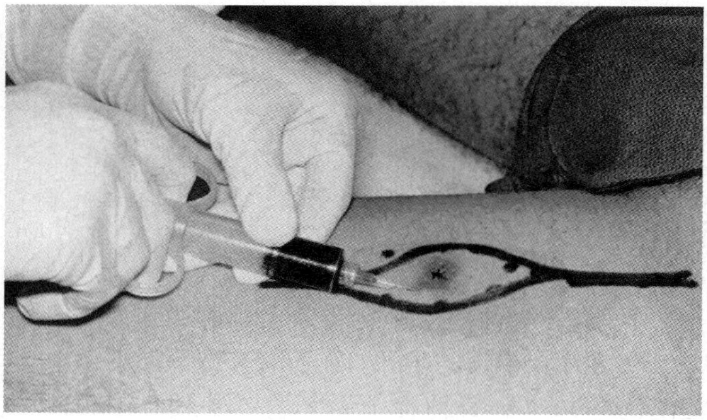
B

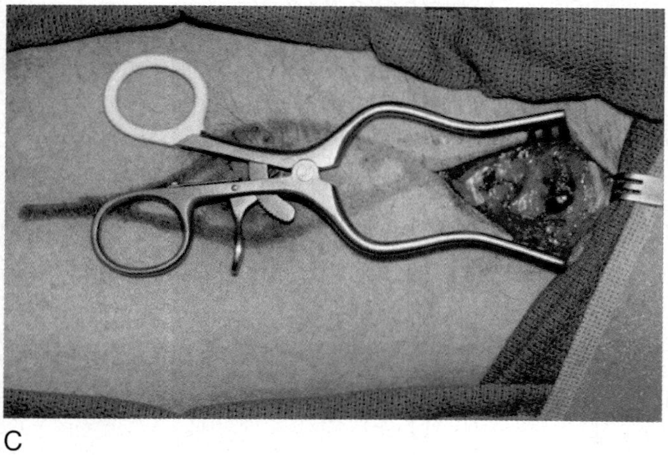
C

图 33–1 A. 左下肢上皮样肉瘤。注意推荐的切口与四肢呈纵向，以便必要时可以进行更广泛的切除术。B. 在切除术前将异硫蓝注入病灶。C. 含有染料的引流淋巴结。(Courtesy of Dr. Bhaskar Rao, St. Jude Children's Research Hospital, Memphis, Tenn.)

的切除手术野中。

当四肢肿瘤怀疑淋巴结浸润时，可以在手术时对病灶注射异硫蓝染料来进行检查。在这种情况下，染料被摄取进入引流病灶的淋巴结中(图 33–1)。

Mandell 等人[68]检查了 34 例肢体横纹肌肉瘤患者，其中 27 例进行区域淋巴结引流的检查，13 例患者（48%）有淋巴结受累征象，只有 1 例存活。相反，在 14 例没有淋巴结浸润的患者中，有 12 例存活。甚至当排除有远处转移的患者后，12 例没有淋巴结浸润的患者中仍有 11 例存活。在所有四肢横纹肌肉瘤患者中，进行淋巴结检查的重要性在横纹肌肉瘤国际协作组研究 -III的分析中得到认可[2]。

肢体保留手术后的功能结局

在过去的 25 年中，肢体保留手术加辅助放疗作为治疗的最佳方法，已经在一定数量的患者中实施。虽然这种联合治疗主要出于对美容的考虑，但在幼儿，特别是骨骼发育未成熟的儿童中，必须给予重视的不仅为生活的质量，而且有相关的局部并发症，包括肢体僵硬、疼痛、肢体缩短、肢体变形或骨骼脱钙引起的骨折[9,54,56,120]。患儿必须接受积极的物理治疗以使肢体挛缩降至最低。肌肉骨骼肿瘤协会用的功能性效果评估在大多数成人文献中都有详细描述。在 75%～80%的患者中获得优良至好的结果，75%以上患者

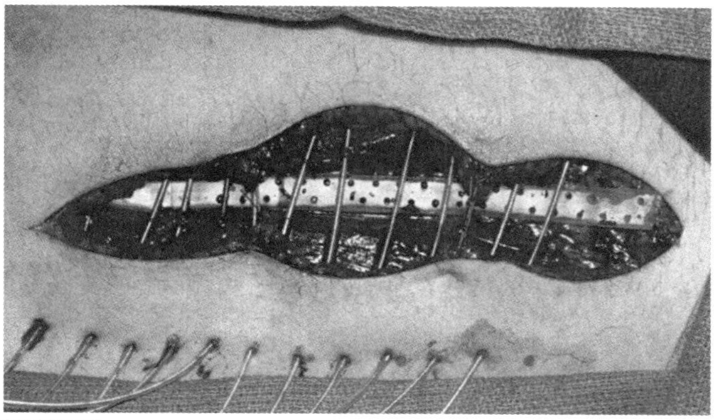

图 33–2 放置后装源导管用于图 33–1 所示上皮样肉瘤患者的近距离放射治疗。（Courtesy of Dr. Bhaskar Rao, St. Jude Children's Research Hospital, Memphis, Tenn.）

恢复了全部功能。在儿科文献中尚无类似的详细研究。在我的经验里，接受联合治疗后长期生存的患者中，50 例长期生存的四肢肉瘤患儿中有 7 例出现了下述的并发症，包括需要骺骨干固定术的肢体缩短、屈曲畸形、纤维化、慢性水肿、骨折和继发骨肉瘤。550
这些患儿均随访了 12～104 个月（中位数 36 个月）。

躯干软组织肉瘤

当需要胸壁切除术时，需要进行标准的开胸术切口。前锯肌或胸肌在与肿瘤合适的距离处被切开。应该进行仔细的触诊以度量切除的程度，可能包括切除骨膜并放置后装源导管用于近距离放射疗法。然而，如果影像学检查或手术时肉眼可见肋间肌浸润或胸廓内扩散，意味着需要完全的胸壁切除。在结扎肋间血管后，肋间肌在合适的部位被分离。仔细进行胸廓内触诊，以决定切除的程度和需要切除的肋骨数量。前壁和后壁切除的程度应该为 2.5～5cm。上面和后面的程度一般是原发病灶的上下各一个肋骨。任何在肺实质和肿瘤间的粘连用腔镜直线型切割吻合器来切除，以使标本能被整块切除。出现的缺损能用一个双层纱布和邻近的肌肉或肌皮瓣来封闭。

腹壁原发肿瘤是罕见的。准确的术前影像学检查能确定肿瘤能否切除。整个肿瘤被切除以获得满意的切缘。只要可能，切除的深度应该包括切除腹膜。腹膜的缺损能用网膜补片或可吸收纱布来关闭。应该避免不可吸收纱布和肠道的直接接触以减少肠瘘的风险。原则是通过可吸收纱布把肠袢放置于术后放疗野之外，特别是对下腹壁肿瘤患者，并至少把部分放疗剂量以近距离放射疗法进行。近距离放射疗法提高了局部控制，与外照射放疗比较还减少了晚期并发症（特别是骨骼和器官生长的改变）的可能性(图33–2)。低能量放射性核素和远距离后装源技术使婴、幼儿能接受治疗，同时可减少患儿、家属和医疗人员的放射物接触[78]。

（叶启东译 王耀平校）

参考文献

1. Al-gahtany M, Shroft M, Bouffet E, et al: Primary central nervous system sarcomas in children: Clinical, radiological, and pathological features. Childs Nerv Syst 2003;19: 808-817.
2. Andrassy RJ, Corpron CA, Hays D, et al: Extremity sarcomas: An analysis of prognostic factors from the Intergroup Rhabdomyosarcoma Study III. J Pediatr Surg 1996;31: 191-196.
3. Argani P, Ladanyi M: Recent advances in pediatric renal neoplasia. Adv Anat Pathol 2003;10:243-260.
4. Atkinson JB, Mahour JB, Isaacs H, et al: Hemangiopericytoma in infants and children: A report of six patients. Am J Surg 1984;148:372-374.
5. Atra A, Pinkerton R: High-dose chemotherapy in soft tissue sarcoma in children. Crit Rev Oncol Hematol 2002;41: 191-196.
6. Bailey PV, Webber TR, Tracy TF, et al: Congenital hemangiopericytoma: An unusual vascular neoplasm of infancy. Surgery 1993;114:936-941.
7. Bastiaannet E, Groen H, Jager PL, et al: The value of FDG-PET in the detection, grading and response to therapy of soft tissue and bone sarcomas: A systematic review and meta-analysis. Cancer Treat Rev 2004;30:83-101.
8. Bauernhofer T, Stoger H, Schmid M, et al: Sequential treatment of recurrent mesenteric desmoid tumor. Cancer 1996;77:1061-1065.
9. Bell RS, O'Sullivan B, Davis A, et al: Functional outcome in patients treated with surgery and irradiation for soft tissue tumours. J Surg Oncol 1 991;48:224-231.
10. Bisogno G, Roganovich J, Sotti G, et al: Desmoplastic small round cell tumour in children and adolescents. Med Pediatr Oncol 2000;34:338-342.
11. Bisogno G, Sotti G, Nowicki Y, et al: Soft tissue sarcoma as a second malignant neoplasm in the pediatric age group. Cancer 2004;100:1758-1765.
12. Brennan MF: Management of soft tissue sarcoma. Aust N Z J Surg 1990;60:419-428.
13. Brennan MF: The enigma of local recurrence. Ann Surg Oncol 1997;4:1-12.
14. Brennan MF, Casper ES, Harrison L, et al: The role of multimodality therapy in soft-tissue sarcoma. Ann Surg 1991; 214:328-338.
15. Brien EW, Terek RM, Geer RJ, et al: Treatment of soft-tissue sarcomas of the hand. J Bone Joint Surg Am 1995;77:564-571.
16. Casanova M, Ferrari A, Bisogno G, et al: Alveolar soft part sarcoma in children and adolescents: A report from the Soft-Tissue Italian Cooperative Group. Ann Oncol 2000;11:1445-1449.
17. Casanova M, Ferrari A, Spreafico F, et al: Malignant peripheral nerve sheath tumors in children: A single-institution twenty-year experience. J Pediatr Hematol Oncol 1999; 21:509-513.
18. Castillo BV, Kaufman L: Pediatric tumors of the eye and orbit. Pediatr Clin North Am 2003;50:1-20.
19. Castleberry RP, Kelly DR, Wilson ER, et al: Childhood liposarcoma: Report of a case and review of the literature. Cancer 1984;54:579-584.
20. Chang HR, Hajdu SI, Collin C, et al: The prognostic value of histologic subtypes in primary extremity liposarcoma. Cancer 1989;64:1514-1520.
21. Chen KT, Kassel SH, Medrano VA: Congenital hemangiopericytoma. J Surg Oncol 1986;31:127-129.
22. Cheng EY, Dusenbery KE, Winters MR, et al: Soft tissue sarcomas: Preoperative versus postoperative radiotherapy. J Surg Oncol 1996;61:90-99.
23. Chung EB, Enzinger FM: Infantile fibrosarcoma. Cancer 1976;38:729-739.
24. Chung EB, Enzinger FM: Infantile myofibromatosis. Cancer 1981;48:1807-1818.
25. Chung EB, Enzinger FM: Malignant melanoma of soft parts. Am J Surg Pathol 1983;7:405-413.
26. Cionini L, Marzano S, Olmi P: Soft tissue sarcomas: Experience with intraoperative brachytherapy in the conservative management. Ann Oncol 1992;3:S63-S66.
27. DeCou JM, Rao BN, Parham DM, et al: Malignant peripheral nerve sheath tumors: The St Jude Children's Research Hospital experience. Ann Surg Oncol 1995;2:524-529.
28. Dehner LP, Hill DA, Deschryver K: Pathology of the breast in children, adolescents and young adults. Semin Diagn Pathol 1999;16:235-247.
29. Demetri GD, Elias AD: Results of single agent and combination chemotherapy for advanced stage soft tissue sarcomas: Implications for decision making in the clinic. Hematol Oncol Clin North Am 1995;9:765-783.
30. de Oliveira-Filho AG, Miranda ML, Diz FL, et al: Use of radiofrequency for ablation of unresectable hepatic metastasis in desmoplastic small round cell tumor. Med Pediatr Oncol 2003;41:476-477.
31. Dominguez Malagon HR, Alfeiran Ruiz A, Chavarriaxicotencatl P, et al: Clinical and cellular effects of colchicine in fibromatosis. Cancer 1992;69:2478-2483.
32. Ducatman BS, Scheithouer BW, Peipgras DG, et al: Malignant peripheral nerve sheath tumors in childhood. J Neurooncol 1984;2:241-248.
33. Ducatman BS, Scheithouer BW, Peipgras DG, et al: Malignant peripheral nerve sheath tumors: A clinicopathologic study of 120 cases. Cancer 1986;57:2006-2021.
34. Enzinger FM: Hemangiopericytoma. In Weiss SW (ed): Soft Tissue Tumors, 2nd ed. St Louis, Mosby, 1988, pp 596-613.
35. Enzinger FM, Weiss SW: Soft Tissue Tumors, 3rd ed. St Louis, Mosby, 1995.
36. Farhat F, Culine S, Lhomme C, et al: Desmoplastic small round cell tumors: Results of a four-drug chemotherapy regimen in five adult patients. Cancer 1996;7:1363-1366.
37. Ferguson WS: Advances in the adjuvant treatment of infantile fibrosarcoma. Expert Rev Anticancer Ther 2003;3: 185-191.
38. Ferrari A, Casanova M, Massimino M, et al: Synovial sarcoma: Report of a series of 25 consecutive children from a single institution. Med Pediatr Oncol 1999;32:32-37.
39. Ferrari A, Casanova M, Spreafico F, et al: Childhood liposarcoma: A single-institution twenty year experience. Pediatr Hematol Oncol 1999;16:415-421.
40. Ferrari A, Gronchi A, Casanova M, et al: Synovial sarcoma: A retrospective analysis of 271 patients of all ages treated at a single institution. Cancer 2004;101:627-634.
41. Fontanesi J, Pappo AS, Parham DM, et al: Role of irradiation in management of synovial sarcoma: St Jude Children's Research Hospital experience. Med Pediatr Oncol 1996;26:264-267.
42. Frezza G, Barbieri E, Ammendolia I, et al: Surgery and radiation therapy in the treatment of soft tissue sarcomas of extremities. Ann Oncol 1992;3:S93-S95.
43. Fritsch MK, Bridge JA, Schuster AE, et al: Performance characteristics of a reverse transcriptase-polymerase chain reaction assay for the detection of tumor-specific fusion transcripts from archival tissue. Pediatr Dev Pathol

2003;6:43-53.
44. Gandolfo N, Marinoli C, Cafiero F, et al: Malignant melanoma of soft tissues (clear cell sarcoma) of the foot: Is MRI able to perform a specific diagnosis? Report of one case and review of the radiological literature. Anticancer Res 2000;20:3993-3998.
45. Gerald WL, Ladanyi M, de Alava E, et al: Clinical, pathological, and molecular spectrum of tumors associated with t(11:22)(p13:q12): Desmoplastic small round-cell tumor and its variants. J Clin Oncol 1998;16:3026-3036.
46. Gonzalez-Crussi F, Crawford SE, Sun CC: Intraabdominal desmoplastic small tumors with divergent differentiation: Observations on three cases of childhood. Am J Surg Pathol 1990;14:633-642.
47. Goodlad JR, Fletcher CD, Smith MA: Surgical resection of primary soft-tissue sarcoma: Incidence of residual tumour in 95 patients needing re-excision after local resection. J Bone Joint Surg Br 1996;78:658-661.
48. Gross E, Rao BN, Bowman L, et al: Outcome of treatment for pediatric sarcoma of the foot: A retrospective review over a 20-year period. J Pediatr Surg 1997;32:1181-1184.
49. Gross E, Rao BN, Pappo AS, et al: Soft tissue sarcoma of the hand in children: Clinical outcome and management. J Pediatr Surg 1997;32:698-702.
50. Gupta A, Maddalozzo J, Win Htin T, et al: Spindle cell rhabdomyosarcoma of the tongue in an infant: A case report with emphasis on differential diagnosis of childhood spindle cell lesions. Pathol Res Pract 2004;200:537-543.
51. Harjai MM, Bal RK, Hagpal BM, et al: Synovial sarcoma of the hand. Indian Pediatr 1999;36:194-197.
52. Heslin MJ, Lewis JJ, Woodruff JM, et al: Core needle biopsy for diagnosis of extremity soft tissue sarcoma. Ann Surg Oncol 1997;4:425-431.
53. Jaffe KA, Morris SG: Resection and reconstruction for soft-tissue sarcomas of the extremity. Orthop Clin North Am 1991;22:161-176.
54. Johnstone PA, Wexler LH, Venzon DJ, et al: Sarcomas of the hand and foot: Analysis of local control and functional result with combined modality therapy in extremity preservation. Int J Radiat Oncol Biol Phys 1994;29:735-745.
55. Karakousis CP, Proimakis C, Walsh DL: Primary soft tissue sarcoma of the extremities in adults. Br J Surg 1995;82: 1208-1212.
56. Karasek K, Constine LS, Rosier R: Sarcoma therapy: Functional outcome and relationship to treatment parameters. Int J Radiat Oncol Biol Phys 1992;24:651-656.
57. Kauffman SL, Stout AP: Hemangiopericytoma in children. Cancer 1960;13:695-710.
58. Keus RB, Rutgers EJ, Ho GH, et al: Limb-sparing therapy of extremity soft tissue sarcomas: Treatment outcome and long-term functional results. Eur J Cancer 1994;30A: 1459-1463.
59. Koutcher KA, Ballon D, Grahan M, et al: ^{31}P NMR spectra of extremity sarcomas: Diversity of metabolic profiles and changes in response to chemotherapy. Magn Reson Med 1990;16:19-34.
60. Kurkchubasche AG, Halvorson EG, Forman EN, et al: The role of preoperative chemotherapy in the treatment of infantile fibrosarcoma. J Pediatr Surg 2000;35:880-883.
61. Kushner BH, LaQuaglia MP, Wollner N, et al: Desmoplastic small round cell tumor: Prolonged progression-free survival with aggressive multimodal therapy. J Clin Oncol 1996;14:1526-1531.
62. Ladanyi M, Antonescu CR, Leung DH, et al: Impact of SYT-SSX fusion type on the clinical behavior of synovial sarcoma: A multi-institutional retrospective study of 243 patients. Cancer Res 2002;62:135-140.
63. Ladenstein R, Treuner J, Koscielniak E, et al: Synovial sarcoma in childhood and adolescents: Report of the German CWS-81 study. Cancer 1993;71:3647-3655.
64. LaQuaglia MP, Spiro SA, Ghavimi F, et al: Liposarcoma in patients younger than or equal to 22 years of age. Cancer 1999;72:3114-3119.
65. Lawrence W, Neifield JP: Soft tissue sarcomas. Curr Probl Surg 1989;2:753-827.
66. Lieberman PH, Brennan MF, Kimmel M, et al: Alveolar soft-part sarcoma: A clinico-pathologic study of half a century. Cancer 1989;63:1-13.
67. Madden NP, Spicer RD, Allibone EB, et al: Spontaneous regression of neonatal fibrosarcoma. Br J Cancer Suppl 1992;18:S72-S75.
68. Mandell L, Ghavimi F, LaQuaglia M, et al: Prognostic significance of regional lymph node involvement in childhood extremity rhabdomyosarcoma. Med Pediatr Oncol 1990;18:466-471.
69. Mazeron JJ, Suit HD: Lymph nodes as sites of metastasis from sarcomas of soft tissue. Cancer 1987;60:1800-1808.
70. McClain KL, Leach CT, Jenson HB, et al: Association of Epstein-Barr virus with leiomyosarcomas in children with AIDS. N Engl J Med 1995;332:12.
71. Meis JM, Enzinger FM, Martz KL, et al: Malignant peripheral nerve sheath tumors (malignant schwannoma) in children. Am J Surg Pathol 1992;16:694-707.
72. Merens WC, Bramwell VH: Adjuvant chemotherapy for soft tissue sarcomas. Hematol Oncol Clin North Am 1995; 9:801-815.
73. Meterissian SH, Reilly JA, Murphy A, et al: Soft-tissue sarcomas of the shoulder girdle: Factors influencing local recurrence, distant metastases, and survival. Ann Surg Oncol 1995;2:530-536.
74. Miller RW, Young JL, Novakovic B: Childhood cancer. Cancer 1995;75:395-405.
75. Miser JS, Triche TJ, Kinsella TJ, et al: Other soft tissue sarcomas of childhood. In Pizzo PA, Poplack DG (eds): Principles and Practice of Pediatric Oncology. Philadelphia, Lippincott-Raven, 1997, pp 865-888.
76. Mounayer C, Benndorf G, Bisdorff A, et al: Facial infantile hemangiopericytoma resembling an arteriovenous malformation. J Neuroradiol 2004;31:227-230.
77. Nag S, Olson T, Ruymann F, et al: High-dose-rate brachytherapy in childhood sarcomas: A local control strategy preserving bone growth and function. Med Pediatr Oncol 1995;25:463-469.
78. Nag S, Tippin DB: Brachytherapy for pediatric tumors. Brachytherapy 2003;2:131-138.
79. Neifeld J, Maurer H, Dillon P, et al: Non-rhabdomyosarcoma soft tissue sarcomas (NRSTS) in children. Society of Surgical Oncology, 1994.
80. Newton WA Jr, Soule EH, Hamoudi AB, et al: Histopathology of childhood sarcomas, Intergroup Rhabdomyosarcoma Studies I and II: Clinicopathologic correlation. J Clin Oncol 1988;6:67-75.
81. Nielsen OS, Cummings B, O'Sullivan B, et al: Preoperative and postoperative irradiation of soft tissue sarcomas: Effect of radiation field size. Int J Radiat Oncol Biol Phys 1991;21:1595-1599.
82. Okeu MF, Despa S, Choroszy M, et al: Synovial sarcoma in children and adolescents: Thirty three years of experience with multimodal therapy. Med Pediatr Oncol 2001;37:90-96.

83. Ordonez NG: Alveolor soft part sarcoma: A review and update. Adv Academ Pathol 1999;6:125-139.
84. Pappo AS, Fontanesi J, Luo X, et al: Synovial sarcoma in children and adolescents: The St Jude Children's Research Hospital experience. J Clin Oncol 1994;12: 2360-2366.
85. Pappo AS, Parham D, Cain A, et al: Alveolar soft part sarcoma in children and adolescents: Clinical features and outcomes in 11 patients. Med Pediatr Oncol 1996;26:81-84.
86. Pappo AS, Parham D, Lobe TE: Soft tissue sarcomas in children. Semin Surg Oncol 1999;16:121-143.
87. Pappo AS, Shapiro DN, Crist WM, et al: Biology and therapy of pediatric rhabdomyosarcoma. J Clin Oncol 1995;13:2123-2139.
88. Parham DM, Webber BL, Jenkins JJ III, et al: Nonrhabdomyosarcomatous soft tissue sarcomas of childhood: Formulation of a simplified system for grading. Mod Pathol 1995;8:705-710.
89. Paulino AC: Late effects of radiotherapy for pediatric extremity sarcomas. Int J Radiat Oncol Biol Phys 2004;60:265-274.
90. Philippe PG, Rao BN, Rogers DA, et al: Sarcomas of the flexor fossae in children: Is amputation necessary? J Pediatr Surg 1992;27:964-967.
91. Picard E, Udassin R, Ramu N, et al: Pulmonary fibrosarcoma in childhood: Fiber-optic bronchoscopic diagnosis and review of the literature. Pediatr Pulmonol 1999;27:347-350.
92. Pitcher ME, Thomas JM: Functional compartmental resection for soft tissue sarcomas. Eur J Surg Oncol 1994; 20:441-445.
93. Postovsky S, Peleg H, Ben-Itzhak O, et al: Fibrosarcoma of the trachea in a child: Case report and review of the literature. Am J Otolaryngol 1999;20:332-335.
94. Pratt CB, Kun LE: Soft Tissue Sarcomas of Children. Boston, Kluwer, 1993.
95. Pratt CB, Maurer HM, Salzberg A, et al: Treatment of unresectable or metastatic pediatric soft tissue sarcomas with surgery, irradiation and chemotherapy: A Pediatric Oncology Group study. Med Pediatr Oncol 1998;4: 201-209.
96. Pratt CB, Pappo AS, Gieser P: Role of adjuvant chemotherapy in the treatment of surgically resected pediatric nonrhabdomyosarcomatous soft tissue sarcomas: A Pediatric Oncology Group Study. J Clin Oncol 1999; 17:1219-1226.
97. Raney RB, Kollath J, Anderson J, et al: Late effects of therapy for patients with primary orbital rhabdomyosarcoma: A report from the Intergroup Rhabdomyosarcoma Study (IRS-III), 1984-1991. Med Pediatr Oncol 1997;29:425.
98. Rao BN: Malignant lesions of the chest and chest wall in childhood. Chest Surg Clin North Am 1993;3:461-475.
99. Rao BN: Nonrhabdomyosarcoma in children: Prognostic factors influencing survival. Semin Surg Oncol 1993;9: 524-531.
100. Rao BN: Present day concepts of thoracoscopy as a modality in pediatric cancer management. Int Surg 1997;82: 123-126.
101. Rao BN, Etcubanas EE, Green AA: Present-day concepts in the management of sarcomas in children. Cancer Invest 1989;7:349-356.
102. Rao BN, Santana VM, Parham D, et al: Pediatric nonrhabdomyosarcomas of the extremities: Influence of size, invasiveness, and grade on outcome. Arch Surg 1991;126: 1490-1495.
103. Rosen G, Forscher C, Lowenbraun S, et al: Synovial sarcoma: Uniform response of metastasis to high dose ifosfamide. Cancer 1994;73:2506-2511.
104. Rosoff PM, Bayliff S: Successful clinical response to irinotecan in desmoplastic round blue cell tumor. Med Pediatr Oncol 1999;33:500-503.
105. Rydholm A, Gustafson P, Rooser B: Limb-sparing surgery without radiotherapy based on anatomic location of soft tissue sarcoma. J Clin Oncol 1991;9:1757-1765.
106. Sara AS, Evans HL, Benjamin RS: Malignant melanoma of soft parts (clear cell sarcoma): A study of 17 cases, with emphasis on prognostic factors. Cancer 1990;65:367-374.
107. Schmidt D, Thum P, Harms D, et al: Synovial sarcoma in children and adolescents: A report from the Kiel Pediatric Tumor Registry. Cancer 1991;67:1667-1672.
108. Schwartz HS, Spengler DM: Needle tract recurrences after closed biopsy for sarcoma: Three cases and review of the literature. Ann Surg Oncol 1997;4:228-236.
109. Serpell JW, Ball AB, Robinson MH, et al: Factors influencing local recurrence and survival in patients with soft tissue sarcoma of the upper limb. Br J Surg 1991;78:1368-1372.
110. Shetty AK, Yu LC, Gardner RV, et al: Role of chemotherapy in the treatment of infantile fibrosarcoma. Med Pediatr Oncol 1999;33:425-427.
111. Shmookler BM, Enzinger FM: Liposarcoma occurring in children: An analysis of 17 cases and review of the literature. Cancer 1983;52:567-574.
112. Sorensen SA, Mulvihill JJ, Nielsen A: Long-term follow-up of von Recklinghausen neurofibromatosis: Survival and malignant neoplasms. N Engl J Med 1986;314:1010-1015.
113. Soule EH, Pritchard DJ: Fibrosarcoma in infants and children. Cancer 1977;40:1711-1721.
114. Spunt SL, Poquette CA, Hurt YS, et al: Prognostic factors for children and adolescents with surgically resected nonrhabdomyosarcomatous soft-tissue sarcoma: An analysis of 121 patients treated at St Jude Children's Research Hospital. J Clin Oncol 1999;17:3697-3707.
115. Stark AM, Buhl R, Hugo HH, et al: Malignant peripheral nerve sheath tumors: Report of 8 cases and review of the literature. Acta Neurochir 2001;143:357-364.
116. Taylor SR, Nunez C: Fine-needle aspiration biopsy in a pediatric population: Report of 64 consecutive cases. Cancer 1984;54:1449-1453.
117. Vadlamani I, Ma E, Brink DS, et al: Trisomy 15 in a case of pediatric hemangiopericytoma and review of the literature. Cancer Genet Cytogenet 2002;138:116-119.
118. Vaiday SJ, Payne GS, Leach MO, et al: Potential role of magnetic resonance spectroscopy in assessment of tumour response in childhood cancer. Eur J Cancer 2003;39:728-735.
119. Valle AA, Kraybill WG: Management of soft tissue sarcomas of the extremity in adults. J Surg Oncol 1996;63: 271-279.
120. Wall JE, Kaste SC, Greenwald CA, et al: Fractures in children treated with radiotherapy for soft tissue sarcoma. Orthopedics 1996;19:657-664.
121. Wexler LH, Helman LJ: Rhabdomyosarcoma and the undifferentiated sarcomas. In Pizzo PA, Poplack DG (eds): Principles and Practice of Pediatric Oncology. Philadelphia, Lippincott-Raven, 1997, pp 799-829.
122. Wiklund T, Huuhtanen R, Blomqvist C, et al: The importance of a multidisciplinary group in the treatment of soft tissue sarcomas. Eur J Cancer 1996;32A:269-273.
123. Willett CG, Suit HD, Tepper JE, et al: Intraoperative electron beam radiation therapy for retroperitoneal soft

tissue sarcoma. Cancer 1991;68:278-283.
124. Williard WC, Collin C, Casper ES, et al: The changing role of amputation for soft tissue sarcoma of the extremity in adults. Surg Gynecol Obstet 1992;175:389-396.
125. Wilson AN, Davis A, Bell RS, et al: Local control of soft tissue sarcoma of the extremity: The experience of a multidisciplinary sarcoma group with definitive surgery and radiotherapy. Eur J Cancer 1994;30A:746-751.
126. Wong WW, Hirose T, Scheithauer BW, et al: Malignant peripheral nerve sheath tumor: Analysis of treatment outcome. Int J Radiat Oncol Biol Phys 1998;42:351-360.
127. Zalupski MM, Baker LH: Systemic adjuvant chemotherapy for soft tissue sarcomas. Hematol Oncol Clin North Am 1995;9:787-800.
128. Zornig C, Peiper M, Schroder S: Re-excision of soft tissue sarcoma after inadequate initial operation. Br J Surg 1995;82:278-279.

第 34 章

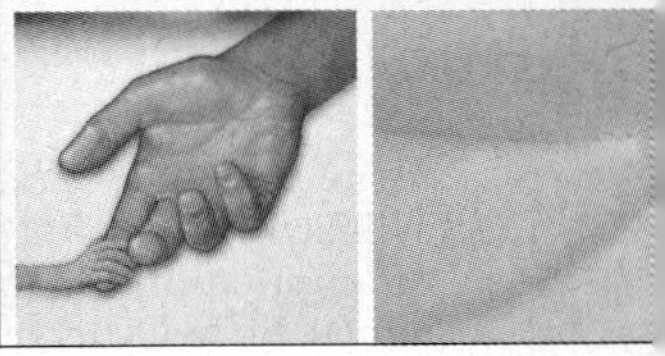

畸胎瘤和其他胚芽细胞肿瘤

Richard G. Azizkhan

554 小儿胚芽细胞肿瘤（GCT）是一种由不同种类肿瘤组成的较少见的肿瘤。其发生率为每百万儿童中 2.4 例，在小于 15 岁被诊断为癌症的儿童中约占 1%[195]。这些肿瘤可发生在性腺和性腺外部位，性腺外和睾丸的这类肿瘤主要出现于小于 3 岁的儿童，性腺肿瘤主要发生在青春期和青春期后的年龄。胚芽细胞肿瘤可出现各种临床表现和各种组织病理学特征，并根据病变类型有恶性风险。除了有这些特点外，这种肿瘤被推测源于原始胚细胞。临床和病理变化因在胚细胞发育阶段受到肿瘤发生、性别和瘤源性的影响而不同[36]。在胚胎发生早期，胚芽细胞开始沿着后肠中线嵴肠系膜定向移位并最终合并进入胚胎性腺组织。如果这一移行过程被扰乱，胚芽细胞可停滞于异常的部位，因此胚芽细胞肿瘤可发生于骶尾部、纵隔、腹膜后、脑松果体、卵巢和睾丸。恶性变化可发生在这些区域的任何部位。在不同解剖部位的多种胚芽细胞肿瘤和组织类型的多样性反映出胚芽细胞的全能性质，特殊肿瘤类型与细胞分化程度不同有关。

多数胚芽细胞肿瘤有许多生物标志物，有助于识别这些肿瘤和处理及评估肿瘤是否复发。肿瘤的治疗取决于多种因素，包括特殊的病理类型、解剖部位、肿瘤分级、组织学改变和肿瘤的可切除性。获得理想的治疗效果与彻底的手术切除、精确的组织学检查和选择性使用化疗有关。特别重要的是，在 20 世纪 70 年代后期，化疗中引入顺铂使复发和转移病变在治疗生存率上发生了显著提高[46]。目前，病理分级低的性腺外肿瘤和各分级的性腺肿瘤的生存率根据部位为 90%～100%。性腺外病理分级高的肿瘤生存率近 75%[148]。

本章重点介绍多数常见的性腺外胚芽细胞肿瘤、畸胎瘤和小儿外科见到的典型恶性性腺外胚芽细胞肿瘤。本章对卵巢、睾丸和颅内肿瘤仅做简单讨论，第 36 章、37 章和 41 章将分别做更详细的介绍。

胚胎学

原始胚芽细胞来源于胚胎卵黄囊内胚层接近尿囊处，并在妊娠第 4 周逐渐明显。至第 5 周，这些细胞通过肠系膜移行到性腺嵴[94]并最终成为性腺。这一移行似乎由 c-kit 受体和干细胞因子调节。随着胚芽细胞出现转移，干细胞因子从卵黄囊到性生殖嵴呈现一增加的梯度[108,171]。细胞从头部向性腺嵴的移行到妊娠第 6 周完成。在这一阶段，生殖嵴从颈部水平延伸到发育中的脊柱两侧的下腰椎水平[67]。

在动物模型中，在原始胚芽细胞中 c-kit 受体表达缺失与移行失败与性腺形成失败有关[36]。主要的假设是：性腺外胚芽细胞肿瘤由异常的移行引起，或在移行途中由胚芽细胞的残留引起[65]，细胞可移行到达非正常途径的区域（如松果腺部和骶尾部），或可残留在性腺组织以外的部位。

组织病理学分类和分级

虽然各种已发表的分类方法有少许不同，胚芽细胞肿瘤一般被认为有七种主要组织类型：无性细胞瘤（或精原细胞瘤）、卵黄囊瘤（内胚窦瘤）、胚胎癌、 55
多胚癌、绒毛膜癌、畸胎瘤和混合性胚芽细胞瘤。大多数恶性胚芽细胞瘤以单一形式出现，但在 10%的病例，可含有两种或更多种肿瘤类型[161]。按常见的发生频率排序依次为：畸胎瘤、内胚窦瘤、生殖细胞瘤和混合性胚芽细胞瘤。绒毛膜癌、胚胎癌和多胚癌少见。

表 34-1　恶性性腺外胚芽细胞肿瘤的分期

Ⅰ期：肿瘤局限，各部位肿瘤可完全切除（骶尾部肿瘤带尾骨切除）；肿瘤边缘完整；肿瘤标志物阳性或阴性

Ⅱ期：肿瘤有镜下残留；肿瘤囊壁侵犯；淋巴结阴性或镜下淋巴结累及；肿瘤标志物阳性或阴性

Ⅲ期：肉眼肿瘤残留；肉眼淋巴结累及；腹水或胸水细胞学检查可找到肿瘤细胞；肿瘤标志物阳性或阴性

Ⅳ期：远处转移（肺、肝、脑、骨、远处淋巴结或其他部位转移）

Adapted from staging systems of the Children's Oncology Group and the National Cancer Institute.

与其他器官特殊恶性肿瘤比较，由于存在多种肿瘤类型和多个来源部位，同一分级系统的应用受到了影响。

然而，儿童肿瘤组织和国家癌症研究所已采用了一针对性腺外恶性胚芽细胞肿瘤总的分级系统（表 34-1）。（女性和男性性腺肿瘤的分级见第 36 章和第 37 章。）

主要生物标志物

甲胎蛋白

在过去的几十年中，在诊断和处理胚芽细胞肿瘤中使用的许多生物标志物都曾是重点研究课目[25]，这些标志物的临床重要性已被很好地确定。许多胚芽细胞肿瘤分泌甲胎蛋白（AFP）或 β-人绒毛膜促性腺素（β-HCG）；最好在手术切除怀疑的肿瘤前测定 AFP 和 β-HCG 水平，以建立一个基准并确定治疗的效果。

AFP 最早被认为是一种肝脏肿瘤的血清标志物，是一种主要的胎儿血清结合蛋白。胎儿和新生儿肝脏可分泌大量的 AFP，正常新生儿的血清 AFP 水平为 50 000ng/ml；早产儿的水平更高。在妊娠 12～14 周时 AFP 达到其峰值，至出生后 8 个月至 1 岁时逐渐降到正常成人水平（10ng/dL）[62]。出生后的第一年中，婴儿的 AFP 必须在正常范围内，如果 AFP 明显高于特定年龄段的正常范围则有临床意义（图 34-1）。AFP 水平升高或针对 AFP 的胚芽细胞肿瘤免疫组化染色阳性表明存在恶性成分，尤其是卵黄囊瘤或胚胎癌。

手术切除肿瘤通常可使血清 AFP 恢复到正常；AFP 的血清半衰期为 5～7 天[109]。在大多数病例，通过治疗可消除 AFP 分泌的来源。术后检测 AFP 水平有助于在出现临床症状前早期发现肿瘤复发。如果因为 AFP 没有像期望的那样下降而怀疑有肿瘤残留或转移，可应用诊断性影像学仔细检查，并可能需要手术。然而，AFP 升高并不一定提示肿瘤进展。化疗导致肿瘤减小，能引起短暂的 AFP 突然升高[187]。肝功能异常也可伴有 AFP 异常，如良性肝脏病变、肝脏和胃肠道恶性肿瘤、病毒性肝炎、麻醉后继发性胆汁

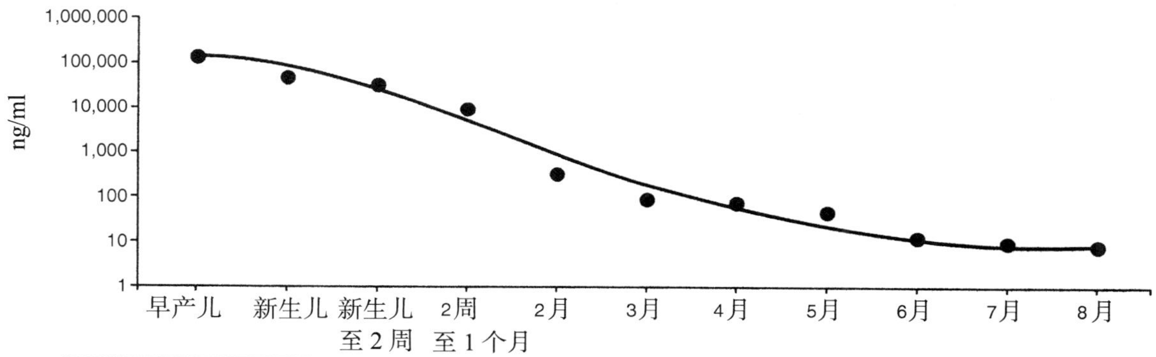

平均值	134 734	48 406	33 113	9 452	323	88	74	46.5	12.5	9.7	8.5
标准差	±41 444	±34 718	±32 503	±12 610	±278	±87	±56	±19.0	±9.8	±7.1	±5.5

图 34-1　正常新生儿血清 AFP 的衰退情况。（Adapted Wu JT, Sudar K: Serum alpha fetoprotein (AFP) levels in normal infants. Pediatr Res.91981:15:50.）

淤滞或药物引起的肝脏胆汁淤滞均可导致持续性 AFP 水平升高[15,60,96]。其他伴有 AFP 升高的疾病包括：甲状腺功能减退、毛细血管扩张症和遗传性酪氨酸血症[194]。虽然，这些异常容易与胚芽细胞肿瘤
556 区别，但当解释 AFP 水平升高时应当考虑到。

β－人绒毛膜促性腺素（β－HCG）

β-HCG 是一种糖蛋白，被认为由胚胎合体滋养层产生，是由 α 和 β 亚单位组成，后者能被可靠地检测出。β-HCG 升高提示有合体滋养层成分存在，如在绒毛膜癌、精原细胞瘤或无性细胞瘤中见到的，偶尔在胚胎癌中也可见到[73]。对照半衰期较长的 AFP，HCG 的 β 亚单位的半衰期仅为 24～36 小时[106]，它消失很快。β-HCG 维持阴性表明肿瘤被完全切除，监测 β-HCG 水平有助于评估分泌 β-HCG 的肿瘤患者的预后。

如同 AFP，血清 β-HCG 突然升高可发生在继发于化疗后肿瘤细胞消退时[187]。同样，这些标志物的升高可伴发于双侧睾丸切除或双侧卵巢切除后的黄体化激素升高。其发生是由于黄体化激素的 α 亚单位和绒毛膜促性腺素的 α 亚单位之间的交叉免疫反应所致[60]。虽然其他一些肿瘤（如多发性骨髓瘤、胰腺、胃肠道、乳腺、肺和膀胱恶性肿瘤）也可伴有一定程度的血清 β-HCG 升高，这些变化主要是在成人中见到。

观察和警惕

在过去 12 年中，关于血清 AFP 和 β-HCG 水平的解释有过激烈的争论。现今，由 Trigo 等人[180]完成的一项研究比较中肯地指出，肿瘤标志物没有升高并不总是当时不存在病灶的确凿而可信的依据。作者建议，虽然肿瘤标志物作为评估指标应被包括在治疗随访中，但早期发现肿瘤复发不应仅依赖这一指标。

许多研究已把焦点集中到 AFP 和 β-HCG 的半衰期延长并将其作为显著的预兆，但这些还没有得到多数人的认同或至少还有一些疑问。Christensen 等人[34]提出了一个固定的 β-HCG 半衰期的概念，提示化疗后期伴有半衰期延长，并不总是表示有病灶持续存在，这种延迟与半衰期内标志物清除的两个阶段的模式有关，与化疗后发生较慢的合成有关。其他临床医生的发现[125,131]提出：标志物在化疗早期的下降率通过风险分组有预后评估价值。Bosl 和 Head[26]报告：治疗前的风险情况和治疗后标志物的清除是各自独立的，有相同的预后价值。半衰期延长在没有治疗前和治疗后的患者都是重要参数。Morre 和 Bosl[130]报告了 6 例在治疗后存在稳定的、轻度的血清标志物升高，但没有病灶持续存在的临床和影像学迹象病例，经过密切随访，患者无需额外的化疗。虽然，肿瘤标志物水平和标志物清除的半衰期有预后价值，但在化疗后阶段，将标志物轻到中度的升高作为病灶持续存在的指标其可信度可能很低。

其他标志物

在胚芽细胞肿瘤患儿已观察到血清中乳酸脱氢酶（LDH）水平升高，其为肝脏糖分解酶，可能是一种预后指标[90]。LDH 是一种非特异性标志物，虽然与任何类型的胚芽细胞肿瘤没有特殊的关联，但被认为与肿瘤的生长和衰退有关[36,111]。在无性细胞肿瘤患者中，血清 LDH 同工酶增加 1 个单位，肿瘤的负荷相应增加，这在手术处理中也有意义[160]。LDH 假性增高可出现在病毒性疾病、肝脏疾病、化疗中和化疗后[111]。

胎盘碱性磷酸酶（PLAP）是一种区别胚芽细胞肿瘤的可靠标志物[93]。PLAP 的组化免疫染色可用于确定无法区分的胚芽细胞肿瘤的组织学来源[106]。事实上，PLAP 在所有晚期精原细胞瘤患者的血清中都升高，在 30% 的Ⅰ期精原细胞患者中升高[103,151]。PLAP 也可用于分析其他不能确定组织来源的肿瘤，尤其是当对精原细胞瘤和淋巴瘤很难做出诊断时[25]。

两项最近的研究显示，脑脊液中 s-kit（c-kit 的可溶性异构体）浓度可作为中枢神经系统生殖细胞瘤的有效临床标志物，尤其是可用于检测肿瘤复发或蛛网膜下播散[129,174]。其他研究表明，结合性 CD117（c-kit）和 CD30（Ki-1 抗原）免疫组化可能对于从胚胎癌中区别精原细胞瘤是一种有用的工具[113]。

血管内皮生长因子的表达在睾丸胚芽细胞肿瘤中高于在正常睾丸中并与微血管数量和全身转移有关[58]。表皮生长因子受体对于识别睾丸胚芽细胞肿瘤中合体滋养层细胞是一有用的标志物[81]。

研究者还在继续寻找有助于区别胚芽细胞肿瘤类型和不同患者的生物和免疫组织化学标志物[5,59,96,114,124,188]。虽然已经得到许多有意义的结果，但还需进一步在大样本病例研究中进行验证。重要的是要认识到，大多数研究来自于成人而非来自于儿童。

细胞遗传学

目前，细胞遗传学技术已能让我们理解包括胚芽细胞肿瘤发生在内的遗传学和分子学机制。遗传学改变也许与临床结果有关，是值得认真研究的课题。流式细胞计数已证实，儿童胚芽细胞肿瘤有不同的
557 DNA 整倍体，与成人胚芽细胞肿瘤不同，成人胚芽细胞肿瘤倾向于为非整倍体 DNA[168]。大多数小于 4 岁儿童的畸胎瘤是双倍体，有正常的染色体组型。如果不考虑病变来源部位，具有良性生物学行为[28,85,98]。恶性胚芽细胞在这一年龄组几乎都是卵黄囊瘤，一般是双倍体或四倍体[145,170]。多数常见的细胞遗传学异常涉及 1 号、3 号和 6 号染色体。研究已证明，在来自睾丸和性腺外的儿童恶性胚芽细胞肿瘤中，80%～100%有 1p36 的缺失[145,170]，其中极少数显示有 c-*myc* 或 n-*myc* 扩增的证据， 这些主要致癌基因可能具有预后意义[144]。

在大龄儿童和青少年中，中枢神经系统畸胎瘤的细胞遗传学分析显示，它们有较高频率的性染色体异常，最常见 X 染色体复制增加[32,197]。虽然在所有类型的成人胚芽细胞肿瘤中，12p 或 i（12p）等臂染色体相当常见，但在儿童胚芽细胞肿瘤中并不常见。这些等臂染色体的三次或更多次复制常与治疗无效有关，被认为可用来判断预后[86]。这一异常已在松果体生殖细胞肿瘤中描述过，但在松果体畸胎瘤中没有见到[38,165,191]。在成人和青少年的卵巢肿瘤中也已证实有 12p 等臂染色体[4]。

畸胎瘤

畸胎瘤是最常见的胚芽细胞肿瘤。其来自于性腺或性腺外部位，与原始全能细胞在胚胎期停留的部位一致。畸胎瘤的表现与年龄和解剖部位有关。出现在新生儿期和幼儿期的畸胎瘤常为性腺外畸胎瘤，年长儿童中卵巢或睾丸畸胎瘤更常见[154]。超过一半的畸胎瘤在出生时被发现；肿瘤可发生在各个部位，但最常见于骶尾部（图 34-2）。在青春期前儿童中，约 75%的畸胎瘤发生在骶尾部，诊断常在 1 岁前做出。虽然，超过 1/3 的睾丸畸胎瘤在 1 岁前被发现，但这些肿瘤极少在新生儿期被诊断[99,176]。如果不考虑年龄，骶尾部也是最常见的性腺外肿瘤部位（45%～65%）

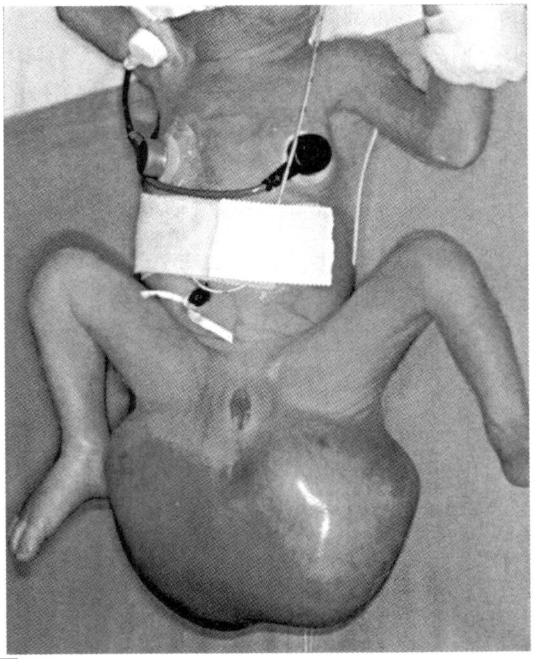

图 34-2　一位有 30 周胎龄的骶尾部畸胎瘤新生儿，肿瘤被成功地切除，患者现已是一位青年人。

表 34-2　肿瘤发生的部位

部位	发生率（%）
骶尾部	45～65
前纵隔	10～12
性腺（卵巢和睾丸）	10～35
腹膜后	3～5
颈部	3～6
骶前	3～5
中枢神经系统	2～4
其他少见部位（如肝脏、肾脏、阴道、胃）	＜1

From Shamberger RC: Teratomas and germ cell tumors. In O'Neill JA Jr, Grosfeld JL, Fonkalsrud EW, et al (eds): Principles of Pediatric Surgery, 2nd ed. St Louis, Mosby, 2004.

(表 34–2)。颈面部畸胎瘤和颅腔内畸胎瘤较为少见。出现在纵隔、心脏、腹膜后和肝脏的畸胎瘤则更少见。除了睾丸畸胎瘤，75%～80%的畸胎瘤发生在女性，约 20%的肿瘤含有恶性成分，最常见的为内胚窦瘤。

与畸胎瘤伴发的先天性异常疾病谱中[8,87,142]，异常的类型常与肿瘤的部位和大小有关。在严重的骶尾部畸胎瘤患者中，有时可见到单一的或多发的泌尿生殖道、直肠、肛门、椎骨、脊索远端畸形[10,112,138,142]。在新生儿巨大头颅和鼻咽部畸胎瘤中可伴有腭裂[65,146]。

畸胎瘤可表现为实质性、囊性或实质性囊性的混合性病变。确切地说，这些肿瘤是由来源于胚胎三胚层（中胚层、内胚层和外胚层）中各胚层的组织组成，并常包含有对原发解剖部位来说是异物的组织[40]。肿瘤可以以一个胚层的组织为主，偶尔畸胎瘤可以是单一胚层的组织。大多数在出生时发现的畸胎瘤包含有中胚层和外胚层成分。经常出现表皮和真皮样结构，如毛发、脂肪和汗腺，并可出现发育完好的牙齿。也可见胰腺组织、肾上腺组织和甲状腺组织。
558 事实上，所有畸胎瘤都有外胚层成分，包括脂肪、软骨、骨和肌肉。常可见到的内胚层成分包括：肠上皮细胞和由鳞状上皮、立方上皮或扁平上皮排列的囊性结构[36]。成熟和非成熟的神经上皮和神经胶质组织也经常可见。

肿瘤组织可显示不同的成熟程度，在组织学上被分为成熟畸胎瘤和非成熟畸胎瘤（图 34–3）。多数儿童畸胎瘤是成熟畸胎瘤，肿瘤内没有共存的恶性肿瘤细胞，极少或没有肿瘤恶变倾向。性腺成熟畸胎瘤有单囊性和多囊性肿瘤或实体瘤，而性腺外畸胎瘤并没有清晰明显的外囊[41,77,78]。虽然某一成熟畸胎瘤从组织学上观察可以是良性的，但重要的是要注意到，如果肿瘤压迫气道或侵犯重要的结构，如脑或心脏，也可以是致命的。更有甚者，根据肿瘤的部位和大小，即使是良性肿瘤可能也无法手术，且无法适应宫外生存。

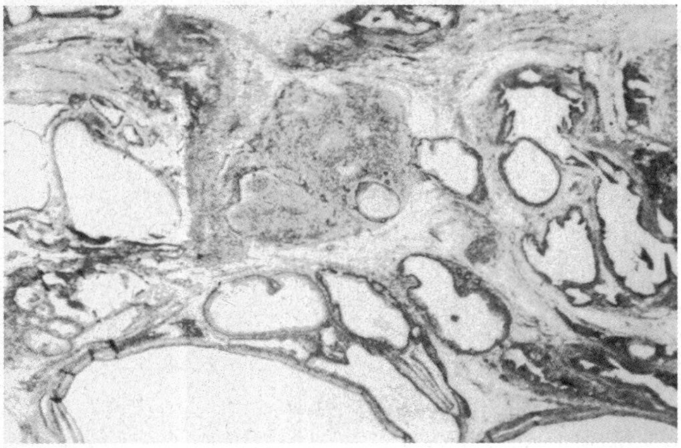

图 34–3 骶尾部畸胎瘤的组织学改变，苏木素–伊红染色证实，成熟的囊性上皮成分围绕着一个中心密集的未成熟神经上皮组织灶。

未成熟畸胎瘤常比成熟畸胎瘤瘤体更大，更多为实体瘤。在各种未成熟组织中，未成熟畸胎瘤有不同的组织学表现，出现在瘤体中的通常为神经上皮细胞。许多作者为未成熟畸胎瘤设计和改良了分级系统[137,153]，一般考虑肿瘤的未成熟程度和神经上皮成分的存在及数量。虽然分级仅对成人卵巢未成熟畸胎瘤有预后意义[36]，但在青少年患者的处理中也提供了临床医生有用的提示：这些肿瘤可能有恶性转化倾向，因此，需要密切观察。分级系统在胎儿和新生儿中没有意义，因为对于发育成熟阶段的胎儿和新生儿，出现未成熟成分也可以是正常的[92,184]，在这些患者中不考虑肿瘤的分级。未成熟畸胎瘤常有良好的预后，仅在极少的病例中，未成熟的神经胶质瘤组织从未成熟的原发部位转移至邻近的淋巴结、肺和其他远处器官[17,43,66,179]。

儿童未成熟畸胎瘤中最重要的肿瘤复发现象是出现微小的卵黄囊瘤转移结节[84]。由于在混合性肿瘤中卵黄囊瘤成分较小，它们可在病理取样操作中被遗漏。这可解释未成熟畸胎瘤切除后出现卵黄囊瘤转移现象。

一般来说，预后取决于患者的年龄、肿瘤的可切除性和是否存在转移或是否有转移的可能。

寄生胎

寄生胎和畸胎瘤之间的关系仍不清楚并有争议，两者的区分仍不清晰[2,48,65,83,134]。有连续的椎骨、肌肉骨骼和器官结构是寄生胎的特征，这些可类似于胎儿（图 34–4）。寄生胎可在产前和产后被发现，腹膜后肿块是最常见的临床部位[48]。目前认为，寄生胎是畸胎瘤高度变异的一种少见形式。根据 WHO 的分类，寄生胎目前被归类为一种成熟畸胎瘤[161]。

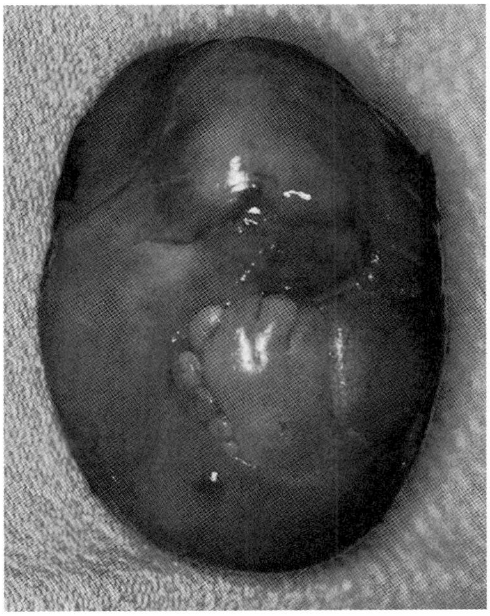

图 34-4　从一位 9 个月的女婴腹中取出的腹膜后寄生胎。这一无脑畸胎瘤，有手足、脊柱和原始的面部结构。

骶尾部畸胎瘤

临床表现和诊断

骶尾部畸胎瘤（SCT）是一种显性畸胎瘤，是胎儿和新生儿最常见的肿瘤，估计发生率为每 2～4 万活产儿中有 1 例，女性居多，男女比例约为 1∶2～
59 1∶4[10,39,117,158]。大多数骶尾部畸胎瘤组织学呈良性；然而约 17%呈现恶性组织学或临床特征[3,20]。大多数骶尾部畸胎瘤病例为散在发生，10%的病例有双胞胎家族史。

10%～20%的骶尾部畸胎瘤患者有伴发异常，如气管食管瘘、无肛、肛直肠狭窄、脊柱裂、泌尿生殖道畸形、脊髓脊膜膨出和无脑儿[10,68,142,150,191]。许多患者也可由于大的畸胎瘤推压导致邻近器官有显著的结构异常。

由 Altman 等人[3]提出的分类系统将骶尾部畸胎瘤分为四种不同的解剖类型，各型的区别在于肿瘤在骨盆内和骨盆外延伸的程度。Ⅰ型（46.7%）为显著外露型，仅有很小部分向骶前延伸；Ⅱ型（34.7%）的肿瘤主要部分外露，骶前盆腔内也有部分肿瘤；Ⅲ型（8.8%）原发于盆腔和腹腔，但有明显的外突部分；Ⅳ型（9.8%）为骶前肿瘤，没有外露的表现（图 34-5）。这些作者观察到：恶性成分发生率不仅与解剖类型相关（Ⅰ型中 8%，Ⅳ型 38%），也与诊断时的年龄与性别有关，而与肿瘤的大小无关[3,79]。肿瘤恶性变在年龄稍大的婴儿（大于 6 个月）和儿童中明显高于肿瘤显著外突的新生儿。恶性变似乎在男孩更为常见[3,30,57]。与复合性或囊性肿瘤相比，实体瘤中恶性变更为多见[157]。在骶尾部肿瘤中，最常见的恶性畸胎瘤是卵黄囊瘤和胚胎癌[80]。

许多大的骶尾部畸胎瘤在子宫内就出现，并能在产前获得诊断。至今，已有 60 多例报告[24,69]。虽然诊断常常在妊娠 22～34 周之间做出，但最早也有在妊娠 13 周时做出。子宫大于正常妊娠日期（羊水过多或因肿瘤增大）是做母婴超声检查最常见的产科指征。超声检查可提示来自胎儿骶部的外突性肿瘤（图 34-6A）。后者由囊性和实性组成，有时出现钙化灶。多数产前诊断的骶尾部畸胎瘤在彩色多普勒检查中能

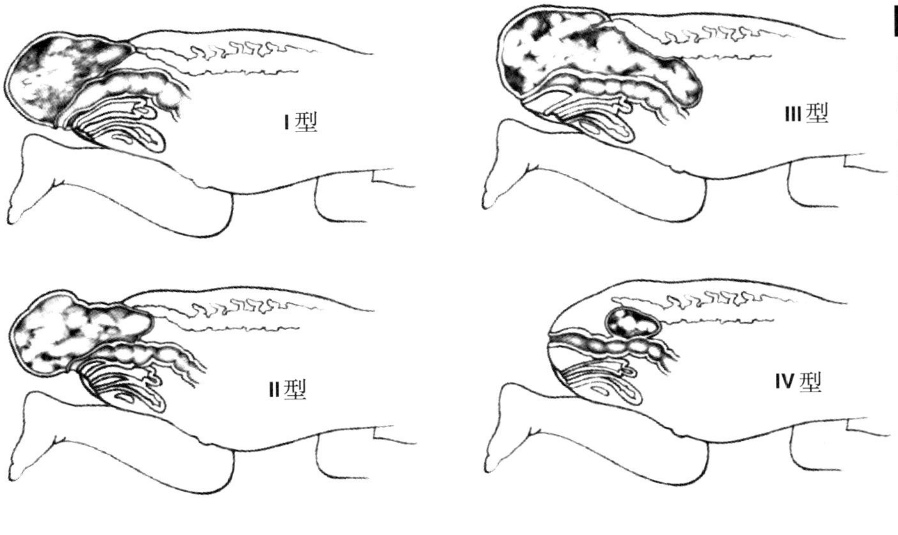

图 34-5　骶尾部畸胎瘤分型。(From Altman RP, Randolph JG, Lilly JR: Sacrococcygeal teratoma: American Academy of Pediatrics Surgical Section Survey-1973. J Pediatr Surg 1974;9:389.)

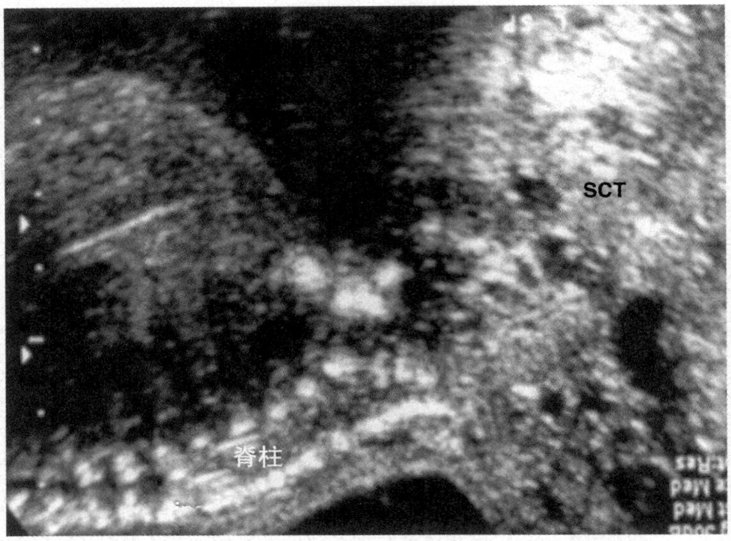

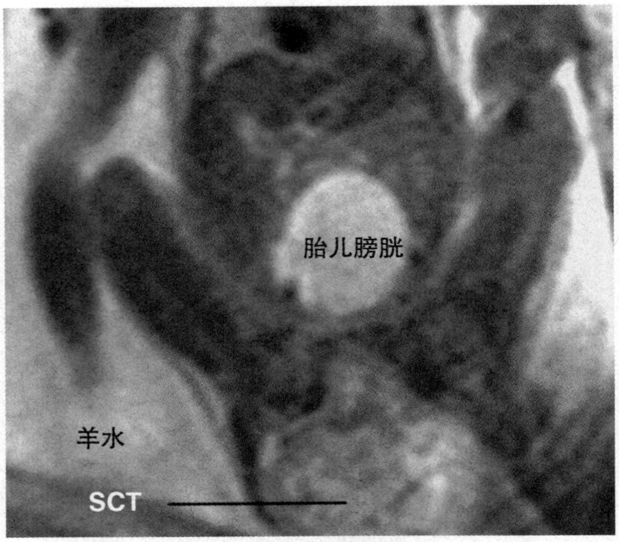

图 34-6 骶尾部畸胎瘤胎儿的影像学检查。A. 产前母体-胎儿超声检查显示：胎儿患有骶尾部畸胎瘤（SCT）。B. 20 周龄胎儿，母亲-胎儿磁共振检查显示一相当大的骶尾部畸胎瘤。（Courtesy of Dr. Timothy Crombleholme.）

见到丰富的血管[21]。

腰骶部脊髓脊膜膨出最容易与骶尾部畸胎瘤相混淆。这类脊髓脊膜膨出和囊性骶尾部畸胎瘤在超声检查中表现相似。因为两者都可伴有孕妇 AFP 水平升高，这两种疾病无法根据 AFP 来区分。其他从超声检查可得到的信息包括：可能出现的腹腔或盆腔扩张，肠道或尿路梗阻的证据，以及对胎儿脊椎完整性和胎儿下肢功能的评估[163]。对胎儿颅脑的影像检查有助于建立诊断，因为多数胎儿脊髓脊膜膨出有头颅征象，如 Arnold-Chiari 畸形[21]。当有怀疑时，胎儿磁共振检查对区别胎儿解剖结构和做出确切的诊断是极有价值的（图 34-6B）。其他与骶尾部畸胎瘤相似的软组织肿块包括：神经母细胞瘤、血管瘤、平滑肌瘤和淋巴瘤[21]。

肿瘤能以不可预见的速度生长至巨大肿块，并可向腹膜后延伸，推压盆腔或腹腔内结构。巨大的肿瘤可引起巨大胎盘、非免疫性胎儿水肿和“镜子”综合征（mirror syndrome）[53,155]，这些情况被认为是由于畸胎瘤中血管的低阻力引起的高动力状态[7]。如果不对胎儿进行干预，高输出性心衰和水肿导致胎儿死亡几乎是必然的。因此，选择部分符合严格标准的胎儿，通过宫内外科手术减少畸胎瘤体积，可使胎儿恢复正常生理功能[82]。

因肿瘤破裂、早产、难产等产科并发症可导致新生儿死亡[24,54,71,132]，对因肿瘤引起的羊水过多或子宫过大而有早产倾向的孕妇可通过减少羊水或囊肿穿刺抽液进行治疗。可通过对肿瘤大于 5cm 的胎儿做计划性剖宫产来避免难产和肿瘤破裂[164]。 56

与产时做出诊断的病例相比，产前诊断的病例预后明显稍差。目前骶尾部畸胎瘤分类系统中的预后因素分析还没应用于胎儿病例[3,24]。诊断为骶尾部畸胎瘤的新生儿其死亡率最高为 5%，而胎儿骶尾部畸胎瘤的死亡率接近 50%[24,53,54]。大多数临床资料结果表明，胎儿水肿、羊水过多和胎盘巨大预示着不良预后。母体-胎儿超声指标也是一种预后因素[24]。如果骶尾部畸胎瘤是在常规产前超声检查中偶尔发现的，在任何妊娠期，预后都要稍好。许多肿瘤以囊性为主，血管相对较少，并能在产后通过手术切除进行治疗。如果由于母亲出现症状的原因而进行超声检查，预后要差得多。另外，在孕 30～32 周前施行剖宫产或羊水过多的早产儿死亡率增加[164]。根据这些因素，产前诊断的患者应推荐至高危产科中心，以便产后能立即获得新生儿重症监护和小儿外科、麻醉科专科处理。

产后可通过体格检查中的临床发现、AFP 和 β-HCG 水平以及许多放射影像学检查来确定诊断。90%的骶尾部畸胎瘤在出生时可发现尾骨区域有一凸出肿块。虽然不常见，但这些肿瘤很容易认出，通常仅通过体格检查就能做出可靠的诊断。骶前肿块可通过直肠指检进行诊断。出生时发现的骶尾部畸胎瘤大多数呈良性，许多患儿没有功能性症状。

骶前病灶可有产后迟发性的症状[3,53,155]，典型的可在新生儿期和 4 个月至 4 岁间发现。与新生儿外露的骶尾部畸胎瘤相比，这些肿瘤位于盆腔，没有外露部分。超过 1/3 的病例可伴有恶性成分。临床表现可包括便秘、肛门狭窄、肿瘤压迫膀胱或直肠引起的相关症状和可触及的肿块。骶前肿瘤可伴有骶骨缺损、肛直肠畸形（Currarino's triad）（图 34-7）。

561 骨盆 X 线检查能识别各种骶骨缺陷或肿瘤钙化。CT 增强扫描和直肠造影能确定盆腔内肿瘤的范围，辨别各种结节或远处转移，确定可能存在的尿路压迫移位或梗阻。CT 也能辨认肝脏转移灶和主动脉周围的淋巴结增大。当怀疑脊椎浸润或者诊断可疑时应用磁共振检查（MRI）是有效的。胸部 X 线检查可用于明显的肺转移，而胸部 CT 在辨认小的转移病灶时更为可靠，当有高度怀疑时应做 CT 检查。

恶性肿瘤的发生率与诊断时的年龄有关[3]，出生时发现的骶尾部畸胎瘤约 8%为恶性。出生 2个月后恶性发生率迅速上升。到 6 个月时，骶尾部畸胎瘤的恶性率为 40%～80%，最常见的恶性类型是卵黄囊瘤。由于骶前畸胎瘤（Ⅳ型）常在较大年龄时获得诊断，其恶性率上升。

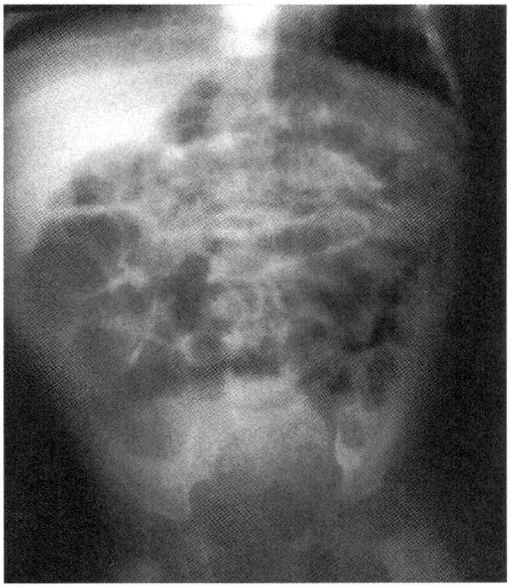

图 34-7 患有 Currarino 三联症的女婴 9 个月腹部 X 片，见到一盆腔肿块，肠管向头偏移，也能显现一半月形骶骨。

手术治疗

对新生儿骶尾部畸胎瘤的治疗选择是肿瘤完全手术切除。除了肿瘤破裂或出血严重影响新生儿血流动力学需急诊手术外，手术干预可在新生儿早期选择性进行。肿瘤的解剖位置决定手术途径。盆腔内大范围延伸或腹腔部分为主体的肿瘤（Ⅲ型或Ⅳ型）开始就需经腹途径。大多数Ⅰ型和Ⅱ型肿瘤骶后途径足以处理（图 34-8）。

手术的目的包括：（1）肿瘤完全和迅速地切除；（2）切除尾骨以防肿瘤复发；（3）控制肛直肠的肌肉重建；（4）恢复会阴部和臀部外观[6,51]。手术过度延迟可导致严重并发症，包括压迫坏死、肿瘤出血和恶性变。

对于一些虚弱的新生儿，为了安全切除肿瘤，需要首先控制骶中和髂内动脉。手术应在在环境温度控制下施行，新生儿要适时地测量体温，防止热量丢失。留置导尿管，一般手术时患者取俯卧臀高位，垫一消
562 毒的海绵环（见图 34-8A）。在皮肤准备和消毒后，沿肿瘤上缘做一眉形或倒“V”形切口（见图 34-8B）。这一切口可提供很好的暴露并在关闭伤口时距肛门开口有一些距离。为了发现直肠，术者可用手指或 Hegar 扩张器插入肛门 3cm。将皮瓣从肿瘤翻起后，仔细辨认和保护已被削弱的直肠后肌肉。紧贴囊壁游离肿瘤，电灼和缝扎血管止血是安全的。为防止热量丢失，用温纱布覆盖暴露的创面和肿瘤。肿瘤的主要血供通常来自于骶中动脉或髂内动脉分支。将尾骨从骶骨切除后，可见到从骶前间隙腹侧发出到尾骨的血管（见图 34-8C）。肿瘤特别大的病例或瘤体内血液潴留由于可使大量体液转移或出血，可导致术中死亡，外科医生偶尔可以使用体外人工膜式氧合（ECMO）并结合降低体温和降低灌注在术中更好地控制出血[116]。

因为不切除尾骨术后复发率高达 37%[70]，所以需将与肿瘤相连的尾骨切除。将肿瘤从直肠壁游离，并做肛直肠肌重建（见图 34-8D 和 E）。肛提肌向上牵拉，为直肠提供支持并使肛门保持在正常位置。在皮瓣下可放置一负压引流管。伤口用间断可吸收线做分层关闭（见图 34-8F）。留置导尿管数天。保持伤口清洁，术后几天患者保持俯卧位。

对伴有巨大畸胎瘤的早产新生儿的处理具有挑战性。由于肺未成熟，肿瘤血管丰富，失血耐受性差，手术风险高[154]。为避免血液大量丢失，对这些患者可

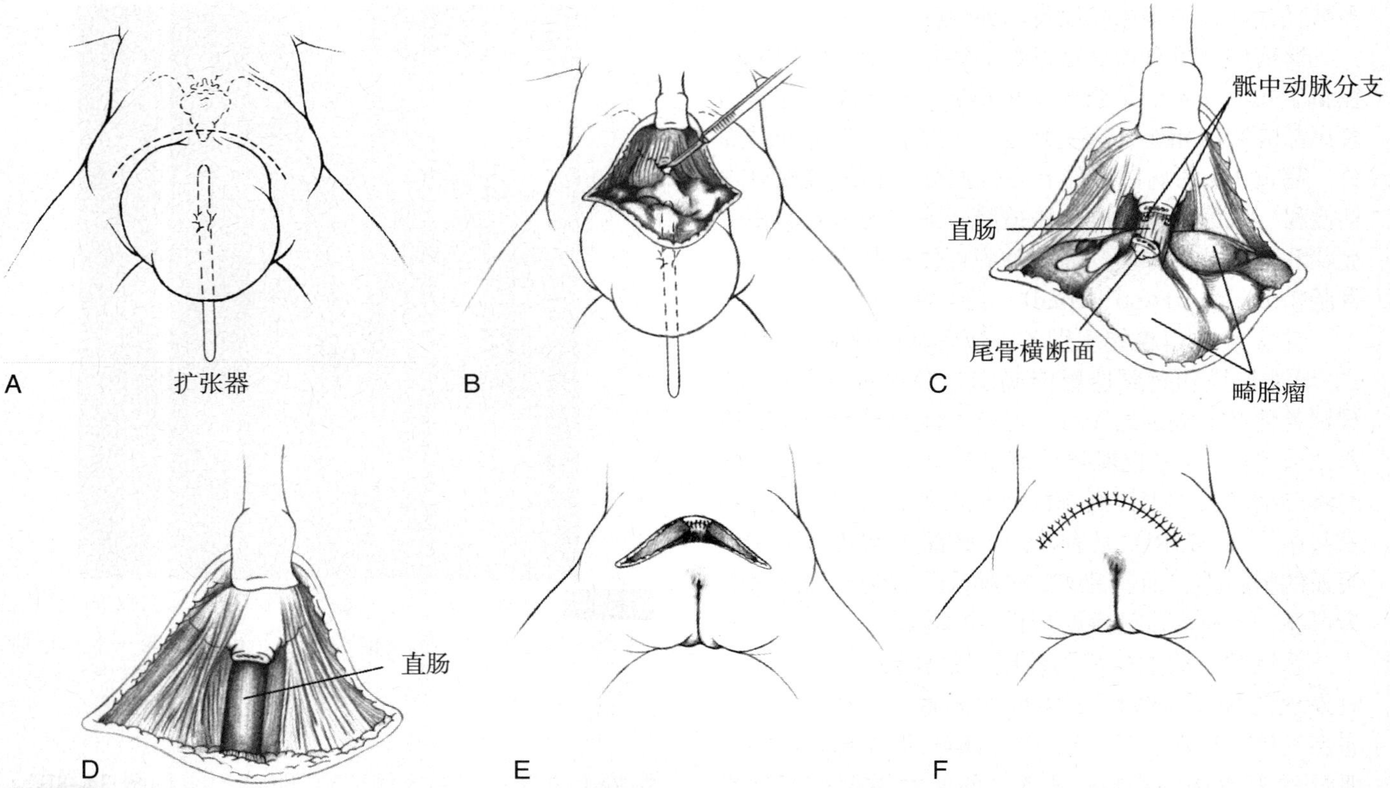

图 34-8 骶尾部畸胎瘤的手术治疗。A. 婴儿前倾体位，有助于将 Hegar 扩张器部分插入直肠，也便于在肿瘤切除过程中辨认直肠。B. 一“眉形”或倒“V”形后切口，便于接近被分离的肿瘤和尾骨。C. 分离尾骨后的骶中血管，一旦这些血管被结扎和分离，肿瘤即能从直肠上游离并与臀肌和肛提肌分离。D. 肿瘤已经被切除，能见到直肠后缘和盆腔肌肉。E. 将肛直肠肌做解剖上重建。F. 最后关闭切口。

考虑血流阻断和分期切除。胎儿巨大骶尾部畸胎瘤在处理上具有更大的挑战性。如前所述，胎儿水肿和巨大胎盘常可导致胎儿死亡。

肿瘤切除术最严重的并发症是术中出血，死亡的主要原因是出血性休克。为了稳定肿瘤血流丰富和明显出血的患者，可用一弹力绑带绕畸胎瘤包扎作为术前处理。为了抢救危及生命的急性大出血，Teitelbaum 等人[177]报告施行紧急剖腹探查，并临时钳夹远端腹主动脉。

与任何一种外科手术类同，可出现伤口并发症。明显向盆腔和腹腔内伸展的畸胎瘤切除后可伴发临时或持久的术后尿潴留，但这些症状一般会缓解。虽然，肿瘤较小的患者都有正常的肛直肠节制，但 30%～40%的巨大骶尾部畸胎瘤早产婴儿其肛提肌和臀部肌肉被严重削弱，有排便失禁。长期的肠道处理策略使大多数患者能达到被社会接受的肠道功能。

长期结局

过去几十年的研究表明，诊断时的年龄是骶尾部畸胎瘤主要的预后因素。妊娠 30 周后诊断出的骶尾部畸胎瘤胎儿比更早期被发现的畸胎瘤胎儿倾向于有更好的预后[54,104,157]。出生 2 个月后做出诊断或 4 个月后进行肿瘤切除的患儿，其恶性率是 5%～10%[44,189]。另外，囊性肿瘤一般来说是成熟的肿瘤，预后较好。涉及出血、肿瘤窃血和恶变的并发症在实体瘤患者中更常见。

新生儿骶尾部畸胎瘤的长期预后总的来说很好。小儿肿瘤组织–儿童癌症组织的研究报告：未成熟畸胎瘤甚至当显微镜下发现卵黄囊瘤成分时，仅做肿瘤完全切除，生存率达 100%，其中 80%可达治愈[120]。然而，因为所有的骶尾部畸胎瘤都具有局部或远处复发风险，必须进行 3～4 年每隔 3 个月 1 次的随访。

根据 Rescorla 等人[150]报道，一儿童癌症组织的研究提到成熟畸胎瘤的肿瘤复发率为 11%，未成熟畸胎瘤的复发率为 4%。尽管这些复发中 43%～50%是恶性的，由于卵黄囊瘤（内胚窦瘤）对化疗敏感，其有较高的生存率。应监测血清 AFP 指标并做体检。特别注意应进行直肠指检，这样可及时发现骶尾部肿瘤复发。当 APF 水平没有出现应有的下降时，应做腹部超声检查。当有怀疑时，做盆腔 CT 或 MIR 和肺部 CT 检查。复发性肿瘤可以是良性的，但应做再次手术切除以减少恶性转移的长期风险。

辅助治疗

发现恶性成分后要进行多种药物辅助化疗。最有效的抗肿瘤药物包括顺铂、鬼臼乙叉甙、博莱霉素。目前的报告显示，在有局部浸润和转移灶的患者中采用强化疗后生存率会有很大提高[63,64,149]，甚至在骶尾部畸胎瘤恶性变后。Misra 等人[128]报告：局限性病变的生存率为 88%，有远处转移的生存率为 75%。此外，以顺铂为主治疗患儿时似乎对分期、转移的程度和侵及骨骼没有预后意义[29]。

对原发性恶性肿瘤不能切除的患者，给予联合化疗以便于后期肿瘤切除。如果血清 APF 水平下降和 CT、胸部 X 片检查提示肿瘤对化疗反应好，在几个
563 疗程的化疗后进行切除手术。

对局部恶性肿瘤复发的患者，完全切除病灶仍是治疗的主要手段，并辅以联合化疗。化疗对治疗有肺和肝脏转移灶的病例也是有效的。然而，为了确保消除所有恶性成分，必须清除残留灶。虽然在选择性患者中不常用放疗，但放疗对控制未能完全切除的病灶复发有一定作用。

头颈部畸胎瘤

头颈部畸胎瘤占所有新生儿畸胎瘤的 5%。这些少见的肿瘤可发生在脑内、眼眶、口咽、鼻咽或颈部。

颅内畸胎瘤

颅内畸胎瘤（在第 41 章进行详细描述）有两个高峰年龄，占婴儿早期所有脑肿瘤的比例近 50%，并在 12～16 岁青少年中有一发病高峰。新生儿颅内畸胎瘤发病在性别之间没有区别；但在大龄儿童中，颅内畸胎瘤在男性中更为多见（男∶女= 2∶1）。虽然畸胎瘤在视丘下部、脑室、蝶鞍上和小脑区域也有发现，但松果体是最常见的发生部位。在新生儿发生的颅内畸胎瘤一般是良性的，而在大龄儿童和十几岁的患儿中见到的则几乎都是恶性的。所有的组织类型都能见到，但颅内畸胎瘤大致可被分成两类：近 50%为生殖细胞瘤，余下的为非生殖细胞瘤。然而，在许多病例中，肿瘤可显示为混合性组织类型。在婴儿中，最常见的表现是阻塞性脑积水引起的颅内压力增高。年长儿童和青少年表现为严重的头痛、癫痫样发作、嗜睡、视物模糊及呕吐。患有能产生 β-HCG 的肿瘤的男孩出现青春期性早熟。

颅骨 X 片、头颅 CT 或 MRI 显示中线或幕上近轴线存在病灶并常有钙化可支持诊断。治疗选择手术切除肿瘤，但许多新生儿颅内畸胎瘤无法切除。减压分流对于减轻颅内压力和减轻脑积水在短期内有明显疗效，但对恶性畸胎瘤患者并不一定延长生存期。此外，在一些婴儿中，分流可导致肿瘤颅外播散。

化疗和放疗已被组合成目前的治疗方案。用放疗治疗儿童生殖细胞瘤已产生很好的 5 年生存率，为 80%～90%[13,76,156]。然而，在非生殖细胞性胚芽细胞瘤患者中，手术和放疗效果均不佳，5 年生存率为 0～33%[76,141]。针对这些患者的化疗还没有很好地建立，这已成为目前的研究重点，以努力降低放疗伴发的长期并发症，尤其是在小年龄儿童。另外，化疗和放疗也用于治疗不同特征的晚期患者[11,12,127]。一些作者认为，将化疗加入儿童生殖细胞瘤治疗方案中可能并不能提高已有的较高的生存率，但可通过减少照射面和放射量或在低龄儿童中延迟放射治疗来减少放射导致的损害[13,76,156]。进一步理想的处理生殖细胞瘤的方案应是：结合小剂量和小范围的照射和较少侵袭性的化疗。作为对照，高风险的非生殖细胞性胚芽细胞瘤患者可从更具侵袭性的方案中获得疗效提高，包括大剂量化疗、放疗和手术。鉴于颅内畸胎瘤的少见性和治疗相关的副作用，通过前瞻性随机研究来取得证据是一个长期目标。

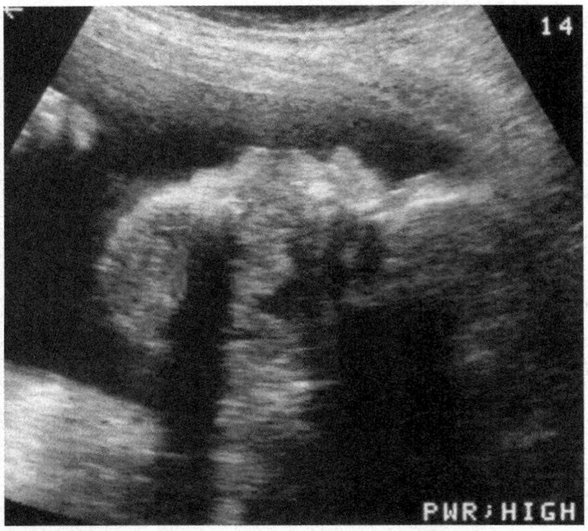

图 34-9 产前超声显示一大的颈部畸胎瘤。

颈面部畸胎瘤

颈面部畸胎瘤是极少见的肿瘤。虽然这些肿瘤大多数在组织学上呈良性，但肿瘤常常在围生期引起显著的气道和食管梗阻，因此，有潜在的致命性。肿瘤原发部位可包括舌部、鼻咽部、上腭、窦部、下颌部、扁桃体、前颈部和甲状腺。如同骶尾部畸胎瘤，颈面部畸胎瘤在发生上以先天性为主，男女发生率相当。

产前超声检查对发现这些子宫内病灶是一种可靠的手段，产前获诊的病例可被仔细地安排分娩的时间、方式和地点。当产前超声检查发现一大的颈
564 部不规则的有囊实性成分的肿块时常提示为畸胎瘤（图 34-9）[72]。为了更清楚地显示解剖结构，可选择胎儿 MRI 做诊断性检查。在产前发现的病例中，淋巴管畸形（囊性水瘤）最容易与颈部畸胎瘤相混淆。其肿块大小、超声检查特点、临床特征、部位、发现时的妊娠年龄都与畸胎瘤相似，使其区别非常困难[16]。在鉴别诊断中要考虑的其他病变包括大的鳃裂囊肿和先天性甲状腺肿大。因伴有血清 AFP 升高的颈部畸胎瘤病例不到 30%，因此，血清 AFP 水平在胎儿颈部肿块的鉴别诊断中没有特殊的帮助[21]。近 1/3 的产前获得诊断的病例伴有羊水过多，羊水过多被认为是由于食管梗阻或胎儿吞咽受影响所致。因羊水过多和肿瘤导致子宫增大，可继发早产，因此这类患儿有较高的早产发生率。

颈部畸胎瘤通常体积较大，直径常在 5～12cm（图 34-10）[16,167]。有肿瘤大于胎儿头部的报道[16,95,140]。肿瘤可累及口底、突入口腔（上颌寄生胎），并可延伸入上纵隔[95]。巨大的病灶可引起难产，需剖宫产分娩患儿。有各种不同的畸形伴发颈部畸胎瘤的报告。这些畸形包括颅面部和中枢神经系统异常[8]、左心室发育不全、13 三体，并有软骨营养障碍和肛门闭锁各 1 例报告。也已见到因在下颌骨发育中受到肿瘤影响直接导致下颌骨发育不良[21]。

高达 50%的颈部畸胎瘤含有钙化灶[72,100]，常在产后 X 线平片中很清晰的见到[74,172]。当钙化出现在部分囊性和部分实性的颈部肿块时，颈部畸胎瘤的诊断已能成立[72]。在描述肿瘤的解剖范围和精确浸润程度时，产后患儿 CT 特别有用。

如 Azizkhan 等人[8]所提出的，出生时气道梗阻可危及生命，伴有很高的死亡率。一些产前获得诊断的胎儿巨大颈部肿瘤患儿在出生后通常开放气道延迟，不能有效通气。延迟通气可导致组织缺氧和酸中毒，气道开放延迟超过 5 分钟能导致缺氧性损害。鉴于这些问题，大多数颈面部畸胎瘤在分娩后需做决定性的处理，分娩应在具有包括小儿外科医生在内的围生期专家队伍的特殊的监护中心。理想的是，如果做剖宫产，母体-胎儿的胎盘血循环应当保持到新生儿获得可靠的通气。可通过腹部同一切口完成（不包括分娩期子宫的处理），以便有时间完成一些必要的操作，如直接的喉部检查、支气管检查、气管切开、表面活化剂的应用和囊肿减压这些对于保证气道通畅可能需要的操作[21]。由于肿瘤内出血可发生紧急气道梗阻[16,72,89]，不管出现或未出现症状，所有病例都有气管插管的指征。

在有些病例[110,179]，新生儿在出生后几小时或几天内发生急性气道梗阻或失去了原先通畅的气道。生命体征稳定后早期肿瘤切除是获得整个气道控制的最有效的方法，因此是治疗的首选。延迟手术可发生其他衍生出来的严重问题，包括分泌物潴留、肺膨胀不全或吞咽受影响而引起吸入性肺炎[16,65]。肿瘤切除也排除了肿瘤恶化的风险，在没有获得诊断或直到青少年后期或成人才治疗的颈部畸胎瘤病例中，恶性病变的发生率相当高（＞90%）[27]。

为了减少手术并发症，肿瘤的解剖应远离重要的神经部位。颈部畸胎瘤常有一假性包膜，可使肿瘤较为容易的被提出颈部。如果肿瘤来自甲状腺，将畸胎瘤连同受累的一叶甲状腺一起切除。任何肿大的淋巴

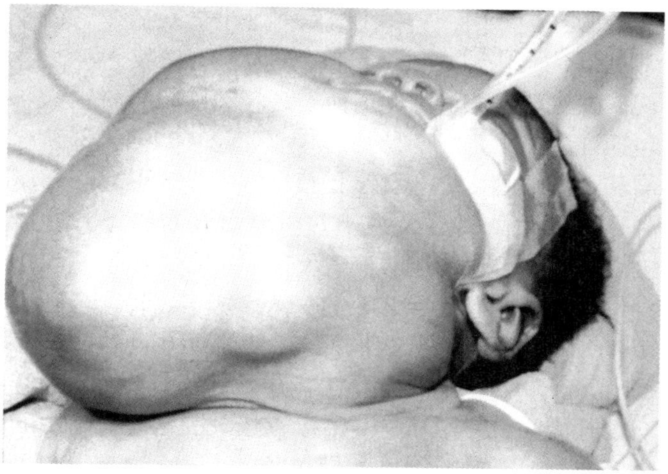

图 34–10 一位 34 周早产患儿的巨大颈部畸胎瘤，该患儿在出生时有明显气道梗阻，在产房内成功进行了气管插管。

结应与肿瘤一起切除，因为可发生神经胶质转移。肿瘤切除后，留置引流管 24～48 小时。因为这些肿瘤通常较大，包绕重要的颈部解剖结构是常见的。在一些病例中，只有通过分期手术才能将肿瘤完全切除并得到可以接受的功能和美容效果[8]。

与成人肿瘤恶变的发生率（>60%）相比，新生儿恶性颈面部畸胎瘤伴转移的相对少见。Azizkhan 等人[8]报告的发生率为 20%。尽管在原发性肿瘤中存在很难区分或无法区分的组织，但许多婴儿在颈部畸胎瘤完全切除后的随访中并没有复发。这些病例提示在这一人群中，肿瘤的恶性生物学行为是不常见的[16,45,72]。报告显示许多组织学类型相一致[8]。神经外胚层成分和未成熟的神经组织是转移灶中最常见的组织。在接近 1/3 的病例中，需要进一步区分的转移灶被证实为局部结节。有孤立性局部转移性结节的患者手术切除原发肿瘤后一般可无瘤生存。这也支持了这样一种概念，即出现的转移灶仅包含可以鉴别的肿瘤常常与好的预后相关。

目前，对于新生儿恶性颈部畸胎瘤还没有统一的化疗方案。然而，根据一项病例研究的结果，Azizkhan 等人[8]推荐对有播散性病灶的（没有鉴别过）新生儿和具有浸润性肿瘤以及术后有残留病灶的病例保留化疗方式。

虽然颈部畸胎瘤一般为良性肿瘤，但有恶性转化的可能性，需要对肿瘤的复发做密切监测。在婴儿期，应对血清 AFP 每 3 个月做一次监测，随后再每年复查一次。如 AFP 升高，提示临床医生注意有肿瘤复发的可能性。正如本章前面讨论的，对血清 AFP 水平的升高需要谨慎分析，要注意到其自然的半衰期。建议作为监测项目，影像学检查每年 2 次，连续 3 年。因在肿瘤切除中可能切除或影响到甲状腺或甲状旁腺，必须考虑到一过性的或永久性的甲状腺功能低下风险[8]。如果发生，必须对这些并发症进行监测并做适当的处理。

纵隔畸胎瘤

纵隔畸胎瘤约占所有儿童纵隔肿瘤的 20%，在性腺外畸胎瘤中列为第二常见部位，男女发生率相近。虽然不常见，但其他各种组织类型的恶性纵隔胚芽细胞肿瘤也有发生。纵隔畸胎瘤常常发生在前纵隔，但也可在心包内或心脏见到，偶尔也可发生在后纵隔。少于 50%的儿童纵隔畸胎瘤发生在新生儿期。虽然，青年和少年患者常没有症状，但婴儿和儿童常有因肺或气管受压引起的症状，从急性呼吸窘迫到慢性咳嗽、胸痛或喘息。前纵隔和心包肿瘤可伴发上腔静脉综合征。一些含有分泌 β–HCG 的肿瘤成分的良性或恶性纵隔畸胎瘤男性患儿可出现青春期性早熟。因这些肿瘤可伴有 Klinefeiter 综合征，应做染色体组型分析。

已有 30 多例病例在产前获得诊断。可伴有羊水过多、胎儿水肿和其他许多严重情况影响胎儿的后果。虽然有 2 例尝试未能成功，但在选择性患者中做开放性胎儿外科手术可能有效果。产后胸部 X 片检查可提示一纵隔肿块；在近 1/3 的病例中，肿块有钙化。胸部超声检查可显示有一囊性和实性成分的肿块，并有助于判断肿块来自于纵隔还是来自于心包和心脏。CT 常能显示肿瘤的范围和肿瘤与周围解剖结构的关系。鉴别诊断包括胸腺瘤、胸腺囊肿、淋巴管畸形、纵隔非 Hodgkin 淋巴瘤、食管重复畸形和支气管源性囊肿。当有怀疑指征时，可做骨扫描以发现骨转移。血清 AFP、β–HCG、LDH 和 PLAP 水平可升高[52]。

在儿童年龄组，已有报告总的恶性率为 15%的报道[40]。许多研究已显示，在新生儿和婴儿期切除的成熟和未成熟畸胎瘤具有良好的生物学行为[31,107,176]，这一年龄组已显示较青少年和成人有更好的预后。

不管是良性还是恶性，手术完全切除肿瘤是治疗首选。因为前纵隔肿块常压迫气道，麻醉处理比较关键。静脉应用肌松剂后一旦自主呼吸消失，患者可失去呼吸能力，应及时做气管内插管。胸骨切开或开胸能提供很好的手术暴露。应小心避免损伤膈神经。

在低年龄儿童中，接近20%的纵隔肿瘤的组织学研究提示有未成熟细胞成分。虽然在这些儿童中，未成熟成分几乎并不增加恶变的风险，但在少年及青年成人中，未成熟组织出现因为进展性肿瘤伴有较高的死亡率。因此，这些患者应给予辅助化疗。在已侵及重要结构的恶性肿瘤病例，如肿瘤切除已不可能，则需要化疗使畸胎瘤缩小以便于后期手术切除。因恶性肿瘤的治疗不仅仅依靠手术切除，所有的患者都需要术后辅助化疗来预防肿瘤复发和进展。

虽然，多药联合化疗的效果不像在骶尾部病灶那样突出，但还是相当不错。在最近的一组病例中[22]，36例经活检后给予化疗的病例中，18例随后肿瘤被切除。6例肿瘤大小不变或增大，12例肿瘤平均缩小57%。儿童应用以鬼臼乙叉甙、博莱霉素和顺铂为主的化疗总的4年生存率为71%；无瘤生存率为69%。作者认为，15岁以上的男孩因肿瘤的侵袭性导致的较高死亡率，他们是一高危人群。

心脏畸胎瘤

虽然心脏畸胎瘤可来自于心脏，但非常罕见，并几乎仅发生在女孩。典型的心脏畸胎瘤表现为充血性
566 心衰的症状和体征，右侧心脏受限。通过心脏超声发现多囊性心内肿块可以怀疑该诊断。心电图可出现心律失常和心室内阻滞。常能见到伴发的先天性心脏病，如房间隔缺损和室间隔缺损。为了避免发生完全性输出阻塞或致命的心律失常，需要及时切除肿瘤。恶性畸胎瘤（25%）需要给予化疗。对于良性肿瘤患者，可切除心脏畸胎瘤，心脏移植提供了一种可行的治疗选择。

腹膜后畸胎瘤

腹膜后是性腺外畸胎瘤第三个好发部位，占所有畸胎瘤的5%[118]。多数肿瘤在婴儿早期被发现，50%的病例在1岁内，75%在5岁前发生。女孩较男孩更常见（2∶1）。患者常常出现一大的可触及的腹部肿块，肿块可因压迫消化道而出现相关症状。鉴别诊断包括许多在儿童早期见到的其他肿瘤（如神经母细胞瘤和肾母细胞瘤）和囊性腹膜后淋巴管畸形、网膜囊肿、寄生胎。腹部X线平片可显示肠管移位和肿瘤内钙化。当出现钙化时，其形态较特殊，需注意与在神经母细胞瘤中见到的散在点状钙化区别，腹部CT或MRI有助于区别这种肿瘤和其他更常见的儿童肿瘤。

开腹完全肿瘤切除是治疗首选。因这些肿瘤中的大多数为良性肿瘤，手术常能获得成功。在诊断时，接近20%的腹膜后畸胎瘤是恶性肿瘤，30%～40%可以有未成熟组织。偶尔，可见到良性神经胶质种植，表明这些转移灶的一个成熟过程。因为有报道在含有未成熟成分的良性畸胎瘤患者中出现恶性复发，对恶性肿瘤和含有高度未成熟成分的患者应给予术后化疗[155]。

其他少见的性腺外畸胎瘤

胃畸胎瘤

胃畸胎瘤极其少见，这些肿瘤可出现一可触及的上腹部肿块和胃排出梗阻症状或在婴儿期出现上消化道出血。肿瘤通常较大，并常呈多囊性。腹部X线平片常显示有钙化灶。上消化道造影可明确胃和肿瘤的关系。胃镜检查可显示一外来的肿块压迫胃腔或肿瘤侵蚀胃壁的证据。组织学检查显示这些病变由成熟组织组成，常包含有未成熟的神经胶质成分。治疗首选手术切除肿瘤。畸胎瘤的预后通常良好[47,91,162]。

阴道畸胎瘤

这些少见的肿瘤发生在1岁内，常出现在新生儿期。检查可显示容易看到的来自于阴道肿瘤的少量出血。多数肿瘤为卵黄囊瘤。胸部X线片可以排除肺转移，CT可描述肿瘤的范围。如果肿瘤局限，治疗包括手术肿瘤切除和低剂量的多药联合化疗。手术时应将肿瘤原发部位的部分阴道一起切除。如侵及子宫，需做子宫切除，先期辅助化疗可减少需要切除的范围[164]。

性腺畸胎瘤

卵巢畸胎瘤

畸胎瘤是最常见的儿童卵巢肿瘤，超过所有儿童卵巢肿瘤的 50%并占总的儿童畸胎瘤的 25%。多数卵巢畸胎瘤发生在 5～16 岁，2～3 岁以内不常见。疼痛是最常出现的症状，可在超过 50%的患者中见到。25%的患者中因肿瘤扭转发生急腹痛。因多数肿瘤较大（10～15cm），患儿的另一常见表现为腹部出现一无症状的肿块。在近一半的病例中，腹部 X 片中可在腹腔和盆腔内见到类似于牙齿的钙化灶。左右侧卵巢发生肿瘤的概率相同，5%～10%的病例出现双侧卵巢畸胎瘤。虽然盆腹腔超声显示肿瘤由囊性和实质性成分组成，并有对侧正常卵巢结构，对于术前分期，CT 是理想的影像学检查。应测定血清 AFP 和 HCG 水平。如果升高，提示肿瘤有恶性可能。

对于有完整包膜并在组织学检查中为成熟成分的良性肿瘤，单纯卵巢切除或输卵管-卵巢切除是治疗的首选。在手术时，应收集所有腹水做细胞学分析。如果没有腹水，可通过腹腔灌洗来获得并对存在的肿瘤细胞做评估。检查所有的腹膜表面，包括膈面有无肿瘤种植。如果见到腹膜肿瘤种植，应取得活检标本。如果大网膜有肉眼肿瘤，应沿结肠下方做大网膜切除。一些外科医生已经提倡对良性囊性卵巢畸胎瘤做保留卵巢的肿瘤切除。但长期随访资料有限，这一手术仍有争议[135]。

有卵巢外腹膜浸润的未成熟卵巢畸胎瘤的处理较复杂。幸运的是，多数患者为成熟的神经胶质种植。他们不需要化疗并有很好的预后[155]。组织学分级较高的肿瘤（Ⅱ级和Ⅲ级）有恶变的风险，需要辅助多药联合化疗。采用目前的化疗方案治疗已取得接近 90%的生存率[97]（更详细的讨论参考第 36 章）。

睾丸畸胎瘤

睾丸畸胎瘤是儿童最常见的睾丸肿瘤。肿瘤有两个高发年龄段，小于 2 岁的婴儿和十几岁的青少年和青年最常受到影响。婴儿通常出现无痛性阴囊肿块。15%的患者也可出现阴囊积水。获取术前血清 AFP 和 HCG 水平。胸部 X 线检查和腹部 CT 扫描可评估有无淋巴结和内脏转移。

通过肿瘤的可切除性和是否出现淋巴结和远处转移来进行肿瘤分期。Ⅰ期（占 80%）治疗由经腹股沟做根治性睾丸切除，包括至内环口的精索切除。婴儿Ⅰ期病例仅做根治性睾丸切除 5 年生存率超过 90%。

多数恶性肿瘤为卵黄囊瘤，很少转移到腹膜后淋巴结。因此，对于小于 2 岁的Ⅰ期肿瘤，术前腹部 CT 正常的婴儿不需做后腹膜淋巴结清扫。如果升高的血清肿瘤标志物术后不能恢复到正常（20%的病例），应做重新分期，随后做腹膜后淋巴结清扫和应用辅助化疗。通常做单侧腹膜后淋巴结切除，使用神经保护技术来防止精液倒射。对可疑的对侧淋巴结应做活检。淋巴结切除后的复发率是 10%～15%，转移复发常出现在肺部或纵隔。多数肿瘤转移的患者通过联合化疗取得疗效（进一步的详细讨论见第 37 章）。

卵黄囊瘤

卵黄囊瘤是从婴儿到青少年影响儿童的最常见的恶性胚芽细胞肿瘤。在新生儿和低龄儿童中，发现这些肿瘤主要位于性腺外部位，尤其是骶尾部区域。然而其在婴儿和低龄男孩的睾丸中也较常见[196]。卵黄囊瘤是累及睾丸的主要儿童恶性胚芽细胞肿瘤。在年长儿童和青少年中，卵巢是最常见的发病部位。其次的原发部位包括纵隔、腹膜后、松果体区域和阴道。在青少年中，这些肿瘤很少在性腺外以单纯卵黄囊瘤的形式出现，但能见到作为混合性恶性胚芽细胞肿瘤的一种组成成分出现[42,49]。儿童卵黄囊瘤与成人同类肿瘤在细胞遗传学和生物学上截然不同。检查儿童肿瘤组织显示有 1 号染色体短臂（1p）和 6 号染色体长臂（6q）缺失，但没有在成人胚芽细胞肿瘤中见到的 i（12p）缺失的证据[143]。

大体标本上，卵黄囊瘤呈灰白色到黄色，组织脆弱易碎，囊肿的中央有黏液样组织和坏死[36,73]。一个相对新的可信的理论提出，这些肿瘤源自于原始卵黄囊[136]——胚胎中早期形成的结构。卵黄囊有多种潜能，可分化成原肠和其衍生组织，包括肝脏。因此，导致多样的组织学类型。假乳头状（花菜样）和微囊型（网状型）是最常见的并被广泛认识的类型。二者常显示涉及内胚窦结构的血管周围细胞鞘或 Schiller-Duval 体。多数容易区别的卵黄囊瘤也含有细胞内和细胞外玻璃质样沉淀，后者能对抗周期性酸性 Schiff

淀粉酵素染色并对AFP呈阳性。然而，微囊型很难区别，其常与嗜曙红细胞小球相关，AFP阳性染色很少，难于区别。然而，内胚窦瘤更多呈实质性，并很难与胚胎癌区别。一些肿瘤可呈肝脏型，类似于胎儿肝细胞[73]。组织学形态的变化并不与预后相关，多药联合化疗被认为具有疗效。然而，儿童肿瘤研究（1971—1984年）提供的证据表明[79]，新生儿骶尾部畸胎瘤可以像卵黄囊瘤一样复发，由于肿瘤的浸润性质，卵黄囊瘤预后较差。

胚胎癌

虽然比卵黄囊瘤少得多，但胚胎癌也可发生在1岁内的患儿。在儿童中，它极少以单纯胚胎癌形式出现；更常见的是混合性胚芽细胞肿瘤中的一种组成成分。其主要的组织类型是伴有不同数量中心坏死的大的细胞巢组成的上皮。然而，假小管型和乳突状型常可与卵黄囊瘤混淆。细胞呈AFP阴性，肿瘤一般缺乏有些卵黄囊瘤的特征性嗜酸细胞透明小球。与其他胚芽细胞肿瘤，胚胎癌在免疫组织化疗染色中细胞角蛋白呈阳性[36]。

生殖细胞瘤

生殖细胞瘤一词目前用于涉及一组具有共同组织学特征的肿瘤。以前如果病灶发生在睾丸称为精原细胞瘤，发生在卵巢称为无性细胞瘤，在性腺外部位称为生殖细胞瘤。这些肿瘤被认为来源于在性腺发育的未分化阶段。肿瘤常出现在卵巢、前纵隔和松果体区域，是儿童中在卵巢和中枢神经系统最常见的单一恶性胚芽细胞肿瘤[49,175]。儿童中，生殖细胞瘤占所有卵巢肿瘤的10%，占全身各部位胚芽细胞肿瘤的比例近15%。这些肿瘤很少在婴幼儿中见到，最常发生在青春期女孩和年轻妇女，44%的病例发生在20岁前[73]。生殖细胞瘤是出现在发育不良的性腺和下降不全的睾
568 丸中的主要恶性肿瘤。

在大体检查中，生殖细胞瘤呈实质性，有包膜，呈粉红色或棕褐色，偶尔有出血性小结节和坏死灶及呈橡胶样密度。肿瘤细胞排列成巢状，由纤维组织囊带分隔，伴有不同程度的淋巴细胞浸润。细胞增大，轻度嗜曙红细胞细胞质，细胞膜明显，细胞核大而圆并有1～2个分叶的核仁[36]。虽然可以出现有巨细胞和合滋养层的肉芽肿，但仅当绒癌病灶中伴有细胞滋养层时，它们才可改变肿瘤的预后。生殖细胞瘤细胞对胎盘碱性磷酸酶（PLAP）呈强染色，而合滋养层对β-HCG染色。正如Scully等人[161]提到的，生殖细胞瘤也对波形蛋白有免疫反应。在有些病例中，乳酸脱氢酶（LDH）、特殊神经烯醇酶、Leu-7、细胞角蛋白、肌间线蛋白和神经胶质原纤维酸蛋白呈阳性。在一项研究中[183]，在92%的生殖细胞瘤中发现c-kit定位。

绒癌

绒癌是一种罕见的高度恶性肿瘤，主要在女性患者见到。典型的肿瘤作为一恶性混合性胚芽细胞肿瘤的一种成分发生。如同卵黄囊瘤和胚胎癌，这一肿瘤能发生在1岁内患儿，可以作为继发于胎盘绒癌的转移灶[33,37]，也可作为一来源于不同部位的原发性肿瘤，如肝脏、肺、脑、肾或上颌骨[101,166]，最常见的部位是松果腺部位[56,166]。肿瘤出现于青春期前和少年阶段，主要发生在性腺，少数在纵隔。在小婴儿，单纯性绒癌几乎总是表现为来自母体或胎盘妊娠期滋养层肿瘤的播散转移[19,55]。

在大体检查中，单纯绒癌的特点为实质性、出血灶和脆弱易碎。镜下检查呈现细胞滋养层和合体滋养层。细胞滋养层典型地表现为紧密堆积相对一致的中等大小的细胞巢，细胞质清晰、细胞边界清楚并有小泡的细胞核，而合体滋养层表现为巨大的多核合体滋养层细胞[36]。两种细胞类型都对细胞角蛋白有典型的免疫反应。合体滋养层细胞也对HCG、人胎盘催乳素和妊娠期特殊β_1-糖蛋白有免疫反应。另外，在一些肿瘤中见到对PLAP、上皮膜抗原、神经特殊烯醇酶、α_1-胰岛素拮抗剂和癌抗原均有免疫反应[161]。

多胚瘤

多胚瘤是一种极其少见的卵巢恶性肿瘤。在过去40多年中报道不到10例[161]。据报道，其常与其他肿

瘤成分结合在一起[18,102]。典型的患者为儿童或年轻妇女，相关的临床症状和体征提示出现一大的盆腔肿块。极个别的患者在表达中有相关卵巢外肿瘤播散的症状[182]。肿瘤的组织学表现特点是以胚胎结构为主，这些结构类似于在不同发育阶段的正常早期胚胎。由卵黄囊、胚芽、肝脏成分和绒毛膜成分（如合体滋养层的巨大细胞）组成。成熟和未成熟的畸胎瘤成分、以内胚层来源的为主的结构也常常出现[161]。在许多病例中，已注意到有血清 AFP 和 β-HCG 水平升高。在组织学上，卵黄囊和肝脏成分对 AFP 和 α_1-胰岛素拮抗剂有免疫反应。合体成分对 HCG 有免疫反应[102,133,147,173]。

性腺胚细胞瘤

性腺胚细胞瘤是一种相当罕见的肿瘤，由胚芽细胞与基质细胞混合组成[139,185,186]。它被认为是形成恶性胚芽细胞肿瘤的前期表现。性腺胚细胞瘤最常见于至少有一 Y 染色体片段的女性表型的发育不良的性腺中[181]。患者一般为年龄较大的青少年或三十几岁的成人，并从未有过月经史。她们可表现为第二性征缺乏，出现促性腺激素水平升高和条状性腺[50,139,190]。这些肿瘤通常相对较小，质地从软到硬不等，色泽呈灰茶色到褐色，稍呈分叶状。显微镜下特征包括胚芽细胞和性腺性索细胞增生。胚芽细胞对 PLAP 呈阳性[36]。

多数性腺胚细胞瘤呈良性肿瘤的表现形式，虽然 30%有恶性胚芽细胞成分过度生长的风险[185]。肿瘤可出现不同的恶性成分。其中，生殖细胞瘤最常见，在接近 50%的病例中出现[188,189]。由潜在的恶性成分确定了这些肿瘤的潜在恶性倾向。对于混合有性腺发育不全的年轻患者，建议做性腺切除术，因为残留的发育不良的性腺可增加发生性腺胚细胞瘤和生殖细胞瘤的机会，并且，可因残留的睾丸组织使女性男性化[152]。

混合性胚芽细胞瘤

胚芽细胞肿瘤常由两种或更多的组织类型组成。良性可能恶变的胚芽细胞肿瘤如未成熟畸胎瘤，可与真正的恶性胚芽细胞肿瘤共存。10%～40%的恶性肿瘤患者具有混合性的组织学表现[1,61,105,121]，这些患者中，40%在青春期前被诊断[105]。混合性胚芽细胞瘤最常见的组织成分是无性细胞瘤（生殖细胞瘤），虽然未成熟畸胎瘤、内胚窦瘤和胚胎癌也可在不同的部分发现[36]。同样，混合性胚芽细胞瘤占卵巢的恶性原发性胚芽细胞肿瘤的 8%～10%[105,159]。

面对这些肿瘤，仔细进行大体检查并谨慎地选择
肿瘤组织样本是重要的。混合性胚芽细胞肿瘤患者的 569
预后一般认为要根据肿瘤中恶性度最高的成分确定，但一些调查者已报道，如果高度恶性成分很少，没有肿瘤内占主要部分的成分对预后影响大[105]。

治疗上总的现状和前景

外科手术治疗的进步和包含使用铂在内的多药联合化疗方案已使儿童恶性胚芽细胞肿瘤的预后有了显著性的提高。使用整体多种模式治疗策略的国际性研究已将生存率大幅提高了 75%～90%[14,63,121,149,178,193]，这些研究中化疗方案有些不同。在美国针对儿童恶性性腺外胚芽细胞肿瘤的标准化化疗方案包括顺铂、鬼臼乙叉甙、博莱霉素（PEB）。然而，这一方案伴有较高的后期影响风险，尤其是顺铂的肾毒性和耳毒性[35,75]。有关这些副作用越来越大的影响已激励研究者在用长期毒副作用更小的方案来替代。在英国，用卡铂、鬼臼乙叉甙和博莱霉素（JEB）联合化疗已在小于 16 岁的患儿做临床研究。作者报告，与 PEB 方案相比，可获得无瘤生存且耳毒性和肾毒性更小[119]。因这些发现的确认，一份来自于美国的最近的前瞻性研究推断：卡铂能替代顺铂，但还没有提供对药物的反应和生存率，总的生存率和无瘤生存率分别是 91%和 87%[169]。作为对照，在成人组研究中用标准剂量的卡铂代替顺铂仅联合用鬼臼乙叉甙[9]或联合用鬼臼乙叉甙和小剂量博莱霉素[88]证明：在恶性胚芽细胞肿瘤中总的生存率和无瘤生存率都较差。到目前为止，在儿童中还没有做 PEB 与 JEB 方案的随机比较研究。

因儿童性腺外胚芽细胞肿瘤少见，并且治疗有效，复发的患者数量少，在 20%～30%的范围。有在手术切除后恶性肿瘤复发的患儿可用标准化的 PEB方案治疗。对于用顺铂难以控制或反应差的肿瘤患儿，

在阿米斯丁保护下进一步加大顺铂剂量，在美国正在评估中的有关毒性的结果还未得出。来自德国的方案结果显示，特定局部高热疗法提供了一个吸引人的选择，因为顺铂是一种好的热感受剂，高热可提高顺铂的敏感性[192]。另外，作者预见，特定区域的高热比增大顺铂剂量更有益于减少全身的副作用。

虽然异环磷酰胺没有被用作一线治疗，但它已被组合进不同的治疗方案用于成人复发性或难以控制的肿瘤[115,126]，并且与顺铂和鬼臼乙叉甙联合（ICE）已用于少量的儿童病例[122,123]。然而，这种药物组合对儿童的肾毒性增加了人们的关注。另外正在进行的研究，尤其是对大龄青少年和青年中的高风险胚芽细胞肿瘤领域的研究，是大剂量化疗和周围血干细胞移植[23]，结果还不明确。

在一项为了进一步减少治疗的晚期毒性影响的研究中，儿童肿瘤组织和儿童癌症组织合作发展了分类方案，这一方案使化疗强度降低，并使治疗方法更加个体化。根据他们的研究结果，患者被分成三个不同的风险组：

低风险组——Ⅰ期恶性性腺和性腺外胚芽细胞肿瘤患者，包括Ⅰ期未成熟畸胎瘤；

中等风险组——Ⅱ期到Ⅳ期性腺胚芽细胞肿瘤患者和Ⅱ期性腺外胚芽细胞肿瘤患者；

高风险组——Ⅲ期和Ⅳ期性腺外胚芽细胞肿瘤患者。

根据这一新的方案，儿童肿瘤组织现在正在发展一套特殊的风险治疗策略。对于所有的Ⅰ期肿瘤患者，在手术切除肿瘤后不用辅助化疗进行观察这一策略正在考虑中[63,119]。为了保证早期发现复发的肿瘤，将要求有一个对这些患者随访和评估的严格方案。对于中等风险的肿瘤患者，正在考虑给予一个改良的标准化的 PEB 治疗方案以缩短治疗时间。对于高风险组的性腺外胚芽细胞肿瘤患儿，前面引用的使用大剂量 PEB 结合阿米斯丁的研究正在进行中。

（吴晔明译　董其刚校）

参考文献

1. Ablin A, Krailo M, Ramsey N, et al: Results of treatment of malignant germ cell tumors in 93 children: A report from the Children's Cancer Study Group. J Clin Oncol 1991;9:1782.
2. Alpers CE, Harrison MR: Fetus in fetu associated with an undescended testis. Pediatr Pathol 1985;4:37.
3. Altman RP, Randolph JG, Lilly JR: Sacrococcygeal teratoma: American Academy of Pediatrics Surgical Section Survey—1973. J Pediatr Surg 1974;9:389.
4. Atkin NB, Baker MC: Abnormal chromosomes including small metacentrics in 14 ovarian cancers. Cancer Genet Cytogenet 1987;26:355.
5. Aubry F, Satie AP, Rioux-Leclercq N, et al: MAGE-A4, a germ cell specific marker, is expressed differentially in testicular tumors. Cancer 2001;92:2778.
6. Azizkhan RG: Neonatal tumors. In Carachi R, Azmy A, Grosfeld JL (eds): The Surgery of Childhood Tumors. New York, Oxford University Press, 1999, ch 8.
7. Azizkhan RG, Caty MG: Teratomas in childhood. Curr Opin Pediatr 1996;8:287.
8. Azizkhan RG, Haase GM, Applebaum H, et al: Diagnosis, management, and outcome of cervicofacial teratomas in neonates: A Children's Cancer Group study. J Pediatr Surg 1995;30:312.
9. Bajorin DF, Sarosdy MF, Pfister DG, et al: Randomized trial of etoposide and cisplatin versus etoposide and carboplatin in patients with good-risk germ cell tumors: A multi-institutional study. J Clin Oncol 1993;11:598.
10. Bale PM: Sacrococcygeal developmental abnormalities and tumors in children. Perspect Pediatr Pathol 1984;8:9.
11. Balmaceda C, Diez B, Villablanca J, et al: Chemotherapy the only strategy in primary central nervous system germ cell tumours: Results of an international study. J Neurooncol 1993;15:S3.
12. Balmaceda C, Heller G, Rosenblum M, et al: Chemotherapy without irradiation: A novel approach for newly diagnosed CNS germ cell tumours: Results of an international cooperative trial. J Clin Oncol 1996;14:2908.
13. Balmaceda C, Modak S, Finlay J: Central nervous system germ cell tumours. Semin Oncol 1998;25:243.
14. Baranzelli MC, Patte C: The French experience in paediatric malignant germ cell tumours. In Jones WG, Appleyard I, Harnden T, et al (eds): Germ Cell Tumours, 4th ed. London, John Libbey & Co, 1998, p 219.
15. Bartlett NL, Freiha FS, Torti FM: Serum markers in germ cell neoplasms. Hematol Oncol Clin North Am 1991;5:1245.
16. Batsakis JG, Littler ER, Oberman HA: Teratomas of the neck. A clinicopathologic appraisal. Arch Otolaryngol 1964;79:619.
17. Baumann FR, Nerlich A: Metastasizing cervical teratoma of the fetus. Pediatr Pathol 1993;13:21.
18. Beck JS, Fulmer HF, Lee ST: Solid malignant ovarian teratoma with "embryoid bodies" and trophoblastic differentiation. J Pathol 1969;99:67.
19. Belchis DA, Mowry J, Davis JH: Infantile choriocarcinoma: Re-examination of a potentially curable entity. Cancer 1993;72:2028.
20. Berry CL, Keeling J, Hilton C: Teratomata in infancy and childhood: A review of 91 cases. J Pathol 1969;98:241.
21. Bianchi DW, Crombleholme TM, D'Alton ME: Fetology: Diagnosis and Management of the Fetal Patient. New York, McGraw-Hill, 2000, chs 111, 116.
22. Billmire D, Vinocur C, Rescorla F, et al: Malignant mediastinal germ cell tumors: An intergroup study. J Pediatr

astinal germ cell tumors: An intergroup study. J Pediatr Surg 2001;36:18.
23. Bokemeyer C, Kollmannsberger C, Meisner C, et al: First-line high-dose chemotherapy compared with standard-dose PEB/VIP chemotherapy in patients with advanced germ cell tumors: A multivariate and matched-pair analysis. J Clin Oncol 1999;17:3450.
24. Bond SJ, Harrison MR, Schmidt KG, et al: Death due to high-output cardiac failure in fetal sacrococcygeal teratoma. J Pediatr Surg 1990;25:1287.
25. Bosl GJ, Chaganti RS: The use of tumor markers in germ cell malignancies. Hematol Oncol Clin North Am 1994;8:573.
26. Bosl GJ, Head MD: Serum tumor marker half-life during chemotherapy in patients with germ cell tumors. Int J Biol Markers 1994;9:25.
27. Buckley NJ, Burch WM, Leight GS: Malignant teratoma in the thyroid gland of an adult: A case report and a review of the literature. Surgery 1986;100:932.
28. Bussey KJ, Lawce HJ, Olson SB, et al: Chromosome abnormalities of eighty-one pediatric germ cell tumors: Sex-, age-, site-, and histopathology-related differences—a Children's Cancer Group study. Genes Chromosomes Cancer 1999; 25:134.
29. Calaminus G, Schneider DT, Bokkerink JP, et al: Prognostic value of tumor size, metastases, extension into bone, and increased tumor marker in children with malignant sacrococcygeal germ cell tumors: A prospective evaluation of 71 patients treated in the German cooperative protocols Maligne Keimzelltumoren (MAKEI) 83/86 and MAKEI 89. J Clin Oncol 2003;21:781.
30. Carney JA, Thompson DP, Johnson CL, et al: Teratomas in children: Clinical and pathologic aspects. J Pediatr Surg 1972;7:271.
31. Carter D, Bibro MC, Touloukian RJ: Benign clinical behavior of immature mediastinal teratoma in infancy and childhood. Cancer 1982;49:398.
32. Casalone R, Righi R, Granata P, et al: Cerebral germ cell tumor and XXY karyotype. Cancer Genet Cytogenet 1994; 74:25.
33. Chandra SA, Gilbert EF, Viseskul C, et al: Neonatal intracranial choriocarcinoma. Arch Pathol Lab Med 1990; 114:1079.
34. Christensen TB, Engbaek F, Marqversen J, et al: ^{125}I-labelled human chorionic gonadotrophin (hCG) as an elimination marker in the evaluation of hCG decline during chemotherapy in patients with testicular cancer. Br J Cancer 1999; 80:1577.
35. Cushing B, Giller R, Lauer S, et al: Comparison of high dose or standard dose cisplatin with etoposide and bleomycin (HDPEB vs PEB) in children with stage I-IV extragonadal malignant germ cell tumors (MGCT): A Pediatric Intergroup report (POG9049/CCG8882) [abstract]. Proc Am Soc Clin Oncol 1998;17:525a.
36. Cushing B, Perlman E, Marina N, et al: Germ cell tumors. In Pizzo PA, Poplock DG (eds): Principles and Practice of Pediatric Oncology, 2nd ed. Philadelphia, JB Lippincott, 1993, ch 36.
37. Dautenhahn L, Babyn PS, Smith CR: Metastatic choriocarcinoma in an infant: Imaging appearance. Pediatr Radiol 1993;23:597.
38. deBruin TW, Slater RM, Defferari R, et al: Isochromosome 12p-positive pineal germ cell tumor. Cancer Res 1994; 54:1542.
39. Dehner LP: Neoplasms of the fetus and neonate. In Naeye RL, Kissane JM, Kaufman N (eds): Perinatal Diseases. International Academy of Pathology, Monograph No. 22. Baltimore, Williams & Wilkins, 1981, p 286.
40. Dehner LP: Gonadal and extragonadal germ cell neoplasia of childhood. Hum Pathol 1983;14:493.
41. Dehner LP: Gonadal and extragonadal germ cell neoplasms: Teratomas in childhood. In Finegold MJ, Bennington J (eds): Pathology of Neoplasia in Children and Adolescents. Philadelphia, WB Saunders, 1986, p 282.
42. Dehner LP: Germ cell tumors of the mediastinum. Semin Diagn Pathol 1990;7:266.
43. Dehner LP, Mills A, Talerman A, et al: Germ cell neoplasms of head and neck soft tissues: A pathologic spectrum of teratomatous and endodermal sinus tumors. Hum Pathol 1990;21:309.
44. Donnellan WA, Swenson O: Benign and malignant sacrococcygeal teratomas. Pediatr Surg 1988;64:834.
45. Dunn CJ, Nguyen DL, Leonard JC: Ultrasound diagnosis of immature cervical teratoma: A case report. Am J Perinatol 1992;9:445.
46. Einhorn LH, Donohue J: Cis-diamminedichloroplatinum, vinblastine, and bleomycin combination chemotherapy in disseminated testicular cancer. Ann Intern Med 1977;87:293.
47. Esposito G, Cigliano B, Paludetto R: Abdominothoracic gastric teratoma in a female newborn infant. J Pediatr Surg 1983;18:304.
48. Federici S, Ceccarelli PL, Ferrari M, et al: Fetus in fetu: Report of three cases and review of the literature. Pediatr Surg Int 1991;6:60.
49. Felix I, Becker LE: Intracranial germ cell tumors in children: An immunohistochemical and electron microscopic study. Pediatr Neurosurg 1990;16:156.
50. Fisher RA, Salm R, Spencer RW: Bilateral gonadoblastoma/dysgerminoma in a 46XY individual: Case report with hormonal studies. J Clin Pathol 1982;35:420.
51. Fishman SJ, Jennings RW, Johnson SM, et al: Contouring buttock reconstruction after sacrococcygeal teratoma resection. J Pediatr Surg 2004;39:439.
52. Fishman WH: Alkaline phosphatase isoenzymes: Recent progress. Clin Biochem 1990;23:94.
53. Flake AW: Fetal sacrococcygeal teratoma. Semin Pediatr Surg 1993;2:113.
54. Flake AW, Harrison MR, Adzick NS, et al: Fetal sacrococcygeal teratoma. J Pediatr Surg 1986;21:563.
55. Flam F, Lundstrom V, Silfversward C: Choriocarcinoma in mother and child: Case report. Br J Obstet Gynaecol 1989; 96:241.
56. Fraser GC, Blair GK, Hemming A, et al: The treatment of simultaneous choriocarcinoma in mother and baby. J Pediatr Surg 1992;27:1318.
57. Fraumeni JF Jr, Li FP, Dalager N: Teratomas in children: Epidemiologic features. J Natl Cancer Inst 1973; 51:1425.
58. Fukuda S, Shirahama T, Imazono Y, et al: Expression of vascular endothelial growth factor in patients with testicular germ cell tumors as an indicator of metastatic disease. Cancer 1999;85:1323.
59. Gels ME, Marrink J, Visser P, et al: Importance of a new tumor marker TRA-1-60 in the follow-up of patients with clinical stage 1 nonseminomatous testicular germ cell tumors. Ann Surg Oncol 1997;4:321.
60. Germa JR, Llanos M, Tabernero JM, et al: False elevations of alpha-fetoprotein associated with liver dysfunction in germ cell tumors. Cancer 1993;72:2491.
61. Gershenson DM, Del Junco G, Copeland LJ, et al: Mixed germ cell tumors of the ovary. Obstet Gynecol 1984; 64:200.

62. Gitlin D, Perricelli A, Gillin GM: Synthesis of fetoprotein by liver, yolk sac, and gastrointestinal tract of the human conceptus. Cancer Res 1972;32:979.
63. Göbel U, Calaminus G, Schneider DT, et al: Management of germ cell tumors in children: Approaches to cure. Onkologie 2002;25:14.
64. Göbel U, Schneider DT, Calaminus G, et al: Multimodal treatment of malignant sacrococcygeal germ cell tumors: A prospective analysis of 66 patients of the German cooperative protocols MAKEI 83/86 and 89. J Clin Oncol 2001;19:1943.
65. Gonzalez-Crussi F: Extragonadal teratomas. In Atlas of Tumor Pathology, 2nd ser, fascicle 18. Washington, DC, Armed Forces Institute of Pathology, 1982.
66. Gonzalez-Crussi F, Winkler RF, Mirkin DL: Sacrococcygeal teratomas in infants and children: Relationship of histology and prognosis in 40 cases. Arch Pathol Lab Med 1978; 102:420.
67. Gornall P: Malignant germ cell tumors. In Carachi R, Azmy A, Grosfeld JL (eds): The Surgery of Childhood Tumors. New York, Oxford University Press, 1999, ch 12.
68. Goto M, Makino Y, Tamura R, et al: Sacrococcygeal teratoma with hydrops fetalis and bilateral hydronephrosis. J Perinat Med 2000;28:414.
69. Grisoni ER, Gauderer MWL, Wolfson RN, et al: Antenatal diagnosis of sacrococcygeal teratomas: Prognostic features. Pediatr Surg Int 1988;3:173.
70. Gross RE, Clatworthy HW, Meeker IA: Sacrococcygeal teratoma in infants and children. Surg Gynecol Obstet 1951; 92:341.
71. Gross SJ, Benzie RJ, Sermer M, et al: Sacrococcygeal teratoma: Prenatal diagnosis and management. Am J Obstet Gynecol 1987;156:393.
72. Gundry SR, Wesley JR, Klein MD, et al: Cervical teratomas in the newborn. J Pediatr Surg 1983;18:382.
73. Haase GM, Vinocur CD: Ovarian tumors. In O'Neill JA Jr, Rowe MI, Grosfeld JL, et al (eds): Pediatric Surgery, vol 1, 5th ed. St Louis, Mosby, 1998, ch 33.
74. Hajdu SI, Faruque AA, Hajdu E, et al: Teratoma of the neck in infants. Am J Dis Child 1966;3:412.
75. Hale GA, Marina NM, Jones-Wallace D, et al: Late effects of treatment for germ cell tumors during childhood and adolescence. J Pediatr Hematol Oncol 1999;21:115.
76. Halperin EC, Constine LS, Tarbell NJ, Kun LE (eds): Supratentorial brain tumours. In Paediatric Radiation Oncology, 3rd ed. Philadelphia, Lippincott Williams & Wilkins, 1999, p 67.
77. Harms D, Janig U: Germ cell tumors of childhood: Report of 170 cases including 59 pure and partial yolk-sac tumors. Virchows Arch A Pathol Anat Histopathol 1986;409:223.
78. Hawkins EP: Pathology of germ cell tumors in children. Crit Rev Oncol Hematol 1990;10:165.
79. Hawkins EP, Finegold MJ, Hawkins HK, et al: Nongerminomatous malignant germ cell tumors in children: A review of 89 cases from the Pediatric Oncology Group, 1971-1984. Cancer 1986;58:2579.
80. Hawkins EP, Perlman EJ: Germ cell tumors in childhood: Morphology and biology. In Parham DM (ed): Pediatric Neoplasia: Morphology and Biology. New York, Raven Press, 1996, p 297.
81. Hechelhammer L, Storkel S, Odermatt B, et al: Epidermal growth factor receptor is a marker for syncytiotrophoblastic cells in testicular germ cell tumors. Virchows Arch 2003; 443:28.
82. Hedrick HL, Flake AW, Crombleholme TM, et al: Sacrococcygeal teratoma: Prenatal assessment, fetal intervention, and outcome. J Pediatr Surg 2004;39:430.
83. Heifetz SA, Alrabeeah A, Brown BS, et al: Fetus in fetu: A fetiform teratoma. Pediatr Pathol 1988;8:215.
84. Heifetz SA, Cushing B, Biller R, et al: Immature teratomas in children: Pathologic considerations. Am J Surg Pathol 1998;22:1115.
85. Hoffner L, Deka R, Chakravarti A: Cytogenetics and origins of pediatric germ cell tumors. Cancer Genet Cytogenet 1994;74:54.
86. Hoffner L, Shen-Schwartz S, Deka R, et al: Genetics and biology of human ovarian teratomas. III. Cytogenetics and origins of malignant ovarian germ cell tumors. Cancer Genet Cytogenet 1992;62:58.
87. Holzgreve W, Miny P, Anderson R, et al: Experience with 8 cases of prenatally diagnosed sacrococcygeal teratomas. Fetal Ther 1987;2:88.
88. Horwich A, Sleijfer DT, Fossa SD, et al: Randomized trial of bleomycin, etoposide, and cisplatin compared with bleomycin, etoposide, and carboplatin in good-prognosis metastatic nonseminomatous germ cell cancer: A multi-institutional Medical Research Council/European Organization for Research and Treatment of Cancer trial. J Clin Oncol 1997;15:1844.
89. Hurlbut HJ, Webb HW, Moseley T: Cervical teratoma in infant siblings. J Pediatr Surg 1967;2:424.
90. International Germ Cell Consensus Classification: A prognostic factor-based staging system for metastatic germ cell cancers. International Germ Cell Cancer Collaborative Group. J Clin Oncol 1997;15:594.
91. Isaacs H Jr: Tumors of the Newborn and Infant. St Louis, Mosby–Year Book, 1991.
92. Isaacs H Jr: Germ cell tumors. In Tumors of the Fetus and Newborn, vol 35 in Major Problems in Pathology. Philadelphia, WB Saunders, 1997, p 15.
93. Jacobsen GK, Norgaard-Pedersen B: Placental alkaline phosphatase in testicular germ cell tumours and in carcinoma in-situ of the testis: An immunohistochemical study. Acta Pathol Microbiol Immunol Scand (A) 1984;92:323.
94. Jirasek JE: Morphogenesis of the genital system in the human. Birth Defects Orig Artic Ser 1977;13:13.
95. Jordan RB, Gauderer MW: Cervical teratomas: An analysis, literature review and proposed classification. J Pediatr Surg 1988;23:583.
96. Kamoto T, Satomura S, Yoshiki T, et al: Lectin-reactive alpha-fetoprotein (AFP-L3%) curability and prediction of clinical course after treatment of non-seminomatous germ cell tumors. Jpn J Clin Oncol 2002;32:472.
97. Kapoor G, Advani SH, Nair CN, et al: Pediatric germ cell tumor: An experience with BEP. J Pediatr Hematol Oncol 1995;17:318.
98. Kashiwagi A, Nagamori S, Toyota K, et al: DNA ploidy of testicular germ cell tumors in childhood: Difference from adult testicular tumors. Nippon Hinyokika Gakkai Zasshi 1993;84:1655.
99. Kay R: Prepubertal testicular tumor registry. Urol Clin North Am 1993;20:1.
100. Kelly MF, Berenholz L, Rizzo KA, et al: Approach for oxygenation of the newborn with airway obstruction due to a cervical mass. Ann Otol Rhinol Laryngol 1990;99:179.
101. Kim SN, Chi JG, Kim YW, et al: Neonatal choriocarcinoma of the liver. Pediatr Pathol 1993;13:723.
102. King ME, Hubbell MJ, Talerman A: Mixed germ cell tumor of the ovary with a prominent polyembryoma component. Int J Gynecol Pathol 1991;10:88.
103. Koshida K, Nishino A, Yamamoto H, et al: The role of alkaline phosphatase isoenzymes as tumor markers for

testicular germ cell tumors. J Urol 1991;146:57.
104. Kuhlmann RS, Warsof SL, Levy DL, et al: Fetal sacrococcygeal teratoma. Fetal Ther 1987;2:95.
105. Kurman RJ, Norris HJ: Malignant mixed germ cell tumors of the ovary: A clinical and pathologic analysis of 30 cases. Obstet Gynecol 1976;48:579.
106. Lachman MF, Kim K, Koo BC: Mediastinal teratoma associated with Klinefelter's syndrome. Arch Pathol Lab Med 1986;110:1067.
107. Lakhoo K, Boyle M, Drake DP: Mediastinal teratomas: Review of 15 pediatric cases. J Pediatr Surg 1993;28:1161.
108. Lamb DJ: Growth factors and testicular development. J Urol 1993;150:583.
109. Lange PH, Vogelzang NJ, Goldman A, et al: Marker half-life analysis as a prognostic tool in testicular cancer. J Urol 1982;128:708.
110. Langer JC, Tabb T, Thompson P, et al: Management of prenatally diagnosed tracheal obstruction: Access to the airway in utero prior to delivery. Fetal Diagn Ther 1992;7:12.
111. Lawton AJ, Mead GM: Staging and prognostic factors in testicular cancer. Semin Surg Oncol 1999;17:223.
112. Lemire RG, Beckwith JB: Pathogenesis of congenital tumors and malformations of the sacrococcygeal region. Teratology 1982;25:201.
113. Leroy X, Augusto D, Leteurtre E, et al: CD30 and CD117 (c-kit) used in combination are useful for distinguishing embryonal carcinoma from seminoma. J Histochem Cytochem 2002;50:283.
114. Lifschitz-Mercer B, Elliott DJ, Leider-Trejo L, et al: Absence of RBM expression as a marker of intratubular (in situ) germ cell neoplasia of the testis. Hum Pathol 2000;31:1116.
115. Loehrer PJ Sr, Gonin R, Nichols CR, et al: Vinblastine plus ifosfamide plus cisplatin as initial salvage therapy in recurrent germ cell tumor. J Clin Oncol 1998;16:2500.
116. Lund DP, Soriano SG, Fauza D, et al: Resection of a massive sacrococcygeal teratoma using hypothermic hypoperfusion: A novel use of extracorporeal membrane oxygenation. J Pediatr Surg 1995;30:1557.
117. Magee JF, McFadden DE, Pantzar JT: Congenital tumors. In Dimmick JE, Kalousek DK (eds): Developmental Pathology of the Embryo and Fetus. Philadelphia, JB Lippincott, 1992, p 235.
118. Mahour GH, Landing BH, Woolley MM: Teratomas in children: Clinicopathologic studies in 133 patients. Z Kinderchir 1978;23:365.
119. Mann JR, Raafat F, Robinson K, et al: The United Kingdom Children's Cancer Study Group's second germ cell tumor study: Carboplatin, etoposide, and bleomycin are effective treatment for children with malignant extracranial germ cell tumors, with acceptable toxicity. J Clin Oncol 2000;18:3809.
120. Marina NM, Cushing B, Giller R, et al: Complete surgical excision is effective treatment for children with immature teratomas with or without malignant elements: A Pediatric Oncology Group/Children's Cancer Group Intergroup Study. J Clin Oncol 1999;17:2137.
121. Marina NM, Fontanesi J, Kun L, et al: Treatment of childhood germ cell tumors: Review of the St Jude experience from 1979 to 1988. Cancer 1992;70:2568.
122. Marina NM, Rodman JH, Murry DJ, et al: Phase I study of escalating targeted doses of carboplatin combined with ifosfamide and etoposide in treatment of newly diagnosed pediatric solid tumors. J Natl Cancer Inst 1994;86:544.
123. Marina NM, Shema SJ, Bowman LC, et al: Failure of granulocyte-macrophage colony-stimulating factor to reduce febrile neutropenia in children with recurrent solid tumors treated with ifosfamide, carboplatin, and etoposide chemotherapy. Med Pediatr Oncol 1994;23:328.
124. Mazumdar M, Bacik J, Tickoo SK, et al: Cluster analysis of p53 and Ki67 expression, apoptosis, alpha-fetoprotein, and human chorionic gonadotrophin indicates a favorable prognostic subgroup within the embryonal carcinoma germ cell tumor. J Clin Oncol 2003;21:2679.
125. Mazumdar M, Bajorin DF, Bacik J, et al: Predicting outcome to chemotherapy in patients with germ cell tumors: The value of the rate of decline of human chorionic gonadotrophin and alpha-fetoprotein during therapy. J Clin Oncol 2001;19:2534.
126. McCaffrey JA, Mazumdar M, Bajorin DF, et al: Ifosfamide- and cisplatin-containing chemotherapy as first-line salvage therapy in germ cell tumors: Response and survival. J Clin Oncol 1997;15:2559.
127. Merchant TE, Davis BJ, Sheldon JM, et al: Radiation therapy for relapsed CNS germinoma after primary chemotherapy. J Clin Oncol 1998;16:204.
128. Misra D, Pritchard J, Drake DP, et al: Markedly improved survival in malignant sacrococcygeal teratomas—16 years' experience. Eur J Pediatr Surg 1997;7:152.
129. Miyanohara O, Takeshima H, Kaji M, et al: Diagnostic significance of soluble c-kit in the cerebrospinal fluid of patients with germ cell tumors. J Neurosurg 2002; 97:177.
130. Morris MJ, Bosl GJ: Recognizing abnormal marker results that do not reflect disease in patients with germ cell tumors. J Urol 2000;163:796.
131. Murphy BA, Motzer RJ, Mazumdar M, et al: Serum tumor marker decline is an early predictor of treatment outcome in germ cell tumor patients treated with cisplatin and ifosfamide salvage chemotherapy. Cancer 1994; 73:2520.
132. Musci MN Jr, Clark MJ, Ayres RE, et al: Management of dystocia caused by a large sacrococcygeal teratoma. Obstet Gynecol 1983;62(3 Suppl):10s.
133. Nakashima N, Fukatsu T, Nagasaka T, et al: The frequency and histology of hepatic tissue in germ cell tumors. Am J Surg Pathol 1987;11:682.
134. Naudin Ten Cate L, Vermeij-Keers C, Smit DA, et al: Intracranial teratoma with multiple fetuses: Pre- and postnatal appearance. Hum Pathol 1995;26:804.
135. Nirasawa Y, Ito Y: Reproduction-preserving technique for benign cystic teratoma of the ovary. Pediatr Surg Int 1995; 10:126.
136. Nogales FF: Embryologic clues to human yolk sac tumors: A review. Int J Gynecol Pathol 1993;12:101.
137. Norris HJ, Zirkin HJ, Benson WL: Immature (malignant) teratoma of the ovary: A clinical and pathologic study of 58 cases. Cancer 1976;37:2359.
138. Noseworthy J, Lack EE, Kozakewich HP, et al: Sacrococcygeal germ cell tumors in childhood: An updated experience with 118 patients. J Pediatr Surg 1981;16:358.
139. Olsen MM, Caldamone AA, Jackson CL, et al: Gonadoblastoma in infancy: Indications for early gonadectomy in 46XY gonadal dysgenesis. J Pediatr Surg 1988;23:270.
140. Owor R, Master SP: Cervical teratomas in the newborn. East Afr Med J 1974;51:376.
141. Packer RJ, Sutton LN, Rosenstock JG, et al: Pineal region tumors of childhood. Pediatrics 1984;74:97.
142. Parkes SE, Muir KR, Southern L, et al: Neonatal tumours: A thirty-year population based study. Med Pediatr Oncol 1994;22:309.

143. Perlman EJ, Cushing B, Hawkins E, et al: Cytogenetic analysis of childhood endodermal sinus tumors: A Pediatric Oncology Group study. Pediatr Pathol 1994;14:695.
144. Perlman EJ, Hu J, Ho D, et al: Genetic analysis of childhood endodermal sinus tumors by comparative genomic hybridization. J Pediatr Hematol Oncol 2000;22:100.
145. Perlman EJ, Valentine MB, Look AT, et al: Deletion of the short arm of chromosome 1 in childhood endodermal sinus tumor by two color fluorescence in situ hybridization. Lab Invest 1995;72:5.
146. Potter EL, Craig JM: Pathology of the Fetus and the Infant, 3rd ed. Chicago, Year Book Medical Publishers, 1975, p 177.
147. Prat J, Matias-Guiu X, Scully RE: Hepatic yolk sac differentiation in an ovarian polyembryoma. Surg Pathol 1989;2:147.
148. Rescorla FJ: Pediatric germ cell tumors. Semin Surg Oncol 1999;16:144.
149. Rescorla FJ, Billmire D, Stolar C, et al: The effect of cisplatin dose and surgical resection in children with malignant germ cell tumors at the sacrococcygeal region: A pediatric intergroup trial (POG 9049/CCG 8882). J Pediatr Surg 2001;36:12.
150. Rescorla FJ, Sawin RS, Coran AG, et al: Long-term outcome for infants and children with sacrococcygeal teratoma: A report from the Children's Cancer Group. J Pediatr Surg 1998;33:171.
151. Richie JP: Neoplasms of the testis. In Walsh PC, Retik AB, Stamey TA, et al (eds): Campbell's Urology, 6th ed. Philadelphia, WB Saunders, 1992, p 1222.
152. Robboy SJ, Miller T, Donahoe PK, et al: Dysgenesis of testicular and streak gonads in syndrome of mixed gonadal dysgenesis: Perspective derived from a clinicopathologic analysis of twenty one cases. Hum Pathol 1982; 13:700.
153. Robboy SJ, Scully RE: Ovarian teratoma with glial implants on the peritoneum: An analysis of 12 cases. Hum Pathol 1970;1:643.
154. Robertson FM, Crombleholme TM, Frantz ID, et al: Devascularization and staged resection of giant sacrococcygeal teratoma in the premature infant. J Pediatr Surg 1995;30:309.
155. Rowe MI, O'Neill JA, Grosfeld JL, et al: Teratomas and germ cell tumors. In Essentials of Pediatric Surgery. St Louis, Mosby, 1995, p 296.
156. Sawamura Y, Ikeda J, Shirato H, et al: Germ cell tumours of the central nervous system: Treatment considerations based on 111 cases and their long-term clinical outcomes. Eur J Cancer 1998;34:104.
157. Schey WL, Shkolnik A, White H: Clinical and radiographic considerations of sacrococcygeal teratomas: An analysis of 26 new cases and review of the literature. Radiology 1977;125:189.
158. Schropp KP, Lobe TE, Rao B, et al: Sacrococcygeal teratoma: The experience of four decades. J Pediatr Surg 1992;27:1075.
159. Schwartz PE, Chambers SK, Chambers JT, et al: Ovarian germ cell malignancies: The Yale University experience. Gynecol Oncol 1992;45:26.
160. Schwartz PE, Morris JM: Serum lactic dehydrogenase: A tumor marker for dysgerminoma. Obstet Gynecol 1988;72:511.
161. Scully RE, Young RH, Clement PB: Atlas of Tumor Pathology, 3rd ser, fascicle 23. Washington, DC, Armed Forces Institute of Pathology, 1998, ch 13.
162. Senocak ME, Kale G, Buyukpamukcu N, et al: Gastric teratoma in children including the third reported female case. J Pediatr Surg 1990;25:681.
163. Shaaban AF, Kim HB, Flake AW: Fetal surgery, diagnosis, and intervention. In Ziegler MM, Azizkhan RG, Weber TR (eds): Operative Pediatric Surgery. New York, McGraw-Hill, 2003, ch 3.
164. Shamberger RC: Teratomas and germ cell tumors. In O'Neill JA, Grosfeld JL, Fonkalsrud EW, et al (eds): Principles of Pediatric Surgery, 2nd ed. St Louis, Mosby, 2004, ch 24.
165. Shen V, Chaparro M, Choi BH, et al: Absence of isochromosome 12p in a pineal region malignant germ cell tumor. Cancer Genet Cytogenet 1990;50:153.
166. Shitara T, Oshima Y, Yugami S, et al: Choriocarcinoma in children. Am J Pediatr Hematol Oncol 1993;15:268.
167. Silberman R, Mendelson IR: Teratoma of the neck: Report of 2 cases and review of the literature. Arch Dis Child 1960;35:159.
168. Silver SA, Wiley JM, Perlman EJ: DNA ploidy analysis of pediatric germ cell tumors. Mod Pathol 1994;7:951.
169. Stern JW, Bunin N: Prospective study of carboplatin-based chemotherapy for pediatric germ cell tumors. Med Pediatr Oncol 2002;39:163.
170. Stock C, Ambros IM, Lion T, et al: Detection of numerical and structural chromosome abnormalities in pediatric germ cell tumors by means of interphase cytogenetics. Cancer 1994;11:40.
171. Strohmeyer T, Reese D, Press M, et al: Expression of the c-kit proto-oncogene and its ligand stem cell factor (SCF) in normal and malignant human testicular tissue. J Urol 1995;153:511.
172. Suita S, Ikeda K, Nakano H, et al: Teratoma of the neck in a newborn infant—a case report. Z Kinderchir 1982;35:9.
173. Takeda A, Ishizuka T, Goto T, et al: Polyembryoma of ovary producing alpha-fetoprotein and HCG: Immunoperoxidase and electron microscopic study. Cancer 1982;49:1878.
174. Takeshima H, Kuratsu J: A review of soluble c-kit (s-kit) as a novel tumor marker and possible molecular target for the treatment of CNS germinoma. Surg Neurol 2003; 60:321.
175. Talerman A: Germ cell tumors of the ovary. In Kurman RJ (ed): Blaustein's Pathology of the Female Genital Tract, 4th ed. New York, Springer-Verlag, 1994, p 849.
176. Tapper D, Lack EE: Teratomas in infancy and childhood: A 54-year experience at the Children's Hospital Medical Center. Ann Surg 1983;198:398.
177. Teitelbaum D, Teich S, Cassidy S, et al: Highly vascularized sacrococcygeal teratoma: Description of this atypical variant and its operative management. J Pediatr Surg 1994;29:98.
178. Toner GC, Stockler MR, Boyer MJ, et al: Comparison of two standard chemotherapy regimens for good prognosis germ cell tumors: A randomized trial. Lancet 2001;357:739.
179. Touran T, Applebaum H, Frost DB, et al: Congenital metastatic cervical teratoma: Diagnostic and management considerations. J Pediatr Surg 1989;24:21.
180. Trigo JM, Tabernero JM, Paz-Ares L, et al: Tumor markers at the time of recurrence in patients with germ cell tumors. Cancer 2000;88:162.
181. Troche V, Hernandez E: Neoplasia arising in dysgenetic gonads: A review. Obstet Gynecol Surv 1986;41:74.
182. Tsukahara Y, Fukuta T, Yamada T, et al: Retroperitoneal giant tumor formed by migrating polyembryoma with numerous embryoid bodies from an ovarian mixed germ cell tumor. Gynecol Obstet Invest 1991;31:58.

183. Tsuura Y, Hiraki H, Watanabe K, et al: Preferential localization of c-kit product in tissue mast cells, basal cells of skin, epithelial cells of breast, small cell lung carcinoma and seminoma/dysgerminoma in human: Immunohistochemical study on formalin-fixed, paraffin-embedded tissues. Virchows Arch 1994;424:135.
184. Valdiserri RO, Yunis EJ: Sacrococcygeal teratomas: A review of 68 cases. Cancer 1981;48:217.
185. Verp MS, Simpson JL: Abnormal sexual differentiation and neoplasia. Cancer Genet Cytogenet 1987; 25:191.
186. Vilain E, Jaubert F, Fellous M, et al: Pathology of 46,XY pure gonadal dysgenesis: Absence of testis differentiation associated with mutations in the testis-determining factor. Differentiation 1993;52:151.
187. Vogelzang NJ, Lange PH, Goldman A, et al: Acute changes of alpha-fetoprotein and human chorionic gonadotropin during induction chemotherapy of germ cell tumors. Cancer Res 1982;42:4855.
188. von Eyben FE, Madsen EL, Blaabjerg O, et al: Serum lactate dehydrogenase isoenzyme 1 and relapse in patients with nonseminomatous testicular germ cell tumors clinical stage I. Acta Oncol 2001;40:536.
189. Waldhausen JA, Kolman JW, Vellios F, et al: Sacrococcygeal teratoma. Pediatr Surg 1963;54:933.
190. Warner BA, Monsaert RP, Stumpf PG, et al: 46,XY gonadal dysgenesis: Is oncogenesis related to H-Y phenotype or breast development? Hum Genet 1985;69:79.
191. Werb P, Scurry J, Ostor A, et al: Survey of congenital tumors in perinatal necropsies. Pathology 1992;24:247.
192. Wessalowski R, Kruck H, Pape H, et al: Hyperthermia for the treatment of patients with malignant germ cell tumors: A phase I/II study in ten children and adolescents with recurrent or refractory tumors. Cancer 1998;82:793.
193. Wollner N, Ghavimi F, Wachtel A, et al: Germ cell tumors in children: Gonadal and extragonadal. Med Pediatr Oncol 1991;19:228.
194. Wu JT, Book L, Sudar K: Serum alpha fetoprotein (AFP) levels in normal infants. Pediatr Res 1981;15:50.
195. Young JL Jr, Ries LG, Silverberg E, et al: Cancer incidence, survival and mortality for children younger than age 15 years. Cancer 1986;58(2 Suppl):598.
196. Young R, Scully R: Germ cell tumors: Nonseminomatous Tumors, Occult Tumors, Effects of Chemotherapy in Testicular Tumors. Chicago: ASCP Press, 1990, p 37.
197. Yu IT, Griffin CA, Phillips PC, et al: Numerical sex chromosomal abnormalities in pineal teratomas by cytogenetic analysis and fluorescence in situ hybridization. Lab Invest 1995;72:419.

第 35 章

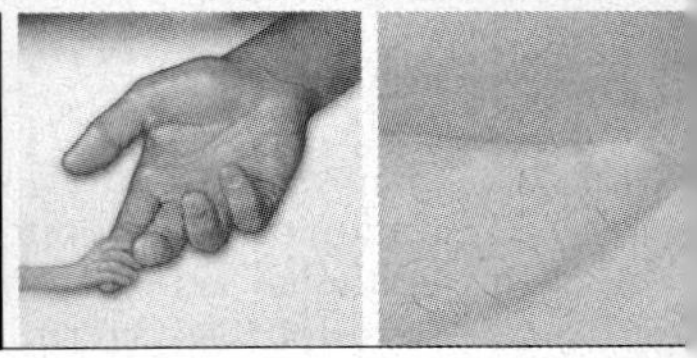

Hodgkin病和非 Hodgkin淋巴瘤

Michael P. La Quaglia 和 Wendy T. Su

575 ## Hodgkin病

Hodgkin 于 1832 年首先根据解剖学上的观察报道了 Hodgkin 病。原文是“淋巴结和脾脏的一些病态表现”[44]。随着显微组织学的发展，Sternberg 和 Reed 分别于 1898 年和 1902 年描述了该病的组织病理学特征[110,121]。他们强调了 Hodgkin 病与结核的显著区别在于其独特形态并具有大核仁的多核巨细胞。1902 和 1903 年初次报道了通过放疗来治疗 Hodgkin 病[98]。Gilbert 报道了治愈 Hodgkin 病所需遵循的一些放疗原则[33]。多伦多的 Peters[94]随后报道了一系列 Hodgkin 病无病生存 20 年的病例。在 20 世纪 60 年代末期出现了分期剖腹手术来明确转移扩散的途径并用于研究[34]。斯坦福大学的 Kaplan 等人[13,51,103]则为现代超高电压治疗 Hodgkin 病奠定了基础。1946 年出现了用氮芥的衍生物治疗淋巴肉瘤和 Hodgkin 病的报道[36]，而 1967 年出现多药联合治疗的方案 MOPP（氮芥、长春新碱、丙卡巴肼和泼尼松）[22]。随着生存率的提高，人们发现了药物治疗的一些副反应，如继发肿瘤和不育。20 世纪 70 年代出现了无交叉耐药的 ABVD 方案（阿霉素、博来霉素、长春碱和达卡巴嗪），该方案出现继发性髓系白血病和不育的危险较少。在 20 世纪 80 年代，更多的研究者认识到标准剂量放疗和化疗的长期后遗症，特别是针对儿童肿瘤患者。至 20 世纪 90 年代，在部分患者中采用了联合治疗方案，首先分期剖腹探查手术，然后进行影像学诊断。这 10 年期间研究者的精力主要在于研究按危险度分级和个体化治疗，其目的在于找到最佳疗效和最轻毒副作用的联合治疗方案。

发生率和流行病学

Hodgkin 病（HD）在年龄分布上有双峰特征，第一个峰出现于 15 岁到 20 岁末，第二个峰出现于 50 岁以上。流行病学研究发现 HD 有三个类型。儿童型出现于 14 岁以下，青年型出现于 15～34 岁，老年型出现于 55～74 岁。儿童和青少年病例在 HD 中约占 15%，十几岁患儿的 HD 发生率是 10 岁以下患儿的 2 倍。HD 在儿童恶性肿瘤中占 5%，发生率约为 6 例 /1 百万。不同年龄组其组织学类型也不同。混合细胞型在年幼儿中较多见，而结节硬化型在青少年中更多见。

HD 发病是很多原因造成的，但在 10 岁以下患儿中，EB 病毒暴露与疾病的相关性最为明显。病毒感染似乎先于肿瘤细胞的扩增，且 EB 病毒可以单独或和其他致癌物质发挥作用。直到最近，镜影细胞（Reed-Sternberg 细胞）的起源仍然未明。免疫组化和分子生物学研究显示了这些细胞的克隆特性。HD 中的镜影细胞、淋巴细胞和组织细胞来源于经过克隆性扩增转化的 B 细胞。已经证实，HD 细胞的免疫表型为 B 细胞抗原。HD 细胞也有许多产生细胞因子和应答的细胞特征，这些特征与该肿瘤的一些非特异性症状和体征相关。

临床表现

无痛性的颈部和锁骨上淋巴结肿大是 HD 最常见的症状（80%）。原发于腋窝或腹股沟淋巴结的肿大相对较为少见（30%），而原发腹股沟的病例不到 576

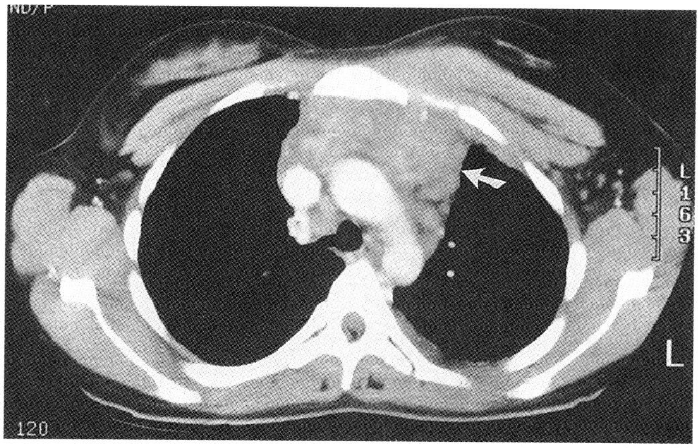

图 35-1　胸部 CT 扫描显示 1 例 IIB 期的 Hodgkin 病患者位于纵隔的肿瘤（箭头所示）。这些检查在手术前必须完成以识别有无气管支气管梗阻。

5%。通常淋巴结质硬，有弹性但无触痛，2/3 以上患者在诊断时已经侵犯纵隔，因此在做任何侵袭性手术前应该拍一个清晰的前后位的胸片来评估纵隔及排除气道梗阻。当胸部平片检查发现纵隔肿块时，建议做胸部 CT 平扫加增强检查以评估气道和获得更多的解剖学资料（图 35-1 和 35-2）。在全身麻醉前，临床医生应该想到气道被肿瘤压迫的可能性。上腔静脉综合征表现为面部水肿、颈静脉怒张和面部充血，这些高度提示纵隔肿瘤压迫上腔静脉导致梗阻。

大约 1/3 患者出现全身症状（B 亚期症状，见后），可能包括在过去 6 个月中体重减轻大于 10%，夜间盗汗，或发热高于 38℃。瘙痒症在 HD 患者中也较为常见，但并无判断预后价值。HD 患者的免疫状况会发生改变，其特征是全面的免疫功能下降、无效的宿主自动免疫反应和皮肤应变力缺乏[123]。

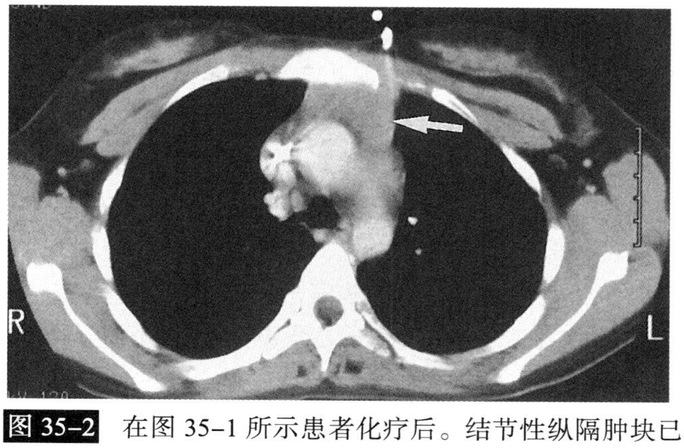

图 35-2　在图 35-1 所示患者化疗后。结节性纵隔肿块已经缩小（箭头所示），但同时胸腺出现均一性增大。这种胸腺反弹性增生可能与肿瘤持续存在或复发相混淆。

诊断

可疑 HD 患者的诊断必须从病史和体格检查开始。所有淋巴结区都应该检查，并测量肿大淋巴结的大小。组成 Waldeyer 环的淋巴组织（扁桃腺及腺样体）也应该检查。HD 的确诊需要有淋巴结活检做病理检查。镜影细胞出现对 HD 有确诊意义（图 35-3）。Rye 分类把 HD 分成四种组织学类型：淋巴细胞为主型、结节硬化型、混合细胞型和淋巴细胞减少型，每种类型都有特异的免疫表型[40]。儿童中最常见的是结节硬化型（＞65%），其次分别是混合细胞型和淋巴细胞为主型。淋巴细胞为主型的预后最佳。然而，随着有效的联合化疗和多学科联合治疗方案的发展，所有类型 HD 的治疗都有效果。

实验室检查必须包括血常规、ESR、肝肾功能和电解质。诊断时的血清铜和 LDH 水平与肿瘤负荷相关，但无特异的肿瘤标记。

分期

HD 可以有临床或病理分期。临床分期基于成熟的 Ann Arbor 分期系统（表 35-1），并需病史、体格 576
检查和诊断相关影像学检查资料。亚型 A、B 和 E 根

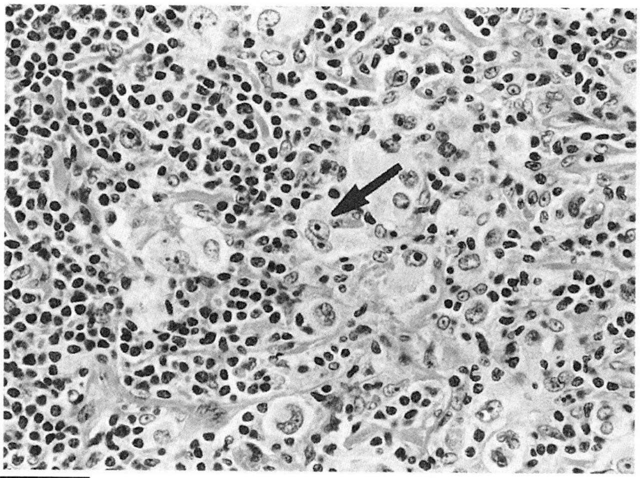

图 35-3　结节性硬化型 Hodgkin 病的组织病理切片。箭头显示一个镜影细胞。

表 35-1　Hodgkin 病的 Ann Arbor 标准分期

分期	标准
Ⅰ期	一个淋巴结区（I）或一个结外器官或部位受累（IE）
Ⅱ期	横膈同侧 2 个或 2 个以上淋巴结区（II）或一个结外病变伴局部淋巴结受累（IIE）
Ⅲ期	横膈两侧淋巴结区受累（III）；可同时伴脾脏浸润（IIIS）、或局部的结外器官（IIIE）或结外部位（IIIES）受累
Ⅳ期	一个或多个结外部位的播散性受累，伴或不伴淋巴结受累

据临床特征来划分。亚型 A 是临床上无症状，亚型 B 症状是严格定义为在过去 6 个月中体重减轻 10%，夜间盗汗，或持续 3 天高于 38℃的发热。亚型 E 表示有微小淋巴结外疾病。

影像学资料是临床分期的重要组成部分。胸片往往能提示是否有纵隔肿块，而胸部后前位片上肿块最大直径和胸腔直径的比例对判断预后有重要意义。当该比例大于 1∶3 时属于巨大纵隔肿块，预后较差，需要足量全身的化疗。胸腹部 CT 检查能够提供更为精确的疾病程度的评价，如果上颈部淋巴结受累，需做颈部 CT 检查以评估 Waldeyer 环受累情况。胸部 CT 能提供最好的反映纵隔病变程度的资料，同时能评估肺实质、胸膜、心包和胸壁的情况。在评估横隔下肿瘤时，必须同时使用静脉和口服的造影剂，以更好地将淋巴结肿块和其他组织区别。由于儿童腹膜后脂肪量少以及该年龄段良性淋巴结肿大常见，故 CT 扫描在儿童的作用有限。在这些情况下，用 CT 扫描评估脾脏或主动脉周围淋巴结受累是不够准确的，和剖腹探查术比较，其准确率约为 71%～74%。由于 MRI 能更好地发现脂肪包绕的腹膜后淋巴结，故与 CT 比较，能更准确的评估横膈下肿块。由于技术的难度，淋巴管造影术在儿童很少进行。

镓[67]扫描的特异性较低，不能区分炎症和恶性肿瘤，但若持续阳性可能意味着肿瘤残留。虽然在儿童中资料有限，但正电子断层扫描技术最近已经在成人用于检测不能被 CT 识别的肿块[30]。

除非在骨骼、骨髓、肝脏或肺活检中发现转移病，否则病理分期理论上需要外科参与评价，包括脾切除术。然而，现在的 HD 治疗基本上都是全身的化疗，因此病理分期并不影响治疗，故现在基本不再用脾切除术做外科分期。唯一非常少见的例外是对于只有局部 HD 而只需要放疗的男性青少年。

治疗

外科

所有 HD 患者需要对累及的淋巴结做活检以建立诊断和组织类型。对于诊断，冰冻切片是不够的，必须做苏木精-伊红染色切片。此外，对组织切片做详细的研究更重要，如免疫组化、免疫表型和细胞遗传学等。应该从最容易接近的部位做活检。如果患者病变只有累及纵隔，可以通过纵隔镜、Chamberlain 法或胸腔镜检查获得活检组织[35]。后腹膜淋巴结肿块一般可以通过腹腔镜获得活检。用细针抽吸物细胞学方法来检测出稀少的镜影细胞是不够的，有研究显示，20%的介入放射检查法诊断 HD 会出现假阴性的结果[32]。淋巴结切除活检、巨大或融合淋巴结的部分切除活检对于准确诊断是必不可少的。应该做各种努力来取得未经压碾和腐蚀并保持细胞结构的标本。

随着治疗 HD 方法规范的变化，外科分期的作用已经发生了改变。剖腹手术的分期最初由放射肿瘤专家设计，以确定疾病的病理程度和准确的超高电压放疗区域，假使要治愈疾病，必须所有的受累淋巴结都得到放疗。颈部低分期的 HD 常随着一个可预测的进展过程恶化，而这种进展过程则可通过腹膜后淋巴结取样及切除脾脏来明确。如果疾病范围超过了放疗允许的标准，将有必要采用化疗。HD 患者做剖腹手术和脾脏切除术的目的是明确疾病的范围以决定需要接受放疗的淋巴结梯次。因此，这不是一种治疗方法。随着化疗在 HD 所有分期的应用[25,62]，外科分期对于治疗不能提供有用的信息来改变治疗而不再应用。就像前面所说，例外的是少数男性青少年 HD 患者中，若病灶局限可能只需要放疗。

传统上，外科分期需要剖腹手术、脾脏切除、双叶肝脏穿刺和楔形活检以及彻底的多个淋巴结区（脾门、肝门、胰腺上方、主动脉两侧和肠系膜）的活检。女孩还需做双侧卵巢区域淋巴结活检。剖腹探查可以减少术后死亡率[110,116,117,129]，包括术后肠道梗阻的发生[27]。然而，由于脾脏切除所致的感染风险没有改变。

化疗

HD 的有效化疗方案包含单用有效和一些不同作用机制的药物，连用可以破坏肿瘤细胞内的稳定状态同时使耐药降到最低限（表 35-2）。这些药物的毒性不能重叠，以使每一种药物的剂量都能用到足量。MOPP 方案能够达到这些要求，是第一个对 HD 有效的联合化疗方案。NCI 对 188 例用 MOPP 方案治疗的患者进行了长期跟踪，完全缓解率为 89%，10 年的无病生存率为 54%[67]。这组患者诊断时的平均年龄为 32 岁（12～69 岁）。在该项研究中，95%患者为Ⅲ或Ⅳ期，89%有 B 症状。维持治疗对缓解率无影响，因此，维持治疗对 HD 患者似无必要。

表 35-2 HD 的化疗方案

方案	药物
ABVD[9]	阿霉素、博来霉素、长春新碱、达卡巴嗪
ABVE（DBVE）	阿霉素、博来霉素、长春新碱、鬼臼乙叉甙
VAMP[23]	长春新碱、阿霉素、甲氨蝶呤、泼尼松
OPPA ± COPP（女性）[107]	长春新碱、泼尼松、丙卡巴肼、阿霉素、环磷酰胺、长春新碱、泼尼松、丙卡巴肼
OEPA ± COPP（男性）[107]	长春新碱、鬼臼乙叉甙、泼尼松、阿霉素、环磷酰胺、长春新碱、泼尼松、丙卡巴肼
COPP/ABV[84]	环磷酰氨、长春新碱、泼尼松、丙卡巴肼、阿霉素、博来霉素、长春碱
BEACOPP（晚期）[54]	博来霉素、鬼臼乙叉甙、阿霉素、环磷酰胺、长春新碱、泼尼松、丙卡巴肼
COPP	环磷酰胺、长春新碱、泼尼松、丙卡巴肼
CHOP	环磷酰胺、阿霉素、长春新碱、泼尼松
ABVE-PC（DBVE-PC）[12]	阿霉素、博来霉素、长春新碱、鬼臼乙叉甙、泼尼松、环磷酰胺

ABVD 是应用于 HD 患者的第二个化疗方案[11]。该方案为那些 MOPP 治疗失败的患者而设计，包含了单药治疗有效而无交叉毒性的药物。由于 MOPP 和 ABVD 方案均有效，而且两者毒性无重叠，有研究把两个方案合并使用，并获得较好的初步治疗效果[10]。这些方案在门诊使用，急性毒副作用容易处理。然而，它们的长期毒副作用促使研究者去设计 MOPP-ABVD 的交替方案，以避免累积剂量相关的药物毒副作用的出现。

目前的趋势是基于疾病的反应而采用“量体裁衣式的化疗”。这个方案通过限制累积剂量，以使化疗毒性降至最低同时保持疗效。儿童肿瘤协作组最近报道了基于反应的治疗研究的结果[114]。对于晚期 HD，早期反应的患者只需接受 3 个疗程的 ABVE-PC（阿霉素、多柔比星、长春新碱、表鬼臼乙叉甙、泼尼松和环磷酰胺），而不需接受 5 个疗程，随后做 25Gy 的放疗，早期反应者和晚期反应者两组的 2 年无病生存率分别是 90.8%和 87.7%。低分期的早期反应者和晚期反应者分别接受 2 个或 4 个 ABVE 化疗，随后做放疗，两组的治疗效果无显著性差异。关于药物剂量和给药时间强化应用方面的研究目前正在进行。

放疗

在历史上，应用放疗的概念基于邻近淋巴结区的浸润。理想的话，最好用 4～8MeV 的直线加速器做治疗。中电压技术治疗是无指征的，钴 60 有明显的放射散射，这在儿童中需避免。如果给予 3500 到 4400cGy 的照射剂量，复发的风险为 10%以下。因此，临床上受累区域的照射剂量通常为 4000～4400cGy，而亚临床区的预防性治疗可以用 3000～4000cGy。化疗和放疗的联合使用是有效的，局部病灶控制率达 97%。然而，考虑到治疗的远期毒性，促使上世纪 80 年代设计出新的研究方案，包括六个疗程的化疗及低剂量（1500～2500cGy）的局部放疗。研究发现疾病的控制良好，同时减少了肌肉骨骼畸形发生[25,87]。

按危险度分级的联合化疗已经取得很好的无病生存率和总存活率。最近的研究显示，对于那些对化疗反应良好的患者，增加小剂量局部放疗提高了无病生存率，但对总存活率无影响[84]。目前，对于儿童和青少年 HD 患者，采用按危险度分级的联合治疗，包括小剂量、受累野放疗和联合多药化疗。

并发症

治疗毒性

治疗的远期不良作用包括手术并发症、软组织和骨骼生长异常、心肺作用、内分泌后遗症和第二肿
579 瘤。在中轴骨骼放疗的患者，已经注意到有坐高和站高比例的异常[97]。男孩似乎比女孩受到的影响更严重。还有锁骨的缩短、锁骨间距的减少、颈部软组织的纤维化和颈后毛发的变细。接受治疗时骨龄 14～15 岁的患儿，其生长所受的影响不明显。

治疗可能发生放疗导致的显著肺损伤，这与放疗区的容积、照射剂量和每天的分次量有关。对于接受大剂量斗篷式放疗的患者，有症状的肺损伤发生率为 3.6%。博来霉素也可以导致严重的肺功能异常。

放疗对心肌的损伤也与剂量、每次照射量和照射野有关。接受大剂量斗篷式放疗的患者中，大约 13% 出现心脏损害。冠状动脉和大血管也可能受影响。已知阿霉素也可产生心脏损害。也有报道使用长春新碱和博来霉素患者出现雷诺综合征。

内分泌影响包括甲状腺功能减退、不育和其他生殖异常。用促甲状腺素作为甲状腺功能减退的标记，4%～79%的患者出现这种并发症[19]。甲状腺异常与颈部接受的放疗剂量有关；放疗剂量小于 26Gy 的患者，有 17%出现甲状腺异常，而放疗剂量大于或等于 26Gy 的患者，78%出现甲状腺功能减退。

HD 治疗后还可出现生殖腺（包括卵巢和睾丸）功能异常[111]。骨盆照射导致卵巢功能消除的可能性极高。卵巢移位，即将卵巢移动到照射野以外，能够保存卵巢的功能和生殖能力[31]。卵巢可以移动到中线子宫后或双侧腰部。在放置卵巢区域的腹膜上必须放置一个小夹子以使放疗科医生可以识别。在男性，生殖能力是一个更重要的问题，30%～40%的患者在初诊时就存在性腺功能异常[15,88,127]。在年长患者必须考虑在治疗前冷冻精子。

第二肿瘤

第二肿瘤包括急性非淋巴细胞白血病、非 Hodgkin 淋巴瘤、甲状腺癌（通常是分化型）、乳腺癌（见于放疗患者）[8,17,59,73,125]和骨骼或软组织肉瘤。预先接受脾脏切除的患者也有可能发生白血病。MOPP 方案比 ABVD 方案出现第二肿瘤的可能性大。需要再次治疗者，由于剂量的直接作用，发生第二肿瘤的危险性较高[49]。初次接受 MOPP 方案治疗的患者其继发肿瘤的发生率为 5%～7%；如果加用了放疗则该发生率升至 10%。10 年后，白血病发生率下降，而非 Hodgkin 淋巴瘤的发生率随时间而增加，这说明持续跟踪随访的重要性。约 4%的患者会发生实体瘤。

剖腹手术并发症

分期剖腹手术并发症按时间可以分成三种：（1）早期术后并发症（术后＜6 周）；（2）远期并发症（术后＞6 月）；（3）脾切除相关败血症。Hays 等[42,43]回顾性研究了儿童 HD 国际研究协作组的 234 例分期性剖腹探查病例；在最初的报道中，55%的患儿至少随访了 2 年，在最近的报告中，随访的中位数为 5 年。在剖腹探查术后的最初 6 周中出现了 3 例肺部和 3 例腹部并发症，其总的发生率为 2.6%。这些患者包括 1 例继发手术瘢痕形成的尿路梗阻，需要手术来松解；1 例粘连导致的肠道梗阻，需要再次手术；1 例表浅伤口感染；1 例肺膨胀不全性肺炎。没有术后死亡的病例。5 例患者出现晚期术后并发症（2.1%）。4 例肠梗阻需要手术粘连松解，其中 1 例因为粘连肠段周围出现肠扭转继发穿孔需要修补。第 5 例患者由于右侧卵巢扭转继发坏死需要做切除术。这个卵巢原来在剖腹探查时被移至协腹以避免放疗的损伤。这样，剖腹探查术时出现的早期和远期并发症的总发生率是 4.7%，包括临床上明显的肺膨胀不全。

Schneeberger 和 Girvan[112]报道了 39 例做分期剖腹探查的 HD 患儿。没有手术相关的死亡，没有轻微并发症，如肺膨胀不全。有 5 例（12.8%）出现小肠梗阻，其中 4 例通过胃肠减压的非手术治疗好转，1 例在术后 11 年由于小肠粘连导致扭转而做了再次剖腹探查。Donaldson 和 Kaplan[24]报道，在儿童做剖腹探查术后早期出现明显的非致死的并发症的发生率为 1%。此研究中明显的并发症包括：伤口感染和裂开、膈下脓肿、肺部感染、腹膜后血肿、胰腺炎和明显的术后出血。一般的术后轻度肺膨胀不全没有包括在其中。在其他研究中，远期并发症如粘连性的肠道梗阻

的发生率为 3%～12%，甚至在未接受腹部放疗的患儿中也有发生[50]。

脾脏切除的并发症

King 和 Shumacker[56]在 1952 年最早注意到脾切除术后的感染易感性增加，从那以后，许多报道证实了这一说法[29,119]。在幼儿中脾切除术后败血症发生率增高，特别是那些年龄小于 10 岁的患儿。在解释 HD 患儿接受脾切除的临床资料时，应该牢记疾病本身和化疗药物的免疫抑制作用。

随着 Chilcote 等人[16]在 1976 年的报道，脾切除在 HD 患儿中的使用受到严厉的质疑。这是一项针对儿童肿瘤研究协作组各合作单位中 200 例 19 岁及以下患儿的回顾性研究。该研究发现，18 例患儿出现 20 次败血症，脾切除至出现败血症的间隔时间为 8 天至 3 年。出现败血症的中位年龄为 10 岁。除 3 例外均接受过或正在接受化疗，除了 2 例外均接受过放疗。病源包括肺炎双球菌、流感嗜血杆菌、链球菌和脑膜炎球菌。其中 10 例死于败血症，大多数为一个暴发性发病过程。值得注意的是，只有两个合作单位使用预防性抗生素，而他们均没有严重感染病例的报道。整个随访时间间隔并没提及。

儿童 HD 国际研究协作组随后对脾切除后败血症发生率的分析显示，随着疫苗和预防性抗生素的使用，这已不再是一个问题[42]。在这个协作组的第 1 次报告中，55%患者随访时间大于 2 年，只有 2 例患者出现明确的败血症。另 2 例患者在复发后进行化疗中出现败血症。另有 3 例可疑的败血症，但血培养是阴性的。最重要的是，这组研究没死亡病例。值得注意的是，83%患儿在脾切除前进行肺炎双球菌疫苗接种，74%患儿使用预防性抗生素。该研究的进一步中位随访时间为 5.5 年，败血症患儿总数达 5 例，但仍没有死亡病例。其中 2 例患儿血中分离到肺炎双球菌，其余 3 例为流感嗜血杆菌。出现败血症的 5 例患儿，4 例曾使用肺炎双球菌疫苗，但只有 3 例在术前接种。4 例患儿在出现败血症前曾使用抗生素不规则或曾停止使用。出现败血症患儿组诊断时的年龄范围是 4～14 岁，中位年龄 9 岁。另有 5 例患儿病情较重，由于对抗生素效应良好被认为有败血症；这些患儿的血培养为阴性，没有死亡病例。该项研究随访时间超过 5 年，发现 5 例（2.1%）确诊和 5 例可疑败血症患儿，该并发症的死亡率为[0]。

由脾切除导致的体液免疫缺陷是永久性的，然而，在做过剖腹探查的 HD 存活患儿中，可以预测将出现脾切除后感染的病例[105]。从儿童 HD 研究协作组的资料（5.5 年中的发生率为 2.1%）可推算出：每年败血症的发生率为 0.38%，根据推算，在 50 年中约 20%的脾切除的 HD 患儿将出现该并发症[96]。而成人的败血症发生率将下降，并随年龄增加而下降，因此这个发生率或许是高估的。患儿生存期间的败血症累积风险目前未知。

肿瘤转移和复发的治疗

难治性和复发病例的补救治疗有赖于发病时初次治疗方案。最初单纯接受放疗的患者 50%～80%能通过化疗和联合治疗方案治愈。早期患儿接受联合治疗，晚期患儿按危险度分级接受治疗方案，近 90% Hodgkin 淋巴瘤可以通过初始治疗方案治愈。然而，对于难治性和复发病例，加大治疗剂量和自体干细胞移植是最佳的选择。外周血干细胞的使用使移植相关的死亡率下降至 3%以下，但长期无疾病进展存活率没有明显提高[77-79]。

预后因素

目前 HD 的治疗方案是按危险度调整的治疗。诊断时的危险因素有 B 症状、年龄、分期、淋巴结大小和受累淋巴结区的数量。只有局部淋巴结受累和没有 B 症状的患儿临床预后较好。那些有 B 症状、纵隔或外周淋巴结巨大肿块、结外浸润、和晚期患者（IIIB 到Ⅳ期）临床预后较差。预后较差患者接受标准的无交叉耐药化疗，随后给予低剂量受累野部位的巩固性放疗。此外，也有简化的大剂量的联合化疗加放疗方案正在评估之中。早期效应与预后有关，并反映出肿瘤的负荷和生物学特性[12]。

结果

单独采用按危险度调整的化疗方案，其 5 年存活率高于 90%，无病生存率大于 85%。选择合适治疗方案的目标是保持高存活率，减少复发率，并将长期副作用降低到最小。

非 Hodgkin淋巴瘤

非 Hodgkin 淋巴瘤分为 Burkitt 和 Burkitt 样淋巴瘤、淋巴母细胞性淋巴瘤、弥漫性大 B 细胞淋巴瘤、和间变性大细胞性淋巴瘤。对这些肿瘤的解剖学分布至少部分能通过正常的 B 和 T 细胞的个体发育来理解。

发生率和流行病学

在美国，每年有 750～800 例初发非 Hodgkin 淋
581 巴瘤患者[93]。在 20 岁以下人群中，Burkitt 和 Burkitt 样淋巴瘤在男性中的发病率比女性高 5 倍（1 百万人群中发病率分别为 3.3 和 0.7）。5 岁后，Burkitt 淋巴瘤的发生率上升，15 岁后发生率下降。相反的是，弥漫性大细胞淋巴瘤随着年龄增长而上升，男女发病率的比为 1.4。淋巴母细胞性淋巴瘤在 20 岁以下人群中的发生率相似，男女发病率的比为 2.5。

生物学

淋巴细胞个体发育和分化

虽然关于淋巴细胞发育的详细过程讨论不在本章节范围内，但简单的介绍有助于我们理解各种组织学亚型和它们独特的临床表现。我们目前对正常和病理的免疫系统的理解的基础是基于这样一个认识，即 B 和 T 细胞有功能上独立的部分[68,76,130]。第二个重要概念是成熟的淋巴细胞不是终末期细胞，在有抗原存在时，能经过转化而成为效应细胞。淋巴系发育的概念可以理解像是从干细胞到活性细胞的分化过程。当有合适的刺激因子时，细胞随后经转化而成为效应表型。B 细胞分化的简化图解见图 35-4。B 细胞在骨髓中起源于多能干细胞，通过许多中间相的分化最终成为产生抗体的浆细胞。在分化过程的任何点上都可以发生恶性转化，这样产生了一些临床上可识别的综合征或组织病理亚型。对于小儿外科感兴趣的是 B 细胞，在可以检测到免疫球蛋白 M（IgM）（见图 35-4）的发育阶段，它可以经过恶性转化成为未分化淋巴瘤。由于它们在光学显微镜下的表现，也被称为小无裂细胞淋巴瘤。Burkitt 淋巴瘤就是这些未分化淋巴瘤的一个亚型。由于 B 细胞在骨髓中发育，然后迁移入次级淋巴器官（淋巴结、脾脏、Peyer 结和肝脏），可以想象到在这些解剖结构中肿瘤发育时的临床定位。作为一个推论，B 细胞淋巴瘤应该不会出现在前纵隔胸腺的区域，因为正常的 B 细胞不是胸腺依赖的。通常这个解剖学分布与临床观察到的还是一致的，但并不全是这样。在美国，Burkitt 淋巴瘤好发于腹部（在非洲赤道西部，Burkitt 淋巴瘤常出现于下颚，但腹部淋巴瘤也在这些患者中占到 20%以上）。扁桃腺和睾丸的 Burkitt 淋巴瘤（复发部位）也有报道，但前纵隔的 Burkitt 淋巴瘤是极为罕见的[53,57]。

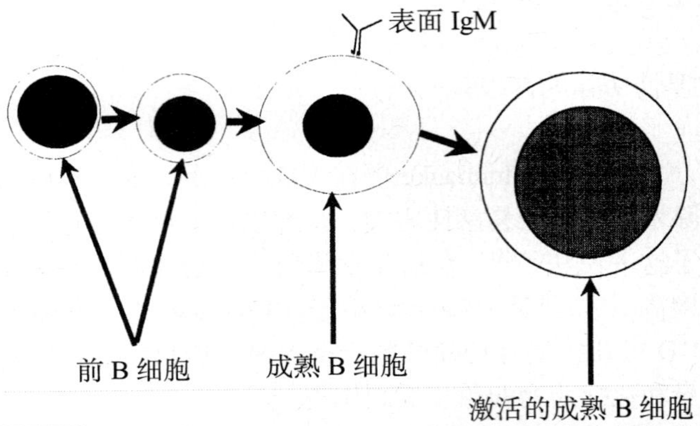

图 35-4 B 细胞分化途径简图。未分化淋巴细胞在细胞表达表面 IgM 后出现。

T 细胞分化的简化图示见图 35-5。由于胸腺是 T 细胞发育必要的部位，大多数前纵隔淋巴瘤起源于 T 细胞系。50%～70%的淋巴母细胞性淋巴瘤（T 细胞）表现为胸廓内肿瘤，通常为前纵隔肿块；表现为腹部肿块的少见。一般，淋巴瘤好发于 T 细胞或 B 细胞依赖的淋巴系统解剖区域，而淋巴瘤也表达他们各自特异的 T 或 B 淋巴细胞表面标记。有意思的是，发现胸腺摘除阻止了小鼠的 T 淋巴瘤，而法氏囊摘除阻止了鸡的 B 淋巴瘤[92,105]。

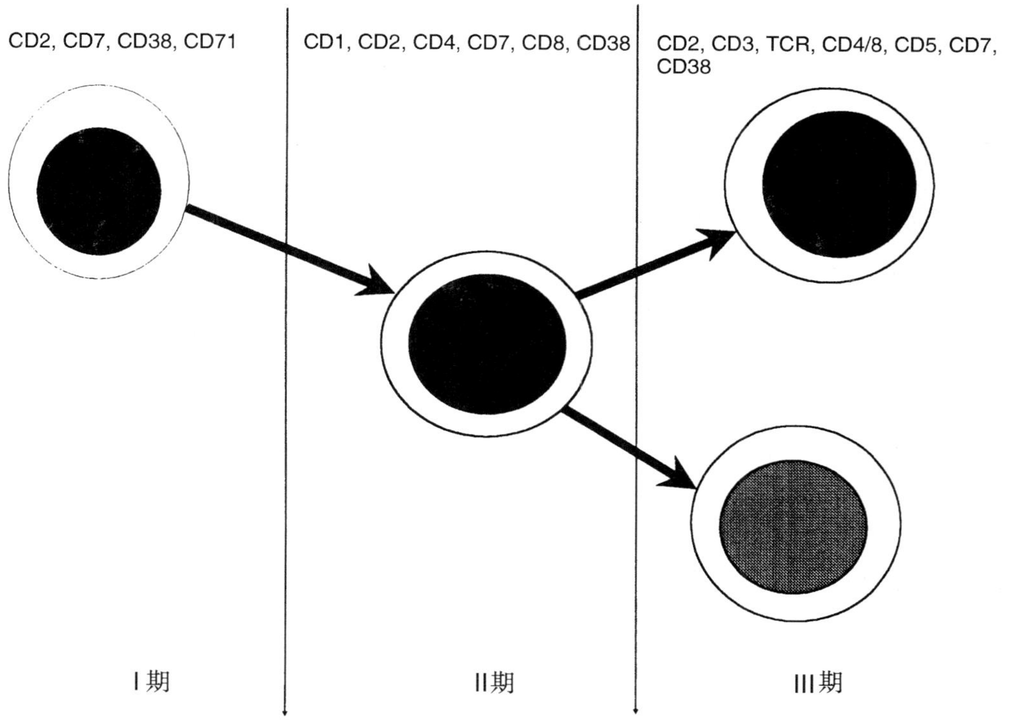

图 35-5　T 细胞分化简图。淋巴母细胞性淋巴瘤通常表达末端脱氧核苷酸转移酶。T 细胞在分化过程中必须经过胸腺。

细胞遗传学和分子生物学发现

1976 年，在 Burkitt 淋巴瘤中发现了特征性的涉及 8 和 14 号染色体的易位。随后研究显示，8 号染色体的 c-myc 原癌基因转位到 14 号染色体的免疫球蛋白重链[135]。最后，研究发现在少数 Burkitt 淋巴瘤中，8;14 易位被 8;22 或 2;8 易位代替[99]。这仍涉及 8 号染色体的 c-myc 基因。这些少见病例的异常是 2 号染色体的 κ 轻链或 22 号染色体的 λ 轻链取代了免疫球蛋白重链。这样，一个原癌基因始终与一个免疫球蛋白编码序列并列。由于 Burkitt 淋巴瘤是 B 细胞源性的，因此认为这些涉及已知的原癌基因和免疫球蛋白编码序列的细胞遗传学异常不是巧合性的，而是有病理生理学基础的。随后的研究显示，易位的 c-myc 基因通过连接到免疫球蛋白编码区域而被激活[6]。这可能导致这个分化阶段的 B 淋巴细胞的 c-myc RNA 和蛋白的异常表达[72]。

与小无裂细胞淋巴瘤的大量细胞遗传学信息相反的是，大多数淋巴母细胞性淋巴瘤没有特异的非随机性的突变类型[58]。小部分 T 细胞源性的淋巴母细胞淋巴瘤有染色体易位，大多数涉及 14 号染色体（14q11）的 T cc 区域和 8 受体基因（T 细胞受体），或靠近 Tβ 的 7 号染色体[21]。这与 B 细胞淋巴瘤涉及的免疫球蛋白编码区域类似。细胞遗传学和分子生物学分析资料提供了重要的淋巴细胞肿瘤性恶变的分子机制。

淋巴瘤亚型和病理组织学

关于免疫系统个体发育的简述是为了对三种儿童非 Hodgkin 淋巴瘤亚型的理解奠定基础：（1）未分化型的，也称之为小无裂细胞淋巴瘤；（2）淋巴母细胞型；（3）大细胞型（弥漫性大 B 细胞和间变性大细胞淋巴瘤）。与其他在成年患者中出现的类型相反的是这三种类型均被认为是高危型。例外的是某些有中心滤泡细胞类型的大细胞淋巴瘤，被认为是中危的，但在儿童和青少年中少见。未分化型淋巴瘤原发于腹部，起源于 B 系祖细胞。恶性变发生于分化时细胞核裂解前。根据光镜下形态学不同分为 Burkitt 淋巴瘤和非 Burkitt 淋巴瘤。Burkitt 淋巴瘤的特征是核大小中等，与中间穿插的良性组织细胞核大小相当，这提供了一个简便的测量方法，并被称为“星空”现象（图 35-6）。通常有 2～5 个明显的嗜碱性

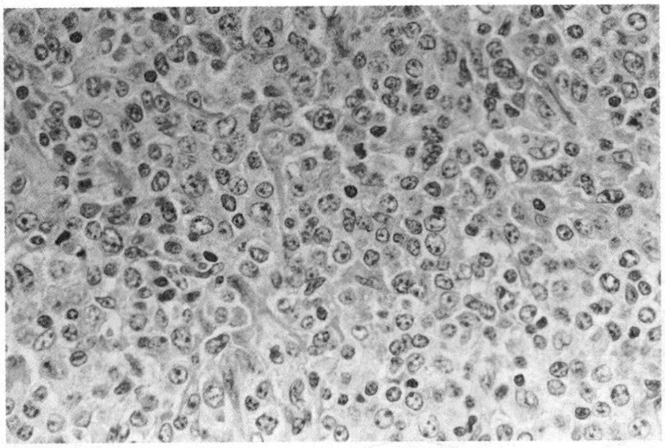

图 35–6　1 例 Burkitt 淋巴瘤患者的组织病理切片，显示多个明显的核仁。

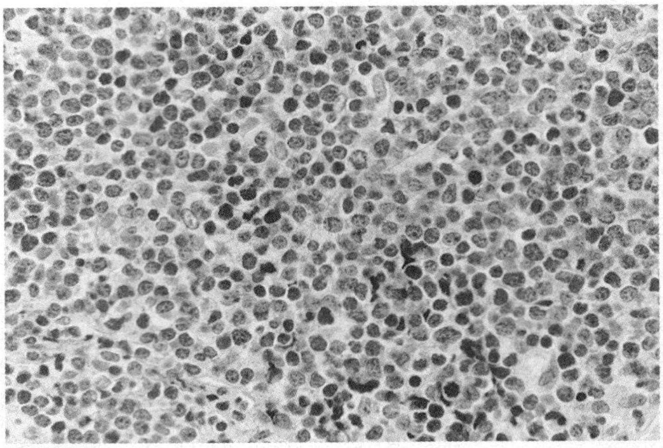

图 35–7　典型的淋巴母细胞性淋巴瘤切片。黑染细胞是正常淋巴细胞。

核仁。核 / 浆比例高。非 Burkitt 淋巴瘤常表现为单个大细胞核，在核仁的大小和形状上变化更多。非 Burkitt 小无裂细胞淋巴瘤往往发病年龄晚，外周淋巴结或骨髓浸润发生率高。两者之间无细胞遗传学、免疫组化或分子生物学标记的区别。
583 小无裂细胞淋巴瘤表达 IgM 的表面免疫球蛋白和可以被单克隆抗体 CD19 和 CD20 检测的表面抗原[109]。它们不含末端脱氧核苷酸转移酶，而在淋巴母细胞型淋巴瘤常能发现这种酶。小无裂细胞淋巴瘤必须与小细胞结节性淋巴瘤相区别，后者见于成人并有更缓慢的病程。

淋巴母细胞性淋巴瘤主要位于前纵隔，特征为淋巴结结构的弥漫性消失。由于肿瘤细胞沿正常组织延伸，可以出现小叶表现。细胞学上，核比散在的组织细胞要小，而核仁不明显（图 35–7）。可以看到“星空”现象，核 / 浆比例比小无裂细胞淋巴瘤还要高。半数病例的核膜是卷绕或裂开的。总能发现末端脱氧核苷酸转移酶，大多数淋巴母细胞性淋巴瘤表达 T 细胞标记，包括 CD7 或 CD5[65]。

大细胞性淋巴瘤（弥漫性大细胞淋巴瘤）通常是高危的。就像前面提及的，中心滤泡细胞类型的大细胞淋巴瘤被认为是中危，但有侵袭性生物行为。正常的淋巴结结构被核大胞浆少的瘤细胞所取代（图 35–8）。细胞核比侵袭性组织细胞要大。这些细胞较大并开裂，有裂开的细胞核，而核仁不明显。另一种细胞类型是大的开裂的细胞，有较窄的环形细胞浆，可以看见明显的固缩核仁。这两种细胞类型可以同时在一个肿瘤中出现。儿童肿瘤协作组所做的一项研究把大细胞淋巴瘤分成两种亚型[85]。第一种是大细

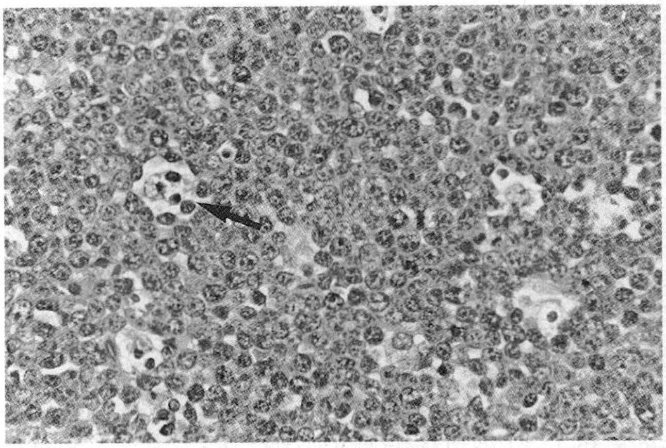

图 35–8　典型的弥漫性大细胞淋巴瘤切片。数个巨噬细胞（箭头所示）正在吞噬肿瘤细胞。

胞的、开裂或未开裂的淋巴瘤，起自淋巴滤泡的生发中心，来源于 B 细胞。第二种大细胞淋巴瘤是免疫母细胞性，大多数起源于 T 系前体细胞。免疫母细胞性大细胞淋巴瘤的类浆细胞亚型被认为是 B 细胞起源。大多数大细胞淋巴瘤表达 Ki–1 抗原，该抗原也见于镜影细胞，是 T 细胞源性的[4,104,113]。

应该强调，所有儿童非 Burkitt 淋巴瘤是弥散性的，生长很快。这与成人淋巴瘤的结节性和生长缓慢型的淋巴瘤相反。因此，儿童淋巴瘤从诊断开始，应该按照全身性疾病治疗，早期进行多药联合化疗。据估计，部分儿童淋巴瘤的生长分数达 100%，若不考虑到细胞自然死亡（凋亡），则未修正的倍增时间慢至 12 小时至数天。在皮下注射小无裂细胞淋巴瘤的小鼠中，考虑到细胞死亡的因素前提下得到的倍增时

间平均为 3 天。据估计，非洲 Burkitt 淋巴瘤的细胞死亡率占细胞的 70%。儿童未分化 B 细胞淋巴瘤的生长分数最高，流式细胞仪检测约 27%的细胞处于 S 期[47,48]。

临床表现

未分化淋巴瘤

在美国，非 Hodgkin 淋巴瘤患儿表现出少数特定的综合征，这和细胞类型有关。小无裂细胞性淋巴瘤 90%以上表现为腹部可触及的肿块[7,132]。肿瘤可以导致腹部疼痛、腹胀、排便习惯改变、恶心、呕吐、肠梗阻、肠套迭、肠道出血、腹水或肠穿孔。通常，这种淋巴瘤表现为右髂窝肿块，易和阑尾炎或阑尾脓肿混淆。患者可以有腹股沟或髂窝淋巴结肿大。腹腔内广泛浸润的患者可以出现乏力、倦怠和体重减轻。图 35-9 显示了 1 例肝脏几乎全部被移位肿瘤替代的广泛性腹部 Burkitt 淋巴瘤。有意思的是，赤道非洲的 Burkitt 淋巴瘤虽然常表现为弥漫性下颌部肿瘤，但 50%以上患者也有腹部肿块。在美国，起病时其他受累部位包括骨髓、胸膜渗出液、脑脊液、中枢神经系统、外周淋巴结、肾脏和咽部[57,132]。美国和非洲患者中卵巢也是经常发病的部位[80]。

临床实际应用中，腹部非 Hodgkin 淋巴瘤患者可以被分成两组。第一组的疾病局限于腹部。肿瘤常浸润肠壁，许多患儿表现为阑尾炎或肠套迭等急腹症。大多数可以做肿瘤的完全切除，一般只要做简单的肠道切除和吻合术，基本上极少致死。第二组为腹部肿瘤广泛浸润，很可能表现为腹部巨大肿块而无急腹症。肠系膜根部和后腹膜重度浸润，完全切除后并发症的发生率更高。

淋巴母细胞性淋巴瘤

50%～70%的淋巴母细胞性淋巴瘤患者表现为前纵隔或胸廓内（或两者均有）肿块。图 35-10 显示为 1 例纵隔淋巴母细胞性淋巴瘤患者的胸部 CT 扫描。这些肿瘤可以与 HD 的中纵隔肿块相鉴别，但这往往是不可行的，特别是出现纵隔内巨大肿块的时候。50%～80%患者有横膈上淋巴结病，包括颈部、锁骨上和腋窝等区域。腹部受累并不常见，但当出现时常有肝脾肿大。该型的骨髓浸润较为常见，难以与急性淋巴细胞性白血病鉴别。这些患者按照淋巴细胞性白血病方案治疗的效果会更好。胸膜渗出较为常见，患者可能会主诉呼吸困难、胸痛或吞咽困难。腔静脉综合征，即面部、胸部和上肢水肿、躯干上部和肩部浅表静脉扩张，或气道压迫出现严重的呼吸困难或端坐呼吸（或两者均有），常意味着要紧急进行化疗或放疗[1,132]。诊断时，中枢神经系统受累罕见。

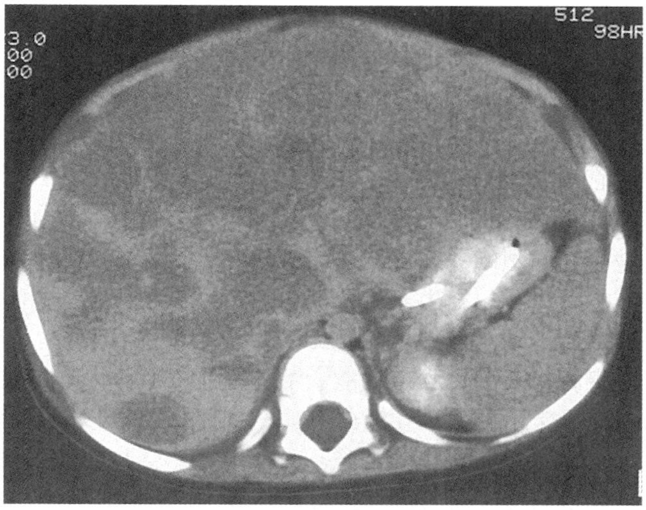

图 35-9　1 例 Burkitt 淋巴瘤患者的腹部 CT 扫描显示几乎整个肝脏被肿瘤取代。通过骨穿做出诊断。

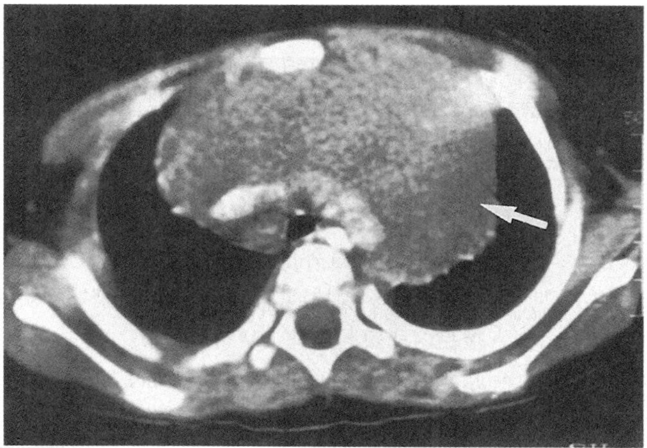

图 35-10　1 例淋巴母细胞性淋巴瘤患者的胸部 CT 扫描发现一个大的前纵隔肿块（箭头所示）。气管发生移位但未受压迫。

大细胞淋巴瘤

大细胞淋巴瘤的原发部位与小无裂细胞淋巴瘤相似。然而，一些少见的部位也可能会出现，例如 B 细胞大细胞淋巴瘤出现于前纵隔。Ki-1 阳性（间变性，通常是 T 细胞源性的）大细胞淋巴瘤除了胃肠道外，还常累及皮肤、中枢神经系统、淋巴结、肺部、睾丸和肌肉。大细胞淋巴瘤更可能原发于肺部、面部和颅内[86,106,108]。临床最常见的表现是肿块的进行性增大。

移植后淋巴组织增生病

移植后淋巴组织增生病（PTLD）是同种异基因移植后发生的并发症，可以不断进展危及生命。实体器官和骨髓移植都可以发生。在做 T 细胞去除的骨髓移植、无关供体移植、发生 GVHD 的患者，尤其是接受强烈的免疫抑制剂方案治疗（包括接受抗胸腺球蛋白）后，发生 PLTD 的可能性在增加。做骨髓移植后由于供体 B 细胞被 EBV 转化而发生 PTLD。这
585 些患者常表现胃肠道功能紊乱，如恶心和呕吐，或肝功能异常。原发消化道的肿瘤，内镜活检可以明确诊断。为了寻找转化的细胞，常需取多个活检组织。肝脏病变可以通过腹腔镜或经皮活检来明确[38,45,92,120,122]。

PLTD 的治疗包括停止使用免疫抑制剂和给予抗 CD-20 单克隆抗体（美罗华）。此外，已经开发了多种针对抗 EBV 转化细胞的靶向细胞治疗策略，包括再次输注少量供体淋巴细胞。外科切除是不起作用的。

诊断

非 Hodgkin 淋巴瘤可疑患者的检查包括详细的病史和体格检查。随后做血常规、肝功能（包括 LDH、电解质、尿素氮、肌苷和尿酸）、胸片、骨穿和腰穿做脑脊液甩片行细胞学检查。常需做四个部位的骨穿和两个部位的骨髓活检以了解骨髓受累情况，骨髓受累导致严重的并发症对预后影响很大。镓-67 扫描和胸腹部口服及静脉造影剂 CT 增强检查能够提供有用的关于肿瘤部位和分布的资料。镓能被恶性淋巴细胞（特别是小无裂细胞）摄取，而能较好的做全身扫描。骨扫描能发现可疑的骨骼受累。MRI 可以发挥作用，特别是评估硬膜外肿瘤，但可能不是非常必要的检查。正电子发射 X 线断层摄影术的作用仍在研究中。

分期

在非 Hodgkin 淋巴瘤患者中不做分期性剖腹探查术，因为所有患者均要求做全身性化疗。由于腹部并发症，如肠套迭、出血或为了得到诊断用的组织，许多患者也要做外科干预。小儿外科医生必须意识到儿童淋巴瘤是一个全身性疾病，手术必须不能耽搁化疗。HD 的 Ann Arbor 分期不适用于非 Hodgkin 淋巴

表 35-3　St. Jude 儿童研究医院的非 Hodgkin 淋巴瘤的分期系统 *

分期	未分化型	分期	淋巴母细胞型
I	单个腹腔以外肿块	I	单个胸腔以外肿块
IR	切除的（>90%）腹腔肿块	II	除 BM 和 CNS 外的多个胸腔以外肿块
II	除 BM 和 CNS 外的多个腹腔以外肿块	IIIA	单个胸腺肿块
IIIA	腹腔未切除肿块或非 IV 期的硬脑膜外肿块	IIIB	有胸水的纵隔肿块
IIIB	腹腔内和腹腔外除 BM 外的肿块	IVA	有胸腔外延伸的纵隔肿块（无 BM 或 CNS 浸润）
IVA	原发 BM，没有腹部或 CNS 浸润	IVB	BM 和胸腔内肿块，没有 CNS 或其他胸腔外浸润
IVB	BM 和腹部肿瘤，没有 CNS 浸润	IVC	BM 和胸腔外肿块，没有 CNS 浸润
IVC	CNS 肿瘤（肿瘤细胞出现于脑脊	IVD	BM 和 CNS 疾病

* 在诊断时检查肿瘤负荷，这是预后的主要判断指标。

BM：骨髓；CNS：中枢神经系统。

瘤，许多协作组试图建立更合适的分期[5,82]。目前，尚没有令人满意的分期标准，更重要的是测量发病时肿瘤的体积，而不是急着把肿瘤归类到分期中。非 Hodgkin 淋巴瘤患儿中最广泛应用的分期体系是来自 St. Jude 儿童研究医院（表 35–3）。儿童肿瘤协作组把非 Hodgkin 淋巴瘤分成两类：局限的和广泛的。前者与 St. Jude 体系的 I 和 II 期相应，后者与 III 和 IV 期相应[81]。

治疗

手术治疗

Magrath 等[70]基于他们对治疗乌干达腹部 Burkitt 淋巴瘤患者的丰富经验，认为减瘤手术对存活有较好的影响。回顾性研究发现这个结论存在几个问题。首先，没有评估诊断时疾病的程度对预后的影响。随后的研究发现，对预后影响最大的因素是疾病的程度。其次，实际上 68 个病例中只有 9 例做了肿瘤的完全切除（定义为切除范围＞90%切除）。绝大多数仅做了活检（63%）或次全切除术（24%）。这个研究强烈建议对完全切除术患者做生物学选择。此外，患者只受到单药化疗（环磷酰胺），而目前标准的是多药联合并根据组织病理选择针对性的方案。最后，该研
86 究报道的手术死亡率为 10%，在目前条件下这是过高的。

Kemeny 等人[55]评价了在美国 Burkitt 淋巴瘤患者中，手术对原发肿瘤和其并发症的治疗作用。他们认为完全切除有好处，但也指出疾病的程度没有被作为一个独立变量分析。他们也提倡手术作为非 Hodgkin 淋巴瘤的支持治疗。前面讲到过，小无裂细胞淋巴瘤有特别高的生长分数。因尿酸性肾病导致的肾衰竭是真正的危险，当后腹膜肿块导致机械性尿路梗阻时，亦可并发肾衰竭。此外，可能发生肿瘤溶解综合征，特别是在小无裂细胞淋巴瘤的诱导化疗期间[18,126]。最后，多种消化道并发症，包括出血、梗阻或穿孔，可能发生。作者指出，手术可以提供血管通道以用于透析或水化、及在梗阻部位做输尿管内支架和为消化道并发症做根治性的手术。

除了小的容易切除的肿块，最初的外科治疗应该仅用于诊断的切开性活检，随后进行强化的联合化疗。关于手术对腹部 Burkitt 淋巴瘤的作用研究资料显示，疾病的程度与手术切除程度相比是一个更有意义的预后预测因素[115]。广泛腹部浸润的肿瘤患者做手术治疗是不可能完全切除肿块的，并可能使并发症发生率增加，从而导致化疗的延迟[115]。

同样，儿童癌症协作组（CCG）的外科委员会在 CCG-551 研究中评估了 68 例非 Hodgkin 淋巴瘤患者手术治疗的作用[60]。分析的变量包括：（1）诊断时疾病程度；（2）手术切除程度；（3）原发部位的放疗；（4）性别、年龄和种族。67 例患者（99%）做了剖腹手术，其中 28 例（42%）做了完全整体切除。诊断时的年龄、性别和种族对无病生存率无影响。肿瘤负荷是最重要的预后因素。肿瘤的完全切除也是一项重要的无病生存预测因素，但没有肿瘤负荷显得重要。10 个出现手术并发症的患者，8 例肿瘤分布广泛而切除不完全。这些资料支持完全切除在肿瘤局限时有用，尤其当肿瘤局限于肠道时。在这些情况下，肿瘤切除通过减少肿瘤负荷和防止某些并发症，如肠道穿孔，而对治疗有益[75]。由于可导致明显的出血或败

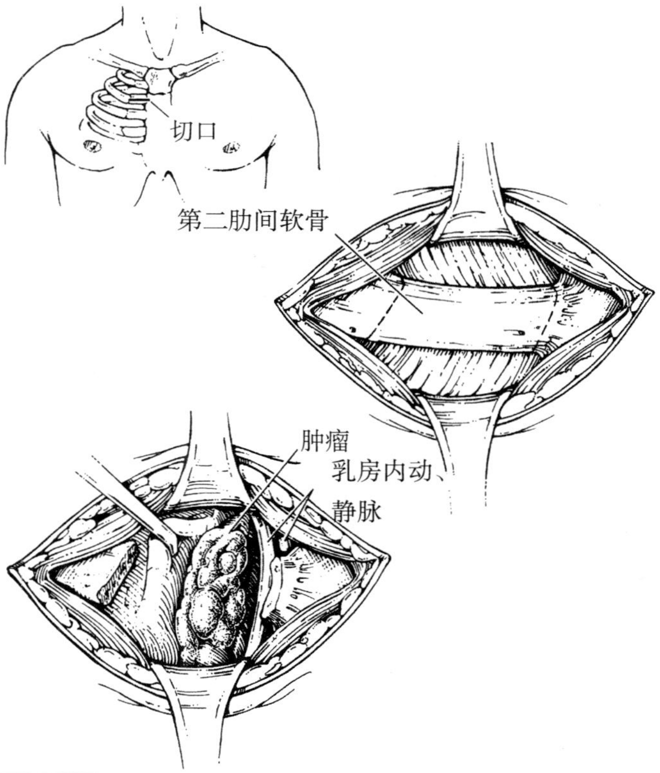

图 35–11　前纵隔切开术，或称 Chamberlain 法。当较低损伤的诊断技术如淋巴结活检、骨穿或胸腔穿刺术不能明确淋巴瘤诊断时，这是一个有用的方法。

血症等并发症，所以避免做后腹膜广泛探查，因此化疗应迅速开始。

巨大后腹膜肿块或肝脏巨大淋巴瘤切除的尝试使并发症发生率增加，并使化疗延期。由于未分化淋巴瘤生长如此迅速，所以这是特别有害的。腹部肿瘤分布广泛的患儿，常能通过骨穿做诊断，因为临床上至少 20%患者有明显的骨髓受累（症状，骨扫描阳性），另有 20%的患者临床上未怀疑，但有显微镜下受累表现。其他可用于诊断的组织包括腹水和胸腔积液、外周淋巴结或局部骨病变活检，有时可用穿刺针做活检。肿瘤可以侵入肠壁并发生坏疽，导致穿孔和腹膜炎或严重的出血。通常，Burkitt 淋巴瘤位于右下腹肠道集合淋巴结区域，症状与急性阑尾炎相似。在这种情况下，切除回盲部和临近的肠系膜常可以达到完全切除。

有纵隔巨大肿块的患者在术前需要仔细的评估；术前通过临床和影像学检查做气道的评估是至关紧要的。胸部平片和 CT 扫描能够显示气道压迫的程度。由于颈部、锁骨上和腋窝淋巴结浸润接近 50%，在局麻下做诊断性活检避免了麻醉和气道处理中的风险。恶性胸腔积液的穿刺也可以为诊断提供标本。如果要
587 做胸腔内活检，可能需要改变麻醉技术以使患者能安全插管。在肿瘤治疗前，通常不能行术后拔管，患儿应该置于 ICU 中[29]。图 35-11 描述了纵隔肿瘤切开术或 Chamberlain 前纵隔切开术。这个方法对纵隔巨大肿块但没有可接近的淋巴结可用于活检的情况有用。根据 CT 结果，它可以从纵隔任何一侧进入，一般不需放置胸腔引流。目前，关于纵隔淋巴瘤手术切除的作用尚没有定论，故没有做手术切除的指征。

很少有纵隔淋巴母细胞性淋巴瘤的患者出现恶性心包积液和心脏填塞。如果临床表现明显，包括心动过速、呼吸急促、颈静脉怒张、奇脉和心音遥远，则必须做急诊心脏超声检查。通过心包穿刺引流。大量心包积液都能通过心包穿刺置管排出[74]。

能够更彻底的探查胸腔和腹部而没有大手术的相关并发症，且损伤最少的技术，可能在非 Hodgkin 淋巴瘤患儿的诊断、分期和治疗中是最理想的状况。虽然前瞻性或随机研究发现这种手术的作用仍是不确定的，但儿童肿瘤协作组和 CCG 均正在研究其在疾病过程中的最终作用。对于淋巴增殖性疾病，腹腔镜在以下情况中是可以选择的方法：（1）与肝脏或脾脏的局灶性病变鉴别；（2）经皮穿刺活检失败或需要做遗传学分析以指导治疗；（3）对于因没有外周淋巴结受累的后腹膜弥漫性病变需要初步诊断和分期的患者；（4）放化疗后需要重新分期的患者和怀疑复发的患者技术上不能施行经皮穿刺活检时；（5）以及淋巴增殖性疾病患者需要做脾脏切除时仍然是最佳的方法[110,116,117,129]。

明显的骨髓转移能够导致严重的血小板减少症；因此，术前应该做血常规检查及血小板计数。肝脏浸润将影响血清凝血因子的产生，因此手术前准备时应该做全套的凝血功能筛查。

非 Hodgkin 淋巴瘤患者在其他途径无法获得标本时，外科手术能取得足够的活检组织。如果骨穿能够获得足够的诊断性标本，则没必要再行损伤性手术。当出现急腹症或其他手段无法获取足够用于诊断的组织时，则需行剖腹手术。类似的，胸腔或纵隔手术，例如 Chamberlain 前纵隔切开术，在设计和施行时应该尽量减少手术损伤以尽早进行全身性化疗。术前必须排除危及生命的代谢和血液学问题，并确保气道通畅。外科医生必须确保组织保存运送的安全以用于免疫组化、免疫分型和细胞遗传学检查。腹部肿块局限的患儿，特别是当肿瘤局限于部分肠段时，如果能迅速完成且并发症很少，应该做完全性切除。患者如果出现肠系膜或后腹膜的广泛受累，或表现为巨大实质性肿块，则最好用损伤最小的办法来取得活检组织，并尽快开始合适的联合化疗。纵隔或颈部肿块应该做诊断性活检，而避免做肿块的完全切除。采用腹腔镜和胸腔镜诊断和治疗非 Hodgkin 淋巴瘤可能是有用的办法。由于这些技术损伤很小，全身的治疗能很快开始，不会耽搁，因此将是有用的办法。已经有一些协作组在评价实体瘤患者中使用微创手术的研究。

化疗

儿童非 Hodgkin 淋巴瘤在诊断时就已出现播散。发现肿瘤局限的患儿经过完全切除后总是会在远处（如骨髓和脑脊液）复发，这点支持了以上这个概念[46,131]。因此，有效的治疗方案必须是全身性的，化疗就是最基本的治疗形式。历史上，在 Wollner 等人的开创性工作前，非 Hodgkin 淋巴瘤患者 5 年存活率只有 20%～30%[28,133,134]。在 1975 年，借鉴急性淋巴细胞白血病的治疗方案，LSA2-L2 取得了 73%的存活率。与此同时，Ziegler 等人[71,136]报道了用 COMP 方案

（环磷酰胺、长春新碱、甲氨蝶呤和泼尼松）成功的治疗了非 Hodgkin 淋巴瘤患者。儿童癌症研究协作组在 1977 年开始了一项随机研究（CCG-551）[3]，通过在诊断时随机分组的方法来比较这两个大剂量化疗方案的治疗效果。研究结果显示，儿童非 Hodgkin 淋巴瘤的治疗必须考虑到组织病理类型。下面对这个研究做了简单的归纳。CCG-551 研究的 2 年无病生存率是 60%。非局限性肿瘤和淋巴母细胞性组织类型的患儿接受 LSA2-L2 方案治疗后，其 2 年无病生存率为 76%，而接受 COMP 方案的类似患儿的 2 年无病生存率只有 26%（P =0.00002）。相反的是，在非局限性、未分化（小无裂细胞）非 Hodgkin 淋巴瘤中，COMP 方案的无病生存率为 57%，LSA2-L2 方案的无病生存率为 28%（P =0.02）。淋巴母细胞性非 Hodgkin 淋巴瘤接受 LSA2-L2 方案化疗的效果明显更好，而 COMP 方案对于未分化类型的非 Hodgkin 淋巴瘤更有效。

对于各个分期和组织病理类型的非 Hodgkin 淋巴瘤来说，化疗是最主要的治疗形式。考虑到高生长分
88 数，特别是未分化的非 Hodgkin 淋巴瘤，尽早开始化疗是至关紧要的。

非 Hodgkin 淋巴瘤的化疗方案不断取得进展，部分方案列于表 35-4。许多局限性肿块类型的淋巴瘤仍接受 COMP 化疗。纵隔 T 细胞性淋巴瘤的方案与淋巴母细胞性淋巴瘤相似或相同，而 LSA2-L2 方案不再广泛应用。小无裂细胞淋巴瘤，包括 Burkitt 淋巴瘤的方案强度更强但耐受性更差。支持性的 G-CSF 使用能够缩短中心粒细胞减少所致发热的再住院时间[61,66,91]。抗 CD20 单克隆抗体已经被应用于难治性或复发的 B 细胞淋巴瘤[118]。但尚无关于儿童淋巴瘤的研究报道。

放疗

在局限性的非 Hodgkin 淋巴瘤治疗中，放疗增加了毒性而对治疗无益[26,83]。相反的，体外放射治疗不能用于治疗多个解剖部位广泛浸润的患者。目前，放疗保留用于一些特定的紧急情况，如纵隔浸润伴气道梗阻或睾丸巨大浸润。通过鞘注 MTX 和 Ara-C 能达到常规中枢神经系统的预防[69]。最近大量的研究一直表明，非 Hodgkin 淋巴瘤通过化疗取得满意的疗效，而无需放疗[37,63,101]。

并发症

表 35-4　非 Hodgkin 淋巴瘤的治疗方案

淋巴母细胞性淋巴瘤		小无裂淋巴瘤	
I、II 期	**III、IV 期**	**I、II 期**	**III、IV 期**
长春新碱、阿霉素、环磷酰胺、泼尼松、巯基嘌呤、甲氨蝶呤[64]	BFM-NHL90：泼尼松、地塞米松、长春新碱、柔红霉素、阿霉素、L-Asp、环磷酰胺、阿糖胞苷、甲氨蝶呤、6-MP、6-TG、CNS 放疗[37]	COMP 法国 LMB-89：大剂量环磷酰胺、长春新碱、泼尼松、阿霉素[89]	法国 LMB-89
CHOP＋MTX（NCI-POB-7704）：环磷酰胺、阿霉素、长春新碱和泼尼松，交替用甲氨蝶呤静滴[69] COMP：环磷酰胺、长春新碱、甲氨蝶呤、泼尼松[3]	LMTB1：LSA2L2 方案，补充 10 个疗程大剂量甲氨蝶呤[90]	CHOP CHOP＋MTX（NCI-POB-7704） NHL-BFM90：泼尼松、地塞米松、长春新碱、阿霉素、环磷酰胺、异环磷酰胺、鬼臼乙叉甙、阿糖胞苷、甲氨蝶玲[102]	NHL-BFM90 NCI-89-C-0041F：环磷酰胺、长春新碱阿霉素 和甲氨蝶呤（Codox-M），与阿糖胞苷、鬼臼乙叉甙和异环磷（IVAC）方案交替[2]

就像前面提到的，儿童非 Hodgkin 淋巴瘤，特别是小无裂细胞类型，有非常高的生长分数和很快的细胞更新率。导致大量肿瘤细胞的更新，或者因为它们生长过快而超出血液供应，或者因为其他一些原因出现细胞死亡和溶解。根据肿瘤大小，这使肾脏产生巨大的代谢负荷，包括磷酸、钾、嘌呤和蛋白。患者血清可出现尿酸、乳酸盐和钾的升高。这个综合征在化疗后大量细胞裂解的过程中将进一步加重。其结果就是肿瘤溶解综合征，将导致高尿酸肾病和肾衰竭[41]。很明显，在术前应该监测患者的代谢和血液学状态。术前必须检查电解质系列，以及肌苷和尿素氮，而且为了纠正电解质异常，术前还可能要做血液透析。所有患者在化疗前必须给予别嘌呤醇并碱化尿液。

手术的其他作用包括为化疗建立静脉通路，必要时也可用于血液透析。腹部巨大肿块导致尿路梗阻时也可能需要手术治疗使尿路通畅。膀胱镜放置输尿管导管（双 J 管）可以显著改善排尿和肾功能。在化疗后粒细胞计数下降时，与经皮穿刺术相比应优先选择这项技术，既能使患者感觉舒适，又能避免经皮置管的感染。

预后因素

临床的预后依赖于诊断时肿瘤的负荷。这可以反映在临床分期上，但目前的临床分期体系与肿瘤负荷
589 没有线性相关性[18,69]。许多血清指标能够用于估计肿瘤负荷，因为这些物质由肿瘤细胞分泌或脱落。这些指标包括 LDH、IL–2 受体、β2 微球蛋白、尿酸、乳酸和多胺[20,39,128]。血清 LDH 较为稳定且容易检测。LDH 水平高于 250mg/（U·L）意味着肿瘤负荷明显，而高于 500 时预后往往较差。

总结

非 Hodgkin 淋巴瘤是异质性的淋巴细胞恶性肿瘤，可以通过正常淋巴细胞的个体发育过程来分类。大多数腹部淋巴瘤是未分化型组织病理类型（也称为小无裂细胞），Burkitt 淋巴瘤也是该类型。目前的资料显示，只有在保证并发症很小且不延误化疗时才考虑做腹部淋巴瘤的完全切除。大多数纵隔淋巴瘤是 T 细胞源性的，不能做手术切除。手术干预可用于一些并发症治疗，如巨大肿瘤的溶解、肠穿孔、消化道出血和尿路梗阻。

（叶启东译 王耀平校）

参考文献

1. Abruzzo LV, Jaffe ES, Cotelingam JD, et al: T-cell lymphoblastic lymphoma with eosinophilia associated with subsequent myeloid malignancy. Am J Surg Pathol 1992;16:236-245.
2. Adde M, Shad A, Venzon D, et al: Additional chemotherapy agents improve treatment outcome for children and adults with advanced B-cell lymphomas. Semin Oncol 1998;25 (Suppl 4):33-39; discussion 45-48.
3. Anderson JR, Jenkin RD, Wilson JF, et al: Long-term follow-up of patients treated with COMP or LSA2l2 therapy for childhood non-Hodgkin's lymphoma: A report of CCG-551 from the Children's Cancer Group. J Clin Oncol 1993;11:1024-1032 (see comments).
4. Anderson MM, Ross CW, Singleton TP, et al: Ki-1 anaplastic large cell lymphoma with a prominent leukemic phase. Hum Pathol 1996;27:1093-1095.
5. Anderson T, Chabner BA, Young RC, et al: Malignant lymphoma. 1. The histology and staging of 473 patients at the National Cancer Institute: Validity of the Ann Arbor staging classification for the non-Hodgkin's lymphomas. Cancer 1982;50:2699-2707.
6. ar-Rushdi A, Nishikura K, Erikson J, et al: Differential expression of the translocated and the untranslocated c-myc oncogene in Burkitt lymphoma. Science 1983;222:390-393.
7. Arseneau JC, Canellos GP, Banks PM, et al: American Burkitt's lymphoma: A clinicopathologic study of 30 cases. I. Clinical factors relating to prolonged survival. Am J Med 1975;58:314-321.
8. Beaty O 3rd, Hudson MM, Greenwald C, et al: Subsequent malignancies in children and adolescents after treatment for Hodgkin's disease. J Clin Oncol 1995;13:603-609 (see comments).
9. Behrendt H, Brinkhuis M, Van Leeuwen EF: Treatment of childhood Hodgkin's disease with ABVD without radiotherapy. Med Pediatr Oncol 1996;26:244-248.
10. Bonadonna G, Valagussa P, Santoro A: Alternating non-cross-resistant combination chemotherapy or MOPP in stage IV Hodgkin's disease. A report of 8-year results. Ann Intern Med 1986;104:739-746.
11. Bonadonna G, Zucali R, Monfardini S, et al: Combination chemotherapy of Hodgkin's disease with Adriamycin, bleomycin, vinblastine, and imidazole carboxamide versus MOPP. Cancer 1975;36:252-259.
12. Carde P, Koscielny S, Franklin J, et al: Early response to chemotherapy: A surrogate for final outcome of Hodgkin's disease patients that should influence initial treatment length and intensity? Ann Oncol 2002;13(Suppl 1):86-91.
13. Castellino RA, Dunnick NR, Goffinet DR, et al: Predictive value of lymphography for sites of subdiaphragmatic disease encountered at staging laparotomy in newly diagnosed

Hodgkin's disease and non-Hodgkin's lymphoma. J Clin Oncol 1993;1:532-536.
14. Castellino RA, Hoppe RT, Blank N, et al: Computed tomography, lymphography, and staging laparotomy: Correlations in initial staging of Hodgkin disease. AJR Am J Roentgenol 1984;143:37-41.
15. Chapman RM, Sutcliffe SB, Malpas JS: Male gonadal dysfunction in Hodgkin's disease: A prospective study. JAMA 1981;245:1323-1328.
16. Chilcote RR, Baehner RL, Hammond D: Septicemia and meningitis in children splenectomized for Hodgkin's disease. N Engl J Med 1976;295:798-800.
17. Chung CT, Bogart JA, Adams JF, et al: Increased risk of breast cancer in splenectomized patients undergoing radiation therapy for Hodgkin's disease. Int J Radiat Oncol Biol Phys 1997;37:405-409.
18. Cohen LF, Balow JE, Magrath IT, et al: Acute tumor lysis syndrome: A review of 37 patients with Burkitt's lymphoma. Am J Med 1980;68:486-491.
19. Constine LS, Donaldson SS, McDougall IR, et al: Thyroid dysfunction after radiotherapy in children with Hodgkin's disease. Cancer 1984;53:878-883.
20. Csako G, Magrath IT, Elin RJ: Serum total and isoenzyme lactate dehydrogenase activity in American Burkitt's lymphoma patients. Am J Clin Pathol 1982;78:712-717.
21. Denny CT, Yoshikai Y, Mak TW, et al: A chromosome 14 inversion in a T-cell lymphoma is caused by site-specific recombination between immunoglobulin and T-cell receptor loci. Nature 1986;320:549-551.
22. DeVita VTJ, Serpick A, Carbone PP: Combination chemotherapy in the treatment of advanced Hodgkin's disease. Ann Intern Med 1970;73:881-895.
23. Donaldson SS, Hudson MM, Lamborn KR, et al: VAMP and low-dose, involved-field radiation for children and adolescents with favorable, early-stage Hodgkin's disease: Results of a prospective clinical trial. J Clin Oncol 2002; 20:3081-3087.
24. Donaldson SS, Kaplan HS: Complications of treatment of Hodgkin's disease in children. Cancer Treat Rep 1982; 66:977-989.
25. Donaldson SS, Link MP: Combined modality treatment with low-dose radiation and MOPP chemotherapy for children with Hodgkin's disease. J Clin Oncol 1987;5: 742-749.
26. Donaldson SS, Whitaker SJ, Plowman PN, et al: Stage I-II pediatric Hodgkin's disease: Long-term follow-up demonstrates equivalent survival rates following different management schemes. J Clin Oncol 1990;8:1128-1137 (see comments).
27. Duepree HJ, Senagore AJ, Delaney CP, Fazio VW: Does means of access affect the incidence of small bowel obstruction and ventral hernia after bowel resection? Laparoscopy versus laparotomy. J Am Coll Surg 2003; 197:177-181.
28. Duque-Hammershaimb L, Wollner N, Miller DR: LSA2-l2 protocol treatment of stage IV non-Hodgkin's lymphoma in children with partial and extensive bone marrow involvement. Cancer 1983;52:39-43.
29. Eraklis AJ, Filler RM: Splenectomy in childhood: A review of 1413 cases. J Pediatr Surg 1972;7:382-388.
30. Franzius C, Schober O: Assessment of therapy response by FDG PET in pediatric patients. Q J Nucl Med 2003;47:41-45.
31. Gaetini A, De Simone M, Urgesi A, et al: Lateral high abdominal ovariopexy: An original surgical technique for protection of the ovaries during curative radiotherapy for Hodgkin's disease. J Surg Oncol 1988;39:22-28.
32. Garrett KM, Hoffer FA, Behm FG, et al: Interventional radiology techniques for the diagnosis of lymphoma or leukemia. Pediatr Radiol 2002;32:653-662.
33. Gilbert R: Radiotherapy in Hodgkin's disease (malignant granulomatosis): Anatomic and clinical foundations, governing principles, results. AJR Am J Roentgenol 1939;41: 198-241.
34. Glatstein E, Guernsey JM, Rosenberg SA, et al: The value of laparotomy and splenectomy in the staging of Hodgkin's disease. Cancer 1969;24:709-718.
35. Glick RD, La Quaglia MP: Lymphomas of the anterior mediastinum. Semin Pediatr Surg 1999;8:69-77.
36. Goodman LS, Wintrobe MM, Dameshek W, et al: Nitrogen mustard therapy: Use of methyl-bis(-chlorethyl)amine hydrochloride for Hodgkin's disease, lymphosarcoma, leukemia, and certain allied diseases and miscellaneous disorders. JAMA 1946;132:126-132.
37. Grenzebach J, Schrappe M, Ludwig WD, et al: Favorable outcome for children and adolescents with T-cell lymphoblastic lymphoma with an intensive ALL-type therapy without local radiotherapy. Ann Hematol 2001;80(Suppl 3): B73-B76.
38. Gross TG, Filipovich AH, Conley ME, et al: Cure of X-linked lymphoproliferative disease (XLP) with allogeneic hematopoietic stem cell transplantation (HSCT): Report from the XLP Registry. Bone Marrow Transplant 1996;17: 741-744.
39. Hagberg H, Killander A, Simonsson B: Serum beta 2-microglobulin in malignant lymphoma. Cancer 1983;51: 2220-2225.
40. Haluska FG, Brufsky AM, Canellos GP: The cellular biology of the Reed-Sternberg cell. Blood 1994;84:1005-1019.
41. Hande KR, Garrow GC: Acute tumor lysis syndrome in patients with high-grade non-Hodgkin's lymphoma. Am J Med 1993;94:133-139.
42. Hays DM: Malignant solid tumors of childhood. Curr Probl Surg 1986;23:161-242.
43. Hays DM, Ternberg JL, Chen TT, et al: Complications related to 234 staging laparotomies performed in the Intergroup Hodgkin's Disease in Childhood Study. Surgery 1984;96:471-478.
44. Hodgkin T: On some morbid appearances of the absorbent glands and spleen. Med Chir Trans Soc Lond 1832;17: 68-114.
45. Hurwitz M, Desai DM, Cox KL, et al: Complete immunosuppressive withdrawal as a uniform approach to post-transplant lymphoproliferative disease in pediatric liver transplantation. Pediatr Transplant 2004;8:267-272.
46. Hutter JJ Jr, Favara BE, Nelson M, Holton CP: Non-Hodgkin's lymphoma in children: Correlation of CNS disease with initial presentation. Cancer 1975;36:2132-2137.
47. Iversen OH, Bjerknes R, Iversen U, et al: Cell kinetics in Burkitt's lymphoma. In Drewinko B, Humphrey RM (eds): Growth Kinetics and Biochemical. 1997, pp 675-686.
48. Iversen OH, Iversen U, Ziegler JL, Bluming AZ: Cell kinetics in Burkitt lymphoma. Eur J Cancer 1974;10:155-163.
49. Jenkin D, Greenberg M, Fitzgerald A: Second malignant tumours in childhood Hodgkin's disease. Med Pediatr Oncol 1996;26:373-379.
50. Jenkin RD, Brown TC, Peters MV, Sonley MJ: Hodgkin's disease in children: A retrospective analysis: 1958-73. Cancer 1975;35:979-990.
51. Kaplan HS: Long-term results of palliative and radical radiotherapy of Hodgkin's disease. Cancer Res 1966;26: 1250-1252.
52. Kaufman BH, Burgert EO Jr, Banks PM: Abdominal

Burkitt's lymphoma: Role of early aggressive surgery. J Pediatr Surg 1987;22:671-674.
53. Kellie SJ, Pui CH, Murphy SB: Childhood non-Hodgkin's lymphoma involving the testis: Clinical features and treatment outcome. J Clin Oncol 1989;7:1066-1070.
54. Kelly KM, Hutchinson RJ, Sposto R, et al: Feasibility of upfront dose-intensive chemotherapy in children with advanced-stage Hodgkin's lymphoma: Preliminary results from the Children's Cancer Group Study CCG-59704. Ann Oncol 2002;13(Suppl 1):107-111.
55. Kemeny MM, Magrath IT, Brennan MF: The role of surgery in the management of American Burkitt's lymphoma and its treatment. Ann Surg 1982;196:82-86.
56. King H, Shumacker HBJ: Splenic studies. I. Susceptibility to infection after splenectomy performed in infancy. Ann Surg 1952;136:239-242.
57. Kraus M, Fliss DM, Argov S, et al: Burkitt's lymphoma of the tonsil. J Laryngol Otol 1990;104:991-994.
58. Kristoffersson U, Heim S, Mandahl N, et al: Trisomy 5 and t(5;14)(q11;q32) as the sole abnormalities in two different clones from a centroblastic non-Hodgkin's lymphoma. Cancer Genet Cytogenet 1988;36:173-176.
59. Kushner BH, Zauber A, Tan CT: Second malignancies after childhood Hodgkin's disease: The Memorial Sloan-Kettering Cancer Center experience. Cancer 1988;62:1364-1370.
60. La Quaglia MP, Stolar CJ, Krailo M, et al: The role of surgery in abdominal non-Hodgkin's lymphoma: Experience from the Children's Cancer Study Group. J Pediatr Surg 1992;27: 230-235.
61. Laver J, Amylon M, Desai S, et al: Randomized trial of r-metHu granulocyte colony-stimulating factor in an intensive treatment for T-cell leukemia and advanced-stage lymphoblastic lymphoma of childhood: A Pediatric Oncology Group pilot study. J Clin Oncol 1998;16:522-526.
62. Leventhal BG, Kato GJ: Childhood Hodgkin and non-Hodgkin lymphomas. Pediatr Rev 1990;12:171-179.
63. Link MP, Donaldson SS, Berard CW, et al: Results of treatment of childhood localized non-Hodgkin's lymphoma with combination chemotherapy with or without radiotherapy. N Engl J Med 1990;322:1169-1174.
64. Link MP, Shuster JJ, Donaldson SS, et al: Treatment of children and young adults with early-stage non-Hodgkin's lymphoma. N Engl J Med 1997;337:1259-1266.
65. Link MP, Warnke R, Finlay J, et al: A single monoclonal antibody identifies T-cell lineage of childhood lymphoid malignancies. Blood 1983;62:722-728.
66. Little MA, Morland B, Chisholm J, et al: A randomised study of prophylactic G-CSF following MRC UKALL XI intensification regimen in childhood ALL and T-NHL. Med Pediatr Oncol 2002;38:98-103.
67. Longo DL, Young RC, Wesley M, et al: Twenty years of MOPP therapy for Hodgkin's disease. J Clin Oncol 1986; 4:1295-1306.
68. Magrath IT: Lymphocyte differentiation: An essential basis for the comprehension of lymphoid neoplasia. J Natl Cancer Inst 1981;67:501-514.
69. Magrath IT, Janus C, Edwards BK, et al: An effective therapy for both undifferentiated (including Burkitt's) lymphomas and lymphoblastic lymphomas in children and young adults. Blood 1984;63:1102-1111.
70. Magrath IT, Lwanga S, Carswell W, Harrison N: Surgical reduction of tumour bulk in management of abdominal Burkitt's lymphoma. BMJ 1974;2:308-312.
71. Magrath IT, Ziegler JL: Failure of BCG immunostimulation to affect the clinical course of Burkitt's lymphoma. BMJ 1976;1:615-618.
72. Maguire RT, Robins TS, Thorgeirsson SS, Heilman CA: Expression of cellular myc and mos genes in undifferentiated B cell lymphomas of Burkitt and non-Burkitt types. Proc Natl Acad Sci U S A 1983;80:1947-1950.
73. Mauch PM, Kalish LA, Marcus KC, et al: Second malignancies after treatment for laparotomy staged IA-IIIB Hodgkin's disease: Long-term analysis of risk factors and outcome. Blood 1996;87:3625-3632.
74. Medary I, Steinherz LJ, Aronson DC, La Quaglia MP: Cardiac tamponade in the pediatric oncology population: Treatment by percutaneous catheter drainage. J Pediatr Surg 1996;31: 197-199.
75. Meyers PA, Potter VP, Wollner N, Exelby P: Bowel perforation during initial treatment for childhood non-Hodgkin's lymphoma. Cancer 1985;56:259-261.
76. Miller JF: Immunologic functions of the thymus. Lancet 1961;2:748-749.
77. Moskowitz C: Risk-adapted therapy for relapsed and refractory lymphoma using ICE chemotherapy. Cancer Chemother Pharmacol 2002;49(Suppl 1):S9-S12.
78. Moskowitz C: An update on the management of relapsed and primary refractory Hodgkin's disease. Semin Oncol 2004;31(2 Suppl 4):54-59.
79. Moskowitz CH, Kewalramani T, Nimer SD, et al: Effectiveness of high dose chemoradiotherapy and autologous stem cell transplantation for patients with biopsy-proven primary refractory Hodgkin's disease. Br J Haematol 2004;124:645-652.
80. Mukhtar AU, Mugerwa B: Burkitt's lymphoma of the ovary. Cent Afr J Med 1999;45:104-105.
81. Murphy SB, Fairclough DL, Hutchison RE, Berard CW: Non-Hodgkin's lymphomas of childhood: An analysis of the histology, staging, and response to treatment of 338 cases at a single institution. J Clin Oncol 1989;7:186-193.
82. Murphy SB, Frizzera G, Evans AE: A study of childhood non-Hodgkin's lymphoma. Cancer 1975;36:2121-2131.
83. Murphy SB, Hustu HO: A randomized trial of combined modality therapy of childhood non-Hodgkin's lymphoma. Cancer 1980;45:630-637.
84. Nachman JB, Sposto R, Herzog P, et al: Randomized comparison of low-dose involved-field radiotherapy and no radiotherapy for children with Hodgkin's disease who achieve a complete response to chemotherapy. J Clin Oncol 2002;20:3765-3771.
85. Nathwani BN, Griffith RC, Kelly DR: A morphological study of childhood lymphoma of the diffuse histiocytic type: The Pediatric Oncology Group experience. Cancer 1976;38: 964-983.
86. Nathwani BN, Griffith RC, Kelly DR, et al: A morphologic study of childhood lymphoma of the diffuse "histiocytic" type: The Pediatric Oncology Group experience. Cancer 1987;59: 1138-1142.
87. Oberlin O, Leverger G, Pacquement H, et al: Low-dose radiation therapy and reduced chemotherapy in childhood Hodgkin's disease: The experience of the French Society of Pediatric Oncology. J Clin Oncol 1992;10:1602-1608.
88. Ortin TT, Shostak CA, Donaldson SS: Gonadal status and reproductive function following treatment for Hodgkin's disease in childhood: The Stanford experience. Int J Radiat Oncol Biol Phys 1990;19:873-880.
89. Patte C, Auperin A, Michon J, et al: The Societe Francaise d'Oncologie Pediatrique LMB89 protocol: Highly effective multiagent chemotherapy tailored to the tumor burden and initial response in 561 unselected children with B-cell lymphomas and L3 leukemia. Blood 2001;97: 3370-3379.

90. Patte C, Kalifa C, Flamant F, et al: Results of the LMT81 protocol, a modified LSA2L2 protocol with high dose methotrexate, on 84 children with non-B-cell (lymphoblastic) lymphoma. Med Pediatr Oncol 1992;20:105-113.
91. Patte C, Laplanche A, Bertozzi AI, et al: Granulocyte colony-stimulating factor in induction treatment of children with non-Hodgkin's lymphoma: A randomized study of the French Society of Pediatric Oncology. J Clin Oncol 2002;20:441-448.
92. Penn I: De novo malignances in pediatric organ transplant recipients. Pediatr Transplant 1998;2:56-63.
93. Percy CL, Smith MA, Linet M, et al: Lymphomas and reticuloendothelial neoplasms. In Ries LAG, Smith MA, Gurney JG, et al (eds): Cancer Incidence and Survival among Children and Adolescents: United States SEER Program 1975-1995. NIH Pub. No. 99-4649. Bethesda, Md, National Cancer Institute, SEER Program, 1999.
94. Peters MV: A study of survival in Hodgkin's disease treated radiologically. AJR Am J Roentgenol 1950;63: 299-311.
95. Pondarre C, Kebaili K, Dijoud F, et al: Epstein-Barr virus-related lymphoproliferative disease complicating childhood acute lymphoblastic leukemia: No recurrence after unrelated donor bone marrow transplantation. Bone Marrow Transplant 2001;27:93-95.
96. Pringle KC, Rowley D, Burrington JD: Immunologic response in splenectomized and partially splenectomized rats. J Pediatr Surg 1980;15:531-536.
97. Probert JC, Parker BR: The effects of radiation therapy on bone growth. Radiology 1975;114:155-162.
98. Pusey WA: Cases of sarcoma and Hodgkin's disease treated by exposure to x-rays: A preliminary report. JAMA 1902;38:166-169.
99. Rappold GA, Hameister H, Cremer T, et al: C-myc and immunoglobulin kappa light chain constant genes are on the 8q+ chromosome of three Burkitt lymphoma lines with t(2;8) translocations. EMBO J 1984;3:2951-2955.
100. Reed DM: On the pathological changes in Hodgkin's disease with especial reference to its relation to tuberculosis. Johns Hopkins Hosp Rep 1902;10:133-196.
101. Reiter A, Schrappe M, Ludwig WD, et al: Intensive ALL-type therapy without local radiotherapy provides a 90% event-free survival for children with T-cell lymphoblastic lymphoma: A BFM group report. Blood 2000; 92:416-421.
102. Reiter A, Schrappe M, Tiemann M, et al: Improved treatment results in childhood B-cell neoplasms with tailored intensification of therapy: A report of the Berlin-Frankfurt-Munster Group Trial NHL-BFM 90. Blood 1999;94:3294-3306.
103. Rosenberg SA, Kaplan HS: Evidence for an orderly progression in the spread of Hodgkin's disease. Cancer Res 1966;26:1225-1231.
104. Ross CW, Hanson CA, Schnitzer B: CD30 (Ki-1)-positive, anaplastic large cell lymphoma mimicking gastrointestinal carcinoma. Cancer 1992;70:2517-2523.
105. Rowley DA: The formation of circulating antibody in the splenectomized human being following intravenous injection of heterologous erythrocytes. J Immunol 1950;65: 515-521.
106. Rubie H, Gladieff L, Robert A, et al: Childhood anaplastic large cell lymphoma Ki-1/CD30: Clinicopathologic features of 19 cases. Med Pediatr Oncol 1994;22:155-161.
107. Ruhl U, Albrecht M, Dieckmann K, et al: Response-adapted radiotherapy in the treatment of pediatric Hodgkin's disease: An interim report at 5 years of the German GPOH-HD 95 trial. Int J Radiat Oncol Biol Phys 2001;51: 1209-1218.
108. Samuelsson BO, Ridell B, Rockert L, et al: Non-Hodgkin lymphoma in children: A 20-year population-based epidemiologic study in western Sweden. J Pediatr Hematol Oncol 1999;21:103-110.
109. Sandlund JT, Downing JR, Crist WM: Non-Hodgkin's lymphoma in childhood. N Engl J Med 1996;334:1238-1248.
110. Sandoval C, Strom K, Stringel G: Laparoscopy in the management of pediatric intraabdominal tumors. JSLS 2004;8: 115-118.
111. Schellong G, Bramswig JH, Hornig-Franz I, et al: Hodgkin's disease in children: Combined modality treatment for stages IA, IB, and IIA. Results in 356 patients of the German/Austrian Pediatric Study Group. Ann Oncol 1994;5(Suppl 2):113-115.
112. Schneeberger AL, Girvan DP: Staging laparotomy for Hodgkin's disease in children. J Pediatr Surg 1988;23: 714-717.
113. Schnitzer B, Roth MS, Hyder DM, Ginsburg D: Ki-1 lymphomas in children. Cancer 1988;61:1213-1221.
114. Schwartz CL: Prognostic factors in pediatric Hodgkin disease. Curr Oncol Rep 2003;5:498-504.
115. Shamberger RC, Weinstein HJ: The role of surgery in abdominal Burkitt's lymphoma. J Pediatr Surg 1992;27: 236-240.
116. Silecchia G, Fantini A, Raparelli L, et al: Management of abdominal lymphoproliferative diseases in the era of laparoscopy. Am J Surg 1999;177:325-330.
117. Silecchia G, Raparelli L, Perrotta N, et al: Accuracy of laparoscopy in the diagnosis and staging of lymphoproliferative diseases. World J Surg 2003;27:653-658.
118. Silverman DH, Delpassand ES, Torabi F, et al: Radiolabeled antibody therapy in non-Hodgkins lymphoma: Radiation protection, isotope comparisons and quality of life issues. Cancer Treat Rev 2004;30:165-172.
119. Singer DB: Postsplenectomy sepsis. Perspect Pediatr Pathol 1973;1:285-311.
120. Socie G, Curtis RE, Deeg HJ, et al: New malignant diseases after allogeneic marrow transplantation for childhood acute leukemia. J Clin Oncol 2000;18:348-357.
121. Sternberg C: Uber eine Eigenartige unter dem Bilde der Pseudoleukamie verlaufende Tuberculose des lymphatischen Apparates. Z Heilk 1898;19:21-90.
122. Su IJ, Wang CH, Cheng AL, Chen RL: Hemophagocytic syndrome in Epstein-Barr virus-associated T-lymphoproliferative disorders: Disease spectrum, pathogenesis, and management. Leuk Lymphoma 1995;19:401-406.
123. Tan CT, De Sousa M, Good RA: Distinguishing features of the immunology of Hodgkin's disease in children. Cancer Treat Rep 1982;66:969-975.
124. Taub R, Moulding C, Battey J, et al: Activation and somatic mutation of the translocated c-myc gene in Burkitt lymphoma cells. Cell 1984;36:339-348.
125. Thomson AB, Wallace WH: Treatment of paediatric Hodgkin's disease: A balance of risks. Eur J Cancer 2002;38: 468-477.
126. Tsokos GC, Balow JE, Spiegel RJ, Magrath IT: Renal and metabolic complications of undifferentiated and lymphoblastic lymphomas. Medicine (Baltimore) 1981; 60:218-229.
127. Vigersky RA, Chapman RM, Berenberg J, Glass AR: Testicular dysfunction in untreated Hodgkin's disease. Am J Med 1982;73:482-486.
128. Wagner DK, Kiwanuka J, Edwards BK, et al: Soluble interleukin-2 receptor levels in patients with undifferentiated

and lymphoblastic lymphomas: Correlation with survival. J Clin Oncol 1987;5:1262-1274.
129. Walsh RM, Heniford BT: Role of laparoscopy for Hodgkin's and non-Hodgkin's lymphoma. Semin Surg Oncol 1999;16:284-292.
130. Warner NL, Szenberg A, Burnet FM: The immunological role of different lymphoid organs in the chicken. I. Dissociation of immunological responsiveness. Aust J Exp Biol Med Sci 1962;40:373-388.
131. Watanabe A, Sullivan MP, Sutow WW, Wilbur JR: Undifferentiated lymphoma, non-Burkitt's type: Meningeal and bone marrow involvement in children. Am J Dis Child 1973; 125:57-61.
132. White L, Siegel SE, Quah TC: Non-Hodgkin's lymphomas in children. I. Patterns of disease and classification. Crit Rev Oncol Hematol 1992;13:55-71.
133. Wollner N: Non-Hodgkin's lymphoma in children. Pediatr Clin North Am 1976;23:371-378.
134. Wollner N, Burchenal JH, Lieberman PH, et al: Non-Hodgkin's lymphoma in children: A comparative study of two modalities of therapy. Cancer 1976;37:123-134.
135. Zech L, Haglund U, Nilsson K, Klein G: Characteristic chromosomal abnormalities in biopsies and lymphoid-cell lines from patients with Burkitt and non-Burkitt lymphomas. Int J Cancer 1976;17:47-56.
136. Ziegler JL: Treatment results of 54 American patients with Burkitt's lymphoma are similar to the African experience. N Engl J Med 1977;297:75-80.

第 36 章

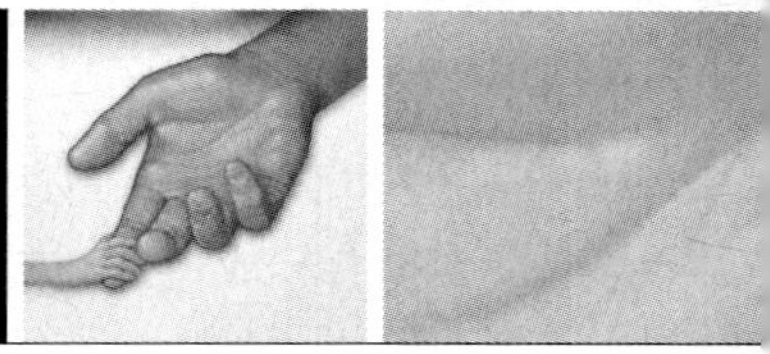

卵巢肿瘤

Claire L. Templeman 和 Mary E. Fallat

93 ## 发生率

儿童原发性卵巢囊肿和肿瘤并不常见，而且大多数都是良性的[64]。大约 2%的儿童肿瘤与妇科的恶性疾病相关，而这些与妇科相关的恶性肿瘤中有 60%～70%是卵巢肿瘤[158]。最近，北美联合癌症登记中心（North American Association of Central Cancer Registries）的一项数据显示，在 1992—1997 年间，超过 160 万的妇女和儿童被确诊为癌症[233]。报道显示其中 1.2%的卵巢肿瘤发生在小于 19 岁的女孩中[233]。Lindfors[47]分析了一些儿童常见的卵巢肿瘤，估计每年在 10 万个小于 15 岁的女孩中就有 2.6 例良性或者恶性卵巢肿瘤发生。

一些特殊的卵巢肿瘤的发生率和患儿的年龄分布有关。Lack 等[112]回顾了波士顿儿童医院 50 年间的 157 例原发性卵巢肿瘤病例。成熟的囊性畸胎瘤在 5 岁以后相对稳定，颗粒细胞肿瘤在 9 岁之后迅速减少，卵黄囊瘤的高发期在 10～14 岁，在这之后发生率迅速下降，而卵巢上皮肿瘤只在大于 10 岁的女孩中发生。

卵巢恶性肿瘤最容易发生在幼儿中的概念已经被重新评定。新的影像诊断技术提高了所有生殖腺肿块的发现率，而卵巢肿瘤的发生率已经相对下降。Gribbon 等[77]在 1992 年发表的 43 年回顾文章中提出，卵巢恶性肿瘤更容易（70%）在十几岁的青少年中发生。

先前的报告指出，55%～67%的卵巢肿瘤是恶性的[78,142]。而 1993 年发表的费城儿童医院对 11 年间 91 例卵巢肿瘤的回顾文章提出，只有 21%是恶性的[26]。小于 8 岁儿童的卵巢肿瘤 97%是良性的，而年长儿童中的比例为 33%。Imai 等[96]收集了日本医院的 114 例卵巢肿瘤病例后报告，其中 20%是恶性的。其他一些研究报告指出，儿童和青少年中卵巢恶性肿瘤的发生率大约在 10%～40%[48,53,190]。

流行病学

一些综合征或疾病可同时存在有卵巢的病变。Peutz-Jeghers 综合征与颗粒细胞瘤、卵巢囊腺瘤和性索-间质环状小管瘤相关[161]。幼年型颗粒细胞瘤见于 Ollier 病（多发性内生软骨瘤病）[11]和 Maffucci 综合征（内生软骨瘤病和血管瘤）[201]。支持-间质细胞瘤可见于 Ollier 病[3]，纤维肉瘤可见于 Maffucci 综合征[32]。硬化性间质瘤可见于 Chédiak-Higashi 综合征（眼皮肤白化病、化脓性感染和白细胞颗粒变性导致的吞噬不足）[97]。卵巢囊肿可见于各种同质异形的综合征，有些综合征同时还可以有颅面部、喉部和指（趾）部的畸形[126]。McCune-Albright 综合征（咖啡牛奶斑、多发性骨纤维性发育不良和自主内分泌亢进）主要表现为反复卵巢滤泡形成和周期性雌二醇分泌导致的绒毛膜促性腺激素依赖的性早熟[224]。纤维瘤常见于基底细胞痣综合征。

未产妇发生卵巢恶性肿瘤的可能性是经产妇的 1.5～3.2 倍。从未使用过口服避孕药的妇女发生卵巢恶性肿瘤的可能性是使用过口服避孕药的妇女的 1.4～2.5 倍。其他潜在性的但尚有争议的因素有：使用诱发排卵药物但未受孕、饮食中含有较多肉类、动物脂肪、乳制品和乳糖。输卵管结扎术和子宫切除术可以减少卵巢恶性肿瘤的发生率[136,184]。

大约有 5%～10%的患有乳房和卵巢恶性肿瘤的妇女有遗传性基因缺陷。大多数遗传性乳房和卵巢恶性肿瘤都是由肿瘤抑制基因 *BRCA1* 和 *BRCA2* 突变引起的。大约 70%的家族性卵巢肿瘤是由于 *BRCA1* 594
突变引起的，20%是由于 *BRCA2* 突变引起。这些突变是以常染色体显性遗传的方式遗传的。如果一个妇女是其中一种突变基因的携带者，那么她一生患卵巢恶性肿瘤的概率高达60%[51,130]。

对未成年人进行基因检测还存在争议[185,222]。Kodish[107]认为，医生必须尊重“最早发病原则”，尽量推迟到疾病发生时再检测。对有乳房和卵巢恶性肿瘤高危因素的成年妇女有必要告之将来可能需要的手术或药物介入的功效，但是对未成年人也许还不恰当。大多数情况下，外科介入是在35岁以后或者分娩后。口服避孕药被认为对大多数人都有减少卵巢恶性肿瘤危险的作用。但是对存在*BRCA*畸变的年轻妇女是否有作用还有待证实[130]。

美国人类基因学会和美国医学基因学院在1995年联合公布了儿童和青少年的基因检测报告[107]。如果对儿童的基因检测的最初目的是为了促进儿童更好地成长，也只有当有可以指导预防性措施或治疗医学价值时，基因检测才可以被接受。目前，预防性手术或者对未成年患者增加检测的必要性还没有评估或检测过，也没有确切的证据表明对18岁以下未成年人的*BRCA*检测有任何医学价值。Elger和Harding[56]认为，如果对一些年轻妇女告之基因突变的情况，也许会减轻她们的心理负担，并利用这些信息对她们的生育问题和健康问题作出抉择。

临床表现

卵巢肿瘤可以有各种临床症状和体征。一般卵巢良性和恶性肿瘤的临床表现差异并不是很大。腹痛是最常见的症状[26,96,190]。卵巢囊肿或其他非新生物，一般以急性腹痛起病，如果出现扭转、破裂或出血，腹痛可明显加重。整个临床症状类似于阑尾炎[39]。

其他表现有慢性隐匿性腹痛、腹围增大和几周到几个月时间内腹部明显膨隆。继发症状包括食欲下降、恶心、呕吐和尿频尿急。体检时最容易发现的体征是腹部高张力性或低张力性肿块，超过60%的卵巢肿瘤患者腹部都可以触及肿块[26,190]。这些肿块一般是可活动的，位置要高于骨盆上缘。下腹部–直肠双合诊有利于发现小病变。虽然阴道视诊对所有患者都是有价值的，但是一般阴道检查只适用于有性活动的患者。越来越多的卵巢病变是因其他原因行腹立位平片或腹部超声时偶然发现的。

大约10%的卵巢新生物和非新生物病变可以出现内分泌作用[26,92,112]。卵巢单纯的滤泡性或黄体来源的囊肿由于分泌雌激素可能会引起同性假性性早熟。这些卵巢病变具有自主分泌功能，患儿一般可有绒毛膜促性腺激素的增高。囊肿退化或者切除后，患儿雌激素水平下降并可有阴道出血，这一点可以与中枢性性早熟（骨骼加速发育）以及乳房过早发育（单独的乳房发育）相鉴别。一些患生殖细胞肿瘤如无性细胞瘤、卵黄囊瘤和绒毛膜癌的患儿可能由于其分泌的人绒毛膜促性腺激素的作用而出现青春期提前。性早熟在性索–间质肿瘤如幼年型颗粒细胞瘤和支持–间质细胞瘤患儿中最易发生，因为它们能加速雌激素循环的进行。

支持–间质细胞瘤患儿如果雄激素分泌过多可导致男性第二性征出现，含有合体滋养层巨细胞的无性细胞瘤的年长女孩偶尔也会出现男性化表现。卵黄囊瘤、类固醇细胞瘤和多囊卵巢也会导致男性第二性征出现。

诊断

实验室检查

很多卵巢肿瘤都能分泌特异的肿瘤标志物或激素，表36–1和36–2中列出了这些肿瘤标志物和激

表36–1 卵巢肿瘤和肿瘤标志物

组织学亚型	CA–125	CA–19.9	AFP	β–HCG	LDH
子宫肌腺瘤	+				
上皮来源					
交界性肿瘤	+				
恶性肿瘤	+				
生殖细胞来源*					
无性细胞瘤				+	+
卵黄囊瘤			+	+	
未成熟畸胎瘤					
绒毛膜癌				+	
胚胎性			+	+	
内胚窦瘤			+		
支持–间质细胞瘤			+		

* 标志物表明在单纯性肿瘤中升高；混合肿瘤可分泌各种标志物。

AFP：甲胎蛋白；HCG：绒毛膜促性腺激素；LDH：乳酸脱氢酶。

表 36-2　卵巢肿瘤和激素

组织学亚型	雌二醇	睾丸酮	尿 17 酮类固醇	绒毛膜促性腺激素
卵巢囊肿				
单纯性	↑			
滤泡性	↑			
黄体来源	↑			
性索-间质肿瘤				
幼年型颗粒细胞瘤	↑	↑ *		↓
支持-间质细胞肿瘤	↑ †	↑ ‡		↓
黄体化的泡膜细胞瘤	↑	↑ *		
环状小管性索瘤	↑			
类固醇细胞瘤		↑	↑	
性腺母细胞瘤	↑ *	↑	↑	↓
绒毛膜癌	↑			↑

* 表明罕见的肿瘤变异。
† 功能性支持细胞为主。
‡ 功能性间质细胞为主。

素，在后面对各个肿瘤的讨论中还会进一步论述。

肿瘤标志物

生殖细胞肿瘤具有很多生物活性的标志物，对诊
5 断和处理这一类肿瘤很有帮助[48]。蛋白标志物，包括甲胎蛋白（AFP）、β-人绒毛膜促性腺激素（β-HCG）和乳酸脱氢酶（LDH）是最常用的标志物。通常通过血清测定或对石蜡固定或冰冻的肿瘤组织行免疫组化染色而测得。

甲胎蛋白（AFP）

AFP 和生殖细胞肿瘤的关系最早由 Abelev 等人提出的[1]。因为在人类胚胎发生过程中，胎儿卵黄囊是 AFP 的最早来源，卵黄囊肿瘤可伴有 AFP 增高[207]。同时，肝母细胞瘤、肝细胞癌和恶性畸胎瘤也会出现 AFP 增高[200]。AFP 增高反映出现了胚胎组织，正常条件下这些胚胎组织可以发育为各种组织结构。

从出生到 1 周岁，人体 AFP 水平会发生很大的变化[230]，AFP 在早产儿和正常新生儿中特别高（表 36-3）。所以不能在出生后第一个月用 AFP 诊断卵黄囊瘤或胚胎性癌[66,71]。在其他任一年龄段，如果出现 AFP 显著增高，就提示有肿瘤存在。正常血清 AFP 半衰期是 5～7 天。AFP 相关肿瘤切除后可导致血液中 AFP 的明显下降。任何治疗的目的就是将 AFP 降至正常水平。如果出现 AFP 水平突然再次上升常提示有肿瘤的复发。

β-人绒毛膜促性腺激素（β-HCG）

β-HCG 是由胎盘合体滋养层分泌的糖蛋白。它含有两个亚基；α 亚基和 β 亚基；只有 β 亚基可以被可靠地检测到[214]。生殖细胞肿瘤如精原细胞瘤、无性细胞瘤、绒毛膜癌和少见的胚胎性癌患者出现 β-HCG 增高，提示肿瘤中含有合体滋养层细胞[152]。β-HCG 超过 100ng/ml 比较少见，通常暗示绒毛膜

表 36-3　婴儿平均正常甲胎蛋白含量

年龄	样本数	平均数 ± 标准差（ng/ml）
未成熟儿	11	134 734 ± 41 444
新生儿	55	48 406 ± 34 718
新生至 2 周	16	33 113 ± 32 503
2 周至 1 个月	12	9452 ± 12 610
2 个月	40	323 ± 278
3个月	5	88 ± 87
4个月	31	74 ± 56
5个月	6	46.5 ± 19
6个月	9	12.5 ± 9.8
7个月	5	9.7 ± 7.1
8个月	3	8.5 ± 5.5

瘤[154]。相比 AFP，β 亚基的半衰期只有 20～30 小时[154]。当完全切除肿瘤后，β-HCG 可完全消失。

血清乳酸脱氢酶（LDH）

血清 LDH 是一种非特异性标志物，广泛存在于人体各组织，对诊断肿瘤类型和反应治疗效果作用有限。然而，LDH 增高提示细胞增殖加快，可以作为诊断恶性肿瘤的非特异性标记[145]。LDH 也是判断淋巴瘤和神经母细胞瘤预后最有价值的标志物。LDH 同工酶基因位于 12p 染色体，所有亚型的生殖细胞肿瘤都可以发现 12 号染色体的非随机性结构改变。

癌基因

卵巢生殖细胞肿瘤和性染色体畸变有关。与一些
596 报告的结论不同，在一项对 78 名卵巢生殖细胞肿瘤患者的 456 名直系或旁系女性亲属的大型研究中，并没有显示出发生卵巢肿瘤的危险性增加[8,188,219]。

新的细胞遗传学技术的应用增加了我们对生殖细胞肿瘤发生发展中基因学和分子学机制的了解。经常有报道称，发现在 1 号、12 号以及其他染色体中的非随机性分子结构改变[37,88,128]。比如，许多间质肿瘤细胞中经常可以发现 12 号染色体三体畸变[199]。等臂染色体是一种由一条染色体的两臂在着丝点分裂后经复制后形成的具有两条相同臂的染色体。在所有类型的生殖细胞肿瘤中，包括男性的精原细胞瘤[21,172,196]，均可以发现等臂染色体 12p[i(12p)][137,172,191]。三倍及以上的等臂染色体 i(12p)的存在被认为与治疗失败有关[88]。非随机性研究发现，内胚窦瘤患儿存在 1p 和 6q 染色体片段的缺失。1p 终端位点片段的缺失也出现在其他肿瘤的患儿中，提示该部位存在某些目前尚未证实的一种或多种肿瘤抑制性基因。在青春期和成人卵巢肿瘤患者中，已经证实有等臂染色体 12p 存在[12]。儿童内胚窦瘤患者与成人存在细胞遗传学差异，没有发现等臂染色体 i(12p)，但是存在 1p、3q 和 6q 的基因缺失[153]。在一些内胚窦瘤患者中发现有癌基因 c-*myc* 存在，目前儿童肿瘤学工作组的研究成果认为，它与肿瘤患者最终的存活以及对治疗的反应直接相关[31]。需要更进一步的深入研究来确立这些研究成果的重要意义。很多儿童的生殖细胞肿瘤表达 P-糖蛋白，这是一种能够降低肿瘤对化学治疗反应的膜结合蛋白；它可以解释为什么这些肿瘤经常对治疗产生耐受[221]。

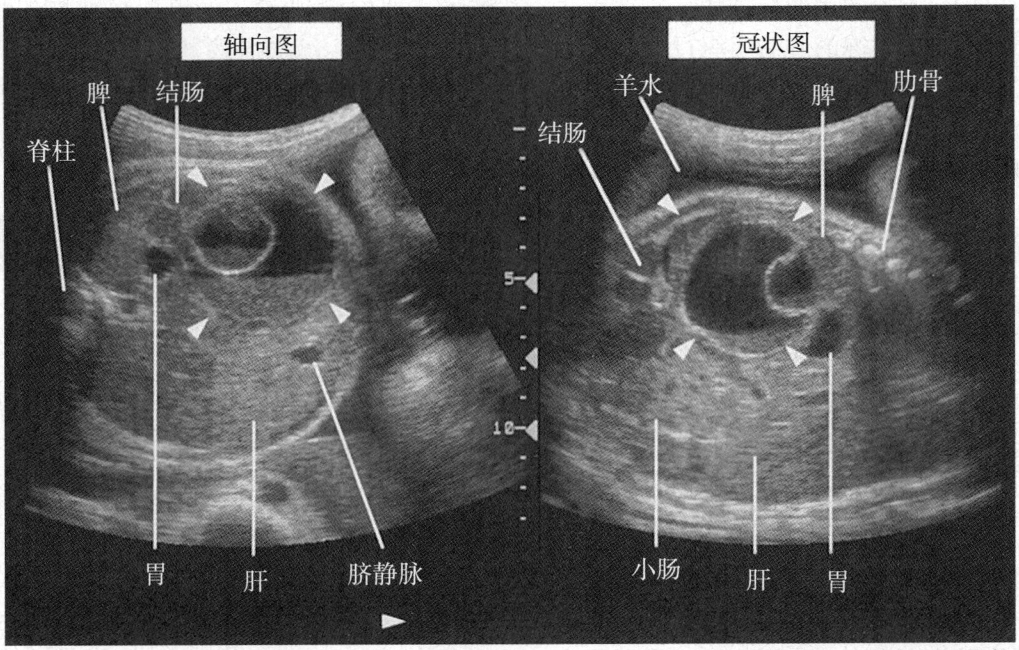

图 36-1 A 和 B. 是两张妊娠末期胎儿的超声图像，可以看到一个巨大的混合性卵巢囊肿，囊内可见液体、碎片、隔膜以及一些固体成分。患儿出生后手术证实存在卵巢肿瘤。（Courtesy of Gary A. Thieme, MD, Prenatal Diagnosis Center, University of Colorado School of Medicine.）

影像学技术

各种影像学技术对儿童卵巢疾病的鉴别有很重要的临床应用价值。产前超声可以将卵巢疾病与肠重复畸形、肾积水、十二指肠闭锁、胆总管囊肿、脐尿管残留、子宫阴道积水和肠梗阻相鉴别（图 36–1）。因为婴儿期卵巢还是一个腹腔器官而不是盆腔器官，所以肠系膜和大网膜囊肿与单纯性卵巢囊肿较难鉴别。

在任一年龄组对怀疑卵巢病变的患者中，超声检查都是首选的检查手段。检查时要求膀胱憋尿保持膀胱足够的扩张，将充气的肠袢推出盆腔，以便有足够的声波能够通过卵巢。随着年龄的增长，卵巢大小由小于 2 岁时的不足 0.7cm² 增加到青春期后的 1.8～5.7cm³[197]。同时，形态学上也发生改变。小于 8 岁儿童的卵巢一般是实性的器官，在超声检查时显示等回声的结构。而在青春期及之后，随着卵巢滤泡形成并开始排卵，卵巢的超声图像出现囊性改变。卵巢囊肿的超声表现一般为均一无回声、薄壁的占位肿块，当发生扭转时可见液体碎片和隔膜[189]。大多数良性卵巢肿瘤表现为复合性的占位，中央呈低回声区，外周可见高回声的附壁肿瘤，部分可能存在声影。恶性卵巢肿瘤直径常大于 10cm，超声表现为复合性的软组织团块影，边界不清、不规则，中心坏死，可见厚的隔膜或乳头状结构。彩色多普勒超声检查和经阴道超声检查对鉴别诊断青春期后卵巢病变的形态学改变也有一定价值[21,169,215]。

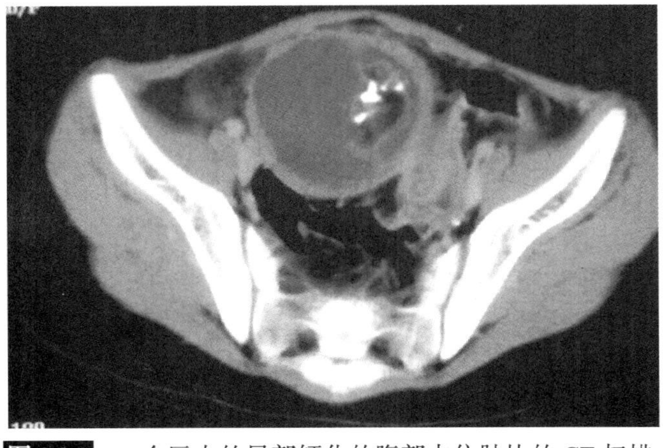

图 36–2　一个巨大的局部钙化的腹部占位肿块的 CT 扫描。肿块表现为一个巨大的囊性成分，囊壁实性、较厚、稍有偏心。肿瘤为一个薄壁的纤维囊肿，整个纤维囊壁都由出血性血栓形成。组织学检查证实为一良性囊性畸胎瘤。

当超声检查不能明确盆腔占位肿块的来源或者有必要对卵巢非囊性占位进行范围评估时，就需要进行计算机断层扫描（CT）和核磁共振成像（MRI）检查。良性肿瘤的 CT 的特征性表现是囊性的占位，局部可见脂肪和钙化灶[99]。经常可见肿瘤壁局部形成实性的结构（图 36–2）。恶性肿瘤体积巨大，主要为实性结构，偶尔出现囊性区域和（或）细小或粗大的钙化灶。CT检查也可发现肿瘤对附近盆腔结构或者肝、肺的直接浸润，CT 对肿瘤的分期比超声检查更准确。卵巢肿瘤伴发附件扭转的 CT 表现不同，一般需要加入造影剂后动态观察。主要特点是缺少附壁肿瘤的强化，显示血流中断，并可见粗大充盈的血管包绕在肿瘤周围，扭转部位的远端静脉显著充血。

MRI 不受皮下脂肪的影响，并能利用软组织提供很高的对比分辨率，很适于盆腔病变的检查[15]，特别是鉴别盆腔占位是卵巢来源还是泌尿系统来源，而且它具有特殊的信号表现，能够鉴别皮样囊肿、子宫肌腺瘤和子宫内膜植入片[106,194]。子宫内膜异位症患者在腹腔镜活检后用 MRI 对病变的程度进行检查有助于监测治疗效果[60]。MRI 同时还能对囊液的性质如单纯血性还是混合性进行鉴别[65]。MRI 成像时间较长，身体的移动和呼吸运动可能会引起腹膜和肠表面图像模糊，而且幼儿需要给予适当的镇静。卵巢扭转伴出血性血栓形成在 MRI T1 加权图像的特点是在病变外周形成高密度的边缘[104]。

表 36–4　世界卫生组织对卵巢非肿瘤性病变的组织学分类

单发性滤泡囊肿
多发性滤泡囊肿（卵巢多囊病，多囊性卵巢）
妊娠期和产褥期巨大单发性黄体滤泡性囊肿
高反应性黄体（多发性黄体滤泡性囊肿）
黄体囊肿
妊娠期黄体瘤
异位妊娠
间质性增生
卵泡膜细胞增殖症
重度水肿
纤维瘤病
子宫内膜异位
未分类囊肿（单纯性囊肿）
炎性病变

疾病分类和分期

卵巢病变大致可以分为非新生物性病变和新生物性病变；前者主要包括一些功能性的囊肿，后者包括一些良恶性的肿瘤。目前临床上应用的分类系统改良自最近的世界卫生组织对疾病的组织学分类以及特别针对肿瘤的修订（表 36–4 和 36–5）[184]。非肿瘤性病变和新生物性病变均可起源于上皮组织、生殖细胞成分和间质成分。列出的新生物性病变根据起源的组织不同而分类。

卵巢肿瘤的处理需要首先对疾病进展的程度进行准确的分期。近来对卵巢恶性肿瘤的治疗进展主要体现在生存率的提高和生育能力的保留。必须将根据组织学检查结果的外科分期作为对疾病的临床评估的一部分。精确的临床分期主要根据临床检查结果、手术探查结果、组织学检查结果和体液细胞学检查结果，国际妇产科联合会癌症委员会（FIGO）曾提出过详细的分期标准（表 36–6）[62]。

卵巢肿瘤是一种相对少见的疾病，由多专业机构合作研究得出的肿瘤评估和处理意见有很大的利用价值。儿童癌症组织（CCG）、儿科肿瘤学组（POG）和妇科肿瘤学组（GOG）曾对间质和生殖细胞肿瘤进行评估[31,41,69,167]。在儿童，组间 POG 9048/9049 和 CCG 8882/8891 对儿童的研究评分标准结合了手术和病理的检查结果。儿童肿瘤学组（COG）曾提出过类似的评分标准（表 36–7）[31]。

虽然目前对卵巢肿瘤的处理越来越倾向于保守性的手术治疗，但还是需要制订统一的针对这些病变的外科处理方案[208,209]。术前评估需要通过肿瘤标志物的检查排除明显恶性的卵巢肿瘤，通过盆腔超声检查判断卵巢肿瘤的结构是单一性还是混合性。

肿瘤标志物含量增高以及超声显示一混合性占位病变提示存在恶性肿瘤的可能，需要行腹部和盆腔 CT 扫描检查。对于可能恶性的病变，手术时需要有足够长的腹部切口，并严禁切开肿瘤包膜。相反，如果肿瘤标志物阴性，一般考虑为良性肿瘤（如成熟囊性畸胎瘤），可以考虑行腹腔镜下肿瘤切除术（图 36–3）。

儿童的初次手术治疗一般相对保守。盆腔灌洗、单侧卵巢囊肿切除、术中冰冻切片和对侧卵巢的仔细观察在对良性卵巢病变和低度恶性肿瘤的初次处理中是很必要的。盆腔灌洗也是卵巢肿瘤分期的一部分，

表 36–5 卵巢肿瘤的世界卫生组织分类

1. 表皮–间质肿瘤
   - 1.1. 浆液性瘤
   - 1.2. 黏液性瘤
   - 1.3. 内膜样瘤
   - 1.4. 透明细胞瘤
   - 1.5. 移行细胞瘤
   - 1.6. 鳞状上皮肿瘤
   - 1.7. 混合性上皮肿瘤
   - 1.8. 未分化及未分类的肿瘤
2. 性索–间质肿瘤
   - 2.1. 颗粒间质细胞瘤
     - 2.1.1. 颗粒细胞瘤
       - 2.1.1.1. 成人型
       - 2.1.1.2. 幼年型
     - 2.1.2. 泡膜–纤维瘤
   - 2.2. 支持间质细胞瘤
   - 2.3. 混合性或未分类的性索–间质肿瘤
     - 2.3.1. 环状小管性索瘤
     - 2.3.2. 两性胚细胞瘤
   - 2.4. 类固醇细胞瘤
3. 生殖细胞肿瘤
   - 3.1. 初级生殖细胞肿瘤
     - 3.1.1. 无性细胞瘤
     - 3.1.2. 卵黄囊瘤（内胚窦瘤）
     - 3.1.3. 胚胎性癌
     - 3.1.4. 多胚癌
     - 3.1.5. 非妊娠性绒毛膜癌
     - 3.1.6. 混合性生殖细胞肿瘤(特定成分)
   - 3.2 双胚层或三胚层畸胎瘤
     - 3.2.1. 未成熟
     - 3.2.2. 成熟
   - 3.3 单胚层畸胎瘤
4. 生殖细胞性索–间质肿瘤
   - 4.1. 性腺母细胞瘤
   - 4.2. 非成性腺细胞的混合性生殖细胞性索–间质肿瘤
5. 卵巢网肿瘤
6. 混合性肿瘤
   - 6.1. 小细胞癌，高血钙型
   - 6.2. 妊娠性绒毛膜癌
   - 6.3. 非卵巢特异性软组织肿瘤
7. 肿瘤样改变
8. 淋巴瘤和血管瘤
9. 继发性肿瘤

表 36-6 国际妇产科联合会癌症委员会（FIGO）的卵巢恶性肿瘤分期标准

分期	疾病程度
0	无证据显示原发性肿瘤
I	肿瘤局限于卵巢
IA	肿瘤局限于一侧卵巢，包膜完整，卵巢表面无肿瘤浸润，腹水及腹腔灌洗液中无恶性肿瘤细胞
IB	肿瘤局限于两侧卵巢，包膜完整，卵巢表面无肿瘤浸润，腹水及腹腔灌洗液中无恶性肿瘤细胞
IC	肿瘤局限于一侧或两侧卵巢，同时有下列任一种情况：包膜破裂，卵巢表面肿瘤浸润，腹水及腹腔灌洗液中发现恶性肿瘤细胞
II	一侧或两侧卵巢肿瘤同时有盆腔浸润
IIA	浸润或种植于子宫、输卵管或两者，腹水及腹腔灌洗液中无恶性肿瘤细胞
IIB	浸润到其他盆腔器官，腹水及腹腔灌洗液中无恶性肿瘤细胞
IIC	IIA 或 IIB 同时腹水及腹腔灌洗液中发现恶性肿瘤细胞
III	一侧或两侧卵巢肿瘤同时显微镜发现有盆腔外的腹腔转移或局部淋巴结转移
IIIA	显微镜发现有盆腔外的腹腔转移
IIIB	肉眼发现腹腔转移最大距离超出盆腔不足 2cm
IIIC	肉眼发现腹腔转移最大距离超出盆腔大于 2cm 或有局部淋巴结转移
IV	超出腹腔的远处转移

在进入腹腔（通过腹腔镜或通过腹部切口）的同时需要进行盆腔灌洗，以避免术中肿瘤破裂引起污染。最终的病理结果必须要等到冰冻切片或石蜡包埋组织切片的组织学检查结果出来后才能揭晓，为了避免遗漏潜在的恶性肿瘤，对于所有的混合性附件占位的患者都需要行腹腔灌洗。如果腹腔没有游离液体，可以用乳酸林格液灌洗盆腔和结肠旁沟，并抽取灌洗液送检。

恶性生殖细胞和间质肿瘤在疾病早期基本上都是单侧的，所以初次手术处理时行单侧的输卵管卵巢切除术就已经足够。有报道称化疗疗效出色，甚至对儿童进展期肿瘤的效果也不错，并且保留了生育能力。对于两侧卵巢浸润甚至更严重的卵巢浸润肿瘤，目前试管内受精技术的成功开展使得越来越多的初次肿瘤切除手术考虑保留子宫[14,202]。肿瘤的生物学表现和对辅助治疗的反应直接影响到手术的最终效果。

腹腔镜检查评估盆腔疾病有相当高的利用价值（见图 36-3）。Elsheikh 等[57]报道 54 名 14～20 岁的卵巢占位患者成功进行腹腔镜检查的病例。最终的病理结果显示，22 例为成熟囊性畸胎瘤，12 例为子宫内膜异位，8 例为浆液性囊腺瘤，5 例为黏液性囊腺瘤，3 例为交界性肿瘤，3 例为纤维-泡膜细胞瘤。Heloury 等[86]对 28 名有附件疾患的儿童进行了腹腔镜检查，在其中 25 名只以检查为目的的患儿中发现了一些非卵巢的病变。另外，对 4 名患有卵巢肿瘤的患儿进行了肿瘤的组织学检查，对 9 名功能性囊肿的患儿进行了诊断性的穿刺。有 1 例由于盆腔粘连而导致腹腔镜检查失败，有 1 例由于术后并发症而需要进行开腹手术。 600

美国妇科腹腔镜学会回顾了超过 13 000 例腹腔镜检查持续性卵巢占位的病例[93]。其中 0.4%的病例

表 36-7 儿童肿瘤学组（COG）对卵巢生殖细胞肿瘤的临床病理学分期

I	局限于卵巢（腹腔无转移）；没有临床、影像学、组织学证据显示肿瘤范围超出卵巢（注意：腹膜神经胶质瘤病的存在并不影响肿瘤 I 期的分期）
II	镜下残余病灶，腹腔无转移（注意：腹膜神经胶质瘤病的存在并不影响肿瘤 II 期的分期）
III	淋巴结转移（转移性小结）；大体残余病灶或活检发现；相邻脏器浸润（大网膜、肠、膀胱）；腹腔发现恶性肿瘤细胞
IV	远处转移，包括肝脏

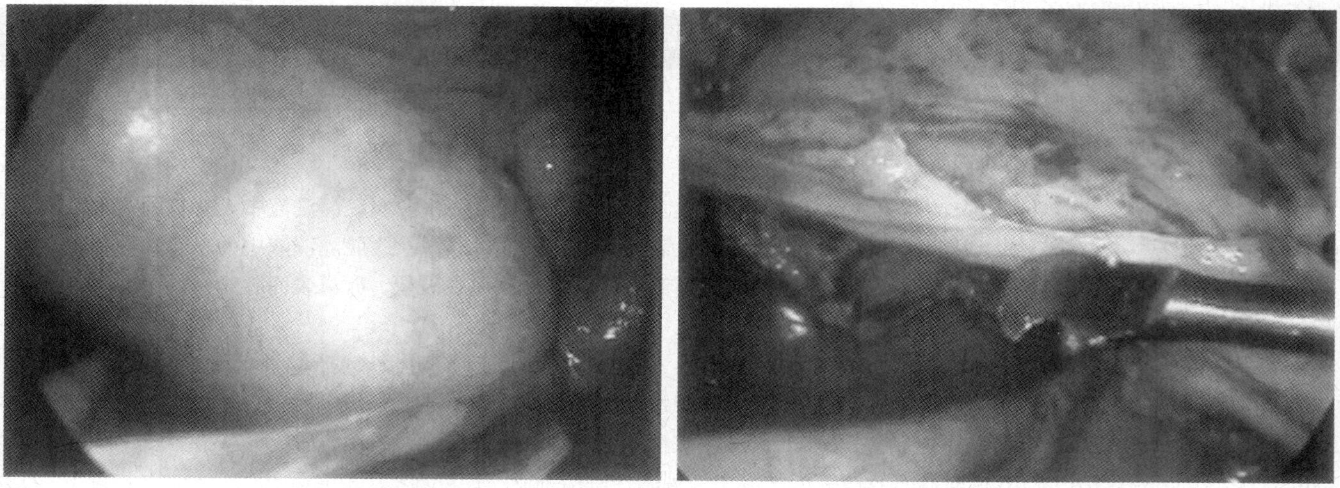

图 36-3　A. 儿童常规体检时触诊发现的腹部肿块的腹腔镜图像。行腹部和盆腔 CT 检查证实左侧卵巢巨大囊性占位。B. 用 Harmonic 解剖刀从肿块的中部和腰部剥除囊肿，保留卵巢。

为Ⅰ期卵巢癌。虽然在成年妇女中这一结果是鼓舞人心的，但是在儿童中，因为缺少相关的经验，用肉眼观察卵巢肿瘤来确定卵巢肿瘤的性质还是相当困难的。尽管如此，腹腔镜技术可以防止肿瘤细胞的漏出，适用范围可相对扩大。另外，一些经验丰富的外科医生已经开始在腹腔镜下进行更晚期的肿瘤处理和淋巴结分离[87]。

治疗

非肿瘤性卵巢肿瘤

卵巢囊肿来源于成熟的卵巢滤泡。对青春期前女童的尸检报告表明，在所有年龄的女童中都有卵巢滤泡的生长，并可以看到卵母细胞、颗粒细胞和不同退化程度的卵巢囊泡[155,156]。一般来说，生理性滤泡和病理性卵巢囊肿可以从大小上加以区分：直径大于 2cm 的病变一般不再认为是成熟的卵巢滤泡。

非肿瘤性卵巢囊肿大多是良性的，一般无症状，大约占儿童和青少年所有外科治疗的卵巢病变的 35%[24]。外科手段鉴别非肿瘤性卵巢囊肿和肿瘤性卵巢肿瘤比较困难，前者由于大小和一些功能性活动导致偶尔出现临床症状，以此可与后者鉴别。当必须行手术治疗时，也应该采用相对保守的手术方案。很多情况下，可以只切除囊肿而保留周围正常的卵巢组织。

滤泡囊肿

滤泡囊肿大约占所有非肿瘤性卵巢病变的 50%。这些病变都为单侧、单腔、组织学良性，并且含有稀薄的黄色清亮液体。目前发现这些改变在新生儿和婴儿中很常见。Cohen 等[34]研究了 77 名从出生到 24 个月大的患儿的卵巢影像，其中 84%的病例为囊肿。按每 3 个月为一组，每组的患病率是相似的。另一项对 2～12 岁初潮前女孩的研究也有类似的发现[34]。其中 68%的患者有囊肿，而这些囊肿患者基本上平均分布在各个年龄组中。其他一切正常的儿童初潮前卵巢出现囊肿并不一定意味着内分泌或者其他系统的疾病。偶尔，卵巢囊肿持续不消退甚至扩大并可分泌雌二醇，可导致同性假性性早熟[118]。

卵巢滤泡囊肿的大小是决定临床治疗方案的主要因素。Millar 等[129]统计了 99 名 5 岁的患儿，17 例卵巢囊肿直径大于 2cm。其中 7 例仅给予临床观察，并没有不良的预后；而另外 10 例滤泡性或黄体性的囊肿均予以手术切除，其中 2 例（直径在 5～10cm）已经发生附件扭转而看不到明显的卵巢组织。在另一组 28 名同时有性早熟的卵巢囊肿患者中，12 例仅有乳房过早发育，4 例有阴道出血，7 例为真性中枢性性早熟。在这 23 人中，没有一例卵巢囊肿的直径大于 2cm[63]。乳房过早发育的女孩经常会有卵巢微囊肿形成。剩下 5 名同性假性性早熟的患儿有巨大的卵巢囊肿。尽管其中 2 例自发退化，其他 3 例黄体滤泡囊肿还需要外科手术切除。

随着产前超声的运用，一些卵巢囊肿经常可以在产前就被发现[23]。胎儿卵巢囊肿的确切原因还不是很清楚，它们大概是由于胎儿滤泡刺激激素、母体雌二醇、胎盘绒毛膜促性腺激素和不成熟的下丘脑-垂体-卵巢轴的联合作用的结果。胎儿产出后，由于激素刺激下降，往往可以导致囊肿自限性消退。

产前和围生期发现的卵巢囊肿可以在 1 岁以内自行消退，不推荐子宫内治疗[85,125]。即使存在巨大卵巢囊肿，也应该根据产科指征决定是否采用剖宫产[85,171]。这些囊肿偶尔会导致蒂扭转、肠梗阻、肠穿孔和囊肿破裂。Bagolan[15]和 Giorlandino[70]等认为，卵巢囊肿患者超声检查发现液体碎片、血凝块或者隔膜的需要进行手术治疗，因为这些发现往往提示蒂扭转或者囊内出血[195]。在这一年龄组，一般在产前就已经发生附件扭转，即使出生后立即予以手术治疗，也基本上不能保存有活力的卵巢组织（图 36-4）[6,23]。胎儿期的囊肿大多都是黄体细胞囊肿，而年长儿童更多的是颗粒细胞囊肿[154]。

目前大多数的学者提倡对新生儿卵巢病变行保守治疗。小的、无症状的囊肿主要予以超声随访，等待自行消退；直径达到或超过 5cm 以及长蒂囊肿容易发生蒂扭转，需要行保留卵巢的囊肿切除术[23]或穿刺抽液[6,129,171]。超声引导下的囊肿穿刺抽液复发率低，几乎没有并发症[43,52]。除非出现临床症状、复发或持续几个月后仍不消退，小的单纯性囊肿一般仅予观察随访[30]。

在青春期前儿童中，急性症状和内分泌活动的出现增加了处理的难度。Warner[218]等描述了 92 名卵巢巨大囊肿患儿的处理结果。90%的囊肿自行消退或萎缩。在 23 名外科手术治疗的患儿中，17 例是由于急性剧烈腹痛而紧急手术。囊肿大小和超声特点并不是处理方案的决定因素。症状在 24 小时内不缓解，或者巨大占位造成了腹内并发症，或者影像学检查发现肿瘤性病变存在，这些情况下需要行开腹手术。那些进行性增大的囊肿或者超声随访下持续不消退的囊肿也需要手术治疗。

大约 75%的青少年甲状腺功能减退的女孩同时存

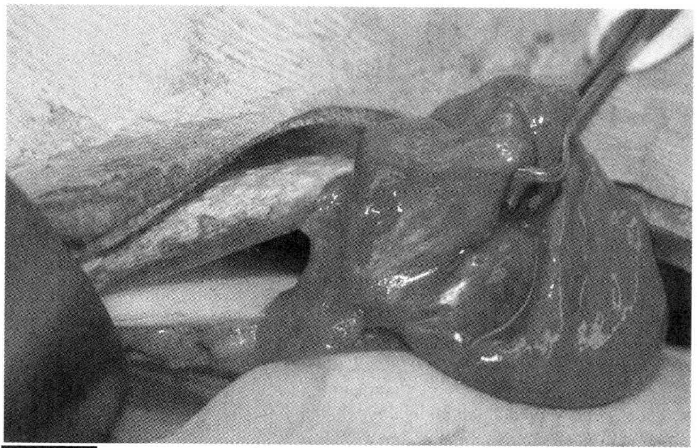

图 36-4　这个新生女婴产前检查发现腹内囊性占位，产后影像学检查发现低衰减的囊性结构和囊壁的不规则钙化。经腹手术分离扭转的囊肿和卵巢后发现两者间仅有一个小蒂相连。输卵管予以保留，病理显示薄壁的囊肿伴有营养不良性钙化灶。

在多发性卵巢囊肿，并由于垂体促性腺激素和催乳素分泌增加，表现为不同程度的性早熟和溢乳[154]。多发性卵巢囊肿也需要与多囊卵巢综合征相鉴别，后者可导致青春期女孩发育延迟、严重的无排卵性功血[170]。

在一项对初潮后患者的随机研究中，针对囊肿直径达到或超过 5cm 以及影像学检查有混合性表现的患者用盆腔超声进行了短期随访。发现这些囊肿自行消退的比率仍相当高[192]。2～3 个月随访中囊肿未消退甚至增大[192]，并伴发急性或严重慢性腹痛或腹内并发症的患者，需要进行开腹或者腹腔镜下手术探查。

外科手术治疗非肿瘤性卵巢囊肿，应该以尽可能保留更多的正常卵巢组织为前提。用细针在脏层腹膜下注射生理盐水可以在切面上清楚地区分正常卵巢组织和囊肿组织。如果手术完整切除囊肿会对有活力的卵巢组织造成损伤，就需要剪去部分囊壁，抽空囊液，在保护卵巢的前提下尽可能剥离囊壁。只有在有确切证据显示没有有活力的卵巢组织可以保留时才可以行单侧卵巢切除。同侧的输卵管予以保留，因为还有可能成为对侧卵巢排卵后的受孕场所。

黄体囊肿

真性功能性黄体囊肿只出现在活跃排卵期的青

少年。虽然这些囊肿有可能发生在两侧卵巢并形成巨大囊肿，但是大多数能够随着体内血清黄体酮下降自发退化。黄体囊肿大体外观呈金黄色，部分由于囊内充血可能会出现血色。囊内含有黄体化的颗粒细胞和泡膜细胞，并能分泌雌激素和孕激素。当囊肿破裂时或发生蒂扭转时会引起急性盆腔疼痛，不能自发退化的囊肿有可能引起月经紊乱和功能障碍性功血。

黄体囊肿的手术目的和其他卵巢滤泡性病变的手术目的相同，如果囊肿发生急性病变或者在超声随访4～6周后囊肿持续不退就需要手术介入。Hasson[83]在19名卵巢黄体囊肿患儿中选择了17名进行腹腔镜下抽吸囊液、开窗或囊壁剥除治疗。术后16名患儿症状消退。卵巢黄体囊肿的复发率是很低的。

卵巢冠囊肿

卵巢冠囊肿通常很小，而且没有症状，它们并非起源于卵巢组织，只因与卵巢组织相当接近而被归类到卵巢囊肿中。卵巢冠囊肿起源于卵巢冠，一般生长在输卵管系膜上。卵巢冠囊肿和其他卵巢滤泡性囊肿不能通过影像学手段鉴别。即使在手术中，两者的大体外观也相同，但是由于它们的解剖位置不同，往往可以比较准确地加以鉴别。当需要外科手术介入时，常规开腹手术和微创手术都可以采用[83,179]。大的卵巢冠囊肿（＞3cm）应该在保护输卵管和卵巢不受损伤的情况下将其从输卵管系膜上完全剥除，处理直径＜3cm的囊肿可以用穿刺和对囊壁双极电凝的方法[42]。

子宫内膜异位症

子宫内膜异位症表现为子宫内膜腺体和基质种植到子宫外的腹膜表面，它的病理机制一般认为包括月经排出受阻引起月经逆行、机械性转移、子宫内膜成分的种植和体腔细胞化生[81,105,144]。从初潮到子宫内膜异位症的发生有可能只有1个月的时间，20岁以下的女孩中子宫内膜异位的发生率要远远高于预先估计和文献记载的比率[165]。青少年中该病进一步进展的可能较小，除非患儿还并发有梗阻性 müller 管畸形。

据报道，子宫内膜异位症的发生率在年幼女孩中约为1%，而在年长女孩中约为47%[73,89,124]。典型的临床表现包括慢性的周期性或非周期性的盆腔疼痛和痛经[13]。早期诊断相当重要，因为早期治疗可以预防腹腔内的炎症扩散，包括广泛粘连和子宫腺肌瘤的形成。种植在腹膜表面的早期病变一般表现为小淤点，厚度不超过1mm。近来发现部分子宫内膜异位症可能会有不典型的外观表现，包括水泡、白斑、火药灼伤样改变和粘连[216]。

美国生育协会修订的子宫内膜异位症分类标准已经广泛应用于该病的分期并作为因该病导致不孕的患者预测预后的工具[7]。然而，四期的划分并不是依据临床疼痛的程度，而是与疾病的严重程度相关[108]。对于有盆腔疼痛并怀疑子宫内膜异位症的患者，应该考虑给予非固醇类抗炎药或者口服避孕药治疗。这两种药物都能抑制前列腺素，而前列腺素是引起痛经的重要原因。药物治疗子宫内膜异位症一般同时还需要加用绒毛膜促性腺激素对抗剂，并维持6个月。

虽然子宫内膜异位症可以通过超声发现，但是目前对可疑病变做腹腔镜活检仍是可行的方法。对子宫内膜异位症的病变部位做组织学检查相当重要，一些病例显示，幼儿的微小病理改变随着年龄的增长可能演变成严重的病变[109]。如果外科医生对子宫内膜异位症的手术处理相当熟悉，那么通过手术切除所有可见病变对于治疗子宫内膜异位症引起的盆腔疼痛的效果要优于对照组[198]。

单纯性囊肿

大多数学者认为单纯性囊肿来源于滤泡囊肿。它们的解剖结构大多是体积小、单腔、薄壁的病变，与滤泡囊肿比较类似。大多数是良性的，不分泌激素。对于大的、引起临床症状的单纯性囊肿，处理方案与滤泡性囊肿的相似。有人在1990年对腹腔镜检、细针穿刺、开窗术、组织活检以及行囊肿内壁切除和没有行囊肿内壁切除的病例进行了评估[83]。56例功能性单纯性囊肿或卵巢冠囊肿中只有1例在腹腔镜术后复发。

肿瘤性卵巢肿瘤

大多数肿瘤性卵巢肿瘤来源于三层组织之一的细

胞：尿生殖嵴表面的生殖上皮细胞、其下方的间质细胞和卵黄囊来源的生殖细胞。这些来源的细胞通过失分化、异常增殖并最终恶变形成卵巢肿瘤[190]。恶性卵巢肿瘤有可能是由某些良性肿瘤在直接或间接的激素刺激下恶变形成。已经发现在组织学上和生物学上介于良性和恶性病变之间的中间类型，它们是一群具有低恶性度的肿瘤。

各种类型卵巢肿瘤的发生频率随着患者年龄的不同而不同。成年人中，大多数卵巢肿瘤来源于上皮层，以腺癌占多数；而儿童中，生殖细胞肿瘤最为常见，占大约 60%[47,190]。上皮来源的肿瘤在较小年龄组中只占大约 15%（表 36–8）[36,47]。虽然在未成年人中的各个年龄组，生殖细胞肿瘤均占优势，但是性索–间质细胞肿瘤的高发阶段为 4 岁之前，上皮性肿瘤更多见于较年长的青少年。儿童中比较少见的卵巢肿瘤包括恶性的，如子宫内膜样瘤、透明细胞瘤，以及良性的，如 Brenner 瘤。同时，播散性恶性淋巴瘤和卵巢转移瘤也不多见。

表 36–8　不同类型卵巢肿瘤的年龄分布（%）

组织学类型	0～4 岁	5～9 岁	10～14 岁	15～19 岁	所有年龄
生殖细胞肿瘤	48	59	68	47	62.2
性索–间质肿瘤	40	17	5	12	9.7
上皮细胞肿瘤	6	4	13	34	19.3
混合性肿瘤	8	20	14	6	8.7

表皮 – 间质肿瘤

上皮来源的卵巢肿瘤占所有卵巢肿瘤的 70%，但是在儿童中并不常见。最近的一项统计显示，它们只占到所有需要手术切除的卵巢占位性病变的 16%[134]。在 Norris 和 Jensen[142]报道的 353 名卵巢肿瘤患儿中，有 67 例（19%）为上皮来源的肿瘤，其中 12%为恶性。上皮来源的卵巢肿瘤大多数为浆液性或黏液性[112]。20%的浆液性肿瘤可以同时发生在双侧卵巢，其中很少是恶性的[112,132]。黏液性肿瘤通常只发生于单侧卵巢，其中 10%为恶性[112]。Deprest 等[47]统计了超过 1700 例各种类型的卵巢肿瘤患儿的病例后提出，上皮来源的卵巢肿瘤的恶性率为 16%。这些恶性肿瘤的类型在儿童中和在成人中是不同的。儿童中黏液性的恶性肿瘤占所有上皮来源的卵巢恶性肿瘤的 40%，而在成人这一比例为 12%；儿童中有 30%为交界性低恶性度的肿瘤，而在成人这一相对乐观的病变只占到不足 10%。

血清 CA–125 是监测上皮来源的卵巢恶性肿瘤常用的肿瘤标志物。但是在一些绝经前的患者中，一些良性的妇科疾病包括子宫内膜异位、盆腔炎、纤维瘤和妊娠，也会导致 CA–125 的增高。目前应用于研究领域的免疫闪烁成像术在将来有可能成为临床上常规的诊断方法。它通过使用单克隆抗体技术定位 CA–125[51]，也有助于定位化疗后的活动性病变以及监测肿瘤的复发[101]。

上皮来源的卵巢肿瘤根据国际妇产科协会 FIGO 分期[62]。IA 期的卵巢肿瘤需要行单侧输卵管卵巢切除术。并仔细检查对侧卵巢，任何异常的部位都需要做病理活检。大多数 IB 期卵巢肿瘤（肿瘤局限于两侧卵巢）的患者需要行双侧卵巢切除术，保留子宫供将来人工授精胚胎的植入[14,146]。对于更进展期的卵巢肿瘤，尽可能多地缩减细胞相当重要，与良好的预后直接相关[217]。可以行经腹的子宫全切和双侧输卵管卵巢 603 切除术。同时行大网膜切除以及腹腔内所有可见病变的切除。对于进展期的卵巢恶性肿瘤，手术后的辅助化疗相当重要。卡铂和环磷酰胺 6 个周期的化疗临床有效率达 60%～70%，患者的 5 年生存率为 10%～20%[146]。最近有人尝试用顺铂和紫杉醇作为术后化疗用药，效果值得期待。放疗、二次手术和二次减灭细胞术对于进展期卵巢恶性肿瘤也有一定作用，但是目前尚存在争议。

混合性肿瘤

卵巢小细胞癌非常少见，但是预后极差[61]。这种肿瘤侵袭性高，是儿童中最主要的低分化卵巢恶性肿瘤。卵巢小细胞癌的患者年龄在 9～44 岁之间，平均年龄为 23 岁[163,183]。2/3 的患者可以因旁分泌而引起高钙血症，但是很少有临床表现。患者的血清甲状旁腺激素水平正常。基本上所有的卵巢小细胞癌发生在单侧，大约只有 40%能在 IA 期被发现。肿瘤的大体外观常为肉色到灰褐色；并经常可以见到大面积的出血或坏死。小细胞癌的组织发生不明，所以往往需要电镜下检查以最终确立诊断。IA 期的患者只有三分之一能存活较长时间，更进展期的患者的存活率更低[112]。单侧的输卵管卵巢切除术是使一些 IA 期患者长期存活的手术治疗方法。但是在一些患者中发现对侧保留的卵巢中存在非同步表现的小细胞癌，所以手术选择双侧附件切除术更为合适。虽然治疗方法多种多样，包括手术切除、放疗和增强化疗，卵巢小细胞癌患儿的存活时间还是相当短，平均为 18 个月[163]。

低度恶性肿瘤

卵巢上皮来源的低度恶性肿瘤与上皮来源的恶性肿瘤有两点不同：第一是前者发生在更为年幼的患儿中，第二是前者的预后要好于后者。卵巢低度恶性肿瘤可见于所有卵巢恶性肿瘤的亚型[47]。浆液性和黏液性低度恶性肿瘤最为常见，而且与良性病变很相似。这些交界性肿瘤与腺癌的区别主要是它们的肿瘤性上皮成分尚未侵入间质中（图 36-5）。高达 60
50%的低恶性度肿瘤发生于双侧卵巢，临床上表现为特征性的无痛性病变。这些肿瘤在手术切除 10～15 年后有可能会复发，并且进展为侵袭性的恶性肿瘤[38]。

最近的成人病例统计中，将浆液性和黏液性卵巢交界性肿瘤患者的长期生存率做了比较。浆液性卵巢交界性肿瘤和恶性肿瘤的 10 年生存率分别为 96%和 30.4%；黏液性卵巢交界性肿瘤和恶性肿瘤的 10 年生存率分别为 94%和 64%[187]。成人中，91%的黏液性卵巢交界性肿瘤为 I 期肿瘤，5 年生存率为 98%。浆液性交界性肿瘤的生存率也与此类似。Massad 等[122]的

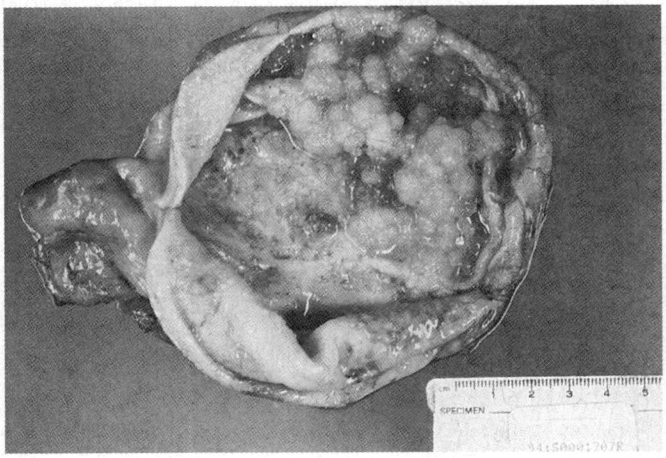

A

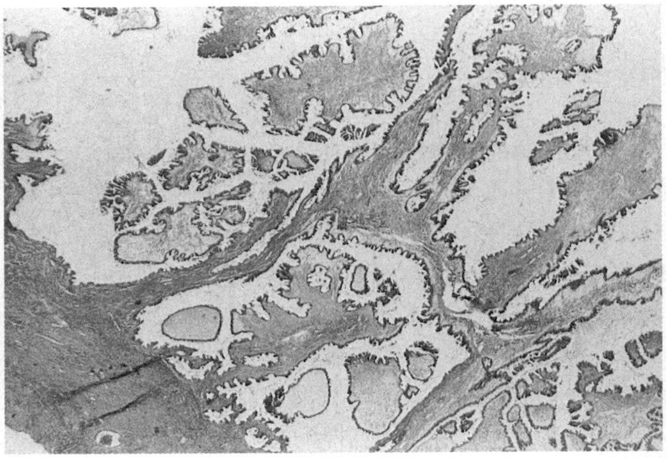

B

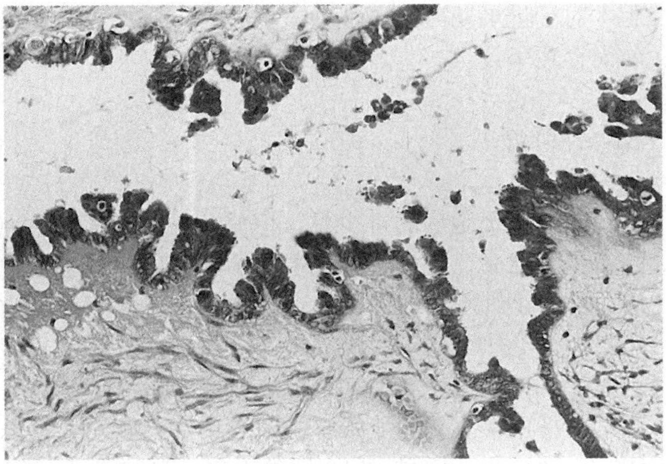

C

图 36-5 A. 一位 17 岁女孩的巨大双侧卵巢肿块切除术后的卵巢肿瘤。切开的样本显示了充满清亮液体的囊腔，囊壁可见大量小瘤和乳头状隆起物。B. 病理组织切片显示浆液性乳头状低度恶性肿瘤（HE 染色，40 倍）。C. 组织切片的高倍显微照片显示，乳头中纤维血管束和上皮细胞分层排列，没有侵入间质（HE 染色，400 倍）。

大量回访资料显示，卵巢交界性 I 期肿瘤的生存率为 98%，II 期为 94%，III 期和 IV 为 79%。儿童中，Morris 等[135]报告，75%的卵巢交界性肿瘤为 I 期肿瘤，生存率为 100%。临床各期的总的 10 年生存率为 73%。

手术是首选的治疗方案。早期的交界性肿瘤只需行单侧的输卵管卵巢切除术，并可以作为标准的处理方案。然而，最近的研究提出，幼儿如果有严格随访条件的，可以仅行卵巢囊肿切除术。术后每 3～6 个月需进行一次盆腔检查、CA-125 测定和超声检查，因为仅行卵巢囊肿切除术的患儿复发的危险性要高于行其他更为侵袭性手术的患儿。Morice 等[133]报告，卵巢囊肿切除术、卵巢切除术和双侧卵巢切除加子宫全切术术后复发率分别为 36.3%、15.1%和 5.7%。虽然复发率不同，但是并不影响患儿最终的生存率；因为所有复发的患儿都可以通过进一步的手术来治疗。所以，对于如果要求保留生育功能并能保证按时随访的患儿，可以采用保守疗法。如果超声显示对侧卵巢无异常[16]，常规的对侧卵巢楔形切除活检是不必要的[132]。

双侧的交界性肿瘤需要行双侧的卵巢囊肿切除术或输卵管卵巢切除术。如果是更为晚期的病变，则需要加行子宫切除术。提示预后不良的病理改变尚在论证中[38]，目前还没有这方面的明确的报告。目前，外科手术仍然是治疗这一类肿瘤的最有效的方法，还没有人提出有效的辅助治疗手段[16,113]。虽然还没有个体化的治疗方案能够提供稳定的良好预后，但是这一类肿瘤的良好的生物学特性弥补了辅助治疗临床作用有限的不足。

性索－间质肿瘤

性索–间质肿瘤很可能起源于尿生殖嵴表面上皮下方的未定型的间充质干细胞[164]。这些全能的组织可以分化成不同的细胞系，包括卵巢的颗粒–泡膜细胞和睾丸间质的支持–间质细胞。性索–间质肿瘤被认为是功能性的卵巢肿瘤，它们能引起全身的激素反应。性索–间质肿瘤大约占 Boston 儿童医院所有卵巢肿瘤的 13%[112]，在另一项统计中大约占所有儿童卵巢肿瘤的 17%。大多数 9 岁以前的性索–间质患儿有雌性化表现；而 9 岁以后则以男性化表现占优势。

颗粒–泡膜细胞瘤

颗粒 - 泡膜细胞瘤是最常见的性索–间质肿瘤，也是最常见的功能性卵巢肿瘤。幼年型颗粒细胞瘤是其中的一种特殊的亚型；大约 44%发生在十几岁前儿童，97%发生在 30 岁以前[162]。大多数患有这种肿瘤的初潮前女孩可以出现同性假性性早熟（图 36–6）[164]。大多数患儿血清和尿液中雌二醇的含量增高。而绒毛膜促性腺激素的水平不高，凭这一点可以将幼年型颗粒细胞瘤和真性性早熟、绒毛膜促性腺激素分泌性疾病以及女性化肾上腺瘤鉴别开来。血清抑制素，一种卵巢颗粒细胞分泌的糖蛋白，是有价值的肿瘤标志物[114,140]。在一些颗粒–泡膜细胞瘤患儿中，副中肾管抑制因子水平增高，提示也可以作为预测肿瘤的标志物[80]。

临床表现包括乳房过早发育、阴道溢液或出血、阴唇肥厚、阴毛或腋毛出现、身体发育加快和骨龄超前。阴蒂增大是少见的男性化表现，是肿瘤分泌雄激素作用的结果。青春期后的女孩一般表现为腹部肿块、相对非特异性腹痛或者腹围增加。肿瘤破裂致腹腔积血虽然很少见，却是需要立即手术的外科急症。另外青春期后的女孩还会出现闭经以及其他月经紊乱。临床急症也可出现在幼儿，表现为急剧加重的胸腔积液和腹水，导致严重的腹部膨隆和呼吸窘迫[95]。

除了临床表现上的区别，幼年型颗粒细胞瘤和成人型颗粒细胞瘤还有组织学和生物学表现的不同。幼年型颗粒细胞瘤相对比较大，平均直径在 12.5cm[234]。腹腔镜下可见实性部分一般为黄褐色或灰色，囊性部分含有血性液体。与成人型颗粒细胞瘤细胞相比，幼年型颗粒细胞瘤细胞含有大量嗜酸性或黄体化的胞浆，胞核不典型，有丝分裂比例较高。DNA 含量测定和流式细胞仪细胞周期核型分析对判断成人患者的预后有一定相关性，而在儿童两者不一定相关[199]。

成人型颗粒细胞瘤一般是一种无痛的缓慢生长的肿瘤，潜在恶性程度相对较低，而幼年型颗粒细胞瘤则相对更具侵袭性，其生物学表现与肿瘤的大小、疾病的分期、是否发生破裂、胞核异形的程度以及有丝分裂活跃性相关。在 Young 等[236]报告的 125 例病例中，122 例累及单侧卵巢。成人型颗粒细胞瘤的复发间隔时间一般超过诊断后 5 年。而幼年型恶性颗粒细胞瘤的复发间隔时间明显较短。 605

颗粒细胞瘤的分期方法与其他卵巢肿瘤类似（见表 36–6）。儿童颗粒细胞瘤的预后相对良好，因为超过 90%的患儿为 I 期肿瘤。IA 期肿瘤的生存率大约在 95%，IC 期肿瘤的生存率大约在 80%。II 期或更晚期肿瘤的患儿死亡与治疗无关。Plantaz 等[159]分析了法国多个中心 39 例幼年型颗粒细胞瘤病例。患儿的平均年龄为 6 岁；52%出现了同性假性性早熟，10%的患儿青春期后出现内分泌紊乱。3 例因肿瘤破裂造成外科急症。5 例死亡患儿中有 4 例是 6 个月以内的 III 期或 IV 期女性肿瘤患儿。

因为较少出现累及双侧卵巢的颗粒–泡膜细胞瘤，而且 I 期肿瘤的预后良好，如果要求保留生育功能，手术时可以仅行单侧的卵巢切除术或输卵管卵巢切除术。而因为晚期颗粒–泡膜细胞瘤患儿的预后很差，所以虽然确切疗效还不是很明确，治疗上需要多学科手段的介入。对于 III 期肿瘤的患儿，出现肿瘤破裂或者肉眼可见的肿瘤扩散时，需要行子宫全切加双侧输卵管卵巢切除，并进行 3000cGy 强度的全腹腔照射和残余病灶追加照射[159]。多种药物联合化疗，包括甲氨蝶呤、放线菌素 D、环磷酰胺、博来霉素和长春花生物碱，也取得了一定的疗效。然而，大多数晚期的患儿复发并死亡。目前，制定用于治疗进展期颗粒–泡膜细胞瘤患儿的特定的化疗方案必须作为一项研究项目开展起来。

纤维瘤和泡膜瘤

纤维瘤和泡膜瘤大约占儿童性索–间质肿瘤的 14%[112]。虽然纤维瘤在 20 岁以下的女孩中相当少见，但是可以引起基底细胞痣综合征，肿瘤通常累及两侧卵巢，呈多中心，并有局部钙化。大多数泡膜瘤发生于绝经后妇女；只有两种类型曾报道在二十几岁的女孩中出现。一种为钙化泡膜瘤，可以引起闭经或其他月经紊乱以及多毛症[235]；另一种为黄体化的泡膜瘤，因为肿瘤内含有大量的黄体细胞，这种肿瘤可见于更为年幼的女孩中，并可造成男性化表现。

从大体上检查，纤维瘤比较硬，是实性的肿块，横切面可见同心圆和小梁结构。而泡膜瘤的液体成分

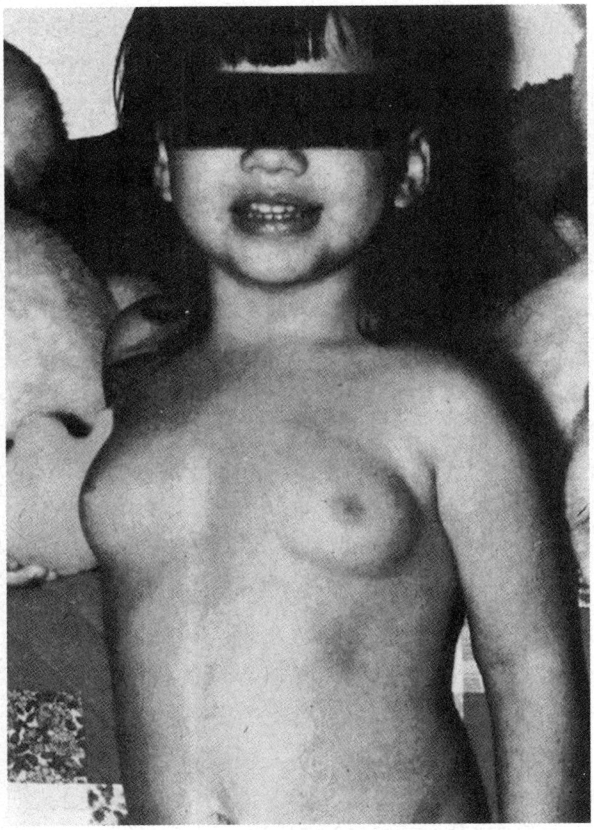
A

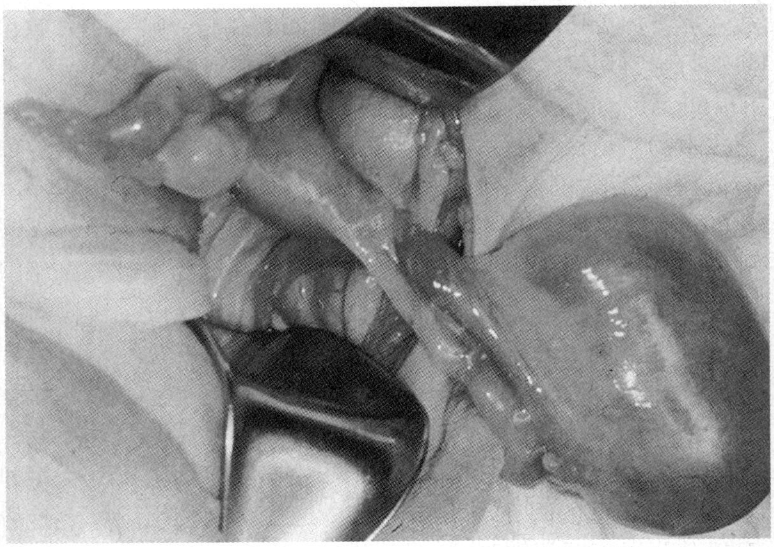
B

图 36–6 A. 一位 3 岁的女孩，表现为同性假性性早熟。B. 手术发现良性的幼年型颗粒细胞瘤，行单侧的输卵管卵巢切除术切除肿瘤。

使它呈现黄白色到橘黄色外观。这些肿瘤都是良性的，治疗上只需行单侧的卵巢切除术。对于累及双侧卵巢的纤维瘤，在分离肉眼可见的肿瘤组织的同时，
606 特别要注意保留正常的卵巢组织[90]。肿瘤复发比较少见，可通过再次手术解决。男性化的症状通常在肿瘤切除后就会缓解。

硬化性间质瘤

硬化性间质瘤是最近发现的与纤维瘤和泡膜瘤不同的实体肿瘤。据报道，这种肿瘤主要发生于女孩，30%的硬化性间质瘤发生在 20 岁以前。偶尔可见硬化性间质瘤分泌雌激素的报道，而有关男性化表现的报道更少见。典型的临床表现包括盆腔肿块、年轻患者有盆腔疼痛以及月经紊乱。这种肿瘤也与 Chédiak-Higashi 综合征有关[97]。

硬化性间质瘤通常累及单侧卵巢，为直径大于 5cm 的良性肿瘤。开腹手术中可以看到这些肿瘤为局限的、实性的、黄白色的肿块，可见边界清楚的水肿区和囊肿形成。组织学检查可以发现这些肿瘤组织存在假小叶结构，在水肿区和胶原区内有边界清晰的细胞聚集[91]。手术治疗一般只需切除肉眼可见的肿瘤组织即可。

支持–间质细胞瘤

支持–间质细胞瘤占所有卵巢肿瘤不足 0.5%，但是占所有性索–间质肿瘤的 10%～30%[112]。这些肿瘤大多数具有男性化的功能，也有一些是无功能的，甚至有一些具有雌激素的作用。所以，以往使用的名称“卵巢男性细胞瘤”或“睾丸母细胞瘤”已经不再适用。1/3 的支持–间质肿瘤发生在小于 20 岁的患者。大多数累及一侧卵巢，诊断时肿瘤多为 IA 期。这些患儿的预后相当良好，肿瘤相关的死亡率只有 5%左右[154]。同颗粒细胞瘤一样，支持–间质细胞瘤的大体外观也各有不同，但是很少会含有血性液体，也不大会表现出单腔、薄壁的囊肿外观。

现行的分类标准根据细胞分化程度和有无异源性、内胚层或间质的成分将支持–间质细胞瘤分为五种组织学类型。肿瘤的分期和组织学表现是影响预后的重要因子。具有异源性成分的支持–间质细胞瘤在幼儿中很常见，很难与不成熟畸胎瘤相鉴别[154]。关于肿瘤过度分泌雄激素导致男性化的过程可以分为两期：首先是失女性化期，表现为闭经、乳房萎缩和失去女性体型；然后紧接着或者重叠发生的是男性化期，表现为多毛、阴蒂肥大和声音低沉。青春期前女孩一般以男性化以及生长发育加速为主；青春期后女孩多表现为月经紊乱、痤疮、男性化体型和多毛。男性化过程是由于分解代谢的酶缺乏导致的睾酮累积引起的。绒毛膜促性腺激素水平低，尿液中 17–酮类固醇和孕三醇的含量正常。睾酮水平和肿瘤组织的大小直接相关，所以睾酮可以用来作为监测肿瘤的生物学指标[49]。肿瘤标志物 AFP 和 CA–125 通常会增高[115]。而 LDH 可能增高或正常。支持–间质细胞瘤的激素改变有助于将其与外源性雄激素增多、肾上腺肿瘤、真两性畸形和多囊卵巢相鉴别。同颗粒细胞瘤一样，支持–间质细胞瘤也与非遗传性中胚层发育不良导致的多发性内生软骨瘤（Ollien 病）有关[223]。

对于早期的支持–间质细胞瘤，手术处理应相对保守，可以行单侧的卵巢切除术或附件切除术，保留患儿将来的生育能力。如果肿瘤累及两侧卵巢、低分化、已经破裂或者有恶性表现，与颗粒细胞瘤的处理一样，需要采用更为侵袭性的手术方案[50]。Gershenson等[67]观察了最初诊断时被认为预后不良的支持–间质细胞瘤手术以及化疗后的反应。在四个周期的博来霉素–依托泊苷–顺铂的化疗后，50%的患者在治疗后 28 个月还没有出现临床症状或恶化迹象，总有效率可以达到 83%。很少有关于化疗后卵巢功能保留情况的资料，口服避孕药或者绒毛膜促性腺激素释放激素激动剂可能在化疗中或者化疗后对卵巢功能起到一些保护作用[28]。

环状小管性索瘤

环状小管性索瘤很少见，是性索–间质肿瘤的不同变异类型。它有朝两个方向分化成为颗粒细胞或支持细胞瘤的趋势[112]。这种肿瘤经常发生于 Peutz–Jeghers 综合征患者。这种情况下病变一般较小，多病灶，常常累及双侧卵巢。肿瘤通常会钙化，往往在尸检或因其他原因行卵巢切除后才意外地发现。虽然部分患者偶尔会出现月经紊乱，提示雌激素过多，但这种环状小管性索瘤一般不需要手术介入。

如果环状小管性索瘤出现在非 Peutz–Jeghers 综合征患者，临床上的差异就相当明显。虽然曾报道这

种患者的年龄分布可以在 6～76 岁之间，但是平均的发病年龄为 34 岁。在年轻的患者中，这种环状小管性索瘤一般累及单侧卵巢，直径大于 5cm，20%为恶性的。即使采取积极的治疗，50%的这种恶性环状小管性索瘤的患者因治疗无效而死亡[234]。

类固醇细胞瘤

类固醇细胞瘤以前称为脂肪细胞瘤。因为这类肿瘤的形态学特点以及倾向于分泌类固醇激素，这类肿瘤很少或者不含有脂肪成分，所以称为类固醇细胞瘤更为合适。这一类肿瘤根据细胞来源的不同主要可以分为三个亚型：（1）间质黄素瘤，是一类卵巢小类固醇细胞瘤，来源于间质黄体细胞；（2）间质细胞
607 瘤，细胞胞浆内含有典型的 Reinke 结晶，来源于与卵巢部位组织学相似的前体细胞；（3）其他的类固醇细胞瘤，大约占 60%左右，主要发生于年轻的患者。

第一类和第二类的类固醇细胞瘤主要发生于绝经后妇女，很少有小于 30 岁患者的报道。而大多数第三类的类固醇细胞瘤发生于青春期前，可以造成男性化和异性假性性早熟[82]。这种肿瘤很少分泌雌激素，但也有同性假性性早熟的报道[45]。这种造成男性化的肿瘤能够提高睾酮和雄烯二酮的水平，增加尿液中 17–酮类固醇排出并降低绒毛膜促性腺激素水平。

这些肿瘤一般为边界清晰的实性肿块，外观为亮黄色到棕黄色，偶尔可见小块出血或坏死灶。在成年患者中，25%可能患有第三类的恶性类固醇细胞瘤，辅助治疗往往无效，所以需要采用积极的手术治疗[84]。发生在儿童的类固醇细胞瘤常常是良性的早期肿瘤。仅需行单侧的输卵管卵巢切除术，术后密切随访。大多数激素症状会在肿瘤切除后逐渐消退，但是也有一部分患儿因为雄激素的长期作用导致下丘脑早熟而在手术切除肿瘤后出现真性性早熟[182]。

生殖细胞肿瘤

原始生殖细胞下行的途径是有缺陷的，部分生殖细胞在下行过程中偶尔会因为失去方向而停留在迁移路线的任何一个部位。所以在很多部位都可以找到生殖细胞，包括脑部的松果体、纵隔、腹膜后腔、骶尾部以及卵巢和睾丸。任何部位的生殖细胞发生恶变，都可以造成生殖腺的或生殖腺外的肿瘤。因为这些细胞是全能的，所以可以形成各种不同类型的肿瘤。Telium[205]曾提出，肿瘤特定的类型取决于肿瘤细胞的分化程度，如果没有分化，则形成生殖细胞瘤；如果出现分化，则可以形成胚胎性癌；如果出现胚外分化，则形成绒毛膜癌或者内胚窦瘤；如果出现胚胎分化，则形成畸胎瘤——最为成熟的生殖细胞肿瘤。

生殖细胞肿瘤在儿童和青少年中比较少见，如果发生，性腺是最常累及的部位。一份对 13 篇综述中共计 1491 例儿童良性或恶性生殖细胞肿瘤病例的总结报告提出，41%的生殖细胞肿瘤发生于性腺[2]，而这些发生于性腺的生殖细胞肿瘤中有 71%为卵巢生殖细胞肿瘤。上皮和间质性卵巢肿瘤多发于成人；而生殖细胞肿瘤则常发生于儿童中。一些有关卵巢肿瘤的大型报告显示，生殖细胞肿瘤在儿童卵巢肿瘤中的比例占 48%～62%[92,96,142]。这一类的肿瘤都来源于相同的全能原始生殖细胞，但是每一种肿瘤都可以造成不同的特殊行为，接下来将分别讨论这些肿瘤的不同特点，然后再讨论对这一类肿瘤的处理方案。

生殖细胞瘤

生殖细胞瘤是指一组具有相同组织学特性的肿瘤。它是发生于异常性腺组织的原发恶性肿瘤。这一类肿瘤包括睾丸的精原细胞瘤、卵巢的无性细胞瘤和性腺外的生殖细胞瘤。生殖细胞瘤被认为来源于性腺发育中未分化的全能生殖细胞[220]，是儿童和成人中最常见的卵巢恶性肿瘤[154]，大约占所有良性和恶性卵巢肿瘤的 10%[44]。

生殖细胞瘤最常见于青春期前的女孩或年轻妇女，44%的病例发生于 20 岁前，87%的病例发生于 30 岁前[9]。典型的患者具有正常的基因型和表型。在巨大的肿瘤作用下可以出现腹痛、盆腔高压症状或胃肠道、尿路梗阻症状。偶尔由于肿瘤扭转、破裂或瘤内出血而出现急腹症表现（图 36–7）[25]。部分患者也可出现腹水。因为生殖细胞瘤一般无内分泌活性，所以如果出现远距离内分泌效应则暗示为混合性生殖细胞瘤。95%的单纯生殖细胞瘤患者 LDH 水平升高，而其他肿瘤标志物阴性[102]。而混合性生殖细胞瘤患者的肿瘤标志物则可以为阳性或阴性，取决于肿瘤的组成成分。

从大体上观察，生殖细胞瘤一般为体积巨大、有完整包膜、实性的黄色肿瘤（见图 36–7），5%～30% 的病例可以累及双侧卵巢[25,46,220]。生殖细胞瘤的镜下表现相对单一，一般为具有泡状核和嗜酸性胞浆的大圆细胞，类似于原始生殖细胞，常常还可以见到淋巴细胞浸润。

生殖细胞肿瘤的处理首先是外科的手术切除。保守的单侧输卵管卵巢切除术、对侧卵巢的彻底检查，包括对可疑部位的活检以及仔细的临床分期（在手术部分强调的）是必需的。虽然过去的文献不赞成[75]，

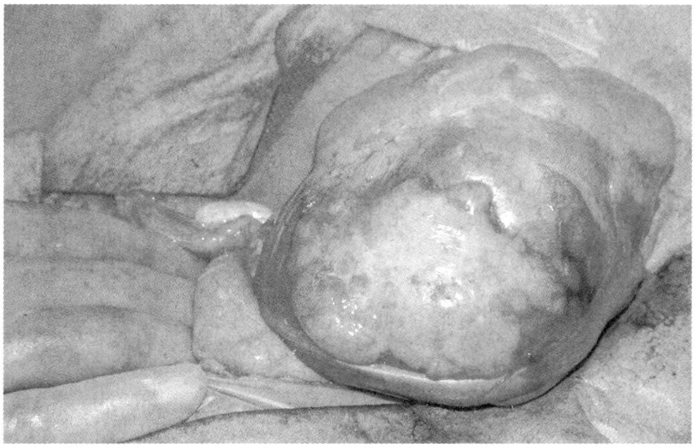

A

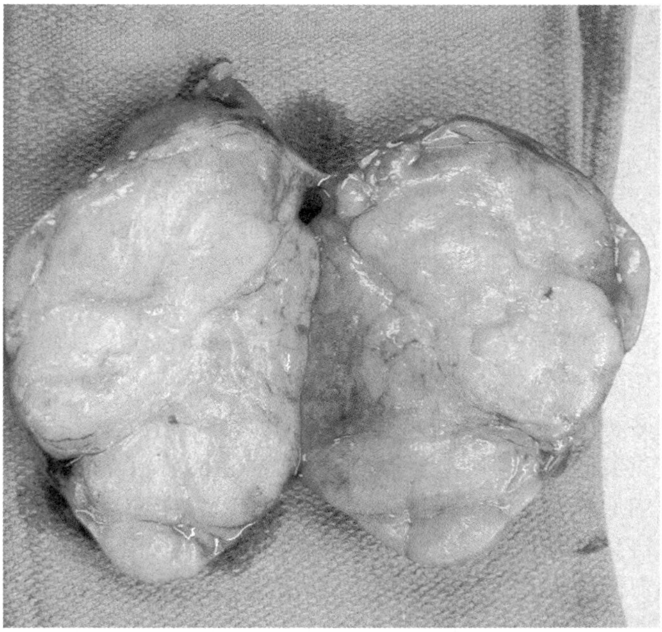

B

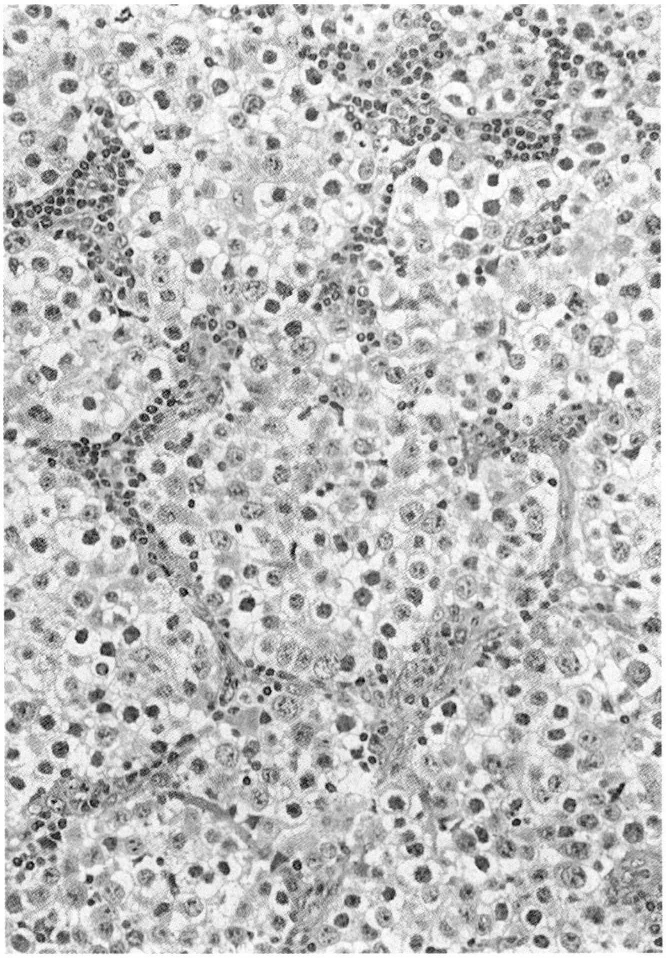

C

图 36–7　A. 从一名 5 岁急性腹痛的女孩体内切除的有完整包膜的肿块，证实为无性细胞瘤。术中发现患儿对侧的输卵管和卵巢靠近肿瘤左侧。术后的标本中包含有小部分同侧的输卵管和子宫，发现无肿瘤浸润。B. 肿瘤的切面可见由薄的纤维中隔分成的小叶。C. 无性细胞瘤的显微照片，可见多边形的透明肿瘤细胞被纤维中隔分割成小叶，其中可见散在的淋巴细胞（A 和 B 也见彩图）。

但是对于 IA 期的肿瘤，仅仅手术治疗就已经足够了。生殖细胞肿瘤对放疗相当敏感，但是由于会影响生育功能，这样代价又未免太高[66]。对于儿童，必须考虑到其他方面的长期影响，如生长发育异常或者继发性肿瘤。自从有效的联合化疗方案实行以来，放疗已经被摒弃，联合的化疗药物包括铂类、依托泊苷和博来霉素，目前已经成为标准的治疗方案[31,76,225]。

内胚窦瘤

内胚窦瘤或卵黄囊瘤以及含有两种成分的混合性
608 肿瘤都是恶性程度很高的肿瘤，它们是儿童和青少年卵巢恶性生殖细胞肿瘤中第二常见的组织学亚型[154]。在新生儿和婴幼儿，这种肿瘤的好发部位为骶尾部。而在年长儿童和青少年，则更多见于卵巢。关于这类肿瘤的来源还存有争议[177,204,205]，这类肿瘤的镜下表现也多种多样。Nogales[141]提出这一类肿瘤来源于初级卵黄囊—— 一种出现于胚胎发生早期、由多潜能原始内胚层成分组成的结构。它能分化为体腔上皮组织、次级卵黄囊（胚胎发生终末期一过性结构，分化能力低）和间质组织。只含有内胚窦结构的卵黄囊瘤亚型要比含有分化的腺体或者肝样结构的亚型分化程
609 度更低[175]。

这一类肿瘤生长迅速，是儿童中第二常见的生殖细胞肿瘤[59]。临床症状大多在肿瘤发生后的一个月内出现，同时可以发现腹内肿块。75%的患儿有腹痛和腹围增加表现[160]。AFP 增高是这一类肿瘤的标志。

手术中可以看到这一类肿瘤的大体外观呈黄白色到棕褐色，表面附有黏液，可以看到囊性区和坏死区[2]，触之柔软且容易破裂。大多数肿瘤具有不同的组织学亚型，可以看到部分分化为卵黄样或卵黄囊样的结构[111]。镜下观察，可以看到许多乳头样结构，称为内胚窦结构（Schiller-Duval 小体）或者血管旁细胞鞘。很多分化的卵黄囊瘤细胞内外还可以看到很多对过碘酸希夫染色抵抗并 AFP 阳性的小体。

胚胎性癌

胚胎性癌类似于具有大片坏死的未分化癌，单独发生相对少见。更常见于其他生殖细胞肿瘤中而构成混合性生殖细胞肿瘤。胚胎性癌的其中一种亚型，多胚瘤，能够产生 AFP 和 β-HCG，可以导致临床内分泌症状，如月经紊乱和同性假性性早熟。这种肿瘤的组织学特点为：可以发现很多类似于小胚胎的小体结构[206]。

这种肿瘤的检查和手术方式和内胚窦瘤相似，孤立的单侧肿瘤可以行单侧输卵管卵巢切除。局部浸润的肿瘤需要加行全子宫切除术，同时还需要联合化疗和放射治疗。

绒毛膜癌

绒毛膜癌比较少见，是一种发生于女孩和妇女的高度恶性的生殖细胞肿瘤，具有内分泌活性。肿瘤本身能够释放雌激素，也能通过释放绒毛膜促性腺激素刺激卵巢释放雌激素。患者的 β-HCG 增高，AFP 一般正常。

临床表现和患者的年龄有关。青春期前的儿童主要表现为同性假性性早熟和肿瘤迅速增大的征象。巨大的实性肿瘤往往会黏附于周围组织，而且还会引起远处转移性疾病。即使采取积极的手术治疗和多学科的联合治疗，患儿也常会出现恶病质而迅速死亡。在青少年患者中，肿瘤生长也相当迅速，但是激素反应主要导致月经紊乱，并可以刺激怀孕，但是怀孕期胎盘内可以形成妊娠期的绒毛膜癌[33]。

这种肿瘤容易破裂且血管丰富，极易浸润周围组织，所以手术切除相当困难[92]。如果病变局限，可以仅行单侧的输卵管卵巢切除术，但是这种情况鲜有发生。多数情况需要行扩大手术来切除肿瘤，切除范围包括对侧卵巢、子宫和尽可能多的转移组织。

大体上观察这种肿瘤为结节状，容易破裂，呈紫色，并可见因出血和坏死而造成的深褐色和黄色的斑点状区域。镜下观察可以看到细胞滋养层和合体滋养层结构，以及大片的出血和坏死区。转移灶的大体和镜下表现和原发灶相似。多种药物联合化疗是常采用的治疗手段。

畸胎瘤

畸胎瘤是一类由不同于其发生的器官或解剖部位的组织构成的肿瘤[74]。这种肿瘤的经典定义为肿瘤含有三个胚层的结构：外胚层、中胚层和内胚层。三个胚层的结构不一定同时出现在某一个畸胎瘤中，但是一定有胚胎组织出现在非正常部位。这些组织结构混

乱，具有不同程度的分化水平，所以畸胎瘤在组织学上可以分成成熟畸胎瘤、不成熟畸胎瘤和具有恶性成分的畸胎瘤[19]。儿童畸胎瘤中出现恶性成分比较少见，一般认为来源于分化的畸胎瘤成分而并非来源于全能胚胎细胞[154]。

成熟畸胎瘤：儿童的大多数畸胎瘤为成熟畸胎瘤。大多数成熟卵巢畸胎瘤被发现并没有完全减数分裂，提示它们来源于中止于减数分裂 I 期的生殖细胞[154]。很少或者没有迹象显示成熟畸胎瘤的良性成分会发生恶变或者良性畸胎瘤中同时存在恶性细胞[36]。新生儿成熟畸胎瘤主要发生于骶尾部，然后是头部和颈部[98,119,203]。卵巢是年长儿童特别是青少年畸胎瘤的好发部位。卵巢畸胎瘤多数为囊性[36]。总的说来，良性的囊性畸胎瘤是儿童最常见的卵巢肿瘤[92]，而且约 10%的患儿可累及双侧卵巢[36,193]。

成熟畸胎瘤的临床症状可以呈急性或慢性。当肿瘤发生扭转、出血或破裂时，患者可以出现类似于阑尾炎的急性症状。而慢性症状主要由腹内附件区肿块压迫周围组织造成。偶尔可由于畸胎瘤破裂引起慢性炎症而导致肠管、大网膜和前腹壁广泛粘连，这种情况也可见于盆腔腺病，是一种类似于恶性肿瘤的疾病[55]。

临床检查主要可以发现肿块。在婴儿和幼儿肿块位于腹部，在青少年肿块位于盆腔。巨大畸胎瘤触诊 610
时可以在腹部触及，质地较软。

高达 67%的病例可以通过腹部立位平片发现钙化灶（图 36–8）[4]。超声检查是常用的诊断手段。如果发现两个或以上的特征性改变，如声影和局部高回声，就可以 100%明确诊断[150]。MRI 在诊断成熟囊性畸胎瘤上要优于 CT，因为 MRI 能够清晰显示软组织结构[212]。

对于儿童和青少年的成熟囊性畸胎瘤，手术治疗宜相对保守，以保证正常发育和今后的生育功能。但是也必须与完全切除肿瘤相权衡（图 36–9）。传统的成熟囊性畸胎瘤手术为经腹的卵巢切除术。然而有经验的腹腔镜医生施行的腹腔镜下囊肿切除或卵巢切除术也是安全的选择（见图 36–3）[209]。Campo 和 Garcea[27]在一项随机的对照试验中提出，在腹腔镜下成熟囊性畸胎瘤切除术中使用取物袋可以使肿瘤溢出的发生率从 46%下降到 3.7%。

对于巨大的囊性畸胎瘤，为了“减瘤”而行单纯的穿刺抽液是不可行的，因为囊液有可能会含有恶性的成分。即使肿瘤很巨大或者累及双侧卵巢，为了保留内分泌和生育功能，也应该尽量保留卵巢（见图 36–8 和 36–9）[100]。如果卵巢无法保留，除非输卵管也因为附件扭转已经发生坏死，否则在切除卵巢和肿瘤后，应该保留输卵管。

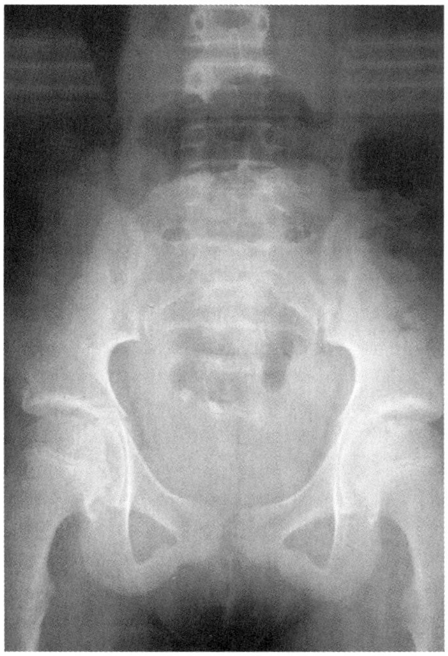

A

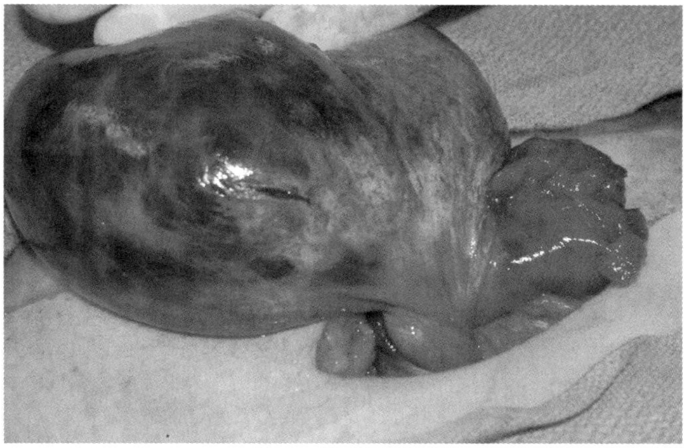

B

图 36–8　A. 一位患有单侧卵巢畸胎瘤的 16 岁女孩的腹部立位平片，可见盆腔肿块含有牙齿样的钙化灶。B. 该患儿由于腹痛数日，发现卵巢良性畸胎瘤扭转并破裂而急诊手术，通过解除扭转，囊肿切除，保留了卵巢。术后 6 月，患儿超声检查，双侧卵巢正常。

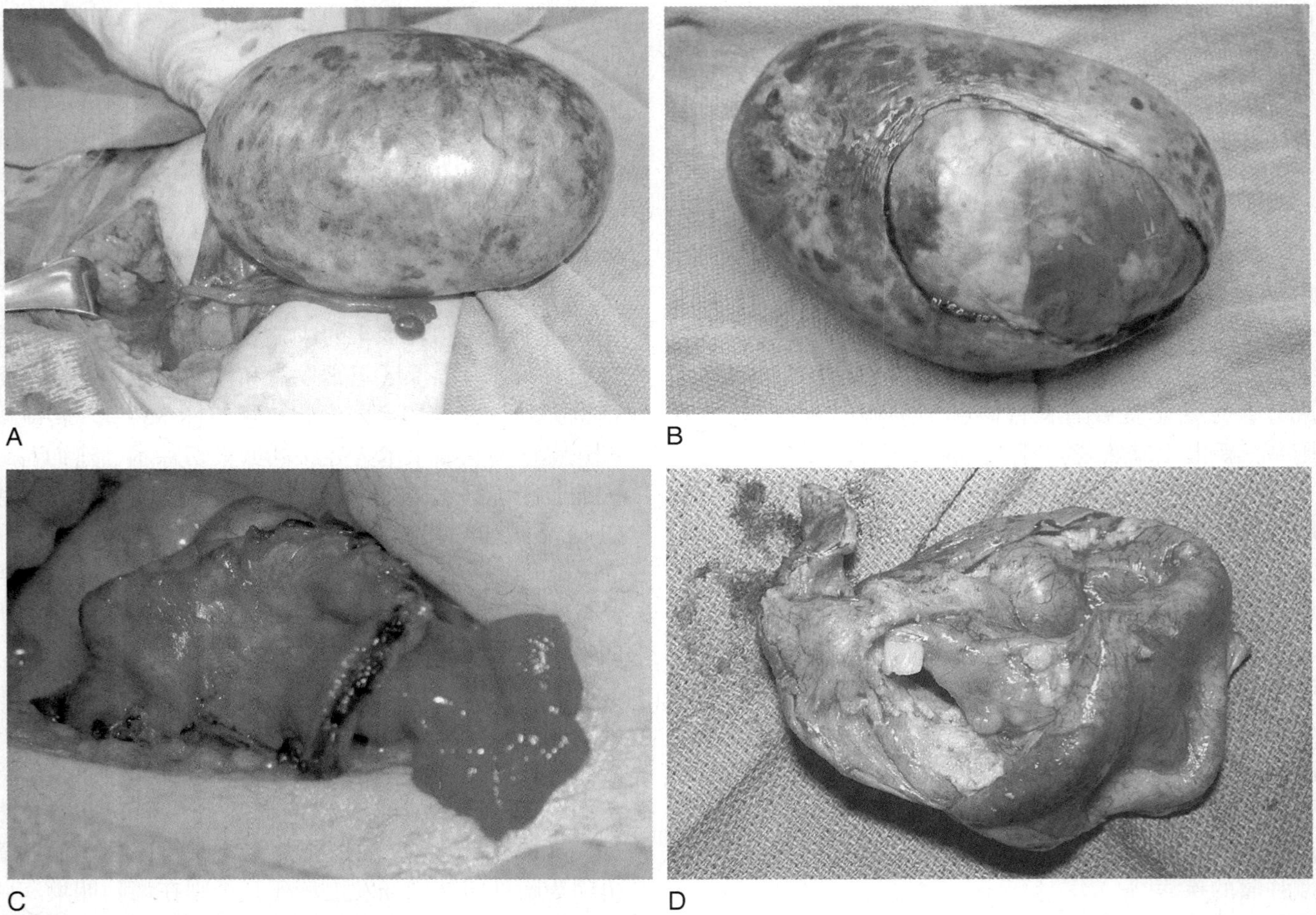

图 36−9 A. 一位醒来时突发剧烈腹痛的 14 岁女孩的巨大卵巢畸胎瘤，肿瘤下方可以看到输卵管。B. 肿瘤切除后，可以看到囊肿剥离后的卵巢表面。C. 肿瘤切除后，卵巢组织（左侧）和输卵管（右侧）仍然保留。D. 卵巢畸胎瘤的大体切面可以看到大量牙齿样和下巴样的钙化（A、B 和 C 也见彩图）。

据报道，成人成熟囊性畸胎瘤囊肿切除后的复发率在 3%～4%[8,29]，而且大多在 40 岁之前[8]。多发性或双侧成熟囊性畸胎瘤的患儿也有 2%～3%的可能性再发生殖细胞肿瘤[8,20,232]。目前还没有特别关于儿童畸胎瘤复发情况调查的文献，所有对术后情况的评论都是经验性的。鉴于超声检查对成熟囊性畸胎瘤的高敏感性，有必要对青春期前和青春期早期的儿童行每年的超声检查，和对青春期后期的青少年行每年的盆腔检查。

成熟畸胎瘤患者偶尔也可出现腹腔内粟粒状胶质种植灶（0 级）[58]。但是一般到手术时才会被发现。这些种植灶一般表现为白色或灰色的结节，直径在 1～3mm，最常见的种植部位为大网膜、盆腔腹膜或者肿瘤附近甚至肿瘤表面。关于种植的机制有很多种理论[166]，其中最被广泛认可的理论认为：原发性肿瘤的包裹缺损，畸胎瘤成分在压力作用下穿透包膜而发生种植。如果缺损部位附近的肿瘤成分为成熟畸胎瘤，那么种植性转移灶的成分也为成熟性畸胎瘤。Robboy 和 Scully[166]报告的 12 例病例中，有 11 例发生了原发肿瘤包膜的破裂或者大网膜或附件结构与肿瘤发生了粘连。大体上看，种植灶有可能相当触目惊心，但是如果它们分化良好，就不需要特别处理，它们的存在也不影响原发肿瘤的治疗方案。不过如果包膜缺损部位附近的肿瘤组织为不成熟的畸胎瘤成分，那么种植灶有可能恶变，需要辅助治疗。

未成熟畸胎瘤：未成熟畸胎瘤是由三个胚层组织组成的生殖细胞肿瘤。由于含有未成熟的神经上皮成分（图 36–10）。临床上不同于良性或恶性畸胎瘤。未成熟畸胎瘤可以同成熟的囊性或实性畸胎瘤或者恶性畸胎瘤同时存在，治疗方案根据恶性成分而定。

未成熟畸胎瘤的分级根据肿瘤未成熟的程度和神经上皮成分存在与否及其量的多少。原发肿瘤的分级相当重要，而且是肿瘤是否容易发生卵巢外转移的决定因素之一。现行的未成熟畸胎瘤分级系统由 Thurlbech 和 Scully[211]提出，由 Norris[143]等和 Ihara[44]等修订。

Ⅰ级：局限于卵巢（腹腔无转移）；没有临床、影像学、组织学证据显示肿瘤范围超出卵巢（腹膜神经胶质瘤病灶的存在并不影响肿瘤Ⅰ级的分级）。

Ⅱ级：镜下残余病灶，腹腔无转移（腹膜神经胶质瘤病灶的存在并不影响肿瘤Ⅱ级的分级）。

Ⅲ级：淋巴结转移（转移性结节）；大体残余病灶或活检发现；相邻脏器浸润（大网膜、肠、膀胱）；腹腔发现恶性肿瘤细胞。

Ⅳ级：远处转移，包括肝脏。

涉及多学科的治疗方案可以改善未成熟畸胎瘤的预后。1976 年 Norris[143]等的研究显示，经联合治疗后Ⅰ级未成熟畸胎瘤患者的生存率为 82%，Ⅱ级为 62%，Ⅲ级为 30%。Anderson 肿瘤中心 1986 年的报告显示，16 名只行手术治疗的患者有 15 名出现了肿瘤的复发，而 11 名经过术后化疗的患者有 10 名预后良好[68]。21 名接受长春新碱、放线菌素 D 和环磷酰 612
胺（VAC）联合化疗的患者中有 18 名存活下来。

基于生存率的提高，目前对未成熟畸胎瘤的处理要求在保证生存率的同时保留患者的生育能力[121]。1989 年 Koulos[110]等回顾了康涅狄格州肿瘤登记的 25 个病例，23 名Ⅰ期肿瘤的患者中有 18 名保留了对侧的附件，进行或没有进行辅助化疗。他们得出结论是：如果可以保证密切随访肿瘤的复发，对临床Ⅰ期组织学Ⅰ级和Ⅱ级的未成熟畸胎瘤患者在行保守性手术之后可以不进行化疗。如果肿瘤复发，可以再进一步采取挽救性措施。Kawai 等[103]认为，对于临床Ⅰ期的未成熟畸胎瘤，如果组织学分级为Ⅰ级，仅行单侧输卵管卵巢切除术就已经足够；而组织学分级为Ⅱ级或Ⅲ级的肿瘤，则需要同时给予 VAC 或者 VAC 联合顺铂化疗。在他们的研究报告中，19 名随访了 62 个月的患者有 18 名仍无病存活。Bonazzi 等通过对 32 名卵巢未成熟畸胎瘤患者进行的 10 年前瞻性研究也提出过类似的结论。临床Ⅰ期或Ⅱ期、组织学Ⅰ级或Ⅱ级的肿瘤患者可以行保留生育功能的手术，并可以不予化疗；而对临床Ⅲ期或组织学Ⅲ级的肿瘤患者

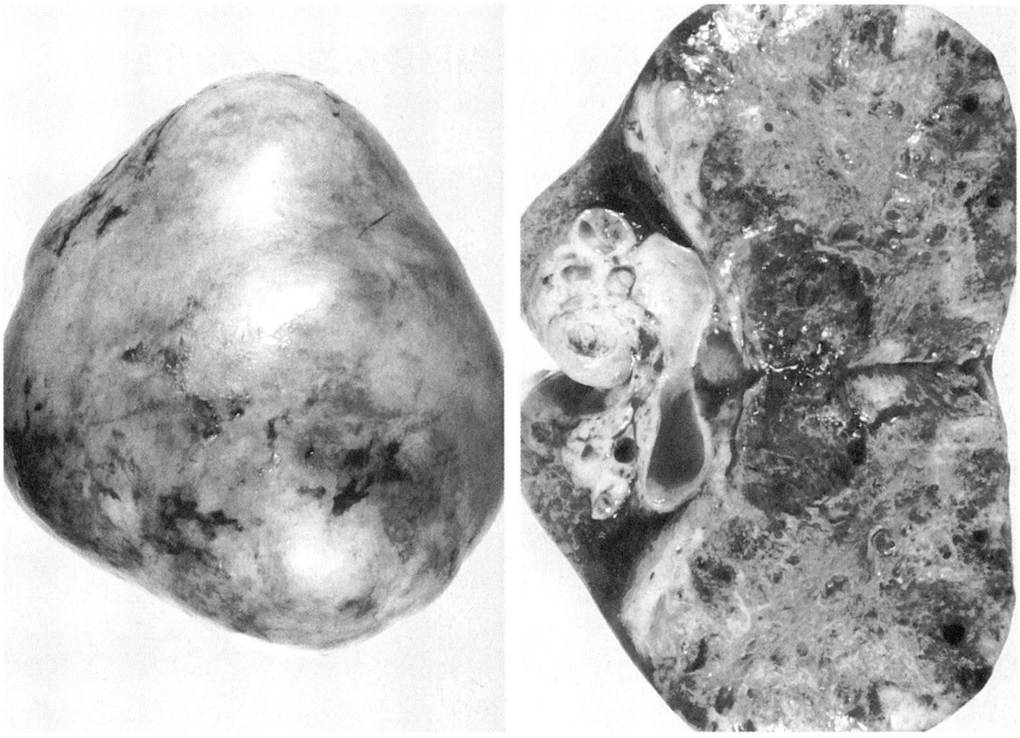

A　B

图 36-10 A. 一位表现为左侧卵巢肿块的 5 岁女孩的未成熟畸胎瘤的特征性大体外观。肿瘤为实性和囊性的球状肿块，表面光滑、有光泽。B. 未成熟畸胎瘤斑驳的囊实性切面，局部可见出血灶。

以及复发患者，需要行铂类药物的化疗。在他们的研究中，所有 32 名患者在平均 47 个月的随访中都保持无病存活。

未成熟畸胎瘤很少累及双侧卵巢[40]，如果对侧卵巢外观正常就不需要进行活检[68]。为了保留患儿将来的生育能力，对临床Ⅰ期组织学Ⅰ级的肿瘤患儿行单侧的输卵管卵巢切除术就已足够[41,121]。组织学Ⅱ级或Ⅲ级肿瘤患儿需要同时给予铂类药物化疗。对于临床Ⅱ期或更晚期肿瘤的患儿，在手术以及化疗中，也应该尽量以保留患儿的生育能力为重。也有人建议，对组织学Ⅱ级或Ⅲ级以及临床Ⅱ期或更晚期肿瘤的患者行诱导化疗后手术，化疗直至完全消除组织学Ⅰ级或以上的肿瘤[68]。

单胚层畸胎瘤：单胚层畸胎瘤是指只有或者基本上只有外胚层或中胚层或内胚层细胞构成的卵巢肿瘤，如神经外胚层瘤[5]。

性腺母细胞瘤

性腺母细胞瘤由 Scully[180]于 1953 年第一个报道，相对罕见，主要发生于性腺发育不良的患者。大多数患者表型为女性，可以伴有或不伴有男性化表现。在唯一一项有关该肿瘤的大型报告中，Scully[181]回顾了 74 个病例，其中有 89%染色体呈阴性，最主要的核型为 46XY 或 45X/46XY。Troche 和 Hernandez[213]在一篇报道中回顾了 140 例性腺发育不良伴发肿瘤的病例，发现 80%的患者是这两种核型。性腺母细胞瘤的患者大多为青春期后期或者三十几岁的女性，常有原发性闭经的病史。肿瘤释放的雄激素可以造成男性化
613 表现。如果对闭经或者有男性化表现的患者行染色体检查，90%左右的患者核型异常，可以出现 Y 染色体或者 Y 染色体片段[213]。这种肿瘤一般较小，可以在检查或是手术探查中被发现。有的是在手术切除条索状性腺或者发育不良性腺时才偶然被发现[136,229]。这种肿瘤早期就可以发生浸润，所以一旦核型为 46XY 的性腺发育不良被诊断，就需要尽早行性腺切除术[139,181,213]。

性腺母细胞瘤由生殖细胞和性索衍生物构成，后者类似于颗粒细胞和支持细胞，可以通过免疫组化和超微结构检查加以区分[168]。大约 2/3 的肿瘤可以看到类似于黄体或者间质细胞的间质细胞，提示肿瘤在绒毛膜促性腺激素作用下的间质反应[168]。因为在超过一半的患者中，性腺母细胞瘤和性腺发育不良或者其他生殖细胞肿瘤同时存在，所以性腺母细胞瘤一般被认为是生殖细胞肿瘤的前体[213]。这种肿瘤从大体上很难鉴定，因为它的恶性成分生长迅速，其他成分也会发生变化，包括钙化、纤维化或者两者。事实上，钙化有可能是性腺母细胞瘤唯一的残迹，如果无性细胞瘤出现钙化灶，就要怀疑性腺母细胞瘤存在的可能。肿瘤的恶性度决定于潜在的恶性成分，需要给予相应的处理。由于异常性早熟症状促进了肿瘤的早期发现和早期诊断，目前患者的预后有所提高。同时，博来霉素、依托泊苷和顺铂的联合化疗也使得非生殖细胞瘤型生殖细胞肿瘤预后得到改善，据报道患者的生存率提高到 70%～90%[154]。

混合性生殖细胞肿瘤

儿童生殖细胞肿瘤一般由一种以上的组织类型构成，可以含有疑似恶性的肿瘤（不成熟畸胎瘤）和恶性的肿瘤（生殖细胞瘤、绒毛膜癌、内胚窦瘤和胚胎性癌）成分。混合性生殖细胞肿瘤的处理根据恶性程度最高的成分的处理措施而定。

卵巢生殖细胞肿瘤的手术治疗原则

手术的目的是对疾病进展程度进行的完整评估、安全完整地切除肿瘤和保留所有未被浸润的生殖器官。手术治疗儿童卵巢病变的一个重要前提是保留生育能力。越来越多的腹腔镜检查已经被运用于对盆腔肿块的评估中。一些针对成人的有关腹腔镜手术术后恢复快、住院时间短的报告同样适用于儿童[209,210]。如果腹腔镜检查怀疑卵巢恶性肿瘤，通常需要进行完整的外科分期，并进行传统的开腹切除术。而良性的病变只需要行卵巢囊肿切除或单侧的输卵管切除术。

单从大体上很难分辨良性肿瘤、恶性肿瘤和组织学混合性肿瘤。如果不能确定，就需要对肿瘤进行分期，因为恶性肿瘤的处理和预后判断都是根据准确的分期而定的。现行的儿童肿瘤学组（COG）协议认为，准确分期的依据必须包括彻底的观察、触诊以及对腹膜、肝脏可疑性结节的活检（包括膈下间隙）[31]。双侧卵巢都必须仔细检查。如果肿瘤仅累

及一侧卵巢，可以仅行单侧卵巢切除术，对侧卵巢需要仔细检查，结节或者可疑性区域需要切除并活检。如果双侧卵巢均被累及，则需要行双侧输卵管卵巢切除术。

需要收集腹水做细胞学检查。如果没有出现腹水，可以用乳酸林格液冲洗腹腔后的冲洗液。对怀疑病变的大网膜需要做活检。如果肿瘤累及大网膜，则需要行大网膜切除术。对腹膜后淋巴结进行触诊，对怀疑的或增大的淋巴结做活检，包括所有的腹膜后淋巴结范围，并去除任何腹腔内巨大的转移组织。如果肿瘤浸润已经超过了一般的安全的非致残性手术所能清除的程度，外科手术切除肿瘤就需要被推迟到有效化疗之后。在治疗的第 12 周，对肿瘤标志物持续增高以及体检或影像学检查显示腹腔残留肿瘤的患者，可以进行诱导化疗后手术。诱导化疗后手术包括活检或切除可见组织、取淋巴结标本以及对肾活检评估顺铂毒性。

卵巢生殖细胞肿瘤的化疗

40 年前，对生殖细胞肿瘤没有有效的化疗方案。自从对睾丸生殖细胞肿瘤采用铂类为基础的多药联合化疗取得成功之后，对卵巢肿瘤的化疗方案也开始进行类似的探索。成人卵巢生殖细胞肿瘤患者在手术切除肿瘤后加用化疗可以减少肿瘤复发的可能性[226]。VAC 很早就运用于术后化疗[226]，由于顺铂在治疗睾丸生殖细胞肿瘤中取得了不错的效果，最近也被加入了很多化疗方案中，顺铂、依托泊苷和博来霉素（PEB）联合化疗已经成为首选的化疗方案。妇科肿瘤学组（GOG）一项于 1992 年结束的历时 8 年的 PEB 方案研究显示，93 名生殖细胞肿瘤患者在治疗后的平均 38.6 个月的中期随访中，有 91 名没有发生肿瘤的复发[228]。

曾经进行过很多化疗药物治疗效果的儿童试验，其中治疗效果最好的是 PEB 方案[116,120]。Pinkerton 等[157]在一项初步研究中用毒性较小的卡铂代替顺铂，与博来霉素、依托泊苷合用。8 名卵巢生殖细胞肿瘤患者全部存活。Gobel 等[72]进行的一项欧洲的铂类药物化疗效果试验显示，17 名根据 FIGO 分期标准为临床 IA 期的卵巢非精原细胞瘤性生殖细胞肿瘤患儿在手术切除肿瘤后使用铂类药物化疗；只有 1 名患儿复发[72]。

1991 年，在一项儿童癌症组织（CCG）对 93 名恶性生殖细胞肿瘤患儿的研究中，有 30 例为卵巢肿瘤[3]。根据研究设计，未成熟畸胎瘤和无性细胞瘤未包括在内。使用顺铂为基础药物的化疗方案，患儿 4 年无病生存率为 63%。肿瘤的大小影响预后，如果肿瘤的直径大于 16cm，预后就比较差。在初次手术中不能完全切除肿瘤的患儿要比初次手术能完全切除肿瘤的患儿预后更差（$P = 0.08$）。1994 年，Nair 等[138]报道的 107 名生殖细胞肿瘤患儿中，有 43 名为卵巢肿瘤患儿，其中 22 名接受了多药联合化疗。11 名用铂、长春碱和博来霉素治疗的患儿中有 6 名完全显效，而 11 名用 PEB 方案（用依托泊苷代替长春碱）治疗的患儿中完全显效者为 10 名。与 PEB 方案的效果相比，化疗相关副作用则相对较次要[227]。

目前有一项儿童肿瘤学组（COG-AGCT0132）启动于 2003 年 11 月 3 日的有关治疗儿童低危和中危颅外生殖细胞肿瘤简化治疗的Ⅲ期研究。基于儿科肿瘤学组（POG）和儿童癌症组织（CCG）的联合研究，恶性生殖细胞肿瘤患者根据临床分期和手术原发部位可以分成三组（高危、中危和低危）。根据儿科肿瘤学组（POG）的 9048 例病例和儿童癌症组织（CCG）的 8891 例病例的数据，I 期卵巢和卵巢外的含有恶性成分的未成熟畸胎瘤在完全手术切除肿瘤后预后良好[41]。在目前的研究中，所有的 I 期肿瘤患者都被列为低危组，外科手术后只需密切观察和监测。而中危组的患者主要为临床Ⅱ期和Ⅲ期的性腺肿瘤患者，这些患者在接受标准剂量的 PEB 治疗后 3 年无病生存率大约为 90%[31,167]。这些患者需要给予修正的 PEB 方案治疗，一个周期 21 天，治疗 3 个周期。Saxman 等[176]报告男性生殖细胞癌患者在接受 3 个或者 4 个周期的PEB 方案治疗后长期生存率相同。对于只有部分反应的患者，可以行手术切除残余肿瘤。当病理检查显示阴性、肿瘤标志物恢复正常后可以结束化疗，对于只有部分反应的儿童，可以再进行第 2 次 3 个周期的化疗。对复发生殖细胞肿瘤的患者可以给予高剂量化疗，并行自体干细胞移植。

未分类的良性肿瘤

卵巢血供丰富，但是卵巢血管瘤非常少见，到目前为止仅报道过 40 例[79]。这些卵巢血管瘤主要分布在婴儿和绝经后妇女中。病变一般较小，无临床症状，只是偶然的发现。很少累及双侧卵巢，而且肿瘤一般为海绵状血管瘤。超声检查可以显示良性肿瘤表现[148]。如果肿瘤体积较大，那么临床上可以出现相关症状，包括腹痛、腹胀以及血性腹水；如果肿瘤发生扭转或破裂，可以引起外科急症。还没有发现过恶性卵巢血管瘤，一般治疗只需行卵巢切除术或者附件切除术。

原发性卵巢淋巴瘤也非常少见，只报道过出现在一些十几岁女孩中[174]。这些患者一般临床无症状，部分肿瘤巨大的患者可以出现腹围增大和盆腔疼痛等表现。肿瘤标志物指标一般正常，影像学检查很难将这种良性实体肿瘤与恶性肿瘤区别开来。治疗上一般采用单侧的输卵管卵巢切除术。

卵巢黏液瘤也是少见的卵巢良性肿瘤，以明显的血管、间质增生为特点，治疗上只需行保守的手术治疗[54]。

未分类的恶性肿瘤

原发性卵巢肉瘤是一类组成不同的恶性肿瘤，预后很差。大多数患者为年纪较大的女性，但是一项对 151 名患者的回顾显示，29 名横纹肌肉瘤的患者中有 10 名患者的年龄小于 20 岁[186]。这些患者无特异性症状，仅表现为腹部不适或腹胀，偶尔可有继发性的泌尿道和胃肠道不适。准确的分期相当重要。手术治疗要求行双侧输卵管卵巢切除加子宫全切术，并尽可能多地切除腹腔内转移的病灶。然后对盆腔残留病灶行放射治疗，并可采用一些化疗方案。与一些其他部位的横纹肌肉瘤相比，卵巢横纹肌肉瘤患者的预后相对更差，可能是由于诊断明确时大多已经位于肿瘤进展期。尽管如此，最近，对手术患者同时给予化疗药物治疗的一项研究中，显示出了较好的疗效，可以想象不久后对于这种罕见的肿瘤，只需行相对保守的手术就可以达到同样的治疗目的。

偶尔在二十几岁的青年中可以发现卵巢间质肉瘤和分级低的子宫内膜性间质肉瘤。这些肿瘤被认为来源于卵巢子宫内膜异位、体腔间质细胞或者卵巢间质细胞的化生。患者常由于非特异性盆腔不适或者由于肿瘤早期浸润周围组织而引起肠道或泌尿道梗阻而被发现。肿瘤浸润在大体上常不明显，所以初次手术治疗时需要行扩大手术，包括双侧输卵管卵巢切除加子宫全切术。黄体酮是有效的辅助治疗药物，但是需要持续使用的时间尚不确定，因为一旦停止用药，间质肿瘤有可能复发并且迅速扩展。对局部残余灶可以行 615
放射治疗，但还是经常会出现复发。目前尚不明确化疗的疗效。

儿童卵巢纤维肉瘤的报道非常少。患儿一般表现为盆腔疼痛和可触及的肿块。纤维肉瘤与 Maffucci 综合征有关[32]。虽然对于年纪较大的卵巢纤维肉瘤患者，预后均较差，但是也有年轻患者经过扩大性手术治疗，包括双侧输卵管卵巢切除加子宫全切术后存活的报道。目前尚没有有关放疗和化疗成功的报道。

儿童原发性卵巢平滑肌肉瘤也非常少见。这些肿瘤可以来源于卵巢任何含有平滑肌的部位，也可以由良性的平滑肌瘤恶变形成[131]。大多数这种罕见的肿瘤患者都没有特异性临床症状，发现时一般已经为进展期。一般需要行扩大的手术治疗，尚没有发现有效的辅助治疗。

继发性肿瘤

卵巢继发性恶性肿瘤比较少见，但是卵巢是各种儿童恶性肿瘤容易转移的部位（表 36–9）[123,238]。区别原发性肿瘤和继发性肿瘤相当重要，可以避免不恰当的治疗和不良的预后。卵巢继发性肿瘤的转移来源主要有四种：（1）血行转移；（2）淋巴结转移；(3) 通过体腔途径种植于卵巢表面；（4）直接浸润[123]。最容易转移到盆腔部位的腹部高度恶性肿瘤是结缔组织增生性小圆细胞肿瘤[232]。

Pais 等[147]回顾了 23 名白血病复发累及卵巢的患者。最常见的症状为腹痛，腹部可触及肿块。虽然大多数白血病治疗无效的患者主要表现为全身症状而不是局部症状，超声检查可以明确显示局部病变，所以超声检查是检测疾病是否累及卵巢的有效手段[17]。患者的生存率决定于积极的全身联合化疗的有效性，而不是对卵巢病变外科手术切除的多少。常规的盆腔放疗没有明显的治疗效果。

有一些关于急性骨髓性白血病急性期或者复发期患者继发卵巢绿色瘤的报道[231]。虽然积极的全身化疗对患者的存活率相当重要，但是也需要立即对卵巢肿

表 36–9 儿童继发性（转移性）卵巢肿瘤

结直肠肿瘤
乳腺肿瘤
胃癌
类癌瘤（肝、肺）
恶性黑色素瘤
Burkitt 淋巴瘤
横纹肌肉瘤
Wilm 瘤
神经母细胞瘤
视网膜母细胞瘤
Ewing 肉瘤
肾脏杆状瘤
髓母细胞瘤
骨肉瘤
软骨肉瘤
白血病

块进行活检以明确它的性质（也就是良性还是恶性，以及确切的细胞型）。这种情况下，需要手术切除卵巢和其他所有肿瘤累及的妇科器官和盆腔组织，并对盆腔残留病灶行放射治疗。虽然绿色瘤的最终预后与化疗的有效性有关，然而一旦发现，对局部肿瘤的处理也不能忽视。

总结

婴儿和儿童卵巢病变具有各种不同的病理结构，其中一些非常罕见，对婴儿和儿童卵巢病变的诊断和处理相当具有挑战性。非肿瘤性卵巢病变随着影像学技术的持续进步变得越来越容易发现，而肿瘤性卵巢病变的诊断和完全定性则有赖于生化、免疫组化和细胞学技术的进步。

儿童卵巢肿瘤相对少见，临床处理方案一般根据成人类似疾病的处理经验而得来。然而必须认识到很多这些幼稚型实体肿瘤的不同特点，它们大多临床分期较早，组织学特性较有利，对治疗反应好。在治疗婴儿和儿童卵巢病变时，保留卵巢生育功能和内分泌功能是首要任务。很多非肿瘤性病变只需密切观察或非手术治疗，大多良性肿瘤，只需行保守的手术治疗，即使是对恶性肿瘤也越来越倾向于多学科联合治疗，以减少扩展性侵袭性手术，同样也能保证长期生存率，并能保留患儿的生育能力。放射治疗有利于某些特殊病例的局部病灶治疗，但是由于缺乏这方面的资料，还不明确它对提高生存率的贡献。

（张　震译 吴晔明校）

致谢

The authors would like to thank Drs. Catheryn Yashar and Alexandra Cheerva for their kind review of the chapter.

参考文献

1. Abelev GI, Assecritova IV, Kraevsky NA, et al: Embryonal serum alpha-globulin in cancer patients: Diagnostic value. Int J Cancer 1967;2:551-558.
2. Ablin A, Isaacs H Jr: Germ cell tumors. In Pizzo PA, Poplack DG (eds): Principles and Practice of Pediatric Oncology, 2nd ed. Philadelphia, JB Lippincott, 1993, pp 867-887.
3. Ablin AR, Krailo MD, Ramsay NKC, et al: Results of treatment of malignant germ cell tumors in 93 children: A report from the Children's Cancer Study Group. J Clin Oncol 1991;9:1782-1792.
4. Adelman S, Benson CD, Hertzler JH: Surgical lesions of the ovary in infancy and childhood. Surg Gynecol Obstet 1975;141:219-222.
5. Aguirre P, Scully R: Malignant neuroectodermal tumor of the ovary, a distinctive form of monodermal teratoma: Report of five cases. Am J Surg Pathol 1982;6:283-292.
6. Alrabeeah A, Galliani CA, Giacomantonio M, et al: Neonatal ovarian torsion: Report of three cases and review of the literature. Pediatr Pathol 1988;8:143-149.
7. American Fertility Society: Revised American Fertility Society classification of endometriosis 1985. Fertil Steril 1985;43:351-352.
8. Anteby E, Ron M, Revel A, et al: Germ cell tumors of the ovary arising after dermoid cyst resection: A long term follow-up study. Obstet Gynecol 1994;83:605-608.
9. Asadourian LA, Taylor HB: Dysgerminoma, an analysis of 105 cases. Obstet Gynecol 1969;33:370-379.
10. ASHG/ACMG Report: Points to consider: Ethical, legal, and psychological implications of genetic testing in children and adolescents. Am J Hum Genet 1995;57:1233-1241.
11. Asirvatham R, Rooney RJ, Watts HG: Ollier's disease with secondary chondrosarcoma associated with ovarian tumour. Int Orthop (SICOT) 1991;15:393-395.
12. Atkin NB, Baker MC: Abnormal chromosomes including small metacentrics in 14 ovarian cancers. Cancer Genet Cytogenet 1987;26:355-361.
13. Attaran M, Gidwani GP: Adolescent endometriosis. Obstet Gynecol Clin North Am 2003;30:379-390.
14. Ayhan A, et al: Oncologic and reproductive outcome after fertility-saving surgery in ovarian cancer. Eur J Gynaecol Oncol 2003;24:223-232.
15. Bagolan P, Rivosecchi M, Giorlandino C, et al: Prenatal

diagnosis and clinical outcome of ovarian cysts. J Pediatr Surg 1992;27:879-881.
16. Barakat RR: Borderline tumors of the ovary. Obstet Gynecol Clin North Am 1994;21:93-104.
17. Bickers GH, Siebert JJ, Anderson JC, et al: Sonography of ovarian involvement in childhood acute lymphocytic leukemia. Am J Res 1981;137:399-401.
18. Blake KI, Gerrard MR: Malignant germ cell tumours in two siblings. Med Pediatr Oncol 1993;21:299-300.
19. Bonazzi C, Pecctori F, Colombo N, et al: Pure ovarian immature teratoma, a unique and curable disease: 10 years' experience of 32 prospectively treated patients. Obstet Gynecol 1994;84:598-604.
20. Borenstein R, Czernobilsky B, Lancet M: Immature ovarian teratoma, an unusual case. Int J Obstet Gynecol 1982;20: 159-162.
21. Bosl GJ, Dmitrovsky E, Reuter VE, et al: Isochromosome of chromosome 12: Clinically useful marker for male germ cell tumors. J Natl Cancer Inst 1989;81:1874-1878.
22. Bourne T, Campbell S, Steer C, et al: Transvaginal color flow imaging: A possible new screening technique for ovarian cancer. BMJ 1989;299:1367-1370.
23. Brandt ML, Luks FI, Filiatrault D, et al: Surgical indications in antenatally diagnosed ovarian cysts. J Pediatr Surg 1991; 26:276-282.
24. Breen JL, Maxson WS: Ovarian tumors in children and adolescents. Clin Obstet Gynecol 1977;20:607-623.
25. Brody S: Clinical aspects of dysgerminoma of the ovary. Acta Radiol 1961;56:209-230.
26. Brown MF, Hebra A, McGeehin K, et al: Ovarian masses in children: A review of 91 cases of malignant and benign masses. J Pediatr Surg 1993;28:930-932.
27. Campo S, Garcea N: Laparoscopic conservative excision of ovarian dermoid cysts with and without an endobag. J Am Assoc Gynecol Laparosc 1998;5:165-170.
28. Chao H, Wang H: Gonadotropin-releasing hormone-agonist as a neoadjunctive therapy for Sertoli-Leydig cell tumors of the ovary. Int J Gynaecol Obstet 1999;66:189-190.
29. Chapron C, Dubuisson JB, Samouh N, et al: Treatment of ovarian dermoid cysts. Surg Endosc 1994;8:1092-1095.
30. Chiaramonte C, Piscopo A, Cataliotto F: Ovarian cysts in newborns. Pediatr Surg Int 2001;17:171-174.
31. Children's Oncology Group AGCT0132: A phase III study of reduced therapy in the treatment of children with low and intermediate risk extracranial germ cell tumors. (Activated November 3, 2003; version date, March 10, 2004.)
32. Christman JE, Ballon SC: Ovarian fibrosarcoma associated with Maffucci's syndrome. Gynecol Oncol 1990;37:290-291.
33. Christopherson WA, Kanbour A, Szulman A: Case report: Choriocarcinoma in a term placenta with maternal metastases. Gynecol Oncol 1992;46:239-245.
34. Cohen HL, Eisenberg P, Mandel FS, et al: Ovarian cysts are common in premenarchal girls: A sonographic study of 101 children 2-12 years old. Am J Res 1992;159:89-91.
35. Cohen HL, Shapiro MA, Manel FS, et al: Normal ovaries in neonates and infants: A sonographic study of 77 patients 1 day to 24 months old. Am J Res 1993;160:583-586.
36. Comerci JT, Licciardi F, Bergh PA et al: Mature cystic teratoma: A clinicopathologic evaluation of 517 cases and a review of the literature. Obstet Gynecol 1994;84:22-28.
37. Craig I, Rawlings C: Human gene mapping 10.5 Oxford conference. Cytogenet Cell Genet 1990;55:5-76.
38. Crispens MA: Borderline ovarian tumours: A review of the recent literature. Curr Opin Obstet Gynecol 2004;15:39-43.
39. Cronen PW, Nagaraj HS: Ovarian tumors in children. South Med J 1988;81:464-468.
40. Curry SL, Smite JP, Gallagher HS: Malignant teratoma of the ovary: Prognostic factors and treatment. Am J Obstet Gynecol 1978;131:845-849.
41. Cushing B, Giller R, Ablin A, et al: Surgical resection alone is effective treatment for ovarian immature teratoma in children and adolescents: A report of the Pediatric Oncology Group and the Children's Cancer Group. Am J Obstet Gynecol 1999;181:353-358.
42. Darwish AM, Amin AF, Mohamad SA: Laparoscopic management of paratubal and paraovarian cysts. JSLS 2003; 7:101-106.
43. DeCrespigny LC, Robinson H, Davoren RA, et al: The "simple" ovarian cyst: Aspirate or operate? Br J Obstet Gynaecol 1989;96:1035-1039.
44. Dehner LP: Gonadal and extragonadal germ cell neoplasia in childhood. Hum Pathol 1983;14:493-511.
45. Dengg K, Fink FM, Heitger A, et al: Precocious puberty due to a lipid-cell tumour of the ovary. Eur J Pediatr 1993;152:12-14.
46. DePalo G, Pilotti S, Kenda R, et al: Natural history of dysgerminoma. Am J Obstet Gynecol 1982;143:799-807.
47. Deprest J, Moerman P, Corneillie P, et al: Ovarian borderline mucinous tumor in a premenarchal girl: Review on ovarian epithelial cancer in young girls. Gynecol Oncol 1992;45:219- 224.
48. Diamond MP, Baxter JW, Peerman CG, et al: Occurrence of ovarian malignancy in childhood and adolescence: A community-wide evaluation. Obstet Gynecol 1988;71: 858-860.
49. Dicker D, Dekel A, Feldberg D, et al: Bilateral Sertoli-Leydig cell tumor with heterologous elements: Report of an unusual case and review of the literature. Eur J Obstet Gynecol Reprod Biol 1986;22:175-181.
50. Dietrich J, Kaplan A, Lopez H, et al: Clinical pathologic correlation: A case of poorly differentiated Sertoli-Leydig tumor of the ovary. J Pediatr Adolesc Gynecol 2004;17: 49-52.
51. Easton DF, Ford D, Bishop T, Breast Cancer Linkage Consortium: Breast and ovarian cancer incidence in BRCA1-mutation carriers. Am J Hum Genet 1995;56: 265-271.
52. Eggermont E, Lecoutere D, Devlieger H, et al: Ovarian cysts in newborn infants. Am J Dis Child 1988;142:702.
53. Ehren IM, Mahour GH, Isaacs H: Benign and malignant ovarian tumors in children and adolescents. Am J Surg 1984;147:339-344.
54. Eichhorn JH, Scully RE: Ovarian myxoma: Clinicopathologic and immunocytologic analysis of five cases and a review of the literature. Int J Gynecol Pathol 1991;10:156-169.
55. Ein SH, Darte JMM, Stephens CA: Cystic and solid ovarian tumors in children: A 44-year review. J Pediatr Surg 1970; 5:148-156.
56. Elger BS, Harding TW: Testing adolescents for a hereditary breast cancer gene (BRCA1): Respecting their autonomy is in their best interest. Arch Pediatr Adolesc Med 2000;154: 113-119.
57. Elsheikh A, Milingos S, Kallipolitis G, et al: Ovarian tumors in young females: A laparoscopic approach. Eur J Gynaecol Oncol 2001;22:243-244.
58. Fanning J, Bates J: Mature solid teratoma associated with gliomatosis peritonei. Am J Obstet Gynecol 1986;155: 661-662.
59. Farahmand SM, Marchetti DL, Asirwatham JE, et al: Ovarian endodermal sinus tumor associated with pregnancy: Case report and review of the literature. Gynecol Oncol 1991;41: 156-160.

60. Fedele L, Dorta M, Brioschi D, et al: Magnetic resonance evaluation of gynecologic masses in adolescents. Adolesc Pediatr Gynecol 1990;3:83-88.
61. Ferrera PC, Whitman MCW: Ovarian small cell carcinoma: A rare neoplasm in a 15-year-old female. Pediatr Emerg Care 2000;16:170-172.
62. FIGO Committee on Gynecologic Oncology: Staging classifications and clinical practice guidelines of gynaecologic cancers. Int J Gynecol Obstet 2000;70:207-312.
63. Freedman SM, Kreitzer PM, Elkowitz SS, et al: Ovarian microcysts in girls with isolated premature thelarche. J Pediatr Surg 1993;122:246-251.
64. Gallup DG, Talledo OE: Benign and malignant tumors. Clin Obstet Gynecol 1987;30:662-670.
65. Gedeit RG, Jay MS, Ross SP: The role of MRI in evaluation of an adolescent with a pelvic mass. J Adolesc Health Care 1990;11:516-518.
66. Gershenson DM, Del Junco G, Silva EG, et al: Immature teratoma of the ovary. Obstet Gynecol 1986;68:624-629.
67. Gershenson DM, Morris M, Burke T, et al: Treatment of poor-prognosis sex cord-stromal tumors of the ovary with a combination of bleomycin, etoposide and cisplatin. Obstet Gynecol 1996;87:527-531.
68. Gershenson DM, Morris M, Cangir A, et al: Treatment of malignant germ cell tumors of the ovary with bleomycin, etoposide and cisplatin. J Clin Oncol 1990;8: 715-720.
69. Giller R, Cushing B, Lauer S, et al: Comparison of high-dose or standard-dose cisplatin with etoposide and bleomycin (HDPEB vs PEB) in children with stage III or IV malignant germ cell tumors (MGCT) at gonadal primary site: A Pediatric Intergroup trial (POG 9049/CCG 8882). Proc Am Soc Clin Oncol 1998;17:525.
70. Giorlandino C, Bilancioni E, Bagolan P, et al: Antenatal ultrasonographic diagnosis and management of fetal ovarian cysts. Int J Gynecol Obstet 1993;44:27-31.
71. Gitlin D, Perricelli A, Gillin GM: Synthesis of fetoprotein by liver, yolk sac, and gastrointestinal tract of the human conceptus. Cancer Res 1972;32:979-982.
72. Göbel U, Haas RJ, Calaminus G, et al: Treatment of germ cell tumors in children: Results of European trials for testicular and non-testicular primary sites. Crit Rev Oncol Hematol 1990;10:89-98.
73. Goldstein D, deCholonoky C, Emans SJ: Adolescent endometriosis. J Adolesc Health 1980;1:37-41.
74. Gonzales-Crussi F: Extragonadal teratomas. In Atlas of Tumor Pathology, 2nd ser, fascicle 18. Washington, DC, Armed Forces Institute of Pathology, 1982, pp 1-43.
75. Gordon A, Lipton D, Woodruff D: Dysgerminoma: A review of 158 cases from the Emil Novak Ovarian Tumor Registry. Obstet Gynecol 1981;58:497-504.
76. Greist A, Roth B, Einhorn L, et al: Cisplatin-combination chemotherapy for disseminated germ cell tumors: Long-term follow-up. Proc Am Soc Clin Oncol 1985;4:100.
77. Gribbon M, Ein SH, Mancer K: Pediatric malignant ovarian tumors: A 43-year review. J Pediatr Surg 1992;27: 480-484.
78. Groeber WR: Ovarian tumors during infancy and childhood. Am J Obstet Gynecol 1963;86:1027-1035.
79. Gunes HA, Egilmez R, Dulger M: Ovarian haemangioma. Br J Clin Pract 1990;44:734-735.
80. Gustafson ML, Lee MM, Scully RE, et al: Mullerian inhibitory substance as a marker for ovarian sex cord tumor. N Engl J Med 1992;326:466-471.
81. Halme J, Hammond MG, Hulka JF, et al: Retrograde menstruation in healthy women and in patients with endometriosis. Obstet Gynecol 1984;64:151-154.
82. Harris AC, Wakely PE, Kaplowitz PB, et al: Steroid cell tumor of the ovary in a child. Arch Pathol Lab Med 1991;115:150-154.
83. Hasson HM: Laparoscopic management of ovarian cysts. J Reprod Med 1990;35:863-867.
84. Hayes MC, Scully RE: Ovarian steroid cell tumors (not otherwise specified): A clinicopathological analysis of 63 cases. Am J Surg Pathol 1987;11:835-845.
85. Heling K, Chaoui R, Kirchmair F, et al: Fetal ovarian cysts: Prenatal diagnosis, management and postnatal outcome. Ultrasound Obstet Gynecol 2002;20:47-50.
86. Héloury Y, Guiberteau V, Sagot P, et al: Laparoscopy in adnexal pathology in the child: A study of 28 cases. Eur J Pediatr Surg 1993;3:75-78.
87. Herd J, Fowler JM, Shenson D, et al: Laparoscopic paraaortic lymph node sampling: Development of a technique. Gynecol Oncol 1992;44:271-276.
88. Hoffner L, Shen-Schwarz S, Deka R, et al: Genetics and biology of human ovarian teratomas. III. Cytogenetics and origins of malignant ovarian germ cell tumors. Cancer Genet Cytogenet 1992;62:58-65.
89. Hoshiai H, Ishikawa M, Sawatari Y, et al: Laparoscopic evaluation of the onset and progression of endometriosis. Am J Obstet Gynecol 1993;169:714-719.
90. Howell CG Jr, Rogers DA, Gable DS, et al: Bilateral ovarian fibromas in children. J Pediatr Surg 1990;25: 690-691.
91. Hsu C, Ma L, Mak L: Sclerosing stromal tumor of the ovary: Case report and review of the literature. Int J Gynecol Pathol 1983;2:192-200.
92. Huffman JW: Ovarian tumors in children and adolescents. In Huffman JW, et al (eds): The Gynecology of Childhood and Adolescence, 2nd ed. Philadelphia, WB Saunders, 1981, pp 277-349.
93. Hulka JF, Parker WH, Surrey MW, et al: Management of ovarian masses: AAGL 1990 survey. J Reprod Med 1992; 37:599-602.
94. Ihara T, Ohama K, Satoh H: Histologic grade and karyotype of immature teratoma of the ovary. Cancer 1984;54: 2988-2994.
95. Imai A, Furui T, Shimokawa K, et al: Juvenile granulosa cell tumor in a 2-year-old infant: Report of a case complicated with ascites and acute respiratory distress. Gynecol Oncol 1992;46:397-400.
96. Imai A, Furui T, Tamaya T: Gynecologic tumors and symptoms in childhood and adolescence: 10-years' experience. Int J Gynecol Obstet 1994;5:227-234.
97. Inoue R, Kondo N, Motoyoshi F, et al: Chediak-Higashi syndrome: Report of a case with an ovarian tumor. Clin Genet 1991;39:316-318.
98. Issacs H Jr: Perinatal (congenital and neonatal) neoplasms: A report of 110 cases. Pediatr Pathol 1985;3:165-216.
99. Jabra AA, Fishman EK, Taylor GA: Primary ovarian tumors in the pediatric patient: CT evaluation. Clin Imaging 1993;17:199-203.
100. Jona JZ, Burchby K, Vitamvas G: Castration-sparing management of an adolescent with high bilateral cystic teratomas of the ovaries. J Pediatr Surg 1988;23:973-974.
101. Kalofonos HP, Karamouzis MV, Epenetos AA: Radioimmunoscintigraphy in patients with ovarian cancer. Acta Oncol 2001;40:549-557.
102. Kawai M, Kano T, Furuhashi Y, et al: Immature teratoma of the ovary. Gynecol Oncol 1991;40:133-137.
103. Kawai M, Kano T, Kikkawa F, et al: Seven tumor markers in benign and malignant germ cell tumors of the ovary.

Gynecol Oncol 1992;45:248-253.

104. Kawakami K, Murata K, Kawaguchi N, et al: Hemorrhagic infarction of the diseased ovary: A common MR finding in two cases. Magn Reson Imaging 1993;11:595-597.
105. Kerner H, Gaton E, Czemobilsky B: Unusual ovarian, tubal and pelvic mesothelial inclusions in patients with endometriosis. Histopathology 1981;5:277-283.
106. Kier R, Smith RC, McCarthy SM: Value of lipid- and water-suppression MR images in distinguishing between blood and lipid within ovarian masses. Am J Res 1992;158:321-325.
107. Kodish ED: Testing children for cancer genes: The rule of earliest onset. J Pediatr 1999;135:390-395.
108. Koninckx PR, Meulman C, Demeyere S, et al: Suggestive evidence that pelvic endometriosis is a progressive disease, whereas deeply infiltrating endometriosis is associated with pelvic pain. Fertil Steril 1991;55:759-765.
109. Koninckx PR, Oosterlynck D, D'Hooghe T, et al: Deeply infiltrating endometriosis is a disease whereas mild endometriosis could be considered a non-disease. Ann N Y Acad Sci 1994;734:333-341.
110. Koulos JP, Hoffman JS, Steinhoff MM: Immature teratoma of the ovary. Gynecol Oncol 1989;34:46-49.
111. Kurman RJ, Norris HJ: Endodermal sinus tumor of the ovary: A clinical and pathologic analysis of 71 cases. Cancer 1976;38:2404-2419.
112. Lack EE, Young RH, Scully RE: Pathology of ovarian neoplasms in childhood and adolescence. Pathol Annu 1992; 27:281-356.
113. Lackman F, Carey MS, Kirk ME, et al: Surgery as sole treatment for serous borderline tumors of the ovary with non-invasive implants. Gynceol Oncol 2003;90:407-412.
114. Lappohn RE, Burger HG, Bouma J, et al: Inhibin as a marker for granulosa cell tumor. Acta Obstet Gynecol Scand 1992;71(Suppl 155):61-65.
115. Larsen WG, Felmar EA, Wallace ME, et al: Sertoli-Leydig cell tumor of the ovary: A rare cause of amenorrhea. Obstet Gynecol 1992;79:831-833.
116. LaVecchia C, Morris HB, Draper GJ: Malignant ovarian tumours in childhood in Britain, 1962-78. Br J Cancer 1983;48:363-374.
117. Lindfors O: Primary ovarian neoplasms in infants and children: A study of 81 cases diagnosed in Finland and Sweden. Ann Chir Gynaecol Fenn 1971;177(Suppl): 1-66.
118. Low LCK, Wang C, Leung A, et al: Undetectable levels of serum FSH immunoactivity and bioactivity in girls with sexual precocity due to ovarian cysts. Acta Paediatr 1994;83:623-626.
119. Mahour GH, Landing HB, Woolley MM: Teratomas in children: Clinicopathologic studies in 133 patients. Z Kinderchir 1978;23:365-380.
120. Mann JR, Pearson D, Barrett A, et al: Results of the United Kingdom Children's Cancer Study Group's germ cell tumor studies. Cancer 1989;63:1657-1667.
121. Marina NM, Cushing B, Giller R, et al: Complete surgical excision is effective treatment for children with immature teratomas with or without malignant elements: A Pediatric Oncology Group/Children's Cancer Group Intergroup Study. J Clin Oncol 1999;17:2137-2143.
122. Massad LS Jr, Hunter VJ, Szpak CA, et al: Epithelial ovarian tumors of low malignant potential. Obstet Gynecol 1991; 78:1027-1032.
123. McCarville MB, Hill DA, Miller BE, et al: Secondary ovarian neoplasms in children: Imaging features with histopathologic correlation. Pediatr Radiol 2001;31:358-364.
124. Meigs JV: Endometriosis. Ann Surg 1948;127:795-809.
125. Meizner I, Levy A, Katz M, et al: Fetal ovarian cysts: Prenatal ultrasonographic detection and postnatal evaluation and treatment. Am J Obstet Gynecol 1991;164:874-878.
126. Mena W, Krassikoff N, Philips JB III: Fused eyelids, airway anomalies, ovarian cysts, and digital abnormalities in siblings: A new autosomal recessive syndrome or a variant of Fraser syndrome? Am J Med Genet 1991;40:377-382.
127. Millar DM, Blake JM, Stringer DA, et al: Prepubertal ovarian cyst formation: 5 years' experience. Obstet Gynecol 1993; 81:434-438.
128. Mitelman F: Catalog of chromosomal aberrations. In Cancer, 4th ed. New York, Wiley-Liss, 1991.
129. Mittermayer C, Blaicher W, Grassauer D, et al: Fetal ovarian cysts: Development and neonatal outcome. Ultraschall Med 2003;24:21-26.
130. Modan B, Hartge P, Hirsh-Yechezkel G, et al: Parity, oral contraceptives, and the risk of ovarian cancer among carriers and noncarriers of a BRCA1 and BRCA2 mutation. N Engl J Med 2001;345:235-240.
131. Monk BJ, Nieberg R, Berek JS: Primary leiomyosarcoma of the ovary in a perimenarchal female. Gynecol Oncol 1993;48:389-393.
132. Moore DT: Ovarian epithelial tumor of low malignant potential in an adolescent. J Tenn Med Assoc 1992;85: 557-558.
133. Morice PCS, Camatte S, Hassan J, et al: Clinical outcomes and fertility after conservative treatment of borderline ovarian tumors. Fertil Steril 2001;75:92-96.
134. Morowitz M, Huff D, von Allmen D: Epithelial ovarian tumors in children: A retrospective analysis. J Pediatr Surg 2003;38:331-335.
135. Morris HB, LaVecchia C, Draper GJ: Malignant epithelial tumors of the ovary in childhood: A clinicopathological study of 13 cases in Great Britain 1962-1978. Gynecol Oncol 1984;19:290-297.
136. Müller J, Visfeldt J, Philip J, et al: Carcinoma in situ, gonadoblastoma, and early invasive neoplasia in a nine-year-old girl with 46,XY gonadal dysgenesis. APMIS 1992; 100:170-174.
137. Murty VV, Dmitrovsky E, Bosl GJ, et al: Nonrandom chromosome abnormalities in testicular and ovarian germ cell tumor lines. Cancer Genet Cytogenet 1990;50:67-73.
138. Nair R, Pai SK, Nair CN, et al: Malignant germ cell tumors in childhood. J Surg Oncol 1994;56:186-190.
139. Narod SA, Risch H, Moslehi R, et al: Oral contraceptives and the risk of hereditary ovarian cancer. N Engl J Med 1998;339:424-428.
140. Nishida M, Jimi S, Haji M, et al: Juvenile granulosa cell tumor in association with a high serum inhibin level. Gynecol Oncol 1991;40:90-94.
141. Nogales FF: Embryologic clues to human yolk sac tumors: A review. Int J Gynecol Pathol 1993;12:101-107.
142. Norris HJ, Jensen RD: Relative frequency of ovarian neoplasms in children and adolescents. Cancer 1972;30: 713-719.
143. Norris HJ, Zirkin HJ, Benson WL: Immature (malignant) teratoma of the ovary: A clinical and pathologic study of 58 cases. Cancer 1976;37:2359-2372.
144. Olive DL, Hammond CB: Endometriosis: Pathogenesis and mechanisms of infertility. Postgrad Obstet Gynecol 1985;5:1-6.
145. Ortega JA, Siegel SE: Biologic markers in pediatric solid tumors. In Pizzo P, Poplack DG (eds): Principles and Practice of Pediatric Oncology, 2nd ed. Philadelphia, JB Lippincott, 1993, pp 179-194.
146. Ovarian cancer: Screening, treatment, and followup.

NIH Consensus Statement 1994;12:1-30.
147. Pais RC, Kim TH, Zwiren GT, et al: Ovarian tumors in relapsing acute lymphoblastic leukemia: A review of 23 cases. J Pediatr Surg 1991;26:70-74.
148. Paladini D, Di Meglio A, Esposito A, et al: Ultrasonic features of an ovarian cystohemangioma: A case report. Eur J Obstet Gynecol Reprod Biol 1991;40:239-240.
149. Parham DM, Bugg FM, Pratt CB: Carcinomas, adenomas, precursor lesions, and second malignancies. In Parham DM (ed): Pediatric Neoplasia: Morphology and Biology. Philadelphia, Lippincott-Raven, 1996, pp 385-390.
150. Patel MD, Feldstein VA, Lipson SD, et al: Cystic teratomas of the ovary: Diagnostic value of sonography. AJR Am J Roentgenol 1998;171:1061-1065.
151. Perkins AC, Powell MC, Wastie ML, et al: A prospective evaluation of OC125 and magnetic resonance imaging in patients with ovarian carcinoma. Eur J Nucl Med 1990; 16:311-316.
152. Perlin E, Engeler JE, Edson M, et al: The value of serial measurement of both human chorionic gonadotropin and alpha-fetoprotein for monitoring germ cell tumors. Cancer 1976;37:215-219.
153. Perlman EJ, Cushing B, Hawkins E, et al: Cytogenetic analysis of childhood endodermal sinus tumors: A Pediatric Oncology Group study. Pediatr Pathol 1994; 14:695-708.
154. Perlman EJ, Fritsch MK: The female reproductive system. In Stocker JT, Dehner LP (eds): Pediatric Pathology, 2nd ed. Philadelphia, Lippincott Williams & Wilkins, 2001, pp 920-938.
155. Peters H, Byskov AG, Grinsted J: Follicular growth in fetal and prepubertal ovaries in humans and other primates. Clin Endocrinol Metab 1978;7:469-485.
156. Peters H, Himelstein-Braun R, Faber M: The normal development of the ovary in childhood. Acta Endocrinol 1976;82:617-630.
157. Pinkerton CR, Broadbent V, Horwich A, et al: "JEB"—a carboplatin based regimen for malignant germ cell tumours in children. Br J Cancer 1990;62:257-262.
158. Piver MS, Patton T: Ovarian cancer in children. Semin Surg Oncol 1986;2:163-169.
159. Plantaz D, Flamant F, Vassal G, et al: Juvenile granulosa cell tumor in children: A clinical study of 39 cases [abstract]. Med Pediatr Oncol 1991;19:396.
160. Pliskow S: Endodermal sinus tumor of the ovary: Review of 10 cases. South Med J 1993;86:187-189.
161. Podczaski E, Kaminski PF, Pees RC, et al: Peutz-Jeghers syndrome with ovarian sex cord tumor with annular tubules and cervical adenoma malignum. Gynecol Oncol 1991;42:74-78.
162. Powell JL, Johnson NA, Bailey CL, et al: Management of advanced juvenile granulosa cell tumor of the ovary. Gynecol Oncol 1993;48:119-123.
163. Powell JL, McAfee RD, McCoy RC, et al: Uterine and ovarian conservation in advanced small cell carcinoma of the ovary. Obstet Gynecol 1998;91:846-848.
164. Raafat F, Klys H, Rylance G: Juvenile granulosa cell tumor. Pediatr Pathol 1990;10:617-623.
165. Ranney B: Etiology, prevention and inhibition of endometriosis. Clin Obstet Gynecol 1980;23:875-883.
166. Robboy SJ, Scully RE: Ovarian teratoma with glial implants on the peritoneum: An analysis of 12 cases. Hum Pathol 1970;1:643-653.
167. Rogers PC, Olson TA, Cullen JW, et al: Treatment of children and adolescents with stage II testicular and stages I and II ovarian malignant germ cell tumors: A Pediatric Intergroup study—Pediatric Oncology Group 9048 and Children's Cancer Group 8891. J Clin Oncol 2004;22: 3563-3569.
168. Roth LM, Eglen DE: Gonadoblastoma: Immunohistochemical and ultrastructural observations. Int J Gynecol Pathol 1989;8:72-81.
169. Rottem S, Levit N, Thaler I, et al: Classification of ovarian lesions by high frequency transvaginal sonography. J Clin Ultrasound 1990;18:359-363.
170. Rotterdam ESHRE/ASRM, Sponsored PCOS Consensus Workshop Group: Revised 2003 consensus on diagnosis criteria and long-term health risks related to polycystic ovary syndrome. Fertil Steril 2004;81:19-25.
171. Sakala EP, Leon ZA, Rouse GA: Management of antenatally diagnosed fetal ovarian cysts. Obstet Gynecol Surv 1991;46:407-414.
172. Samaniego F, Rodriquez E, Houldsworth J, et al: Cytogenetic and molecular analysis of human male germ cell tumors: Chromosome 12 abnormalities and gene amplification. Genes Chromosomes Cancer 1990;4:239-300.
173. Sanfilippo JS, Wakim NG, Schikler K, et al: Endometriosis in association with uterine anomaly. Am J Obstet Gynecol 1986;154:39-43.
174. SanMarco L, Londero F, Stefanutti V, et al: Ovarian leiomyoma. Clin Exp Obstet Gynecol 1991;18:145-148.
175. Sasaki H, Furusato M, Kiyokawa T, et al: Prognostic significance of histopathological subtypes in state I pure yolk sac tumors of the ovary. Br J Cancer 1994;69:529-536.
176. Saxman SB, Finch D, Gonin R, et al: Long term follow-up of a phase III study of three versus four cycles of bleomycin, etoposide, and cisplatin in favorable-prognosis germ-cell tumors: The Indiana University experience. J Clin Oncol 1998;16:702-706.
177. Schiller W: Mesonephroma ovarii. Am J Cancer 1939;35: 1-21.
178. Scholz PM, Key L, Filston HC: Large ovarian cyst causing cecal perforation in a newborn infant. J Pediatr Surg 1982;17:91-92.
179. Schwobel MG, Stauffer UG: Surgical treatment of ovarian tumors in childhood. Prog Pediatr Surg 1991;26:112-123.
180. Scully RE: Gonadoblastoma: A gonadal tumor related to the dysgerminoma (seminoma) and capable of sex-hormone production. Cancer 1953;6:455-463.
181. Scully RE: Gonadoblastoma: A review of 74 cases. Cancer 1970;25:1340-1356.
182. Scully RE: Weekly clinicopathological exercises: Case 22-1982. N Engl J Med 1982;306:1348-1355.
183. Scully RE: Small cell carcinoma of hypercalcemic type. Int J Gynecol Pathol 1993;2:148-152.
184. Scully RE, Young RH, Clement PB: Atlas of Tumor Pathology, Tumors of the Ovary, Maldeveloped Gonads, Fallopian Tube and Broad Ligaments, 3rd ser, fascicle 23. Washington, DC, American Registry of Pathology, Armed Forces Institute of Pathology, 1998.
185. Seeber B, Driscoll D: Hereditary breast and ovarian cancer syndrome: Should we test adolescents? J Pediatr Adolesc Gynecol 2004;17:161-167.
186. Shakfeh SM, Woodruff JD: Primary ovarian sarcomas: Report of 46 cases and review of the literature. Obstet Gynecol Surv 1987;42:331-349.
187. Sherman ME, Mink PJ, Curtis R, et al: Survival among women with borderline ovarian tumors and ovarian carcinoma: A population-based analysis. Cancer 2004;100: 1045-1052.
188. Shulman LP, Muram D, Marina N, et al: Lack of heritability in ovarian germ cell malignancies. Am J Obstet Gynecol

1994;170:1803-1808.
189. Siegel MJ, Surratt JT: Pediatric gynecologic imaging. Obstet Gynecol Clin North Am 1992;19:103-126.
190. Skinner MA, Schlatter MG, Heifetz SA, et al: Ovarian neoplasms in children. Arch Surg 1993;128:849-854.
191. Speleman F, DePotter C, Dal Cin P, et al: i(12p) in a malignant ovarian tumor. Cancer Genet Cytogenet 1990;45: 49-53.
192. Steinkampf MP, Hammond KR, Blackwell RE: Hormonal treatment of functional ovarian cysts: A randomized, prospective study. Fertil Steril 1990;54:775-777.
193. Stern JK, Buscema J, Rosenshein NB, et al: Spontaneous rupture of benign cystic teratomas. Obstet Gynecol 1981; 57:363-366.
194. Stevens SK, Hricak H, Stern JL: Ovarian lesions: Detection and characterization with gadolinium-enhanced MR imaging at 1.5T[1]. Radiology 1991;181:481-488.
195. Stickland JL: Ovarian cysts in neonates, children and adolescents. Curr Opin Obstet Gynecol 2002;14:459-465.
196. Suijkerbuijk RF, van de Veen Y, van Echten J, et al: Demonstration of the genuine i(12p) character of the standard marker chromosome of testicular germ cell tumors and identification of further chromosome 12 aberrations by competitive in situ hybridization. Am J Hum Genet 1991;489:269-401.
197. Surratt JT, Siegel MJ: Imaging of pediatric ovarian masses. Radiographics 1991;11:533-548.
198. Sutton CJ, Ewen SP, Whitelaw N, et al: Prospective, randomized, double-blind, controlled trial of laser laparoscopy in the treatment of pelvic pain associated with minimal, mild, and moderate endometriosis. Fertil Steril 1994;62:696-700.
199. Swanson SA, Norris HJ, Kelsten ML, et al: DNA content of juvenile granulosa tumors determined by flow cytometry. Int J Gynecol Pathol 1990;9:101-109.
200. Talerman A, Haije WG, Baggerman L: Serum alpha-feto protein (AFP) in patients with germ cell tumors of the gonads and extragonadal sites: Correlation between endodermal sinus (yolk sac) tumor and raised serum AFP. Cancer 1980;46:380-385.
201. Tanaka Y, Sasaki Y, Nishihira H, et al: Ovarian juvenile granulosa cell tumor associated with Maffucci's syndrome. Am J Clin Pathol 1992;97:523-527.
202. Tangir J, Zelterman D, Wenging M, et al: Reproductive function after conservative surgery and chemotherapy for malignant germ cell tumors of the ovary. Obstet Gynecol 2003;101:251-257.
203. Tapper D, Lack E: Teratomas in infancy and childhood, a 54 year experience at the Children's Hospital Medical Center. Ann Surg 1983;198:398-410.
204. Teilum G: Endodermal sinus tumor of the ovary and testis. Cancer 1959;12:1092-1105.
205. Teilum G: Classification of endodermal sinus tumor (meloblastoma vitellinum) and so-called embryonal carcinoma of the ovary. Acta Pathol Microbiol Scand 1965;64: 407-429.
206. Teilum G: Special Tumors of Ovary and Testis, 2nd ed. Copenhagen, Munksgaard, 1976.
207. Teilum G, Albrechtsen R, Norgaard-Pedersen B: The histogenetic-embryologic basis for reappearance of AFP in endodermal sinus tumors (yolk sac tumors) and teratomas. Acta Pathol Microbiol Scand 1975;83:80-86.
208. Templeman C, Blenshevsky A, Fallat ME, et al: Noninflammatory ovarian masses in girls and young women. Obstet Gynecol 2000;96:229-233.
209. Templeman CL, Hertweck SP, Scheetz JP, et al: The management of mature cystic teratomas in children and adolescents: A retrospective analysis. Hum Reprod 2000;15: 2669-2672.
210. Templeman CL, Reynolds AM, Hertweck SP, et al: Laparoscopic management of neonatal ovarian cysts. J Am Assoc Gynecol Laparosc 2000;7:401-404.
211. Thurlbeck W, Scully RE: Solid teratoma of the ovary: A clinico-pathologic analysis of 9 cases. Cancer 1960;13: 801-811.
212. Togashi K: Ovarian cancer: The clinical role of US, CT, and MRI. Eur Radiol 2003;13(Suppl 4):L87-L104.
213. Troche V, Hernandez E: Neoplasia arising in dysgenetic gonads: A review. Obstet Gynecol Surv 1986;41: 74-79.
214. Vaitukaitis JK, Braunstein GC, Ross GT: A radioimmunoassay which specifically measures human chorionic gonadotropin in the presence of human luteinizing hormone. Am J Obstet Gynecol 1972;113:751-758.
215. Van Voorhis BJ, Schwaiger J, Syrop CH, et al: Early diagnosis of ovarian torsion by color Doppler ultrasonography. Fertil Steril 1992;58:215-217.
216. Vercellini P, Bocciolone L, Vendola N, et al: Peritoneal endometriosis: Morphologic appearance in women with chronic pelvic pain. J Reprod Med 1991;36:533-536.
217. Vergote IB: Surgery for gynecologic malignancies. Curr Opin Oncol 1993;5:877-884.
218. Warner BW, Kuhn JC, Barr LL: Conservative management of large ovarian cysts in children: The value of serial pelvic ultrasonography. Surgery 1992;112:749-755.
219. Weinblatt M, Kochen J: An unusual family cancer syndrome manifested in young siblings. Cancer 1991;68: 1068-1070.
220. Weinblatt ME, Ortega JA: Treatment of children with dysgerminoma of the ovary. Cancer 1982;49:2608-2611.
221. Weinstein RS, Kuszak JR, Kluskens LF: P-glycoproteins in pathology: The multidrug resistance gene family in humans. Hum Pathol 1990;21:34-48.
222. Wertz DC, Fanos JH, Reilly PR: Genetic testing for children and adolescents: Who decides? JAMA 1994;272: 875-881.
223. Weyl-Ben Arush M, Oslander L: Ollier's disease associated with ovarian Sertoli-Leydig cell tumor and breast adenoma. Am J Pediatr Hematol Oncol 1991;13:49-51.
224. Wierman ME, Beardsworth DE, Mansfield MJ, et al: Puberty without gonadotropins: A unique mechanism of sexual development. N Engl J Med 1985;312:65-72.
225. Williams SD, Birch R, Einhorn LH, et al: Treatment of disseminated germ cell tumors with cisplatin, bleomycin, and either vinblastine or etoposide. N Engl J Med 1987;316:1435-1440.
226. Williams SD, Blessing JA, Liao SY, et al: Adjuvant therapy of ovarian germ cell tumors with cisplatin, etoposide, and bleomycin: A trial of the Gynecologic Oncology Group. J Clin Oncol 1994;12:701-706.
227. Williams SD, Blessing J, Slayton R, et al: Ovarian germ cell tumors: Adjuvant trials of the Gynecologic Oncology Group [abstract 584]. Proc Am Soc Clin Oncol 1989; 8:150.
228. Williams SD, Gershenson DM, Horowitz CJ, et al: Ovarian germ cell and stromal tumors. In Hoskins W, Perez CA, Young RC (eds): Principles and Practice of Gynecologic Oncology. Philadelphia, JB Lippincott, 1992, pp 715-730.
229. Wilson E, Vuitch F, Carr B: Laparoscopic removal of dysgenetic gonads containing a gonadoblastoma in a patient with Swyer syndrome. Obstet Gynecol 1992;79: 842-844.

230. Wu JT, Book L, Sudar K: Serum a-fetoprotein (AFP) levels in normal infants. Pediatr Res 1981;15:50-52.
231. Yamamoto K, Akiyama H, Maruyama T, et al: Granulocytic sarcoma of the ovary in patients with acute myelogenous leukemia. Am J Hematol 1991;38:223-225.
232. Yanai-Inbar ISR: Relation of ovarian dermoid cysts and immature teratomas: An analysis of 350 cases of immature teratoma and 10 cases of dermoid cyst with microscopic foci of immature tissue. Int J Gynecol Pathol 1987;6: 203-212.
233. Young JL Jr, Wu XC, Roffers SD, et al: Ovarian cancer in children and young adults in the United States 1992-1997. Cancer 2003;97(10 Suppl):2694-2700.
234. Young RH: Ovarian tumors other than those of surface epithelial-stromal type. Hum Pathol 1991;22: 763-775.
235. Young RH, Clement PB, Scully RE: Calcified thecomas in young women: A report of four cases. Int J Gynecol Pathol 1988;7:343-350.
236. Young RH, Dickersin GR, Scully RE: Juvenile granulosa cell tumor of the ovary: A clinicopathological analysis of 125 cases. Am J Surg Pathol 1984;8:575-596.
237. Young RH, Eichhorn JH, Dickersin GR, et al: Ovarian involvement by the intraabdominal desmoplastic small round cell tumor with divergent differentiation: A report of three cases. Hum Pathol 1992;23:454-464.
238. Young RH, Kozakewich HPW, Scully RE: Metastatic ovarian tumors in children: A report of 14 cases and review of the literature. Int J Gynecol Pathol 1993;12:8-19.
239. Zanetta GRS, Rota S, Chiari S, et al: Behaviour of borderline tumors with particular interest to persistence, recurrence, and progression to invasive carcinoma: A prospective study. J Clin Oncol 2001;19:2658-2664.

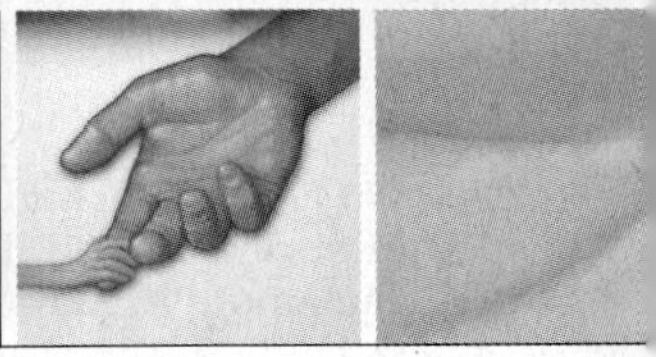

睾丸肿瘤

Hsi-Yang Wu 和 Eugene Wiener

602 发生于青春期前儿童中的睾丸肿瘤与成人比较，其病理特点和转移倾向完全不同。这一不同特点使得在年龄较小的儿童中允许更加大胆地采取保留睾丸的手术方式，而针对年龄稍长的儿童则需要仔细对其发育状态做详细的评价。睾丸肿瘤的发病高峰年龄介于2～4岁[13]，占儿童实体肿瘤的1%，而在非洲裔美国人和亚洲人群中十分罕见。发病年龄较晚的睾丸肿瘤通常合并存在隐睾和混合性腺发育不良。青春期后，腹股沟隐睾恶性变的发生率是1%，而腹腔内隐睾恶变的发生率是5%[6]。从病理角度看，未行手术纠正的隐睾易恶变成精原细胞瘤，手术纠正后的隐睾更易恶变成胚胎源性或畸胎瘤。睾丸下降固定术并不能降低睾丸肿瘤的发生[2]。由于在发育成熟前的睾丸组织中很少有肿瘤组织发现，因此，对于隐睾患儿，睾丸病理发现正常间质并不能够预测今后肿瘤的发生。

临床表现

睾丸肿瘤通常表现为阴囊内质地偏硬的实质性肿块。病史经常是由于意外的创伤引起注意，而这常常会误导患儿或家长对原先就存在的无痛性缓慢增大的睾丸的认识，混淆因果。鉴别诊断包括睾丸扭转和附睾炎，但是只要不存在疼痛、排尿困难或炎症，肿瘤通常最先考虑。然而，由于被误认为睾丸扭转进行手术的肿瘤患儿并不在少数。体格检查应当区分附睾肿胀（附睾炎）和睾丸肿胀（睾丸炎或肿瘤）。其中常常合并存在积液，由于肿瘤和积液可以同时存在，因此透光试验阳性并不能够排除肿瘤的诊断。睾丸基质肿瘤可以表现出早熟（间质细胞）或女性化倾向（支持细胞）。

诊断

影像学

如果由于鞘膜积液的张力使睾丸难以触及或者是由于体格检查不明确，阴囊超声检查有助于确定睾丸的结构和回声性质。正常睾丸的回声性质成同源性质地，而肿瘤则表现出与相邻正常睾丸间质组织异质性质地。如果在睾丸内存在囊性区域，则可能为畸胎瘤或是皮样囊肿，可考虑保留睾丸的手术方式。目前尚不清楚睾丸内多发性细小钙化灶（小结石样病变）是否存在显著性意义。成人多见于睾丸肿瘤患者。如果在对侧被认为是正常的睾丸内发现存在小结石，必须做影像学随访，因为这侧睾丸存在罹患睾丸肿瘤的可能[11]。

一旦睾丸恶性肿瘤的诊断确认，应立即做出肿瘤是否转移的评价。首选胸部CT，因为卵黄囊瘤容易向胸部转移，肺部要高于后腹膜。术后腹部和盆腔CT可以探明后腹膜淋巴结是否存在转移。

肿瘤标志物

血清甲胎蛋白（AFP）和β-人绒毛膜促性腺激素（β-HCG）水平在所有怀疑罹患睾丸肿瘤的患者术前均应做检查。虽然有时其浓度水平增高有助于诊断，但它们通常被用于术后随访检测肿瘤是否复发。AFP（卵黄囊肿瘤标志物）正常情况下在出生至8个月的婴儿中都可以增高[27]，包括存在肝功能异常的患者，因此，对睾丸切除患者，AFP检查应当系列化。由于AFP的半衰期为5天，所以，如果肿瘤被完全切除，其浓度水平应当在25天后下降至正常。

表 37-1　美国儿童睾丸肿瘤学会登记，2002

肿瘤类型	百分比（%）
卵黄囊瘤	62
畸胎瘤	23
性腺基质细胞瘤	4
表皮样囊肿	3
幼年性粒层细胞瘤	3
睾丸支持细胞瘤	3
睾丸间质细胞瘤	1
性腺母细胞瘤	1

β-HCG 在精原细胞瘤中偶然可以升高，它通常在绒毛膜癌中升高，两者都很少在青春期前的人群中发
23 病。β-HCG 的半衰期为 1 天，因此通常在术后 1 周降至正常水平。

分期和分级

表 37-1 列举了 2002 年全美儿童睾丸肿瘤登记的病理学分配比例。卵黄囊肿瘤的突出地位可能反映了传报偏倚，因为许多单中心报告提示畸胎瘤更为多见，而由于其良性肿瘤的性质，并没有被传报至上述睾丸肿瘤登记中[1,14,23,26]。表 37-2 是儿童肿瘤组织（COG）应用于睾丸肿瘤的分期系统。

表 37-2　儿童肿瘤组织（COG）青春期前睾丸肿瘤分期方案（from AGCT0132）

分期	特点
I	局限于睾丸，经腹股沟行高位睾丸完全切除术；无临床、放射影像学或病理组织学依据提示存在睾丸外病灶；对于术前诊断存在正常或不确定睾丸标志物的患者，如果影像学提示后腹膜淋巴结直径＞2cm，术中必须做同侧后腹膜淋巴结活检以确认肿瘤分期为 I 期。
II	经阴囊行肿瘤活检，镜下阴囊肿瘤累及或肿瘤累及精索高位（离精索近段≤5cm）。
III	累及后腹膜淋巴结，但无内脏或腹腔外累及；CT 检查提示淋巴结直径＞4cm 或病理活检证实淋巴结直径＞2cm 而＜4cm。
IV	远处转移，包括肝脏转移。

根据肿瘤类型的治疗

畸胎瘤

畸胎瘤起源于外胚层、中胚层和内胚层三个胚层，因此包含有囊性和实质性成分。皮样囊肿可以被看做是单胚层的畸胎瘤，仅仅起源于外胚层。青春期前，睾丸畸胎瘤均能实施保留睾丸的手术[20,21,24]，因为肿瘤均为良性，即便是病理检查发现其中存在发育未成熟的成分[8]。完全发育成熟的患者，畸胎瘤的处理方法与成人相同，因其存在恶性肿瘤的组织学行为，需要做彻底的经腹股沟睾丸切除术。

如果血清 AFP 浓度高于对应的年龄水平，应当考虑瘤体内含有卵黄囊成分而不能实施保留睾丸的手术；如果阴囊超声提示睾丸内存在钙化灶和异质性肿块，伴有正常水平的 AFP，则首先考虑畸胎瘤；手术通常采用腹股沟切口提出睾丸，在内环口水平控制精索血流后，畸胎瘤可以从睾丸内剥离，冰冻病理切片能够明确肿瘤性质[21]。即使术中发现瘤体严重压迫正常睾丸间质，术后超声检查通常都发现良好的睾丸组织恢复，从而提示保留有功能[14]。

对于冰冻病理切片的应用有两种意见。经典的意见认为可以通过冰冻病理探查明确畸胎瘤的病理性质以及相邻正常睾丸间质尚无成熟改变[20]；另一种意见认为，通过超声影像及正常水平的 AFP 已经足以在术前做出畸胎瘤的诊断。他们同时提出，在成熟发育中的任何患儿不适合实施睾丸保留手术[14,23]。而多数青春期前的畸胎瘤患儿在实施睾丸保留的手术后得以保留良好的性功能。

生殖细胞肿瘤

60%发育成熟前的睾丸肿瘤是生殖细胞肿瘤。儿童期的卵黄囊瘤与成人相比有着截然不同的转移模式。在儿童中有近 20%的病例存在血行胸部转移，而扩散转移到后腹膜淋巴结的仅占所有病例的 4%～6%；相反，在成人中，多数转移至后腹膜淋巴结。大多数的卵黄囊瘤发病于出生后 2 年内，治疗可采

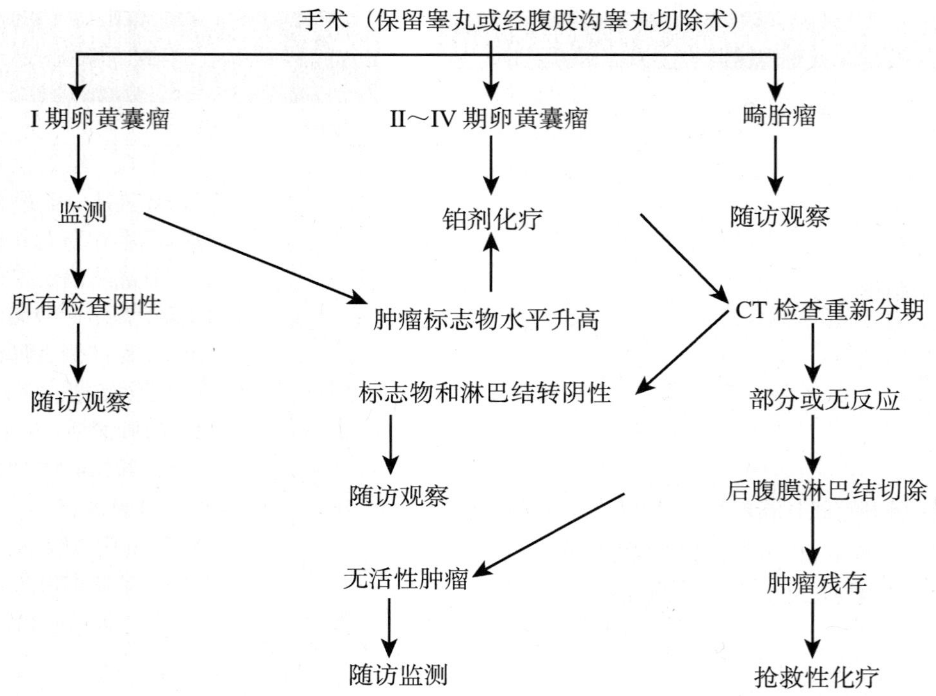

随访内容：

肿瘤标志物第一年每月复查，第二年每 2 月复查一次。

胸片第一年每 2 月复查一次，第二年每 3 月复查一次。

CT 第一年每 3 月复查一次，第二年每 6 月复查一次。

图 37-1 生殖细胞肿瘤术后随访方案。（Adapted from POG 9048/CCSG 8891.）

用经腹股沟切口睾丸切除术，病理可发现存在 Schiller-Duval 小体。如果属于 I 期（无胸部转移或后腹膜淋巴结肿大，术后 AFP 水平相应下降），则无需化疗[20]。后续治疗方案可以参考图 37-1。II 期患儿（经阴囊行睾丸切除术，镜下肿瘤残留或 AFP 水平术后仍持续增高）需要接受含铂剂的化疗方案（顺铂，依托泊苷，博莱霉素）而无需放疗。

经阴囊行睾丸切除术是否需要同时做半侧阴囊切除术，目前仍存在争议[22]，因为虽然在儿童中尚未做过相应的调查，但在成人中发现，同时做局部治疗并不能影响接受化疗方案的患者的疗效[7]。因此，目前 COG 提供的方案中已无需半侧阴囊切除。II 期肿瘤患者如果在化疗后仍持续存在后腹膜肿块或是血清 AFP 水平增高，则应当行后腹膜淋巴结切除术（RPLND）。如果肿瘤性质有改变，则相应的化疗方案也需要做修改。对于III期肿瘤患儿（后腹膜淋巴结直径＞2cm）和IV期患儿（肿瘤转移），需在化疗后
624 行 RPLND 手术清除后腹膜残存的任何肿块。各期肿瘤患儿的总体存活率接近 100%。

对于罕见的性腺外生殖细胞肿瘤（后腹膜或腹腔内），最佳的治疗方案是先行肿块活检（可能的话行完全切除），化疗后再切除残留的肿块，6 年无复发存活率达 83%[4]。

性腺基质细胞瘤

睾丸间质细胞瘤是成人和儿童中最为常见的性腺基质细胞瘤[25]。经典的三联症表现为早熟（10%）、单侧睾丸肿块（90%）和 17-酮类固醇的升高。与神经垂体损伤（促黄体激素、促卵泡激素和睾酮水平升高）引起的早熟不同，睾丸间质细胞瘤表现出低水平的促黄体激素、促卵泡激素和睾酮浓度升高。肿瘤切除后早熟症状并不一定能够消除，但也不足以证明有肿瘤的残余。由于先天性肾上腺增生所导致的结节倾向于双侧同时发生（80%），也存在有低水平的促黄

体激素和促卵泡激素以及高水平的睾酮。而这些增生的结节能够被地塞米松和肾上腺皮质激素所抑制并在注射糖皮质激素后消退。而在成人睾丸基质细胞中作为病理学标志的基质细胞晶体在儿童中甚为罕见。睾丸基质细胞瘤同样可以通过保留睾丸的手术进行治疗，这与畸胎瘤相同，因为它们在儿童期都是良性肿瘤[12,24,25]。

睾丸支持细胞瘤在儿童中罕见，通常是良性的，因此通过保留睾丸手术治疗是安全的[17,24,25]。临床可表现出男性乳腺发育。术后 2 年需要 CT 检查后腹膜，因为病理结果并不总能预示预后。虽然这一肿瘤通常都是良性的，但是由于在未发育成熟的患儿中表现出恶性倾向的仅有几例报道，所以患儿罹患后腹膜淋巴结反应的发病率尚不知晓[25]。

性腺母细胞瘤

性腺母细胞瘤通常见于混合性腺发育不良（45, X/46,XY）或者是伴有 Y 染色体发育不良的雌雄间体的患者。瘤体小，其中 33%为双侧发病，10%为恶性，通常在青春期后发病。病理改变涉及生殖细胞和基质细胞。虽然性腺发育不良为低度恶性疾病，但仍主张早期切除，因为其随着患儿生长易退化成精原细胞瘤。

最近，有人建议对混合性腺发育不良患者做双侧性腺切除[9]。由于意识到新生儿睾酮水平将影响大脑，对该肿瘤的治疗变得越发复杂。因此，双侧性腺切除后并将患儿作为女性进行抚养并不一定符合其事实上的性别作用。如果选择保留一侧性腺于阴囊中，则在患儿完全发育成熟前需要每年做阴囊检查和超声随访，并且在患儿进入及结束青春期的两个时段进行睾丸病理活检以排除睾丸肿瘤的发生[15]。

继发性肿瘤

睾丸继发性瘤多来源于淋巴瘤或白血病，在超声影像上呈低回声信号。虽然对于完成化疗的淋巴瘤或白血病患儿行睾丸活检曾经非常普遍，但是由于并没有发现对预后有任何影响，故而已经不再作为常规[16]。对于完成治疗后的淋巴瘤或白血病患者，如被发现存在睾丸增大，则需要行睾丸活检并行放疗，而由于在睾丸这一全身防护最为严密的器官之一存在转移，常提示在机体其余部位存在肿瘤残余，因此，额外的化疗也是必需的。

附睾的横纹肌肉瘤的详细描述见第 32 章。

治疗方法

保留睾丸的手术通常经腹股沟切口进行。睾丸由切口提出，将一根烟卷式引流在内环口水平环绕精索以闭塞血供。将肿瘤部位的睾丸鞘膜直接打开。如果肿瘤位于睾丸实质的深部，有时术中超声有利于做瘤体定位。手术中可以用刀锋的边缘使肿瘤脱壳，此举有利于保护邻近的睾丸实质，而少量的睾丸实质组织能够帮助病理医生明确患儿有无进入青春期的成熟发

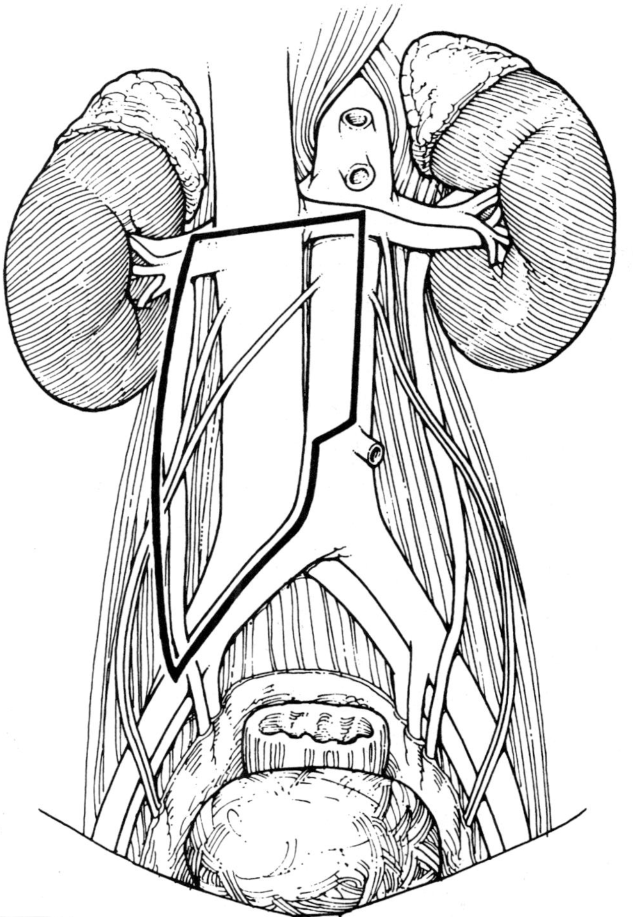

图 37-2 右侧改良保全神经的后腹膜淋巴结清扫范围。（From Marshall FF [ed]: Textbook of Operative Urology. Philadephia, WB Saunders, 1996, pp 368-369.）

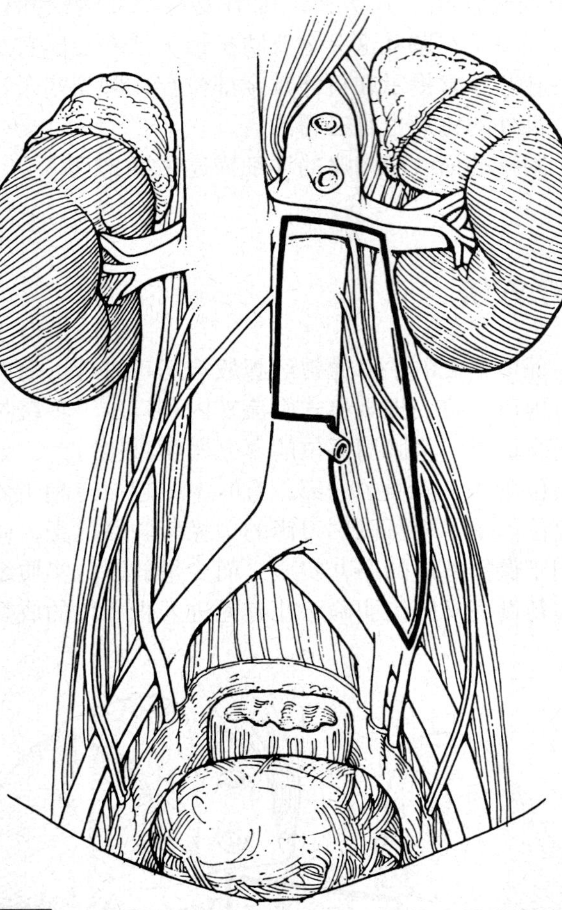

图 37-3　左侧改良保全神经的后腹膜淋巴结清扫范围。(From Marshall FF [ed]: Textbook of Operative Urology. Philadephia, WB Saunders, 1996, pp 368-369.)

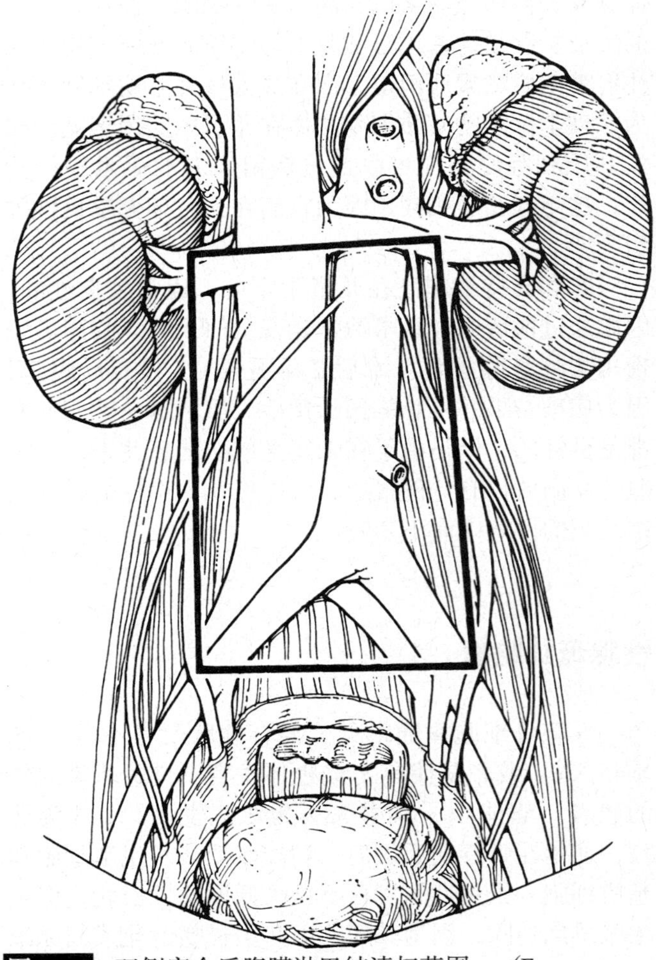

图 37-4　双侧完全后腹膜淋巴结清扫范围。(From Marshall FF [ed]: Textbook of Operative Urology. Philadephia, WB Saunders, 1996, pp 368-369.)

育状态。术中止血应当由双极电凝实施。鞘膜则由可吸收线缝合关闭后回纳入阴囊。

彻底的睾丸切除术则是在内环口水平高位结扎切除所有的精索组织。如果肿瘤巨大而不能拖出阴囊，可以将腹股沟切口延长至阴囊前面以防止瘤体破裂。

RPLND 术可以通过经腹切口、胸腹联合切口或腹腔镜方式施行。其手术步骤是基于成人睾丸肿瘤切除术[10]。右侧肿瘤淋巴转移的好发部位为主动脉腔静脉间和腔静脉旁淋巴结，而左侧肿瘤的淋巴转移好发于主动脉旁和主动脉腔静脉间淋巴结。淋巴结清扫的边界取决于肿瘤的最初分期。如果是Ⅱ期肿瘤，则可采用改良的单侧清扫方案（图 37-2 和 37-3）。对Ⅲ期或Ⅳ期肿瘤则需要实施双侧淋巴结清扫（图
526 37-4）。大血管前的淋巴结组通常是分散的，而经由髂静脉前的交感神经节需要保留以保留射精功能。应用 5 枚经腹孔做腹腔镜 RPLND 同样可以实施淋巴结清扫。由于在成人中也仅限于Ⅰ期和Ⅱ期肿瘤中小的残留肿块，因此儿童中行腹腔镜 RPLND 可能也仅适于Ⅰ期和小的Ⅱ期转移瘤患儿。

并发症

不育和睾丸退化是主要的两个远期并发症。虽然在成人患者中可以在治疗前预先选择精子库做精子保存，但这显然不适用于未发育成熟的儿童。因儿童期生殖器肿瘤而存活的男性仅 45%能保存生殖能力[5]。而如果在 RPLND 手术中损伤交感神经，将

不能保留射精功能。睾丸肿瘤化疗常用的但不是常规使用的烷化剂如环磷酰胺易影响精子。睾丸间细胞对化疗拥有较强的抵抗作用，因此通常不需要实施雄激素替代[19]。

总结

对于青春期前的患儿，如果术前评价提示病理分型可能是非生殖细胞肿瘤，就应当考虑行保留睾丸的肿瘤切除术；而如果由于 AFP 水平升高而考虑肿瘤病理为卵黄囊来源，则完全睾丸切除术及基于术后肿瘤分期的相应治疗也能够获得良好的存活率。

（潘伟华译　吴晔明校）

参考文献

1. Andrassy RJ, Copron C, Ritchey M: Testicular tumors. In O'Neill JA, Rowe MI, Grosfeld JL, et al (eds): Pediatric Surgery, 5th ed. Philadelphia, WB Saunders, 1998, p 542.
2. Batata MA, Whitmore WF, Chu FCH, et al: Cryptorchidism and testicular cancer. J Urol 1980;124:382.
3. Bhayani SB, Ong A, Oh WK, et al: Laparoscopic retroperitoneal lymph node dissection for clinical stage I nonseminomatous germ cell testicular cancer: A long-term update. Urology 2003;62:324.
4. Billmire D, Vinocur C, Rescorla F, et al: Malignant retroperitoneal and abdominal germ cell tumors: An intergroup study. J Pediatr Surg 2003;38:315.
5. Byrne J, Fears TR, Gail MH, et al: Effects of treatment on fertility in long-term survivors of testicular cancer. N Engl J Med 1987;3178:1315.
6. Campbell HE: Incidence of malignant growth of the undescended testicle: A critical and statistical study. Arch Surg 1942;44:353.
7. Capelouto CC, Clark PE, Ransil BJ, et al: A review of scrotal violation in testicular cancer: Is adjuvant local therapy necessary? J Urol 1995;153:981.
8. Carney JA, Thompson DP, Johnson CL, et al: Teratomas in children: Clinical and pathologic aspects. J Pediatr Surg 1972;7:271.
9. Donahoe PK, Crawford JD, Hendren WH: Mixed gonadal dysgenesis, pathogenesis, and management. J Pediatr Surg 1979;14:287.
10. Donohue JP, Foster RS, Rowland RG, et al: Nerve-sparing retroperitoneal lymphadenectomy with preservation of ejaculation. J Urol 1990;144:287.
11. Furness PD III, Husmann DA, Brock JW III, et al: Multi-institutional study of testicular microlithiasis in childhood: A benign or premalignant condition? J Urol 1998;160:1151.
12. Konrad D, Schoenle EJ: Ten-year follow-up in a boy with Leydig cell tumor after selective surgery. Horm Res 1999; 51:96.
13. Li FP, Fraumeni JF Jr: Testicular cancers in children: Epidemiologic characteristics. J Natl Cancer Inst 1972; 48:1575.
14. Metcalfe PD, Farivar-Mosheni H, Farhat W, et al: Pediatric testicular tumors: Contemporary incidence and efficacy of testicular preserving surgery. J Urol 2003;170:2412.
15. Muller J, Ritzen EM, Ivarsson SA, et al: Management of males with 45,X/46,XY gonadal dysgenesis. Horm Res 1999;52:11.
16. Nachman J, Palmer NF, Sather HN, et al: Open-wedge testicular biopsy in childhood acute lymphoblastic leukemia after two years of maintenance therapy: Diagnostic accuracy and influence on outcome—a report from Children's Cancer Study Group. Blood 1990;75:1051.
17. Nonomura K, Koyama T, Kakizaki H, et al: Testicular-sparing surgery for the prepubertal testicular tumor: Experience of two cases with large cell calcifying Sertoli cell tumors. Eur Urol 2001;40:699.
18. Palese MA, Su LM, Kavoussi LR: Laparoscopic retroperitoneal lymph node dissection after chemotherapy. Urology 2002;60:130.
19. Relander T, Cavallin-Stahl E, Garwicz S, et al: Gonadal and sexual function in men treated for childhood cancer. Med Pediatr Oncol 2000;34:52.
20. Ross JH, Rybicki L, Kay R: Clinical behavior and a contemporary management algorithm for prepubertal testis tumors: A summary of the prepubertal testis tumor registry. J Urol 2002;168:1675.
21. Rushton HG, Belman AB, Sesterhenn I, et al: Testicular sparing surgery for prepubertal teratoma of the testis: A clinical and pathological study. J Urol 1990;144:726.
22. Schlatter M, Rescorla F, Giller R, et al: Excellent outcome in patients with stage I germ cell tumors of the testes: A study of the Children's Cancer Group/Pediatric Oncology Group. J Pediatr Surg 2003;38:319.
23. Shukla AR, Woodard C, Carr MC, et al: Experience with testis sparing surgery for testicular teratoma. J Urol 2004;171:161.
24. Sugita Y, Clarnette TD, Cooke-Yarborough C, et al: Testicular and paratesticular tumours in children: 30 years' experience. Aust N Z J Surg 1999;69:505.
25. Thomas JC, Ross JH, Kay R: Stromal testis tumors in children: A report from the Prepubertal Testis Tumor Registry. J Urol 2001;166:2338.
26. Walsh C, Rushton HG: Diagnosis and management of teratomas and epidermoid cysts. Urol Clin North Am 2000; 27:509.
27. Wu JT, Book L, Sudar K: Serum alpha fetoprotein (AFP) levels in normal infants. Pediatr Res 1981;15:50.

第 38 章

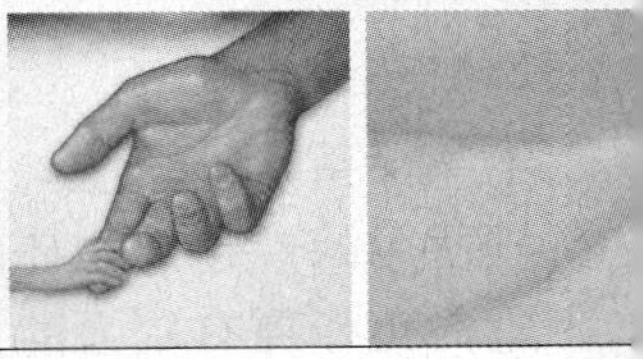

肾上腺肿瘤

Stanley T. Lau 和 Michael G. Caty

628 解剖学

从它的拉丁词根来分析，adrenal 的意思是“肾脏附近”。双侧肾上腺位于肾脏上极的正前方，被肾周脂肪覆盖，包绕着肾筋膜。成人的每个肾上腺重约 5 克。右侧肾上腺邻近下腔静脉和肝脏，位于横膈膜后延伸处，左侧肾上腺邻近脾动脉和胰尾。

虽然肾上腺的血流供应是多变的，但一般有三个来源：膈下动脉上支、主动脉中间支和肾动脉下支。静脉并不与动脉平行；而是每个肾上腺有一个大的肾上腺静脉。右侧肾上腺静脉丛后方汇入下腔静脉，左侧汇入左肾静脉。

肾上腺淋巴管一个来自肾上腺包膜下丛，另一个来自髓质丛。右侧肾上腺淋巴管引流到横膈角附近的主动脉旁淋巴结，左侧肾上腺淋巴管引流到左肾动脉出口附近的淋巴结。

肾上腺的神经来源于腹丛和胸腔内脏大神经。神经节前的交感神经纤维进入肾上腺门，终止于髓质内的神经节。

肾上腺包含两个不同的部分：皮质和髓质。这两个部分不但肉眼检查不同，而且在胚层起源、结构和功能上均不同。髓质起源于神经嵴的外胚层细胞。这些早期细胞形成嗜铬细胞系统和神经元系统，这说明可能发生两种不同的髓质肿瘤：嗜铬细胞瘤和神经母细胞瘤。神经节前交感神经细胞控制嗜铬细胞的分泌，这些细胞合成去甲肾上腺素和肾上腺素。

皮质组成肾上腺的外层，分泌性激素、盐皮质激素和糖皮质激素。它分成三个分别有不同的合成激素功能的独立区域。球状带是皮质最外层区域，产生醛固酮和相关盐皮质激素。束状带位于球状带下方，分泌氢化可的松和肾上腺性激素。最内层的网状带储备胆固醇作为类固醇生成的前体和分泌氢化可的松、雄激素和雌激素。

胚胎学

最早在孕 4 周就能看到肾上腺皮质的原基，在孕 6 周就能清晰看到。在出生前的超声检查中，最早在孕 20 周能看到肾上腺，在大多数胎儿，在孕 30 周时可以识别[30]。在孕 4～6 周，肾上腺生殖嵴的后腹膜中胚层细胞变成柱状，侵入上皮表面下的间充质，最终形成胎儿的肾上腺皮质。上皮细胞的另一种增生继后形成覆盖在皮质细胞表面的“帽”，而成为皮质的球状带。肾上腺髓质的外胚层嗜铬细胞起源于神经嵴，最早出现于第 5 周，来源于第 6～12 的胸神经祖细胞侵入腺体形成髓质。这些原始的髓质细胞在孕 3 月开始分化成为嗜铬细胞，最后导致细胞产生肾上腺素和去甲肾上腺素。

胎儿的肾上腺皮质区在孕 6 周左右出现。这个区不断扩大并占据腺体的大部分。事实上，由于胎儿皮质区体积大，在孕 4 月时，胎儿的肾上腺体积是肾脏的 4 倍。随后，这个胎儿皮质区体积逐渐缩小，在婴儿期消失。

在胎儿发育过程中，异位的髓质和皮质组织，出生后可能依然保留。肾上腺髓质异位通常发现于主动脉和其分支附近。主动脉旁嗜铬体（Zuckerkandl 器）是嗜铬细胞肿块的一个例子，起源于肠系膜下动脉。大多数肾上腺外嗜铬细胞异位在出生后消失；髓质内 6
嗜铬细胞发生分化。

肾上腺外皮质异位在儿童多见，发现于肾脏、肝脏或沿性腺迁移过程中通道上的疝囊或性腺本身。约 50%的新生儿有肾上腺皮质异位，但这些异位残余在生后数周萎缩消失[30]。

生理学

肾上腺髓质功能

肾上腺髓质合成和释放儿茶酚胺——多巴胺、肾上腺素和去甲肾上腺素。儿茶酚胺的合成从非必需氨基酸的酪氨酸开始。酪氨酸羟化酶转化酪氨酸成二羟基苯基丙氨酸（DOPA），这是合成途径的限速酶。DOPA 脱羧酶转化 DOPA 为多巴胺。苯丙氨酸 β-羟化酶转化多巴胺为去甲肾上腺素。最后，苯乙胺 N-甲基转移酶转化去甲肾上腺素为肾上腺素。

髓质内的嗜铬细胞含有储存着儿茶酚胺的胞浆颗粒。神经节前交感神经末梢释放乙酰胆碱，它能导致这些胞浆存储颗粒的钙依赖的胞吐作用并释放儿茶酚胺。肾上腺髓质的儿茶酚胺释放的调控通过去甲肾上腺素的反馈抑制调节机制来实现。去甲肾上腺素抑制乙酰胆碱从突触前 α_2 受体释放，当去甲肾上腺素浓度高时也抑制酪氨酸羟化酶活性。

肾上腺皮质功能

肾上腺皮质合成三种激素：糖皮质激素、盐皮质激素和性激素。这些激素的调控通过下丘脑-垂体-肾上腺轴来实现。下丘脑产生促肾上腺皮质激素释放激素（CRH）；它将被转运至腺垂体，在这里它将刺激促肾上腺皮质激素（ACTH）的释放。ACTH 然后刺激肾上腺皮质产生肾上腺激素。

CRH 释放的每天生理性波动导致 ACTH 和它调控的激素周期性变化。血清峰浓度出现在晨起时，随后在白天逐渐下降。氢化可的松和 ACTH 均抑制 CRH 释放，产生负反馈调控。

肾上腺皮质的糖皮质激素的产生从底物胆固醇开始，受 ACTH 调控。大部分血清中的氢化可的松与氢化可的松结合蛋白（90%）和白蛋白（6%）结合在一起，只留下小部分（4%）呈有活性的游离状态。与多数类固醇相似，未结合氢化可的松部分是亲脂性的，因此能够稳定穿过靶细胞的细胞膜。特异的受体然后与氢化可的松结合，在细胞核内调控 mRNA 的合成。

氢化可的松主要通过对抗胰岛素影响代谢。通过增加糖原异生所必需的蛋白质水解和诱导肝脏糖异生的酶而导致高血糖。氢化可的松也使外周组织减少糖的摄取；抑制脂肪细胞摄取糖和通过胰岛素敏感组织的结合来降低胰岛素量。

氢化可的松也降低炎症反应和免疫功能，而影响伤口愈合。氢化可的松通过降低淋巴细胞对抗原刺激的反应，及影响趋化做用和白细胞的噬菌作用而降低淋巴细胞和粒细胞的免疫效应。这两个免疫功能是伤口早期愈合的一个重要部分；这样，伤口的张力强度下降，并在氢化可的松过多时影响愈合。

醛固酮是一种盐皮质激素，在球状带合成，主要在肝脏内代谢。肾素-血管紧张素系统调控大多数醛固酮的释放，而 ACTH 只起着较小的作用。肾球旁器的致密斑在肾灌注下降或低血钠时释放肾素。肾素使肝内产生的血管紧张素原转化为血管紧张素 I。肺部的血管紧张素转化酶转化血管紧张素 I 为血管紧张素 II。血管紧张素 II 通过直接做用于肾上腺球状带的细胞刺激醛固酮的合成；它也是血管收缩剂。通过增加肾脏对钠的滞留，醛固酮增加血压和纠正低血钠，从而减少肾素的释放。

血清钾浓度也对醛固酮调控发挥一点作用。高钾通过直接做用于球状带细胞，以及增加近肾小球细胞释放肾素而增加醛固酮的产生。醛固酮促使肾脏排钾增加，从而减少醛固酮的产生和提供另一个反馈调节机制。

肾上腺雄激素在网状带合成，主要由 ACTH 调控。这些激素以周期性方式释放，与氢化可的松和 ACTH 的释放相关。肾上腺雄激素只有微弱的活性，但被外周组织转化为活性更强的形式，如睾酮和二氢睾酮。这些激素的代谢发生在肝脏。

肾上腺的影像学

在儿童，当发现腹部肿块或出现肾上腺功能亢进的继发表现时，有必要进行肾上腺影像学检查。腹部和后腹膜影像检查能识别组织来源、发现转移性肿瘤和证明两侧是否对称。核医学检查能用于确定肾上腺源性肿瘤定位和证实是否为肾上腺外肿瘤。特异性放射药物的使用可以预测肾上腺肿瘤的细胞类型。

腹部平片对于评估肾上腺肿块的临床价值极低。630 它无法发现小的肾上腺功能性肿块，虽然大的肿块，如神经母细胞瘤，将表现出钙化和肿块的表现，但通常可以触及，通过体格检查更容易被诊断。

腹部肿块的初筛检查经常选择超声。超声的优点是能提供与体格检查相关的影像而无电离辐射。腹部超声目的是识别发病的器官、了解肿块的特性和大小以及明确肿块的血管分布。由于邻近器官，如肾脏的压迫，对于大的肿块，要明确肾上腺是发病器官是比较困难的。

在生后第一周超声能容易的发现肾上腺。随后肾上腺很快退化，而皮质和髓质的区别也消失。在新生儿，肾上腺出血可以表现为肾上腺肿块，这可能有一些诱发因素，如窒息或难产。肾上腺出血后会有不同表现，可能为等回声或低回声影像、或两者兼而有之[41]。肾上腺出血可能与神经母细胞瘤混淆。尿儿茶酚胺水平正常，并存在肾上腺出血的危险因素的患者，需重复做超声检查。通过超声很难鉴别肾上腺腺瘤和肾癌；此外，两者均类似嗜铬细胞瘤。超声显示恶性肿瘤的特征是由于快速生长而导致的中心性坏死。生化检测，以及 CT、MRI 和核医学等手段的使用均使疾病的可能范围缩小。

当超声发现后腹膜实质性肿块时，影像学检查来明确发病器官和手术切除的可能性。两个可以立即选择的方法是 CT 和 MRI。虽然 CT 是一个诊断肾上腺疾病的准确的方法，在幼儿，由于后腹膜脂肪缺乏，CT 的准确性不高。CT 的其他缺点是需要经脉使用增强剂和需要暴露于电离辐射。但 CT 的一个优点是对疑似肾上腺癌的患者可以同时做胸部扫描以排除肺部转移灶。用 MRI 检查肾上腺疾病的优点是可以做多切面的影像，冠状面能够很好地区别肾上腺肿块和邻近的肾脏，反之亦然[27,33,38]。嗜铬细胞瘤在 T1 影像中呈现出中或低密度信号，用 DTPA 增强后强化[20]。

肾上腺肿瘤细胞的单一属性使放射性药物影像诊断成为可能。利用选择性吸收特异药物的属性能够鉴别肾上腺和肾上腺外嗜铬细胞瘤，以及肾上腺腺瘤和它们的定位。

肾上腺和嗜铬细胞瘤细胞有去甲肾上腺素转运系统。间碘苯甲胍（MIBG）的结构和去甲肾上腺素相似，能够被去甲肾上腺素转运系统摄取进入胞浆内的小泡中。通过 MIBG 的苯环后位与两个同位素碘之一的结合来获得核素成像。放射性 ^{131}I 的半衰期为 8.2 天，能发射高能射线。而放射性 ^{123}I 的半衰期较短，放射能量更低[15]。做 MIBG 扫描的患者必须给予饱和量的碘化钾以阻止甲状腺吸收游离的放射性碘。在 24 和 48 小时做闪烁扫描。MIBG 扫描对于检测肾上腺外及转移性嗜铬细胞瘤是有价值的。它也能确定尿儿茶酚胺试验阳性患者的嗜铬细胞瘤在肾上腺的位置。

正电子发射 X 线断层扫描术（PET）在不久的将来将成为嗜铬细胞瘤诊断的重要技术。PET 扫描利用短效的正电子发射药剂来识别体内特异的摄取区域。由于肿瘤的高代谢，放射标记的葡萄糖能被用于识别恶性肿瘤组织。PET 扫描中最常用的放射标记葡萄糖是[^{18}F]–氟化脱氧葡萄糖（FDG）。然而，FDG PET 不是最理想的判定嗜铬细胞瘤和区别良恶性嗜铬细胞瘤的手段。更有用的药物是 6–[^{18}F]–氟化多巴胺（DA）。去甲肾上腺素和 DA 的相似性使其能被交感肾上腺髓质组织选择性摄取[32]。有研究显示，FDG PET 比 MIBG 扫描能更好地显示转移性肿块[37]。PET 检查暴露于放射性的强度比常规闪烁扫描要低。当特异的药物，如 DA，能轻易获得时，它可能将成为可选的影像学检查。

另一个有用的放射性药物是 N–59（^{131}I–iodomethyl–19–norcholesterol）。这个胆固醇类似物像胆固醇一样被摄取进入肾上腺皮质的类固醇途径。它被用于识别肾上腺皮质和鉴别肾上腺腺瘤与肾上腺皮质增生。

肾上腺髓质病变

嗜铬细胞瘤

来自德国弗赖堡的 Frankel 在 1886 年首次描述了双侧嗜铬细胞瘤，是在对一个患有焦虑、心悸和头痛症状的 18 岁女孩尸检时发现的[44]。Pick 在 1912 年以肿瘤主要的细胞类型——嗜铬细胞命名了该肿瘤，但是，直到 1922 年 Labbe 等才首次清晰地报道了嗜铬细胞瘤和阵发性高血压的关系。在 1927 年，Mayo 首次成功地对 1 例阵发性高血压患者摘除了嗜铬细胞瘤，该患者在手术探查前并没有明确的术前诊断。在 1929 年，Pincoffs 首次做了正确的术前诊断，并由

表 38-1 儿童和成人嗜铬细胞瘤的比较

	儿童	成人
发生率	1∶500 000	1∶50 000
家族史（%）	10	2～3
双侧（%）	24～70	10
肾上腺外部位（%）	30	10
恶性（%）	3	10

Shipley 成功地施行了手术[14]。从此，嗜铬细胞瘤的行为得到更好的理解，特别是对于儿童患者。

嗜铬细胞瘤在儿童中是少见的，与成人比较存在
31 几个明显的特点。儿童的嗜铬细胞瘤发生率是成人的10%，约为 1∶500 000，而成人为 1∶50 000[34]。约10%的儿童嗜铬细胞瘤有家族史，这是成人的 4 倍。只有 7%的成人嗜铬细胞瘤是双侧的，而报道的儿童双侧嗜铬细胞瘤发生率的范围是 24%～70%。儿童肾上腺外嗜铬细胞瘤大约是成人的 2 倍[11,36]（表 38-1）。

嗜铬细胞瘤起源于肾上腺髓质的嗜铬细胞，它产生导致肿瘤症状的儿茶酚胺。这些细胞沿主动脉迁徙，通常保留在主动脉分支附近。

症状

嗜铬细胞瘤能在任何年龄发病，儿童嗜铬细胞瘤就诊的平均年龄是 11 岁。半数以上患儿出现头痛、发热、心悸、口渴、多尿、多汗、恶心和体重减轻，但最常见的表现是持续性高血压[4,34,36]。在儿童，高血压的最常见原因是继发性的，最多见的病因为肾功能异常（78%），其次是肾动脉疾病（12%），及主动脉缩窄（2%）等[23]。嗜铬细胞瘤导致的高血压约占儿童高血压的 0.5%，一旦当其他原因被排除后，必须考虑本病可能。在嗜铬细胞瘤患儿，70%～90%病例有持续性高血压，只有一小部分病例表现为阵发性高血压。相反，成人的嗜铬细胞瘤患者 50%有阵发性高血压[36]。

诊断

嗜铬细胞瘤的诊断有赖于血和尿儿茶酚胺和其代谢物水平的升高。24 小时尿儿茶酚胺、甲基肾上腺素和香草杏仁酸（VMA）是最好的诊断性检查[18,43]。约 95%患者尿甲基肾上腺素升高，而约 90%患者尿香草基杏仁酸和儿茶酚胺水平升高[43]。甚至在香草基杏仁酸和嗜铬细胞瘤大小之间存在线性相关[10]。正常人 24 小时尿中游离儿茶酚胺、尿香草基杏仁酸和甲基肾上腺素的量分别小于 100mg、7mg 和 1.3mg。血浆儿茶酚胺也能通过放射酶学实验来测定。然而，患者在采血时必须保持仰卧和安静，这在儿童有一定难度。当高血压发作期血浆儿茶酚胺水平正常则可能不是嗜铬细胞瘤，但高于 2000pg/ml 时可以诊断为嗜铬细胞瘤。血浆儿茶酚胺在 500～1000pg/ml 之间需考虑嗜铬细胞瘤可能，应进行进一步检查[36]。

在获得生化检测诊断为嗜铬细胞瘤后，必须进行肿瘤定位。虽然大的肿块如神经母细胞瘤可以在腹部平片上看到，但大多数肾上腺肿块在不使用其他影像学方法时是无法看到的。几乎所有嗜铬细胞瘤发生于腹腔或盆腔，虽然肾上腺是最常见的部位，但 43%以上的患者部位为多发[36]。最初用于婴儿和儿童的检查一般是超声，这在鉴别实体瘤和囊性肿块时较有用，但不能发现小的肾上腺肿块。CT 和 MRI 可以提供更
好的分辨率和敏感度，特别是 MRI（图 38-1）。另 632
外一个有用的影像学技术是 ^{131}I 标记的 MIBG 扫描；这种同位素能在摄取去甲肾上腺素的部位积聚而用于检测肿瘤。这在肾上腺外嗜铬细胞瘤的定位特别有用，但儿童的肾上腺外嗜铬细胞瘤少见。与成人比较，儿童的头部和颈部嗜铬细胞瘤更为多见，其次是后腹膜[42]。

治疗

嗜铬细胞瘤的治疗方法是手术切除，但内科治疗是术前准备必不可少的一部分。高水平的儿茶酚胺增加了术中突发严重高血压的风险，以及一旦肿块切除后儿茶酚胺释放停止而出现的明显的低血压。事实上，这些并发症是过去手术切除相关的高死亡率的原因[36]。术前和术中处理的改进已经使手术死亡率从过去的 24%～45%下降到目前的 10%以下[9]。术前使用 α-肾上腺素能阻滞剂，如酚苄明和酚妥拉明，通过阻滞 α-肾上腺素受体而将肾上腺素和去甲肾上腺素的作用减至最低。这些药物应该至少在手术 3～7 天前开始使用以将术中风险降至最低。

β-肾上腺素能阻滞剂，如普萘洛尔和拉贝洛尔，可以在 α-肾上腺素能阻滞剂作用达到后使用，特别

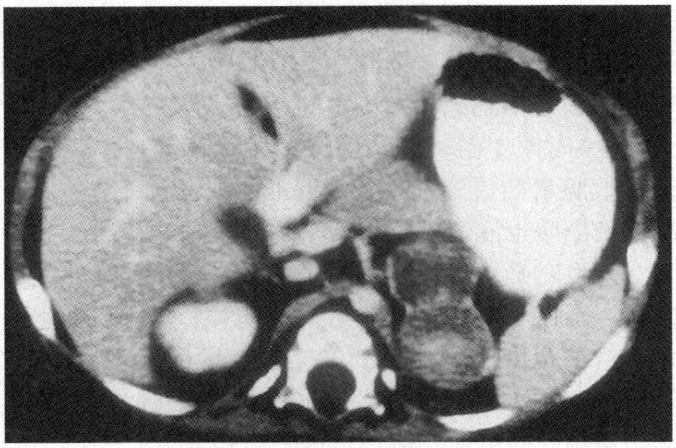

A

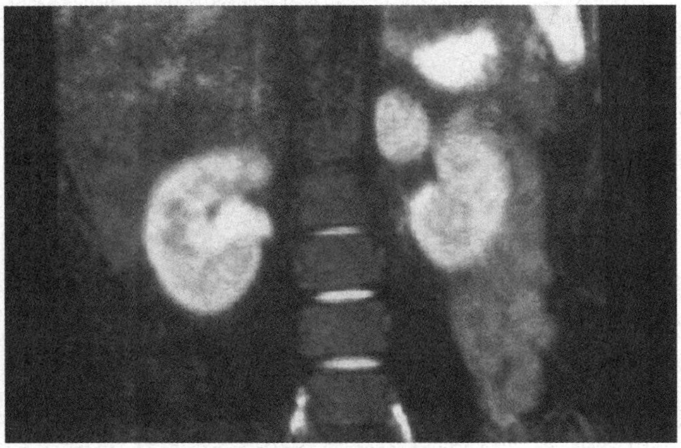

B

图 38–1 A. 一个患有左侧肾上腺肿块伴高血压的 10 岁女孩的腹部 CT。B. MRI 发现一个左侧肾上腺嗜铬细胞瘤。没有发现其他肿块。不需要用增强剂。

是出现静息心动过速时使用。如果使用这些药物，关键的是必须首先使用 α–肾上腺素能阻滞剂。

嗜铬细胞瘤患者易于在基础状态时出现轻度的低血容量，血容量平均约减少 15%。随着术前建立了药理学阻滞作用，必要可使用静脉补液。这种容量再扩张也有助于减少术中血压的波动和心律失常。

尽管良好的术前准备使血压正常，但麻醉医生必须准备应付突发的血压波动。术中风险主要出现在麻醉诱导和插管、术中处理肿块时，以及结扎肿瘤静脉的瞬间[7]。放置动脉和中心静脉导管监测血压和液体状况是必不可少的。麻醉医生还必须准备快速起效的升压和降压药物在必要时调整血压。硝普钠和硝酸甘油是很好的可作为静脉给药的升压药物。心律失常可以通过使用普萘洛尔、艾司洛尔和利多卡因来控制。

传统的手术方法是经腹腔切除，通常是经肋下切口，通过这种方法能够看到双侧肾上腺以及主动脉周围的交感神经节、小肠肠系膜和骨盆。95%以上的儿童嗜铬细胞瘤位于腹部，因此这种手术方法能发现大多数肿瘤。外科医生在肿块切除时必须努力减少对肿块的直接操作。当肿块切除时，早期的控制和结扎肾上腺静脉可限制儿茶酚胺的释放。

外科医生通过将横结肠往下折并将十二指肠推向中间能暴露右侧肾上腺。这能暴露右肾上半部分以及右肾上腺。翻开肝脏上缘和将下腔静脉推向中间而更好的暴露肾上腺。由于右侧肾上腺静脉较短，剥离的风险更大，因此右侧比左侧出血的风险要大。

通过切开后腹膜至脾曲并把结肠推向中间，能暴露左侧肾上腺。然后切开肾周围筋膜暴露左肾上腺。另外，外科医生也可以分离胃结肠韧带，将胃和横结肠分别向上和向下推。然后沿胰腺下缘剪开后腹膜，推动胰尾可暴露肾上腺静脉。

典型的肾上腺嗜铬细胞瘤是有包膜的，虽然可能有小部分正常组织，但必须切除整个肾上腺。因为肿瘤一般不与肾脏粘连，很少需要做肾切除术。

就像前面提及的，一旦肾上腺静脉被结扎以及肿瘤被切除，患者可能由于过多儿茶酚胺的清除而出现低血压。事实上，血压恢复正常需要数天时间。如果术后高血压重新出现，需考虑存在第二个嗜铬细胞瘤。所有患者均必须随访以确认儿茶酚胺水平恢复正常。因为多灶性嗜铬细胞瘤存在异时性发生的可能，患者应做长期随访[7,36]。

相关的疾病

家族性嗜铬细胞瘤可能在几种综合征中出现。最常见的综合征是 II 型多发性内分泌肿瘤（MEN–2）和 von Hippel–Lindau 病。I 型神经纤维瘤病和没有其他任何异常的患者其家族性嗜铬细胞瘤的发生率更低。

MEN–2 是由于 10 号染色体上 *RET* 原癌基因发生突变导致的常染色体显性遗传性疾病。患者易于出现髓样甲状腺癌，高达 50%的患者将出现肾上腺嗜铬细胞瘤。这些肿瘤基本上都是双侧性的，而且基本都不是恶性的。MEN–2A 患者也易于出现甲状旁腺功能亢进，而 MEN–2B 患者易于出现 Marfan 综合征样体型或黏膜神经节瘤。

3 号染色体上的 von Hippel-Lindau 基因突变导致 von Hippel-Lindau 病。它的特征是视网膜血管瘤、中枢神经系统的成血管细胞瘤、肾脏囊肿、肾细胞癌、胰腺囊肿和嗜铬细胞瘤。这些嗜铬细胞瘤通常是多灶性的，而且往往是位于肾上腺外组织
33 （图 38-2）。

恶性肿瘤

据报道，10%的儿童嗜铬细胞瘤患者是恶性的，嗜铬细胞瘤的组织学检查不能准确的判定良恶性[4]。恶性嗜铬细胞瘤的诊断一般与肿瘤的临床表现相关。恶性嗜铬细胞瘤可以有局部浸润或远处转移，主要发生于骨骼、肝脏、淋巴结、肺和中枢神经系统。同时或异时发生的嗜铬细胞瘤可以出现于交感神经链的任何部位。虽然手术切除仍然是可以选择的治疗，但长期缓解需通过多学科协作方法来实现，包括局部切除、放疗和化疗[8]。

肾上腺皮质病变

肾上腺皮质肿瘤在儿童中少见，在所有儿童肿瘤中的比例少于 0.2%，在儿童肾上腺肿瘤中的比例少于 6%[6]。该肿瘤在美国的发生率约为每年 25 例，其中 75%是肾上腺皮质癌[35,45]。肾上腺皮质肿瘤更多的见于女孩，男女比例约为 1∶2～1∶3[26]。与嗜铬细胞瘤类似，肾上腺皮质肿瘤的表现在儿童与成人间存在差异。在儿童大约 85%～95%的肾上腺皮质肿瘤有激素活性，而在成人该比例少于 50%。此外，尽管成人恶性肿瘤有明确的病理学标准，这些标准在儿童人群中并不全部适用。由于这些肿瘤的临床表现并不与病理表现完全相关，恶性肿瘤的诊断必须基于临床表现。在肾上腺皮质肿瘤，诊断时年龄少于 3.5 岁及诊断前症状持续时间少于 6 个月者预后良好。对这些儿童，早期发现是很重要的，因为诊断的延误将影响临床预后[30]。

肾上腺皮质肿瘤与数种先天性异常相关，包括单侧肥大症；与单侧肥大症相关的其他肿瘤包括肾母细胞瘤和肝母细胞瘤。Beckwith-Wiedemann 综合征患者（脐突出、巨舌和巨人症）也比一般人的肾上腺皮质肿瘤发生率要高[21]。然而，大多数肾上腺皮质肿瘤是散发的[30]。

Cushing 综合征

在 1932 年，Cushing 首先对一个垂体腺瘤患者报道了以他的名字为命名的综合征。从此，对其病理生理和病因的理解取得相当大的发展。

内源性的 Cushing 综合征在儿童少见。总的来说，自发性 Cushing 综合征的发生率在每百万人口约有 5 人；主要见于年轻的成年女性，女性和男性比例为 9∶1。10%患者为儿童和青少年[24]。

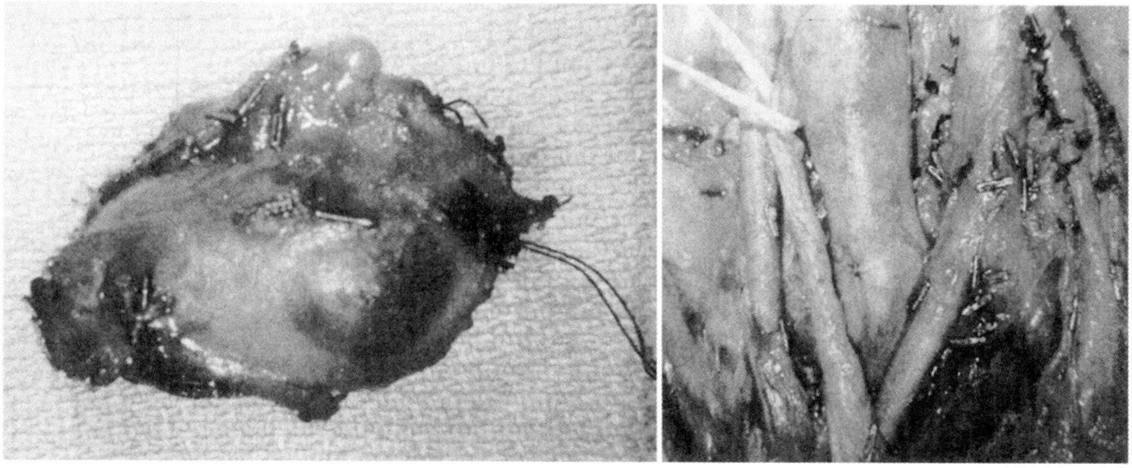

A　　B

图 38-2　A. 一个 13 岁女孩出现相对小的生长于椎旁交感神经节的肾上腺外嗜铬细胞瘤，她在骑马时出现了突发性高血压和严重的头痛。B. 肿瘤切除后的手术野显示腔静脉和主动脉分支。环绕输尿管的是一个血管环。

典型的儿童 Cushing 综合征表现一般是全身性肥胖和长骨生长迟缓[24]。其他症状包括高血压、乏力、皮肤出现条纹并易出现淤斑、粉刺、月经不规则、骨质疏松及糖耐量减低。与成人 Cushing 综合征不同，肌肉乏力、睡眠不佳和精神改变（情绪易变、易怒和抑郁）在儿童少见[24]。

CRH 由下丘脑分泌，是腺垂体释放 ACTH 的最
634 主要刺激物。ACTH 然后刺激肾上腺皮质产生糖皮质激素、盐皮质激素和性激素。Cushing 综合征可以被分为 ACTH 依赖的和非 ACTH 依赖两种类型。前者过高的 ACTH 水平刺激肾上腺皮质产生过多的皮质醇。而在非 ACTH 依赖类型中，异常的肾上腺组织产生过多的皮质醇而与 ACTH 水平无关。

Cushing 病指由垂体肿瘤导致的 ACTH 产生过多而出现的 Cushing 综合征。这些肿瘤典型的是小腺瘤，在直径上小于 1cm；然而也可能出现大的、有侵袭性的垂体腺瘤。这些肿瘤使双侧肾上腺皮质增生，同时糖皮质激素相应增加。随着患者年龄增加，垂体肿瘤导致 Cushing 综合征的可能性更高。

在 6 岁以下患儿中，导致内源性 Cushing 综合征的最可能原因为肾上腺肿瘤。虽然肾上腺皮质癌只占所有儿童恶性肿瘤的 0.2%和肾上腺肿瘤的 6%，但大约 60%～80%的 Cushing 综合征儿童由肾上腺皮质癌所致[5]。

肾上腺功能亢进的临床诊断必须通过生化检查诊断 Cushing 综合征来确诊。此外，必须定位该综合征

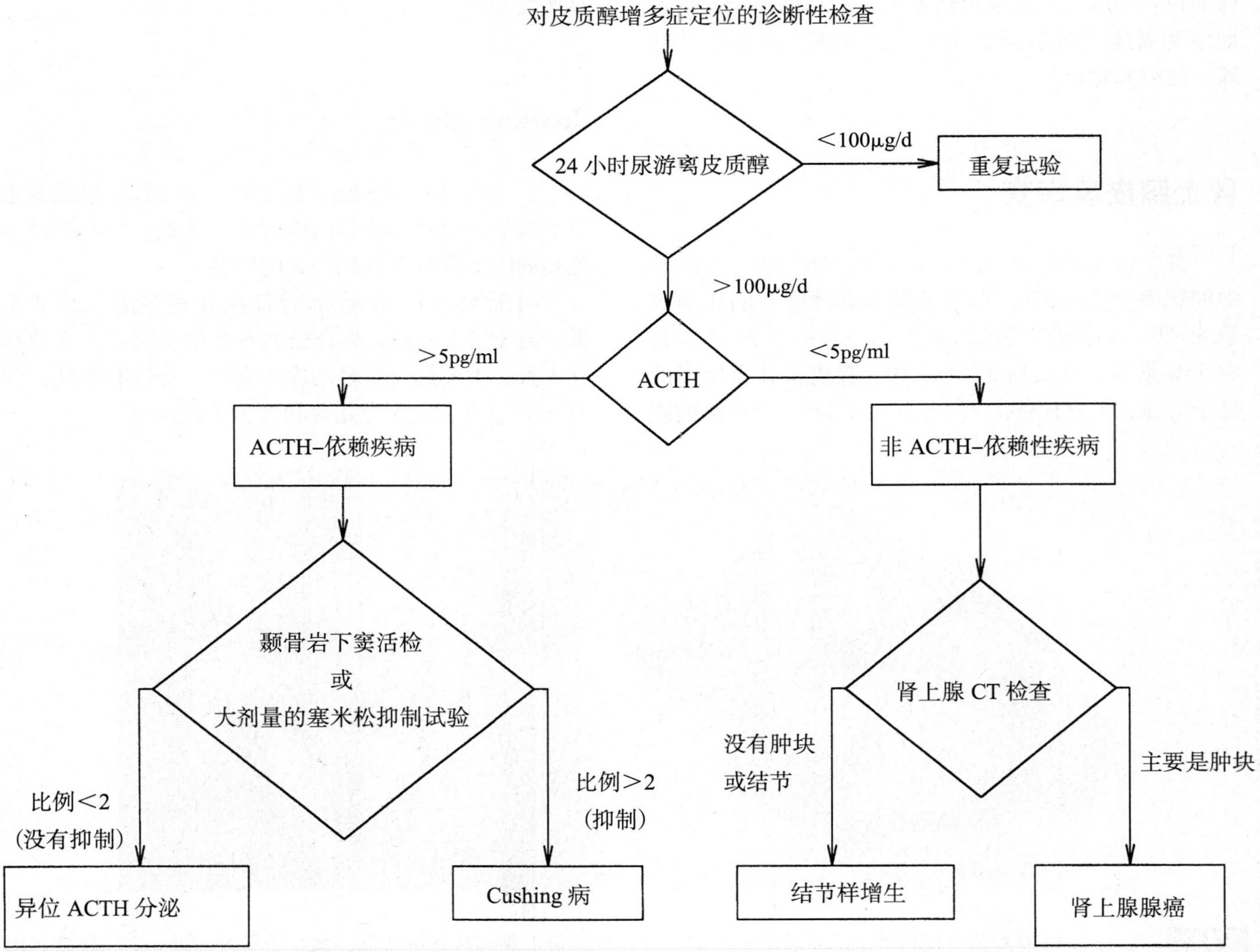

图 38–3 有可疑 Cushing 综合征的儿童皮质醇增多症病因的定位过程。

的特异来源（图 38–3）。因为皮质醇分泌的正常生理节奏在 Cushing 综合征患者中消失，所以随机的血清皮质醇水平的价值有限。检测早晨和晚间血清皮质醇浓度来评估一天的变化敏感性较低。取而代之，24 小时尿游离皮质醇水平是诊断肾上腺功能亢进的最好办法，其敏感性达 98%[16]。在儿童中，这个值需根据体表面积来调整。正常值每天小于 70μg/m²；Cushing 综合征时该值升高。另一个有用的检测是 24 小时尿 17–羟基类固醇的排泄；这是一个间接测定皮质醇分泌的方法，在肾上腺功能亢进时升高。一旦根据肌苷排泄纠正后，正常值为每天每克肌苷的尿 17–羟基类固醇在 2～7mg 间。另一个有用的筛查检测是隔夜 1-mg 地塞米松抑制实验（或在儿童用 0.3mg/m²）。在给予地塞米松后，晨起皮质醇浓度大于 5μg/dL 意味着皮质醇分泌未受抑制，这与 Cushing 综合征是一致的。

一旦 Cushing 综合征的诊断明确，下一步是查找肾上腺功能亢进的发病原因。如图 38–3 显示的，测定 ACTH 水平能够区别 ACTH 依赖和非 ACTH 依赖性的病因。如果 ACTH 水平高于 5pg/ml，则病因是 ACTH 依赖的；如果低于 5pg/ml，则病因是非 ACTH 依赖的。

ACTH 依赖性肾上腺皮质亢进症的病因包括垂体和异位的 ACTH 分泌性肿瘤。虽然 ACTH 的异位分泌在儿童少见，但肾母细胞瘤和胸腺、胰腺或神经系统肿瘤能够产生 ACTH。大多数 ACTH 分泌性肿瘤患者有 Cushing 病（由垂体肿瘤导致的 Cushing 综合征）。虽然大剂量地塞米松抑制实验或颞骨岩下窦活检能够鉴别垂体和异位源性 ACTH 分泌，但 MRI 检查也能显示垂体肿瘤。产生 CRH 的异位肿瘤是另一个导致 Cushing 综合征的 ACTH 依赖性病因，但这个情况尚未在儿童中有报道[3,16]。

在成人和儿童中，Cushing 病的治疗选择是经蝶窦手术切除垂体腺瘤。患者术后若无改善或复发，通过垂体钴 60 放疗可能获得部分缓解。

如果通过检查提示有异位 ACTH 分泌性肿瘤，患者必须做甲状腺髓样癌（血清降钙素水平）和嗜铬细胞瘤（测定 24 小时尿儿茶酚胺、间甲肾上腺素和尿香草基杏仁酸）的筛查。其他异位的部位如支气管、胸腺或肠道类癌可以在胸部和腹部 CT 上看到。如果可能，异位的 ACTH 分泌性肿瘤应该切除。如果无法切除，双侧肾上腺切除对 Cushing 综合征能提供有效的治疗。

Cushing 综合征的非 ACTH 依赖性病因包括肾上腺肿瘤和肾上腺结性增生。非 ACTH 依赖的 Cushing 综合征在儿童比成人相对更多见[16]。在儿童，肾上腺皮质肿瘤在男性化综合征中最为多见，大多数患儿出现男性化症状。这些患者大约 33% 有 Cushing 综合征；10% 以下单纯出现 Cushing 综合征而没有男性化表现[28,35]。

肾上腺结性增生是一个少见病，发生于儿童和青年。该病通常在 20 岁以下出现，主要见于女孩。虽然该结节可以是散发性的，但许多病例有家族史并主要以常染色体显性遗传方式出现[16]。肾上腺出现多个大约 3～5mm 大小的结节。组织学检查显示皮质淋巴细胞浸润，提示该病为自身免疫性疾病。这种病因的 Cushing 综合征治疗是双侧肾上腺切除[16]。该手术伴有明显的致残率，并需要术后一直做盐皮质激素和糖皮质激素的长期替代治疗。

性激素分泌性肿瘤

肾上腺皮质病变可能导致男性化或女性化肿瘤。就像前面提及的，大多数儿童肾上腺皮质肿瘤是有激素活性的。伴有或无皮质醇增多症的女性男性化是最常见的表现[22,28,40,45]。这些男性化肿瘤可能在男孩中比女孩更难识别。男孩可能出现青春期性早熟，包括阴茎增大、痤疮及阴毛、腋毛和面毛的过早出现。女孩可能出现阴蒂肥大、多毛和痤疮（图 38–4）。可以选择的治疗方式是肾上腺切除术。

虽然女性化肾上腺皮质肿瘤在儿童少见，但它们通常是恶性的。在正常肾上腺中，雌激素的分泌量很少。然而在肾上腺皮质肿瘤中，可能出现雌激素特别是雌二醇的过多分泌。在女孩，这些肿瘤出现同性性早熟，包括乳房过早增大、生长过快和骨龄过高。在男孩，这些肿瘤导致双侧女性型乳房、生长加速和性发育延迟；也有精子产生缺乏。

肾上腺皮质肿瘤的治疗

手术切除是治疗肾上腺皮质肿瘤的主要方法。良性肾上腺腺瘤的治疗是肾上腺切除。然而肾上腺皮质癌需要做充分的剖腹探查以发现并切除转移灶。对于任何患者，均需要术后类固醇替代治疗，直到对侧肾上腺从抑制状态恢复。

CT 或 MRI 有助于肾上腺增生和肾上腺肿瘤的鉴别。NP-59 闪烁扫描可能有助于评估肾上腺的病变。肾上腺腺瘤通常摄取 NP-59 增加，而典型的肾上腺皮质癌并不摄取该同位素。双侧摄取 NP-59 意味着双侧肾上腺增生，这可能是 ACTH 过度分泌的结果。

肾上腺皮质癌转移的最常见部位是肺、肝脏、淋巴结、对侧肾上腺、骨骼、肾脏和脑。如果无法做完全切除，减瘤术可能能也有一些益处。用米托坦的内科治疗也可以对病灶无法切除的患者发挥作用。米托坦作为抑肾上腺素药物，是通过改变线粒体功能、阻断肾上腺类固醇羟基化和改变皮质醇和雄激素的肾上腺外代谢来发挥作用的。尚无资料清晰显示化疗的作
636 用，但很明确的是，完全切除是唯一使患者生存明显改善的治疗方法[31]。

醛固酮增多症

醛固酮产生过多或醛固酮增多症可能是因为肾上腺功能异常或肾素分泌过多。原发性醛固酮增多症指肾上腺功能异常，例如分泌醛固酮的肿瘤或双侧肾上腺增生。继发性醛固酮增多症指肾素的分泌过多，这可能由肝硬化、充血性心力衰竭、分泌肾素的近肾小球球细胞肿瘤或肾血管异常（如肾动脉狭窄）所致。

醛固酮增多症的症状包括头痛、乏力、虚弱、嗜睡、体重轻、多尿、烦渴和夜尿症。水钠重吸收增加导致出现高血压。软弱是因为低血钾，这是实验室检查中最常见的异常，而由于尿中氢离子丢失可以观察到代谢性碱中毒。醛固酮增多症的生化诊断通过肾素分泌受抑制时分泌过多的醛固酮来确诊。一旦原发性醛固酮增多症诊断成立，必须区分分泌醛固酮的肾上腺肿瘤和更常见的双侧肾上腺皮质增生。双侧肾上腺皮质增生患者中，给予地塞米松能使异常的高醛固酮和低肾素水平正常[43]。

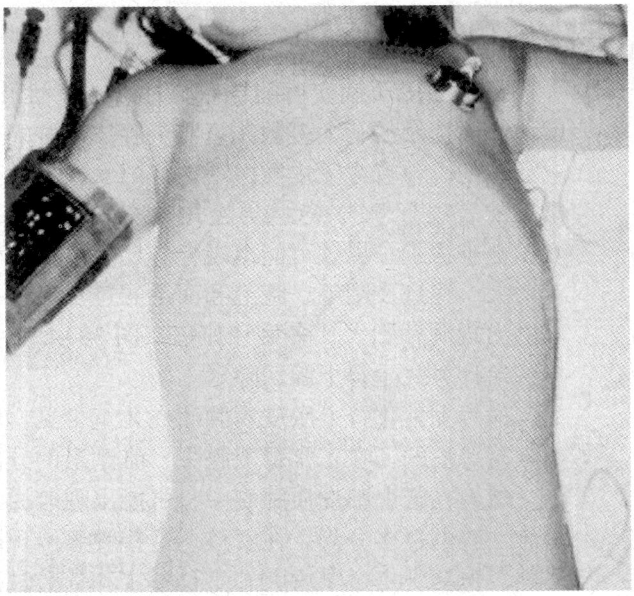

A

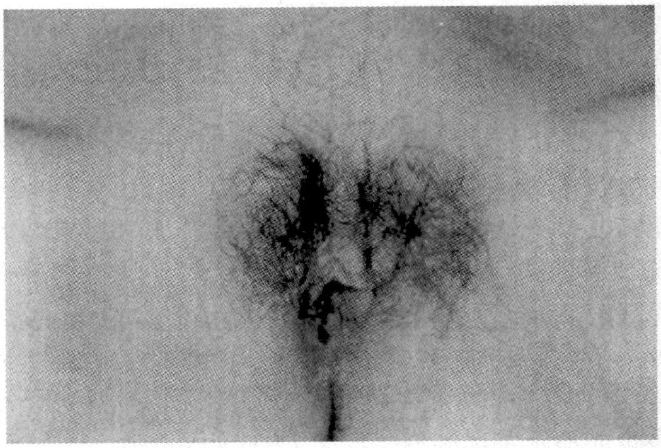

B

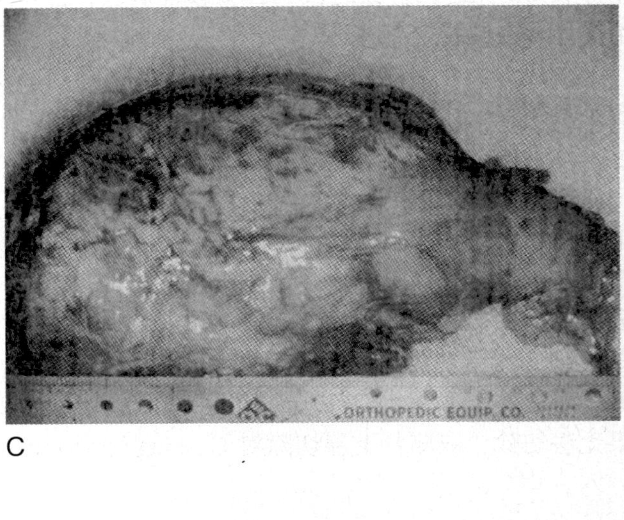

C

图 38-4 A. 该 3 岁女孩表现右上腹巨大肿块。B. 查体发现有阴毛。C. 肿块是一个能使女孩男性化的肾上腺皮质癌。尽管肿块完全切除并进行化疗，患儿出现转移并最后死亡。

在儿童中，导致原发性醛固酮增多症的醛固酮腺瘤或肾上腺腺瘤发生率非常低。只有少数文献报道了该类病例。就像前面提及的，最常见的原发性醛固酮增多症病因是双侧肾上腺皮质增生[1]。醛固酮腺瘤最好做单侧肾上腺切除。手术治疗双侧肾上腺皮质增生的患者效果不佳，最好用螺内酯和氨洛林做内科治疗[43]。双侧肾上腺切除导致的肾上腺功能不全比醛固酮增多症的治疗还要难。

Addison 病

类固醇激素（糖皮质激素或盐皮质激素）产生不足能导致 Addison 病。Addison 病患儿有许多症状，包括虚弱、厌食、体重减轻、疲乏、恶心、呕吐和腹泻。如果患儿 ACTH 水平升高，由于 ACTH 可刺激黑色素细胞，而致出现皮肤色素过度沉着。肾上腺危象时发生低血糖从而可出现惊厥。

许多原因能导致儿童出现肾上腺功能不全。先天性肾上腺发育不全可因为常染色体隐性遗传异常或 X 性染色体异常（见于男孩）所致。类固醇代谢异常也能导致肾上腺功能不全。最常见的先天性异常包括糖皮质激素合成缺陷，统称为先天性肾上腺增生症。累及视丘下部或垂体的病变也能通过 CRH 或 ACTH 分泌减少，而导致获得性肾上腺功能不全。

肾上腺破坏也能导致肾上腺功能不全。导致肾上腺崩解的原因包括出血、感染、肾上腺脑白质营养不良和自身免疫性疾病。在老年患者中，重症感染能导致肾上腺出血。结核病过去常是感染性肾上腺破坏的病因；但现在这种情况的发生率已经下降到中等水平。急性肾上腺功能不全的最常见原因之一是长期外源性糖皮质激素给药的终止。

在新生儿，肾上腺出血不是一个少见病。事实上，肾上腺是新生儿中第二位最常见的腹腔出血来源[39]。新生儿的肾上腺出血发病机制并不完全明确。相关的因素包括产伤、窒息、母亲低血压、重症感染或出血性疾病[19,30]。肾上腺出血的发生率几乎每 1000 个活产儿中有 2 例[30]，但随着影像技术敏感度的提高，该数字将增加。右侧肾上腺出血比左侧高 3～4 倍，在 8%～10%患者中为双侧性[19]。这种偏向于右侧可能是由于右侧肾上腺静脉直接进入下腔静脉，这使右侧肾上腺更易于受静脉压力变化影响。左侧肾上腺静脉进入肾静脉而能够稍微得到保护。胎儿皮质由于他的大小和后期的内卷而易于出现胎儿和新生儿肾上腺出血。胎儿皮质较大从而使肾上腺相对较大，增加了受攻击时的易损伤性。胎儿皮质的生理性内卷可能会非常快，从而撕裂了未受支撑的肾上腺中心静脉[39]。

在产前超声中，肾上腺出血表现为一个强回声肿块。该肿块回声越来越低，常常在随后的声像图中消失。这种病变可以完全消退，只留下残留的钙化。然而，病变也可能不会消退，可能需要手术切除来进行肿块与囊性神经母细胞瘤的鉴别。

Addison 病的治疗是缺乏的类固醇激素替代疗法。这可以用盐皮质激素（如氟氢可的松）或糖皮质激素（如氢化可的松或泼尼松）来实现。在急性应激期间，如感染或手术，需要增加糖皮质激素的剂量。

偶发性肾上腺肿块

在由于其他原因做影像学检查时偶然发现肾上腺病变的情况在儿童和成人中均不断增加，可能由于影像学检查的频率增加及影像学检查方式的灵敏度增加。在成人，目前认为有激素活性的肿瘤，不管肿瘤大小均应切除。而对于无功能的肾上腺肿块，认为其小于 4cm 时进行观察是安全的[2,13,25]。然而在儿童人群中，尚无明确的关于偶发、无功能的肾上腺肿块的治疗规范。由于儿童肾上腺功能性肿瘤和恶性肿瘤的发病率更高，许多外科医生推荐在这种情况下做肾上腺切除[25]。

肾上腺切除术

肾上腺手术的目的是完全切除肿瘤，使内分泌功能正常并治愈恶性肿瘤。围术期准备包括纠正电解质异常、在嗜铬细胞瘤中使用 α 和 β 受体阻断剂和进行局部影像学检查指导手术入路。手术入路基于肾上腺肿块可能的组织学类型、双侧肾上腺病变和外科医生的偏爱。用腹腔镜做肾上腺切除为许多儿童肾上腺肿块切除提供了一个吸引人的选择性方法。

肾上腺切除的传统入路包括前位、后位、和胸腹联合入路。肾上腺切除的前位入路允许切除左侧或右

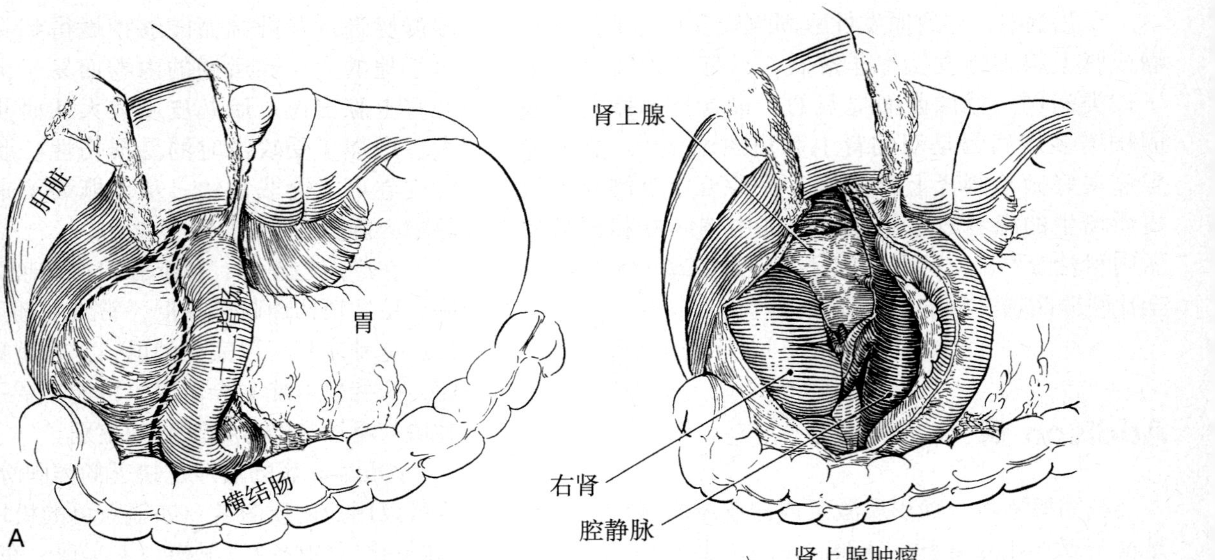

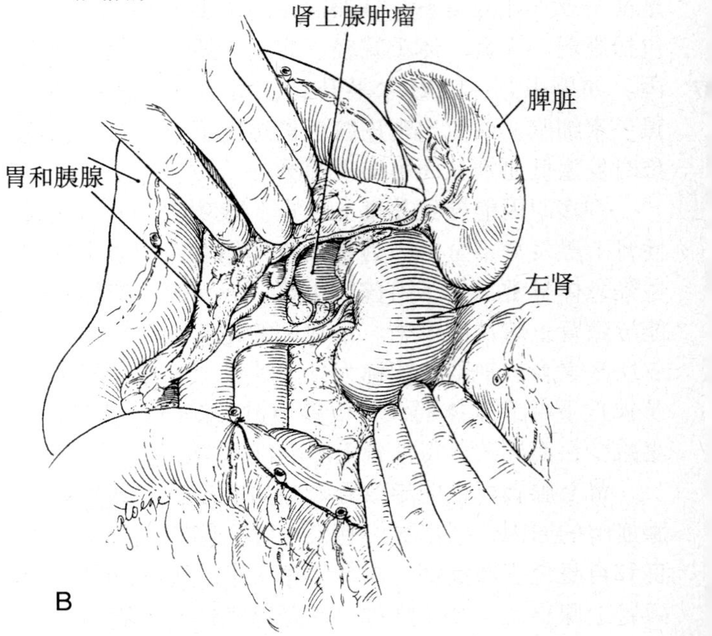

图 38-5 经腹入路切除肾上腺肿瘤。A.右侧肾上腺的暴露可以通过向下牵拉横结肠、Kocher 手法将十二指肠推向中间、和切开后方筋膜暴露横膈膜、肾上腺、和右肾上极。B.左侧肾上腺的暴露可以通过分离胃结肠韧带和将胃向上反折。结肠向下牵拉和胰腺向上反折，从而暴露肾上腺和左侧进入肾静脉的肾上腺静脉。

侧肾上腺。它也能通过单个切口进行双侧肾上腺切除。在前位入路切除右侧肾上腺时，十二指肠可以通过 Kocher 手法来游离（图 38–5）。打开肾周筋膜(Gerota 筋膜)，肝右叶向头侧翻转。手术中最重要的步骤是分离肾上腺肿块的中线缘和下腔静脉侧壁。该平面向头部方向推进，直到相对较短的肾上腺静脉进入腔静脉部分得到分离。可能出现多个静脉，这时必须及时发现以防止意外撕裂。在前位入路切除左肾上腺时，最初的手法是游离结肠的脾曲。胰腺和脾脏向上反折，打开肾周筋膜。左肾上腺静脉进入肾静脉上极，可以在此平面进行结扎。数条动脉从主动脉侧壁进入肾上腺中间表面；这些动脉在肾上腺切除前需要被分离。最常用的肾上腺切除后位入路是通过第 11 肋骨间隙。该方法避免腹膜内探查、消除了术后粘连、和减少术后肠梗阻。后位如不能用于双侧肾上腺
病变、恶性肿瘤或血供丰富的肿瘤。胸腹联合入路常 6
用于非常大的单侧肾上腺肿瘤切除。虽然该方法能很好暴露血供丰富的肿瘤，但术后疼痛和通气受到影响等因素限制了它的应用。

首例腹腔镜切除肾上腺的报道见于 1991 年，用于一个成人患者[12]。自此，已发表了大量关于在儿童中腹腔镜切除肾上腺的研究[17,29]，证明了该方法的可行性和安全性。腹腔镜切除肾上腺最常见的是侧位进行。一个肾支架用来提升肾上腺病变的相对面。4 或

5 个 trocar 被放置于肋下待切除的肾上腺侧。在右侧，通过分离肝脏三角韧带来扩大暴露。分离左侧的脾结肠韧带扩大左侧肾上腺的暴露。可能时，在切开出的肾上腺静脉用夹子进行夹闭。因为可能为恶性肿瘤，肾上腺标本必须移入标本袋内再拿出。大多数儿童肾上腺病变较小且为良性，因此腹腔镜切除对大多数患者来说是一个合适的选择。虽然没有腹腔镜切除的绝对禁忌证存在，但那些有巨大肿瘤、有可能淋巴结受累的恶性肿瘤和血供丰富的嗜铬细胞瘤的患者必须做开放性手术。

（叶启东译 王耀平校）

参考文献

1. Agarwala S, Mitra DK, Bhatnagar V, et al: Aldosteronoma in childhood: A review of clinical features and management. J Pediatr Surg 1994;29:1388-1391.
2. Arnaldi G, Masini AM, Giachetti G, et al: Adrenal incidentaloma. Braz J Med Biol Res 2000;33:1177-1189.
3. Bickler SW, McMahon TJ, Campbell JR, et al: Preoperative diagnostic evaluation of children with Cushing's syndrome. J Pediatr Surg 1994;29:671-676.
4. Caty MG, Coran AG, Geagan M, Thompson NW: Current diagnosis and treatment of pheochromocytoma in children: Experience with 22 consecutive tumors in 14 patients. Arch Surg 1990;125:978-981.
5. Chudler RM, Kay R: Adrenocortical carcinoma in children. Urol Clin North Am 1989;16:469-479.
6. Ciftci AO, Senocak ME, Tanyel FC, et al: Adrenocortical tumors in children. J Pediatr Surg 2001;36:549-554.
7. Ein SH, Pullerits J, Creighton R, Balfe JW: Pediatric pheochromocytoma: A 36-year review. Pediatr Surg Int 1997; 2:595-598.
8. Ein SH, Weitzman S, Thorner P, et al: Pediatric malignant pheochromocytoma. J Pediatr Surg 1994;29:1197-1201.
9. Ellis D, Gartner JC: The intraoperative medical management of childhood pheochromocytoma. J Pediatr Surg 1980;15:655-659.
10. Farndon JR, Davidson HA, Johnston ID, Well SA Jr: VMA excretion in patients with pheochromocytoma. Ann Surg 1980;191:259-263.
11. Fonkalsrud EW: Pheochromocytoma in childhood. Prog Pediatr Surg 1991;26:103-111.
12. Gagner M, LaCroix A, Bolte E: Laparoscopic adrenalectomy in Cushing's syndrome and pheochromocytoma. N Engl J Med 1992;327:1033.
13. Grumbach MM, Biller BM, Braunstein GD, et al: Management of the clinically inapparent adrenal mass ("incidentaloma"). Ann Intern Med 2003;138:424-429.
14. Hume DM: Pheochromocytoma in the adult and in the child. Am J Surg 1960;99:458-496.
15. Ilias I, Pacak K: Current approaches and recommended algorithm for the diagnostic localization of pheochromocytoma. J Clin Endocrinol Metab 2004;89:479-491.
16. Jones KL: The Cushing syndromes. Pediatr Clin North Am 1990;37:1313-1332.
17. Kadamba P, Habib Z, Rossi L: Experience with laparoscopic adrenalectomy in children. J Pediatr Surg 2004;39:764-767.
18. Kaufman BH, Telander RL, vanHeerden JA, et al: Pheochromocytoma in the pediatric age group: Current status. J Pediatr Surg 1983;18:879-884.
19. Khuri FJ, Alton DJ, Hardy BE, et al: Adrenal hemorrhage in neonates: Report of 5 cases and review of the literature. J Urol 1980;124:684-687.
20. Krestin GP, Steinbrich W, Friedmann G, et al: Adrenal masses: Evaluation with fast gradient-echo MR imaging and Gd-DTPA-enhanced dynamic studies. Radiology 1989; 171:675-680.
21. Lack EE, Mulvihill JJ, Travis WD, Kozakewich HP: Adrenal cortical neoplasms in the pediatric and adolescent age group: Clinicopathologic study of 30 cases with emphasis on epidemiological and prognostic factors. Pathol Annu 1992; 27(Pt 1):1-53.
22. Lee PD, Winter RJ, Green OC: Virilizing adrenocortical tumors in childhood: Eight cases and a review of the literature. Pediatrics 1985;76:437-444.
23. Londe S: Causes of hypertension in the young. Pediatr Clin North Am 1978;25:55-65.
24. Magiakou MA, Mastorakos G, Oldfield EH, et al: Cushing's syndrome in children and adolescents: Presentation, diagnosis, and therapy. N Engl J Med 1994;331:629-636.
25. Masiakos PT, Gerstle JT, Cheang T, et al: Is surgery necessary for incidentally discovered adrenal masses in children? J Pediatr Surg 2004;39:754-758.
26. Mayer SK, Oligny LL, Deal C, et al: Childhood adrenocortical tumors: Case series and reevaluation of prognosis—a 24-year experience. J Pediatr Surg 1997;32:911-915.
27. Meyer JS: Retroperitoneal MR imaging in children. Magn Reson Imaging Clin North Am 1996;4:657-678.
28. Michalkiewicz E, Sandrini R, Figueiredo B, et al: Clinical and outcome characteristics of children with adrenocortical tumors: A report from the International Pediatric Adrenocortical Tumor Registry. J Clin Oncol 2004;22: 838-845.
29. Miller KA, Albanese C, Harrison M, et al: Experience with laparoscopic adrenalectomy in pediatric patients. J Pediatr Surg 2002;37:979-982.
30. Nadler EP, Barksdale EM: Adrenal masses in the newborn. Semin Pediatr Surg 2000;9:156-164.
31. Ng L, Libertino JM: Adrenocortical carcinoma: Diagnosis, evaluation and treatment. J Urol 2003;169:5-11.
32. Pacak K, Eisenhofer G, Carrasquillo JA, et al: Diagnostic localization of pheochromocytoma: The coming of age of positron emission tomography. Ann N Y Acad Sci 2002; 970:170-176.
33. Petrus LV, Hall TR, Boechat MI, et al: The pediatric patient with suspected adrenal neoplasm: Which radiological test to use? Med Pediatr Oncol 1992;20:53-57.
34. Reddy VS, O'Neill JA Jr, Holcomb GW III, et al: Twenty-five-year surgical experience with pheochromocytoma in children. Am Surg 2000;66:1085-1091.
35. Ribeiro RC, Michalkiewicz EL, Figueiredo BC, et al: Adrenocortical tumors in children. Braz J Med Biol Res 2000;33:1225-1234.
36. Ross JH: Pheochromocytoma: Special considerations in children. Urol Clin North Am 2000;27:393-402.
37. Shulkin BL, Thompson NW, Shapiro B, et al: Pheochromocytomas: Imaging with 2-[fluorine-18]fluoro-2-deoxy-D-glucose PET. Radiology 1999;212:35-41.
38. Siegel MJ: MR imaging of the pediatric abdomen. Magn

Reson Imaging Clin North Am 1995;3:161-182.
39. Skandalakis J, et al: The suprarenal glands. In Skandalakis J, Gray S: Embryology for Surgeons, 2nd ed. Baltimore, Williams & Wilkins, 1994.
40. Stewart JN, Flageole H, Kavan P: A surgical approach to adrenocortical tumors in children: The mainstay of treatment. J Pediatr Surg 2004;39:759-763.
41. Teele R: Abdominal masses. In Share J, Teele R: Ultrasonography of Infants and Children. Philadelphia, WB Saunders, 1991.
42. Tekautz TM, Pratt CB, Jenkins JJ, Spunt SL: Pediatric extraadrenal paraganglioma. J Pediatr Surg 2003;38: 1317-1321.
43. Telander RL, Zimmerman D, Kaufman BH, vanHeerden JA: Pediatric endocrine surgery. Surg Clin North Am 1985;65:1551-1587.
44. Welbourn RB: Early surgical history of phaeochromocytoma. Br J Surg 1987;4:594-596.
45. Wieneke JA, Thompson LD, Heffess CS: Adrenal cortical neoplasms in the pediatric population: A clinicopathologic and immunophenotypic analysis of 83 patients. Am J Surg Pathol 2003;27:867-881.

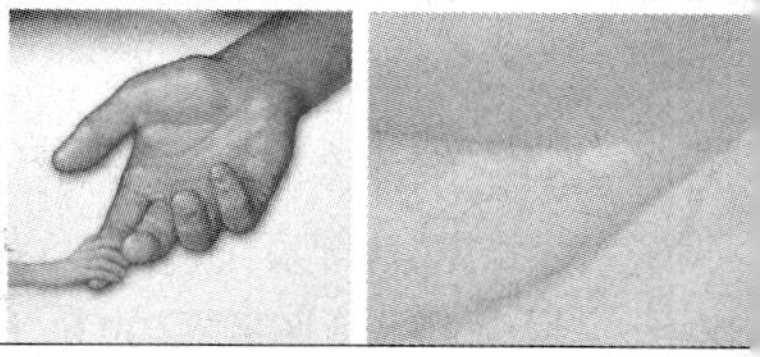

第 39 章

肺部肿瘤

Stephen J. Shochat

大部分儿童肺部肿瘤是转移性疾病；然而，原发性肺部肿瘤确实可能发生于儿童。原发性肺部肿瘤、转移性肺部肿瘤与肺部非肿瘤性病变的大概比例为 1 ：5 ：60[13,15]。虽然原发性肺部肿瘤在儿童罕见，但这些肿瘤绝大多数是恶性的。在 Hancock 等人[29]对 383 例儿童原发性肺肿瘤的回顾中发现，76%是恶性的，24%是良性的。这与先前 Hartman 和 Shochat 报道的发生率相似。表 39-1 说明儿童原发性肺肿瘤的不同类型。本章节阐述了儿童较为常见的肺部原发良、恶性肿瘤，并讨论了儿童肺转移性肿瘤的治疗。

良性肿瘤

浆细胞性肉芽肿（炎性假瘤）

浆细胞性肉芽肿也被称为炎性肌纤维母细胞瘤、纤维黄色瘤、组织细胞瘤、和纤维组织细胞瘤。该病在成人常见，在年龄小于 10 岁的儿童中（约占 8%）罕见。浆细胞性肉芽肿是儿童中最常见的良性肿瘤，占所有良性病变中 50%以上，在原发性肺部肿瘤中约占 20%[31]。这些肿瘤通常表现为外周肺的块影，但偶尔表现为息肉样气管内肿瘤[3,5]。浆细胞性肉芽肿的病因学尚不明，但在约 30%病例中曾有先前的肺部感染。儿童起病的平均年龄是 7 岁，35%的患儿在 1～15 岁之间发病[2,5,81]。许多儿童就诊时是无症状的，但可以出现发热、咳嗽、疼痛、咯血、肺炎、和吞咽困难。自然病程是缓慢生长的肿块，开始时是一个机化的肺炎病灶，伴有局部侵袭倾向。常见肿瘤的生长超出肺部。至少已经有四个死亡病例报道是由于气道梗阻或肿块侵犯纵隔所致。

治疗包括保守性肺切除并尽可能切除所有可见病灶。不管组织切片是否像恶性肿瘤，都可以表现为原发性肺门淋巴结肿大和局部侵袭。常见的难题是如何识别这些肿块的良性特征。然而，通常冰冻切片就能

表 39-1　儿童肺部原发性肿瘤

肿瘤类型	患儿数量（%）*
良性（n=92）	
浆细胞性肉芽肿	48（52.2）
错构瘤	22（23.9）
神经源性肿瘤	9（9.8）
平滑肌瘤	6（6.5）
黏液腺腺瘤	3（3.3）
成肌细胞瘤	3（3.3）
良性畸胎瘤	1（1.1）
恶性（n=291）	
支气管“腺瘤”	118（40.5）
支气管腺泡癌	49（16.8）
肺母细胞瘤	45（15.5）
纤维肉瘤	28（9.6）
横纹肌肉瘤	17（5.8）
平滑肌肉瘤	11（3.8）
肉瘤	6（2.1）
血管外皮瘤	4（1.4）
浆细胞瘤	4（1.4）
淋巴瘤	3（1.0）
畸胎瘤	3（1.0）
间充质瘤	2（1.7）
黏液肉瘤	1（0.3）

* 良恶性肿瘤的百分比。

Modified from Hancock BJ, DiLorenzo M, Youssef S, et al: Childhood primary pulmonary neoplasms. J Pediatr Surg 1993; 28: 1133.

明确诊断。肺恶性纤维组织细胞瘤在儿童中极为少见，与浆细胞性肉芽肿类似，必须在鉴别诊断时考虑到[53]。切除后的复发少见，但也有报道。非类固醇消炎药已经用于治疗大的无法手术的病变，并取得令人鼓舞的结果[72]。

错构瘤

肺部错构瘤是儿童肺部第二常见的良性肿瘤。该病通常表现为实质性病变，病变可以很大。约 1/4 有钙化，“爆米花样”钙化是其特征性改变[21]。已经有 2 例发病于气管内的报道。4 例发生于新生儿期的肿瘤非常大，并伴有明显的呼吸窘迫；均是致命的。有意思的三联症表现为肺部错构瘤、肾上腺外副神经节节细胞瘤和胃平滑肌肿瘤；这些患者大多数是年轻女性。治疗的选择是保守性的肺切除；然而，也可能需要肺叶切除术或全肺切除术，特别是病灶较大和气管内病变而无法做袖式切除术时。

恶性肿瘤

支气管腺瘤

最常见的肺部原发性恶性肿瘤是支气管腺瘤。该病是原发性支气管内的异源性肿瘤。虽然腺瘤意味着一个良性病变，但各种支气管腺瘤常有恶性肿瘤的表现。有三种组织学类型：类癌肿瘤（最常见）、黏液上皮样癌和腺样囊性癌。在儿童中，类癌占所有支气管腺瘤的 80%～85%。表现的症状通常是由于不完全性支气管堵塞所致，可以有咳嗽、反复发作肺炎和咯血。由于诊断困难，症状常持续数月；偶尔，喘息的患儿会被诊断为哮喘，而延误诊断达 4～5 年。6%的患者有转移性病变，2%的患者出现复发。只有 1 例个案报道了一个类癌伴转移的患儿出现典型的类癌综合征[43]。在儿童中，即使出现局部侵袭，所有组织类型的支气管腺瘤的预后都很好[68]。

支气管腺瘤的治疗尚存在争议，大多数是内镜中可见的病灶。该病做活检是危险的，因为有出血的风险，也不推荐做内镜下切除。支气管造影术或 CT 检查对于确定堵塞的远端支气管扩张的程度有帮助，因为肺梗阻的程度将影响手术治疗[3]。然而，Tagge 等人[76]报道了一项用于尽管存在明显的远端肺膨胀不全也能施行的肺保留手术。保守性肺切除术加受累淋巴结清除是一种治疗的选择。袖套型节段性支气管切除在儿童中是可能的，当可行也是治疗的一种选择[24,38]。圆柱瘤有在黏膜下播散的趋势，已经有晚期局部复发或播散的报道。除了肺门淋巴结完全切除术外，在儿童中尚需做支气管边缘的冰冻切片检查。

支气管癌

虽然支气管癌在儿童很少见，但 Hancock 等人[29]报道该肿瘤是第二常见的恶性肿瘤。有意思的是，鳞状细胞癌很少见，大多数肿瘤是未分化癌或腺癌。大多数均用“支气管肺泡细胞癌”这个名称[45]。这些肿瘤与囊状腺瘤样畸形和肺内支气管囊肿均有关系（表 39–2）[7,19,22,27,37,40,45,51,58,59,73]。报道只有很少数患者存活，死亡率超过 90%。大多数患儿为播散性表现，平均生存期只有 7 个月。局限性的肿瘤可以通过完全切除来治疗，随后进行辅助治疗。也有报道提到支气管黏液上皮样癌见于年仅 4 岁的患儿中（图 39–1）[66]。

肺母细胞瘤

肺母细胞瘤是一种少见恶性肿瘤，主要见于成人，起源于间叶细胞胚基。该肿瘤是一种侵袭性疾病，约 20%病例在起病时有转移[17,29]。该病可以出现于肺、胸膜和纵隔[56]。偶尔，该肿瘤可以出现于叶外肺隔离症或以前的肺囊肿中（表 39–3）[1,11,23,36,47,57,64,65,71,74,80,84]。大多数病例出现于右半胸（图 39–2）。常见的转移部位是肝脏、脑和脊髓。局部复发常见，死亡率约为 40%[6,29]。大多数患儿在 4 岁前发病，症状包括持续的咳嗽、胸痛、抗生素治疗无效的反复发作的肺炎和咯血。可以通过胸部 CT、支气管镜和检发现并诊断。因为该肿瘤大多数位于肺外周部分，通常可通过节段性或肺叶切除肿瘤。对于病变广泛和播散的患者，手术切除后的综合新辅助化疗和放疗已经表现出前景很好的结果[56,67]。已经在使用的化疗药物包括放线菌素

表 39-2　与先天性囊性肺部畸形相关的支气管腺泡癌

作者	发表时间	肺部囊肿类型	诊断时年龄（岁）	备注
Prichard[58]	1984	1 型 CCAM	30	死于疾病的转移
Hurley[37]	1985	1 型 CCAM		
Benjamin[7]	1991	1 型 CCAM	19	19 岁时在同一节段性切除的肺叶中诊断出 BAC，死于 23 岁
Morresi[51]	1995	1 型 CCAM	20	
Ribet[59]	1995	1 型 CCAM	42	
Kaslovsky[40]	1997	1 型 CCAM	11	在新生儿期不完全切除 CCAM
Granata[27]	1998	1 型 CCAM	11	对于反复感染行肺叶切除；发现 BAC
Endo[22]	1982	支气管源性的（肺内）	37	10 年前发现 CXR 异常；有呼吸困难表现，偶然发现 BAC，3mm×1mm
De Perrot[19]	2001	支气管源性的（肺内）	79	长期肺部囊肿感染病史
MacSweeney[45]	2003	1 型 CCAM 0.5、13、18、30、36		一例复发肺囊肿中发现 BAC；另有一例患者有典型的腺瘤增生（2 例患者均做肺叶节段切除）
Sudou[73]	2003	1 型 CCAM	17	10 年前发现 CXR 异常

BAC：支气管腺泡状癌；CCAM：先天性囊性肺部畸形；CXR：胸片。

Adapted from LaBerge JM, Puligandla P, Flageole H: Asymptomatic congenital lung malformations. Semin Pediatr Surg 2005;14:16.

D、长春新碱、环磷酰胺与阿霉素和顺铂方案的交替应用。组织学检查主要表现为间叶组分，包括原始小管、未成熟胚基、和梭形细胞基质。某些病例在多囊性病变中出现胚胎性横纹肌肉瘤成分。

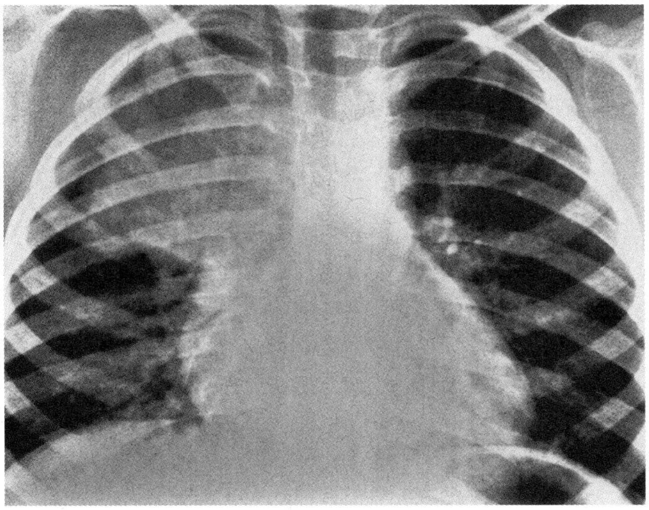

图 39-1　在一位 4 岁女孩的胸部正位片中发现右上肺叶病变。肿瘤通过右上肺叶切除术而被切除，显示为黏液表皮样癌。（Courtesy of Jay L. Grosfeld, MD.）

横纹肌肉瘤

肺部横纹肌肉瘤很少见，只占所有儿童横纹肌肉瘤的 0.5%（见第 32 章）[9]。许多病变是支气管内源性的（图 39-3）；然而，数个病例明显起源于先天性囊泡异常（见表 39-3）[4,8,10,16,33,41,49,52,54,67,79,86]。这是一个重要的问题，因为列举于表 39-1的 4%良性肿瘤和 8.6%恶性肿瘤与先前有据可查的囊泡畸形有关[29]。在这些畸形中发育的肿瘤包括：11 例肉瘤、9 例肺母细胞瘤、3 例支气管癌和 2 例间充质瘤。

评论

虽然儿童原发性肺部肿瘤为一组异质性疾病，但对报道病例的分析表明，大多数患者的评估和治疗是相似的。许多患儿是无症状的，特别是那些良性肿瘤；然而，咳嗽、反复发作性肺炎和不典型支气管哮喘可以是最初的表现。胸部平片常表现出孤立的肿块或气道梗阻所致的肺膨胀不全和肺炎。因为这些肿瘤 644
许多可以通过支气管镜看见，所以应该进行支气管镜

表 39-3 间充质细胞性恶性肿瘤和囊性肺部畸形

作者	时间	肺部囊肿类型	恶性肿瘤类型	诊断时年龄（月）
Stephanopoulos[70]	1963	“囊性错构瘤”	黏液肉瘤	
Ueda[79]	1977	CCAM	RMS	18
Martinez[47]	1978	“多囊肺”	肺母细胞瘤	24
Valderrama[80]	1978	肺叶外肺隔离	肺母细胞瘤	
Sumner[74]	1979	末梢囊肿	肺母细胞瘤	48
Weinbera[83]	1980	先天性肺囊肿	混合性间质细胞肉瘤	108
Krous[41]	1980	支气管原性囊肿（肺内）	胚胎型 RMS	30
Weiblatt[84]	1982	“肺囊肿”	肺母细胞瘤	30
Holland-Moritz[36]	1984	“肺膨出”	PPB	48
Morales[50]	1986	先天性囊肿	肺母细胞瘤	
Williams[86]	1986	CCAM	胚胎型 RMS	21
Allan[4]	1987	“先天性不明原性囊肿”	RMS	21，30
Shariff[67]	1988	1 型 CCAM	RMS	15
Hedlund[33]	1989	“囊性错构瘤”	RMS	18，22
Cairoli[10]	1990	CCAM	RMS	36
Domizio[20]	1990	“先天性囊肿”	恶性间质细胞瘤	48
Senac[65]	1991		PPB	
Murphy[52]	1992	支气管原性囊肿，CCAM（2）	胚胎型 RMS	24，36，42
Bogers[8]	1993	肺叶气肿	RMS	18
Calabria[11]	1993	“肺膨出”	肺母细胞瘤	
McDermott[49]	1993	先天性囊肿	胚胎型 RMS	36
Paupe[57]	1994	囊性肺部病变	肺母细胞瘤	
Seballos[64]	1994	CCAM	肺母细胞瘤	22
Tagge[75]	1996	双侧肺膨出	PPB	45
Adirim[1]	1997	1 型 CCAM	肺母细胞瘤	
D'Agostino[16]	1997	2 型 CCAM	胚胎型 RMS	22
Federici[23]	2001	1 型 CCAM	PPB	36
Ozcan[54]	2001	CCAM	胚胎型 RMS	13
Papagiannopoulos[55]	2001	4 型 CCAM	PPB	30
Stocker[71]	2002	4 型 CCAM	PPB	48

CCAM：先天性囊性腺瘤样畸形；CPAM：先天性肺气道畸形；PPB：胸膜肺母细胞瘤；RMS：横纹肌肉瘤。

Adapted from LaBerge JM, Puligandla P, Flageole H: Asymptomatic congenital lung malformations. Semin Pediatr Surg 2005;14:16.

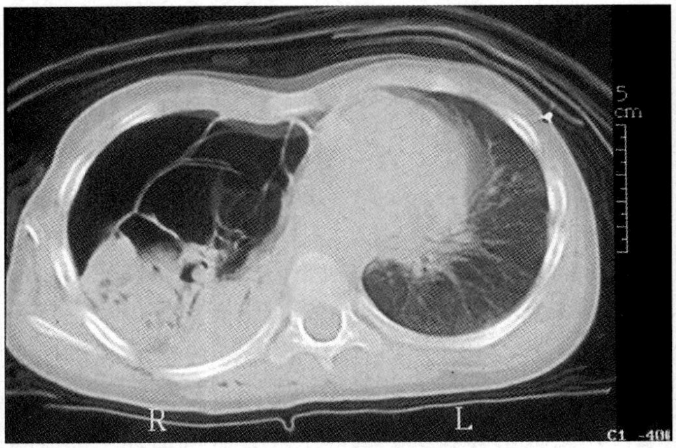

A

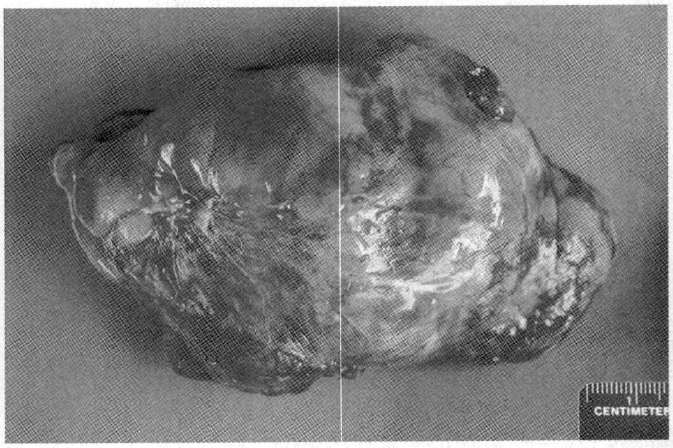

B

图 39-2 A. 胸部 CT 扫描发现右半侧胸廓囊性病变。B. 肿瘤被切除（肺叶切除术），组织学切片显示为胸膜肺母细胞瘤。（Courtesy of Jay L. Grosfeld, MD.）

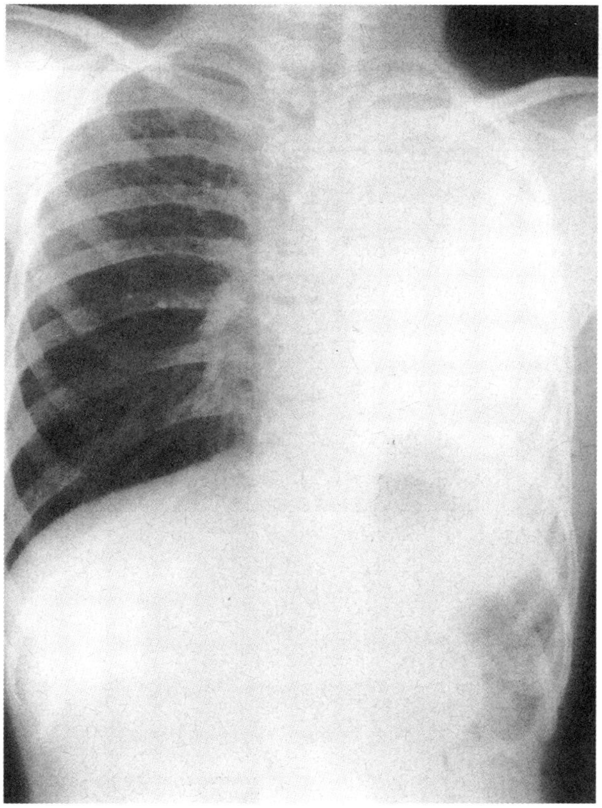

A

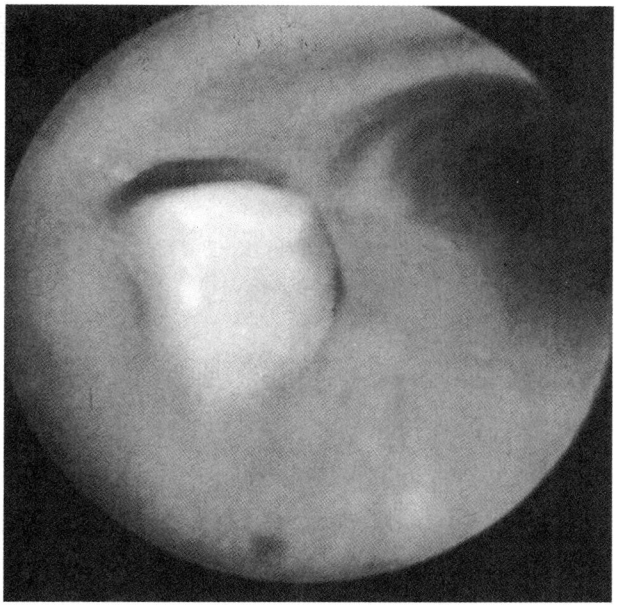

B

图 39–3 继发于横纹肌肉瘤的左肺完全性肺膨胀不全和左主支气管梗阻的患者。

检查。纤维支气管镜技术可能对诊断有帮助，但如果准备做内镜活检，则有必要在全麻下用具有现代放大作用的硬支气管镜检查。在支气管镜检查时必须做急诊开胸的准备以抢救危及生命的出血。

可以尝试对一些孤立的病灶行支气管镜切除，但由于复发的发生率高和可能有严重的出血，该项技术必须有选择性的应用。保守的手术切除是良性肺部肿瘤的治疗选方法，以获得组织学诊断和尽可能保留有功能的肺组织。对这些儿童，胸腔镜切除也是一个选择[35]。对于有大的占位病灶的儿童应该做 CT 和 MRI 影像检查以确定切除的可能性。行细针抽吸活检做细胞学检查或芯针穿刺活检可以作为一些有条件的病例诊断时的最初方法。恶性肿瘤的治疗因部位和组织学的不同而变化。对于支气管腺瘤应该考虑做袖式切除。恶性肿瘤必须考虑切除受累的淋巴结组织。对有大的原发恶性肿瘤或播散的患儿，联合辅助化疗和可能情况下的放疗似乎是有益的。

需要考虑的重要一点是原发性肺部肿瘤和先天性囊性肺部畸形的关系。这些病变可能是无症状的，常偶然被发现。在某些病例中，肺部囊肿的自然病程是不清楚的，少部分可能消退[42]。虽然一些作者推荐简单的随访，但大多数小儿外科医生反对囊性病变长期随访，因为可能导致感染、气胸、囊肿突然增大导致呼吸困难、和相关恶性肿瘤的风险增加[1,11,42,47,55,57,65,75]。如果无症状的肺囊性畸形患者未进行切除而随访，他们应该受到密切跟踪和频繁检查。

转移性肿瘤的治疗

在儿童，肺部转移性肿瘤远比原发性肿瘤多见，手术治疗方法有赖于原发肿瘤的病史和原发部位对多学科协做治疗的效应。除非原发肿瘤清除后没有复发并排除其他部位的转移可能，否则肺转移灶不考虑切除。最需要考虑肺部转移灶切除的是骨肉瘤、软组织
肉瘤和肾母细胞瘤的肺转移灶[39]。 645

骨肉瘤

骨肉瘤患儿一旦原发灶得到控制，应该考虑做肺

表 39-4 肺部骨源性转移瘤切除术

作者	病例数	平均复发间期（范围）（月）	手术例数（病灶数）	无病生存例数（%）	存活者中位随访时间 / 月（范围）
Martini[48]	22	10（2～25）	59（113）	7（32）	33（15～234）
Spanos[69]	29	15.7（4～30）	52（124）	11（37）	36（9～234）
Telander[77]	28	9/6（2～34）	60（173）	13（46）	25（6～48）
Giritsky[25]	12	9（1～21）	19	6（50）	17（9～39）
Rosenberg[60]	18	—	—	7（39）	—
Burgers[9]	12	13（2～20）	9	5（42）	（36～72）
Schller[63]	17	—	34	7（41）	（12～192）
Goorin[26]	32	12.5（4～59）	26（>63）	9（28）	55（19～101）
Carter[12]	43	13（1～83）	—	4（10）	69（59～80）

From LaQuaglia MP: The surgical management of metastases in pediatric cancer. Semin Pediatr Surg 1993;2:75.

部转移灶的切除。在出现异时肺部转移肿瘤的儿童，总的无病生存率是约 40%。多个因素，如肺部结节数量和复发时间等，在骨肉瘤肺部转移患儿中有重要的影响[32,78]。Roth 等人[61]表明肺部结节少于 4 个的患者比结节多于 4 个的患者生存率要好。根据 Goorin 等人[26]研究，完全切除所有肺部结节是预后的一个重要决定因素，而胸膜腔穿刺与预后差有关。虽然有些争议，但如果能完全切除所有转移病灶，即使是有肺部转移的患者情况似乎也能得到些改善[46]。Harris 等人[30]报道 17 例肺部转移灶少于 8 个的患者，在化疗、切除原发灶和肺部转移灶后，其生存率为 68%。表 39-4 的数据表明对于骨肉瘤应进行侵袭性的手术来切除肺部转移灶，而不应考虑转移灶的数量或出现转移的间隔时间。

软组织肉瘤

软组织肉瘤患者切除肺部转移灶的应用取决于其组织学亚型。横纹肌肉瘤很少需要切除转移灶，Ewing 肉瘤的肺部转移灶切除没有任何效果[34]。其余的肉瘤类型，如果可能做转移灶完全切除且原发肿瘤灶已控制，则应考虑切除。出现肺部转移的时间、转移灶的数量、和肿瘤倍增时间在软组织肉瘤中均是重要的预后影响因素。在过去，大约 10%～20%这些患者能通过切除肺部转移灶被挽救[44]。

肾母细胞瘤

肾母细胞瘤患儿很少需要切除肺转移灶。Green 等人[28]在美国全国肾母细胞瘤研究组的回顾性研究中发现，与单独化疗和放疗比较，肺部转移灶切除没有任何益处。为了避免肺部放疗，deKraker 等人[18]推荐了一个方案，对肺部转移灶在化疗后进行肺部切除。总的结果并不令人兴奋，很少有患者在化疗后最后需进行肺部转移灶的切除。因为在有肺部转移的肾母细胞瘤患儿中化疗和全肺放疗的效果很好，所以肺部转移灶的切除只应用于有条件的病例进行（见第 27 章）。

评论

儿童肺部转移灶的手术有赖于原发肿瘤的组织类型、转移的程度、和转移性肿瘤是否对化疗敏感。手术方法根据肿瘤的病程和患者的年龄而变化。侧面胸腔切开术和胸骨正中切开术在生存率比较上没有差别，但后者在年长的骨肉瘤患者中更可取。完全切除所有转移灶是一个重要的需考虑的事项，且使用自动缝合设备会有所帮助。骨肉瘤患儿做楔形切除术通常是可行的。然而，可能需要考虑做肺叶切除术或节段性肺切除以完全切除所有肿瘤，特别是当原发肿瘤对化疗或放疗不敏感的时候[6]。需要做侧后胸腔切开术的患儿可做保留胸肌的手术（Muscle-sparing technigues），而某些病例也适合做胸腔镜手术[55]。然而，已经有报道在胸腔镜切除肺部转移灶后在切口部位出现复发[62,85]。

（叶启东译 王耀平校）

参考文献

1. Adirim AD, King R, Klein BL: Radiologic case of the month: Congenital cystic adenomatoid malformation of the lung and pulmonary blastoma. Arch Pediatr Adolesc Med 1997;151:1053.
2. Agrons GA, Rosado-de-Christenson ML, Kirejczyk WM, et al: Pulmonary inflammatory pscudotumor: Radiologic features. Radiology 1998;206:51.
3. Ahel V, Zubovic I, Rozmanic V: Bronchial adenoid cystic carcinoma with saccular bronchiectasis as a cause of recurrent pneumonia in children. Pediatr Pulmonol 1992:12:160.
4. Allan BT, Day DL, Dehner LP: Primary pulmonary rhabdomyosarcoma of the lung in children: Report of two cases presenting with spontaneous pneumothorax. Cancer 1987;59:1005.
5. Bahadoni M, Liebow AA: Plasma cell granulomas of the lung. Cancer 1973;31:191.
6. Ballantine TVN, Wiseman NE, Filler RM: Assessment of pulmonary wedge resection for the treatment of lung metastases. J Pediatr Surg 1975;10:671.
7. Benjamin DR, Cahill JL: Bronchioalveolar carcinoma of the lung and congenital cystic adenomatoid malformation. Am J Clin Pathol 1991;95:889.
8. Bogers AJ, Hazebroek FW, Molenaar J, et al: Surgical treatment of congenital bronchopulmonary disease in children. Eur J Cardiothorac Surg 1993;7:117.
9. Burgers JM, Brear K, van Dobbenburgh OA, et al: Role of metastasectomy without chemotherapy in the management of osteosarcoma in children. Cancer 1980;45:1664.
10. Cairoli G, Bertana S, Giuntoli M, et al: Cystic adenomatoid malformation of the lung: Experience in four operated cases. Pediatr Med Chir 1990;12:681.
11. Calabria R, Srikanth MS, Chamberlin K, et al: Management of pulmonary blastoma in children. Am Surg 1993;59:192.
12. Carter SR, Grimer RJ, Sneath RS, et al: Results of thoracotomy in osteogenic sarcoma with pulmonary metastases. Thorax 1991;46:727.
13. Crisei KL, Greenberg SB, Wolfson BJ: Cardiopulmonary and thoracic tumors of childhood. Radiol Clin North Am 1997;35:1341.
14. Crist WM, Raney RB, Newton W, et al: Intrathoracic soft tissue sarcomas in children. Cancer 1982;50:598.
15. Cohen MC, Kaschula ROC: Primary pulmonary tumors in childhood: A review of 31 years' experience and the literature. Pediatr Pulmonol 1992;40:222.
16. D'Agostino S, Bonoldi E, Dante S, et al: Embryonal rhabdomyosarcoma of the lung arising in cystic adenomatoid malformation: Case report and review of the literature. J Pediatr Surg 1997;32:1381.
17. Dehner LP: Pleuropulmonary blastoma is the pulmonary blastoma of childhood. Semin Diagn Pathol 1994;11:144.
18. deKraker J, Lemerle J, Voute PA, et al: Wilms' tumor with pulmonary metastases at diagnosis: The significance of primary chemotherapy. J Clin Oncol 1990;8:1187.
19. De Perrot M, Pache JC, Spiliopoulous A: Carcinoma arising in congenital lung cysts. Thorac Cardiovasc Surg 2001;49:184.
20. Domizio P, Liesner RL, Dicks-Mireaux C, et al: Malignant mesenchymoma associated with a congenital lung cyst in a child: Case report and review of the literature. Pediatr Pathol 1990;10:785.
21. Eggli KD, Newman B: Nodules, masses and pseudomasses in the pediatric lung. Radiol Clin North Am 1993;31:651.
22. Endo T, Inoue M, Waatanabe N, et al: Two operative cases of pulmonary blastoma. Kyobu Geka 1982;35:219.
23. Federici S, Domenichelli V, Tani G: Pleuropulmonary blastoma in congenital cystic adenomatoid malformation: Report of a case. Eur J Pediatr Surg 2001;11:196.
24. Gaissert HA, Mathisen DJ, Grillo HC, et al: Tracheobronchial sleeve resection in children and adolescents. J Pediatr Surg 1994;29:192.
25. Giritsky AS, Etcubawas E, Mark JBD: Pulmonary resection in children with metastatic osteogenic sarcoma. J Thorac Cardiovas Surg 1978;75:354.
26. Goorin AM, DeCorey MJ, Lack EE, et al: Prognostic significance of complete surgical resection of pulmonary metastases in patients with osteogenic sarcoma: Analyses of 32 patients. J Clin Oncol 1984;2:425.
27. Granata C, Gambini C, Balducci T, et al: Bronchioalveolar carcinoma arising in a cystic adenomatoid malformation in a child: A case report and review on malignancies originating in congenital adenomatoid malformations. Pediatr Pulmonol 1998;25:62.
28. Green DM, Breslow N, Ii Y, et al: The role of surgical excision in the management of relapsed Wilms' tumor patients with pulmonary metastases: A report from the National Wilms' Tumor Study. J Pediatr Surg 1991;26:728.
29. Hancock BJ, DiLorenzo M, Youssef S, et al: Childhood primary pulmonary neoplasms. J Pediatr Surg 1993;28:1133.
30. Harris M, Gieser P, Goorin AM, et al: Treatment of metastatic osteosarcoma at diagnosis: A Pediatric Oncology Group study. J Clin Oncol 1998;11:3641.
31. Hartman GE, Shochat SJ: Primary pulmonary neoplasms of childhood: A review. Ann Thorac Surg 1983;36:108.
32. Hawkins DS, Arndt CA: Pattern of disease recurrence and prognostic factors in patients with osteosarcoma treated with contemporary chemotherapy. Cancer 2003;98:2447.
33. Hedlund GL, Bisset GS III, Bove KE: Malignant neoplasms arising in cystic hamartomas of the lung in childhood. Radiology 1989;173:77.
34. Heij HA, Vos A, deKraker J, et al: Prognostic factors in surgery for pulmonary metastases in children. Surgery 1994;115:687.
35. Holcomb GW III, Tomita SS, Haase GM, et al: Minimally invasive surgery in children with cancer. Cancer 1995;76:121.
36. Holland-Moritz RM, Heyn RM: Pulmonary blastoma associ-

ated with cystic lesions in children. Med Pediatr Oncol 1984;12:85.
37. Hurley P, Corbishsley C, Pepper J: Bronchoalveolar carcinoma arising in longstanding lung cysts. Thorax 1985; 40:960.
38. Jalal A, Jeyasingham K: Bronchoplasty for malignant and benign conditions: A retrospective study of 44 cases. Eur J Cardiothorac Surg 2000;17:370.
39. Karnak I, Senocak ME, Kutluk T, et al: Pulmonary metastases in children: An analysis of surgical spectrum. Eur J Pediatr Surg 2002;12:15.
40. Kaslovsky RA, Purdy S, Dangman BC, et al: Bronchioalveolar carcinoma in a child with congenital cystic adenomatoid malformation. Chest 1997;112:548.
41. Krous HF, Harper PE, Perlman M: Congenital cystic adenomatoid malformation in bilateral renal agenesis: Its mitigation of Potter's syndrome. Arch Pathol Lab Med 1980;104:368.
42. LaBerge JM, Puligandla P, Flageole H: Asymptomatic congenital lung malformations. Semin Pediatr Surg 2005; 14:16.
43. Lack EE, Harris GBC, Eraklis AJ, et al: Primary bronchial tumors in childhood: A clinicopathologic study of six cases. Cancer 1983;51:492.
44. LaQuaglia MP: The surgical management of metastases in pediatric cancer. Semin Pediatr Surg 1993;2:75.
45. MacSweeney F, Papagiannopoulos K, Goldstraw P, et al: Assessment of the expanded classification of congenital cystic adenomatoid malformations and their relationship to malignant transformation. Am J Surg Pathol 2003; 27:1139.
46. Marina NM, Pratt CB, Rao BN, et al: Improved prognosis of children with osteosarcoma metastatic to the lung(s) at the time of diagnosis. Cancer 1992;70:2722.
47. Martinez JC, Pecero FC, Gutierrez de la Pena C, et al: Pulmonary blastoma: Report of a case. J Pediatr Surg 1978;13:93.
48. Martini N, Havos AG, Mike V, et al: Multiple pulmonary resections in the treatment of osteogenic sarcoma. Ann Thorac Surg 1971;12:271.
49. McDermott VG, MacKenzie S, Hendry GM: Case report: Primary intrathoracic rhabdomyosarcoma: A rare childhood malignancy. Br J Radiol 1993;66:937.
50. Morales L, Julia V, Tardio E, et al: Pulmonary blastoma at the site of a congenital pulmonary cyst. Chir Pediatr 1986; 27:53.
51. Morresi A, Wockel W, Karg O: Adenomatoid cystic lung abnormality in adults with associated bronchioalveolar carcinoma. Pathologe 1995;16:292.
52. Murphy JJ, Blair GK, Fraser GC, et al: Rhabdomyosarcoma arising within congenital pulmonary cysts: Report of three cases. J Pediatr Surg 1992;27:1364.
53. Nistal M, Jimenez-Hefferman JA, Hardisson D, et al: Malignant fibrous histiocytoma of the lung in a child. Eur J Pediatr 1997;156:107.
54. Ozcan C, Celik A, Ural Z, et al: Primary pulmonary rhabdomyosarcoma arising within cystic adenomatoid malformation: A case report and review of the literature. J Pediatr Surg 2001;36:1062.
55. Papagiannopolous KA, Sheppard M, Bush AP, et al: Pleuropulmonary blastoma: Is prophylactic resection of congenital lung cysts effective? Ann Thorac Surg 2001; 72:604.
56. Parsons SK, Fishman SJ, Hoorntje LE, et al: Aggressive multimodal treatment of pleuropulmonary blastoma. Ann Thorac Surg 2001:72:939.
57. Paupe A, Martelli H, Lenclen R, et al: Pneumothorax revealing pneumoblastoma in an infant. Arch Pediatr 1994;1:919.
58. Prichard MG, Brown PJ, Sterrett GF: Bronchioalveolar carcinoma arising in longstanding lung cysts. Thorax 1984;39:545.
59. Ribet ME, Copin MC, Soots JG, et al: Bronchalveolar carcinoma and cystic adenomatoid malformation. Ann Thorac Surg 1995;60:1126.
60. Rosenberg SA, Flye MW, Conkle D, et al: Treatment of osteogenic sarcoma. II. Aggressive resection of pulmonary metastases. Cancer Treat Rep 1979;63:753.
61. Roth JA, Putnam JB, Wesley MN, et al: Differing determinants of prognosis following resection of pulmonary metastases from osteogenic and soft tissue sarcoma patients. Cancer 1985;55:1361.
62. Sartorelli KH, Patrick D, Meagher DP Jr: Port-site recurrence after thoracoscopic resection of pulmonary metastasis owing to osteogenic sarcoma. J Pediatr Surg 1996;31:1443.
63. Schaller RT Jr, Haas J, Schaller J, et al: Improved survival in children with osteosarcoma following resection of pulmonary metastases. J Pediatr Surg 1982;17:546.
64. Seballos RM, Klein RL: Pulmonary blastoma in children: Report of two cases and review of the literature. J Pediatr Surg 1994;29:1553.
65. Senac MO Jr, Wood BP, Isaacs H, et al: Pulmonary blastoma, a rare childhood malignancy. Radiology 1991;179:743.
66. Seo IS, Warren M, Mirkin LD, et al: Mucoepidermoid carcinoma of the bronchus in a four year old child. Cancer 1984;53:1600.
67. Shariff S, Thomas JA, Shetty N, et al: Primary pulmonary rhabdomyosarcoma in a child with a review of the literature. J Surg Oncol 1988;38:261.
68. Soga J, Yakuwa Y: Bronchopulmonary carcinoids: An analysis of 1875 reported cases with special reference to a comparison between typical carcinoids and atypical varieties. Ann Thorac Cardiovasc Surg 1999;5:211.
69. Spanos PK, Payne WS, Ivins JC, Pritchard DJ: Pulmonary resection for metastatic osteogenic sarcoma. J Bone Joint Surg Am 1976;58:624.
70. Stephanopoulos C, Catsaras H: Myxosarcoma complicating a cystic hamartoma of the lung. Thorax 1963;18:144.
71. Stocker JT: Congenital pulmonary airway malformations—a new name for and an expanded classification of congenital cystic adenomatoid malformation of the lung. Histopathology 2002;41(Suppl):S424.
72. Su W, Ko A, O'Connell TX, et al: Treatment of pseudotumors with nonsteroidal anti-inflammatory drugs. J Pediatr Surg 2000;35:1635.
73. Sudou M, Sugi K, Murakami T: Bronchioalveolar carcinoma arising from a congenital cystic adenomatoid malformation in an adolescent: The first case in the Orient. J Thorac Cardiovasc Surg 2003;126:902.
74. Sumner TE, Phelps CR, Crowe JE, et al: Pulmonary blastoma in a child. AJR Am J Roentgenol 1979; 133:147.
75. Tagge EP, Mulvihill D, Chandler JC, et al: Childhood pleuropulmonary blastoma: Caution against nonoperative management of congenital lung cysts. J Pediatr Surg 1996; 31:187.
76. Tagge EP, Yanis E, Chopy KJ, et al: Obstructing endobronchial fibrous histiocytoma: Potential for lung salvage. J Pediatr Surg 1991;26:1067.
77. Telander RL, Pairolero PC, Pritchard DJ, et al: Resection of pulmonary metastatic osteogenic sarcoma in children.

Surgery 1978;84:335H.
78. Thompson RC Jr, Cheng EY, Clohisy DR, et al: Results of treatment for metastatic osteosarcoma with neoadjuvant chemotherapy and surgery. Clin Orthop 2002;397:240.
79. Ueda K, Gruppo R, Unger F, et al: Rhabdomyosarcoma of lung arising in congenital cystic adenomatoid malformation. Cancer 1977;40:383.
80. Valderrama E, Salija G, Shende A, et al: Pulmonary blastoma: Report of two cases in children. Am J Surg Pathol 1978;2:415.
81. Verbeke JIML, Verberne AAPH, Den Hollander JC, Robben SGF: Inflammatory myofibroblastic tumor of the lung manifesting as progressive atelectasis. Pediatr Radiol 1999;29:816.
82. Vujanic GM, Dojcinov D: Inflammatory pseudotumor of the lung in children. Pediatr Hematol Oncol 1991;8:121.
83. Weinberg AG, Currarino G, Moore GC, Votteler TP: Mesenchymal neoplasia and congenital pulmonary cysts. Pediatr Radiol 1980;9:179.
84. Weinblatt ME, Siegel SE, Isaacs H: Pulmonary blastoma associated with cystic lung disease. Cancer 1982;49:669.
85. Wille GA, Gregory R, Guernsey JM: Tumor implantation at port site of video-assisted thoracoscopic resection of pulmonary metastasis. West J Med 1997;166:65.
86. Williams RA: Embryonal rhabdomysosarcoma occurring in cystic adenomatoid malformation. Pediatr Pathol 1986;5:118.
87. Zaidi A, Zamvar V, Macbeth F, et al: Pulmonary blastoma: Medium-term results from a regional center. Ann Thorac Surg 2002;73:1572.

第 40 章

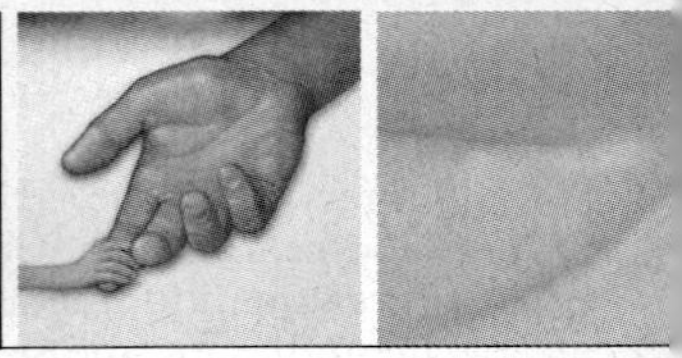

骨肿瘤

Saminathan S. Nathan 和 John H. Healey

649 骨肿瘤是罕见的。在美国，2000 年有 166 487 例乳腺癌病例，164 753 例前列腺癌病例[28]。与之相比，各种类型的骨肉瘤仅有 2051 例，大部分发生于儿童。一项调查数据显示，骨恶性肿瘤 26.8% 发生于儿童时期。由于没有良性骨肿瘤的统计资料，所以骨良性肿瘤的发生率不得而知。恶性肿瘤的有关数据多来源于临床三期药物试验，而良性肿瘤多为无症状的，因此无法做出具体统计。然而有研究显示，在儿童骨发育过程中，约有 43%的儿童会出现骨病变[18]。这意味着多数骨病变是良性的。

由于多种原因，小儿外科医生经常会参与骨肿瘤患儿的处理中。在无关疾病的随访过程中，年幼儿可能可能表现为白血病或骨髓炎继发骨缺损而被发现。有转移的骨源性恶性肿瘤的年长儿童可能需要儿童胸外科医生进行肺部肿块的切除。在有单纯性骨囊肿或非骨化性纤维瘤青少年，病理性骨折可能外科医生接诊时的首诊表现。

这类少见疾病通过细致的临床检查通常可以获得诊断。但是平片非常重要。它们使首诊医生确定是否需要将患儿转至专科中心由专科医生进行治疗。尽管随后进行的其他影像学检查有重要价值，但是平片是决定外科治疗计划的重要组成部分。

本章内容对于小儿外科医生很重要。为避免对病理学的冗长论述，本章采用了一些现有的表格[62,67,128,135]。格式则采用解决这些问题的实用方法。而对一些有争议和特殊的地方也做了深入探讨以激发人们的兴趣。

一般情况

病理生理学

本章的主要目的是阐明骨肿瘤的病理生理学及其与软组织肿瘤鉴别的特殊方面。

首先，应判断骨肿瘤是良性的还是恶性的。传统的有关大多数骨性良性病变的治疗方法一直是一种良性忽略，如果这些病变无临床症状，那么骨良性病变的处理可能由于潜在的骨骼结构的完整性而变得复杂化。皮质缺损、骨强度降低可以采取适当的治疗以避免骨折。如果罕见，则谨慎地考虑其症状表现以防其向恶性转化。这些原则也适用于恶性病变。然而恶性病变以生存率为评价标准。骨的继发性恶性病变在儿童时期不多见，它们的病理生理学特征可能表现为结构性或诊断性的。

在儿童时期，良性病变的发生率远高于原发性恶性病变，而原发恶性高于继发骨转移者。由于良性病变的临床表现多种多样，因此在体检时无明确征象。有关它们的自然史和潜在的恶性可能性的结论因此难于确定[67]。在本章中，我们讨论在儿童人群中最常见发生的骨病理性疾病。在儿童人群中，最常见的良性肿瘤是单房性骨囊肿、动脉瘤样骨囊肿、内生软骨瘤、骨软骨瘤、非骨化性纤维瘤和骨样骨瘤。常见的骨恶性肿瘤是骨母细胞瘤和 Ewing 家族肉瘤（表 40-1）。在这里，我们主要讨论每一肿瘤的特异性表现。如若读者想对其病理学有更全面了解，可以参阅更多的专业书籍[62,67,128,135]。

表 40–1　不同年龄段常见肿瘤

年龄	良性肿瘤	恶性肿瘤	类肿瘤样疾病
出生至 5 岁	嗜酸性粒细胞肉芽肿	白血病	骨髓炎
		转移性成神经细胞瘤	非外伤性损伤
5～15 岁	单房性骨囊肿	Ewing 家族肉瘤	纤维结构不良
	骨软骨瘤	骨肉瘤	骨髓炎
	动脉瘤样骨囊肿		骨纤维结构不良
	骨样骨瘤		应力骨折
	内生软骨瘤		
	非骨化性纤维瘤		
	软骨肌瘤		
	成软骨细胞瘤		
15～20 岁	单房性骨囊肿	骨肉瘤	纤维结构不良
	骨软骨瘤	Ewing 家族肉瘤	应力骨折
	骨样骨瘤		
	动脉瘤样骨囊肿		
	非骨化性纤维瘤		
	巨细胞瘤		
	内生软骨瘤		
	成软骨细胞瘤		
	软骨肌纤维瘤		

考虑患儿的年龄、发病率以及病变位于长骨的位置（见图 40–3），绝大多数病例都可以做出诊断。对小于 5 岁的不健谈的儿童，要考虑创伤的可能性，非偶发性的外伤可能是其病因。

650 良性病变

儿童人群组的典型的良性病变以其发生率排序（表 40–2）。这些病变很少导致临床症状，常常是家长注意到有包块或畸形（例如骨软骨瘤），或患儿因其他疾病拍 X 线片时偶然发现的（如非骨化性纤维瘤）。在这些病例中，有两个重要的手术指征：通过活检明确诊断或骨发生骨折后或可能发生骨折的情况下为获得骨的稳定，尤其是在一些不稳定的部位。如股骨颈部位的骨囊肿需要考虑早期手术治疗，因为如此处发生骨折，可能导致股骨头的缺血性坏死。活检本身无损害，但是活检会降低骨的强度，需要复位或夹板固定。良性骨病变通常为无症状的，而活检可能诱发坏死。从活检结果区分良、恶性肿瘤其难度正在逐日增加。

表 40–2　常见的骨肿瘤的发生率

肿瘤	所有骨肿瘤（%）	20 岁以内的骨肿瘤
良性		
骨软骨瘤	7.86	4.69
动脉瘤样骨囊肿	2.60	1.96
骨样骨瘤	2.99	1.94
非骨化性纤维瘤	1.13	0.99
内生软骨瘤	3.02	0.98
巨细胞瘤	5.10	0.80
成软骨细胞瘤	1.07	0.66
软骨肌纤维瘤	0.41	0.14
单房性骨囊肿	未知	未知
恶性		
骨肉瘤	14.9	7.53
Ewing 家族肉瘤	4.6	3.50

使用这张表格需记注很多条件。大多数良性病变常无症状，只有有症状的才会被发现。这些病例大多在初级保健机构处理。恶性病变通常在转诊中心治疗。因此对于人群发生率，这些数字是不可靠的。相对而言，对提示其流行率有一定作用。单房性骨囊肿被列于表内用以提示其发生频率。

肿瘤的大小

肿瘤的大小是重要的考虑因素。例如，超过 4cm

的软骨瘤在有软骨性肋骨病变的患儿中发生恶性变的可能性大[62]。由于巨大软骨瘤的侵袭性恶性特征，尽管组织学可能无恶性表现，但是仍然需要广泛切除（图 40–1）。巨大的肿瘤可以侵犯邻近组织并导致关节功能受限。尽管这种情况在上肢关节并不多见，但是在脊柱和下肢通常会引起关节功能障碍和疼痛。由
651 于病变骨强度减低，骨小梁塌陷。因此，超过骨横截面 50%的病变要进行治疗[45,46,58]。这些病变能够增加骨折的危险性，并且有向恶性转化的可能，有可能导致潜在的肢体不等长而不是截肢。

良性病变骨折

良性病变发生骨折最常见的是单房性骨囊肿。它表现为侵袭性，但是详细的病史、体格检查以及放射学检查经常能够明确诊断（图 40–2）。单房性骨囊肿骨折可以自发愈合，但是它们在儿童时期可以发生再骨折以及残疾[98]。一般来讲，应采用手术治疗，尤其是对有症状的患儿。

手术治疗的时间非常严格，早期活检可以发现有骨痂形成，难于与恶性病变鉴别。因此在骨折愈合期间，应观察 1 个月左右再行活检并明确诊断。

与骺板的关系

与成人相比，在对儿童的肿瘤进行评价和治疗时，其部位与骺板的关系是非常重要的（图 40–3）。“骨干续连症”是指一种多发性骨软骨瘤疾病，其原发于骺板，可导致长骨线形生长紊乱[135]。这些病例常常为家族性的，但功能受限少见。上肢关节通常可以耐受一定的畸形，功能障碍不明显。但是在偶发病例，特别是在下肢，可能引起退行性关节炎而需要早期手术治疗。

骨肿瘤的多样性

多发性骨病变通常是有症状的，并且可能恶性变发生率高[67,128,135]。多发性骨软骨瘤发生于多种遗传性骨疣——一种常染色体显性遗传病，由常染色体 8、11 和 19 上的 *EXT1*、*EXT2* 和 *EXT3* 基因异常所致[30,74,142]。有基因异常的患儿其退变为软骨肉瘤的发生率在 10%～27.6%。与之相比，孤立的骨软骨瘤的恶性变率为 1%[62,67,128]。由于仅仅有症状的病例才会去

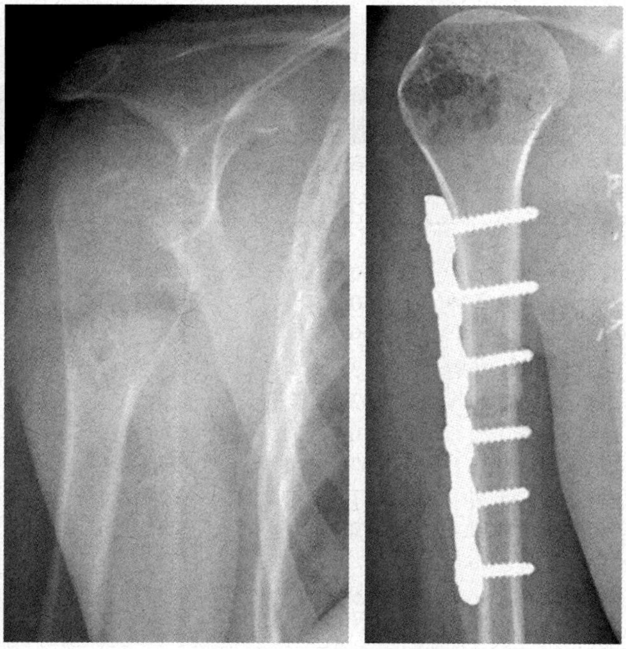

A B

图 40–1 A. 13 岁男孩肱骨近端软骨肉瘤。这是在这一年龄段极少见的肿瘤。B. 肱骨近端切除，同种异体骨重建。在儿童，现有的假体太大，因此同种异体移植是唯一的选择。

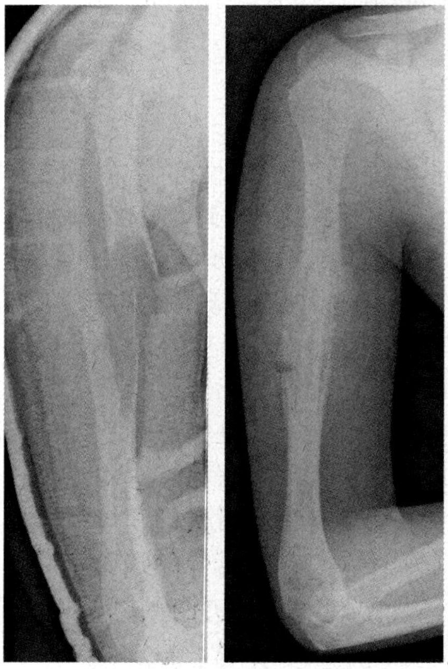

A B

图 40–2 A. 巨大的肱骨近端单房性骨囊肿，已发生病理性骨折。其侵袭性过程容易使人怀疑恶性肿瘤，但是仔细观察病变边缘没有出现骨膜反应。B. 骨折后 1 个月，刮除囊肿，同种异体骨充填，髓内腓骨移植以提高稳定性，同时骨移植。

看医生，孤立性病变的恶性变的发生率难以准确确定。多发性内生软骨瘤是一种散发疾病，在受累骨，其向恶性转化率达 50%[67]。肢体不等长和畸形常见，Ollier 病，就是其中一种，典型者可以影响肢体的肢
652 芽。Maffucci 综合征，是一种变异，表现为广泛的多发性内生软骨瘤，伴有手部的血管瘤。多发性非骨化性纤维瘤伴智力障碍、牛奶咖啡斑、内分泌紊乱、心血管畸形和眼部异常，称为 Jaffe–Campanacci 综合征，并无恶性表现[67,94]。

累及的部位

良性软骨性病变有很强的恶性转化潜能。手部指端病变恶性转化率低，而中轴骨即使其组织学表现为良性，向恶性转化的可能性大[62,67,86,94,128,135]。负重关节周围骨的病变应当给予重视，在儿童时期，这些病变多为软骨纤维瘤。它们向骺板方向生长会导致软骨下骨强度降低，最终向关节内延伸或引起骨折，甚至引起骨软骨缺损。在肉瘤病例，皮质相对保守切除与关节周围截肢有差异。

转移潜能

良性骨肿瘤的一个特异性特征是这些病变的转移可能性小。约 1.7%成软骨细胞瘤和 3%巨细胞瘤[56,61,72,128]会发生转移。实际上，对于一些病变是否一开始即为恶性这一点尚存争议[73]。然而真正良性的肿瘤其表现不典型，经过手术处理，可能会激活肿瘤细胞。当随访时，一些转移性病变，起初位于肺，可能呈静止状态而不发展。因此有可能只是有转移的表象而不是真正的转移，真正的转移要求在最后种植前发生大量的突变[62,128]。

恶性病变

流行病学

骨肿瘤的主要组织学表型是骨源性肉瘤、Ewing 家族肉瘤、软骨肉瘤和其他肉瘤，它们在儿童中的发病率是 6∶3∶2∶1[28,128]。

骨源性肉瘤（骨肉瘤）是骨形成的恶性肿瘤，可发生于任何年龄，但是多发于青少年的四肢长骨。它们有多种亚型，其生存率各不相同。一般来讲，可能除了毛细血管扩张型骨肉瘤，各亚型表现相似，该型比较特殊。在化疗前时代，预后很差[91]。现在预后有很大改善[63]。这些肿瘤的溶骨特性可以降低骨的强度，导致病理性骨折。越来越多的罕见类型的骨肉瘤

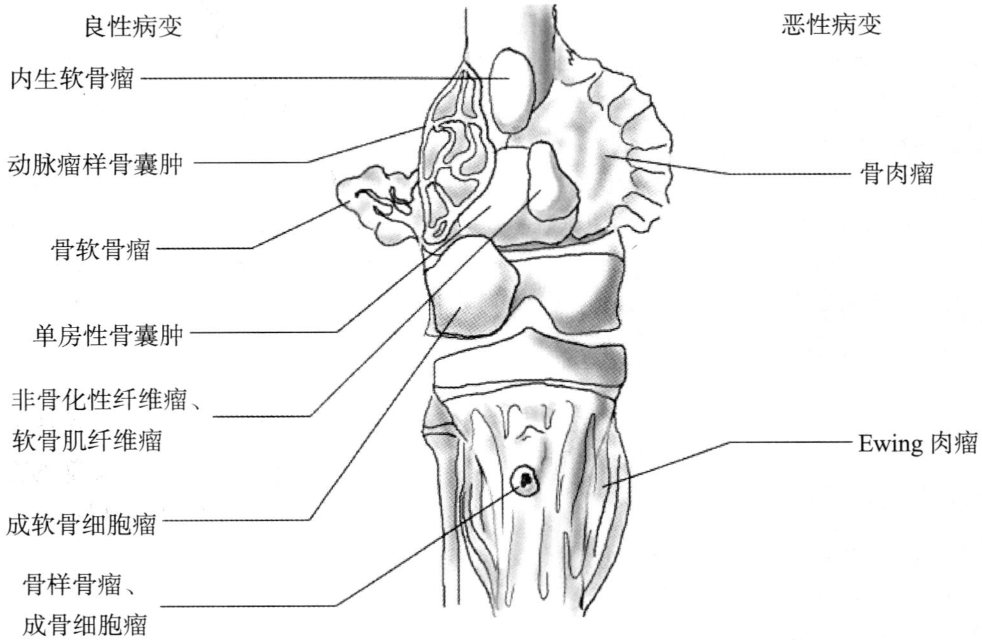

图 40–3　骨骺附近病变的常见部位可给诊断提供帮助。多数患者通过 X 线就可以做出诊断，还可以进行进一步的影像学检查为手术做准备。

开始已被发现。其中两种是小细胞肉瘤和巨细胞性骨
653 肉瘤。前者易与 Esing 家族肉瘤相混淆，因此经常以相似的化疗方案来治疗[90,116]。后者可能与骨巨细胞——一种良性肿瘤——混淆[12,13,141]。

Ewing 肉瘤患儿年龄较小（见表 40–1），可能累及任何骨，尤其是股骨、骨盆和肱骨。它是骨盆、肋骨、足和腓骨最常见的癌症。本病曾被认为应与神经内皮细胞肿瘤鉴别，但后来认为两者具有相同的基因特性。目前认为后者与 Ewing 家族肉瘤为同一家族[62,135]。

软骨肉瘤在儿童时期少见，可发生于身体的各个部位，较成人范围广。

基因组学

骨肉瘤几乎没有一致的基因组学或症状学相关性。Li–Fraumeni 综合征患者[77]在 9p21 位点有 *TP53* 种系的突变[78,81]，对骨肉瘤、乳腺癌和淋巴瘤易感（表 40–4）。2%～3%的骨肉瘤患儿出现在 Li–Fraumeni 疾病家族[124]。另一个基因突变是 13q14，遗传性眼癌患者易发生骨肉瘤[11]。因眼癌、Hodgkin 淋巴瘤、Ewing 家族肉瘤和其他癌症接受放疗的儿童有 5%～10%的可能发生骨肉瘤。*RB* 基因缺失的患儿以及由于恶性疾病接受过烷基化药物治疗的患儿也容易发生骨肉瘤这种并发症[127]。5%的所有骨肉瘤是作为一种放疗后肉瘤出现[65]。

Ewing 家族肉瘤是一种恶性肿瘤，有一定的转移率。导致 EWS–FLI1 融合转录的 11 与 22 易位是最常见的变异，1 型的预后最好 15。其他易位包括 2 型 EWS–FLI1、EWS–ERG 的 21、22 转位，以及 EWS–ETV1 的 7、22 转位。对这些少见的突变尚无深入研究但其预后不良[15]。进一步的涉及细胞周期基因的其他突变可进一步加剧这些肿瘤的预后。Ewing 家族肉瘤是最常见的可发生脑转移的实体肿瘤[32]。

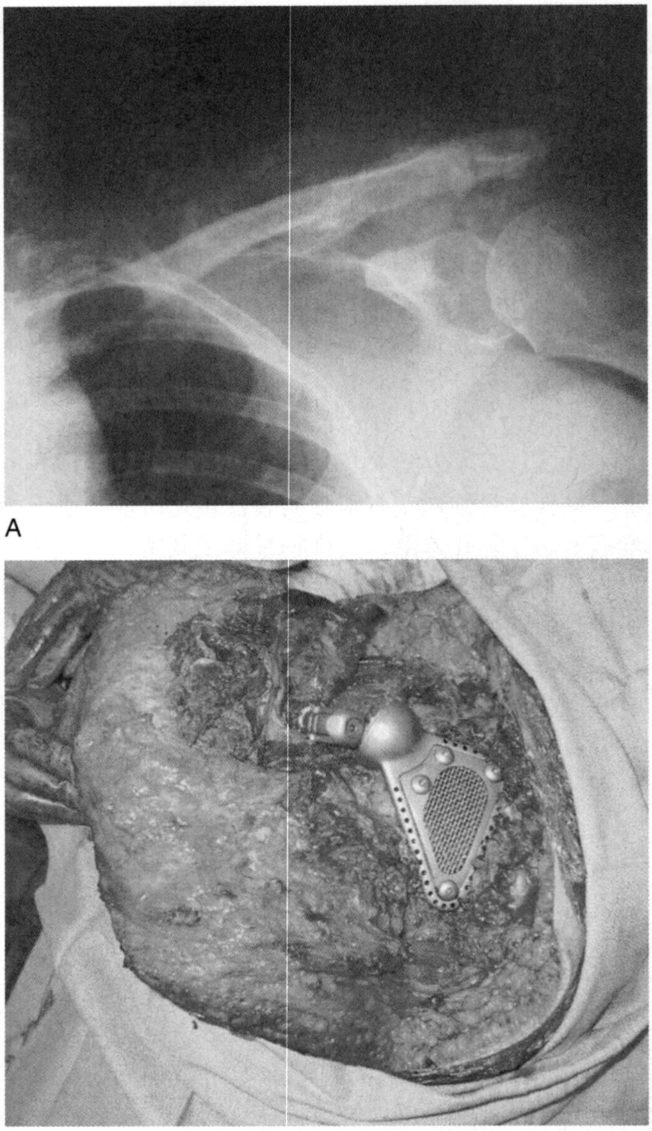

图 40–4 A. 一位 Li–Fraumeni 综合征女性患者的左肩胛骨骨肉瘤。该患者有骨肉瘤家族史。在对骨肉瘤进行分级时，CT 发现其乳房内有病变，随后发现是腺癌。B. 对患者行肩胛骨切除术，背阔肌皮瓣用于覆盖。

诊断和分期

骨肿瘤的诊断是建立在详细询问病史、体格检查和实验室检查基础上的。在临床诊断后、活检进行之前，应行影像学的检查并进行分型。术前分型有利于制订较为准确的手术方案和确定手术切口。另外在活检后，病变部位会发生一定变化，可能难于与影像学上面的肿瘤鉴别。而且在麻醉下肺部的变化（如肺膨胀不全）难以与转移性肿块相鉴别。

临床评估

尽管不能做出完善的评价，但是病史和体格检查

是骨肿瘤患儿临床评价的重要组成部分。疾病发病率和肿瘤部位可以将诊断和鉴别诊断的范围缩小，更容易确定诊断。

患儿的年龄非常重要（见表 40-2）。多数恶性病变发生在 11～20 岁[62,67,128,135]。在儿童，在不同的年龄
654 之间，疾病的分布有一些不同（见表 40-1）。从统计学上讲，非洲儿童极少发生 Ewing 家族肉瘤[135]。

静息痛是最重要的症状，可发生在肿瘤和其他一些原发性疾病，如感染和骨梗死。它与活动痛可以区别，后者在活动时发生。多数恶性肿瘤可有疼痛，疼痛是骨样骨瘤的特征性表现，非甾体类抗炎药可以[59]缓解。骨样骨瘤可以发生于任何年龄，当发生于脊柱时，可表现为疼痛性脊柱侧弯。

恶性肿瘤的家族史尤其应与 Li-Fraumeni 综合征的病例鉴别[77,78,81]。这样的患儿应当 进行系统检查以排除其他疾病，包括放射性骨扫描、正电子辐射断层扫描。

如先前所述，外科医生对有畸形的患儿应当特别注意。神经纤维瘤 | 纤维性发育不良和 Jaffe-Campanacci 综合征的患儿其皮肤有红斑[94]。多发性内生软骨瘤患儿可出现肢体不等长和多样性外生骨疣[119]。

每一个病例都需要与感染鉴别。肿瘤的流行病学资料非常有效，例如，儿童的淋巴细胞瘤的发生率是 Ewing 家族肉瘤的 10 倍，淋巴细胞瘤的表现不具有特征性，与 Ewing 家族肉瘤相比表现不显著。

骨重建的特征也需要选择的方法与患儿的要求相匹配。例如，患儿的期望值应当被重视。

影像学检查

首诊时对于有疑问的患儿，病变部位应拍摄两个平面的放射线片。放射线检查仍然是最具特异性的诊断学检查，也是唯一一个“完形“检查，可以对骨的生物学和力学进行总的评价。通过分析肿瘤的部位（见图 40-3）及对其良、恶性进行鉴别，在多数患儿可以明确诊断[62,67,128,135]。

良性病变边界清晰，有良好的皮质性边界，无软组织水肿。恶性病变机制模糊不清，边界浸润。在脂肪线上水肿通常表现明显。

通常引用的专业名词对于特异性恶性肿瘤来讲并不是特异的。Codman 三角是指在骨源性骨肉瘤的边界出现骨膜骨化和升高。由于肿瘤穿通皮质向外蔓延，日光放射表现是由于纤维和骨膜下血管的骨化。皮质洋葱样变是骨皮质周期性的骨化和骨膜的扩展。在生长足够快的情况下，这些表现中任何一种或几种都可以在肿瘤或感染中见到。

在图表中，骨骺的病变是软骨细胞瘤或巨细胞瘤中的典型表现；骺板病变是骨软骨瘤的典型病变；干骺端为骨肉瘤、单房性骨囊肿、动脉瘤样骨囊肿和非骨化性纤维瘤的典型病变；Esing 家族肉瘤，纤维性发育不良和内生型软骨瘤多发生在骨干部位。

实验室检查

主要的血液学指标是乳酸脱氢酶和碱性磷酸酶[50,76,123]。乳酸脱氢酶水平可以用来判断肿瘤的大小，且在 Esing 家族肉瘤病例与生存率相关[50]。血清碱性磷酸酶升高是骨源性肉瘤的特异性表现，与肿瘤预后不良相关[76,123]。糖耐量试验与软骨性肉瘤有关[48,85]。红细胞沉降率、C 反应蛋白、白细胞计数及分类可以用来排除感染。

术前计划

病变的 MRI 检查可以提供肿瘤的区室评价。区室是一个抽象的概念，是指给邻接的扩展提供筋膜或皮质骨屏障的任一平面。其对手术范围有意义，因为肿瘤必须在区室外才能根治（见下文）[37]。此外，有了基线评估就可在进行新辅助治疗时，对化疗的反应做出初步评价[60]。其次，在提供准确诊断方面也有其重要性。在个别病例，还可用于组织学诊断。动脉瘤样骨囊肿在 MRI 上表现为液-液平面。色素沉着性绒毛膜滑膜炎在 T1 和 T2 加权图像上表现为高密度影（黑色），这是由于含铁血黄素的沉积。在 T_2 加权图像上，软骨性病变是低强度影（白色）。矿化和高密度纤维组织在 T1 和 T2 加权图像上均为黑色[4,96]。

分级

分级意味着评价疾病的扩散程度。在骨肿瘤中，骨肌肉肿瘤协会和美国关节肿瘤协会应用两个系统：Enneking 系统或手术分级系统（SSS）[39]，正在修订第 6 版[53]。Ewing 家族肉瘤应用一种来源于 Enneking

的分类方法[36]。

在 SSS，肿瘤被划分为 G0、G1 和 G2，分别区分良性、低度恶性和高度恶性肿瘤。良性（G0）分类为潜在的、活跃的或侵袭性的，以阿拉伯数字 1、2 和 3 代表。恶性病变如果为低度的则划为Ⅰ，如果为高度的则为Ⅱ。进一步以 A 或 B 区分间室内或间室外。Ⅲ级是转移性疾病。在此分类中，分级、间室和转移是分类的主要指标。

在 AJCC 系统，Ⅰ和Ⅱ简单代表低度和高度病变。A 和 B 各自表示肿瘤小于和大于 8cm。Ⅲ代表多中心疾病，Ⅳ是指肿瘤已有转移。ⅣA 代表肺部转移，ⅣB 代表指肺外转移。这种分类方法是以分级、
655 大小、多中心和转移为诊断的指标。

在 Ewing 家族肉瘤的 Enneking 分型系统中，Ⅰ是指实性的骨内病变，Ⅱ为有骨内向骨外扩散，Ⅲ为多发性病变，Ⅳ为转移性病变。如何分级独立的骨性病灶和光化学显微镜证实有肿瘤细胞转移（Enneking 分级Ⅲ或Ⅳ）并不清楚。现代病理学分析将这些概念延伸至包括免疫组织化学和反转录聚合酶链反应（RT–PCR）。

骨扫描和胸部 CT 形态学检查可以用来进行分级[39]。正电子发射断层扫描可以用于始发性或转移性病变的基础评价[16]。对 Ewing 家族肉瘤病例，在试图确诊多部位发病的患儿时可进行骨髓活检。这种方法

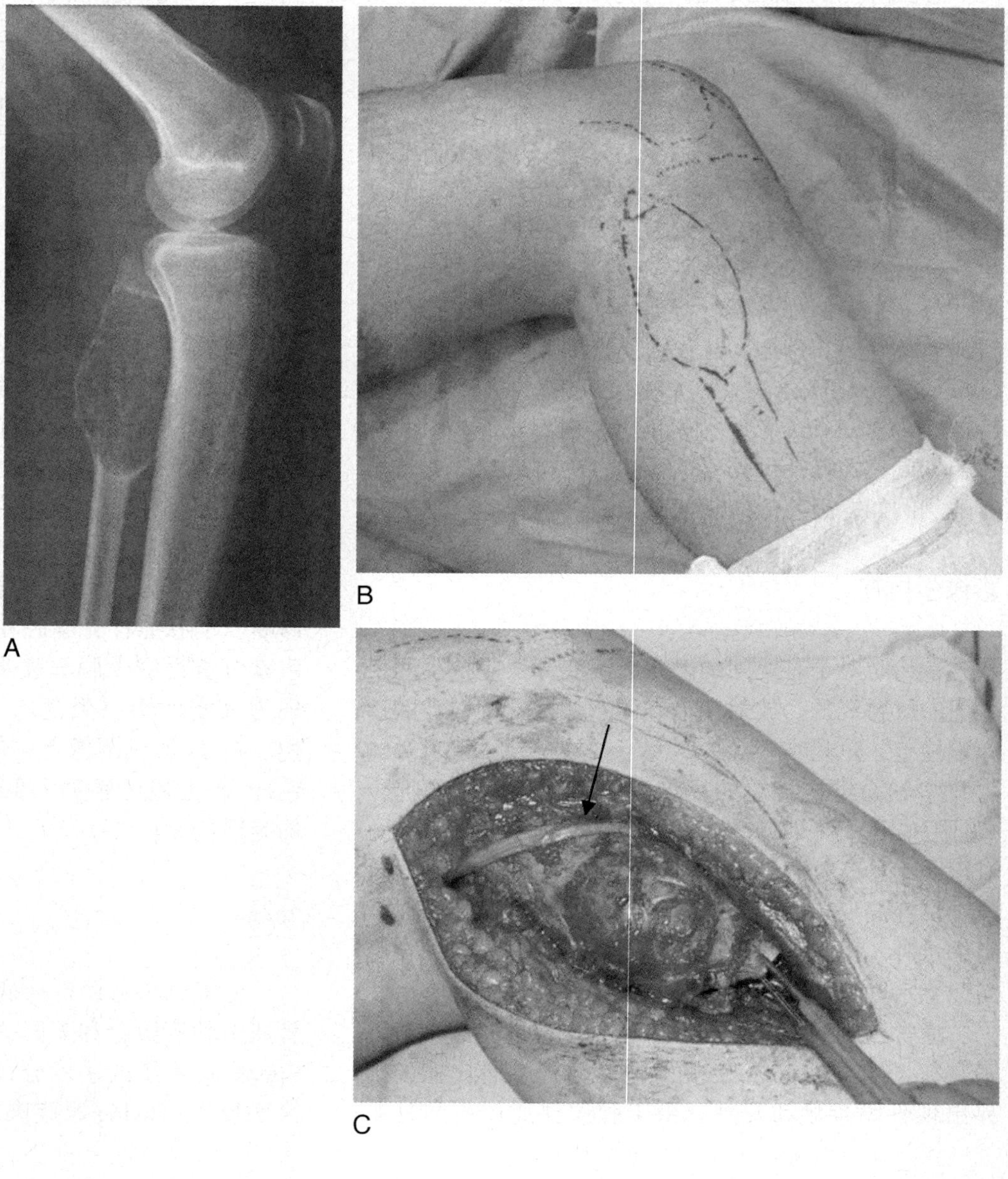

图 40–5 A 和 B. 一位 17 岁男孩的右腓骨近端动脉瘤样骨囊肿。C. 在这个病例进行了广泛的病灶切除，因为骨是可以切除的，可避免腓总神经受累。

的适用性需要进一步验证。

活检

活检是一个关键的步骤，但是如果不能适当采用的话，会使处理变得更复杂。不适当的切口会导致能够被再次切除的肿瘤被遮蔽而不能够行保肢治疗[37,84]。处理骨组织有经验的病理学家对这个过程要求非常严格。在合适的病例，还取出额外的组织做细胞基因学研究。Ewing 家族肉瘤组织易碎，活检样本在处理过程中要非常小心仔细。

术前考虑因素

作为一项常规，所有的影像学和分级应当在活检前完成。有活检指征的病变应考虑初期广泛切除。这种方法尤其适用于小的不超过 3cm 的病变、可以消耗的骨的病变（如远端指骨）、远端尺骨病变和胫骨
656 近段，有可能累及邻近的尺神经（图 40–5）。

病变应当在专科医院由专科医生按照既定的程序进行取样。当与结果不符时可以重复做以达到最后的结果[88,84]。

有时可以采用针吸活检，例如对骨盆或脊柱的病变，因为这些部位如果做切开活检所需切口大，可能使肿瘤扩散。

病理学家必须对骨组织的处理过程非常熟悉，并能够对活检进行即时的判断。如果肿瘤组织能够被刀切动，那么可以用切片机。冰冻切片分析主要用来判断组织的量是否足够以及评价切除的组织是否具有代表性，其次用来做明确的诊断。

在活检前应避免使用抗生素，活检时可以使用止血带以避免出血和肿瘤向邻近组织扩散。当应用止血带时，轻度抬高患处以驱血。由于可能将肿瘤撕裂，压力性驱血应当避免。在任何时候，都应当保护肢体、防止骨折，因为这有可能会导致疾病的局部播散。

手术考虑因素

设计的用于某一例手术的切口应当进行标记，一般应遵循广泛暴露，沿标记的切口纵向切开。切口应当直接位于病变上方，避免皮瓣和过多的分离。

切口应当能够直达肿瘤，如果肿瘤中有软组织成分，对这些软组织需要单独进行病理检查。如果必须先行骨活检，那么活检的样本边缘应为圆形以降低压力。冷冻切片分析可以证实活检取的组织是否足够。同时进行培养，放松止血带，给予抗生素。手术结束后绝对止血，防止肿瘤细胞随血液播散。

切口应分层缝合，如果必须引流，将其放置在切口内，在进行完全切除术时可将其切除。

术后处理

患儿应避免负重，至少至活检愈合或肿瘤骨化，作为对新辅助化疗的反应。通常需要 6 周。

骨肉瘤骨折一般不再行保肢手术。近来研究显示，保肢只适用于某些选择性病例[2,7,113,114]。在这些病例中需要进行特异性的治疗计划。

辅助治疗

这部分的重点是指放疗和化疗的应用。一般来讲，这两种方法并不用来治疗良性病变，当良性病变进行放射治疗时，恶变发生率高达 10%[19,62,65,67,127,128,135]。

在恶性肿瘤的治疗中，化疗和放疗可以用于新辅助疗法（术前）或辅助疗法（术后）部分。新辅助疗法的优点是使肿瘤“缩小”，并提供更为清晰的边界，理论上可以将病变局限化。在化疗中，在假体修复前，常规新辅助疗法是必须的。这项技术已显示与第一次手术同样有效。虽然如此，有一项对术前术后均行化疗者和仅术后行化疗者的生存率进行的随机试验显示，两者无明显差异。因此，在选择性病例，合理而谨慎的方式是先行手术治疗[92]。

化疗

历史上，在化疗时代之前，骨肉瘤的生存率不超过 20%。在 1972—1981 年，骨肉瘤治疗化疗的方案的制订使治疗发生了革命性的变化，现在 5 年生存率达 60%～76%[6,55,64,87,92,106]。

目前，骨肉瘤治疗的标准方法是新辅助疗法，可以治疗一些尚不能辨别的微观疾病，随后进行明确的

切除和辅助化疗。这种方法比依据经验更明智。最后切除时的组织学结果对于预后的判断非常重要。

在切除样本中化疗相关性坏死已进行分级。Ⅰ级坏死是指坏死组织总量少于肿瘤的 50%。Ⅱ级是坏死组织总量占肿瘤的 50%～90%。Ⅲ级坏死占到肿瘤超过 90%，Ⅳ级坏死是指肿瘤几乎全部坏死。Ⅰ和Ⅱ级坏死进一步被列为一组作为标准反应，Ⅲ和Ⅳ级坏死列为反应良好。反应良好在骨肉瘤和 Esing 家族肉瘤切除后是重要的预后因素，表示预后良好[92,143]。

应该想到以前有 20%的患儿可仅通过手术治愈，而现在仍有 24%～40%的患者是不能治愈的。这意味着约有 44%～64%的患者在治疗中无任何变化。然而，他们仍然可以从化疗中受益，获得较长时间的生存期、病灶的局限化和高的保肢率[92]。

常用的药物可以分为细胞周期特异性和非细胞周期特异性药物。细胞周期特异性药物包括甲氨蝶呤和阿霉素。它们可以干扰细胞分裂而影响细胞增殖。任何细胞群都有静止期细胞。这些细胞不受细胞周期特异性药物的影响。因此，非细胞周期特异性药物可以
657 起到一定作用。顺铂和烷基化物（如环磷酰胺和异环磷酰胺）可以直接损伤细胞的 DNA，所以静止期细胞也可以被杀灭。在骨肉瘤和 Esing 家族肉瘤的治疗中，通常采用 Goldie–Coldman 化疗模型[51]。

多种药物联合化疗在治疗骨肉瘤的过程中也常采用。在欧洲，骨肉瘤合作研究协会（COSS）报道了 10 年的实际生存率为 64%[14]。Rizzoli 机构报道 8 年的无病生存率为 59%[43]。因此，显示了多种药物联合化疗的效果，从而使得外科手术治疗处于停滞状态，在过去的 20 年里。新的方法和药物在不断的发展之中。

传统的药物包括顺铂，阿霉素和大剂量的甲氨蝶呤联合应用环磷酰胺，在多个治疗中心中采用。初步的效果良好，Rizzoli 机构，是意大利肉瘤组织 / 斯堪的纳维亚肉瘤组织的一部分，报道联合用药 5 年的生存率可达 87%，5 年的无病生存率为 73%，较先前的研究有所升高[8,43]。异环磷酰胺在本中心使用的疗效多样，化疗相关性坏死并不是灾难性的，与患者生存率的升高也没有相关性。

化疗作为一项独立的治疗在骨肉瘤的治疗中也有其缺点[68]。并发症包括局部复发率和转移率升高，治愈率完全成功的只有 10%[70]。

近来有研究发现，二磷酸盐可能在抗肿瘤方面有重要的作用，动脉内应用新辅助化疗药物顺铂或静脉内应用阿霉素，而后行肿瘤手术治疗，并且彻底化疗，可以达到 10 年无瘤生存率 84%。术前应用血管造影监测坏死，手术仅在 90%或更多的新生血管形成后方实行。在切除以及对坏死进行评价后，辅助化疗根据切除组织对于化疗的反应进行调整。这种方法达到了目前已发展的多种治疗技术的顶点，并且也说明了多种方法联合治疗的必要性[137]。

放疗

放疗在新辅助治疗和辅助治疗在 Ewing 家族肉瘤中均有应用。对化疗反应不佳的骨肉瘤患儿仅是有选择应用[34,75]。

治疗 Ewing 家族肉瘤时，根据肿瘤的部位和中心剂量有所不同。放疗一般是有效的，但是与手术治疗相比，局部复发率高。当单独应用时，剂量大 6600cGy 对于局部局限化是必须的[122]。与之相比，3000～4000cGy 分次使用对于手术联合化疗时[89]。因为放疗可能导致骺板早闭和骨坏死[52,97]，因此附加放疗在肉瘤的治疗中也有所发展，在烷化剂应用后这些患儿的基因学会发生一定的改变[19,34,52,65,127]，一些机构的研究中认为，放疗在肿瘤局限化方面的作用在脊柱和骨盆的病变受到一定的限制。在这些病例中，应当单独应用放疗或在手术中与手术联合应用（图 40–6）。在治疗四肢的病变时，单纯的手术治疗会有

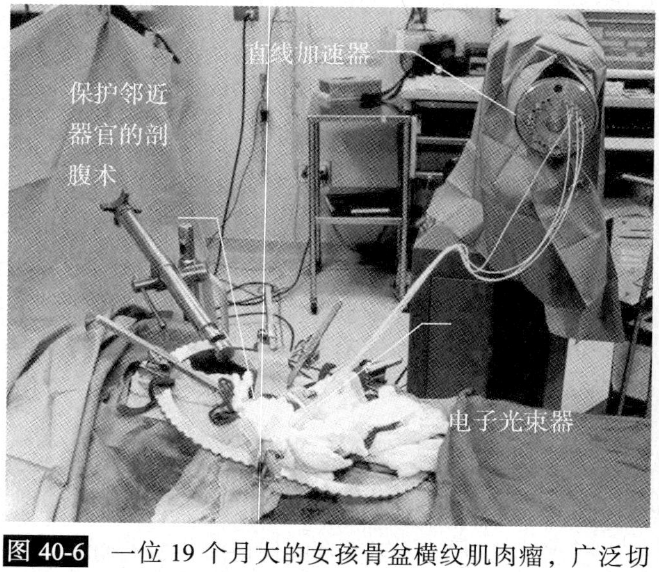

图 40-6 一位 19 个月大的女孩骨盆横纹肌肉瘤，广泛切除加淋巴结清扫后术中放疗。

一定效果，保守量的放疗对无法切除的部位或术前化疗反应不良时可以起到一定控制作用[89,108,143]。

尽管在儿童组中并未进行这方面的专门研究，但是放疗显示在围术期可以增加伤口的并发症，如果患儿要进行化疗时，这就是另外一个需要考虑的因素[102]。因此，一般来讲这种方法的应用需严格把握指征。

在 Langerhans 组织细胞增生症，为避免骨骼的边界受到放疗影响时，低剂量的放疗，总量少于 1000rads 可以起到很好的将疾病局限化的作用[115]。

手术治疗

对骨肿瘤，切除和重建这两个方面可互为补充，但偶尔有所冲突（如对于扩展要切除肿瘤的边界冷冻
658 疗法非常有效，但是会降低骨的强度）。因此尽管切除的目的在于完整切除，使边界尽量清晰（如治愈），但重建的目的通常只是中庸的，尤其在恶性肿瘤。在良性肿瘤，重建倾向于尽量保留其功能。在本节，我们提出一些手术中需要考虑和特别注意的几点。

尽量小的切口

小切口通常用于良性病变。其存在两个处理上的冲突，一方面希望将病变局限化，另一方面犹豫产生的病变是否会比原发病变更多。无论选择何种药物，组织学诊断非常重要。

射频切除

射频切除是利用高密度的热能作用于病变处引起病变部位的坏死。可以应用于多种实体肿瘤。在骨肿瘤，主要用于骨样骨瘤。骨样骨瘤的症状以疼痛为主，多为逐渐加重的夜间痛，应用非甾体类抗炎药物可以缓解。骨样骨瘤多为良性，多发于股骨近段。在这些部位，手术切除可能诱发坏死，因此诸如射频切除这样的方法非常理想，尽管与手术相比，其可以有 10%～15%的复发率[33,107]，而手术的复发率几乎是 0[23]。但是射频切除不适用于脊柱，因为高热能产生后对周围组织的作用是没有选择性的。

注射

这种技术原则上用于治疗单房性骨囊肿。临床上明显的骨囊肿有一种诱发骨折的趋势，需要治疗[98]。它们虽然没有恶性潜能，但可以生长[67,98]。对于皮质醇注射是否是必须的治疗尚存争议，因为囊肿的单纯性减压对于减轻症状已经足够了[126]。治愈率据报道可以达到 50%，需要注射 1～9 次，平均注射 3 次[22,110]。每次注射均需在麻醉下进行，因此，这种治疗方法并未得到广泛接受。

有多种减压方法，效果各有差异。一种是骨髓注射治疗[35,71,79,109,144]，治愈率可达 50%～70%。但是，必须要重复注射，需要多次麻醉并可发生供区的坏死。

刮除法是经典的治疗方法，复发率 5%～50%[98]。因此，在对该疾病的治疗中并无某种特异性的方法。

非甾体类药物治疗

尽管不是一种手术方式，在骨样骨瘤的治疗中，非甾体类药物治疗（NSAID）也用于有选择的病例。在病灶位于脊柱或髋臼的患儿，手术或射频切除可能导致生长紊乱而需要进行脊柱融合或髋关节矫形手术。在这些病例中，NSAID 治疗可以改善症状。只要不存在胃肠道或泌尿系统的副作用，均可以持续用药，治愈率可达到 45%，但是需要持续服药约 30 个月[96]。

切除术

手术计划是建立在肿瘤与间室的关系上的（图 40-7）。间室相当于屏障，可以限制肿瘤的扩展。间室在确定广泛切除的边界或需要同时切除周围一部分正常组织时有重要作用：如果切除边界位于间室外，那么它可以形成一个间隔，使肿瘤局限，不至于向外扩展[39]。我们认识到，这种理论在许多方面有瑕疵。例如，多数骨肉瘤穿出了皮质，与未穿破的骨肉瘤有明显差别。在肢末端，累及股直肌的肿瘤位于一个间室，从前内方的骨盆髂前上棘延伸至胫骨结节。显然，进行股后部及臀部的切除并不可行。最后，尤其在股骨嵴区域，有大量的血管穿过，它们经过外侧肌间隔部——能够形成连续的屏障阻止肿瘤的扩散。

间室化的概念在描述病变内的、边缘性的、广泛

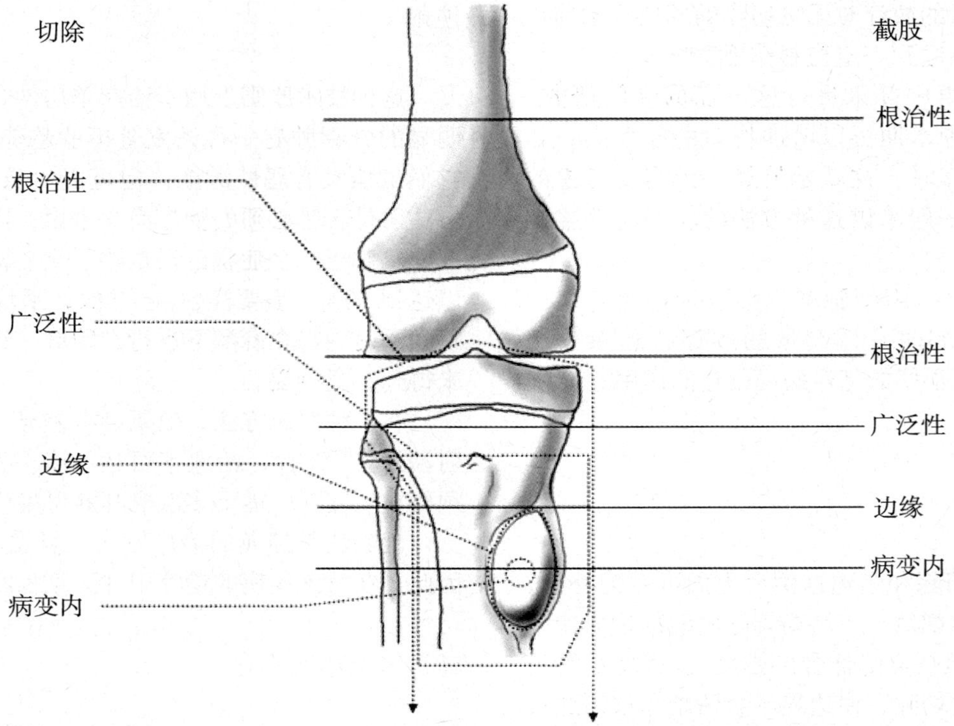

图 40–7 与间室累及有关的外科手术范围。左边是切除范围，右边是截肢范围。很大程度上这些分类是学术性的，因为除了根治性切除和广泛切除或根治性截肢术，多数病例是行切除术。根治性切除包括包容肿瘤的间室，因此在这个病例，应截去胫骨（箭头所示）。在脊柱和骨盆，由于邻近组织可能在疾病控制中起到重要作用，边界的限定要慎重考虑（见图 40–6）。病变内切除在肿瘤的手术治疗中是非治疗性的，但是为完整性起见包括在内。在儿童，腔内切除不可取，因为残余部分可以通过生长传播。为了避免这种并发症，可能需要跨关节截肢。

的和根治性的手术操作时仍然是非常有用的[37]。尽管在截肢时并不常用，但是这些原则适用。病变内部的操作过程，顾名思义，是明显有残留组织的操作。活检或病变内部注射是病变内部操作的过程。边缘性操作停留在肿瘤最大扩展边界的水平。刮除法即是这样一种方法。广泛性切除手术操作超过了肿瘤的反应区。当首次描述时，反应区是指肿瘤周围炎症反应的范围（即充血水肿）[36,37]。这些评价应当在手术时做出。现在更精细的影像学检查可以将这个区的范围延伸。因此，反应区的概念与实际相比更为抽象。作为常规原则，应切除肿瘤包囊，在那里其血管可以发生扭曲，可以有水肿。目前受到影像学进步的影响，切除的范围较以前又有所增加。多数恶性肿瘤要被广泛切除。基底部切除是指从肿瘤的发生部位进行彻底的
659 切除。膝关节上方截肢术治疗胫骨肿瘤即是彻底根治术。

有大量的外科辅助疗法可以应用。有多种形式，包括热能（如氩气凝固器）或冷冻治疗（如液氮冷冻疗法）[80,88]。另外，化学药物也可以应用（如苯酚、聚甲基苯稀酸甲酯接合剂）[25,103]。在个别病例，放疗的特殊形式（如近距离放射疗法、术中放射治疗）可以应用，尤其在骨盆（见图 40–6）。这些手术辅助疗法的目的在于将切除的边缘延伸至超过能够被切除的范围。这些还可以使肿瘤局限化。

良性病变

对病变与周围组织的连接部位进行分级有一定作用。可以分为良性、活动性和侵袭性。处理按照不同的性质进行。良性骨病变可以采用刮除、高热量烧灼囊壁、新辅助疗法以及广泛切除[25,80]。采用的方法根据病变的侵袭性不同而不同。

在良性病变，广泛的切除偶尔用于非承重骨（如肋骨、指骨末节）或骨的末端（如尺骨远端或腓骨近端）。在这些部位，几乎是没有重建价值，实际上，还可能成为许多疾病的来源。此外，在棘手的复发性

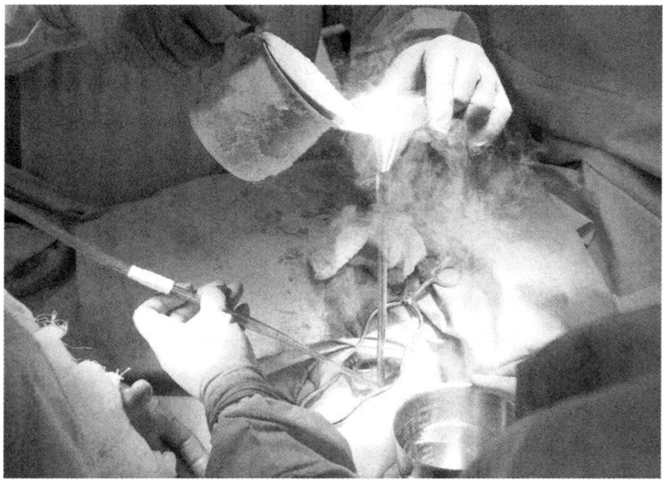

图 40-8　软骨肉瘤冷冻治疗。液氮通过管道直接注入病变，同时避免与周围皮肤接触。冷冻效果可以导致坏死的边缘超过外科医生感觉的部分，从病变内或边缘切除到广泛切除，可有效地扩展手术范围。

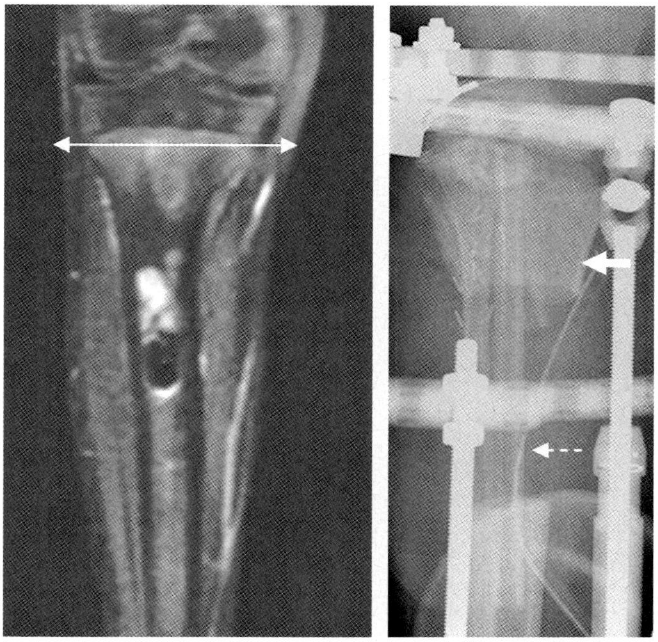

A　B

图 40-9　A. 一位 11 岁男孩的胫骨 Ewing 肉瘤。病变从骺板延伸了 1cm。其对化疗反应良好，没有软组织累及。在放射线引导下，小心地行保留骨骺的切除术（两个箭头之间所示）。B. 应用固定支架进行固定，可以防止近端小的骨块旋转。残余的间隙可以用胫骨近端同种异体移植重建（实心箭头），并带血供的皮瓣腓骨移植（虚线箭头）提供皮肤覆盖。

良性或恶性进展性病变情况下，可诉满于这种方法。用这种方法可以切除的典型的病变有骨巨细胞瘤、动脉瘤样骨囊肿或纤维结构不良。

病变周围切除技术理论上与软组织的脂肪瘤切除相同。这样的手术在大多数骨病变中技术上并不可行。骨软骨瘤和骨膜软骨瘤也可以用这种方法切除。

在良性肿瘤中病变内切除更常用。典型的方法有刮除病变、高速灼烧囊壁。对于多数潜在的或活动性良性骨病变（如单房性骨囊肿），这种方法大量使用。热、冷冻（图 40-8）或化学疗法都能增加这种治疗方法的有效性，可更有效地清除病变，常常应用于活动性或侵袭性肿瘤（如巨细胞瘤、成软骨细胞瘤）。

恶性病变

原则是在一个小的切口内做广泛的切除。但是，在有些情况下，这样做是不可能的。（如肿瘤已扩展至椎管内或已侵犯盆腔）。在这些病例，预后通常不容乐观。

新的延长骨骺辅助器械使在生长期的儿童进行骨骺-分离成为可能（图 40-9）。尽管通常认为骺板是阻隔肿瘤传播的一道屏障，显示邻近骺板的肿瘤仍有 80% 发生了播散[38,69,99,118]。因此，骨骺-分离方法必须要小心使用，观察对化疗的反应后再决定是否可行。

作为一种变异，偶尔有可能通过骨骺延长术在生长板区域进行延长来挽救骨骺及邻近的关节。这样可有效地增加正常组织与肿瘤之间的间隙。然后通过延长的部分行切除术[24]。

另一种保留关节的方法是行 VanNes 旋转成形术（图 40-10）[133]。这种方法多用于膝关节高分化肿瘤，包含广泛的关节周围切除手术，将远端的腿和脚与残留的股近端连接。在这一过程中，坐骨神经保留，节段性切除股动脉，建立股-腘动脉循环。将脚进行旋转，足跟向前。远端外旋，将坐骨神经和血管向前内侧移位。这些在手术中应记录以利于术后进一步治疗。踝关节功能因此类似于膝关节。这种方法由于外观的原因在患者中很难被接受，但是功能和持续时间非常理想[20]。相似的 Winkelmann 手术是将近端胫骨与髋关节连接。在儿童，这些部位骨可以看到明显的再塑形，随着时间的演唱可以逐渐形成稳定的形态[139,140]。

放疗和截肢由于其破坏了外观而使其应用受到限

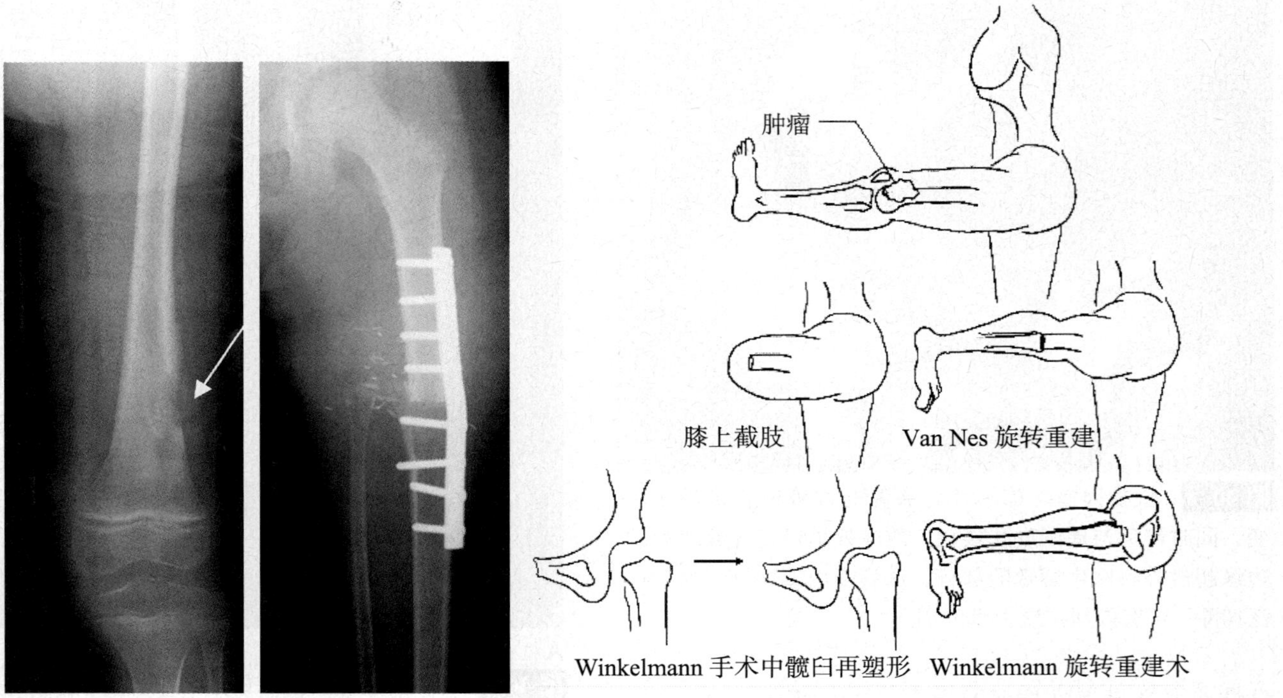

A B C

图 40–10 A. 一位 8 岁儿童的骨肉瘤（箭头所示），伴有巨大的软组织延伸。患儿的尺寸较小和高位的活动性不适合行内源性假体重建。B. 已行 Van Nes 旋转成形术。C. 多种成形术式与膝上截肢的比较。最下方显示了在 Winkelmann 手术中，胫骨近端与髋臼如何相互适应后再塑形。

制。研究显示，保肢患者可以保留更多的功能并节省费用[54,104]。尽管从表面上看是如此，但是深层次分析显示，这些研究种类过于混杂，不能获得准确的结论。随着现代假肢技术的发展，截肢患者能够获得相当高水平的活动能力。而且，保肢手术并发症的发生率是截肢手术的 3～4 倍。尽管多数研究并没有显示截肢和保肢治疗的生存率是否有明显差异，但这些研究不够权威，或截肢患者本身曾经接受过保肢治疗[47,92,117]。主要的问题是：在截肢和阶段性控制组中，生存率和功能改善是否有差异。回答这个问题需要进行病例对照研究，但这种研究不可能进行，因为没有安全保障。

截肢依然有作用，尤其是当肿瘤位于肢体远端时，新辅助化疗无效，或重建手术由于神经、血管或
661 软组织等问题而不能解决。

恶性病变局部复发力是预后不良的重要因素，其死亡率为 90%。这通常是对局部姑息性治疗的反应，尽管有研究显示，局部良好的化疗反应可以使复发率明显降低[47]。尤其是，当骨肉瘤进行病变内手术时，即便是化疗反应良好，其复发率仍然是广泛切除手术的 14 倍，因此需要进行完整的手术切除和有效的化疗。

重建

在多数病例，良性肿瘤切除后，小的缺损会残余。可以简单应用多种充填物解决。对于良性病变的修复，需要一定的创造性。由于相关病例的缺乏和这些操作的危险性，决定采用哪一种技术最为有效变得非常困难。本节中我们列出多种现有的方法，并且给出了每种方法的应用范围。

良性病变

在这些病变切除后，通常会遗留小的缺损。潜在的或活动的条件下，其局部复发率低。因此，治疗目标是骨的重建。许多骨移植的方法和骨的替代物。一般来讲，自体移植其效果最好，但是会发生供体部位坏死的危险，甚至出现供体部位肿瘤的种植。异体移植疾病转移的和免疫学反应危险性小[10,125]。合成的移

植物相容性不佳[31,132]。

在侵袭性更强的病变，其局部复发率升高。在这些部位，骨的替代物能够在疾病过程中完全吸收，延长了随后影像学检查之间的间隔，能够区分术后的改变还是复发。在这种情况下，骨水泥是一种好的替代品。并且，水泥不透光可以作为对照物。骨水泥边缘部分的复发可以很容易地判断并进行治疗。

恶性病变

解决的方法包括在肿瘤切除后解决残余复杂的骨、关节和软组织缺陷，这些形成了技术上的盲点，涵盖了所有骨科和矫形外科手术。这里不可能将所有的治疗方法一一论述。我们将对特殊部位的重建进行一些原则性的讨论。

所有的方法中首要一点是填充缺损和闭合皮肤。没有这两点，就不能继续化疗，患者也不能存活。如 662
果有足够的皮肤用来关闭伤口，大多数解决方法都提供了缺损的充填。如果皮肤不能闭合，则可进行局部皮瓣或带血供的植皮。在一些病例，尤其是有中段切除时，提供稳定性的能力与其上皮肤闭合可通过带血供的腓骨瓣移植做到。腓骨瓣的另一个优点是可以观察皮瓣的活性。旋转成形术和其他改良术明显地能够解决功能方面的问题，但是由于外观问题难于被接受。与之类似，对于这个问题截肢术是即时解决方法，但是在一些情况下仍然不被接受[104]。

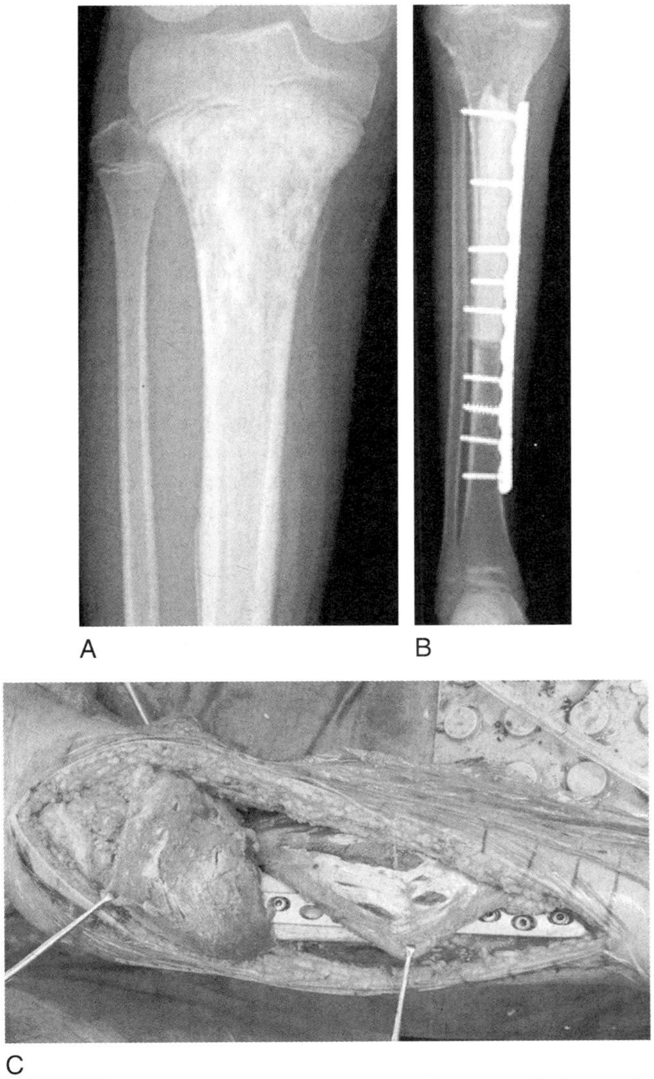

图 40-11 A. 一位 11 岁儿童的胫骨近端 Ewing 肉瘤。B 和 C. 这是广泛切除后用胫骨带关节的同种异体移植重建。腓肠肌皮瓣提供移植物软组织覆盖。

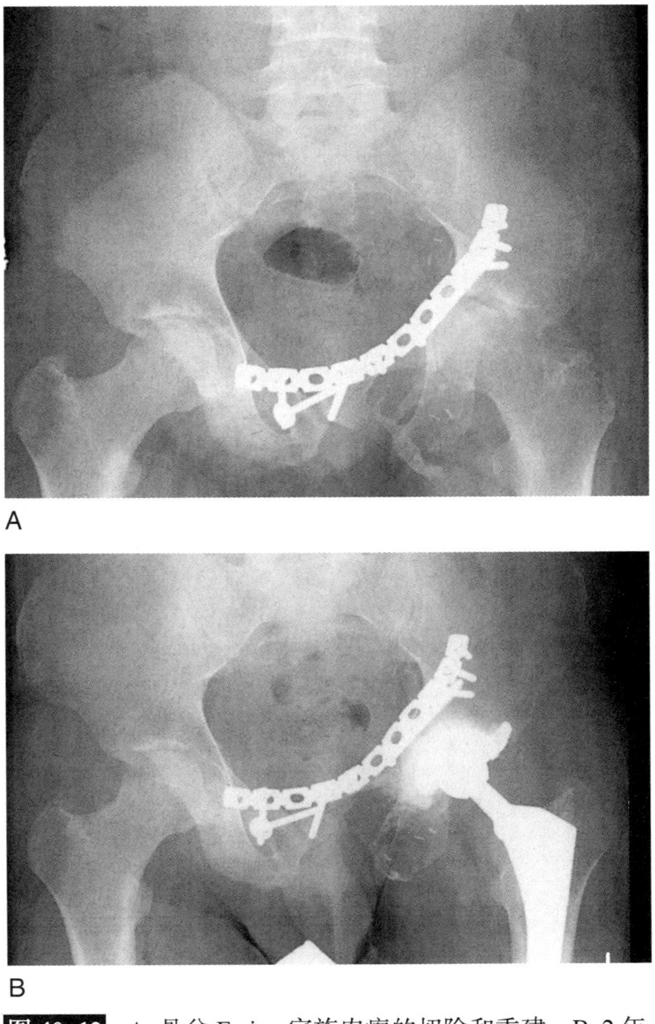

图 40-12 A. 骨盆 Ewing 家族肉瘤的切除和重建。B. 2 年后髋关节的退行性变化，需要行髋关节置换。

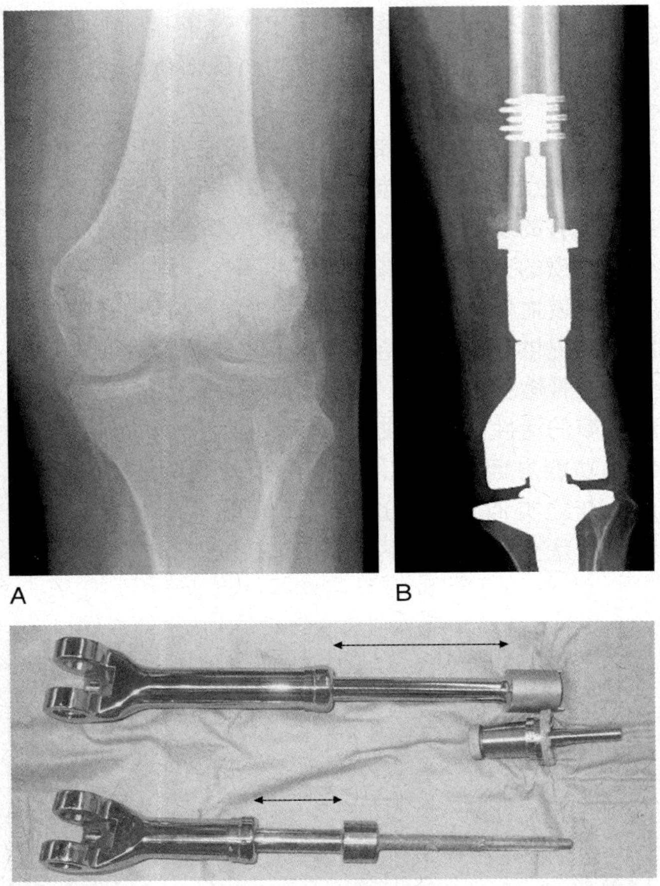

A　　B

C

图 40-13 A. 一位 16 岁女孩的骨肉瘤。B. 切除病变后置入内置假体。C. 随着患儿的生长，逐步延长假体。

关节重建是一种具有挑战的手术。生物学方法包括应用整体的异体移植（图 40-11）。它们的优点在于能够与身体相容[82]。缺点是骨折率高达 19%，骨不连达 17%，感染达 11%。骨关节异体移植也可以发生关节炎 16%。然而从理论上讲，好的相容性可以使患者完成日常的活动而不是关节替代后的强制性活动（图 40-12）。内置式假体修复容易，但是回弹性差，容易随时间的延长而发生撕裂或松弛[57,130,145]。随着技术的进步，放置时间更长的植入物可以通过更好的设计做出（图 40-13）。异体移植假体复合物是另一种方法，其重点是延长假体的放置时间、软组织关节囊附着以及假体的简化（图 40-14）。对于幼儿，现有的内置式假体太大，可以采用整体异体移植（见图 40-1）。小号的儿童植入物于成人不适用，需要进行修正，否则一定会失败而（图 40-15）。假体重建的优点在于可以立即负重，在患儿生活质量的恢复方面非常重要。实际上，多联合应用多种方法而不是单独使用。

在处理这些患儿时，生长是一个复杂问题。患儿在接受化疗期间常会出现生长滞后。但是在这之后，患儿可以恢复生长。有多种方法可以预测此种生长[3,95]。主要的原则是，股骨远端每年生长 1cm，胫骨近段每年生长 7mm。女孩一般在 14 岁停止生长，男孩在 16 岁停止生长。因此，在 10 岁男孩，关节外离断术者还有 10cm 的生长潜能。一般来讲，肢

图 40-14 A. 一位 16 岁男孩的肱骨近端骨肉瘤。B. 肱骨近端切除，同种异体假体复合物移植重建缺损。

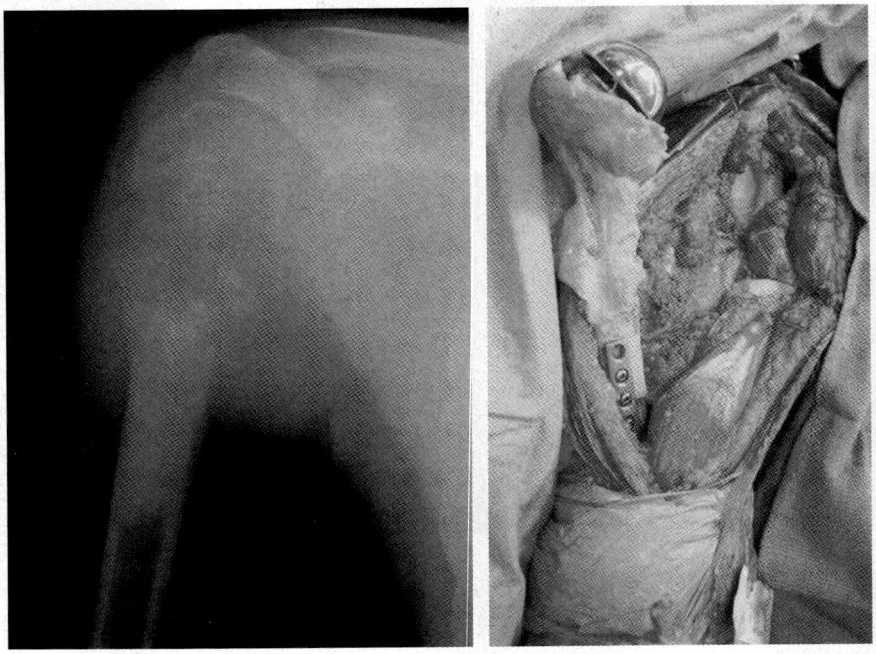

A　　B

体相差 2cm 可以自行校正而不用进行治疗。因此在这种病例中，仅需矫正 8cm 的差异。

现有的改良的方法包括对侧骺骨干固定术。这种方法是切除对侧膝关节的生长板，手术介入时机要求高，一般在患儿接近生长停止时进行。

骨延长是另一种选择。这种方法效果好，但是患儿佩戴支架时间必须较长。每天延长 1mm，短缩 8cm 的儿童佩戴支架至少要 3 个月，然后要再固定 3 个月（图 40–16）。若在化疗时段内，这一持续时间需要 2 倍。针道感染的危险甚至在健康的儿童也会有，在延长过程中发生率高达 90%[17]。在接受化疗的恶性肿瘤患儿，必须要考虑到这一点[105]。另外，其再生能力弱，易骨折（图 40–17）。化疗患儿通常骨质疏松，骨折的危险性高。

可延长假体是现代科学进步的结果，其正处于初始应用阶段[111,112,130,134]。人工设计需要重复手术以使肢
64 体周期性地延长，以便患侧肢体与正常肢体生长一致（图 40-13C）。Stanmore 植入物已应用了近 20 年，返修率为 23%[130]。但是存活率分析显示 10 年存活率接近 0[129]。自体延长的设计是通过电磁连接器或加热线圈、由动力或热量使弹簧放松而延长植入物时间。Phenix 装置在美国正在进行临床试验[138]。预试验的结果显示，并发症的发生率高达 44%[49]，需要进行改进。Repiphysis 系统应用外固定电磁场使弹簧在锁定的位置进行控制性释放。这一装置植入物的返修率达到 44%。一般地说，这些装置中的主干过于狭窄，机械应力不足，固定技术也有待改进。因此，所有这些装置的长期效果均不理想，但是短期内手术的并发症（如感染）减少。同时也能够被患者和家长所接受。

目前有许多方法来解决这些问题，但是没有哪一种方法是最好的。因此，外科医生必须根据患者的情况来具体分析具体处理，选择适当的方法。有一些方法之间可以互相补充。

特殊的考虑因素

这一部分讨论需要特别强调的各个患者的特点及其影响治疗决策的方式。在充分了解患者具体问题的基础上，讨论选择适合的治疗而不是机械地使用一种治疗方法。

年龄

诊断

在幼儿，小于 5 岁者，表现为骨缺损的患儿可能是诊断中的一个（表 40–1）。在这一年龄段的患儿中，主要考虑感染或全身性恶性肿瘤（如白血病）的局部表现。应考虑到转移疾病，在这一年龄段中，成神经细胞瘤最多见。在 5～10 岁的患儿，需要考虑 Ewing 家族肉瘤。在 11～20 岁的青少年，随着其活动增加，在评价意外创伤时，影像学应用越来越多，
许多良性疾病可以做出诊断。另外，骨肉瘤和 Ewing 665

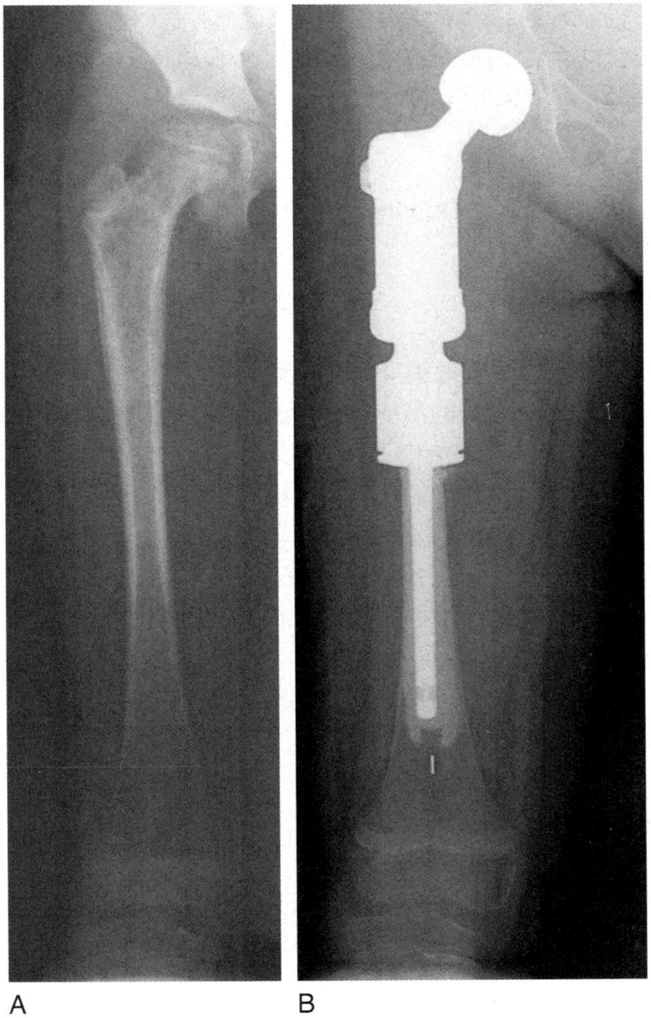

图 40–15　A. 一位 14 岁女孩的股骨近端骨肉瘤。B. 广泛切除，两极半关节置换术，同时股骨近端替代。注意股骨头与髋臼相容，因此不需要行髋臼的置换。

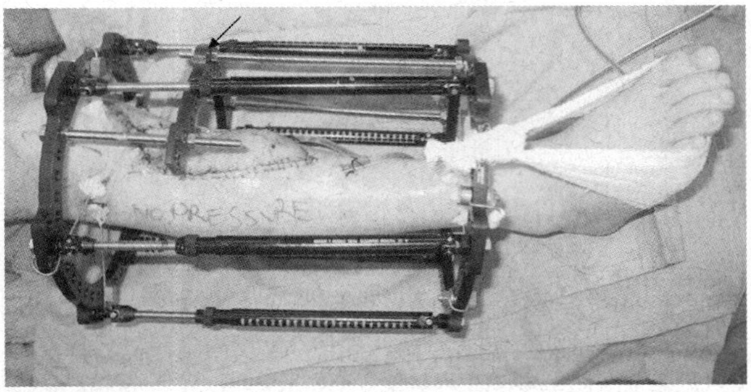

图 40-16 胫骨 Ewing 肉瘤。患者已行广泛切除及骨移植。中间的环（箭头所示）用来固定一段切除后剩余骨。5 天后临时骨痂形成。以 1mm/d 的速度将环向远端渐渐移动，骨块逐渐延长以填补骨缺损，同时与胫骨近端保持连接。这种再生比较微弱，并且延长骨的牢固需要相当长的时间。例如，80mm 的缺损需要 5 天形成临时骨痂，延长需要 80 天，牢固移去固定支架需要 80 天。在肢体延长过程中，必须忍受这种笨拙的装置。

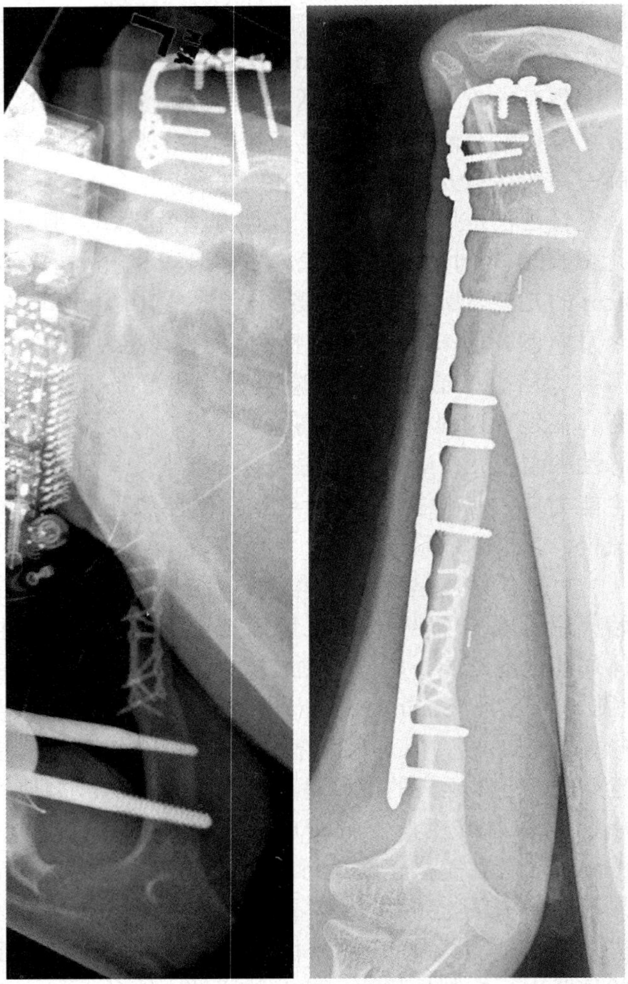

图 40-17 A. 一位 6 岁肱骨近端骨肉瘤患儿切除术后带血供的腓骨移植重建使肩关节固定。成年后肱骨短缩，后行延长术。B. 延长术后钢板保护再生。

家族肉瘤的发病逐渐增加。

生长发育

线性生长问题很早既已触及。在治疗邻近骺板的病变时，未来生长的潜能应当考虑在内。在良性病例中，当可能的非手术治疗不会造成不良预后，应当特别谨慎。因此，在典型的邻近生长板的单房性骨囊肿患者，应小心不要刮伤骺板，但是这样可能会增加复发率。然而在倾向于生长较快的骨软骨瘤患儿，生长板的损伤可能是不可避免的，需要进行局部的辅助化疗（如冷冻疗法）。与之相比，在恶性肿瘤，通过牺牲生长板而达到好的外科手术边缘也是可以接受的方法（见图 40-13）。

部位

病变部位与病理和病理生理学相关的内容已经在早些章节中叙述，这里的重点是病变部位与缺损重建的关系。

上肢

一般来讲，上肢的负重要求与下肢的负重要求有很大差异。在上肢，捕握和自理能力是手术要达到的主要目的。在下肢，负重是主要的。因此对上肢的重建，就耐久力而言要求并不是太高，但是对活动能力的要求高。下面主要讨论对大的骨缺损的治疗。腔性缺损要用适当的骨充填材料（见骨移植和骨移植的替代物）。

在肩关节，好的功能通过关节周围切除术和重建可以恢复[26,101,141]。重建的选择包括关节成形悬吊术或肩胛骨置换术（见图 40-4）。外展受限，但捕握功能好。肱骨切除术一般较容易，但是由于潜在的病理变化，仅适用于分级较低的病变。骨关节异体移植（见图 40-1）或异体假体替代（见图 40-13）可以达到较好的功能。在分级较低的病变，三角肌和旋转袖应当保留，外展通常可以接受。

肘关节由于软组织覆盖少，所以选择有限[120,131,136]。异体骨关节移植和内置式假体可以提供理想的屈伸能力以及旋前和旋后。前臂骨切除要求较高，需要处理骨间膜以及带血管的腓骨瓣移植。腕关节破坏的病例需要进行融合手术。前臂的多条神经使肌腱转移必须进行。在分析需要牺牲桡动脉还是尺动脉时，需要记录手掌的循环这一重要的指征。

手远端缺损如果是良性的很少需要治疗，但是如果视恶性的，有多种截肢术可以进行选择。

下肢

在下肢，骨盆切除可以分为髋臼上方的 I 型切除、髋臼周围部分的 II 型切除以及髋臼下方的III型切除[1,21,100]。这些手术的并发症发生率高，主要是因为内侧髂骨供给臀部后方皮瓣的血供经常在切除的过程中被破坏及手术时间长。另外，由于骨有限，重建过程非常具有挑战性。

在 I 型切除术，需要用小的支撑杆扩展剩余的半骨盆至骶骨。通常应用异体移植或自体腓骨瓣移植。有时移植是不可能的，在局部可能残留骨缺损。在 II 型切除，需要进行关节置换。通过假体植入、异体假体复合物（见图 40–12）或关节融合可以达到。III型切除通常较稳定并可以遗留骨缺损。联合缺损，尤其是在 I – II 型手术后，非常具有挑战性。治疗方法包括异体假体复合物和支撑物。偶尔后 1/4 截肢术还是有必要的。

在股骨近端病变，关节累及需要进行 II 型样关节外骨盆切除和重建。包含股骨近端病变应用假体或异体假体复合物。股骨中间和胫骨缺损处一般应用异体移植或带血供的腓骨瓣移植或两者联合使用。骨延长是另一种方法，但是如前所述，需要较长的时间，而且并发症的发生率高。近来的研究显示，针的固定装置是安全的，即使在患儿在接受化疗时。

膝关节切除术一般可以用内置式假体重建[111,130,145]。整体的骨关节移植也在应用且可以提供较良好的功能（见图 40–11）。骨关节炎可能会发生[82]。但在此处，相对传统的关节置换术可能更好。关节固定术一般不采用，尽管在适合的情况下这种方法也是一种好的替代方法[104]。

在踝关节，可以进行多种腓骨的切除术，功能恢复较好。一般来讲，做胫骨切除时，需要实关节固定施[27,29,104]。与手相似，在足推荐使用多种类型的截肢术。

转移性疾病

有关良性肿瘤的侵袭性特点和恶性肿瘤的间室化早期既已触及。这里的讨论局限于转移性骨肉瘤和 Ewing 家族肉瘤。

转移性骨肉瘤有两方面表现：病灶已经开始转移，以及尽管病情有所减轻但已经发生了转移。在诊断 2 年内出现单侧肺部转移灶者其对侧发病率较高，应择期行双侧开胸手术[121]。晚期单侧肺转移灶倾向于与对侧疾病无关。

有转移的患儿在早期其生存率为 11%～36%[9,93]。处理这类患儿要行渐进性化疗来治疗一些未能发现的微小的病灶，以及行手术介入切除微小病变。这众多学科的方法应在专科治疗中心进行。患儿可能需要在行部分肺切除术的同时切除肿瘤。

发生转移的患儿在病情减轻后可有多种预后，在不同的研究中存活率在 0～26%[42,44]。对于这些患儿，尽管处理的原则相似，但预后不同。手术介入在这些患儿仍然不失为一种有效的方法，并且是决定生存率的一项主要因素[44]。部分患儿需要进行双侧的胸腔切开术和部分实体骨肿瘤切除术[5,121]。

矛盾的是，由于预后不佳，保肢手术具有相对的治疗指征。但是，必须将手术后至化疗前的恢复时间考虑在内。医生应当选择恢复最快的手术方法。例如，可以应用粘固剂假体而不是非粘固剂植入物治疗患儿局部病变。

手术时机较为复杂。肺转移发生在原发病灶切除后者应在恢复期间行肺转移灶的切除手术。病变在化疗期间有所发展者应在一个疗程的化疗结束后行手术切除术。转移发生在化疗后者应逐渐切除，如果发生较早，可以考虑进行阶段性双侧胸腔切开术。

在这些病例，处理的目的并非是一定要治愈。医生需要通过判断预后来选择合适的治疗措施，下面是两个具体的病例。

病例 1

患儿有胫骨侵袭性骨肉瘤，皮肤表面有真菌样改变，伴有肺部多发性转移灶和淋巴结肿大。在 AJCC 分型系统中，患儿为ⅣB 型。该患儿在化疗前行截肢手术。

有几个问题，为什么该患儿不能行保肢手术。在这例患儿保肢手术要求将一个异体或带血供的腓骨瓣植入缺损处，这可能诱发明显的皮肤破损和感染的危险，从而需要游离肌瓣覆盖。同时，转移灶可能会继续进展，患儿有可能发生死亡。当行胸腔切开术切除肺部转移灶时，必须考虑到需要游离的宽大的皮瓣，因此肌肉可能不够。

第二个问题是新辅助化疗的应用。这里，由于感染伤口出现，患儿可能已有免疫受损。在这种情况下，最好的方法是截肢术。

病例 2

有左股骨远端骨肉瘤病史的患儿已经进行了肿瘤切除和重建，化疗后 2 年，现在患儿右股骨远端和胫骨近段出现了转移灶。该患儿行病灶清除术的同时性内置式假体重建。

在该患儿，截肢术不能起到治愈的效果，因为其他部位可能也存在转移灶。然而必须行手术介入使其症状减轻，因为该患儿在化疗后不久就发生了转移，可能对化疗有抵抗。

这两个病例说明，对这些患儿的处理相当复杂，只有认真考虑所有因素，才能制定合适的处理方法。

（葛翼华译　赵　黎校）

参考文献

1. Aboulafia AJ, Buch R, Mathews J, et al: Reconstruction using the saddle prosthesis following excision of primary and metastatic periacetabular tumors. Clin Orthop Relat Res 1995;(314):203-213.
2. Abudu A, Sferopoulos NK, Tillman RM, et al: The surgical treatment and outcome of pathological fractures in localised osteosarcoma. J Bone Joint Surg Br 1996;78:694-698.
3. Anderson M, Green WT, Messner MB: Growth and predictions of growth in the lower extremities. Am J Orthop 1963; 45A:1-14.
4. Araki Y, Tanaka H, Yamamoto H, et al: MR imaging of pigmented villonodular synovitis of the knee. Radiat Med 1994;12:11-15.
5. Aung L, Gorlick R, Healey JH, et al: Metachronous skeletal osteosarcoma in patients treated with adjuvant and neoadjuvant chemotherapy for nonmetastatic osteosarcoma. J Clin Oncol 2003;21:342-348.
6. Bacci G, Briccoli A, Ferrari S, et al: Neoadjuvant chemotherapy for osteosarcoma of the extremity: Long-term results of the Rizzoli's 4th protocol. Eur J Cancer 2001;37:2030-2039.
7. Bacci G, Ferrari S, Longhi A, et al: Nonmetastatic osteosarcoma of the extremity with pathologic fracture at presentation: Local and systemic control by amputation or limb salvage after preoperative chemotherapy. Acta Orthop Scand 2003;74:449-454.
8. Bacci G, Ferrari S, Longhi A, et al: High dose ifosfamide in combination with high dose methotrexate, Adriamycin and cisplatin in the neoadjuvant treatment of extremity osteosarcoma: Preliminary results of an Italian Sarcoma Group/Scandinavian Sarcoma Group pilot study. J Chemother 2002;14:198-206.
9. Bacci G, Picci P, Briccoli A, et al: Osteosarcoma of the extremity metastatic at presentation: Results achieved in 26 patients treated with combined therapy (primary chemotherapy followed by simultaneous resection of the primary and metastatic lesions). Tumori 1992;78:200-206.
10. Bauer TW, Muschler GF: Bone graft materials: An overview of the basic science. Clin Orthop Relat Res 2000;(371):10-27.
11. Berg HL, Weiland AJ: Multiple osteogenic sarcoma following bilateral retinoblastoma: A case report. J Bone Joint Surg Am 1978;60:251-253.
12. Bertoni F, Bacchini P, Staals EL: Malignancy in giant cell tumor. Skeletal Radiol 2003;32:143-146.
13. Bertoni F, Bacchini P, Staals EL: Malignancy in giant cell tumor of bone. Cancer 2003;97:2520-2529.
14. Bielack SS, Kempf-Bielack B, Delling G, et al: Prognostic factors in high-grade osteosarcoma of the extremities or trunk: An analysis of 1,702 patients treated on neoadjuvant cooperative osteosarcoma study group protocols. J Clin Oncol 2002;20:776-790.
15. Bonin G, Scamps C, Turc-Carel C, Lipinski M: Chimeric EWS-FLI1 transcript in a Ewing cell line with a complex t(11;22;14) translocation. Cancer Res 1993;53:3655-3657.
16. Brenner W, Bohuslavizki KH, Eary JF: PET imaging of osteosarcoma. J Nucl Med 2003;44:930-942.
17. Brownlow HC, Simpson AH: Complications of distraction osteogenesis: A changing pattern. Am J Orthop 2002;31:31-36.
18. Caffey J: On fibrous defects in cortical walls of growing tubular bones: Their radiologic appearance, structure, prevalence, natural course, and diagnostic significance. Adv Pediatr 1955;7:13-51.
19. Cahan WG, Woodard HQ, Higinbotham NL, et al: Sarcoma arising in irradiated bone: Report of eleven cases: 1948. Cancer 1998;82:8-34.
20. Cammisa FP Jr, Glasser DB, Otis JC, et al: The Van Nes tibial rotationplasty: A functionally viable reconstructive procedure in children who have a tumor of the distal end of the femur. J Bone Joint Surg Am 1990;72:1541-1547.
21. Campanacci M, Capanna R: Pelvic resections: The Rizzoli Institute experience. Orthop Clin North Am 1991;22:65-86.
22. Campanacci M, De Sessa L, Trentani C: Scaglietti's method for conservative treatment of simple bone cysts with local injections of methylprednisolone acetate. Ital J Orthop

Traumatol 1977;3:27-36.
23. Campanacci M, Ruggieri P, Gasbarrini A, et al: Osteoid osteoma: Direct visual identification and intralesional excision of the nidus with minimal removal of bone. J Bone Joint Surg Br 1999;81:814-820.
24. Canadell J, Forriol F, Cara JA: Removal of metaphyseal bone tumours with preservation of the epiphysis: Physeal distraction before excision. J Bone Joint Surg Br 1994; 76:127-132.
25. Capanna R, Sudanese A, Baldini N, Campanacci M: Phenol as an adjuvant in the control of local recurrence of benign neoplasms of bone treated by curettage. Ital J Orthop Traumatol 1985;11:381-388.
26. Capanna R, van Horn JR, Biagini R, et al: The Tikhoff-Linberg procedure for bone tumors of the proximal humerus: The classical "extensive" technique versus a modified "transglenoid" resection. Arch Orthop Trauma Surg 1990;109:63-67.
27. Casadei R, Ruggieri P, Giuseppe T, et al: Ankle resection arthrodesis in patients with bone tumors. Foot Ankle Int 1994;15:242-249.
28. Centers for Disease Control and Prevention, National Cancer Institute, and North American Association of Central Cancer Registries: United States Cancer Statistics: 2000 Incidence. 2000.
29. Chou LB, Malawer MM: Analysis of surgical treatment of 33 foot and ankle tumors. Foot Ankle Int 1994;15: 175-181.
30. Cook A, Raskind W, Blanton SH, et al: Genetic heterogeneity in families with hereditary multiple exostoses. Am J Hum Genet 1993;53:71-79.
31. Damien CJ, Parsons JR: Bone graft and bone graft substitutes: A review of current technology and applications. J Appl Biomater 1991;2:187-208.
32. de Alava E, Antonescu CR, Panizo A, et al: Prognostic impact of P53 status in Ewing sarcoma. Cancer 2000;89:783-792.
33. de Berg JC, Pattynama PM, Obermann WR, et al: Percutaneous computed-tomography-guided thermocoagulation for osteoid osteomas. Lancet 1995;346:350-351.
34. de Moor NG: Osteosarcoma: A review of 72 cases treated by megavoltage radiation therapy, with or without surgery. S Afr J Surg 1975;13:137-146.
35. Docquier PL, Delloye C: Treatment of simple bone cysts with aspiration and a single bone marrow injection. J Pediatr Orthop 2003;23:766-773.
36. Enneking WF: Musculoskeletal Tumor Surgery. New York: Churchill Livingstone, 1983, vol 2, p 1351.
37. Enneking, WF. Musculoskeletal Tumor Surgery. New York: Churchill Livingstone, 1983, vol 1, pp 89–122.
38. Enneking WF, Kagan A: Transepiphyseal extension of osteosarcoma: Incidence, mechanism, and implications. Cancer 1978;41:1526-1537.
39. Enneking WF, Spanier SS, Goodman MA: A system for the surgical staging of musculoskeletal sarcoma. Clin Orthop Relat Res 1980;(153):106-120.
40. Fagnou C, Michon J, Peter M, et al: Presence of tumor cells in bone marrow but not in blood is associated with adverse prognosis in patients with Ewing's tumor. Société Française d'Oncologie Pediatrique. J Clin Oncol 1998; 16:1707-1711.
41. Fain JS, Unni KK, Beabout JW, Rock MG: Nonepiphyseal giant cell tumor of the long bones: Clinical, radiologic, and pathologic study. Cancer 1993;71:3514-3519.
42. Ferrari S, Bacci G, Picci P, et al: Long-term follow-up and post-relapse survival in patients with non-metastatic osteosarcoma of the extremity treated with neoadjuvant chemotherapy. Ann Oncol 1997;8:765-771.
43. Ferrari S, Bertoni F, Mercuri M, et al: Predictive factors of disease-free survival for non-metastatic osteosarcoma of the extremity: An analysis of 300 patients treated at the Rizzoli Institute. Ann Oncol 2001;12:1145-1150.
44. Ferrari S, Briccoli A, Mercuri M, et al: Postrelapse survival in osteosarcoma of the extremities: Prognostic factors for long-term survival. J Clin Oncol 2003;21:710-715.
45. Fidler M: Prophylactic internal fixation of secondary neoplastic deposits in long bones. BMJ 1973;1:341-343.
46. Fidler M: Incidence of fracture through metastases in long bones. Acta Orthop Scand 1981;52:623-627.
47. Gherlinzoni F, Picci P, Bacci G, Campanacci D: Limb sparing versus amputation in osteosarcoma: Correlation between local control, surgical margins and tumor necrosis: Istituto Rizzoli experience. Ann Oncol 1992;3(Suppl 2): S23-S27.
48. Ghosh L, Huvos AG, Mike V: The pancreatic islets in chondrosarcoma: A qualitative and quantitative study in humans. Am J Pathol 1973;71:23-32.
49. Gitelis S, Neel MD, Wilkins RM, et al: The use of a closed expandable prosthesis for pediatric sarcomas. Chir Organi Mov 2003;88:327-333.
50. Glaubiger DL, Makuch R, Schwarz J, et al: Determination of prognostic factors and their influence on therapeutic results in patients with Ewing's sarcoma. Cancer 1980;45:2213-2219.
51. Goldie JH, Coldman AJ, Gudauskas GA: Rationale for the use of alternating non-cross-resistant chemotherapy. Cancer Treat Rep 1982;66:439-449.
52. Goldwein JW: Effects of radiation therapy on skeletal growth in childhood. Clin Orthop Relat Res 1991;(262):101-107.
53. Greene FL: AJCC Cancer Staging Manual, 6th ed. New York, Springer-Verlag, 2002.
54. Grimer RJ, Carter SR, Pynsent PB: The cost-effectiveness of limb salvage for bone tumours. J Bone Joint Surg Br 1997; 79:558-561.
55. Grimer RJ, Taminiau AM, Cannon SR: Surgical outcomes in osteosarcoma. J Bone Joint Surg Br 2002;84:395-400.
56. Haas A, Ritter SA: Benign giant-cell tumor of femur with embolic metastasis in prepuce of penis. Am J Surg 1955; 89:573-578.
57. Ham SJ, Schraffordt KH, Veth RP, et al: Limb salvage surgery for primary bone sarcoma of the lower extremities: Long-term consequences of endoprosthetic reconstructions. Ann Surg Oncol 1998;5:423-436.
58. Harrington KD: The role of surgery in the management of pathologic fractures. Orthop Clin North Am 1977; 8:841.
59. Hasegawa T, Hirose T, Sakamoto R, et al: Mechanism of pain in osteoid osteomas: An immunohistochemical study. Histopathology 1993;22:487-491.
60. Hogeboom WR, Hoekstra HJ, Mooyaart EL, et al: Magnetic resonance imaging (MRI) in evaluating in vivo response to neoadjuvant chemotherapy for osteosarcomas of the extremities. Eur J Surg Oncol 1989;15:424-430.
61. Huvos AG: "Benign" metastasis in giant cell tumor of bone. Hum Pathol 1981;12:1151.
62. Huvos AG: Bone Tumors—Diagnosis, Treatment & Prognosis, 2nd ed. Philadelphia, WB Saunders, 1991.
63. Huvos AG, Rosen G, Bretsky SS, Butler A: Telangiectatic osteogenic sarcoma: A clinicopathologic study of 124 patients. Cancer 1982;49:1679-1689.
64. Huvos AG, Rosen G, Marcove RC: Primary osteogenic sarcoma: Pathologic aspects in 20 patients after treatment

with chemotherapy en bloc resection, and prosthetic bone replacement. Arch Pathol Lab Med 1977;101:14-18.
65. Huvos AG, Woodard HQ, Cahan WG, et al: Postradiation osteogenic sarcoma of bone and soft tissues: A clinicopathologic study of 66 patients. Cancer 1985;55:1244-1255.
66. Ilyas I, Younge DA: Medical management of osteoid osteoma. Can J Surg 2002;45:435-437.
67. Jaffe HL: Tumors and Tumorous Conditions of the Bones and Joints. Philadelphia, Lea & Febiger, 1958.
68. Jaffe N, Carrasco H, Raymond K, et al: Can cure in patients with osteosarcoma be achieved exclusively with chemotherapy and abrogation of surgery? Cancer 2002;95:2202-2210.
69. Jesus-Garcia R, Seixas MT, Costa SR, et al: Epiphyseal plate involvement in osteosarcoma. Clin Orthop Relat Res 2000;(373):32-38.
70. Klenner T, Wingen F, Keppler BK, et al: Anticancer-agent-linked phosphonates with antiosteolytic and antineoplastic properties: A promising perspective in the treatment of bone-related malignancies? J Cancer Res Clin Oncol 1990;116:341-350.
71. Kose N, Gokturk E, Turgut A, et al: Percutaneous autologous bone marrow grafting for simple bone cysts. Bull Hosp Jt Dis 1999;58:105-110.
72. Kyriakos M, Land VJ, Penning HL, Parker SG: Metastatic chondroblastoma: Report of a fatal case with a review of the literature on atypical, aggressive, and malignant chondroblastoma. Cancer 1985;55:1770-1789.
73. Ladanyi M, Traganos F, Huvos AG: Benign metastasizing giant cell tumors of bone: A DNA flow cytometric study. Cancer 1989;64:1521-1526.
74. Le Merrer M, Legeai-Mallet L, Jeannin PM, et al: A gene for hereditary multiple exostoses maps to chromosome 19p. Hum Mol Genet 1994;3:717-722.
75. Lee ES: Osteosarcoma: A reconnaissance. Clin Radiol 1975; 26:5-25.
76. Levine AM, Rosenberg SA: Alkaline phosphatase levels in osteosarcoma tissue are related to prognosis. Cancer 1979;44:2291-2293.
77. Li FP, Fraumeni JF Jr: Soft-tissue sarcomas, breast cancer, and other neoplasms: A familial syndrome? Ann Intern Med 1969;71:747-752.
78. Li FP, Garber JE, Friend SH, et al: Recommendations on predictive testing for germ line p53 mutations among cancer-prone individuals. J Natl Cancer Inst 1992;84:1156-1160.
79. Lokiec F, Ezra E, Khermosh O, Wientroub S: Simple bone cysts treated by percutaneous autologous marrow grafting: A preliminary report. J Bone Joint Surg Br 1996;78:934-937.
80. Malawer MM, Dunham W: Cryosurgery and acrylic cementation as surgical adjuncts in the treatment of aggressive (benign) bone tumors: Analysis of 25 patients below the age of 21. Clin Orthop Relat Res 1991;(262):42-57.
81. Malkin D, Jolly KW, Barbier N, et al: Germline mutations of the p53 tumor-suppressor gene in children and young adults with second malignant neoplasms. N Engl J Med 1992;326:1309-1315.
82. Mankin HJ, Gebhardt MC, Jennings LC, et al: Long-term results of allograft replacement in the management of bone tumors. Clin Orthop Relat Res 1996;(324):86-97.
83. Mankin HJ, Lange TA, Spanier SS: The hazards of biopsy in patients with malignant primary bone and soft-tissue tumors. J Bone Joint Surg Am 1982;64:1121-1127.
84. Mankin HJ, Mankin CJ, Simon MA: The hazards of the biopsy, revisited. Members of the Musculoskeletal Tumor Society. J Bone Joint Surg Am 1996;78:656-663.
85. Marcove RC, Francis KC: Chondrosarcoma and altered carbohydrate metabolism. N Engl J Med 1963;268: 1399-1400.
86. Marcove RC, Huvos AG: Cartilaginous tumors of the ribs. Cancer 1971;27:794-801.
87. Marcove RC, Mike V, Hajek JV, et al: Osteogenic sarcoma under the age of twenty-one: A review of one hundred and forty-five operative cases. J Bone Joint Surg Am 1970;52:411-423.
88. Marcove RC, Miller TR: Treatment of primary and metastatic bone tumors by cryosurgery. JAMA 1969;207: 1890-1894.
89. Marcove RC, Rosen G: Radical en bloc excision of Ewing's sarcoma. Clin Orthop Relat Res 1980;(153):86-91.
90. Martin SE, Dwyer A, Kissane JM, Costa J: Small-cell osteosarcoma. Cancer 1982;50:990-996.
91. Matsuno T, Unni KK, McLeod RA, Dahlin DC: Telangiectatic osteogenic sarcoma. Cancer 1976;38:2538-2547.
92. Meyers PA, Heller G, Healey J, et al: Chemotherapy for nonmetastatic osteogenic sarcoma: The Memorial Sloan-Kettering experience. J Clin Oncol 1992;10:5-15.
93. Meyers PA, Heller G, Healey JH, et al: Osteogenic sarcoma with clinically detectable metastasis at initial presentation. J Clin Oncol 1993;11:449-453.
94. Mirra JM, Gold RH, Rand F: Disseminated nonossifying fibromas in association with cafe-au-lait spots (Jaffe-Campanacci syndrome). Clin Orthop 1982;(168):192-205.
95. Moseley CF: A straight-line graph for leg-length discrepancies. J Bone Joint Surg Am 1977;59:174-179.
96. Moser RP Jr, Madewell JE: An approach to primary bone tumors. Radiol Clin North Am 1987;25:1049-1093.
97. Mould JJ, Adam NM: The problem of avascular necrosis of bone in patients treated for Hodgkin's disease. Clin Radiol 1983;34:231-236.
98. Neer CS, Francis KC, Johnston AD, Kiernan HA Jr: Current concepts on the treatment of solitary unicameral bone cyst. Clin Orthop Relat Res 1973;(97):40-51.
99. Norton KI, Hermann G, Abdelwahab IF, et al: Epiphyseal involvement in osteosarcoma. Radiology 1991;180:813-816.
100. O'Connor MI, Sim FH: Salvage of the limb in the treatment of malignant pelvic tumors. J Bone Joint Surg Am 1989;71:481-494.
101. O'Connor MI, Sim FH, Chao EY: Limb salvage for neoplasms of the shoulder girdle: Intermediate reconstructive and functional results. J Bone Joint Surg Am 1996;78: 1872-1888.
102. Peat BG, Bell RS, Davis A, et al: Wound-healing complications after soft-tissue sarcoma surgery. Plast Reconstr Surg 1994;93:980-987.
103. Persson BM, Wouters HW: Curettage and acrylic cementation in surgery of giant cell tumors of bone. Clin Orthop Relat Res 1976;(120):125-133.
104. Renard AJ, Veth RP, Schreuder HW, et al: Function and complications after ablative and limb-salvage therapy in lower extremity sarcoma of bone. J Surg Oncol 2000;73: 198-205.
105. Rodl R, Gosheger G, Leidinger B, et al: Correction of leg-length discrepancy after hip transposition. Clin Orthop Relat Res 2003;(416):271-277.
106. Rosen G, Nirenberg A, Caparros B, et al: Osteogenic sarcoma: Eight-percent, three-year, disease-free survival with combination chemotherapy (T-7). Natl Cancer Inst Monogr 1981;(56):213-220.
107. Rosenthal DI, Hornicek FJ, Wolfe MW, et al: Percutaneous radiofrequency coagulation of osteoid osteoma compared with operative treatment. J Bone Joint Surg Am 1998;80:815-821.
108. Rosito P, Mancini AF, Rondelli R, et al: Italian Cooperative

Study for the treatment of children and young adults with localized Ewing sarcoma of bone: A preliminary report of 6 years of experience. Cancer 1999;86:421-428.
109. Rougraff BT, Kling TJ: Treatment of active unicameral bone cysts with percutaneous injection of demineralized bone matrix and autogenous bone marrow. J Bone Joint Surg Am 2002;84:921-929.
110. Scaglietti O, Marchetti PG, Bartolozzi P: The effects of methylprednisolone acetate in the treatment of bone cysts: Results of three years follow-up. J Bone Joint Surg Br 1979;61:200-204.
111. Schiller C, Windhager R, Fellinger EJ, et al: Extendable tumour endoprostheses for the leg in children. J Bone Joint Surg Br 1995;77:608-614.
112. Schindler OS, Cannon SR, Briggs TW, et al: Use of extendable total femoral replacements in children with malignant bone tumors. Clin Orthop Relat Res 1998;(357): 157-170.
113. Scully SP, Ghert MA, Zurakowski D, et al: Pathologic fracture in osteosarcoma: Prognostic importance and treatment implications. J Bone Joint Surg Am 2002;84:49-57.
114. Scully SP, Temple HT, O'Keefe RJ, et al: The surgical treatment of patients with osteosarcoma who sustain a pathologic fracture. Clin Orthop Relat Res 1996;(324):227-232.
115. Selch MT, Parker RG: Radiation therapy in the management of Langerhans cell histiocytosis. Med Pediatr Oncol 1990;18:97-102.
116. Sim FH, Unni KK, Beabout JW, Dahlin DC: Osteosarcoma with small cells simulating Ewing's tumor. J Bone Joint Surg Am 1979;61:207-215.
117. Simon MA, Aschliman MA, Thomas N, Mankin HJ: Limb-salvage treatment versus amputation for osteosarcoma of the distal end of the femur. J Bone Joint Surg Am 1986; 68:1331-1337.
118. Simon MA, Bos GD: Epiphyseal extension of metaphyseal osteosarcoma in skeletally immature individuals. J Bone Joint Surg Am 1980;62:195-204.
119. Solomon L: Bone growth in diaphysial aclasis. J Bone Joint Surg Br 1961;43:700-716.
120. Sperling JW, Pritchard DJ, Morrey BF: Total elbow arthroplasty after resection of tumors at the elbow. Clin Orthop Relat Res 1999;(367):256-261.
121. Su WT, Chewning J, Abramson S, et al: Surgical management and outcome of osteosarcoma patients with unilateral pulmonary metastases. J Pediatr Surg 2004;39:418-423.
122. Suit HD: Role of therapeutic radiology in cancer of bone. Cancer 1975;35:930-935.
123. Thorpe WP, Reilly JJ, Rosenberg SA: Prognostic significance of alkaline phosphatase measurements in patients with osteogenic sarcoma receiving chemotherapy. Cancer 1979;43:2178-2181.
124. Toguchida J, Yamaguchi T, Dayton SH, et al: Prevalence and spectrum of germline mutations of the p53 gene among patients with sarcoma. N Engl J Med 1992;326:1301-1308.
125. Tomford WW: Bone allografts: Past, present and future. Cell Tissue Bank 2000;1:105-109.
126. Tsuchiya H, Abdel-Wanis ME, Uehara K, et al: Cannulation of simple bone cysts. J Bone Joint Surg Br 2002;84:245-248.
127. Tucker MA, D'Angio GJ, Boice JD Jr, et al: Bone sarcomas linked to radiotherapy and chemotherapy in children. N Engl J Med 1987;317:588-593.
128. Unni KK: Dahlin's Bone Tumors—General Aspects and Data on 11,087 Cases, 5th ed. Philadelphia, Lippincott-Raven, 1996.
129. Unwin PS, Blunn GW: Advances in the design of extendible replacements: An analysis of 597 replacements. In: Proceedings of the Musculoskeletal Tumor Society, Long Beach, CA: Musculosketal Tumor Society, 2004, p 51.
130. Unwin PS, Walker PS: Extendible endoprostheses for the skeletally immature. Clin Orthop Relat Res 1996;(322): 179-193.
131. Urbaniak JR, Aitken M: Clinical use of bone allografts in the elbow. Orthop Clin North Am 1987;18:311-321.
132. Vaccaro AR, Chiba K, Heller JG, et al: Bone grafting alternatives in spinal surgery. Spine J 2002;2:206-215.
133. Van Nes CP: Rotation-plasty for congenital defects of the femur: Making use of the shortened limb to control the knee joint of a prosthesis. J Bone Joint Surg Br 1950;32:12-16.
134. Verkerke GJ, Schraffordt KH, Veth RP, et al: An extendable modular endoprosthetic system for bone tumour management in the leg. J Biomed Eng 1990;12:91-96.
135. Vigorita VJ: Orthopaedic Pathology. Philadelphia, Lippincott Williams & Wilkins, 1999.
136. Weber KL, Lin PP, Yasko AW: Complex segmental elbow reconstruction after tumor resection. Clin Orthop Relat Res 2003;(415):31-44.
137. Wilkins RM, Cullen JW, Odom L, et al: Superior survival in treatment of primary nonmetastatic pediatric osteosarcoma of the extremity. Ann Surg Oncol 2003;10: 498-507.
138. Wilkins RM, Soubeiran A: The Phenix expandable prosthesis: Early American experience. Clin Orthop Relat Res 2001;(382):51-58.
139. Winkelmann WW: Hip rotationplasty for malignant tumors of the proximal part of the femur. J Bone Joint Surg Am 1986;68:362-369.
140. Winkelmann WW: Type-B-IIIa hip rotationplasty: An alternative operation for the treatment of malignant tumors of the femur in early childhood. J Bone Joint Surg Am 2000;82:814-828.
141. Wittig JC, Bickels J, Kellar-Graney KL, et al: Osteosarcoma of the proximal humerus: Long-term results with limb-sparing surgery. Clin Orthop Relat Res 2002;397:156-176.
142. Wu YQ, Heutink P, de Vries BB, et al: Assignment of a second locus for multiple exostoses to the pericentromeric region of chromosome 11. Hum Mol Genet 1994;3: 167-171.
143. Wunder JS, Paulian G, Huvos AG, et al: The histological response to chemotherapy as a predictor of the oncological outcome of operative treatment of Ewing sarcoma. J Bone Joint Surg Am 1998;80:1020-1033.
144. Yandow SM, Lundeen GA, Scott SM, Coffin C: Autogenic bone marrow injections as a treatment for simple bone cyst. J Pediatr Orthop 1998;18:616-620.
145. Zeegen EN, Aponte-Tinao LA, Hornicek FJ, et al: Survivorship analysis of 141 modular metallic endoprostheses at early followup. Clin Orthop Relat Res 2004; 420:239-250.

第 41 章

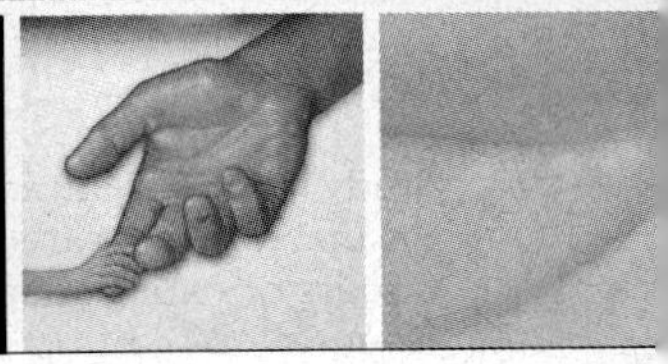

脑肿瘤

Phillip B. Storm 和 Leslie N. Sutton

除了外伤以外，肿瘤是 15 岁以下儿童的最为常见的死亡原因。儿童实体肿瘤中最为常见的发生部位是中枢神经系统，死亡率在所有肿瘤死亡率中占 20%，是继白血病后第二大好发肿瘤[20,22,70]。儿童脑肿瘤每年被诊断出的约为 1700 例，在儿童中的发生率约为 3.1/100 000[10]。

脑肿瘤诊断的重要因素是部位、年龄和细胞类型。发生部位在影像学上最为重要，其次是年龄。颅脑被天幕分成上下两个部分。天幕的上方（幕上）有大脑半球、基底节和丘脑。天幕的下方（幕下）有松果体、顶盖、脑桥、延髓和小脑。与成人脑肿瘤多发生在幕上不同，儿童脑肿瘤幕上、幕下分布比较平均。另外，肿瘤的分布还与年龄有关。小于 2 岁的婴幼儿脑肿瘤多分布在幕上，而 3～15 岁儿童的脑肿瘤多分布在幕下（表 41–1）[15,20]。除了脉络丛乳头状瘤以外，1 岁以下儿童脑肿瘤的预后很差[8]。

随着免疫组化技术的发展，使得儿童脑肿瘤能够按照组织学类型进行分类。颅内任何类型的细胞都能转变成肿瘤。脑组织由神经元和胶质细胞组成。胶质细胞提供营养和支持，数量远多于神经元。胶质细胞主要由三种组成：星形细胞、少突胶质细胞和室管膜细胞，胶质瘤即由这些细胞转变而来。再细分的话，这些细胞可各自转变成星形细胞瘤、少突胶质瘤和室管膜瘤。同时涉及神经元和胶质细胞的肿瘤称为神经节细胞瘤，包括神经节神经胶质瘤、促结缔组织生成的婴儿型神经节神经胶质瘤和神经节细胞瘤。另外一种混合型的神经元和神经胶质细胞来源的肿瘤是胚胎期发育不良神经上皮瘤（DNET）。最后一种是胚胎性肿瘤或称原始神经外胚层肿瘤（PNET）。胚胎性肿瘤包括髓母细胞瘤、髓上皮瘤、神经母细胞瘤、婴儿黑色素神经外胚层瘤和非典型畸胎样 / 杆状瘤（ATRT）。

临床表现

儿童脑肿瘤的症状和体征因肿瘤的类型、部位、年龄不同而表现不一。如果没有癫痫和局灶性的神经损害，如第 6 对颅神经麻痹引起的复视，脑肿瘤引起的大多数症状是非特异性的，早期往往考虑是那些常见的不严重的疾病所引起。常见的症状有头痛、恶心、呕吐、昏睡、明显的性格改变以及学习成绩下降。这些症状常被认为是胃肠道疾病、抑郁、上学焦虑症、偏头痛、鼻窦炎或是配戴眼镜引起的。甚至一个长期存在的癫痫病最终可能是由一个幕上肿瘤所引起。婴儿典型的症状为活动减少、摄入量减低、头围增大和昏睡。

表 41–1　儿童脑肿瘤

年龄（岁）	肿瘤组织学类型
0～2	畸胎瘤
	原发性神经外胚层肿瘤
	星形细胞瘤（高度）
	脉络丛乳头状瘤
2～15	幕上肿瘤（50%）
	星形细胞瘤（低分级）
	颅咽管瘤
	下丘脑胶质瘤
	原发性神经外胚层肿瘤
	室管膜瘤
	脉络丛乳头状瘤
	幕下肿瘤（50%）
	原发性神经外胚层肿瘤（髓母细胞瘤）
	小脑星形细胞瘤
	室管膜瘤
	脑干胶质瘤

72 2～14 岁儿童典型的脑肿瘤症状为头痛、恶心、呕吐、步态不稳和（或）复视，发作时间为几天到几周，核磁共振（MRI）显示后颅窝中线处有一个强化的肿瘤灶伴脑积水。实际上，这些症状是因为发生脑积水的缘故，而不是肿瘤本身。儿童头痛在病毒感染时很常见，但是，如果经常每天早晨都发生的头痛，常需警惕有颅内占位性病变发生的可能，特别是在没有发热和病毒感染后遗症的情况下。颅内压升高的患者常常在清晨症状加重，因为与直立位相比，躺着过夜的体位更能引起颅内压的升高。另外，睡眠时呼吸减慢、PCO_2 升高，同样也能引起颅内压的升高。颅内压升高还能引起小脑扁桃体疝入到枕骨大孔，导致后枕部疼痛和颈部疼痛。

这里有两种肿瘤引起恶心和呕吐的机制：一种是颅内压升高，另一种是肿瘤对呕吐中枢的直接刺激或浸润。呕吐中枢位于第四脑室底部，容易受大的后颅窝肿瘤压迫或者直接受到脑干肿瘤浸润的影响，从而出现呕吐。因为延髓内的肿瘤可以在没有出现其他神经系统症状以前仅引起呕吐，所以持续的呕吐应该怀疑到有后颅窝肿瘤的可能性，在没有进行详细病史和神经系统检查时而不应该归咎为如反流性胃肠道疾病。运动共济失调症的孩子常常被其父母描述成走路笨拙，“像喝醉酒一样的走路”，走路的时候头斜向或倒向一侧。

后颅窝肿瘤引起的视觉症状，最常见的是复视及两眼向上看困难（两眼落日征），偶尔伴有视力减退。同样，这些症状也是脑积水的表现。视力减退是由于视乳头水肿的关系。视觉缺失更常见于鞍上肿瘤，是由于肿瘤的直接压迫导致视神经萎缩。后颅窝肿瘤的患者由于在视觉症状出现以前还可以有其他症状，所以常常行 MRI 检查以确诊。因此缺乏视觉症状和体征的患者并不能排除肿瘤。然而，仍然也有一些患者在体检时发现有视觉缺失从而被查出有后颅窝肿瘤。

虽然儿童典型的肿瘤多发生在后颅窝，但还是有很多幕上肿瘤，尤其是在 2 岁以下儿童中。2 岁以下儿童的症状多表现为运动减少、偏瘫、癫痫或前囟饱满、头围增大[18,35,43]。2 岁以上儿童的症状与成人相似，有头痛和（或）癫痫。肿瘤内出血常可引起患者有突然发作的严重头痛和（或）快速的精神状况恶化。偶尔，阻塞性脑积水也能引起症状快速的恶化，但是由于肿瘤的生长速度相对较慢，肿瘤所表现的症状常常比阻塞性脑积水发生晚一些。

较少见的症状和体征为内分泌异常，如体重增加、体重减轻、糖尿病发作，身材矮小、身材高大，青春期延迟。肿瘤侵及下丘脑垂体轴可引起乳房发育分泌。邻近部位肿瘤压迫视神经和视交叉常引起视力减退、视野缺失，但很多情况下是没有症状的。

放射学评价

怀疑有脑肿瘤的患者需要进行 MRI 平扫或 MRI 平扫 + 增强。虽然 MRI 检查是金标准，但是有脑肿瘤症状和体征的患者在进入急诊室时需行 CT 平扫检查无需造影剂。CT 对诊断脑积水和脑出血这两个可引起神经功能快速恶化的主要原因是很有效的。另外，CT 检查在几分钟内即可完成，常常不需要用镇静剂，价格便宜，能显出很好的详细的影像学信息。如果患者情况快速恶化，通常需要急诊手术，需要进行 CT 对比增强扫描，以便让放射科医生和神经外科医生了解更多的肿瘤信息。如果患者病情稳定，CT 对比增强扫描可以省略，取而代之的是 MRI 平扫或 MRI 平扫 + 增强。至于选择哪种方法，需要根据患者的临床表现来决定。

MRI 能提供更好的颅内结构分辨率，以及矢状面、冠状面和横断面的图像。同时，运用新的图像序列和光谱，甚至可以做出特殊的组织学诊断[62]。这些特点明显优于仅能提供横断面的 CT 扫描。另外，由于颅底骨伪影的影响，CT 扫描很难评价低位脑干的情况。MRI 的缺陷是不能够很好的显示瘤内的钙化，所以，偶尔患者需要 CT、MRI 同时检查以帮助做出准确的诊断。

造影剂能够提供更多的肿瘤信息。由衬在脑毛细血管上的内皮细胞紧密连接组成的血脑屏障，能阻止包括造影剂在内的大多数血液内的物质进入脑组织。某些脑肿瘤能破坏血脑屏障，允许造影剂进入肿瘤内，在增强的 T1 加权像上显示有强化。一般而言，特别是在成人，中轴线内占位性病变的强化意味着肿瘤更具有侵犯性，预后更差。然而儿童肿瘤却不完全相同，也有强化的肿瘤没有浸润性，完全可以切除并治愈。一般来说，不强化的肿瘤，很少有浸润性的生长。

在 MRI 读片时，需要考虑的重要因素有：（1）肿瘤的部位（幕上、幕下、松果体区、鞍上）；（2）

肿瘤是在中轴线内（脑组织内）还是在中轴线外（脑
673 组织外）；（3）患儿年龄；（4）是否有强化；（5）单个还是多个。综合以上几点因素，通过全面的读片，可以缩小诊断范围，为制定手术计划提供有效的帮助。

如果是脑内多发性占位，或者根据部位及强化怀疑是转移性肿瘤或者是肿瘤可能椎管内种植的，此时需要做脊髓的 MRI 平扫或 MRI 平扫加增强扫描。在颅脑肿瘤手术前最好是能够先做脊髓 MRI，但是往往由于临床体检阴性而没有做这方面检查。

所有脑肿瘤患者术后 48 小时内需做 MRI 检查以评估肿瘤切除的范围，是否有脑积水、出血或缺血。强调在 48 小时内做 MRI 检查非常重要，因为 48 小时后脑组织瘢痕形成，强化的瘢痕和残留的肿瘤组织就很难区分。如果患者术前没有做脊髓的 MRI 检查，组织学诊断肿瘤有可能椎管内种植，那么手术后 2 周内应该做 MRI 检查。

手术治疗

手术治疗的目的是在安全的前提下，尽量多的切除肿瘤，获取组织学诊断，重新建立正常的脑脊液通路或分流脑脊液。肿瘤的部位常常决定着肿瘤被切除的程度。事实上，有些肿瘤由于生长部位的特殊性以及 MRI 有能力进行确诊，因此，可以不需要手术获取标本。例如，脑桥区的胶质瘤，一种脑干内的星形细胞瘤，手术风险很大，无法完全切除，而 MRI 又能明确诊断。这些患者可以交给神经肿瘤科医生处理，而不需手术确诊。另外一种不需要手术获取样本就能确诊的例子是松果体区肿瘤。松果体区肿瘤的患者需要做血清绒毛膜促性腺激素（β-HCG）、α-胎蛋白（AFP）和胎盘碱性磷酸酶（PLAP）测定。如果结果是阴性，还需要做脑脊液检查。阳性结果即可获得松果体区生殖细胞瘤的诊断。治疗方法是立体定向放射治疗，不需要组织学诊断。对于生殖细胞瘤的治愈率可达 100%。

然而，大多数的肿瘤需要手术干预，包括立体定向活检或颅脑开放手术。制定手术计划的最重要工具是 MRI。丘脑和基底节区的浸润性肿瘤通常采取立体定向活检。这需要在患者颅骨上安装一个 MRI 相兼容的硬性头架，然后患者行 MRI 检查，并调整 X，Y，Z 的位置。头架上 X，Y，Z 位置的调整，能使穿刺针精确地进入到脑组织预定位置。立体定向手术的优点是手术时间短，术后 1 天即可出院，对于那些风险大，死亡率及并发症高，无法进行开颅手术部位的肿瘤，可用立体定向手术取代以获取组织学诊断。立体定向的缺点是给予病理诊断的肿瘤组织量少；术中如果出血有时很难发现，直到术后病情恶化才发现；如果立体定向手术后还不能确诊，需要神外科医生开颅手术获取诊断，患者面临第二次手术，并且得到的肿瘤组织可能因为前次手术而不能真正代表肿瘤的实际级别。

绝大多数儿童肿瘤需要开颅手术切除或活检，争取通过显微外科的手术方式尽量将肿瘤完全切除，因为许多肿瘤的预后与术后肿瘤残余量关系非常密切[59]。大脑半球的肿瘤可通过开颅手术切除。手术方案的制订可通过 MRI 及无头架立体定向导航技术进行。导航技术能够使神经外科医生在手术室内通过冠状面、矢状面、横断面观察肿瘤，制定手术切口并找到肿瘤。该技术的不足之处是肿瘤的观察和定位是在手术前不是实时的，当脑组织被牵开、囊液或脑脊液被引流后，脑组织移位，肿瘤发生偏移，术前的肿瘤定位出现偏差。此时，可通过手术中超声寻找肿瘤以弥补上述不足。术中 MRI 可以在手术中重新定位，从而纠正术前导航的偏差。然而，术中 MRI 最大限制在于分辨率差，因为磁场与传统的 MRI 相比相当弱。但是仍旧是令人鼓舞的技术，一旦分辨率问题得到解决，将可用于所有肿瘤病例，是神外科医生的很有价值的工具。功能性 MRI 技术能用来定位语言和运动皮层，当肿瘤和这些部位有关时，功能性 MRI 能帮助医生选择一个最安全的地方切开大脑皮层，切除肿瘤[48]。功能性 MRI 需要患者在清醒状态下合作，这对于小儿神经外科是一个挑战。电生理记录和刺激有时对定位运动区有帮助。

虽然这些先进技术可给予神经外科医生足够重要的帮助，但是神外科医生仍旧需要有扎实的颅脑三维立体解剖的概念。在选择手术路径时，如果可能应选择解剖面进入，如大脑半球裂、大脑侧裂以及颅底以避免切开正常脑组织。如果没有解剖平面可利用，则选择切开最少量的脑组织入路，当然应该避开功能区皮层如语言和运动皮层。

中线部位的肿瘤（下丘脑肿瘤、丘脑肿瘤、基底节肿瘤和脑干肿瘤）曾经被认为是不能够手术的部位。然而，现在显微外科技术和导航设备的发展，使得这些部位的肿瘤也能够被切除。同时，化疗、单剂量和分级放射手术的发展也给这些部位的肿瘤的治疗提供了多种方法。但是还不清楚是其中某一个环节还是联合治疗起了最有效的作用。松果体区肿瘤可以从后颅窝入路，将小脑从天幕上牵开；或者通过幕上入路，经两个大脑半球之间通过后胼胝体入路或者直接打开天幕。松果体肿瘤与天幕的关系决定着手术入
74 路。

小脑半球和低位脑干的肿瘤是由小脑入路进行开颅手术。第四脑室中线处肿瘤常伴有阻塞性脑积水。虽然有些神经外科医生喜欢在肿瘤切除以前放置分流管，但是现在多数医生倾向于给予患者激素以及在肿瘤切除术中打通四脑室，术后根据需要，或者去除或者转换分流管。20%～40%的儿童最终需要安置分流管[33]。患者俯卧位，去除小脑骨瓣，偶尔也需要切除 C1 环的后部。剪开硬脑膜后，垂直切开小脑蚓部，进入第四脑室，用双极电凝、吸引器或超声吸引器将肿瘤切除。侧面的桥小脑角的肿瘤需要牵开小脑内侧面，沿着颅神经分离，用电生理监测仪测定分离Ⅴ、Ⅶ、Ⅷ、Ⅸ、Ⅹ、Ⅺ和Ⅻ颅神经。脑干肿瘤如果是低位的，位于背侧并向外生长组织学分级低，也有可能大块切除，缝合硬膜后，再用神经补片覆盖，并用胶原产物加强硬膜，颅骨缺损的替补品可以不用。术后的问题有急性脑积水、假性脑膜膨出、无菌性脑膜炎、缄默症、假性延髓瘫痪、颅神经或脑干功能障碍、胃肠道出血和脊柱不稳定[58]。有吞咽困难和呼吸困难的患者需要行气管切开和胃造瘘进食。

肿瘤类型

小脑星形细胞瘤

这些肿瘤在组织学上通常为良性肿瘤，并且能通过手术完全切除而治愈。发病的平均时间为 9 岁，患者表现为恶性呕吐、间断性早晨头痛发作和平衡障碍，常持续几个月。典型的 CT 表现[71]为一个低密度囊性小脑肿块，靠近蚓部，强化非常明显，呈腔壁结节样强化。然而有约 1/4 的肿瘤是完全实质性的。MRI 检查有助于确定手术解剖界面，特别是肿瘤与脑干的关系以及囊肿壁的特性。典型的小脑星形细胞瘤在 MRI 上的表现为 T1 像呈低密度信号，T2 像信号增强，静脉注射造影剂后肿瘤实质部分强化（图 41–1）。常可同时伴有阻塞性脑积水。

组织学上，肿瘤常由良性外观的星形细胞组成。亚型有幼稚的纤维状细胞型（60%）和原纤维型（30%）。也有呈浸润型的，这可能预示着预后很差[21]。详细的检查能显示细胞的多形性和肿瘤向蛛网膜下腔蔓延，但是这些肿瘤很少有播散。恶性肿瘤很少见，常需要进一步放射治疗[57]。

治疗的方法是手术完全切除肿瘤。这在大多数没有侵及脑干的病例中是可以做到的。影像学证实肿瘤完全切除的病例很少有复发，也不需要做其他的辅助治疗[1]。所以，如果术后影像学检查发现有残余肿瘤，建议再次手术完全切除肿瘤。如果是多次复发或肿瘤侵及脑干不能完全切除者，则考虑行放射治疗，但即使在这种情况下，残余肿瘤仍能够保持多年不发生变化而不需要特殊治疗。对怀疑有残留肿瘤的患者，需术后定期影像学随访。如果条件允许，复发的肿瘤还需要再次手术。

原发性神经外胚层肿瘤和髓母细胞瘤

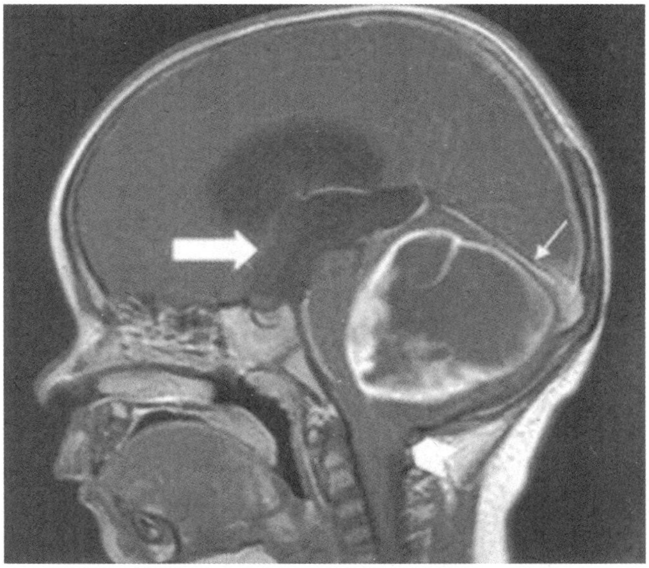

图 41–1 一位 2 岁的女孩，呕吐和昏睡数天。轴位 T1 像增强 MRI 显示一个大的后颅窝肿瘤，位于小脑底部（小箭头所示）。病人有脑积水（大箭头显示扩张的第三脑室）。她还有小脑扁桃体疝入到枕骨大孔（星状箭头所示）。术中诊断小脑星形细胞瘤。

后颅窝原发性神经外胚层肿瘤（PNET）称为髓母细胞瘤。髓母细胞瘤是儿童最常见的恶性肿瘤。组织学上，典型的髓母细胞瘤由致密的包裹细胞组成，核深染，胞浆小，苏木精和伊红组织学切片染色为蓝色。当肿瘤位于后颅窝时，就称为髓母细胞瘤或后颅窝原发性外胚层肿瘤。这种肿瘤也可以发生在大脑半球，称为幕上原发性神经外胚层肿瘤。髓母细胞瘤的儿童典型症状为头痛、呕吐和短时昏睡；确诊时的平
675 均年龄比小脑星形细胞瘤要小。婴儿表现为萎靡。幕上的原发性神经外胚层肿瘤表现为颅内压增高以及肿瘤压迫引起的局部神经损害症状。

典型的髓母细胞瘤 CT 扫描显示边界清楚的等密度的肿块，充填于第四脑室，并引起阻塞性脑积水；然而与室管膜瘤不同的是这种肿瘤没有钙化。肿瘤强化明显。MRI 显示各种信号的特征。T1 像呈略低密度影，在液体衰减转化回复序列上变得明亮，T2 像可能明亮也可能灰暗，注入造影剂通常显示强化（图 41–2）。术前或术后有必要做脊柱 MRI 检查，以判断有无脊髓转移（种植转移）。

治疗的第一步是手术切除并获得病理诊断。单靠手术是不能治愈这些肿瘤的。在肿瘤有转移或肿瘤广泛侵犯脑干的情况下，虽然可以将肿瘤大块切除，但不要试图将生命中枢内的肿瘤切除。手术后需行全颅脑和脊髓的放射治疗肿瘤基底部需大剂量强化照射。婴幼儿放射治疗的后遗症是认识障碍这是由根据年龄和剂量进行的全脑放射治疗造成的[38]。由于化疗已被证明对新发现的和复发的髓母细胞瘤都有效[14,30,40,63]，近期系列报道在试图减少、取消或延迟放疗，而由化疗取代，特别是在婴幼儿组[12]。为了制定最佳治疗方案，很有必要制定分期标准以确定高危组。过去，运用 Chang 体系评价高危组，即通过外科医生术中评估肿瘤的大小以及术后通过影像学判断转移程度[9]。现在，在绝大多数的临床中心，高危组的划定是根据小年龄、术后肿瘤残余以及肿瘤转移而定[31,39,40]。

肿瘤的 5 年生存率为 70%以上，某些高危组则不到 30%[14]。近期的一些报道显示，与低危组单独使用放疗相比，高危组的患者在辅助化疗后生存率有了提高[40]。

患者需要神经肿瘤多学科的长期支持和关爱。随访扫描被证明没有价值，因为经过第一次治疗后复发的肿瘤患者几乎都不可避免地最后死亡[64]。治疗的远期并发症有垂体功能障碍[11]、生长延迟[47]、心肌病[28]、

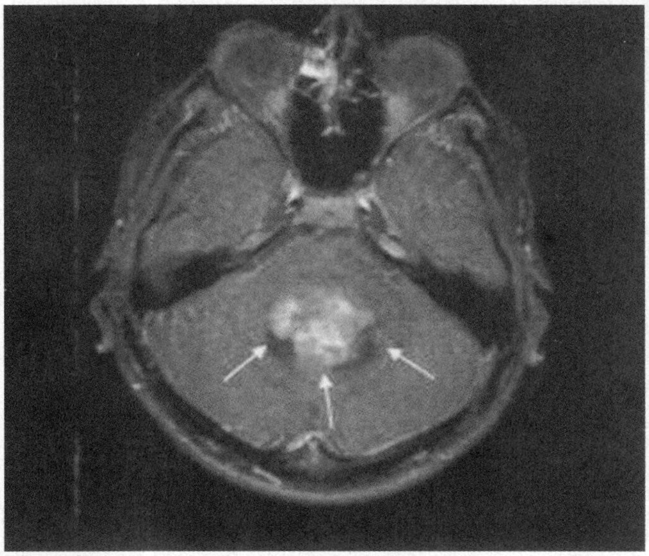

图 41–2 一位 8 岁的男孩，表现为几个星期晨间头痛和呕吐。轴位 T1 加权图像增强 MRI 扫描显示一个不均匀强化的第四脑室内占位性病变（箭头所示）。肿瘤像室管膜瘤一样阻塞了 CSF 通路（Luschka 孔）。病理诊断为髓母细胞瘤。

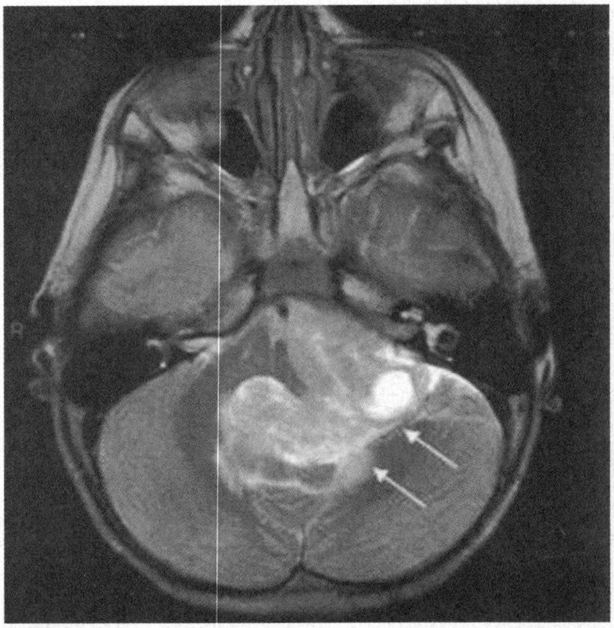

图 41–3 一位 18 个月的男孩，表现为头痛伴呕吐 3 天，步态不稳 2 天。入院当天，在家出现意识丧失。急诊 MRI 显示一个很大的后颅窝肿瘤。轴位 T2 加权图像 MRI 显示肿瘤占据第四脑室，阻塞 Luschka 孔，侵入脑桥小脑角，侵犯所有的后颅窝颅神经（箭头所示）。肿瘤为室管膜瘤。

认识延迟[49]、社会心理调节和家庭问题，以及放疗引起的脑膜瘤、星形细胞瘤和肉瘤[25]。

室管膜瘤

脑管瘤可以发生在第四脑室或桥小脑角（图
76 41–3），脊髓或幕上。组织学类型大多数为良性，但是尽管如此，它们仍旧归类为最差的儿童脑肿瘤范围。它们在局部肿瘤基底部有复发的倾向，也能够沿着神经轴转移。平均确诊年龄在 3～5 岁[23]，但是在婴幼儿和成年人却不多见。当肿瘤发生在后颅窝时（75%的病例），引起的症状与在该部位的其他肿瘤相似。当有颅神经及脑干功能障碍时，常提示肿瘤已向这些部位侵犯。室管膜瘤的特征是不伴有脑积水的呕吐，这是因为肿瘤侵及呕吐中枢的缘故。儿童室管膜瘤发生在幕上时，通常都非常大，尽管起源于室管膜，也有可能与脑室不相连。

CT 的典型表现为等密度肿块伴有斑点状钙化以及不均一的强化。后颅窝的占位能够通过第四脑室出口（Luschka）进入到桥小脑角。室管膜瘤的核磁共振表现为 T1 加权图像的等密度到低密度影和 T2 加权图像的高密度影[55]。增强后呈不均匀强化。

治疗的第一步是手术。预后与手术肿瘤切除的程度关系非常密切，肿瘤切除的程度需要靠术后影像学确定。完全切除后的 5 年生存率为 60%～80%，而未完全切除的 5 年生存率则不到 30%[26]。放射手术切除会引起永久性的神经损伤，某些病例除外。术后针对肿瘤部位进行大范围放疗，除非肿瘤已经转移。辅助化疗作用甚微，甚至没有益处[36]，但是最近研究表明化疗能够改善预后[19,52]。某些医疗中心正在研究对于没能够完全切除的肿瘤进行放射手术的效果。

脑干胶质瘤

现在认识到某些类型的脑干胶质瘤可以有完全不同的结果[13]。最常见的类型是脑桥内在的浸润型胶质瘤，是无法手术切除的。这些肿瘤的典型表现为颅神经损伤而不是脑积水。患者通常是年龄小的儿童，伴有第 6 对颅神经麻痹、面肌无力和共济失调。确诊靠 MRI，能显示肿胀的脑干伴有一个浸润性的异常信号（见图 41–3）。没有手术指征。放疗能缓解全身症状，但大多数儿童在 1 年内死亡。颈延髓星形细胞瘤被认为是脊髓内部的肿瘤向延髓生长，预后相对较好。症状和体征有：呕吐、头颈歪斜、慢性进展的肌力减退或脑积水的症状。MRI 显示上段颈髓扩大，并向上延伸。在枕大池内也能看到扩大的颈髓。这类肿瘤常能手术切除；如果是良性肿瘤，可以推迟辅助性放疗。顶盖胶质瘤现在认为也是一个引起脑积水的并不少见的疾病[46]。他们所表现的症状与脑室阻塞有关，通常治疗采取脑室腹腔分流手术或内镜下三脑室造瘘术。由于肿瘤可以长期不生长，所以不需手术切除，除非肿瘤进行性增大时，再考虑治疗肿瘤。

下丘脑 / 视交叉星形细胞瘤

鞍上星形细胞瘤通常是低度恶性肿瘤，可以和神经纤维瘤 I 型有关，也可以单独发生。这类肿瘤的病因学还不十分清楚，但关于神经纤维瘤病 I 型的病因定位在染色体 17q，推测这类肿瘤的病因学为基因变异。临床表现为原发性视觉异常（视野缺陷或肿瘤侵犯相应的视神经导致视神经萎缩而产生的不对称性视力下降）或下丘脑功能障碍（青春期早熟、生长落后、肥胖、间脑综合征即体重不能增长伴皮下组织损失）。通常视觉和下丘脑症状同时存在。

影像学检查常常不能把下丘脑肿瘤与那些从视觉器官来的肿瘤相区别开。典型的肿瘤没有钙化，这有助于和颅咽管瘤相鉴别，在 CT 或 MRI T1 加权像上呈现一低密度的实质性肿块，增强后有强化。沿着视放射生长或长入到眶内视神经是这类肿瘤的特点，可借此区别于颅咽管瘤、生殖细胞瘤或其他肿瘤（图 41–4）。

治疗存在争议。传统的方法是手术活检，然后放射治疗。最近放线菌素 D 和长春新碱或其他药物的联合化疗提供了另外一种可选择的方法，特别是对婴 677
幼儿，放射治疗对他们的颅脑有损伤[45]。也有报道用放射性手术切除的方法作为治疗的首选[88]。

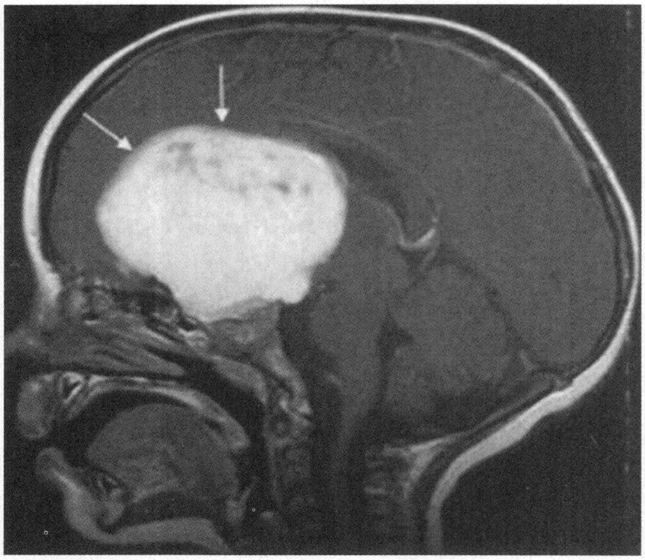

图 41-4　一位 14 个月大的男孩，表现为昏睡一个星期，呕吐 2 天。矢状位 T1 加权图像增强 MRI 显示一个大的强化的鞍上和额叶肿瘤，起源于视交叉和下丘脑（箭头所示）。术中诊断为下丘脑星形细胞瘤。

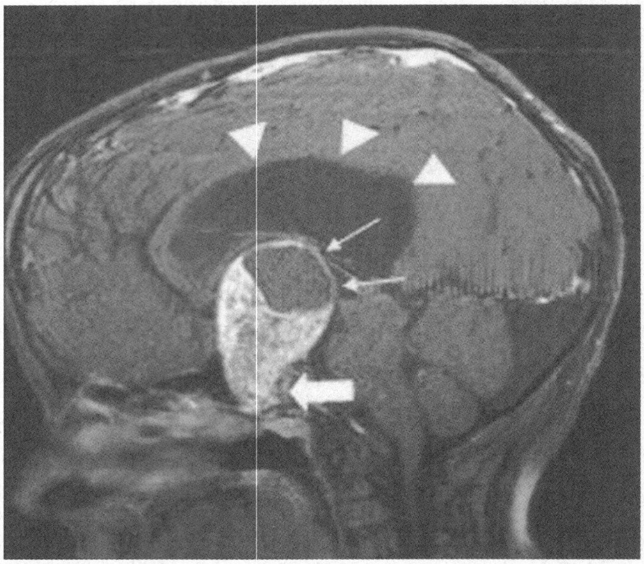

图 41-5　一位 11 岁的男孩，表现为几个月的头痛和昏睡，伴有极度口渴和多尿。矢状位 T1 加权图像增强 MRI 扫描显示一个强化的鞍内肿瘤，鞍区扩大（箭头所示）。肿瘤占据着第三脑室并有囊性变（小箭头所示）。病人还有阻塞性脑积水，表现为侧脑室扩张和薄薄的胼胝体（星状箭头所示）。

颅咽管瘤

颅咽管瘤组织学类型为良性肿瘤，已确诊为由垂体-咽管道退化而来的胚胎残留物。症状有视交叉或视神经压迫症、垂体功能减退、下丘脑功能障碍或脑积水引起的颅内压升高。肿瘤也可以发生在成人，但儿童的肿瘤有自己的特征如肿瘤通常很大伴有广泛钙化。颅咽管有两种类型：成釉细胞型和乳头状型。儿童最常见是的成釉细胞型。组织学上，它们由鳞状上皮囊壁组成，囊液内充满了胆固醇结晶和钙化物。他们通常和垂体腺相连，又和下丘脑上方有一犬牙交错状胶质带。这些特性使得难以保证肿瘤被完全切除。因为在上述界面肿瘤切得少可能引起残留，切得过多可能造成下丘脑功能障碍。

放射学上，CT 显示一个或者边像强化伴基底钙化的囊性肿块或者是一个完全实质性的肿瘤。MRI 能够很好地显示矢状面的解剖，但对钙化显示不清（图 41-5）[24]。在某些情况下，影像学很难分辨出颅咽管瘤和下丘脑胶质瘤。

治疗方法是通过开颅手术将肿瘤完全切除，这在大多数情况下是可以做到的[27]。在肿瘤无法完全切除的情况下，放疗是一个有效的辅助性治疗[66]。治疗后产生的遗留问题可有全垂体功能减

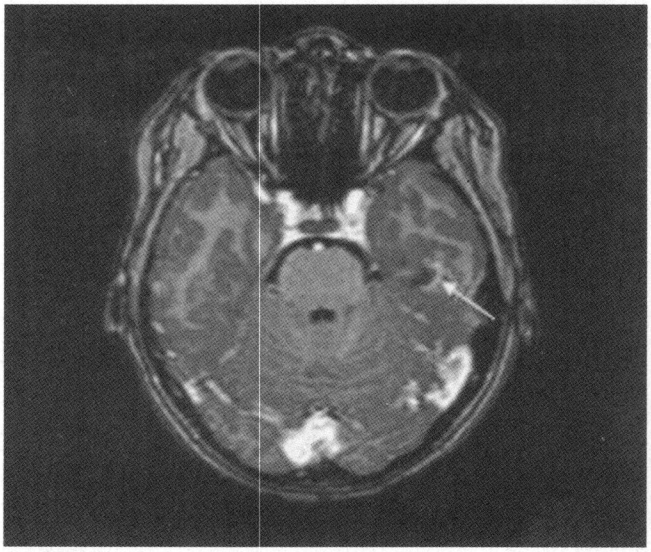

图 41-6　一位 9 岁的男孩，表现为难治性癫痫。轴位 T_1 加权图像增强 MRI 显示左颞叶有一个稍强化的肿瘤（箭头所示）。病理显示为神经节神经胶质细胞瘤。肿瘤完全切除后，癫痫消失。

退、肥胖、视觉障碍、情感不稳定[54]和颈动脉假性动脉瘤[60]。10 年生存率达到 90%[53]，但局部复发也并不少见。肿瘤复发的治疗有再手术切除[67]、

囊腔内放置胶体 32P 或放射手术。

低度恶性幕上星形细胞瘤

发生在皮层区域和颞叶的低度恶性幕上星形细胞瘤和神经节神经胶质瘤常引起难治性癫痫。CT 显示一个低密度的肿块，可以强化也可以不强化。MRI 常显示一个在 T_1 加权像低信号，T_2 加权像高信号的肿块。

手术的目的是完全切除肿瘤，但是有时很难做到，因为肿瘤邻近功能区或肿瘤边界难以确定。有助于解决这一问题的方法有用埋置滤线栅绘制语言和运动图，或者术中电生理监测技术[2]，功能性 MRI 技术，以及影像学引导下的肿瘤切除[29]。颞叶的肿瘤常行颞叶切除以减少儿童期癫痫，也可以用癫痫图技术，但是有时单纯把肿瘤切除也能达到好的癫痫控制效果[41]，这些方法的价值还不确定。

需要监测扫描，但低度恶性的星形细胞瘤[59]，神经节神经胶质瘤[61]（图 41-6）和 DNET（图 41-7）
78 完全切除后的预后是良好的。约 70%的儿童能够长期生存。复发性肿瘤的治疗包括再手术切除或再手术后辅以放疗[32]。

松果体区肿瘤

松果体区的肿瘤有许多种组织学类型，包括生殖细胞瘤（畸胎瘤、绒毛膜癌、胚组织瘤、胚胎细胞癌、卵黄囊肿瘤）、松果体实质肿瘤（松果体细胞肿瘤、成松果体细胞肿瘤）、周围结构肿瘤（星形细胞瘤、脑膜瘤）和其他良性肿块（囊肿、血管畸形）。以前的松果体瘤称呼已不再沿用。

患者有脑积水的症状和体征，眼上视麻痹，以及少见的青春期早熟。MRI 能够证实肿瘤的存在，并排除其他病变的可能，但是无法确定肿瘤的组织学类型。特殊的生殖细胞瘤会分泌特殊的肿瘤标志物，这些标志物可通过腰穿或脑室穿刺留取脑脊液或从血液中检测到。绒毛膜癌可有 β-HCG 升高（>50.0 IU/L），内胚层窦瘤和胚胎细胞癌可有 AFP 的升高（>25.0 IU/L），PLAP 的升高见于胚细胞瘤。

在过去，松果体区的肿瘤是手术的反指征，因为风险很大，肿瘤的治疗常常是在不知其组织学类型的情况下进行。现在许多医疗中心能够通过幕下 / 小脑上入路或者大脑半球间经胼胝体入路获取肿瘤标本，并发症非常少。在鞍上部位松果体区的单纯的胚组织瘤经放疗后有较好的预后，即使肿瘤有转移，经过全脑和脊髓放疗照射效果仍比较好[34]。单独化疗在某些医疗中心也得到推崇。别的恶性生殖细胞常常导致死亡[42]。成松果体细胞肿瘤治疗方法与其他部位的 PNET 相似。松果体细胞瘤如果能被完全切除则仅需要观察即可，如果有残留，再给予局部放射治疗。

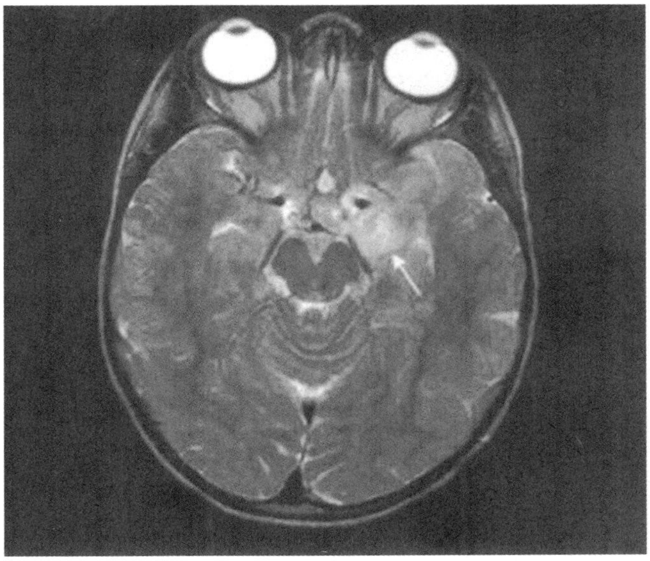

图 41-7 一位 14 岁的男孩，表现为几个月的头痛和癫痫。轴位 T2 加权像 MRI 显示一个颞叶中央高信号占位，侵犯到皮层（箭头所示）。占位性病变在 T1 加权像为低信号，没有强化。诊断为胚胎期发育不良的神经上皮瘤（DNET）。

杆状 / 非典型畸胎样瘤

这类肿瘤只是在最近才被确定。它们是高度恶性的肿瘤，组织学上与肾脏的杆状瘤相似。它们通常发生在婴幼儿的后颅窝，但也有可能在脊髓或幕上。过去，许多这些肿瘤可能被错误地归类到 PNET 中，但与 PNET 不同的是，这些肿瘤细胞大，胞浆粉红，并显示平滑肌肌动细胞和上皮膜抗原免疫组织化学染色阳性。染色体分析显示在大多数病例呈 22 染色单体[5]。在较大儿童治疗方法是手术切除、化疗和放疗，但实际上所有被报道的病例均死亡。

恶性幕上星形细胞瘤

间变型星形细胞瘤和多型性恶性胶质瘤只占儿童肿瘤的6%，与成人相比，发生率低。肿瘤部位不同产生不同的临床症状和体征。影像学特征与成人的肿瘤相似，肿块通常很大、环形强化和中央坏死。肿瘤转移发生率约10%[65]。

治疗方法是最大限度地切除肿瘤并辅以放疗，但预后仍旧很差。虽然大范围的肿瘤切除能有较好的结果，但说明一个事实即越良好的肿瘤越需积极手术切除。对于高度星形细胞瘤，化疗能延长儿童的生命，但是所有5年的生存率仅为33%[17]。目前正在研究大剂量化疗伴自身骨髓移植的作用[16]。

脉络丛瘤

脉络丛瘤被分成良性脉络丛乳头状瘤和恶性脉络丛癌。在儿童，它们倾向于起源于侧脑室三角，在婴儿常伴有脑积水。影像学特征为脑室内一个均匀强化的分成小叶状的肿块。典型的乳头状癌很大，可能转移。肿瘤血供来自脉络丛动脉，通过高分辨率的MRI可以显示出。

治疗方法是手术切除，乳头状瘤可以治愈。手术风险很大，因为这些肿瘤的血供可能非常丰富而患者
679 年龄又很小。脉络丛癌特别难切除，因为血供特别丰富。因而有人建议活检，随后给予化疗，最后再行肿瘤切除[56]。恶性脉络丛癌如果能够被完全切除，长期的存活甚至治愈还是有可能的。

脑膜瘤

脑膜瘤在儿童中不常见，约占2%。它们可能与神经纤维瘤病有关。脑膜瘤可发生在眼眶、蝶骨翼或事实上可发生在颅内任何部位，并且可不发生硬膜粘连。典型的脑膜瘤影像学上可见强化并有可能呈现一个非常大的肿瘤。治疗方法是手术切除。若能完全切除则可以治愈。对于复发性肿瘤或者不能完全切除的肿瘤，放疗是有帮助的[44]。

转移性瘤

脑转移性肿瘤在儿童不多见。能转移到脑的原发性肿瘤有肾母细胞瘤、骨肉瘤和胚胎性横纹肌肉瘤。起病急，由于出血的原因，常会引起严重的神经症状。

肿瘤遗传学

尽管影像学技术、导航系统以及手术器械和技术有了飞速发展，许多肿瘤，特别是高度恶性的肿瘤，单靠手术还是无法治愈，需与放疗、化疗联合治疗。未来的脑肿瘤治疗建立在对肿瘤的生物学、分子生物学更好的理解基础上。这些技术已使我们更好地了解了与儿童脑膜瘤和听神经瘤发展相关的神经纤维瘤2型。在22染色体上找到了基因位点[51]，在不伴有神经纤维瘤2型的儿童脑膜瘤上也找到了同样的染色体[4]。遗传学上的异常，导致了肿瘤抑制基因的缺失。22染色单体已发现与杆状、非典型性畸胎样肿瘤有关[5]。神经纤维瘤1型与儿童的胶质瘤，特别是下丘脑、脑干和视交叉的胶质瘤有关。负责编码神经纤维蛋白的基因位点在17q11.2。神经纤维瘤是*RAS*致肿瘤基因的关闭开关。星形细胞瘤组织常有17染色体异常，原发病是在短臂（*P*）上。17染色体的短臂就是*TP53*肿瘤抑制基因所在之处。可能存在有控制基因的突变导致脑肿瘤的发生，而且如果基因的拷贝功能障碍，就像神经纤维瘤1型一样，产生肿瘤的可能就增大。17染色体的异常在髓母细胞瘤中也有发现[6]，但一些研究显示其位点与*TP53*抑制基因不同。在成神经细胞瘤，*N-MYC*的扩增与肿瘤的生长和侵袭有关。

在与儿童脑肿瘤的斗争不断取得胜利的过程中，非常有必要需要神经外科医生、肿瘤科医生、放射科医生和分子生物学家之间的持续合作。

（鲍　南译　金惠明校）

参考文献

1. Abdollahzadeh M, Hoffman HJ, Blazer SI, et al: Benign cerebellar astrocytoma in childhood: Experience at the Hospital for Sick Children 1980-1992. Childs Nerv Syst 1994;10:380.
2. Berger MS, Ojemann GA, Lettich E: Neurophysiological monitoring during astrocytoma surgery. Neurosurg Clin N Am 1990;1:65.
3. Biegel JA, Burk CD, Barr FG, Emmanuel BS: Evidence for a 17p tumor related locus distinct from p53 in pediatric primitive neuroectodermal tumors. Cancer Res 1992;52:3391.
4. Biegel JA, Parmiter AH, Sutton LN, et al: Abnormalities of chromosome 22 in pediatric meningiomas. Genes Chromosomes Cancer 1994;9:81.
5. Biegel JA, Rorke LB, Packer RJ, Emanuel BS: Monosomy 22 in rhabdoid or atypical tumors of the brain. J Neurosurg 1990;73:710.
6. Biegel JA, Rorke LB, Packer RJ, et al: Isochromosome 17q in primitive neuroectodermal tumors of the central nervous system. Genes Chromosomes Cancer 1989;1:139.
7. Bourne JP, Geyer R, Berger M, et al: The prognostic significance of postoperative residual contrast enhancement on CT scan in pediatric patients with medulloblastoma. J Neurooncol 1992;14:263.
8. Buetow PC, Smirniotopoulos JG, Done S: Congenital brain tumors: A review of 45 cases, AJNR Am J Neuroradiol 1990; 11:793.
9. Chang CH, Housepian EM, Herbert C Jr: An operative staging system and a megavoltage radiotherapeutic technic for cerebellar medulloblastomas. Radiology 1969;93:1351.
10. Crist WM, Kun LE: Common solid tumors of childhood. N Engl J Med 1991;324:461.
11. Duffner PK, Cohen ME, Voorhess ML, et al: Long-term effects of cranial irradiation on endocrine function in children with brain tumors: A prospective study. Cancer 1985; 56:2189.
12. Duffner PK, Horowitz ME, Krischer JP, et al: Postoperative chemotherapy and delayed radiation in children less than three years of age with malignant brain tumors. N Engl J Med 1993;328:1725.
13. Epstein FJ, Farmer JP: Brain-stem glioma growth patterns. J Neurosurg 1993;78:408.
14. Evans AE, Jenkin RD, Sposto R, et al: The treatment of medulloblastoma: Results of a prospective randomized trial of radiation therapy with and without CCNU, vincristine, and prednisone. J Neurosurg 1990;72:572.
15. Farwell JR, Dohrmann GJ, Flannery JT: Central nervous system tumors in children. Cancer 1977;40:3123.
16. Finlay JL, August C, Packer R, et al: High-dose multi-agent chemotherapy followed by bone marrow 'rescue' for malignant astrocytomas of childhood and adolescence. J Neurooncol 1990;9:239.
17. Finlay JL, Boyett JM, Yates AJ, et al: Randomized phase III trial in childhood high-grade astrocytoma comparing vincristine, lomustine, and prednisone with the eight-drugs-in-1-day regimen. Children's Cancer Group. J Clin Oncol 1995;13:112.
18. Freeman CR, Farmer JP, Montes J: Low-grade astrocytomas in children: Evolving management strategies. Int J Radiat Oncol Biol Phys 1998;41:979.
19. Geyer JR, Sposto R, Jennings M, et al: Children's Cancer Group. Multiagent chemotherapy and deferred radiotherapy in infants with malignant brain tumors: a report from the Children's Cancer Group. J Clin Oncol 2005;23:7621.
20. Giuffre R: Biological aspects of brain tumors in infancy and childhood. Childs Nerv Syst 1989;5:55.
21. Gjerris F, Klinken L: Long-term prognosis in children with benign cerebellar astrocytoma. J Neurosurg 1978; 49:179.
22. Gold EB, Leviton A, Lopez R, et al: Parental smoking and risk of childhood brain tumors. Am J Epidemiol 1993; 137:620.
23. Goldwein JW, Leahy JM, Packer RJ, et al: Intracranial ependymomas in children. Int J Radiat Oncol Biol Phys 1990;19:1497.
24. Harwood-Nash DC: Neuroimaging of childhood craniopharyngioma. Pediatr Neurosurg 1994;21(Suppl 1):2.
25. Hawkins MM, Draper GJ, Kingston JE: Incidence of second primary tumours among childhood cancer survivors. Br J Cancer 1987;56:339.
26. Healey EA, Barnes PD, Kupsky WJ, et al: The prognostic significance of postoperative residual tumor in ependymoma. Neurosurgery 1991;28:666.
27. Hoffman HJ, De Silva M, Humphreys RP, et al: Aggressive surgical management of craniopharyngiomas in children. J Neurosurg 1992;76:47.
28. Jakacki RI, Goldwein JW, Larsen RL, et al: Cardiac dysfunction following spinal irradiation during childhood. J Clin Oncol 1993;11:1033.
29. Kelly PJ: Image-directed tumor resection. Neurosurg Clin North Am 1990;1:81.
30. Krischer JP, Ragab AH, Kun L, et al: Nitrogen mustard, vincristine, procarbazine, and prednisone as adjuvant chemotherapy in the treatment of medulloblastoma. A Pediatric Oncology Group study. J Neurosurg 1991; 74:905.
31. Laurent JP, Chang CH, Cohen ME: A classification system for primitive neuroectodermal tumors (medulloblastoma) of the posterior fossa. Cancer 1985;56:1807.
32. Laws ER Jr, Taylor WF, Clifton MB, Okazaki H: Neurosurgical management of low-grade astrocytoma of the cerebral hemispheres. J Neurosurg 1984;61:665.
33. Lee M, Wisoff JH, Abbott R, et al: Management of hydrocephalus in children with medulloblastoma: Prognostic factors for shunting. Pediatr Neurosurg 1994;20:240.
34. Legido A, Packer RJ, Sutton LN, et al: Suprasellar germinomas in childhood: A reappraisal. Cancer 1989;63:340.
35. Loftus CM, Copeland BR, Carmel PW: Cystic supratentorial gliomas: Natural history and evaluation of modes of surgical therapy. Neurosurgery 1985;17:19.
36. Nazar GB, Hoffman HJ, Becker LE, et al: Infratentorial ependymomas in childhood: Prognostic factors and treatment. J Neurosurg 1990;72:408.
37. Packer RJ, Allen JC, Goldwein JL, et al: Hyperfractionated radiotherapy for children with brainstem gliomas: A pilot study using 7,200 cGy. Ann Neurol 1990;27:167.
38. Packer RJ, Sutton LN, Atkins TE, et al: A prospective study of cognitive function in children receiving whole-brain radiotherapy and chemotherapy: 2-year results. J Neurosurg 1989;70:707.
39. Packer RJ, Sutton LN, D'Angio G, et al: Management of children with primitive neuroectodermal tumors of the posterior fossa/medulloblastoma. Pediatr Neurosci 1985;12:272.
40. Packer RJ, Sutton LN, Elterman R, et al: Outcome for children with medulloblastoma treated with radiation and cisplatin, CCNU, and vincristine chemotherapy. J Neurosurg 1994;81:690.
41. Packer RJ, Sutton LN, Patel KM, et al: Seizure control fol-

lowing tumor surgery for childhood cortical low-grade gliomas. J Neurosurg 1994;80:998.

42. Packer RJ, Sutton LN, Rorke LB, et al: Intracranial embryonal cell carcinoma. Cancer 1984;54:520.
43. Palma L, Russo A, Mercuri S: Cystic cerebral astrocytomas in infancy and childhood: Long-term results. Childs Brain 1983;10:79.
44. Perilongo G, Sutton LN, Goldwein JW, et al: Childhood meningiomas: Experience in the modern imaging era. Pediatr Neurosurg 1992;18:16.
45. Petronio J, Edwards MS, Prados M, et al: Management of chiasmal and hypothalamic gliomas of infancy and childhood with chemotherapy. J Neurosurg 1991;74:701.
46. Pollack IF, Pang D, Albright AL: The long-term outcome in children with late-onset aqueductal stenosis resulting from benign intrinsic tectal tumors. J Neurosurg 1994;80:681.
47. Probert JC, Parker BR, Kaplan HS: Growth retardation in children after megavoltage irradiation of the spine. Cancer 1973;32:634.
48. Puce A, Constable RT, Luby ML, et al: Functional magnetic resonance imaging of sensory and motor cortex: Comparison with electrophysiological localization. J Neurosurg 1995; 83:262.
49. Radcliffe J, Bunin GR, Sutton LN, et al: Cognitive deficits in long-term survivors of childhood medulloblastoma and other noncortical tumors: Age-dependent effects of whole brain radiation. Int J Dev Neurosci 1994;12:327.
50. Ross AJ 3rd, Siegel KR, Bell W, et al: Massive gastrointestinal hemorrhage in children with posterior fossa tumors. J Pediatr Surg 1987;22:633.
51. Rouleau GA, Wertelecki W, Haines JL, et al: Genetic linkage of bilateral acoustic neurofibromatosis to a DNA marker on chromosome 22. Nature 1987;329:246.
52. Sandri A, Massimino M, Mastrodicasa L, et al: Treatment with oral etoposide for childhood recurrent ependymomas. J Pediatr Hematol Oncol 2005;27:486.
53. Scott RM, Hetelekidis S, Barnes PD, et al: Surgery, radiation, and combination therapy in the treatment of childhood craniopharyngioma—a 20-year experience. Pediatr Neurosurg 1994;21(Suppl 1):75.
54. Shiminski-Maher T: Patient/family preparation and education for complications and late sequelae of craniopharyngiomas. Pediatr Neurosurg 1994;21(Suppl 1):114.
55. Spoto GP, Press GA, Hesselink JR, Solomon M: Intracranial ependymoma and subependymoma: MR manifestations. AJR Am J Roentgenol 1990;154:837.
56. St. Clair SK, Humphreys RP, Pillary RK, et al: Current management of choroid plexus carcinoma in children. Pediatr Neurosurg 1991;17:225.
57. Steinberg GK, Shuer LM, Conley FK, Hanbery JW: Evolution and outcome in malignant astroglial neoplasms of the cerebellum. J Neurosurg 1985;62:9.
58. Steinbok P, Boyd M, Cochrane D: Cervical spinal deformity following craniotomy and upper cervical laminectomy for posterior fossa tumors in children. Childs Nerv Syst 1989;5:25.
59. Sutton LN: Current management of low-grade astrocytomas of childhood. Pediatr Neurosci 1987;13:98.
60. Sutton LN, Gusnard D, Bruce DA, et al: Fusiform dilatations of the carotid artery following radical surgery of childhood craniopharyngiomas. J Neurosurg 1991;74:695.
61. Sutton LN, Packer RJ, Rorke LB, et al: Cerebral gangliogliomas during childhood. Neurosurgery 1983;13:124.
62. Sutton LN, Wang Z, Gusnard D, et al: Proton magnetic resonance spectroscopy of pediatric brain tumors. Neurosurgery 1992;31:195.
63. Tait DM, Thomton-Jones H, Bloom HJ, et al: Adjuvant chemotherapy for medulloblastoma: The first multi-centre control trial of the International Society of Paediatric Oncology (SIOP I). Eur J Cancer 1990;26:464.
64. Torres CF, Rebsamen S, Silber JH, et al: Surveillance scanning of children with medulloblastoma. N Engl J Med 1994; 330:892.
65. Vertosick FT Jr, Selker RG: Brain stem and spinal metastases of supratentorial glioblastoma multiforme: A clinical series. Neurosurgery 1990;27:516.
66. Weiss M, Sutton L, Marcial V, et al: The role of radiation therapy in the management of childhood craniopharyngioma. Int J Radiat Oncol Biol Phys 1989;17:1313.
67. Wisoff JH: Surgical management of recurrent craniopharyngiomas. Pediatr Neurosurg 1994;21(Suppl 1):108.
68. Wisoff JH, Abbott R, Epstein F: Surgical management of exophytic chiasmatic-hypothalamic tumors of childhood. J Neurosurg 1990;73:661.
69. Wisoff JH, Epstein FJ: Pseudobulbar palsy after posterior fossa operation in children. Neurosurgery 1984;15:707.
70. Young JL Jr, Percy CL, Asire AJ, et al: Cancer incidence and mortality in the United States, 1973-77. Natl Cancer Inst Monogr 1981;(57):1.
71. Zimmerman RA, Bilaniuk LT, Bruno L, Rosenstock J: Computed tomography of cerebellar astrocytoma. AJR Am J Roentgenol 1978;130:929.

第四部分

移　植

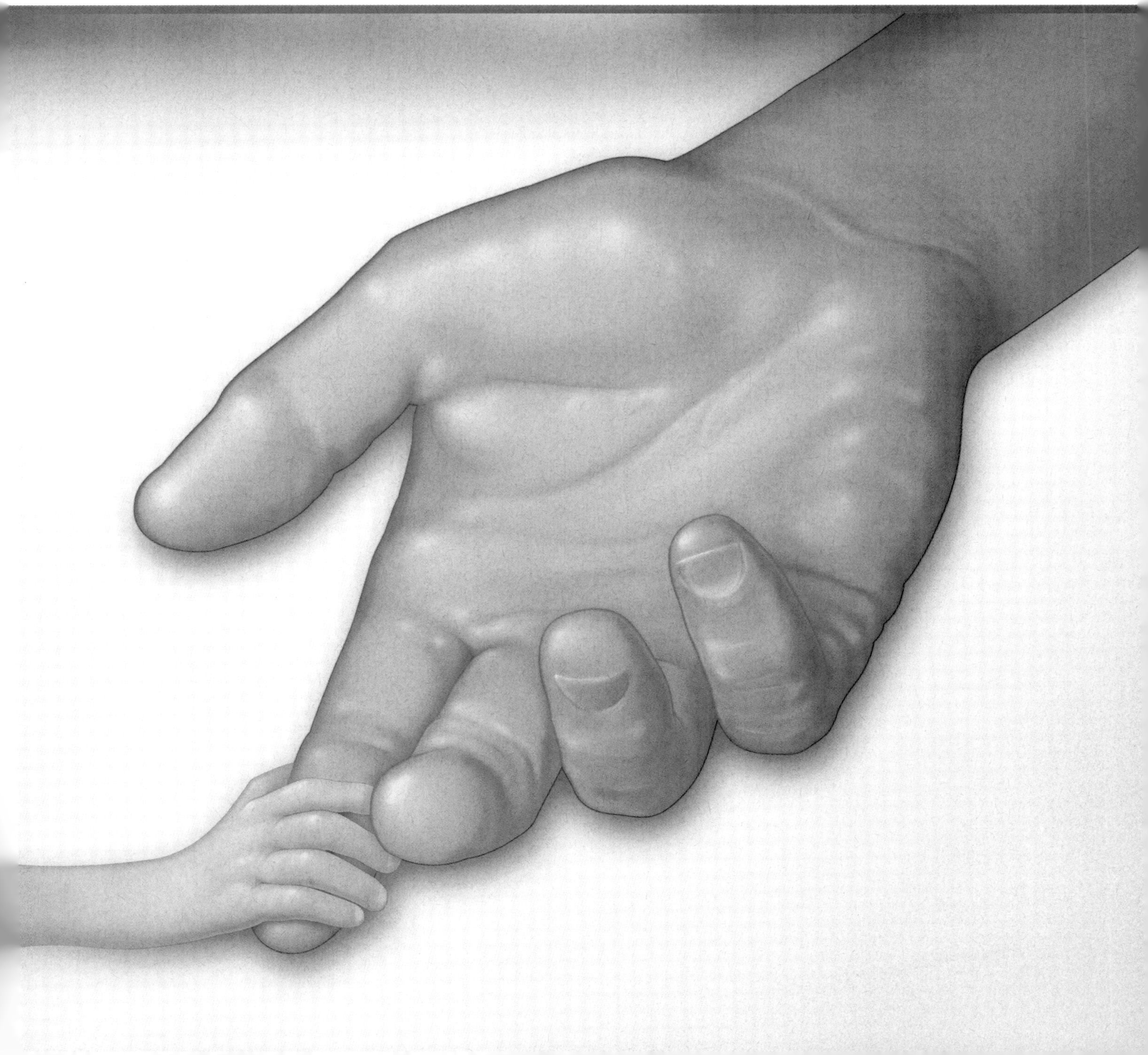

第 42 章

移植原则

Jorge Reyes、Noriko Murase 和 Thomas E. Starzl

685 组织相容性、免疫抑制、组织保存、植入技术被认为是器官和骨髓细胞移植的最重要的问题。然而，若非器官本身有不同程度的供体特异不反应性（耐受），移植就不能作为一种临床服务开展。如这第五个因素不解决，而一直使用移植初期的大量免疫抑制剂治疗，移植受体也不可能长期存活。

获得性耐受之谜

移植所依赖的各种获得性耐受是生物学中最神秘、最有争议的问题之一。这个问题一部分是由意想不到的早年器官移植成功引起的（比骨髓移植成功早10 年，表面上违反了原则，但即将给普通免疫学带来变革）。所以临床器官移植是凭经验发展，而不仅仅作为经典免疫学的一个分支。这形成四个明显的阶段，每阶段持续时间超过十年。只有到最后才最终解释了器官移植，并解开移植的奥秘。

第一阶段：1953—1968 年

第一阶段在 1953～1956 年之间，证明新生小鼠[8,9]和受辐射的成年小鼠在成功植入供体的血淋巴源性细胞后能够产生供体特异性耐受。主要发现耐受供体细胞的小鼠（供体白细胞嵌合状态）能接受原来供体同一品系小鼠的皮肤移植，但不能接受其他品系（图 42-1）。如今行骨髓移植的免疫缺陷和细胞去除者，分别与嵌合的新生小鼠和受辐射的成年小鼠类似。因为好的组织相容性配型能够避免移植物抗宿主疾病（GVHD）以及排异反应，故必须等人类白细胞抗原（HLA）发现以后再进行骨髓移植的临床应用。这完成以后[3,21,99]，1968 年骨髓移植成功的人类受体如同放大的嵌合体耐受小鼠。

1968 年临床骨髓移植取得突破时，肾移植[22, 23, 29, 42, 48 ,49, 64]虽然有缺陷，但已用于临床。另外，首批肝移植、心脏移植的长期存活者也相继出现。随后的 1968—1969 年，肺移植和胰腺移植的首例长期存活者也出现了（表 42-1）。所有这些成功的移植都无白细胞嵌合状态、未进行 HLA 配型，也没有
GVHD 的证据。这些超越了通过小鼠耐受模型建 686
立的白细胞嵌合的界限，器官移植进入非理想的状况。

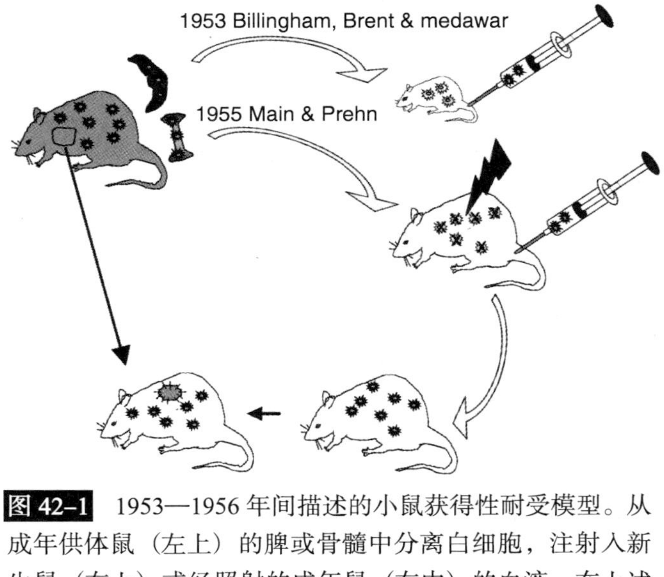

图 42-1 1953—1956 年间描述的小鼠获得性耐受模型。从成年供体鼠（左上）的脾或骨髓中分离白细胞，注射入新生鼠（右上）或经照射的成年鼠（右中）的血液。在上述两种情况下，受体免疫系统太虚弱，无法排斥外来的白细胞（黑色阴影）。植入注射细胞后（即供体白细胞嵌合状态），受体鼠可自由接受白细胞供体的组织和器官，但不能接受来自其他供体的（左下）。

表 42-1 人类同种异体移植物的首次成功移植（存活＞1 年）

器官	城市	日期	医生	参考文献
肾	波士顿	1959.1.24	Merrill, Murray	42,48
肝	丹佛	1967.7.23	Starzl	72
心	开普敦	1968.1.2.	Barnard	5
肺	根特	1968.11.14	Derom	18
胰	明尼阿波利斯	1969.6.3	Lillehei	34

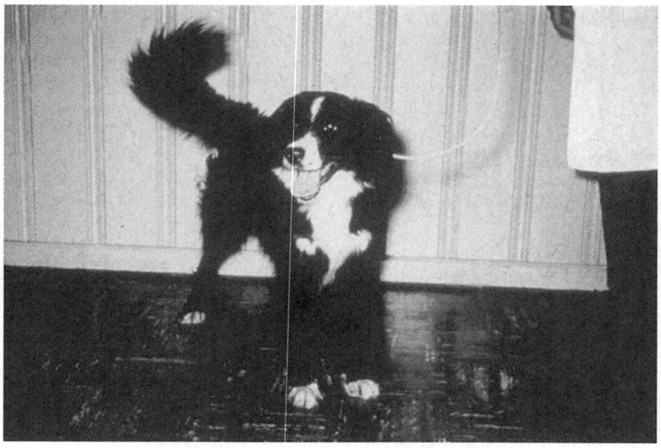

A

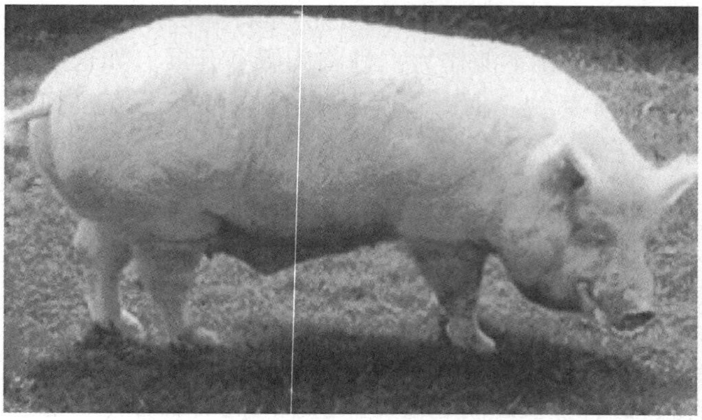

B

图 42-2 A. 原位同种肝移植术后 5 年的受体犬。1964年 3 月 23 日进行手术，该犬仅接受 120 天硫唑嘌呤治疗，13 年后死于高龄。B. Calne[12] 描述的自发性耐受的受体猪。

“假耐受”的器官受体

同种免疫反应的两种不清楚的特征使器官移植得以前进。[64]第一种是器官排斥的高度可逆性。第二种是如果同种异体器官被非特异性免疫抑制保护，可以诱导其自身被接受。1959 年在两个异卵双胎肾移植受体身上首次观察到“自身诱导的植入”，首先是波士顿的 Joseph Murray 报道，接着是巴黎的 Jean Hamburger[22]。这是所有物种的同种异体器官移植的首次成功。两个患者在移植前都接受了 450 R 亚致死量的全身照射。在没有使用药物维持治疗（实际上当时也没有）的情况下移植的肾脏工作超过 20 年。

接着，在杂种狗肾移植后（肝移植后更多见）偶然发现了类似的不需用药状态，之前这些狗都使用单一免疫抑制剂：6-巯嘌呤（6-MP）[55,112]、硫唑嘌呤[50,66]、泼尼松[113]，或抗淋巴细胞球蛋白 (antilymphocyte globulin, ALG)[70]。停用药物后，一些动物不再出现排异反应（图 42-2A）。但这样的结果非常罕见，直到 1962 年夏天，在使用 6-MP 和硫唑嘌呤的犬肾实验中出现此结果的少于 1%。然而，人类经验提示器官可能具有内在耐受性，1963 年一篇报道的标题将其概括为：“人类肾移植排异逆转，随后产生同种移植物耐受”，此报道介绍了一组在丹佛治疗的活体供肾受者[64]。这些受者在肾移植前后均使用硫唑嘌呤，监测血清肌酐观察有无排异，如发生排异则加用大剂量泼尼松（图 42-3A）。几乎所有的病例都出现排异反应，25%的移植物因无法控制的急性排异反应而丧失。然而在 1962—1963 年的 16 个月中，从家族供体取得供体器官的 46 例同种异体移植物的 1 年存活率达到史无前例的 75%。

许多存活者在排异逆转后所需治疗迅速减少，据此可推断产生了部分耐受（图 42-3A）。19%（9/46）的移植物在之后的 40 年里仍然有功能，每例在图 42-4 用水平条表示。此外，9 例中的 7 例最终停止使用所有免疫抑制剂而没有出现排斥，时间从 6 年到 40 年不等（水平条的实心部分）。9 例中的 8 例仍然存活，拥有世界上存活时间最长的同种异体移植器官[92]。

小鼠耐受模型、波士顿和巴黎的经照射后异卵双胎肾移植受者、最终无需药物的器官移植犬（见图 42-2A）和丹佛的人类“假耐受”肾移植受者独特群体间存在什么联系？1966 年，法国[16]、英国[11,12,53]、美国[74]证明，20%的远系杂交猪肝移植后不需任何治疗（见图 42-2B），使其更为神秘。无论免疫抑制是

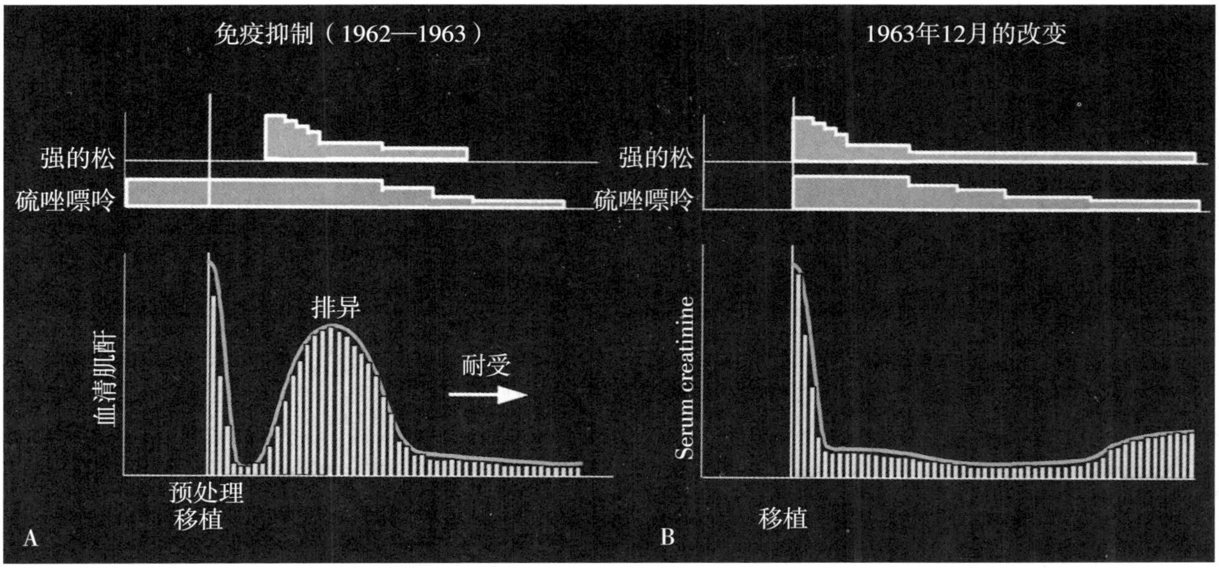

图 42-3 A. 1962—1963 年经验性开展的用于肾移植受者的免疫抑制。注意硫唑嘌呤加用泼尼松后的排异逆转。1/3 世纪后才意识到药物使用的时机与免疫抑制的致耐受性原则相关（见正文）。B. 1963 年 12 月科罗拉多大学修改免疫抑制的方案，无意间违反了致耐受性免疫抑制原则。不再强调或取消了预处理，大剂量预防性使用泼尼松而不是根据需要。虽然急性排异反应减少了，但不再出现图 42-4 所示的无需药物耐受。

否维持，这些动物或人类器官受体都没有供体白细胞嵌合状态。

687 ## 第一阶段：错误前提

器官移植的很早就与白细胞嵌合状态的科学依据分离，后者由小鼠模型建立并被人类骨髓移植例证。两种移植理论的分离（图 42-5）在第一阶段未引起争论，并代代相传。

第一阶段还有一项黑暗的遗留，就是对硫唑嘌呤和泼尼松治疗策略的修改（见图 42-3B）。主要的改变是手术时就大剂量预防性使用泼尼松，而不是只在需要时才使用皮质类固醇。第二次修改后，不再强调预处理（见图 42-3B）。做了这些改变后，急性排异反应的发生率明显降低。然而，世界各地都见不到图 42-4 所示的无需用药的肾移植受者。35 年以后才认识到是这些修改的远期免疫学后果。

图 42-4 1962 年秋起科罗拉多大学在 18 个月时间内治疗的 46 例活供体肾移植受体中的 9 例（19%）。水平条的实心部分代表不用免疫抑制的时间。注意除 1 例以外，其余病例目前血清肌酐浓度正常。

* 被谋杀：尸检发现移植肾正常。

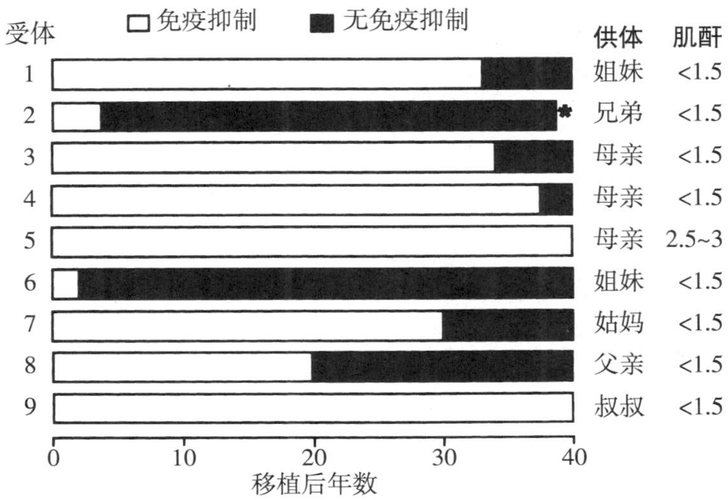

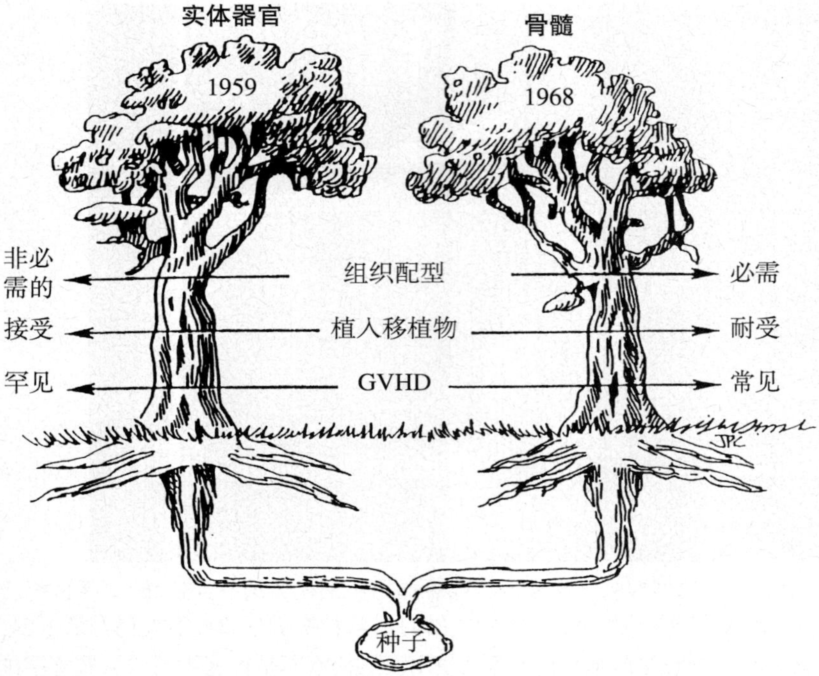

图 42-5 排异反应被证明是一种免疫应答后，骨髓（右）和器官（左）移植发展的树。GVHD：移植物抗宿主疾病。

688 第二阶段：1969—1979 年

1969 年开始的第二阶段中，贯穿于此阶段的器官移植的免疫抑制是基于硫唑嘌呤和预防性的大剂量强的松的，1966 年后[70,71]约 15% 的中心开始加用 ALG。第二阶段是黯淡的时期。在批评家看来，皮质类固醇依赖引起的高死亡率、特别是灾难性的发病，使得器官移植（甚至是肾移植）成为一种治疗的同时也是一种疾病。之前由于起初几例成功而对其抱有很大乐观的肝脏和心脏移植项目大多数都关闭了。

但在少数中心，像图 42-6 所示的患儿成为此移植技术在将来某天大量完成的见证人。她 4 岁的时候（1969 年）由于胆道闭锁和肝脏肿瘤而接受肝移植，她是肾外器官移植后存活时间最长的人。

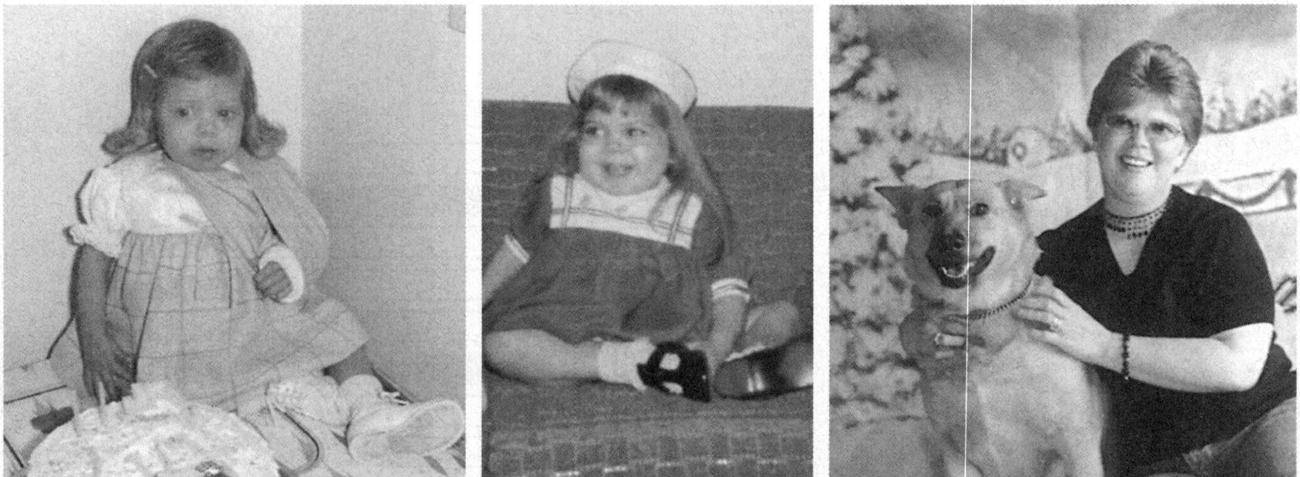

A B C

图 42-6 一位女孩因胆道闭锁和肝癌在 4 岁时进行肝移植，目前已是她移植后的 35 年。她是存活时间最长的肾外器官受者。

689 第三阶段：1980—1991 年

事实上，肾外器官移植似乎开始没落的时候正是第三阶段的起步，临床引入环孢素[13,14,77,78]以及 10 年后的他克莫司[20,81,82,102]是此阶段的开始。这些药物的应用使各种器官移植的效果逐步改善，但在肝脏、心脏移植中它们的效果得到结论性地证明。图 42–7 所示的肝移植结果所使用的免疫抑制是硫唑嘌呤、环孢素和他克莫司，呈现于 1994 年 4 月的美国外科协会会议[103]。当时，在基于他克莫司的免疫抑制帮助下，肠移植已经开展[104,105]。

这些新药物出现之后，它们被简单归入从第一、第二阶段继承的预防性使用重度免疫抑制的改良方案中。由于这些更好药物的加入，从手术时开始的各种多药联用，使得 20 世纪 80 年代至 90 年代早期成为移植的黄金年代。急性排异反应几乎不再是问题。但此时未解决的问题是慢性排异反应、长期免疫抑制的风险（例如感染和新生恶性肿瘤）和药物毒性（例如环孢素和他克莫司的肾毒性）。

第四阶段：1992 年至今

很明显，只有阐明同种移植和获得性耐受的机制，才能解除终身免疫抑制的负担。为了解决植入机制的研究开始于 20 世纪 90 年代早期，在如今的第四阶段占主要地位。

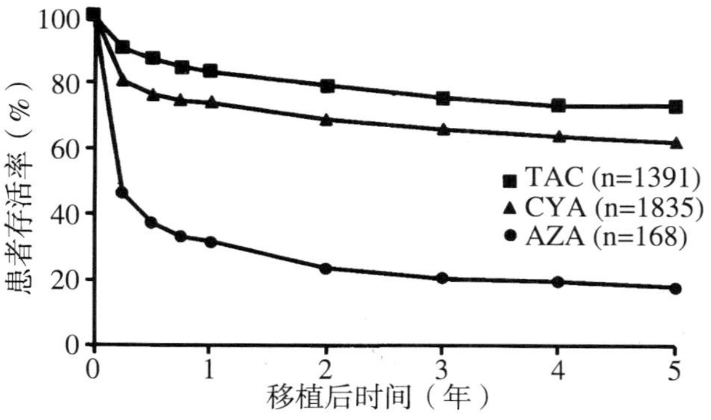

图 42–7　以硫唑嘌呤（AZA）、环孢素（CYA）和他克莫司（TAC）为基础划分的免疫抑制时期中，科罗拉多大学（1963—1980）和匹兹堡大学（1981—1993）原位肝移植患者的存活率。随着这些药物的问世，效果逐步改善，这也见于其他种类的器官移植。

历史教条

直到目前，器官移植机制中仍未涉及或包含白细胞嵌合状态。虽然移植器官中有大量过客白细胞，但这些供体细胞大多能被受体白细胞取代，如图 42–8A 所示。丢失的供体细胞认为被免疫破坏，特异性的实质细胞则被选择性保留。发现骨髓移植（见图 42–8B）的理想结果是受体的免疫细胞完全被替代（即完全血淋巴细胞生成嵌合状态）。

微嵌合状态的发现

在 20 世纪 90 年代初期，此历史教条的缺点开始暴露。西雅图和赫尔辛基[107]令人迷惑的观察都发现患者体内有少量残留的受者血淋巴增生细胞，而之前都认为其完全被骨髓替代（见图 42–8D）。1992 年在长期存活的人类器官移植受者体内发现供体白细胞微嵌合状态。很明显器官植入（见图 42–8C）和骨髓细胞植入（见图 42–8D）是白细胞嵌合状态的反映形式，区别在于供体和受体细胞的细胞逆转的比例。

器官移植受体微嵌合状态的发现是通过一个很简单的临床研究实现的[83-87]。通过敏感的检测技术，在 30 例器官维持功能达 30 年的肝或肾移植受者的血液、淋巴结、皮肤或其他组织中均发现供体不同谱系的血淋巴增生细胞（包括树突状细胞）。这些供体的白细胞明显是供体的前体或多能血淋巴造血干细胞的后代，后者经历了假设的移植后的双重免疫反应后存活并从器官迁移至受者，这发生于移植后几年或几十年或更早[35,45,57,94]。

结论是器官植入是“供体和受体细胞共存、引起相互的耗竭、随后发生外周克隆清除的应答”的结果[83,85]。宿主的应答（图 42–9 的直立曲线）在大多数器官移植中占主导地位，但 GVHD 例外。经传统治疗的骨髓移植受者中，宿主细胞去除使免疫优势从宿主转向移植物（图 42–9 的倒置曲线），这可解释 GVHD 的高发生风险。两种移植的主要区别都由受体的细胞清除引起。经过 1/3 世纪以上辩论，骨髓和器官移植的知识分离终于结束（图 42–10）。

抗原迁移、定位中的免疫调节

但在第一批迁移的白细胞急性诱导后，图 42–9

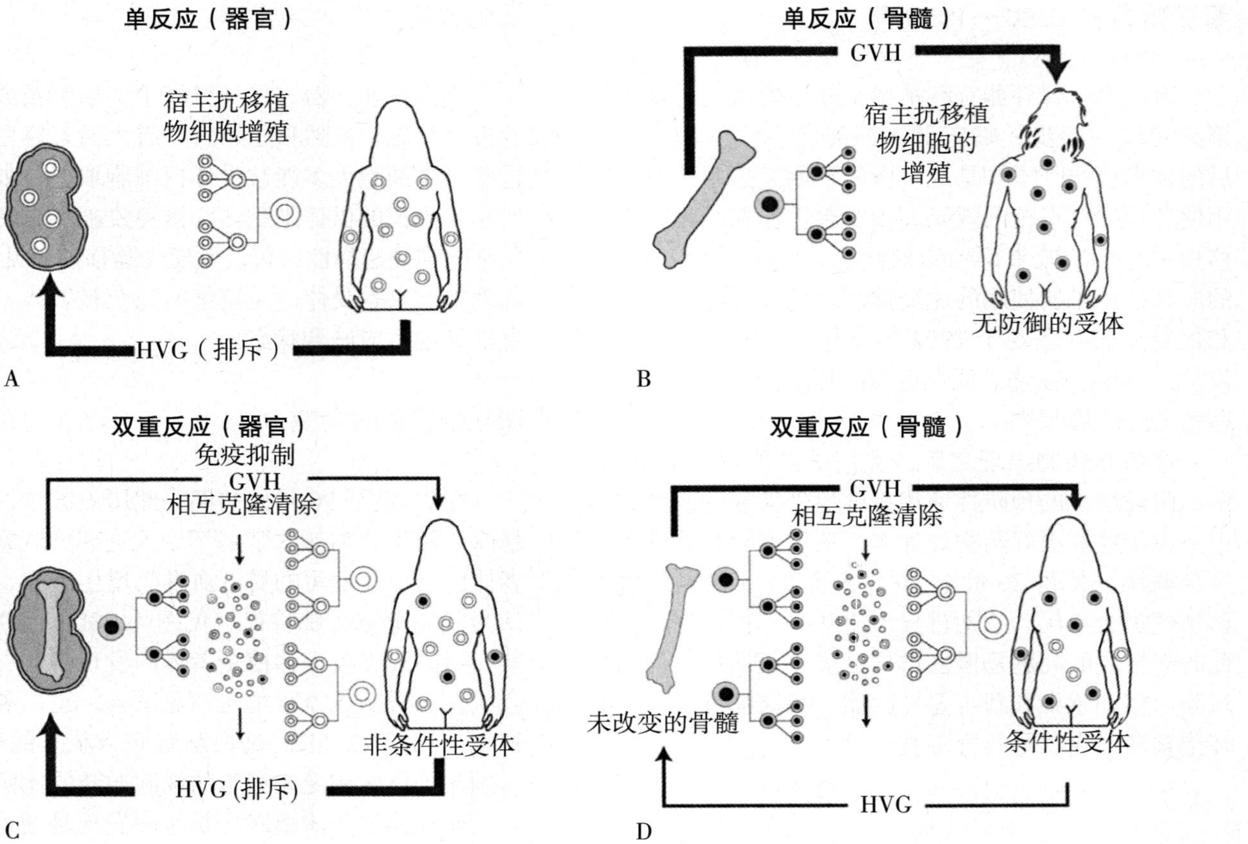

图 42-8 关于移植受体的新（C 和 D）和旧（A 和 B）观点。A. 单向性宿主抗移植物反应是器官移植免疫机制的早期概念。虽然这易于解释器官排斥，但限制了器官植入的可能解释。B. 是 A 图的镜像，描述了对成功骨髓移植的早期认识，认为受体的免疫系统完全被供体替代，致命的非对抗单向性移植物抗宿主反应，即移植物排斥受体，是其潜在并发症。C. 现在的观点认为这是共存免疫活性细胞群双向调节的免疫应答。由于清除性耐受的可变性相互诱导，即使常发生以 HVG 为主导的反应，器官植入仍是可行的。移植物内的骨轮廓代表骨髓来源的过客白细胞。D.目前设想的成功骨髓移植机制，是 C 图的镜像。受体细胞清除引起供体和受体免疫细胞群的比例逆转。HVG：宿主抗移植物；GVH：移植物抗宿主。

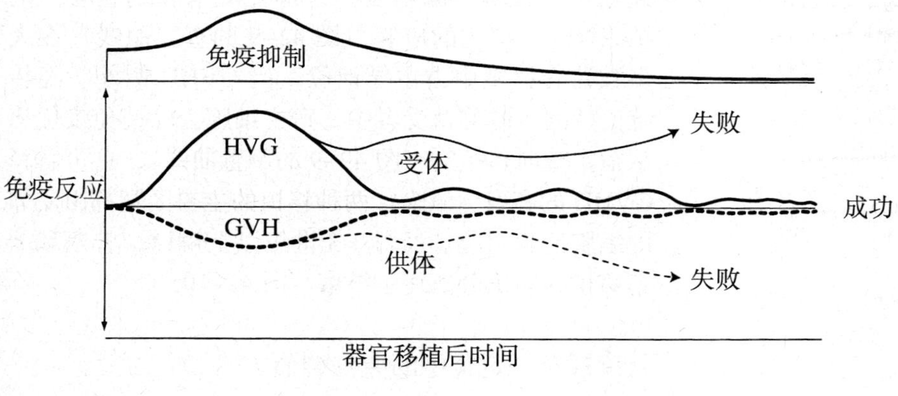

图 42-9 移植术后同时发生的 HVG（直立曲线）和 GVH（倒置曲线）反应。与器官移植中 HVG 反应占主导不同，对受照射或免疫抑制受体进行骨髓移植后 GVH 反应常占主导。任一类型的移植失败说明保护性免疫抑制无法控制其中一种反应，或两种都不能控制。（Starzl TE, Zinkernagel R: Antigen localization and migration in immunity and tolerance. N Engl J Med 1998; 339: 1905-1913.）

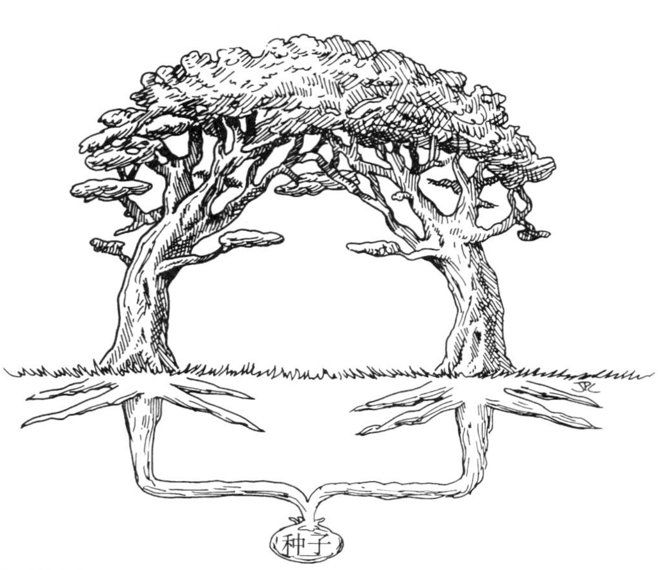

图 42–10 器官移植和骨髓移植的统一（见正文）。

691 所示的双重免疫反应的耗竭–清除如何维持？20 世纪 90 年代，Rolf Zinkernagel 在苏黎世（图 42–11）在无应答的实验研究中提出了这个问题，无应答可引起细胞内微生物感染，如结核杆菌和致病性病毒[43,109-111]。由这些感染性因素引起的综合征与移植

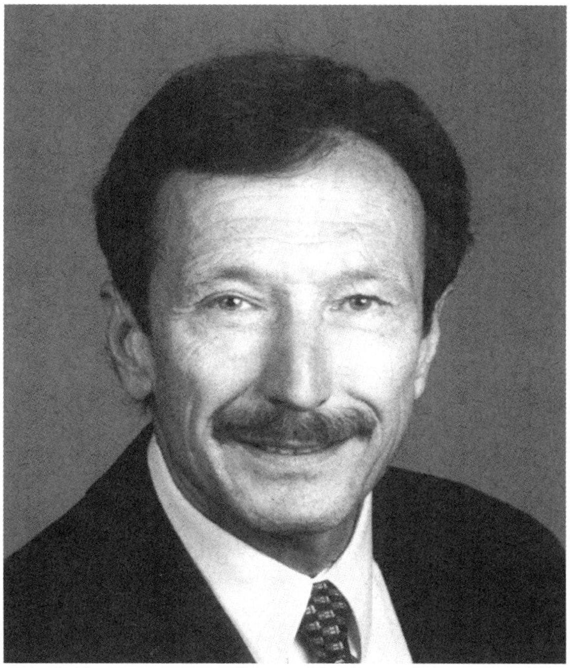

图 42–11 Rolf Zinkernagel（1944—），瑞士内科医生、免疫学家，他和 Peter Doherty 一起发现了对非细胞病变性微生物的适应性免疫应答的机制，获得 1996 年诺贝尔奖。

后的事件的类似之处，在 1998 年 Zinkernagel 发表于新英格兰医学杂志的联合综述中做了描述[89]。

过去，由于移植的特征性双重免疫反应及免疫抑制的复杂因素，移植和感染的类似之处比较模糊。而现在已经清楚。抗供体应答由移植物白细胞开始选择性迁移至宿主淋巴器官引起（图 42–12，左）[17,32,44,51]，这与传播性的细胞内病原体引起的应答相似。不论这些细胞从器官移出或作为骨髓细胞注入，供体白细胞的迁移模式相同。从抗供体应答中存活下来的细胞在几天内开始进入（见图 42–12，右）保护性非淋巴环境，如此免疫系统便不能探测（免疫忽视[4,27,30,31,89]）。这也是非细胞病变性微生物的生存策略。

供体白细胞的迁移在图 42–13（左）中用离心箭头显示：首先经血液途径进入淋巴器官，几周后达非淋巴区域（外环）。图 42–13（右）向内的短箭头描述了供体细胞随后从保护性非淋巴环境逆行迁移至宿主淋巴器官。逆行迁移是一把双刃剑。一方面，这些细胞可维持最初的克隆衰竭–清除，常需免疫抑制的保护。但另一方面，这些细胞保存了同种免疫，方式如同残留的微生物保存保护性免疫。因此，微嵌合状态的另一种结果是产生高反应性抗体（意味着对 HLA 抗原致敏），这常发生于不成功的移植之后[25,61]。

治疗的含意

这些新的观察结果如何应用到临床？抗移植物反应衰退与供体白细胞诱导的克隆清除相关，此机会只存在于移植后的最初几周[46,47,57,95]。显然，术后过度的免疫抑制会阻止此现象产生（见图 42–14，中图）。随着起初过度免疫抑制的不断减少，可使低效清除的克隆恢复，导致延迟的急性排异反应或慢性排异反应，这见于很多移植中心。即使在效果最好的情况下，患者也注定要终身依赖免疫抑制。而过少的免疫抑制会导致无法控制的排异反应（见图 42–14，右图）。

临床医生面对的问题是如何掌握适度的移植后免疫抑制。2001 年，有人建议通过续贯应用两大历史上的治疗原则来解决此困境：对受体进行预处理，移植后使用最低量的免疫抑制[90]。经过预处理，在暴露于供体抗原前受者的免疫应答降低，从而使供体特异 692
性应答降低至更易消除的范围（图 42–15）。在 1959 年的异卵双胎移植病例中（例如亚致死量全身照射或

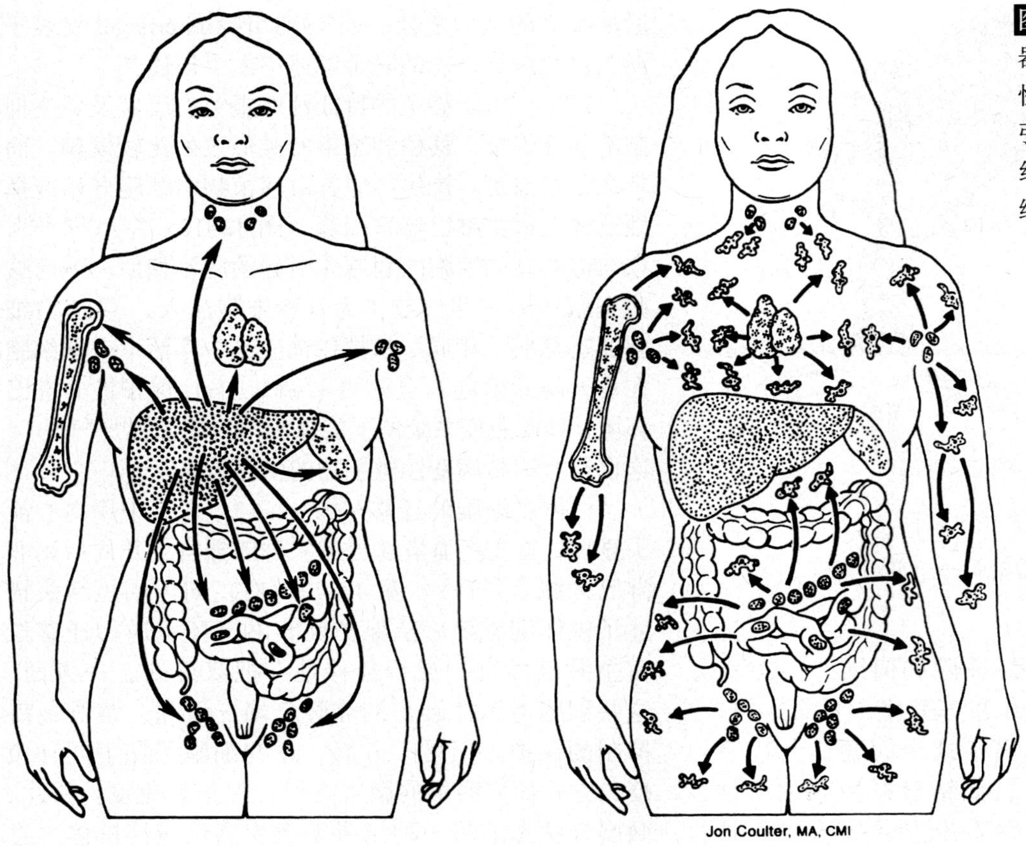

图 42-12 过客白细胞起初从器官移植物（这里是肝）选择性迁移至宿主淋巴器官（左），引起供体特异性免疫反应。大约 30 天后，许多幸存的细胞继续迁移至非淋巴区域（右）。

骨髓毒性药物），仅亚致死量的照射无疑已经取得肾脏过客白细胞克隆清除的作用[22,48]。事实上，受者细胞清除的根治性预处理方式最终成为传统骨髓移植必要的治疗步骤。由于发生 GVHD 的高风险性，这种方式过于危险并应用过于受限，故在器官移植中并不实用。

然而，20 世纪 60 年代以来，较缓和的用 ALG 或其他方式进行淋巴耗竭（所谓的非去髓性清除）一再被证明是有效的，不会引起 GVHD[71]（见图 42-15）。

经目前有效的抗淋巴抗体预处理后，预先削弱的 693

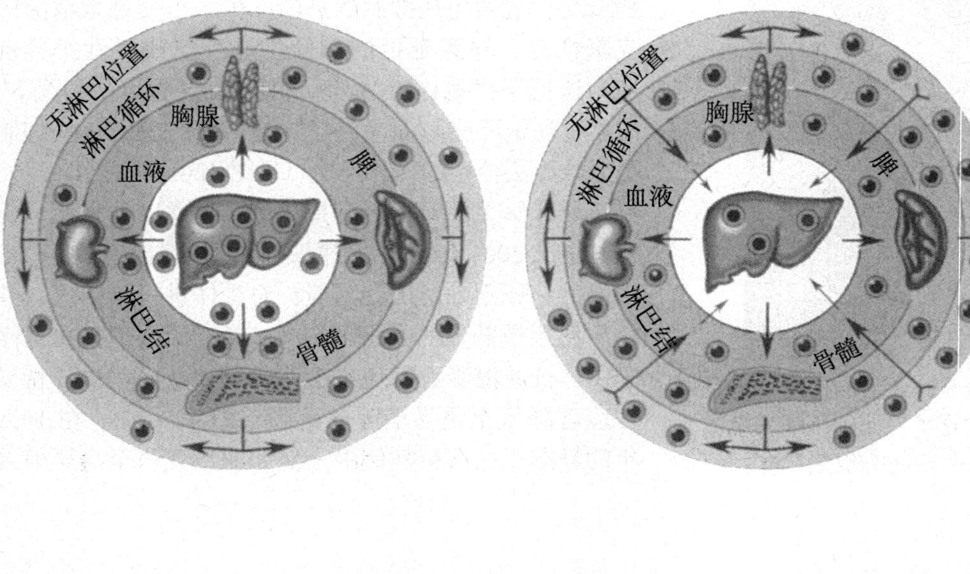

图 42-13 移植器官的过客白细胞迁移路线与输注的骨髓细胞类似。左图，首先向宿主淋巴器官选择性迁移。15～30 天后幸存的细胞再迁移至非淋巴区域。右图：反向迁移使起初诱导的耗竭性清除得以维持。

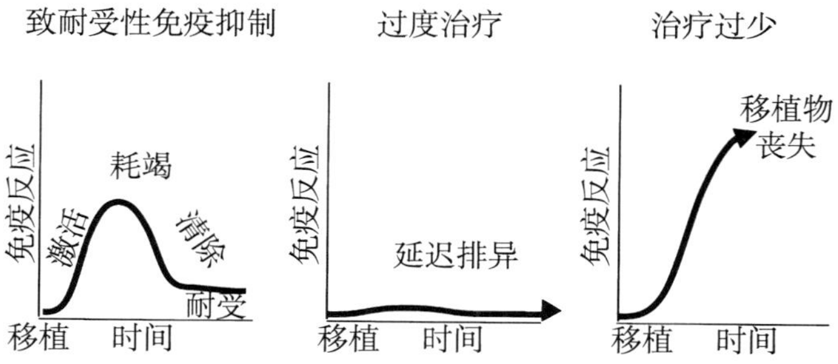

图 42-14 移植后免疫抑制对克隆耗竭清除机制的影响。左图：免疫抑制适当。中图：免疫抑制过多。右图：免疫抑制过少。

克隆激活可在最低量短期或长期维持免疫抑制治疗中进行有效的克隆清除（图 42-16）。2001 年 7 月，我们在成人器官受体中制定了双原则策略。单次 5mg/kg 注射抗人胸腺球蛋白进行预处理。2002 开始，在大多数成人病例中以单次使用 30mg Campath 代替抗人胸腺球蛋白。在任一方式的淋巴耗竭后，给予单一药物（通常是他克莫司）的保守性每日剂量进行移植后处理，只有发生暴发性排异时才加用其他药物，并且使用时间尽可能短。此策略于 2002 年推广至肠移植的婴儿和儿童，2003 年 4 月后用于所有肾移植患儿。

4～8 个月后，对于器官功能稳定的成人患者，将单一疗法减至不需每日用药：隔日用药，然后每周 3 次、每周 2 次，很多患者移植后 1 年减至每周 1 次（图 42-17）。此策略已应用于 1000 多例的成人肾、肝、肠、胰腺、肺移植受者[40,59,91]。此经验证明移植受者的生活质量能够得到改善。首次考虑对儿童进行间隔停药。

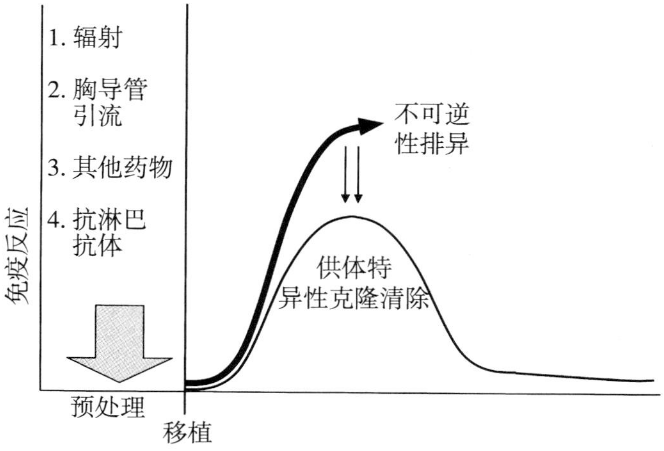

图 42-15 移植前受体免疫应答减弱时（预处理原则），对移植物的供体特异性免疫应答可被耗竭并清除（细曲线起初升高，随后降低），而不产生排异（粗的黑箭头）。

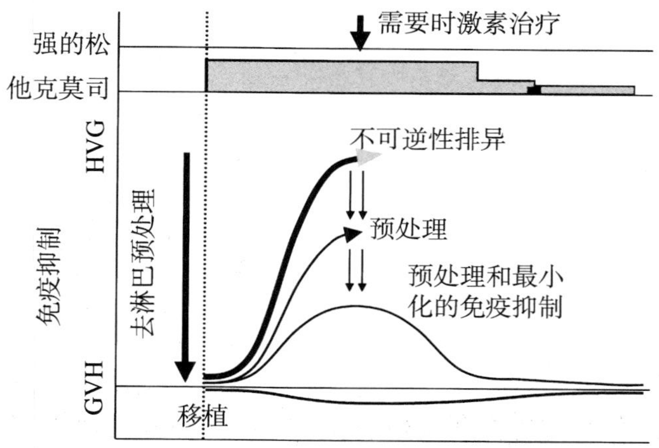

图 42-16 排异反应（粗的黑箭头）向免疫应答转变，可通过预处理和移植后最小化的免疫抑制使后者耗竭并清除。

器官保存

获取

20 世纪 60 年代早期的突破使移植具有临床实用性，这是始料未及的，那时对移植器官的保存几乎没有正规的准备。1950 年起心脏外科医生开心手术时使用低体温方法，知道降低膈以下器官的温度可减少主动脉横跨钳闭水平以下的缺血性损伤[58]。在一份早期的报道中，Lillehei 和他的同事等[33]报道在自体肠移植前将肠浸入冰盐水。Sicular 和 Moore[60]在波士顿报道在冷的肝切片中酶降解大大减慢。

尽管意识到低温作用，但直到 1963 年前，肾仍是常规移植，未在器官转运时做热缺血的保护。那时 694

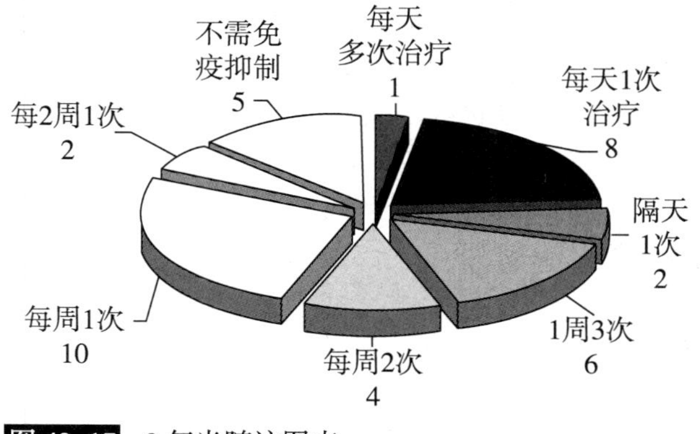

图 42-17 2 年半随访图表。

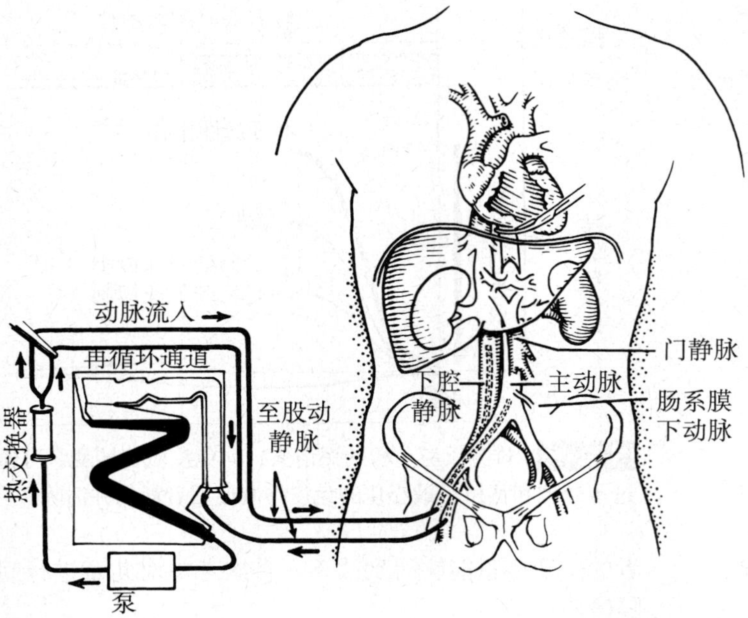

图 42-18 通过体外低温灌注进行原位冷却的初始技术。在供体死后，尽快经股血管向主动脉和腔静脉插入导管。通过热交换器进行体温控制。横形钳闭胸主动脉，限制躯体下部的灌注。在脑死亡标准被接受以前，1962—1969 年使用此方法获取尸体器官。此方法为之后的原位灌注技术打下基础。

仅有的使肾冷却的尝试是将活供体浸入装有冰水的浴缸内（全身低体温，胸外科医生开心手术时使用此方法），而这具有潜在危险性[63]。这种麻烦的冷却方法很快被供体肾切除后[67]向肾动脉内注射低温溶液的方法代替，利用了几年前实验性肝移植时就已标准化的中心降温（经血管）原则[62]。

原位中心降温是所有尸体完整器官保存中的首要步骤，如今的技术与 1963 年 Marchioro 及其同事们描述的有了改变[37]，使得原位冷却得以实施（图 42-18）[68]。Ackerman 和 Snell[1]、Merkel 及其同事[41]推广了经供体股动脉或远端主动脉注入冷电解质溶液的尸肾降温方法。获得技术最终得以完善，可摘除包括肝在内的所有胸腹腔器官而不危及个体器官（图 42-19）[79]。这个可变通的手术经改良后已用于情况不稳定甚至心脏已经停跳的供体[80]。1980～1985 的 5 年中，此技术在世界各地已具有通用性，使器官得以可靠地分享。切除冷却的器官后，原型策略使随后的保存成为可能：简单的冷冻或持续灌注（见下文）。

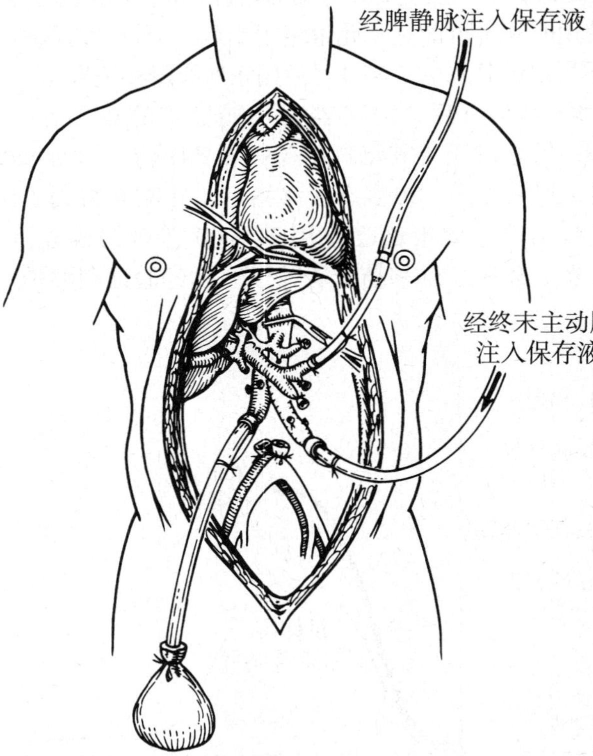

图 42-19 用于多器官获取的原位冷却原则。预先局部解剖主动脉和大的内脏静脉（此例为脾静脉）后，用冷的灌注液原位冷却器官。此例中肾和肝被切除。注意在腹腔干以上横跨钳闭主动脉。

保存方式的延伸

持续血管灌注

离体器官的持续灌注被证明是困难的。Ackerman

和 Barnard[2] 使用装有血液的常温灌注液，血液在高
695 压舱内氧合。Brettschneider 等人[10]改良了设备，使犬肝能保存 2 天，这是史无前例的成绩。Belzer 等去除了血红蛋白和高压舱部件，他们的血液低温灌注很快被临床肾移植接受，但后来知道其保存 2 天的质量并不明显优于更简单更廉价的输注及雪泥疗法（见下文）后，大多数中心慢慢摒弃了这种方法。然而，灌注技术的改进可能在某天使器官银行成为现实。

静态保存

有了“雪泥技术”后，可在预冷及分离后将特殊溶液（例如 Collins 等人[15]描述的）注入肾或其他器官的血管系统。原先的 Collins 液及其改良溶液被使用了将近 20 年，后来被威斯康星大学溶液代替，后者由 Folkert Belzer 的团队开发。虽然 UW 液首选用于肝移植[7,26,101]，但也给肾及其他器官提供了好的保存条件[24,106]。UW 液使肾（2 天）和肝（18 小时）的保存更长更安全、移植物存活率更高、初期原发无功能发生率更低。有了 UW 液，国家器官共享变得更经济可行。

组织配型

抗原配型

首次前瞻性抗原配型试验开始于 1964 年，由 Terasaki 等和科罗拉多大学肾移植组[97]合作开展。虽然当肾供体是高度适合的家族成员（完全配型）时[75]，此血清学技术的价值得到证明[75]，但较低程度的配型与肾移植预后相关性差[88]。此矛盾的原因不明，直到发现受体的嵌合状态之后才搞清楚（图 42-20）。尽管如此，配型是移植成功的首要决定性因素使其成为美国尸肾分配最重要的因素。

此肾分配方案的妥当性在近 1/3 世纪中反复受到伦理和科学的挑战。支持 HLA 配型分级者引用美国和欧洲的多中心病例并发症统计，显示组织相容性移植肾在移植存活率上有小的获益，而许多单个的捐献中心在他们的工作中未看到此趋势[19,38,58,93]。在一项强制性研究中，Terasaki 等人[98]报道，随机配对、非亲属活体供肾的早期存活、半寿期和亲代-后代（一个

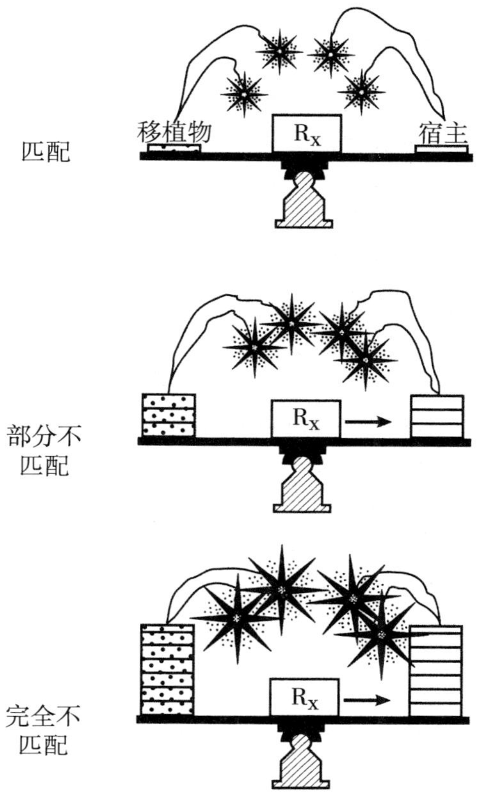

图 42-20　当器官植入免疫系统未去细胞化反应的受体时，同时产生 HVG 和 GVH 反应失效。共存细胞群相互诱导耐受解释了器官移植后 HLA 配型和结局相关性差的原因。

单倍体配对）肾移植相同。结论自然是改善完整器官移植效果的首要方式是免疫抑制治疗的有效时机和剂量，而不是组织配型及器官共享的改进。

交叉配型

目前没有一种免疫抑制方式能防止肾及其他器官移植物的立即破坏，即所谓的的超急性排异反应。这种并发症首次见于 ABO 血型不相配供体的肾植入带有抗供体同种凝集素的受体中的时候[69]。Terasaki 等人[96]描述了一名带有抗供体的淋巴细胞毒性抗体的受者发生超急性肾排异反应之后，Kissmeyer Nielsen 等人[28]以及其他人[73,76,100,108]证实，超急性排异反应与这些抗移植物抗体有关。虽然超急性排异反应常可通过
Terasaki 等推荐的淋巴细胞毒交叉配型来避免，但其 696
确切的发病原因 30 年来一直至之甚少，直到 30 年后补体激活综合征的认识才得以突破[73,76]。

展望

用药时机和剂量控制的修改可促进克隆耗竭一清除和免疫忽视机制，使全面减少在慢性免疫抑制风险中的暴露成为可能。我们的预测是大部分可实现不用药的完全耐受，但仅限于HLA匹配的器官，故不能完全实现。通过开发更好的药物，更重要的是基于机制使用已有的药物，大多数未实现完全耐受的患者常可获得不同程度的部分耐受。异种移植将在相同的免疫学框架下发展。原则性的问题是通过转基因修饰创造一种更好的种间组织匹配。虽然和更高级灵长类动物超急性排斥猪器官[54]有关的α-1,3GT基因已被敲除，但尚不知在猪器官应用于临床前还需做何进一步改变。目前仍未知干细胞生物学将适用于何处，但其也需遵守相同的免疫学规则。

（许 恩译 董其刚校）

参考文献

1. Ackermann JR, Snell MR: Cadaveric renal transplantation. Br J Urol 1963;40:515.
2. Ackermann JR, Barnard CN: Successful storage of kidneys. Br J Surg 1966;53:525-532.
3. Bach FH: Bone-marrow transplantation in a patient with the Wiskott-Aldrich syndrome. Lancet 1968;2:1364-1366.
4. Barker CF, Billingham RE: The role of afferent lymphatics in the rejection of skin homografts. J Exp Med 1968;128:197-221.
5. Barnard CN: What we have learned about heart transplants. J Thorac Cardiovasc Surg 1968;56:457-468.
6. Belzer FO, Ashby BS, Dunphy JE: 24-hour and 72-hour preservation of canine kidneys. Lancet 1967;2:536-538.
7. Belzer FO, Southard JH: Principles of solid-organ preservation by cold storage. Transplantation 1988;45:673-676.
8. Billingham RE, Brent L, Medawar PB: "Actively acquired tolerance" of foreign cells. Nature 1953;172:603-606.
9. Billingham R, Brent L, Medawar P: Quantitative studies on tissue transplantation immunity: III. Actively acquired tolerance. Philos Trans R Soc Lond (Biol) 1956;239:357-412.
10. Brettschneider L, Daloze PM, Huguet C, et al: The use of combined preservation techniques for extended storage of orthotopic liver homografts. Surg Gynecol Obstet 1968;126:263-274.
11. Calne RY, White HJO, Yoffa DE, et al: Prolonged survival of liver transplants in the pig. BMJ 1967;4:645-648.
12. Calne RY, Sells RA, Pena JR, et al: Induction of immunological tolerance by porcine liver allografts. Nature 1969;223:472-474.
13. Calne RY, White DJG, Thiru S, et al: Cyclosporin A in patients receiving renal allografts from cadaver donors. Lancet 1978;2:1323-1327.
14. Calne RY, Rolles K, White DJG, et al: Cyclosporin A initially as the only immunosuppressant in 34 recipients of cadaveric organs; 32 kidneys, 2 pancreases, and 2 livers. Lancet 1979;2:1033-1036.
15. Collins GM, Bravo-Shugarman M, Terasaki PI: Kidney preservation for transportation: Initial perfusion and 30 hours ice storage. Lancet 1969;2:1219-1224.
16. Cordier G, Garnier H, Clot JP, et al: La greffe de foie orthotopique chez le porc. Mem Acad Chir (Paris) 1966;92:799-807.
17. Demetris AJ, Qian S, Sun H, et al: Early events in liver allograft rejection. Am J Pathol 1991;138:609-618.
18. Derom F, Barbier F, Ringoir S, et al: Ten-month survival after lung homotransplantation in man. J Thorac Cardiovasc Surg 1971;61:835-846.
19. Ferguson R: For the Transplant Information Share Group (TISG): A multicenter experience with sequential ALG/cyclosporine therapy in renal transplantation. Clin Transpl 1988;2:285.
20. Fung JJ, Todo S, Tzakis A, et al: Conversion of liver allograft recipients from cyclosporine to FK506-based immunosuppression: Benefits and pitfalls. Transplant Proc 1991;23:14-21.
21. Gatti RA, Meuwissen HJ, Allen HD, et al: Immunological reconstitution of sex-linked lymphopenic immunological deficiency. Lancet 1968;2:1366-1369.
22. Hamburger J, Vaysse J, Crosnier J, et al: Transplantation of a kidney between nonmonozygotic twins after irradiation of the receiver: Good function at the fourth month. Presse Med 1959;67:1771-1775.
23. Hamburger J, Vaysse J, Crosnier J, et al: Renal homotransplantation in man after radiation of the recipient. Am J Med 1962;32:854-871.
24. Hoffman B, Sollinger H, Kalayoglu M, Belzer FO: Use of UW solution for kidney transplantation. Transplantation 1988;46:338-339.
25. Inman B, Halloran B, Melk A, et al: Microchimerism in sensitized renal patients. Transplantation 1999;67:1381-1383.
26. Kalayoglu M, Sollinger HW, Stratta RJ, et al: Extended preservation of the liver for clinical transplantation. Lancet 1988;1:617-619.
27. Karrer U, Althage A, Odermatt B, et al: On the key role of secondary lymphoid organs in antiviral immune responses studied in alymphoplastic (aly/aly) and spleenless (Hox11(-)/-) mutant mice. J Exp Med 1997;185:2157-2170.
28. Kissmeyer-Nielsen F, Olsen S, Peterson VP, Fjeldborg O: Hyperacute rejection of kidney allografts, associated with preexisting humoral antibodies against donor cells. Lancet 1966;2:622.
29. Kuss R, Legrain M, Mathe G, et al: Homologous human kidney transplantation: Experience with six patients. Postgrad Med J 1962;38:528-531.
30. Lafferty KJ, Prowse SJ, Simeonovic CJ: Immunobiology of tissue transplantation: A return to the passenger leukocyte concept. Ann Rev Immunol 1983;1:143-173.
31. Lakkis FG, Arakelov A, Konieczny BT, Inoue Y: Immunologic ignorance of vascularized organ transplants in the absence of secondary lymphoid tissue. Nature Med 2000;6:686-688.
32. Larsen CP, Morris PJ, Austyn JM: Migration of dendritic leukocytes from cardiac allografts into host spleens: A novel route for initiation of rejection. J Exp Med 1990;171:307-314.
33. Lillehei RC, Goott B, Miller FA: The physiological response of the small bowel of the dog to ischemia including prolonged in vitro preservation of the bowel with successful replacement and survival. Ann Surg 1959;150:543-560.
34. Lillehei RC, Simmons RL, Najarian JS, et al: Pancreaticoduodenal allotransplantation: Experimental and clinical observations. Ann Surg 1970;172:405-436.

35. Lu L, Rudert WA, Qian S, et al: Growth of donor-derived dendritic cells from the bone marrow of murine liver allograft recipients in response to granulocyte/macrophage colony-stimulating factor. J Exp Med 1995;182:379-387.
36. Main JM, Prehn RT: Successful skin homografts after the administration of high dosage X radiation and homologous bone marrow. J Natl Cancer Inst 1955;15:1023-1029.
37. Marchioro TL, Waddell WR, Starzl TE: Use of extracorporeal cadaver perfusion for preparation of organ homografts. Surg Forum 1963;14:174-176.
38. Matas AJ, Sutherland DER, Najarian JS: The impact of HLA matching on graft survival. Transplantation 1992;54: 568-569.
39. Mathe G, Amiel JL, Schwarzenberg L, et al: Haematopoietic chimera in man after allogeneic (homologous) bone-marrow transplantation. BMJ 1963;2:1633-1635.
40. McCurry K, Iacono A, Zeevi A, et al: Early outcomes in human lung transplantation utilizing thymoglobulin or campath 1H for recipient pretreatment followed by post-transplant tacrolimus near-monotherapy. J Thorac Cardiovasc Surg, 2005;2:528-537.
41. Merkel FK, Jonasson O, Bergan JJ: Procurement of cadaver donor organs: Evisceration technique. Transplant Proc 1972;4:585-589.
42. Merrill JP, Murray JE, Harrison JH, et al: Successful homotransplantation of the kidney between non-identical twins. N Engl J Med 1960;262:1251-1260.
43. Moskophidis D, Lechner F, Pircher H, Zinkernagel RM: Virus persistence in acutely infected immunocompetent mice by exhaustion of antiviral cytotoxic effector T cells. Nature 1993;362:758-761.
44. Murase N, Demetris AJ, Woo J, et al: Lymphocyte traffic and graft-versus-host disease after fully allogeneic small bowel transplantation. Transplant Proc 1991;23:3246-3247.
45. Murase N, Starzl TE, Ye Q, et al: Multilineage hematopoietic reconstitution of supralethally irradiated rats by syngeneic whole organ transplantation: with particular reference to the liver. Transplantation 1996;61:1-4.
46. Murase N, Demetris A, Woo J, et al: Graft versus host disease (GVHD) after BN to LEW compared to LEW to BN rat intestinal transplantation under FK 506. Transplantation 1993;55:1-7.
47. Murase N, Starzl TE, Tanabe M, et al: Variable chimerism, graft versus host disease, and tolerance after different kinds of cell and whole organ transplantation from Lewis to Brown-Norway rats. Transplantation 1995;60:158-171.
48. Murray JE, Merrill JP, Dammin GJ, et al: Study of transplantation immunity after total body irradiation: Clinical and experimental investigation. Surgery 1960;48:272-284.
49. Murray JE, Merrill JP, Harrison JH, et al: Prolonged survival of human-kidney homografts by immunosuppressive drug therapy. N Engl J Med 1963;268:1315-1323.
50. Murray JE, Sheil AGR, Moseley R, et al: Analysis of mechanism of immunosuppressive drugs in renal homotransplantation. Ann Surg 1964;160:449-473.
51. Nemlander A, Soots A, von Willebrand E, et al: Redistribution of renal allograft-responding leukocytes during rejection: II. Kinetics and specificity. J Exp Med 1982;156:1087-1100.
52. Peacock JH, Terblanche J: Orthotopic homotransplantation of the liver in the pig. In Read AE (ed): The Liver. London, Butterworth, 1967, p 333.
53. Phelps CJ, Koike C, Vaught TD, et al: Production of α1,3-galactosyltransferase-deficient pigs. Science 2003;299: 411-414.
54. Pierce JC, Varco RL: Induction of tolerance to a canine renal homotransplant with 6-mercaptopurine. Lancet 1962;1:781-782.
55. Przepiorka D, Thomas ED, Durham DM, Fisher L: Use of a probe to repeat sequence of the Y chromosome for detection of host cells in peripheral blood of bone marrow transplant recipients. Am J Clin Pathol 1991;95:201-206.
56. Sakamoto T, Ye Q, Lu L, et al: Donor hematopoietic progenitor cells in non-myeloablated rat recipients of allogeneic bone marrow and liver grafts. Transplantation 1999; 67:833-840.
57. Owens JC, Prevedel AE, Swan H: Prolonged experimental occlusion of thoracic aorta during hypothermia. Arch Surg 1955;70:95-97.
58. Salvatierra O Jr: Optimal use of organs for transplantation. N Engl J Med 1988;318:1329-1331.
59. Shapiro R, Jordan M, Basu A, et al: Kidney transplantation under a tolerogenic regimen of recipient pre-treatment and low-dose postoperative immunosuppression, with subsequent weaning. Ann Surg 2003;238:520-527.
60. Sicular A, Moore FD: The postmortem survival of tissues. J Surg Res 1961;1:16.
61. SivaSai KS, Jendrisak M, Duffy BF, et al: Chimerism in peripheral blood of sensitized patients waiting for renal transplantation: Clinical implications. Transplantation 2000;69:538-544.
62. Starzl TE, Kaupp HA Jr, Brock DR, et al: Reconstructive problems in canine liver homotransplantation with special reference to the postoperative role of hepatic venous flow. Surg Gynecol Obstet 1960;111:733-743.
63. Starzl TE, Brittain RS, Stonnington OG, et al: Renal transplantation in identical twins. Arch Surg 1963;86:600-607.
64. Starzl TE, Marchioro TL, Waddell WR: The reversal of rejection in human renal homografts with subsequent development of homograft tolerance. Surg Gynecol Obstet 1963;117:385-395.
65. Starzl TE: Experience in Renal Transplantation. Philadelphia, WB Saunders, 1964.
66. Starzl TE: Host-graft adaptation. In Starzl TE: Experience in Renal Transplantation. Philadelphia, WB Saunders, 1964, pp 164-170.
67. Starzl TE: Donor nephrectomy. In Starzl TE: Experience in Renal Transplantation. Philadelphia, WB Saunders, 1964, pp 68-82.
68. Starzl TE: The role of cadaveric donors in homotransplantation. In Starzl TE: Experience in Renal Transplantation. Philadelphia, WB Saunders, 1964, pp 54-58.
69. Starzl TE: Patterns of permissible donor-recipient tissue transfer in relation to ABO blood groups. In Starzl TE: Experience in Renal Transplantation. Philadelphia, WB Saunders, 1964, pp 37-46.
70. Starzl TE, Marchioro TL, Porter KA, et al: The use of heterologous antilymphoid agents in canine renal and liver homotransplantation and in human renal homotransplantation. Surg Gynecol Obstet 1967;124:301-318.
71. Starzl TE, Porter KA, Iwasaki Y, et al: The use of antilymphocyte globulin in human renal homotransplantation. In Wolstenholme GEW, O'Connor M (eds): Antilymphocytic Serum. London, J & A Churchill, 1967, pp 4-34.
72. Starzl TE, Groth CG, Brettschneider L, et al: Orthotopic homotransplantation of the human liver. Ann Surg 1968; 168:392-415.
73. Starzl TE, Lerner RA, Dixon FJ, et al: Shwartzman reaction after human renal transplantation. N Engl J Med 1968;278: 642-648.
74. Starzl TE: Rejection in unmodified animals. In Starzl TE: Experience in Renal Transplantation. Philadelphia, WB Saunders, 1964, p 184.
75. Starzl TE, Porter KA, Andres G, et al: Long-term survival after renal transplantation in humans: With special reference to histocompatibility matching, thymectomy, homograft

glomerulonephritis, heterologous ALG, and recipient malignancy. Ann Surg 1970;172:437-472.
76. Starzl TE, Boehmig HJ, Amemiya H, et al: Clotting changes, including disseminated intravascular coagulation, during rapid renal-homograft rejection. N Engl J Med 1970;283:383-390.
77. Starzl TE, Weil R III, Iwatsuki S, et al: The use of cyclosporin A and prednisone in cadaver kidney transplantation. Surg Gynecol Obstet 1980;151:17-26.
78. Starzl TE, Klintmalm GBG, Porter KA, et al: Liver transplantation with use of cyclosporin A and prednisone. N Engl J Med 1981;305:266-269.
79. Starzl TE, Hakala TR, Shaw BW Jr, et al: A flexible procedure for multiple cadaveric organ procurement. Surg Gynecol Obstet 1984;158:223-230.
80. Starzl TE, Miller C, Broznick B, Makowka L: An improved technique for multiple organ harvesting. Surg Gynecol Obstet 1987;165:343-348.
81. Starzl TE, Todo S, Fung J, et al: FK 506 for human liver, kidney and pancreas transplantation. Lancet 1989;2: 1000-1004.
82. Starzl TE, Fung J, Jordan M, et al: Kidney transplantation under FK 506. JAMA 1990;264:63-67.
83. Starzl TE, Demetris AJ, Murase N, et al: Cell migration, chimerism, and graft acceptance. Lancet 1992;339:1579-1582.
84. Starzl TE, Demetris AJ, Trucco M, et al: Systemic chimerism in human female recipients of male livers. Lancet 1992;340: 876-877.
85. Starzl TE, Demetris AJ, Trucco M, et al: Cell migration and chimerism after whole-organ transplantation: The basis of graft acceptance. Hepatology 1993;17:1127-1152.
86. Starzl TE, Demetris AJ, Trucco M, et al: Chimerism after liver transplantation for type IV glycogen storage disease and type I Gaucher's disease. N Engl J Med 1993;328:745-749.
87. Starzl TE, Demetris AJ, Trucco M, et al: Chimerism and donor-specific nonreactivity 27 to 29 years after kidney allotransplantation. Transplantation 1993;55:1272-1277.
88. Starzl TE, Eliasziw M, Gjertson M, et al: HLA and cross reactive antigen group (CREG) matching for cadaver kidney allocation. Transplantation 1997;64:983-991.
89. Starzl TE, Zinkernagel R: Antigen localization and migration in immunity and tolerance. N Engl J Med 1998;339: 1905-1913.
90. Starzl TE, Zinkernagel R: Transplantation tolerance from a historical perspective. Nature Rev Immunol 2001;1:233-239.
91. Starzl TE, Murase N, Abu-Elmagd K, et al: Tolerogenic immunosuppression for organ transplantation. Lancet 2003;361:1502-1510.
92. Starzl TE, Murase N, Demetris AJ, et al: Lessons of organ-induced tolerance learned from historical clinical experience. Transplantation 2004;77:926-929.
93. Takemoto S Terasaki PI, Cecka JM, et al: Survival of nationally shared HLA-matched kidney transplants from cadaveric donors. N Engl J Med 1992;327:834-839.
94. Taniguchi H, Toyoshima T, Fukao K, Nakauchi H: Presence of hematopoietic stem cells in the adult liver. Nat Med 1996;2:198-203.
95. Terakura M, Murase N, Demetris AJ, et al: Lymphoid/non-lymphoid compartmentalization of donor leukocyte chimerism in rat recipients of heart allografts, with or without adjunct bone marrow. Transplantation 1998;66: 350-357.
96. Terasaki PI, Marchioro TL, Starzl TE: Sero-typing of human lymphocyte antigens: Preliminary trials on long-term kidney homograft survivors. In Russel PS, Winn HJ, Amos DB (eds): Histocompatibility Testing. Washington, DC, National Academy of Science—National Research Council, 1965.
97. Terasaki PI, Vredevoe DL, Mickey MR, et al: Serotyping for homotransplantation: VII. Selection of kidney donors for thirty-two recipients. Ann N Y Acad Sci 1966;129:500.
98. Terasaki PI, Cecka JM, Gjertson DW, Takemoto S: High survival rates of kidney transplants from spousal and living unrelated donors. N Engl J Med 1995;333:333-336.
99. Thomas ED, Storb R, Clift RA, et al: Bone marrow transplantation. N Engl J Med 1975;292:832, 895-902 (2 parts).
100. Ting A: The lymphocytotoxic crossmatch test in clinical renal transplantation. Transplantation 1983;35:403-407.
101. Todo S, Nery J, Yanaga K, et al: Extended preservation of human liver grafts with UW solution. JAMA 1989;261: 711-714.
102. Todo S, Fung JJ, Starzl TE, et al: Liver, kidney, and thoracic organ transplantation under FK 506. Ann Surg 1990; 212:295-305.
103. Todo S, Fung JJ, Starzl TE, et al: Single center experience with primary orthotopic liver transplantation under FK506 immunosuppression. Ann Surg 1994;220:297-309.
104. Todo S, Tzakis A, Reyes J, et al: Small intestinal transplantation in humans with or without colon. Transplantation 1994;57:840-848.
105. Todo S, Reyes J, Furukawa H, et al: Outcome analysis of 71 clinical intestinal transplantations. Ann Surg 1995;222: 270-282.
106. Ueda Y, Todo S, Imventarza O, et al: The UW solution for canine kidney preservation: Its specific effect on renal hemodynamics and microvasculature. Transplantation 1989;48:913-918.
107. Wessman M, Popp S, Ruutu T, et al: Detection of residual host cells after bone marrow transplantation using non-isotopic in situ hybridization and karyotype analysis. Bone Marrow Transplant 1993;11:279-284.
108. Williams GM, et al: Studies in hyperacute and chronic renal homograft rejection in man. Surgery 1967;62:204.
109. Zinkernagel RM, Ehl S, Aichele P, et al: Antigen localization regulates immune responses in a dose- and time-dependent fashion: A geographical view of immune reactivity. Immunol Rev 1997;156:199-209.
110. Zinkernagel RM, Hengartner H: Antiviral immunity. Immunol Today 1997;18:258-260.
111. Zinkernagel RM, Bachmann MF, Kundig TM, et al: On immunologic memory. Annu Rev Immunol 1996;14: 333-367.
112. Zukoski CF, Callaway JM: Adult tolerance induced by 6-methyl mercaptopurine to canine renal homografts. Nature (London) 1963;198:706-707.
113. Zukoski CF, Callaway JM, Rhea WG Jr: Tolerance to a canine renal homograft induced by prednisolone. Surg Forum 1963;14:208-210.

第 43 章

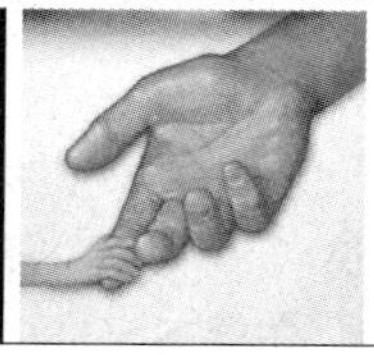

肾移植

John C. Magee 和 Darrell A. Campbell, Jr.

699 肾移植对于终末期肾病（ESRD）的儿童是首选的治疗选择，因为其给儿童的健康、生长发育提供最好的机会。儿科移植不断进步，目前儿童肾移植受者及器官的存活率非常高。效果的改善反映出移植前护理、供体选择、外科技术及围术期管理的进步，以及对儿童受者免疫抑制认识的加深。一些单中心记录的治疗结果非常好，甚至在小年龄儿童也很好[34,42,47,57]。

虽然单中心的知识给很多移植问题提供很好的见解，但更多的登记资料能更好地反应全国的移植情况从而得到广泛的认可。创立于 1987 年的北美儿童肾移植合作研究学会（NAPRTCS）是这些信息的主要来源之一[6,59,80]。此外，美国的资料从器官获取移植网（OPTN）收集，定期由移植受体科学登记处（SRTR）分析。

儿童终末期肾病

根据美国肾脏资料系统统计，2002 年有 1216 名 19 岁及以下的个体开始 ESRD 的治疗[96]。这个年龄组 ESRD 的发病率为每年 14.5/100 万。由于儿童的 ESRD 较成人罕见，此发病率明显低于整个国家每年 333/100 万的发病率。

表 43-1 概括了儿童肾移植群体中肾病的病因。根据 NAPRTCS 的数据，前五位病因分别为：梗阻性尿路病变、肾不发育 / 发育不全 / 发育异常、局灶节段性肾小球硬化（FSGS）、反流性肾病和慢性肾小球肾炎。这些病因占肾移植的一半以上。儿童肾衰的病因与成人明显不同，先天性畸形、梗阻性尿路病变是儿童肾移植的主要原因为主。此外，FSGS 是最常见的获得性肾病，儿童远多于成人。

儿童人群中，病因随年龄、性别、人种而不同。700
小年龄儿童先天性原因较多，大年龄儿童获得性原因

表 43-1　20 岁及以下肾移植受体（n=7939）的原发疾病诊断

疾病	%
梗阻性尿路病变	16.1
肾不发育 / 发育不全 / 发育不良	16.0
局灶节段性肾小球硬化	11.4
反流性肾病	5.2
慢性肾小球肾炎	3.5
髓质囊性病	2.8
溶血尿毒症综合征	2.8
多囊肾	2.7
梅干腹综合征	2.6
先天性肾病综合征	2.5
家族性肾炎	2.3
胱氨酸贮积症	2.1
特发性新月体性肾小球肾炎	1.9
Ⅰ型膜增生性肾小球肾炎	1.9
肾盂 / 间质性肾炎	1.9
系统性红斑狼疮性肾炎	1.7
肾梗死	1.5
过敏性紫癜肾炎	1.3
Berger（IgA）肾炎	1.3
Ⅱ型性增生性肾小球肾炎	0.9
肾母细胞瘤	0.6
Denys-Drash 综合征	0.6
草酸盐沉积症	0.5
Wegener 肉芽肿病	0.5
膜性肾病	0.5
其他全身免疫性疾病	0.4
镰状细胞肾病	0.2
糖尿病性肾小球肾炎	0.1
其他	8.0
不明原因	6.2

From North American Pediatric Renal Transplant Cooperative Study, (NAPRTCS) 2004 annual report. Available at www.naprtcs.org.

较多。总体上，60%的受者为男性，男性占梗阻性尿路病变（86%）、肾不发育/发育不全/发育异常（62%）、FSGS（58%）受者的大多数。反流性肾病、慢性肾小球肾炎、狼疮性肾炎更多见于女性受者，女性分别占55%、59%和81%。种族分布上，黑人儿童最常见的是FSGS（23%），其次是梗阻性尿路病变（16%）、肾不发育/发育不全/发育异常（14%）、慢性肾小球肾炎（4%）和狼疮性肾炎（4%）。白人受者中梗阻性尿路病变（17%）最常见，其次是肾不发育/发育不全/发育异常（17%）、FSGS（9%），反流性肾病（6%）和肾髓质囊性病（4%）。

受体评估

任何一名ESRD患儿都应考虑行肾移植。绝对禁忌证很少，包括未经治疗的恶性肿瘤或全身败血症。相对禁忌证包括严重缩短患儿生命的全身性疾病，或社会原因导致完全无法进行移植后护理及免疫抑制治疗的情况。有时，决定是否对一名生活质量差或有严重脏器损害的患儿进行移植是很困难的。此时没有明显正确的答案。在这种情况下，应进行深入讨论，考虑对患儿的期望和目标。

所有进行性慢性肾功能不全的患儿应该由一个多学科的儿科肾移植团队评估，包括一名小儿肾病学家、一名移植手术医生、一名社会工作者和一名营养学家。此外，许多团队中还包括小儿泌尿科医生和临床心理学家，如需要还可有其他专家。最好在透析前对患儿进行充分评估，以便于评估潜在的活体供者，并为移植做好所有准备。理想的情况是早期评估后提前移植，从而避免透析。对于婴儿的大小，可对小至6kg的小婴儿进行成功的肾移植，但我们及其他作者[57]认为在不损害患儿健康的情况下，10kg是理想体重。

表43-2概括了我们的标准化评估。应该努力完善ESRD患儿的内科治疗，包括骨病治疗、营养优化、完成免疫接种。对儿童受者的一些评估有别于成人，需要特别注意。其一是膀胱功能的评估和治疗。许多患儿有下极的畸形，膀胱状况可能不适于移植。很多患儿之前已做了泌尿系手术。此时专家的意见或与小儿泌尿外科的密切合作是必要的。营养对于儿童的生长发育是首要的。最后，评估并解决儿童及其护理者的

表43-2 儿童肾移植候选人的评估

病史和体格检查
实验室检查：
血液学（包括血小板的全血细胞计数、凝血酶原时间/部分凝血活酶时间）
生化（肾功能、电解质、肝功能）
血清学（乙肝、丙肝、疱疹病毒、巨细胞病毒、EB病毒、水痘-带状疱疹病毒、人免疫缺陷病毒）
ABO血型
组织分型（人白细胞抗原分型；同种异体抗体筛查）
尿液分析
胸片
心电图
社会心理学评估
可选的检查：
排泄性膀胱尿道造影
血管造影

心理状态非常重要。足够的社会支持也很重要的。患有慢性疾病、接受过复杂治疗的患儿压力很大，对其进行教育和安慰使其放心非常重要。对于年长儿童需保证让其积极参与治疗过程。青少年群体特别具有挑战性，因为无论术前术后，其不配合的风险是最大的。

除了上述因素，其他一些问题也需特别关注。其一是评估患儿的脉管系统的潜在必要性。随着肾替代治疗的进步，目前能够对越来越小的患儿进行血液透析，包括新生儿。但这些治疗需留置导管，这与髂静脉及腔静脉血栓发生率增高有关。静脉流量不足使得移植变得困难，并限制标准手术的选择。Thomas等人总结了关于静脉血栓的经验，提出一种利用放射学影像对风险患儿（尤其是有股静脉置管史和炎症相关的腹腔内操作史的患儿）进行筛查的方式[92]。

原肾切除的必要性常是评估中的一个问题。儿童原肾切除较成人移植群体多。23%的儿童受者在移植前已完全切除自体肾组织[72]。原肾切除的可能指征包括：反流性肾病导致的反复严重感染、无法控制的高血压和先天性肾病综合征。肾病综合征患儿因严重的蛋白尿可促血栓形成而许行原肾切除。多囊肾患儿因出血、反复感染或疼痛而需行原肾切除。有时因自体肾过大危及移植肾而需切除。有人主张小婴儿严重多尿也是原肾切除指征，因为如此便于术后液体管理，减少移植物灌注不足的风险。但这是在肤浅的水平呼

吁，仔细的术后管理常可使之避免成为肾切除的单独指征。另外，一些人认为 FSGS 患儿需行原肾切除，因为这便于疾病复发的诊断，如出现蛋白反映了移植物疾病而不是来自自体肾。这些情况下，可考虑尝试非激素疗法的“药物性肾切除”。

除了考虑原肾切除的指征，肾切除时机也是重要的。对于已接受肾替代治疗的患儿，如需做双侧原肾切除，则在移植前几周完成是安全便利的。对于没有肾替代治疗的患儿，问题更为复杂。在肾移植时我们不推荐同时做双侧肾切除，因为两者结合是一个大手术。此外，即使是小婴儿也可经腹膜后径路做移植，此路径不能暴露对侧原肾。需切除双侧原肾、未接受肾替代治疗的患儿中，许多在移植前有足够的肾储备、可耐受单侧左肾切除，而不需透析。在此情况下，移植时可做标准腹膜后切口并略向头侧延伸，从而可做右侧原肾切除。对于移植前做单侧原肾切除后需肾替代治疗的病例，可在移植时切除同侧原肾。如需要可在移植后数月切除对侧肾。

何时做肾移植？只要有合适的活体供体或尸体器官，需尽快为最近接受肾替代治疗的患儿做移植手术。对于未行透析治疗的患儿，应在尿毒症出现前手术。应注意 ESRD 对儿童生长发育的影响。对于 FSGS 或狼疮性肾炎患儿，移植需推迟到疾病静止期进行，这样就无法提前移植。在多数情况下，提前移植可让患儿避免透析而无肾损害[24]。但目前接受活供体器官移植的患儿中仅有 33% 患儿在透析前提前移植，而在接受尸体器官的患儿中仅为 13% [6]。

泌尿系问题

ESRD 患儿中的泌尿系问题高发，因此在移植前需仔细评估膀胱功能。除了发育异常、膀胱出口梗阻，还可因为神经病变、获得性排尿功能障碍及获得性膀胱病变而引起膀胱功能异常。之前任何膀胱扩大术都会损害正常膀胱功能。对于有尿失禁史、反复尿路感染、以前做过泌尿系手术以及需留置导尿管的患儿，都应进一步检查评估。如怀疑膀胱功能异常，应进行排泄性膀胱尿道造影（VCUG）和尿流动力学检测。VCUG 充盈期压力低于 30cmH_2O 一般提示膀胱功能良好。

应慎重考虑任何手术干预的时机。一些无尿或少尿患儿，其膀胱可能功能不佳，但此时难以判断是否最终可恢复正常功能。如施行膀胱扩大术，需长期留置导尿管，因为此时膀胱无正常功能。因此，应慎行使原肾功能保留多年的泌尿系手术，做移植前干预时需仔细考虑手术的风险和益处，充分认识其对接下来的移植及远期治疗的影响。

透析通路

对于未接受提前移植或早期发生 ESRD 的患儿，建立足够的透析通路非常重要。适当的透析通路对充分透析是必要的，后者与患儿的生活质量和健康直接相关。 血液透析、腹膜透析都是可以选择的。根据 USRDS 的资料，截止 2002 年底，19 岁及以下儿童中，61%接受血液透析，39%接受腹膜透析[96]。选择血透或腹透最好因人而异，需考虑患儿及家庭的意愿、技术水平及当地可以获得的医疗资源。

对于血液透析，首先应尝试一期建立动静脉瘘。如果患儿无合适的静脉，则需用聚四氟乙烯植入物。自体动静脉瘘需要合适的静脉，这是首选的透析通路，因为它的通畅率高。此外，术后几周自体瘘才能成熟并使用。因此但对于急需血透但没有通路的患儿，只能选用临时导管。约 3/4 的患儿开始透析使用临时导管[61]。使用导管后感染风险增加，透析清除率低。此外，导管可引起中心静脉狭窄及血栓形成，造成将来永久性的上肢血管通路建立困难。因此颈静脉 702
置管优于锁骨下静脉置管。

腹膜透析需置入 Tenckhoff 导管。在全麻下通过开放性手术置入双套囊腹膜透析导管。导管环放入骨盆。置管的关键是确定液体能自由地进出。使用双套囊导管并使导管的出口向下可减少感染[61]。

供体选择

活体肾移植对所有 ESRD 患儿是首选的。与尸体肾移植相比，活体肾移植的效果更好。此外，活体肾移植在找到合适的供体后马上可以施行，不需在移植名单上等待尸体供者。活供体与受体在遗传学上可相关或无关。两种活供体的移植效果相同，都优于尸体供者。虽然不需要遗传学的匹配，但几乎所有活供体和预期受体之间都有亲近的亲属关系。可能的活供体需经过有经验的移植中心进行充分评估。供体必须自愿、健康并有两个正常肾。此外，供、受体必须 ABO 血型匹配。虽然跨越此壁垒的方法越来越得到注意，但这些努力仍处于早期阶段并且对儿童群体的经验有限[66,83]。此外，受体和供体的淋巴细胞毒交叉配型试验应为阴性。交叉配型试验用于确定受体是否产生抗供体人类白细胞抗原（HLA）的抗体，此抗体可能导致超急性排异反应及移植物迅速丧失。此过程产生迅速，并且几乎不可能逆转。已开始研究处理抗供体抗体活性的方法，包括静脉内使用免疫球蛋白及血浆去除术。受体产生抗 HLA 抗体的主要原因有输血、先期的移植病史和妊娠。

表 43–3 活体肾供体评估

病史和体格检查
实验室检查：
血液学（包括血小板的全血细胞计数、凝血酶原时间 / 部分凝血活酶时间）
生化（肾功能、电解质、肝功能）
血清学（乙肝、丙肝、疱疹病毒、巨细胞病毒、EB 病毒、水痘–带状疱疹病毒、人免疫缺陷病毒）
ABO 血型
组织分型（人白细胞抗原分型）
尿液分析
胸片
心电图
社会心理学评估
螺旋 CT 扫描

活体供体的评估

活供体的评估应和受体评估分开，把供体的安全放在首位。表 43–3 概括了我们的标准化评估。虽然传统上 HLA 配型对活供体评估的挑选很重要，但目前免疫抑制剂已把配型的影响降到最低，我们认为因此最好的供体是最主动捐助的人。如这方面没有区别，其他条件也相同，应选择 HLA 最匹配的供体。考虑每个供体的其他问题也很重要，包括社会心理问题，如需要照顾其他儿童或受者，需考虑何种选择对家庭的干扰是最小的。与患儿家庭讨论情况时，需考虑将来可能需要肾移植的其他家庭成员，因为这将有助于决定哪个供体移植给哪个受体。很少使用 18 岁以下的活供体，也不鼓励这么做[16,44]。

活体肾捐献是安全的，已实施了 50 年，手术死亡率为 3/10 000[50]。术后供体可保持长期正常生活。腹腔镜下供体肾切除的引入对于考虑捐肾者是一个重要进步。腹腔镜手术恢复更快，并与开放性肾切除一样安全[93,100]。虽然有人担心腹腔镜下捐献的效果不如开放性供体肾切除，特别对于小婴儿，但此问题未被研究中心的研究证实[41,95]。然而，无论使用何种方法，施行供体肾切除的手术团队应是这方面的专家。

死亡供体的评估

对于无合适的活供体的患儿，尸体肾移植是唯一的选择。死亡供体可能为脑死亡或心脏不可逆性停跳者，后者常被称为“无心跳供体”。在美国器官分配按照 OPTN 制定的政策管理。这些政策根据出现更公平合理的分配方法而会进行不断改进。目前，尸体肾在国家和地方水平接受分配。如有潜在 703
的死亡供体被确定，其血型、HLA 类型及其他相关的供体因素将进入器官共享联合网络（UNOS）维护的国家数据库。如找到 ABO 血型匹配、HLA 相同的受体，则会向此个体提供肾源。零抗原误配的肾在国家水平共享。虽然此方法有一定益处，但由于需将肾转运至受者所在的中心，常使冷缺血时间增加。如未找到零抗原误配的受体，肾通常在当地移植。肾的分配由一个积分系统指导，后者根据 DR 位点 HLA 匹配程度及受者等待时间计算。给抗 HLA 抗体水平高的受者加分，因为其难以寻找适当的供体。如果透析时患儿情况不佳，会根据其年龄额外加分。进一步的优先分配给予列入候选名单后未能在规定年龄内施行移植的儿童候选人：出生至 5 岁、列入名单达 6 个月者；6～10 岁列入名单达 12 个月者；11～17 岁列入名单达 1 个月者。总之，这些分配方案使儿童候选人在移植名单上的等待时间短于成人。然而许多患儿的等待时间比预计的长。在过去的 2004 年，分配方案进一步修订，将 35 岁以下的尸肾优先供给儿童候选人。

死亡供体的总数每年相对稳定，但可做供体的评估标准扩大了。供体的年龄较前增大，高血压及其他类似疾病比例较高，这可能影响器官的质量。为了改善高风险组供体肾的利用率，其被定义为扩大标准供体（ECD），按照便于利用这些器官的原则进行分配[55,69]。ECD 标准包括任何 60 岁以上的死亡供体或 50 岁以上有以下两种情况者：有高血压史且捐献前血清肌酐大于等于 1.5mg/dL 或死于脑血管意外（中风）。这些肾移植失败的相对风险比理想的死亡供体参照组高 1.7 倍。ECD 肾将使许多成年候选人获益。由于儿童候选人已得到分配优先权，所以不需要使用 ECD 肾。所以，大多数儿童不出现在 ECD 肾源的等待名单上。

由于供体器官的严重短缺，心源性死亡后捐献（DCD）（以前被称作无心跳器官捐献）再次兴起，使可获得器官数量明显增加。符合严格脑死亡标准的患者只占所有住院死亡患者的一小部分。大部分患者在心跳停止前未经历脑死亡。患有严重的不可恢复性神经损害、但不符合脑死亡标准的患者可能捐献器官，只要照看此患者的法定近亲和医生都做出撤出重症监护病房（ICU）的决定。DCD 使这些患者及其家庭实现器官捐献的愿望。2002 年 DCD 仅占所有移植的死亡供体肾的 3.3%，与 1994 年的 1.2%相比略有增加[67]。虽然使用 DCD 肾的起初效果好，但迟发性功能不良的风险较高[12,15]。

考虑给患儿移植哪个供体的器官时，移植医生必须在获得“理想肾”（例如供体质量、HLA 匹配程度）的愿望和使患儿摆脱透析间权衡利弊。器官分配制度的优化使得此过程变得更简单。儿童受者希望获得长期有功能的肾，因此这限制了接受年老或边缘性供体的器官。总之，ECD 或 DCD 供体肾一般不用于儿童。另外，小年龄死亡儿童的肾移植效果不佳，且这些供体肾很少适合儿童候选人。但经长时间等待但无适合供体的高致敏受者是个例外。此时应根据具体情况分析，权衡各种风险及其益处。

移植

移植前准备

一旦有合适的供体肾，死亡供体的移植受者就收治入院。虽然若透析治疗稳定或不行透析治疗，受者可在手术当天入院，但目前我们仍将提前接受活体供体的小儿受者收治入院。入院时需评估透析的必要性。询问最近一次就诊之后患儿有无健康问题，并检查有无感染迹象。

麻醉

与麻醉医生的密切合作对于任何手术都很重要，小婴儿肾移植时更是如此。维持足够的血容量很关键。因为肾来源于成人供体，进入肾的血流量常等于受者的心输出量，因此容易产生低血压的问题。许多患儿有强制性多尿，如不仔细监测可能引起血容量不 704
足。恢复灌注后移植肾可容纳几百毫升血液，这进一步加重了血容量不足。

手术过程

患儿入手术室后全麻诱导。建立足够的静脉通路。对于 20kg 以上的儿童如能建立足够的外周静脉通路，则不开放中心静脉。对于较小的患儿，中心静脉是有用的，可用于液体管理及监测中心静脉压。同时应放置动脉导管以便连续监测动脉压。患儿仰卧位，将 Foley 导尿管插入膀胱。我们将导尿管连于注有盐水稀释聚维酮碘（Betadine）的三通冲洗装置，其他中心可能更喜欢使用抗生素溶液。如此可在手术区域以外使膀胱充盈或排空。然后腹部消毒铺巾。应密切监测患儿体温，特别对较小儿童，因为液体复苏或冷肾脏灌注可能造成低体温。应保持手术室的温度并使用加热毯。除了常规的麻醉监测，需时常注意血容量状况。当肾再灌注时，重要的是维持足够的动脉血压、中心静脉压。婴儿和小年龄儿童中心静脉压应维持在 12.0～18.0cmH_2O，必要时补充晶体和（或）胶体。血管吻合快完成时，0.5mg/kg 静脉使用甘露醇,而不常规使用袢利尿剂。

手术技巧

小年龄儿童（＜20kg）

过去许多人经正中切口给婴儿或小年龄儿童进行

肾移植。1998 年以来，我们使用和成人类似的腹膜后入路。对小年龄儿童，首选将肾置于右侧，这样最易接近腔静脉。右下腹做弧形切口，分离腹壁肌肉，进入腹膜前间隙，解剖分离在腹膜外进行，用固定拉钩暴露。男性需游离精索并保护，女性则常规切断圆韧带。向内侧解剖，直至看见髂总血管、远端主动脉及腔静脉。若需要可在此时切除右侧原肾，沿输尿管向上到肾脏。

根据肾脏及患儿的大小决定血管吻合的确切部位。一般小年龄儿童的肾静脉与腔静脉吻合，肾动脉与远端主动脉或髂总动脉吻合。用丝线结扎血管表面的淋巴管，从而使术后发生囊性淋巴管瘤的风险降至最低。行主动脉吻合时，需从肠系膜下动脉以下游离至主动脉分叉处。腰部分支用 Pott 带控制而不结扎。做主动脉吻合时，在主动脉分叉远端控制左右髂总动脉。游离腔静脉以便放置侧壁钳，这还需要结扎一些腰静脉。在游离时常用套圈轻柔地控制血管。当受者的血管暴露后将供体肾置入手术区域。检查肾有无未被发现的病变并检查肾血管。准备供肾后，仔细考虑如何将其植入受者体腔内。特别注意肾血管的长度和方向。重要的是考虑再灌注后、去除拉钩关闭切口后肾的最终静息位。

首先做静脉吻合。用侧壁钳控制腔静脉或髂静脉，沿前外侧或侧方将静脉纵向切开。考虑好肾的植入位置后将肾静脉切至合适长度，因为过长的肾静脉易致血栓形成。用 5-0 Prolene 线缝住两个角做连续吻合，保证血管是通畅的。接着做供体动脉和受体远端主动脉或髂总动脉的端侧吻合。用轻柔的弹簧夹或小血管钳控制受者的血管。纵向切开动脉，注意肾动脉的最终方向。我们 4mm 的主动脉钻孔器扩大动脉切开处。用 6-0 Prolene 线连续缝合，端侧吻合肾动脉。放大镜下操作可缝合更加精确。

如果有两根肾动脉，可分别植入，也可在移植前合并后再植入。因为血管合并将使两根血管在二维平面上相对固定，故合并时重要的是考虑能否使血管在手术结束时处于好的位置。这可能对适当吻合位置的选择造成限制，如果预期的最终肾静息位不恰当，可导致供体动脉的一根或两根扭结。

完成动脉吻合前，最好与麻醉医生讨论患儿的血
705 流动力学状态。术中可直接通过腔静脉评估血管容量。此时也需给予甘露醇。由于成人肾体积和正常儿童血容量之间的差异，可使肾灌注减慢并隔离大量血液。麻醉医生必须在需要时迅速补充容量。此时放开静脉的血管钳，查看有无出血。接下来，轻柔地关闭肾动脉后，从受者血管上撤去血管钳，恢复远端血流。几秒钟后，肾脏血流建立。对于小年龄儿童，有时我们会短暂地重复钳夹吻合口远端的血管，使肾得到更多血流。仔细检查手术野，查看有无出血。评估肾的颜色和充盈情况。肾动脉应有良好的搏动，常可感觉到震颤。应评估肾上下极的灌注情况。肾静脉应饱满但不紧张，充盈程度如同腔静脉，再次检查肾的位置。

接着行输尿管膀胱吻合术。我们通常用膀胱外输尿管膀胱吻合的方法做输尿管吻合[47,64]，也有人使用经膀胱 Politano-Leadbetter 吻合方法[42,57]。钳闭 Foley 导尿管使膀胱充盈。在膀胱顶部选择吻合部位，避免成角。分离膀胱肌层，暴露并切开黏膜。修剪供体输尿管至合适长度，使之能与膀胱行无张力吻合，避免过长，因为远端输尿管灌注不足会造成输尿管梗阻或狭窄。将输尿管末端修剪为铲型，使用 5-0 PDS 线做黏膜-黏膜的连续吻合，此处用连续缝合就足够，但注意避免打结过紧，这会造成荷包效应，导致吻合口狭窄。为了避免膀胱输尿管反流，需用 4-0 PDS 线间断吻合使膀胱肌层覆盖在输尿管吻合口之上。这使得输尿管在膀胱壁内呈切线位，排尿时，输尿管的经膀胱段受到膀胱壁的压迫。如果膀胱正常、输尿管远端血供良好，不常规放置支撑管。如果担心输尿管吻合（不管对供体输尿管还是受者的膀胱功能），需放置双 J 管，这将在移植数周后于门诊拔除。

完成输尿管吻合后，再次检查肾血管及去除拉钩后肾的位置。吻合前的仔细规划以及对细节的注意常在此时看出成效。去除拉钩，用连续缝合的方式分一层或两层关闭筋膜，用可吸收线连续缝合关闭皮肤。用生理盐水冲洗导尿管，去除可能阻塞导管的血块，将导尿管接于集尿袋。对于小婴儿，为保证好的肾灌注，需结合肾的体积进行容量复苏，如此会引起呼吸幅度减小，故术后立即进行通气支持是必需的。如果患儿氧饱和度及肺功能好，可在手术室拔管。

大年龄儿童（＞20kg）

大年龄儿童肾移植方法与成人类似。我们偏向于将肾置于盆腔右侧。做右下腹切口，从耻骨上一至两指宽处向上延长切口至腹直肌鞘外侧。暴露腹膜前间

隙，游离髂血管。同样，结扎血管表面的淋巴管，以期使术后发生囊性淋巴管瘤的风险降至最低。像小年龄儿童一样，动静脉吻合的方式取决于患儿的大小和肾血管的粗细。静脉吻合可选用腔静脉、髂总静脉或髂外静脉。动脉吻合可采用远端主动脉、髂总动脉、或髂外动脉。十多年来我们未使用过髂内动脉。在重建肾血管后，经膀胱外途径进行输尿管膀胱吻合。手术完成后拔管。

有泌尿系手术史患儿的输尿管重建

理想的尿液贮藏器可以在低压力下储存一定量的尿液，不漏，排尿后几乎完全排空[24]。大多数病例中理想的贮藏器是患儿的膀胱。如果在出现少尿前膀胱功能正常，移植术后膀胱就可能有良好的功能。然而，30%的患儿无正常膀胱功能，移植前常做过扩大切除术或其他泌尿系手术。

当自身膀胱功能障碍或缺如时，将移植肾产生的尿液引流至扩大的膀胱或代膀胱是合适的治疗策略[10,26]。如有必要，可在移植前重新建立一个适于使用的尿液贮藏器。术中对扩大的膀胱进行输尿管膀胱吻合时，要考虑扩大部分的血供，使之在移植中不受损伤。最好对自身膀胱进行吻合，如此可在大多数情况下完成吻合。我们认为要给所有患儿做抗反流的输尿管膀胱吻合，利用膀胱壁可容易地完成此操作。

将尿液引流入扩大的膀胱或代膀胱的患儿尿路感染风险增加。但与历史对照比较后，移植物存活率未受到负面影响[32]。与输尿管吻合相关的手术并发症发生率在此类患儿中较高，约为 20% [25,32,43]。不管膀胱功能障碍病因如何，这些患儿在移植后需定期做间歇性清洁导尿。

后尿道瓣膜引起梗阻性尿路病变的患儿无正常的膀胱功能，可导致移植后肾功能障碍[26]。需意识到这些问题的重要性，对排尿障碍的患儿需要进行尿流动力学的随访评估。膀胱功能障碍，如低顺应性和（或）高反流需药物或手术治疗[76]。

术后处理

对术后细节问题的关注是必要的。必须关心水、电解质平衡状况。移植前许多患儿有多尿，这种强制性尿丧失将会在术后一段时间内持续存在。经静脉补液，需将尿量及非显性失水计算在内。定期监测血清电解质，根据需要调节补液的成分。密切观察血清钠、钾、钙的水平，根据需要补充。仔细监测心率、血压和中心静脉压。评估血管内容量时单个因素是不可靠的，有些结果不能反映患儿的真实情况。

对于少尿或移植前已切除原肾的患儿，如移植物迅速发挥功能，尿量是监测移植物功能很好的手段。如患儿术前多尿或移植物功能延迟，则评估较为困难。患儿术前有尿的情况下，术后尿量的多少能反映移植物功能。另外，血清肌酐应持续下降。少尿患儿需仔细检查。用少量无菌生理盐水冲洗导尿管。患儿的容量状况需仔细评估。通常补液试验是正确的，既可作为诊断性试验，也可作为治疗干预措施。多普勒超声可以明确移植肾是否有足够的动脉血供和静脉流出。此外，超声还可显示肾周是否积液或积血，以及可能的输尿管梗阻。如患儿似乎血容量充足、血流动力学稳定，可使用一剂利尿剂观察反应。但需谨慎，因为大量的尿液排出可使血管内血容量明显下降，引起肾灌注不足。如患儿血容量过多或电解质严重异常时需透析。

术后如需机械通气，小年龄儿童一般于术后 24 小时内脱离呼吸机。经腹膜外手术后可马上给予少量肠道进食。对于移植前用导管喂养的婴儿，术后应予恢复，因为术后短时间内尚不能经口喂养。高血压也可以是一个问题。手术相关的血容量补充、用于免疫抑制的神经钙调蛋白抑制剂均可引起严重的高血压，需积极治疗，防止癫痫和其他后遗症。

为了每小时监测尿量并予补充，一般需把患儿置于 ICU。如外科病房能做到这些，大一点的患儿可住在肾移植的专门监护区。送入 ICU 的患儿 1～2 天后可转回普通病房。只要患儿能够进食、家长熟悉免疫抑制治疗方案后，大多数患儿可于术后 5～7 天出院。

移植物早期功能障碍的评估

理想状态下，供体肾在血管接通后很快产生尿液。但这取决于多种因素，首先是供体器官的质量。活供体肾因供体健康状况良好且冷缺血时间短，一般可立即产生功能。尸肾的冷缺血时间一般较长。此外，更重要的是有多种与供体死亡有关的因素，包括低血压、可能需要大剂量的血管加压药及其他与供体整体健康状况有关的问题。

不考虑供体来源，手术室内就应对移植物进行评估，检查肾的颜色、充盈及动静脉吻合情况。尤其要注意关腹后肾的位置及其对脉管系统的影响。肾动脉常有震颤，说明血流灌注良好，肾内阻力低。假定手术操作满意，给肾补充额外的容量而不产生尿液是最好的选择。一旦患儿有足够的容量负荷，应使用袢利尿剂缓和的利尿。对于术前无尿、移植后仍无排尿的患儿，应行床边多普勒超声检查。对于术前有尿的患儿，确定移植肾是否排尿较为困难，有时尿量是肾产
707 生功能的标志之一。术后 24 小时血清肌酐水平应下降。如果仍担心肾功能，应做多普勒超声检查，若显示动静脉有问题，应立即回手术室再次手术。超声结果正常，但有时可发现血流中度减少，提示肾内阻力增加，最常见是由急性肾小管坏死引起。这种情况无特殊处理也能解决。其他诊断性检查较少应用。很少需做肾动脉造影。一些中心使用放射性核素扫描，但我们发现这并不比超声有更多益处。放射性核素扫描可能对在经皮肾造瘘前发现可疑尿漏有帮助。

输尿管吻合的并发症包括漏和梗阻。输尿管并发症的发生率约为 9%[57]。输尿管吻合口漏一般在移植后的最初几天逐渐凸显。尿漏一般可通过经皮放置肾造瘘管的非手术方式治疗。随后此导管可通过吻合口进入膀胱并转变为常规支撑管。支撑管通常开放，此后几天进行体位性外引流，尿漏愈合后可将其封闭。如果出现大的尿囊肿，则需引流肾周积液。

泌尿系统梗阻可发生在任何时候。早期梗阻和供体输尿管吻合的技术问题或其他机械性问题（如吻合前输尿管扭转导致的吻合后输尿管扭转）有关。因为输尿管血供来源于肾下极的小滋养动脉，故不能将输尿管留得太长。移植后较长时间发生的输尿管狭窄一般需手术治疗，切除狭窄段并做输尿管重新吻合。

腹膜后肾移植术后的另一并发症是囊性淋巴管瘤。囊性淋巴管瘤可引起不适或移植物功能障碍。超声引导下经皮穿刺得肌酐浓度与血清相同的清澈液体后可诊断。经皮引流的复发率很高，最好做腹膜开窗。可在腹腔镜下完成，或做一小的开放性切口将囊性淋巴管瘤引流入腹腔。

如出现肾静脉血栓，移植物一般不可挽救。肾静脉血栓的原因不明，但更可能由免疫因素及受者的高凝状态引起，而非技术问题。

免疫抑制治疗

在过去的几十年中，对免疫应答的认识有了明显进步，一些新的免疫抑制剂被应用到临床。现有几种免疫抑制药物，但均需在防止排异和不利的副作用间取得平衡[87]。有的中心对所有受者采用标准化方案，另一些则对每个受者采用个体化方案治疗。免疫抑制剂用于排异反应发作的诱导、维持和治疗。

抗体准备

需制备多克隆和单克隆抗体用来备用。抗体准备可在诱导免疫抑制和治疗排异反应时发挥作用。

抗淋巴细胞抗体

抗淋巴细胞抗体包括多克隆制备，如马抗胸腺细胞球蛋白（ATGAM）、兔抗胸腺细胞球蛋白（即复宁）和单克隆抗体莫罗单抗–CD3（OKT3）。这些药物通过使淋巴耗竭及细胞受体相互作用而产生作用。过去诱导方案中常规使用抗淋巴细胞制备物，但随着时间推移其使用已迅速减少[6]。目前我们将这些药物的使用限定于有较大免疫性移植物丧失风险的受体，如需再次移植或高度致敏者，或黑人受体。

抗白介素–2 受体单克隆抗体

已经开发了两种可与白介素–2 受体（CD25）α 亚单位结合并抑制白介素–2 介导的淋巴细胞增殖的单克隆抗体。两者都于 1998 年获得美国食品药品管理局（FDA）的批准。巴利昔单抗（Simulect）是一种人 / 鼠单克隆嵌合抗体[39]。达珠单抗（赛尼哌）是一种人源化鼠单克隆抗体[99]。两者均可有效减少急性细胞排斥的发生率，有良好的远期效果，且无感染或恶性肿瘤风险增加的证据[8,63,88]。白介素–2 受体抗体可用于免疫抑制的诱导方案，但对治疗排异反应无效。

神经钙蛋白抑制剂

自从 1983 年被 FDA 批准后，环孢素的应用被广

泛认为是移植最重要的进步之一。它对儿童肾移植同样有效[31]。1994 年他克莫司被 FDA 批准。这两种药都是通过抑制神经钙蛋白活性而起效。

药物首先进入细胞，与特异性细胞质蛋白结合。环孢素与 cyclophilin 结合，他克莫司与他克莫司结合蛋白（也称作 FK 结合蛋白）结合。然后两种药物蛋白质复合体与神经钙蛋白结合，后者是一种能控制转录调节因子跨核膜转运的磷酸酶。通过抑制这些因子转运进入细胞核，两种药物都可抑制一些早期 T 细胞激活基因（最主要是白介素-2）的转录。

两种药物都可有效防止排异[40]。在欧洲儿童肾移植受者中进行的开放性前瞻性随机试验将他克莫司和环孢素（与硫唑嘌呤和类固醇一起使用）进行比较。他克莫司组的急性排异反应发生率（36.9%）较环孢素组（59.1%）更低[94]。与此观察不同，对 NAPRTCS 的资料进行回顾性分析，比较他克莫司和环孢素（与麦考酚酸莫酯和皮质类固醇一起使用）后发现两者排异反应率和移植物存活率相似。虽然排异反应率相似，他克莫司治疗者移植后 1～2 年移植物功能更好。对 OPTN 资料的新近分析表明，与环孢素相比，大多数儿童受者出院时使用他克莫司（71.4% 对 22.5%）[46]。

环孢霉素的副作用包括多毛症和牙龈增生，而他克莫司与移植后糖尿病发生率增高及神经毒性有关。两者都有明显的神经毒性，并且对神经钙蛋白抑制剂在肾和非肾移植中引起神经毒性的认识正在增加。需权衡每种药物的副作用以及对每个患儿的利弊[40]。如患儿对一种药物产生副作用，应换用另一种。

麦考酚酸莫酯

麦考酚酸莫酯（MMF，麦考酚酸）能抑制嘌呤合成，已代替硫唑嘌呤作为首选抗增殖药物[6,46]。MMF 在体内转化为麦考酚酸——肌苷酸脱氢酶（IMPDH）的非竞争性抑制剂，肌苷酸脱氢酶是嘌呤从头合成的关键酶。虽然大多数细胞可通过从头合成途径或补救途径合成嘌呤，但 B 淋巴细胞和 T 淋巴细胞缺乏补救途径。因此 MMF 是淋巴细胞增殖的选择性抑制剂。已证明它可在儿童中安全有效地使用[9,37]。其主要副作用为白细胞减少和胃肠道不耐受。已开发出作用及副作用相似的肠溶性麦考酚酯（Myfortic）。

泼尼松

从移植的最早期开始糖皮质激素在大多数免疫抑制方案中是必需的。它主要通过转录调节发挥作用。糖皮质激素先经质膜扩散，与细胞质类固醇受体结合。此复合体被转运至细胞核，与特定的基因启动子及其他调节区结合，从而抑制细胞因子合成。皮质类固醇还具有淋巴毒性及明显的抗炎活性，可抑制巨噬细胞功能及炎症反应的其他非特异性作用。

长期使用皮质类固醇可引起高血压、高脂血症、糖尿病、骨质疏松、容貌受损及白内障。即使使用最小剂量也不能避免这些副作用，故现在正试图避免使用该药。虽然一直以来在考虑不用皮质类固醇，但这似乎会使急性和慢性排异反应的风险增高[73]。一些研究者认为不用该药可防止以后的依赖反应。无皮质类固醇的免疫抑制方案已被使用，且回顾性研究发现效果令人乐观[7]。Sarwal 等人在无皮质类固醇方案中使用达珠单抗、他克莫司及酶酚酸酯延长诱导，取得很好的初期效果[78]。平均随访 20 个月，移植物和患者的总体存活率为 98%，第 1 年的急性排异反应率为 8%。基于此前驱研究，目前已准备开展多中心的前瞻性随机研究。

西罗莫司

西罗莫司或称雷帕霉素，是具有免疫抑制作用的大环内酯类抗生素。它可抑制雷帕霉素靶向（TOR）的蛋白质，这是一种可控制细胞因子介导的细胞增殖的关键调节性激酶。西罗莫司在肾移植中的潜在作用已被肯定[30,38]。我们已有使用西罗莫司而避免使用神经钙蛋白抑制剂或皮质类固醇的想法。此外，如其他药物产生并发症，可改用西罗莫司。西罗莫司可与神经钙蛋白抑制剂（特别是环孢素）产生相互作用，故需仔细监测。和其他许多免疫抑制剂一样，有证据表明西罗莫司在儿童体内代谢较成人快[79]。此药物族的另一种药物依维莫司已在开发中[36]。目前使用西罗莫司的经验有限，需注意长期使用的风险。

排异反应的治疗

如怀疑发生排异反应应，立即做活检确诊。急性细胞排斥的一线治疗是皮质类固醇冲击疗法。可静脉使用甲泼尼龙 3 天，剂量根据不同的方案而不同，为每天 5.0～25.0mg/kg（最大剂量为 1.0g）。我们中心通常对于 6 岁以下儿童，使用 10.0mg/kg，6 岁及以上儿童则为 5.0mg/kg，最大剂量为 500mg/d。对于严重排异或对皮质类固醇冲击疗法耐受的排异，可使用
709 多克隆抗淋巴细胞球蛋白或单克隆 OKT3 抗体；我们偏向于使用前者。白介素-2 受体抗体对治疗排异反应无效。虽然急性排异反应的治疗通常能够成功，但迟发的排异反应对药物治疗反应不佳。治疗成功后，许多中心会考虑改变免疫抑制的维持治疗方案，包括换用另一种神经钙蛋白抑制剂，或用西罗莫司代替 MMF；然而这种方法缺少证据支持。我们需评估是否坚持原免疫抑制方案。如治疗后患儿的肌酐水平不能下降至基线值，必须考虑随访再次活检。

预后

移植物和患儿的存活

美国每年约有 800 例儿童进行肾移植。2002 年，有 769 例移植，57%为活体肾，43%为尸体肾[46]。过去 10 年中，移植物存活率不断上升（图 43-1）。所有儿童受者中，尸肾的 1 年存活率从 1993 年的 83%上升至 2002 年的 91%。同样的，同时期内活体肾的存活率从 90%上升至 97%。目前肾移植后移植物及患儿存活率很高。2001 年 1 月 1 日至 2003 年 6 月 30 日，38 例在我们中心移植的患儿存活率为 100%。全国范围内，移植物和患儿的存活率同期分别为 94.5%和 98.9%。图 43-2 显示了目前儿童活体肾及尸肾移植的器官存活率。图 43-3 总结了不同年龄组受者存活率。虽然患儿存活率高，但要意识到即使做了移

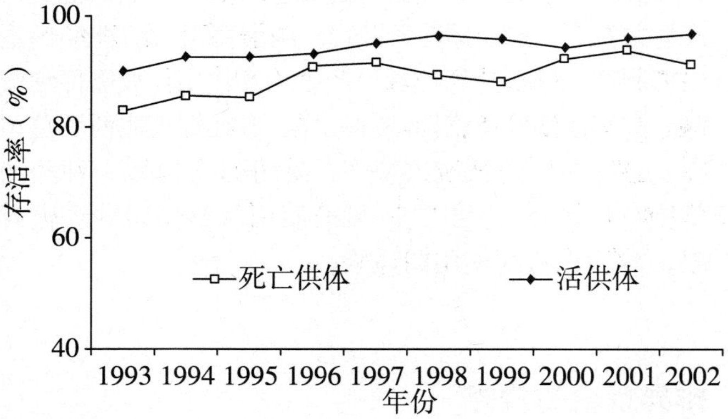

图 43-1 儿童肾移植受体移植物 1 年存活率，1993—2002 年。(From SRTR analysis, August 2004.)

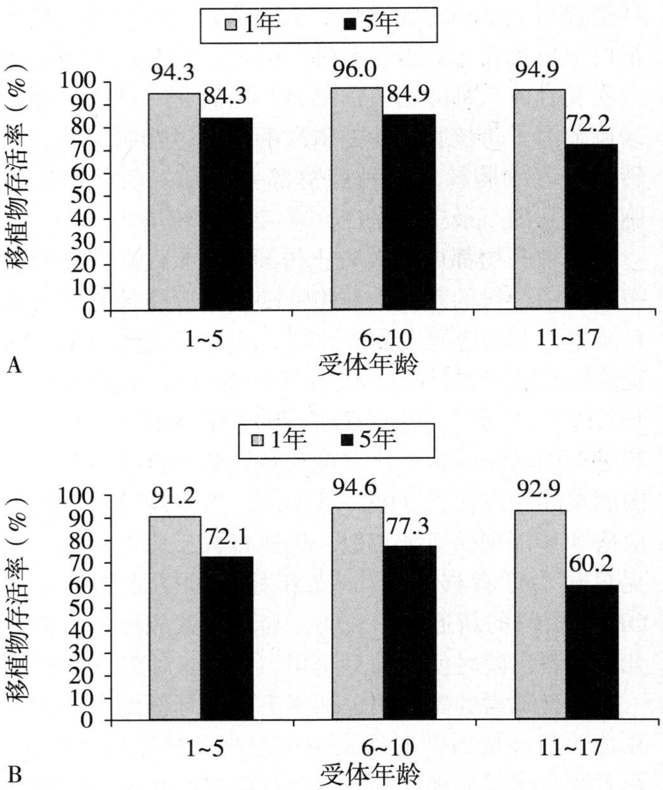

图 43-2 A. 不同年龄组活体肾移植 1 年及 5 年移植物存活率。B. 不同年龄组尸肾移植 1 年及 5 年移植物存活率。(From OPTN/SRTR: 2003 OPTN/SRTR Annual Report: Transplant Data 1993-2002. HHS/HRSA/SPB/DOT; UNOS; URREA. Available online at: www.ustransplant.org.)

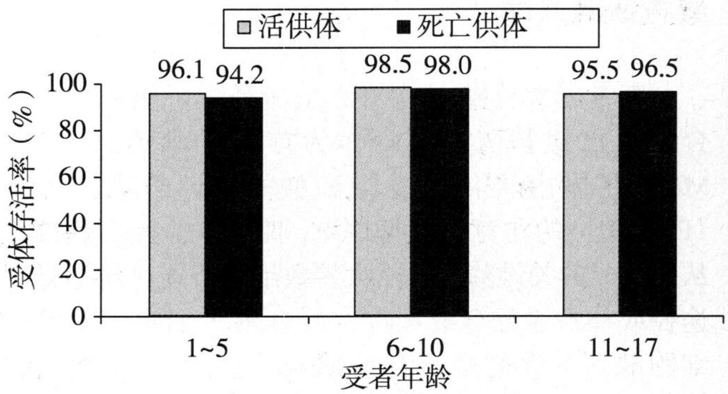

图 43-3 不同受体年龄组活体和尸体肾移植患儿的 5 年存活率。(From OPTN/SRTR: 2003 OPTN/SRTR Annual Report: Transplant Data 1993-2002. HHS/HRSA/SPB/DOT; UNOS; URREA. Available online at: www.ustransplant.org.)

植，这些儿童的死亡风险仍明显高于普通人群[54]。

过去 10 年中，各年龄组儿童的存活率都有改善。特别是 2 岁以下的儿童存活率改善显著，之前此组儿童效果较差，而现在其效果已等同于其他年龄组[6,46]。近期报道显示年龄最小的受者移植半寿期最长，特别是儿童受者接受了能立即产生功能的成人肾[11,77]。这些结果的改善反映了更好的供体选择、手术技术的改善、免疫抑制剂的进步及对儿童免疫抑制治疗的认识改善。

虽然目前在儿童中的短期成功令人鼓舞，但应意识到青少年组（11～17 岁）的移植物远期存活率很低（见图 43-2）。此年龄组的移植物存活率只高于 65 岁以上组[46]。如此高的移植物丧失的原因不明，可能与患儿的依从性差有关[85]。复发性 FSGS 的高发生率也可能与移植物丧失有关[5]。不论原因如何，改善此年龄组患儿的远期移植效果是儿科移植最大的挑战之一。

移植后预后及与移植物丧失有关的危险因素

Benfield 等报道 NAPRTCS 记录的 1605 例一期移植失败最常见的原因为：慢性排异反应（32.4%）、急性排异反应（15.2%）、血栓形成（11.6%）、受者死亡但移植物有功能（10.1%）以及原发疾病复发（5.9%）[6]。对大型单中心经验及登记数据的分析揭示了与特异性移植后预后有关的危险因素。对于某些特定的儿童人群，一些危险因素是不可变的，如种族、年龄及原发疾病。其他因素是可能改变的，可能的话应努力使危险度降低。

移植肾的类型和时机可影响预后。活体移植的移植物存活率高于尸体移植[28]，但此差异在近来的受者人群中已经变得更小了[6]。提前移植的移植物存活率高于透析期间的移植[98]。对于接受透析的患儿，透析类型不影响移植物的存活率，但腹膜透析发生血栓形成引起移植物丧失的概率高于血液透析。

移植物功能延迟

移植物功能延迟（DGF）指移植后第 1 周内需要透析，是急性肾小管坏死（ATN）的表现。与活体移植相比，DGF 在尸肾受者中更常见。对 5000 多例儿童肾移植受者分析后证明 DGF 是移植物丧失的一个独立危险因素[91]。DGF 也使急、慢性排异反应的危险增加。这反映了 DGF 后的免疫应答对肾的损伤。DGF 引起的肾功能障碍与急性排斥反应相混淆，故排异的诊断可能延迟。我们认为如 DGF 超过 5～7 天应进行活检，对排异反应发生危险性高的患儿更应及早进行。

由于 DGF 可影响移植物的存活率，应尽量降低 ATN 发生的风险。在过去的 10 年中，尸肾移植后 DGF 发生率从 16%降至 2002 年的 12.5% [46]。此结果反映了受体治疗和供体选择上的进步。儿童受者的 DGF 发生率为成人的一半（23.4%），反映了器官分配系统造成的供体选择差异。

血管内血栓形成

血栓形成是移植物丧失的第三常见原因[6]。发生血栓的危险因素包括：供体年龄小于 6 岁，冷缺血时间超过 24 小时，之前有移植史、移植前做过腹膜透析。仔细考虑供体的质量，保证移植物的充分灌注，是降低血栓形成风险的对策。ESRD 患儿高凝状态发生率较高，任何的血栓形成史，包括反复或无法解释的血液透析通路血栓，故需进行更深入地评估。

急性排异反应

虽然急性排异反应可发生于任何时间，但实际上常发生于移植后 1 周至 3 月。血清肌酐升高通常为排异反应的首发征象。其他发现包括低热、移植物触痛、高血压，可伴有或不伴有尿量减少。如出现任何肾功能障碍的征象，应立即检查。经皮肾穿刺活检可明确诊断，因为其他许多情况也可引起移植物功能障碍，包括神经钙蛋白毒性、输尿管梗阻、感染、肾动脉狭窄及原疾病复发。急性排异反应可用之前描述的皮质类固醇冲击或抗淋巴细胞抗体治疗。

急性排异反应，特别是移植 1 年余后发生的迟发性急性排异反应，是慢性排异反应引起移植物丧失的独立危险因素[90]。急性排异反应发作一次使慢性排异反应引起移植物丧失的风险增加 3 倍，发作两次使该风险增加 12 倍。急性排异反应的发生率已逐渐降低，这可能是移植物存活率改善的主要因素[6]。分析
711 NAPRTCS 数据发现，移植后第 1 年内的急性排异反应发生率从 1987—1989 年的 71%降至 1997—1999 年的 40% [52]。目前该比率为 20%～30%。

即使治疗成功，急性排异反应也会严重影响移植物存活，所以应尽量降低该风险。遗憾的是，仅加强免疫抑制会造成非特异性全身免疫抑制的不利后果。保证患儿维持治疗性免疫抑制很重要，患儿的不依从会引起灾难性的后果。提高对排异的认识并治疗排异是另一个重要原则。由于血清肌酐是一个反映肾功能障碍相对不灵敏的指标（特别对于接受成人肾的小儿），有人提倡进行常规术后肾活检来检测亚临床排异，这可能对及时治疗有益。

慢性移植物肾病

虽然短期效果很好，但慢性移植物肾病是移植物功能衰竭最常见的原因，可引起进行性肾功能障碍。慢性移植物肾病常被称作“慢性排异反应”，发生因素包括免疫及非免疫因素。虽然急性排异反应是慢性移植物肾病发生的主要危险因素，但其他因素也可参与发病[49]。对该过程的认识不足限制了对其的预防和治疗。除了最终导致移植物丧失，慢性移植物肾病引起的肾功能障碍也对患儿的全身健康和发育造成不利影响。

不依从

药物治疗的依从性是成功移植所必需的。不依从被认为与所有患儿的移植物丧失有关，很大程度上也与青少年受者移植物远期存活率低有关。Shaw 等对 112 例儿童肾移植受者进行回顾，发现 1/3 患儿有明显的不能坚持服药的时期[82]。与小年龄受体相比，不坚持服药者在青少年中更常见。不依从与急慢性排异反应和移植物丧失相关。父母更好地参与、讨论患儿–家长关系可改善患儿的依从性。

疾病复发

患儿原发疾病复发是复杂多样的，复发会 / 不会引起移植物失功。由于 ESRD 病因的诊断水平，以及与复发相关的移植物失去功能发生率上升，疾病复发是患儿的一个重要问题[81]。

FSGS 是最多见、临床上最重要的肾移植后复发疾病[4]。儿童中复发率高达 40% [3]。它可在移植后立即复发，但多数在 1 个月内发生。FSGS 患儿应于术后密切监测尿蛋白。FSGS 复发的青少年移植物存活率常较低，丧失率达 38% [62]。循环渗透性因素被认为在 FSGS 发病中起到关键作用。尽管循证对照试验发现其效果有限，但血浆置换是疾病复发后最常用的治疗方式[62]。早期的血浆置换疗法得到较好的效果，[70]有人提出术前血浆置换可降低复发的风险[65]。还有人建议加强免疫抑制治疗[13]。除了 FSGS，与疾病复发及移植物丧失有关的其他原发性肾疾病包括1 型及 2 型膜性增生性肾小球性肾炎和 IgA 肾病[81]。移植物丧失的风险时不同的，这并不构成移植的绝对禁忌证。

除了这些原发性肾小球疾病，还有其他复发性疾病不同程度地影响着这一儿童群体。溶血性尿毒症综合征可在移植后复发。不典型非腹泻相关性溶血性尿毒症综合征患儿复发风险最高、最易发生移植物丧失[45,71]。过敏性紫癜移植后也可复发[56]。其肾病复发的 5 年危险率为 35%，随后的移植物丧失发生率为 11% [56]。开始向 ESRD 进展者复发率更高，可在紫癜消失一年后复发。

草酸盐沉积症（原发性高草酸盐尿症 1 型）是一种肝丙氨酸过氧化物酶–乙醛酸转氨酶缺乏引起的代谢性疾病，可导致草酸盐合成及分泌增加。过多的草酸盐可引起尿石病、骨髓钙质沉积及 ESRD。另外还有明显的肾外草酸盐沉积。肾移植不能纠正原发性代谢缺陷，移植后持续的草酸盐沉积可移植物丧失。持续肾外草酸盐沉积与患儿早期死亡相关。因此对于这样的自然病史，提倡将肝肾联合移植作为该病的首要治疗方式[21,27,35]。这种方式风险很大，对一些特定的患儿可只行肾移植，特别是对维生素 B6 敏感或草酸盐负担较低的患儿[74]。

内科并发症

感染

感染是免疫抑制的常见危险，也是免疫抑制过度和不足之间平衡不稳定的临床表现。在移植后或治疗
12 排异期间使用重度免疫抑制时需保持高度警惕。在这些高度危险的时期内需预防感染。

目前移植后感染的住院率高于急性排异反应，甚至在移植后 6 个月内也是如此[18]。移植后感染主要为细菌及病毒感染。虽然真菌感染只占感染相关住院患者的 0.2%～2.7%，但非常危险。一些病毒病原体值得讨论。儿童受者的危险性更高，因为与大多数人群相比，他们对某种特殊病原体无防范的可能性更大。

巨细胞病毒（CMV）

CMV 是移植后最常见的病毒感染。CMV 感染可能发生于任何受者，但血清 CMV 阴性受者接受 CMV 阳性供体的肾时感染危险最大。CMV 阳性受者发生感染是由于潜伏病毒被激活。通过更有效的预防，CMV 感染的发生率及程度已有所降低。CMV 感染的程度可以从无症状至器官受累甚至死亡。典型症状出现在移植后 1～3 个月，表现为患儿感觉尚可但有发热，或有时表现出流感样症状。白细胞减少是常见的实验室发现。组织侵袭性 CMV 病患儿表现为中毒症状和终末期器官功能障碍。目前，依靠 CMV pp65 抗原试验或 CMV 聚合酶链反应（PCR）试验可诊断。二者都可监测对治疗的反应。治疗上应用更昔洛韦或缬更昔洛韦。对于严重病例，CMV 高效价免疫球蛋白可能会有效。但不幸的是。对更昔洛韦耐药的 CMV 株已经出现。

水痘-带状疱疹病毒（VZV）

儿童受者发生原发水痘感染的风险较高。治疗应为静脉使用阿昔洛韦直至皮损结痂，后改为口服。原发感染可能非常严重。移植前我们对血清 VZV 阴性患儿进行免疫接种。有明确暴露史的血清 VZV 阴性受者，我们使用 VZV 免疫球蛋白给予主动免疫。

BK 病毒

BK 病毒是一种普遍存在的多瘤病毒，目前确定其对肾移植有严重危害[97]。儿童晚期血清转换率较高（60%～100%），病毒静止于肾上皮直至再次活化。近来对此病原体认识增加将对目前的免疫抑制方案造成强烈的冲击。早期报道（主要在有关成人的文献中）指出 BK 病毒是移植肾功能障碍的一个重要原因，BK 间质性肾炎造成被感染的移植物丧失率达 45%～70%。

评价移植肾功能障碍时需考虑 BK 肾病。活检后免疫组化可确诊该病，但急性排异反应有时可使组织学混淆。加用免疫抑制剂不能改善肾功能，相反常引起病情恶化。治疗该病首先应减少免疫抑制的程度。可用小剂量西多福韦或静脉使用免疫球蛋白。目前正越来越广泛地使用 PCR 检测 BK 病毒，可用于诊断及监测疗效。

令人担心的是，BK 血清阳性可能性较小的患儿 BK 的感染危险增加。在一项包括 18 例儿童受者的研究中，BK 血清阳性率为 56%，BK 病毒尿症发生率为 33% [33]。这些数据与在成人移植受者中观察到的血清阳性率及病毒活化率相似。BK 病毒相关性移植肾病的发生率估计为 4%～7% [97]。在一项对此问题最大规模的儿童群体调查中，Smith 等评估了单中心 173 例肾移植儿童，确定 6 人（3.5%）患 BK 肾病[86]。他们通过移植后平均 15 个月时的活检建立诊断。治疗措施为降低基线免疫抑制治疗，经过中位数 25 个月的随访，所有移植物功能稳定。此外，Smith 等还证实 BK 肾病和血清阴性之间有密切联系[86]。通过提高认识、快速诊断及治疗可减少此疾病相关的移植物丧失。

恶性肿瘤

移植受者发生免疫抑制相关性新生恶性肿瘤的危险增加。淋巴瘤，特别是移植后淋巴细胞增生性疾病（PTLD）最常见。肾移植中发生率约为 1% [19,20]。实际上 PTLD 代表了是一大类疾病。EB 病毒（EBV）被认为是 PTLD 的诱因，特别是 B 细胞淋巴瘤[2]。PTLD 的治疗和预后取决于组织病理学[29]。有许多高危因素，包括抗淋巴细胞诱导治疗、EBV 血清阴性受者、移植年代和 EBV 感染，但在儿童中这些联系未经证实。PTLD 与免疫抑制过度有关[17,19]。最近

的分析显示，PTLD 的发生率在升高，似乎年轻的白人男性危险性最大[20]。

儿童受者中第二常见的癌症是皮肤癌。鳞状细胞癌占皮肤新生物的大多数，其次是恶性黑色素瘤和基
713 底细胞癌。最好的治疗方法是防晒乳和避免阳光照射。针对此风险，所有移植受者应定期做皮肤随访。长期免疫抑制后发生颈部、外阴部及肛门癌症的危险也增高。

其他内科问题

除了感染和恶性肿瘤，移植受者还面临其他许多风险，这是由 ESRD、基础肾病以及药物治疗引起的个体风险的。

肾移植受者发生心血管疾病的风险较高。原来的肾功能不全、透析时间及移植后免疫抑制治疗都与此风险相关。此外，儿童受者高血压的发生率为 50%～80% [58]。许多受者还有其他一些心血管病的危险因素，包括高脂血症、高半胱氨酸血症、贫血、营养不良及慢性炎症[84]。Matteucci 等人检查了 28 例儿童肾移植受者后发现 82%的患儿有左心室肥厚[51]。虽然评估儿童中此危险度的数据很少，但 ESRD 的年轻成人患者因心血管疾病死亡的风险比正常人群高 1000 倍。虽然与透析相比，成功肾移植可降低心血管疾病死亡的风险，但仍不正常[68]。除了心血管风险以外，高血压还使得移植物功能障碍及丧失的危险增高[89]。应尽量减少心血管病的危险因素，以促进健康、延长生命。

移植受者还面临骨代谢及生长的严重问题[22]。部分是因为慢性肾功能不全、营养不良、术后移植物功能障碍及免疫抑制治疗而产生。肾性骨营养不良是一个严重问题，但经钙、维生素 D 的补充及其他药物治疗后可改善骨的健康。随着时间推移，骨并发症的风险正在改善，与透析相比，移植后此风险降低[75]。使用重组人生长激素被证实是安全有效的。虽然该药能地促进骨骼线性生长，但许多患儿最终仍不能取得满意的成人身高。

认知和社会心理发育

近些年来，由于药物治疗提高和肾替代治疗的进步，ESRD 对儿童认知发展的负面影响已减少[23]。现在认为，接受移植的 ESRD 患儿可达到或接近健康儿童的认知水平。虽然肾移植儿童的前景优于透析儿童，但患儿的社会心理发育仍低于正常。与透析相比，肾移植患儿及其家庭的总体生活质量更好，但与正常人群仍有差距[23,48,72]。

（许 恩译 董其刚校）

参考文献

1. Acott PD, Pernica JM: Growth hormone therapy before and after pediatric renal transplant. Pediatr Transplant 2003;7:426-440.
2. ASTS/AST: Epstein-Barr virus and lymphoproliferative disorders after transplantation. Am J Transplant 2004;4:59-65.
3. Baqi N, Tejani A: Recurrence of the original disease in pediatric renal transplantation. J Nephrol 1997;10:85-92.
4. Baum MA: Outcomes after renal transplantation for FSGS in children. Pediatr Transplant 2004;8:329-333.
5. Baum MA, Ho M, Stablein D, et al: Outcome of renal transplantation in adolescents with focal segmental glomerulosclerosis. Pediatr Transplant 2002;6:488-492.
6. Benfield MR, McDonald RA, Bartosh S, et al: Changing trends in pediatric transplantation: 2001 Annual Report of the North American Pediatric Renal Transplant Cooperative Study. Pediatr Transplant 2003;7:321-335.
7. Birkeland SA: Steroid-free immunosuppression in renal transplantation: A long-term follow-up of 100 consecutive patients. Transplantation 2001;71:1089-1090.
8. Bumgardner GL, Hardie I, Johnson RW, et al: Results of 3-year phase III clinical trials with daclizumab prophylaxis for prevention of acute rejection after renal transplantation. Transplantation 2001;72:839-845.
9. Bunchman T, Navarro M, Broyer M, et al: The use of mycophenolate mofetil suspension in pediatric renal allograft recipients. Pediatr Nephrol 2001;16:978-984.
10. Capizzi A, Zanon GF, Zacchello G, Rigamonti W: Kidney transplantation in children with reconstructed bladder. Transplantation 2004;77:1113-1116.
11. Cecka JM, Gjertson DW, Terasaki PI: Pediatric renal transplantation: A review of the UNOS data. United Network for Organ Sharing. Pediatr Transplant 1997;1:55-64.
12. Cho YW, Terasaki PI, Cecka JM, Gjertson DW: Transplantation of kidneys from donors whose hearts have stopped beating. N Engl J Med 1998;338:221-225.
13. Cochat P, Schell M, Ranchin B, et al: Management of recurrent nephrotic syndrome after kidney transplantation in children. Clin Nephrol 1996;46:17-20.
14. Colombani PM, Dunn SP, Harmon WE, et al: Pediatric transplantation. Am J Transplant 2003;3(Suppl 4):S53-S63.
15. Cooper JT, Chin LT, Krieger NR, et al: Donation after cardiac death: The University of Wisconsin experience with renal transplantation. Am J Transplant 2004;4:1490-1494.
16. Delmonico FL, Harmon WE: The use of a minor as a live kidney donor. Am J Transplant 2002;2:333-336.
17. Dharnidharka VR, Ho PL, Stablein DM, et al: Mycophenolate, tacrolimus and post-transplant lymphoproliferative disorder: A report of the North American Pediatric Renal Transplant Cooperative Study. Pediatr Transplant 2002;6:396-399.
18. Dharnidharka VR, Stablein DM, Harmon WE: Post-transplant infections now exceed acute rejection as cause for hospitalization: A report of the NAPRTCS. Am J Transplant 2004;4:384-389.
19. Dharnidharka VR, Sullivan EK, Stablein DM, et al: Risk factors for posttransplant lymphoproliferative disorder (PTLD) in

pediatric kidney transplantation: A report of the North American Pediatric Renal Transplant Cooperative Study (NAPRTCS). Transplantation 2001;71:1065-1068.
20. Dharnidharka VR, Tejani AH, Ho PL, Harmon WE: Post-transplant lymphoproliferative disorder in the United States: Young Caucasian males are at highest risk. Am J Transplant 2002;2:993-998.
21. Ellis SR, Hulton SA, McKiernan PJ, et al: Combined liver-kidney transplantation for primary hyperoxaluria type 1 in young children. Nephrol Dial Transplant 2001;16:348-354.
22. Fine RN: Growth following solid-organ transplantation. Pediatr Transplant 2002;6:47-52.
23. Fine RN, Alonso EM, Fischel JE, et al: Pediatric transplantation of the kidney, liver and heart: Summary report. Pediatr Transplant 2004;8:75-86.
24. Fine RN, Tejani A, Sullivan EK: Pre-emptive renal transplantation in children: Report of the North American Pediatric Renal Transplant Cooperative Study (NAPRTCS). Clin Transplant 1994;8:474-478.
25. Fontaine E, Gagnadoux MF, Niaudet P, et al: Renal transplantation in children with augmentation cystoplasty: Long-term results. J Urol 1998;159:2110-2113.
26. Franc-Guimond J, Gonzalez R: Renal transplantation in children with reconstructed bladders. Transplantation 2004;77:1116-1120.
27. Gagnadoux MF, Lacaille F, Niaudet P, et al: Long term results of liver-kidney transplantation in children with primary hyperoxaluria. Pediatr Nephrol 2001;16:946-950.
28. Gjertson DW, Cecka JM: Determinants of long-term survival of pediatric kidney grafts reported to the United Network for Organ Sharing kidney transplant registry. Pediatr Transplant 2001;5:5-15.
29. Green M, Webber S: Posttransplantation lymphoproliferative disorders. Pediatr Clin North Am 2003;50:1471-1491.
30. Groth CG, Backman L, Morales JM, et al: Sirolimus (rapamycin)-based therapy in human renal transplantation: Similar efficacy and different toxicity compared with cyclosporine. Sirolimus European Renal Transplant Study Group. Transplantation 1999;67:1036-1042.
31. Harmon WE, Sullivan EK: Cyclosporine dosing and its relationship to outcome in pediatric renal transplantation. Kidney Int Suppl 1993;43:S50-S55.
32. Hatch DA, Koyle MA, Baskin LS, et al: Kidney transplantation in children with urinary diversion or bladder augmentation. J Urol 2001;165 (Suppl):2265-2268.
33. Haysom L, Rosenberg AR, Kainer G, et al: BK viral infection in an Australian pediatric renal transplant population. Pediatr Transplant 2004;8:480-484.
34. Healey PJ, McDonald R, Waldhausen JH, et al: Transplantation of adult living donor kidneys into infants and small children. Arch Surg 2000;135:1035-1041.
35. Hoppe B, Langman CB: A United States survey on diagnosis, treatment, and outcome of primary hyperoxaluria. Pediatr Nephrol 2003;18:986-991.
36. Hoyer PF, Ettenger R, Kovarik JM, et al: Everolimus in pediatric de nova renal transplant patients. Transplantation 2003;75:2082-2085.
37. Jungraithmayr T, Staskewitz A, Kirste G, et al: Pediatric renal transplantation with mycophenolate mofetil-based immunosuppression without induction: Results after three years. Transplantation 2003;75:454-461.
38. Kahan BD, Julian BA, Pescovitz MD, et al: Sirolimus reduces the incidence of acute rejection episodes despite lower cyclosporine doses in Caucasian recipients of mismatched primary renal allografts: A phase II trial. Rapamune Study Group. Transplantation 1999;68:1526-1532.
39. Kahan BD, Rajagopalan PR, Hall M: Reduction of the occurrence of acute cellular rejection among renal allograft recipients treated with basiliximab, a chimeric anti-interleukin-2-receptor monoclonal antibody. United States Simulect Renal Study Group. Transplantation 1999;67:276-284.
40. Kari JA, Trompeter RS: What is the calcineurin inhibitor of choice for pediatric renal transplantation? Pediatr Transplant 2004;8:437-444.
41. Kayler LK, Merion RM, Maraschio MA, et al: Outcomes of pediatric living donor renal transplant after laparoscopic versus open donor nephrectomy. Transplant Proc 2002;34:3097-3098.
42. Khwaja K, Humar A, Najarian JS: Kidney transplants for children under 1 year of age—a single-center experience. Pediatr Transplant 2003;7:163-167.
43. Koo HP, Bunchman TE, Flynn JT, et al: Renal transplantation in children with severe lower urinary tract dysfunction. J Urol 1999;161:240-245.
44. Live Organ Donor Consensus Group. Consensus statement on the live organ donor. JAMA 2000;284:2919-2926.
45. Loirat C, Niaudet P: The risk of recurrence of hemolytic uremic syndrome after renal transplantation in children. Pediatr Nephrol 2003;18:1095-1101.
46. Magee JC, Bucuvalas JC, Farmer DG, et al: Pediatric transplantation. Am J Transplant 2004;4(Suppl 9):S54-S71.
47. Magee JC, Sung RS, Turcotte JG, et al: Renal transplantation at the University of Michigan 1964 to 1999. In Cecka JM, Terasaki PI, eds: Clinical Transplants 1999, Los Angeles: UCLA Tissue Typing Laboratory, 2000, pp 139-148.
48. Manificat S, Dazord A, Cochat P, et al: Quality of life of children and adolescents after kidney or liver transplantation: Child, parents and caregiver's point of view. Pediatr Transplant 2003;7:228-235.
49. Matas AJ: Impact of acute rejection on development of chronic rejection in pediatric renal transplant recipients. Pediatr Transplant 2000;4:92-99.
50. Matas AJ, Bartlett ST, Leichtman AB, Delmonico FL: Morbidity and mortality after living kidney donation, 1999-2001: Survey of United States transplant centers. Am J Transplant 2003;3:830-834.
51. Matteucci MC, Giordano U, Calzolari A, et al: Left ventricular hypertrophy, treadmill tests, and 24-hour blood pressure in pediatric transplant patients. Kidney Int 1999;56:1566-1570.
52. McDonald R, Ho PL, Stablein DM, et al: Rejection profile of recent pediatric renal transplant recipients compared with historical controls: A report of the North American Pediatric Renal Transplant Cooperative Study (NAPRTCS). Am J Transplant 2001;1:55-60.
53. McDonald RA, Smith JM, Stablein D, Harmon WE: Pretransplant peritoneal dialysis and graft thrombosis following pediatric kidney transplantation: A NAPRTCS report. Pediatr Transplant 2003;7:204-208.
54. McDonald SP, Craig JC, Australian and New Zealand Paediatric Nephrology A: Long-term survival of children with end-stage renal disease. N Engl J Med 2004;350:2654-2662.
55. Metzger RA, Delmonico FL, Feng S, et al: Expanded criteria donors for kidney transplantation. Am J Transplant 2003; 3(Suppl 4):S114-S125.
56. Meulders Q, Pirson Y, Cosyns JP, et al: Course of Henoch-Schönlein nephritis after renal transplantation: Report on ten patients and review of the literature. Transplantation 1994;58:1179-1186.
57. Millan MT, Sarwal MM, Lemley KV, et al: A 100% 2-year graft survival can be attained in high-risk 15-kg or smaller infant recipients of kidney allografts. Arch Surg 2000; 135:1063-1068; discussion 1068-1069.
58. Mitsnefes MM: Hypertension and end-organ damage in pediatric renal transplantation. Pediatr Transplant 2004; 8:394-399.

59. NAPRTCS: North American Pediatric Renal Transplant Cooperative Study (NAPRTCS) 2004 Annual Report. Available online at www.naprtcs.org.
60. Neu AM, Ho PL, Fine RN, et al: Tacrolimus vs. cyclosporine A as primary immunosuppression in pediatric renal transplantation: A NAPRTCS study. Pediatr Transplant 2003; 7:217-222.
61. Neu AM, Ho PL, McDonald RA, Warady BA: Chronic dialysis in children and adolescents. The 2001 NAPRTCS Annual Report. Pediatr Nephrol 2002;17:656-663.
62. Newstead CG: Recurrent disease in renal transplants. Nephrol Dial Transplant 2003;18(Suppl 6):vi68-74.
63. Offner G, Broyer M, Niaudet P, et al: A multicenter, open-label, pharmacokinetic/pharmacodynamic safety, and tolerability study of basiliximab (Simulect) in pediatric de novo renal transplant recipients. Transplantation 2002; 74:961-966.
64. Ohl DA, Konnak JW, Campbell DA, et al: Extravesical ureteroneocystostomy in renal transplantation. J Urol 1988;139: 499-502.
65. Ohta T, Kawaguchi H, Hattori M, et al: Effect of pre- and postoperative plasmapheresis on posttransplant recurrence of focal segmental glomerulosclerosis in children. Transplantation 2001;71:628-633.
66. Ohta T, Kawaguchi H, Hattori M, et al: ABO-incompatible pediatric kidney transplantation in a single-center trial. Pediatr Nephrol 2000;14:1-5.
67. OPTN/SRTR: 2003 OPTN/SRTR Annual Report: Transplant Data 1993-2002. HHS/HRSA/SPB/DOT; UNOS; URREA. Available online at: www.ustransplant.org.
68. Parekh RS, Carroll CE, Wolfe RA, Port FK: Cardiovascular mortality in children and young adults with end-stage kidney disease. J Pediatr 2002;141:191-197.
69. Port FK, Bragg-Gresham JL, Metzger RA, et al: Donor characteristics associated with reduced graft survival: An approach to expanding the pool of kidney donors. Transplantation 2002;74:1281-1286.
70. Pradhan M, Petro J, Palmer J, et al: Early use of plasmapheresis for recurrent post-transplant FSGS. Pediatr Nephrol 2003; 18:934-938.
71. Quan A, Sullivan EK, Alexander SR: Recurrence of hemolytic uremic syndrome after renal transplantation in children: A report of the North American Pediatric Renal Transplant Cooperative Study. Transplantation 2001;72: 742-745.
72. Qvist E, Narhi V, Apajasalo M, et al: Psychosocial adjustment and quality of life after renal transplantation in early childhood. Pediatr Transplant 2004;8:120-125.
73. Roberti I, Reisman L, Lieberman KV, Burrows L: Risk of steroid withdrawal in pediatric renal allograft recipients (a 5-year follow-up). Clin Transplant 1994;8:405-408.
74. Saborio P, Scheinman JI: Transplantation for primary hyperoxaluria in the United States. Kidney Int 1999; 56:1094-1100.
75. Saland JM: Osseous complications of pediatric transplantation. Pediatr Transplant 2004;8:400-415.
76. Salomon L, Fontaine E, Guest G, et al: Role of the bladder in delayed failure of kidney transplants in boys with posterior urethral valves. J Urol 2000;163:1282-1285.
77. Sarwal MM, Cecka JM, Millan MT, Salvatierra O Jr: Adult-size kidneys without acute tubular necrosis provide exceedingly superior long-term graft outcomes for infants and small children: A single center and UNOS analysis. United Network for Organ Sharing. Transplantation 2000;70: 1728-1736.
78. Sarwal MM, Vidhun JR, Alexander SR, et al: Continued superior outcomes with modification and lengthened follow-up of a steroid-avoidance pilot with extended daclizumab induction in pediatric renal transplantation. Transplantation 2003;76:1331-1339.
79. Schachter AD, Meyers KE, Spaneas LD, et al: Short sirolimus half-life in pediatric renal transplant recipients on a calcineurin inhibitor-free protocol. Pediatr Transplant 2004;8:171-177.
80. Seikaly MG: Recurrence of primary disease in children after renal transplantation: An evidence-based update. Pediatr Transplant 2004;8:113-119.
81. Seikaly M, Ho PL, Emmett L, Tejani A: The 12th Annual Report of the North American Pediatric Renal Transplant Cooperative Study: Renal transplantation from 1987 through 1998. Pediatr Transplant 2001;5:215-231.
82. Shaw RJ, Palmer L, Blasey C, Sarwal M: A typology of non-adherence in pediatric renal transplant recipients. Pediatr Transplant 2003;7:489-493.
83. Shishido S, Asanuma H, Tajima E, et al: ABO-incompatible living-donor kidney transplantation in children. Transplantation 2001;72:1037-1042.
84. Silverstein DM: Risk factors for cardiovascular disease in pediatric renal transplant recipients. Pediatr Transplant 2004;8:386-393.
85. Smith JM, Ho PL, McDonald RA, et al: Renal transplant outcomes in adolescents: A report of the North American Pediatric Renal Transplant Cooperative Study. Pediatr Transplant 2002;6:493-499.
86. Smith JM, McDonald RA, Finn LS, et al: Polyomavirus nephropathy in pediatric kidney transplant recipients. Am J Transplant 2004;4:2109-2117.
87. Smith JM, McDonald RA, Nemeth TL: Current immunosuppressive agents in pediatric renal transplantation: Efficacy, side-effects and utilization. Pediatr Transplant 2004;8:445-453.
88. Sollinger H, Kaplan B, Pescovitz MD, et al: Basiliximab versus antithymocyte globulin for prevention of acute renal allograft rejection. Transplantation 2001;72:1915-1919.
89. Sorof JM, Sullivan EK, Tejani A, Portman RJ: Antihypertensive medication and renal allograft failure: A North American Pediatric Renal Transplant Cooperative Study report. J Am Soc Nephrol 1999;10:1324-1330.
90. Tejani A, Sullivan EK: The impact of acute rejection on chronic rejection: A report of the North American Pediatric Renal Transplant Cooperative Study. Pediatr Transplant 2000;4:107-111.
91. Tejani AH, Sullivan EK, Alexander SR, et al: Predictive factors for delayed graft function (DGF) and its impact on renal graft survival in children: A report of the North American Pediatric Renal Transplant Cooperative Study (NAPRTCS). Pediatr Transplant 1999;3:293-300.
92. Thomas SE, Hickman RO, Tapper D, et al: Asymptomatic inferior vena cava abnormalities in three children with end-stage renal disease: Risk factors and screening guidelines for pretransplant diagnosis. Pediatr Transplant 2000; 4:28-34.
93. Tooher RL, Rao MM, Scott DF, et al: A systematic review of laparoscopic live-donor nephrectomy. Transplantation 2004;78:404-414.
94. Trompeter R, Filler G, Webb NJ, et al: Randomized trial of tacrolimus versus cyclosporin microemulsion in renal transplantation. Pediatr Nephrol 2002;17:141-149.
95. Troppmann C, Pierce JL, Wiesmann KM, et al: Early and late recipient graft function and donor outcome after laparoscopic vs open adult live donor nephrectomy for pediatric renal transplantation. Arch Surg 2002;137: 908-915; discussion 915-916.
96. U.S. Renal Data System: USRDS 2004 Annual Data Report: Atlas of End-Stage Renal Disease in the United States, National Institutes of Health, National Institute of Diabetes and Digestive and Kidney Diseases, Bethesda, MD, 2004. Available at www.usrds.org.

97. Vats A: BK virus-associated transplant nephropathy: Need for increased awareness in children. Pediatr Transplant 2004;8:421-425.
98. Vats AN, Donaldson L, Fine RN, Chavers BM: Pretransplant dialysis status and outcome of renal transplantation in North American children: A NAPRTCS Study. North American Pediatric Renal Transplant Cooperative Study. Transplantation 2000;69:1414-1419.
99. Vincenti F, Kirkman R, Light S, et al: Interleukin-2-receptor blockade with daclizumab to prevent acute rejection in renal transplantation. Daclizumab Triple Therapy Study Group. N Engl J Med 1998;338:161-165.
100. Wolf JS Jr, Merion RM, Leichtman AB, et al: Randomized controlled trial of hand-assisted laparoscopic versus open surgical live donor nephrectomy. Transplantation 2001;72:284-290.

第 44 章

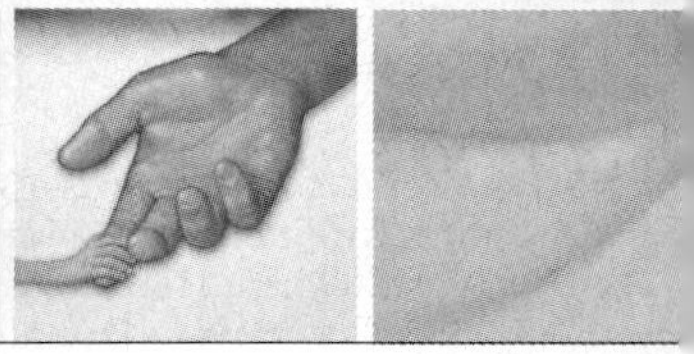

胰腺和胰岛细胞移植

David E. R. Sutherland、Angelika C. Gruessner、Bernhard J. Hering
和 Rainer W. G. Gruessner

717 1 型糖尿病多发生于儿童期，到目前为止，其治疗仍面临挑战。在发病 20 年以上的患者中，糖尿病并发症的发生率达到 30%～50%，通常会导致患者生活质量下降、过早死亡以及卫生保健开支增加[54]。无时不在的高血糖风险是导致这些严重并发症的最根本因素[1]。因此，建立一种安全有效的方法来控制并维持正常的血糖水平是对糖尿病患者的健康和生活质量最有意义的措施。

糖尿病控制和并发症研究组（DCCT）的研究表明，如果给予糖尿病患者合理的护理和胰岛素强化治疗，能够达到接近正常的血糖水平并维持数年。然而尽管这种疗法能很好地控制血糖水平，但会加重患者每日治疗的负担，从而难以推广，因为与临床常规疗法相比它需要耗费更多精力和医疗资源[6]，而且会增加严重低血糖的发生率[1]。目前能维持正常血糖水平且没有继发低血糖风险的唯一方法是置换具有血糖感应和胰岛素分泌功能的胰岛 β 细胞，一般借助带血管胰腺移植或者输注分离纯化的胰岛来实现[81]。因为需要应用免疫抑制来防止异体组织的排斥，所以胰腺或胰岛移植的受体大多选择成人。然而，有些在发病早期就已有进行移植的潜在需求，尤其是因为其他适应证已经应用免疫抑制剂治疗的糖尿病儿童患者[3]。

胰腺移植

历史

1966 年 William Kelly 和 Richard Lillehei 医生在明尼苏达州立大学对一名发生尿毒症的糖尿病患者同时进行了肾移植和胰腺移植，这成为全世界第一个完成临床胰腺移植的病例[46]。不久以后胰腺移植在世界各地的研究机构陆续开展起来，有关内容其他文献已有详细报道[84]。

最初胰腺移植的成功率（长期脱离胰岛素）较低，20 世纪 80 年代开始显著提高，因此胰腺移植得以广泛开展（图 44-1）。移植成功率的提高主要得益于外科技术和免疫抑制两方面的革新。

第 1 例胰腺移植采取的是带导管的节段性（体部和尾部）移植[46]，但这种术式会产生较多的并发症。1966—1973 年，Lillehei 在明尼苏达州立大学又相继 718
进行了 13 例胰腺移植[48,49]，从而设计出了全胰十二指肠移植到髂血管的术式，该术式通过十二指肠小肠吻合来引流肠液，成为大多数移植中心的常规术式。该方法最初的效果并不如现在好，因此在 70 年代和 80

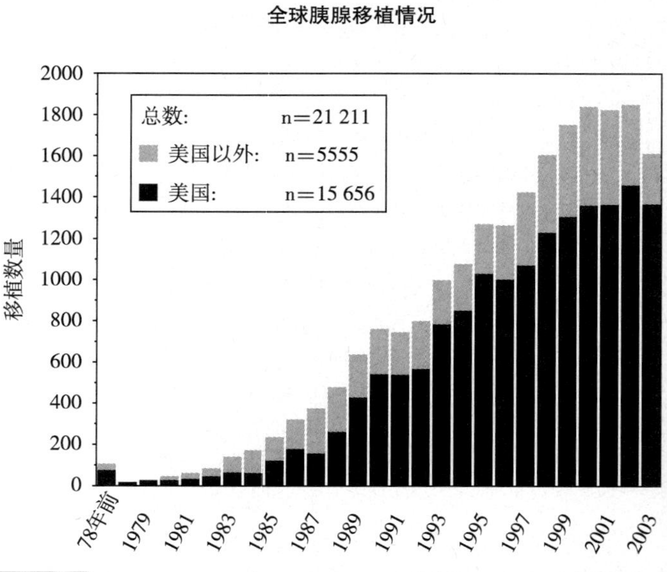

图 44-1 1978—2003 年美国和美国以外国际胰腺移植登记（IPTR）的年度胰腺移植例数。

年代早期另外几位外科医生设计了一些其他术式[84]。法国里昂的 Dubernard 采取导管内注射合成高分子物质的方法来封闭移植物的分泌使其外分泌部纤维化，同时保留一定的内分泌部分[19]，该方法曾经被许多开拓性的移植中心采纳，但现在已经很少应用。Gliedman 通过输尿管胰管吻合创立了节段性移植胰腺经尿路引流的术式[23]， Sollinger 不久后对这一方法进行了改进，将移植的部分十二指肠全胰腺和受者的膀胱直接进行吻合[70]。Dai Nghiem 和 Robert Corry 医生对经尿路引流做了进一步的改良[57]，保留了十二指肠球部，行十二指肠膀胱吻合术来代替 Lillehei 术式的十二指肠小肠吻合[49]。从 80 年代到 90 年代中期，十二指肠膀胱吻合进行膀胱引流成为胰腺移植的主要术式。膀胱引流术式早期并发症的发生率低，并且便于通过尿淀粉酶活性的变化来监测排斥反应，但长期并发症比较常见，例如反复的尿路感染或者由于胰腺外分泌引起体液丢失而造成脱水。因此在 90 年代中期情况发生了变化，正如 Lillehei 及其同事[49]所描述的，肠道引流从未完全过时，并且超过膀胱引流成为主要的引流途径[72,79]。另外，一些研究小组在进行经肠道引流的全胰腺十二指肠移植时采取了门静脉而非腔静脉回流[65]。门静脉回流术式由 Calne 于 1984 年首创并应用于节段性胰腺移植，该术式更符合生理[12]要求，多年来也有一些小组有过报道[84]。

免疫抑制方面的进展，包括 Calne 小组于 1979 年应用的环孢霉素[13]、Starzl 小组于 1989 年应用的他克莫司[73]和 Sollinger 小组于 1995 年应用的麦考酚酸莫酯[61]，这一系列免疫抑制剂的应用，使得借助膀胱引流来监测排斥反应不再那么重要。另外，对于接受同一供体器官的胰腺肾脏联合移植病例，肾脏可以用来监测排斥反应（肌酐的升高），从而在胰腺受损导致高血糖之前就有替代指标来监测胰腺的排斥。当然对于单独胰腺移植的病例来说，血肌酐不能作为监测排斥反应的指标，此时尿路引流仍有其优势并一直得以应用[84]。

手术技巧的细节

正如前面历史部分提到的那样，为了处理移植胰腺的外分泌液和静脉回流，人们设计了多种术式。胰腺供体大多取自多器官衰竭而死亡的尸体捐献者。由于肝脏和胰腺的动脉供血属于同一来源，因此全胰腺移植往往需要血管重建[8,52]。胰尾的血供来自腹腔干的分支——脾动脉，胰头的血供来自由肠系膜上动脉和肝动脉发出的胰十二指肠血管弓。因为肝动脉沿腹腔干与肝脏伴行，通常的方法是从供体髂血管选取一段 Y 型动脉，将其髂内动脉端与移植脾动脉吻合，髂外动脉端与移植肠系膜上动脉吻合，剩下的 Y 型髂总动脉端与受体的动脉系统（一般选取右髂总动脉）做吻合。供体胰腺的门静脉可选择与腔静脉或受体的肠系膜上静脉吻合。

如果考虑静脉回流至受体的髂静脉，完整移植胰腺的胰头可以选择朝向盆腔或者上腹部。如果胰头方向朝上，肠道引流是唯一的选择。而如果胰头方向朝下，十二指肠既可以选择与膀胱（图 44–2），也可与小肠（图 44–3）吻合。图 44–2 所示为膀胱引流术式和同时进行的左侧髂血管内肾移植。如前文所述，如果同时进行肾移植，较多选用肠道引流术式。

关于膀胱引流术式，吻合可用手工缝合或者借助 EEA 吻合器，吻合器柄伸入远端十二指肠（随后将被闭合器闭合），铁砧通过膀胱前壁切开置入膀胱，其接头穿过后壁，完成十二指肠与膀胱吻合（见图 44–2）。内层再用可吸收缝线连续缝合进行加强，目的是止血和包埋黏膜下层的吻合钉。

关于肠道引流或体静脉回流术式，可以手工行端侧吻合（图 44–3），也可以手工或借助 EEA 吻合器行侧侧吻合[22a]。吻合器柄伸入供体十二指肠末端，接头穿出肠道侧壁。铁砧通过肠切开置入受体小肠，接头周围行荷包缝合以保安全。将两接头紧靠，扣动吻合器扳机完成吻合，最后用闭合器闭合十二指肠末端。肠吻合可以就近选择最便利的受体近端小肠肠袢，也可以选择同时进行 Roux–en–Y 吻合。但结果分析显示后者并无统计学意义上的优势。

如果移植胰腺血流经门静脉回流（图 44–4）其胰头和十二指肠朝上，移植门静脉可直接与受体肠系膜上静脉吻合。在插图中，移植胰腺的腹侧朝向受体小肠系膜，因此静脉吻合口位于静脉的腹侧，移植动脉的 Y 段如果与受体主动脉或髂动脉吻合必须穿过肠系膜孔。移植十二指肠与受体小肠的吻合采取与前述髂静脉回流术式相同的方法，受体小肠可 719
行 Roux–en–Y 吻合或直接吻合（如前述）。

经门静脉引流的另一方法由 Boggi 及其同事提出[7,9]，翻转右半结肠至左侧并暴露肠系膜上静脉的背

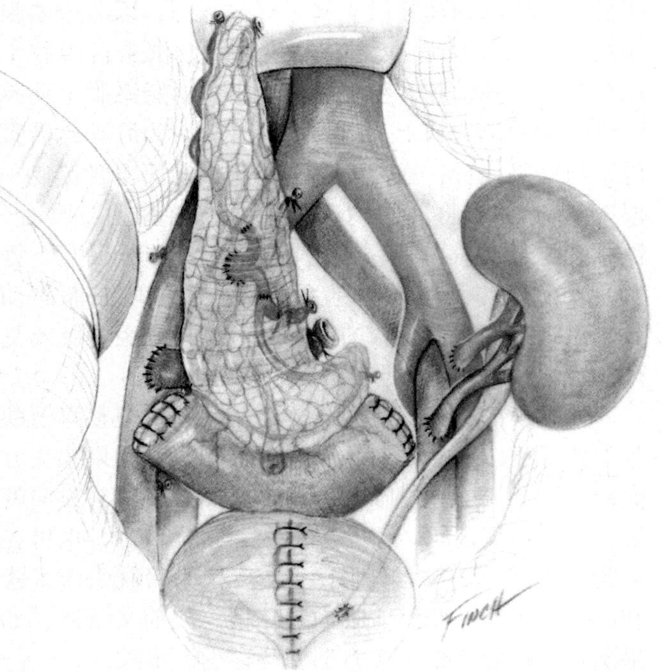

图 44-2 从尸体捐献者获取全胰腺或十二指肠供体，经右髂静脉引流血液，借助十二指肠膀胱吻合使胰腺外分泌液经膀胱引流的胰肾联合（SPK）移植。胰腺和膀胱均经腹部正中切口植入腹腔。胰尾由供体脾动脉供血，胰头由供体肠系膜上动脉供血，截取供体髂总和髂内或外动脉分叉处的Y型血管段来连接前述两支动脉，其主干段与受者髂总动脉吻合。十二指肠中段与膀胱后壁吻合，残端对缝闭合。移植肾可以取自活体捐献或者与移植胰腺同一尸体，不管哪种情况，均应优先植于左侧髂血管，以便游离的右侧髂血管用于移植胰腺。该图中供体输尿管采用经膀胱前壁切开 Politano-Leadbetter 术式植入膀胱，此术式可使用 EEA 吻合器行十二指肠膀胱吻合，吻合口内壁再用可吸收线对缝包埋吻合钉，最后关闭膀胱切口。此外，在用肠道引流术式行 SPK 移植时，腔外输尿管膀胱吻合很常用。(Reproduced from Gruessner RWG, Sutherland DER [eds]: Transplantation of the Pancreas. New York, Springer-Verlag, 2004.)

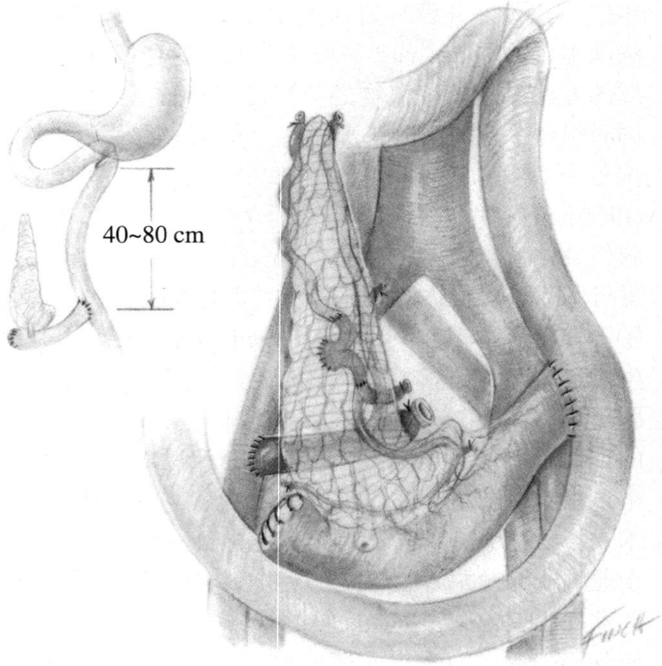

图 44-3 使用尸体捐献者的供体，经腔静脉引流血液，肠道引流供体外分泌液至受体近端空肠袢的胰十二指肠移植。该图所示为供体十二指肠远端与受者空肠行双层十二指肠空肠端侧吻合，吻合口距离屈氏韧带 40～80cm（嵌图）。类似的十二指肠空肠侧侧吻合术式可选择手工或吻合器吻合，可行直接吻合或 Roux-en-Y 吻合。(Reproduced from Gruessner RWG, Sutherland DER [eds]: Transplantation of the Pancreas. New York, Springer-Verlag, 2004.)

面使胰腺置于腹膜后，这样 Y 型动脉段就能直接与右髂总动脉吻合，但该方法要求受体小肠留有 Roux-en-Y 肠袢穿过小肠或横结肠的系膜行十二指肠小肠吻合。

还可以使用其他一些术式，例如导管注射节段移植。节段性移植很少被使用，仅见于很少的几例活体胰腺移植[4,33,82]，这几例病例中，外分泌液大多通过胰管小肠吻合引流至受体小肠的 Roux-en-Y 段或者胰管膀胱吻合引流至受体膀胱（图 44-5）。活体节段性胰腺移植或胰肾联合移植特别适用于需长时间等待捐赠尸体器官的患者，例如人类白细胞抗原（HLA）抗体水平很高而与活体志愿者交叉配型阴性的患者。有关胰腺供体（尸体和活体）和受体各种外科技术的更多细节，读者可以参阅 Benedetti 及其同事的著作[5]。

概述、胰腺移植分类和免疫抑制

据国际胰腺移植登记（IPTR）的统计，到 20 世纪 90 年代中期，全世界每年有 1 500 例以上的胰腺移植（见图 44-1）。截止到 2003 年，累计有超过 720

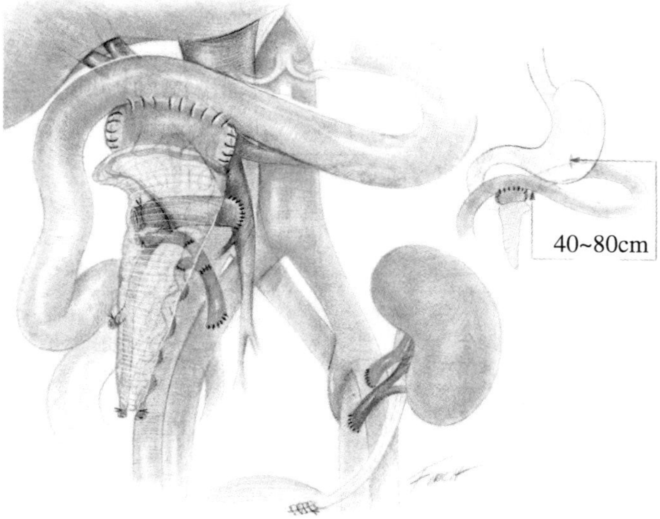

图 44-4 使用尸体捐献者的供体，经门静脉引流血液的全胰十二指肠移植。受体肠系膜上静脉通过端侧吻合收集供体血液再与脾静脉一道汇入门静脉。外分泌液通过十二指肠空肠侧侧吻合来引流，吻合口距离屈氏韧带 40～80cm。注意在门静脉引流术式胰头的方向是朝头侧的，与腔静脉引流术式可能出现的胰头朝尾侧相反，而与膀胱引流时对方向的要求相同。该图中移植胰腺覆于小肠系膜根部之上，供体十二指肠位于横结肠之下，Y 型动脉段穿过系膜孔与受体髂总动脉吻合。当然也可选择右半结肠下的腹膜后入路，这样 Y 型动脉段就能直接跟受体髂动脉吻合，但十二指肠必须穿过系膜与受体 Roux-en-Y 段吻合。如果同时在左侧髂血管行肾移植，可通过前述膀胱外输尿管膀胱吻合（Lich 术式）将输尿管植入膀胱。(Reproduced from Gruessner RWG, Sutherland DER [eds]: Transplantation of the Pancreas. New York, Springer-Verlag, 2004.)

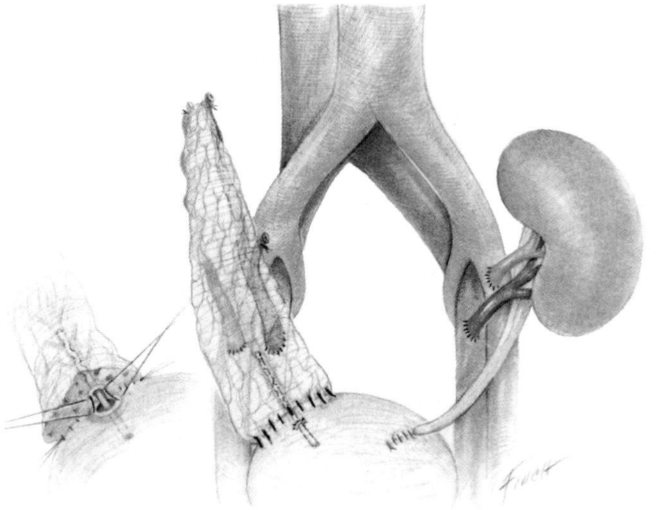

图 44-5 活体节段性（体尾部）胰腺移植至右侧髂血管（血液经腔静脉引流），经腹膜内径路的胰管膀胱吻合使胰腺外分泌液经膀胱引流。结扎和游离下腹部静脉尽量暴露主要静脉后将供体脾动脉和脾静脉分别与受者髂外动静脉行端侧吻合。脾动脉吻合口位于脾静脉吻合口的外侧。胰管膀胱采取双层吻合，用 7-0 可吸收线借助内支架（嵌图）将胰管与膀胱上皮层（内层）对合。如果同时进行肾移植，可通过膀胱外输尿管膀胱吻合（Lich 术式）将供体输尿管植入膀胱。(Reproduced from Gruessner RWG, Sutherland DER [eds]: Transplantation of the Pancreas. New York, Springer-Verlag, 2004.)

21 000 例的患者进行了带血管胰腺移植，其中约 3/4 在美国完成，同时进行了大量的系列性研究[79]。大多数移植应用于原发的 1 型糖尿病患者，使其摆脱胰岛素治疗的依赖，但有些肠道引流的胰腺移植是为了同时纠正全胰切除患者的内分泌和外分泌缺陷[31,34]，或者用来治疗胰腺囊性纤维化等其他病变[74]。

美国有 120 个以上的从事胰腺移植研究的机构，美国以外的机构数目与之相当[29]。为了进行病例的统计分析，1980 年成立了 IPTR[80]。1987 年起，美国的病例报告必须通过器官共享联合网（UNOS），从那以后每年都会发布年报[28-30]。

接受胰腺移植的患者分为三种：（1）尿毒症糖尿病患者同时行 SPK 尸体或活体移植[33]；（2）肾功能不全已得到纠正的肾脏疾病患者，通常已经接受了活体肾移植，再进行肾移植后胰腺（PAK）移植；（3）非尿毒症患者单独进行胰腺移植（PTA）。胰腺移植登记处对各个时期这三种移植的治疗结果进行了比较[28-30]。

一直以来胰腺移植以 SPK 移植为主，但近年来提倡对合并肾脏疾病的糖尿病患者行活体肾移植以先解决其透析的需要，因此 PAK 移植的数量上升而 SPK 移植的数量呈下降趋势（图 44-6）。随之而来的是，PTA 移植的数量也出现了上升，用于治疗不伴有严重肾脏疾病并证实有免疫抑制的难治性糖尿病患者，或者用来治疗能满足后述条件也适用胰岛移植的部分患者。

大多数胰腺移植受体接受的免疫抑制治疗方法与肾移植等其他实体器官移植相似。利用单克隆或多克

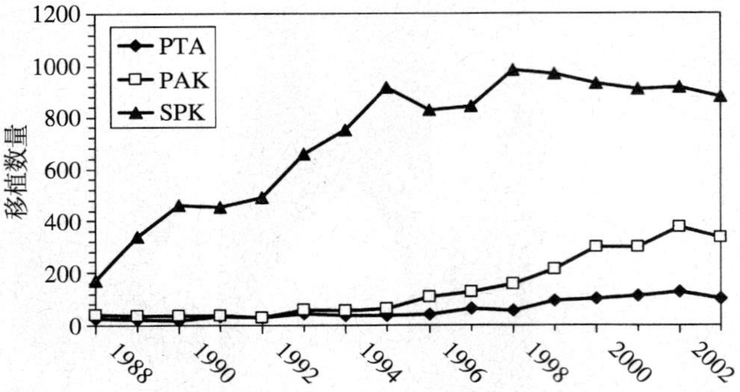

图 44-6 美国 1998—2003 年间各年度各类受体胰腺移植数。PTA：单独胰腺移植；SPK：胰腺肾脏同时移植；PAK：肾脏移植后胰腺移植。

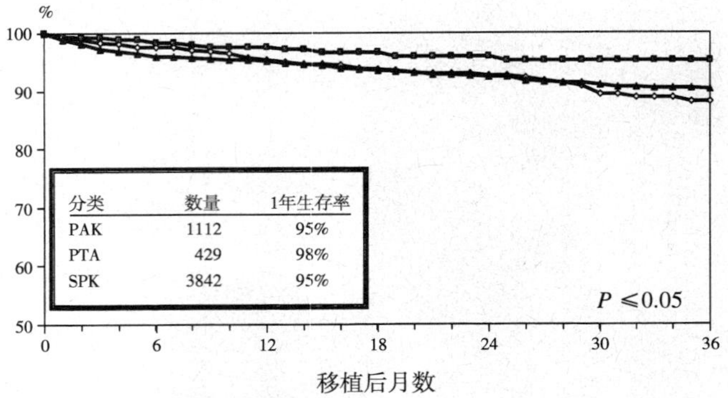

图 44-7 2000—2004 年间美国各受体组的首次尸体移植生存率。PTA：单独胰腺移植；SPK：胰腺肾脏同时移植；PAK：肾脏移植后胰腺移植。

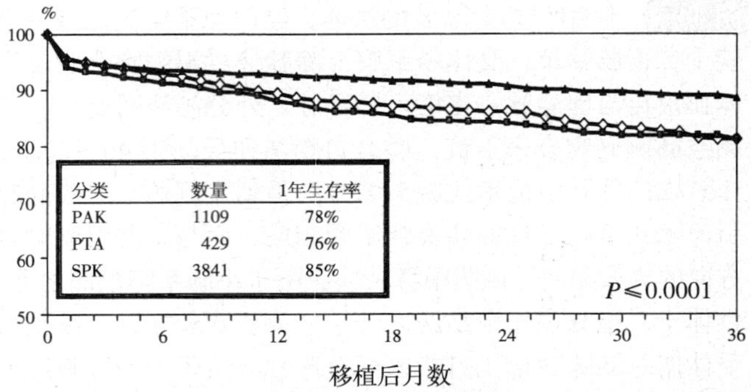

图 44-8 2000—2004 年间美国各受体组首次尸体移植的胰腺功能性存活率（胰岛素不依赖）。PTA：单独胰腺移植；SPK：胰腺肾脏同时移植；PAK：肾脏移植后胰腺移植。

隆的 T 细胞抗体作为 T 细胞的消耗或非消耗因子诱
721 导免疫抑制，可以治疗或预防排斥的发作。维持免疫抑制的药物通常包括神经钙蛋白抑制剂（环孢霉素或他克莫司）的复合物，调整剂量和血药浓度使肾脏毒性降到最小，也可使用增殖抑制剂（麦考酚酸莫酯或西罗莫司），单用或者联用泼尼松。不包括无皮质激素的用药方案已经普遍应用于所有器官移植，包括胰腺移植在内[45]。

胰腺移植的结果

这里对 2000 年 1 月至 2004 年 6 月间 UNOS 报告的美国尸体胰腺移植结果按其受体类型、外科术式和免疫抑制方案的不同而进行了总结。这期间 UNOS 共报告了 5800 多例胰腺移植，其中包括 3800 多例 SPK 移植、1300 多例 PAK 移植和 400 多例 PTA 移植。

三种受体类型胰腺移植的首次移植患者生存率见图 44-7。SPK、PAK 和 PTA 的 1 年生存率分别是 95%、95%和 98%；3 年生存率分别是 90%、88%和 95%（$P=0.05$）。PTA 组的患者生存率最高，推测其原因可能是这组患者移植之前严重并发症较少。

三种受体类型胰腺首次移植的移植物存活率见图 44-8。SPK、PAK 和 PTA 的 1 年胰岛素不依赖率分别是 85%、78%和 76%；3 年胰岛素不依赖率分别是 77%、62%和 62%（$P<0.001$）。SPK 组的移植物存活率最高，推测可能是因为对供体肾（通常与胰腺来自同一供体）的监测比仅对胰腺监测的另两组能更早发现排斥反应。登记处的数据表明各组之间的技术性失败率无显著差异，而排斥性失败率差异显著，从而为以上假说提供了支持。

2000—2004 年间的首次移植当中，8%的失败源于技术原因，血栓形成是导致技术性失败的最大因素（5%）；其他原因包括感染、胰腺炎和吻合口瘘。关于技术性失败各组之间无显著差异。

排斥导致的首次移植失败率见图 44-9。1 年后 2%的 SPK、8%的 PAK 和 10%的 PTA 受者尽管技术上移植成功，但仍必须重新使用外源性胰岛素治疗（SPK 组明显较低；$P=0.0001$）。

有关 2000—2004 年间病例中胰管外分泌的处理，SPK 移植组肠道引流占绝大多数（81%）；PAK 和 PTA 组肠道引流的比例要略低（分别为 67%和 56%）。总体来说，肠道引流的技术性失败率要略高于膀胱引流（8%对 6%）。而关于移植胰腺的存活率，

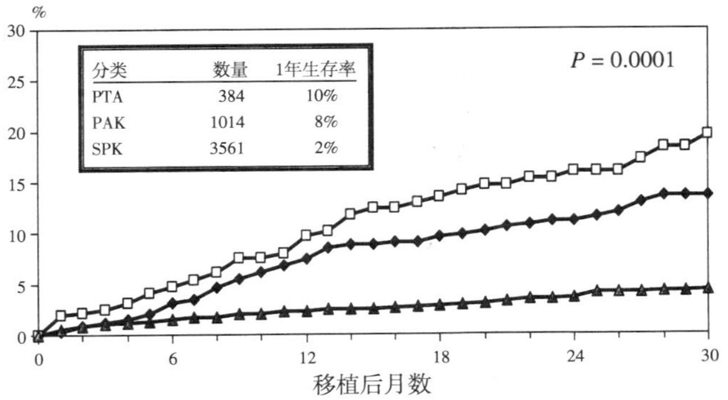

图 44-9 2000—2004 年间美国各受体组的首次尸体胰腺移植中技术成功者的免疫性失败率（重新使用外源性胰岛素）。PTA：单独胰腺移植；SPK：胰腺肾脏同时移植；PAK：肾脏移植后胰腺移植。

在任何一组中肠道引流与膀胱引流比较均没有显著差异：1 年存活率 SPK 组为 85%（n=3047）对 87%（n=707）；PAK 组为 77%（n=733）对 80%（n=364）；
722 PTA 组为 72%（n=238）对 79%（n=184）。在 PTA 组中，与肠道引流相比，膀胱引流技术成功的移植胰腺因排斥反应导致的失败率明显要低：1 年失败率分别为 5%（n=161）和 15%（n=216）（$P = 0.03$）。

在 SPK 组中，膀胱引流和肠道引流理应得到相近的结果：因为大多数病例的供体取自同一捐献者，血清肌酐可以作为监测胰腺移植后排斥反应指标，从而能够早期发现排斥反应并通过治疗来逆转。相反，单独胰腺移植（PAK 和 PTA）中血清肌酐却不能作为监测胰腺排斥反应的指标，排斥反应的高糖血症出现较晚，因而必须利用外分泌指标来判断。尽管发生排斥反应者时血清淀粉酶和脂肪酶会升高，但并非所有病例都升高；而膀胱引流者发生排斥反应者都伴有尿淀粉酶逐渐下降（100%敏感，尽管并非特异）且几乎都发生在高糖血症之前，因此排斥反应在膀胱引流者更容易被诊断进而获得治疗和逆转。

众所周知，肠道引流的各类胰腺移植中，移植小肠吻合采用 Roux-en-Y 袢时移植物的存活率要略低[29]。UNOS 报告中肠道引流的胰腺移植中大约 1/3 采用了 Roux-en-Y 袢，但这一步骤并未改善移植的结果，至少在 PTA 组中使用 Roux-en-Y 袢时技术性失败率反而上升[29]。

术式的另一变化是肠道引流的移植物静脉血流经门静脉引流[64]。该术式符合正常生理，理论上比腔静脉引流更具代谢优势，有些研究小组曾报道门静脉肠道引流移植的排斥倾向较低于腔静脉肠道引流移植[58,78]。登记处最近的分析表明有 1/5 的肠道引流移植采用了门静脉引流，移植胰腺的存活率与腔静脉肠道引流移植相比在任一组内均无显著差异：1 年存活率 SPK 组为 85%（n=610）对 85%（n=2437）；PAK 组为 78%（n=168）对 77%（n=564）；PTA 组为 71%（n=85）对 72%（n=153）。

关于免疫抑制，根据登记处最新的分析，在美国 2000－2004 年各组大约有 3/4 的受者使用 T 细胞抑制剂进行诱导治疗[30]。维持用药最常用的方案（每组中 2/3 的受者）是他克莫司和麦考酚酸莫酯二联或加用泼尼松三联用药。使用 T 细胞抑制剂诱导免疫抑制并用他克莫司和麦考酚酸莫酯维持时（图 44-10），首次胰腺尸体移植的胰腺移植物 1 年存活率分别为：SPK 88%（n=2500）、PAK 82%（n=712）和 PTA 81%（n=278）。每组大约有 1/6 的受者使用西罗莫司作为维持免疫抑制用药（图 44-11），对比数据为：SPK、PAK 和 PTA 组的胰腺移植物 1 年存活率分别为 87%（n=675）、82%（n=184）和 83%（n=67）。
与之对照的是，另外 1/6 患者采用其他免疫抑制方案 723
的胰腺移植物存活率明显低：SPK、PAK 和 PTA 的一年存活率分别为 63%（n=666）、61%（n=213）和 54%（n=84）。中心效应可能会对登记处根据免疫抑制方案进行分析得到的结果产生一定的影响。

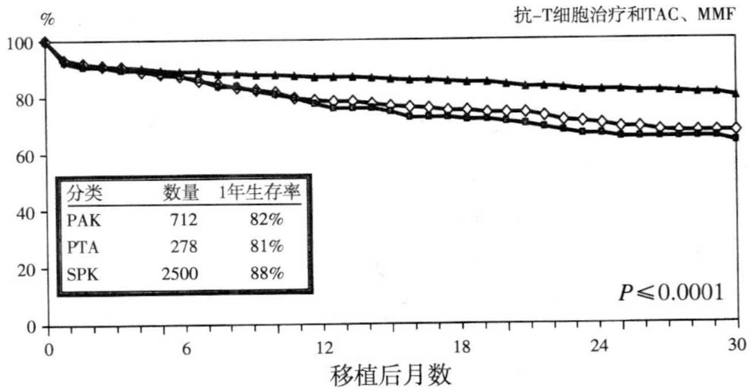

图 44-10 在应用 T 细胞抑制剂诱导免疫抑制、他克莫司（TAC）和麦考酚酸莫酯（MMF）维持免疫抑制时，2000—2004 年间美国不同受者组的首次尸体胰腺移植的移植物功能性存活率（胰岛素不依赖）。PTA：单独胰腺移植；SPK：胰腺肾脏同时移植；PAK：肾脏移植后胰腺移植。

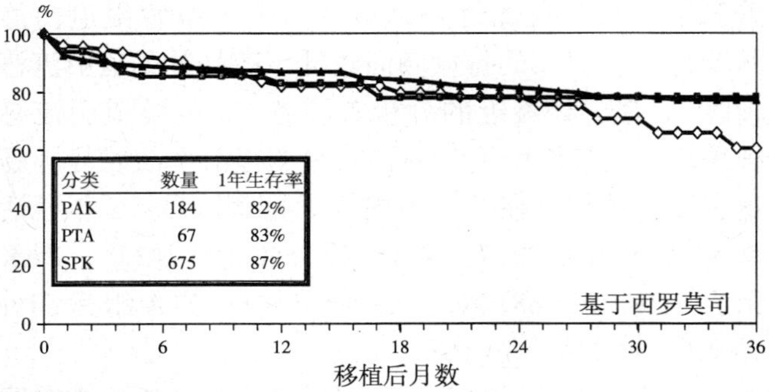

图 44-11 在应用西罗莫司维持免疫抑制时，2000—2004 年间美国不同受者组的首次尸体胰腺移植的移植物功能性存活率（胰岛素不依赖）。PTA：单独胰腺移植；SPK：胰腺肾脏同时移植；PAK：肾脏移植后胰腺移植。

关于胰腺移植的术前准备，登记处最近的数据表明，随着供体保存时间的延长，技术性失败率略有上升，而移植物存活率略有下降[30]。例如在 SPK 组，保存时间为 4～7 小时的胰腺移植物 1 年存活率为 86%，而保存时间为 28～31 小时的胰腺移植物 1 年存活率为 81%。HLA 配型对 SPK 移植的存活率并无实质影响，而对 PAK 和 PTA 组的影响至少在 1 级地区是有益的。

关于胰腺受者的年龄，登记处 2000—2004 年的数据分析表明，其主要对 PTA 受者的预后产生影响，年轻患者更容易发生排斥反应。在 PAK 组，所有受体均超过 20 岁，每 10 岁做一个排斥率分析，1 年排斥率为 4%～7%。在 SPK 组，20 岁以上各年龄段患者的 1 年排斥率为 2%～4%，而 20 岁以下患者（n=4）的 1 年排斥率为 0%。相反，在 PTA 组，20 岁以下（n=14）的 1 年排斥率为 50%；20～29 岁患者的 1 年排斥率为 13%；30 岁以上患者的 1 年排斥率为 4%～6%，这与另两组的数据相近。因此，年轻的尿毒症糖尿病患者具有较高的免疫活性而更容易对移植胰腺产生排斥反应，这也与 1988—1999 年美国小儿胰腺移植的结果分析相符[27]。分析的对象包括 8000 多例的胰腺移植病例，其中仅有 49 例受者年龄小于 21 岁（＜1%），包括 34 例 SPK、2 例 PAK 和 13 例 PTA；两例节段性 PTA 移植采用活体供体，其余均为尸体移植。小儿胰腺移植中少于 50%的受者年龄小于 19 岁。其中 PTA 患者的移植物 1 年存活率只有 15%，除 1 例外均因排斥反应而在 1 年内失败。登记处的资料没有小儿 PTA 移植的适应证，假设他们患有非常不稳定的糖尿病，则应该尝试通过免疫抑制来进行控制。小儿 SPK 受者中，患者、胰腺和肾脏移植物的 1 年存活率分别为 96%、78%和 71%，这一结果可与各时期成人 SPK 相比较。多数小儿 SPK 受者患有糖尿病肾病之外的肾脏疾病。

因此，在小儿年龄组的胰腺移植并不普遍，其中多数为合并肾衰竭，需要肾移植而必须接受免疫抑制治疗的糖尿病儿童。这组儿童至少可以获得这样的结果，如果采用联合胰腺移植，患者就能因免疫抑制而脱离胰岛素依赖和脱离透析，因此是值得推荐的。对无尿毒症的不稳定型糖尿病患儿来说，成功的胰腺移植是恰当的治疗，抗排斥策略需要优化以获得比过去更高的移植物存活率。

关于接受胰腺移植的 1 型糖尿病患者，除胰岛素不依赖之外的效果评价指标，其他如继发并发症的预防和逆转、生活质量的提高、寿命的延长和每年维持生活质量所需保健费用的降低等均有所改善[18,20,26,56,76,88,97]。对于容易发生不自觉低血糖的不稳定型糖尿病患者，胰腺移植能够解决一些棘手和威胁生命的疑难问题[47,55,63]。

胰腺移植对移植候选者的糖尿病患者生存率的影响仍存在争论。两组来自 UNOS 和器官获取和移植网络（OPTN）的数据分析收集了 1995—2000 年间美国的胰腺移植候选者和受者的情况，对等待移植名单中患者和已经接受某类移植的患者的生存率进行了比较[32,90]。第一个分析研究中，SPK 受者生存率明显高于等待移植者，但进行单独移植（PAK 或 PTA）的受者结果却相反[90]。第二个分析研究中，SPK 受者具有较高的生存率是可以肯定的，此外单独胰腺移植受者的总体生存率与等待移植甚至 1 年后仍适合移植者相当[32]。第二个分析研究中，患者在多个中心的登记处被确认并只计数 1 次，更换类别的患者将被更正信息并提供长期随访。因此，对那些等待接受移植的患者，单独及联合胰腺移植并不比继续使用外源性胰岛素风险更高，并且有可能提高生存率。

胰岛移植

除胰腺移植或带血管胰腺移植之外，还有另一种侵入性较低的方法可以置换 β 细胞，即把分离的胰岛作为单体进行移植[39,41,59,94]。1974 年对 1 名做过肾移植的糖尿病患者进行了第一例临床同种异体胰岛移植[53]，此后共开展了 700 多例同种胰岛移植。同种胰岛移植的成功率一直较低，直到近来（始于 2000 年）情况才发生了变化。但是对全胰切除术后 20 年以上的患者进行胰岛自体移植具有相对较高的成功率，因此在综述胰岛同种移植在 1 型和手术后糖尿病中的应用现状之前简单介绍一下。

胰岛自体移植在胰腺良性疾病切除后的应用

24 自从 20 世纪 70 年代第 1 例胰岛自体移植成功以来，已经通过其来成功预防因良性疾病，如慢性胰腺炎行全胰切除术后继发性糖尿病的发生，但却受限于移植胰岛的数量[83,85,92]。患有慢性胰腺炎，并有顽固性疼痛的儿童需要行胰腺切除术来解除麻醉剂依赖，胰岛自体移植防止了这些儿童发生糖尿病[83,91]。图 44–12 展示了保留幽门的全胰及十二指肠切除的术式。手术可以分步进行，但当胰体和胰尾被切除时通常必须进行胰岛分离处理以便进行经门静脉的自体移植（图 44–13A）。

如果先行胰腺末端切除，而且 Whipple 式（完全）胰腺切除是必需的时候，将利用初始胰岛自体移植来预防糖尿病。如果先行 Whipple 式手术后疼痛仍持续，且胰腺远端（体和尾）必须完全切除时，那么切除术应在一个能够从切除胰腺分离自体移植所需胰岛的医院中进行。

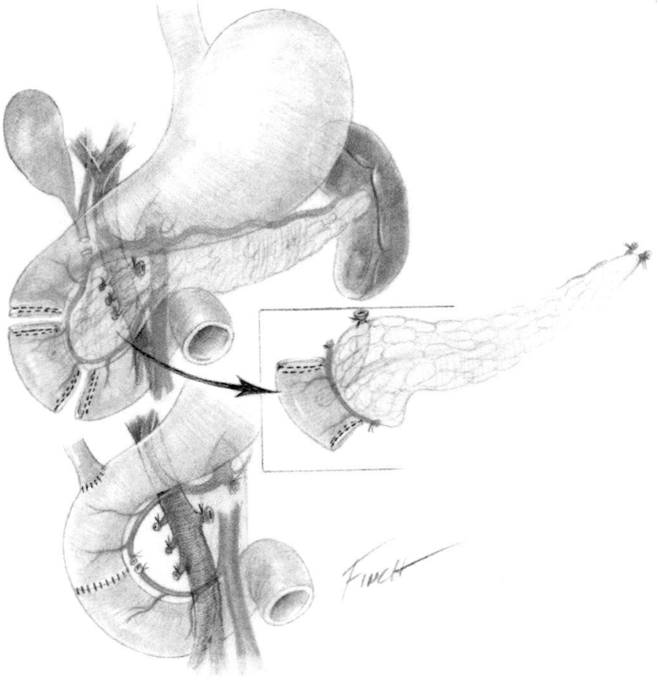

图 44–12 保留幽门的全胰及部分十二指肠切除的术式，用于拟行胰岛自体移植的慢性胰腺炎患者。将胆总管横断并再植于十二指肠，该图示再植于十二指肠或十二指肠空肠吻合口的近端，但更普遍的是位于肠吻合口的远端，主要取决于个体的解剖结构。如果可能，仅切除十二指肠的第二段并行十二指肠十二指肠端端吻合；但如果活力不够，整个远端十二指肠必须切除并行十二指肠空肠端端或端侧吻合。胃短血管和胃网膜动脉尽可能保留，如脾有活力，则不需切除。(Reproduced from Gruessner RWG, Sutherland DER [eds]: Transplantation of the Pancreas. New York, Springer-Verlag, 2004.)

胰岛同种移植

对手术后糖尿病患者进行胰岛同种移植已经具有很高的成功率[62,89]。对自身免疫性 1 型糖尿病患者进行胰岛同种移植则更具挑战性，即使是在无基础对照的情况下，直到 20 世纪 90 年代早期这组患者的胰岛素不依赖才得以实现[11,24,67,68,93]。

胰岛同种移植及自体移植通常是将胰岛细胞团经门静脉注射入肝脏，在肝内至少有部分胰岛通过营养的弥散而存活直至血管再形成（见图 44–13B）。与胰腺移植相比，同种胰岛移植的缺点在于 β 细胞团的减少，更多的研究已经致力于如何补偿这种损耗的发生。

近来，通过增加移植胰岛细胞团数量和选择抗排斥药联用减少免疫抑制剂导致的糖尿病并发症，胰岛同种移植的成功率已得到显著提高。Shapiro 及其同事报道，对 7 名 1 型糖尿病患者进行重复移植（相继多个供体），并采用由达克珠单抗、西罗莫司和相对低剂量的他克莫司组成的无糖皮质激素免疫抑制治疗方案，全部实现了胰岛素不依赖[69]。

皮质激素具有较强的致糖尿病特性，是所有类型同种器官移植受者发生移植后糖尿病的一个众所周知的危险因素。药物引起的糖尿病在胰腺同种移植受者的发生率低，这是因为完整的正常胰腺拥有大量的 β

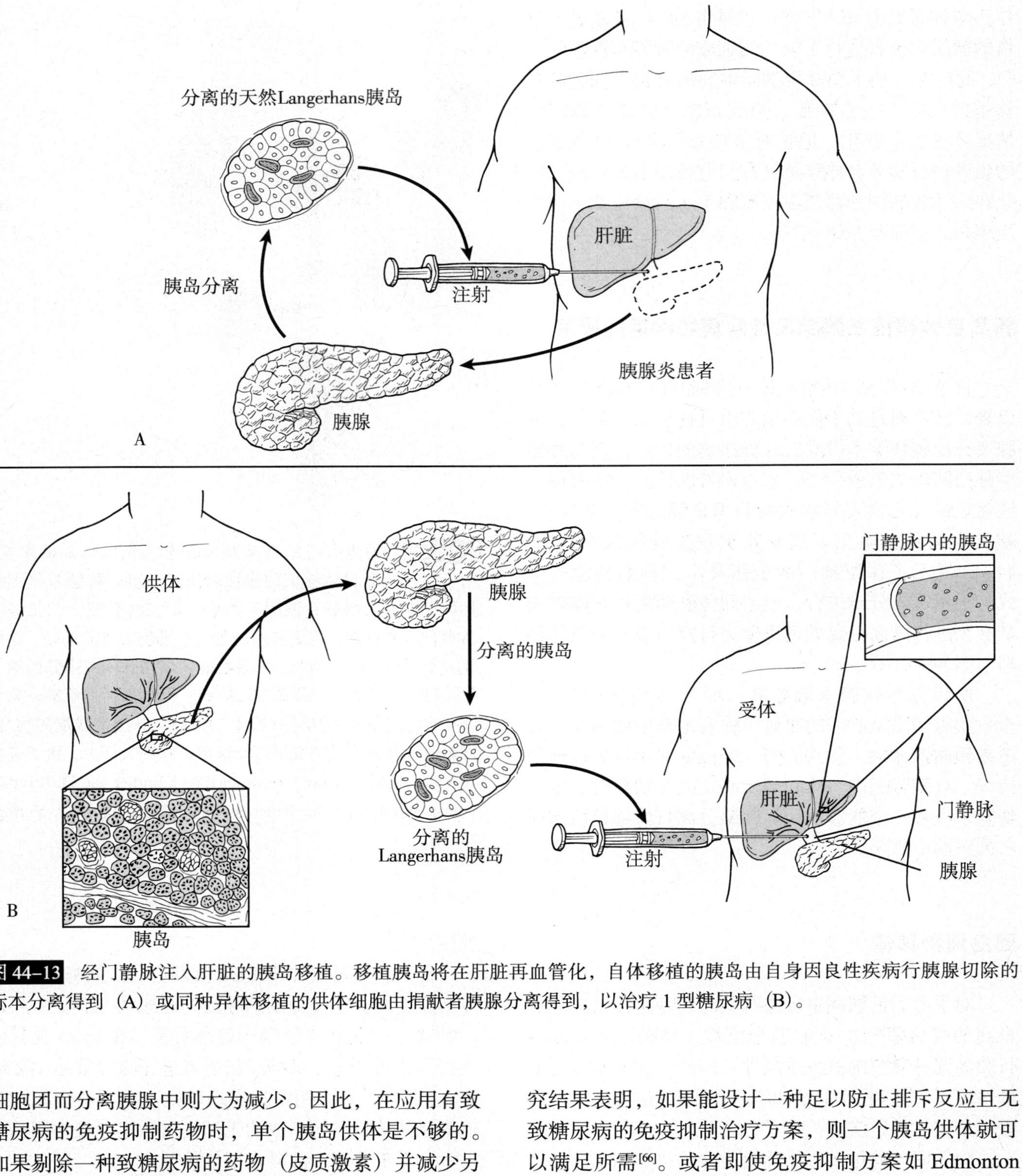

图 44-13 经门静脉注入肝脏的胰岛移植。移植胰岛将在肝脏再血管化，自体移植的胰岛由自身因良性疾病行胰腺切除的标本分离得到（A）或同种异体移植的供体细胞由捐献者胰腺分离得到，以治疗 1 型糖尿病（B）。

细胞团而分离胰腺中则大为减少。因此，在应用有致糖尿病的免疫抑制药物时，单个胰岛供体是不够的。如果剔除一种致糖尿病的药物（皮质激素）并减少另一种能导致糖尿病但免疫抑制效果不错的他克莫司的剂量，再加用西罗莫司（致糖尿病性较轻而免疫抑制效果与他克莫司相当），则 β 细胞团就足以解决广大患者对外源性胰岛素的需求[66]。Edmonton 小组的研究结果表明，如果能设计一种足以防止排斥反应且无致糖尿病的免疫抑制治疗方案，则一个胰岛供体就可以满足所需[66]。或者即使免疫抑制方案如 Edmonton 方案的病例那样并非完全无致糖尿病，但如果提高从胰岛细胞分离出活性 β 细胞团的效率，也能够使单个供体满足所需。

早期的传统免疫抑制治疗所具有的致糖尿病并发

症是胰岛同种移植成功率不高的一个原因。通常胰岛的分离率低于 50%，并且胰岛 β 细胞的植入率也低于 50% [17]。文献中已经证明[15]。免疫抑制剂具有致糖尿病性（不仅皮质激素，还包括神经钙蛋白抑制剂他克莫司和环孢霉素），大剂量时更为明显，使得胰岛素用量增加同时也抑制了胰岛素分泌。直接带血管胰腺移植供体的完整胰岛群能够克服药物造成的胰岛
725 素抵抗，而目前单个胰岛供体很难达到所需的 β 细胞团数量。幸运的是，新一代免疫抑制剂的出现已使大多数临床移植的受体不再需要使用泼尼松，神经钙蛋白抑制剂的用量也得以减少，其致糖尿病性也得以降低[21,22]。

Edmonton 小组报道了首例通过胰岛移植获得持续胰岛素不依赖的糖尿病病例[69]，并已经得到其他研究机构的证实[25,36,37,44,51]。大多数研究中受者都需要来自两个或两个以上胰腺供体的胰岛[25,44,51,69]。胰岛移植取代胰腺移植成为临床大规模治疗糖尿病的重要手段还需要更多的改进，包括尽可能提高胰岛提取的数量和质量，降低免疫移植的并发症和风险。

明尼苏达州立大学最近的两个胰岛移植实验对提高移植胰岛细胞效能、植入率和功能性存活率的方法
726 进行了研究：（1）排除了年龄超过 50 岁的供体；（2）限制胰腺保存过程中胰岛的缺血性损伤；（3）胰岛处理过程中避免使用对胰岛有害的试剂；（4）进行胰岛培养使移植前就能启动免疫抑制；（5）移植前后给予有效的预防性抗凝和胰岛素治疗；（6）增加免疫诱导的免疫抑制和抗炎效应；（7）免疫抑制的维持避免使用皮质激素，并尽量降低神经钙蛋白抑制剂用量[36,37]。在伴有不自觉低血糖的 1 型糖尿病患者中进行了两项先导性试验，接受单供体胰岛移植的 14 名 1 型糖尿病患者中有 12 人实现了胰岛素不依赖，且糖化血红蛋白（HbA_{1c}）水平正常。该结果表明，单胰腺供体的胰岛移植治疗 1 型糖尿病时，以上 7 条措施中的部分或全部有助于糖尿病的长期逆转。其中以下三条尤其重要：

首先，延长移植前胰腺冷藏时间的保存方法适用于带血管胰腺移植，却不适用于胰岛移植，即使胰岛分离和移植前小段时间的冷藏也不行。供体胰腺前任何冷缺血损伤都会加重胰岛分离过程中的细胞应激，并且，这种应激程度超过带血管胰腺移植后胰岛再灌注损伤引起的应激[38]。试验结果表明，联用两种保存液（全氟萘烷 / 威斯康星大学液）的保存方法既能增加胰岛分离率，又能保留分离胰岛逆转糖尿病的能力[42,87]。

其次，经门静脉移植的胰岛在血管内定植，使得移植物立即暴露于已经对胰岛 β 细胞致敏的自体反应性 T 细胞。这种定植也加快了同种异体免疫反应的发生。移植前对胰岛进行预培养能使其在注射前处于适当的免疫抑制状态，进而减少移植后自身免疫、同种异体免疫和先天性免疫导致的胰岛细胞团损耗[35]。1 型糖尿病患者同种异体移植后期望达到胰岛素不依赖所需的胰岛数量要大于手术后糖尿病患者。这一差异表明，异体胰岛的植入和存活在自身免疫的环境中会得到削弱[39]。Edmonton 的试验中需要一个以上的胰腺供体[69]，反映了抗 IL-2R 单克隆抗体（mAb）不足以消除持续自身免疫介导的早期效应物反应。因此，围移植期针对自体反应性 T 细胞我们采用抗 CD3 抗体或多克隆 T 细胞抗体，这也是极少数被证实能够有效抑制活化的自体反应性 T 细胞方法中的两种[14,50,96]。

最后，移植前的胰岛培养是我们研究中的重要环节。胰岛培养能够在胰岛注入前对受体 T 细胞进行定向免疫抑制，可能对抑制胰岛定向免疫反应具有重要意义，该反应是由自体反应性致敏 T 细胞介导的，植入血管内的胰岛将直接接触这种 T 细胞。T 细胞清除性抗体治疗后 2 天再行移植，能阻止移植胰岛暴露于初次和二次抗体注射引起的不同程度的细胞因子释放。移植前培养还能进行注射前的质量控制研究，这样就能避免移植的组织不能达到严格的释放标准。动物研究表明培养后（与新鲜胰岛相对）胰岛代谢效率提高[43]。最近的临床试验结果与实验研究一致，说明移植前胰岛培养除存在免疫学优势之外，对代谢没有不良影响，甚至可能有益。

因此，综合应用几种胰岛移植的改进手段能选择性改善受者的移植结果。新的无皮质激素、无神经钙蛋白抑制剂及无致糖尿病性的免疫抑制治疗方案已经在相关灵长类动物的胰岛移植模型中被证明是安全有效的，并有望使胰岛移植的结果得到更显著的改善[2,95]。

但是，在供体分配和胰岛分离率问题解决之前，胰腺移植仍将是大多数供体器官最高效的利用途径。显然，为了治疗糖尿病，简单的细胞移植肯定优于整个胰腺的移植，但胰岛分离需要特定的设备，而胰腺移植只需医院能开展移植并拥有经适当训练的医生。

建立人胰岛处理技术的控制和统一规范、通过胰岛产品的效价测定来预测移植后的胰岛功能以及整理胰岛移植临床应用的安全性和有效性资料，都需要分离人胰岛的生物制品生产许可执照。这一执照对第三方赔偿责任来说至关重要，后者将极大地推动胰腺供体利用率。胰腺保存技术的进步和区域性胰岛加工中心的建立可能将改变胰腺供体的分配格局，克服供应和技术障碍，从而提高胰岛移植的可行性。

目前，普通免疫抑制治疗的目的是防止对直接带血管胰腺或新形成血管的胰岛移植物的排斥。然而，为了诱导对供体的免疫耐受设计出多种方案，在胰岛受者检测这些方案要比在实质器官受者更为容易：手术操作的强度和排斥引起的后果都较小[40]。因此，采用新的免疫监测和抗排斥策略推进胰岛异体移植极为重要，尽管目前因 1 型糖尿病而进行 β 细胞置换的临床模式仍以胰腺移植为主。

尽管在几年之后 β 细胞置换疗法的主流形式可能使胰腺移植向胰岛移植转变，但胰腺移植也不会彻底消失。对移植前高胰岛素依赖的患者，利用胰岛移
727 植来逆转糖尿病并不合适，最好采用带血管胰腺移植。而且，伴有外分泌不足的糖尿病患者最好采用肠道引流的胰腺移植。另外，在有高胰岛素需求或胰岛素抵抗（2 型糖尿病）的患者出现胰岛素抵抗时，可能需要单个供体的完整器官以便获取足够的胰岛细胞团来恢复胰岛素不依赖。

组织获取将是决定 β 细胞置换治疗影响力的限制因素。每年美国能提供 6000 个尸体供体，但据估计只有一半适合胰腺移植。因此，假设每个尸体胰腺能劈裂供应两个受体[86]，活体节段性胰腺移植能达到肾移植开展的程度[33]（美国目前是大约每年 6000），美国每年最多能完成 12 000 例胰腺移植。这一假想尚未实现，但潜在需要移植的患者已接近每年新发生的 1 型糖尿病患者（30000/ 年，美国）的一半。如果一个供体能分离足够的胰岛以供应两个以上的受者，移植的数量将增加。尽管胰岛移植方案的效果持续改进，相关的技术和免疫抑制风险也持续降低，胰岛移植仍不会成为糖尿病治疗的终极手段。正如胰腺移植为胰岛移植搭建了平台，胰岛移植的真正价值将在于为异种和干或前体细胞源的胰岛 β 细胞治疗[10,60,71]的发展提供了契机，后者将使得细胞置换成为糖尿病的常规治疗。

从胰腺移植到胰岛移植，应该成为每个移植中心治疗糖尿病患者的全套配备。同样，每个内分泌医生都应该考虑对并发低血糖相关的血糖自主节律丧失和（或）进展性微血管并发症的 1 型糖尿病患者进行 β 细胞替代治疗[16]。必须对胰腺和胰岛移植进行长期的临床研究，以便确定最适宜接受移植的人群、糖尿病病程中最佳移植时间和患者的移植方式。胰腺和胰岛移植的施行都应该尽可能更经济[77]。对胰肾联合移植受者的研究已经表明，移植对复杂糖尿病的治疗也有效果[18]，胰岛移植受者也需要进行类似的研究。目前，β 细胞置换治疗对伴有不能耐受的低血糖性意识丧失的成年患者已有明确的临床疗效，并且也适用于因肾移植等其他需要而接受免疫抑制治疗的儿童和成人。随着抗排斥手段安全性的提高和并发症减少，小儿 β 细胞置换治疗的适应证也将放宽。

（王 浩译 李民驹校）

致 谢

We are indebted to Heather Nelson for assistance in preparing the manuscript.

参考文献

1. The effect of intensive treatment of diabetes on the development and progression of long-term complications in insulin-dependent diabetes mellitus. The Diabetes Control and Complications Trial Research Group. N Engl J Med 1993;329:977-986.
2. Adams AB, Shirasugi N, Durham MM, et al: Calcineurin inhibitor-free CD28 blockade-based protocol protects allogeneic islets in nonhuman primates. Diabetes 2002;51: 265-270.
3. Bendel-Stenzel MR, Kashtan CE, Sutherland DER, Chavers BM: Simultaneous pancreas-kidney transplant in two children with hemolytic-uremic symptoms. Pediatr Nephrol 1997;11:485-487.
4. Benedetti E, Dunn T, Massad MG, et al: Successful living related simultaneous pancreas-kidney transplant between identical twins. Transplantation 1999;67:915-918.
5. Benedetti E, Sileri P, Kandaswamy R, et al: Surgical aspects of pancreas transplantation. In Gruessner RW, Sutherland DER (eds): Transplantation of the Pancreas. New York, Springer-Verlag, 2004, pp 111-178.
6. Bloomgarden ZT: American Diabetes Association Postgraduate Course, 1996: treatment and prevention of diabetes. Diabetes Care 1996;19:784-786.

7. Boggi U, Vistoli F, Del Chiaro M, et al: Portal enteric-drained solitary pancreas transplantation without surveillance biopsy: Is it safe? Transplant Proc 2004;36:1090-1092.
8. Boggi U, Vistoli F, Del Chiaro M, et al: A simplified technique for the en bloc procurement of abdominal organs that is suitable for pancreas and small-bowel transplantation. Surgery 2004;135:629-641.
9. Boggi U, Vistoli F, Signori S, et al: A new technique for retroperitoneal pancreas transplantation with portal-enteric drainage. Transplantation 2005;79:1137-1142.
10. Bonner-Weir S, Sharma A: Pancreatic stem cells. J Pathol 2002;197:519-526.
11. Bretzel RG, Hering BJ, Federlin KF: Islet cell transplantation in diabetes mellitus—from bench to bedside. Exp Clin Endocrinol Diabetes 2004;103(Suppl 2):143-159.
12. Calne RY: Paratopic segmental pancreas grafting: A technique with portal venous drainage. Lancet 1984;1:595-597.
13. Calne RY, Rolles K, White DJ, et al: Cyclosporin A initially as the only immunosuppressant in 34 recipients of cadaveric organs: 32 kidneys, 2 pancreases, and 2 livers. Lancet 1979;2:1033-1036.
14. Chatenoud L, Thervet E, Primo J, Bach JF: Anti-CD3 antibody induces long-term remission of overt autoimmunity in nonobese diabetic mice. Proc Natl Acad Sci U S A 1994;91:123-127.
15. Christiansen E, Andersen HB, Rasmussen K, et al: Pancreatic beta-cell function and glucose metabolism in human segmental pancreas and kidney transplantation. Am J Physiol 1993;264(3 Pt 1):E441-E449.
16. Cryer PE: Banting lecture. Hypoglycemia: The limiting factor in the management of IDDM. Diabetes 1994;43:1378-1389.
17. Davalli AM, Ogawa Y, Scaglia L, et al: Function, mass, and replication of porcine and rat islets transplanted into diabetic nude mice. Diabetes 1995;44:104-111.
18. Douzdjian V, Ferrara D, Silvestri G: Treatment strategies for insulin-dependent diabetics with ESRD: A cost-effectiveness decision analysis model. Am J Kidney Dis 1998;31:794-802.
19. Dubernard JM, Traeger J, Neyra P, et al: A new method of preparation of segmental pancreatic grafts for transplantation: Trials in dogs and in man. Surgery 1978;84:633-640.
20. Fioretto P, Steffes MW, Sutherland DER, et al: Reversal of lesions of diabetic nephropathy after pancreas transplantation. N Engl J Med 1998;339:69-75.
21. First MR: Immunosuppressive agents and their actions. Transplant Proc 2002;34:1369-1371.
22. First MR, Gerber DA, Hariharan S, et al: Posttransplant diabetes mellitus in kidney allograft recipients: Incidence, risk factors, and management. Transplantation 2002;73:379-386.
22a. Fridell JA, Milgrom M, Henson S, et al: Use of the end-to-end anastomotic circular stapler for creation of the duodenoenterostomy for enteric drainage of the pancreas allograft. J Am Coll Surg 2004;198:495-497.
23. Gliedman ML, Gold M, Whittaker J, et al: Clinical segmental pancreatic transplantation with ureter-pancreatic duct anastomosis for exocrine drainage. Surgery 1973;74:171-180.
24. Gores PF, Najarian JS, Stephanian E, et al: Insulin independence in type I diabetes after transplantation of unpurified islets from a single donor using 15-deoxyspergualin. Lancet 1993;341:19-21.
25. Goss JA, Schock AP, Brunicardi FC, et al: Achievement of insulin independence in three consecutive type-1 diabetic patients via pancreatic islet transplantation using islets isolated at a remote islet isolation center. Transplantation 2002;74:1761-1766.
26. Gross CR, Limwattananon C, Matthees BJ: Quality of life after pancreas transplantation: A review. Clin Transplant 1998;12:351-361.
27. Gruessner AC: Pediatric pancreas transplants in the USA 1988-2000. Pediatr Transplant 2000;4:100.
28. Gruessner AC, Sutherland DER: Pancreas transplant outcomes for United States and non-US cases as reported to the United Network for Organ Sharing and the International Pancreas Transplant Registry as of October 2002. In Cecka JM, Terasaki PI (eds): Clinical Transplants 2002. Los Angeles, UCLA Immunogenetics Center, 2003.
29. Gruessner AC, Sutherland DER: Pancreas transplant outcomes for United States (US) and non-US cases as reported to the United Network for Organ Sharing (UNOS) and the International Pancreas Transplant Registry (IPTR) as of May 2003. In Cecka JM, Terasaki PI (eds): Clinical Transplants 2003. Los Angeles, UCLA Immunogenetics Center, 2004.
30. Gruessner AC, Sutherland DER: Pancreas Transplantation Analyses of United States (US) and non-US cases as reported to the United Network for Organ Sharing (UNOS) and the International Pancreas Transplant Registry (IPTR) as of June 2004. In Cecka JM, Terasaki PI (eds): Clinical Transplants 2004. Los Angeles, UCLA Immunogenetics Center, 2005.
31. Gruessner RW, Sutherland DE, Dunn DL, et al: Transplant options for patients undergoing total pancreatectomy for chronic pancreatitis. J Am Coll Surg 2004;198:559-567.
32. Gruessner RW, Sutherland DE, Gruessner AC: Mortality assessment for pancreas transplants. Am J Transplant 2004;4:2018-2026.
33. Gruessner RWG, Kendall DM, Drangstveit MB, et al: Simultaneous pancreas-kidney transplantation from live donors. Ann Surg 1997;226:471-482.
34. Gruessner RWG, Manivel DC, Dunn DL, Sutherland DER: Pancreaticoduodenal transplantation with enteric drainage following native total pancreatectomy for chronic pancreatitis: A case report. Pancreas 1991;6:479-488.
35. Hering BJ, Bretzel RG, Hopt UT, et al: New protocol toward prevention of early human islet allograft failure. Transplant Proc 1994;26:570-571.
36. Hering BJ, Kandaswamy R, Ansite JD, et al: Successful single donor islet transplantation in type 1 diabetes. Am J Transplant 2003;3(Suppl 5):296.
37. Hering BJ, Kandaswamy R, Harmon JV, et al: Transplantation of cultured islets from two-layer preserved pancreases in type 1 diabetes with anti-CD3 antibody. Am J Transplant 2004;4:390-401.
38. Hering BJ, Matsumoto I, Sawada T, et al: Impact of two-layer pancreas preservation on islet isolation and transplantation. Transplantation 2002;74:1813-1816.
39. Hering BJ, Ricordi C: Islet transplantation for patients with type I diabetes. Graft 1999;2:12-27.
40. Hering BJ, Ricordi C, Sutherland DER, Bluestone JA: Islet transplantation: At the forefront of clinical research on immune tolerance. In Norman DJ, Suki WN (eds): Primer on Transplantation. Thorofare, NJ, American Society of Transplant Physicians, 2000.
41. Hering BJ, Wijkstrom M, Eckman PM: Islet transplantation. In Gruessner RW, Sutherland DER (eds): Transplantation of the Pancreas. New York, Springer-Verlag, 2004.
42. Hiraoka K, Trexler A, Fujioka B, et al: Optimal temperature in pancreas preservation by the two-layer cold storage

method before islet isolation. Transplant Proc 2001;33(1-2): 891-892.
43. Jahr H, Hussmann B, Eckhardt T, Bretzel RG: Successful single donor islet allotransplantation in the streptozotocin diabetes rat model. Cell Transplant 2002;11:513-518.
44. Kaufman DB, Baker MS, Chen X, et al: Sequential kidney/islet transplantation using prednisone-free immunosuppression. Am J Transplant 2002;2:674-677.
45. Kaufman DB, Leventhal JR, Koffron AJ, et al: A prospective study of rapid corticosteroid elimination in simultaneous pancreas-kidney transplantation: Comparison of two maintenance immunosuppression protocols: Tacrolimus/mycophenolate mofetil versus tacrolimus/sirolimus. Transplantation 2002;73:169-177.
46. Kelly WD, Lillehei RC, Merkel FK: Allotransplantation of the pancreas and duodenum along with the kidney in diabetic nephropathy. Surgery 1967;61:827-835.
47. Kendall DM, Rooney DP, Smets YF, et al: Pancreas transplantation restores epinephrine response and symptom recognition during hypoglycemia in patients with longstanding type I diabetes and autonomic neuropathy. Diabetes 2000;46:249-257.
48. Lillehei RC, Ruiz JO, Aquino C, Goetz FC: Transplantation of the pancreas. Acta Endocrinol 1976;83(Suppl 205): 303-320.
49. Lillehei RC, Simmons RL, Najarian JS, et al: Pancreaticoduodenal allotransplantation: Experimental and clinical experience. Ann Surg 1970;172:405-436.
50. Maki T, Ichikawa T, Blanco R, Porter J: Long-term abrogation of autoimmune diabetes in nonobese diabetic mice by immunotherapy with anti-lymphocyte serum. Proc Natl Acad Sci U S A 1992;89:3434-3438.
51. Markmann JF, Deng S, Huang X, et al: Insulin independence following isolated islet transplantation and single islet infusions. Ann Surg 2003;237:741-749.
52. Marsh CL, Perkins JD, Sutherland DER, et al: Combined hepatic and pancreaticoduodenal procurement for transplantation. Surg Gynecol Obstet 1989;168:254-258.
53. Najarian JS, Sutherland DER, Matas AJ, et al: Human islet transplantation: A preliminary experience. Transplant Proc 1977;9:233-236.
54. Nathan DM: Long-term complications of diabetes mellitus. N Engl J Med 1993;328:1676-1685.
55. Navarro X, Kennedy WR, Aeppli D, Sutherland DER: Neuropathy and mortality in diabetes: Influence of pancreas transplantation. Muscle Nerve 1996;19:1009-1016.
56. Navarro X, Sutherland DER, Kennedy WR: Long-term effects of pancreatic transplantation on diabetic neuropathy. Ann Neurol 1997;42:727-736.
57. Nghiem DD, Corry RJ: Technique of simultaneous pancreaticoduodenal transplantation with urinary drainage of pancreatic secretion. Am J Surg 1987;153:405-406.
58. Philosophe B, Farney AC, Schweitzer EJ, et al: Superiority of portal venous drainage over systemic venous drainage in pancreas transplantation: A retrospective study. Ann Surg 2001;234:689-696.
59. Pileggi A, Ricordi C, Alessiani M, Inverardi L: Factors influencing islet of Langerhans graft function and monitoring. Clin Chim Acta 2001;310:3-16.
60. Poggioli R, Inverardi L, Ricordi C: Islet xenotransplantation. Cell Transplant 2002;11:89-94.
61. Rayhill SC, Kirk AD, Odorico JS, et al: Simultaneous pancreas-kidney transplantation at the University of Wisconsin. In Cecka JM, Terasaki PI (eds): Clinical Transplants 1995. Los Angeles, UCLA Tissue Typing Laboratory, 1996.
62. Ricordi C, Tzakis A, Carroll PB, et al: Human islet isolation and allotransplantation in 22 consecutive cases. Transplantation 1992;53:407-414.
63. Robertson RP, Sutherland DE, Kendall DM, et al: Metabolic characterization of long-term successful pancreas transplants in type I diabetes. J Investig Med 1996;44: 549-555.
64. Rosenlof LK, Earnhardt RC, Pruett TL, et al: Pancreas transplantation: An initial experience with systemic and portal drainage of pancreatic allografts. Ann Surg 1992; 215:586-595.
65. Rosenlof LK, Earnhardt RC, Pruett TL, et al: Pancreas transplantation: An initial experience with systemic and portal drainage of pancreatic allografts. Ann Surg 1992; 215:586-595.
66. Ryan EA, Lakey JR, Paty BW, et al: Successful islet transplantation: Continued insulin reserve provides long-term glycemic control. Diabetes 2002;51:2148-2157.
67. Scharp DW, Lacy PE, Santiago JV, et al: Insulin independence after islet transplantation into type I diabetic patient. Diabetes 1990;39:515-518.
68. Secchi A, Socci C, Maffi P, et al: Islet transplantation in IDDM patients. Diabetologia 1997;40:225-231.
69. Shapiro AM, Lakey JR, Ryan EA, et al: Islet transplantation in seven patients with type 1 diabetes mellitus using a glucocorticoid-free immunosuppressive regimen [see comments]. N Engl J Med 2000;343:230-238.
70. Sollinger HW, Cook K, Kamps D: Clinical and experimental experience with pancreaticocystostomy for exocrine pancreatic drainage in pancreas transplantation. Transplant Proc 1984;16:749-751.
71. Soria B, Roche E, Berna G, et al: Insulin-secreting cells derived from embryonic stem cells normalize glycemia in streptozotocin-induced diabetic mice. Diabetes 2000;49: 157-162.
72. Starzl TE, Iwatsuki S, Shaw BW Jr, et al: Pancreaticoduodenal transplantation in humans. Surg Gynecol Obstet 1984; 159:265-272.
73. Starzl TE, Todo S, Fung J, et al: FK 506 for liver, kidney, and pancreas transplantation. Lancet 1989;2:1000-1004.
74. Stern RC, Mayes JT, Weber FL Jr, et al: Restoration of exocrine pancreatic function following pancreas-liver-kidney transplantation in a cystic fibrosis patient. Clin Transplant 1994;8:1-4.
75. Stock PG, Bluestone JA: Beta-cell replacement for type I diabetes. Annu Rev Med 2004;55:133-156.
76. Stratta RJ: The economics of pancreas transplantation. Graft 2000;3:19.
77. Stratta RJ, Cushing KA, Frisbie K, Miller SA: Analysis of hospital charges after simultaneous pancreas-kidney transplantation in the era of managed care. Transplantation 1997;64:287-292.
78. Stratta RJ, Shokouh-Amiri MH, Egidi MF, et al: A prospective comparison of simultaneous kidney-pancreas transplantation with systemic-enteric versus portal-enteric drainage. Ann Surg 2001;233:740-751.
79. Sutherland DE, Gruessner RW, Dunn DL, et al: Lessons learned from more than 1,000 pancreas transplants at a single institution. Ann Surg 2001;233:463-501.
80. Sutherland DER: International human pancreas and islet transplant registry. Transplant Proc 1980;12(No 4, Suppl 2):229-236.
81. Sutherland DER: Pancreas and islet transplant population. In Gruessner RWG, Sutherland DER (eds): Transplantation of the Pancreas. New York, Springer-Verlag, 2004.

82. Sutherland DER, Goetz FC, Najarian JS: Pancreas transplants from living related donors. Transplantation 1984;38: 625-633.
83. Sutherland DER, Gruessner RG, Jie T, et al: Pancreatic islet auto-transplantation for chronic pancreatitis. Clin Transplant 2004;18(Suppl 13):17-18.
84. Sutherland DER, Gruessner RWG: History of pancreas transplantation. In Gruessner RWG, Sutherland DER (eds): Transplantation of the Pancreas. New York, Springer-Verlag, 2004.
85. Sutherland DER, Matas AJ, Najarian JS: Pancreatic islet cell transplantation. Surg Clin North Am 1978;58:365-382.
86. Sutherland DER, Morel P, Gruessner RWG: Transplantation of two diabetic patients with one divided cadaver donor pancreas. Transplant Proc 1990;22:585.
87. Tanioka Y, Sutherland DER, Kuroda Y, et al: Excellence of the two-layer method (University of Wisconsin solution/perfluorochemical) in pancreas preservation before islet isolation. Surgery 1997;122:435-442.
88. Tyden G, Bolinder J, Solders G, et al: Improved survival in patients with insulin-dependent diabetes mellitus and end-stage diabetic nephropathy 10 years after combined pancreas and kidney transplantation. Transplantation 1999;67:645-648.
89. Tzakis A, Ricordi C, Alejandro R, et al: Pancreatic islet transplantation after upper abdominal exenteration and liver replacement. Lancet 1990;336:402-405.
90. Venstrom JM, McBride MA, Rother KI, et al: Survival after pancreas transplantation in patients with diabetes and preserved kidney function. JAMA 2003;290:2817-2823.
91. Wahoff DC, Papalois B, Najarian JS, et al: Islet autotransplantation after total pancreatectomy in a child. J Pediatr Surg 1996;31:1-6.
92. Wahoff DC, Papalois B, Najarian JS, et al: Autologous islet transplantation to prevent diabetes after pancreatic resection. Ann Surg 1995;222:562-579.
93. Warnock GL, Kneteman NM, Ryan E, et al: Normoglycaemia after transplantation of freshly isolated and cryopreserved pancreatic islets in type 1 (insulin-dependent) diabetes mellitus. Diabetologia 1991;34:55-58.
94. White SA, James RF, Swift SM, et al: Human islet cell transplantation—future prospects. Diabet Med 2001;18:78-103.
95. Wijkstrom M, Kenyon NS, Kirchhof N, et al: Islet allograft survival in nonhuman primates immunosuppressed with basiliximab, RAD, and FTY720.Transplantation 2004;77: 827-835.
96. Woodle ES, Xu D, Zivin RA, et al: Phase I trial of a humanized, Fc receptor nonbinding OKT3 antibody, huOKT3gamma1(Ala-Ala), in the treatment of acute renal allograft rejection. Transplantation 1999;68:608-616.
97. Zehrer CL, Gross CR: Quality of life of pancreas transplant recipients. Diabetologia 1991;34 (Suppl 1):S145-S149.

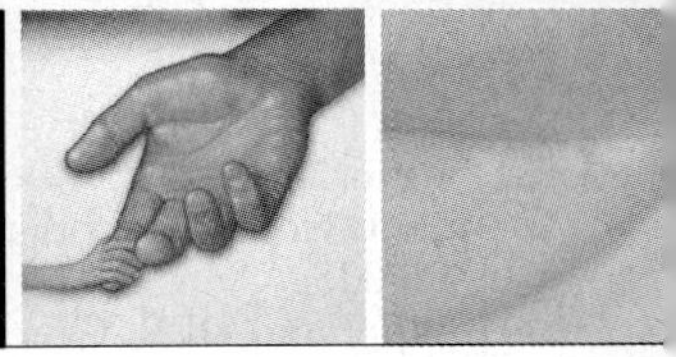

第 45 章

肝脏移植

Bob H. Saggi、Douglas G. Farmer 和 Ronald W. Busuttil

731 通过移植治疗小儿肝脏疾病的方法源于成人肝脏移植，最初的病例是由 Thomas E. Starzl 于 1963 和 1968 年对两名儿童进行的肝脏移植[19]。尽管早期的结果并不令人满意，经过随后 20 年的发展，肝脏移植已经成为终末期肝脏疾病（end-stage liver disease，ESLD）、某些肝胆恶性肿瘤、急性肝衰竭和许多代谢紊乱疾病的标准治疗方法。1983 年美国国家卫生研究院发展会议正式确认了这一点，并于 1987 年通过国家器官移植法建立了统一分配器官的规范系统。器官共享联合网（UNOS）由此创建并根据同行评议程序来统一调度。在 2003 年，共进行了 5600 多例肝脏移植，其中包括 546 例患儿[21]。20 世纪 90 年代中期以来，开展移植的例数已经相对稳定，但无论尸体还是活体供体的利用，均出现了“部分肝脏移植”增多的变化趋势。小儿肝脏移植在体积、可能的高免疫反应性和器官相对缺乏等方面都面临特有的挑战。约 2/3 的小儿肝脏移植受体的年龄小于 5 岁，但 5 岁以下的小儿尸体供体仅占 26% [21]（图 45-1）。因此，小儿的肝脏成功移植需要完美的技术，无论是从获取合适供体的角度还是进行精细的移植手术方面。随着移植等待时间的缩短和免疫抑制、手术技巧及移植后长期监护的进步，患者生存率已显著提高，目前 1 年生存率达 90%，5 年生存率达 80%，许多儿童存活至青春期甚至成年，并有着良好的生活质量[3]。在这一章，我们综述了儿童肝脏移植的主要适应证，肝衰竭的基本病理生理和临床表现，肝移植的手术方式、术后处理以及结果分析，其中手术方式重点介绍儿童独有的术式选择，术后处理侧重于对手术并发症

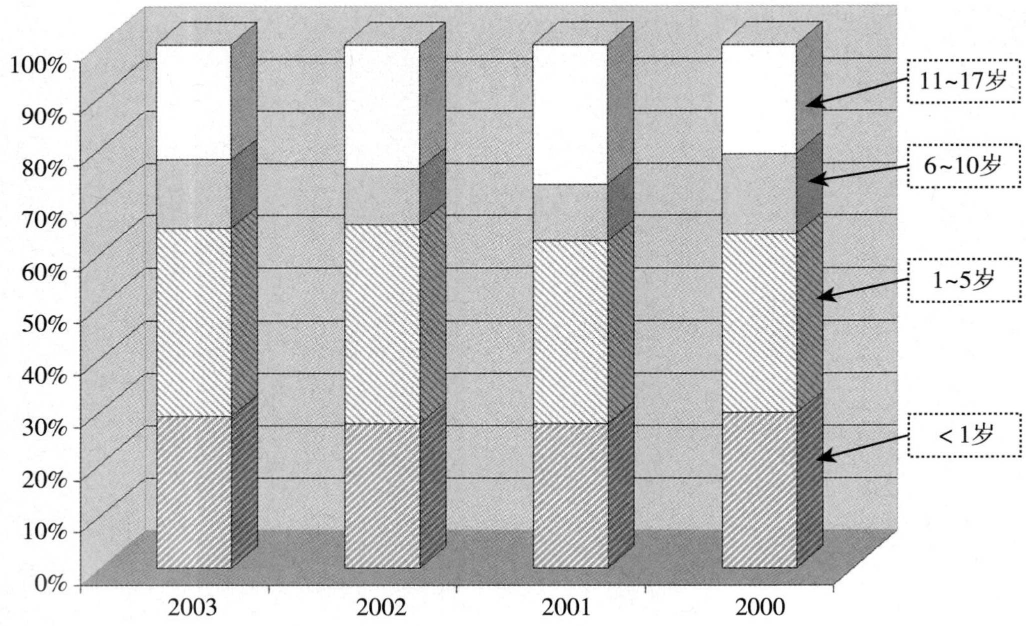

图 45-1 小儿肝脏移植的年龄分布。(Data from www.unos.org)

的处理。

732 ## 适应证

目前儿童肝脏移植适用于包括胆汁淤积和非胆汁淤积性肝硬化、急性肝衰竭、某些代谢性肝病、特定肿瘤引起的 ESLD 以及其他各种适应证（图 45–2）。儿童肝脏移植的一般适应证为影响长期存活或生活质量以及严重损害正常生长发育的肝脏疾病。单纯的肝硬化并非移植的指征，因为许多这种患者在失代偿前能够用药物维持较长时间。在急性肝衰竭时，随着顽固性凝血障碍、酸中毒和脑水肿等肝脏廓清功能的进展，肝功能很难自然恢复，往往预后不良，因此是肝脏移植的适应证。但对那些预后较好的患者应给予内科支持治疗直至肝功能恢复正常[5]。

长期肝硬化，随着肝细胞功能或门静脉高压失代偿等一系列症候群的出现提示需要进行移植。这些症候群包括进展性黄疸、凝血功能紊乱、蛋白质–热量营养不良和生长迟缓、认知障碍、脑病、脾功能亢进、静脉曲张出血和大量或顽固性腹水。这一群体中接受移植的大多数患者都有重度黄疸，原因是长期肝内和（或）肝外胆道梗阻引起继发或原发性胆汁性肝硬化。这些患者的体格检查往往表现为肌肉萎缩、脾大、可触及的质硬肝脏、腹水引起的腹胀和外周水肿。在不进行肝脏移植的情况下，失代偿患者很难长期存活，因此必须在失代偿之前进行移植[3,12]。

胆汁淤积性肝病

肝移植最常见的适应证是胆汁淤积性肝脏疾病，其中以胆道闭锁尤为常见。该病因大约占 2003 年儿童肝脏移植总数的 50%，而胆道闭锁又占到胆汁淤积组的 70% [21]（见图 45–2）。胆道闭锁的治疗依赖早期诊断，大多数病例通过手术探查取活检组织来确诊。具体的诊断步骤见于本书其他章节。通常月龄小于 3 个月时患儿尚未发生肝硬化，如果在之前即明确诊断，首选肝门肠吻合术，但远期效果最理想的手术时机为 8 周以内[22]。这一手术对肝脏疾病向肝硬化和门静脉高压进展具有重要的减缓作用，在某些病例甚至有阻止的作用。不幸的是，尽管经过有效的胆道引流，仍有 70%以上的患者在 5 岁之前进展为终末期肝脏疾病而需要进行移植[4,22]。无论如何，有许多例肝门肠道吻合术可使患儿生长发育到一定年龄后再接受移植。胆道闭锁后期行初次肝门肠道吻合和胆道引流失败后的再次探查术往往失败，只能进行移植。因此，一旦肝门肠道吻合失败，患者就应该行肝脏移植评估。当诊断明确时患儿年龄已大于 3 个月、任何年龄或肝门肠道吻合失败后出现终末期肝脏疾病，均是肝脏移植的适应证。当胆道闭锁患者出现肝脏失代偿

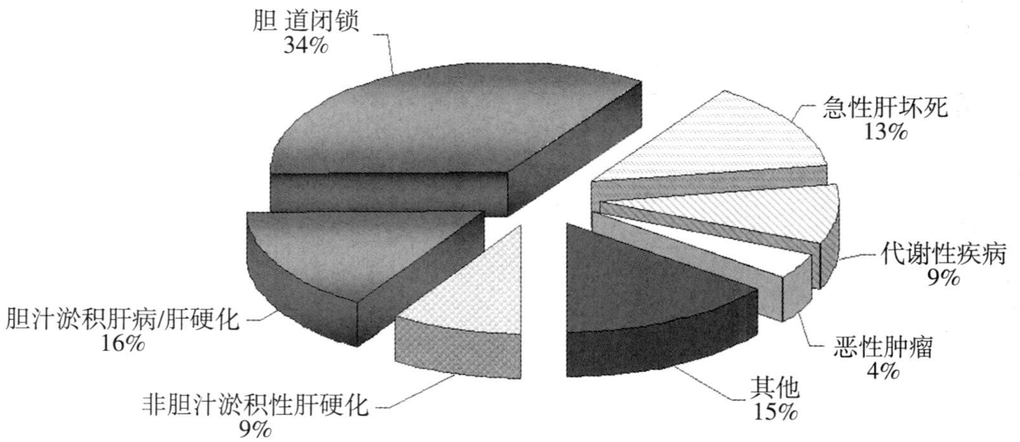

图 45–2　小儿肝脏移植的适应证。(Data obtained from www.unos.org, based on 2003 transplants.)

征象时，应该让富有肝移植经验的小儿肝病专家来决定是否行早期移植。

其他罕见的胆汁淤积性肝病和肝硬化原因包括家族性肝内胆管缺乏症，其包括综合征（Alagille 综合征）和非综合征两种形式；家族性胆汁淤积综合征、原发或继发的硬化性胆管炎以及包括 Caroli 病在内的难治性胆总管囊肿疾病。囊性病变有一部分表现为难治性肝外梗阻，另一部分囊性病变源于肝内胆管和
733 （或）动脉系统的畸形和破坏。以上情况通常都有一个可变而难以预料的进展，最后发展为严重纤维化、肝硬化和门静脉高压，出现典型进行性黄疸的年龄要大于胆道闭锁者。这些患儿并不一定要行肝门肠道吻合术，但基于与胆道闭锁相同的理由而具备肝脏移植的指征。

非胆汁淤积性肝硬化

这是儿童肝脏移植中并不常见的适应证，不到 2003 年移植病例总数的 10%（见图 45–2）[21]。这些儿童发病通常晚于胆汁淤积性疾病。引起这些患儿肝硬化和终末期肝脏疾病的原因包括慢性自身免疫性肝炎、新生儿肝炎、慢性病毒性（乙型或丙型）肝炎和病因不明的肝硬化。

急性肝衰竭

暴发性肝功能衰竭定义通常为急性肝衰竭且无慢性肝脏疾病证据的患者在黄疸出现 28 天内发生脑病。急性肝衰竭的标志包括广泛的凝血紊乱、酸中毒、低血糖和进行性高胆红素血症。这类患者可能发展为急性肾衰竭、多器官衰竭综合征或脑水肿甚至进展为脑疝。早期的治疗原则是避免病情发展到禁忌移植的阶段。欧洲各中心制定了许多标准来决定是否移植，在那里这些患者接受有组织的和集中的治疗[15]。儿童最常见的病因是病毒性肝炎、对乙酰氨基酚及其他药物的毒性损害和 Wilson 病。但仍有接近 2/3 的患者病因不明。对符合暴发性肝功能衰竭诊断标准的患者，肝移植是唯一有效的治疗方案，并且对所有急性肝功能衰竭患者进行早期干预都是必需的[5]。

代谢性肝病

这类疾病通常是因为酶缺乏或肝细胞功能的其他缺陷。这些疾病能够引起进行性肝纤维化或硬化（例如囊性纤维化、慢性 Wilsons 病和新生儿铁贮积病）并有典型终末期肝脏疾病表现。另外有些病例肝脏结构正常，但有毒的代谢产物蓄积会导致神经系统损害（例如 Crigler–Najjar 综合征、鸟氨酸氨甲酰转移酶缺乏症和 Wilson 病）、心血管疾病（家族性高胆固醇血症）或肾脏损害（家族性高草酸尿症）。某些代谢紊乱与恶性肿瘤的进展相关（例如酪氨酸血症），应该优先考虑进行移植。所有代谢紊乱患者的移植评估均应包括肝外器官功能的全面评估。这样才能确保进行肝脏移植患者能够由此获益并阻止肝外疾病的进展。某些患者可能需要同时或相继的双器官移植（例如肺、肾及心脏）。

肿瘤

儿童最常见的肝脏恶性肿瘤为肝母细胞瘤[16]。而肝细胞癌只有散发病例的报告，主要见于患有病毒性肝炎和酪氨酸血症的年长儿，或与其他原因引起的肝硬化相关。小儿非转移性恶性肿瘤的治疗一般采取手术切除，除非肿瘤的大小和（或）部位不宜切除。大量文献报道了新辅助治疗和（或）辅助化疗及少数放疗对肝母细胞瘤的疗效，但其对肝细胞癌却没有确切的疗效[17,20]。术前进行动脉栓塞化疗和（或）射频消融可能也有一定效果[1]。如果肿瘤无法切除，在排除肝外疾病之后可以考虑进行移植[14]。肝母细胞瘤患者肝移植后长期生存率大约 50%，而肝细胞癌的结果还不及前者[14,17]。仍待解决的主要问题是，针对巨大肝母细胞瘤，移植应该作为首选治疗还是手术切除后复发的补救措施。欧洲的数据表明作为补救措施的肝移植效果较差。肝脏最常见的良性肿瘤是血管内皮瘤，尽管多数随着生长和内科治疗而消退，但偶尔也会因心力衰竭或体积效应的进展而需要移植治疗[16]。

其他疾病

其他疾病包括 Budd–Chiari 综合征、创伤以及继

发于肠衰竭和长期全肠外营养的胆汁性肝硬化等，将在第 46 章详述。

器官分配和移植前监护

有终末期肝脏疾病证据的患者是进行肝脏移植的合适人选。然而，小儿患者的体格较小，而且相对于等待名单中患者的数量来说存在全国性的器官短缺，使得及时移植成为一个难题。2003 年共进行了 546 例小儿肝脏移植。同一年中可提供的小儿尸体供体数量为 800。6 岁以下年龄组的问题和矛盾尤其突出，肝脏受者 354 例，而供体仅 207 例。另一个问题当然是时机：当有小儿供体提供时，未必同时就有与之大小匹配的小儿受者。因此 18 岁以上的成人可作为小儿的供体以解决小儿供体不足问题[21]（见图 45–1）。
734 上述原因造成器官的相对短缺，因此需要有一个分配系统来将有限的器官分给那些可能受益最多的患者。2002 年起，建立了基于这种“病重优先”模式的小儿终末期肝脏疾病（PELD）评分系统[12]。PELD 评分包括 5 个参数：国际标准化率、血清总胆红素、血清白蛋白水平、生长迟缓（＝低于相应年龄中位身高或体重 2 倍标准差）以及低龄（<1 岁或 1～2 岁）。状态 I 通常指发生暴发性肝功能衰竭、原发性移植后移植物无功能、早期肝动脉血栓形成和其他出现急性状况的患者。与成人不同的是，小儿 ESLD 患者尽管 PELD 评分变化很小，但如出现状态 I 所列的任何情况都需要在重症监护病房监护，因为其死亡率很高。为了尽量缓解可供移植器官的短缺，所有 18 岁及以下的供体均优先分配给小儿受者。劈裂式肝移植（见下文）的广泛应用，显著缩短了等待时间，并且对等待移植者的死亡率也有积极的影响[7,25]。

供体获取和肝胆管解剖学

肝胆管解剖学

供体肝切除或移植手术的进行均需要对解剖学有透彻的理解。此外，详尽的了解该解剖位置的结构对节段性肝移植领域是至关重要的，甚至影响到整个肝胆外科。肝脏的血供基于高度变异的肝动脉和门静脉系统。静脉回流通过右、中和左肝静脉汇入下腔静脉，后者由肝脏背侧表面穿过（肝后腔静脉）。肝脏根据其外部标志主要分为左右两叶，进一步可以细分为右前、后，左内及外段。这一命名体系仍被沿用于描述大多数肝脏结构的解剖。然而，外科解剖学的先驱 Couinaud 运用其高超的解剖技巧发现肝脏的解剖结构要复杂得多（图 45–3）。“Couinaud 命名法”基于门静脉的分支与横断面（位于肝静脉“中点”的横断层面）及各肝静脉的纵断面的关系（见图 45–3）。每个节段都有单独的门静脉和肝动脉分支供血，并且有单独的胆管分支引流胆汁。胆道系统的变异性仅次于动脉系统。肝脏的静脉回流是跨节段的。其他著作有对肝脏解剖更详尽的描述，对其的讨论已超出本章涉及范围。

供体的手术

利用尸体供给器官进行的小儿肝脏移植包括：选择功能良好和大小匹配的供体、组织有经验的器官摘取小组以及进行精细的手术操作以便辨认动脉解剖的变异使能够进行多器官的摘取。节段性肝脏移植的出现使供体年龄范围扩大到约 40 岁。器官摘取前供体的治疗重点在于用适当但不过度的容量负荷来维持血

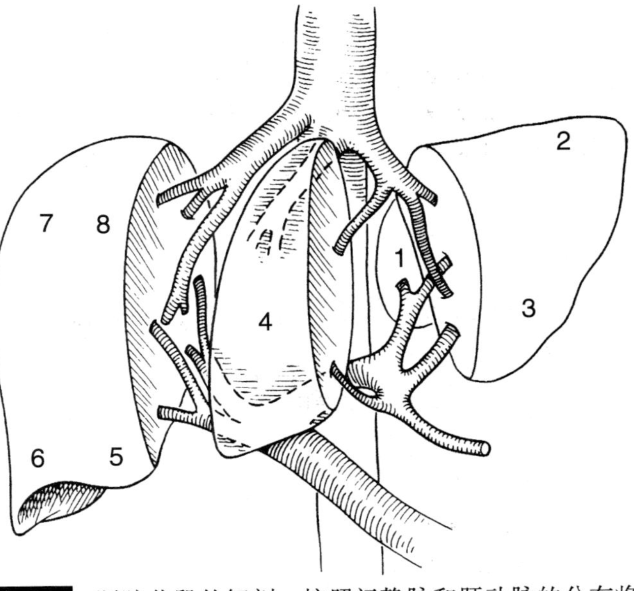

图 45–3 肝脏节段的解剖。按照门静脉和肝动脉的分布将肝脏分成具有独立血供和回流的节段。

流动力学稳定、尽可能少使用升压药、不过度使用呼气末正压通气（PEEP）而获得最佳氧合以及纠正糖尿病性尿崩而引起的高钠血症。一旦供体状况稳定达到这些目标，即可进行器官摘取手术。对于合理挑选出的不稳定供体，应该避免不必要的时间拖延，因为作为权宜之计的低温灌注和冷保存仅能帮助减少手术进行中的器官缺血。

供体手术采取腹正中及胸骨正中切开以获得良好的暴露。翻转右半结肠和小肠暴露腹腔大血管，在主动脉和肠系膜下静脉插管。然后评估肝脏功能，通过胆囊进行胆道系统灌洗。全身肝素化之后，横跨钳闭上端腹主动脉，并切开心包内下腔静脉给供体放血。通过预留的插管开始进行器官冷灌注，并且用冰
735 块浸渍腹腔使得肝脏深部温度达到 4℃。1987 年 Belzer 和 Southhard 成功研制了威斯康星大学（UW）液，从此 UW 液就成为了美国的标准保存液。在此之前器官保存超过 12～18 小时之后，原发性移植失败的机会就会增加，而 UW 液突破了这一保存时间限制。当然，合适的保存时间取决于供体和受体很多的参数，并且应该尽可能缩短，这在减体积或劈裂式肝移植中尤为重要。UW 液是一种高钾、高渗溶液，能够防止细胞肿胀，通过阻止保存过程中细胞内钾外流来维持再灌注后跨膜电位的稳定，并且含多种氧自由基清除成分。近来，一些中心采用了组氨酸-色氨酸-酮戊二酸溶液，因为其具有较低的钾含量和黏滞度[2]。但这一保存液尚未通过长期对照试验来评估，在得到这些数据前，UW 液仍然是器官保存的金标准。一旦获取供体器官，摘取小组应立即将移植肝脏送抵移植中心并行移植前准备，以便另外的受体手术小组进行移植手术。

活体、减体积和劈裂式节段性肝移植

小儿器官的短缺和等待者较高的死亡率使得人们去寻找其他器官的来源。有三种利用完整器官之外的选择：活体、减体积和劈裂式移植[6,7,24,25]。完整器官供体的缺乏使活体移植成为另外的选择得以发展，典型的活体移植利用供肝的 2、3 段（左外侧段，LLS）。健康供体的安全风险尽管较小但也存在，因此减体积移植也同时发展起来，其方法是器官冷灌注之前或之后切除供肝的 LLS，而将剩余部分丢弃。显然，这样能够使小儿受者获益，但却浪费了一个本可用于成人受者的器官。1988 年 Pichlmayr 在德国 Hanover 首先报道了将完整肝脏劈裂为右侧段和 LLS 段分别用于成人和小儿受者。劈裂术的进行可以在器官冷灌注之前（原位技术）（图 45-4），也可在冷灌注及从供体移除肝脏之后（离体技术）[24]。这一技术为小儿患者提供了合适的供体，却并不加重已存在的成人器官的短缺问题。最初的结果并不是很令人满意，但随着经验的积累，患者和移植物存活率已经接近完整器官移植和活体移植，但血管和胆道并发症略高些[8,25]。作者所在的洛杉矶加利福尼亚大学（UCLA）在不能及时得到全肝或劈裂式移植供体或在特殊的适应证时仅进行活体肝脏移植。自从该方案常规应用于节段性移植物后，移植等待时间已经大大缩短[7,25]。

肝移植的手术操作

过去 20 年中尸体完整肝脏移植的手术过程变化很少。尽管在具体技巧的应用上存在许多个人和机构间的微妙差别，移植的主要步骤还是相同的。下面描述的是 UCLA 目前常用的肝脏移植步骤，已经在 800 例以上的小儿患者中得到应用[13]。该手术大致分为四

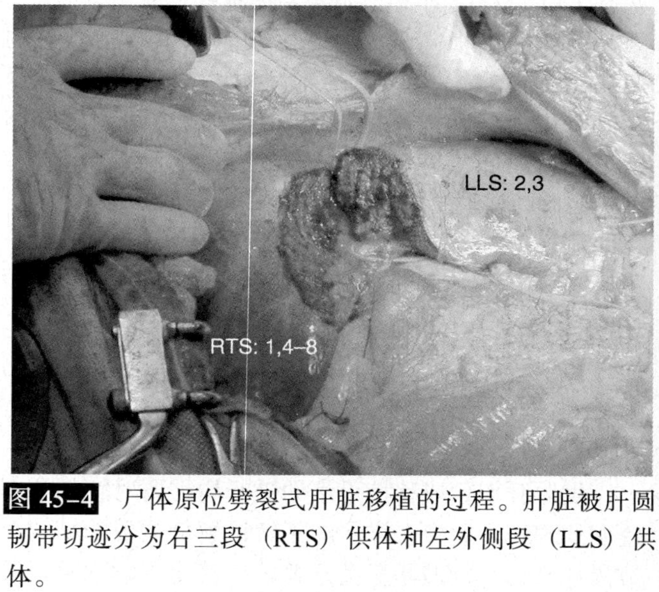

图 45-4 尸体原位劈裂式肝脏移植的过程。肝脏被肝圆韧带切迹分为右三段（RTS）供体和左外侧段（LLS）供体。

个主要阶段：肝切除期、供体植入无肝期、动脉开放再灌注以及胆道重建期，每阶段都有其解剖和生理上的难点。可能肝脏移植中最具挑战的步骤是肝切除。凝血功能紊乱、门静脉高压和肝肾功能不全导致了一个可能出血不止的手术环境。在这一阶段，麻醉师起了关键的作用，需要快速输液以维持血容量、纠正凝血和纤溶紊乱以及维持体温。这一阶段的目标是通过结扎和分离肝动脉和门静脉并且动员肝上和肝下腔静脉来排空肝脏血液以便切除。当受者各血管留下合适的长度以便后续的供体植入，这些目标就算达到了。多数小儿肝脏移植中，通过分离肝右叶和尾状叶的分支将肝脏从腔静脉切离时，均保留肝后腔静脉，并且通常仅需部分阻断腔静脉。肝切除时仔细而简便的手术技巧是至关重要的，以确保患者获得最佳效果。在无肝期，麻醉师必须提供部分肝功能支持以预防或治疗酸中毒、低体温、凝血紊乱和偶发的纤溶。此外，还必须保证合适的循环血容量并维持血流动力学的稳定。静脉-静脉体外转流很少用于
736 儿童。

受者肝切除后供肝从低温保存液转移并置入受者体内。移植物的置入按照肝上腔静脉、肝下腔静脉和门静脉的吻合依次进行。如果保留了肝后腔静脉，可采用“背驼”式，方法是将供体的肝上下腔静脉与受体肝静脉共干吻合，并结扎供体肝下下腔静脉（图 45-5）。在再灌注之前，用冷胶体和白蛋白溶液经供体门静脉灌洗肝脏，目的是降低发生再灌注相关性损伤的风险。

然后用可控的方式行再灌注。手术医生和麻醉医生之间的沟通是十分重要的，以便麻醉师有时间制定准备和预防措施。再灌注的步骤是依次去除肝上下腔静脉、肝下下腔静脉和门静脉的血管夹。当血液重新进入移植肝脏并回流至右心房时，会发生许多严重可能危及生命的并发症。此时麻醉师面临的主要问题是威胁生命的高钾血症、酸中毒、心律不齐和血流动力学不稳定，后者可能伴有外科性或凝血障碍性出血。其中一个原因就是冰冷、偏酸且高钾的血液直接回流入右心房。此时，前几个阶段手术医生和麻醉师对生理状态稳定的维持情况、受者的术前状态以及移植物的功能状况等共同决定了移植物早期功能和手术的效果。毫无疑问，这是整个肝脏移植过程中最危险的部分之一。

接下来进行肝动脉的吻合。通常动脉来源取自腹腔干的某个分支。然而在某些情况下没有合适的血管，不得不利用主动脉导管。导管一般置于上腹或肾下主动脉。有些病例，动脉管径很细（<3mm），必须在再灌注之前行动脉吻合。然后，通过胆总管对口吻合或 Roux-en-Y 胆总管空肠吻合行胆道重建，后者较常用于低龄儿童，而且仅用于部分肝脏移植的供体胆管（见图 45-5）。确认充分止血后，放置引流管并关闭腹腔。然后患者直接被转至重症监护病房。关于节段性移植，无论是劈裂式、减体积或者活体移植，虽然在吻合的操作方式上有所不同，但基本步骤是相似的（图 45-6）。

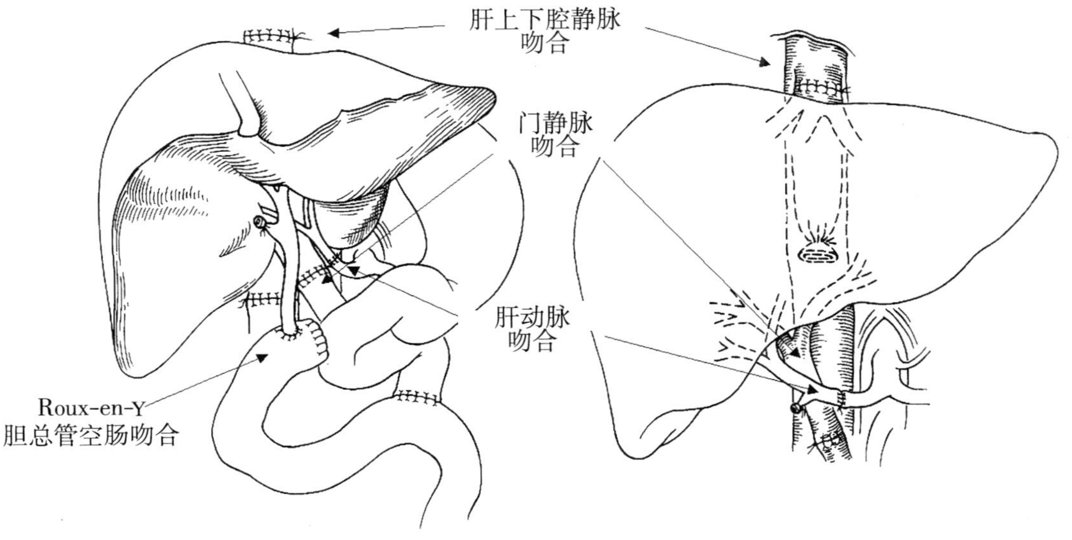

图 45-5 完整器官的植入。经典原位和“背驼”式示意图。

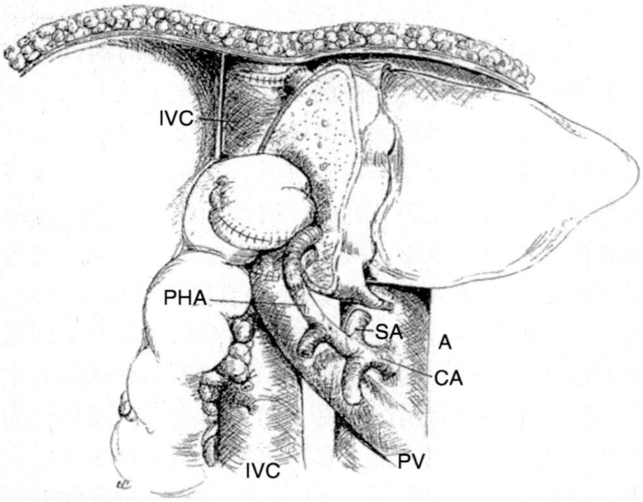

图 45-6 肝左外段的植入。IVC：下腔静脉；PHA：肝固有动脉；SA：脾动脉；CA：腹腔动脉；A：主动脉；PV：门静脉。（Reprinted with permission from Goss J, Yersiz H, Shackleton CR, et al: In situ splitting of the cadaveric liver for transplantation. Transplantation 1997;64:871-877.）

737 ## 移植后的监护

肝脏移植受体接受早期和长期的术后监护对确保最佳结果的重要性几乎等同于手术技术操作。早期术后监护的目的是评估移植物功能、为受者提供支持性治疗以及早期发现并发症。评估移植物功能有多种途径。温暖、可唤醒、血流动力学稳定、标志着移植物有肝脏分泌功能的“金黄色”胆汁（少数病例会放置胆道引流管）出现的患者，几乎可以立即做出生理和临床评估。然后移植物功能可以通过反映合成和代谢功能（例如凝血酶原时间的纠正和酸血症的纠正）的生化指标的检查得到确认。保存器官的损伤程度可以通过酶水平来检测，与移植物功能并非呈线性相关，损伤严重的移植物可能表现为功能恢复延迟或无功能。非血管因素的移植物无功能（原发性肝无功能）几乎都需要再次移植，再次移植的时间直接关系到结果。在小儿患者原发性肝无功能的发生率为 5%～10% [6,10,25]。

技术性并发症

技术性并发症可以分为血管、胆道和一般手术性并发症。在术后早期，肝脏移植后发生的感染及常见手术并发症与其他腹部手术相似。但是真菌感染发生率较高，并且在一些移植组小儿受体肠穿孔的发生率高达 19%[23]。

血管性并发症

血管性并发症主要包括肝动脉血栓、门静脉血栓及腔静脉血栓或狭窄。常规静脉给予小剂量普通肝素或联用低分子量右旋糖酐来预防血栓。超声显像和 CT 联合或者常规血管造影是可接受的诊断方法。肝动脉血栓形成是最常见的血管性并发症，因患者年龄和移植类型的不同发生率在 5%～18%不等[6,10,23,25]。早期的血管性并发症往往是因为技术本身的问题，而移植后数月才发生的血管性并发症与免疫和感染（例如巨细胞病毒成果）因素有关。移植术后一周内发生的肝动脉血栓常常伴有移植物无功能和胆道坏死或渗漏，而发生较晚的血栓并不一定会立即影响移植物功能，但会引起胆道并发症，包括肝内胆道脓肿、胆道吻合口狭窄以及伴有脓毒症的硬化性胆管炎，且都会导致病死率明显上升。如果早期获得诊断，一些患者可以采取血栓切除术和手术修正。但多数早期肝动脉血栓的患者需要紧急行再次移植。移植物仍有功能的迟发型肝动脉血栓可以利用放射介入技术来处理，并且患者可以在首次移植后稍久一点时间行再次移植。小儿肝脏移植的门静脉血栓发生率为 2%～4%，并且通常伴有移植物的功能丧失，需要立即进行再次移植挽救患者生命。迟发的门静脉血栓通常表现为反复静脉曲张破裂出血或者腹水，可以通过药物、内镜以及手术分流或再次移植治疗。小儿肝脏移植的腔静脉、肝静脉血栓或狭窄的发生率为 3%～6%，最佳的处理方法是在放射介入下行球囊扩张术[6,10,23,25]。

胆道并发症

因移植类型的不同和是否行胆总管空肠吻合，非肝动脉血栓相关性胆道并发症的发生率为 3%～20%不等。通常由于技术错误，但有时也可能与热缺血或者免疫和感染因素有关（例如巨细胞病毒感染）。通过胆道造影可进行诊断，可通过内镜、放射介入或手术治疗[6,10,23,25]。

免疫抑制治疗和排斥

现代移植的免疫抑制治疗依赖神经钙蛋白抑制剂（CNI）类药物，其原型就是环孢霉素 A（表 45-1）。环孢霉素 A，尤其是其生物利用度更高、治疗浓度更稳定的微乳剂型，减少了所有实质脏器移植的排斥发生率，从而引发了器官移植的革命。20 世纪 90 年代第二代 CNI——他克莫司首先在临床应用。其具有更强的效，使肝脏移植后早期排斥率进一步降低，也使得早期就可以停用皮质激素治疗。最初报告的机会感染发生率升高和移植后淋巴增生性障碍的问题已经被新的数据所否定。当前，大多数肝脏移植中心使用基于他克莫司的免疫抑制治疗方案，联合应用皮质激素，有时选择联用辅助药物。环孢霉素 A 和他克莫司有一些共同的急性或远期并发症，而有些并发症是它们各自所独有的。最重要的并发症就是肾毒性，表现为可逆的入球小动脉收缩，以及一些慢性改变，表现为肾小管萎缩、间质纤维化和肾小球硬化。这些慢性改变具有不同程度的可逆性，取决于其严重程度。为了减少早期 CNI
39 用量使急性肾毒性降到最低，尤其是对移植前就有肾功能不全的患者，一种嘌呤代谢拮抗剂麦考酚酸莫酯被用作辅助用药（见表 45-1）。最新的一类免疫抑制剂是哺乳动物类西罗莫司靶抑制剂，其原型就是西罗莫司。这类药物很少用于小儿肝脏移植，关于其疗效仅有早期的资料。尽管不存在肾毒性，但有其他远期并发症，例如高胆固醇血症。到目前为止尚没有免疫副作用极小的理想的抑制剂（如并发症最少的药物）。

小儿肝脏移植急性排斥反应比较常见，高发于最初的 6 个月，30%～50%的患者至少发作 1 次[6,10,25]。移植 1 年之后的急性排斥反应不太常见，发生率低于 10%。当发现天冬氨酸或丙氨酸转氨酶水平升高，或者碱性磷酸酶和 γ-谷氨酰转移酶水平升高，就应考虑诊断为急性排斥反应。急性排斥反应是一种抗原特异性、T 细胞介导的炎症反应过程，其靶点是血管内皮和胆道上皮细胞而非肝细胞。这与前两种细胞较多表达供体人类白细胞抗原有关。急性排斥反应的组织学特征是门管三联区的混合性炎症细胞浸润（多形核细胞、淋巴细胞和嗜酸性粒细胞）伴有明显的血管内皮炎和（或）胆道上皮的损伤。根据门管三联区的受侵比例、浸润和损伤程度以及是否有中心静脉内皮炎（重度急性排斥反应的征兆），排斥反应可分为轻、中、重三级。急性排斥反应的治疗以大剂量甲泼尼龙冲击治疗为主，但激素无反应者可能需要使用抗体治疗（OKT-3, ATG；见表 45-1）。无论成人或儿童，急性排斥反应一般不影响移植物的长期存活，除非出现多器官排斥或皮质激素抵抗[6,9]。在所有死亡患者或移植物无功能病例中发生急性排斥反应的不到 3%。但是对发生巨细胞病毒和 EB 病毒感染的儿童来说，急性排斥反应的治疗是一重要的危险因素。病毒感染者有发生移植后淋巴增生性障碍的危险。因此，需要在适当的免疫抑制预防急性排斥反应和过度抑制之间寻找平衡以避免毒性。目前，免疫抑制药物治疗引发的远期病变是对实质脏器移植儿童长期存活和生活质量的主要挑战。

慢性排斥反应是儿童迟发性移植物失去功能的常见原因，但复发并不常见。慢性排斥反应并不完全由异体抗原引起，可能是许多因素共同作用导致了移植物损伤的结局。其标志是肝内胆管的消失，这是活检中一个著名的组织学发现，因此又被称为“*胆管消失综合征*”。当出现进行性黄疸和血清碱性磷酸酶水平升高时，就该考虑是否发生慢性排斥反应。目前尚没有有效预防或治疗慢性排斥反应的药物，尽管根据动物实验资料发现西罗莫司能阻止移植物的纤维化[11]。当发生移植物功能失代偿时，唯一可行的治疗是再次移植。

感染性并发症

移植后感染是影响肝移植并发症发生率和移植后死亡率的最常见原因。移植后第 1 个月内细菌和真菌感染的发生率最高。发生于数月甚至数年后的真菌感染并不常见，且一般是非典型或特异菌属，例如隐球菌属、毛霉菌属、芽生菌或球孢子菌属。病毒感染是移植后早期最常见的感染。巨细胞病毒和 EB 病毒感染是主要的条件致病性病毒感染。免疫抑制剂的减量和其他选择性，以及预防性应用更昔洛韦，已降低了病毒感染的发病率和死亡率。感染性并发症还有其他的致病因素，关于它们的介

表 45-1 应用于肝脏移植的现代免疫抑制剂

名称	作用机制	主要应用	常见毒性作用
神经钙蛋白抑制剂（CNI） 环孢霉素 A 他克莫司	具体而完整的机制尚不清楚。抑制 IL-2 及其他细胞因子的转录，从而阻止 T 辅助细胞增殖。	免疫抑制的诱导和长期维持。他克莫司是唯一可以单用的制剂，而环孢霉素 A 必须和其他制剂长期联用。	共有的：肾毒性、高血压、高血糖及神经毒性（癫痫、肌阵挛和特发性震颤） 环孢霉素 A：多毛症、牙龈增生和糖尿病多见 他克莫司：腹泻、食欲减退、神经毒性和高血压多见
糖皮质激素 甲泼尼松龙 泼尼松	通过抗炎作用，尤其是抑制 IL-1 的作用，广泛作用于免疫系统	免疫抑制的诱导和维持。 有些患者不能长期应用。	高脂血症、骨质减少、高血压、糖尿病、伤口愈合不良、生长迟缓、Cushing 面容、嗅纹及痤疮
麦考酚酸莫酯	嘌呤代谢拮抗药，为补救途径的可供选择性用药，主要作用于淋巴细胞	作为一种辅助用药，以减小 CNI 和皮质类固醇的剂量	骨髓抑制、腹泻、食欲减退、恶心，呕吐及胃肠道黏膜溃疡?
哺乳动物雷帕霉素靶抑制剂 雷帕霉素 RAD	抑制被活化的细胞进入细胞分裂周期，从而抑制活化的 T 细胞和 B 细胞的克隆扩增	不明确，用于儿童患者的初步试验，可以用于 CNI 发生毒性反应、抵抗或慢性的同种异体移植物排斥时，以尽可能减少 CNI 的用量	高脂血症、伤口愈合不良、肺炎及口腔溃疡
OKT-3 单克隆抗体	$CD3^{+}$ T 细胞的克隆排除	严重的或顽固的急性同种异体移植物排斥	全身炎症反应综合征（SIRS）及输液反应、病毒感染和移植后淋巴增生障碍风险增加
抗淋巴细胞免疫球蛋白（复宁）	具体而完整的机制尚不清楚，但可以引起中央及周围性淋巴样细胞的清除	严重的或顽固的急性同种异体移植物排斥	病毒感染和移植后淋巴增生障碍的风险增加、输液反应发生较 OKT-3 低率和血小板减少症
IL-2 受体拮抗剂 巴利昔单抗 达（克）珠单抗	竞争性抑制 IL-2 受体	作为 CNI 的辅助用药来诱导免疫抑制。用于减少其他免疫抑制用量（CNI 和皮质类固醇）	病毒感染的风险增加、可能引起移植后淋巴增生障碍及偶有输液反应

表 45-2 肝脏移植后的感染性并发症

病原体	表现	诊断	对策
巨细胞病毒（CMV）	感染途径：病毒再活化、输血及受感染的移植器官 温和的病毒性感冒样症候群 侵袭性组织感染（视网膜炎、肺炎、心肌炎、小肠结肠炎、肝炎、中枢神经系统感染）	定量的 CMV-DNA PCR P-65 抗原 组织培养 血液或体液培养 免疫染色活检	预防：静脉注射更昔洛韦、口服更昔洛韦 治疗：静脉注射更昔洛韦单用或联用 CMV 免疫球蛋白
EB 病毒（EBV）	疾病谱，从传染性单核细胞增多症到淋巴细胞增多症，再到淋巴瘤，再到 EB 病毒相关性软组织肿瘤 见于有 EB 病毒和免疫抑制者，肝脏移植后婴儿的 10%～15% 胃肠道、颈部、胸腔及中枢神经系统	定量的 EBV-DNA PCR 血涂片 免疫染色活检 可疑部位的 CT 扫描	预防：静脉注射更昔洛韦，口服更昔洛韦 治疗：阿昔洛韦，免疫抑制剂减量或停药 可以运用全身化疗治疗淋巴增生性障碍或淋巴瘤
单纯疱疹病毒（HSV）	皮肤损害、胃肠道播散性疱疹、发热、乏力、肝功能异常、肝炎和肺炎	HSV-1 和 HSV-2 抗体 活检组织病毒培养	阿昔洛韦
肺囊虫	非典型性肺炎，可进展为危及生命的肺炎	支气管肺泡灌洗，肺组织活检	预防：口服小剂量甲氧苄啶或磺胺甲基异噁唑、氨苯砜或喷他脒 治疗：大剂量静脉注射甲氧苄啶 / 磺胺甲基异噁唑
念珠菌	局部黏膜、侵袭性组织感染，真菌血症	血液、体液和组织培养，眼底检查	预防：氟康唑，风险很大，患者可用两性霉素 B 脂质体 治疗：氟康唑(用于敏感的念珠菌株)或两性霉素 B 脂质体及卡泊芬净或伏立康唑(不敏感的念珠菌属或曲霉)
曲霉菌	通过上呼吸道或下呼吸侵入并播散（中枢神经系统、腹腔内及实质性脏器）	血液、体液和组织培养、支气管肺泡灌洗和 CT 扫描	
细菌	革兰阴性菌：肠杆菌科、大肠杆菌和假单胞菌 革兰阳性菌：肠球菌和葡糖球菌	血液、体液和组织培养 支气管肺泡灌洗，CT 扫描，外科探查	多种方法

绍、诊断和治疗见表 45-2。对儿童来说，预防和有效治疗 EB 病毒尤其重要。因为 EB 病毒感染与很多不良结果相关。其中最常见的就是淋巴样组织的弥漫性增生，即所谓的移植后淋巴增生障碍，可以表现为广泛淋巴结病变的单核细胞增生症样综合征，或者表现为发生于任何器官的淋巴瘤。很多其他肿瘤的发生也与 EB 病毒感染相关[9]。移植后淋巴增生障碍的一般疗法是减少或停用免疫抑制剂，偶尔也可行外科手术治疗和（或）化疗。对这类疾病的全面讨论不属于本章节的范畴，在 Holmes 和 Sokol 的报道中有详尽的阐述[9]。

预后

许多已知因素能影响儿童肝脏移植后患者及移植物的存活率[3,6,10,23,25]。总的来说生存率已得到提高，在18岁以下患儿当中，患者的1年和5年生存率分别接近90%和80%[3]。年龄、营养状况、移植的紧迫性，移植适应证和是否有肾功能不全都是决定预后的主要因素。早期的数据提示胆道闭锁的患儿预后较差，因为他们往往营养不良，年龄偏低甚至有既往手术史，但是近来的资料表明其预后与其他患儿并无显著差异[4]。代谢性疾病的患者预后很好，因为他们通常年龄较大，没有肝衰竭及其并发症，也没有既往腹部手术史。最后，肿瘤患儿移植后的生存率虽然明显低于移植患儿的平均水平，但仍比自然病程者即非移植者高得多。各种文献有大量报道，详细介绍了其预
741 后改善的经验[6,10]。

虽然预后已有所改善，但仍然存在着很多需要解决的问题。首当便是器官的缺乏。需要移植的患者数呈直线上升趋势，但合适供体的数目，即使算上节段性肝脏移植的供体数量，根本的解决方法在于扩大供体库，并且将器官分配给那些通过移植可以明显改善生存率也只能算是平稳趋势且移植后效果最佳的患者。关于有效鉴定供体是否应该劈裂和发展劈裂器官的本地、区域及全国共享的国家政策还有待进一步改进。最后，随着基因治疗的发展和替代性全肝脏移植治疗代谢性疾病的肝细胞移植的优化，可能将部分缓解目前的供体器官短缺压力。

肝脏移植面临的另一个重要挑战就是免疫抑制治疗方案的进一步完善。目前，所有免疫抑制剂均有长期的并发症，导致生长发育受抑、感染性疾病和恶性肿瘤的发生以及肾衰。研制并发症少甚至无并发症出现的药物极为必要。此外，更深刻理解外周T细胞耐受和慢性排斥反应的免疫机制也很重要。尽管在过去10年中我们在肝脏移植的技术和免疫抑制治疗方面取得了无可置疑的进步，未来十年要想提高生存率和生活质量仍要坚定依靠从细胞和分子水平来更深刻理解我们的免疫系统。对免疫耐受的探索仍有许多疑问亟待解决。

（王 浩译 李民驹校）

参考文献

1. Arcement CM, Towbin RB, Meza MP, et al: Intrahepatic chemoembolization in unresectable pediatric liver malignancies. Pediatr Radiol 2000;30:779-785.
2. Canelo R, Hakim NS, Ringe B: Experience with histidine tryptophan ketoglutarate versus University Wisconsin preservation solutions in transplantation. Int Surg 2003;88:145-151.
3. Colombani PM, Dunn SP, Harmon WE, et al: Pediatric transplantation. Am J Transplant 2003;3(Suppl 4):53-63.
4. Diem HV, Evrard V, Vinh HT, et al: Pediatric liver transplantation for biliary atresia: Results of primary grafts in 328 recipients. Transplantation 2003;75:1692-1697.
5. Farmer DG, Anselmo DM, Ghobrial RM, et al: Liver transplantation for fulminant hepatic failure: Experience with more than 200 patients over a 17-year period. Ann Surg 2003;237:666-675.
6. Goss JA, Shackleton CR, McDiarmid SV, et al: Long-term results of pediatric liver transplantation: An analysis of 569 transplants. Ann Surg 1998;228:411-420.
7. Gridelli B, Spada M, Petz W, et al: Split-liver transplantation eliminates the need for living-donor liver transplantation in children with end-stage cholestatic liver disease. Transplantation 2003;75:1197-1203.
8. Heffron TG, Pillen T, Welch D, et al: Biliary complications after pediatric liver transplantation revisited. Transplant Proc 2003;35:1461-1462.
9. Holmes RD, Sokol RJ: Epstein-Barr virus and post-transplant lymphoproliferative disease. Pediatr Transplant 2002;6:456-464.
10. Jain A, Mazariegos G, Kashyap R, et al: Pediatric liver transplantation in 808 consecutive children: 20-years experience from a single center. Transplant Proc 2002;34:1955-1957.
11. Markiewicz M, Kalicinski J, Teisseyre J, et al: Rapamycin in children after liver transplantation. Transplant Proc 2003;35:2284-2286.
12. McDiarmid SV, Anand R, Lindblad AS; Principal investigators and Institutions of the Studies of Pediatric Liver Transplantation (SPLIT) Research Group. Development of a pediatric end-stage liver disease score to predict poor outcome in children awaiting liver transplantation. Transplantation 2002;74:173-181.
13. Klintmalm GB, Busuttil RW: The recipient hepatectomy and grafting. In Busuttil RW, Klintmalm GB (eds): Transplantation of the Liver. Philadelphia, WB Saunders, 1996, pp 405-418.
14. Molmenti EP, Wilkinson K, Molmenti H, et al: Treatment of unresectable hepatoblastoma with liver transplantation in the pediatric population. Am J Transplant 2002;2:535-538.
15. O'Grady JG, Alexander GJ, Hayllar KM, et al: Early indicators of prognosis in fulminant hepatic failure. Gastroenterology 1989;97:439-445.
16. Reynolds M: Pediatric liver tumors. Semin Surg Oncol 1999;16:159-172.
17. Schnater JM, Aronson DC, Plaschkes J, et al: Surgical view of the treatment of patients with hepatoblastoma: Results from the first prospective trial of the International Society of Pediatric Oncology Liver Tumor Study Group. Cancer 2002;94:1111-1120.
18. Sieders E, Peeters PM, TenVergert EM, et al: Early vascular complications after pediatric liver transplantation. Liver Transpl 2000;6:326-332.

19. Starzl TE, Groth CG, Brettschneider L, et al: Orthotopic homotransplantation of the human liver. Ann Surg 1968;168:392-415.
20. Suita S, Tajiri T, Takamatsu H, et al: Improved survival outcome for hepatoblastoma based on an optimal chemotherapeutic regimen—a report from the study group for pediatric solid malignant tumors in the Kyushu area. J Pediatr Surg 2004;39:195-198.
21. United Network for Organ Sharing: http://www.unos.org/data/about/viewDataReports.asp
22. Wildhaber BE, Coran AG, Drongowski RA, et al: The Kasai portoenterostomy for biliary atresia: A review of a 27-year experience with 81 patients. Transplantation 2003;75:1692-1697.
23. Yamanaka J, Lynch SV, Ong TH, et al: Surgical complications and long-term outcome in pediatric liver transplantation. Hepatogastroenterology 2000;47:1371-1374.
24. Yersiz H, Renz JF, Hisatake GM, et al: The conventional technique in in-situ split-liver transplantation. J Hepatobiliary Pancreat Surg 2003;10:11-15.
25. Yersiz H, Renz JF, Farmer DG, et al: One hundred in situ split-liver transplantations: A single-center experience. Ann Surg 2003;238:496-505; discussion 506-507.

第 46 章

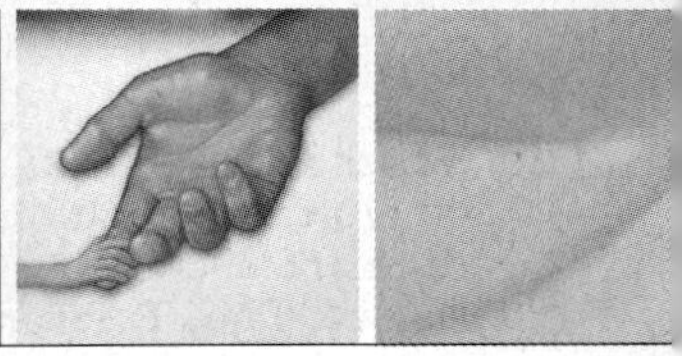

小肠移植

Douglas G. Farmer 和 Sherilyn A. Gordon

在过去的 10～15 年，小肠移植（ITx）领域已有巨大的发展。从 20 世纪 60 年代尝试小肠移植失败至今，目前部分患者的生存率接近 80%～90%。外科技术的进步无疑起到了重要的作用。然而，真正的飞跃来自新的有效的免疫抑制剂的发展。本章将回顾发展历程，讨论该领域的手术指征和技术。结果及更大的手术成功所面临的挑战也进行了回顾。

历史

20 世纪 50 年代后期，Lillehei[34]和 Starzl[46]首先开始小肠移植的实验研究，并成功建立了犬的小肠移植模型。在这些模型和人肾移植成功的推动下，有 9 例人小肠移植报道（表 46–1）[35]。这些临床病例采取了当时标准的免疫抑制疗法（类固醇、硫唑嘌呤、抗淋巴细胞球蛋白或这些药物的任意组合），由于严重和无法控制的排异或技术方面的缺陷，结果令人沮丧。显然，在临床应用之前，淋巴组织丰富的小肠移植的长期生存需要特殊的免疫抑制剂和更先进的手术技术的进步。几乎同时，Wilmore 和 Dudrick[16]研究的全肠外营养（TPN）和 Broviac[6]在 1968 年和 1972 年的长期中心静脉置管补液，为胃肠功能障碍患者提供短期或长期的液体、电解质和营养，明显改善这些患者的预后。这些临床技术的进步使小肠移植一直陷于研究阶段，发展晚了 15 年。

随着环孢霉素的开发以及在其他实质性器官移植中的成功应用[5,10]，使人们对小肠移植又重新发生了兴趣。之后出现几个重要的标志性个案报道，包括 1987 年 Starzl[49] 等人首次成功进行人体多器官移植，1987 年 Deltz[13]等人进行的单独小肠移植，以及 1988 年 Grant 等人施行的肝肠联合移植（表 46–2）[35]。然而成功仅限于个案报道，排异仍然是移植物长期存活的主要障碍。

20 世纪 90 年代随着免疫抑制剂 FK–506（他克莫司；普乐可复；非正式使用）的应用，近代移植技术飞速发展[31]。随着这些药物的应用，首次出现了一系列成功小肠移植病例报道[35]（个人报道，W. Burns，

表 46–1　人类早期小肠移植的尝试

年份	中心	移植物	存活时间	失败原因
1964	波士顿 Floating 医院	活体小肠	12 小时	小肠坏死
1964	波士顿 Floating 医院	小肠	2 天	小肠坏死
1967	明尼苏达大学	小肠、结肠	12 小时	肺栓塞
1968	圣保罗大学	小肠	12 天	排异
1969	巴黎大学	小肠、结肠	23 天	排异
1969	密西西比大学	活体小肠	32 天	排异
1969	圣保罗大学	小肠	5 天	排异
1969	艾伯特爱因斯坦医院	小肠	18 小时	患儿低血容量性休克
1970	康乃尔大学医院	活体小肠	79 天	排异

表 46-2　临床小肠移植首次使用环孢霉素免疫抑制剂的结果

年份	作者	移植物	存活时间	失败原因
1985	Cohen	小肠	12 天	排异
1987	Goulet	小肠	3 小时	血栓
1987	Goulet	小肠	211 天	排异
1987	Deltz	小肠	12 天	排异
1987	Starzl	多脏器	192 天	多器官功能衰竭
1988	Grant	肝、小肠	5 年	不明

43 2003）。如今，他克莫司已成为小肠移植的主要免疫抑制剂，并成为推动将小肠移植作为儿童和成人小肠衰竭以及危及生命的 TPN 相关并发症标准疗法的重要因素之一。

受体选择

肠衰竭儿童进行小肠移植的选择基于是否存在 TPN 相关并发症，肠道适应性和手术治疗适应性。为了进一步了解小肠移植候选人的选择，在这里需要简短描述短肠综合征、肠功能衰竭及肠道适应。通常，短肠综合征是指患者胃肠道吸收力不足导致无法满足患者日常液体、电解质及营养吸收需要。各种先天性、手术及功能性因素都可引起此病发生并需进行小肠移植（表 46-3）[25]。在 TPN 出现前，短肠综合征患者预后极差，多数因脱水、分解代谢过多及饥饿而过早死亡（图 46-1）[23]。

TPN 不仅提供了足够的水、电解质及营养来维持生命，还促进肠道进行适应。残余肠道的适应经过肥大、扩张及活力增强这一复杂的过程，使单位长度的肠段净吸收能力有效地增强。尽管有个案报道肠道完全适应需要更长时间[14]，但通常该过程于小肠切除后 24小时内开始，2～3 年后最活跃。其他章节提到的适应的关键因素包括 TPN 提供足够的热量和营养支持以及肠道内营养。TPN 肠道完全适应的预后与下列因素有关：剩余肠段长度、是否留有回盲瓣、剩余结肠长度、患者年龄、短肠综合征出现时间长短及剩余肠段的疾病[43]。适应不良或无法适应的患儿即被认为肠衰竭并需终身应用 TPN。据估计，西方国家百万活产新生儿中有 2 例肠衰竭[2]。

表 46-3　儿童小肠移植指征

指征	施行 ITX 比例（%）
腹裂畸形	21
肠扭转	18
坏死性肠炎	12
假性梗阻	9
肠闭锁	7
首次移植失败	7
先天性巨结肠	7
微绒毛病	6
短肠综合征	6
吸收不良	4
畸形	2
肿瘤	1

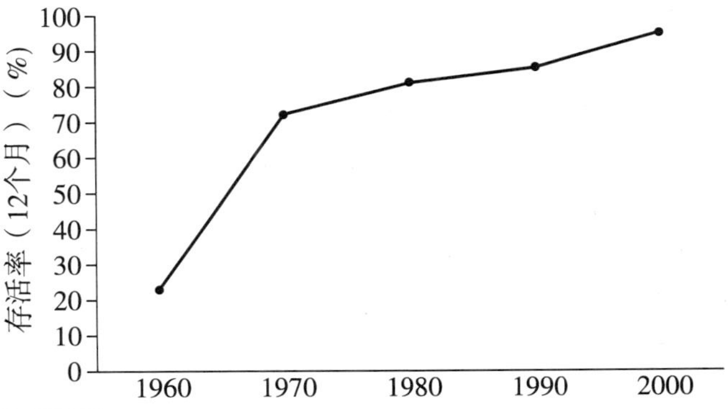

图 46-1　使用 TPN 前后的短肠综合征的存活率[11,15,50,59]

加强肠道适应能力包括使用药物如肠内谷氨酰胺、谷胱甘肽、短链脂肪酸及生长激素等。遗憾的是，这只能在特定的肠康复中心进行，且只对部分患者有效[7,43]。外科手术，如狭窄肠道成形术、人工瓣 744

膜以及抗蠕动或促蠕动的结肠间置手术，也作为增强肠道适应的方法被应用[12]。然而同药物治疗一样，这些干预措施只对部分患者有效，似乎不能广泛推广[7]。近来，横向肠成形术被提倡作为增长肠段的手术方法[56]。但不幸的是，患者数量太少且随访时间过短，因此目前无法得出结论。最终近 50%肠衰竭患儿无法形成肠道适应状态[29]。

对长期家庭 TPN 疗法维持患者的分析显示，总体效果良好，少有严重的并发症。但并非全部患者能耐受 TPN，除生活方式受限的疾病外，还会发生各种致命性并发症。最常见的危及生命的并发症包括 TPN 相关肝病、中心血管通路丧失、反复中心血管感染、水、电解质紊乱、骨质疏松、直立生长受限以及死亡[29]。事实上，许多 TPN 系列报道 5 年存活率仅 80% [59]，远低于正常同龄人群。

手术指征

简而言之，小肠移植指征是肠衰竭患者发生一种或多种 TPN 相关的致命并发症或存在高发的风险。统计上来说，该策略是成功的，因为当肠衰竭患者发生这些并发症时，其使用长期 TPN 的生存率低于小肠移植术后的患者。美国移植协会的 Kaufman 等人首次发表了儿童小肠移植的明确指征，总结如下[27]。

第一类指征范围较广，包括肠衰竭或发生 / 即将发生危及生命的 TPN 相关并发症，如肝衰竭、反复中心静脉脓毒血症和中心静脉通路丧失。继发于 TPN 的进行性肝病也许是最有必要手术的，因为如果不进行移植，死亡是不可避免的结果[29,59]。但早期肝功能障碍指征并不确定，因为尚不能预知进行性肝病的发生[30]。不过，单独小肠移植能逆转早期肝功能障碍已被报道，应考虑作为这些患者的疗法，因为肝脏供体的紧缺增加了等待肝肠移植患者的病死率。

反复的中心静脉脓毒血症也是小肠移植指征。通常该指征不包括偶尔感染的患者，而是指多重反复感染、伴转移灶如心内膜炎的感染，感染相关的多器官功能衰竭综合征及多重耐药微生物的感染。

最后，发生肠衰竭且血管通路建立受限的患者也应该考虑小肠移植。通路受限指丧失半数正常颈、锁骨下及髂静脉通路且不是极端情况，后者即肝内静脉、心房内或胸腔内通路是唯一可供选择的。

第二类考虑小肠移植的是发生早期死亡或 TPN 失败的高危人群。包括小婴儿，残留肠道过短（肠道＜10cm、无结肠、近端空肠造瘘等），胃结肠不连续（整个空回肠缺失，需要分别引流前肠和后肠分泌物），以及因先天性上皮性疾病如微绒毛包体疾病、簇状肠病、先天性绒毛萎缩而无法进行肠道适应的患者。

第三类伴有高病死率和低生活质量的功能障碍引起肠衰竭的患者应考虑小肠移植。包括不能很好地进行补充水和电解质而长期滞留在医院。肠蠕动不良如假性慢性肠梗阻，以及严重运动障碍伴剧烈疼痛的患者也包括在内。

评估 / 排队

为了达到最佳小肠移植术前管理和术后预后，肠恢复和小肠移植医疗中心的早期治疗至关重要。特别是由于所患疾病不能进行肠恢复治疗的患儿，如胃结肠不连续和微绒毛包体疾病，必须立即治疗，由移植小组严密监测，早期评估并排队等待移植。另外，因排队等待而生存率下降的高危患者也应迅速评估，包括 1 岁以内的婴儿、桥接纤维化或肝硬化、胆红素＞3mg/dL 以及血小板减少[9]。

能够肠功能恢复的患儿先由小肠移植小组进行粗略评估，之后如果要满足移植标准则需完整评估。否则首先尝试肠道康复治疗。在将患者列入小肠移植名单前，必须评估所有重要器官。表 46-4 是我们中心的评估方案。这个方案包括了许多利于手术的细节，如移植手术类型、目标血管通路、移植物流入流出血管、病变脏器的切除以及胃肠道重建部位。小肠移植的禁忌证包括严重的神经系统损伤，不能控制的全身感染，非消化系统相关的不能纠正的全身性疾病，严重的免疫缺陷以及不能切除的恶性肿瘤。

一旦符合小肠移植的条件，患儿就被列入器官分享网络系统（UNOS）根据器官类型要求和紧急程度等待移植。关于小肠移植排队等待状态有三种：状态 1（紧急）、状态 2（不紧急）以及状态 7（因

表 46–4　加利福尼亚、洛杉矶大学儿童进入小肠移植受体等待名单前的评估

实验室检查	影像学检查
分型和筛查：HLA 分型、细胞毒性抗体筛查	上 / 下消化道钡餐
血清生化：肝功能、白蛋白、前白蛋白、转铁蛋白、胆固醇	腹部 CT 或 MRI
锌、铁、铜、硒、铬、叶酸、VitB12、A、D、E	中心静脉彩超或 MRI
全血细胞计数、PT/APTT、纤维蛋白原	同位素肾小球率过滤
尿液分析	同位素胃排空检查
病毒血清学：EBV、CMV、HIV、HBV、HCV	超声心动图（化疗史、先天性缺陷、心内膜炎）

APTT：活化部分凝血激酶时间 PT：凝血酶原时间。

感染活动期暂时不能移植）。如需肝小肠移植，则根据儿童终末期肝病评分系统排队[36]。如需胰小肠移植，将启用第三个排队系统。

包括肝脏在内的同种异体移植的列入和等待策略是有根据的。小肠移植受者单独根据儿童终末期肝病评分系统排队等待移植物的进行肝小肠移植。但这一系统只针对最常见的儿童肝病，即胆道闭锁，而不包括胃肠外营养相关肝病。在该系统实行后，UNOS 年报报道了令人惊讶的高死亡率。Fryer[19]等人在 2003 年报道了因肝衰竭等待多器官移植患者的情况。根据回顾分析，这些高死亡率是由于疾病的自然进程和 TPN 相关肝病恶化引起，但其他类型的肝病与前者不同，许多用于肝脏疾病评分的指标其 PT 时间和国际标准化比率直到肝衰后期才出现异常。因此 UNOS 已经采取措施以保证患有肝病的多器官移植受体更具移植物竞争力。由于该措施最近才实施，因此判断该措施对小肠移植受者因排队等待引起的病死率的影响为时尚早。

移植物的选择

根据残留肠段的完整性和其他脏器的状态，有五种可供选择的移植方案：（1）包括全部或部分空回肠的单独肠段移植（图 46–2A）；（2）肝小肠移植（图 46–2B）；（3）包括肝、胃、胰、十二指肠或空肠的多脏器移植（图 46–2C）；（4）改良的多脏器移植（不包括肝的第 3 种选择）；（5）独立的肝移植[18]。

肠衰竭合并可逆性 / 无其他脏器疾病（诸如胃、肝及胰腺）的患者可施行单独的小肠移植。肠衰竭合并不可逆肝病（先天或后天性）患儿施行肝小肠移植。多脏器疾病患儿，如全消化道或不可逆性肝病患儿，可施行多脏器联合移植。胰胃肠动力疾病是此类移植的常见指征。另外，儿童低度恶性肿瘤，如硬纤维瘤侵及肠系膜根部，需切除肠系膜上动脉和髂动脉，这也是多脏器移植的指征。多脏器移植时，如果肝脏疾病是可逆的，这些患者可实行改良多脏器移植。最后，单独肝移植是小肠移植患者可选择的治疗措施。只有当移植患者有进行性肝病且肠道康复预后较好的情况下才进行单独肝移植。这种情况最常见于有足够残留肠段但肝病末期进展迅速的小婴儿。但该方法对于肠衰竭合并进展性肝功能障碍患者不是合适的选择。对于合适的病例，单独肝移植可纠正肝病并使受体逐渐脱离 TPN。但病例选择非常严格，因为肠衰竭患者单独肝移植术后如果无法进行肠道适应且需持续应用 TPN，其预后极差。

供体选择

除标准选取尸肝的规范如包括近期无全身性病
毒、细菌或真菌感染或恶性肿瘤，小肠移植供体选择 747
还基于长短的选择。通常小肠移植受者已进行多次腹腔手术，损失部分肠道并且发生瘢痕化，这些都可导致“空间减少”效应，即对于与患者年龄体形相似的供体器官，相应受体腹腔内容量偏小。要解决这个问题，供体大小比预期小 25%～30% 为最佳。此外，由于肠黏膜对缺血敏感，因此应严格评估供体的死亡机

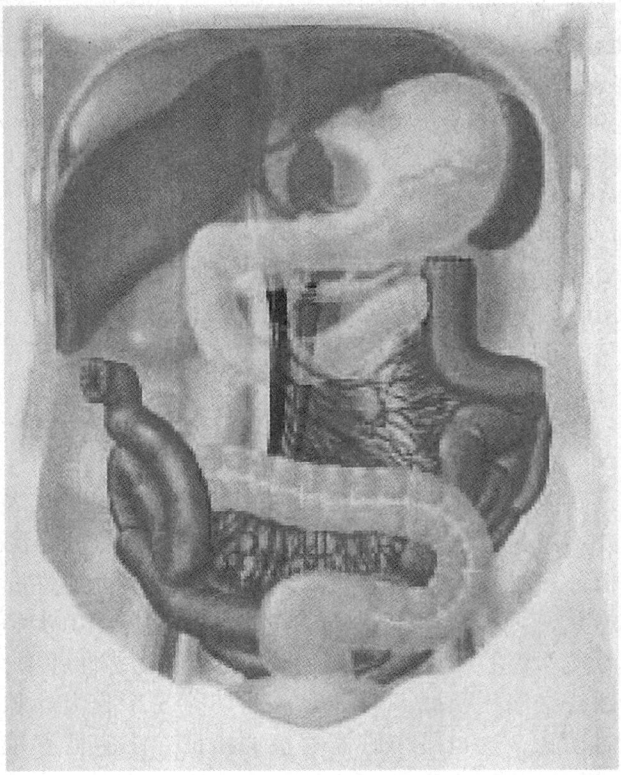

A

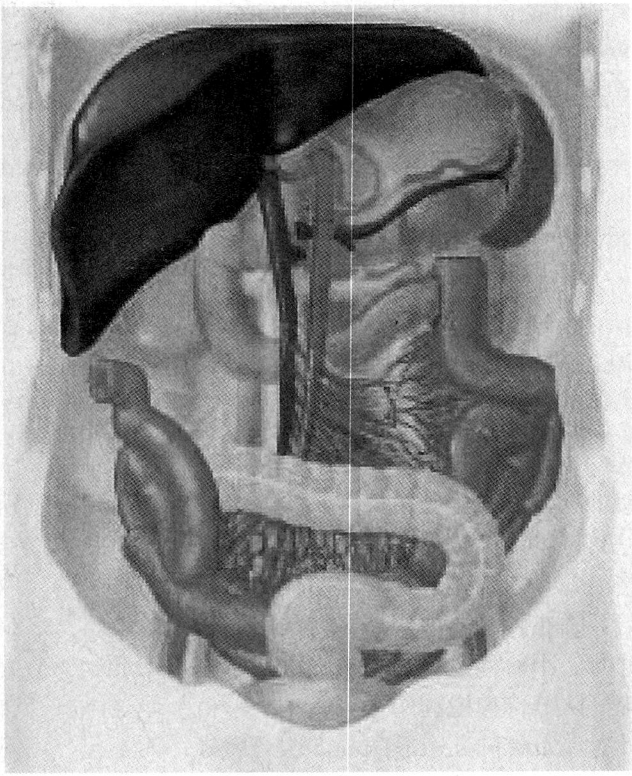

B

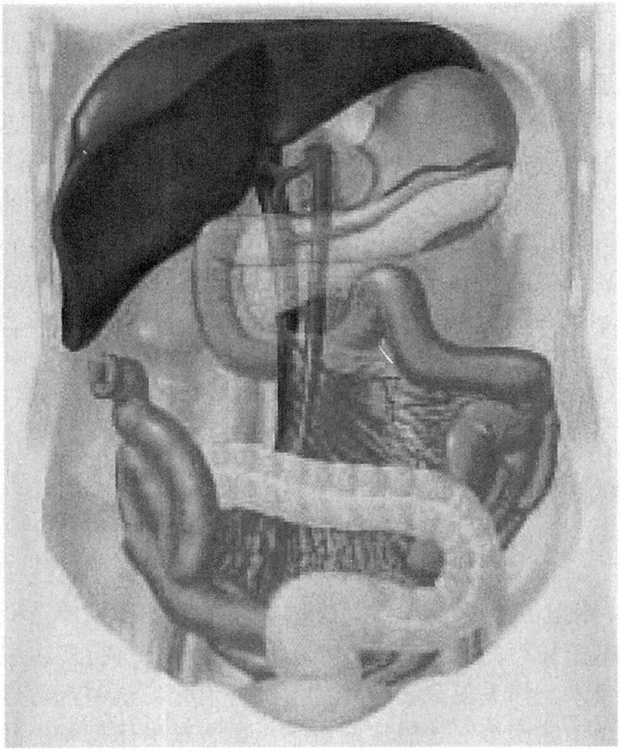

C

图 46-2 A. 单独的肠移植。B. 肝肠联合移植。C. 多脏器移植。（也见彩图）（From Fishbein TM, Gondolesi GE, Kaufman SS: Intestinal transplantation for gut failure. Gastroenterology 2003; 126:1615.）

制，包括脏器缺血时间、延长复苏时间以及应用大剂量血管加压素使血液流出肠道血管外的情况。供受体需血型相同或相配。一些专家不主张用 CMV 阳性的供体[39]；但这样会明显减少供体数量，特别是对于血清阴性的婴儿。多数中心要求进行 HLA 和细胞毒素交叉配型，但这不是供体选择中决定性的因素，因为等待配型结果导致冷缺血时间的延长对移植物功能有很大影响。此外，供体所在地理位置也和冷缺血时间有关，多数肠移植小组希望缺血时间少于 8～12 小时。

理论上由于亲属间 HLA 相似，活体肠移植具有缩短缺血时间、减少免疫并发症的优势，单独活体肠移植也开展过[41,57]。遗憾的是，虽然单中心报道肯定了活体移植的效果，但肠移植登记库记录显示迄今为止活体和尸体肠移植的生存率无明显区别（图 46-3）[25]。除非未来数据反映出活体移植的优势，否则就目前的记录和肠移植供受体之间明显的差距（2003 年美国有 5500 名尸体供体，而肠移植受体只有 120 名）将限制活体肠移植的应用。

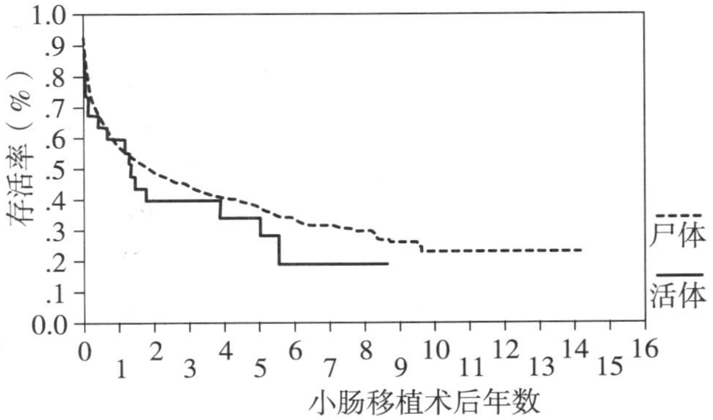

图 46-3　不同供体类型的移植物存活率。（From International Transplant Registry. Available at http://www.intestinaltransplant.org）

移植手术

供体

所有多脏器摘取技术都源自最初 Starzl 等人提出的技术[45]。Grant[22]、Starzl[47,51,52]、Bueno[9]和 Abu-Elmagd[1]等人在之后做了改进。这些技术共同之处在于不预先去除胸腔和肾区器官，只进行小的调整以获得之前提及的各种移植器官。根据过去文献[61]总结的基本原则包括应用正中切口、在髂上动脉及肾下区域取得供体主动脉血管控制，游离靶器官的同时进行供体灌注（图 46-4A 和 B）。 748

移除胸腔脏器后，将腹腔内靶器官全部切除。单独小肠移植情况下，肝、胰、肠可分别移植于不同受体[1]。取器官时，通常流入血管（从腹腔至肠系膜上动脉）以及流出血管（经肝上腔静脉）连同全部空肠一起获取。获取肝肠移植物时保留十二指肠

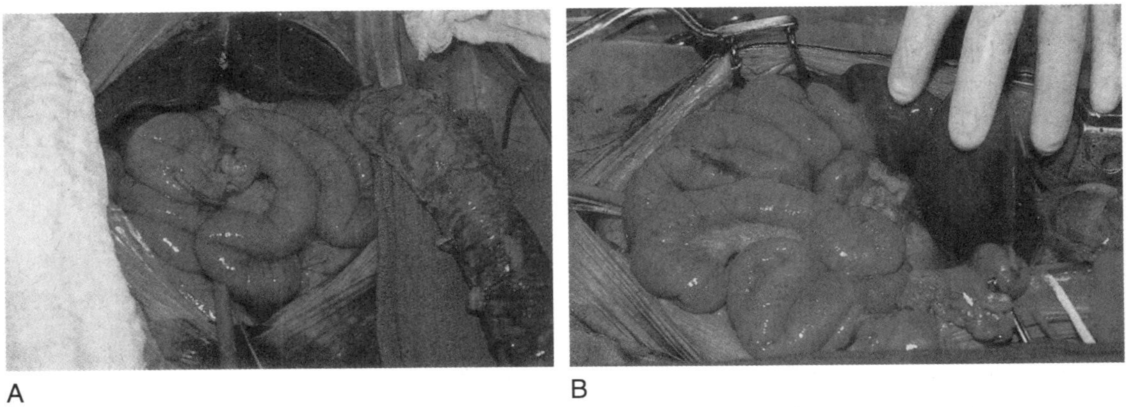

图 46-4　多脏器移植的手术入路。A. 肝圆韧带和镰状韧带已分离，肝完全游离，另外，左侧结肠移到脾曲，末端回肠已缝合（左下角），主动脉插管位置暴露。B. 插管位置在脐带周围的腹主动脉（右下）。供体进行肝素准备，然后钳夹，灌注器官（也见彩图）。(From Yersiz H, Renz J, Histaki G, et al: Multivisceral and isolated intestinal procurement techniques. Liver Transpl 2003;9:881.)

(Omaha 技术)[55]代表了一种改进，该技术可保留供体的十二指肠和胰头，因此受体不必施行胆道重建。许多中心已采用这项技术。最终，多脏器移植物与其他所有器官重新相连，血液再次从腹腔和肠系膜上动脉流入，经肝上上腔静脉流出。多脏器移植物体外准备包括准备胸主动脉导管和对缝缝合横断的胰腺以及远端腔静脉，可通过扩大解剖范围方便摘取器官以缩短准备时间。这样可减少总体冷冻缺血时间，避免不慎复温。

受体

受体手术有一定挑战性，需要进行精确的术前评估和制定手术计划。手术计划的制订非常严格，包括原靶器官移除、明确流入流出血管、器官植入及剩余脏器的胃肠道重建。通常，手术计划根据患者个体的病情和解剖结构而定。对于一般患者，特别是进行性肝病患者，多次手术史、瘢痕粘连、凝血功能障碍 / 门静脉高压很常见。

受体手术根据移植类型分五步。第一步，建立足够的补液通路，供术中及术后胃肠外营养和药物的治疗。特别值得注意的是，术前应行血管造影以避免使用已闭塞的血管。我们的标准是在移植评估期间应用磁共振静脉显像来确立静脉通路。

第二步为打开腹腔切除病变脏器。对于单独肠移植受体，采用正中切口，在结肠系膜下松解粘连并切除病变空肠是安全的。对于肝肠移植，我们更倾向于双侧肋缘下切口，首先分离肝周区域。全肝切除时保留下腔静脉，不使用静脉旁路。最后，完成多脏器移植患者整个前肠的切除，包括部分胃切除、全肝切除、全胰十二指肠切除、脾切除及残留肠段切除。

在切除脏器之后，开始植入前，需要寻找移植物流入、流出血管通道并充分游离。血管重建需要精巧的吻合技术。需要注意的是单独肠移植的流出血管倾向于选用受体门静脉系统分支或下腔静脉。肝肠移植时，要找到受体本身门静脉系统供血的前肠脏器。以我们的经验，施行受体门腔分流手术可能最容易，但也可以使用供体门静脉与受体门静脉端侧吻合。

第三步为植入（图 46–5）。单独肠移植的病例通过将供体肠系膜上动脉和受体肾下动脉吻合重建肠道血供。包括肝在内的多脏器移植时，流入动脉来源于髂上动脉。我们更倾向于施行背驮式肝移植，这样可以避免下腔静脉在肝下吻合。某些改良多脏器移植病例原则同单独的肠移植一样，但其他病例需切除更多的病变脏器如胃和十二指肠 / 胰腺。

第四步，恢复胃肠道的连续性。单独肠移植时，通常进行残留空肠近端吻合，但有时也需要与胃直接吻合。可以通过各种技术行远端回肠造口术以便移植术后监测移植物。如受体有合适的残留结肠，也可将其与供体回肠吻合。多脏器移植患者整个前肠都被切除，只保留少量近端胃和结肠。因此将移植的胃或空肠与受体残留的胃 / 食管吻合，远端吻
合同前所述。如胃存在需做幽门成形术。肝肠移 749
植患者，我们在移植灌注后才切除病变肠段。我们这样做可以避免受体在门脉高压、凝血障碍的条件下切除更多的器官。我们已对此类移植的复杂病例成功进行“分级”[44]。尤其对于凝血障碍需大量输血的移植患者，我们在这步就中止移植手术，引流远端肠管并关闭腹腔，而非进行下一步移植手术。当患者在重症监护室稳定后再行二期手术完成整个移植手术。不管使用什么方法，肝肠移植患者都需像前面描述的一样切除病变肠段，恢复肠道的完整性。

手术的最后一步为建立肠道通路。各大医疗中心使用方法各异。无论使用何种技术，建立移植肠道的

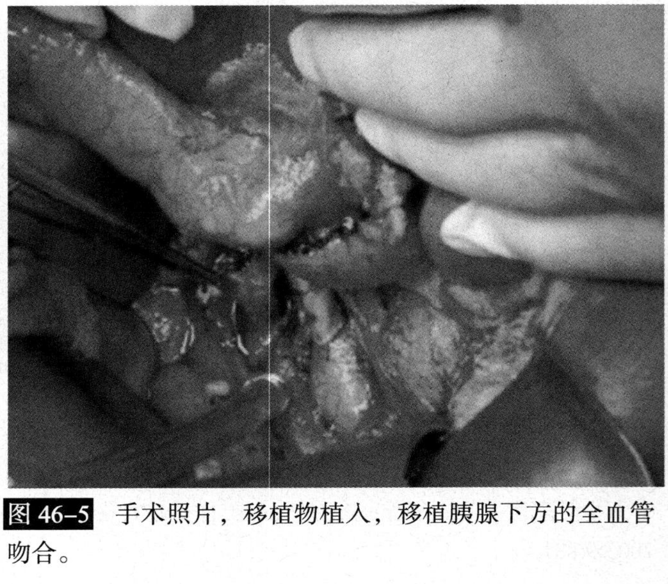

图 46–5 手术照片，移植物植入，移植胰腺下方的全血管吻合。

通路以应用营养和药物治疗对于良好预后是必须的。我们倾向于使用 2 合 1 的胃空肠造瘘管。该技术只需建立一个造瘘口（胃造瘘），用手将胃空肠造瘘管的空肠部分放入移植的空肠内。其他有报道使用单独的胃造瘘管和空肠造瘘管。

关腹时，由于腹腔容量限制和腹壁缺损，有时需行脾切除、肝切除及部分移植肠道切除。目前赞成使用供体劈离式肝移植。关腹压力过高可导致移植物坏死或血管血栓，或两者同时发生，因此需避免。如出现这种情况，可使用补片或先关闭皮肤后延期重建腹壁。迈阿密大学对肠移植后的腹壁移植进行报道，效果良好[33]。

术后处理

药物治疗

术后患儿送入儿童重症监护病房，在接下来的几天内需监测血容量、胃肠道丢失、肾功能，移植物的灌注指标，包括血清乳酸盐及其他化学成分、肝功能及动脉血气分析。由于儿童血浆容量少，所以其血浓度和凝血因子浓度变化较成人大[24]。对于肝移植患儿由于其早期肝功能波动使该反应更加强烈。我们使用前列腺素、多巴胺、右旋糖酐及小剂量肝素来增加脾灌注，避免血栓形成。另外，患儿需预先使用 TPN 直到移植肠道吸收功能恢复，其指标为能耐受逐渐增量的稀释食物并彻底经口喂养。

免疫抑制剂

由于目前的免疫抑制剂更有效、更特异性，经证实移植物和患者的存活率已提高。虽然各种治疗方案存在差异，但许多医疗中心都应用诱导剂诱导 T 细胞或其产物减少，促使达到微嵌合状态或免疫耐受。诱导剂包括抗胸腺细胞球胆白[48]、阿伦单抗（处方药，可适应证外使用）[58]、供体骨髓源性细胞[32]以及 IL-2 受体阻断药[17,53]。他克莫司加激素是主要的维持治疗药物。我们的治疗方案包括术前、术后应用达株单抗（赛尼哌，罗氏药业实验室，Nutley，NJ；可适应证外使用），肠移植的最初 24 小时肠道内维持应用他克莫司。在移植肠道吸收功能恢复后，我们也用二线、三线的免疫抑制剂，包括激素冲击后减量和麦考酚酸吗乙酯（骁悉，罗氏药业实验室；适应证外使用）。我们发现这个方案可以明显增加患者和移植肠道存活率，降低排异和感染的发生。对于他克莫司不耐受以及排异高风险的患者（或同时具备两种情况），不管对于成人或儿童，我们改用西罗莫司（Rapamune，Wyeth；适应证外使用）进行补救[21]。

小肠移植发病和死亡的首要原因是败血症。Beath 等人根据注册登记资料报道败血症为移植患者主要死因（50%）[4]。因此多数医疗中心过渡期及长期免疫抑制的目标包括停用激素和减少用量来降低他克莫司血清浓度以避免败血症发生。免疫抑制剂不但会引起感染，长期使用激素的副作用如骨质疏松、肾上腺功能不全、胃溃疡、精神疾病、白内障、生长障碍及糖耐量异常等，也会因肠移植中同时使用的其他免疫抑制剂的毒性而增强。他克莫司有神经毒性、肾毒性、糖耐量异常及高血压等；霉酚酸酯有骨髓移植、黏膜溃疡、胃肠道功能紊乱；西罗莫司有骨髓抑制、口腔炎、高脂血症。停用免疫抑制剂以避免这些并发症的发生需要担负发生排异的长期风险，这在肠移植患者中是一个显著问题。

并发症

排异

排异是继败血症引起肠移植术后死亡的第二大原因，但却是导致移植物衰竭的首要原因[4]。因为没有
特异性临床症状、体征，所以发现排异较为困难。排 750
异症状各异，包括发热、大量胃肠液丧失、腹痛及便血。少数以梗阻症状为主。另外，由于移植肝较晚发生排异，因此检测肝功能对临床判断肠排异通常不可靠。血清指标如肠脂肪酸结合蛋白[28]，瓜氨酸[20]和粒酶 B[37]可被作为排异反应的标志，但由于缺乏肠道特异性且其他肠道感染时也会发生相似改变，因此没有临床应用。

内镜和活检是肠移植急性排异早期诊断的金标准。排异时内镜表现包括水肿、充血、黏膜颗粒状、良好的黏膜血管形态丧失、蠕动减少、黏膜溃疡。排异时的组织学改变包括单核细胞浸润、隐窝损伤、细

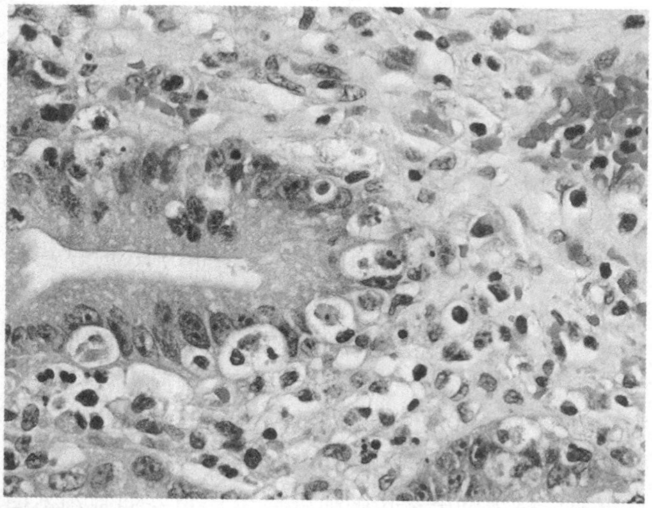

图 46-6　小肠移植物急性细胞排异反应的组织学表现，包括隐窝变形、凋亡，广泛的炎性细胞浸润（又见彩图）。

胞核增大、浓染、细胞严重减少、粘蛋白减少、隐窝凋亡、绒毛及隐窝结构变形（图 46-6）[60]。最近提倡使用聚焦电视内镜，因其能更精确地观察黏膜、诊断排异[26]。但目前还未广泛应用。

内镜随访频率应根据各中心而定。通常，多数中心在术后 1～2 周开始常规内镜随访，以后每周 1 次，直至术后 6～8 周。当临床症状和体征怀疑有排异时，不论何时应立即施行内镜检查和活检。

排异治疗基于临床和组织学的严重程度。严重排异反应可使用单克隆抗淋巴细胞抗体疗法，常暗示有很大风险发生移植物失功能。抗淋巴细胞疗法需要经验性抗病毒治疗，并有可能发生移植后淋巴细胞增生病（PTLD）。轻中程度的排异反应可通过增加免疫抑制剂或 / 和激素的冲击来治疗。对于治疗困难的患者应立即行肠切除，停用免疫抑制剂，以避免败血症和死亡发生。

感染

如前所述，感染是肠移植患者死亡的首要原因。感染 / 败血症发生率通常因免疫抑制剂用量而异。肠移植患者无疑是使用免疫抑制剂最多的人群之一，而且长时间复杂的腹部手术使患者更易感染。感染灶通常位于腹腔内和肺部。当临床出现症状、体征时，必须予以评估和治疗。

虽然移植术后可发生典型腹腔内和肺部感染且很严重，但这不是肠移植患者所特有的。该人群可发生其他特征性的感染，值得探讨。感染性肠炎作为肠移植后并发症，已被人们已不断认识[62]。该病不仅发作时类似排异反应（许多时候治疗不正确），而且可导致排异和移植失功。以我们的经验，主要病原体为病毒，主要为腺病毒和轮状病毒，但也包括其他病原体如孢子虫、兰伯贾第虫和艰难梭菌。

CMV 和 EB 病毒（EBV）也可导致肠移植术后特异性感染。事实上肠移植术后 CMV 和 EBV 感染率可高达 40% [62]——比其他任何实体器官移植后的发生率都高得多。两种病毒均可直接引起肠道感染并引发其他疾病甚至死亡。有几种疗法可用于控制术后病毒的复制。在洛杉矶加利福尼亚大学，我们使用标准化预防性治疗，包括在肠移植术后前 100 天静脉用更昔洛韦，之后改为口服阿昔洛韦。另外，我们应用预防性监测和药物治疗，包括反复应用 PCR 检测血液中 EBV、CMV 病毒 DNA 含量。如查出病毒 DNA 复制增多，则迅速应用预防性疗法，包括静脉使用更昔洛韦或（和）CMV 免疫球蛋白治疗。我们使用该疗法显著降低了肠移植术后 CMV、EBV 的病毒血症和感染率[62]。

移植后淋巴增生性疾病（PTLD）

PTLD 是一种 B 细胞恶性肿瘤，许多病例由 EBV 感染引起。肠移植登记库资料显示 PTLD 可导致 1.6%移植物失功及 6.1%小儿肠移植死亡[4]。及时诊断和治疗对改善预后是必要的。需要对患者进行全面评估，包括体格检查和完整影像学检查。怀疑有腺体病变应尽快活检和骨髓取样。治疗上包括应用更昔洛韦、CMV 免疫球蛋白和减少使用免疫抑制剂。早期针对移植物和患者抢救的资料显示人抗 CD20 单克隆抗体（利妥昔单抗）替代化疗治疗 PTLD 的效果是肯定的[38]。严重耐药或 EBV 阴性 PTLD 患者需化疗。使用前面提到的早期预防性监测可使治疗成功率上升。我们中心的患者 PTLD 的发生率低于 2%。

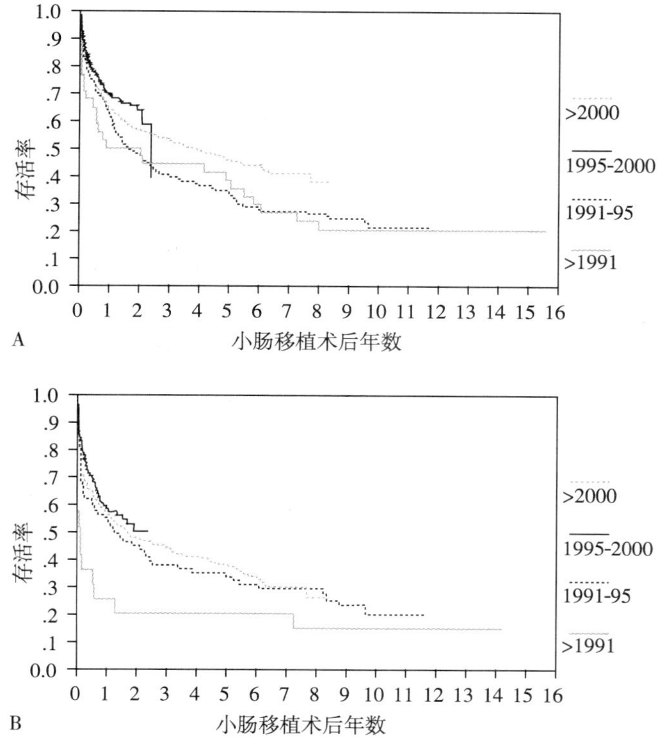

图 46-7 不同时期肠移植患者（A）和移植物（B）的存活率。(From International Transplant Registry. Available at http://www.intestinaltransplant.org. Accessed 2004.)

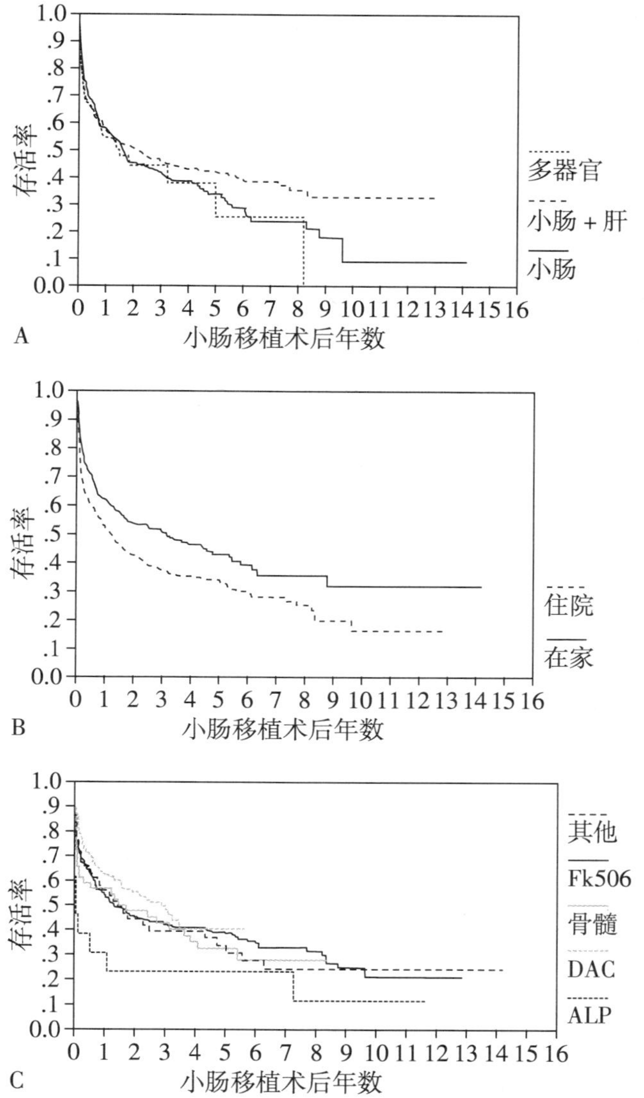

图 46-8 A. 不同移植物类型的肠移植后移植物存活率（多器官移植、肝肠移植、单独肠移植）。B. 肠移植前所处不同地点的患者移植物存活率。C. 不同免疫诱导剂的移植物生存率。ALP：抗淋巴细胞抗体；DAC：达（克）珠单抗；髓：骨髓。(From International Transplant Registry. Available at http://www.intestinaltransplant.org. Accessed 2004.)

结果

有几个资料来源可用于评估结果。有来自单中心的匹兹堡、迈阿密、内布拉斯、加利福尼亚和西奈山大学的资料。另外还有两个：一个是肠移植登记资料库，它记录了所有人类肠移植的资料，因此分析价值很高。另一个可通过 UNOS 进行美国移植受体年报搜集。预后资料将反应在这些主要的数据库上。

如前所述，肠移植预后与不同时期使用的免疫抑制剂相关。肠移植登记库显示部分患者和移植物 1 年存活率已分别超过 75% 和 65%（图 46-7A 和 B）[25]。进一步观察包括不同肠移植的类型、受体的地理方位及诱导治疗药物（图 46-8A 至 C）[25]。特别注意的是，成功的肠移植患者 90% 能够脱离 TPN[25]。

另一种预后是评估术后生活质量。Sudan 等人报道，肠移植患儿术后生活质量与同龄正常儿童 752
无显著差异[54]，因此在这点上小肠移植优于其他移植。但这些数据需要谨慎解释，因为长期在家应用 TPN 没有并发症的患者可得到相似的生活质量评价。

结论

经过试验性的 20 世纪 50 年代、60 年代、70 年代，小肠移植领域发生了巨大变化。如今，小肠移植手术已在一些专业移植中心广泛开展。患者移植成功率获得前所未有的提高。这归功于外科手术技巧的提高、免疫抑制剂的改善及经验的积累。遗憾的是，该技术仅限于一些专业移植中心开展，且仅针对肠衰竭和合并有威胁生命的 TPN 并发症的患者进行。广泛开展此项技术需减少术后死亡率、感染率、免疫抑制剂相关并发症及住院时间和费用。随着这个领域的发展，这些目标将在不久的将来得以实现。

（许 恩译 董其刚校）

参考文献

1. Abu-Elmagd K, Fung J, Bueno J, et al: Logistics and technique for procurement of intestinal, pancreatic, and hepatic grafts from the same donor. Ann Surg 2000;232:680.
2. American Gastroenterological Association Clinical Practice Committee: AGA technical review on short bowel syndrome and intestinal transplantation. Gastroenterology 2003;125:1111.
3. Asfar S, Atkinson P, Ghent C, et al: Small bowel transplantation, a life-saving option for selected patients with intestinal failure. Dig Dis Sci 1996;441:875.
4. Beath S, deVille Goyet J, Kelly D: Risk factors for death and graft loss after small bowel transplantation. Curr Opin Organ Transplant 2003;8:195.
5. Borel J, Feurer C, Magnee C, et al: Effects of the new antilymphocytic peptide cyclosporine A in animals. Immunology 1977;32:1017.
6. Broviac J, Cole J, Scribner B: A silicone rubber atrial catheter for prolonged parenteral nutrition. Surg Gynecol Obstet 1974;139:24.
7. Byrne T, Cox S, Karimbakas M, et al: Bowel rehabilitation: An alternative to long-term parenteral nutrition and intestinal transplantation for some patients with short bowel syndrome. Transplant Proc 2002;34:887.
8. Bueno J, Abu-Elmagd K, Mazariegos G, et al: Composite liver–small bowel allografts with preservation of donor duodenum and hepatic biliary system in children. J Pediatr Surg 2000;35:291.
9. Bueno J, Ohwada S, Kocoshis S, et al: Factors impacting the survival of children with intestinal failure referred for intestinal transplantation. J Pediatr Surg 1999;34:27.
10. Calne R, Rolles K, White D, et al: Cyclosporin-A in clinical organ grafting. Transplant Proc 1981;13:349.
11. Caniano D, Starr J, Ginn-Pease M, et al: Extensive short-bowel syndrome in neonates: Outcome in the 1980's. Surgery 1989;105:119.
12. Carlson G: Surgical management of intestinal failure. Proc Nutr Soc 2003;62:711.
13. Deltz E, Schroeder P, Gebhard H, et al: Successful clinical small bowel transplantation: A report of a case. Clin Transpl 1989;21:89.
14. DiBaise J, Young R, Vanderhoof J: Intestinal rehabilitation and the short bowel syndrome: Part 2. Am J Gastroenterol 2004;99:1823.
15. Dorney S, Ament M, Berquist W, et al: Improved survival in very short small bowel of infancy with use of long-term parenteral nutrition. J Pediatr 1985;107:521.
16. Dudrick S, Wilmore D, Rhoads J: Long-term total parenteral nutrition with growth, development and positive nitrogen balance. Surgery 1968;64:138.
17. Farmer D, McDiarmid S, Edelstein S, et al: Induction therapy with interleukin-2 receptor antagonist after intestinal transplantation is associated with reduced acute cellular rejection and improved renal function. Transplant Proc 2004;36:331.
18. Fishbein TM, Gondolesi GE, Kaufman SS: Intestinal transplantation for gut failure. Gastroenterology 2003;126:1615.
19. Fryer J, Pellar S, Osmond D, et al: Mortality in candidates waiting for combined liver-intestine transplants exceeds that for other candidates waiting for liver transplants. Liver Transpl 2003;9:748.
20. Gondolesi G, Fishbein T, Chehade M, et al: Serum citrulline is a potential marker for rejection of intestinal allografts. Transplant Proc 2002;34:918.
21. Gordon S, Yersiz H, McDiarmid S, et al: Rescue immunotherapy using sirolimus after small bowel transplantation. Presented at the IXth International Small Bowel Transplantation symposium, 2005.
22. Grant D, Wall W, Mineualt R, et al: Successful small bowel/liver transplantation. Lancet 1990;335:181.
23. Hancock B, Wiseman N: Lethal short-bowel syndrome. J Pediatr Surg 1990;25:1131.
24. Harper P, Luddington R, Carrell R, et al: Protein C deficiency and portal thrombosis in liver transplantation in children. Lancet 1988;2:924.
25. International Transplant Registry. Available at http: www.intestinaltransplants.org. Accessed 2004.
26. Kato T, O'Brien CB, Nishida S, et al: The first case report of the use of a zoom videoendoscope for the evaluation of small bowel graft mucosa in a human after intestinal transplantation. Gastrointest Endosc 1999;50:257.
27. Kaufman S, Atkinson J, Bianchi A, et al: Indications for pediatric intestinal transplantation: A position paper of the American Society of Transplantation. Pediatr Transplant 2001;5:80.
28. Kaufman S, Lyden E, Marks W, et al: Lack of utility of intestinal fatty acid binding protein levels in predicting intestinal allograft rejection. Transplantation 2001;71:1058.
29. Kaufman SS: Prevention of parenteral nutrition–associated liver disease in children. Pediatr Transplant 2002;6:37.
30. Kelly D: Liver complications of pediatric parenteral nutrition—epidemiology. Nutrition 1998;14:153.
31. Kino T, Hatanaka H, Miyata S, et al: FK-506, a novel immunosuppressant isolated from a *Streptomyces*. II. Immunosuppressive effect of FK-506 in vitro. J Antibiot (Tokyo) 40:1256, 1987.
32. Levi D, Tzakis A, Kato T, et al: Immune responses and their regulation by donor bone marrow cells in clinical organ transplantation. Transpl Immunol 2003;11:307.

33. Levi D, Tzakis A, Madariaga J, et al: Transplantation of the abdominal wall. Lancet 2003;361:2173.
34. Lillehei R, Goot B, Miller F: The physiologic response of the small bowel of the dog to ischemia including prolonged in vitro preservation of the bowel with successful replacement and survival. Ann Surg 1959;150:543.
35. McAllister V, Grant DR: Clinical small bowel transplantation. In Grant DR, Rim (eds): Small Bowel Transplantation. London, Edward Arnold, 1994, pp 121-132.
36. McDiarmid SV, Anand R, Lindblad AS: Principal Investigators and Institutions of the Studies of Pediatric Liver Transplantation (SPLIT) Research Group. Development of a pediatric end-stage liver disease score to predict poor outcome in children awaiting liver transplantation. Transplantation 2002;74:173.
37. McDiarmid S, Farmer D, Kuniyoshi J, et al: Perforin and granzyme B. Cytolytic proteins up-regulated during rejection of rat small intestine allografts. Transplantation 1995; 69:762.
38. McGhee W, Mazariegos G, Sindhi R, et al: Rituximab in the treatment of pediatric small bowel transplant patients with post transplant lymphoproliferative disorder unresponsive to standard treatment. Transplant Proc 2002; 34:955.
39. Manez R, Kusne S, Green M, et al: Incidence and risk factors associated with the development of cytomegalovirus disease after intestinal transplantation. Transplantation 1995;59:1010.
40. The Organ Procurement and Transplantation Network: Available at http://www.optn.org. Accessed 2004.
41. Pollard S: Intestinal transplantation: Living related. Br Med Bull 1997;53:868.
42. Potts W: Pediatric surgery. JAMA 1955;157:627.
43. Quiros-Tejeira R, Ament M, Reyen L: Long-term parenteral nutritional support and intestinal adaptation in children with short bowel syndrome: A 25-year experience. J Pediatr 2004;145:157.
44. Renz J, McDiarmid S, Edelstein S, et al: Application of combined liver-intestinal transplantation as a staged procedure. Transpant Proc 2004;36:314.
45. Starzl T, Hakala T, Shaw B, et al: A flexible procedure for multiple cadaveric organ procurement. Surg Gynecol Obstet 1984;158:228.
46. Starzl T, Kaupp H: Mass homotransplantations of abdominal organs in dogs. Surg Forum 1960;11:28.
47. Starzl T, Miller C, Bronznick B, et al: An improved technique for multiple organ harvesting. Surg Gynecol Obstet 1987;165:343.
48. Starzl T, Murase N, Abu-Elmagd K, et al: Tolerogenic immunosuppression for organ transplantation. Lancet 2003; 361:1502.
49. Starzl T, Rowe M, Todo S, et al: Transplantation of multiple abdominal viscera. JAMA 1989;261:1449.
50. Starzl T, Todo S, Fung J, et al: FK 506 for liver, kidney, and pancreas transplantation. Lancet 1989;2:1000.
51. Starzl T, Todo S, Tzakis A, et al: Abdominal organ cluster transplantation for the treatment of upper abdominal malignancies. Ann Surg 1989;210:374.
52. Starzl T, Todo S, Tzakis A, et al: The many faces of multivisceral transplantation. Surg Gynecol Obstet 1991;172:335.
53. Sudan D, Chinnakotla S, Horslen S, et al: Basiliximab decreases the incidence of acute rejection after intestinal transplantation. Transplant Proc 2002;34:940.
54. Sudan D, Horslen S, Botha J, et al: Quality of life after pediatric intestinal transplantation: The perception of pediatric recipients and their parents. Am J Transplant 2004;4:407.
55. Sudan D, Iyer K, Deroover A, et al: A new technique for combined liver-intestinal transplantation. Transplantation 2001;72:1846.
56. Tannuri U: Serial transverse tapering enteroplasty (STEP): A novel bowel lengthening procedure, and serial transverse enteroplasty for short bowel syndrome. J Pediatr Surg 2003;38:1845.
57. Tesi R, Beck R, Lambiase L, et al: Living-related small bowel transplantation: Donor evaluation and outcome. Transplant Proc 1997;29:686.
58. Tzakis A, Dato T, Nishida S, et al: Alemtuzumab (Campath 1-H) combined with tacrolimus in intestinal and multivisceral transplantation. Transplantation 2001;75:1512.
59. Vantini I, Benini L, Bonfante F, et al: Survival rate and prognostic factors in patients with intestinal failure. Dig Liver Dis 2004;36:46.
60. Wu T, Abu-Elmagd K, Bond G, et al: A schema for histologic grading of small intestine allograft acute rejection. Transplantation 2002;75:1241.
61. Yersiz H, Renz J, Hisatake G, et al: Multivisceral and isolated intestinal procurement techniques. Liver Transpl 2003;9:881.
62. Ziring D, Tran R, Edelstein S, et al: Infectious enteritis after intestinal transplantation: Incidence, timing, and outcome. Transplantation 2005;79:702.

第 47 章

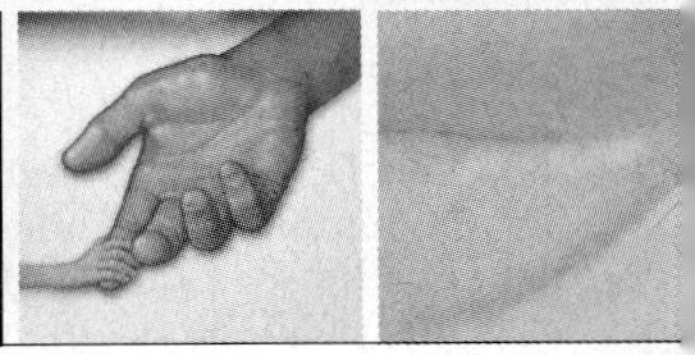

心脏移植

Thomas L. Spray 和 Stephanie M. P. Fuller

754 自 20 世纪 80 年代中期以来，已经成功地对儿科患者实施了胸部器官移植，目前这已作为一个治疗儿童先天性和终末期心肺疾病的重要手段。美国每年大约有 350 例儿科心脏移植，或大约占总数[4,15]的 10% 的患者进行了全胸部器官移植[4,15]。尽管儿童心脏和肺移植在临床上取得了成功，但是可用的供体有限，使这一治疗手段无法广泛地得到运用。急性和慢性排斥，植入心冠状动脉病变（CAD）和梗阻性细支气管炎等并发症，以及目前的免疫抑制方法引起的感染和肿瘤并发症都对移植物的寿命产生威胁。本章的重点是婴儿和儿童心脏移植包括适应证、术前评估、手术技术、术后管理、并发症和效果。

历史要点

Kantrowitz 等在 1967 年实施了首例儿科心脏移植手术，当时他们将一个无脑儿的心脏植入一个出生后 3 周的三尖瓣闭锁的婴儿体内。次年，Cooley 将一个无脑新生儿的心脏和肺移植给一个 3 个月的房室间隔缺损伴肺动脉高压的婴儿。虽然由于同种异体移植物排斥，这些婴儿没人存活超过几个小时，但这些探索性手术证明了儿童胸部器官移植的技术可行性。直到 1980 年，环孢霉素 A 作为免疫抑制剂开始使用，才使得真正意义上的临床成功成为可能。1985 年 11 月，Bailey 在 Loma Linda 大学为 1 个出生后 4 天的左心发育不良综合征（HLHS）新生儿实施了第一例成功的心脏移植手术[1]。在此后的 20 年中，随着技术的进步、免疫抑制治疗方案的完善、包括减少类固醇的使用和伴随而来的诱导分化治疗，排斥发生率的降低、对病毒感染预防治疗的注意和对移植后淋巴瘤与其他移植后并发症的有力治疗，使疗效得到了提高。

适应证

2004 年 5 月的第七次官方儿科报道中，国际心脏和肺移植协会公布的登记资料显示，最近 10 年中，儿科心脏移植的数量相对保持在稳定水平（图 47–1）[4]。儿科患者中心脏移植的最常见适应证仍是先天性心脏病和心肌病，图 47–2 到图 47–4 说明了这一点。根据年龄分布，先天性心脏病在婴儿中更多见，大多数年龄低于 2 个月；而心肌病在年长儿中的发生率更高一些。如同所预计的，随着患者年龄的增长，再次移植的发生率也升高。

婴儿期心脏移植的主要适应证仍是无法有效进行根治或者姑息手术的复杂性先天性心脏病。在这些情况中，最常见的通过心脏移植治疗的畸形是 HLHS，其特征是主动脉瓣或二尖瓣闭锁或狭窄和一个小型左心室。起初采用分期姑息方法治疗 HLHS 的效果不 755
好，使得一些中心将原位心脏移植作为这一畸形的主

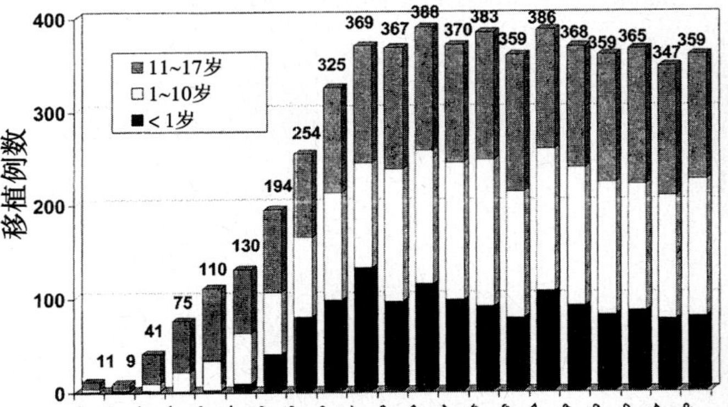

图 47–1 从 1996 年 1 月到 2003 年 6 月，各年实施的儿科心脏移植的年龄分布。(Reprinted from Journal of Heart and Lung Transplantation, August 2004, with permission from International Society of Heart and Lung Transplantation.)

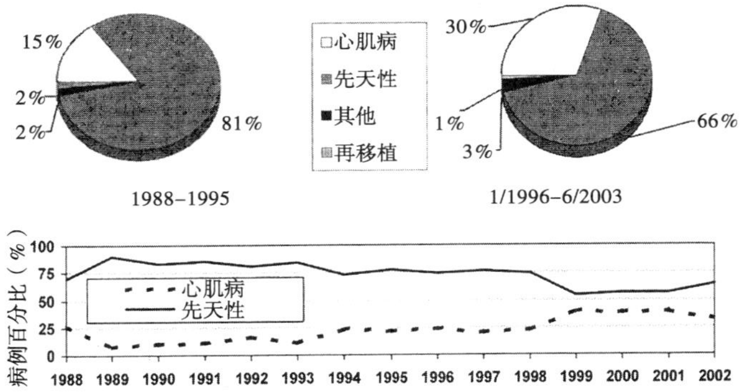

图 47–2 儿科心脏移植受体的诊断（年龄<1 岁）。
（Reprinted from Journal of Heart and Lung Transplantation, August 2004, with permission from International Society of Heart and Lung Transplantation.）

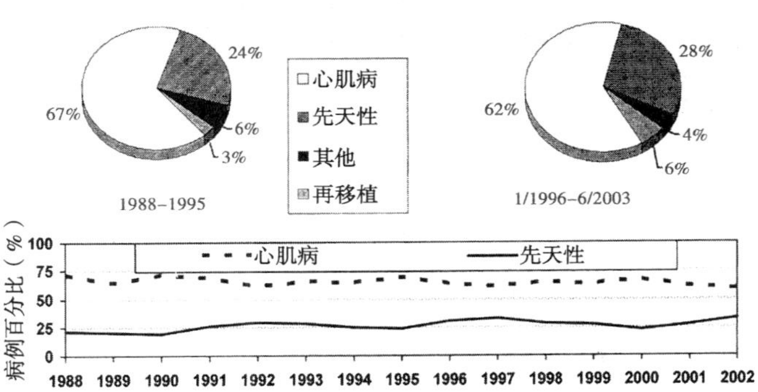

图 47–4 儿科心脏移植受体的诊断（年龄为 11～17 岁）。
(Reprinted from Journal of Heart and Lung Transplantation, August 2004, with permission from International Society of Heart and Lung Transplantation.)

要治疗方法。等待移植的患者很多，使得其他单位支持先实施 I 期姑息手术（Norwood 或 Sano 手术）来帮助患者保持病情稳定，然后再将患者列入移植等待名单中[5]。但是，随着先行 Norwood 手术，再行 Fontan 手术后的早期存活率的提高，大部分中心已经放弃了将 1 期心脏移植作为 HLHS 的首选治疗手段。将移植作为面临非同高风险的患者的治疗选择，包括主动脉闭锁合并降主动脉细小和重症三尖瓣反流[6]。

在新生儿期通过心脏移植治疗的其他先天性心脏病包括不平衡性房室通道、单心室、复杂性永存动脉干、右心室双出口、Ebstein 畸形、L 大动脉转位和室间隔完整的肺动脉闭锁[3]。甚至最复杂的先天性心脏病，如内脏异位综合征合并体循环和静脉引流异常的，都可以通过心脏移植和适当的重建手术加以治疗[14]。其他适于进行心脏移植的儿科患者包括既往已经接受了根治或者姑息手术，但仍存在由左心室衰竭引起的残余的或进行性心脏功能不全，而最终需要心脏移植的患者。在这些病例中，术后心功能不全通常与房室瓣或半月瓣关闭不全及最终引起的扩张性心肌病有关。众所周知，既往多次的姑息手术并不妨碍心脏移植[12]手术的成功。

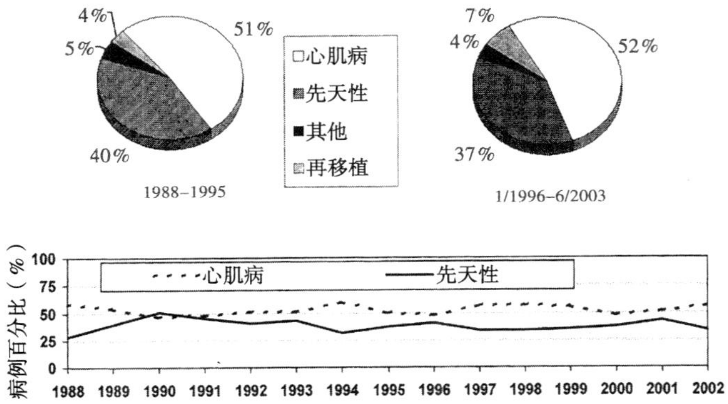

图 47–3 儿科心脏移植受体的诊断（年龄为 1～10 岁）。
(Reprinted from Journal of Heart and Lung Transplantation, August 2004, with permission from International Society of Heart and Lung Transplantation.)

心肌病是另一个婴儿期和儿童期的心脏移植最常见适应证。除婴儿期以外，实施的大部分心脏移植是为了治疗特发性心肌病。其他引起心肌病的原因包括病毒性、家族性和肥厚性。引起心肌病的原因有不同种类，一些种类的预后很差，包括左心室舒张末压非常高、左心室射血分数低于 20%、室性心律失常和有心肌病家族史[18,30]。而由炎症或心律失常引起的心肌病预后可能会好一些，在进行心脏移植之前，应该对这些患者进行尽可能长时间的支持治疗，以便有可能让他们自行康复。其他较不常见的心脏移植适应证是肿瘤化疗使用的阿霉素引起的心脏毒性，以及诸如纤维瘤和横纹肌瘤等无法手术切除的梗阻性心脏肿瘤。

术前评估

移植前的评估是一个多学科的筛选过程，这是器官移植成功的关键（表 47–1）。对可能的接受者进行彻底的生理和心理评估，包括仔细检查心脏、肺、神经、肾脏、感染和社会经济系统等方面。有正确的家庭支持系统对术后存活率是至关重要的。父母必须证

表 47–1 心脏移植候选人的评估

病史和体格检查
血型
集合抗体
全血计数及分类
生化试验及电解质
肝功能检测
脂类物质指标
水痘、CMV、EBV、单纯疱疹、麻疹、甲乙丙丁型肝炎、HIV 和弓形体病抗体的血清学检查
胸部 X 光影像
胸部计算机断层扫描
肺功能测试
通过心电图、超声心动图、MUGA——心室射血分数、心导管和运动耐受试验来进行心脏评估
儿科心脏科医师、移植协调人、感染性疾病学家、肺病学家、营养学家、心理学家、社会工作者和牙科医生进行会诊咨询

CMV：巨细胞病毒；EBV：EB 病毒；HIV：人类免疫缺陷病毒；MUGA：放射性核素活动血管成像。

明有能力和财力应对复杂的药物治疗和甚至移植后长期或频繁住院。作为这些多学科评估的一部分，患者要接受实验室筛选试验，包括病毒血清学试验（如人类免疫缺陷病毒、巨细胞病毒、人 EB 病毒和肝炎病毒）。

主要通过超声心动图和心导管来进行心脏评估，可以精确鉴别心脏和肺的体静脉和肺静脉是否存在异位连接畸形。重要的血流动力学数据，包括以患者体表面积为指数的体循环心排出量和肺血管阻力（PVR），都是通过心导管检查获得，并用来筛选候选人。这些数据非常重要，因为大部分的移植候选人都存在对肺血管扩张药物无反应的顽固性肺动脉高压。使用肺血管扩张药物对 PVR 升高（>4～6 Wood 单位）患者进行测试，包括硝普钠、氧（FiO_2 100%）和吸入性一氧化氮，以评价肺血管床是否有反应。通常，PVR 固定在 6～8 Wood 单位以上的话，就属于原位心脏移植的禁忌证了，因为供体心脏无法耐受因肺阻力高引起的右心扩张。那些血管扩张药物能改善肺阻力的患者，实施心脏移植手术后的存活率与那些肺阻力正常患者的存活率相当[12]。虽然有顽固性肺动脉高压的患者成功实施了移植手术，但死亡率很高，通常是因为术后的右心室衰竭。其他心脏移植的禁忌证包括多发性先天性心外畸形、恶性肿瘤活动期、感染、重症代谢性疾病（如糖尿病）、多器官衰竭、多发性先天性畸形和缺乏正确的家庭支持系统，除此之外还存在引起无法进行药物治疗和随访治疗的社会经济因素。

患有心肌病的儿童和慢性充血性心力衰竭症状明显而导致活动受限或心律失常无法控制的儿童，通常首选心脏移植，特别对药物治疗无效的患者。这些儿童的移植时机不是很明确，特别是有肥厚性心肌病的患者，因为有些患者在药物治疗和保守治疗之后有所改善。

如前所述，儿童特发性扩张性心肌病在诊断后 1 年内的死亡率是最高的，且主要取决于左心室衰竭的程度。

心脏移植候选儿童应给给予密切监护，直到进行心脏移植为止，如果条件允许可以在门诊就诊，也可以住院监护。应该保持良好的营养状态，如果需要可以给予管饲或者全胃肠外营养进行支持治疗。对感染并发症的密切关注也很重要，任何细微的感染症候都应给予彻底检查。严重感染时，需把患者的移植手术推迟，直到对他们进行了正确的治疗。应该优化使用地高辛、利尿药物和卡托普利或其他血管紧张素转化酶抑制剂来降低后负荷，以进行抗充血性心力衰竭的治疗。如果心力衰竭程度恶化，可能需要住院应用多巴酚丁胺或诸如米力农之类的磷酸二酯酶抑制剂等变力性药物的支持治疗。长期治疗可能需要放置静脉内通路装置，诸如 Broviac 导管。体外膜式氧合（ECMO）作为危重儿童等待心脏移植的过渡措施，大多数仅限于那些心脏切开术后心室衰竭的患者。虽然一些研究显示，当把 ECMO 作为心脏移植过渡措施时存活率为 45%～73%，但总的来说，效果很差[13,16]。虽然年长儿和青少年使用长时间心室支持装置作为移植过渡措施的效果很好，但是由于尺寸的限制，无法在婴儿人群中应用。

对要进行心脏移植的新生儿，还需要考虑其他一些因素。患有诸如 HLHS 之类复杂性先天性心脏病的婴儿，大部分处于新生儿重症监护病房内，并且如果处于动脉导管依赖性生理状态时，通常给予连续输注前列腺素 E1 维持治疗，以防止动脉导管闭合。在动脉导管内置入可扩张性支架，可能可以替代前列腺素的治疗。如果开放的卵圆孔是限制性的，那么采用球囊房间隔切开术加用或不加用支架来增加氧合血和脱氧合血的混合，以减压左心房，可能是有帮助的。其他重要措施是对这些脆弱的婴儿维持合理的营养支持，避免肾脏和代谢性并发症，并迅速和彻底治疗任何感染并发症，特别是各种输液管路引起的败血症。常见的新生儿并发症也可出现于在这些患者，诸如癫痫发作、坏死性小肠结肠炎和脑室内出血。最少有 10%～20%的婴儿在等待供体心脏的过程中死去。
757 如有所述，在长期等待供体时，可以实施 Norwood 手术作为初期姑息手术治疗；对于那些动脉导管依赖性肺血流的病变采用 Blalock–Taussig 分流作为初期姑息手术治疗。

器官共享联合网络决定器官的分配，且在 2002 年修订了等待心脏移植的儿科患者的分类。1A 级是指需要通气或者机械循环支持（如左心室支持装置、ECMO 或者球囊泵）、需要多种或高剂量变力性药物支持，年龄小于 6 个月，合并肺动脉压高于体循环压 50%以上的婴儿患者，或任何不进行心脏移植预期寿命低于 14 天的患者。1B 级指需要单次剂量变力性药物支持的患者，或者年龄低于 6 个月的，显著生长不良的婴儿（体重或身高低于第 5 百分位数，或低于预期生长值 1.5 个标准差）。所有那些迫切度稍低的患者都划入 2 级分类。一个患者的分类可能会根据其临床状况的变化而变化，或患者可能因为感染、恶性肿瘤或其他并发症而处于暂停状态（7 级状态），其状态以后可再次激活。

供体评估和器官获取

理想的器官供体的标准如下：达到了脑死亡的标准、最近血亲的同意、年长儿童的 ABO 相容性、体重相容性（受体体重的 1～3 倍）、正常的超声心动图、年龄低于 35 岁和在获取心脏时目视检查表现正常。对于儿科受者来说，心肺复苏不是一个心脏供体的绝对禁忌证。对所有可能供体都要仔细评估其死亡原因，包括是否存在胸部创伤、是否需要心肺复苏和死前的心脏功能。对于新生儿，大多数供体都是死于婴儿猝死综合征或出生窒息，而年长的供体可能是由于暴力或者车祸的死亡者。

由于适合的供体短缺，尤其是对于新生儿受者，致使人们进行了诸多努力来扩展供体范围。超声心动图证实的中度心室功能受损（左心室缩短分数高于 25%及无重大室壁运动异常）的供体心脏也可成功地置入婴儿受者中[14]。在婴儿中运用的供体–受者的体重比率最高为 4∶1。Tamisier 及其同事证实了 PVR 越高，成功移植所需的供体心脏就越大，且对于 PVR 高于正常的心脏也是可以用的[78]。虽然理想供体的缺血时间为 2～4 小时，但是缺血时间已经成功地被延长到 9 小时。“理想”供体标准的偏移应该是个体化的，甚至使用来自依靠 ECMO 维持生命的濒死婴儿的边缘化供体心脏也可能证明是合理的，而使用那些病情稳定的门诊儿童患者的心脏就不一定合理。

ABO 不相容移植也被作为一种减少受者等待时间和降低等待移植者死亡率的方法[29]。因为新生儿没有对 T 细胞抗原产生抗体的能力，包括主要的血型抗原。ABO 不相容性就成为一个可以忽略不计的并发症。美国不常用 ABO 不相容移植，什么年龄就不能实施不相容移植，现在仍未明确定义。

良好的供体管理是器官移植成功的重要部分。主要目的是维持正常温度、维持等量体液，适当的组织灌注和防止感染。通常，初始评估心功能差的供体应该对容量负荷和低剂量的变力性药物支持有反应，并在心脏获取后有功能显著改善，这是多器官获取手术的一部分。所有供体都要进行可能引起免疫抑制宿主发生严重感染因素的筛查，诸如 CMV、EBV、HIV、肝炎和弓形虫。CMV、EBV 和弓形虫抗体阴性并非移植的禁忌证，但有助于指导移植后的治疗。

获取供体心脏的四个主要目的是：（1）与其他小组一起有效工作以确保每一相关器官的良好状态；（2）评估患者的血流动力学状态和目视检查心脏的大体功能；（3）使用有效的心脏停搏和排空措施，最大限度地保护心脏；（4）熟练地移出心脏及与相邻的血管连接部分，以确保植入时所需的解剖特征。通过正中胸骨切口获取心脏。留取供体血液，用于病毒滴度试验和回顾性 HLA 配型。最初的剥离是将主动脉与肺动脉分开，以便阻断。认真地目视检查心脏，患者全身肝素化。当主动脉阻断时，就开始分离心脏。通过主动脉根部灌注停搏液，通过右心耳或右侧上腔静脉和上肺静脉或左侧的左心耳排空心脏。将上腔静脉从其心包附着部位游离，一直向上到无名静脉高度，结扎奇静脉并断开。右上肺静脉和下腔静脉周围的心包反折处进行锐性断开。心脏切除术首先从下

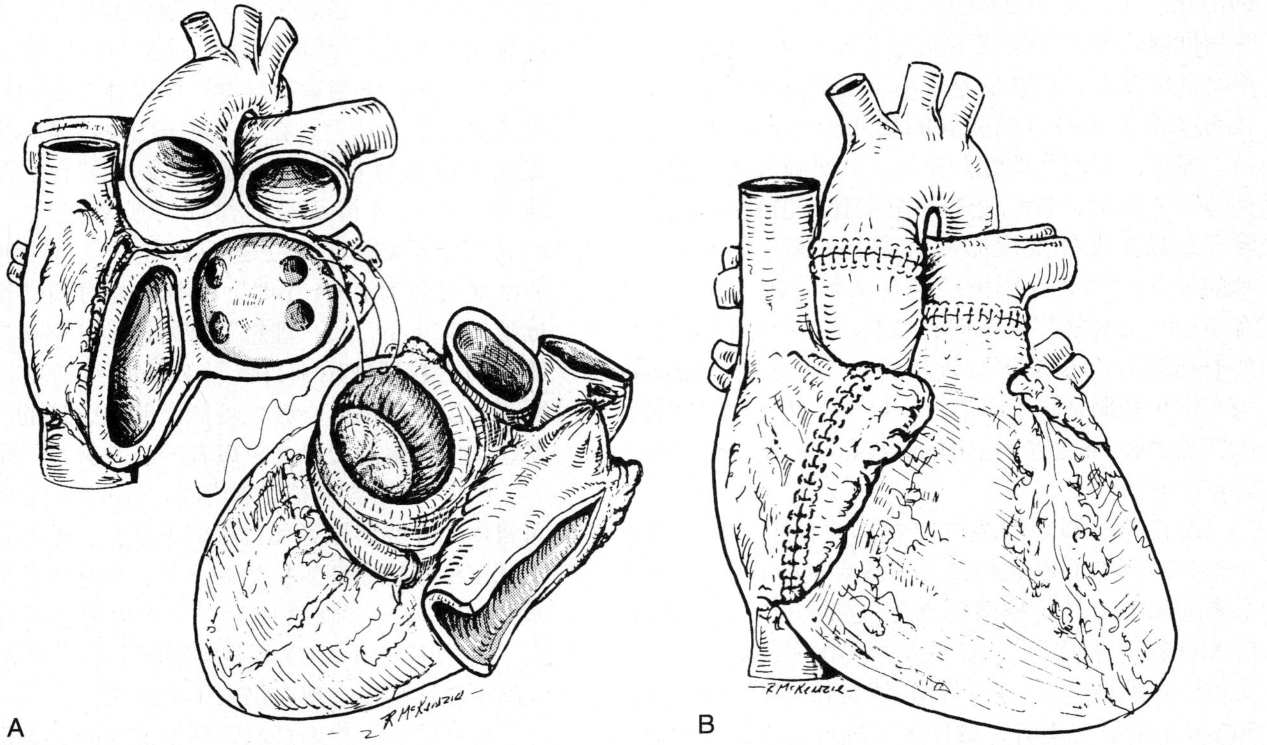

图 47–5　使用双心房吻合的标准心脏移植。A. 受体心室完整切除，开始左心房吻合。B. 所有吻合口完成后的最后外观。

腔静脉横断开始，接着在心包反折处横断右和左肺静脉。断开肺总动脉，再断开后方的心包附着和上腔静脉。最后，在无名动脉高度横断主动脉，如果受者需要更长的主动脉，则在更远端横断。供体心脏浸没在冷（4℃）的无菌盐水中，然后用三层无菌袋包装进行运送。通常，冷缺血时间应该限制在 4～5 小时以内。

受体准备和植入技术

Lower 和 Shumway 在 1960 年首次描述了原位心
758 脏移植的标准术式和双侧心房吻合，因此要避免单独的腔静脉和肺静脉连接（图 47–5）[19]。但是，目前大部分心脏移植中心采用的是双腔静脉吻合技术，因为这保持了心房的形态和运动，且在既往先天性心脏病手术后进行再次重建时，操作相对简单。一旦建立起合理的血流动力学监测和对受体进行合理的麻醉之后，行正中胸骨切口，将心脏悬吊于一个心包支架上。如果以前做过胸骨切口，应采取适当的预防措施，包括暴露腹股沟的无菌手术野，以便进行股动静脉转流。一旦进胸，将肺总动脉从其汇合部远端的主动脉上游离下来，松解主动脉弓部的心包反折。正常情况下，使用主动脉和上下腔静脉插管。

HLHS 的受体病例中，向近端游离其主动脉弓部血管，并圈套器控制住，胸部降主动脉移植游离到动脉导管连接处水平以下 2～3 cm。松解游离左右肺动脉，并用圈套器控制，做好心肺转流的准备。肝素化以后，肺总动脉插管作为动脉血流入口，单根静脉插管放置在右心房，因为可能需要使用停循环技术。一旦开始心肺转流，即刻将肺动脉紧紧地圈套控制住，这样可以通过未闭的动脉导管进行身体灌注。受者降温到 18℃，准备停循环。

一旦供体器官在手术室内准备好，且患者也已经正确降温，并停循环后，主动脉弓血管勒紧，患者的血液被放入静脉储血器。在主动脉瓣上方断开主动脉，并延主动脉弓的小弧纵行切开到动脉导管连接到降主动脉处以上的 1～2 cm 处。靠肺动脉处结扎动脉导管并切断，然后肺总动脉在其分叉处下方横断。从心耳根部做从上方开始的右心房切口，这一切口一直延伸到冠状窦，并跨过房间隔进入左心房。右心房上面切口也随后跨过房间隔，打开左心房根部。在左肺静脉上方切开左心房侧壁，左心耳保留在切下的心脏上。

供体器官置于后台的冷生理盐水中备用。右心房从下腔静脉侧面切开到心耳的基底部；如果做心房吻合而不是腔静脉吻合时，要避免切到窦房结区域。在左心房背侧切下肺静脉汇合点，保留开口与受体左心房残口比较尺寸大小。在分叉下方横断肺动脉，以提供一个宽阔的吻合口。主动脉的修剪取决于受者需要的长度。必须仔细检查并关闭卵圆孔，时常存在未闭的卵圆孔，特别是婴儿心脏。如果未能关闭卵圆孔的话，在面临肺动脉高压时，可能会导致显著的术后右向左分流。

植入时先从左心耳下缘开始进行左心房侧壁的吻
759 合。经右上肺静脉放置左心室引流，通过重建心房内分隔来完成左心房吻合。然后重建主动脉弓。从下腔静脉开口开始进行右心房吻合，然后沿心房内分隔向上吻合。一旦完成右心房吻合，移去供体心脏的上腔静脉结扎线，经腔静脉残端放置静脉插管。然后在升主动脉上做新的荷包缝线，进行插管，排出气体，重新恢复心肺转流。移去头部血管的圈套器，开始升温。然后再以端端吻合的方式完成肺动脉吻合。如果时间允许，这一步骤可以在停循环期间的无血手术野内完成。在适当升温后，患者脱离心肺转流，移去插管（图 47-6）[19]。心肺转流停止前，在右心房，左心房放置测压管，测压管从皮肤切口下方穿出，有时也放置肺动脉测压管。

760 对于心肌病的年长儿或没有主动脉弓畸形的婴儿，受者手术与成人的步骤相同。升主动脉一直游离松解到心包反折，用来进行主动脉插管。儿童降温到 28℃～34℃，因为是在主动脉阻断下进行植入手术，而不是停循环。在完成左心房吻合后，可以直接吻合完成右心房连接；如果以往接受过腔肺连接手术者，则可使用双腔静脉技术完成连接。这可能可以降低特定患者的三尖瓣反流发生率。然后采用端端吻合的方式，在升主动脉中部的高度，完成升主动脉吻合口。肺动脉吻合口可以在主动脉阻断期间完成，也可以不在主动脉阻断期间完成，这取决于植入手术时间的长短。

其他很多有所变化的植入手术方法也能加以使用，这取决于受者的解剖特征。针对左上腔静脉残存，以往接受过腔肺分流或 Fontan 手术，大动脉错位的纠正，完全性内脏反位手术的改良都已经阐明。

术后管理

受者从手术室返回到重症监护病房的一个隔离房间内。起初需要机械通气，但要尽快脱离机械通气。持续给予抗生素，直到拔除所有测压管和胸腔引流管。

事实上，所有心脏移植受者都需要一定程度的变力性药物支持。异丙肾上腺素由于有肺动脉血管扩张效应，及其变力性和变时性效应，通常是一个理想的选择，因为很多患者起初的心率都比理想心率慢。这一短暂的窦房结功能不全罕有变为永久性的。多巴酚丁胺和多巴胺也常用于提高心室收缩功能，特别是以“肾脏剂量”使用时。肾上腺素和去甲肾上腺素通常仅在移植心功能较差时使用。输注硝普钠或磷酸二酯酶抑制剂可用于术后早期降低后负荷。诸如米力农之类的磷酸二酯酶抑制剂可能对肺动脉高压引起的右心室功能不全有效。吸入一氧化氮是一种有效的选择性肺血管扩张药物，其对体循环系统的作用小，并对肺动脉高压的心脏移植受者有用。

移植免疫抑制

免疫药物联合疗法是用于预防和治疗排斥。由泼尼松、环孢霉素 A 和硫唑嘌呤组成的标准三联药物免疫抑制治疗治疗已成功地用于儿科心脏移植受者患者，并成为最常用的药物疗法[11]。表 47-2 列出了费城儿童医院用于免疫移植治疗的药物起始剂量和维持剂量。由于皮质类固醇存在并发症，因此通常在移植术后 6 个月尝试泼尼松撤药。高达 80%的受者患者可成功地停服类固醇，这些患者中仅有 1/4 在移植后头 6 个月内发生排斥[10]。显示他克莫司[27]（以前叫做 FK-506）是一种有效的儿童免疫抑制药物。近 5 年来，使用较多，在所有儿科心脏移植患者中，约 40%在移植后 1 年，将其作为代替环孢霉素 A 的免疫抑制维持药物[4]。总的来说，使用他克莫司的患者排斥的发生率并发症较低。硫唑嘌呤治疗存在并发症，如 761

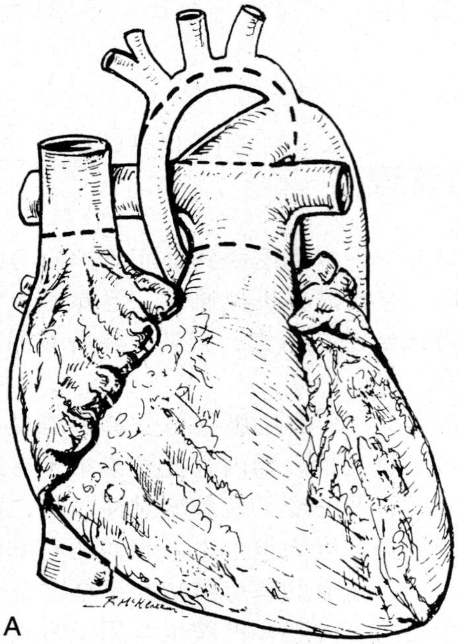
A

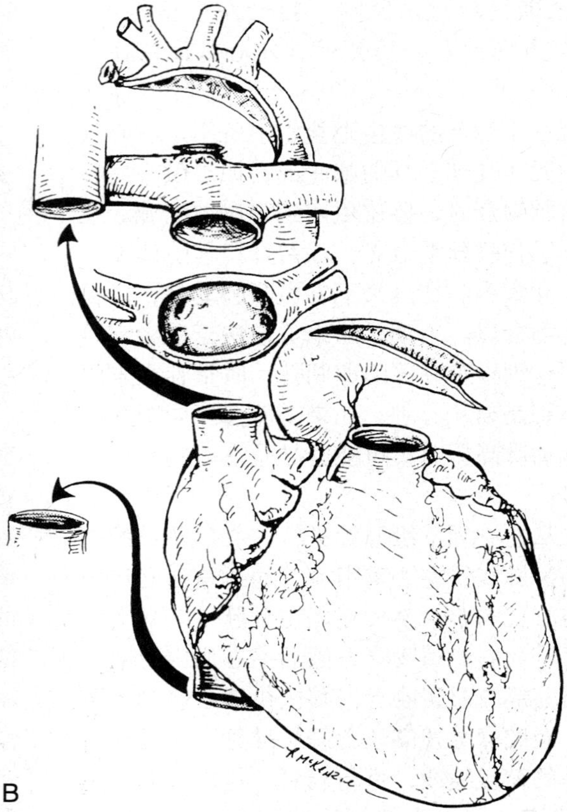
B

图 47-6 左心发育不良综合征的移植技术（使用双腔静脉吻合技术）。A. 心脏切除前的受体解剖特征。B. 心脏切除后的受体解剖特征。注意主动脉切口必须延伸入降主动脉，到动脉导管水平上方。C. 所有吻合口完成后的最后外观。

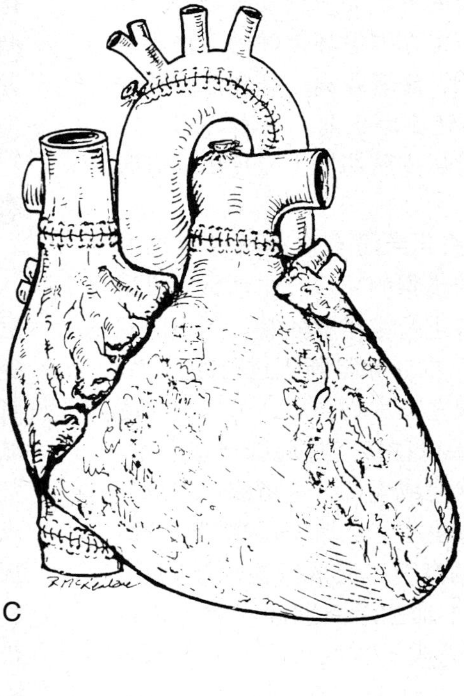
C

表 47-2　费城儿童医院心脏移植的免疫抑制疗法

药物	剂量
硫唑嘌呤 / 麦考酚酸吗乙酯（MMF）	移植前，手术室内静脉使用 2 mg/kg
	此后静脉使用 2 mg/kg，每日 1 次，新生儿使用 5 天，婴儿使用 7 天，青少年使用 9 天
	在完成硫唑嘌呤疗程后，改用 MMF，静脉使用每天 120 mg/kg，每日 2 次（靶浓度，2.5～3.0）
	胃肠道功能恢复后，改用口服 MMF
环孢霉素 A	移植前，在手术室内开始静脉使用，0.02 mg/kg/h
	此后静脉使用每小时 0.02 mg/kg，维持 24 小时（靶浓度，100）术后 3 天改用 ATG，静脉使用 1.5 mg/kg，每日 1 次，新生儿使用 3 天，婴儿使用 5 天，青少年使用 7 天
	ATG 疗程完成后，改回口服环孢霉素 A，新生儿出院时维持量靶浓度约为 125，年长儿为 150～175
	在之后的 2 个月内，应仔细调整剂量，新生儿达到浓度为 125～150，婴儿为 175～200，6～12 岁儿童为 250，青少年为 250～300
甲泼尼龙	移植前，手术室内静脉使用 10～15 mg/kg
	此后静脉使用 3 mg/kg，每日 2 次，共使用 3 个疗程

ATG：免抗胸腺细胞球蛋白；IV：静脉内用。

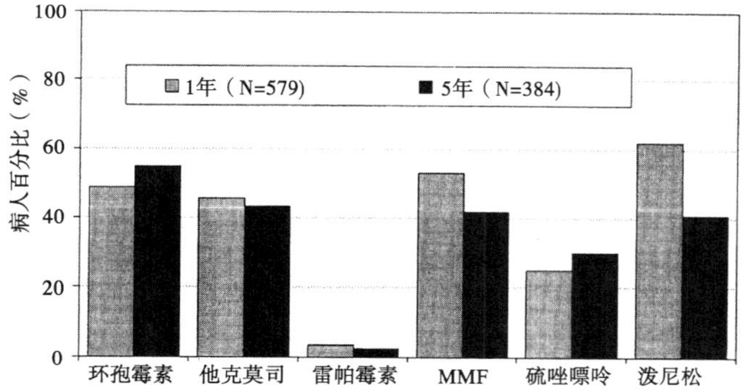

图 47-7 儿科心脏移植受者患者：从 2000 年 1 月到 2003 年 6 月之间随访时的维持免疫抑制在术后 1 年和 5 年对不同患者进行分析。MMF：麦考酚酸吗乙酯。(Reprinted from Journal of Heart and Lung Transplantation, August 2004, with permission from International Society of Heart and Lung Transplantation.)

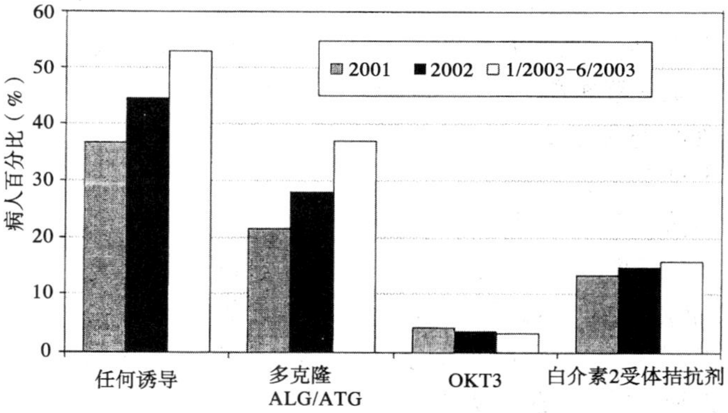

图 47-8 儿科心脏移植受者患者：诱导免疫抑制（从 2001 年 1 月随访到 2003 年 6 月）。ALG：抗淋巴细胞抗体；ATG：抗胸腺细胞抗体；IL-2R：白介素-2 受体。(Reprinted from Journal of Heart and Lung Transplantation, August 2004, with permission from International Society of Heart and Lung Transplantation.)

骨髓抑制，因此促进使用麦考酚酯来取而代之。其并发症可耐受，且在大型临床试验中显示出有益于生存率和治疗排斥反应的优势（图 47-7）[17]。更多中心推荐对儿科心脏移植受者患者使用诱导免疫抑制，目前接近 40%的患者在移植后即刻接受多克隆抗 T 细胞制剂，OKT3（一种鼠单克隆 CD3 抗体），或白介素 2 受体抗体（图 47-8）。然而，无论使用何种诱导药物，在抗排斥治疗患者中的平均排斥反应发生次数无显著差异[4]。

预防感染包括口服制霉菌素预防真菌和每周 3 次口服复方新诺明。如果出现骨髓抑制，吸入性戊氧苯咪治疗是一种有效的复方新诺明的替代疗法，用来治疗卡氏肺囊虫。在我们单位，心脏移植受者患者并不常规进行巨细胞病毒的预防治疗。

早期并发症

急性排斥和感染是心脏移植术后最常见的早期并发症。约 60%～75%的患者至少发生过一次排斥，应该可以预期约 1/3 的人将在移植后头 3 个月内发生排斥，而 50%的人将在 1 年内发生排斥[7]。一些研究提示婴儿的排斥可能比年长儿稍晚一点。排斥的监测基于临床评估，包括超声心动图和心内膜心肌活检。临床评估包括观察患者活动和胃口的变化。出现心房或心室异位节律，包括心动过速时，要怀疑排斥并进行评估。超声心动图对新生儿特别有用，因为新生儿的体形小，对新生儿进行活检存在技术困难且风险高。移植后第 1 个月内要每周做 1 次超声心动图评估，移植后 1 年内要每月做 1 次超声心动图评估。显示超声心动图引导的经颈静脉心内膜心肌活检是一种监测儿科心脏移植受者患者排斥的有效手段，并依然是发现排斥的金标准[9]。更积极的方法包括在移植后头 1 个月内，每周常规做心内膜心肌活检，第 2 个月内每两周 1 次，然后在这 1 年剩余的时间中，每月做 1 次，费城儿童医院采用这一方法来进行排斥监测。随后的活检是每年 2 次，或者当临床怀疑排斥时进行活检。大部分活检都是在门诊完成的。表 47-3 显示了心脏移植排斥的国际分级系统。

通常静脉内使用 3 天一个疗程的甲泼尼龙（10 mg/kg）来治疗急性排斥事件。对类固醇疗效不显著或反复发生排斥的患者，给予 OKT3 和抗胸腺细胞抗体。在治疗后 1～2 周通过随访性活检来证实疗效。

762 虽然在心脏移植受者患者中，感染性并发症常见，但是并没有出现过感染引起的死亡。细菌性感染后最多见于移植后早期，但是也可以在移植后晚期发生，通常对合理的抗生素治疗有效。在病毒感染中，巨细胞病毒可能是最常见的，可通过静脉内使用羟甲基阿昔洛韦来治疗。呼吸道病毒性感染的发生率通常与正常儿童相似，且可以被受者患者良好地耐受。

表 47-3 国际心脏和肺移植协会的急性排斥分级

0级	无细胞排斥证据
1A 级	局部血管周围或间质浸润，无肌细胞损伤
1B 级	多发性或弥漫性稀疏浸润，无肌细胞损伤
2 级	单发性或致密浸润，有肌细胞损伤
3A 级	多发性致密浸润，有肌细胞损伤
3B 级	弥漫性，致密浸润，有肌细胞损伤
4 级	弥漫性和广泛性多形性浸润，有肌细胞损伤——可能有出血、水肿和微血管侵犯

From Rodriguez ER: The pathology of heart transplant biopsy specimens: Revisiting the 1990 ISHLT working formulation. J Heart Lung Transplant 2003;22:3.

除排斥和感染之外，心脏移植术后即刻发生的术后并发症有高血压、癫痫、肾功能障碍和糖尿病。约 10%的心脏移植受者婴儿需要围术期的腹膜透析。在新生儿中，10%～15%需要使用苯巴比妥来治疗术后癫痫，这可能是由于对这些患者使用了停循环技术造成的[2]。

晚期并发症

儿科心脏移植受者患者的主要晚期并发症是慢性排斥、淋巴组织增生性疾病（PTLD）和慢性移植物功能减退（CAD）。心脏移植术后的死亡中，高达 40%的是由排斥引起的[4]。目前通常采用降低免疫抑制剂、阿昔洛韦和化疗来治疗淋巴组织增生性疾病。

出现移植物功能减退的发生率为 10%～15%，受者患者出现充血性心力衰竭症状可能提示该并发症。心脏移植受者患者随访就诊时，常规进行超声心动图检查，且心室功能恶化是移植物功能减退的一个标志。移植后新出现的心律失常，特别是室性心律失常，可能也是一个存在移植物功能减退的提示[23]。此外，常规的随访性心导管或冠状动脉内超声检查也可能发现移植物的功能减退，且可以没有既往的发病史。很多原因都与移植物功能减退有关，包括慢性细胞排斥、高脂血症、血管排斥和巨细胞病毒感染。与成人心脏移植受者患者不同，儿科患者相对在移植后早期发生移植物功能减退，一个系列研究证实，移植后 2 年的发生率为 35% [8]。一个针对 815 例儿科移植患者的研究，通过血管造影或活检结果，发现约 8%的显著移植物功能减退[22]。移植后的平均诊断时间是 2.2 年，其中有 1 个患者在移植后 2 月就出现了显著的移植物功能减退。仅有 20%的移植物功能减退患者得以诊断并继续存活，大多数的死亡都是突发或意料之外的。对这些患者，再次移植可能是唯一的存活之道，虽然总的来说结果并不令人满意，1 年和 3 年生存率分别为 71%和 47%，且 20%的再移植患者会发生二次移植物功能减退[20]。但是，Loma Linda 大学的小组报道了对那些初次移植年龄小于 6 个月的婴儿进行再次移植的良好经验[14]。在这组患者中，再次移植后观察到的 10 年实际存活率为 91%，可能与该中心早期采用非类固醇免疫抑制疗法有关。此外，针对胆固醇的药物治疗和降低脂质的治疗目前仍在研究之中[25]。

结果

文献中所报道的最大例数的婴儿心脏移植受者患者组来自 Loma Linda 大学，有 233 例年龄低于 6 个月的婴儿进行了心脏移植手术[14]。约 65% 的是 HLHS，其余的是复杂性先天畸形（29%）或心肌病或肿瘤（8%）。手术存活率（30 天）为 89%，造成死亡的主要原因是移植物衰竭、技术问题、肺炎或急性排斥。总体的 1 年存活率为 84%，5 年和 10 年的实际存活率分别为 73%和 68%。此外，接受移植时年龄低于 30 天的患者，其预后显著地比年长婴儿好，其 5 年和 10 年的实际存活率为 80%和 77%，可能与年幼组患者的免疫耐受性改善有关。

斯坦福大学[24]报道了一组自 1977 年以来的 72 例年龄低于 18 岁的心脏移植患者。仅有 25%的人年龄小于 1 岁（平均年龄 9 岁），约 2/3 的患者为与先天性心脏病无关的心肌病。手术存活率为 87.5%，主要由于肺动脉高压或右心室衰竭和急性排斥死亡。有 20 例晚期死亡，其中 24%是由于排斥，17%是移植物功能减退。1，5 和 10 年的实际存活率分别为 75%，60%和 50%。

在圣路易斯儿童医院，1983—1993 年，对 45 例患者进行了心脏移植，约 50%的婴儿是 HLHS[26]。婴儿组的存活率（92%）和 Loma Linda 大学的研究相同，而儿科组（年龄低于 1 岁）的早期存活率为 80%。

来自国际心脏和肺移植协会登记资料的结果显示，婴儿的围术期死亡率比年长儿的高（图 47-9）[4]。尽管早期死亡率非常高，但是 13.3 岁的半寿期比儿童或青少年存活者要长的多。对于 1～10 岁的儿童年龄组，其半寿期为 17.5 岁；而青少年组的半寿期是 13.7 岁，因此证实了年龄越小的患者其生存率的优势越明显。根据 15 年的平均值，婴儿受体患者每年的死亡率风险约 2%，而对年长儿童来说是约 4%，再次提示了年幼的心脏移植受体患者的长期生存率更具优势。最可预见的儿科人群的 1 年死亡率的风险因素仍是先天性心脏病、再次移植、供体年龄、肺动脉收缩压高于 35 mmHg 和在等待移植时需要机械通气和住院治疗。5 年死亡率的最显著的风险因素是透析、先天性心脏病和女性。死亡原因包括移植物功能减退、急性排斥、淋巴瘤、移植物衰竭和感染。移植后存活者的并发症包括高血压（45%），肾功能障碍（5.4%），高脂血症（9.9%）和糖尿病（3.2%）[4]。

除存活率以外，可以证实移植给儿童的心脏可以随着时间推移而正常生长，且左心室肌肉质量也增加，以保持正常的左心室质量-容量比率。年长儿童的运动试验显示最高心率和氧耗量始终为心脏移植受者患者预期值的 2/3。婴儿在心脏移植后的躯体生长发育也接近正常，通常神经系统发育也得以保持，虽然在长期随访过程中，高达 20%的新生儿受者患者可能存在一些神经病学畸形[4]。

结论

尽管外科技术、免疫抑制、围术期管理和排斥监测都得到了进一步的发展，但是儿科心脏移植患者的长期效果变化很小，15 年生存率约为 50%（见图 47-9）。心脏移植作为复杂性先天性心脏病的主要治疗手段，而慢性排斥、移植物慢性功能减退和类固醇使用对生长的长期影响，都会对移植的疗效产生持续的影响。但是，对于多数终末期心肌病和无法采用手术根治的结构性心脏病的儿童来说，心脏移植是唯一选择。未

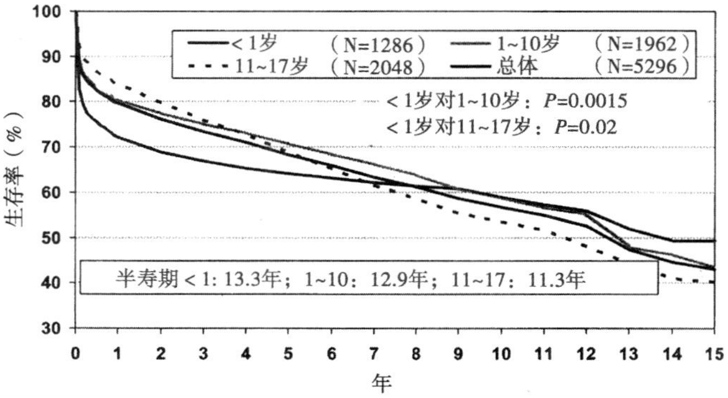

图 47-9　儿科心脏移植：Kaplan-Meier 生存率（1982 年 1 月到 2002 年 6 月）。(Reprinted from Journal of Heart and Lung Transplantation, August 2004, with permission from International Society of Heart and Lung Transplantation.)

来的探索领域包括异种移植、ABO 非匹配移植、永久性机械支持和采用更小型化和更易于接受的辅助装置来拓宽心脏移植的过渡手段。

(孙彦隽译 刘锦纷校)

参考文献

1. Bailey LL: Role of cardiac replacement in the neonate. J Heart Lung Transplant 1985;4:506.
2. Bailey LL, Gundry SR, Razzouk AJ, et al: Bless the babies: One hundred fifteen late survivors of heart transplantation during the first year of life. J Thorac Cardiovasc Surg 1993;105:805.
3. Boucek MM, Bernstein D: Heart transplantation in infancy. Prog Pediatr Cardiol 1993;2(4):20.
4. Boucek MM, Edwards LB, Keck BM, et al: The Registry of the International Society for Heart and Lung Transplantation: Seventh Official Pediatric Report—2004. J Heart Lung Transplant 2004;23:933.
5. Bove EL: Transplantation after first-stage reconstruction for hypoplastic left heart syndrome. Ann Thorac Surg 1991; 52:701.
6. Bove EL: Surgical treatment for hypoplastic left heart syndrome. Jpn J Thorac Cardiovasc Surg 1999;47(2):47.
7. Braunlin EA, Canter CE, Olivari MT, et al: Rejection and infection after pediatric cardiac transplantation. Ann Thorac Surg 1990;49:385.
8. Braunlin EA, Hunter DW, Canter CE, et al: Coronary artery disease in pediatric cardiac transplant recipients receiving triple-drug immunosuppression. Circulation 1991;84(Suppl):III303.
9. Canter CE, Appleton RS, Soffitz JE, et al: Surveillance for rejection by echocardiographically guided endomyocardial biopsy in the infant heart transplant recipient. Circulation 1991;84(Suppl III)III-310.
10. Canter CE, Moorehead S, Soffitz JE, et al: Steroid withdrawal in the pediatric heart transplant recipient initially treated with triple immunosuppression. J Heart Lung Transplant 1994;13:74.
11. Canter CE, Soffitz JE, Moorehead S, et al: Early results after pediatric cardiac transplantation with triple immunosuppression therapy. Am J Cardiol 1993;71:971.
12. Cooper MM, Fuzesi L, Addonizio LI, et al: Pediatric heart transplantation after operations involving the pulmonary arteries. J Thorac Cardiovascular Surg 1991;102:386.
13. del Nido PJ, Armitage JM, Fricker FJ, et al: Extracorporeal membrane oxygenation support as a bridge to pediatric heart transplantation. Circulation 1994;90(5 Pt 2, Suppl):II66.
14. Fortuna KS, Chinnock RE, Bailey LL, et al: Heart transplantation among 233 infants during the first six months of life: The Loma Linda experience. Loma Linda Pediatric Heart Transplant Group. Clin Transpl 1999;263.
15. Hosenpud JD, Bennen LE, Keck BM, et al: The Registry of the International Society for Heart and Lung Transplantation: Eighteenth Official Report—2001. J Heart Lung Transplant 2001;20:805.
16. Kirshborn PM, Bridges ND, Myung RJ, et al: Use of extracorporeal membrane oxygenation in pediatric thoracic organ transplantation. J Thorac Cardiovasc Surg 2002;123:130.
17. Kobashigawa JA: Mycophenolate mofetil in cardiac transplantation. Curr Opin Cardiol 1998;13:117.
18. Lewis AB: Prognostic value of echocardiography in children with idiopathic dilated cardiomyopathy. Am Heart J 1994;128:133.
19. Lower RR, Shumway NE: Studies on orthotopic homotransplantations of the canine heart. Surg Forum 1960;11:18.
20. Michler RE, Edward NM, Hsu D, et al: Pediatric retransplantation. J Heart Lung Transplant 1993;12:5319.
21. Nixon PA, Fricker FJ, Noyes BE, et al: Exercise testing in pediatric heart, heart-lung and lung recipients. Chest 1995; 107:1328.
22. Pahl E, Zalos VR, Ficker FI, et al: Posttransplant coronary artery disease in children: A multicenter national survey. Circulation 1994;9(5 Pt 2, Suppl):II56.
23. Park JK, Hus DT, Hordof AI, et al: Arrhythmias in pediatric heart transplant recipients: Prevalence and association with death, coronary artery disease, and rejection. J Heart Lung Transplant 1993;12:596.
24. Sarris CE, Smith JA, Bernstin D, et al: Pediatric cardiac transplantation: The Stanford experience. Circulation 1994;90(5 Pt 2, Suppl):II51.
25. Seipelt IM, Crawford SE, Rodgers S, et al: Hypercholesterolemia is common after pediatric heart transplantation: Initial experience with pravastatin. J Heart Lung Transplant 2004;23:317.
26. Spray TL: Transplantation of the heart and lungs in children. Annu Rev Med 1994;45:139.
27. Swenson JM, Fricker FJ, Armitage JM: Immunosuppression switch in pediatric heart transplant recipients: Cyclosporine to FK506. J Am Coll Cardiol 1995;25:1183.
28. Tamisier D, Vouhe P, Le Bidois J, et al: Donor-recipient size matching in pediatric heart transplantation; a word of caution about small grafts. J Heart Lung Transplant 1996; 15:190.
29. West LJ, Pollock-Barziv SM, Dipchand AI, et al: ABO-incompatible heart transplantation in infants. N Engl J Med 2001;344:793.
30. Wiles HB: Prognostic features of children with idiopathic dilated cardiomyopathy. Am J Cardiol 1991;68:1372.
31. Zales VR, Wright KL, Pahl E, et al: Normal left ventricular muscle mass and mass/volume ratio after pediatric cardiac transplantation. Circulation 1994;90(5 Pt 2, Suppl):II61.

第 48 章

肺移植

Charles B. Huddleston 和 Joel Cooper

765 1963 年报道世界上首例肺移植手术由密西西比医疗中心的 James Hardy 完成[27]。该患者于术后 18 天在医院内死亡。此后几年有多位医生尝试过几次，但是都以失败告终，其中大多数失败是由于气管吻合口的愈合不良。在 Hardy 医生失败后 20 年，由加拿大多伦多 Joel Cooper 带领的医疗小组首次成功完成了肺移植。该患者因肺纤维化进行了单侧肺移植，术后存活了 6 年，最后因肾衰竭而死亡[8]。数年后，特别是在 20 世纪 90 年代后期，逐渐开展了儿童肺移植手术，并成为儿童终末期肺实质性疾病和肺血管疾病的一种可行的治疗手段。即使如此，自 1989 年以来在全世界范围内实施的儿童肺移植手术仍然数量有限，仅占全部肺移植手术的 4% [67]。本章仅介绍独立的儿童移植术，而不包括心肺联合移植。

指征

单独的肺移植在儿童中主要适用于危及生命并且进行性发展的肺实质或肺血管疾病。通常而言，该手术的目的是为了延长生命而不仅仅是改善生活质量。目前肺移植手术后 5 年存活率约为 50%。因此，患者的选择和手术的时机显得非常重要。需要准确的预计出如果患儿不接受治疗，是否会在 2 年以内死亡，显然这是非常困难的事情。儿童需要进行肺移植手术的主要适应证有肺囊性纤维化、肺间质疾病伴纤维化、原发性肺高压、先天性心脏病继发肺高压、肺再移植以及其他一些疾病（表 48–1）。而在成人中最常见的肺移植指征慢性肺阻塞性疾病在儿童中却非常罕见[67]。

肺囊性纤维化

肺囊性纤维化是 18 岁以下需要进行肺移植的最常见疾病，它是北美最为常见的危及生命的遗传性疾病。虽然该疾病患者的平均生存时间已经延长到 29 岁，但是仍有 1/3 的患者在儿童期死亡。毫无疑问，导致死亡的最常见原因是呼吸问题。大约每年有 100 例该疾病患者在美国接受肺移植手术[13]。虽然该数字增长缓慢，但是供体的缺乏依然是主要的制约因素。

就像其他疾病一样，对于慢性疾病选择合适的移植时机是非常重要的。Kerem 在 20 世纪 90 年代早期证实如果 FEV_1 低于正常的 30%，PaO_2 低于 55mmHg 和（或）$PaCO_2$ 超过 50mmHg，那么该患者生存时间超过 2 年的机会不超过 50% [39]。这些指标对儿童患者尤其是女童的影响更大。不过，对于罹患肺囊性纤维化患者自然病程的最新研究表明，对于严重肺功能受损的患者仅仅测量 FEV_1 对于预测自然病程是不够的。FEV_1 降低的速度更有助于预测患者的生存时 766
间[47,58]。其他相对因素还包括需要持续给氧治疗、住院频率增加以及体重相对于身高的比值下降（低于 80 百分位）[39]。

表 48–1　儿童肺移植的适应证

- 肺囊性纤维化
- 肺纤维化
- 肺血管疾病
  - 原发性肺动脉高压
  - Eisenmenger 综合征
- 梗阻性细支气管炎
- 再移植
- 其他

痰液中存在有耐药的微生物是肺移植的一个相对禁忌证。通过联合应用抗生素可以判断是否存在耐药性的细菌感染，然后考虑是否进行移植手术。只要联合应用抗生素具有协同作用，那么即使有耐药细菌的存在，进行移植手术也是可以接受的。不过，洋葱伯尔霍尔德菌预示着预后不良，因此需要特别关注[24,61]。肺囊性纤维化患者中有5%～10%的患者存在门脉高压伴肝纤维化，这些患儿存在静脉曲张出血以及代谢紊乱的危险性。一般情况下，只要代谢功能正常，用经皮的方法降低门静脉的压力能够把相应的危险性降低到一个可以接受的水平[44]。但是，一旦存在肝脏代谢紊乱，那么联合的肝和肺移植是唯一正确的选择[11]。除非存在血管病理改变，否则糖尿病一般不被视为肺移植的禁忌证。不过应当意识到手术以后控制血糖水平会更加困难[19]。大约10%～15%的肺囊性纤维化患者在肺移植手术前有开胸手术史，这些手术可能包括治疗气胸或者肺叶切除等。虽然有手术史的患者肺部的粘连确实增加手术的难度和术后出血量[18]，但是大多数医疗中心并不将其作为移植手术的禁忌证。使用呼吸机或者气管切开的患者也不是移植手术的禁忌证，但是对于这些患者应当仔细评估其全身状态。

肺血管疾病

这类患者的范围比较大，包括原发性肺动脉高压（PPH）和因先天性心脏病引起的肺动脉高压（PH/CHD）。后一类患者中包括患有Eisenmenger综合征的患者及其他一些患者，这些患者一般因渐进性的右心衰竭、心律失常或致命的咯血而死亡。预测患者何时会出现致命的心律失常或咯血是很困难的，不过大多数患者的死亡原因是慢性渐进性右心衰竭[15]。在过去的几年中，有多种肺血管扩张药物开始应用临床，其中有静脉使用的前列环素[1]、前列环素衍生物伊洛前列腺素（吸入）[29]、β前列腺素（口服）[50]和内皮素受体拮抗剂波生坦[5]等。这些药物可以使患者接受移植手术的时间推迟数年。而事实上，近年来因肺血管疾病而接受移植手术的患者也确实明显减少。

对于罹患肺血管疾病的患者进行肺移植手术的时机很大程度上与该患者药物治疗的效果和肺血管疾病的原因有关。原发性肺动脉高压和Eisenmenger综合征都可以导致独特的肺血管组织变化，但后者长期的预后较前者为优。霍普金斯医院对100位Eisenmenger综合征或原发性肺动脉高压患者的回顾性研究结果显示，在没有进行移植手术的情况下Eisenmenger综合征患者1年生存率为97%，2年是89%，3年为77%；而原发性肺动脉高压患者的相关数据则为77%，69%，35%[30]。据推测是因为心内缺损的存在使右心室在肺血管床严重病变，后负荷过高的时候得以减压。基于类似的一些研究，通过心导管手术进行房间隔造孔手术有助于原发性肺动脉高压的患者[41]。一个有关原发性肺动脉高压的多中心研究显示在前列环素长期静脉使用以前，该类患者从诊断到死亡的平均时间是2.8年。在该研究中，还建立了一个计算公式利用血流动力学指标来帮助估算2年内的死亡率[15]。当超过50%时，该患者就应当列在等待移植的患者名单中。这些对成人的研究结果也应用中儿童患者，但是不清楚的是是否这些疾病在儿童中的自然病程和成人一样。Clabby等回顾了50名PPH患儿并给出了一种估计存活时间的方法[6]。这种方法通过平均右房压和肺动脉阻力来估计生存时间[6]。但随着人们对PPH潜在机制认识的深入和治疗上的进步，比如选择性肺血管扩张剂的发现，这些估计生存时间的公式已经过时。对于肺动脉高压进行治疗多长的时间尚不清楚，这些治疗手段如何应用于继发性肺动脉高压，如Eisenmenger综合征的患者也不清楚。

对于Eisenmenger综合征或者PH/CHD患者的肺移植，有两个方面非常重要，其一是列入移植名单的时间，其二是心脏畸形的复杂程度。如前所述，这类患者在明确诊断后的存活时间较PPH的患者长[30]。这类患者的死亡往往是因为渐进性的心衰、肺出血、脑血管意外或由于心律失常导致的猝死[6]。当症状进展，单侧肺出血或者处于30岁后期应当将患者列为等待移植的人选。大多数PH/CHD患者是房间隔缺损、室间隔缺损或者动脉导管未闭，这些畸形经过一般的手术治疗即可纠正。但是对于那些患有房室间隔缺损、大动脉转位、永存动脉干等复杂畸形的患者，手术就比较复杂。有一个选择就是进行心肺联合移植，不过根据胸腔器官的分配原则，超过40kg的患者同时获得心肺的机会很小。此外，心肺联合移植的长期生存率并不高（5年存活率仅40%）[67]。在决定是进行危险性比较高的肺移植合并复杂心脏畸形纠治手术还是进行心肺联合移植，上述两个因素也应考虑在内。

有些先天性心脏病的患儿即使接受了手术纠治，肺血管阻力也不能下降，有时是因为手术纠治的时机较晚所致，但确实有些患者即使在恰当的时机接受治疗仍然出现严重的肺动脉高压。如何分辨这些患者还不清楚，一般而言，这些患者比原发性肺动脉高压和 Eisenmenger 综合征的患者更少。这些患者的病情发展和治疗手段可能和 PPH 的患者类似[30]。

另一类肺血管疾病是指肺血管床不正常，比如肺动脉闭锁伴室间隔缺损和多发的体肺动脉侧支，先天性膈疝伴有肺实质缺陷。对于前一类患者，手术纠治（关闭室间隔缺损，外管道连接重建右室流出道和汇合的体肺动脉侧支）虽然危险性很大，但是可以救治大多数患者。不过，当体肺动脉侧支无法汇总或者汇总后肺血管树的生长不好，其结果就会导致渐进性发绀或渐进性肺动脉高压。肺移植以及残余心内解剖畸形纠治是这些患者唯一的选择。对于先天性膈疝的患儿，即使手术成功，其肺实质仍然可能存在缺陷，血管床不能承受所有的心排出量。由此引起的肺动脉高压是该类患者的常见死亡原因，也是肺移植的指征之一。但这些患者在围术期往往需接受体外膜肺氧合（ECMO）的治疗，这就限制了患者等待可供供体的时间。此类患者只需要对患肺进行单肺移植。对于这些患者而言，如果患儿长大，可以将移植的一侧肺取出，仅需要一侧健康肺就可以维持正常的呼吸功能。实际上，如果发现这些患者肺储备功能不足，就应当在早期将移植作为一种治疗手段考虑在内。不过，即使供体合适，该类患者的死亡率仍然很高。

在前面述及的这些情形中，只要患者的左心室功能正常，那么单独的肺移植都是可行的。但当左心室功能很差的时候，由于左心室舒张末期压力上升，会引起肺水肿和早期的移植物功能衰竭。而右心室功能在这些患者中，特别是在 PPH 的患者中通常都是较差的。但这并不影响进行肺移植的决定，因为右心室功能一般会在较短的时间内恢复正常[53]。

虽然在肺实质疾病的患者中，胸部手术史不是肺移植的禁忌证，但是对于有肺血管疾病的患者就不相同了，特别是发绀型先天性心脏病手术以后的患者都需要另外考虑。发绀型心脏病姑息手术所形成的粘连包含了很多血管，如肋间血管和乳房内血管会直接通过胸膜和肺实质内血管相连，这是一种增加肺内血流的补偿机制。因此，当进行移植手术时由于肺切除所引起的出血往往是非常严重甚至致命的[53]。

肺纤维化

这类患者占儿童肺移植患者的 5%～10%。患者包括“普通”的肺间质纤维化、辐射引起的纤维化、支气管肺发育不良以及继发于慢性吸入的肺纤维化。这些疾病的发展过程各不相同。通常情况下，当患者出现明显的正常活动受限或者由于轻微的病毒感染就导致严重后果时应当将其列在等待移植的名单中。大多数患者会出现氧依赖以及同时存在肺高压的征象。对于由于慢性吸入所引起病症的儿童，必须去除吸入源。

儿童原发性肺纤维化患者的预后尚不明确，其原因可能是因为在儿童中没有“常见的肺间质纤维化”，每个患者的病因都是独特而且不常见的，因此决定是否等待移植是比较困难的。以前认为婴儿期出现的肺纤维化预后不佳，但是最近的研究显示使用大剂量激素治疗以后其生存率显著提高[51]。成人患者肺总容量低于正常的 60%时预后很差，基本所有患者都在 2 年内死亡[37]，但这一结果不能简单的应用到儿童患者中。肺动脉高压往往伴随着疾病进程而发展，当患者表现出临床症状时就应当进行评估判断是否应列在等待移植的名单上。如果患者对激素治疗反应良好，可以通过标准（年龄＞5 岁）或婴儿（年龄＜5 岁）肺功能测定进行随访。患者通常随着病情的发 768
展接受大剂量激素治疗，因而在移植手术时表现出明显的类 Cushing 综合征样体态，这不能作为移植的禁忌证。

梗阻性细支气管炎和再移植

梗阻性细支气管炎不是一个特定的疾病，而是一种组织学变化，以远端气道的阻塞和结构破坏为特征。可以发生于任何严重肺损伤之后，比如病毒感染、骨髓移植后移植物抗宿主反应、自身免疫性疾病、化学损伤和 Stevens-Johnson 综合征等。这是肺移植中较为常见的远期并发症（详见下文），其发病原因目前尚未明确。“原发性”梗阻性细支气管炎（和肺移植无关）是肺移植的适应证：这是一种慢性渐进性疾病，迄今为止没有任何已知的有效治疗方法。任何一种肺损伤后发生该病症，可以直接作出肺移植的决定。但是，对于曾经进行骨髓移植（通常因为白血病）[54]的患者则需要特别处理。其一是白血病治愈的标准是缓解时间超过 5 年，但是这些患者往往出现在骨髓移植后 2～3 年，另一个问题是骨髓移植后的免疫失调，而肺移植手术以后免疫抑制剂的使用会加重免疫失调的情况。我们发现对这些患者来说手术以后较少发生急性排斥反应，但是发生机会性感染的几率则较高[54]。不过这类患者较少。因为免疫损伤如自身免疫性疾病而出现梗阻性细支气管炎的患者，移植后仍然存在的原发疾病有再次累及移植肺的可能，因此在移植时应当确定原发疾病已经完全消除。

肺移植后出现急性移植物功能衰竭而进行再次移植的预后非常差[49]，而且从现实的角度而言，由于等待移植的患者非常多，所以再次移植并不是一个很合适的选择。有时，由于婴儿患者等待供体的时间明显较成人短，所以对于婴幼儿而言再移植是一个可行的选择。对于梗阻性细支气管炎的患者进行再移植仍然存在争议，肺移植手术 90 天以上的患者死亡大多与梗阻性细支气管炎有关[67]，这一数据是我们对儿童患者的研究所得到的结果[65]。虽然再次移植手术以后的早期死亡率高于首次移植手术，但是如果度过这一时期，长期存活率两者相似[49]。再移植手术后早期死亡的危险因素有卧床不起、首次移植手术后时间较短、在经验不足的医院进行手术以及呼吸机依赖。我们还进一步观察到低肾小球滤过率是一个独立的危险因素。由于等待移植的患者在等待期间有可能死亡，所以有人认为不应该进行再次移植手术，因为那样有可能剥夺一位低危因素患者及时获得供体的机会，在当前的情况下，这个问题还无法解决。我们只能建议当出现再次移植的情况时，采用合适的选择方法，只选择最佳的患者。

其他

其他很多种疾病都可以列在这个条目下。先天性肺实质疾病是其中的一大类，典型的如足月新生儿伴有严重呼吸窘迫而不存在如胎粪吸入、败血症或持续胎儿循环等明显原因的。这些疾病包括表面活性物质蛋白 B 缺乏、肺泡表面蛋白沉积、肺泡–毛细血管发育不良、肺发育不成熟、先天性间质性肺炎以及其他一些疾病。这些婴儿通常表现为严重呼吸衰竭需要高强度的呼吸支持治疗。有的还已经或正在使用 ECMO 治疗，一般需要做开胸肺活检来明确诊断或排除其他可能性。对于表面活性物质蛋白 B 缺乏的患者可以通过外周血的基因突变检查以及分析气道分泌物来诊断[25]。患儿即使经过积极治疗仍可能在 3 个月之内死亡。而且，由于表面活性物质蛋白仅在肺部表达，其他脏器功能很少累及。目前肺移植仍是唯一的治疗方法。除非今后出现其他治疗方式，同样，表面活性物质蛋白 C 基因编码异常也被发现与婴儿肺间质疾病有关，该疾病也可能进展到需要肺移植治疗[26]。通常情况下，婴儿器官供体的等待时间相对较短，因此对于一个有 3 个月生存预期时间的婴儿来说足以等待到合适的供体。当其使用 ECMO 支持时，应当努力争取使其脱离机械支持，包括高频通气使用和（或）一氧化氮吸入等方法。虽然 ECMO 不是器官移植的绝对禁忌证，但是这类患者出现其他脏器功能不全的几率很高。

禁忌证

儿童肺移植的禁忌证是从成人患者的经验上总结的（表 48–2）。绝对禁忌证包括机体疾病并伴有除肺脏外主要器官的表现或其他脏器严重功能不全。因此，广泛转移的恶性肿瘤、血管胶原病、人类免疫缺陷病毒感染和严重神经肌肉病都是绝对禁忌证。有些一般程度的肾功能不全是可以进行移植的。由于几乎所有的免疫抑制剂都是以环孢霉素和他克莫司为基础，且两者具有肾毒性，所以当血清肌酐超过 2.0mg/dL 时可能在手术后需要透析治疗，因此就认为不宜移植。肾小球滤过率低于 50ml/min 时，会 76
影响移植效果。严重的肝脏合成功能紊乱的患者除非可同时进行肝脏移植，否则也不宜进行肺移植。比较复杂的情况有严重营养不良、控制不好的糖尿病、骨质减少、椎体压缩性骨折以及需要呼吸机支持的病例。以上这些因素虽不是绝对禁忌证，但是都需要慎重考虑，根据患者全身状况评估移植以后的成功率。患者在移植手术前长期服用激素也会影响移植手术，应当降低每日剂量或者更换为隔天服用方案。以前认为激素会对气道的愈合，特别是双肺移植患者气管的愈合产生不良影响，现在通过引用支气管吻合对双侧肺先后进行移植已经在很大程度上缓解了这个问题。患者或者儿童患者的监护人有严重精神疾病是一个严重的相对禁忌证。最后，具有不配合医疗行为记录或

表 48–2 肺移植禁忌证

绝对禁忌证
恶性肿瘤
人免疫缺陷病毒感染
多器官功能衰竭
左心室功能不全
活动性血管胶原病
严重神经肌肉病
相对禁忌证
肾功能不全
肝功能损害
营养不良
痰液中有耐药微生物
糖尿病控制不佳
骨质疏松
因肺血管疾病曾经行开胸手术
曾有肺叶切除史导致纵隔偏移
极度早产儿
肺顺应性差
心理社会支持不恰当

不能保持随访的患者也是移植的禁忌证之一。由于缺乏恰当的治疗而引起移植物衰竭不仅会导致患者的死亡而且会使应当接受移植的患者拖延手术时机或移植手术错失[26]。

特殊情况

一些孕周很小的早产儿虽然出生后得以生存但是在出生 1 年以内会出现严重的肺支气管发育不良而导致呼吸功能衰竭。这组患者中脑损伤的发生率很高，约 50%的患者存在不同程度的残疾。我们只能推测，在这些人群中有较为严重的肺部残留疾患而需要进行肺移植的患者较多。要评估这些患者的神经系统功能是很困难的，因为婴儿的体型比较小而且通常需要镇静和肌松药物维持才能维持满意的机械通气。因此除非能精确评价神经系统功能，否则对一个孕 25～28 周的婴儿进行肺移植是不合适的。影像学检查可以提供一些信息帮助诊断，但是并不能仅靠影像学结果来得到结论。另一种比较少见但也可以考虑肺移植的情况是儿童罹患严重的急性呼吸窘迫综合征。这些患儿处于急性期时，往往伴有其他脏器功能损伤，病情也不稳定，不适合立即进行肺移植手术，而度过急性期以后则需要通过评估肺纤维化程度和呼吸支持程度来判断是否需要移植。最后，偶尔有做过肺叶切除的患者需要做肺移植，这些患者的纵隔偏向患侧，肺门结构扭曲，所以双侧肺移植和单侧肺移植无法进行。如果将来有条件的话，这些肺叶切除患者进行肺移植之后，最好有一个人造的支架以保持移植侧纵隔的正常几何结构。

供体评估和器官获取

供体数量仍然是终末期肺部疾病进行肺移植的主要限制。供体必须符合 ABO 血型并且体积和受者基本相符。身高通常是评估肺体积的最精确指标。供者身高超过受者身高 25%以内一般是合适的，即使高于这个限度也可以接受，因为可以通过修剪边缘而减少肺叶体积或甚至仅使用肺下叶。但是低于这个标准就需要谨慎考虑——由于移植肺如不能充满胸腔会导致其更容易发生肺水肿。供者本身存在 HIV 感染、活动性肝炎、哮喘史、结核或者其他明显的肺部疾患则不适宜。其他指标都合适时，少量吸烟史是可以接受的。一般要求供者年龄不超过 55 岁，胸片检查没有明显渗出，在合适潮气量、5cmH_2O 呼气末正压和 100%吸入氧浓度下血氧分压超过 300mmHg。只要符合上述标准，轻度肺挫伤或者部分肺节段肺不张不影
响供体肺的使用。准备移植前，应进行支气管镜检 770
查，并探查气道是否有红斑，这提示是否有胃内容物吸入。此外也可以帮助判断肺分泌物的情况。如果有脓性分泌物，即使胸片清晰，氧合正常也应把该供体排除在外。

取供体肺通过胸骨正中切口进行，术者应打开双侧胸腔直视肺脏并局部应用冰冻盐水和冰屑。在主动脉和上腔静脉之间游离气管。解剖房间沟可能会有助于供体取出，并且在大多数情况下也有利于其他人取出心脏作为供体。上述处理的原则有：（1）大剂量（300U/kg）肝素抗凝；（2）主肺动脉一次性注入前列腺素 E_1（50～70μg/kg）；（3）切开下腔静脉对右心系统进行减压；（4）截断左心耳对左心系统减压；（5）大剂量（50ml/kg），低压灌注冷（4℃）肺保护液；（6）肺表面局部应用冰盐水和冰屑；（7）持续

对肺进行低容量低压通气，吸入氧浓度 0.4。所有肺保护液灌完以后，将全肺和后纵隔组织一起切除下来，其中包括食管和降主动脉。用 U 型钉将食管分离以防止污染。切断气管时保持肺轻微膨胀（压力约 20cmH$_2$O），吸入氧浓度 0.4。然后取下肺，保存在保护液中，冷藏运输。

一直有许多研究致力于研制“理想”的肺保护液以延长肺缺血时间并避免再灌注损伤[35]。该话题全面讨论超出了本章的范畴。现在最常用的保护液是 Euro-Collins 液、威斯康星大学保护液、Perfadex 液和 Celsior 液。这些保护液效果良好没有明显的区别。但是也没有一个保护液可以将肺保存超过 8 个小时，也不能完全避免再灌注损伤。

移植技术

除了儿童手术中必须使用体外循环，而成人则不一定需要外。儿童肺移植手术技术和成人手术基本相似，如果不使用体外循环，则移植手术中需要使用单肺通气，由于在小儿中气道很小，要使用双腔气管插管保持单肺通气是非常困难的。由于考虑到移植肺后的生长，所以几乎所有的儿童都是接受双肺移植。经第四肋间隙横跨胸骨的双前外侧切口（称之为“蛤壳”切口）可以很清楚的暴露心脏和肺门结构。所有的吻合都应采用可吸收缝线以保证最大的组织生长潜能[20]。对于气道吻合，我们建议使用简单的端端吻合技术而不宜采用内镜吻合，因为后者更容易引起术后狭窄[17,32]。如果患者同时需要纠治心内畸形（比如 Eisenmenger 综合征患者），那么心内操作最好在肺切除后或供体肺植入之前。许多肺移植患者由于存在大量的体肺循环侧支，所以体外循环中有很多肺静脉血液回流至心脏，当受者的肺脏切除以后，也同时去除了支气管动脉和其他侧支的回流，为心内畸形的纠治提供无血的手术野。其后进行的同种肺移植手术也为心脏在脱离体外循环前提供了适应再灌注的充分时间。

由于供体缺乏，目前活体肺叶移植，即使用供体的部分肺叶移植替代全肺移植的手段已经越来越常见[62]。虽然有仅使用肺上叶的，不过从解剖角度而言，单叶肺之中下叶肺更适合替代单侧肺脏。当肺叶是从活体身上取出时，支气管和血管比较少，需要保留受者较多的支气管、肺动脉和静脉以供手术。目前已经有技术将单侧左肺分离，其中上叶肺用在右侧，而下叶则用在左侧[12]。这种情况非常少见，只有当获得一个大供体的左侧肺应用在小儿身上时才可行。不过，这也是解决供体不足的一个方法。

免疫抑制

虽然各医院免疫抑制药物使用的方案并不完全相同，但是大多数还是采用三药联合的方案。联合用药方式既可以获得更好的免疫抑制效果，又可以降低各自的毒性效应（表 48-3）。一般药物包括环孢霉素或他克莫司，联合咪唑硫嘌呤和泼尼松。从疗效和并发症角度而言，没有明确证据表明环孢霉素和他克莫司两者何者更好。对于用抗胸腺球蛋白或 OKT3 进行溶细胞治疗仍然存在争议，不过一般不建议使用，主要因为该方法会导致感染的并发症。达珠单抗（Daclizumab）和巴利昔单抗（basiliximab）是两种白介素 2 的特异性单克隆抗体，可作为溶细胞治疗的一种替代疗法，用以诱导免疫耐受[4]。与溶细胞疗法不同，这些药物通过 771

表 48-3　免疫抑制剂

药物分类	副作用
白介素 2 合成抑制剂	
环胞素	高血压，癫痫发作，肾毒性，多毛症，牙龈增生
他克莫司	高血糖，癫痫发作，肾毒性
淋巴细胞增殖抑制剂	
硫唑嘌呤	白细胞减少，恶心
麦考酚酸莫酯	白细胞减少，恶心，腹泻，肝酶升高
西罗莫司	高三酰甘油血症，伤口愈合延迟
皮质激素	高血压，高血糖，Cushing 综合征外观
诱导剂	
抗胸腺细胞球蛋白	发热，寒战，白细胞减少，巨细胞病毒感染，移植后淋巴组织增生性疾病
OKT3	发热、寒战、巨细胞病毒感染、移植后淋巴细胞、增生性疾病
达珠单抗、巴利昔单抗	恶心，腹泻

阻断淋巴细胞激活途径中的关键步骤来减轻细胞排斥反应。这种单克隆抗体降低了感染的几率，促进了肺移植手术后早期进行诱导治疗的使用[3]。

使用环孢霉素的初始目标是将其血药浓度维持到300～400ng/ml（全血单克隆检验）。而当使用他克莫司时，其目标血药浓度为 10～15 ng/ml。激素的初始剂量为泼尼松或者甲泼尼龙每天 0.5mg/kg。硫唑嘌呤（azathioprine）的剂量是每天 2.5～3.0 mg/kg。发生急性排斥反应时应连续 3 天静脉使用甲泼尼龙10mg/kg。若甲泼尼龙效果不佳，应换用抗胸腺球蛋白 7～10 天。复发的急性排斥提示各种药物如环孢霉素、硫唑嘌呤、他克莫司和霉酚酸酯（mycophenolate mofetil）等免疫抑制反应的基值改变。虽然激素的使用剂量逐渐降低，但我们仍不确定停止使用激素是否合适。免疫抑制剂的并发症在儿童中和成人类似，只是环孢霉素所引起的多毛症在女性儿童中更为多见。此并发症有时足以使用药更改为他克莫司。西罗莫司（Sirolimus）（雷帕霉素 rapamycin）在化学结构上类似于他克莫司，作用在于抑制白介素-2 刺激淋巴细胞所引起的增殖反应[63]，但其没有他克莫司的神经毒性，目前，该药物用于其他免疫抑制剂失效以后。该药物不宜作为移植手术后首选的免疫抑制剂是因为其影响伤口和气管的愈合，有可能导致严重的并发症[43]。

所有患者都需口服磺胺甲基异恶唑-甲氧苄啶，一周 3 次预防肺孢子虫感染性肺炎，如果有磺胺药物过敏或耐受则改为戊烷脒气雾剂 1 个月治疗。同时还要预防皮肤或黏膜的念珠菌感染。

移植术后检查

移植手术后的检查基于定期测量肺活量、支气管镜进行活检及支气管肺泡灌洗术。出院以前，患者应配备家用的肺活量测量仪，至少每天测量 1 次，如果 FEV_1 较基值下降 10%，就需要就诊。所有患者，不论年龄体重，都需要定期进行支气管镜检以判断是否存在下呼吸道感染、亚临床状态的排斥反应以及气管吻合口的并发症等。事实上，一旦怀疑存在排斥反应，都要通过支气管镜活检来确诊。对于婴儿来说，进行活检主要的障碍是足以容纳活检钳子纤维支气管镜，很有可能阻塞气道[48]。最近，正在研究一种不用支气管镜的“非直视下”肺活检技术，该技术使用特殊的吸引管导引活检钳到达指定位置进行组织活检。支气管镜活检应在移植术后 10～14 天、6 周以及 3、6、9、12、18 和 24 个月进行。呼吸功能下降、胸片显示渗出影和临床情况恶化比如发热或需要吸氧都提示应当进行支气管镜活检。支气管肺泡灌洗也应同时进行，通过培养判断是否有细菌、病毒或真菌感染。

术后并发症

外科并发症

吻合口并发症

吻合口并发症包括气道吻合口和血管吻合口两方面。当还采用气管吻合时，气道裂开是移植手术后早期主要的并发症和引起死亡的原因。此后虽然采用网膜包住吻合口也没有很好的解决这个问题[9]。现在，虽然不再采用网膜，但是吻合口裂开的情况已很少见，主要是由于采用了供体和受者支气管周围组织加固吻合口。气道裂开可以是全部，也可以是局部。局 772
部裂开一般可以治愈，但是增加了术后气道狭窄的可能性[56]。完全裂开可危及生命必须进行急诊手术。虽然这种情况有时可以尝试再次吻合，但是失败的几率相当高，所以大多数时候要将移植的肺切除。由于儿童气道口径狭小，所以支气管狭窄的发生率高，而且吻合口能否继续生长也是至关重要的。现有的资料显示气道吻合口可以生长，而且狭窄的发生也和手术的年龄或气道大小无关[31,57]。狭窄的支气管通常使用逐渐增粗的支气管内镜或血管造影的气囊进行扩张。气囊扩张可能优于内镜，因为后者有可能损伤远端气道。扩张后 10～14 天应进行支气管镜检查，来评估扩张的效果以及是否有复发。需要根据狭窄严重程度和速度来决定是否安放支架。有两种支架可供选择，其一是硅橡胶，另一种是金属网状支架。后者容易放置，但放置后难以取出，而前者正好相反。除了支架外，还可以进行袖状切除（支气管或上肺叶）或再次移植。袖状切除在成人中疗效满意，但是在小儿中非常困难[59]。只有当狭窄蔓延超过支气管分支并且不能采用内镜或局部切除等技术时，才考虑进行再次移植。

血管吻合口并发症

不论是动脉还是静脉吻合口，并发症都非常少见。大多数情况下，吻合口狭窄继发于供体肺动脉或左房壁过长，或者两者在吻合时发生扭曲。肺动脉吻合口狭窄可以表现为右室高压，也有的表现不明显。由于肺动脉测压管在儿童中较少使用，所以体外循环以后应当进行直接的右心室穿刺来测定压力。如果有升高，应通过直接穿刺测量所有吻合口远端的压力。单侧肺动脉轻或中度狭窄不一定导致右心室压力升高。术后24小时以内应当进行肺灌洗检查以排除肺血管吻合口的机械性梗阻，一旦有明显的两肺灌洗差异，就应当再次进行手术探查或血管造影。单侧或双侧肺静脉狭窄表现为肺动脉高压，会产生大量的粉红色泡沫痰，胸片显示肺部渗出。这些情况也可能由于严重的再灌注损伤和弥漫性肺泡损伤所致。但是，肺毛细血管嵌压在后两种情况中不会升高，而在肺静脉狭窄时会升高。食管超声检查对于肺静脉吻合口的诊断是很有帮助的。明确诊断，特别在婴儿中需要直接测量肺静脉和左心房压力。早期纠治是必须的。

出血

在移植手术中，很多因素使患者出血的危险性增加。所有的儿童在手术时都需要长时间的体外循环支持，以切除受者肺脏并植入供体。此外，很多患者有胸部手术史。抑肽酶可以较有效地预防出血的发生[38]。如前所述，患有发绀型先天性心脏病以及有胸部手术史的患者出血的危险性最大。

膈神经损伤

约20%的肺移植患者会发生膈神经损伤，该并发症是由于肺门组织牵拉的损伤所致，右侧多见[60]。通常膈肌功能在手术后6个月以内恢复。右侧多见的原因可能是因为右侧膈神经更接近肺动脉而且上腔静脉也位于右侧。上腔静脉（以及膈神经）需要拉开以暴露近端右肺动脉。有胸部手术史的患者膈神经损伤更容易发生，这是因为组织粘连使膈神经难以分辨。

声嘶

喉返神经损伤所致的声带麻痹发生率约为10%，可通过纤维支气管镜检查直接观察到声带麻痹而确诊。即使无直接治疗，大多数声带不对称也会在6个月内有所改善。一般累及左侧声带，这是因为在动脉韧带区域分离左肺动脉时引起的。

胃肠道并发症

肺移植手术后发生胃食管反流几乎仅见于婴儿。在我们的病例中，术后存活超过30天的婴儿50%发生这一并发症。诊断手段包括上消化道造影、24小时连续食管pH监测或者在支气管肺泡灌洗中发现有充满脂肪的巨噬细胞[34]。虽然发生率很高，但是胃食管反流的病因并不清楚，可能是因为切除受体肺时损伤了双侧迷走神经所致。肠道蠕动减弱也是一个所有 773
年龄段患者都比较多见的并发症。胃食管反流在肺移植手术后的成人中也有较高的发生率。有人认为可能和毛细支气管炎有关[16]。肺囊性纤维病变的患者有发生远端肠道梗阻综合征的危险。在移植手术后积极使用高渗泻药可以防止该并发症。如果口服泻药没有疗效，应当进行泛影葡胺灌肠。

房颤

房性心律失常在肺移植手术后也比较常见，发生率约10%，其中以房颤最多，许多患者还需要长期治疗[21]。最近的研究显示左房吻合口处在外来刺激的情况下会成为房颤发生的原因[22]。

移植物并发症

由再灌注损伤引起的移植物功能衰竭伴随有胸片上渗出影、粉红色泡沫痰和血液氧合程度低，这是肺移植手术后早期最常见的移植物并发症，发生率约为20%～30%。这也是移植手术以后30天内死亡的最常见原因[67]。其原因往往是多因素的，和供体及受者的状态都有关系。最佳预防措施包括谨慎、仔细地评估和收集供体器官，避免受者存在活动性感染及其他急性病。而一个顺利的移植过程也是非常重要的。虽然一氧化氮[14]和前列环素[46]的治疗对于出现再灌注损伤的患者有一定的疗效，但是对于再灌注损伤的治疗往往是以支持性治疗为主。

排斥反应在肺移植手术后是比较多见的，比其他实质性脏器移植后的发生率要高（图 48–1）。由于体内主要的组织相容性抗原表达在内皮细胞表面，该抗原参与最初的免疫识别，而肺内的血管内皮细胞表面积远大于其他脏器，因此肺是最不容易逃避免疫识别的脏器。而且肺移植物往往还伴有支气管等软组织所携带的淋巴细胞和巨噬细胞，这些细胞将逐渐被受者的同类细胞所取代。这些具有相当强烈免疫活性的细胞增加了排斥反应的危险性。移植手术早期的排斥反应没有很明显的特征性表现，因此任何可能的症状都应当通过气管镜或开胸手术取肺组织进行组织学检查。大多数急性排斥反应发生在手术后 6 个月内[36]。虽然急性排斥反应在儿童中的发生率和成人相似，不过在婴儿中发生率比较低。这一现象的原因目前尚不清楚，不过有可能和婴儿的免疫系统尚未成熟有关。

大多数临床医生认为梗阻性细支气管炎是慢性排斥反应的一种表现，并且该现象在约 50%的长期存活的患者中发生[64]。虽然目前认为供体缺血时间长和早期急性排斥反应可增加其发生几率，但是其确切原因至今尚不明确[33]。梗阻性细支气管炎的表现是无其他明显原因的 FEV_1 显著下降。胸片检查一般显示肺野清晰，CT 检查也不能发现明显渗出。肺通气或血流
774 扫描可显示血流灌注区和气体存贮区互相交杂。此时需要进行支气管镜活检以及支气管肺泡灌洗以排除如急性排斥反应或感染等其他原因，并评估气道内活性淋巴细胞浸润程度。梗阻性细支气管炎的组织学切片显示为膜性支气管和呼吸性细支气管由一片致密的瘢痕组织所覆盖（图 48–2）。也可以根据活检组织中没有可以辨认的细支气管的情况来推断梗阻性细支气管炎的发生。要根据组织学检查和支气管镜活检结果来诊断梗阻性细支气管炎是非常困难的，不过许多医生认为不一定需要明确诊断。目前已经根据 FEV_1 值下降程度建立了一个分期系统：一期下降 20%～35%，二期下降 35%～50%，三期下降超过 50% [10]。目前推荐的对梗阻性细支气管炎的治疗方法是采用加强的免疫抑制治疗，通常是每天使用抗胸腺球蛋白，连续 7～10 天，但是临床疗效各不相同。抗增生药物可能是更有效的方法，但是尚未证实。另一个可以尝试的方法就是采用全身淋巴结放射治疗。对以上治疗方法都没有效果的患者可以作为再次移植的候选对象。但是如前文所述，由于供体的短缺以及再移植的效果不如首次接受移植的患者，因此对于再移植仍然有相当的争议。不过，如果患者还能够走动，并没有呼吸机依赖，那么在经验丰富的移植中心，再移植的结果和首次肺移植的效果近似[49]。

肺移植手术以后约 5%～10%的患者会发生移植后淋巴增生病（PTLD）。有原发性 EB 病毒感染的患者该病症发生率高[68]。由于儿童在移植时血清内没有相应抗体，所以在移植手术后更有可能感染 EB 病

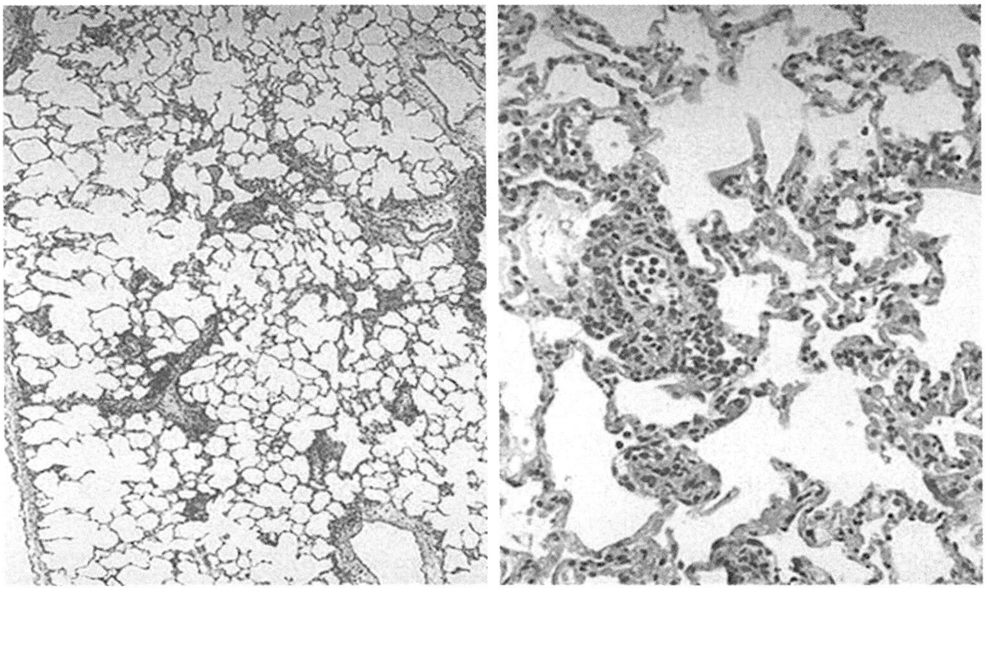

图 48–1　急性排斥反应。在许多血管周围存在大量淋巴细胞浸润，在高倍镜下显示更清楚。该图列为 A2 级急性排斥反应。

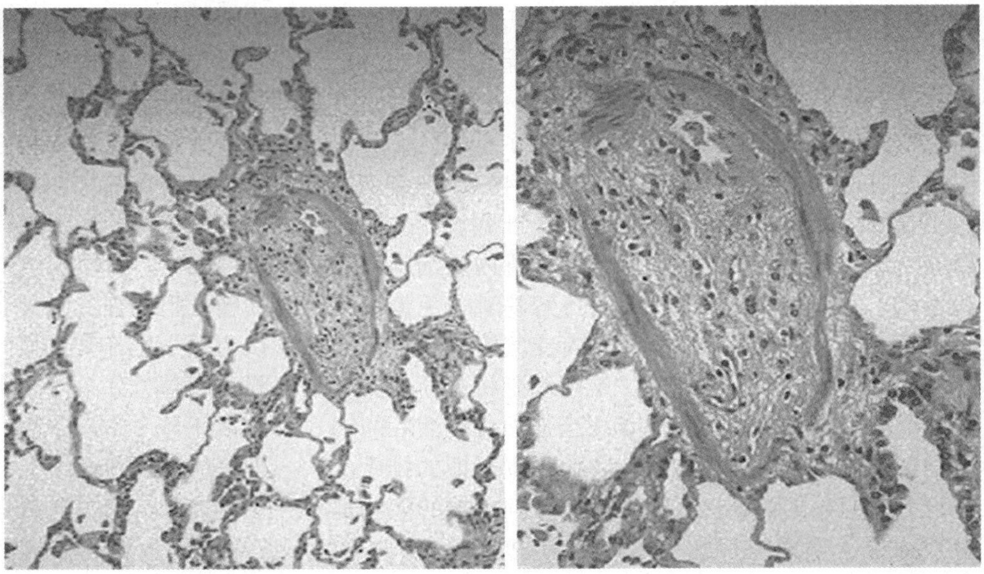

图 48-2 因梗阻性细支气管炎而进行再次肺移植的患者的组织学图像。小气道被纤维组织所覆盖。

毒，所以发生该并发症的几率高于成人。降低免疫抑制的程度是早期治疗的主要方法，虽然这样有可能会导致免疫抑制不足，但一般并不会引起继发的梗阻性细支气管炎。利妥昔（Rituximab），一种[66]CD20 单克隆抗体，可以有效地治疗 PTLD[64]。其他治疗方式包括传统化疗、放疗[20]以及注射人粒细胞抗原匹配的 T 细胞[52]。

感染

虽然实质性脏器移植术后感染是常见的并发症，但是肺移植手术以后感染的危险性更大。供者都接受呼吸机辅助，导致呼吸道内可能有监护室里的细菌生长。除了肠道以外，肺脏是唯一和外界环境接触的实质性脏器。移植手术后气管插管，必然影响呼吸道的自然防御能力。移植手术中切断神经也使得咳嗽反射明显减弱甚至缺失。这些以及其他许多因素都要求肺移植手术患者的看护人员必须高度注意呼吸道感染的诊断和治疗，并应当加强肺部冲洗。

所有接受移植手术的候选患者都要接受气道微生物检查以确定是否存在感染征象。是否存在病毒感染则采用血清学检查来检测巨细胞病毒，单纯性疱疹，水痘，EB 病毒，甲、乙、丙型肝炎病毒以及人免疫缺陷病毒的抗体。但是在婴儿中病毒血清学检查所提供的信息有限，这是因为其体内的免疫球蛋白来自于母体。移植手术后早期所使用的抗微生物治疗部分是直接根据移植前的检查结果所确定的。不论是
供体还是受者的巨细胞病毒血清学检查结果阳性， 775
都要使用更昔洛韦（Ganciclovir）每天 5mg/kg，连续使用 6 周。如果患者有曲霉菌感染或感染史，应静脉使用两性霉素 B（每天 3.0mg/kg）5～10 天，并根据临床症状继续使用两性霉素 B 雾化吸入（10mg，每日 3 次）。

在儿童患者中呼吸道病毒感染是很常见的。如腺病毒和副流感病毒感染，其处理特别棘手。至于巨细胞病毒，原发疾病通常较反应性疾病严重。而 EB 病毒感染则出现前面已经提到的 PTLD 危险因素。

真菌感染虽然比较少见但是后果可能是致命性的。口服制霉菌素可以降低念珠菌属的感染危险。事实上所有由念珠菌属所引起的感染都可以通过口服或静脉输注三唑抗真菌药物控制。而曲霉菌感染的处理就较麻烦，如果没有采取及时合适的抗真菌治疗会导致感染扩散至全身。

细菌感染是肺移植手术以后最常见的严重并发症。大多数患者手术以后会发生下呼吸道细菌感染，包括化脓性支气管炎和肺炎。其中囊性纤维化的患者最有可能发生，感染的微生物往往和术前呼吸道培养结果相同。对于囊性纤维化的患者可以使用抗生素（妥布霉素或黏菌素）雾化吸入来预防下呼吸道感染。

其他并发症

高血压是移植手术后比较常见的并发症，其原因是使用磷脂酶抑制剂——环孢霉素（Calcineurin）、他克莫司和甲泼尼龙治疗。肾功能不全的发生率随着手术后时间延长而增加，其发生和服用环孢霉素及他克莫司有关。移植手术后约 15%的患者出现糖尿病，主要发生在囊性纤维化的患者中[8]。使用他克莫司可增加高血糖症的发生率。

存活率

根据世界心肺移植协会的统计数据，儿童肺移植手术后 3 年和 5 年的存活率分别为 54%和 45%（图 48-3）[67]。急性排斥反应在移植后最初 30 天内是最主要的死亡原因。出院 1 年以内死亡的患者中 50%是因为感染导致。而 1 年以后的死亡病例中 50%是由梗阻性细支气管炎导致的，而且也是影响肺移植患者长期存活的主要因素[49]。

肺功能及其生长

目前尚不清楚移植以后肺的生长是肺泡体积扩大还是数量增加，相关研究也仍没有确定的结果。测量肺的生长受到许多复杂因素的干扰。肺功能测量的结果和由胸片或 CT 检查的肺体积是不能被采用的，因为这些结果受到许多因素的影响不能精确显示肺泡的数量和体积。肺的生长问题对婴儿尤为重要，因为所移植的肺必须生长以满足今后生活的生理需要。这些患儿往往太小，不能进行标准的儿童肺功能测试以确定功能残气量，而功能残气量可以较好地替代肺容量指标。儿童移植手术后 3 个月的平均功能残气量是每 776
厘米身高 2.3ml，术后 15 个月大约是 2.1～2.8ml。在此期间，儿童的生长是非常显著的[7]。因此，只要没有大气道或外周小气道梗阻，那么以上数据用来显示肺部的生长对于整个身体而言是合适的。但是我们还尚不清楚究竟是肺泡数量增加了还是原有肺泡的体积扩大了。

活体供者的肺移植

使用活体供者的肺进行移植（LDLTx）是受到肾脏和肝脏活体移植的成功（特别是肾脏）启发而开展的。其原则是一个健康的成人捐献出左或右侧肺的下叶，将其作为儿童（或体型较小的成人）的一侧全肺[62]。供体必须有足够的功能贮备。丧失 20%～25%的肺容量不会引起任何功能的缺失以及影响今后的日常生活。LDLTx 和活体供肾或肝相比，前者要两个供者接受开胸手术，开胸手术的危险性较腹腔手术为高。这样，两个健康人为了一个人而经历手术风险，这首先要面对的就是伦理问题，特别是目前肺移植手术的生存率还不十分理想。但是，该方法较从死者身上取器官有一些明显的优点，比如供肺缺血时间短，可以在术前对供者进行全面评估确定肺脏是否正常；移植时间的选择较随意，可以考虑到各方面的因

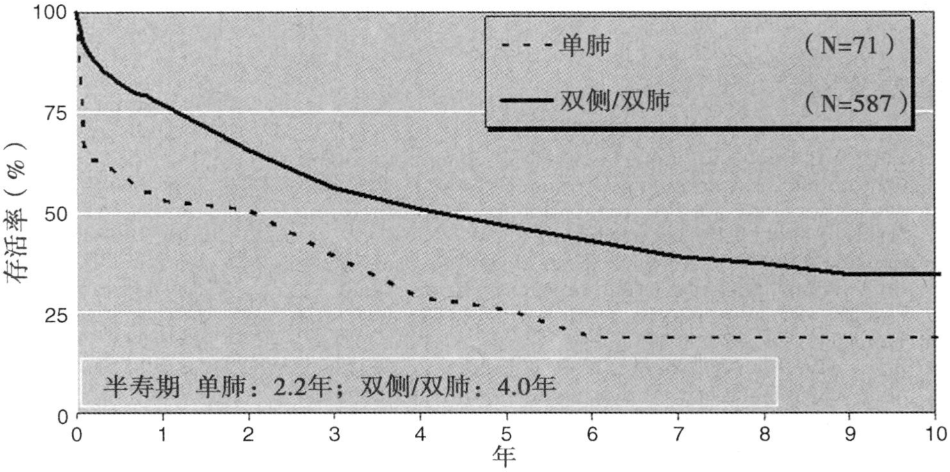

图 48-3 儿童肺移植手术以后的 Kaplan-Meier 存活曲线。（From Boucek MM, Faro A, Novick RJ, et al: The Registry of the International Society for Heart and Lung Transplantation: Fourth official pediatric report-2000. J Heart Lung Transplant 2001;20:39-52.）

素；人白细胞抗原的吻合程度也较好。这一手术在技术上更具有挑战性，只对那些无法继续等待供体的患者才可以实施 LDLTx。这一类患者和从死者身上取肺的患者移植手术后存活率相似。一个比较有趣的现象就是在此类患者中，梗阻性细支气管炎的发生率很低[69]。这可能和缺血时间短有关，因为供体获得是在邻近的医院。其他可能的原因是由于供体大都为亲属，免疫方面可能有一定优势。

未来的展望

在儿童中限制肺移植成功的因素和成人类似：供体缺乏、免疫抑制和预防感染之间的平衡及梗阻性细支气管炎的发生等。作为供体缺乏的解决办法之一，LDLTx 可能会在今后几年内更多被采用，但是该方法不能根本上改变供体缺乏的现象和缩短等待器官的时间。异种移植可能是另一个解决方法，但是事实上离实际应用还是有相当大的差距。直接针对特定脏器以及特定抗体的新免疫抑制药物是必须要研究的。梗阻性细支气管炎仍然是肺移植后影响长期存活的主要因素。虽然至今没有定论，但是大多数学者认为其和慢性排斥反应有关。因此对于该领域的临床和基础研究以了解梗阻性细支气管炎的发病原因和病情进程是非常重要的。由于气道易于接受评估和治疗，梗阻性细支气管炎可能提供了一个慢性排斥反应的模型，对它的研究同样会涉及心、肾、肝等其他脏器移植中所遇到的问题，有助于这些问题的了解和解决。

（王　炜译　吕志葆校）

参考文献

1. Barst RJ, Rubin LJ, Long WA, et al: A comparison of continuous intravenous epoprostenol (prostacyclin) with conventional therapy for primary pulmonary hypertension. N Engl J Med 1996;334:296-302.
2. Boucek MM, Faro A, Novick RJ, et al: The Registry of the International Society for Heart and Lung Transplantation: Fourth official pediatric report—2000. J Heart Lung Transplant 2001;20:39-52.
3. Brock MV, Borja MC, Ferber L, et al: Induction therapy in lung transplantation: A prospective, controlled clinical trial comparing OKT3, anti-thymocyte globulin, and daclizumab. J Heart Lung Transplant 2001;20:1282-1290.
4. Bumgardner GL, Hardie I, Johnson RW, et al: Phase III Daclizumab Study Group: Results of 3-year phase III clinical trials with daclizumab prophylaxis for prevention of acute rejection after renal transplantation. Transplantation 2001;72:839-845.
5. Channick RN, Simonneau G, Sitbon O, et al: Effects of the dual endothelin-receptor antagonist bosentan in patients with pulmonary hypertension: A randomised placebo-controlled study. Lancet 2001;358:1119-1123.
6. Clabby ML, Canter CE, Moller JH, Bridges ND: Hemodynamic data and survival in children with pulmonary hypertension. J Am Coll Cardiol 1997;30:554-560.
7. Cohen AH, Mallory GB, Ross K, et al: Growth of lungs after transplantation in infants and in children younger than 3 years of age. Am J Respir Crit Care Med 1999;159:1747-1751.
8. Cooper JD, Ginsberg RJ, Goldberg M, the Toronto Lung Transplant Group: Unilateral transplantation for pulmonary fibrosis. N Engl J Med 1986;314:1140-1145.
9. Cooper JD, Pearson FG, Patterson GA, et al: Technique of successful lung transplantation in humans. J Thorac Cardiovasc Surg 1987;93:173-181.
10. Cooper JD, Billingham M, Egan T, et al: A working formulation for the standardization of nomenclature and for clinical staging of chronic dysfunction in lung allografts. J Heart Lung Transplant 1993;12:713-716.
11. Couetil JP, Houssin DP, Soubrane O, et al:. Combined lung and liver transplantation in patients with cystic fibrosis: A 4½-year experience. J Thorac Cardiovasc Surg 1995; 110:1415-1422.
12. Couetil J-P, Achkar A, Chevalier P, et al: Split lung with bilateral lobar transplantation: A two-year experience. J Heart Lung Transplant 1995;14(Suppl):S60.
13. Cystic Fibrosis Foundation: Patient Registry 1999 Annual Report. Bethesda, MD, September 2000.
14. Date H, Triantafillou AN, Trulock EP, et al: Inhaled nitric oxide reduces human lung allograft dysfunction. J Thorac Cardiovasc Surg 1996;111:913-919.
15. D' Alonzo GE, Barst RJ, Ayres SM, et al: Survival in patients with primary pulmonary hypertension: Results from a national prospective registry. Ann Intern Med 1991;115: 343-349.
16. Davis RD, Lau CL, Eubanks S, et al: Improved lung allograft function after fundoplication in patients with gastroesophageal reflux disease undergoing lung transplantation. J Thorac Cardiovasc Surg 2003;125:533-542.
17. Egan TM, Westerman JH, Lambert CJ, et al: Isolated lung transplantation for end-stage lung disease: A viable therapy. Ann Thorac Surg 1992;53:590-596.
18. Egan TM, Detterbeck FC, Mill MR, et al: Improved results of lung transplantation for patients with cystic fibrosis. J Thorac Cardiovasc Surg 1995;109:224-235.
19. Finkelstein SM, Wielinski CL, Elliott GR, et al: Diabetes mellitus associated with cystic fibrosis. J Pediatr 1988;112: 373-377.
20. Friedman E, Perez-Atayde AR, Silvera M, Jonas RA: Growth of tracheal anastomoses in lambs. J Thorac Cardiovasc Surg 1990;100:188-193.
21. Gandhi SK, Bromberg BI, Mallory GB, Huddleston CB: Atrial flutter—a newly recognized complication of pediatric lung transplantation. J Thorac Cardiovasc Surg 1996;112: 984-991.
22. Gandhi SK, Bromberg BI, Schuessler RB, et al: Left sided atrial flutter—characterization of a novel complication of pediatric lung transplantation in an acute canine model. J Thorac Cardiovasc Surg 1996;112:992-1001.

23. Ganne V, Siddiqi N, Kamaplath B, et al: Humanized anti-CD20 monoclonal antibody (Rituximab) treatment for post-transplant lymphoproliferative disorder. Clin Transplant 2003;17:417-422.
24. Gilligan PH, Neuringer IP, Gott KK, et al: The effects of panresistant bacteria in cystic fibrosis patients on lung transplant outcome. Am J Respir Crit Care Med 1997; 155:1699-1704.
25. Hamvas A, Mallory GB, Spray TL, et al: Lung transplantation for treatment of infants with surfactant protein B deficiency. J Pediatr 1997;130:231-239.
26. Hamvas A, Nogee LM, White FV, et al: Progressive lung disease and surfactant dysfunction with a deletion in surfactant protein C gene. Am J Respir Cell Mol Biol 2004; 30:771-776.
27. Hardy JD, Webb WR, Dalton ML, et al: Lung homotransplantation in man. JAMA 1963;186:1065-1074.
28. Hislop AA, Odom NJ, McGregor CGA, Haworth SG: Growth potential of the immature transplanted lung: An experimental study. J Thorac Cardiovasc Surg 1990;100: 360-370.
29. Hoeper MM, Schwarze M, Ehlerding S, et al: Long-term treatment of primary pulmonary hypertension with aerosolized iloprost, a prostacyclin analogue. N Engl J Med 2000;342:1866-1870.
30. Hopkins WE, Ochoe LL, Richardson GW, Trulock EP: Comparison of the hemodynamics and survival of adults with severe primary pulmonary hypertension or Eisenmenger syndrome. J Heart Lung Transplant 1996;15:100-105.
31. Huddleston CB, Spray TL, Mallory GB: Airway complications following pediatric lung transplant. J Heart Lung Transplant 1995;14 (Suppl):S60.
32. Huddleston CB: Airway complications in children following lung transplantation. In Cooper DKC, Miller L, Patterson GA (eds): The Transplantation and Replacement of Thoracic Organs. Lancaster, UK, Kluwer, 1996, pp 581-588.
33. Huddleston CB, Sweet SC, Cohen AH, et al: Bronchiolitis obliterans after pediatric lung transplantation. J Heart Lung Transplant 1998;17:65.
34. Huddleston CB, Sweet SC, Mallory GB, et al: Lung transplantation in very young infants. J Thorac Cardiovasc Surg 1999;118:796-804.
35. Huddleston CB, Mendeloff EN: Heart and lung preservation for transplantation. J Cardiac Surg 2000;15:108-121.
36. Ibrahim JE, Sweet SC, Flippin MC, et al: Rejection is reduced in thoracic organ recipients when transplanted in the first year of life. J Heart Lung Transplant 2002;21: 311-318.
37. Jackson LK: Idiopathic pulmonary fibrosis. Clin Chest Med 1982;3:579.
38. Jaquiss RDB, Huddleston CB, Spray TL: Use of aprotinin in pediatric lung transplantation. J Heart Lung Transplant 1995;14:302-307.
39. Kerem E, Reisman J, Corey M, et al: Prediction of mortality in patients with cystic fibrosis. N Engl J Med 1992;326: 1187-1191.
40. Kern JA, Tribble CG, Flanagan TL, et al: Growth potential of porcine reduced-size mature pulmonary lobar transplants. J Thorac Cardiovasc Surg 1992;104:1329-1332.
41. Kerstein D, Levy PS, Hsu DT, et al: Blade balloon atrial septostomy in patients with severe primary pulmonary hypertension. Circulation 1995;91:2028-2035.
42. King RC, Binns OAR, Rodriguz F, et al: Reperfusion injury significantly impacts clinical outcome after pulmonary transplantation. Ann Thorac Surg 2000;69:1681-1685.
43. King-Biggs MB, Dunitz JM, Park SJ, et al: Airway anastomotic dehiscence associated with use of sirolimus immediately after lung transplantation. Transplantation 2003;75:1437-1443.
44. Klima LD, Kowdley KV, Lewis SL, et al: Successful lung transplantation in spite of cystic fibrosis-associated liver disease: A case series. J Heart Lung Transplant 1997;16:934-938.
45. Kurland G: Pediatric lung transplantation: Indications and contraindications. Semin Thorac Cardiovasc Surg 1996;8: 277-285.
46. Matsuzaki Y, Waddell TK, Puskas JD, et al: Amelioration of post-ischemic lung reperfusion injury by prostaglandin E_1. Am Rev Respir Dis 1993;148:882-889.
47. Milla CE, Warwick WJ: Risk of death in cystic fibrosis patients with severely compromised lung function. Chest 1998;113:1230-1234.
48. Mullins D, Livne M, Mallory GB, Kemp JS: A new technique for transbronchial biopsy in infants and small children. Pediatr Pulmonol 1995;20:253-257.
49. Novick RJ, Stitt LW, Al-Kattan K, et al: Pulmonary retransplantation: Predictors of graft function and survival in 230 patients. Ann Thorac Surg 1998;65:227-234.
50. Okano Y, Yoshioka T, Shimouchi A, et al: Orally active prostacyclin analogue in primary pulmonary hypertension. Lancet 1997;349:1365.
51. Osika E, Muller MH, Boccon-Gibod L, et al: Idiopathic pulmonary fibrosis in infants. Pediatr Pulmonol 1997;23:49-54.
52. Papadopoulos EB, Ladanyi M, Emanuel D, et al: Infusions of donor leukocytes to treat Epstein-Barr virus-associated lymphoproliferative disorders after allogeneic bone marrow transplantation. N Engl J Med 1994;330:1185-1191.
53. Pasque MK, Trulock EP, Cooper JD, et al: Single lung transplantation of pulmonary hypertension: Single institution experience in 34 patients. Circulation 1995;92:2252-2258.
54. Pechet TV, de la Morena MT, Mendeloff EN, et al: Lung transplantation in children following treatment for malignancy. J Heart Lung Transplant 2003;22:154-160.
55. Ramirez J, Patterson GA: Airway complications after lung transplantation. Semin Thorac Cardiovasc Surg 1992;4: 147-153.
56. Rand KH, Pollard RB, Merigan TC: Increased pulmonary superinfections—cardiac transplant recipients undergoing primary cytomegalovirus infection. N Engl J Med 1987; 298:951-953.
57. Ro PS, Bush DM, Kramer SS, et al: Airway growth after pediatric lung transplantation. J Heart Lung Transplant 2001;20:619-624.
58. Robinson W, Waltz DA: FEV_1 as a guide to lung transplant referral in young patients with cystic fibrosis. Pediatr Pulmonol 2000;30:198-202.
59. Schafers HJ, Schafer CM, Zink C, et al: Surgical treatment of airway complications after lung transplantation. J Thorac Cardiovasc Surg 1994;107:1476-1480.
60. Sheridan PH, Cheriyan A, Doud J, et al: Incidence of phrenic neuropathy after isolated lung transplantation. J Heart Lung Transplant 1995;14:684-691.
61. Snell GI, de Hoyos A, Krajden M, et al: *Pseudomonas cepacia* in lung transplant recipients with cystic fibrosis. Chest 1993;103:466-471.
62. Starnes VA, Barr ML, Cohen RG: Lobar transplantation: Indications, technique, and outcome. J Thorac Cardiovasc Surg 1994;108:403-411.
63. Stepkowski SM, Chen H, Daloze P, Kahan BD: Rapamycin, a potent immunosuppressive drug for vascularized heart, kidney and small bowel transplantation in the rat. Transplantation 1991;51:22-26.

64. Sundaresan S, Trulock EP, Mohanakumar T, et al: Prevalence and outcome of bronchiolitis syndrome after lung transplantation. Ann Thorac Surg 1995;60: 1341-1346.
65. Sweet SC, Spray TL, Huddleston CB, et al: Pediatric lung transplantation at St. Louis Children's Hospital 1990-1995. Am J Respir Crit Care Med 1997;155:1027-1035.
66. Swinnen LJ, Mullen GM, Carr TJ, et al: Aggressive treatment for postcardiac transplant lymphoproliferation. Blood 1995;86:3333-3340.
67. Trulock EP, Edwards LB, Taylor DO, et al: The Registry of the International Society for Heart and Lung Transplantation: Twentieth official adult lung and heart-lung transplant report—2003. J Heart Lung Transplant 2003;22: 625-635.
68. Walker RC, Paya CV, Marshall WF, et al: Pretransplantation sero-negative Epstein-Barr virus status is the primary risk factor for post-transplantation lymphoproliferative disease in adult heart, lung and other solid organ transplantation. J Heart Lung Transplant 1995;14:214-221.
69. Woo MS, MacLaughlin EF, Horn MV, et al: Bronchiolitis obliterans is not the primary cause of death in pediatric living donor lobar lung transplant recipients. J Heart Lung Transplant 2001;20:491-496.
70. Wood NS, Marlow N, Costeloe K, et al: Neurologic and developmental disability after extremely preterm birth. N Engl J Med 2000;343:378-384.
71. Wood P: The Eisenmenger syndrome or pulmonary hypertension with reversed central shunt. BMJ 1958;2:701-762.

第 49 章

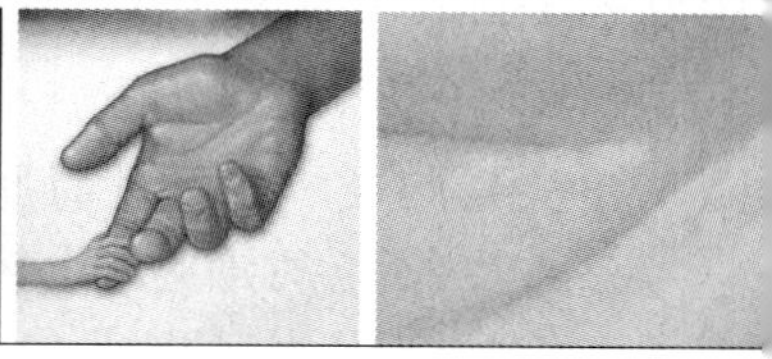

骨髓移植相关的外科并发症

Paul M. Colombani 和 Mark L. Kayton

79 骨髓移植(BMT)现在被用于治疗许多儿童疾病，包括血液系统恶性肿瘤、实体瘤、和免疫性疾病。小儿外科医生常被叫去以提供血管通道及解决BMT患者发生的并发症。儿外科医生了解与BMT的病程、适应证和可能出现的问题能使小儿外科医生在日益增多的患者的医疗处理中发挥重要的作用。

术语“*骨髓移植*”包含所有各种目前所用的重建造血干细胞的方法，但实际上，干细胞来源可以是脐带血、外周血干细胞或骨髓本身[25]。细胞可以是自体的（当患者病情缓解时收集）或异体的（例如来源于亲属，其人类白细胞抗原（HLA）相合者）。移植的受体接受化疗加 / 不加全身放疗作为预处理方案，目的是清除血液的恶性肿瘤及造血祖细胞，这样就为应用供体细胞进行血液重建铺平道路。免疫抑制方案以及预防方案是用来消除移植物抗宿主病（GVHD）。就像预期的一样，这个过程中的任何一个阶段的并发症，包括细胞采集、免疫系统清除、免疫抑制或GVHD都常规需要小儿外科医生的介入。

干细胞采集和血管通路问题

在我们的医疗机构中，当需要建立一次性静脉通路来采集血液细胞时，我们在腹股沟或颈部使用各种临时性管道，但我们正越来越多的放置带套囊的双腔锁骨下静脉管（8 F Medcomp 导管用于儿童，13.5 F Hickmen 导管用于青少年），它能用于采集，然后可以长期放置用于中心静脉通路。

BMT患者可能还需要临时性的通路用于透析或血液过滤。例如，在明尼苏达大学，在12年间有5%的儿童BMT患者因急性肾衰竭需要透析[13]。在BMT受体发生肾功能不全与环孢霉素A、两性霉素B和全身放疗的应用有关[33]。

在重症监护病房（ICU）中可能需要紧急建立血管通路。为了改善急性呼吸窘迫综合征患儿的疗效，斯坦福大学的研究组对出现急性呼吸窘迫综合征（ARDS）的10例儿童肿瘤患者，在插管后进行了早期持续静脉–静脉血液过滤（CVVH）治疗[4]。其中的6例做过BMT。8例（80%）患者存活；虽然没有对照组，该存活率与文献报道的存在显著差异。例如，Great Ormond Street 医院对BMT患者做的回顾性研究发现在出现呼吸衰竭的BMT患者中只有40%存活[10]。如果这种早期CVVH能够更广泛的应用，则对外科医生建立血管通路的需求将增加。

可能还会出现更奇怪的建立血管通路的需求。费城儿童医院的Leahey和同事提供了一个关于BMT后3天使用体外膜肺（ECMO）的病例报道[15]。该患儿是一个年龄8个月的联合免疫缺陷综合征（SCID）女孩，因呼吸道合胞病毒和A型流感病毒感染出现毛细支气管炎，她在使用了15天的ECMO和经受一次打击后，来源于她的一个HLA相合同胞的骨髓成功植入，恢复了足够数量的淋巴细胞来对抗感染。她后来存活并出院了。

免疫系统清除和免疫抑制的并发症 780

肠道并发症

出现腹泻、腹痛的BMT受体患儿的鉴别诊断必须包括GVHD、继发于药物治疗的黏膜炎、细菌性胃肠炎、病毒性胃肠炎（包括腺病毒、轮状病毒和巨细胞病毒）、难辨梭状芽胞杆菌感染和阿米巴病。因为其中部分病因在儿外科少见，故需要仔细鉴别。

特别是考虑到消化道 GVHD 将经常需要立即请儿外科医生会诊以获得上或下消化道的活检，处理随后可能发生的并发症。上消化道的活检可以在内镜检查食管、胃或十二指肠时获得。Ramakrishna 和 Treem 的报道[23]建议，在血小板减少患者慎做十二指肠活检，他们在 2 例骨髓移植患儿中发现十二指肠血肿，其血小板计数分别是 55 000/mm^3 和 65 000/mm^3 [23]。然而，胃和十二指肠仍然是活检的重要部位，我们已经通过直肠针吸活检枪收集的直肠标本成功地诊断了 GVHD，该技术可以在病房中无需镇静即可操作，避免了到手术室进行全麻。

在已经出现 GVHD 损害的肠道中，可能要注意意想不到的病理过程。例如，智利在两例并发 GVHD 接受皮质类固醇治疗后已获得部分缓解的患者中发现了痢疾阿米巴滋养体[21]。在一个相似的肠道 GVHD 患者中发现腺病毒小肠结肠炎[27]。

艰难梭状芽胞杆菌结肠炎在该类患儿中能有惊人的临床表现。有个案报道描述了在一个 13 岁的 BMT 受体出现的艰难梭状芽胞杆菌结肠炎，在降结肠部位出现梗阻性的结肠炎后狭窄，需要做横结肠造口术[12]。

虽然很少见，但盲肠炎（中性粒细胞减少性肠病）确实在 BMT 受体中发生过（图 49–1）。临床上，盲肠炎表现为发热、腹痛或触痛，以及中性粒细胞减少[9]。Hobson 和同事发现在盲肠炎患者中经常能观察到腹泻[9]。在加拿大 Alberta 做的一项回顾性研究中，142 例 BMT 患者中的 5 例出现盲肠炎。他们均接受了禁食、肠道外营养和广谱抗生素治疗（包括全身性的抗真菌药物），最后均存活并出院。这与成人盲肠炎的经典外科学说惊人的相反，后者的死亡率达 50%。盲肠炎预后的改善反映了早期诊断、积极使用粒细胞集落刺激因子、更好的使用抗生素或所有这些因素的重要性。令人惊讶的是并不是所有患者需要做 CT 检查来确诊盲肠炎。5 例患者中的 1 例患者通过腹部平片、2 例患者通过超声检查作出诊断[1]。盲肠炎患儿的 CT 中可见盲肠壁的异常增厚以及周围炎症性改变。

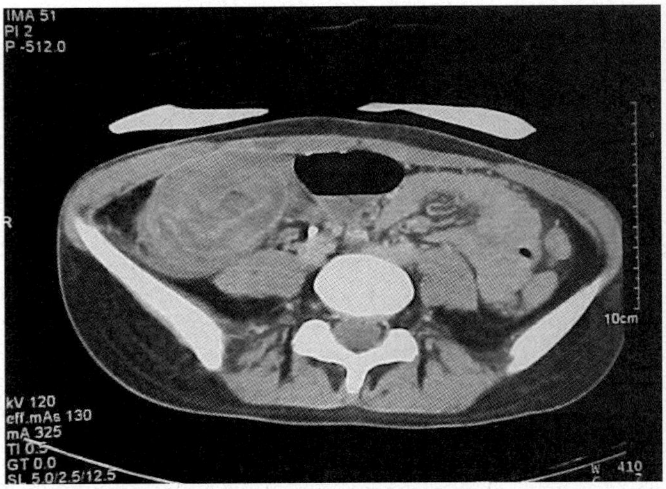

图 49–1　1 例因急性粒细胞性白血病而做 BMT 的少年发生盲肠炎。注意盲肠壁增厚的、葱皮样表现和微小的内腔。该患儿经过右半结肠切除术加回肠造口术和黏膜瘘管成形术；1 年后，仍然处于白血病缓解，她的病情被成功控制。大多数盲肠炎做非手术性治疗。

肝胆问题

肝功能异常在 BMT 患者中常见，经常需要请外科医生鉴别梗阻性黄疸和肝细胞性黄疸。Safford 和同事已经分析了 BMT 患儿中胆结石的发生率和病史的回顾性资料[24]。在接受移植后超声检查的 235 例患儿中，20 例（8.5%）有胆结石。将这些患儿根据移植病因进行分组，Safford 和同事发现在因为肿瘤、遗传性代谢异常、或免疫疾病接受移植的患儿中 7% 出现胆结石，而因为各种贫血和原发骨髓异常接受移植的患儿中 27%出现胆结石，这表明溶血等因素导致胆石症在后者中更多见。但是在 20 例有胆结石的 BMT 受体中，只有 3 例需要手术干预（平均在诊断胆石症 1.9 年后），而 5 例在超声上发现胆结石溶解（平均在诊断胆结石后 150 天）。虽然这不是一个前瞻性的研究，但它能给外科医生一些提示，不必急着试图切除无症状性胆结石的胆囊。

另一个影响 BMT 患者肝脏的令人烦恼的问题是肝静脉闭塞病。这是指 BMT 后第一个月内经常出现的一个综合征，这可能是移植时的清髓和预处理治疗方案的毒性反应。 78

肝静脉闭塞病的特征是肝窦和小静脉的充血和纤

维变性闭塞。3 区肝细胞和内皮细胞的损伤被认为是诱发原因。高凝状态和细胞因子（如肿瘤坏死因子-α）的释放也可能发挥作用[29]。

根据 McDonald 的诊断标准[18]，在 BMT 后不久出现以下三项中的任何两项时即可做出临床诊断：（1）出现腹水，同时体重增加 2%；（2）肝大或右上腹触痛；（3）血清总胆红素超过 2mg/dl。预防性使用肝素来改善该病未获得令人信服的结果。虽然没有做有效的对照性研究，但仍有报道的一些其他方法，包括与肝素联用的组织纤溶酶原激活剂[14]，以及一个儿童案例报道的做肝脏移植[3]。

静脉闭塞病也出现于肺，可以表现出肺高压，这在几乎所有病例中都是致命的[32]。心彩超能够作出诊断，但不幸的是大多数病例都是通过尸检获得诊断，也有部分通过肺活检诊断。

肺部并发症

比静脉闭塞病更常见的许多病情能通过肺活检获得诊断。感染的病源包括细菌、病毒、真菌、军团菌、分枝杆菌和肺囊虫。在病毒感染中，巨细胞病毒、呼吸道合胞病毒、腺病毒和疱疹病毒较为多见。非感染性疾病包括出血、恶性肿瘤、药物毒性和间质性肺炎，最后一项指观察到炎症反应但病源微生物培养阴性的肺炎[30]。最后，亦可见到闭塞性细支气管机化的肺炎（BOOP），这是呼吸道末端肉芽组织沉积的皮质类固醇敏感限制性肺病[16]。

肺活检在 BMT 中心常见。关于他们对预后的影响存在激烈的讨论。Shorter 和同事重新评估了 1976～1986 年间费城儿童医院的资料，发现尽管做了肺活检，21 例中的 13 例患儿仍持续恶化并在 11 周内死亡，只有 2 例指导治疗做明显改变使患儿存活[28]。Dunn 和同事[5]统计了 15 例干细胞移植受体。在活检时需要机械通气的 9 例患者中有 8 例死亡。15 例中根据活检结果改变治疗的只有 1 例。Hayes-Jordan 和同事在最近做的一个回顾性研究再次有以下一些发现：大部分（19 例中的 7 例，37%）在肺活检后 30 天内死亡，只有 3 例改变了治疗从而长期生存[8]。

能够通过开放肺活检获得更多益处的一组患者是曲霉菌病患者，如果病变区域能被完全切除的话。St. Jude 研究组报导 43 例曲霉菌病患者中的 27 例做了 BMT[6]。与未做切除的患儿相比，那些将累及的所有肺实质切除的患儿存活方面明显受益。这不是随机或前瞻性的研究，所有 4 例存活的患儿（随访期从 1.7 到 43 个月）均有需要做楔形切除的指征，其中 1 例做肺叶切除。然而，肺曲霉菌病在免疫抑制患儿中基本上是 100%致死。这意味着在这些病例中考虑做手术切除是合理的。

软组织并发症

皮肤和深部软组织感染包括坏死性筋膜炎、坏死性肌炎和皮肤毛霉菌感染可以发生于 BMT 患者，特别是在中心粒细胞低下的时候。一些案例报导描述了中心粒细胞低下的肿瘤患儿软组织感染，其中包括了一些移植受体[11, 19]。值得注意的是，肠道微生物——包括埃希氏菌、假单胞菌和肠球菌——出现于 BMT 受体的分泌物培养中。据推测系细菌从胃肠道移位，从而导致血源性播散的结果。与之相反的传统假设则认为软组织感染源于皮肤屏障破坏后在软组织中生存的革兰阳性菌或厌氧菌引起的。在 BMT 人群中，需要用广谱抗生素，包括那些对革兰阴性菌有效的药物。BMT 人群的手术清创与其他患者一样需要紧急处理，如果清髓已经耗尽所有血小板则手术会变得更具挑战性。在中性粒细胞低下患者中需考虑用粒细胞集落刺激因子和粒细胞输注。Johnston 和同事[11]认为发热、心动过速以及剧烈局限性的疼痛是有用的诊断性特征和症状。如果诊断不能确定，在时间和患者临床条件允许时做 MRI 检查可能会有帮助。

在任何皮肤和软组织感染时，皮肤毛霉菌感染必须在鉴别诊断时考虑到。这种真菌感染与细菌性软组织感染一样，通常需要做早期清创。在年轻 BMT 受体中，皮肤毛霉菌感染可表现为触痛性硬结，并能发展为坏死。显微镜检查侵犯的软组织和血管时可发现菌丝[20, 31]。

出血性膀胱炎

膀胱上皮的出血对 BMT 受体可能是一个严重的

临床问题。出血性膀胱炎可能与预处理化疗方案（如环磷酰胺和马利兰）的毒性[26]或者病毒感染有关。782 临床表现从镜下血尿到肉眼血尿（血凝块可导致膀胱出口阻塞）都有。超声显示膀胱壁增厚；彩色多普勒可以发现局部充血和活动性出血，常需要膀胱镜检查以确诊[17]。根据临床上出血性膀胱炎的严重性，患者可以通过静脉水化以强制利尿、使用 Foley 管导尿来进行持续膀胱冲洗、或用膀胱镜清除血凝块和电灼膀胱上皮治疗。幼儿的尿道可能无法通过足够粗的 Foley导管来阻止血凝块重新阻塞尿道。这些患儿可能需要通过手术在耻骨联合上放置大的导管[34]。

血小板减少症

难治性的血小板减少症可以在 BMT 后出现，并常常需要考虑短时间内行脾脏切除。血小板减少症可能与药物治疗、骨髓巨核细胞生成下降、或血小板滞留在脾脏内相关。然而，血小板可能滞留于其他部位，故脾脏切除并不是对所有血小板滞留患者中有用。Hammersmith 和同事报道了用一种核医学技术来确认脾脏内是否有血小板滞留，这能用来决定是否需做脾脏切除术[7]。血小板用铟-111 标记后输注；血小板在脾脏的滞留能通过输注后不同时间点脾脏和肝脏同位素标记密度的比值来证实。脾肝比值大于 1.9 提示脾脏异常滞留。然而该项技术还未能得到广泛应用，而且没有资料表明是否阳性扫描预示着脾脏切除后预后良好。因此，临床上考虑难治性血小板减少症的处理仍然需要根据经验来决定是否做脾脏切除。

罕见问题

急性化脓性甲状腺炎已经有个案报道，见于 1 例做二次 BMT 的慢性粒单细胞性白血病的 3 岁患儿[22]。虽然患儿接受全身放疗，该项治疗意味着将引起甲状腺功能障碍，但他在移植后不久出现了甲状腺肿胀和甲状腺功能减退。在此病例中，作者认为疾病与放疗无关。超声显示在甲状腺中出现“半透明”区，需要手术引流脓性分泌物。

输血并发症

因为外科医生和手术室成员经常需要在围术期输血，所以重要的是要记住输血本身能引起 GVHD。过客 T 淋巴细胞能污染红细胞、血浆或血小板制品，从而介导针对免疫抑制 BMT 受体的免疫反应。输血相关的 GVHD 表现为皮疹、肝功能异常、全血细胞减少，以及 84%受累患者死亡[2]。两项技术——白细胞过滤和血制品照射——分别用于减少血制品中的白细胞负荷和使白细胞失活。因此，BMT 患者的血制品必须同时做白细胞过滤和照射。

慢性 GVHD

慢性 GVHD 的特征是全身皮肤和软组织结构的硬化症和胆汁郁积性黄疸。甚至在一个 13 岁的晚期男孩中因继发性包茎而需做包皮环切术。

结论

鉴于 BMT 的发展传统上属于内科、儿科和肿瘤科专业，本章突出讨论 BMT 后许多器官系统表现出的外科的病理过程。肺、消化道、肝脏、脾脏、膀胱、软组织和血液系统都与各种外科并发症相关。此外，实际上每位 BMT 患者均需建立血管通路以用于用药、营养、透析或细胞采集。这些可能出现的 BMT 并发症表明每一个做儿童 BMT 的医院需配备儿外科医生。同时，儿外科医生必须训练和使得自己能向同事提供意见、与专家一起处理这些问题、以及为这个不断扩展的移植领域的发展作出贡献。

（叶启东译　王耀平校）

参考文献

1. Al Otaibi A, Barker C, Anderson R, et al: Neutropenic enterocolitis (typhlitis) after pediatric bone marrow transplant. J Pediatr Surg 2002;37:770-772.
2. Anderson KC, Weinstein HJ: Transfusion-associated graft-versus-host disease. N Engl J Med 1990;323:315-321.
3. Bunin N, Leahey A, Dunn S: Related donor liver transplant for veno-occlusive disease following T-depleted unrelated donor bone marrow transplantation. Transplantation 1996; 61:664-666.
4. DiCarlo JV, Alexander SR, Agarwal R, et al: Continuous veno-venous hemofiltration may improve survival from acute respiratory distress syndrome after bone marrow transplantation or chemotherapy. J Pediatr Hematol Oncol 2003;25:801-805.
5. Dunn JC, West KW, Resurla FJ, et al: The utility of lung biopsy in recipients of stem-cell transplantation. J Pediatr Surg 2001;36:1302-1303.
6. Gow KW, Hayes-Jordan AA, Billups CA, et al: Benefit of surgical resection of invasive pulmonary aspergillosis in pediatric patients undergoing treatment for malignancies and immunodeficiency syndromes. J Pediatr Surg 2003;38: 1354-1360.
7. Hammersmith SM, Jacobson AF, Mankoff DA: Scintigraphy with indium-111 labeled homologous (donor) platelets in the platelet transfusion refractory bone marrow transplant patient. J Nucl Med 1997;38:1135-1138.
8. Hayes-Jordan A, Benaim E, Richardson S, et al: Open lung biopsy in pediatric bone marrow transplant patients. J Pediatr Surg 2002;37:446-452.
9. Hobson MJ, Carney DE, Molik KA, et al: Appendicitis in childhood hematological malignancies: Analysis and comparison with typhlitis. J Pediatr Surg 2005;40:214-219; discussion 219-220.
10. Jacobe SJ, Hassan A, Veys P, et al: Outcome of children requiring admission to an intensive care unit after bone marrow transplantation. Crit Care Med 2003;31:1299-1305.
11. Johnston DL, Waldhausen JHT, Park JR: Deep soft tissue infections in the neutropenic pediatric oncology patient. J Pediatr Hematol Oncol 2001;23:443-447.
12. Kavan P, Sochor M, Nyc O, et al: Pseudomembranous *Clostridium* after autologous bone marrow transplantation. Bone Marrow Transplant 1998;21:521-523.
13. Lane PH, Mauer SM, Blazar BR, et al: Outcome of dialysis for acute renal failure in pediatric bone marrow transplant patients. Bone Marrow Transplant 1994;13:613-617.
14. Leahey AM, Bunin NJ: Recombinant human tissue plasminogen activator for the treatment of severe hepatic veno-occlusive disease in pediatric bone marrow transplant patients. Bone Marrow Transplant 1996;17:1101-1104.
15. Leahey AM, Bunin NJ, Schears GJ, et al: Successful use of extracorporeal membrane oxygenation (ECMO) during BMT for SCID. Bone Marrow Transplant 1998;21:839-840.
16. Mathew P, Bozeman P, Krance RA, et al: Bronchiolitis obliterans organizing pneumonia (BOOP) in children after allogeneic bone marrow transplantation. Bone Marrow Transplant 1994;13:221-223.
17. McCarville MB, Hoffer FA, Gingrich JR, et al: Imaging findings of hemorrhagic cystitis in pediatric oncology patients. Pediatr Radiol 2000;30:131-138.
18. McDonald GB, Sharma P, Matthews DE, et al: Veno-occlusive disease of the liver after bone marrow transplantation: Diagnosis, incidence, and predisposing factors. Hepatology 1984;4:116-122.
19. Murphy JJ, Granger R, Blair GK, et al: Necrotizing fasciitis in childhood. J Pediatr Surg 1995;30:1131-1134.
20. Nomura J, Ruskin J, Sahebi F, et al: Mucormycosis of the vulva following bone marrow transplantation. Bone Marrow Transplant 1997;19:859-860.
21. Perret C, Harris PR, Rivera M, et al: Refractory enteric amebiasis in pediatric patients with acute graft-versus-host disease after allogeneic bone marrow transplantation. J Pediatr Gastroenterol Nutr 2000;31:86-90.
22. Poelman M, Benoit Y, Laureys G, et al: Acute suppurative thyroiditis complicating second allogeneic transplant for juvenile CMML. Bone Marrow Transplant 1992;10: 547-548.
23. Ramakrishna J, Treem WR: Duodenal hematoma as a complication of endoscopic biopsy in pediatric bone marrow transplant recipients. J Pediatr Gastroenterol Nutr 1997; 25:426-429.
24. Safford SD, Safford KM, Martin P, et al: Management of cholelithiasis in pediatric patients who undergo bone marrow transplantation. J Pediatr Surg 2001;36:86-90.
25. Sanders JE: Bone marrow transplantation for pediatric malignancies. Pediatr Clin North Am 1997;44:1005-1020.
26. Seber A, Shu XO, Defor T, et al: Risk factors for hemorrhagic cystitis following BMT. Bone Marrow Transplant 1999;23:35-40.
27. Shayan K, Saunders F, Roberts E, et al: Adenovirus enterocolitis in pediatric patients following bone marrow transplantation. Arch Pathol Lab Med 2003;127: 1615-1618.
28. Shorter NA, Ross AJ III, August C, et al: The usefulness of open-lung biopsy in the pediatric bone marrow transplant population. J Pediatr Surg 1988;23:533-537.
29. Shulman HM, Hinterberger W: Hepatic veno-occlusive disease—liver toxicity syndrome after bone marrow transplantation. Bone Marrow Transplant 1992;10:197-214.
30. Stokes DC: Pulmonary complications of tissue transplantation in children. Curr Opin Pediatr 1994;6:272-279.
31. Trigg ME, Comito MA, Rumelhart SL: Cutaneous *Mucor* infection treated with wide excision in two children who underwent marrow transplantation. J Pediatr Surg 1996; 31:976-977.
32. Trobaugh-Lotrario AD, Greffe B, Deterding R, et al: Pulmonary veno-occlusive disease after autologous bone marrow transplant in a child with stage IV neuroblastoma: Case report and literature review. J Pediatr Hematol Oncol 2003;25:405-409.
33. Van Why SK, Friedman AL, Wei LJ, et al: Renal insufficiency after bone marrow transplantation in children. Bone Marrow Transplant 1991;7:383-388.
34. Vogeli TA, Peinemann F, Burdach S, et al: Urological treatment and clinical course of BK polyomavirus-associated hemorrhagic cystitis in children after bone marrow transplantation. Eur Urol 1999;36:252-257.

第五部分

头　颈　部

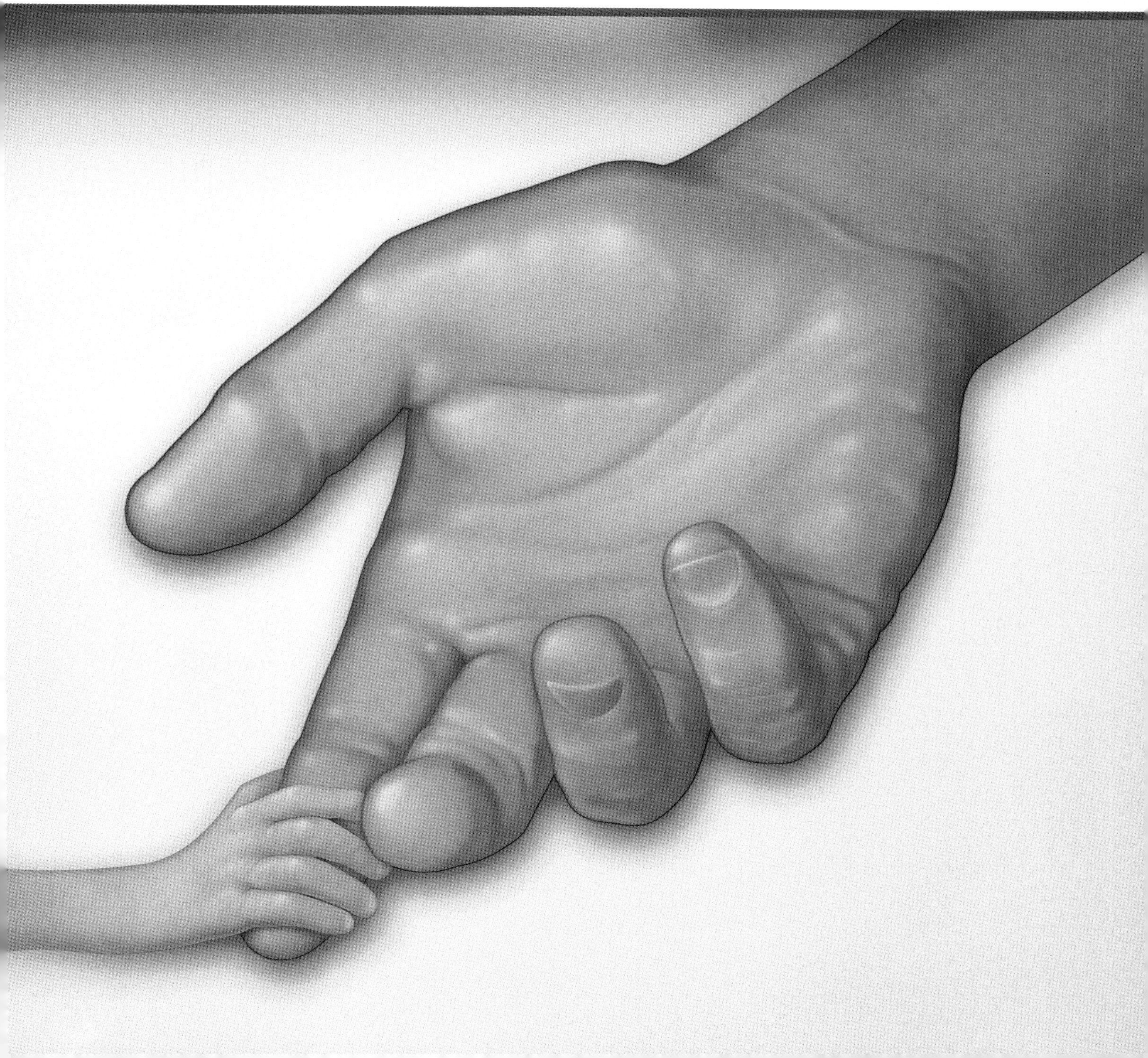

第 50 章

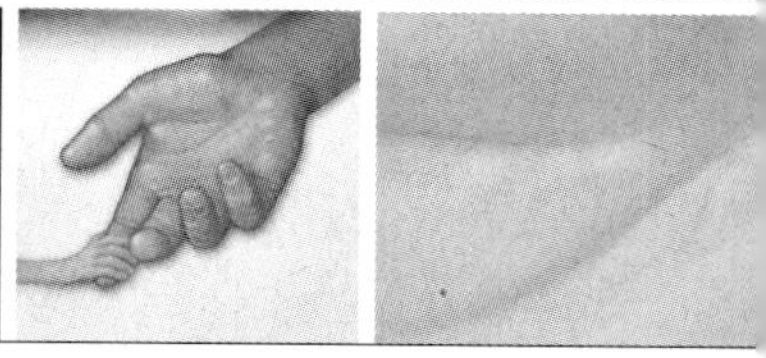

颅面部畸形

Henry K. Kawamoto, Jr.

787 颅面部畸形发生时是破坏性的。初次看到会留下持久的印象且照顾时会产生困惑。有些畸形比较常见，如唇腭裂，还有一些非常罕见，一个临床医生在其职业生涯中可能一例也碰不到。尽管如此，颅面部畸形儿童总数还是巨大的。

提及颅面外科这个名词，就会自然提到它的创始者 Paul L. Tessier。20 世纪 60 年代末期，当他们初期工作的消息传开时，只有诸如绷带包扎那样的技术可以用于纠正这些畸形[54]。Tessier 和他同事们通过充分暴露歪曲的颅面部骨骼，用截开术恢复解剖学上的排列，用自生组织取代缺失部分，提供稳定的固定，以及必要时采用颅内方法等进行解剖学纠正。抗生素的运用使传统意义上的避免污染的教条受到了挑战（如将无菌的颅内环境暴露于鼻、口腔污染的情况下）。这一新的专业并没有带来感染和其他不健康因素。

在以后的 25 年里，去巴黎学习 Tessier 医生的工作成了想精通这一领域技术的外科医生的必经途径。知识被迅速地传播开来。全世界范围内，现在大多数主要的医学中心都拥有颅面畸形治疗组，其成员包括麻醉医生、语音学医生、遗传学医生、神经外科医生、眼科医生、口腔颌面外科医生、正畸医生、耳鼻喉科医生、儿科医生、整形外科医生、放射科医生、社会工作者和语音病理学家。这些成员共同为复杂性畸形患者进行综合性治疗。

虽然颅面部畸形多种多样，但可以简单地分成两大类：（1）颅面部裂；（2）颅缝早闭。后者可再分为综合征型和非综合征畸形。所有的教科书都描述了这些畸形，还有些书详述了手术方法。但在手术时机和技术方面存在差异。以下是对一些畸形以及它们的整复方法的主要共同点的概述。由肿瘤和外伤引起的后天畸形和缺损也是这个领域里的一部分。但对于它们的讨论不在本章范围内。

颅面部手术的基本原则

儿童外表及面部的多种多样表情下隐藏着复杂的终末器官，可产生视力、嗅觉、听力、语言和咀嚼功能。颅面部畸形患儿在社会交往中存在严重障碍。他们应该得到专业人员的长期精心治疗，以满足他们各种复杂的需求。进行这类修复的外科医生必须经过特殊的训练，具有足够的经验，稍有疏忽就会永远毁掉复原的机会。

手术介入时机的选择，首先要考虑保存和恢复功能。满足这些要求后，就应关注使手术与面部生长发育及孩子的社会心理需求相协调。正常的个体解剖差异和畸形的完全异常发育都必须加以考虑。手术治疗通常以各区域结构的最终生长形态为标准。采用隐蔽切口到达畸形区域，通过不易察觉的冠状、眼睑和口内切口来充分暴露需要整复的颅面部骨骼（图 50-1）。如果可见的瘢痕不可避免，手术切口必须设计得与正常解剖特征相似或者落在符合美学观点的面部连接上。

必须使异常的面部骨骼尽可能恢复到接近正常。任何方案都一样，应先建立好的基础，其次是细节。因此，应首先重建面部骨骼的完整性。病变部分的解剖学重置是基础，要尽可能采用自生组织代替缺失部分。骨的重建用分离的颅骨是普遍选择，因为
后者接近于主要手术区域、吸收率低、发病率低且 788
与植骨区域的骨骼的胚胎起源相似。异质替代物很难取代自身组织，在生长性骨骼中的运用尤其应该避免。

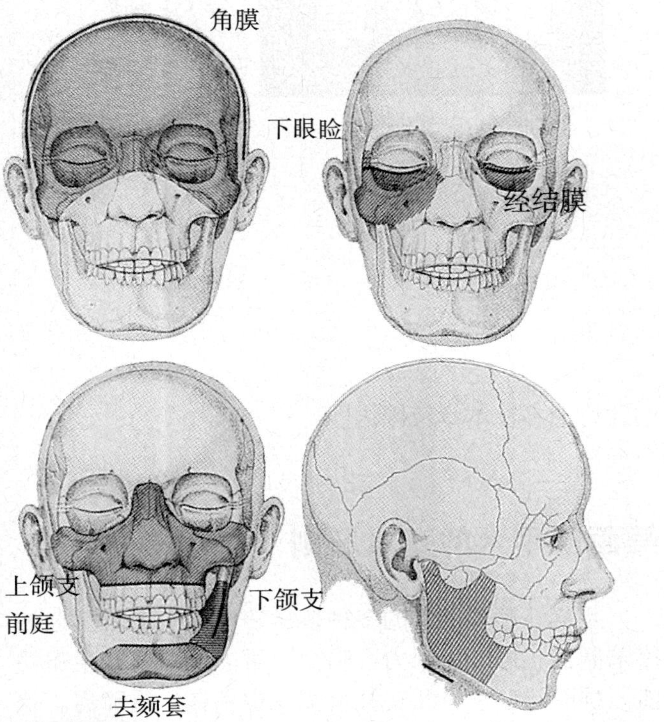

图 50-1 暴露颅面部骨骼的手术切口。阴影区表示每一种切口提供的暴露范围。

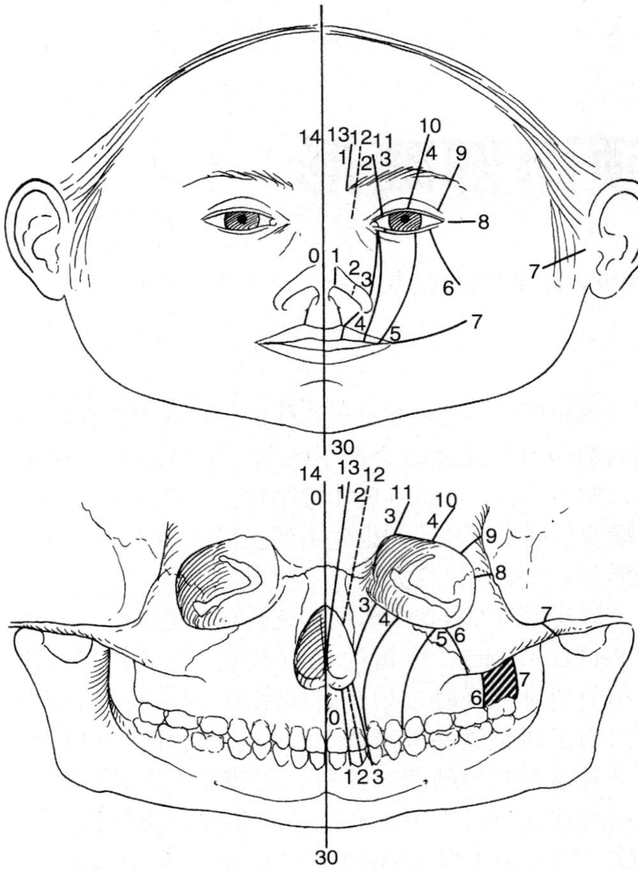

图 50-2 Tessier 分类。经线表示颅面裂的病理走向及其与面部解剖特征的关系。二者同时出现时，面裂（0～7 型）常随其对应的颅骨（9～4 型）沿相同经线顺延。

颅面部裂

颅面部裂第一眼看来令人困惑，同万花筒一样，稍稍改变一部分的表现，就是一种不同的畸形。改变更多，就会产生更奇异的改变或产生一种全新的类型。

各种各样的分类法尝试着把纷乱复杂的畸形表现进行归类，其中 Tessier 分类法[26,53]被广泛接受（图 50-2）。这个分类法的基础是来源于 Tessier 个人的临床观察。分类图上的线条促使人们去研究各种面部骨骼的潜在缺陷。颅面裂分类图中，第 8 型裂居于中纬线，0～7 型描绘了面裂，9～14 型描绘了 0～7 型裂的颅骨延伸裂。虽然裂缝可能只表现在颅部和面部的半球上，但是沿着子午线仔细地检查往往会有细微甚至重要发现。

一些颅面裂极其罕见，只有大量接触颅面裂患者的外科医生才会注意到，所以本章只关注常见的类型。

唇腭裂

详见第 51 章。

颅面部短小

颅面部短小也被称为第一和第二鳃弓综合征、半面短小和耳下颌骨发育不全。在 Tessier 分类中，描绘为 7 型裂（见图 50-2）。这种畸形最早记载于公元前 2000 年美索不达米亚占星术师记录的畸形学图表上[4]。1869 年[46]，Reissman 第一个用语言报告。颅面部短小的罹患率大约在 1/3000[42]和 1/5642[19]之间。

通常为单侧表现，不过有接近 10%为双侧累及，且表现不对称[10,48]。受影响的结构都起源于第一和第二鳃弓，常见起始于扩大的口联合（巨口）的凹槽，延伸至耳，路径有附耳（图 50-3），常发生外耳的部分缺损导致传导性听力丧失。下颌骨、颧骨和上颌骨的一部分发育不良（图 50-4）。下颌骨升支发育不全程度差异很大，从完全缺如到骨关节、下颌 789

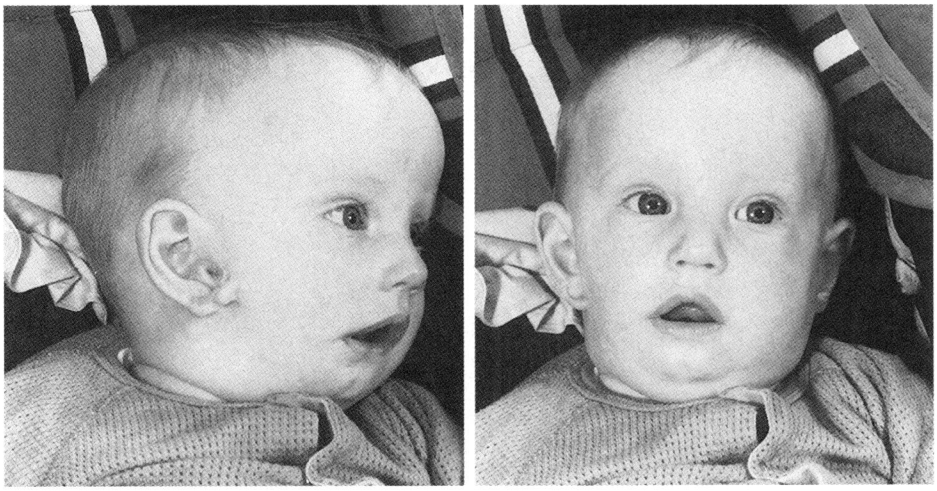

图 50-3　颅面部短小（Tessier 7 型裂）。注意横裂、附耳和走向小耳的浅沟。

支的小缺陷不等。

由于同样起源于第一和第二鳃弓，面部表情肌（Möbius 综合征）和咀嚼肌群也不同程度地累及。也可见腮腺发育不全或缺失。

根据畸形严重程度的不同，治疗亦不同。通常较大的裂隙需要尽早干预。用局部皮瓣修复巨口以及去除附耳通常在 1 岁内完成。对完全的下颌支缺失，可用肋软骨移植。在加州大学洛杉矶分校，我们在患者 6 岁时进行这个手术。用肋软骨重建外耳的手术也在这个年龄进行。下颌支尚存较多时，应用 Ilizarov 原则的牵拉骨生成术可延长已有的下颌骨或之前插入肋软骨移植物[33]。下颌支绝大部分存在时，颌面骨畸形的修复可以延期至青春期晚期，面部发育停止后。作为一个必要的准备步骤，上下颌的牙列要进行矫正，上颌骨做 LeFort 型截骨术，下颌骨做口内双侧下颌支劈开术（图 50-5）。所有的骨断片用具有生物相容性的微型片和钉固定。这样不需要进行颌间固定，极大地简化了术后过程。

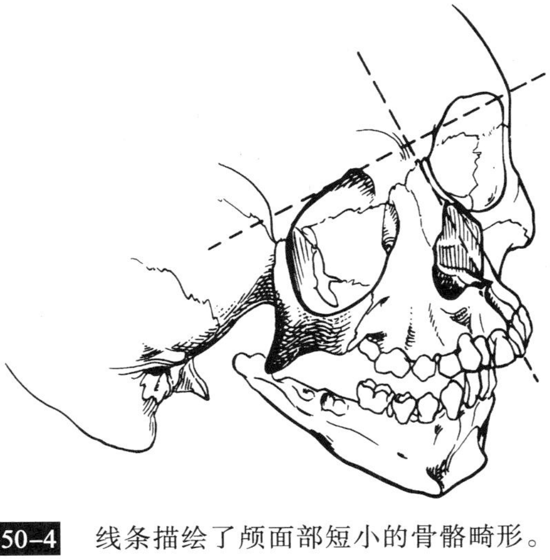

图 50-4　线条描绘了颅面部短小的骨骼畸形。下颌支、颧弓部分缺失，上颌骨发育不全。

Treacher Collins 综合征

Tessier 分类法第 6、7 和 8 型裂的混合形态表现为 Treacher Collins 畸形（见图 50-2）Tompson 在 1847 年最先报道了这种畸形[43]。在 Treacher Collins 记录了二例颧骨发育不全后[56]，Berry[6]第一个描述了眼睑的畸形，这种综合征也称为下颌面部骨发育不全。Rogers 综合了 200 个这一系列的病例[49]。

这类畸形的发生率大约是 1/10 000，遗传方式为常染色体显性遗传。有着较高但不确定的外显率和表达性。家族型畸形中明确了 TCOFI 基因的突变[12,13]。

临床上，畸形对称地累及双侧眼睑、耳颧骨、上颌骨和下颌骨（图 50-6）。睑裂呈反先天愚型样倾斜，下眼睑缺损，其内 2/3 无睫毛。颧骨发育不全，外观塌陷。有不同程度的小耳畸形，伴传导性 791
听力下降。耳前区的头发可向前覆盖至面颊部，上颌骨后端高度的缩短限制了鼻后孔和通过空气。下颌骨也同样存在着下颌骨支高度不足和下颌骨体长度不足。中间的角前切迹明显，颏部明显后移。

畸形的严重性决定了手术介入的时机。下颌后缩

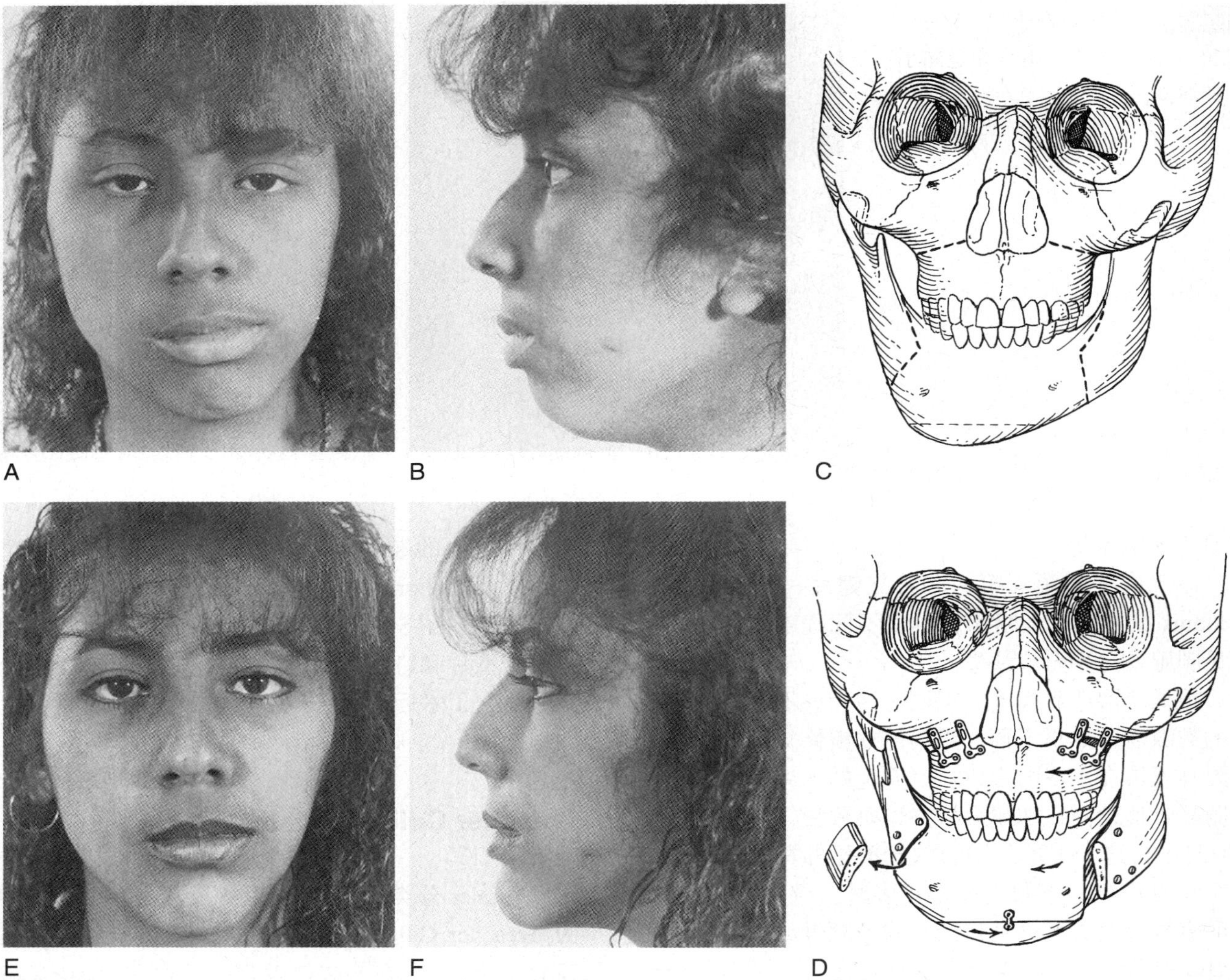

图 50–5 颅面部短小患者。A. 术前正面观。B. 侧面观显示下颌后缩。C. 线条描绘了 LeFort I（上颌）术，下颌支矢状劈开截骨术和颏成形术。D. 重置骨片和固定后的外观。E 和 F. 术后观。

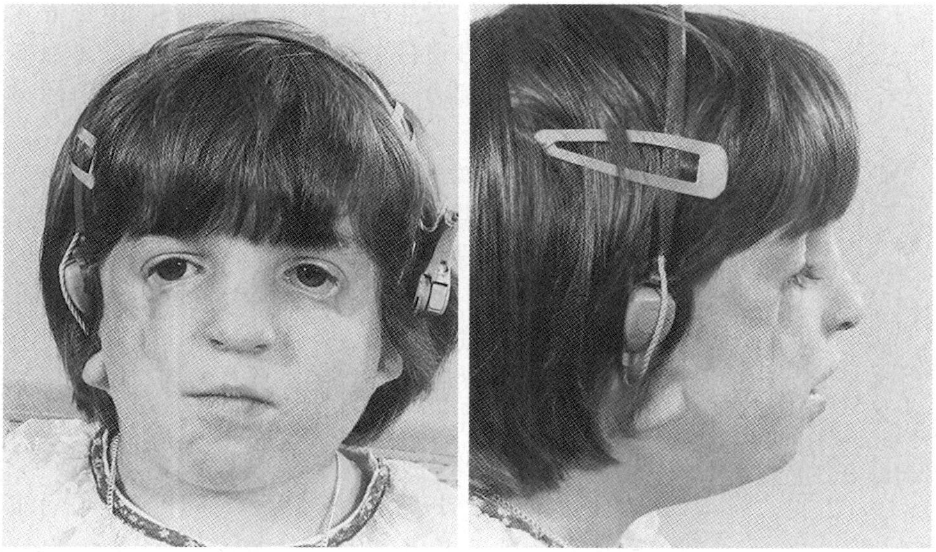

图 50–6 Treacher Collins 综合征患者。注意双侧睑裂呈反先天愚型样倾斜、颧骨突出缺失、小耳畸形和后缩的下颌骨和颏部。

甚至能危及气道畅通，必要时要行气管切开术。早期的牵拉骨生成技术能增大气道，避免气管造瘘或可及早拔除。

用肋软骨重建外耳通常在 6 岁左右开始，这时耳廓的发育已近成人的 95%。用异体移植物或外部假体来制作耳廓的方法较少采用。同期，用颅盖骨移植重建颧骨和眼眶，同时用局部皮瓣修整下眼睑缺损和睑裂的反先天愚型样倾斜。青春期末，运用同治疗颅面短小相似的技术处理上下颌骨畸形（图 50–7）。

颅裂

侧面的 9～14 型颅裂类型比较罕见。越接近中线，发生率越大。尽管如此，由于这类病例数量稀少，确切的发病率不明。 792

位于眼眶内侧的裂（11～14 型裂）增加了眶间距使眼眶移位，眶间距过大就这样产生了。本质上这是个特征，而不是综合征。出生缺陷和肿瘤侵犯眼眶能引起同样的畸形。眼眶内侧壁（泪点距离）常被用来测量眶间距。女性的正常距离是 25mm，13 岁时可达到，男性 21 岁时达到最大值 28mm[21]。

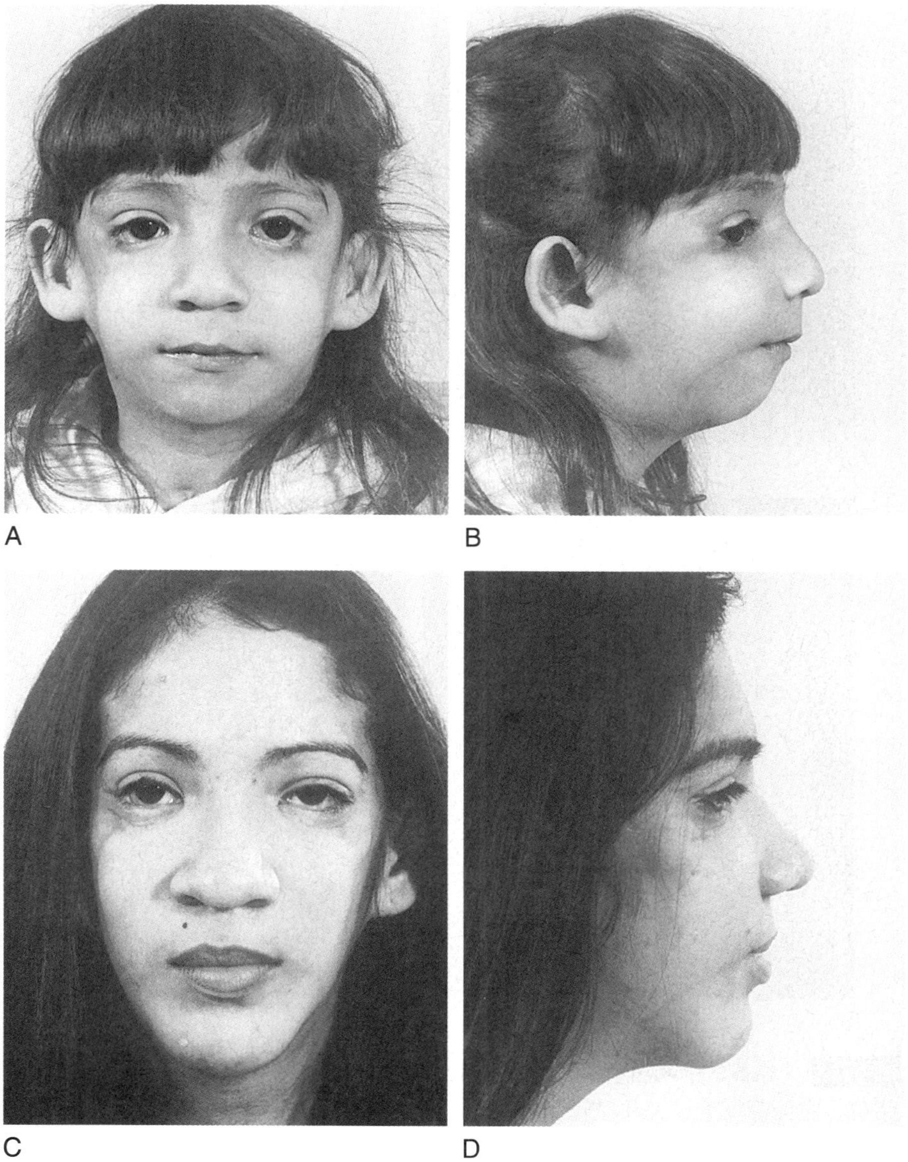

图 50–7　Treacher Collins 综合征患者。A 和 B. 术前外貌。C 和 D. 颧骨、眶侧缘、外眦、从上至下外侧皮瓣重建后的外观。

Tessier 把眶距过大分为三个等级：（1）30～34mm；（2）大于 34mm 但形态及眶位置正常；（3）大于 40mm[52]。根据分离程度选择颅外径路或颅外颅内联合径路，前者用于移位较小者。

择期手术纠治。没有证据显示早期的手术介入可预防弱视或改变视力。这样，手术治疗主要针对恢复正常的面部特征。大多数医疗机构认为 5～7 岁这个阶段最适合进行整复。患儿开始上学时，上部分脸也生长了大部分。还有一些医疗机构主张 2 岁时施行手术。对任何病例，复杂的畸形矫治最好由常规治疗此类患儿的专业组处理。偶尔治疗的外科生还不能做此类手术。

基本上需做颅内和颅外联合径路。由神经外科医生通过前颅骨切开术来暴露眼眶顶，由 Tessier[52,54]最先提出的传统的眶周盒形截骨术基本已被面中线二等分代替（图 50-8）[50]。

基本步骤包括，沿冠部和上颌骨前庭切口暴露颅面部骨骼（见图 50-1），进行前颅骨切开术，用传统的盒形截骨或面部双分技术游离眼眶，从鼻中线处去除多余的骨。合并眼眶骨体，关闭空隙，固定断骨，

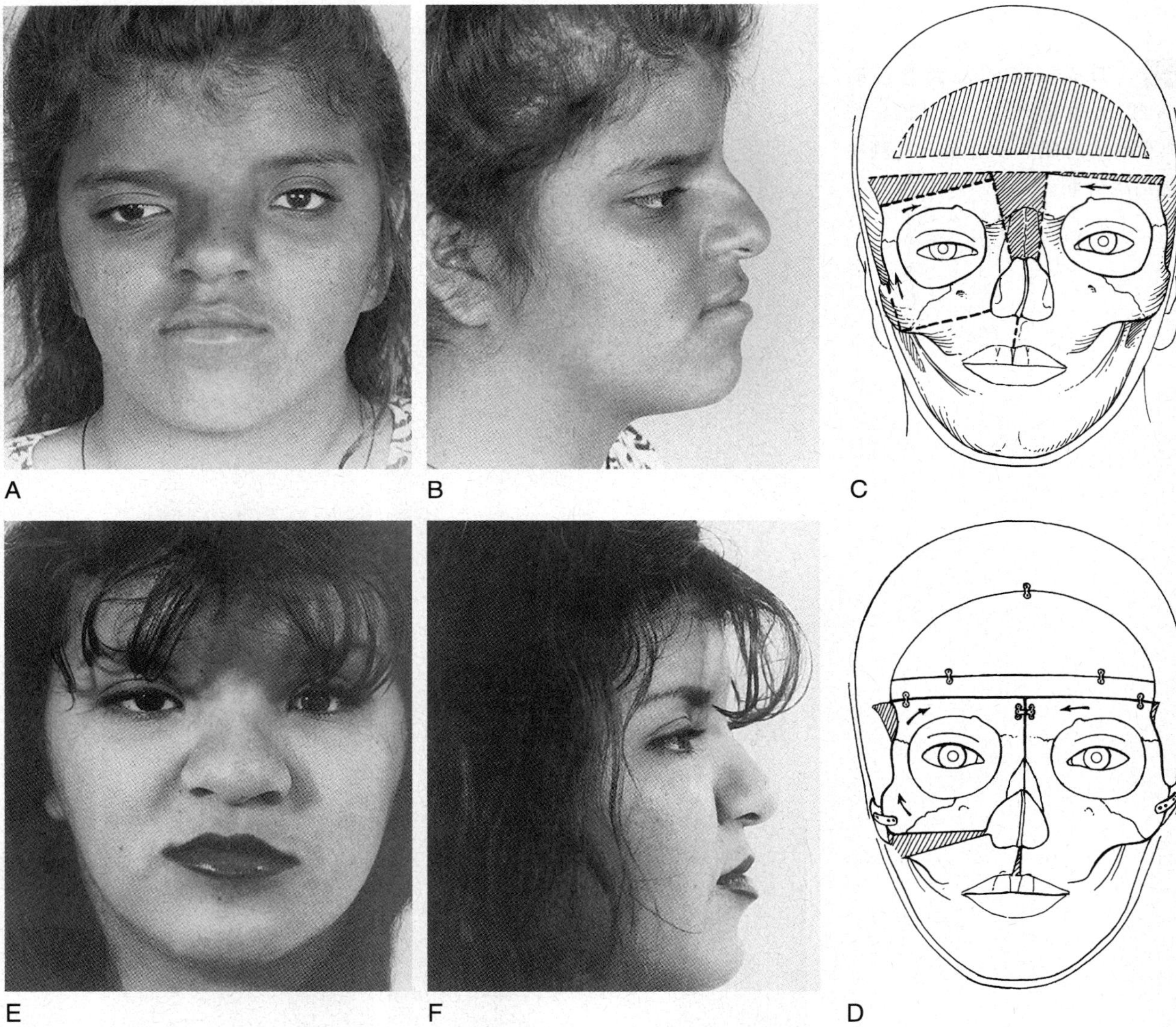

图 50-8 患者由于额鼻部发育异常和左侧冠状骨性连结导致不对称的眶距过大。A 和 B. 术前外观显示增大的眶距，眼眶错位，左面部高度过大和左侧前额平坦。C. 线条表示骨骼畸形和截骨术。D. 骨骼重建和固定断片。E 和 F. 术后外观。

关闭手术创口。如一切顺利，患儿在重症监护室观察
793 几天，通常大约一周就能出院。

颅缝早闭

出生后一年时间内，大脑体积增大超过 1 倍，重量达到成人的 60%[8]。若非颅顶骨缝的特殊性，大脑无法耐受密闭环境，在不断增加的颅内压下会产生不可逆的损伤。过去认为骨缝部位是主动生长的位置，会推开骨板。但进一步的研究显示，它们是被动生长的。为适应快速增大的大脑，硬脑膜表面的颅骨吸收时，骨在边缘及头盖处沉积[14,36]。

正常情况下，颅缝出生时很明显，到幼儿早期发展成易弯曲的纤维联合时允许颅骨持续生长。6 岁时颅骨达到了成人的 90%[8]，但骨缝完全的骨性闭合至少到 50 岁才会出现[31,32]。若骨缝关闭过早，垂直于闭合骨缝方向的颅骨生长停止，但平行于颅缝的平面上发生代偿性扩张（Virchow 法则）。头骨变形扭曲的结果取决于颅缝或关闭的颅缝。

颅缝早闭的两个亚类与遗传以及远期生长有关。一般而言，非综合征型畸形散发，而综合征型畸形有遗传因素。此外，手术整复后，非综合征型患者颅面部发育必定正常，而综合征型患者颅面部发育不良。

非综合征型颅缝早闭

非综合征型颅骨缝早闭的总发病率是 1/1000[7]，包括所有类型的单一颅缝闭锁。最常累及矢状缝，其次依次累及单侧冠状缝、额缝及人字缝。双侧冠状缝及多颅缝早闭也可发生。

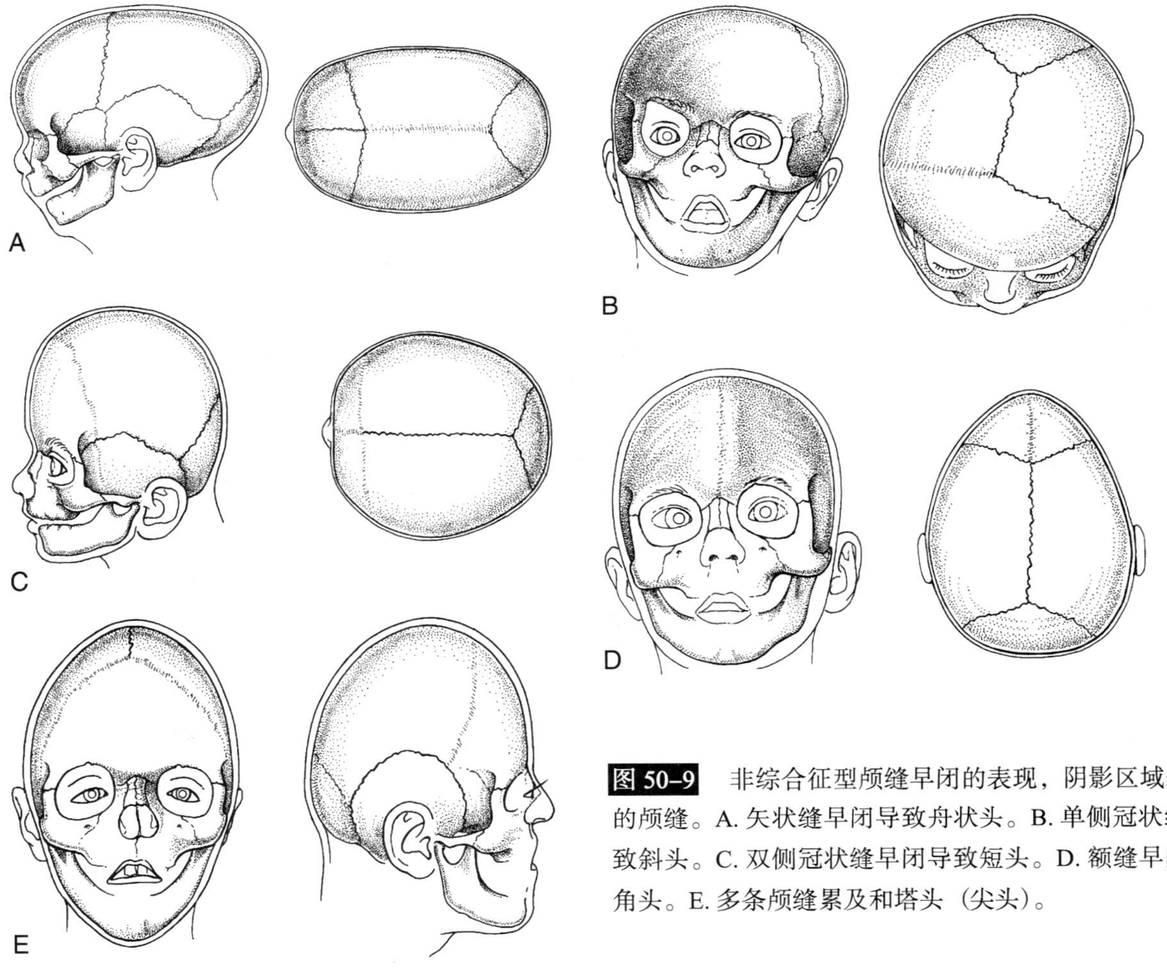

图 50–9　非综合征型颅缝早闭的表现，阴影区域表示早闭的颅缝。A. 矢状缝早闭导致舟状头。B. 单侧冠状缝早闭导致斜头。C. 双侧冠状缝早闭导致短头。D. 额缝早闭产生三角头。E. 多条颅缝累及和塔头（尖头）。

如使用颅缝闭合的特定名称描述头颅畸形，可减少混淆。以下这些名称已广泛得到认同：舟状头——矢状缝；斜头——单侧冠状缝；短头——双侧冠状缝；三角头——额缝；尖头或塔头——多颅缝（图50–9）。

由于颅骨的畸形特征及触摸颅缝闭合形成的骨嵴，大多数病例通过临床检查便能做出诊断。拍摄头颅X光片有助于确定临床诊断。在X光片上一条不
794 透明的线代替了光亮透明的颅缝。在单侧冠状缝早闭中，由于同侧蝶骨小翼抬高而表现为典型的小丑眼特征，在头颅正位片中可见。虽然CT检查对诊断不是很有帮助，通常不需要，除非要进行三维重建。

不能过分强调建立明确论断的重要性，颅面部骨骼畸形可以是次要的，肌性斜颈、颈椎畸形和睡姿均能产生位置性畸形。在这类情形下，颅缝是明显的。治疗应首先关注位置性畸形的原因，而不是头骨的歪曲。颅缝开放时，早期运用婴幼儿塑型头帽能恢复正常的头颅轮廓，但把它作为真正的颅缝早闭引起的颅骨扭曲进行治疗是错误的。

为减少婴儿猝死综合征的发生，美国儿科学会在1992年的6月推行一个“仰睡”计划[1]。所有的颅面部畸形治疗中心体检到的婴儿单侧或双侧枕骨畸形数量已大大增加[3,57]。这些位置性畸形有时被误诊，当X片不能证明颅缝不透明时就被认为是颅缝粘连。故

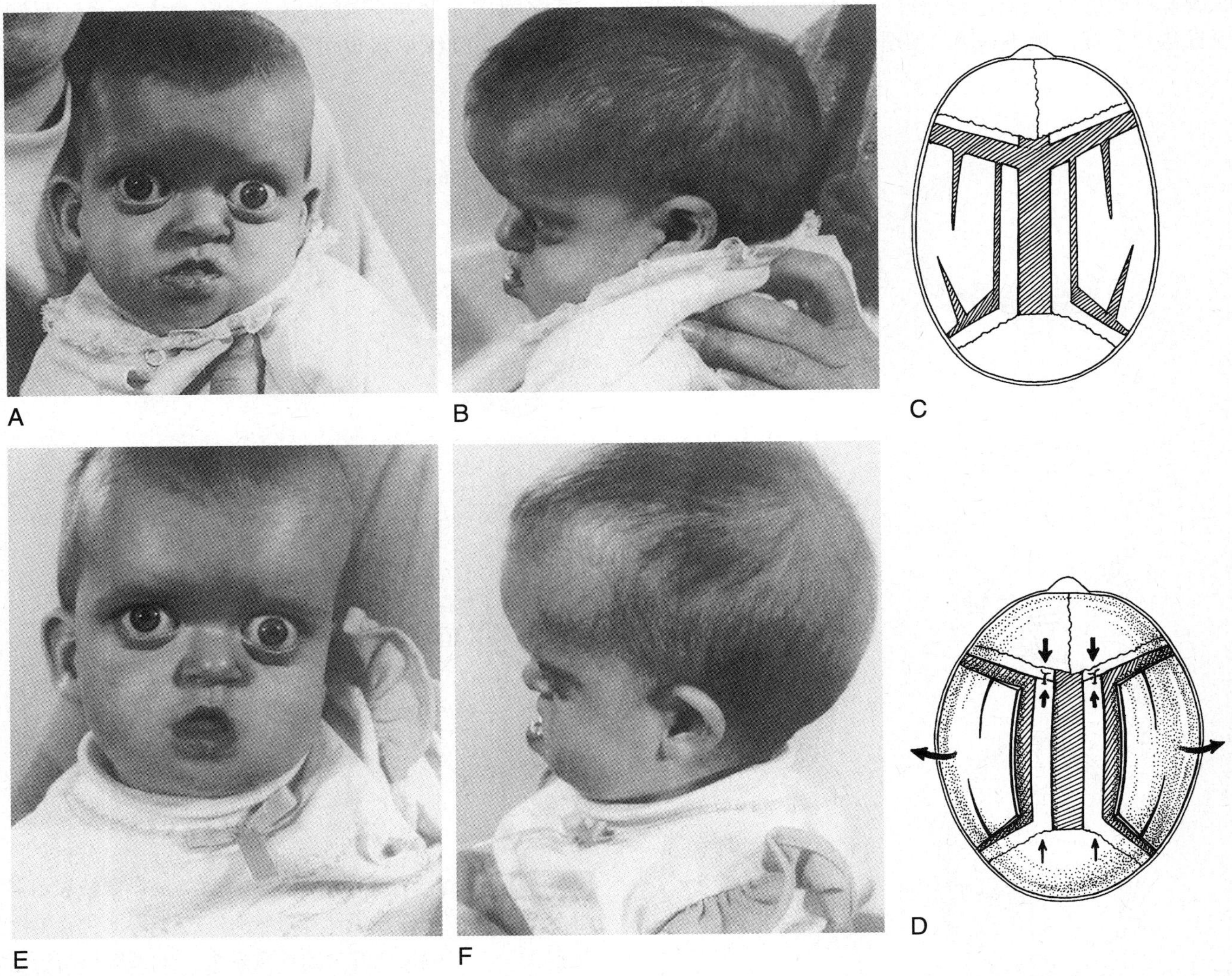

图 50–10 矢状缝早闭患儿（舟状头）。A和B.术前外貌，显示头颅前后径增加，双侧宽度减小，耳朵位置靠前，后方距离增大。C.π形截骨术的图示，阴影区表示切除区域。D.缩短前后径尺寸和将颞顶骨片向外移位。E和F.术后观。

进行不必要的后颅重建被施行，而如果观察到了鉴别性的临床特征，这完全是可以避免的。从头顶看，位置性的后方斜头畸形，头盖倾斜，患侧耳朵被推向前方，远离变平的后侧。相反，真性的单侧人字缝早闭表现为梯形畸形，畸形侧耳朵向缺陷的颅缝移位[20]。幸运的是，对畸形的意识的加强已极大地减少了位置性畸形的手术，几乎为零。

因为严重的畸形反映在面部，非综合征型颅缝早闭必须整复。其他原因在于可能引起功能方面的障
795 碍，都与颅内压增高有关。Renier 和他的同事发现，13%的单颅缝早闭婴儿颅内压增高，累及多颅缝的可达 42%[47]。可发生视觉损伤，但单颅缝早闭时非常罕见[35]。高颅内压是否与发育迟缓有关一直有争论。有的研究显示有联系[47]，有的则认为没有[29]。

在颅面部手术时代之前，传统的治疗方法是对病理性骨缝的条状颅骨切除术。然而，再融合和持续畸形的发生率很高。Shillito 和 Matson 在回顾 519 例病例时发现[50]，取得满意外观的只有 52%，单独矢状缝早闭效果最好。1965 年，Powiertowsky 和 Matlosz 提出一种完全移动颅顶和眼眶顶的不寻常的技术[44]，但由于存在不可预期的再骨化导致的全层缺损及轮廓不规则风险，这个方法被废止。

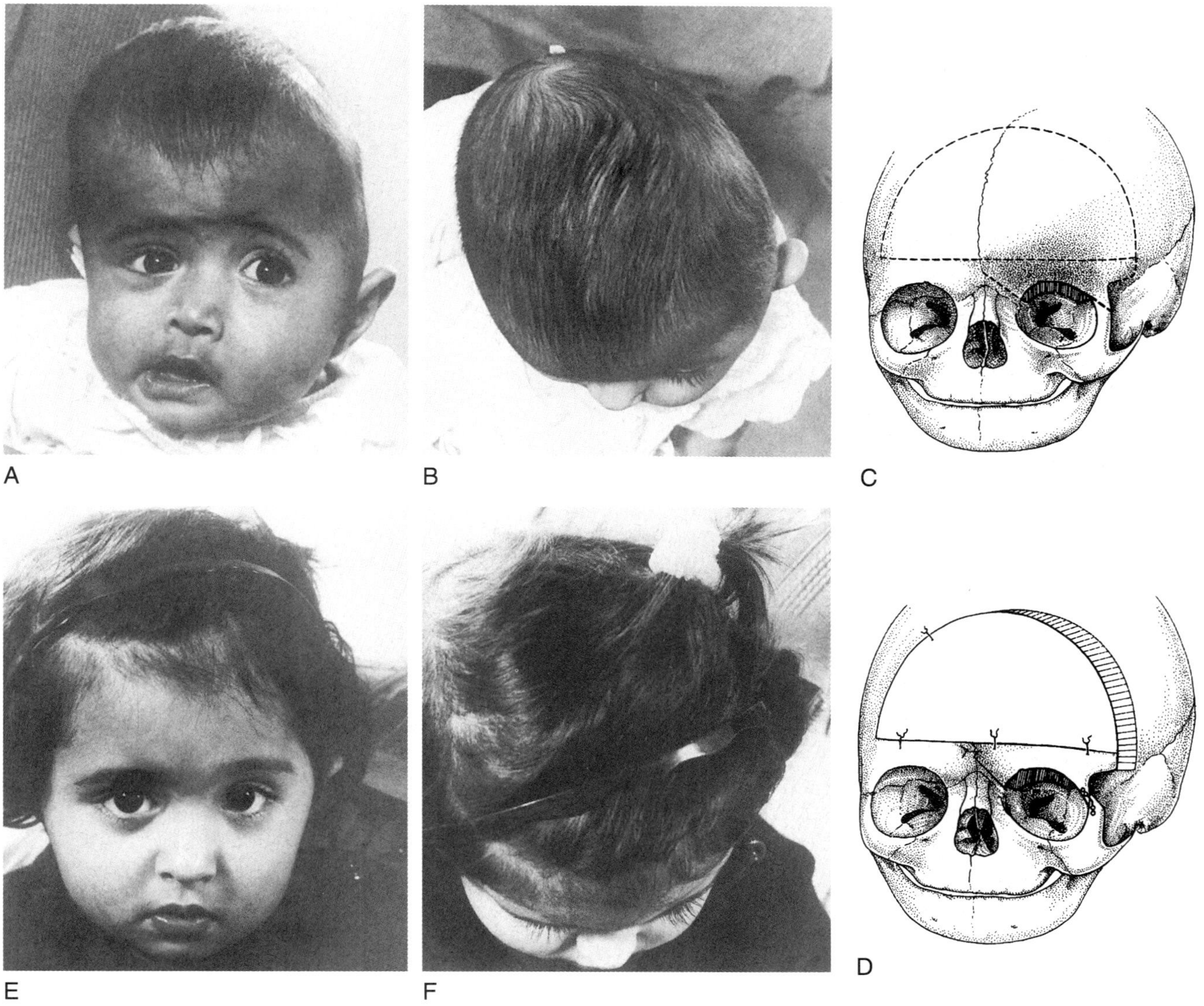

图 50-11 单侧冠状缝早闭病例。A 和 B. 术前外观。注意左右侧面部高度不对称，一侧较高，面中线弯曲，对侧下颌偏斜，前额一侧平坦，一侧隆起。C. 线条描绘畸形截骨术。D. 恢复轮廓，固定移动骨片。E 和 F. 术后外观。

为利用婴幼儿脑组织快速扩大的优势，建议早期手术干预。大多数治疗中心建议在3～6个月间进行，还有一些建议稍大再手术。但1岁以内必须进行手术是共识。在一份对额缝早闭患者治疗的长期研究中，早期整复产生了较好的术后效果[15]。

由于条状颅骨切除术令人失望，治疗原则随之改变。不论何种类型的颅缝早闭，强调释放关闭的骨缝，重置修整畸形骨骼轮廓，立即恢复正常的结构形态（图50–10和50–11）。Hoffman和Mohr[22]在治疗单侧冠状缝早闭中运用了这些措施。Marchac和Renier[31,32]完善了方法，运用了众多几何学设计和固定方法。受生物相容性金属片和金属钉进行牢固固定的益 796
处所吸引，外科医生随后将其应用于生长中的颅骨后发现，它们可从头盖骨移位到硬脑膜[16]。虽然，最初的反应是一种警告，但有害的后果并没有观察到[27]。不过，金属固定装置还是被可生物降解的片和钉所取代。

内镜手术技术的应用再加上头颅塑型帽的使用，

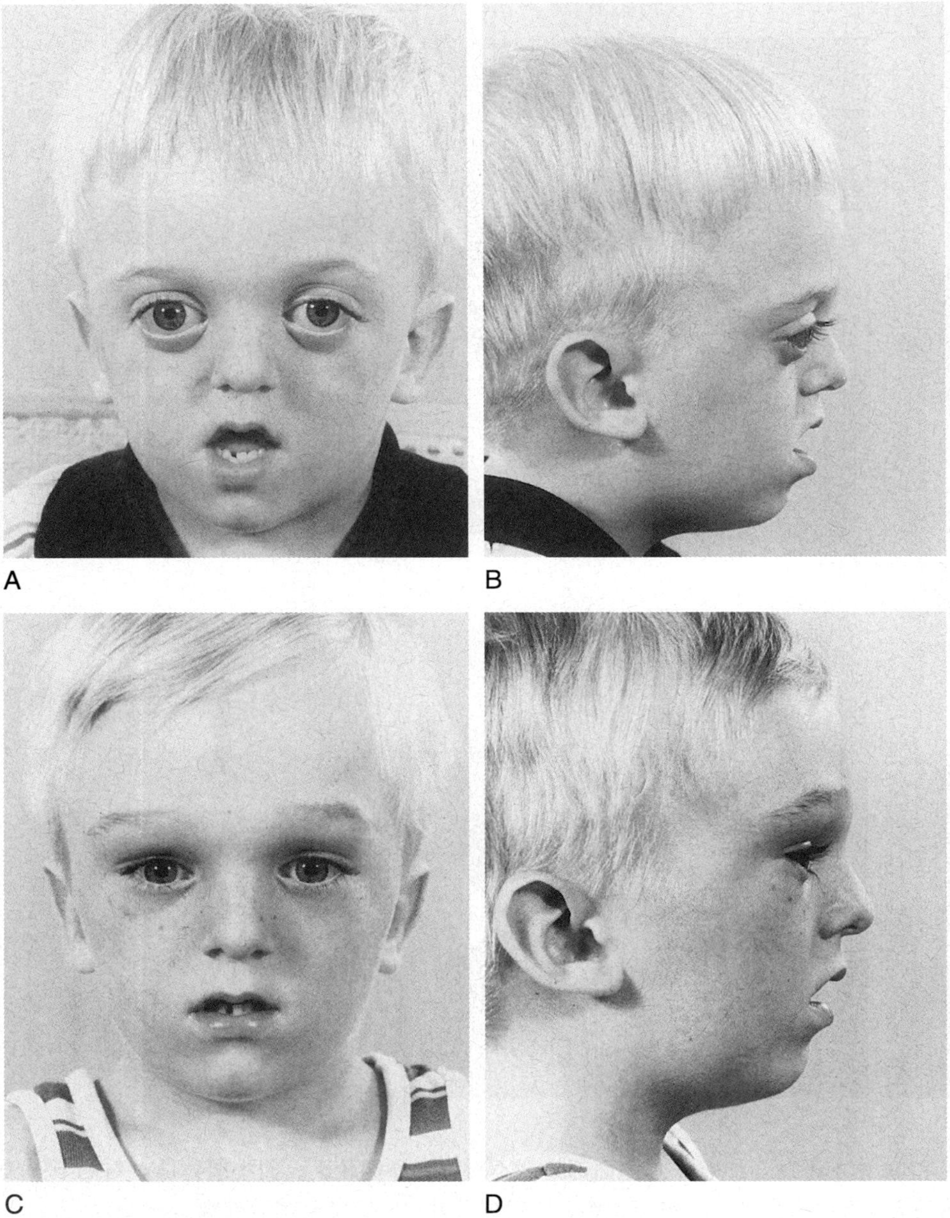

图50–12 Crouzon综合征患者。A和B. 术前外貌，患儿突眼，面中部后缩。下颌假性前突。C和D. 前额面部整体前移术后外观，前移前额，使眼球位置正常，矫正面中部后缩。

使得线状颅骨切开术获得了新生[5,25]。颅缝骨性连结在内镜帮助下除去，根据颅缝累及情况进行颅骨切除术。接着，应用定型头帽来保持期望的轮廓。这种手术方法的优点在于侵入步骤较少、失血量少和住院时间短。缺点在于定型头帽的额外手术以及增加了术后调整的回访次数。此外，为获得令人满意的结果，这种方法的运用只限于出生后 5 个月内。

综合征型颅缝早闭

与非综合征型颅骨骨缝融合相反，综合征型颅缝早闭连结表现各异。由于牵涉到遗传因素，早期分离融合的骨缝并不能导致随后颅面部骨骼的正常生长。因此患儿发育成熟后需要另行手术。和零星发生的非综合征型相反，这类畸形已经明确了遗传方式。

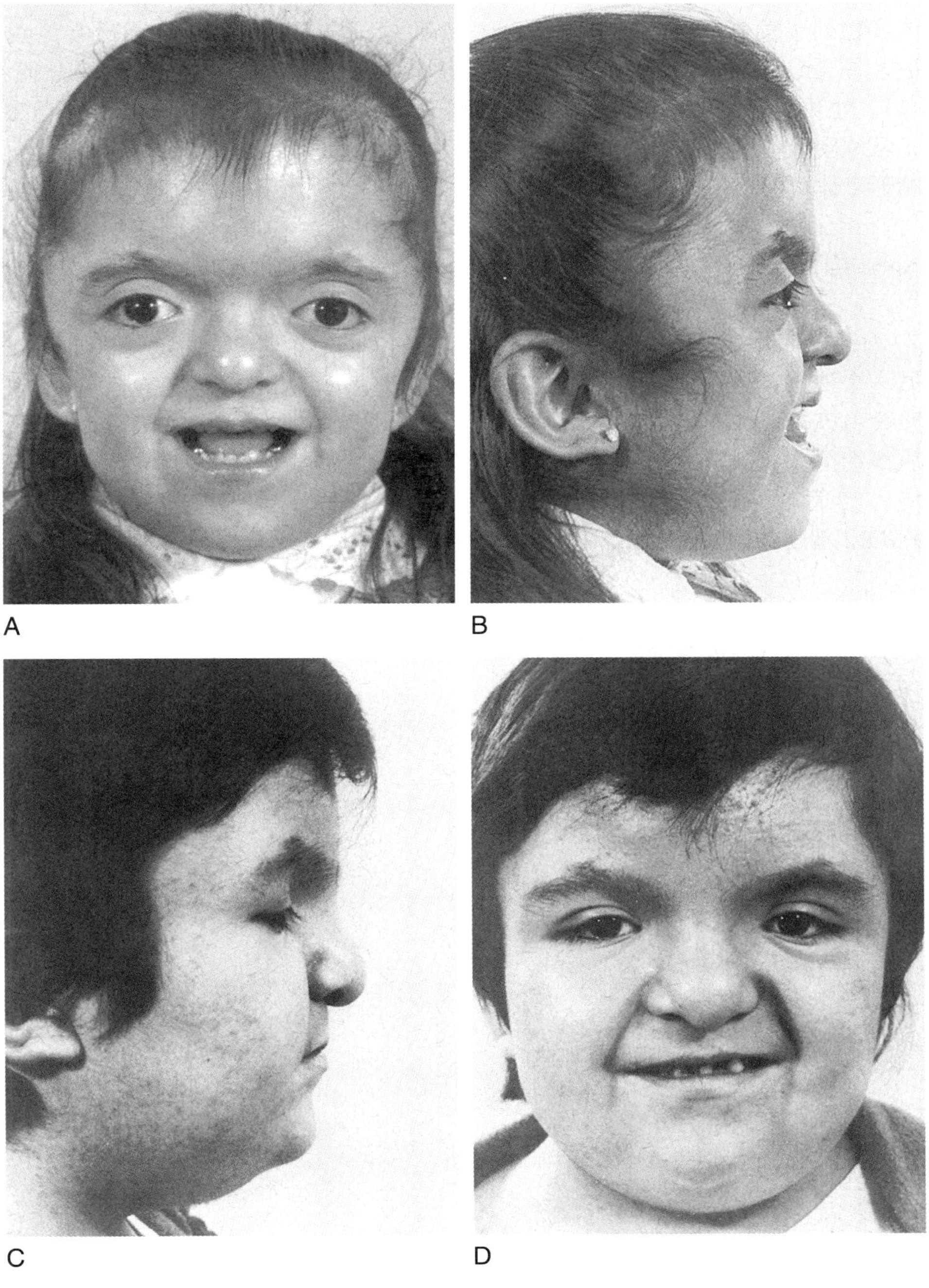

图 50–13 Apert 综合征患儿。A 和 B. 扁平脸、后缩的前额和面中部后移、突眼和眶间距过大纠正之前的外貌。C 和 D. 前额面整体前移术纠正面部后缩和面部曲度，恢复面部弯曲和减小眶间距。

Crouzon 综合征

具有讽刺意味的是法国外科医生 Panl Tessier 创建的颅面部畸形专业起源于半个世纪前一个法国神经科医
797 生的描述[11]。Crouzon 综合征是最常见的综合征型颅缝早闭畸形。估计它的发生率为 1/100 000[17]，其遗传方式为常染色体完全显性遗传，几乎完全外显，*FGFR2* 基因的突变在此综合征患者中已被确定[18,24,28,38,45]。

尽管可累及任何或全部颅缝，双侧冠状缝早闭是最常见的。主要的面部特征包括，突眼（正常的眼眶内容物处于发育不全的眼眶中）、面中部后缩、塌陷的上颌骨、假性下颌骨突出和鹦鹉嘴状鼻（图 50-12）。也可见轻度的眶间距过大。智力下降，但处于正常范围。其他的躯体特征正常，与此类疾病中其他畸形个体可发现手指畸形不同。

Apert 综合征

由 Wheaton 在 1894 年最初描述[59]。在 12 年后，另一个法国神经病学家描述了 4 例病例并以他的名字命名该畸形并使用"尖头并指综合征"一词[2]。发病率约为 1/160 000[17]，遗传方式为常染色体显性遗传，尽管趋向于散发。同 Crouzon 综合征一样，*FGFR2* 基因的缺失已被识别[30,41,60]。

突眼、上颌骨收缩引起的面中部后缩和假性下颌突出的表现和 Crouzon 综合征相同（图 50-13）。
中度突眼且不对称。眶间距较大，面部横向扁平。 798
最主要的辨别特征是对称的手和脚的并趾现象，指节间关节的融合严重到产生连指手套样畸形。此外，青春期时面部、躯干、肢体分布粉刺样皮疹。另一个独特的表现是轻度的智力发育迟缓。

其他综合征

除了最常见的 Crouzon 和 Apert 综合征外，有超过 50 种综合征和颅缝早闭有关[9]。因为其数量非常稀少，发病率还没有确定。Pfeiffer、Carpenter 和 Saethre-Chotzen 综合征属于这类：宽大的脚趾和大拇指（Pfeiffer），多指、短指伴软组织并指（Carpenter），第二和第三指的软组织蹼（Saethr-Chotzen）可以分别辨别以上三种综合征。Pfeiffer 和 Saethre-Carpenter 综合征的遗传方式为常染色体显性遗传，而 Carpenter 综合征为常染色体隐性遗传。

只要见过一次，罕见的 Kleeblattschädel 畸形（三叶草形头骨）就不会忘记。头盖骨呈现头顶突出，两侧膨隆的三叶特征（图 50-14）。

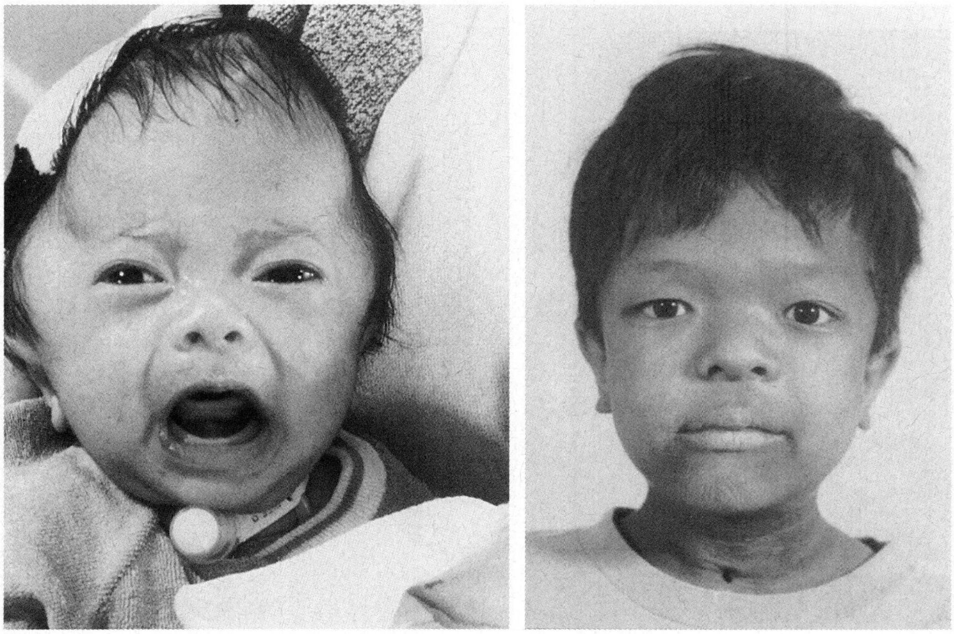

A B

图 50-14 由多颅缝早闭引起的 Kleeblatfschädel 畸形（三叶草）的病例。A. 注意头颅的三叶形状及前额和面中部后缩。B. 在婴儿时进行前额眼眶前移术 8 年后外观，6 岁时还进行过整体前移术。

治疗

所有综合征型颅缝早闭畸形的手术处理一般分为3个年龄段。与非综合征型相反，对这类畸形手术干预后，不能实现面部正常生长。治疗只针对当时的问题。这样，只能采用阶段性的方法。必须考虑的要点是缓解由于骨缝早闭引起的颅内压升高、严重的面中部后缩引起的气道损害及保护突眼的角膜。在1岁内，松解早闭的骨缝和进行前额–眼眶前移术（图50–15）。这可使快速扩大的脑组织自由生长，获得相对正常的头盖轮廓，更好地保护角膜。

治疗方案和时机因外科医生的经验和习惯而不同。加州大学洛杉矶分校的处理方案是较流行的一种。第二次手术在6岁左右进行，这时，眼眶和头盖骨的发育已达到了成人尺寸的90%。如果前额形态正常，进行传统的LeFort III面中部前移术把整个

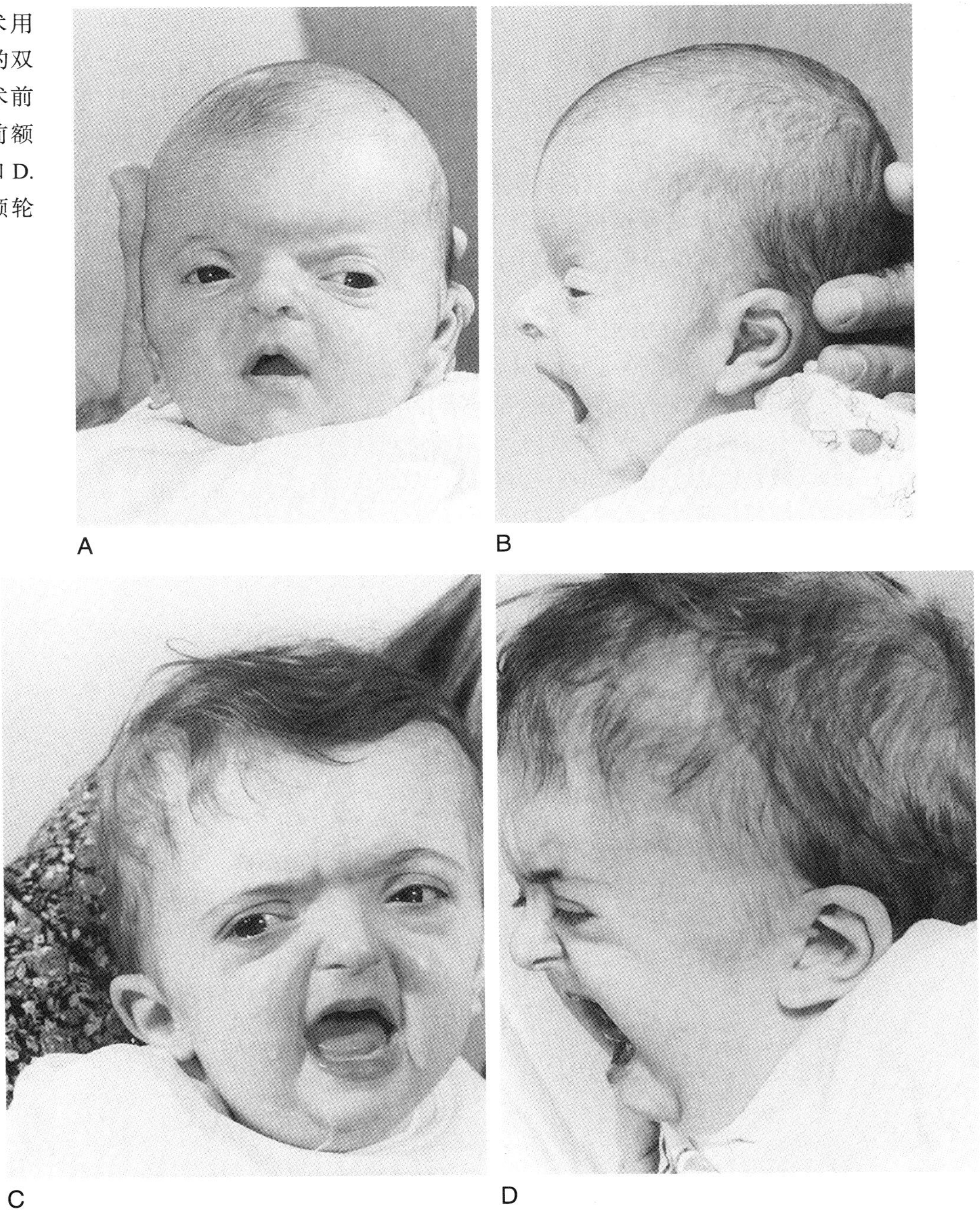

图 50–15　额、眶前移术用以矫治Apert综合征患儿的双侧冠状缝早闭。A和B. 术前外观照片显示眶上缘和前额退缩以及眼球突出。C和D. 术后外观显示正常的前额轮廓和眼眶关系。

面中部推向前方。因为知道将来面中部发育会受限制，上颌骨被有意置于一个过度矫正的前方位置（图50–16）。这样就能开放拥挤的鼻咽部和矫正突眼。

799 如果前额有凹陷（这种病例常见）有两种治疗方式可选择。作为初步手术，进行第二次额眶前移术。大约 6 个月后，再进行 LEFORT II 前移进术。由于把清洁环境下的颅内治疗和有污染的颅外面中部前移术分开进行，无菌性得到了保障，所以这种方法是安全的。与婴儿期相比，这一年龄段患儿的硬脑膜扩张缓慢，待脑组织增大、填满额眶前移术产生的硬脑膜外无效腔需更长一段时间。

另一种方法是整体额眶前移术[40]。其优势在于只需要进行一次手术复位前额和面中部骨骼。常能得到最佳的美观效果[61]。但是感染的风险增加。如存在分流，最好避免行此手术，因为分流会抑制脑扩张，延
800 长死腔存在的时间[28]。通过牵拉骨生成技术，使额面部以每天 1mm 的速度缓慢前移，减少了很多急性前移的危险[51]。

眶距过大时，除 LeFort III 或额面整体前移术外，还要进行面部等分术（见图 50–8）。尤其是用在整复以前额和面中部扁平为特征的 Apert 综合征患者中[54]。最后的步骤必须等待面部发育完成再进行。术前矫正牙列后，用 LeFort I（上额）前移术纠正假性的下颌前突。常需要同时行颏前移成形术纠正后缩的颏部。

（徐建民译 董其刚校）

参考文献

1. American Academy of Pediatrics Task Force on Infant Positioning and SIDS: Positioning and SIDS. Pediatrics 1992;89:1120-1126.
2. Apert E: De l'acrocephalosyndactylie. Bull Soc Med Hôp Paris 1906;23:1310.
3. Argenta LC, David LR, Wilson JA, et al: An increase in infant cranial deformity with supine sleeping position. J Craniofac Surg 1996;7:5-11.
4. Ballatyne JW: The teratological records of Chaldea. Teratologia 1894;1:127.
5. Barone CM, Jimenez EF: Endoscopic craniectomy for early correction of craniosynostosis. Plast Reconstr Surg 1999; 104:1965-1973.
6. Berry GA: Note on a congenital defect (? coloboma) of the lower lid. Roy Lond Ophth Hosp Rep 1889;12:255.
7. Bertelson TL: The premature synostosis of the cranial sutures. Acta Ophthalmol Suppl 1958;51:47.
8. Blinkov SM, Glezer II: The Human Brain in Figures and Tables: A Quantitative Handbook. New York, Plenum Press, 1968.
9. Cohen MM Jr: Craniosynostosis and syndromes with craniosynostosis: Incidence, genetics, penetrance, variability, and new syndrome updating. Birth Defects 1979; 15:13-63.
10. Converse JM, Coccaro PJ, Becker M, Wood-Smith D: On hemifacial microsomia: The first and second branchial arch syndrome. Plast Reconstr Surg 1973;51: 268-279.
11. Crouzon O: Dysotose, cranio-faciale héréditaire. Bull Soc Med Hôp Paris 1912;33:545.
12. Dixon MJ, Hann E, Baker E, et al: Association of Treacher

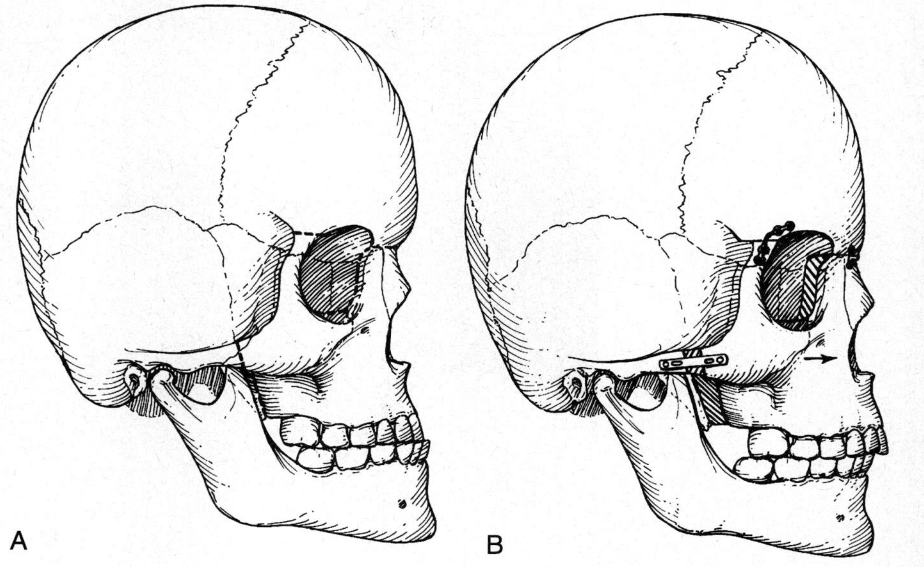

图 50–16 Lefort III 面中部推进术的说明。A. 描述了面中部后缩，假性下颌骨突出和骨切开术的设计。B. 移动后，过矫正的前伸和固定。

Collins syndrome and translocation 6p21.31/16p13.11: Exclusion of the locus from these candidate regions. J Hum Genet 1991;48:274-280.
13. Dixon MJ: Treacher Collins syndrome. Hum Mol Genet 1996;5(Spec):1391-1396.
14. Enlow DH, Azuma M: Functional growth boundaries in the human and mammalian face. Birth Defects 1975;11: 217-230.
15. Fearon JA, Kolar JC, Munro IR: Trigonocephaly—associated hypotelorbitism: Is treatment necessary? Plast Reconstr Surg 1996;97:503-509.
16. Fearon JA, Munro IA, Bruce DA: Observations on the use of rigid fixation for craniofacial deformities in infants and young children. Plast Reconstr Surg 1995;95: 634-637.
17. Gorlin RJ, Pindborg JH, Cohen MM Jr: Syndromes of the Head and Neck, 2nd ed. New York, McGraw-Hill, 1976, pp 220-224.
18. Gorry MC, Preston RA, White GJ, et al: Crouzon syndrome: Mutations in two spliceoforms of FGFR2 and a common point mutation shared with Jackson-Weiss syndrome. Hum Mol Genet 1995;4:1387-1390.
19. Grabb WC: The first and second branchial arch syndrome. Plast Reconstr Surg 1965;36:485-508.
20. Gruss JS: The diagnosis of plagiocephaly due to lambdoid suture synostosis: Clinical, radiological and operative findings. Craniofacial Surgery: State of the Art Symposium. New York, March 20, 1996.
21. Hangman CB: Growth of interorbital distance and skull thickness as observed in roentgenographic measurements. Radiology 1966;86:87.
22. Hoffman HJ, Mohr G: Lateral canthal advancement of the supraorbital margin. J Neurosurg 1976;45: 376-381.
23. Hollway GE, Phillip HA, Ades LC, et al: Localization of craniosynostosis Adelaide type to 4p16. Hum Mol Genet 1995;4:681-683.
24. Jabs EW, Li X, Scott AF, et al: Jackson-Weiss and Crouzon syndromes are allelic with mutations in fibroblast growth factor receptor. Nat Genet 1994;8:275-279.
25. Jimenez DF, Barone CM, McGee ME, et al: Endoscopy-assisted wide-vertex craniectomy, barrel stave osteotomies, and postoperative helmet molding therapy in the management of sagittal suture craniosynostosis. J Neurosurg Spine 2004;100:407-417.
26. Kawamoto HK: The kaleidoscopic world of rare craniofacial clefts: Order out of chaos (Tessier classification). Clin Plast Surg 1976;3:529-572.
27. Kawamoto HK, McCarthy JG: Discussion of Fearon JR, et al: Observation on the use of rigid fixation for craniofacial deformities in infants and young children. Plast Reconstr Surg 1995;95:638.
28. Kawamoto HK Jr, Stuzin JM: Complication associated with the monobloc-frontofacial advancement. Presented before the American Association of Plastic Surgeons meeting, Palm Beach, May 3, 1988.
29. Kapp-Simon KA, Figueroa A, Jocher A, Schafer M: Longitudinal assessment of mental development in infants with nonsyndromic craniosynostosis with and without cranial release and reconstruction. Plast Reconstr Surg 1993;92: 831-839.
30. Lewanda AF, Cohen MM Jr, Hood J, et al: Cytogenetic survey of Apert syndrome: Reevaluation of translocation (2;9)(p11.2;q34.2) in patient suggests the breakpoints are not related to the disorder. Am J Dis Child 1993;147: 1306-1308.
31. Marchac D: Radical forehead remodeling for craniostenosis. Plast Reconstr Surg 1978;61:823-835.
32. Marchac D, Renier D: Craniofacial Surgery for Craniosynostosis. Boston, Little Brown, 1982.
33. McCarthy JG: The role of distraction osteogenesis in the reconstruction of the mandible in unilateral craniofacial microsomia. Clin Plast Surg 1994;21:625-631.
34. Molina F, Ortiz-Monasterio F: Mandibular elongation and remodeling by distraction: A farewell to major osteotomies. Plast Reconstr Surg 1995;96:825-840.
35. Montaut J, Stricker M: Dysmorphies Craniofaciales: Les Synostoses Prematuries (Craniostenosis et Faciostenosis). Paris, Masson, 1977.
36. Moss ML: New studies of cranial growth. Birth Defects 1975;11:283-295.
37. Murray DJ, Kaban LP, Mulliken JB: Analysis and treatment of hemifacial microsomia. Plast Reconstr Surg 1984;74: 186-199.
38. Neilson KM, Friesel RE: Constitutive activation of fibroblast growth factor receptor-2 by a point mutation associated with Crouzon syndrome. J Biol Chem 1995;270: 26037-26040.
39. Oldridge M, Wilkie AO, Slaney SF, et al: Mutations in the third immunoglobulin domain of the fibroblast growth factor receptor-2 gene in Crouzon syndrome. Hum Mol Genet 1995;4:1077-1082.
40. Ortiz-Monasterio F, Fuente del Campo A, Carrillo A: Advancement of the orbits and the midface in one piece, combined with frontal repositioning for the correction of Crouzon's deformities. Plast Reconstr Surg 1978;61: 507-516.
41. Park W-J, Theda C, Maestri NE, et al: Analysis of phenotypic features and FGFR2 mutations in Apert syndrome. Am J Hum Genet 1995;57:321-328.
42. Poswillo D: Orofacial malformations. Proc R Soc Med 1974;67:343-349.
43. Poswillo D: The pathogenesis of the Treacher Collins syndrome (mandibulofacial dysostosis). Br J Oral Surg 1975;13:1-26.
44. Powiertowsky H, Matlosz Z: The treatment of craniostenosis by a method of extensive resection of the vault of the skull. In: Proceedings of the Third International Congress on Neurosurgery. Excerpta Med Int Cong Ser 1965;110:834.
45. Readon W, Winter RM, Rutland P, et al: Mutations in the fibroblast growth factor receptor 2 gene cause Crouzon syndrome. Nat Genet 1994;8:98-103.
46. Reissmann H: Ein Fall von Makrostoma. Arch Minerva Chir 1869;6:858.
47. Renier D, Sainte-Rose C, Marchac D, Hirsh JF: Intracranial pressure in craniosynostosis. J Neurosurg 1982;57:370-377.
48. Renier D, Marchac D.: Craniofacial surgery for craniosynostosis: Functional and morphologic results. Ann Acad Med Singapore 1988;17:415.
49. Rogers BO: Berry–Treacher Collins syndrome: A review of 200 cases. Br J Plast Surg 1964;17:109-137.
50. Shillito J, Matson DD: Craniosynostosis: A review of 519 surgical patients. Pediatrics 1968;41:829-853.
51. Taub PJ, Bradley JP, Stuzin JM, Kawamoto HK: Decreased morbidity in monobloc advancement with distraction osteogenesis. Presented before the 71st annual meeting of the American Society of Plastic Surgery, San Antonio, TX, November 4, 2002.
52. Tessier P: Orbital hypertelorism: I. Successive surgical attempts, materials and methods, causes and mechanisms. Scand J Plast Reconstr Surg 1972;6:133-155.

53. Tessier P: Anatomical classification of facial, craniofacial and laterofacial clefts. J Maxillofac Surg 1976;4:69-92.
54. Tessier PL: Apert's syndrome: Acrocephalosyndactyly type I. In Caronni E (ed): Craniofacial Surgery. Boston, Little Brown, 1985, p 280.
55. Tessier P, Guiot B, Rougerie J, et al: Ostéotomies cranio-naso-orbito-faciales hypertélorisme. Ann Chir Plast 1967; 12:103-118.
56. Treacher Collins E: Case with symmetrical congenital notches in the outer part of each lower lid and defective development of the malar bones. Trans Ophthalmol Soc UK 1900;20:190.
57. Turk AE, McCarthy JG, Thorne CHM, et al: The "Back to Sleep" campaign and deformational plagiocephaly: Is there cause for concern? J Craniofac Surg 1996;7:12-18.
58. van der Meulen JC: Medial faciotomy. Br J Plast Surg 1979;32:339.
59. Wheaton SW: Two specimens of congenital cranial deformities in infants in association with fusion of the fingers and toes. In Smith DW (ed): Major Problems in Clinical Pediatrics, Vol 7, Recognizable Patterns of Human Malformation. Philadelphia, WB Saunders, 1982, p 308.
60. Wilkie AOM, Slaney SF, Oldridge M, et al: Apert syndrome results from localized mutations of FGFR2 and is allelic with Crouzon syndrome. Nat Genet 1995;9: 165-172.
61. Wolfe SA, Morrison G, Page LK, et al: The monobloc frontofacial advancement: Do the pluses outweigh the minuses? Plast Reconstr Surg 1993;91:977-987.

第 51 章

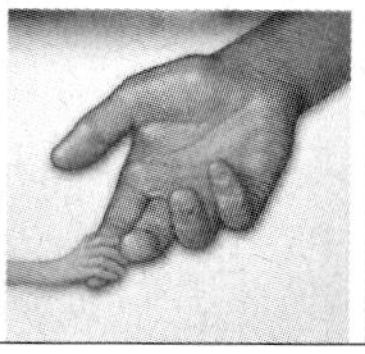

唇腭裂

A. Michael Sadove 和 Barry L. Eppley

803 唇裂和腭裂是最常见的先天性面部缺陷。绝大多数先天性面部畸形和大多数口腔颌面部面裂类型都包含在内。唇裂可伴有切牙孔前的齿槽缺损，被归类为前腭裂。累及切牙孔后方的软硬腭裂归类为次生腭裂。唇腭裂可以表现为多种不同的形态，从程度最轻的不完全性单纯唇裂到最严重的完全性双侧唇腭裂不等。

各人种发生率不同，这是因为宫内胎儿面部融合的时机和协调性不同。这可能由于不同人种面部组织的厚度不同所致。由于这些差异，在亚洲人和美国本土人，唇裂的发生率是每 500 个活产儿中有 1 例，而在非洲裔美国人则是每 1500～2000 个活产儿中有 1 例，在白种人平均是每 750～900 个活产儿中有 1 例。左侧唇裂多于右侧唇裂，原因尚不清楚。与上述不同的是，单纯腭裂的发生率各人种之间基本相同（大约每 1000 个活产儿中有 0.50 例）。

唇裂的形成

神经嵴间质迁移和随后增殖形成面突，大约在人胚胎发育到 30 天，面突逐渐融合形成原始的唇和腭，建立了口鼻腔间的初始分隔，最终形成上唇和上颌。事实上所有唇裂都是由中鼻（球状）突未连接或侧鼻突及上颌突保持连接引起。面突面中会聚时任何结构接触时未能融合或未能粘连（不能保持接触）都可导致面裂（图 51–1）。

腭裂的形成

硬软腭的发育由原腭（前腭）和次生腭（后腭）组成。原腭的发育与切牙孔前（如面部、唇、前颌骨上面 4 个切牙）有关。它与面部融合过程（已于唇裂处描述）有密切关系，开始于胚胎第 4 周，结束于第 7 周。因为这个原因，唇腭裂意味着一个从唇经牙槽向后到软腭的完全的残缺畸形（图 51–2A）。

次生腭的发育与切牙孔后的结构（如硬腭、软腭、上颌齿）相关。此区域从腭突或上颌骨板开始发育，胚胎 6～7 周时变得明显。它们从原腭延伸至扁桃弓，垂直悬在舌旁。胚胎第 8～9 周时腭突开始改变位置，从垂直变为水平。腭架一度与舌分开，但随着舌降至口底并移向前方，两侧腭板融合。舌不能下降引起腭裂（见图 51–2B）。此相互关联的过程最好的例子是 Pierre Robin 综合征，存在软腭裂、舌下垂及下颌骨发育不良，易致潜在性的气道阻塞。

不常见的面裂

之前描述的唇腭裂是面裂的传统类型，其他不常见的类型可发生于口面区[58]。可为经上唇的中线（Tessier 0）、围绕鼻部斜向眼（Tessier 4、5 和 6）或 805
从口角向外（Tessier 7）。这此类型的面裂较罕见，累及不同的解剖结构，需要新的修补技术。常伴有更广泛的面部缺损和（或）缺陷。出现这些面裂时，需对面部和脑进行仔细评估，因为正中的唇裂应评估有无额鼻及脑畸形，而斜向及外侧口裂可累及眼、耳及下颌畸形。

面裂的病因学

唇腭裂的病因是多因素的，包括遗传和环境因素。虽然面裂发生在多种遗传综合征中（约 15%的面

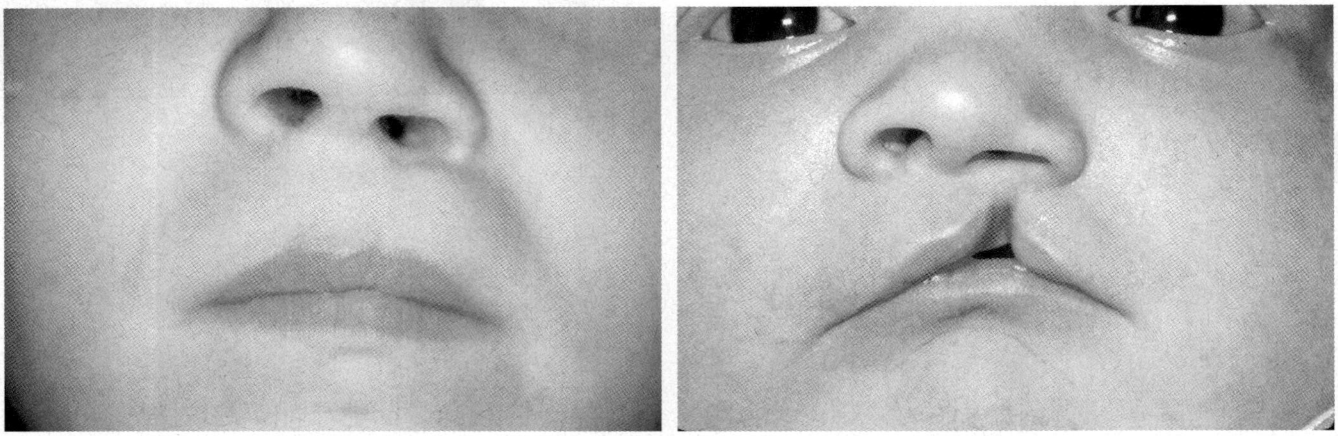

A B

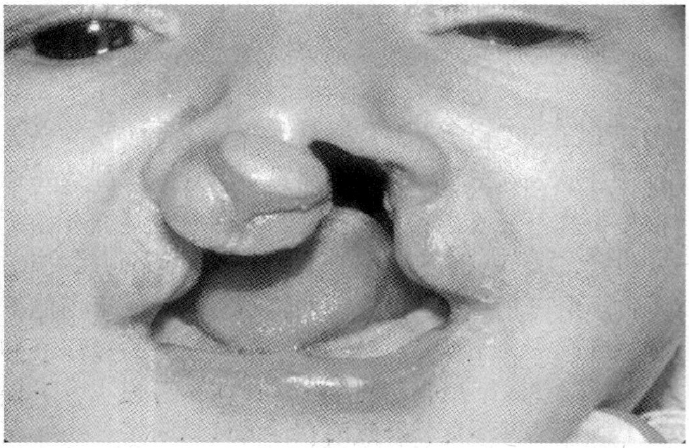

C

图 51-1 唇裂的多种表现。A. 小唇裂（不完全型）。B. 不完全性单侧唇裂。C. 双侧完全性唇裂。

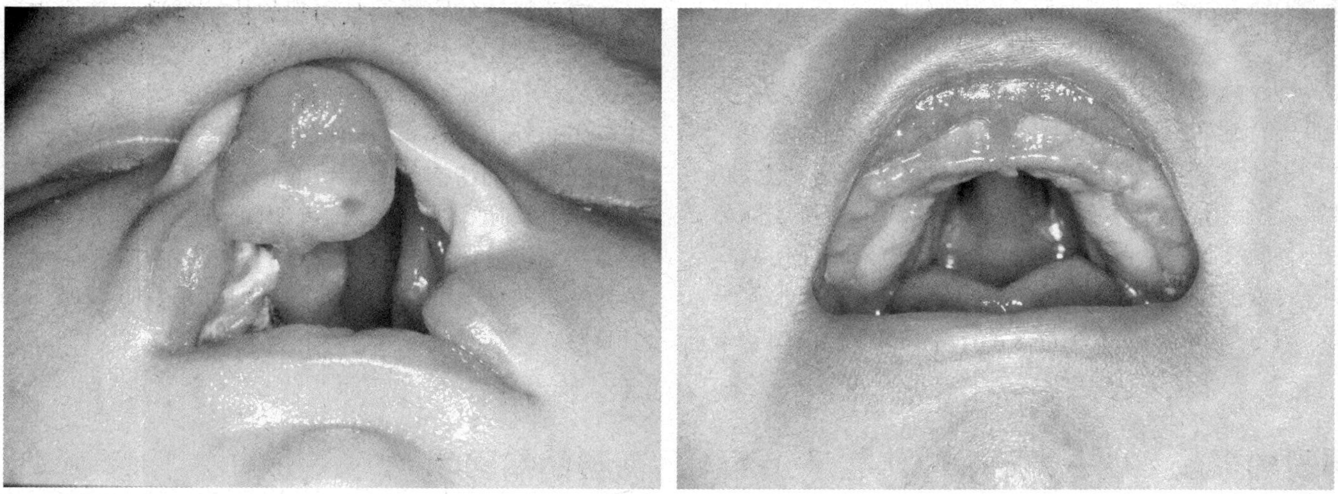

A B

图 51-2 腭裂的多种表现。A.完全性腭裂伴唇裂。B. 仅有软腭裂。

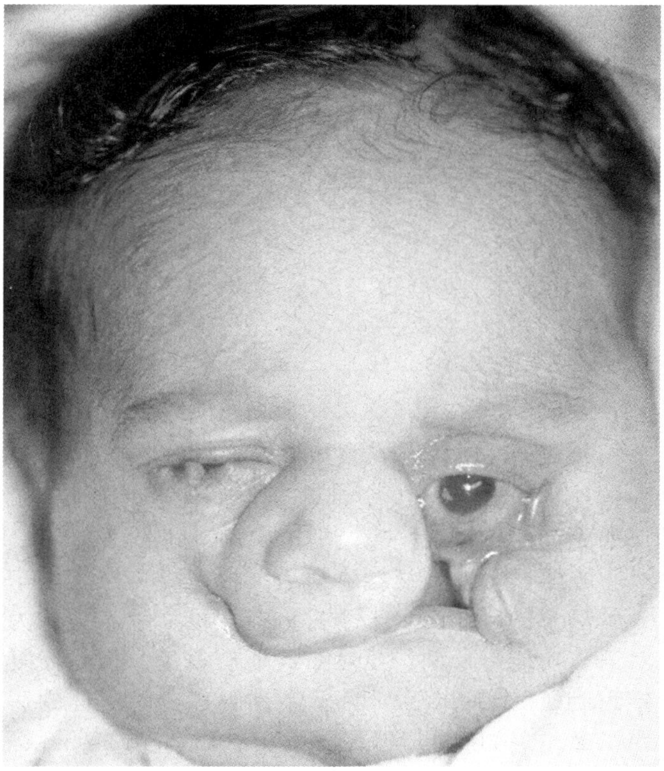

A

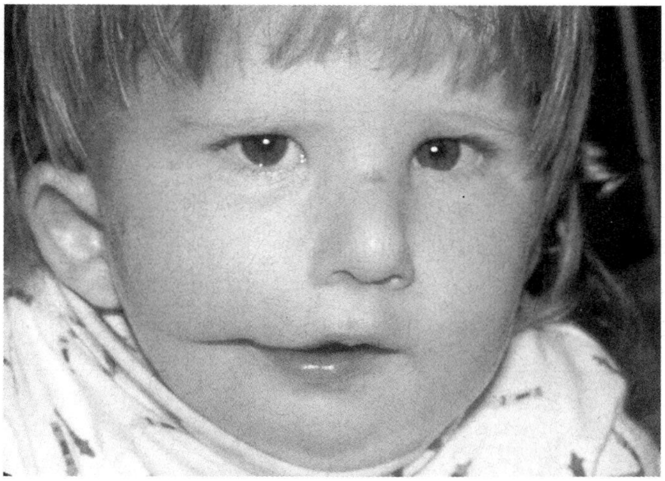

B

图 51-3　非典型面裂。A. Tessier 4 面斜裂。B. Tessier 7 外侧面裂。

裂为综合征性，超过 170 种综合征有面裂现象），但控制唇腭裂发病的单独基因尚未发现[18,24]。面裂基因已被确认存在于 1、2、4、6、11、14、17 和 19 号染色体上。可见到某种特定的染色体异常（如 D 三体综合征伴中央唇裂），或唇裂伴有下唇凹陷（Vander Woude 综合征）。因为常伴有综合征，寻找其他先天性缺陷就很重要，畸形常发生于头颅其他部分及颈部、心脏和肢体。只有一些环境因素被发现与面裂有关，包括怀孕期服用某些药物（如苯妥英、维甲酸、叶酸拮抗剂）。母亲吸烟可增加面裂发生率[3]。孕期头 4 个月补充复合维生素，特别是叶酸，被认为可起到预防保护作用[17]。

外科修复面裂

团队治疗

面裂畸形解剖复杂，影响到多种口面功能（面部生长，出牙和口腔卫生，下颌发育、听力、语言）以及对口面部生长发育，必须要建立一个团队去诊疗面裂患儿。面裂治疗组由整形外科、牙科（儿童牙科、正畸科和口腔外科）、听力学、语言病理学、耳鼻喉科和遗传学专家组成。这样的治疗组能提供各种专业知识，将治疗干预和生长发育结合起来，提供更有效及成本–效益更好的服务[1]。

新生儿治疗

父母

以前面裂儿的出生可能是意外的，但现在产前超声检查能早期发现面部缺陷[13]。这就能让现在的 806
父母有机会在孩子出生前去寻求产前咨询和请教面裂治疗团队，为将来的外科手术重建打好基础。父母常为没能预防面裂畸形的发生而内疚。遗传学咨询可以讨论下一胎的危险性，这样可以让父母放心（表 51–1）。

表 51-1 唇腭裂遗传风险

	唇裂伴或不伴腭裂（%）	腭裂（%）
普通人群发病率	0.08	0.02
第二胎风险		
(a) 父母均正常	3.7	2.5
(b) 父母一方与患儿有相似的唇腭裂	19.4	14.3
第三胎风险（a 和 b）	9.0	0.90
如父母一方有唇腭裂，第一胎的风险	4.04	5.82

孩子

除了外部唇裂引起的明显面部缺陷外，功能上的担忧是气道是否通畅和进食的能力。某些面裂畸形（如 Pirre Robin 综合征）除腭裂外，还有气道阻塞，需要不同形式的处理。由于舌与裂开的腭部不能产生负压，唇和硬腭的分裂可导致吮吸困难，患儿要用舌头挤开裂开的腭。因此，常见液体从鼻腔回流。需改变喂养方法，包括应用十字形开口的奶嘴和腭填充器来产生有效吸吮进食。

新生儿上颌骨整形

完全性唇腭裂畸形中，上颌骨和硬腭裂开，提倡在修复唇裂前运用各种各样的口内和口外的正畸装置来复位错位的牙槽骨片段。包括简单的方法，如用胶带粘合唇裂和圆形的弹性牵引。鼻齿槽塑形矫治装置越来越普及，因为它是把鼻、唇和牙槽骨塑形到手术前最佳位置的最有效方法。由于减小了唇裂的宽度，唇裂修复变得更简单，在双侧唇裂的病例中更有价值，这类病例中唇缘裂片包括了切牙骨，中唇位置较前。很多机械方式如口内固定装置已在一些患者中的使用，但同时也增加了损伤发育中牙齿的危险性，因为这类装置要植入牙槽骨中，而牙槽骨中都是发育中的牙齿。

手术时机

唇裂常在出生后 3～4 个月间修复。虽然出生几周做修复技术上可行，但传统的修复需等患儿再大些。著名的 10 规则是比较好的手术指标：10 周龄、10 克血色素和 10 磅体重。这些指标下对婴儿的创伤愈合和麻醉安全都适合。如伴有其他畸形，例如先天性心脏病，建议推迟手术时间。

传统上腭裂修复在唇裂后，根据外科医生的个人看法，一般在 9～15 个月进行。早期手术被认为对语言功能有帮助。虽然对此还有争论，但是修复推迟到 18 个月以后，明显伴有语言功能不佳的后果。患儿有早期的呼吸困难病史（如 Pierre Robin 综合征）是一个例外。这类患儿有必要把修复时间推迟到 18 个月以后，使鼻咽气道增大，来减少术后鼻咽气道缩小后气道阻塞的风险。

牙槽裂（上颌长牙齿的部分）通常在 5～8 岁间用自生骨移植修复。这不仅建立上颌弓的连接性，而且使牙齿能够萌出并改善裂开鼻底的支持。一些中心主张在腭裂修复前做早期骨移植。如果上颌骨片段端端对齐，就可在大约 9～12 个月时施行手术，使上颌骨及早稳定并关闭口鼻瘘。

唇裂修复

唇裂修复方法有很多种，因为不是所有的唇裂都一样。不同点在于相邻解剖中断的数量和程度。因此，要找出一种手术方法来解决所有唇裂病例是非常困难的。尽管如此，Millard 旋转前进法唇裂修复术成为修复单侧唇裂的最常用方法[21]。它能有效地把错位的唇和鼻结构复位到正常位置。因为术后瘢痕线基本在解剖边界上且最小限度地切除组织，所以术后瘢痕不明显。其要点包括：内侧唇片段下方旋转，外侧 807
唇片段前移至鼻小柱下空间，与内侧唇片片段连接（图 51-4）。此手术可延人中线、延长唇重建唇裂周

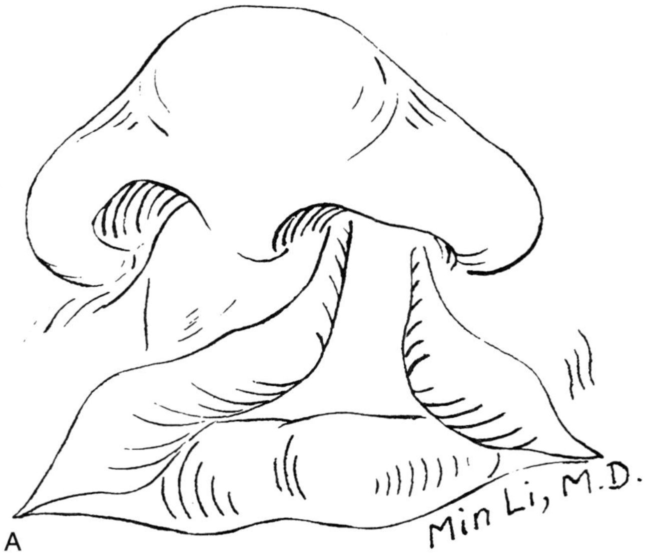

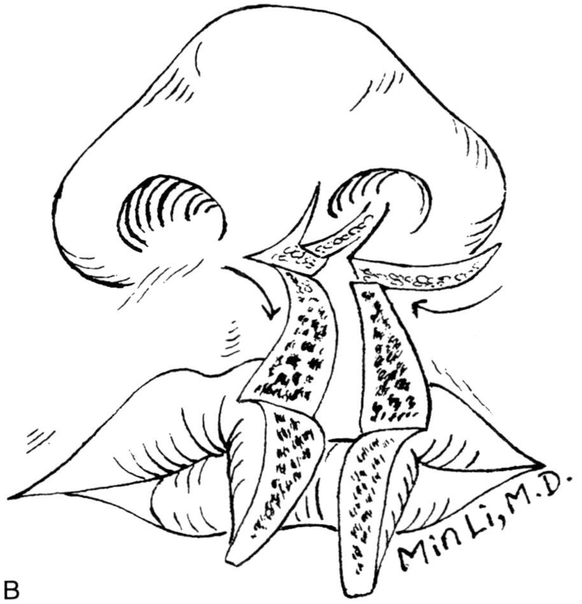

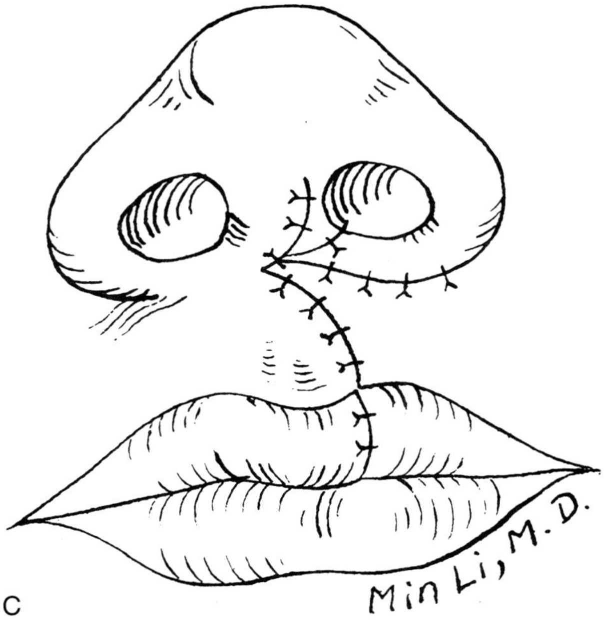

图 51–4　单侧唇裂的旋转前进法修复。A. 过宽的鼻底部，唇裂和过短的内侧外侧唇瓣的原始形态。B. 沿鼻底部和外侧唇切开分离唇瓣，跨过鼻柱基底至对侧人中嵴，同时上提双侧唇红瓣。箭头表示向下旋转内侧唇瓣和向鼻中柱推进侧唇瓣。C. 跨过缺损对合轮匝肌后，缝合皮肤。

围轮匝肌、向内侧旋转移位的鼻底，轻度延长轮匝肌，建立唇沟。概念简单、修复可裁身调整是这种唇裂修复方式的主要优势之一。另外，最小限度切除组织，以及瘢痕线所在的位置对二次手术修改（经常需要二次修改）有利。除此之外，围绕着鼻同时操作，移动同侧下部鼻翼软骨及鼻底。

修复双侧唇裂比单侧唇裂所遇到的困难更多。鼻小柱的缺失，敞开的鼻翼软骨和鼻底部，突出的切牙骨不仅使起初的唇裂修复与单侧唇裂修复不同，而且必须进行后继手术。作出修复双侧唇裂的决定包括是同时修复双侧唇裂还是分步骤修复、在最终唇修复之前是否粘合唇瓣、怎么样解决切牙骨突出的问题。所有这些问题都是有争议的，方法步骤每个唇腭裂治疗组不尽相同。我们的方法是：如果唇裂和切牙骨的宽度可使唇裂关闭后唇环状肌和皮肤缝合处的张力适当，那么就做同步的双侧唇裂修复[22]。Millart 旋转前进法能有效地重塑弓形唇线和双侧人中嵴（图 51–5）。当切牙骨太突出，对唇 808

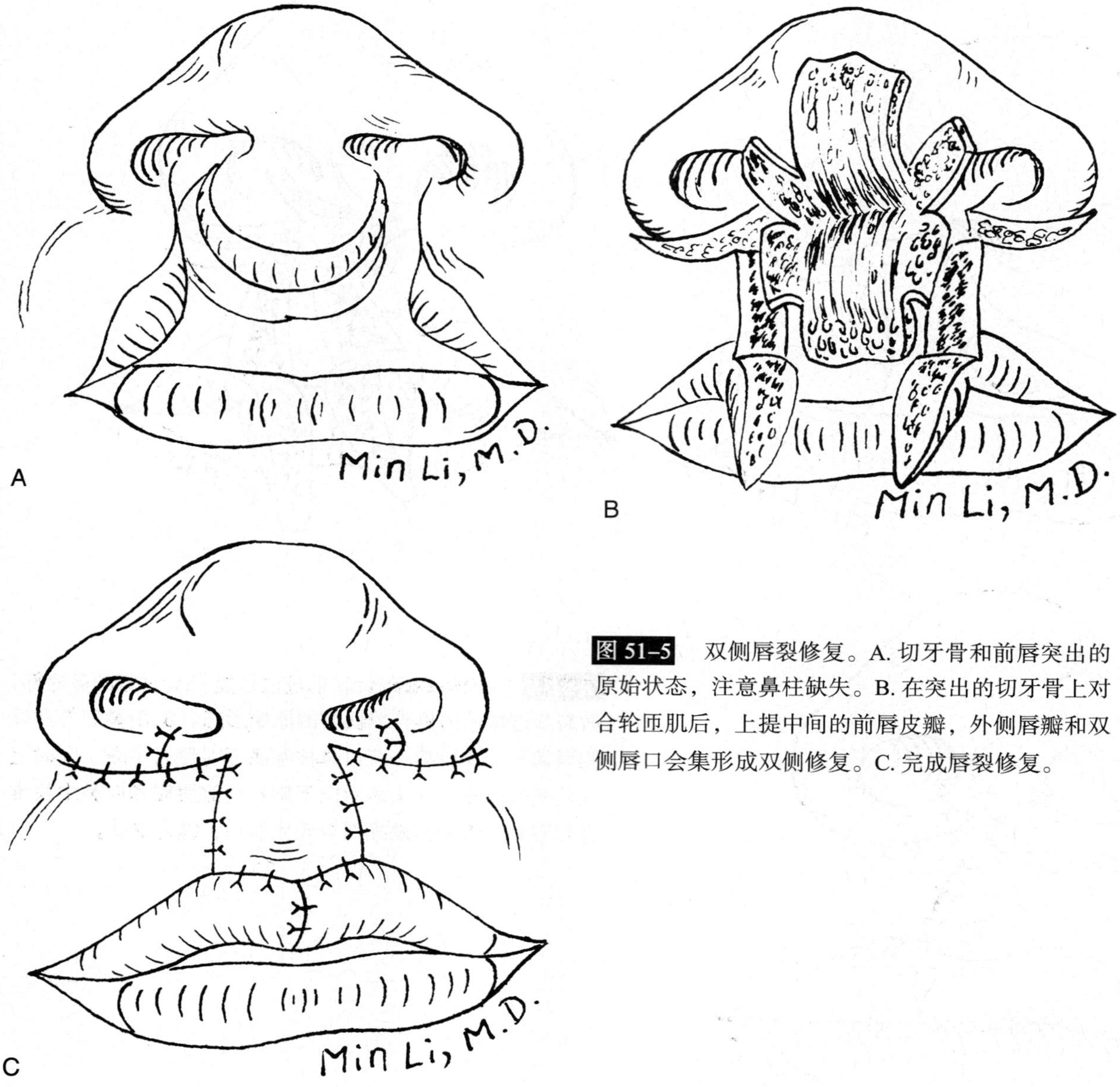

图 51–5　双侧唇裂修复。A. 切牙骨和前唇突出的原始状态，注意鼻柱缺失。B. 在突出的切牙骨上对合轮匝肌后，上提中间的前唇皮瓣，外侧唇瓣和双侧唇口会集形成双侧修复。C. 完成唇裂修复。

裂修复的完整性有潜在的威胁时，在 8 到 10 周龄时先进行简单的唇粘合，2～3 个月后待前颌骨稍后退再行最后的唇裂修复。

腭裂修复

尽管有很长的历史，外科的腭裂整复仍在争论哪种外科修复方法会影响语言和面部骨骼发育[25]。腭裂手术因干预时间、分期或完全修复采用哪种组织瓣来关闭腭裂而不同。基本目标是软腭肌肉的重建，双层（鼻腔和口腔）关闭硬软腭和合适的腭长度。虽然没有统一的腭裂修复技术或方式，但手术采用三种基本类型：直线关闭、V–Y 延长关闭或 Z 形整形重排。

沿腭裂边缘切开黏膜，在骨膜下水平松解组织， 809
向内侧移动腭瓣，使两层的直线修复得以完成。这种技术，称为 Von Langenbeck 修复法。但不能提供足够的软腭长度。通过在前面建立斜形切口，改良直线修复。腭瓣松解后，向后向内移动，形成 V–Y 重排（图 51–6）。这种技术称为后推术或称 Veau–Wardill–Kilner 修复法。以上两种方法，都可使腭提肌和腭张

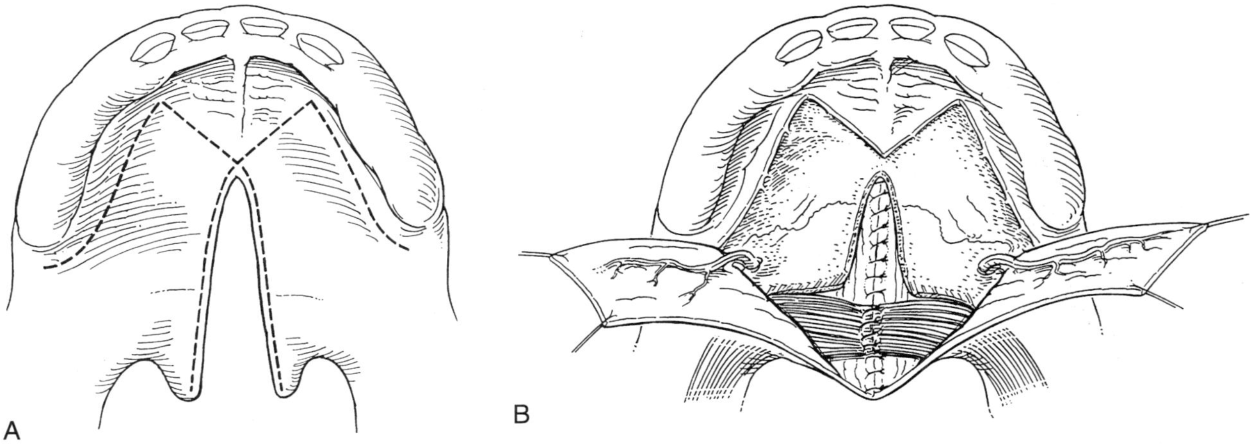

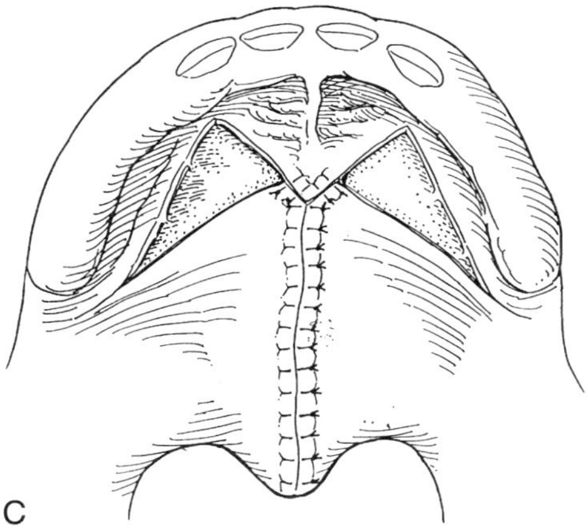

图 51-6 V-Y 后推腭裂修复术。A. 切口位置轮廓。B. 翻起，腭大血管表面的黏膜骨膜瓣，关闭黏膜的鼻层，对合软腭。C. 通过腭黏膜组织后方复位，延长；腭长度，关闭口腔层，留下腭前骨开放区域。

肌的异常粘连从后方及腭架的内侧边缘分开，并在软腭关闭的中线上将其缝合（腭帆为软腭成形术）：一种新的腭修复技术，灵活运用了 Z 形整形原则、双重反转口和鼻组织的肌黏膜瓣，被称为 Furlar 腭修复术[4,7]。这种方法不仅能有效地使软腭肌肉纤维再定位，而且增加了腭的长度（图 51-7）。大量的临床证据指出，这种肌肉修复方法能改善远期的语言功能[15]，另外，术后瘘的风险也减小了，因为口腔层和鼻腔层的缝合线不直接重叠。

牙槽骨移植

上颌骨生长牙齿部分（牙槽骨）进行骨移植后，最初的腭裂畸形就完成了一期修复。此手术不但可使上颌骨联成一体，消除了残留的口鼻瘘，而且可提供适当的组织以支持牙齿萌出。自生骨是移植材料的通常选择。大多数医疗中心在患儿 5～8 岁时进行骨移植[6,11]。这时，尖牙牙根发育较充分，移植能提供支持使得后继牙齿萌出在正常的牙弓位置。少数医疗中心偏向于在 1 岁以内进行早期的牙槽骨移植，认为这样能预防上颌骨塌陷和减少将来的广泛正畸[27]。这项技术的长期评估显示，面部发育良好，改善了上颌弓形态，在远期能减少随后上颌截骨术和骨移植的需要[28]。去骨牙槽骨移植物（通过胫骨骨膜移植物，跨裂口关闭骨膜，即骨膜整形）已被尝试，但还未显示一致明显的骨再生。

二期唇腭裂处理

唇和鼻的修整

尽管一期实施了理想的面部修复，大多数唇腭裂
还需要二期修整唇或（和）鼻，包括各种手术，瘢痕 810
修整、唇红重排、人中延长、鼻底旋转或鼻尖软骨纠

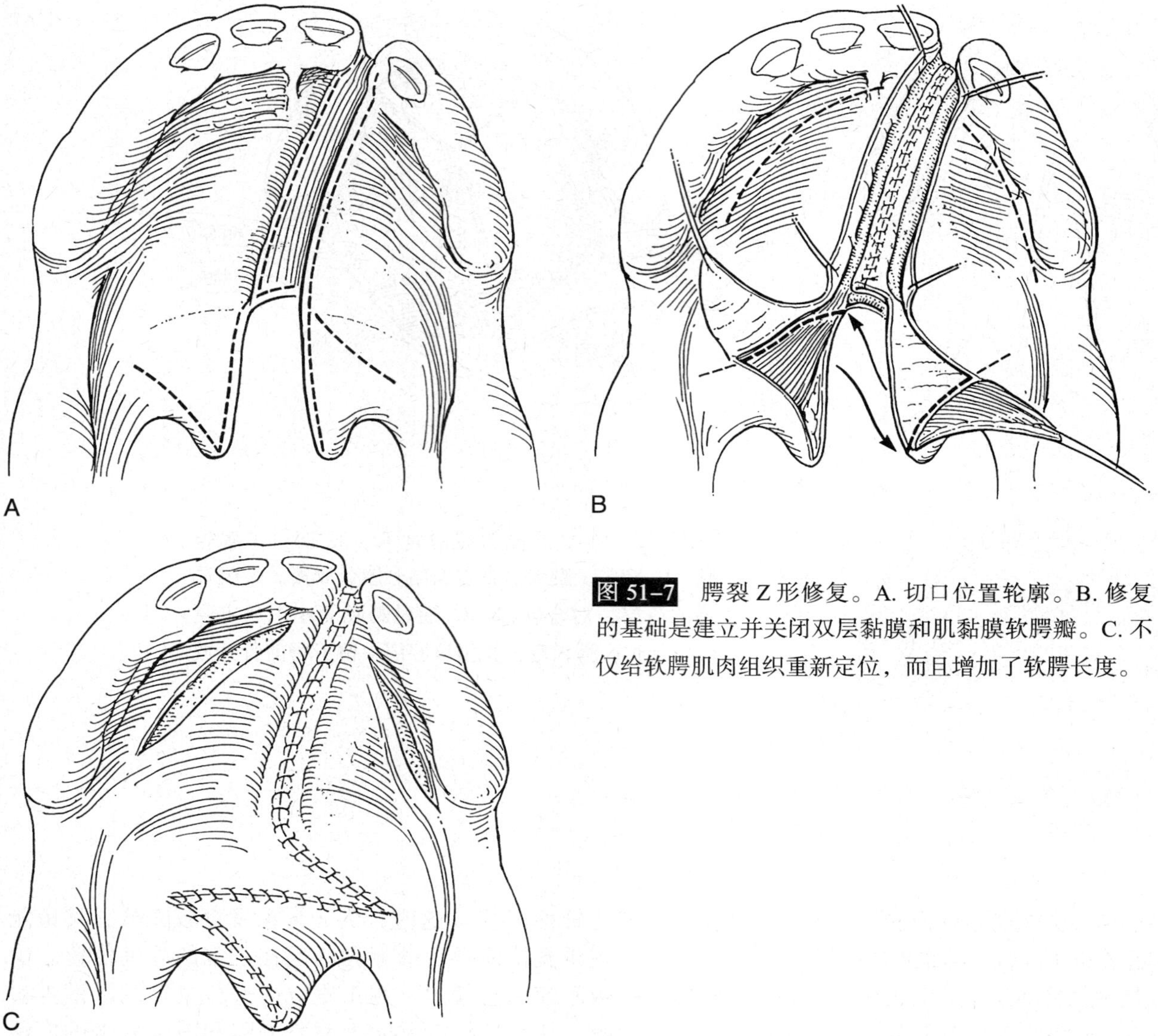

图 51-7 腭裂 Z 形修复。A. 切口位置轮廓。B. 修复的基础是建立并关闭双层黏膜和肌黏膜软腭瓣。C. 不仅给软腭肌肉组织重新定位，而且增加了软腭长度。

正[31]。需要强调的是，双侧唇裂患儿鼻小柱二期成形是必要的。因为在这类畸形病例中，这个鼻部结构通常缺失[23]。大多数唇和鼻的二期修整在 2～4 岁年龄范围内完成，使得瘢痕成熟，进入学校环境[14]。青春期进一步的唇裂修整就像青春期的社会心理需求一样逐步增多，大多数患者在青春期发育期最终需要进行一次完全的鼻中隔鼻成形术[5]。

腭裂修整

腭裂一期修整术后，瘘的发生率较高，即使手术经验丰富的医生其发生率也平均为 10%～20%，通常发生在硬软腭连接处或切牙骨和上颌骨连接处。根据伴随症状的程度，大的鼻液反流、鼻腔漏气影响说话等，决定是否需使用局部组织关闭腭瘘。大的瘘或出现在上切牙后的瘘，需要使用带蒂重建技术从舌取下 811
组织进行局部覆盖。

发音时，如果软腭不能适当地与咽后壁接触，气流就会从鼻腔中逃逸，产生重鼻音。大约有 15%的患者会出现累及次生腭的腭裂。这种腭咽功能障碍需要基于鼻内镜评估腭及咽壁运动的外科处理。重排咽侧壁、咽后壁组织使腭咽括约肌紧张度提高[16]，或将咽后壁黏膜肌瓣附于软腭咽瓣来缩小腭咽气道横截面[2]，以此来改善腭咽功能（图 51-8）。手术的成功与否取决于手术类型与术前鼻内镜评估腭咽功能障碍是否匹配。

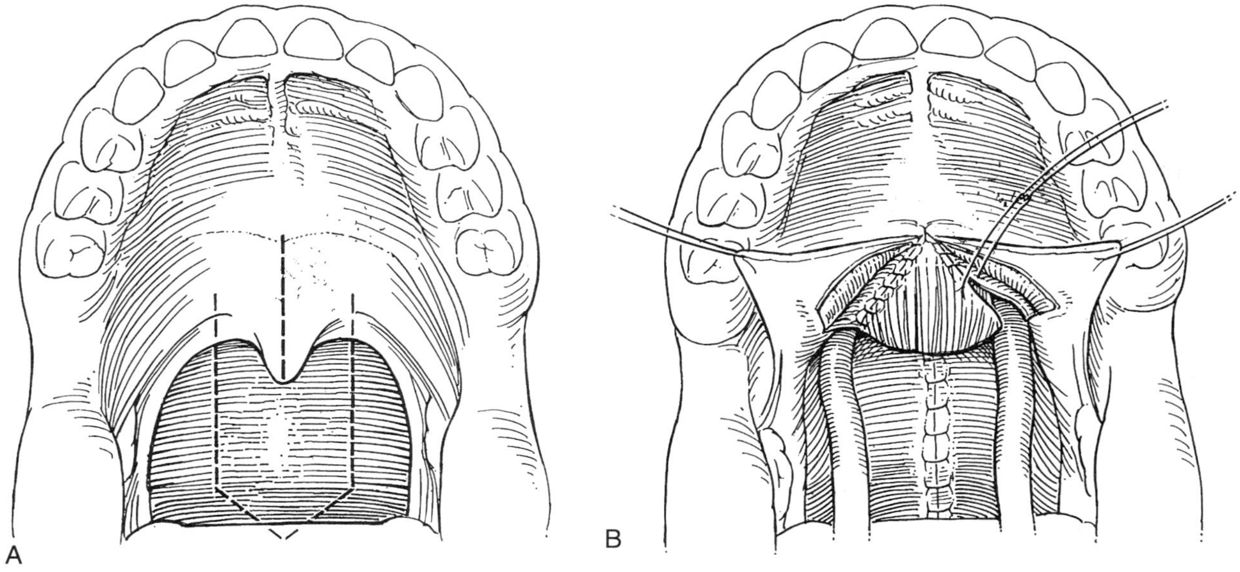

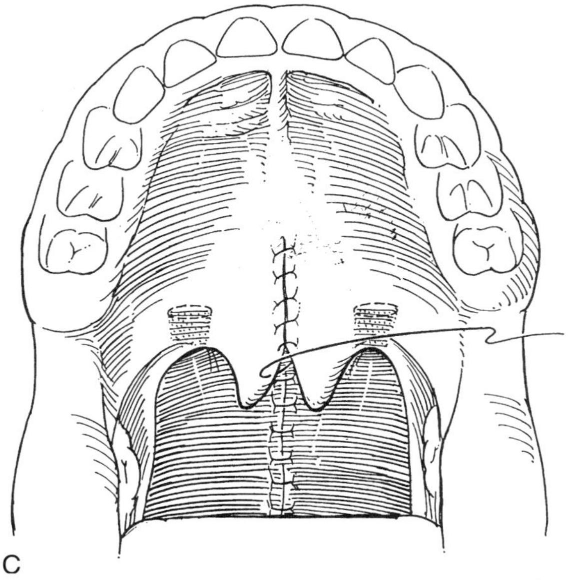

图 51-8 腭咽功能障碍手术的咽皮瓣。A. 切口轮廓，包括切开软腭以获得手术进路及皮瓣插入，以及基底左上方的咽后壁肌黏膜瓣。B. 用小导管来定型两旁空隙，提起咽皮瓣插入软腭，关闭咽后壁供瓣侧。C. 关闭软腭，皮瓣有效地把腭咽口分成两个两侧的小口，以减少说话时鼻腔气体流失。

正颌手术

上颌骨裂开的不良影响显著表现在限制了骨的向前及横向发育。形成面中部外观缺陷及错牙颌和反牙颌。需要进行矫正牙列和截骨术来使上颌骨与下颌骨形成正常骨骼和牙合关系。20%～30%的腭裂患者需要进行 Lefort I 前移术[10]。双侧腭裂患者可出现严重的面中部后缩，需要行截骨术移动面中部骨骼，术后还要用牵引装置使明显移动后的骨骼保持稳定[20]。

相关的先天性畸形

唇瘘（凹陷）

这种现象常是遗传的，可伴有或不伴有唇腭裂。 812
对称的盲端瘘或凹陷发生在下方唇红的中央部分被称为 Vander Woude 综合征。治疗为 1～3 岁间切除黏膜组织和邻近的腺体组织[26]。

黏膜下腭裂

这种看上去严重性最小的腭裂常常逃过检查，直到语言发育时才发现。仔细的口内检查有三个发现：硬腭内侧凹陷或切迹、悬雍垂分裂和软腭肌肉在中线上未连接，即便上覆的黏膜完整。可导致腭咽功能障碍，并需要手术治疗[30]。

Pierre Robin 综合征

Pierre Robin 综合征有软腭裂、舌后移（舌下垂）和下颌骨发育不全三个经典表现。这种病症并不罕见，当发现只有软腭裂时必须排除这种疾病。显著的下颌骨后移经常能在出生后立即引起气道问题，需根据其严重度给予不同类型的处理，包括手术[19]。这些患者的腭裂修复通常推迟至 1 岁后，以减少继发性气道并发症的风险。此时，下颌骨的生长使得舌体前移。

（徐建民译　董其刚校）

参考文献

1. American Cleft Palate/Craniofacial Association: Parameters for the evaluation and treatment of patients with cleft lip/palate or other craniofacial anomalies. Cleft Palate Craniofac J 1993;30(suppl 1):4.
2. Cable BB, Canady JW, Karnell MP, et al: Pharyngeal flap surgery: Long-term outcomes at the University of Iowa. Plast Reconstr Surg 2004;113:475.
3. Chung KC, Kowalski CP, Kim HM, Buchman SR: Maternal cigarette smoking during pregnancy and the risk of having a child with cleft lip/palate. Plast Reconstr Surg 2000; 105:485.
4. Cohen M: Cleft lip and palate. Clin Plast Surg 2004;31:57.
5. Cutting C: Secondary cleft lip nasal reconstruction: State of the art. Cleft Palate Craniofac J 2000;37:538.
6. Dempf R, Telzrow T, Kramer FJ, Hausamen JE: Alveolar bone grafting in patients with complete clefts: A comparative study between secondary and tertiary bone grafting. Cleft Palate Craniofac J 2002;39:18.
7. Eppley BL: Pediatric plastic surgery revisited. Clin Plast Surg 2001;28:731.
8. Eppley BL, van Aalst J, Robey A: The spectrum of orofacial clefting. Plast Reconstr Surg 2005;115:101e-114e.
9. Grayson BH, Cutting CB: Presurgical nasoalveolar orthopedic molding in primary correction of the nose, lip, and alveolus of infants born with unilateral and bilateral clefts. Cleft Palate Craniofac J 2001;38:193.
10. Heliovaara A, Ranta R, Hukki J, Rintala A: Skeletal stability of LeFort I osteotomy in patients with isolated cleft palate and bilateral cleft lip and palate. Int J Oral Maxillofac Surg 2002;31:358.
11. Horswell BB, Henderson JM: Secondary osteoplasty of the alveolar cleft defect. J Oral Maxillofac Surg 2003;61:1082.
12. Johns DF, Rohrich RJ, Awada M: Velopharyngeal incompetence: A guide for clinical evaluation. Plast Reconstr Surg 2003;112:1890.
13. Johnson N, Sandy J: Prenatal diagnosis of cleft lip and palate. Cleft Palate Craniofac J 2003;40:186.
14. Kane AA, Pilgram TK, Moshiri M, Marsh JL: Long-term outcome of cleft lip nasal reconstruction in childhood. Plast Reconstr Surg 2000;105:1600.
15. LaRossa D, Jackson OH, Kirschner RE, et al: The Children's Hospital of Philadelphia modification of the Furlow double-opposing Z-palatoplasty: Long-term speech and growth results. Clin Plast Surg 2004;31:243.
16. Losken A, Williams JK, Burstein FD, et al: An outcome evaluation of sphincter pharyngoplasty for the management of velopharyngeal insufficiency. Plast Reconstr Surg 2003; 112:1755.
17. Loffredo LC, Souza JM, Freitas JA, Mossey PA: Oral clefts and vitamin supplementation. Cleft Palate Craniofac J 2001; 38:76.
18. Marazita ML, Mooney MP: Current concepts in the embryology and genetics of cleft lip and palate. Clin Plast Surg 2004;31:125.
19. Matsas R, Thomson A, Goodacre T: Management of infants with Pierre Robin sequence. Cleft Palate Craniofac J 2004; 41:219.
20. Molina F: Distraction osteogenesis for the cleft lip and palate patient. Clin Plast Surg 2004;31:291.
21. Mulliken JB, Martinez-Perez D: The principle of rotation advancement for repair of unilateral complete cleft lip and nasal deformity: Technical variations and analysis of results. Plast Reconstr Surg 1999;104:1247.
22. Mulliken JB: Primary repair of bilateral cleft lip and nasal deformity. Plast Reconstr Surg 2001;108:181.
23. Mulliken JB, Wu JK, Padwa BL: Repair of bilateral cleft lip: Review, revisions, and reflections. J Craniofac Surg 2003; 14:609.
24. Murray JC: Gene/environment causes of cleft lip and/or palate. Clin Genet 2002;61:248.
25. Pigott RW, Albery EH, Hathorn IS, et al: A comparison of three methods of repairing the hard palate. Cleft Palate Craniofac J 2002;39:383.
26. Rizos M, Spyropoulos MN: Van der Woude syndrome: A review. Cardinal signs, epidemiology, associated features, differential diagnosis, expressivity, genetic counseling and treatment. Eur J Orthod 2004;26:17.
27. Rosenstein SW: Early bone grafting of alveolar cleft deformities. J Oral Maxillofac Surg 2003;61:1078.
28. Rosenstein SW, Grasseschi M, Dado DV: A long-term retrospective outcome assessment of facial growth, secondary surgical need, and maxillary lateral incisor status is a surgical-orthodontic protocol for complete clefts. Plast Reconstr Surg 2003;111:1.
29. Salyer KE, Genecov ER, Genecov DG: Unilateral cleft lip-nose repair: A 33-year experience. J Craniofac Surg 2003; 14:549.
30. Sommerlad BC, Fenn C, Harland K, et al: Submucous cleft palate: A grading system and review of 40 consecutive submucous cleft palate repairs. Cleft Palate Craniofac J 2004; 41:114.
31. Stal S, Hollier L: Correction of secondary cleft lip deformities. Plast Reconstr Surg 2002;109:1672.

第 52 章

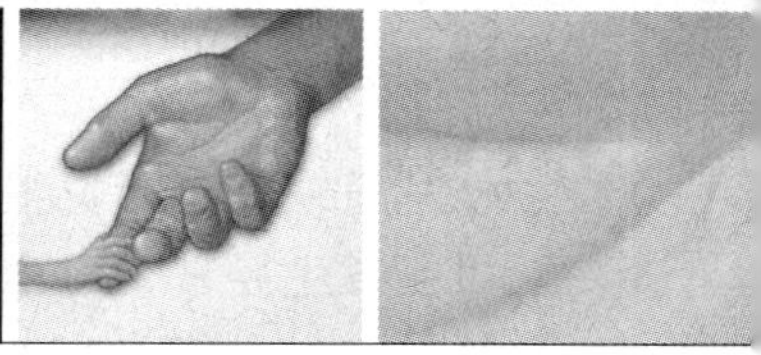

耳鼻喉疾病

William P. Potsic 和 Ralph F. Wetmore

耳

解剖学

813 耳分为三个解剖功能区：外耳、中耳和内耳。外耳包括耳廓、外耳道和鼓膜的外侧面。耳廓是复杂的纤维弹性组织支架，表面覆盖皮肤和皮下组织，耳廓的功能是传导声音入耳道。

外耳道在上下长轴方向上是椭圆形的。新生儿的外耳道几乎都是由柔软的有弹性的软骨组织所支持。颞骨经过几年的生长，外耳道的骨性部分增多，占外耳道的内侧 1/3，外侧 2/3 外耳道由坚实的软骨组织支持。毛囊和耵聍腺都位于外耳道的外 2/3 部分。外耳道皮肤与鼓膜外侧相延续，它的神经支配来自颅神经第Ⅴ、Ⅶ和Ⅹ支以及颈神经第Ⅲ支。

鼓膜分离外耳道和中耳。它有三层结构：外层皮肤层；中层纤维组织层，与外侧的中耳听小骨锤骨相连；内层黏膜层，与中耳的黏膜衬里相延续。纤维层通过一条粗纤维环带固定于颞骨。

中耳是位于颞骨中的充满空气的腔隙，腔内覆盖纤毛柱状呼吸上皮。中耳向后与覆盖同种黏膜的乳突小房系统相连通。中耳向前通过咽鼓管与鼻咽部相连通。中耳的黏液纤维运输系统可把黏液和分泌物运送至鼻咽部被吞噬。分泌细胞并非均等地分布于中耳和乳突结构中，而更多分布于前部近咽鼓管处。中耳内有三块小骨：锤骨、砧骨和镫骨。声音通过鼓膜的振动传送至镫骨底。镫骨在内耳产生流动波传送至圆窗膜，圆窗膜往复运动使流动波消失。

中耳有两种横纹肌。鼓膜张肌沿咽鼓管走行而分布，肌腱附于镫骨柄上端。镫骨肌沿面神经位于中耳后上部的垂直部分分布，肌腱附于镫骨头。这两种肌肉能使听骨链在受到持续高声噪音时得到保护。

面神经的水平部分横过中耳，位于镫骨上方。在镫骨后方，面神经垂直向下转，离开面神经管到达乳突尖部。面神经的一支分支鼓索神经支配舌前 2/3 的味觉。鼓索在面神经的垂直段发出，经鼓膜上后面的下方，穿过鼓膜的中耳侧到达砧骨长脚和锤骨之间。面神经分布于中耳的部分位于一保护性骨管中，但多达 30%的患者的骨管可能缺失（垂直段）。脑神经Ⅸ支配中耳的感觉。

内耳包括耳蜗、半规管和前庭。耳蜗是一个充满液体的螺旋管，它 11/4 圈螺旋被密质骨所包绕，螺旋膜上有螺旋器。螺旋器上的毛细胞通过镫骨底的振动感受到液体波。毛细胞产生神统冲动，经听神经（脑神经Ⅷ）传送至脑，从而产生听觉。三对半规管（水平向，前垂直向，后垂直向）也充满液体，被密质骨包绕。每个半规管包含一个毛细胞结构（壶腹），它感受运动的刺激。前庭的椭圆囊和球囊也有毛细胞结构，感受加速度运动引起的刺激[26]。

814

胚胎发生

外耳在孕 6 周发生，到孕 20 周发育完全。六个突起融合形成耳廓的基本单位。这些突起融合过程中出现任何差错将会导致耳前副耳和耳前瘘管。外耳道由第一咽裂发育，孕 3 月，固体上皮栓形成。孕 7 月时上皮栓穿通形成外耳道。

中耳由第一咽囊发育。听小骨由第一和第二咽裂发育。内耳来源于听基板的神经外胚层组织。听基板形成听窝[26]。

任何异常的联合都有可能发生。耳发育过程中的异常可能导致耳廓、外耳道、中耳内耳的畸形。外耳和中耳的一种畸形是先天性听力丧失（外耳道缺失）。

外耳道缺失可能发生于正常或异常的外耳。听小骨也可能发生异常，三个听小骨可能互相融合。面神经经过颞骨时可能改变走行。闭锁管道的重建，骨性鼓室板的去除，融合听小骨的分离，新耳鼓的重建是一项复杂的外科手术，可能改善听力。内耳很少出现发育畸形。最常见的耳蜗发育障碍其严重程度也不一，可导致感音神经性耳聋[6,12]。

检查

耳部的检查常需从耳及其周围结构开始。外耳道结构畸形可能预示着其他畸形的存在，如第一鳃裂瘘管。第一鳃裂瘘管往往发生于耳垂以下靠近下颌角处。瘘管可能与外耳道相连通，但几乎不与中耳相通。

外耳道与鼓膜可通过带有光纤光源的便携式耳镜检查。最大尺寸的反射镜正好适合外耳道的大小，可提高可见度，减轻疼痛。一种非常小的反射镜能较深地插入外耳道，但它可能划破外耳，降低鼓膜的可见度。通过耳镜能够观察到耳道和鼓膜。若鼓膜是透明的，还能观察到中耳内容物。

耳道内如果有耳垢，有可能妨碍鼓膜的观察。可用内耳手术耳镜头和耳匙去除耳垢。如果使用照明灯或手术显微镜，可同时使用双手检查，得到较好的可见度。要避免儿童突然移动，同时应轻柔地使用耳匙以免引起疼痛和划破耳道。

对有较明显的耳疾的儿童的检查，常需通过听力测检法对听力做客观评估。当前的科技和专业知识使我们能对任何年龄的儿童进行检测。

行为听力检测法可通过音域测试准确地检测6个月以上的儿童。让年龄稍大点的孩子戴上耳机，给予250～8000Hz范围内的声音用于耳特异性检测。在第10个频率记录听力阈值，此值可代表空气传导阈值。声音传过耳道、鼓膜、中耳，内耳产生电冲动把声音信号传送至脑部。儿童的正常阈值小于20dB。骨传导阈值用于检测听力的感觉神经部分。骨振荡器通过对颅骨振动的检测，检测一定频率范围的声音，它直接刺激内耳，不经外耳、中耳途径。通常空气传导阈值比骨传导的阈值低。如果骨传导阈比空气传导阈需要更小的声音强度，则儿童可能患传导性耳聋。如果空气传导阈值和骨传导阈值升高但二者阈值相同，儿童可患感音神经性耳聋。大多数患感音神经性耳聋患儿是由螺旋器的毛细胞功能障碍引起的。听力丧失可能是传导性的、感音神经性的或混合性的。电生理检测如脑干听力诱发反应和声音发射检测，能衡量来自内耳的内源性声音（耳声发射），可用于婴儿和不能接受行为听力检测法的儿童。一种对鼓膜韧性的机械测试（鼓室压测量）也可用于听力测评。所有检测方法都由儿科听力学家应用[23]。

描述听力丧失程度方面，阈值20～40dB为轻度，40～65dB为中度，55～70dB为较严重，70～90dB为严重，大于90dB为极严重。4‰的儿童有先天性耳聋，其中1‰的患儿耳聋程度在严重与极严重之间。

传导性听力丧失可能与耳科手术有关。助听器和FM系统可以帮助有传导性和感音神经性耳聋的患儿。可通过听力训练、语言治疗和培训最大限度地提高他们的交流能力。如果患有极严重的感音神经性耳聋，助听器不能起到作用时，植入耳蜗也是值得考虑的。

耳蜗植入是指把一种电设备植入耳后头皮下。这种电设备的处理程序可将声音转化为电冲动。电缆通过乳突和面神经隐窝到达中耳，以电极阵式经耳蜗上的孔插入耳蜗。

耳蜗的植入直接刺激耳蜗神经元绕开了毛细胞。815
因为大多数儿童感音神经性耳聋是由于毛细胞的功能障碍，几乎所有的患儿都能通过耳蜗植入而得到声音的感知。耳蜗植入对一些罕见疾病，如听神经缺失或耳蜗缺失是起不到作用的。

在实施耳蜗植入术前，耳蜗植入研究组需对患儿进行多学科评估，主要通过颞骨CT扫描和（或）MRI对耳蜗和听力神经作出评估。

先天性耳聋或3岁以下患儿，以及在听力丧失之前已具备沟通交流能力和语言表达能力的患儿，在耳蜗植入后获益最大。美国食品和药物管理机构规定耳蜗植入术适用于12个月大及以上的患儿。耳蜗植入后，需进行大量的听力口语训练，以提高患儿听力技能，表达能力和语言能力。已经丧失听力声音感知多年的患儿改善程度不会太大[33]。

炎性分泌性中耳炎

分泌性中耳炎是儿童最常见的耳部慢性疾病。部分儿童先天性咽鼓管过小，过小的咽鼓管不能把乳突和中耳分泌的黏液清除干净。

上呼吸道感染时黏液可能在中耳积聚。随着上呼吸感染的缓解，黏液可在几周内被吸收。颅面部畸形的儿童如腭裂和 Down 综合征患儿，也易发生中耳黏液渗出。还没有完全有效的治疗方法解决渗出问题。

持续渗出可能导致在 20～40dB 范围内的传导性耳聋。中耳渗出液还可能成为病原菌的培养基，导致儿童反复发作急性化脓性中耳炎（ASOM）。

黏液积聚于中耳达 3～4 个月时，可导致听力丧失伴急性化脓性中耳炎。鼓膜切开术和鼓膜造孔置管术有助于减轻听力丧失和减少反复严重的感染。全身麻醉下使用手术显微镜行鼓膜切开术和鼓膜置管术。除了鼓膜的后上象限部分，可以在鼓膜的任一象限做小切口，因为在后上象限做切口有可能损伤听小骨。从耳中吸出黏液，并在中耳置入硅橡胶管，可使中耳空气流通时间延长。橡胶管通常取出，而鼓膜造孔将在 6 个月至 1 年时间内愈合。当中耳不再需要通过橡胶管流通空气，咽鼓管将为中耳开通气孔。如果液体反复持续渗出，则需再次手术。随着咽鼓管的发育，大多数患儿将不再发病。有时，鼻咽部的淋巴组织可能导致中耳的持续性渗出，在置管时也可同时将鼻咽淋巴组织切除。

急性化脓性中耳炎

急性化脓性中耳炎（ASPOM）是除急性上呼吸道感染之外儿童最常见的感染疾病。急性化脓性中耳炎的病原菌包括肺炎链球菌、流感嗜血杆菌和卡他莫拉菌[25]。

急性化脓性中耳炎常引起剧烈的耳痛、发热、患侧耳传导性耳聋。中耳脓液常会影响乳突小房，因为两者是相连通的。

急性化脓性中耳炎可使用广谱口服抗生素治疗。但是，滥用抗生素导致的细菌抗药性已越来越引起关注，所以，在使用抗生素前要通过耳镜明确诊断。

有时广谱抗生素对 ASOM 不能达到预期效果。这时，耳道用酒精消毒后，取 22 号细针通过鼓膜穿刺鼓膜后上或前上象限，用小注射器将液体吸出，并作细菌培养及药敏试验。

如果正确使用抗生素，ASOM 的并发症是很少见的。随着中耳渗出液的清除，传导性听力丧失也逐渐减轻。但是感染会使鼓膜坏死，引起自发穿孔。小的穿孔常在 7 天以内愈合，但大的穿孔可能持续，并引起传导性听力丧失，需要鼓膜修复术来修补。砧骨的长期坏死也可能破坏听骨链，需要听骨重建以恢复听觉。

当感染侵袭乳突皮质骨，破坏乳突骨隔膜时，就会发生联合性的急性乳突炎。并出现骨膜下脓肿。常有耳后红斑和水肿在乳突区。耳廓被推向前、外方（图 52-1）。耳镜能向前放置，显示耳道的后上方皮肤。

除了抗生素，治疗方法还包括，从前上象限到后上象限的大范围鼓膜切开术，鼓膜置管引流中耳，及耳后乳突切除术引流骨膜下脓肿，排尽乳突部脓液。

急性化脓性中耳炎如果炎症累及面神经，可能发生面神经麻痹。注射抗生素、耳道内滴注抗生素、广 816
泛的鼓膜切开术或鼓膜造孔置管术可使面部功能完全恢复，面神经的恢复需要几周到几个月时间。

ASOM 的颅内并发症包括脑膜炎、硬脑膜外脓肿、脑脓肿、耳源性脑积水和旁窦血栓。脑膜炎是 ASOM 最常见的颅内并发症，它可与严重的感音神经

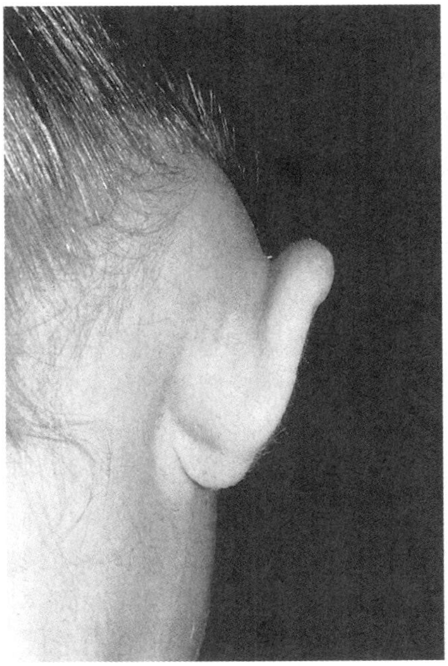

图 52-1　急性乳突炎。急性炎症过程从中耳和乳突小房向上延伸至覆盖的软组织，在头部的一侧向下向两侧推挤耳廓。乳突皮质触诊有波动感。经常可见皮质骨的缺损。需要进行乳突切除的手术引流。

性耳聋和前庭功能丧失相伴。ASOM 颅内并发症的治疗，除了对患耳进行广泛的鼓膜切开术和鼓膜造孔置管术外，正确处理颅内病情更为重要[2]。

慢性中耳炎

慢性中耳炎表现为鼓膜长期穿孔或中耳胆酯瘤。表皮样瘤是一囊性结构，囊内壁为鳞状上皮，可先天性或后天性。先天性表皮样瘤来源于颞骨发育过程中遗留于中耳的上皮剩余。它在完整的鼓膜后，表现为中耳的白色光滑团块。表皮样瘤随时间而不断扩展，并产生鳞状上皮残屑，可能侵蚀听骨链和乳突。

后天性表皮样瘤可由鼓膜穿孔继而表皮组织进入中耳形成，或咽鼓管功能不良使鼓膜袋口回缩。

表皮样瘤常为无痛性的，会引起传导性耳聋，在特定条件下，会引起耳漏。耳漏应用抗生素滴耳剂治疗。但是表皮样瘤唯一的治疗方法是彻底切除病变组织、鼓膜乳突根治术及听力重建[27][pp18–59]。表皮样瘤的潜在并发症与 ASOM 相同。

外伤

外物如毛线针、涂药器刺入耳道可能引起鼓膜穿孔，常引起剧痛、出血、传导性耳聋。如果听骨链未受损，大部分的穿孔将在 2 周内自行愈合。如果鼓膜穿孔且有水入中耳，则需口服抗生素。

耳廓撕裂伤应尽早清创以防感染，尽可能对位缝合皮肤和软组织以恢复耳部轮廓。软骨通常不需要缝合。部分或全部撕裂组织都应复位。如果组织已坏死，则不能再利用。一些严重的耳廓外伤，可口服抗生素，以预防软骨炎和软骨结构丧失。

耳部钝挫伤常由摔跤引起或见于神经肌肉系统发育不全的儿童、有自残行为的儿童。耳部出现钝挫伤时，血液和浆液聚集在骨膜与耳软骨间。如果软骨有挫伤，液体将积聚于两侧软骨与骨膜间。需引流积聚液以恢复耳轮廓，预防感染防止结疤形成，形成“菜花耳”。曾尝试引流积聚液并在乳突区放置敷料加压，但未起作用。最有效的处理方法是切开排出血液和浆液，在耳两侧放置引流棉条及褥式缝合。引流条需连续放置 7～10 天，在此期间，患者仍需口服抗生素。切口处不需要覆盖敷料[27][pp106–109]。

头部钝挫伤可能损伤内耳膜，引起感音神经性耳聋和眩晕。不需治疗，症状会自动减轻，但感音神经性耳聋可能仍会持续。严重的头部外伤可能引起颞骨骨折。颞骨骨折可分为纵行骨折、横行骨折和混合性骨折（图 52–2）。但大多数骨折类型较复杂，而不能完全归类。高分辨的断层 CT 扫描可对骨折情况作较全面的描述。骨折发生时中耳和乳突将被血液充满。血液积聚引起的传导性耳聋将随耳部积血的清除而缓解。 817

用耳镜检查颞骨骨折患儿可观察到耳道及鼓膜的撕裂伤。血液充满耳道时，鼓膜为深蓝色，因为此时中耳充满了血液，有淤血存在于乳突区（Battle 征）。

患者失去知觉时，在检查颅骨及颞骨骨折时观察记录面神经的功能是很重要的。面神经麻痹的症状可立即出现或较晚才表现。延迟性面瘫预后好，可自行恢复。即刻性面瘫可能提示神经断裂或被骨碎片压迫。如果出现即刻性面瘫，在患者病情稳定并出现好转时，应进行探查和修复。应在乳突区、中耳、颅中窝对面神经解压。应清除压迫面神经的骨碎片，将面神经缝合或接合起来。所有颞骨骨折患者一旦病情稳定，应进行听力图检测。若骨折引起听骨链断离，那么即使中耳乳突区血液被清除掉，患者的传导性耳聋仍得不到改善。

颞骨骨折的骨折线可能穿过耳蜗与前庭器。这种骨折可引起患侧严重的感音神经性耳聋和前庭功能丧失。严重的头外伤，还可引起健侧耳的耳蜗的震荡性损伤。

颞骨骨折可引起脑脊液漏入中耳及乳突。脑脊液经撕裂的鼓膜流出，引起脑脊液耳漏。脑脊液漏常可自行停止，但持续性的脑脊液耳漏则需行腰椎穿刺减压以促进愈合。极少数情况下，需行鼓膜乳突探查以关闭漏口。持续性脑脊液漏有引起脑膜炎之虑。

肿瘤

耳部良恶性肿瘤较少见。鼓膜血管瘤和面神经瘤可发生于中耳。另外颞骨结构可发生白细胞肉芽肿和横纹肌肉瘤[5,13]。

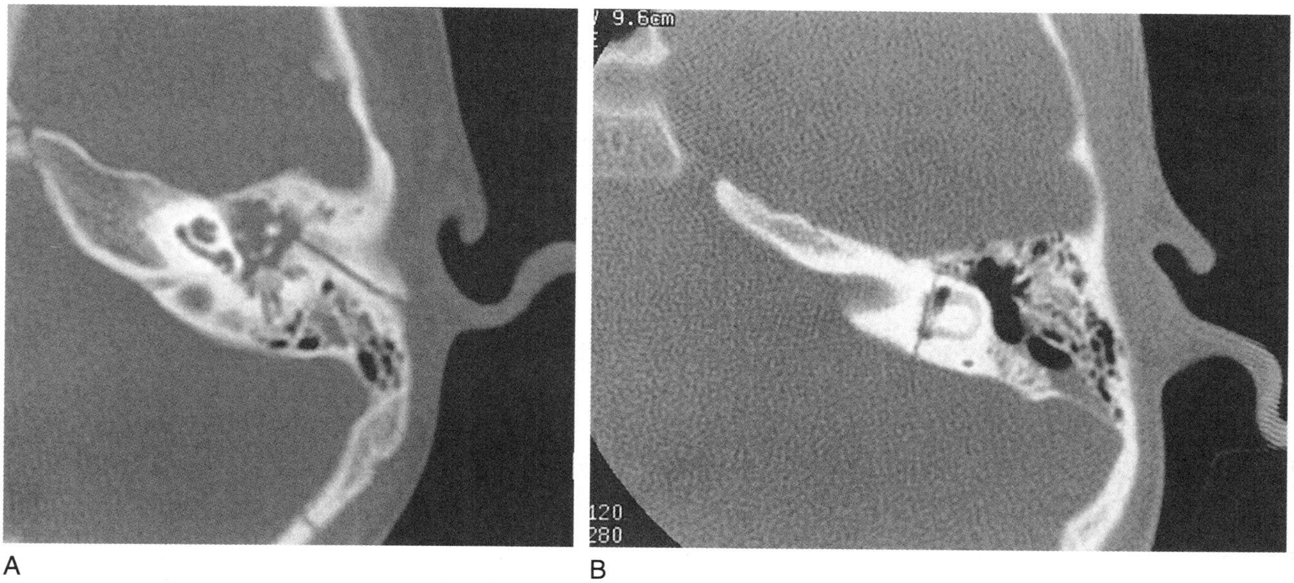

图 52-2 A. 纵向颞骨骨折。骨折平行于颞骨岩部，平衡、听力及面部功能均保持完好。B. 横向颞骨骨折。通常延伸过耳蜗和面神经管，立即导致耳聋，眩晕和面神经瘫痪。在这类病例中都必须考虑进行面神经探查修复。

鼻

解剖学

鼻可分为三个解剖部分，鼻腔是鼻的不可活动部分，包括一对鼻骨、上颌骨额突、额骨鼻突。软骨腔由上外侧的软骨与鼻中隔软骨支持。鼻小柱由下外侧的软骨和鼻中隔软骨支持。前部鼻中隔由四边形的软骨组成，后部鼻中隔由犁骨、筛骨、垂直板、上颌骨
818 鼻突和腭骨组成。

颈内、颈外动脉系统都为鼻部提供血供。鼻腔顶部和上外侧壁由筛前、后动脉、蝶腭动脉、腭大动脉供血，鼻中隔是由筛前、筛后动脉、腭动脉、上唇动脉供血。这些血管汇聚于鼻前部 Kiesselbach 动脉丛或 Little 区处。静脉回流主要是通过眼静脉、面前静脉、蝶腭静脉。嗅球位于鼻腔上壁，负责嗅觉功能。感官信息经神经传递穿过筛板，经脑神经 I（嗅神经）到达脑部。嗅觉对味觉也起到重要作用。

骨性结构、鼻甲形成鼻侧壁显著增加了鼻表面积，可对空气进行更有效的润湿加温作用，可加温至 36℃。三个鼻甲为上、中、下鼻甲。最上鼻甲也常常存在，它对于黏膜的振动是必要的。鼻甲可形成紊乱的气流，产生的阻力占呼吸道总阻力的 50%。鼻毛和鼻黏膜可对空气进行清洁过滤。鼻前部为复层鳞状上皮，至鼻甲前部移行为呼吸上皮，被捕捉到的异物颗粒通过黏膜纤毛运输机制被向后运往鼻咽部。

发音也受鼻部解剖和病理状态的影响。鼻腔阻塞可引起低鼻音，过多空气通过鼻腔（因腭咽部关闭不全）可引起鼻音过强，影响发音和语言的可理解度。

胚胎发生

鼻旁窦开口于鼻腔。鼻道是位于鼻甲侧方与鼻腔外侧壁之间的间隙，分别称为上、中、下鼻道。上颌窦、额窦、前组筛窦开口于中鼻道。后组筛窦开口于上鼻道。蝶窦开口于位于上鼻道后上方的蝶筛隐窝。鼻泪管开口于上鼻道。胚胎第 4 周形成鼻凹，鼻凹内陷并向中央移行形成鼻腔，口鼻膜分隔口腔和鼻腔。口鼻膜在胚胎第 7 周打开，连通鼻与鼻咽部。

胚胎 3～4 个月，鼻外侧壁外翻形成鼻旁窦。上颌窦和筛窦在出生时已完成发育。额窦和蝶窦 7 岁时开始发育，但直到成年才发育完全[1]。

炎性疾病

病毒性鼻窦炎占鼻及鼻窦感染性疾病的绝大部分。常由各种病毒引起。该病有自限性。发热、鼻充血、头痛、鼻涕等症状常在 5～7 天内缓解。可对症治疗。

细菌性鼻窦炎

急性呼吸道感染可诱发急性细菌性鼻窦炎，最常见的致病菌是肺炎链球菌、流感嗜血杆菌、卡他球菌。急性鼻窦炎引起周身不适、头痛、鼻塞。还可出现鼻窦区疼痛或上颌窦、额窦压痛。慢性鼻窦炎常由急性迁延所致，病程超过 30 天。

诊断鼻窦炎的“金标准”是 CT 检查，但是完整病史和鼻检查对诊断急性鼻窦炎很有效。检查鼻腔可用耳镜头上的反射镜。后鼻腔可用直杆内镜或柔软的光纤鼻咽镜。

治疗包括口服抗生素、短期局部使用减充血剂（如麻黄碱）和鼻喷雾。局部使用类固醇激素类喷雾对慢性鼻窦炎有效。

如果患有食管反流性疾病、自身免疫性疾病、黏液纤毛功能障碍和更常见的上呼吸道敏感症，则该患儿慢性鼻窦炎可以恶化。因此在治疗鼻窦感染的同时要注意这些疾病的控制。如果慢性鼻窦感染症状和体征持续，需作 CT 评估窦黏膜情况及引流途径，必要时做鼻窦内镜手术解除引流障碍。

鼻及鼻窦黏膜的慢性炎症导致息肉形成，阻塞鼻及鼻窦。上颌窦后鼻孔息肉是一种较大的息肉，来源于上颌窦壁，通过鼻腔向鼻咽部发展。鼻息肉可通过内镜手术切除，但大的上颌窦后鼻孔息肉需打开上颌窦切除。儿童鼻息肉可引起囊性纤维化。

鼻窦炎并发症

鼻窦围绕着眼眶，故常见鼻源性眶内并发症。表
819 现为红斑、眼睑水肿，球结膜水肿少见。但若感染鼻窦附近，眶周骨膜下脓肿形成，则有可能出现眼球突出、球结膜水肿、眼肌麻痹及视力丧失。筛窦感染最易引起这些并发症。眶周骨膜下脓肿最好的检查手段是鼻窦 CT。首先要静注抗生素，一些病例需内镜或外部引流。

颅内并发症包括大脑炎、海绵窦血栓性静脉炎、硬脑膜外脓肿、硬脑膜下脓肿、脑脓肿。治疗可手术使脓液引流，同时，颅内病灶应请神经外科合作手术[30]。

真菌性鼻窦炎

真菌性鼻窦炎常发生于有免疫缺陷的儿童，特别是严重糖尿病、接受化疗的儿童、及骨髓移植接受者。治疗包括鼻窦引流和静脉抗真菌治疗。

但是，变态反应性鼻窦炎是真菌鼻窦炎的慢性形式。这种患者常有过敏表现，如哮喘。治疗使用类固醇激素和鼻窦清创术，通过 CT 检查和鼻窦分泌物中查有真菌和嗜伊红白细胞以诊断[11]。

先天畸形

梨状孔狭窄

先天性前鼻孔狭窄可引起鼻部分阻塞，导致进食困难、呼吸障碍、生长发育障碍，鼻窥镜检查显示两侧狭窄鼻孔，鼻 CT 检查可见明显的梨状孔狭窄。新生儿依靠鼻呼吸，严重的梨状孔狭窄需行手术以解除阻塞。由于狭窄的部位位于鼻腔前部，而鼻腔剩余部分正常，故手术可从唇下方入路用钻去除阻塞。在鼻孔放置 3mm 气管套管并缝合固定，几周后去除。

鼻后孔闭锁

鼻后孔闭锁可为单侧或双侧性。大多为骨性闭锁，但也有少数为膜性闭锁。单侧鼻后孔闭锁表现为一侧慢性鼻液溢，没有明显的呼吸困难。但因为新生儿只依靠鼻进行呼吸，所以双侧鼻后孔闭锁会引起严重的呼吸困难，进食障碍以至生命危险。用导管试通，如果不能经鼻进入咽部，则可诊断为鼻后孔闭锁。将黏液从鼻腔中吸出，并用鼻减充血剂收缩鼻黏膜后，可使用细的柔软的鼻咽内镜检查。最好的诊断方法是鼻腔 CT。CT 显示闭锁区，辨别组织性质（骨

性或膜性）和整个鼻腔的构造。

鼻后孔闭锁可经鼻切除闭锁部分而得到有效治疗。耳匙、骨钻可有效去除闭锁部。但当闭锁骨板很厚或鼻腔后部极狭窄时，则需直接经腭手术。经腭手术入路可较好地切除骨板和后鼻中隔（图 52–3）。移植组织片来源于气管，置入鼻部并与鼻中隔缝合，几周后去除。移植片需经过生理盐水润湿，并每天抽吸清洁，以防止黏液栓形成和急性呼吸困难。经腭手术的再狭窄率较低 [27[pp196–205]]。

鼻皮样囊肿

鼻皮样囊肿或鼻瘘管一般发生于鼻背中线区（图 52–4）。表现为圆形肿块或带毛发的凹陷（图 52–5），可并发感染。鼻瘘管可经鼻骨到达鼻额区和颅内。CT 和 MRI 可显示病变范围。手术切除可防止感染及
820 复发，要在感染发生前 3～5 年进行手术。局限于鼻部的病灶可在鼻中线处做围绕窦道的椭圆形切口完全切除 [27[pp188–191]]。窦道必须完全切除，必要时需分离鼻骨。如果病变波及颅内，则需与神经外科医生合作行联合颅骨切开术。

鼻神经胶质瘤和脑膨出

鼻神经胶质瘤表现为鼻内肿块，可与鼻息肉相混

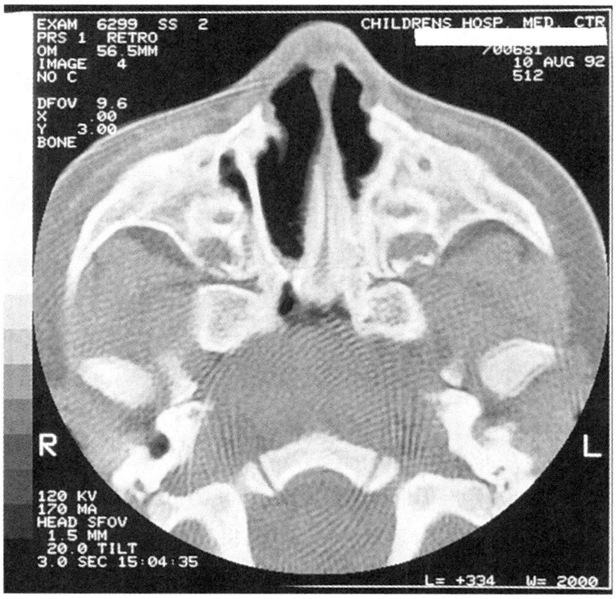

图 52–3　鼻后孔闭锁。这一异常表现为出生时呼吸吸窘迫。

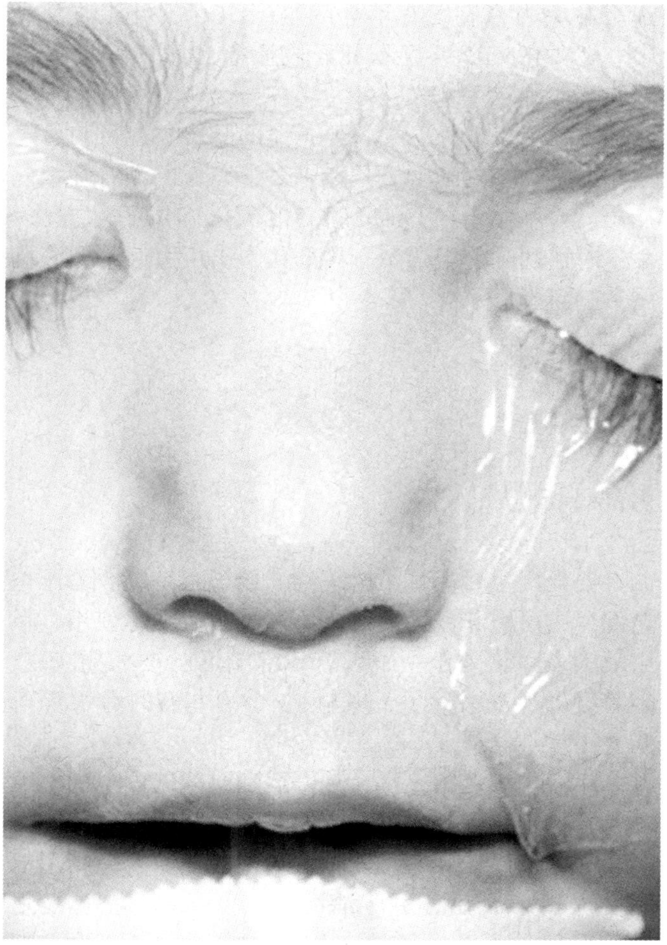

图 52–4　鼻皮样囊肿表现为正中线上的一个凹陷。

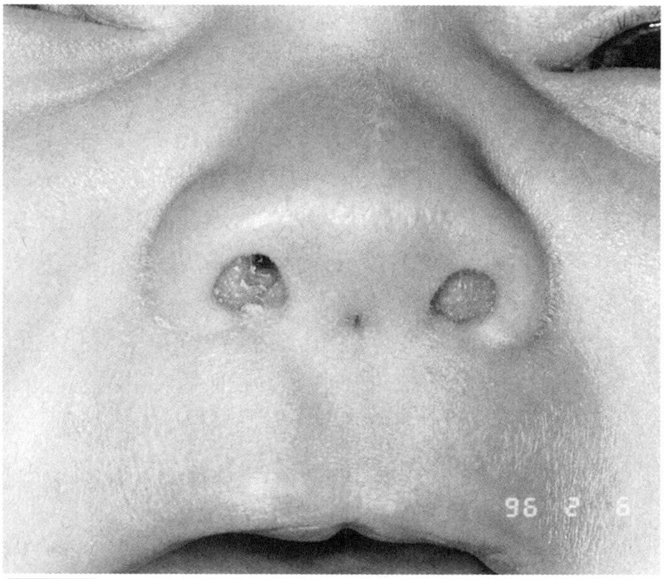

图 52–5　鼻皮样囊肿。损害的典型表现是单一的鼻背中线上的凹陷，凹陷深处有毛发可挤出。凹陷也可在鼻小柱上发生。

淆。肿块内含有发育不全的脑组织，还可能波及颅内。CT 和 MRI 可显示神经胶质瘤和颅内病变的范围，从而确定手术入路。

脑膨出表现为一柔软可压缩的肿块，也可与鼻息肉相混淆。鼻内脑膨出是指未发育完善的颅骨筛板外疝出。CT、MRI 可确定病变范围以确定手术方法。手术时需切除前组筛窦。鼻部脑膨出可引起脑脊液鼻漏和脑膜炎。

外伤

鼻部骨折

婴儿出生时鼻骨柔软，难产或子宫持续收缩压迫鼻部，则可引起鼻中隔偏离。通过指法熟练使用，鼻中隔大多可恢复至中线。若鼻部畸形已被部分恢复，随着婴儿生长发育，1 岁至 18 个月左右时鼻中隔可恢复正常。

年龄稍大点的儿童，常因运动时撞击面部而引起鼻骨及鼻中隔骨折，表现为短时鼻出血和鼻背偏向一侧，并即刻出现肿胀，此时很难确定需要复位畸形的程度。4～6 天后，肿胀消退，方可确定需把鼻畸形复位至何种程度。鼻骨 X 线检查诊断意义不大，畸形的复位只依据临床检查。有效的骨折复位可在伤后两周进行。闭合复位需在全身麻醉下进行，并可服抗生素预防感染，鼻腔内加以填塞以支持鼻骨。鼻部骨折不需立即复位，但首诊医生须首先排除鼻中隔血肿的可能。鼻中隔血肿如果未得到及时治疗可导致鼻软骨坏死、鼻支持结构丧失、以致形成马鞍鼻畸形。治疗主要是切开并清除血凝块，黏膜软骨瓣应通过鼻中隔褥式缝合。放置细橡皮引流条 12～24 小时，并给予抗生素。

儿童鼻出血常发生在 Little 区。压迫鼻翼出血可
821 停止。极少数情况需在全麻下灼烧血管以止血。

鼻异物

儿童可发生异物刺入鼻腔，患儿可能向父母诉说此类事件。大多数患儿表现为一侧鼻流脓伴恶臭，并拒绝将物体放入鼻中。

大多数鼻部异物为无痛性的，对鼻无不利影响，但鼻部会出现恶臭排出物。此外，圆形电池，可引起鼻腔迅速碱烧伤和疼痛。必须尽快取出电池，否则化学性烧伤将在几分钟至几小内出现。若出现大面积组织坏死，会导致鼻狭窄。

去除鼻异物时要使用鼻减充血剂以减轻鼻黏膜充血，并借助照明装置观察异物。可使用镊子或钩子。如果异物位于鼻深部，最好在麻醉下取出。如果异物被推入鼻咽部，应行气管镜以防止异物被吸入支气管。

鼻撕裂伤

鼻撕裂伤处理时应小心对齐撕裂边缘以恢复鼻部轮廓。标准化伤口闭合术也被应用。若无大皮瓣代替，不必缝合鼻黏膜。

鼻部肿瘤

横纹肌肉瘤、淋巴瘤、鳞状上皮癌和鼻腔神经胶质瘤可发生于儿童的鼻腔及鼻窦。幸运的是，这些恶性肿瘤在儿童中的发病率很低。对鼻及鼻窦性肿瘤患儿的治疗方法是多学科性、多模式的。

青少年鼻咽部血管纤维瘤是发生于青春期男性的一种良性肿瘤，它来源于鼻侧壁和鼻咽部。肿瘤可完全阻塞鼻腔及鼻咽部。这种血管纤维瘤可经颅底侵及颅内，患者表现为鼻阻塞，复发性鼻出血和鼻液溢。在减轻鼻黏膜充血后，肿瘤可借助于柔软的光纤鼻咽内镜观察，可见光滑的红色肿块。应避免活检以免形成大出血。CT 和 MRI 可确定肿瘤部位及范围。从 MRI 血管造影术显示肿瘤的血液供应，可来自于颈内和颈外动脉。对比血管造影术有助于术前制订计划。青春期鼻咽部血管纤维瘤的治疗主要是术前栓塞和完整的手术切除。根据使用材料的不同，栓塞有效期可持续几天至几周。有多种手术方法可供选择，包括内镜下切除小肿瘤。大范围肿瘤则需行面中部颅内联合术[29]。

许多文章提出放疗是青春期鼻咽部血管纤维瘤的主要治疗方法，但很多外科医生更关心放疗对患儿的长期疗效，包括对恶性肿瘤的诱导。

口腔 / 咽

解剖学

口腔边界为：前界为唇，侧方边界是颊，上边界是腭部，后边界是一从软腭到舌前 1/3 与舌后 2/3 交汇处连接而形成的平面。口腔包括口腔前庭（即唇颊部与牙槽突间的潜在间隙）和固有口腔。牙槽突和牙列将口腔前庭与固有口腔分隔开。口腔前庭在中线处被上下唇系带分为两部分。牙槽突与硬腭相连接。腮腺导管（Stensen 导管）开口于上颌第二磨牙相对应的颊黏膜上。颌下腺导管 Wharton 导管开口底舌系带附近。

腭部由前方的原发腭突与中部的继发腭突融合而成。硬腭分隔口腔和鼻腔。硬腭由前颌骨和腭骨垂直板组成。软腭由腭帆张肌腱膜形成，有五种肌肉插入腱膜，包括腭帆张肌、腭帆提肌、腭舌肌、腭咽肌和腭垂。硬腭和（或）软腭形成过程中的任何障碍可导致腭裂。腭部的感觉和运动受三叉神经和咽丛支配。

轮廓乳头将舌分为位于口腔的前 2/3 和位于口咽部的后 1/3。舌的两大不同的神经支配和血供反应了他们不同的胚胎来源。舌前 2/3 来源于第一鳃弓（三叉神经），而舌后 1/3 则起源于第三、四鳃弓（咽丛）。舌下神经支配舌内肌的运动。除了舌内肌，四条舌外肌的协同运动变换舌的位置。颏舌肌收缩，使舌向前向下；舌骨舌肌收缩，使舌向后向下；茎突舌骨肌收缩，使舌向后；腭舌肌收缩，使舌向上下运动。除了轮廓乳头，舌面其他味蕾分布于锥状乳头、
822 丝状乳头、菌状乳头和叶状乳头。

咽为纤维黏膜性管道，上端附于颅底，下端位于喉环状软骨水平。可分为三部分。鼻咽部位于颅底与软腭之间，口咽部位于软腭与舌根之间，喉咽部位于舌根与环状软骨之间。三组收缩肌联合形成了咽的肌肉部分：咽上缩肌、咽中缩肌、咽下缩肌。Passavant 隆起是咽缩肌的一部分，参与腭咽闭合。咽下缩肌下部纤维参与上部食管括约肌的形成。咽的运动和感觉神经支配来源于经过咽丛的舌咽神经和迷走神经。

咽部的淋巴组织聚集成 Waldeyer 环，包括腭扁桃体、腺样体（咽扁桃体）、咽侧索和咽后壁的淋巴滤泡。

急性咽扁桃体炎

除了突然出现的咽痛外，病毒性咽炎一般表现为发热和周身不适。体征包括咽部充血和颈部淋巴结肿大。按不同种病毒感染，还可表现为鼻阻塞和鼻液溢。主要致病原是鼻病毒、冠状病毒、副流感病毒、呼吸性多核心病毒、腺病毒和流感病毒。

原发性疱疹龈口炎由疱疹病毒 I 型或 II 型引起，表现为发热、淋巴结肿大、唇、舌、颊黏膜、软腭、咽黏膜的水疱、溃疡。疱疹性咽峡炎和手足口病是口咽部的病毒感染。EBV 感染（传染性单核细胞增多症）表现为急性咽扁桃体炎、发热、全身多发性淋巴结肿大、周身不适和脾大。全血细胞计数，有超过 10% 的异常淋巴细胞，Monospot 试验阳性可以用来诊断。EBV 感染需以 EBV 定量来确诊。

溶血性链球菌 A 组（GABHS，即 S 化脓菌）主要感染咽部。除了咽痛，伴发症状还包括发热，头痛和腹痛。体征有咽部红肿、口臭、扁桃体有渗出物和轻度淋巴结肿大。确诊主要依据快速链球菌抗原检侧。因为快速抗原检测比正规血琼脂培养基涂片培养更加敏感。检测为阴性并不能排除链球菌感染，但是检测阳性加上涂片培养结果就可确诊。其他引起急性咽炎的细菌性病原体包括流感嗜血杆菌，β 溶血性链球菌 C 组和 G 组。有时，抗青霉素的金黄色葡萄球菌与链球菌的同时感染可能干扰对 GABHS 感染的治疗[28]。虽然许多 GABHS 感染病例使用青霉素或阿莫西林可有疗效，对一些缺少依从性的患者可使用苄星青霉素或头孢曲松。

复发性扁桃体炎

咽部的复发性感染可由病毒或细菌引起。GABHS 是最令人不安的细菌，因为复发感染可能引起并发症，如猩红热、急性风湿热、脓毒性关节炎和急性血管球性肾炎。除了有 S 化脓菌多次培养阳性病史外，升高的抗链球菌溶血素 O 滴度可以确定。一些无症状的儿童可能是 GABHS 的慢性携带者，升高的 ASO 滴度可能不是区分感染活动期与慢性期的可靠指标。

对反复链球菌感染或儿童携带者的治疗包括试验性的抗生素治疗并已显示出一定疗效（如克林霉素、

万古霉素、利福平），内科治疗无效或并发症引起的儿童复发性咽扁桃体炎，则需考虑外科治疗。对于每个儿童的治疗应个体化，外科治疗的指征为 1 年感染 7 次，每年或每两年感染五次以上，或每年或每三年感染三次以上者[24]。是否选择外科治疗的其他考虑因素，还包括感染的严重程度，是否对抗生素治疗有效，失学的时间及住院治疗的需要。

慢性咽扁桃体炎

慢性感染可发生于咽部特别是扁桃体。儿童患者主诉慢性咽痛、口臭、扁桃体隐窝有白色点状物。体征为：扁桃体充血、隐蔽的白色点状物和颈淋巴结慢性肿大。咽部感染可由多种病毒和细菌引起。患者的细菌培养可能为阳性或阴性，因为表面组织培养可能是阴性但深处组织细菌培养为阳性。针对厌氧微生物或金黄色葡萄球菌的抗生素有助于顽固性病例的治疗。内科治疗无效的儿童可考虑扁桃体切除术。

扁桃体周蜂窝织炎 / 脓肿

扁桃体炎症局部扩散可引起扁桃体周蜂窝织炎，
823 致病菌相同。除了剧烈的咽痛，症状和体征还有流涎、牙关紧密、声音含糊不清、（疼痛向同侧耳部放射）身体同侧的放射性耳痛和轻度淋巴结肿大。扁桃体周蜂窝组织炎进一步发展可形成扁桃体周脓肿。早期扁桃体周蜂窝织炎可口服抗生素治疗，如青霉素、头孢菌素、红霉素或林可霉素。治疗效果不佳的蜂窝织炎或脓肿应给予静脉内抗生素治疗。儿童脓肿形成后，需行引流排脓，穿刺或切开排脓有同样的效果[15]。对多次脓肿发作者或需在普通麻醉下排脓的儿童，应考虑行扁桃体切除术（扁桃体周脓肿切除术）。

咽后 / 咽旁间隙感染

颈深间隙（咽后 / 咽旁）感染表现为发热、流涎、烦躁、食欲缺乏、斜颈或和（或）牙关紧闭。常有病毒感染病史。喘鸣音或上呼吸道阻塞症状可见于一半患者[32]。局部感染引起颈部肿块或颈淋巴结肿大。常见病原菌包括凝固酶阳性的葡萄球菌和 GABHS（β–溶血性链球菌 A 组）。50%病例中可检测到厌氧菌[32]。颈深间隙感染并发症包括呼吸道阻塞、菌血症、脓肿破裂脓液涌入咽部、炎症扩散引起纵隔炎、颈静脉血栓形成和颈动脉破裂。

对于疑似病例，可通过高对比度 CT 或 MRI 确诊咽后 / 咽旁间隙感染。颈侧 X 光片显示咽后间隙变宽提示咽后间隙感染。超声可检测脓腔是否形成，CT 或 MRI 可有效。显示感染范围和周围重要结构的分布，尤其是大血管。心血管高对比度 CT 对于区分蜂窝织炎和脓肿非常有效。92%的病例脓肿表现为低密度区中心围绕密度高的边缘区（图 52–6）。

颈深间隙感染的主要治疗首先要静脉抗炎，包括新青霉素、林可霉素、头孢唑啉、β–内酰胺酶青霉素或联合应用。手术引流可应用于病情有改善的儿童或 CT 显示脓肿已形成者，如果脓肿位于大血管内侧手术入路通常从口内入路，如果脓肿位于大血管外侧则从口外入路。

对并发症应积极治疗。大多数纵隔感染需立即外科引流，感染性静脉血栓（Lemierre 综合征）可作为败血症栓子成为转移性的感染源。症状体征包括寒战、发热和对抗炎治疗无效的颈部肿块，对感染血栓

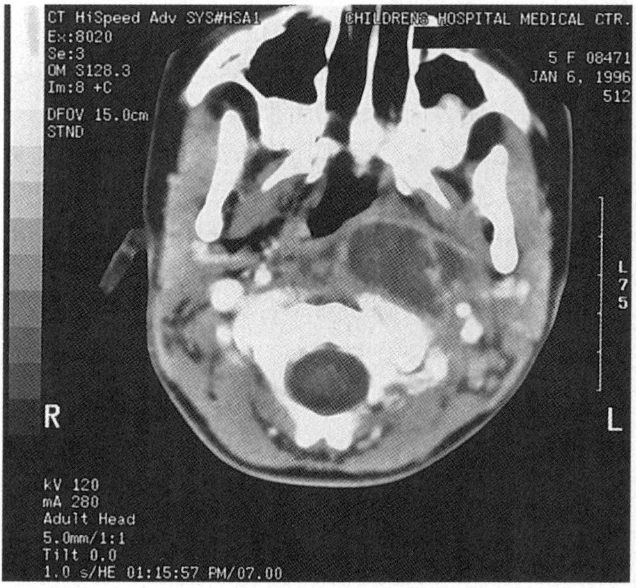

图 52–6 咽后脓肿。颈部 CT 示咽后间隙液体腔形成。典型的脓肿是单侧的，经常蔓延至咽旁间隙的中间区域，在没有并发症的情况下，可以进行口内引流。

进行结扎或切除以清除感染。

睡眠障碍性呼吸（SDB）

最近十年，从 Marous 和他的同事们对标准睡眠数据的报道开始，SDB 对儿童健康的影响已被广泛报告[20]。儿童表现为短暂高频的呼吸微弱和完全呼吸暂停。因为儿童呼吸暂停少于 10 秒可引起气息错乱。大多数病例阻塞部分发生在咽部。成年患者阻塞原因主要是咽肌肉周围的脂肪组织，而儿童的主要原因是扁桃腺肥大。

呼吸暂停指数指 1 小时呼吸暂停的次数，儿童正常值小于 1。因为大多数儿童与成人相比部分梗阻的频率增加，所以对于呼吸不足的治疗更加重要。呼吸
824 不足可表现为气流量减少、呼吸急促、氧饱和度不足或同时出现。呼吸阻塞 RDI 指数，是对呼吸暂停和不足 1 小时内的测量，可以更好反应儿童 SDB。RDI 大于 5 次为异常。上呼吸道阻塞表现为呼吸障碍而呼吸指数正常，但有睡眠中断及脑电描记器显示睡眠紊乱。

SDB 的高危人群包括扁桃体肥大的儿童，其次是淋巴过度增生的儿童（图 52–7 和 52–8）。儿童发病年龄为 2 岁至青少年时期。而在 2～6 岁，儿童的扁桃体和淋巴组织达到最大体积。其他高危人群包括 Down 综合征的患儿、颅面畸形的儿童和腭裂患者（Hunter、 Hurler 综合征）。儿童阻塞性呼吸暂停的不利影响包括学习成绩下降、发育不良、面部及牙齿发育不良和罕见的心脏损害，包括高血压、心律失常和肺源性心脏病。

日间症状包括口呼吸、鼻阻塞充血、鼻音和呼吸困难。与成人相比，儿童的嗜睡情况较少，因为儿童较少发生气体交换异常，特别是高碳酸血症。儿童可能主述头痛、烦躁、学习成绩下降。夜间症状更加明显，包括打鼾、气促和其他表现包括梦游、说梦话、磨牙。遗尿可出现在呼吸道阻塞的儿童，经手术治疗，遗尿可减轻。除了扁桃体肥大，体征还有腭裂患者的咽后瓣、颅面畸形、腺病面容和少见的右心衰。

SDB 可通过病史和体格检查进行诊断。确诊可依据整夜睡眠时连续血氧测定和视频或音频监测。诊断阻塞性睡眠暂停的“金标准”是多种睡眠描记法，包括鼻和口气流测定、胸壁运动的测量、心电图、眼外肌运动测定、胃 pH 监测。在可疑阻塞部位，可用辅助检查如颈侧区 X 线、头颈部 CT、上呼吸道内镜。

SDB 的非手术治疗包括肥胖患者减重、过敏疾病和胃食管反流的治疗。使用鼻和口腔器械维持呼吸

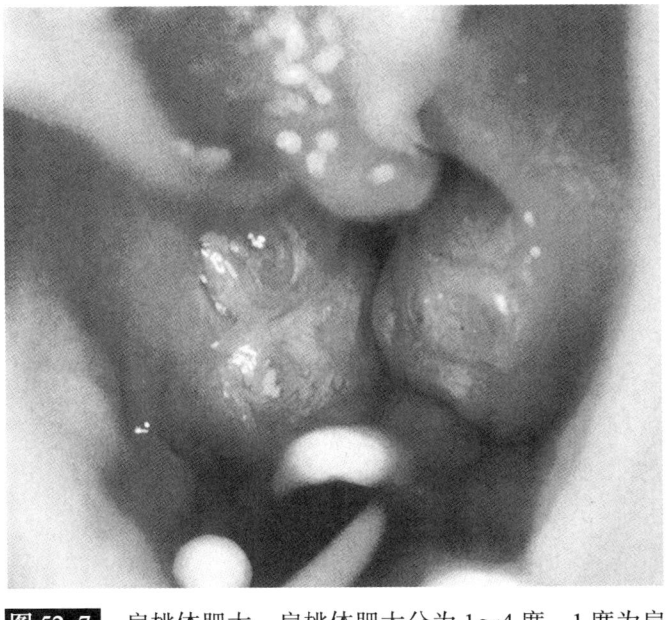

图 52–7　扁桃体肥大。扁桃体肥大分为 1～4 度，1 度为扁桃体肥大，2 度为扁桃体轻度越过扁桃体弓，3 度，扁桃体向中线方向越过扁桃体前弓，4 度为扁桃体肥大至中线。

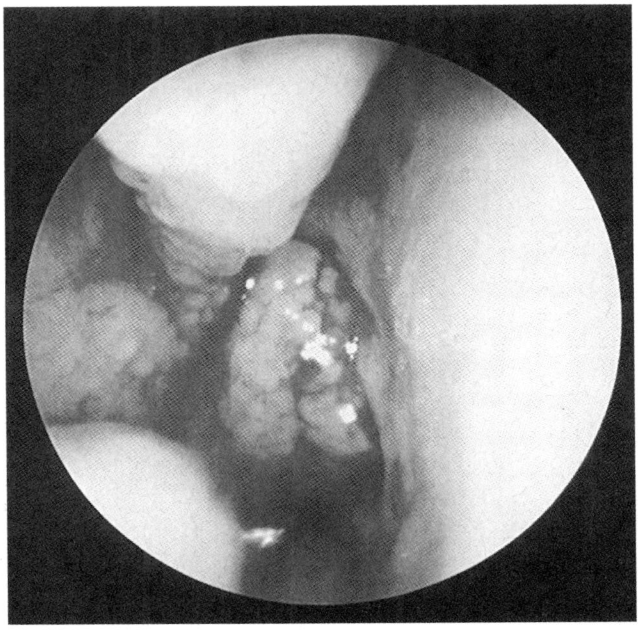

图 52–8　腺样体肥大。腺样体肥大能引起鼻咽阻塞。照片显示小的增生组织长入后鼻孔亦能引起鼻腔呼吸阻塞。

道开放可能对成人患者有效，但儿童常难以耐受，鼻持续性正压通气法是成人的主要治疗方法，特别是对其他治疗方法无效的患者。

大多儿童 SDB 患者的最初的外科治疗是扁桃体切除和腺样体切除术。通常，这是一种可治愈的措施。
825 对于有睡眠呼吸暂停或睡眠障碍的患儿，即使扁桃体小，也应该行这两种手术。扁桃体及腺样体切除术数十年来已经成为标准，但在一些机构已被新技术取代，包括等离子低温射频消融、谐波手术刀和微型整复器的应用。但这些新技术的效果还未被证实。

扁桃体及淋巴结切除术后并发症包括呼吸道损伤和急性或延迟性出血。自从有了现代儿童麻醉术，呼吸道并发症如吸入性肺炎和肺脓肿已很少见。保持湿润环境、使用类固醇激素和抗生素可以改善术后并发症。儿童最易受并发症的影响，在大多数机构，4 岁以下儿童需进行夜间监护以防脱水和呼吸道并发症。

SDB 的辅助性手术治疗包括对合适患者颅面修复或腭裂后皮瓣修复术。面中部下颌和舌骨修复在特定患者已取得疗效，鼻部手术有鼻中隔成形术，部分上鼻甲切除术，或鼻甲切除术。气管造口术对于其他治疗无效的患者来说是最后的治疗方法。

舌粘连

舌粘连或舌系带过短是发生在舌系带的常见的先天性疾病（图 52-9）。新生儿因为舌系带过短引起舌活动度减少，可导致吮吸进食障碍。新生儿和婴儿的舌系带较细且没有血管，手术可常规切开。大一点的儿童，舌系带过短主要对发音有影响。因为舌尖向上向侧方卷曲受到限制，可影响发音。这种患者的手术治疗，如果系带较粗且含血管较多，需在短时普通麻醉下手术。手术矫正可简单切开加或不加 Z 成形术。

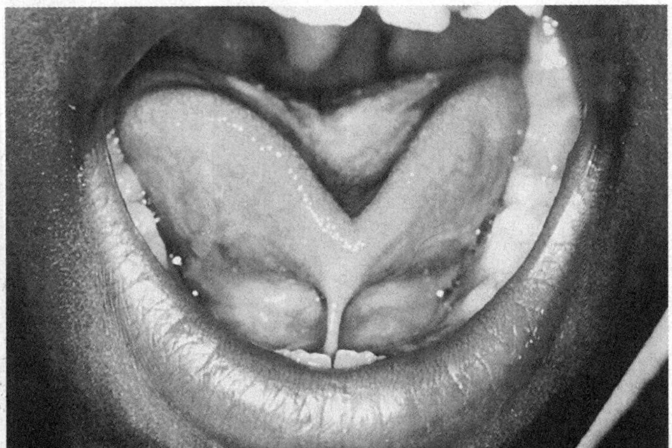

图 52-9 舌粘连。舌系带的不正常发育限制了舌尖向下颌骨前区的伸展，经常引起发音障碍必须矫正。

巨舌症

巨舌较少见。巨舌症常伴脐膨出、内脏巨大、肾上腺和肾脏疾病（Beckwith Wiedemann 综合征），或与糖原贮积病同时存在（Hunter 和 Harler 综合征），或伴甲状腺功能减退，较少见。巨舌症并不十分常见，但多见于 Down 综合征患者。最严重的并发症是呼吸道阻塞。婴儿巨舌症需与淋巴畸形或血管瘤引起的舌局部肿大区别。舌下垂、正常大小的舌后移常见于腭裂和小颌畸形的婴儿。由舌肿大或易位引起的婴儿呼吸道阻塞需行气管切开术，大一点的儿童巨舌可影响美观、干扰发音、引起流涎，则需行舌体缩小。

良性病变

龈瘤是一种先天性颗粒细胞肿瘤，表现为上颌牙

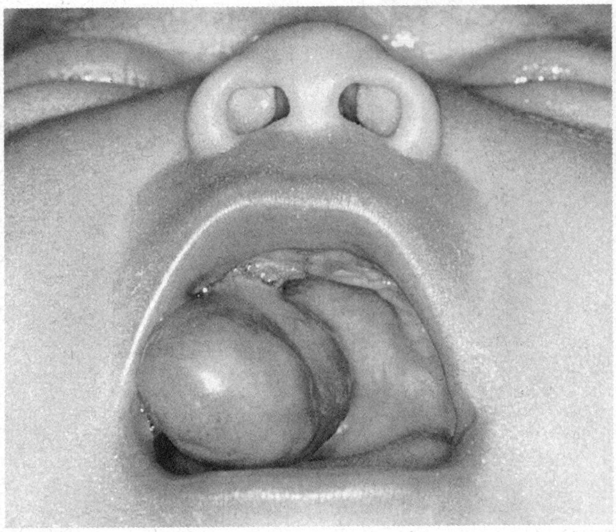

图 52-10 先天性龈瘤。先天性龈瘤是一种罕见的良性病变。常起于上颌前部牙槽嵴上。比较大的病变常引起通气道和喂食困难，需要手术切除。

槽嵴前部的黏膜下柔软粉红肿块（图 52–10）。多发生在女性，影响进食，可手术切除。

826 舌下囊肿是一种位于口底区的假囊肿，可为先天性的或由口内创伤引起的（图 52–11），大的舌下囊肿可穿过颌舌骨肌伸展到颈部。治疗方法为切除囊肿或假囊肿袋形缝术，常连舌下腺一同切除。黏液囊肿也是一种假囊肿，发生于小涎腺，常可自行破溃。复发或有症状的黏液囊肿可手术切除。

血管瘤是常发生于头颈部的内皮增生性疾病，在出生后第一年增大，之后可自行消退。对于引起溃疡、出血、呼吸道阻塞、心血管损害或凝血病（Kasabach–Merritt 综合征）的血管瘤来说，手术切除或类固醇治疗是必要的。血管畸形，包括静脉、动脉或动静脉畸形，很少发生在口腔和咽部，能引起疼痛、出血、溃疡、心衰。治疗方法可手术切除或对低流量病变（静脉）行硬化疗法，高流量（动脉）行血管造影栓塞。

淋巴畸形以前称为淋巴管瘤或囊性水瘤，为先天性疾病，常在 2 岁以前发病。病理上，淋巴畸形含有大量膨胀的淋巴管，或含有毛细血管或静脉成分。淋巴畸形可发生在颈部的任何位置。累及舌、口底、下颌骨或喉可引起功能障碍。淋巴畸形的切除十分困难，因为缺少包膜而且为浸润性的。切除过程中应避免损伤邻近重要结构。术后引流可有效预防皮下淋巴再次排出。CO_2 激光治疗已应用于舌表浅淋巴畸形，大的囊性病变可使用硬化疗法。

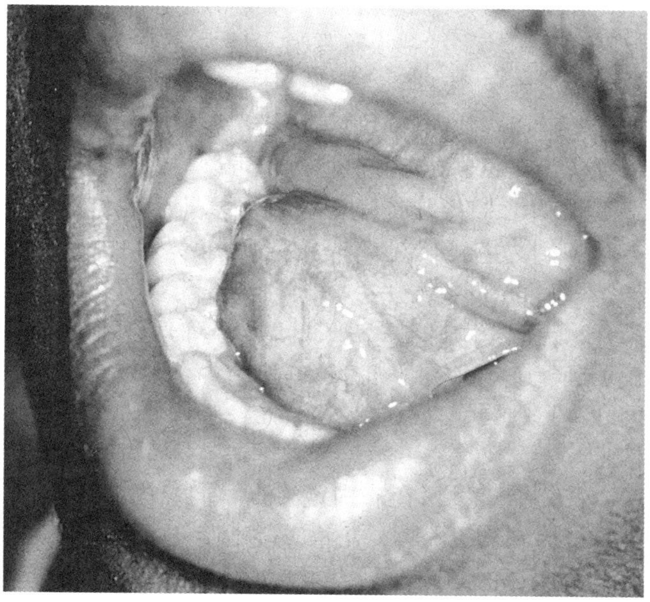

图 52–11 舌下囊肿是由于舌下腺阻塞而引起的假性囊肿。通常表现为口底单侧的无痛性肿胀。

前肠囊肿是真性囊肿，囊壁内衬呼吸上皮。发生在口底的应与皮样囊肿相鉴别，皮样囊肿囊壁上皮为复层鳞状上皮，还可在此找到皮肤附属器。甲状舌管囊肿很少位于舌根部。而异位甲状腺，即舌甲状腺，表现为舌根部的紫色肿块。异位甲状腺组织往往功能低下，儿童患者需补充甲状腺素。其他异位组织迷芽瘤包括组织结构正常的胃肠神经组织异位。

第二鳃裂衍生物很少表现为扁桃体上端的囊性肿块，MRI 可清楚显示它的范围。Tornwaldt 囊肿是位于鼻咽部的盲袋，为胚胎发育时期原始脊索与咽部连接而衍生的。其他良性鼻咽部肿块包括鼻咽畸形瘤、表样病变和鼻咽部脑膨出。这些疾病多数可由 CT 或 MRI 确定病变范围以及与颅内联系路径。手术切除对大多数病例有治疗效果。

鳞状乳头瘤是一种生长缓慢的良性肿瘤，常发生于软腭、悬雍垂和扁桃体，由 HPV（乳头状瘤病毒）6、4 或 22 血清型感染引起。疾病可扩展至咽和气管，所以应完整外科切除。多形性腺瘤（混合瘤）是发生于小涎腺的良性肿瘤，好发于腭，也可见于唇、颊黏膜。治疗需手术切除。

恶性病变

横纹肌肉瘤，儿童最常见的软组织恶性肿瘤，发生于 2～6 岁，来源于间叶组织[4,18]。在口腔和口咽部表现为发生于舌、腭、悬雍垂和颊部的快速生长的肿块。肿瘤早期转移至局部，淋巴结、肺、骨。手术治疗只适用于活检病变范围较小和晚期患者的姑息治疗。常用治疗方法是化疗和放疗联合治疗。

口腔和咽部的淋巴瘤常发病于 Waldeyer 环的淋 827
巴组织，表现为扁桃体或鼻咽部的肿块[8]。可根据颈部肿大淋巴结诊断，但确诊需活检。一般为放化疗联合治疗。

其他口腔咽部恶性肿瘤包括恶性涎腺肿瘤（黏液表皮样癌）和表皮样或鳞状细胞癌，据报道后者见于器官移植患者和吸鼻烟或嚼烟叶的青少年[19]。手术治疗要根据病变部位和范围。

喉

解剖学

除了舌骨，咽的主要支持结构包括软骨和软组织。舌骨位于咽上方，并通过甲状舌骨膜与之相连。舌骨来源于第二、三鳃弓。咽的软骨组织由透明软骨组成，除了会厌软骨是由弹性软骨组成的。咽的软骨结构来源于4、5、6鳃弓。有9个咽软骨，三个为单一软骨（甲状软骨、环状、会厌），6个成对（杓状软骨、楔状软骨和小角软骨）。甲状软骨由两块四边形的软骨组成，形成咽的前部支持结构。环状软骨是呼吸道唯一呈完整环状的软骨，是支持环杓关节和环甲关节的基础。

环甲肌是成对的喉外肌，收缩时使喉向下、向前，使声带紧张。成对的喉内肌——甲杓肌、甲状会厌肌和杓会厌肌，是关闭喉入口的括约肌。声带肌由甲杓肌的内侧肌纤维组成，连接于声带。声带肌的收缩可调节发音的调。其他成对肌还有环杓后肌、环杓侧肌和杓内肌。环杓后肌使声门变大，杓内肌和环杓肌使声门关闭。

四边形的弹性纤维组织膜覆盖于咽上方，止于喉前庭韧带侧缘。喉弹性圆锥是一弹性组织膜，向下附于环状软骨上缘，组成对声韧带及声门的支持结构。

咽的血供来自喉上、喉下动脉。喉上动脉是甲状腺上动脉的分支，喉下动脉是甲状腺下动脉的分支。喉内肌由喉返神经支配。喉返神经发出感觉神经分支至喉上部。喉上神经有两个分支，外支支配环甲肌，内支支配咽上部的感觉。

咽位于呼吸道上部，有多种呼吸功能，通过调整声门裂大小以调节气流量，吸气时，在横膈下降以前环杓后肌收缩以外展声带。咽的保护功能有两种反射，咳嗽反射和关闭反射。咳嗽可以有效排出黏液和异物。关闭反射可防止吸入异物，除了关闭反射，吞咽时喉部上升。吞咽食物时，喉入口关闭和喉部上升与环咽肌舒张同时发生。最后，咽部对发声也起重要作用，通过覆盖于声带肌上的黏膜的振动发声。声音调和音域与声带肌和声带的张力长度有关。

小儿喉位置较成人为高，环状软骨高度相当于第4颈椎水平，会厌位于第1颈椎水平。会厌与软腭距离较近，所以小儿主要为鼻呼吸。2岁时，咽下降至第5颈椎水平，成年则下降至6～7颈椎水平。新生儿的声门前后径为7mm，左右径为4mm，婴儿呼吸道的最狭区是声门下区直径约4mm。

上呼吸道阻塞

急性呼吸道阻塞症状有呼吸困难、咳嗽、声音改变、吞咽困难、咽痛。呼吸困难和劳力性呼吸困难提示通气不足，可由 PCO_2 和 PO_2 改变引起。呼吸道任何部位的刺激物都引起咳嗽。从咳嗽的性质很难定位刺激物的位置。儿童声音改变如嘶哑、声音模糊不清或哭声减弱，有助于定位阻塞。固体和（或）液体吞咽困难与呼吸道阻塞有关，因为阻塞，患者常主诉咽痛。

小儿的面部表现是呼吸道阻塞的首要征象，因为呼吸道的状态可指示进一步的治疗措施。应判断患者的意识态，如果失去知觉或意识模糊的患者应立即行气管切开。非发绀性心脏病患者出现发绀、焦虑、烦躁多动、出汗都预示急性气管病变。其他症状还有气促、胸骨下凹。儿童有心动过速、心动过缓提示缺氧症。哭闹声嘶提示阻塞部位在喉部，而犬吠样咳嗽与喉炎症水肿有关。鼾声来源于喉部的喷鼻息声。喘鸣音是由咽部或气管的湍流引起。吸气性喘鸣提示湍流位于会厌或会厌以上。呼气性喘鸣由气管远端或小支气管的湍流引起。声音的大小不一定与阻塞程度成正比，在完全阻塞前喘鸣音会变小。其他重要体征还有流涎和使用辅助性呼吸肌呼吸。

除了确定儿童阻塞部位，还要估计呼吸道阻塞程度，包括通气状况。脉血氧定量法可以快速测定动脉氧化作用。CO_2 的经皮肤监测定可以较好测定供氧情况。颈侧位X线片仍是对呼吸阻塞儿童的最好检查方法，因为它可以显示从鼻尖到胸部入口的解剖结构。颈后前位X线片可以确定狭窄区域，如尖塔征象提示声门下水肿。胸片对于确定异物和其他病变如单侧肺气肿、肺不张和肺炎的诊断也有帮助。如果时间允许，钡餐检查或呼吸道荧光检查仪可以提供更多信息。

其他检查手段还有内镜检查，向鼻内喷入2%的利多卡因和氧甲唑啉，儿童应轻微制动。可检查从鼻孔到会厌部的呼吸道。应避免把内镜穿过儿童会厌。另外，有声门上炎的儿童应避免使内镜，因为有引起气道完全阻塞的可能。

急性呼吸道阻塞的儿童的非手术治疗可在高度监护室监护观察。通过面罩输送湿润氧气可改善 PO_2 和清除分泌物。喷塞器给予补消旋肾上腺素可以减轻黏膜水肿，对喉气管支气管炎（感染性哮喘）也有效。因为它的作用时间可持续 30～60 分钟。患者在治疗后 4～6 小时应继续观察以防病情反复。类固醇激素对 EBV 感染引起的扁桃腺肥大、过敏性水肿和痉挛性哮喘也有一定疗效[10,16]。

辅助治疗包括抗生素或吸入氦氧混合气。虽然咽气管炎症多由病毒引起，细菌双重感染也很常见。因为青霉素抵抗性的生物越来越多，广谱抗生素，包括新代头孢菌素、青霉素酶抵抗的青霉素或 β 内酰胺酶青霉素被用来预防或治疗感染。氦氧混合气是一种用氦代替氮的混合气体，其优点是它的低密度可减少气流紊乱和气体阻力，改善呼吸道阻塞患者的氧气输送。

非手术治疗包括经鼻或口通气、气管内插管和较少用的经气管供氧。经鼻通气在使用水溶性润滑剂后，使用橡胶或其他合成材料可以很容易地插入鼻内。最适合用于阻塞部位在喉部的患者。经口通气，小儿往往难以忍受，通常只作为简单处理方法。20 世纪 70 年代，使用聚氯乙烯管行气管内插管是治疗声门上炎的一次改革。直到今天，插管仍是儿童严重呼吸道阻塞的主要治疗方法。使用气管内插管的大小与儿童年龄有关。声门下区，小儿呼吸道最狭窄处，可容纳内径 3.5～4mm 的管子。1 岁以上儿童使用的插管大小可用以下公式粗略估算，管尺寸 =（16 + 年龄）÷ 4。一旦呼吸道建立，应保护好管子，使用镇静剂和（或）限制其活动，以避免脱落。其他治疗方法应考虑儿童颈脊柱的不稳定和口、颈部外伤降低可见性。经气管供氧，从环甲膜插入 16 号针以输送氧气，一般只是紧急情况下使用，而且要在能得到稳定通气情况下才能使用。

小儿急性呼吸道阻塞的手术治疗首先可使用内镜。喉部检查可使用儿科喉内镜，尺寸合适的儿科通气气管镜可保持呼吸道通畅。一旦呼吸道通畅，可使用更稳定的治疗方法。较少见的小儿急性呼吸道阻塞，不能建立呼吸道，则需行环甲膜切开。在成人，这种方法可避免发生于紧急气管切开中的出血和气胸。气管造口置管，管子经切口插入环甲膜，但尽快应建立更稳定的呼吸道。气管造口术对于经咽建立气管通道失败或不能经咽建立气管通道的急性阻塞患者是更好的方法。紧急气管造口。应尽量避免以减少并发症如出血、肺气肿、周围组织损伤。手术技巧、良好照明、充足的协助可以减少并发症发生率。 829

先天喉畸形

喉软骨软化是新生儿喘鸣最常见的原因。它由声门上结构（杓状软骨杓会厌襞）在吸气时的下垂引起（图 52–12），典型症状在出生后不久即可出现，包括吸气性喘鸣、进食困难和少见的呼吸暂停或严重呼吸道阻塞体征。胃食管反流性疾病可能加重喉软骨化的症状。确诊可通过喉内镜，其他病理学排除可依靠颈侧、胸和锁餐 X 线片。在大多数病例，喉软骨软化有自限性，18 个月以后常能自愈。改变体位和进食，治疗反流性疾病，新生儿使用监护可能是必要的。对严重病例，可行声门上成形术（手术分离杓会厌襞）或气管切开术。

气管支气管软化，定义为气管支气管呼吸道结构倒塌。可能是先天性的或获得性的（长期插管或感染）。可发生于部分气管支气管或累及全部。根据病变的程度及部位，可表现为低音调的两阶段的喘鸣和吸气困难征。通常使用内镜进行诊断，虽然呼吸道荧光检查也可证实。对大多数患者可先观察病情，一些严重患者需行气管插管和正压供氧。

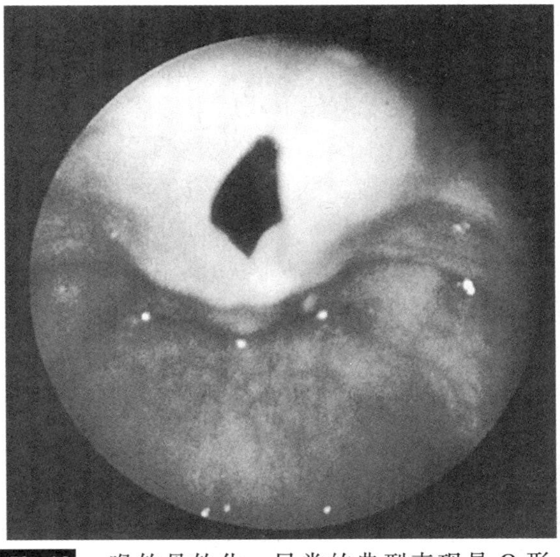

图 52–12　喉软骨软化。异常的典型表现是 Ω 形会厌。杓状软骨黏膜多余，杓会厌襞逐渐聚拢，造成的结果是组织覆盖物嵌入声门，导致呼吸时气道阻塞。

声带麻痹是第二常见的先天喉畸形（仅次于喉软骨软化）可能为单侧或双侧性的。先天声带麻痹可能由神经异常（脑积水，Arnold–Chiari 畸形），出生时外伤或少见的喉颈部肿瘤引起，双侧声带麻痹的新生儿典型表现为高音调的吸气性或呼、吸气两阶段的喘鸣，但哭未受影响。呼吸困难及进食困难可伴喘鸣。单侧声带麻痹的婴儿，可能不会出现呼吸困难，但一少部分婴儿会表现出明显的呼吸困难，特别是在进食时。哭声通常为嘶哑或带呼吸声的。获得性声带麻痹可能来源于外伤或胸部颈部肿瘤或医源性的，特别是在颈部或主动脉弓手术后。单、双侧声带麻痹的诊断主要依据内镜检查，其他检查方法还包括颈侧部、胸部 X 线片、钡餐试验、头颈部 MRI、CT。大多数单侧麻痹患者可暂不处理，留待观察，但是双侧声带麻痹的婴儿则需行气管切开术。另外，进食困难的婴儿需行胃造口术。大于 4 或 5 岁的儿童可考虑行脊髓前侧柱切断术或杓状软骨切除术以改善通气。

先天性声门下狭窄在先天性喉畸形中发病率为第三位。表现为新生儿喉部允许进入直径 3.5mm 的气管内管，但却没有气管内手术或插管的病史（图 52–13）。主要畸形是环状软骨过小或变形。先天性声门下狭窄的婴儿表现为吸气性或吸气，呼气两阶段的喘鸣，犬吠样咳嗽，和呼吸道阻塞的其他症状。诊断可依据狭窄部的颈侧区 X 线片，确诊则依据内镜检查。治疗方法随症状严重程度不同。可选用观察、喉重建术或气管切开术。

830 声门下血管瘤的儿童表现为从出生后前几个月开始的渐进性的喘鸣（图 52–14）。血管瘤是增生性的内皮病变，可形成于声门下区后方的黏膜下。有时，也可表现为环绕声门下区一周的病变形式。约 50%的患者伴有皮肤血管瘤。临床表现依据呼吸道受累程度，可表现为两阶段喘鸣、犬吠样咳嗽、进食困难或呼吸道阻塞的其他症状体征。诊断参考颈侧 X 线检查，但确诊主要依据内镜检查。声门下血管瘤婴儿的非手术治疗包括继续观察或全身使用类固醇激素。手术治疗包括激光切除、喉正中切开术切除血管瘤或气管切开术。

喉囊肿为喉室小囊异常扩张，内有气体，可表现为向后上方的假声带突出或以甲状软骨膜向外突出，囊肿内含液体，在真性、假性声带之间突出。诊断依靠内镜。喉 CT 有助于确定病变范围和囊肿内含物为液体或气体。治疗为内镜造袋术或喉正中切开切除术。

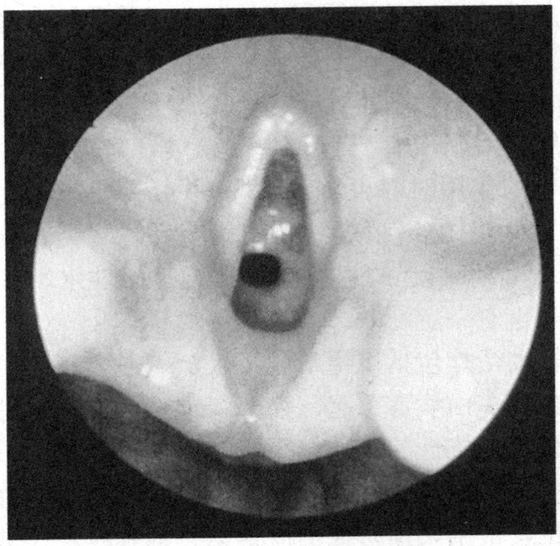

图 52–13 声门下狭窄。先天性和获得性狭窄引起气道阻塞，取决于严重度和狭窄类型。各种类型的重建都有效（见第 63 章）。

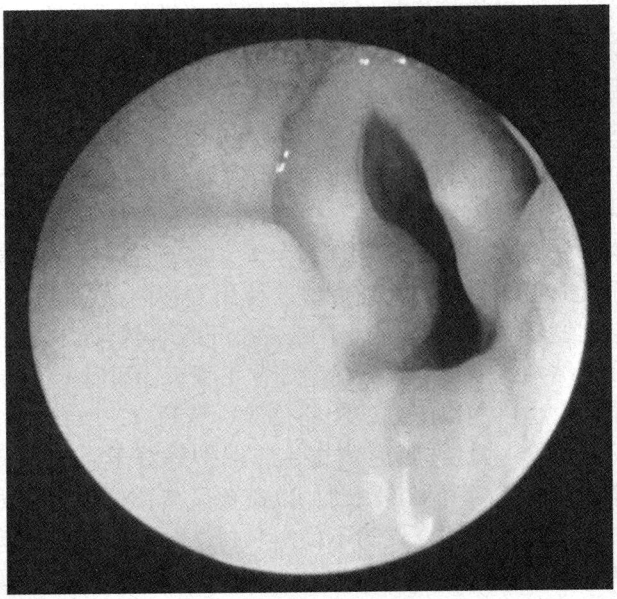

图 52–14 声门下血管瘤典型起于喉的后侧方，较小的病变可保守治疗，然而有渐进性生长的病变需要气管切开术以绕开喉头阻塞。

上呼吸道炎症性疾病

喉气管支气管炎（病毒性喉炎）是声门下区呼吸道的炎症性疾病。由多种副流感和流感病毒引起，炎症可累及整个声门区并向气管支气管扩散。1～3 岁的儿童易受感染，男性比女性易受感染。临床表现有阶段的喘鸣，犬吠样咳嗽和声嘶，常有上呼吸道感染的前驱症状。诊断主要依据临床表现，但内镜检查有助于排除其他病变。不应使用声门区的各种器械检查，这样会导致进一步的肿胀和炎症引起急性阻塞。颈侧区 X 线片显示声门下区狭窄，颈后前位 X 线片显示“尖塔征”，是由声门下水肿引起的。治疗选用皮质激素仍有争议。在急诊室或病房使用肾上腺素喷雾可缓解症状。但是几小时后病情可有反复，因此，儿童需监测。严重感染儿童需行插管以缓解呼吸衰竭，应使用比正常插管稍小的管子。如果炎症没有得到控制少数病例可能需行气管切开术。

有复发性喉炎的 1 岁以下儿童应怀疑可能有先天性声门下狭窄或血管瘤。痉挛性喉炎指儿童哮吼样症状反复发作，而儿童无其他疾病。很少出现发热，常在夜间发作。胃食管反流性疾病可能是刺激因素。痉挛性喉炎的治疗通常为密切观察，虽然使用皮质激素类药或治疗药物也有一定帮助。

声门上炎（会厌炎）是发生于声门上区的感染性疾病。儿童常见病原菌为 B 型流感嗜血杆菌（HIB）。青少年和成年人可见其他病原菌。儿童声门上炎发病率自从 20 世纪 90 年代早期 HIB 疫苗的引入后已显著降低[17]。发病年龄晚于喉炎，在 3～6 岁左右发病。临床表现为发病急，快速进展为呼吸道阻塞，喘鸣、呼吸困难、发热、发音含糊不清和全身中毒症状。患儿坐立不安，反复调整体位以减轻呼吸困难。疑似患者应避免口内或内镜检查以免引起呼吸道完全阻塞。颈侧 X 线片显示典型的会厌“拇纹征”。

儿童声门上炎患者需行紧急治疗，不论是在急诊室还是手术室。治疗医生需包括儿科医生、麻醉医生、急诊医生、耳鼻喉科医生、小儿外科医生或小儿呼吸科医生。儿童经全身麻醉后行气管插管术，应检查声门上区，获得咽部组织及血培养材料。气管切开术的设备应容易得到。儿童需插管 24～72 小时并持续静脉输液和使用针对抗生素抵抗的嗜血杆菌的抗生
831 素（第三代头孢菌素、氯霉素）。

细菌性气管炎（假膜性喉炎）常发生在其他感染的并发症，如麻疹、水痘和其他病毒感染。最常见的致病菌包括金黄色葡萄球菌、β 溶血性链球菌 A 组、或流感嗜血杆菌。它可发生于任何年龄的儿童，表现为喘鸣、犬吠样咳嗽和低热。病情进展中表现为高热、进行性呼吸道阻塞和中毒症状。诊断可参考胸片上气管阴影的弥散性狭窄。确诊需在手术室作内镜检查。同时可去除化脓性分泌物质和假膜。分泌物和假膜培养有助于指导静脉抗生素治疗，抗生素治疗主要应针对常见病原菌。应行气管内插管或较少用的气管切开术以保持呼吸道通畅。应行呼吸道内镜复查以继续清创和决定气管拔管的可行性。

慢性呼吸道阻塞

声门下狭窄和其他呼吸道慢性疾病的长期治疗在第 63 章讨论。

喉良性肿瘤

复发性呼吸性多发性乳头状瘤是儿童喉部最常见的良性肿瘤。鳞状上皮乳头状瘤发生于喉部，有时可发生于气管和下呼吸道，表现为外生性病损。因为它的易复发性，常可引起患者病态，少数恶变病例可导致死亡。此病可发生于任何年龄人群，但更常见于儿童。人类乳头状瘤病毒 6、11、16 和 18 亚型都已在乳头状瘤组织中发现。6、11 亚型与生殖器疣有关，16、18 亚型与颈、喉部癌症有关。人类乳头状瘤病毒感染喉部的确切机制未明。许多病例可能是病毒有生殖器疣的母亲传染至儿童引起的，但是没有具体证据支持这种说法。

此病的儿童患者主要表现为声音嘶哑，但也可能有呼吸道阻塞的症状和体征，包括喘鸣，颈侧区 X 线片可显示喉部病变，但确诊主要依据直接喉内镜检查和活检（图 52–15）。除了气管和支气管，鳞状上皮性乳头状瘤也可能发生于口腔。

手术切除是主要治疗方法。过去，乳头状瘤使用 CO_2 激光器切除。最近，喉微创手术已成为许多机构更常用的切除方法。频繁发作的和伴发呼吸道阻塞的病例需行气管切开术，虽然气管切开术已应用于累及气管和下呼吸道的病例中。药物辅助治疗已被应用，如干扰素、用双血卟啉乙醚行光能治疗、吲哚–3–甲醇或抗病毒药物，如西多福韦。

喉部其他良性肿瘤较少见，包括结缔组织肿瘤如软骨瘤或纤维瘤，神经组织肿瘤如神经纤维瘤或粒细胞肿瘤或其他细胞类型如错构瘤或纤维组织细胞瘤。喉恶性肿瘤也很少见，包括鳞状细胞癌和和各种上皮

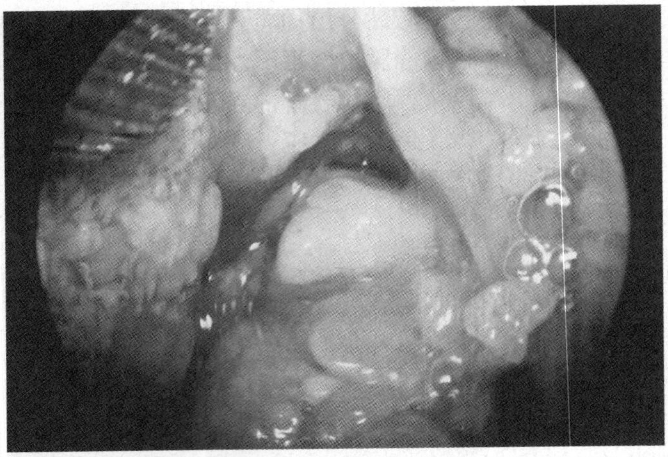

图 52-15 复发性呼吸道多发性乳头状瘤。严重的多发性乳头状瘤能完全阻塞喉。乳头状瘤的特征是恶性化和渐进性生长。

及结缔组织恶性肿瘤如梭形细胞癌、横纹肌肉瘤和软骨肉瘤。转移性肿瘤和淋巴瘤也较少见于儿童喉部。诊断可参考突然出现的喘鸣、声嘶和呼吸道阻塞。确诊则依据活检。根据细胞类型不同选择不同治疗方法，可包括手术切除，放疗和（或）化疗。

颈

解剖学

颈部解剖及胚胎发生在第 56 章讨论。

临床评估

颈部疾病或异常的检查首先要有一份完整的病史。根据详细的病史记录常可作出颈部疾病的不同诊
832 断。儿童的年龄是首要考虑因素。婴儿颈部肿块常常提示先天性疾病，而青少年突然出现的颈部肿块可能为恶性病变。颈炎症性疾病可发生于任何年龄，但多见于儿童上呼吸道感染。肿块生长快慢有助于诊断。快速生长的颈部肿块可能为炎症或恶性肿瘤，生长缓慢的肿块一般为良性病变。身体其他部位感染的病史或最近接触过动物常提示肿块为炎症性的。颈部外伤病史可解释颈部突然出现的肿块。另外，肿块大小随进食而改变，可提示为涎腺疾病。血管病变在用力或哭泣时增大。全身症状如发热、体重减轻、盗汗或疲劳与突然增大的颈部肿块同时出现则可能为恶性肿瘤。

对有颈部肿块的儿童体检应从整个头颈部全面检查开始。因为头部的血管，神经和淋巴都汇集到颈部，颈部疾病可能来源于头部。依据不同的诊断，需要对整个身体进行检查，包括腹股沟及腋窝的淋巴结，脾、肝大。儿童颈部触诊常可触及淋巴结。正常增生的淋巴结一般不超过 2cm，若超过 2cm 则需密切观察和探究。颈后区或锁骨上区淋巴结突然增大提示恶性肿瘤[31]。颈部肿块的特征有助于诊断肿块的性质。质硬的肿块往往为炎症性病变或恶性肿瘤。颈部肿块固定于皮肤或周围结构也提示为恶性肿瘤。囊肿或脓肿在触诊时也有其特征。

根据病史和体格检查可做出不同的诊断，而放射检查可能有助于诊断。颈侧区 X 线片可显示鼻咽部、咽后区、颈椎的异常。另外，胸片可确定恶性肿瘤，结节病或结核病。鼻窦部的炎症或肿瘤性病变可表现在鼻窦部 X 线片上。CT 和 MRI 有助于颈部肿块的诊断。CT 低密度影像提示炎症或肿瘤性病变。CT 扫描图像上低密度区的外周环状高密度增强区为脓肿征象。MRI 可以较好的显示软组织细微结构和颈部血管病变。最后，超声检查有助于区分固体肿块和囊性肿块。触诊不明显的甲状舌管囊肿患者术前行 B 超检查是显示正常甲状腺组织的一种经济有效的方法。超声和甲状腺扫描可用于诊断任何甲状腺肿块。

实验室检查有助于诊断儿童颈部疾病。全血血细胞分类计数可区分恶性肿瘤和全身感染。对 EB 病毒，巨细胞病毒感染、弓形体病或猫抓病行血清学检查是有一定诊断价值。儿童疑似患甲状腺疾病需行甲状腺功能检测。最后，小便收集检测儿茶酚胺代谢物（香草扁桃酸）有助于神经母细胞瘤的诊断。

如果通过以上检查诊断仍未明确，可行切取活检或切除活检。活检可为病理检查、组织培养和为其他更复杂精密的检测提供材料。对疑似恶性肿瘤的儿童行颈部肿块细针吸取活检的诊断可靠性不及成人患者。

先天性瘘管和囊肿

先天性瘘管和囊肿的讨论见第 56 章。

炎症性和感染性肿块

病毒性淋巴结炎是儿童最常见的颈部感染性疾病。淋巴结肿大或增生，常由上呼吸道病毒感染引起。常见病原菌包括鼻病毒、腺病毒和肠道病毒，但麻疹、流行性腮腺炎、风疹、水痘、EBV 和巨细胞病毒也可引起淋巴结肿大。诊断可参考病史和体格检查，但确诊需依据血清学检查。HIV 急性感染与其他病毒感染的症状相似，发热头痛、周身不适、胃肠道症状和颈部肿块。

细菌性淋巴结炎最常见的感染源来自咽部。病原菌常为链球菌属或葡萄球菌属。患者颈部肿块表现为弥散性肿胀，质软，伴有红斑，另外还有全身症状发热和周身不适。病毒性淋巴结炎多为双侧发病，而颈部细菌感染多为单侧。高对比度 CT 有助于诊断大的可能包含脓腔的颈部肿块，细针吸取可疑感染肿块可为细菌培养提供材料及肿块减压。口服或静脉使用广谱抗生素可有疗效，但对范围较大的肿块必要时行切开排脓。

猫抓病由巴尔通氏体感染引起。临床表现包括被猫抓后突然出现的单侧淋巴结肿大，大多数病例可伴发热和周身不适。巴尔通氏体抗体血清学检查有诊断价值。猫抓病有自限性，虽然红霉素和其他抗生素有一定疗效[21]。

过去，多数分枝杆菌感染由非典型病原菌引起，如鸟胞内分枝杆菌瘰疬分枝杆菌，牛分枝杆菌或堪
833 萨斯分枝杆菌。过去几十年，随着颈部感染分枝杆菌，分枝杆菌结核病又逐渐复苏。非典型分枝杆菌感染表现为耳前区，腮腺区或颈后三角区的质硬肿块。淋巴结外的皮肤为紫色，很少出现全身症状。如果怀疑结核分枝杆菌感染，应拍胸片。细针吸取病变组织切开引流或切除病变淋巴结以抗酸染色和细胞培养来辅助诊断。手术刮除或整体切除对非典型病变有一定疗效。结核病应使用合适的抗结核药物治疗。

少数情况下，一些感染性疾病可波及颈部，如兔热病、布氏菌病、放线菌病、鼠疫、组织浆菌病或弓形体病。可能累及颈部的炎症性疾病包括 Kawasaki 综合征，结节病，鼻窦组织细胞增多症（Rosai–Dorfman 病）、Kikuchi–Fujimoto 病和 PFAPA 综合征（周期性反复发热）。

恶性肿瘤

甲状腺恶性肿瘤在青少年中较少见，10%的甲状腺癌发生于 21 岁以下患者[3]。分化良好的肿瘤多为乳头状癌，占肿瘤的大多数。囊性、混合性和髓状肿瘤较少见。大多数患者表现为颈中线区的无痛性肿块。大多数患者颈部可触及淋巴结肿大，反映了经淋巴结转移的乳头状疾病的高发病率[9]。其他重要症状体征包括肿块生长迅速、疼痛、声嘶和呼吸困难。以前接受过放射治疗的儿童是甲状腺恶性肿瘤的高危人群。甲状腺恶性肿瘤可伴发碘缺乏、Hashimoto 甲状腺炎和 Graves 病[9,22]。术前应行甲状腺核素扫描以区分冷结节（功能低下）和热结节（功能亢进）。1/3 的冷结节可为恶性，而热结节较少为恶性[12]。超声波检查可区分实性或囊性病变，细针吸取活检是另一种诊断方法。手术方法包括甲状腺大部切除术或全甲状腺切除术，必要时行颈淋巴结清扫术，术后行 ^{131}I 消融。

淋巴瘤是儿童常见恶性肿瘤，表现为颈部无痛性淋巴结肿大。Hodgkin 病多发病于青春期，可分为 4 种组织学类型：淋巴细胞为主型，结节硬化型，混合细胞型和淋巴细胞耗尽型。大多数病例为淋巴细胞为主型和结节硬化型。Hodgkin 病的临床分期主要依据受累淋巴结的数量和部位，以及是否伴有全身或 B 症状（发热、盗汗、体重减轻），治疗主要是联合化疗加局部放疗。非 Hodgkin 淋巴瘤可分为低度恶性组，中度恶性组，高度恶性组。高度恶性组可分为大细胞型，淋巴母细胞型和小细胞型。非 Hodgkm 淋巴瘤的临床分期依据受累淋巴结部位及范围。治疗主要是联合化疗。

Langerhans 细胞组织细胞增多症（组织细胞增多症 X）即一种疾病实体包括嗜伊红细胞肉芽肿，Hand–Schüller–Christian 综合征和 Letterer–Siwe 病。这种疾病的确切机制仍未明。可表现为肿瘤或超免疫反应[7]。临床表现包括：淋巴结肿大、皮疹、耳漏、口腔病变和肝脾肿大。诊断依靠病理样本中的朗格汉斯细胞。治疗方法可选择刮除术，或全身皮质激素类化学药物治疗和放疗。

神经系统的两种多见肿瘤可发生于颈部。神经纤维瘤是一种良性肿瘤，但某种分型（丛状型）可浸润周围组织，所以，术前行 CT 和（或）MRI 检查是很重要的。手术切除是主要治疗方法。神经母细胞瘤是一种恶性肿瘤，来源于神经嵴细胞，表现为单发性肿

瘤或淋巴结肿大。临床分期决定治疗方法，包括手术切除、化疗和放疗。

横纹肌肉瘤最初很少表现为颈部肿瘤，而更常表现为眼眶、颞骨、鼻咽部的肿瘤。诊断主要依据活检。临床分期依据病变范围大小。治疗包括手术切除，化疗和放疗。

发生于任何部位的各种恶性肿瘤，大部分可转移至颈部，最常见的是甲状腺恶性肿瘤。青少年的癌症，特别是来源于鼻咽部的癌，可能转移至颈部淋巴结。

（徐建民译 董其刚校）

参考文献

1. Anon JB, Rontal M, Zinreich SJ: Anatomy and Embryology of the Paranasal Sinuses. New York, Thieme, 1996.
2. Bluestone CD, Klein JO: Otitis media and eustachian tube dysfunction. In Bluestone CD, Stool SE, Alper CM, et al (eds): Pediatric Otolaryngology, 4th ed. Philadelphia, WB Saunders, 2003, pp 474-686.
3. Buckwalter JA, Guril NJ, Thomas CG Jr: Cancer of the thyroid in youth. World J Surg 1981;5:15-25.
4. Cole RR, Cotton RT: Pediatric malignancies. In Bailey BJ, Johnson JT, Kohut RI, et al (eds): Head and Neck Surgery—Otolaryngology. Philadelphia, JB Lippincott, 1993, p 1388.
5. Cunningham MJ: Neoplasms of the ear and temporal bone. In Wetmore RF, Muntz HR, McGill TJ, et al (eds): Pediatric Otolaryngology: Principles and Practice Pathways. New York, Thieme, 2000, pp 385-408.
6. De la Cruz A, Chandrasekhar SS: Congenital malformations of the temporal bone. In Brackman DE, Shelton C, Arriaga MA (eds): Otologic Surgery. Philadelphia, WB Saunders, 1994, pp 69-84.
7. Devaney KO, Putzi MJ, Ferlito A, et al: Head and neck Langerhans' cell histiocytosis. Ann Otol Rhinol Laryngol 1997;106:526-532.
8. Fierstein J, Thawley S: Lymphomas of the head and neck. Laryngoscope 1978;88:582-593.
9. Geiger JD, Thompson NW: Thyroid tumors in children. Otolaryngol Clin North Am 1996;4:711-719.
10. Hawkins DB, Crockett DM, Shum TK: Corticosteroids in airway management. Otolaryngol Head Neck Surg 1983; 91:593-596.
11. Houser SM, Corey JP: Allergic fungal sinusitis: Pathophysiology, epidemiology and diagnosis. Otolaryngol Clin North Am 2000;33:399.
12. Hung W, Anderson KD, Chandra R: Solitary thyroid nodules in 71 children and adolescents. J Pediatr Surg 1992;27: 1407-1409.
13. Jacobs IN, Potsic WP: Glomus tympanicum in infancy. Arch Otolaryngol Head Neck Surg 1994;120:203-205.
14. Jahrsdoerfer RA, Yeakley JW, Aguilar EA, et al: Grading system for the selection of patients with congenital aural atresia. Am J Otol 1992;13:6-12.
15. Johnson RF, Stewart MG, Wright CC: An evidence-based review of the treatment of peritonsillar abscess. Otolaryngol Head Neck Surg 2003;128:332-343.
16. Kairys SW, Olmstead EM, O'Connor GT: Steroid treatment of laryngotracheitis: A meta-analysis of the evidence from randomized trials. Pediatrics 1989;83:683-693.
17. Kessler A, Wetmore RF, Marsh RR: Childhood epiglottitis in recent years. Int J Pediatr Otorhinolaryngol 1993;25:155-162.
18. Kodet R, Fajstavr J, Kabelka Z, et al: Is fetal cellular rhabdomyoma an entity or a differentiated rhabdomyosarcoma? A study of patients with rhabdomyoma of the tongue and sarcoma of the tongue enrolled in the intergroup rhabdomyosarcoma studies I, II and III. Cancer 1991;67: 2907-2913.
19. Lee YW, Gisser SD: Squamous cell carcinoma of the tongue in a nine-year renal transplant survivor: A case report with a discussion of the risk of development of epithelial carcinoma in renal transplant survivors. Cancer 1978;41:1-6.
20. Marcus CL, Omlin KJ, Basinki DJ, et al: Normal polysomnographic values for children and adolescents. Am Rev Respir Dis 1992;146:1235-1239.
21. Maurin M, Birtles R, Raoult D: Current knowledge of *Bartonella* species. Eur J Clin Microbiol Infect Dis 1997; 16:487-506.
22. Millman B, Pellitteri PK: Thyroid carcinoma in children and adolescents. Arch Otolaryngol Head Neck Surg 1995; 121:1261-1264.
23. Neault MW: Pediatric audiology. In Wetmore RF, Muntz HR, McGill TJ, et al (eds): Pediatric Otolaryngology: Principles and Practice Pathways. New York, Thieme, 2000, pp 183-202.
24. Paradise JL, Bluestone CD, Bachman RZ, et al: Efficacy of tonsillectomy for recurrent throat infection in severely affected children: Results of parallel randomized and nonrandomized clinical trials. N Engl J Med 1984;310: 674-683.
25. Pichichero ME: First-line treatment of otitis media. In Alper CM, Bluestone CD, Casselbrant ML, et al (eds): Advanced Therapy of Otitis Media. Hamilton, ON, BC Decker, 2004, p 32.
26. Poje CP, Rechtweg JS: Structure and function of the temporal bone. In Wetmore RF, Muntz HR, McGill TJ, et al (eds): Pediatric Otolaryngology: Principles and Practice Pathways. New York, Thieme, 2000, pp 127-146.
27. Potsic WP, Cotton RT, Handler SD (eds): Surgical Pediatric Otolaryngology. New York, Thieme, 1997, pp 18-59, 106-109, 188-191, 196-205.
28. Quie PG, Pierce HC, Wannamaker LW: Influence of penicillin-producing staphylococci and the eradication of group A streptococci from the upper respiratory tract by penicillin treatments. Pediatrics 1966;37:467-476.
29. Radkowski D, McGill TJ, Healhy GB, et al: Angiofibroma: Changes in staging and treatment. Arch Otolaryngol Head Neck Surg 1996;122:122-129.
30. Richardson MA: Regional and intracranial complications of sinuses. In Wetmore RF, Muntz HR, McGill TJ, et al (eds): Pediatric Otolaryngology: Principles and Practice Pathways. New York, Thieme, 2000, pp 487-496.
31. Torsiglieri AJ, Tom LWC, Ross A, et al: Pediatric neck masses: Guidelines for evaluation. Int J Pediatr Otorhinolaryngol 1988;16:199-210.
32. Wetmore RF, Mahboubi S, Soyupak SK: Computed tomography in the evaluation of pediatric neck infections. Otolaryngol Head Neck Surg 1998;119:624-627.
33. Woolley AL, Lusk RP: Pediatric cochlear implantation. In Wetmore RF, Muntz HR, McGill TJ, et al (eds): Pediatric Otolaryngology: Principles and Practice Pathways. New York, Thieme, 2000, pp 359-370.

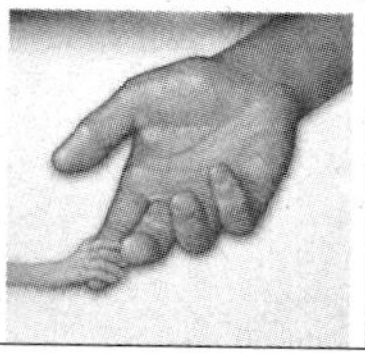

第 53 章

唾 液 腺

Nina L. Shapiro

唾液腺疾病在儿童中很少见，常表现为疼痛，少数情况下表现为受累腺体的无痛性肿胀。唾液腺疾病可能为感染性的、炎症性的、全身性疾病来源的、先天性疾病、肿瘤或外伤性的[6]。要依据不同性质唾液腺疾病的特点制定药物和手术治疗方案。

分类

唾液腺可分为大唾液腺和小唾液腺。大唾液腺包括腮腺、颌下腺、舌下腺，这三种大唾液腺是成对存在的，各有明确的解剖结构，包括血液供应、排泄导管。小唾液腺可辅助大唾液腺行使功能。小唾液腺包括分布于颊黏膜、腭部、唇黏膜面和口底的黏液分泌组织。

胚胎学

胚胎第 6 个月时，来自发育中的口腔的外胚层的实性上皮芽套入周围的间充质。此套入部的一条沟发育为隧道，随后形成涎导管组织的分支。而间充质发育为唾液腺被膜及结缔组织。实性上皮条索末端中央变空，发育为分泌腺泡。三种大唾液腺的胚胎发育过程基本相同[9]。胚胎发育早期，腮腺导管围绕面神经及其分支发育，这一点具有重要的临床意义及手术意义，因为腮腺损伤可能会压迫或损伤面神经，腮腺手术也有可能损伤面神经分支[28]。

解剖学和生理学

腮腺位于外耳道与下颌骨之间。腮腺主导管（Stensen 导管）在咬肌浅面走行，开口于上颌第二磨牙相对应的颊黏膜上。腮腺深叶位于面神经分支和下颌骨之间。腮腺深叶也可能向咽旁间隙伸展而来，表现为向口内生长。颌下腺位于颈部的下颌下三角。颌下腺主导管 Wharton 导管从腺体发出时形成一定角度，开口于舌系带两侧。舌下腺位于口底的侧方[6]。

唾液腺受多种刺激物刺激行使生理功能，这些刺激可能来自于脑部、视觉、嗅觉、味觉，唾液腺受刺激后促使唾液分泌，从而润湿口腔，有利于保持口腔卫生、发音、吞咽，对食物进行润湿以利于品尝和咀嚼，此外，唾液中的 α 淀粉酶开始对淀粉的初步消化[6]。

病理学

唾液腺的病理反应表现为肿胀，也可能伴有其他症状，如疼痛、压痛、红斑或导管开口处异常。唾液腺疾病可能为先天性的，也可能为后天性的[62]。先天性疾病包括血管瘤、淋巴畸形。儿童唾液腺疾病多为先天性血管畸形伴血管瘤，可占唾液腺疾病的 50%～60%，而淋巴畸形约占 25%[3]。后天获得性疾病可为炎症性、感染性、自身免疫性、外伤性疾病或肿瘤。大多数唾液腺疾病最初表现为腺体及周围组织的肿胀，随着病情进展，可累及颅神经导致神经不全麻痹或完全麻痹。

诊断

病史

应详细记录病史，特别是疾病的持续时间，双侧
836 或单侧病变，是否有与进食有关的症状波动。一份完整的病史是很重要的，因为唾液腺疾病可能是一些全身疾病的表现。

体格检查

体格检查应对浅表皮肤进行检查，包括病变局部的皮肤和较远处的皮肤，以诊断皮肤血管瘤。检查口腔黏膜以确定肿块是否侵及口内，对腮腺和颌下腺行双手检查有助于确定病变的性质。沿导管走行触诊导管以检查导管是否阻塞及唾液中是否有脓性分泌物。唾液腺良性病变一般可活动、柔软有弹性，而恶性病变多较固定、触诊质硬。

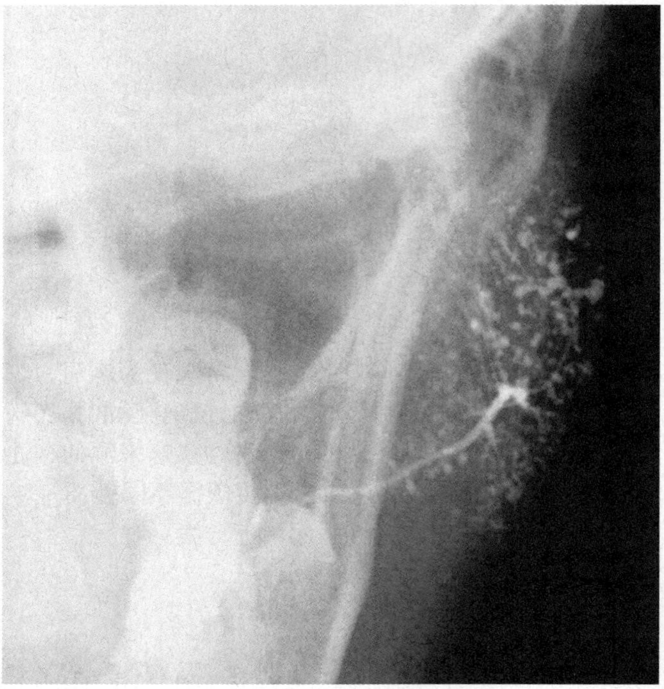

图 53-1 涎管造影 X 线片显示腮腺的囊状涎石病。

放射成像

唾液腺 X 线平片可用于检查导管结石或弥散性腺体钙化[6]。唾液腺造影术是通过细小的聚乙烯管向唾液腺导管（Stensen 导管或 Wharton 导管）内注入放射性对比物。这种技术在诊断导管狭窄、导管扩张、结石或囊性扩张等病变上有较好效果（图 53-1）[33]，但主要缺点是可能会引起疼痛，年龄较小的儿童需在麻醉和服用镇静剂条件下才能行唾液腺造影术。

高分辨率超声波扫描术对诊断唾液腺导管扩张和唾液腺结石是一种有效的无创性的检查技术[19]。而彩色多普勒成像技术可提供准确的病变范围、血管类型及血流方向（图 53-2）[66]。

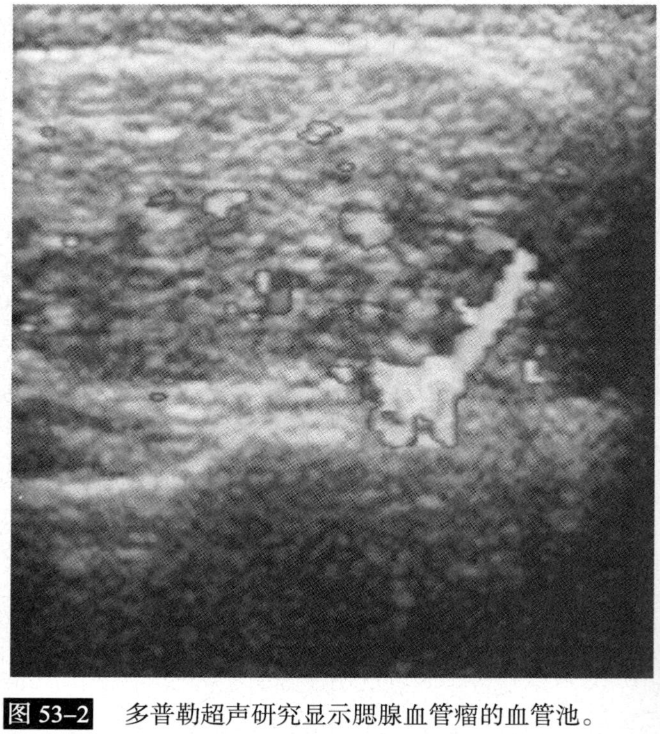

图 53-2 多普勒超声研究显示腮腺血管瘤的血管池。

计算机断层扫描

CT 可以较好地显示疾病的病理状态和解剖形态，可确定脓肿的形态。静脉滴注对比性介质可判断脓肿是否形成、描绘先天性血管分布和后天性血管病变[6]。通过这些检查手段有助于制定治疗及手术方案[10,16]。

磁共振成像（MRI）

MRI 是唾液软组织最好的检查方法。它是唯一能显示面神经在腮腺中解剖形态的成像技术。MRI 信号密度变化（T1 成像和 T2 成像）能提供有关疾病性质的有用信号[24,58]。例如，腮腺最常见的肿块血管瘤具有特征性的 MRI 表现。T1 成像为中密度，T2 成像
337 为高密度[6]。

活检

细针吸取活检是一种判断唾液腺肿块性质的较好方法[8,21]，可用于局麻下门诊患者或配合性较好的儿童。诊断准确率为 84%[1,40]。合适的活检样本可能免除手术切除的必要，更多的有助于制定手术计划。唾液腺深部肿瘤，细针吸取活检应在 B 超、CT 或 MRI 引导下进行。开放性切除活检可以确诊并有治疗效果。如果病变较易切除，手术可从口内或口外入路，活检样本应配备完整的临床记录以便作出病理诊断。大多数情况下不能从冰冻切片中得出确切诊断。在行大范围手术切除之前，要考虑病史报告结果。如果病变的大小、部位确定，可完整切除整个肿瘤，切口应做在病变周围的正常组织上。干燥综合征的诊断可依据唇黏膜 小唾液腺切取活检或腮腺切除活检[39]。

炎症性疾病

病毒性唾液腺炎

唾液腺急性炎症 85%以上由病毒引起。病毒性唾液腺炎多发生于腮腺。病毒感染多为良性的自限性的，病程超过 2～3 周。可服用解热镇痛药、止痛药和消炎药以缓解症状。病因包括柯萨奇病毒 A 和埃可病毒。在流行性腮腺炎疫苗研制出来之前，流行性腮腺炎病毒（副黏病毒）是儿童急性腮腺炎的最常见病因[13]。在美国，由于开始于 1967 年的流行性腮腺炎免疫预防针的普及，流行性腮腺炎已很少见了[12,43,50]。病毒性唾液腺炎的其他可能病因还有巨细胞病毒和 EB 病毒。巨细胞病毒在婴儿及幼儿[59]中的传播感染很常见。在健康儿童，EB 病毒与传染性单核细胞增多症有关；患慢性疾病的儿童，EBV 与 HIV 感染有关[14,60]。

细菌性化脓性唾液腺炎

急性化脓性唾液腺炎常表现为迅速发展的肿胀、疼痛、伴发热和食欲缺乏。可有脓性物质从感染腺体的导管中排出。多见于腮腺，其次是颌下腺和舌下腺。病因多为金黄色葡萄球菌、草绿色链球菌[49]。急性唾液腺炎多发生于脱水的患者，因为脱水后唾液量减少，口腔黏膜干燥。大多数病例经过抗葡萄球菌抗生素治疗、补液、漱口水漱口保持口腔卫生、局部热敷和促唾液分泌剂（如用酸柠檬刺激唾液分泌）可得到较好疗效。少数情况治疗对急性唾液腺炎无效，感染组织形成脓肿。唾液腺脓肿的治疗包括静滴抗生素和切开引流[52]。如果脓肿在腮腺内扩散，则需行腮腺切除以排净脓液，切口应与面神经走向相平行；如果术前已发生面神经麻痹，切开引流有利于面神经功能的恢复[6]。

慢性唾液腺炎

慢性唾液腺炎是儿童中最常见的唾液腺感染性疾病（图 53-3）。反复感染将导致腺体渐进性结构改变，包括涎管扩张及郁滞，以及随后的腺泡破坏。区别疾病为阻塞性或非阻塞性是很重要的。阻塞性是由导管狭窄引起的。狭窄可为先天性的或结石引起的。咀嚼或咬到导管开口可引起内源性损伤。在这种情况下，应用细直径的鼻泪管探针探查唾液腺导管并使导管口开放以持续引流。非阻塞性慢性唾液腺炎可发生于代谢性疾病如干燥综合征、慢性肉芽肿病如结节病、结核病或非典型分枝杆菌病。

阻塞性唾液腺炎主要是保守治疗，包括热敷和使用消炎药。顽固性的可使用导管扩张术或袋形缝合术，一般不需腺体切除。

涎石病（唾液腺或导管结石）在儿童中很少见，如果发生，80%发生于颌下腺。结石如果位于导管远端且在口内可见或探查到，可在导管口处切除。暂时性导管内置管可预防结疤或导管狭窄。罕见的大结石位于导管近端或腺体实质内，如果引起慢性炎性，则需完全切除腺体和含有结石的导管。

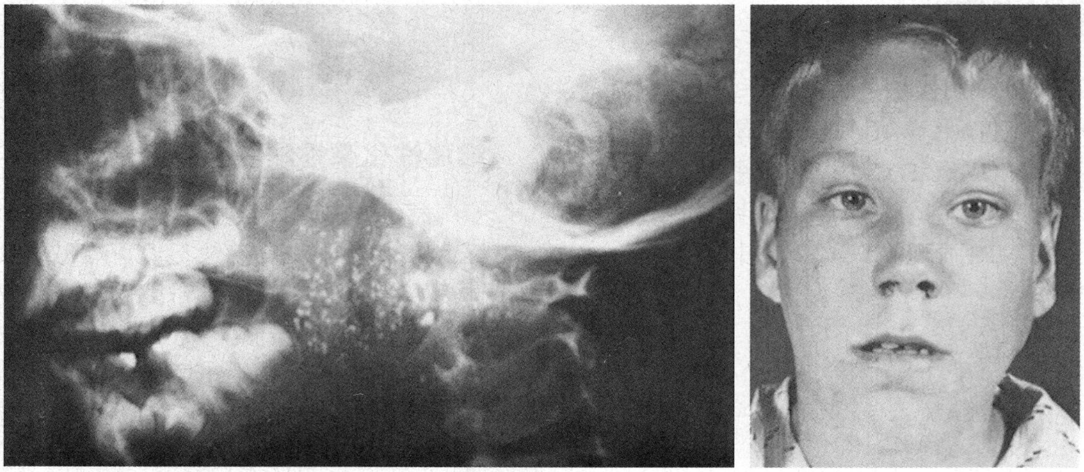

A B

图 53-3 A. 有复发性腮腺肿大病史的患者的唾液腺造影。注意导管系统早期的散布斑点状的涎管扩张。B. 急性炎症性的腮腺肿大。

囊性疾病

囊性疾病可为后天的、先天的或外伤性的，常发生于较小唾液腺或腮腺[64]。先天性囊性疾病可发生在
838 唾液腺，但不来源于唾液腺。第一、第二鳃裂囊肿可表现为腮腺肿块[65]。先天性淋巴畸形也表现于腮腺、颌下腺或舌下腺。大的双侧性腮腺内淋巴上皮是 HIV 感染的表现[6]。

小的黏液潴留囊肿可发病于唇小唾液腺或颊黏膜小唾液腺。这些囊肿常由小唾液腺的一次或反复外伤引起，可导致复发性局部黏膜肿胀，如果他们没有自动消退，则需完整切除。局部切开引流或袋形缝合术会有复发。

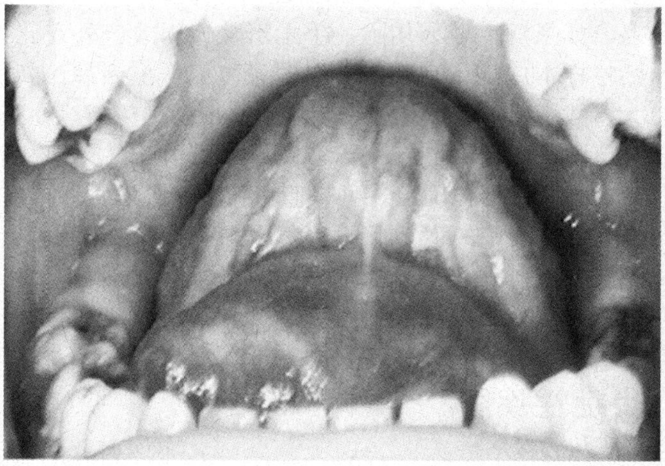

图 53-4 中底部的舌下囊肿使舌呈后上位。

舌下囊肿

舌下囊肿是舌下腺的黏液渗出性囊肿。最初表现为口底的蓝色囊性肿块，可引起舌抬高和吞咽困难（图 53-4）。舌下腺囊肿的手术治疗方法仍有争论。虽然一些人认为袋形缝合术是最合适的治疗方法[31,44]，但其他人却提出前者的高复发率和随后经下颌舌骨肌向颈部扩展，他们主张完整切除舌下腺[35,48]。切除过程中要避免损伤 Wharton 导管。术前在导管内放置一探针可避免术中误伤导管。舌下腺深部的舌神经必须小心解剖。

肿瘤

唾液腺肿瘤在儿童中极少见[3,51]，只有不到 5%的唾液腺肿瘤发生在 16 岁以上的患者[4,34]，但一旦发生必须经检查以排除恶性[7,47,54]。

良性肿瘤及畸形

良性肿瘤占儿童唾液腺肿瘤的 60%，大多数来源于血管[3]。血管病变包括血管瘤和淋巴畸形，两者都为先天性的（图 53–5）。

血管瘤

血管瘤是儿童中最常见的唾液腺（主要在腮腺内）肿瘤之一。它主要表现为腮腺的质软的肿胀，伴或不伴有皮肤着色[45]。常使用多普勒彩超或 MRI 来确诊[38]。几乎不对可疑唾液腺血管瘤进行活检[15]。腮
339 腺血管瘤常可自行消退。如迅速生成则引起功能性损害，如面神经损害、外耳道阻塞或皮肤破坏，需系统治疗，如使用皮质类固醇类、干扰素 α–2a 或 α–2b。这是一种可抑制血管生长及促进肿瘤萎缩的方法[5,30]。

一种更少见的血管性肿瘤是 Kaposi 样血管内皮瘤，是一种良性肿瘤。虽具有局部侵袭性，但触诊较硬，呈紫色结节性生长方式。对它的治疗方法仍有争议，可包括系统性使用皮质类固醇类激素，INF–α 或手术切除[42]。

淋巴畸形

淋巴畸形与血管瘤相比较少见。先天性脉管畸形的生物学特性导致它不同于其他血管瘤的病程[45]。它不会自行消退，出生时或出生后不久即可发生，随孩子的生长而长大。它不是确切的唾液腺疾病，但常见于婴儿与较小儿童的颈部和腮腺区[46]。因为是淋巴系统疾病，他们易受感染，有可能发展为蜂窝织炎。病灶内出血、脓肿形成或淋巴液外溢至口底或气管。治疗方法仍在探索之中[23,29]。手术必须完整切除以防止复发，但通常很难做到，因为肿瘤壁脆弱易破，而且邻近有大血管和面神经分支。为避免手术并发症，病灶内硬化疗法已成功应用，可减小肿瘤体积，减少创伤和复发[57]。

多形性腺瘤

多形性腺瘤（良性混合瘤）是儿童最常见的非血管性良性唾液腺肿瘤（图 53–6）[57,54]，表现为固定的有弹性的肿块，多发生于腮腺。在儿童中平均发病率年龄是 9.5 岁[26,51]。肿瘤为无痛性缓慢生长的肿块[22]，没有浸润性腮腺浅叶肿瘤的治疗包括腮腺浅叶切除术，解剖并保留面神经。据报道复发率达 40%，所以建议长期随访[36,55]。偶尔复发性多形性腺病可发生恶变[11]。

颌下腺、小唾液腺、舌、软腭也可发生多形性腺瘤，但很少见[3]。

单形性腺瘤

单形性腺瘤在儿童中少见。镜下表现类似腺样囊性癌——是一种高度侵袭性的恶性唾液腺肿瘤[37]，治

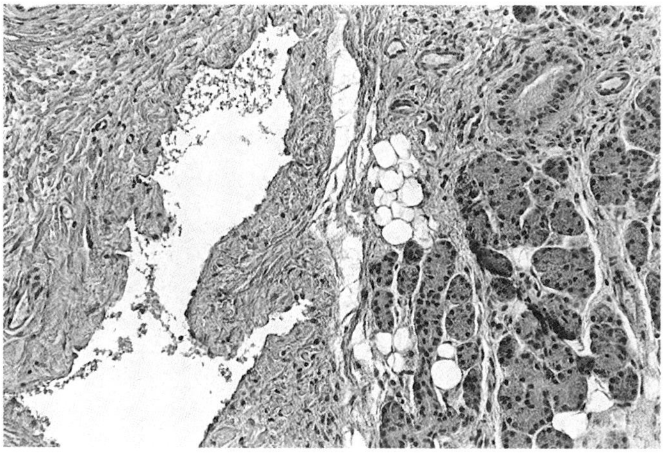

图 53–5 腮腺的血管畸形。显示大而不规则的血管池。（苏木素伊红染色，50 倍。）

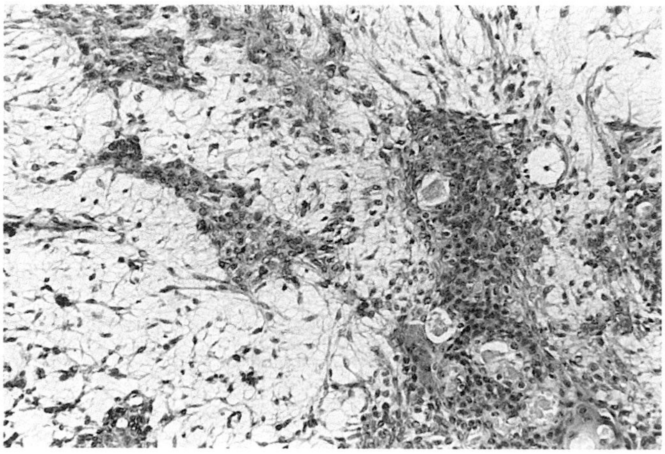

图 53–6 腮腺多形性腺瘤（混合瘤）。上皮区域混杂着黏液样和软骨样基质（苏木精伊红染色，50 倍）。

疗包括手术完全切除和长期密切随访。

乳头状囊腺淋巴瘤（Warthin 瘤）

这种肿瘤多见于男性，累及双侧腮腺。偶尔作为儿童良性腮腺肿瘤出现[6]。治疗方法与多形性腺瘤相似。

恶性肿瘤

唾液腺恶性肿瘤极少见于儿童。若发生则常为低度恶性型的，多发生于腮腺，女性多见[51]。诊断依据包括 CT、MRI 和细针吸取活检。治疗方法为：有清楚边界的肿瘤完整切除。侵袭性恶性肿瘤可能需切除
840 部分面神经分支，神经接合以恢复面部肌肉功能。高度恶性型建议术后放疗[27,41]。

黏液表皮样癌

黏液表皮样癌是最常见的儿童唾液腺恶性肿瘤，通常是腮腺的低度恶性肿瘤。手术治疗可选择腮腺浅叶切除或全腮腺切除，这取决于肿瘤累及的范围。手术治疗通常有效[32,34]。对于高度恶性黏液表皮样癌或累及颌下腺、小唾液腺的黏液表皮样癌，许多机构建议行颈淋巴清扫术和辅助性放疗[17,25,53]。

腺泡细胞癌

腺泡细胞癌的表现与黏液表皮样癌相似，多为低度恶性，治疗方法也与黏液表皮样癌相同（图 53–7）。

腺样囊性癌

腺样囊性癌是一种少见的，高度恶性的唾液腺肿瘤，它的神经浸润性可引起面瘫，发生于颌下腺的肿瘤可侵袭舌神经、舌下神经和面神经下颌缘支。区域性淋巴结转移发生率很高，远距离可转移至肺、肝和骨。治疗包括扩大切除术、颈淋巴清扫术，并辅以放疗[27]。

横纹肌肉瘤

横纹肌肉瘤表现为腮腺肿块。组织学分型包括未分化型和胚胎型（图 53–8），治疗方法及疗效取决于肿瘤的进展进程，可行局部扩大切除术，辅以放、化疗。

手术方法

Davis 及其同事[20]对其解剖结构的研究以及 Beahrs 和 Chong[2]的研究成果奠定了腮腺手术的基础。通过面神经监控设备，可以加强术中面神经解剖的精细程度而提供更好的保护[63]。手术开始时，与麻痹医生合作，关注肌肉麻痹的逆转是重要的。

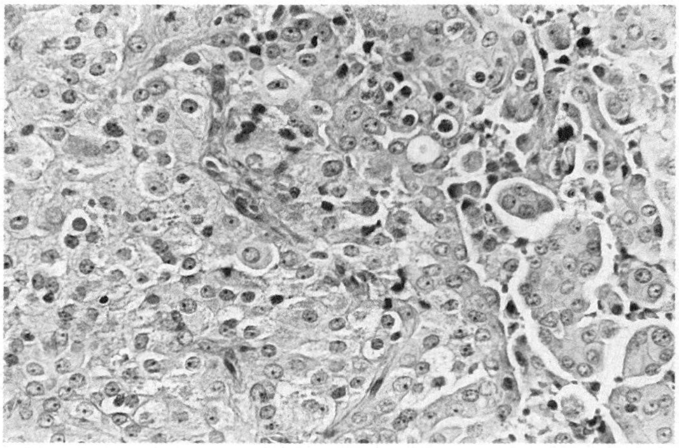

图 53–7 腮腺腺泡细胞癌显示侵犯性增殖。（苏木素伊红染色，100 倍）

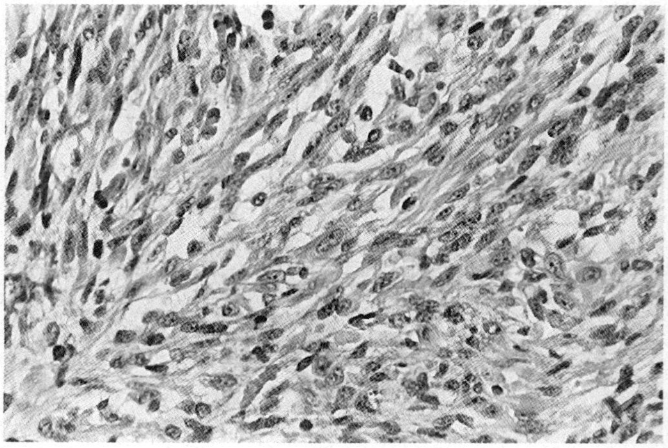

图 53–8 腮腺横纹肌肉瘤显示梭形细胞肉瘤，伴肌肉分化（苏木素伊红染色，100 倍）。

腮腺

做 S 形切口，从耳前皱褶开始，切口线呈曲线形并延伸至耳后区，接着向下延伸至下颌角以下两横指（图 53–9）。皮瓣厚度应深达皮下组织和腮腺筋膜浅部。在后方，将皮瓣提高至颈阔肌下平面，直至看见

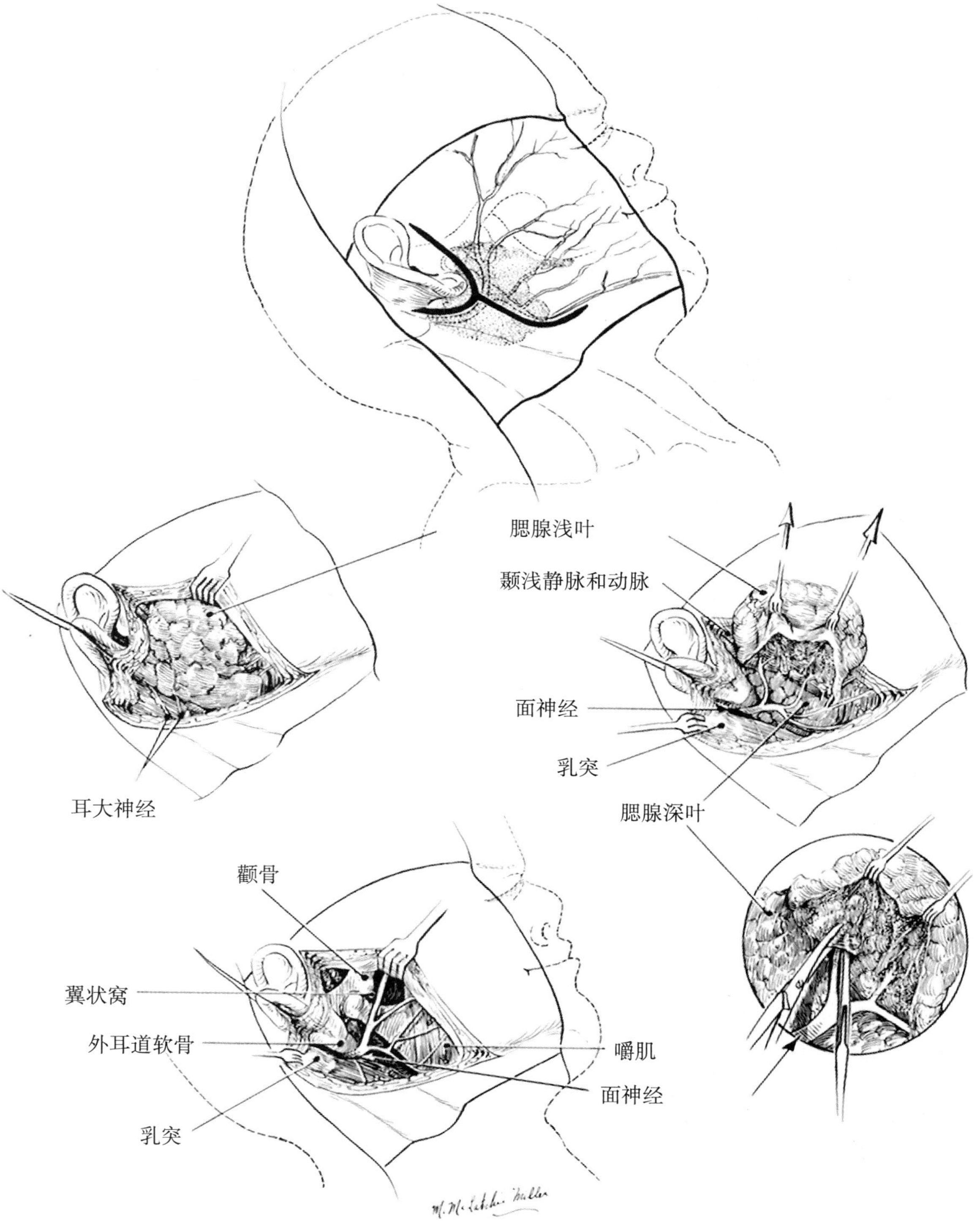

图 53–9　腮腺切除技术。

胸锁乳突肌前缘。确认耳大神经及面后静脉，可能需要切断两者，从而暴露腮腺后缘。面神经主干将腮的浅叶分开。为了确认面神经主干，必须将耳垂向上牵引，并将腮腺向前牵引。沿耳屏和乳突解剖可见到面神经主干，后者从茎乳孔中发生。沿面神经分支向前精细地解剖可使腮腺浅叶抬起。如需解剖深叶，必须轻柔地牵开神经分支，从而进入肿瘤的深处。仔细地
841 钝性分离，使用双极电凝和面神经监测仪，可使神经损伤降至最低，获得最好的手术效果[18]。

颌下腺

颌下腺切除，应在下颌骨下方二横指处皮肤做水平切口，分离深度在皮下组织和颈阔肌之下的颌下腺
842 筋膜。手术视野暴露范围向前至茎突舌骨肌，向后至胸锁乳突肌，上至二腹肌。鉴别并分离颌下腺筋膜深面的面前静脉，以保护面神经下颌缘支。舌下神经走行于二腹肌深面。向前牵拉舌骨肌，下拉颌下腺，可辨认舌神经和 Wharton 导管，分离导管，可使舌神经从腺体分离，并可完整钝性分离颌下腺[18]。

并发症

唾液腺疾病很少发生于儿童，外科医生对大唾液腺的解剖知识和对系统生理、肿瘤生理机制的理解对正确的治疗是非常重要的。唾液腺肿瘤很少见于儿童，且多为良性[56]。无论是全身性疾病还是肿瘤，诊断和治疗方法要依据每个患者的不同情况来制定。诊断方法有许多种，包括放射性检查或病理学检查。

炎症感染性疾病可用药物治疗，肿瘤则需手术治疗。外科医生必须具有面神经解剖的经验，还需了解婴儿、儿童面神经解剖变异情况。手术中如果不慎断离或切除面神经，可导致长期并发症。如果牵拉面神经，则可导致短期并发症。患者及家属要被告知面神经损伤后可能的长期、短期并发症。

尽管对腮腺及颌下腺手术有严格的要求，但凭借医生丰富的手术经验，适当的监测设备，谨慎的解剖和严格止血，会取得很好的手术效果[61]。

（徐建民译　陈其民校）

参考文献

1. Al-Khafaiji BM, Nestok BR, Katz RL: Fine needle aspiration of 154 parotid masses with histologic correlation: Ten year experience at the University of Texas MD Anderson Cancer Center. Cancer 1998;84:153.
2. Beahrs OH, Chong GC: Management of the facial nerve in parotidectomy. Am J Surg 1972;124:473.
3. Bentz BG, Hughes A, Ludemann JP, Maddalozzo J: Masses of the salivary gland region in children. Arch Otolaryngol Head Neck Surg 2000;126:1435-1439.
4. Bianchi A, Cudmore RE: Salivary gland tumors in childhood. J Pediatr Surg 1978;13:512.
5. Blei F, Isakoff M, Deb G: The response of parotid hemangiomas to the use of systemic interferon alfa-2a or corticosteroids. Arch Otolaryngol Head Neck Surg 1997; 123:841-844.
6. Bower CM, Dyleski RA: Diseases of the salivary glands. In Bluestone CD, Stool SE, Kenna M (eds): Textbook of Pediatric Otolaryngology. Philadelphia, WB Saunders, 2004, pp 1251-1267.
7. Camacho AE, Goodman ML, Eavey RD: Pathologic correlation of the unknown solid parotid mass in children. Otolaryngol Head Neck Surg 1989;101:566-571.
8. Candel A, Gattuso P, Reddy V, et al: Is fine needle aspiration biopsy of salivary gland masses really necessary? Ear Nose Throat J 1993;72:485.
9. Carlson GW: The salivary glands: Embryology, anatomy, and surgical applications. Surg Clin North Am 2000;80:261-273.
10. Casselman JW, Mancuso AA: Major salivary gland masses: comparison of MR imaging and CT. Radiology 1987; 165:183.
11. Castro EB, Huvos AG, Atrong EW, Foote FW Jr: Tumors of the major salivary glands in children. Cancer 1972;29:312.
12. Centers for Disease Control: Mumps prevention. MMWR Morb Mortal Wkly Rep 1989;38:338-392, 397-400.
13. Cherry JD: Mumps virus. In Feigen RD, Cherry JD, Demmler GJ, Kaplan SL (eds): Textbook of Pediatric Infectious Diseases, 5th ed. Philadelphia, WB Saunders, 2004, pp 2305-2314.
14. Chetty R, Vaithilingum M, Thejpal R: Epstein-Barr virus status and the histopathological changes of parotid gland lymphoid infiltrates in HIV-positive children. Pathology 1999;31:413-417.
15. Childers EL, Furlong MA, Fanburg-Smith JC: Hemangioma of the salivary gland: A study of ten cases of a rarely biopsied/excised lesion. Ann Diagn Pathol 2002;6:339-344.
16. Corr P, Cheng P, Metrweli C: The role of ultrasound and computed tomography in the evaluation of parotid masses. Aust Radiol 1993;37:195.
17. Conley J, Tinsley PP Jr: Treatment and prognosis of mucoepidermoid carcinoma in the pediatric age group. Arch Otolaryngol 1985;111:322-324.
18. Cunningham MJ: Tumors of the head and neck. In Bluestone CD, Stool SE (eds): Atlas of Pediatric Otolaryngology. Philadelphia, WB Saunders, 1995, pp 530-570.
19. Cvetinovic M, Jovic N, Mijatovic D: Evaluation of ultrasound in the diagnosis of pathologic processes in the parotid gland. J Oral Maxillofac Surg 1991;49;147.
20. Davis RA, Anson BJ, Budinger JM, Kurth LR: Surgical anatomy of the facial nerve and parotid gland based on 350 cervicofacial halves. Surg Gynecol Obstet 1956;102:358.
21. Dean GT, Briggs K, Spence RAG: An audit of surgery of the parotid gland. Ann R Coll Surg Engl 1995;77:188.

22. Ethunandan M, Ethunandan A, Macpherson D, et al: Parotid neoplasms in children: Experience of diagnosis and management in a district general hospital. Int J Oral Maxillofac Surg 2003;32:373-377.
23. Fageeh N, Manoukian J, Tewfik T, et al: Management of head and neck lymphatic malformations in children. J Otolaryngol 1997;26:253-258.
24. Freling NJ, Molenaar WM, Verney A: Malignant parotid tumors: Clinical use of MR imaging and histological correlation. Radiology 1992;185:691.
25. Friedman M, Levin B, Grybauskas V, et al: Malignant tumors of the major salivary glands. Otolaryngol Clin North Am 1986;19:625-636.
26. Galick R: Salivary gland neoplasms in children. Arch Otolaryngol 1969;89:878.
27. Garden AS, el-Naggar AK, Morrison WH, et al: Postoperative radiotherapy for malignant tumors of the parotid gland. Int J Radiat Oncol Biol Phys 1997;37:79.
28. Gasser RF: The early development of the parotid gland around the facial nerve branches. Anat Rec 1992;15:244.
29. Giguere CM, Bauman NM, Smith RJ: New treatment options for lymphangioma in infants and children. Ann Otol Rhinol Laryngol 2002;111:1066-1075.
30. Greene AK, Rogers GF, Mulliken JB: Management of parotid hemangioma in 100 children. Plast Reconstr Surg 2004;113:53-60.
31. Haberal I, Gocmen H, Samim E: Surgical management of pediatric ranula. Int J Pediatr Otorhinolaryngol 2004;68: 161-163.
32. Hicks J, Flaitz C: Mucoepidermoid carcinoma of the salivary glands in children and adolescents: Assessment and proliferation of markers. Oral Oncol 2000;36:454-460.
33. Ilgit ET, et al: Digital subtraction sialography techniques: Advantages and results in 107 cases. Eur J Radiol 1992;15:44.
34. Jaques DA, Krolls SO, Chambers RG: Parotid tumors in children. Am J Surg 1976;132:469-471.
35. Kobayashi T, Ochi K, Komatsuzaki Y, et al: Blanket removal of the sublingual gland for treatment of plunging ranula. Laryngoscope 2003;113:386-388.
36. Koral K, Sayre J, Bhuta S, et al: Recurrent pleomorphic adenoma of the parotid gland in pediatric and adult patients: Value of multiple lesions as a diagnostic indicator. AJR Am J Roentgenol 2003;180:1171-1174.
37. Krolls SO, Trodahl JN, Boyers R: Salivary gland lesions in children. Cancer 1972;30:459.
38. Lowe LH, Stokes LS, Johnson JE, et al: Swelling at the angle of the mandible: Imaging of the pediatric parotid gland and periparotid region. Radiographics 2001;21:1211-1227.
39. McGuirt WF, Whang C, Moreland W: The role of parotid biopsy in the diagnosis of pediatric Sjögren syndrome. Arch Otolaryngol Head Neck Surg 2002;128:1279-1281.
40. Megerian CA, Maniglia AJ: Parotidectomy: A ten-year experience with fine needle aspiration and frozen section biopsy correlation. Ear Nose Throat J 1994;73:377.
41. Mendenhall WM, Morris CG, Amdur RJ, et al: Radiotherapy alone or combined with carbogen breathing for squamous cell carcinoma of the head and neck: A prospective, randomized trial. Cancer 2005;104:332-337.
42. Metry DW, Hebert AA: Benign cutaneous vascular tumors of infancy: When to worry, what to do. Arch Dermatol 2000;136:905-914.
43. Modlin JF: Current status of mumps in the United States. Infection 1975;132:106.
44. Morita Y, Sato K, Kawana M, et al: Treatment of ranula—excision of the sublingual gland versus marsupialization. Auris Nasus Larynx 2003;30:311-314.
45. Mulliken JB, Glowacki J: Hemangiomas and vascular malformations in infants and children: A classification based on endothelial characteristics. Plast Reconstr Surg 1982;69: 412-420.
46. Orvidas LJ, Kasperbauer JL: Pediatric lymphangiomas of the head and neck. Ann Otol Rhinol Laryngol 2000;109:411-421.
47. Orvidas LJ, Kasperbauer JL, Lewis JE, et al: Pediatric parotid masses. Arch Otolaryngol Head Neck Surg 2000;126:177-184.
48. Pandit RT, Park AH: Management of pediatric ranula. Otolaryngol Head Neck Surg 2002;127:115-118.
49. Pershall KE, Koopman CF, Coultard SW: Sialadenitis in children. J Pediatr Otolaryngol 1986;11:199.
50. Peter G (ed): 1997 Red Book: Report of the Committee on Infectious Diseases, 24th ed. Elk Grove Village, IL, American Academy of Pediatrics, 1997, pp 366-369.
51. Ribeiro Kde C, Kowalski LP, Saba LM, de Camargo B: Epithelial salivary gland neoplasms in children and adolescents: A forty-four year experience. Med Pediatr Oncol 2002;39:504-600.
52. Rice DH: Non-neoplastic diseases of the salivary glands. In Paparella MM, et al (eds): Otolaryngology. Philadelphia, WB Saunders, 1991.
53. Rogers DA, Rao BN, Bowman L, et al: Primary malignancy of the salivary gland in children. J Pediatr Surg 1994;29: 44-47.
54. Schuller DE, McCabe BF: Salivary gland neoplasms in childhood. Otolaryngol Clin North Am 1977;10:39.
55. Shikani AH, Johns ME: Tumors of the major salivary glands in children. Head Neck Surg 1998;10:257.
56. Siefert G, Sobin LH: The World Health Organization's Histological classification of salivary gland tumours: A commentary on the second edition. Cancer 1992;70:379.
57. Sung MW, Lee DW, Kim DY, et al: Sclerotherapy with picibinal (OK-432) for congenital lymphatic malformation in the head and neck. Laryngoscope 2001;111:1430-1433.
58. Tabor EK, Curtin HD: MR of the salivary glands. Radiol Clin North Am 1989;379:27.
59. Variend S, O'Neill D, Arnold P: The possible significance of cytomegaloviral parotitis in infant and early childhood deaths. Arch Pathol Lab Med 1997;121:1272.
60. Venkateswaran L, Gan YJ, Sixbey JW, Santana VM: Epstein-Barr virus infection in salivary gland tumors in children and young adults. Cancer 2000;89:463-466.
61. Watanabe Y, et al: Facial nerve palsy as a complication of parotid surgery and its prevention. Acta Otolaryngol Suppl (Stockh) 1993;504:137.
62. White AK: Salivary gland diseases in infancy and childhood. J Otorhinolaryngol 1992;21:422.
63. Woods JE: Parotidectomy: Points of technique for a brief and safe operation. Am J Surg 1983;145:678.
64. Work WP: Cysts and congenital lesions of the parotid gland. Otorhinolaryngol Clin North Am 1977;10:339.
65. Work WP: Newer concepts of first branchial cleft defects. Laryngoscope 1972;82:1581.
66. Yang WT, Ahuja A, Metreweli C: Sonographic features of head and neck hemangiomas and vascular malformations: Review of 23 patients. J Ultrasound Med 1997;16:39.

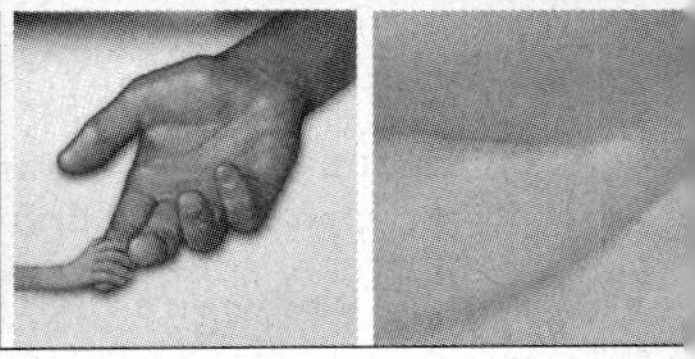

第 54 章

淋巴结病

Kurt D. Newman 和 Andrea A. Hayes-Jordan

844 ## 淋巴结病基本知识

儿童颈部的持续肿大的肿块可引起家长与儿科医生的关注，也是转诊至外科医生的常见原因。大多数儿童颈部肿块是先天性病变（如甲状舌管、鳃裂来源）或淋巴结肿大。临床上表现为明显的颈部淋巴结肿大，常见于儿童。据流行病学报告，淋巴结病在婴儿和儿童比例为 28%～55%[23,32]。虽然大多数颈部淋巴结病是由感染引起的反应性增生，但较为慢性的或经抗生素治疗后仍然持续存在的病例，则必须考虑恶性病变的可能[19]。一些特殊感染病例，如非典型分枝杆菌性淋巴结炎，需行外科治疗。同样，对化脓性或有瘘管形成的复杂病例，或对适当的药物治疗抵抗的淋巴结炎病，可行手术治疗。抗生素治疗 2 周后仍持续的淋巴结病，仅累及单侧锁骨上或颈后三角的淋巴结病，以及目前诊断不明确的淋巴结病，最好行活组织检查以排除恶性的可能。影像学检查有助于鉴别囊性、突性或固体病变和混合性病变[16]。

解剖学

图 54-1 展示了头颈部区域的淋巴结组。淋巴池的引流遵循可预测的解剖路径，命名反映了淋巴结的位置。面部和口咽部淋巴主要汇入耳前、颌下和颏下淋巴结，头后部汇入枕淋巴结组，口、舌、扁桃腺、咽和鼻咽部汇入颈前浅淋巴结组和颈前深淋巴结组。Shah 和他的同事们提出了一个用于颈部淋巴结分组的分类系统（图 54-2）[49]。该表描述的淋巴结组如下：Ⅰ级——颏下三角淋巴结组；Ⅱ、Ⅲ、Ⅳ级——颈内上组、颈内中组、颈内下组；Ⅴ级——颈后三角淋巴结组；Ⅵ级——气管食管沟淋巴结组；Ⅶ级——上纵隔淋巴结组。

急性淋巴结病

急性自限性炎症性淋巴结肿大的常见病因是病毒感染[5]。急性双侧颈淋巴结病常由呼吸道病毒感染或链球菌性咽炎引起。而占病例 40%～80%的单侧颈淋巴结炎常由链球菌或葡萄球菌感染引起[29]。病毒感染引起的双侧淋巴结病常可自行好转。急性化脓性淋巴结炎的常见病因是耐青霉素的葡萄球菌或 A 组链球菌感染或两者混合感染[3]。葡萄球菌性淋巴 845
结炎多见于婴儿[25]。厌氧菌、B 型链球菌和 B 型嗜血杆菌不是常见的致病微生物[8,20,47]。最近，一种新的耐药模式被识别。已从儿童浅脓肿和化脓性淋巴

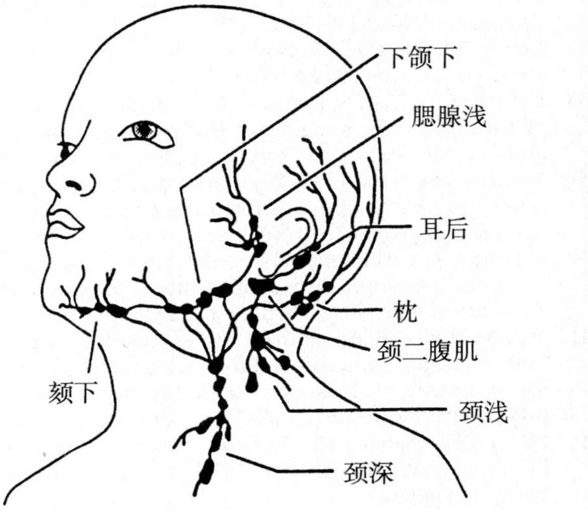

图 54-1 头颈部区域性淋巴结组。(From Bodenstein L, Altman RP: Cervical lymphadenitis in infants and children. Semin Pediatr Surg 1994;3:134. Used with permission.)

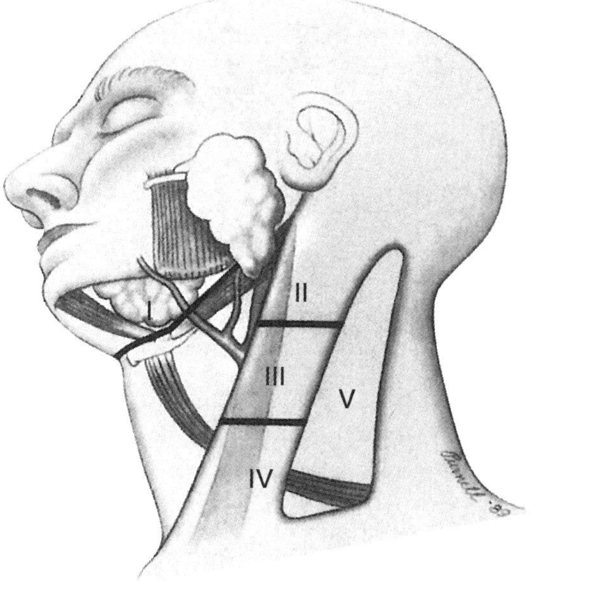

图 54-2　颈部淋巴结系统。Ⅵ级水平（气管食管沟）和Ⅲ(上纵隔）淋巴结组未显示。(From Shah JP, Medina JE, Shaha AR, et al: Cervical lymph node metastasis. Curr Prob Surg 1993;30:273. Used with permission.)

结炎病例中分离出社区获得性耐甲氧西林、对氯可霉素敏感的金黄色葡萄球菌（MRSA）[29,41]。不考虑致病菌，化脓性淋巴结炎的局部炎症体征可强烈提示诊断。儿童多表现为单侧轻度淋巴结肿大（累及引流口咽的颌下或颈内淋巴结）。皮肤表面可能出现红斑。可出现不同程度的发热、不适和全身症状。应详细检查头颈部的原发感染，包括口咽和中耳并进行治疗。

无并发症的颈部淋巴结炎的主要治疗方法为：5～10 天的经验性使用口服抗 β 内酰胺酶抗生素。绝大多数患者在门诊能得到安全有效的治疗。对于出现全身症状的感染（包括蜂窝织炎），或发生于小婴儿的感染，静脉应用抗生素可能更有临床疗效。治疗的第一个 72 小时应有显著疗效。若未出现好转，则需进一步诊断检查，包括肿块的超声检查和细针穿刺[6]。针吸活检确定病原菌可指导选择针对特定致病菌的抗生素治疗。但在儿童患者行细针穿刺需服镇静剂或在麻醉下进行。穿刺吸取物应送检，行需氧菌、厌氧菌和耐酸菌的染色和培养检测。治疗应基于穿刺结果进行。如果穿刺结果提示金黄色葡萄球菌感染，则应使用氯林可霉素治疗[29,41]。

超声检查有助于区分颈部实性肿块或囊性肿块。此外，肿大的炎性淋巴结液体性质有助于决定是否需要手术切开引流。其他诊断方法如 CT 和 MRI对大多数疑似淋巴结病病例不必使用（图 54-3）。适当的抗菌治疗一般会对增大的淋巴结起作用，淋巴结突会迅速消退。反复穿刺、抗生素治疗[7]或切开引流能有效治疗有波动感的化脓性淋巴结炎。在对 110 名患儿的回顾性研究中，95 名患儿的 107 个颈部感染点行手术引流。余下的 15 名患儿经内科治疗后好转。仅在 81 个病例（76%）中，CT 准确预测了手术发现。另外 26 例的 CT 检查结果和手术发现有差异。18 例有假阳性结果，CT 显示为脓肿，而手术中确认为蜂窝织炎[16]。

非典型分枝杆菌淋巴结炎（又称非结核分枝杆菌）

这些分枝杆菌属是在光学显微镜下具有浓密脂滴
的杆菌。脂滴着色后能抗酸性乙醇脱色，因此被称为 846

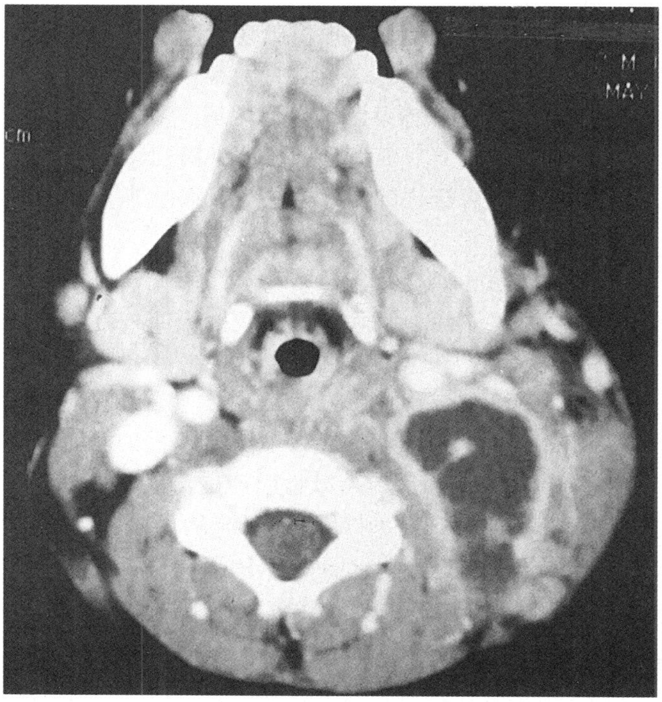

图 54-3　尽管在大多数病例中不必采用 CT 检查，这张 CT 扫描显示了化脓性淋巴结炎引起的颈深部脓肿。这位 2 岁患儿有弥漫性单侧颈部水肿进而脓肿，位于左侧颈动脉鞘后方。

抗酸杆菌[1]。非典型分枝杆菌是分枝杆菌淋巴结炎最常见的病原。最常见的非典型分枝杆菌包括：鸟胞内分枝杆菌，瘰疬分枝杆菌、偶发分枝杆菌、龟分枝杆菌[1]。与结核性淋巴结炎相反，非典型（或非结核）分枝杆菌淋巴结炎通常被认为是一种局限性感染，对具有免疫能力的宿主无全身累及[35]。据观察，获得性或先天性免疫缺陷的患者有全身散布性淋巴结炎的可能。非典型分枝杆菌淋巴结炎无接触传染性。在健康儿童，它从口咽部入侵人体[2]。

非典型分枝杆菌淋巴结炎常发生于1～5岁的儿童。常见症状为：局限性累及单侧颈二腹肌淋巴结组、耳前淋巴结组或颌下淋巴结组。与急性化脓性淋巴结炎相比，非典型分枝杆菌病累及的淋巴结组表现为：触诊坚实、有弹性，与下方结构粘连。虽然肿块不柔软，但偶尔有引流窦道[36]。通常很少或不出现全身感染症状。胸片一般正常。

由于交叉反应，非典型分枝杆菌淋巴结炎患者进行纯化蛋白衍生的结核菌素或旧结核菌素皮肤试验可以产生中度反应[58]。应用非典型分枝杆菌的特定抗原进行的皮肤试验已在开发[5,26]，但未广泛应用于临床。据文献记录，体外全血化验发现，非典型分枝杆菌淋巴结炎患者的淋巴细胞产物 γ-干扰素增加[15]。细针穿刺可发现抗酸杆菌，以提供确切诊断。但术前区分结核性和非结核性淋巴结炎常有困难。结核性和非结核性分枝杆菌混合感染已有报道但极少见[35]。与结核性淋巴结炎不同，非典型分枝杆菌性淋巴结炎一般对化疗无反应。可选择的治疗方法是彻底手术切除、一期关闭创口。

回顾儿童非典型分枝杆菌性淋巴结炎外科治疗的文献：切除、引流、刮除术和穿刺抽吸四种方法的疗效在16项研究中进行了比较，治愈率分别为92%、10%、86%和41%。在510例行手术切除的患者中，11例出现暂时性面神经麻痹；1例出现永久性面神经瘫痪；13例全切除后有持续性引流的患者中，7例在切口底部复发[18]；70例行切开引流的患者中，至少15例形成流液的窦道。四种不同研究中，在35例行刮除术的患者中，2例延迟愈合，1例须行二次刮除，1例复发[1]。

因此应避免仅仅行切开引流。椭圆形切除皮肤、皮下组织及受累淋巴结，不需行正式的淋巴结清除术。只有无条件进行手术切除时，方考虑刮除术。对于下颌角处的病变，神经刺激器有助于避免损伤面神经分支。对于确诊的、已行足够局部切除的非典型分枝杆菌性淋巴结炎患者，不需抗结核化疗和患者隔离。

分枝杆菌淋巴结炎

在发达国家，结核杆菌几乎是结核性淋巴结炎（淋巴结核）的唯一病原菌（图54-4）。在牛结核病控制之前，结核性淋巴结炎的主要原因是牛分枝杆菌。有时可在来自不发达地区的、饮用受污染的生牛奶的患者中发现牛分枝杆菌。人结核性淋巴炎患者常主诉之前露暴于已知的肺结核携带者[48]，但多数患者的胸片无活动性病变迹象[44]。结核性淋巴结炎常有其他症状和表现，包括：结核菌素皮肤试验呈强阳性，胸片显示有肺门淋巴结病或钙化[56]。研究表明，满足下列三项标准中的两项的人群中，92%患该病。三项标准为：结核菌素皮肤试验阳性、胸片异常、与已知传染性肺结核患者的接触史[44]。通常认为，结核 847
性淋巴结炎是系统性疾病的局部表现，而不是结核

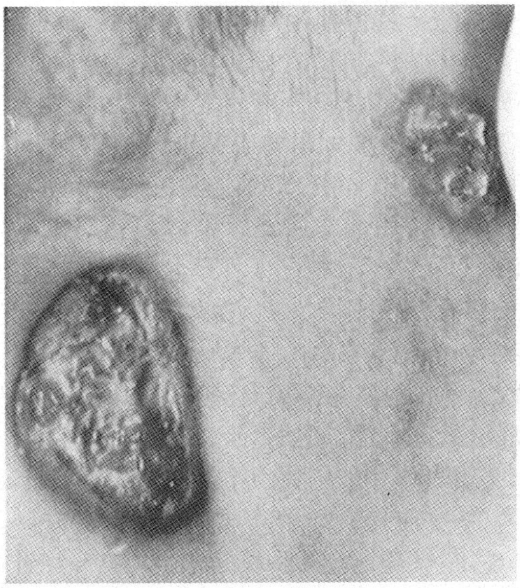

图 54-4 颈部淋巴结核（耳朵在照片的右侧）。有家族性接触史，结核菌素皮试阳性的7岁男孩患者的颈部淋巴结。经过7个月的使用两种药物的抗结核治疗，完全康复。(From Jones PG: Glands of the neck. In Welch KJ, et al (eds): Pediatric Surgery, 4th ed. St. Louis, Mosby-Year Book, 1986. Used with permission.)

感染的最初原发病灶[5,10]。临床上，结核性淋巴结炎患者通常是发生于较年长儿童和青少年的非化脓性淋巴结炎[31]（可能为双侧的）。对 24 例具有免疫能力的结核性淋巴结炎患儿进行的回顾性研究表明，仅 29%累及颌下区淋巴结，71%仅累及颈前淋巴结[44]，但颈后三角区淋巴结累及确有发生[34]。

有相关病史、疑似淋巴结病，伴结核菌素皮肤试验强阳性，淋巴组织染色或培养后发现抗酸菌，可诊断为结核性淋巴结炎。确诊可通过穿刺活检进行培养和细胞学检查[14,33]。有报道称可通过聚合酶链反应技术扩增淋巴结组织的 DNA 来进行结核性淋巴结炎的快速诊断[42]。相反，结核菌素试验阴性则基本可排除结核性淋巴结炎。如诊断不明确，可在患者全麻状态下，在手术室行淋巴结完整切除送活组织检查。应避免行切开活组织检查或切开引流，以防慢性流液性窦道形成[5,51,56]。结核感染的淋巴结切开引流后，几乎 100%有瘘管和瘢痕瘤[44]。

结核性淋巴结炎的治疗一般采用联合化疗药物治疗。如果直接观察到结核菌感染，世界卫生组织提倡应用短期疗法，起初 2 个月使用异烟肼、利福平和吡嗪酰胺，接着再使用异烟肼和利福平 4 个月[60]。尽管抗结核化疗是必要的，但完整切除受累及的淋巴结存在争议[6,12]。当需行活检进行诊断，或当内科治疗期间有慢性瘘管形成，或积极的内科治疗无效时完整切除是明智的。

猫抓病

猫抓病是儿童淋巴结炎的常见原因。据估计，每年美国儿童及成年人猫抓病发病率为 9.3/100 000[27]，发病率最高的年龄段是 10 岁以下的儿童[32]。当前的微生物分析和 PCR 技术进行的 DNA 分析表明：多形性革兰阴性杆菌——汉赛巴尔通体是猫抓病的病原微生物[4,13,22]。绝大多数患者有猫接触史，常见感染部位是肢体。随后的淋巴结炎发生于区域淋巴引流池（腹股沟、腋窝、滑车上淋巴结）[11]。同样，头颈部有抓痕时，常可观察到颈淋巴结病（图 54–5）。虽然汉赛巴尔通体感染的主要表现是淋巴结病，但一些病例研究报道称，近 25%的病例出现严重的系统性疾病[30]。

感染最初发生于皮肤创口（如抓痕或咬痕）。3～5 天内感染部位丘疹形成，1～2 周内，区域淋巴引流池的淋巴结出现亚急性淋巴结炎。常见的最初全身症状为：全身不适、肌痛和厌食。尽管绝大多数病例累及肢体淋巴结，但约 25%的病例感染部位累及颈部淋巴结[11]。诊断基于猫接触史、有病变区域（可在淋巴结病出现时好转）及局部淋巴结病。Warthin–Starrly 嗜银染色曾被用于鉴定受累淋巴结中的巴尔通体，但最近这种方法被认为不可靠且缺乏特异性[40]。用淋巴结或其他组织的石蜡切片进行巴尔通体的聚合酶链反应更可靠快速[40]。由于为良性、自限性的，故多数病例的淋巴结病不需特殊治疗即可在 6～8 周内痊愈[39]。化脓性淋巴结炎不常见，所以通常不需行切除活组织检查，但如果窦道形成或诊断不明且不能排除恶性肿瘤，可行切除活检。

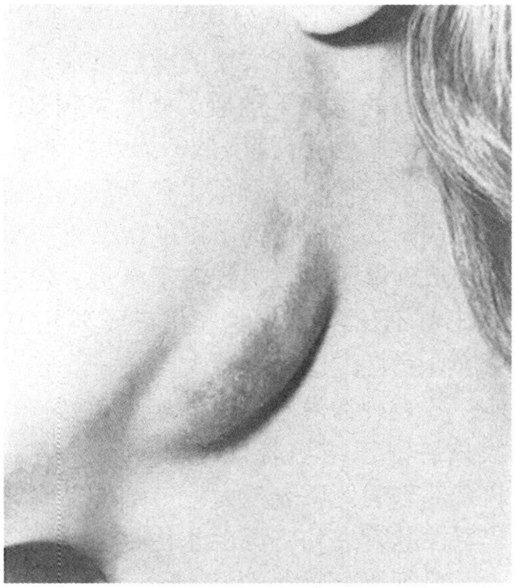

图 54–5　一个猫抓病患者的颈部淋巴结感染。感染的病原体是多形性革兰阴性杆菌——汉赛巴尔通体。(From Jones PG: Glands of the neck. In Welch KJ, et al [eds]: Pediatric Surgery, 4th ed. St. Louis, Mosby-Year Book, 1986.Used with permission.)

其他病变

婴儿或儿童的其他多种感染或炎症能导致淋巴结病。多数患者不需手术治疗，特别是切除性活检组织检查。患者病情的全面评估方法包括：完整的病史、物理检查和诊断性试验，通常能做出正确诊断。外科治疗应用于以下情况：（1）诊断不明确；（2）锁骨

上或颈后三角等可疑区域出现淋巴结病；或（3）经
848 多次适当内科治疗仍有持续性的淋巴结病。

淋巴结病的病原因子包括：弓形体病（由弓形虫引起）、兔热病（土拉菌引起）、单核细胞增多症（EB 病毒引起）[28,53,57]。头颈部以色列放线菌感染可引起头颈部放线菌病，表现为质硬的结节性颈部肿块和慢性瘘管形成。淋巴结直接受累不常见，但这种硬结会加大临床鉴别诊断的难度。儿童或婴儿 HIV 感染一般会引起全身性淋巴结病[17]。

其他一些表现为淋巴结病的疾病包括：Kawasaki 病和黏膜皮肤淋巴结综合征。Kawasaki 病是儿童发热性疾病，部分病例可表现为：口咽部黏膜突然出现的红斑、急性脉管炎和广泛性非化脓性硬质颈部淋巴结病[24]。组织细胞坏死性淋巴结炎（Kikuchi 病）可表现为可自行消退的颈部淋巴结病。该病临床上易与恶性淋巴结病相混淆，患者适合行诊断性淋巴结切除活组织检查[21]。Castleman 病（巨型淋巴结增生）有时亦可表现为实性增大的颈淋巴结[45]，不需淋巴结活检或切除。

淋巴瘤是一种更为多见的儿童恶性疾病。表现为原发性颈淋巴结病，抗生素治疗后不消退或肿块持续增大。先天或后天获得性免疫缺陷的患者，是并发恶性淋巴组织增生症的高危人群[17]。Hodgkin 病和非 Hodgkin 淋巴瘤手术治疗将于第 35 章详细讨论。必须重申，虽然绝大多数儿童颈部肿块为良性，但在采用适当治疗后肿块仍然存在时，须考虑其他可能。这些肿块在行切除活检前需考虑恶性的可能。

虽然淋巴瘤最常见的表现为颈淋巴结病，但神经母细胞瘤和甲状腺癌也是可表现为颈淋巴结肿大的儿童癌症。神经母细胞瘤患儿的颈淋巴结肿大为双侧性，其病程可分为 4 期。腹部肾上腺原发灶可能无法触及。胸、腹、盆腔做影像学检查，如发现腹部原发肿瘤，则可行颈淋巴结切除活检以诊断 4 期神经母细胞瘤（见第 28 章）。转移性甲状腺癌患儿可表现为单侧颈淋巴结肿大，不应误认为是异位甲状腺。如果彻底的颈部检查未发现甲状腺结节，且无颈部放射史或其他患病的高危因素，则可使用甲状腺超声检查以评估颈淋巴结病。

（徐建民译　陈其民校）

参考文献

1. Albright JT, Pransky SM: Nontuberculous mycobacterial infections of the head and neck. Pediatr Clin North Am 2003;50:503-514.
2. Altman RP, Margileth AM: Cervical lymphadenopathy from atypical mycobacteria: Diagnosis and surgical treatment. J Pediatr Surg 1975;10:419.
3. Barton LL, Feigin RD: Childhood cervical lymphadenitis: A reappraisal. J Pediatr 1974;84:846.
4. Bergmans AM, Groothedde JW, Schellekens JF, et al: Etiology of cat-scratch disease: Comparison of polymerase chain reaction detection of *Bartonella* (formerly *Rochalimaea*) and *Afipia felis* DNA with serology and skin tests. J Infect Dis 1995;171:916.
5. Bodenstein L, Altman RP: Cervical lymphadenitis in infants and children. Semin Pediatr Surg 1994;3:134.
6. British Thoracic Society Research Committee: Short course chemotherapy for tuberculosis of lymph nodes: A controlled trial. BMJ 1985;290:1106.
7. Brodsky L, Belles W, Broday A, et al: Needle aspiration of neck masses in infants and children. Clin Pediatr 1992; 31:71.
8. Brook I: Aerobic and anaerobic bacteriology of cervical adenitis in children. Clin Pediatr 1980;19:693.
9. Burden P: Actinomycosis. J Infect 1989;19:95.
10. Cantrell RW, Jensen JH, Reid D: Diagnosis and management of tuberculous cervical adenitis. Arch Otolaryngol 1975;101:53.
11. Carithers HA: Cat-scratch disease: An overview based on the study of 1,200 patients. Am J Dis Child 1985;139:1124.
12. Castro DJ, Hoover L, Zuckerbraun L: Cervical mycobacterial lymphadenitis: Medical vs. surgical management. Arch Otolaryngol 1985;111:816.
13. Dalton MJ, Robinson LE, Cooper J, et al: Use of *Bartonella* antigens for serologic diagnosis of cat-scratch disease at a national referral center. Arch Intern Med 1995;155:1670.
14. Dasgupta A, Ghosh RN, Poddar AK, et al: Fine needle aspiration of cervical lymphadenopathy with special reference to tuberculosis. J Indian Med Assoc 1994;92:44.
15. Davidson PM, Creati K, Wood PR, et al: Lymphocyte production of gamma-interferon as a test for non-tuberculous mycobacterial lymphadenitis in childhood. Eur J Pediatr 1993;152:31.
16. Elden LM, Grundfast KM, Vezina G: Accuracy and usefulness of radiographic assessment of cervical neck infections in children. J Otolaryngol 2001;30:82.
17. Falloon J, Eddy J, Weinter K, Pizzo PA: Human immunodeficiency virus infection in children. J Pediatr 1989; 114:1.
18. Fergusson JAE, Simpson E: Surgical treatment of atypical mycobacterial cervicofacial adenitis in children. Aust NZ J Surg 1999;69:426.
19. Filston HC: Common lumps and bumps of the head and neck in infants and children. Pediatr Ann 1989;18:180.
20. Fishaut JM, Mokrohisky ST: Cervical lymphadenitis caused by *Haemophilus influenzae* type B. Am J Dis Child 1977; 131:925.
21. Fulcher AS: Cervical lymphadenopathy due to Kikuchi disease: US and CT appearance. J Comput Assist Tomogr 1993;17:131.

22. Goral S, Anderson B, Hager C, et al: Detection of *Rochalimaea henselae* DNA by polymerase chain reaction from suppurative nodes of children with cat-scratch disease. Pediatr Infect Dis J 1994;13:994.
23. Hartzog LW: Prevalence of lymphadenopathy of the head and neck in infants and children. Clin Pediatr 1983;22:485.
24. Hicks RV, Melish ME: Kawasaki syndrome. Pediatr Clin North Am 1986;33:1151.
25. Hieber JP, Davis AT: Staphylococcal cervical adenitis in young infants. Pediatrics 1976;57:424.
26. Huebner RE, Schein MF, Cauthern GM, et al: Usefulness of skin testing with mycobacterial antigens in children with cervical lymphadenopathy. Pediatr Infect Dis J 1992;11:450.
27. Jackson LA, Perkins BA, Wenger JD: Cat-scratch disease in the United States: An analysis of three national databases. Am J Public Health 1993;83:1707.
28. Jacobs RF, Condrey YM, Yamauchi T: Tularemia in adults and children: A changing presentation. Pediatrics 1985;76:818.
29. Johnigan RH, Periera KD, Poole MD: Community-acquired methicillin-resistant *Staphylococcus aureus* in children and adolescents: Changing trends. Arch Otolaryngol Head Neck Surg 2003;129:1049.
30. Kaplan S, Rawlings J, Paddock C, et al: Cat-scratch disease in children. MMWR 2002;51:212.
31. Lai KK, Stottmeier KD, Sherman IH, McCabe WR: Mycobacterial cervical lymphadenopathy: Relation of etiologic agents to age. JAMA 1984;251:1286.
32. Larsson LO, Bentzon MW, BergKelly K, Mellander L: Palpable lymph nodes of the neck in Swedish school children. Acta Paediatr 1994;83:1091.
33. Lau SK, Wei WI, Kwan S, Yew WW: Combined use of fine-needle aspiration cytologic examination and tuberculin skin test in the diagnosis of cervical tuberculous lymphadenitis. Arch Otolaryngol Head Neck Surg 1991;117:87.
34. Leung AK, Robson WL: Childhood cervical lymphadenopathy. J Pediatr Health Care 2004;18:3.
35. Lincoln EM, Gilbert LA: Disease in children due to mycobacteria other than *Mycobacterium tuberculosis*. Am Rev Respir Dis 1972;105:683.
36. Mair IWS, Elverland HH: Cervical mycobacterial infection. J Laryngol 1975;89:933.
37. Margileth AW: Management of nontuberculous (atypical) mycobacterial infections in children and adolescents. Pediatr Infect Dis 1985;4:119.
38. Margileth AM: Cat-scratch disease: No longer a diagnostic dilemma. Semin Vet Med Surg 1991;6:199.
39. Margileth AM: Antibiotic therapy for cat-scratch disease: Clinical study of therapeutic outcome in 268 patients and a review of the literature. Pediatr Infect Dis J 1992;11:474.
40. Margolis B, Kuzu I, Herrmann M, et al: Rapid polymerase chain reaction–based confirmation of cat-scratch disease and *Bartonella henselae* infection. Arch Pathol Lab Med 2003;127:706-710.
41. Martinez-Aguilar G, Hammerman WA, Mason EO Jr, Kaplan SL: Clindamycin treatment of invasive infections caused by community-acquired methicillin-resistant and methicillin-susceptible *Staphylococcus aureus* in children. Pediatr Infect Dis J 2003;22:593.
42. Narita M, Shibata M, Togashi T, Kobayashi H: Polymerase chain reaction for detection of *Mycobacterium tuberculosis*. Acta Pediatr 1992;81:141.
43. Ord RJ, Matz GJ: Tuberculosis cervical lymphadenitis. Arch Otolaryngol 1974;99:327.
44. Panagiotis S, Maltezou HC, Hantzakos A, et al: Mycobacterial cervical lymphadenitis in children: Clinical and laboratory factors of importance for differential diagnosis. Scand J Infect Dis 2001;33:362.
45. Penfold CN, Cottrell BJ, Talbot R: Neonatal giant lymph node hyperplasia (Castleman's disease) presenting in the head and neck. Br J Oral Maxillofac Surg 1991;29:110.
46. Piersimoni C, Felici L, Giorgi P, et al: Mixed mycobacterial infection of the cervical lymph nodes. Pediatr Infect Dis 1991;10:544.
47. Rathmore MH: Group B streptococcal cellulitis and adenitis concurrent with meningitis. Clin Pediatr 1989;28:411.
48. Schuit KE, Powell DA: Mycobacterial lymphadenitis in childhood. Am J Dis Child 1978;132:675.
49. Shah JP, Mdina JE, Shaha AR, et al: Cervical lymph node metastasis. Curr Prob Surg 1993;30:273.
50. Sigalet D, Lees G, Fanning A: Atypical tuberculosis in the pediatric patient: Implications for the pediatric surgeon. J Pediatr Surg 1992;27:1381.
51. Siu KF, Ng A, Wong J: Tuberculous lymphadenopathy: A review of results of surgical treatment. Aust NZ J Surg 1983;53:253.
52. Speck WT: Tuberculosis. In Behrman RE, et al (eds): Nelson Textbook of Pediatrics, 14th ed. Philadelphia, WB Saunders, 1992.
53. Sumaya CV, Ench Y: Epstein-Barr virus infectious mononucleosis in children: I. Clinical and laboratory findings. Pediatrics 1985;75:1003.
54. Taha AM, Davidson PT, Bailey WC: Surgical treatment of atypical mycobacterial lymphadenitis in children. Pediatr Infect Dis 1985;4:664.
55. Talmi YP, Cohen AH, Finkelstein Y, et al: *Mycobacterium tuberculosis* cervical adenitis: Diagnosis and management. Clin Pediatr 1989;28:408.
56. Telander RL, Filston HC: Review of head and neck lesions in infancy and childhood. Surg Clin North Am 1992; 72:1429.
57. Thomaidis T, Anastassea-Vlachou K, Mandalenaki-Lambrou C, et al: Chronic lymphoglandular enlargement and toxoplasmosis in children. Arch Dis Child 1977;52:403.
58. Tomblin JL, Roberts FJ: Tuberculous cervical lymphadenitis. Can Med Assoc J 1979;121:324.
59. Wear DJ, Margileth AM, Hadfield TL, et al: Cat-scratch disease: A bacterial infection. Science 1983;221:1403.
60. World Health Organization: Global Tuberculosis Program: Global Tuberculosis Control. WHO report 1997, publication WHO/TB/225. Geneva, World Health Organization, 1997.

第 55 章

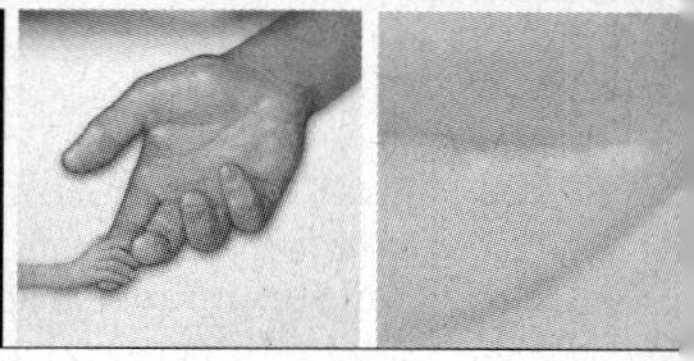

甲状腺和甲状旁腺的外科疾病

Michael A. Skinner

850 在儿童这个年龄阶段，甲状腺和甲状旁腺的疾病并不常见。在美国的一次基于人口普查的研究表明，学龄儿童甲状腺疾病的发病率是 36.7‰[36]。弥漫性甲状腺肥大（甲状腺肿）是最常见的诊断，约占了该类疾病的一半。甲状腺炎是第二位最多见的疾病。甲状腺结节和甲状腺激素水平异常比较少见，甲状腺恶性肿瘤就更为罕见了。在这些人群的临床观察中，3 年里在 5000 个儿童中只发生了 2 例甲状腺乳头样癌。

对于患有甲状腺良性或者恶性肿块的患者，或者在儿童期间就表现出生理功能上异常（如甲状腺素分泌增加）的患儿，必须进行外科评估或相应的治疗。

胚胎学

在胚胎发育过程中，甲状腺是最先成熟的内分泌器官，大约在妊娠 24 天，在胚胎消化道的原始咽底部形成一个外翻袋状甲状腺始基。随着胚胎的增长，发育中的甲状腺逐渐从舌的根部下降到颈部，从舌骨和喉软骨的腹侧穿过，其经过路径形成一个管道与舌部相连，称为甲状舌管。该管道在舌根部的开口端称为舌盲孔。典型的情况下，甲状舌管逐渐从一个中空的管道变成一个实性的憩室；在舌咽底部的原始开口最后残留一个小凹陷样的盲端。甲状腺一般在妊娠第 7 周下降到最终目的地。来源于甲状舌管的残留组织可以出现在舌根或甲状腺发育下降路径中的任何部位。如果腺体不能下降，则导致甲状腺异位。对外科来说这很重要。下降不完全时甲状腺会出现在颈部较高的位置或舌骨周围。

妊娠第 10 周时，组织学上可以看到原始的甲状腺细胞开始形成不连续的束状物，这些束状物进一步分化成小细胞群体。胶质开始形成，在第 11 周胚胎内会出现甲状腺素。在甲状腺发育的早期，第四咽裂（囊）的腹侧会发育成后鳃体，这些结构含有神经嵴细胞，它们会融合进入甲状腺胚胎然后转化成滤泡旁细胞或者 C 细胞。

甲状旁腺在妊娠第 5 周时从第 3、4 咽裂（囊）分离出来，第 6 周时，甲状旁腺连同第三咽（裂）囊和胸腺始基一起向尾端迁移，最后停留在甲状腺背侧表面，位于颈部低位。第 4 咽裂（囊）来源的甲状旁腺也下降到颈部，最后停留的位置比来源于第三咽裂（囊）的甲状旁腺要高。其中主要细胞功能在胎儿发育期就起到调节钙代谢的作用。

生理学

甲状腺素产生于滤泡细胞和甲状腺球蛋白或胶质的交界面，甲状腺素合成第一步就是碘和酪氨酸分子结合，如果结合了一个碘分子称为一碘酪氨酸，如果结合了两个碘分子称为二碘酪氨酸。结合后酪氨酸分子再相互结合形成甲状腺素三碘甲腺原氨酸（T_3）和甲状腺氨酸（T_4）。一碘酪氨酸和二碘酪氨酸结合形成 T_3，二碘酪氨酸和二碘酪氨酸结合形成 T_4。

甲状腺主要分泌 T_4；在血液循环中 80% 的 T_3 是 T_4 的代谢产物——是在肝脏、肾脏以及其他周围组织经过部分脱碘而形成。在循环中甲状腺素和血清中的 851
蛋白结合可增加它们的可溶性。最丰富的甲状腺素载体是甲状腺素结合球蛋白（TBG），其他一些载体包括前白蛋白以及白蛋白。因为甲状腺素和蛋白结合状态时无生理学活性，所以在评价甲状腺分泌功能异常时要考虑血清蛋白水平的影响。然而血清中的 T_4 浓度约比 T_3 高 50 倍，其余部分与甲状腺素受体紧密连接在一起，产生甲状腺素的主要生理功能。

T_3 和 T_4 的产生主要受促甲状腺激素刺激激素（TSH）调控。这种蛋白由腺垂体分泌，受下丘脑分泌的促甲状腺激素释放激素（TRH）调控。在 TSH 影响下腺细胞活跃起来，伸出伪足进入胶质并包围形成甲状球蛋白的胶质小滴并吞饮入腺细胞内，随即与溶酶体融合而形成吞噬体。在溶酶体蛋白水解酶的作用下，甲状腺球蛋白被水解、蛋白解离，甲状腺素游离并释放入循环。

非肿瘤性甲状腺疾病

对儿童甲状腺疾病进行评估前首先要对颈部进行体检，评估甲状腺的大小和质地。弥漫性甲状腺肿大最有可能的诊断是单纯性胶样甲状腺肿；如果同时合并甲状腺功能亢进，则还应考虑 Graves 病。如果触摸甲状腺有颗粒感和结节感，则要考虑慢性淋巴细胞性甲状腺炎（桥本甲状腺炎）；如果腺体触之有韧性，则腺体可能处于炎症浸润过程；如腺体触摸非常坚硬，则肿瘤可能性大；如果腺体有触痛，可能处于急性炎症状态；最后要注意颈部肿大的淋巴结，甲状腺癌在局部尚未触及肿块时就可能出现局部转移。

在评价甲状腺功能改变时，实验室检查是最基本和必要的。在甲状腺功能低下时，TSH 水平上升，血清游离 T_4 水平是最精确测量激素生物学活性的指标，因为它一般不受血清蛋白水平的影响。与之相反，测量血中总 T_3、T_4 时就必须考虑到血中 TBG 的水平，这样才能估计出甲状腺的生物学功能，因为只有不与蛋白结合的才会发挥生物学功能。血清中 TBG 在很多情况下会发生变化而影响总的甲状腺素的水平。比如说，在新生儿期 TBG 的水平是上升的，而在存在外源性糖皮质激素时，存在雄激素和合成的皮质激素时，它的水平会出现下降。其他一些药物也可以影响甲状腺素的代谢，如苯妥英钠和苯巴比妥，它们一方面可以增加肝脏对 T_4 的降解，另一方面可以降低激素与 TGB 的结合力。另外还有一些罕见的情况也可以引起 TGB 水平先天性改变。

通过几种影像学检查可以获得甲状腺影像学资料。超声波成像已越来越多地应用于甲状腺检查，特别是对甲状腺囊肿和多发性结节的检查。这种方法对于非手术治疗的甲状腺结节的评价非常有效。放射性核素闪烁扫描是另一种常用的检查手段。最常用的三种核素是碘-123（^{123}I）、碘-131（^{131}I）和锝-99m（^{99m}Tc），放射性核素检查对于了解异位甲状腺和甲状腺癌的转移病灶是最有效的手段。同时有些放射科专家认为，放射性高锝酸（^{99m}Tc）可以获得甲状腺结节和肿瘤的高质量图像。

甲状腺功能减退

甲状腺功能低下之类的疾病很少在外科治疗，一般都是下丘脑-垂体-甲状腺轴出现问题所造成。对甲状腺激素无反应所导致的甲状腺功能减低很罕见，例如甲状腺素受体基因出现缺陷时，通常血清甲状腺素水平上升。

通过对新生儿筛查可以发现先天性甲减患儿，这些孩子大约 90%是由于甲状腺发育异常造成的，其中大约有 1/3 的患儿放射性核素检查未见甲状腺组织显影，其余患儿往往在舌底部可以发现发育不全的异位甲状腺组织。完全性甲状腺发育不良的患儿出生时往往无任何症状，因为患儿体内还有从胎盘传送过来的来源于母体的甲状腺素。在一些患儿中，异位甲状腺可以多年提供足够的甲状腺素，也可能因出现异位甲状腺减小引起激素供给不足而导致甲减。以上这些情况最可能是由于舌下肿块和颈部正中肿块引起临床上的注意，外科医生遇到此类肿块时要小心有无异位甲状腺。在切除舌下和颈部正中的肿块之前要进行甲状腺核素扫描，以避免有功能的甲状腺被意外切除。

甲状腺肿和甲状腺炎

在因甲状腺异常进行检查的儿童中，3%是甲状腺肿[36]。甲状腺肿分为两种，分别是弥漫性甲状腺肿和结节性甲状腺肿。通常甲状腺素分泌是正常的或是甲状腺毒症。常见的弥漫性甲状腺肿的诊断见表 55-1。从生理上来说，弥漫性甲状腺肿可以是由自身免疫性疾病引起的，也可以是非自身免疫性炎症造成，还有可能是激素分泌障碍造成的腺体增大。大多数甲状腺肿儿童其甲状腺功能正常，很少需要进行甲状腺切除。

表 55-1 儿童甲状腺肿的诊断

自身免疫介导

慢性淋巴细胞性（桥本）甲状腺炎
Graves 病
单纯性胶样甲状腺肿

代偿性的

缺碘型甲状腺肿
药物性甲状腺肿
致甲状腺肿物质
激素或者受体缺陷

炎症导致肿大

急性甲状腺炎
亚急性甲状腺炎

一项对克罗埃西亚地区 5000 多位学龄期儿童的人口调查表明，有 2.78%的儿童出现甲状腺增大[19]，在这个人群中引起甲状腺肿大的病因见表 55-2。在其他有足够碘摄入的人群中，最常见的甲状腺肿大是单纯性胶样甲状腺肿，通常称为青春期甲状腺肿或者
852 非毒性甲状腺肿。诊断基于影像学检查（放射性核素检查或超声波检查）存在甲状腺肿大，同时 TSH 和甲状腺素在正常范围。胶样甲状腺肿的自然病程目前尚不清楚，但有一项研究表明，青春期甲状腺肿的患儿 20 年后将近 60%甲状腺恢复正常大小[36]。患儿服用甲状腺素甲状腺肿自行缓解的比率和未服用的无明显差异，所以单纯性胶样甲状腺肿无需进行任何治疗。在一些少见的患者，因为肿块较大、怀疑有肿瘤或因为美容方面的原因才进行手术。

表 55-2 5462 例克罗埃西亚学龄儿童甲状腺肿的流行病学调查

诊断	频率(%)
单纯性甲状腺肿	2.3
慢性淋巴细胞性甲状腺肿	0.35
Graves 病	0.07
良性腺瘤	0.04
囊肿	0.02
总计	2.78

Adapted from Jaksic J, Dumic M, Filipovic B, et al: Thyroid disease in a school population with thyromegaly. Arch Dis Child 1994;70:103-103.

慢性淋巴细胞性甲状腺炎，就是我们所称的桥本甲状腺炎，是另一种引起儿童甲状腺弥漫性肿大的常见原因，好发于女孩，是一种甲状腺的自身免疫性疾病，实际上通常伴随着其他自身免疫性疾病，如青春期风湿性关节炎、Addison 病以及 I 型糖尿病。患者通常会缓慢地由甲状腺功能正常转变成甲状腺功能低下。大约有 10%的患者表现是甲状腺功能亢进，这种情况被称为桥本中毒。慢性淋巴细胞性甲状腺炎患者的特点是循环中有高滴度的甲状腺球蛋白抗体和甲状腺微粒体抗体这两种自身抗体，这被认为是导致组织学上腺体内 B 淋巴细胞浸润的原因。

患有慢性淋巴细胞性甲状腺炎的儿童去医院就诊的原因一般是甲状腺肿大，这时候腺体通常有结节感或颗粒感，有时候有轻度的触痛。当患儿血中有高滴度的抗甲状腺抗体，同时有相应的临床症状和实验室检查结果时，就可以明确诊断了。血清中甲状腺素水平对于诊断帮助不大，但 70%的患者有 TSH 水平上升。超声波检查提示甲状腺弥漫性的低回声，同位素扫描显示斑片状的核素摄取增高。在很少一些患者中没有发现自身抗体时，需要进行细针穿刺活检（FNA）以明确诊断。慢性淋巴细胞性甲状腺炎患儿治疗一般采取观察策略，大约 1/3 的青少年患者将来可以自然缓解，最后甲状腺恢复正常大小，抗甲状腺抗体消失。甲状腺功能正常的患儿服用甲状腺激素对减小甲状腺肿大没有作用，这时候没有使用甲状腺素的指征[39]。甲状腺功能必须每 6 个月检测一次，一旦出现甲状腺功能减退，就需要使用外源性的激素。

亚急性甲状腺炎（de Quervain）在儿童非常少见，是一种由病毒感染引起的疾病。体检发现包括甲状腺肿大，伴有疼痛和触痛。通常有轻度的甲状腺功能亢进，一般是由于甲状腺滤泡破坏导致的甲状腺素释放入血。甲状腺滤泡细胞功能障碍可导致甲状腺对放射性碘的吸收减少；这些表现可以很容易与 Grave 病区分开来。组织学上可以见到肉芽肿细胞和上皮样细胞。治疗上主要是对症治疗，使用非甾体抗炎药物和皮质类固醇药物。病程一般为 2～9 个月，可以获得痊愈。

急性化脓性甲状腺炎是由于腺体细菌感染造成

的，患者一般有败血症的症状和甲状腺急性炎症表现。患者的甲状腺功能一般是正常的，侵犯腺体的微生物一般是葡萄球菌或需氧菌和厌氧菌混合感染，有可能是先天性咽窦道导致的感染。治疗包括使用抗生素，如果出现脓肿，应该切开引流，甲状腺可以获得完全的恢复。

甲状腺功能亢进

儿童期甲状腺功能亢进基本上都是由 Graves 病引起，Graves 病亦称为弥漫性毒性甲状腺肿，其他可能导致甲状腺功能亢进的原因见表 55-3。在这些患者中，甲亢的表现可能延迟至出生后 2～3 周。女
853 孩 Graves 病发病率是男孩的 5 倍，而且发病率随着年龄的增加逐渐增加，在青春期达到高峰。在病情隐匿的情况下常常要发展好几个月，开始的症状包括神经过敏、情绪不稳定以及在学校的表现下降。然后出现体重减轻、容易出汗、心悸、怕热以及不适等症状。真正的突眼征在儿童不是很常见，但可以见到明显的凝视。体检中超过 95%的患儿可以发现甲状腺肿大，光滑、质地较硬，没有触痛；有可能听到局部杂音。实验室检查通常可见游离 T_4 水平上升，TSH 水平下降；在 10%～20%的患者仅可见 T_3 水平上升，这就是我们所称的 T_3 中毒。如果发现血中出现 TSH 刺激性免疫球蛋白，则可以进一步支持 Graves 病的诊断。

Graves 病是一种自身免疫性疾病，主要是由于体内产生了 TSH 受体的抗体所致。后者能够刺激甲状腺滤泡对碘的摄取，增加甲状腺素的生成和释放。有人提出，在一些革兰阳性和革兰阴性细菌中存在一些 TSH 结合蛋白，因此在感染了这些细菌时有可能会产生与 TSH 受体有交叉反应的抗体[47]。有些流行病报告显示，Graves 病有群集发作特点，进一步证实感染是其病因[33]。

目前治疗 Graves 病通常使用抗甲状腺药物或者通过放射性 ^{131}I 或者外科手术切除甲状腺[17]。大多数儿科内分泌医生把药物治疗作为最初的治疗，不过现在越来越多的医生把放射性内切除作为一线治疗手段[26]。最常用的治疗药物是甲巯咪唑或丙硫氧嘧啶（PTU），它们可以通过抑制滤泡细胞对碘的有机化及碘化酪氨酸偶联减少而减少甲状腺素的产生。甲巯咪唑半衰期较长、作用强，因而较常使用。初始剂量一般为每天 30mg，如果患者年龄较小，则剂量要相对降低。血清 TSH 水平要仔细监测，水平上升提示抑制过度，可导致腺体进一步增大。当患者的甲状腺功能正常，血清中 T_3、T_4 水平在正常范围时，甲巯咪唑可减少到 10mg 并保持在这个水平以确保患者的甲状腺素在正常水平。

甲巯咪唑的最严重的副作用是特发性粒细胞减少，可以发生在药物治疗的任何时候，甚至在第二疗程。如在治疗中患者出现咽痛、体温上升，则要考虑该病，需进行血中性粒细胞计数。典型情况下停药 2～3 周，粒细胞计数就会上升。但有报道表明，在罕见的情况下会出现致命的机会性感染，因而主张在恢复期使用抗生素。其他副作用包括恶心、轻微皮肤反应、风疹、关节疼痛、关节炎以及发热。

在药物治疗的疗程上存在争议。通常药物治疗要持续 3～4 年，Graves 病药物治疗 2 年后停药大约有 20%可以缓解，以后每 2 年的缓解率大约是 25%。大多数儿童 Graves 病患者停药 6 月内可以获得缓解。治疗中或者治疗后血中可持续检测到 TSH 受体抗体者缓解率会下降。当 Graves 病患儿对药物治疗无反应或者出现严重副作用时，则应施行有限度的甲状腺切除。目前流行的切除方法是外科切除或是通过放射性 ^{131}I 切除部分甲状腺。这两种治疗模式都有一定的并发症，放射性 I^{131} 治疗有效，但缓解率低，大约有 50%～80%的患者在该治疗后会出现长期甲状腺功能减退。有些患者使用大剂量的放射性碘可以造成甲状腺组织全部破坏，导致永久性甲状腺功能减退。最近的研究显示，没有证据表明年轻患者使用放射性 ^{131}I 治疗有致畸和致癌作用[9,22]。

表 55-3 儿童甲状腺功能亢进的病因
Graves 病（毒性甲状腺肿）
毒性甲状腺结节
亚急性甲状腺炎
慢性淋巴细胞性甲状腺炎
新生儿甲状腺炎
有甲状腺素分泌激素分泌的垂体肿瘤
McCune-Albright 综合征
促甲状腺激素受体变异

对于药物治疗无效的 Graves 病儿童患者，可以使用外科手术治疗，于对不愿使用 ^{131}I 治疗的患者以及对药物治疗无效且甲状腺体积大以致产生压迫症状的患者，选择甲状腺次全切除术是合适的。在进行外科手术前必须使用甲巯咪唑。此外还可以使用 β-肾上腺素能阻滞药物如心得安（普萘洛尔）来减轻甲亢的肾上腺素能症状；另外还要服用含碘的 Lugol 液补充碘剂，在外科手术前 4～7 天开始，每天 5～10 滴，以减少腺体的血供。对成人的大规模研究表明，Graves 病行甲状腺次全切除的患者随访 10 年时，甲亢的复发率大约有 6%～10%。术后 25 年大约有 30%会出现甲亢复发。同时手术患者确实存在永久性甲减的风险，约有 5%患者在外科手术后一年出现
854 甲减，而到术后 25 年，大约有 50%的患者出现甲减。这些发现表明，术后仔细检测这些患者的甲状腺功能状态非常重要。

甲状腺肿瘤

甲状腺结节

在儿童，甲状腺结节少见，但常常是甲状腺癌的表现。最近的儿科研究表明，甲状腺恶性结节大约占 20%或者更低[2,8,16,53]，这比 10 年前癌症的发病率更低，反映了近年来颈部暴露在放射线下的儿童数量下降。因为该病可能处在可以治愈的阶段，所以正确的评价和处理非常重要。表 55-4 是近期对儿童甲状腺结节病理学研究结果的总结。

表 55-5 是甲状腺实性单发结节的不同诊断，在最大规模的儿科病例研究中，有甲状腺结节的女孩数量超过男孩的 2 倍[53]。颈部包块是引起大多数患者注意的主要临床症状。这时要进行仔细的甲状腺检查，当怀疑颈部有进展期癌症时，特别要注意局部有无肿大的淋巴结。当患者因存在自主分泌功能的甲状腺结节而造成明确的甲状腺素毒性症状时，应该进行血清 TSH 检查。影像学检查对于鉴别肿块的良恶性是不可靠的。举例来说，恶性肿块在甲状腺扫描上既可以是无功能的也可以是有功能的；超声波同样也不能区分恶性肿瘤，因为实性的和囊性的都可能是恶性的；所以在用影像学手段评价儿童甲状腺结节时要非常小心。不建议使用外源性甲状腺素对甲状腺结节进行诊断性治疗以诱导肿块的消退。

表 55-4 儿童甲状腺结节外科切除术后诊断

	Yip 等人 1994	Lafferty 和 Batch，1997
患者数量	122	52
恶性比率（%）	16*（13）	17（33）
组织学分型		
乳头状癌	12	7
滤泡状癌	3	7
混合型癌	0	0
未分化癌	0	0
髓样癌	0	0
良性病变比率（%）	106（87）	35（67）
诊断		
甲状腺炎	17	1
甲状腺舌骨囊肿	0	2
滤泡状腺瘤	26	16
胶样结节	57	2
气管囊肿	0	0
其他	6	14

* 在这个病例研究中有一个患者为甲状腺淋巴瘤。

Data from Yip FWK, Reeve TS, Poole AG, Delbridge L: Thyroid nodules in childhood and adolescence. Aust NZ J Surg 1994;64:676-678; and Lafferty AR, Batch JA: Thyroid nodules in childhood and adolescence—thirty years of experience. J Pediatr Endocrinol Metab 1997;10:479-486.

表 55-5 儿童实性甲状腺肿瘤的鉴别诊断

腺瘤
癌症
甲状腺囊肿
异位甲状腺
水囊状淋巴管瘤
甲状舌管残留
生殖细胞瘤

在成人中普遍使用的细针穿刺（FNA）细胞学检查这项技术在儿童中是否有效尚没有明确。儿童比成

人更难诊断和评价，主要因为：一方面结节一般比较小，另一方面经常要使用镇静剂以保证安全和穿刺抽吸的精确。任何诊断性检查的有效性部分取决于检查之前阳性结果的可能性。与成人相比，婴幼儿甲状腺结节的恶性可能性较高，而其细胞学检查结果阴性的比率比成人稍有增加，这种错误的阴性细胞学结果往往会延误诊断和治疗。然而由于儿童各种甲状腺肿瘤的预后都是不错的，应该承认，这种诊断和延迟对生存率无明显影响。

在青少年患者中，FNA 诊断安全。青少年期甲状腺疾病的发病形式与成年人类似，这些患者可以安全地进行 FNA 检查。在一项大型病例研究中，13～18 岁甲状腺结节患儿中，恶性的比率只有 11%[53]。在另一项研究中，57 例患儿通过 FNA 对甲状腺结节进行评价，恶性的比率为 18%[34]，只有一个乳头状癌开始被误诊为良性病变，后来在临床观察中被认定为癌。还有一组 57 例患儿用 FNA 进行甲状腺结节的评价，癌症的发病率类似，初诊误诊为阴性者为 1 例，在接下来的 6 个月其肿块增大，切除活检提示为
855 Hürthle 细胞肿瘤[20]。因此，对多数青少年患者的研究证明，FNA 在这个年龄段是安全有效的。

FNA 细胞学结果可明确是癌或良性病变，或癌肿有待于确诊。如果判断是良性的，那么应该通过一系列的体检和超声波检查来随访；当结节为恶性的或者不能明确诊断以及为良性病变但体积逐渐增时，应该行外科手术。有些内分泌科医生通过外源性的甲状腺素来抑制良性结节，但这种治疗目前没有显示能够改变这些良性结节的自然病程。如果囊性病变在穿刺抽吸后消失，那么外科手术也许应该延迟，如果明确复发则需切除。对囊液可进行细胞学分析，但这项检查的癌检出率较低[25]。

青春期前的儿童细胞学检查难度有所增加，而且良性病变的发病类型与成人不同；同时这些疾病的自然病程是不明确的，非手术治疗的安全性不得而知。因此建议对于所有 13 岁以下儿童的甲状腺结节，都给予切除。有些外科医生通过术前超声波检查以及甲状腺放射显像来决定手术[16,27]。不能过分相信细胞学检查结果，如果对细胞学检查有任何的疑问，无论患者的年龄如何，对所有的结节均应进行切除活检。

甲状腺癌

儿童甲状腺癌是比较少见的，基于威尔士和洛杉矶人口调查的研究表明，每年甲状腺癌的发病率在低于 20 岁的人群中为 1～2 例 / 百万[14,32]，在所有儿童恶性肿瘤中占 3%，发病高峰年龄在 10～18 岁，女孩和男孩比率 2∶1。大约有 10%的甲状腺癌出现在儿童，最近 20 年儿童甲状腺肿瘤的发病率明显下降，这主要由于放疗已经较少用于治疗良性病变。近期重新强调放射线是导致甲状腺癌发病的重要病因，因为在 1986 年切尔诺贝利核电站灾难之后，甲状腺癌发病率明显增加。放射线暴露后甲状腺癌的潜伏期是 4～6 年。在切尔诺贝利事故后，白俄罗斯甲状腺癌发病率增加了 62 倍。

甲状腺癌同样也发生在因其他恶性肿瘤接受治疗的患儿中。一项研究表明，在儿童期因肿瘤接受治疗后再次患恶性肿瘤的患者中，甲状腺癌占 9% [45]。最常见的初发肿瘤为 Hodgkin 淋巴瘤，接受过颈部放疗的患儿，即使单独使用烷化剂治疗，其对甲状腺癌的易感性也有所增加。放疗后出现甲状腺疾病的中位时间是 12 年[1]。所以强调对成功治愈肿瘤的儿童要小心监测他们患第二种肿瘤的可能性，这是非常重要的。

近期的研究表明，一些基因改变与甲状腺肿瘤的进程有关。*RET* 癌基因编码酪氨酸激酶受体分子，位于第 10 对染色体，乳头状癌常常出现染色体重排，在细胞内该基因和一些固定表达的基因并列，形成的融合基因，称为 *RET/PTC* 基因，产生的融合蛋白表达酪氨酸激酶活性增高，这种基因重排在放射诱导的甲状腺癌较常出现。在白俄罗斯切尔诺贝利事故后，该地儿童甲状腺癌超过 62%出现 *RET* 融合基因表达[35]。其他的一些研究表明，特定的 *RET* 融合基因与肿瘤组织亚型有关[41]。

在甲状腺髓样癌（MTC）发生发展中，*RET* 基因也起很重要的作用，各种不同的 *RET* 变异与多发性内分泌腺瘤病 2 型（MEN 2A，MEN 2B）和家族性甲状腺髓样癌（FMTC）有关。MTC 通常是这些患者的首发肿瘤。此外，有多达 40%的散发性非家族性 MTC 伴有 *RET* 变异[10]。易感组织 *RET* 变异感染细胞间的信号传导系统可产生神经嵴细胞来源的组织细胞增殖和分化异常，导致 MEN2 综合征。

甲状腺癌的典型症状是甲状腺包块、颈部淋巴结

肿大或者两者都有。在一项大规模的儿童甲状腺癌的临床研究中，近期诊断为甲状腺癌的患者中有少部分在初次诊断时出现颈部淋巴结肿大[13]。表 55-6 列出了近期几项大规模儿童患者临床病例研究中不同病理类型患者的临床表现。病理结果可以通过术前 FNA 细胞学检查和术中冰冻切片获得。近期的多项研究表明，术中冰冻切片在评价滤泡状病变时准确性稍低。如表 55-6 所示，乳头状癌最多见。在手术前大多数患儿需要进行甲状腺扫描以明确肿块中是否存在有功能的甲状腺组织。有些研究者还强调，进行术前的超声波检查、鉴别肿块是否是囊性的，对手术有一定的指导作用[27]。由于甲状腺癌常有肺部转移，所以术前应行胸片或胸部 CT 检查。

儿童甲状腺癌的外科治疗方式尚存争议，因为目前还没有对大范围根治术和非扩大根治术进行前瞻性比较研究。正如表 55-6 所示，对有些患者施行甲状腺部分切除后，该病的长期预后通常很好。外科医生

表 55-6 不同大型病例研究的儿童甲状腺癌分型的临床表现

患者总数	329
平均年龄	15.2
女性%	76
组织学	
乳头状癌	297
滤泡状癌	32
髓样癌	0
其他	0
转移的百分比（%）	74
外科处理方式	
甲状腺全切	178
甲状腺次全切除	55
腺叶切除或其他	96
淋巴结清扫	255
接受放射性治疗的%	43
中位随访时间（年）	11.3
癌症死亡率（%）	0.7

Data from Newman KD, Black T, Heller G, et al: Differentiated thyroid cancer: Determinants of disease progression in patients <21 years of age at diagnosis: A report of the Surgical Discipline Committee of the Children's Cancer Group.Ann Surg 1998;227:533-541.

856 在局部有淋巴结侵犯的时候提倡采取甲状腺全切加上淋巴结清扫，这是获得肿瘤局部控制最成功的方式[5,13,28,42]。而且切除整个甲状腺可使辅助放射性碘内照射治疗更为有效，因为几乎没有功能的甲状腺组织和剩余的肿瘤组织竞争摄取放射性碘。最后当甲状腺全切之后，可以通过检测血中甲状腺球蛋白来监视肿瘤有无复发。

外科医生不认为大范围甲状腺切除有益，因为儿童分化型甲状腺癌恶性程度不高，且其治愈率与甲状腺切除的程度无关[24,54]，而且甲状腺全切可使相应外科并发症的发生率升高。例如喉返神经损伤的比率是0～24%[18]，永久性低钙血症的比率是 6%～27%[7,13,24]，这些并发症的发生率在近期的病例研究报道中有所下降[13]。

一项对 329 例分化型甲状腺癌患儿进行的回顾性研究对疾病早期复发的一些指标进行了多变量分析，预示疾病复发的最显著特点是：确诊时年龄小和手术后颈部有肿瘤残留[28]。患儿确诊时年龄大于 15 岁其复发率比低龄的患者低。经过中位时间为 11.3 年的随访，治疗后的复发率为 32%，只有 2 例死亡与肿瘤有关。分化型甲状腺癌初次诊断后 10 年的无进展性生存率为 67%，20 年无进展性生存率是 60%。不影响无进展性生存率的因素包括甲状腺切除范围、原发肿瘤的大小、肿瘤的甲状腺外浸润、局部淋巴结侵犯、远处转移、在最初治疗时应用 ^{131}I 放疗以及放射线暴露病史[28]。总而言之，在儿童分化型甲状腺癌的临床预后决定因素中，肿瘤本身的因素比治疗因素更为重要。

因此，由于缺乏对比性的前瞻研究，所以很难确定外科治疗手段在儿童甲状腺癌治疗上的可取之处，而公认的方法是应该采用大范围切除术。外科医生和儿科内分泌科医生越来越推荐采用甲状腺全切或甲状腺次全切除术加上后续使用 ^{131}I 将残余的肿瘤放射性切除[17]，同时长期服用甲状腺素作为抑制性治疗。如果局部有淋巴结肿大提示有局部转移可能时，在切除病变的甲状腺的同时，还应进行改良的颈部淋巴结清扫。对于局部为进展期的患者，尽可能地切除所有的甲状腺是非常重要的，这样当患者出现复发时，使用放射性碘扫描和再次治疗才成为可能。当肿瘤侵犯喉返神经时，无需进行广泛切除去牺牲神经，因为残留在神经上的肿瘤细胞可以通过放射性碘得到充分的治疗。

随着手术范围的扩大，出现外科手术并发症的风

险亦增加[24]，且年龄越小，发生并发症的风险越大。最常见的严重并发症为喉返神经损伤和永久性的甲状旁腺功能低下。为了减少术后甲状旁腺功能低下的可能性，术中结扎甲状腺下动脉时要靠近甲状腺被膜[46]。保留甲状旁腺功能的方法就是在将术中确认的 1～2 个甲状旁腺移植到胸锁乳突肌或运动较少的前臂内[44,52]。如果在切除肿瘤的过程中甲状旁腺的血供被破坏，则应立即将其移植到邻近的胸锁乳突肌内。为了在术中确认和保护喉返神经，术中可应用神经刺激仪，已经有一篇文献报道了该技术在儿童中的应用[4]。

儿童中甲状腺癌初次诊断时即存在肺部转移的比率大约是 6%[50,54]，这些患者几乎都有明显的颈部淋巴结转移，术后必须行放射性碘治疗。在这些患者中只有 60%能通过普通胸片发现病变[50]，所以需要进行放射性碘扫描来明确转移病灶的位置。但是需注意的是，当颈部残留有较多的甲状腺组织时，放射性碘扫描可能出现假阴性，因此对儿童中分化性甲状腺癌需施行扩大的甲状腺切除术[17]。

经过 20 年随访，甲状腺癌的复发率大约是 30%[24,28,42]，这更强调了早期积极治疗的重要性，以及需要相对频繁和长期的随访。甲状腺切除术后大约 6 周进行放射性 ^{131}I 全身扫描和肺部 CT 检查[17]，以检
857 测颈部和肺部残留的肿瘤。多数患者使用治疗剂量的放射性碘可以清除残留的肿瘤组织[13]，必要时对于残留的转移性肿瘤可行重复治疗。为了检测术后有无复发，每年都要进行诊断性放射性碘扫描。最近研究表明甲状腺球蛋白是检测甲状腺肿瘤残留和转移很有效的标志物，每年都要测定血清中甲状腺球蛋白水平，如果出现上升，则要怀疑有肿瘤复发。该项检查在患者有残留的甲状腺组织和使用甲状腺素补充治疗的时候准确性明显下降，通过产生短暂的医源性甲状腺功能低下或使用重组人 TSH 使血中 TSH 升高可以增加甲状腺球蛋白，作为检测肿瘤残留和复发的敏感性指标[17]。

儿童甲状腺肿瘤中大约有 5%是从甲状腺滤泡旁 C 细胞来源的髓样癌，MTC 可以是散发的，也可以表现为家族性肿瘤出现在患有多发性内分泌腺瘤病 2 型（MEN 2A，MEN 2B）和家族性甲状腺髓样癌（FMTC）的患者中。在 MEN 患者中，MTC 通常是第一个发生的肿瘤，在 MEN 2B 患者中，这种肿瘤是致命的，已有在婴儿期发病的报道[30,40]。和其他甲状腺癌一样，MTC 通常在肿瘤已经出现明显的颈部淋巴结播散和远处转移时才能作出临床诊断[12]。

外科手术切除是治疗 MTC 唯一有效的方法，在转移发生之前的早期诊断和治疗尤为重要。因此对于家族性 MEN 2 综合征患儿，目前 MTC 治疗策略是基于临床症状出现前导致本病原癌基因 *RET* 变异的检测。患儿约 5 岁时施行预防性甲状腺全切除，可以防肿瘤播散出甲状腺之外[5]。在单单因为 *RET* 基因变异而施行甲状腺切除的患儿中，约有 80%甲状腺中已经存在 MTC 病灶[43]。由于在 MEN 2B 患者中 MTC 更为致命，因此在婴儿期施行甲状腺切除可能更为合适。

甲状旁腺

甲状旁腺调节机体钙磷代谢。甲状旁腺素（PTH）是以 84 个氨基酸的蛋白质形式分泌，在代谢过程中转变成碳末端和氨基末端等中间段，被肝脏和肾脏清除。在肾脏里，PTH 与其受体结合发挥作用，刺激产生活化维生素 D 的代谢物 1,25-二羟胆钙化醇，即二羟维生素 D_3。后者作用于肠黏膜增加钙的吸收。PTH 直接刺激骨骼的钙动员，这个过程也需要通过维生素 D。

PTH 的生物学活性存在于氨基末端片断，但是血浆中这部分的含量很低，这主要是因为它在循环中的半衰期很短。大多数临床上对 PTH 的检测是测量碳末端片断的水平，在血浆中它的浓度是氨基末端片断的 50～500 倍，这些检测对评价甲状旁腺功能亢进是相当有效的，但值得注意的是由于碳末端片断是由肾脏清除的，所以当存在肾功能损害时该蛋白血浆水平出现上升。甲状旁腺功能亢进的实验室特点是：血浆 PTH 升高伴高钙血症。对 PTH 水平缓慢升高患者进行放射学检查，临床上有一定的意义，但骨骼特征性的变化并不是很快出现。

评价高钙血症的第一步就是进行 24 小时尿钙测定，以排除家族性低尿钙性高血钙症。后者是众所周知的家族性良性高钙血症，儿童一般无症状，唯一引起临床上注意的是血清钙增高。一般血镁的水平也会出现上升。家庭中的其他成员也有可能会发病，这种情况是因为遗传性的编码血清钙离子敏感受体基因变异所致，可导致细胞水平的钙离子变化不敏感。这是一种常染色体显性遗传疾病。但此时血中 PTH 水平

和甲状旁腺正常，甲状旁腺切除通常对此没有益处。偶尔，刚出生的新生儿可表现出严重的、致命性高钙血症。这是由于两个等位基因同时发生变异导致。这些婴儿通常会出现甲状旁腺增生，行甲状旁腺切除有效。

儿童高钙血症的不同诊断详见表 55–7。与成人不同，儿童很少由于肿瘤引起血钙水平异常。然而，有些儿童肿瘤可能分泌出甲状旁腺相关性多肽也可以引起血钙上升，例如恶性横纹肌样肉瘤、转移性肾瘤、横纹肌肉瘤、神经母细胞瘤以及淋巴瘤。在这些
858 患者中 PTH 水平一般正常或下降。

如图 55–1 所示，儿童原发性甲状旁腺亢进最常见的是由于单发性高功能腺瘤所致。所有 4 个腺体弥漫性增生很少见[37]，由所有 4 个腺体弥漫性增生所引起的甲状旁腺功能亢进是 MEN 综合征的特点之一。大约有 30%的 MEN 2A 会出现弥漫性甲状旁腺肿大，但该综合征很少在儿童期出现低血钙[15]。原发性甲状旁腺功能亢进在婴儿期非常罕见，约有一半的患者是家族性发病，常常是致命的[23,38]。通常在出生后 3 个月内发病，临床表现为肌张力下降、呼吸困难、发育停滞、嗜睡以及多尿。婴儿原发性甲状旁腺功能亢进的早期诊断和治疗对患儿正常发育和生长有重要意义，病理学上常常表现为弥漫性甲状旁腺肿大。

没有药物能够治疗原发性甲状旁腺功能亢进，一旦明确诊断，该腺体组织应该被切除。最近影像学和实时 PTH 测定的发展已使微创技术得到应用[18,49]。目前值得推荐的是对该疾病患者术前进行 ^{99m}TC–sestamibi（司他比锝）扫描定位病灶[6]。如果扫描显示病变累及单一甲状旁腺，则可行微创手术。通过手持针式 γ 探测器定位切除病变的腺体。为了确定病变的甲状旁腺已经切除，可以在孩子没有清醒之前行快速的甲状旁腺素测定来证实病变的腺体

表 55–7 儿童高钙血症的鉴别诊断

甲状旁腺激素水平上升
原发性甲状旁腺功能亢进
继发性甲状旁腺亢进
三发性甲状旁腺功能功能亢进
异位甲状旁腺素的产生
维生素 D 过多
肉样瘤病
皮下脂肪坏死
家族性低尿钙性高血钙症
婴儿期特发性高钙血症
甲状腺毒症
维生素 A 过多
低磷酸酶症
长期制动
噻嗪类利尿剂使用

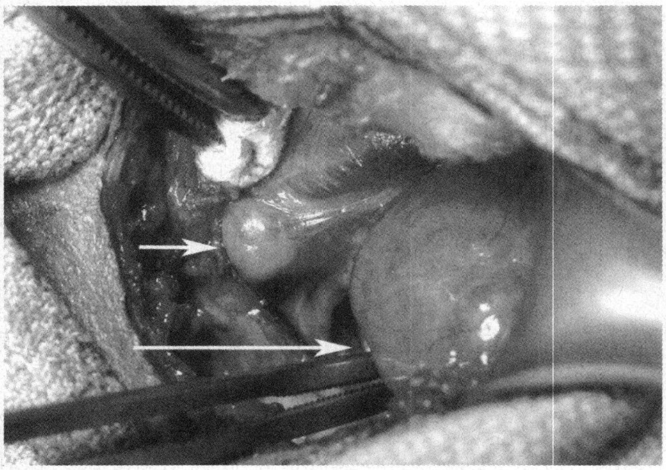

A

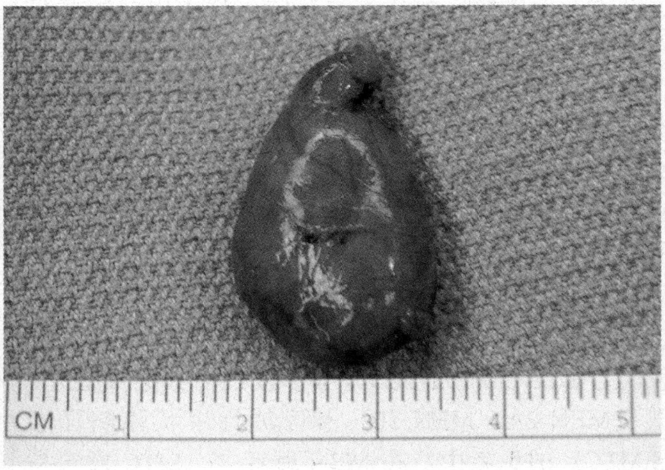

B

图 55–1 A. 导致高血钙的甲状旁腺瘤，大箭头指向增大的上部腺体，小箭头指向正常大小的下部腺体。B. 切除后的甲状旁腺瘤。

已经切除。这种模式在儿科领域应用并不广泛，但其在成人中的应用已显示出可以减少病死率和住院时间以及费用[49]。

首选外科手术切除所有腺体治疗甲状旁腺功能亢进存在争议。有些外科医生提倡切除三个半腺体，有些则提倡将所有的腺体全部切除，将部分腺体组织自体移植到非优势的前臂内[38]。后一种措施在甲状旁腺功能亢进复发的时候，可以避免再次进行颈部探查，这在儿童和婴儿中是安全的[43]。而且，有证据表明，甲状旁腺全切除同时行自体移植可以提高婴儿中严重高钙血症患儿的生存率[38]。

继发性甲状旁腺功能亢进是由于血钙降低刺激甲状旁腺造成 PTH 分泌增加所致，这最常见于肾功能不全的患者，但有时可能是吸收不良综合征造成的。继发性甲状旁腺亢进一般对减少肠道磷吸收的药物治疗有效。在很罕见的病例中，患儿会出现严重的肾性骨营养不良，表现为骨折和转移性钙化；这些患儿有指征行三个半甲状旁腺切除或甲状旁腺全切，同时自体甲状旁腺移植。在一些慢性肾衰和继发性甲状旁腺功能亢进已行肾移植的患者中，甚至在由于肾衰所致的低钙血症这一刺激因素去除之后，甲状旁腺高功能状态仍可持续存在，这称为第三型甲状旁腺功能亢进，是由于四个甲状旁腺处于增生状态所致；处于这种状况的患儿也是进行甲状旁腺全切除和自体移植的候选者。

（李巍松译　王　俊校）

参考文献

1. Acharya S, Sarafoglou K, LaQuaglia MP, et al: Thyroid neoplasms after therapeutic radiation for malignancies during childhood or adolescence. Cancer 2003;97:2397-2403.
2. Al-Shaikh A, Ngan B, Daneman A, et al: Fine-needle aspiration biopsy in the management of thyroid nodules in children and adolescents. J Pediatr 2001;138:140-142.
3. Berglund J, Christensen SB, Dymling JF, et al: The incidence of recurrence and hypothyroidism following treatment with antithyroid drugs, surgery, or radioiodine in all patients with thyrotoxicosis in Malmo during the period 1970-1974. J Intern Med 1991;229:435-442.
4. Brauckhoff M, Gimm O, Thanh PN, et al: First experience in intraoperative neurostimulation of the recurrent laryngeal nerve during thyroid surgery in children and adolescents. J Pediatr Surg 2002;37:1414-1418.
5. Ceccarelli C, Pacini F, Lippi F, et al: Thyroid cancer in children and adolescents. Surgery 1988;104:1143-1148.
6. Chen H: Surgery for primary hyperparathyroidism: What is the best approach? Ann Surg 2002;236:552-553.
7. de Roy van Zuidewijn DBW, Songun I, Kievit J, et al: Complications of thyroid surgery. Ann Surg Oncol 1995;2:56-60.
8. Desjardins JG, Khan AH, Montupet P, et al: Management of thyroid nodules in children: A 20-year experience. J Pediatr Surg 1987;22:736-739.
9. Dickman PW, Holm L-E, Lundell G, et al: Thyroid cancer risk after thyroid examination with ^{131}I: A population-based cohort study in Sweden. Int J Cancer 2003;106:580-587.
10. Eng C, Smith DP, Mulligan LM, et al: Point mutation within the tyrosine kinase domain of the *RET* proto-oncogene in multiple endocrine neoplasia type 2B and related sporadic tumours. Hum Mol Genet 1994;3:237-241.
11. Franklyn JA: The management of hyperthyroidism. N Engl J Med 1994;330:1731-1738.
12. Gorlin JB, Sallan SE: Thyroid cancer in childhood. Endocrinol Metab Clin North Am 1990;19:649-662.
13. Harness JA, Thompson NW, McLeod MK, et al: Differentiated thyroid carcinoma in children and adolescents. World J Surg 1992;16:547-554.
14. Haselkorn T, Bernstein L, Preston-Martin S, et al: Descriptive epidemiology of thyroid cancer in Los Angeles County, 1972-1995. Cancer Causes Control 2000;11:163-170.
15. Howe JR, Norton JA, Wells SA Jr: Prevalence of pheochromocytoma and hyperparathyroidism in multiple endocrine neoplasia type 2A: Results of long-term follow-up. Surgery 1993;114:1070-1077.
16. Hung W, Anderson KD, Chandra RS, et al: Solitary thyroid nodules in 71 children and adolescents. J Pediatr Surg 1992;27:1407-1409.
17. Hung W, Sarlis NJ: Current controversies in the management of pediatric patients with well-differentiated nonmedullary thyroid cancer: A review. Thyroid 2002;12:683-702.
18. Irvin GL III, Molinari AS, Figueroa C, et al: Improved success rate in reoperative parathyroidectomy with intraoperative PTH assay. Ann Surg 1999;229:874-879.
19. Jaksic J, Dumic M, Filipovic B, et al: Thyroid disease in a school population with thyromegaly. Arch Dis Child 1994;70:103-106.
20. Khurana KK, Labrador E, Izquierdo R, et al: The role of fine-needle aspiration biopsy in the management of thyroid nodules in children, adolescents, and young adults: A multi-institutional study. Thyroid 1999;9:383-386.
21. Kirk JM, Mort C, Grant DB, et al: The usefulness of serum thyroglobulin in the follow-up of differentiated thyroid carcinoma in children. Med Pediatr Oncol 1992;20:201-208.
22. Klein I, Becker DV, Levey GS: Treatment of hyperthyroid disease. Ann Intern Med 1994;121:281-288.
23. Kulczycka H, Kaminski W, Wozniewicz B, et al: Primary hyperparathyroidism in infancy: Diagnostic and therapeutic difficulties. Klin Padiatr 1991;203:116-118.
24. La Quaglia MP, Corbally MT, Heller G, et al: Recurrence and morbidity in differentiated thyroid carcinoma in children. Surgery 1988;104:1149-1156.
25. Mazzaferri EL: Management of a solitary thyroid nodule. N Engl J Med 1993;328:553-559.
26. Nebesio TD, Siddiqui AR, Pescovitz OH, et al: Time course to hypothyroidism after fixed-dose radioablation therapy of Graves' disease in children. J Pediatr 2002;141:99-103.
27. Newman KD: The current management of thyroid tumors in childhood. Semin Pediatr Surg 1993;2:69-74.
28. Newman KD, Black T, Heller G, et al: Differentiated thyroid

cancer: Determinants of disease progression in patients < 21 years of age at diagnosis. Ann Surg 1998;227:533-541.
29. Nikiforov Y, Gnepp DR: Pediatric thyroid cancer after the Chernobyl disaster: Pathomorphologic study of 84 cases (1991-1992) from the Republic of Belarus. Cancer 1994;74: 748-765.
30. Norton JA, Froome LC, Farrell RE, et al: Multiple endocrine neoplasia type IIb: The most aggressive form of medullary thyroid carcinoma. Surg Clin North Am 1979;59:109-118.
31. Pacini F, Vorontsova T, Molinaro E, et al: Thyroid consequences of the Chernobyl nuclear accident. Acta Paediatr Suppl 1999;433:23-27.
32. Paterson ICM, Greenlee R, Adams Jones D: Thyroid cancer in Wales 1985-1996: A cancer registry-based study. Clin Oncol 1999;11:245-251.
33. Phillips DI, Barker DJ, Rees Smith B, et al: The geographical distribution of thyrotoxicosis in England according to the presence or absence of TSH-receptor antibodies. Clin Endocrinol 1985;23:283-287.
34. Raab SS, Silverman JF, Elsheikh TM, et al: Pediatric thyroid nodules: Disease demographics and clinical management by fine needle aspiration biopsy. Pediatrics 1995;95:46-49.
35. Rabes HM, Demidchik EP, Siderow JD, et al: Pattern of radiation-induced RET and NTRK1 rearrangement in 191 post-Chernobyl papillary thyroid carcinomas: Biological, phenotypic, and clinical implications. Clin Cancer Res 2000; 6:1093-1103.
36. Rallison ML, Dobyns BM, Meikle AW, et al: Natural history of thyroid abnormalities: Prevalence, incidence, and regression of thyroid diseases in adolescents and young adults. Am J Med 1991;91:363-370.
37. Ross AJ III: Parathyroid surgery in children. Prog Pediatr Surg 1991;26:48-59.
38. Ross AJ III, Cooper A, Attie MF, et al: Primary hyperparathyroidism in infancy. J Pediatr Surg 1986;21:493-499.
39. Rother KI, Zimmerman D, Schwenk WF: Effect of thyroid hormone treatment on thyromegaly in children and adolescents with Hashimoto disease. J Pediatr 1994;124: 599-601.
40. Samaan NA, Draznin MB, Halpin RE, et al: Multiple endocrine syndrome type IIb in early childhood. Cancer 1991;68:1832-1834.
41. Santoro M, Thomas GA, Vecchio G, et al: Gene rearrangement and Chernobyl related thyroid cancers. Br J Cancer 2000;82:315-322.
42. Schlumberger M, De Vathaire F, Travagli JP, et al: Differentiated thyroid carcinoma in childhood: Long term follow-up in 72 patients. J Clin Endocrinol Metab 1987;65:1088-1094.
43. Skinner MA, DeBenedetti MK, Moley JF, et al: Medullary thyroid carcinoma in children with multiple endocrine neoplasia types 2A and 2B. J Pediatr Surg 1996;31:177-182.
44. Skinner MA, Norton JA, Moley JF, et al: Heterotopic autotransplantation of parathyroid tissue in children undergoing total thyroidectomy. J Pediatr Surg 1997;32:510-513.
45. Smith MB, Xue H, Strong L, et al: Forty-year experience with second malignancies after treatment of childhood cancer: Analysis of outcome following the development of the second malignancy. J Pediatr Surg 1993;28:1342-1349.
46. Thomusch O, Machens A, Sekulla C, et al: The impact of surgical technique on postoperative hypoparathyroidism in bilateral thyroid surgery: A multivariate analysis of 5846 consecutive patients. Surgery 2003;133:180-185.
47. Tomer Y, Davies TF: Infection, thyroid disease, and autoimmunity. Endocrine Rev 1993;14:107-120.
48. Udelsman R, Aruny JE, Donovan PI, et al: Rapid parathyroid hormone analysis during venous localization. Ann Surg 2003;237:714-721.
49. Udelsman R, Donovan PI, Sokoll LJ: One hundred consecutive minimally invasive parathyroid explorations. Ann Surg 2000;232:331-339.
50. Vassilopoulou-Sellin R, Klein MJ, Smith TH, et al: Pulmonary metastases in children and young adults with differentiated thyroid cancer. Cancer 1993;71:1348-1352.
51. Wells SA Jr, Chi DD, Toshima K, et al: Predictive DNA testing and prophylactic thyroidectomy in patients at risk for multiple endocrine neoplasia type 2A. Ann Surg 1994;220: 237-250.
52. Wells SA Jr, Farndon JR, Dale JK, et al: Long term evaluation of patients with primary parathyroid hyperplasia managed by total parathyroidectomy and heterotopic autotransplantation. Ann Surg 1980;192:451-458.
53. Yip FWK, Reeve TS, Poole AG, et al: Thyroid nodules in childhood and adolescence. Aust NZ J Surg 1994;64: 676-678.
54. Zimmerman D, Hay ID, Gough IR, et al: Papillary thyroid carcinoma in children and adults: Long-term follow-up of 1039 patients conservatively treated at one institution during three decades. Surgery 1988;104:1157-1163.

第 56 章

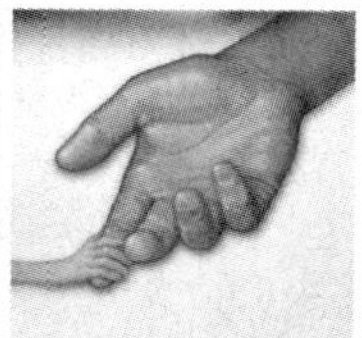

颈部囊肿和窦道

C. D. Smith

颈部的囊肿和窦道构成儿科病理学上有趣的一部分。尽管病因是先天性的，但可以直到成年才出现临床症状并被认识。在成人期它可能会伪装成癌肿[5,8]。而在儿童期通常是良性的，只在很罕见的情况下方潜伏恶性病变[5,8]。儿童最常见的是甲状舌管囊肿和第二鳃裂畸形[7,29]，通常很容易通过体检明确诊断，不需要其他的检查。常可通过日间手术切除。该病的诊治存在很多误区，对于外科医生来说如果忽视解剖上的变异或者没有具备良好的外科技能可能会给患者带来多次复发的痛苦或者损伤神经，了解这些囊肿和窦道在胚胎学上的来源以及它们与颈部正常解剖结构的关系，是成功治疗的前提，也是完全切除所需要的。另外，一些不常见的表现，例如：急性化脓性甲状腺炎（来源于第三、第四鳃裂畸形造成的梨状隐窝）、耳漏（第一鳃裂畸形）、严重的呼吸困难或者婴儿期猝死（甲状舌管囊肿、鳃裂畸形），或者是异位甲状腺误认为甲状舌管囊肿会导致不合适的治疗措施。本章节重点在于有关颈部的胚胎学，描述每个疾病常见和不常见的表现，讨论原发性病变和复发性病变的外科处理策略，突出挑战传统治疗原则的新手段，以及使用微创手段治疗这些颈部病变的初步尝试。

胚胎学

原始胚胎的 6 对鳃弓由 6 对主动脉弓滋养，后者直接通向成对的背侧和腹侧主动脉（图 56–1）。第五鳃弓的出现是一过性的，最后消失得毫无踪迹。每对鳃弓外面覆盖着外胚层，内衬内胚层，充满中胚层，包含有动脉、神经、软骨和肌肉，在鳃弓之间凹陷外面的称为裂，内部的称为囊，外胚层排列于裂，内胚层排列于囊（图 56–2）。这些相对的点称为封闭膜，在人类这些膜最终不会像鱼那样发育成鳃。

表 56–1 总结了每个弓、裂、窝对于颈部和颌的形成的作用，颈部囊肿和窦道起源的理论是建立于这些畸形和周围的动脉、肌肉、神经的关系基础上以及已知的甲状腺、甲状旁腺、胸腺胚胎迁移途径，此外还有各种畸形的内皮层类型。

图 56–1 显示动脉弓和大动脉转变成明确的血管结构的过程，三个例子说明对此过程的知识已被用来推测鳃裂畸形的来源。第一，可以表明梨状窦管（第三、四鳃裂病变）通往颈内动脉之后的鳃弓结构，不是位于颈外动脉和颈内动脉之间，第二鳃裂畸形的病例也是如此（图 56–3）；第二，外窦的开口位于胸锁乳突肌的前面以及颈部的下方，这对于第二、三、四鳃裂残留是无法区分的，在胚胎期这些裂在颈部有共同出口，HIS 颈窦形成于第二鳃弓过度生长于这些裂的开口时（图 56–4A）。囊肿、窦道或瘘管到颈动脉杈、舌下神经、茎突舌骨肌、二腹肌等颈部结构的关系决定了这些病变的起源，而不是取决于它们开口的位置[76]。第三，完全性第四鳃裂瘘仍有待确认，推测其过程在两侧颈部不同。在左侧瘘管会在主动脉弓（来源于胚胎期左侧第四主动脉弓）下方进入上纵隔。由于右侧第四主动脉弓转变成锁骨下动脉，所以右侧瘘管会从其下方穿过（图 56–1 和图 56–5）。

与这些弓相关的神经是非常重要的标志，不仅用于推测各种鳃裂畸形的来源，而且是术中的风险因素，在第一鳃裂瘘，瘘管可能通过面神经分支的下方、上方以及从其中穿过[46]，所以在切除时最重要的原则是辨认出神经的分支。在低位不复杂的鳃裂瘘中造成邻近神经的损伤并非是常见的临床问题，而当有炎症存在之前有手术史导致正常解剖的异常会使神经损伤的风险明显增加，图 56–3 和 56–5 显示了第二、

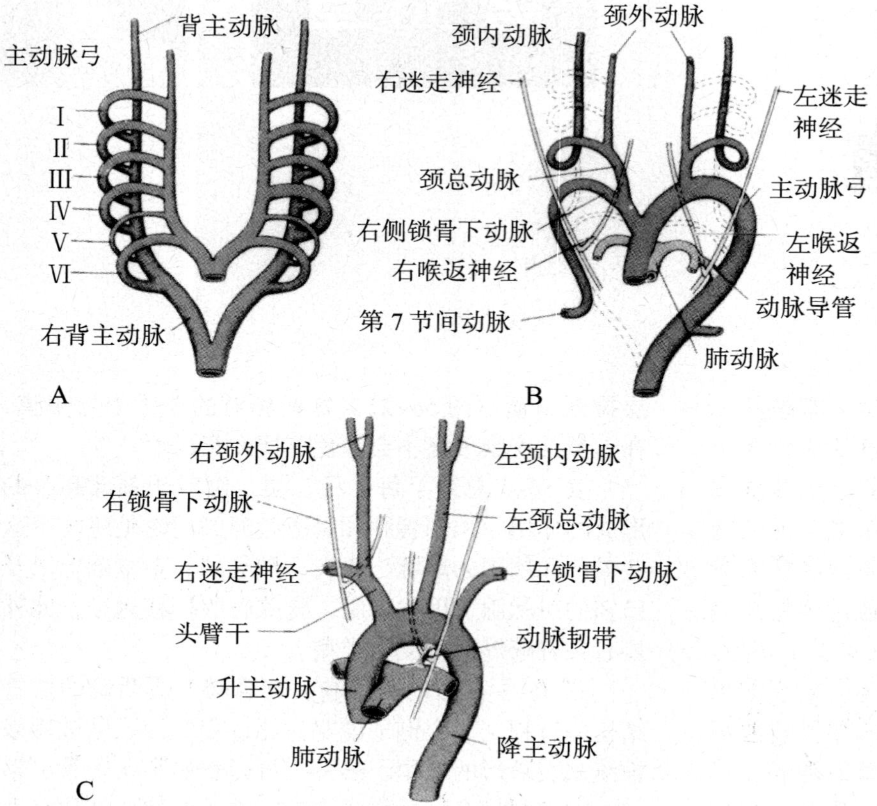

图 56-1 A. 主动脉弓和背主动脉转化成具体血管结构之前的图示。B. 主动脉弓和背主动脉转化之后的图示。擦去的部分通过间断线表示。注意动脉导管的开放和左侧的第七节间动脉的位置。C. 成人的大动脉。比较 B 和 C中左侧颈总动脉起源位置和左锁骨下动脉之间的距离。在第六动脉弓消失之后（第五动脉弓从来没有完全形成），右侧的喉返神经呈钩状围绕右侧锁骨下动脉。在左侧神经保留在原位呈钩状围绕动脉导管。(From Sadler TW: Head and neck. In Langman ' s Medical Embryology, 7th ed. Baltimore, Williams & Wilkins, 1995.)

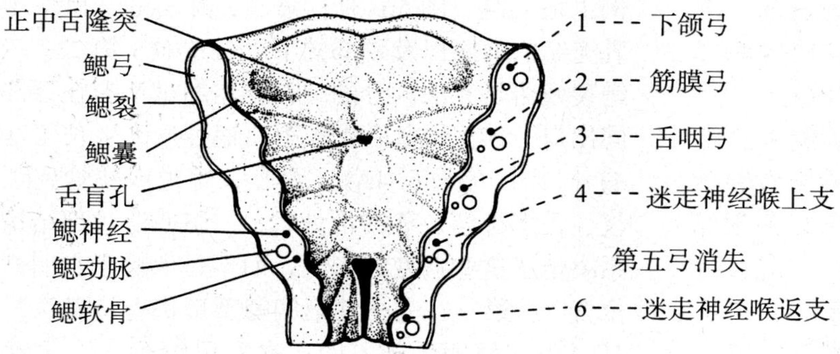

图 56-2 鳃器官的早期发育。(From Donegan JO: Congenital neck masses. In Cummings CW,et al [eds]:Otolaryngology—Head and Neck Surgery, 2nd ed. St Louis, Mosby Year Book, 1993.)

第三、第四鳃裂瘘和舌咽神经（Ⅸ）、喉上神经、迷走神经（X）喉返神经支和舌下神经（Ⅻ）。

对鳃裂瘘内口的了解对于诊断和治疗均有帮助，第一鳃裂畸形通常进入外耳道（很少见于中耳）。第
863 二鳃裂畸形通常进入扁桃体窝。第三和第四鳃裂畸形通常经过梨状隐窝进后在喉上神经处上升，第四鳃裂瘘从顶（下部）进入然后在喉上神经处下降[24]。

首先需要鳃囊、封闭膜 / 裂复合物的存留才可成为咽鼓管、外耳道、鼓膜（图 56-4A），剩下的鳃囊发育成扁桃体、胸腺、甲状旁腺、甲状腺的 C 细胞，这些裂的出口逐渐退化（图 56-4B 和 56-6），所有这些腺体只有扁桃体是起源于鳃裂，第三鳃囊慢慢延长最终失去和咽喉的交通。其背侧分化成将来的下甲状旁腺（III），紧靠甲状腺下极，腹侧进入上纵隔胸腺同侧腺叶，胚胎学家已经确认甲状旁腺来源于第四鳃囊，但他们不认为后鳃体（甲状腺后角和分泌降钙素的 C 细胞）来源于第四鳃囊或者是退化的第五鳃囊（图 56-4）。建立在对 15 例患者甲状腺和瘘管切除标本的免疫组化研究基础上，Miyauchi和其同事令人信服的提出这些瘘管是残留的后鳃体[52]。

表 56-1 鳃弓、鳃裂和鳃囊的分化

	背侧	腹侧	咽的中线板
Ⅰ			
弓	砧骨体	Meckel 软骨	舌体
外颚动脉	锤骨头	锤骨	
神经 Ⅴ	耳廓		
裂	外耳道		
囊	咽鼓管		
	中耳		
	乳突气房		
Ⅱ			
弓	镫骨	茎突	舌根
镫骨动脉		舌骨（小角和部分体部）	舌盲孔
神经Ⅶ和Ⅷ			甲状腺中部始基
囊	腭扁桃体		
	扁桃体上窝		
Ⅲ			
弓		舌骨（小角和部分体部）	
颈内动脉		部分会厌	
神经Ⅸ		甲状腺	
囊	下甲状旁腺		
	梨状窝		
Ⅳ			
弓		甲状软骨	
主动脉弓（左）		楔状软骨	
部分锁骨下动脉（右）		会厌	
神经Ⅹ			
囊	上甲状旁腺（甲状腺的后角）	甲状腺	
Ⅴ			
弓	后鳃体（甲状腺的后角）		
囊			
Ⅵ			
弓		环状软骨	
肺动脉		杓状软骨	
动脉导管（左侧）		小角状软骨	
神经Ⅹ（喉返神经）			

From Skandalakis JE, Gray SW, Todd NW: The pharynx and its derivatives. In Skandalakis JE, Gray SW (eds): Embryology for Surgeons, 2nd ed. Baltimore, Williams & Wilkins, 1994.

Himi 和 Kataura 对梨状窦瘘的甲状腺中 C 细胞分布
364 的研究支持了这一解释[34]。

第四鳃囊结构迁移程度要比第三鳃囊的衍生物轻，甲状旁腺组织通常位于甲状腺上部的背侧表面，C 细胞有他们自己通向甲状腺的途径。颈侧区域的囊肿和窦道可能来源于第二、第三、第四鳃囊自身持续

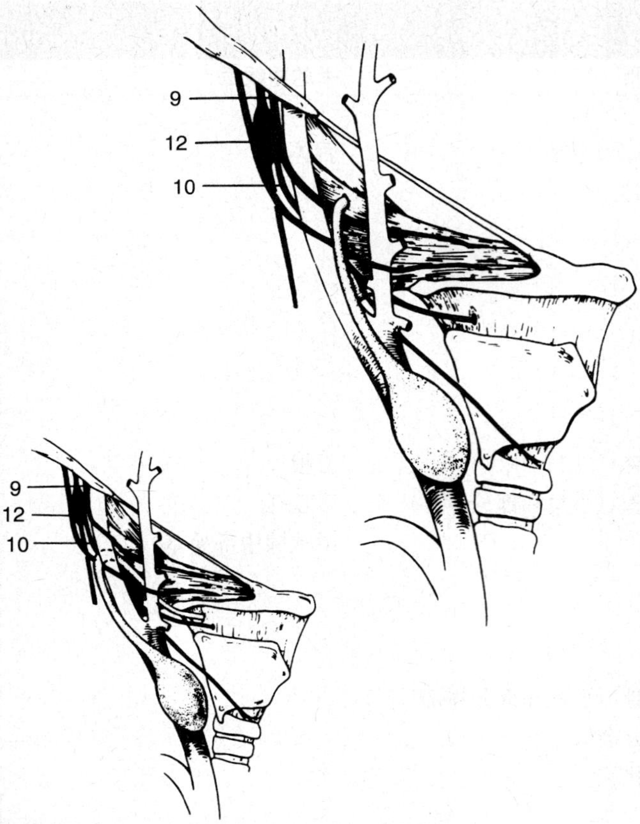

图 56-3 第二鳃裂囊肿和瘘管（右侧）；第三鳃裂囊肿和瘘管（左侧）。(From Donegan JO: Congenital neck masses. In Cummings CW, et al [eds]: Otolaryngology—Head and Neck Surgery, 2nd ed. St Louis,Mosby Year Book, 1993.)

存在，也可能来源于甲状腺和甲状旁腺的残留，后者可能遗留在它们迁移途径中的任何一个部位，在囊肿壁中有甲状腺组织并不能表明它们的来源，因为第三和第四鳃囊通常均含有甲状腺组织。

甲状腺发育自舌前部和后部肌肉前体之间的双叶憩室，处于舌盲孔的位置（图 56–6）， 腺体从中线向下从舌骨前方下降到颈的下部，它临时性地和其起源点有细胞索相连，这就是甲状舌管，其末端常成为甲状腺的锥状叶，当甲状舌管持续存在时作为外科医生需要认识其与舌骨的关系，以及舌骨和舌盲孔之间还有其残留。Horisawa 通过手术标本三维重建甲状舌管，显示了舌骨中部也含有核心组织通向舌盲孔，所以在术中需要切除舌骨中段避免复发（图 56–7）[35]。

在很少的情况下甲状腺不能完全下降，通常保
留在舌根部，有时会下降到颈根部更远处。该畸形不 865
仅和外科有关，还和法医学有关，在术前告知、术前准备和术中处理时都要注意[62]。

发病率

在费城儿童医院的资料中，5 年中对 445 例患儿进行了 481 例颈部肿块切除手术，244 例（55%）为先天性颈部肿块，其中 78 例（32%）为鳃裂畸形，

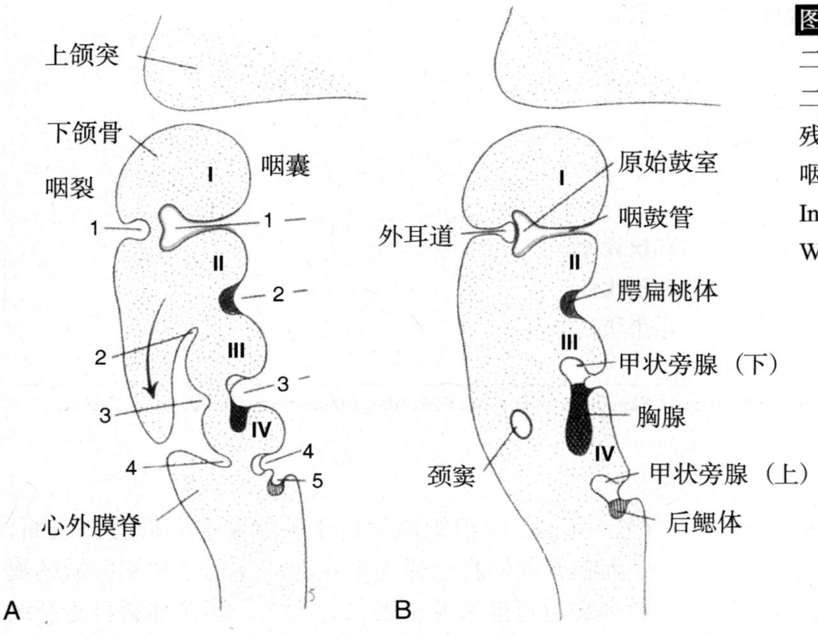

图 56-4 A. 咽裂和咽囊的发育示意图。请注意第二弓是在第三弓和第四弓之上生长，然后埋藏了第二、第三和第四咽裂。B. 第二、第三和第四咽裂的残余部分形成颈窦，这通常是闭塞的。注意不同的咽囊形成的结构。(From Sadler TW: Head and neck. In Langman's Medical Embryology, 7th ed. Baltimore, Williams & Wilkins,1995.)

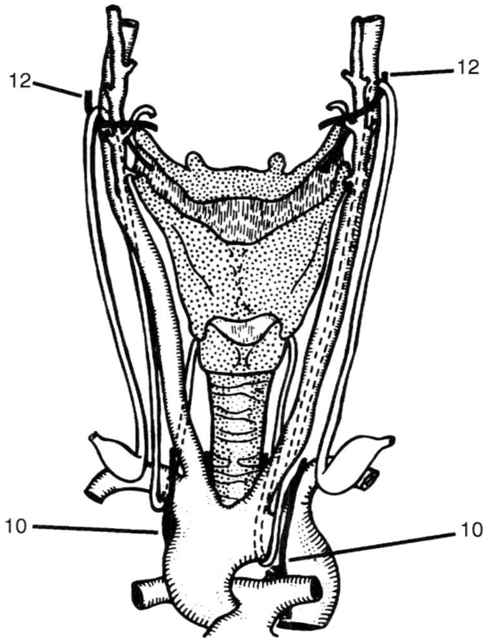

图 56-5　可能的第四鳃裂瘘和周围的解剖关系。(From Liston SL: Fourth branchial fistula. Otolaryngol Head Neck Surg 1981;89:520.)

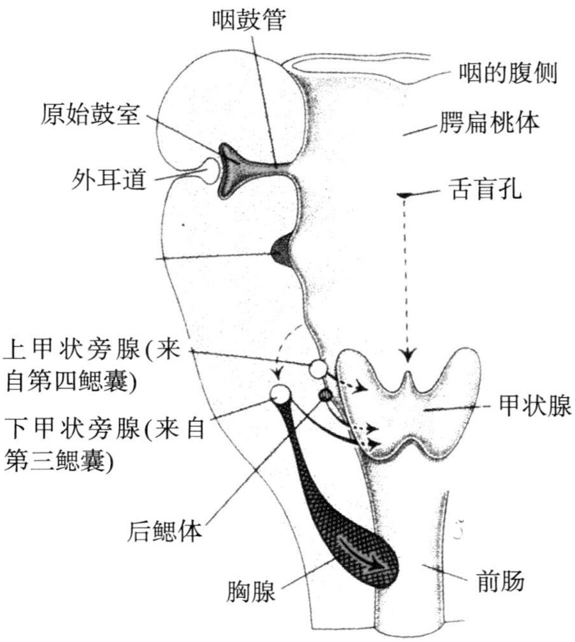

图 56-6　图示表明甲状腺、甲状旁腺、后鳃体的迁移。甲状腺来源于舌盲孔中线部位下降到第一气管环的位置。(From Sadler TW: Head and neck. In Langman's Medical Embryology, 7th ed. Baltimore, Williams & Wilkins, 1995.)

73 例（30%）为甲状舌管囊肿。43 例（18%）为皮样囊肿[78]。甲状舌管囊肿比鳃裂病变更为常见，在 Mayo 临床系列中有 612 例，成人和儿童比例为 55%对 45%[72]。在法国 15 年的病例中，191 例儿童中中线关闭异常多于鳃迁移异常，其中 53%为甲状舌管囊肿，11%为皮样囊肿，19%为第二鳃裂畸形，10%为第一鳃裂畸形，4%为第四鳃囊畸形，2%为甲状腺囊肿[57]。

第二鳃裂异常

据估计大约超过 90%的鳃裂畸形来源于第二鳃裂结构，大约有 8%为第一鳃裂畸形，剩下的第三和第四鳃裂结构畸形比较少见[11]。男性和女性的比例相同。大多数的鳃裂畸形在出生后 10 年内被诊断，当没有外源性的窦道时可至成人期才被诊断，Mayo 临 866
床系列中 74%为囊肿，25%为瘘管，1%为皮赘和软骨[72]。令人惊奇的是在伦敦儿童医院的资料回顾中，在 32 年间 98 例中有 92 例为第二鳃裂 / 囊畸形，在颈部均有开放性的窦道，这解释了为什么在所有的病例中只有 2 例在 10 岁才被诊断，78%在 5 岁之前被诊断[23]，6 例患者没有窦道开口，只有局部软骨残留（图 56-8），6 例（6%）为双侧病变，其他人的报道双侧为 2%～10%[26]。

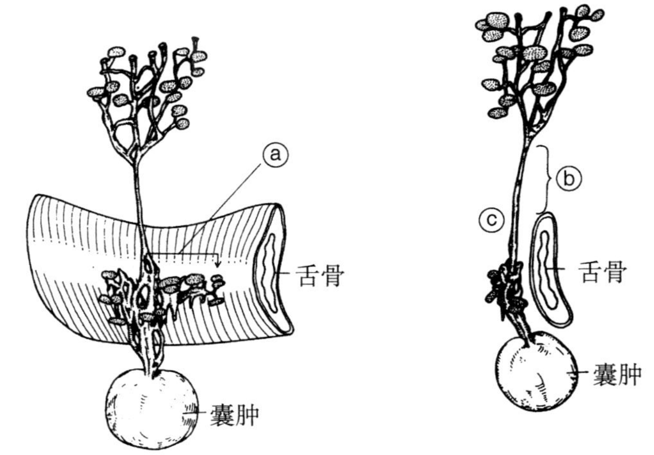

图 56-7　基于解剖学重建的甲状舌管的走向。a. 从中线至最远处甲状舌管的水平距离；b. 舌骨上方单一管道的长度；c. 测量管道直径的点。(From Horisawa M, Niinomi N, Ito T: What is the optimal depth for core-out toward the foramen cecum in a thyroglossal duct cyst operation? J Pediatr Surg 1992;27:710.)

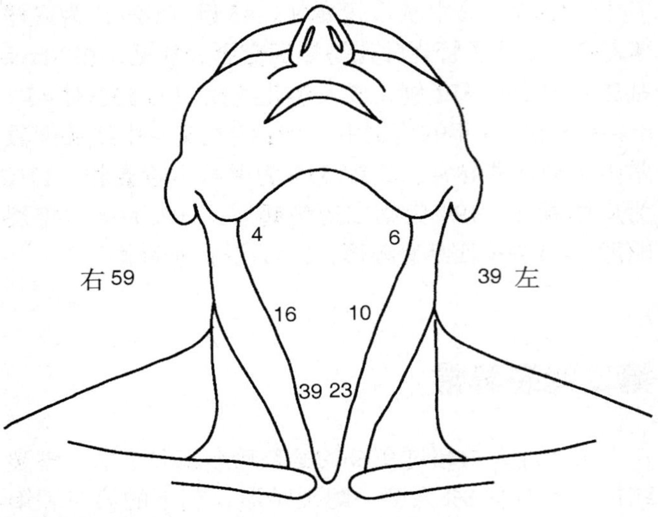

图 56-8 鳃裂囊肿的位置。(From Ford GR, et al: Branchial cleft and pouch anomalies. J Laryngol Otol 1992;106:137.)

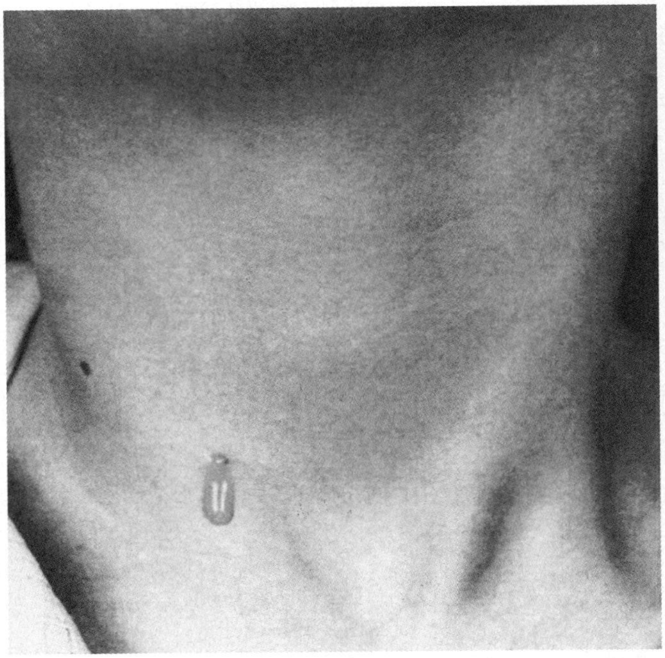

图 56-9 单侧第二鳃裂瘘的引流。(From Ford GR, et al: Branchial cleft and pouch anomalies. J Laryngol Otol 1992; 106:137.)

典型情况下在胸锁乳突肌下三分之一前出现皮肤小凹陷同时伴有液体流出，提示有第二鳃裂窦或瘘的存在（图 56-9），从颈部瘘口的上方可以触摸到向上的条索，挤压和剥脱管道可以导致黏液流出，囊肿在胸锁乳突肌上三分之一的部位成为囊性肿块。该部位突然出现痛性肿块为该类病变的首发表现。

不常见的表现包括喘鸣、咽喉部囊肿导致喉部疼痛、喉部充实感、发音时鼻音减少、吞咽困难、吞咽疼痛、甲状腺扫描为冷结节[70]、热结节[70]，舌下神经麻痹[25]，或者多发性颅神经麻痹[18]。鳃裂异常也可以是鳃颜面综合征的一部分[44]；由鳃发生的癌在成人有过报道，在儿童未有过诊断[27]。

因为任何鳃裂瘘均存在感染的可能性，所以最好是在未发生感染之前给予切除，婴儿通常在 3～6 月之后手术。在发生感染之后，手术需要延迟，可能情况下最好采用抗生素和穿刺抽吸，最好避免切开引流因为这会扰乱正常的组织结构从而导致复发率的上升，在 Mayo 临床系列分析中三分之二的术后复发者曾有感染史、手术史或者两者均有[72]。

在儿童第二鳃裂异常伴有颈部瘘口者可沿瘘口周围做一切口进行切除。在青少年和成人可能需要两级阶梯切口。相对于甲状舌管囊肿，该瘘管相对较好辨认，术中可沿瘘管壁进行操作，在瘘管内插入导管、Prolene 缝线、或者金属探子对于手术均有帮助。术中注射美兰如果有溢出可能使操作变得复杂；术前瘘管造影可能会有帮助，但不作为常规[10]。手术目的是切除所有病变，但不损伤周围重要结构，这些结构包括颈内动脉、颈动脉、舌下神经和舌咽神经（图 56-3），切口可以选择在囊肿表面，也可采用在颈动脉分叉处切口。

颈部手术的微创技术一直在动物模型和尸体模型的探索中发展[73,74]，使用一个内镜孔和两个操作孔，从颈部下方戳孔，通过皮下扩张产生一个可以进行外科操作的空间，皮下测得充气二氧化碳压力为 4mmHg，避免皮下血肿、气胸、纵隔气肿和空气栓塞等并发症[32]。这些研究者使用 DaVinci 系统在动物模型中进行实验已取得进步，使用关节内镜和运动定位系统有以下优点：增加外科手术的精确性和灵活性，减少了三维图像的抖动。目前仅应用于颈部淋巴结切除，应用于颈部鳃裂疾病还需要设备和技术的进一步发展[1]。

第一鳃裂异常

第一鳃裂畸形少见，诊断困难，特别当其出现于合并有感染的颌下腺及皮脂腺的相同区域时（图 56-10）。有一些迹象提示临床上有第一鳃裂异常存在的可能性：在感染发生前有下颌角流液病史；没有深部硬结；相对非脓性的耳道引流液；鼓膜和中耳的囊性病灶，伴有舌骨上方的窦道和脓肿[16,77]。显然进行仔细的耳科检查是发现此类疾病的一个非常重要的部分。如同第二鳃裂异常，各年龄组中表现为囊肿的病例比窦道和瘘管要多，而且出现症状的年龄相对较迟，从 1950 年到 1978 年 Mayo 临床中心治疗了 460 例鳃裂异常，其中 38 例（8%）为第一鳃裂病变，其中 26 例（68%）为囊肿，17 例（65%）发生于女性，囊肿病例的平均年龄为 15 岁（13～18 岁）。作为对照组，有窦道和瘘管的病例在诊断或第一次治疗时的年龄相对较小，性别相同[59]，感染一般发生在明确诊断之前，这导致瘢痕的形成并干扰了正常的解剖标志。

Arnot[6]和 Work[83]描述了两种类型的病变，其中 I 型较少见，被认为是膜性外耳道的重复畸形，一般出现在大龄儿童，位于面神经的侧面，具有外胚层内衬（鳞状上皮），和外耳道平行，位于耳前方或者后方。II 型被认为是膜性外耳道和耳廓的重复畸形，病变中包括外胚层和中胚层（软骨）组织（图 56-11）。Olsen 和其同事坚持把病变分成孤立性囊肿、窦道或瘘管，更精确地描述了病变的解剖学发现，使之能更好地理解适当的诊断和治疗措施[59]。当怀疑有第一鳃裂病变时，超声检查和 CT 检查有助于确定管道的走向以及和面神经和中耳的关系。

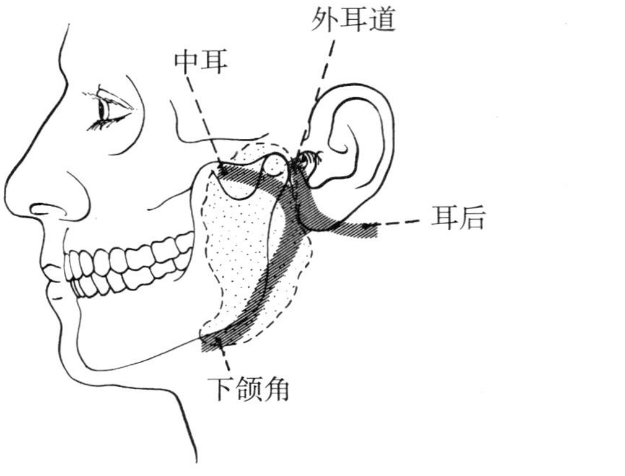

图 56-10　第一鳃裂病变的通常位置。(From Olsen KD, Maragos NE, Weiland LH: First branchial cleft anomalies. Laryngoscope 1980;90:423.)

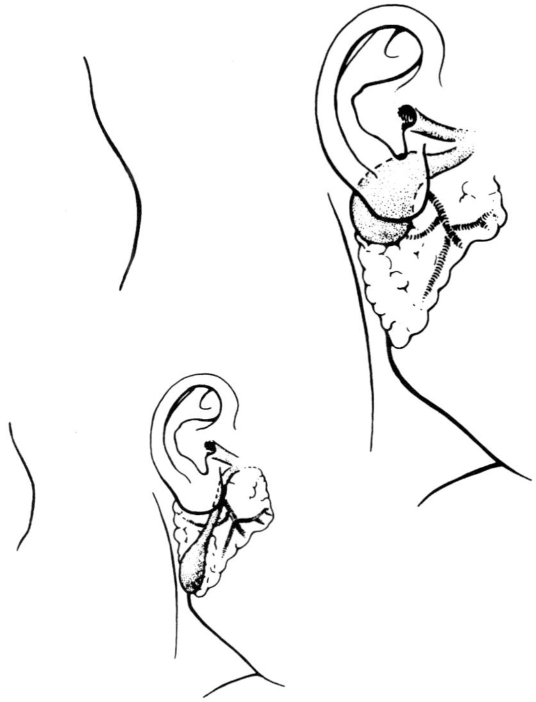

图 56-11　I 型的第一鳃裂异常（右侧）；II 型的第一鳃裂异常（右侧）。(From Donegan JO: Congenital neck masses. In Cummings CW, et al [eds]: Otolaryngology—Head and Neck Surgery, 2nd ed. St Louis, Mosby-Year Book, 1993.)

第一鳃裂瘘很难修补，特别是在幼年患者。手术中最重要的是首先要显露面神经主干，然后暴露所有的周围分支[40]，特别要强调的是在腮腺手术时面神经损伤是引起儿童面神经瘫痪最常见的原因之一。通过对婴儿的尸体解剖，Farrior 和 Santini 指出儿童面神经较细、更表浅、并更难以辨认[2,42]，是由于周围结构没有充分发育的缘故[22]。他们和另一些人[55]推荐通 868
过耳后切口先暴露从茎突孔传出的神经而不是耳前切口，并辨认通过胸锁乳突肌、二腹肌后腹侧以及软骨耳道形成的三角地带的神经（图 56-12）。在有些病例术前的感染造成颞骨外的面神经辨认困难。Todd 推荐在乳突部位寻找面神经，然后沿着它到茎突孔[76]。神经的主干暴露后，解剖其周围分支并切除腮腺的浅叶。当瘘管位于面神经深部，进行腮腺全切。然后将瘘管从面神经分支中游离，并沿着瘘管分到和耳道相通处。即使瘘管没有进入耳道，部分附近的软骨和耳道的内衬皮肤需要切除以避免复发，造成的耳道缺损可通过再次手术关闭，很少引起狭窄。窦道进入中耳和鼓膜很少见，但当出现时

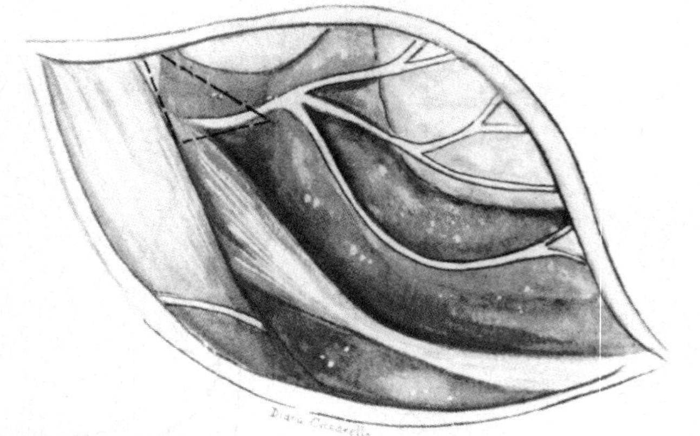

图 56-12 面神经的主干经软骨耳道、胸锁乳突肌和二腹肌（点线标志）形成的三角出茎乳孔。在婴儿面神经腮腺丛位于颚骨分支的后方。(From Farrior JB, Santini H: Facial nerve identification in children. Otolaryngol Head Neck Surg 1985;93:173.)

需要进行部分鼓膜切除、鼓膜成形以及刮除经过颞骨的管道[77]。Ikarashi 和同事指出外科医生在切除这些病变时，术者应认识到这些管道可能和咽鼓管平行延伸到鼻咽部[37]。如果管道和下颌腺紧密粘连，那么在切除时需要同时切除腺体[59]。

在 I 型鳃裂囊肿切除中，已有采用面神经电生理定位，使手术可采用更小的切口，避开面神经干，安全地完全切除病灶。在一个经历 9 年涉及 11 例儿童的报道中，Isaacson 和 Martin 强调当病变位于茎乳孔上方、术前没有感染或先前没有手术时这项技术较为适用[38]。

梨状隐窝瘘

梨状隐窝瘘是鳃器官异常中最为少见的，是由于第三和第四鳃裂及复合体的残留导致，有可能引起两种严重的临床情况：新生儿期[12,24,45,51,54]致命的呼吸窘迫和急性甲状腺炎[51,53]。因为两种情况都非常少见，经常发生诊断延误，可导致明显错误的切除术和引流术，这使后期处理更复杂。在梨状隐窝瘘的患儿常有反复的上呼吸道感染和咽喉疼痛病史，常有甲状腺疼痛和触痛，可伴有化脓和不伴有化脓。有这种病变的成人常常回忆起幼年期常有类似发作。声音嘶哑是常见症状，吞咽常有疼痛和头部可保持于伸展位[51]。

正确诊断的关键是想到和证实口腔梨状隐窝处瘘管。如前面指出的现在认为第三鳃裂异常瘘管进入梨状隐窝的基底部(上部)，第四鳃裂异常进入其顶部（后部）[24]。据报道，这种病变的大多数和所有的新生儿病例发生在颈部左侧。目前在宫内也能获得诊断[65]，在该报道中由于有发生先天性高位呼吸道梗阻综合征（CHAOS）的可能性，在分娩时需要多专业的团队来处理可能发生的致命的呼吸道梗阻，幸运的是它并非总是发生[65]。产前检查有囊肿而出生后没有，一旦喂养就出现是本病的证据[12]。

除了新生儿期，诊断常延迟到当患者发生左侧颈部靠近甲状腺上极部位发生感染和肿胀时才能作出，在这之前有可能被诊断为单侧甲状腺炎或者化脓性淋巴结炎。由于切开和引流能使后期治疗复杂化，所以重要的是要认识到潜在的梨状隐窝瘘可能是感染的根源。内镜和影像学检查能用于诊断，在一份回顾性研究中，比较了钡剂食管造影、CT、磁共振检查（MRI）和 B 超的效果，其中 CT 是最可靠的显示窦道或瘘管的方法。在出现急性感染时，食管钡剂造影可能不显示瘘管，但感染恢复后可以显示病变。

在确定手术时，直接使用 Fogaty 导管、导丝或鼻泪管探子明确管道的走向，比使用软的内镜更容易操作，有助于术中切除，放置食管探条去协助触摸管道[20,43,58,79]。Nonomura 和其同事建议采用甲状软骨翼水平状切口，然后沿带状肌向中线延长，垂直切开咽缩肌，使环甲关节脱位，从而使甲状软骨翼向前回缩[58]。也有人喜欢暴露甲状腺接近上极部位上方解剖[51]或者在切开环状软骨前方的皮肤后在甲状软骨下缘辨认瘘管，向侧方牵开甲状腺，然后暴露环甲肌和环咽肌（图 56-13）[53]。Enepekides 强调注意喉返神经从深部和中间进入病灶，必须注意辨认和保护，部分切除甲状软骨可获得足够的暴露。喉上神经的外侧支在解剖时同样也有损伤的危险（图 56-14）[20]。切除管道及附近的瘢痕组织，当瘘管粘连时作部分甲状腺或者一侧甲状腺切除，并在接近梨状隐窝处结扎，以上被认为是手术中的基本步骤，可完全清除病变，并将复发机会降低到最小。

对于梨状隐窝瘘来说，第四鳃裂疾病的治疗，有可能即使完全切除也不能完全预防复发。第四鳃裂病变的走向仍是理论上的，完整的管道如图 56-5 显示那样，在右侧绕过锁骨下动脉，在左侧绕过主动脉。Shugar 和 Healy 建议不要过度侵袭性地试图切除纵隔

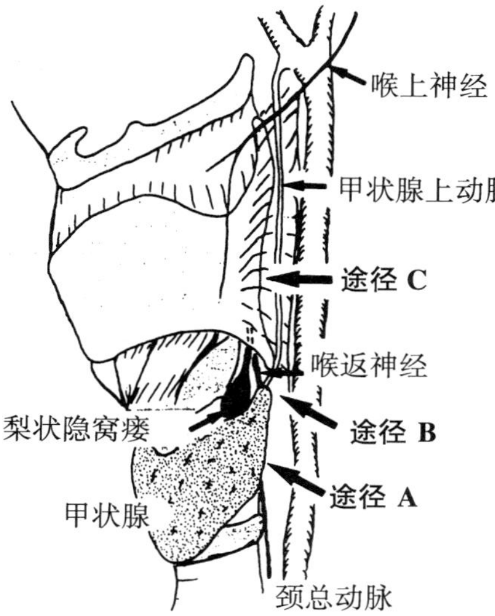

图 56-13　梨状窝瘘的外科操作途径。途径 C 是 Nonomura 和其同事推荐。(From Nonomura N, et al: Surgical approach to piriform sinus fistula. Am J Otolaryngol 1993;14:111.)

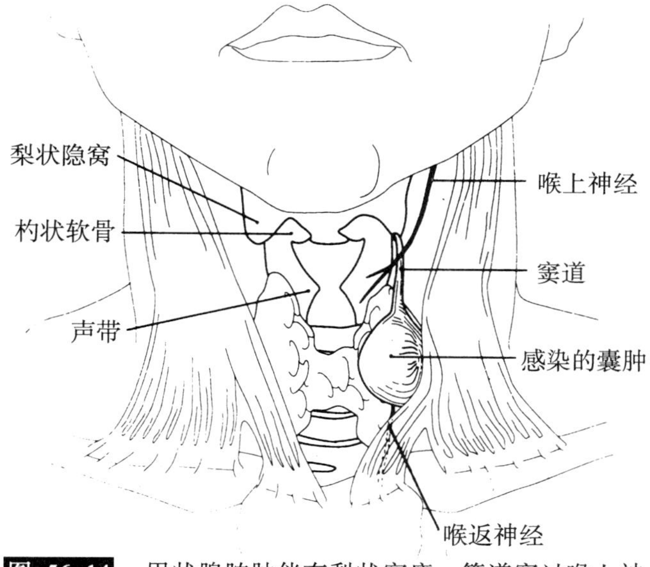

图 56-14　甲状腺脓肿伴有梨状窝瘘，管道穿过喉上神经上方到达喉返神经的上面。注意这相对应的第四鳃裂瘘的走向是从梨状窝顶点开口，下降到喉上神经的深部。

内管道。资料表明，对可疑的深达锁骨的第 10 鳃裂瘘管的解剖可从颈部操作，不必暴露主动脉，也无复发报道[28,67,71]。此外，目前有报道使用内镜下电烧灼[39]或三氯乙酸[60]消除瘘管。这样治疗的患者数量有限，随访时间短，最长的随访时间仅 6 年，另外这些技术的经验可支持它们被应用于那些有反复感染和以前有手术史的患者，在完整切除有危险时作进一步的尝试。

甲状舌管囊肿

外科医生对术前颈部中线位置的肿块的诊断可能很少有疑问，但他们常常犯错误。Knight 和其同事发现 28 位外科医生在 10 年间对 146 例患者做出的术前诊断中只有 61%的诊断是正确的[41]，外科医生作出的术后诊断和最终的诊断符合率为 83%；稍超过 50%的病例为甲状舌管囊肿，25%为皮样囊肿，15%为增大的淋巴结，1.4%为异位的甲状腺，还有 5%为不明原因的感染。同样 Torsiglieri 和其同事发现 97 例甲状舌管囊肿患儿中只有 70%术前获得正确诊断[72]。在 Mayo 临床系列中 263 例患者 78%表现为囊肿，剩下的均为自发形成的引流口或者外科手术造成的窦道，40%位于中线稍偏[72]。在一组 381 例报告中，60%与舌骨相连，24%在舌骨上方，13%在其下方，8%位于舌内，其中 1/3 有感染史，1/4 以前有外科处理的经历。多种需氧和厌氧菌从中分离出来，流感嗜血杆菌和金黄色葡萄球菌是最常见的细菌[69]。在大多数的研究系列中男性和女性患病率基本相同。

大多数病例开始为相对良性的表现如无痛性肿块、流液的窦道、或者是触痛性包块，偶尔患者出现口腔异味伴有自发性的囊肿减压。囊肿随吞咽上下活动常常作为可靠的诊断体征，但在低龄儿童很多靠近
舌骨的病变也会随之运动。不常见的表现包括，当病 870
变位于舌根部位[9,66]时严重的呼吸窘迫或婴儿猝死、甲状腺冷小结[48,70]、在甲状舌管囊肿切除后发现舌根部的甲状腺[3]、一侧颈部肿块[70]、前舌瘘管[56]、甲状舌管的放线菌病[13]、舌下附近的甲状舌管囊肿和皮样囊肿[17]、Hodgkin 病[29]以及同时存在的甲状舌管和鳃裂囊肿[72]。

当怀疑有甲状舌管囊肿时最好尽可能在术前明确诊断，而更重要的是确定何时不宜手术和在手术中何时应改变原来的手术计划。

对怀疑有甲状舌管囊肿的患儿术前进行何种检查是个复杂和有争议问题，有些专家认为所有的患者在术前均要进行甲状腺扫描以排除异位甲状腺，这样可避免因患者仅有的有功能甲状腺组织被切除后导致的

甲状腺功能减退，虽然如 Enepekides 指出的大多数颈部异位甲状腺患者有甲状腺功能减退[20]。这些患者使用外源性的甲状腺素可以减小因为增加的代谢需要导致异位甲状腺代偿性增生，这些患者要避免外科手术。也有内科医生成功的“切除”异位甲状腺的有趣报道[62]。

给所有的颈部正中包块的患者进行核素扫描使费用明显增加，也有提出处理这些问题的其他方法，异位甲状腺被误诊为甲状舌管囊肿的发生率在 1%～2%[4]，如果包括皮样囊肿和颈前淋巴结，这些被误诊为甲状舌管囊肿的病例比例更低。因此，理论上为了分辨出一个异位甲状腺要进行超过 100 次以上的阴性扫描是一种浪费，更不用提倡百位患者暴露于不必要的放射性辐射。对 1978～1987 年在 Boston 儿童医院和 Cleveland's Rainbow 儿童医院做过甲状腺扫描的儿童的回顾性研究后，Radkowski 和其同事建议只对经仔细的病史询问和体检或者有异常甲状腺功能指标提示甲状腺功能减退（例如慢性便秘、生长和发育迟缓、过度嗜睡，尽管喂养差但体重增加，以及促甲状腺激素上升）[64]。其他人建议，当术前 B 超提示颈部肿块为实性包块，或正常位置不能明确甲状腺组织时进行核素扫描[78,81]。当术中发现未预料的实性包块可以冰冻活检切片以证实诊断，然后做出决定是否通过自体移植方式保留腺体或者切除异源性的腺体。这两组病例中常需要终身使用外源性甲状腺素，尽管在一些存在正常甲状腺组织的病例不是必需的[30]。最好在术前对家长告知这些可能性。

CT[21]、MRI[47]、瘘管造影、细针穿刺[63]加血清甲状腺素水平测定、超声和核素扫描都被建议用于颈部正中肿块的术前检查，除了那些缺乏相关病理性腺病、怀疑有喉部结构损伤或反复复发的病变很少需要，然而在合适的指征下它们非常有用（图 56–15 和 56–16）。

感染的甲状舌管囊肿应先给以抗生素治疗，如果需要则行针刺抽吸。切开和引流会导致管道上皮的种植，因此应尽可能避免，以减少以后切除病变后的复发，对有感染病史的病例进行 Sistrunk 手术时建议使用抗生素，术后如果没有呼吸或者吞咽困难，以及家庭环境可靠的情况下无需住院过夜[33]。

很多文章报道了复发性甲状舌管囊肿的治疗[19,36,50,61,75]，尽管多数复发被早期发现，但也有术后间

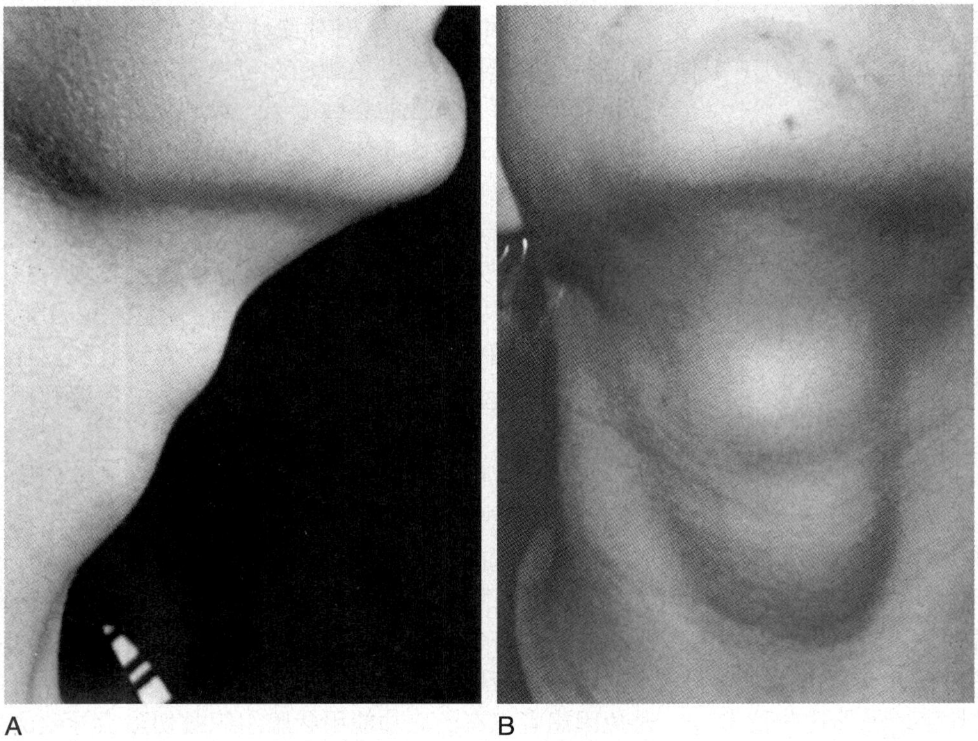

图 56–15 侧面（A）和前后位（B）可以见到两个颈前的包块，这是临床上 1 例 14 岁的儿童，上方的肿块存在有 1 年，下方的 2～3 月出现而且逐渐增大。

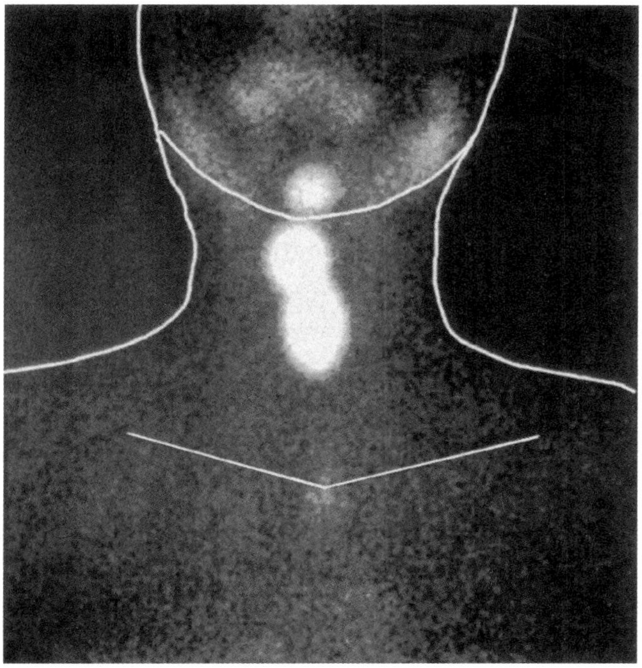

图 56-16　超声波检查发现的颈部实性肿块用甲状腺 ^{99m}Tc 扫描获得的正位图像，促甲状腺激素水平处于正常上限。临床上发现的两个颈部肿块具有放射性活性，之前未发现的位于舌根部的肿块也有放射性活性，而颈部下方无放射性活性，这些发现提示在三个位置有异位甲状腺。该患儿在儿童放疗科医生的建议下通过 ^{131}I 内放射性治疗，肿块消失。9 年之后该患者成为药学学生，继续研究甲状腺素替代治疗。

隔 39 年复发的报道[36]。患者的年龄、侵及皮肤、感染病史或者当时存在感染、分叶状囊肿、术中囊肿破裂以及没有切除舌骨中段、没有切除舌骨前的核心组织均是导致复发的危险因素。再次手术的原则包括广泛切除可能存在的向下延伸的锥状叶、切除中央 3～4cm 的带状肌肉直到气管前筋膜水平，并再稍宽地切除舌骨中段，以及切除深达舌盲孔的条索组织。据报道按照这些原则再次手术后可以减少 25%～35%的复发率[50,69]。

据估计少于 1%的甲状舌管囊肿会发展成癌[4]，自 1994 年以来在成人共有 158 例被报道，但有一例 6 岁儿童也被报道[14,80]，80%为乳头状癌，但除了髓样癌所有类型的甲状腺恶性肿瘤都有出现[80]。对于没有包膜侵犯、无局部和远处转移时，Sistrunk术被认为是适当的。对于乳头状癌这种手术的治愈率有望达到 95%，对于其他类型的癌肿需要更广泛的手术和术后放疗[80]。

皮样囊肿

皮样囊肿的诊断是建立在病理发现囊壁内存在带有上皮附件的上皮，如毛囊、毛发、皮脂腺，这些囊
肿在颈前部沿着胚胎融合线形成[14]。它们术前常和甲 871
状舌管囊肿混淆，因为它们有相同的分布，并可出现感染。同样当病变接近舌骨时，在术中也会混淆。当有疑问时，目前推荐采用 Sistrunk 术[15,76]。穿刺或切开这些囊肿可导致囊内容物溢出，可导致感染或复发。

耳前囊肿

耳前囊肿在此讨论不是因为它们真正表现为颈部囊肿和窦道，而是因为它们需要与第一鳃裂囊肿相区别。耳前囊肿较常见，通常是双侧的，有遗传倾向，只有很罕见情况下会因感染牵涉面神经或进入外耳道导致复杂化[49]。它们被认为是外耳形成中的异常导致，外耳来自于位于前 2 个鳃弓上背侧末端三个突起中的两个。Singer 强调典型情况下发现这类囊肿均有与皮肤相通的窦道[68]。可以通过倒 L 型切口切除所有的管道成功切除，当以前有过感染形成瘢痕时切除比较困难。一般认为有症状的病例有外科手术指征，但仍并不清楚没有症状的是否需要切除，很多病例可终
身不引起临床问题。 872

胸腺囊肿

颈部低位的实质性肿块在儿童罕见，Wagner 和其同事收集了至 1988 年的 75 例 20 岁以下胸腺囊肿病例和 10 例其他病例[82]，诊断是建立在出现纺锤状细胞、螺旋性细胞或者柱状细胞、胆固醇结晶、Hassall 小体和巨细胞反应，所有的这些均可发生在低位鳃裂异常。它们表现为可移动的囊性包块，位于前方但是延伸到胸锁乳突肌下三分之一后方。尽管通常无症状，10%的患者可出现明显的呼吸道症状和吞咽困

难、颈部疼痛或声音嘶哑[31]。它们最有可能是第三或第四鳃裂的残留物。

（李巍松译 吴晔明校）

参考文献

1. Adams A: First endoscopic neck surgery deemed a success. Stanford Hosp Clin Med Staff Update Online 2002;26:1.
2. Alberti PW, Biagioni E: Facial paralysis in children: A review of 150 cases. Laryngoscope 1972;82:1013.
3. Alderson DJ, Lannigan FJ: Lingual thyroid presenting after previous thyroglossal cyst excision. J Laryngol Otol 1994; 108:341.
4. Allard RH: The thyroglossal cyst. Head Neck Surg 1982; 5:134.
5. Androulakis M, Johnson JT, Wagner RL: Thyroglossal duct and second branchial cleft anomalies in adults. Ear Nose Throat J 1990;69:318.
6. Arnot RS: Defects of the first branchial cleft. S Afr J Surg 1971;9:93.
7. Borger JA, Bercu BB: Papillary-follicular carcinoma arising in a thyroglossal duct cyst in a 12-year-old child. J Pediatr Surg 1988;23:362.
8. Burgess KL, Hartwick RW, Bedard YC: Metastatic squamous carcinoma presenting as a neck cyst: Differential diagnosis from inflamed branchial cleft cyst in fine needle aspirates. Acta Cytol 1993;37:494.
9. Byard RW, Bourne AJ, Silver MM: The association of lingual thyroglossal duct remnants with sudden death in infancy. Int J Pediatr Otorhinolaryngol 1990;20:107.
10. Celis I, Bijnens E, Peene P, Cleeren P: The use of preoperative fistulography in patients with a second branchial cleft anomaly. Eur Radiol 1998;8:1179.
11. Chandler JR, Mitchell B: Branchial cleft cysts, sinuses, and fistulas. Otolaryngol Clin North Am 1981;14:175.
12. Chin AC, Radhakrishnan J, Slatton D, Geissler G: Congenital cysts of the third and fourth pharyngeal pouches or pyriform sinus cysts. J Pediatr Surg 2000;35:1252.
13. Cobb RA, Ross HB: Actinomycosis in a persistent thyroglossal duct. Br J Surg 1986;73:751.
14. Cunningham MJ: The management of congenital neck masses. Am J Otolaryngol 1992;13:78.
15. deMello DE, Lima JA, Liapis H: Midline cervical cysts in children: Thyroglossal anomalies. Arch Otolaryngol Head Neck Surg 1987;113:418.
16. Dougall AJ: Anomalies of the first branchial cleft. J Pediatr Surg 1974;9:203.
17. Drucker C, Gerson CR: Sublingual contiguous thyroglossal and dermoid cysts in a neonate. Int J Pediatr Otorhinolaryngol 1992;23:181.
18. Durrant TJ, Sevick RJ, Lauryssen C, MacRae ME: Parapharyngeal branchial cleft cyst presenting with cranial nerve palsies. Can Assoc Radiol J 1994;45:134.
19. Ein SH, Shandling B, Stephens CA, Mancer K: The problem of recurrent thyroglossal duct remnants. J Pediatr Surg 1984;19:437.
20. Enepekides DJ: Management of congenital anomalies of the neck. Facial Plast Surg Clin North Am 2001;9:131.
21. Faerber EN, Swartz JD: Imaging of neck masses in infants and children. Crit Rev Diagn Imaging 1991;31:283.
22. Farrior JB, Santini H: Facial nerve identification in children. Otolaryngol Head Neck Surg 1985;93:173.
23. Ford GR, Balakrishnan A, Evans JN, Bailey CM: Branchial cleft and pouch anomalies. J Laryngol Otol 1992;106:137.
24. Franciosi JP, Sell LL, Conley SF, Bolender DL: Pyriform sinus malformations: A cadaveric representation. J Pediatr Surg 2002;37:533.
25. Gatot A, Tovi F, Fliss DM, Yanai-Inbar I: Branchial cleft cyst manifesting as hypoglossal nerve palsy. Head Neck 1991; 13:249.
26. Gatti WM, Zimm J: Bilateral branchial cleft fistulas: Diagnosis and management of two cases. Ear Nose Throat J 1988;67:256.
27. Girvigian MR, Rechdouni AK, Zeger GD, et al: Squamous cell carcinoma arising in a second branchial cleft cyst. Am J Clin Oncol 2004;27:96.
28. Godin MS, Kearns DB, Pransky SM, et al: Fourth branchial pouch sinus: Principles of diagnosis and management. Laryngoscope 1990;100:174.
29. Good GM, Isaacson G: Hodgkin's disease simulating a pediatric thyroglossal duct cyst. Am J Otolaryngol 2000; 21:277.
30. Grant DB, Hulse JA, Jackson DB, et al: Ectopic thyroid: Residual function after withdrawal of treatment in infancy and later childhood. Acta Paediatr Scand 1989;78:889.
31. Guba AM Jr, Adam AE, Jaques DA, Chambers RG: Cervical presentation of thymic cysts. Am J Surg 1978;136:430.
32. Haus BM, Kambham N, Le D, et al: Surgical robotic applications in otolaryngology. Laryngoscope 2003;113:1139.
33. Helmus C, Grin M, Westfall R: Same-day-stay head and neck surgery. Laryngoscope 1992;102:1331.
34. Himi T, Kataura A: Distribution of C cells in the thyroid gland with pyriform sinus fistula. Otolaryngol Head Neck Surg 1995;112:268.
35. Horisawa M, Niinomi N, Ito T: Anatomical reconstruction of the thyroglossal duct. J Pediatr Surg 1991;26:766.
36. Howard DJ, Lund VJ: Thyroglossal ducts, cysts and sinuses: A recurrent problem. Ann R Coll Surg Engl 1986;68:137.
37. Ikarashi F, Nakano Y, Nonomura N, et al: Clinical features of first branchial cleft anomalies. Am J Otolaryngol 1996; 17:233.
38. Isaacson G, Martin WH: First branchial cleft cyst excision with electrophysiological facial nerve localization. Arch Otolaryngol Head Neck Surg 2000;126:513.
39. Jordan JA, Graves JE, Manning SC, et al: Endoscopic cauterization for treatment of fourth branchial cleft sinuses. Arch Otolaryngol Head Neck Surg 1998;124:1021.
40. Kaneko T, Kitamura T, Asano H: Anomalies of the first branchial cleft (fistula and cyst). J Laryngol Otol 1974;88:1213.
41. Knight PJ, Hamoudi AB, Vassy LE: The diagnosis and treatment of midline neck masses in children. Surgery 1983;93:603.
42. Kornblut AD: Traumatic facial nerve injuries in children. Adv Otorhinolaryngol 1977;22:171.
43. Kubota M, Suita S, Kamimura T, Zaizen Y: Surgical strategy for the treatment of pyriform sinus fistula. J Pediatr Surg 1997;32:34.

44. Lin AE, Losken HW, Jaffe R, Biglan AW: The branchio-oculo-facial syndrome. Cleft Palate Craniofac J 1991;28:96.
45. Lin JN, Wang KL: Persistent third branchial apparatus. J Pediatr Surg 1991;26:663.
46. Liston SL: The relationship of the facial nerve and first branchial cleft anomalies—embryologic considerations. Laryngoscope 1982;92:1308.
47. Massoud TF, Schnetler JF: Case report: Taste of success in thyroglossal fistulography. Clin Radiol 1992;45:281.
48. McHenry CR, Danish R, Murphy T, Marty JJ: Atypical thyroglossal duct cyst: A rare cause for a solitary cold thyroid nodule in childhood. Am Surg 1993;59:223.
49. Melnick M, Myrianthopoulos NC, Paul NW: External ear malformations: Epidemiology, genetics, and natural history. Birth Defects Orig Artic Ser 1979;15:i.
50. Mickel RA, Calcaterra TC: Management of recurrent thyroglossal duct cysts. Arch Otolaryngol 1983;109:34.
51. Miller D, Hill JL, Sun CC, et al: The diagnosis and management of pyriform sinus fistulae in infants and young children. J Pediatr Surg 1983;18:377.
52. Miyauchi A, Matsuzuka F, Kuma K, Katayama S: Piriform sinus fistula and the ultimobranchial body. Histopathology 1992;20:221.
53. Miyauchi A, Matsuzuka F, Kuma K, Takai S: Piriform sinus fistula: An underlying abnormality common in patients with acute suppurative thyroiditis. World J Surg 1990;14:400.
54. Mouri N, Muraji T, Nishijima E, Tsugawa C: Reappraisal of lateral cervical cysts in neonates: Pyriform sinus cysts as an anatomy-based nomenclature. J Pediatr Surg 1998; 33:1141.
55. Murthy P, Shenoy P, Khan NA: First cleft branchial fistula in a child—a modified surgical technique. J Laryngol Otol 1994;108:1078.
56. Ngo HH, Frenkiel S, Satin R: Thyroglossal duct cyst presenting as an anterior tongue fistula, J Otolaryngol 1988; 17:227.
57. Nicollas R, Guelfucci B, Roman S, Triglia JM: Congenital cysts and fistulas of the neck. Int J Pediatr Otorhinolaryngol 2000;55:117.
58. Nonomura N, Ikarashi F, Fujisaki T, Nakano Y: Surgical approach to pyriform sinus fistula. Am J Otolaryngol 1993;14:111.
59. Olsen KD, Maragos NE, Weiland LH: First branchial cleft anomalies. Laryngoscope 1980;90:423.
60. Park SW, Han MH, Sung MH et al: Neck infection associated with pyriform sinus fistula: Imaging findings. AJNR Am J Neuroradiol 2000;21:817.
61. Pelausa ME, Forte V: Sistrunk revisited: A 10-year review of revision thyroglossal duct surgery at Toronto's Hospital for Sick Children. J Otolaryngol 1989;18:325.
62. Pinczower E, Crockett DM, Atkinson JB, Kun S: Preoperative thyroid scanning in presumed thyroglossal duct cysts. Arch Otolaryngol Head Neck Surg 1992;118:985.
63. Pitts WC, Tani EM, Skoog L: Papillary carcinoma in fine needle aspiration smears of a thyroglossal duct lesion. Acta Cytol 1988;32:599.
64. Radkowski D, Arnold J, Healy GB, et al: Thyroglossal duct remnants: Preoperative evaluation and management. Arch Otolaryngol Head Neck Surg 1991;117:1378.
65. Robichaud J, Papsin BC, Forte V: Third branchial cleft anomaly detected in utero. J Otolaryngol 2000;29:185.
66. Samuel M, Freeman NV, Sajwany MJ: Lingual thyroglossal duct cyst presenting in infancy. J Pediatr Surg 1993;28:891.
67. Shugar MA, Healy GB: The fourth branchial cleft anomaly. Head Neck Surg 1980;3:72.
68. Singer R: A new technic for extirpation of preauricular cysts. Am J Surg 1966;111:291.
69. Solomon JR, Rangecroft L: Thyroglossal-duct lesions in childhood. J Pediatr Surg 1984;19:555.
70. Sonnino RE, Spigland N, Laberge JM, et al: Unusual patterns of congenital neck masses in children. J Pediatr Surg 1989;24:966.
71. Takimoto T, Yoshizaki T, Ohoka H, Sakashita H: Fourth branchial pouch anomaly. J Laryngol Otol 1990;104:905.
72. Telander RL, Deane SA: Thyroglossal and branchial cleft cysts and sinuses. Surg Clin North Am 1977;57:779.
73. Terris DJ, Haus BM, Gourin CG: Endoscopic neck surgery: Resection of the submandibular gland in a cadaver model. Laryngoscope 2004;114:407.
74. Terris DJ, Monfared A, Thomas A, et al: Endoscopic selective neck dissection in a porcine model. Arch Otolaryngol Head Neck Surg 2003;129:613.
75. Tetteroo GW, Snellen JP, Knegt P, Jeekel J: Operative treatment of median cervical cysts. Br J Surg 1988;75:382.
76. Todd NW: Common congenital anomalies of the neck: Embryology and surgical anatomy, Surg Clin North Am 1993;73:599.
77. Tom LW, Kenealy JF, Torsiglieri AJ Jr: First branchial cleft anomalies involving the tympanic membrane and middle ear. Otolaryngol Head Neck Surg 1991;105:473.
78. Torsiglieri AJ Jr, Tom LW, Ross AJ 3rd, et al: Pediatric neck masses: Guidelines for evaluation. Int J Pediatr Otorhinolaryngol 1988;16:199.
79. Tyler D, Effmann E, Shorter N: Pyriform sinus cyst and fistula in the newborn: The value of endoscopic cannulation. J Pediatr Surg 1992;27:1500.
80. Van Vuuren PA, Balm AJ, Gregor RT, et al: Carcinoma arising in thyroglossal remnants. Clin Otolaryngol 1994;19:509.
81. Wadsworth DT, Siegel MJ: Thyroglossal duct cysts: Variability of sonographic findings. AJR Am J Roentgenol 1994;163:1475.
82. Wagner CW, Vinocur CD, Weintraub WH, Golladay ES: Respiratory complications in cervical thymic cysts. J Pediatr Surg 1988;23:657.
83. Work WP: Newer concepts of first branchial cleft defects. Laryngoscope 1972;82:1581.

第 57 章

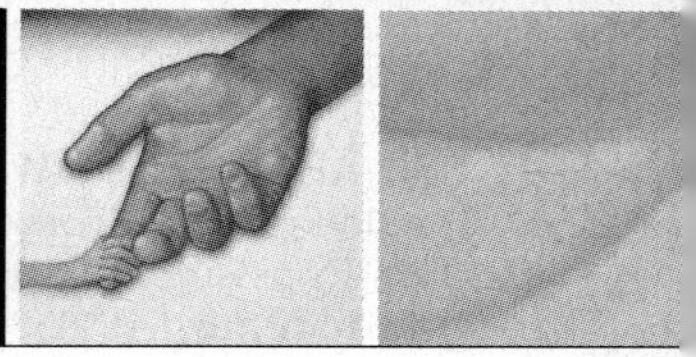

斜　颈

Spencer Beasley

875 有很多原因可引起儿童斜颈（表 57-1），但大多数原因是罕见的。最常见的原因是一侧的胸锁乳突肌紧缩和变短，这种情况在所有出生小儿中的发生率为 0.4%。典型的情况下，在出生后大约 3 周可以触摸或看到部分或全部胸锁乳突肌肿胀；这种肿胀称为胸锁乳突肌瘤。后者发生在右侧者占 60%[31]，双侧者占 2%～8%[43,45]，通常持续一年。年长的儿童会出现纤维化和缩短的胸锁乳突肌，在许多病例中，一般认为是先前没有被注意到的胸锁乳突肌瘤遗留所致。

历史

亚历山大大帝可能患有斜颈，这归功于希腊的历史学家 Plutarch[38]。据说 Antyllus 在公元前 350 年施行过肌腱切断术，但是第一次证实的胸锁乳突肌分离是 1641 年 Minnus 在阿姆斯特丹施行的。1826 年 Heusinger 首次描述了胸锁乳突肌瘤[23]，斜颈也是 Dupuybren 感兴趣的一个课题[18]。

表 57-1　导致儿童和婴儿斜颈的原因

病因	注释
胸锁乳突肌瘤	常见；通常在出生后 3 周出现
宫内位置异常	随着年龄会好转
颈部淋巴结炎 / 脓肿	急性；通常在出生后 2 岁以内
咽后壁脓肿	急性；有中毒症状
后颅凹肿瘤	罕见；有其他神经系统症状
急性寰枕关节半脱位	可能发生在扁桃体切除术后[2]
寰枕关节旋转半脱位	其重要性有争议[25]，通过动态 CT 诊断
痉挛伴有胃食管反流	Sanifer 综合征
体位性	家族性

病因学

尽管曾提出过几种理论来解释这种情况，但对乳突肌纤维化的病因目前知之甚少。其可能与宫内特定的胚胎发育异常有关[29]，或可能是胎位异常造成的胸锁乳突肌分隔综合征的表现[25]。高比率的难产，如臀先露等需要助产[10,11]，可能是胸锁乳突肌变短的结果，而不是其原因。至今没有报道表明，产前 B 超检查会发现胸锁乳突肌瘤[49]。伴随有臀部的异常较为常见[10]。

病理学

最基本的组织学异常是肌束被纤维代替[34]。Jones[29]曾经描述肌肉内膜纤维化，胶原和成纤维细胞在每个肌纤维周围沉积可导致肌肉萎缩。肌浆核压缩在一起形成巨大的细胞，看上去像多核细胞。这些纤维在新生儿期的成熟度提示，这些病变发生在出生之前[17,29,32]，可能引起分娩困难。据报道，有臀先露的发生率约为 20%～30%[14]，较正常出生者的高很多。大约 60%的斜颈婴儿在出生时会遇到复杂的情况[14]，提示肌肉的纤维化会导致胎儿在宫内胎位的异常，并可能会造成胎头入盆的困难。

未处理的胸锁乳突肌纤维化 50%～70%在出生后 6 个月可完全消退。大约 10%的患儿的肿块和胸锁乳突肌缩短会持续到 12 个月[15,43]。纤维化程度和分布各异，导致多种分类。分类是基于可触及的胸锁乳突肌 876
局部肿块，或整块肌肉增厚缩短，或基于超声发现。

系统的分级有很重要的预后提示作用：病变位于肌肉之内无论是临床还是 B 超诊断[27,42]，一般比整个肌肉完全受累者容易自行缓解。在有斜颈的较大年龄儿童中，纤维降解的表现，更伴有肌肉失用性萎缩，这是由于纤维化导致活动受限造成。

临床特征

肌源性斜颈

肿块通常为坚硬的、纺锤状的、孤立无痛的肿块，直径大约 1～3cm，位于胸锁乳突肌内。90%出现在出生后的 3 个月以内[10]。通常出现在出生后的 3 个星期。明显的斜颈和头部歪斜在其后发生[49]。在婴儿期，头部旋转向肿块的对侧，头部向病变侧少许弯曲（图 57–1）。

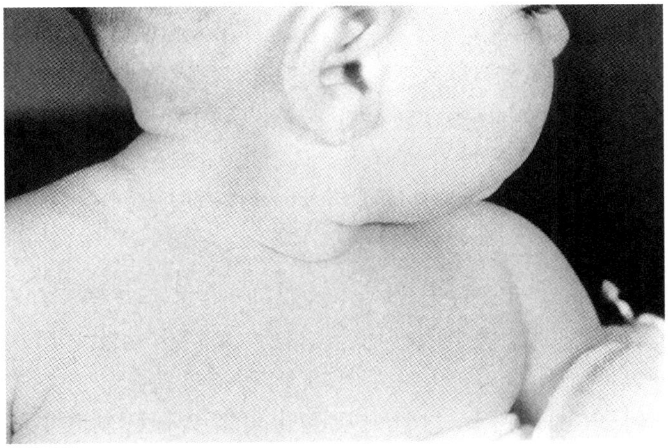

图 57–1 婴儿右侧胸锁乳突肌瘤的表现；头偏向对侧。

在其他患者，胸锁乳突肌肌瘤是不连续的，看上去为胸锁乳突肌整个增厚变紧。这些变化限制了头部的旋转和侧曲（图 57–2）。在头旋转过程中胸锁乳突肌的动作是很容易测量的，可以通过站在患儿的后方在两手之间旋转其头部来评价。当把患儿的头部向患侧旋转时，病变的胸锁乳突肌伸展到其最大长度。如果肌肉发生纤维化，则不能伸展到其最大长度，所以头部向同侧的旋转受到限制。

有斜颈的年长儿童会通过抬高一侧肩膀使眼睛尽可能保持水平来弥补明显的倾斜。年幼的婴儿没有这种变化，因为只有到他们能站起来的时候才需要保持视线的水平[28]。而且大龄的孩子不把他们的头向对侧旋转过多，而是通过扭转脖子和背部来使他们的眼睛向前看。

鉴别诊断

最初的临床评估需要了解斜颈是由于一侧胸锁乳突肌变短造成的，还是由于其他原因造成的。在胸锁乳突肌纤维化的患者，肌肉的前缘突起像拉紧的带子，虽然有些小婴儿脖子比较短，肌肉很难轻易看到。此时需要对肌肉的全长进行触诊，明确有无胸锁乳突肌部分或全部变厚、纤维化。大约 2/3 的患儿有明确的局部肿块，而其他患儿则为整个胸锁乳突肌病变。B 超检查对于诊断不是必需的，但是 B 超的典型表现可以提供能否自行缓解的线索[19,31,42]。斜颈还可以通过核磁共振（MRI）[19]和 CT[33]来诊断。当患儿的肌肉无明显的突起和缩短的时候，要考虑非胸锁乳突肌病变，需要寻找其他造成斜颈的原因（见表 57–1，877
图 57–4）[3,28]。

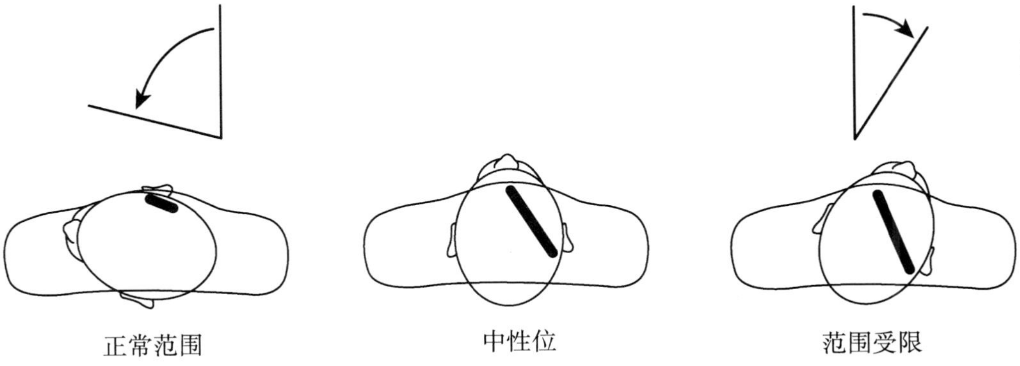

图 57–2 从头顶观察，由于胸锁乳突肌缩短造成头部的旋转限制，黑色的棒表示右侧胸锁乳突肌，表明如果不能延长，会限制向该侧的旋转。

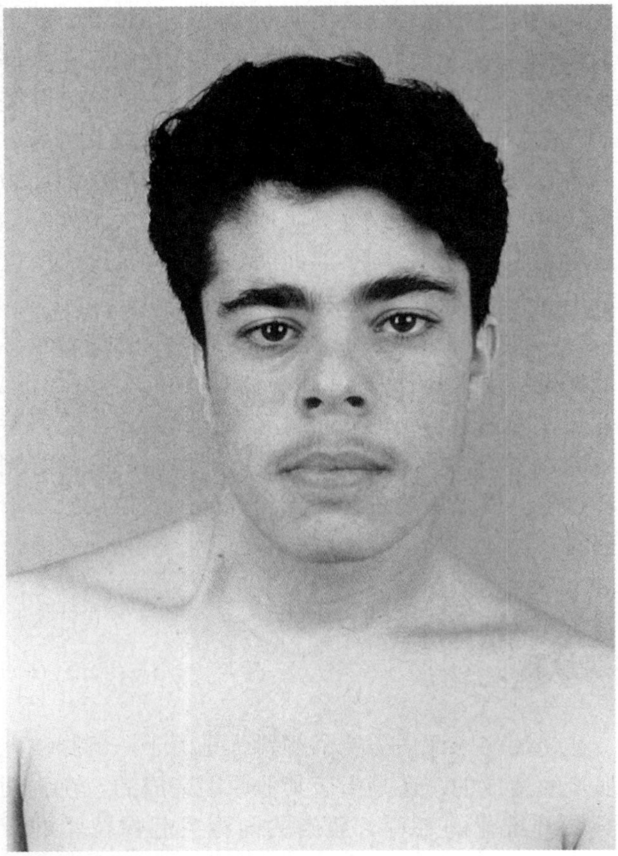

图 57-3 一位大龄儿童由于胸锁乳突肌纤维化造成的斜颈表现。眼睛保持水平，但是变短的胸锁乳突肌导致补偿性的肩膀抬高。(From Beasley SW: Pediatric Diagnosis. London, Chapman & Hall, 1994.)

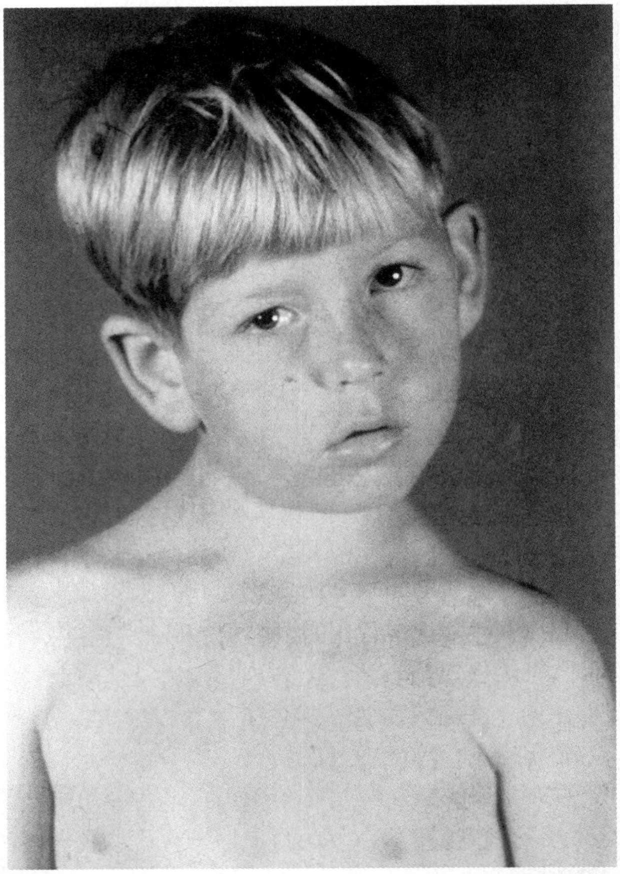

图 57-4 扁桃腺切除术后寰枕关节半脱位造成的斜颈。注意到两次均没有胸锁乳突肌紧张。(From Beasley SW: Pediatric Diagnosis. London, Chapman & Hall, 1994.)

斜视患儿为了平衡眼球的旋转也会斜颈，开始斜视不一定很明显，因为斜颈可以补偿

眼球位置的异常。如使头竖直，斜视会变得明显。有时候胸锁乳突肌的纤维化同时会伴有眼性斜颈。

后颅凹肿瘤有可能会在枕骨大孔压迫脑干，导致颈部的僵硬，使头向一侧偏斜。此时颈部会被固定在一个位置并出现运动困难。中枢神经系统肿瘤可能是已知的，偶尔斜颈可为其首发症状。仔细的神经系统检查有可能显示低位颅神经异常和小脑功能异常，具体的病因可以通过 CT 或 MRI 来明确。

累及颈椎的半锥体可导致头部偏斜，这从出生后就会出现，一般不会进展。脊柱的病变可以通过对脊柱背侧的检查和触摸来获得临床诊断，并可通过拍摄颈部的平片来明确。

急性斜颈可能由寰枕关节脱位造成，通过动态的 CT 可以明确诊断[36,37]，但是有人认为，当症状和体征非常明确时无需一开始就进行 CT 检查[24]。有报告表明，寰枕半脱位可能出现在扁桃体切除之后[2]，急性斜颈有可能是由颈部炎症和感染造成，包括咽后壁的脓肿[21]，急性淋巴瘤也可能会导致斜颈的发生[39]。

继发性斜颈

878

表 57-2 列出了继发性斜颈的表现。

表 57-2 继发于斜颈的表现

婴儿	斜形头
	半侧面部发育不良
大龄儿童	补偿性的脊柱侧凸

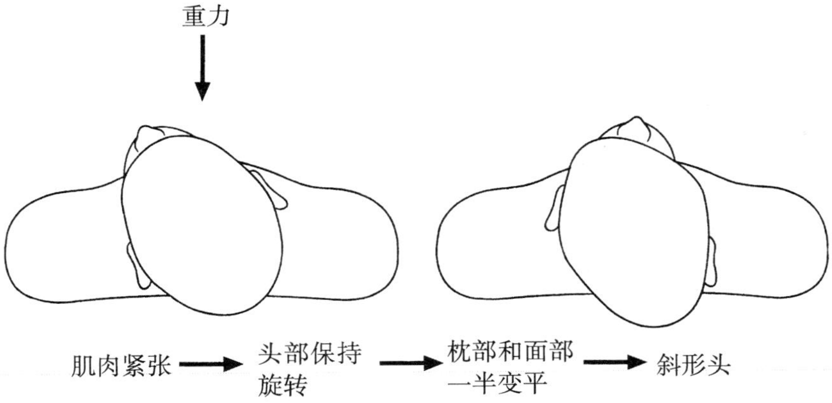

图 57-5 斜形头。

斜形头

在有斜颈和头部相对位置固定的小婴儿，重力会导致相应软的头部变形，这是因为其头部长期位于同样位置造成的。一侧枕部变平会导致对侧额部继发性变平（图 57-5）。这种不对称的颅骨变形称为斜形头，在出生后最初的几个月里会逐渐发展[26]。这种变化从头的上方观察最为明显。当患儿开始站立或斜颈问题解决后，斜形头会自行缓解[35]。斜形头可能需要几年才能消失，极少数孩子会有轻微的永久变形。

面部的发育不良

当胸锁乳突肌使面部长期固定时会出现进行性面部变形。纤维化的胸锁乳突肌固定侧的颧突生长较正常侧缓慢[25]，这会导致进行性不对称（图 57-6）。这种下颌骨和颚骨的生长抑制体现了儿科一个重要的理论：正常骨的发育是建立在正常肌肉运动基础上。

半侧面部发育不良的程度取决于眼平面和嘴平面的夹角。正常情况下两者是平行的，当面部不对称时，两者成角，出现半侧面部发育不良是外科手术的指征之一；分离紧张的胸锁乳突肌会解决骨骼异常并获得正常生长[25]。

明显的半侧面部发育不良在 8 个月大小时就会出现[29]，但经常要到 3～4 岁才被认识[15]。当斜颈被解除之后，其可逐渐变得不明显。

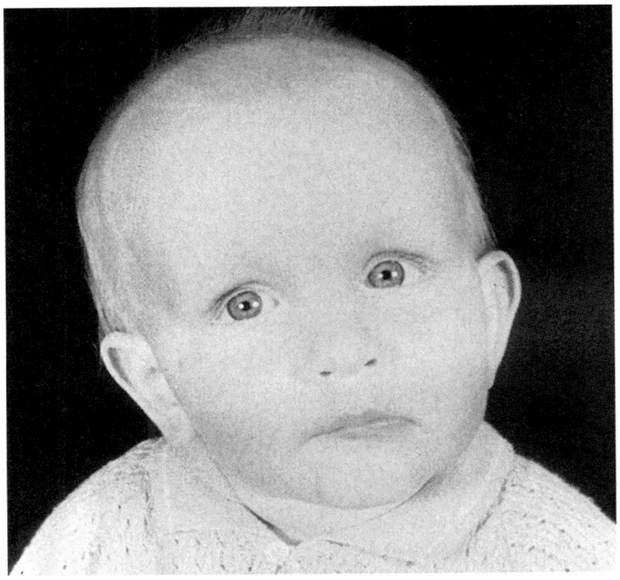

图 57-6 半侧面部发育不良。

体位的补偿

当孩子足够大能够行走时，眼睛要保持水平以有利于保持平衡和眼睛的水平运动。患儿为了补偿纤维化而短缩的胸锁乳突肌而抬高同侧的肩膀（见图 57-3）。另外患儿还可能会通过颈椎和胸椎的侧凸来补偿。相邻的肌肉如斜方肌会因为不活动而失用性萎缩[29]。

保守治疗

很多患儿的胸锁乳突肌纤维化会出现自行缓解，因此很少需要手术治疗[12]。对于在 1 岁以内头部和颈部处理的价值目前没有得到证明[49]，虽然目前的广泛应用可能有益处。理疗和经常性的颈部锻炼是安全的[12]，这只是让患者家属感到给孩子做了治疗。在治疗中无意识的猛拉已经证明对预后改观没有明显的意义[8]。有些临床工作者提倡的早期开始的强力牵拉被报告有较高的缓解率[5,6,25,41]，但没有确实的证
879 据表明这些措施会改变疾病的自然病程。

有些人认为把玩具或其他患儿想要的东西放在对侧、鼓励婴儿向患病的对侧转动很重要[29]。然而实际上这种策略与其说对患儿有好处倒不如说家长有帮助，但这是无害的。试图让孩子在睡眠时面对患侧总是会失败，特别是肌肉很紧的时候。在大多数情况下所要做的只是让家长安心。

手术治疗

手术指征

手术指征包括：

1. 持续性的胸锁乳突肌紧缩限制了头部的运动，且孩子年龄超过 12～15 个月[47]。
2. 持续性的胸锁乳突肌紧缩伴有进行性的半侧面部发育不良。
3. 诊断时患儿年龄超过 1 岁[16]。

手术治疗技巧

手术操作在一般性麻醉下、喉插管或气管插管下进行，这要根据儿科麻醉医生的经验和操作习惯而定。患儿取仰卧位、肩部垫高、颈部转向对侧。肌肉最好在最下端分离切断[25,38]，虽然也可在上端[30]或两端同时[1,7,22]、或在中部切断[20,29]，都有文献描述。内镜下切断也是可行的[4,13,40]。

在病变胸锁乳突肌侧的胸骨和锁骨头上方 1cm 处切开皮肤 3～4cm（图 57–7）。在切开处分离颈阔肌。如果在手术视野中见到颈外静脉，可以牵开。胸锁乳突肌的两个头都必须完全切断，可以通过透热电疗仪切开肌肉以避免出血。肌肉前方、后方以及周围的浅筋膜直到颈后三角同样也要分离（图 57–8）。在

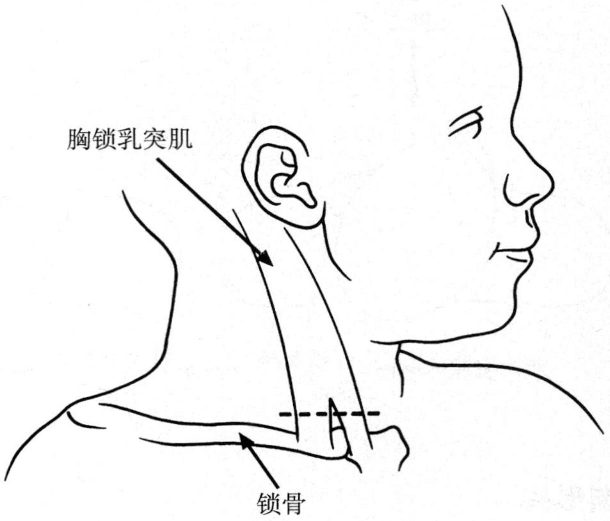

图 57–7 低位切断胸锁乳突肌皮肤切口。

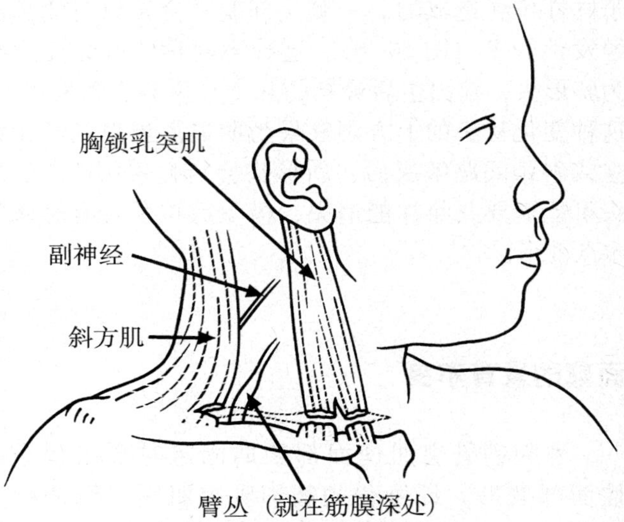

图 57–8 切断胸锁乳突肌和周围的颈筋膜直到斜方肌的前缘。

胸锁乳突肌和斜方肌之间，紧张的颈筋膜可以触摸到，必须在直视下分离，避免造成其他结构损伤，特别是副神经和颈丛神经损伤。

伤口可以用丁哌卡因或其他局部麻醉药局部浸润麻醉，颈阔肌采用 4–0 的可吸收缝线缝合，皮肤采用 5–0 的单股可吸收缝线皮内缝合，不需放置引流管。

该手术可以在一日手术中施行，术后无需限制患儿的活动。术后一周内颈部可以全范围活动。术后的物理治疗通常不是必需的，尽管有些人建议术后延长

一段时间的物理治疗[1]。在大龄儿童，纠正需要更长时间，最后的美容效果不是很确定[9]。

并发症

手术中止血不彻底时会出现血肿。热疗仪可以使出血减少到最小。大的表面血管如果不能牵拉时，需要分离结扎。

如果胸锁乳突肌两个头分离不完全、颈浅筋膜没有完全分离至颈后三角，均会造成持续性斜颈。在术中仔细检查和触摸颈部残留的紧张和束带可以预防这种情况发生。术后斜颈复发是罕见的，发生率低于
880 3%[48]。

随访

术后患儿需要监测直到以下几种情况：（1）斜颈完全解除；（2）头部和颈部能全范围运动；（3）触摸胸锁乳突肌是正常的。大龄儿童合并有继发性脊柱侧凸时，随访中需要进行放射线检查，如果需要，随访可直到脊柱侧凸缓解。

（李巍松译　吴晔明校）

参考文献

1. Arslan H, Gunduz S, Subasy M, et al: Frontal cephalometric analysis in the evaluation of facial asymmetry in torticollis, and outcomes of bipolar release in patients over six years of age. Arch Orthop Trauma Surg 2002;122:489.
2. Bedi HS, Angliss RD, Williams SA, Connelly DP: Torticollis following adenotonsillectomy. Aust N Z J Surg 1999; 69:63.
3. Bredenkamp JK, Hoover LA, Berke GS, Shaw A: Congenital muscular torticollis. A spectrum of disease. Arch Otolaryngol Head Neck Surg 1990;116:212.
4. Burstein FD, Cohen SR: Endoscopic surgical treatment for congenital muscular torticollis. Plast Reconstr Surg 1998;101:20.
5. Cameron BH, Langer JC, Cameron GS: Success of non-operative treatment for congenital muscular torticollis is dependent on early therapy. Pediatr Surg Int 1994; 9:391.
6. Celayir AC: Congenital muscular torticollis: Early and intensive treatment is critical. A prospective study. Pediatr Int 2000;42:504.
7. Chen CE, Ko JY: Surgical treatment of muscular torticollis for patients above six years of age. Arch Orthop Trauma Surg 2000;120:149.
8. Cheng JC, Chen TM, Tang SP, et al: Snapping during manual stretching in congenital muscular torticollis. Clin Orthop 2001;384:237.
9. Cheng JC, Tang SP: Outcome of surgical treatment of congenital muscular torticollis. Clin Orthop 1999;362:190.
10. Cheng JC, Tang SP, Chen TM: Sternocleidomastoid pseudotumor and congenital muscular torticollis in infants: A prospective study of 510 cases. J Pediatr 1999;134:712.
11. Cheng JC, Tang SP, Chen TM, et al: The clinical presentation and outcome of treatment of congenital muscular torticollis in infants—a study of 1,086 cases. J Pediatr Surg 2000;35:1091.
12. Cheng JC, Wong MW, Tang SP, et al: Clinical determinants of the outcome of manual stretching in the treatment of congenital muscular torticollis in infants. A prospective study of 821 cases. J Bone Joint Surg Am 2001;83:679.
13. Cole R: Endoscopic surgical treatment for congenital muscular torticollis. Plast Reconstr Surg 1998;102:579.
14. Davids JR, Wenger DR, Mubarak SJ: Congenital muscular torticollis: Sequela of intrauterine or perinatal compartment syndrome. J Pediatr Orthop 1993;13:141.
15. de Chalain TM, Katz A: Idiopathic muscular torticollis in children: The Cape Town experience. Br J Plast Surg 1992;45:297.
16. Demirbilek S, Atayurt HF: Congenital muscular torticollis and sternomastoid tumour: Results of non-operative treatment. J Pediatr Surg 1999;34:549.
17. Dunn PM: Congenital sternomastoid torticollis: An intrauterine postural deformity. J Bone Joint Surg Br 1973;55:877.
18. Dupuytren G: Lecons Orales de Clinique Chirurgicale. Paris, JB Bailliere et Fils, 1839.
19. Entel RJ, Carolan FJ: Congenital muscular torticollis: Magnetic resonance imaging and ultrasound diagnosis. J Neuroimaging 1997;7:128.
20. Gurpinar A, Kiristioglu I, Balkan E, Dogruyol H: Surgical correction of muscular torticollis in older children with Peter G. Jones technique. J Pediatr Orthop 1998;18:98.
21. Harries PG: Retropharyngeal abscess and acute torticollis. J Laryngol Otol 1997;111:1183.
22. Hellstadius A: Torticollis congenita. Acta Chir Scand 1972;62:586.
23. Heusinger KP: Berichte von konighlichen, anthropanatomischen Anstalt zur Wurtzburg, Ber F D Schuljahr 1824/25, Etlinger, Wurtzburg 1826;4:43.
24. Hicazi A, Acaroglu E, Alanay A, et al: Atlantoaxial rotatory fixation-subluxation revisited: A computed tomographic analysis of acute torticollis in pediatric patients. Spine 2002;27:2771.
25. Hirschl RB: Sternocleidomastoid torticollis. In Spitz L, Coran A (eds): Rob & Smith's Operative Surgery: Pediatric Surgery, 5th ed. London, Chapman & Hall, 1995.
26. Hollier L, Kim J, Grayson BH, McCarthy JG: Congenital muscular torticollis and the associated craniofacial changes. Plast Reconstr Surg 2000;105:827.
27. Hsu TC, Wang CL, Wong MK, et al: Correlation of clinical and ultrasonographic features in congenital muscular torticollis. Arch Phys Med Rehabil 1999;80:637.
28. Hutson JM, Beasley SW: The Surgical Examination of Children. London, Heinemann, 1988.
29. Jones PG: Torticollis in Infancy and Childhood. Springfield IL, Charles C Thomas, 1967.
30. Lange C: Zur Behandlung des Schiefhalses. Wochenschr Orthop Chir 1910;27:440.

31. Lin JN, Chou ML: Ultrasonographic study of the sternocleidomastoid muscle in the management of congenital muscular torticollis. J Pediatr Surg 1997;32:1648.
32. MacDonald D: Sternomastoid tumour and muscular torticollis. J Bone Joint Surg Br 1969;41:432.
33. McGuire KJ, Silber J, Flynn JM, et al: Torticollis in children: Can dynamic computed tomography help determine severity and treatment? J Pediatr Orthop 2002;22:766.
34. Middleton DS: The pathology of congenital torticollis, Br J Surg 1930;18:188.
35. Morrison DL, Macewan GD: Congenital muscular torticollis: Observations regarding clinical findings, associated conditions and results of treatment. J Pediatr Orthop 1982;2:500.
36. Muniz AE, Belfer RA: Atlantoaxial rotary subluxation in children. Pediatr Emerg Care 1999;15:25.
37. Nicholson P, Higgins T, Fogarty E, et al: Three-dimensional spiral CT scanning in children with acute torticollis. Int Orthop 1999;23:47.
38. Peterson F: Zur Frage des Kopfnickerhamatoms bei Neugeborenen. Zentralbl Gynzkol 1886;10:777.
39. Rauch R, Jungert J, Rupprecht T, Greil J: Torticollis revealing as a symptom of acute lymphoblastic leukaemia in a 14 month old girl. Acta Paediatr 2002;90:587.
40. Sasaki S, Yamamoto Y, Sugihara T, et al: Endoscopic tenotomy of the sternocleidomastoid muscle: New method for surgical correction of muscular torticollis. Plast Reconstr Surg 2000;105:1764.
41. Stassen LF, Kerawala CJ: New surgical technique for the correction of congenital muscular torticollis (wry neck). Br J Oral Maxillofac Surg 2000;38:142.
42. Tang SF, Hsu KH, Wong AM, et al: Longitudinal followup study of ultrasonography in congenital muscular torticollis. Clin Orthop 2002;403:179.
43. Thomsen JR, Koltai PJ: Sternomastoid tumour of infancy. Ann Otol Rhinol Laryngol 1989;98:955.
44. Tubby AH: Deformities, 2nd ed. London, Macmillan, 1912.
45. Tufano RP, Tom LW, Austin MB: Bilateral sternocleidomastoid tumors of infancy. Int J Pediatr Otorhinolaryngol 1999;51:41.
46. Turgut M: Torticollis secondary to posterior fossa tumors. J Pediatr Orthop 1998;18:415.
47. Wei JL, Schwartz KM, Weaver AL, Orvidas LJ: Pseudotumor of infancy and congenital muscular torticollis: 170 cases. Laryngoscope 2001;111:688.
48. Wirth CJ, Hagena FW, Wuelker N, Siebert WE: Biterminal tenotomy for the treatment of congenital muscular torticollis. Long-term results. J Bone Joint Surg Am 1992;74:427.
49. Wright JE: Sternomastoid tumour and torticollis in infancy and childhood. Paediatr Surg Int 1994;9:172.

第六部分

胸部疾病

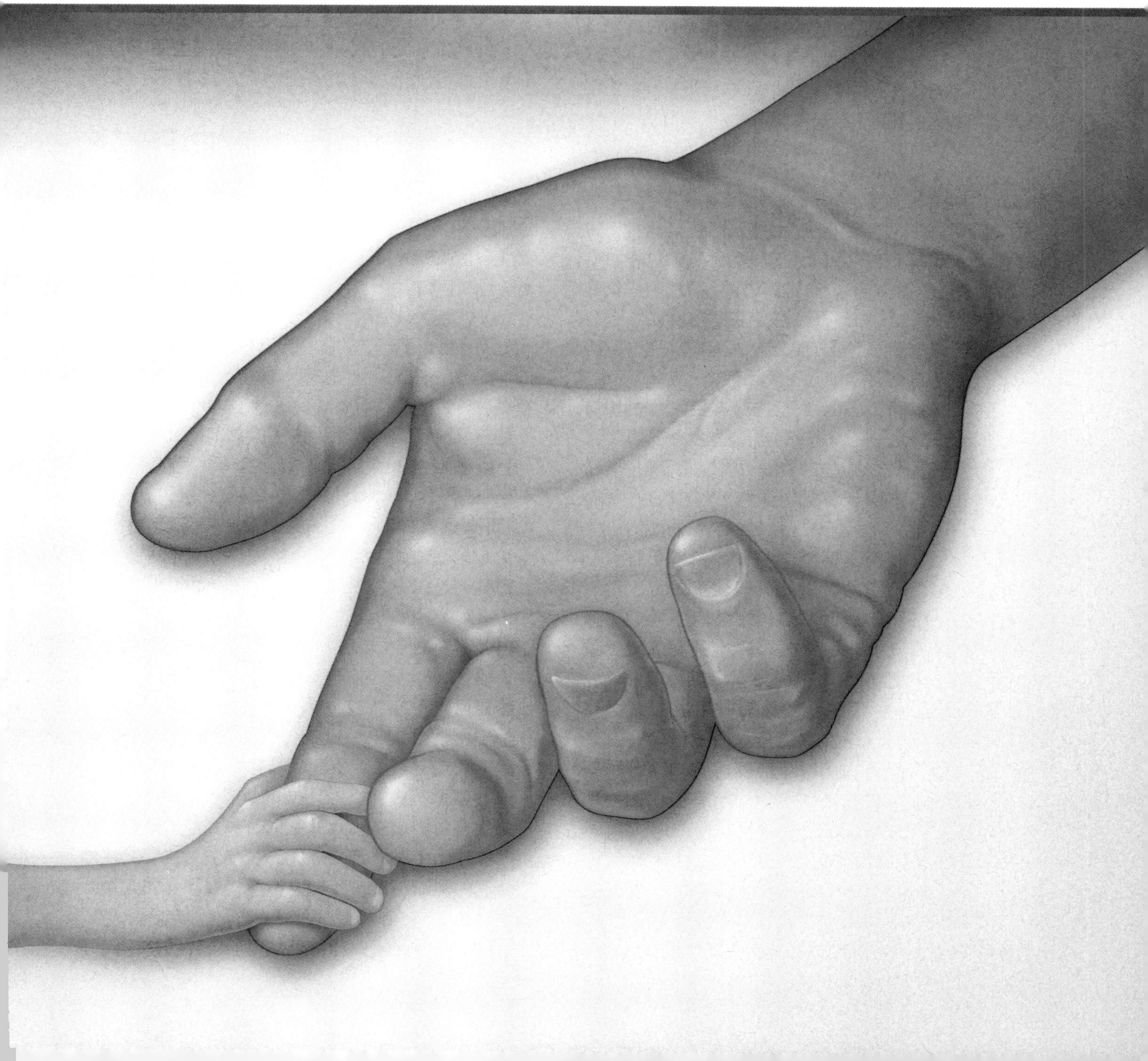

第 58 章

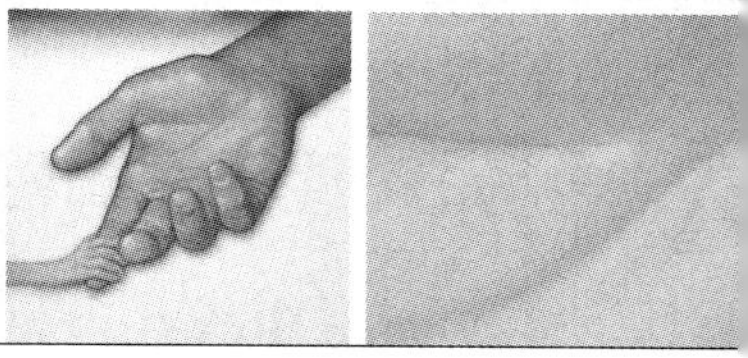

乳房疾病

Mary L. Brandt

在妊娠 35 天左右，当身体前壁的外胚层增厚形成被称为乳房线、乳线或者 Hughes 线[20]的皱褶时，乳房开始发育。这一皱褶组织从发育中的腋窝区域开始向发育中的腹股沟管延伸。足月婴儿的，乳线延伸进入腋窝，并向下延伸到腹股沟区域的大腿内侧。胸肌区域上下的乳线在妊娠第 10 周左右消退，留下乳腺原基，这是输乳管的起源[12,41]。在妊娠 10～20 周之间，原始管道形成，并散布进入发育中的间充质，间充质形成乳房的纤维和脂肪部分[12]。乳房芽在妊娠 34 周时可触及[12]。乳头出现得更晚一些，在妊娠第 8 月时出现。最初是一个凹窝，后来变得隆起[41]。

8～13 岁之间，乳房初发育、或青春期乳房发育开始，平均年龄是 11～11.5 岁[50]。到 13 岁还没有发育得话，就要考虑发育迟缓，并确保进行内分泌学评估[48]。正常的乳房发育是激素介导的[19]。脂肪组织和输乳管在雌激素的作用下生长。黄体酮的刺激导致小叶生长和腺泡出芽[19,50]。乳房的正常发育在乳房初发育后的 2～4 年内发生，根据 Tanner 系统分为五个阶段（表 58–1）。月经初潮通常约在 Tanner 第二期后 2 年出现。

乳房过早发育

正常的乳房初发育发生在 8～13 岁之间，但是有些 1～3 岁的婴儿也会有乳房芽出现，现在有报道表明，有些婴儿在出生时就存在乳房芽[47]。虽然大部分乳房过早发育的患者没有并发的医学问题，但是甲状腺功能减退作为一个乳房过早发育的罕见病因，应该加以考虑[19]。乳房过早发育通常是一个孤立的情况，但可能会是性早熟的第一症状，尤其是那些 2 岁以上的女孩。有报道表明，对乳房过早发育的女孩进行的随访发现，高达 18%的人有性早熟[44]。一系列特别强调生长速度和第二性征（如阴毛的生长和阴唇或乳晕的色素沉着）的检查，通常足以鉴别乳房过早发育女孩的性早熟[12,47]。如果怀疑有性早熟，可用放射影像来评估某些患者的骨龄[44]。除非乳房发育患者合并性早熟体征，否则应消除父母的疑虑并对患者进行随访[50]。90%的孤立性乳房过早发育的患者，在诊断后的 6 个月到 6 年内，其乳房增大会消退[46]。不对称的乳房过早发育，其消退也可能是不对称的[47]。长期随访表明，孤立性乳房过早发育患者，在青春期乳房发育正常，且并无乳房疾病或肿瘤风险的升高[46]。

表 58–1　乳房发育的 Tanner 分期

Tanner 分期	特征
1（青春期前）	仅有乳头隆起
2	乳芽和乳头隆起，如同一个小山丘 乳晕直径增大 乳晕颜色更加粉红
3	乳房和乳晕进一步增大，其轮廓无分别 出现蒙氏结节
4	进一步增大，乳晕和乳头凸出形成在乳房水平上的第二个小丘
5（成熟期）	仅有乳头凸出，这是乳晕退缩进入乳房的整体轮廓引起的 乳晕组织能够勃起

From Duflos D, et al: Breast diseases in adolescents. In Sultan C (ed): Pediatric and Adolescent Gynecology. Basel, Karger, 2004; and Templeman C, Hertweck SP: Breast disorders in the pediatric and adolescent patient. Obstet Gynecol Clin North Am 2000;27:19-34.

886 先天性乳房畸形

乳房缺如或乳房过小

乳房完全缺失，或乳房缺如罕见，且被认为是由于乳线未形成或消失造成的[41]。乳房缺如可合并一些更广泛的外胚层畸形综合征，如先天性外胚层发育不良[29,41]。也可合并下方中胚层的畸形，如 Poland 综合征（胸肌缺失–并指(趾)综合征）中的胸肌畸形[14,41]。40%的患者双侧乳房缺如合并其他的先天畸形[29]。无乳头畸形的定义是有乳房组织的外观但缺少乳头。这在副乳中并不少见，但是在正常位置却非常罕见[41]。胸廓切开术、放置胸腔引流管、不适当的乳芽活检、放疗或严重烧伤引起的持续性损伤，都会导致乳房缺如或乳房过小[12]。因为乳头复合体正常情况下要到妊娠第 8 月才发育，所以在早产婴儿中就难以鉴别。因此，放置胸腔引流管或中心导管时不注意，会损伤发育中的乳房（图 58–1）。

多乳房和多乳头

大约 1%～2%的人有额外的乳房组织，最常见的是副乳头[19,20,41]。这种位置异常的组织几乎都位于腋区或沿胚胎期乳线在位置正常的乳房下方[41]。不应将乳房组织向腋部的正常延伸（Spence 尾：乳腺组织生长突出于腋区的部分）与额外的乳房组织相混淆。65%有额外乳房组织的儿童有 1 个副乳头或副乳，30%～35%有 2 个[41]。已报道的额外结构的最大数量是 10 个[41]。完整的副乳房称为多乳房（图 58–2）。额外的乳头称为多乳头。一些研究提示多乳头与尿路畸形及先天性心脏病之间存在关联，虽然其他人对此也有质疑[12,20,29,45]。真正异位的乳房组织，或在正常乳线以外发现的乳房组织是极其罕见的，但是有位于脸面、背部和会阴，以及在躯干前正中线上的报道[24,26,41]。女孩的多乳房需要外科手术切除，以防止妊娠期的疼痛肿胀。通常为了美观的原因而需要切除副乳头。

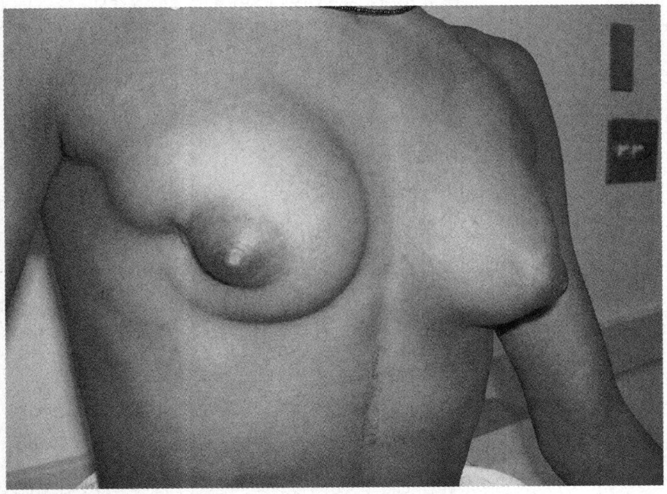

图 58–1 放置新生儿胸腔引流管引起的乳房变形。

先天性乳头畸形

乳头内陷的患者可能易发生感染，对内陷区域的卫生多加注意的话，通常可以预防感染[19]。手术矫正也是可能的，但是提升乳头会不可避免地造成输乳管的断裂以及将来母乳喂养的问题，这也不是不可能的。其他乳头畸形包括分叉乳头和乳晕内多乳头，也可以称作分裂乳头（图 58–3）[19,29]。

乳房不对称和乳房过小

妇女乳房一定程度的不对称是正常的，在青春期

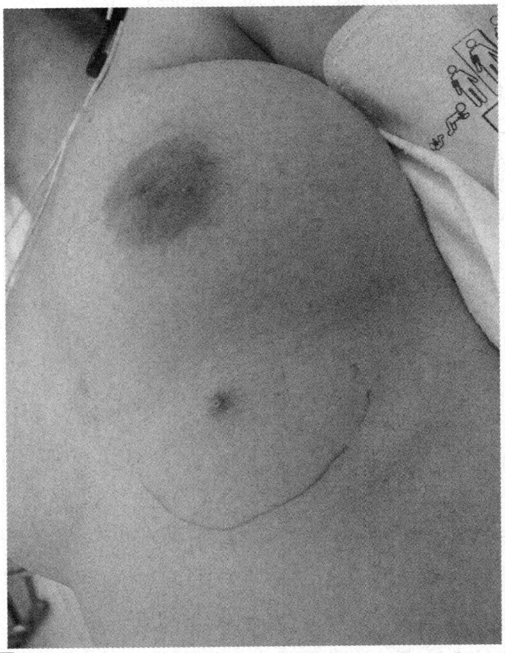

图 58–2 多乳房。这个有乳头复合体的完整乳房，是位于最常见的部位，在正常乳房下方。

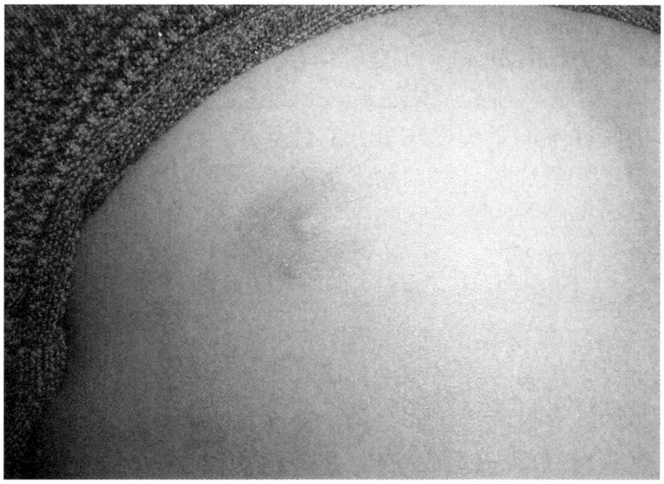

图 58-3 乳晕内多乳头，也称作发育不良的乳头分裂。

乳房发育的时候可能更显著[19,44]。乳房明显过小可能合并结缔组织病或二尖瓣脱垂[19]。乳房过小经常多是家族性的[12]。有报道发现单侧发育不良合并乳房 Becker 痣（由松散成簇的棕色斑构成的痣，多发于青春期末），在检查时呈现一个明显的棕色色素斑[12]。据报道这种痣的雄性性征受体增多，这就可以解释为何乳房过小[12]。胸壁放疗之后也会发生乳房过小。对于双侧乳房发育不良的女孩，应该评估她的卵巢功能障碍、甲状腺功能减退或产生雄激素的肿瘤的状况[19]。发育不良的乳房组织也会合并异常的结节状乳房。在这种情况下，乳房底部受限，发育不良的乳房组织会“脱”入乳晕复合体[19,44]。可以采用整形手术矫正乳晕复合体并增大发育不良的乳房。

887 # 乳房增大

巨乳房

极其大的乳房称为巨乳房。青少年巨乳房的鉴别诊断包括青少年乳房增大、妊娠、乳房肿瘤以及内源性或外源性的雌激素或黄体酮水平超量或两者兼有（表 58-2）[32]。有报道 D-青霉胺和大麻也是引起巨乳房的外源性病因。

表 58-2 巨乳房的鉴别诊断

青少年增大
乳房肿瘤
巨型纤维腺瘤
错构瘤[49]
叶状囊肉瘤
癌
激素活性肿瘤
卵巢颗粒细胞瘤
卵巢卵泡细胞瘤
肾上腺皮质瘤
外源性激素
雌激素
睾酮
促性腺素
皮质酮
药物
D-青霉胺
大麻

青少年或处女乳房增大

青少年单侧或者双侧乳房的自发性大型生长被认为是靶器官对性腺激素过度敏感所致[32]。增大的乳房组织的激素受体数量正常，血浆中雌二醇的水平也正常[12,32]。因为偶尔会合并一些自身免疫性疾病，如桥本甲状腺炎、风湿性关节炎和肌无力，一些作者提出了自身免疫因素[12]。青少年乳房增大患者的乳房生长迅速，在乳房初发育后迅速开始增大，可能是非常令人注目的，导致每个乳房可重达 50 磅[19,44]。自发性消退非常罕见[32]。在迅速生长期，可能会有皮肤变化，出现橘皮样变，甚至坏死[32]。治疗取决于乳房生长是否已经结束。如果患者仍在生长，可使用黄体酮或抗雌激素药物来控制乳房生长[44]。如果药物治疗没有成功，或者乳房生长结束，则需要进行乳房缩小术[32]。应该告知患者，青少年乳房增大可能会影响哺乳，特别在乳房减容手术之后，但是发生乳癌的风险不会增加[32]。

乳房感染

新生儿乳腺炎是一种罕见的感染，通常发生在足月婴儿或接近足月的婴儿中[13]。感染对女性婴儿的影响是男性婴儿的两倍[13]。约 50%的新生儿乳腺炎患儿发展为乳房脓肿[13]。青少年出现非产褥期乳腺炎或乳房脓肿，是由皮肤、异物或表皮囊肿感染刺激所致[44]。所有乳房感染的初始治疗是抗生素和止痛剂[13]。患乳腺炎的青少年女孩，采取乳房支撑后症状可能会缓解[44]。虽然几乎所有的病例中，大多数致病微生物都是金黄色葡萄球菌，但是在婴儿中，也有志贺菌、大肠杆菌和克雷白菌感染的报道[13]。在大多数社区，耐甲氧苯青霉素金黄色葡萄球菌的发生率很显著，以至于要使用长达 10 天的克林霉素或万古霉素。只有在取得培养结果之后，才能显示出革兰阴性菌的覆盖度。不论是婴儿还是年长儿童的小脓肿，都应该采用针刺抽吸，如果有必要，则采用超声引导，随后继续采用抗生素治疗[44]。较大的脓肿可能需要切开和引流，但是一些作者建议最初用针刺抽吸，如果抽吸失败再进行外科治疗[44]。如果进行切开和引流，小的乳晕周边切口较为合适。对于青春期前的儿童，探查和分离组织时，应采取最小限度，以免伤及下方的乳
888 芽。

乳头溢液

血性溢液

儿童和青少年血性溢液的鉴别诊断包括乳腺管扩张、慢性囊性乳腺炎、乳腺管内乳房囊肿和乳腺管内乳头状瘤。乳腺管扩张是感染和纤维化引起的乳晕下乳腺管的良性扩张。这被认为是一种乳腺管发育异常，由乳腺管腔内的上皮细胞“褶”堵塞管腔引起的[12,42]。这种梗阻会造成细菌滋生和脓肿，最常见的是金黄色葡萄球菌[50]。其他可能的原因包括乳腺管周间质的慢性炎症、创伤和自身免疫反应[42]。乳腺管扩张的婴儿一般出现血性溢液。青少年的典型体征是乳晕后肿块，通常呈青蓝色，可能会有血性或褐色溢液。对于所有血性溢液的患儿，应该留取溢液进行培养，并开始适当的抗生素治疗[50]。乳腺导管扩张通常可以自行消退[12,30,50]。也可能复发，但是通常都是在保守治疗后复发的。对于持续症状或复发症状，或者合并持续性囊肿者，可能需要进行手术切除[50]。对于女孩，切除范围应局限在任一已经鉴别明确的囊肿，要极其仔细地避免损伤下方的乳芽。对于有这种情况的男孩，单纯的乳房切除术可以治愈[50]。

乳腺管内乳头状瘤是罕见的乳晕下病变，而且通常难以触及[19]。25%的患者为双侧病变[19]。血性溢液的细胞学检查显示有乳腺导管细胞[19]。经乳晕周边切口的局部切除，可以治愈[19]。乳头腺瘤是非常罕见的，可能也存在乳头糜烂或乳头溢液。在青少年运动员中，血性溢液可能是由于慢性乳头刺激（慢跑者的乳头）或冷冻创伤（自行车手的乳头）所致[27]。

溢乳

新生儿乳房的乳汁溢出是对胎儿催乳素水平的正常反应，催乳素在出生是达到高峰（图 58–4）[38]。青少年的非产褥期泌乳，根据其原因可分为神经性、下丘脑、脑垂体、内分泌、药物引起或特发性[38]。胸壁、胸腔或乳房疾病可引起神经性泌乳。有报道显示在胸廓切开术、胸壁烧伤或损伤、带状疱疹或乳头慢性刺激后发生神经性泌乳[38]。脑垂体肿瘤，尤其是催乳素瘤，是引起溢乳的最常见的下丘脑或脑垂体因素[38]。青少年最常见的乳溢原因是甲状腺功能减退[38]。很多药物都可以造成溢乳，包括多巴胺受体阻断药和降低儿茶酚胺功效的药物[38,44]。需要对溢乳患者乳溢的可能原因进行仔细的病史回顾和体格检

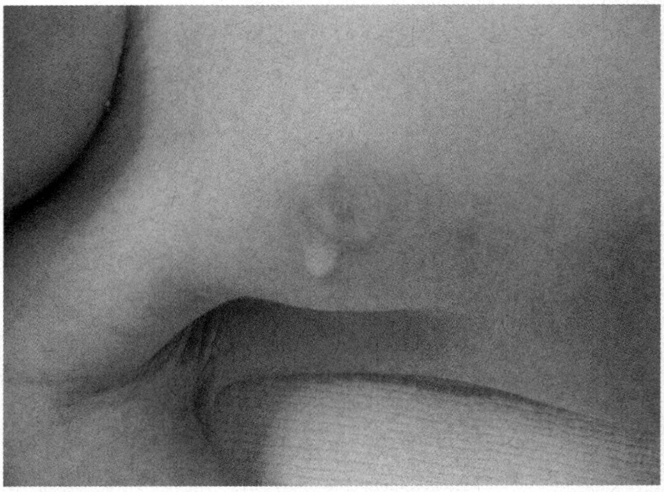

图 58–4　新生儿正常的乳芽和乳性溢液。

查。如果对溢液是否为真性溢乳有疑问，应该将液体送去进行脂肪染色。实验室检查应该包括对血清催乳素、促卵泡激素、黄体生成素和甲状腺功能的检查[38]。青少年乳晕的蒙氏腺溢液可能是正常的，不应与溢乳相混淆[19]。

乳房肿块

青春期前乳房肿块

出生后第一周的男女新生儿乳房增大是对母体雌激素的正常反应[19]。类似试图挤压乳房来促进排液的刺激，可能会引起持久性的组织增大。新生儿乳房增大会自行消退，且无需治疗。

乳房初发育的乳房发育始于乳晕复合体下方一个坚实的蝶形组织，可误认为是肿块。通常最初是单侧的[50]。这几乎是一个完全正常的生理过程，但有报道单侧乳房初发育是使用西咪替丁的副作用，在停药之后可以逆转[6]。为活检的禁忌证，因为会对发育中的乳房造成损伤[48]。

发育中的乳房可能出现血管瘤和淋巴管瘤（图 58–5）。虽然血管瘤会在最初的生长高峰后消退，但是其快速生长会压迫乳芽而引起损伤和相应的乳房畸形。通常可通过体格检查建立诊断，但是要通过超声波图像检查和磁共振影像（MRI）才能确诊。如果对诊断有质疑，可能需要细针穿刺活检。迅速生长的血管瘤可能需要切除（如果技术上可能的话）或使用类

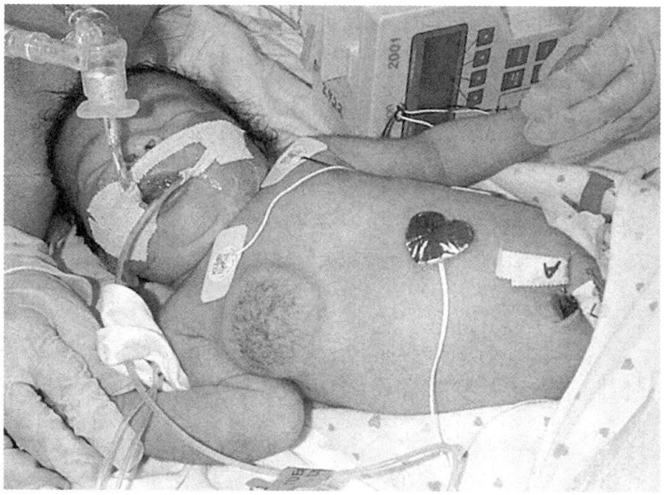

图 58–5　新生婴儿的乳房血管瘤。

固醇治疗[1,50]。对于女孩，必须在手术引起乳芽损伤和血管瘤或淋巴管瘤快速生长引起乳芽损伤的风险间加以权衡。MRI 可能有助于判定病变的可治愈程度，从而判断相应的手术切除的利弊。出现溃疡或出血等 889
并发症时，成为手术切除病灶的适应证，以保护正常的乳房组织[50]。

乳房其他的软组织或转移性肿瘤是罕见的，但在青春期前儿童中也可能出现（图 58–3）。大部分的病变是良性的，但是如果诊断不确定，那么可以进行细针穿刺或切开活检[50]。

青少年女孩的肿块

纤维腺瘤

青少年女孩中最常见的肿块是纤维腺瘤。这些肿块通常在青春期晚期出现，但是最早可在月经初潮前 1～2 年就发生[19]。纤维腺瘤大多位于乳房上外四分之一的区域，且在非洲裔的美国患者中更常见[50]。平均大小是 2～3 cm，但也能变得很大（图 58–6）[44]。10%的患者为双侧病变[44]。高达 25%的患者有多发性纤维腺瘤，这种情况称为纤维腺瘤病。[12,19]这种病灶在月经周期中可能轻微增大[50]。体格检查通常可以诊断；这些病灶为局限性的、“橡胶样有弹性的”，可移动，无触痛。在可疑病例中，超声图像检查有助于建立诊断[15]。青少年患者无乳房造影的适应证，因为大量的纤维腺体组织使得影像判读有困难[50]。

因为雌激素刺激可以导致局部增大，所以纤维腺瘤被认为是会发展的[50]。这些病变的自然病史通常是在最初的生长期时，肿块的大小在 6～12 月内增加一

表 58–3　青春期前乳房肿块的鉴别诊断
单侧乳芽发育（乳房过早发育）
出血性囊肿[50]
脓肿[50]
淋巴管瘤[50]
血管瘤[50]
淋巴瘤[50]
转移性肿瘤
乳腺囊肿[4]

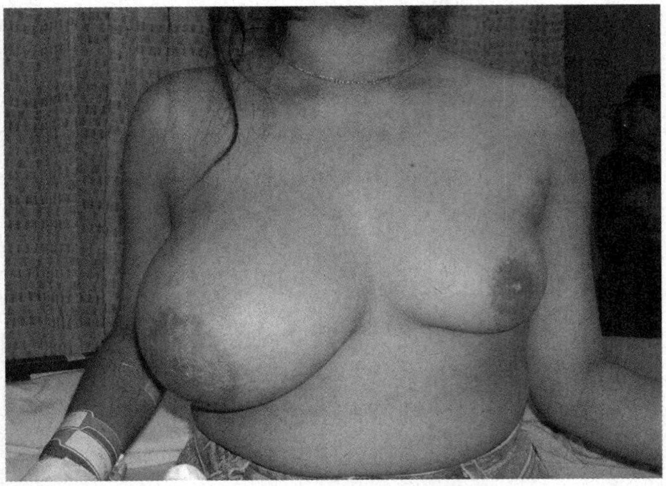

图 58-6 青春期女孩的巨大纤维腺瘤，类似青少年肥大。

倍，然后就保持稳定。仅有 5%的纤维腺瘤生长地更迅速[21]。有报道显示纤维腺瘤存在自发性消退[7,50]。在 40 岁以上的女性患者的这些病灶中发现硬化支持了这一点[10]。对 99 名 14～55 岁（年龄中值为 20 岁）女性进行的 7～9 年的随访发现，107 个临床诊断的纤维腺瘤中，有 38%自行消退[7]。某研究小组报道在 2 年的随访期内，40%的纤维腺瘤成年疑似病例的肿块缩小[33]。即使其中一些病变并非真正的纤维腺瘤，这些发现仍然支持对纤维腺瘤的疑似病例进行观察，而不是进行早期切除。所有小于 5 cm 的疑似纤维腺瘤都可以安全地观察至少 1 或 2 个月经周期。如果病灶有生长，则需要进行切开活检[33]。如果病灶稳定的话，则需要同患者和家属讨论两个要点：

1. 观察，进行或不进行细针穿刺。大约在 200 例纤维腺瘤成年患者中有乳房癌的报道[36]。没有青少年恶性纤维腺瘤的报道。检查时发现患典型的纤维腺瘤的青少年女孩，其恶性肿瘤的风险非常低。如果进行了标准检查，且无肿瘤生长，那基本上对这些病变进行观察就没有风险。
2. 切除活检。许多作者推荐切除成人期仍然存在的所有病灶，所以患者在青春期持续存在的纤维腺瘤会被全数切除[50]。应该告知患者活检可能会影响乳房的美观。也有报道显示在切除纤维腺瘤后有持续性的局部疼痛[40]。

巨大纤维腺瘤 890

大于 5 cm 的纤维腺瘤称为巨大纤维腺瘤。在检查中，可能比典型的纤维腺瘤更柔软，甚至类似周围正常的乳房组织[44]。在表面可能有扩张的静脉，而且肿块上方的皮肤触摸时较为温暖（见图 58-6）[44]。巨大纤维腺瘤应该切除，因为无法通过体格检查、乳房造影或超声检查与囊性肉瘤相鉴别[8]。此外，有报道称极少数患者的肿瘤在短短的 3 个月内就增大一倍[19]。如果组织学上倾向于确诊为叶状囊肉瘤时，细针穿刺抽吸和空心针活检有助于设计手术方案。但是，穿刺抽吸和穿刺活检难以区别纤维腺瘤和叶状囊性肉瘤，所以阴性结果也不应该影响手术决定。

切除巨大纤维腺瘤可能存在问题。一旦有可能的话，应该使用环乳晕切口。大型病灶可通过环乳晕切口切除，在移出前将其放入一个袋中，并切碎[39]。如果肿块靠近乳房下皱褶，这就提供了另外一个美观的路径。切除大型纤维腺瘤可引起明显的乳房畸形。不推荐放置引流，因为这会造成皮肤对胸壁的粘连。但是，让血浆或血液渗满这一空隙也不是很好；这也可能引起此空隙的收缩和皮肤粘连。使用静脉内导管针的“Z”形穿刺，将盐水和局部麻醉药的混合液注满此空隙。对于大部分患者，这种做法防止血浆的快速注入，并降低了皮肤粘连的风险。

叶状肿瘤

1838 年 Muller 首次描述了叶状肿瘤，他将其称为叶状囊肉瘤。但是，这个名称使人产生误解，因为这些肿瘤很少是囊性的，而且没有大多数肉瘤的恶性潜质[33]。因此，最好将它们称作叶状肿瘤。

叶状肿瘤是间质肿瘤，在组织学上分为良性、中间性或恶性[50]。因为良性的叶状病灶会转移并可能在局部复发，所以在说法上有很大差异。发生叶状肿瘤的年龄中值为 45 岁；但是有报道在 10 岁女孩中也有发生[2,33]。这些肿瘤可能在非洲裔美国青少年中更常规[19]。

不通过活检难以诊断。在检查时，肿瘤类似巨大纤维腺瘤。大型肿瘤可能引起皮肤扩张和溃疡，以及静脉曲张[19]。如果乳头复合体受累，可能出现血性溢液[19]。对于叶状肿瘤，超声结果有提示作用，但是并非诊断性的，包括分叶、非均质回声模式和无微钙化[8]。

良性叶状肿瘤的治疗是完全手术切除，包含 1 cm 厚的正常组织边缘[34]。组织学恶性叶状肿瘤的患者应该接受乳房切除术[8]。一些作者报道了恶性叶状肿瘤的青少年患者的病程比成人更“良性”，并建议可以保留这些患者的乳房[33]。约 20%的患者仅有临床上可以触诊到的结节，也应该进行切除[28]。对这些肿瘤而言，前哨淋巴结活检的作用尚不明了。大部分淋巴结因肿瘤坏死和炎症而增大；通过血源性途径发生转移，而不是淋巴性、播散性的[19]。如果初次手术没有切除足够的边缘，则有进行再次切除的适应证[28]。如果无法在胸壁上切除足够的边缘，则应该考虑进行局部放疗[28]。

高达 20%的叶状肿瘤患者在局部复发，采用再次切除或乳房切除术进行治疗[33]。14%～15%的患者报告有全身性复发[28]。肺、胸膜、软组织、骨骼、胰腺和中枢神经系统都可能发生转移，通常不累及淋巴结[28,33]。有采用单一或多种化疗药物缓解病症的单独报道，但是总的来说，辅助治疗对于成功治疗叶状肿瘤来说，作用有限[33]。

成人良性、临界性和恶性叶状肿瘤的 5 年生存率分别为 96%、74%和 66%[33]。成人恶性叶状肿瘤的 5 年总体生存率约为 80%[33]。因为青少年叶状肿瘤的生物学侵袭性比成人要低，所以其预后可能较好[33]。

乳晕后囊肿

蒙氏结节是在乳晕边缘上的小丘形突起，并与蒙氏腺相连，泌乳时发挥重要作用[44]。青少年的这些腺体可能被堵塞，出现急性炎症（62%）或无症状肿块（38%）[22]。乳晕后囊肿的诊断也就是指蒙氏囊肿，主要是临床诊断，但可以通过超声图像检查确诊，大多数超声图像显示有一个单一的囊性病灶，通常为单房性的，位于预期的乳晕后位置。乳晕后囊肿患者最常见的表现是急性炎症，合并局部触痛、红斑和乳晕下肿胀，并延伸到乳房组织[22]。使用针对葡萄球菌的口服抗生素和非类固醇类抗炎药物，通常可在 7 天内消除急性炎症[22]。仅在持续脓肿时才进行引流，这比较少见。非手术治疗之后，通常会存在一个无症状的肿块。乳晕后囊肿的患者可能会报告某个蒙氏结节流出褐色溢液，特别在压迫肿块时。没有持续感染或其他并发症时，应该对乳晕后囊肿进行观察，并采取一系列体格检查，而且如果需要，再次进行超声图像检
查。80%以上的囊肿可自行消退，但是这可能需要长 891
达 2 年的时间[22]。应该告诉患者不要压迫此区，因为这可能会妨碍肿块的消退。如果肿块持续存在或对诊断有争议的话，可能需要切除[44]。

纤维囊性变

乳房的纤维囊性变可能会引起双侧乳房的局限性肿块和疼痛，或乳腺疼痛。应该消除患者的疑虑，告诉她们这是女性生理的正常变化，而且 50%的育龄妇女和 90%的女性尸检中都有这些变化[44]。通常单凭体格检查足以得出诊断，因为在月经周期的不同时间进行的一系列检查通常有显著的变化。如果诊断不明确，超声图像检查可能有助于做出诊断，但是并无乳房造影适应证。采用硬质乳罩和非类固醇类抗炎药物治疗乳腺疼痛[19]。有报道口服避孕药可改善 70%～90%妇女的症状[44]。采用维生素 E 或月见草油进行治疗，并避免接触咖啡因的疗效并未得到证实，但却是普遍采用的方法[19,44]。

其他良性乳房肿块

青少年和年轻成人有很多良性乳房肿块（表 58–4）。由正常乳房成分构成的乳房错构瘤是罕见的肿瘤，会引起单侧巨乳房[49]。也被称为脂肪纤维瘤、腺脂瘤和纤维腺脂瘤[49]。仅有 8 例年龄低于 20 岁的女性病例的报道[49]。错构瘤的治疗是全切除术。

乳头腺瘤极其罕见，但是有报道在儿童和青少年中发生。其治疗是局部切除[43]。根据病史或体格检查无法区分管状腺瘤和纤维腺瘤，因此通常根据病理学评估来作出诊断[10]。在局部切除后，无需进一步治疗。

侵蚀性腺瘤病一种罕见的良性肿瘤，表现为红斑、糜烂和乳头结痂[3]。可能发生血清血液性溢液，可触及小结、或未触及小结[3]。通过局部切除病灶进行治疗，治疗可推迟到乳房生长完全后进行；有采用冷冻手术成功治疗的报道[3]。

少年型乳头状瘤病是一种良性、局限性的分化病灶，通常见于年龄大于 10 岁的女孩，但是也有青春期前男孩发病的报道[35]。少年型乳头状瘤病在体检时通常发现与纤维腺瘤相似的肿块，位于一侧乳房上。

表 58-4 女孩青春期后乳房肿块的鉴别诊断
纤维腺瘤
蒙氏囊肿
乳腺管扩张
脂肪坏死
血管脂肪瘤[50]
乳晕下神经瘤[50]
错构瘤[40]
脓肿[50]
淋巴管瘤[50]
血管瘤[50]
脂肪瘤[50]
少年型分泌性癌
导管癌
转移性疾病

切除时，可见一个分界完全、由纤维间质分隔的多囊性的肿块，外观呈“瑞士奶酪”样[10]。少年型乳头状瘤病被认为是家族成员中乳房癌风险升高的标志，但是对患者来说不是必然的，除非复发[35]。但是，高达15%的少年型乳头状瘤病患者报道有原位癌和侵袭性癌（通常为少年型分泌性癌）[10]。少年型乳头状瘤病的治疗是全切除术，并保留正常乳房[35]。

创伤可造成青少年出现类似感染或肿块的病灶。特别是创伤后的脂肪坏死与乳房的实质性肿块相类似[19]。有报道在汽车坐椅安全带造成损伤和其他乳房直接打击损伤后会有这类症状[51]。

乳房恶性肿瘤

据报道，39 例 3～19 岁的儿童有原发性乳房癌[31,50]。80%以上的患者被诊断为少年型分泌性癌，余下的是导管内癌。有少年型分泌性癌合并少年型乳头状瘤病的报道[50]。少年型分泌性癌通常有一个厚壁的被膜，这使得病灶在超声图像检查时呈现囊性[31]。儿童原发乳房癌的治疗是手术完全切除，通常是乳房切除术[50]。前哨淋巴结定位在儿童中的作用尚不明确。应该判定雌激素和黄体酮的受体。通过再次切除或乳房全切除术来治疗局部复发。少年型分泌性癌很少使用辅助治疗，局部切除之后，这些患者的预后良好。导管内癌的辅助治疗取决于淋巴结状况和激素受体，大多数肿瘤学家使用改良的成人方案来治疗患此肿瘤的儿童。

胸壁放疗通常用于治疗 Hodgkin 淋巴瘤，这增加了乳房癌的风险。年龄在 10～16 岁的女孩接受放疗时更是如此，因为这是乳房快速生长的时期[18]。患 Hodgkin 病而需要胸壁放疗的女孩患乳房癌的风险升高 82 倍，大约 40%的患者最终发展成乳房癌[18]。从放疗到诊断乳房癌之间的平均间隔是 20 年。
如果有明显的家族史，乳房癌的风险也会升高。在 892
所有乳房癌病例中，7%～9%发现存在 *BRCA1* 和 *BRCA2* 基因突变[44]。这些基因中任何一个有突变的女孩，30 岁时患乳房癌的风险为 3.2%，70 岁前为 85%[44]。

乳房肉瘤在所有年龄组中罕见，在儿童中更是少见。横纹肌肉瘤作为乳房原发性肿瘤，通常发生在青少年女孩中[5]。这些肿瘤的典型表现为快速生长的可移动肿块，而不累及皮肤；在组织学上它们通常为小泡型横纹肌肉瘤[5]。有报道成年妇女在为了保留乳房而进行的外线束放疗后出现乳房血管肉瘤[2]。这种罕见的肿瘤在青少年中也有报道[34]。治疗方法是乳房切除术，而无需常规的腋窝清扫[34]。有青少年患者乳房叶状肿瘤中出现脂肪肉瘤的报道[23]。这些肿瘤外观上有被膜，但是应该通过局部扩大切除加以治疗[2]。纤维肉瘤和恶性纤维组织细胞瘤可能是最常见的乳房软组织肉瘤；其他罕见的乳房原发肉瘤包括平滑肌肉瘤和骨肉瘤[2]。有儿童患乳房原发性非霍奇金淋巴瘤的报道[37]。这些罕见的乳房恶性原发性肿瘤的治疗建立在原有的针对儿童期常见肿瘤的方案基础之上。

在儿童原发性肝细胞癌、Hodgkin 淋巴瘤、非 Hodgkin 淋巴瘤、神经母细胞瘤和横纹肌肉瘤，特别是小泡变异型横纹肌肉瘤中，有乳房转移癌的报道[9,37,50]。在儿童期报道有乳房转移的其他较不常见的肿瘤包括组织细胞增多病、髓母细胞瘤、肾癌和神经母细胞瘤[9]。横纹肌肉瘤转移到乳房的儿童中，30%为双侧乳房病变[9]。超声图像检查是可供选择的诊断工具，因为它通常可将这些病灶与其他更常见的良性病灶进行鉴别[9]。

男性乳腺发育

高达 70%的男孩在青春期有男性乳腺发育[19,25]。

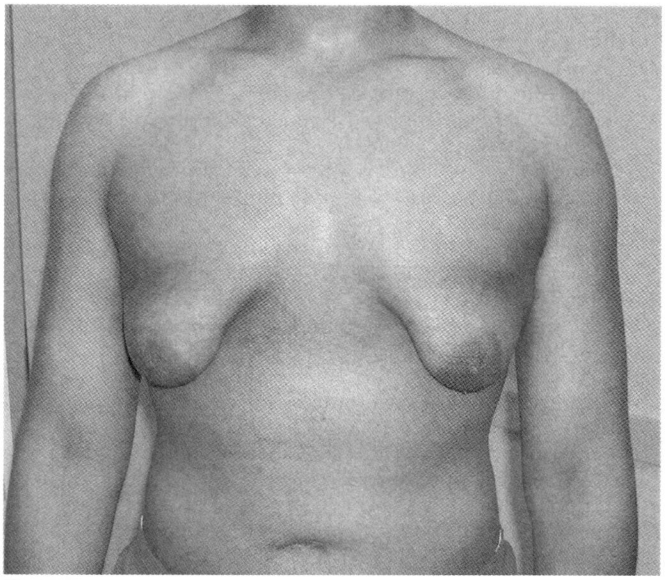

图 58-7 一个青春期男孩的第 5 期男性乳房发育。

大部分的男孩为双侧男性乳腺发育，仅 10%为单侧乳房增大。应该获取患者的药物服用史，因为有报道在使用促蛋白合成类固醇、洋地黄、异烟肼、三环类抗抑郁药、螺内酯和大麻后会出现男性乳腺发育[50]。通常使用 Nydick 定义的分级方法对男性乳腺发育进行分类，此分级方法类似女孩乳房发育的 Tanner 分期方法。1 期局限在乳晕下区域，而不达到乳晕边缘；2 期扩展到乳晕边缘（B2）或超过乳晕边缘（B3）。男性乳腺发育到 4 期和 5 期时，乳房类似女性乳房的特征[11]。睾丸检查也是很重要的。男性乳腺发育合并性腺发育不全提示 Klinefelter 综合征（男性乳房发育-精子生成缺乏综合征）的诊断。在大多数男孩中，生理性的男性乳腺发育在青春期过程中自行消退，但这可能需要几年的时间。但是，一些男孩会因为乳房的增大而使自尊心受到伤害（图 58-7）。这些男孩需要手术来获取正常的心理成长和发育。虽然整形外科医生将抽脂术发展为代替切除的方法，但是大多数的儿童外科医生乐于采取切口途径进行手术[16,17]。通过环乳晕切口进行单纯乳房切除术。对于乳房组织明显的病例，通常需要引流，以防止术后发生血清肿。在乳头后方应保留一个乳房组织“垫”，以防止乳头和胸壁产生粘连[50]。

（孙彦隽译 刘锦纷校）

参考文献

1. Akyuz C, et al: Management of cutaneous hemangiomas: A retrospective analysis of 1109 cases and comparison of conventional dose prednisolone with high-dose methylprednisolone therapy. Pediatr Hematol Oncol 2001;18:47-55.
2. Alabassi A, Fentiman IS: Sarcomas of the breast. Int J Clin Pract 2003;57:886-889.
3. Albers SE, et al: Erosive adenomatosis of the nipple in an eight-year-old girl. J Am Acad Dermatol 1999;40:834-837.
4. Al Salem AH, Al Nazer M: An unusual cause of breast enlargement in a 5-year-old boy. Pediatr Pathol Mol Med 2002;21:485-489.
5. Binokay F, et al: Primary and metastatic rhabdomyosarcoma in the breast: Report of two pediatric cases. Eur J Radiol 2003;48:282-284.
6. Bosman JM, Bax NM, Wit JM: Premature thelarche: A possible adverse effect of cimetidine treatment. Eur J Pediatr 1990;149:534-535.
7. Cant PJ, et al: Non-operative management of breast masses diagnosed as fibroadenoma. Br J Surg 1995;82:792-794.
8. Chao TC, et al: Sonographic features of phyllodes tumors of the breast. Ultrasound Obstet Gynecol 2002;20:64-71.
9. Chateil JF, et al: Breast metastases in adolescent girls: US findings. Pediatr Radiol 1998;28:832-835.
10. Dehner LP, Hill DA, Deschryver K: Pathology of the breast in children, adolescents, and young adults. Semin Diagn Pathol 1999;16:235-247.
11. De Sanctis V, et al: Pubertal gynecomastia. Minerva Pediatr 2002;54:357-361.
12. Duflos D, et al: Breast diseases in adolescents. In Sultan C (ed): Pediatric and Adolescent Gynecology. Basel, Karger, 2004.
13. Efrat M, et al: Neonatal mastitis—diagnosis and treatment. Isr J Med Sci 1995;31:558-560.
14. Fokin AA, Robicsek F: Poland's syndrome revisited. Ann Thorac Surg 2002;74:2218-2225.
15. Fornage BD, Lorigan JG, Andry E: Fibroadenoma of the breast: Sonographic appearance. Radiology 1989;172: 671-675.
16. Fruhstorfer BH, Malata CM: A systematic approach to the surgical treatment of gynaecomastia. Br J Plast Surg 2003; 56:237-246.
17. Gabra HO, et al: Gynaecomastia in the adolescent: A surgically relevant condition. Eur J Pediatr Surg 2004;14:3-6.
18. Gold DG, Neglia JP, Dusenbery KE: Second neoplasms after megavoltage radiation for pediatric tumors. Cancer 2003;97:2588-2596.
19. Greydanus DE, Parks DS, Farrell EG: Breast disorders in children and adolescents. Pediatr Clin North Am 1989; 36:601-638.
20. Grossl NA: Supernumerary breast tissue: Historical perspectives and clinical features. South Med J 2000;93: 29-32.
21. Hanna RM, Ashebu SD: Giant fibroadenoma of the breast in an Arab population. Australas Radiol 2002;46:252-256.
22. Huneeus A, et al: Retroareolar cysts in the adolescent. J Pediatr Adolesc Gynecol 2003;16:45-49.
23. Jimenez JF, et al: Liposarcoma arising within a cystosarcoma phyllodes. J Surg Oncol 1986;31:294-298.
24. Koltuksuz U, Aydin E: Supernumerary breast tissue: A case of pseudomamma on the face. J Pediatr Surg 1997;32: 1377-1378.
25. Lazala C, Saenger P: Pubertal gynecomastia. J Pediatr Endocrinol Metab 2002;15:553-560.
26. Leung W, Heaton JP, Morales A: An uncommon urologic

presentation of a supernumerary breast. Urology 1997; 50:122-124.
27. Loud KJ, Micheli LJ: Common athletic injuries in adolescent girls. Curr Opin Pediatr 2001;13:317-322.
28. Mangi AA, et al: Surgical management of phyllodes tumors. Arch Surg 1999;134:487-492.
29. Merlob P: Congenital malformations and developmental changes of the breast: A neonatological view. J Pediatr Endocrinol Metab 2003;16:471-485.
30. Miller JD, Brownell MD, Shaw A: Bilateral breast masses and bloody nipple discharge in a 4-year-old boy. J Pediatr 1990;116:744-747.
31. Murphy JJ, et al: Breast cancer in a 6-year-old child. J Pediatr Surg 2000;35:765-767.
32. O'Hare PM, Frieden IJ: Virginal breast hypertrophy. Pediatr Dermatol 2000;17:277-281.
33. Parker SJ, Harries SA: Phyllodes tumours. Postgrad Med J 2001;77:428-435.
34. Rainwater LM, et al: Angiosarcoma of the breast. Arch Surg 1986;121:669-672.
35. Rice HE, et al: Juvenile papillomatosis of the breast in male infants: Two case reports. Pediatr Surg Int 2000;16: 104-106.
36. Rivera-Hueto F, et al: Long-term prognosis of teenagers with breast cancer. Int J Surg Pathol 2002;10:273-279.
37. Rogers DA, et al: Breast malignancy in children. J Pediatr Surg 1994;29:48-51.
38. Rohn RD: Galactorrhea in the adolescent. J Adolesc Health Care 1984;5:37-49.
39. Rojananin S, Ratanawichitrasin A: Limited incision with plastic bag removal for a large fibroadenoma. Br J Surg 2002;89:787-788.
40. Siegal A, Kaufman Z, Siegal G: Breast masses in adolescent females. J Surg Oncol 1992;51:169-173.
41. Skandalakis J, et al: The anterior body wall. In Gray S (ed): Embryology for Surgeons: The Embryologic Basis for the Treatment of Congenital Anomalies. Baltimore, Williams & Wilkins, 1994, pp 539-593.
42. Stringel G, Perelman A, Jimenez C: Infantile mammary duct ectasia: A cause of bloody nipple discharge. J Pediatr Surg 1986;21:671-674.
43. Sugai M, et al: Adenoma of the nipple in an adolescent. Breast Cancer 2002;9:254-256.
44. Templeman C, Hertweck SP: Breast disorders in the pediatric and adolescent patient. Obstet Gynecol Clin North Am 2000;27:19-34.
45. Urbani CE, Betti R: Accessory mammary tissue associated with congenital and hereditary nephrourinary malformations. Int J Dermatol 1996;35:349-352.
46. Van Winter JT, et al: Natural history of premature thelarche in Olmsted County, Minnesota, 1940 to 1984. J Pediatr 1990; 116:278-280.
47. Verrotti A, et al: Premature thelarche: A long-term follow-up. Gynecol Endocrinol 1996;10:241-247.
48. Weinstein SP, et al: Spectrum of US findings in pediatric and adolescent patients with palpable breast masses. Radiographics 2000;20:1613-1621.
49. Weinzweig N, Botts J, Marcus E: Giant hamartoma of the breast. Plast Reconstr Surg 2001;107:1216-1220.
50. West KW, et al: Diagnosis and treatment of symptomatic breast masses in the pediatric population. J Pediatr Surg 1995;30:182-186.
51. Williams HJ, et al: Imaging features of breast trauma: A pictorial review. Breast 2002;11:107-115.

第 59 章

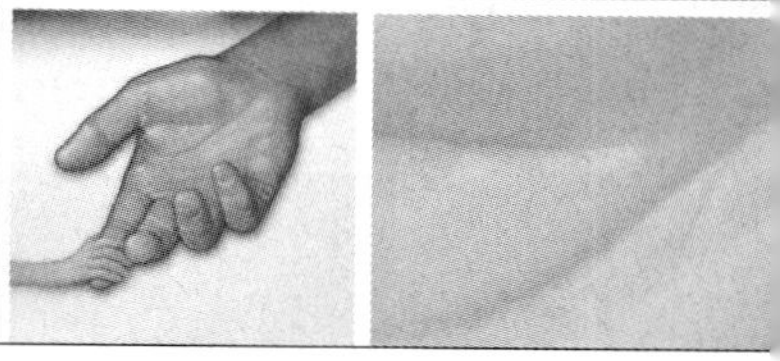

先天性胸壁畸形

Robert C. Shamberger

894 先天性胸壁畸形通常分为五类：漏斗胸、鸡胸、Poland 综合征、胸骨缺陷和其他发育异常或见于广泛性骨病的胸部畸形。大多数病变不威胁生命，但造成一些功能异常。但是，诸如胸部的心脏体外异位和 Jeune 窒息性胸廓发育不良等少数罕见病变几乎都是致命的。

压迫畸形：漏斗胸

漏斗胸（漏斗样胸、漏斗状胸或胸部前凹）是最常见的前胸壁畸形，包括胸骨和下方肋软骨的向后压迫。男孩比女孩更常见，发生率比例高达 3∶1。90% 的病例是在出生后第一年内发现的[125]。虽然有自发性缓解的病例，但非常罕见，因此给予孩子“这种胸部压迫会自己恢复”的建议时应该非常谨慎。漏斗胸的儿童除中央胸骨压迫以外，通常身材瘦高，体态较弱，且整体的胸部前后径（AP）长度减少[100,118]。

病因

漏斗胸的病因尚未明了。假设的理论包括子宫内压、佝偻病和横膈异常导致胸骨向后拉[15,16,22]。在横膈发育不全或先天性膈疝修补术后发生漏斗胸的报道为最后的这一理论提供了支持[136]。漏斗胸和其他肌肉骨骼异常之间的关联提示了结缔组织异常是重要因素，特别是脊柱侧弯（15%的发病率）和 Marfan 综合征（表 59–1）。研究证实有肋软骨畸形，包括锌浓度降低和钙、镁浓度升高。生物力学分析提示漏斗胸患者肋软骨的弹性增高，但是未证实受累个体和对照组之间的蛋白聚糖或胶原分布存在异常[35]。37%的病例有

表 59–1　704 例漏斗胸患者中查出的肌肉骨骼异常

异常	患者人数
脊柱侧弯	107
脊柱后凸	4
肌病	3
Poland 综合征	3
Marfan 综合征	2
Pierre Robin 综合征	2
Prune-belly 综合征	2
神经纤维瘤病	3
脑瘫	4
结节性硬化症	1
先天性膈疝	2

From Shamberger RC, Welch KJ: Surgical repair of pectus excavatum. J Pediatr Surg 1988;23:615-622.

胸壁畸形的家族史，支持了基因遗传因素[125]。

临床表现

儿童表现出一系列压迫畸形（表 59–1），从轻度的胸骨压迫到胸骨几乎压迫到椎体的重度压迫。压迫由两个因素所致：（1）胸骨体向后成角，通常从第二肋软骨连接处开始；（2）肋软骨向后成角与胸骨相连。在年长青少年和成人中，骨性肋骨的前端大部分向后成角。右侧的压迫可能比左侧深，胸骨也可能 895
发生旋转。两侧肋骨的前后深度可能有差异，而且许多患儿胸部的前后深度比正常儿童窄[100]。患儿可能有一个宽而浅的缺损或形成一个较窄的中央袋性缺损。通常同时发现患儿身材瘦弱和体态无力。在一个研究

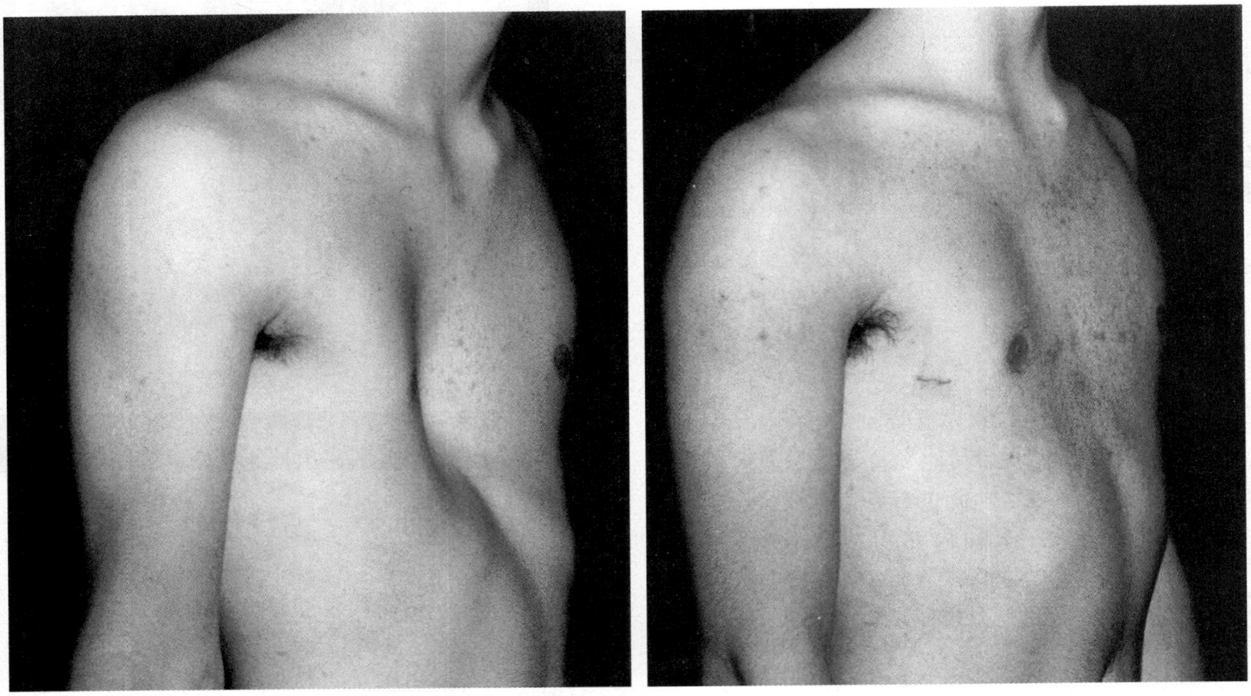

A B

图 59-1 A．一个有对称性漏斗胸畸形的 14 岁半的男孩在手术之前的临床照片。B．进行胸骨后支撑手术后 1 年的临床照片，显示畸形被完全纠正。

中，1.5%的接受胸壁矫正手术的患儿合并先天性心脏病，而且先天性心脏病儿童中合并胸壁畸形的发生率为 0.17%[126]。

已经发展出许多评估压迫严重程度的方法。大部分方法将胸骨和脊柱的距离作为首要因素。Willital[148]和Klinke 等人使用压迫深度和胸部前后径的比例[72]。Welch[143]使用胸骨脊柱间距与 Louis 角水平的胸骨前后深度的比值表示，如果心胸比率高于 50%或肋骨角超过水平线 25 度，则考虑额外增加的缝线因素。Backer 等人[5]使用椎体直径与剑突胸骨连接到椎体后缘距离的比值来表示压迫的严重程度。Haller 等人提出了一种分级方法，对胸部计算机断层扫描（CT）取得的横径和前后径进行测量，但是对标准胸部放射影像也要进行相似的测量[50]。

在婴儿期和儿童期，漏斗胸耐受良好。扁桃体和腺样体肥大引起的慢性上气道梗阻，可能会加重胸部弯曲婴儿的压迫，但是这并非病因。年长儿童可能有在软骨畸形区域疼痛或持久运动后心前区疼痛的主诉。偶尔会发生心悸，可能由一过性房性心律失常引起，并可能合并二尖瓣脱垂。经常发现漏斗胸患者有收缩期杂音。胸骨后侧与肺动脉靠得很近，引起血流杂音的传导[45]。

漏斗胸的生理学影响是许多报道的主题，并有所争论。一些作者坚称漏斗胸对心血管或肺没有影响。而这种情况又与临床上许多患者在手术修复后耐力和运动耐受性增加的情况完全相反。广泛研究了漏斗胸对心血管的影响，结果各不相同。尽管在此领域工作了 60 年，但这种重常见的胸壁畸形对心肺影响的程度未达成共识。针对漏斗胸患者的早期病理学研究证实位于脊柱和凹陷胸骨之间的心脏受到了压迫。左肺也受到压迫，程度超过右肺，因为胸壁畸形多不对称。后来许多研究的目的是解释这些解剖所见的生理学发现。1988 的一个综述对这一系列的长期研究进行了整合[123]。

肺功能评估

胸壁畸形使早期许多作者将漏斗胸术后的症状改善归功于肺功能的改善。在一项早期研究中，Brown[17]在术前和术后对患者进行了呼吸研究。这些患者的肺活量正常，但是在 11 例患者中，有 9 例的最大换气量明显降低（大于等于 50%）。最大换气量在术后平均上升 31%。

Orzalesi 和 Cook[102]对 12 例严重的漏斗胸畸形儿童进行了研究。来自不同患者的数据都在身高正常值的两个标准差之内，但有 3 位患者的肺活量低，1 位患者的最大换气量低。但是，总的来看，该组肺活量、肺总容量和最大换气量与身高匹配的正常儿童相比，明显降低（P＜0.001）。Weg 等人[141]评估了 25 名空军新兵以采集呼吸症状和漏斗胸的数据，并将他们与 50 名未经选择的新兵进行比较。虽然两组的平均肺活量和最大通气量相当，但是其最好地反映了胸壁功能、肌肉活力和患者的作用，结果显示与期望的正常值有显著差异（P = 0.005）。

Liese 和 Bühlmann[81]采用直立位自行车测力计对 12 例严重的漏斗胸成人进行了术前和术后的肺容量和体力劳动能力的测定。手术校正后进行了 3～11 年（平均 8 年）的术后研究。仅那些在术后长高的患者的绝对肺容量增加。10 例患者中有 9 人的劳动能力增强，但难以评估，因为测试之间都有时间间隔。Godfrey[44]报道选择了一组 5 例漏斗胸和节段性支气管软化的患者，包括左侧主支气管软化。放射核素肺扫描证实 2 例患者的左肺有严重的气井，而第三位患者左肺通气不足和灌注不足。这好像是一个特别的临床组，且所有病例的支气管软化都通过支气管镜加以证实。胸部畸形引起支气管软化的原因尚未明确。

Castile 等人[21]对 8 例患者进行了全面评估，7 例为漏斗胸，1 例为鸡胸。5 例患者在运动后有症状，其余无症状。进行了全面的肺动力学研究，包括标准肺容量、最大肺活量（FVC）、静息压力–容量曲线和自行车测力计的递增稳定状态运动试验。1 例鸡胸患者的气流和容量正常。漏斗胸患者的平均肺总容量为预期值的 79%，有轻度的限制性通气不足。气流容量图正常，并未提示有气道梗阻。运动负荷试验显示运动时的无效腔正常；潮气量比率和肺泡–动脉氧差异并未提示有症状的患者有显著的通气–灌注异常。但是，在运动负荷最大时测定的氧摄取量显著超过预期值；与呈线性反应的正常情况相比，这是一个显著的差异。有症状的患者在最大做功时的平均氧摄取量超过预期值的 25.4%。3 例无症状的患者在运动时显示出正常的线性的氧摄取。尽管其肺活量正常或轻度降低，但这 3 例患者的氧摄取增加提示呼吸做工增加。漏斗胸患者在运动时的潮气量增加普通受限。对这些方面未进行手术后的研究。

Cahill 等人[19]对 19 例 6～17 岁鸡胸（5 例）和漏斗胸（14 例）患者进行了术前和术后（术后 3～9 月）研究。对于鸡胸患者，未证实有术前异常或术后改变。漏斗胸患者肺活量低于正常，术后也没有变化。但是，通过手术校正，患者的肺总容量得到了小幅提升（术前 3.21 ± 1.12，术后 3.49 ± 1.07；P＜0.02），最大主动通气量有显著改善（术前 65.1 ± 31.5 L，术后 78.9 ± 31.5 L；P＜0.001）。通过总运动时间和最大氧耗量（术前 1.26 ± 0.44 L/min，术后 1.46 ± 0.42 L/min；P＜0.001）显示出术后运动耐力也有改善，但是这些因素有明显的相关性。在术前和术后研究中，评估每一位患者在三个不同功率的状态下的心率。在漏斗胸患者的术后研究中，如果给定输出功率，心率相应降低（配对 t 检验显示 P＜0.02），但是鸡胸患者未观察到心率降低。术后不同功率的氧耗量无差异，这支持了做功效能的改善。所观察到的每一运动负荷水平的心率降低，支持了一些关于心脏每搏输出量升高导致运动能力改善的假说。Mead 等[90]通过评估腹内压研究肋架的移动率，发现漏斗胸患者腹压正常，提示其肋架的移动率也是正常水平。

Derveaux 等[30]使用肺功能试验，在手术前和手术后 1～20 年（平均 8 年）评估了 88 例经过相对广泛的胸壁游离修复手术的漏斗胸和鸡胸患者。除那些脊柱侧弯合并漏斗胸的患者外，术前研究值均在正常范围内（即大于预期值的 80%）。所有患者术后的第一秒末用力呼气量（FEV_1）和肺活量都降低，降低程度用预期值的百分比表示，但是随访的绝对数值高于手术前评估的数值。这些患者的放射影像评估证实胸壁轮廓的改善，因此，肺功能恶化不是胸部畸形复发引起的。研究发现患者术前和术后的功能间存在负性相 897
关。那些术前功能低于期望值 75%的人，术后功能有改善，如果术前功能数值高于 75%，则术后结果更差。Morshuis 等[95]的一项研究中发现了相同的结果，他对 152 例漏斗胸患者进行了术前评估和术后平均 8 年的随访。这些生理学结果与患者自述症状和胸壁轮廓的改善相悖。术后研究中的肺功能降低与手术有关，因为在一系列研究中，不管初次手术时年龄如何，术前病损是稳定的。由于明显缺少一个年龄和严重程度匹配的未手术对照组，这些研究都是有问题的。

Derveaux 等人[31]评估了 17 例漏斗胸患者在肺总容量下的经肺压力和经横膈压力。术前和术后长期随访评估之间平均相隔 12 年。经肺和经横膈压力显示，肺外因素比肺部因素引起的限制性病变更大，提示手术增加了胸壁的硬度。

Wynn 等[120]评估了 12 例漏斗胸患者的肺功能测试和运动试验。8 例手术患者进行手术修复并在术前和术后评估。4 例评估了 2 次但未手术。结果发现手术患者的肺总容量减少，而对照组的此数值稳定。两组术前和术后心排量和每搏输出量随运动而增加，认为手术对运动无明显的生理学影响。

Kaguraoka 等[71]评估了 138 例漏斗胸患者术前和术后的肺功能。术后头 2 个月之内的肺活量降低，在术后 1 年恢复到术前水平。术后 42 个月时，尽管胸壁轮廓有明显改善，但是该数值还是维持在基线水平。Tanaka 等[132]得到相似的结果，并证实进行过更大范围的胸骨翻转手术的患者的肺活量在远期显著降低。

Morshuis 等[96]评估了 35 例经过手术的青少年或青年漏斗胸患者（年龄为 17.9 ± 5.6 岁）。术前评估一次，术后 1 年再评估一次。术前肺总容量（预期值的 86.0 ± 14.4%）和肺活量（79.7 ± 16.2%）均显著低于期望值，手术后进一步降低（–9.2 ± 9.27% 和–6.6 ± 10.7%）。最大运动状态下的呼吸效能在术后有显著的改善。43%的患者术后运动时通气受限，而在术后又有改善的趋势。但是，无通气受限组在术后开始表现出受限，并有氧耗量显著升高。

Haller 等[31]评估了 36 例漏斗胸患者和 10 例正常对照。术后 6 个月，对 15 例患者和 6 例对照组再次进行了研究。在手术校正前，漏斗胸组 FVC 降低，而在术后没有变化。虽然 58%的患者主诉运动受限，但其中 66%在术后有改善，他们可承受与对照组相同的运动负荷。两组运动时的呼吸参数相近，提示限制性疾病并不限制运动。手术以后，患者的运动时间比术前长，脉氧水平比术前高，而对照组无变化。运动耐力的增强是由于心功能的改善，脉氧水平增高和肺功能参数无变化证明了这一点。

Borowitz 等[12]对接受微创漏斗胸纠正术（MIRPE）的患者进行早期评估。在 10 例患者的研究中，证实术前和术后肺功能正常。Sigalet 等[129]也报道了 11 例 MIRPE 患者的早期效果，此报道建立在肺功能评估、运动耐力和超声心动图评估心功能的基础上。虽然报道患者的运动耐力有明显改善，但是术后 3 月时的肺功能（FVC 和肺活量）显著降低；同样，最大氧摄取量也降低。相反，心功能增强，每搏输出量升高。

Malek 等人[84]评估了 21 例漏斗胸患者的生理运动。FVC、FEV_1、最大通气量和肺二氧化碳弥散能力的观察值都显著低于正常值，但是肺总容量和残气量却并非如此。运动试验显示，最大氧摄取和氧张力显著低于正常对照组。认为对这些患者而言最大运动受限的心血管因素比肺因素大得多，乳酸集聚的代谢阈值异常降低证实了这一点。在最严重的漏斗胸患者中，这种损害也是最大。

总的来说，过去 40 年的肺功能研究未能证实手术校正能改善肺功能。实际上，许多研究证实，远期评估中的肺功能是恶化的，这是因为术后胸壁硬度增加。尽管有这一发现，但是一些运动负荷试验显示术后运动耐力改善。

心血管功能

胸骨后置引起心脏畸形，特别是右心室前凹。Garusi[42]使用血管造影显示心脏向左侧移位，并在右心室前壁有胸骨压痕。

Bevegård[9]在 1962 年采用右心导管和运动负荷试验研究了 16 例漏斗胸患者。给定心率时，坐位的生 898
理运动能力明显低于仰卧位。那些坐位生理运动能力比仰卧位低 20%以上的人，其胸骨到脊柱的距离比那些运动能力降低在 20%以内的人要短。从仰卧位变为坐位时，静息每搏输出量平均降低 40.3%，与正常人相似。仰卧位时，运动后每搏输出量增加 13.2%。坐位时，从静息到运动后的每搏输出量增加 18.5%，显著低于正常人 51%的增幅（$P<0.001$）。因此，尽管每搏输出量受限，但可通过增加心率来提高心排出量。这解释了坐位时，任何给定心率的运动能力较低。尽管心室容量明显受限，但是所有患者在静息和运动时的心内压都正常。

Beiser 等[8]提供了直立运动时心功能减弱，而在仰卧位相对正常的进一步证据。对 6 例中度漏斗胸患者进行了心导管检查。在静息仰卧位时测得的右心房压、右心室压、肺动脉压和肺毛细血管楔压均正常。虽然有 2 例患者直立运动时的心指数低于期望值，并有 3 例患者位于正常低限，但是中等运动时的心指数正常。漏斗胸患者直立位的心功能差异，主要是由于每搏输出量较小引起的。直立位运动比仰卧位运动的每搏输出量低 31%，心排出量低 28%。对 3 例患者进行了术后研究；2 例手术后运动水平增高。心指数的平均增幅为 38%。因为术后最大运动时的心率没有增加，所以是每搏输出量的反应引起了这一增长。

Peterson 等[104]使用放射核素血管造影评估了 13 例漏斗胸患者的心脏容量和心排出量。7 例患者在术前有症状，但症状的程度与解剖畸形的严重程度无关。使用自行车测力计进行直立位运动，直至达到根据年龄预测的最大心率的 85%，或患者由于疲劳或呼吸困难而无法继续运动为止。13 例患者中术前有 10 人可达到目标心率，但仅 4 人在完成检查时未出现症状。手术后，除 1 人外的所有人在运动试验中达到目标心率，13 例患者中有 9 人在完成检查时未出现症状。漏斗胸矫正术后，在常规运动模式下症状明显改善的证据，证实了早年许多无对照报道中症状改善的情况。难以评价这种变化的作用和对手术的主要反应。在患者静息时，然后在目标心率时或运动终末点时注入放射核素。这个研究未能证实漏斗胸矫正后患者在静息状态或运动状态时，左心室射血分数有任何显著的变化。术后静息状态的左心室舒张末容量相应增加，而且术后平均每搏排出量增加 19%，但在运动时无相应增加。术后静息状态或运动时的心指数未有显著上升。Kowalewski 等[73]对 42 例漏斗胸患者进行研究，通过超声心动图评估了术前和术后 6 月时的心功能。术后右心室容量指数（收缩期、舒张期和每搏排出量）有显著的统计学变化。胸指数和心脏变化之间无相关。这些结果支持了早期 Haller 等[51]、Sigalet 等[129]和 Malek 等[84]引用的数据，均提示右心室压迫造成了每搏排出量受限。

需要进行附加研究来判定漏斗胸和心肺功能之间的关系。动力或运动试验是这一领域内最有前景的研究方法。需要更好的方法评估术前的心肺功能来鉴别哪些儿童可能在手术以后得到症状和生理学的改善。

超声心动图检查

Udoshi 等人[134]对成年漏斗胸患者的前瞻性超声心动图研究证实了 33 例患者中 6 例有二尖瓣脱垂（18%），Saint-Mezard 等人[113]也发现 17 例患者中 11 例有二尖瓣脱垂。胸骨凹陷造成的心脏前部压迫可能是二尖瓣瓣环或心室腔变形的原因，并引起这些患者的二尖瓣脱垂。23 例儿童和青少年患者中，有 10 例的二尖瓣脱垂在术后缓解。

治疗

Meyer[90]在 1911 年，Sauerbruch[115]在 1913 年首次提出了漏斗胸的手术治疗。随着经验的增加和对疾病基本因素的明确，手术方法有了显著的变化。1939年 Ochsner 和 DeBakey[98]总结了早期手术许多重要的经验。Ravitch[108]在 1949 年报道了一种技术，此技术包括切除所有畸形肋软骨和软骨膜，将剑突从胸骨上断开，从胸骨上断开肋间肌束，并做胸骨横向截骨，最初 2 例患者采用的 Kirschner 钢针向前固定胸骨的技术，以及以后病例采用的丝线固定胸骨。他的技术后来被改良，以保留软骨膜鞘，但是仍然将肋间肌束和软骨膜鞘与胸骨分离[109]。在 1957 和 1958 年，Baronofsky[7]和 Welch[42]分别报道了相似的技术，并强调了完全保留肋 899
软骨的软骨膜鞘、保留上部的肋间肌束、胸骨截骨和采用丝线向前固定胸骨。Haller 等[52]随后发展出一种技术，称为三脚架固定，对畸形软骨做软骨膜下切除和胸骨后截骨。然后将大部分头侧的正常软骨延后外侧方向进行斜形断开。提升胸骨时，软骨的胸骨端保留在软骨断端上，以提供胸骨进一步的前向支撑。

一些作者将肋骨或软骨放在胸骨后方进行支撑，但是这个技术从未被广泛接受[27,109]。该技术有一种变型，就是采用带血管的肋骨[54]。许多作者也采用外支架对胸骨进行支撑，将支架用缝线或钢丝与松解游离的胸骨固定在一起，但是使用时间必须加以限制，以避免引起手术伤口的感染[16,80,98,149,151]。许多作者对支撑胸骨的金属支撑杆进行了改进[36,53]。Rehbein[110]发明一种支撑杆，放在肋骨软骨连接处的肋骨骨髓腔中。这种支撑杆向前固定在胸骨上形成一个弓，胸骨与此弓相连接。Paltia[103]在胸骨的尾端放置一个横向的支撑杆，用肋骨来支撑此杆的两端，并紧紧固定其位置。Adkins 和 Blades[1]和后来的 Jensen 等人[66]使用了一个胸骨后的金属支撑杆来提升胸骨。Willital[148]对肋软骨进行了多重软骨切开术，为胸骨和胸壁提供柔韧度，再采用一个相似的胸骨后支撑杆。对于这些方法的改革包括使用生物吸收性支撑杆，采用 Marlex 聚乙烯网或 Dacron 人造血管作为支撑体，或采用小型化的金属板。但是，并没有证据证明这些技术比传统方法好[29,43,76,78,87,90,97]。

1954 年和 1956 年，Judet[69]和 Jung[70]分别在法语文献中提出了胸骨翻转的假说。这种方法最初在日本使用，Wada 等[138]报道了大量系列病例。这一技术采用一块游离的自体胸骨，翻转 180 度后，向后固定在原来切下它的肋软骨位置。这个方法严重并发症的发病率高，包括伤口感染、开裂和胸骨坏死。Taguchi[131]改良了此方法，保留乳内动脉，以防止骨坏死和伤口感染。其他人阐述了对乳内动脉进行微血管吻合，以保留胸骨的血供[133]。胸骨翻转是一种儿童漏斗胸畸形的根治方法，给治疗增加了一个选择。

最后一种修复方法是在皮下间隙注入硅胶来填满畸形的地方。虽然这种方法能改善胸部轮廓，但是不能增加胸廓内容积，通常会并发早期血清肿或形成血肿。

Nuss 阐述的 MIRPE 技术见本章附录。

手术技术

图 59–2 描绘的是手术技术。对女性患者要特别注意将切口定位在乳房下的皱褶处，以避免损伤乳芽或形成的瘢痕延伸到乳房[60]。目前使用胸骨后支撑杆将胸骨紧紧地向前固定。避免进行胸骨截骨；但是，在获取胸骨的游离度以便缝合固定时需要这么做。保留肋间肌束、软骨膜和直肌剑的连接，以提供更正常的胸部轮廓。

围术期使用抗生素，在即将手术前给予一剂，术后给予三剂。告诫所有患者在术前 2 周内不要服用阿司匹林或含有布洛芬的复方药物，以免造成血小板功能异常。当引流量降低到每 8 小时 15 ml 以下时，去除 Hemovac 引流器。术后 6 个月移去 Rehbein 支撑杆或胸骨后支撑杆，以使胸骨坚实固定。在胸骨后支撑杆一端做小切口将其取出。

并发症

应限制术后并发症的发生，包括伤口感染和气胸。大多数病例采用电灼止血来避免输血。除非影响了肺功能，大多数气胸只需要观察。复发是手术的缺点，且无论使用何种技术都有可能发生。转而将支撑杆固定在胸骨上来改善早期效果，将手术推迟到儿童即将进入青春期发育时再进行。胸部的生长为胸壁重构和随后的复发提供了机会。没有支撑杆固定和无支撑杆固定的随机化研究，因为对这样一个研究能否完成还存在疑问。在随访良好的大型研究中，报道有 5%～15% 的病例复发。术后随时间推移而逐渐恶化的病例已有详细的报道，特别是在青春期的快速生长期内发生的[11,62,74]。对 Marfan 综合征患者都应实施牢固固定，因为已经完全认识到这种患者的复发风险高[117]。

已经注意到，早年接受手术的儿童有一个严重的并发症，特别是 4 岁以下进行手术的儿童：切除肋软骨后，肋骨的生长受损，造成了胸廓中部的束带样狭窄（图 59–3）。在一些病例中，第一和第二肋骨生长相对过度，造成胸骨上部向前凸出。1990 年，Martinez[86]首先提出了在学龄前进行漏斗胸手术后，胸廓生长存在这种缺陷。1995 年，Haller[48]报道了 3 例早年手术切除肋软骨的男孩，在十几岁时出现了这种问题，将这种并发症称为获得性青少年病。Haller 等[48]将这种并 90
发症归咎于手术时损伤了肋骨软骨连接处，纵行生长就会以肋骨为中心。

Martinez[86]通过实验切除了 6 周大的正常兔子的肋软骨，在 5 个半月的观察期内，证实对胸部生长，特别是前后径的发育造成了明显损害。如果仅切除四分之三的肋软骨，造成的损害会稍微减轻，因为这样就保留了以肋骨软骨连接处为中心的生长。该损害是由软骨膜鞘内纤维化和瘢痕形成引起的。由于形成了横跨胸部的束带样狭窄，所以软骨膜鞘、骨或其他无法生长的前体组织不能在胸骨后方联合。将手术推迟到儿童年长期再进行可避免这种并发症。通过在肋骨的骨性部分保留一段软骨来保存肋骨软骨连接处，可以部分减少生长受损。Weber[139]描述了一种改善严重肺部损害的方法，用于治疗 1 例获得性青少年患者。进行胸骨切开，使用肋骨支撑杆将其永久撑开。双侧胸膜打开，同时在 6 对肋骨上做软骨膜下切除。术后 90
肺功能改善。

有报道支撑杆断裂后长期存留体内，侵犯心肌的案例[101]。由于这个原因，大多数支撑杆应该在一个合适的时期后取出，以便胸壁完全愈合。

图 59-2 漏斗胸修复的手术技术。A．在乳房下皱褶水平的两乳头线之间做横向皮肤切口。采用电刀游离松解皮瓣，主要沿中线；向上到 Louis 角，向下到剑突水平。将胸大肌从胸骨上提起，同时提起胸小肌和前锯肌。B．使用电刀掀起肌肉的内缘之后，将一把空刀柄直接伸到肋软骨前方来确定正确的胸肌瓣分离平面。接着用一个直角拉钩代替刀柄，向前拉起。然后在毗邻的肋软骨前方重复此过程。肌肉分离和提升的两侧边界是到第三至第五肋的肋软骨连接处。分离时向前拉开肌肉，以便确定无血管的间隙平面，避免进入肋间肌束。

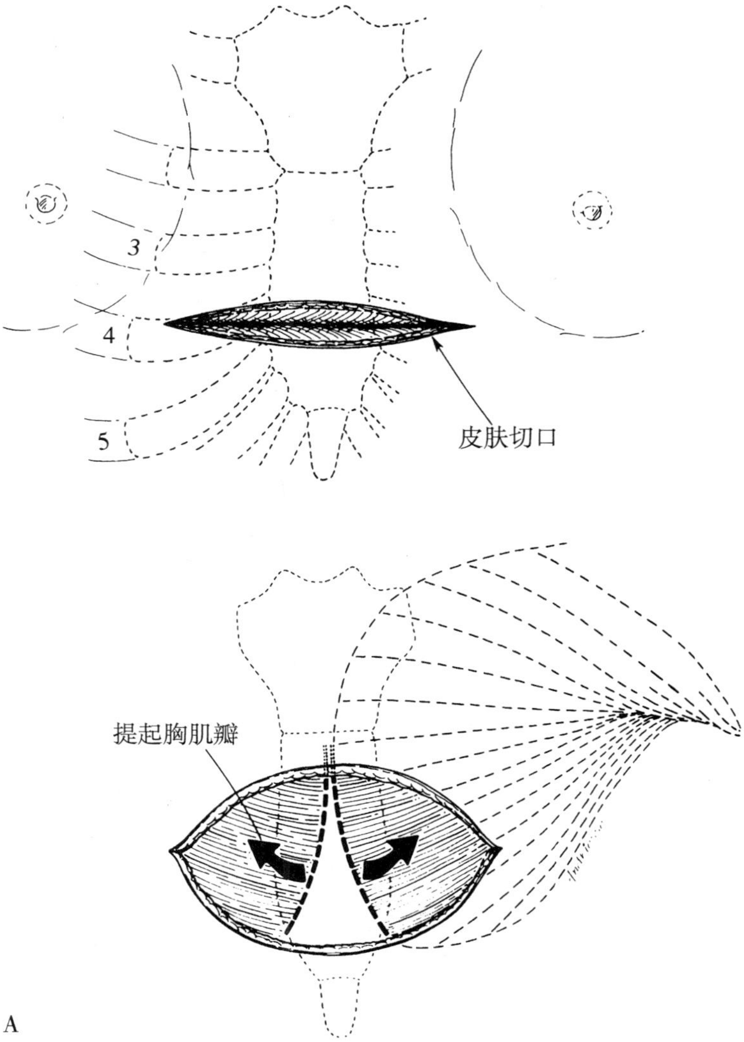

A

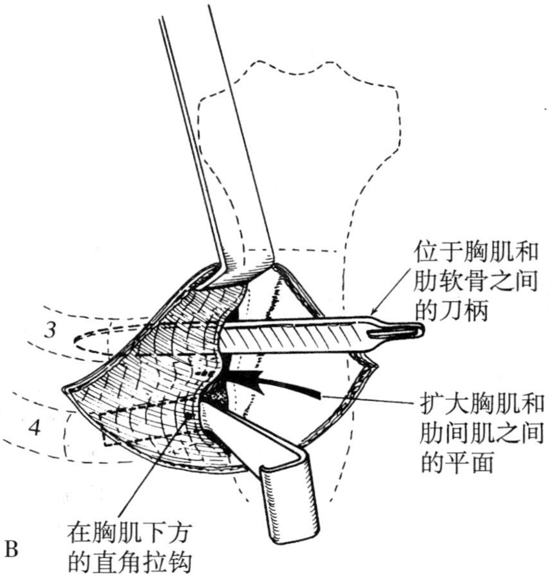

B

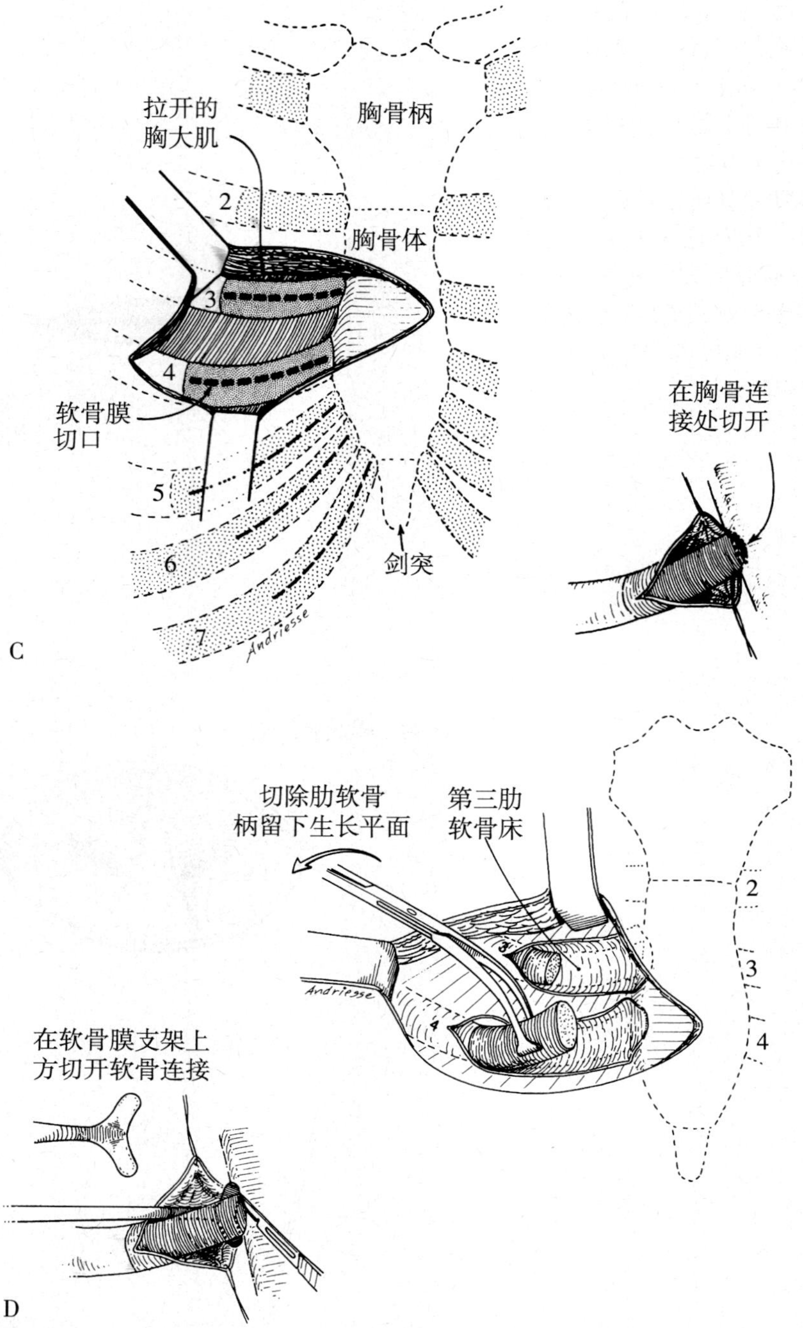

图 59–2　（续）C．切开前方的软骨膜，对肋软骨进行软骨膜下切除。然后在软骨膜和肋软骨之间的无血管平面上分离肋软骨。在每一个软骨膜与胸骨连接（插图）处，延 90° 方向向后切开软骨膜，以获取肋软骨后壁的视野。D．用刀在胸骨连接处切断软骨。将一个 Welch 软骨膜支架放在肋骨后方，以保护纵隔（插图）。然后用 Allis 钳夹住已切断的软骨，并提起，切除肋软骨，在肋骨上要保留 5～10 mm 的边缘，以保护肋骨软骨连接和纵行生长平面。第六和第七肋软骨做节段切除，一直切到它们平直地进入肋弓的位置。熟悉肋软骨内侧端的横截面有利于对它们的切除。第二和第三软骨扁而宽，第四和第五为圆形，第六和第七窄而深。

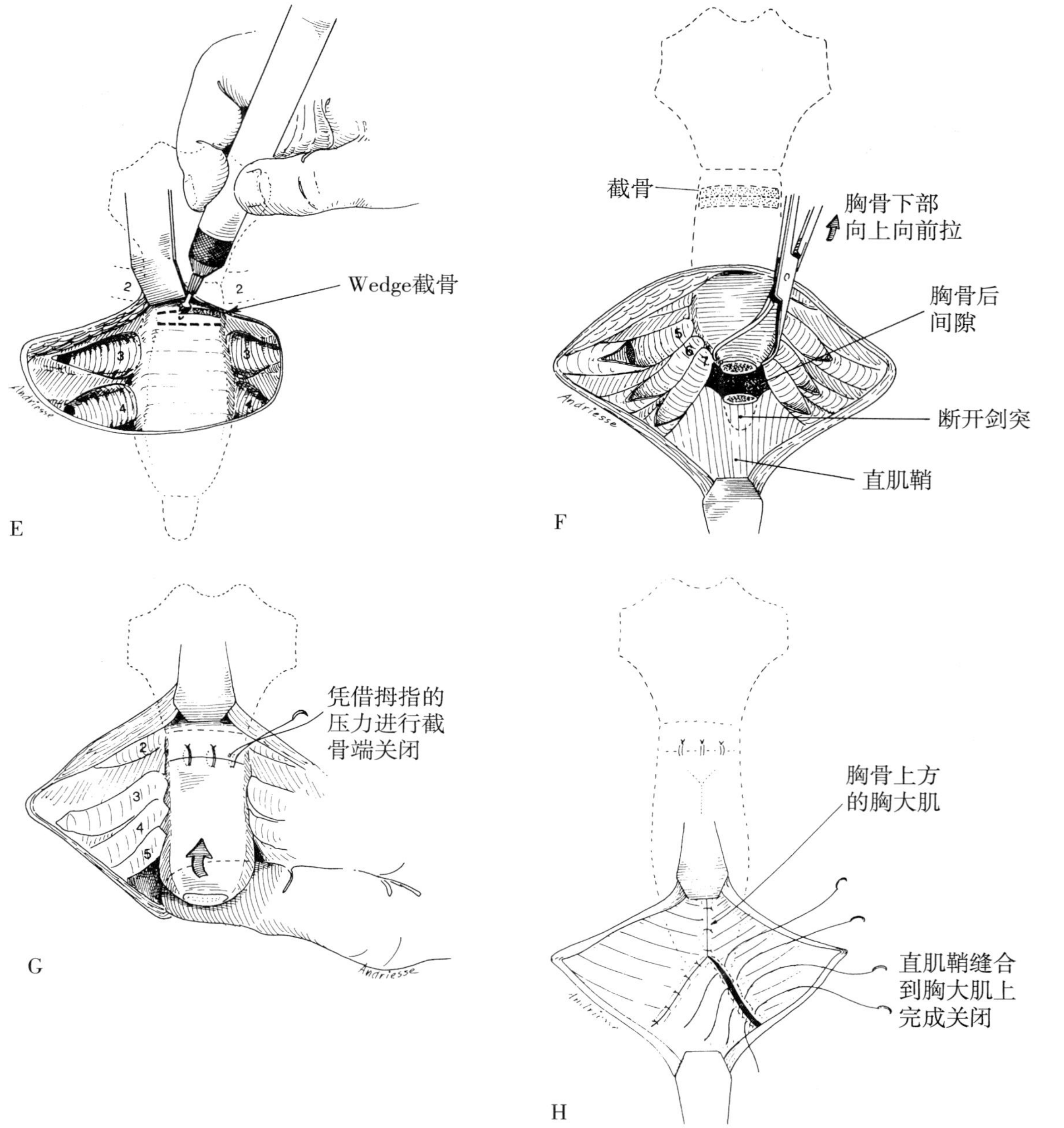

图 59–2　（续）E．在最后一根畸形软骨的上方进行胸骨截骨，截骨位于胸骨向后成角处。通常位于第三肋软骨连接处的上方，偶尔是第二肋软骨。在胸骨的前皮质用手持式钻孔机（Zimmer USA, Inc., Warsaw, Ind.）进行两次横向胸骨截骨，两次截骨距离 2～4 cm。去除之间的前皮质短节段，和下方的网状骨质。F．胸骨基底部和直肌瓣用两个巾钳提起，打断胸骨后板。用电刀将剑突从胸骨上离断下来，进入胸骨后间隙。如果使用胸骨后支撑杆的话，就不需要这一步骤。保留鞘和剑突的附着，避免胸骨下方可能发生的丑陋压迫。G．不使用支撑杆时，助手用拇指将胸骨提升到过度矫正的位置，用几根粗丝线对截骨部位进行缝合关闭。H．在皮瓣下方将单腔中型 Hemovac 引流器（Snyder Laboratories, Inc., New Philadelphia, Ohio）放到胸骨左侧，并放置在正确的胸骨旁位置，向上到最高的肋软骨切除点的水平。胸肌瓣固定到胸骨中线，向前拉拢以完全覆盖胸骨。直肌瓣如果也离断过的话，就和胸肌瓣缝在一起。

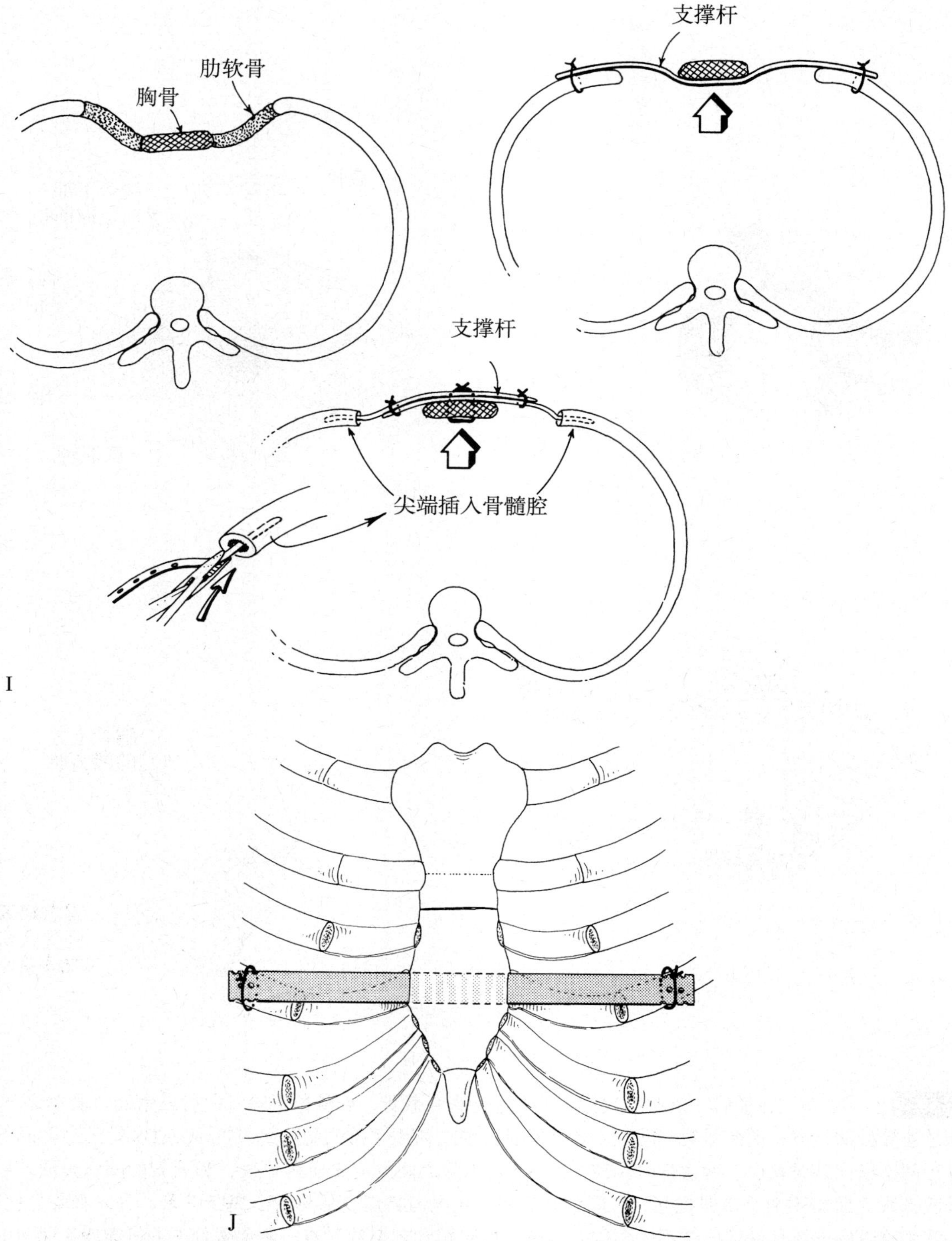

图 59-2　（续）I. 使用胸骨后支撑杆和Rehbein支撑杆。将 Rehbein 支撑杆插入第三或第四肋骨的骨髓腔（插图），然后将两部分向中间靠拢，以形成一个位于胸骨前的弓形金属结构。将胸骨固定在这个弓上，保持前倾位。胸骨后支撑杆放置在胸骨后方，并固定在两侧肋骨骨端上防止移位。J. 胸骨后支撑杆的前面观。第三或第四肋的软骨膜鞘在胸骨连接处离断，胸骨后间隙进行钝性分离，以便在胸骨后方穿过支撑杆。必须获得一个足够的空间，以免损伤心包。用两道环绕肋骨的缝线固定于支撑杆两侧，以防移位。（A to H, From Shamberger RC, Welch KJ: Surgical repair of pectus excavatum. J Pediatr Surg 1988;23:615-622. I and J, From Shamberger RC: Chest wall deformities. In Shields TW [ed]: General Thoracic Surgery, 5th ed. Philadelphia, Lippincott Williams & Wilkins, 2000.）

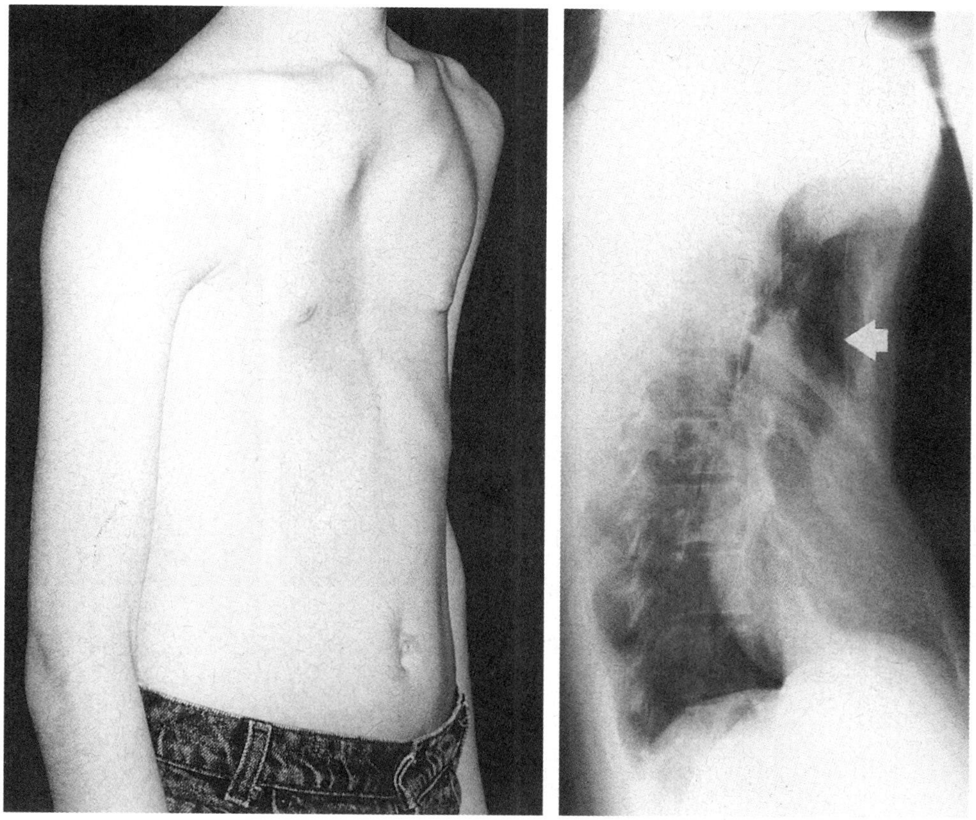
A　B

图 59-3　A. 18 岁男性，漏斗胸术后 15 年，中央广泛复发，并有上方未切除之肋软骨和肋骨的过度生长。B. 侧位放射影像证实胸骨（箭头处）与脊柱平行，且上方肋骨相对凸出。

凸出畸形：鸡胸

鸡胸由一组畸形组成，其发生率略低于漏斗胸，与漏斗胸的发病率比值为 1∶5[122]。男孩比女孩更多见，男女比例为 4∶1，这和漏斗胸相似。几乎半数的儿童在 11 岁前未表现出畸形。出生时或童年早期发现的轻度畸形通常随着儿童的生长发育有所恶化，特别在青春期。因此，大多数儿童在十几岁时寻求治疗。

病因

鸡胸的病因没有漏斗胸明确。早期的研究认为与横膈的发育异常有关，但是却从未肯定[14,22]。还有人提出，由于肋骨或肋软骨的生长过度造成了鸡胸或漏斗胸[128]。两种关联为病因提供了一些线索：（1）26%的患者有胸壁畸形的家族史，提示有遗传学因素；（2）15%的患者有脊柱侧弯，提示广泛的结缔组织发育异常。

临床表现

鸡胸最常见的形态是胸骨体和肋软骨的对称性凸出，称为软骨胸骨凸出（图 59-4）。通常合并肋骨侧面凹陷（Harrison 沟），胸部两侧如同遭受大掌挤压一般[61]。凸出也可是不对称的，局限于胸骨的一侧和肋骨，造成一种龙骨样的凸出（图 59-5）。也会发生凸出和凹陷同时存在的混合性畸形。胸骨通常朝凹陷侧向后旋转。这种变异多见于 Poland 综合征。鸡胸最罕见的形态是软骨胸骨柄凸出，由胸骨柄和上方肋软骨凸出所致，同时胸骨体相对凹陷（图 59-6）。多合并胸骨缝的过早融合，而且胸骨呈逗号样或 Z 形。发现这些儿童合并先天性心脏病的比率很高[25]。Lees 和 Caldicott[79]在 1915 个儿童中发现 135 例胸骨融合畸形

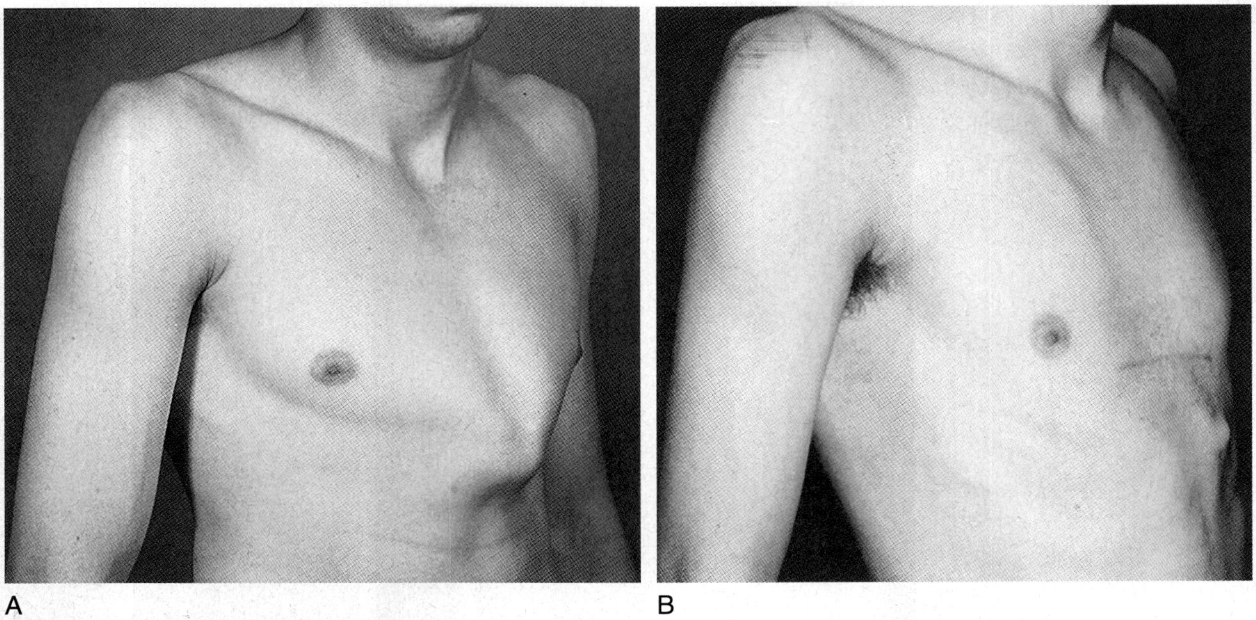

图 59-4 A．对称性软骨胸骨体鸡胸的 19 岁男性患者。B．术后照片显示凸出的胸骨和肋软骨矫正良好。

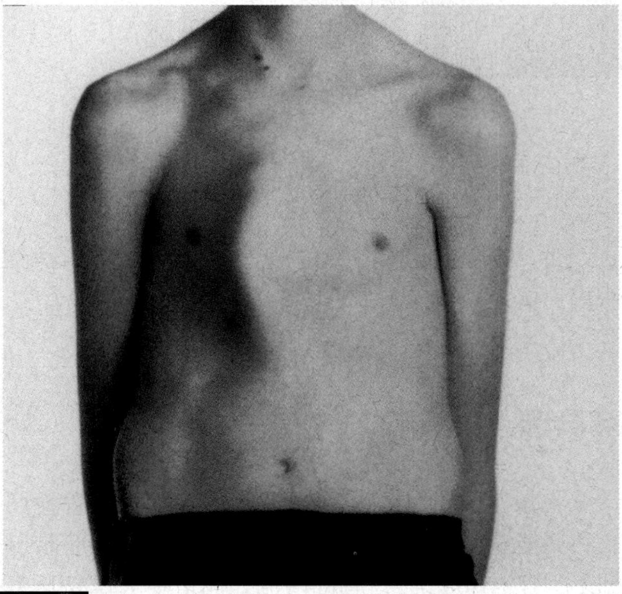

图 59-5 非对称性鸡胸的 12 岁男孩，肋软骨向右侧凸出，形成龙骨样畸形。

病例。20%胸骨融合的患者中，患有先天性心脏病。

治疗

已有文献回顾了鸡胸手术治疗的历史[122]。1973 年 Welch 和 Vos[144]报道了他们治疗 26 例此类畸形患者的方法。他们强调需要保留软骨膜鞘并通过设计截骨来获取胸骨的合理位置。Pickard 等人[105]也采用了类似的方法。采用矫形支具治疗鸡胸的案例也有所报道，并在年幼儿童中取得了成功[33,46,93]。年长儿童对支具的依从性较差，主要是因为会引起不适。

手术技术

最初与漏斗胸手术一样，通过横切口进行鸡胸手术的暴露，然后再进行皮肤和胸肌瓣的松解游离。许多作者强调需要去除全部或部分畸形的软骨[114,122]，因为随着生长继续，轻度畸形会恶化并变得明显。在软骨胸骨体畸形中，通过单次或偶尔二次截骨打断胸骨后板，将胸骨恢复到正常位置（图 59-7A）。切口放置引流，并采用和漏斗胸手术一样的方法进行关闭。

混合畸形的胸骨倾斜必须加以矫正，凹陷和凸出的肋软骨也必须矫正。对异常的肋软骨做软骨膜下切除后，在胸骨前板做楔形截骨，楔形宽边朝向胸骨凹陷一侧（图 59-7B）。关闭截骨点能将胸骨提升并旋转到矫正位置。用缝线加固关闭截骨点或使用支撑杆加固。

对于软骨胸骨柄畸形和混合畸形，处理胸骨时要

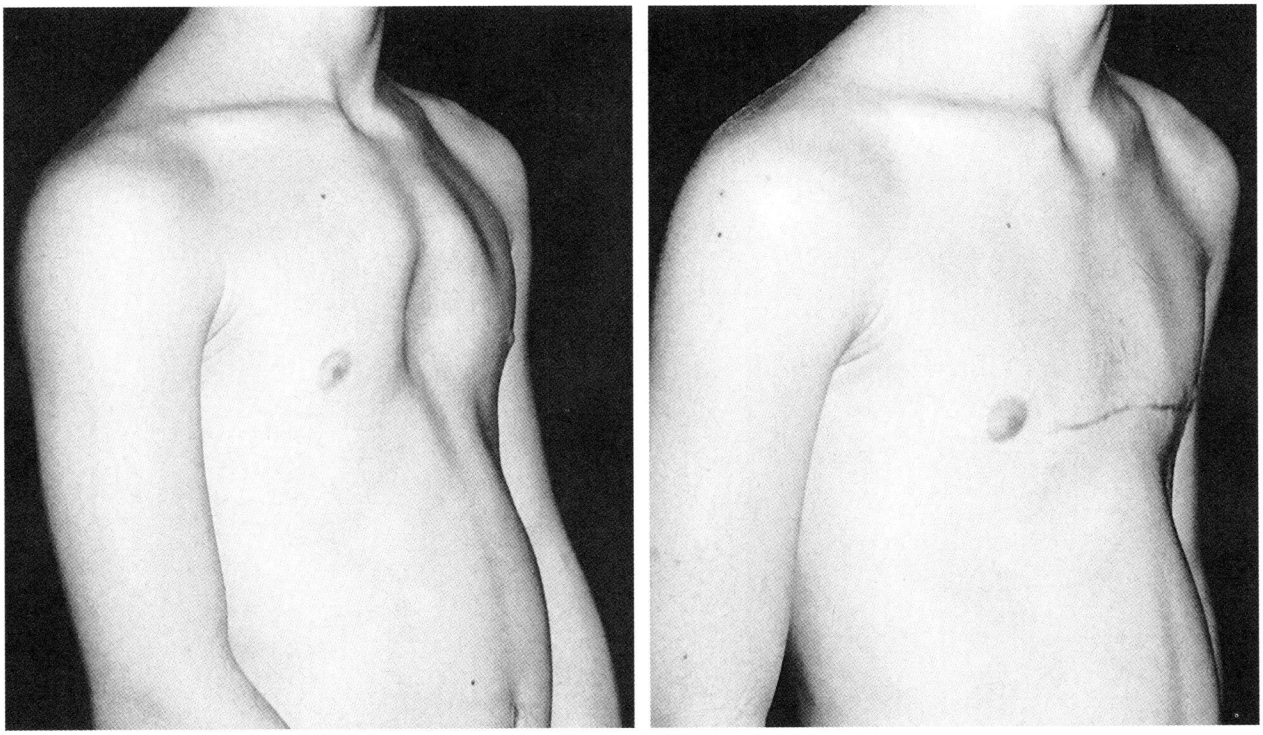

A B

图 59-6 A．软骨胸骨柄畸形的 15 岁男孩。注意第二和第三肋软骨向前的弓状凸出加重了下部胸骨的向后凹陷。B．术后，胸骨轮廓改善，肋软骨重新塑形到更合理的部位。

907 特别注意。软骨胸部柄畸形时，胸骨上部凸出，下部向脊柱成角。Ravitch[108]在对此畸形的矫正手术进行首次报道时指出，他在胸骨凸出程度最大的地方，将胸骨前板切除一块楔形骨质，并在 Z 形胸骨的第二弯曲点进行了二次截骨。根据我的经验，将胸骨截短并塑造成逗号的形状，就无需进行二次截骨了 (图 59–7C)。当截骨端关闭后，胸骨的下部后凹和胸骨柄的向前成角就得以矫正，胸骨柄在其与第一肋软骨的连接点位置向后旋转。

并发症

手术的并发症很少见，包括感染、气胸、肺炎或伤口裂开。使用电刀止血就很少需要输血。矫正的效果是极其成功的，罕有复发。畸形矫正不完全和在幼年畸形发育完全之前进行手术，都是再次手术的主要原因。

Poland 综合征

虽然德国和法国有更早的病例报道[41,128]，但对 Poland 综合征的最初描述出现在 1841 年的英语文献中[106]。Poland 在他还是个医学生的时候，就报道了一例他进行解剖的病例。他描述了一组畸形，包括胸大肌和胸小肌缺如以及并指（趾）畸形。随后的报道补充了该综合征的其他畸形，包括肋骨缺如、胸壁凹陷、无乳头或无乳房、无腋毛以及皮下脂肪有限。Thompson 在 1895 年最早对所有的畸形进行了总结[128]。虽然以前其他人对此病进行过描述，但是 1962 年后，Clarkson[23]首次对这组患者进行命名时，将此病称为 Poland 综合征。

胚胎学

Poland 综合征呈散发发病，每 30 000～32 000 例

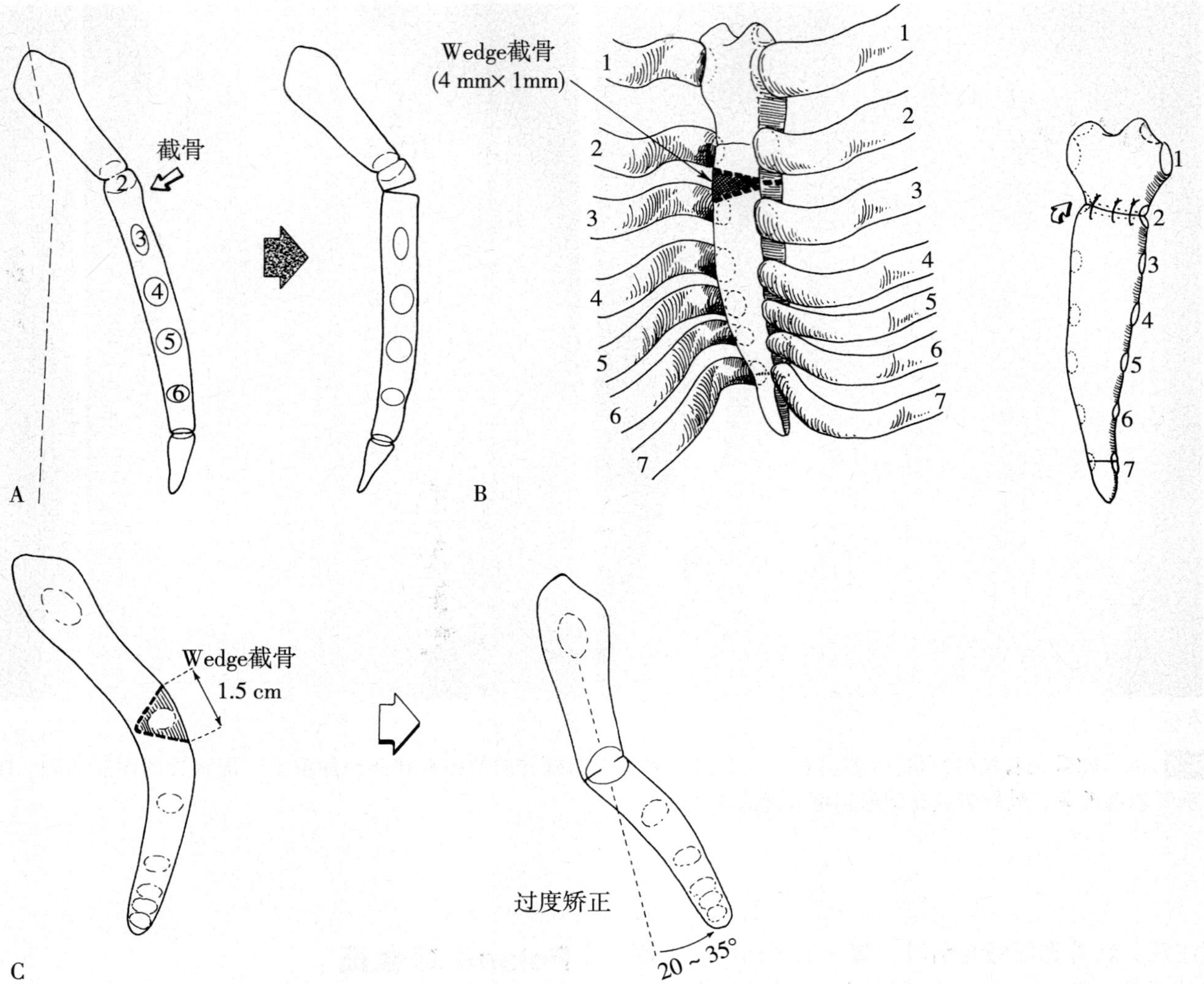

图 59-7 A. 切除肋软骨后的单次或二次截骨，将向后异位的胸骨恢复到正常位置。B. 通过全部和对称切除第三至第七肋软骨，并做横向偏转的楔形胸骨截骨，来矫正混合性胸部畸形。关闭此缺损使胸骨前移并旋转。C. 在闭合的胸骨柄连接处的前皮质进行宽楔形胸骨截骨，来矫正软骨胸骨畸形。打断胸骨后皮质后关闭截骨点，使胸骨前部向后移，此时胸骨仅通过与第一肋骨的连接来确保定位。胸骨下部过度矫正 20～35°。(B, From Shamberger RC, Welch KJ: Surgical correction of pectus carinatum. J Pediatr Surg 1987;22:48-53. C, From Shamberger RC, Welch KJ: Surgical correction of chondromanubrial deformity (Currarino-Silverman syndrome). J Pediatr Surg 1988;34:319-322.)

活产婴儿中有 1 例；家族性罕见[40,88]。已经提出不少发病因素，包括形成胸肌的胚胎组织移行异常、锁骨下动脉发育不良和试图流产造成的宫内损伤，但是这些理论均没有得到广泛接受[13,28]。虽然一些并指（趾）畸形被认为是染色体显性性状，但是 Poland 综合征的患者却没有发现有相同的模式：此病通常为散发。Poland 综合征会合并第二种罕见的综合征，Möbius 综合征，包括双侧或单侧面瘫和眼外直肌瘫痪。Fontaine 和 Ovlaque[39]鉴别出 19 例这种患者，但缺乏一致的发病原因。Boaz 等人[10]报道了 Poland 综合征与儿童期白血病之间非同寻常的关联。

临床表现

该综合征患儿的临床表现存在显著的多样性（图 59-8）。显著的缺陷存在不同，取决于不同部位的受累程度。根据定义，所有的 Poland 综合征儿童有胸

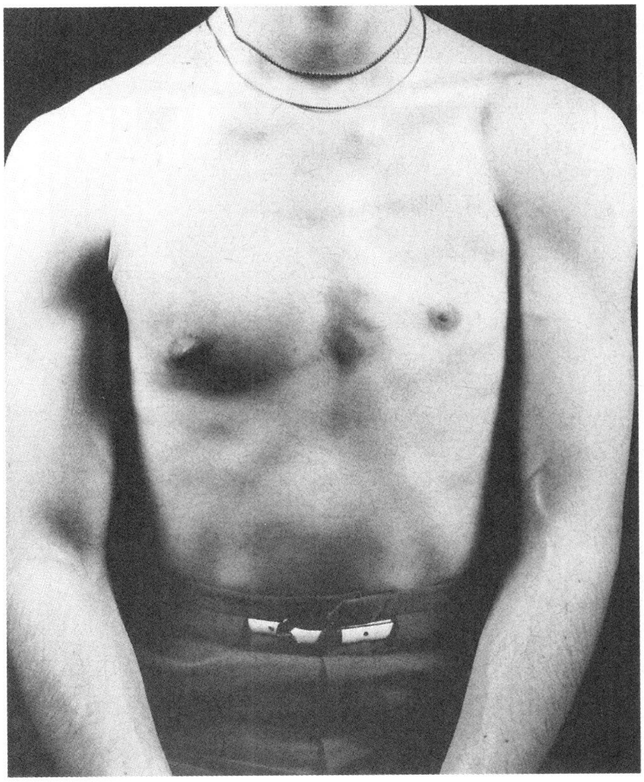

A

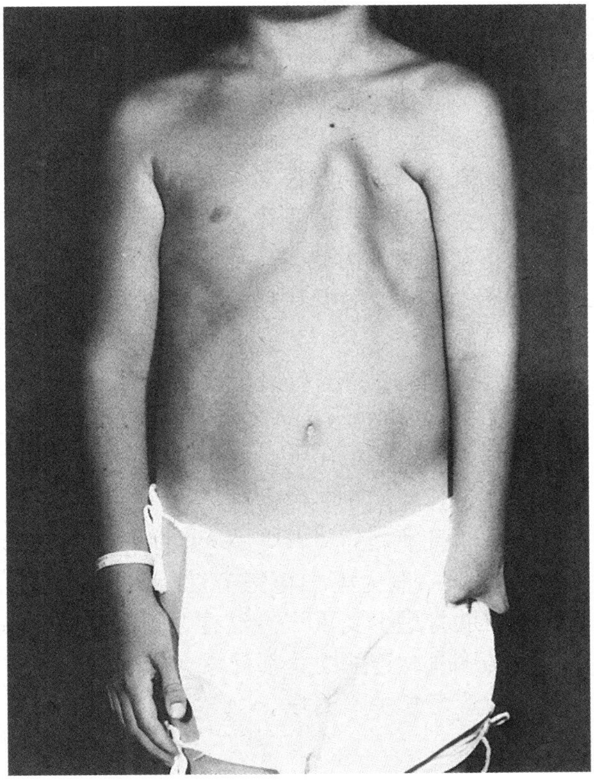

B

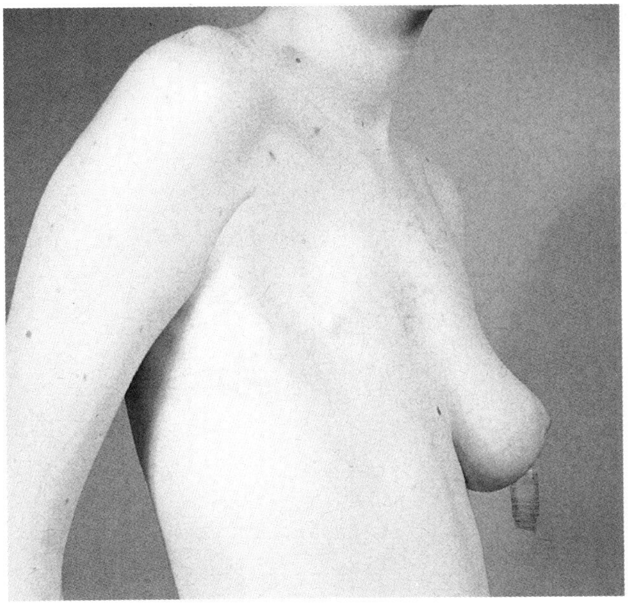

C

图 59-8　Poland 综合征。A．健壮的 15 岁男孩，左胸轻度发育不良，胸小肌和胸大肌的软骨胸骨柄部分缺如，造成腋前皱褶缺失。B．8 岁儿童，左侧第三至第五肋骨发育不全，胸骨向左旋转，左侧肋骨凹陷畸形。注意同时有左乳头发育不良和手的缺肢畸形。C．14 岁女孩，右侧胸壁中度凹陷，发育不良的高位乳头和无乳房畸形。第二至第四肋骨前部发育不全。（From Shamberger RC, Welch KJ, Upton J III: Surgical treatment of thoracic deformity in Poland's syndrome. J Pediatr Surg 1989;24:760.）

大肌、胸骨、软骨部分的发育不全或发育不良，并至少合并一种其他病变。手、乳房或胸壁畸形的程度存在很大的变异。Thompson[128]早年对此综合征进行总结时发现，20 例患者的胸大肌完全缺如，63 例部分缺陷；胸骨软骨部分是普遍的缺失部分。53 例患者的胸小肌缺如，许多其他病例也有部分缺陷。无一病例是正常的。但是，患儿同侧的手臂不会出现功能障碍，因为他们对缺失的胸肌有良好的代偿。手部的畸形变化很广泛。在 Ireland 等人[64]的报道中，所有的患者都有并指（趾）和不同程度的短指（趾），作者对患者的选择和参照的模式造成了这一明显的结果。在另一组对 75 例 Poland 综合征儿童的研究中，50 例有手部畸形，37 例有乳房或乳头的缺如或发育不良[120]。许多患者的乳头有轻度的色素沉积，并比对侧正常的乳头高出胸壁很多。胸壁和手部畸形的严重程度之间无相关性。这些儿童胸部畸形的变异程度很大，从正常的肋骨构型到二至三根肋骨发育不全（表 59-2；图 59-9）。很少有儿童严重到需要手术来治疗胸壁畸形。

已经证实 CT 扫描有助于评估胸壁的构型以及是否需要重建（图 59-10）[6]。CT 扫描也可以评估肌肉受累的程度。有一例患者，由于没有发现背阔肌发育不良，而导致背阔肌肌皮瓣衰竭[24]。

所有肋骨缺如的患者应该考虑进行手术修复。肋骨发育不全一般为第二至第五肋骨的复合性发育不
908 全，第二肋骨最少受累[128]。仅有 2 例报道在第一肋以下所有与胸骨相连的肋骨都受累。同侧胸壁严重凹陷的患者，应考虑手术治疗。

表 59-2 75 例 Poland 综合征患者的胸壁畸形

畸形	患者人数
无畸形	41
肋骨发育不良，无凹陷	10
肋骨凹陷畸形	
重大	11
轻微	5
肋骨发育不全	8

From Shamberger RC, Welch KJ, Upton J III: Surgical treatment of thoracic deformity in Poland's syndrome. J Pediatr Surg 1989;24:760.

治疗

Ravitch[109]和其他人报道了采用自体肋骨移植来重建发育不全的肋骨。使用背阔肌覆盖肋骨来改善外

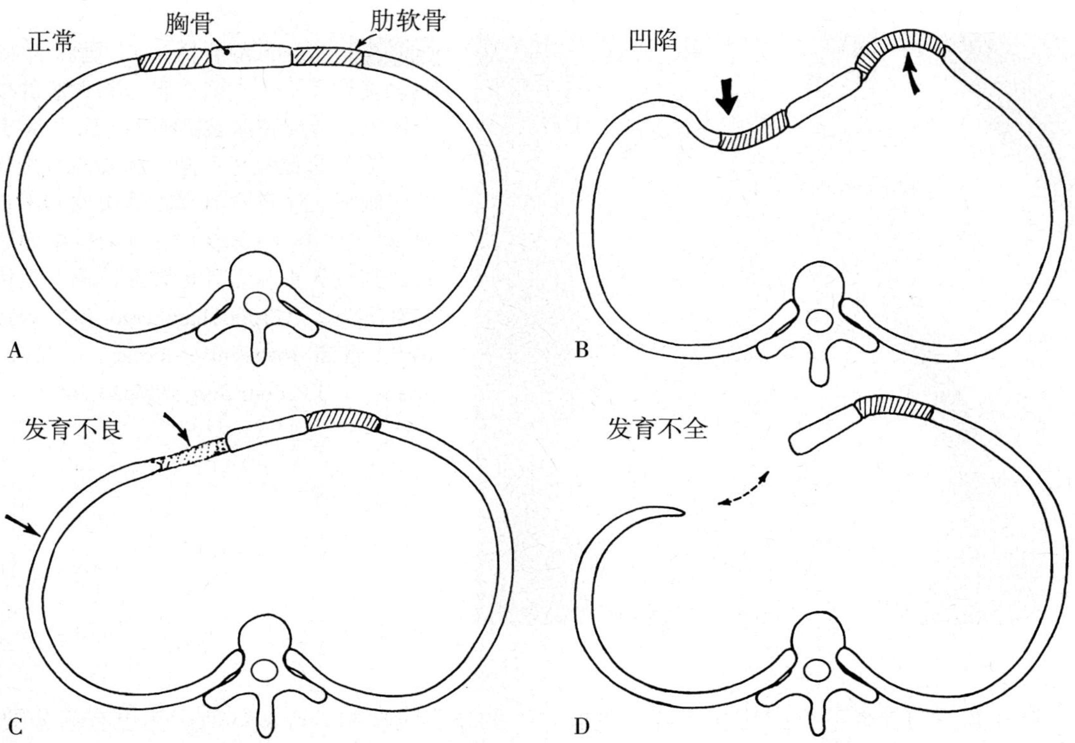

图 59-9 Poland 综合征的一系列肋架畸形。A. 最常见的，肋架正常，仅胸肌缺如。B. 胸壁受累侧凹陷，胸骨有旋转和常见的凹陷畸形。对侧常有龙骨状凸出。C. 受累侧肋骨发育不良，但无显著凹陷。这通常不需要手术矫正。D. 受累侧有一根或多根肋骨发育不全，合并相邻肋骨的凹陷和胸骨旋转。（From Shamberger RC, Welch KJ, Upton J III: Surgical treatment of thoracic deformity in Poland's syndrome. J Pediatr Surg 1989;24:760.）

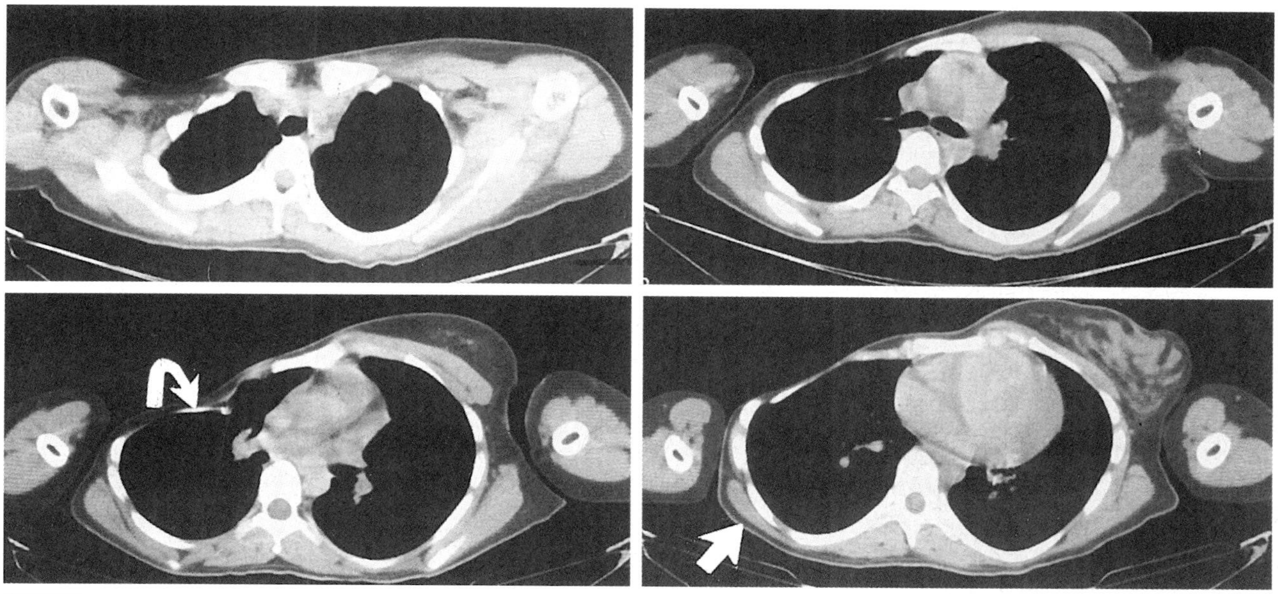

图 59-10 图 59-8C 患者的计算机断层扫描。肋骨凹陷明显（弯箭头处），下方两幅图像上有肋骨发育不全。注意在右下方一幅图像上的背阔肌发育不良(直箭头)。(From Shamberger RC, Welch KJ, Upton J III: Surgical treatment of thoracic deformity in Poland's syndrome. J Pediatr Surg 1989;24:760.)

观，但是如果背阔肌也发育不良的话，就会导致背阔肌的功能丧失[37,58,99]。使用背阔肌瓣进行乳房重建可能对女性较合适，但是在男性中的使用还有质疑——虽然背阔肌瓣和埋植体一起使用可纠正胸壁畸形，但是男性手臂的力量更重要。Haller 等人[49]和 Urschel 等人[135]在 1984 年各自独立的报道中，同时使用了背
910 阔肌瓣和放置肋骨移植体或 Marlex 网片。胸部修复的重要部分包括纠正胸骨畸形的位置和旋转，同时替换发育不全的肋骨。Haller 等人[47]报道对侧肋骨常有龙骨状的凸起畸形，需要切除以优化效果。切除也可纠正胸骨的凹陷和旋转。无局部凹陷的肋骨发育不良无需手术矫正（见图 59-9C）。

手术技术

同漏斗胸手术一样，通过一个横切口初步暴露胸壁（图 59-11A）。对于需要手术矫正的患者，患侧常有严重的凹陷（偶尔有肋骨缺如）和胸骨旋转，通常在对侧形成龙骨状的凸出（图 59-11B）。存在
911 肋骨缺如时，一定要小心分离，因为在皮瓣和胸内筋膜之间只有一层薄且脆的胸膜（图 59-11C）。应避免侵犯该层，以防突入胸腔。双侧肋软骨进行软骨膜下切除，去除直至肋骨软骨连接的全部第三、第四和第五肋软骨，肋骨软骨连接予以保留。第六和第七肋软骨也进行切除，直到能平直与肋弓连接的位置。为纠正胸骨的旋转畸形并缓解受累肋骨的压迫，采取同治疗混合性鸡胸一样的横向楔形截骨（图 59-11D）。关闭截骨点，纠正胸骨位置异常的部
分。对于第二、第三和第四肋骨缺如的患者，经手 912
术切口获取对侧的第五或第六肋骨作为肋骨移植体；骨膜留在原位以利肋骨再生。普遍采用劈开肋骨体来促进移植体骨髓腔的血管重建。通常仅需要采集一根肋骨进行移植就可以纠正缺损（图 59-11E）。在将胸骨向前移动前，将肋骨移植体固定于在胸骨切迹上，并在肋骨移植体和周围的自身肋骨上钻孔，用钢丝将它们固定在一起。如果需要进一步对肋骨移植体进行加固的话，可使用人造材料的网片加以覆盖支持。

大多数女孩需要乳房重建，但是最好推迟到青春期晚期进行，以优化对侧乳房和重建乳房的相互匹配。一般需要植入物，通常与背阔肌瓣一起植入。采用专用的植入物来矫正发育不良的胸壁和缺如的乳房组织，但并不是总能获得成功的。

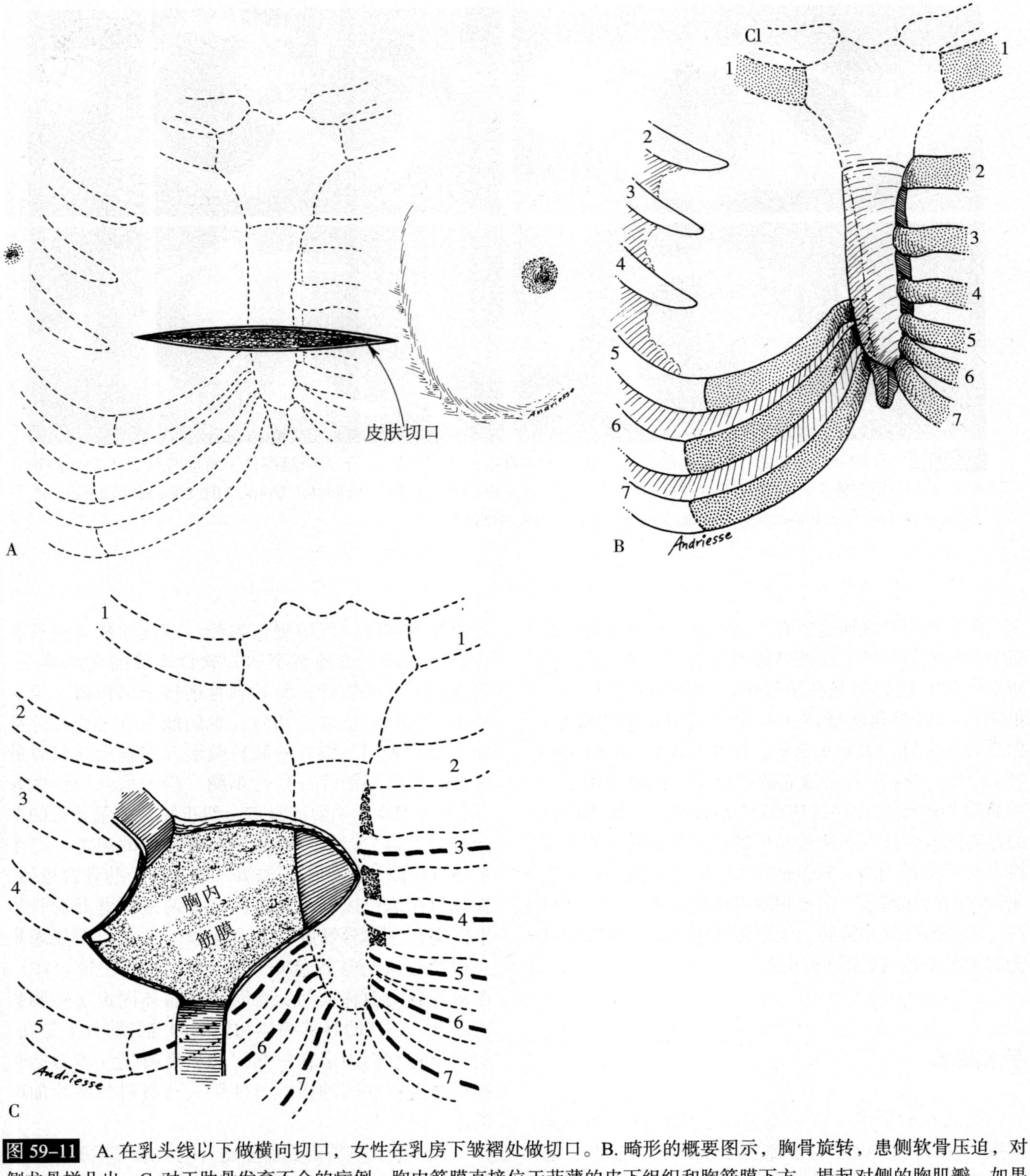

图 59-11 A. 在乳头线以下做横向切口，女性在乳房下皱褶处做切口。B. 畸形的概要图示，胸骨旋转，患侧软骨压迫，对侧龙骨样凸出。C. 对于肋骨发育不全的病例，胸内筋膜直接位于菲薄的皮下组织和胸筋膜下方。提起对侧的胸肌瓣，如果患侧有胸筋膜的话，也一并提起。然后进行软骨膜下的肋软骨切除，如虚线所示。很少有必须切到第二肋软骨水平的情况。

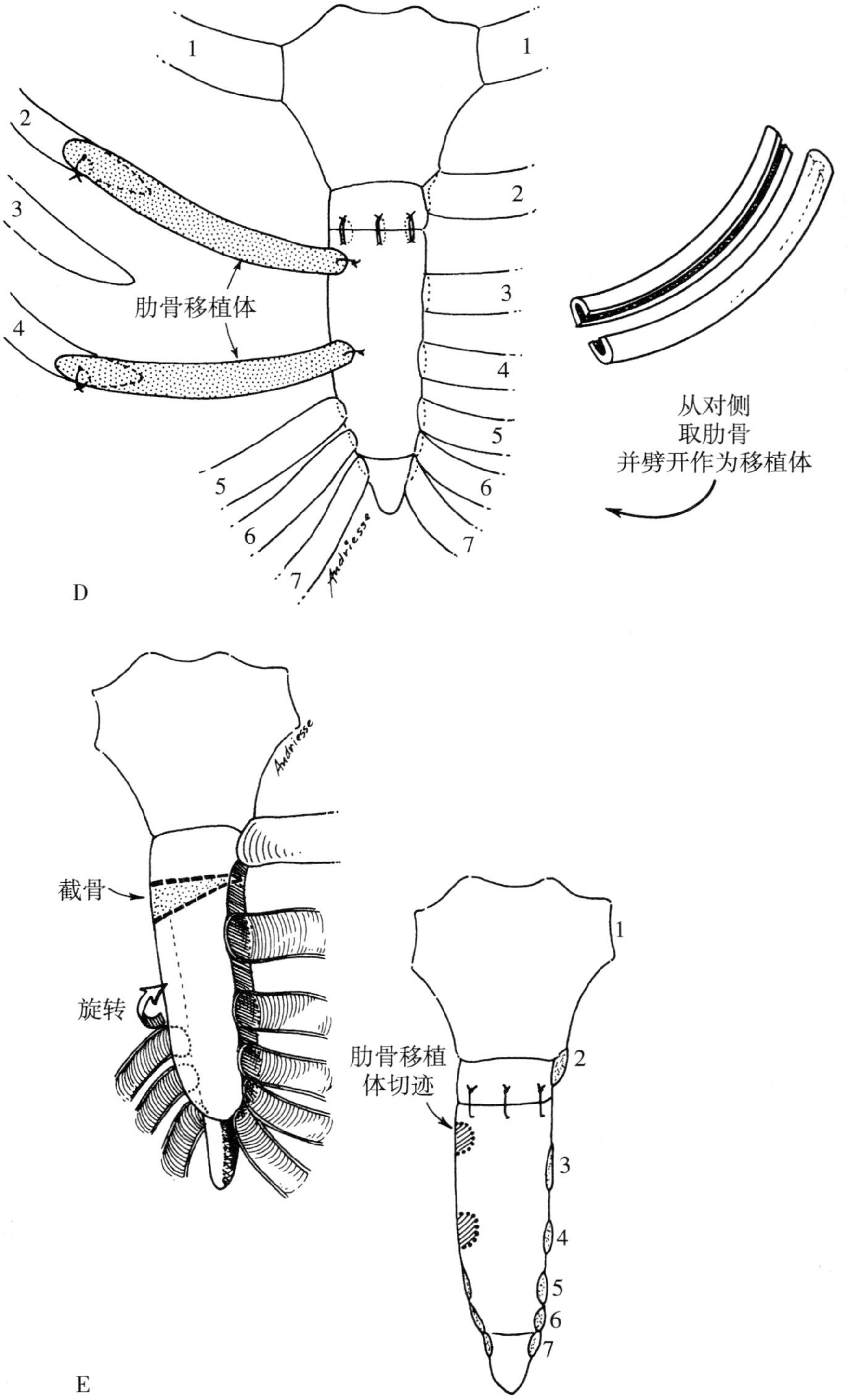

图 59-11 （续） D. 在第二肋软骨下方进行偏置的楔形截骨。采用粗丝线缝合或支撑杆支撑来此截骨端，矫正胸骨的后向异位和旋转。E. 对于肋骨发育不全的病例，获得对劈的肋骨移植体并用钢丝缝合到内侧先前形成的胸骨切迹上，外侧也用钢丝缝合到发育不良的肋骨上。沿肋骨短轴进行对劈，以保持最大的机械强度。（From Shamberger RC, Welch KJ, Upton J III: Surgical treatment of thoracic deformity in Poland's syndrome. J Pediatr Surg 1989;24:760.）

并发症和结果

患者及其父母和外科医生必须共同参与畸形的矫正，并设定现实合理的期望。必须明确胸壁缺损的部分，以明确矫正因素。无凹陷的广泛性肋骨发育不良不用矫正。同侧压迫和对侧凸出合并胸骨旋转通常可以改善，肋骨发育不全也可以改善。胸大肌发育不良造成的肋骨下的凹陷对女孩来说大都是令人烦恼的，因为在穿游泳衣或睡衣时，该区域就很明显。在乳房重建时，进行背阔肌瓣翻转可部分矫正这一问题，但是已经注意到这些肌瓣会随时间而萎缩[85]。

胸骨缺损

与漏斗胸和鸡胸相比，胸骨缺损很少见，但是医学文献还是非常重视此病的。事实上，在 Nineveh 皇家图书馆的古代楔形文字板中就有对该病的记载[125]。对这些楔形字板进行了翻译，显示古代人相信那些出生时“心脏外露，无皮肤覆盖”的婴儿预示着灾难。从那时起，一直到现代的医学文献中，对此畸形的特殊表现有许多孤立性的病例报道，特别还包括心脏直接裸露在体外的报道，同时也有一些优秀的综述报道。

Weese[128]在 1818 年给出了第一种胸骨缺损的解剖分类，将其分成胸骨裂心脏异位、胸上异位和胸下异位。Breschet[128]在 1826 年给出了三种比较分类：心脏胸部异位、腹部异位和向头端异位。Roth[128]在 1939 年将这类畸形分为胸部心脏胸外异位、心脏腹部异位和心脏胸上（颈部）异位；第一种分类进一步细分为胸骨柄缺损、胸骨体缺损和腹上角胸肌缺损性心脏体外异位。同样，Shao-tsu[128]将胸骨缺损分为：颈部心脏异位，心脏在颈部；胸部心脏异位，心脏在胸壁以外，并有胸骨裂缝；心脏胸腹异位；心脏腹部异位。尽管有这些分类，后续病例报道经常混淆分类，并将早期作者已经明确定义的领域搞得混淆不堪。有一种胸骨缺损未列入这些分类中，那就是胸骨分叉或胸骨分裂。在这种畸形中心脏位于胸腔的正常位置，但是胸骨有裂隙或在心脏上方部分融合。有正常的皮肤覆盖，或上方仅有一个浅表的皮肤溃疡。

在这些描述和分类的一个多世纪以后，Cantrell 和 Ravitch[20]总结了一组心脏胸下异位或心脏腹部异位畸形，患者合并横膈、心包、腹壁和心脏缺损。因此，后来这些患者通常被称为患有 Cantrell 五联症，更加重了混淆。最近的一篇报道对世界文献进行了总结，并对这些婴儿和儿童存在的并发畸形进行了整理[121]。对这一主题的综述根据心脏的组织覆盖程度，给出了四种胸骨缺损的基本类型，有些分类略有交叉。进一步的分类似乎人为因素过多，而没有阐明解剖结构或缺少明显的预后意义。

胸部心脏异位

胸部心脏异位包括 Weese 的胸骨裂心脏异位和 Breschet 的心脏胸部异位。这些病性是典型的心脏裸露，且无躯干组织覆盖。心尖向前，且经常向上（图 59-12）。多数存在心脏内的畸形，对合并的病损已经有所总结[121]。因为主要注重心脏的外观，所以许多病例报道未提供心脏自身解剖的信息。胸骨在上部的胸骨柄处可能是完整的，或者是完全分裂的；有些罕见病例的心脏可能就通过一个胸骨中央部位的缺损而凸出体外。由于躯干中线的组织严重缺乏，一些一期关闭的努力都失败了。CT 评估证实这些婴儿的胸腔内容积低于正常。多数成功修复的案例是胸腹心脏异位，而并非真性胸部心脏异位。1925 年，Cutler 和 Wilens[26]首先尝试使用皮瓣覆盖来进行修补手术，但是由于心脏功能崩溃而宣告失败，可能是由于压迫心脏而造成了心力衰竭。29 次手术尝试中，只有 4 个病例存活[32,77,94,116]。

1975 年，如 Saxena 的报告 Koop 获得了第一例心脏异位手术的成功[116]。一例出生时心脏正常、上有皮瓣覆盖的婴儿，在出生后 5 小时，横膈的前附着点向下移动。胸骨有 2 英寸宽度的裂开带，而且无法在 913
不引起心脏压迫和窘迫的情况下将其合拢。在 7 个月大时，在胸骨裂缝中插入 Dacron 涤纶丙烯酸树脂和 Marlex 网片，进行扩张，并将皮肤一期缝合关闭。术后出现皮瓣坏死的并发症，人造材料的感染必须将皮瓣去除。这个孩子一直活到 18 岁，据报道身体整体状况良好。Dobell 等人[32]的病例值得注意，因为手术矫正分两期进行：在新生儿期进行皮瓣覆盖；19 个月大时，在胸骨缺损处放置肋骨支撑杆移植体，并用胸肌瓣加以覆盖。将心包前部与胸壁的附着点分离，使心脏部分后退入胸腔。只有 Amato 等人[4]和

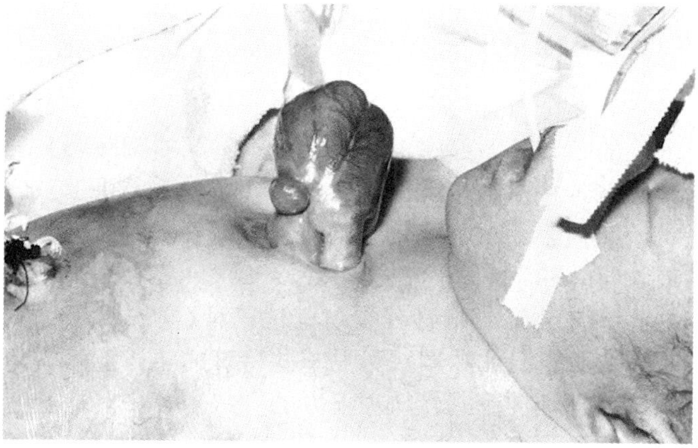

A

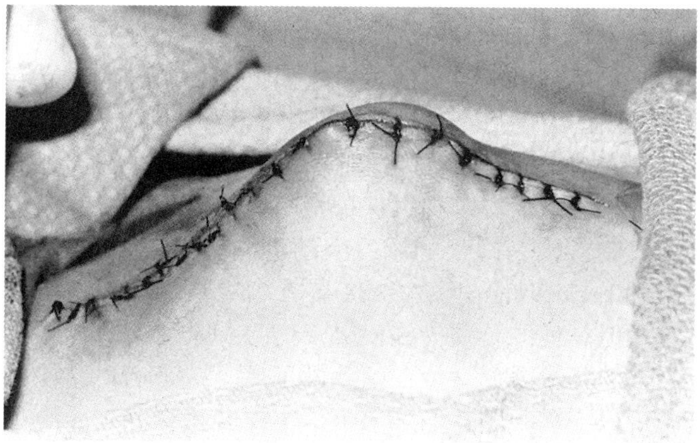

B

图 59-12 A. 胸部心脏异位的婴儿，无明显的腹部缺损。B. 在出生当天，通过向侧方进行皮瓣广泛分离来完成皮瓣覆盖修复。心内缺损的修复——法洛四联症合并长段肺动脉闭锁——以后通过经皮瓣切口再进行手术。(Courtesy of Craig W. Lillehei, M.D.)

Morales 等人[94]成功完成了一期完整的软组织覆盖。成功治疗的一致主题是在心脏周围部分重建前部胸腔以及避免将心脏纳回正常位置（见图 59-12B）。请注意，在成功的病例中，没有心脏自身病变和并发的腹部缺损，除了 Morales[94]的病例中有肌部室间隔缺损和心室憩室；这些特征对病例的成功与失败造成的影响，远远超过手术技术造成的差异。在需要使用自身组织移植体（骨或软骨）或人造材料的病例中，常会发生移植体感染和突出。可通过仅用组织覆盖异位心脏来获取最终的成功，这样避免了将心脏向后压迫入一个已经容量受限的胸腔中去。这种覆盖方式需要使用距离前胸壁很远的组织或者对局部组织进行广泛游离。严重的心内缺损合并胸部心脏异位也造成了最终存活的困难。遗憾的是，这种病变治疗上的唯一进步就是出生前超声影像学检查，包括明确心内畸形和父母是否需要终止妊娠[145]。

上腹壁缺损在这些患者中也非常常见，包括脐膨出、腹直肌分离和罕见的腹腔内脏凸出。但是，与胸部心脏异位同时存在的腹壁缺损却会将这些病变的分类变成胸腹心脏异位；这一术语应该用于那些出生时心脏表面有覆盖的病例。

颈部心脏异位

历史上根据心脏向上异位的程度，将颈部心脏异位（Weese 的胸上异位和 Breschet 的头端异位）定义成与胸部心脏异位不同的一个单独的分类。心尖和口腔常有融合，存在严重的颅面畸形。与胸部心脏异位相比，这种病变相对罕见，但是患者的预后同样恶劣。Shao-tsu[128]的总结中，仅有 5 例为颈部心脏异位，而 121 例婴儿为胸部异位。该组严重畸形的婴儿未有存活或尝试对其进行手术的报道。

胸腹心脏异位

胸腹心脏异位包括那些 Weese 定义为胸下异位和 Breschet 定义为腹部异位的病变。这整合了一些很人为化的分类，包括 Roth 的胸部心脏胸外异位和颈部异位；以及 Shao-tsu 的腹部心脏异位。该病的患者中，心脏表面有一层薄膜覆盖，通常是有色素沉着的皮肤覆盖在下部分裂的胸骨上（图 59-13）。心脏没有胸部心脏异位时严重的前旋。Wilson[77]在 1789
年报道了这一病变，明确定义了合并的腹壁、横膈和 914
心包缺损，以及心脏内部畸形，这比 Major[83]和 Cantrell 与 Ravitch[20]的报道要早 150 多年。这些患者几乎都合并有腹壁缺损（脐膨出、腹直肌分离或腹疝），以及横膈和心包前部的半月形缺损。这些患者大都有心脏内部畸形，并已经有所总结。[121]心脏的位置存在变异：它可能位于胸腔之内，仅有下方的横膈和心包缺损；或可能完全位于腹腔内，发出的大血管穿过横膈的缺损。该畸形合并左心室憩室的发生率惊人的高。许多病例的憩室通过横膈和心包缺损

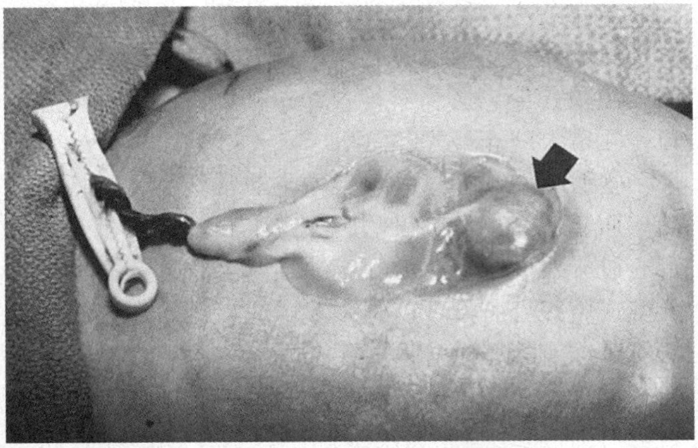

图 59-13 胸腹心脏异位的婴儿显示腹壁有小缺损，并由位于肋弓下的脐膨出加以覆盖。婴儿头部向右，可见心脏（箭头所示）就在缺损上缘的下方，有一层薄膜覆盖。在初步手术中，完成了一期皮肤覆盖，以后再修复心脏缺损。

突入腹腔。

胸腹心脏异位手术的成功率和长期生存率要高于胸部心脏异位。Arndt[3]在 1896 年进行了第一例手术尝试，但是将心脏纳回胸腔造成了死亡。Wieting[146]在 1912 年实施了第一例成功的手术修复，一期关闭了横膈和腹壁筋膜。初步手术干预必须找到心脏和腹腔上方的皮肤缺损。虽然通过局部使用收敛剂可以实现上皮的二次形成，成功地治疗了一些病例，但优先进行一期脐膨出切除并关闭皮肤可避免感染和纵隔炎。一些早期病例证明当腹腔内的心脏上有完整的皮肤覆盖时，胸腹心脏异位患者具有生存能力。

随着儿科心脏手术的进步，现在可对以往通常致命的心脏内部畸形进行修补。这些婴儿需要进行积极的治疗。可通过一期关闭缺损或采用人造网片来关闭腹壁缺损或扩张。通常难以进行一期关闭，因为两侧附着于上方肋弓的腹直肌之间的距离过宽，限制了中线结构的移动度。有一种改良的关闭方法将肋软骨断开，向内侧旋转[68]。在心脏外放置任何人造材料之前，最好完成对心内缺损的修复。一旦可以进行皮肤覆盖，关闭此缺损就非常重要，主要为心脏提供机械性的保护。一些这类畸形的婴儿有致命的肺发育不良[121]。

胸骨分叉或胸骨分裂

胸骨分叉或胸骨分裂是第四种，也是严重程度最低的胸骨畸形。这组婴儿的心脏位置正常，有正常的皮肤覆盖，完整的心包和部分或完全分裂的胸骨（图 59-14）。胸骨分裂不合并脐膨出。如果胸骨缺损是部分性的，涉及上部胸骨和胸骨柄；胸部或胸腹心脏异位的胸骨缺损则相反，这部分胸骨缺损主要是下部胸骨的缺损。大多数病例是部分裂开（图 59-3），剑突或胸骨体的下三分之一完整。

胸骨分叉或胸骨分裂与其他三种胸骨缺损不同，罕有心脏自身的缺损。可见一些特殊的躯体症状，包括从脐部延伸到胸骨缺损下方的带状瘢痕。其他儿童有向上到颈部或者下颚的瘢痕样延伸；胸骨柄分裂非常罕见。1879 年 Fischer[36]报道了与颅面血管瘤之间存在原因不明的关联，后来 Ingelrans 和 Debeugny[63]报道术后发生了致命的出血，据推测是胸骨缺损术后气管内的血管瘤产生了出血。

大多数病例中，这些婴儿的胸骨缺损是无症状的。进行修复是为心脏提供保护性的覆盖。也可能改善呼吸机制，因为缺损的矛盾运动可能会损害呼吸机制。据说 Lannelongue[77]在 1888 年首次对胸骨分裂进行修复，但是他的干预措施仅限于切除一个位于胸骨缺损上方的环形溃疡。他在两侧做了两个减张切口，使皮肤可以一期关闭，但是忽略了主要的胸骨分裂。第一例胸骨分裂完全矫正手术是通过在缺损上放置从肋弓取得的软骨移植体来完成的[18]。Maier 和 Bortone[82]在 1949 年完成了第一例 6 周婴儿的一期关闭。以后的方法包括通过双侧跨肋弓斜切口获得更大的长度，并使两侧胸骨向中线对合（Sabiston[112]的滑动软骨切开术）；离断周围的软骨，向中央旋转覆盖缺损（Meissner[91]的翼形活门成形术）；用不同的自体移植物加以覆盖（肋软骨、肋骨、颅顶骨）；和用人造材 915

表 59-3 109 例胸骨分裂患者的胸骨缺损

缺损	患者人数
上部分裂	46
剑突以上分裂	33
完全分裂	23
下部分裂，胸骨柄或中段完整	5
中央分裂，胸骨柄和剑突完整	2
仅发现皮肤溃疡	3

From Shamberger R, Welch KJ: Sternal defects. Pediatr Surg Int 1990; 5:156-164.

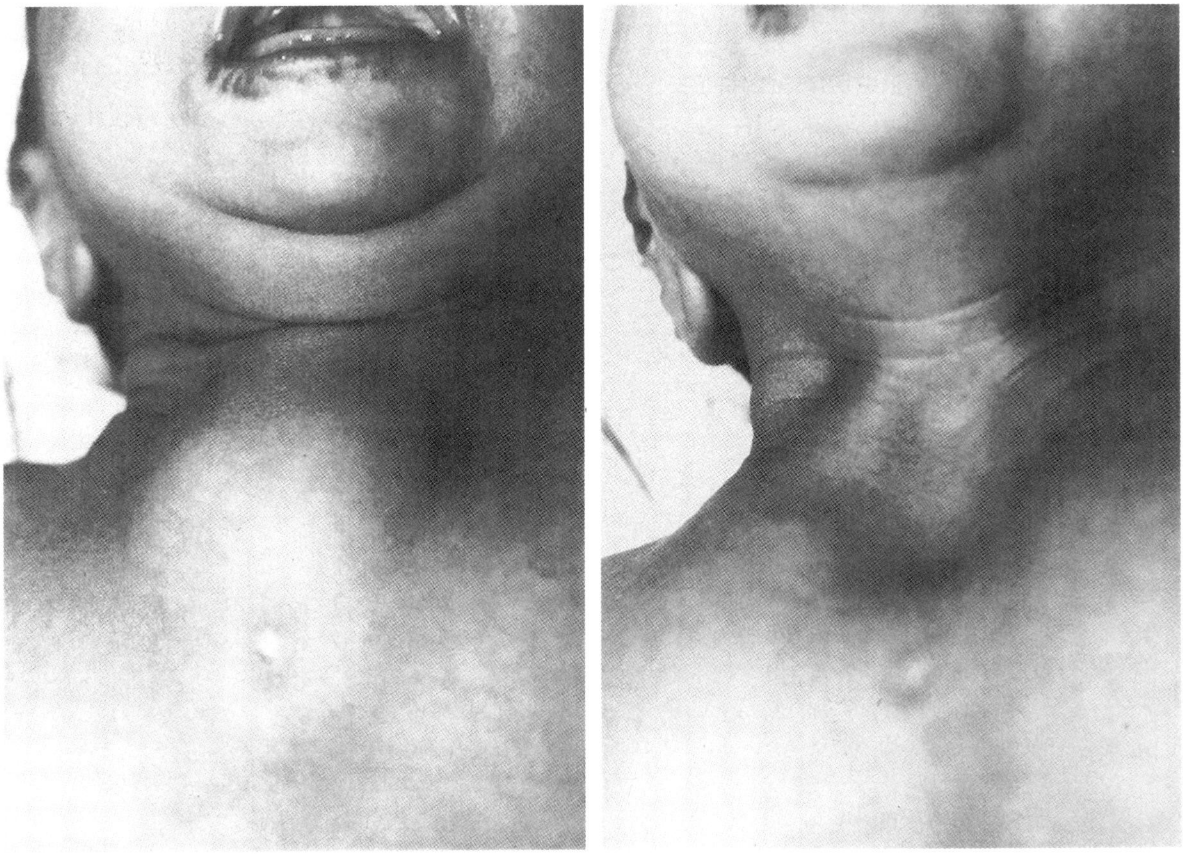

A　　B

图 59-14 一位年龄为 6 周的胸骨分叉的婴儿。注意当啼哭时，从缺损凸出的组织（A）和吸气时缺损部位的凹陷（B）。也可在嘴唇上看见有毛细血管瘤。

料覆盖。Maier 和 Bortone[82]首先强调了在婴儿期进行早期修复的重要性，此时胸壁柔软度好，可进行一期关闭（图 59-15）。大多数报道的一期修复的病例是在出生后头 3 个月内进行矫正的（22 例中的 18 例），很少在 1 岁后进行矫正（2 例）[121]。相反，在 22 例患者中，需进行软骨切开术的患者有 8 例是大于 1 岁的。通常必须在两侧胸骨可无张力合拢的地方进行软骨的楔形切除。

散发的骨骼病中的胸廓畸形

窒息性胸廓萎缩：Jeune 综合征

1954 年，Jeune 等人[67]报道了一个胸部狭窄、僵硬，并有多发软骨畸形的新生儿。因为呼吸功能障碍，患者在围生期早期死亡。随后的作者进一步描述了这种骨软骨营养不良的特征，不同的骨骼受累。这是一种常染色体隐性遗传模式，与染色体异常无关。最凸出的特征是狭窄的钟形胸和腹部凸出。胸廓在横轴和矢状轴上狭窄，只有一些呼吸运动，因为肋骨呈水平状（图 59-16）。肋骨短而宽，八字形的肋骨软骨连接仅仅到达腋前线。肋软骨数量多而不规则，与佝偻病性串珠肋相似。肋骨软骨连接部分的显微镜检查显示了发育不良的软骨内成骨异常，造成了肋骨长度的减小。 916

该综合征并发的骨骼畸形包括肢体粗短，骨骼相对短而宽。锁骨处于固定的提升位置，骨盆小而发育不良，髂骨呈方形。

该综合征的表达形式不一，并有肺损害的倾

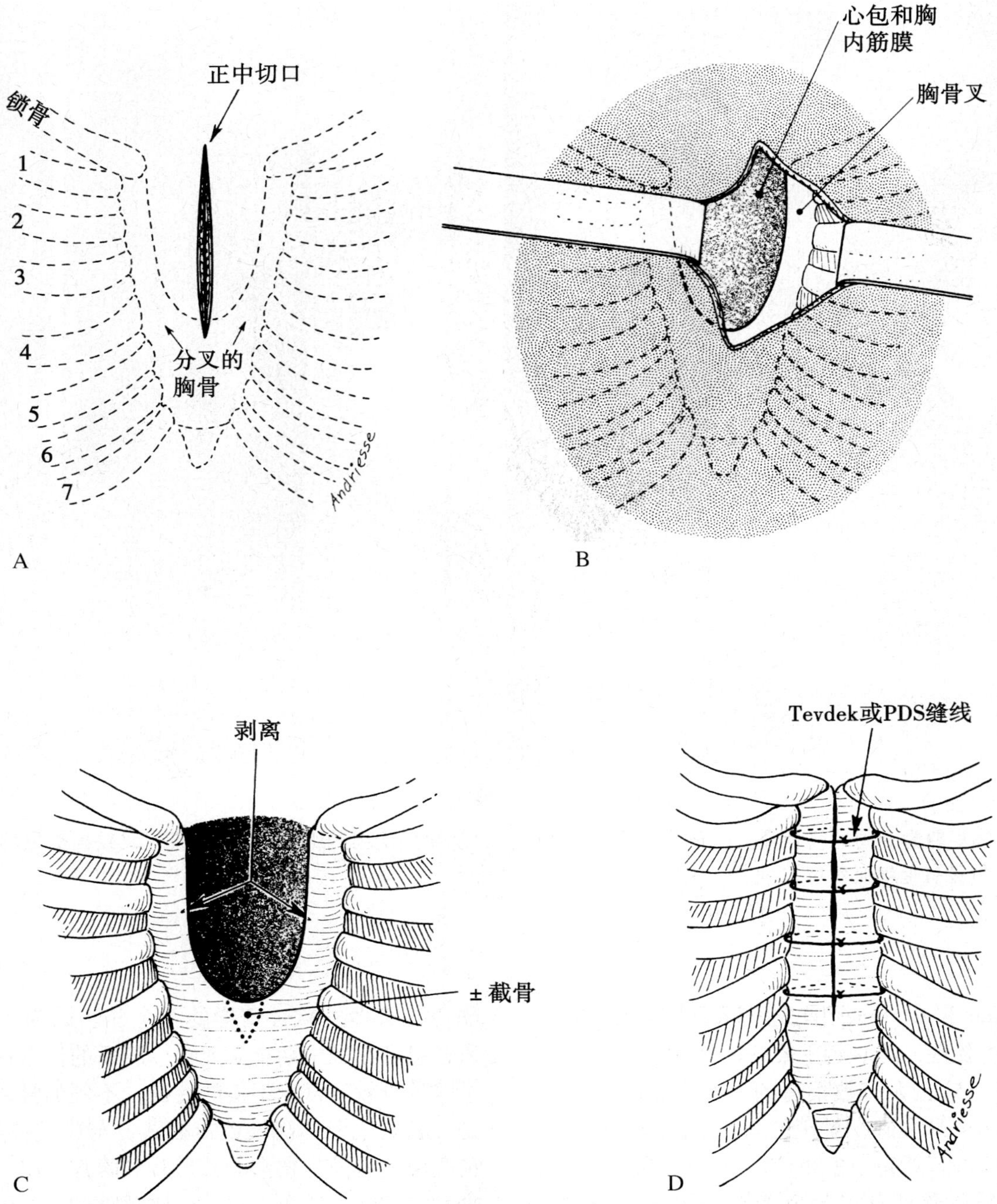

图 59-15 A. 最好经跨缺损长度的纵向切口来进行胸骨分叉的修复。B. 直接在皮下组织下进行胸骨叉的对合，胸肌在胸骨叉的外侧。胸内筋膜和心包就位于这些结构下方。C. 采用钝性分离将胸内筋膜从胸骨叉后方分离下来，以便安全地放置缝线。在下方进行楔形截骨可能更容易将胸骨叉合拢。最好在新生儿期完成修复手术，因为那时胸壁的柔软度最好。D. 采用非吸收缝线来完成缺损的关闭。（From Shamberger RC, Welch KJ: Sternal defects. Pediatr Surg Int 1990;5:156-164.）

向。虽然最初报道的病例都在新生儿期死亡，但是随后的报道证实了这种综合征的患者有一定的生存率[75]。尸体解剖的病理学发现不尽相同，显示有一系列的肺发育异常。但是，大多数的病例中，支气管发育是正常的，Williams 等[147]描述的肺泡分隔的情况更少。手术扩大胸腔的尝试基本上都失败了，延长了住院时间和最终的呼吸衰竭与死亡。

917

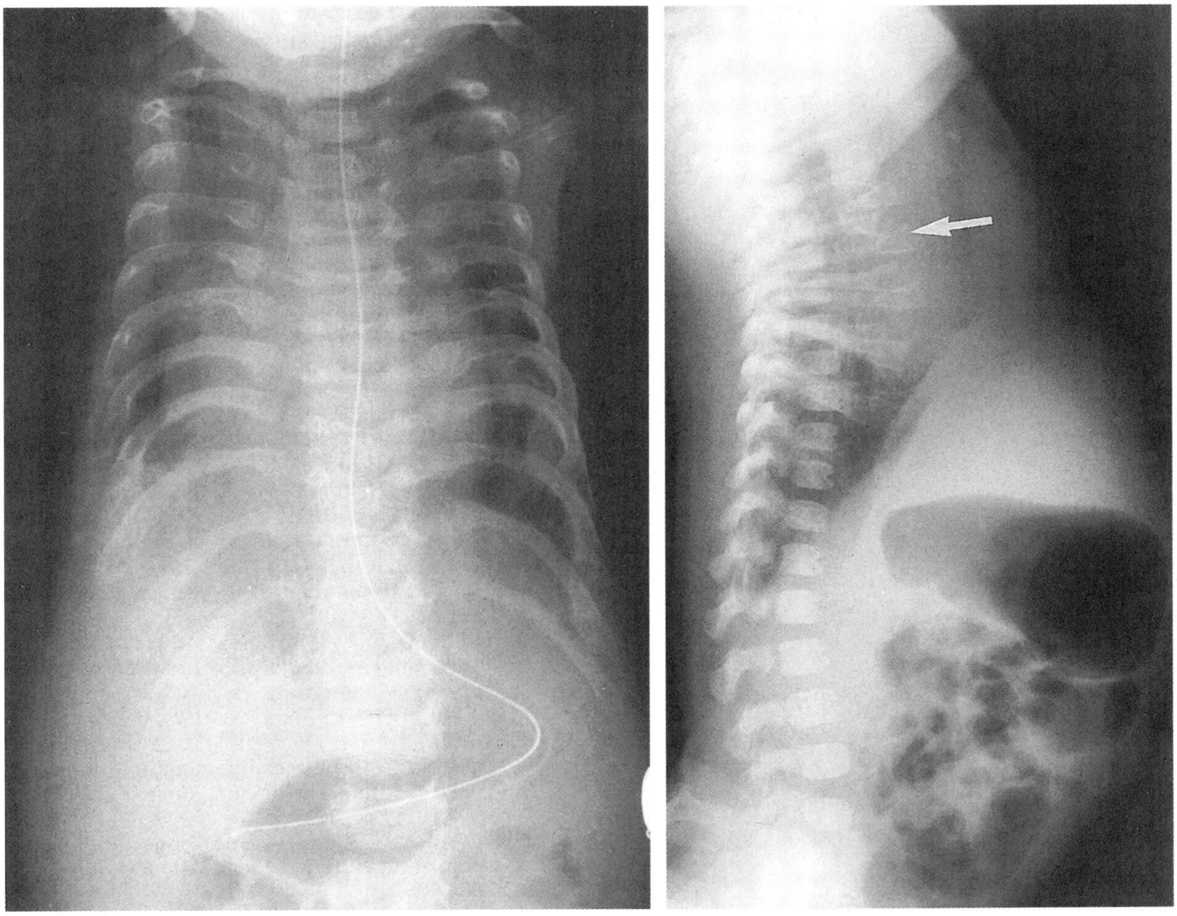

图 59-16 A．前后位放射影像显示 Jeune 综合征婴儿的肋骨短而呈水平位和狭窄的胸部（窒息性胸廓萎缩）B．侧位放射影像显示缩短的肋骨端终止于腋前线（箭头所示）且在肋骨软骨连接处呈不正常的喇叭状。婴儿在 1 个月时死于渐进性呼吸功能障碍，死后检查发现有肺泡发育不良。

脊椎胸廓结构不良：Jarcho-Levin 综合征

Jarcho 和 Levin[65]在 1938 年阐述的脊椎胸廓结构不良是一种常染色体隐性畸形，合并多发的脊椎骨和肋骨畸形。通常在婴儿早期因呼吸衰竭和肺炎而死亡。患者有交替出现的多发半椎体，可能影响大部分或全部的胸椎和腰椎。椎体的骨化中心很少跨过中线。多发的肋骨后部融合和胸椎明显的缩短使胸部在放射影像学上呈蟹形表现（图 59-17）。三分之一的此综合征患者合并其他畸形，包括先天性心脏病和肾畸形。Heilbronner 和 Renshaw[57]报道此综合征多发生在波多黎各人的家族中。这些患者的骨骼形成是正常的。

胸廓畸形继发于脊柱畸形，造成后方肋骨起源部位的靠拢。大多数这类畸形的婴儿在 15 个月前死亡，未有手术的建议或尝试。

大脑 -肋骨 -下颌综合征

1966 年 Smith 等人[130]首先描述了严重肋骨缺损、小颌畸形和其他畸形之间的关系，后来 McNicholl 等人[89]也有所描述。有这组畸形的婴儿在后部肋骨角不远处有节段性发育不全的骨化肋骨。他们也有小颌畸形、异常的气管软骨和软腭及硬腭缺损。出生后头一年内生存下来的婴儿中，50%有轻到中度的智力低下[130]。肋骨缺损的程度变化不一，受累肋骨的数量和缺损的范围也有不同，从狭窄的缝隙到发育不全的肋骨。最多见的是第三肋到第七肋骨受累。肋骨缝隙可

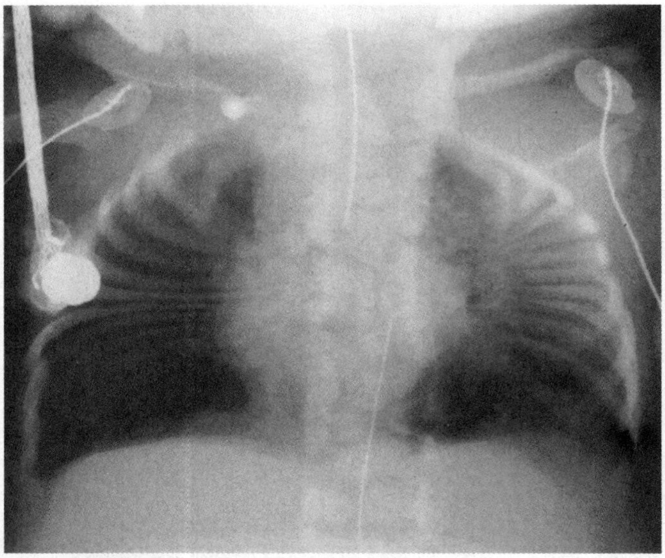

图 59-17 脊椎胸廓结构不良婴儿的胸片。可见明显的脊椎严重畸形、多发性交替半椎体和蟹状的肋骨。

918 能包含纤维组织、骨骼肌或钙化程度不同的软骨。肋骨缝隙造成连枷胸，而且这些婴儿的预后差。40%的人在出生后头一年内死于呼吸衰竭。主要病因和遗传模式不明，其染色体检查正常。

（孙彦隽译 刘锦纷校）

参考文献

1. Adkins PC, Blades B: A stainless steel strut for correction of pectus excavatum. Suvr Med (Sofiia) 1961;113:111-113.
2. Allen RG, Douglas M: Cosmetic improvement of thoracic wall defects using a rapid setting Silastic mold: A special technique. J Pediatr Surg 1979;14:745-749.
3. Arndt C: Nabelschnurbruch mit Herzhernie. Operation durch Laparotomie mit Tödlichern Ausgang. Centralbl Gynäkol 1896;20:632-633.
4. Amato JT, Cotroneo JV, Gladiere R: Repair of complete ectopia cordis (film). Presented at the American College of Surgeons Clinical Congress, Chicago, October 23-28, 1988.
5. Backer OG, Brünner S, Larsen V: The surgical treatment of funnel chest: Initial and follow-up results. Acta Chir Scand 1961;121:253-261.
6. Bainbridge LC, Wright AR, Kanthan R: Computed tomography in the preoperative assessment of Poland's syndrome. Br J Plast Surg 1991;44:604-607.
7. Baronofsky I: Technique for the correction of pectus excavatum. Surgery 1957;42:884-890.
8. Beiser GD, Epstein SE, Stampfer M, et al: Impairment of cardiac function in patients with pectus excavatum, with improvement after operative correction. N Engl J Med 1972;287:267-272.
9. Bevegård S: Postural circulatory changes at rest and during exercise in patients with pectus excavatum. Acta Med Scand 1962;171:695-713.
10. Boaz D, Mace J, Gotlin RW: Poland's syndrome and leukemia. Lancet 1971;1:349-350.
11. Borgeskov S, Raahave D: Long-term result after operative correction of funnel chest. Thorax 1971;26:74-76.
12. Borowitz D, Cerny F, Zallen G, et al: Pulmonary function and exercise response in patients with pectus excavatum after Nuss repair. J Pediatr Surg 2003;38:544-547.
13. Bouvet J: Vascular origin of Poland syndrome? A comparative rheographic study of the vascularization of the arms in eight patients. Eur J Pediatr 1978;128:17-26.
14. Brodkin H: Congenital chondrosternal prominence (pigeon breast): A new interpretation. Pediatrics 1949;3:286-295.
15. Brodkin HA: Congenital anterior chest wall deformities of diaphragmatic origin. Dis Chest 1953;24:259-277.
16. Brown A: Pectus excavatum (funnel chest): Anatomic basis; surgical treatment of the incipient stage in infancy; and correction of the deformity in the fully developed stage. J Thorac Surg 1939;9:164-184.
17. Brown A: Cardio-respiratory studies in pre and postoperative funnel chest. Dis Chest 1951;20:378-391.
18. Burton JF: Method of correction of ectopia cordis. Arch Surg 1947;54:79-84.
19. Cahill JL, Lees GM, Robertson HT: A summary of preoperative and postoperative cardiorespiratory performance in patients undergoing pectus excavatum and carinatum repair. J Pediatr Surg 1984;19:430-433.
20. Cantrell HJ Jr, Ravitch MM: A syndrome of congenital defects involving the abdominal wall, sternum, diaphragm, pericardium, and heart. Surg Gynecol Obstet 1958; 107:602-614.
21. Castile RG, Staats BA, Westbrook PR: Symptomatic pectus deformities of the chest. Am Rev Respir Dis 1982;126: 564-568.
22. Chin E: Surgery of funnel chest and congenital sternal prominence. Br J Surg 1957;44:360-376.
23. Clarkson P: Poland's syndactyly. Guy Hosp Rep 1962; 111:335-346.
24. Cochran JH Jr, Pauly TJ, Edstrom LE, et al: Hypoplasia of the latissimus dorsi muscle complicating breast reconstruction in Poland's syndrome. Ann Plast Surg 1981;6:402-404.
25. Currarino G, Silverman FN: Premature obliteration of the sternal sutures and pigeon-breast deformity. Radiology 1958;70:532-540.
26. Cutler GD, Wilens G: Ectopia cordis: Report of a case. Am J Dis Child 1925;30:76-81.
27. Dailey JE: Repair of funnel chest using sub-sternal osteoperiosteal rib graft strut: Report of a case with four year follow-up. JAMA 1952;150:1203-1204.
28. David TJ: Nature and etiology of the Poland anomaly. N Engl J Med 1972;287:487-489.
29. de Agustin-Asensio JC, Banuelos C, Vazquez JJ: Titanium miniplates for the surgical correction of pectus excavatum. J Am Coll Surg 1999;188:455-458.
30. Derveaux L, Clarysse I, Ivanoff I, et al: Preoperative and postoperative abnormalities in chest x-ray indices and in lung function in pectus deformities. Chest 1989;95:850-856.
31. Derveaux L, Ivanoff I, Rochette F, et al: Mechanism of pulmonary function changes after surgical correction for funnel chest. Eur Respir J 1988;1:823-825.
32. Dobell ARC, Williams H, Long R: Staged repair of ectopia cordis. J Pediatr Surg 1982;17:353-358.
33. Egan JC, DuBois JJ, Morphy M, et al: Compressive orthotics in the treatment of asymmetric pectus carinatum: A preliminary report with an objective radiographic marker. J Pediatr Surg 2000;35:1183-1186.

34. Erbella J Jr, Behmand R, Cederna PS: Endoscopically assisted pectus excavatum repair. Surg Laparosc Endosc Percutan Tech 2001;11:213-216.
35. Feng J, Hu T, Liu W, et al: The biomechanical, morphologic, and histochemical properties of the costal cartilages in children with pectus excavatum. J Pediatr Surg 2001; 36:1770-1776.
36. Fischer H: Fissura sterno congenita mit partieller Bauchspalte. Dtsch Z Chir 1879;12:367-369.
37. Fodor PB, Khoury F: Latissimus dorsi muscle flap in reconstruction of congenitally absent breast and pectoralis muscle. Ann Plast Surg 1980;4:422-425.
38. Fonkalsrud EW, Salman T, Guo W, et al: Repair of pectus deformities with sternal support. J Thorac Cardiovasc Surg 1994;107:37-42.
39. Fontaine G, Ovlaque S: Le syndrome de Poland-Mobius. Arch Fr Pediatr 1984;41:351-352.
40. Freire-Maia N, et al: The Poland syndrome: Clinical and geneaological data, dermatoglyphic analysis, and incidence. Hum Hered 1973;23:97-104.
41. Froriep R: Beobachtung eines Falles Von Mangel der Brustdruse. Notizen aus dem Gebiete der Naturund Heilkunde 1839;10:9-14.
42. Garusi G: Angiocardiographic patterns in funnel chest. Cardiologia 1964;45:312-330.
43. Genc A, Mutaf O: Polytetrafluoroethylene bars in stabilizing the reconstructed sternum for pectus excavatum operations in children. Plast Reconstr Surg 2002;110:54-57.
44. Godfrey S: Association between pectus excavatum and segmental bronchomalacia. J Pediatr 1980;96:649-652.
45. Guller B, Hable K: Cardiac findings in pectus excavatum in children: Review and differential diagnosis. Chest 1974;66:165-171.
46. Haje SA, Bowen JR: Preliminary results of orthotic treatment of pectus deformities in children and adolescents. J Pediatr Orthop 1992;12:795-800.
47. Haller JA Jr: Severe chest wall construction from growth retardation after too extensive and too early (<4 years) pectus excavatum repair: An alert. Ann Thorac Surg 1995; 60:1857-1858.
48. Haller JA Jr, Colombani PM, Humphries CT, et al: Chest wall constriction after too extensive and too early operations for pectus excavatum. Ann Thorac Surg 1996;61:1618-1624.
49. Haller JA Jr, Colombani PM, Miller D, et al: Early reconstruction of Poland's syndrome using autologous rib grafts combined with a latissimus muscle flap. J Pediatr Surg 1984;19:423-429.
50. Hallen JAJ Jr, Kramen SS, Lietman SA: Use of CT scans in selection of patients for pectus excavatum surgery: a preliminary report. J Pediatr Surg 1987;22:904-906.
51. Haller JA Jr, Loughlin GM: Cardiorespiratory function is significantly improved following corrective surgery for severe pectus excavatum: Proposed treatment guidelines. J Cardiovasc Surg (Torino) 2000;41:125-130.
52. Haller JA Jr, Peters GN, Mazur D, et al: Pectus excavatum: A 20 year surgical experience. J Thorac Cardiovasc Surg 1970;60:375-383.
53. Haller JA Jr, Scherer LR, Turner CS, et al: Evolving management of pectus excavatum based on a single institutional experience of 664 patients. Ann Surg 1989;209:578-582.
54. Hayashi A, Maruyama Y: Vascularized rib strut technique for repair of pectus excavatum. Ann Thorac Surg 1992; 53:346-348.
55. Haynor DR, Shuman WP, Brewers DK, et al: Imaging of fetal ectopia cordis: Roles of sonography and computed tomography. J Ultrasound Med 1984;3:25-27.
56. Hecker WC, Procher G, Dietz HG: [Results of operative correction of pigeon and funnel chest following a modified procedure of Ravitch and Haller]. Z Kinderchir 1981;34:220-227.
57. Heilbronner DM, Renshaw TS: Spondylothoracic dysplasia: A case report. J Bone Joint Surg Am 1984;66:302-303.
58. Hester TR Jr, Bostwick J 3rd: Poland's syndrome: Correction with latissimus muscle transposition. Plast Reconstr Surg 1982;69:226-233.
59. Hochberg J, Ardenghy M, Graeber GM, et al: Complex reconstruction of the chest wall and breast utilizing a customized silicone implant. Ann Plast Surg 1994;32:524-528.
60. Hougaard K, Arendrup H: Deformities of the female breasts after surgery for funnel chest. Scand J Thorac Cardiovasc Surg 1983;17:171-174.
61. Howard R: Pigeon chest (protrusion deformity of the sternum). Med J Aust 1958;45:664-666.
62. Humphreys GH 2nd, Jaretzki A 3rd: Pectus excavatum: Late results with and without operation. J Thorac Cardiovasc Surg 1980;80:686-695.
63. Ingelrans P, Debeugny P: [Case of bifidity of the sternum associated with tracheal angiomatosis]. Ann Chir Infant 1965;6:123-128.
64. Ireland DC, Takayama N, Flatt AE: Poland's syndrome. J Bone Joint Surg Am 1976;58:52-58.
65. Jarcho S, Levin P: Hereditary malformation of the vertebral bodies. Bull Johns Hopkins Hosp 1938;62:216-262.
66. Jensen NK, Schmidt WR, Garamella JJ, et al: Pectus excavatum and carinatum: The how, when, and why of surgical correction. J Pediatr Surg 1970;5:4-13.
67. Jeune M, Carron R, Beraud C, et al: Polychondrodystrophie avec blocage thoracique d'evolution fatale. Pediatrie 1954;9:390-392.
68. Jona JZ: The surgical approach for reconstruction of the sternal and epigastric defects in children with Cantrell's deformity. J Pediatr Surg 1991;26:702-706.
69. Judet J: Thorax en entonnoir: Un procede operatoire. Rev Orthop 1954;40:248-257.
70. Jung A: Le traitement du thorax en entoinnoir par le "retournement pedicule" de la cuvette sterno-chondrale. Mem Acad Chir 1956;82:242-249.
71. Kaguraoka H, Ohnuki T, Itaoka T, et al: Degree of severity of pectus excavatum and pulmonary function in preoperative and postoperative periods. J Thorac Cardiovasc Surg 1992;104:1483-1488.
72. Klinke F, Dittrich H, Kujat R: [Scoring system for indication for operative correction of funnel chest]. Z Kinderchir 1981;33:237-243.
73. Kowalewski J, Brocki M, Dryjanski T, et al: Pectus excavatum: Increase of right ventricular systolic, diastolic, and stroke volumes after surgical repair. J Thorac Cardiovasc Surg 1999;118:87-92.
74. Kowalewski J, Brocki M, Zolynski K: Long-term observation in 68 patients operated on for pectus excavatum: Surgical repair of funnel chest. Ann Thorac Surg 1999;67:821-824.
75. Kozlowski K, Masel J: Asphyxiating thoracic dystrophy without respiratory disease: Report of two cases of the latent form. Pediatr Radiol 1976;5:30-33.
76. Lane-Smith DM, Gillis DA, Roy PD: Repair of pectus excavatum using a Dacron vascular graft strut. J Pediatr Surg 1994;29:1179-1182.
77. Lannelongue: De l'ectocardie et de sa cure par l'autoplastie. Ann Medico-Chirurgicales 1888;4:101-107.
78. Lansman S, Serlo W, Linna O, et al: Treatment of pectus excavatum with bioabsorbable polylactide plates: Preliminary results. J Pediatr Surg 2002;37:1281-1286.
79. Lees RF, Caldicott JH: Sternal anomalies and congenital heart disease. Am J Roentgenol Radium Ther Nucl Med 1975;124:423-427.

80. Lester C: The surgical treatment of funnel chest. Ann Surg 1946;123:1003-1022.
81. Liese W, Bühlmann A: Arbeitskapazitat und lungenvolumina vor und nach chirurgischer korrektur einer trichterbruszt. Schweiz Med Wochenschr 1974;104:83-86.
82. Maier HC, Bortone F: Complete failure of sternal fusion with herniation of pericardium. J Thorac Surg 1949; 18:851-859.
83. Major JW: Thoracoabdominal ectopia cordis. J Thorac Surg 1953;26:309-317.
84. Malek MH, Fonkalsrud EW, Cooper CB: Ventilatory and cardiovascular responses to exercise in patients with pectus excavatum. Chest 2003;124:870-882.
85. Marks MW, Argenta LC, Izenberg PH, et al: Management of the chest-wall deformity in male patients with Poland's syndrome. Plast Reconstr Surg 1991;87:674-678.
86. Martinez D: The effect of costal cartilage resection on chest wall development. Pediatr Surg Int 1990;5:170-173.
87. Matsui T, Kitano M, Nakamura T, et al: Bioabsorbable struts made from poly-L-lactide and their application for treatment of chest deformity. J Thorac Cardiovasc Surg 1994;108:162-168.
88. McGillivray BC, Lowry RB: Poland syndrome in British Columbia: Incidence and reproductive experience of affected persons. Am J Med Genet 1977;1:65-74.
89. McNicholl B, Egan-Mitchell B, Murray JP, et al: Cerebro-costo-mandibular syndrome: A new familial developmental disorder. Arch Dis Child 1970;45:421-424.
90. Mead J, Sly P, Le Souef P, et al: Rib cage mobility in pectus excavatum. Am Rev Respir Dis 1985;132:1223-1228.
91. Meissner F: Fissura sterni congenita. Zentralbl Chir 1964;89:1832-1839.
92. Meyer L: Zur chirurgischen behandlung der angeborenen trichterbrust. Verh Berliner Med Gesellschaft 1911; 42:364-373.
93. Mielke CH, Winter RB: Pectus carinatum successfully treated with bracing: A case report. Int Orthop 1993; 17:350-352.
94. Morales JM, Patel SG, Duff JA, et al: Ectopia cordis and other midline defects. Ann Thorac Surg 2000;70:111-114.
95. Morshuis W, Folgering H, Barentsz J, et al: Pulmonary function before surgery for pectus excavatum and at long-term follow-up. Chest 1994;105:1646-1652.
96. Morshuis WJ, Folgering HT, Barentsz JO, et al: Exercise cardiorespiratory function before and one year after operation for pectus excavatum. J Thorac Cardiovasc Surg 1994;107:1403-1409.
97. Nakajima H, Chang H: A new method of reconstruction for pectus excavatum that preserves blood supply and costal cartilage. Plast Reconstr Surg 1999;103:1661-1666.
98. Ochsner A, Debakey M: Chone-chondrosternon: Report of a case and review of the literature. J Thorac Surg 1939; 8:469-511.
99. Ohmori K, Takada H: Correction of Poland's pectoralis major muscle anomaly with latissimus dorsi musculocutaneous flaps. Plast Reconstr Surg 1980;65:400-404.
100. Ohno K, Nakahira M, Takeuchi S, et al: Indications for surgical treatment of funnel chest by chest radiograph. Pediatr Surg Int 2001;17:591-595.
101. Onursal E, Toker A, Vostanci K, et al: A complication of pectus excavatum operation: Endomyocardial steel strut. Ann Thorac Surg 1999;68:1082-1083.
102. Orzalesi MM, Cook CD: Pulmonary function in children with pectus excavatum. J Pediatr 1965;66:898-900.
103. Paltia V: Operative technique in funnel chest: Experience in 81 cases. Acta Chir Scand 1958;116:90-98.
104. Peterson RJ, Young WG Jr, Godwin JD, et al: Noninvasive assessment of exercise cardiac function before and after pectus excavatum repair. J Thorac Cardiovasc Surg 1985;90:251-260.
105. Pickard LR, Tepas JJ, Shermeta DW, et al: Pectus carinatum: Results of surgical therapy. J Pediatr Surg 1979; 14:228-230.
106. Poland A: Deficiency of the pectoralis muscles. Guys Hosp Rep 1841;6:191-193.
107. Prevot J: Treatment of sternocostal wall malformations of the child: A series of 210 surgical corrections since 1975. Eur J Pediatr Surg 1994;4:131-136.
108. Ravitch M: The operative treatment of pectus excavatum. Ann Surg 1949;129:429-444.
109. Ravitch MM: Operative treatment of congenital deformities of the chest. Am J Surg 1961;101:588-597.
110. Rehbein F: The operative treatment of the funnel chest. Arch Dis Child 1957;32:5-8.
111. Roberts A: Spondylothoracic and spondylocostal dysostosis: Hereditary forms of spinal deformity. J Bone Joint Surg Br 1988;70:123-126.
112. Sabiston DC Jr: The surgical management of congenital bifid sternum with partial ectopia cordis. J Thorac Surg 1958;35:118-122.
113. Saint-Mezard G, Duret JC, Chanudet X, et al: Mitral valve prolapse and pectus excavatum: Fortuitous association or syndrome? Presse Med 1986;15:439.
114. Sanger PW, Taylor FH, Robicsek F: Deformities of the anterior wall of the chest. Surg Gynecol Obstet 1963; 116:515-522.
115. Sauerbruch F: Die Chirurgie der Brustorgane. Berlin, Springer, 1920.
116. Saxena NC: Ectopia cordis child surviving: Prosthesis fails. Pediatr News 1976;10:3.
117. Scherer LR, Arn PH, Dressel DA, et al: Surgical management of children and young adults with Marfan syndrome and pectus excavatum. J Pediatr Surg 1988;23:1169-1172.
118. Schoenmakers MA, Gulmans VA, Bax NM, et al: Physiotherapy as an adjuvant to the surgical treatment of anterior chest wall deformities: A necessity? A prospective descriptive study in 21 patients. J Pediatr Surg 2000; 35:1440-1443.
119. Seyfer AE, Icochea R, Graeber GM: Poland's anomaly: Natural history and long-term results of chest wall reconstruction in 33 patients. Ann Surg 1988;208:776-782.
120. Shamberger R: Surgical treatment of thoracic deformity in Poland's syndrome. J Pediatr Surg 1989;24:760-765.
121. Shamberger R, Welch KJ: Sternal defects. Pediatr Surg Int 1990;5:156-164.
122. Shamberger RC, Welch KJ: Surgical correction of pectus carinatum. J Pediatr Surg 1987;22:48-53.
123. Shamberger RC, Welch KJ: Cardiopulmonary function in pectus excavatum. Surg Gynecol Obstet 1988;166: 383-391.
124. Shamberger RC, Welch KJ: Surgical correction of chondromanubrial deformity (Currarino-Silverman syndrome). J Pediatr Surg 1988;23:319-322.
125. Shamberger RC, Welch KJ: Surgical repair of pectus excavatum. J Pediatr Surg 1988;23:615-622.
126. Shamberger RC, Welch KJ, Castaneda AR, et al: Anterior chest wall deformities and congenital heart disease. J Thorac Cardiovasc Surg 1988;96:427-432.
127. Shamberger RC, Welch KJ, Sanders SP: Mitral valve prolapse associated with pectus excavatum. J Pediatr 1987; 111:404-407.
128. Shao-tsu L: Ectopia cordis congenita. Thoraxchirurgie 1957;5:197-212.
129. Sigalet DL, Montgomery M, Harder J: Cardiopulmonary effects of closed repair of pectus excavatum. J Pediatr Surg 2003;38:380-385.

130. Smith KG, Sekar KC: Cerebrocostomandibular syndrome: Case report and literature review. Clin Pediatr (Phila) 1985;24:223-225.
131. Taguchi K: A new plastic operation for pectus excavatum: Sternal turnover surgical procedure with preserved internal mammary vessels. Chest 1975;67:606-608.
132. Tanaka F, Kitano M, Shindo T, et al: [Postoperative lung function in patients with funnel chest]. Nippon Kyobu Geka Gakkai Zasshi 1993;41:2161-2165.
133. Tang Chen YB, Chen JS, Lee YC, et al: Revascularization of turnover sternum: A definitive treatment for intractable funnel chest. Microsurgery 1999;19:296-302.
134. Udoshi MB, Shah A, Fisher VJ, et al: Incidence of mitral valve prolapse in subjects with thoracic skeletal abnormalities—a prospective study. Am Heart J 1979;97:303-311.
135. Urschel HC Jr, Byrd HS, Sethi SM, et al: Poland's syndrome: Improved surgical management. Ann Thorac Surg 1984;37:204-211.
136. Vanamo K, Peltonen J, Rintala R, et al: Chest wall and spinal deformities in adults with congenital diaphragmatic defects. J Pediatr Surg 1996;31:851-854.
137. von der Oelsnitz G: [Anomalies of the chest]. Z Kinderchir 1981;33:229-236.
138. Wada J, Ikeda K, Ishida T, et al: Results of 271 funnel chest operations. Ann Thorac Surg 1970;10:526-532.
139. Weber TR, Kurkchubasche AG: Operative management of asphyxiating thoracic dystrophy after pectus repair. J Pediatr Surg 1998;33:262-265.
140. Wechselberger G, Ohlbauer M, Haslinger J, Schoeller T: Silicone implant correction of pectus excavatum. Ann Plast Surg 2001;47:489-493.
141. Weg JG, Krumholz RA, Harkleroad LE: Pulmonary dysfunction in pectus excavatum. Am Rev Respir Dis 1967;96:936-945.
142. Welch K: Satisfactory surgical correction of pectus excavatum deformity in childhood: A limited opportunity. J Thorac Surg 1958;36:697-713.
143. Welch K: Chest Wall Deformities. Philadelphia, WB Saunders, 1980.
144. Welch KJ, Vos A: Surgical correction of pectus carinatum (pigeon breast). J Pediatr Surg 1973;8:659-667.
145. Wicks JD, Levine MD, Mettler FA Jr: Intrauterine sonography of thoracic ectopia cordis. AJR Am J Roentgenol 1981; 137:619-621.
146. Wieting R: Eine operative behandelte Herzmissbildung. Dtsch Z Chir 1912;114:293-295.
147. Williams AJ, Vauter G, Reid LM: Lung structure in asphyxiating thoracic dystrophy. Arch Pathol Lab Med 1984; 108:658-661.
148. Willital GH: [Indication and operative technique in chest deformities]. Z Kinderchir 1981;33:244-252.
149. Wolf WM, Fischer MD, Saltzman DA, et al: Surgical correction of pectus excavatum and carinatum. Minn Med 1987;70:447-453.
150. Wynn SR, Driscoll DJ, Ostrom NK, et al: Exercise cardiorespiratory function in adolescents with pectus excavatum: Observations before and after operation. J Thorac Cardiovasc Surg 1990;99:41-47.
151. Yamaguchi M, Tsukube T, Ohashi H, et al: [Early and long-term results of sternocostal elevation combined with bridge external traction for funnel chest in children]. Nippon Kyobu Geka Gakkai Zasshi 1993;41:2341-2348.

漏斗胸的 Nuss 手术

Donald Nuss 和 Robert E. Kelly, Jr.

微创手术

漏斗胸的微创手术由两部分组成：手术矫正和锻炼与体态调整过程。

漏斗胸的手术矫正是在胸骨下置入一根带有凸面的钢条，并使钢条的凸面向后。当钢条到位以后，将其翻转 180°，以此来矫正畸形（见图 59-18 至 59-27）。这个技术是可能的，因为前胸壁具有伸展性和柔软度；不需要切开或切除软骨，也不需要胸骨截骨。因为这类患者都喜欢坐着，并有典型的“胸部体态”，这进一步加重了畸形，也要让他们每天进行一系列的呼吸和体态锻炼，并鼓励他们参与有氧运动。

分类和治疗原则

第一次对漏斗胸患者进行评估时，可将他们分为轻度、中度和重度畸形。轻度或中度的患者一开始就进行锻炼和体态调整过程，并在 12 月之后再次评估，以确定他们已经进行了常规锻炼并正确地进行了锻 922
炼。约 66%的患者可进行保守治疗。对重度畸形患者进行一套评估以判定是否适宜手术。评估工作包括：肺功能测试；心电图和超声心动图在内的心血管评估；CT 扫描。为了取得一致的结果，放射学家建议在安静呼吸状态下进行胸部 CT 检查，而不是在最大吸气状态下进行检查。如果患者符合以下两条及两条

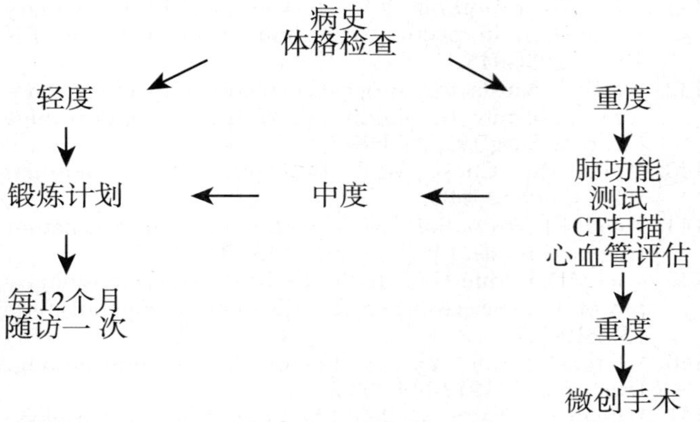

图 59-18 漏斗胸患者的临床治疗途径。

以上标准，则可进行手术矫正：（1）渐进性或有症状的漏斗胸；（2）限制性病变，可通过肺功能测试确定；（3）CT 扫描显示心脏压迫或异位，肺不张，Haller CT 指数大于 3.25；（4）心脏畸形，包括二尖瓣脱垂或束枝传导阻滞；（5）手术失败后的漏斗胸复发。

手术技术

术前检查列表：术前日

1. 对过敏反应进行回顾和检查，包括对金属物质的过敏反应。
2. 计算漏斗胸钢条所需的长度，测量左右腋中线之间的距离，并在此测量值上减去 2 cm。支撑条的行程比卷尺测量时的行程要短，所以长度也需要比测量值短一些（图 59-19）。

患者的麻醉、准备和体位

1. 气管内全身麻醉。
2. 麻醉医生置入胸部硬膜外麻醉导管。硬膜外麻醉要持续 3～5 天（平均 3 天）。
3. 置入导尿管。术后第一天，患者苏醒并有方向感时拔除导尿管。
4. 手术过程中要经鼻或经口置入胃管，手术结束时拔除。

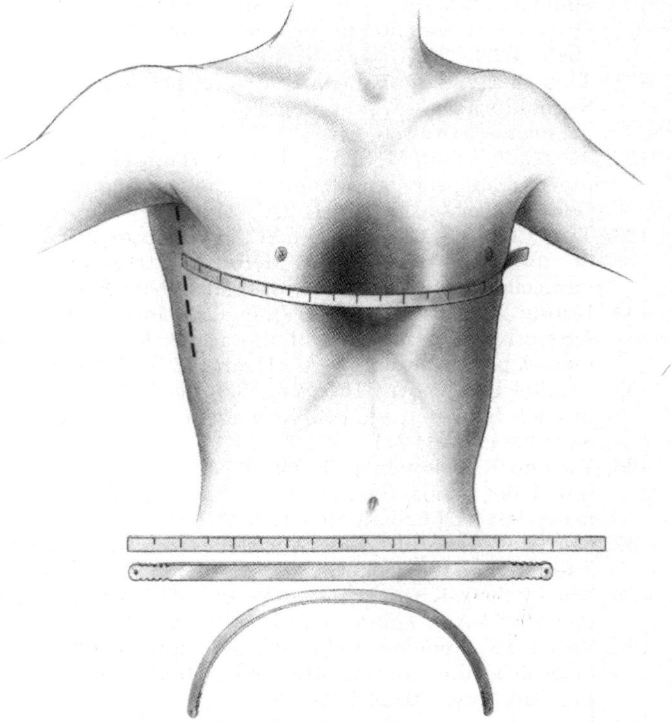

图 59-19 测量右侧腋前线到左侧腋前线之间的距离。支撑条应该比测量数值短 2 cm。将支撑条弯成如图所示的形状，在中部保留 2～4 cm 的平直段以支撑胸骨。

5. 需要进行抗生素覆盖疗法（例如，头孢唑啉用 5 天）来降低肺炎和支撑钢条的感染。
6. 双臂在肩部取外展位，下垫胶垫防止臂丛损伤（见图 59-19），肘部稍屈曲。
7. 铺巾后，将 Lorenz 胸部支撑条弯成半圆形，中部保持 2 cm 长度的平直段以用来支撑胸骨（图 59-19）。将支撑条弯成弓形，使支撑条所受负荷均匀。如果中部的平直段过长，那会导致矫正不够。

患者的标记

1. 用记号笔在漏斗胸最深点画一个圆形标记（图 59-20）。如果胸部最深点在胸骨以下，那就在胸骨的最下端做一个标记。该点是放置支撑条后平直面所处的位置。
2. 在漏斗胸最深点同一水平面的肋间隙做一个 X 形标记。胸骨两侧的出入点应该位于胸（肋软骨）脊最高点的内侧（见图 59-20）。

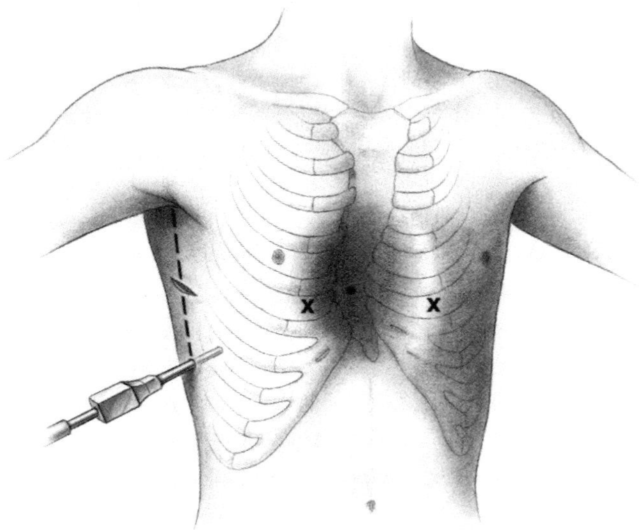

图 59–20　在压迫的最深点画一个圆圈的记号，在胸脊顶点内侧的肋间隙上画一个 X 记号，并用线标出切口位置。这些标记应在同一水平面上。在切口下方两个肋间隙的位置插入胸腔镜。

3．在胸壁两侧同一水平面上画线，明确预定的切口位（见图 59–20）。

胸腔镜和建立隧道

1．在设定的皮肤切口下两个肋间隙处的右下侧胸壁插入胸腔镜（见图 59–20）。对右侧胸腔和纵隔进行彻底检查，确认无手术禁忌证。然后在标定要置入支撑条的肋间隙上施压，确定外部标志线确实在内部解剖结构的上方。

2．在经胸腔镜确认内部和外部解剖完全匹配后，在双侧胸部做皮肤切开，皮下深部隧道向前延伸到标注 X 记号的肋间隙，该点位于胸脊顶部内侧（图 59–21）。同样，在胸骨支撑杆远端和固定器所处部位做一个皮袋。

3．在胸腔镜的监视下，经胸脊顶端以前做好的 X 形标记的右侧肋间隙穿入尺寸合适的 Lorenz 引导器（图 59–22）。将心电图音量调高，以便能通过声音来表示心电图的变化。

4．轻柔地将心包从胸骨的后侧面分离下来（见图 59–22）。在胸腔镜的引导下，慢慢向前推送引导器，并跨过纵隔，头端通常向前与胸骨相贴。

5．建立胸骨下隧道后，将引导器推向对侧肋间隙上原先标注好 X 的地方，并向前穿出皮肤切口（图 59–23）。

提升胸骨和置入支撑条

1．用引导器提升胸骨。主刀在右侧提起引导器，助手在左侧提起引导器（见图 59–33）。反复进行提升动作，直至将胸骨提出受压位置，这样漏斗胸就纠正过来了。将一根脐带线系到引导器上， 925

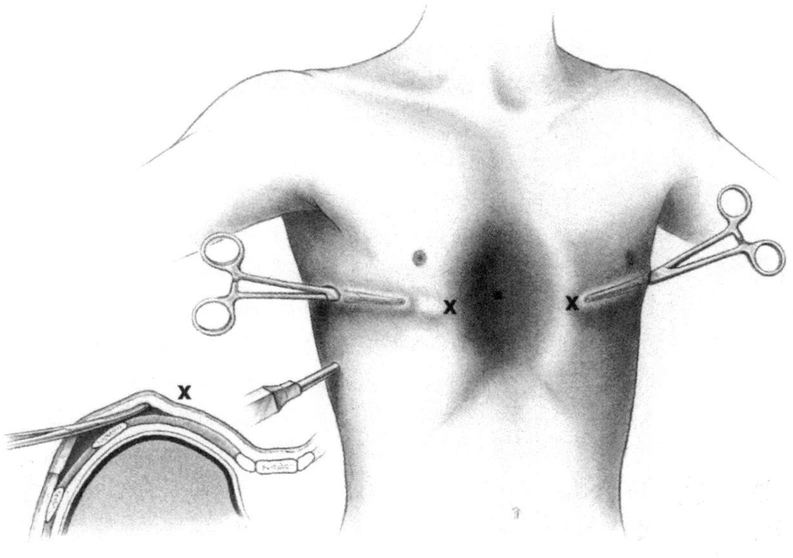

图 59–21　在每侧做一个从胸部侧切口前面到有 X 记号的肋间隙的皮下深隧道，X 记号位于胸脊顶点的内侧。

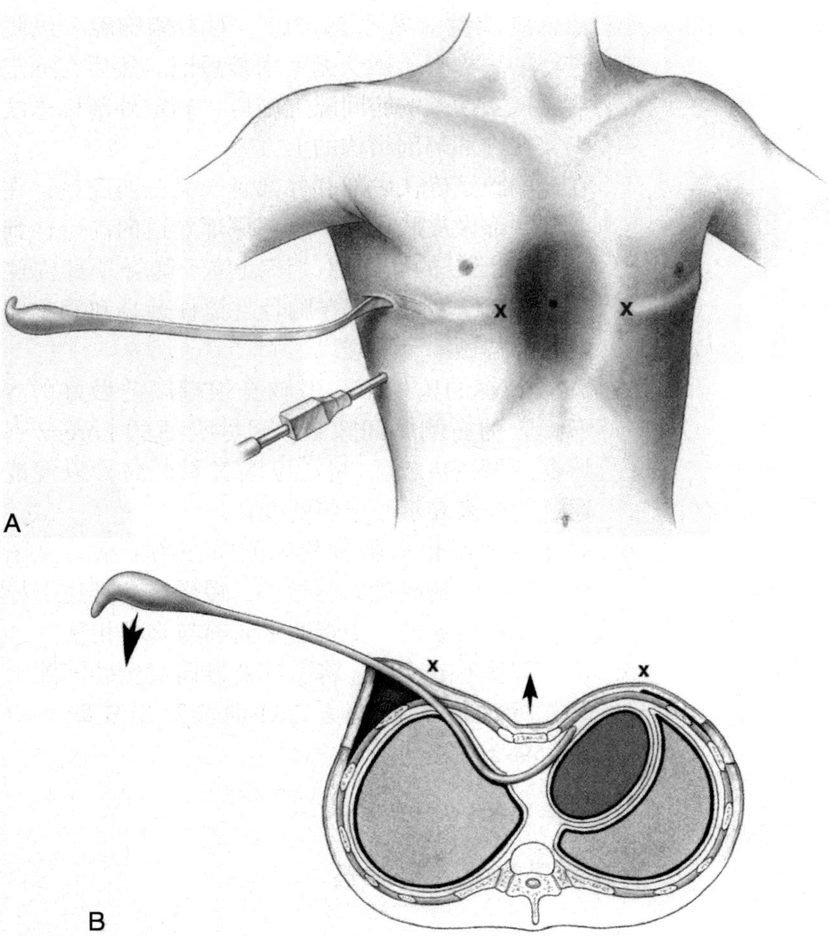

图 59-22 A. 将 Lorenz 引导器从右侧的皮下隧道插入。在胸腔镜的引导下，将其推入有 X 标记的右侧肋间隙。B. 在胸腔镜的引导下，用引导器将胸膜和心包从胸骨的后侧面上分离下来，以此经胸建立胸骨后隧道。前推引导器，从 X 标记处的左侧肋间隙穿过，然后从左侧胸切口穿出。

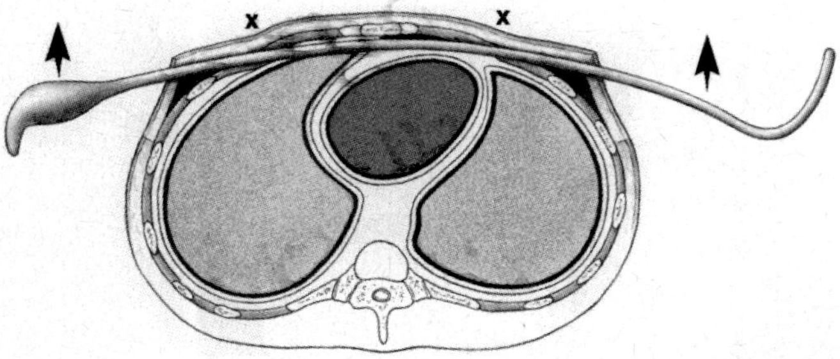

图 59-23 在下方肋弓上施压，从两侧提起引导器，将胸骨从其凹陷位置提出。重复抬起动作，直到漏斗胸被矫正。

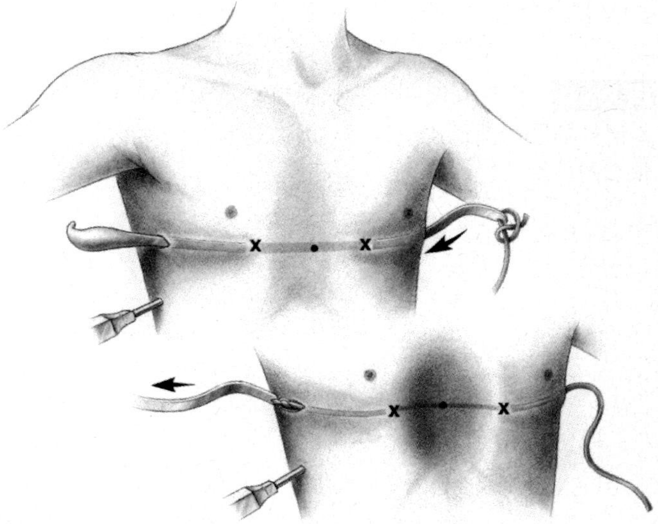

图 59-24 漏斗胸矫正后，将一根脐带线系到引导器一端，再慢慢回抽过胸腔，因此将脐带线抽过经胸隧道。

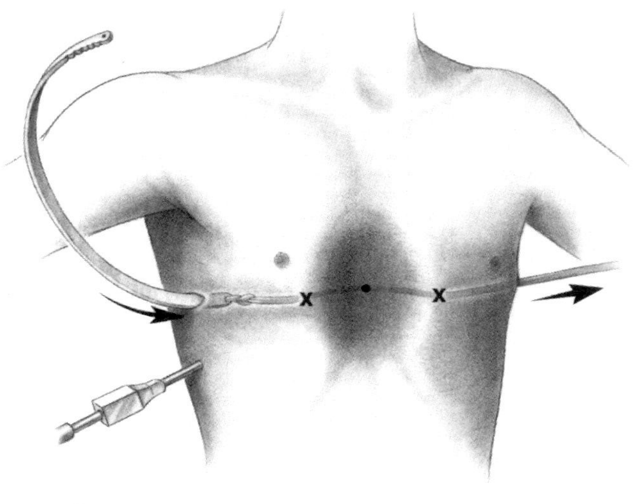

图 59-25　将预先准备好的胸部支撑条系在脐带线上，在胸腔镜的引导下，拉过胸腔，凸面保持向后。

并将引导器慢慢展平，将脐带线从胸骨下隧道内拉出（图 59-24）。

2. 将预先准备好的胸部支撑条系到脐带系上，并在胸腔镜的监视下，回抽脐带线将其拉过胸骨后隧道。插入此支撑条的时候，使其凸面向后（图 59-25）。
3. 支撑条到位后，将其翻转 180°（图 59-26）。
4. 如果支撑条需要进一步弯曲的话，将其翻过来，在需要的地方用 Lorenz 支撑条弯曲器进行重新塑形。
5. 如果一根支撑条不够，可以在上或下一个肋间隙置入第二根支撑条。特别对于年长患者，两根支撑条可提供更好和更稳定的矫正。
6. 必须稍稍的过度矫正一些，以防去除支撑条后病情复发（图 59-27 和 59-28）。
7. 一些外科医生喜欢从左侧建立纵隔隧道，而不是在右侧。其他外科医生在剑突下做第三个切口，然后使用一把巾钳来提起胸骨；其他人在穿入引 926
导器前，用手指进行胸骨后分离。

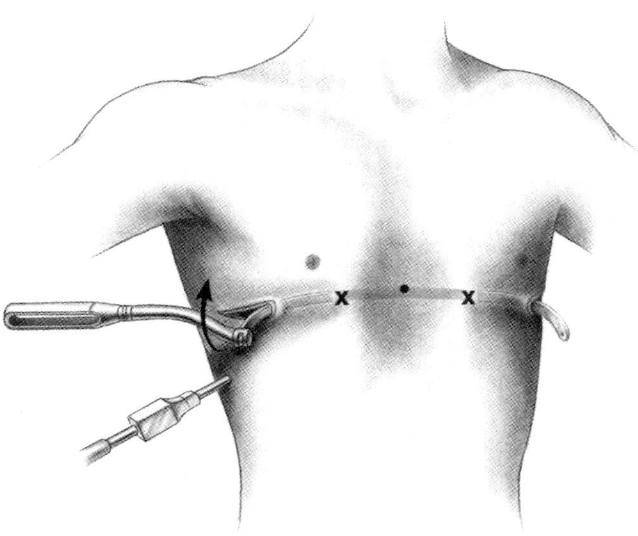

图 59-26　当支撑条到位后，再用支撑条手柄将其翻转 180°。

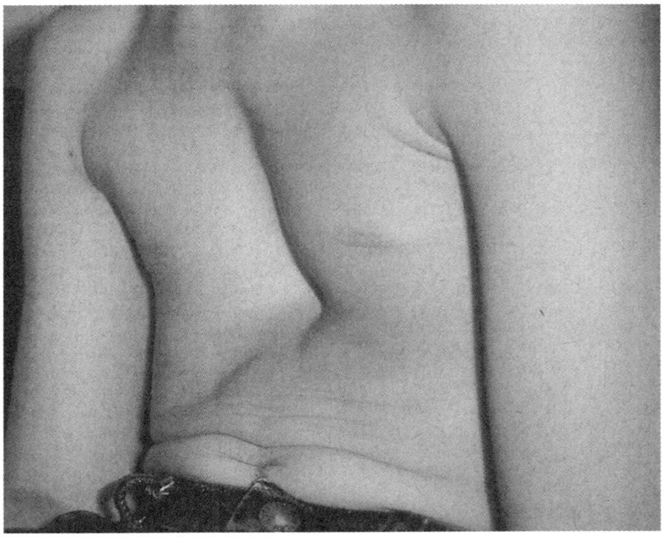

图 59-27　重度漏斗胸，术前。

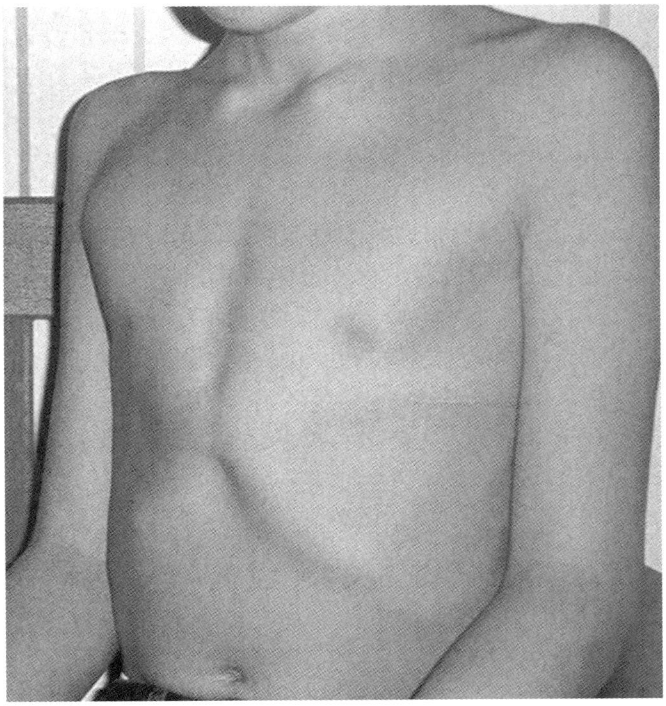

图 59-28　图 59-27 的患者术后显示有轻微的过度矫正。

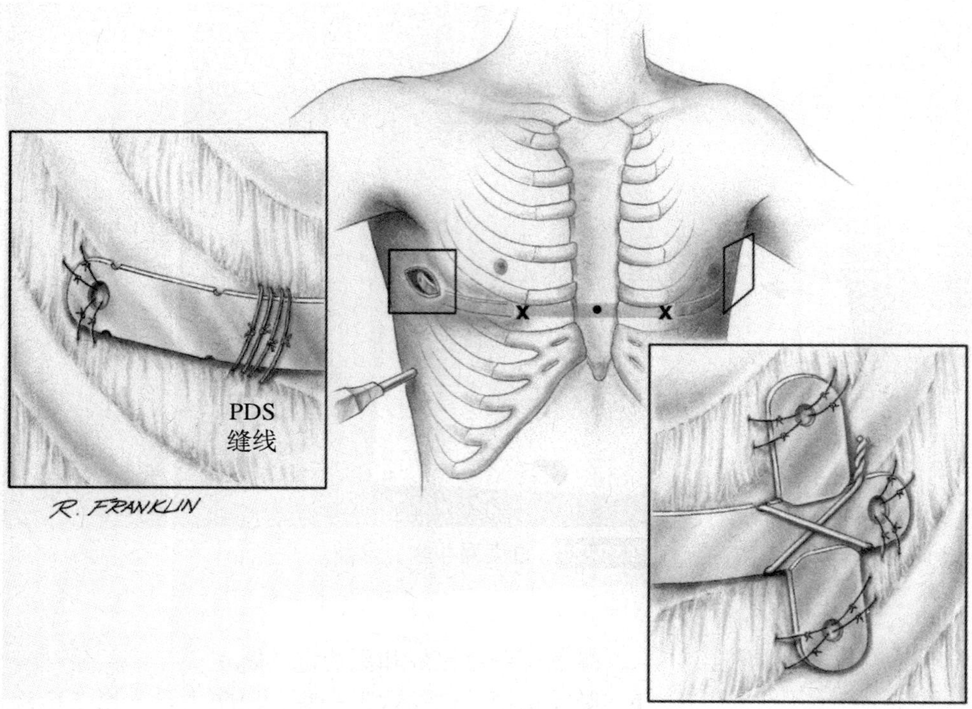

图 59-29 为了防止支撑条移位，在左侧用钢丝缝线和固定器进行固定。在右侧用粗的吸收线（0号或1号 PDS 线）将支撑条和下面的肋骨缝合在一起。此外，将缝线穿过支撑条和固定器的孔，并与下方的筋膜缝在一起。

支撑条的固定

1. 固定对成功手术来说是绝对必要的。在支撑条的左端装上一个固定器，并用3号手术钢丝将其与支撑条绑在一起（图 59-29）。如果支撑条似乎还不稳定的话，可能需要第二根支撑条进行支撑，而不是再加一个固定器。
2. 在胸腔镜监视下，在右侧采用腹腔镜的内缝合针，将粗的0号或1号 PDS 吸收线环绕支撑条和下方肋骨进行缝合（见图 59-29）。Hebra 等[5]建议在邻近胸骨的地方也缝一针。
3. 一旦支撑条固定好，逐层关闭切口，用套管和连接管排气消除气胸，也可放置一根带“水封”系统的胸引管。
4. 在患者出手术室之前，拍一张胸片，以检查是否还有残余气胸。

术后治疗

1. 在康复室内，患者镇静1～2小时，使其从麻醉状态下平稳复苏。
2. 硬膜外套管保留3～5天。
3. 术后第四～第五天患者出院回家。
4. 患者2周后可以上学，但是术后6周内不要参加运动。
5. 6周后，鼓励患者恢复胸部呼吸和体态训练，并参加有氧运动（例如，足球、棒球、游泳）。
6. 在去除支撑条之前，不要参加对抗强烈的运动（例如，拳击、橄榄球、冰球）。

支撑条取出技术（植入后2～4年）

1. 气管内全身麻醉，给予5～6cmH_2O的呼气末正压。
2. 患者取仰卧位，双臂在肩部外展。
3. 查看放射影像学图片，确定固定器的位置。
4. 触诊检查是否可以触及支撑条和固定器及他们与陈旧瘢痕的距离。如果无法触及，采用C形臂透视机来判断这些装置的确切位置。
5. 如果可能，在原先的瘢痕上做切口。大多数的患者，如果仅用了一个固定器的话，只需要做一个切口。

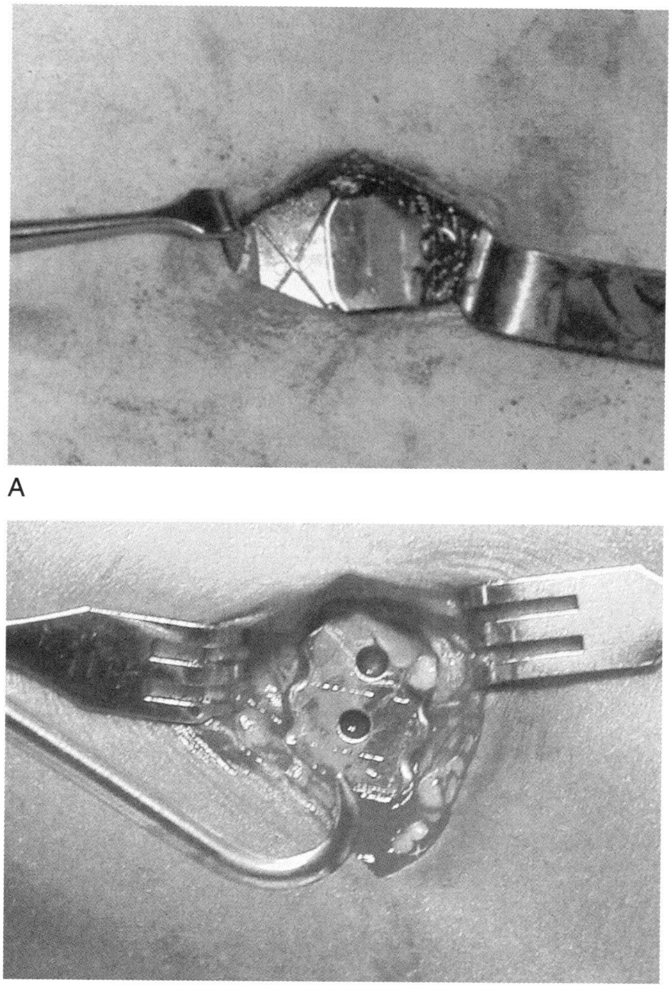

A

B

图 59-30　A. 松解支撑条和固定器，并将之从切口取出。B. 将固定器从支撑条上卸下，并取出。

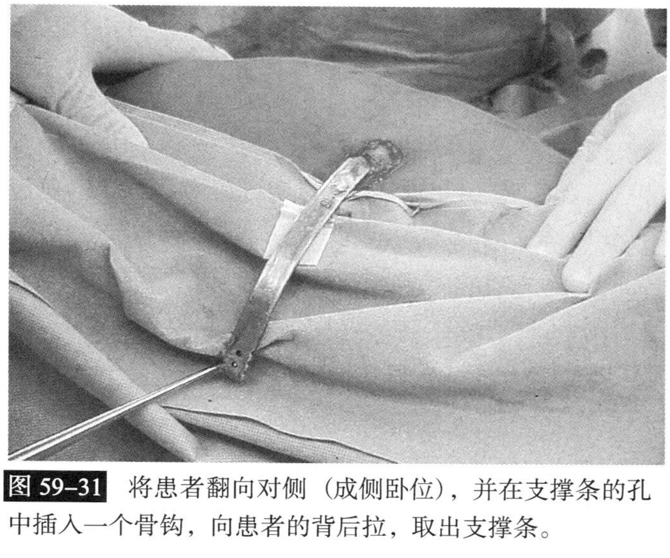

图 59-31　将患者翻向对侧（成侧卧位），并在支撑条的孔中插入一个骨钩，向患者的背后拉，取出支撑条。

6. 松解支撑条的末端和固定器。切断两处的钢丝并取出。
7. 当支撑条和固定器从周围瘢痕组织中分离出来后，在固定器下段的孔内插入一个骨钩，并将其从切口中拉出。然后拉住固定器上段的孔，将支撑条的末端拉出。从支撑条上卸下固定器。
8. 在支撑条末端的孔内插入一个矫形外科用的骨钩，并轻轻拉抽（图 59-30 和 59-31）。如果支撑条有所活动，将患者翻至侧卧位，将支撑条向患者背后放下向下拉出。将患者翻回仰卧位，然后关闭切口。
9. 使患者保持呼气末正压通气，直到切口关闭。
10. 目前发展出一种支撑条“伸直器”，对于那些采用两个固定器且需要做左右两侧切口的患者很有用。

取出支撑条的时机

我们建议将支撑条在患者体内保留 2～4 年（平均 3 年）。患者每年评估一次，监测他们的生长和活动水平。鼓励他们进行胸部锻炼并参加有氧运动。6～10 岁之间的患者生长通常不是很迅速，他们对支撑条可以有 3 年甚至 4 年的良好耐受。相反，青少年的生长很快，可能需要在 2 年后就取出支撑条。

我们认为运动锻炼和手术同样重要。许多儿童和成人的生活方式过于安静，从不进行有氧运动；因此必须对其心肺系统进行刺激，因为潮气量只有肺总容量的 10%。大力鼓励进行深呼吸并屏气 10～15 秒钟和诸如奔跑（如足球、棒球）和游泳的有氧运动。

效果

人口统计学

到 2005 年 12 月，在我们单位共有 785 例患者接受了 Nuss 手术；473 例患者取出了支撑条，387 例患者取出支撑条超过 1 年（图 59-32）。自此技术问世以来[14]，在手术技术（例如，常规使用胸腔镜）和微创器械及胸骨后支撑条的植入和固定方面有了诸多重大改良[3]。这些极大地降低了手术风险和并发症，并在其他文献中有详细的报道[7,13]。

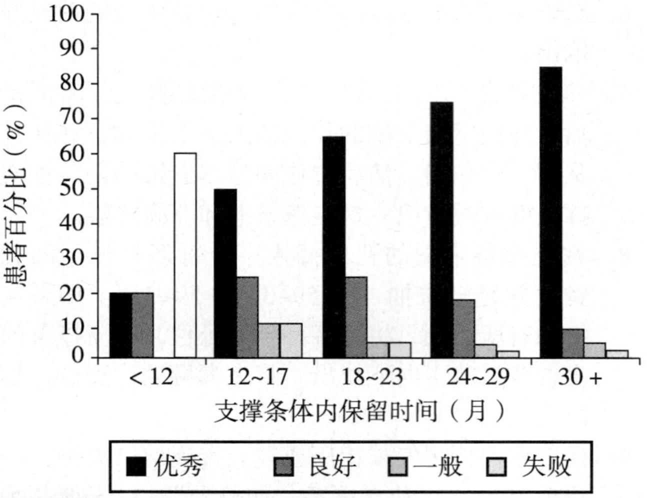

928

图 59-32 支撑条在患者体内保留 1 年或 1 年以上，取出支撑条后的效果（N＝387）。

表 59-5 Nuss 手术术后早期并发症

并发症	患者人数（%）
死亡	0
心脏穿孔	0
气胸	481（51.2）
需要放置胸引管	20（2.5）
需要抽气	3（0.3）
胸腔积液需要引流	3（0.3）
心包炎	4（0.5）
血胸（手术造成的）	7（0.9）
肺炎	2（0.2）
药物反应	32（4.0）
Horner 综合征	166（21.1）

从 1987 年到 2005 年 12 月的 17 年中，共有 1511 例患者进行了胸壁畸形的评估（表 59-4）；785 例在我们中心进行了初期微创手术（一期矫正），67 例进行了再次手术（初期手术是在别处进行的）。

手术患者的男女比例为 4.7∶1。平均年龄为 14.2 岁，年龄跨度为 22 个月～29 岁。平均 CT Haller 指数为 4.6（2.4～31）。785 例患者中有 654 例（83%）经超声心动图或 CT 扫描发现有心脏压迫。785 例患者中有 117 例（14.9%）有二尖瓣脱垂。692 例患者进行静息肺功能测试，证实高达 42.3%的患者有异常。

手术操作、麻醉和住院时间

584 例（74.4%）患者植入了一根支撑条；197 例（25.1%）患者植入了两根支撑条。大多数患者出血很少（≤10 ml），除了一例出现血胸，但是不需要输血治疗。绝大多数患者的硬膜外麻醉使用 3 天。住院天数的中值为 5 天。

表 59-4 Nuss 手术患者的人口统计学

评估的患者总数	1278
微创（Nuss）手术患者总数	685
一期手术总例数	633
再次手术总例数	52
前次为 Ravitch 手术	28
前次为 Nuss 手术	24
前次为 Leonard 手术	2*

* Leonard 手术也是一种 Ravitch 手术，只是在统计中我们将其单独列开。

并发症

早期并发症[4,6,7]

我们单位手术的 785 例患者中没有死亡和心脏穿孔（表 59-5）。20 例（2.5%）患者发生气胸并需要放置胸引管；仅 3 例（0.4%）患者需要经皮穿刺抽气。7 例（0.9%）患者发生血胸，需要进行引流。3 例（0.3%）胸腔积液需要放置胸引管或穿刺抽液。

4 例（0.5%）术后出现心包炎需要用吲哚美辛治疗，1 例需要心包穿刺放液。2 例（0.2%）术后出现肺炎，32 例（4.0%）术后有药物反应。共 166 例患者在胸部硬膜外麻醉过程中，有不同时间的一过性 Horner 综合征。 929

远期并发症

51 例（6.5%）患者的支撑条移位（表 59-6）；但是，仅有 28 例（3.5%）患者需要再次固定。这组 28

表 59-6 Nuss 手术术后晚期并发症

并发症	患者人数（%）
支撑条移位	51/785（6.5%）
需要矫正	28/785（3.5%）
使用固定器之前发生的移位	10/113（8.8%）
用了固定器后的移位	18/672（2.6%）
固定器钢丝加固后的移位	9/360（2.5%）
PDS 缝线加固后的移位	1/237（0.4%）
血胸	2/785（0.2%）
伤口感染	7/785（0.9%）
支撑条感染	6/785（0.7%）
需要早期取出	2/785（0.2%）
支撑条过敏	19/785（2.4%）
矫正过度	22/785（2.8%）
复发	8/785（1.0%）

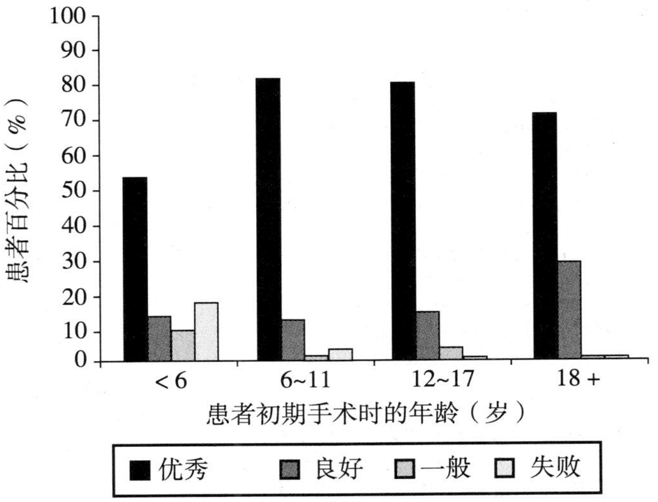

图 59-33 取出支撑条后 1 年或超过 1 年时的患者，根据手术年龄来判定的疗效（N=276）。

例移位患者中，10 例是在固定器问世之前发生的，我们在固定器问世之前的时间内，对最初的 113 例患者进行了手术。在固定器问世之后，支撑条移位的发生率从 8.8%降至 2.6%。当用钢丝将固定器和支撑条捆绑固定后，支撑条移位的发生率降至 2.5%。自我们开始采用左侧放置固定器和在右侧把支撑条和下方肋骨用 PDS 线捆绑缝合的附加固定策略之后，仅有 1 例（0.4%）的支撑条移位。6 例（0.7%）患者发生支撑条感染，2 例（0.2%）需要早期取出。

19 例患者对支撑条产生过敏反应。在放置支撑条或固定器的区域产生红斑，切口位置产生无菌性脓肿、胸腔和（或）心包积液。

785 例患者中，22 例（2.8%）出现中度的过度矫正畸形，4 例（0.5%）发展成真正的鸡胸畸形。

整体效果和长期随访

患者术后 6 个月随访一次，然后每年随访一次。在长期评估中，将术后效果分为优秀、良好、一般和失败。如果患者的胸骨完全得以矫正并无任何并发症状的话，效果即为优秀。胸部畸形明显改善，但为达到完全正常的胸壁外观，且无任何并发症状，效果即为良好。有轻度残余漏斗胸，且症状未完全消除的效果为一般。手术失败就是漏斗胸复发，并有合并症状或在支撑条取出后需要再次进行其他手术。

718 例（91%）患者初期手术的美观和功能效果为优秀，64 例（8%）为良好，1 例（0.2%）为一般，2 例（0.25%）失败。共 385 例患者在植入超过 1 年后再将支撑条取出，88 例在 1 年内取出。那些支撑条取出 1 年或 1 年以上的患者，79.8%为优秀，14.9%为良好，2.3%为一般，2.0%为失败。不进行锻炼的和在青春期前取出支撑条的患者，复发率高。支撑条体内保留时间对远期效果有直接影响。支撑条保留的时间越长，效果越好（见图 59-32）。患者的年龄也影响远期疗效，7～12 岁和 13～18 岁患者的手术效果最好（图 59-33）[2]。在 785 例一期手术以外，还成功进行了 67 例微创漏斗胸再次矫正手术。

结论

90%的患者通过微创手术获得了良好或优秀的漏斗胸矫正，无需切除肋骨，无需胸骨截骨，出血最少，可迅速恢复正常活动[1,4,6,10-12]。研究表明，患者的体形有显著的改善[8,15]，同时肺功能测试的结果也有改善[1,9]。

（孙彦隽译　刘锦纷校）

参考文献

1. Borowitz D, Cemy F, Zallen G, et al: Pulmonary function and exercise response in patients with pectus excavatum after Nuss repair. J Pediatr Surg 2003;38:544-547.
2. Coln D, Gunning T, Ramsey M: Early experience with the Nuss minimally invasive procedure. World J Surg 2002;26:1217-1221.
3. Croitoru DP, Kelly RE Jr, Nuss D, et al: Experience and modification update for the minimally invasive Nuss technique for pectus excavatum repair in 303 patients. J Pediatr Surg 2002;37:437-445.
4. Fonkalsrud EW, Beanes S, Hebra A, et al: Comparison of minimally invasive and modified Ravitch pectus excavatum repair. J Pediatr Surg 2002;37:413-417.
5. Hebra A, Gauderer MW, Tagge EP: A simple technique for preventing bar displacement with the Nuss repair of pectus excavatum. J Pediatr Surg 2001;36:1266-1268.
6. Hebra A, Swoveland B, Egbert M, et al: Outcome analysis of minimally invasive repair of pectus excavatum: Review of 251 cases. J Pediatr Surg 2000;35:252-257.
7. Hyung JP, Seock Y, Cheol SL: Complications associated with the Nuss procedure: Analysis of risk factors and suggested measures for prevention of complications. J Pediatr Surg 2004;39:391-395.
8. Lawson ML, Cash TF, Akers RA, et al: A pilot study of the impact of surgical repair on disease-specific quality of life among patients with pectus excavatum. J Pediatr Surg 2003;38:916-918.
9. Lawson M, Mellins R, Tabangin M, et al: Impact of pectus excavatum on pulmonary function before and after repair with the Nuss procedure. J Pediatr Surg (submitted for publication).
10. Miller KA, Woods RK, Sharp RJ, et al: Minimally invasive repair of pectus excavatum: A single institution's experience. Surgery 2001;130:652-657.
11. Miller RA: Minimally invasive bar repair for redo correction. J Pediatr Surg 2002;37:1090-1092.
12. Molik KA, Engum SA, Rescorla FJ, et al: Pectus excavatum repair: Experience with standard and minimally invasive techniques. J Pediatr Surg 2001;36:324-328.
13. Nuss D, Kelly RE Jr, et al: Repair of pectus excavatum. Pediatr Endosurg Innovat Techn 1998;2:205-221.
14. Nuss D, Kelly RE Jr, et al: A 10-year review of a minimally invasive technique for the correction of pectus excavatum. J Pediatr 1998;33:545-552.
15. Roberts J, Hayashi A, Anderson JO, et al: Quality of life of patients who have undergone the Nuss procedure for pectus excavatum: Preliminary findings. J Pediatr Surg 2003;38:779-783.
16. Saitoh C, Yamada A, Kosaka K, et al: Allergy to pectus bar for funnel chest. Plast Reconstr Surg 2002;110:719-721.

第 60 章

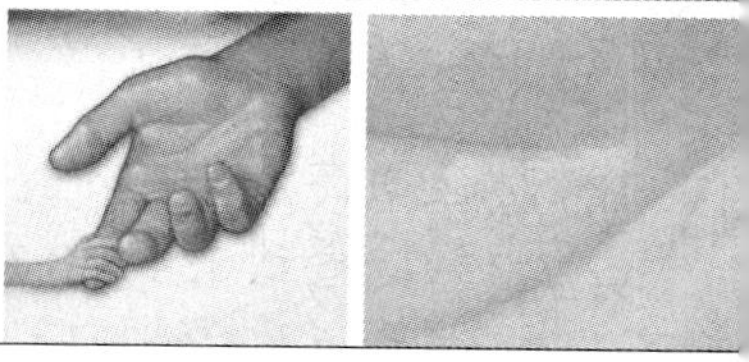

先天性膈疝和膈膨升

Charles J. H. Stolar 和 Peter W. Dillon

历史

931 在 1754 年的《皇家医师协会期刊》(Proceeding of Royal College of Physicans)[203]中，Hunter 的同事 McCauley 描述了有关新生儿先天性膈疝（CDH）的大体解剖和病理生理学，这是英文文献中最早的有关报道。

> 1752 年的 8 月 24 日，一名出生于 Brownlow 街医院的男婴，发育完全，非常的丰满并富有肉感。他是一名健康的年轻产妇生下的第 5 个孩子，在母亲怀孕期间一切情况都很好。这名婴儿在刚出生时，有些发抖，护士以为他将要昏死过去。他的呼吸也有困难，需要停顿一段时间才能哭出来；当他哭的时候声调有一些特别的特征。大约半个小时以后，这名婴儿似乎恢复了一点精神，呼吸更加通畅了：但是就在他出生以后一个半小时，症状很快反复并死亡。在这名婴儿的母亲、护士长和护士告诉我这些细节以后，我希望能够解剖这名婴儿的尸体……打开该婴儿的腹部，发现在腹腔内除了一部分含有胎粪的膨胀结肠以外，没有看到小肠。在我开始进一步的解剖以前，我派人通知了我机灵的朋友 Hunter 医生。我们一起进行了解剖，检查了这种古怪的疾病，同时忠实的记录下最值得注意的解剖发现。
>
> 当胸骨提升以后，我们就发现胃和绝大部分的小肠、脾脏、部分的胰腺都位于左侧胸腔，这些脏器通过一个膈肌的中断，或者更正确地的说是一个膈肌的小孔，在距离食管的自然通道大约有 1 英寸（2.54 厘米）的地方，进入胸腔中。
>
> 由于特别多的脏器进入了左侧胸腔中，纵隔、心脏、食管和降主动脉都被迫压迫而明显地移向胸腔的右侧；因为裂口边缘没有发现破裂或炎症的痕迹，可能是逐渐受到疝入胸腔的腹腔脏器的影响，左叶肺的体积减小，心脏和纵隔被推到右侧。
>
> 由于食管被胃和肠道推到右侧，食管在胸腔内的走行不变但没有在通常的地方穿透膈肌，而是显著偏到了右侧。食管穿透膈肌的位置偏向后侧，在胸腔下腔静脉的右侧。
>
> 我保存了心脏和肺以显示肺叶大小的不成比例。我烘干并制作了膈肌和脊柱及胸骨连接部的标本，以显示肠道进入胸腔而穿过的异常裂孔，也显示出食管穿过膈肌右侧的部位。这些标本也同时展示给整个医生协会。

Cooper[59]在 1827 年，Laennec[177]在 1834 年，不仅报道了先天性膈疝的临床症状和大体的病理学研究，也提出剖腹手术可能是一种正确的办法，可以复位并纠治膈疝。Bowditch[34]在 1847 年首次做出了先天性膈疝的床边诊断，进一步强调了临床诊断的标准。虽然 Bochdalek 对胚胎学的理解不正确，但是这种先天性缺陷仍然继续沿用他的名字[23]。他推测先天性膈疝是由分隔胸腔、腹腔的隔膜后外侧的破裂所致。他也错误地推测修补先天性膈疝缺损的最佳通路是通过第 12 肋床的位置。至于这种方法，事实上是否曾经尝试过，记录显示并不清楚。最早的手术修补先天性膈疝的尝试，是由 Nauman[220]在 1888 年和 O'Dwyer 在 1890 年进行的，但是这种努力并没有获得成功[227]。最早成功修补成年人膈疝的记录是由 Aue[12]在 1901 年报道的，而最早成功修补儿童膈疝是由 Heidenhain[132]在 1905 年报道的。

在新生儿时期，治疗先天性膈疝的基础是由 Hedblom[128]打下的，他回顾了到 1925 年为止所报道的病例，显示 44 例在新生儿时期被诊断为先天性膈疝的婴幼儿的死亡率为 75%。他建议早期的干预可能 932

会提高生存率。成功修补先天性膈疝的病例非常罕见，直到 1940 年 Ladd 和 Gross[176]报道了 16 例先天性膈疝手术修补后有 9 例得以存活，最小的为出生后 40 个小时。直到 1946 年，Gross[113]才报道了第 1 例出生后不到 24 小时的婴儿被成功进行先天性膈疝修补手术以后存活的病例。一直到 20 世纪 80 年代，治疗标准还是即刻进行新生儿膈疝修补术，并在术后进行复苏治疗（图 60–1）。

流行病学和遗传学

报道的先天性膈疝的发病率估计在新生儿的 1/2000～1/5000 之间[46,107,120,238]。在美国，每年有接近 1000 例新生儿患有这种疾病；最近，一项来自亚特兰大的研究显示，发生率为每 10 000 个新生儿中有 2.4 例[84]。先天性膈疝在死产儿中的发病率没有很好

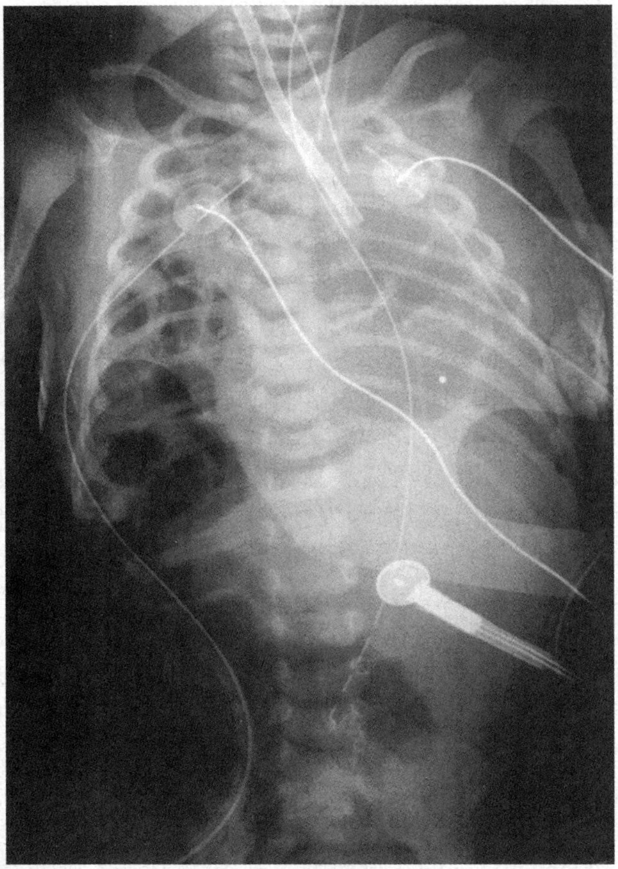

图 60–1 右侧先天性膈疝婴儿的胸部平片，显示在右侧胸腔有空气充盈的小肠袢，纵隔向对侧移位。婴儿已经插管以便进行体外膜肺氧合器的支持。

的记载。患有先天性膈疝的婴儿中接近 1/3 为死产儿，但是这些死亡通常是由合并的致命性先天性畸形所致[110,238,312]。当死产儿与活产儿一起统计时，女性似乎比男性更常受累[46,104,238]。

先天性膈疝更常见于左侧，接近 80%的病例发生在左侧，20%发生在右侧。双侧的先天性膈疝比较罕见，合并相关畸形的发生率较高[222]。单纯的先天性膈疝的婴儿更容易是早产儿、巨大儿、和男性婴儿；大约三分之一的受累婴儿可能会合并的主要缺陷[84]。瘦小的或者相对身高是低体重的妇女，生出单纯的先天性膈疝婴儿的风险可能会升高[305]。先天性膈疝被认为是呈现为一种散发性的发育性畸形，但是也有许多家族性病例的报道[46,111,208]。在直系亲属中，预期的复发风险估计为 1/45 或者接近 2%[193]。9%～34%的先天性膈疝婴儿中，鉴定出有结构性的染色体异常，包括三体畸形、缺失和易位[140,321]。有基因缺失或者易位的特异性染色体，可能是发生先天性膈疝的候选部位[13,42,197]。先天性膈疝和异常染色体组型的结合，与不良的结果有关[112]。

先天性膈疝的病因还不清楚。如同其他的胚胎性疾病一样，不断有证据表明先天性膈疝可能是由于遗传学上有发病倾向或者遗传易感性的个体暴露于环境因素中所导致的。在它的发生过程中，涉及暴露于多种药物和环境危害因素。这些因素包括杀虫剂和药物，如维洛沙秦、反应停、奎宁、镉、铅和除草醚[65,138,149,232,307]。在先天性膈疝患儿中，维生素 A 缺乏的临床发现和服用维生素 A 在除草醚诱导的肺发育不全患儿中的作用，都强压了这种进化的假设，类维生素 A 调控的靶基因的改变，可能是发生先天性膈疝的原因[112]。

合并的畸形

任何有大的先天性畸形的新生儿，包括新生儿先天性膈疝，与一般人群相比其他畸形的发生率明显增多。虽然以前认为发生率较低，先天性膈疝的婴儿合并其他畸形的发生率在 10%～50%之间[65,95,110,194,207,226,296,312]，32%的先天性膈疝婴儿发现存在骨骼畸形，包括肢体缩小和肋椎缺陷[207,226,285]。24%的膈疝婴儿发现存在心脏畸形。经常有报道称累及左心室的心脏发育不全经常合并主动脉弓的发育不全，

并可能与心脏发育不全综合征相混淆。然而，其临床意义是有限的。大多数的心血管畸形会涉及心脏流出道，例如室间隔缺损、法洛四联症、大血管转位、右心室双出口、主动脉缩窄[88,206,284]。18%的先天性膈疝患儿中，发现存在气管支气管树的解剖异常，包括先天性气管狭窄、气管支气管、分成三叉的气管[226]。在先天性膈疝的死产儿中，合并畸形的发生率甚至更高。一项研究显示，先天性膈疝的死产儿中 100%合并有致死性的畸形[238]。在这个死产儿组中发现的畸形主要是神经管缺损，包括无脑畸形、脊髓脊膜膨出、脑积水和脑膨出。甚至在出生时仍存活但是随后很快
933 就死去的婴儿中，发现神经管缺损是最为常见的畸形。心脏缺陷是第二常见的畸形，包括室间隔缺损、血管环和主动脉缩窄[284]。其他中线发育畸形也已经有所报道，包括食管闭锁、脐膨出和腭裂。许多综合征都有先天性膈疝的病理性发现。这些综合征包括 21 三体、18 三体、13 三体、Frey 综合征、Beckwith-Wiedemann 综合征、Goldenhar 综合征、Coffin-Siris 综合征、Fryns 综合征、Meacham 综合征和 Kabuki 综合征。

胚胎学

膈的发育

膈的胚胎发育还不完全清楚，其中涉及多种复杂的细胞和组织间的相互作用。发育完全的横膈膜起源于四个特异性的成分：（1）原始横隔形成前的中心腱；（2）胸腹隔膜形成背外侧部分；（3）发育自食管肠系膜的背侧膈肌脚；（4）发育自胸廓肋间肌群的横膈膜的肌性部分。在妊娠第 4 周，膈结构的前体开始形成，并在侧面的间充质组织中出现腹膜反折。同时，从心包腔的下方开始形成原始横隔。原始横膈用以分隔胸腔和腹腔，最终形成发育完全的横隔中心腱部分。横隔中心腱部分定义为原始的胸腹膜管，使间充质组织在这些通道内得以建立，最终导致肺实质的发育。

胸腹膜管的关闭以及胸腹隔膜的形成发生在妊娠第 8 周。已经有多个理论来解释这种胸腹隔膜的形成和膈结构的随后发育。有人认为胸腹隔膜的进行性生长是胸腹膜管关闭的一种机制[62,152]。其他的研究者提出，同时发生的肝和肾的器官形成对这个过程起到了至关重要的作用[41,43,311]。有人提出横膈的形成涉及肝后间充质板[149]。

从体壁侧延伸过来的胸腹膜反折向中间和前侧生长，直到妊娠第 6 周，与横膈膜和食管的背侧肠系膜发生融合。胸腹膜管的完全关闭发生在妊娠第 8 周。在解剖学上，右侧胸腹膜管的关闭要早于左侧[212]。虽然有学者提出肝后间充质板是肌肉组织的一个可能来源，但是横膈的肌性化似乎来自胸腔最里面的肌肉层[41,149]。后侧面上，在腰椎和肋间肌群的连接处，纤维化的腰肋三角区仍然是一小块胸腹膈膜的残留，在发育的终末期依靠两组肌群的融合来获得自己的强度。肌群融合的延迟或者融合障碍就留下了这片薄弱区域，也许是容易形成疝的薄弱部位。Bochdalek 首先在 1848 年描述了横膈后侧面上的这片区域，出于这个原因，先天性膈疝最常见的部位就以他的名字命名。

肺的发育

胎儿肺的发育可以分为五个阶段：胚胎期、假腺体期、微管期、囊状期和肺泡期[79]。妊娠第 3 周，胚胎肺开始发育，它作为前肠的一种衍生物，以喉气管凹槽尾侧末端的憩室形成标记[35]。到妊娠第 4 周，这个憩室形成气管和两支主要的原始肺芽。妊娠第 6 周时，这些肺芽进一步发育成为清晰的肺叶结构。肺发育的假腺体期发生在妊娠第 7～16 周，其中包括肺气道的分化。在这个时期，所有的支气管气道开始发育。从妊娠第 16～24周，胎儿肺的发育进入到微管期。在此期间，气体空间发育开始，就是未成熟的肺泡空气囊开始形成。1型肺细胞开始分化，最终，产生表面活性物质的 2 型肺细胞前体开始出现。在这个时期，功能性的气体交换变为可能。

未成熟的肺泡空间继续发育成熟发生在肺发育的囊状期，就是从妊娠的第 24 周持续到足月分娩。在这段时期，肺泡空间大小持续进行重塑，合成表面活性物质的能力不断成熟[115]。成熟的成人样的肺泡在出生后不久便开始出现[36,37]。出生以后便开始出现广泛的肺泡成熟和数量增加，直到接近 8 周岁时，功能性肺泡的数量增加了 10 倍[66,87,309]。研究者提出肺泡的形成可能到 2 岁时就已经完成[290]。

在气道和肺泡的生长期之后，肺部血管开始发育，根据相关的气道结构可分为两组解剖单位。术语腺泡指的是肺的功能性单位，包括呼吸性细支气管、肺泡导管、和肺泡——所有的结构都是在肺发育的微管期或者以后发育的。在这个区域，血管发育与肺泡的生长和数量的增加同时发生。腺泡前的结构包括气管、主支气管、小叶支气管一直到终末细支气管。腺泡前的血管发育到妊娠第 16 周的时候完成[136,137,243]。

现在已经认识到，肺的发育是以一系列的程序性事件为标记，并由主宰基因所调控，例如同位序列基因、核转录因子、激素和生长因子。这些过程涉及基因调控性的上皮细胞和内皮细胞间的相互作用，以及数个激素和生长因子之间时间和空间上的相互作用。
934 早期发育性的转录因子，例如肝细胞核因子-3β 和甲状腺转录因子-1，从前肠的间充质开始调控肺的发育。其他肺发育刺激物包括转化生长因子-β 途径、信号蛋白 sonic hedgehog 途径、Notch-delta 途径、Wingless-Int 通道和细胞因子受体途径。随后的器官发生的信号转导调控包括细胞凋亡途径、细胞核受体途径、和白介素途径。激素例如糖皮质激素、甲状腺素、和维甲酸调控数个重要的细胞间相互作用，以满足适当的肺器官发生和分化的需要[49]。

虽然正常的肺发育途径已经变得越来越清晰，但是关于基因表达的改变，生长因子的相互作用，与先天性膈疝的肺发育不良相关的激素水平还知之甚少。在先天性膈疝肺标本中，发现许多因子水平都升高，包括表皮生长因子、转移生长因子-α、血管内皮细胞生长因子、胰岛素样生长因子、肿瘤坏死因子-α、和糖皮质激素受体基因的表达[114,210,229,263,272]。其他的因子，例如信号蛋白 sonic hedgehog 的表达、血红素加氧酶-1 和内皮型一氧化氮水平都降低。这些发现的重要性还有待于确定[271,294]。

近来，通过大鼠除草醚动物模型加深了对与先天性膈疝相关的哺乳动物的肺形成发育缺陷的理解[50]。实验型先天性膈疝的除草醚动物模型的采用，与认为许多发育缺陷，包括先天性膈疝，都是由于毒素暴露所导致的胚胎病理理论一致。除草醚是一种环境毒素，将它应用于妊娠的老鼠可导致下一代的肺发育不全、膈疝缺陷、气道分支减少、肺血管过度肌化、表面活性物质缺乏以及出生时的呼吸衰竭。由除草醚诱导的肺发育不全，伴有胚胎老鼠许多生长因子和胚的发育途径的改变[49,50]。先天性膈疝形成的除草醚动物模型，戏剧性地改变了对这种疾病过程的理解，即它是一种膈肌形成的单纯机械缺陷，导致了肺的压缩和呼吸衰竭。现在多个研究提示，肺发育不全可能发生在膈疝形成之前，其中涉及肺胚胎期发育的许多基本途径[153]。

许多物理因素也可能会影响肺的生长和发育[79]。足够的胸腔内空间是肺正常生长的先决条件。任何可导致胸腔内空间减小和肺实质压缩的胸腔内或胸腔外的变化，都可导致肺结构上的发育不成熟[69,78,121,190,235,315]。在肺的生长发育中，其他重要的物理因素包括维持正常的胎儿肺液和羊水动力[4,75,96,211]。

病理学

虽然先天性膈疝的病因还不能确定，但是它在肺的发育和功能方面的结果有很多的文献记载。在横膈的早期发育过程中，中肠疝出并进入卵黄囊。如果在妊娠的第 9～10 周，中肠回到腹腔内时胸腹膜管还没有完成关闭，腹腔内脏就通过腰肋三角区疝入同侧的胸腔。因此肠道的异常位置妨碍了肠道正常的逆时针旋转和固定。如果内脏疝出发生在胸腹膜管完全关闭以前，就不存在疝囊，但是在 10%～15% 的先天性膈疝患者中，非肌性的隔膜形成了疝囊[189]。虽然一些学者声称膈疝可发生在妊娠的晚期，或者由于动态变化而间歇地出现，但是大多数的病例在妊娠第 12 周时，膈疝就已经存在了[3]。后来的出生以后的问题，与疝出的内脏对发育中的心脏和肺的作用有关。

经典的左侧先天性膈疝的特征是一个直径为 2.0～4.0cm 的膈肌后外侧缺损，通过这个缺损腹腔内脏器可疝出并进入半侧胸廓（图 60-2）。疝出的内容物经常包括肝脏的左叶、脾脏、几乎全部的胃肠道。胃经常位于胸腔内，可导致某种程度的胃食管连接处梗阻。这种梗阻可导致食管的扩张和膨胀。肾脏在肾 935
血管允许的限度内偶尔可能会疝出进入胸腔。发生右侧先天性膈疝时，除了其他腹腔内的脏器疝出以外，较大的肝脏右叶也可以占据半侧胸腔的大部分空间。肝静脉可异位回流入右心房，肝肺之间发生纤维性融合也有报道。这些解剖学上的异常都会使得外科手术修补膈肌缺损变得异常的复杂[158,163]。

膈肌缺损通常的特征是在胸腹之间有一个完全开

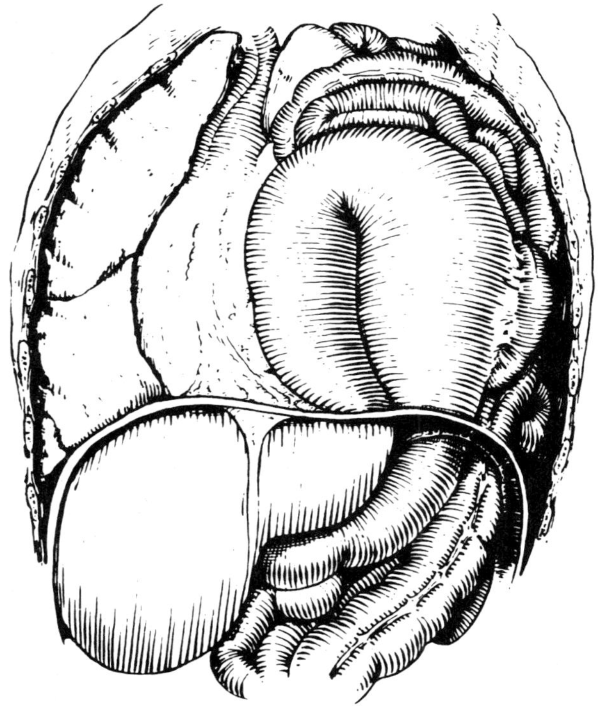

图 60–2 左侧先天性膈疝的图解，显示腹部内脏通过后外侧裂孔疝进入胸腔。（From Spitz L,Coran AG (eds): Rob & Smith's Pediatric Surgery. London, Chapman & Hall, 1996.）

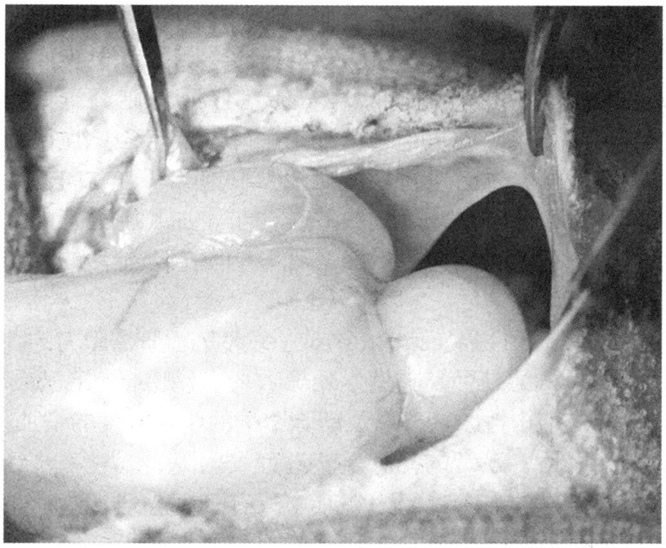

图 60–3 胎羊动物模型左侧先天性膈疝的术中照片。可以看到从腹腔进入胸腔的后外侧膈肌缺损。(From Spitz L, Coran AG (eds): Rob & Smith' s Pediatric Surgery.London, Chapman & Hall, 1996.)

放的空间，但是有些婴儿具有由壁层胸膜和腹膜构成疝囊。这可以用来区别膈膨升，膈膨升是由膈神经或者前角细胞变性所致。膈肌的肌纤维通常存在。

由 de Lorimier 和 Harrison 制作的一流的动物模型已经显示，腹腔内容物疝入胸腔长期压迫发育中的胎肺，可引起肺发育不良和肺发育不全[69,121]（图 60–3）。单侧的内脏疝入可同时影响同侧及对侧的肺发育，但是同侧肺的发育不全可能更为严重。在人类尸体解剖标本和动物模型中，通过分析肺的体积和重量可以证实这一点[10,69,121,235]。因为在先天性膈疝中，内脏疝出的过程发生在支气管细分的时候，因此就在这个时期肺的发育受到损害。在先天性膈疝的肺中，虽然所有主要的支气管芽都已经存在，但是在受累肺中支气管分支的数量极大地减小。这种发现同时出现在同侧以及对侧的肺标本中[10]。肺泡的发育严重受损，有报道称，在足月时，肺中只有很少的正常肺泡存在[234]。另外，气道结构的改变相当的多样化。在治疗期间需要低流量辅助机械通气的婴儿具有与对照组相同的气道肌肉层，而进行长时间机械通气支持的婴儿其整个气道都有显著的肌肉层增厚[44]。

在先天性膈疝患者的肺中，肺血管床存在明显的畸形。已经有报道称在同侧和对侧的肺实质中，动脉分支减少[170,187]。在结构上，先天性膈疝肺中，所有尺寸的肺动脉都存在动脉壁外层和中层的显著增厚，伴有小的腺泡前动脉和腺泡内动脉的异常肌化[26,216,325]。这种异常的动脉肌化的生理学结果，可能增加了发生固定的和难处理的肺动脉高压的易感性。在肺静脉结构上没有发现先天性膈疝所致的显著变化。在先天性膈疝婴儿中，已经发现有肺静脉外层的增厚，但这种增厚似乎是出生以后发生的，可能是由于治疗或者是继发于肺动脉高压的结果[206]。

在正常胎儿的发育期间，肺血流量只占心脏输出量的 7%，肺血管的阻力依然很高。胎儿通过卵圆孔和动脉导管优先分流来自胎盘的氧合血，以从右至左方向进入体循环中。出生时，新生儿发生了许多血流动力学的改变，极大地改变了这种胎儿循环模式。随着呼吸的开始，肺血管阻力下降，肺动脉的压力也随之下降，使肺血流量增加。体循环血管阻力和左心房压力上升，导致卵圆孔关闭。动脉血氧分压的增加可导致动脉导管的自然关闭。从胎儿循环到成人循环模式的转变就完成了。如果这个过程被打断，就可能发生持续胎儿循环。出生以后随着胎盘血循环支持的打断，肺血管阻力的持续升高可导致肺动脉压力的升高和肺血管血流量的减少。血管阻力的升高可导致在心房或动脉导管的水平发生右向左分流，未经氧饱和的血液进入体循环中。随着右向左分流中血流量的增加，体循环中的氧饱和度开始下降，混合静脉血回流到右心房，发生进行性的血液去氧饱和。当右向左分流增加时，随之产生的缺氧进一步增加了肺血管的阻力，减少了肺血流量。随之就可能发生进行性的重度呼吸衰竭。

在先天性膈疝肺中，造成持续性肺血管高阻力的因
936 素，被认为是受累肺发生的导致所有动脉横切面面积下降的结构性改变，以及动脉结构的肌化程度的增加。出生以后，正常的动脉重塑过程发生障碍，进一步维持了异常的血管高阻力，其中只有一部分通过治疗干预可能逆转[264]。另外，肺血管阻力的加剧可能是由已知的肺动脉高压的刺激因素所致，包括缺氧、酸中毒、低体温和应激[295]。多种前列腺素、白三烯、儿茶酚胺和肾素–血管紧张素系统水平的改变，提示这些物质是这个复杂过程的介质。现在，只能推测，先天性膈疝肺的异常血管结构对这些刺激是否存在夸大反应。

诊断

先天性膈疝的诊断经常是通过产前超声检查得出的，准确率为 40%～90%[188]。虽然已经报道的发现率存在较大的差别，但是发现先天性膈疝时的平均妊娠时间为 24 周，也有报道最早在妊娠第 11 周就可发现[105]。超声检查多用于常规的产科检查，或者是因为出现羊水过多而怀疑。有报道称 80%的先天性膈疝在妊娠中都可出现羊水过多[3]。羊水过多的机制被认为是由于胃疝入胸腔而出现胃食管连接处的纽结所导致的前肠梗阻。发现胃或者是充满液体的肠袢位于与胎儿心脏同一横断层面的胸腔,就可提示先天性膈疝的诊断（图 60–4A 和 B）。另外提示先天性膈疝的其他超声检查发现包括：在腹腔内缺乏胃的声影、在胸腔内出现肝脏或其他实质性内脏。因为胎儿的吞咽受到影响，所以胃可能较小。如果膈缺损位于右侧，肝脏就可填塞膈疝的位置，使诊断变得困难。有报道称，因为腹腔内脏器间歇性地疝出到胸腔内，所以先天性膈疝的诊断有可能会被遗漏[3]。其他诊断，例如食管闭锁和肺囊性畸形，也可能会引起对胎儿超声检查的误解。在进行胎儿超声检查时，关于胎儿呼吸的功能性信息，可以通过多普勒超声检查胎儿鼻孔处的羊水来获知。通过这个方法可以确定胎儿的潮气量 / 每分通气量，该指标与胎儿的预后有关[15]。

产前超声检查除了应用于产前诊断，也可以通过定量技术评估先天性膈疝胎儿肺发育不全的严重程度，有助于对结果的预测。三维估算胎肺的体积，计算右肺面积 / 胸腔面积的比例，计算肺 / 胸腔的圆周比例，这是与新生儿结果相关的三个不同的检测指标[17,218,250]。在胎儿肺和疝出的内脏做超声检查时会受到鉴别不良的声学对比、胎儿的位置和操作者的经验

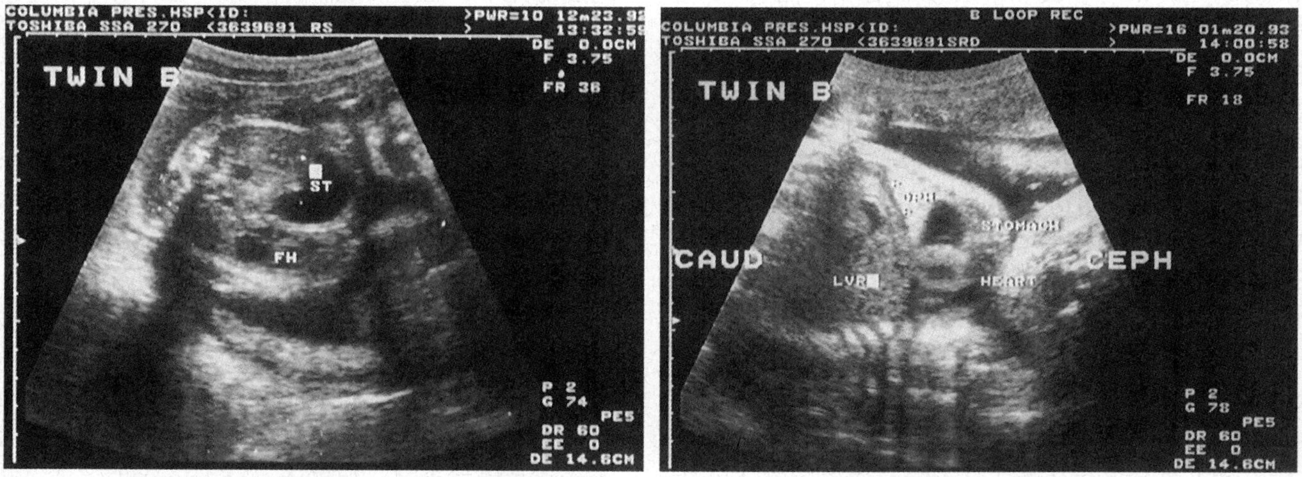

A　B

图 60–4　A. 一名妊娠 28 周的胎儿（双胞胎 B）的超声检查，横截面显示出胎儿的心脏（FH）和胃（ST）位于同一平面。B. 同一胎儿的超声检查，但是在矢状面显示出胃、肝脏和心脏的关系。

的限制。这样，当产科超声检查已经发现复杂的胎儿畸形时，应用产前核磁共振（MRI）检查的频率逐渐增多，这是适用于先天性膈疝胎儿的理想检查[142,186]。MRI 可以轻易地确定肝脏与横膈的相对位置，发现疝出的肝脏进入任何一侧的胸腔。MRI 也可以用于更加精确地评估肺体积，以便于确定肺发育不全的程度以及由此引发的相关结果[199,230,306]。

出生以后，先天性膈疝婴儿的呼吸系统症状取决于肺发育不全的程度和反应性的肺高压。尽管大部分
937 呼吸道症状出现在出生后最初的 24 小时内，但是最为严重的受累婴儿可在出生即刻便发生呼吸窘迫。这些婴儿有典型的舟状腹和胸部的不对称扩张。当吞咽的空气进入胃肠道时，胸部可能会变得更加扩张。胃肠道的扩张进一步压迫了肺实质，影响了肺实质的通气特性。这可能会导致纵隔压迫和对侧肺的损伤。因为新生儿胸部体积较小，在膈肌缺损侧可能或者不会听到呼吸音。纵隔压迫伴移位进入对侧胸腔，可能会导致气管偏离发生膈疝的一侧，也可能会导致静脉回流的梗阻和低血压，以及外周灌注不足的血流动力学结果。呼吸窘迫的体征可包括发绀、喘息、胸骨凹陷和呼吸运动障碍。

先天性膈疝的诊断可以通过胸部平片来证实，可以显示胸腔内有肠袢的存在。也应该注意观察胃泡，胃泡的位置可以通过放置胃管来证实。少数情况下需要进行上消化道造影。胸部平片可显示纵隔成角和心脏轮廓偏移到对侧胸腔。虽然可能会发现同侧极少量的肺实质充气，但是胸部平片对于肺发育不全程度的估计是不可靠的[52,140]。

一旦先天性膈疝的诊断得到证实，就应该进行其他影像学和超声检查以寻找合并的畸形。超声心动图和肾脏以及头颅超声检查都应该进行。

虽然大多数的先天性膈疝发生在出生后最初的 24 小时内，但是有 10%～20%的膈疝患者出现症状的时间较晚[201]。这些晚期发生的膈疝婴儿可表现为反复发作的轻度呼吸道疾病、慢性肺病、肺炎、渗出、脓胸、或者胃扭结。

鉴别诊断

先天性膈疝的诊断可能会与其他许多先天性胸部疾病相混淆，包括膈膨升、Morgagni 前膈疝、先天性食管裂孔疝、先天性肺囊性疾病、原发性肺发育不全。膈膨升有许多病因，但可见于有产伤或者 Werdnig-Hoffmann 病的新生儿中。膈膨升中的横膈可以抬高至第三肋间隙的高度，具有与先天性膈疝一样的生理结果。它也可以完全没有症状。膈膨升可以通过荧光透视或者实时超声检查来显示膈肌的矛盾运动。MRI 也可用于确定膈肌的结构。Morgagni 疝发生在乳内动脉的裂缝，远不如 Bochdalek 疝常见。受累婴儿可表现为胃肠道危象，可因为结肠或者小肠的钳闭或者扭转而需要即刻进行手术治疗。

预后因素

寻找临床上相关的确定预后的因素以预测先天性膈疝婴儿的结果，这是一个非常复杂且相互矛盾的过程，因为绝大部分的努力都没有取得成功。许多的研究试图检测与存活相关的解剖学及生理参数，但是由于新的治疗方法不断进展，每一个研究都局限于回顾性分析。考虑到多个因素都可能会影响到人们对先天性膈疝婴儿存活潜力的临床印象，这样的一种印象不可能来自于一个单独的测定。

解剖学因素

随着产前超声检查使用的增多，进行子宫内先天性膈疝诊断的能力确定，研究显示在妊娠 24 周以前的产前检查诊断出的先天性膈疝的死亡率较高。其他研究也显示：不论产前诊断的时间，单纯的先天性膈疝没有其他相关畸形并不是预测结果的一个指标[317]。先天性膈疝合并其他显著畸形时预后仍然不良。如果先天性膈疝并不是通过产前超声检查发现的，而是在出生后检查得出诊断的，那么存活率就可能非常好。也有报道称出现羊水增多则可能提示预后不良[119]。然而，许多的研究反驳了这种观点，提出羊水增多的出现对先天性膈疝婴儿的最终结果并没有预测价值[61,261,278]。

许多研究者提出胃的位置可以作为一项预后指标。有报道称在得出诊断时胃的位置完全位于膈肌下方时，先天性膈疝婴儿的存活率可高达 100%，但是当胃疝出并进入胸腔时的存活率只有 30%[45,61,123]。其他研究显示胃的位置没有预测预后的价值[289]。膈肌缺

损发生的部位可能在某种程度上对结果有预测意义。有报道称右侧膈疝的患儿比左侧膈疝的预后要更差[106,291]。近期的一个研究报道两侧膈疝在结果方面没有差别[129]。然而，右侧的膈肌缺损在新生儿期可能不会那么明显，而在随后的年龄增长期间可能会表现出非常轻微的呼吸道症状[64]。

似乎具有预测相关性的产前解剖学参数是肺和头比例（LHR）的测定。在同时进行肺脏和头部超声检查的时候检测肺和头比例，肺和头比例小于 1.0 与预后不良有关[164,183,192]。肺和头比例与结果的相关性并不依赖于妊娠时间。并不是所有的围生期人群都发现肺和头比例对临床诊断有用[133]。

心肺结构的分析包括产前或者产后心室和大血管的直径，以及在产后功能方面的检测，这也可能是重
938 要的决定预后的指标[61,124]。已经报道了许多指数，包括心室指数（左心室 / 右心室）、心血管指数（Ao/PA）和改良的 McGoon 指数（肺门动脉结合直径 / 降主动脉的指数）的计算[282,287]。改良的 McGoon 指数小于或者等于 1.3 时，预测死亡率有 85%的敏感性，100%的特异性。左心室肿块的分析结合同时测定的心室短轴缩短分数也已经用于预测结果，指数为 1.2 时预测存活率为 0[273]。无论在子宫内或者出生后这些测量都难以进行，而且主要依赖于研究者。另外，在先天性膈疝的新生儿中，没有一项测定结果可以给出足够的信息来完全评估心肺的状态[288]。

生理学参数

不幸的是，在评估新生儿肺功能的时候，除了 PO_2、PCO_2 和 pH 外，很少有生理学参数可以使用。因此，动脉血气分析已经成为建立临床预测标准的基础。早期研究显示，存活儿和非存活儿的 pH 和 PCO_2 对当时可采用的治疗措施的反应存在差别[30,209]。PCO_2 较低、PO_2 最初正常或者通过机械通气可以改善的患儿的结果良好，而那些 PCO_2 水平较高，对机械通气无反应的患儿则预后不良。这些作者提出了同时检测动脉导管前后血气的重要性，可用于评估左向右分流的程度。

自从这些最初的报道出现以后，研究者们获得了许多公式，采用不同的血气成分来预测结果。最为基本的概念是肺泡-动脉血氧分压差（$AadO_2$）。它通过以下公式来进行计算：

$$AadO_2 = [(713 \times FiO_2 - PaCO_2)/0.8] - PaO_2$$

虽然肺泡-动脉血氧分压差刚开始用于确定体外膜肺氧合（ECMO）的准入标准，但是它的应用已经为其他指数的发展所取代。采用血气分析和 PCO_2 水平结合通气的数据，就可以确定参数以预测采用传统的通气技术治疗的先天性膈疝婴儿的结果。为此，需要计算通气指数（VI）：

$$VI = (RR \times MAP \times PaCO_2)$$

当 PCO_2 水平能够减少到小于 40mmHg，并且通气指数小于 1000 的时候，所有的患儿都可以存活。改良的通气指数（MVI）是通过采用峰值吸气压（PIP）而不是平均气道压力（MAP）来计算：

$$MVI = (RR \times PIP \times PaCO_2) \div 1000$$

在改良通气指数小于 40 的婴儿中，采用传统治疗的存活率为 96%。如果改良通气指数大于 80，则所有的婴儿都会死亡[225]。

最常用的计算公式是氧合指数（OI）。它通过以下公式计算：

$$OI = (MAP \times FiO_2 / PaO_2)$$

采用传统的通气治疗，氧合指数小于 0.06 时先天性膈疝患儿的存活率为 98%，而氧合指数大于 0.175 时则存活率为 0[225]。这些因素的预测能力，在采用一些治疗措施例如：体外膜肺氧合（ECMO）、高频振荡通气（HFO）、表面活性物质和一氧化氮（NO）时，还没有得到确定。

肺功能测试

有报道称对术前和术后肺功能测试的分析，在鉴定婴儿可能需要 ECMO 治疗以及确定存活者方面，具有预测的价值。针对先天性膈疝婴儿呼吸功能的初期研究揭示了手术修补损伤了肺的顺应性，因而支持了医疗稳定和延迟进行手术治疗的假说[219,252]。适时采用延迟手术修补和 ECMO 的治疗策略，当患儿初始的术前肺顺应性大于每公斤 0.25ml/cmH_2O 而初始潮气量大于 3.5ml /kg 时，就不要进行 ECMO 治疗。膈

疝修补术后潮气量为 4ml /kg 时存活率得到改善[292]。

研究显示术前测定功能性残气量可以预测致死性肺发育不全[8]。另外，已经发现针对全肺顺应性的一系列测定有助于高风险婴儿的结果预测[159]。

虽然在治疗先天性膈疝的婴儿时，没有单独的某个参数被证实足以作为决定预后的因素，但是近期的多中心研究显示重要的总死亡率的非依赖性预测指标包括：产前诊断、出生体重、较低的 1 分钟和 5 分钟 Apgar 评分和右侧膈疝。

治疗

1929 年 Greenwald 和 Steiner[111]写道“对于这个出生时就出现膈疝的患者，从外科的角度很少甚至没有可以做的事情。”但是从那时起先天性膈疝的治疗成功率就已得到显著提高。虽然对于总体的存活率难以获得一致性的效果，但当时许多创新的治疗策略都得到了应用。

产前治疗

通过产前超声检查的使用，得出先天性膈疝诊断的频率正在不断增加。在胎儿大小和妊娠时间发生差异的时候，就要开始进行产前超声检查。产前诊断先天性膈疝时应该要仔细寻找其他先天性畸形，尤其是
939 那些影响到心血管和神经系统的畸形。胎儿染色体组型的检测，应该通过羊膜穿刺或者绒膜绒毛或胎儿血采样完成。目前标准的治疗是支持胎儿和母亲，保证尽可能接近足月时才进行分娩。产前诊断的优势在于能够进行适当的准备，通知父母亲可能进行的治疗和结果。胎儿和母亲应该到适当的第 III 期的围生期医学中心就诊，那儿随时都有成套的呼吸治疗策略备用，包括 NO、高频振荡通气和 ECMO。任何的不足都有可能影响到可能的最佳结果[262]。除非发生了产科问题自发的经阴道分娩是首选方式。仅有先天性膈疝的诊断并不是选择性剖宫产的手术指征。

在这个时候，试图在子宫内纠正膈肌缺损的胚胎干预只是研究性和高度实验性的。近期对于先天性膈疝胎儿进行胎儿气管堵塞以促进产前胎肺生长的试验已经被放弃，因为没有研究显示采用这种技术治疗的患儿的存活率比同期的传统治疗有更好的效果[73,98,122,123]。气管堵塞可导致肺的增大，但是没有逆转肺发育不全的相关病理过程。如在结果部分中所讨论的，单纯性先天性膈疝的预后并不是普遍所认为的前景黯淡，因此对于危害母亲和胎儿的基本原则首先就可能需要进行再次评估。

虽然在未成熟的婴儿中，产前应用皮质类固醇可以提高肺的发育，但是在先天性膈疝婴儿中产前皮质类固醇治疗的作用还不能确定。在发育不全的肺中，这些治疗的原理是诱导发育不良肺的成熟，这是建立在动物实验研究和孤立的病例报道的基础之上[100,161,200]。反对这些观点的是不断有早产儿研究报道显示，这些药物也可能会有围生期和长期的不良作用[160,270]。在改善先天性膈疝预后中，这种治疗潜在的真正意义有待于随机化前瞻性研究的结果。

术前治疗

复苏

婴儿出生以后，一旦先天性膈疝的诊断得到证实，所有的努力都应该是稳定心肺系统，减少因治疗干预而产生的医源性损伤。重要的是要考虑到先天性膈疝是一种生理学急症，而不是一种外科急症。新生儿先天性膈疝呈现的呼吸窘迫，是由于前面所讨论的两种因素联合作用所导致的：不可纠正的肺发育不全和潜在可逆性的肺高压。这两种因素之间的平衡决定了对治疗的反应和最终的结果。在临床上，两者都表现为肺血管阻力的增加、肺动脉压力的增高、动脉导管和卵圆孔水平右向左分流以及进展性的低氧血症。因为此时还没有证实可以促进肺生长的治疗，所以治疗干预的目的在于控制肺血管的张力。

复苏从气管内插管和置入鼻胃管开始。为了避免可能位于胸腔内的胃和小肠的扩张，禁用面罩通气和急救袋。通过脐血管获得动脉和静脉的通路。如果脐静脉导管能够经过肝脏进入右心房，它就可以用于监测中心静脉压力，同时可以获得混合静脉血气的采样。虽然脐动脉可以很好地监测体循环的血压，获得动脉导管后动脉血气的标本，但是在动脉导管前的位置通过右侧桡动脉插管或是经皮氧饱和度探头就可以监测动脉氧饱和度来获得其他信息。治疗工作步骤中

一个重要的部分就是评估婴儿是否有足够的肺容量来进行有意义的气体交换。重要的是要在婴儿及其家庭实施治疗策略以前考虑到这个事实。

同任何新生儿复苏一样，必须要注意维持适当的温度调节、葡萄糖的稳态、新生儿的体液状态以维持足够的氧输送。任何应激刺激都可以恶化已经升高的肺动脉压力，导致血液分流的增加和全身氧饱和度的进一步下降。应适当的给予婴儿镇静剂和任何混合制剂，包括咪达唑仑、芬太尼或者吗啡。肌肉麻痹的结果是非常令人气馁的，因为它可造成通气机制的不良后果和潜在的并发症。对机械通气治疗不"耐受"的婴儿，一般需要注意他们的不适，而不是肌肉麻痹。可能会发现低血压和组织灌注不足，可以通过静脉补液来逆转，包括晶体液、血制品和胶体液。可能会需要强心剂类药物，例如多巴胺或者多巴酚丁胺。

代谢性酸碱平衡紊乱通常与组织灌注不足有关，可以通过补液或者应用重碳酸盐来纠正。如果能够进行适当的机械通气管理，代谢性酸中毒就可以通过应用重碳酸盐来纠正。重度的血碳酸过多症（PCO_2＞70mmHg）就应该通过改变通气治疗策略来纠正。

机械通气

先天性膈疝婴儿所需要的机械通气的类型，由个人或医院的喜好所决定。大多数婴儿通过简单的压力循环模式就可以成功地进行机械通气管理，采用的模式为高频通气（呼吸 100 次 / 分钟）和适度的峰值气道压力（8～22cmH_2O 和非呼气末正压[PEEP]）模式，或者是低频通气（呼吸 20～40 次 / 分钟）和较高的气道压力（22～35cmH_2O 和 3～5cmPEEP）模式。这种通气支持的目的是维持每分钟通气达到动脉导管前 PO_2 大于 60mmHg（Sao_2 90%～100%），而相
940 应的 PCO_2 小于 60mmHg。已经显示 pH 和 PCO_2 的水平在调节肺血管张力中具有重要作用[251]。在治疗有持续性肺动脉高压的新生儿时，临床上成功地处理这些参数就是一种初始的治疗策略[86]。然而，现在已经明确，应该要避免极度的强力呼吸以及由此产生的呼吸性碱中毒，因为这样的治疗加上肺部原有疾病便可产生严重的医源性损伤[162]。呼吸治疗的策略是基于允许的高碳酸血症和自主呼吸，已经证实该策略是非常成功的[31]。如果传统的机械通气技术不能够逆转低氧血症或者高碳酸血症，就可能需要采用高频振荡通气技术。在重度呼吸窘迫婴儿中，这种技术可以有效地去除二氧化碳且暂时稳定婴儿的状态。当这种技术用作初始的治疗时，存活率相当不错[25]。

药物治疗

对先天性膈疝和呼吸衰竭的婴儿，已经应用广谱抗生素和抗高血压药物以调节肺血管的阻力。已经从新生儿持续性肺动脉高压（PPHN）和其他类型的新生儿呼吸衰竭的婴幼儿临床试验中获得了经验。

过去，面对低氧血症和呼吸衰竭的时候，一些药物，例如妥拉唑啉，通过阻断 α 受体发挥作用，被用来降低肺血管的阻力[236,271]。它在先天性膈疝婴儿中的功效不是主要的。其他药物，例如硝普盐、异丙肾上腺素、硝酸甘油和卡托普利，并不是有效药物[38]。应用不同的前列腺素衍生物，包括前列腺素 D_2（PGD_2）、前列腺素 E_1（PGE_1）和前列腺环素、环氧化酶抑制剂吲哚美辛，治疗效果也都令人失望[198,293]。

至于治疗持续性肺动脉高压的治疗新策略，现在正在进行临床评估，包括各种钙离子通道阻滞剂、前列腺环素衍生物、内皮受体拮抗剂、磷酸二酯酶-5阻滞剂，例如西地那非[92,240]。

表面活性物质

动物模型已经显示，实验诱导的先天性膈疝肺缺乏表面活性物质，但是这些结果并没有在人类研究中得到重复。先天性膈疝婴儿的早期报道显示表面活性物质的水平和成分发生了改变[277,314]。然而，近期的研究已经表明，先天性膈疝婴儿的表面活性物质池与对照组患儿没有差别，甚至与需要 ECMO 支持的婴幼儿也没有差别[54,147,151]。可能在个别成分的合成和代谢动力学方面存在区别[53]。在改善呼吸功能和结果方面，应用表面活性物质的临床和实验研究已经在同步进行[32,108,195,256]。一项先天性膈疝患儿应用表面活性物质的多中心回顾分析表明，它的应用并不是全部都有效，相对于足月儿来说，早产儿显示出较低的存活率[178]。此时，在先天性膈疝婴儿的治疗中，没有临床数据支持应该应用表面活性物质。

一氧化氮

一氧化氮是一种有效的血管舒张调节剂，最初被认为是血管内皮源性舒张因子[145,289]。因为一氧化氮是一种高度扩散性的气体，通过结合血红蛋白而快速失活，所以它尤其适合于使用机械通气技术支持下的肺血管。在临床研究中，一氧化氮的作用是提高 PPHN 所致的呼吸衰竭新生儿的氧饱和度[169,249]。在 PPHN 的动物模型中，一氧化氮降低了肺动脉的压力，增加了动脉氧饱和度，没有出现明显的副作用[103]。不幸的是，它在先天性膈疝合并呼吸衰竭的婴儿中的作用是复杂的[1,80,91,157,167]。没有数据表明应用一氧化氮可提高存活率或者降低对 ECMO的需求[97]。在这些婴儿中对一氧化氮不同的生理反应可能与应用的方法有关[155]。通过鼻导管使用一氧化氮已经应用于拔管后的肺动脉高压的晚期治疗[168]。尽管一氧化氮已经得到了广泛应用，但是在先天性膈疝婴儿中，一氧化氮在治疗肺动脉高压和呼吸衰竭中的确切作用还没有被证实。

手术治疗

手术修补的时机

在历史上，先天性膈疝被认为是一种外科急症。婴儿在出生以后立即被送到手术室进行手术，因为坚信还纳胸腔内的腹部内容物可以减轻对肺的压迫。而经常发生的情况是，短暂的术后蜜月期期间有足够的气体交换，紧接着婴儿的呼吸状态出现进行性恶化，表现为肺血管阻力升高、右向左分流增加、低氧血症和最终由于呼吸衰竭而死亡。

随着新生儿呼吸衰竭治疗技术的发展，学者们提出进行一段时间的内科稳定治疗和延迟手术修补的技术以改善先天性膈疝婴儿的总体情况[26,181]。与此同时，早期手术修补对呼吸功能存在潜在危害的证据不断增多[252]。从此以后，多个单独研究报道了将延迟手术修补作为他们治疗方案的一部分，先天性膈疝婴儿的生存率得到提高，而其他研究者发现总体的结果并没有发生改变*。重要的是，没有研究显示使用这种技术后，先天性膈疝婴儿的存活率下降。虽然延迟手术修补现在已经被广泛的应用，但是直到目前，还是没有统计学的证据来支持这种延迟手术修补技术而不是即刻进行手术[214]。 941

应用延迟手术修补时，手术修补的最佳时机还没有得到确定。术前稳定的时间从数天到数周不等[40,224,240,323]。一些学者报道手术时机要等到婴儿成功地脱离机械呼吸机的支持，只需要较低的通气设定时。而其他学者则根据，肺动脉高压和的一系列心动超声检查的严重程度，等到肺动脉高压得以减轻或者至少稳定以后才进行手术[81,126]。

手术修补

虽然也可以通过胸廓切口来进行膈疝修补手术，但是大多数外科医生通过肋缘下切口来暴露膈肌缺损。对于因为肝或者脾的异常形状而使疝内容物复位困难的罕见病例，可能会采用胸腹联合切口。胸腔镜和胸腔镜手术技术都已经应用于这些缺损的修补手术[21,173,228,245,259,324]。微创技术非常适合于有迟发性表现的年龄较大的婴幼儿，而在新生儿中使用微创技术出现技术性和生理性后果的发生率可能更高[9]。

分开腹壁肌层并进入到腹腔以后，轻柔的将从缺损处疝出的内脏复位，并将内脏拖出切口以获得足够清楚的视野。位于左侧的脾脏和位于右侧的肝脏通常是最后需要从胸腔内搬出的器官（图 60-5A 和 B）。搬动器官可能是困难的，操作时不要损伤任何一个器官。在右侧，肾脏和肾上腺也可能位于胸腔内。任何 942
一侧的肝静脉异常回流都使得肝脏的搬动变得复杂。

一旦腹腔内容物复位以后，就能够看到后外侧的膈肌缺损。在 20% 的病例中，存在由胸膜壁层和腹膜形成的疝囊，必须给予切除以减少复发的机会[237]。通常会有大小不一的膈肌前缘。必须在腹膜后的组织中寻找膈肌的后缘，因为它可能被腹膜卷起成窗户的形状。必须在这个腹膜折叠处打开腹膜，游离膈肌组织。当组织足够时，采用不可吸收缝线间断缝合进行一期手术修补膈疝缺损（见图 60-5C）。在一些病例中，沿着侧胸膜的膈肌后缘可能消失。如果前方有足够的膈肌组织时，就可以直接缝合到体壁，围绕肋骨缝合。

如果膈肌缺损太大而不能进行一期关闭的话，就可以利用各种邻近结构进行重建，例如肾前筋膜、肋骨、各种胸壁和腹壁的肌瓣[22,139,255,266,304,310]。然而，在

---

* 见参考文献 6,31,40,48,101,109,127,224,241,246,260,313 和 320。

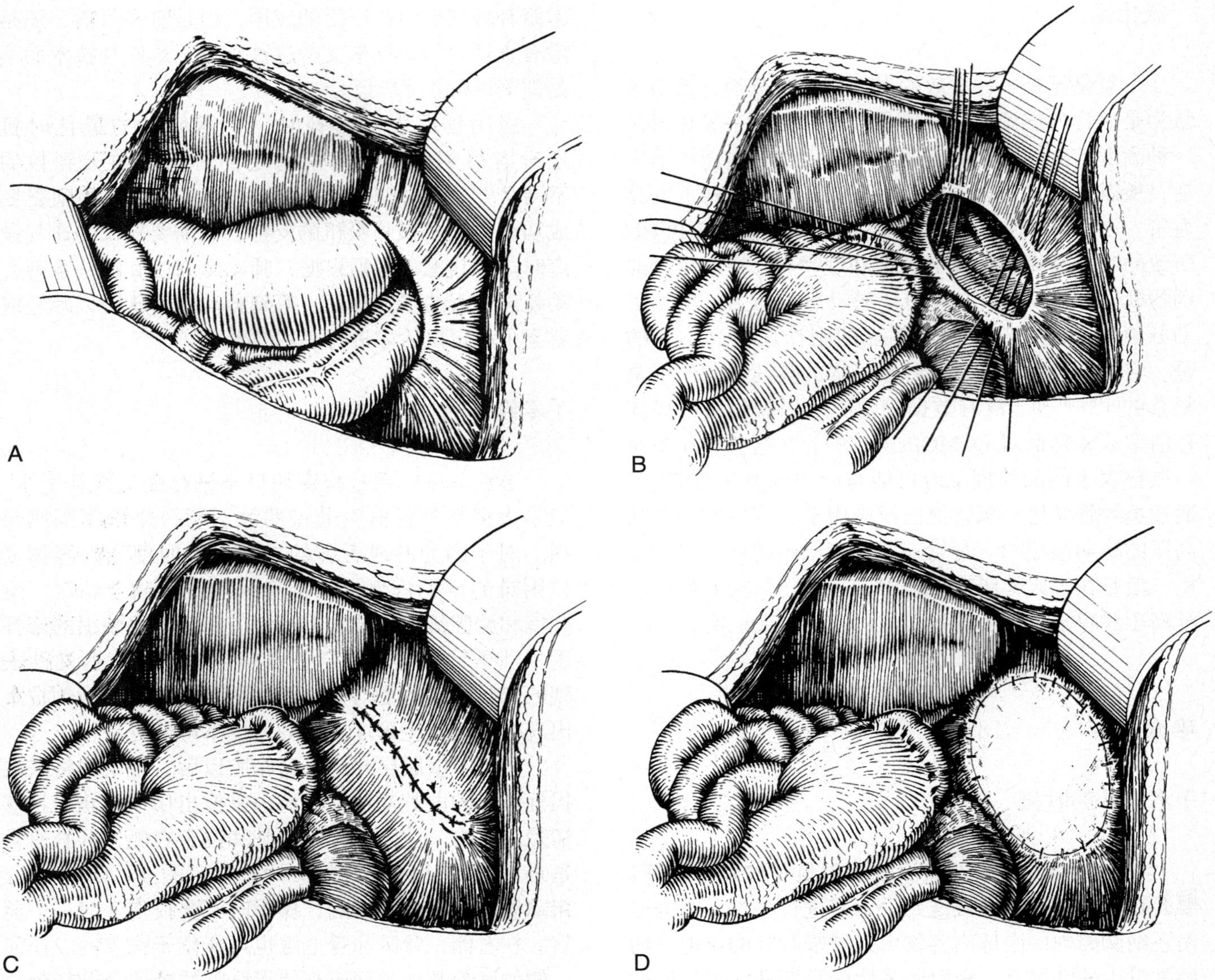

图 60-5　A. 未经复位的左侧先天性膈疝，从腹腔观察的示意图。B. 同一个膈疝患儿复位以后，显示脾脏通常是最后从胸腔回纳的器官。放置缝线以便进行一期修补。C. 左侧先天性膈疝一期完全修补以后。D. 采用假体材料修补以后的左侧先天性膈疝。

先天性膈疝婴儿的治疗中，如果需要 ECMO 支持的可能存在，则需要广泛组织分离的复杂的重建技术是一种禁忌证，因为存在出血的风险。使用假体材料以完成膈肌的关闭已经得到了广泛的认同（见图 60-5D）。它可以完成松软的没有张力的膈肌修补，减少关闭腹壁时腹腔内压力的程度[19]。除了感染的风险，应用假体材料关闭膈肌缺损的主要缺点是假体材料的移动以及膈疝复发的风险[11]。在接近 10%至几乎 50%的病例中，都可发生假体补片修补膈疝的并发症。膈疝复发的患儿，可表现为小肠梗阻或是呼吸窘迫或者可能没有症状[68,213]。

由于腹腔内空间减小，即使在广泛的腹壁伸展之后，腹壁关闭可能根本无法进行，或者可能会导致不可接受的腹腔内压力（即发生腹腔间隔综合征）。在这些情况下，可实行单纯的皮肤关闭并在数月后完成腹壁缺损修补手术。如果不能成功的关闭皮肤，就可采用假体材料，例如 silo，进行暂时性的关闭。术后，一旦可以安全地进行手术，就应该进行生物学上的关闭。并不建议在膈疝修补手术一侧的胸腔行胸廓置管引流，除非有活动性的出血或者是不可控制的空气泄漏。已经有学者提出，在发育不全的肺中进行机械通气时，利用这样一根引流管，甚至采用低负压吸引，都可能增加气压性创伤和肺高压[323]。在手术修补时，并不建议进行额外的手术步骤，例如纠正肠旋转不良以及阑尾切除术，如果考虑行 ECMO 时都应该避免这些额外手术。

复发性膈疝的修补呈现为一个令人敬畏的手术挑战。由于复发性膈疝所涉及的最为常见的器官是小肠或结肠，肠道黏附到破裂的膈肌或是胸腔内的器官上，可能会影响到关闭手术。修补手术最为常见的是通过腹部切口完成，但也可以通过胸廓切口来完成。如果有足够的膈肌组织，就应该尝试进行一期的缝合。另外，可以试用网孔置入等多种不同的技术[68,248,254]。

麻醉

在送往手术室的途中，为了避免转运时应激反应和机械通气参数的突然改变，一些医学中心已经采用在新生儿重症监护病房中对先天性膈疝婴儿进行手术修补的策略。这种手术地点的改变可以最大限度地降低对新生儿环境的干扰。通过静脉内应用镇静剂和肌松剂进行麻醉。采用静脉内麻醉以后，就可以持续使用婴儿呼吸机，而不是传统的麻醉机。

术后管理

术后管理应该继续术前制定的倾向和目标。通气支持应该用以保持动脉导管前 PO_2 水平至少大于 80mmHg，PCO_2 水平小于 30～35mmHg。应该常规进行心动超声检查，评估肺动脉高压、血液分流流速和左心室的功能。如果发生呼吸失代偿，就可能会用到以前所讨论的治疗干预措施。应该缓慢小心地脱离呼吸机的支持，当婴儿呼吸耐受以后，就做好准备脱离呼吸机支持。

必须注意保持体液平衡，尤其是在术后的一小段时间内。作为手术修补的结果，这些婴儿经常会出现血容量的降低，而需要额外补充液体。

体外膜肺氧合（ECMO）

即使采用最先进的治疗策略，在先天性膈疝婴儿中，需要 ECMO 支持的无法抵抗的呼吸衰竭的发生率为 15%～45%[14,57,81,241]。最初，急诊行膈疝缺损的手术修补术后，婴儿发生呼吸衰竭需要进行 ECMO 支持。随着延迟手术修补技术的发展，现在考虑把 ECMO 作为术前稳定支持治疗的一个部分。

确定在先天性膈疝婴儿中使用 ECMO 的临床标准是，基于预测机械通气至少有 80%的死亡率等一些因素。已经有学者提出了许多参数，包括氧合指数（OI）和肺泡-动脉血氧分压差[$(A-a)DO_2$]的计算。对于先天性膈疝患儿，开始行 ECMO 支持 943
的最为常见的原因是氧合指数大于等于 40，氧合指数低至 25 时也经常考虑 ECMO 支持[57]。基于[$(A-a)$ DO_2]标准的新生儿呼吸衰竭，开始进行 ECMO 支持的通常接受的标准为：尽管进行了 8 个小时最大限度的内科治疗，但是数值仍然大于等于 610。必须要认识到这些标准仍然是学院特异性的，而且没有哪项计算能够替代临床判断和定期的床边评估。尽管进行了最大限度的内科治疗，重度肺动脉高压和进行性低氧血症的患儿病情不能获得改善，仍然是进行 ECMO 支持治疗的有效的应用标准。

至于是否所有的先天性膈疝和呼吸衰竭婴儿都应该应用 ECMO 支持治疗仍然存在争论。当考虑进行 ECMO 支持的时候，必须要记住，重度肺发育不全与生命不相容的问题。当采用措施支持婴儿可使肺动脉高压逆转时，这种治疗就获得成功。然而，这种治疗并不是针对那些患有不可逆的肺发育不全的婴儿。根据临床指标来鉴别这些婴儿可能相当的困难。先天性膈疝的新生儿，其动脉导管前氧饱和度不能达到90%，或者是有显著升高的 PCO_2 水平，在进行 ECMO 支持以前对任何一种类型的机械通气治疗都没有反应，那么他就很有可能存在不可逆的肺发育不全。另一方面，其他学者提出，所有的婴儿都应该是 ECMO 支持的候选者。

虽然 ECMO 作为先天性膈疝伴呼吸衰竭的一种治疗措施而得到广泛的接受，但是 ECMO 对改善总体存活率的效果一直存在争论。在过去的十年间，许多研究显示采用 ECMO 支持作为治疗策略的一部分以后，先天性膈疝婴儿的存活率得到了提高[57,101,302]。然而，其他研究或者没有发现 ECMO 导致的任何存活率的提高，或者是一些不用 ECMO治疗的患儿同样可以获得成功[6,25,165]。采用ECMO治疗的婴儿总体存活率为34%～87%不等，明显依赖于许多变量，包括妊娠时间和出生体重、呼吸功能、肺发育以及相关的肺动脉高压的程度[81,90,165,185,276]。由于传统的治疗策略在持续改善，ECMO的应用以及伴随的存活率可能会下降[14]。

对先天性膈疝的婴儿进行ECMO治疗时会涉及许多外科问题。已经有报道称，在进行体外循环支持时，静脉-静脉通路和静脉-动脉通路技术同样的有效[82,174]。应用静脉-静脉通路技术时，重度的右侧心力衰竭可以通过临时灌注PGE_1，保持动脉导管的开放，直到肺动脉高压得到解决，或者是转换到静脉-动脉通路进行体外循环支持。与ECMO支持相关的外科修补先天性膈疝缺损的时机还没有确定。作为一种治疗策略，接受延迟手术修补的结果是，有超过90%的需要ECMO支持的先天性膈疝婴儿，在进行手术修补之前就先进行了体外循环支持[180]。在有ECMO支持时就可以完成膈疝的手术修补，但是在60%的患儿中可能会出现出血的并发症[179,301]。ECMO支持的手术后的存活率从43%～80%不等[58,313,316]。为了减少出血并发症的风险，已经提出了多种技术，包括包被肝素的ECMO导管的应用，就在预期拔管前进行手术修补，积极处理婴儿的抗凝状态，还包括抗纤维蛋白溶解治疗的应用。因为血液凝固的问题，只有不到20%的患儿在ECMO支持下进行修补手术[51]。大多数病例是在结束ECMO支持以后才进行修补手术的。有时候要在ECMO拔管数天以后才进行修补手术，这种延迟手术的办法非常成功，存活率几乎可以达到80%或者更高[1,81,265]。然而，目前还没有比较这两种方法的研究。

结果

对于单纯性先天性膈疝婴儿的存活率（出院回家），与历史上接近50%的数值相比，在过去的十年内得到了显著提高[3,116,185,261,319]。采用目前的治疗策略后，膈疝患儿的存活率可高达80%～93%[7,31,85,182,305]。不过，膈疝患儿的存活率变化仍然较大，在治疗策略和患儿的受益中表现出具有显著的医院之间的差别[14,275]。大多数研究的更为复杂的解释是呼吸监护和内科治疗策略的不断进展。另外，合并畸形的出现，例如先天性心脏病，在这些婴儿中还是提示不良预后的一个显著的高危因素[55,154,267]。随着总体存活率的提高，一大部分有生理损伤的婴儿都活过了新生儿时期，有报道称，初期存活的患儿中有接近10%的患儿在后期死亡了，大多数是由于持续性肺动脉高压或者是医源性的并发症所致[150,248,257]。

在ECMO和新的治疗策略得到广泛应用以前，据报道传统机械通气的长期存活儿健康状态良好，临床上没有明显的呼吸系统疾病。研究显示，先天性膈疝的存活儿可能处于许多长期的病态风险之中，例如慢性肺病、生长迟缓、神经系统发育迟滞、胃肠道和整形外科的问题。呼吸、营养和骨骼肌系统发病的可能性，在采用ECMO支持的先天性膈疝婴儿中会更高[50]。

到目前为止，在活过了新生儿时期的膈疝患儿中，肺的问题是最为常见的远期问题。肺发育的研究显示，肺泡的繁殖在出生以后会持续数年。然而，在先天性膈疝患儿中，发育不全的肺永远达不到一个正常的数值。随着时间的流逝，肺泡变得气肿，肺床逐 944
渐进行重构[20]。气肿性改变可能会影响到双侧的肺野，因为对侧肺可经纵隔疝出。研究表明，即使新生儿时期有重度呼吸窘迫的婴儿，肺的体积也会随着时间而增加。然而，肺血流与对侧相比仍然是显著的下降，这表明在重症病例中，肺血管的生长并不与肺泡的生长相匹配[217]。肺功能试验对长期存活儿是最为有用的检测指标，因为胸部平片和通气灌注研究几乎总是异常的，因此很少影响到治疗。虽然许多婴儿在其病程早期就可以显示出肺顺应性下降，但是随着时间的过去，伴随着真正的肺生长，一系列肺功能试验显示肺的顺应性会得到改善[172]。在存活儿的长期研究中，许多存活儿有正常的肺功能试验，甚至是运动试验[202,215,300,322]。在30%～50%的存活儿中，可能会有梗阻性或限制性通气损伤[215,242,300]。也有学者发现支气管高反应性的增加[146,269]。对于这些患者的治疗策略包括应用吸氧、支气管扩张治疗、皮质类固醇和利尿剂。

临床上，在先天性膈疝存活儿中有慢性肺病的报道，尤其是在那些需要ECMO支持的患儿中[63,196,215]。这些发现是否与该病的病理基础有关，或者是否与由于通气技术所致的医源性因素有关，目前还不清楚[253]。无论如何，不论是肺发育不全还是支气管肺发育不全所致的长时间肺动脉压升高，都会影响长期的存活率。到 3 周龄时，在所有患儿中有接近 50%的病例肺动脉压力是正常的，但是仍然有 1/3 的存活儿肺动脉高压会持续数月时间[81,148,258]。随着时间的过去，这种状态会得到改善，大多数的存活儿可以不受影响地生活[172,196]。

研究表明，神经系统发育异常的肺健全的先天性膈疝存活儿最为常见。有报道称，许多存活的婴儿呈现生长发育迟缓[196]。在运动和认知能力方面都有异常[63,279]。其他神经系统障碍包括视力障碍、听力丧失、癫痫、异常的头颅 CT 和 MRI 改变，以及异常的脑电图改变。大多数的研究表明，在这些神经系统疾病中 ECMO 是一个发病因素，但是没有进行 ECMO 支持治疗的先天性膈疝存活儿也处于神经系统疾病的风险之中[5,33,204,239]。

胃食管反流和前肠蠕动障碍的较高的发生率可见于先天性膈疝的存活儿中（图 60–6）[63,93,196,281,299]。大多数婴儿通过改变喂养方式和促肠胃蠕动药物来治疗。抗反流手术适用于内科治疗无效的患儿，或者是那些需要放置胃造口导管以便于喂养的患儿。在这些存活儿中，绝大多数患儿都存在营养和生长发育相关的问题[20]。对于这些婴儿，需要进行长期的监督和积极的营养治疗。令人不安的无对照报告描述了 Barrett 食管炎和继发于慢性胃食管反流的慢性肺病。

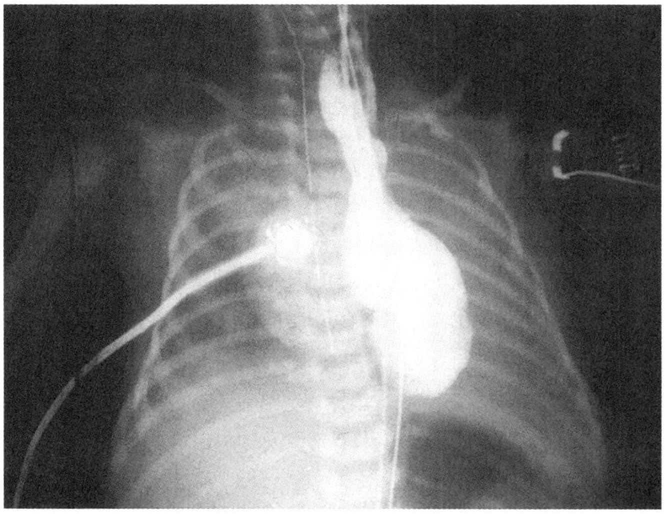

图 60–6　左侧先天性膈疝患儿硫酸钡食管造影，显示出一个扩张膨胀的食管。胃呈垂直朝向，排空缓慢。

也有学者已经有报道了许多骨骼异常，包括胸壁缺损（漏斗胸）和脊柱侧凸[63,249,298]。这些疾病的治疗包括早期的支撑治疗，以及随后的手术纠正。

随着干预治疗的发展，出现了一组新的具有不同类型的远期疾病的存活儿。在生理上受到不同程度损害的患儿大量存活。正如我们试图决定和判断治疗策略对生存率和生活质量的影响时一样，这些婴儿资源管理在将来也是至关紧要的[231]。

未来的治疗

尽管先天性膈疝的治疗取得了很大的进展，但是它仍然表现为一个使人受挫的复杂的临床问题。由于在证明存活率上没有达成一致，所以目前所采用的治疗干预或处理策略还没有成功地得到广泛应用。目前治疗策略包括许可的高碳酸血症、延迟手术修补、抗高血压药物、先进的通气技术等。即使这些策略的成功率并不新增加，但一大部分婴儿的病情不能被这些治疗控制，继续成为新奇治疗的受试者。

胚胎手术干预的概念来自于对羔羊的实验观察，在羔羊中降低对肺的压力可导致持续的肺生长和发育[2,118]。虽然在技术上和理论上令人兴奋，但是胎儿膈疝修补的临床试验还是令人失望[117]。

遇到的主要问题是患者的选择和术后母亲的治
疗。这些在子宫内修补膈疝手术的直接扩展是，在 945
胎羊和胎鼠的先天性膈疝动物模型中，观察到气管韧带加速了胎儿肺的生长，逆转了肺泡的发育不全和异常的肺血管形式[77,78,171,315]。当与未经治疗的对照组进行比较时，气管阻塞或者 PLUG 治疗（堵塞肺脏直至肺生长）可以改善出生后的氧合状态和通气状态[130]。这些观察最后导致了一个随机化的临床试验，来比较内镜下胎儿气管阻塞与目前标准的出生后治疗重度先天性膈疝之间的效果[122]。如果妊娠时间为 22～27 周，肝脏疝出进入左侧胸腔且 LHR 小于 1.4 时，胎儿就具有入选资格。气管阻塞组的 90 天存活率为 73%，而对照组则为 77%。因为两组在存活率之间没有差异，该研究在治疗了 24 位患儿以后就停止了。虽然如此，在欧洲的医疗中心有持续应用这种治疗措施的报道[72]。将来的研究将确定胎儿外科干预在先天性膈疝的治

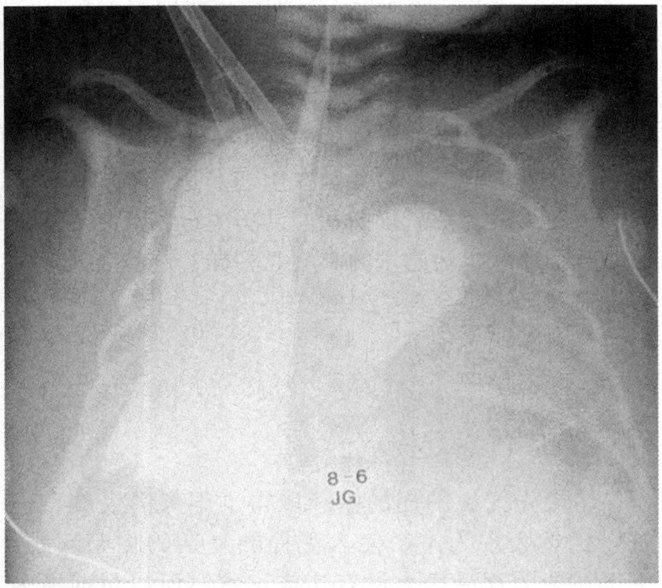

图 60-7 在体外膜肺氧合器支持下的左侧先天性膈疝的胸部平片。肺已经被全氟碳药物所占据以便进行液体通气。肺发育不全可以改善。(Courtesy of R. B. Hirschl, MD.)

疗中是否真的有效。

液体通气技术已经应用于 ECMO 支持下的先天性膈疝患儿（图 60-7）[233]。应用全氟碳药物以后，报道称可显著增加 PaO_2 水平和全肺静态顺应性，显著降低 $PaCO_2$ 水平。没有观察到不良反应。在能够判断它的效果以前，需要进行广泛的研究来检测这种最新的通气方式。

基于气管阻塞可促使胎儿肺生长的现象，也开始了在出生后采用静态肺膨胀诱导肺生长的研究。在进行液体通气的实验期间，可以观察到应用全氟碳药物可导致肺的膨胀。于是就有报道称，全氟碳药物可以作为先天性膈疝患儿出生以后诱导肺生长的一种潜在的治疗手段[94,135,303]。初步的研究结果显示，肺在影像学检查中显著增大，气体交换功能得到改善。在肺泡内应用白蛋白也可以达到同样的效果[67,175]。这种潜在的治疗措施需要进行进一步的研究。

也有采用肺移植的方法手术治疗先天性膈疝[184,297]。已经尝试了进行单侧肺移植和双侧肺移植的办法。目前，还没有足够的经验来推荐这种治疗方式。

药物促进肺的生长和发育的潜在作用目前正在研究当中。联合应用促甲状腺素释放激素和糖皮质激素的研究，已经应用于化学诱导的大鼠先天性膈疝动物模型之中，在促进肺的生长方面有阳性的结果[283]。众所周知，有许多生长因子对肺脏正常的生长发育是至关重要的。有人提出，也许选择性的应用一种或者多种药物制剂或生长因子就可以逆转先天性膈疝中的肺发育不全[39,283]。持续使用除草醚制作的先天性膈疝动物模型进行实验研究，可能会揭示一些新的方法，在产前或产后促进肺的生长和发育的方法。

最后，由于各个不同的医院目前提供的存活率范围较广，就必须深入研究并评价目前的治疗技术及结果。先天性膈疝研究组努力解释每一个遗传基因数据是一个令人鼓舞的开始。这样的研究可能会使目前的治疗措施更为精致，成为一种广泛有效的治疗策略。

Morgagni 疝的疝囊口

Morgagni 前膈疝是位于任何一侧横膈膜和胸壁连接处的前中部。缺损发生在 Larrey 胚胎空间。偶尔，双侧的 Morgagni 膈疝会在中线汇合，构成一个巨大的前膈缺损，从右至左穿过中线。典型的 Morgagni 膈疝有疝囊，通常会发现结肠和小肠疝出到中线的右侧或者左侧。Morgagni 膈疝只占到膈肌缺损的不到 2%。虽然这种缺损可见于新生儿中，但是通常在年长儿和成年人中更为常见。可能会存在合并畸形，其中包括肠旋转不良。膈肌的前中线缺乏，伴有或者不伴有 Cantrell 五联征中的其他缺陷，心包和腹膜自由交通，可能会使得疝出的小肠进入到心包膜中。这种疝经常是在胸部平片中作为一个肿块或者气液平而偶尔被发现。钡剂灌肠造影或者是 CT 扫描可以证实诊断。

上腹部横切口方便地进行手术纠治。在回纳疝内容物和切除疝囊以后，膈肌缝合到肋缘水平的腹直肌后鞘下侧。腹腔镜和胸腔镜技术也可以应用于这种膈肌缺损的修补之中[70,144,191,221]。 946

膈膨升

膈膨升可能是先天性的，也可能是获得性的。先天性膈膨升可能与有疝囊的先天性膈疝难以鉴别，症状通常相似。获得性膈膨升可能是由于膈神经麻痹所致，可发生在先天性心脏病的手术修补中，一些所谓的先天性膈膨升可能是产伤（Erb 瘫痪）造成的。膈肌分布通常是正常的，但是薄弱且没有活性。如果具有膈肌边缘，中央缺乏胸膜和腹膜的覆盖，这种缺损很可能就是膈疝，但是这样的区别可能需要讨论。

虽然可能出现哮喘、频繁的呼吸道感染、不能耐受锻炼，甚至是极度的呼吸窘迫，但是即使在巨大的膈膨中，也可能不表现出任何症状。通常通过胸部荧光透视法得出诊断。在这些病例中，膈肌运动与呼吸动作相反。这种矛盾运动可能是非常显著的，以至于导致严重的气体交换障碍。虽然在过去经常用气腹来诊断，但是现在更为常用的是 CT 和 MRI。

小型的膈膨升可能不需要治疗。在同侧肺功能的通气 / 血流灌注研究中，没有明显症状的患儿出现巨大的功能性缺陷时就有手术修补的指征。在这些病例中，被压迫的肺不可能生长良好。由于相同的原因，即使是没有出现症状，巨大的膈膨升应该进行修补。修补手术可以通过腹部或者胸部切口来完成，但是，在大多数病例中，推荐采用低位的胸部切口。通过这种切口，可以很好地折叠膈肌，并用 2/0 不可吸收缝线间断缝合。在膈肌上也可以做放射状或是外周切口，边缘进行折叠并缝合。重要的是收起并折叠膈肌，以便拉紧膈肌，稍微过度矫正，因为膈肌总是会伸展，如果不这么做膈膨升将会复发。对于获得性膈膨升，常需要进行膈肌折叠以便使婴儿脱离呼吸机的支持。膈肌折叠术也可以通过腹腔镜或者是胸腔镜技术来完成。

（顾 松译 陈永卫校）

参考文献

1. Adolph V, Flageole H, Perreault T, et al: Repair of congenital diaphragmatic hernia after weaning from extracorporeal membrane oxygenation. J Pediatr Surg 1995;30:349.
2. Adzick NS, Outwater KM, Harrison MR, et al: Correction of congenital diaphragmatic hernia in utero: IV. An early gestational fetal lamb model for pulmonary vascular morphometric analysis. J Pediatr Surg 1985;20:673.
3. Adzick NS, Harrison MR, Glick PL, et al: Diaphragmatic hernia in the fetus: Prenatal diagnosis and outcome in 94 cases. J Pediatr Surg 1985;20:357.
4. Adzick NS, Harrison MR, Glick PL, et al: Experimental pulmonary hypoplasia and oligohydramnios: Relative contributions of lung fluid and fetal breathing movements. J Pediatr Surg 1984;19:658.
5. Ahmad A, Gangitano E, Odell RM, et al: Survival, intracranial lesions, and neurodevelopmental outcome in infants with congenital diaphragmatic hernia treated with extracorporeal membrane oxygenation. J Perinatol 1999;19 (6 Pt 1):436.
6. Al-Hathal M, Crankson SH, al-Hargi F, et al: Congenital diaphragmatic hernia: Experience with preoperative stabilization and delayed surgery without ECMO and inhaled nitric oxide. Am J Perinatal 1998;15:487.
7. Al-Shanafey S, Giacomantonio M, Henteleff H: Congenital diaphragmatic hernia: Experience without extracorporeal membrane oxygenation. Pediatr Surg Int 2002;18:28.
8. Antunes MJ, Greenspan JS, Cullen JA, et al: Prognosis with preoperative pulmonary function and lung volume assessment in infants with congenital diaphragmatic hernia. Pediatrics 1995;96:1117.
9. Arca MJ, Barnhart DC, Lelli JL Jr, et al: Early experience with minimally invasive repair of congenital diaphragmatic hernias: Results and lessons learned. J Pediatr Surg 2003;38:1563.
10. Areechon W, Eid L: Hypoplasia of the lung with congenital diaphragmatic hernia. BMJ 1963;5325:230.
11. Atkinson JB, Poon MW: ECMO and the management of congenital diaghragmatic hernia with large diaphragmatic defects requiring a prosthetic patch. J Pediatr Surg 1992; 27:754.
12. Aue O: Uber angeborene Zwerfellhernien. Dtsch Z Chir 1920;160:14.
13. Aviram-Goldring A, Daniely M, Frydman M, et al: Congenital diaphragmatic hernia in a family segregating a reciprocal translocation t(5;15)(p15.3;q24). Am J Med Genet 2000;90:120.
14. Azarow K, Messineo A, Pearl R, et al: Congenital diaphragmatic hernia—a tale of two cities: Toronto experience. J Pediatr Surg 1997;32:395.
15. Badalian SS, Fox HE, Chao CR, et al: Fetal breathing characteristics and postnatal outcome in cases of congenital diaphragmatic hernia. Am J Obstet Gynecol 1994;171:970.
16. Bae JO, Wung JT, Stolar CJ: ECMO is unlikely to rescue CDH inborn CDH infants refractory to permissive hypercapnea/spontaneous ventilation. Pediatrics, in press.
17. Bahlmann F, Merz E, Hallermann C, et al: Congenital diaphragmatic hernia: Ultrasonic measurement of fetal lungs to predict pulmonary hypoplasia. Ultrasound Obstet Gynecol 1999;14:162.
18. Bartlett RH, Gazzaniga AB, Toomasian J, et al: Extracorporeal membrane oxygenation (ECMO) in neonatal respiratory failure: 100 cases. Ann Surg 1986;204:236.
19. Bax NM, Collins DL: The advantages of reconstruction of the dome of the diaphragm in congenital posterolateral diaphragmatic defects. J Pediatr Surg 1984;19:484.
20. Beals DA, Schloo BL, Vacanti JP, et al: Pulmonary growth and remodeling in infants with high-risk congenital diaphragmatic hernia. J Pediatr Surg 1992;27:997.
21. Becmeur F, Jamali RR, Moog R, et al: Thoracoscopic treatment for delayed presentation of congenital diaphragmatic hernia in the infant: A report of three cases. Surg Endosc 2001;15:1163.
22. Bianchi A, Doig CM, Cohen SJ: The reverse latissimus dorsi flap for congenital diaphragmatic hernia repair. J Pediatr Surg 1983;18:560.

23. Bochdalek VA: Einige Betrachtungen uber die Enstehung des angeborenen Zwerfekkbruches. Als Bietrag Zur pathologischen Anatomie der Hernien vjscher. Prakt Heilk 1848;18:89.
24. Bohn D: Blood gas and ventilatory parameters in predicting survival in congenital diaphragmatic hernia. Pediatr Surg Int 1987;2:336.
25. Bohn D: Congenital diaphragmatic hernia. Am J Respir Crit Care Med 2002;166:911.
26. Bohn D, Tamura M, Perrin D, et al: Ventilatory predictors of pulmonary hypoplasia in congenital diaphragmatic hernia, confirmed by morphologic assessment. J Pediatr 1987; 111:423.
27. Bohn DJ: Ventilatory management of blood gas changes in congenital diaphragmatic hernia. In Puri P (ed): Congenital Diaphragmatic Hernia. New York, Karger, 1989.
28. Bohn DJ, James I, Filler RM, et al: The relationship between $PaCO_2$ and ventilation parameters in predicting survival in congenital daphragmatic hernia. J Pediatr Surg 1984;19:666.
29. Bohn DJ, Pearl R, Irish M, et al: Postnatal management of congenital diaphragmatic hernia. Clin Perinatol 1996; 23:843.
30. Boix-Ochoa J, Peguero G, Seijo G, et al: Acid-base balance and blood gases in prognosis and therapy of congenital diaphragmatic hernia. J Pediatr Surg 1974;9:49.
31. Boloker J, Bateman DA, Wung JT, et al: Congenital diaphragmatic hernia in 120 infants treated consecutively with permissive hypercapnea/spontaneous respiration/ elective repair. J Pediatr Surg 2002;37:357.
32. Bos AP, Tibboel D, Hazebroek FW, et al: Surfactant replacement therapy in high-risk congenital diaphragmatic hernia. Lancet 1991;338:1279.
33. Bouman NH, Koot HM, Tibboel D, et al: Children with congenital diaphragmatic hernia are at risk for lower levels of cognitive functioning and increased emotional and behavioral problems. Eur J Pediatr Surg 2000;10:3.
34. Bowditch HI: Peculiar case of diaphragmatic hernia. Buffalo Med J 1853;9:65.
35. Boyden EA: Development and growth of the airways. In Hodson WA (ed): Development of the Lung. New York, Marcel Dekker, 1977.
36. Boyden EA: The pattern of terminal air spaces in a premature infant of 30-32 weeks that lived nineteen and a quarter hours. Am J Anat 1969;126:31.
37. Boyden EA: The terminal air sacs and their blood supply in a 37-day infant lung. Am J Anat 1965;116:413.
38. Brands W, Kachel W, Wirth H, et al: Indication for using extracorporeal membrane oxygenation in congenital diaphragmatic hernias and pulmonary hypoplasia. Eur J Pediatr Surg 1992;2:81.
39. Brandsma AE, Tenbrinck R, Ijsselstijn H, et al: Congenital diaphragmatic hernia: New models, new ideas. Pediatr Surg Int 1995;10:10.
40. Breaux CW Jr, Rouse TM, Cain WS, et al: Improvement in survival of patients with congenital diaphragmatic hernia utilizing a strategy of delayed repair after medical and/or extracorporeal membrane oxygenation stabilization. J Pediatr Surg 1991;26:333.
41. Bremer JL: The diaphragm and diaphragmatic hernia. Arch Pathol 1943;36:539.
42. Brennan P, Croaker GD, Heath M: Congenital diaphragmatic hernia and interstitial deletion of chromosome 3. J Med Genet 2001;38:556.
43. Broman I: Uber die entwicklung der swerchfells beim menschen. Verh Anat Gres 1902;21:9.
44. Broughton AR, Thibeault DW, Mabry SM, Truog WE: Airway muscle in infants with congenital diaphragmatic hernia: Response to treatment. J Pediatr Surg 1998; 33:1471.
45. Burge DM, Atwell JD, Freeman NV: Could the stomach site help predict outcome in babies with left sided congenital diaphragmatic hernia diagnosed antenatally? J Pediatr Surg 1989;24:567.
46. Butler N, Claireaux AE: Congenital diaphragmatic hernia as a cause of perinatal mortality. Lancet 1962;1:659.
47. Cacciari A, Ruggeri G, Mordenti M, et al: High frequency oscillatory ventilation versus conventional mechanical ventilation in congenital diaphragmatic hernia. Eur J Pediatr Surg 2001;11:3.
48. Charlton AJ, Bruce J, Davenport M: Timing of surgery in congenital diaphragmatic hernia: Low mortality after pre-operative stabilization. Anaesthesia 1991;46:820.
49. Chinoy MR: Lung growth and development. Front Biosci 2003;8:d392.
50. Chinoy MR: Pulmonary hypoplasia and congenital diaphragmatic hernia: Advances in the pathogenetics and regulation of lung development. J Surg Res 2002;106:209.
51. Clark RH, Hardin WD Jr, Hirschl RB, et al: Current surgical management of congenital diaphragmatic hernia: A report from the congenital diaphragmatic hernia study group. J Pediatr Surg 1998;33:1004.
52. Cloutier R, Allard V, Fournier L, et al: Estimation of lungs' hypoplasia on postoperative chest x-rays in congenital diaphragmatic hernia. J Pediatr Surg 1993;28:1086.
53. Cogo PE, Zimmerman LJ, Meneghini L, et al: Pulmonary surfactant disaturated-phosphatidylcholine (DSPC) turnover and pool size in newborn infants with congenital diaphragmatic hernia (CDH). Pediatr Res 2003;54:653.
54. Cogo PE, Zimmerman LJ, Rosso F, et al: Surfactant synthesis and kinetics in infants with congenital diaphragmatic hernia. Am J Respir Crit Care Med 2002;166:154.
55. Cohen MS, Rychik J, Bush DM, et al: Influence of congenital heart disease on survival in children with congenital diaphragmatic hernia. J Pediatr 2002;141:25.
56. Congenital Diaphragmatic Hernia Study Group: Estimating disease severity of congenital diaphragmatic hernia in the first 5 minutes of life. J Pediatr Surg 2001; 36:141.
57. Congenital Diaphragmatic Hernia Study Group: Does extracorporeal membrane oxygenation improve survival in neonates with congenital diaphragmatic hernia? J Pediatr Surg 1999;34:720.
58. Connors RH, Tracy T Jr, Bailey PV, et al: Congenital diaphragmatic hernia repair on ECMO. J Pediatr Surg 1990;25:1043.
59. Cooper AP: The Anatomy and Surgical Treatment of Abdominal Hernia. London, Longman, Rees, Orme, Brown and Green, 1827.
60. Coppola CP, Gosche JR: Oxygen-induced vasodilatation is blunted in pulmonary arterioles from fetal rats with nitrofen-induced congenital diaphragmatic hernia. J Pediatr Surg 2001;36:593.
61. Crawford DC, Wright VM, Drake DP, et al: Fetal diaphragmatic hernia: The value of fetal echocardiography in the prediction of postnatal outcome. Br J Obstet Gynaecol 1989;96:705.
62. Crosser O, Ottmann R: Grundiss der Entwicklungsgenchickle des Manchen, 7th ed. Berlin, Springer, 1970.
63. D'Agostino JA, Bernbaum JC, Gerdes M, et al: Outcome for infants with congenital diaphragmatic hernia requiring extracorporeal membrane oxygenation: The first year. J Pediatr Surg 1995;30:10.
64. Daher P, Zeidan S, Azar E, et al: Right congenital diaphragmatic hernia: A well-known pathology? Pediatr Surg Int 2003;19:293.

65. David TJ, Illingsworth CA: Diaphragmatic hernia in the south-west of England. J Med Genet 1976;13:253.
66. Davies G, Reid L: Growth of the alveoli and pulmonary arteries in childhood. Thorax 1970;25:669.
67. Davis C, et al: Post-natal trophic effects of perfluorcarbons on lung growth with congenital diaphragmatic hernia. J Pediatr Surg, in press.
68. de Kort LM, Bax KM: Prosthetic patches used to close congenital diaphragmatic defects behave well: A long-term follow-up study. Eur J Pediatr Surg 1996;6:136.
69. de Lorimier AA, Tierney DF, Parker HR: Hypoplastic lungs in fetal lambs with surgically produced congenital diaphragmatic hernia. Surgery 1967;62:12.
70. Del Castillo D, Sanchez J, Hernandez M, et al: Morgagni's hernia resolved by laparoscopic surgery. J Laparoendosc Surg Tech A 1998;8:105.
71. Delvaux V, Moerman P, Fryns JP: Diaphragmatic hernia in the Coffin-Siris syndrome. Genet Couns 1998;9:45.
72. Deprest J, Gratacos E, Nicolaides KH: The FETO Task Group. Fetoscopic tracheal occlusion (FETO) for severe congenital diaphragmatic hernia: Evolution of a technique and preliminary results. Obstet Gynecol Surv 2005;60:85.
73. Deprest J, Gratacos E, Nicolaides KH, et al: FETO Task Group: Fetoscopic tracheal occlusion (FETO) for severe congenital diaphragmatic hernia: Evolution of a technique and preliminary results. Ultrasound Obstet Gynecol 2004; 24:121.
74. Desfrere L, Jarreau PH, Dommergues M, et al: Impact of delayed repair and elective high-frequency oscillatory ventilation on survival of antenatally diagnosed congenital diaphragmatic hernia: First application of these strategies in the more "severe" subgroup of antenatally diagnosed newborns. Intensive Care Med 2000;26:934.
75. Dickson KA, Harding R: Decline in lung liquid volume and secretion rate during oligohydramnios in fetal sheep. J Appl Physiol 1989;67:2401.
76. Dickson KA, Maloney JE, Berger PJ: State-related changes in lung liquid secretion and tracheal flow rate in fetal lambs. J Appl Physiol 1987;62:34.
77. DiFiore JW, Fauza DO, Slavin R, et al: Experimental fetal tracheal ligation and congenital diaphragmatic hernia: A pulmonary vascular morphometric analysis. J Pediatr Surg 1995;30:917.
78. DiFiore JW, Fauza DO, Slavin R, et al: Experimental fetal tracheal ligation reverses the structural and physiological effects of pulmonary hypoplasia in congenital diaphragmatic hernia. J Pediatr Surg 1994;29:248.
79. DiFiore JW, Wilson JM: Lung development. Semin Pediatr Surg 1994;3:221.
80. Dillon PW, Cilley RE, Hudome SM, et al: Nitric oxide reversal of recurrent pulmonary hypertension and respiratory failure in an infant with CDH after successful ECMO therapy. J Pediatr Surg 1995;30:743.
81. Dillon PW, Cilley RE, Mauger D, et al: The relationship of pulmonary artery pressure and survival in congenital diaphragmatic hernia. J Pediatr Surg 2004;39:307.
82. Dimmitt RA, Moss RL, Rhine WD, et al: Venoarterial versus venovenous extracorporeal membrane oxygenation in congenital diaphragmatic hernia: The extracorporeal life support organization registry, 1990-1999. J Pediatr Surg 2001;36:1199.
83. Donadio A, Garavelli L, Banchini G, et al: Kabuki syndrome and diaphragmatic defects: A frequent association in non-Asian patients? Am J Med Genet 2000;91:164.
84. Dott MM, Wong LY, Rasmussen SA: Population-based study of congenital diaphragmatic hernia: Risk factors and survival in Metropolitan Atlanta, 1968-1999. Birth Defects Res A Clin Mol Teratol 2003;67:261.
85. Downard CD, Jaksic T, Garza JJ, et al: Analysis of an improved survival rate for congenital diaphragmatic hernia. J Pediatr Surg 2003;38:729.
86. Drummond WH, Gregory GA, Heymann MA, et al: The independent effects of hyperventilation, tolazoline and dopamine in infants with persistent pulmonary hypertension. J Pediatr Surg 1981;98:603.
87. Dunhill MS: Postnatal growth of the lung. Thorax 1962;17:329.
88. Eghtesady P, Skarsgard ED, Smith BM, et al: Congenital diaphragmatic hernia associated with aortic coarctation. J Pediatr Surg 1998;33:943.
89. Erenberg A, Rhodes ML, Weinstein MM, et al: The effect of thyroidectomy on ovine fetal lung maturation. Pediatr Res 1979;13(4 pt 1):230.
90. Extracorporeal Life Support Organization: 2004 ECMO Registry Data. Ann Arbor, Extracorporeal Life Support Organization, 2004.
91. Fackler JC, et al: Nitric oxide has no effect on hypoxia associated with congenital diaphragmatic hernia: Preliminary data. Children's National Medical Center ECMO Symposium 1993;9:35.
92. Farber HW, Loscalzo J: Pulmonary arterial hypertension. N Engl J Med 2004;351:1655.
93. Fasching G, Huber A, Uray E, et al: Gastroesophageal reflux and diaphragmatic motility after repair of congenital diaphragmatic hernia. Eur J Pediatr Surg 2000; 10:360.
94. Fauza DO, Hirschl RB, Wilson JM: Continuous intrapulmonary distension with perfluorocarbon accelerates lung growth in infants with congenital diaphragmatic hernia: Initial experience. J Pediatr Surg 2001;36:1237.
95. Fauza DO, Wilson JM: Congenital diaphragmatic hernia and associated anomalies: Their incidence, identification, and impact on prognosis. J Pediatr Surg 1994;29:1113.
96. Fewell JE, Hislop AA, Kitterman JA, et al: Effect of tracheostomy on lung development in fetal lambs. J Appl Physiol 1983;55:1103.
97. Finer NN, Barrington KJ: Nitric oxide for respiratory failure in infants born at or near term. Cochrane Database Syst Rev 2001;(4):CD 000399.
98. Flake AW, Crombleholme TM, Johnson MP, et al: Treatment of severe congenital diaphragmatic hernia by fetal tracheal occlusion: Clinical experience with fifteen cases. Am J Obstet Gynecol 2000;183:1059.
99. Ford WD, James MJ, Walsh JA: Congenital diaphragmatic hernia: Association between pulmonary vascular resistance and plasma thromboxane concentrations. Arch Dis Child 1984;59:143.
100. Ford WD, Kirby CP, Wilkinson CS, et al: Antenatal betamethasone and favourable outcomes in fetuses with 'poor prognosis' diaphragmatic hernia. Pediatr Surg Int 2002;18:244.
101. Frenckner B, Ehren H, Granholm T, et al: Improved results in patients who have congenital diaphragmatic hernia using preoperative stabilization, extracorporeal membrane oxygenation, and delayed surgery. J Pediatr Surg 1997;32:1185.
102. Frenckner B, Freyschsuss U: Long-term effects on lung function after repair of congenital diaphragmatic hernia. In Puri P (ed): Congenital Diaphragmatic Hernia. New York, Karger, 1989.
103. Frostell C, Fratacci MD, Wain JC, et al: Inhaled nitric oxide: A selective pulmonary vasodilator reversing hypoxic pulmonary vasoconstriction. Circulation 1991;83:2038.
104. Furuta Y, Nakamura Y, Miyamoto K: Bilateral congenital posterolateral diaphragmatic hernia. J Pediatr Surg 1987; 22:182.

105. Garne E, Haeusler M, Barisic I, et al: Congenital diaphragmatic hernia: Evaluation of prenatal diagnosis in 20 European regions. Ultrasound Obstet Gynecol 2002; 19:329.
106. Gibson C, Fonkalsrud EW: Iatrogenic pneumothorax and mortality in congenital diaphragmatic hernia. J Pediatr Surg 1983;18:555.
107. Gleeson F, Spitz L: Pitfalls in the diagnosis of congenital diaphragmatic hernia. Arch Dis Child 1991;66:670.
108. Glick PL, Leach CL, Besner GE, et al: Pathophysiology of congenital diaphragmatic hernia: III. Exogenous surfactant therapy for the high-risk neonate with CDH. J Pediatr Surg 1992;27:866.
109. Goh DW, Drake DP, Brereton RJ, et al: Delayed surgery for congenital diaphragmatic hernia. Br J Surg 1992; 79:644.
110. Green PW, Kreismer PT: Registry of fetal defects in Minnesota, incidence of congenital diaphragmatic hernia. Presented at annual meeting of the Extracorporeal Life Support Organization, Ann Arbor, Michigan, September 1990.
111. Greenwald HM, Steiner M: Diaphragmatic hernia in infancy and childhood. Am J Dis Child 1929;38:361.
112. Green JJ, Babiuk RP, Thebaud B: Etiology of congenital diaphragmatic hernia: The retinoid hypothesis. Pediatr Res 2003;53:726.
113. Gross RE: Congenital hernia of the diaphragm. Am J Dis Child 1946;71:579.
114. Guarino N, Solari V, Shima H, et al: Upregulated expression of EGF and TGF-alpha in the proximal respiratory epithelium in the human hypoplastic lung in congenital diaphragmatic hernia. Pediatr Surg Int 2004; 19:755.
115. Hallman M, Kulovich M, Kirkpatrick E, et al: Phosphatidylinositol and phosphatidylgylcerol in amniotic fluid: Indices of lung maturity. Am J Obstet Gynecol 1976;125:613.
116. Harrison MR, Adzick NS, Estes JM, et al: A prospective study of the outcome for fetuses with diaphragmatic hernia. JAMA 1994;271:382.
117. Harrison MR, Adzick NS, Flake AW, et al: Correction of congenital diaphragmatic hernia in utero: VI. Hard-earned lessons. J Pediatr Surg 1993;28:1411.
118. Harrison MR, Bressack MA, Churg AM, et al: Corrections of congenital diaphragmatic hernia in utero: II. Simulated correction permits fetal lung growth with survival at birth. Surgery 1980;88:260.
119. Harrison MR, Adzick NS, Nakayama DK, et al: Fetal diaphragmatic hernia: Fatal but fixable. Semin Perinatol 1985;9:103.
120. Harrison MR, de Lorimier AA: Congenital diaphragmatic hernia. Surg Clin North Am 1981;61:1023.
121. Harrison MR, Jester JA, Ross NA: Correction of congenital diaphragmatic hernia in utero: I. The model: Intrathoracic balloon produces fatal pulmonary hypoplasia. Surgery 1980;88:174.
122. Harrison MR, Keller RL, Hawgood SB, et al: A randomized trial of fetal endoscopic tracheal occlusion for severe fetal congenital diaphragmatic hernia. N Engl J Med 2003;349:1916.
123. Harrison MR, Sydorak RM, Farrell JA, et al: Fetoscopic temporary tracheal occlusion for congenital diaphragmatic hernia: Prelude to a randomized, controlled trial. J Pediatr Surg 2003;38:1012.
124. Hasegawa S, Kohno S, Sugiyama T, et al: Usefulness of echocardiographic measurement of bilateral pulmonary artery dimensions in congenital diaphragmatic hernia. J Pediatr Surg 1994;29:622.
125. Hatch EI Jr, Kendall J, Blumhagen J: Stomach position as in utero predictor of neonatal outcome in left sided diaphragmatic hernia. J Pediatr Surg 1992;27:778.
126. Haugen SE, Linker D, Eik-Nes S, et al: Congenital diaphragmatic hernia: Determination of the optimal time for operation by echocardiographic monitoring of the pulmonary arterial pressure. J Pediatr Surg 1991;26:560.
127. Hazebroek FW, Tibboel D, Bos AP, et al: Congenital diaphragmatic hernia: Impact of preoperative stabilization. A prospective pilot study in 13 patients. J Pediatr Surg 1988;23:1139.
128. Hedblom CA: Diaphragmatic hernia: A study of 378 cases in which an operation was performed. JAMA 1925;85:947.
129. Hedrick HL, Crumbleholme TM, Flake AW, et al: Right congenital diaphragmatic hernia: Prenatal assessment and outcome. J Pediatr Surg 2004;39:319.
130. Hedrick MH, Estes JM, Sullivan KM, et al: Plug the lung until it grows (PLUG): A new method to treat congenital diaphragmatic hernia in utero. J Pediatr Surg 1994; 29:612.
131. Heerema AE, Rabban JT, Sydorak RM, et al: Lung pathology in patients with congenital diaphragmatic hernia treated with fetal surgical intervention, including tracheal occlusion. Pediatr Dev Pathol 2003;6:536.
132. Heidenhain L: Geisichte eines Falles von chronisher: Incarceration des Mageus in einer angehorenen Zwerchfellhernie welcher durcher Laparotomie geheilt wurde, mitansheissenden Bermerkungen uber die Moglichkot, das Kardiacarconom der Speiserhre zzu reseciren. Dtsch Z Chir 1905;76:394.
133. Heling KS, Wauer RR, Hammer H, et al: Reliability of the lung-to-head ratio in predicting outcome and neonatal ventilation parameters in fetuses with congenital diaphragmatic hernia. Ultrasound Obstet Gynecol 2005; 25:112.
134. Hilfiker ML, Karamanoukian HL, Hudak M, et al: Congenital diaphragmatic hernia and chromosomal abnormalities: Report of a lethal association. Pediatr Surg Int 1998;13:550.
135. Hirschl RB, Philip WF, Glick L, et al: A prospective, randomized pilot trial of perfluorocarbon-induced lung growth in newborns with congenital diaphragmatic hernia. J Pediatr Surg 2003;38:283.
136. Hislop A, Reid L: Intra-pulmonary arterial development during fetal life: Branching pattern and structure. J Anat 1972;113:35.
137. Hislop A, Reid L: Pulmonary arterial development during childhood: Branching pattern and structure. Thorax 1973;28:129.
138. Hobolth N: Drugs and congenital abnormalities. Lancet 1962;2:1332.
139. Holcomb GW Jr: A new technique for repair of congenital diaphragmatic hernia with absence of the left hemidiaphragm. Surgery 1962;51:534.
140. Holt PD, Arkovitz MS, Berdon WE, et al: Newborns with diaphragmatic hernia: Initial chest radiography does not have a role in predicting clinical outcome. Pediatr Radiol 2003;34:462.
141. Howe DT, Kilby MD, Sirry H, et al: Structural chromosome anomalies in congenital diaphragmatic hernia. Prenat Diagn 1996;16:1003.
142. Hubbard AM, Crombleholme TM, Adzick NS, et al: Prenatal MRI evaluation of congenital diaphragmatic hernia. Am J Perinatol 1999;16:407.
143. Hunt RW, Kean MJ, Stewart MJ, et al: Patterns of cerebral injury in a series of infants with congenital diaphragmatic hernia utilizing magnetic resonance imaging. J Pediatr Surg 2004;39:31.

144. Hussong RL Jr, Landreneau RJ, Cole FH Jr: Diagnosis and repair of a Morgagni hernia with video-assisted thoracic surgery. Ann Thorac Surg 1997;63:1474.
145. Ignarro LJ, Buga GM, Wood KS, et al: Endothelium-derived relaxing factor produced and released from artery and vein is nitric oxide. Proc Natl Acad Sci U S A 1987;84:9265.
146. Ijsselstijn H, Tibboel D, Hop WJ, et al: Long-term pulmonary sequelae in children with congenital diaphragmatic hernia. Am J Respir Crit Care Med 1997;155:174.
147. Ijsselstijn H, Zimmerman LJ, Bunt JE, et al: Prospective evaluation of surfactant composition in bronchoalveolar lavage fluid of infants with congenital diaphragmatic hernia and of age-matched controls. Crit Care Med 1998;26:573.
148. Iocono JA, Cilley RE, Mauger DT, et al: Postnatal pulmonary hypertension after repair of congenital diaphragmatic hernia: Predicting risk and outcome. J Pediatr Surg 1999; 34:349.
149. Iritani I: Experimental study on embryogenesis of congenital diaphragmatic hernia. Anat Embryol (Berl) 1984; 169:133.
150. Jaillard SM, Pierrat V, Dubois A, et al: Outcome at 2 years of infants with congenital diaphragmatic hernia: A population-based study. Ann Thorac Surg 2003;75:250.
151. Janssen DJ, Tibboel D, Carnielli VP, et al: Surfactant phosphatidylcholine pool size in human neonates with congenital diaphragmatic hernia requiring ECMO. J Pediatr 2003;142:247.
152. Jenkinson EL: Absence of half of the diaphragm (thoracic stomach; diaphragmatic hernia). AJR Am J Roentgenol 1931:26:899.
153. Jesudason EC: Challenging embryological theories on congenital diaphragmatic hernia: Future therapeutic implications for paediatric surgery. Ann R Coll Surg Engl 2002;84:252.
154. Kaiser JR, Rosenfeld CR: A population-based study of congenital diaphragmatic hernia: Impact of associated anomalies and preoperative blood gases on survival. J Pediatr Surg 1999;34:1196.
155. Karamanoukian HL, Glick PL, Wilcox DT, et al: Pathophysiology of congenital diaphragmatic hernia: VIII. Inhaled nitric oxide requires exogenous surfactant therapy in the lamb model of congenital diaphragmatic hernia. J Pediatr Surg 1995;30:1.
156. Karamanoukian HL, Glick PL, Wilcox DT, et al: Pathophysiology of congenital diaphragmatic hernia: X: Localization of nitric oxide synthase in the intima of pulmonary artery trunks of lambs with surgically created congenital diaphragmatic hernia. J Pediatr Surg 1995;30:5.
157. Karamanoukian HL, Glick PL, Zayek M, et al: Inhaled nitric oxide in congenital hypoplasia of the lungs due to diaphragmatic hernia or oligohydramnios. Pediatrics 1994; 94:715.
158. Katz S, Kidron D, Litmanovitz I, et al: Fibrous fusion between the liver and the lung: An unusual complication of right congenital diaphragmatic hernia. J Pediatr Surg 1998;33:766.
159. Kavvadia V, Greenough A, Laubscher B, et al: Perioperative assessment of respiratory compliance and lung volume in infants with congenital diaphragmatic hernia: Prediction of outcome. J Pediatr Surg 1997;32:1665.
160. Kay HH, Bird IM, Coe CL, et al: Antenatal steroid treatment and adverse fetal effects: What is the evidence? J Soc Gynecol Invest 2000;7:269.
161. Kay S, Laberge JM, Flageole H, et al: Use of antenatal steroids to counteract the negative effects of tracheal occlusion in the fetal lamb model. Pediatr Res 2001;50:495.
162. Kays DW, Langham MR Jr, Ledbetter DJ, et al: Detrimental effects of standard medical therapy in congenital diaphragmatic hernia. Ann Surg 1999;230:340.
163. Keller RL, Aaroz PA, Hawgood S, et al: MR Imaging of hepatic pulmonary fusion in neonates. AJR Am J Roentgenol 2003;180:438.
164. Keller RL, Glidden DV, Paek BW, et al: The lung-to-head ratio and fetoscopic temporary tracheal occlusion: Prediction of survival in severe left congenital diaphragmatic hernia. Ultrasound Obstet Gynecol 2003;21:244.
165. Keshen TH, Gursoy M, Shew SB, et al: Does extracorporeal membrane oxygenation benefit neonates with congenital diaphragmatic hernia? Application of a predictive equation. J Pediatr Surg 1997;32:818.
166. Killeen OG, Kelehan P, Reardon W: Double vagina with sex reversal, congenital diaphragmatic hernia, pulmonary and cardiac malformations—another case of Meacham syndrome. Clin Dysmorphol 2002;11:25.
167. Kinsella JP, Neish SR, Ivy DD, et al: Clinical responses to prolonged treatment of persistent pulmonary hypertension with low doses of inhaled nitric oxide. J Pediatr 1993;123:103.
168. Kinsella JP, Parker TA, Ivy DD, et al: Noninvasive delivery of inhaled nitric oxide therapy for late pulmonary hypertension in newborn infants with congenital diaphragmatic hernia. J Pediatr 2003;142:397.
169. Kinsella JP, Neish SR, Shaffer E, et al: Low-dose inhalational nitric oxide in persistent pulmonary hypertension of the newborn. Lancet 1992;340:819.
170. Kitagawa M, Hislop A, Boyden EA, et al: Lung hypoplasia in congenital diaphragmatic hernia: A quantitative study of airway, artery, and alveolar development. Br J Surg 1971;58:342.
171. Kitano Y, Kanai M, Davies P, et al: Lung growth induced by prenatal tracheal occlusion and its modifying factors: A study in the rat model of congenital diaphragmatic hernia. J Pediatr Surg 2001;36:251.
172. Koumbourlis AC, Stolar CJ, Stylianos S: Lung function in infants after repair of congenital diaphragmatic hernia [abstract]. Am Rev Respir Dis 1994;148:A548.
173. Krishna A, Zargar N: Laparoscopic repair of a congenital diaphragmatic hernia. Pediatr Surg Int 2002;18:491.
174. Kugelman A, Gangitano E, Pincros J, et al: Venovenous versus venoarterial extracorporeal membrane oxygenation in congenital diaphragmatic hernia. J Pediatr Surg 2003; 38:1131.
175. Kunaisaki SM, Chanh R, Fauza D, et al: Hypertonic enhancement of fetal pulmonary growth after tracheal occlusion. J Pediatr Surg, in press.
176. Ladd WE, Gross RE: Congenital diaphragmatic hernia. N Engl J Med 1940;223:917.
177. Laennec RTH, 1834, cited in Ravitch MM: Congenital diaphragmatic hernia. In Nyhus LM (ed): Hernia. Philadelphia, JB Lippincott, 1964.
178. Lally KP, Lally PA, Langham MR, et al: Congenital Diaphragmatic Hernia Study Group: Surfactant does not improve survival rate in preterm infants with congenital diaphragmatic hernia. J Pediatr Surg 2004;39:829.
179. Lally KP, Paranka MS, Roden J, et al: Congenital diaphragmatic hernia: Stabilization and repair on ECMO. Ann Surg 1992;216:569.
180. Lally KP, The CDH Study Group. The use of ECMO for stabilization of infants with congenital diaphragmatic hernia—a report of the CDH Study Group. Presented at the 20th annual meeting of the Surgical Section of the American Academy of Pediatrics, Boston, October 2002.

181. Langer JC, Filler RM, Bohn DJ, et al: Timing of surgery for congenital diaphragmatic hernia: Is emergency operation necessary? J Pediatr Surg 1988;23:731.
182. Langham MR Jr, Kays DW, Beierle EA, et al: Twenty years of progress in congenital diaphragmatic hernia at the University of Florida. Am Surg 2003;69:45.
183. Laudy JA, Van Gucht M, Van Dooren MF, et al: Congenital diaphragmatic hernia: Evaluation of the prognostic value of the lung-to-head ratio and other prenatal parameters. Prenat Diagn 2003;23:634.
184. Lee R, Mendeloff EN, Huddleston C, et al: Bilateral lung transplantation for pulmonary hypoplasia caused by congenital diaphragmatic hernia. J Thorac Cardiovasc Surg 2003;126:295.
185. Lessin MS, Thompson IM, Deprez MF, et al: Congenital diaphragmatic hernia with or without extracorporeal membrane oxygenation: Are we making progress? J Am Coll Surg 1995;181:65.
186. Leung JW, Coakley FV, Hricak H, et al: Prenatal MR imaging of congenital diaphragmatic hernia. AJR Am J Roentgenol 2000;174:1607.
187. Levin DL: Morphologic analysis of the pulmonary vascular bed in congenital left-sided diaphragmatic hernia. J Pediatr 1978;92:805.
188. Lewis DA, Reickert C, Bowerman R, et al: Prenatal ultrasonography frequently fails to diagnose congenital diaphragmatic hernia. J Pediatr Surg 1997;32:352.
189. Lewis WH: The development of the muscular system. In Keibel F, Mall FP (eds): Manual of Human Embryology. Philadelphia, JB Lippincott, 1910.
190. Liggins GC, Vilos GA, Campos GA, et al: The effect of bilateral thoracoplasty on lung development in fetal sheep. J Dev Physiol 1981;3:275.
191. Lima M, Domini M, Libri M, et al: Laparoscopic repair of Morgagni-Larrey hernia in a child. J Pediatr Surg 2000; 35:1266.
192. Lipshutz GS, Albanese CT, Feldstein VA, et al: Prospective analysis of lung-to-head ratio predicts survival for patients with prenatally diagnosed congenital diaphragmatic hernia. J Pediatr Surg 1997;32:1634.
193. Lipson AH, Williams G: Congenital diaphragmatic hernia in half sibs. J Med Genet 1985;22:145.
194. Losty PD, Vanamo K, Rintala RJ, et al: Congenital diaphragmatic hernia—does the side of the defect influence the incidence of associated malformations? J Pediatr Surg 1998;33:507.
195. Lotze A, Knight GR, Anderson KD, et al: Surfactant (beractant) therapy for infants with congenital diaphragmatic hernia on ECMO: Evidence for persistent surfactant deficiency. J Pediatr Surg 1994;29:407.
196. Lund DP, Mitchell J, Kharasch V, et al: Congenital diaphragmatic hernia: The hidden morbidity. J Pediatr Surg 1994;29:258.
197. Lurie IW: Where to look for genes related to diaphragmatic hernia? Genet Couns 2003;14:75.
198. Lyrene RK, Phillips JB 3rd: Control of pulmonary vascular resistance in the fetus and the newborn. Clin Perinatol 1984;11:551.
199. Mahieu-Caputo D, Sonigo P, Dommergues M, et al: Fetal lung volume measurement by magnetic resonance imaging in congenital diaphragmatic hernia. Br J Obstet Gynaecol 2001;108:863.
200. Mann O, Huppertz C, Langwieler TE, et al: Effect of prenatal glucocorticoids and postnatal nitric oxide inhalation on survival of newborn rats with nitrofen-induced congenital diaphragmatic hernia. J Pediatr Surg 2002; 37:730.
201. Manning PB, Murphy JP, Raynor SC, et al: Congenital diaphragmatic hernia presenting due to gastrointestinal complications. J Pediatr Surg 1992;27:1225.
202. Marven SS, Smith CM, Claxton D, et al: Pulmonary function, exercise performance, and growth in survivors of congenital diaphragmatic hernia. Arch Dis Child 1998;78:137.
203. McCauley G: An account of viscera herniation. Phil Trans R Coll Phys 1754;6:25.
204. McGahren ED, Malik K, Rodgers BM: Neurologic outcome is diminished in survivors of congenital diaphragmatic hernia requiring extracorporeal membrane oxygenation. J Pediatr Surg 1997;32:1216.
205. Metkus AP, Filly RA, Stringer MD, et al: Sonographic predictors of survival in fetal diaphragmatic hernia. J Pediatr Surg 1996;31:148.
206. Migliazza L, Otten C, Xia H, et al: Cardiovascular malformations in congenital diaphragmatic hernia: Human and experimental studies. J Pediatr Surg 1999;34:1352.
207. Migliazza L, Xia H, Diez-Pardo JA, et al: Skeletal malformations associated with congenital diaphragmatic hernia: Experimental and human studies. J Pediatr Surg 1999; 34:1624.
208. Mishalany H, Gordo J: Congenital diaphragmatic hernia in monozygotic twins. J Pediatr Surg 1986;21:372.
209. Mishalany HG, Nakada K, Wooley MM: Congenital diaphragmatic hernias: Eleven years' experience. Arch Surg 1979;114:1118.
210. Miyazaki E, Ohshiro K, Tiara Y, et al: Altered insulin-like growth factor I mRNA expression in human hypoplastic lung in congenital diaphragmatic hernia. J Pediatr Surg 1998;33:1476.
211. Moessinger AC, Harding R, Adamson TM, et al: Role of lung fluid volume in growth and maturation of the fetal sheep lung. J Clin Invest 1990;86:1270.
212. Moore KL: The Developing Human: Clinically Oriented Embryology, 3rd ed. Philadelphia, WB Saunders, 1982.
213. Moss RL, Chen CM, Harrison MR: Prosthetic patch durability in congenital diaphragmatic hernia: A long term follow-up study. J Pediatr Surg 2001;36:152.
214. Moyer V, Moya F, Tibboel R, et al: Late versus early surgical correction for congenital diaphragmatic hernia in newborn infants. Cochrane Database Syst Rev 2002;CD001695.
215. Muratore CS, Kharasch V, Lund DP, et al: Pulmonary morbidity in 100 survivors of congenital diaphragmatic hernia monitored in a multidisciplinary clinic. J Pediatr Surg 2001; 36:133.
216. Naeye RL, Shochat SJ, Whitman V, et al: Unsuspected pulmonary vascular abnormalities associated with diaphragmatic hernia. Pediatrics 1976;58:902.
217. Nagaya M, Akatsuka H, Kato J, et al: Development in lung function of the affected side after repair of congenital diaphragmatic hernia. J Pediatr Surg 1996;31:349.
218. Nakata M, Sase M, Anno K, et al: Prenatal sonographic chest and lung measurements for predicting severe pulmonary hypoplasia in left-sided congenital diaphragmatic hernia. Early Hum Dev 2003;72:75.
219. Nakayama DK, Motoyama EK, Tagge EM: Effect of preoperative stabilization on respiratory system compliance and outcome in newborn infants with congenital diaphragmatic hernia. J Pediatr 1991;118:793.
220. Nauman G: Hernia diaphragmatic: Laparotomie dod. Hygeia 1888;50:524.
221. Nawaz A, Matta H, Jacobsz A, et al: Congenital Morgagni's hernia in infants and children. Int Surg 2000;85:158.
222. Neville HL, Jaksic T, Wilson JM, et al: Congenital Diaphragmatic Hernia Study Group: Bilateral congenital diaphragmatic hernia. J Pediatr Surg 2003;38:522.

223. Neville HL, Jaksic T, Wilson, JM, et al: Congenital Diaphragmatic Hernia Study Group: Fryns syndrome in children with congenital diaphragmatic hernia. J Pediatr Surg 2002;37:1685.
224. Nio M, Haase G, Kennaugh J, et al: A prospective randomized trial of delayed versus immediate repair of congenital diaphragmatic hernia. J Pediatr Surg 1994;29:618.
225. Norden MA, Butt W, McDougall P: Predictors of survival for infants with congenital diaphragmatic hernia. J Pediatr Surg 1994;29:1442.
226. Nose K, Kamata S, Sawai T, et al: Airway anomalies in patients with congenital diaphragmatic hernia. J Pediatr Surg 2000;35:1562.
227. O'Dwyer J: Operation for relief of congenital diaphragmatic hernia. Ann Surg 1890;11:124.
228. Ochoa de Castro A, Ramos MR, Calonge WM, et al: Congenital left-sided Bochdalek diaphragmatic hernia thoracoscopic repair—case report. Eur J Pediatr Surg 2003; 13:407.
229. Ohshiro K, Miyazaki E, Taira Y, et al: Upregulated tumor necrosis factor-alpha gene expression in the hypoplastic lung in patients with congenital diaphragmatic hernia. Pediatr Surg Int 1998;14:21.
230. Paek BW, Coakley FV, Lu Y, et al: Congenital diaphragmatic hernia: Prenatal evaluation with MR lung volumetry—preliminary experience. Radiology 2001;220:63.
231. Poley MJ, Stolk EA, Tibboel D, et al: The cost-effectiveness of treatment for congenital diaphragmatic hernia. J Pediatr Surg 2002;37:1245.
232. Powell PD, Johnstone JM: Phenmetrazine and fetal abnormalities. BMJ 1962;17:1327.
233. Pranikoff T, Gauger PG, Hirschl RB: Partial liquid ventilation in newborn patients with congenital diaphragmatic hernia. J Pediatr Surg 1996;31:613.
234. Pringle KC: Lung development in congenital diaphragmatic hernia. In Puri P (ed): Congenital Diaphragmatic Hernia. Basel, Karger, 1989.
235. Pringle KC, Turner JW, Schofield JC, et al: Creation and repair of diaphragmatic hernia in the fetal lamb: Lung development and morphology. J Pediatr Surg 1984; 19:131.
236. Purohit DM, Pais S, Levkoff AH: Effect of tolazoline on hypoxemia in neonatal respiratory distress. Crit Care Med 1978;6:14.
237. Puri P: Congenital diaphragmatic hernia. Curr Probl Surg 1994;31:787.
238. Puri P, Gorman WA: Natural history of congenital diaphragmatic hernia: Implication for management. Pediatr Surg Int 1987;2:327.
239. Rasheed A, Tindall S, Cueny DL, et al: Neurodevelopmental outcome after congenital diaphragmatic hernia: Extracorporeal membrane oxygenation before and after surgery. J Pediatr Surg 2001;36:539.
240. Rashid A, Ivy D: Severe paediatric pulmonary hypertension: New management strategies. Arch Dis Child 2005; 90:92.
241. Reickert CA, Hirschl RB, Schumacher R, et al: Effect of very delayed repair of congenital diaphragmatic hernia on survival and extracorporeal life support use. Surgery 1996;120:766.
242. Reid IS, Hutcherson RJ: Long-term follow-up of patients with congenital diaphragmatic hernia. J Pediatr Surg 1976; 11:939.
243. Reid L: Structural and functional reappraisal of the pulmonary artery system. In Scientific Basis of Medicine Annual Reviews. University of London, Athlone Press, 1968.
244. Reyes C, Chang LK, Waffarn F, et al: Delayed repair of congenital diaphragmatic hernia with early high-frequency oscillatory ventilation during preoperative stabilization. J Pediatr Surg 1998;33:1010.
245. Richardson WS, Bolton JS: Laparoscopic repair of congenital diaphragmatic hernias. J Laparoendosc Adv Surg Tech A 2002;12:277.
246. Roberts JP, Burge DM, Griffiths DM: High-risk congenital diaphragmatic hernia: How long should surgery be delayed? Pediatr Surg Int 1994;9:555.
247. Roberts JD, Polaner DM, Lang P: Inhaled nitric oxide in persistent pulmonary hypertension of the newborn. Lancet 1992;340:818.
248. Rowe DH, Stolar CJ: Recurrent diaphragmatic hernia. Semin Pediatr Surg 2003;12:107.
249. Roye DP: Personal communication, 1992.
250. Ruano R, Benachi A, Martinovic J, et al: Can three-dimensional ultrasound be used for the assessment of the fetal lung volume in cases of congenital diaphragmatic hernia? Fetal Diagn Ther 2004;19:87.
251. Rudolph AM, Yuan S: Response of the pulmonary vasculature to hypoxia and H^+ ion concentration changes. J Clin Invest 1966;45:399.
252. Sakai H, Tamura M, Hosokawa Y, et al: Effect of surgical repair on respiratory mechanics in congenital diaphragmatic hernia. J Pediatr 1987;111:432.
253. Sakurai Y, Azarow K, Cutz E, et al: Pulmonary barotrauma in congenital diaphragmatic hernia: A clinicopathological correlation. J Pediatr Surg 1999;34:1813.
254. Saltzman DA, Ennis JS, Mehall JR, et al: Recurrent congenital diaphragmatic hernia: A novel repair. J Pediatr Surg 2001;36:1768.
255. Scaife ER, Johnson DG, Meyers RL, et al: The split abdominal wall muscle flap—a simple, mesh-free approach to repair large diaphragmatic hernia. J Pediatr Surg 2003;38:1748.
256. Scheffers EC, Ijsselstijn H, Tenbrinck R, et al: Evaluation of lung function changes before and after surfactant application during artificial ventilation in newborn rats with congenital diaphragmatic hernia. J Pediatr Surg 1994;29:820.
257. Schoeman L, Pierro A, Macrae D, et al: Late death after extracorporeal membrane oxygenation for congenital diaphragmatic hernia. J Pediatr Surg 1999;34:357.
258. Schwartz IP, Bernbaum JC, Rychik J, et al: Pulmonary hypertension in children following extracorporeal membrane oxygenation therapy and repair of congenital diaphragmatic hernia. J Perinatol 1999;19:220.
259. Shah AV, Shah AA: Laparoscopic approach to surgical management of congenital diaphragmatic hernia in the newborn. J Pediatr Surg 2002;37:548.
260. Shanbhogue LK, Tam PK, Ninan G, et al: Preoperative stabilisation in congenital diaphragmatic hernia. Arch Dis Child 1990;65(10 spec no):1043.
261. Sharland GK, Lockhart SM, Heward AJ, et al: Prognosis in fetal diaphragmatic hernia. Am J Obstet Gynecol 1992;166(1 pt 1):9.
262. Shaw KS, Filiatrault D, Yazbeck S, et al: Improved survival for congenital diaphragmatic hernia, based on prenatal ultrasound diagnosis and referral to a combined obstetric-pediatric surgical center. J Pediatr Surg 1994;29:1268.
263. Shehata SM, Mooi WJ, Okazaki T, et al: Enhanced expression of vascular endothelial growth factor in lungs of newborn infants with congenital diaphragmatic hernia and pulmonary hypertension. Thorax 1999;54:427.
264. Shehata SM, Sharma HS, van der Staak FH, et al: Remodeling of pulmonary arteries in human congenital diaphragmatic hernia with or without extracorporeal membrane oxygenation. J Pediatr Surg 2000;35:208.
265. Sigalet DL, Tierney A, Adolph V, et al: Timing of repair of congenital diaphragmatic hernia requiring extracorporeal membrane oxygenation support. J Pediatr Surg 1995; 30:1183.

266. Simpson JS, Gossage JD: Use of abdominal wall muscle flap in repair of large congenital diaphragmatic hernia. J Pediatr Surg 1971;6:42.
267. Skari H, Bjornland K, Frenckner B, et al: Congenital diaphragmatic hernia in Scandinavia from 1995 to 1998: Predictors of mortality. J Pediatr Surg 2002;37:1269.
268. Skari H, Bjornland K, Haugen G, et al: Congenital diaphragmatic hernia: A meta-analysis of mortality factors. J Pediatr Surg 2000;35:1187.
269. Skousgaard SG: Severe bronchial hyperreactivity as a sequel to congenital diaphragmatic hernia. Paediatr Anaesth 1998; 8:503.
270. Smith GN, Kingdom JC, Penning DH, et al: Antenatal corticosteroids: Is more better? Lancet 2000;355:251.
271. Solari V, Piotrowska AP, Puri P: Expression of heme oxygenase-1 and endothelial nitric oxide synthase in the lung of newborns with congenital diaphragmatic hernia and persistent pulmonary hypertension. J Pediatr Surg 2003;38:808.
272. Solari V, Puri P: Glucocorticoid receptor gene expression in the hypoplastic lung of newborns with congenital diaphragmatic hernia. J Pediatr Surg 2002;37:715.
273. Springer SC, Fleming D, Hulsey TC: A statistical model to predict nonsurvival in congenital diaphragmatic hernia. J Perinatol 2002;22:263.
274. Sreenan C, Etches P, Osiovich H: The western Canadian experience with congenital diaphragmatic hernia: Perinatal factors predictive of extracorporeal membrane oxygenation and death. Pediatr Surg Int 2001;17:196.
275. Stege G, Fenton A, Jaffray B: Nihilism in the 1990s: The true mortality of congenital diaphragmatic hernia. Pediatrics 2003;112:532.
276. Stevens TP, Chess PR, McConnochie KM, et al: Survival in early and late-term infants with congenital diaphragmatic hernia treated with extracorporeal membrane oxygenation. Pediatrics 2002;110:590.
277. Stevens DC, Schreiner RL, Bull MJ, et al: An analysis of tolazoline therapy in the critically-ill neonate. J Pediatr Surg 1980;15:964.
278. Stolar C, Dillon P, Reyes C: Selective use of extracorporeal membrane oxygenation in the management of congenital diaphragmatic hernia. J Pediatr Surg 1988;23:207.
279. Stolar CJ, Crisafi MA, Discoll YT: Neurocognitive outcome for infants treated with extracorporeal membrane oxygenation: Are infants with congenital diaphragmatic hernia different? J Pediatr Surg 1995;30:366.
280. Stolar CJ, Dillon PW, Stalcup SA: Extracorporeal membrane oxygenation and congenital diaphragmatic hernia: Modification of the pulmonary vasoactive profile. J Pediatr Surg 1985;20:681.
281. Stolar CJ, Levy JP, Dillon PW, et al: Anatomic and functional abnormalities of the esophagus in infants surviving congenital diaphragmatic hernia. Am J Surg 1990; 159:204.
282. Suda K, Bigras JL, Bohn D, et al: Echocardiographic predictors of outcome in newborns with congenital diaphragmatic hernia. Pediatrics 2000;105:1106.
283. Suen HC, Losty P, Donahoe PK, et al: Combined antenatal thyrotropin-releasing hormone and low-dose glucocorticoid therapy improves the pulmonary biochemical immaturity in congenital diaphragmatic hernia. J Pediatr Surg 1994;29:359.
284. Sweed Y, Puri P: Congenital diaphragmatic hernia: Influence of associated malformations on survival. Arch Dis Child 1993;69(1 spec no):68.
285. Swietlinski J, Swist-Szulik K, Maruniak-Chudek I, et al: Spondylothoracic dysostosis associated with diaphragmatic hernia and camptodactyly. Genet Couns 2002; 13:309.
286. Taira Y, Yamataka T, Miyazaki E, et al: Comparison of the pulmonary vasculature in newborn and stillborns with congenital diaphragmatic hernia. Pediatr Surg Int 1998;14:30.
287. Thebaud B, Azancot A, de Lagausie P, et al: Congenital diaphragmatic hernia: Antenatal prognostic factors. Does cardiac ventricular disproportion in utero predict outcome and pulmonary hypoplasia? Intensive Care Med 1997;23:10062.
288. Thibeault DW, Olsen SL, Truog WE, Hubbell MM: Pre-ECMO predictors of nonsurvival in congenital diaphragmatic hernia. J Perinatol 2002;22:682.
289. Thorpe-Beeston JG, Gosden CM, Nicolaides KH: Prenatal diagnosis of congenital diaphragmatic hernia: Associated malformations and chromosomal defects. Fetal Ther 1989;4:21.
290. Thurlbeck WM: Postnatal human lung growth. Thorax 1982;37:564.
291. Touloukian RJ, Markowitz RI: A preoperative x-ray scoring system for risk assessment of newborns with congenital diaphragmatic hernia. J Pediatr Surg 1984;19:252.
292. Tracy TF Jr, Bailey PV, Sadiq F, et al: Predictive capabilities of preoperative and postoperative pulmonary function tests in delayed repair of congenital diaphragmatic hernia. J Pediatr Surg 1994;29:265.
293. Turner GR, Levin DL: Prostaglandin synthesis inhibition in persistent pulmonary hypertension of the newborn. Clin Perinatol 1984;11:581.
294. Unger S, Copland I, Tibboel D, et al: Down-regulation of sonic hedgehog expression in pulmonary hypoplasia is associated with congenital diaphragmatic hernia. Am J Pathol 2003;162:547.
295. Vacanti JP, Crone RK, Murphy JD, et al: The pulmonary hemodynamic response to perioperative anesthesia in the treatment of high-risk infants with congenital diaphragmatic hernia. J Pediatr Surg 1984;19:672.
296. van Dooren MF, Brooks AS, Tibboel D, et al: Association of congenital diaphragmatic hernia with limb-reduction defects. Birth Defects Res A Clin Mol Teratol 2003;67:578.
297. Van Meurs KP, Rhine WD, Benitz WE, et al: Lobar lung transplantation as a treatment for congenital diaphragmatic hernia. J Pediatr Surg 1994;29:1557.
298. Vanamo K, Peltonen J, Rintala R, et al: Chest wall and spinal deformities in adults with congenital diaphragmatic defects. J Pediatr Surg 1996;31:851.
299. Vanamo K, Rintala RJ, Lindahl H, et al: Long-term gastrointestinal morbidity in patients with congenital diaphragmatic defects. J Pediatr Surg 1996;31:551.
300. Vanamo K, Rintala R, Sovijarvi A, et al: Long-term pulmonary sequelae in survivors of congenital diaphragmatic defects. J Pediatr Surg 1996;31:1096.
301. Vazquez WD, Cheu HW: Hemorrhagic complications and repair of congenital diaphragmatic hernias: Does timing of the repair make a difference? Data from the Extracorporeal Life Support Organization. J Pediatr Surg 1994;29:1002.
302. von Staak FH, de Haan AF, Geven WB, et al: Improving survival for patients with high-risk congenital diaphragmatic hernia by using extracorporeal membrane oxygenation. J Pediatr Surg 1995;30:1463.
303. Walker GM, Kasem KF, O'Toole SJ, et al: Early perfluorodecalin lung distension in infants with congenital diaphragmatic hernia. J Pediatr Surg 2003;38:17.
304. Wallace CA, Roden JS: Reverse, innervated latissimus dorsi flap reconstruction of congenital diaphragmatic absence. Plast Reconstr Surg 1995;96:761.
305. Waller DK, Tita AT, Werler MM, et al: Association between prepregnancy maternal body mass index and the risk of having an infant with a congenital diaphragmatic hernia. Birth Defects Res A Clin Mol Teratol 2003;67:73.

306. Walsh DS, Hubbard AM, Olutoye OO, et al: Assessment of fetal lung volumes and liver herniation with magnetic resonance imaging in congenital diaphragmatic hernia. Am J Obstet Gynecol 2000;183:1067.
307. Warkany J, Roth CB: Malformations induced in rats by maternal vitamin A deficiency. J Nutr 1948;35:1.
308. Weber TR, Kountzman B, Dillon PA, et al: Improved survival in congenital diaphragmatic hernia with evolving therapeutic strategies. Arch Surg 1998;133:498.
309. Weibel ER, Gomez DM: A principle for counting tissue structures on random sections. J Appl Physiol 1962;17:343.
310. Weinberg J: Diaphragmatic hernia in infants: Surgical treatment with use of renal fascia. Surgery 1938;3(4):78.
311. Wells LJ: Development of the human diaphragm and pleural sacs. Contr Embryol Carnegie Inst 1954;35:107.
312. Wenstrom KD, Weiner CP, Hanson JW, et al: A five year statewide experience with congenital diaphragmatic hernia. Am J Obstet Gynecol 1991;165:838.
313. West KW, Bengston K, Rescorla FJ, et al: Delayed surgical repair and ECMO improves survival in congenital diaphragmatic hernia. Ann Surg 1992;216:454.
314. Wigglesworth JS, Desai R, Guerrini P: Fetal lung hypoplasia: Biochemical and structural variations and their possible significance. Arch Dis Child 1981;56:606.
315. Wilson JM, Difiore JW, Peters CA: Experimental fetal tracheal ligation prevents the pulmonary hypoplasia associated with fetal nephrectomy: Possible application for congenital diaphragmatic hernia. J Pediatr Surg 1993;28:1433.
316. Wilson JM, Bower LK, Lund DP: Evolution of the technique of congenital diaphragmatic hernia repair on ECMO. J Pediatr Surg 1994;29:1109.
317. Wilson JM, Fauza DO, Lund DP, et al: Antenatal diagnosis of isolated congenital diaphragmatic hernia is not an indicator of outcome. J Pediatr Surg 1994;29:815.
318. Wilson JM, Lund DP, Lillehei CW, et al: Congenital diaphragmatic hernia—a tale of two cities: Boston experience. J Pediatr Surg 1997;32:401.
319. Wilson JM, Lund DP, Lillehei CW, et al: Congenital diaphragmatic hernia: Predictors of severity in the ECMO era. J Pediatr Surg 1991;26:1028.
320. Wilson JM, Lund DP, Lillehei CW, et al: Delayed repair and preoperative ECMO does not improve survival in high-risk congenital diaphragmatic hernia. J Pediatr Surg 1992;27:368.
321. Witters I, Legius E, Moerman P, et al: Associated malformations and chromosomal anomalies in 42 cases of prenatally diagnosed diaphragmatic hernia. Am J Med Genet 2001; 103:278.
322. Wohl ME, Griscom NT, Streider DJ, et al: The lung following repair of congenital diaphragmatic hernia. J Pediatr 1977;90:405.
323. Wung JT, Sahni R, Moffitt ST, et al: Congenital diaphragmatic hernia: Survival treated with very delayed surgery, spontaneous respiration, and no chest tube. J Pediatr Surg 1995;30:406.
324. Yamaguchi M, Kuwano H, Hashizume M, et al: Thoracoscopic treatment of Bochdalek hernia in the adult: Report of a case. Ann Thorac Cardiovasc Surg 2002; 8:106.
325. Yamataka T, Puri P: Pulmonary artery structural changes in pulmonary hypertension complicating congenital diaphragmatic hernia. J Pediatr Surg 1997;32:387.

第 61 章

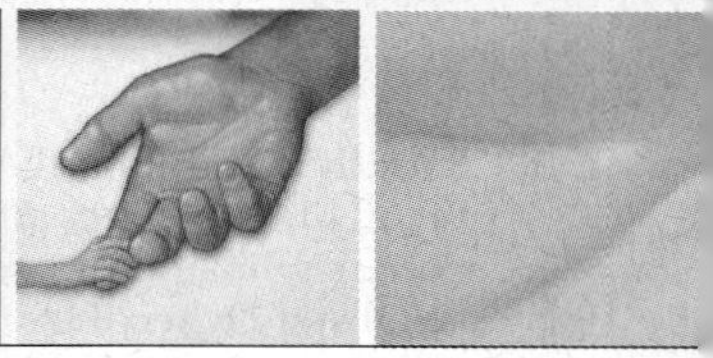

肺和纵隔囊肿

N. Scott Adzick 和 Diana L. Farmer

955 熟悉肺和纵隔的正常变异及潜在的病理畸形是必需的，因为在评价胸部平片时经常会出现问题。纵隔或肺部有囊性肿块的儿童，由于病变占据了胸腔空间，有发生肺部感染、呼吸困难和气道阻塞的可能，必须进行迅速的评价和治疗。在大多数儿童中，肺和纵隔囊肿的预后良好。

胚胎学

肺和纵隔囊肿在起源上是由发育性因素所致。纵隔肿块的胚胎发育，大多数情况下与前肠和胸腺有关。前肠最初可辨认的部分是覆盖有上皮的管腔，在妊娠第三周晚期，此时可以看到呼吸凹槽（气管芽）。在之后的 2 周时间内，食管和气管通过从头到尾的结构生长、前肠侧面包绕、从尾到头的分离这样一个过程，完成了分隔。在此期间，前肠上皮细胞增殖，在随后进行的管道化以前，增殖的前肠上皮细胞几乎完全湮没了食管腔。食管和气管上皮细胞之间的差别，可以在妊娠第 4 周时辨认。这个过程主要在妊娠第 32～34 天完成。可以推定在上皮细胞增殖期以后，不完全的管道在可导致前肠重复畸形囊肿。

作为成对出现的原基器官，胸腺从腹侧的第三个咽囊开始发育。在妊娠的第 7 周，原基器官向后向腹内侧延长，达到它们正常的位置，即主动脉弓的前方。这个时候，两个胸腺小叶通过结缔组织而不是实质相互连接在一起。在完全下降以前，胸腺原基含有一个胸腺咽导管，在胸腺完全下降以后就退化了。胸腺的不完全下降可能会导致颈部实质性的或囊性的肿块。胸腺咽导管没有退化可导致先天性的胸腺囊肿[118]。

产前的肺发育已经在第 60 章“先天性膈疝和膈膨升”中进行了描述。同时出现包括支气管源性囊肿、支气管肺隔离症、和先天性囊腺瘤样畸形的混合性的肺部病变，则提示了这些畸形的常见的胚胎联系，但是胚胎学上的精确病因还不清楚[81]。

肺囊性病变

诊断和治疗

囊性肺病变确切的发生率还不清楚，因为在文献中还没有基于人群进行的研究。先天性囊腺瘤样畸形最初是由 Chin 和 Tang 在 1949 年描述的一种独特的病理性疾病[27]。在这以前，先天性囊腺瘤样畸形连同支气管肺隔离症、先天性小叶性肺气肿和支气管源性囊肿一起，被归在先天性囊性肺疾病的总体诊断下面。

产前诊断提供了在子宫内观察胎儿肺部病变发展的机会，例如先天性囊腺瘤样畸形（CCAM）、支气管肺隔离症（BPS）和先天性小叶性肺气肿。对有肺部病变的胎儿进行一系列超声检查，有助于详细说明这些病变的自然病程，确定影响临床结果的病理生理学特征，并建立基于预后的治疗措施[1,34,86,112,128,131]。来自费城儿童医院、加利福尼亚大学、和旧金山的一组超过 175 例的产前诊断病例，发现预后整体上取决于肺部肿块的大小和继发性的生理紊乱：巨大的肿块可导致纵隔移位、正常肺组织的发育不全、羊水过多以及可以导致胎儿水肿和死亡的心血管损伤（图 61-1）[2]。

巨大的胎儿肺部病变对胎儿的发育具有可再生性 956
的病理生理学作用。胸腔肿块对食管的压迫妨碍到胎儿吞咽羊水，从而造成羊水过多。羊水过多是进行超声检查的常见的产科指征，因此对于许多巨大的胎儿

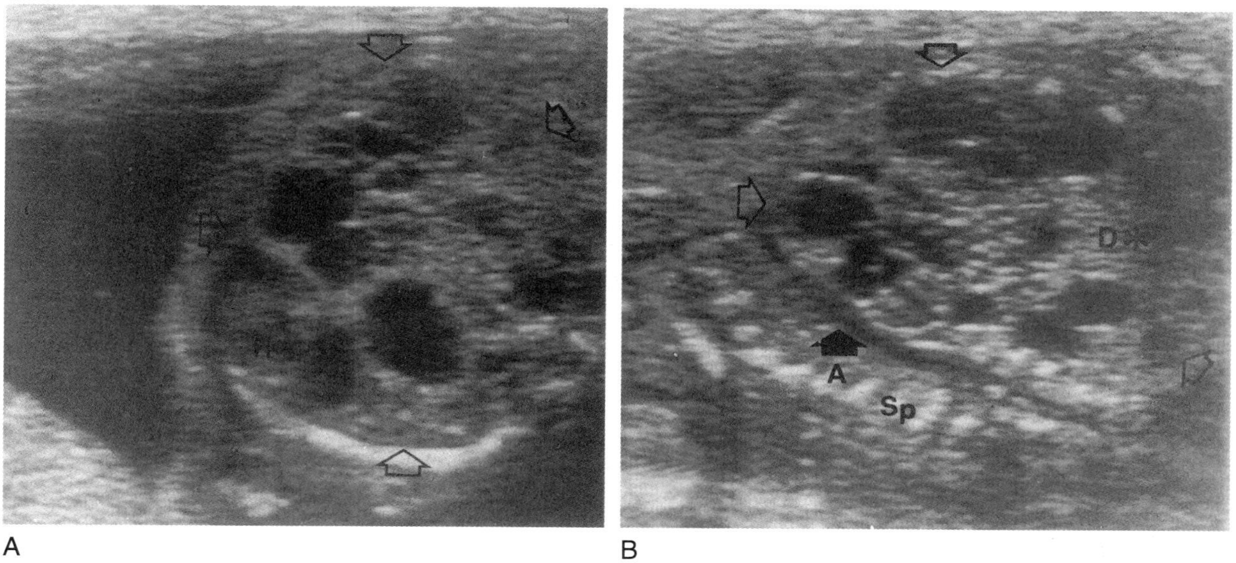

图 61-1　A. 妊娠第 22 周时胎儿胸部超声检查的横断面图像。一个巨大的多囊性肿块位于左半侧胸腔（空心箭头），将纵隔压迫到右侧。H：心脏；B. 胎儿胸部和腹部超声检查的矢状位图像显示，左半侧胸腔内有回波发生的肿块（空心箭头）压平了左侧的膈肌(D)。A：主动脉；Sp：脊柱。这种病变的生长可导致胎儿水肿。妊娠第 23 周时成功进行了受累侧肺叶的胎儿外科手术切除，妊娠第 35 周分娩，婴儿存活。

肺肿瘤具有产前诊断的标记意义。在羊水过多的病例中有一些胎儿的胃中缺乏液体支持了这一概念，经过有效的胎儿治疗后羊水过多就缓解了[2]。水肿继发于巨大肿瘤引起的极度纵隔移位所致的腔静脉阻塞和心脏压迫。就像先天性囊腺瘤样畸形一样，胎儿的支气管肺隔离症也可以导致胎儿水肿，可能是由于肿块压迫，或是胸膜积水的压力所致，这种胸腔积水是支气管肺隔离症分泌的液体或淋巴液导致的结果[2]。水肿是胎儿或新生儿将要死亡的一种预兆，表现为胎儿腹水、胸膜和心包渗出、皮肤和头皮的水肿。虽然羊水过多和水肿都与胎儿肺部病变之间存在有一些联系，但是经验表明任何一种情况都可以独立发生。

在新生儿时期，较小的胸腔病变可以导致呼吸窘迫，而最小的肿块可能没有症状，直到童年后期发生感染、气胸，或恶变的时候才出现症状。一系列的产前超声检查发现，巨大的胎儿肺肿瘤可以消退变小，这就说明了情况在胎儿时期可以改善[70,80,113]。尤其是，许多非囊性的支气管肺隔离症在出生以前大大缩小，出生以后不再需要治疗[2]。然而，在产前超声检查中似乎就已经消失并且不能在新生儿胸部平片中看到的胎儿肺肿瘤，仍然需要胸部 CT 扫描进行评估，因为 CT 扫描常常可发现病变[135]。

近来，胎儿先天性囊腺瘤样畸形的体积已经可以通过超声测量的方法来确定，采用计算扁长椭圆形的公式（长度 × 厚度 × 宽度 × 0.52）。头围可校正胎儿的大小，再除以先天性囊腺瘤样畸形的体积可得到先天性囊腺瘤样畸形体积比例（CVR）。CVR 大于 1.6 就预示着发生积水的风险较高，这些先天性囊腺瘤样畸形的胎儿中有 80%的病例会发生积水。CVR 可用于筛选有发生积水风险的胎儿，因此需要密切的超声观察和可能的胎儿干预[30]。连续的 CVR 检测显示，先天性囊腺瘤样畸形的生长通常到妊娠第 28 周达到一个平台。对于妊娠小于 28 周的胎儿，以及对于 CVR 数值较小的胎儿，开始时每周 1 次胎儿超声检查，如果 CVR 大于 1.6 则推荐每周 2 次超声检查。

发现水肿的胎儿发生胎儿或新生儿死亡的风险极高，所以对于囊性或实质性的肺部病变，需要进行胎儿外科手术切除大块增大的肺叶（胎儿肺叶切除术），或对主要是囊性病变的病例进行胸腔羊水分流[2,3,52]。在妊娠后期得出诊断的水肿性病变，可以通过采用子宫外产房外科治疗技术的病变切除手术改善。有肺部肿块但没有水肿的胎儿，可通过母亲转运、计划性分娩、新生儿评估和外科手术获得极好的机会得以存活。

对因肺部囊性病变而呼吸功能受损的新生儿，需要即刻进行手术切除囊性病变，通常是进行肺叶切除术。对大多数严重的病例，可能需要采用高频振荡通
957 气或体外膜肺氧合器来进行通气支持。在没有症状的囊性肺部病变的新生儿中，我们相信选择性切除手术是有理由的，因为囊性肺部病变有发生感染和潜在的发生恶变的风险[71]。在新生儿和幼儿中，恶性肿瘤主要是肺母细胞瘤和横纹肌肉瘤，而在年长儿和成年人中主要是支气管肺泡癌[15,31,89,106,132]。通过产后胸部静脉造影增强的 CT 扫描证实了先天性囊腺瘤样畸形（CCAM）的病变位置以后，我们推荐在出生后 1 个月或更晚一点时进行选择性的切除手术。一名有经验的小儿外科医生可以安全地进行胸廓切开和肺叶切除术而很少发生并发症，胸腔镜肺叶切除术也已经出现了[4]。早期的肺叶切除术也最大地补偿了肺的生长，长期随访显示术后患儿具有正常的肺功能[66,71]。与此相反的是，如果我们确信基于产后影像学检查得出的诊断正确，我们通常对一些没有症状的小的非囊性的小叶间支气管肺隔离症患者进行随访。我们不赞成采用插管和进行栓塞而不是选择手术切除的办法来治疗大的支气管肺隔离症。

先天性囊腺瘤样畸形

先天性囊腺瘤样畸形的特征是形成不同大小囊泡，造成终末细支气管“腺瘤样”的增加。先天性囊腺瘤样畸形是肺内部极度不连续的囊性肿块，直径从小于 1.0mm 到超过 10.0cm 不等。在组织学上，先天性囊腺瘤样畸形可通过以下几点区别于其他病变和正常的肺组织：（1）黏膜层的息肉样突出物；（2）在囊壁内平滑肌和弹性组织增厚；（3）缺乏软骨（除了在“残存的”正常支气管中发现的软骨）；（4）出现黏液分泌细胞；（5）没有炎症[122]。虽然在这些畸形的肺泡组织中没有正常的气体交换功能，但是与气管支气管树之间有交通，就如在出生后复苏过程中可能产生气体残存所证实的一般。Cha 已经鉴定出胎儿先天性囊腺瘤样畸形的两种组织学类型：假性腺体型和微管型[26]。Stocker 主要根据囊肿的大小定义了三种类型的先天性囊腺瘤样畸形（I～III 型）[122,123]，但是这种分类没有临床相关性。根据大体解剖和超声检查的发现，产前诊断的先天性囊腺瘤样畸形可以分为两个类型[1]。巨型囊肿病变包含了单囊性和多囊性病变，在产前超声检查中直径在 50mm 以上；而微囊性的病变在超声检查中显示为实质性回声的肿块。

产前诊断的先天性囊腺瘤样畸形的总体预后，主要取决于病变的大小而不是病变的类型，潜在的生长特性可能是重要的。手术切除的胎儿巨大先天性囊腺瘤样畸形的标本显示，与妊娠周数相匹配的正常胎儿的肺组织相比，细胞增殖增多，细胞凋亡显著下降[24]。在先天性囊腺瘤样畸形中，增加的细胞增殖或下调的细胞凋亡的因素分析，可以进一步认识这种肿瘤的发病机制，并可能提出新的治疗性措施。快速生长、进展出现水肿、需要在子宫内进行切除手术的胎儿先天性囊腺瘤样畸形，与正常胎儿的肺组织或是足月儿的先天性囊腺瘤样畸形的标本相比较，血小板衍生生长因子（PDGF）的基因表达和 PDGF 蛋白产物增多[76]。

先天性囊腺瘤样畸形通常源于肺的一叶，肺下叶是最为常见的发病部位。累及双侧肺叶的病变罕见。先天性囊腺瘤样畸形在左侧和右侧的发病率相当。对于那些没有在胎儿或新生儿时期得出诊断的患儿，通常的临床表现是发生先天性囊腺瘤样畸形区域的肺部感染，可能是由于病变处的细菌性病原体清除障碍所致。其他表现包括气胸、反应性气道疾病、生长发育迟滞。发病率没有性别之间的差异。在我们的经验中，相关的畸形非常罕见。

支气管肺隔离症

支气管肺隔离症是非功能性的肺组织肿块，由异常的体循环动脉提供血供，与天然的气管支气管树没有支气管连接。有两种类型的支气管肺隔离症：叶间型和叶内型。叶间型支气管肺隔离症完全独立于正常的肺，由单独的胸膜包裹，而叶内型的支气管肺隔离症与周围正常的肺组织混合。叶间型的支气管肺隔离症可以位于胸部、膈肌内部或膈下部。叶内型和叶间型支气管肺隔离症可以同时发生。整个肺都可以被隔离，双侧的支气管肺隔离症有报道，但是非常的罕见[89]。因为支气管肺隔离症起源于前肠，所以可能会发生食管或胃与支气管肺隔离症之间的交通，如果怀疑存在这种交通，就应该通过上消化道钡餐造影检查在术前进行排除[121]。支气管肺

隔离症的动脉血供，来源于膈下动脉膈上动脉，静脉回流可以到肺静脉或体循环静脉。异常的血液供应可能会因为通过支气管肺隔离症实质中大量的动脉静脉分流[104]或大量的咯血性失血或胸腔积血，导致高排性的心力衰竭[109]。

在产前超声检查中，支气管肺隔离症呈现为边界清晰、回声致密的均一性肿块。通过彩色血流多普勒探查后发现体循环动脉，或是来自主动脉到胎儿肺部病变的动脉，是胎儿支气管肺隔离症的诊断特征（图 61–2）[55]。然而，如果这种多普勒特征没有被探测到，那么一种回声致密的微囊性先天性囊腺瘤样畸形和支气管肺隔离症就可能有同样的产前超声检查的改变。超快速的胎儿磁共振成像有助于鉴别先天性囊腺瘤样畸形和支气管肺隔离症[102]。而且，产前得出诊断的胎儿肺部肿块，显示出先天性囊腺瘤样畸形和支气管肺隔离症的临床病理学特征（混合型病变），则提示有些肺部肿块具有共同的胚胎学基础[25,29,56]。在出生以前鉴别叶内型和叶间型支气管肺隔离症的能力是有限的，除非叶间型支气管肺隔离症通过胸膜渗出得到增强，或是位于腹腔内（通常紧靠左侧肾上腺）。叶内型支气管肺隔离症的特异性产前诊断，不具有诊断学意义的特征。

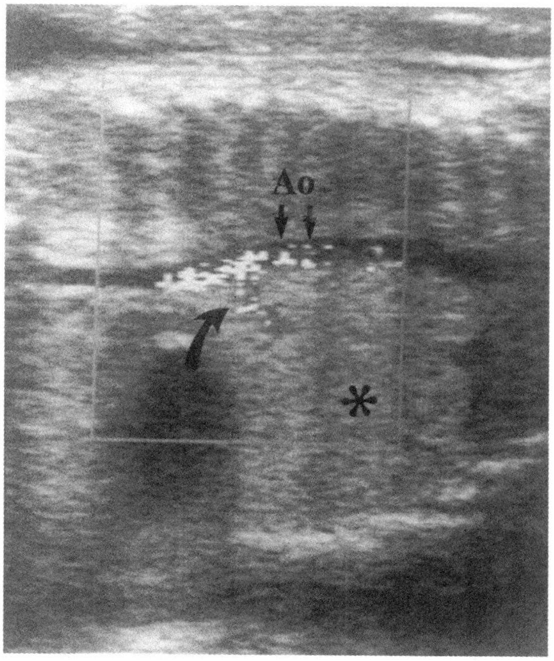

图 61–2 通过多普勒超声检查，起源于降主动脉（Ao）的体循环动脉（弯曲箭头）来供应肿块（*），符合肺隔离症的产前诊断。

叶间型支气管肺隔离症在男性多好发（男女比例 3∶1），以左侧更为常见，可以与一些疾病并发，例
如先天性膈疝、脊椎畸形和先天性心脏病。在先天性 958
膈疝的新生儿中，有接近 5%的病例伴有叶间型的支气管肺隔离症，其通常是在手术中偶然发现的。孤立而微小的非囊性叶间型支气管肺隔离症很少需要进行手术治疗。大多数叶内型支气管肺隔离症常见于肺下叶的中央基底段后侧基底段，左侧比右侧更为常见。累及肺上叶的支气管肺隔离症只出现在 10%～15%的病例中。对于那些没有在产前得出诊断的病例，叶内型支气管肺隔离症在出生以后通常的表现是反复发作性肺炎，甚至是在支气管肺隔离症中形成脓肿；因此需要进行手术切除（通常是肺叶切除术）。必须要识别和结扎来自体循环动脉的滋养血管，通常在肺下叶的韧带中发现。

先天性小叶型肺气肿

对于先天性小叶型肺气肿的数种病因已经进行了描述[79]，但是基本的发病机制是受累支气管允许吸入的空气通过，但是只限制呼气时空气的排出，这就导致了肺叶的过度膨胀。气体困在肺气肿性肺叶中可能是由于：（1）发育不良的支气管软骨产生了一种球阀效应，或是完全的支气管闭锁[35,133]；（2）浓缩的黏液[130]或是广泛的黏膜增殖和折叠，形成了支气管内的梗阻[54]；（3）异常的心肺血管或是增大的心室腔，对支气管造成了外在的压迫[44]；（4）弥漫性的支气管异常，可能与或不与感染有关[74]。术前进行仔细的支气管镜检查，有助于排除支气管内的梗阻性病变[35]。先天性小叶型肺气肿最常见的病变部位是左肺上叶（40%～50%）、其次是右肺中叶（30%～40%）、右肺上叶（20%）、肺下叶（1%），剩余的发生在多个不同的部位。

在早产儿中，与支气管肺发育不良治疗相关的气压性创伤可以导致获得性肺气肿，可以在多个区域出现充气过度[11]。因为气管内插管位置的关系，在这些病例中累及右肺下叶的肺气肿比较常见，有助于鉴别获得性肺气肿和先天性肺气肿。首先由 Hislop 和 Reid 描述的多泡的和多泡性肺叶，见于先天性小叶型肺气肿的一些病例中[57]。在这种疾病中，肺泡总量

增长了数倍，但是气道和动脉在数量、大小和结构上与年龄相符合。因为受累肺叶的气体交换受到损害，这种多泡性肺叶在胸片中就变得过度膨胀和过于透亮。

在产前超声检查中，先天性小叶型肺气肿可以区别于其他囊性的肺部病变，相对于微小囊性的先天性囊腺瘤样畸形，回声深度和声波反射性都有所增加；相对于支气管肺隔离症，缺乏来自体循环动脉的血液供应[8,92]。在妊娠 28 周以前，这些病变进行性增大，可能是由于胎儿肺液滞留在肺叶中，类似于出生以后所见到的空气滞留。在妊娠晚期，小叶型肺气肿可能在大小和肿块的特征上发生消退，不能与周围正常的胎儿肺组织进行鉴别[92]。出生以后进行评估是非常重要的，因为在肺气肿性肺叶中存在出生后空气滞留的风险。在出生的时候，因为胎儿肺液清除延迟，受累肺叶在胸片上可能是不透X射线的。产前诊断的主干型支气管闭锁可导致大面积的肺增大、水肿和胎儿死亡；超快速的胎儿磁共振可以显示出整个肺脏受累，主干闭锁远端的支气管扩张[65]。

在大约 25%的病例中，先天性小叶型肺气肿是在出生时得出的诊断，到出生后 1 个月时大约有 50%的病例可以做出诊断。在出生 6 个月以后得出诊断的病例是偶尔发生的。越早出现症状，越有可能发生进行性的小叶型肺气肿，需要进行手术切除。不过，一些婴幼儿只有非常轻微的症状，没有发生进展，肺气肿性肺叶持续稳定，不会侵占周围正常的肺组织，所以对这些病例不需要进行手术切除[93]。除了胸片和 CT（图 61–3），通气–血流扫描可以显示氙放射性同位素在受累肺叶中的摄取和洗净被延迟，很少有血流经过。如果出现呼吸窘迫和肺叶的过度膨胀，那么主流的治疗措施是手术切除肺气肿性肺叶。正压通气可以导致肺叶内突发性的大量空气滞留并伴有心肺功能不全，所以对于外科医生来说，重要的是在麻醉诱导期间要在场，以防需要进行急诊胸廓切开术。手术过程中，受累肺叶将特征性地“突出” 到胸廓切开术的切口外。高频振荡通气[45]、选择性支气管插管[42]、和内镜下肺气肿性肺
959 叶[96]减压术，在呼吸窘迫患者的术前处理中可能是有效的措施。先天性小叶型肺气肿行肺叶切除后，远期的肺生长和肺功能都很好。

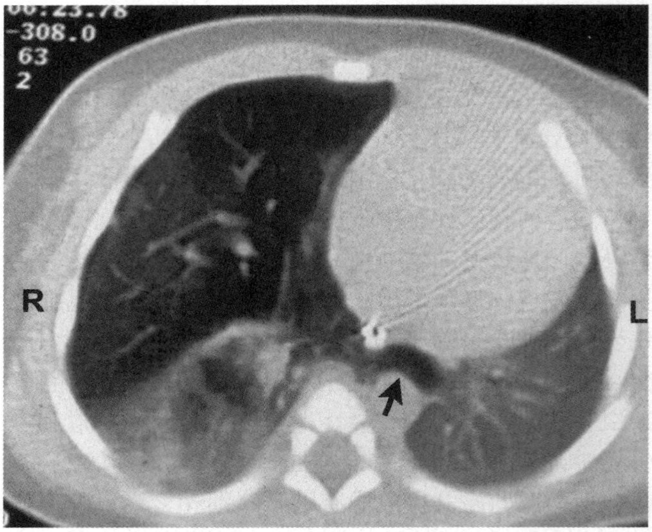

图 61–3 先天性小叶型肺气肿累及右肺中叶的新生儿的胸部 CT 扫描图像。右肺中叶的空气体积发生膨胀，伴有压迫性的右肺下叶的肺膨胀不全。纵隔移位到左侧，肺气肿性肺叶经中线疝出到心脏的后方（箭头所示）。

囊性纵隔病变

临床特征

纵隔内病变的临床表现主要是肿块作用的结果，可受到胸腔内病变位置的影响。许多纵隔内病变是没有症状的，但是在前、中纵隔肿块的最为重要的症状是呼吸窘迫，尤其是在婴幼儿开始吵闹的时候，在喂养时可看到患儿出现喘鸣的呼吸音或是发绀[67]。年长儿童，可发生咳嗽、胸痛、呼吸困难、端坐呼吸，或是罕见的咯血[20]。在所有的年龄组中，呼吸窘迫可能是致命性的症状[9,10,61,98,108]。呼吸窘迫或上腔静脉梗阻急性发作提示为淋巴瘤[67,100]。虽然罕见，但是有报道感染性的畸胎瘤可以破裂并进入支气管、胸膜、肺动脉和心包中[20,94,110]。后纵隔肿块可以非常大而没有症状，经常是因为其他原因拍摄胸片时偶尔发现的。较少见的情况是，因疼痛或脊髓压迫症状而被发现[75,115]。

来自个别医疗中心的关于纵隔肿块的报道可能会有选择性的结果偏倚。如果将最近的一系列病例与那些在 1967 年以前（表 61–1）发表的病例进行比较，恶性肿瘤有所增加，尤其是淋巴瘤和神经母细胞瘤有明显的增加[19,48,49,51,67,100,110,114,115]。就如来自 Walter Reed

表 61-1 不同的纵隔肿瘤的发生率

囊肿/肿瘤	King 等，1982 年[67]	Simpson 和 Campbell，1991 年[116]	Saenz 等，1993 年[111]	Cohen 等，1991 年[28]	Grosfeld，1994 年[49]	总数	%
神经源性肿瘤							
神经母细胞瘤 / 神经节神经母细胞瘤	20	16	32	13	50	277	33
神经节瘤	17	9	14	8	14		
神经纤维瘤	4	4	3		2		
神经鞘瘤 /schwann 细胞瘤	6	1	3	1	5		
副神经节瘤（嗜铬细胞瘤）	1		2				
原发性神经外胚层的肿瘤 / 神经肉瘤			2				
淋巴瘤							
Hodgkin 病	33	29	34	1	49	281	41
非 Hodgkin 病	54	34	6	3	38		
生殖细胞肿瘤							
畸胎瘤样皮样囊肿							
良性	8	7	2	4	18	50	7
恶性	7						
精原细胞瘤 / 胚胎癌	1				3		
间叶细胞肿瘤							
淋巴管瘤（囊性）/ 囊性水囊瘤	3	3	1	3	11	50	7
血管瘤	2				1		
纤维瘤 / 纤维肉瘤	1				1		
脂肪瘤 / 脂肪肉瘤 / 肉瘤	12		3	1	3		
横纹肌肉瘤	5						
囊肿							
心包囊肿		1		1		35	7
支气管源性囊肿	6	7		7			
肠源性囊肿	2	3		5			
神经管原肠性 / 其他				3			
胸腺的病变				2		17	2.5
胸腺囊肿	2	1		3			
胸腺增生				2	3		
胸腺瘤	2			1			
胸腺癌		1					
其他混合性病变							
肉芽肿、脓肿、纤维化	2	5	3	4	3	17	
总数	188	121	105	62	201	677	

军队医院[28]的一个大型报告，其中的回顾性综述比较了 1970 年前后 60 年的治疗经验。纵隔肿块流行病学的最佳评估，是由来自澳大利亚维多利亚的纵隔肿块回顾性病理研究所提供的，评估了 900 000 名儿童。在那组病例中，50%的纵隔肿块是淋巴瘤，20%的纵隔肿块是神经源性的，8%的病例是前肠重复畸形性囊肿，6%的病例是畸胎瘤[116]。这个流行病学数据类似于美国近来的一组流行病学调查数据（见表 61–1）。

解剖学因素

清楚理解纵隔的亚解剖结构有助于鉴别诊断和诊断性检查的选择。纵隔是胸腔中央的空间，侧面的界限是右侧和左侧的壁层胸膜，前面是胸骨，后面是椎体，包括横突，上面是胸廓入口，下面是膈肌。虽然有多种将纵隔分成亚区的分类方法，但是这里采用的是经典的解剖学描述[82]。任何解剖亚结构分类系统的价值是为了提供对那个区域的内容物的认识，简化了鉴别诊断。

上纵隔定界为上面到胸廓入口，下面到第四胸椎下限和胸骨柄连接处的平面。侧面的边界是壁层胸膜。这个亚区的正常解剖学内容物是胸腺、其他淋巴结结构、间叶细胞来源的组织，包括脉管系统，遍及整个纵隔都可以广泛地见到。

前纵隔的区域后面到心包，前面到胸骨，下面到膈肌，上面到平胸骨柄连接处水平。这个空间内正常情况下含有间叶细胞来源的组织、脂肪、和结缔组织。

中纵隔由心包和大血管起端定界。因此，它的正常内容物是心包、心脏、大血管、淋巴管和间叶细胞来源的组织。

后纵隔的轮廓为前面是心包和大血管，后面为脊柱，就如在前面每一个亚区一样，侧面为壁层胸膜。它的内容物包括气管、主支气管、食管、广泛分布的淋巴结构、交感神经的神经节、降主动脉、奇静脉系统和胸导管。

巨大的肿块或弥漫性病变可能越过多个亚区的边界。鉴别诊断中有帮助的另外一个条件是年龄。除了后纵隔的神经母细胞瘤以外，幼儿的纵隔肿块最可能是原位生长。也会提及非囊性的纵隔肿块。

诊断和治疗

对囊性纵隔肿块的认识最初可能开始于胎儿的
超声检查[69,83,88]。发生进展性非免疫性水肿、心力衰 960
竭，或纵隔移位伴有对正常发育的肺组织压迫的胎儿，可能会从子宫内减压术或手术切除囊性纵隔病变中受益[84]。

对于囊性纵隔肿块，出生后最初的诊断性检查应该是前后位和侧位的胸部 X 光片。经常可以基于胸部平片上病变的位置得出假定性的诊断。作为术前评估的一部分，现在 CT 扫描已经在很大程度上替代了内镜和食管 X 光片检查。造影剂增强 CT 扫描和 MRI 的多个比较研究显示，CT 比较优越，有能力在肿块中间确定钙化斑[13,59]。如果怀疑累及到脊髓，或考虑到可能有血管病变，MRI 检查就比较有效。食管 X 光片检查揭示了前肠重复畸形性囊肿的外在特征性的肿块效应，但是 CT 扫描可能是对这种诊断最为有效的检查。超声心动描记术在确定心包轮廓增大[47]的新生儿是否有罕见的心包内畸胎瘤方面具有很大的价值，还可以发现先天性心脏病。

术前诊断小组的目标是帮助确定最佳的手术方式。当纵隔肿块的性质还不清楚，或存在潜在恶变的时候，应该抽取术前血清标本以测定甲胎蛋白或 β–人类绒毛膜促性腺激素的水平，尤其是在前纵隔肿瘤的病例中。类似的，怀疑后纵隔肿块时，应该要检查尿液中儿茶酚胺的分解代谢产物。

在诊断的同时进行手术切除是良性纵隔囊肿和肿瘤的首选治疗方法。有手术指征时，可以进行胸腔镜切除或活检，具有良好的结果和较少的致病率[32,64,78]。巨大的前纵隔肿块最佳的手术途径是胸骨正中切开
术，中纵隔和后纵隔肿块最佳的手术途径是后外侧的 961
胸廓切开术。

前纵隔和上纵隔

前纵隔和上纵隔中包含了胸腺、大血管和淋巴网络结构，同时还有结缔组织和脂肪组织。淋巴瘤是最为常见的肿瘤，其次是畸胎瘤、生殖细胞肿瘤、水囊状淋巴管瘤和胸腺的病变（图 61–4）。在婴幼儿中，前纵隔的肿块通常是畸胎瘤或是增大的胸腺。

在评估前纵隔的肿块时，首先评估的是恶性肿瘤

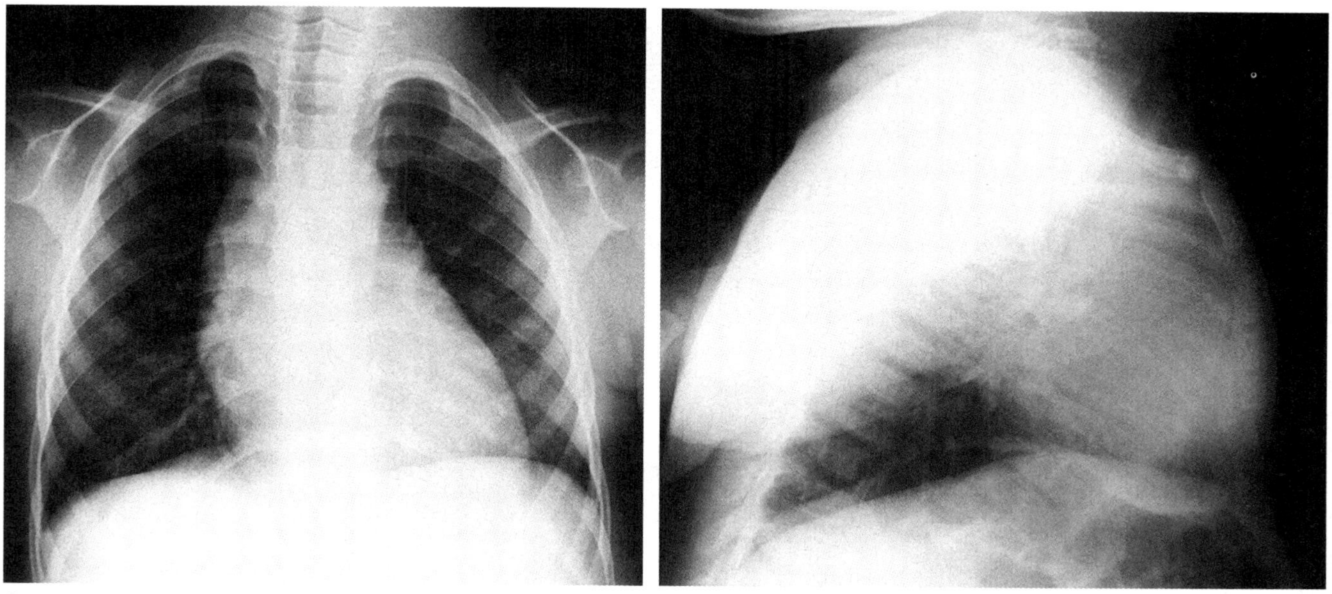

A B

图 61-4 一名 5 岁大的男孩出现前上纵隔肿块，在前后位胸部平片（A）中显示出与心包的轮廓是分开的。侧位胸片（B）揭示胸骨柄突出，肿块位于气管前方。该肿块证实为畸胎瘤。

发生的风险。恶性疾病如淋巴瘤，一般出现在较年长的儿童中，经常伴有全身症状和别处的淋巴结增大，通常有气道受累症状。只要有可能，诊断应该从非纵隔来源开始寻找，例如骨髓、胸水，或其他结节样组织，因此避免进行全身麻醉[6,49,84]。如果气道受累时仍然没有得出诊断，应用皮质类固醇可以减少手术活检的风险而不会影响诊断的精确性。淋巴瘤在第 35 章中进行讨论。

胸腺

胸腺囊肿可见于前纵隔和颈部（图 61-5 和 61-6）。它们通常没有症状，但是也可以发生感染或出血，或因为肿块的作用而产生症状，可能会造成不可接受的外观。囊肿内衬有纤毛、呼吸上皮细胞；含有淋巴细胞以及正常的胸腺组织；经常显示出有炎症和肉芽肿性改变。胸腺脂肪瘤是一种良性的肿瘤，可能是一种错构瘤，混合有脂肪和胸腺组织。手术切除可以得出诊断，并治愈。

胸腺瘤在儿童中罕见，占到纵隔肿瘤的不到 1%，在文献中只有 20 例记录完好的儿童恶性胸腺瘤的病例。这些肿瘤起源于胸腺上皮细胞，通常是侵袭性生长[21]。治疗可有多种方式，但是疗效不佳。

虽然胸腺位于前纵隔和上纵隔，但是异位的胸腺组织可见于颈部和后纵隔[7,12,119]。良性的胸腺组织增生是胸腺的一种生理性增大，不再被认为可导致呼吸阻碍，但是对于快速的胸腺增大，有些学者还是建议进行手术切除[77,107]。如果有必要的话，短期内给予泼尼松治疗可以使正常的胸腺缩小，有助于与非淋巴来源的纵隔肿块相鉴别。MRI 也是一种有效的鉴别诊断手段[17,119]。纵隔放射疗法在历史上曾经是热点，只是因为它与甲状腺癌有不可接受的高度相关而被放弃。只有当恶性肿瘤不能被排除时才推荐进行纵隔探查，就像良性的结节样胸腺增生一样。结节样胸腺增生通常没有症状，在偶尔进行的胸片检查中经常作为上纵隔的肿块被发现。CT 扫描显示为胸腺小叶中的一种实质性不对称的没有增强的肿块。外周血和骨髓检查都正常。在这些情况下手术探查揭示为胸腺小叶内的一种淋巴样肿块，组织上会压迫邻近正常的胸腺。分析肿块中的淋巴细胞可显示，T淋巴细胞和 B 细胞的比 962
例正常。现在，大多数的胸腺病变都可以采用胸腔镜技术进行切除。

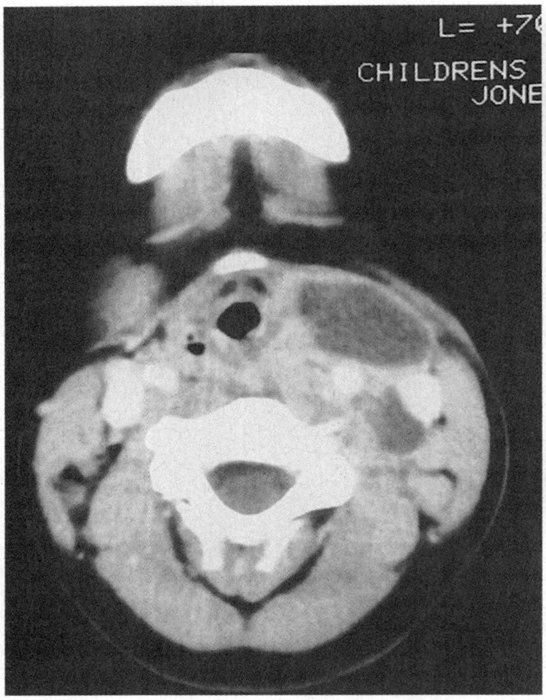

A

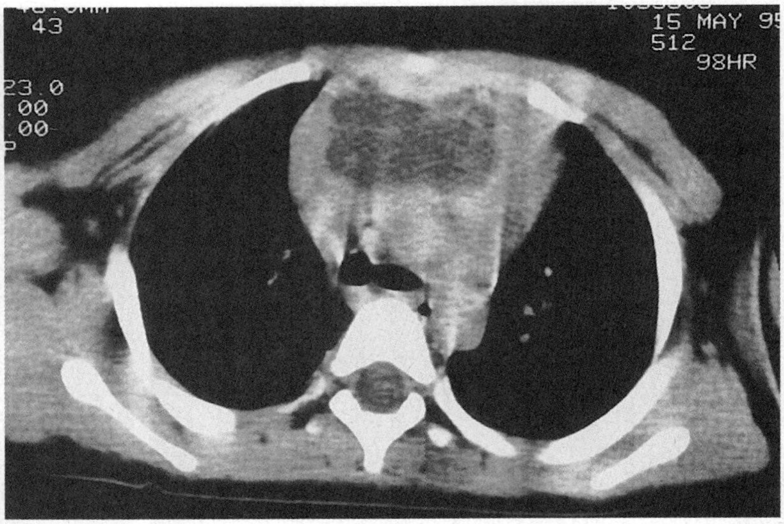

B

图 61-5 因左侧颈部饱满而进行 CT 扫描，显示出左侧一个胸腺囊肿位于颈部血管的前方，并且延伸到前纵隔隆凸水平（A）和隆凸以下（B）。

畸胎瘤、皮样囊肿和生殖细胞肿瘤

在淋巴瘤之后，畸胎瘤是最为常见的前纵隔肿瘤。也有报道称可在纵隔的其他亚区发现这些肿瘤[62]。畸胎瘤的特征是同时具有囊性和实质性的成分，起源于至少两个胚层，大多数情况下通常是来源于全部的三个生殖细胞胚层[22]。关于畸胎瘤的起源存在一些争论，因为它们可以发生在从大脑到肛门的中线或中线附近。一种观点是畸胎瘤表现为性腺外生殖细胞肿瘤的一种成熟的类型[32]。另一种观点是畸胎瘤来源于未分化的胚胎细胞。世界卫生组织将畸胎瘤归类为生殖细胞肿瘤[75]。根据定义，皮样囊肿只是外胚层和中胚层起源的肿块。皮样囊肿是成熟的、良性肿块，经常包裹在一种纤维性的厚壁囊内，包含有各种不同的皮肤附属物，包括毛发和牙齿。真正的畸胎瘤可以是某些最大的、最为罕见的肿瘤，其中有恶性的成分，尤其是当诊断被延误时会发现有恶性的成分。

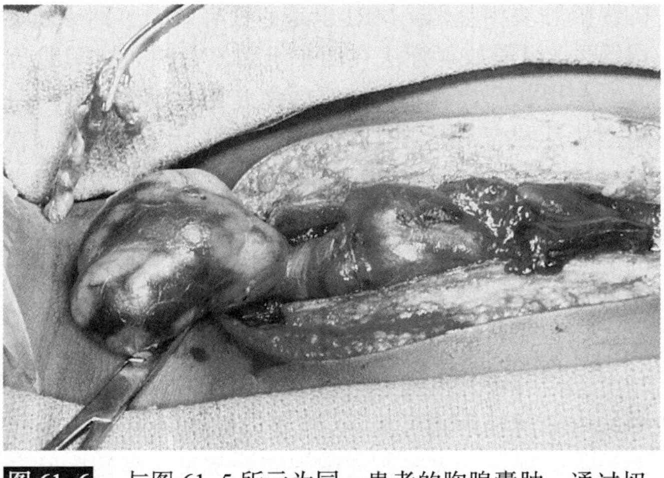

图 61-6 与图 61-5 所示为同一患者的胸腺囊肿，通过切开胸骨从纵隔游离，此图为切除颈部延伸肿瘤的图像。

在年轻的患者中，畸胎瘤通常是良性肿瘤。在所有的年龄组中，只有 25%的畸胎瘤是恶性的[129]。因为并不总是能够在术前就确定畸胎瘤是否完全成熟，所以在所有患者中都应该检测甲胎蛋白或 β-人类绒毛膜促性腺激素的水平。如果出现恶性成分，则最为常见的是卵黄囊源性的，目前术语中称作“内胚窦肿瘤”[36]。

心包外畸胎瘤的症状和体征可以是任何压迫性前纵隔肿块的表现，例如呼吸促迫或喘鸣。虽然有报道称畸胎瘤破裂后可进入邻近的结构，但是这是一种罕见的事件[94,129]。心包内畸胎瘤在新生儿和婴幼儿中更为常见，表现为心排出量下降。心包内畸胎瘤总是为良性的，起源于主动脉根与主肺动脉之间的动脉沟内。

在胸部平片和 CT 扫描中，肿块通常不对称，位于前纵隔内，经常扩展到右半胸或左半胸。经常可以看到柔毛状的钙化斑。前纵隔的畸胎瘤通常最好通过进入。尽管畸胎瘤体积较大，但是血液供应经常是不充分的。具有恶性成分的肿瘤例外，术前主动脉造影可
963 以显示出后纵隔的畸胎瘤动脉血供起源于主动脉[60,62]。

中纵隔

在经典的解剖学描述中，中纵隔是以心包为界的区域[82]。因而，心包囊肿可能是唯一真正常见的中纵隔囊肿。心包囊肿是良性的，薄壁而含有液体的囊肿内衬间皮细胞。有一种假说认为心包起源于间充质中一系列不连续的腔隙，后来发生联合并形成心包囊。偶然情况下，这些腔隙中的一个腔隙作为心包囊肿而持续存在。心包囊肿几乎总是没有症状，经常是在常规的胸片或尸体解剖中发现。经典的描述是位于前胸部任何一个心膈沟内的囊性肿块，但右侧更为常见。以前，胸廓切开术是推荐的确定最终诊断的方法。目前，CT 扫描提供了足够的特征性改变，可以进行精确诊断，因此除非心包囊肿巨大，可以不进行干预。如果心包囊肿诊断没有明确，也可以在胸腔镜下进行切除或除去顶。

后纵隔

后纵隔位于气管分叉前平面的后方，向后伸展至脊椎旁沟[82]。后纵隔是儿童发生各种囊肿、肿瘤、和炎症病变的部位。这些病变中最为常见的是交感神经系统的肿瘤，从良性到恶性的各种不同的神经源性肿瘤。在年幼儿童中，最为常见的肿瘤是恶性神经母细胞瘤，在年长的儿童中最为常见的肿瘤则是良性的神经节瘤；这两种肿瘤都在第 28 章中进行讨论。

前肠重复畸形性囊肿

前肠重复畸形性囊肿在儿童医学中心中相当常见。这些病变的名称显著不同。在临床上和病理学上可以分为以下几类：（1）小肠重复畸形和囊肿（内衬小肠上皮）；（2）支气管源性的囊肿（内衬呼吸上皮）；（3）神经肠源性囊肿（伴脊椎畸形，或与神经系统有联系）。肠源性是一个历史上易被混淆的术语，在各种不同的报道中包括了上述每一种分类。共同的名称前肠重复畸形性囊肿是一种更为精确的胚胎学描述，根据囊壁黏膜层的组织学，再分为支气管源性或小肠重复畸形性囊肿。事实上，所有的三种内胚层起源的囊肿都可以见于偶尔发现的前肠重复畸形中，这就支持了前肠重复畸形性囊肿是一种常见的胚胎源性囊肿。

支气管源性的囊肿

支气管源性的囊肿（图 61–7）起源于气管憩室
或前肠腹侧的异常出芽。这些囊肿可见于各种不同的 964
部位，从食管旁到气管旁、肺门周围或肺实质内[91]，发生的部位取决于前肠或气管支气管树发育过程中异常出芽的水平。已经有报道称，大约 2/3 的支气管源性囊肿位于肺实质内，余下的囊肿位于纵隔中；但是这种分布在不同的报道中有所不同。罕见情况是，它们也可见于距离较远的部位，例如舌头、颈部、背部，甚至是在膈下[18,40,51,101,127]。

组织学上，支气管源性的囊肿是一种薄壁的、内衬支气管上皮的、充满黏液的囊肿。它们可以单发或多发，呈白色或略带桃色。有报道这些囊肿的壁中有软骨成分，可能会存在气液平面。左侧或右侧囊肿的发生率相当。虽然支气管源性的囊肿与气管支气管树之间通常没有交通，但是有可能从一开始就有交通，或可能是重复感染所引起的后天性交通。

年长儿童的诊断，经常是在非相关疾病拍摄的胸片中偶尔发现肿块。婴幼儿经常表现为呼吸道症状，因为并发肺膨胀不全和感染，所以囊肿在胸片上可能是模糊不清的（图 61–8 和 61–9）[37,73,120]。在这种情况下，诊断可能被耽误，但是 CT 扫描通常可以证实诊断。支气管源性的囊肿也可以在产前超声检查，以及因其他疾病行食管造影检查中被发现。鉴别诊断包括异物、小叶性肺气肿、肺炎、支气管狭窄和气胸。

支气管源性的囊肿应该进行切除以避免感染、出血、或是在压力下快速膨胀而导致突然死亡等并发

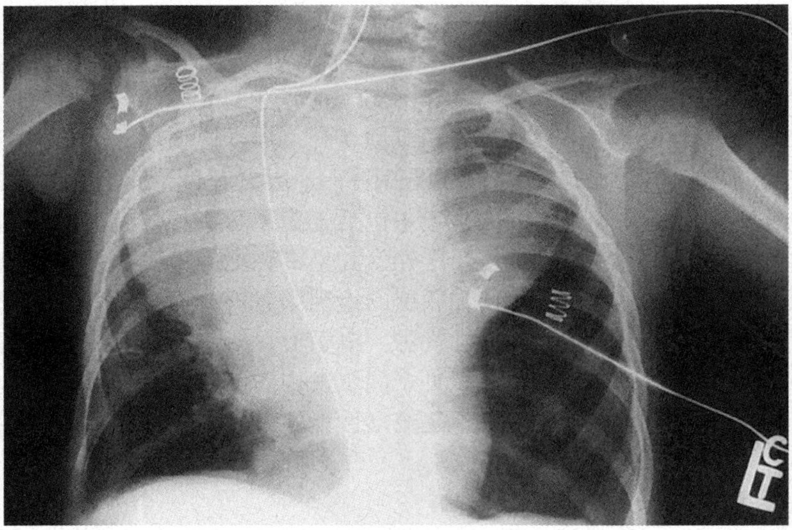

A

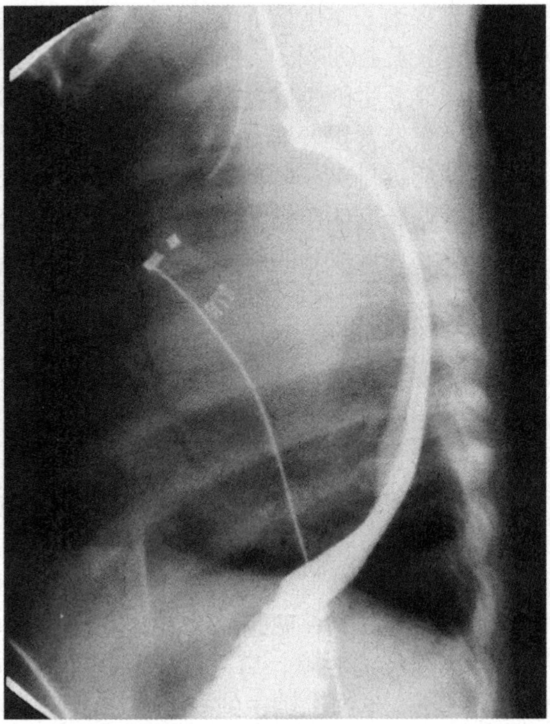

B

图 61–7 A. 支气管源性的囊肿。这名 15 个月大的男婴因病情紧急而转移到重症监护病房，显示出中央气管支气管受压迫伴有呼吸窘迫。他因为哮喘症状已经治疗了一年。B. 侧位图像显示出明显的气管压迫伴有气管食管的分离，通过食管内造影得到证实。

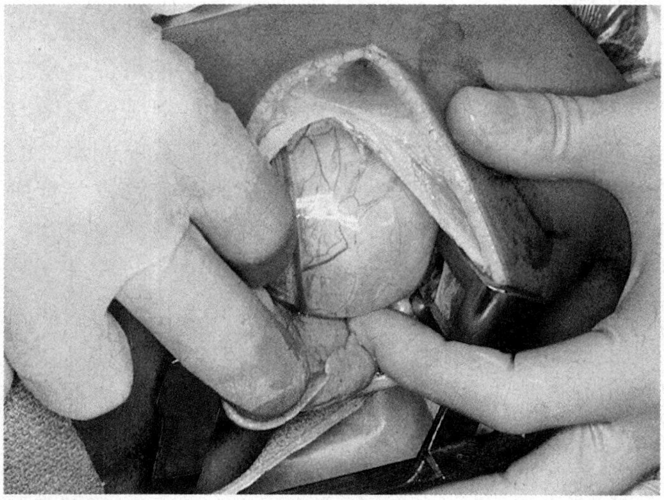

图 61–8 为图 61–7 所示的同一患者，行急诊胸廓切开术显示有巨大的单房性囊肿。吸引出感染性的黏液以缓解心动过慢，然后从其气管后侧的粘连处切除。显微镜检查的图像显示在图 61–9 中。

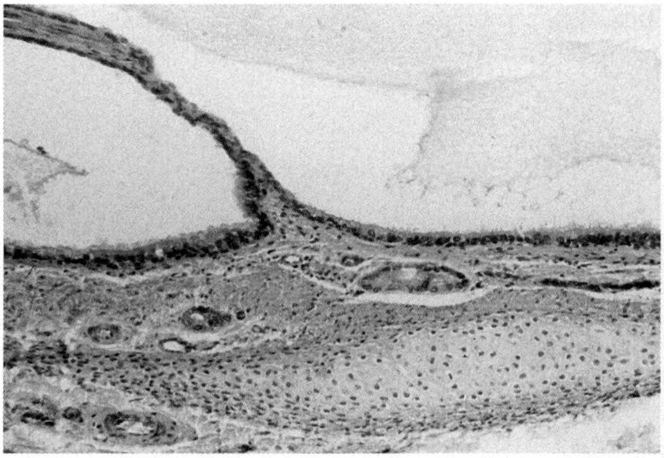

图 61–9 显微镜下，这种支气管源性囊肿壁内衬有纤毛的呼吸上皮，含有支气管软骨，支气管源性囊肿的特征和证据显示，它们是中央支气管发育畸形（与囊腺瘤样畸形不同的是，它是一种外周实质性病变）。

症。恶变的风险确实存在，就如有报道称，2 例成年支气管源性囊肿患者出现恶变，1 例 8 岁大的女孩的支气管源性囊肿变成了腺癌[125]。手术切除囊肿不能损伤到支气管或食管。肺门处的小型囊肿直到纵隔胸膜被打开以后才会被看到。通常是直接切除囊肿，但是偶尔可能需要进行局限性肺实质切除或肺叶切除术。对大多数患者，支气管源性囊肿可以进行胸腔镜下囊肿切除术[33,64]。由于诊断的错误可能会导致不必要的气肿性肺组织切除，而不是导致支气管梗阻的囊肿切除。推荐进行完整的囊肿切除术，有报道称不完全切除囊肿以后 25 年仍然有复发[105]。虽然有经支气管进行引流手术的报道，但是我们不推荐这种手术方式[95]。

肠重复畸形性囊肿

肠重复畸形性囊肿起源于在前肠发育早期出现的空泡融合障碍。这些囊肿内衬食管上皮或胃上皮，周围有平滑肌包绕。它们曾经被认为是各种不同的肠源性或小肠源性囊肿、食管囊肿、肠囊肿和食管重复畸形。经常可以看到胃黏膜，也有壁内残留肾上腺皮质的报道[136]。肠源性囊肿可位于整个后纵隔和颈部。虽然最常见的是与食管共壁，它们可以与食管腔有完全的交通，或是完全隔离于起源结构的囊肿。已经报道了许多巨大的胸腹部肠源性囊肿，或是一个盲端位于
965 腹腔内，或者是与胃、空肠、回肠或胰管有交通[51,99]。有报道称 1 个小肠重复畸形的病例，在支气管镜检查时发生了胆汁反流，囊肿穿透了膈肌，使隆凸与胆管树交通[73]。肠重复畸形性囊肿合并畸形的发生率为 12%。这种病例中大多数是其他的小肠重复畸形[58]。2 例产前诊断的胸腔内小肠重复畸形性囊肿合并有积水的病例，采用在子宫内放置胸腔羊水分流管来治疗[39]。

在大多数病例中，肠源性囊肿在出生时没有症状。胸片和 CT 扫描是诊断的主要方式（图 61–10 至 61–12）。虽然 ^{99m}Tc 高锝酸盐、腹部超声检查、吞钡检查或 MRI 偶尔都可能有助于诊断，但是术前检查的目标不是为了尽量得出最终的诊断，而是为了提供足够的信息以便制订手术计划。治疗措施是完整的手术切除，或是通过胸廓切开术，或是通过胸腔镜。如有必要，就如在长管状重复畸形中一般，前肠重复畸形的内衬黏膜可以剥除，留下完整的共同肌肉壁[124]。不再推荐进行袋形缝合术。这些囊肿是良性病变，应该保证食管的完整性。

神经管原肠性囊肿

神经管原肠性囊肿是罕见的、与脊髓管（有时候是硬脑膜）有交通的前肠重复畸形。虽然它们以最常见的胸廓内肿块的形式出现，但是也可能以脊髓腔内肿块的形式出现。囊性后纵隔肿块和邻近的半椎体共存时，应该提高警惕，小心神经肠管性囊肿以及前面的脊髓脊膜突出[14]。神经肠管性囊肿被认为是在发育早期形成的，当时脊索和前肠在一起，或是完全性的分离障碍，或是前肠内胚层疝出到背侧的外胚层所致[68,97]。

在组织学上，神经肠管性囊肿具有消化道黏膜和发育完好的肌层管壁，没有浆膜层。可能存在胃黏膜，因此可以出现炎症和溃疡的体征[68]。症状经常包括疼痛或神经系统症状（或同时发生）。当后纵隔肿 966
块伴有椎体畸形时，建议进行 MRI 检查。需要即刻进行手术切除。由于脑膜炎而导致的截瘫和死亡也有报道[97]。虽然有些作者报道了手术中可留下神经交通管道，但是大多数的学者推荐进行完整的切除，如果有必要的话同时进行椎板切除术[14,16,38]。

其他各种各样的病变都是罕见的后纵隔囊性肿块的诊断。前面的胸段脑(脊)膜膨出可见于年长儿，被认为是脊椎畸形有关的进展性退行性病变[134]。MRI应该可以鉴别这种病变和神经肠管性囊肿。

其他间叶细胞来源的囊性肿瘤

间叶细胞来源性肿瘤可以发生在整个纵隔中，可能会妨碍到气道。它们起源于结缔组织、淋巴组织、平滑肌和横纹肌、脂肪和血管。作为一组肿瘤，它们只占儿童纵隔肿块的不到 5%。

起源于血管和淋巴管的间叶细胞肿瘤在儿童中最为常见，尤其是淋巴管瘤（囊性水囊瘤）。在大多数患者中，淋巴管瘤表现为延伸到上纵隔或后纵隔的颈部病变；然而，也可以发生纵隔的淋巴管瘤[43,87]。这些肿瘤在组织平面内通过内衬内皮细胞的出芽增殖生

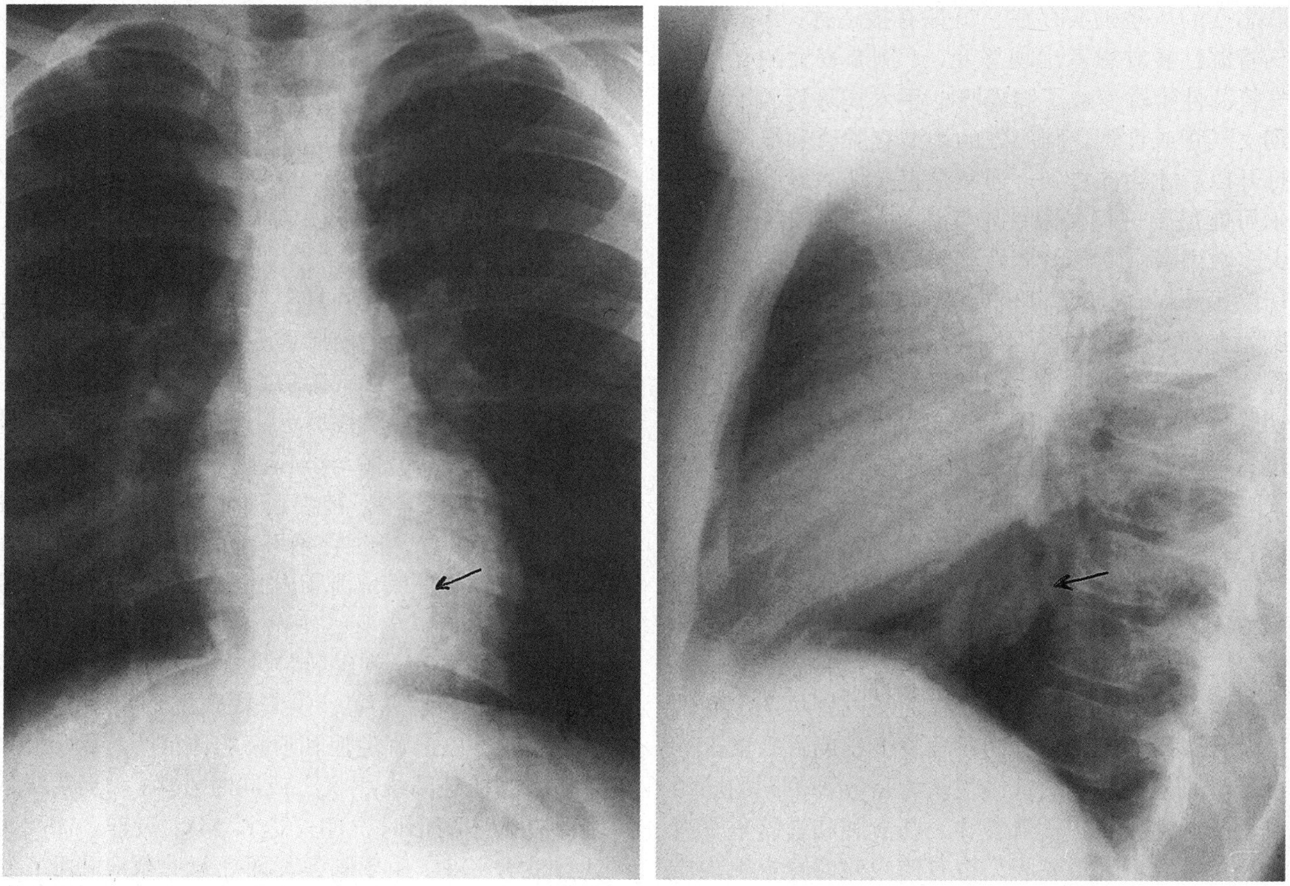

A B

图 61–10 A. 前后位胸部平片中，偶然发现的没有症状的纵隔肿块，位于心脏轮廓后方（箭头所示）。B. 侧位片上，病变位于心底部的正下方和后方（箭头所示），毗邻食管。

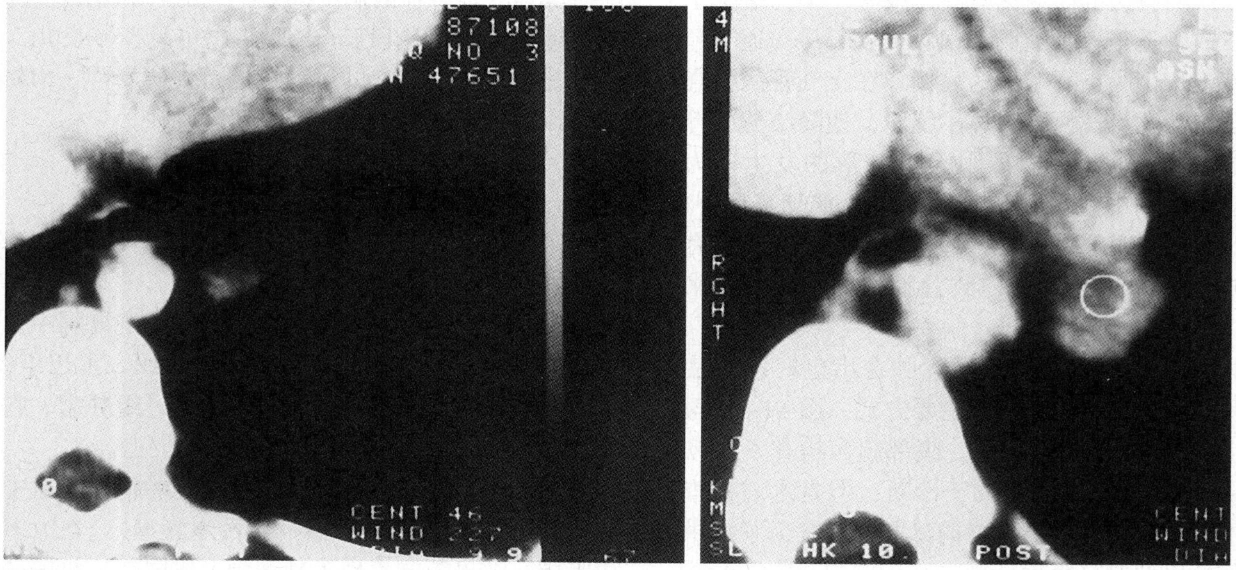

A B

图 61–11 A 和 B. CT 扫描进一步揭示出图 61–10（环状标记处）所示的患者的病变。对于纵隔肿瘤，CT 扫描可能是最为有效的影像学诊断办法。

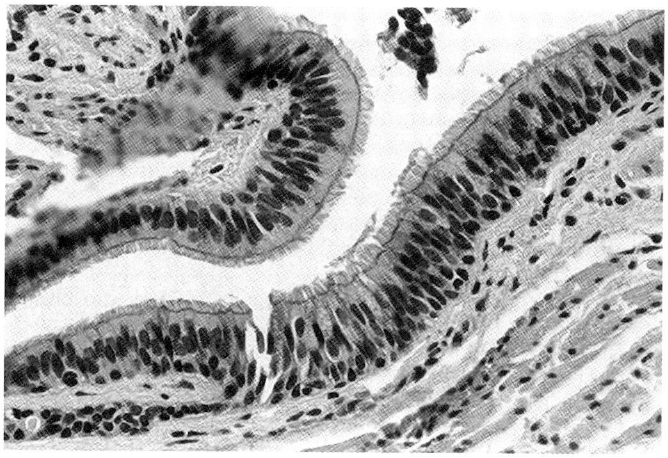

图 61-12　手术探查显示内衬食管黏膜的孤立囊肿，显微镜检查证实存在有食管黏膜。

长。症状与肿瘤的大小和侵袭性生长有关，或与感染有关[85,87]。淋巴管瘤内出血可以因体积的快速增大而导致梗阻症状。诊断性检查包括静脉造影 CT或 MRI 扫描。纤维性的反应和新生血管化可能使得手术切除比较困难，但是手术切除仍然是最佳的治疗方式。采用 OK-432 的硬化剂治疗在美国还在试验中，在其他国家已经显示出了神奇的疗效。纵隔淋巴管瘤手术切除以后，最为常见的并发症是淋巴液渗漏。这种并发症的治疗措施是抽吸、胸腔引流、应用纤维蛋白胶（如果单纯引流失败的话），通常都是有效的方法。在手术切除以后至少有 15%的病例会发生淋巴管瘤复发，所以长期随访是重要的。纵隔血管瘤的报道罕见。只要有可能，血管瘤首选的治疗措施是非手术治疗，包括应用皮质类固醇冲击治疗或是 α-干扰素治疗。

（顾　松译　陈永卫校）

参考文献

1. Adzick NS, Harrison MR, Glick PL, et al: Fetal cystic adenomatoid malformation: Prenatal diagnosis and natural history. J Pediatr Surg 1985;20:483-488.
2. Adzick NS, Harrison MR, Crombleholme TM, et al: Fetal lung lesions: Management and outcome. Am J Obstet Gynecol 1998;179:884-889.
3. Adzick NS, Harrison MR, Flake AW, et al: Fetal surgery for cystic adenomatoid malformation of the lung. J Pediatr Surg 1993;28:806-812.
4. Albanese CT, Sydorak RM, Tsao K: Thoracoscopic lobectomy for prenatally diagnosed lung lesions. J Pediatr Surg 2003:38:553-555.
5. Albright EB, Crane JP, Shackelford GD: Prenatal diagnosis of a bronchogenic cyst. J Ultrasound Med 1988;7: 91-95.
6. Aldousany AW, Joyner JC, Priam RA, et al: Diagnosis and treatment of intrapericardial teratoma. Pediatr Cardiol 1987;8:51-53.
7. al-Salem AH: Ectopic thymic tissue simulating a posterior mediastinal mass. Eur J Pediatr Surg 1992;2: 106-107.
8. Ankermann T, Oppermann HC, Engler S, et al: Congenital masses of the lung, cystic adenomatoid malformation versus congenital lobar emphysema. J Ultrasound Med 2004; 23:1379-1384.
9. Azarow KS, Pearl RH, Zurcher R, et al: Primary mediastinal masses. J Thorac Cardiovasc Surg 1993;106:67-72.
10. Azizkhan RG, Dudgeon DL, Buck JR, et al: Life-threatening airway obstruction as a complication to the management of mediastinal masses in children. J Pediatr Surg 1985;20: 816-819.
11. Azizkhan RG, Grimmer DL, Askin FB, et al: Acquired lobar emphysema (over-inflation): Clinical and pathologic evaluation of infants requiring lobectomy. J Pediatr Surg 1992; 27:1145-1151.
12. Bale PM, Sotelo-Avila C: Maldescent of the thymus: 34 necropsy and 10 surgical cases, including 7 thymuses medial to the mandible. Pediatr Pathol 1993;13: 889-892.
13. Batra P, Brown K, Collins JD, et al: Mediastinal masses: Magnetic resonance imaging in comparison with computed tomography. J Natl Med Assoc 1991;83:969-974.
14. Beardmore HE, Wigglesworth FW: Vertebral anomalies and alimentary duplication. Pediatr Clin North Am 1958; 5:457-462.
15. Benjamin DR, Cahill JL: Bronchoalveolar carcinoma of the lung and congenital cystic adenomatoid malformation. Am J Clin Pathol 1991;95:889-892.
16. Bilik R, Ginzberg H, Superina RA: Unconventional treatment of neurenteric cyst in a newborn. J Pediatr Surg 1995; 30:115-117.
17. Boothroyd AE, Hall-Craggs MA, Dicks-Mireauz C, et al: The magnetic resonance appearances of the normal thymus in children. Clin Radiol 1992;45:378-381.
18. Boue DR, Smith GA, Krous HF: Lingual bronchogenic cyst in a child: An unusual site of presentation. Pediatr Pathol 1994;14:201-202.
19. Bower RJ, Kiesewetter WB: Mediastinal masses in infants and children. Arch Surg 1977;112:1003-1008.
20. Burgner DP, Carachi R, Beattie TJ: Foregut duplication cyst presenting as neonatal respiratory distress and hemoptysis. Thorax 1994;49:287-290.
21. Cajal SR, Suster S: Primary thymic epithelial neoplasm in children. Am J Surg Pathol 1991;15:466-467.
22. Carney JA, Thompson DP, Johnson CL, et al: Teratomas in children: Clinical and pathologic aspects. J Pediatr Surg 1972;7:271-282.
23. Cartagena AM: Pericardial effusion and cardiac hemangioma in the neonate. Pediatr Radiol l993;23:384-385.
24. Cass DL, Quinn TM, Yang EY, et al: Increased cell proliferation and decreased apoptosis characterizes congenital cystic adenomatoid malformation. J Pediatr Surg 1998;33: 1043-1047.
25. Cass DL, Crombleholme TM, Howell LJ, et al: Cystic lung lesions with systemic arterial blood supply: A hybrid of congenital cystic adenomatoid malformation and bron-

congenital cystic adenomatoid malformation and bronchopulmonary sequestration. J Pediatr Surg 1997;32: 986-990.
26. Cha I, Adzick NS, Harrison MR, et al: Fetal congenital cystic adenomatoid malformations of the lung: A clinicopathologic study of eleven cases. Am J Surg Pathol 1997; 21:537-544.
27. Chin KY, Tang MY: Congenital adenomatoid malformation of one lobe of a lung with general anasarca. Arch Pathol 1949;48:221-229.
28. Cohen AJ, Thompson L, Edwards FH, et al: Primary cysts and tumors of the mediastinum. Ann Thorac Surg 1991; 51:378-384.
29. Conran RM, Stocker JT: Extralobar sequestration with frequently associated congenital cystic adenomatoid malformation, type 2: Report of 50 cases. Pediatr Dev Pathol 1999;2:454-463.
30. Crombleholme TM, Coleman BG, Howell LJ, et al: Elevated cystic adenomatoid malformation volume ratio (CVR) predicts outcome in prenatal diagnosis of cystic adenomatoid malformation of the lung. J Pediatr Surg 2002;37:331-338.
31. d'Agnostino S, Bonoldi E, Dante S, et al: Embryonal rhabdomyosarcoma of the lung arising in cystic adenomatoid malformation. J Pediatr Surg 1997;32:1381-1383.
32. Dehner LP: Germ cell tumors of the mediastinum. Semin Diagn Pathol 1990;7:266-270.
33. Dillon PW, Cilley RE, Krummel TM: Video-assisted thoracoscopic excision of intrathoracic masses in children: Report of two cases. Surg Laparosc Endosc 1993;3:433-435.
34. Dommergues M, Louis-Sylvestre C, Mandelbrot L, et al. Congenital adenomatoid malformation of the lung: When is active fetal therapy indicated? Am J Obstet Gynecol 1997;177:953-958.
35. Doull IJ, Connett GJ, Warner JO: Bronchoscopic appearances of congenital lobar emphysema. Pediatr Pulmonol 1996;21:195-198.
36. Englund AT, Geffner ME, Nagel RA, et al: Pediatric germ cell and human chorionic gonadotropin producing tumors. Am J Dis Child 1991;145:1294-1297.
37. Eraklis AL, Griscom NT, McGovern JB: Bronchogenic cysts of the mediastinum in infancy. N Engl J Med 1969;281: 1150-1153.
38. Fallon M, Gordon ARG, Lendrum AD: Mediastinal cysts of foregut origin associated with vertebral anomalies. Br J Surg 1954;41:520-524.
39. Ferro MM, Milner R, Cannizzaro C, et al: Intrathoracic alimentary tract duplication cysts treated in utero by thoracoamniotic shunting. Fetal Diagn Ther 1998;13: 343-347.
40. Fischbach R, Benz-Bohm G, Berthold F, et al: Infradiaphragmatic bronchogenic cyst with high CT numbers in a boy with primitive neuroectodermal tumor. Pediatr Radiol 1994;24:504-505.
41. Frenckner B, Freyschuss U: Pulmonary function after lobectomy for congenital lobar emphysema and congenital cystic adenomatoid malformation: A follow-up study. Scand J Thorac Cardiovasc Surg 1982;16:293-297.
42. Gienski JA, Thibeault DW, Hall FK, et al: Selective bronchial intubation in infants with lobar emphysema: Indications, complications, and long-term outcome. Am J Perinatol 1986;3:199-204.
43. Goetch E: Hygroma colli cysticum and hygroma axillae. Arch Surg 1938;36:395-399.
44. Gordon I, Dempsey JE: Infantile lobar emphysema in association with congenital heart disease. Clin Radiol 1990; 41:48-53.
45. Goto H, Boozalis ST, Benson KI, et al: High-frequency jet ventilation for resection of congenital lobar emphysema. Anesth Analg 1987;66:684-686.
46. Granata C, Gambini C, Balducci T, et al: Bronchioloalveolar carcinoma arising in a congenital cystic adenomatoid malformation in a child: Case report and review of the literature. Pediatr Pulmonol 1996;25:62-66.
47. Grosfeld JL: Primary tumors of the chest wall and mediastinum in children. Semin Thorac Cardiovasc Surg 1994; 6:235-239.
48. Grosfeld JL, Billmire DF: Teratomas in infancy and childhood. Curr Probl Cancer 1985;11:3-34.
49. Grosfeld JL, Skinner MA, Rescorla FJ, et al: Mediastinal tumors in children: Experience with 196 cases. Ann Surg Oncol 1994;1:121-127.
50. Gross RE: The Surgery of Infancy and Childhood: Its Principles and Techniques. Philadelphia, WB Saunders, 1953.
51. Gross RE, Neuhauser ED, Longino LA: Thoracic diverticula which originate from the intestine. Ann Surg 1950; 131:363-365.
52. Harrison MR, Adzick NS, Jennings RW, et al: Antenatal intervention for congenital cystic adenomatoid malformation. Lancet 1990;336:965-966.
53. Hedrick HL, Flake AW, Crombleholme TM, et al: The EXIT procedure for high risk fetal lung lesions. J Pediatr Surg 2005;40:1038-1043.
54. Hendren WH, McKee DM: Lobar emphysema in infancy. J Pediatr Surg 1966;1:24-32.
55. Hemanz-Schulman M, Stein SM, Neblett WW, et al: Pulmonary sequestration: Diagnosis with color Doppler sonography and a new theory of associated hydrothorax. Radiology 1991;180:817-821.
56. Hirose R, Suita S, Taguchi T, et al: Extralobar pulmonary sequestration mimicking cystic adenomatoid malformation in prenatal sonographic appearance and histologic findings. J Pediatr Surg 1995;30:1390-1394.
57. Hislop A, Reid L: New pathologic findings in emphysema of childhood: I. Polyalveolar lobe with emphysema. Thorax 1970;25:682-690.
58. Holcomb GW III, Gheissari A, O'Neill JA Jr, et al: Surgical management of alimentary tract duplications. Ann Surg 1989;209:167-174.
59. Ikezoe J, Takeuch N, Johkoh T, et al: MRI of anterior mediastinal tumors. Radiat Med 1992;10:176-183.
60. John LC, Kingston J, Edmondson ST: Teratoma associated with endodermal sinus tumor. Pediatr Hematol Oncol 1993; 10:49-53.
61. Kaplinsky C, Mor C, Cohen IJ, et al: Childhood malignant thymoma: Clinical, therapeutic, and immunohistochemical considerations. Pediatr Hematol Oncol 1992;9: 261-268.
62. Karl SR, Dunn J: Posterior mediastinal teratomas. J Pediatr Surg 1985;5:508-511.
63. Keon TP: Death on induction of anesthesia for cervical node biopsy. Anesthesiology 1981;55:471-473.
64. Kern JA, Daniel TM, Tribble C, et al: Thoracoscopic diagnosis and treatment of mediastinal masses. Ann Thorac Surg 1993;56:92-96.
65. Keswani SG, Crombleholme TM, Pawel BR, et al: Prenatal diagnosis and management of mainstem bronchial atresia. Fetal Diagn Ther 2005;20:74-78.
66. Khosa JK, Leong SL, Borzi PA: Congenital cystic adenomatoid malformation of the lung: Indications and timing of surgery. Pediatr Surg Int 2004;20:505-508.

67. King RM, Telander RL, Smithson KA, et al: Primary mediastinal tumors in children. J Pediatr Surg 1982;5:512-520.
68. Kropp J, Emons D, Winkler C: Neurenteric cyst diagnosed by technetium-99m pertechnetate sequential scintigraphy. J Nucl Med 1987;28:1218-1221.
69. Kuller JA, Laifer JA, Martin JG, et al: Unusual presentations of fetal teratoma. J Perinatol 1991;11:294-296.
70. Laberge JM, Flageole H, Pugash D, et al: Outcome of the prenatally diagnosed congenital cystic adenomatoid lung malformation: A Canadian experience. Fetal Diagn Ther 2001;16:178-186.
71. Laberge JM, Bratu I, Flageole H: The management of asymptomatic congenital lung malformations. Paediatr Respir Rev 2004;5(Suppl):S305-S312.
72. Lam WW, Chan FL, Lau YL, et al: Paediatric thymoma: Unusual occurrence in two siblings. Pediatr Radiol 1993;23: 124-126.
73. Lazar RH, Younis RT, Bassila MN: Bronchogenic cysts: A cause of stridor in the neonate, Am J Otolaryngol 1991; 12:117-120.
74. Leape LL, Longino LA: Infantile lobar emphysema. Pediatrics 1964;34:246-251.
75. Lemoine G, Montupet P: Mediastinal tumors in infancy and childhood. In Fallis JC, Filler FM, Lemoine G (eds): Pediatric Thoracic Surgery. New York, Elsevier, 1991, pp 103-110.
76. Liechty KW, Quinn TM, Cass DL, et al: Elevated PDGF-β in congenital cystic adenomatoid malformations requiring fetal resection. J Pediatr Surg 1999;34:805-810.
77. Linegar AG, Odell JA, Fennell WM, et al: Massive thymic hyperplasia. Ann Thorac Surg 1993;55:1197-1199.
78. Lobe TE: Pediatric thoracoscopy. Semin Thorac Cardiovasc Surg 1993;5:298-302.
79. Mani H, Suarez E, Stocker JT: The morphologic spectrum of infantile lobar emphysema: A study of 33 cases. Paediatr Respir Rev 2004;5(Suppl):S313-S320.
80. MacGillivray TE, Harrison MR, Goldstein RB, et al: Disappearing fetal lung lesions. J Pediatr Surg 1993;28: 1321-1324.
81. MacKenzie TC, Guttenberg ME, Nissenbaum HL, et al: A fetal lung lesion consisting of bronchogenic cyst, bronchopulmonary sequestration, and congenital cystic adenomatoid malformation: The missing link? Fetal Diagn Ther 2001;16:193-195.
82. McVay CB: Mediastinum. In Anson BJ, McVay CB (eds): Surgical Anatomy, 6th ed. Philadelphia, WB Saunders, 1984, pp 296-308.
83. Meizner I, Levy A: A survey of non-cardiac fetal intrathoracic malformations diagnosed by ultrasound. Arch Gynecol Obstet 1994;255:31-37.
84. Merchant AM, Hedrick HL, Crombleholme TM, et al: Management of fetal mediastinal teratoma: A report of two cases. J Pediatr Surg 2005;40:228-231.
85. Messineo A, Wesson DE, Filler RA, et al: Juvenile hemangiomas involving the thoracic trachea in children: Report of two cases. J Pediatr Surg 1992;27:1291-1295.
86. Miller JA, Corteville JE, Langer JC: Congenital cystic adenomatoid malformation in the fetus: Natural history and predictors of outcome. J Pediatr Surg 1996;31:805-808.
87. Moran CA, Suster S: Mediastinal hemangiomas: A study of 18 cases with emphasis on the spectrum of morphological features. Hum Pathol 1995;26:416-420.
88. Muraskas JK, Gianopoulos JG, Husain A, Black PR: Mediastinal cystic hygroma: Prenatal decompression with neonatal resection and recurrence at 19 months of age. J Perinatol 1993;13:381-383.
89. Murphy JJ, Blair GK, Fraser GC, et al: Rhabdomyosarcoma arising within congenital pulmonary cysts: Report of three cases. J Pediatr Surg 1992;27:1364-1367.
90. Murray ME: Bilateral communicating bronchopulmonary foregut malformation in an infant with multiple congenital anomalies. Pediatr Radiol 1994;24:128-132.
91. Nuchtern JG, Harberg FJ: Congenital lung cysts. Semin Pediatr Surg 3:233, 1994.
92. Olutoye O, Coleman B, Hubbard AM, et al: Prenatal diagnosis and management of congenital lobar emphysema. J Pediatr Surg 2000;35:792-795.
93. Ozcelik U, Gocmen A, Kiper N, et al: Congenital lobar emphysema: Evaluation and long-term followup of thirty cases at a single center. Pediatr Pulmonol 2003;35:384-391.
94. Paterson IM, Cockburn JS: Acute pericarditis due to perforation of a benign mediastinal teratodermoid into the pericardial sac. Thorax 1982;37:863-865.
95. Philippart AI: On foregut duplications. J Pediatr Pulm 1994;18:45.
96. Phillipos EZ, Libsekal K: Flexible bronchoscopy in the management of congenital lobar emphysema in the neonate. Can Resp J 1998;5:219-221.
97. Piramoon AN, Abbassioun K: Mediastinal enterogenic cyst with spinal cord compression. J Pediatr Surg 1974;9: 543-545.
98. Pokomy WJ: Mediastinal tumors. In Ashcraft KW, Holder TM (eds): Pediatric Surgery, 2nd ed. Philadelphia, WB Saunders, 1993, pp 218-227.
99. Pokorny WJ, Goldstein IR: Enteric thoracoabdominal duplications in children. J Thorac Cardiovasc Surg 1984; 87:821-825.
100. Pokorny WJ, Sherman JO: Mediastinal masses in infants and children. J Thorac Cardiovasc Surg 1974;68: 869-873.
101. Pul N, Pul M: Bronchogenic cyst of the scapular area in an infant: Case report and review of the literature. J Am Acad Dermatol 1994;3:120-122.
102. Quinn TM, Hubbard AM, Adzick NS: Prenatal magnetic resonance imaging enhances prenatal diagnosis. J Pediatr Surg 1998;33:312-316.
103. Ramon Y, Cajal S, Suster S: Primary thymic epithelial neoplasms in children. Am J Surg Pathol 1991;15:466-471.
104. Ransom JM, Norton JB: Pulmonary sequestration presenting as congestive heart failure. J Thorac Cardiovasc Surg 1978;76:378-381.
105. Read CA, Moront M, Carangelo R, et al: Recurrent bronchogenic cyst: An argument for complete surgical excision. Arch Surg 1991;126:1306-1308.
106. Ribet ME, Copin MC, Soots JG, et al: Bronchioloalveolar carcinoma and congenital cystic adenomatoid malformation. Ann Thorac Surg 1995;60:1126-1128.
107. Rice HE, Flake AW, Hori T, et al: Massive thymic hyperplasia: Characterization of a rare mediastinal mass. J Pediatr Surg 1994;29:1561-1564.
108. Robie DK, Gursoy MH, Pokorny WJ: Mediastinal tumors: Airway obstruction and management. Semin Pediatr Surg 1994;3:259-263.
109. Rubin EM, Garciatt C, Horowitz MD, et al: Fatal massive hemoptysis secondary to intralobar sequestration. Chest 1994;106:954-955.
110. Rubush JL, Gardner IR, Boyd WC, et al: Mediastinal tumors: Review of 186 cases. J Thorac Cardiovasc Surg 1973;65:216-222.
111. Saenz NC, Schnitzer JJ, Eraklis AE, et al: Posterior mediastinal masses. J Pediatr Surg 1993;28:172-176.
112. Sakala EP, Perrott WS, Grube GL: Sonographic characteristics of antenatally diagnosed extralobar pulmonary

sequestration and congenital cystic adenomatoid malformation. Obstet Gynecol Surv 1994;49:647-655.
113. Saltzman DH, Adzick NS, Benacerraf BR: Fetal cystic adenomatoid malformation of the lung: Apparent improvement in utero. Obstet Gynecol 1988;71:1000-1003.
114. Shamberger RC, Holzman RS, Griscom NT, et al: CT quantification of tracheal cross-sectional area as a guide to the surgical and anesthetic management of children with anterior mediastinal masses. J Pediatr Surg 1991;26: 138-142.
115. Shields TW: Primary Tumors and Cysts of the Mediastinum. Philadelphia, Lea & Febiger, 1972, p 32.
116. Simpson I, Campbell PE: Mediastinal masses in childhood: A review from a paediatric pathologist's point of view. Prog Pediatr Surg 1991;27:92-96.
117. Skandalakis JE, Gray SW, Ricketts R: The esophagus. In Skandalakis JE, Gray SW (eds): Embryology for Surgeons. Philadelphia, WB Saunders, 1994, pp 65-112.
118. Skandalakis JE, Gray SW, Todd NW: The pharynx and its derivatives. In Skandalakis JE, Gray SW (eds): Embryology for Surgeons. Philadelphia, WB Saunders, 1994, pp 17-64.
119. Slovis TL, Meza M, Kuhn JP: Aberrant thymus--MR assessment. Pediatr Radiol 1992;22:490-494.
120. Snyder ME, Luck SR, Hernandez R, et al: Diagnostic dilemmas of mediastinal cysts. J Pediatr Surg 1985;20: 810-815.
121. Srikanth MS, Ford EG, Stanley P, et al: Communicating bronchopulmonary foregut malformations: Classification and embryogenesis. J Pediatr Surg 1992;27:732-736.
122. Stocker JT, Manewell JE, Drake RM: Congenital cystic adenomatoid malformation of the lung: Classification and morphologic spectrum. Hum Pathol 1977;8:155-161.
123. Stocker JT: Congenital pulmonary airway malformation: A new name and an expanded classification of congenital cystic adenomatoid malformations of the lung. Histopathology 2002;41:424-431.
124. Stringer MD, Spitz L, Abel R, et al: Management of alimentary tract duplications in children. Br J Surg 1995; 82:74-78.
125. Suen HC, Mathisen DJ, Grillo HC, et al: Surgical management and radiological characteristics of bronchogenic cysts. Ann Thorac Surg 1993;55:476-481.
126. Suster S, Rosai J: Thymic carcinoma. Cancer 1991;67: 1025-1028.
127. Swanson SJ 3d, Skoog SJ, Garcia V, et al: Pseudoadrenal mass: Unusual presentation of bronchogenic cyst. J Pediatr Surg 1991;26:1401-1403.
128. Taguchi T, Suita S, Yamanouchi T, et al: Antenatal diagnosis and surgical management of congenital cystic adenomatoid malformation of the lung. Fetal Diagn Ther 1995;10:400-404.
129. Thompson DP, Moore TC: Acute thoracic distress in childhood due to spontaneous rupture of a large mediastinal teratoma. J Pediatr Surg 1969;4:416-419.
130. Thompson J, Forfar JO: Regional obstructive emphysema in infancy. Arch Dis Child 1958;33:97-101.
131. Thorpe-Veeston JG, Nicolaides KH: Cystic adenomatoid malformation of the lung: Prenatal diagnosis and outcome. Prenat Diagn 1994;14:677-681.
132. Ueda K, Gruppo R, Martin L, et al: Rhabdomyosarcoma arising in a congenital cystic adenomatoid malformation. Cancer 1977;40:383-388.
133. Warner JO, Rubin S, Heard BE: Congenital lobar emphysema: A case with bronchial atresia and abnormal bronchial cartilages. Br J Dis Chest 1982;76:177-181.
134. Weimann RB, Hallman GL, Bahar D, et al: Intrathoracic meningocele: A case report and review of the literature. J Thorac Cardiovasc Surg 1963;46:40-49.
135. Winters WD, Effmann EL, Nghien HV, et al: Disappearing fetal lung masses: Importance of postnatal imaging studies. Pediatr Radiol 1997;27:535-539.
136. Wright JR Jr, Gillis DA: Mediastinal foregut cyst containing an intramural adrenal cortical rest: A case report and review of supradiaphragmatic adrenal rests. Pediatr Pathol 1993;13:407-409.

第 62 章

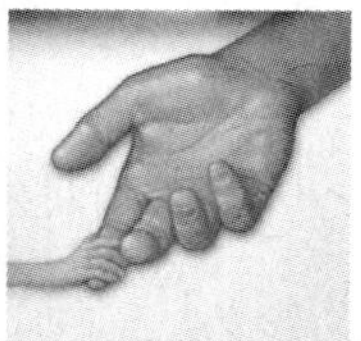

喉镜检查术、支气管镜检查术和胸腔镜检查术

Bradley M. Rodgers 和 Eugene D. McGahren III

长久以来能够在活体上观察喉和气管一直是内科医生的兴趣所在。1806 年，Bozzini 因第一个设计了一种专门用来观察喉和上呼吸道的仪器而获得殊荣[5]。他的空心管借助一根蜡烛照明，蜡烛发出的光通过沿仪器轴的镜子反射。1829 年，Babington 发明了利用反射光的喉镜。随后几个内科医生发明了一种带有反射光的硬管，用来观察食管和胃的近端部分。然而，内镜演变的最大的突破出现在 1879 年，当时 Nitze 开发了一种带有一个远端透镜的通过加热的白金线圈照明的膀胱镜[40]。后来不久，Nitze 利用 Thomas Edison 发明的白炽灯泡来改进他的内镜装置，在管的末端放置一个带有微型灯丝的灯泡。Kirstein 发展了带镜片的一种喉镜，类似于我们现在的 Miller 镜片，是通过手柄上的白炽灯泡照明。Chevalier Jeckson 改良了这种仪器，把灯泡置于镜片的远端，并给喉镜加了一个可移动的底部[27]。

硬管内镜技术最终的重要进展是 Hopkins 斯柱状透镜系统的发展。Hopkins 构造了一个带有一系列透镜的硬管内镜镜身，透镜用石英玻璃分隔，极大地改善了光在仪器内的传导，并且得到了比以往更好的图像清晰率。其次，这种发展使内镜微型化，适用于儿童，并且可在胶片或电视上记录高清晰率的图像。

Hopkins 也促进了早期可弯曲光导纤维内镜的发展。1930 年，Lamm 发现影像可以通过这种玻璃纤维线传导，这些细的玻璃纤维线可定向并紧紧绑在一起[29]。1954 年，Hopkins 利用这种光导纤维技术发展了可弯曲胃镜的原型，并在 1958 年由 Hirschowitz 等人第一次在临床运用。Ikeda 在 1970 年修改了这项技术，发展了可弯曲光导纤维支气管镜[21]。这项技术随后的改进使得真正微型的可弯曲光导纤维喉镜和支气管镜得到发展，适用于大小不同的婴儿和儿童。

在很大程度上，胸腔镜的发展史与气道和胃肠道内镜的发展是平行的。1910 年，Hans Jacobaeus 利用 Nitze 膀胱镜观察肺结核患者的胸腔[22]。在那个时代，人工气胸被认为可以有效地治疗许多伴空洞型结核，很快 Jacobaeus 完善了这项技术，用膀胱镜和一个电灼器进行“闭合的胸膜腔内肺松解术”。Jacobaeus 创造了术语“胸腔镜”并且在 1921 年显示这种方式即借助观察和直接活检可用于胸腔内肿瘤的诊断[23]。Rodgers 和 Talbert 利用 Hopkins 柱状透镜望远镜行胸腔镜检，并且建议这一技术用于肺组织的活检，以在免疫抑制儿童中诊断肺浸润，并在 1976 年报道了在临床环境中的成功应用[59]。

喉镜技术

适应证

喉镜可以用于诊断和治疗儿科患者。喉镜在婴儿和儿童中最常见的适应证是对于喘鸣的评估[17,37]。术语喘鸣是指气道内气体的湍流所致的高音调的呼吸音。喉和声门上的病变通常会产生吸气性喘鸣，这种喘鸣的性质可以随着不同位置或是某种活动而改变。气管狭窄通常表现为呼气性喘鸣。大多数有持续性吸气性喘鸣的婴儿和儿童应该做喉镜检查以建立一个准确的解剖诊断。儿童的其他诊断性喉镜检查的适应证包括哭声和声音的改变、急性呼吸困难或重复的误吸

972 发作。儿童治疗性喉镜的适应证包括先天性或获得性声门狭窄、喉蹼、喉异物和喉乳头状瘤。喉异物虽然并不多见，但可能造成突然呼吸困难，因此是急诊喉镜检查的重要适应证。

仪器操作

对婴儿和儿童实施喉镜的外科医生必须能熟练地应用柔韧的和硬管的内镜，并且有各种型号的仪器可用。经常，硬管和可弯曲内镜相互结合使用，因为它们在某些特定的临床状况下有各自的优缺点。在儿科操作中标准的硬管内镜是开放式的带有长度在 8～13.5cm 之间的镜片。照明由一高强度的光源提供，从仪器柄上的棱镜射向镜片（图 62-1）。一些特殊的喉镜例如儿科 Dedo 喉镜，允许悬挂喉镜用于更复杂的操作步骤。前方联合的内镜有一个 11cm 长的镜片，远端部分有一个龙骨结构（图 62-2）。这种喉镜有助于暴露小婴儿喉的前部。另外，镜片的构型允许外展声带以诊断喉气管裂。

用于婴儿和儿童喉镜的可弯曲仪器的尺寸不同，从外直径为 2.0mm 的超细支气管镜到外直径为 3.6mm 的儿科支气管镜。超细内镜没有器械和吸引通道，尖端仅能双向偏转，这样就限制了它在诊断检查中的应用。标准的儿科可弯曲支气管镜有双向头端偏转和吸引管或是器械通道。这种内镜可以用来很好地显示除了极小早产儿（<1000g）以外的所有婴儿喉部并可以用来取活检标本[10]。可弯曲的光纤维鼻咽镜是一种专门设计用于咽和喉评估的仪器。这种仪器的外套管直径是 3.9mm，长度仅 25cm[66]。然而，考虑到可弯曲仪器的费用，尽管它们的长度短，大多数内科医生仍喜欢用小的支气管镜来评估喉部[11]。

外科医生在准备进行喉镜检查时必须肯定所有这些仪器都处在功能状态，且附属的器械如活检和异物

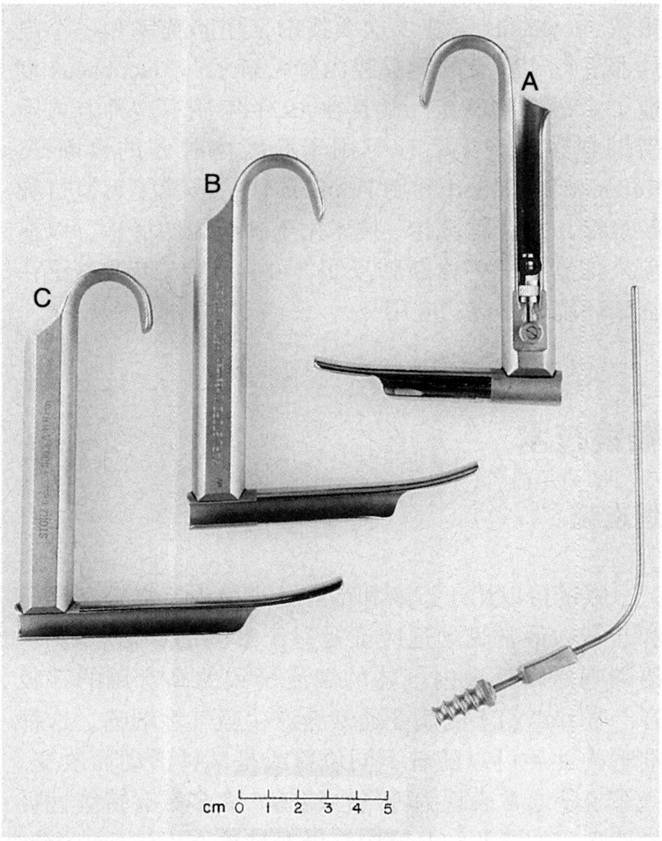

图 62-1 儿科硬管喉镜。这些设备有范围 8cm（A）至 13.5cm（C）长的镜片。照明是由仪器柄上的光棱镜提供。这些仪器可以被悬吊。

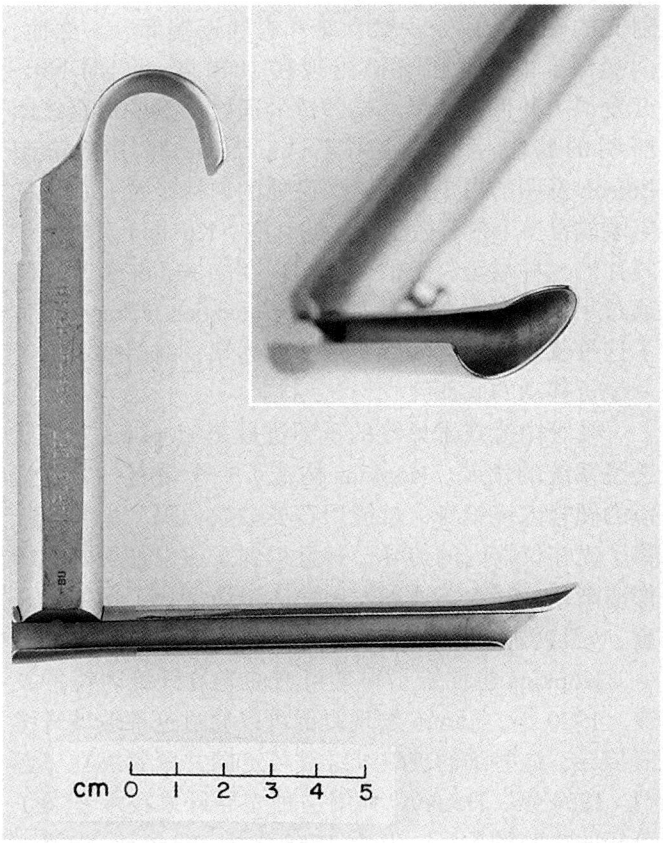

图 62-2 前联合内镜。该仪器有一个 11cm 长的镜片，远端部分有一龙骨结构（插页）。照明通过仪器柄上的棱镜提供。这一仪器可以悬吊。

钳也处在可用和功能状态。

973 **步骤**

婴幼儿和儿童诊断性喉镜检查时可以用镇静剂、局部麻醉或全身麻醉。通常，患者进行硬式喉镜检查时采用全身麻醉。所有患者在内镜操作中必须被完全监护。应进行持续心电图（ECG）和脉氧监护以探测偶尔由上述操作导致的缺氧症或心动过缓。如果可能的话，用面罩进行麻醉诱导，在直接喉镜检查前患者不插管，然后患者放置在颈部伸展和颌微曲的位置。在气道检查时所有要使用到的器械必须消毒并备在手术室里。硬管支气管镜沿着舌的右缘进入直到看到会厌。支气管镜的镜片在会厌下方通过，抬高会厌可以看到声门上的喉和声带。通常，声门下的病变可以利用这种优势进行鉴别。内镜在该位置时，可以观察到随用力呼吸的喉的运动。有喉软化的患者，会厌的基底部通常是狭窄的（“Ω 形”），随着用力吸气杓状软骨在中线处接合（图 62-3）。常常，这些患者吸气时完全看不到声带。在声带麻痹的病例，可以看到受累的声带处在中间的位置，且不随着吸气外展。声带抬高后，余下检查可以在会厌气道内喷雾利多卡因（4mg/kg）以减少喉痉挛。应用前部连合的内镜通常可以更好地看到喉的前面，尤其是在小婴儿中。内镜窄的尖端通过会厌口允许用力外展声带并可观察到声带和后部的喉隔膜，喉食管裂的部位。

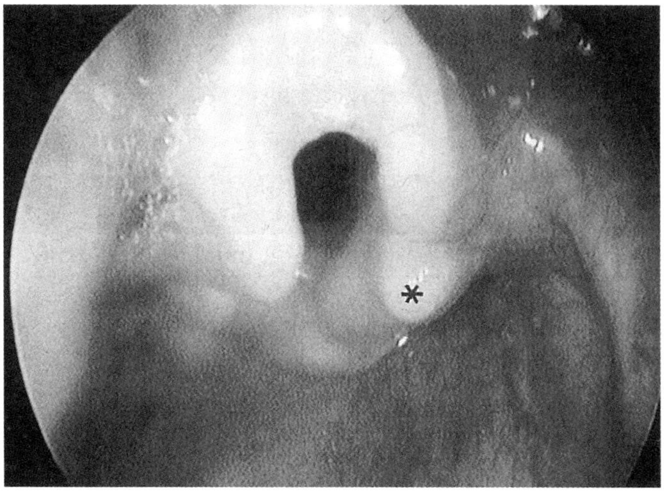

图 62-3　一喉软化患儿声门上区域内镜外观图。注意“Ω 形”会厌伴有一个非常狭窄的基底部。随吸气杓状软骨（星号）在中线处塌陷。

在喉的许多治疗性操作中，应用支撑式喉镜至关重要，因为它允许双目镜放大喉部，无受阻地应用喉外科器械。支撑式喉镜的直角镜片在会厌的下部通过，尖端抬高以暴露喉部和声门上气道。支撑装置由一个放在患者胸部上的 Mayo 架支持。对于涉及喉前面的操作，前连合内镜可以相似的方式悬挂。

如果术前的诊断是喉软化，这种检查通常开始用可弯曲的内镜。仪器通过鼻进入咽的后部，缓慢前进直到确定会厌。将内镜的尖端放置在刚好超过会厌在咽喉的后壁，能很好地观察喉部的气道和评估其在用力呼吸时的动态功能。用可弯曲内镜评估喉的运动要优于硬管内镜，因为不会有仪器本身所造成的喉和声门上的气道扭曲[15]。可弯曲内镜在全麻的患者可以通过喉罩通气道（LMA）来观察声门[2]。在许多情况下，完成喉和声门上气道评估后，会做一个支气管镜检查以排除相关的远端病变。

并发症

除了继发的喉水肿加剧气道梗阻，诊断性喉镜的并发症罕见。给有严重的呼吸道阻塞的患者行诊断性喉镜检查时，应该准备好紧急气管切开的装备。同样地，在与麻醉师的术前讨论中应该强调可能需要用小号的气管内套管（2.5mm）插管用于紧急的通气。治疗性喉镜检查所致的并发症依赖于操作的步骤。用力进行喉扩张或是激光或冷冻疗法治疗喉或声门下狭窄后，喉或咽穿孔是一个可能发生但不常见的并发症。在可弯曲喉镜检查时通过吸引通道送入氧气或在用硬管内镜时嘴角放置一小管子直接送入氧气以避免喉镜检查时可能发生的低氧血症。Hoeve 等对行硬质喉支气管镜检查的儿童患者的并发症进行了记录，整体并发症率为 1.9%[19]。小于三个月的婴幼儿的并发症发生率为 0.5%。并发症包括出血（0.5%）、心律失常（0.6%），声门下水肿（0.3%）和气胸（1.2%）。用脉氧仪监护患者可以消灭心律失常的发生。在接受可弯曲喉支气管镜检查的大批儿童中，Wood 报道并发症为 2.9%，没有死亡[74]。

974 支气管镜

适应证

在婴幼儿和儿童中，支气管镜可以用作诊断的治疗目的。适应证包括喘鸣、持续肺不张、持续咳嗽、反复或持续性肺炎、怀疑气道内有异物、插管中的辅助、评价气管内导管的放置、支气管的冲洗、气道出血和术后或拔管后声嘶或喘鸣[47,56,76]。在支气管镜下的介入可能包括气管内异物或分泌物的清除、气管切除术的护理、支气管肺泡的灌洗、药物的滴入、激光治疗、针对梗阻病变的球形扩张或放置支架和经支气管活检[8,39,51,57,63,77]。支气管镜检查的相对禁忌证包括出血素质、血流动力学不稳定、心律失常、低氧血症、肺动脉高压、或潜在的气道阻塞[37,42]。通过支气管镜检查获得的信息价值通常必须与操作的潜在危险相权衡。

仪器设备

可弯曲的和硬质设备均可作为儿科支气管镜使用。最初的和仍然是儿科标准的可弯曲支气管镜有一个 3.5～3.7mm 外径并带有一个 1.2mm 吸引设备的端口。尖端的移动是双向的，范围在 180～220°，吸引端允许滴入液体或氧气，也可以吸引气道内的黏液。然而，由于吸引通道尺寸小，吸引黏稠的黏液较困难，经气管内活检也不容易。这种内镜可以通过的最小的气管内导管直径是 4.5mm。然而，在没有气管内导管的患者，这种支气管镜通常可以经鼻通过，甚至可用于 700 克重的小婴儿[10,74,75,77]。也有一种 2.8mm 的可弯曲支气管镜伴一个 1.2mm 的吸引端，具有 3.5mm 镜的能力，多用于更小的儿童。现在普遍运用的外套管直径为 2.7、2.2、2.0 和 1.8mm 的小的、超细的支气管镜。在 2.7 和 2.2 mm 内镜中，可用 0.7～0.8mm 的吸引管[16,65,77,78]。1.8mm 的内镜缺乏一个双向的尖端。2.2mm 和更小的内镜可以通过 2.5mm 气管内导管[41]。

硬管的儿科支气管镜由一个硬管的柱状透镜内镜组成，通过一个外鞘进入。这个外鞘有一个 3.5～7.5mm 的内径，长约 23cm 或 30cm（图 62-4）。对任何特殊鞘，必须选择能达到最大的视觉效果和最小的气道阻力的望远镜尺寸[35]。一个特别的接头允许直接通过鞘通气。另外，仪器端口允许通过一个用于冲洗或吸引的导管。抓取和活检的设备直接与硬管望远镜
接合以产生能通过鞘的光学钳（图 62-5）。即使硬管 975
的支气管镜的鞘根据其最小内径做了标记，这些尺寸不需要与实际工作的尺寸相对。表 62-1 所示为 Storz 硬管支气管镜的实际尺寸。必须仔细选择适合于婴儿或儿童检查的支气管镜，在鞘内能有足够的空间放置望远镜设备或在需要时放入导管。

步骤

在任何支气管镜检查前，应做彻底的病史和体格检查。特别的注意应放在任何使支气管镜通过困难的颈或脊柱畸形、颈部的气管位置和任何呼吸音的不对称。所有的患者应该有正位和侧位的胸片，以明确胸腔内的解剖和病理。如果怀疑有血管压迫或是胃食管反流，吞钡检查可能有帮助。电影荧光镜透视检查或吸气-呼气胸片有助于确定气管内异物的存在以及位置。在一些情况下，胸部 CT 可以帮助评估胸腔内气道和周围结构。一旦开始支气管镜操作，必须准备通过气管插管或是气管切开术紧急进入气道。

准备做支气管镜的外科医生必须熟悉所有可用的设备，并且所有的设备处在工作状态。还必须仔细维护支气管镜的设备，因为不合适的清洗或是仪器有裂缝发生可能发生细菌污染[39]。必须根据儿童尺寸和需
要使用型号合适的仪器。如果要移出一气管内异物， 976
在进行操作前在一个疑似物样本上检测一下抓握的设备是有价值的[71]。实际上现在所有支气管镜检查都在视频监视下进行的并且有放大的记录。这样便于解剖

表 62-1 Storz 支气管镜尺寸

正常尺寸	内径（mm）	外径（mm）	长度（cm）
2.5 × 20	3.5	4.2	20
3.0 × 20/26/30	4.3	5.0	20/26/30
3.5 × 20/26/30	5.0	5.7	20/26/30
4.0 × 30	6.0	6.7	30
5.0 × 30	7.1	7.8	30
6.0 × 30	7.5	8.2	30

Adapted from Marzo SJ, Hotaling AJ: Trade-off between airway resistance and optical resolution in pediatric rigid bronchoscopy. Ann Otol Rhinol Laryngol 1995;104:282.

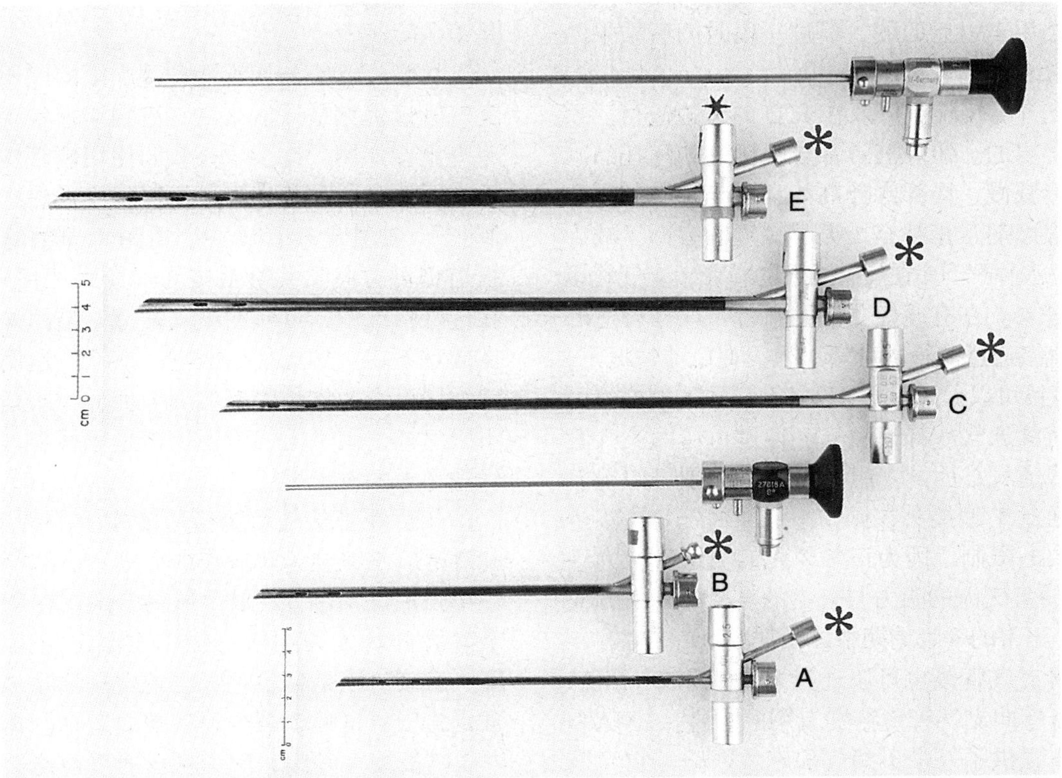

图 62-4　儿科硬管支气管镜。这些仪器尺寸不同，2.5cm × 20cm（A）～6cm × 30cm（E）。这些仪器杆直接通过柱状透镜的望远镜。操作的侧通道（星标）允许通过吸引器和操作器械。通气的侧通道（星号）允许操作中持续通气。

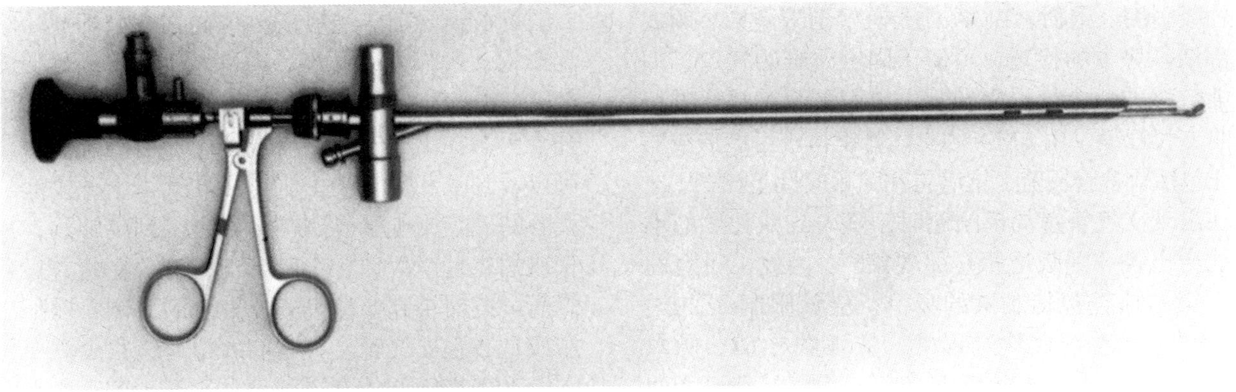

A

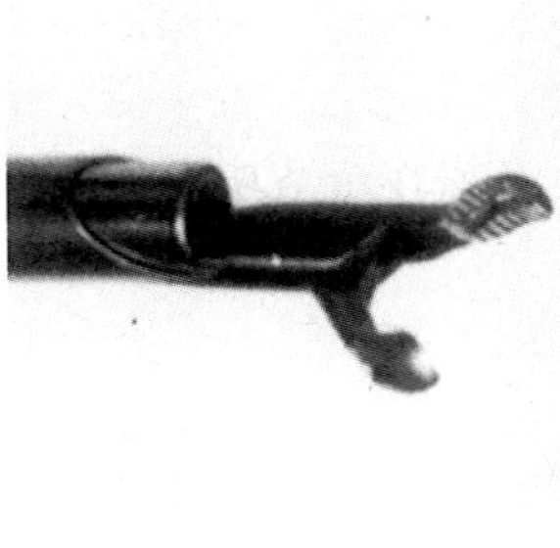

B

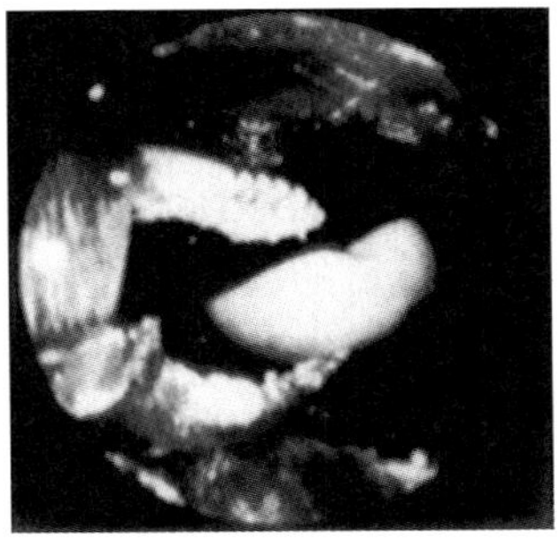

C

图 62-5　A. 光学钳。B. 花生抓紧器与一长的内镜望远镜结合用于直接放大观察及异物的取出。C. 放大的图像可精确放置抓紧钳以保证安全取出异物。

的观察、存档用于以后回顾、经过一段时间后结果的比较和与家长及护理人员的讨论[39]。

可弯曲支气管镜检查可以在ICU的床边进行。预先充氧法是必要的。镇静剂常常与止涎剂如阿托品减少反应性心律减慢、局部麻醉剂如利多卡因麻醉喉和上气道和抗焦虑剂互相补充。类固醇可以有助于减少操作后的喉头水肿[37,41,47]。在没有插管的患者，支气管镜可以通过鼻进入。在有通气支持的患者，尺寸合适的支气管镜可直接通过气管内套管进入。在一些情况下，可弯曲支气管镜可以通过一个T型接头引入，这样就可以在操作中持续通气或补充氧气。通过可弯曲支气管镜不可能完成通气；因此，患者必须能够围绕内镜自主呼吸或是通过T型接头在操作中机械通气。这不是一个无关紧要的限制，因为正常婴儿的气道直径大约只有5mm，并且气流的阻力与气道的半径的四次方成反比。另外，正常的呼吸周期中，吸呼比为1∶2。

虽然硬管支气管镜也可以通过LMA完成，LMA已被证明是可弯曲支气管镜特别有用的附件。LMA为支气管镜检查提供了一个不漏气的麻醉回路。它允许气道用正压支持、CO_2监测、辅助通气和麻醉的递送不会泄漏到周围环境。LMA也允许应用可能比经鼻或支气管内途径大的光导纤维设备。由此，也可以允许用更大的吸引腔。最后，LMA便于有解剖限制如小颌症和颈部僵硬患者的检查，可便于固定困难的气道，即在可能放置的一个气管内导管上允许更简易地通过一可弯曲支气管镜。用LMA的支气管镜检查可能造成的禁忌证包括胃食管反流、饱满胃和肺顺应性差[2,43,64,70]。

在出现支气管镜局部闭塞时，随着二氧化碳的堆积可能会出现“呼吸堆积”的现象[25]。因此，可弯曲支气管镜的检查包括黏液的吸引，应该限制在30～45秒内[76]。在整个操作过程中，应该做ECG、脉氧监护和可能的话呼气末CO_2监测[39]。为了补偿可弯曲支气管镜的闭塞效应，可通过吸引端口补充氧气，或应用没有吸引端口的超细可弯曲支气管镜检时可通过另一个鼻孔导管供氧。在清除黏液的部位，可通过吸引端口滴入盐水或是黏液溶解剂以允许清除较稠厚的分泌物。如果黏液栓特别的顽固并且不能够通过吸引端口吸引出来，有时可以顶住支气管镜的尖端，并且仔细地从气道内拔出内镜来去除分泌物。除了支气管镜检的专家，非常重要的是团队的成员应专心监测儿童进程，因为“支气管镜检查者催眠状态”（即专注于支气管镜检查的发现而忽视了对患者状态的关注）是很危险的[75]。

尽管可弯曲支气管镜日益广泛的应用，但是硬管支气管镜仍然是评估儿童气道和治疗各种气道病变的一个重要仪器。许多中心依旧使用硬管支气管镜，几乎专用于婴儿和儿童，儿科医生应该熟悉其能力和限制[12,50]。硬管支气管镜特别适用于异物的取出。已有报道将可弯曲支气管镜作为辅助来评估异物的存在。在这些情况中，可弯曲支气管镜只是用来确定异物存在或是不在。如果找到异物，那么应运用硬管支气管镜。用可弯曲支气管镜实际取回异物报道很有限[68,73]。不管怎样，硬管支气管镜依然是取回吸入的气道异物优先考虑的技术[8,77]。

儿童硬管支气管镜检通常在手术室全麻下进行。麻醉师应是完全了解操作的方案。麻醉师作用的重要性再强调也不过分，就是维持合适的麻醉水平并且完全熟悉外科大夫的所有操作方案。根据检查的适应证，患者可以是自主呼吸或是控制呼吸。自主呼吸通常是希望评价喉、声带和咽壁的运动。在异物的取出时也需要自主呼吸，因为正压通气可能会使异物压入远端的支气管。在病情很严重的婴儿或儿童中，支气管镜可以在有适当的人员和设备的ICU环境中安全地进行[38]。

麻醉诱导后，患者的体位是在其肩下放一个小的卷形物，颈部稍许伸展。通过左手拿着的喉镜看到喉部，Miller喉镜片最有用，因为它可在喉镜前进时移开会厌。在支气管镜沿着喉镜的右侧轻轻进入气管时可以看到喉和声带。由于小儿的气道十分柔润，合适型号的硬管支气管镜通常可以进入到足够远，用一个直接的望远镜评估各个肺叶支气管。在检查过程中可以通过把头转到要检查的支气管的对侧，以便于伸直左或是右主支气管。有角度的望远镜很少需要，尽管
它们对于特别低的气道的评估有帮助[71]。检查完气道 977
后，任何适当的操作也就完成了。通气变得困难时，可以把望远镜拿掉，可以持续通过无阻塞的支气管镜套管通气。通过在望远镜的目镜上放置一摄影机可以把图像投影到监视器上。在操作过程中，必须注意评估气道的动力学和解剖变异。

取出各种大小和类型的异物需要有各种类型的抓取设备可用[4]。通常，从气道取出异物需要取出全部支气管镜，因为异物并不能够通过支气管镜的鞘。如果异物特别脆，例如一颗吸入的花生，在异物外经进入端口或鞘放入Fogarty球囊导管是有帮助的，必须

小心不要弄破球囊。球囊充气膨胀，异物被拉入支气管镜鞘，然后将整个装置一同取出[28]。必须再次检查气道，排除残留的异物碎片并吸引出异物外气道内积累的黏液和分泌物。

虽然所有的操作都是以一种非常有效的方式进行，但时间通常并不像可弯曲支气管镜检那样是一个限制因素，因为硬管支气管镜可以通过镜鞘通气。操作结束时，在直视下取出内镜。如果需要的话可以放置气管内导管，先前存在的气管切开导管可以被替换，或观察到患者的自主呼吸。

并发症

可弯曲支气管镜或是硬管支气管镜的明显并发症并不常见，但可包括低氧、高碳酸血症、心动过缓、喉痉挛、气胸、声门下的或其他气道的水肿、出血、发热和院内感染[42,48,71,75]。最严重的并发症出现在接受支气管镜检查的小婴儿上。一组 132 名小于 1 个月的婴儿，接受硬管支气管镜检查，其中 5 例出现气胸，1 例支气管破裂，1 例肺动脉破裂，所有这些损伤都得到成功治疗[31]。

胸腔镜

适应证

胸腔镜在儿童中最初的用途是作为一种获取的免疫抑制的患者肺活检样本的方法[59]。随着技术的进一步改良和仪器设备更好的发展，现在儿童胸腔镜有了更多的诊断和治疗的适应证。在我们自己的系列中，胸腔镜最常见的适应证是用于治疗脓胸的胸膜清创术[14,26,55]。这种操作依然是我们对纵隔病变尤其是淋巴瘤活检选择的技术[52]。一些纵隔疾病如支气管源性的或是重复畸形可以通过胸腔镜完全切除，这些患者因此可以避免胸廓切开术[46,55]。这一技术对免疫抑制和诊断不明的肺渗出和结节的正常儿童的肺活检依旧非常有用[6]。它在许多胸膜病变如自发性气胸或乳糜胸的治疗中也很有用[13,44]。最近报道显示了胸腔镜在儿童肺叶解剖切除时的有用性和安全性[61]。目前，有几个作者描述用胸腔镜技术修补伴有或是不伴有气管食管瘘的食管闭锁[3,33,62]。这一技术已经被发展用于膈疝的关闭和闭合未闭的动脉导管[30,62]。心包开窗可以用来引流慢性心包渗出。胸腔镜已经被用于胸部脊柱侧弯儿童的椎间盘切除术的暴露[49]。机器人在儿童胸腔镜中的作用还处于界定的早期阶段[9,20]。带机器人的设备的运动范围可便于在很小的空间进行工作。

仪器设备

儿童胸腔镜可以用 3，5 或 10mm 的霍普金斯柱状透镜望远镜。尽管其他作者介绍在某些情况下用 30°和 70°内镜，我们倾向于用 0°镜[54]。在小婴儿中，3mm 内镜望远镜可能有用（图 62–6）。望远镜和操作仪器通过套管针进入胸腔，可以像腹腔镜一样有阀或没有阀。我们发现 Innerdyne 可扩张 trocar 在儿童有用，因为它的放射状扩张允许在小的儿童中放置一个 5mm 或 10mm 套管针而不危害肋间血管和损伤神经（图 62–7）。操作仪器，绝大部分是直径为 3mm 或 5mm带有一个用于烧灼的绝缘杆状物。我们喜欢用可再度使用的仪器，并且用它们复制成开胸可能用得到的仪器类型（图 62–8）。内镜 GIA 吻合器用于获取肺活检标本或是切除肺囊肿，但是这种器械必须通过直径为 12mm 的套管针，在胸腔中要有 5cm 的空间来完全打开触点，这样就限制了这种仪器在小儿童中的应用。

步骤

成功地实施儿童胸腔镜需要注意的是患者的选择和术前的影像。在有纵隔疾病的儿童，特殊的影像检查，如 CT 或是核磁共振，在确定病变与其他纵隔结构的关系和进入病变的最直接途径是很有帮助的。对 978
于肺活检，正侧位片通常足以确定病变的位置。必须根据术前 CT 扫描仔细挑选行胸腔镜活检的实质性结节患者脏层胸膜上 1cm 大的结节在胸腔镜下很难确定，术前定位技术例如经胸腔放置金属丝或是纹身可能非常有帮助[45,59,72]。在有胸膜渗出或是脓胸考虑用胸腔镜做引流和清创术的患者中，经胸超声或胸部 CT 可以帮助定位一个最大的区域，在这个区域内应放置最初的套管针。

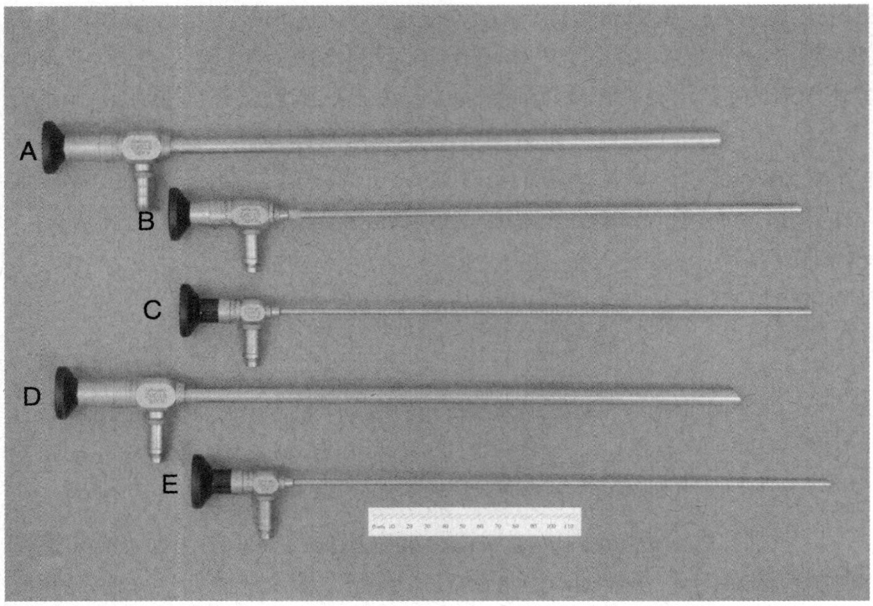

图 62-6 内镜的望远镜。可用的内镜的望远镜的直径范围是 3~10mm：A. 10mm，0°；B. 5mm，0°；C. 3mm，0°；D. 10mm，30°；E. 3mm，30°。

979 儿童胸腔镜的操作可以用镇静剂、局部麻醉或全身麻醉[36]。快速手术操作和对脏层胸膜的较少操作如滑石粉胸膜固定术和肺活检可以在由肋间神经阻滞诱导的局部麻醉下成功地完成。更长和更复杂的手术最好在全身麻醉下进行。单侧通气，对侧主支气管插管，对于需要广泛纵隔解剖的病例是有帮助的。在这些操作过程中，应对患者进行连续的 ECG 和脉氧仪监护。手术室应备有用于紧急胸廓切开术的器械，以

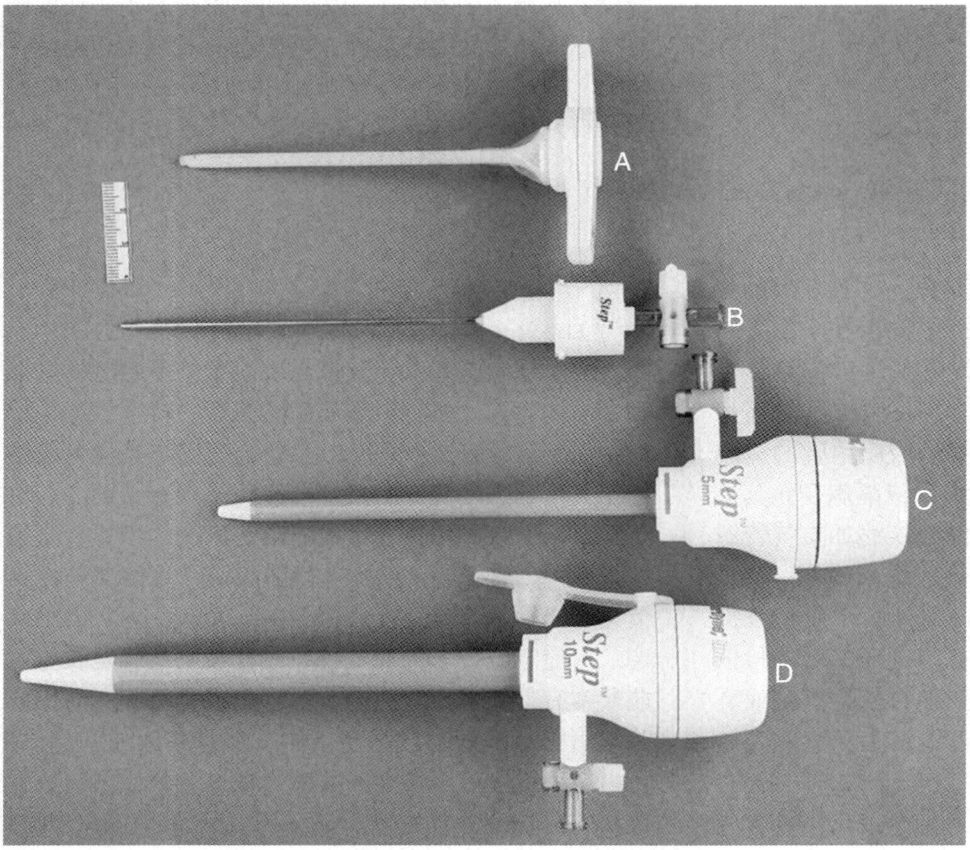

图 62-7 可扩张的 trocar 装置。可扩张的 trocar（A）用一个 Veress 针（B）插入通过胸壁。trocar 借助套管通过扩张的鞘能扩张到 5mm（C）或 10mm（D）。

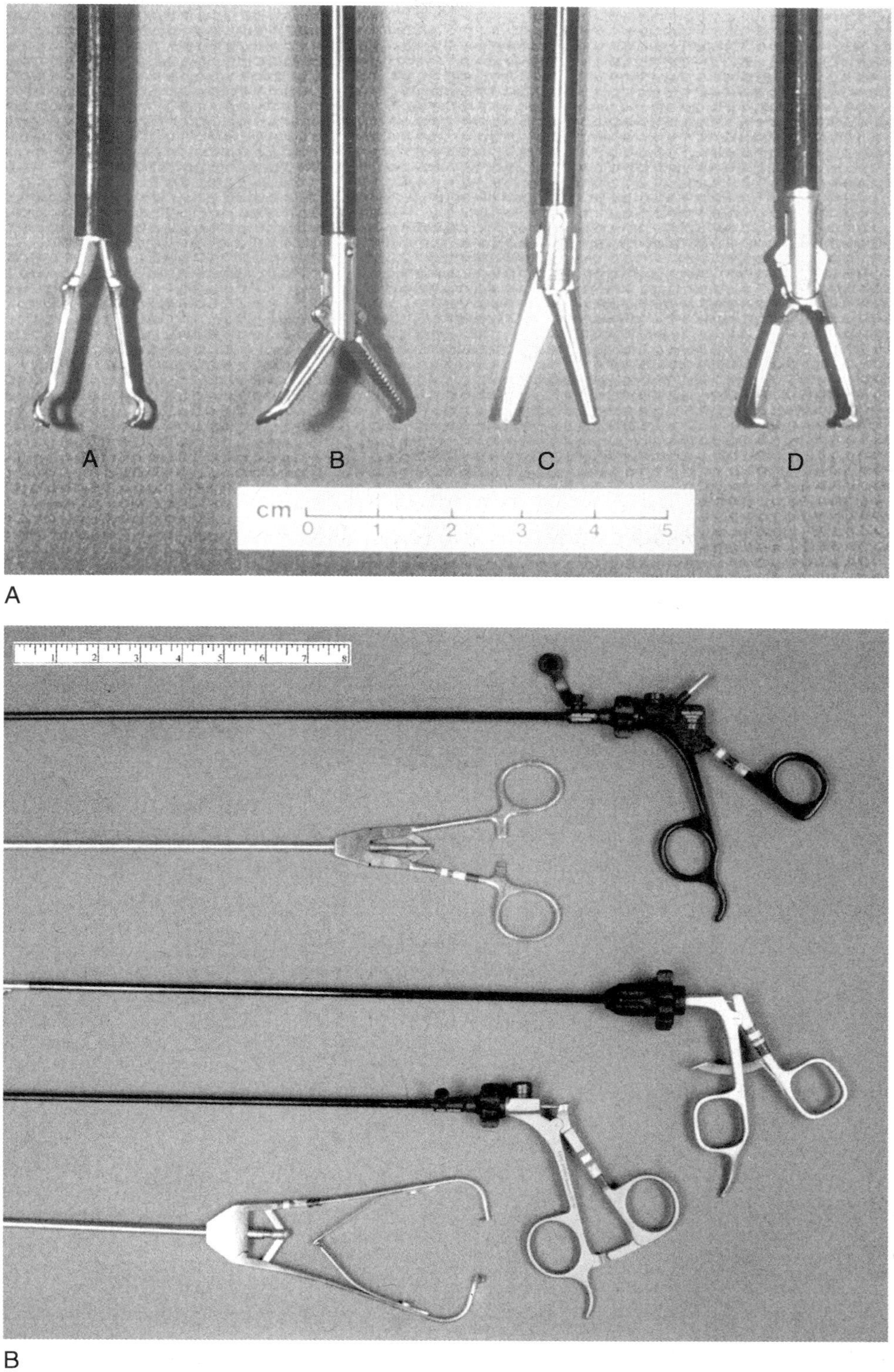

图 62-8　胸腔镜的仪器。A. 下列所有的仪器均有 5mm 的绝缘杆：A：Babcock 钳；B：直角解剖器；C：Metzenbaum 剪；D：Allis 钳。B. 不同手柄结构，根据它们预期的用途和操作者的喜爱可用于所有仪器。

980 便必要时控制出血。

将患者置于手术台上以便于接近病变的部位。手术包括肺活检或肺切除术的患者处于完全侧卧位，这样允许接触到所有肺叶和裂隙。位于后纵隔的病变最好通过把患者从真正的侧卧位向前滚动而进入，而前纵隔病变最好是通过真正的侧卧位向后滚动进入。最初的套管针通常置于腋中线第五或第六肋间隙。接下来的套管针的放置根据病变的可接近性。

而是一般采取一种三角形的结构，用于手术操作的套管针放在望远镜的任意一侧，把望远镜置于顶点。

脓胸的清创术需要大的抓握钳和压力灌洗完成。致密的粘连用烧灼术分离。肺活检标本最初是用杯状的活检钳获得，当钳子从套管针中退出时剪下一块肺实质。然而，这种技术不提供肺郁滞或止血。组织凝固设备现在在 5mm 的内镜中可用，在肺活检时能提供很好的肺郁滞和止血[69]。在大一些的儿童中，运用内镜 GIA 吻合器可以安全地获得大的楔形活检标本。纵隔病变可以通过打开附着于病变上的壁层胸膜和用钝性及锐性技术解剖病变来取活检或切除。低压下（4～6mmHg）胸腔内注入 CO_2 使同侧肺萎陷可以改善考虑要切除的纵隔病变的暴露。虽然金属夹子可以用于大血管，通常用电灼来止血。在用杯形钳取得纵隔淋巴结表浅部分活检后，我们用芯针直接穿过胸壁，在直视下得到深部的样本。乳糜胸的患者可以通过结扎或夹闭胸导管及连同一起的主动脉裂孔处食管后的邻近组织来治疗[7,24,67]。导管也可以单独分离并用金属夹闭合。在出现大量弥漫的淋巴漏的时候，结扎胸导管后紧接着在漏的区域运用纤维蛋白胶[13]。因气胸而采用胸腔镜的患者在电灼下分离腹膜粘连后，可以有一个完全的胸膜摩擦。我们用抓握钳夹住一块聚乙烯纤维的织物后进行摩擦。在一些病例通过第六肋侧方的壁胸膜切开和钝性分离上半胸膜行顶端胸膜切除术。在经过选择的患者可以通过在全部胸壁的壁层胸膜和脏层胸膜表面撒 USP 纯滑石粉进行滑石粉胸膜固定术。在取出套管针后，我们喜欢在原位留一根胸腔导管，即使有些作者在手术过程中如果壁胸膜没有损伤的话不会这么做。

并发症

胸腔镜的并发症大部分是由操作的程序和患者的医学情况决定的。报道的儿童胸腔镜的大部分并发症和所有的死亡率出现机械通气下为弥漫性肺渗出做胸腔镜肺活检的患者[53]。延长的支气管胸膜瘘在这组患者中的发病率最高，使得他们的呼吸处理更复杂。需要输血的出血是胸腔镜检查罕见的并发症，即使在由于化疗导致血小板减少的患者。术前纠正凝血异常可减少这种并发症的风险。与任何活检操作一样，偶尔有报道胸腔镜活检的假阳性结果。我们相信对浅表瘤的活检加上直视下直接芯针活检已经减少了这一问题的发生。偶尔，影像学检查看到的病变在胸腔镜下并不能定位，尤其是肺实质性结节。进行胸腔镜检查的外科医生“触摸”肺表面的能力有限，并且经常难于定位位于肺实质深部的病变。偶尔，在同侧肺塌陷单侧肺通气下可使这些深部病变更明显。已介绍用各种技术对这些病变进行术前标记这些病变以帮助定位。总体来讲，胸腔镜检查已经证实是一种高度准确和安全的操作。总体结果与开放的胸廓切开术相当，但是术后发病率更少。

用于观察气道和胸腔内结构的内镜技术在儿童治疗中被认为起到至关重要的作用。随着技术的改良，这些技术新的应用得到了发展。小儿外科医生熟悉这些技术并灵活地操作是义不容辞的。

（汪　健译　朱锦祥校）

参考文献

1. Arca MJ, Barnhart DC, Lelli JL, et al: Early experience with minimally invasive repair of congenital diaphragmatic hernias: Results and lessons learned. J Pediatr Surg 2003;38:1563.
2. Badr A, Tobias J, Rasmussen GE, et al: Bronchoscopic evaluation facilitated by the laryngeal mask airway in pediatric patients. Pediatr Pulmonol 1996;21:57.
3. Bax KN, van der Zee DC: Feasibility of thoracoscopic repair of esophageal atresia with distal fistula. J Pediatr Surg 2002; 37:192.
4. Black RE, Johnson DG, Matlak ME: Bronchoscopic removal of aspirated foreign bodies in children. J Pediatr Surg 1994; 29:682.
5. Bozzini PH: Lichteiter, eine Erfindung zur Anschauung innerer Teile und Krankheiten. J Prak Heilk 1806; 24:107.
6. Burns RC, McGahren ED, Rodgers BM: Thoracoscopic approach to pulmonary parenchymal lesions. Pediatr Endosurg Innov Tech 2001;5:141.
7. Burns RC, McGahren ED, Rodgers BM: Thoracoscopy in the management of chylothorax. Pediatr Endosurg Innov Tech 2001;5:153.
8. Cohen S, Pine H, Drake A: Use of rigid and flexible bronchoscopy among pediatric otolaryngologists. Arch Otolaryngol Head Neck Surg 2001;127:505.
9. Drasin T, Gracia C, Atkinson J: Pediatric applications of robotic surgery. Pediatr Endosurg Innov Tech 2003; 7:377.
10. Fan LL, Sparks LM, Fix EJ: Flexible fiberoptic endoscopy for airway problems in a pediatric intensive care unit. Chest 1988;93:556.
11. Gaafar HA: The fiberoptic bronchoscope in the diagnosis and investigation of laryngeal disorders. Clin Otolaryngol

1983;8:103.
12. Godfrey S, Springer C, Maayan C, et al: Is there a place for rigid bronchoscopy in the management of pediatric lung disease? Pediatr Pulmonol 1987;3:179.
13. Graham DD, McGahren ED, Tribble CG, et al: Use of video-assisted thoracic surgery in the treatment of chylothorax. Ann Thorac Surg 1994;57:1507.
14. Grewal H, Jackson RJ, Wagner CW, Smith SD: Early video-assisted thoracic surgery in the management of empyema. Pediatrics 1999;103:63.
15. Handler SD: Direct laryngoscopy in children: Rigid and flexible fiberoptic. Ear Nose Throat J 1995;74:100.
16. Hasagawa S, Hitomi S, Murakawa M, et al: Development of an ultrathin fiberscope with a built-in channel for bronchoscopy in infants. Chest 1996;110:1543.
17. Hawkins DB, Clark RW: Flexible laryngoscopy in neonates, infants, and young children. Ann Otol Rhinol Laryngol 1987;96:81.
18. Hirschowitz BI, Curtis LE, Peters CW, et al: Demonstration of a new gastroscope, the fibergastroscope. Gastroenterology 1958;35:50.
19. Hoeve LJ, Rombout J, Meursing AEE: Complications of rigid laryngobronchoscopy in children. Int J Pediatr Otorhinolaryngol 1993;26:47.
20. Hollands CM, Dixey LN: Robotic-assisted esophago-esophagostomy. J Pediatr Surg 2002;37:983.
21. Ikeda S: Flexible bronchofiberscope. Ann Otol Rhinol Laryngol 1970;79:916.
22. Jacobaeus HC: Über die Moglichkeit die Zystoskopie bei Untersuchung seroser hohzungen Anzuwenden. Munch Med Wochenschr 1910;40:2090.
23. Jacobaeus HC, Key E: Some experiences of intrathoracic tumors, their diagnosis and their operative treatment. Acta Chir Scand 1921;53:573.
24. Kent RB III, Pinson TW: Thoracoscopic ligation of the thoracic duct. Surg Endosc 1993;7:52.
25. Keohane JD, Forte V, MacPherson B: Pressure, flow, and resistance characteristics of the pediatric Storz-Hopkins bronchoscopes. Otology 1991;20:155.
26. Kern JA, Rodgers BM: Thoracoscopy in the management of empyema in children. J Pediatr Surg 1993;28:1128.
27. Koltai PJ, Nixon RE: The story of the laryngoscope. Ear Nose Throat J 1989;68:494.
28. Kosloske AM: The Fogarty balloon technique for the removal of foreign bodies from the tracheobronchial tree. Surg Gynecol Obstet 1982;155:72.
29. Lamm H: Biegsame optische Cerate. Z Instrumentenkunde 1930;30:579.
30. LeBret E, Folliquet TA, Laborde F: Videothoracoscopic surgical interruption of patent ductus arteriosus. Ann Thorac Surg 1997;64:1492.
31. Lindahl H, Rintala R, Malinen L, et al: Bronchoscopy during the first month of life. J Pediatr Surg 1992;27:548.
32. Lis G, Szczerbinski T, Cichocka-Jarosz E: Congenital stridor. Pediatr Pulmonol 1995;20:220.
33. Lobe TE, Rothenberg SS, Waldschmidt J, et al: Thoracoscopic repair of esophageal atresia in an infant: A surgical first. Pediatr Endosurg Innov Tech 1999;3:141.
34. Martinot A, Closset M, Marquette CH, et al: Indications for flexible versus rigid bronchoscopy in children with suspected foreign-body aspiration. Am J Respir Crit Care Med 1997;155:1676.
35. Marzo SJ, Hotaling AJ: Trade-off between airway resistance and optical resolution in pediatric rigid bronchoscopy. Ann Otol Rhinol Laryngol 1995;104:282.
36. McGahren ED, Kern JA, Rodgers BM: Anesthetic techniques for pediatric thoracoscopy. Ann Thorac Surg 1995; 60:927.
37. Mehrishi S, Raoof S, Mehta AC: Therapeutic flexible bronchoscopy. Chest Surg Clin North Am 2001;11:657.
38. Muntz HR: Therapeutic rigid bronchoscopy in the neonatal intensive care unit. Ann Otol Rhinol Laryngol 1985;94:462.
39. Nicolai T: Pediatric bronchoscopy. Pediatr Pulmonol 2001; 31:150.
40. Nitze M: Eine neue Boebachtungs und Untersuchungsmethode fur Harnblase. Wien Med Wochenschr 1879; 24:650.
41. Nussbaum E: Usefulness of miniature flexible fiberoptic bronchoscopy in children. Chest 1994;106:1438.
42. Nussbaum E: Pediatric fiberoptic bronchoscopy. Clin Pediatr (Phila) 1995;34:430.
43. Nussbaum E, Zagnoev M: Pediatric fiberoptic bronchoscopy with a laryngeal mask airway. Chest 2001;120:614.
44. Ozcan C, McGahren ED, Rodgers BM: Thoracoscopic treatment of spontaneous pneumothorax in children. J Pediatr Surg 2003;38:1459.
45. Partrick DA, Bensard DD, Teitelbaum DH, et al: Successful thoracoscopic lung biopsy in children utilizing preoperative CT-guided localization. J Pediatr Surg 2002;37:970.
46. Partrick DA, Rothenberg SS: Thoracoscopic resection of mediastinal masses in infants and children: An evaluation of techniques and results. J Pediatr Surg 2001;36:1165.
47. Perez CR, Wood RE: Update on pediatric flexible bronchoscopy. Pediatr Clin North Am 1994;41:85.
48. Picard E, Schwartz S, Goldberg S, et al: A prospective study of fever and bacteremia after flexible fiberoptic bronchoscopy in children. Chest 2000;117:573.
49. Pollock ME, O'Neal KO, Picetti G, Blackman R: Results of video-assisted exposure of the anterior thoracic spine in idiopathic scoliosis. Ann Thorac Surg 1996;62:818.
50. Puhakka H, Kero P, Valli P, et al: Pediatric bronchoscopy—a report of methodology and results. Clin Pediatr (Phila) 1989;28:253-257.
51. Rimell FL, Shapiro AM, Mitskavich MT, et al: Pediatric fiberoptic laser rigid bronchoscopy. Otol Head Neck Surg 1996;114:413.
52. Rodgers BM: Thoracoscopy. In Holcomb GE (ed): Pediatric Endoscopic Surgery. Norwalk, CT, Appleton & Lange, 1993.
53. Rodgers BM: Pediatric thoracoscopy: Where have we come and what have we learned. Ann Thorac Surg 1994;56:704.
54. Rodgers BM: Instrumentation and technique for pediatric thoracoscopy. Pediatr Endosurg Innov Tech 2001;5:93.
55. Rodgers BM: The role of thoracoscopy in pediatric surgical practice. Semin Pediatr Surg 2003;12:62.
56. Rodgers BM, McGahren ED: Endoscopy in children. Chest Surg Clin North Am 1993;3:405.
57. Rodgers BM, Moazam R, Talbert JL: Endotracheal cryotherapy in the treatment of refractory airway strictures. Ann Thorac Surg 1983;35:52.
58. Rogers DA, Philippe PG, Lobe TE, et al: Thoracoscopy in children: An initial experience with an evolving technique. J Laparoendosc Surg 1992;2:7.
59. Rodgers BM, Talbert JL: Thoracoscopy for diagnosis of intrathoracic lesions in children. J Pediatr Surg 1976; 11:703.
60. Rothenberg SS: Thoracoscopic repair of tracheoesophageal fistula in newborns. J Pediatr Surg 2002;37:869.
61. Rothenberg SS: Experience with thoracoscopic lobectomy in infants and children. J Pediatr Surg 2003;38:102.
62. Rothenberg SS, Chang JH, Toews WH, Washington RL: Thoracoscopic closure of patent ductus arteriosus: A less

traumatic and more cost-effective technique. J Pediatr Surg 1995;30:1057.
63. Schellhase D: Pediatric flexible airway bronchoscopy. Curr Opin Pediatr 2002;14:327.
64. Selim M, Mowafi H, Al-Ghamdi A, et al: Intubation via LMA in pediatric patients with difficult airways. Can J Anaesth 1999;46:891-893.
65. Shinwell ES: Ultrathin fiberoptic bronchoscopy for airway toilet in neonatal pulmonary atelectasis. Pediatr Pulmonol 1992;13:48.
66. Silberman HD: The use of flexible fiberoptic nasopharyngolaryngoscope in the pediatric upper airway. Otolaryngol Clin North Am 1978;11:365.
67. Stringel G, Teixcira JA: Thoracoscopic ligation of the thoracic duct. J Soc Laparoendosc Surg 2000;4:239.
68. Swanson KL, Prakash UB, Midthun DE, et al: Flexible bronchoscopic management of airway foreign bodies in children. Chest 2002;121:1695.
69. Tirabassi MV, Banever GT, Tashjian DB, et al: Use of energy devices in thoracoscopy: Quantification of lung-sealing capacity. Pediatr Endosurg Innov Tech 2003;7:267.
70. Tunkel DE, Fisher QA: Pediatric flexible fiberoptic bronchoscopy through the laryngeal mask airway. Arch Otolarygol Head Neck Surg 1996;122:1364.
71. Wain G: Rigid bronchoscopy: The value of a venerable procedure. Chest Surg Clin North Am 2001;11:691.
72. Waldhausen JH, Shaw DW, Hall DG, et al: Needle localization for thoracoscopic resection of small pulmonary nodules in children. J Pediatr Surg 1997;32:1624.
73. Wong K, Lai S, Lien R, et al: Retrieval of bronchial foreign body with central lumen using a flexible bronchoscope. Int J Pediatr Otorhinolaryngol 2002;28:253.
74. Wood RE: Spelunking in the pediatric airways: Explorations with the flexible fiberoptic bronchoscope. Pediatr Clin North Am 1984;31:785.
75. Wood RE: Pitfalls in the use of the flexible bronchoscope in pediatric patients. Chest 1990;97:99.
76. Wood RE: Flexible bronchoscopy in infants. Int Anesthesiol Clin 1992;30:125.
77. Wood RE: The emerging role of flexible bronchoscopy in infants. Clin Chest Med 2001;22:311.
78. Wood RE, Azizkhan RG, Lacey SR, et al: Surgical applications of ultrathin flexible bronchoscopes in infants. Ann Otol Rhinol Laryngol 1991;100:116.
79. Wood RE, Gauderer MWL: Flexible fiberoptic bronchoscopy in the management of tracheobronchial foreign bodies in children: The value of a combined approach with open tube bronchoscopy. J Pediatr Surg 1984;19:693.

第 63 章

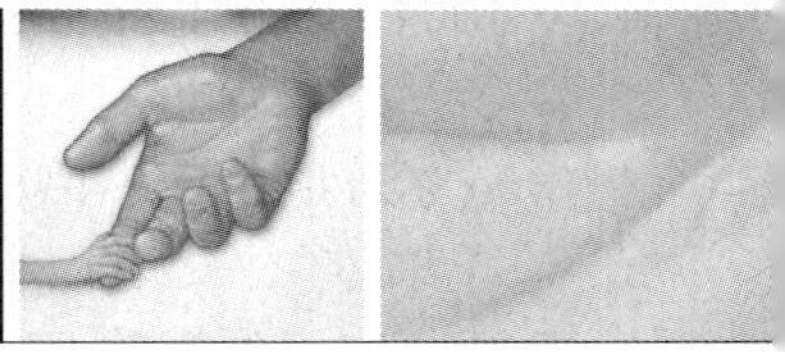

喉、气管和上呼吸道病变

Dana Mara Thompson 和 Robin T. Cotton

983 上呼吸道病变，即喉和气管的病变，能够引起致命的呼吸道梗阻。梗阻性气道疾病的病因通常是多因素的，包括解剖的、先天性的和炎症性的问题，而多数处理需要外科的介入。多样化的临床体征和症状与气道梗阻相关联。急性气道梗阻的体征有喘鸣、呼吸窘迫、呼吸暂停、发绀、苍白、呼吸急促、呼吸和回缩辅助肌的运用以及精神状况的改变。慢性气道梗阻可以有相似的症状和体征，出现气道梗阻和缺氧的长期并发症如生长延迟、体重不增、肺动脉高压和胸廓凹陷。不管是急性还是慢性梗阻，在确定气道梗阻部位的非创伤性临床体检中，喘鸣是最有用的发现。喘鸣的出现是由于紊流的气流通过狭窄的管腔所致，除了那些处于完全窒息边缘的孩子，它实际上出现在所有气道梗阻的患儿中。听到的喘鸣所处的呼吸时相可以帮助一个机敏的检查者更好地确定病变位置。典型的吸气性喘鸣出现于声门以上的梗阻性病变，如喉软化和声带麻痹。双相性喘鸣出现于声门以下（声门下或气管）的、固定的梗阻性病变。呼气性喘鸣通常代表了一种胸腔内气道的梗阻，如气管软化。在呼吸性“哮鸣”的基础上，气道的梗阻性病变可以误诊为哮喘。因此，高度怀疑指标并结合其他临床检查发现对于不忽视具有潜在危险性或外科可矫治的气道梗阻原因是必要的。

气道的内镜评估彻底改变了梗阻性气道的诊断和处理。内镜评估的实施分为清醒状态下和镇静状态或全麻下两种。可弯曲的光纤鼻喉镜和喉镜在小儿清醒状态下实施。尽管年龄小或缺乏合作，这种技术事实上可以在所有儿童在中安全快速地检查鼻、咽下部、声门上和声门。清醒状态使得我们能够评估声门上音调的动力学、声带的活动度和喉固定性梗阻病变的影响。镇静或全麻下的检查可以改变结果，因此，一种气道梗阻的重要原因特别是咽软化、喉软化和声带麻痹可能被忽视。在全麻或镇静下的气道直接检查仍然是气道梗阻的诊断和病变确诊的主要依据，特别是那些声门下的、清醒下光纤镜检不能够做出准确评估的病变。气道的内镜检查可以证实有怀疑的喉气管病变，如声门上的狭窄和气管狭窄。

任何由喉或气管疾病引起的呼吸道梗阻的评估和处理的目标是建立并保持一个安全稳定的呼吸道。因呼吸道梗阻而需要外科介入的儿童数量进一步增加，部分是因为 1960 年长期插管法和通气技术的发展使危重早产儿的生存率得以增加。由于长期插管法，这些婴儿能够生存，但是，一个全新的领域出现了，即长期健康问题，包括呼吸道、特别是喉和气管的问题。

呼吸道病理生理学和诊断考虑

喉是空气进入气管支气管树和呼吸系统的入口。没有一个能够发挥功能的喉，呼吸系统的剩余部分就会受到损害。喉系统发育的目的是呼吸和保护下呼吸道以防误吸。声音是喉的进化和继发的功能。儿童的呼吸道与成人在结构和功能上均存在差异。一个婴儿的喉大约为成人的 1/3，矢状面的尺寸大约为 7mm，984 冠状面为 4mm。声带长为 6～8mm。声门下空间的横径大约为 4.5mm；它以上呼吸道唯一完整的软骨环–环状软骨为界，同时是上呼吸道最狭窄的部分。因此，在婴幼儿呼吸道的这一部分，只要 1mm 的黏膜水肿就可以阻塞 40%的呼吸道。呼吸道空间随着年龄的增长，黏膜水肿引起的呼吸道损害也随之减小。婴幼儿喉和气管的软骨框架更加柔软且易曲折。这就导致在外界压力或空气的压力梯度下出现塌陷的倾向，导致我们在喉软化和气管软化时看到呼吸道梗阻。随着婴幼儿的生长和软骨的成熟，这些情况的症状通常自发改善，没有干预而消失。在婴幼儿，喉的位置较高，位于颈椎的 C2 和 C3 水平，直接在鼻的后方，接近缘膜、舌和声门上（功能上将呼吸道和吞咽分开）。由于对呼吸道起保护作用的神经肌肉功能在这期间没有完全发育好，这种故意的解剖关系允许婴儿安全地呼吸和进食，同时又不会引起误吸。然而，由于这一解剖关系，任何鼻腔的阻塞可以引起明显的呼吸道梗阻，也可导致进食困难。随着神经肌肉的成熟，喉在颈部的位置下降，2 周岁时降到 C4，呼吸和吞咽的功能性分离作用减弱；6 周岁时，喉下降至成人水平，直接在 C6 的后方。假如神经肌肉功能受损或随着喉的下降，神经肌肉没有成熟，呼吸道和吞咽的症状就会加剧。

气管切开术

气管切开术是处理本章讨论的几乎所有的呼吸道病变引起的严重呼吸道阻塞的一种手段。正如较早提到的，因呼吸道阻塞而需要外科干预的患儿数量增加，部分是因为 1960 年长期插管法和通气技术的发展使得危重早产儿的生存率增加。由于它是建立上呼吸道梗阻旁路不可缺少的操作，我们在回顾特定的阻塞性喉气管疾病前先讨论气管切开术的适应证、技术和并发症。儿童期最主要的三个适应证是呼吸道梗阻、通气支持和肺冲洗。许多因呼吸道梗阻而放置气管导管的儿童在非常幼小的时候经历了气管切开术，或者是因为长期气管插管导致了获得性声门下狭窄，或者是先天性病变损害了呼吸道。由于气管切开术的发病率和心理社会及发育的并发症，在实施气管切开术前应探索所有可能的替代方法。

气管切开技术

作者推荐的小儿气管切开术的技术如下。患者被带至手术室，呼吸道的安全性由气管内插管予以保证。由于喉和环状软骨的尺寸较小，典型的气管切开术的标记很难确定，紧急气管切开最好在有呼吸道保证（插管或刚性支气管镜）的情况下实施。取颈部正中垂直切口，上界到达环状软骨。皮下脂肪用电刀除去，中线处分离筋膜。带状肌在咽缝处分离，甲状腺峡用电刀分离。通过第 3 和第 4 气管软骨环在左右两侧靠近中线处垂直放置 4–0 不可吸收牵引线，松松地打结。给予牵引线轻微的张力抬高气管环，用尖刀在气管前正中线切开气管的第 3～4（或 4～5）软骨环。如图 63–1 所示，通过气管的切缘放置 4–0 的铬肠线并与皮肤缝合以产生气孔。有些作者认为这种技术形 985
成了一种更加永久的“气孔”以及取管后可导致持续的气管皮肤瘘没有被证实。由于行气管切开术的患儿死亡主要来源于意外脱管或不能更换阻塞的管道，作者相信，加上一个安全的界限，特别是在头几天，是有正当理由的。另外，儿科的气管切开术很少是短期的，即使没有皮肤的线结，随着时间的推移，管道也会上皮化。

拔除气管内导管（或支气管镜），插入大小适合的气管套管，保证双侧通气。如图 63–2 所示，以前

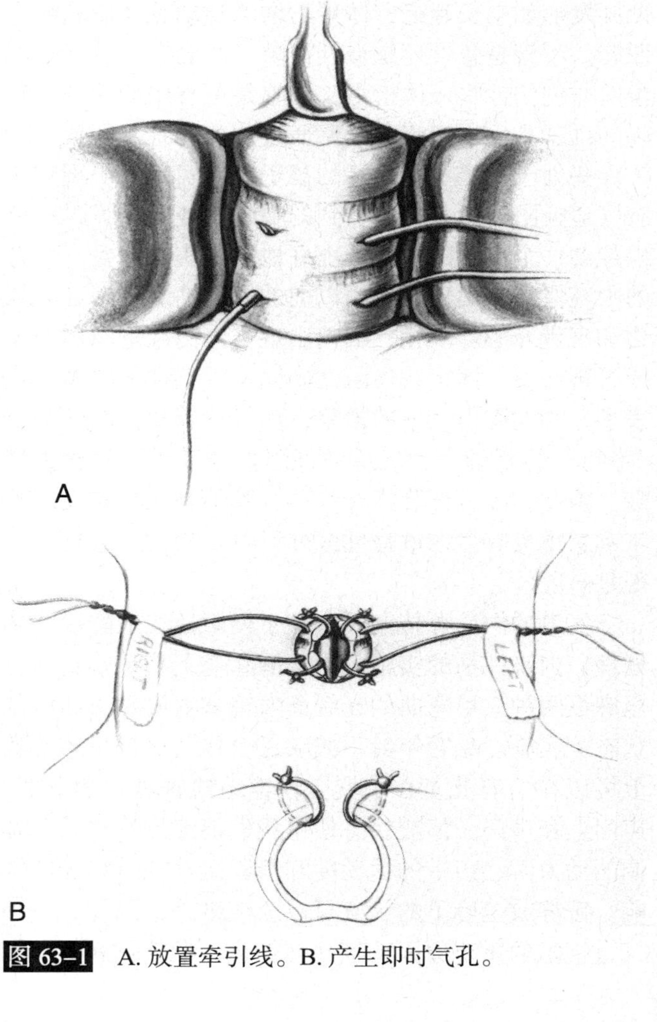

图 63–1 A. 放置牵引线。B. 产生即时气孔。

放置的牵引线分别作为左边和右边的标记，然后用胶带固定在前胸壁，作为意外脱管紧急情况下的牵引线。气管套管用斜纹棉固定带绕过颈后固定。气管套管，特别是没有内管的，不要直接缝合至小儿的皮肤。假如有明显威胁生命的黏液栓阻塞了气管套管，特别是在术后早期管道尚未完全建立时，有一固定于皮肤的套管延误紧急去除和用通畅的清洁套管替代。理论上，可以借助内镜通过声门，沿着气管套管对其位置做出评估。这允许外科医生能够保证气管套管接近隆凸。这种技术也允许外科医生估计气管套管在气管腔内的位置是否合适。理想的是同一直线和同心圆的关系，在气管的前壁或后壁没有任何摩擦或侵占。假如这种评估方法不能实施的话，可以将一可弯曲的支气管镜穿过气管套管以保证它的尖端接近隆凸。一旦管道建立，更换气管套管，牵引线 5 天内去除。这些患者应该在有监护的医院内实施气管切开术，至少应等到管道已建立、能顺利地更换气管套管，而且至少有 2 名护理人员接受教育并能理解如何护理。

气管切开术的并发症

气管切开术可发生围术期、术后和远期并发症，只要放置气管套管就可能出现。气管套管放置后的围术期并发症包括气胸和大血管出血，特别是来自无名动脉的出血。在手术操作结束时应行 X 线检查以排除气胸或纵隔气肿的可能性。最常见的手术后早期并发症可能危及生命，包括黏液栓和意外脱管。儿童气管套管的直径明显小于成人，任何由黏液引起的管腔堵塞都可以导致呼吸道的完全阻塞，特别是那些完全依靠气管切开术呼吸的小儿。同样，放置气管套管的气孔在小儿更小。假如套管意外移位，增加的呼吸负担引起进一步的塌陷，“吸吮”引起气孔的关闭，使得呼吸困难，对更换套管也是一种挑战。这种影响在术后早期特别引人注目，因为气孔还没有完全成熟。因为这些并发症是危及生命的，应采取预防措施保证气管套管通畅，仔细吸引，同时注意绕过颈部的固定以防止意外脱管。

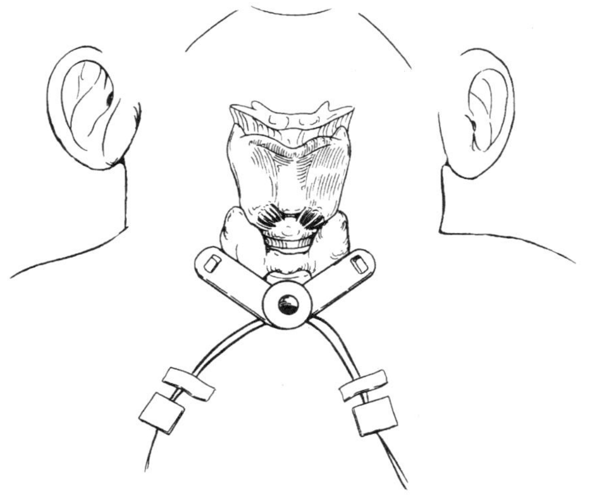

图 63–2　标记牵引线。

任何长期佩戴气管套管的小儿都存在发生轻微的和严重并发症的危险。术后早期，黏液栓和意外脱管是可能出现的最严重的、危及生命的并发症。只要气管套管还在，意外脱管始终是一个主要关心的问题。当幼小的患儿能够灵巧地用手拔出气管套管时更应特别关注。气管套管以上的呼吸道几乎完全阻塞的儿童，意外脱管被证明是致命的。尽管没有普遍使用，许多护理人员推荐一种家庭呼吸暂停监测仪或脉氧仪来帮助护理人员发现这种情况。在许多病例中，儿童仍能通过气孔舒服地呼吸，但应立即快速且安全地更换套管。慌忙地插入气管套管可能导致将套管放在假道中，导致呼吸道损害。我们推荐小尺寸的套管以方便护理人员使用。

可能出现与局部感染有关的并发症，可能是围绕气孔的皮肤或软组织（蜂窝织炎）、气管黏膜（气管炎）或气管软骨（软骨炎）。随着皮肤与气管软骨切缘的接触，管道的上皮化加速，促进愈合。然而，围术期后的局部感染在有些患者中可以发展。有代表性的 986
是，这些个体有一些潜在的因素容易导致衰弱和细菌侵入，如药物诱导的免疫抑制、原发性的免疫性疾病和糖尿病。治疗包括局部的抗生素包裹、经常更换敷料和导管以及全身应用抗生素。依照培养的结果选择抗生素。金黄色葡萄球菌感染和假单胞菌感染通常出现在重症监护病房。侵袭性的感染可导致软骨炎伴随伤口裂开、大血管暴露和感染向纵隔延伸，但少见。

气孔上方塌陷和肉芽形成是气管切开插管的普遍后果，但是阻塞程度的差异很大。虽然有些作者推荐定期地常规清除这些组织，但不是所有患者都需要。过分激进地清除肉芽组织可导致更加频繁的复发，常规切除的争论还将继续[82]。完全阻塞气孔上方呼吸道的肉芽肿需要清除，因为如果管道封闭或移位，有潜在的呼吸道完全阻塞的可能，同时可以保护发声。父母通常第一个注意到明显的气孔上方肉芽形成的症状或发现。最常见的是进行性失声和更换气管插管困难。失声的出现是因为肉芽肿阻止了空气沿气管切开插管周围通过，而这对于振动声带产生声音是需要的。

气管切开术更加致命的远期并发症是穿过气管前壁水平的无名动脉的腐蚀。这一并发症的出现是由于气管切开插管的尖端对前气管壁的压力增大的结果，导致肉芽组织形成、软骨变弱以及最终的腐蚀，如果没有提前发现。硬的和弧度不合适的导管促进这一并发症的发生，因此强调选择合适的气管切开插管的重要性。通常，医生在警惕鲜红色的出血，提示动脉即将破裂。因此，即使吸引小量的血液也应该借助可弯曲的内镜进行全面评估。

气管前壁由于连续的气管套管压力而腐蚀，以同样的方式，后壁也可以破裂。这作为一个远期并发症很罕见，尽管插入鼻胃管，喉部陷于两个硬的异物之间可以使情况更加恶化。患者出现无法解释的再发肺炎或肺纵隔炎，应怀疑此诊断。呼吸通气的患者，随出每一次吸气将出现嗳气。对这一并发症，传统是采用开放手术处理，在气管和食管之间插入健康的肌肉。

随着手术经验的增加、手术技术的改进、影响预后的共病情况的确定和处理以及术后护理的改善，气道扩张手术的适应证已经扩展到喉气管狭窄的一期明确手术，因此避免了对许多气道疾病行气管切开术，传统上，在最初的处理中需要气管切开术[29,34,101,105]。

喉和声门下病变

喉软骨软化病

喉软骨软化病是婴幼儿喉部异常和喘鸣最常见的原因。临床表现为吸气性的喘鸣，随进食、骚动和仰卧位加重。症状通常出现在出生时或出生后不久，高峰在 6～8 个月，通常在 18～24 个月消退[44]。轻型的特点是仅有吸气性喘鸣。因为那些呼吸道梗阻的婴幼儿，很难协调“吸吮-吞咽-呼吸”的顺序，所以中等程度的病变通常表现为进食困难。许多这些婴幼儿伴有胃食管反流（GERD），需要抗反流处理和其他措施治疗[30,79]。几个因素解释这种情况：第一，近端的呼吸道阻塞增加了胸腔内的气道压力促进反流；第二，调节食管运动的反射不成熟引起食管的排空不足；第三，像其他患有呼吸道疾病和呼吸暂停的婴幼儿一样，这些婴幼儿的 GERD 可能与下食管括约肌的频繁松弛有关[83]。

患有严重喉软骨软化病的婴幼儿经历了危及生命的呼吸道梗阻并发症，可能导致漏斗胸、生长延迟、慢性缺氧、肺动脉高压和肺源性心脏病。这些患者需要外科干预[43,77,81,110]。

如果听诊有喘鸣，应怀疑喉软骨软化病的可能，但必须得到纤维喉镜检查的证实。这一检查必须在婴幼儿清醒的状态下进行，以显示周期性塌陷至喉入口的声门上组织。全身麻醉可能遮盖这些发现。其他典型的发现是 Ω 形的会厌和向前脱垂的杓状软骨阻塞了气流以及声带的完整视野。这个检查也可以排除其他明显的声门上病变。这种情况的病因是多因素的。提出的理论包括异常的呼吸道解剖[6,65]、软骨形成的不成熟和神经疾患。

喉软骨软化病通常是一个自限性疾病，很少需要外科干预。对那些危及生命的呼吸道梗阻或发生低氧并发症的婴幼儿，推荐外科干预。直到 80 年代中期，在声门上成形技术被引入之前，气管切开术一直都是该情况的治疗选择[54,87,110]。气管切开术作为呼吸道梗阻部位的旁路直至这种情况自发缓解，一般在 18～24 个月后。行声门上成形术可避免气管切开术。这 987
一手术是通过显微外科除去楔状软骨区域多余的脱垂组织并松解束缚会厌部位的杓状会厌襞（图 63-3）[110]。这一处理的长期结果一般说来是不错的，80%～100%的病例症状逆转[43,51,61,63,81,96,110]。有些作者报道多达 50%的患者需要另外的呼吸道手术，或是修正的声门上成形术，或是气管切开术[63,96]。声门上狭窄是手术后最严重的并发症，可能由于过分去除组织或对酸反流性疾病控制的失败所致。尽管声门上成形术是一个优先于气管切开术的选择，但在许多情况下，有些伴有复杂的共病情况的儿童，特别是那些有严重的神经系统损害或涉及呼吸道的并发症，最初的处理最好还是气管切开术[22]。

喉闭锁和喉蹼

喉蹼是先天性的（图 63-4）或获得性的（图 63-5）。

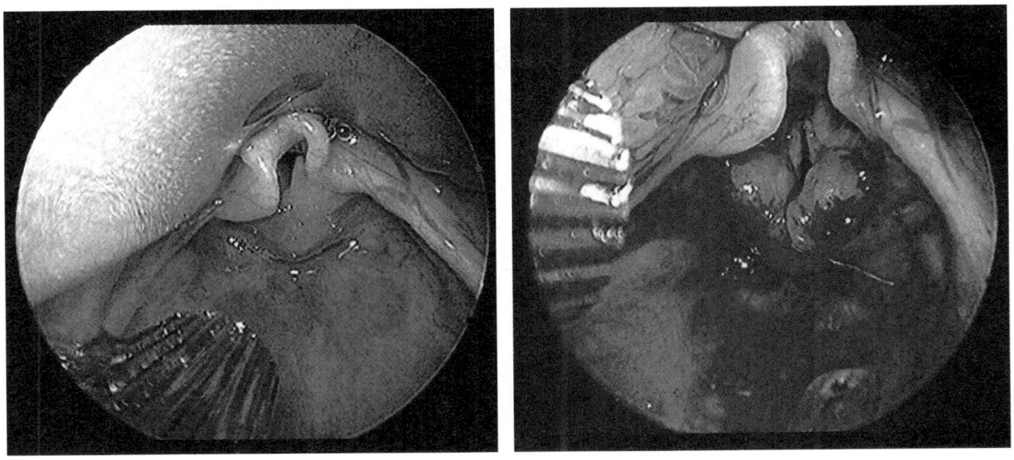

A　　B

图 63-3　声门上成形术前（A）和后（B）的喉软化。

先天性喉蹼和闭锁少见，可能与软腭-心-面综合征有关。胚胎学的原因是产前发育期间，闭锁或喉管的再通失败。如果没有及时发现，闭锁或足够大小的喉蹼在出生时将表现为失声和快速窒息。残余狭窄呼吸道的细薄喉蹼在插管时可以破裂。即使不是完全不可能，厚的喉蹼和闭锁使得标准技术的紧急插管变得困难。在这种情况下，婴幼儿的生存可能依靠紧急气管切开术以保证呼吸道通畅。厚的喉蹼和闭锁的外科处理需要气管切开插管直到外科干预完成[67]。外科矫正通常需要喉正中切开术，打开呼吸道，分离闭锁区域，切除多余的环状软骨环的软骨。需要将肋软骨移植到前环状软骨，类似于治疗声门下狭窄的喉气管再建术。再建的时间取决于许多因素，包括儿童的年龄和外科医生的经验。

细薄和中等厚度的前蹼表现为失声或出生时哭声
微弱，没有呼吸道梗阻的症状。处理的主要目标是提 988
供一个开放的呼吸道并达到良好的声音质量。这是一种挑战，因为手术干预后声带有纤维化和形成肉芽组织的倾向。传统上，如果外科医生认为小儿生长适当，一般在 12 个月后，选择喉正中切开术和放置支架来治疗薄的和中等厚度的前蹼。最近的报道建议，某些喉蹼可以用内镜松解和局部应用丝裂霉素 C来处理，即使患儿小于 1 周岁。这种技术使得先天性喉蹼能够在很小的年纪得到成功的治疗。然而，这种技术的长期预后还不知道，而且也不清楚接受这种方法治疗的婴幼儿最终是否仍需要喉气管再建以保持一个通

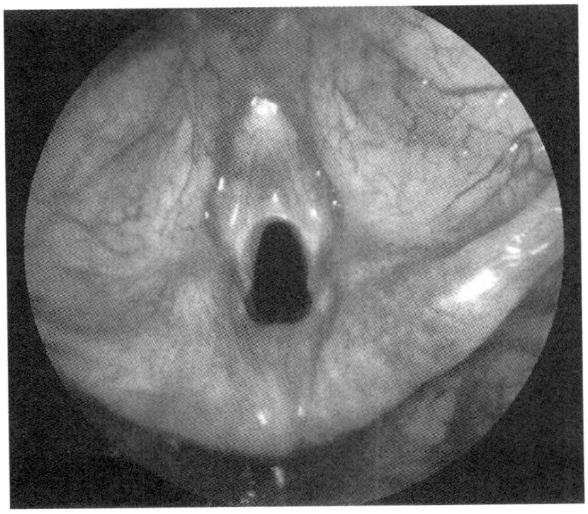

图 63-4　先天性喉蹼。

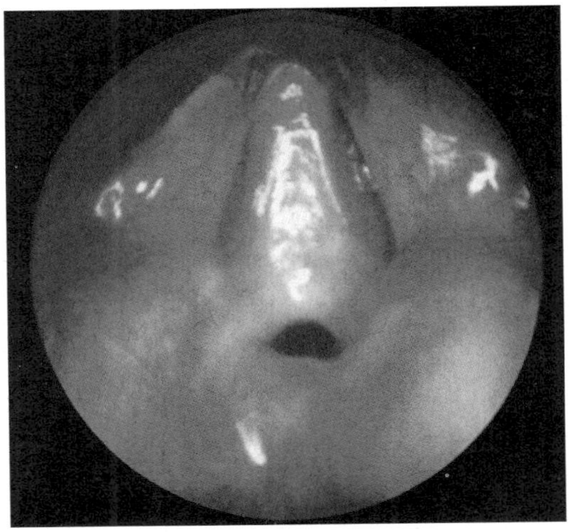

图 63-5　获得性喉蹼。

畅的呼吸道。喉蹼治疗的长期结果依据原发病情的严重程度。经过外科处理的细小喉蹼通常可以痊愈，伴随轻微的发声破裂，而有声门下狭窄的厚的喉蹼很少有满意的结果[7]。

获得性喉蹼不常见，通常由直接的喉外伤引起，两侧声带的近中心面破裂，愈合后形成了蹼。在喉乳头状瘤的处理和治疗中经常遇到，特别是在喉咽反流的情况下[42]。

声带不动：声带麻痹和声带固定

声带的运动需要完整的迷走神经功能和环杓关节的自由转动。声带从中线外展打开会厌的入口以便气流进入气管支气管树。假如没有出现声带的外展，气流就会受限。声带不动由声带外展失败所致。声带不动的两个主要原因是声带麻痹和声带固定，两者可能是先天性的或后天性的。从颅神经核至胸腔走行的迷走神经任何地方的损伤都可以引起神经源性的声带麻痹。后天性的声带不动通常由牵拉损伤、压力侵入、炎症发作和外伤或神经本身的切割伤所致；环杓关节是灵活的，但是神经肌肉功能受损。环杓关节的先天疾患、外伤和炎症都可以引起声带固定；环杓关节固定，但神经肌肉功能是完整的。固定和麻痹可以同时存在。不论声带不动的病因如何，一侧或两侧声带的外展失败能够导致喘鸣和呼吸道梗阻。

单侧声带不动引起喘鸣但通常不会造成呼吸道阻塞。双侧声带不动限制了通过声门的气流，通常引起严重的呼吸道梗阻，需要人工通气。有些婴幼儿和儿童有轻微的症状仅仅出现在上呼吸道感染期间，可能不需要气管切开术。许多双侧声带固定的儿童在疾病病程的早期、明确的外科治疗之前需要进行气管切开术。由于双侧声带不动多数可引起呼吸道梗阻，外科治疗仅限制在双侧不动的处理上。

双侧声带麻痹（BVCP）的呼吸道症状的处理依据病因和迷走神经的受累位置进行。在新生儿和婴幼儿中，BVCP可能是中枢原因的，最常见与Chiari畸形或脑积水相关。在Chiari畸形可以看到的脑干尾侧移位引起脑干、迷走神经及迷走神经核的受压。对这种压迫的认识加上明确诊断对于防止Chiari畸形的其他并发症是十分重要的。一旦Chiari畸形的压力减小，BVCP即可以缓解。除了压迫迷走神经及其核以外，脑积水导致第四脑室的压力增加。放置分流管降低颅内压经常能达到治愈[76,106]。有中枢病因的BVCP婴幼儿，不能从中枢减压的措施中得到改善，为了呼吸道的安全需要行气管切开术。这组患儿最终也容易出现其他下颅神经问题和误吸，保持对气管切开插管的依赖，也不是通过外科手术实现成功拔管的候选人。如果迷走神经完整且BVCP的原因局限于迷走神经的损害，如产伤、感染或外部压迫所造成的神经牵拉，如果没有急性的呼吸道梗阻现象，应当观察一定的时间。对这些患儿来说，麻痹是暂时性的，他们在其他方面是健康的。如果声带麻痹的原因是直接神经损伤之类的外伤，功能没有恢复的希望，需要气管切开术直至能采取另外的步骤以扩大声门的开口。这种情况可以在伴有神经损伤的"固定线"颈部外伤[57]或者在甲状腺或心胸手术并发症的患者中看到。

继发于固定的双侧声带不动出现在环杓关节的滑液关节面变得固定时，因为此时阻止了声带的外展或内收。在这种情况下，迷走神经通常在功能和结构上是完全完整的。关节固定最常见的原因是某些类型的直接针对关节区域本身的外伤，如插管或颈部外伤导致环杓关节脱位。一旦关节损伤，炎症出现，引起关节的固定。青少年风湿性关节炎也能导致双侧固定。先天性少见。

不论声带固定的原因如何，处理的外科方法在儿童中是相似的。事实上，有很多的外科方法可供使用意味着没有一个单一的步骤是理想的。处理的目标是充分打开声门后的呼吸道允许足够的气流通过，而又不增加患者暴露于误吸并发症或声音变弱的危险。在气管切开插管保证了呼吸道安全和稳定后，通常实施 989
前面描述的步骤，尽管外科手术的基本目标是避免气管切开。做出一期明确手术的决定依据于呼吸道梗阻的程度、儿童的年龄和保护呼吸道避免误吸的能力。

复位和清除声门后的结构和组织，换句话说，杓状软骨和黏膜，是一种在双侧声门固定情况下打开呼吸道的技术。该技术包括杓状软骨侧偏、杓状软骨固定、杓状软骨部分切除和脊髓丘脑外侧束切断术[10,28,73,97]。这些步骤可以单独使用，也可以联合实施。外科方法从外面可以通过喉正中切开术，内镜用CO_2激光，或两者结合使用。已有用内镜CO_2激光成功除去杓状软骨声带突和部分后声带的病例报道[28]。用这种技术处理的挑战是手术后肉芽组织的治疗，而肉芽的形成可以导致呼吸道阻塞[80]。最近的评估小儿 BVCP 手术治疗预后的无分析和回顾性研究提示，与 CO_2 激光杓状软骨切除术和脊髓丘脑外侧束切断术或单独的杓状软骨的固定术相比，带有部分杓状软骨切除术的喉正中切开术，结合声带的侧偏步骤带来最高的脱管率[11,39]。这些相同的研究推断，开放的手术作为儿科 BVCP 的一线治疗似乎更加有效，杓状软骨固定术伴或不伴杓状软骨切除术提供了一种有吸引力的一线手术选择。他们也得出结论，作为原始的步骤，CO_2 激光尽管不太成功，但在修正的时候有效。尽管这些步骤在成功脱管和保持呼吸道开放上有效，但有关误吸和声音的长期预后没有资料证明。

后部嫁接的喉气管成形术是另外一种开放后声门的有效技术[32,108]。通过喉正中切开术，并延伸至气管的前两个环，切开并分离后方的环状软骨板以分开杓状软骨。将肋软骨移植至分开的环状软骨后板处以稳定杓状软骨的位置。尽管这一技术的报道较少，脱管率都接近 100%[39]。内镜后环状软骨劈开和插入肋骨移植物已经在少数声门后和声门下狭窄的儿童中成功完成。

复发性呼吸道乳头状瘤病

复发性呼吸道乳头状瘤病（RRP）是人乳头瘤病毒（HPV）感染上呼吸消化道黏膜的一种表达形式。涉及喉的乳头状瘤是儿童最常见的喉肿瘤，喉是呼吸消化道最常发的部位（图 63–6）。儿童期的 RRP 以簇状出现，有难以置信的复发倾向。喉乳头状瘤的临床表现是进行性的气道梗阻和发声困难，甚至发展到失声。RRP 最常与 HPV–6 和 HPV–11 相关联。16 和 18 亚型很少与 RRP 有关联，一旦出现，有恶变的高度危险。这些病毒颗粒出现在接近呼吸道临床正常的位置，但是主要是在靠近上皮的解剖位置表达，因此声带特别好发[53]。另一个常见的部位是黏膜损伤处，如气管切开的部位[53]。带菌传播具有争议。儿科 RRP 和阴道尖锐湿疣都是由 HPV–6 和–11 亚型引起，因此大多数的研究者认为，大多数病例为母婴垂直传播。尽管不常见，已有报道患有阴道软疣的母亲垂直传播给剖宫产出生的儿童[90]。

RRP 的自然病程变化极多，没有明显的患者相关的危险因素对预测预后有帮助。每位患儿的平均手

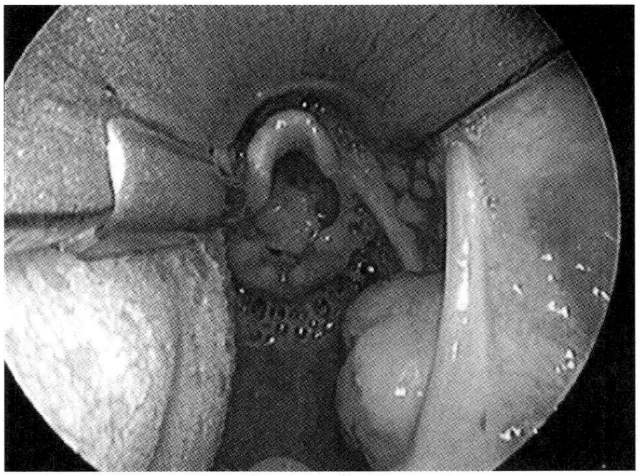

图 63–6　喉乳头状瘤阻塞会厌。

术次数估计为 19.7 次，每年平均为 4.4 次。已看到许多病例的症状在青春期自然消退，但另外一些进展至涉及气管和肺实质的广泛性疾病，伴有不可治疗的气道梗阻或肺部并发症，病死率高。即使更加不常遇见，乳头状瘤可以恶变为鳞状细胞癌。出于这个原因，定期切除组织的组织学检查很重要。

儿科 RRP 继续成为一个极难处理的问题。外科处理的目标是保持一个通畅的气道，同时还要提供一个可用的声音并且防止疾病扩散至远端气道。

尽管传统的外科处理主要依靠的是 CO_2 激光，新的外科技术包括动力仪器、喉刮刀[75]和脉冲染料激光[23]，已经显示有效。不管用何种外科技术，尽管通过内镜仔细的清除病变，并发症仍然存在，包括喉部的
瘢痕、狭窄和蹼的形成。乳头状瘤的切除应下至声带黏 990
膜的水平，但声带本身不应该切开。在前联合处操作时，不要做双侧切开以避免蹼的形成。即使是有经验的医生，前声门轻微瘢痕的发生率也高达 25%[104]。超过上述范围的激进切除需要保持一个安全的气道，长期的预后中没有明显的缓和，但晚期死亡率可能下降。

气管切开术在喉乳头状瘤外科处理中的作用是有争议的。可能的话，许多外科医生试图避免气管切开术。气管切开位置的黏膜损伤促进了乳头状瘤向喉外生长，可能增加了该病向远端扩散的可能性。据报道需要气管切开的患者，其气管播散率高达 50%[16]。假设 RRP 的侵蚀程度不同，有疾病远端播散的患者代表了一种播散，超过喉的具有播散倾向的亚型，不管怎样都需要气管切开，这是很可能的。对于喉内或超过喉的病变进展所致的危及生命的气道梗阻，而内镜

治疗又不能处理的患者，应该实行气管切开直到疾病被进一步的外科干预和辅助治疗控制。假如实行了气管切开，临床医生应该尽一切努力，只要有可能就要脱管。

许多用于 RRP 治疗的辅助治疗没有一个确信能够改变病程的结局。最常见的用于儿科 RRP 的辅助性内科疗法是干扰素 α-2a、视黄酸、吲哚-3-甲醇/二吲哚甲烷（I3C/DIM）。最近引入的辅助治疗是西多福韦，一种有抗病毒作用的非周期性膦酸盐腺苷，用于 AIDS 患者巨细胞病毒视网膜炎的治疗。对某些患者，清除喉乳头状瘤后局部直接注射西多福韦显示有效。而且，有希望发展一种针对儿科 RRP 疫苗的研究正在进行。

喉气管和声门下的狭窄

喉气管的狭窄以病因学和累及的区域为特点。累及的区域包括声门上、声门、声门下和气管的上部。单一的或多个区域可能被累及。喉狭窄是先天性的（图 63-7）或后天性的（图 63-8）。先天性狭窄被认为是孕 10 周时喉腔的再通失败或不完全所致。先天性声门下狭窄在组织学上分为膜性和软骨性狭窄（表 63-1）。

足月儿气道环状软骨区域的内腔小于 4mm，早产儿小于 3mm 且没有插管病史，考虑为先天性狭窄。如图 63-7 所示，先天性软骨性狭窄的典型表现为椭

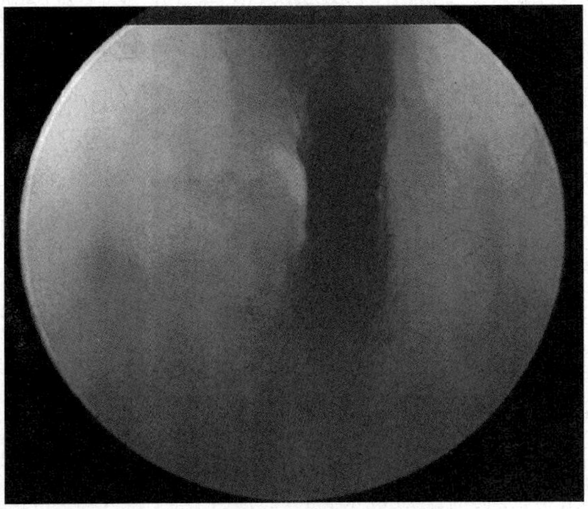

图 63-7 先天性声门下狭窄伴椭圆形的环状软骨。

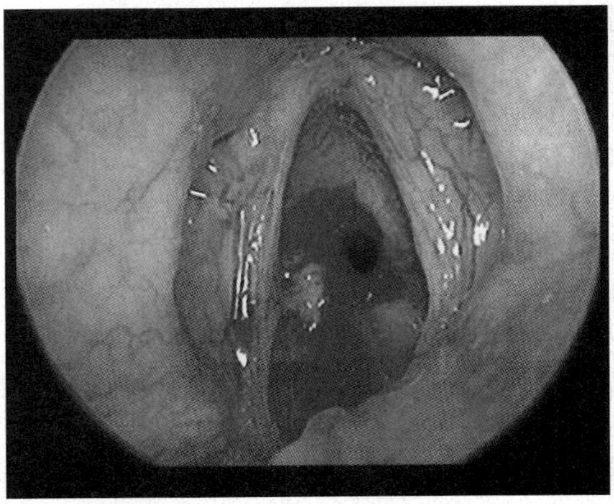

图 63-8 获得性声门下狭窄。

圆形的环状软骨。先天性或后天性的定义可能有些任意，因为继发于损伤的软组织狭窄和瘢痕可以在先天性声门下狭窄的患儿中发生，导致后天性的狭窄。这最常出现在持续很长时间的插管中，所以先天性声门狭窄的真正的发生率很难确定。在狭窄累及的区域中，声门下最常见。许多需要外科处理的声门下狭窄都是后天性的。后天性狭窄的例子如图 63-8 所示。讨论的外科处理原则可应用于先天性和后天性疾病。

后天性的声门下狭窄从 1965 年新生儿长时间气管内插管和通气支持的引入后变得更常见[64]。随着极低出生体重儿生存率的增加，继发性喉气管狭窄的患者数亦随之增加。已经认识到，后天性狭窄比先天性声门下狭窄更严重，也是一个更难处理的问题[45]。幸运的是，气管内插管技术的进步和导管固定以及柔软材料在管的应用已经使生存的新生儿气管/喉气管狭 991
窄的发生率降至 0.9%～8.3%[78]。随着药物和手术挽救生命的技术进展，作为治疗的结果，发生了其他慢性疾病，声门狭窄就是其中之一。目前患有喉狭窄的幼儿、儿童和青少年的数量已经有所增加，但确切的百分率还不知道。狭窄可以是柔软的或坚硬的，常见的是两者兼有。软组织狭窄的原因是黏膜下的黏液腺增生、导管囊肿、纤维和肉芽组织以及胃酸咽喉反流引起的黏膜水肿。坚硬的狭窄通常与环状软骨的畸形发育或增厚或瘢痕组织有关。Cotton-Myer 分级系统是使用最广泛的梗阻程度的评估文件（图 63-9）。气管内导管的尺寸成为分级和估计狭窄程度应用最广泛的工具[71]。

表 63-1　先天性声门下狭窄的分类

软骨性狭窄	软组织狭窄
环状软骨畸形	肉芽组织
正常形状	黏膜下纤维化
小于婴幼儿尺寸	黏膜下腺体增生
异常形状	
大的前板	
大的后板	
弥漫性增厚	
椭圆形	
黏膜下裂	
其他先天性环状软骨狭窄	
受困的第一气管环	

成功的喉气管再造手术需要一个仔细的公式化的计划，包括鉴别和处理对不良预后有影响的重要的内科共病情况。该计划也需要准确地鉴别狭窄的类型和累及的所有的喉和上气管区域，因为狭窄可能是多水平的且需要超过一种类型的手术。治疗计划依据特殊的患者以及患者的内科共病情况和解剖位置而制定。治疗计划最好由多学科团队来共同制定，包括小儿耳鼻喉科医生、小儿外科医生、肺脏学家、胃肠学家、麻醉师和合适的辅助健康人员。

任何喉狭窄都可以通过气管切开术而得到有效的处理。与气管导管放置有关的发病率和死亡率鼓励了

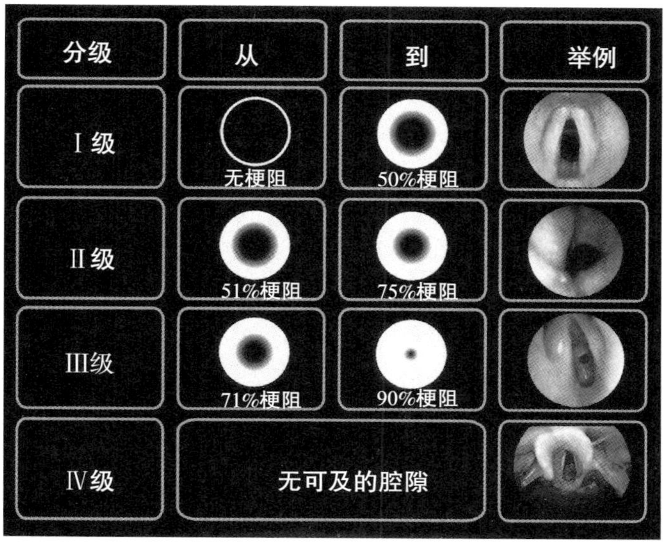

图 63-9　Cotton-Myer 声门下狭窄分级系统 。

喉气管再造方法的进步，以避免气管导管的放置或实现套管的成功去除。

在考虑外科干预前，必须注意有关的内科共病情况特别是心肺疾病和 GERD，稳定且处理。需要明显的通气或内科支持的儿童不是喉气管再造的好的候选人。吞咽功能的评估对于帮助确定保护气道的能力和误吸的危险是必需的，以便在术前和围术期能做出调节将误吸的并发症减至最小。有明显误吸的患者通常不是喉气管再造的好的候选人。

必须强调胃食管反流对喉气管狭窄和损伤的影响。GERD 是获得性声门下狭窄的病因性因素。临床和动物研究显示喉区出现酸类物质妨碍愈合[31, 36, 58, 62, 95, 107]。喉气管再造手术的围术期和术后推荐积极的内科治疗，有时甚至是外科抗反流治疗[95]。尚没有前瞻性和回顾性研究评估这种手术控制反流的长期预后。

喉气管狭窄的外科处理是针对患者的个性化处理，没有手术步骤对所有的病例来说是完全相同的。每一个个体患者有多个变量需要考虑，包括狭窄区域的位置和程度、内科共病情况、气道保护及吞咽功能、年龄和体重。外科的选择包括内镜技术、扩张手术和切除手术。根据狭窄的程度和部位选择使用的方法。一般而言，Ⅰ级狭窄通常用内镜技术处理。Ⅱ级狭窄根据病变的部位和程度采用内镜技术或开放手术。Ⅲ和Ⅳ狭窄几乎总是需要开放手术重建。

Ⅰ级和Ⅱ级狭窄可以通过内镜技术治疗。由于它们精确的组织特点，CO_2 和磷钛钾晶体（KTP）激光是应用最广泛的方法。激光在治疗早期插管损伤伴肉
芽组织形成、声门下囊肿、细的环状面蹼和月牙形的 992
束带是有用的。导致声门下狭窄内镜激光治疗失败的因素是先前内镜步骤的失败、软骨构架的明显丢失、垂直方向上大于 1cm 的厚的环形瘢痕、累及后连合。激光治疗声门下狭窄的并发症是软骨膜或软骨的暴露，接着是软骨膜炎和软骨炎，可导致进一步的瘢痕形成。

当内镜方法建立的开放气道不合适或失败时，推荐开放的手术重建。前方的环状软骨劈开是扩张的手术技术之一。它主要用于前声门下狭窄的新生儿，尽管有足够的肺储备但多次试图除管失败。在这种情况下,喉气管的问题是环状软骨水平的狭窄所致，一旦前环状软骨在中线处分开，气道腔扩张并解压。气管内导管留在原位 5～10 天。在除管前 24 小时开始应

用地塞米松磷酸钠，除管后继续应用 5 天。这一技术帮助 66%～78%的患者成功除管[19]。如表 63–2 所示，新生儿在考虑应用这一技术前，必须满足几个临床标准以增加前环状软骨分离后成功除管的可能性。

表 63–2 行前环状软骨分离的标准

至少两个继发于声门下喉病变情况下的拔管失败
体重大于 1500g
在修补前没有通气支持至少 10 天
增补的氧气需要量少于 30%
修补前至少 1 个月没有充血性心力衰竭
没有急性呼吸道感染
修补前没有用抗高血压的药 10 天以上

对作者来说，这一技术已经被前环状软骨分离和放置小的耳软骨移植物，然后气管内插管 7 天所取代。还没有正式的综述比较环状软骨分离和环状软骨分离加上耳软骨移植物这两种方法除管率的结果。

许多扩张狭窄气道的开放步骤已被描述。这些步骤和它们的应用在过去的 30 年中得到发展。自从 1972 年采用喉气管再造和在分离的前环状软骨及上气管之间置软骨移植物以来[19]，这种方法已成为扩张狭窄气道最常见的技术之一。单独的前方移植物通常应用于没有累及后声门和声门下的Ⅱ级和Ⅲ级狭窄。如果前狭窄同时累及后声门或声门下，则根据狭窄的程度，选择后环状软骨板劈开放置或不放置间置的移植物。这一问题在Ⅲ和Ⅳ级狭窄中更常看到。

部分环状软骨气管切除已经进展到成为某些Ⅲ级和Ⅳ级狭窄外科处理的另一个选择[38,39,85,93,98,102]。在这一手术中，前环状软骨板狭窄的区域和任何被累及的气管狭窄部分被切除，气管游离容许端端吻合。后部的气管和气管肌被吻合到后环状软骨板及其黏膜上。然后将前方松解的气管缝在环状软骨移去的部分并固定在甲状软骨上（图 63–10 和 63–11）[38,85,93,98]。

喉气管再建手术的传统方法包括再造的几个阶段[17,18,20,109]，当实施扩张手术时，放置一支架（塑料板或特氟纶）以稳定重建。支架留在气管切开导管的上方（气孔上支架）1～6 周。支架除去后，一旦手术部位愈合，声门开放，减小气管导管的尺寸直到患儿能够耐受且围绕塞紧的气管导管能够呼吸。一旦这一过程完成，移除气管切开导管。这个再建和除管的过程可能要花几周到几个月的时间。与气管切开导管有关的发病率和潜在的死亡率儿童中已得到充分的认识，并已在本章节的早前面讨论过。随着分期重建和支架放置，患儿的气管切开导管的上方仅有很少或没有气道留下，如果导管意外脱落或阻塞将威胁生命。长期支架带来了肉芽组织形成、感染、支架移位、吞咽困难和误吸的额外发病率。针对这些危险并防止这些问题发生，发展了一期喉气管再建（SSLTR）。对于伴有肺储备受损、伴有复杂的多水平狭窄需要延长支架的患儿或镇静成为问题的患儿作者仍采用分期的步骤。 993

SSLTR 包括外科纠正狭窄的气道和短期的气管内插管，因此避免了延长喉气管支架的需要和气管切开导管的依赖。考虑 SSLTR 作为手术选择时，气道必须要有合适的软骨支撑。SSLTR 需要全面理解气

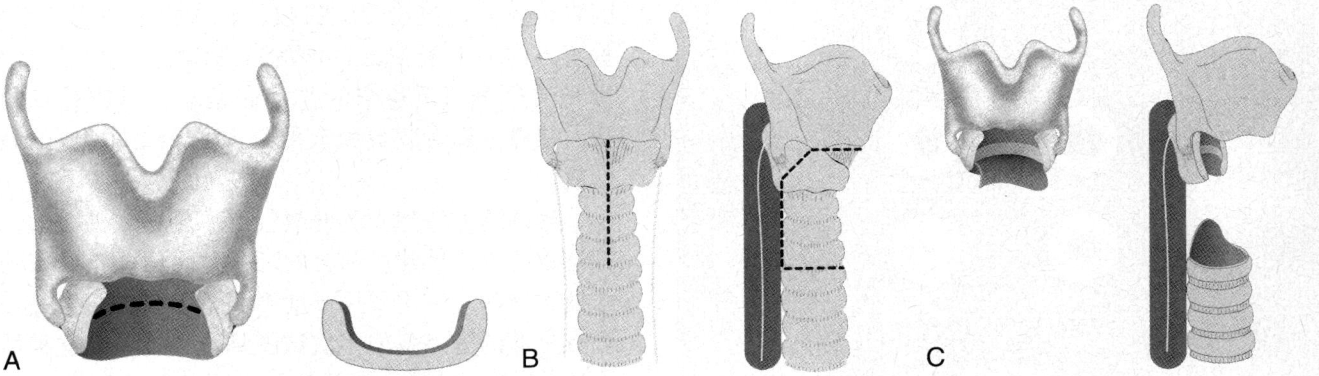

图 63–10 气管环状软骨的切除。A．后环状软骨黏膜切口切除前面的环状软骨。B．保留喉返神经的瘢痕气道切除示意。C．包括后气管黏膜套的完全切除。

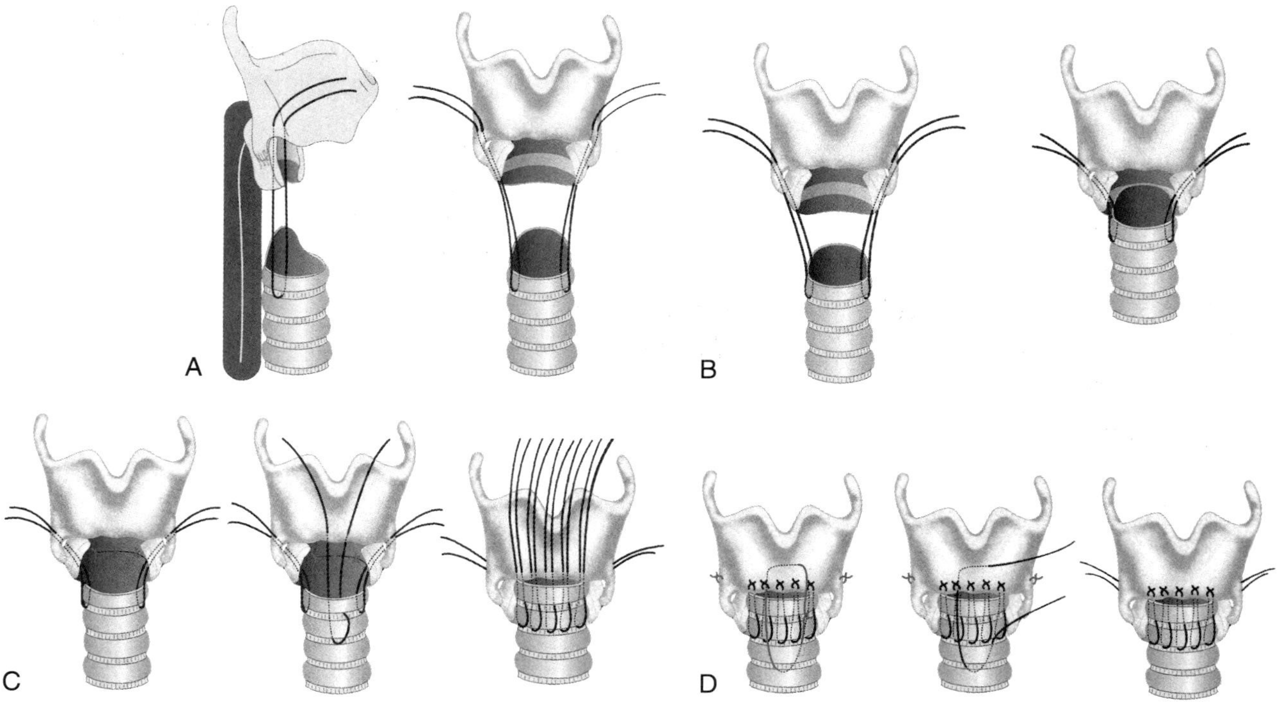

图 63–11 切除气道的再吻合。A．放松的线结。B．气管松解。C．后面完全吻合，前面放置吻合线。D．完全吻合。

道再建的原则，外科医生、麻醉师、ICU 专科医生和护理人员应有多方面的经验。这些患者的术后护理可能是复杂的[34,37,48]。我们医院 200 例 SSLTR 病例的经验显示，29%需要再插管，15%术后需要气管切开术。总的去管率为 96%。同时也发现，前肋或后肋软骨移植物的使用、年龄大于 4 岁、镇静剂超过 48 小时、沿气管内导管周围漏出压大于 20cmH$_2$O 和中或重度的气管软化显著增加再插管率。支架的时间不影响预后。有前后移植物的患儿和那些有中度或严重气管软化的患儿可能更需要术后的气管切开。SSLTR 能够有效用于儿科喉气管狭窄的治疗。然而，患儿共病情况和细心的气道术前评估、术后护理、外科技术及经验对于手术的成功非常重要。

喉气管再造的最终目的是气管切开术的去管或防止。去管率随狭窄的严重度和再建的方法而不同。儿科声门下狭窄的外科处理极具挑战性。为了达到最后除管或除套管的成功，需要多个手术，没有特别的模型来预测儿科气道再建手术的预后。回顾我们医院的经验显示，对 Cotton–Myer 分级 Ⅱ 、Ⅲ和Ⅳ级行二期喉气管再建后的去管率分别为 95%、74%和 86%。我们的经验是 Cotton–Myer 分级Ⅲ或Ⅳ级的患儿代表了一种明显的挑战，针对这群患儿需要采用精致的技术。

Ⅳ级狭窄的儿童是手术处理最难取得良好结果的一组。我们发现，外科技术的改进和环状软骨气管的切除作为Ⅳ级狭窄的根本手术，去管率从 80 年代的 67%提高到 20 世纪 90 年代的 86%[33]。我们的经验还显示，行环状软骨气管切除的患儿的去管率（92%）比那些行喉气管再建和前后肋软骨移植的患儿
（81%）要高。环状软骨气管切除的患者很少需要另 994
外的开放手术来达到除管（18%：46%）[33]。累及喉和气管其他区域的Ⅳ级狭窄患儿通常需要扩大的环状软骨气管切除并应用软骨移植物或喉环状软骨和杓状软骨的步骤。

血管瘤

声门下和气管血管瘤是来自中胚层的先天性良性血管畸形。病变相对不常见，占所有先天性喉畸形的 1.5%，性别比例 2：1，女性较多[44]。出生时患儿通常无症状，但是在生后的头几个月出现喘鸣，85%的

患者在头 6 个月内确诊[14]，50%在诊断时出现皮肤血管瘤[56]。在软组织的颈部 X 线片上不对称的声门下狭窄是典型的发现。通常采用内镜诊断而不需要活检，因为病变的典型表现为声门下后外侧区域的带有蓝色或红色点状的可压缩的、不对称的、黏膜下肿块（图 63–12）。

声门下和气管的血管瘤有一个快速的生长期，到 12 个月时减慢，在接下来的数月至数年慢慢消退，大多数显示在 5 年内完全消退。然而，如果声门下血管瘤不处理的话，有 30%～70%的死亡率[56]。这一问题的治疗和手术处理是针对保持气道通畅同时减少治疗本身的长期后遗症。当前的处理选择包括部分激光切除、开放手术切除、全身或病变内激素治疗、全身干扰素 α–2a 治疗和气管切开术。

应用气管切开术绕过病变部位同时等待预期的退化提供了最理想的解剖结果，许多人认为可以作为治疗的标准，衡量其他所有选题。然而，正如本章节先前讨论的，气管切开术存在危险，而且儿童在年幼时气管切开，一般会出现说话和语言的延迟。早期的治疗方法包括外源性光辐射、镭、金的植入物和硬化剂，但因为相关的发病率而不再使用。

1969 年，Cohen[15]引入了全身皮质类固醇治疗，用于声门下血管瘤的基础和辅助治疗。激素以未知的机制减小血管瘤的尺寸并加速退化。它们被认为是通过阻止雌二醇诱导的生长[40]或直接增加毛细血管对血管收缩药的敏感性来减小血管瘤的大小。皮质类固醇治疗伴或不伴气管切开术已在 82%～97%的病例中获得成功，然而，气管切开套管插入的时期是否缩短还不知道[91]。与长期应用激素有关的危险包括生长延迟、柯兴氏面容、感染易感性的增加，包括威胁生命的卡氏肺囊虫肺炎[3]。采用隔天、最小剂量的方法可以降低这些影响。最近的报道提示，诊断性支气管镜检查后，全身激素治疗伴随短期插管可以作为治疗阻塞性儿童声门下血管瘤的一种安全有效的选择[2]。还有人[66]报告采用内镜血管瘤内注入激素伴或不伴短期插管成功地避免了气管切开术。

CO_2 激光的内镜手术处理由 Healy 及同事在 1980 年第一次报道[41]。自从被引入以来，CO_2 激光单独或结合激素或气管切开术已经变成了标准治疗。孤立的单侧声门下血管瘤通常是 CO_2 激光治疗的最佳类型和部位。用 CO_2 激光部分切除血管瘤，用或不用全身皮质类固醇，在仔细选择的病例是成功的[92]。最近的报道显示 KTP 激光是一种处理声门下血管瘤的良好手段，并发症的发生率低。KTP 激光被血红蛋白优先吸收，因此使得这种激光系统适于治疗血管瘤等血管肿瘤。这种技术的长期预后尚未获得。 995

干扰素 α–2a 最近已被用于对激光或皮质类固醇治疗（或两者）无反应的阻塞性血管瘤患儿，73%的患者达到 50%以上的病变消退[74]。干扰素 α–2a 需要长期应用，因为它不能促进退化但是通过阻止血管形成的不同步骤来抑制增生。潜在的副作用包括神经肌肉损害、皮肤脱落、发热和肝酶增高[74]，限制了它用于巨大的、潜在致命的病变。

尽管激素和其他治疗方法的应用更广泛，在过去

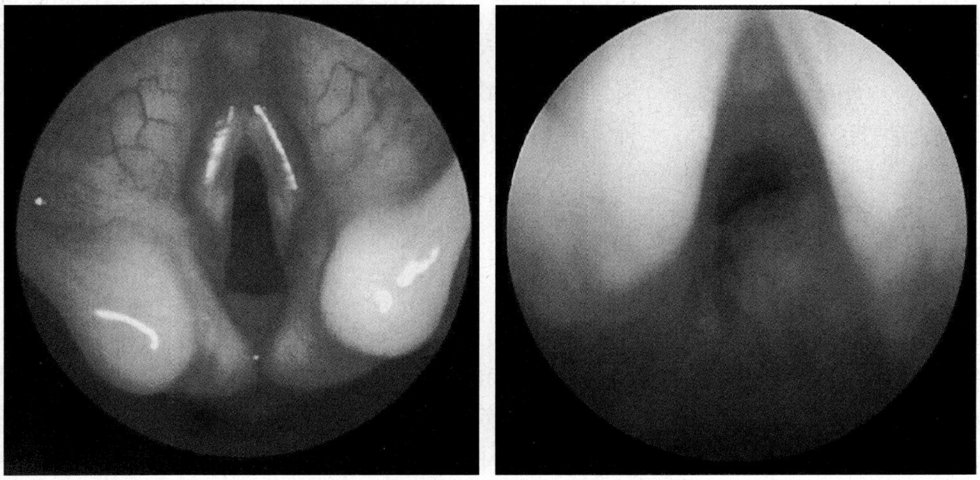

A B

图 63–12 声门下血管瘤。

20 多年，对气管切开术的需要仍没有改变。激光治疗的应用似乎并没有带来任何超过单独行气管切开术使声门下血管瘤消退的额外好处。全身类固醇可以减小血管瘤的大小但与许多副反应有关。因此，决定用上述技术时必须依据这些观察[13]。为了避免并发症和提供更确定的治疗，开放手术切除的话题被再次提起[13,29,72,88,89,101,105]。手术技术与 SSLTR 相似。在环状软骨水平打开气道，然后黏膜下分离，切除血管瘤。由于经常出现关联的中度声门下狭窄，通常放置前方的软骨移植物，患者插管 2～3 天。最近的研究得出结论，在经过挑选的患者中，手术对于严重的声门下血管瘤是一种可靠的技术，皮质激素抵抗和皮质激素依赖、环状或双侧血管瘤[101]和威胁生命的巨大血管瘤应考虑手术治疗[29]。一期切除的早期经验提示，这一技术是一项令人激动的、有希望的外科选择，它的更加广泛的使用可能是进一步改善声门下血管瘤预后的最佳方法。

喉和喉气管食管裂

先天性的喉和喉气管食管裂（LTEC）是罕见的畸形，表现为喉和气管与下咽部和食管在中线处的分隔缺陷（图 63-13），发生率小于 0.1%，大多数病例散发或与综合征有关。与其他畸形存在牢固的联系（56%），最常见的是气管食管瘘（20%～27%）[26]。6%的气管食管瘘患儿有并存的喉裂，3/4 的患儿没有发现喉裂，直到成功地修补了气管食管瘘后仍继续发为误吸，促使进一步检查时才发现[26]。喉裂或 LTEC 常与一个综合征有关，最常见的是 Opitz-G 综合征、VATER 联合（椎骨缺损、无肛、气管食管瘘、桡骨和肾发育异常）、VACTERL 联合（椎体、肛门、心脏、气管、肾和肢体畸形）和 Pallister-Hall 综合征。

裂隙的程度可能相对较轻，只累及杓状软骨肌的发育停滞，或者可以延伸至隆突，甚至进入主支气管。多元分类系统被用于描述喉裂。独立于已用的编号系统，它有助于区分裂隙的长度是喉（只有杓状软骨肌、部分环状软骨或完全的环状软骨）还是喉气管食管（进入颈部的气管段和胸腔的气管段）的。

喉裂或 LTEC 患儿有先天性的吸气性喘鸣、进食有关的发绀发作、误吸和反复的肺部感染。随着裂隙长度的增加，症状的严重性亦增加，LTEC 患者

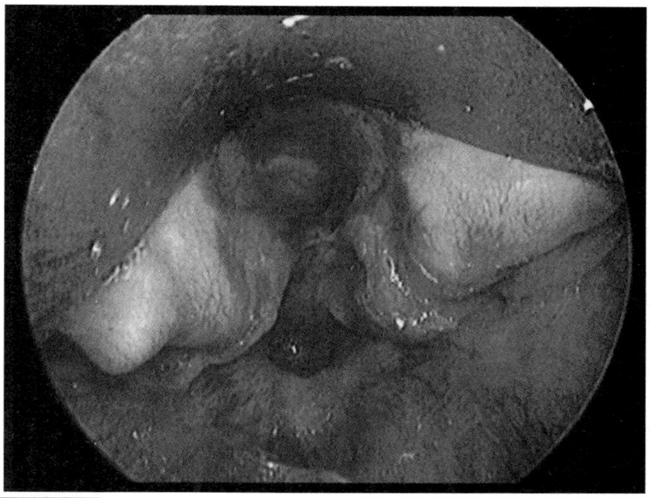

图 63-13　喉裂。

100%出现误吸。尽管造影检查可以提示误吸，但确定喉裂的最佳的单一检查是内镜仔细检查高度怀疑的部分。需要断开杓状软骨以获得足够的视野，因为裂隙可能被多余的食管黏膜脱垂到声门和声门下而变得模糊不清。许多裂隙局限在上声门喉部，不需要外科干预。这些小裂隙的解剖深度达到杓状软骨水平和止在声带突，治疗方法包括胃食管反流的评估和治疗以及吞咽治疗。当需要外科干预时，作者更喜欢开放修补，尽管有些人提倡内镜修补[8,26]。

所有延伸至声带下的喉裂都要手术修补。通过喉正中切开的路径是标准技术，它很好地暴露整个缺损而不会对喉的神经支配造成危险。延伸到隆突的完全 LTEC 可能需要后外侧路径以允许两层关闭或需要带有心肺旁路或体外循环的前路径。在许多情况下，气管切开术在术前或再建手术时实行。然而，一期修复伴气管内插管作为短期支架的使用正在增加，作者认为延伸到 Midtrachea 的裂隙更适用。

气管病变 996

气管软化

气管软化是气管壁软骨柔软的一种病变。气管软化的主要症状是随呼吸努力增加而出现的喘鸣，导致气道的动力塌陷。气管软化可以是原发的也可以是继发的，原发性气管软化的病因未知。它是婴幼儿喘鸣

常见的原因。原发性气管软化与喉软化不同，喘鸣出现在呼气期，然而，喉软化与气管软化可以同时存在，患儿可以同时有吸气性和呼气性喘鸣。许多原发性的或独立的气管软化患儿到 18 个月时可以摆脱这种情况。继发性的气管软化是另外的共病情况的结果。继发性气管软化最常见的先天性病因是血管畸形如血管环或无名动脉的外部压迫（图 63–14），和气管食管瘘，软化位于瘘的对侧、后气管壁上。气管软化也可以发生在需要用高压气管内套管或带袖套的气管切开导管作长期通气支持的婴幼儿。对于严重的或威胁生命的气管软化，除了用气管切开导管绕过并支撑软化区域外，没有更好的治疗方法。气管内放置支架（用血管成形术和 Palmaz 支架）的方法已被尝试并获得了不同的成功，作者更喜欢用气管切开导管。

先天性气管狭窄

先天性气管狭窄是一种罕见的、威胁生命的畸形，它通常累及全部的软骨气管环，经过数年被证实很难处理。1964 年，Cantrell 和 Guild 将先天性喉狭窄分成三类：长段型的狭窄伴弥漫性的发育不全（22%）、漏斗样狭窄（37%）和节段性狭窄（41%）。先天性气管狭窄的患儿常有联合畸形，24%与心血管畸形共存，包括肺动脉系带[9]。

伴有先天性气管狭窄的患儿通常有二相性喘鸣和可能的急性呼吸困难病史。前后位的 X 片在最初的评估中被强烈推荐，但确定性的诊断最好是用内镜获得（图 63–15）。新发展的三维磁共振为诊断和随访提供了一个选择。另外，磁共振、增强 CT 或超声心动通常需要用来确定相关的心血管畸形。最近几年，先天性气管狭窄的治疗有了巨大的进步。节段切除同时一期吻合已成为治疗 50%的气管狭窄的选择。然而，大量的手术步骤用于治疗长段型狭窄，并获得支持，说明没有一种被证明是普遍成功的。我们医院的发现重申，完全气管环的非手术治疗在选定的患者中是适当的。一个回顾性的研究[86]估计 10%的伴有完全气管环的患者不需要气管成形术。选定的患者必须是无症状的或仅有轻微症状，在连续的检查中显示出气管生长。带有心包的前气管成形术由 Idriss 及其同事在 1984 年第一次描写[46]。从那时起，这一技术的结果显示在大系列中的生存率为 47%～76%[24]。在少数量的患者中，肋软骨移植物有相似的结果[103]。已经尝 997
试的其他加入材料包括食管壁、肋骨、硬膜和骨膜。

Tsang 及其同事[99]描述的错位气管成形术包括在狭窄的中线处横向分离气管，在一端纵向切开前壁，另一端纵向切开后壁；两端互相错位，因此长度减半，口径增加一倍。在原始描写中，错位气管成形术用于漏斗样狭窄。这一技术已经进展，现在已成为气管狭窄（不管狭窄的长度）优先考虑的方法（图 63–16）[21,64]。只有当其他方法都不能用时，才考虑气管同种移植重建。据报道此项技术的成功率和生存率为 83%[49,50]但还没有经过时间的考验。

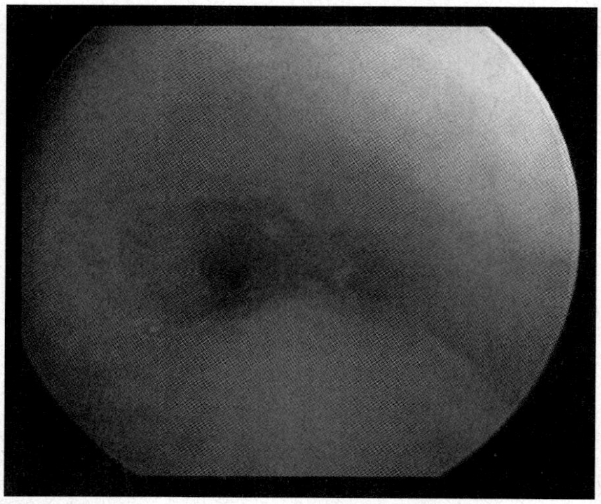

图 63–14 继发于无名动脉压迫的气管软化。

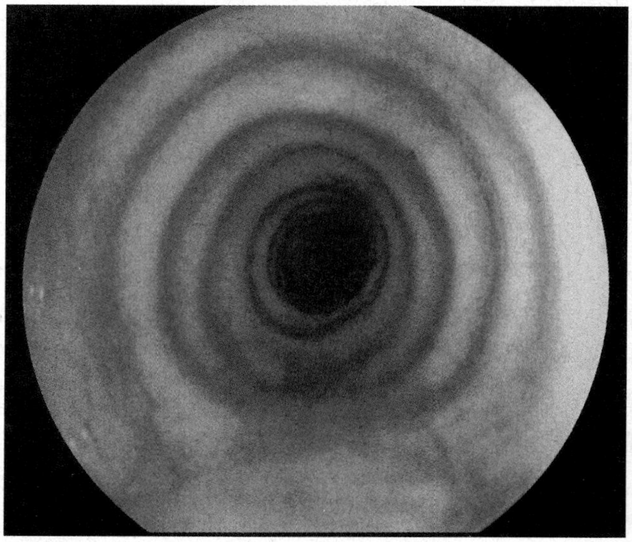

图 63–15 完全气管环。

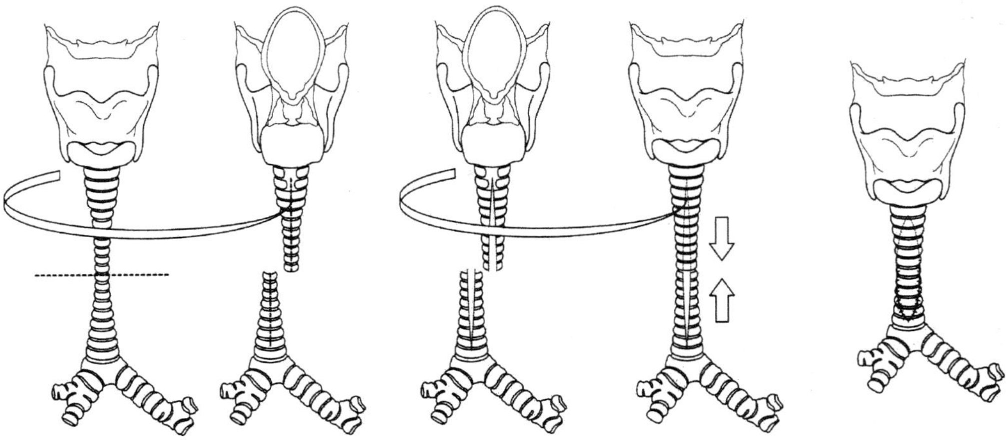

图 63-16　错位气管成形术：横断气管，近端部分向后错位，远端部分向前错位。错位的两部分接合后周长增加一倍，长度缩短一半。

气管支气管血管压迫

自 1945 年报告的第一例双主动脉弓手术成功以来，气管支气管血管压迫已经成为许多讨论的主题。一份 1963 年的报告[27]回顾了 104 个案例并创造了术语“反射性呼吸暂停”描述与气道血管压迫有关的发作性呼吸暂停。这一系列在 1969 年回顾并更新[70]，报告的 285 病例中有 86.3%内科处理成功。

最初的手术适应证包括反射性呼吸暂停和反复的支气管肺感染，这些适应证被扩展成绝对和相对标准[59]。相对标准包括内科处理失败、大于 50%的气管腔压迫及有关的气道和肺部异常。进一步的适应证定义出现在 1975 年，60 名儿童因为无名动脉压迫气管而接受手术，同时与 30 个没有手术的儿童进行比较，应该注意的是，手术干预的适合程度不是根据内镜和影像学看到的压迫的严重程度而是依据症状的严重程度[68]。1981 年建议停用“异常”一词，当时报道无名动脉部分或完全在气管的左侧起源是儿童的正常发现，在 96%的患者主动脉造影中看到[94]。

气管支气管树血管压迫的总发生率为 3%。最常见症状性真性血管环是双主动脉弓，如果第四鳃弓和背侧的主动脉根两侧都存在就会发生。右侧的弓和右降主动脉不会引起气道压迫。然而，假如存在一相关的左导管或异常的左锁骨下动脉，可以形成松弛的血管环，导致的气道压迫一般要比真性双主动脉弓小得多。由于相关的下气管和右主支气管的气道压迫，肺动脉系带是最有症状的非环形的血管畸形，出现时左第六弓消融，左肺动脉作为起源于右肺动脉的一个大的侧支动脉在食管与气管之间穿过去灌注左肺。这一畸形通常导致右主支气管的明显受损和气道症状。另外，30%有肺动脉系带的患者存在相关的完全气管环[4]。异常的右锁骨下动脉是最常见的纵隔血管畸形。然而，由于它的食管后走行，受累的个体可以出现吞咽困难，但很少有呼吸道受损的症状。无名动脉压迫气管与真正的血管畸形无关。正常情况下，无名动脉从位于中线左侧的主动脉弓起源，跨越气管的前表面，到达右侧。有人假设，表现出症状的患者的无名动脉比正常人紧张，气管软骨顺应性异乎寻常，更容易受压，或者其他结构如心脏、食管或胸腺扩张引起纵隔拥挤。

来自气管支气管血管压迫的呼吸道损害可以威胁生命但症状不明显。高度怀疑时需要做出诊断。由于出现喘鸣、慢性咳嗽、反复的支气管炎和肺炎、进食困难和生长停滞以及偶尔的反射性呼吸暂停，有明显血管压迫的患者通常较早识别。反射性呼吸暂停已被描述为一种反射性的持续时间不定的呼吸停止，继发 998
于吞咽时和其他形式的短暂的胸腔压力改变对迷走传入神经纤维的刺激，可能是致命的。

胸片可以提供气管受压的证据，钡餐食管造影可显示与血管压迫各种类型相符的相对特征性充盈缺损。然而，一旦血管压迫被怀疑，首选的诊断模式是磁共振，它可以清楚地显示纵隔血管畸形和下气道的尺寸。螺旋 CT 可能有用，作为磁共振的辅助或替代方法[35,55]。尽管今天血管压迫的诊断在内镜检查前通常已经获得，根据血管环或系带的类型，支气管镜也可以显示压迫的特征性发现。支气管镜为压迫缓解手术的结果和残留的气管软化程度提供即时视觉评估。

对于大多数无名动脉压迫和有轻度症状的血管环

或系带松弛的病例，非手术治疗可能是有效的。相对的，中重度症状的患者通常需要手术修补。手术治疗的绝对适应证包括反射性的呼吸暂停、严重的呼吸困难、内科治疗 48 小时后失败和延长的插管。相对适应证包括反复发作的下呼吸道感染、锻炼不耐受、吞咽困难伴生长停滞、或共存声门下狭窄、哮喘、囊性纤维化或气管食管瘘的修补史。

无名动脉压迫可以通过主动脉固定术或再植术缓解，成功率为 93～100%，没有手术死亡率或长期发病率的报道。偶尔，主动脉固定术的线结可能松脱，需要再次手术。

血管环手术处理的结果也是令人鼓舞的，70%～92%的患者的症状完全解决[5]。双主动脉弓需要外科分离成两个较小的弓。如果右主动脉弓伴左动脉导管未闭或异常的左锁骨下动脉，分离动脉导管未闭或异常的锁骨下动脉。有严重气管支气管压迫的患者，残余的气管软化可能持续一段时间，长短不定，偶尔，需要气管切开术来支撑软化的节段。

对肺动脉系带，通过在它的起始部分离异常的左肺动脉，再把它移植到气管的前面来纠正。共存的完全气管环需要在同一手术中，通过切除和端端吻合或错位气管成形术处理。

（汪 健译 朱锦祥校）

参考文献

1. Adler SC, Isaacson G, Balsara RK: Innominate artery compression of the trachea: Diagnosis and treatment by anterior suspension. A 25-year experience. Ann Otol Rhinol Laryngol 1995;104:924-927.
2. Al-Sebeih K, Manoukian J: Systemic steroids for the management of obstructive subglottic hemangioma. J Otolaryngol 2000;29:361-366.
3. Aviles R, Boyce TG, Thompson DM: *Pneumocystis carinii* pneumonia in a 3-month-old infant receiving high-dose corticosteroid therapy for airway hemangiomas. Mayo Clin Proc 2004;79:243-245.
4. Backer CL: Vascular rings, slings, and tracheal rings. Mayo Clin Proc 1993;68:1131-1133.
5. Backer CL, Ilbawi MN, Idriss FS, et al: Vascular anomalies causing tracheoesophageal compression. Review of experience in children. J Thorac Cardiovasc Surg 1989;97:725-731.
6. Baxter MR: Congenital laryngomalacia. Can J Anaesth 1994; 41:332-339.
7. Benjamin B: Chevalier Jackson Lecture. Congenital laryngeal webs. Ann Otol Rhinol Laryngol 1983;92:317-326.
8. Bent JP 3rd, Bauman NM, Smith RJ: Endoscopic repair of type IA laryngeal clefts. Laryngoscope 1997;107:282-286.
9. Blumer JR, Bauman NM, Kearns DP, et al: Distal tracheal stenosis in neonates and infants. Otolaryngol Head Neck Surg 1992;107:583-590.
10. Bower CM, Choi SS, Cotton RT: Arytenoidectomy in children. Ann Otol Rhinol Laryngol 1994;103:271-278.
11. Brigger MT, Hartnick CJ: Surgery for pediatric vocal cord paralysis: A meta-analysis. Otolaryngol Head Neck Surg 2002; 126:349-355.
12. Cantrell JR, Guild HG: Congenital stenosis of the trachea. Am J Surg 1964;108:297-305.
13. Chatrath P, Black M, Jani P, et al: A review of the current management of infantile subglottic haemangioma, including a comparison of CO_2 laser therapy versus tracheostomy. Int J Pediatr Otorhinolaryngol 2002;64:143-157.
14. Choa DI, Smith MC, Evans JN, et al: Subglottic haemangioma in children. J Laryngol Otol 1986;100:447-454.
15. Cohen SR: Unusual lesions of the larynx, trachea and bronchial tree. Ann Otol Rhinol Laryngol 1969;78: 476-489.
16. Cole RR, Myer CM 3rd, Cotton RT: Tracheotomy in children with recurrent respiratory papillomatosis. Head Neck 1989;11:226-230.
17. Cotton RT: Pediatric laryngotracheal stenosis. J Pediatr Surg 1984;19:699-704.
18. Cotton RT, Myer CM 3rd: Contemporary surgical management of laryngeal stenosis in children. Am J Otolaryngol 1984;5:360-368.
19. Cotton RT, Myer CM 3rd, Bratcher GO, et al: Anterior cricoid split, 1977-1987. Evolution of a technique. Arch Otolaryngol Head Neck Surg 1988;114:1300-1302.
20. Cotton RT, Gray SD, Miller RP: Update of the Cincinnati experience in pediatric laryngotracheal reconstruction. Laryngoscope 1989;99:1111-1116.
21. Cunningham MJ, Eavey RD, Vlahakes GJ, et al: Slide tracheoplasty for long-segment tracheal stenosis. Arch Otolaryngol Head Neck Surg 1998;124:98-103.
22. Denoyelle F, Mondain M, Gresillon N, et al: Failures and complications of supraglottoplasty in children. Arch Otolaryngol Head Neck Surg 2003;129:1077-1080, discussion 1080.
23. Derkay CS, Darrow DH: Recurrent respiratory papillomatosis of the larynx: Current diagnosis and treatment. Otolaryngol Clin North Am 2000;33:1127-1142.
24. Dunham ME, Holinger LD, Backer CL, et al: Management of severe congenital tracheal stenosis. Ann Otol Rhinol Laryngol 1994;103:351-356.
25. Eriksen C, Zwillenberg D, Robinson N: Diagnosis and management of cleft larynx. Literature review and case report. Ann Otol Rhinol Laryngol 1990;99:703-708.
26. Evans KL, Courteney-Harris R, Bailey CM, et al: Management of posterior laryngeal and laryngotracheoesophageal clefts. Arch Otolaryngol Head Neck Surg 1995;121:1380-1385.
27. Fearon B, Shortreed R: Tracheobronchial compression by congenital cardiovascular anomalies in children. Syndrome of apnea. Ann Otol Rhinol Laryngol 1963;72:949-969.
28. Friedman EM, de Jong AL, Sulek M: Pediatric bilateral vocal fold immobility: The role of carbon dioxide laser posterior transverse partial cordectomy. Ann Otol Rhinol Laryngol 2001;110:723-728.
29. Froehlich P, Seid AB, Morgon A: Contrasting strategic approaches to the management of subglottic hemangiomas. Int J Pediatr Otorhinolaryngol 1996;36:137-146.
30. Giannoni C, Sulek M, Friedman EM, et al: Gastroesophageal reflux association with laryngomalacia: A prospective study. Int J Pediatr Otorhinolaryngol 1998;43: 11-20.

31. Gilger MA: Pediatric otolaryngologic manifestations of gastroesophageal reflux disease. Curr Gastroenterol Rep 2003; 5:247-252.
32. Gray SD, Kelly SM, Dove H: Arytenoid separation for impaired pediatric vocal fold mobility. Ann Otol Rhinol Laryngol 1994;103:510-515.
33. Gustafson LM, Hartley BE, Cotton RT: Acquired total (grade 4) subglottic stenosis in children. Ann Otol Rhinol Laryngol 2001;110:16-19.
34. Gustafson LM, Hartley BE, Liu JH, et al: Single-stage laryngotracheal reconstruction in children: A review of 200 cases. Otolaryngol Head Neck Surg 2000;123:430-434.
35. Gustafson LM, Liu JH, Link DT, et al: Spiral CT versus MRI in neonatal airway evaluation. Int J Pediatr Otorhinolaryngol 2000;52:197-201.
36. Halstead LA: Gastroesophageal reflux: A critical factor in pediatric subglottic stenosis. Otolaryngol Head Neck Surg 1999;120:683-688.
37. Hartley BE, Gustafson LM, Liu JH, et al: Duration of stenting in single-stage laryngotracheal reconstruction with anterior costal cartilage grafts. Ann Otol Rhinol Laryngol 2001;110:413-416.
38. Hartley BE, Rutter MJ, Cotton RT: Cricotracheal resection as a primary procedure for laryngotracheal stenosis in children. Int J Pediatr Otorhinolaryngol 2000;54:133-136.
39. Hartnick CJ, Brigger MT, Willging JP, et al: Surgery for pediatric vocal cord paralysis: A retrospective review. Ann Otol Rhinol Laryngol 2003;112:1-6.
40. Hawkins DB, Crockett DM, Kahlstrom EJ, et al: Corticosteroid management of airway hemangiomas: Long-term follow-up. Laryngoscope 1984;94:633-637.
41. Healy GB, Fearon B, French R, et al: Treatment of subglottic hemangioma with the carbon dioxide laser. Laryngoscope 1980;90:809-813.
42. Holland BW, Koufman JA, Postma GN, et al: Laryngopharyngeal reflux and laryngeal web formation in patients with pediatric recurrent respiratory papillomas. Laryngoscope 2002;112:1926-1929.
43. Holinger LD, Konior RJ: Surgical management of severe laryngomalacia. Laryngoscope 1989;99:136-142.
44. Holinger PH, Brown WT: Congenital webs, cysts, laryngoceles and other anomalies of the larynx. Ann Otol Rhinol Laryngol 1967;76:744-752.
45. Holinger PH, Kutnick SL, Schild JA, et al: Subglottic stenosis in infants and children. Ann Otol Rhinol Laryngol 1976; 85:591-599.
46. Idriss FS, DeLeon SY, Ilbawi MN, et al: Tracheoplasty with pericardial patch for extensive tracheal stenosis in infants and children. J Thorac Cardiovasc Surg 1984;88:527-536.
47. Inglis AF Jr, Perkins JA, Manning SC, et al: Endoscopic posterior cricoid split and rib grafting in 10 children. Laryngoscope 2003;113:2004-2009.
48. Jacobs BR, Salman BA, Cotton RT, et al: Postoperative management of children after single-stage laryngotracheal reconstruction. Crit Care Med 2001;29:164-168.
49. Jacobs JP, Elliott MJ, Haw MP, et al: Pediatric tracheal homograft reconstruction: A novel approach to complex tracheal stenoses in children. J Thorac Cardiovasc Surg 1996;112:1549-1558, discussion 1559-1560.
50. Jacobs JP, Haw MP, Motbey JA, et al: Successful complete tracheal resection in a three-month-old infant. Ann Thorac Surg 1996;61:1824-1826, discussion 1827.
51. Jani P, Koltai P, Ochi JW, et al: Surgical treatment of laryngomalacia. J Laryngol Otol 1991;105:1040-1045.
52. Kacker A, April M, Ward RF: Use of potassium titanyl phosphate (KTP) laser in management of subglottic hemangiomas. Int J Pediatr Otorhinolaryngol 2001;59:15-21.
53. Kashima H, Mounts P, Leventhal B, et al: Sites of predilection in recurrent respiratory papillomatosis. Ann Otol Rhinol Laryngol 1993;102:580-583.
54. Lane RW, Weider DJ, Steinem C, et al: Laryngomalacia. A review and case report of surgical treatment with resolution of pectus excavatum. Arch Otolaryngol 1984;110:546-551.
55. Lee KH, Yoon CS, Choe KO, et al: Use of imaging for assessing anatomical relationships of tracheobronchial anomalies associated with left pulmonary artery sling. Pediatr Radiol 2001;31:269-278.
56. Leikensohn JR, Benton C, Cotton R: Subglottic hemangioma. J Otolaryngol 1976;5:487-492.
57. Link DT, Cotton R: The laryngotracheal complex in pediatric head and neck trauma: Securing the airway and management of external laryngeal injury. Facial Plast Surg Clin North Am 1999;7:133-144.
58. Little FB, Koufman JA, Kohut RI, et al: Effect of gastric acid on the pathogenesis of subglottic stenosis. Ann Otol Rhinol Laryngol 1985;94:516-519.
59. Macdonald RE, Fearon B: Innominate artery compression syndrome in children. Ann Otol Rhinol Laryngol 1971; 80:535-540.
60. Madgy D, Ahsan SF, Kest D, et al: The application of the potassium-titanyl-phosphate (KTP) laser in the management of subglottic hemangioma. Arch Otolaryngol Head Neck Surg 2001;127:47-50.
61. Marcus CL, Crockett DM, Ward SL: Evaluation of epiglottoplasty as treatment for severe laryngomalacia. J Pediatr 1990;117:706-710.
62. Maronian NC, Azadeh H, Waugh P, et al: Association of laryngopharyngeal reflux disease and subglottic stenosis. Ann Otol Rhinol Laryngol 2001;110:606-612.
63. McClurg FL, Evans DA: Laser laryngoplasty for laryngomalacia. Laryngoscope 1994;104:247-252.
64. McDonald IH, Stocks JG: Prolonged nasotracheal intubation. A review of its development in a paediatric hospital. Br J Anaesth 1965;37:161-173.
65. McSwiney PF, Cavanagh NP, Languth P: Outcome in congenital stridor (laryngomalacia). Arch Dis Child 1977;52: 215-218.
66. Meeuwis J, Bos CE, Hoeve LJ, et al: Subglottic hemangiomas in infants: Treatment with intralesional corticosteroid injection and intubation. Int J Pediatr Otorhinolaryngol 1990; 19:145-150.
67. Milczuk HA, Smith JD, Everts EC: Congenital laryngeal webs: Surgical management and clinical embryology. Int J Pediatr Otorhinolaryngol 2000;52:1-9.
68. Moes CA, Izukawa T, Trusler GA: Innominate artery compression of the trachea. Arch Otolaryngol 1975;101: 733-738.
69. Monnier P, Lang F, Savary M: Partial cricotracheal resection for pediatric subglottic stenosis: A single institution's experience in 60 cases. Eur Arch Otorhinolaryngol 2003; 260:295-297.
70. Mustard WT, Bayliss CE, Fearon B, et al: Tracheal compression by the innominate artery in children. Ann Thorac Surg 1969;8:312-319.
71. Myer CM 3rd, O'Connor DM, Cotton RT: Proposed grading system for subglottic stenosis based on endotracheal tube sizes. Ann Otol Rhinol Laryngol 1994;103: 319-323.
72. Naiman AN, Ayari S, Froehlich P: Controlled risk of stenosis after surgical excision of laryngeal hemangioma. Arch Otolaryngol Head Neck Surg 2003;129:1291-1295.
73. Narcy P, Contencin P, Viala P: Surgical treatment for laryn-

geal paralysis in infants and children. Ann Otol Rhinol Laryngol 1990;99:124-128.
74. Ohlms LA, Jones DT, McGill TJ, et al: Interferon alfa-2a therapy for airway hemangiomas. Ann Otol Rhinol Laryngol 1994;103:1-8.
75. Parsons DS, Bothwell MR: Powered instrument papilloma excision: An alternative to laser therapy for recurrent respiratory papilloma. Laryngoscope 2001;111:1494-1496.
76. Pollack IF, Kinnunen D, Albright AL: The effect of early craniocervical decompression on functional outcome in neonates and young infants with myelodysplasia and symptomatic Chiari II malformations: Results from a prospective series. Neurosurgery 1996;38:703-710, discussion 710.
77. Polonovski JM, Contencin P, Francois M, et al: Aryepiglottic fold excision for the treatment of severe laryngomalacia. Ann Otol Rhinol Laryngol 1990;99:625-627.
78. Ratner I, Whitfield J: Acquired subglottic stenosis in the very-low-birth-weight infant. Am J Dis Child 1983;137: 40-43.
79. Remacle M, Bodart E, Lawson G, et al: Use of the CO_2-laser micropoint micromanipulator for the treatment of laryngomalacia. Eur Arch Otorhinolaryngol 1996;253:401-404.
80. Rimell FL, Dohar JE: Endoscopic management of pediatric posterior glottic stenosis. Ann Otol Rhinol Laryngol 1998; 107:285-290.
81. Roger G, Denoyelle F, Triglia JM, et al: Severe laryngomalacia: Surgical indications and results in 115 patients. Laryngoscope 1995;105:1111-1117.
82. Rosenfeld RM, Stool SE: Should granulomas be excised in children with long-term tracheotomy? Arch Otolaryngol Head Neck Surg 1992;118:1323-1327.
83. Rudolph CD, Mazur LJ, Liptak GS, et al: Guidelines for evaluation and treatment of gastroesophageal reflux in infants and children: Recommendations of the North American Society for Pediatric Gastroenterology and Nutrition. J Pediatr Gastroenterol Nutr 2001;32(Suppl 2): S1-S31.
84. Rutter MJ, Cotton RT, Azizkhan RG, et al: Slide tracheoplasty for the management of complete tracheal rings. J Pediatr Surg 2003;38:928-934.
85. Rutter MJ, Hartley BE, Cotton RT: Cricotracheal resection in children. Arch Otolaryngol Head Neck Surg 2001;127: 289-292.
86. Rutter MJ, Willging JP, Cotton RT: Nonoperative management of complete tracheal rings. Arch Otolaryngol Head Neck Surg 2004;130:450-452.
87. Seid AB, Park SM, Kearns MJ, et al: Laser division of the aryepiglottic folds for severe laryngomalacia. Int J Pediatr Otorhinolaryngol 1985;10:153-158.
88. Seid AB, Pransky SM, Kearns DB: The open surgical approach to subglottic hemangioma. Int J Pediatr Otorhinolaryngol 1991;22:85-90.
89. Seid AB, Pransky SM, Kearns DB: The open surgical approach to subglottic hemangioma. Int J Pediatr Otorhinolaryngol 1993;26:95-96.
90. Shah K, Kashima H, Polk BF, et al: Rarity of cesarean delivery in cases of juvenile-onset respiratory papillomatosis. Obstet Gynecol 1986;68:795-799.
91. Shikhani AH, Jones MM, Marsh BR, et al: Infantile subglottic hemangiomas. An update. Ann Otol Rhinol Laryngol 1986;95:336-347.
92. Sie KC, McGill T, Healy GB: Subglottic hemangioma: Ten years' experience with the carbon dioxide laser. Ann Otol Rhinol Laryngol 1994;103:167-172.
93. Stern Y, Gerber ME, Walner DL, et al: Partial cricotracheal resection with primary anastomosis in the pediatric age group. Ann Otol Rhinol Laryngol 1997;106:891-896.
94. Strife JL, Baumel AS, Dunbar JS: Tracheal compression by the innominate artery in infancy and childhood. Radiology 1981;139:73-75.
95. Suskind DL, Zeringue GP 3rd, Kluka EA, et al: Gastroesophageal reflux and pediatric otolaryngologic disease: The role of antireflux surgery. Arch Otolaryngol Head Neck Surg 2001;127:511-514.
96. Toynton SC, Saunders MW, Bailey CM: Aryepiglottoplasty for laryngomalacia: 100 consecutive cases. J Laryngol Otol 2001;115:35-38.
97. Triglia JM, Belus JF, Nicollas R: Arytenoidopexy for bilateral vocal fold paralysis in young children. J Laryngol Otol 1996;110:1027-1030.
98. Triglia JM, Nicollas R, Roman S: Primary cricotracheal resection in children: Indications, technique and outcome. Int J Pediatr Otorhinolaryngol 2001;58:17-25.
99. Tsang V, Murday A, Gillbe C, et al: Slide tracheoplasty for congenital funnel-shaped tracheal stenosis. Ann Thorac Surg 1989;48:632-635.
100. Unal M: The successful management of congenital laryngeal web with endoscopic lysis and topical mitomycin-C. Int J Pediatr Otorhinolaryngol 2004;68:231-235.
101. Van Den Abbeele T, Triglia JM, Lescanne E, et al: Surgical removal of subglottic hemangiomas in children. Laryngoscope 1999;109:1281-1286.
102. Walner DL, Stern Y, Cotton RT: Margins of partial cricotracheal resection in children. Laryngoscope 1999;109: 1607-1610.
103. Weber TR, Eigen H, Scott PH, et al: Resection of congenital tracheal stenosis involving the carina. J Thorac Cardiovasc Surg 1982;84:200-203.
104. Wetmore SJ, Key JM, Suen JY: Complications of laser surgery for laryngeal papillomatosis. Laryngoscope 1985;95: 798-801.
105. Wiatrak BJ, Reilly JS, Seid AB, et al: Open surgical excision of subglottic hemangioma in children. Int J Pediatr Otorhinolaryngol 1996;34:191-206.
106. Yamada H, Tanaka Y, Nakamura S: Laryngeal stridor associated with the Chiari II malformation. Childs Nerv Syst 1985;1:312-318.
107. Yellon RF, Goldberg H: Update on gastroesophageal reflux disease in pediatric airway disorders. Am J Med 2001;111(Suppl 8A):78S-84S.
108. Younis RT, Lazar RH, Astor F: Posterior cartilage graft in single-stage laryngotracheal reconstruction. Otolaryngol Head Neck Surg 2003;129:168-175.
109. Zalzal GH, Cotton RT, McAdams AJ: Cartilage grafts—present status. Head Neck Surg 1986;8:363-374.
110. Zalzal GH, Anon JB, Cotton RT: Epiglottoplasty for the treatment of laryngomalacia. Ann Otol Rhinol Laryngol 1987;96:72-76.

第 64 章

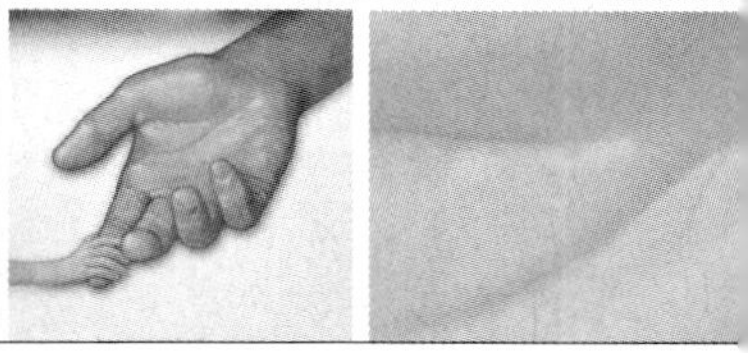

肺部、胸膜和纵隔的感染及疾病

Pramod S. Puligandla 和 Jean-Martin Laberge

肺部感染

1001 所有年龄段的儿童皆可罹患肺部感染。尽管大多数轻中度感染可在门诊得到有效治疗，但仍有一些患者需要住院治疗。接种疫苗和大量备选抗生素的应用可减少严重肺部感染和并发症的发生。事实上，目前肺部感染造成的脓胸和肺脓肿确实不常见。然而，随着使用免疫抑制药物和高强度化疗的增加，这一人群发生肺部感染的风险也增加。免疫功能障碍的患者更常需要如支气管肺泡灌洗和肺活检等辅助技术，以指导治疗和直接处理。

流行病学

先前的呼吸道感染的发病率估计依据的是欧洲和美国 20 世纪 80 年代和 90 年代初期的资料[160,208,265]。这些报道显示，呼吸道感染的发生率以年幼儿童最高（6 个月～5 岁），以后随年龄增加而降低。目前更多近期的资料支持之前的发现[25,247,,253,408]。5 岁前儿童的呼吸道感染发病率为 3.0%～3.6%。从病因来看，一些研究发现，肺炎链球菌和病毒是呼吸道感染最常见的病原。依据发病年龄，呼吸道合胞病毒（RSV）在幼儿（<2 岁）中流行，而大部分 2 岁以上的儿童罹患肺炎链球菌引起的社区获得性肺炎[247,253,341]。高达 40%～60%的社区获得性肺炎没有确定的病原体[158]。

社区获得性细菌性肺炎

肺炎链球菌

肺炎链球菌是全世界致病和致死的主要原因。它是婴儿和儿童最常见的病原体，在美国，每年大约引起 50 万例肺炎[356]。全世界每年由于肺炎死亡的人数高达 300 万，且多数发生在发展中国家，由肺炎链球菌感染所致[116,143]。这个菌种的耐药性在过去几年中日益增加，使经验治疗未必有效[185,260,358]。

肺炎链球菌是一种革兰阳性球菌，是儿童和成人正常菌群的一部分。其定殖速率，尤其在鼻咽部黏膜处，随着年龄增加而降低，它是感染发展的一个重要因素[356]。感染的症状包括发热、排痰性咳嗽、呼吸急促、呼吸困难、全身乏力和偶尔呕吐。体格检查，患者有缺氧表现和炎症累及区域的呼吸音降低伴啰音。放射学检查方面，肺部感染可为一叶、多叶感染，有时为节段性的（图 64-1），这些患者中 40%以上会引起胸腔积液。这种感染的治疗最常在门诊进行，因细菌耐药而变得复杂[37,185,358]。患者感染了低中度的抗药性菌株时，青霉素和其他 β-内酰胺抗生素仍然有效。头孢菌素可用于高度耐药菌株感染或经常规疗法临床没有改善者[185,358]。引进新的七价结合疫苗可影响疾病的严重程度[60,287]。这些疫苗似乎是安全有效的，潜在性地减少肺炎病例每年达 5～30 万[357]。 1002

流感嗜血杆菌

这种有荚膜的小型革兰阴性菌是社区获得性肺炎的常见病原[137,253,408]。嗜血杆菌引起的侵袭病例 95%是由 B 型引起的。嗜血杆菌感染通常发生在冬季和春季。临床表现包括发热、呼吸急促、白细胞计数升高以及胸片上的单侧实变和胸膜渗出影。肺外表现，如脑膜炎和会厌炎，是这一病原体感染的常见病灶。治疗依赖于这些细菌对 β-内酰胺抗生素的敏感性。头孢菌素可用于治疗产生 β-内酰胺酶的菌株[277]。随着嗜血杆菌疫苗的应用，这一菌种的整

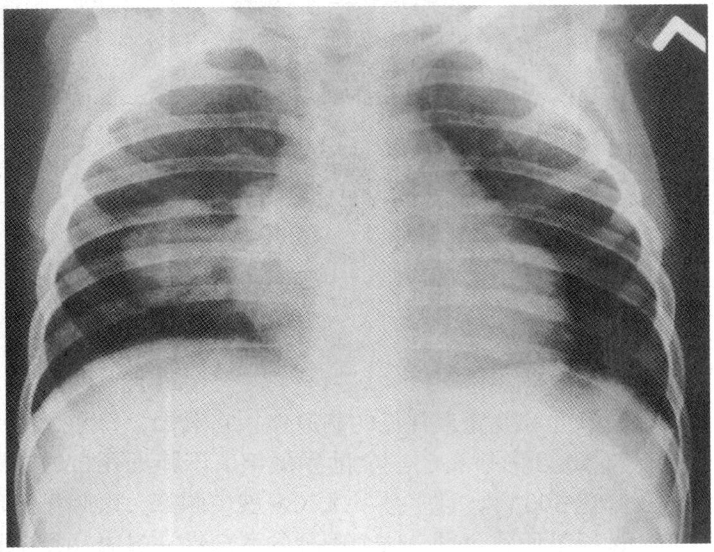

A

图 64-1 一名 1 岁半的男孩有发热和呼吸困难，胸片表现出下肺叶上段典型的圆形的肺炎病灶；在不透明区内可见空气支气管征。A. 前后位片。B. 侧位片。

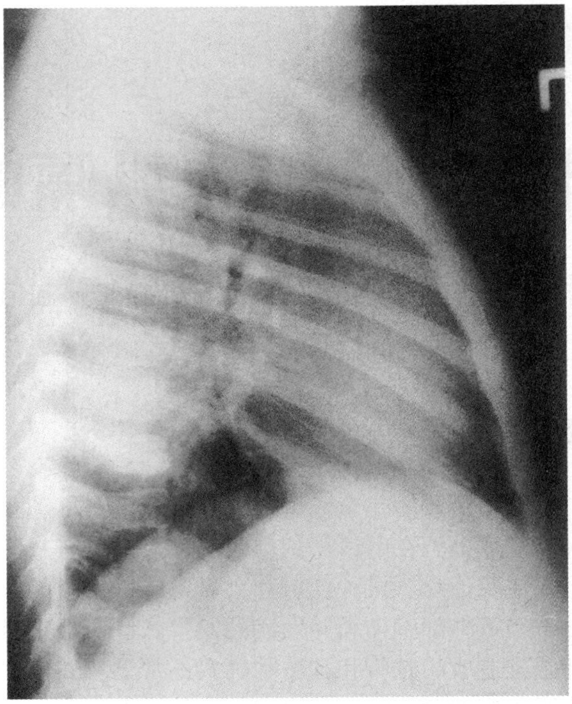

B

体发病率大幅度降低，但最近有一份报告提示，这种免疫接种与儿童 I 型糖尿病有关联[75]。侵袭性嗜血杆菌的次级传播仍可能发生在家庭或日托所[81]。因此，对高危儿童或者希望消除鼻咽部带菌时可给予利福平预防用药[81]。

金黄色葡萄球菌

这些无所不在的革兰阳性球菌常见于皮肤和鼻黏膜处，人群中 20%～30%是本菌的正常携带者[81]。金黄色葡萄球菌产生的毒素和酶形成了这种病原体的病变基础——脓性渗出或脓肿[81,114]。葡萄球菌感染通常是进行性的，发生在婴儿期和儿童早期。原发性肺炎发生在冬季和春季。患者常表现为发热和迅速出现呼吸道症状。若感染未经治疗，临床和放射检查结果很快恶化。X 线检查中，原发性肺炎显示为单侧肺实变。继发性感染 / 肺炎通常造成长期的发热性疾病，葡萄球菌肺炎常在康复期合并发生胸腔积液[58,319]、脓胸[63,175,182]、肺脓肿[114,405]或肺膨出[203,405]。这些病损常需要随访，直至炎症彻底消散（见下文）。治疗措施包括选用适当的抗葡萄球菌抗生素。如果患者对青霉素过敏，其他药物如万古霉素、克林霉素和大环内酯类也可使用。开始治疗后发热最多持续 2 周，疗程通常为 3～4 周。

支原体和衣原体

肺炎支原体和肺炎衣原体是能引起所有年龄段呼吸道感染的少见的病原体。但是，这些感染常见于学龄期儿童和年长儿[153,267,297]。这些微生物是临床上非典型肺炎的重要病原。肺炎支原体和肺炎衣原体有类似的血清学特征[267,296,383]。感染传播方式是人与人接触传 1003
染，通常有 1～2 周的潜伏期。由此引起的非典型肺炎与 RSV 感染很相似。其症状逐步发生，包括喉部痛、声音沙哑和鼻炎，伴有或不伴有发热。这些上呼吸道症状在数天内进展为下呼吸道症状，包括咳嗽、胸痛、湿啰音和干啰音。支原体也能引起发烧、畏寒、头痛和肌痛。这些感染的典型表现为单侧节段性间质浸润，但具有高度变异性[121]。诊断通常依赖以病史和体格检为基础的临床背景资料。其他辅助检查包括聚合酶链反应（PCR），培养和血清学检查也有助于确诊[82,133,156]。大环内酯类药物（红霉素、克拉霉素）是治疗这些感染的主要药物[135,153,26]。新氮杂内酯类（阿奇霉素）药物经多项研究已被列为标准的大环内酯类抗生素，而且疗程更短，通常是 5 天[157,219]。

结核分枝杆菌

儿童肺结核感染几乎都是从活跃的成年肺病患者那里传染的[99,100,183]。在成人结核病得到适当控制后，儿童结核病发病率也大幅降低[100,146]。的确，疾病初期积极的抗感染治疗，对发病和以后的感染传播有重大影响[183,354]。在北美，有效的药物治疗和积极的随访大大减少结核病的并发症。最近发达国家的结核病流行病学报告[120,136,191]有共同主题如下：(1) 移民及其子女的结核病发病率最高；(2) 幼儿感染表现更严重；(3) 皮肤试验和筛查对鉴别儿童肺结核起重要作用。结核病抗药菌株的出现是今后存在的问题，并反映这一微生物在整个社会里的变化。[4,190,272,328]

儿童结核病不同于成人肺结核之处在于：原发性肺结核是淋巴系统疾病，即“原发复合征”[99]。原发性肺结核造成肺部阻塞或损害大气道的继发损伤，导致肺不张、慢性感染和支气管扩张。许多原发感染治愈后无肺部残留病损，这与 Ghon 综合征（钙沉积在纵隔或肺门淋巴结）不同。目前认为，原发病灶的愈合与宿主–微生物的正平衡有关，即与宿主强有力的自然抵抗力或小剂量的初次接种有关[173]。如果防御机制不能控制原发感染，结核性肺炎进一步发展为干酪样变，并常合并胸腔积液。临床表现包括发热、呼吸困难和咳嗽。对任何慢性咳嗽、有成人肺结核接触史、发育迟缓或经适当治疗感染无法痊愈的儿童，都应怀疑为肺结核[100,171]。

确定结核病诊断依靠从痰、支气管冲洗液、胃液、或其他感染物质中培养出结核分枝杆菌[230,231,320]。近期引进一种可靠的 PCR 方法可从尿液检验肺结核[231,302]。儿童的结核菌素皮肤试验阳性显示患儿需要抗结核治疗[115]。免疫抑制儿童、严重营养不良者或播散性肺结核患者的结核菌素试验常常因没有免疫反应能力而为阴性[115,250]。其他可能导致误诊的因素包括：观察者之间对皮试结果解释的可靠性、重复进行皮肤试验，特别是在高发人群以及皮试期间使用类固醇者[99,173]。由于培养可能需要数周，对于存在以上怀疑的患者可立即开始抗结核治疗。现已证明，不论患者的免疫状况如何，成人抗结核药物的吸收可能都受包括食物消耗的多种因素影响[138,284,304]。尚缺乏这方面的儿童数据，但药物监测能确保适当的组织药物浓度。此外，标准药品如利福平、异烟肼、乙硫异烟肼、乙胺丁醇和吡嗪酰胺有肝脏毒性[173]。

目前，手术只适用于肺局部严重损害的肺结核患者。与成人不同的是，这种情况在儿童常见于下肺叶。应采取保守的手术方法，通常是楔形切除、节段性切除或肺叶切除。儿童期肺结核的外科干预指征包括：(1) 支气管外淋巴结阻塞大气道；(2) 慢性呼吸道病变；(3) 支气管内物质阻塞气道；(4) 肺结核后肺损坏，伴有或不伴有真菌感染；(5) 慢性空洞病变；(6) 结核病导致支气管扩张。

非典型分枝杆菌

20 世纪 50 年代首次鉴别出非典型分枝杆菌属[72]。直到 20 世纪 80 年代人类免疫缺陷病毒（HIV）流行之前，这些疾病的发病率相当稳定[243]。由于有更先进的培养技术以及免疫功能降低的患者增加，更多微生物被鉴别出来[2,316]。非典型分枝杆菌感染最常见的表现是颈部淋巴结炎[2,22,313]。具有免疫活性的患者较少发生非典型分枝杆菌引起的肺部感染，但囊性纤维化[110,145,239,278]和 HIV 感染[96,180,184,295]患者经常发生这一感染（见下文）。引起肺部感染的最常见亚型包括鸟分枝杆菌复合群。其他重要的菌属包括堪萨斯分枝杆菌、脓肿分枝杆菌、非洲蟾蜍分枝杆菌和玛尔 1004
摩分枝杆菌[2]。临床上，有免疫活性的患者可能有轻微症状或表现出疲劳和伴喘鸣的慢性咳嗽。如果胸片与高解析度电脑断层扫描（CT）[2,154,178]显示肺部纤维空洞性病变，特别是在肺尖，应怀疑该诊断。也可出现肺结节、肺间质病变，甚至可出现支气管扩张症[154]。非典型分枝杆菌的实验室诊断依靠痰液 PCR 检查[57]、高效液相色谱[61]或 DNA 探针技术[69,345]。在应用大环内酯类药物之前，此类感染治疗后复燃是屡见不鲜的，因为抗结核药物对非典型分枝杆菌的治疗效果不及对肺结核的。因此，许多患者需要手术切除受累的肺部区域。然而，随着大环内酯类（红霉素、克拉霉素）、氮杂内酯类（阿奇霉素）和新型非大环内酯类抗生素（环丙沙星）的发展，这种肺部疾病已很少需要手术治疗[2]。相比之下，非典型分枝杆菌引起的颈部淋巴结炎最好以手术切除受累的淋巴结，抗生素治疗可用于经手术切除病灶或疾病播散期的患者。

病毒感染

支气管炎

支气管炎是幼儿住院的主要原因。RSV 是引起支气管炎的最常见病原体，在美国每年因此住院的有 12.5 万人，并造成 200～500 人死亡[333]。其他可致支气管炎的病原体包括副流感病毒、流感病毒和腺病毒[347]。感染的高发期在初冬至次年春天，传播方式为直接接触。感染的好发年龄是 2～6 个月月龄[392]。以流鼻涕、咳嗽和低热的上呼吸道感染起病，在 24～48 小时迅速进展，出现下呼吸道症状。此时，患者可表现为气促、吸凹和喘息。高热不常见，小婴儿可出现呼吸暂停。经皮氧饱和度可下降，低于 95%，但是这些测量不必与临床发现相关。患者的胸片检查显示肺过度膨胀、间质性肺炎，偶尔有胸膜增厚。偶发获得性肺气肿（图 64–2）。很少有患者需要肺切除，但许多患者的肺过度膨胀会随时间的推移而缓解。

多个患者群感染 RSV 的风险增高，包括早产儿、6 周龄之内的患儿以及慢性肺部疾病或先天性心脏病患儿。土著居民也是高危人群[236]。有症状和无症状的儿童都可携带 RSV[152]，携带率随年龄的增加而降低[151]。但是，免疫功能降低的患者无论多大年龄都可长期携带病毒。总之，RSV 感染的死亡率约为 1%，但一些高危患者的死亡率可升至 4%[167,333,347]。支气管炎的假设的诊断依据临床表现做出，并由 X 线影像帮助诊断。证实感染需要快速免疫吸附实验检测鼻咽部吸出物[19,49,163]。支气管炎的治疗包括吸氧支持、维持体液和密切监护[198,281]。严重感染者，尤其是高危人群，可能需要机械通气。在医院病房，切断传播对防止疫情极为关键[246]；因此，严格洗手和隔离感染患者也是非常重要的。支气管扩张剂和吸入类固醇药物在总体治疗方案中的作用有限，但可暂时缓解症状[322]。抗病毒治疗并不如期望的那样成功，但在免疫功能降低患者中仍可应用[176,202,393]。高危儿童应接种抗
1005 RSV 疫苗[288]。大多数感染是自限性的，但是越来越多的证据支持，RSV 既往感染史与儿童哮喘的发病有关[244,369]。

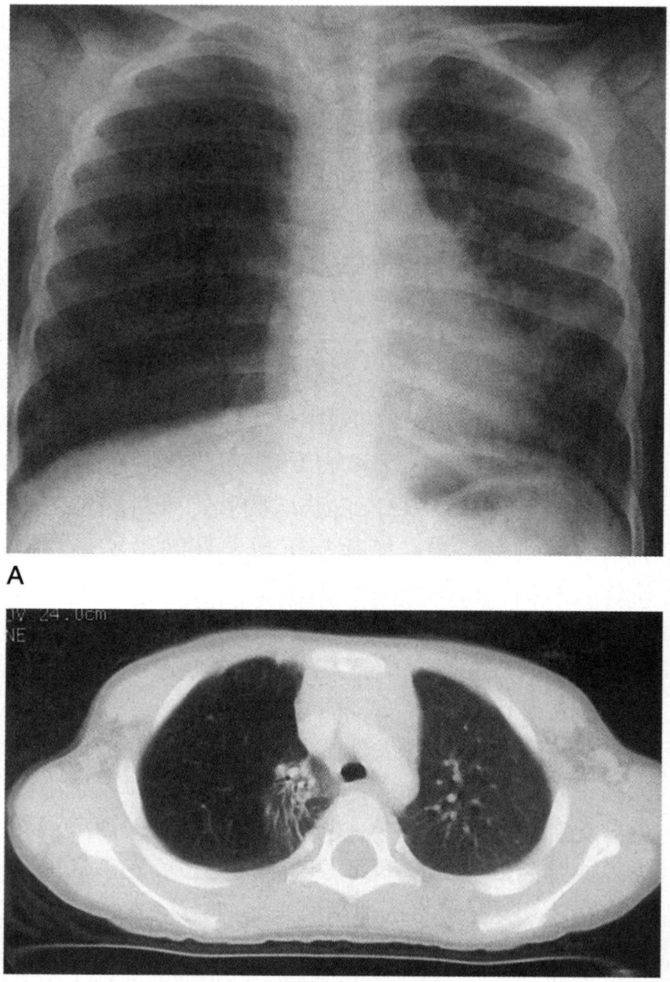

A

B

图 64–2 A. 一名 3 岁儿童患呼吸道合胞病毒性肺炎，并继发获得性叶性肺气肿。B. 胸部 CT 平扫显示萎陷的肺上叶和气肿的肺中叶。

寄生虫感染

棘球绦虫

包虫病是绦虫寄生感染羊和犬，并传染给人类所致。常见于埃及、中东和澳大利亚。以前在北美很少见，但在美国西南部[102]和加拿大北部已诊断出数例患者[216,258]。肝脏、脾脏和肺部可出现包囊。发生肺部疾病的患者多为儿童。30%的病损最终破裂[35]，导致胸腔积液[18]、支气管种植，偶有急性过敏反应，因此需切除这些包囊[186,196,365]。一些有肺部包虫病的患儿没有症状，而另一些则有干咳。典型胸片显示单个

大型肺结节或一至数个大囊肿伴有大的气液平面（图 64–3）。CT 和核磁共振（MRI）也可用来提供更多细节，或当患者症状明显而常规放射检查未见异常，需要找出偶发病灶时。经放射检查不能明确诊断者，可行血清酶联免疫吸附试验确定诊断。甲苯达唑药物治疗可用于小囊肿或无症状的患者[192]。对存在继发感染或症状性 / 囊肿增大的患者需行肺切除术[35,196,317,372]。目前有证据显示，一期外科切除大型或复杂的包虫包囊可减少术后并发症并缩短住院天数[192]。包虫病的手术治疗要求对肺组织的操作轻柔，严格控制囊肿内容物，避免溢出，并推荐使用肺实质保留方法。已有包囊经皮引流的报道，但只获得部分成功[21]。

免疫受损的患者

儿科癌症患者

总体而言，所有类型的儿童期癌症的治愈率超过 60%[269]。这一明显提高是完善化疗方案、改进药物和提高治疗强度的结果。然而，这些患者的长期障碍是并发感染的威胁。事实上，唯一重要的感染因素是粒细胞减少的程度。中性粒细胞计数低于 1006
0.5×10^9/L 的患者，其细菌感染的风险明显增加[181,318]。如果粒细胞减少持续的时间延长，真菌感染的风险也会增加[200,388,389]。

免疫功能降低的癌症患者发生机会感染最常见部位是肺部[269]。这一人群的肺炎发生率为 0.5%～10%[123]。感染机制可以是病原体从上呼吸道吸入气管支气管树或由血行传播。免疫系统受许多不同方式的影响，取决于种类、时间和化疗强度。的确，联合化疗能破坏多种不同层面的免疫反应，是这些药物的不同作用机制的结果。

细菌感染

化疗早期，肺部感染最常见的原因是细菌感染。一些因素，包括菌血症、吸入、纤毛功能障碍、肺清除功能降低、黏膜屏障受损和气管插管都使癌症患儿容易发生肺部感染[70,380]。免疫抑制造成免疫球蛋白不

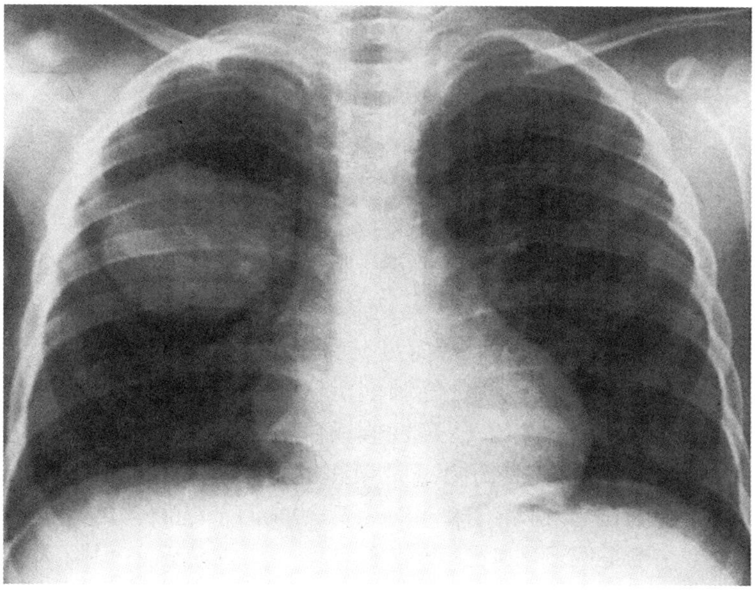

A

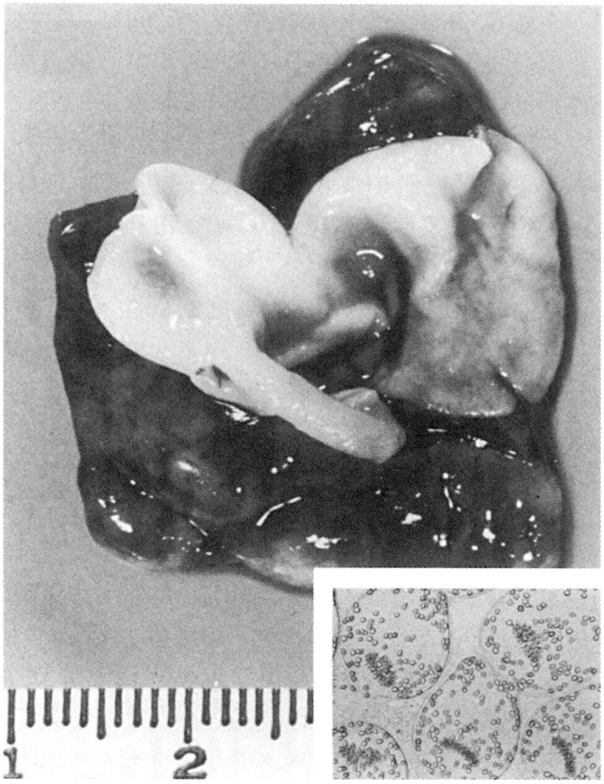

B

图 64–3　一名患有包虫病的 4 岁美籍印第安男孩，他住在牧羊区，并养了几只狗。在后前位片上可见右肺有一个大的均一的球形团块影（A）。行楔形切除术（B），打开囊肿可见内有头节和小钩的节片。男孩术后恢复健康，无并发症。（插图，400 倍）

足，使这些患者成为荚膜细菌感染的高风险者，例如肺炎链球菌和嗜血杆菌，这是由于调理作用不当导致的[225]。骨髓移植患者的感染发生率为 12%～15%，多在移植后 100 天内发生[54,87,235]。

总体而言，革兰阴性菌是引起儿科癌症患者肺部感染的最常见的病原体。最常见的革兰阴性菌种包括假单胞菌、克雷白菌和肠杆菌。革兰阴性菌感染的患者可表现为早期肺部渗出，此时应用 β–内酰胺类、头孢菌素和（或）氨基糖苷类药物有效。假单胞菌感染一般需要合用两种敏感抗生素。治疗 7 天后仍有持续渗出者，通常是由于这一菌种中的天然抗生素耐药属所致，需要改变治疗常规。革兰阳性菌感染通常包括葡萄球菌、肺炎链球菌和 A 组链球菌[389]，β–内酰胺类、头孢菌素和万古霉素治疗有效。李斯特菌常引起晚期和复发性渗出。诺卡菌的感染并不常见，但因其感染可扩散到中枢神经系统而可使病情非常严重[289]。可选用磺胺类治疗这一微生物引起的感染。

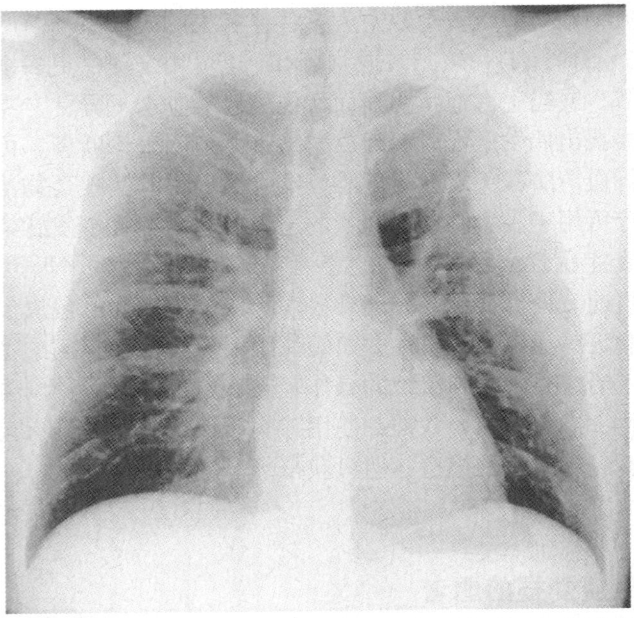

图 64–4 一名 17 岁接受强烈化疗的急性淋巴母细胞性白血病患者，左上肺叶曲霉病，伴弥漫性双侧肺浸润。

真菌感染

真菌感染是导致重度免疫功能降低患者死亡的一个常见原因，尤其在粒细胞长时间减少、长期接受皮质类固醇或抗生素治疗的患者中。侵入性真菌感染的发生率有所升高[226,291]。真菌感染的两个主要模式为：（1）曲霉菌和假丝酵母菌引起的机会感染，它们是侵犯免疫功能降低患者的最常见的真菌；（2）组织胞浆菌属、球孢子菌属和芽生菌的潜伏感染再激活[79]。

曲霉菌侵入性感染最常见的部位是肺部[291,335]。上呼吸道是此真菌进入机体最常见的入口。的确，医院中传播的疫情是继发于吸入从受污染的空调管路和邻近建筑物或重新翻修场所释放出来的孢子[20]。使用层流和高效过滤器可减少这类疾病的发病[44]。

曲霉菌感染可以迅速侵入。肺动脉和肺静脉受侵袭且形成血栓可导致坏死和出血。继而引起空洞病变。胸部 X 线平片不如 CT 平扫敏感，这是因为这些感染既可表现为弥漫性渗出，也可表现为结节性病变（图 64–4）[74]。可选用两性霉素 B 治疗[350]，疗效标准为白细胞和粒细胞的恢复。由于肺曲霉病对单用两性霉素 B 的有效性低至 5%[70]，因此临床无改善者可行局部病灶手术切除[95,404]。新型两性霉素脂质体的疗效可能优于标准制剂[228]。骨髓移植患者中曲霉菌感染的发生率可高达 10%[384]。对这些患者的曲霉病做出诊断较困难，因为此时可合并存在如移植物抗宿主病（GVHD）的问题。骨髓移植患者的痰液标本中出现
曲霉菌即高度提示被感染，但对可疑病例需要进行肺 1007
部活检以确诊。

假丝酵母菌是引起免疫功能降低患者感染最常见的真菌体[291]。感染发生的主要部位是口腔。肺部虽不常见假丝酵母菌感染，但它是侵入性感染的最常见部位[113,161,344]。感染可经血源播散或吸入受污染的口咽分泌物而蔓延到肺部。胸部 X 线平片常无特异性。支气管肺泡灌洗可以帮助确诊，但往往需行肺活检。侵袭性假丝酵母菌感染的治疗已有进展[283]。唑类药物氟康唑和伊曲康唑是对抗大多数假丝酵母菌感染的标准药物[282]，但某些假丝酵母菌仍较特殊，对唑类药物和（或）两性霉素 B 具有天然抗药性。新的抗真菌药物，如棘白菌素，能影响真菌壁的合成，在标准治疗无效或者标准药物的副作用限制了治疗时，治疗有抗药性的菌种有效[94,282]。目前已明确，如果患者的假丝酵母菌感染不经治疗，预后均差[289]。

病毒感染

癌症患者除非免疫功能严重降低，否则发生病毒感染并不常见。病毒感染的易感性取决于宿主防御机制受影响的程度。例如，细胞免疫功能紊乱者较易感染疱疹病毒家族，如巨细胞病毒（CMV）。CMV 感染的发病率随潜在疾病的进程发生变化。这一感染在同种异体骨髓移植患者中，比在自体骨髓移植者中更普遍[269]。它常是潜在感染的再激活，表现为发热、头痛、全身乏力和肌痛，这些表现可在肺炎前 1～2 周出现。X 线表现无特异性，显示肺部弥漫、结节或肺膨胀不全等变化[79]。CMV 感染确诊依靠细胞学或 PCR 方法对支气管肺泡灌洗液标本进行分析[361,374]。治疗包括应用更昔洛韦和免疫球蛋白[374,411]。骨髓移植患者的间质性肺炎由 CMV 感染造成的多达 50%[252]。并发 GVHD、接受频繁输血或接受氨甲蝶呤或抗胸腺细胞药物治疗的患者，CMV 感染的危险性增加[79]。

免疫功能有活性的患者很少发生水痘肺炎。30% 有内脏受累的患者可出现肺炎[269]。如果同时接受化疗，其肺炎发生率可达 80%。这些患者的 X 线表现为模糊的双侧弥漫性渗出影。如果患者有水痘接触史，应在隔离观察期内停止化疗（约 21 天）。此时，应给予水痘–带状疱疹免疫球蛋白被动免疫接种。感染活动期的治疗包括阿昔洛韦。疱疹病毒一般罕见，除非合并口腔炎。RSV 感染在骨髓移植患者中可成为棘手的问题，因为它降低了 T 细胞介导的免疫反应。高达 80%的免疫功能降低并感染 RSV 病毒的患者，其感染可进展到危及生命。此时，只能提供支持治疗；因此，高危患者应推荐接受预防接种[393]。

卡氏肺囊虫

这个不同寻常的微生物具有原生动物（甲氧苄啶敏感）和真菌（基于 RNA 研究）的特性，且几乎是免疫功能降低患者特有的感染。常规预防可明显降低这种病毒感染的发病率[79]。肺孢子虫感染往往是潜在疾病再次激活造成的。感染的风险取决于免疫抑制的程度，而骨髓移植患者和接受皮质类固醇治疗的患者感染风险尤高。患者通常主诉有发烧、干咳和呼吸困难。疾病进展期可出现缺氧和呼吸窘迫。疾病暴发期的 X 线表现为双侧肺门浸润，并扩展到外侧带（图 64–5）。确诊依靠组织学及细胞学方法在支气管肺泡灌洗液中鉴别出滋养体包囊[269]。甲氧苄啶 / 磺胺甲基异噁唑（TMP/SMX）是此症治疗和预防的主要药物[172]。皮质类固醇激素和供氧均有助于治疗重症感染患者。如治疗 72 小时无反应，需行肺活检。感染未经治疗者 1008
的死亡率接近 100%。如出现骨髓抑制或 TMP/SMX 用药有继发皮疹者，可应用戊烷脒气雾剂[266]。

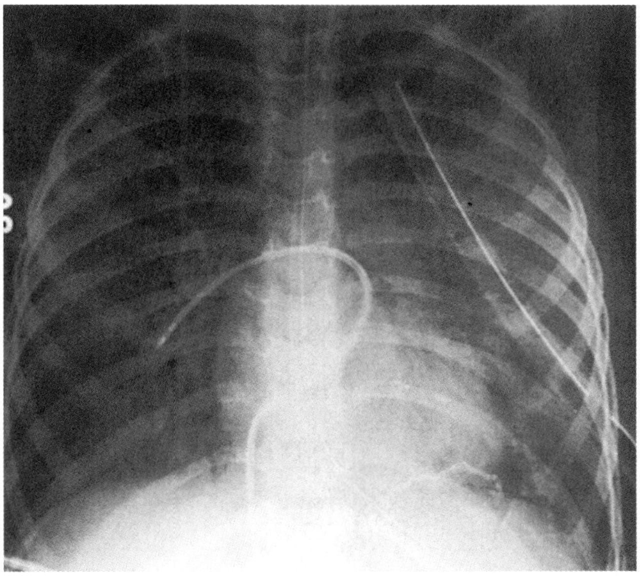

图 64–5　一名患急性淋巴母细胞性白血病的 5 岁女孩，正在接受化疗时的卡氏肺囊虫性肺炎。双肺均见弥漫性间质浸润。舌叶活组织检查（U 形钉标注）提示卡氏肺囊虫。一根 SWAN–GANZ 漂浮导管置入右下肺动脉。虽然白血病得到缓解，但患儿死于肺部疾病引起的呼吸衰竭。（现在应用抗生素预防治疗，早期开始经验治疗，并进行支气管肺泡灌洗以确诊，像她这样的预后已经罕见。）

HIV 儿科患者

HIV 感染如能早期诊断则可延长存活期[286]。在美国，儿童 HIV 感染者最常见的严重感染是急性肺炎[286]。在发展中国家，尤其是在非洲撒哈拉以南的沙漠区域，呼吸道感染是儿童 HIV 感染者患病、住院和死亡的最常见原因之一[141]。在 1997 年引进的高效抗反转录病毒疗法（HAART）通过“免疫系统重建”已大幅改善发达国家成人 HIV 感染患者[8]的存活[223]。

这一疗法对儿童也有效果，尤其是对严重的免疫抑制患儿[375]。有趣的是，尽管 HAART 对 HIV 感染的自然病程有效，但也有证据显示，它具有增加细菌性肺炎发病的作用[353,403]。

引起 HIV 感染患者罹患细菌性肺炎的最常见的微生物是肺炎链球菌、金黄色葡萄球菌和 A 组 β 溶血性链球菌、流感嗜血杆菌 b 型、沙门杆菌和假单胞菌[141]。HIV 患儿呼吸道感染的临床特点与免疫系统正常的儿童相似。但 CD4+ 计数减少、严重的免疫抑制和先前有过获得性免疫功能缺陷综合征（AIDS）相关呼吸道感染的患儿更易发生急性肺炎[14,256]。此外，这些患者易反复感染，后遗症包括支气管扩张、肺实质结构异常、肺大泡性疾病[286]。儿童 HIV 感染者的肺炎诊断依靠临床和 X 线检查发现。但对这一组患者，应重视排除机会性和非典型性感染。此外，这些患者肺部渗出病变的鉴别诊断还应包括非感染因素，如非 Hodgkin 病，经 HAART 治疗者此症发生率增高[141,403]。肺活检有助于确诊。预防感染对于这些患者的治疗很重要，方法包括嗜血杆菌和肺炎球菌的常规免疫接种以及应用 TMP/SMX 预防肺孢虫病[5,7]。针对特定病原体的治疗应尽快开始，但在等待培养结果之前仍可进行经验治疗（头孢他啶或头孢曲松）。

肺孢子虫

肺孢子虫感染是 1 岁以内的 AIDS 患者最常见的特征性疾病。即使患儿的 CD4+ 计数高，儿童期发生此感染的死亡率较成人高[13]。但肺孢子虫性肺炎的发生率已随 TMP/SMX 预防性治疗而降低[1]。尽管现有的儿童资料不全，近期的成人系列资料显示，对 HAART 疗法反应好的患者很少发生肺孢子虫性肺炎[323,395]。目前，在下列情况仍推荐对肺囊虫病以进行预防：（1）有 HIV 接触史的婴儿，可在 4～6 周时开始治疗直至证明感染诊断不成立；（2）不论其 CD4+ 计数，所有 1 岁内的婴儿 HIV 感染者；（3）所有 CD4+ 计数低于年龄分组阈值的儿童 HIV 感染者。肺孢子虫性肺炎的临床表现包括：迅速发作的呼吸困难、气促和缺氧，伴有咳嗽和发热。血清乳酸脱氢酶升高可支持诊断。X 线片通常显示充气过度和支气管周围影增厚，并可进展为肺泡渗出。经支气管肺泡灌洗和用气囊导管行深部气管抽吸术常可确诊肺孢子虫性肺炎，但有时需要肺活检。TMP/SMX 联合皮质类固醇和给严重病例供氧是主要的治疗方法。

淋巴样间质性肺炎

淋巴细胞或淋巴样间质性肺炎（LIP）是一种慢性淋巴浸润，可见于 2 岁以上的 HIV 患儿，是另一种 AIDS 特征性疾病。EB 病毒是致病因子。据估计，在美国和欧洲的 HIV 垂直传播病例中，LIP 发生率为 20%～30%[331]。患者常以呼吸道症状隐匿起病，易与肺结核混淆。其他临床症状包括发热、杵状指、无症状的腮喉痈、对称的淋巴结病和肝大。临床过程为良性，但可使患者易发生细菌性和病毒性肺炎、支气管扩张和肺大泡病变[141,286]。X 线平片显示持续网状结节样浸润和肺门淋巴结肿大，CT 检查更清晰（图 64–6）。确诊通常需要进行肺活检，浸润病变 4～6 周时可发现明显的肺组织结构改变，后者通常使浸润消退。HAART 可改善 LIP 的临床进程，并减少相关的慢性肺病的流行。

肺结核

发达国家儿童结核病发病率的升高与成年 HIV 感染者此症发病率的增加平行，后者是传播给儿童的主要来源[349]。儿童 HIV 感染者肺结核的临床特征类似于有免疫能力的患者，但病情更易迅速进展，出现 1009
肺外和（或）播散性病变[66]。X 线片常提示肺叶或弥漫性渗出以及肿大的肺门淋巴结压迫支气管造成的肺不张。如果发现儿童感染肺结核，应着手进行 HIV 测试。肺结核的诊断基于所获得的临床的、流行病学的和影像学的资料[6]。清晨胃液抽吸物中保留有前晚的分泌物，是肺结核最好的无创培养技术，它比许多有创操作如支气管肺泡灌洗和支气管镜检查法更有辅助诊断价值[11]。结核菌素皮肤试验仍是用于所有儿童 HIV 感染者的有价值的辅助诊断方法，每 9～12 个月应进行一次[5,115]。预防是关键，明确家庭中所有成年人的结核病情况是必要的。目前在美国，儿童 HIV 感染者禁忌接种卡介苗，因为可增加播散性病变的风险[80]。但在疾病流行区，世界卫生组织推荐无症状的儿童 HIV 感染者接种疫苗[286]。如果在 3 个月时重复 PPD 试验为阴性，即可停药。感染活动期的治疗为一个多因素疗法[337,348]。必须注意观察抗反转录病毒药物

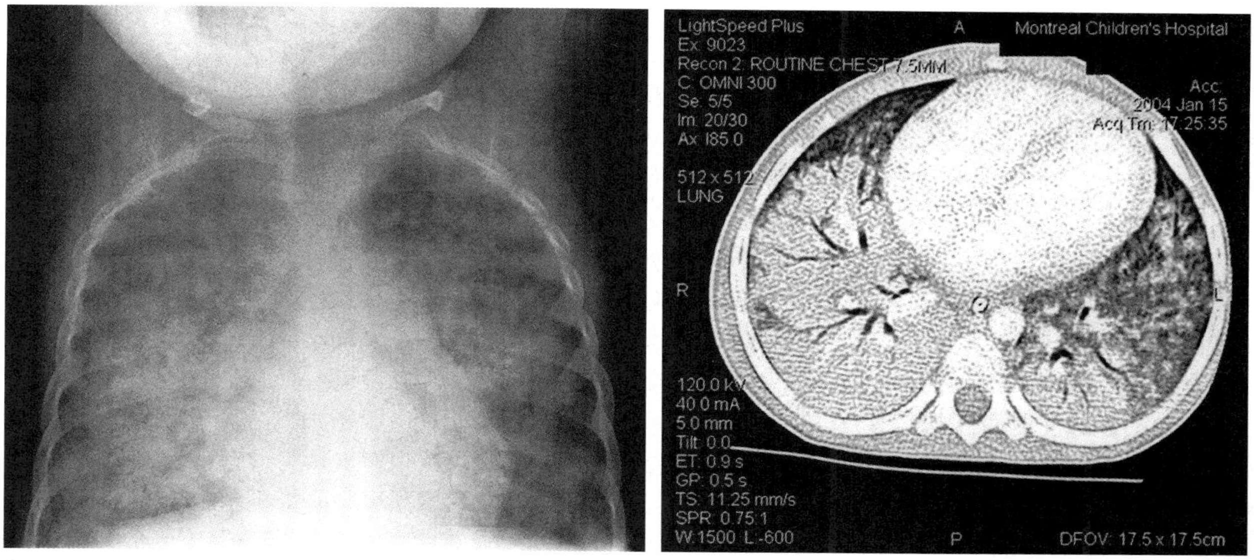

A　B

图 64-6　一名刚从非洲移民来的 3 岁儿童有虚弱和咳嗽症状，并在之前的 2 年开始抗肺结核治疗。其临床表现为呼吸窘迫恶化，并需要气管插管。A. X 线平片显示肺泡型肺浸润。B. CT 提示弥漫性肺实变伴空气支气管征，尤其在右下肺叶。怀疑为HIV 感染，稍后得到证实。支气管镜检查和支气管肺泡灌洗没有诊断意义。肺活检提示淋巴样间质性肺炎。他接受了皮质类固醇和三联抗反转录病毒治疗，并很快康复。

和抗结核药物之间的相互作用[9]。

非典型分枝杆菌感染

多种非典型分枝杆菌对 HIV 患者有重大的临床意义。包括鸟分枝杆菌、胞内分枝杆菌、鼠麻风分枝杆菌和淋巴结分枝杆菌。这些细菌是儿童 HIV 感染者发病的主要来源，常引起 AIDS 病程晚期的全身感染。此前，感染非典型分枝杆菌的患者有 9～11 个月的预期寿命[170,312]，但随着更有效的治疗 HIV 和非典型分枝杆菌感染方法的出现，此症已不太常见，且预后改善。的确，播散性非结核分枝杆菌感染的发病率在成人 HAART 时代呈下降趋势[96,218,370]。存在的争议是对这种疗法有反应的患者，是否应停止针对机会感染的预防性治疗[200,370]。在儿科，评价 HAART 对非典型分枝杆菌感染效应的临床试验尚未进行。所以，对患有播散性疾病的儿科患者仍推荐进行预防[3]。

这些患者的临床症状通常是生长发育停滞、腹痛和疲劳，而非呼吸道症状。患者也可能有白细胞减少、血小板减少和血清乳酸脱氢酶升高。诊断方法是血培养或正常无菌部位的活检，包括骨髓和淋巴结。检查还必须排除感染肺结核的可能性。预防感染是通过保护免疫系统及有效的抗反转录病毒疗法来完成。根据按年龄分组的 CD4$^+$ 计数，选用克拉霉素或阿奇霉素进行初级预防[5]。感染活动期可以用克拉霉素、乙胺丁醇、环丙沙星或阿奇霉素治疗。大环内酯类药物抑制许多抗反转录病毒药物的代谢。

病毒感染

CMV 感染可表现为慢性间质性肺炎，且常伴发视网膜炎、肝炎或结肠炎。它经常发生于严重的免疫抑制患者。呼吸系统症状包括干咳、呼吸困难和 1010
低氧血症。肺炎可能与并发的肺孢子虫感染有关。X线检查发现包括弥漫的间质性浸润。CMV 感染的诊断依靠从尿液、支气管肺泡灌洗或活检标本中识别出病毒。然而，区分 HIV 患者是处于感染活动期还是无症状排毒期较困难，这使治疗方案错综复杂[396]。更昔洛韦是首选治疗，特别是在证实病毒侵及胃肠道或视网膜者。

真菌感染

全身性真菌感染在 HIV 患者中并不常见，因为真菌感染更常累及皮肤或黏膜。肺真菌病在儿童 HIV 患者中有一定的发病率，是由于 T 细胞免疫受损所致。组织胞浆菌病的报道在这组患者中不常见。原发性肺部病灶可能迅速进展为播散性病变，如未经处理可致命。严重时，可出现发热、肝脾肿大、全血细胞减少症、网状结节状肺叶浸润，偶尔进展为感染性休克。可根据支气管肺泡灌洗物培养或肺活检进行诊断。治疗包括静脉注射两性霉素 B。小儿原发性肺部疾病患者应接受伊曲康唑的预防性治疗，以防止播散性病变。

隐球菌和球孢子菌感染通常引起播散性感染，而且这些患者中的 50%并发肺部感染。隐球菌感染表现为发烧、头痛、肺部浸润，可与播散性疾病混淆。诊断靠痰、血液或脑脊液培养，以及用印度墨汁或乳胶凝集反应直接进行脑脊液检查。治疗包括两性霉素 B，2 周后用氟康唑继续治疗。球孢子菌病常表现为播散性疾病，累及肺、脑组织和皮肤。常见发烧、体重减轻、咳嗽和不同程度的意识改变。诊断是从痰、支气管肺泡或肺活检标本中获得证据。急性感染可用两性霉素 B 治疗，但常复发，因而要求进行氟康唑的预防性治疗。曲霉菌病是另一种不常见的真菌感染，通常引起肺部疾病和鼻窦炎。这些患者可出现发热、咳嗽、呼吸困难和胸膜炎性胸痛。确诊需要痰液分析、支气管肺泡灌洗，有时进行肺活检。虽然新的唑类和棘球白素已证明有效，此症治疗仍选用两性霉素 B[188,305]。还可应用伊曲康唑进行长期抑菌治疗[335,336]。

免疫功能降低的患儿在感染的持续威胁下，需要不断监护和积极管理的治疗策略。对有肺部浸润的患者，应立即开始使用广谱抗生素。若在治疗后 48～72 小时无反应，就应更换抗生素，并提示可能需增加两性霉素 B 和 TMP/SMX。对于持续肺部浸润者，可进行支气管肺泡灌洗，但更应施行肺活检。已表明，长期肺浸润患者的肺活检结果会对高达 90%的患者的当前治疗产生影响[206]。

囊性纤维化

囊性纤维化（CF）是白人中最常见的常染色体隐性遗传病，发生率约为 1/ 3400 活产新生儿[259]。在美国，将近 30 000 人受此病影响[298]。此症的预后在过去 30 年中已大大改善，但自 20 世纪 90 年代中期以来保持平稳。目前，CF 患者的预期寿命超过 30 岁。它的特点是不舒服的浓稠黏液、慢性感染和以中性粒细胞为主的气道炎症[298]。囊性纤维化跨膜传导调节体（CFTR）是环磷酸腺苷依赖性氯离子通道，位于染色体 7q21–31[193]。*CFTR* 突变导致此病的临床表现。关于这一点，现已提出若干假说。有一个假说指出，CF 中 *CFTR* 作为一种离子通道丢失，使得液体生成减少、钠吸收增强[51]。这导致纤毛功能和黏液运输过程受损。也有人认为，气道表层的钠增加会抑制抗菌防御素且损害肺防御机制，包括腔内杀死摄入的细菌[147]。在此病的纯合子患者中，还发现钠可增加黏附在气道上皮细胞上的细菌量，尤其是绿脓杆菌。此外，CF 患者似乎还存在炎症级联反应失调而导致的慢性炎症[26]。

CF 的临床症状和体征有很大差异。患者可能相对无症状，表现为慢性疾患和生长发育停滞，或主诉急性、反复加重的肺病。不过，常见症状是逐渐加重的干咳，发展为伴有脓性分泌物的疏松咳痰性咳嗽。典型的体格检查结果包括桶状胸、湿啰音、干啰音和杵状指，偶尔伴有发绀。虽然初期肺功能检查提示为阻塞性病变，病情进展可导致限制性肺病。CF 的确诊依靠汗液测试（氯升高）或 *CFTR* 的突变鉴定，最常见的是△*F508*。

在人生的第一个十年中，CF 患者最常见的病原微生物是金黄色葡萄球菌（40%），其次是流感嗜血杆菌（15%）[299]。绿脓杆菌通常是在 1 岁以内患儿分离到的第一个病原体，而有超过 80%的 18 岁左右的患者感染此菌。临床上，绿脓杆菌是 CF 中最重要的病原体。这些细菌能形成生物膜而逃避正常的清除机制和抗生素的渗透作用[59]。绿脓杆菌还能产生外毒素 1011
增加其致病性、增加分泌物黏度并进一步损害纤毛运输[346]。洋葱假单胞菌是一种具有天然抗药性的生物体。患者感染这种细菌后出现高热、肺部病变迅速恶化，有时致死。病毒感染可能构成一个特殊问题，尤其在幼儿中，因为它们更容易发生继发感染、需要机械通气和出现氧气依赖[12]。对这些婴儿要求进行 RSV 预防[31]。

CF 患者肺部病变的内科治疗基础是积极使用静脉内、口腔和雾化吸入的抗生素。实际上，CF 患者寿命的增加可直接归功于抗绿脓杆菌有效药物的发展。维持治疗旨在延长绿脓杆菌感染加重肺部病变的间隔期。最近的III期临床试验已证实雾化吸入妥布霉素的有效性。大环内酯类药物也有治疗效果，因为它们具备抗炎特性且有助于防止生物膜形成[301]。清除异常分泌物是极为重要的，包括规则的胸部物理治疗和体位引流。雾化剂，如 N-乙酰半胱氨酸和 DNA 酶，能够帮助 CF 患者咳出浓稠分泌物[299,300]。试图用皮质类固醇或其他消炎药减少炎症反应时，可合并出现这些药物的副作用。

充足的营养支持和胰腺功能不全的早期治疗是 CF 患者内科治疗的另一个关键领域。即使无其他症状的新生儿及幼儿，在获得诊断时可能已有重度营养不良。婴儿成长所需的能量增加与他们摄入足够营养的能力受损之间的失衡使他们容易出现肺部并发症[205,324]。的确，经早期治疗的胰腺功能不全患儿的远期身高和体重增长情况均已得到证实[119]，据此指导临床医生应重视囊性纤维化患儿的营养需求和监督[50]。

这些患者长大后，小儿外科医生可能参与几个方面的工作。植入式的输液港导管可以为经常需要抗生素治疗肺部病变恶化的患者提供静脉通道。营养管理需要进行胃造口术。CF 的肺部并发症如支气管扩张、大量咯血和气胸在本章稍后部分再做讨论，而胃肠道和肝脏并发症在本书其他章节讨论。

肺移植仍是末期肺部疾病患者最终的治疗手段。大约 1200 名来自美国、加拿大、英国和法国的患者接受了移植[298]。结果显示双侧肺移植是 CF 患儿的首选处理。已有报告此症 1～2 年生存率在 65%～85%之间，但长期存活率仍是大部分患者的问题[32,112,249,351]。不过，可带来最大裨益的最佳移植时间还不清楚。不幸的是，尽管致病基因 10 多年以前已被确定，但基因治疗并没有超越 I 期试验阶段[193]。研究的主要限制因素在于，脂质炎性反应的发生发展和用来传送 *CFTR* 功能基因到达气道上皮细胞的病毒载体[189]。现正积极进行更多的涉及此病适当治疗方法的研究。

慢性和复发性肺炎

肺炎是一种儿童常见的疾病和住院原因。复发性或持续性肺炎的差别往往难以判断。的确，对于这些类型的肺炎并无统一定义，而且在疾病真正消散前，X 线检查异常也可能持续数个星期至数月。诊断复发性肺炎最好在标准感染完全消退之后，但这很困难。顾名思义，复发性肺炎是一年中发生两次肺部感染或任何时间段内发作三次[385]。几位作者曾试图找出最常见的小儿复发性肺炎的原因[16,159,232,279]。有趣的是，此症不同于急性肺炎，多达 92%的慢性或复发性肺炎能确定出一个根本原因。在众多病因之中，哮喘是复发性肺炎最常见的原因，其次为吸入。

广义上，肺炎可分为累及单个肺区和多个肺区。累及单个肺区的异常情况包括病程进展造成的气道腔内梗阻（异物、支气管肿瘤）、腔外受压（肺结核、肉样瘤病、肿瘤和血管环）或肺结构异常（气管延续性支气管、局部支气管扩张、先天性囊性腺瘤样畸形）[379]。累及多个肺区的异常情况包括反复发生微小异物吸入、哮喘、免疫缺陷综合征、黏液纤毛功能障碍（囊性纤维化）、结构异常（支气管软化、Williams-Campbell 综合征即支气管软骨缺失-支气管扩张综合征）、支气管肺发育不良以及其他罕见疾病，如 Wegener 肉芽肿病和特发性肺纤维化[379]。其他造成反复肺部浸润的病因也存在，如镰状细胞病患者的急性胸部综合征（图 64-7）。

慢性或复发性肺炎的临床评定要求细致的病史和体检。必须详细描述先前感染的发生频率、持续时间和严重程度，以及当时的外周环境。其相关症状如喘鸣、体重减轻和发烧也是重要的细节。症状出现的时间，特别是对先天畸形或遗传病，如囊性纤维化，有助于缩小鉴别诊断的范围。家族史也可提供有价值的资料。体检时，有必要全面评估患儿的生长和发育。近期的胸部 X 线评价以及以前肺炎发作时 X 线片回 1012
顾可提供一些细节并直接指导治疗和检查。患儿的临床状况将决定后继检查的紧急程度。患儿是否需要补充氧气或呼吸支持常可通过体检结合脉氧饱和度监测和血气分析进行评价。局灶性肺炎患者可能需要接受支气管镜检查以除去异物或评估支气管肿瘤和结构畸形。胸部高分辨 CT 可有助于找出肺实质病变以及支气管阻塞的内部因素和外在原因。多灶性肺炎患者可能需要进行上消化道检查和 pH探头以排除吸入、评估哮喘的肺功能检查或免疫缺陷和其他全身性疾病的检查。

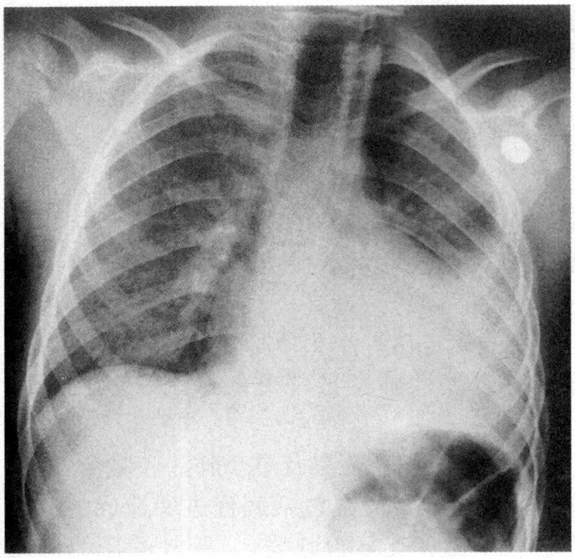

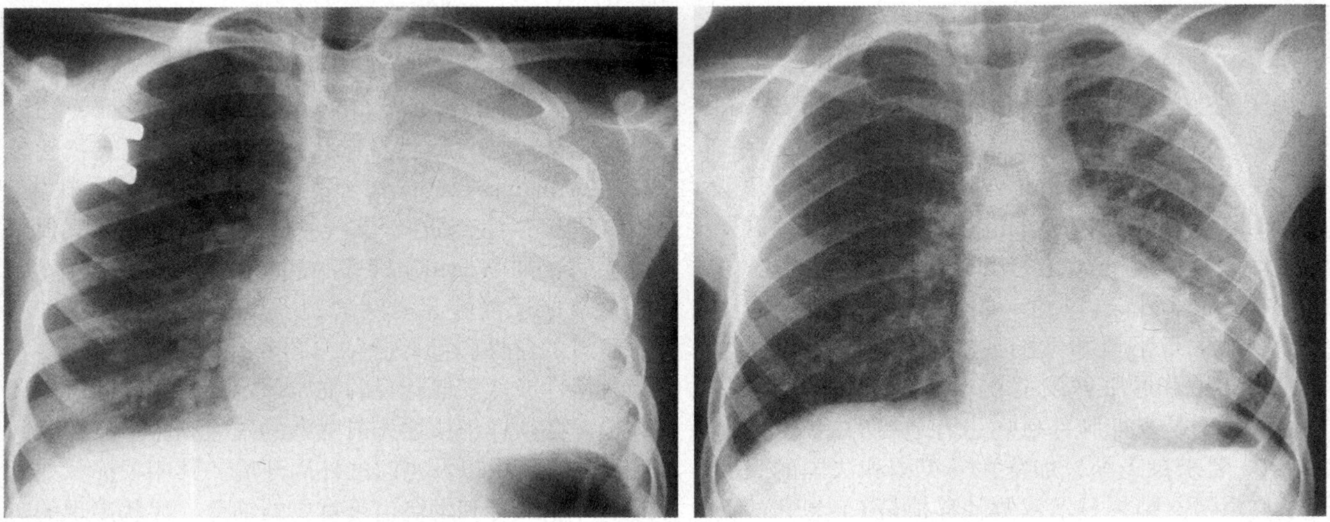

图 64–7 图示为镰状细胞病的急性胸部综合征。一名已知有血红蛋白 S、被诊断为 β-地中海贫血的 5 岁女孩，表现为鼻充血、咳嗽和胸痛。起初胸片正常（未出示）。住院接受静脉注射和止痛治疗。当她出现发热时，开始接受抗生素治疗。但她的呼吸越来越急促并缺氧。A. 入院后 2 天，胸片显示气腔病变，左下肺叶最明显。B. 住院第 5 天，整个左侧胸廓出现模糊影，而右肺底气腔病变加重。C. 在接受输血治疗后 4 天，胸片表现明显改善。

支气管扩张

1819 年，Laennec 首次描述了[56]支气管扩张是继发于支气管及支气管周围组织炎症破坏的不可逆转的气道扩张。在 20 世纪 40 和 50 年代，支气管扩张是导致儿童肺切除的首要原因[306]。目前，在发达国家它已成为一种少见病，主要限于儿科患者。但是，支气管扩张的发病率和继发疾病的发生率仍是发展中国家和某些发达国家土著居民（阿拉斯加和澳大利亚土著
1013 和萨摩亚人）的一个问题[303]。此症总体发病率和死亡率的下降是由于抗生素治疗的进步和针对常见病原体（如肺炎链球菌）的疫苗改进的结果。

发病机制和病因学

支气管扩张症的发病机制包括三个进展阶段。最初是纤毛上皮的破坏，被立方鳞状上皮取代。疾病早期（圆柱状支气管扩张）是气道弹性组织的局部损坏伴水肿和炎症。疾病后期（囊状支气管扩张）病变累及气道肌肉层及软骨，而且囊性扩张区域的肺动脉与支气管动脉之间形成吻合支。还有证据支持宿主介导成分引起局部组织损伤。

关于支气管扩张症的发生，目前已有众多不同的假说[91,398]。显然，支气管扩张症最常见的原因是感染，而且是唯一得到动物研究支持的理论（图 64–8）[56]。支气管扩张可能不是由标准感染造成的，而常由伴随感染或随后并发的多病因感染（如肺结核和组织胞浆菌病[309]、病毒[41,330]、某些真菌[262]和偶见支原体）引起[397]。历史上，麻疹和百日咳感染与继而发生的支气管扩张有关联[187,330]。囊性纤维化是支气管扩张最常见的遗传原因；此时是继发于感染和黏液浓稠的支气管阻塞。其他原因包括先天性气管软骨支持缺陷（Williams–Campbell 综合征）[400]、气管扩张、Marfan 综合征[406]、α_1 抗胰蛋白酶缺乏症[378]、异物吸入[212]、纤毛异常（Kartagener 综合征）[43,368]、免疫缺陷（IgA）[164]、哮喘[108]和右肺中叶综合征[33,382]。

临床表现和检查

大部分患者在学龄前期出现咳嗽、多痰、喘鸣和胸痛。多达 50% 的病儿可有杵状指，但可逆。支气管扩张症在 X 线平片上显示出支气管扩张、支气管增厚或印戒征。有人认为对于支气管扩张症患者，肺闪烁成像术是一种有价值的辅助检查[29,377]。这一技术能确定胸部 X 线检查没有显示出的肺部病变范围，并取代支气管造影术用以设计支气管切除术方案[257]。而胸部高分辨 CT 已取代支气管造影术用以描述疾病类型和严重程度[155,343]。检查发现包括：支气管呈圆柱状或囊状扩张、分泌物汇集和支气管增厚（图 64–9）。但是，急性化脓性肺部感染可引起可逆性支气管扩张，与支气管扩张症混淆[306]。支气管扩张症的病灶分布有助于洞察根本原因。肺结核患者通常累及单侧肺，而 CF 患者和病毒诱导患病者分别累及肺上叶和肺下叶。

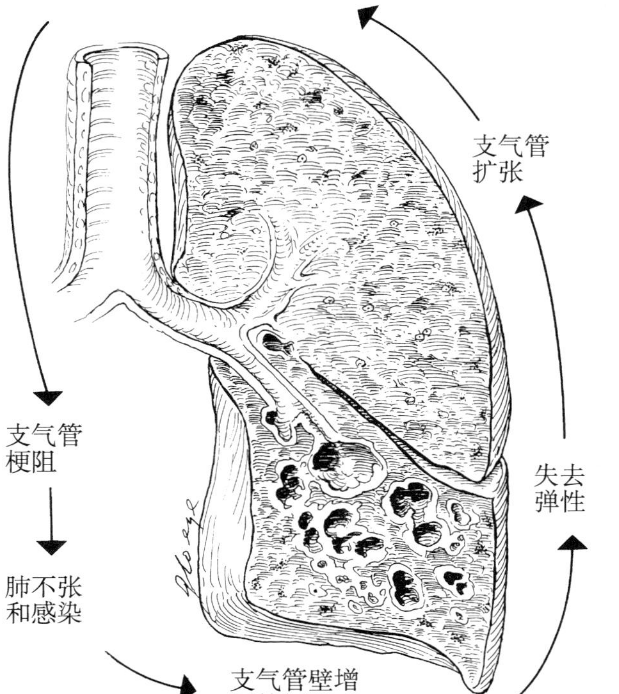

图 64–8　支气管扩张症发病机制的影响因素的图解说明。

治疗

支气管扩张症的治疗重点是找出并治疗根本原因，辅以体位引流和胸部物理治疗。急性加重时必须应用抗生素治疗，而对囊性纤维化患者给予适当的营养支持和胰酶替代治疗可用于防止复发感染和肺病恶化导致的生长发育停滞。支气管镜检查也可用以暂时缓解因异物[97]或浓稠分泌物[342]引起的支气管阻塞，或者用于慢性肺部感染术前或诊断的辅助评估[68,131]。 1014

虽然，过去几年来手术治疗支气管扩张症的频率有所下降，但还是有患者对药物治疗无反应而从手术切除中获益。主要手术适应证包括[401]：（1）伴严重和衰弱症状的局部性疾病，如多痰、呼吸臭味和明显影响生活质量的严重咳嗽；（2）局灶性疾病的致命出血；（3）可致生长发育停滞的可切除病灶；（4）

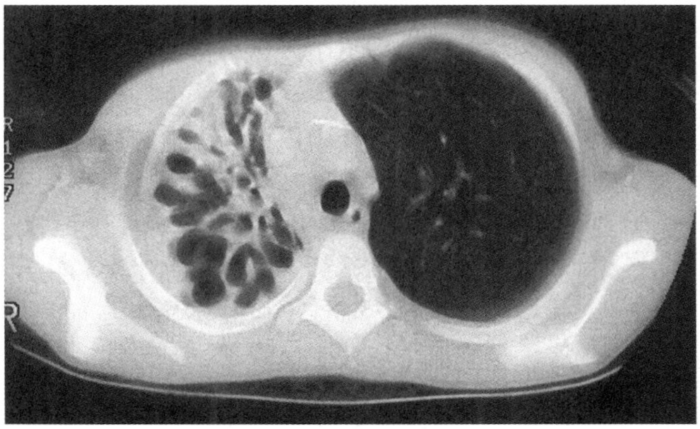

图 64–9　图示为一名患囊性纤维化的 10 岁女孩的胸部 CT 图像。术前的通气–灌注扫描检查显示这一支气管扩张的肺叶已无功能。患者接受了上肺叶切除术。

复发性下呼吸道感染所在区域的可切除病灶。次要手术适应证包括双侧或非局灶性病变，或仅有轻中度症状的患者。

大多数儿科患者在接受手术切除后，临床症状消失或得到改善。的确，年长儿童的病例研究资料显示 3/4 的患者术后改善，且疾病发生率降到最低程度[355,390,401]。这一成功结果也反映在最近评估儿童与成人患者的联合报告中，这些患者为非局灶性和双侧病变[30,36,131,213]。在这些病例手术中，已进行过肺段切除术、肺叶切除术和肺切除术（伴或不伴肺段切除术或肺叶切除术）。联合累积有 581 名患者接受了这些手术，超过 80% 的患者在术后 4 年的中期随访中没有症状或症状改善。手术死亡率为 0～1.7%，手术并发症包括肺不张、持续气漏、脓胸、支气管胸膜瘘和术后出血，发生率为 8%～17%。在一份 33 例小儿病例手术的报告中[150]，相似类型手术的死亡率和发病率分别为 2.8% 和 17.6%。此报告中只有 11.7% 的患儿未从手术操作中获益。2003 年，Rothenberg 报告了他在 7 年中经胸腔镜对 45 例婴儿和儿童[311]实施肺切除手术的经验。其中 12 例患儿为重症局灶性支气管扩张。在这一系列手术中，无手术死亡和仅有 1 例发生术中并发症（一名左下叶支气管扩张症患者），表明这种手术在儿童中可行。对成功进行支气管扩张症手术治疗的常见问题是认真选择手术患者、术前评估和手术技巧，以及试着彻底切除所有病变的肺组织。

肺出血和咯血

肺出血和咯血的原因很广泛，可按照患者年龄或者根据潜在的肺病进行分类。在新生儿中，早产、肺水肿、呼吸窘迫综合征、脑内出血、凝血障碍和代谢异常可导致肺出血。对于慢性肺病患者而言，继发于囊性纤维化的支气管扩张症是儿科患者最常见的原因。不过，空洞性肺病变、肺结核、肿瘤、固定的异物和频繁的气道操作可导致症状性出血。在其他方面正常的患者中，大量咯血可继发于血管瘤、先天性动静脉畸形、叶内型肺隔离、支气管肺前肠畸形、单侧肺动脉发育不全（由于分支发育）和 Ehlers-Danlos 综合征（即遗传性结缔组织疾病，可有夹层动脉瘤、主动脉缩窄和二尖瓣关闭不全等）。

儿童大量咯血定义为 24 小时内咳出物中至少有 240 ml 血液或在数天至数周的时间内经常发作实质性出血（>100ml/d）[362]。约 1% 的 CF 患者可发生咯血，而伴有严重肺病的 CF 患者则更频繁[124]。这些患者大多在 10 岁以上。发病机制与支气管动脉扩大和迂曲以及这些血管与肺动脉之间形成多个吻合支（图 64-10）有关[407]。非支气管动脉也可发自与支气管循环伴行的血管，或经肉芽组织进入肺部。大多数大量咯血可自行缓解，但应注意镇静和停止使用损害凝血功能的药物。咯血通常表明肺功能恶化，因此在这个时候可以使用抗生素来治疗潜在感染。还可应用加压素、支气管气囊填塞、选择性主干道插管和局部使用 α-肾上腺素激动剂[321]。

支气管动脉栓塞术已成为一个非常成功的、能短期控制咯血的非手术干预方法[177]。但是，这些患者中多达 20%的人需要反复栓塞。栓塞失败的主要原因是非支气管分支血管[85,409]。支气管镜有助于出血灶的术前定位。肺叶切除术可挽救栓塞术失败的或呈暴发性大量咯血患者的生命。

肺炎并发症

肺膨出

肺膨出是一种细小的薄壁结构，由单一或多发性囊肿组成，腔内含空气，主要继发于肺泡和细支气管坏死。这些异常病变通常是金黄色葡萄球菌、A 组链球菌及偶尔的流感嗜血杆菌感染导致的后果。金黄色葡萄球菌感染继发的肺囊肿可在病程早期发现，发生率高达 80%[203]。感染的肺囊肿破裂可并发气胸和脓气胸[334]。这些病损较难与先天性肺囊肿鉴别。但是，肺膨出有自愈倾向，而先天性异常不应消失。在肺膨出消散之前应随访胸片，如有可疑情况行 CT 扫描检查（图 64-11）。 1015

肺部脓肿

当肺实质的局部感染灶发生坏死时即可发生肺脓肿，继而形成空洞。肺脓肿可分为原发性（发生于健康儿童）或继发性（其他方面有异常的儿童）[242]。目前已明确，肺脓肿几乎专门发生在肺炎区域。如

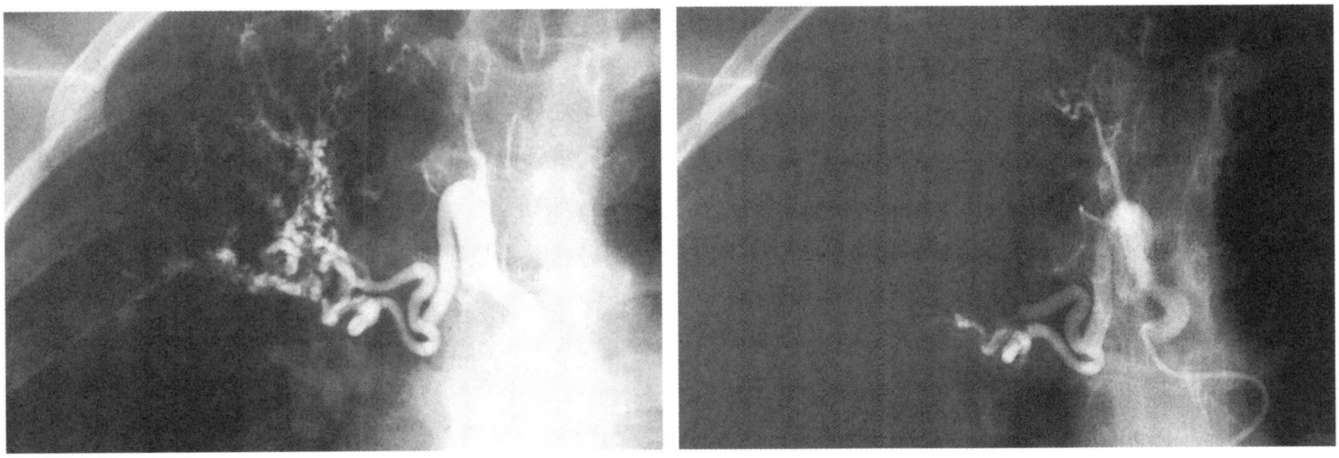

图 64-10 A. 通过动脉造影术确定一名患囊性纤维化的 10 岁女孩咯血的原因。注意图中迂曲的支气管动脉。B. 成功施行吸收性明胶海绵栓塞术后，动脉的周围分支不见了。

果早期开始适当的抗生素治疗，则肺脓肿发生率大大降低。近年来，免疫功能下降、重症患者或有时非常年幼患儿的肺脓肿成为越来越常见的难题。先天性支气管或肺囊肿偶尔出现继发感染。这些病变的胸片表现可能较难与肺脓肿区分（见图 64-11C 和 64-12）。

历史

在 17 世纪，Bonet 报道了他用体外引流治愈的 2 例肺脓肿患者[165]。在 20 世纪 30 年代，Neuhoff和Touroff[268]报告一期外科引流术成功治疗急性腐烂性肺脓肿。Welch[391]采用二期手术程序，第一步诱导胸膜腔愈合，死亡率为 40%。在 20 世纪 40 年代初期，肺脓肿切除手术几乎完全被依赖抗生素的疗法所替代，后者仍是目前的治疗方法。

发病机制

吸入胃内容物是儿童慢性肺炎和肺脓肿的主要病因[27]，特别是在神经功能缺损的患儿[360]。外伤、麻醉、癫痫发作或重症胃食管反流患儿可发生急性吸入。食管闭锁或食管运动障碍修补术后的患者也是吸入的危险人群[306]。吸入的异物，包括血液或扁桃腺切除术后的扁桃体组织，是以前常见的肺脓肿来源物[27,306]。这些脓肿现在已不常见，因为及时的支气管镜检查能清除外来异物，而且气管内插管和咽部填塞法可在口咽手术时防止发生吸入。

肺脓肿不是常见的细菌性肺炎并发症，儿科患者较成年患者少见[360]。最常见的致病菌是厌氧菌[55]，其次是金黄色葡萄球菌、绿脓杆菌、链球菌属和肺炎双球菌，偶见流感嗜血杆菌。其他引起肺脓肿的细菌包括克雷白菌、大肠杆菌、消化球菌属和消化链球菌属。细胞或体液免疫缺陷患儿，无论先天性或获得性，有时即便选用了适当的抗生素也无法根除肺部感染，可导致炎症、肺实质崩解，并最终形成脓肿。从组织学上确认肺脓肿，需在促发事件后 18～36 小时，但胸片表现只有在 7 天之后才出现[27]。婴儿发生肺脓肿，应怀疑是否存在一种潜在的先天性异常，例如支气管囊肿或先天性囊腺瘤样畸形（见图 64-11）[84]。这些病变需要切除，但初步治疗可用抗生素加（或不加）引流术。

患儿吸入时的体位决定肺脓肿的发生部位[306]。仰卧患者中，最常见的累及部位是肺下叶上段。如果孩子为右侧卧位，其右上肺叶发病风险高；如果孩子为左侧卧位，其肺尖左上肺叶后段有可能发病。直立体位孩子的吸入发生在肺下叶基底段。小儿肺脓肿在不同肺叶和节段的分布情况与成人的相似。肺脓肿常发生在一个节段或肺叶的边缘区域，这使该病适合做外 1016

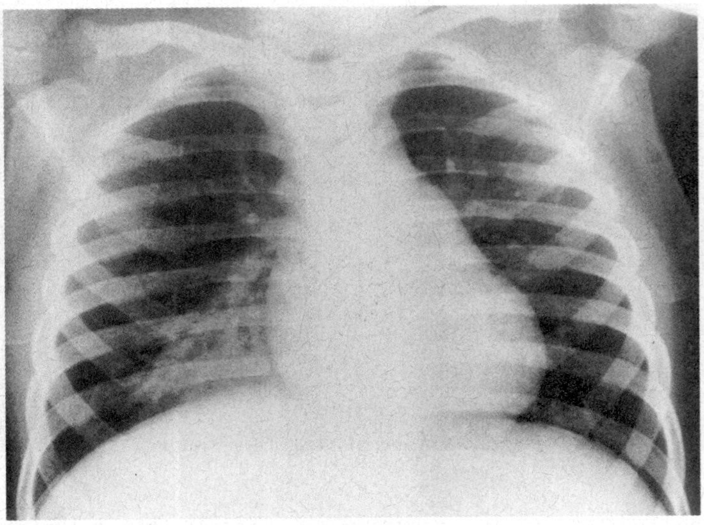

A

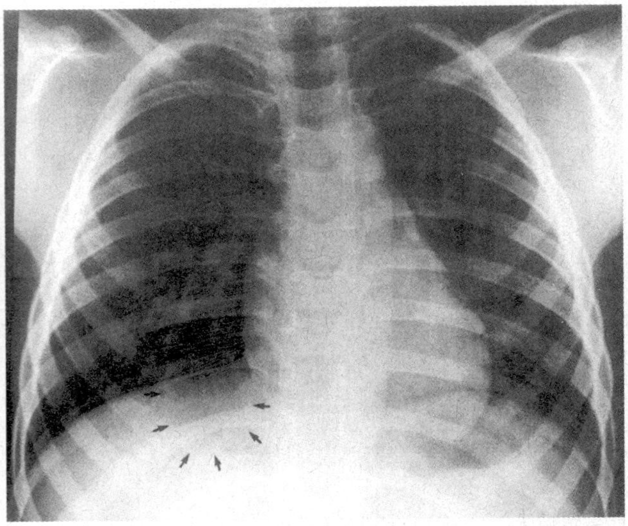

B

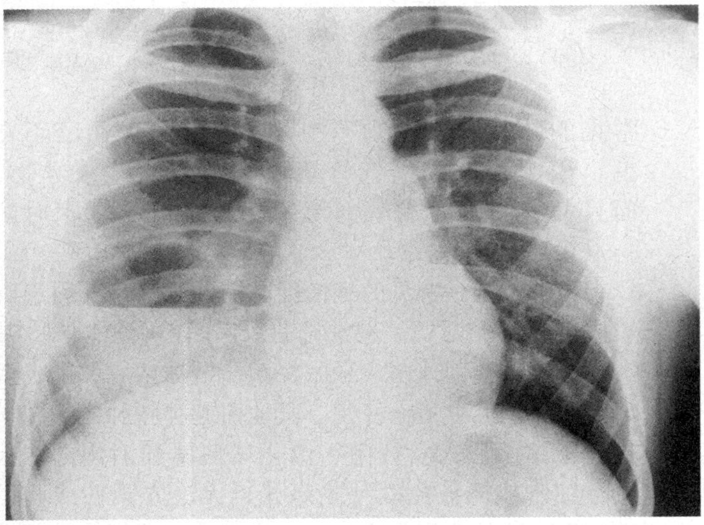

C

图 64–11 A. 一名 5 岁儿童表现为右下肺炎，对静脉抗生素有反应。B. 在门诊观察期间，于 6 周后出现小囊肿，并在这张摄于开始研究后 11 周的平片中融合产生较大的肺膨出。对患者进行随访。C. 在 14 岁时，此患者又出现一次新的感染，伴有一个大的和一些较小的气液平面。应用静脉抗生素需超过 2 周。经 CT 检查确定有三个囊肿。6 周后，患者接受右下肺叶切除术，并经显微镜检查确诊为Ⅰ型先天性囊性腺瘤样畸形。

分流术。

诊断

肺脓肿最常见的症状包括发烧、咳嗽、胸痛、食欲缺乏、生痰、体重减轻、全身乏力、咯血和畏寒。从年长儿中较易获得脓痰，有助于细菌学诊断；年幼病儿通常会吞下自己的分泌物。厌氧菌性肺脓肿的痰液特点是具有腐败味。受累部位的胸壁叩诊声音发闷，且呼吸音减少。常见白细胞增多症。脓肿增大的患者还可表现为限制性肺部疾病，或可继发胸膜炎性胸痛。

肺脓肿的诊断依靠胸部 X 线检查显示的空洞，通常具有气液平面（见图 64–12）。肺脓肿应与肺膨出鉴别，后者表现为局部的肺内空气集聚，通常没有气液平，但脓胸有气液平面。在诊断合并肺炎的肺部疾病中，CT 已成为有价值的辅助方法，并能描绘出病变特征，可揭示胸部平片中不能表现的病理学改变。

治疗

应尽可能在治疗前获得明确的细菌学诊断。应该使用诊断性支气管镜直接从患者支气管中抽吸出脓痰进行检查，除了在能排出满意痰液样本的年长儿。在

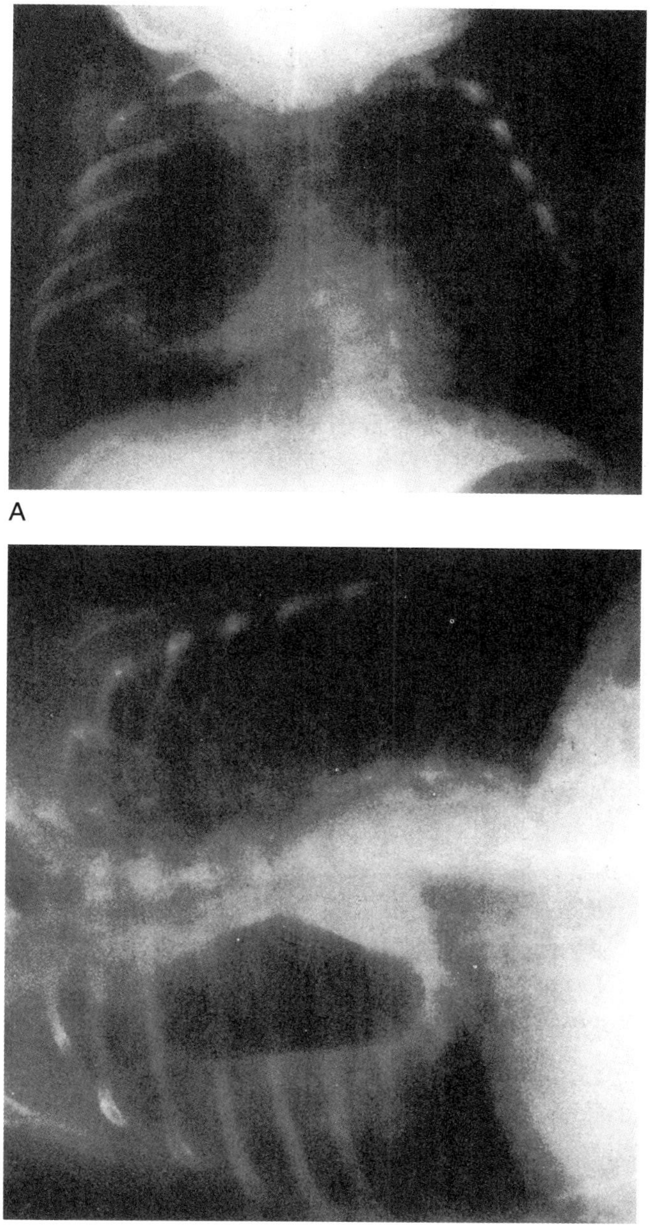

A

B

图 64-12　图示为一名婴儿吸入后导致的肺脓肿。A. 卧位前后位片中表现为一个厚壁空洞。B. 侧卧位片中可见气液平面。

影像引导下，针刺抽吸边缘型脓肿空洞以分离细菌菌株和引流脓液的操作已获得稳定成效[285]。即使对正在接受抗生素治疗的患者，也可以使用这种技术分离病
017 原体。

肺脓肿的首选治疗是适当的静脉内抗生素治疗及引流。通过胸部体位引流和叩诊可获得满意的引流效果，偶尔也可通过支气管镜抽吸术。无法充分咳嗽的儿童，可能需要进行治疗性支气管镜或经支气管引流，静脉抗生素使用 2～4 周，然后口服抗生素 6～8 周。患儿症状消失且胸片清晰后即可停止使用抗生素。这可能需要 1～6 个月[28]。治疗肺脓肿最有效的抗生素是克林霉素。大肠杆菌感染时，通常推荐使用氨基糖苷类抗生素。如果强烈怀疑假单胞菌感染，那么推荐使用合适的 β-内酰胺类抗生素与氨基糖苷类抗生素合用[360]。

内科治疗新生儿和免疫功能降低患儿的肺脓肿通常不成功，死亡率达 20%[391]。脓肿经皮导管引流有助于改善急性期患儿的病情[38,209,386,412]，特别是对尽管已接受最大剂量的抗生素治疗但疾病仍快速进展的患儿。经皮操作技术偶尔会出现并发症，包括气胸、血胸、引流不畅和支气管胸膜瘘[201,386]。肺脓肿手术切除方法中，对于慢性、大型和腔壁增厚的肺脓肿患者或者接受增强抗生素治疗或经皮穿刺引流术疗效不佳的少数患者，推荐施行肺段或肺叶切除术[84,274]。其他脓肿切除的指征包括病程超过 3 个月的慢性脓肿、持续大量咯血、支气管狭窄、明显的支气管扩张和大片肺坏死。

脓胸

历史

即使在希波克拉底、埃吉纳的保罗和 Fabricius 时代，已认识到脓胸是肺部感染的并发症，并需要外部引流治疗。早在 16 世纪，Pare 就为一位法国军人手工剥离胸膜腔中的一个腐烂血肿[165]。在 1889 年和 1891 年，Kuster 和 Fowler 分别完成正式的皮质剥除术[125]。直到抗生素时代，脓胸治疗的讨论才主要集中在开放引流的相对优势、各类闭式引流和这些措施的最佳使用时机[93]。

定义和发病机制

脓胸是脓液积聚在胸膜腔，高达 30%的儿童合并肺炎[359]。它也可能发生于创伤、肿瘤进展、胸腔食管穿孔或胸部手术之后。正常情况下，胸膜对液体有通透性，并且少量液体存在于胸膜脏层和壁层之间可以减少呼吸摩擦。当毗邻的肺组织健康，胸膜腔一般能

抵抗感染。脓胸一经确定，可表现为三个特征性阶段[67,314]：（1）渗出阶段或早期，此时渗出液稀薄、细胞内容物少；（2）中期或脓性纤维蛋白阶段，其间大量多形核细胞和纤维蛋白沉积在胸膜腔中，逐步削弱肺部膨胀并导致液体小腔的形成；以及（3）终末期或脓胸形成阶段，此期渗出物稠厚并有纤维蛋白侵
1018 入纤维素表层。脓胸可能弥漫并累及整个胸膜腔，或者可以局限并包裹于叶间、横膈或纵隔旁部位。

目前，儿童脓胸最常见的病原体是肺炎链球菌、金黄色葡萄球菌和流感嗜血杆菌[128]。与脓胸发生有关的经典的病原体还有其他链球菌、混合口腔菌群和厌氧菌。细菌学的变化可能是由于抗生素耐药模式的转变。不过，脓胸的发病率可能上升[109,292]，而病原微生物的致病力会影响自然病程，并最终影响对这类患者的治疗[241]。结核性脓胸明显比结核性胸腔积液少见，它与胸膜腔内高细菌接种量有关。在这种情况下，结核菌抗药性是一个难题，这是由于标准化学治疗药物对胸膜的渗透性差[174]。

临床表现和诊断

小儿脓胸的症状通常是在短期肺部感染史后出现呼吸窘迫、发烧和咳嗽。胸部或肩部疼痛伴随腹痛、腹胀和肠梗阻可加重呼吸困难。X 线表现为双侧肺部受累，可有肺膨出，偶尔为肺内型。半侧胸廓肺野模糊既可能为肺实变，也可能为胸水的表现。在早期渗出阶段，卧位影像可见胸水沿着胸壁侧面自由流动（图 64-13）。晚期脓胸，渗出物为实质性纤维蛋白团块，且不随体位改变而移动。在中期的脓性纤维蛋白阶段出现典型的小腔（见图 64-13C）。小腔内的气液平提示在胸膜中有厌氧菌驻留。胸腔穿刺术可以提供有价值的关于胸水性质的资料。经诊断性胸腔穿刺术得到的患者胸水具有以下任何一个特点者，应怀疑病变已发展到晚期脓胸：（1）肉眼可见的脓液；（2）pH <7.0；（3）乳酸脱氢酶 >1000 U/ml；（4）糖 <40 mg/dL；以及（5）革兰染色可见细菌。

治疗

脓胸主要的治疗方法是给予高剂量的静脉内抗生素。有效的胸腔引流也可加快脓胸的消散。卧位时见液体层者适合单独应用胸管引流。这种方式对分房积液者不能充分引流，而这些患者的最佳治疗措施仍在讨论中。早在 20 世纪 40 年代，就推荐采用纤维蛋白溶解疗法改善胸水的引流[364]。目前，对使用纤溶剂仍然有争议。Cameron 和 Davies[64]对四项已完成的、患者年龄超过 14 岁的随机研究进行了评价，得出的结论是：纤维蛋白溶解疗法与盐水对照组相比具有明显的益处（胸管引流留置时间缩短，引流量增加），且无并发症。然而，由于这项分析包含的病例数较少，所以不推荐该疗法作为常规治疗。一些回顾性的儿童病例研究也显示，使用尿激酶[207,211]和链激酶[161,280]可增加胸腔引流量，平均治疗失败率为 20%。重组组织型纤维蛋白酶原激活剂（阿替普酶）可以使引流更有效，但迄今未获得广泛评估[394]。至今只有 Thomson 及其同事进行了一项小儿随机试验，评估了尿激酶对 60 例脓胸患儿的疗效[363]。虽然，治疗组的住院时间大大缩短，但对照组患者住院前的疾病天数较长（9 天对 5 天）。有趣的是，这项研究也提示，应用小口径胸管引流的这些患者住院时间缩短。最后，有证据支持使用纤维蛋白溶解作为儿童复杂性胸腔积液或脓胸的辅助治疗。已报道的纤维蛋白溶解疗法的主要并发症包括：过敏反应 / 变态反应（对链激酶）、胸痛、出血和支气管胸膜瘘，在这些病例报告偶有发生。市场上已不再供应尿激酶，而阿替普酶的价格非常昂贵。

在复杂的胸腔积液及脓胸的治疗中，对内科治疗无效和尝试胸腔引流失败者推荐采取皮质剥除术。的确，Hoff 及其同事对开胸术患者进行脓胸评分显示，可缩短住院时间并减少住院并发症，尤其对重症患者[166]。此症治疗中，电视辅助胸腔镜手术（VATS）是一个很好的替代开胸术的方法，许多人主张将它作为儿科患者的主要干预手法[77,104,144,204,229,352]。鉴于非分房积液（1 期）患者在接受适当的抗生素治疗和胸管引流后可康复[67]，因此，VATS 可在晚期脓胸中发挥更大的作用。Chen 及其同事[71]指出，这些患者中的 70% 最终都需要手术治疗，延误手术会增加住院天数。在这一研究的患者中，经 VATS 治疗者尽管接受干预稍晚，但其住院天数最短。Gates 及其同事系统回顾了自 1987—2002 年的英语和西班牙语文献以确定小儿脓胸最有效的治疗策略。他们对 44 项研究的分析涉及 1369 例患者，在统计上显示只有经开胸术或 VATS 治疗的患儿的住院时间缩短。

成人的脓胸治疗指南由美国胸内科医生学会制

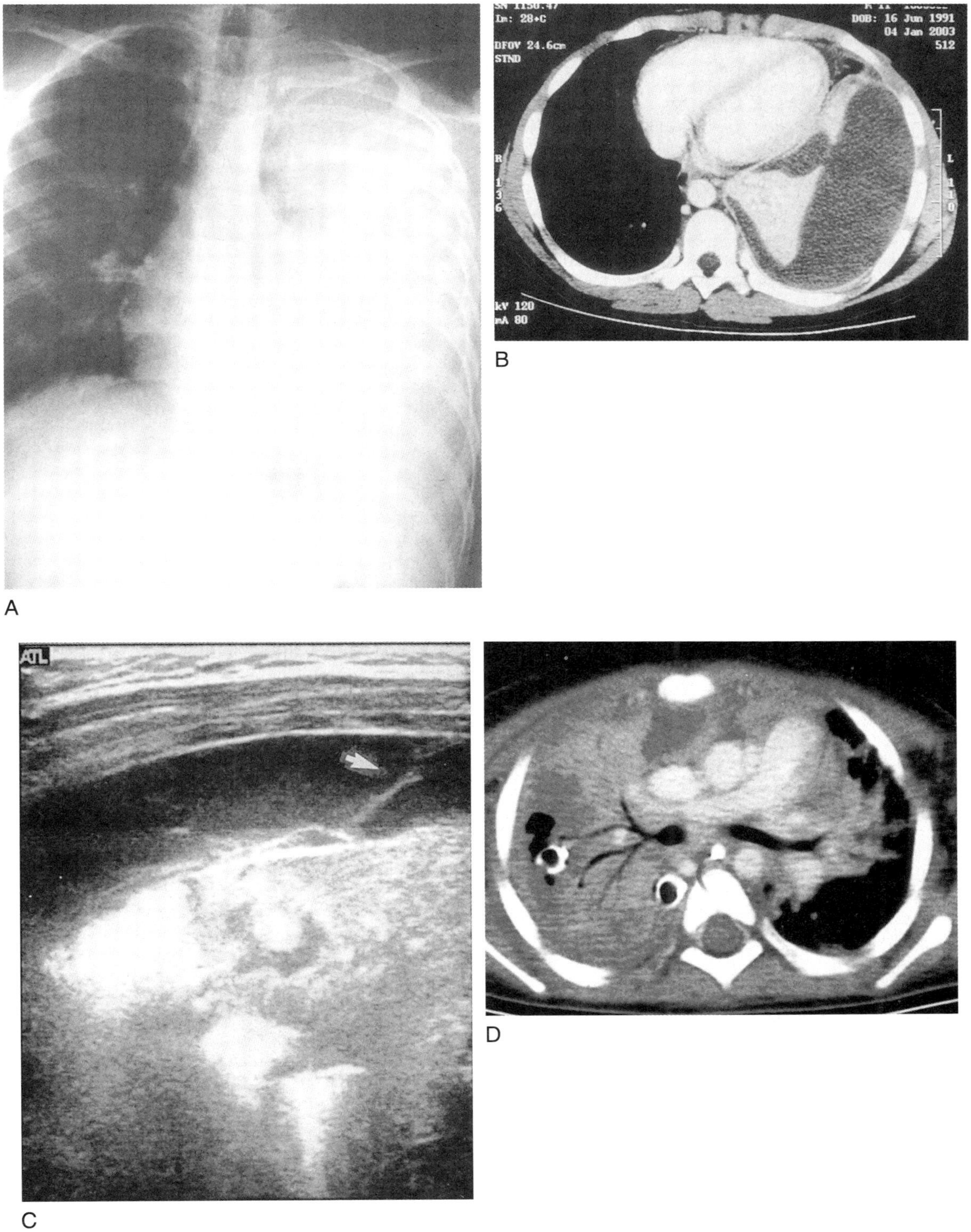

图 64-13　A 和 B. 一名表现为左侧胸膜痛和发热的 11 岁男孩。A. 胸片表现为左侧大量胸腔积液伴纵隔移位。B. 因考虑到可能有潜在的恶性肿瘤，所以进行一次 CT 扫描，显示一个大型非房性积液，伴下叶塌陷；叶间裂中可见液体。置入一根胸管，并引流出 400ml 血性液体，其乳酸脱氢酶为 4000U/L，因而认定为脓性纤维蛋白性脓胸。革兰染色未见细菌，但培养中有链球菌生长。应用静脉抗生素治疗后病情改善，并于 8 天后拔掉胸管。C 和 D. 是一名相对暴发起病的 3 岁女孩。C. 超声证实胸腔积液中的小腔（箭头）和碎屑。尽管早期经胸腔镜引流，她仍进展为肺坏死（见 D 中 CT 检查的静脉造影）伴持续气漏，留在重症监护病房中 10 天，住院 1 个月。

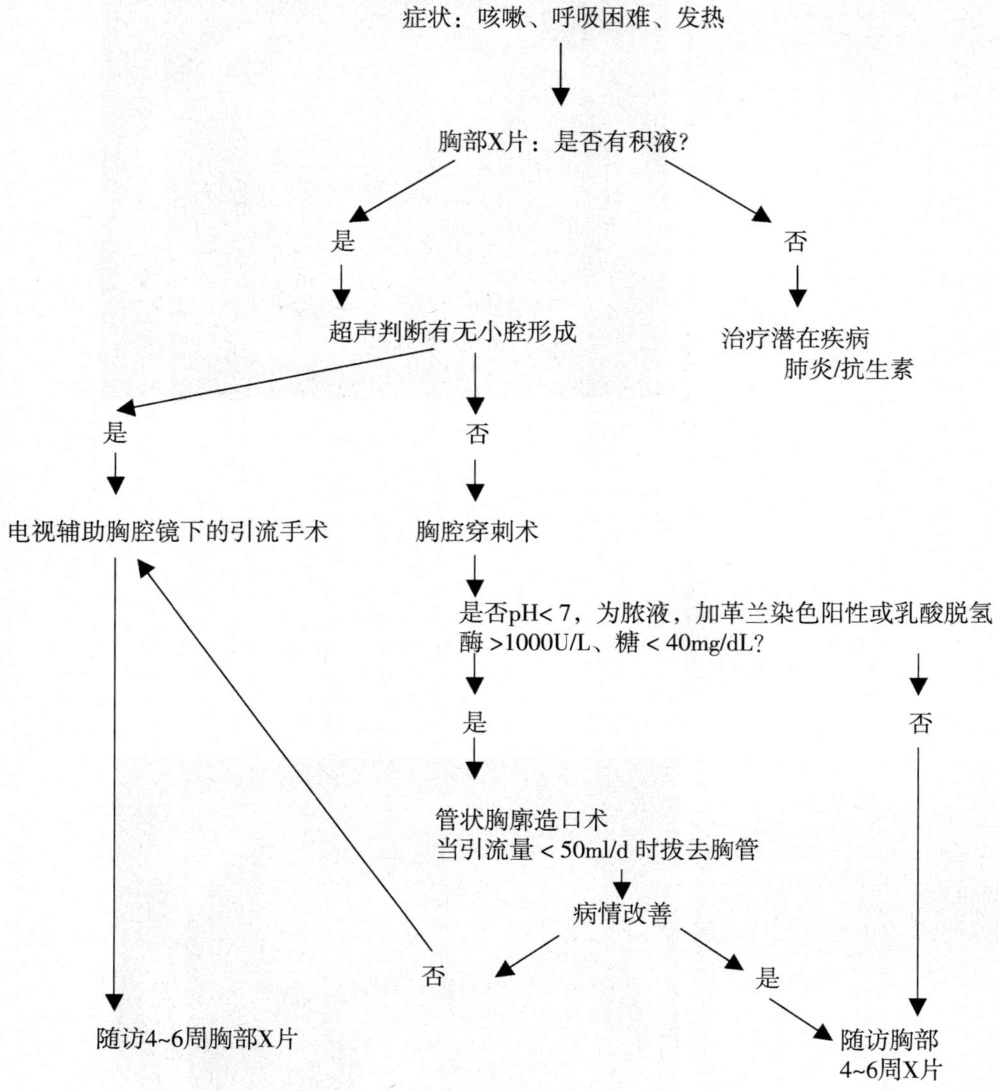

图 64-14 儿童脓胸治疗的关键途径。(From Finck C, Wagner C, Jackson R, Smith S: Empyema: Development of a critical pathway. Semin Pediatr Surg 2002;11:25-28, with permission.)

定[78]，不同的是，小儿脓胸治疗指南各不相同，往往是由各机构自行制定。有趣的是，从阿肯色州儿童医院的一项研究[122]中发展出适当治疗小儿脓胸的临床途径（图 64-14）。此草案提示，如果经胸片确定为脓胸者，则以超声评估是否存在小腔。如果发现小腔，主张尽早接受 VATS 治疗。与全国儿童数据库比较的结果表明，这一治疗途径大大缩短了患儿的住院时间并降低了住院费用。但是，其他作者认为，抗生素治疗和胸管引流仍然是最有效的脓胸治疗策略[248]。由于没有前瞻性研究，所以需要有一项多中心的前瞻
1020 性随机试验以解答进行中的有关小儿脓胸患者最佳治疗方法的问题。

小儿自发性气胸

原发的自发性气胸是指继发于肺尖气泡或肺大泡的气胸，而无其他的肺部的病理学证据[293,332,399]。它也可以发生在没有任何危险因素的足月新生儿。相反，再发的自发性气胸多有潜在的肺部疾病背景，如囊性纤维化或肺孢子虫性肺炎。其他的肺部感染、毛细支气管炎、哮喘（甚至轻度）、结缔组织疾病、先天性囊性腺瘤样畸形和创伤性肺挫伤也都是危险因素[89,214,332]。在美国，原发的自发性气胸的发病率估计在每 100 000 名男孩中有 7.4～18 例，而每 100 000 名女孩中有 1.2～6.0 例[149,315]。典型病例为身材单薄、

消瘦的青少年，表现为急性发作性患侧胸膜炎性胸痛和干咳。大多数患者在初步评估后临床情况稳定。但是，也有少数可能暴发危重症，包括继发于张力性气胸的低血压和呼吸衰竭。气胸患者的其他临床表现包括呼吸急促和心动过速。胸片可确诊，并可确定肺内继发的病理过程。呼气相摄片有助于识别小型气胸。气胸大小的定量方法各不相同，因为定量可影响之后的处理。的确，光线指数可作为气胸大小的定量方法，它可以比较患侧肺与同半侧胸廓的直径[227,275]。

急性气胸患者需要补充供氧并建立静脉通道。对于少数有张力性气胸的患者，应立即在第二肋间隙
1021 （锁骨中线）穿刺减压，甚至于在拍摄胸片确诊之前进行，然后迅速放置胸管。气胸量小于 15%者常可在供氧或不供氧的情况下继续观察，尤其是对初期症状超过 24 小时后发病的患者。也可用针刺抽吸和插入小型胸腔引流管的方法[293]，但 Delphi 共识声明（2001）不支持在此症中常规使用针刺减压[10]。将胸腔引流管与 Heimlich 阀门连通可以门诊治疗依从性好的小型气胸患者。对大型气胸患者需留置水下密封的胸管，并引流气体。气漏持续超过 5～7 天者可能需要进一步干预，或者至少应证实所置胸管的运作正常[245]。大多数幼儿（<8 岁）和患有哮喘病的儿童较易发病，应用胸管引流足以治疗。但是，有报道称，青少年自发性气胸患者的复发率高达 40%～60%[80,293,332]。有趣的是，在一项成人病例研究报告中，小型引流者的气胸复发率较高（33%），比单纯观察组（17%）或大口径胸管引流组（6%）都高[381]。最后应对症状直接进行进一步的检查和治疗。对发现气泡和肺大泡，CT 比平片敏感，但尚不清楚在自发性气胸中常规使用该检查最终是否会改变此症的治疗方法[255,332,338]。有些作者主张在出现标准症状后即行 CT 检查，而其他人认为可等待复发后再做进一步检查[197]。对自发性气胸的影像学检查的作用尚未建立明确共识。

手术治疗的适应证包括复发、持续气漏、双侧病变以及可能存在肺大泡。数个病例研究报道提示，VATS 在术后疼痛和并发症方面似乎优于标准开胸术[168,387]。经腋前线的小型开胸术可替代 VATS，它具有一定优势，特别是显影不良和存在致密粘连时[169,332,339]。对于胸膜剥脱术，经胸腔镜施行的胸膜磨损法和滑石粉撒粉法都是有效技术[65,367]。经腋前线切开可轻易地完成肺尖胸膜部分切除术。对双侧病变者，VATS 和经腋前线的小型开胸术都有效，而且可以作为一期手术[217,332]。尽管治疗结果相似，VATS 在治疗自发性气胸中越来越受到外科医生的欢迎，即使存在一些争论[98,111,197,387]。VATS 术后复发率为 2%～14%，虽然随着经验的增加，此值已有所下降[105,169,179,263]。有报道经腋前线的小型开胸术的复发率低至 2%[105,197]。总之，VATS 和经腋前线的小型开胸术都能有效治疗自发性气胸。此外，小儿自发性气胸的治疗指南常自成人病例标准中推定，因此应进行儿科患者的随机试验。

囊性纤维化患者的气胸很难治疗，因其气漏常持续存在。使用高负压（20～25 cmH_2O）可能有所帮助。如果此法失败，经胸腔镜施行的滑石粉撒粉法[367]或投入其他硬化剂[238]可完成胸膜剥离术并防止复发。胸膜部分切除术通常可避免进行肺切除术，后者术后需要接受肺移植。

建立胸腔内通路及其操作

新生儿气胸的胸管置入

准备插入胸管前，将婴儿置于氧气罩内，对已插入喉管者仍以呼吸机通气维持，同时制动，并监测脉氧饱和度和心电图。应备有手术者头上戴的小型照明灯或高于手术者头顶的装置提供类似性质的照明光源。其过程为无菌技术操作（口罩、帽子、手术衣和手套）。除了无菌器械（手术刀、蚊式止血钳、Adson 镊子、持针器、精细手术剪）和布帘，8 号和 10 号法式导管、无菌接头、穿上 3–0 和 4–0 不吸收缝线的弯曲缝线针头，以及婴儿型水下密封引流系统要一应俱全。胸壁用碘附溶液消毒，并铺上无菌巾。25 号注射针在乳头外侧的腋前线、第四肋骨上方用利多卡因进行皮肤浸润麻醉。应避免损伤乳头和乳腺组织。用 11 号手术刀片做一个 3～4mm 的切口。将蚊式止血钳放入切口用来分离皮下组织。在肋骨上方继续向上进行分离，并分离切口处的肋间肌肉，这需要有较强的压力，然后就可进入胸膜腔。这种方法产生一个“隧道”，使进入胸膜腔的入口在皮肤切口水平的上方。阻力减少预示进入胸膜腔，然后通常有空气逸出声。用弯式蚊式止血钳夹住 8 号法式胸管的尖端，将其伸入胸膜腔（图 64–15）。另一种方法是将套管针

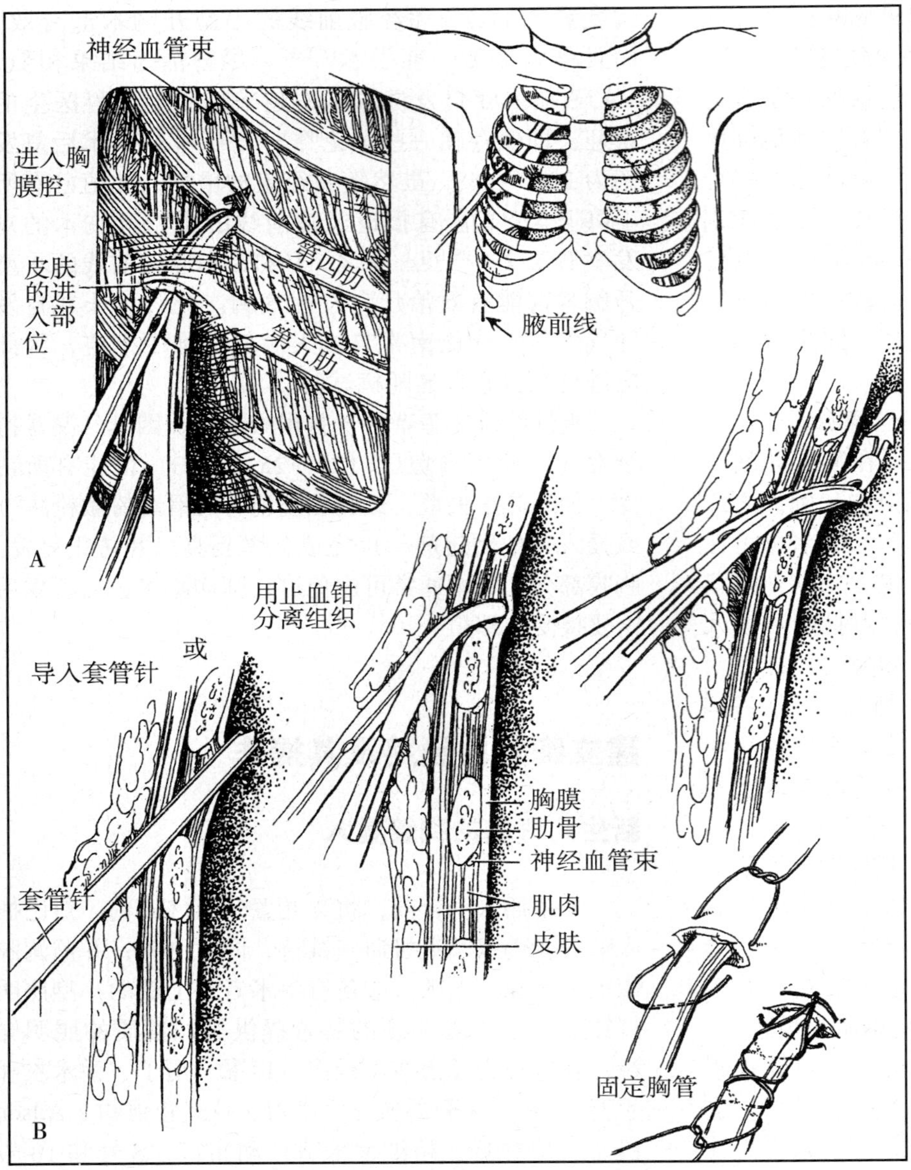

图 64-15 新生儿气胸置入胸管。A. 可取小的止血钳插入腋前线或腋中线的小切口，并向上形成隧道，在下一个肋骨上缘进入胸腔。插入胸管，并缝合结扎固定。缝线每绕一圈都应打几个结以防止滑脱。B. 套管针可替代胸管插入，只要套管针置入的长度为在导管内退出数毫米；这一技巧可以更容易地引导导管，比如，必须向后向下引流积液时。

放入胸管中，并引导后者进入隧道。使用这种技术时，较安全的做法是内置套管针的尖端应撤出数毫米，并在导管近端 5cm 处放置一个大夹子，这样可避免无节制地伸入胸管造成的穿透伤或损伤纵隔结构。将胸管向上向前伸入 3～4cm，确定导管上的孔洞都已在胸膜腔内，还要避免置管太深、抵达纵隔后纽结。然后可用 3～0 非吸收缝线将胸管固定并作荷包缝合。将碘附软膏涂于胸管-皮肤的交界处以确保其密闭。连接管道通到水下密封，并观察呼吸时水面是否随之波动。如有需要，该系统可设置为 10 cm
1022 H_2O 的负压，应记住高负压适用于正压呼吸机通气时，并可能造成气压伤。在新生儿重症监护病房中，一次性婴儿 Pleur-Evac 胸腔闭式引流系统高效且易于管理。

拍摄胸片可确定胸管的位置，以确保所有的孔洞都在胸膜腔内，并检查所置胸管是否可有效地使塌陷的肺组织扩张。拍摄胸部侧位片可确定胸管在前部还是后部。上端和前部的置管能最有效地排出气胸。过多气泡提示有持续漏气，来自受损肺组织、肺支气管瘘，或最常见的是系统漏气。

插入胸管最常见的并发症为：（1）插管时损伤肋间血管；（2）钳子和胸管造成肺穿孔。如果有大量出血和持续的明显漏气，就需进行手术矫治。也有报道，在操作中损伤纵隔淋巴管、静脉和神经结构。

现有手术器械包可应用 Seldinger 技术（经股动脉穿刺术）迅速且安全地完成婴儿小型胸管的置入。穿刺针插入胸膜腔，并引导导线进入。拿走穿刺针，将扩张器穿到导线上，然后置入猪尾导管。

胸管护理和拔除

气胸时插入的胸管通常在引流出气体后会有少量液体排出。对于不需要机械通气的婴儿，当水封闭腔内没有水泡出现且肺充分扩张持续 24～48 小时，如
1023 果使用了抽吸的就可停止抽吸，只留水下密封的胸管。观察 12～24 小时，如气胸没有再出现，可安全地拔管。胸管应迅速拔出，同时置管部位应用纱布敷料压迫以防止空气进入胸部。通常可再次拍摄胸片以确定气胸没有复发。对于需要机械通气的婴儿，比较安全的做法是延长胸管留置时间，尤其是需要高吸气峰压和（或）呼气末正压者。

年长儿的胸管置入

年长儿气胸患者通常是肺大泡自然破裂、哮喘、囊性纤维化、胸壁钝击伤或偶尔为胸壁穿透伤引起的。有症状的患者需要接受管状胸廓造口术。年龄稍大的婴儿和儿童的胸管插入也应用于各种原因造成的胸腔积液，包括乳糜胸，外伤性血胸，淋巴瘤，细菌、真菌、病毒性肺炎导致的炎症，脓胸，以及其他原因。

表 64-1　胸管型号的选择指导。

患者体重（kg）	型号（法式）		
	气胸	漏出	渗出
＜3	8～10	8～10	10～12
3～8	10～12	10～12	12～16
8～15	12～16	12～16	16～20
16～40	16～20	16～20	20～28
＞40	20～24	24～28	28～36

为这些患者插入胸管的无菌技术和准备工作模式与新生儿的相同。婴儿和幼儿可先期使用静脉注射芬太尼（1.0μg/kg）和咪哒唑仑（0.1mg/kg）作为镇静剂。或者，选择氯胺酮（1.0mg/kg）和（或）无咪哒唑仑，可用以提供良好的止痛和镇静作用，同时在整个操作中维护呼吸反射和心脏参数。儿童保持仰卧位，在患侧胸廓下垫一小布卷以抬高受累区域。同侧手臂上抬，置于体侧。胸管的大小取决于患儿的体重和病理问题是气胸、漏出还是渗出（表 64-1）。在无菌准备后，行局部麻醉。对于气胸患者，在第三或第四肋间隙的腋中线前方做小皮肤切口，向上向前置入适当大小的导管。如果患者有积液，导管置入的部位应根据相关体检（例如叩诊浊音和触觉语颤减弱），结合胸片、超声和（或）胸部 CT 检查的结果确定。插入 20 号注射针或血管导管至叩诊音过渡的水平（从鼓音到浊音）以勘定积液。胸管便可依先前的标记插入，并向下向后置管。胸管不应低于第七肋骨的水平，以免伤及脾脏、肝脏或膈肌。

肺活检

开胸肺活检通常应用在儿童弥漫性肺疾病的早期诊断评价，并且在确定诊断时，整体效果要优于经皮胸廓针吸活检。针吸肺活检相当可靠且准确；然而，大约 1/3 的患者会发生气胸或血胸。开胸肺活检时可获取大量标本进行培养和组织学研究，进行特殊染色和偶尔的电子显微镜检查。开胸楔形活检术可较轻易地避免气漏，并保证充分止血。常规放置胸管可防止发生气胸。术后死亡很少是由操作引起的；当发生患者死亡时，几乎都是其潜在疾病造成的。开胸肺活检后几乎所有患者都能获得一个组织诊断，并影响超过 90%的患者以后的治疗[206]。大约 60%的患者的术前诊断得到证实，而超过 35%的患者的术前诊断得到纠正。此外，鉴别诊断常包括传染性疾病、肿瘤或炎症性过程，如闭塞性细支气管炎伴机化性肺炎（BOOP）或淋巴样间质性肺炎。由于炎症性过程需要获取组织进行诊断，且需应用皮质激素治疗，因此肺活检确诊是必不可少（图 64-16；也见图 64-6）。

必须接受开胸肺活检的儿童可能是手术和麻醉的

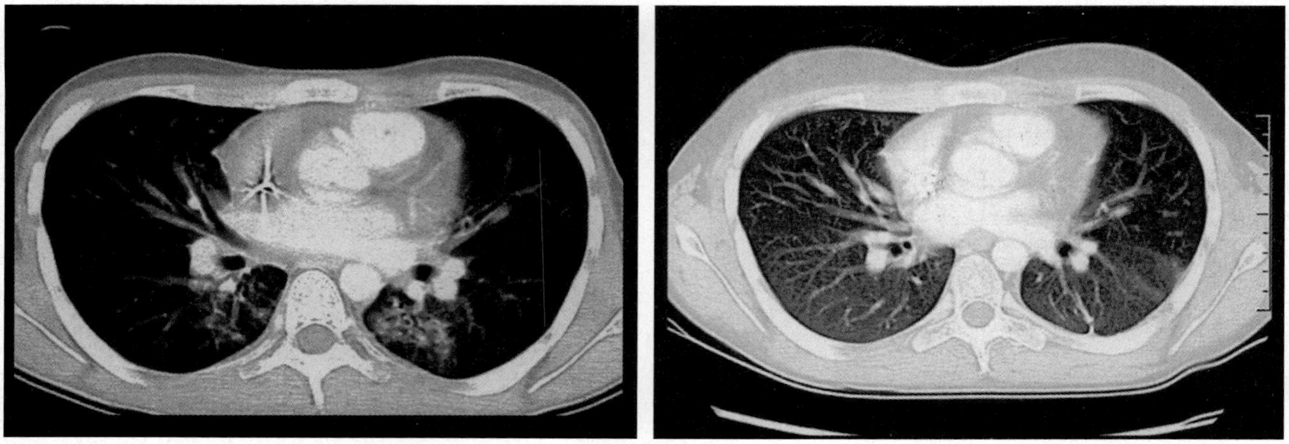

图 64-16 一名患Ⅳ期 Hodgkin病的 17 岁男孩，接受过放射治疗和自体骨髓移植。A. 常规 CT 检查显示双侧局部的气腔病变，大部分位于下肺叶的上段。肺活检提示梗阻性细支气管炎。他接受了皮质激素治疗，3 个月后复查 CT 扫描（B）显示病灶几乎彻底吸收。

中度危险人群。他们往往有免疫抑制并伴有弥漫性肺部浸润和急性呼吸衰竭。当有指征时应及早进行活检，不要等到患儿并发呼吸衰竭和依赖呼吸机通气时。不过，即使是持续的或不能诊断的呼吸衰竭患者，肺活检仍可导致其治疗发生重大变化，尽管此时的并发症——主要是气漏（45%）——的发生率较高。术前认真检查胸片对确定最佳活检部位很重要；有时应在两个不同区域取样，其中之一是严重浸润区域。而另一个是受累较轻的区域。与病理学家进行术前讨论是非常有价值的。活检时做一个小的前侧剖胸术切口，并选用吻合器既安全又快捷；在较小的儿童中，使用 Lahey 钳可从小切口中取出足够的活检标本，尤其是在肺实质僵硬且无法通过切口运出获得肺活检标本时（图 64-17）。另外，经腋前线的切口可获取希望得到的、足够的肺组织进行肺活检。无论什么患者群体，熟练术者操作的开胸肺活检术的死亡率
1024 或发病率是最低的。大到足以使用内镜 U 形钉固定装置的患者，可经胸腔镜进行肺活检，其风险和并发症与开胸操作相似（见第 62 章）。

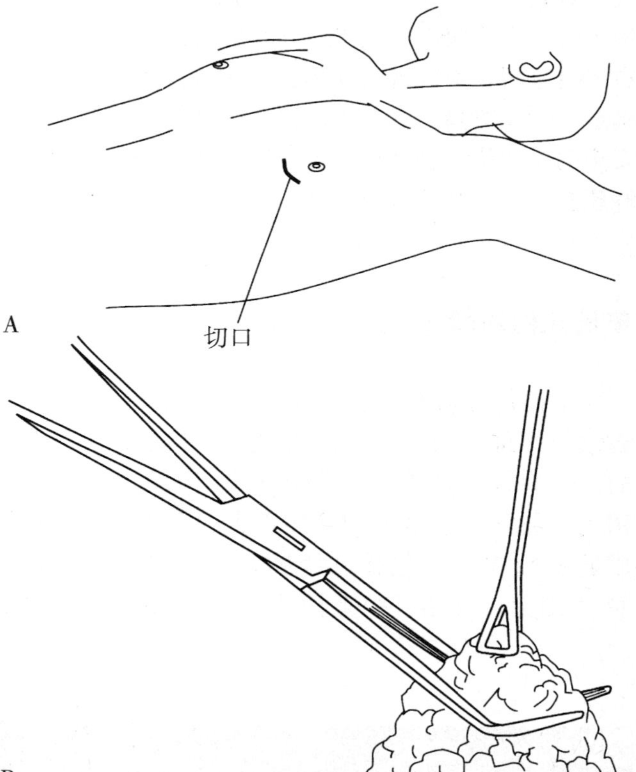

图 64-17 A. 应用前侧剖胸术进行开胸肺活检可将手术并发症的发生率降至最低。B. 轻松抓紧舌叶，并从弥漫性肺浸润患者的肺部获取足够的样本；在一些小婴儿（或当肺组织僵硬不能从胸壁取出时）中可用 Lahey 钳取代直线型吻合器提取活检样本。用手术刀整齐切下 Lahey 钳上部的肺组织后，在钳子底下做连续的 U 形缝合，然后拿掉钳子，再加固缝合，并复原肺组织做单纯的连续缝合。这样可很好地止血和防止气漏。

乳糜胸

此症的实质被描述为乳糜从破损的胸导管溢入纵隔，因而进入一侧或双侧胸膜腔。乳糜胸及其治疗的

历史观点包括胸导管解剖学和生理学知识的演化、营养科学的发展和胸外科的进展。值得注意的是，在 1937 年 Blalock 的实验报告显示，实验性上腔静脉阻塞可产生乳糜胸，而先期结扎胸导管可阻止其发生[45]。10 年后，Lampson 首先将这种治疗用于临床[215]。治疗着重考虑诱发因素，还包括饮食变更和使用奥曲肽降低胸导管流量，进行胸部穿刺术和（或）胸廓造口术引流以减轻呼吸窘迫和促进胸膜密封，以及当保守疗法失败时采用断裂胸导管结扎手术或胸腹分流术。

病因学

新生儿乳糜液进入胸腔产生积液可能为自发性，常由先天性胸导管畸形或生产时的创伤引起。但是，在多数情况下乳糜胸的发生与产程或产式无关，而且可能在产前就发现淋巴积液[118,233]。乳糜胸是造成新生儿胸腔积液的主要原因[92]。

1025 年长儿的乳糜胸很少为自发性，几乎总是在创伤或心胸外科术后出现；但有些胸部淋巴管瘤患者也可见于年长儿组中（图 64–18）[42,48,215,261]。手术损伤可能导致部分胸导管的解剖变异。外伤可导致脊椎伸展过度，在伸展时引起胸导管破裂，有报道如高空跳水、摔跤和其他这样的活动时发生[215,327]。已有报道，多次发作性咳嗽能引起胸导管破裂，胸导管在一顿丰富的脂肪膳食后特别容易受损[310]。有人指出肿瘤，尤其是淋巴瘤和神经母细胞瘤，有时也会造成胸导管阻塞[107,254]。淋巴管瘤病或弥漫性淋巴管扩张可产生乳糜性胸腔积液和腹水。其他原因包括纵隔炎症、锁骨下静脉或上腔静脉血栓、中央静脉导管错位和虐待儿童[42,62,92,148,251,373]。

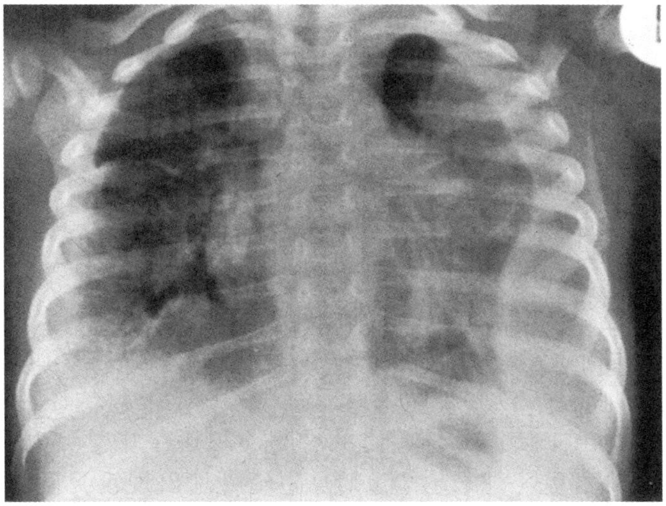

图 64–18　图示为一名 4 岁女孩的胸片，她患有双侧弥漫性淋巴管瘤和乳糜胸。注意液体的模糊表现和左肺大部分被压缩。

解剖学和病理生理学

胸导管源自于向外生长的颈淋巴囊和乳糜池。在胚胎期，存在双侧胸部淋巴隙，各自在颈部汇入相应的颈淋巴囊。在发育过程中，右侧胸导管的上三分之一和左侧胸导管的下三分之二退化关闭。最终总导管系统的解剖结构有较大变异，证明组成淋巴系统的小管之间有众多的交通支。胸导管起源于腹部的乳糜池，位于第二腰椎上方（图 64–19）。导管通过主动脉裂孔延伸到胸部，接着向上进入右侧后纵隔，然后在第五胸椎水平转向左侧。随后，向上伴行于主动脉弓后面进入后颈部，与锁骨下静脉和颈内静脉连接。

整个导管系统有很多变异，仅有大约 50%的个体有典型的胸导管路径[90,310]。最常见的变异是起自乳糜池的双套系统或横膈水平的多导管结构。在胸部丰富的侧支系统来源于肋间隙、后纵隔和内脏淋巴管，这些侧支经集合干与总导管自由连通。

胸导管壁包含的平滑肌收缩能产生足够的力量，以 50～200ml/h 的速度推动淋巴液向上朝着颈静脉连接处流动[15]。胸导管内淋巴液的流动速率差异颇大，与脂肪摄取量、纵隔的瘢痕组织、门脉高压的存在和其他因素有关。向上汇入锁骨下静脉的乳糜液流量可因胸导管内瓣膜、门脉压力以及胸腔内负压与腹内正 1026
压之间压力梯度的存在而增加[45,139]。反之，研究表明，在使用呼气末正压时，升高的胸内压可因胸导管内乳糜液流量减半而降低。

胸导管内的乳糜液运载来自肠道摄入的大约四分之三的脂肪向体循环流转。乳糜液的脂肪含量为 0.4～4.0g/dL[45,310]。自肠道乳糜管吸收的大型脂肪分子流经乳糜池，并向上流经胸导管[127]。胸导管淋巴液的总蛋白质含量也很高。在肠外营养之前，营养并发症是乳糜胸致死的主要来源。除营养素之外，胸导管还运送 2000～20 000 个 / 毫升白细胞（主要是淋巴细胞[T 细胞]）。嗜酸性粒细胞的比例也较循

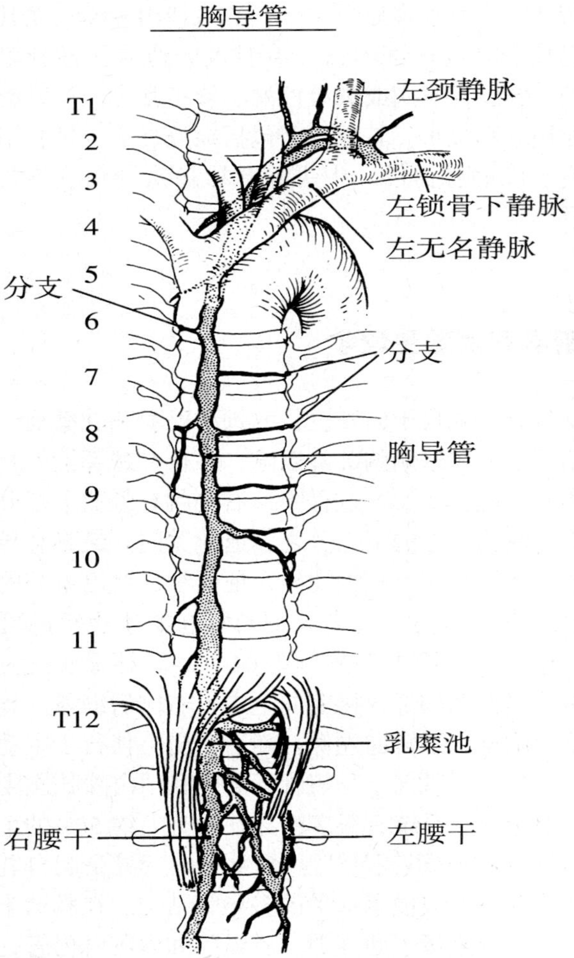

图 64-19 最常见的胸导管解剖排列图解说明。(From DeMeester R, Lafontaine E: The pleura. In Sabiston DC, Spencer FC [eds]: Gibbon' s Surgery of the Chest, 4th ed. Philadelphia, WB Saunders, 1983, reprinted with permission.)

环血液中的高。经胸导管瘘丢失的淋巴细胞可能导致免疫功能降低[139]；事实上，在早期器官移植时代胸导管外分流术就被用作免疫抑制的辅助方法。乳糜似乎具有抑菌特性，这解释了为什么乳糜胸很少并发感染。

临床表现

以往认为产伤是造成许多新生儿乳糜胸的原因，但日益增多的产前超声检查改变了这一观点。幼儿非医源性乳糜胸常与先天性乳糜管、乳糜池或胸导管本身的畸形有关。这种乳糜胸大多数是由扩张的和薄壁的肋间、横膈或从属的纵隔淋巴系统漏出液体到胸膜内引起的。当出现淋巴液超载时，这些交汇的淋巴系统可明显扩张，最终形成漏出性淋巴管曲张。在其他情况下，如在某些心脏畸形时（例如，完全性肺静脉异位引流），胸膜下淋巴系统破裂使液体流入胸膜腔。

从胸导管漏出的乳糜液可迅速在胸膜腔内积聚，并产生压力压迫胸部其他结构，引起急性呼吸窘迫、呼吸困难和发绀伴呼吸急促。在胎儿期，胸腔积液可能继发于全身水肿，但原发性淋巴积液（特发性，继发于胸膜细淋巴管扩张、肺隔离症或与综合征有关联，如 Down、Turner 和 Noonan 综合征）可引起纵隔移位并导致水肿或肺发育不良。出生后，乳糜胸和长期丢失乳糜液对新生儿的影响包括营养不良、低蛋白血症、水电解质失衡、代谢性酸中毒和免疫缺陷。

在新生儿中，如观察到呼吸窘迫症状合并胸腔积液者强烈提示为乳糜胸。与胸腔积液有关的其他特征性表现有呼吸迟缓、叩诊为浊音、呼吸声减弱和纵隔移位。发烧并不常见。典型胸片显示患侧胸部大量积液，伴肺部受压和纵隔移位。双侧积液亦可发生。禁食患者抽出的胸水为清亮的稻草色液体，而进食后则为乳状胸水。乳糜液的分析一般提示总脂肪含量超过 400mg/dL （或三酰甘油浓度高于 110mg/dL），且蛋白质含量超过 5g/dL。在胎儿或禁食新生儿中，最有用且简单的测试是进行胸水的全血细胞计数和分类；当淋巴细胞超过白细胞的 80% 或 90%，可证实为淋巴积液；这一细胞分类可与所得的血细胞计数相比，血中淋巴细胞比例很少超过血白细胞的 70%以上。

外伤性乳糜胸多数发生在胸部手术后，尤其是动脉导管未闭修复术、主动脉缩窄纠治术和 Blalock-Taussig 分流术[217]。在矫正降主动脉病变的二次开胸术或紧贴主动脉弓后方的食管手术中，左侧胸腔内的胸导管损伤尤为常见。如果手术记录有淋巴引流时，胸导管的近端和远端都应结扎[217]。外伤或手术与症状性乳糜胸的发病可相隔几天或几周的时间。

由于从胸导管漏出的乳糜液积聚在胸膜腔内，当肺部受压越来越严重时就进行性地出现较明显的呼吸道症状，可表现为呼吸困难、呼吸急促，并最终发生动脉去饱和伴发绀。营养缺乏是乳糜液枯竭的一种晚期表现，发生在饮食摄入不足代替胸导管液体丢失时。

治疗

80%～90%由肠道吸收的脂肪经胸导管以乳糜微粒的形式转运，而少量短链脂肪酸经门静脉系统吸收。因此，限制饮食中的中链或短链三酰甘油理论上可相应减少胸导管的淋巴流量，从而加强胸导管瘘的自愈[168,210]。但事实证明，任何摄入体内的食物，甚至是清水也会明显增加胸导管流量[221]。因此，大量乳糜液丢失的患者应禁止经口喂养，并首选接受全肠外营养[24]。对已经依靠机械通气的患者，施加额外的呼气末正压可进一步减少淋巴液流量。最近有些报告认为，生长抑素或其类似物奥曲肽有治疗作用[73,83,221]。这些药物减少胃、胰腺和肠分泌，已成为治疗胰瘘和肠瘘的重要工具。由于其半衰期短，生长抑素需要连续静脉滴注，而合成的类似物奥曲肽每 8 小时经皮下
1027 注射给药一次，起始剂量为每天 10～20μg/kg[73]。1～4μg/（kg·h）连续输注奥曲肽可能更有效。它已被作为手术失败后的抢救用药[83]，甚至成为未经饮食纠正的一线治疗[224]。如果非手术治疗有效，应重新开始经口摄入，先从中链三酰甘油开始，2 周后可依据年龄正常饮食。乳糜液培养结果很少阳性；没必要在胸管引流全程长期使用抗生素。

胸腔穿刺术可用于此症的诊断，而且偶尔可结合饮食措施以减轻婴儿的自发性乳糜胸；不过，大多数病例仍需胸管引流。另外，导管引流可对每天漏出的乳糜液定量，并促进肺部复张，加强愈合。新生儿乳糜胸通常能自然停止[233,329,376]。由于确定液体漏出的部位很难，手术往往被拖延数周。同样，多数情况下的胸导管创伤性损伤可通过胸管引流以及蛋白质和脂肪丢失的替代疗法而成功治愈[271]。若引流量持续超出婴儿或儿童的耐受量且没有逐渐减少的证据，或者持续 2～3 周而无减少者，就需要结扎积液侧胸腔的胸导管。标准对照的淋巴管造影术已不再进行，但使用锝-99m 胶体或其他标志物的同位素淋巴管造影术有助于查明管瘘部位[194]。

乳糜液有时可进入心包，并引起乳糜性心包炎，在这种情况下应立即进行心包穿刺放液术以缓解病情。尽管新生儿双侧自发性乳糜胸并不常见，但对此症如不迅速识别并行引流，会引起致命的呼吸窘迫。

长时间胸管引流及全肠外营养下乳糜胸仍然存在时，可能需要在患侧进行开胸术或胸腔镜检查[48,329]。决定是继续保守治疗还是进行手术干预应根据潜在疾病的性质、漏出的持续时间、每日的引流量以及营养和（或）免疫耗竭的严重程度决定。一些作者曾建议，对胸管引流量超过每天每岁 100ml 或每天 10ml/kg，且 10～20 天后无缓解的患者应考虑手术治疗。虽然，这不是绝对指征，但我们应该记住淋巴细胞丢失可导致严重的细菌或真菌感染，这是当前因乳糜胸死亡的主要原因[23,221,222]。术前 30 分钟吃下 60ml 奶油有助于确认胸导管和瘘管部位。当术中确认后，应缝合结扎漏出部位以上及以下的引流淋巴管，并用一部分胸膜或肋间肌肌瓣加固。精细解剖胸导管并分离出瘘管常常不可行。在无法肯定漏出部位或多个漏出点源于纵隔时，在主动脉裂孔水平结扎所有的主动脉周围组织可得到最好的治疗效果。纤维蛋白胶和氩气束凝结物也被作为漏出区域不清或淋巴管瘤不全切除的辅助药剂[270]。

胸腔镜检查可用于较大的患者以避免进行开胸术[140]。术中看见漏出部位，即可以结扎、钳夹或用纤维蛋白胶密封。如果无法鉴定漏出部位，透过胸腔镜在直视下用滑石粉或其他硬化剂完成胸膜剥脱术，但这种技术应避免在婴儿中进行，因为它会影响肺和胸壁的发育。如果合并乳糜性心包积液，可做一个心包窗。由于胸腔镜的微创性，有些外科医生提倡可于 5～10 天时作为早期干预手法。这一方法可用于保守治疗失败率较高的情况，如上腔静脉血栓形成或右侧心腔压力升高的相关问题。

胸腹分流术已用于难治性乳糜胸，即漏出部位尚未查明以及对初步的非手术治疗无反应的患者，尤其是有较高的手术风险时[264]。这种方法已在先天性胸导管畸形或淋巴管瘤患者或在心脏手术后需持续引流的患者中获得成功[307]。一种名为 Denver 双阀分流系统是最常用的；在局部麻醉下完全植入，让患者或家长上下按压阀门使胸水减压流入腹腔并在此处重吸收。在小婴儿的皮肤表面有外置泵室[402]。它可提供侵袭性最小的治疗，用于新生儿或婴儿在复杂心脏畸形手术后的难治性乳糜胸，只要右侧心腔压力低于 25cm H_2O。

总体而言，大多数乳糜胸患者可经保守措施、营养支持和偶尔的手术介入治愈。而治疗弥漫性淋巴管畸形患者仍是一项挑战。

纵隔感染

急性纵隔炎

急性纵隔炎是由于纵隔腔被污染和（或）弄脏的结果，继发于气管或食管创伤或穿孔。少数情况下，纵隔炎由下行的咽后或颈部脓肿[195]或化脓的纵隔淋巴结破裂发展而来。纵隔感染可迅速播散，这是因为此空间内没有阻挡感染扩散的解剖屏障。临床上，急性纵隔炎表现为高烧、胸痛、呼吸困难、发绀和明显的心动过速，以及白细胞明显增高。新生儿的体征和症状可能较不明显，包括嗜睡、发烧、呼吸暂停、体温
1028 不稳定和白细胞减少。纵隔炎的治疗包括血流动力学支持治疗、立即给予静脉内抗生素和纵隔引流。引流对纵隔脓肿或来自食管穿孔的持续漏出 / 污染特别重要。颈部、经胸腔、胸膜腔后或前路手术都可用以促成引流，视脓肿或漏出的位置而定。

正中胸骨切开术后的感染

虽然正中胸骨切开术后胸骨伤口和纵隔感染的发生率很低，但这些感染对术后患者可产生破坏性影响。成人系列资料中，胸骨伤口感染的发生率多达20%[234]，而纵隔炎的发生率为1%～2%[308]。Tortoriello及其同事综述了自己15年来在德州儿童医院经历的小儿心脏手术后的纵隔炎病例[366]。总计7616例的系列资料中仅15例儿科患者发生纵隔炎（0.2%）。这一系列中，只有1例在原位心脏移植术后死于继发的暴发性真菌纵隔炎。最常见的病原感染是金黄色葡萄球菌，这也得到其他综述的支持[237]。其他病原体包括绿脓杆菌和假丝酵母。胸骨深部感染也可由革兰阴性的肠道菌群和厌氧菌所致。

纵隔感染需要及早发现、积极治疗。临床上，患者表现为局部红斑、局部波动感、脓性引流液、胸骨不稳定、发烧和白细胞增多。这些特点可能在术后一周才出现。的确，在德州儿童医院的系列资料中诊断胸骨伤口感染的中数时间是术后14天[366]。CT和镓扫描可用于确认胸骨深部感染和胸骨骨髓炎。关于胸骨切开术后纵隔炎的最佳治疗方式仍然存在争议。包括清创术和抗生素冲洗在内的规范治疗策略已演变为大量使用网膜和旋转肌瓣[34,117,142]。这些新技术的成效一般都很好，对于胸骨伤口并发症建议采取积极的治疗方法。

肉芽肿性和硬化性纵隔炎

这个侵袭性的压迫过程是由纵隔和肺门淋巴结增大引起的，后者继发于肺结核或真菌病如组织胞浆菌病[106]。在一个180例患者的综述报告中，Schowengerdt指出这些淋巴结的进行性增大或化脓将导致压迫、侵犯和纵隔结构纤维化[325]。上腔静脉综合征以及肺血管和支气管阻塞也是由这个过程所致。CT和MRI常可用以充分划定病变范围[276]，但往往需要活检确诊。这个疾病的进程一般比较平缓，并可用药物治疗。潜在的结核性或真菌性感染得到控制后，纵隔结构受压的有关症状常可缓解。

（李 菁译 黄 萍校）

参考文献

1. 1995 Revised guidelines for prophylaxis against *Pneumocystis carinii* pneumonia for children infected with or perinatally exposed to human immunodeficiency virus. MMWR Recomm Rep 1995;44:1.
2. Diagnosis and treatment of disease caused by nontuberculous mycobacteria. Am J Respir Crit Care Med 1997;156 (Suppl):S1.
3. Antiretroviral therapy and medical management of pediatric HIV infection. Pediatrics 1998;102:1005.
4. Guidelines for surveillance of drug resistance in tuberculosis. Int J Tuberc Lung Dis 1998;2:72.
5. 1999 USPHS/IDSA guidelines for the prevention of opportunistic infections in persons infected with human immunodeficiency virus. MMWR Recomm Rep 1999;48:1.
6. Diagnostic standards and classification of tuberculosis in adults and children. Am J Respir Crit Care Med 2000; 161:1376.
7. Policy statement: Recommendations for the prevention of pneumococcal infections, including the use of pneumococcal conjugate vaccine (Prevnar), pneumococcal polysaccharide vaccine, and antibiotic prophylaxis. Pediatrics 2000;106:362.
8. Survival after introduction of HAART in people with known duration of HIV-1 infection. Lancet 2000;355:1158.
9. Updated guidelines for the use of rifabutin or rifampin for the treatment and prevention of tuberculosis among HIV-infected patients taking protease inhibitors or nonnucleoside reverse transcriptase inhibitors. Centers for Disease Control and Prevention. MMWR 2000;49:185.
10. American College of Chest Physicians Delphi consensus statement on management of spontaneous pneumothorax.

Chest 2001;119:148.
11. Abadco DL, Steiner P: Gastric lavage is better than bronchoalveolar lavage for isolation of *Mycobacterium tuberculosis* in childhood pulmonary tuberculosis. Pediatr Infect Dis J 1992;11:735.
12. Abman SH, Ogle JW, Butler-Simon N, et al: Role of respiratory syncytial virus in early hospitalizations for respiratory distress of young infants with cystic fibrosis. J Pediatr 1988; 113:826.
13. Abrams EJ: Opportunistic infections and other clinical manifestations of HIV disease in children. Pediatr Clin North Am 2000;47:79.
14. Abuzaitoun OR, Hanson IC: Organ-specific manifestations of HIV disease in children. Pediatr Clin North Am 2000;47:109.
15. Acevedo D: Motor control of the thoracic duct. Am J Physiol 1943;139:600.
16. Adam KA: Persistent or recurrent pneumonia in Saudi children seen at King Khalid University Hospital, Riyadh: Clinical profile and some predisposing factors. Ann Trop Paediatr 1991;11:129.
17. Aeba R, Katogi T, Moro K, et al: Omental flap for mediastinitis after median sternotomy in asplenia syndrome and gut malrotation. Thorac Cardiovasc Surg 2000;48:243.
18. Agrawal RL, Jain SK, Gupta SC, et al: Hydropneumothorax secondary to hydatid lung disease. Indian J Chest Dis Allied Sci 1993;35:93.
19. Ahluwalia GS, Hammond GW: Comparison of cell culture and three enzyme-linked immunosorbent assays for the rapid diagnosis of respiratory syncytial virus from nasopharyngeal aspirate and tracheal secretion specimens. Diagn Microbiol Infect Dis 1988;9:187.
20. Aisner J, Schimpff SC, Bennett JE, et al: *Aspergillus* infections in cancer patients: Association with fireproofing materials in a new hospital. JAMA 1976;235:411.
21. Akhan O, Ozmen MN, Dincer A, et al: Percutaneous treatment of pulmonary hydatid cysts. Cardiovasc Intervent Radiol 1994;17:271.
22. Albright JT, Pransky SM: Nontuberculous mycobacterial infections of the head and neck. Pediatr Clin North Am 2003;50:503.
23. Allen EM, van Heeckeren DW, Spector ML, et al: Management of nutritional and infectious complications of postoperative chylothorax in children. J Pediatr Surg 1991;26:1169.
24. Alvarez JRF, Kalache KD, Grauel EL: Management of spontaneous congenital chylothorax: Oral medium-chain triglycerides versus total parenteral nutrition. Am J Perinatal 1999;16:415.
25. Andrews J, Nadjm B, Gant V, et al: Community-acquired pneumonia. Curr Opin Pulm Med 2003;9:175.
26. Armstrong DS, Grimwood K, Carlin JB, et al: Lower airway inflammation in infants and young children with cystic fibrosis. Am J Respir Crit Care Med 1997;156:1197.
27. Asher MI, Leversha AM: Lung abscess. In Chernick V, Boat TF (eds): Kendig's Disorders of the Respiratory Tract in Children, 6th ed. Philadelphia, WB Saunders, 1998.
28. Asher MI, Spier S, Beland M, et al: Primary lung abscess in childhood: The long-term outcome of conservative management. Am J Dis Child 1982;136:491.
29. Ashford NS, Buxton-Thomas MS, Flower CD, et al: Aerosol lung scintigraphy in the detection of bronchiectasis. Clin Radiol 1988;39:29.
30. Ashour M, Al Kattan K, Rafay MA, et al: Current surgical therapy for bronchiectasis. World J Surg 1999;23:1096.
31. Aujard Y, Fauroux B: Risk factors for severe respiratory syncytial virus infection in infants. Respir Med 2002; 96(Suppl B):S9.
32. Aurora P, Whitehead B, Wade A, et al: Lung transplantation and life extension in children with cystic fibrosis. Lancet 1999;354:1591.
33. Ayed AK: Resection of the right middle lobe and lingula in children for middle lobe/lingula syndrome. Chest 2004; 125:38.
34. Backer CL, Pensler JM, Tobin GR, et al: Vascularized muscle flaps for life-threatening mediastinal wounds in children. Ann Thorac Surg 1994;57:797.
35. Balci AE, Eren N, Eren S, et al: Ruptured hydatid cysts of the lung in children: Clinical review and results of surgery. Ann Thorac Surg 2002;74:889.
36. Balkanli K, Genc O, Dakak M, et al: Surgical management of bronchiectasis: Analysis and short-term results in 238 patients. Eur J Cardiothorac Surg 2003;24:699.
37. Ball P: Therapy for pneumococcal infection at the millennium: Doubts and certainties. Am J Med 1999;107(Suppl):77S.
38. Ball WS Jr, Bisset GS III, Towbin RB: Percutaneous drainage of chest abscesses in children. Radiology 1989; 171:431.
39. Barben J, Robertson D, Olinsky A, et al: Bronchial artery embolization for hemoptysis in young patients with cystic fibrosis. Radiology 2002;224:124.
40. Bass JB Jr, Farer LS, Hopewell PC, et al: Treatment of tuberculosis and tuberculosis infection in adults and children. American Thoracic Society and the Centers for Disease Control and Prevention. Am J Respir Crit Care Med 1994;149:1359.
41. Bateman ED, Hayashi S, Kuwano K, et al: Latent adenoviral infection in follicular bronchiectasis. Am J Respir Crit Care Med 1995;151:170.
42. Beghetti M, La Scala G, Belli D, et al: Etiology and management of pediatric chylothorax. J Pediatr 2000;136:653.
43. Berdon WE, Willi U: Situs inversus, bronchiectasis, and sinusitis and its relation to immotile cilia: History of the diseases and their discoverers—Manes Kartagener and Bjorn Afzelius. Pediatr Radiol 2004;34:38.
44. Bergen GA, Shelhamer JH: Pulmonary infiltrates in the cancer patient: New approaches to an old problem. Infect Dis Clin North Am 1996;10:297.
45. Blalock A, Robinson CS, Cunningham RS: Experimental studies in lymphatic blockage. Arch Surg 1937;34:1049.
46. Boat TF: Pulmonary hemorrhage and hemoptysis. In Chernick V, Boat TF (eds): Kendig's Disorders of the Respiratory Tract in Children, 6th ed. Philadelphia, WB Saunders, 1998.
47. Boles ET, Izant RJ: Spontaneous chylothorax in the neonatal period. Am J Surg 1960;99:870.
48. Bond S, et al: Management of pediatric postoperative chylothorax. Ann Thorac Surg 1993;56:469.
49. Bordley WC, Viswanathan M, King VJ, et al: Diagnosis and testing in bronchiolitis: A systematic review. Arch Pediatr Adolesc Med 2004;158:119.
50. Borowitz D, Baker RD, Stallings V: Consensus report on nutrition for pediatric patients with cystic fibrosis. J Pediatr Gastroenterol Nutr 2002;35:246.
51. Boucher RC: Human airway ion transport: II. Am J Respir Crit Care Med 1994;150:581.
52. Bouros D, Schiza S, Patsourakis G, et al: Intrapleural streptokinase versus urokinase in the treatment of complicated parapneumonic effusions: A prospective, double-blind study. Am J Respir Crit Care Med 1997;155:291.
53. Bouros D, Schiza S, Tzanakis N, et al: Intrapleural uroki-

nase versus normal saline in the treatment of complicated parapneumonic effusions and empyema: A randomized, double-blind study. Am J Respir Crit Care Med 1999; 159:37.
54. Breuer R, Lossos IS, Berkman N, et al: Pulmonary complications of bone marrow transplantation. Respir Med 1993; 87:571.
55. Brook I, Finegold SM: Bacteriology of aspiration pneumonia in children. Pediatrics 1980;65:1115.
56. Brown RA, Lemen RJ: Bronchiectasis. In Chernick V, Boat TF (eds): Kendig's Disorders of the Respiratory Tract in Children, 6th ed. Philadelphia, WB Saunders, 1998.
57. Brown-Elliott BA, Griffith DE, Wallace RJ Jr: Diagnosis of nontuberculous mycobacterial infections. Clin Lab Med 2002;22:911.
58. Buckingham SC, King MD, Miller ML: Incidence and etiologies of complicated parapneumonic effusions in children, 1996 to 2001. Pediatr Infect Dis J 2003;22:499.
59. Burns JL, Emerson J, Stapp JR, et al: Microbiology of sputum from patients at cystic fibrosis centers in the United States. Clin Infect Dis 1998;27:158.
60. Butler JC, Shapiro ED, Carlone GM: Pneumococcal vaccines: History, current status, and future directions. Am J Med 1999;107(Suppl):69S.
61. Butler WR, Guthertz LS: Mycolic acid analysis by high-performance liquid chromatography for identification of *Mycobacterium* species. Clin Microbiol Rev 2001;14:704.
62. Buttiker V, Fanconi S, Burger R: Chylothorax in children: Guidelines for diagnosis and management. Chest 1999; 116:682.
63. Caksen H, Ozturk MK, Uzum K, et al: Pulmonary complications in patients with staphylococcal sepsis. Pediatr Int 2000;42:268.
64. Cameron R, Davies HR: Intra-pleural fibrinolytic therapy versus conservative management in the treatment of parapneumonic effusions and empyema. Cochrane Database Syst Rev 2004;CD002312.
65. Cardillo G, Facciolo F, Giunti R, et al: Videothoracoscopic treatment of primary spontaneous pneumothorax. Ann Thorac Surg 2000;69:357.
66. Chan SP, Birnbaum J, Rao M, et al: Clinical manifestation and outcome of tuberculosis in children with acquired immunodeficiency syndrome. Pediatr Infect Dis J 1996;15:443.
67. Chan W, Keyser-Gauvin E, Davis GM, et al: Empyema thoracis in children: A 26-year review of the Montreal Children's Hospital experience. J Pediatr Surg 1997;32:870.
68. Chang AB, Boyce NC, Masters IB, et al: Bronchoscopic findings in children with non-cystic fibrosis chronic suppurative lung disease. Thorax 2002;57:935.
69. Chang CT, Wang LY, Liao CY, et al: Identification of nontuberculous mycobacteria existing in tap water by PCR-restriction fragment length polymorphism. Appl Environ Microbiol 2002;68:3159.
70. Chanock SJ, Pizzo PA: Infectious complications of patients undergoing therapy for acute leukemia: Current status and future prospects. Semin Oncol 1997;24:132.
71. Chen CF, Soong WJ, Lee YS, et al: Thoracic empyema in children: Early surgical intervention hastens recovery. Acta Paediatr Taiwan 2003;44:93.
72. Chesney PJ: Nontuberculous mycobacteria. Pediatr Rev 2002;23:300.
73. Cheung Y, Leung MP, Yip M: Octreotide for treatment of postoperative chylothorax. J Pediatr 2001;139:157.
74. Choi YH, Leung AN: Radiologic findings: Pulmonary infections after bone marrow transplantation. J Thorac Imaging 1999;14:201.
75. Classen JB, Classen DC: Clustering of cases of insulin dependent diabetes (IDDM) occurring three years after *Haemophilus influenzae* B (HiB) immunization support causal relationship between immunization and IDDM. Autoimmunity 2002; 35:247.
76. Cochran JB, Tecklenburg FW, Turner RB: Intrapleural instillation of fibrinolytic agents for treatment of pleural empyema. Pediatr Crit Care Med 2003;4:39.
77. Cohen G, Hjortdal V, Ricci M, et al: Primary thoracoscopic treatment of empyema in children. J Thorac Cardiovasc Surg 2003;125:79.
78. Colice GL, Curtis A, Deslauriers J, et al: Medical and surgical treatment of parapneumonic effusions: An evidence-based guideline. Chest 2000;118:1158.
79. Collin BA, Ramphal R: Pneumonia in the compromised host including cancer patients and transplant patients. Infect Dis Clin North Am 1998;12:781.
80. Cook CH, Melvin WS, Groner JI, et al: A cost-effective thoracoscopic treatment strategy for pediatric spontaneous pneumothorax. Surg Endosc 1999;13:1208.
81. Correa AG, Starke JR: Bacterial pneumonias. In Chernick V, Boat TF (eds): Kendig's Disorders of the Respiratory Tract in Children, 6th ed. Philadelphia, WB Saunders, 1998.
82. Corsaro D, Valassina M, Venditti D, et al: Multiplex PCR for rapid and differential diagnosis of *Mycoplasma pneumoniae* and *Chlamydia pneumoniae* in respiratory infections. Diagn Microbiol Infect Dis 1999;35:105.
83. Coulter DM: Successful treatment with octreotide of spontaneous chylothorax in a premature infant. J Perinatol 2004;24:194.
84. Cowles RA, Lelli JL Jr, Takayasu J, et al: Lung resection in infants and children with pulmonary infections refractory to medical therapy. J Pediatr Surg 2002;37:643.
85. Cowling MG, Belli AM: A potential pitfall in bronchial artery embolization. Clin Radiol 1995;50:105.
86. Cremaschi P, Nascimbene C, Vitulo P, et al: Therapeutic embolization of bronchial artery: A successful treatment in 209 cases of relapse hemoptysis. Angiology 1993;44:295.
87. Cunningham I: Pulmonary infections after bone marrow transplant. Semin Respir Infect 1992;7:132.
88. Davies RJ, Traill ZC, Gleeson FV: Randomised controlled trial of intrapleural streptokinase in community acquired pleural infection. Thorax 1997;52:416.
89. Davis AM, Wensley DF, Phelan PD: Spontaneous pneumothorax in pediatric patients. Respir Med 1993;87:531.
90. Davis H: A statistical study of the thoracic duct in man. Am J Anat 1915;17:211.
91. Davis PB, Hubbard VS, McCoy K, et al: Familial bronchiectasis. J Pediatr 1983;102:177.
92. de Beer HG, Mol MJ, Janseen JP: Chylothorax. Neth J Med 2000;56:25.
93. de la Rocha AG: Empyema thoracis. Surg Gynecol Obstet 1982;155:839.
94. Denning DW: Echinocandin antifungal drugs. Lancet 2003;362:1142.
95. Denning DW, Stevens DA: Antifungal and surgical treatment of invasive aspergillosis: Review of 2,121 published cases. Rev Infect Dis 1990;12:1147.
96. Desimone JA Jr, Babinchak TJ, Kaulback KR, et al: Treatment of *Mycobacterium avium* complex immune reconstitution disease in HIV-1–infected individuals. AIDS Patient Care STDS 2003;17:617.
97. Dikensoy O, Usalan C, Filiz A: Foreign body aspiration: Clinical utility of flexible bronchoscopy. Postgrad Med J

2002;78:399.
98. Donahue DM, Wright CD, Viale G, Mathisen DJ: Resection of pulmonary blebs and pleurodesis for spontaneous pneumothorax. Chest 1993;104:1767.
99. Donald PR: Childhood tuberculosis. Curr Opin Pulm Med 2000;6:187.
100. Donald PR: Preventing tuberculosis in childhood. Indian J Pediatr 2000;67:383.
101. Donnelly LF, Klosterman LA: The yield of CT of children who have complicated pneumonia and noncontributory chest radiography. AJR Am J Roentgenol 1998;170:1627.
102. Donovan SM, Mickiewicz N, Meyer RD, et al: Imported echinococcosis in southern California. Am J Trop Med Hyg 1995;53:668.
103. Dore ND, LeSouef PN, Masters B, et al: Atypical mycobacterial pulmonary disease and bronchial obstruction in HIV-negative children. Pediatr Pulmonol 1998;26:380.
104. Doski JJ, Lou D, Hicks BA, et al: Management of parapneumonic collections in infants and children. J Pediatr Surg 2000;35:265.
105. Dumont P, Diemont F, Massard G, et al: Does a thoracoscopic approach for surgical treatment of spontaneous pneumothorax represent progress? Eur J Cardiothorac Surg 1997;11:27.
106. Dunn EJ, Ulicny KS Jr, Wright CB, et al: Surgical implications of sclerosing mediastinitis: A report of six cases and review of the literature. Chest 1990;97:338.
107. Easa D, Balaraman V, Ash K, et al: Congenital chylothorax and mediastinal neuroblastoma. J Pediatr Surg 1991;26:96.
108. Eastham KM, Fall AJ, Mitchell L, et al: The need to redefine non-cystic fibrosis bronchiectasis in childhood. Thorax 2004;59:324.
109. Eastham KM, Freeman R, Kearns AM, et al: Clinical features, aetiology and outcome of empyema in children in the north east of England. Thorax 2004;59:522.
110. Ebert DL, Olivier KN: Nontuberculous mycobacteria in the setting of cystic fibrosis. Clin Chest Med 2002;23:655.
111. Efeldt RJ, Shroder DW, Thies J: Long-term follow up of different therapy procedures in spontaneous pneumothorax. J Cardiovasc Surg 1994;35:229.
112. Egan TM, Detterbeck FC, Mill MR, et al: Long term results of lung transplantation for cystic fibrosis. Eur J Cardiothorac Surg 2002;22:602.
113. Eggimann P, Garbino J, Pittet D: Management of *Candida* species infections in critically ill patients. Lancet Infect Dis 2003;3:772.
114. Emanuel B, Shulman ST: Lung abscess in infants and children. Clin Pediatr (Phila) 1995;34:2.
115. Enarson DA: Use of the tuberculin skin test in children. Paediatr Respir Rev 2004;5(Suppl A):S135.
116. English M: Impact of bacterial pneumonias on world child health. Paediatr Resp Rev 2000;1:21.
117. Erez E, Katz M, Sharoni E, et al: Pectoralis major muscle flap for deep sternal wound infection in neonates. Ann Thorac Surg 2000;69:572.
118. Farmer DL, Albanese CT: Fetal hydrothorax. In Harrison MR, Evans MI, Adzick NS, Holzgreve W (eds): The Unborn Patient, 3rd ed. Philadelphia, WB Saunders, 2001.
119. Farrell PM, Mischler EH: Newborn screening for cystic fibrosis. The Cystic Fibrosis Neonatal Screening Study Group. Adv Pediatr 1992;39:35.
120. Felten MK, Rath T, Magdorf K, et al: Childhood tuberculosis in Germany between 1985 and 1994: Comparison of three selected patient groups. Int J Tuberc Lung Dis 1998;2:797.
121. Fernald GW: Infections of the Respiratory Tract due to *Mycoplasma pneumoniae*. In Chernick V, Boat TF (eds): Kendig's Disorders of the Respiratory Tract in Children, 6th ed. Philadelphia, WB Saunders, 1998.
122. Finck C, Wagner C, Jackson R, et al: Empyema: Development of a critical pathway. Semin Pediatr Surg 2002;11:25.
123. Fishman JA, Rubin RH: Infection in organ-transplant recipients. N Engl J Med 1998;338:1741.
124. FitzSimmons SC: The changing epidemiology of cystic fibrosis. J Pediatr 1993;122:1.
125. Fowler GR: A case of thoracoplasty for removal of a large cicatricial fibrous growth from the interior chest, the result of an old empyema. Med Rec 1893;44:838.
126. Frank AL, Marcinak JF, Mangat PD, et al: Clindamycin treatment of methicillin-resistant *Staphylococcus aureus* infections in children. Pediatr Infect Dis J 2002;21:530.
127. Frazer A: Differentiation in the absorption of olive oil and oleic acid in the rat. J Physiol 1943;102:306.
128. Freij BJ, Kusmiesz H, Nelson JD, et al: Parapneumonic effusions and empyema in hospitalized children: A retrospective review of 227 cases. Pediatr Infect Dis J 1984;3:578.
129. Freixinet J: Surgical indications for treatment of pulmonary tuberculosis. World J Surg 1997;21:475.
130. Freixinet J, Varela A, Lopez RL, et al: Surgical treatment of childhood mediastinal tuberculous lymphadenitis. Ann Thorac Surg 1995;59:644.
131. Fujimoto T, Hillejan L, Stamatis G: Current strategy for surgical management of bronchiectasis. Ann Thorac Surg 2001;72:1711.
132. Gates RL, Caniano DA, Hayes JR, et al: Does VATS provide optimal treatment of empyema in children? A systematic review. J Pediatr Surg 2004;39:381.
133. Gaydos CA, Roblin PM, Hammerschlag MR, et al: Diagnostic utility of PCR-enzyme immunoassay, culture, and serology for detection of *Chlamydia pneumoniae* in symptomatic and asymptomatic patients. J Clin Microbiol 1994;32:903.
134. Gaylor AS, Reilly JC: Therapy with macrolides in patients with cystic fibrosis. Pharmacotherapy 2002;22:227.
135. Gendrel D: Antibiotic treatment of *Mycoplasma pneumoniae* infections. Pediatr Pulmonol Suppl 1997;16:46.
136. Gessner BD: Incidence rates, clinical features and case identification of pediatric tuberculosis in Alaska. Int J Tuberc Lung Dis 1998;2:378.
137. Gilbert K, Fine MJ: Assessing prognosis and predicting patient outcomes in community-acquired pneumonia. Semin Respir Infect 1994;9:140.
138. Gilljam M, Berning SE, Peloquin CA, et al: Therapeutic drug monitoring in patients with cystic fibrosis and mycobacterial disease. Eur Respir J 1999;14:347.
139. Glenn W: The lymphatic system, some surgical considerations. Arch Surg 1981;116:989.
140. Graham DD, McGahren ED, Tribble CG, et al: Use of video-assisted thoracic surgery in the treatment of chylothorax. Ann Thorac Surg 1994;57:1507.
141. Graham SM: HIV and respiratory infections in children. Curr Opin Pulm Med 2003;9:215.
142. Grant RT, Breitbart AS, Parnell V: Muscle flap reconstruction of pediatric poststernotomy wound infections. Ann Plast Surg 1997;38:365.
143. Greenwood B: The epidemiology of pneumococcal infection in children in the developing world. Philos Trans R Soc Lond B Biol Sci 1999;354:777.
144. Grewal H, Jackson RJ, Wagner CW, et al: Early video-assisted thoracic surgery in the management of empyema. Pediatrics 1999;103:e63.

145. Griffith DE: Emergence of nontuberculous mycobacteria as pathogens in cystic fibrosis. Am J Respir Crit Care Med 2003;167:810.
146. Grzybowski S: Tuberculosis. Chest 1983;84:756.
147. Guggino WB: Cystic fibrosis and the salt controversy. Cell 1999;96:607.
148. Guleserian KJ, Gilchrist BF, Luks FI, et al: Child abuse as a cause of traumatic chylothorax. J Pediatr Surg 1996;31:1696.
149. Gupta D, Hansell A, Nichols T, et al: Epidemiology of pneumothorax in England. Thorax 2000;55:666.
150. Haciibrahimoglu G, Fazlioglu M, Olcmen A, et al: Surgical management of childhood bronchiectasis due to infectious disease. J Thorac Cardiovasc Surg 2004;127:1361.
151. Hall CB, Douglas RG Jr, Geiman JM: Quantitative shedding patterns of respiratory syncytial virus in infants. J Infect Dis 1975;132:151.
152. Hall CB, Douglas RG Jr, Geiman JM: Respiratory syncytial virus infections in infants: Quantitation and duration of shedding. J Pediatr 1976;89:11.
153. Hammerschlag MR: Pneumonia due to *Chlamydia pneumoniae* in children: Epidemiology, diagnosis, and treatment. Pediatr Pulmonol 2003;36:384.
154. Han D, Lee KS, Koh WJ, et al: Radiographic and CT findings of nontuberculous mycobacterial pulmonary infection caused by *Mycobacterium abscessus.* AJR Am J Roentgenol 2003;181:513.
155. Hansell DM: Bronchiectasis. Radiol Clin North Am 1998; 36:107.
156. Hardegger D, Nadal D, Bossart W, et al: Rapid detection of *Mycoplasma pneumoniae* in clinical samples by real-time PCR. J Microbiol Methods 2000;41:45.
157. Harris JA, Kolokathis A, Campbell M, et al: Safety and efficacy of azithromycin in the treatment of community-acquired pneumonia in children. Pediatr Infect Dis J 1998;17:865.
158. Heath PT: Epidemiology and bacteriology of bacterial pneumonias. Paediatr Resp Rev 2000;1:4.
159. Heffelfinger JD, Davis TE, Gebrian B, et al: Evaluation of children with recurrent pneumonia diagnosed by World Health Organization criteria. Pediatr Infect Dis J 2002;21:108.
160. Heiskanen-Kosma T, Korppi M, Jokinen C, et al: Etiology of childhood pneumonia: Serologic results of a prospective, population-based study. Pediatr Infect Dis J 1998;17:986.
161. Heurlin N, Bergstrom SE, Winiarski J, et al: Fungal pneumonia: The predominant lung infection causing death in children undergoing bone marrow transplantation. Acta Paediatr 1996;85:168.
162. Hewitson JP, Von Oppell UO: Role of thoracic surgery for childhood tuberculosis. World J Surg 1997;21:468.
163. Hierholzer JC, Bingham PG, Coombs RA, et al: Comparison of monoclonal antibody time-resolved fluoroimmunoassay with monoclonal antibody capture-biotinylated detector enzyme immunoassay for respiratory syncytial virus and parainfluenza virus antigen detection. J Clin Microbiol 1989;27:1243.
164. Hilton AM, Doyle L: Immunological abnormalities in bronchiectasis with chronic bronchial suppuration. Br J Dis Chest 1978;72:207.
165. Hochberg LA: Thoracic Surgery Before the 20th Century. New York, Vantage Press, 1960.
166. Hoff SJ, Neblett WW, Edwards KM, et al: Parapneumonic empyema in children: Decortication hastens recovery in patients with severe pleural infections. Pediatr Infect Dis J 1991;10:194.
167. Holman RC, Shay DK, Curns AT, et al: Risk factors for bronchiolitis-associated deaths among infants in the United States. Pediatr Infect Dis J 2003;22:483.
168. Holt P: Studies of medium chain triglycerides in patients with differing mechanisms for fat malabsorption. In Senior JR (ed): Medium Chain Triglycerides. Philadelphia, University of Pennsylvania Press, 1968.
169. Horio H, Nomori H, Fuyuno G, et al: Limited axillary thoracotomy vs video-assisted thoracoscopic surgery for spontaneous pneumothorax. Surg Endosc 1998;12:1155.
170. Horsburgh CR Jr, Caldwell MB, Simonds RJ: Epidemiology of disseminated nontuberculous mycobacterial disease in children with acquired immunodeficiency syndrome. Pediatr Infect Dis J 1993;12:219.
171. Huebner RE, Castro KG: The changing face of tuberculosis. Annu Rev Med 1995;46:47.
172. Hughes WT, Rivera GK, Schell MJ, et al: Successful intermittent chemoprophylaxis for *Pneumocystis carinii* pneumonitis. N Engl J Med 1987;316:1627.
173. Inselman LS, Kendig EL: Tuberculosis. In Chernick V, Boat TF (eds): Kendig's Disorders of the Respiratory Tract in Children, 6th ed. Philadelphia, WB Saunders, 1998.
174. Iseman MD, Madsen LA: Chronic tuberculous empyema with bronchopleural fistula resulting in treatment failure and progressive drug resistance. Chest 1991;100:124.
175. Jaffe A, Cohen G: Thoracic empyema. Arch Dis Child 2003;88:839.
176. Jafri HS: Treatment of respiratory syncytial virus: Antiviral therapies. Pediatr Infect Dis J 2003;22(Suppl):S89.
177. Jean-Baptiste E: Clinical assessment and management of massive hemoptysis. Crit Care Med 2000;28:1642.
178. Jeong YJ, Lee KS, Koh WJ, et al: Nontuberculous mycobacterial pulmonary infection in immunocompetent patients: Comparison of thin-section CT and histopathologic findings. Radiology 2004;231:880.
179. Jimenez-Mercàn R, Garcia-Diaz F, Arenas-Linàres C, et al: Comparative retrospective study of surgical treatment of spontaneous pneumothorax. Surg Endosc 1997;11:919.
180. Jones D, Havlir DV: Nontuberculous mycobacteria in the HIV infected patient. Clin Chest Med 2002;23:665.
181. Jones GR, Konsler GK, Dunaway RP, et al: Infection risk factors in febrile, neutropenic children and adolescents. Pediatr Hematol Oncol 1996;13:217.
182. Joosten KF, Hazelzet JA, Tiddens HA, et al: Staphylococcal pneumonia in childhood: Will early surgical intervention lower mortality? Pediatr Pulmonol 1995;20:83.
183. Kabra SK, Lodha R, Seth V: Tuberculosis in children—what has changed in last 20 years? Indian J Pediatr 2002;69(Suppl 1):S5.
184. Kaplan JE, Hanson D, Dworkin MS, et al: Epidemiology of human immunodeficiency virus-associated opportunistic infections in the United States in the era of highly active antiretroviral therapy. Clin Infect Dis 2000; 30(Suppl 1):S5.
185. Kaplan SL: Review of antibiotic resistance, antibiotic treatment and prevention of pneumococcal pneumonia. Paediatr Respir Rev 2004;5(Suppl A):S153.
186. Karaoglanoglu N, Kurkcuoglu IC, Gorguner M, et al: Giant hydatid lung cysts. Eur J Cardiothorac Surg 2001;19:914.
187. Kaschula RO, Druker J, Kipps A: Late morphologic consequences of measles: A lethal and debilitating lung disease among the poor. Rev Infect Dis 1983;5:395.
188. Keating G, Figgitt D: Caspofungin: A review of its use in oesophageal candidiasis, invasive candidiasis and invasive aspergillosis. Drugs 2003;63:2235.

189. Kennedy MJ: Current status of gene therapy for cystic fibrosis pulmonary disease. Am J Respir Med 2002;1:349.
190. Kent JH: The epidemiology of multidrug-resistant tuberculosis in the United States. Med Clin North Am 1993;77:1391.
191. Kenyon TA, Driver C, Haas E, et al: Immigration and tuberculosis among children on the United States–Mexico border, county of San Diego, California. Pediatrics 1998;104:103.
192. Keramidas D, Mavridis G, Soutis M, et al: Medical treatment of pulmonary hydatidosis: Complications and surgical management. Pediatr Surg Int 2004;19:774.
193. Kerem B, Rommens JM, Buchanan JA, et al: Identification of the cystic fibrosis gene: Genetic analysis. Science 1989;245:1073.
194. Kettner BI, Aurisch R, Ruckert JC, et al: Scintigraphic localization of lymphatic leakage site after oral administration of iodine-123 IPPA. J Nucl Med 1998;39:2141.
195. Kiernan PD, Hernandez A, Byrne WD, et al: Descending cervical mediastinitis. Ann Thorac Surg 1998;65:1483.
196. Kilani T, El Hammami S: Pulmonary hydatid and other lung parasitic infections. Curr Opin Pulm Med 2002;8:218.
197. Kim J, Kim K, Shim YM, et al: Video-assisted thoracic surgery as a primary therapy for primary spontaneous pneumothorax. Surg Endosc 1998;12:1290.
198. Kimpen JL: Management of respiratory syncytial virus infection. Curr Opin Infect Dis 2001;14:323.
199. King JC Jr, Burke AR, Clemens JD, et al: Respiratory syncytial virus illnesses in human immunodeficiency virus- and noninfected children. Pediatr Infect Dis J 1993;12:733.
200. Kirk O, Reiss P, Uberti-Foppa C, et al: Safe interruption of maintenance therapy against previous infection with four common HIV-associated opportunistic pathogens during potent antiretroviral therapy. Ann Intern Med 2002;137:239.
201. Klein JS, Schultz S, Heffner JE: Interventional radiology of the chest: Image-guided percutaneous drainage of pleural effusions, lung abscess, and pneumothorax. AJR Am J Roentgenol 1995;164:581.
202. Kneyber MC, Kimpen JL: Current concepts on active immunization against respiratory syncytial virus for infants and young children. Pediatr Infect Dis J 2002;21:685.
203. Knight GJ, Carman PG: Primary staphylococcal pneumonia in childhood: A review of 69 cases. J Paediatr Child Health 1992;28:447.
204. Knudtson J, Grewal H: Pediatric empyema—an algorithm for early thoracoscopic intervention. JSLS 2004;8:31.
205. Koletzko S, Reinhardt D: Nutritional challenges of infants with cystic fibrosis. Early Hum Dev 2001;65(Suppl):S53.
206. Kornecki A, Shemie SD: Open lung biopsy in children with respiratory failure. Crit Care Med 2001;29:1247.
207. Kornecki A, Sivan Y: Treatment of loculated pleural effusion with intrapleural urokinase in children. J Pediatr Surg 1997;32:1473.
208. Korppi M, Heiskanen-Kosma T, Kleemola M: *Mycoplasma pneumoniae* causes over 50% of community-acquired pneumonia in school-aged children. Scand J Infect Dis 2003;35:294.
209. Kosloske AM, Ball WS Jr, Butler C, et al: Drainage of pediatric lung abscess by cough, catheter, or complete resection. J Pediatr Surg 1986;21:596.
210. Kosloske A, Martin L, Schubert W: Management of chylothorax in children by thoracentesis and medium-chain triglyceride feedings. J Pediatr Surg 1974;9:365.
211. Krishnan S, Amin N, Dozor AJ, et al: Urokinase in the management of complicated parapneumonic effusions in children. Chest 1997;112:1579.
212. Kurklu EU, Williams MA, Le Roux BT: Bronchiectasis consequent upon foreign body retention. Thorax 1973;28:601.
213. Kutlay H, Cangir AK, Enon S, et al: Surgical treatment in bronchiectasis: Analysis of 166 patients. Eur J Cardiothorac Surg 2002;21:634.
214. Laberge J-M, Bratu I, Flageole H: The management of asymptomatic congenital lung malformations. Paediatr Resp Rev 2004;5(Suppl):S305.
215. Lampson RS: Traumatic chylothorax—a review of the literature and report of a case treated by mediastinal ligation of the thoracic duct. J Thorac Surg 1948;17:778.
216. Lamy AL, Cameron BH, LeBlanc JG, et al: Giant hydatid lung cysts in the Canadian northwest: Outcome of conservative treatment in three children. J Pediatr Surg 1993;28:1140.
217. Lang-Lazdunski L, Kerangal X, Pons F, et al: Primary spontaneous pneumothorax: One-stage treatment by bilateral video-thoracoscopy. Ann Thorac Surg 2000;70:412.
218. Lange CG, Woolley IJ, Brodt RH: Disseminated mycobacterium avium-intracellulare complex (MAC) infection in the era of effective antiretroviral therapy: Is prophylaxis still indicated? Drugs 2004;64:679.
219. Langtry HD, Balfour JA: Azithromycin: A review of its use in paediatric infectious diseases. Drugs 1998;56:273.
220. Langtry HD, Brogden RN: Clarithromycin: A review of its efficacy in the treatment of respiratory tract infections in immunocompetent patients. Drugs 1997;53:973.
221. Le Coultre C: Chylothorax. In Ziegler MM, Azizkhan RG, Weber TR (eds): Operative Pediatric Surgery. New York, McGraw-Hill, 2003.
222. Le Coultre C, Oberhänsli I, Mossaz A, et al: Postoperative chylothorax in children: Differences between vascular and traumatic origin. J Pediatr Surg 1991;26:519.
223. Lederman MM, Valdez H: Immune restoration with antiretroviral therapies: Implications for clinical management. JAMA 2000;284:223.
224. Leelahanon S, Petlek W, Sontimuang W, et al: Can octreotide be the first line treatment for chylothorax? J Med Assoc Thai 2003;86(Suppl 3):S741.
225. Lehrnbecher T, Foster C, Vazquez N, et al: Therapy-induced alterations in host defense in children receiving therapy for cancer. J Pediatr Hematol Oncol 1997;19:399.
226. Lehrnbecher T, Groll AH, Chanock SJ: Treatment of fungal infections in neutropenic children. Curr Opin Pediatr 1999;11:47.
227. Light PW, O'Hara VS, Moritz TE, et al: Intrapleural tetracycline or the prevention of recurrent spontaneous pneumothorax. JAMA 1990;264:2224.
228. Linden PK: Amphotericin B lipid complex for the treatment of invasive fungal infections. Expert Opin Pharmacother 2003;4:2099.
229. Liu HP, Hsieh MJ, Lu HI, et al: Thoracoscopic-assisted management of postpneumonic empyema in children refractory to medical response. Surg Endosc 2002;16:1612.
230. Lobato MN, Loeffler AM, Furst K, et al: Detection of *Mycobacterium tuberculosis* in gastric aspirates collected from children: Hospitalization is not necessary. Pediatrics 1998;102:E40.
231. Lodha R, Kabra SK: Newer diagnostic modalities for tuberculosis. Indian J Pediatr 2004;71:221.

232. Lodha R, Puranik M, Natchu UC, et al: Recurrent pneumonia in children: Clinical profile and underlying causes. Acta Paediatr 2002;91:1170.
233. Longaker MT, Laberge J-M, Danserau J, et al: Primary fetal hydrothorax: Natural history and management. J Pediatr Surg 1989;24:573.
234. Loop FD, Lytle BW, Cosgrove DM, et al: J. Maxwell Chamberlain memorial paper. Sternal wound complications after isolated coronary artery bypass grafting: Early and late mortality, morbidity, and cost of care. Ann Thorac Surg 1990;49:179.
235. Lossos IS, Breuer R, Or R, et al: Bacterial pneumonia in recipients of bone marrow transplantation: A five-year prospective study. Transplantation 1995;60:672.
236. Lowther SA, Shay DK, Holman RC, et al: Bronchiolitis-associated hospitalizations among American Indian and Alaska Native children. Pediatr Infect Dis J 2000;19:11.
237. Lowy FD, Waldhausen JA, Miller M, et al: Report of the National Heart, Lung and Blood Institute-National Institute of Allergy and Infectious Diseases working group on antimicrobial strategies and cardiothoracic surgery. Am Heart J 2004;147:575.
238. Luck SR, Raffensperger JG, Sullivan HJ, et al: Management of pneumothorax in children with chronic pulmonary diseases. J Thorac Cardiovasc Surg 1997;74:834.
239. Maiz-Carro L, Navas-Elorza E: Nontuberculous mycobacterial pulmonary infection in patients with cystic fibrosis: Diagnosis and treatment. Am J Respir Med 2002;1:107.
240. Marcinak JF, Frank AL: Treatment of community-acquired methicillin-resistant *Staphylococcus aureus* in children. Curr Opin Infect Dis 2003;16:265.
241. Margenthaler JA, Weber TR, Keller MS: Predictors of surgical outcome for complicated pneumonia in children: Impact of bacterial virulence. World J Surg 2004;28:87.
242. Mark PH, Turner JA: Lung abscess in childhood. Thorax 1968;23:216.
243. Marras TK, Daley CL: Epidemiology of human pulmonary infection with nontuberculous mycobacteria. Clin Chest Med 2002;23:553.
244. Martinez FD: Respiratory syncytial virus bronchiolitis and the pathogenesis of childhood asthma. Pediatr Infect Dis J 2003;22(Suppl):S76.
245. Mathur R, Cullen J, Kinnear WJ, et al: Time course of resolution of persistent air leak in spontaneous pneumothorax. Respir Med 1995;89:129.
246. McCarthy CA, Hall CB: Respiratory syncytial virus: Concerns and control. Pediatr Rev 2003;24:301.
247. McCracken GH Jr: Etiology and treatment of pneumonia. Pediatr Infect Dis J 2000;19:373.
248. Meier AH, Smith B, Raghavan A, et al: Rational treatment of empyema in children. Arch Surg 2000;135:907.
249. Mendeloff EN: Lung transplantation for cystic fibrosis. Semin Thorac Cardiovasc Surg 1998;10:202.
250. Menzies D: Interpretation of repeated tuberculin tests: Boosting, conversion and reversion. Am J Respir Crit Care Med 1999;159:15.
251. Merrigan BA, Winter DC, O'Sullivan GC: Chylothorax. Br J Surg 1997;84:15.
252. Meyers JD, McGuffin RW, Bryson YJ, et al: Treatment of cytomegalovirus pneumonia after marrow transplant with combined vidarabine and human leukocyte interferon. J Infect Dis 1982;146:80.
253. Michelow IC, Olsen K, Lozano J, et al: Epidemiology and clinical characteristics of community-acquired pneumonia in hospitalized children. Pediatrics 2004;113:701.
254. Miller JI Jr: Diagnosis and management of chylothorax. Chest Surg Clin North Am 1996;6:139.
255. Mitlehner W, Friedrich M, Dissmann W: Value of computed tomography in the detection of bullae and blebs in patients with primary spontaneous pneumothorax. Respiration 1992;59:221.
256. Mofenson LM, Yogev R, Korelitz J, et al: Characteristics of acute pneumonia in human immunodeficiency virus-infected children and association with long term mortality risk. National Institute of Child Health and Human Development Intravenous Immunoglobulin Clinical Trial Study Group. Pediatr Infect Dis J 1998;17:872.
257. Mohamadiyeh MK, Ashour M, el Desouki M, et al: Contribution of ventilation and perfusion lung imaging to the management of patients with bronchiectasis. Clin Nucl Med 1994;19:292.
258. Moore RD, Urschel JD, Fraser RE, et al: Cystic hydatid lung disease in northwest Canada. Can J Surg 1994;37:20.
259. Morgan WJ, Butler SM, Johnson CA, et al: Epidemiologic study of cystic fibrosis: Design and implementation of a prospective, multicenter, observational study of patients with cystic fibrosis in the U.S. and Canada. Pediatr Pulmonol 1999;28:231.
260. Moroney JF, Fiore AE, Harrison LH, et al: Clinical outcomes of bacteremic pneumococcal pneumonia in the era of antibiotic resistance. Clin Infect Dis 2001;33:797.
261. Morphis GL, Arcinne EL, Krause JR: Generalized lymphangioma in infancy with chylothorax. Pediatrics 1970;46:566.
262. Morrissey BM, Evans SJ: Severe bronchiectasis. Clin Rev Allergy Immunol 2003;25:233.
263. Moureux J, Elkaim D, Padovani B, et al: Video-assisted thoracoscopic treatment of spontaneous pneumothorax: Technique and results of one hundred cases. J Thorac Cardiovasc Surg 1996;112:385.
264. Murphy MC, Newman BM, Rodgers BM: Pleuroperitoneal shunts in the management of persistent chylothorax. Ann Thorac Surg 1989;48:195.
265. Murphy TF, Henderson FW, Clyde WA Jr, et al: Pneumonia: An eleven-year study in a pediatric practice. Am J Epidemiol 1981;113:12.
266. Mustafa MM, Pappo A, Cash J, et al: Aerosolized pentamidine for the prevention of *Pneumocystis* pneumonia in children with cancer intolerant or allergic to trimethoprim/sulfamethoxazole. J Clin Oncol 1994;12:258.
267. Nelson CT: *Mycoplasma* and *Chlamydia* pneumonia in pediatrics. Semin Respir Infect 2002;17:10.
268. Neuhoff H, Touroff ASW: Acute putrid abscess of the lung: Principles of operative treatment. Surg Gynecol Obstet 1936;63:353.
269. Neville K, Renbarger J, Dreyer Z: Pneumonia in the immunocompromised pediatric cancer patient. Semin Respir Infect 2002;17:21.
270. Nguyen D, Tchervenkov CI: Successful management of postoperative chylothorax with fibrin glue in a premature neonate. Can J Surg 1994;37:158.
271. Nguyen DM, Shum-Tim D, Dobell AR, et al: The management of chylothorax/chylopericardium following pediatric cardiac surgery: A 10-year experience. J Card Surg 1995; 10:302.
272. Nolan CM, Goldberg SV: Treatment of isoniazid-resistant tuberculosis with isoniazid, rifampin, ethambutol, and pyrazinamide for 6 months. Int J Tuberc Lung Dis 2002;6:952.
273. Nolt D, Michaels MG, Wald ER: Intrathoracic disease from nontuberculous mycobacteria in children: Two cases and a review of the literature. Pediatrics 2003;112:e434.
274. Nonoyama A, Tanaka K, Osako T, et al: Surgical treatment

of pulmonary abscess in children under ten years of age. Chest 1984;85:358.
275. Noppen M, Alexander P, Driesen P, et al: Quantification of primary spontaneous pneumothorax: Accuracy of the Light index. Respiration 2001;68:396.
276. Odev K, Ozer F, Ceran S, et al: CT diagnosis of granulomatous mediastinitis due to tuberculosis. Eur J Radiol 1996;23:241.
277. Olivier C: Clinical use of cefuroxime in paediatric community-acquired pneumonia. Paediatr Drugs 2000; 2:331.
278. Olivier KN, Weber DJ, Wallace RJ Jr, et al: Nontuberculous mycobacteria: I: Multicenter prevalence study in cystic fibrosis. Am J Respir Crit Care Med 2003;167:828.
279. Owayed AF, Campbell DM, Wang EE: Underlying causes of recurrent pneumonia in children. Arch Pediatr Adolesc Med 2000;154:190.
280. Ozcelik C, Inci I, Nizam O, et al: Intrapleural fibrinolytic treatment of multiloculated postpneumonic pediatric empyemas. Ann Thorac Surg 2003;76:1849.
281. Panitch HB: Respiratory syncytial virus bronchiolitis: Supportive care and therapies designed to overcome airway obstruction. Pediatr Infect Dis J 2003;22(Suppl):S83.
282. Pappas PG, Rex JH: Therapeutic approach to *Candida* sepsis. Curr Infect Dis Rep 1999;1:245.
283. Pappas PG, Rex JH, Sobel JD, et al: Guidelines for treatment of candidiasis. Clin Infect Dis 2004;38:161.
284. Peloquin CA: Therapeutic drug monitoring in the treatment of tuberculosis. Drugs 2002;62:2169.
285. Pena GN, Munoz LF, Vargas RJ, et al: Yield of percutaneous needle lung aspiration in lung abscess. Chest 1990;97:69.
286. Perez MS,Van Dyke RB: Pulmonary infections in children with HIV infection. Semin Respir Infect 2002;17:33.
287. Peters TR, Edwards KM: The pneumococcal protein conjugate vaccines. J Pediatr 2000;137:416.
288. Piedra PA: Clinical experience with respiratory syncytial virus vaccines. Pediatr Infect Dis J 2003;22(Suppl):S94.
289. Pizzo PA: Infectious complications in the child with cancer: II. Management of specific infectious organisms. J Pediatr 1981;98:513.
290. Pizzo PA, Rubin M, Freifeld A, et al: The child with cancer and infection: II. Nonbacterial infections. J Pediatr 1991;119:845.
291. Pizzo PA, Walsh TJ: Fungal infections in the pediatric cancer patient. Semin Oncol 1990;17:6.
292. Playfor SD, Smyth AR, Stewart RJ: Increase in incidence of childhood empyema. Thorax 1997;52:932.
293. Poenaru D, Yazbeck S, Murphy S: Primary spontaneous pneumothorax in children. J Pediatr Surg 1994;29:1183.
294. Pomerantz M, Brown J: The surgical management of tuberculosis. Semin Thorac Cardiovasc Surg 1995;7:108.
295. Pozniak A: Mycobacterial diseases and HIV. J HIV Ther 2002;7:13.
296. Principi N, Esposito S: Emerging role of *Mycoplasma pneumoniae* and *Chlamydia pneumoniae* in paediatric respiratory-tract infections. Lancet Infect Dis 2001;1:334.
297. Principi N, Esposito S: *Mycoplasma pneumoniae* and *Chlamydia pneumoniae* cause lower respiratory tract disease in paediatric patients. Curr Opin Infect Dis 2002;15:295.
298. Rajan S, Saiman L: Pulmonary infections in patients with cystic fibrosis. Semin Respir Infect 2002;17:47.
299. Ramsey BW: Management of pulmonary disease in patients with cystic fibrosis. N Engl J Med 1996;335:179.
300. Ramsey BW, Dorkin HL: Consensus conference: Practical applications of Pulmozyme. September 22, 1993. Pediatr Pulmonol 1994;17:404.
301. Ramsey BW, Pepe MS, Quan JM, et al: Intermittent administration of inhaled tobramycin in patients with cystic fibrosis. Cystic Fibrosis Inhaled Tobramycin Study Group. N Engl J Med 1999;340:23.
302. Rattan A: Diagnosis of tuberculosis by polymerase chain reaction. Indian J Pediatr 1990;57:673.
303. Redding G, Singleton R, Lewis T, et al: Early radiographic and clinical features associated with bronchiectasis in children. Pediatr Pulmonol 2004;37:297.
304. Reid J, Marciniuk D, Peloquin CA, et al: Pharmacokinetics of antituberculosis medications delivered via percutaneous gastrojejunostomy tube. Chest 2002;121:281.
305. Rex JH, Walsh TJ, Sobel JD, et al: Practice guidelines for the treatment of candidiasis. Infectious Diseases Society of America. Clin Infect Dis 2000;30:662.
306. Reynolds M: Disorders of the thoracic cavity and pleura and infections of the lung, pleura and mediastinum. In O'Neill JAJ, Rowe MI, Grosfeld JL, et al (eds): Pediatric Surgery, 5th ed. St. Louis, Mosby–Year Book, 1998.
307. Rheuban KS, Kron IL, Carpenter MA, et al: Pleuroperitoneal shunts for refractory chylothorax after operation for congenital heart disease. Ann Thorac Surg 1992;53:85.
308. Ridderstolpe L, Gill H, Granfeldt H, et al: Superficial and deep sternal wound complications: Incidence, risk factors and mortality. Eur J Cardiothorac Surg 2001;20:1168.
309. Rosenzweig DY, Stead WW: The role of tuberculosis and other forms of bronchopulmonary necrosis in the pathogenesis of bronchiectasis. Am Rev Respir Dis 1966;93:769.
310. Ross JK: A review of the surgery of the thoracic duct. Thorax 1961;16:12.
311. Rothenberg SS: Experience with thoracoscopic lobectomy in infants and children. J Pediatr Surg 2003;38:102.
312. Rutstein RM, Cobb P, McGowan KL, et al: *Mycobacterium avium-intracellulare* complex infection in HIV-infected children. AIDS 1993;7:507.
313. Saggese D, Compadretti GC, Burnelli R: Nontuberculous mycobacterial adenitis in children: Diagnostic and therapeutic management. Am J Otolaryngol 2003;24:79.
314. Sahn SA: Management of complicated parapneumonic effusions. Am Rev Respir Dis 1993;148:813.
315. Sahn SA, Heffner JE: Spontaneous pneumothorax. N Engl J Med 2000;342:868.
316. Saiman L: The mycobacteriology of non-tuberculous mycobacteria. Paediatr Respir Rev 2004;5(Suppl A):S221.
317. Salih OK, Topcuoglu MS, Celik SK, et al: Surgical treatment of hydatid cysts of the lung: Analysis of 405 patients. Can J Surg 1998;41:131.
318. Santolaya ME, Alvarez AM, Aviles CL, et al: Prospective evaluation of a model of prediction of invasive bacterial infection risk among children with cancer, fever, and neutropenia. Clin Infect Dis 2002;35:678.
319. Sarihan H, Cay A, Aynaci M, et al: Empyema in children. J Cardiovasc Surg (Torino) 1998;39:113.
320. Schaaf HS, Shean K, Donald PR: Culture confirmed multidrug resistant tuberculosis: Diagnostic delay, clinical features, and outcome. Arch Dis Child 2003;88:1106.
321. Schidlow DV, Taussig LM, Knowles MR: Cystic Fibrosis Foundation consensus conference report on pulmonary complications of cystic fibrosis. Pediatr Pulmonol 1993; 15:187.
322. Schlesinger C, Koss MN: Bronchiolitis: Update 2001. Curr Opin Pulm Med 2002;8:112.
323. Schneider MM, Borleffs JC, Stolk RP, et al: Discontinuation of prophylaxis for *Pneumocystis carinii* pneumonia in HIV-1-infected patients treated with highly active antiretroviral therapy. Lancet 1999;353:201.

324. Schoni MH, Casaulta-Aebischer C: Nutrition and lung function in cystic fibrosis patients: Review. Clin Nutr 2000;19:79.
325. Schowengerdt CG, Suyemoto R, Main FB: Granulomatous and fibrous mediastinitis: A review and analysis of 180 cases. J Thorac Cardiovasc Surg 1969;57:365.
326. Schultz MJ: Macrolide activities beyond their antimicrobial effects: Macrolides in diffuse panbronchiolitis and cystic fibrosis. J Antimicrob Chemother 2004;54:21.
327. Schumacker HP, Moore TC: Surgical management of traumatic chylothorax. Surg Gynecol Obstet 1951;93:46.
328. Schwoebel V, Lambregts-van Weezenbeek CS, Moro ML, et al: Standardization of antituberculosis drug resistance surveillance in Europe. Recommendations of a World Health Organization (WHO) and International Union Against Tuberculosis and Lung Disease (IUATLD) Working Group. Eur Respir J 2000;16:364.
329. Selle JG, Snyder WH, Schreiber JT: Chylothorax: Indications for surgery. Ann Surg 1973;177:245.
330. Severien C, Teig N, Riedel F, et al: Severe pneumonia and chronic lung disease in a young child with adenovirus and *Bordetella pertussis* infection. Pediatr Infect Dis J 1995;14:400.
331. Sharland M, Gibb DM, Holland F: Respiratory morbidity from lymphocytic interstitial pneumonitis (LIP) in vertically acquired HIV infection. Arch Dis Child 1997;76:334.
332. Shaw KS, Prasil P, Nguyen LT, et al: Pediatric spontaneous pneumothorax. Semin Pediatr Surg 2003;12:55.
333. Shay DK, Holman RC, Roosevelt GE, et al: Bronchiolitis-associated mortality and estimates of respiratory syncytial virus-associated deaths among US children, 1979-1997. J Infect Dis 2001;183:16.
334. Shen HN, Lu FL, Wu HD, et al: Management of tension pneumatocele with high-frequency oscillatory ventilation. Chest 2002;121:284.
335. Shenep JL, Flynn PM: Pulmonary fungal infections in immunocompromised children. Curr Opin Pediatr 1997; 9:213.
336. Shetty D, Giri N, Gonzalez CE, et al: Invasive aspergillosis in human immunodeficiency virus-infected children. Pediatr Infect Dis J 1997;16:216.
337. Shingadia D, Novelli V: Diagnosis and treatment of tuberculosis in children. Lancet Infect Dis 2003;3:624.
338. Sihoe AD, Yim APC, Lee TW, et al: Can CT scanning be used to select patients with unilateral primary spontaneous pneumothorax for bilateral surgery? Chest 2000; 118:380.
339. Simansky DA, Yellin A: Pleural abrasion via axillary thoracotomy in the era of video-assisted thoracic surgery. Thorax 1994;49:922.
340. Simonds RJ, Orejas G: *Pneumocystis carinii* pneumonia and toxoplasmosis. In Pizzo PA, Wilfert C (eds): Pediatric AIDS: The Challenge of HIV Infection in Infants, Children and Adolescents, 3rd ed. Baltimore, Williams & Wilkins, 1998.
341. Sinaniotis CA: Viral pneumoniae in children: Incidence and aetiology. Paediatr Respir Rev 2004;5(Suppl A):S197.
342. Slattery DM, Waltz DA, Denham B, et al: Bronchoscopically administered recombinant human DNase for lobar atelectasis in cystic fibrosis. Pediatr Pulmonol 2001;31:383.
343. Smevik B: Complementary investigations in bronchiectasis in children. Monaldi Arch Chest Dis 2000;55:420.
344. Sobel JD, Vazquez J: Candidemia and systemic candidiasis. Semin Respir Infect 1990;5:123.
345. Somoskovi A, Mester J, Hale YM, et al: Laboratory diagnosis of nontuberculous mycobacteria. Clin Chest Med 2003; 23:585.
346. Sorensen RU, Waller RL, Klinger JD: Cystic fibrosis: Infection and immunity to *Pseudomonas*. Clin Rev Allergy 1991;9:47.
347. Staat MA: Respiratory syncytial virus infections in children. Semin Respir Infect 2002;17:15.
348. Starke JR: Childhood tuberculosis: Treatment strategies and recent advances. Paediatr Respir Rev 2001;2:103.
349. Starke JR, Jacobs RF, Jereb J: Resurgence of tuberculosis in children. J Pediatr 1992;120:839.
350. Stevens DA, Kan VL, Judson MA, et al: Practice guidelines for diseases caused by *Aspergillus*. Infectious Diseases Society of America. Clin Infect Dis 2000;30:696.
351. Stillwell PC, Mallory GB Jr: Pediatric lung transplantation. Clin Chest Med 1997;18:405.
352. Subramaniam R, Joseph VT, Tan GM, et al: Experience with video-assisted thoracoscopic surgery in the management of complicated pneumonia in children. J Pediatr Surg 2001;36:316.
353. Sullivan JH, Moore RD, Keruly JC, et al: Effect of antiretroviral therapy on the incidence of bacterial pneumonia in patients with advanced HIV infection. Am J Respir Crit Care Med 2000;162:64.
354. Swaminathan S: Basic concepts in the treatment of tuberculosis. Indian J Pediatr 2002;69(Suppl 1):S44.
355. Tabachnik NF: Surgical treatment and the patient with cystic fibrosis. Surg Gynecol Obstet 1981;152:837.
356. Tan TQ: Pneumococcal infections in children. Pediatr Ann 2002;31:241.
357. Tan TQ: Update on pneumococcal infections of the respiratory tract. Semin Respir Infect 2002;17:3.
358. Tan TQ: Antibiotic resistant infections due to *Streptococcus pneumoniae:* Impact on therapeutic options and clinical outcome. Curr Opin Infect Dis 2003;16:271.
359. Tan TQ, Mason EO Jr, Wald ER, et al: Clinical characteristics of children with complicated pneumonia caused by *Streptococcus pneumoniae.* Pediatrics 2002;110:1.
360. Tan TQ, Seilheimer DK, Kaplan SL: Pediatric lung abscess: Clinical management and outcome. Pediatr Infect Dis J 1995;14:51.
361. Tendero DT: Laboratory diagnosis of cytomegalovirus (CMV) infections in immunodepressed patients, mainly in patients with AIDS. Clin Lab 2001;47:169.
362. Thompson AB, Teschler H, Rennard SI: Pathogenesis, evaluation, and therapy for massive hemoptysis. Clin Chest Med 1992;13:69.
363. Thomson AH, Hull J, Kumar MR, et al: Randomised trial of intrapleural urokinase in the treatment of childhood empyema. Thorax 2002;57:343.
364. Tillet WS, Sherry S: The effect in patients of streptococcal fibrinolysin (streptokinase) and streptococcal deoxyribonuclease on fibrinous, purulent and sanguineous pleural exudations. J Clin Invest 1949;23:173.
365. Tor M, Atasalihi A, Altuntas N, et al: Review of cases with cystic hydatid lung disease in a tertiary referral hospital located in an endemic region: A 10 years' experience. Respiration 2000;67:539.
366. Tortoriello TA, Friedman JD, McKenzie ED, et al: Mediastinitis after pediatric cardiac surgery: A 15-year experience at a single institution. Ann Thorac Surg 2003; 76:1655.
367. Tribble CG: Talc poudrage in the treatment of spontaneous pneumothoraces in patients with cystic fibrosis. Ann Surg 1986;204:677.
368. Tsang KW, Zheng L, Tipoe G: Ciliary assessment in bronchiectasis. Respirology 2000;5:91.
369. Tuffaha A, Gern JE, Lemanske RF Jr: The role of respiratory viruses in acute and chronic asthma. Clin Chest Med

2000;21:289.
370. Tumbarello M, Tacconelli E, de Donati KG, et al: Changes in incidence and risk factors of *Mycobacterium avium complex* infections in patients with AIDS in the era of new antiretroviral therapies. Eur J Clin Microbiol Infect Dis 2001;20:498.
371. Tuncozgur B, Ustunsoy H, Sivrikoz MC, et al: Intrapleural urokinase in the management of parapneumonic empyema: A randomised controlled trial. Int J Clin Pract 2001; 55:658.
372. Turna A, Yilmaz MA, Haciibrahimoglu G, et al: Surgical treatment of pulmonary hydatid cysts: Is capitonnage necessary? Ann Thorac Surg 2002;74:191.
373. Vain NE, Swarner OW, Cha CC: Neonatal chylothorax. J Pediatr Surg 1980;15:261.
374. van der Meer JT, Drew WL, Bowden RA, et al: Summary of the International Consensus Symposium on Advances in the Diagnosis, Treatment and Prophylaxis of Cytomegalovirus Infection. Antiviral Res 1996;32:119.
375. van Rossum AM, Fraaij PL, de Groot R: Efficacy of highly active antiretroviral therapy in HIV-1 infected children. Lancet Infect Dis 2002;2:93.
376. van Straaten HL, Gerards LJ, Krediet TG: Chylothorax in the neonatal period. Eur J Pediatr 1993;152:2.
377. Vandevivere J, Spehl M, Dab I, et al: Bronchiectasis in childhood: Comparison of chest roentgenograms, bronchography and lung scintigraphy. Pediatr Radiol 1980; 9:193.
378. Varpela E, Koistinen J, Korhola O, et al: Deficiency of alpha1-antitrypsin and bronchiectasis. Ann Clin Res 1978;10:79.
379. Vaughan D, Katkin JP: Chronic and recurrent pneumonias in children. Semin Respir Infect 2002;17:72.
380. Vento S, Cainelli F: Infections in patients with cancer undergoing chemotherapy: Aetiology, prevention, and treatment. Lancet Oncol 2003;4:595.
381. Vernejoux JM, Raherison C, Combe P, et al: Spontaneous pneumothorax: Pragmatic management and long-term outcome. Respir Med 2001;95:857.
382. Wagner RB, Johnston MR: Middle lobe syndrome. Ann Thorac Surg 1983;35:679.
383. Waites KB: New concepts of *Mycoplasma pneumoniae* infections in children. Pediatr Pulmonol 2003;36:267.
384. Wald A, Leisenring W, van Burik JA, et al: Epidemiology of *Aspergillus* infections in a large cohort of patients undergoing bone marrow transplantation. J Infect Dis 1997;175:145.
385. Wald ER: Recurrent and nonresolving pneumonia in children. Semin Respir Infect 1993;8:46.
386. Wali SO, Shugaeri A, Samman YS, et al: Percutaneous drainage of pyogenic lung abscess. Scand J Infect Dis 2002;34:673.
387. Waller DA, Forty J, Morritt GN: Video-assisted thoracoscopic surgery versus thoracotomy for spontaneous pneumothorax. Ann Thorac Surg 1994;58:372.
388. Walsh TJ, Lee JW, Roilides E, et al: Recent progress and current problems in management of invasive fungal infections in patients with neoplastic diseases. Curr Opin Oncol 1992;4:647.
389. Walsh TJ, Rubin M, Pizzo PA: Respiratory diseases in patients with malignant neoplasms. In Shelhammer J, Pizzo PA, Parillo JE (eds): Respiratory Disease in the Immunocompromised Host. Philadelphia, JB Lippincott, 1991.
390. Welch KJ: Bronchiectasis. In Ravitch MM, Welch KJ, Benson CA, et al (eds): Pediatric Surgery, 3rd ed. Chicago, Year Book Medical Publishers, 1979.
391. Welch KJ: Lung abscess. In Ravitch MM, Welch KJ, Benson CA, et al (eds): Pediatric Surgery, 3rd ed. Chicago, Year Book Medical Publishers, 1979.
392. Welliver RC: Review of epidemiology and clinical risk factors for severe respiratory syncytial virus (RSV) infection. J Pediatr 2003;143(Suppl):S112.
393. Welliver RC: Respiratory syncytial virus infection: Therapy and prevention. Paediatr Respir Rev 2004;5(Suppl A):S127.
394. Wells RG, Havens PL: Intrapleural fibrinolysis for parapneumonic effusion and empyema in children. Radiology 2003;228:370.
395. Weverling GJ, Mocroft A, Ledergerber B, et al: Discontinuation of *Pneumocystis carinii* pneumonia prophylaxis after start of highly active antiretroviral therapy in HIV-1 infection. EuroSIDA Study Group. Lancet 1999; 353:1293.
396. Whitley RJ, Jacobson MA, Friedberg DN, et al: Guidelines for the treatment of cytomegalovirus diseases in patients with AIDS in the era of potent antiretroviral therapy: Recommendations of an international panel. International AIDS Society-USA. Arch Intern Med 1998;158:957.
397. Whyte KF, Williams GR: Bronchiectasis after mycoplasma pneumonia. Thorax 1984;39:390.
398. Wigglesworth FW: Bronchiectasis: An evaluation of present concepts. McGill Med J 1955;24:189.
399. Wilcox DT, Glick PL, Karamanoukian HL, et al: Spontaneous pneumothorax: A single-institution, 12-year experience in patients under 16 years of age. J Pediatr Surg 1995;30:1452.
400. Williams HE, Landau LI, Phelan PD: Generalized bronchiectasis due to extensive deficiency of bronchial cartilage. Arch Dis Child 1972;47:423.
401. Wilson JF, Decker AM: The surgical management of childhood bronchiectasis: A review of 96 consecutive pulmonary resections in children with nontuberculous bronchiectasis. Ann Surg 1982;195:354.
402. Wolff AB, Silen ML, Kokoska ER, et al: Treatment of refractory chylothorax with externalized pleuroperitoneal shunts in children. Ann Thorac Surg 1999;68:1053.
403. Wolff AJ, O'Donnell AE: Pulmonary manifestations of HIV infection in the era of highly active antiretroviral therapy. Chest 2001;120:1888.
404. Wong K, Waters CM, Walesby RK: Surgical management of invasive pulmonary aspergillosis in immunocompromised patients. Eur J Cardiothorac Surg 1992;6:138.
405. Wong KS, Chiu CH, Yeow KM, et al: Necrotising pneumonitis in children. Eur J Pediatr 2000;159:684.
406. Wood JR, Bellamy D, Child AH, et al: Pulmonary disease in patients with Marfan syndrome. Thorax 1984;39:780.
407. Wood RE: Hemoptysis in cystic fibrosis. Pediatr Pulmonol 1992;8:82.
408. Wubbel L, Muniz L, Ahmed A, et al: Etiology and treatment of community-acquired pneumonia in ambulatory children. Pediatr Infect Dis J 1999;18:98.
409. Yoon W, Kim JK, Kim YH, et al: Bronchial and nonbronchial systemic artery embolization for life-threatening hemoptysis: A comprehensive review. Radiographics 2002;22:1395.
410. Yu-Tang GP, Lin M, Teo N, et al: Embolization for hemoptysis: A six-year review. Cardiovasc Intervent Radiol 2002;25:17.
411. Zaia JA: Prevention and management of CMV-related problems after hematopoietic stem cell transplantation. Bone Marrow Transplant 2002;29:633.
412. Zuhdi MK, Spear RM, Worthen HM, et al: Percutaneous catheter drainage of tension pneumatocele, secondarily infected pneumatocele, and lung abscess in children. Crit Care Med 1996;24:330.

第 65 章

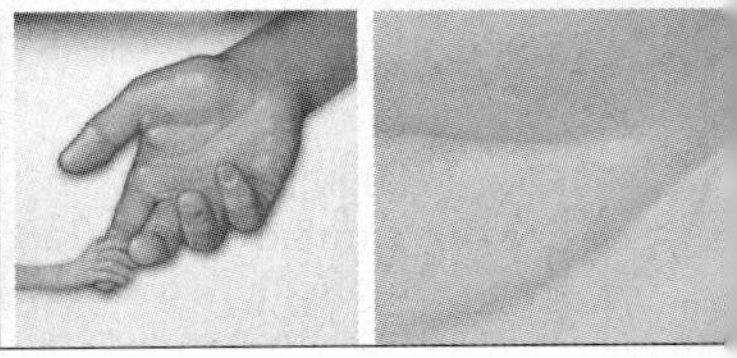

食管镜检查和诊断技术

Harry Lindahl

历史

1038 1870 年，Kussmaul 成为第一个开展食管镜检查者，他使用了一个带有反射光照明的空心硬直管。患者是一名专业吞剑表演者[22]。

1881 年，Mikulicz 介绍了他制造的胃镜，由一些小的光学元件通过关节连接而成。1897 年，Kelling 发明了一种可弯曲的金属食管镜；并且在 1898 年发明了胃镜，后者下三分之一部分可以弯曲 45°。该胃镜具有一个可以旋转 360°的物镜，用一个微小的电灯泡和一个棱镜作为照明。在 1936 年，Schindler 与一名光学物理专家和制造者 Wolf 合作设计了一种半软质胃镜，工作端连接了一个橡皮手指，这个系统包含 48 个透镜，用一个灯泡照明[22]。

1958 年，Hirschowirz 与其合作者发明了用于进行上消化道内镜检查的软式光学纤维胃镜。在过去的 10～15 年中，软式视频内镜已经取代了普通的纤维内镜。目前，制造商可提供用于上消化道检查的各种大小的视频内镜，甚至可用于早产儿[22]。

食管的解剖和功能评估

放射影像学

观察食管的长度、直径和形态最好用腔内钡剂造影的影像学检查。但如果怀疑食管穿孔，则不能用钡剂，而应该用水溶性的造影剂如 Hypaque 或等渗性溶液如 Omnipaque，以免钡剂通过食管的穿孔处漏入纵隔。

食管造影判断食管、胃连接部与横膈食管裂孔相对位置的精确性有限。食管镜检查可更好地确定食管的腹腔段是否存在以及其长度，而食管测压对于评估食管下端括约肌的功能是必要的。

食管镜检查

通过食管镜进行直接观察和黏膜活检是唯一的准确评估食管黏膜改变的方法。正常的食管黏膜表面平滑而有光泽，可见细小的血管。

内镜检查时可观察食管的轮廓，因为食管的曲线可反映正常的胸部脊柱弯曲。在食管的上 1/3 处常可见主动脉弓的搏动。轻轻吹入空气可在食管下端识别食管横膈部的闭合处。正常时，平滑的食管黏膜与颜色更红的天鹅绒状胃黏膜的连接部位于横膈的食管闭合下。胃食管连接部形成一个很容易被确认的波纹状环。

黏膜活检对判断黏膜下和轻微的表面改变是必要的。严重的炎症在食管镜观察下即可确定，并常可推断更深层的改变。

明渠食管镜是有用的，是所有上消化道内镜检查的先驱，但目前仅用于取食管异物。

食管压力监测

腔内测定食管压动力学是当前最精确的评估食管
运动的方法。观察造影剂蠕动的检查方法虽然容易观 1039
察食管的蠕动协调性、食管痉挛和食管收缩完全不协调等情况，但可重复性较差且缺乏定量指标。早期的压力记录技术采用食管内气囊测压法。现在的水灌注导管多压力记录泵技术已取代了气囊测压法，在测压时将带有多个压力记录器的水灌注导管通过食管的全长往回拉。更精确的技术是应用环形泵回拉时进行放射状矢量测压[23]。

食管测压在成人已成为食管疾病的基本检查方法。食管失弛缓症、弥漫性食管痉挛、非特异性食管动力异常等疾病可通过食管测压检查明确诊断，有些外科医生认为，食管测压是选择抗反流手术患者的一个重要方法[24]。

目前，食管测压在婴儿和儿童中的应用还不十分广泛。患儿的合作是需要进一步解决的问题。在不用镇静剂的情况下，婴儿和儿童较少能忍受食管测压探子的插入，而镇静剂本身可能影响对测定结果的判断。此外，在成人可通过食管测压诊断的食管动力异常在儿童中较少见。除了少数的食管失弛缓症外，儿童的食管动力学数据在外科处理中较少具有决定性意义[18]。

18～24 小时的食管 pH 监测

胃酸反流入食管是食管炎症最常见的原因。评估有无反流性食管炎及其严重程度是儿童食管镜检查最普遍的指征。有些情况下需要对反流进行量化，则应进行 24 小时食管 pH 监测[14]。有些学者已介绍了儿童进行食管 pH 监测的技术[3,29]。婴儿和儿童的正常值也已有报道[11,28]。但是，pH 监测仅仅测定了酸的反流，最近有报道认为，连续 pH 监测的结果缺乏可重复性[17]。

食管 pH 监测很少能为儿童食管反流手术提供主要依据，但其数据可对怀疑为反流性疾病而不能确诊的复杂的临床情况提供重要的证据。这些情况主要是可疑为食管反流合并呼吸道并发症而食管钡剂造影或食管镜活检未能确诊。在成人，食管炎是胃食管反流最常见的并发症，但食管反流引起呼吸道并发症而不伴明显的食管炎在婴儿和儿童中更常见。因此，食管 pH 监测在这些患儿的处理中常具有重要的意义[10]。

胆汁反流的探查

胆汁反流至食管已被认为是反流性食管炎形成的促进因素[26]，令人信服的数据表明胆汁协同酸的反流是形成下段食管 Barrett 黏膜发育异常的关键因素[25]。

食管的胆汁检测是困难的，而且用 pH 监测不能确定，因为胃酸与碱性的胆汁混合后常在 pH 监测时表现为中性范围，可掩盖胆汁与酸反流的存在，除非从胃的抽吸物中直接测定胆酸。通过技术的改进，目前已可在食管内不依赖 pH 而直接连续测定胆汁[2]。

食管镜的应用指征

食管镜的应用指征为诊断或治疗。诊断性内镜检查最好用适当大小的软式视频内镜。对于某些治疗操作，开放管腔式硬食管镜仍具有其优势。食管镜检查是一种不适的操作，对小儿最好在气管插管全身麻醉下进行。治疗性食管镜必须在全身麻醉气管插管下进行。如果不能保证安全的麻醉，则不宜进行治疗性的食管镜操作。

诊断评估

怀疑胃食管反流

怀疑胃食管反流可能是小儿行诊断性食管镜检查最常见的原因。该检查用以评估是否发生反流性食管炎及其严重程度。但是，如果内镜下未见黏膜溃疡或糜烂则不能可靠地诊断食管黏膜和黏膜下炎症。单凭食管黏膜的肉眼观很难做出判断，因此食管炎的诊断和分级要依据黏膜活检[20]。

较严重的食管炎容易确认。正常时可见黏膜表层以下细小血管的形态（图 65-1）。无血管形态而伴有红斑、糜烂、溃疡或结节时，通过活检可证实为不同程度的食管炎。食管炎的其他表现有黏膜接触性出血、围绕红斑边缘的不同形态的白斑和黏膜的鹅卵石样改变等。狭窄引起的管腔缩小是严重食管炎长期未愈的并发症。

对怀疑胃食管反流者的食管镜检查必须包括胃十二指肠镜检查，以了解有无胃黏膜损害并排除幽门或十二指肠梗阻。倒退式贲门观察可了解有无食管裂孔

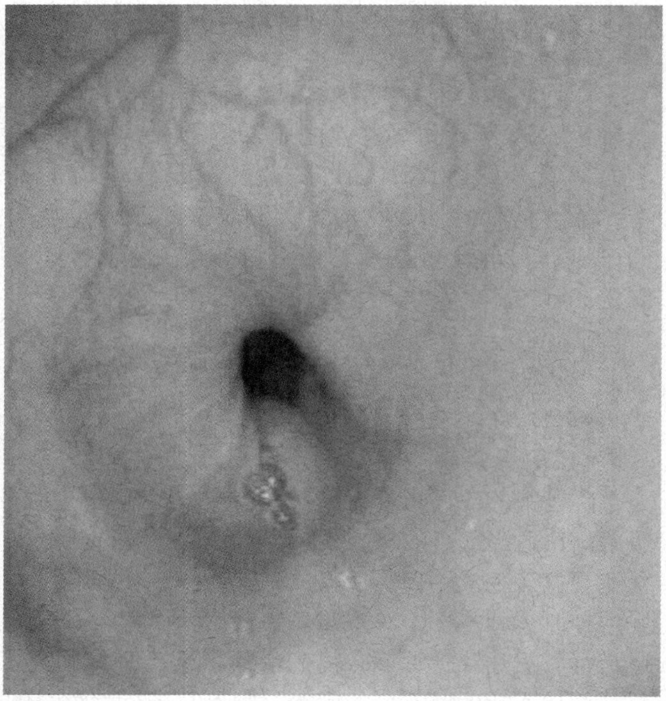

图 65-1 一名正常的 7 个月龄男孩的贲门。可见正常的食管黏膜：黏膜下可看到纤细的血管。

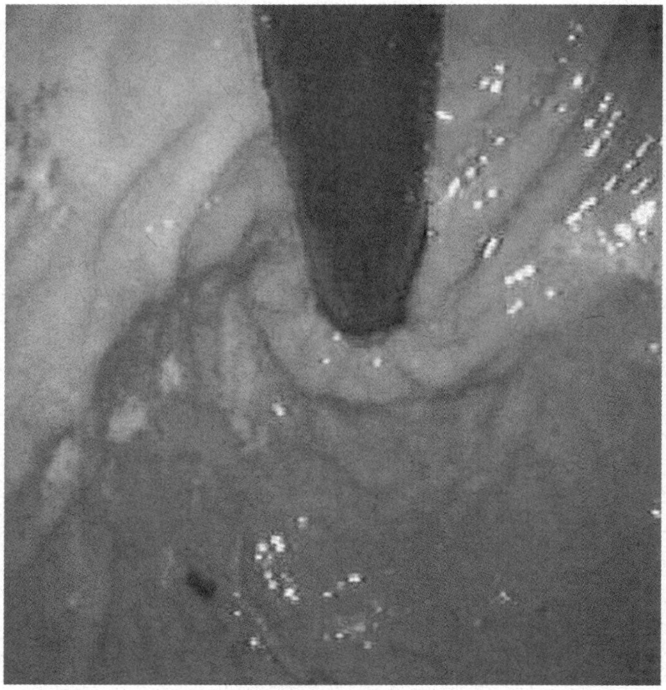

图 65-2 一例 10 岁男孩在成功进行了 Rex 分流后 3 个月开始出现门静脉血栓。可见 His 角正常。10 年的门脉高压后黏膜下静脉仍然突出。

1040 疝和 His 角的情况，这两者是引起胃食管反流的因素（图 65-2 和 65-3）。

吞咽困难

吞咽困难可能与食管炎、食管异物、食管的先天性或获得性狭窄、先天性畸形、良性肿瘤、食管壁结构性疾病或功能性疾病等有关。食管镜检查可提供解剖学异常的信息（如狭窄），但功能性疾病无异常表现。

腐蚀性损伤

对于小儿吞食腐蚀性物质后的食管镜检查指征目前尚有争议，对于食管镜检查的时间也有不同的观点。作者倾向于对吞食腐蚀性液体后有症状的患者在 24 小时内进行食管镜检查。如果没有症状，即没有吞咽困难和疼痛则不必进行内镜检查。

应该用软式食管镜取代硬式食管镜检查黏膜损伤的程度。对严重的病例、甚至较大的儿童也可用直径

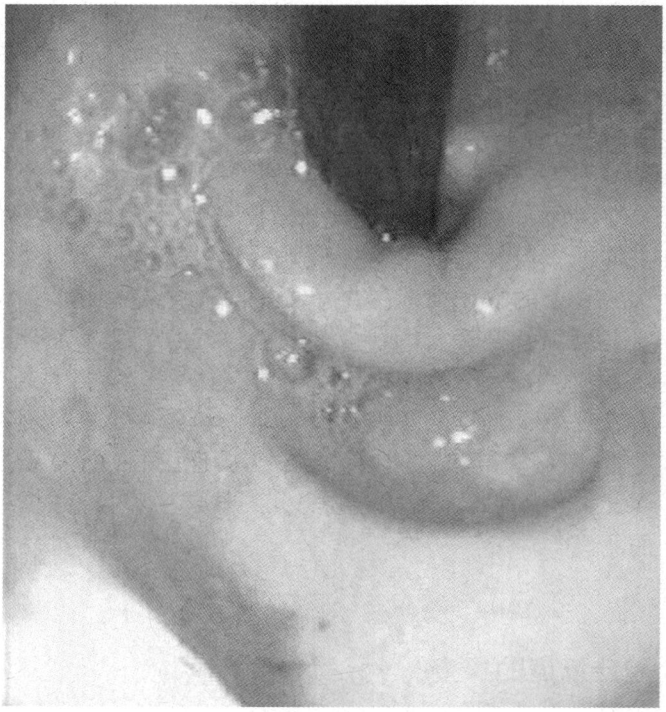

图 65-3 逆行内镜检查时的贲门图像，食管闭锁和胃底折叠术后的 6 岁男孩。胃底的折叠已经部分滑入胸腔。

5～6mm 的新生儿视频内镜，因为这样造成的损伤比大器械的小。内镜检查应始终在完全可视控制下进行。器械绝不能盲目推进，否则可能造成食管穿孔，尤其是全层损伤的患者。如果能在完全可视控制下进行检查，环状损伤不是内镜进入的禁忌证。
1041 对食管有环形损伤的患者，建议将一硅胶管插入胃中，这样可进行肠内营养，也易于在以后发生食管狭窄时进行扩张。

食管的全层损伤不能通过内镜诊断。它是一个临床诊断，根据所吞食的腐蚀物的性质和数量、患者的临床状况和实验室参数等进行判断比内镜所见更重要。

上消化道出血

上消化道出血在儿童中较少见，原因有严重的食管炎、食管静脉曲张出血、Mallory-Weiss 病、胃或十二指肠黏膜病损等。最好的诊断方法是上消化道内镜检查。

对于急性上消化道出血的内镜检查的技术要求较高，应该由经验丰富的内镜医生进行操作。食管静脉曲张出血者常可触及巨大的脾脏，原因可能为门静脉血栓或肝硬化。婴儿肝硬化通常是由胆道闭锁所致。如果怀疑为食管静脉曲张出血，则应做好急诊硬化剂治疗或结扎曲张静脉的准备。

严重的食管炎引起大量失血是非常少见的，但在内镜下易被发现。Mallory-Weiss 撕裂即使在新生儿也可发生，在贲门的胃部用内镜易于见到。常表现为贲门部的局限性血肿而掩盖了实际的撕裂。

外伤

引起食管破裂最常见的原因是医源性损伤。最常发生于食管扩张术或其他治疗性器械操作时[15]。如果在内镜的监视下进行扩张，则穿孔常在当时就可得到诊断。诊断性内镜检查时不会引起穿孔。

钝性或锐性的力量均可能引起食管破裂或穿孔。胸部的压迫性损伤通常只引起气道破裂，但空气充盈食管也可能发生破裂。如果患者清醒且可以进行吞咽试验，则应用水溶性造影剂进行食管造影是诊断食管破裂的最好方法。软式食管镜可发现大的撕裂或完全断裂，但食管狭窄扩张术后小的食管壁破裂可能只有通过食管造影才能发现。

解剖学畸形

食管的解剖学畸形，如先天性狭窄、食管壁内的软骨环畸形、平滑肌瘤和囊性重复畸形等常首先通过影像学检查被发现，然后用内镜进行确诊。用软式食管镜可见到具有软骨环的坚硬且有螺纹的食管壁。气管食管瘘最好用气管镜检查，通常在食管面不能看到。图 65-4 显示食管闭锁患者的吻合口狭窄。

先天性上消化道畸形的随访

先天性上消化道畸形手术后发生晚期并发症的风险较大。曾报道的并发症有胃食管反流、食管炎、胃组织化生、甚至腺癌等。许多患者，甚至在有胃化生时也无症状。为了防止不可逆的恶变前的黏膜改变，应考虑在上消化道畸形手术后常规进行食管镜随访[12,13,19,27]。图 65-5 为 1 例食管闭锁的 3 岁男孩的胃管。图 65-6 为 1 例 22 岁女性在食管闭锁术后的吻合口。

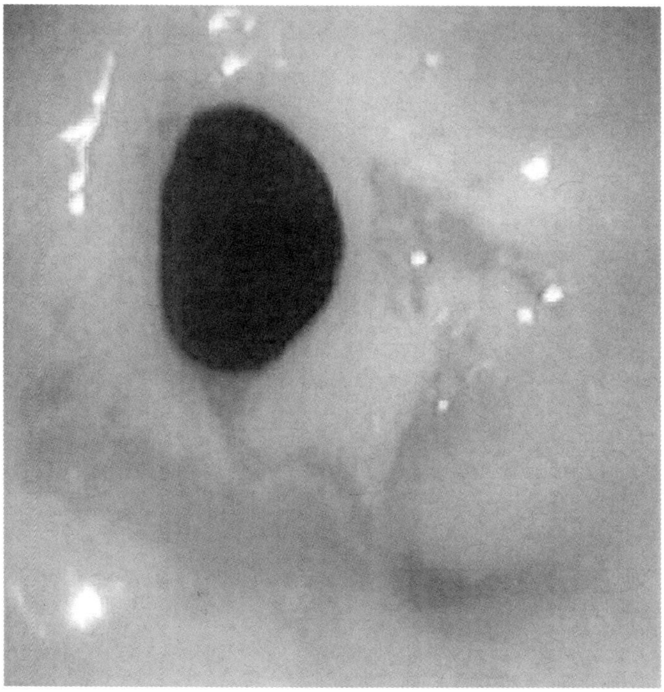

图 65-4　一名 6 个月月龄男孩食管闭锁手术后的吻合口狭窄。

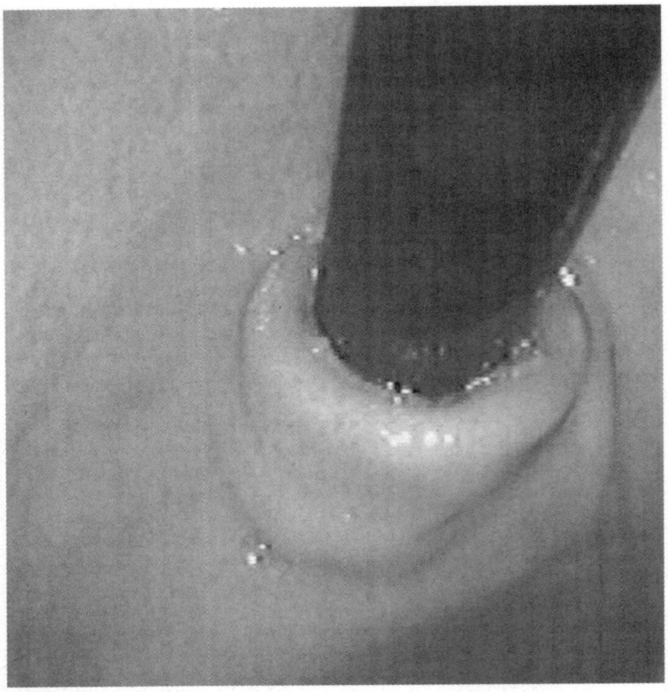

图 65-5 一名食管闭锁患儿的假幽门。已用管状胃组织通过胸骨后翻转重建食管。

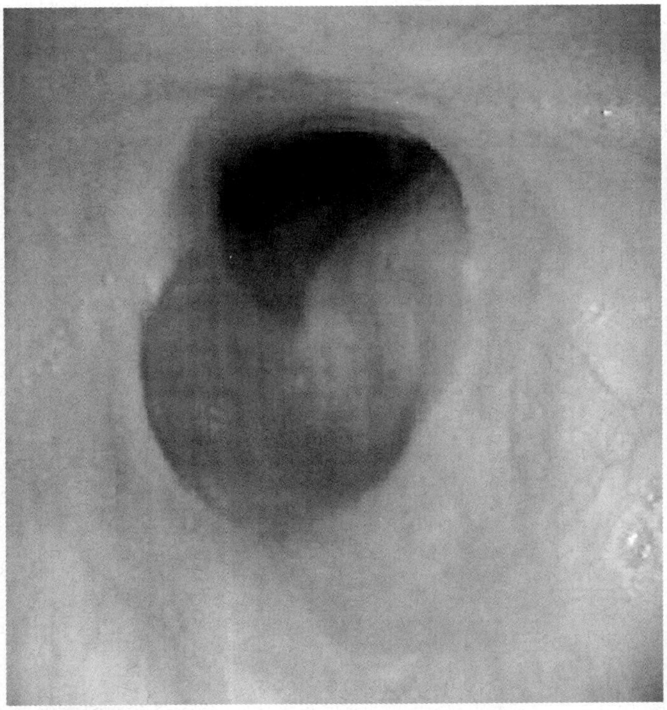

图 65-6 一名 22 岁女性患者的食管闭锁手术后吻合口。

治疗的应用

食管狭窄的扩张

治疗食管狭窄的方法为在荧光屏或内镜的监视下、用或不用导引钢丝的球囊扩张。对局限性的吻合口狭窄，通常在荧光屏的监视或直接的内镜观察下行球囊扩张。长的或紧密曲折的狭窄需要在内镜或荧光屏的监视下进入导丝。选择荧光屏监视或内镜观察下行扩张取决于术者的喜好和经验。硬质金属扩张器、橡胶探针和逆行扩张法目前已经很少采用。 1042

荧光屏监视下的球囊扩张术

高压球囊最早用于血管成型，后来被用于食管扩张技术，可精确地控制最大直径。扩张的球囊穿过一根细的光滑导丝，导丝在荧光屏监视下通过食管进入胃。用适当直径的球囊穿过导丝骑跨于狭窄处。如果轻度的狭窄不是太细，也可不用导丝而直接将带有软头的球囊导入。然后将水溶性造影剂注入球囊，这样可在扩张食管狭窄部时用荧光屏监视球囊腰部的凹痕。

该技术的优点是扩张时可直接观察且形成放射状的力，比纵向锥形的扩张器更安全，力量更集中。

内镜直视下的球囊扩张术

球囊扩张器也可用内镜送入。适合内镜内径的小直径扩张器可直接被送至狭窄部位。直径大的球囊通常需要先将导丝通过内镜的工作管道插入狭窄部，然后取出内镜，将扩张器穿过导丝到达狭窄处进行扩张，扩张的方法与荧光屏监视下的相同。如果内镜可在扩张器旁通过而直接看到狭窄部位，则扩张过程可在内镜中直视。该方法的优点是可估计炎症部位的长度并进行活检，通过可弯曲的食管镜可监视球囊扩张过程，在球囊被拖出后可评估有无黏膜破裂或损伤。图 65-4 为 1 例食管闭锁患者的解剖性狭窄。

留置导丝的食管扩张术

严重的食管狭窄需要多次扩张可应用本技术。该方法需要做胃造瘘。将导丝从食管上端插入，通过软式食管镜进入胃。用内镜通过胃造瘘口将导丝的胃内部分拉出。利用这根导丝可将球囊扩张器从下方或上方推至狭窄部位。扩张以后可用鼻胃管代替导丝，然后将鼻胃管与胃造瘘管绑在一起。下一次扩张时该鼻胃管可引导导丝从鼻部进入，直至胃造瘘口，使反复
1043 扩张变得容易且安全。

胃造瘘导管或纽扣植入

软式胃镜是经皮放置胃造瘘管或胃造瘘纽扣行“倒拉”技术的主要器械[5]。该技术的详细资料已在产品说明书中详述。以前有上腹部手术史的患者是内镜胃造瘘的相对禁忌证，因为胃镜使胃充满空气时可影响胃与前腹壁的附着。由于粘连局限于胃与腹膜壁层直接接触的部位，导管在到达胃时可能已经穿过结肠或小肠。

“拖出”技术是在内镜下将一个经皮置入的导引线或可弯曲导丝从胃内拖出。最简单的方法是用网篮通过胃镜的管腔将导丝经食管从口腔拖出。然后将导管的可穿透肌肉的锥形端联结于导丝，沿食管向下拉，经过胃，然后从前腹壁穿出。应通过胃镜直接监视导管在胃内伞端的最后位置，确保胃壁平整地紧贴壁层腹膜。

我喜欢在内镜监视下做第一个导管或纽扣交换，以确保导管末端或纽扣位于胃内。如果胃壁与前腹壁分离而导致进食时食物进入腹腔，可引起危及生命的并发症。

取食管异物

食管异物处理的要点是需要各种熟练的取异物技巧。

许多食管异物不是尖锐的，并未插入黏膜，长期留存的异物也可用充有造影剂的球囊导管在透视下将其取出。硬币是最常见的异物，有报道 415 例食管异物中 76%为硬币，91%可用球囊导管取出[21]。卡在环咽括约肌部位的异物常可用长叶片的喉镜和 Magill 镊取出[9]。也有其他取硬币的微创技术[4]。当异物可能为嵌入性的，具有尖端或角，或者柔软而易破碎，在球囊拖出时有吸入的危险，必须考虑用食管镜取出异物。但是，根据各医院的经验，明渠食管镜也可用于简单的取硬币。

嵌入的有机物最好用硬质的明渠食管镜取出。大块的肉和其他碎片常卡在食管狭窄的上方，如果用探条将其推入胃比较困难甚至是危险的。大的取物镊可通过硬质食管镜进入，取物镊可在不取出镜鞘的情况下多次进入。大的、尖锐的异物也可较安全地被移入开放管道食管镜的保护鞘中，这样异物与食管镜成为一体，拖出异物时不至于与食管壁接触。用明渠食管镜取异物时可应用硬质儿科支气管镜的光学镊子，因为它可将视野放大。

有时取小的嵌入性异物可用软式食管镜和适当大小的鳄口钳、杯状钳、尖头镊或各种抓物导丝或网篮等。针尖向上的开放型安全别针可用抓钳钳夹其弹簧圈，将整个别针先推入胃，旋转使开口向下，然后与食管镜一并取出。

注射硬化治疗

食管静脉曲张的注射硬化治疗在软式食管镜和可弯曲的注射器下进行。我们用 3%的十四烃基硫酸钠行曲张静脉注射。每条曲张的静脉注入量为 0.5～1.0ml，每次的总量为 2.0～3.0ml。在 25 余年的经验中，作者未见硬化剂导致的并发症，也无因注射治疗而需要输血。关于注射硬化治疗疗效的随机对照研究很少。对 100 例食管静脉曲张儿童进行的预防性硬化治疗的随机研究发现，硬化剂治疗组的静脉曲张明显清除，但是未见生存率提高[7]。

内镜下用小的橡皮带行曲张静脉结扎是对内镜下曲张静脉硬化治疗的一种改进。在成人的随机研究中，这两种治疗方法的有效率和并发症发生率相似[6]。曲张静脉结扎术正在逐渐普及，包括儿童年龄组[1,8]。

管腔内激光治疗

管腔内激光消融已被用于成人的食管病变[30]。用于切割、硬化或消融病变的可弯曲光纤能够穿过纤维镜的测量管道，但至今临床上很少用于婴儿和儿童，大多数小儿外科没有必须的设备和专门技术。内镜激光技术的应用将来会有发展。

仪器

软式光学纤维镜

婴儿和儿童适用的食管镜是可弯曲的视频端口胃镜。现在一些大的内镜制造商已能提供儿童使用的最佳视频内镜。对于常规诊断和治疗应用，内镜至少要
1044 有一个管道用于吸引和置入操作器械。胃镜也包括正压喷射器和能够不取出内镜而冲洗和清洁镜头的设备。标准的胃镜具有四通方向控制的观察端。现代化的设备可用磁带记录视频图像，获得纸质和数码照片。具有这些性能的儿科视频胃镜的外径一般为6.0～9.0mm。

现在对纤维内镜的消毒要求相当严格。制造商可提供自动清洗器以便于清洗和消毒。通过长的内镜工作通道的附件有各种活检钳和取异物钳、抓钳、网兜、可弯曲注射器、磁性材料、电切环和激光光学纤维。

硬质的明渠内镜

硬质的明渠器械在食管的应用仍有一些特殊指征。这种硬质内镜的开放式工作通道较大，可用以安全地取出大而尖锐的异物，因为异物的尖锐边缘可部分拉入内镜中，在拖出时起到对食管的保护作用。大的工作通道可允许较大的取物器械多次进入，进入较大的抓钳可避免异物破碎，避免使用可弯曲器械时复杂操作。为了更好地观察，可应用硬支气管镜的硬质Hopkins光学棒。应用支气管镜的硬质光学异物钳常有助于异物的取出。

患者的准备、镇静和止痛

对于儿童患者，即使用软式食管镜也是一个不舒服的过程。因此，我喜欢在气管插管全身麻醉下进行，这样可较好地控制，而且比用镇静剂做食管镜检查安全。对于儿童患者的食管异物取出、食管狭窄扩张、硬化剂注射或曲张静脉结扎等治疗必须在全身麻醉下进行。全身麻醉看上去似乎会增加患者的危险，但结果常常与此相反。无气道控制情况下的静脉镇静和对烦躁不安或不合作的儿童内镜强行检查可造成呼吸抑制和心血管衰竭。吸入也可增加手术的危险，例如注射硬化治疗或检查急性出血时的冲洗液或血液可反流进入气道。而全身麻醉时心理创伤较小，增加了操作的安全性，使医生行内镜检查更为容易。

我本人没有在无全身麻醉、仅用镇静剂的清醒情况下进行食管镜检查的经验。但是，有些医院仍应用该方法。常用的静脉镇静药物包括短效的中枢神经系统抑制剂苯二氮䓬类联合一种麻醉剂。内镜检查前的喷雾麻醉咽喉部有利于检查。术中必须持续监测心率和氧饱和度，适当的间断性监测血压。氧气、氧气袋、面罩和静脉内麻醉剂拮抗剂在检查过程中必须放在旁边。在不具备复苏和心肺支持设备的内镜室以外的地方不应进行镇静后的食管镜检查。当然，只有一个例外，即在具有上述条件的监护室内。受过培训的人员，适当的器械设备是保证手术成功和安全的关键。

一些合作的十几岁患儿可在无镇静剂的情况下进行内镜检查，仅用咽喉部局部喷雾麻醉。某些患者对该过程比用镇静剂后行内镜检查更配合。

操作技巧

在使用前必须检查所有的器械，确认可以正常工作。纤维内镜的镜头焦距也必须在插入之前被校正。视频内镜必须先调节黑白平衡。将内镜的操作件握于左手拇指和示指之间。示指和中指的指尖控制吸引器和喷射器，无名指和小指稳定内镜。用左手拇指控制向上下运动，右手在患者口部固定内镜的远端，控制内镜的插入，并在内镜旋转时进行横向移动。通过侧向调节转盘可调节内镜尖端转向左、右侧。为了保护纤维内镜，检查时应将一个口腔片插入上下门齿之间。

全麻下的软式内镜检查

全麻下行可弯曲的视频内镜检查，除了插入镜子通过环咽肌外时，其他方面都比较简单。麻醉的患者不能自觉的或不自觉吞咽。患者仰卧。内镜操作者站在患者头端右侧。内镜在视频控制下从喉的后方进入

食管。如果喉部紧靠下咽部后壁，可要求麻醉师轻轻上抬患者的下颌角。在梨状窝水平喷入少量空气以打开咽环肌，然后在观察下将内镜的前端送入开口。一旦通过了环咽肌，调整内镜使前方的食管管腔变直。观察在内镜前进和后退的过程中进行。在评估食管炎
1045 或者腐蚀性损伤时，重要的是应在内镜通过前记录黏膜的情况。

用与不用静脉镇静的软式内镜检查

进行儿童内镜检查时，静脉内注射镇静剂很少能使患儿完全合作。检查必须全面而简短。这需要轻柔而精准的操作，无不必要的或错误的动作，以及内镜操作者丰富的经验。

对未镇静或轻度镇静的年龄较大的患儿，内镜插入时患儿最好取坐位。通常在内镜通过环咽括约肌后使患者呈左侧卧位，头稍后仰。平稳的插入内镜可大大减少患儿的恐惧和对操作的抵抗。很多内镜操作者喜欢盲插通过环咽肌，当吞咽时右手向前推镜子，用左手示指和中指将舌向前压舌完成这个过程。然而，在直视下插入镜子可以更加精确的定位。通过镜头的冲洗系统在喉部喷水有时可使患儿出现吞咽动作。

明渠观察的硬式内镜

硬式内镜用于儿童时均应在气管插管全身麻醉下进行，以减小创伤和穿孔的危险。仰卧位，颈部向前和头部后仰的体位适用于是大多数检查。

明渠硬式食管镜在直视下插入咽后部，斜面部分的唇缘朝向前方。用唇缘轻轻抬起喉部并打开环咽肌。操作者左手托住患者的下颌骨和上颌骨，大拇指和示指像扶住台球杆那样地扶住食管镜。右手像操作台球杆一样操作食管镜。只有清楚看到前方喉或食管的管腔时才能向前推进。如果食管镜前端的唇缘抬起后未能使环咽肌张开，则应通过食管镜管腔插入一个软的吸引管探查，以确定食管的管腔。然后食管镜在直视下沿这个吸引管进入上食管。当食管镜向前通过食管胃连接处进入胃时，应维持食管腔的视野。然后在食管镜后退时可更细微地观察。

并发症

食管镜检查除了直接操作引起咽部、食管或胃的穿孔外，也包括镇静或者麻醉的相关风险。药物反应、气管支气管吸入、缺氧脑损伤等都是潜在的但几乎可完全预防的上消化道内镜检查的相关并发症。仪器引起的穿孔完全可以预防，但是这个并发症仍有发生。

在软式内镜被应用之前，小儿在清醒状态检查时较常见的穿孔部位为咽后壁。食管镜下的食管狭窄扩张术与单纯的诊断性检查相比有较大的穿孔风险，但是儿童器械操作引起穿孔的发生率尚无确切的数据。即使是简单的诊断性检查，在有严重食管炎的患者中，无论是反流或吞食腐蚀剂所致，比没有食管炎的患者有更大的穿孔风险。近年来以软式器械的应用为主，因此儿童的器械所致穿孔明显减少。只要在整个检查过程中保持对食管管腔的放大观察，穿孔就不太可能发生。

在 Helsinki 大学儿童医院，小儿外科医生在 10 年间（1994—2003）进行了 6418 例次食管镜或上消化道内镜检查，386 例次食管扩张术。有 2 例穿孔，都发生于食管闭锁修复术后吻合口狭窄的扩张时，均需要手术治疗。穿孔者均无死亡，但是其中一例做了多次手术才保住了他的食管。在同期行食管镜取异物术 140 例，食管静脉曲张硬化剂注射治疗 102 例。这些过程中没有发生外科并发症，在诊断性内镜操作中无食管穿孔发生。

（胡 明译 李民驹校）

参考文献

1. Celinska-Cedro D, Teisseyre M, Woynarowski M, et al: Endoscopic ligation of esophageal varices for prophylaxis of first bleeding in children and adolescents with portal hypertension: Preliminary results of a prospective study. J Pediatr Surg 2003;38:1008-1011.
2. Champion G, Richter JE, Vaezi MF, et al: Duodenogastroesophageal reflux: Relationship to pH and importance in Barrett's esophagus. Gastroenterology 1994;107:747.
3. Evans DF, Haynes J, Jones JA, et al: Ambulatory esophageal pH monitoring in children as an indicator for surgery. J Pediatr Surg 1986;21:221.
4. Gauderer MW, DeCou JM, Abrams RS, et al: The penny pincher: A new technique for fast and safe removal of

esophageal coins. J Pediatr Surg 2000;35:276-278.
5. Gauderer MW: Percutaneous endoscopic gastrostomy 20-years later: A historical perspective. J Pediatr Surg 2001; 36:217-219.
6. Gimson AE, Ramage JK, Panos MZ, et al: Randomised trial of variceal banding ligation versus injection sclerotherapy for bleeding oesophageal varices. Lancet 1993;342:391.
7. Gonçalves MEP, Cardoso SR, Maksoud JG: Prophylactic sclerotherapy in children with esophageal varices: Long-term results of a controlled prospective randomized trial. J Pediatr Surg 2000;35:401-405.
8. Hall RJ, Lilly JR, Stiegmann GV: Endoscopic esophageal varix ligation: Technique and preliminary results in children. J Pediatr Surg 1988;23:1222.
9. Janik JE, Janik JS: Magill forceps extraction of upper esophageal coins. J Pediatr Surg 2003;38:227-229.
10. Johnson DG, Syme WC, Matlak ME, et al: Gastro-oesophageal reflux and respiratory disease: The place of the surgeon. Aust NZ J Surg 1984;54:405.
11. Jolley SG, Johnson DG, Herbst JJ, et al: An assessment of gastroesophageal reflux in children by extended pH monitoring of the distal esophagus. Surgery 1978;84:16.
12. Koivusalo A, Rintala R, Lindahl H: Gastroesophageal reflux in children with a congenital abdominal wall defect. J Pediatr Surg 1999;34:1127-1129.
13. Lindahl H, Rintala R, Sariola H: Chronic esophagitis and gastric metaplasia are frequent complications of esophageal atresia. J Pediatr Surg 1993;28:1178-1180.
14. Meyers WF, Roberts CC, Johnson DG, et al: Value of tests for evaluation of gastroesophageal reflux in children. J Pediatr Surg 1985;20:515.
15. Moghissi K, Pender D: Instrumental perforations of the oesophagus and their management. Thorax 1988;43:642.
16. Myer CM III, Ball WS Jr, Bisset GS III: Balloon dilatation of esophageal strictures in children. Arch Otolaryngol Head Neck Surg 1991;117:529.
17. Nielsen RG, Kruse-Andersen S, Husby S: Low reproducibility of 2 × 24-hour continuous esophageal pH monitoring in infants and children: A limiting factor for interventional studies. Dig Dis Sci 2003;48:1495-1502.
18. Opie JC, Chaye H, Fraser GC: Fundoplication and pediatric esophageal manometry: Actuarial analysis over 7 years. J Pediatr Surg 1987;22:935.
19. Schalamon J, Lindahl H, Saarikoski H, et al: Endoscopic follow-up in esophageal atresia—for how long is it necessary? J Pediatr Surg 2003;38:702-704.
20. Schapiro M: Flexible fiberoptic esophagoscopy. In Berci G (ed): Endoscopy. New York, Appleton-Century-Crofts, 1976.
21. Schunk JE, Harrison AM, Corneli HM, et al: Fluoroscopic Foley catheter removal of esophageal foreign bodies in children: Experience with 415 episodes. Pediatrics 1994;94:709.
22. Spaner SJ, Warnock GL: A brief history of endoscopy, laparoscopy and laparoscopic surgery. J Laparoendosc Adv Surg Tech A 1997;7:369-373.
23. Stein HJ, DeMeester TR, Naspetti R, et al: Three-dimensional imaging of the lower esophageal sphincter in gastroesophageal reflux disease. Ann Surg 1991;214:374.
24. Stein HJ, DeMeester TR: Indications, technique, and clinical use of ambulatory 24-hour esophageal motility monitoring in a surgical practice. Ann Surg 1993;217:128.
25. Stein HJ, Hoeft S, DeMeester TR: Functional foregut abnormalities in Barrett's esophagus. J Thorac Cardiovasc Surg 1993;105:107.
26. Stoker DL, Williams JG: Alkaline reflux oesophagitis. Gut 1991;32:1090.
27. Vanamo K, Rintala RJ, Lindahl H, et al: Long-term gastrointestinal morbidity in patients with congenital diaphragmatic defects. J Pediatr Surg 1996;31:551-554.
28. Vandenplas Y, Goyvaerts H, Helven R, et al: Gastroesophageal reflux, as measured by 24-hour pH monitoring, in 509 healthy infants screened for risk of sudden infant death syndrome. Pediatrics 1991;88:834.
29. Vandenplas Y: Esophageal pH monitoring: Methodology, indication and interpretation. Eur J Pediatr Surg 1991;1:67.
30. Weston AP: Use of lasers in Barrett's esophagus. Gastrointest Endosc Clin North Am 2003;13:467-481.

第 66 章

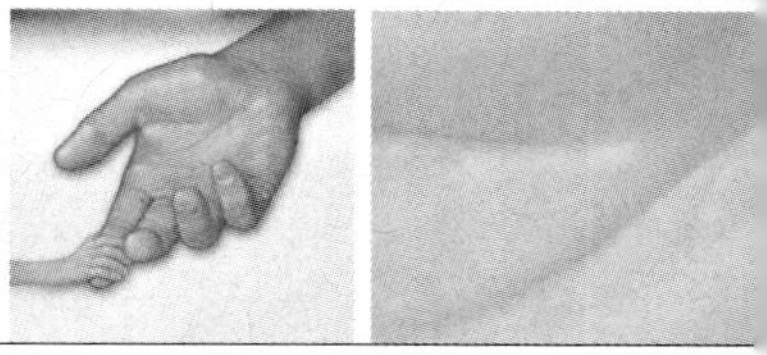

食管破裂和穿孔

Thomas R. Weber

1047 Boerhaave 的经典尸体解剖描述了 1 例名为 Baron Wassenaer 的患者，是第一例自发性的催吐后食管破裂病例的报道。在 1952 年 Fryfogle[12]报道了新生儿自发性食管破裂并通过外科手术成功修补的病例。在 1968 年，Ekdof 等[8]首先报道了新生儿插入导管时发生的医源性颈部食管穿孔。这些作者认为非手术治疗对大多数病例是适当的。

分类和发病率

食管与胸腔或纵隔的异常交通可分为食管破裂或穿孔。食管破裂也被称为自发性穿孔、Boerhaave 综合征、劳累性穿孔和食管卒中。发生这些情况时如果没有食管内使用器械或者插管史，说明食管壁存在严重的解剖学异常或功能紊乱[1,6,7,15,17]。而食管穿孔是物体插入食管腔内所致，这种病变是外伤性的，许多病例是由诊断和治疗操作所致[2,9,10,13,18,23,24]，也可因吞食异物[5,16]、腐蚀性物质、钝性或锐性创伤所致[4,22]。

新生儿和婴儿食管的自发性穿孔很少见，仅占所有病例的 4%[13]。但在试图插入鼻胃管或气管内插管时的医源性食管上段穿孔并非少见，很可能比文献报道的更多[18,19]。此外，食管镜检查和食管扩张过程中引起食管穿孔并发症的发生率为 0.4%～1.2%。因此这些操作的应用是一个重要的风险因素。

临床表现

新生儿自发性食管破裂多数发生于孕期无并发症的足月儿。可以立刻发生或者数小时后发生呼吸窘迫伴发钳[15]。呼吸窘迫常由于右侧气胸压力迅速上升所致。新生儿 Boerhaave 综合征常表现为右侧气胸，这与破裂进入左侧胸腔（常发生与成人）相反，因为婴儿的主动脉与食管左侧紧密粘连，使该侧食管壁得到了额外的支持[11]。如果穿孔未及时得到诊断，呼吸窘迫通常在第一次喂养后加重。有些病例可有呕吐、咳嗽、暂时性窒息和轻度咯血等症状。胸腔穿刺或胸腔造口引流可有血清血液样或全血性的胸腔积液或含有先前喂养物。如果再次喂养则在胸腔引流液中立即出现所进食的液体食物。

与上述情况相反，食管穿孔常与早产儿插入鼻胃管困难相关（占 63%的病例）[18,19]。至少 75%的穿孔患者存在吞咽困难。特征性的表现为流口水、口腔分泌物增多和喂养困难。较大儿童食管穿孔的特征为食管镜检查或者扩张后出现严重的胸部或胸骨下疼痛。发烧，常为高烧，和迅速发生的中毒性进行性休克可出现在任何年龄组，但在大龄儿童的纵隔或开放性胸膜穿孔后更常见。皮下气肿常见于成人食管穿孔，而在婴儿中少见，除非有大量纵隔积气。

诊断

食管破裂或穿孔的早期诊断是根据临床表现做出的，并通过胸片检查证实。自发性食管破裂或广泛性食管创伤的典型表现包括直立位胸片示右侧张力性气胸或气液胸，或纵隔积气（图 66–1）。儿童插管引起的医源性穿孔在胸部平片常表现为鼻胃管移位，通常进入右侧胸腔（图 66–2）。

在其他病例中，引起穿孔的导管可位于黏膜下或者纵隔部，并形成“假憩室”。食管扩张引起的穿孔 1048
常表现为纵隔积气或左侧气胸（图 66–3）。侧位胸片可在早期显示纵隔积气。

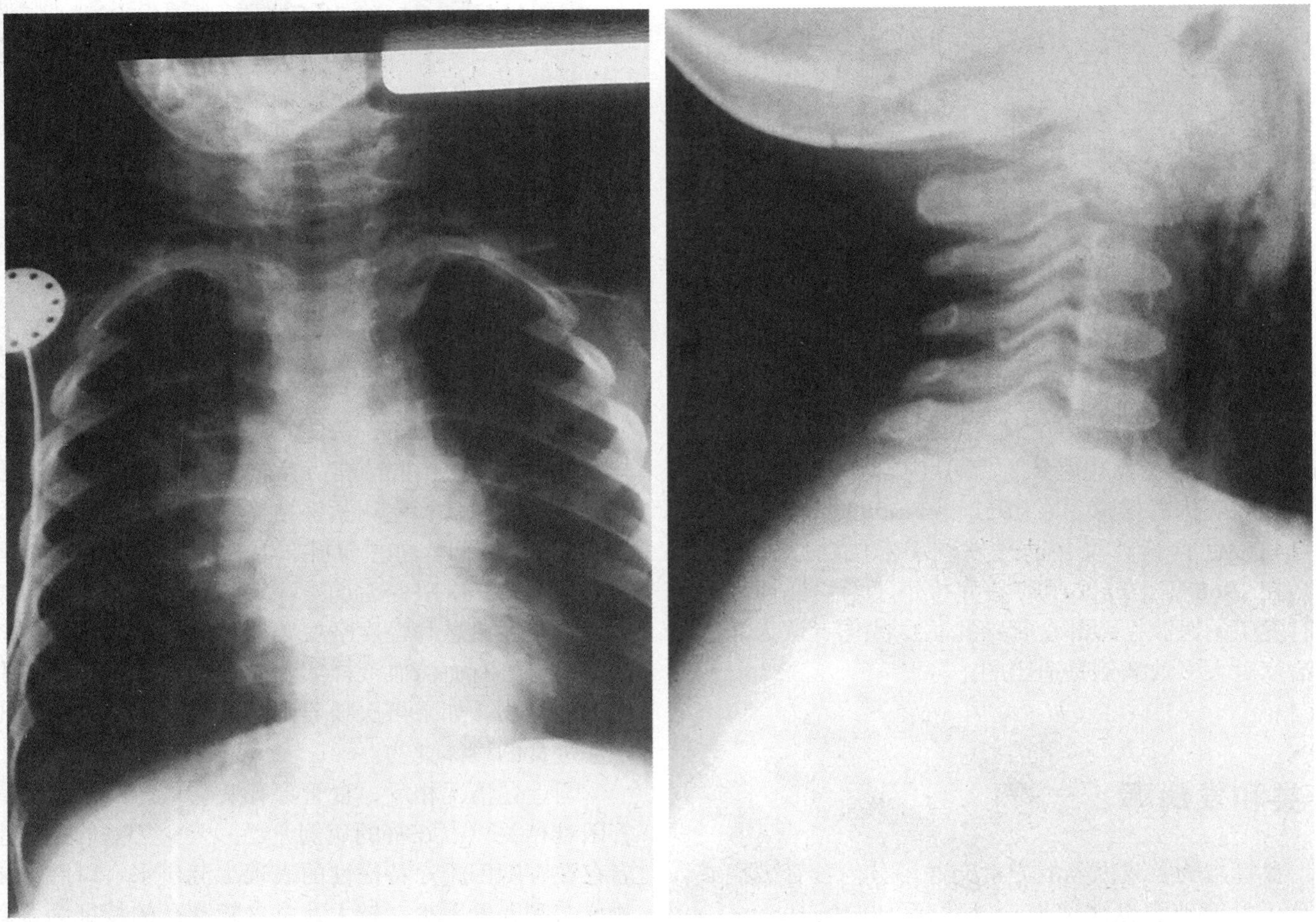

A B

图 66–1 A. 患儿跌倒时口含一支铅笔导致的食管损伤。注意在纵隔的两侧均有大量的纵隔气体。B. 气体也可在颈部软组织中看到，表明颈部食管的损伤。侧位片特别有助于显示颈部或胸部的气体。

对所有的食管穿孔病例，食管造影 X 线检查是明确诊断所必需的操作，可确定穿孔部位并指导治疗[10]。如果怀疑鼻胃管造成食管上段穿孔，可将管子保留原位并通过胃管注入少量的水溶性造影剂。如果胃管已被取出或穿孔为其他操作如喉镜检查或气管内的插管所致，可通过一小管小心注入水溶性造影剂到上段食管进行检查。继发于器械操作的下段食管穿孔在食管造影检查时常可见造影剂进入胸腔或者纵隔。如果水溶性造影剂的食管检查仍然存在问题或解剖定位不确定，可用钡剂重复上述检查。然而，大多数外科医生认为钡剂溢出进入胸腔不好。食管镜检查对于诊断没有优势，而且实际上可能扩大穿孔，使得修补变得更加困难。

治疗

对于食管破裂或穿孔，应根据穿孔的部位、是开放性或包裹性、损伤到诊断的时间间隔，对损伤的全身反应等来决定最适合的治疗方法[3,21]。自发性破裂不涉及器械操作，通常导致纵隔或者胸腔的污染，引起严重的全身性反应，发热、脓毒血症、胸痛，偶尔
发生休克。这类患者需要迅速进行术前准备，包括静 1049
脉补液、抗生素治疗、胸腔穿刺、胸腔造口引流术（如果存在气胸或胸腔积液）以及禁食。应行食管造影 X 线检查明确穿孔部位，并迅速行开胸手术，冲洗胸腔间隙，如果找到破裂口应予以缝合或修补。在探查的过程中应用纤维食管镜可帮助确定穿孔的部

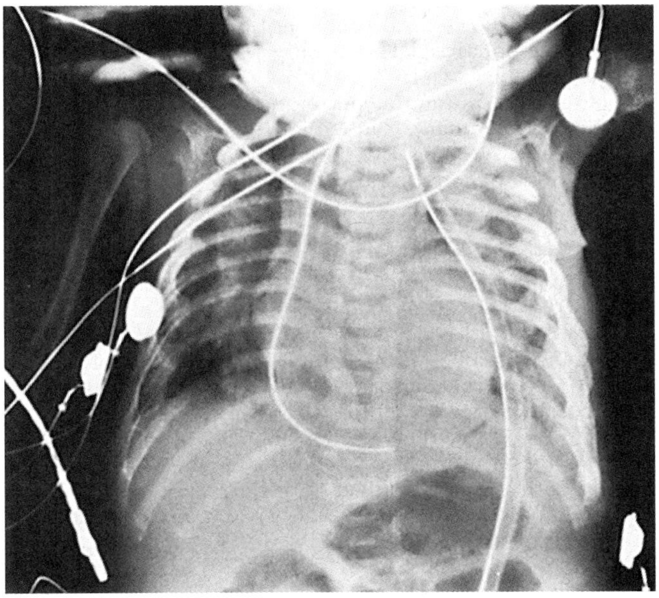

图 66-2 一个早产儿食管上段的穿孔。注意胃管可能位于右侧胸腔。拔出胃管后经非手术治疗完全恢复。

位。也可用一块胸膜或者心包膜加固食管缝合处[14]。手术结束时放置一些大的胸腔引流管。

继发于器械操作的开放性胸膜穿孔应予以相同的处理。因为这些穿孔大多数被早期诊断，很少表现出反应，通常可以进行穿孔的早期修补，或者早期食管切除吻合。应在胸腔行广泛灌洗并留置 1～2 根的胸腔引流管。辅助手术如食管的颈部造口或置导管造口、无吻合口的食管分流、胃造瘘、空肠造口喂养等对于某些病例也可以起到作用。然而这些技术在儿童并未广泛应用。

试图放置鼻胃管或者气管内插管引起的食管上段穿孔通常可以非手术治疗[18,20]。这些穿孔可以仅累及纵隔或扩散到胸膜腔（通常是右侧），应该拔除引起穿孔的管子，在电视内镜指引下插入新的鼻胃管，并注入造影剂确认已经将管子插入到胃内。如有气胸需要放置胸腔引流管。对婴儿应给予广谱抗生素和静脉内营养，禁止经口喂养。几天后，可以开始通过鼻胃管喂养。如果发生胃食管反流，可将胃管通过幽门送入十二指肠进行喂养。如果非手术治疗时发生脓毒血症，应考虑纵隔脓肿的可能，行胸部 CT 检查和胸腔引流术。

不管用什么治疗，都需要在创伤或者手术后 7～10 天进行食管 X 线造影。如果穿孔已经完全愈合，可拔除胸腔或纵隔的引流管并恢复经口喂养。如果发现有溢出，继续保守治疗 7～10 天可以愈合。持续性食管瘘并不常见，提示有远端食管或胃的出口梗阻。

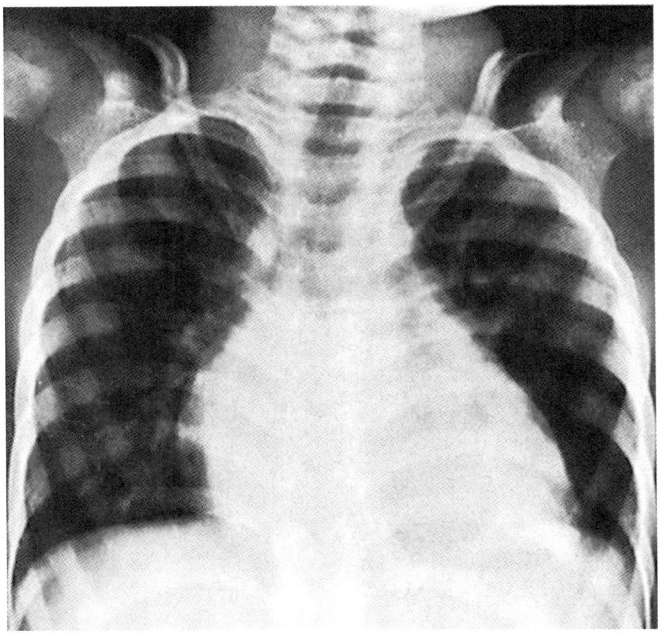

图 66-3 食管扩张术后 1 小时，气体在心脏后方的纵隔内聚集。后来行食管造影显示为远端食管穿孔。

治疗的结果

由于自发性食管破裂在儿童中很少见，所以很难估计外科修补的成功率。Aaronson 等[1]在 13 例患者的回顾分析中提到有 3 例仅用胸腔引流管治疗的患者死亡，而 8 例婴儿中有 7 例通过开胸缝合修补术后得以存活。晚期的修补处食管狭窄偶有发生，扩张术对于这个并发症很有疗效。其他的病例报告强调非手术治疗者均死亡[9]，而开胸修补术得到了满意的结果[6]。对于器械和异物所致的继发性食管穿孔 1050
进入胸膜腔者进行积极的手术修补，可以期望得到相似的结果。

许多作者提倡用非手术方法治疗上段食管的穿孔[2,8,13,17,18,20,21,24]。当选择性地应用于有穿孔而无全身症状的婴儿时，存活率可达到 100%。这通常是黏膜下穿孔或纵隔内包裹的病例，被称为食管的假憩室。如果开放性穿孔进入胸膜腔，如患儿无临床表现仍然可以采取保守治疗；然而必须严密监测生命体征，一旦出现脓毒血症则应行开胸手术。

（胡 明译 李民驹校）

参考文献

1. Aaronson IA, Cywes S, Louw JH: Spontaneous esophageal rupture in the newborn. J Pediatr Surg 1975;10:459.
2. Astley R, Roberts KD: Intubation perforation of the oesophagus in the newborn baby. Br J Radiol 1970;43:219.
3. Attar S, Hankins JR, Suter CM, et al: Esophageal perforation: A therapeutic challenge. Ann Thorac Surg 1991; 50:45.
4. Beal SL, Pottmeyer EV, Pisso S: Esophageal perforation following external blunt trauma. J Trauma 1988;28:1425.
5. Benda TJ: Perforating foreign body of the esophagus. Laryngoscope 1969;79:470.
6. Chunn UD, Geppert LJ: Spontaneous rupture of the esophagus in the newborn. J Pediatr 1962;60:404.
7. Dorsey JM, Hohf RP, Lynn TE: Relationship of peptic esophagitis to spontaneous rupture of the esophagus. Arch Surg 1959;78:878.
8. Eklof O, Lohr G, Okmian L: Submucosal perforation of the esophagus in the neonate. Acta Radiol 1969;8:187.
9. Engum SA, Grosfeld JL, West KW, et al: Improved survival in children with esophageal perforation. Arch Surg 1996; 131:604.
10. Fadoo F, Ruiz DE, Dawn SK, et al: Helical CT esophagography for the evaluation of suspected esophageal perforation or rupture. AJR Am J Roentgenol 2004;182:1177.
11. Fleming PJ, Venugopal S, Lewins M, et al: Esophageal perforation into the right pleural cavity in a neonate. J Pediatr Surg 1980;15:335.
12. Fryfogle JD: Discussion of paper by Anderson RL: Rupture of the esophagus. J Thorac Surg 1952;24:369.
13. Grunebaum M, Horodniceanu C, Wilunsky E, et al: Iatrogenic transmural perforation of the oesophagus in the preterm infant. Clin Radiol 1980;31:257.
14. Grillo HC, Wilkins EW: Esophageal repair following late diagnosis of intrathoracic perforation. Ann Thorac Surg 1975;20:387.
15. Harrell GS, Friedland GW, Daily WJ, et al: Neonatal Boerhaave's syndrome. Radiology 1970;95:665.
16. Kerschner JE, Beste DJ, Conley SF, et al: Mediastinitis associated with foreign body erosion of the esophagus in children. Int J Pediatr Otorhinolaryngol 2001;59:89.
17. Kimura K, Kubo M, Okasora T, et al: Esophageal perforation in a neonate associated with gastroesophageal reflux. J Pediatr Surg 1984;19:191.
18. Krasna IH, Rosenfeld D, Benjamin BG, et al: Esophageal perforation in the neonate: An emerging problem in the newborn nursery. J Pediatr Surg 1987;22:784.
19. Lee HB, Kuhn JP: Esophageal perforation in the neonate. Am J Dis Child 1976;130:325.
20. Lynch FP, Coran AG, Cohen SR, et al: Traumatic esophageal pseudodiverticula in the newborn. J Pediatr Surg 1974;9:675.
21. Martinez L, Rivas S, Hernandez F, et al: Aggressive conservative treatment of esophageal perforations in children. J Pediatr Surg 2003;38:685.
22. Sartorelli KH, McBride WJ, Vane DW: Perforation of the intrathoracic esophagus from blunt trauma in a child: Case report and review of the literature. J Pediatr Surg 1999;34:495.
23. Wychulis AR, Fontana RS, Payne WS: Instrumental perforation of the esophagus. Dis Chest 1969;55:184.
24. Zorzi C, Perale R, Piovesan A, et al: Esophageal perforation in the newborn. Eur J Pediatr 1981;13:113.

第 67 章

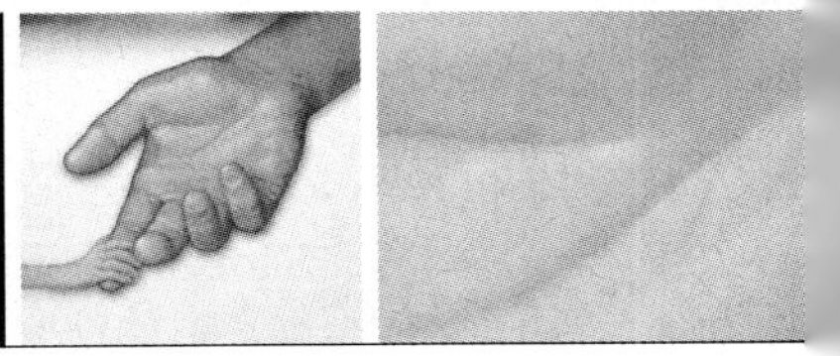

先天性食管异常

Carroll M. Harmon 和 Arnold G. Coran

1057 历史背景

食管闭锁（EA）的历史记载开始于 1670 年，William Durston 报道了“一例出生在普利茅斯的畸形儿”，他描述了一对胸部联体女婴中的一个食管上端呈袋状盲端[66]。首先描述食管闭锁合并典型食管气管瘘（EA-TEF）的是 1679 年 Thomas Gibson 的《人体解剖学》第 5 版[91]。独立的 EA-TEF 病例报道是在 19 世纪，包括 1840 年 Thomas Hill 在《波士顿内科学和外科学期刊》上报道的一个病例，该报道描述了一个有 EA-TEF 的婴儿伴直肠发育不全和直肠尿道瘘[106]。1861 年，哥本哈根的 Harald Hirschsprung 报道了他自己的 4 个病例，并且从文献中收集了 10 个 EA 和远端 TEF 病例[108]。1880 年，19 世纪另一个杰出的医学人物 Morell Mackenzie[165] 报道了 57 例先天性食管畸形和 37 例气管或者支气管食管瘘，还讨论了胚胎期的食管长度和这些畸形的临床诊断，并描述了伴发的畸形，如脊柱分裂、马蹄肾和无肛。E. D. Plass 是 Johns Hopkins 大学的产科学教师，他调查了 1919 年的文献，并报道了 136 例确切的 EA 病例，包括 92 例合并 TEF 的病例[199]。1931 年，Rosenthal 收集了 255 例患者的数据[215]并指出，如 Ladd 在 1944 年强调，“食管闭锁是比我们通常所想象的更为常见的畸形[143]。”

外科治疗 EA-TEF 的历史是值得注意的，自第一个描述和第一个患者存活以来已超过 270 年。1869 年，伦敦的 Timothy Holmes 在其发表的“儿童疾病的外科处理”一文中首先提出对不伴有 TEF 的 EA 婴儿行外科食管吻合是可能的，然而他补充说“我认为不应该进行这个尝试”[113]。第一个不伴有 TEA 的 EA 矫正手术是在 1888 年由伦敦 Charles Steele 进行的，他在题为“食管缺陷病例”的报道被刊登在《柳叶刀》杂志上[257]。在氯仿麻醉下，Steele 进行了胃造瘘，且试图用一细长钢质探子穿过胃造瘘部向上到达食管的下端盲袋，穿破他所怀疑的食管隔膜进入上端盲袋，同时用一个探针在食管内从上往下推[257]。这次尝试没有成功，在尸体解剖时发现食管“上、下各有一个盲端，间距为 1 英寸半（1 英寸 =2.54 厘米），而且两部分之间没有索带和连接”[257]。在 1899 年，Hoffman 完成了第一例 EA 婴儿的永久性胃造瘘术[111]。1913 年，芝加哥的 H. M. Richter 报道了他做的 2 例 EA-TEF 婴儿的手术，但是手术并没有成功。尽管这样，Richter 还是对一期食管修复手术可能取得成功持乐观态度，并强调“我不想放弃一期连接食管两盲端的想法”[214]。然而在同一年，一个在芝加哥与 Richter 一起工作的杰出儿科医生 J. Brennemann 在提到在 2 个婴儿尝试进行外科修补术的死亡结果时，认为“医生在做出了先天性食管闭锁的诊断后，决定让小患者没有干扰地死去是正当的”[20]。尽管 Richter 持乐观态度，但一期食管吻合术和无数的其他手术还是失败了，EA 的死亡率达到 100%。在 1925 年的胸外科教科书中，Lilienthal 指出，手术治疗可能应包括“分离食管气管瘘和在一个橡皮管固定模上缝合两端盲袋，吻合闭锁的食管”[151]。1936 年，新奥尔良和路易斯安那的 Mims Gage 和 Alton Oschner 提出，早期经腹部结扎食管的贲门端、胃造瘘和早期颈部食管造瘘术[86]。Riter 等人指出，“理想的手术是将食管与气管分离，并将食管的上下两部分端端吻合”[86]。“但是这样广泛的胸腔内手术不适用于新生儿，这个手术总是在死后完成。”

第一个报道 EA-TEF 结扎瘘管和一期食管吻合术的是得克萨斯州达拉斯的 Robert Shaw。Shaw 于 1938 年 9 月 25 日进行了该手术，并在 1939 年 12 月进行了报道[234]。他的报道中提到，他曾与 Paul C. Samson进行私人交流经验，后者也做过一个与此“非常相似的手术”。Samson 的患者死于手术后 12 小时。而 Shaw 的患者于手术后的第 12 天死亡，原因明显是输血反应。Shaw 进行手术时不知道 Thomas Lanman 已经于 1936 年 1 月 2 日至 1937 年 1 月 27 日期间在波士顿完成了 4 例 EA–TEF 的胸膜外进路一期食管修补术[146]。在 1940 年的 11 月，Lanman 报道了这 4 个病例，另外还有 1 例一期食管修补和 1929 年 9 月至 1940 年 2 月间在波士顿儿童医院所见的其他 27 例 EA。这 32 例患者相继死亡，然而 Lanman 的第 4 个患者通过结扎瘘管和一期食管修补后存活了 9 天，尸体检查中发现患儿死于补液过量，而不是由于纵隔炎症和肺炎。Lamnan 总结道：“尽管 30 个手术病例最终全部死亡，但是在合理的道路上正在取得巨大的进步。通过手术来治疗这种疾病只不过是一个时间问题。”

根据 Humphreys 和 Ferrer 的报道，第一例非 TEF 先天性食管闭锁存活患者是一位 1935 年 2 月 16 日在纽约出生的男孩，初期仅行胃造瘘术，“至 1946 年才行第一次开胸手术”[115]。最早的 EA–TEF 存活病例是一位 1939 年 11 月 26 日出生于明尼苏达州的男孩和一位第二天出生于马塞诸塞州的女孩。明尼苏达大学的 N. Logan Leven 在经历了多例 EA 婴儿治疗失败后，在 1939 年 11 月 29 日对 1 例 2500g 的 EA–TEF 男婴进行了胃造瘘术。在试图通过气管镜用电凝方法闭合 TEF 失败后，于 1940 年 1 月 5 日采用胸膜外结扎瘘管获得成功。当婴儿的体重增加到 4630g 时，于 1940 年 3 月 27 日进行了颈部的食管造瘘术。这个孩子成长良好，Leven 准备接下来行经胸的食管成形术重建胃肠道的连续性。1939 年 11 月 28 日波士顿的 William Ladd 进行了一例女婴的胃造瘘术，1940 年 3 月 15 日进行了 TEF 的闭合并进行了颈部食管造瘘术。尽管两名患儿都存活了，但是经多次手术，创建了一个用皮肤衬里的胸部新食管才实现了食管胃连续性的重建。

在 1935 年，密歇根州大学的 Cameron Haight 开始对 EA 婴儿进行治疗（图 67–1）。他的第一个患儿仅做了胃造瘘术，但没有成功。1939 年 Haight 第一次尝试 EA 一期修复而以失败告终。接下来尝试一期修补的 4 个患儿也失败了。然而在 1941 年 3 月 15 日 EA 一期修补术第一次取得成功。这是个“极其强壮”的女婴，12 天龄体重 8 磅 4 盎司（约 3118g），从密歇根的 Marquette 转到儿科主任 Harry A. Towsley 处就诊，Towsley 医生和 Haight 医生进行了会诊。

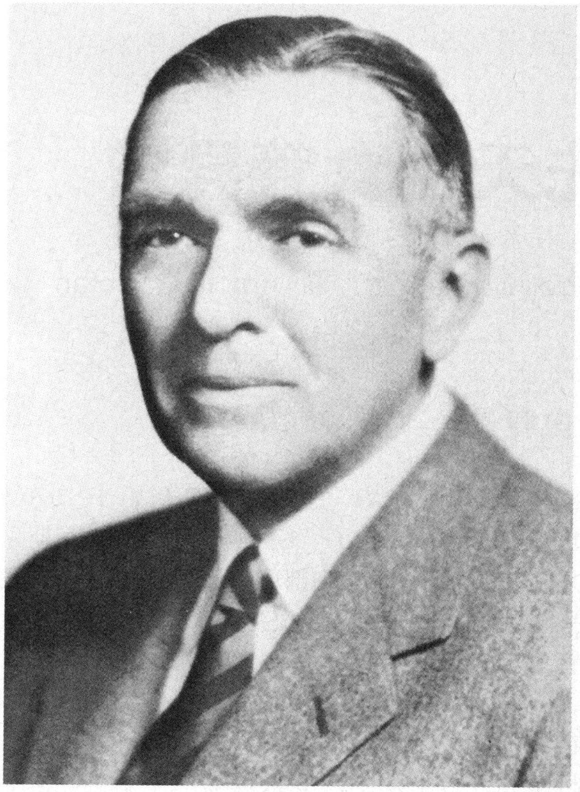

图 67–1 Cameron Haight，MD，在 1941 年 3 月 15 日成功完成第一例食管闭锁伴食管气管瘘的一期修复术。

第一个成功的 EA–TEF 一期修复病例是通过左侧胸膜外途径瘘管结扎和单层食管吻合术完成的。术后第六天出现了吻合口漏，但是没有通过外科手段干预即得到控制，之后形成吻合口狭窄，通过单纯的扩张而治愈。Haight 医生和 Towsley 医生于 1942 年 2 月在芝加哥中心外科协会会议上介绍了这个病例，并在 1943 年发表了报告[101]。在 1943 年，Haight 医生改从右侧胸膜外进路，他认为从该侧可以更好地暴露远端的食管段。他也进行了双层缝合的改良，希望“望远镜式”的吻合可以降低出现漏的风险。在 1939—1969 年，Haight 治疗了 284 例 EA 婴儿，并且总存活率为 52%[100]。自 1941 年 Haight 第一次成功之后，直接行食管吻合术后存活的报道是零星的；然而，很多医疗中心很快开始报道连续的成功案例。1947 年，Longmire（发表了一篇有趣的报道）描述了连续成功的 4 例一期食管吻合术，其中包括 1 例仅重 1.4kg 的婴儿[162]。

在对 EA 分类的过程中所用的术语不同，但是畸

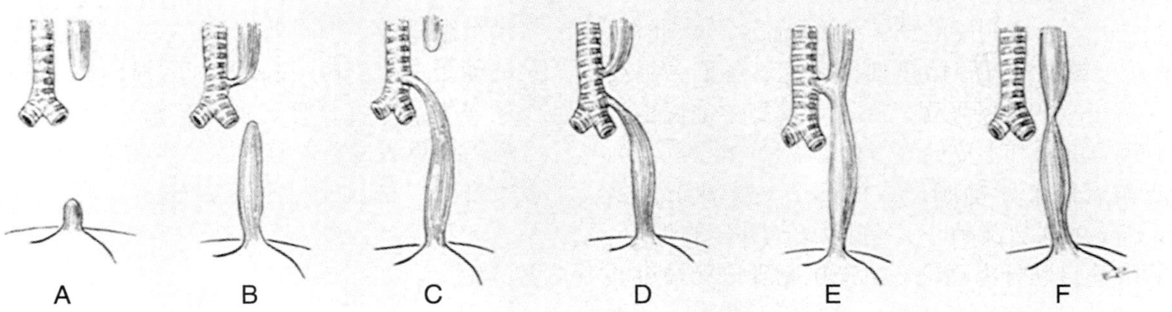

图 67-2 食管闭锁畸形解剖类型的大致分型。A. 食管闭锁且不伴气管食管瘘。该畸形几乎总是连有“长间隙”。B. 食管闭锁伴近端气管食管瘘。这种畸形并不常见；腹腔内无气体，诊断可能被遗漏，除非行造影检查或者内镜检查。C. 食管闭锁伴远端气管食管瘘管，是最常见的食管畸形。D. 食管闭锁伴有双瘘管（近端和远端）。虽然很少见，但这个类型比原本料想的要多见。E. 气管食管瘘不伴有食管闭锁（H 型瘘管）。这个畸形可能在新生儿期被漏诊，因为患儿可以吞咽。它常伴有反复的咳嗽、肺炎和腹胀。F. 食管狭窄。(From Gross RE: Surgery of Infancy and Childhood. Philadelphia, WB Saunders, 1953.)

1053 形的种类并没有区别。1929 年，放射学家 E. C. Vogt 做了以下的畸形分类[290]：1 型，食管缺失；2 型，EA 不伴有 TEF；3 型，EA 合并 TEF；3a 型，EA 合并近段 TEF；3b 型，EA 合并远端 TEF；3c 型，EA 合并 TEF，上下食管段与气管之间都有瘘；4 型，孤立的 TEF 伴完整的食管。随着手术修补的成功，又出现了其他的解剖学分类法。在 1944 年 Ladd 介绍了数字分类法，共分为五种类型，以罗马字母标注[143]。1953，Gross 将这个数字系统改为一个字母顺序系统，至今仍常被应用（图 67-2）[97]。1962 年，Swenson 改回到数字分类，并用阿拉伯数字代替罗马数字[179]。1976 年，Kluth 发表了完整的列表，描述了各种不同的 EA，包括 10 个单独的类别和补充的亚类。

作为解剖学分类的补充，1962 年伦敦儿童医院的 D. J. Waterston、R. E. Bonham Carter 和 Eoin Aberdeen 提出了一种与婴儿 EA 危险因素相关的分类系统[293]，可不同时间和不同医院的病例进行预后比较。该方案基于出生体重、有无肺炎存在和有无相关先天性畸形进行分类，可明确其预后因素并指导手术治疗，这种 EA 畸形的分类法对患儿的治疗有重要的贡献（表 67-1）。

表 67-1 Waterston 风险分组和目前生存率数据

组	生存率（%）	Waterston 分级
A	100	出生体重＞2500g，其他方面健康
B	85	出生体重 2000～2500g 且健康，或体重稍高伴有中度畸形（无心脏畸形加动脉导管未闭，室间隔缺损和房间隔缺损）
C	65	出生体重＜2000g，或体重稍重但伴严重心脏畸形

胚胎学

EA 畸形的发病机制目前还不清楚。尽管有很多的理论来解释 EA、EA-TEF 和 TEF 的病因，但是根据解剖学的分组没有统一的理论。因为大多数 EA 畸形是散发的，它很可能并不是由简单的遗传基因机制所致，因此其发病机制可能是各不相同和多因素的，涉及多个基因和复杂的基因环境之间的相互作用。

由于对正常前肠胚胎学不完全了解，因此仍不能完全解释 EA 畸形的发病机制。Wilhelm His, Sr.是人类胚胎学的奠基人，最早描述了正常呼吸系统的发育[109]。他认为前肠的分开是由于内陷的侧面纵向嵴融合的结果，形成隔膜将前肠分为背侧的消化道和腹侧的呼吸系统。上述所谓的气管食管隔膜是从尾端开始至头端终止而形成的，关于 EA 畸形发病机制的很多理论都在这些描述的基础上的[98,215,240,242,258]。但是，最近一些研究者几乎没有发现能够支持这个前肠分裂和发育理论的证据。卡内基研究所从所收集的胚胎中再

次研究人类标本提示，侧方的前肠壁嵴向内生长，在人类胚胎中并不形成头端的气管食管隔膜[188,302]。此外，
1054 Kluth 等人[133]通过电子显微镜扫描研究了各期的小鸡胚胎以了解正常的前肠发育。在这个模型中他们也没有发现有侧方的嵴和上皮性气管食管隔膜的证据。

最近解释胚胎学前肠形成的几个主要理论是由 Kluth 和 Fiegel 总结出的[132]，包括食管闭合的理论、食管气管隔膜自动分离理论、机械机制理论和最近的致畸剂（阿霉素）在鼠的模型中诱导 EA 畸形的新理论[132]。

在讨论包括食管闭锁在内的肠闭锁发病机制时，前肠闭塞和肠腔再通失败的理论在历史上是卓越的[139,265]。食管上皮的过度增殖可能在罕见的膜性食管闭锁的发育中起着一定的作用，但是如果作为解释典型食管闭锁畸形的理论还不够全面[131]。如上所述，关于气管食管隔膜移行异常的发病学说是非常著名的[98,215,240,242,258]。然而，由于缺乏证据表明正常的前肠形成过程中存在这个结构，所以其理论重要性被降低。关于在前肠发育中受到机械性压迫而导致食管闭锁的胚胎发生这些学说目前仍被继续讨论。

然而 Cozzi 等人[50,176]和其他研究者[192]也提出了另一套理论，他们认为食管闭锁是头端神经嵴病变的组成部分。观察发现，神经嵴相关的心血管畸形（主动脉弓、圆锥动脉干畸形和膜性室间隔缺损）以及胸腺、甲状腺、甲状旁腺和面部畸形等都与食管闭锁有明显的联系，如在 DiGorge 综合征中所见，表明食管闭锁的发病机制可能与鳃弓发育缺陷有关。

在动物模型中用阿霉素作致畸剂导致胚胎出现了各种不同的畸形，比如食管闭锁和食管气管瘘，这种动物模型已有报道，并且有希望为研究食管闭锁的发病机制提供新的视角[60,269]。Merei 和 Hutson 用这个模型发展了一种理论，指出原始的前肠发育成为气管，继而引起食管闭锁和食管气管瘘畸形[173]。Gittes 最近用这个模型和人类的食管气管瘘组织标本对分子学机制进行了研究，该机制在食管闭锁和食管气管瘘的发病机制中可能起到了一定的作用。他提出远端的瘘管和食管来源于呼吸道，肺的形态发育缺陷是导致食管闭锁和食管气管瘘畸形发生的原因[51,245]。

一些分子和途径已经被认为在食管闭锁和食管气管瘘发病机制中起一定的作用。Spitz 提出在肢体和前肠的形成中，基因的 HOX D 组可能和 VACTERL（脊柱、肛门直肠、贲门、气管食管、肾和肢体畸形）连锁[249]。Gittes 报道在鼠的模型[244]和人的气管食管瘘组织[244]中，细胞外信号途径的缺陷、促进器官分化的糖蛋白（Shh）在食管气管瘘的发生中起重要的作用。为了了解食管气管瘘及相关畸形的发病机制，今后需要更清楚地了解细胞、生物化学和基因的信号以及和正常的细胞-细胞与细胞-间质之间的相互关系。

流行病学

有或无 TEF（EA ± TEF）的 EA 发生率差异较大，在芬兰新生儿中为 1/2440[142]，在美国[101]和澳大利亚[180]新生儿中为 1/4500。最近加利福尼亚的出生婴儿缺陷检测项目的数据表明，1983—1988 年间 EA、EA-TEF 和单独 TEF 的总发病率为每 10 000 名新生儿中 2.82 例[274]。欧洲 1980—1988 年间 EA-TEF 的发病率为 10 000 个新生儿 2.86 例，不过其发病率随时间逐年下降[57]。在欧洲的研究中，有 62% 的 EA-TEF 婴儿为男性，而加利福尼亚的数据发现，各种类型食管闭锁的男女比率有很大的不同，仅有 TEF 缺陷的男女比例为 2.29，EA-TEF 的为 1.44，仅有 EA 者为 1.33[274]。非白种人的 EA-TEF 和 TEF 发病率比白种人低[102,274]。也有报道称，第一次怀孕，怀孕年龄小于 20 者[57]或怀孕年龄过大者[19,274]发生 EA-TEF 的风险增高。

多胞胎对于每一种 EA-TEF 类型的发生率都较高（对照组 TEF 3.7%；EA-TEF 4.9%；单纯 EA 8.8%）[102,274]。染色体异常也常见于 EA 的婴儿，6%～10%的婴儿存在某种类型的 EA[57,102]，这些畸形包括染色体 13 三体 和 18 三体综合征，以及常被描述的 VACTERL 多发畸形。

除了上述的阿霉素可引起鼠模型 EA-TRF 以外，环境致畸剂也被提示为 EA ± TEF 的发病机制之一。EA 可发生于母亲长期服用避孕物[263]和在怀孕期间接触雌激素的婴儿[184]。此外据报道，EA 发生在一些母亲患有甲状腺功能亢进[228]、糖尿病以及受孕后用过安眠药物[36]的婴儿中。

虽然 EA 通常是散发性的，但也有报道发生于伴有多种基因综合征的婴儿，包括 DiGeorge 综合征[125]、多脾综合征、Holt-Oram 综合征、Pierre Robin 综合征[200]和 Feingold 综合征[31]。很多研究描述了横向和纵

表 67-2 合并畸形的发病率

心血管	≈35%
泌尿生殖系统	≈24%
消化系统	≈24%
神经系统	≈12%
肌肉骨骼	≈20%
VACTERL 联合畸形	≈20%
总的发生率	50%～70%

注：VACTERL：脊柱、肛门直肠、心脏、气管食管、肾和肢体畸形。

向的家族性 EA 病例。文献报道有一个 EA 患儿的双亲再次生出 EA 患儿的风险为 0.5%～2.0%，如果同胞中有一个以上患有 EA，其双亲再次生出 EA 患儿的风险增至 20%[200]。如父母中有一个 EA 患者，生出 EA 患儿的风险为 3%～4%。

合并畸形

在器官形成的早期，干扰会导致 EA 畸形，无论
1055 确切原因是什么，也会影响其他器官系统。其他先天性畸形常合并 EA，这些合伴畸形常对治疗和生存有重要的影响（表 67-2）。大量报道表明，50%～70%的 EA 患儿至少存在一种合并的先天性畸形。这些畸形最常见于有 EA 而没有 TEF 的病例，而最不常见于 H 型的 TEF 患儿[112]。心血管畸形发生的频率最高（11%～49%）[59,62,148,176]，其次是泌尿生殖系统畸形（24%）[14]、胃肠道畸形（24%）[253]和肌肉骨骼系统畸形（13%～22%）[89,285]。神经系统相关的畸形包括神经管缺陷（2.3%）、脑积水（5.2%）、前脑无裂畸形（2.3%）和无眼畸形或者小眼畸形（3.7%）[102]。其他的畸形有后鼻孔闭锁（5.2%）、面裂（7.2%）、腹壁缺损（4.3%）和膈疝（2.9%）[102]。最近一个报道显示，某些合并畸形的发病率可能因地区而不同，泌尿生殖畸形异常的发生率在欧洲为 26%，而在亚洲只有 4%[285]。

在致死性 EA 合并畸形中，复杂心脏缺陷合并 EA 畸形所导致的死亡最多。相对死亡风险在 EA 畸形合并重要心脏畸形的婴儿中为 3.47（95%置信区间，1.51～7.96）[62,248]。Leonard 等人报道在 153 例 EA 患儿中，先天性心脏病（CHD）患儿的 1 年生存率是 67%，而无先天性心脏病的患儿为 95%[148]。有趣的是，这些作者总结认为，尽管 CHD 伴有 EA 者有较高的死亡率，但这不是直接导致死亡的直接原因[148]。最常见的单纯缺陷是室间隔缺损（19%）和房间隔缺损（20%）[59]，前者的死亡率为 16%。其他常见的心脏畸形包括法洛四联症（5%）和动脉导管未闭（13%）[59]。1%～4%的 EA 畸形婴儿合并存在大动脉缩窄[59,278]。4%的 EA 患儿报告有右位降主动脉[59]。

EA-TEF 合并的胃肠道畸形有肛门直肠畸形（14%）[59]、十二指肠闭锁（2%）[59]、肠旋转不良（4%）[41]、回肠闭锁、环状胰腺、幽门狭窄等。泌尿生殖系统的缺陷包括肾发育不全（1%）、尿道下裂、隐睾、肾囊性病、肾盂积水、膀胱输尿管反流、输尿管重复、肾盂输尿管梗阻和膀胱输尿管梗阻、脐尿管畸形、两性畸形、泄殖腔畸形和膀胱外翻[14,47,102]。典型的骨骼肌肉畸形包括四肢（15%）和脊柱（17%）畸形等[59]。

1973 年，Quan 和 Smith[207]提出了一系列与 EA 并发的畸形。他们将这些并发畸形以首字母缩写词 VATER 命名：脊柱缺陷、肛门闭锁、气管食管瘘、食管闭锁和直肠缺陷。“并发”的定义为“非随机发生在 2 个或 2 个以上个体的多发先天性畸形，而不是多处缺陷、序列或综合征”[48]。患者无畸形的家族史，无明确的致畸剂接触史，无染色体异常。由于表型数目增多，该综合征的缩写改为 VACTERL，包括脊柱、肛门直肠、心脏、食管气管、直肠和四肢的畸形[12]。EA 伴发 VACTERL 的发生率大约为 20%[62]。有 EA-TEF 的婴儿经常有 VACTERL 畸形（脊柱 17%，肛门 12%，心脏 20%，直肠 16%，肢体 10%），以及其他的中线的畸形（唇裂和腭裂 2%，骶部畸形 2%，泌尿生殖系统畸形 5%）[28]。“肾的畸形”中应包括尿道畸形，比如巨输尿管、输尿管重复畸形、输尿管瓣膜、狭窄和尿道下裂等。最近，已描述 VACTERL-H 并发畸形，包括先天性脑积水。EA 畸形患儿合并 VACTERL 的死亡率升高。Iuchtman 等人分析了 313 例 EA、TET 或两者兼有的病例中 46 例出生时有 EA 和合并 VACTERL 特征的婴儿的结果，该组死亡率达 24%。心血管畸形存在于 78%的患者，而且是死亡的主要原因。最近 Driver 等人报道，并发 VACTERL 的病例发生死亡的相对风险为 2.54（95%的置信区间，1.14～4.86）[62]。

关于 EA 畸形合并其他多部位缺陷、序列、综合征或合并症的描述不断增多。其中包括 Down 综合征[18]、DiGeorge 综合征[125]、多脾综合征、Holt-Oram综合

征、Pierre Robin 综合征[200]、Feingold 综合征[31]、Fanconi 综合征、Townes–Brock 综合征、Bartsocas–Papas 综合征、McKusick–Kaufman 综合征、CHARGE 联合（眼缺损、心脏缺陷、后鼻孔闭锁、发育迟缓、生殖器发育不全、耳畸形）和 schisis 联合（脐膨出、神经管缺陷、唇裂腭裂、生殖发育不全）[38,250]。其他严重或致命的联合有 18 三体综合征、脑发育不全、Potter 综合征（双侧肾发育不全）[201,254]。除了上述提到的与 EA 相关的畸形外，很多最近的报道描述了严重的畸形和相关情况。EA–TEF 合并单侧肺发育不全
1055 非常罕见，自 1874 年至今，只有 37 例报道[35,110,130,160,222,246,256]。Usui 等人[281]报道了伴发食管气管畸形的发生率有 47%，如右上肺支气管异位或缺如、先天性支气管狭窄以及环状软骨性气管对膜性气管的比例下降。气管软化和肺膨胀不全伴 EA 等呼吸道畸形有重要的意义。一些报道也提出了 EA 合并有不影响外科食管缺陷修补的迷走神经分布区域异常[54]。

分型

在来自六项大型病例报道的 2200 多例不同类型的食管畸形中，各种畸形类型的发生率列于表 67–3。

如上所述，曾有人提出各种分型方法并将其用于描述 EA。尽管很多医院和外科医生仍用 Gross 分型，但最有效和最实用的分类方法可能是简单的解剖分类法，如表 67–3 所示。值得注意的是，表中的解剖分型描述还有许多其他的变异型。1976 年，Kluth[131]总结并列出了很多上述各种分类法未提到的畸形。

1962 年，Waterston 的分型是基于危险因素根据出生体重、肺炎和合并先天畸形将 EA–TEF 的婴儿进行了分型（图 67–1）。这种分型可决定患者的外科手术治疗。“良好型”风险类别（A）的婴儿可立即手术修补治疗；“中等”风险的婴儿（B）应延期修补，“高”风险婴儿（C）通过分期手术修补。尽管 Waterston 分型仍被用于比较各医院的疗效，但很多研究者对它目前治疗这些婴儿的效度提出了疑问[201,209,253]。随着现代新生儿危重症治疗的进展，越来越多的低体重儿得以存活，并且对先天性多发畸形的婴儿有了更多的治疗方法。因此对生存率现代标准的研究结果产生了一些新的分型方法。

1989 年，Randolph 等人[209]建议在 EA 婴儿的生理学情况的基础上对 Waterston 的分型进行改进。根据分析，39 例婴儿根据生理学情况进行分型处理后，更多病例更早地实施了一期修补术。并与 87 例以前用 Waterston 标准分型的婴儿比较，结果生理学情况稳定的婴儿有非常高的存活率[209]。

最近有人提出其他的预后分型法。Poenaru 等人[201]提出，只有严重的肺功能不全、需要术前机械通气和合并严重畸形才是独立的生存预后因素。Brown 和 Tam[29]提出了测量食管间隙长度进行分型的方法，可预测术后病死率和远期预后。Spitz 等人回顾了 1980—1992 年间伦敦 Great Ormond 大街儿童医院收治的 375 例 EA，发现出生体重和主要心血管疾病是重要的生存率预后因素，分析的结果见表 67–4[116]。Spitz 分类是目前最常用的分类系统[62,135]。最近有人又提出一种新的分类系统，对 Spitz的危险因子补充了术前呼吸道窘迫综合征和肺炎[299]。

表 67–3 各种食管畸形的发生率

类型	发生率（%）	Gross 分型
1. 食管闭锁伴有远端气管食管瘘	85.8	C
2. 食管闭锁不伴有气管食管瘘	7.8	A
3. 气管食管瘘无食管闭锁	4.2	E
4. 食管闭锁，两盲端各有一个瘘管	1.4	D
5. 食管闭锁伴近端食管气管瘘	0.8	B

表 67–4 Spitz 分级：食管畸形病例的生存率预测

分组	生存率（%）
I. 出生体重＞1500g，不伴有严重的先天性心脏病	97
II. 出生体重＜1500g 或伴有严重的先天性心脏病	59
III. 出生体重＜1500g 伴有严重的先天性心脏病	22

诊断和临床表现

与许多先天性小儿外科疾病不同，产前很少可以诊断出 EA。产前超声检查 EA 是根据发现一个小的胃泡或者无胃泡并伴有母亲羊水过多而推断的[76]。然而，根据这些标准，产前超声检查对诊断 EA 的预测价值只有 20%～40%[243,259]。超声检查在胎儿颈中部发现无回声区、合并出现羊水过多和小胃，则可增加产前诊断的准确性[223]。最近有报告表明，胎儿核磁共振成像可能在超声检查怀疑 EA 畸形时提供有效的产前诊断[145,170]。

大多数 EA 的婴儿在出生后数小时出现症状。最早的临床表现通常是进行性流涎，这是由于咽后方分
1057 泌物淤积所致。通常在第一次喂奶后出现反流、窒息和咳嗽。其他特征表现是喂食或不喂食时出现发绀、呼吸窘迫、吞咽困难、不能将经口腔或鼻腔插入的饲养管或吸引管插入胃内。如果存在远端瘘管，吸气时气体通过瘘管进入胃中可引起腹部膨胀。当胃内的液体通过 TEF 流入气管和肺，并继而导致化学性肺炎时，肺的损害可以非常明显。当由于吸入气体引起腹部扩张时，横膈（新生儿呼吸时的主要肌肉）抬高，肺部状况恶化。从上部的盲端吸入唾液进入气管可进一步加重肺的损害。

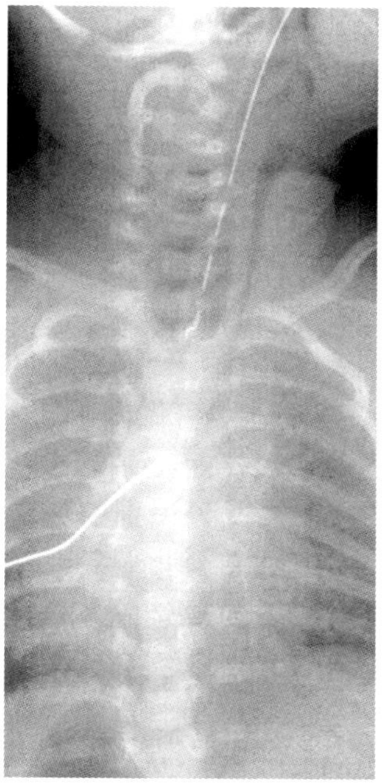

图 67-3 在注入 2ml 的空气后，放射线胸部平片提示“Replogle”管位于上食管盲端内。

EA 的诊断可以通过将导管经口腔插入食管后遇到阻力点得到明确。可通过导管注入几毫升气体，作为造影剂扩张上端食管盲端，并摄下正、侧位片(图 67-3)。必要时可用 0.5～1.0ml 稀释的钡剂作为对比剂注入上方盲端以确定诊断（图 67-4）。仔细控制荧光透视，钡剂也可能发现近端的 TEF。但是在新生儿病

图 67-4 注入 0.5～1.0ml 的稀释钡剂后，前位片（A）和后位片（B）显示上端食管盲端。

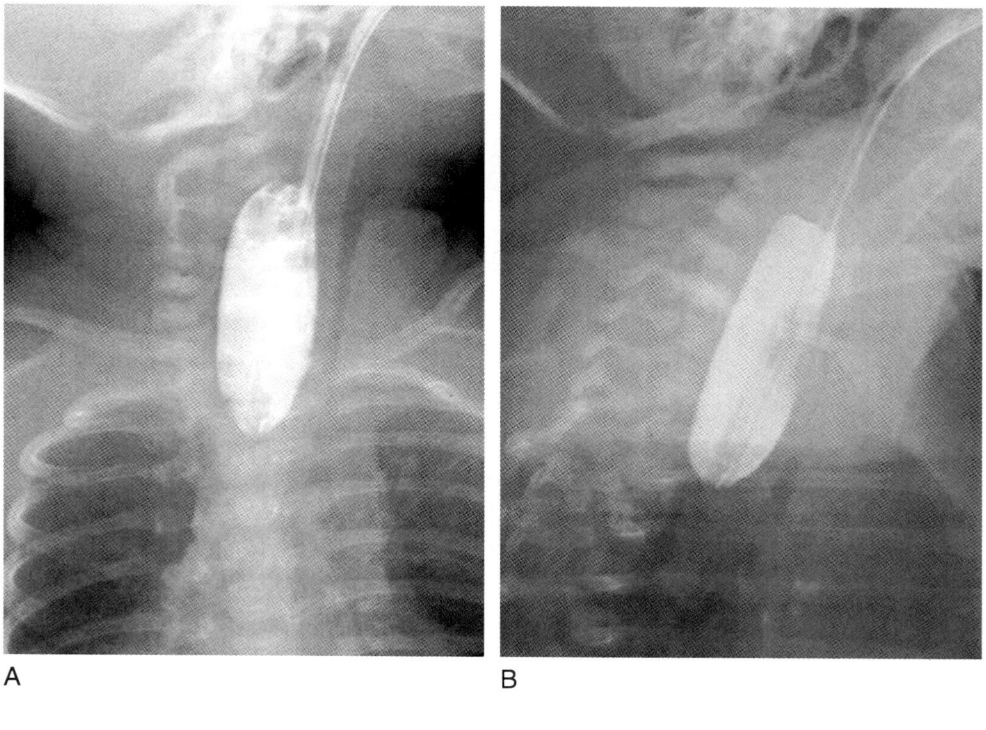

A B

房常用的便携式摄片机下，气管支气管树内的钡剂很像是通过喉部吸入的造影剂所致，而不像通过近端 TEF 吸入所致。小的上端盲袋可以提示存在近端 TEF。胃和肠内有气体可证实存在远端的 TEF。腹腔内无气体是独立 EA 不伴有 TEF 的典型表现（图 67–5）。然而，根据报道描述，在肠道内无气体时行开胸手术可发现存在狭窄或者闭塞的远端瘘管[93,193]。不伴有 TEF的 EA 诊断较困难，应对有临床表现者高度怀疑。通过患儿俯卧位的食管钡剂造影可做出诊断（图 67–6），但
1058 是通常需要通过气管镜或食管镜检查来明确诊断。

如上所述，EA 合并可识别的先天性缺陷的发生率为 50%～70%，因此在诊断性评估 EA 时应考虑有无此类其他畸形的临床证据。除体格检查以外，应注意有无联合畸形（如 VACTERL 联合），其他检查通常包括心脏超声检查、肾脏超声波检查、染色体分析等。实际上，在伴发 EA 的临床表现和症状出现之前，先发现有肛门直肠畸形并不罕见。

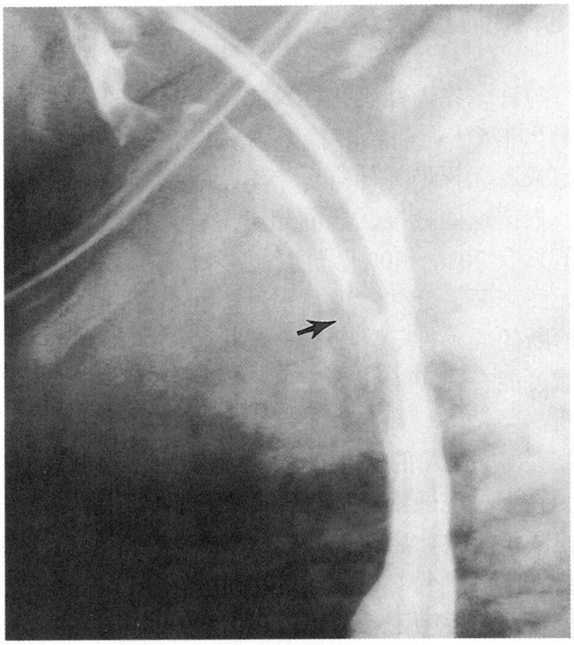

图 67–6 通过鼻食管管注入造影剂后，可见一个 H 型的气管食管瘘。造影剂通过瘘管（箭头所示）进入食管，注入并充盈气管上端和喉部。

术前治疗

有 EA–TEF 的婴儿，上端盲袋分泌物误吸入肺和胃酸通过 TEF 反流而引起肺炎是术前处理中最为关键的问题。即刻处理的措施包括防止进一步吸入和肺炎。应将一导管放入上端的食管盲端，持续低压吸出涎液。双腔 Replogle 型导管是最好的处理管道，因为它仅在导管前端附近的侧方有多个小孔，这样可减少从喉部吸走含氧气的空气。婴儿应取适当的体位以减少胃液向上通过 TEF 反流。通常主张采取竖直坐位（图 67–7），但有一些作者认为抬头俯卧位是降低反流最有效的位置。同样，也需要开始应用广谱抗生素和肺部的理疗。静脉内补液开始应用 10%右旋葡萄糖和低张液体以保持体液、电解质和糖的平衡。术前还应该给以维生素 K 制剂。应该避免常规气管内插管，因为有导致胃穿孔的危险，并且通过 TEF 的通气可引起腹部膨胀继而加重呼吸窘迫。

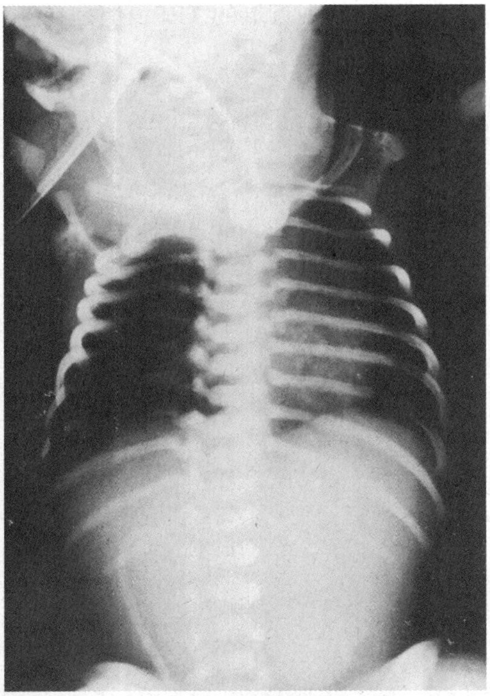

图 67–5 小肠不充气表明存在孤立的食管闭锁且不伴有气管食管瘘管。稀释的钡剂充盈食管上端的盲端。

手术修补

EA 婴儿的手术方法很大程度上取决于所存在畸形的类型和是否已发生合并畸形。

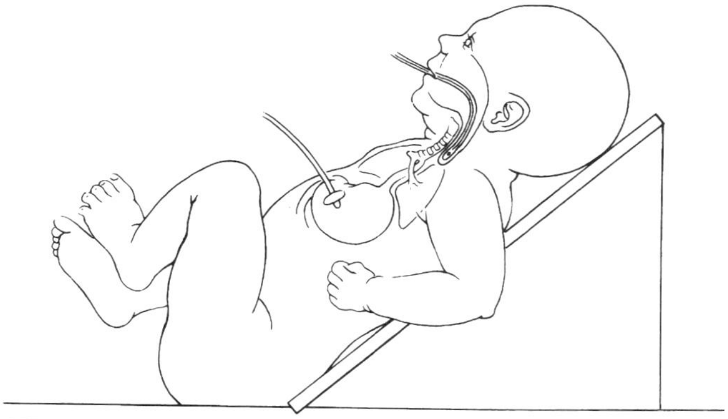

图 67-7　食管闭锁-气管食管瘘的婴儿体位，以尽量减少胃反流和气管上端食管盲端分泌物的吸入。一双腔管被放置在食管上端的盲袋处。个别情况下，在食管闭锁-气管食管瘘修补前放置胃造瘘管。

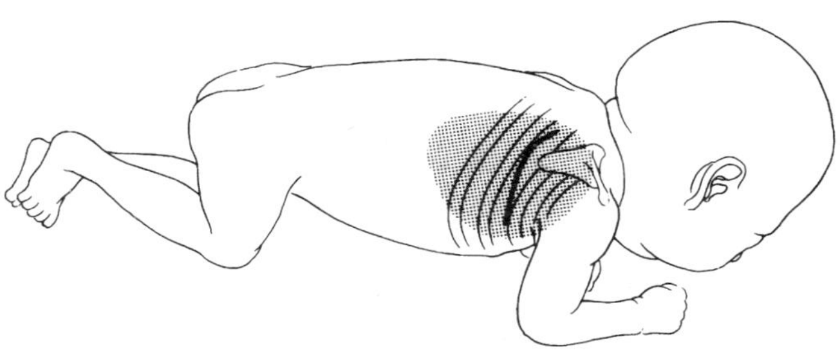

图 67-8　有或者没有气管食管瘘的婴儿食管闭锁手术时的体位。经第 4 肋间隙进入胸腔，开始胸膜外分离。

1059 食管狭窄伴远端气管食管瘘

EA 合并远端 TEF 一般不需要立即手术，做出诊断 24～48 小时后手术可对婴儿进行全面评估并治疗肺功能不全，包括肺不张和肺炎。大多数患儿有手术治疗的适应证，可行瘘管分离和一期食管吻合。

当前的麻醉技术包括少量应用术前用药，小心的气管插管以充分通气同时使通过瘘管的气流量最小，通常手控通气直至瘘管结扎。患儿常取标准的右后外侧开胸术体位，右臂向头侧伸展，头稍屈曲。如果术前心动超声检查时右位主动脉弓（2.5%），则优先采用左侧开胸术。但是，双侧主动脉弓并不少见，从而导致左胸进路也比较困难[9]。先围绕肩胛骨下缘做弧形的皮肤切口，从腋前线向后延伸至脊柱旁区（图 67-8）。用电刀将皮下组织和胸壁肌肉切开，这样可上提肩胛骨和识别第 4 肋间隙。经第 4 肋间切开肋间肌进胸，小心避免切开胸膜。大多数小儿外科医生仍主张行胸膜外 EA-TEF 修补，因为出现吻合口漏不会导致脓胸，而仅会引起食管皮下瘘，通常会在 1～2 周内闭合。采用经胸途径手术的外科医生则认为手术时间可缩短，结合抗生素的应用，吻合口漏引起脓胸的风险很小。采用胸膜外途径手术时，将胸膜轻柔地从胸壁推开，使肋间撑开器可以插入。在肋骨扩张器不断撑开的同时用湿纱布或拭子分离前内侧胸膜（图 67-9）。进一步胸膜后分离，将肺和胸膜轻轻推向内侧，暴露奇静脉并予以结扎离断。后纵隔暴露后，可识别近端盲袋、远端 TEF 气管和迷走神经。在瘘管水平将食管的远端部分行环状游离，并注意保护支配远端食管的迷走神经纤维。用粗丝线、纱布带或血管圈套围绕食管远端进行牵引，避免瘘管中的空气进入胃，并有助于暴露创面以便进行瘘管关闭。闭合瘘管时通常使用 5-0 或 6-0 丝线或者聚丙烯缝线进

图 67-9　胸膜外分离时用湿的纱布或拭子可有助于将壁层胸膜从胸壁和后纵隔上推开。

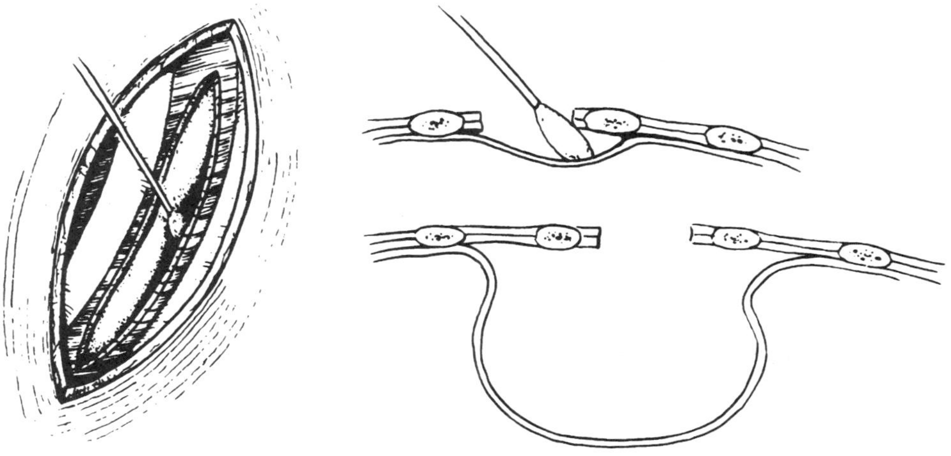

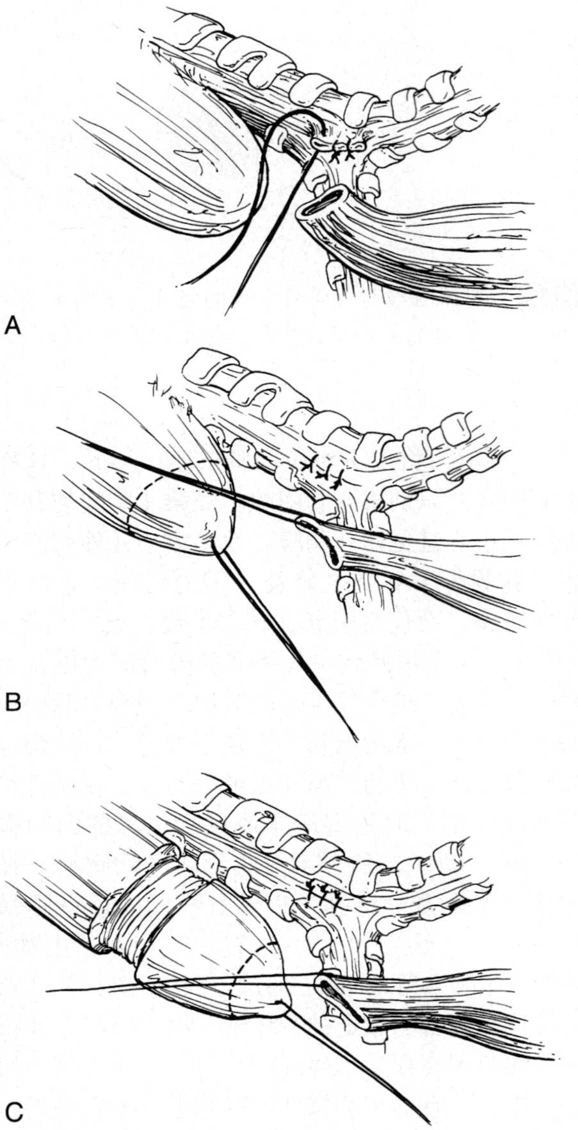

图 67-10 A. 用 5-0 或 6-0 不可吸收线缝合气管食管瘘管开口。B. 评估两个食管段一期吻合的可行性。C. 近端食管肌层切开，使食管延长。(From Rowe M, O'Neill JA, Grosfeld JL, et al: Essentials of Pediatric Surgery. St Louis, Mosby Year Book, 1995.)

行间断缝合（图 67-10）。重要的是瘘管的气管端应保留 1～2mm 的食管，以尽量减少出现术后气管狭窄的可能。关闭气管后的密闭性可通过在胸腔注入生理盐水、观察在正压通气下有无气泡冒出来的试验来检测。

应将一小的导管插入远端食管，以保证管腔大小足够并且畅通无阻，并吸出胃内的空气舒缓胃胀。在远端食管开口处先缝 2 针细的牵引线以便在游离时轻轻牵引，远端食管游离的范围不能过大，以免损伤迷走神经分支和该节段的血供，但为了保证一期吻合的成功，如果有必要，一定要进行远端游离。麻醉师从 1060
口腔插入至近端食管盲端缓慢推动吸引管，可有助于识别食管上端的盲袋。穿过食管盲袋的顶部做一牵引缝线，该牵引线缝合时甚至可穿过吸引管，以辅助近端的切开，并避免由于反复应用血管钳分离近端盲端所造成的损伤。上端食管盲袋应充分游离，使其可下拉抵达远端食管段。通常需要游离到胸廓入口处方可。近端食管盲袋的广泛环状分离也有助于发现有无未明确诊断的近端 TEF（1.4%的病例）。因为近端食管的颈部血供非常好，这种广泛的游离切开没有造成局部血供缺血受损的危险。但是在分离食管和膜状气管时应十分小心，以免意外切开气管。不幸的是，近端解剖越广泛，越容易损伤迷走神经的分支。

上端食管盲袋的末端最低处切予以切除，直径应与远端食管腔直径相当。在两侧进行牵引线缝合，后壁应行端端吻合，用 5-0 或 6-0 缝线进行间断缝合，结打在腔内，应务必注意做到食管壁的全层缝合，包括黏膜和肌肉层（图 67-11）。上端盲端的黏膜通常会回缩，因而手术大夫若不注意则很容易遗漏。除非两个食管端距离非常近，否则最好在后排缝线全部放置好后再一一打结。然后将细的胃管插入，并通过吻合口抵达胃，以保证远端食管的通畅，并在必要时可 1061
术后早期给予喂养[175,230,262]。然后，在胃管的表面进行食管前壁吻合，缝线打结在食管外面。食管吻合术所用缝线材料的类型与术后食管狭窄的关系已成争论的焦点。在对术后形成吻合口狭窄的回顾分析中，Chittmittrapap 等[39]对采用编织丝线与聚丙烯线或聚乙醇酸缝线进行了比较，前者的狭窄发生率较高，且具有统计学显著性意义。

吻合口完成后，如果需要保留胃管在术后给予胃肠减压和喂养，则应保证管道的位置恰当。通常在胸膜后间隙置胸腔引流管或闭式吸引引流，并用宽松的可吸收线缝合固定在侧胸壁。引流管应放置在稍远离吻合口处。有些外科医生在胸膜后分离后并不留置胸壁或胸腔引流管[196]。

在伴有远端 TEF 的 EA 婴儿，另一种处理瘘管和联合食管两端的方法是 Sulamaa 等人[260]创立的端一侧吻合术，该术式后又获得了 Duhamel 和其他人[64,198,275]的支持。这个技术是简单的结扎瘘管，上端的盲袋下移到下端食管段处，做一个宽、斜的端侧吻合。因为

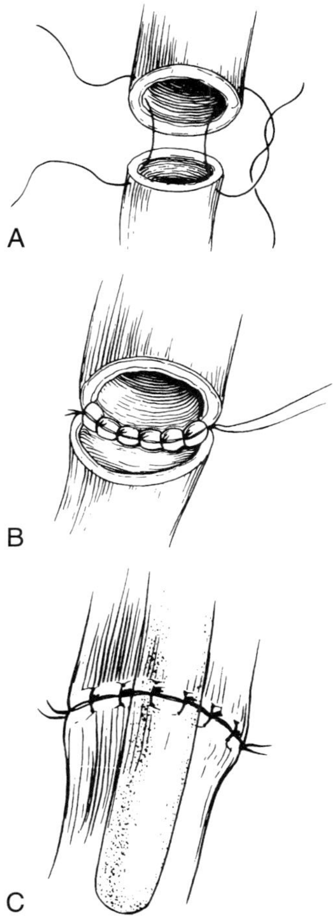

图 67-11　单层食管吻合法。A. 吻合口的两侧各缝一针，将结打在腔外。B. 后排的缝合打结在腔内。C. 前排缝合（在胃管上面），线结打在腔外。(From Rowe M, O'Neill JA, Grosfeld JL, et al: Essentials of Pediatric Surgery. St Louis, Mosby-Year Book, 1995.)

考虑到有 TEF 的复发的可能，所以该方法还没有被广泛接受。然而，Touloukian 等人[275]在 68 例采用该方法治疗的婴儿中发现 TEF 的复发率是 7%，这与大量的端-端吻合重建手术病例的复发率相似或者更低。此外，其他并发症的发生率，如狭窄（5%）、吻合口漏（8%）以及胃食管反流（GRE）（6%）要比其他端-端吻合重建术后相应的发生率都低。

近年来，儿童微创内镜手术被提倡，许多外科医生已建立并提倡胸腔镜下修补 EA-TEF[13,217,218]。该技术通常采用三个 2.5～5mm 的经胸套管针，一个成角的望远镜头、一个视频照相机和一些小直径（2.5～5mm）的操作器械。为明确和结扎 TEF，牵拉近端食管盲袋，用与开胸手术相类似的方法进行端端食管吻合术（图 67-12）。到目前为止，已有一些小婴儿胸腔镜 EA-TEF 修补术的报道，全世界很多的小儿外科医生已经采用了该方法。提倡者认为这个手术的优点是视频清晰可见、切口美观，并且可以减少新生儿开胸手术并发症，包括脊柱侧凸、翼状肩胛骨、慢性疼痛、肩部薄弱、胸廓不对称和畸形等。然而，胸腔镜 EA-TEF 修补术需要熟练的内镜操作技巧。胸腔镜下行端端食管吻合是一个挑战，因为操作空间有限制，器械末端缺少清晰度（特别是缝针的缝合），以及结需要打紧。目前，少数的关于内镜手术修补 EA-TEF 报道如下：手术时间 2～4 小时，食管狭窄的发生率 30%～50%，吻合口漏发生率 12%～15%，需要行胃底折叠术的手术后胃食管反流发生率 30%～50%。随着儿科内镜外科技术提高，更精确食管吻合技术的进步，胸腔镜 EA-TEF 修补术可能成为标准的外科手术方法。然而与传统开胸手术相比，目前这个新的进入后纵隔的方法的优势尚不明显。

对于远端 TEF 合并严重呼吸窘迫综合征的 EA 患儿应给予特别的关注。在这些情况下，进行手术前通常需要气管内插管。然而，高压通气会使肺通气状况更加恶化，而且吸入的气体可能通过 TEF 进入胃引起腹部膨胀，进而加重呼吸困难。患儿可能需要急诊手术治疗来稳定肺功能和避免胃穿孔，后者可能有致命的危险。

一些手术方法已被报道用于处理这个难题，包括胃分流术[210]、胃食管连接处的绑扎[147]，以及将气管内插管的尖端置于瘘管开口的下方等[221]。支气管镜下通过瘘管放置 Fogarty 球囊导管可成功地消除通过瘘管的气流[80]，该方法可用于稳定快速恶化的患儿，但是可能存在的技术困难和球囊膨胀可能损伤食管远端的问题已引起了人们的关注。在这种情况下也可行急症胃造瘘使充满空气的胃和小肠减压，但有可能引起婴儿肺功能衰竭的危险，因为每次呼吸机的通气呼吸量优先通过 TEF 进入低阻力的胃造瘘管，分流肺的通气。采用带水封瓶的胃造瘘管可能会增加空气阻力并减少通过瘘管逸出的气流。

我们和 Templeton 等人[208]及 Spitz[249]一样，建议对需要高压通气的严重呼吸道窘迫综合征患儿行早期开胸瘘管离断手术。我们相信这些技术提供了最迅速有效地改善吸道衰竭的方法。在很多情况下，紧急结扎瘘管后患儿情况可明显改善，从而可以进行一期修

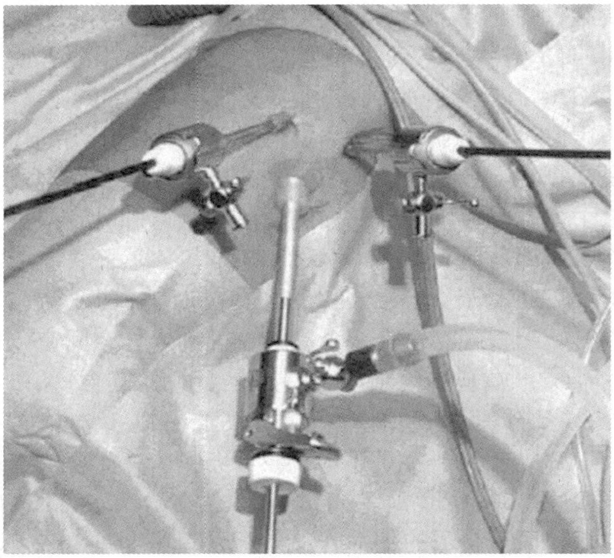

A

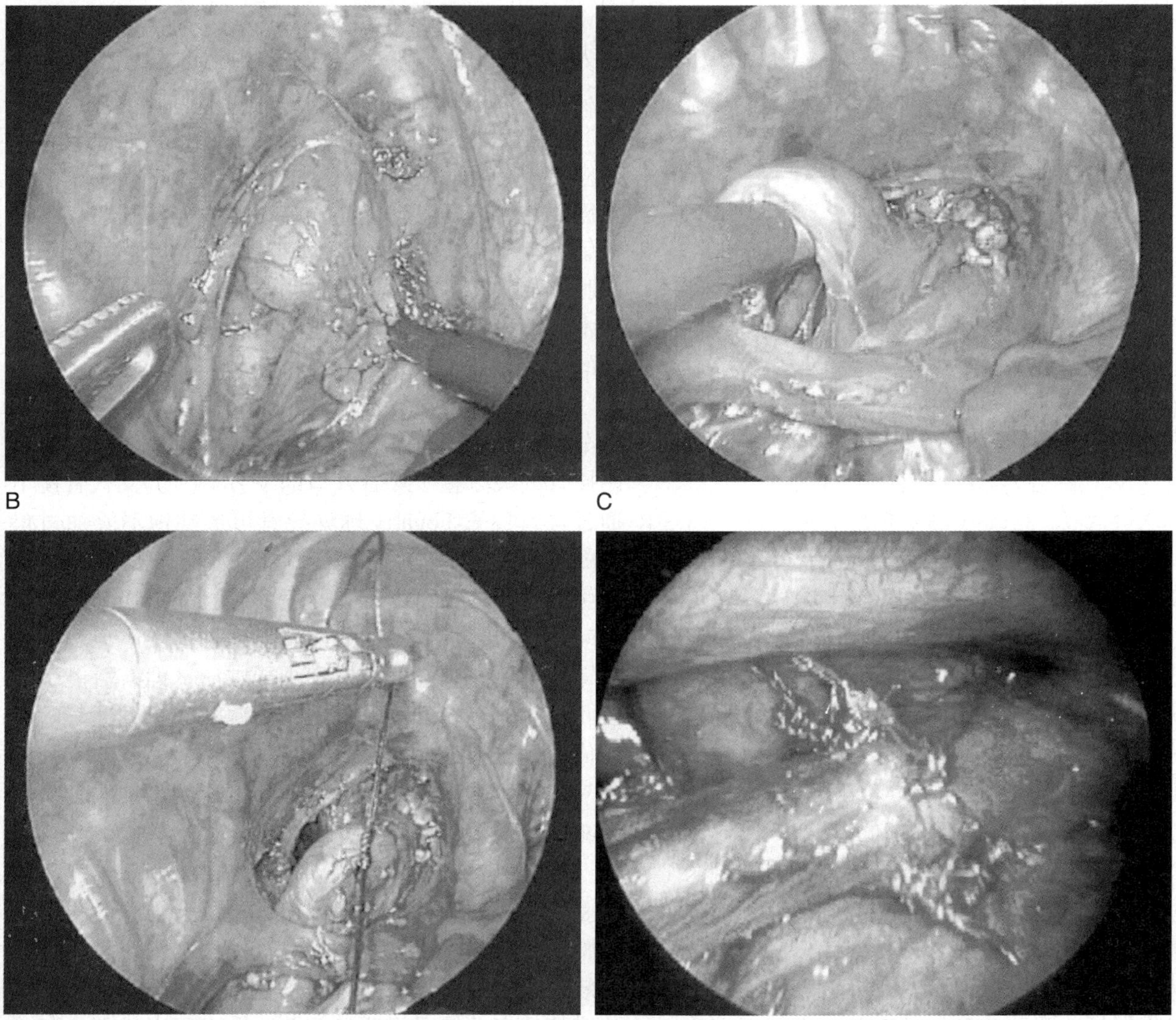

B　C　D　E

图 67–12　胸腔镜修补食管闭锁合并远端气管食管狭窄。A. 套管针，6mm 套管针插入视频头和两个 4mm 器械套管针的位置。B. 切开后侧胸膜，游离上端食管盲端。C. 游离远端瘘管，保持奇静脉完整。D. 紧靠气管结扎闭合瘘管。E. 食管的端端吻合已完成。(From Bax KMA, Van der Zee DC: Feasibility of thoracoscopic repair of esophageal atresia with distal fistula. J Pediatr Surg 2002; 37:192.)

补食管，而无需进行第二次手术。

长间隙的食管闭锁

有时 EA-TEF 的婴儿，通常是单独存在 EA 的患儿，其上端盲袋很高，上、下端食管段之间的距离很长，限制了简单无张力地进行端端食管-食管吻合术的可能。虽然这一问题已受到很大的关注，但“长
1063 间隙”EA 还没有很精确的定义。有些 EA 对于某些医生来说是仍可进行一期吻合的，称为“长间隙”，而其他医生则可能称之为“很长间隙”或“超长间隙”。此外，间隙的距离可因测量方法而出现偏差。有些报道描述了术前通过插入造影剂导管或探条进入上端食管盲袋，通过预置的胃造瘘管注入造影剂或插入可弯内镜进入远端盲袋的方法测量间隙距离的方法[33]。其他定义则是基于术中在游离近端盲袋之前或之后测量间距长度的方法。这些不同的测定方法引起了“长间隙”定义的混淆和争论[45]。

对疑为存在长间隙的单纯性 EA 患儿，大多数小儿外科医生先采用手术放置胃造瘘管，观察一段时间，然后尝试行延期一期修补术（图 67-13）。有报道称，患儿在刚出生后的几个月中，由于自然生长，食管两个末端的间隙会呈现变小的趋势，因而使一期修补更可行[68,206]。此外，很多术前的机械技术也被描述为一种可减小食管间隙的方法。最为常用的是 Howard 和 Myers[114] 在 1965 年首先描述的上端食管探条扩张术，即将一个有重量的探条通过口腔进入上端食管末端，在准备延期修补手术之前，每天 1 次或每天 2 次，维持 6～12 周[168]。采用术前的上下盲端探条减小间距长度的方法也有过报道[249]。1975 年，Hendren 和 Hale 报道了采用电磁场来牵拉放在两个食管末端的金属“子弹”从而使间距缩小的作法。

许多新的手术方法也被提倡用以在外科食管吻合术之前缩短长间隙。1971 年，Rehbein 和 Schweder[212] 描述了采用尼龙线在两个食管的末端做桥连，牵拉位于每个腔内的银的橄榄形探头[249]。探头往前推进，直到两个食管末端互相挤压在一起形成瘘管。Shafer 和 David[229]采用类似的技术对两个已游离的食管末端用桥接丝线进行了简单缝合，在两个食管盲端之间进行造瘘。其他有助于延长食管的方法有多阶段的胸外延伸技术，即先游离食管的上部，最初作为颈部的食管

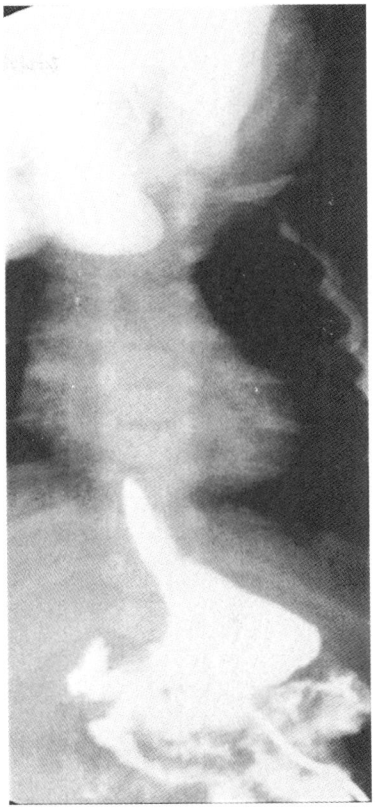

图 67-13 食管上端盲袋造影，同时通过胃造瘘管注入造影剂充盈胃和远端的食管段可见孤立的长间隙食管闭锁。

末端造瘘术。每 2～3 周通过手术游离食管和其皮肤开口一次并向下易位至前胸壁，直至有足够的食管长度行食管的端端吻合术[127,128]。

最近，Foker 报道了一种新的技术，向外牵拉近端和远端的食管盲端的牵拉线通过胸壁，并连续朝相对的方向牵引，直到两个盲端靠近为止（图 67-14）。外部牵引技术被报道可加速盲端的靠近，这样可早期进行一期修补（10～14 天）[4,82]。

除了各种术前延长食管的方法，很多手术技巧也被用于新生儿阶段初期食管吻合术，用上述延长方法后进行的延期食管吻合术。Livaditis 等人[157,159]对 EA 小猪模型采用上端食管部分的环肌切开术来减少端-端吻合的张力，并在 1973 年报道了临床为对长间隙 EA 婴儿行食管一期吻合术时采用了该技术来延长上端食管段（图见 67-10）[158]。此后，在长间隙 EA 患儿行近端食管环肌切开，以延长上端食管盲端，同时一期吻合术得到了广泛的应用。采用球囊管扩张上端食管盲袋，然后行环肌切开术是对该

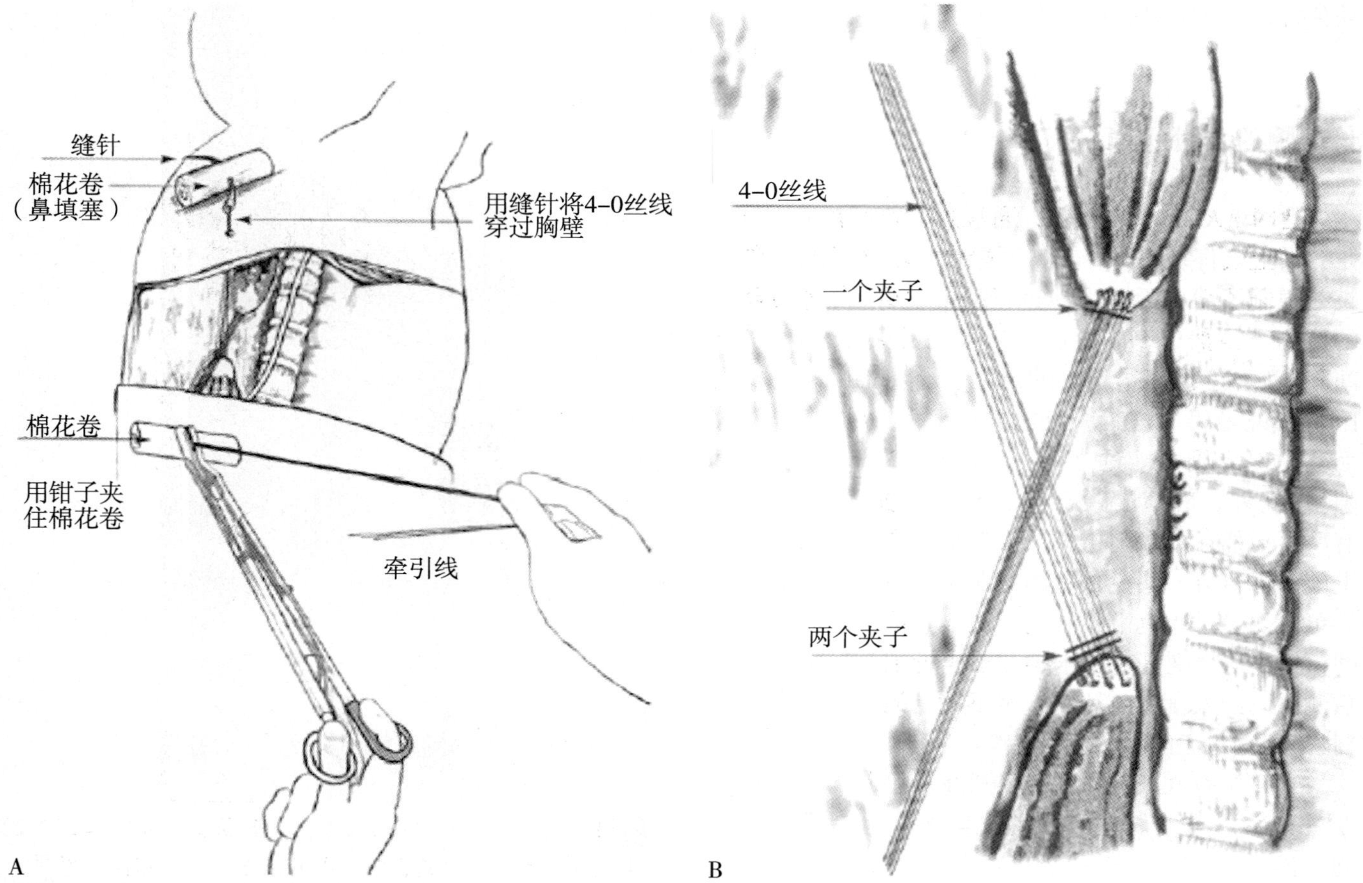

图 67–14 Foker 技术，通过外部牵拉缝线的方法延长上端和下端的食管盲端。A. 交叉牵拉缝线和垫子的外面观。B. 内面观。(From Foker JE, Linden BC, Boyle EM Jr, et al: Development of a true primary repair for the full spectrum of esophageal atresia. Ann Surg 1997;226:533.)

法的改良[55,73,152,226]。我们有时额外进行右侧颈部切口，从而将上端食管盲袋游离并拉出颈部，并行更近端的第二、第三个环肌切开[45]。

然而，环肌切开术的并发症已有报道，对于其安
1064 全性，外科医生间已有争论。并发症包括食管瘘、食管环肌切开段的食物嵌顿[241]，环肌切开段的食管轻度球形扩张等。有报道称，严重的扩张可导致食管假憩室的形成，只有很少的病例可能会出现这种严重并发症，我们最近在一例单纯长间隙 EA 患儿中发现了这种状况。一些报道指出假憩室的形成可能伴有远端吻合口的狭窄[73,191,241]。如果狭窄不予以治疗，假憩室可能扩大，以致引起吞咽困难和威胁生命的呼吸道梗阻等并发症[191]。

除了假性憩室的形成，环肌切开术也可以加重食管运动功能障碍，任何 EA 患儿都可能出现这种情况[65,190,236,296]。不过，这已经成为争论的焦点，对于该手术有人支持[237,241,266]有人反对[150,261]。有些报道建议在远端食管盲端环肌切开术时加用近端食管环肌切开术以达到一期食管吻合[90,144]。建议采用多种改良技术减少环肌切开的严重并发症。采用螺旋形上端食管环肌切开术辅以斜形缝合肌层技术可以将引起憩室的危险降低到最小，并且理论上可以提高存活率[126,216]。另一种改良食管环肌切开术是在上端盲端肌层做环形多排水平位短小切口，这样当向远端拖拉时，可使上端的食管盲端变长变细。该技术更适用于远端食管较细的节段[154]。

其他用来延长上端食管盲端的方法如 Gough描述的包括形成一个上端食管壁的全层前瓣。当向远端折叠时，这个皮瓣可以卷成管状并与下方的食管段接合[94]。1989 年，Bar–Maor 等[11]人强调了这个延长食

管上端盲端方法的技术细节。Davenport 和 Bianchi[53] 报道了 25 例采用这个方法的 EA 患儿，5 年随访结果取得了很好的预后。该技术的改良方法已有描述，包括创造一个 5mm 的食管后皮瓣[233]或者前皮瓣[239]，然后与铲形远端食管行端端斜形吻合。

在尝试一期或者延期一期修补时，有时即使已经尝试了上述一种或多种方法，但两食管段仍未能达到
1065 足够的靠拢。据描述有些附加的技术已被用以辅助进行食管吻合。尽管一直有游离食管可能会引起远端食管末端血供损害的观点，但很多外科医生发现远端食管可以进行游离，以实现与近端的吻合并且他们通常也是这么做的[149]。我们已经通过完全游离远端食管向下直至食管裂孔，甚至通过横膈食管裂孔成功地完成了食管端端吻合术。采用该方法时，有时可将胃底部提升到胸腔以辅助完成吻合[45]。

进一步按照这个概念，Schärli 描述了一个腹腔胸腔联合手术，通过结扎切断胃左动脉，横向或者斜向切开胃小弯，然后将胃的贲门和胃底部游离后移入胸腔完成远端食管的延长，进而取得一期食管吻合术的成功[77,225]。对于有胃食管反流的患者建议进行部分胃底折叠术。毫无疑问，术后胃食管反流为一种严重的术后并发症[284]。通过应用相似的方法，Collis 胃成形术辅以 Nissen 胃底折叠术已经成为延长远端食管末端、避免食管替代术的一种方法[75,122]。

除了应用外科手术技术保留原有的食管作为修补长间隙 EA 的管道外，术后还强烈建议保持头屈曲位，给以松弛剂和机械通气支持，以减少食管高张力吻合后发生吻合口破裂的危险[5,166,249,253]。

这种方法的原理是通过屈颈、麻痹食管近端的横纹肌以防止吻合处的破裂。

食管替代

第 69 章节将进一步对食管替代进行讨论。尽管实现婴儿 EA 的食管连续性已有了很多方法和创新，但如果这些方法失败，食管可能需要被置换。对于 EA 婴儿和腐蚀性食管损伤儿童进行手术治疗的多种方法已有过报道。

是否选择食管替代物要取决于很多因素。结肠或回结肠替代食管已经被广泛应用多年。右结肠或左结肠可置于胸骨后，或左、右侧肺门后方。迷走神经切断术和胃引流术是经典的避免胃结肠吻合口狭窄和溃疡的方法。一些并发症发生在结肠代食管术后，包括颈部吻合口漏（30%～50%病例）、狭窄、胸腔内冗长的结肠淤滞、胃反流、呼吸道并发症和腹泻等。有些外科医生喜欢用翻转的胃管替代食管，该方法是将胃大弯部分做成管状，经胸骨后或肺门后向上提到颈部食管[23,69,204]，其并发症与结肠代食管相似。改良的胃管法是将保留胃网膜右动脉供血的胃大弯一部分做成带蒂“游离”管状移植物[30]。空肠也可用做替代食管，可用 Roux-en-Y 术式或作为游离移植物行微血管吻合[52]。

最近，胃移位术已进一步被确立为一种成功的 EA 婴儿食管替代疗法[107,249,255]。Spitz 等人报道逾 173 例婴儿和儿童（127 例为 EA）采用该术[255]，预后良好与极好者达 90%。生存率达 94.8%，吻合口漏发生率为 12%，需要扩张的狭窄发生率 19.6%，10 年随访中未发现有功能减退者[257]。

不伴有食管气管瘘的食管狭窄

先天性患有单纯食管闭锁（不伴气管食管瘘）的患儿大多胸腔内没有食管。事先明确这一事实对于制定治疗计划和避免无效的开胸探查是非常重要的。这种疾病的术前和术中治疗在本章的长间隙 EA 治疗部分已进行过讨论。Ein 和 Shandling[67]对 50 年中接受治疗的 69 例单纯食管闭锁婴儿进行了回顾，其中早产儿的发生率是 52%，Down 综合征的发生率 10%～20%，十二指肠闭锁的发生率 10%，所有这些发病率都比典型的 EA-TEF 患者要高。

在无法吞咽方面，单纯食管闭锁婴儿的临床表现和 EA-TEF 患儿的表现相似。但前者的腹部通常是舟状腹，腹平片显示消化道内无气体。胃造瘘管应该在出生后 24～48 小时内放置，应尝试采用上述各种不同方法进行延期一期手术修补。放置胃造瘘管后可以早期给予肠道内营养，使得小胃得以扩大（图 67-13）。如果需要，扩大后的胃可作为食管替代。放置胃造瘘管时，用造影检查可能会发现不常见的食管闭锁伴远端食管气管瘘，这样则提示应早期行食管修补[93,193]。对于单纯食管闭锁可观察一段时间，给以肠道内营养支持，同时每天进行或不进行上端食管探条扩张。持续 8～12 周，期间可将金属探子或金属扩张器置于上端或下端的食管段，行放射影像学检

查可监测食管的延长。

当无明显的进一步延长或者食管的两端非常接近时，可行外科手术治疗。开胸后行胸膜后分离，同时游
1066 离近端和远端的食管段，行一期吻合术。如果上述努力后仍不能完成一期吻合术，可采用环肌切开术、贲门游离、近端盲端瓣状成形术或辅以腹部切口来游离部分或全部的胃并将其拉入胸腔（或颈部）。如果食管的两盲端间距过大、不能一期吻合而需要术前延长食管时，我们行一期的胃移位至颈部食管术，而不行开胸。一些外科医生行左侧颈部造瘘术，为将来的食管替代术做准备。术后并发症和EA–TEF修补术后相似（见后面的“结局”部分）。主要的并发症包括吻合口漏和狭窄，吞咽困难和胃食管反流。令人惊奇的是不伴有TEF的EA据报道会有严重的气管软化症。这个发现与EA合并气管支气管异常的发生是一致的[67,281]。

单纯（H型）食管气管瘘

不伴有食管闭锁的先天性气管食管瘘，或称H型TEF（若称为N型更符合解剖结构），在食管畸形中约占4%。这种畸形通常在出生后的数天内表现出来，新生儿会在喂养时出现窒息或不明原因的发绀发作[120]。当婴儿咳嗽或哭闹时，可发现空气通过瘘管进入胃内所致的间断性的腹部膨胀。年龄较大的婴儿和儿童更可能反复出现肺炎，通常会累及右上肺。有上述症状时应高度怀疑本病。

如果胸部平片显示有吸入型肺炎伴胃扩张，应考虑H型TEF的诊断。一个检验诊断可靠的方法是让患儿俯卧位进行食管造影检查，插入一细的鼻胃管至食管远端，回抽鼻胃管时逐渐注入造影剂。进行检查的放射科医生必须熟悉这种诊断方法，因为在常规的食管吞钡检查时50%以上的H型瘘管可能被漏诊（图67–6）。支气管镜辅以食管镜可特异性地确定诊断，如果在赶在手术分离瘘管前进行检查，可将一细小导管或导丝通入瘘管，有助于在后面进行手术探查时识别瘘管[87]。

大多数H型TEF可以成功地通过颈部切口离断瘘管[134]。做右侧下颈部切口，患儿取头部后伸并向左扭的体位，胸锁乳突肌会被拉向后方，必要时可离断其胸骨端，然后逐渐向中央分离至颈动脉鞘。仔细触摸气管内插管和鼻胃管有助于明确气管和食管的位置。暴露食管和气管间的平面时，可能需要离断甲状腺上动脉和甲状腺中静脉。必须识别并保护喉返神经。用吊带环绕食管有助于识别瘘管，但值得注意的是这个过程中可能会损伤对侧喉返神经。一旦明确瘘管（经常比预期的位置较高），在瘘管的上方和下方紧邻食管处置牵引缝线，避免在瘘管离断后造成食管扭转。在气管侧，用5–0的聚乙烯缝线或者丝线在瘘管的上下限位置进行缝扎。紧靠食管处离断瘘管，用5–0的聚乙烯缝线或者丝线在气管侧间断缝合瘘管。瘘管的食管端用细丝线或可吸收聚乙二醇酸线进行间断缝合（图67–15）。一些外科医生主张在两排相对的缝线之间有肌肉组织隔开以减少瘘管复发的可能。如果瘘管完全位于胸腔内或是食管闭锁手术后出现瘘管复发，最好行右侧胸腔切开术。最近有报道用胸腔镜手术修补位于胸部的H型TEF[2]。

术后并发症包括因气管水肿或喉返神经损伤继发引起的呼吸窘迫。先前肺部病变较重者和气管水肿可能者手术后应继续留置几天气管插管。食管漏和H型TEF的复发很少见。

食管闭锁伴有上端食管盲端瘘管

文献报道中关于上端食管盲端和气管之间形成瘘管的概率不一。这种类型瘘管的确切发病率可能被低估了，因为一些最初没有被认识的近端食管盲端瘘在现在的报道中已被作为EA伴远端气管食管瘘修补后的TEF复发[117]，有些病例因遗漏了上端TEF而被诊断为单纯性EA。这种畸形共有两种类型：（1）近端食管盲端瘘管合并远端的TEF（双瘘管）（发生率为1.4%）；（2）近端食管盲端的瘘管，不伴有远端TEF（发病率为0.8%）。这些发生率是根据几次大规模的病例报道所得的平均数。虽然这种类型的瘘管很少见，但是必须能够早期确诊和治疗，以避免发生进行性肺吸入和肺炎复发。

可以通过术前的食管远端盲袋造影检查做出诊断，最好由有经验的儿科放射科医生行荧光透视和视频记录后做出。该项检查可显示小的食管上端盲端，并可辨认出瘘管。不过，由于造影剂会从盲袋向上进入喉部和向下进入气管，因而常会导致结果出现混淆。由于这种潜在的不准确性一些外科医生会根据术前气管镜检查和食管镜检查来诊断是否存在上端盲端的瘘管，但是内镜检查时也可能遗漏近端小的瘘管。 1067

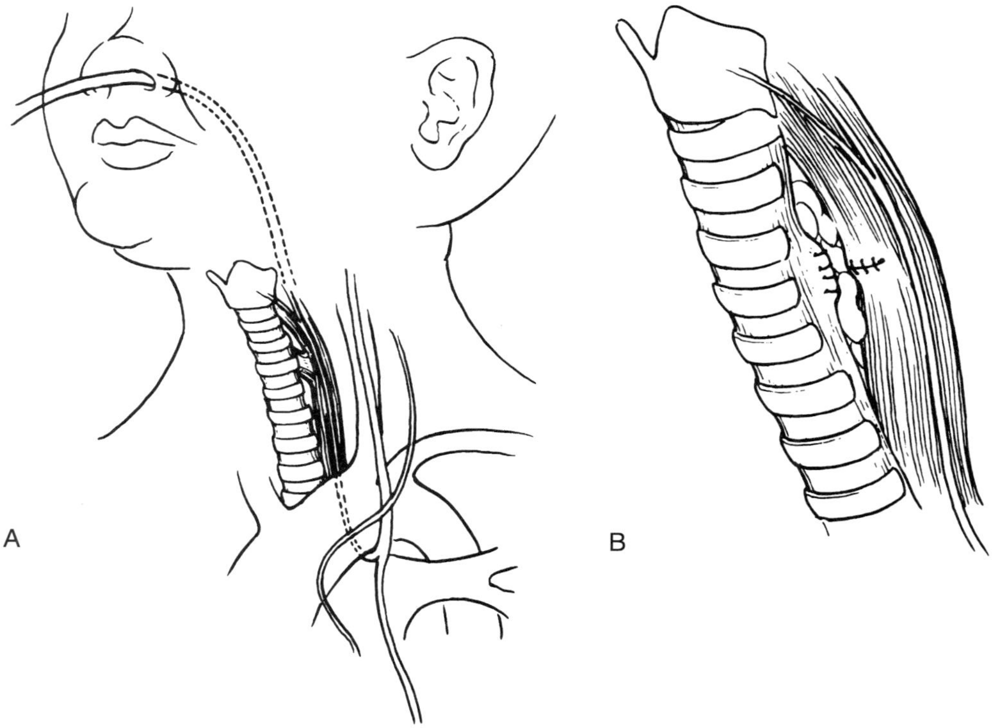

图 67-15　H 型气管食管瘘。A. 瘘管和喉返神经的解剖关系。B. 在切断瘘管后，在气管和食管处行间断缝合。

其他常用的诊断方法是在修补 EA 时完全游离上端食管的盲端，以便定位和修补术前未发现的食管盲端瘘管。与上述其他检查方法一样，外科手术探查中近端盲端的瘘管也可能被忽视，其中一部分是因为某些瘘管位于最近端的部位。如果在术前造影检查时或手术中发现近端盲袋异常狭窄或短小，应怀疑有近端盲袋瘘并仔细寻找，因为这些表现提示通过瘘管有减压。

一旦明确诊断存在瘘管，应像处理远端 TEF 一样进行手术，结扎和离断瘘管。如果在最初的伴有或不伴有远端 TEF 的 EA 修补术后才诊断出上端盲袋瘘管，常可行经颈部切口手术，如上面描述的 H 型 TEF 的手术一样。

结果

伴有或不伴有 TEF 的 EA 患儿生存率在过去的 50 年里都有显著的提高。最近报道总生存率可达 85%～95%，而 20 世纪 50 年代之前，生存率还不到 40%[40,59,62,135,189,232,273]。然而，EA 亚型患儿的预后仍较差。Waterston 的风险分类表历史性地有助于确定 EA 患儿是否为特别预后不良，直接有助于治疗的选择[293]。近年来，也提出了其他的风险分级法。具有以下因素的 EA 婴儿发生死亡和远期并发症风险增高：(1) 低出生体重（<1500g）/ 早产儿[59,249]；(2) 严重的先天性心脏病[40,148,273]；(3) 严重的合并畸形和依赖机械通气者[201]；(4) 食管两个盲端间的距离为长间隙[29]。

并发症

EA 尽管婴儿有很好的长期生存率，但仍可能发生很多严重的并发症。并发症通常被分为早期并发症（包括吻合口漏、吻合口狭窄、气管食管狭窄复发）和晚期并发症（包括胃食管反流、气管软化和食管蠕动障碍）。

早期并发症

吻合口漏

EA 患者发生食管吻合术后吻合口漏的发生率大

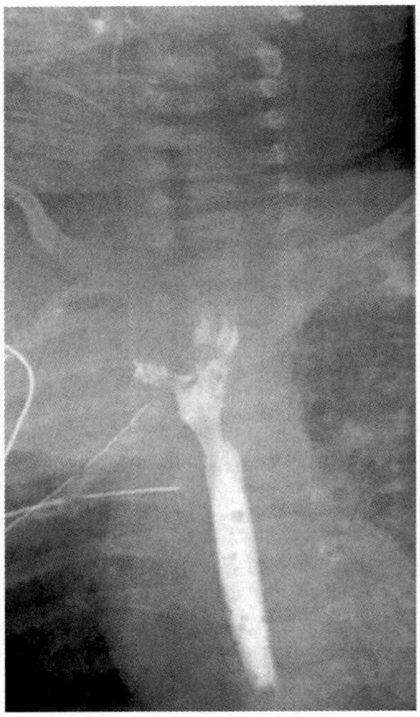

图 67-16 食管食管吻合术后的吻合口漏。漏是包裹性的，已充分引流。右上肺肺不张广泛。

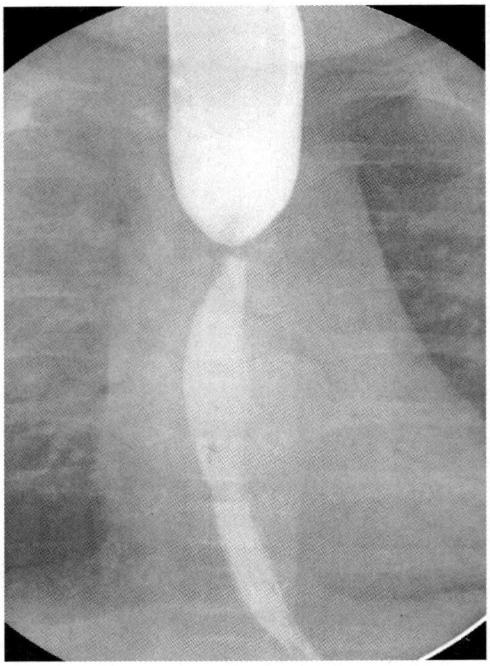

图 67-17 钡餐食管造影可见吻合口狭窄。

约为 14%～16%。大多数在临床上并不严重，可通过充分引流和营养支持进行治疗（图 67-16）。如果行胸膜后开放式纵隔引流，95%的吻合口漏可自然闭合[169]。即使胸腔修补术后发生了吻合口破裂并且胸膜间隙受到污染，也常可通过行充分的引流，进而使漏口 1068 自然关闭。吻合口破裂后常会形成漏口部分狭窄，有时并发反复发作性 TEF。大的食管吻合口破裂所致的术后漏只占 3%～5%，并且经常在第一次修补后早期即被发现（24～48 小时）。患儿常由于发生张力性气胸或纵隔炎经引流和应用抗生素仍不能控制而恶化。可能会引起吻合口漏的因素包括外科手术技术不佳、食管末端缺血、使用环肌切开术以及吻合口张力过大等[288,300]。在这些危急情况下，再次手术控制脓毒血症和充分引流并尝试修补吻合口漏是可靠的。伴有或不伴有肋间肌肉片衬垫的胸膜或者心包膜补片可能有助于确保吻合口的闭合[34,297]。如果食管吻合口无法修补，则可能需要行颈部食管造瘘术和延期食管替代术。

食管狭窄

食管狭窄是 EA 患者常见的并发症，但是据报道，食管狭窄的发生率由于狭窄的定义标准不同而差异很大。最近的大宗报道中，食管患者需要扩张的食管狭窄者超过 80%。Spitz 和 Hitchcock[250]提出狭窄的定义为存在临床症状（吞咽困难、吸入或异物梗阻引起的复发性呼吸障碍）并且通过内镜或者食管造影能够发现存在狭窄（图 67-17）。食管狭窄可能的病理机制包括吻合技术不良（张力过高、两层吻合口、丝线材料）、食管末端的局部缺血、胃食管反流和吻合口漏。伴有或不伴 TEF 的 EA 婴幼儿修补术后出现食管异物的比率达 13%[303]。

对食管吻合口存在明显狭窄者的传统治疗方法是通过向前或者向后回拉探条头进行扩张。我们发现沿导丝通过 Savory 型扩张器的同向运动有很多优点：这种方法可在荧光透视下观察连续的扩张过程；在扩张期间可使用造影剂；通常不必进行硬质食管镜检查。最近有人报道采用 Gruntzig 型球囊扩张管来扩张食管的狭窄部位，其中包括 EA 修补术后发生的食管狭窄。该技术理论上的优势是在狭窄的部位产生一个均衡的和放射状的力，而不是传统探条扩张术的剪轴力[3,92,220,264]。很多狭窄(53%)在食管修复后 1 个月内做 1～3 次扩张可得到缓解。但是，反复扩张无效的狭窄需要行狭窄部切除和重新吻合，甚至有时要做食管替代治疗。通过造影剂食管造影、pH 监测或者联合这些检查来明确食管狭窄是否合并胃食管反流是至关重要的。如果存在严重的胃食管反流而使狭窄部位浸泡在酸中，则往往扩张无效[220]。在抗反
1069 流手术后，狭窄常可通过扩张疗法治疗成功。

复发性食管气管瘘

经初期手术离断或结扎后，食管气管瘘的复发率为 3%～14%[71,72,135,163,169,171,275]。TEF 的复发是由先前 TEF 修补部位的吻合口瘘伴发局部炎症和糜烂所致。减少复发可能性的技术包括应用胸膜片[72]，带血管的心包片[24,44,298]和奇静脉片[136]插入食管和气管缝线之间。虽然复发性 TEF 通常发生在手术后的早期，但也可能需要数月至数年才被发现。临床症状与先天性 H 型 TEF 的典型症状相同，包括在喂养后出现咳嗽、窒息或发绀等表现。然而，不明显的症状更为常见如反复肺部感染。胸部平片上见到空气充盈的食管可提示诊断为本病。常规的造影剂吞咽检查的复发瘘管漏诊率可能会有 50%。可靠的诊断方法与先天性 H 型瘘管的诊断相同，即俯卧位在视频荧光透视下行食管造影检查。支气管镜下用 2-和 3-F 的导管插入瘘管也是一种可靠的诊断方法，而且对术中瘘管的定位具有重要的价值。复发性 TEF 很少能自行闭合，通常需要进行外科手术修补。应选择的手术方法是开胸结扎和离断瘘管。第一次复发 TEF 的患者约占 10%～20%，为了减少复发瘘管的可能性，可将胸膜、肋间肌肉或心包间置于食管和气管之间[251]。内镜下用各种化学或电灼法消除瘘管的方法已有报道[88,202,211]。最近有成功地应用纤维蛋白胶治疗单个病例报道[99]，不过，仍然有应用化学方法失败的报道[27]。

晚期并发症

胃食管反流病

胃食管反流病（GERD）在 EA 修补后的婴儿和儿童中很常见，由于怀疑和诊断检查的普及，其发生率似乎在上升。此外，在本章中已描述过的许多保留自身食管的倾向也促使了胃食管反流病的增多。这个问题的严重性在于文献报道 EA 患者修补术后有 30%～70%出现胃食管反流病[10,72,135,155,169,276,298]。EA 婴儿发生胃食管反流的原因可能与因吻合口牵拉或食管动力障碍引起的食管腹腔部分缩短有关，或者是因为手术操作不当或先天性畸形本身所引起[8,119,276]。胃食管反流病的后果会由于食管的蠕动变得更慢或者缺失，从而使得食管暴露于酸性物质的时间延长而加重。在长期随访的中发现，食管炎常见于患有 EA 的年长儿童和青少年[43,195,270,276,277]。最近在一些长期随访研究中发现，在婴儿期做过 EA 修补术的成人仍有胃食管反流病及其并发症的风险，包括发生 Barrett 食管炎的风险会明显增高，可能会高达 9%[58,140]。有报道一名 20 岁的患者在婴儿期间曾行 TEF 修补术的一位 20 岁病例出现了食管腺癌[1]。

当患者出现呕吐、吞咽困难、复发性的吻合口狭窄（后者有时伴有异物或食物块嵌顿）等症状时，应怀疑为病理性胃食管反流病。此外，喘鸣等呼吸道症状、阵发性发绀、复发性肺炎和反应性呼吸道疾病也都可能提示胃食管反流病的发生，少数可出现气管软化等其他表现。

婴儿和儿童 EA 修补术后胃食管反流病的病理学诊断是通过上消化道的造影检查、24 小时 pH 监测数据（虽然这在儿童已不作为标准诊断检查，而在成人依然是标准检查）和典型的病理性反流记录等做出[276]。但是，大量的食管测压研究一致地记录了 EA 修复术后可出现的异常食管蠕动和食管下括约肌压力下降，因此这个测试可能并不能作为辅助诊断胃食管反流病的依据[272]。

在患有病理性胃食管反流病的婴儿和儿童，积极的医学处理方法通常包括喂养稠的食物，将婴儿保持俯卧位或直立体位，以及给予减少胃酸产生的药物，如组胺-2 阻滞剂（如西咪替丁或雷尼替丁）、质子泵抑制剂（如奥美拉唑）和促进胃动力药（如甲氧氯普胺）等。然而，这些婴儿有 45%～75%因药物治疗失败、慢性呼吸道感染、难治性吻合口狭窄或远端食管狭窄而最终需要行抗反流手术[72,169,298]。对抗反流手术的选择尚存在争议。Nissen 胃底折叠术通常被认为是最好的选择[17,83,119,252]。但是，360 度包绕食管后常发生吞咽困难和其他严重的并发症，如 1/3 患者出现包裹性破裂和复发性胃食管反流病[46,153,169,298]。由于通常这种情况下采取 Nissen 胃底折叠术的效果很差，有些外科医生会采用前侧的 Thal 部分包绕胃底折叠术。但是，由于其他有些外科医生对 Nissen 胃底折叠术

进行了改良，使包绕较短而且宽松（通过大的扩张器1.0～1.5cm），因而这种术式至今仍被普遍应用[17]。此外，由于在EA修补术后食管通常会缩短，有些外科医生会采用Collis-Nissen胃底折叠术来增加食管内的长度[122]。

气管软化

气管软化可引起EA-TEF修补手术后出现的严
1070 重呼吸道症状。在EA-TEF患者的病理标本中发现气管软化的发生率高达75%。然而，EA-TEF婴儿患者中修补术后出现症状的大概占10%～25%，其中大约有一半需要手术纠正[72,79,137,187]。在临床上通常难以与复发性TEF、吻合口漏或胃食管反流的症状相鉴别[56]。气管软化被定义为广泛性的或者局限性的气管薄弱，使得前侧或者后侧的气管壁在呼气或者咳嗽的时候并拢。合并TEF的婴儿中，气管结构异常的发生率在40例婴儿的尸体解剖中达到75%，这表明导致TEF的胚胎学原因可能与气管软化的发生有关[291]。这种患者的气管软骨比正常稍短，因而不能提供保持气道开放所需的支持[291]。在婴儿EA-TEF修补术后，气管也容易被前方的主动脉弓和后方的膨胀的上段食管所压迫，这种压迫被认为是气管软化病理生理学的重要原因。Kimura等人[129]用连续CT对气管软化进行了研究并提出气管软化的原发性病因与气管内先天存在的薄弱因素有关。一系列的研究表明没有证据支持单纯EA的婴儿存在气管软化，这表明EA具有与气管软化不同的发病机制[215]。这已在阿霉素诱导的EA-TEF老鼠模型中得到证实，也有助于对畸形的发病机制进行更深入的了解。气管萎陷的水平通常刚好在TEF形成部位的上方气管的下三分之一段，通常是在主动脉弓的水平。

气管软化的临床表现程度不一，可从轻度患者的“铜锣音”或者“吠鸣”状咳嗽至复发性肺炎或急性致命的呼吸暂停。气管软化的婴儿常会因进食时呼吸困难或发绀发作而不愿进食。这些症状通常在婴儿几个月大时表现出来[24]。Filler等人1992年报道称，32例气管软化儿童中发现27例存在威胁生命的呼吸暂停[78]。这些情况在进食后5～10分钟之内发生，特征表现为发绀性的进行性呼吸暂停、心动过缓，并且如果不给以干预最终可导致心跳呼吸停止。诊断方法是自主呼吸下的气管镜检查，镜下可见病变区域的气管腔呈裂隙状（图67-18）。

对于气管软化的治疗仍有争议。大多数中轻度症状的气管软化婴儿不需要进行手术治疗，因为其症状可以随着时间而缓解。对严重症状的婴儿，包括有急性威胁生命的发作者，应选取的手术方法是主动脉固定术[97,227,287,294]。该手术通常通过左前侧开胸切口进路，将升主动脉和主动脉弓缝合至胸骨后侧的上方。该术式中，上提主动脉提起了气管的前壁，同时打开了气管腔[16,42,124]。当主动脉弓不能在无张力下达到胸骨后方时，建议采用该手术的改良方法，即将主动脉根部的心包瓣缝合在胸骨上[7,138]。最近有人主张经前纵隔入路，通过一个低的颈部横切口行主动脉固定和气管固定[174]。很多外科医生用术中气管镜观察主动脉固定术的适当程度，在缝线打结时观察气管腔的开放情况。最近，采用胸腔镜技术行主动脉固定术已取得了良好的效果[224]。

其他一些手术治疗方法也被用于治疗气管软化合并EA。各种移植片固定支架被用于治疗EA修补术后的气管软化，虽然一些个例报道取得了成功，但要作为为标准治疗方法还有待评估[25,118,267,289]。Filler等人[78]主张对主动脉固定术治疗气管萎陷失败的儿童

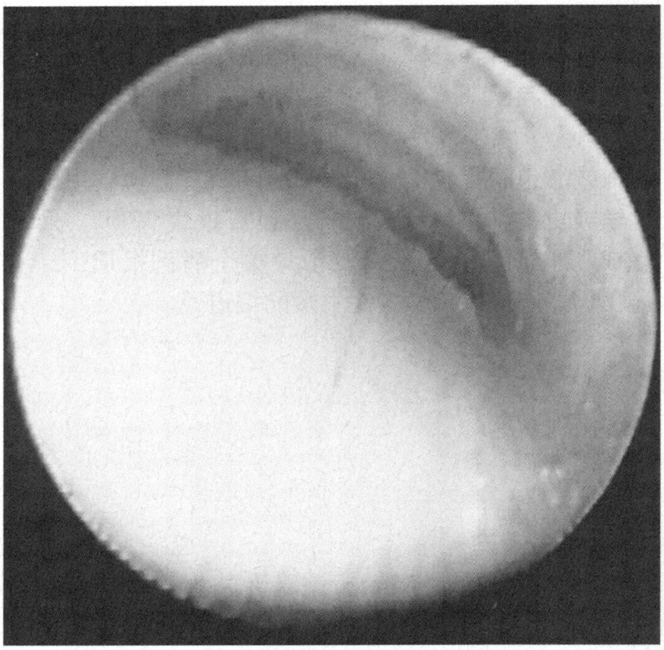

图67-18 修补食管闭锁-气管食管瘘后的气管软化。自主呼吸时用支气管镜观察气管腔显示呼气时气管几乎完全塌陷。

应用气道固定支架。最近，唇舌粘连替代主动脉固定术被提出作为舌后移（舌下垂）婴儿的早期治疗[49]。气管造瘘术是最后的治疗选择。

其他的长期生活质量问题

如上所述，EA 患儿的食管蠕动功能异常，这可能是由于先天性缺陷本身所致，也可能是继发于手术修补。通过对儿童与成人食管测压检查，发现其发生率在 75%～100%。肠管间置替代食管术后会出现严重的吞咽困难。据报道，一过性吞咽困难在成人患者中的发生率达 50%～90%，其中 30%还会有
1071 窒息症状[20,37,137]。该症状具有重要的临床意义，因为它与很多 EA 修补术后的远期症状有关，包括吞咽困难、食管异物梗阻、胃食管反流病和复发性呼吸道病变。尽管这些症状可能会随着时间而改善，早期的喂养不能耐受和食物团块阻塞问题可导致生长弛缓。很多儿童必须缓慢进食并且会挑食。

先天性食管狭窄

真正的先天性食管狭窄（CES）是很少见的情况，在历史上曾与继发于炎症、尤其是胃食管反流的食管狭窄相混淆。据报道，CES 的发生率为每 25 000～50 000 出生儿中 1 例[182,283]。2004 年，全世界文献中所报道的病例不到 600 例。不知什么病因，日本 CES 的发病率似乎高于世界上其他地区[121,183]。其他畸形合并 CES 的发生率被报道为 17%～33%，这些畸形包括 EA 伴或不伴 TEF、H 型 TEF、心脏畸形、肠闭锁、中肠旋转不良、肛门直肠畸形、尿道下裂、头面部和肢体畸形以及染色体异常[182]。除此之外，最近 Vasudevan 等人报道 5%的气管食管畸形患者存在 CES（3 个存在支气管残留），而 Kawahara 等人报道 14%的 EA 患者合并发生 CES[121,286]。

CES 分类方法很多，而且混淆不清，部分是因为难以鉴别先天性与后天获得性病变。Nihoul-Fekete 等人[182]提出的 CES 的定义和分类可能是最清晰的。先天性食管狭窄的定义为：出生时固有的并且是由食管壁结构先天畸形所致的食管狭窄[182]。该分类法将 CES 分为三种类型：（1）膜性食管蹼或隔膜；（2）纤维肌肉性增厚；（3）继发于食管壁内气管支气管残留的狭窄。

据报道，先天性膜性食管蹼或隔膜在这三种类型的 CES 中最为罕见[178]。它被认为是被忽略的一种食管闭锁中形式[131]，并可能与消化道其他部位的隔膜相似。通常引起食管中段或下段的部分性梗阻。膜的两面覆盖有鳞状上皮，并经常有一个偏心的开口。典型的症状发生在数月龄大、开始喂养固体食物的婴儿。

第二个类型的 CES 被称为特发性的肌肉肥厚或纤维肌肉性增厚，在一些报道中它是 CES 中最常见的类型[182]。其组织学特征为平滑肌纤维和纤维结缔组织的黏膜层下增生，表层有正常的鳞状上皮覆盖[182]。有人提出其组织学特征与肥厚性幽门狭窄十分类似，但是并没有明确的胚胎学和发病机制因素能解释这些病变。

在一些报道中认为，气管支气管残留物引起的 CES 是最常见的 CES 类型，这些也是这三种类型中被描述最多的和最了解的。目前认为它是包括 EA-TEF 在内的一类先天性畸形中的一种，这类畸形与胚胎 25 天左右时前肠与呼吸道分离有关[275]。气管支气管组织被隐藏在食管壁内，因为食管的生长速度比气管支气管树的生长快，因此通常位于远端食管的部分。

继发于气管支气管残留的 CES 是由 Frey 和 Dusche[85]在 1936 年首先报道的，这是一位 19 岁的女性，死因被诊断为贲门失迟缓症[275]。1964 年，Holder 等人[112]报道在回顾的 1058 例 EA、TEF 或者 EA-TEF 患儿中，有 3 例具有远端食管狭窄。在其他一些报道发表后[167,279]，1973 年 Spitz[247]首先论证了该病的先天性基础。1991 年，英语和德语文献中共报道了近 50 例由于气管支气管残留物引起的 CES 病例[301]。此外，1981 年，日本文献中已经有 71 例 CES 报道[183]，1987 年，中国报道 6 例（出自总的 76 例 CES）[156]。另有 3 例 CES 最近被报道[208]。

诊断

CES 的症状通常开始于婴儿期，表现为进行性的吞咽困难和呕吐，通常为 6 个月龄左右的婴儿在喂养半流质或者固体食物后开始出现。但有些病例报告中新生儿会出现严重的反流和呼吸窘迫症状[182]。有些患者最早被发现的症状可能是食管内异物[21]。正确的诊

断常十分困难。食管造影检查可特征性地发现突然出现的远端食管狭窄，而这常被误认为是胃食管反流引起的狭窄。继发于肌肉纤维性肥厚的狭窄可以导致更明显的锥形狭窄（图 67-19）。由于食管蹼或肌肉纤维肥厚引起的 CES 可表现为中段食管或者上段食管的狭窄[95]。随着时间的变化，狭窄近端的食管可能会扩张，造影检查结果可能被误认为是失迟缓症[181]。其他有助于鉴别 CES 与失迟缓症和胃食管反流所致狭窄的检查手段包括食管测压和 pH监测。食管镜检查通常可看到 CES 患者在食管狭窄处有正常外观的黏膜。最近，据报道，高频内镜超声检查有助于 CES 的诊断[282]。

治疗

CES 的治疗应该减轻狭窄的症状并维持胃食管连接处的抗反流机制。探条扩张术已经成功用于治疗纤维肌肉肥厚继发性 CES 和有时为食管蹼引起的
1072 CES。向前和向后的锥形扩张器已经成为探条扩张的传统形式，但最近采用静水力学的球囊扩张也取得了成功[6,181,182]。为了解决狭窄的问题，可能需要进行一系列的扩张。膜性食管蹼有时可通过扩张得到足够的治疗，有一例报道了通过内镜成功切除先天性食管蹼的病例[208,231,286]。

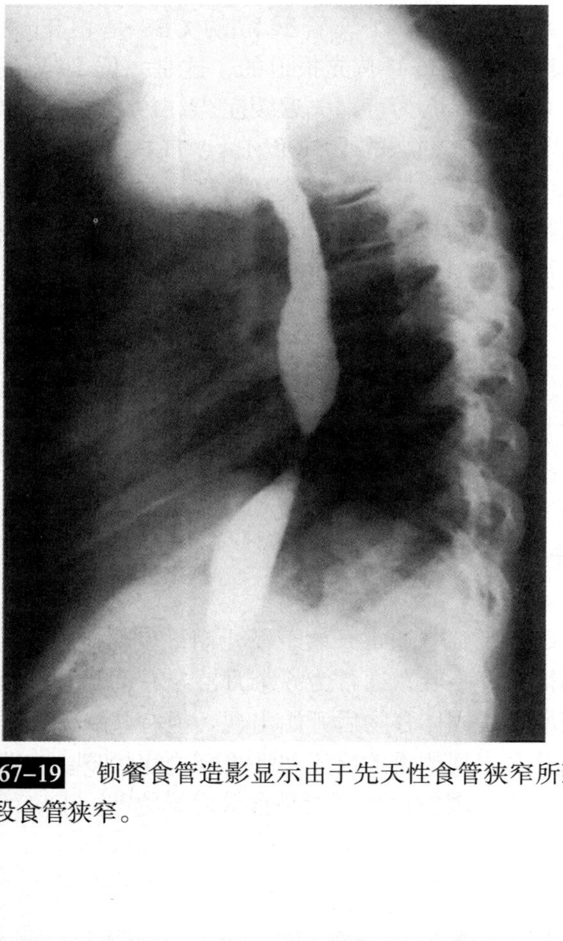

图 67-19 钡餐食管造影显示由于先天性食管狭窄所致的中段食管狭窄。

大多数网膜和继发于气管支气管残留物的 CES 必须通过外科手术，进行治疗有的是作为主要方法，有时在尝试扩张失败之后再进行[6]。术前通过食管造影清楚确定狭窄的位置非常重要，以便确定手术路径。右侧胸廓切开术用于中段食管狭窄，左侧胸廓切开则适用于下段食管狭窄。食管腹腔段 CES 的患者应采用经腹手术。探查中可能很难确定狭窄的范围。将球囊扩张导管通过狭窄段，然后给球囊充气，最后向后拖拉至狭窄部位，这是一项有助于手术的技术[186]。大多数情况下狭窄段的长度小于 3cm，可以完成该节段的切除和行端端食管吻合。术中应注意保护迷走神经。长段的纤维肌肉肥厚狭窄的患者经扩张无效时，可能需要切除并采用结肠、胃或空肠替代手术。如果狭窄部位靠近例胃食管连接部，大多数外科医生主张行节段切除、食管吻合和抗反流手术，以避免术后出现反流。做或者不做幽门成形的改良 Hill 胃固定术和 Nissen 胃底折叠术是最常采用的方法[182,186]。然而，Collis 胃成形术联合 Nissen 胃底折叠术已经被报道可有效治疗食管缩短和术后 GER[6,32,121]。

结果

扩张和手术切除都有良好的长期随访结果[182]。在进行食管远端 CES 切除术后不做抗反流手术的患者中，会有明显的 GER 形成并需要再行抗反流手术[123]。扩张治疗后的并发症包括食管漏和治疗失败。切除和吻合手术的并发症包括食管漏和纵隔炎症，可以通过纵隔引流治愈[121,286]。

喉气管食管裂

喉气管食管裂（LTEC）是一个罕见的先天性畸形，即在喉、气管和食管之间存在中线交通。1792 年，这种畸形可能是在 Richter 的博士论文中第一次被描述，他描述了一例喂养时出现窒息和呕吐的婴儿[213]。婴儿

死亡，但由于未行尸体解剖，因而诊断不能确定。1949 年，LTEC 婴儿再次被 Finlay 描述[81]。在 1955 年，Pettersson[197]首次成功矫正了喉气管食管裂。

像 EA-TEF 一样，LTEC 的胚胎发生尚未完全明了。长期以来，理论认为是由于头颅的气管食管中隔向头侧延伸停滞，使得食管气管被存留下来[22,109,242]。最近的研究表明像 TEF 一样，LTEC 是在起初的正常发育之后发生了广泛的气管和食管融合的结果[188]。虽然没有一致的遗传类型，但有散发的家族性联合发生。据报道，LTEC 合并发“G”综合征和 Pallister-Hall 综合征[96]。LTEC 发病倾向于男性，男女比例为 5∶3.63。

LTCE 可并发多种先天性畸形，包括有胃肠道、泌尿生殖系统和心脏畸形[63]。有 LTEC 患儿伴有 EA 合并 TEF 的发生率在 20%～37%。其他的合并胃肠道畸形包括肛门畸形（21%）、肠旋转和固定异常（13%）、胎粪性肠梗阻（8%）等[63,280]。泌尿生殖系畸形的发生率为 14%～44%，包括尿道下裂、腹股沟斜疝、睾丸未降和肾发育不全[63,280]。心血管畸形的发生率为 16%～33%，包括室间隔缺损、主动脉缩窄、大血管转位等[63]。

为了更好地指导治疗，目前已提出了几种分类方案。在 1955 年，Pettersson 在报道第一例修补手术时描述了三种类型：I 型，局限在喉部和累及部分或者
1073 全部的环状软骨板；II 型，超过环状软骨板延伸至颈部气管；III 型，包括整个气管，向下至气管隆嵴。1991 年，Ryan 等人[219]提出了 IV 型，即裂孔延伸超过气管隆突，累及到单侧或双侧主支气管。

LTEC 的症状根据裂隙扩展的程度而不同，但大多数患者出生后立即出现在喂养后恶化的呼吸窘迫。其他症状可包括特征性的无声或者沙哑的哭声、发绀、窒息、分泌物增多和复发性吸入性肺炎。合并畸形的严重程度掩盖了 LTEC 存在的情况并不少见，尤其如果是极小的 I 型或 II 型病变。根据 LTEC 的常见症状，诊断的思路通常是先怀疑为 EA-TEF 或气管软化症。食管造影可见造影物质迅速在上部食管和气管处融合。但是，常很确定这是否是继发于喉水平的溢出或是造影剂通过裂口所致。内镜是明确诊断 LTCE 的方法，但是仍很难确认裂口位置，除非是怀疑指数非常高，或者在声门下区水平推开黏膜皱褶后发现常见的裂隙（图 67-20）。

LTEC 婴儿的治疗首先是要减少吸入和保持气道通畅。Ryan 等人[219,238]推荐在手术前尽可能避免气管内插管，但是在进行明确的外科修补之前常需要进行气管插管和胃造口术。修补 LTCE 的手术方式由于裂隙的严重程度而不同。无症状的 I 型裂口可能不需要手术干预，有症状的裂隙可以通过内镜下进行修补[63]。II 型 LTEC 可通过咽侧切开术、咽后切开术或喉正中切开术进行治疗。关于侧方暴露的报道最多，这种方法可比较容易地进入裂隙，而且能够不对称地切开黏膜，因此避免了连绵不断的缝合。该方法的主要缺点是存在损伤喉返神经的风险。喉前部途径

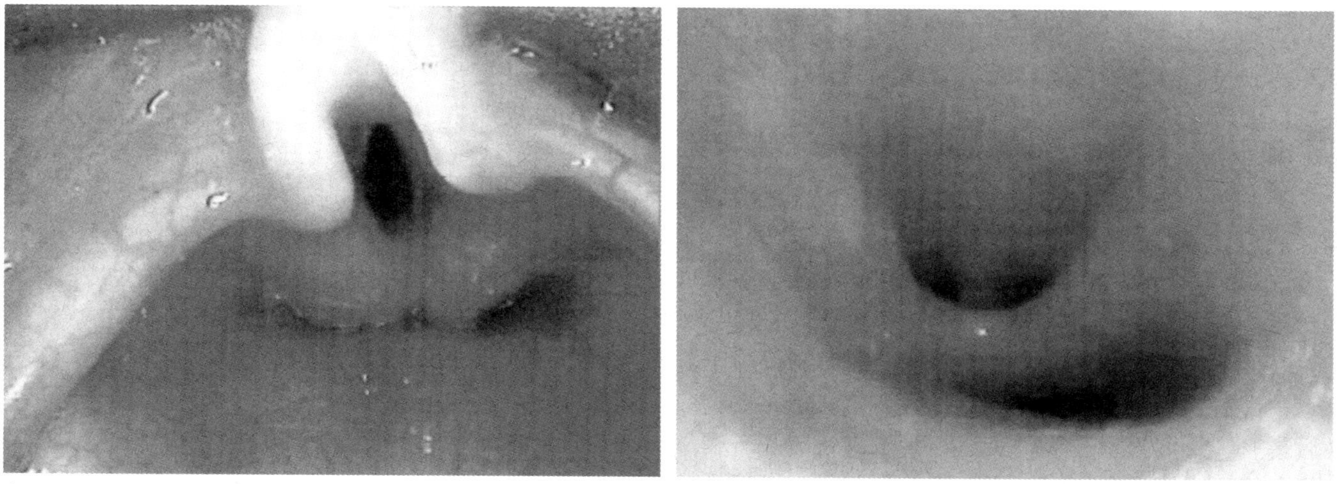

A　　B

图 67-20　内镜所见的 III 型喉气管食管裂。A. 裂的近端可能在很难一眼就发现。B. 裂的远端刚好在气管分叉的近端。

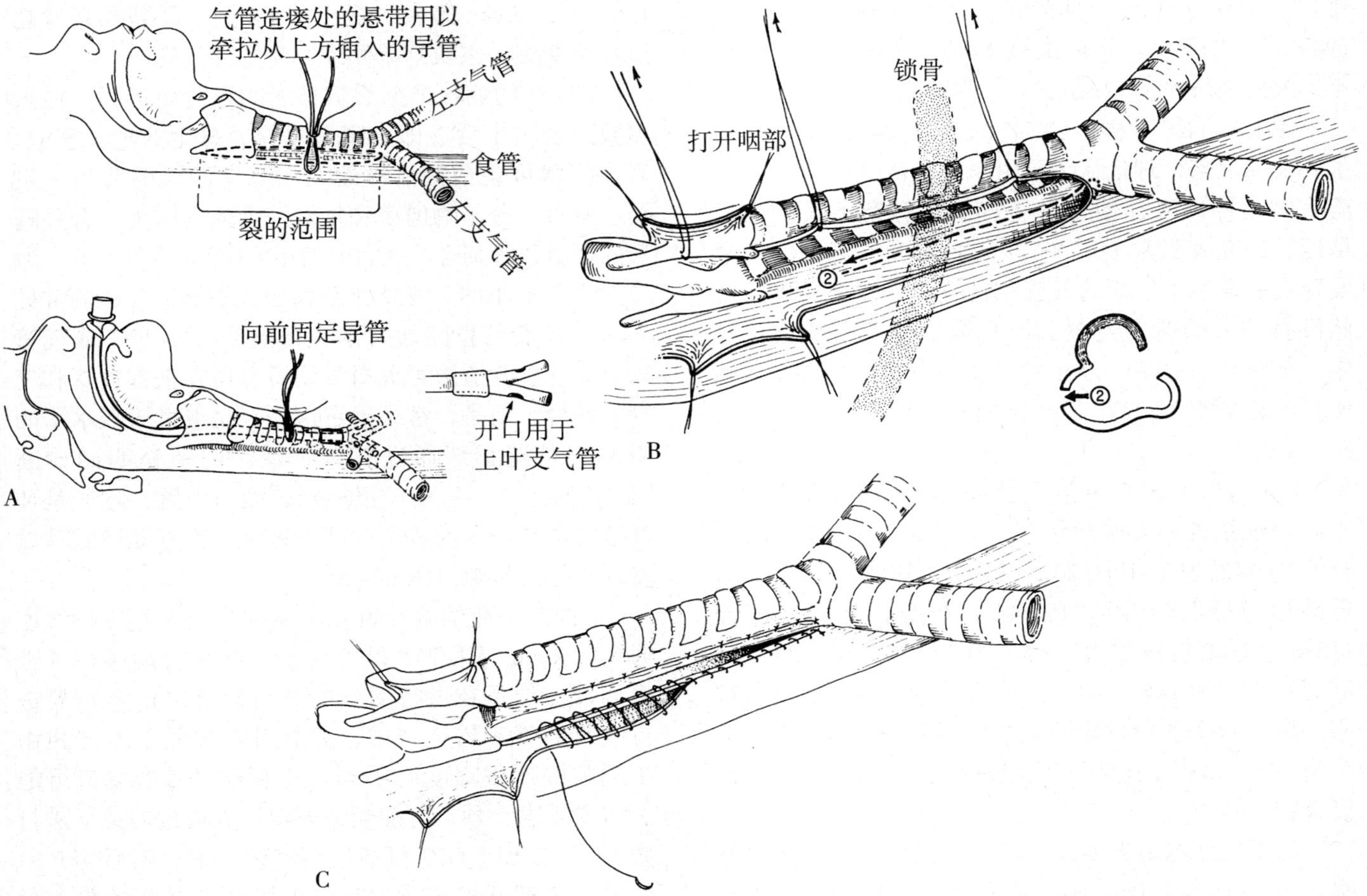

图 67-21 III 型喉气管食管裂的修补。A. 下支气管镜下，通过气管造瘘口置入一用输尿管导管做的悬带，用悬带将气管内导管向前拖拉完成分叉形气管内导管的固定。B. 颈胸部切口，在胸膜暴露喉气管食管裂。在气管环下方的右气管食管沟内做一纵切口。切口向下延伸并跨过食管上方向上至左侧，在气管上保留大约 1cm 宽的食管壁，使得有足够的组织关闭气管。C.间断缝合气管，连续缝合，向上直至胸廓入口闭合食管。喉部裂口和咽侧壁的闭合还没有完成。(From Donahoe PK, Gee PE: Complete laryngotracheal cleft: Management and repair. J Pediatr Surg 1984;19:143.)

可暴露喉和上部气管，而且对于喉返神经没有损伤的风险。术后喉的稳定性已受到越来越多的关注，一些医生推荐在治疗的过程中使用支架[15,63]。

手术治疗 III 型和 IV 型 LTEC 需要做联合颈部和胸部切口。Donahoe 等人[61,219,238]应用了特别设计的有凸缘末端的分叉形气管内导管，它可在支气管镜下置入，然后用一输尿管导管做的悬带将气管向前悬起(图 67-21)。气管内的导管可保证气道的通畅，由于手术中常需要频繁地改变体位。做右胸切口，并在胸膜后暴露气管食管裂。从隆凸至胸廓入口处切开右侧气管食管沟，然后在左侧切开食管气管壁，完成气管与食管的分离。切开时应在气管全长保留约 1.0cm 宽的食管，以便形成新的气管膜性部分。正确测量该食管片的宽度非常重要，可避免气管狭窄或后壁松垂，从而避免造成气管阻塞。当进行分离解剖的时候，推开和保护左侧迷走神经和喉返神经也十分重要。关闭气管和食管时应从尾端至头端进行，并用聚丙烯缝线
连续缝合食管、间断缝合气管这一点也很重要。然后 1074
再做右侧颈部切口，暴露食管的上端部分、气管、咽和喉；喉部行三层连续内翻缝合修补，并放置一根气管造瘘管，该造瘘管可根据患者定制，以避免对后侧的气管修补处产生不适当的压力。有些外科医生喜欢采用前侧入路的方法，并在中线处分离喉和气管，该法与 II 型缺损的手术方法类似[185]。心肺分流术已被

用于前路法修补 IV 型喉气管食管裂[177]和并作为经侧胸和颈部手术患者在体外膜式人工氧合时的支持。

存在这种复杂畸形的患者很少在同一家医院治疗[185,235,238]，术后生存率仍很低，由于畸形的严重程度不同，生存率在 50%～75%不等。据报道，修补术后吻合口漏的发生率大约 50%，需要通过不同的途径再次手术[63]。此外，患者不能脱离呼吸机，咽食管功能异常和胃食管反流是常见的术后并发症。降低术后并发症率和病死率部分要依靠早期诊断，从而预防继发性并发症的发生。目前还没有一致公认的最佳手术方法，然而，治疗很明显是非常复杂的，应该在具有多学科专家的中心内进行。

（胡　明译　李民驹校）

参考文献

1. Adzick NS, Fisher JH, Winter HS, et al: Esophageal adenocarcinoma 20 years after esophageal atresia repair. J Pediatr Surg 1989;24:741.
2. Allal H, Montes-Tapia F, Andina G, et al: Thoracoscopic repair of H-type tracheoesophageal fistula in the newborn: A technical case report. J Pediatr Surg 2004;39:1568.
3. Allmendinger N, Hallisey MJ, Markowitz SK, et al: Balloon dilation of esophageal strictures in children. J Pediatr Surg 1966;31:334.
4. Al-Qahtani AR, Yazbeck S, Rosen NG, et al: Lengthening technique for long gap esophageal atresia and early anastomosis. J Pediatr Surg 2003;38:737.
5. Al-Salem AH, Qaisaruddin S, Abu Srair H, et al: Elective, postoperative ventilation in the management of esophageal atresia and tracheoesophageal fistula. Pediatr Surg Int 1997;12:261.
6. Amae S, Nio M, Kamiyama T, et al: Clinical characteristics and management of congenital esophageal stenosis: A report on 14 cases. J Pediatr Surg 2003;38:565.
7. Applebaum H, Wosley MM: Pericardial flap aortopexy for tracheomalacia. J Pediatr Surg 1990;25:30, discussion 31.
8. Ashcraft KW, Goodwin C, Amoury RA, Holder TM: Early recognition and aggressive treatment of gastroesophageal reflux following repair of esophageal atresia. J Pediatr Surg 1977;12:317.
9. Babu R, Pierro A, Spitz L, et al: The management of oesophageal atresia in neonates with right-sided aortic arch. J Pediatr Surg 2000;35:56.
10. Bagolan P, Iacobelli Bd B, De Angelis P, et al: Long gap esophageal atresia and esophageal replacement: Moving toward a separation? J Pediatr Surg 2004;39:1084.
11. Bar-Maor JA, Shoshany G, Sweed Y: Wide gap esophageal atresia: A new method to elongate the upper pouch. J Pediatr Surg 1989;24:882.
12. Baumann W, Greinacher I, Emmrich P, Sprenger J: [VATER oder VACTERL syndrome.] Klin Padiatr 1976;188:328.
13. Bax KMA, Van der Zee DC: Feasibility of thoracoscopic repair of esophageal atresia with distal fistula. J Pediatr Surg 2002;37:192.
14. Beasley SW, Phelan E, Kelly JH, et al: Urinary tract abnormalities in association with oesophageal atresia: Frequency, significance, and influence on management. Pediatr Surg Int 1992;7:94.
15. Bell DW, Christiansen TW, Smith TE Jr, Stucker FJ: Laryngotracheoesophageal cleft: The anterior approach. Ann Otol Rhinol Laryngol 1977;86:616.
16. Benjamin B, Cohen D, Glasson M: Tracheomalacia in association with congenital tracheoesophageal fistula. Surgery 1976;79:504.
17. Bergmeijer JH, Tibboel D, Hazebroek FW: Nissen fundoplication in the management of gastroesophageal reflux occurring after repair of esophageal atresia. J Pediatr Surg 2000;35:573.
18. Bianca S, Bianca M, Ettore G: Oesophageal atresia and Down syndrome. Down Syndr Res Pract 2002;8:29.
19. Bianca S, Ettore G: Isolated esophageal atresia and perinatal risk factors. Dis Esophagus 2003;16:39.
20. Biller JA, Allen JL, Schuster SR, et al: Long-term evaluation of esophageal and pulmonary function in patients with repaired esophageal atresia and tracheoesophageal fistula. Dig Dis Sci 1987;32:985.
21. Bluestone CD, Kerry R, Sieber WK: Congenital esophageal stenosis. Laryngoscope 1969;79:1095.
22. Blumberg JB, Stevenson JK, Lemire RJ, Boyden EA: Larynogotracheo-esophageal cleft, the embryologic implications: Review of the literature. Surgery 1965;57:559.
23. Borgnon J, Tounian P, Auber F, et al: Esophageal replacement in children by an isoperistaltic gastric tube: A 12-year experience. Pediatr Surg Int 2004;20:829.
24. Botham MJ, Coran AG: The use of pericardium for the management of recurrent tracheoesophageal fistula. J Pediatr Surg 1986;21:164.
25. Bousamra M 2nd, Tweddell JS, Wells RG, et al: Wire sent for tracheomalacia in a five-year-old girl. Ann Thorac Surg 1996;61:1239.
26. Brennemann J: Am J Dis Child 1913;5:143.
27. Broto J, Asensio M, Vernet JM, et al: [Endoscopic treatment of tracheo-esophageal fistulas: Fact or fiction?] Cir Pediatr 2003;16(2):69.
28. Brown AK, Roddam AW, Spitz L, et al: Oesophageal atresia, related malformations, and medical problems: A family study. Am J Med Genet 1999;85:31.
29. Brown AK, Tam P: Measurement of gap length in esophageal atresia: A simple predictor of outcome. J Am Coll Surg 1996;182:41.
30. Burge DM: Gastric tube interposition: A new technique for the management of long-gap oesophageal atresia. Pediatr Surg Int 1995;10:279.
31. Celli J, van Bokhoven H, Brunner HG: Feingold syndrome: Clinical review and genetic mapping. Am J Med Genet 2003;122A:294.
32. Chahine AA, Campbell AB, Hoffman MA: Management of congenital distal esophageal stenosis with combined Collis gastroplasty–Nissen fundoplication. Pediatr Surg Int 1995;10:23.
33. Chan KL, Saing H: Combined flexible endoscopy and fluoroscopy in the assessment of the gap between the two esophageal pouches in esophageal atresia without fistula. J Pediatr Surg 1995;30:668.
34. Chavin K, Field G, Chandler J, et al: Save the child's esophagus: Management of major disruption after repair of esophageal atresia. J Pediatr Surg 1996;31:48.

35. Chen CY, Tsao PN, Chou HC, et al: Esophageal atresia associated with tracheal stenosis and right lung agenesis: Report of one case. Acta Paediatr Taiwan 2002;43:348.
36. Chen H, Goei GS, Hertzler JH: Family studies in congenital esophageal atresia with or without tracheoesophageal fistula. Birth Defects Orig Artic Ser 1979;15(5C):117.
37. Chetcuti P, Myers NA, Phelan PD, Beasley SW: Adults who survived repair of congenital oesophageal atresia and tracheo-oesophageal fistula. BMJ 1988;297:344.
38. Chittmittrapap S, Spitz L, Kiely EM, Bereton RJ: Oesophageal atresia and associated anomalies. Arch Dis Child 1989;64:364.
39. Chittmittrapap S, Spitz L, Kiely EM, Bereton RJ: Anastomotic stricture following repair of esophageal atresia. J Pediatr Surg 1990;25:508.
40. Choudhury SR, Ashcraft KW, Sharp RJ, et al: Survival of patients with esophageal atresia: Influence of birth weight, cardiac anomaly, and late respiratory complications. J Pediatr Surg 1999;34:70, discussion 74.
41. Cieri MV, Arnold GL, Torfs CP: Malrotation in conjunction with esophageal atresia/tracheo-esophageal fistula. Teratology 1999;60(3):114.
42. Cohen D: Tracheopexy—aorto-tracheal suspension for severe tracheomalacia. Aust Paediatr J 1981;17:117.
43. Cooper JE, Spitz L, Wilkins BM: Barrett's esophagus in children: A histologic and histochemical study of 11 cases. J Pediatr Surg 1987;22:191.
44. Coran AG: Pericardioesophagesoplasty. A new operation for partial esophageal replacement. Am J Surg 1973; 125:294.
45. Coran AG: Ultra-long gap esophageal atresia: How long is long? Ann Thorac Surg 1994;57:528.
46. Corbally MT, Muftah M, Gunney EJ: Nissen fundoplication for gastro-esophageal reflux in repaired tracheo-esophageal fistula. Eur J Pediatr Surg 1992;2:332.
47. Cord-Udy CL, Wright VM, Drake DP: Association of ambiguous genitalia with VATER anomalies and its significance in management. Pediatr Surg Int 1996;11:50.
48. Corsello G, Maresi E, Corrao AM, et al: VATER/VACTERL association: Clinical variability and expanding phenotype including laryngeal stenosis. Am J Med Genet 1992:44:813.
49. Cozzi F, Morini F, Casati A, et al: Glossopexy as an alternative to aortopexy in infants with repaired esophageal atresia and upper airway obstruction. J Pediatr Surg 2002; 37:202.
50. Cozzi F, Myers NA, Piacenti S, et al: Maturational dysautonomia and facial anomalies associated with esophageal atresia: Support for neural crest involvement. J Pediatr Surg 1993;28:798.
51. Crisera CA, Connelly PR, Marmureanu AR, et al: TTF-1 and HNF-3beta in the developing tracheoesophageal fistula: Further evidence for the respiratory origin of the distal esophagus. J Pediatr Surg 1999;34:1322.
52. Cusick EL, Batchelor AA, Spicer RD: Development of a technique for jejunal interposition in long-gap esophageal atresia. J Pediatr Surg 1993;28:990.
53. Davenport M, Bianchi A: Early experience with oesophageal flap oesophagoplasty for repair of oesophageal atresia. Pediatr Surg Int 1990;5:332.
54. Davenport M, Mughal M, McCloy RF, Doig CM: Hypogastrinemia and esophageal atresia. J Pediatr Surg 1992;27:568.
55. De Carvalho JL, Maynard J, Hadley GP: An improved technique for in situ esophageal myotomy and proximal pouch mobilization in patients with esophageal atresia. J Pediatr Surg 1989;24:872.
56. Delius RE, Wheatley MJ, Coran AG: Etiology and management of respiratory complications after repair of esophageal atresia with tracheoesophageal fistula. Surgery 1992;112:527.
57. Depaepe A, Dolk H, Lechat MF: The epidemiology of tracheo-oesophageal fistula and oesophageal atresia in Europe. EUROCAT Working Group. Arch Dis Child 1993; 68:743.
58. Deurloo JA, Ekkelkamp S, Bartelsman JF, et al: Gastroesophageal reflux: Prevalence in adults older than 28 years after correction of esophageal atresia. Ann Surg 2003; 238:686.
59. Deurloo JA, Ekkelkamp S, Schoorl M, et al: Esophageal atresia: Historical evolution of management and results in 371 patients. Ann Thorac Surg 2002;73:267.
60. Diez-Pardo JA, Bao-Quan Q, Navarro C, Tovar JA: A new rodent experimental model of esophageal atresia and tracheoesophageal fistula: Preliminary report. J Pediatr Surg 1996;31:498.
61. Donahoe PK, Hendren WH: The surgical management of laryngotracheoesophageal cleft with tracheoesophageal fistula and esophageal atresia. Surgery 1972;71:363.
62. Driver CP, Shankar KR, Jones MO, et al: Phenotypic presentation and outcome of esophageal atresia in the era of the Spitz classification. J Pediatr Surg 2001;36:1419.
63. DuBois JJ, Pokorny WJ, Harberg FJ, et al: Current management of laryngeal and laryngotracheoesophageal clefts. J Pediatr Surg 1990;25:855.
64. Duhamel B: Technique Chirurgicale Infantile. Paris, 1957.
65. Duranceau A, Fisher SR, Flye M, et al: Motor function of the esophagus after repair of esophageal atresia and tracheoesophageal fistula. Surgery 1977;82:116.
66. Durston W: A Narrative of a Monstrous Birth in Plymouth. Philosophical Transactions of the Royal Society. 1670.
67. Ein SH, Shandling B: Pure esophageal atresia: A 50-year review. J Pediatr Surg 1994;29:1208.
68. Ein SH, Shandling B, Heiss K: Pure esophageal atresia: Outlook in the 1990s. J Pediatr Surg 1993;28:1147.
69. Ein SH, Shandling B, Stephens CA: Twenty-one year experience with the pediatric gastric tube. J Pediatr Surg 1987; 22:77.
70. Ein SH, Shandling B, Wesson D, et al: Esophageal atresia with distal tracheoesophageal fistula: Associated anomalies and prognosis in the 1980s. J Pediatr Surg 1989;24:1055.
71. Ein SH, Stringer DA, Stephens CA, et al: Recurrent tracheoesophageal fistulas—seventeen-year review. J Pediatr Surg 1983;18:436.
72. Engum SA, Grosfeld JL, West KW, et al: Analysis of morbidity and mortality in 227 cases of esophageal atresia and/or tracheoesophageal fistula over two decades. Arch Surg 1995; 130:502, discussion 508.
73. Eraklis AJ, Rossello PJ, Ballantine TV: Circular esophagomyotomy of upper pouch in primary repair of long-segment esophageal atresia. J Pediatr Surg 1976;11:709.
74. Erdogan E, Emir H, Eroglu E, et al: Esophageal replacement using the colon: A 15-year review. Pediatr Surg Int 2000;16:546.
75. Evans M: Application of Collis gastroplasty to the management of esophageal atresia. J Pediatr Surg 1995;30:1232.
76. Farrant P: The antenatal diagnosis of oesophageal atresia by ultrasound. Br J Radiol 1980;53:1202.
77. Fernandez MS, Gutierrez C, Ibanez V, et al: Long-gap esophageal atresia: Reconstruction preserving all portions of the esophagus by Scharli's technique. Pediatr Surg Int 1998;14:17.
78. Filler RM, Messineo A, Vinograd I: Severe tracheomalacia associated with esophageal atresia: Results of surgical treat-

ment. J Pediatr Surg 1992;27:1136, discussion 1140.
79. Filler RM, Rossello PJ, Lebowitz RL: Life-threatening anoxic spells caused by tracheal compression after repair of esophageal atresia: Correction by surgery. J Pediatr Surg 1976;11:739.
80. Filston HC, Chitwood WR Jr, Schkolne B, et al: The Fogarty balloon catheter as an aid to management of the infant with esophageal atresia and tracheoesophageal fistula complicated by severe RDS or pneumonia. J Pediatr Surg 1982;17:149.
81. Finlay HVL: Familial congenital stridor. Arch Dis Child 1949;24:219.
82. Foker JE, Linden BC, Boyle EM Jr, et al: Development of a true primary repair for the full spectrum of esophageal atresia. Ann Surg 1997;226:533, discussion 541.
83. Fonkalsrud EW: Gastroesophageal fundoplication for reflux following repair of esophageal atresia. Experience with nine patients. Arch Surg 1979;114:48.
84. Freeman NV, Cass DT: Colon interposition: A modification of the Waterston technique using the normal esophageal route. J Pediatr Surg 1982;17:17.
85. Frey EK, Dusche L: The cardiospasms. Ergeb Chirur Orthop 1936;29:637.
86. Gage M, Oschner A: The surgical treatment of congenital tracheoesophageal fistula in the new-born. Ann Surg 1936;103:725.
87. Garcia NM, Thompson JW, Shaul DB: Definitive localization of isolated tracheoesophageal fistula using bronchoscopy and esophagoscopy for guide wire placement. J Pediatr Surg 1998;33:1645.
88. Gdanietz K, Krause I: Plastic adhesives for closing esophagotracheal fistulae in children. Z Kinderchir 1975;17:137.
89. German JC, Mahour GH, Woolley MM: Esophageal atresia and associated anomalies. J Pediatr Surg 1976;11:299.
90. Giacomoni MA, Tresoldi M, Zamana C, et al: Circular myotomy of the distal esophageal stump for long gap esophageal atresia. J Pediatr Surg 2001;36:855.
91. Gibson T: The Anatomy of Humane Bodies Epitomized. London, Awnsham & Churchill, 1697.
92. Gilchrist BF, Scriven R, Sanchez J, et al: The application of vascular technology to esophageal and airway strictures. J Pediatr Surg 2002;37:47.
93. Goh DW, Brereton RJ: Success and failure with neonatal tracheo-oesophageal anomalies. Br J Surg 1991;78:834.
94. Gough MH: Esophageal atresia—use of an anterior flap in the difficult anastomosis. J Pediatr Surg 1980;15:310.
95. Grabowski ST, Andrews DA: Upper esophageal stenosis: Two case reports. J Pediatr Surg 1996;31:1438.
96. Greenberg CR, Schnaufnagel D: The G syndrome: A case report. Am J Med Genet 1979;3:59.
97. Gross RE: The Surgery of Infancy and Childhood. Philadelphia, WB Saunders, 1953.
98. Grosser O, Lewis FT, McMurrich JP: The development of the intestinal tract and respiratory organs. In Keibel F, Mall FP (eds): Manual of Human Embryology. Philadelphia, JB Lippincott.
99. Gutierrez, C, Barrios JE, Lluna J, et al: Recurrent tracheoesophageal fistula treated with fibrin glue. J Pediatr Surg 1994;29:1567.
100. Haight C: Congenital esophageal atresia and tracheso-phageal fistula. In Mustard W (ed): Pediatric Surgery. Chicago, Year Book.
101. Haight C, Towsley H: Congenital atresia of the esophagus with tracheoesophageal fistula: Extrapleural ligation of fistula and end-to-end anastomosis of esophageal segments. Surg Gynecol Obstet 1943;76:672.
102. Harris J, Kallen B, Robert E: Descriptive epidemiology of alimentary tract atresia. Teratology 1995;52:15.
103. Hendren WH: Esophageal atresia treated by electromagnetic bougienage and subsequent repair. J Pediatr Surg 1975;11:719.
104. Hendren WH, Hale JR: Electromagnetic bougienage to lengthen esophageal segments in congenital esophageal atresia. N Engl J Med 1975;293:428.
105. Hennekam RC, Huber J, Variend D: Bartsocas-Papas syndrome with internal anomalies: Evidence for a more generalized epithelial defect or new syndrome? Am J Med Genet 1994;53:102.
106. Hill TP: Bost Med Surg J 1840;21:320.
107. Hirschl RB, Yardeni D, Oldham K, et al: Gastric transposition for esophageal replacement in children: Experience with 41 consecutive cases with special emphasis on esophageal atresia. Ann Surg 2002;236:531, discussion 539.
108. Hirschsprung H: Den medfordte tillerkning of spieseroret. Medico-Chirurg Rev 31;1861:437.
109. His W: Zur Bildungsgechischte der Lungen beim menschlischen Embryo. Arch Anat 89, 1887.
110. Hoffman MA, Superina R, Wesson DE: Unilateral pulmonary agenesis with esophageal atresia and distal tracheoesophageal fistula: Report of two cases. J Pediatr Surg 1989;24:1084.
111. Hoffman W: Atresia oesophogi congenital et communicato inter oesapgaiu et tracheoni. Griefswald, (Dissertation). University of Griefswald, Germany, 1899.
112. Holder TM, Clout DT, Lewis JE Jr, Pilling GP 4th: Esophageal atresia and tracheoesophageal fistula: A survey of its members by the surgical section of the American Academy of Pediatrics. Pediatrics 1964;34:542.
113. Holmes T: Surgical Management of Children's Diseases. London, Longmans, Green, Reader, & Dyer, 1869.
114. Howard R, Myers N: Esophageal atresia: A technique for elongating the upper pouch. Surgery 1965;58:725.
115. Humphreys GH II, Ferrer JM Jr: Management of esophageal atresia. Am J Surg 1964;107:406.
116. Iuchtman M, Brereton R, Spitz L, et al: Morbidity and mortality in 46 patients with the VACTERL association. Isr J Med Sci 1992;28:281.
117. Johnson AM, Rodgers BM, Alford B, et al: Esophageal atresia with double fistula: The missed anomaly. Ann Thorac Surg 1984;38:195.
118. Johnston MR, Loebner N, Hillyer P, et al: External stent for repair of secondary tracheomalacia. Ann Thorac Surg 1980;30:291.
119. Jolley SG, Johnson DG, Roberts CC, et al: Patterns of gastroesophageal reflux in children following repair of esophageal atresia and distal tracheoesophageal fistula. J Pediatr Surg 1980;15:857.
120. Karnak I, Senocak ME, Hicsonmez A, et al: The diagnosis and treatment of H-type tracheoesophageal fistula. J Pediatr Surg 1997;32:1670.
121. Kawahara H, Imura K, Yagi M, Kubota A: Clinical characteristics of congenital esophageal stenosis distal to associated esophageal atresia. Surgery 2001;127:29.
122. Kawahara H, Imura K, Yagi M, et al: Collis-Nissen procedure in patients with esophageal atresia: Long-term evaluation. World J Surg 2002;26:1222.
123. Kawahara H, Oue T, Okuyama H, et al: Esophageal motor function in congenital esophageal stenosis. J Pediatr Surg 2003;38:1716.
124. Kiely E, Spitz L, Brereton R: Management of tracheomalacia. Pediatr Surg Int 1987;2:13.
125. Kilic SS, Gurpinar A, Yakut T, et al: Esophageal atresia and

tracheo-esophageal fistula in a patient with DiGeorge syndrome. J Pediatr Surg 2003;38:E21.
126. Kimura K, Nishijima E, Tsugawa C, et al: A new approach for the salvage of unsuccessful esophageal atresia repair: A spiral myotomy and delayed definitive operation. J Pediatr Surg 1987;22:981.
127. Kimura K, Nishijima E, Tsugawa C, et al: Multistaged extrathoracic esophageal elongation procedure for long gap esophageal atresia: Experience with 12 patients. J Pediatr Surg 2001;36:1725.
128. Kimura K, Soper RT: Multistaged extrathoracic esophageal elongation for long gap esophageal atresia. J Pediatr Surg 1994;29:566.
129. Kimura K, Soper RT, Kao SC, et al: Aortosternopexy for tracheomalacia following repair of esophageal atresia: Evaluation by cine-CT and technical refinement. J Pediatr Surg 1990;25:769.
130. Kitagawa H, Nakada K, Fujioka T, et al: Unilateral pulmonary agenesis with tracheoesophageal fistula: A case report. J Pediatr Surg 1995;30:1523.
131. Kluth D: Atlas of esophageal atresia. J Pediatr Surg 1976; 11:901.
132. Kluth D, Fiegel DH: The embryology of the foregut. Semin Pediatr Surg 2003;12:3.
133. Kluth D, Steding G, Seidl W: The embryology of foregut malformations. J Pediatr Surg 1987;22:389.
134. Ko BA, Frederic R, DiTirro PA, et al: Simplified access for division of the low cervical/high thoracic H-type tracheoesophageal fistula. J Pediatr Surg 2000;35:1621.
135. Konkin DE, O'Hali AW, Webber EM, Blair GK: Outcomes in esophageal atresia and tracheoesophageal fistula. J Pediatr Surg 2003;38:1726.
136. Kosloske AM: Azygous flap technique for reinforcement of esophageal closure. J Pediatr Surg 1990;25:793.
137. Kovesi T, Rubin T: Long-term complications of congenital esophageal atresia and/or tracheoesophageal fistula. Chest 2004;126:915.
138. Koyluoglu G, Gunay I, Ceran C, Berkan O: Pericardial flap aortopexy: An easy and safe technique in the treatment of tracheomalacia. J Cardiovasc Surg (Torino) 2002; 43:295.
139. Kreuter E: Die angeborenen Verschliebungen und Verengungen des Darmkanals im Lichte der Entwicklungsgeschichte. Dtsch Z Chir 1905;79:1.
140. Krug E, Bergmeijer JH, Dees J, et al: Gastroesophageal reflux and Barrett's esophagus in adults born with esophageal atresia. Am J Gastroenterol 1999;94:2825.
141. Kutiyanawala M, Wyse RK, Brereton RJ, et al: CHARGE and esophageal atresia. J Pediatr Surg 1992;27:558.
142. Kyyronen P, Hemminki K: Gastro-intestinal atresias in Finland in 1970-79, indicating time-place clustering. J Epidemiol Commun Health 1988;42:257.
143. Ladd WE: The surgical treatment of esophageal atresia and tracheoesophageal fistulas. N Engl J Med 1944;230:625.
144. Lai JY, Sheu JC, Chang PY, et al: Experience with distal circular myotomy for long-gap esophageal atresia. J Pediatr Surg 1996;31:1503.
145. Langer JC, Hussain H, Khan A, et al: Prenatal diagnosis of esophageal atresia using sonography and magnetic resonance imaging. J Pediatr Surg 2001;36:804.
146. Lanman TH: Congenital atresia of the esophagus: A study of thirty-two cases. Arch Surg 1940;7:1060.
147. Leininger BJ: Silastic banding of esophagus with subsequent repair of esophageal atresia and tracheosesophageal fistula. J Pediatr Surg 1972;7:404.
148. Leonard H, Barrett AM, Scott JE, et al: The influence of congenital heart disease on survival of infants with oesophageal atresia. Arch Dis Child Fetal Neonat Ed 2001;85:F204.
149. Lessin MS, Wesselhoeft CW, Luks FI, et al: Primary repair of long-gap esophageal atresia by mobilization of the distal esophagus. Eur J Pediatr Surg 1999;9:369.
150. Levine JJ, Shoshany G, Davidson M, et al: Manometric variations following spiral myotomy for long-gap esophageal atresia. J Pediatr Gastroenterol Nutr 1990;10:380.
151. Lilienthal H: Thoracic Surgery. Philadelphia, WB Saunders, 1925.
152. Lindahl H: Esophageal atresia: A simple technical detail aiding the mobilization and circular myotomy of the proximal segment. J Pediatr Surg 1987;22:113.
153. Lindahl H, Rintala R, Louhimo I: Failure of the Nissen fundoplication to control gastroesophageal reflux in esophageal atresia patients. J Pediatr Surg 1989;24:985.
154. Lindell-Iwan L: Modification of Livaditis' myotomy for long gap oesophageal atresia. Ann Chir Gynaecol 1990; 79:101.
155. Little DC, Rescorla FJ, Grosfeld JL, et al: Long-term analysis of children with esophageal atresia and tracheoesophageal fistula. J Pediatr Surg 2003;38:852.
156. Liu YX, Xue F: Congenital esophageal stenosis due to tracheo-bronchial cartilage. Int J Pediatr Otorhinolaryngol 1987;14:95.
157. Livaditis A: End-to-end anastomosis in esophageal atresia. A clinical and experimental study. Scand J Thorac Cardiovasc Surg Suppl 1969;2:7-20.
158. Livaditis A: Esophageal atresia. A method of over-bridging long segmental gaps. Z Kinderchir 1973;13:298.
159. Livaditis A, Radberg L, Odensjo G: Esophageal end-to-end anastomosis. Reduction of anastomotic tension by circular myotomy. Scand J Thorac Cardiovasc Surg 1972;6:206.
160. Lokare RV, Manvi RS: Esophageal atresia with right pulmonary agenesis. Indian Pediatr 1998;35:555.
161. Lomas FE, Dahlstrom JE, Ford JH: VACTERL with hydrocephalus: Family with X-linked VACTERL-H. Am J Med Genet 1998;76:74.
162. Longmire WP: Congenital atresia and tracheo-esophageal fistula. Arch Surg 1947;55:330.
163. Louhimo IH, Lindahl H: Esophageal atresia: Primary results of 500 consecutively treated patients. J Pediatr Surg 1983; 18:217.
164. Lyall P, Bao-Quan Q, Beasley S: The effect of neck flexion on oesophageal tension in the pig and its relevance to repaired oesophageal atresia. Pediatr Surg Int 2001;17:193.
165. Mackenzie M: Malformation of the esophagus. Arch Laryngol 1880;1:301.
166. MacKinlay GA, Burlles R: Oesophageal atresia: Paralysis and ventilation in management of the wide gap. Pediatr Surg Int 1987;2:10.
167. Mahour GH, Johnston PW, Gwinn JL, et al: Congenital esophageal stenosis distal to esophageal atresia. Surgery 1971;69:936.
168. Mahour GH, Woolley MM, Gwinn JL: Elongation of the upper pouch and delayed anatomic reconstruction in esophageal atresia. J Pediatr Surg 1974;9:373.
169. Manning PB, Morgan RA, Coran AG, et al: Fifty years' experience with esophageal atresia and tracheoesophageal fistula. Beginning with Cameron Haight's first operation in 1935. Ann Surg 1986;204:446.
170. Matsuoka S, Takeuchi K, Yamanaka Y, et al: Comparison of magnetic resonance imaging and ultrasonography in the prenatal diagnosis of congenital thoracic abnormalities. Fetal Diagn Ther 2003;18:447.
171. McKinnon LJ, Kosloske AM: Prediction and prevention

of anastomotic complications of esophageal atresia and tracheoesophageal fistula. J Pediatr Surg 1990;25:778.
172. Mee RBB, Beasley SW, Auldist AW, et al: Influence of congenital heart disease on management of oesophageal atresia. Pediatr Surg Int 1992;7:90.
173. Merei JM, Hutson JM: Embryogenesis of tracheoesophageal anomalies: A review. Pediatr Surg Int 2002;18:319.
174. Morabito A, MacKinnon E, Alizai N, et al: The anterior mediastinal approach for management of tracheomalacia. J Pediatr Surg 2000;35:1456.
175. Moriarty KP, Jacir NN, Harris BH, et al: Transanastomotic feeding tubes in repair of esophageal atresia. J Pediatr Surg 1996;31:53, discussion 54.
176. Morini F, Cozzi DA, Ilari M, et al: Pattern of cardiovascular anomalies associated with esophageal atresia: Support for a caudal pharyngeal arch neurocristopathy. Pediatr Res 2001;50:565.
177. Moukheiber AK, Camboulives J, Guys JM, et al: Repair of a type IV laryngotracheoesophageal cleft with cardiopulmonary bypass. Ann Otol Rhinol Laryngol 2002;111:1076.
178. Murphy SG, Yazbeck S, Russo P: Isolated congenital esophageal stenosis. J Pediatr Surg 1995;30:1238.
179. Myers NA: The history of oesophageal atresia and tracheo-oesophageal fistula—1670-1984. Prog Pediatr Surg 1986;20:106.
180. Myers NA: Oesophageal atresia: The epitome of modern surgery. Ann R Coll Surg Engl 1974;54:277.
181. Neilson IR, Croitoru DP, Guttman FM, et al: Distal congenital esophageal stenosis associated with esophageal atresia. J Pediatr Surg 1991;26:478, discussion 481.
182. Nihoul-Fekete C, Backer A, Lortat-Jacob S, et al: Congenital esophageal stenosis. Pediatr Surg Int 1987;2:86.
183. Nishina T, Tsuchida Y, Saito S: Congenital esophageal stenosis due to tracheobronchial remnants and its associated anomalies. J Pediatr Surg 1981;16:190.
184. Nora AH, Nora JJ: A syndrome of multiple congenital anomalies associated with teratogenic exposure. Arch Environ Health 1975;30:17.
185. Obatake M, Tanaka T, Muraoka M, et al: Anterior approach bilateral musculomucosal flaps repair for laryngotracheoesophageal clefts. J Pediatr Surg 2003;38:1720.
186. Ohi R, Tseng SW: Congenital oesophageal stenosis. In Newborn Surgery. Oxford, Butterworth-Heinemann.
187. Okada A, Usui N, Inoue M, et al: Esophageal atresia in Osaka: A review of 39 years' experience. J Pediatr Surg 1997;32:1570.
188. O'Rahilly R, Muller F: Chevalier Jackson lecture. Respiratory and alimentary relations in staged human embryos. New embrological data and congenital anomalies. Ann Otol Rhinol Laryngol 1984;93:421.
189. Orford J, Cass DT, Glasson MJ: Advances in the treatment of oesophageal atresia over three decades: The 1970s and the 1990s. Pediatr Surg Int 2004;20:402.
190. Orringer MB, Kirsh MM, Sloan H: Long-term esophageal function following repair of esophageal atresia. Ann Surg 1977;186:436.
191. Otte JB, Gianello P, Wese FX, et al: Diverticulum formation after circular myotomy for esophageal atresia. J Pediatr Surg 1984;19:68.
192. Otten C, Migliazza L, Xia H, et al: Neural crest–derived defects in experimental esophageal atresia. Pediatr Res 2000;47:178.
193. Pandit SK, Rattan KN, Budhiraja S: Esophageal atresia with blocked distal tracheo-esophageal fistula. Indian J Pediatr 1998;65:763.
194. Parent P, Bensaid M, Le Guern H, et al: [Clinical heterogeneity of Townes-Brock syndrome.] Arch Pediatr 1995;2:551.
195. Parker AF, Christie DL, Cahill JL: Incidence and significance of gastroesophageal reflux following repair of esophageal atresia and tracheoesophageal fistula and the need for anti-reflux procedures. J Pediatr Surg 1979;14:5.
196. Patel SB, Ade-Ajayi N, Kiely EM: Oesophageal atresia: A simplified approach to early management. Pediatr Surg Int 2002;18:87.
197. Pettersson G: Inhibited separation of the larynx and the upper part of the trachea from the esophagus in a newborn: Report of a case successfully operated upon. Acta Chir Scand 1955;10:250.
198. Pietsch JB, Stokes KB, Beardmore HE: Esophageal atresia with tracheoesophageal fistula: End-to-end version versus end-to-side repair. J Pediatr Surg 1978:13:677.
199. Plass E: Congenital atresia of the esophagus with tracheoesophageal fistula: Associated with fused kidney. A case report and a survey of the literature on congenital anomalies of the esophagus. Johns Hopkins Hosp Rep 1919;18:259.
200. Pletcher BA, Friedes JS, Breg WR, et al: Familial occurrence of esophageal atresia with and without tracheoesophagel fistula: Report of two unusual kindreds. Am J Med Genet 1991;39:380.
201. Poenaru D, Laberge JM, Neilson IR, et al: A new prognostic classification for esophageal atresia. Surgery 1993; 113:426.
202. Pompino HJ: Endoscopic closure of tracheo-esophageal fistulae. Z Kinderchir 1979;27:90.
203. Postlethwait R: Clonic interposition for esophageal substitution. Surg Gynecol Obstet 1983;156:377.
204. Postlethwait RW: Technique for isoperistaltic gastric tube for esophageal bypass. Ann Surg 1979;189:673.
205. Pul N, Pul M, Gedik Y: McKusick-Kaufman syndrome associated with esophageal atresia and distal tracheoesophageal fistula: A case report and review of the literature. Am J Med Genet 1994;49:341.
206. Puri P, Ninan GK, Blake NS, et al: Delayed primary anastomosis for esophageal atresia: 18 months' to 11 years' follow-up. J Pediatr Surg 1992;27:1127.
207. Quan LD, Smith W: The VATER association. Vertebral defects, Anal atresia, T-E fistula with esophageal atresia, Radial and Renal dysplasia: A spectrum of associated defects. J Pediatr 1973;82:104.
208. Ramesh JC, Ramanujam TM, Jayaram G: Congenital esophageal stenosis: Report of three cases, literature review, and a proposed classification. Pediatr Surg Int 2001; 17:188.
209. Randolph JG, Newman KD, Anderson KD: Current results in repair of esophageal atresia with tracheoesophageal fistula using physiologic status as a guide to therapy. Ann Surg 1989;209:526, discussion 530.
210. Randolph JG, Tunell WP, Lilly JR: Gastric division in the critically ill infant with esophageal atresia and tracheoesophageal fistula. Surgery 1968;63:496.
211. Rangecroft L, Bush GH, Lister J, et al: Endoscopic diathermy obliteration of recurrent tracheoesophageal fistulae. J Pediatr Surg 1984;19:41.
212. Rehbein F, Schweder N: Reconstruction of the esophagus without colon transplantation in cases of atresia. J Pediatr Surg 1971;6:746.
213. Richter CF: Dissertatio Medica de Infanticido in Artis Obstericae. Leipzig, Germany, 1792.
214. Richter HM: Congenital atresia of the esophagus: An operation designed for its cure. Surg Gynecol Obstet 1913;17:397.

An operation designed for its cure. Surg Gynecol Obstet 1913;17:397.
215. Rosenthal AH: Congenital atresia of the esophagus with tracheoesophageal fistula: Report of eight cases. Arch Pathol 1931;12:756.
216. Rossello PJ, Lebron H, Franco AA: The technique of myotomy in esophageal reconstruction: An experimental study. J Pediatr Surg 1980;15:430.
217. Rothenberg S: Thoracoscopic repair of a tracheoesophageal fistula in a newborn infant. Pediatr Surg Innov Tech 2000;4:289.
218. Rothenberg S: Thoracoscopic repair of tracheoesphageal fistula in newborns. J Pediatr Surg 2002;37:869.
219. Ryan DP, Meuhrcke DD, Doody DP, et al: Laryngotracheoesophageal cleft (type IV): Management and repair of lesions beyond the carina. J Pediatr Surg 1991;26:962, discussion 969.
220. Said M, Mekki M, Golli M, et al: Balloon dilatation of anastomotic strictures secondary to surgical repair of oesophageal atresia. Br J Radiol 2003;76:26.
221. Salem M, Wong AY, Lin YH, et al: Prevention of gastric distention during anesthesia for newborns with tracheoesophageal fistulas. Anesthesiology 1973;38:82.
222. Sarin YK: Esophageal atresia and tracheo-esophageal fistula with right pulmonary agenesis. Indian Pediatr 1996; 33:595.
223. Satoh S, Takashima T, Takeuchi H, et al: Antenatal sonographic detection of the proximal esophageal segment: Specific evidence for congenital esophageal atresia. J Clin Ultrasound 1995;23:419.
224. Schaarschmidt K, Kolberg-Schwerdt A, Bunke K, Strauss J: A technique for thoracoscopic aortopericardiosternopexy. Surg Endosc 2002;16:1639.
225. Schärli AF: Esophageal reconstruction in very long atresias by elongation of the lesser curvature. Pediatr Surg Int 1992;7:101.
226. Schwartz MZ: An improved technique for circular myotomy in long-gap esophageal atresia. J Pediatr Surg 1983;18:833.
227. Schwartz MZ, Filler RM: Tracheal compression as a cause of apnea following repair of tracheoesophageal fistula: Treatment by aortopexy. J Pediatr Surg 1980;15:842.
228. Seoud M, Nassar A, Usta I, et al: Gastrointestinal malformations in two infants born to women with hyperthyroidism untreated in the first trimester. Am J Perinatol 2003;20:59.
229. Shafer AD, David TE: Suture fistula as a means of connecting upper and lower segments in esophageal atresia. J Pediatr Surg 1974;9:669.
230. Shandling B: The insertion of a soft Silastic nasogastric tube at an operation for an esophageal atresia. J Pediatr Surg 1993;28:280.
231. Sharma AK, Sharma KK, Sharma CS, et al: Congenital esophageal obstruction by intraluminal mucosal diaphragm. J Pediatr Surg 1991;26:213.
232. Sharma AK, Shekhawat NS, Agrawal LD, et al: Esophageal atresia and tracheoesophageal fistula: A review of 25 years' experience. Pediatr Surg Int 2000;16:478.
233. Sharma AK, Wakhlu A: Simple technique for proximal pouch mobilization and circular myotomy in cases of esophageal atresia with tracheoesophageal fistula. J Pediatr Surg 1994;29:1402.
234. Shaw R: Surgical correction of congenital atresia of the esophagus with tracheo-esophageal fistula. J Thorac Surg 1939;9:213.
235. Shehab ZP, Bailey CM: Type IV laryngotracheoesophageal clefts—recent 5 year experience at Great Ormond Street Hospital for Children. Int J Pediatr Otorhinolaryngol 2001;60:1.
236. Shepard R, Fenn S, Sieber WK: Evaluation of esophageal function in postoperative esophageal atresia and tracheoesophageal fistula. Surgery 1966;59:608.
237. Siegel MJ, Shackelford GD, McAlister WH, et al: Circular esophageal myotomy simulating a pulmonary or mediastinal pseudocyst. Radiology 1980;136:365.
238. Simpson BB, Ryan DP, Donahoe PK, et al: Type IV laryngotracheoesophageal clefts: Surgical management for long-term survival. J Pediatr Surg 1996;31:1128.
239. Singh S, Shun JA: A new technique of anastomosis to avoid stricture formation in oesophageal atresia. Pediatr Surg Int 2001;17:575.
240. Skandalakis JE, Gray SW: Embrology for Surgeons. Philadelphia, WB Saunders, 1994.
241. Slim MS: Circular myotomy of the esophagus: Clinical application in esophageal atresia. Ann Thorac Surg 1977; 23:62.
242. Smith EI: The early development of the trachea and esophagus in relation to atresia of the esophagus and tracheoesophageal fistula. Embryol Carnegie Inst 1957; 36:41.
243. Sparey C, Jawaheer G, Barrett AM, et al: Esophageal atresia in the Northern Region Congenital Anomaly Survey, 1985-1997: Prenatal diagnosis and outcome. Am J Obstet Gynecol 2000;182:427.
244. Spilde T, Bhatia A, Ostlie D, et al: A role for sonic hedgehog signaling in the pathogenesis of human tracheoesophageal fistula. J Pediatr Surg 2003;38:465.
245. Spilde TL, Bhatia AM, Marosky JK, et al: Complete discontinuity of the distal fistula tract from the developing gut: Direct histologic evidence for the mechanism of tracheoesophageal fistula formation. Anat Rec 2002;267:220.
246. Spilde TL, Bhatia AM, Mehta S, et al: Defective sonic hedgehog signaling in esophageal atresia with tracheoesophageal fistula. Surgery 2003;134:345.
247. Spitz L: Congenital esophageal stenosis distal to associated esophageal atresia. J Pediatr Surg 1973;8:973.
248. Spitz L: Esophageal atresia and tracheoesophageal fistula in children. Curr Opin Pediatr 1993;5:347.
249. Spitz L: Esophageal atresia: Past, present, and future. J Pediatr Surg 1996;31:19.
250. Spitz L, Hitchcock R: Oesophageal atresia and tracheoesophageal fistula. In Burge DM, Griffiths M, Freeman NV (eds): Surgery of the Newborn. New York, Churchill Livingstone.
251. Spitz L, Hitchcock R: Recurrent tracheoesophageal fistula. In Spitz L, Coran AG (eds): Pediatric Surgery. London, Chapman & Hall.
252. Spitz L, Kiely E, Brereton RJ: Esophageal atresia: Five years' experience with 148 cases. J Pediatr Surg 1987;22:103.
253. Spitz L, Kiely E, Brereton RJ, Drake D: Management of esophageal atresia. World J Surg 1993;17:296.
254. Spitz L, Kiely EM, Morecroft JA, Drake DP: Esophageal atresia: At-risk groups for the 1990s. J Pediatr Surg 1994; 29:723.
255. Spitz L, Kiely E, Pierro A: Gastric transposition in children—a 21-year experience. J Pediatr Surg 2004;39:276, discussion 276.
256. Steadland KM, Langham MR Jr, Greene MA, et al: Unilateral pulmonary agenesis, esophageal atresia, and distal tracheoesophageal fistula. Ann Thorac Surg 1995; 59:511.
257. Steele C: Case of deficient oesophagus. Lancet 1888; 2:764.

258. Streeter GL: Development horizons in human embryos: Description of age groups XV, XVI, XVII, XVIII. Contr Embryol Carnegie Inst 1945;32:133.
259. Stringer MD, McKenna KM, Goldstein RB, et al: Prenatal diagnosis of esophageal atresia. J Pediatr Surg 1995; 30:1258.
260. Sulamaa MGL, Alvenainen EK: Prognosis and treatment of congenital atresia of the esophagus. Acta Chir Scand 1951;102:141.
261. Sumitomo K, Ikeda K, Nagasaki A: Esophageal manometrical assessment after esophageal circular myotomy for wide-gap esophageal atresia. Jpn J Surg 1988;18:218.
262. Sweed Y, Bar-Maor JA, Shoshany G: Insertion of a soft Silastic nasogastric tube at operation for esophageal atresia: A new technical method. J Pediatr Surg 1992; 27:650.
263. Szendrey T, Danyi G, Czeizel A: Etiological study on isolated esophageal atresia. Hum Genet 1985;70:51.
264. Tam PK, Sprigg A, Cudmore RE, et al: Endoscopy-guided balloon dilatation of esophageal strictures and anastomotic strictures after esophageal replacement in children. J Pediatr Surg 1991;26:1101.
265. Tandler J: Entwicklungsgeschichte des menschlichen Duodenum in frühen Embryonalstadien. Morph JB 1902;29:187.
266. Tannuri U, Teodoro WR, de Santana Witzel S, et al: Livaditis' circular myotomy does not decrease anastomotic leak rates and induces deleterious changes in anastomotic healing. Eur J Pediatr Surg 2003;13:224.
267. Tazuke Y, Kawahara H, Yagi M, et al: Use of a Palmaz stent for tracheomalacia: Case report of an infant with esophageal atresia. J Pediatr Surg 1999;34:1291.
268. Templeton JM Jr, Templeton JJ, Schnaufer L, et al: Management of esophageal atresia and tracheoesophageal fistula in the neonate with severe respiratory distress syndrome. J Pediatr Surg 1985;20:394.
269. Thompson DJ, Molello JA, Strebing RJ, et al: Teratogenicity of Adriamycin and daunomycin in the rat and rabbit. Teratology 1978;17:151.
270. Tibboel D, Pattenier JW, Krugten RJ, et al: Prospective evaluation of postoperative morbidity in patients with esophageal atresia. Pediatr Surg Int 1988;4:252.
271. Todani T, Watanabe Y, Mizuguchi T, et al: Congenital oesophageal stenosis due to fibromuscular thickening. Z Kinderchir 1984;39:11.
272. Tomaselli V, Volpi ML, Dell'Agnola CA, et al: Long-term evaluation of esophageal function in patients treated at birth for esophageal atresia. Pediatr Surg Int 2003; 19:40.
273. Tonz M, Kohli S, Kaiser G: Oesophageal atresia: What has changed in the last 3 decades? Pediatr Surg Int 2004.
274. Torfs CP, Curry CJ, Bateson TF: Population-based study of tracheoesophageal fistula and esophageal atresia. Teratology 1995;52:220.
275. Touloukian RJ, Seashore JH: Thirty-five-year institutional experience with end-to-side repair for esophageal atresia. Arch Surg 2004;139:371, discussion 374.
276. Tovar JA, Diez Pardo JA, Murcia J, et al: Ambulatory 24-hour manometric and pH metric evidence of permanent impairment of clearance capacity in patients with esophageal atresia. J Pediatr Surg 1995;30:1224.
277. Tovar JA, Gorostiaga L, Escheverry J, et al: Barrett's esophagus in children and adolescents. Pediatr Surg Int 1993; 8:389.
278. Tsang TM, Tam PKH, Westaby S: Management of coexisting coarctation of the aorta and oesophageal atresia. Pediatr Surg Int 1996;11:107.
279. Tuqan NA: Annular stricture of the esophagus distal to the congenital tracheoesophageal fistula. Surgery 1962;52:394.
280. Tyler DC: Laryngeal cleft: Report of eight patients and review of the literature. Am J Genet 1990;21:61.
281. Usui N, Kamata S, Ishikawa S, et al: Anomalies of the tracheobronchial tree in patients with esophageal atresia. J Pediatr Surg 1996;31:258.
282. Usui N, Kamata S, Kawahara H, et al: Usefulness of endoscopic ultrasonography in the diagnosis of congenital esophageal stenosis. J Pediatr Surg 2002;37:1744.
283. Valerio D, Jones PF, Stewart AM: Congenital oesophageal stenosis. Arch Dis Child 1977;52:414.
284. Van Biervliet S, Van Winckel M, Robberecht E, et al: High-dose omeprazole in esophagitis with stenosis after surgical treatment of esophageal atresia. J Pediatr Surg 2001; 36:1416.
285. van Heurn LW, Cheng W, de Vries B, et al: Anomalies associated with oesophageal atresia in Asians and Europeans. Pediatr Surg Int 2002;18:241.
286. Vasudevan SA, Kerendi F, Lee H, Ricketts RR: Management of congenital esophageal stenosis. J Pediatr Surg 2002;37:1024.
287. Vazquez-Jimenez JF, Sachweh JS, Liakopoulos OJ, et al: Aortopexy in severe tracheal instability: Short-term and long-term outcome in 29 infants and children. Ann Thorac Surg 2001;72:1898.
288. Villegas-Alvarez F, Olvera-Duran J, Rodriguez-Aranda E: et al: Esophageal anastomotic failure: An experimental study. Arch Med Res 2003;34:171.
289. Vinograd I, Filler RM, Bahoric A: Long-term functional results of prosthetic airway in tracheomalacia and bronchomalacia. J Pediatr Surg 22:38, 1987.
290. Vogt EC: Congenital atresia of the esophagus. AJR Am J Roentgenol 1929;22:463.
291. Wailoo MP, Emery JL: The trachea in children with tracheo-oesophageal fistula. Histopathology 1979;3:329.
292. Waterston D: Colonic replacement of esophagus (intrathoracic). Surg Clin North Am 1964;44:1441.
293. Waterston DJ, Bonham Carter RE, Aberdeen E: Esophageal atresia: Tracheo-oesophageal fistula. A study of survival in 218 infants. Lancet 1962;1:819.
294. Weber TR, Keller MS, Fiore A: Aortic suspension (aortopexy) for severe tracheomalacia in infants and children. 2002;184:573, discussion 577.
295. Welch RG, Husain OAN: Atresia of the oesophagus with common tracheo-oesophageal tube. Arch Dis Child 1958;33:367.
296. Werlin SL, Dodds WJ, Hogan WJ, et al: Esophageal function in esophageal atresia. Dig Dis Sci 1981;26:796.
297. Wheatley MJ, Coran AG: Pericardial flap interposition for the definitive management of recurrent tracheoesophageal fistula. J Pediatr Surg 1992;27:1122.
298. Wheatley MJ, Coran AG, Wesley JR: Efficacy of the Nissen fundoplication in the management of gastroesophageal reflux following esophageal atresia repair. J Pediatr Surg 1993;28:53.
299. Yagyu M, Gitter H, Richter B, et al: Esophageal atresia in Bremen, Germany—evaluation of preoperative risk classification in esophageal atresia. J Pediatr Surg 2000; 35:584.
300. Yanchar NL, Gordon R, Cooper M, et al: Significance of the clinical course and early upper gastrointestinal studies in predicting complications associated with repair of esophageal atresia. J Pediatr Surg 2001;36:815.
301. Yeung CK, Spitz L, Brereton RJ, et al: Congenital

301. Yeung CK, Spitz L, Brereton RJ, et al: Congenital esophageal stenosis due to tracheobronchial remnants: A rare but important association with esophageal atresia. J Pediatr Surg 1992;27:852.
302. Zaw-Tun HA: The tracheo-esophageal septum—fact or fantasy? Origin and development of the respiratory primordium and esophagus. Acta Anat 1982;114:1.
303. Zigman AS, Yazbeck: Esophageal foreign body obstruction after esophageal atresia repair. J Pediatr Surg 2002; 37:776.

第 68 章

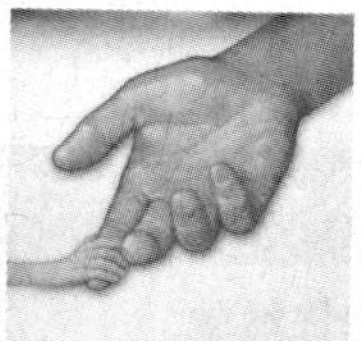

食管腐蚀性狭窄

Alastair J. W. Millar、Alp Numanoglu 和 Heinz Rode

历史记录

1082 吞入腐蚀剂是工业时代的一种疾病[75]。Tucker 等人总结了吞食腐蚀性物质的悲惨结果和治疗方法的演变[119]。食管狭窄扩张最初是盲目地经口探入扩张，现在原则上没有很大改变，但是由于技术的进步，在实践中有了很多变化[95,96]。末端照明食管镜的发明、经胃造口术的索带引导回拉扩张法的应用以及基本药物和营养支持的进步等明显降低了早期死亡率[60,103,119,127]。20 世纪 50 和 60 年代，根据试验结果，广泛应用类固醇和抗生素抑制炎症、瘢痕形成和感染以降低狭窄的发生率[16,18,21,24,52,56,67,70,80,99]。然而，因咽喉烧伤导致的水肿和呼吸道阻塞、吞入大量腐蚀剂引起的穿孔、狭窄扩张或食管不可逆性损伤行改道手术后的并发症仍然能造成死亡[4,9,31,32,48,49,79]。

流行病学

尽管有很多针对儿童和成人的教育课程、预防性标签和包装，甚至立法规定限制了腐蚀性物质的强度和买卖，吞食腐蚀性物质仍是儿童健康的重要威胁[26,75,103,112,119,122,123]。在贫困地区和发展中国家，晶体和液态的腐蚀性苏打用于制造肥皂的家庭产业、果实干燥和农场的容器清洁等。此外，许多可随意购买的腐蚀性清洁剂实际上使儿童继续处于危险之中。最可惜的是大多数腐蚀性吞食发生在 3 岁以下的儿童，而这是完全可以预防的。本病在男孩中较常发生[26,32,75]。吞食毒物发生在 5 岁以上的儿童可能是故意的，而发生在青少年期（女孩居多）则通常是故意的[54,75]。这些病例往往吞食大量的强腐蚀剂和腐蚀性物质。尽管死亡率低，但病损通常是破坏性的，会影响终身。20 世纪 70 年代以来，全面统计学数据表明其发生率在下降，然而，在发展中国家，许多食管替代手术的报道证明，这是严重的世界范围的公共卫生问题[2,11,48,75,86]。这些现象在一些地区特别明显，腐蚀性物质没有放在对儿童安全的容器内出售，或者要从较大的容器中倒出作为家用[75]。目前仍然非常需要成人教育，并立法保证正确的标贴和安全的包装，限制腐蚀性物质的强度和可购买性[26,122,123]。

大约 20%的腐蚀性物质吞食会导致不同程度的食管损伤[54,70,77]。目前已经制定了早期的吞食后处理方案，特别是用纤维光学内镜评估损伤部位的范围和严重程度[1,40,128]。然而，在预防和治疗腐蚀性狭窄中应用类固醇、抗生素和食管支架以及食管扩张的时间、次数、方法等问题上仍有分歧。食管手术或旁路的指征及其手术的形式仍是继续争论的问题[31]。

原因

以液态或颗粒状出售的强碱是严重损伤的主要原因（表 68–1）[26]。家用漂白剂、洗碗机用洗涤剂和其他去污物都是中度碱性的，也是最常见的腐蚀性吞食物。然而这些物质的烧灼通常局限于食管黏膜，无广泛的坏死或继发性狭窄形成[26,72]。许多腐蚀性物质可直接造成活组织的损伤特别是在湿润黏膜，包括腐蚀剂如氢氧化钾、氢氧化钠钠和苯酚，还原剂如氯化氢和硝酸，干燥剂如硫磺酸，氧化剂如铬酸、次氯酸盐和高锰酸钾，以及原生质毒素如乙酸和蚁酸等[61,103,126]。这些被吞食物质的外观和 pH对吞食后食管损伤的部位和类型有重要影响，吞食物 pH超过 12 或小于 1.5 1083
会造成严重的腐蚀性损害[10,52,53,61,75]。晶体状的清洁剂

表 68-1 常见的被吞入的腐蚀性物质

腐蚀性物质	类型	商品形式
酸	硫酸	电池
		工业清洁剂
		金属镀层
	草酸	油漆稀释剂
		清除剂
		金属清洁剂
	盐酸	溶剂
		金属清洁剂
		厕所和下水道清洁剂
		防锈化合物
	磷酸	厕所清洁剂
碱	氢氧化钠	排水沟清洁剂
	氢氧化钾	烤箱清洁剂
		洗衣粉
	碳酸氢钠	肥皂制造成分
		农场的水果干燥剂
氨	商业氨水	家用清洁剂
	氢氧化铵	
清洁剂漂白	次氯酸钠	家用漂白剂
		清洁剂
	多磷酸钠	工业去垢剂
高锰酸钾晶体	高锰酸钾	消毒剂
		染发剂

主要以浓缩的氢氧化钠为主，会黏附在口咽部或者聚集在上段食管，这些部位的损害最严重[52,64,66,90,127]。高浓度的腐蚀性液体通常快速通过口咽部，损伤食管入口、食管中段，并迅速接近胃食管连接处。

不像碱溶液没有很大的味道，强酸是苦的，接触时有烧灼感，通常会咳出来。然而，当吞咽时它们迅速通过食管，在胃窦部造成最严重的损害。当胃空虚时损伤更加严重[51]。十二指肠和近端小肠因幽门括约肌痉挛而相对受到保护[25,62,98,103]。硫酸亚铁片（Clinitest）或胶囊也可以造成食管或胃的腐蚀性损伤[19]。纽扣电池含高浓度的氢氧化钾或者氢氧化钠，但由于它们体积小而很少在食管内嵌顿[76]。如果电池带有电荷，也可由于负极的水解造成邻近黏膜的损伤。

病理生理学

儿童腐蚀性损伤的病理学知识大多数来自于成人的自残性损伤经验和动物实验研究[38,53,57,64,66,69,78,91,106]。黏膜表面的损伤发生在接触强酸或者强碱后数秒钟内[53,66]。酸性或碱性物质造成的损伤性质有很大的不同。吞食酸后黏膜凝固性坏死，形成硬痂，酸通常只穿透黏膜。吞食碱后组织穿孔伴随液化坏死，然后是上皮细胞和黏膜下层破坏，并可深入到肌层[16,53,61]形成一个易碎而浅色的痂，痂下方的组织继续被破坏，直到碱性被中和。食管损伤主要发生在停顿的部位：环咽部、中段食管跨过主动脉弓和左主气管部、和胃食管连接部上方。吞食后发生即刻的痉挛和运动紊乱，可导致排空延迟，甚至出现胃液反流[47]。出血、血栓和显著的炎症伴水肿可在损伤后 24 小时内出现。根据烧灼的程度，炎症可以扩散穿过肌肉层，直至穿孔。48 小时之后，有证据证明黏膜下血管的血栓形成，可导致局部坏死和坏疽。细菌污染可以导致小的壁内脓肿，可以扩散到纵隔，伴食管全层损伤[18]。数天后坏死组织脱落，水肿消退，新的血管形成。从损伤后的第一周末至第二周是早期修复或亚急性阶段。瘢痕的形成在第三周开始，成纤维细胞增殖代替了黏膜和肌肉层并形成狭窄。黏膜再上皮化在第三周内开始，通常在第六周完成。粘连在这个阶段形成，食管腔变得狭窄或闭塞。最终结果可能是食管纤维化和缩短[16]。如果损伤是穿透性的，坏死可能延伸到周围纵隔，导致纵隔炎，或向前到气管，引起气管食管瘘甚至食管大动脉瘘[9,20,79,87]。

类固醇已经被用于缓和烧灼处和深部组织的炎症反应，最终达到减少瘢痕形成的目的[18,30,52,53,90,109]。然而，最初的损伤长度很大程度上决定了损伤愈合的结果，从黏膜的再上皮化、食管腺体缺失和轻度黏膜下纤维化但保留肌层，到食管壁完全由纤维组织替代不等[66,81]。一旦食管肌层被破坏就不能再生，这时纤维替代成熟伴腔面上皮化是唯一的“正性”结果[24]。用山黧豆中毒原和丝裂霉素 C 抑制胶原分子间共价键的形成来减少瘢痕组织的形成已有实验研究，但还未用于临床[21,34,35,44]。

临床表现

大多数吞食腐蚀性物质的婴儿和儿童很少表现出症状和体征[1,29,40,77]。仅有 1/4 的病例有明确的吞食了
1084 腐蚀性物质的客观证据[43,77]。损伤累及的长度和严重程度取决于吞食物质的浓度和性状。晶体碱会黏附于湿润表面，立即引起疼痛，造成口咽部的烧灼和上段食管的损伤。少数食管烧伤患者（≤10%）口咽部没有客观表现，临床医生仍应进行适当的诊断检查。然而，大多数患者的咽喉部表现出广泛损伤伴明确的食管损伤。如果仅仅累及舌和软腭，则食管损伤不太可能发生[1,40,43,77]。

腐蚀性酸的黏性和比重比碱性液体的低，因此吞食酸后会迅速通过食管，大部分食管可能不会损伤。由于幽门接触酸后引起痉挛，吞食下去的酸聚集在幽门近端，损伤主要发生在胃窦部[49,62,97,113]。

损伤后可能出现明显的体征和症状，口咽部的黏膜炎症肿胀和严重的口腔与胸骨后疼痛[29,43]。常伴有焦虑和心动过速。流口水和无法吞咽表明有严重的咽后壁或食管上段损伤[30,90]。溢出的腐蚀性物质进入上呼吸道会引起咽后壁和喉部水肿，导致上呼吸道急性梗阻[54,116]。

浓缩的氨气可以被吸入，导致鼻咽部水肿和呼吸道损伤[54]。食管穿孔伴纵隔炎、腹膜炎和休克虽然很少见，但是可能发生[9,90]。

初期处理和诊断

最初的处理是保证气道畅通和供氧，保证心血管的稳定。部分患者可能立刻需要维持呼吸道畅通的干预。一旦呼吸和血流动力学达到稳定，需要对吞食的有害物质及成分、浓度和周围环境进行调查。虽然家长应该能够确定吞食的物质，但经常缺乏这些信息。很多区域都有中毒中心，可获得详细的物质信息[117]。对吞食了腐蚀性物质的病例，引吐和鼓励吞食任何液体都是禁止的，因为大多数碱已被胃酸中和，而且酸回流的结果可能导致进一步的损伤。吸入呕吐物可导致腐蚀性物质进入上呼吸道，引起急性炎症反应和水肿伴气道阻塞。

因为病史和体检不能可靠地评估食管受累的程度，口咽部和上消化道的内镜检查是非常重要的、光学纤维内镜既准确又安全，特别是在吞食后的 24～48 小时内进行[38,40,95,127,128]。如果食管损伤可以被排除，应避免不必要的治疗。然而，对于有吞食史的患者是否需要内镜检查仍然存在争论。有些人提倡内镜检查仅适用于有症状的患者[50,74]。

锝标记的硫糖铝放射同位素食管扫描作为筛查装置已获得成功应用，缺少硫糖铝黏附的地方说明没有严重的损伤[83]。根据内镜的检查结果对损伤的严重程度进行分级，据此提示远期结果，特别是继发性狭窄的形成；然而有时在实践中也很难获得精确的评估（表 68–2）[37,38,54]。有人尝试用内镜观察整个上消化道来确定环状或三级损伤，为初期治疗提供充分的信息；但试图进一步观察是不必要的，并有潜在的危险[54,81]。穿孔是一个严重的并发症，可能合并纵隔炎症甚至导致死亡。明显的咽部烧灼伴有哮鸣时，早期食管镜检查不适合，因为有加重气道阻塞的危险[123]。间接光学纤维喉镜对于评估上呼吸道是有用的。如果需要插管，可以同时进行食管镜检查，或者等上呼吸道水肿消退后再行食管镜检查。如果怀疑有吸入或呼吸道灼伤，早期 X 线检查应限于颈部、胸部和腹部。如果存在发热、全身性脓毒血症和上腹部体征，则可能存在穿孔，水溶性造影剂食管检查可提供穿孔的证据[40]。食管造影检查通常在 10～14 天后进行，此时全食管和上消化道检查可明确损伤的范围，并有助于选择适当的治疗方法（图 68–1）[71]。

治疗

如果已知吞食的是轻度刺激物，如次氯酸盐的漂白剂，而且无损伤的证据，可以等待观察[43,96,128]。如

表 68–2　内镜下的损伤程度分级

分级	描述
0	正常
I	黏膜水肿和充血
II a	易碎，出血，腐蚀性水疱，分泌物或白色膜，浅表溃疡
II b	比 II a 级深，分散的或环状溃疡
III a	小的分散性坏疽；黑褐色或灰色变色区域
III b	广泛的坏疽

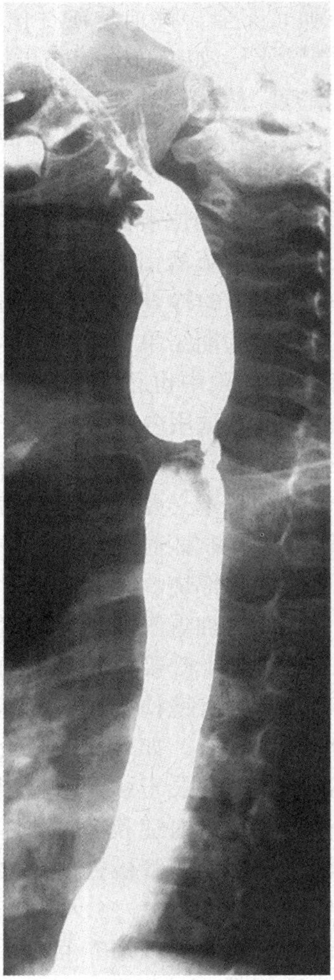

图 68-1 一名 4 岁男孩吞入腐蚀性晶体后，食管的部分狭窄。患儿成功进行了食管局部切除和一期食管吻合术。

果不知道吞食的是什么物质但症状明显，则需要行内镜镜检查[36,37,92,96]。I 度灼伤的患者不需要特殊的治疗。起初进食流体，逐渐改为进食固体食物。如果固体食物可以承受，那么孩子可以出院。临床随访 2～3 周，
1085 如果仍有吞咽困难的临床症状，则造影检查是必要的。

中等程度（Ⅱ度）或重度（IIb 度和 III 度）损伤需要进一步治疗，目的在于防止狭窄的形成[89]。虽然大多数 IIa 度损伤的患者可以完全恢复，但严密的随访是必要的，作为预防措施必须行内镜检和扩张[95,96]。主要的争论围绕重度损伤的治疗选择展开，即类固醇和抗生素、食管支架以及食管扩张的应用[112]。IIIb 度损伤在儿科年龄组中很少见，通常发生在青春期试图自杀的孩子。如果出现广泛的坏死和穿孔，可能立即需要积极的急诊手术，特别是胃部也被累及者[3,38,78]。

全身性类固醇治疗基于其抑制炎症应答反应的作用，这在动物实验中已得到证实[16,18,52,53,111]。然而，临床研究采用的各种不同剂量在预防狭窄形成中无明显的统计学差异[5,120]。广泛的回顾性研究也不能显示类固醇治疗对严重损害的患者有显著的优点[38,90]。最近有人提倡用很大剂量的类固醇（地塞米松 1mg/kg，4～6 周）[22,24,30]。然而该报道的病例数较少，而且副作用如食管真菌感染、骨炎、消化性溃疡和骨质疏松症等明显。

对于严重损伤的患者，出于早期喂养的目的可放置鼻胃管。对于不能吞咽的患者，鼻胃管可用于肠内营养，作为扩张的导引并在一定程度上起到保持食管腔开放的作用。

对于大多数病例，患者一旦能够吞咽唾液就可以开始经口喂养。如果发生吞咽困难，可行食管造影检查明确损伤的范围。同时应用抗真菌药物、抗酸剂和胃酸分泌抑制剂（H_2 受体阻断药或质子泵抑制剂），但是疗效尚未得到证明[95,96,103,123]。

损伤的并发症及其治疗

如果损伤后 10～14 天通过食管造影发现有食管狭窄，那么需要开始扩张治疗（图 68-2）[96]。可以采
用多种不同的方法，包括水银探条、可弯曲的分级探 1086
条、导丝引导的金属橄榄（Edel-Puestow 系统）或不同规格的球囊扩张器*。扩张时应非常小心，最初不应盲目地进入探子。如果狭窄严重或很难看清，放置食管内绳线的方法比较安全，它可引导扩张器成通过胃造瘘口行逆行扩张，或经口行顺行扩张[119]。最好的方法是先通过胃造瘘口插入一个软头的可弯曲导丝进入远端食管[80,114]。从胃造瘘口插入聚氯乙烯气管导管至胃小弯，可将导丝较易地送入胃食管开口[82]。为了得到满意的扩张，在早期需要全身麻醉，以保护气道。

扩张应该至少每周一次，开始用 1～2 F 号扩张器，要小于估计的狭窄部。注意不要扩到比第一次扩张时受阻时的尺寸大 2～3 号。持续扩张直至食管愈合，并注意食管直径的逐渐增大和正常喂养的重建。不良的预后因素是发现较迟、广泛的 III 度损伤、有进行性食管溃疡、致密的纤维化狭窄在扩张时有破裂

* 见参考文献 17,28,32,36,41,63,95,96,104,105,108,114,122,124。

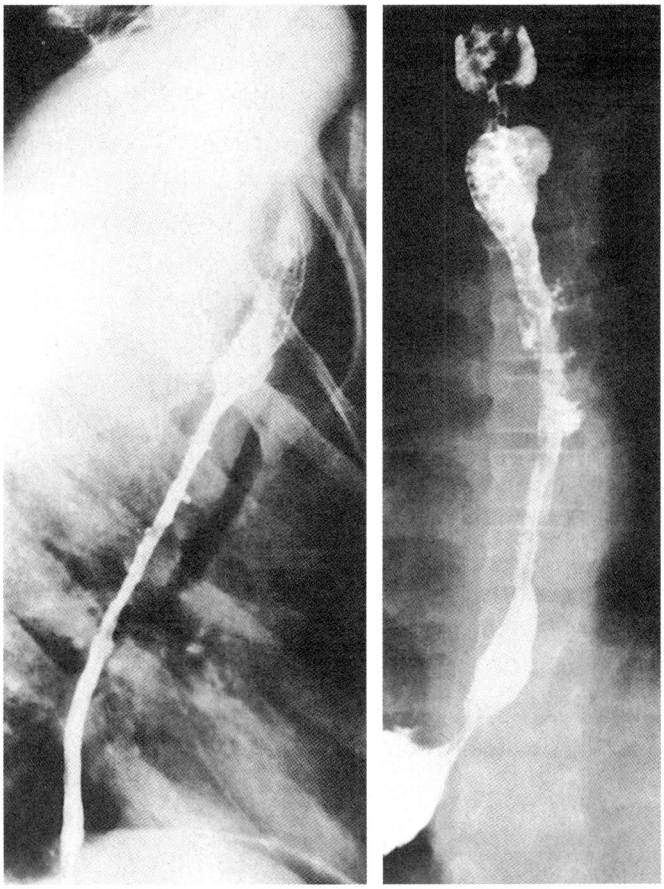

A　B

图 68-2　A. 吞食腐蚀性物质后的早期食管造影。B. 一些区域的全层溃疡进展至广泛狭窄，需要行食管旁路手术。

声、狭窄长度超过 5cm、重复扩张超过 9～12 月仍有明显的管腔开放不足等[9,32]。无数据支持应常规使用预防性抗生素，但如果全身感染或发生透壁性坏死，就应考虑适当的抗生素治疗[41,43,53]。在恢复期间，提供充足的营养十分重要，大多数患者的胃肠道仍可以使用，可通过鼻胃管、胃造瘘管或空肠造瘘管喂养。

如果扩张失败或形成致密的狭窄，需要进一步治疗。像其他良性食管狭窄一样，必须了解有无胃食管反流及其程度，并作为永久性狭窄的原因被排除[23,32,88]。如果需要，在尝试明确的操作前应先手术纠正胃食管反流[101]。局限性狭窄可以切除并作端端吻合。然而，首先必须通过内镜仔细检查整个食管确认狭窄是局限性的，因为纤维化的实际范围可大大超过影像学所显示的范围。[32,86]食管镜下健康的食管黏膜颜色和气体吹入后出现膨大扩张有助于对食管的判断。对短的狭窄局部注射类固醇（1%的曲安西龙醋酸盐）联合应用食管扩张取得了一定的成功，但还没有进行前瞻性的评估。

一些研究人员提倡采用留置鼻胃管的方法作食管支架[27,39,55]。食管腔得到维持，预防食管去上皮区域的粘连，同时可以给予管饲喂养。多年来，不同类型的支架得以应用（如硅胶材料，聚四氟乙烯材料）[14,27,39,84,88,125]。如果使用支架，应该持续放置至少 6 周，在此期间上皮修复完成，纤维化开始成熟。但很多病例对支架管不能很好耐受，可能会引起胃食管反流。如果发生穿过肌肉的广泛炎症，支架必须放置更久的时间才能有效。支架也可用于腐蚀性损伤或扩张治疗引起的食管瘘，主要作为外科修补或食管旁路手术前的暂时性措施（图 68-3）[87]。

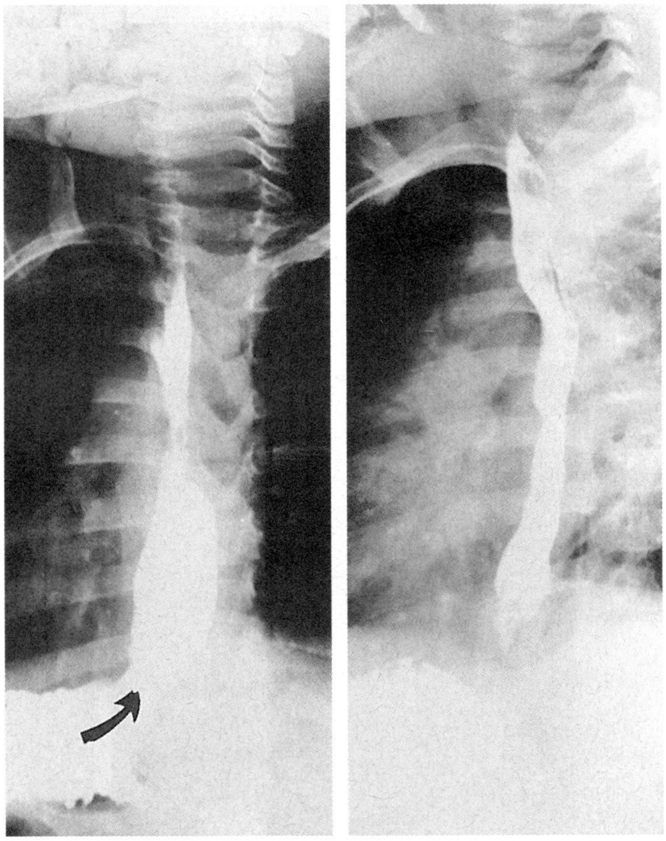

A　B

图 68-3　A. 食管中段持续的腐蚀性狭窄的食管对照造影，食管缩短且有明显的胃食管反流（箭头所示）。B. 在抗反流手术和扩张术后好转。

远期结果

广泛的腐蚀性损伤可以治愈而没有狭窄形成，或可能对上述各种预防性或治疗性措施反应良好。但是可预期有运动功能障碍的残留，也有报道产生食管失弛缓症样表现[33,45,85]。

有食管损伤史者有癌变的危险，但潜伏期可达15～40年[8,12,15,46,58,69,73,96,118]。另外碱性物质损伤后可见
1087 Barrett食管。因此，建议长期的食管内镜监视。在这点上，有两个谨慎的问题：什么情况下应保留损伤的食管？什么时候应放弃扩张的尝试？[59,94]

目前，趋向于对严重的食管损伤采取早期食管旁路，并切除损伤食管段的方法[9,95,109,111]。在已行旁路的食管保留部分的脓肿或囊肿形成等并发症少见，并且未报道有癌变的发生[9,32]。

食管穿孔表现为疼痛、发热和心动过速，是食管扩张术引起的威胁生命的医源性并发症（图68–4）[65,82]。通过内镜或造影剂检查可以及时发现，很多食管穿孔患者可采用全身抗生素和肠道外营养支持的保守治疗[93,107,121]。对于发现较迟或广泛破裂者，确定的治疗方法是胸腔造瘘引流或一期修补近端和远端食管与胃转向。提倡用水冲洗食管，加或不加胸腔引流，作为保守治疗的补充[93]。如果扩张已经失败或食管不能保留，则应行食管旁路或替代手术。目前采用的手术是结肠间置、胃管代食管成形术、空肠间置术和胃上提术（见第69章）等[32,86,92,100,111,115]。结肠补片术也已用于小面积而持久的狭窄[92]。决定采用什么方法和是否需要建立旁路或切除受损食管应根据当地的实际经验和食管切除后并发症的发生率与死亡率而定。显然，切除术的风险比建立旁路保留食管引起癌症的危险性低。

结果

1957—2003年间，327例吞食腐蚀性物质导致食管损伤的儿童在开普敦大学教学医院（红十字Water纪念儿童医院和Groote Schuur医院）接受治疗。平

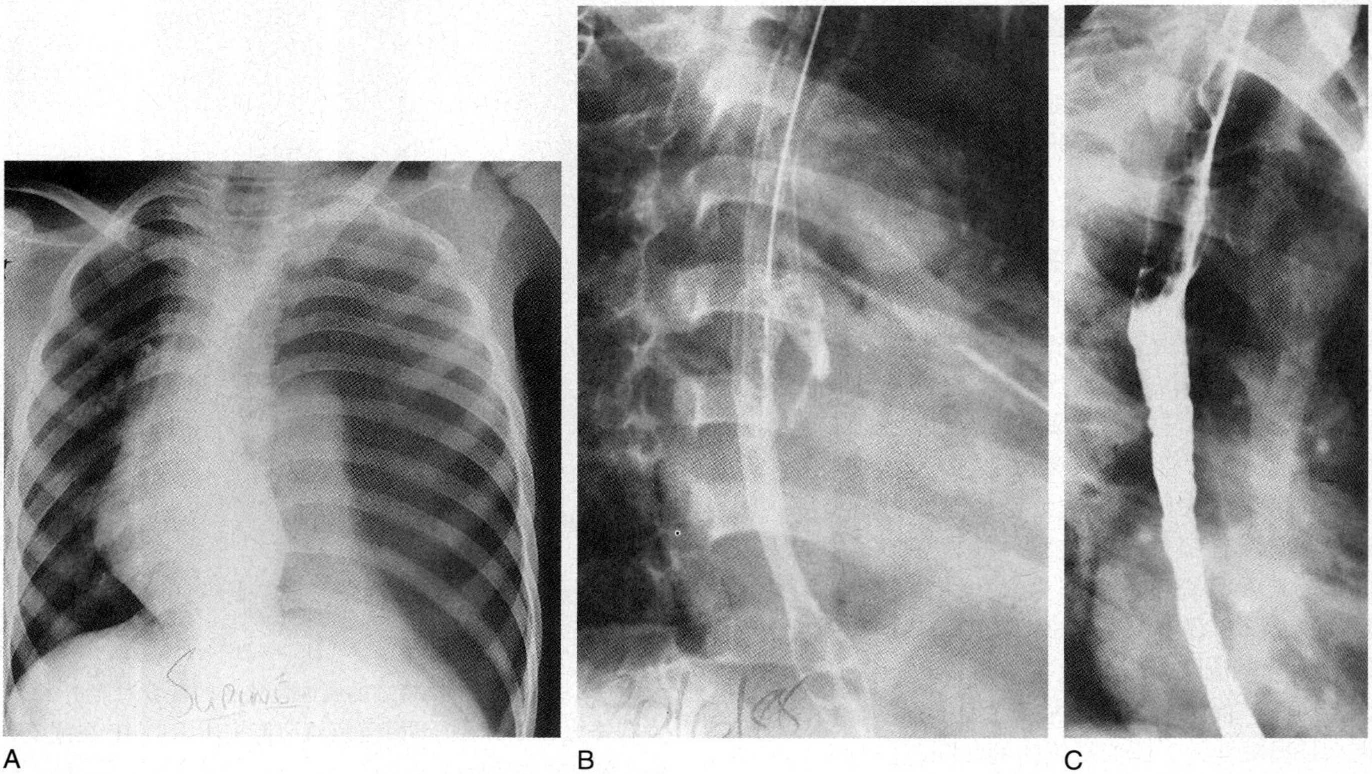

图68–4 左侧张力性气胸，继发于上段食管腐蚀性狭窄行扩张术后所致的穿孔。A. 通过开胸引流治疗。B. 10天后造影检查显示漏洞已受限。C. 穿孔后12周愈合。该患者不需要行食管替代手术。

表 68–3　吞食腐蚀性物质后的住院病例，1990～2003　(N=305)

物质	病例数
酸（厕所、碗清洁剂、焊接溶剂、防锈化合物、电池酸）	7
阴离子表面活性物质和多磷酸盐（家用清洁剂）	9
氢氧化钠（排水沟和烤箱清洁剂）	52
氢氧化铵（漂白剂、清洁剂）	5
2%～3.5%次氯酸钠（漂白剂）	154
3.2%苯酚磺酸盐，2%碱（家用清洁剂和消毒剂）	19
高锰酸钾晶体	44
洗碟清洁颗粒	1
不详	14

均年龄为 35 个月，年龄范围是 9～144 个月。48%的患儿大于 2 岁。近年来（1990—2003 年）吞食腐蚀性物质的患者有增多的趋势（832 例），但仅有 305 例患者（36%）需要住院治疗，其中仅 24 例（8%）形成狭窄。平均年龄为 3.1 岁，男性稍多（58%）。大多数孩子是吞食了家里的清洁剂或消毒剂表（68–3）。

总的来说，327 例患者中有 82 例（25%）形成了食管纤维性狭窄。腐蚀性碳酸氢钠是最常见的腐蚀性物质（82 例中有 78 例），其中吞食结晶态碳酸氢钠的有 31 例。这种形态的腐蚀性碳酸氢钠被广泛用于果园或牧羊农场。酸性烧灼形成狭窄者仅 4 例。一例酸性物质引起食管广泛灼伤的患者形成了胃窦部和上
1088 段空肠的严重狭窄。另一例患者吞食热焊接酸后 8 个月胃窦部几乎完全狭窄。早期治疗不包括类固醇或常规的抗生素治疗，抗生素仅用于感染的病例，通常为呼吸道感染。最近，我们经验性预防应用抗真菌药物（抑制真菌的“制真菌素”）和抗酸性黏膜保护剂（硫糖铝）保护食管防止真菌感染和胃食管反流。大多数采用内镜检查的患者为低于 IIa 度的损伤。

插入鼻胃管至胃，用以喂养和预防食管腔完全阻塞。狭窄首先通过定期的渐进性扩张治疗。食管扩张从损伤后 10～14 天开始，在全身麻醉下进行。最初，顺行扩张通过硬式食管镜的树胶弹性探子进行，但近 20 年已采用带有球囊的光学纤维内镜扩张器、Eder–Puestow 导丝引导的扩张系统或用经食管和胃造瘘口的细绳引导扩张。扩张成功后逐渐延长扩张的间歇时间，并进行吞钡造影检查。过去的十年内我们采用了经口的细绳引导系统，因为我们发现对于大的扩张探子来说胃造瘘口的孔径一般太小。有时候 Eder–Puestow 系统有效，但大部分太硬，不能在有充分的“感觉”下安全扩张。食管扩张球囊对于已经形成的纤维狭窄无效。自从一例患者发生脑脓肿后，我们对食管溃疡需重复扩张者在每次扩张后给予抗生素预防细菌扩散[7]。2 名患者接受了局部注射 1%的类固醇曲安西龙，1 例注入瘢痕化非常严重的声门上方区域，另 1 例注入相当局限的食管狭窄处，但均未获得持久的效果。1 例广泛的Ⅲ度灼伤患者使用食管支架 6 周，但取出后数周食管腔完全闭塞。

82 例狭窄的患者中，38 例（46%）反复扩张有效，而其他 44 例需要手术治疗。44 例中有 10 例除食管瘢痕外还有严重的口咽部烧灼伤，其中 6 例需要气管切开。82 例患者平均扩张 18 次（1～38 次）。38 例扩张有效的患者平均在 15 个月内扩张 17 次（0.5～20 个月）。44 例因狭窄而行食管替代的患儿在 13 个月内（0.5～87 个月）平均扩张 12 次（1～31 次）。灼伤后 1 个月以上才就诊者预后很差，这种患者 10 例中有 8 例需要通过旁路手术治疗。狭窄的长度超过 5cm 的是另一个不利因素，18 例患者中有 17 例对于扩张无明显反应。

最严重的并发症是食管穿孔，发生于 11 例患者（表 68–4）。穿孔发生于平均 6 次扩张之后。2 例穿孔发生在第一次扩张时，其他病例发生在 14 次扩张后，说明穿孔可以发生在任何阶段。早期发现，穿孔后的并发症最少，部分患者仅通过保守地静脉内应用抗生素治疗就能痊愈。如果炎症的范围扩大或穿孔进入纵

表 68–4　食管腐蚀性狭窄的并发症（N=82）

并发症	病例数
穿孔	11
气管食管瘘	1
胃食管反流	7
肺炎	8
脑脓肿	1
出血	1
气管切开	6

隔或胸腔，则这些区域需要引流。一例患者发生了食管气管瘘，手术切除了瘢痕广泛食管段，并在胸骨后行左结肠间置术。保留的食管段未出现囊肿和脓肿形成等并发症。7例患者发生了胃食管反流，其中六例行抗反流手术。4例接着进行食管扩张，而其他的3例需要行食管替代术。从1969年起，我们进行了35例胸骨后的带左结肠血管升支的左横结肠和左侧降结肠顺蠕动间置术和1例局部切除伴端端吻合术，手术过程已被详细报道[32]。结肠间置术已被证实为有效的食管替代术，具有满意的远期疗
1089 效（图68-5，表68-5）。

一些具体的手术操作值得注意并应该强调，因为大多数并发症可以预防。必须小心地选择移植管道的营养血管并保留邻近的肠系膜。通常可保留左结肠动脉的两个上升分支。需要到达上段食管及咽部的结肠段长度应在蒂部被拉张的情况下在肠系膜边缘测量，因为在减压和冲洗之后肠的周径缩小、长度缩短。在胸骨后用手指分离隧道时必须注意避免进入胸腔，因为胸膜撕裂后会将结肠吸入邻近的胸腔，导致移植物的扭转。在行胃食管吻合时，应切除远端多余的间置肠管，以避免造成替代食管的下端冗长。上端吻合口吻合时结肠应呈倒转的U型嵌入近端食管或咽的前侧方，这样可延长吻合口的长度并避免狭窄的发生。应加行幽门形成术，以保证胃的充分排空，防止胃结肠反流或反流进入残留的远端食管。应避免上腹部腹壁鞘的缝合过密[30,32]。最后的程序是用缝线将胃提拉固定于前腹壁或行胃造瘘，以避免移植物下方向后屈曲。

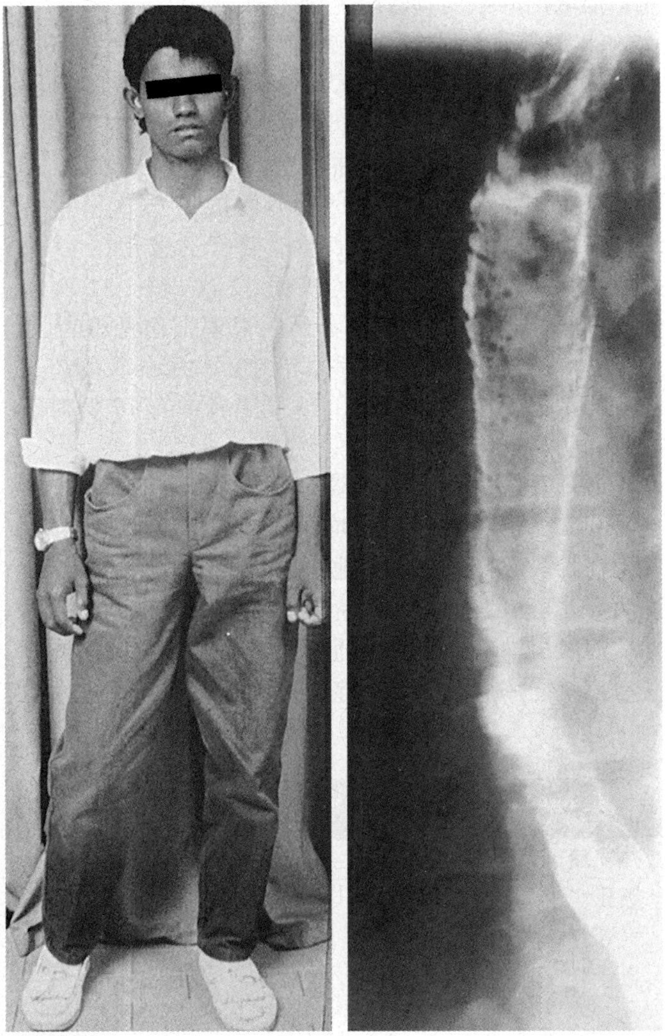

图68-5 一名21岁男青年，腐蚀性食管损伤后行胸骨后左结肠代食管术，及其食管X线片。在腐蚀性吞服损伤近30年后，最近出现了致命的环状软骨鳞状上皮癌。

表68-5 食管腐蚀性狭窄行左结肠间置术后的并发症，1969—1995（N=33）

并发症	病例数
早期并发症	
死亡	2（1例小肠扭转；1例PVC中央线心脏压塞）
漏（上端吻合口）	2
喉返神经瘫痪	1
晚期并发症	
狭窄（上吻合口）	4
重症胃结肠反流	1
肠梗阻（粘连性）	1
消化性溃疡（远端的结肠胃部分）	1

（胡　明译　李民驹校）

参考文献

1. Adams JS, Brick HG: Pediatric caustic ingestion. Ann Otol Rhinolaryngol 1982;91:656.
2. Aghaji MAC, Chuklwu OC: Oesophageal replacement in pediatric patients. J R Coll Surg Edinb 1992;37:101.
3. Allen RE, et al: Corrosive injuries of the stomach. Arch Surg 1970;100:409.
4. Amoury RA, et al: Tracheoesophageal fistula after lye ingestion. J Pediatr Surg 1975;10:273.

5. Anderson KD, Rouse TM, Randolph JG: A controlled trial of corticosteroids in children with corrosive injury of the esophagus. N Engl J Med 1990;323:637.
6. Anderson KD, et al: Long-term follow-up of children with colon and gastric tube interposition for esophageal atresia. Surgery 1992;111:131.
7. Angel C, Wrenn E, Lobe T: Brain abscess: An unusual complication of multiple esophageal dilatations. Pediatr Surg Int 1991;6:42.
8. Appelqvist P, Salmo M: Lye corrosion carcinoma of the esophagus: A review of 63 cases. Cancer 1980;43:2655.
9. Ashcraft KW: Chemical esophageal injuries. In Ashcraft KW, Holder TM (eds): Pediatric Surgery, 2nd ed. Philadelphia, WB Saunders, 1993.
10. Ashcraft KW, Padula RT: The effect of dilute corrosives on the esophagus. Pediatrics 1974;53:226.
11. Bahnassy AF, Bassiouny IE: Esophagocoloplasty for caustic stricture of the esophagus: Changing concepts. Pediatr Surg Int 1993;8:103.
12. Benirschke T: Time bomb of lye ingestion? Am J Dis Child 1981;135:17.
13. Berenson GA, et al: Intralesional steroids in the treatment of refractory esophageal strictures. J Pediatr Gastroenterol Nutr 1994;18:250.
14. Berkovits RN, et al: Caustic injury of the esophagus: Sixteen years' experience, an introduction of a new model oesophageal stent. J Laryngol Otol 1996;110:1041.
15. Bigelow NH: Carcinoma of the esophagus developing at the site of lye stricture. Cancer 1953;6:1159.
16. Bosher LJ Jr, Burford TH, Ackerman L: The pathology of experimentally produced lye burns and strictures of the esophagus. J Thorac Surg 1951;21:483.
17. Broor SL, et al: Long term results of endoscopic dilatation for corrosive oesophageal strictures. Gut 1993;34:1498.
18. Burford TH, Webb WR, Ackerman L: Caustic burns of the esophagus and their surgical management: A clinico-experimental correlation. Ann Surg 1953;138:453.
19. Burrington JD: Clinitest burns of the esophagus. Ann Thorac Surg 1975;20:400.
20. Burrington JD, Raffensberger JG: Surgical management of tracheoesophageal fistula complicating caustic ingestion. Surgery 1978;84:329.
21. Butler C, et al: Morphologic aspects of experimental esophageal lye strictures. II. Effect of steroid hormones, bouginage and induced lathyrism on acute lye burns. Surgery 1977;81:431.
22. Cadranel S, et al: Treatment of esophageal caustic injuries: Experience with high-dose dexamethasone. Pediatr Surg Int 1993;8:97.
23. Capella M, et al: Persistence of corrosive esophageal stricture due to gastroesophageal reflux in children. Pediatr Surg Int 1992;7:180.
24. Cardona JC, Daly JF: Management of corrosive esophagitis: Analysis of treatment, methods and results. N Y State J Med 1964;4:2307.
25. Chodak GW, Paesaro E Jr: Acid ingestion, need for gastric resection. JAMA 1978;239:225.
26. Christensen HBT: Epidemiology and prevention of caustic ingestion. Acta Pediatr 1994;83:212.
27. Coln D, Chang JHT: Experience with esophageal stenting for caustic burns in children. J Pediatr Surg 1986;21:588.
28. Cox JGC, et al: Balloon or bougie for dilatation of benign esophageal stricture. Dig Dis Sci 1994;39:776.
29. Crain EF, Gershel JC, Mezey AP: Caustic ingestions: Symptoms as prediction of esophageal injury. Am J Dis Child 1984;138:863.
30. Curtis JA, et al: Endocrine complications of topical and intralesional corticosteroid therapy. Arch Dis Child 1982; 57:204.
31. Cywes S: Challenges and dilemmas for a pediatric surgeon. J Pediatr Surg 1994;29:957.
32. Cywes S, et al: Corrosive strictures of the esophagus in children. Pediatr Surg Int 1993;8:8.
33. Dantas RO, Mamede RC: Esophageal motility in patients with esophageal caustic injury. Am J Gastroenterol 1996; 91:1157.
34. Davis WM, Madden JW, Peacock EE Jr: A new approach to control of esophageal stenosis. Ann Surg 1972;176:469.
35. Demitbilek S, et al: Effects of estradiol and progesterone on the synthesis of collagen in corrosive esophageal burns in rats. J Pediatr Surg 1994;29:1425.
36. De Peppo F, et al: Conservative treatment of corrosive esophageal strictures: A comparative study of endoscopic dilatations and esophageal stenting. Pediatr Surg Int 1993;8:2.
37. DiConstanzo J, et al: New therapeutic approach to corrosive burns of the upper gastrointestinal tract. Gut 1980;21:370.
38. Estrera A, et al: Corrosive burns of esophagus and stomach: A recommendation for an aggressive surgical approach. Ann Thorac Surg 1986;41:276.
39. Fell SC, et al: The effect of intraluminal splinting in the prevention of caustic stricture of the esophagus. J Thorac Cardiovasc Surg 1966;52:675.
40. Ferguson MK, et al: Early evaluation and therapy for caustic esophageal injury. Am J Surg 1989;157:116.
41. Fyfe AH, Auldist AW: Corrosive ingestion in children. Z Kinderchir 1984;39:229.
42. Gandhi RP, Cooper A, Barlow BA: Successful management of esophageal strictures without resection or replacement. J Pediatr Surg 1989;24:745.
43. Gaudreault P, et al: Predictability of esophageal injury from signs and symptoms: A study of caustic ingestion in 378 children. Pediatrics 1983;71:767.
44. Gehanno P, Guedon C: Inhibition of experimental esophageal lye strictures by penicillamine. Arch Otolaryngol 1981;107:145.
45. Genc A, Mutaf O: Esophageal motility changes in acute and late periods of caustic esophageal burns and their relation to prognosis in children. J Pediatr Surg 1998;37:1526.
46. Gerzic Z, et al: Post corrosive stricture and carcinoma of the esophagus. In Siewert JR, Holsher AH (eds): Diseases of the Esophagus. New York, Springer Verlag, 1988.
47. Guelrud M, Ardeha M: Motor function abnormalities in acute caustic esophagitis. J Clin Gastroenterol 1980;2:247.
48. Gundogdu HZ, et al: Colonic replacement for the treatment of caustic esophageal strictures in children. J Pediatr Surg 1992;27:771.
49. Gupta S: Total obliteration of esophagus and hypopharynx due to corrosives. J Thorac Cardiovasc Surg 1970;60:264.
50. Gupta SK, Croffie JM, Fitzgerald JF: Is esophagogastroduodenoscopy necessary in all caustic ingestions? J Pediatr Gastroenterol Nutr 2001;32:50.
51. Hall RJ, Lilly JR: Treatment of acid burns of the stomach in children by pedicle pyloroplasty. Surg Gynecol Obstet 1988; 167:153.
52. Haller JA Jr, Bachman K: The comparative effect of current therapy on experimental burns of the esophagus. Pediatrics 1964;34:236.
53. Haller JA Jr, et al: Pathophysiology and management of acute corrosive burns of the esophagus: Results and treatment of 285 children. J Pediatr Surg 1971;6:578.
54. Hawkins DB, Demerer MJ, Barnett TE: Caustic ingestion: Controversies in management. A review of 214 cases. Laryngoscope 1980;90:98.

55. Hill JL, et al: Clinical technique and success of the esophageal stent to prevent corrosive strictures. J Pediatr Surg 1976;11:443.
56. Holder TM, Ashcraft KW, Leape L: The treatment of patients with esophageal strictures by local steroid injections. J Pediatr Surg 1969;4:646.
57. Holinger PH: Management of esophageal lesions caused by chemical burns. Ann Otol Rhinolaryngol 1968;77:819.
58. Hopkins RA, Postlethwaite RW: Caustic burns and carcinoma of the esophagus. Ann Surg 1981;194:146.
59. Imre J, Kopp M: Arguments against long term conservative treatment of esophageal strictures due to corrosive burns. Thorax 1972;27:594.
60. Jackson C: Esophageal stenosis following swallowing of caustic alkalis. JAMA 1971;77:22.
61. Jelenko C: Chemicals that "burn." J Trauma 1974;14:65.
62. Jena GP, Lazarus C: A case report: Acid corrosive gastritis. S Afr Med J 1985;67:473.
63. Johnsen A, Jensen LI, Mauritzen K: Balloon-dilatation of esophageal strictures in children. Pediatr Radiol 1986;16:388.
64. Johnson EE: A study of corrosive esophagitis. Laryngoscope 1963;73:1651.
65. Kim I-O, et al: Perforation complicating balloon dilatation of esophageal strictures in infants and children. Radiology 1993;189:741.
66. Kirsch MM, Ritter F: Caustic ingestion and subsequent damage to the oropharyngeal and digestive passages. Ann Thorac Surg 1976;21:74.
67. Kirsch MM, et al: Treatment of caustic injuries of the esophagus. Ann Surg 1978;188:675.
68. Kirsch MM, et al: Intralesional steroid injections for peptic oesophageal strictures. Gastrointest Endosc 1991;37:180.
69. Kiviranta UK: Corrosion carcinoma of the esophagus. Acta Otolaryngol 1952;42:88.
70. Krey H: Treatment of corrosive lesions of the esophagus. Acta Otolaryngol 1952;102(Suppl):1.
71. Kuhn JR, Tunell WP: The role of initial cine-esophagography in caustic esophageal injury. Am J Surg 1983;146:804.
72. Landau G, Saunders W: The effect of chlorine bleach on the esophagus. Laryngol Rhinol Otol 1978;92:499.
73. Lansing PB, Ferrante WA, Ochsner JL: Carcinoma of the esophagus at the site of lye stricture. Am J Surg 1969;118:108.
74. Larimeau T, et al: Accidental caustic injury in children: Is endoscopy always mandatory? J Pediatr Gastroenterol Nutr 2001;33:81.
75. Leape LL, et al: Hazard to health—liquid lye. N Engl J Med 1971;284:578.
76. Litovitz R, Schmitz BF: Ingestion of cylindrical and button batteries: An analysis of 2382 cases. Pediatrics 1992;89:747.
77. Mansson I: Diagnosis of acute corrosive lesions of the esophagus. J Laryngol Otol 1978;92:499.
78. Marshall F: Caustic burns of the esophagus: Ten-year results of aggressive care. South Med J 1979;72:1236.
79. McCabe RE, Scott JR, Knox WC: Fistulation between the esophagus, aorta and trachea as a complication of acute corrosive esophagitis: Report of a case. Ann Surg 1969;35:450.
80. Mendelsohn HJ, Maloney WH: The treatment of benign strictures of the esophagus with cortisone injection. Ann Rhinol Laryngol 1970;79:85.
81. Middlekamp JN, et al: The management and problems of caustic burns in children. J Thorac Cardiovasc Surg 1969; 57:341.
82. Millar AJW, et al: Negotiating the "difficult" oesophageal stricture. Pediatr Surg Int 1993;8:445.
83. Millar AJW, et al: Detection of caustic oesophageal injury with technetium 99m-labelled sucralfate. J Pediatr Surg 2001; 36:262.
84. Mills LJ, Estrera SA, Platt MR: Avoidance of esophageal stricture following severe caustic burns by use of an intraluminal stent. Ann Thorac Surg 1979;28:60.
85. Moody FG, Garrett JM: Esophageal achalasia following lye ingestion. Ann Surg 1969;17:775.
86. Mutaf O: Esophagoplasty for caustic esophageal burns in children. Pediatr Surg Int 1992;7:106.
87. Mutaf O, et al: Management of tracheoesophageal fistula as a complication of esophageal dilatations in caustic esophageal burns. J Pediatr Surg 1995;30:823.
88. Mutaf O, et al: Gastroesophageal reflux: A determinant in the outcome of caustic esophageal burns. J Pediatr Surg 1996; 31:1494.
89. Naef AP, Savary M, Ozzello L: Columnar lined lower esophagus: An acquired lesion with malignant predisposition: Report of 140 cases of Barrett's esophagus with 12 adenocarcinomas. J Thorac Cardiovasc Surg 1975;70:826.
90. Oakes DD, Sherck JP, Mark JBD: Lye ingestion: Clinical patterns and therapeutic implications. J Thorac Cardiovasc Surg 1982;83:194.
91. Orringer MB, Orringer JS, Arbor A: Esophagectomy without thoracotomy: A dangerous operation? J Thorac Cardiovasc Surg 1983;85:72.
92. Othersen BH Jr, Parker EP, Smith CD: The surgical management of esophageal stricture in children. Ann Surg 1988; 207:590.
93. Panieri E, et al: Iatrogenic esophageal perforation in children: Patterns of injury, presentation, management and outcome. J Pediatr Surg 1996;31:890.
94. Panieri E, et al: Oesophageal replacement in the management of corrosive strictures: When is surgery indicated? Pediatr Surg Int 1998;13:336.
95. Pintus C, et al: Caustic ingestion in childhood: Current treatment possibilities and their complications. Pediatr Surg Int 1993;8:109.
96. Rappert P, et al: Diagnosis and therapeutic management of oesophageal and gastric caustic burns in childhood. Eur J Pediatr Surg 1993;3:202.
97. Ray JF, et al: The natural history of liquid lye ingestion. Arch Surg 1974;109:436.
98. Ritter F, Newman MH, Newman DE: A clinical and experimental study of corrosive burns of the stomach. Ann Otol Rhinol Laryngol 1968;77:830.
99. Rivosecchi M: Lye strictures (part 1) [editorial]. Pediatr Surg Int 1993;8:1.
100. Rode H, et al: Colonic oesophageal replacement in children—functional results. Z Kinderchir 1986;41:201.
101. Rode H, et al: Reflux strictures of the esophagus in children. J Pediatr Surg 1992;27:462.
102. Rodgers BM, Ryckman FC, Talbert JL: Blunt transmediastinal esophagectomy with simultaneous substernal colon interposition for esophageal strictures in children. J Pediatr Surg 1981;16:184.
103. Rothstein FC: Caustic injuries to the esophagus in children. Pediatr Clin North Am 1986;33:665.
104. Saeed ZA, Graham DY: Treatment of benign esophageal stricture: Where do we go from here? Dig Dis Sci 1994; 39:2099.
105. Sato Y, et al: Balloon dilatation of esophageal stenosis in children. AJR Am J Roentgenol 1988;150:639.
106. Sellars SL, Spence RAJ: Chemical burns of the oesophagus. J Laryngol Otol 1987;101:1211.
107. Shaffer HA, Valenzuela G, Mittal RK: Esophageal perforation: A reassessment of the criteria for choosing medical or surgical therapy. Arch Intern Med 1992;152:757.

108. Shemesh E, Czerniak A: Comparison between Savary-Gilliard and balloon dilatation of benign esophageal stricture. World J Surg 1990;14:518.
109. Spain DM, Molomut N, Haber A: The effect of cortisone on the formation of granulation tissue in mice. Am J Pathol 1957;26:710.
110. Spechler SJ, et al: Barrett's epithelium complicating lye ingestion with sparing of the distal esophagus. Gastroenterology 1981;81:580.
111. Spitz L: Gastric transposition via the mediastinal route for infants with long-gap esophageal atresia. Pediatr Surg 1984;19:149.
112. Spitz L, Lakhoo K: Caustic ingestion. Arch Dis Child 1993;68:157.
113. Symbas PN, Vlasis SE, Hatcher CR Jr: Esophagitis secondary to ingestion of caustic material. Ann Thorac Surg 1983;36:73.
114. Tanyel FC, Buyukpamukcu NB, Hicsonmez A: An improved stringing method for retrograde dilatations of caustic esophageal strictures. Pediatr Surg Int 1987;2:57.
115. Thomas AN, Dedo HH: Pharyngogastrostomy for treatment of severe stricture of the pharynx and esophagus. J Thorac Cardiovasc Surg 1977;73:817.
116. Thomas AN, et al: Pharyngoesophageal caustic stricture. Am J Surg 1976;132:195.
117. Thompson DF, et al: Evaluation of regional and nonregional poison centers. N Engl J Med 1983;308:191.
118. Ti TK: Esophageal carcinoma associated with corrosive injury—prevention and treatment by esophageal resection. Br J Surg 1983;70:223.
119. Tucker JA, et al: Tucker retrograde esophageal dilatation 1924-1974: A historical review. Ann Otol Rhinol Laryngol 1974;83(Suppl 16):1.
120. Ulman I, Mutaf O: A critique of systemic steroids in the management of esophageal burns in children. Eur J Pediatr Surg 1998;8:71.
121. Van der Zee DC, et al: Management of pediatric esophageal perforation. J Thorac Cardiovasc Surg 1988;95:692.
122. Walton WW: An evaluation of the poison prevention packaging act. Pediatrics 1982;69:363.
123. Wasserman RL, Ginsburg CM: Caustic substance injuries. J Pediatr 1985;107:169.
124. Webb WA: Esophageal dilatation: Personal experience with current instruments and techniques. Am J Gastroenterol 1988;83:471.
125. Wijburg FA, Heymans HAS, Urbanus NAM: Caustic esophageal lesions in childhood: Prevention of stricture formation. J Pediatr Surg 1989;24:171.
126. Yarrington CT Jr: The experimental causticity of sodium hypochloride in the esophagus. Ann Otol Rhinol 1970; 179:895.
127. Zarger SA, et al: Ingestion of strong corrosive alkalis: Spectrum of injury to upper gastrointestinal tract and natural history. Gastroenterology 1989;97:276.
128. Zarger SA, et al: The role of fibreoptic endoscopy in the management of corrosive ingestion and modified endoscopic classification of burns. Gastrointest Endosc 1991; 37:165.

第 69 章

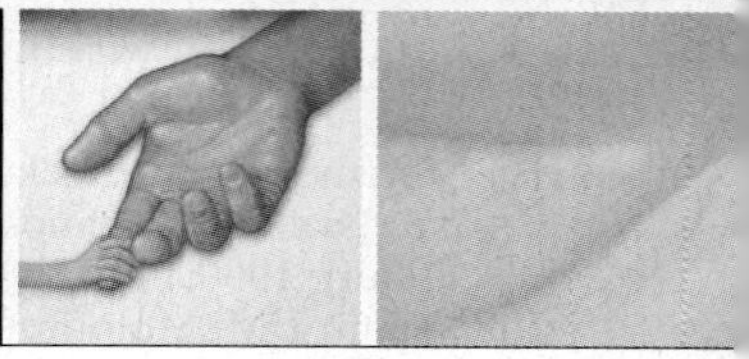

食管替代

Lewis Spitz

1093 食管替代术的需要已越来越少，主要是因为手术方法改进，保留了长间距食管闭锁患儿的原有食管。此外，对难治性胃食管反流危害的普遍认识、导致更积极的抗反流手术方法，并且随着儿童安全容器的使用，减少了碱性和腐蚀性物质损伤食管的发生。然而，仍然有需要进行食管替代治疗的患者，因此小儿外科医生需要了解各种可应用的食管替代方式。

食管替代的适应证

食管闭锁

长间距食管闭锁的患儿因不能成功进行端端吻合，是需要食管替代术的主要人群。许多方法已被用于克服长间距并实现一期食管吻合，保留婴儿自身的食管。这些技术列于表 69–1。对于孤立的食管闭锁，重要的是排除上段盲端的食管气管瘘。如果远端食管仅有很小的残端位于食管裂孔部，或完全没有胸腔内食管，那就显然需要行替代手术，最好能在早期行颈部食管造瘘后让婴儿回家，等待以后的替代手术。这样患儿没有吸入的危险，而且可在家里与家长建立亲密关系。如果在很大的张力下仍不能完成吻合，目前的观点倾向于推迟一期修复术。先通过胃造瘘进行喂养，同时对上端食管盲端吸引 6～12 周。在此期间两个盲端的距离逐渐缩小。如果此时不能行一期吻合术，再拖延也无益，需要行食管替代术。目前可行初期间置手术，如果情况不允许，可先行颈部食管造瘘，以后再行食管替代术。虽然最好能保留患儿自己的食管，但在有严重并发症（如积脓、不可控制的狭窄、反复发生瘘管）的情况下坚持保留原食管的无效尝试可能是有害的。这种情况下，显然对患者最有利的是放弃原有的食管并在以后行食管替代手术。

消化性狭窄

抗反流手术通常在难以控制的狭窄形成之前用于治疗病理性的胃食管反流。然而对于食管有严重瘢痕 1094
和炎症性狭窄的患儿，狭窄大多可通过有效的抗反流手术和术后规律的食管扩张治愈，少数需要狭窄段局部的“袖管”切除，但是有些患者经上述治疗失败仍需要行食管替代术。

表 69–1 纠治长间隙食管闭锁的手术技巧
初期手术
无张力吻合[40,69,112]
减张手术[26,50,65,96]
补片技术[25,36]
瘘管缝合[48,100,103,104]
延迟的一期吻合
采用探条扩张：近端[51,70]，近端和远端[43]，磁力[47]
不用探条扩张[89]
食管延长技术（例如采用补片[22,36]，螺旋形肌层切开术[123]，胃分裂术[101]）
经纵隔的“线”
采用或不采用“橄榄”探条[80,91]
KATO 技术[57]
食管代替手术
结肠间置术[29,115,127]
胃管食管成形术[5,45]
空肠间置术[93]
胃代食管术[73,114]

腐蚀性狭窄

在发达国家，由于盛装腐蚀性物质的容器必须是法律规定的儿童安全器皿，因而本病不多见，但在许多发展中国家的儿童仍遭受腐蚀性食管损伤。大多数病例是轻度损伤，反复扩张治疗有效。但食管的全层损伤除了病变段很短的以外，总是导致难以控制的狭窄，扩张无效而通常需要行替代手术。对于持续的有规律扩张超过 6～12 个月而无效者，是否应切除损伤的食管仍有争议。因为保留食管有恶变的危险，而且儿童的食管切除术较容易实行，所以儿童行食管部分切除和替代术比旁路手术更适宜。关于腐蚀性狭窄在第 68 章有详细讨论。

其他适应证

因食管静脉曲张出血而行食管替代的方法已经过时，因为现在有许多可选用的有效技术，特别是硬化疗法和门静脉分流术。食管肿瘤可能需要切除很长一段的食管，儿童食管肿瘤的例子是弥漫性平滑肌瘤和炎症性假瘤。食管异物长期压迫也可能引起广泛损伤，例如铝质拉环，可透过 X 线，因而常规 X 线检查时可能被遗漏。其他不常见的食管替代术适应证包括不可控制的食管失弛缓症、伴有免疫缺陷的播散性念珠菌病、硬皮病[71]和大疱性表皮松解症等[118]。

理想的食管替代物的特点

1. 替代物必须起到从口腔到胃的管道作用，以满足儿童对营养的需求。
2. 胃酸反流到管腔的可能必须减少到最小，如果发生反流，替代的管道必须可以抵抗胃酸。
3. 替代管道不应影响呼吸和心血管功能。
4. 手术的技术必须完美，并适用于低龄儿童。
5. 管道不引起其他畸形的产生。
6. 管道必须随着儿童的成长而增大，其功能持续到成年[13]。

食管替代物的类型

虽然结肠仍是儿童食管替代最常用的器官，但是有些外科医生仍不满意并已经开始选择其他替代物。最常用的手术方法见图 69–1。

各种替代手术的优点和缺点均列于表 69–2。

一些人工假体已经被用于食管的替代，然而，所有假体的功能仅能维持很短的时间[100]。

食管替代术的途径

对于食管代替，从颈部到腹部最短的距离是后纵

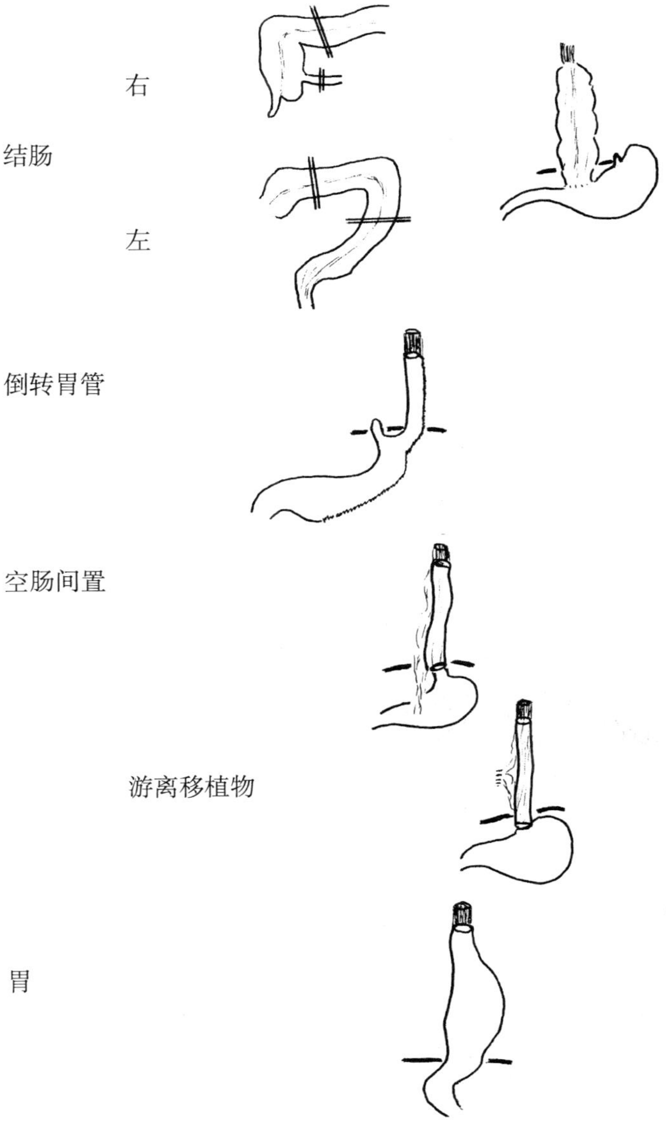

图 69–1　食管替代方法。

表 69–2 食管替代术

方法	优点	缺点
结肠间置术	长度足够 很少发生反流	血供不稳定 移植物坏死 漏和狭窄发生率高 多处吻合 远期易变冗长 食物传输缓慢
胃管食管成形术	长度足够 血供良好 管腔大小适合 传输食物快速	吻合线较长 漏和狭窄的发生率高 反流导致 Barrett 综合征
空肠间置术	管腔大小适合	血供非常不稳定 保留蠕动功能 长度可能不够 三个吻合
游离空肠移植术	管腔大小适合 良好的蠕动功能	需要特殊的微血管吻合技术 手术时间长 血供不稳定 失败率高
胃代食管术	长度足够，容易实现 极丰富的血供 单个吻合口 操作简单	位于胸部的胃体积较大 早期普遍有反流 胃排空不佳 影响呼吸功能？ 影响生长发育？

隔。结肠间置最初置于前胸壁的皮下，但该方法的外观不能接受，已被弃用。其他途径的优点和缺点列于 1095
表 69–3。

手术时机的选择

尽管食管替代可以在新生儿期实施，但是通常这个手术被延期到婴儿长大且体重超过 5kg 时。在此期间重要的是，在规律的胃造口喂养中给予经口假饲以刺激吞咽反射。当食管替代成功接通后，毫无疑问受到良好的吞咽假饲训练的患儿将迅速接受经口营养。对所有病例，适当的肠道机械性准备是十分重要的，因为被选为食管替代的器官可能不适合，而需要改用其他技术。

1969 年 May 和 Samson[74]，1983 年 Postlethwait[87]，都对食管替代治疗的历史做了很好的全面综述。

结肠间置术

结肠间置术仍是儿童食管替代治疗中最常用的手术。目前成人食管癌患者更偏向于胃代食管术，结肠间置术已作为第二选择。

历史

1911 年，Kelling [58]采用横结肠段作为食管旁路。

表 69–3 食管替代术的途径

途径	优点	缺点
胸骨后	操作方便 可用于胸部和后纵隔有炎症或以前有手术史的患者	从颈部到腹部最长的路径 移植物成角不可避免 如需要心脏手术，手术入路困难
经胸	手术操作简便	肺移位 需要开胸手术
后纵隔	最直接的途径 器官在纵隔内 轻度或无肺压迫 不一定需要开胸手术	有手术史、纤维化或炎症患者可能无法经纵隔手术

由于原来计划的空肠间置的肠系膜太短，他使用了带左结肠动脉的结肠段。然而试图连接左颈部食管造口与结肠上端时患者死亡。1911 年，Vulliet[125]在尸体上进行了保留结肠移植物右端肠系膜蒂的移植手术。1914 年，Von Hacker 进行了首例成功的成人结肠间置手术[124]。1921 年，Lundblad 报道了第一例成功的儿童结肠旁路手术[68]。该患儿在 3 岁时做了食管狭窄手术，直至 37 岁因意外事故死亡。1934 年，Ochsner 和 Owens[79]回顾了文献，发现仅有 20 例结肠食管成形术的报道。1951 年，Rudler 和 Monod-Broca[98]描述了胸骨后回结肠间置代食管术。1955 年，Dale 和
1096 Sherman[20]描述了 2 例食管闭锁婴儿在 2 岁时行胃后前纵隔的右结肠间置的食管重建。4 年后，Battersby 和 Moore[10]报道了 5 例先天性食管闭锁的右结肠替代术，3 例进行胸骨后结肠替代的儿童存活，他们建议手术时间推迟到 9 个月龄以上。1957 年，Sherman 和 Waterston[106]，1961 年和 1964 年，Waterston[126]，1965 年，Belsey[12]均报道了结肠代食管术的主要优点。Waterston 和 Belsey 是经胸途径的强烈支持者，采用带左结肠血管的左结肠替代食管。1967 年，Othersen 和 Clatworthy[83]提出，结肠是儿童食管替代的最佳器官，并建议将手术时间延缓至患儿 18～24 个月月龄，这样在直立位时重力可辅助食物通过间置的结肠。1982 年，Freeman 和 Cass[29]建议将结肠置于后纵隔食管原来的位置，并报道了很低的并发症发生率。

手术技术

结肠间置术需要用带回结肠血管的右结肠置于胸骨后，或将带左结肠血管的左结肠置于左胸腔内的肺门后方或后纵隔（图 69-2）。

右结肠胸骨后技术

通过上腹部正中线切口或横断腹直肌的上腹部横切口打开腹腔。必须游离并暴露整个结肠，以便准确详细地评估其血供。Sonneland 等[108]在一个有 600 例标本的研究中报告，只有 24%的标本有教科书所描述

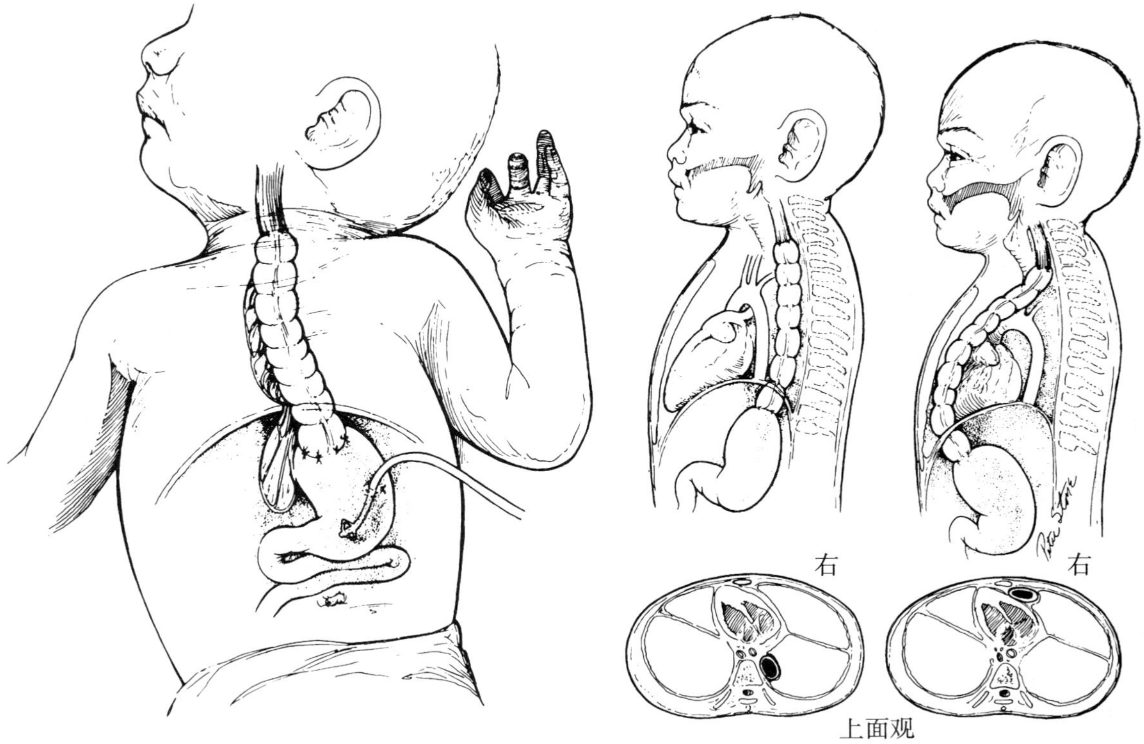

图 69-2　结肠代食管成形术。结肠置于胸骨后或肺门后均可。(From Randolph JG:Surgical problems of the esophagus. In Sabiston D, Spencer F [eds]: Gibbon’s Surgery of the Chest, 3rd ed. Philadelphia, WB Saunders, 1976.)

的典型的从肠系膜上动脉发出三条血管至结肠右侧。3.6%的病例结肠中动脉缺如。边缘动脉有时缺如。血管供应的解剖决定了每个儿童最合适的结肠间置手术方法。右结肠间置的血供来源于结肠中动脉。然而，如果末端回肠的一段被用于间置[119]，如果可能必须保留回结肠血管对移植段的血供。所利用的肠管长度需要仔细估算，用动脉夹夹住所有需要离断的血管。动脉夹至少钳夹 10 分钟以确定拟用于间置插入的结肠段有足够的血供、边缘血管继续搏动且色泽保持正常。可以通过切除阑尾和观察阑尾动脉的血流进一步评估血供状况。如果血供看上去满意，仔细安全地结扎并离断需要切断的血管。重要的是要防止肠系膜血
1097 肿的形成。将回肠在两把血管钳之间切断，远端关闭以准备放置到颈部，然后在结肠中动脉左侧离断横结肠，行回肠横结肠的端端吻合恢复肠管的连续性。

环绕先前的颈部食管造口做颈部横切口。切口应延伸到颈部中线、胸骨柄上方约 1cm 处。分离颈筋膜和胸锁乳突肌起始部，暴露胸骨柄的上缘和后面。必要时扩大切口，切除胸骨柄上部和胸锁关节，进入胸骨后间隙。

胸骨后隧道是从上方通过颈部切口在胸骨后、胸腺和心包前的平面穿通而成，从下方分离横隔的前方附着处。隧道的宽度必须足够容纳 2～3 个手指。

然后游离胃，使结肠及其血管蒂可通过胃的后方，跨过肝脏前表面，通过胸骨后隧道进入颈部。确认移植物无曲折或扭曲是至关重要的，否则会导致血供不足。间置结肠的远端在紧靠胃小弯处与胃前壁吻合。作为预防胃酸反流进入结肠的一种方法，有人设计了在胃黏膜下层做抗反流隧道[39]。移植物的近端，包括升结肠或末端回肠，与颈部食管的远端行端端吻合。在食管吻合的准备期间，必须保证血供并仔细游离食管的全层。间置结肠的长度必须刚好足够连接食管与胃。过多的肠管应在吻合之前切除而保留移植肠管的血供。肠管冗长会导致食物进入的延长和停滞。幽门成形术常用于预防该并发症。

左结肠经胸技术

左结肠经胸膜技术最早由 Waterston 描述[126]。在此方法中，将由左结肠动脉升支供血的左侧横结肠按顺蠕动方向置于肺门后方。在最初的描述中，整个过程是通过左胸部的切口，从胸壁分开横膈附着处进入腹腔。另一种方法是采用腹部和胸部两个切口，或胸腹联合切口[12]。移植的左结肠由左结肠动脉的升支供血。肠管的连续性重建通过结肠端端吻合实现。移植的结肠沿胃后和胰腺后方向，通过横膈后方的一个侧切口进入左侧胸腔。结肠通过左肺肺门后方，穿过 Sibson 筋膜后方沿锁骨下血管和颈动脉鞘外侧的隧道进入颈部。间置结肠的近端与颈部食管行端端吻合，远端与食管远侧盲端（食管闭锁的病例）或者与胃后壁吻合。幽门成形术也是推荐的。Freeman 和 Cass[29] 改良手术过程；将结肠放置在后纵隔正常的食管位置。

结果

随着现代麻醉技术和术后管理的进展，结肠间置术本身的死亡率是不足以考虑的[52]。移植肠段的坏死也极少见，尤其是在术中注意了确保移植段的充足血供以及血管通过胃后时不发生扭曲。静脉阻塞可能会导致间置结肠在术后数周至数月逐渐发生梗死。最常见的并发症是吻合口漏和狭窄形成，特别是颈部食管结肠吻合口漏。漏的原因是近端结肠血供不良或损伤造成食管壁血供不足。大多数漏可在数周内自愈，但有一些病例可进展为狭窄形成。颈部吻合口狭窄通常可通过扩张治愈，但有时需要切除狭窄段并重做吻合口。

文献报道的结肠间置术后并发症发生率列于表 69–4。

可能发生胃食管反流到间置的结肠，有时可导致结肠的消化性溃疡，引起出血，少数情况可发生穿孔并导致脓肿。已有报道由于穿孔和脓肿最后死亡的病例。

旁路手术后保留的食管部分的并发症也有报道[46,81]。Shamberger 等人[105]报道 8 例保留食管发生了慢性炎症，包括 3 例 Barrett 综合征。其他保留食管的并发症有黏液囊肿和脓肿形成等[56]。

间置的结肠段通常没有蠕动，食物借助重力作用通过结肠[53,67,95]。胸廓内的结肠可随着时间而变得过长[64]，导致排空延迟和食物留滞，增加了反流和吸入的危险。必要时需切除结肠的冗长部分，但必须十分注意避免损伤保留结肠的血供。

结肠间置手术后，儿童的营养状况是满意的[42]。原来患有食管闭锁的儿童的身高和体重趋向于较低的

表 69-4　结肠间置术的结果

年份	作者	患者数	死亡	漏（%）	狭窄（%）
1967	Gross 和 Firestone[38]	47	4	6 (13)	7 (15)
1967	Othersen 和 Clatworthy[83]	11	0	4 (36)	3 (27)
1971	Azar 等人[9]	60	5	15 (25)	18 (30)
1972	Soave[107]	32	5	28 (87)	—
1972	Martin[72]	21	2	4 (19)	6 (28)
1978	Rodgers 等人[95]	13	0	5 (38)	3 (23)
1976	German 和 Waterston[34]	32	1	7 (21)	7 (21)
1982	Freeman 和 Cass[29]	33	2	2 (6)	2 (6)
1982	Campbell 等人[15]	23	1	8 (34)	4 (17)
1985	Hendren 和 Hendren[48]	32	1	2 (6)	0
1986	Rode 等人[94]	35	4	8 (23)	5 (14)
1986	West 等人[127]	25	0	10 (40)	11 (44)
1986	Ahmed 和 Spitz[2]	112	15	54 (48)	34 (30)
1989	Mitchell 等人[76]	79	9	23 (29)	17 (22)
1993	Carneiro 和 Doig[16]	11	2	5 (45)	2 (18)
1995	Raffensperger 等人[90]	59	2	11 (19)	13 (22)
1998	Khan 等人[60]	25	0	10 (40)	7 (28)
2000	Erdogan 等人[27]	18	4	11 (61)	3 (17)
2003	Hamza 等人[41]	475	5	47 (10)	25 (5)

百分点，而由于食管腐蚀性狭窄进行食管置换术的孩子处于正常的生理曲线[6,7,34,38,59]。将近一半的结肠间置术患儿存在铁储藏的耗竭[95]。

1098 胃管道化食管成形术

历史

1905 年，Beck 和 Carrel[11]在尸体和狗的实验中建立了胃大弯管道来替代食管，管道从胸前进入颈部。1912 年，Jiauu[55]为两位食管狭窄患者成功地进行了该管道从胸腔内通过的手术。1984 年，Mes[75]报道胃大弯形成的管道可进入颈部。后来，匈牙利的研究员 Gavriliu[31,32,33]和美国的 Heimlich[44,45]普及了这个食管替代的方法。最近支持胃管道食管重建的有：Burrington 与 Stephens[14]、Cohen[18]、Ein 等[24]和 Anderson 等[5,6,7]。

外科技术

经脐上横切口打开腹腔，在胃网膜弓的安全部位分离大网膜（图 69-3 和 69-4）[3]。在胃管的开始部位离断胃网膜右动脉，离断的部位必须仔细选择，以避免幽门口的狭窄。理想的位置通常是距离幽门 2cm 处，在此处垂直切开前、后胃壁。将一根 18～24F 号的胸腔引流管沿胃大弯置于胃内，作为一个导引来确保胃管的大小合适，在距胃大弯 1.5～2.0cm 处应用 GIA 缝合器将胃的前壁和后壁缝合，然后在与胃大弯平行的方向切开胃。通常需要用 GIA 缝合器缝合 3～4 次。离断胃短血管，注意保护脾脏，从不需要做脾切除。胃管和原有胃的缝合线均用 4-0 不吸收缝线行间断的 Lembert 缝合加强。如果胃网膜左动脉先前已被结扎、不能供应逆蠕动的管道，那么可以建立一个由胃网膜右动脉供血的顺蠕动管道。

此时，可选择通往颈部的途径，建立胸骨后通道，或在第六肋间切开左胸。胸骨后通道的颈部切口位于胸骨上窝，胸通道的颈部切口位于左前三角区。用手指分离颈部和胸部，有助于选择在最安全的部位切开 Sibson 筋膜。切开处可在锁骨下血管之前或之后，取决于哪个空间更大。在横膈膜正前方、朝向主动脉裂的方向做一个切口，将胃管从这个切口经胸部拖入颈部。保持蒂部的方向，防止血管扭转或屈曲。与颈部食管的吻合采用单层不可吸收线。在胃管与横膈之间做数针缝合，将胃管固定于胸部。在残余的胃重建胃造口。颈部和胸部做引流，关闭腹腔不做引

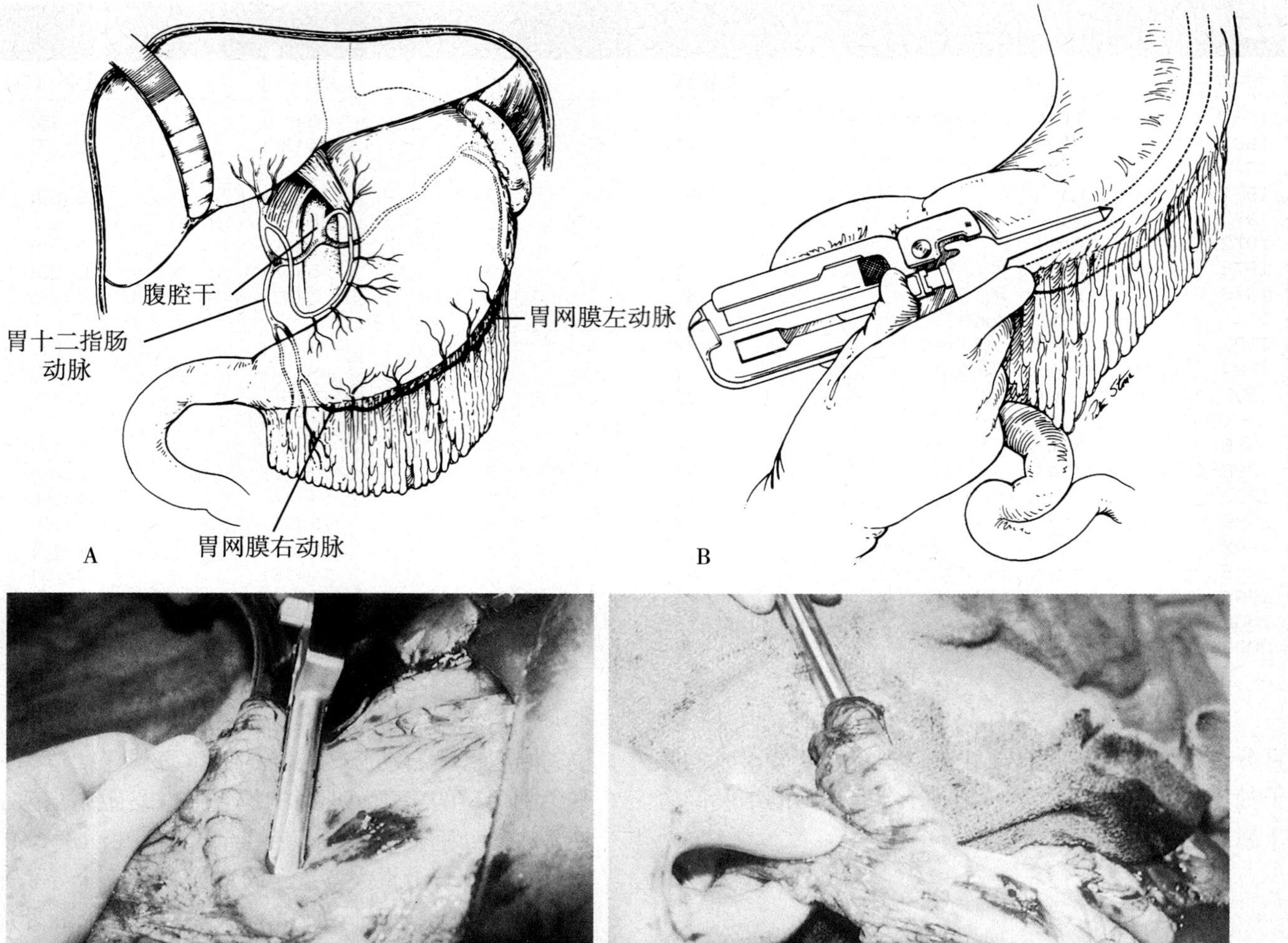

图 69-3 逆行的胃管道化食管成形。A. 管道由胃网膜左动脉供血。可见胃网膜右动脉被分离，小心保护血管弓。B 至 E. 用 GIA 吻合器逐步切开胃。沿胃大弯放置胸腔引流管做引导，确定与胃管道的直径一致。也可见在胃管道和胃的吻合线的缝接。

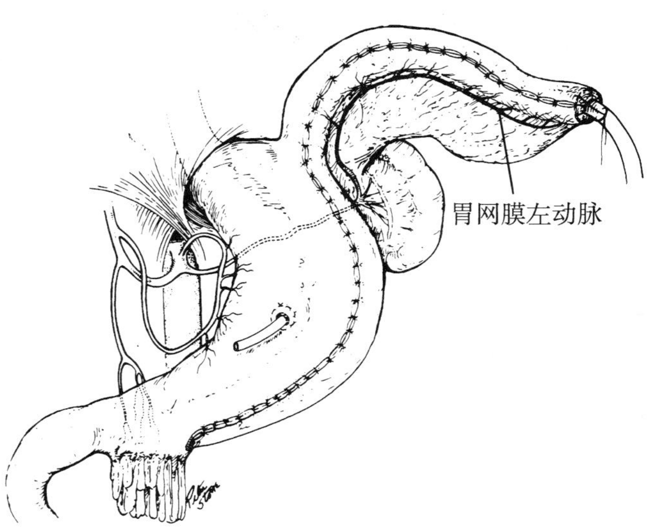

A

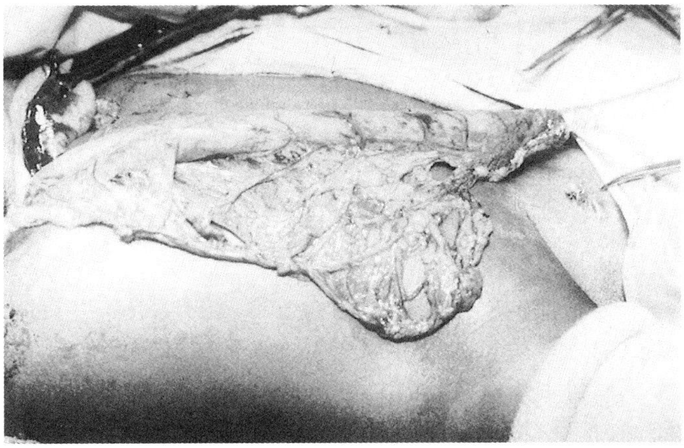

B

图 69-4　倒置的胃管道。A. 脾脏被保留；间断缝合加固吻合器闭合的胃管道和胃。B. 胃制成的管道在胸骨后到达颈部食管造口处，血管钳所指之处。如采用胸腔内途径，则径路更短。

流。如果胃网膜左动脉在先前的手术中已经破坏，可以用胃网膜右动脉供应血管蒂，此时胃管呈倒置（顺蠕动）方向。在这种情况下，胃管建成后胃将向后旋转，使得管道可以被放至颈部。 1100

结果

胃管可保持自己的形态，不会出现结肠移植容易发生的冗长和扩张。但几乎总有反流，可能导致近端食管残端的 Barrett 改变[63]。消化性溃疡是胃管食管成形术的远期并发症[120,121]。夜间咳嗽是常见的问题，可以通过抬高床头、睡前避免进食液体而缓解。胃管食管成形术有良好的营养支持。碱性灼伤所致的食管狭窄的孩子可具有正常的生长曲线，食管闭锁的孩子的体重和身高常较低，但生长满意并能保持良好的营养[4]。

胃管食管成形术的死亡率低，但是漏和狭窄常见，偶尔发生胃管穿孔[102]。通常不存在蠕动，管道的排空依靠重力作用（表 69–5）。

空肠间置术

历史

1906 年，Roux[97]对一位 12 岁的腐蚀性狭窄患儿用空肠做了胸骨前旁路手术。Pirot–Roux 和 Hase 于 1950 年[85]报道了这个患者的随访结果。患者一直很好，直至 1940 年由于创伤导致巨大的瘘管，并且 1941 年发现食管的皮肤部分发生上皮癌，通过放射治疗成功治愈。患者在 53 岁的时候由于不相关的原因死亡。1913 年，Lexer[62]在空肠长度不能到达颈部时，将 Roux 法游离的空肠袢与一个皮肤皮管相连接。大约 20 年后，Ochsner 和 Owens[79]回顾了胸骨前食管替代的文献，发现在 240 名胸骨前食管替代患者中，有 56%采用了空肠的管道。1946 年，Reinhoff[92]

表 69–5　胃管道化食管成形术的结果

年份	作者	患者数	死亡	漏（%）	狭窄（%）
1968	Burrington 和 Stephens[14]	8	1	3 (37)	—
1973	Ein 等人[24]	15	—	7 (47)	9 (60)
1978	Anderson 和 Randolph[6]	15	—	5 (33)	5 (33)
1985	Goon 等人[35]	46	1	35 (76)	27 (59)
1987	Ein 等人[25]	36	3	24 (67)	15 (42)
1998	Ein[23]	11	—	9 (81)	8 (72)

表 69-6 空肠间置代食管术的结果

年份	作者	患者数	死亡	漏（%）	狭窄（%）
1958	Jezioro 和 Kus[54]	14	2	3 (21)	1 (7)
1982	Ring等人[93]	16	0	4 (25)	2 (12)
1988	Saeki等人[99]	19	2	3 (15)	2 (10)
1993	Cusick等人[19]	6	2	1 (17)	2 (33)

进行了第一例胸腔内的空肠替代食管术。他认为胸腔内途径较短，并强调空肠有足够长度可达到颈部。Longmire[66]在 1951 年报道了一例空肠间置术治疗食管腐蚀性狭窄的病例，因空肠上端的血供不足，做乳房内动脉和空肠的肠系膜动脉的吻合。

空肠替代食管的优点是保留了其蠕动性，并且管径与正常的食管相似（表 69-2）。

外科技术

空肠替代食管可以采用两种方法[28,93]：（1）带蒂空肠间置，在屈氏韧带的远端横断空肠，肠袢的
1101 近端向上提穿过胸腔进入颈部，与食管吻合，其远端与胃吻合，通过空肠-空肠吻合重建小肠的连续性；（2）游离的空肠间置，插入一段游离的空肠段，并行空肠蒂的微血管吻合。小宗病例的空肠间置术结果列于表 69-6。

胃代食管术

历史

1922 年，Kummell 报道了对 2 例患者使用了从颈部和腹部创口用手指钝性分离食管的食管游离法[61,78]；然后将胃移植入食管床行食管与胃吻合。虽然这 2 例患者均死亡，但却是第一次尝试通过纵隔途径进行胃代食管术。1938 年，Adams 和 Phemister[1]成功地切除了一位 53 岁患者的下胸段食管癌，并做了胃食管吻合术重建消化道的连续性。1944 年，Garlock 在切除了一位 58 岁男性患者的中 1/3 段食管癌后，成功地重建了食管与胃的连续性[30]。随访中仅有的并发症是侧卧时有反流，这个问题用两个枕头抬高头部就可以解决。1945 年，Sweetm[116]报告了 12 例食管切除术伴主动脉弓上方的食管胃吻合术，并且 1948 年[117]他描述了他的技术在切除上胸段食管癌伴胃与颈部食管吻合的成功应用。不久以后又有成功的咽胃吻合术的报道。胃代食管术是目前成人食管癌的主要手术方式，但用于儿童是有限制的。Atwell 和 Harrison[8]报道了 6 例进行胃代食管手术的儿童，2 例死亡，但是另外 4 例患儿获得了良好的远期疗效。

手术技术

不开胸的经裂孔胃代食管手术是可选择的方式（图 69-5）[82,88,109,111,114]。其禁忌证是广泛存在的先前手术的瘢痕或纵隔炎症[110]。

为了保护胃网膜血管的血管弓，初期喂养性胃造瘘口的理想位置应该在远离胃大弯的胃体前面。

通过上腹部正中切口暴露胃，或者选择左腹外斜肌切口，这样可以扩大为左胸切开，尤其是需要切除纤维化食管或先前曾行结肠间置手术的患者。

仔细切除胃造口，胃的缺损用 4-0 聚乙醇酸线间断缝合，双层关闭。

仔细分离胃和左肝的粘连，避免大血管的损伤。结扎并离断大网膜和胃短血管，游离胃大弯。这些血管的结扎应远离胃壁，以保护胃网膜右血管的血管弓。需要非常小心地避免损伤脾脏。离断幽门到膈食管裂孔之间的小网膜，游离胃小弯。胃右动脉需要仔细识别并小心保留，而将左胃血管在靠近胃处结扎并离断（图 69-5A）。

分离膈食管膜暴露下段食管，确认横膈膜上食管裂孔的边缘。对于单纯性食管闭锁，可通过对横膈食管裂孔的钝性和锐性分离，从后纵隔分离出短的下段食管的盲端。迷走神经通常在此步骤中被分离。胃体和胃底游离后，在胃食管连接处横断食管，断面用 4-0 聚乙醇酸线缝合两层。通常加行 Heineke-Mickulicz 幽门形成术，虽然对幽门形成有无必要尚有争

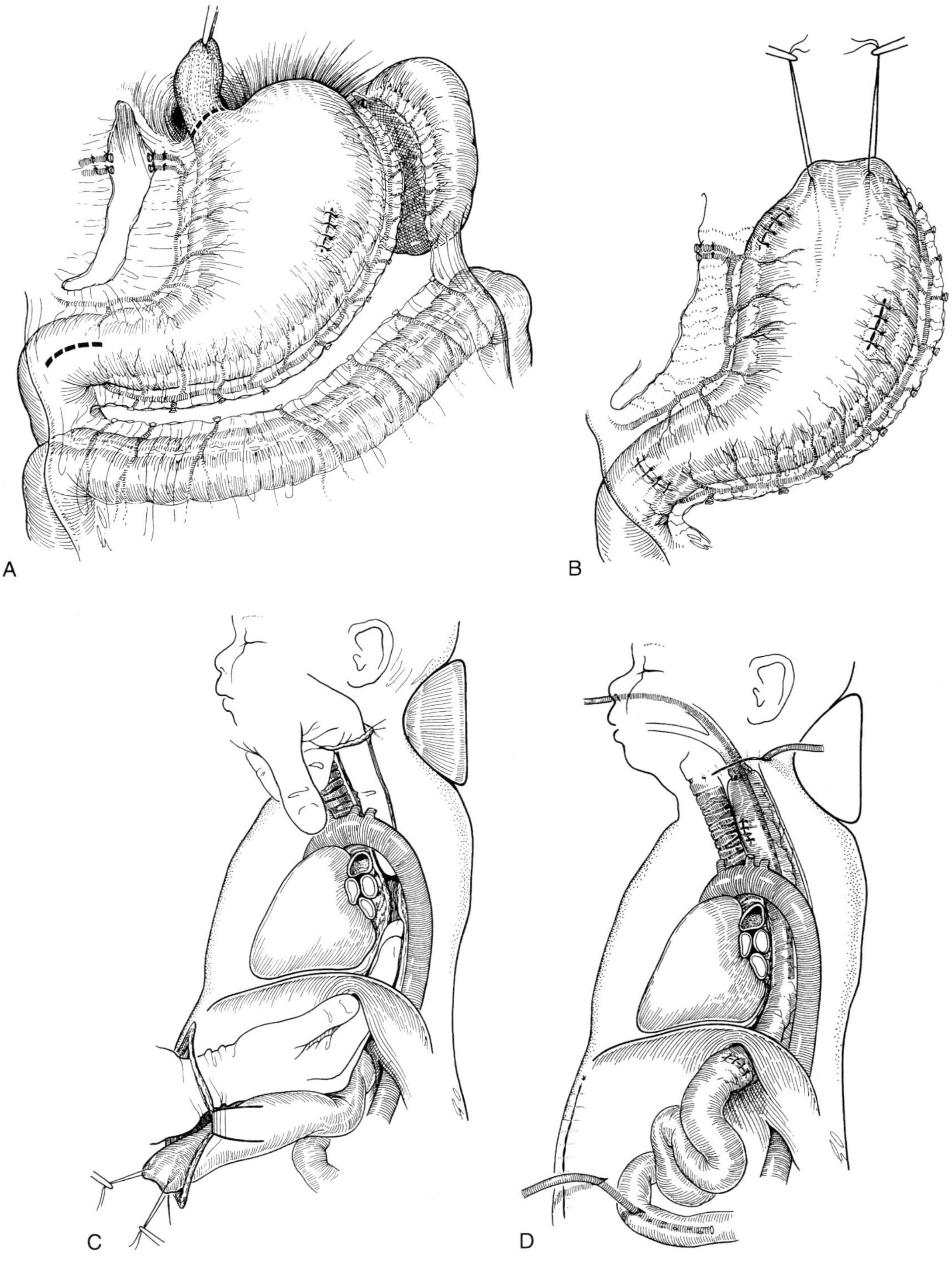

图 69-5 A. 胃管道化食管成形术。胃大弯和小弯被游离，保留胃网膜右血管和胃右血管。仔细离断胃短血管，避免损伤脾脏。胃左血管被结扎并离断；图中指出了十二指肠（已应用 Kocher 技术使十二指肠移动度增大）和幽门成形术的部位。图中示一例单纯性食管闭锁患者的食管短端从横膈的食管裂孔中游离出来。胃造口处已被缝合。B. 幽门成形术已完成，食管远端已被切除。胃底部的两处缝合标记了胃的最高点，该处是胃食管吻合的预期部位。C. 对一例食管灼伤患者，经颈部切口游离食管造口或暴露食管后，从上方钝性分离后纵隔隧道，同时从下方经横膈的食管裂孔向上钝性分离。分离沿正中线椎前平面进行。D. 胃在后纵隔的最终位置，胃食管吻合在下颈部，幽门成形后位于腹腔内的食管裂孔下方。一个空肠造瘘管已被放置，以便术后肠道内营养。

议[17]。在十二指肠第二部分行 Kocher 切开，使幽门获得最大的移动度。

确认胃底最高的部分，在拟做吻合口的左右两侧置牵引缝线，牵引线可由多种材料制成，这些牵引线有助于防止胃在通过后纵隔拖到颈部时发生扭转（图 69–5B）。

现在将注意转向颈部手术，通过一个 3～4cm 的横切口游离先前做好的颈部食管造口。必须注意不要损伤食管的外层肌肉。识别并保护气管后外方上行的
1103 喉返神经。在气管后膜面与椎前筋膜之间进行分离，沿中线行钝性分离建立一个进入上纵隔的隧道。从下面在正常的食管裂孔线上建立一个心脏后、筋膜前的隧道[37]。后纵隔的上下隧道贯通，形成 2～3 指宽的可容纳胃的空间（图 69–5C）。

如需要切开胸腔来切除食管的纤维组织（例如腐蚀性食管灼伤或反流性食管炎）、或切除以前间置的无功能食管，或者当以前的手术或感染导致钝性分离困难时，经胸步骤应在直视下展开，方法与上述的纵隔手法相似。

用长的钝性血管钳从颈部切口进入，穿过后纵隔隧道，提起胃底部的两条牵引缝线。轻轻回拉血管钳，将胃通过食管裂孔和后纵隔隧道拖入颈部切口。调整牵引线的位置，确定胃底的方向。用单层间断的 4–0 聚乙醇酸缝线将食管末端吻合到胃最高的部分。

用一大口径的鼻胃管（12 号）通过胃食管吻合插入胃内。保留鼻胃管使得引流畅通，规律地间断吸引以防止术后早期出现的急性胃扩张。吻合口旁置一软橡皮引流管，逐层闭合创口。

然后回到腹部操作，间断缝合数针，将食管裂孔的边缘与胃窦缝合，使得幽门直接位于横膈下方的中线上。做一个小口径的空肠造口，可在术后几周内、经口营养之前，提供肠内营养（图 69–5D）。

术后处理

术后早期仔细监测生命功能十分重要。术中广泛分离气管后方的软组织，引起的水肿可能会导致呼吸窘迫。经鼻气管插管数日，伴或不伴辅助通气可以简化术后病程，并减少呼吸并发症的发生。

空肠喂养可在术后第二天或第三天开始。空肠喂养最安全的方法是缓慢、持续地灌输，而不是间歇性给予，后者可能会造成“倾倒”效应。术后第 7 天行造影检查，如果确定吻合口无渗漏，可开始小心地经口喂养。证实吻合通畅后可以拔除颈部的引流管。

从 1981 年起，伦敦 Great Ormond Street 医院进行了 173 例胃代食管手术[113]。最常见的食管替代指征是食管闭锁（127 例），其中 70 例的早期修补失败，43 例是无瘘管的食管闭锁。23 例患儿为严重的腐蚀性狭窄。超过 80%的患者来自国外或从英国的其他医院转来。替代手术的方法是经后纵隔的不开胸手术有 90 例（52%），其余患者因原来的损伤（腐蚀性损伤、穿孔）导致致密的纵隔瘢痕或先前食管重建术失败而需要进行开胸手术。所有的患者术后常规使用松弛剂和机械通气至少 48～72 小时。

有 9 例死亡（5.2%），其中 8 例在胃转流术前的病程复杂。12%的病例发生胃食管连接处的吻合口漏，除了一例以外均自行闭合。狭窄发生率 19.6%，除了 3 例以外，食管镜下扩张均有效。这 3 例通过颈部切口成功地进行了狭窄段的切除再吻合。狭窄多见于碱性腐蚀性损伤后（38%）。30%的病例术后出现吞咽困难。

建立经口喂养可能非常困难，尤其是对于没有经过适当假饲的食管闭锁患儿。空肠喂养管的放置大大简化了术后的营养供应，避免了肠道外营养的需要。胆汁性呕吐可能是幽门成形术的结果，在术后早期常见，尤其是孩子处于侧卧位时。

表 69–7 胃代食管术的结果

年份	作者	患者数	死亡	漏（%）	狭窄（%）
1980	Atwell 和 Harrison[8]	6	2 (33)	—	—
1987	Valente 等人[122]	21	1 (4.7)	4 (19)	3 (14)
1991	Marujo 等人[73]	21	1 (4.7)	4 (17)	3 (14)
1995	Spitz[111]	83	6 (7.2)	10 (12)	10 (12)
2002	Hirschl[49]	41	0	15 (36)	20 (49)
2004	Spitz 等人[113]	173	9 (5.2)	21 (12)	34 (19.6)

对 17 例胃转流术后 5 年以上的患儿进行随访，
1104 结果发现，胸内胃的功能是液体和固体的管道而非储存器[21]。82%的患者在进食后 5 分钟之内快速排空液体和固体（>50%）。倾倒症状有时候是早期的特征，但大多数病例的这些症状在数周内可以缓解。这 17 例中，13 例有正常的身高百分比，11 例有正常的体重百分比。铁储量低是各种食管替代手术的共同特征，也发生于所有的胃转流患者术后。除 1 例之外，均有肺功能受限，平均肺总量（TLC）和平均用力肺活量（FVC）分别为预期容量的 68%和 64%。目前仍然不确定这些容量的降低是基本状况的结果还是胃代食管术的直接后果[22]。

在我们的患者中，90%的远期疗效良好或极好，表现为无吞咽困难和倾倒或腹泻等其他消化道症状，胃代食管部分无功能退化。

儿童胃代食管术的结果见表 69-7。

（胡　明译　李民驹校）

参考文献

1. Adams WE, Phemister DB: Carcinoma of the lower thoracic esophagus: Report of a successful resection and esophagogastrostomy. J Thorac Surg 1938;7:621.
2. Ahmed A, Spitz L: The outcome of colonic replacement of the esophagus in children. Prog Pediatr Surg 1986;19:37.
3. Anderson KD: Progress in pediatric surgery. In Wurnick P (ed): Long-Gap Esophageal Atresia—Prenatal Diagnosis of Congenital Malformations. Berlin, Springer-Verlag, 1986.
4. Anderson KD, Noblett H, Belsey R: Long-term follow-up of children with colon and gastric tube interposition for esophageal atresia. Surgery 1992;111:131.
5. Anderson KD, Randolph JG: The gastric tube for esophageal replacement in infants and children. J Thorac Cardiovasc Surg 1973;66:333.
6. Anderson KD, Randolph JG: Gastric tube interposition: A satisfactory alternative to the colon for esophageal replacement in children. Ann Thorac Surg 1978;25:521.
7. Anderson KD, Randolph JG, Lilley JR: Peptic ulcer in children with gastric tube interposition. J Pediatr Surg 1975;10:701.
8. Atwell JD, Harrison GSM: Observations on the role of esophagogastrostomy in infancy and childhood with particular reference to the long-term results and operative mortality. J Pediatr Surg 1980;15:303.
9. Azar H, Chrispin AR, Waterston DJ: Esophageal replacement with transverse colon in infants and children. J Pediatr Surg 1971;6:3.
10. Battersby JS, Moore TC: Esophageal replacement and bypass with the ascending and right half of transverse colon for the treatment of congenital atresia of the esophagus. Surg Gynecol Obstet 1959;109:207.
11. Beck C, Carrel A: Demonstration of specimens illustrating a method of formation of a prethoracic esophagus. Illinois Med J 1905;7:463.
12. Belsey R: Reconstruction of the esophagus with left colon. J Thorac Cardiovasc Surg 1965;49:33.
13. Belsey R: Reconstruction of the oesophagus. Ann R Coll Surg Engl 1983;65:360.
14. Burrington JD, Stephens CA: Esophageal replacement with a gastric tube in infants and children. J Pediatr Surg 1968;3:24.
15. Campbell JR, Webber BR, Harrison MW, Campbell TJ: Esophageal replacement in infants and children by colon interposition. Am J Surg 1982;144:29.
16. Carneiro PM, Doig CM: Colon interposition for wide gap oesophageal atresia. East Afr Med J 1993;70:682.
17. Cheung HC, Siu KG, Wong J: Is pyloroplasty necessary in esophageal replacement by stomach? A prospective randomised, controlled trial. Surgery 1987;102:19.
18. Cohen D: Oesophageal reconstruction using a gastric tube: A preliminary report. Aust Pediatr J 1970;6:22.
19. Cusick EL, Batchelor AAG, Spicer RD: Development of a technique for jejunal interposition in long-gap esophageal atresia. J Pediatr Surg 1993;28:990.
20. Dale WA, Sherman CD: Late reconstruction of congenital esophageal atresia by intrathoracic colon transplantation. J Thorac Surg 1955;29:344.
21. Davenport M, Bianchi A: Early experience with oesophageal flap esophagoplasty for repair of esophageal atresia. Pediatr Surg Int 1990;5:332.
22. Davenport M, Hosie GP, Tasker RC, et al: The long-term effects of gastric transposition in children: A physiological study. J Pediatr Surg 1996;31:588.
23. Ein SH: Gastric tubes in children with caustic esophageal injury. J Pediatr Surg 1998;33:1363.
24. Ein SH, Shandling B, Simpson JS, Stevens CA: A further look at the gastric tube as an esophageal replacement in infants and children. J Pediatr Surg 1973;8:859.
25. Ein SH, Shandling B, Stephens CA: Twenty-one year experience with the pediatric gastric tube. J Pediatr Surg 1987;22:77.
26. Eraklis AJ, Rosello PJ, Ballantine TVN: Circular esophagomyotomy of upper pouch in primary repair of long segment esophageal atresia. J Pediatr Surg 1976;11:709.
27. Erdogan E, Emir H, Eroglu E: Esophageal replacement using the colon: A 15-year review. Pediatr Surg Int 2000;16:546.
28. Foker JE, Ring WS, Varco RL: Technique of jejunal interposition for esophageal replacement. J Thorac Cardiovasc Surg 1982;83:928.
29. Freeman NV, Cass DT: Colon interposition: A modification of the Waterston technique using the normal esophageal route. J Pediatr Surg 1982;17:17.
30. Garlock JH: Reestablishment of esophagogastric continuity following resection of esophagus for carcinoma of middle third. Surg Gynecol Obstet 1944;78:23.
31. Gavriliu D: Etat actual de procede de reconstruction de l'oesophage par tube gastrique. Ann Chir 1965;19:219.
32. Gavriliu D: Aspects of esophageal surgery. Curr Probl Surg 1975;12:1.
33. Gavriliu D, Georgescue L: Esofagoplastie directa cu material gastric. Rev Stiintelor Medicale (Bucurest) 1951;3:33.
34. German JC, Waterston DJ: Colon interposition for replacement of the esophagus in children. J Pediatr Surg 1976;11:227.
35. Goon HK, Cohen DH, Middleton AW: Gastric tube oesophagoplasty—a long-term assessment. Z Kinderchir 1985;40:21.
36. Gough MH: Esophageal atresia—use of an anterior flap in

the difficult anastomosis. J Pediatr Surg 1980;15:310.
37. Gross BH, Asha FP, Galzer GM, Orringer MB: Gastric interposition following transhiatal esophagectomy: CT evaluation. Radiology 1985;155:177.
38. Gross RE, Firestone N: Colonic reconstruction of the esophagus in infants and children. Surgery 1967;61:955.
39. Guzzetta PC, Randolph JG: Antireflux cologastric anastomosis following colonic interposition for esophageal replacement. J Pediatr Surg 1986;21:1137.
40. Hagberg S, Rubenson A, Sillen U, Werkmaster K: Management of long-gap esophagus: Experience with end-to-end anastomosis under maximal tension. Prog Pediatr Surg 1986;19:88-92.
41. Hamza AF, Abdelhay S, Sherif H, et al: Caustic esophageal strictures in children: 30 years' experience. J Pediatr Surg 2003;38:828.
42. Harju E, Isolauri J: Nutritional state after colon interposition for benign oesophageal disease. Eur J Clin Nutr 1988;42:351.
43. Hays DM, Woolley M, Synder WH: Esophageal atresia and tracheoesophageal fistula: Management of the uncommon types. J Pediatr Surg 1966;1:240.
44. Heimlich HJ: Peptic esophagitis with stricture treated by reconstruction of the esophagus with a reversed gastric tube. Surg Gynecol Obstet 1962;114:673.
45. Heimlich HJ: Elective replacement of esophagus. Br J Surg 1966;53:913.
46. Heiss K, Wesson D, Bohn D, et al: Respiratory failure due to retained esophagus: A complication of esophageal replacement. J Pediatr Surg 1991;26:1359.
47. Hendren WH, Hale JR: Electromagnetic bougienage to lengthen esophageal segments in congenital esophageal atresia. N Engl J Med 1975;293:428.
48. Hendren WH, Hendren WG: Colon interposition for esophagus in children. J Pediatr Surg 1985;20:829.
49. Hirschl RB: Gastric transposition for esophageal replacement in children: Experience with 41 consecutive cases with special emphasis on esophageal atresia. Ann Surg 2002;236:531.
50. Hoffman DG, Moazam F: Transcervical myotomy for wide-gap esophageal atresia. J Pediatr Surg 1984;19:680.
51. Howard R, Myers NA: Esophageal atresia: A technique for elongating the upper pouch. Surgery 1965;58:725.
52. Isolauri J: Colonic interposition for benign esophageal disease. Long-term clinical and endoscopic results. Am J Surg 1988;155:498.
53. Isolauri J, Reinikainen P, Markkula H: Functional evaluation of interposed colon in esophagus. Manometric and 24-hour pH observations. Acta Chir Scand 1987;44:84.
54. Jezioro Z, Kus H: Experiences with the retrosternal esophageal replacement employing jejunum or ileum. J Pediatr Surg 1958;44:275.
55. Jianu A: Gastrostomie und Oesophagoplastik. Dtsch Z Chir 1912;11:8.
56. Kamath MV, Ellison RG, Rubin JW, et al: Esophageal mucocele: A complication of blind loop esophagus. Ann Thorac Surg 1987;43:263.
57. Kato T, Hollmann G, Hopper F, et al: Ein neues Instrument zur Faden-legung ohne Thorakotomie in ausgewahlten Fallen von oesophagusatresie. Z Kinderchir 1980;29:20.
58. Kelling G: Oesophagoplastik mit Hilfe des Quercolon. Zentralbl Chir 1911;38:1209.
59. Kelly JP, Shackelford GD, Roper CL: Esophageal replacement with colon in children: Functional results and long-term growth. Ann Thorac Surg 1983;36:634.
60. Khan AR, Stiff G, Mohammed AR, et al: Esophageal replacement with colon in children. Pediatr Surg Int 1998; 13:79.
61. Kummell HJ: Ueber intrathorakale Oesophagus Plastik. Beitr Klin Chir 1922;126:264.
62. Lexer E: Oesophagoplastik. Zentrabl Chir 1914;40:1970.
63. Lindahl H, Louhimo I, Virkola K: Colon interposition or gastric tube? Follow-up study of colon-esophagus and gastric tube–esophagus patients. J Pediatr Surg 1983;18:58.
64. Lindahl H, Rintala R, Sariola H, Louhimo I: Long-term endoscopic and flow cytometric follow-up of colon interposition. J Pediatr Surg 1992;27:859.
65. Lividitis A: Esophageal atresia. A method of over-bridging large segment gaps. Z Kinderchir 1973;13:278.
66. Longmire WP: Antethoracic jejunal transplantation for congenital esophageal atresia with hypoplasia of the lower esophagus. Surg Gynecol Obstet 1951;93:310.
67. Louhimo I, Pasila M, Visa Koepi JK: Late gastrointestinal complications in patients with colonic replacement of the oesophagus. J Pediatr Surg 1969;4:663.
68. Lundblad O: Uber antethorakale Osophagoplastik. Acta Chir Scand 1921;53:535.
69. MacKinlay GA, Burtles R: Oesophageal atresia: Paralysis and ventilation in management of the wide gap. Pediatr Surg Int 1987;2:10.
70. Mahour GH, Woolley MM, Gwinn JL: Elongation of the upper pouch and delayed anatomic reconstruction in esophageal atresia. J Pediatr Surg 1974;9:373.
71. Mansour KA, Malone CE: Surgery for scleroderma of the esophagus: A 12-year experience. Ann Thorac Surg 1988; 46:513.
72. Martin LW: The use of colon for esophageal replacement in children. Aust N Z J Surg 1972;42:160.
73. Marujo WC, Tannuri U, Maksoud JG: Total gastric transposition: An alternative to esophageal replacement in children. J Pediatr Surg 1991;26:676.
74. May IA, Samson PC: Esophageal reconstruction and replacements. Ann Thorac Surg 1969;7:249.
75. Mes GM: New method of esophagoplasty. J Int Coll Surg 1948;11:270.
76. Mitchell IM, Goh DW, Roberts KD, Abrahms CD: Colon interposition in children. Br J Surg 1989;76:681.
77. Ngan SY, Wong J: Lengths of different routes for esophageal replacement. J Thorac Cardiovasc Surg 1986;91:790.
78. Ochsner A, De Bakey M: Surgical aspects of cancer of the esophagus. A review of the literature. J Thorac Surg 1940; 10:401.
79. Ochsner A, Owens N: Antethoracic esophagoplasty for impermeable stricture of the esophagus. Ann Surg 1934; 100:1055.
80. Okmian Z, Booss D, Ekelund I: An endoscopic technique for Rehbein's silver olive method. Z Kinderchir 1975; 16:212.
81. Orringer MB, Kirsh MM, Sloan H: New trends in esophageal replacement for benign disease. Ann Thorac Surg 1977; 23:409.
82. Orringer MB, Sloan H: Esophagectomy without thoracotomy. J Thorac Cardiovasc Surg 1978;76:643.
83. Othersen HB Jr, Clatworthy HW Jr: Functional evaluation of esophageal replacement in children. J Thorac Cardiovasc Surg 1967;53:55.
84. Pierie JP, de Graaf PW, Poen H, et al: Incidence and management of benign anastomotic stricture after cervical oesophagogastrostomy. Br J Surg 1993;80:471.
85. Pirot-Roux L, Hase O: Epicrise de la premiére operatian de l'oesophagoplastie prethoracique faite par le Dr. Cesar Roux en 1906. Rev Med Suisse Romande 1950;90:19.

86. Postlethwait RW: Technique for isoperistaltic gastric tube for esophageal bypass. Ann Surg 1979;189:673.
87. Postlethwait RW: Colonic interposition for esophageal substitution. Surg Gynecol Obstet 1983;156:377.
88. Postlethwait RW: Surgery of the Esophagus, 2nd ed. Norwalk, CT, Appleton-Century-Crofts, 1995.
89. Puri P, Blake N, O'Donnell B, Guiney EJ: Delayed primary anastomosis following spontaneous growth of esophageal segments in esophageal atresia. J Pediatr Surg 1981;6:180.
90. Raffensperger JG, Luck SR, Reynolds M, Schwartz D: Intestinal bypass of the esophagus. J Pediatr Surg 1996; 31:38.
91. Rehbein F, Schweder N: Reconstruction of the esophagus without colon transplantation in cases of atresia. J Pediatr Surg 1971;6:746.
92. Rienhoff WF: Intrathoracic esophagojejunostomy for lesions of the upper third of the esophagus. South Med J 1946;39:928.
93. Ring WS, Varco RL, L'Heureux PR, Foker JE: Esophageal replacement with jejunum in children: An 18 to 33 year follow-up. J Thorac Cardiovasc Surg 1982;83:918.
94. Rode H, Cywes S, Millar AJ, Davies MR: Colonic oesophageal replacement in children—functional results. Z Kinderchir 1986;41:201.
95. Rodgers BM, Talbert JL, Moazarn F, Felman AH: Functional and metabolic evaluation of colon replacement of the esophagus in children. J Pediatr Surg 1978; 13:35.
96. Rossello PJ, Lebron H: The technique of myotomy in esophageal reconstruction: An experimental study. J Pediatr Surg 1980;15:430.
97. Roux C: L'esophago-jejuno-gastrome: Nouvelle operation pour retrecessement infranchissable de l'esophage. Semin Med 1907;27:37.
98. Rudler JC, Monod-Broca P: Uncas d'esophagoplastie palliative retro-sternale avec l'ileocolon droit. Mem Acad Chir (Paris) 1951;77:747.
99. Saeki M, Tsuchida Y, Ogata T, et al: Long-term results of jejunal replacement of the esophagus. J Pediatr Surg 1988;23:483.
100. Salo JA, Heikkila L, Nemlander A, et al: Barrett's oesophagus and perforation of gastric tube ulceration into the pericardium: A late complication after reconstruction of oesophageal atresia. Ann Chir Gynaecol 1995;84:92.
101. Scharli AF: Esophageal reconstruction in very long atresias by elongation of the lesser curvature. Pediatr Surg Int 1992;7:101.
102. Schier F, Schier C, Hoppner D, Willital GH: [Esophageal replacement with resorbable vicryl tubes—an animal experiment study.] Osophagusersatz mit resorbierbaren Vicryl-Schlauchen—Eine tierexperimentelle Untersuchung. Z Kinderchir 1987;42:224.
103. Schullinger JN, Vinocur CD, Santulli T: The suture-fistula technique in the repair of selected cases of esophageal atresia. J Pediatr Surg 1982;17:234.
104. Shafer AD, David TE: Suture fistula as a means of connecting upper and lower segments in oesophageal atresia. J Pediatr Surg 1974;9:669.
105. Shamberger RC, Eraklis AJ, Kosakewich HP, Hendren WH: Fate of the distal esophageal remnant following esophageal replacement. J Pediatr Surg 1988;23:1210.
106. Sherman CD, Waterston DW: Oesophageal reconstruction in children using intrathoracic colon. Arch Dis Child 1957;32:11.
107. Soave F: Intrathoracic transposition of the transverse colon in complicated oesophageal atresia. Proc Pediatr Surg 1972; 4:91.
108. Sonneland J, Anson BJ, Beaton LE: Surgical anatomy of the arterial supply to the colon from the superior mesenteric artery based upon a study of 600 specimens. Surg Gynecol Obstet 1958;106:385.
109. Spitz L: Gastric transposition via the mediastinal route for infants with long-gap esophageal atresia. J Pediatr Surg 1984;19:149.
110. Spitz L: Gastric transposition for esophageal substitution in children. J Pediatr Surg 1992;27:252.
111. Spitz L: Gastric replacement of the esophagus. In Spitz L, Coran AG (eds): Pediatric Surgery, 5th ed. London, Chapman & Hall, 1995.
112. Spitz L, Kiely E, Brereton RJ, Drake D: Management of esophageal atresia. World J Surg 1993;17:296.
113. Spitz L, Kiely E, Pierro A: Gastric transposition in children—a 21-year experience. J Pediatr Surg 2004;39:276.
114. Spitz L, Kiely E, Sparnon T: Gastric transposition for esophageal replacement in children. Ann Surg 1987;206:69.
115. Stone MM, Fonkalsrud EW, Mahour GH, et al: Esophageal replacement with colon interposition in children. Ann Surg 1986;203:346-351.
116. Sweet RH: Transthoracic gastrectomy and esophagectomy for carcinoma of the stomach and esophagus. Clinics 1945;3:1288.
117. Sweet RH: A method of restoring continuity of the alimentary canal in cases of congenital atresia of the esophagus and with tracheo-esophageal fistula not treated by immediate primary anastomosis. Ann Surg 1948;127:757.
118. Touloukian RJ, Schonholz SM, Gryboski JD, et al: Perioperative considerations in esophageal replacement for epidermolysis bullosa: Report of two cases successfully treated by colon interposition. Am J Gastroenterol 1988; 83:857.
119. Touloukian RJ, Tellides G: Retrosternal ileocolic esophageal replacement in children revisited. Antireflux role of the ileocecal valve. J Thorac Cardiovasc Surg 1994;107:1067.
120. Tsujinaka T, Ogawa M, Kido Y, et al: A giant tracheogastric tube fistula caused by a penetrated peptic ulcer after esophageal replacement. Am J Gastroenterol 1988;83:862.
121. Uchida Y, Tomonari K, Murakami S, et al: Occurrence of peptic ulcer in the gastric tube used for esophageal replacement in adults. Jpn J Surg 1987;17:190.
122. Valente A, Brereton RJ, Mackersie A: Esophageal replacement with whole stomach in infants and children. J Pediatr Surg 1987;22:913.
123. Vizas D, Ein SH, Simpson JS: The value of circular myotomy for esophageal atresia. J Pediatr Surg 1978;13:357.
124. Von Hacker V: [On esophagoplasty in general and on the repair of the esophagus by antethoracic construction of a skin-colon tube in particular.] Uber Oesophagoplastic in allgemeinen unter uber den ersatz der Speuserohre durch antethorackle Hauntdickdarmschlauchbildung im besonderen. Arch Klin Chir 1914;105:973.
125. Vulliet H: De l'esophagoplastie et des diverses modifications. Semin Med 1911;31:529.
126. Waterson D: Colonic replacement of esophagus (intrathoracic). Surg Clin North Am 1964;44:1441.
127. West KW, Vane DW, Grosfeld JL: Esophageal replacement in children: Experience with thirty-one cases. Surgery 1986; 100:751.

第 70 章

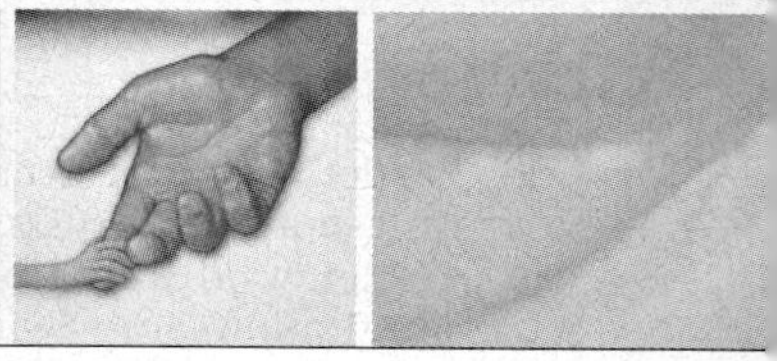

食管功能异常

Juan A. Tovar

1107 食管没有重要的分泌和吸收功能，仅起到从咽到胃的管道作用。所以它的主要功能是推动食物，此功能的异常可导致一些通常反映在成年人的病变，但发生于儿童时也有特殊表现。婴儿和儿童期的这些功能异常常与畸形有关，并且有明显的临床表现。大多数尚不能完全理解，主要是因为我们对消化道运动调节机制的知识有限，而且由于器械的大小和患儿合作性的问题，可用于儿童的诊断工具不足。本章讨论食管的运动功能异常。

历史

小儿内科和外科医生很多年前就认识到胃食管反流（GER）或失弛缓症，其历史将在本书第 71 章介绍。但是，对其他的儿童食管功能异常最近才有认识。除了失弛缓症[63,133]和“食管憩室”外，后者可能与环咽弛缓有关，其他的食管功能异常在最新的小儿外科学教科书里均未提及[63,133,134,164]。这些功能障碍的本质涉及其发病机制，最近只有在必要的诊断工具被发明且小型化以后，其难以捉摸的症状才得以阐明。自对这些疾病进行研究以来，以运动失调为主的新的临床表现已被识别并进行检查。

胚胎学

食管起源于内胚层管的前肠或颅侧部分，在体腔内沿胚体纵轴生长。颅侧起始于咽的下端，尾侧与胃相连，后者是原始前肠扩张而成[92]。前肠的内胚层内层被来源于间叶的双层肌纤维包绕（外层纵形纤维和内层环形纤维）。

约在孕第 26 天时，前肠上部的腹侧出现一个分支，这个基芽逐渐出现分叉直到最后构成气管支气管树[92]。内胚层与间叶之间的相互作用以及各种基因、转录因子和生长因子的影响，促使了肺及其多种类型细胞的形成[30,188]。内胚层内层的改变导致它向食管或者气管支气管的上皮分化[189]。该食管气管分裂期对于正常器官的形成十分重要，严重的食管畸形或者功能障碍来源于这一时点。这些阶段完成后，食管最终的形态是由两层肌肉、一层黏膜下层和一层非角化的黏膜层所构成。一些内胚层分化而来的食管腺体在食管黏膜下层形成，但是它们的碱性分泌物与胃肠道的其他部分相比是很少的。

在胚胎第 8～12 周，起源于颅神经嵴的成神经细胞以头尾方向移至原始前肠，并停留在肌间和黏膜下层，形成纤维连接，通过副交感神经和交感神经系统实现食管功能的神经控制[121]。非肾上腺-非胆碱能或氮能神经的神经支配于第 12 周出现在肠肌丛，第 14 周出现于黏膜下丛，至 22[68]或 23[19]周时发育完全。迷走神经和椎旁交感神经链源自神经嵴，它们的形成与肠壁的神经分布同步。

当体腔被分割为胸腔和腹腔后，横膈与食管远端建立了功能性联系，这对食管的生理功能非常重要：胃和部分食管被定位于横膈下方，而大部分食管仍位 1108
于胸腔内。横膈的肌纤维来自躯干中胚层，其中一部分成肌细胞极可能起源于颈部[2,3]。来源于肝后间叶细胞层的中心腱和其他结缔组织闭合了余留的胸腹通道[88]。

解剖学

食管上端直接与咽喉相连，肌纤维与环咽肌、咽括约肌下部融合，形成食管上括约肌（UES）。食管体位于后纵隔，后方与脊柱、前方与气管和心脏紧邻，两侧为胸腔。迷走神经干紧贴食管表面行走，并发出许多神经分支。新生儿食管的长度小于 10cm，而成人达 35～40cm 。食管下端横贯横膈的食管裂孔，在进入胃之前成为食管腹腔段。该末端没有解剖上可识别的括约肌纤维，但在胃食管连接处水平，右侧食管的环形肌呈水平的 U 形（扣带纤维）。食管左侧的肌纤维排成 U 形越过胃切迹向下进入胃的前、后面（悬带纤维）[98]。来自右膈脚的肌肉形成食管裂孔的膈悬带并与食管远端括约肌重叠，其横纹肌纤维紧贴食管并分隔胸腔与腹腔。所有这些结构组成一个高压区，在高压区中，食管下括约肌（LES）和膈肌脚悬带是主要的功能性结构。与胃肠道的其他节段相反，食管缺乏浆膜层，但在胸腔段食管侧面有一部分紧贴左、右侧纵隔胸膜，短的腹腔段前方与腹膜紧密接触。食管肌层与肠道肌层非常相似，但肌纤维的本质不同，食管的上三分之一是横纹肌，其余部位是平滑肌。

食管肌间和黏膜下的神经丛内含有神经节细胞和广泛的纤维网状结构，后者连接神经丛自身的神经元，并与副交感迷走神经、交感干和腹腔神经丛连接。胆碱能和肾上腺能介质分别对食管发挥阳性和阴性的运动作用。放松通过氮能神经末端介导，其神经元位于肌间神经丛[165]。C-kit 阳性的 Cajal 间质细胞分布在肌纤维中并具有起搏作用[86,141,142,179]。神经控制调节这些细胞的程度尚未阐明[194]。

生理学

食管的功能主要是将食物团从咽喉部输送到胃部，其次是清除从胃反流而来的液体。

为了避免消化液吸入喉或呼吸时食管吸入空气，食管的上括约肌保持收缩状态，只有在关闭声门和停止呼吸吞咽时才会放松[77]。食管在胸腔的负压条件下，要求其在正常时关闭远端以防止反流。个功能通过下端食管括约肌来保证，后者除吞咽以外一直保持张力[178]。胆碱能介质和氮能介质的平衡调节着括约肌的关闭和舒张[171]。

由于食管大部分位于胸腔内而胃位于腹腔内，保持了持续的腹腔胸腔压力梯度。结果，间歇性的吸气胸腔负压与持续性的腹腔正压协同作用，倾向于将胃内容物推回食管[187]。正常的食管下端括约肌静息张力对抗这个压力梯度，并在膈肌脚悬韧带节律收缩的辅助下，可在吸气时闭合食管腔。此时的反压力梯度更大，悬韧带使贲门向下移位，这样使 HIS 角增大和食管腹腔段延长[110]。这种平滑肌和横纹肌结构的协同作用已在动物中广泛研究[112,183,184]，并且具有与肛门直肠括约功能相似的机制，后者的情况是正常的静息张力由内括约肌提供，通过有意识的横纹肌复合体和外括约肌收缩间歇性地增加压力。

吞咽是只有当上下括约肌都松弛的时候才可进行。这种松弛发生在咽部肌肉遇到推动波时，持续松弛直至咽的收缩到达食管下端触发食管体的蠕动。为了使这些推动波发挥作用，食管肌肉在食管全长以协同方式从头侧向尾侧收缩，推动食管内容物进入胃。这些被称为“初始”波。实现这个复杂功能必须具有正常的肌层和神经控制，食管运动障碍则可能是肌层和神经控制异常的结果。

反流是胃内容物逆向进入食管，这在一定程度上说是正常的，因为每天食管下括约肌会有多次不能维持自然张力的时候，特别是在进食和稳定的胃食管压力梯度推动胃液倒退时。在有些患者中，这个括约肌力量可能长期不足，特别是神经受损时[56]，但是现在认识到，大多数的成人和儿童的反流是由于非吞咽的
一时性括约肌松弛[32,83,178,181]。在这松弛过程中，食管 1109
腔充满含有酸性胃液和其他消化物的反流液。黏膜不能抵抗这些化学物质的侵蚀，它必须及时清除这些液体以避免永久性的损伤。为了达到这个目的，食管开始产生与吞咽无关的蠕动性收缩，这些收缩可发生于食管的不同平面，并向前推进，这样可将反流的物质推返入胃，这就是“第二次”波[155]。这一运动功能使得食管摆脱了大量的反流液体，但是黏附在黏膜上的酸只有通过多次吞咽碱性唾液的缓冲作用和通过食管腺的碱性分泌物一定程度上对酸的中和作用才可以完全清除。正常的食管同样可以产生少量同时发生的推进波，闭合食管全长的管腔。这些被称为“第三”波，当它们发生的过于频繁时，可能造成一些食管功能的紊乱[7,8,62,116,175]。

食管功能的评估方法

多年来钡餐一直作为主要的食管检查工具，它不

仅可看到器官解剖上的异常，也可以看到食管上括约肌和下括约肌的收缩和舒张异常。然而，如果需要延长评估，则严重的放射性暴露不可避免，而且这个暴露会随着应用增多而限制其应用。然而，对本章提到的一些情况，该方法仍是必要的。

用液体或固体的放射性标志物餐做闪烁扫描检查已能帮助识别正常的食管清除机制并评估食管的运送、胃和食管的排空等。然而，该方法在儿童中的应用相对有限[42,146,168,177]。

大小合适的纤维内镜可以直接观察食管的管腔和黏膜。一些收缩性疾病可以在检查过程中发现，但其主要功能在于通过对黏膜的观看和活检获取信息。

延期 pH检查主要用于测定食管暴露于酸的程度，但是与清除的动力功能和器官的清除能力有关。因此，pH 测试的结果可能对一些动力性疾病的理解很重要[29,31,32,139,146]。

测压法是常用的检查食管动力功能的方法。该方法建立在 Pascal 理论的基础上，强调压力的向外放射，在液体每个点的各个方向具有相同的力。应用一个尖端封闭、有侧孔的探针，从侧孔恒速注入液体，通过与注入系统“T”形连接的压力传感器记录食管腔内任何一个点的压力。集合数个有间隔小孔的探针，可检测压力波沿着食管传递的过程（图 70–1）。固体传感器可以取代灌注探针，但是其易碎性和高造价限制了使用。

测压法也有助于评估括约肌的功能。采用单个输注探针或集合数个探针，放射状排列小孔，这些记录小孔匀速通过胃食管连接处，可记录食管上括约肌和食管下括约肌的压力[7,14,83,104,166]。食管下括约肌检测的结果显示胃的压力之后是一个“高原期”，即食管下括约肌压力与膈肌脚悬韧带收缩的重叠[69]。除此之外，它可检测食管进入胸腔的位点，因为当正压吸气
1110 转变成负压时，有一个“倒置点”（图 70–2）。将一个孔固定在括约肌水平的固定括约肌测压法可探测并评估舒张的程度。

然而，因为已认识到在正常括约肌压力下也可发生反流，所以较多地注意适当水平的连续括约肌记录探针和持续灌注套管的舒张波[32,83,84,111,178]。这些记录探针与细的硅橡胶探针连接已被用于幼婴和早产儿的胃食管生理学研究[122,123]。

测压法需要庞大、昂贵且灵敏的设备以及患者的合作，在小儿可能很难进行。此外，镇静可能会改变压力的记录[58,172]。

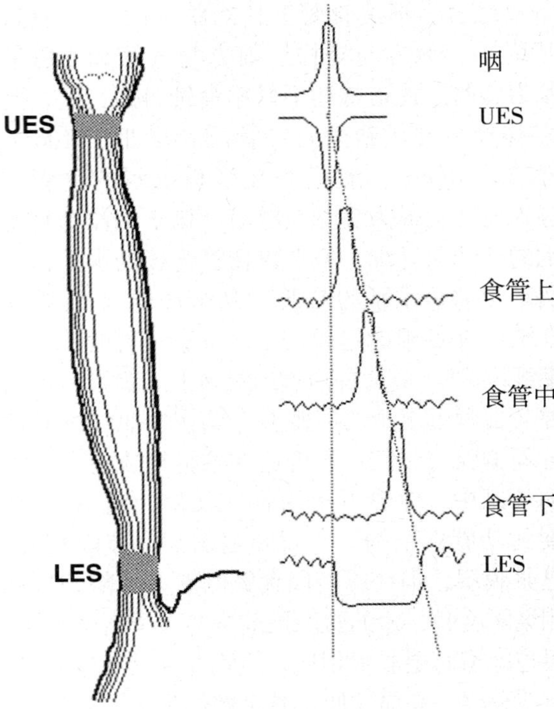

图 70–1 吞咽时食管腔内测压记录示意图。咽括约肌收缩的同时伴有环咽肌或上食管括约肌（UES）的松弛。在食管体产生进行性蠕动波。在整个过程中食管下括约肌（LES）保持松弛，紧接着一个松弛后高峰而关闭。

最近提出 24 小时连续测压，同时进行 pH测定，已经为成人和儿童的一些食管疾病提供了重要的信息[1,5,6,20,50,76,125,150,161]。但是，目前固体传感器探针的大小和设备的体积已限制了对大龄儿童的测试[29,62,174,185]。广泛记录压力或 pH的技术已改为电信号，可通过特殊设计的计算机软件进行分析。这些诊断工具将进一步缩小，在不久的将来可适合在儿童中应用，从而扩大测压研究的范围。

食管上段疾病

咽环肌有时候不能保持其正常的状态，或在吞咽的过程中过度松弛，导致吞咽困难和窒息，可能威胁幼婴生命。

* 见参考文献 7,15,32,33,59,64,83,104,138,154,158,185。

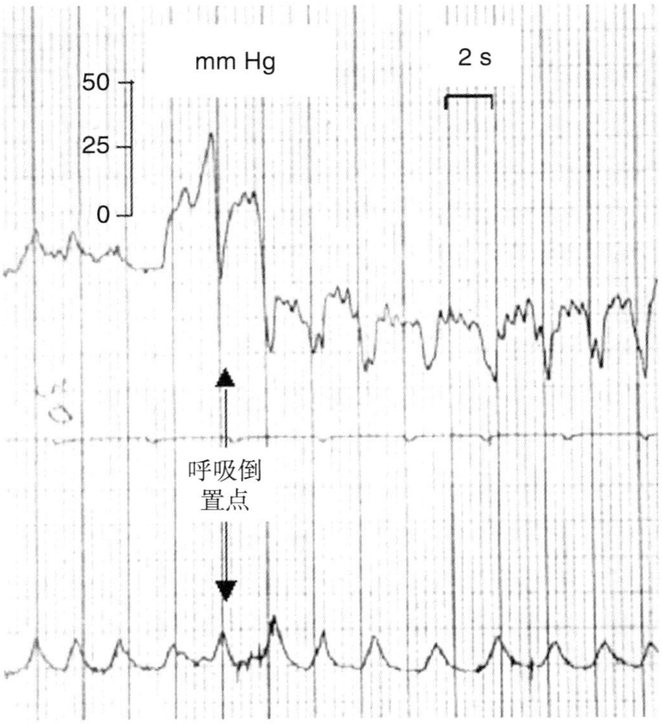

图 70-2　对一个正常儿童采用拖出测压法记录的食管下括约肌（LES）（上轨迹）和同时测得的腹部压力（下轨迹）。胃内压是第一个记录的正吸气偏转。“高原”相当于 LES 的高压区。当探头进入食管胸腔段时，食管腔内的吸气偏转变为阴性（呼吸倒置点）。此后压力的基线较低，吸气记录为阴性波。拖动速度为 1mm/s。垂直标志之间的时间为 2 秒。

持续环咽肌松弛有时可在神经衰弱的患者中发现，患者反复地吸气[159]。延迟松弛或不完全放松可发生于 22q 11.2 缺失[48]的 Chiari 综合征[127,129]患儿，或在给予安定药物后出现[99]。松弛不能（环咽肌失弛缓症）偶见为原发现象，通常继发于神经肌肉疾病[135,159]。在这些条件下，首发症状是幼婴在喂养时的窒息和呼吸窘迫，常需要及时的诊断处理。持续环咽肌松弛者在钡餐检查或射线活动摄影时可见呼吸道和消化道同时不透光。延缓松弛和松弛不能者可见扩大的咽腔伴持续的上食管关闭，偶见造影剂进入气管[89,135]。

测压法有助于诊断环咽肌疾病，因为它可显示吞咽时肌肉的不完全松弛或不松弛[22,129,159]。然而，这在婴儿很难实施，因为在食管上段应用灌注导管对于孩子来说会很不舒服，可引起窒息、咳嗽和不合作。用括约肌套描记松弛缺失的方法更好，而且液体误吸的风险也更小[37]。

对于持续性环咽肌松弛和食管上括约肌失弛缓症患儿需要行胃造瘘术进行喂养[54,127]。肌肉的失弛缓可通过球囊扩张治疗[43,95]但是黏膜外的肌层切开更为有效[22,117]。如果存在胃食管反流，应同时行胃底折叠术，因为上、下食管关闭机制均不全的结果可能是毁灭性的[113]。有报道从环咽肌失弛缓症患者的肌切开术中所获得的肌肉中可见有一些非特异性的组织学改变[93]。

食管体疾病

原发性动力疾病

食管体的运动异常是成人症状的常见原因，在对吞咽困难、非心脏相关性胸痛或怀疑胃食管反流的患者检查时，可能发现弥漫性食管痉挛[10,40,144,161,181]、“胡桃夹”食管[21,82]或其他影响食物团推进的动力异常。 1111
在这些情况下，首先可发现同时发生的无推进收缩或过多的长持续波与正常波交替，其次可发现非常有力的蠕动性或倒退性高振幅波[125,160,161]。“胡桃夹”食管可以发展为失弛缓症[4]。

测压法是主要的诊断工具，自从可进行 24 小时记录后，它的准确性已有明显提高，因为障碍不会持久存在，仅偶尔出现在生理节律循环的某些点上。由于在儿童中进行这些操作过程比较困难，至今尚无关于原发性食管体动力异常的报道，虽然呼吸暂停、心动过缓[57]和奇怪的体位[192]等已经被认为是动力性疾病的症状和表现。然而，较好的测压技术已发现这些动力异常在儿童中也存在。已经发现儿童无食管狭窄时的食物嵌塞的测压波形与成人的胡桃夹食管波形相似（图 70-3），但是这个疾病可能不是原发的，因为大多数患者有反流，而且在食管炎治疗后可好转[26,90,138,185]。

促动力剂或钙通道阻滞剂[17,61]很少在儿童中用于治疗原发性动力疾病[65]。西地那非有助于增加一氧化氮相关的食管体和食管下括约肌的松弛，它已被用于治疗成人的动力性疾病[94,136,196]，但很少用于儿童。球囊扩张或者广泛的肌层切开术有时在成人中采用，但还没有用于儿童。

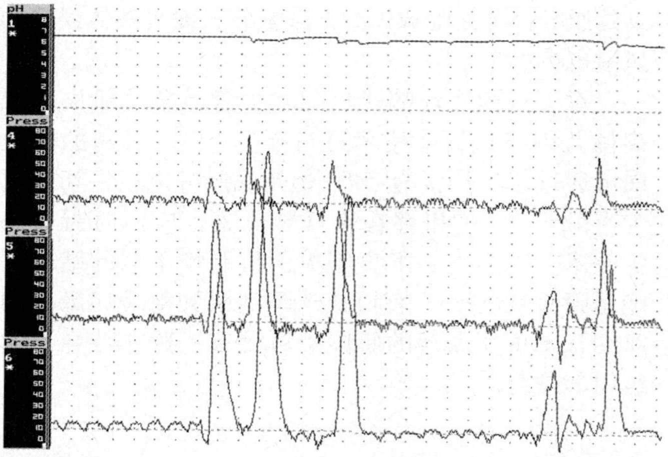

图 70-3 1 例 10 岁男孩反复发作无梗阻性的食物嵌塞，夜间测压记录的下段食管腔内 pH（1）和上段（4）、中段（5）、下段（6）食管压。轨迹提示有持续长时间的胡桃夹食管波形，明显而非常有力的蠕动波，尤其在食管体的下端（超过 200mmHg 或者在正常水平之上 3～4 次）。这发生在睡眠时，pH 测定未见反流。

继发性动力疾病

异常的食管运动已经在一些综合征和染色体疾病中发现。患有 Down 综合征[169,195]、Cornelia de Lange 综合征[23,25,47,103,126]、硬皮病[55,191]、多发肌炎-皮肌炎[192]和狼疮[91]的儿童，有时可有异常的食管蠕动伴反流。这些病常引起成人的食管动力障碍，但儿童时期的发病较少。母亲乳房有硅胶植入者的婴儿在母乳喂养时[96]也可发生食管动力紊乱，与硬皮病时相似。

与小儿外科医生关系更密切的食管动力紊乱，是新生儿期食管闭锁合并食管气管瘘的术后幸存者所经历的食管动力紊乱[44,45,46,168,170,173]。在这个畸形中，肌层结构[198]、外源性[38,130]和内源性[28,131]神经的分布异常，蠕动泵作用降低，而且可能持续终生。这种情况特别有害，因为此时常伴有食管下端括约肌的功能异常，这两种缺陷导致自出生后开始的持续性胃食管反流，不依赖于修补的类型[137,166]。此外，继发于食管吻合术的食管缩短[114]、食管裂孔异常[197]、和可能由手术引起的去神经都会影响食管的运动功能。很多研究表明食管闭锁术后的存活者有食管下括约肌的功能异常[45,166]。一些作者发现食管蠕动有持久性损伤，甚至可在吻合术后持续很多年[170,173]。这些异常的临床影响可能比我们以前所想象的要多。食管闭锁外科手术后的患者很少感到吞咽困难，但在专门检查时几乎都存在[79,173]。这些食管不能防止反流，因为这些动力异常的结构基础，促动力药物的治疗没有很明显的效果。食管闭锁患儿术后的反流不可能随着年龄增长而自行好转，而无食管闭锁者的反流常可自行好转。

食管闭锁患者的胃食管反流如有症状或引起食管炎时应予以治疗。由于持续缺乏动力，需要行宽松的完全性胃底折叠术。重力是食管排空的主要力量，如果折叠宽松，排空应该没有问题，然而远期疗效不好，因为所有导致胃食管反流和缺乏动力的原因仍然存在[56,153]。

其他与食管动力相关的疾病是慢性假性肠梗阻，
这是一组不同种类的肌源性或神经源性的胃肠道功 1112
能失调，其特征为同时发生的短暂性低振幅波的远端食管动力缺乏[18,109,145]。然而，这种动力缺乏是广泛性的，并且食管不是最重要的部分。巨结肠的患者可同时出现双峰食管波。先天性中枢性肺换气不足综合征（Ondine's curse）[53]或 Goldenhar 综合征[148]也有食管的动力缺乏。新生儿时期进行先天性膈疝手术的存活者在影像学和临床检查时表现出食管动力功能异常[105,162,163]，这可能与神经分布异常有关。食管功能紊乱包括括约肌压力降低或食管远端收缩异常，这些已在合并慢性肾衰竭[132]、Noonan 综合征[147]和 Pierre Robin 综合征[12]的儿童中发现。同样的异常已在所谓腹腔病[74]的成人中有报道，但这种病在儿童中尚未发现。

食管腐蚀性损伤的儿童，在损伤急性期[60]和瘢痕形成[13]后都会有食管蠕动功能的降低。这些压力测试的结果已得到放射性核素研究的证实[24]。虽然继发性食管炎可能加重病情，但这种动力异常对于临床经过和预后的影响仍不清楚。

在过去的几年里我们治疗的嗜酸性细胞食管炎的患者增多，这可能是过敏所致，伴有反流或食物积压的症状[36,85,97,124]。通常无反流和狭窄，但内镜下可见典型的 Schatzki 环[120]或多发性环[149]（图 70-4）。可在活检中发现严重的黏膜层嗜酸性细胞浸润。嗜酸性细胞食管炎很少发生狭窄，只有 1 例，经保守治疗痊愈。口服皮质类固醇、氟替卡松或嗜酸性细胞稳定剂，如孟鲁司特，通常对治疗这种病情有帮

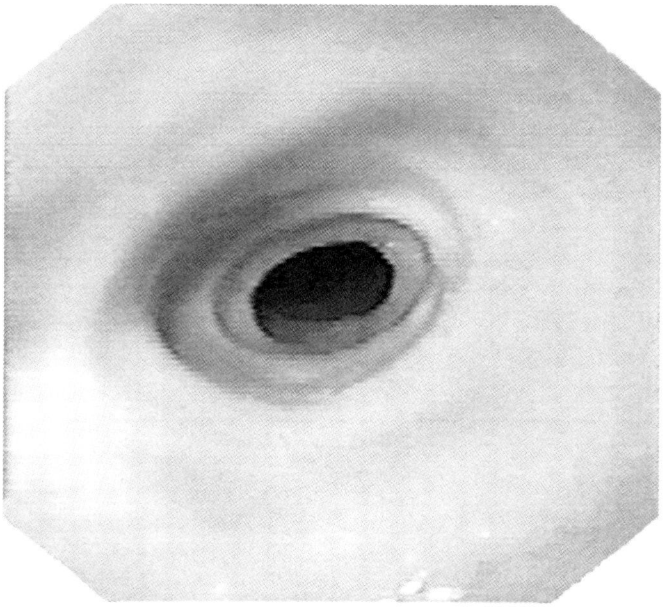

图 70-4 1 例 11 岁女孩继发于嗜酸性细胞食管炎的吞咽困难，纤维内镜下见典型的食管“多环”。pH 水平正常，类固醇治疗效果很好。

助。

远端食管疾病

原发性胃食管反流包括胃食管屏障失效和食管动力异常。食管括约肌功能失效的病因尚未完全了解，但越来越多的证据表明非吞咽松弛延长是主要的发病机制[32,83,178]。这些异常导致“共同腔”现象的形成，使正常的胃食管压力梯度消失。胃液反流进入食管后应该通过蠕动予以清除，但是胃食管反流患者的这第二道防御机制也异常，增加了食管炎的危险。吞咽后成反流蠕动的比例和波的振幅均降低，特别是在食管的下端[7,59,62]。胃食管反流患者的动力障碍是原发现象还是继发于食管炎症仍不清楚。可靠的临床和实验证据表明慢性食管炎会对先前健康的食管蠕动产生负面影响[35,182]，至少在一些病例中可见药物或手术治愈反流和食管炎之后仍有动力异常[7,33,35,108]。

在近 20 年中，广泛应用促动力药物治疗的成功表明了胃食管反流中动力失调的相关性。这些药物通过加强已变弱的括约肌而促进胃排空并加强蠕动。

更有特征的食管下端动力异常是食管失弛缓症，该病的食管下括约肌张力高，而且在吞咽时不松弛。此外，食管扩张和原发的蠕动功能低下形成了一个完全无效的推进功能。这个情况在幼儿中相对少见，尽管有些病例早期发作，但大多数在童年晚期或青春期早期得到诊断。仅有少数的研究包括超过一定数量的病例[16,73,78,80,174,176,180]，而最大的多中心系列研究仅包括 175 例患者[178]。

失弛缓症的病因不清楚，但越来越多的证据表明它与渐进性的内在神经异常以及一氧化氮合酶（NOS）活性的下降或缺失有关[86,165]。该酶与一氧化氮的合成有关，而后者是与平滑肌松弛有关的非肾上腺素能非胆碱能神经介质[165]。NOS 缺失的 nNOS(–/–) 鼠有高张力、不松弛的食管下括约肌[152]。这种内在神经的渐进性退变与 Chagas 病中所见的有些相似，后者是南美洲一种克鲁斯锥虫引起的寄生虫病，可引起神经结构变性，导致巨食管症[41]。

食管失弛缓症可能与 Allgrove 综合征有关，后
者是 AAAS 基因突变[81,143,194]所致的家族性常染色体 1113
隐性遗传病[81,143,194]，其特征为除了食管运动障碍外，还有肾上腺皮质功能低下和泪缺乏，这种联合被称作ALADIN 综合征（泪缺失、失弛缓症、肾上腺素功能低下和神经系统异常）[70]。失弛缓症在男孩中较多见，有时与 Down 综合征伴发[195]。

失弛缓症的症状为渐进性的吞咽困难和停留在食管内食物的反流，这些症状不应与呕吐相混淆。有些失弛缓症患者有胸骨后疼痛并可能十分严重，患者体重下降并常有呼吸受阻和呼吸道症状，如夜间咳嗽或经常由于少量误吸而引起反复发作性肺炎[72,80]。Allgrove 综合征患者也有肾上腺皮质功能不全的症状，如进行性色素沉着、乏力和有时出现泪液缺失（无泪），但是这些症状和其他神经系统疾病的表现[70]可能出现在明显的失弛缓症临床表现之后。

钡餐为常用的诊断手段：可见食管变大（巨食管）和钡剂圆柱上方停滞的液体。出现明显的蠕动停止，胃食管连接处纤细，呈典型的“鸟嘴”状[80]。造影剂在很长一段时间后逐渐进入胃内，大多数造影剂残留在食管内数小时（图 70-5）。

光学纤维内镜检查可排除食管狭窄，食管镜通常可以相对容易地进入胃。食管炎可能发生于滞留的液体被吸入后，但通常继发于滞留液体的发酵。pH 检查在这个阶段没有帮助，而且可能会引起误导。因为液体通常为酸性，探针测试的数据可能提示胃食管反流，但这实际上这是不可能的。放射性核素扫描可见食管内容物停滞不前，而且可较长时间的观察同时受

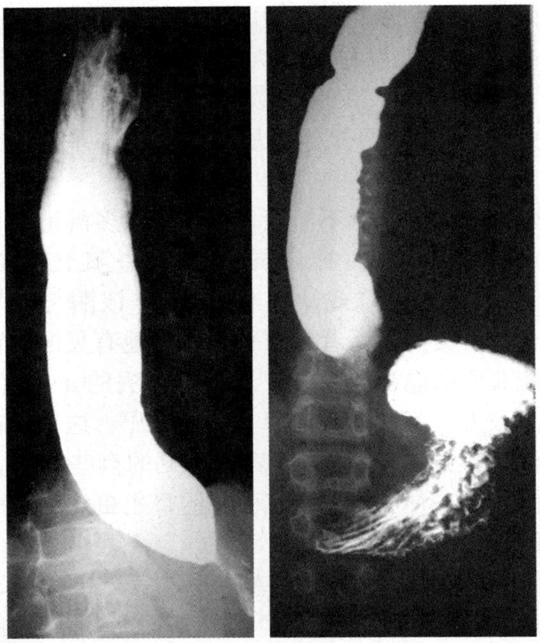

图 70-5 1 例 9 岁食管失弛缓症患儿的钡餐造影。可见食管扩张并在造影剂吞入之前有液体滞留。排空非常慢，贲门呈典型的“胡萝卜”或者“鸟嘴”状（左）。可见一些微弱的食管收缩（右），但是不能蠕动，因为食管壁仍保持很宽的分离状态。

到较少的放射暴露，但在评估食管远端形状时不如钡餐检查[27,195]。

测压检查是对于失弛缓症最为有用的工具：可见括约肌的张力高，在吞咽时不松弛或松弛不全。食管蠕动缺失，很少有压力，尤其是在进食时。这种压力在食管腔内的所有点均可被同时测到，实际上是一个共室（图 70-6）[16,78]。用装有多个晶体传感器的探针进行 24 小时监测可显示食管在整个生理节律循环中缺乏蠕动，包括进食时，而正常情况下，进食时运动波应该更加活跃[174]。

药物治疗，特别是钙通道阻滞剂如硝苯地平在
1114 一些病例中可以减轻痉挛[106]，但是它们不能用于儿童的长期治疗[61]。强力球囊扩张食管末端对成人的失弛缓症常有效，但是这个治疗方法很少对儿童持续有效[16,49,180]。局部注射肉毒素也被试用于儿童，但其效果也有限[71,72,75,87,186]。Heller 黏膜外肌层切开术仍是对儿童治疗的有效方法，手术可从胸部或腹部进入[16,78,80,118,174,180]。后者可能可以更完全切开胃侧的肌层且较易加做胃底折叠术。事实上，如果长远考虑，

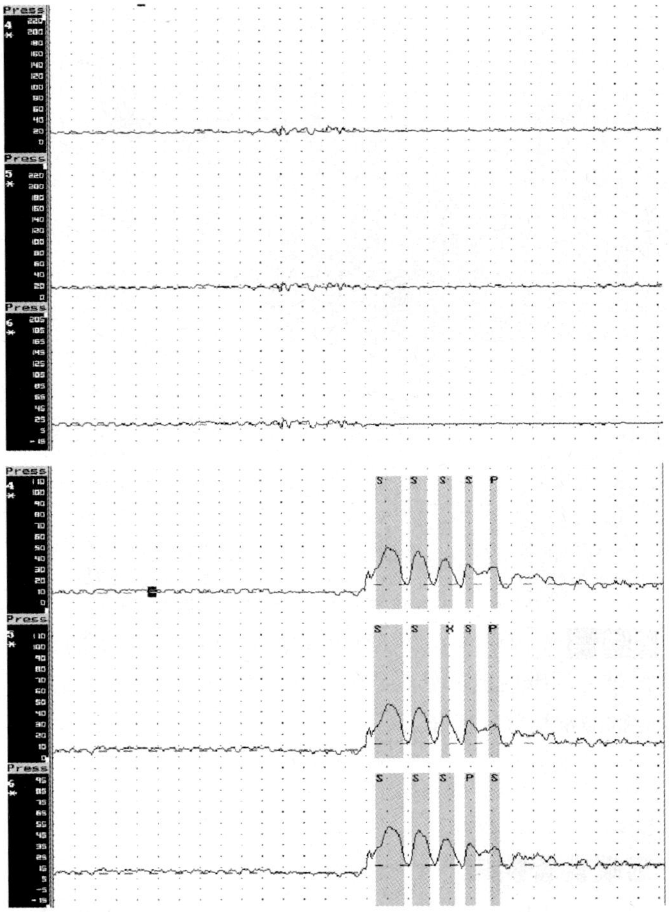

图 70-6 1 例 8 岁失迟缓症患者的移动食管测压记录。在上面的轨迹中，食管上（4）、中（5）、下（6）段的压力相同，未见波动。在下面的轨迹中，对于食物的反应有一些同时发生的、无推进的波（垂直标记之间的时间为 5 秒）。

Heller 肌层切开术后仍有持续性反流，因此对儿童，可能更有理由考虑加作胃底折叠术，以防止胃食管反流[72,73,78,115,140,174,180]。Nissen 抗反流手术可能不适合，因为增厚的食管直径巨大。最好做后侧的 Toupet 或前侧的 Thal-Dor 半胃底折叠术[78,140,174]。所有这些手术均可通过腹腔镜进行，这是目前的金标准[51,52,107,140]。

术后，患者的症状立即缓解，可以进行适当的喂养且体重增加。然而食管仍然会保持扩张数个月甚至几年，仅很少数可以完全恢复正常的食管功能。尽管肌层切开术减少了括约肌的张力（图 70-7），但多数患者的食管蠕动仍很少成无效[100,101,115,174,180]。一些症状较轻的患者，如吞咽困难和进食时常需要吞一些水，

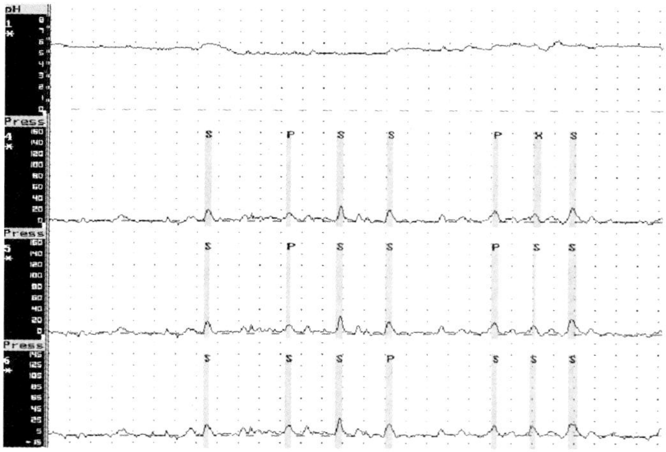

图 70-7 1 例 24 岁女性因失迟缓症行 Heller 肌切开术后 12 年，图示其进食期间的移动食管测压。她无自觉症状，但食管动力非常差。食管上（4）、中（5）和下（6）段的动力波显示有蠕动，但是非常微弱（低于 25mmHg，大概是正常的一半）。图中垂直标记之间的时间为 5 秒。

但食管肌层切开后可获得良好的生活质量。有报道少数失弛缓症病例在其他治疗方法都无效时可采用食管替代术[119,156]。这表明肌层切开术可缓解梗阻，但是不能完全治愈该病。长期的随访是必要的。

（胡　明译　李民驹校）

参考文献

1. Adamek RJ, Wegener M, Wienbeck M, Gielen B: Long-term esophageal manometry in healthy subjects. Evaluation of normal values and influence of age. Dig Dis Sci 1994; 39:2069.
2. Allan DW, Greer JJ: Pathogenesis of nitrofen-induced congenital diaphragmatic hernia in fetal rats. J Appl Physiol 1997;83:338.
3. Allan DW, Greer JJ: Embryogenesis of the phrenic nerve and diaphragm in the fetal rat. J Comp Neurol 1997; 382:459.
4. Anggiansah A, Bright NF, McCullagh M, Owen WJ: Transition from nutcracker esophagus to achalasia. Dig Dis Sci 1990;35:1162.
5. Anggiansah A, Taylor G, Marshall RE, et al: Oesophageal motor responses to gastro-oesophageal reflux in healthy controls and reflux patients. Gut 1997;41:600.
6. Anggiansah A, Taylor G, Marshall RE, et al: What is normal oesophageal motility? An ambulatory study. Scand J Gastroenterol 1998;33:473.
7. Arana J, Tovar JA: Motor efficiency of the refluxing esophagus in basal conditions and after acid challenge. J Pediatr Surg 1989;24:1049.
8. Arana J, Tovar JA, Garay J: Abnormal preoperative and postoperative esophageal peristalsis in gastroesophageal reflux. J Pediatr Surg 1986;21:711.
9. Attwood SE, Lewis CJ, Bronder CS, et al: Eosinophilic oesophagitis: A novel treatment using montelukast. Gut 2003;52:181.
10. Barham CP, Gotley DC, Fowler A, et al: Diffuse oesophageal spasm: Diagnosis by ambulatory 24 hour manometry. Gut 1997;41:151.
11. Batres LA, Liacouras C, Schnaufer L, Mascarenhas MR: Eosinophilic esophagitis associated with anastomotic strictures after esophageal atresia repair. J Pediatr Gastroenterol Nutr 2002;35:224.
12. Baujat G, Faure C, Zaouche A, et al: Oroesophageal motor disorders in Pierre Robin syndrome. J Pediatr Gastroenterol Nutr 2001;32:297.
13. Bautista A, Varela R, Villanueva A, et al: Motor function of the esophagus after caustic burn. Eur J Pediatr Surg 1996; 6:204.
14. Berezin S, Halata MS, Newman LJ, et al: Esophageal manometry in children with esophagitis. Am J Gastroenterol 1993;88:680.
15. Berezin S, Medow MS, Glassman MS, Newman LJ: Esophageal chest pain in children with asthma. J Pediatr Gastroenterol Nutr 1991;12:52.
16. Berquist WE, Byrne WJ, Ament ME, et al: Achalasia: Diagnosis, management, and clinical course in 16 children. Pediatrics 1983;71:798.
17. Blackwell JN, Holt S, Heading RC: Effect of nifedipine on oesophageal motility and gastric emptying. Digestion 1981; 21:50.
18. Boige N, Faure C, Cargill G, et al: Manometrical evaluation in visceral neuropathies in children. J Pediatr Gastroenterol Nutr 1994;19:71.
19. Brandt CT, Tam PK, Gould SJ: Nitrergic innervation of the human gut during early fetal development. J Pediatr Surg 1996;31:661.
20. Bremner RM, Costantini M, DeMeester TR, et al: Normal esophageal body function: A study using ambulatory esophageal manometry. Am J Gastroenterol 1998;93:183.
21. Breumelhof R, Van Wijk HJ, Van Es CD, Smout AJ: Food impaction in nutcracker esophagus. Dig Dis Sci 1990; 35:1167.
22. Brooks A, Millar AJ, Rode H: The surgical management of cricopharyngeal achalasia in children. Int J Pediatr Otorhinolaryngol 2000;56:1.
23. Bull MJ, Fitzgerald JF, Heifetz SA, Brei TJ: Gastrointestinal abnormalities: A significant cause of feeding difficulties and failure to thrive in Brachmann–de Lange syndrome. Am J Med Genet 1993;47:1029.
24. Cadranel S, Di Lorenzo C, Rodesch P, et al: Caustic ingestion and esophageal function. J Pediatr Gastroenterol Nutr 1990;10:164.
25. Cates M, Billmire DF, Bull MJ, Grosfeld JL: Gastroesophageal dysfunction in Cornelia de Lange syndrome. J Pediatr Surg 1989;24:248.
26. Catto-Smith AG, Machida H, Butzner JD, et al: The role of gastroesophageal reflux in pediatric dysphagia. J Pediatr Gastroenterol Nutr 1991;12:159.
27. Chawda SJ, Watura R, Adams H, Smith PM: A comparison of barium swallow and erect esophageal transit scintigraphy following balloon dilatation for achalasia. Dis Esophagus 1998;11:181.
28. Cheng W, Bishop AE, Spitz L, Polak JM: Abnormal enteric nerve morphology in atretic esophagus of fetal rats with Adriamycin-induced esophageal atresia. Pediatr Surg Int 1999;15:8.

29. Chitkara DK, Fortunato C, Nurko S: Prolonged monitoring of esophageal motor function in healthy children. J Pediatr Gastroenterol Nutr 2004;38:192.
30. Costa RH, Kalinichenko VV, Lim L: Transcription factors in mouse lung development and function. Am J Physiol Lung Cell Mol Physiol 2001;280:L823.
31. Cucchiara S, Bortolotti M, Minella R, Auricchio S: Fasting and postprandial mechanisms of gastroesophageal reflux in children with gastroesophageal reflux disease. Dig Dis Sci 1993;38:86.
32. Cucchiara S, Campanozzi A, Greco L, et al: Predictive value of esophageal manometry and gastroesophageal pH monitoring for responsiveness of reflux disease to medical therapy in children. Am J Gastroenterol 1996;91:680.
33. Cucchiara S, Staiano A, Di Lorenzo C, et al: Esophageal motor abnormalities in children with gastroesophageal reflux and peptic esophagitis. J Pediatr 1986;108:907.
34. Cucchiara S, Staiano A, Di Lorenzo C, et al: Pathophysiology of gastroesophageal reflux and distal esophageal motility in children with gastroesophageal reflux disease. J Pediatr Gastroenterol Nutr 1988;7:830.
35. Cucchiara S, Staiano A, Paone FM, Basile P: Esophageal aperistalsis due to reflux esophagitis: A report of two cases. J Pediatr Gastroenterol Nutr 1989;9:388.
36. Cury EK, Schraibman V, Faintuch S: Eosinophilic infiltration of the esophagus: Gastroesophageal reflux versus eosinophilic esophagitis in children—discussion on daily practice. J Pediatr Surg 2004;39:e4.
37. Davidson GP, Dent J, Willing J: Monitoring of upper oesophageal sphincter pressure in children. Gut 1991; 32:607.
38. Davies MRQ: Anatomy of the extrinsic nerve supply of the oesophagus in oesophageal atresia of the common type. Pediatr Surg Int 1996;11:230.
39. De Agustin JC, Sanz N, Canals MJ, et al: Successful medical treatment of two patients with eosinophilic oesophagitis. J Pediatr Surg 2002;37:207.
40. de Caestecker JS, Blackwell JN, Brown J, Heading RC: The oesophagus as a cause of recurrent chest pain: Which patients should be investigated and which tests should be used? Lancet 1985;2:1143.
41. de Oliveira RB, Rezende Filho J, Dantas RO, Iazigi N: The spectrum of esophageal motor disorders in Chagas' disease. Am J Gastroenterol 1995;90:1119.
42. Di Lorenzo C, Piepsz A, Ham H, Cadranel S: Gastric emptying with gastro-oesophageal reflux. Arch Dis Child 1987; 62:449.
43. Dinari G, Danziger Y, Mimouni M, et al: Cricopharyngeal dysfunction in childhood: Treatment by dilatations. J Pediatr Gastroenterol Nutr 1987;6:212.
44. Duranceau A, Fisher SR, Flye M, et al: Motor function of the esophagus after repair of esophageal atresia and tracheoesophageal fistula. Surgery 1977;82:116.
45. Dutta HK, Grover VP, Dwivedi SN, Bhatnagar V: Manometric evaluation of postoperative patients of esophageal atresia and tracheo-esophageal fistula. Eur J Pediatr Surg 2001; 11:371.
46. Dutta HK, Rajani M, Bhatnagar V: Cineradiographic evaluation of postoperative patients with esophageal atresia and tracheoesophageal fistula. Pediatr Surg Int 2000;16:322.
47. DuVall GA, Walden DT: Adenocarcinoma of the esophagus complicating Cornelia de Lange syndrome. J Clin Gastroenterol 1996;22:131.
48. Eicher PS, McDonald-Mcginn DM, Fox CA, et al: Dysphagia in children with a 22q11.2 deletion: Unusual pattern found on modified barium swallow. J Pediatr 2000;137:158.
49. Emblem R, Stringer MD, Hall CM, Spitz L: Current results of surgery for achalasia of the cardia. Arch Dis Child 1993; 68:749.
50. Emde C, Armstrong D, Castiglione F, et al: Reproducibility of long-term ambulatory esophageal combined pH/manometry. Gastroenterology 1991;100:1630.
51. Esposito C, Cucchiara S, Borrelli O, et al: Laparoscopic esophagomyotomy for the treatment of achalasia in children. A preliminary report of eight cases. Surg Endosc 2000; 14:110.
52. Esposito C, Mendoza-Sagaon M, Roblot-Maigret B, et al: Complications of laparoscopic treatment of esophageal achalasia in children. J Pediatr Surg 2000;35:680.
53. Faure C, Viarme F, Cargill G, et al: Abnormal esophageal motility in children with congenital central hypoventilation syndrome. Gastroenterology 2002;122:1258.
54. Fernbach SK, McLone DG: Derangement of swallowing in children with myelomeningocele. Pediatr Radiol 1985; 15:311.
55. Flick JA, Boyle JT, Tuchman DN, et al: Esophageal motor abnormalities in children and adolescents with scleroderma and mixed connective tissue disease. Pediatrics 1988;82:107.
56. Fonkalsrud EW, Ament ME: Gastroesophageal reflux in childhood. Curr Probl Surg 1996;33:1.
57. Fontan JP, Heldt GP, Heyman MB, et al: Esophageal spasm associated with apnea and bradycardia in an infant. Pediatrics 1984;73:52.
58. Fung KP, Math MV, Ho CO, Yap KM: Midazolam as a sedative in esophageal manometry: A study of the effect on esophageal motility. J Pediatr Gastroenterol Nutr 1992; 15:85.
59. Ganatra JV, Medow MS, Berezin S, et al: Esophageal dysmotility elicited by acid perfusion in children with esophagitis. Am J Gastroenterol 1995;90:1080.
60. Genc A, Mutaf O: Esophageal motility changes in acute and late periods of caustic esophageal burns and their relation to prognosis in children. J Pediatr Surg 2002;37:1526.
61. Glassman MS, Medow MS, Berezin S, Newman LJ: Spectrum of esophageal disorders in children with chest pain. Dig Dis Sci 1992;37:663.
62. Godoy J, Tovar JA, Vicente Y, et al: Esophageal motor dysfunction persists in children after surgical cure of reflux: An ambulatory manometric study. J Pediatr Surg 2001; 36:1405.
63. Gross RE: The Surgery of Infancy and Childhood, 1st ed. Philadelphia, WB Saunders, 1953.
64. Gustafsson PM, Tibbling L: Gastro-oesophageal reflux and oesophageal dysfunction in children and adolescents with brain damage. Acta Paediatr 1994;83:1081.
65. Hegar B, de Pont S, Vandemaele K, Vandenplas Y: Effect of prokinetics in children with recurrent nocturnal retrosternal pain. Eur J Gastroenterol Hepatol 1998;10:565.
66. Helm JF: Esophageal acid clearance. J Clin Gastroenterol 1986;8(Suppl 1):5.
67. Helm JF, Dodds WJ, Riedel DR, et al: Determinants of esophageal acid clearance in normal subjects. Gastroenterology 1983;85:607.
68. Hitchcock RJ, Pemble MJ, Bishop AE, et al: The ontogeny and distribution of neuropeptides in the human fetal and infant esophagus. Gastroenterology 1992;102:840.
69. Hollwarth M, Uray E: Physiology and pathophysiology of the esophagus in childhood. Prog Pediatr Surg 1985; 18:1.
70. Houlden H, Smith S, De Carvalho M, et al: Clinical and genetic characterization of families with triple A (Allgrove)

syndrome. Brain 2002;125:2681.
71. Hurwitz M, Bahar RJ, Ament ME, et al: Evaluation of the use of botulinum toxin in children with achalasia. J Pediatr Gastroenterol Nutr 2000;30:509.
72. Hussain SZ, Thomas R, Tolia V: A review of achalasia in 33 children. Dig Dis Sci 2002;47:2538.
73. Illi OE, Stauffer UG: Achalasia in childhood and adolescence. Eur J Pediatr Surg 1994;4:214.
74. Iovino P, Ciacci C, Sabbatini F, et al: Esophageal impairment in adult celiac disease with steatorrhea. Am J Gastroenterol 1998;93:1243.
75. Ip KS, Cameron DJ, Catto-Smith AG, Hardikar W: Botulinum toxin for achalasia in children. J Gastroenterol Hepatol 2000;15:1100.
76. Janssens J, Vantrappen G, Ghillebert G: 24-Hour recording of esophageal pressure and pH in patients with noncardiac chest pain. Gastroenterology 1986;90:1978.
77. Kahrilas PJ: Anatomy, physiology and pathophysiology of dysphagia. Acta Otorhinolaryngol Belg 1994;48:97.
78. Kalicinski P, Dluski E, Drewniak T, Kaminski W: Esophageal manometric studies in children with achalasia before and after operative treatment. Pediatr Surg Int 1997; 12:571.
79. Kapila L, Daniel RD: Foreign body impaction arising in adulthood: A result of neonatal repair of tracheo-oesophageal fistula and oesophageal atresia [letter]. Ann R Coll Surg Engl 1996;78:559.
80. Karnak I, Senocak ME, Tanyel FC, Buyukpamukcu N: Achalasia in childhood: Surgical treatment and outcome. Eur J Pediatr Surg 2001;11:223.
81. Katsumata N, Hirose H, Kagami M, Tanaka T: Analysis of the AAAS gene in a Japanese patient with triple A syndrome. Endocr J 2002;49:49.
82. Katz PO, Castell JA: Nonachalasia motility disorders. In Castell DO, Richter JE (eds): The Esophagus, 3rd ed. Philadelphia, Lippincott Williams & Wilkins, 1999, p 215.
83. Kawahara H, Dent J, Davidson G: Mechanisms responsible for gastroesophageal reflux in children. Gastroenterology 1997;113:399.
84. Kawahara H, Imura K, Yagi M, et al: Mechanisms underlying the antireflux effect of Nissen fundoplication in children. J Pediatr Surg 1998;33:1618.
85. Khan S, Orenstein SR, Di Lorenzo C, et al: Eosinophilic esophagitis: Strictures, impactions, dysphagia. Dig Dis Sci 2003;48:22.
86. Khelif K, De Laet MH, Chaouachi B, et al: Achalasia of the cardia in Allgrove's (triple A) syndrome: Histopathologic study of 10 cases. Am J Surg Pathol 2003;27:667.
87. Khoshoo V, LaGarde DC, Udall JN Jr: Intrasphincteric injection of botulinum toxin for treating achalasia in children. J Pediatr Gastroenterol Nutr 1997;24:439.
88. Kluth D, Keijzer R, Hertl M, Tibboel D: Embryology of congenital diaphragmatic hernia. Semin Pediatr Surg 1996;5:224.
89. Kohda E, Hisazumi H, Hiramatsu K: Swallowing dysfunction and aspiration in neonates and infants. Acta Otolaryngol Suppl 1994;517:11.
90. Lao J, Bostwick HE, Berezin S, et al: Esophageal food impaction in children. Pediatr Emerg Care 2003;19:402.
91. Lapadula G, Muolo P, Semeraro F, et al: Esophageal motility disorders in the rheumatic diseases: A review of 150 patients. Clin Exp Rheumatol 1994;12:515.
92. Larsen WJ: Human Embryology, 2nd ed. New York, Churchill Livingstone, 1997.
93. Laurikainen E, Aitasalo K, Halonen P, et al: Muscle pathology in idiopathic cricopharyngeal dysphagia. Enzyme histochemical and electron microscopic findings. Eur Arch Otorhinolaryngol 1992;249:216.
94. Lee JI, Park H, Kim JH, et al: The effect of sildenafil on oesophageal motor function in healthy subjects and patients with nutcracker oesophagus. Neurogastroenterol Motil 2003;15:617.
95. Lernau OZ, Sherzer E, Mogle P, Nissan S: Congenital cricopharyngeal achalasia treatment by dilatations. J Pediatr Surg 1984;19:202.
96. Levine JJ, Trachtman H, Gold DM, Pettei MJ: Esophageal dysmotility in children breast-fed by mothers with silicone breast implants. Long-term follow-up and response to treatment. Dig Dis Sci 1996;41:1600.
97. Liacouras CA, Wenner WJ, Brown K, Ruchelli E: Primary eosinophilic esophagitis in children: Successful treatment with oral corticosteroids. J Pediatr Gastroenterol Nutr 1998;26:380.
98. Liebermann-Meffert D, Allgöwer M, Schmid P, Blum AL: Muscular equivalent of the lower esophageal sphincter. Gastroenterology 1979;76:31.
99. Lim HC, Nigro MA, Beierwaltes P, et al: Nitrazepam-induced cricopharyngeal dysphagia, abnormal esophageal peristalsis and associated bronchospasm: Probable cause of nitrazepam-related sudden death. Brain Dev 1992; 14:309.
100. Liu HC, Huang BS, Hsu WH, et al: Surgery for achalasia: Long-term results in operated achalasic patients. Ann Thorac Cardiovasc Surg 1998;4:312.
101. Liu JF, Zhang J, Tian ZQ, et al: Long-term outcome of esophageal myotomy for achalasia. World J Gastroenterol 2004;10:287.
102. Long JD, Orlando RC: Esophageal submucosal glands: Structure and function. Am J Gastroenterol 1999; 94:2818.
103. Luzzani S, Macchini F, Valade A, et al: Gastroesophageal reflux and Cornelia de Lange syndrome: Typical and atypical symptoms. Am J Med Genet 2003;119A:283.
104. Mahony MJ, Migliavacca M, Spitz L, Milla PJ: Motor disorders of the oesophagus in gastro-oesophageal reflux. Arch Dis Child 1988;63:1333.
105. Makhoul IR, Shoshany G, Smolkin T, et al: Transient mega-esophagus in a neonate with congenital diaphragmatic hernia. Eur Radiol 2001;11:867.
106. Maksimak M, Perlmutter DH, Winter HS: The use of nifedipine for the treatment of achalasia in children. J Pediatr Gastroenterol Nutr 1986;5:883.
107. Mattioli G, Esposito C, Prato AP, et al: Results of the laparoscopic Heller-Dor procedure for pediatric esophageal achalasia. Surg Endosc 2003;17:1650.
108. McDougall NI, Mooney RB, Ferguson WR, et al: The effect of healing oesophagitis on oesophageal motor function as determined by oesophageal scintigraphy and ambulatory oesophageal motility/pH monitoring. Aliment Pharmacol Ther 1998;12:899.
109. Milla PJ: Intestinal motility during ontogeny and intestinal pseudo-obstruction in children. Pediatr Clin North Am 1996;43:511.
110. Mittal RK, Balaban DH: The esophagogastric junction. N Engl J Med 1997;336:924.
111. Mittal RK, Rochester DF, McCallum RW: Sphincteric action of the diaphragm during a relaxed lower esophageal sphincter in humans. Am J Physiol 1989;256:G139.
112. Mittal RK, Sivri B, Schirmer BD, Heine KJ: Effect of crural myotomy on the incidence and mechanism of gastroesophageal reflux in cats. Gastroenterology 1993;105:740.
113. Mondragon F, Arana J, Tovar JA, et al: Cricopharyngeal

dysphagia and gastro-oesophageal reflux. Z Kinderchir 1985;40:361.
114. Montedonico S, Diez-Pardo JA, Possogel AK, Tovar JA: Effects of esophageal shortening on the gastroesophageal barrier: An experimental study on the causes of reflux in esophageal atresia. J Pediatr Surg 1999;34:300.
115. Morris-Stiff G, Khan R, Foster ME, Lari J: Long-term results of surgery for childhood achalasia. Ann R Coll Surg Engl 1997;79:432.
116. Motil KJ, Schultz RJ, Browning K, et al: Oropharyngeal dysfunction and gastroesophageal dysmotility are present in girls and women with Rett syndrome. J Pediatr Gastroenterol Nutr 1999;29:31.
117. Muraji T, Takamizawa S, Satoh S, et al: Congenital cricopharyngeal achalasia: Diagnosis and surgical management. J Pediatr Surg 2002;37:E12.
118. Myers NA, Jolley SG, Taylor R: Achalasia of the cardia in children: A worldwide survey. J Pediatr Surg 1994;29:1375.
119. Neville WE, Najem AZ: Colon replacement of the esophagus for congenital and benign disease. Ann Thorac Surg 1983;36:626.
120. Nurko S, Teitelbaum JE, Husain K, et al: Association of Schatzki ring with eosinophilic esophagitis in children. J Pediatr Gastroenterol Nutr 2004;38:436.
121. Okamoto E, Ueda T: Embryogenesis of intramural ganglia of the gut and its relationship to Hirschsprung's disease. J Pediatr Surg 1967;2:437.
122. Omari TI, Barnett C, Snel A, et al: Mechanisms of gastroesophageal reflux in healthy premature infants. J Pediatr 1998;133:650.
123. Omari T, Barnett C, Snel A, et al: Mechanism of gastroesophageal reflux in premature infants with chronic lung disease. J Pediatr Surg 1999;34:1795.
124. Orenstein SR, Shalaby TM, Di Lorenzo C, et al: The spectrum of pediatric eosinophilic esophagitis beyond infancy: A clinical series of 30 children. Am J Gastroenterol 2000; 95:1422.
125. Paterson WG, Beck IT, Wang H: Ambulatory esophageal manometry/pH-metry discriminates between patients with different esophageal symptoms. Dig Dis Sci 1996; 41:357.
126. Pei RS, Lin CC, Mak SC, et al: Barrett's esophagus in a child with de Lange syndrome: Report of one case. Acta Paediatr Taiwan 2000;41:155.
127. Pollack IF, Pang D, Kocoshis S, Putnam P: Neurogenic dysphagia resulting from Chiari malformations. Neurosurgery 1992;30:709.
128. Prpic I, Huebner A, Persic M, et al: Triple A syndrome: Genotype-phenotype assessment. Clin Genet 2003;63:415.
129. Putnam PE, Orenstein SR, Pang D, et al: Cricopharyngeal dysfunction associated with Chiari malformations. Pediatrics 1992;89:871.
130. Qi BQ, Merei J, Farmer P, et al: The vagus and recurrent laryngeal nerves in the rodent experimental model of esophageal atresia. J Pediatr Surg 1997;32:1580.
131. Qi BQ, Uemura S, Farmer P, et al: Intrinsic innervation of the oesophagus in fetal rats with oesophageal atresia. Pediatr Surg Int 1999;15:2.
132. Ravelli AM, Ledermann SE, Bisset WM, et al: Foregut motor function in chronic renal failure. Arch Dis Child 1992;67:1343.
133. Ravitch MM: Chalasia and achalasia of the esophagus. In Benson CD, Mustard WT, Ravitch MM, et al (eds): Pediatric Surgery, vol 1, 1st ed. Chicago, Year Book, 1962, p 299.
134. Rehbein F: Kinderchirurgische Operationen, 1st ed. Stuttgart, Germany, Hippokrates Verlag, 1976.
135. Reichert TJ, Bluestone CD, Stool SE, et al: Congenital cricopharyngeal achalasia. Ann Otol Rhinol Laryngol 1977;86:603.
136. Rhee PL, Hyun JG, Lee JH, et al: The effect of sildenafil on lower esophageal sphincter and body motility in normal male adults. Am J Gastroenterol 2001;96:3251.
137. Romeo G, Zuccarello B, Proietto F, Romeo C: Disorders of the esophageal motor activity in atresia of the esophagus. J Pediatr Surg 1987;22:120.
138. Rosario JA, Medow MS, Halata MS, et al: Nonspecific esophageal motility disorders in children without gastroesophageal reflux. J Pediatr Gastroenterol Nutr 1999; 28:480.
139. Ross MN, Haase GM, Reiley TT, Meagher DP Jr: The importance of acid reflux patterns in neurologically damaged children detected by four-channel esophageal pH monitoring. J Pediatr Surg 1988;23:573.
140. Rothenberg SS, Partrick DA, Bealer JF, Chang JH: Evaluation of minimally invasive approaches to achalasia in children. J Pediatr Surg 2001;36:808.
141. Rumessen JJ, de Kerchove d'Exaerde A, Mignon S, et al: Interstitial cells of Cajal in the striated musculature of the mouse esophagus. Cell Tissue Res 2001;306:1.
142. Rumessen JJ, Vanderwinden JM: Interstitial cells in the musculature of the gastrointestinal tract: Cajal and beyond. Int Rev Cytol 2003;229:115.
143. Sandrini F, Farmakidis C, Kirschner LS, et al: Spectrum of mutations of the AAAS gene in Allgrove syndrome: Lack of mutations in six kindreds with isolated resistance to corticotropin. J Clin Endocrinol Metab 2001;86:5433.
144. Schima W, Stacher G, Pokieser P, et al: Esophageal motor disorders: Videofluoroscopic and manometric evaluation—prospective study in 88 symptomatic patients. Radiology 1992;185:487.
145. Schuffler MD, Pope CE 2nd: Studies of idiopathic intestinal pseudoobstruction. II. Hereditary hollow visceral myopathy: Family studies. Gastroenterology 1977; 73:339.
146. Seibert JJ, Byrne WJ, Euler AR, et al: Gastroesophageal reflux—the acid test: Scintigraphy or the pH probe? AJR Am J Roentgenol 1983;140:1087.
147. Shah N, Rodriguez M, Louis DS, et al: Feeding difficulties and foregut dysmotility in Noonan's syndrome. Arch Dis Child 1999;81:28.
148. Shokeir MH: The Goldenhar syndrome: A natural history. Birth Defects Orig Artic Ser 1977;13:67.
149. Siafakas CG, Ryan CK, Brown MR, Miller TL: Multiple esophageal rings: An association with eosinophilic esophagitis: Case report and review of the literature. Am J Gastroenterol 2000;95:1572.
150. Singh S, Stein HJ, DeMeester TR, Hinder RA: Nonobstructive dysphagia in gastroesophageal reflux disease: A study with combined ambulatory pH and motility monitoring. Am J Gastroenterol 1992;87:562.
151. Sinharay R: Eosinophilic oesophagitis: Treatment using montelukast. Gut 2003;52:1228.
152. Sivarao DV, Mashimo HL, Thatte HS, Goyal RK: Lower esophageal sphincter is achalasic in nNOS(−/−) and hypotensive in W/W(v) mutant mice. Gastroenterology 2001;121:34.
153. Snyder CL, Ramachandran V, Kennedy AP, et al: Efficacy of partial wrap fundoplication for gastroesophageal reflux after repair of esophageal atresia. J Pediatr Surg 1997; 32:1089.
154. Sondheimer JM: Gastroesophageal reflux: Update on

pathogenesis and diagnosis. Pediatr Clin North Am 1988; 35:103.
155. Sondheimer JM: Clearance of spontaneous gastroesophageal reflux in awake and sleeping infants. Gastroenterology 1989;97:821.
156. Spitz L: Gastric transposition for esophageal substitution in children. J Pediatr Surg 1992;27:252.
157. Staiano A, Corazziari E, Andreotti MR, Clouse RE: Esophageal motility in children with Hirschsprung's disease. Am J Dis Child 1991;145:310.
158. Staiano A, Cucchiara S, Del Giudice E, et al: Disorders of oesophageal motility in children with psychomotor retardation and gastro-oesophageal reflux. Eur J Pediatr 1991;150:638.
159. Staiano A, Cucchiara S, De Vizia B, et al: Disorders of upper esophageal sphincter motility in children. J Pediatr Gastroenterol Nutr 1987;6:892.
160. Stein HJ, DeMeester TR: Indications, technique, and clinical use of ambulatory 24-hour esophageal motility monitoring in a surgical practice. Ann Surg 1993;217:128.
161. Stein HJ, DeMeester TR, Eypasch EP, Klingman RR: Ambulatory 24-hour esophageal manometry in the evaluation of esophageal motor disorders and noncardiac chest pain. Surgery 1991;110:753.
162. Stolar CJ, Berdon WE, Dillon PW, et al: Esophageal dilatation and reflux in neonates supported by ECMO after diaphragmatic hernia repair. AJR Am J Roentgenol 1988; 151:135.
163. Stolar CJ, Levy JP, Dillon PW, et al: Anatomic and functional abnormalities of the esophagus in infants surviving congenital diaphragmatic hernia. Am J Surg 1990; 159:204.
164. Swenson O: Pediatric Surgery, vol 1, 3rd ed. London, Butterworths, 1969.
165. Takahashi T: Pathophysiological significance of neuronal nitric oxide synthase in the gastrointestinal tract. J Gastroenterol 2003;38:421.
166. Takano K, Iwafuchi M, Uchiyama M, et al: Evaluation of lower esophageal sphincter function in infants and children following esophageal surgery. J Pediatr Surg 1988; 23:410.
167. Teitelbaum JE, Fox VL, Twarog FJ, et al: Eosinophilic esophagitis in children: Immunopathological analysis and response to fluticasone propionate. Gastroenterology 2002; 122:1216.
168. Thomas EJ, Kumar R, Dasan JB, et al: Radionuclide scintigraphy in the evaluation of gastro-oesophageal reflux in post-operative oesophageal atresia and tracheo-oesophageal fistula patients. Nucl Med Commun 2003;24:317.
169. Thompson LD, McElhinney DB, Jue KL, Hodge D: Gastroesophageal reflux after repair of atrioventricular septal defect in infants with trisomy 21: A comparison of medical and surgical therapy. J Pediatr Surg 1999;34:1359.
170. Tomaselli V, Volpi ML, Dell'Agnola CA, et al: Long-term evaluation of esophageal function in patients treated at birth for esophageal atresia. Pediatr Surg Int 2003;19:40.
171. Tomita R, Tanjoh K, Fujisaki S, Fukuzawa M: Physiological studies on nitric oxide in the lower esophageal sphincter of patients with reflux esophagitis. Hepatogastroenterology 2003;50:110.
172. Tovar JA, Arana J, Tapia I: Effects of sedation on motor function of the refluxing esophagus. Pediatr Surg Int 1990;5:418.
173. Tovar JA, Diez Pardo JA, Murcia J, et al: Ambulatory 24-hour manometric and pH metric evidence of permanent impairment of clearance capacity in patients with esophageal atresia. J Pediatr Surg 1995;30:1224.
174. Tovar JA, Prieto G, Molina M, Arana J: Esophageal function in achalasia: Preoperative and postoperative manometric studies. J Pediatr Surg 1998;33:834.
175. Triadafilopoulos G, Castillo T: Nonpropulsive esophageal contractions and gastroesophageal reflux. Am J Gastroenterol 1991;86:153.
176. Tuck JS, Bisset RA, Doig CM: Achalasia of the cardia in childhood and the syndrome of achalasia alacrima and ACTH insensitivity. Clin Radiol 1991;44:260.
177. Vandenplas Y, Derde MP, Piepsz A: Evaluation of reflux episodes during simultaneous esophageal pH monitoring and gastroesophageal reflux scintigraphy in children. J Pediatr Gastroenterol Nutr 1992;14:256.
178. Vandenplas Y, Hassall E: Mechanisms of gastroesophageal reflux and gastroesophageal reflux disease. J Pediatr Gastroenterol Nutr 2002;35:119.
179. Vanderwinden JM: Role of interstitial cells of Cajal and their relationship with the enteric nervous system. Eur J Morphol 1999;37:250.
180. Vane DW, Cosby K, West K, Grosfeld JL: Late results following esophagomyotomy in children with achalasia. J Pediatr Surg 1988;23:515.
181. Vantrappen G, Janssens J, Hellemans J, Coremans G: Achalasia, diffuse esophageal spasm, and related motility disorders. Gastroenterology 1979;76:450.
182. Vicente Y, da Rocha C, Perez-Mies B, et al: Effect of reflux and esophagitis on esophageal volume and acid clearance in piglets. J Pediatr Gastroenterol Nutr 2004;38:328.
183. Vicente Y, Da Rocha C, Yu J, et al: Architecture and function of the gastroesophageal barrier in the piglet. Dig Dis Sci 2001;46:1899.
184. Vicente Y, Da Rocha C, Yu J, et al: Individual inactivation of the sphincteric component of the gastroesophageal barrier causes reflux esophagitis in piglets. J Pediatr Surg 2002;37:40.
185. Vicente Y, Hernandez-Peredo G, Molina M, et al: Acute food bolus impaction without stricture in children with gastroesophageal reflux. J Pediatr Surg 2001; 36:1397.
186. Walton JM, Tougas G: Botulinum toxin use in pediatric esophageal achalasia: A case report. J Pediatr Surg 1997; 32:916.
187. Wang WL, Tovar JA, Eizaguirre I, Aldazabal P: Airway obstruction and gastroesophageal reflux—an experimental study on the pathogenesis of this association. J Pediatr Surg 1993;28:995.
188. Warburton D, Schwarz M, Tefft D, et al: The molecular basis of lung morphogenesis. Mech Dev 2000;92:55.
189. Warburton D, Zhao J, Berberich MA, Bernfield M: Molecular embryology of the lung: Then, now, and in the future. Am J Physiol 1999;276:L697.
190. Watanabe Y, Ando H, Seo T, et al: Attenuated nitrergic inhibitory neurotransmission to interstitial cells of Cajal in the lower esophageal sphincter with esophageal achalasia in children. Pediatr Int 2002;44:145.
191. Weber P, Ganser G, Frosch M, et al: Twenty-four hour intraesophageal pH monitoring in children and adolescents with scleroderma and mixed connective tissue disease. J Rheumatol 2000;27:2692.
192. Weston S, Thumshirn M, Wiste J, Camilleri M: Clinical and upper gastrointestinal motility features in systemic sclerosis and related disorders. Am J Gastroenterol 1998;93:1085.

193. Wyllie E, Wyllie R, Rothner AD, Morris HH: Diffuse esophageal spasm: A cause of paroxysmal posturing and irritability in infants and mentally retarded children. J Pediatr 1989;115:261.
194. Yuksel B, Braun R, Topaloglu AK, et al: Three children with triple A syndrome due to a mutation (R478X) in the AAAS gene. Horm Res 2004;61:3.
195. Zarate N, Mearin F, Hidalgo A, Malagelada JR: Prospective evaluation of esophageal motor dysfunction in Down's syndrome. Am J Gastroenterol 2001;96:1718.
196. Zhang X, Tack J, Janssens J, Sifrim DA: Effect of sildenafil, a phosphodiesterase-5 inhibitor, on oesophageal peristalsis and lower oesophageal sphincter function in cats. Neurogastroenterol Motil 2001;13:325.
197. Zhou B, Hutson JM, Myers NA: Investigation of the intra-abdominal oesophagus and hiatus in fetal rats with oesophageal atresia and tracheo-oesophageal fistula. Pediatr Surg Int 2001;17:97.
198. Zuccarello B, Nicotina PA, Centorrino A, et al: Immunohistochemical study on muscle actinin content of atresic esophageal upper pouch. J Pediatr Surg 1988;2:75.

第 71 章

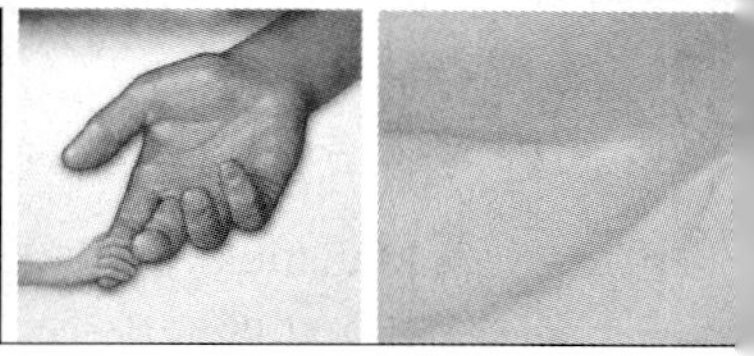

胃食管反流

Keith E. Georgeson 和 Gonca Topuzlu Tekant

历史

1120 胃食管反流（GRE）的症状几百年来已经为人们所熟知，莎士比亚就曾经把婴儿“在护士的怀抱中哺乳和呕吐”描述成人生的第一幕。文艺复兴时期的人体解剖学为源于食管损伤和狭窄以致胃食管反流的病理发展提供了新的研究途径。第 1 例有关儿童胃食管反流疾病（GERD）的描述来自 1928 年的巴黎，尸体解剖发现反复呕吐患儿存在食管溃疡[25]。1836 年，Bright 报道了部分胃疝入胸腔的先天畸形，并将其与胃食管反流联系在一起[37]。1935 年，Winkelstein 提出了消化性食管炎的概念[261]。Allison 则在 1943 年归纳出引起反流性食管炎的潜在病因，并且提供了修补食管裂孔疝的手术方式[6]。同时 Allison 将这一解剖学问题定义为功能不良性胃食管瓣，并且指出，胃灼热感是胃食管反流的首要症状[5]。

首先正式详细报道儿童胃食管反流的文章出自 Neuhauser 和 Berenberg，他们将婴儿期的生理性胃食管反流定义为“食管迟缓”[167]。1960 年，Carré 强调了婴儿期的胃食管反流是一种自限性疾病，并且提出了体位治疗控制症状的方法[42,43]。

Allison 倡导并描述了修补食管裂孔疝控制胃食管反流的方法，之后 Belsey 和 Nissen 分别描述了胃底折叠术能够在大多数患者中有效地控制反流[20,168]。Rossetti 改良了 Nissen 的方法，仅用胃的前壁作包裹[202]，Lucius Hill 着重指出了将胃食管连接部置于横膈以下的重要性[103]。Thal 和 Toupet 推广了部分胃底折叠与完全而紧密地折叠控制反流症状的手术方法[231,237]。

在各种手术方式不断出新的同时，诊断方法也在不断改进。食管钡剂造影[66,205]、pH 监测[119]、内镜检查[244]、闪烁扫描术[22]和食管测压[61]等方法在近几十年里逐渐发展并得以改良。这些检查更优越，同时能够对潜在疾病提供更彻底的了解，并能对疗效进行评价。

所有上述手术方式都已经应用于儿童。Nissen 胃底折叠术已经成为治疗儿童胃食管反流最常用的方法[80,83,117,130]，但是仍有许多部分胃底折叠术的拥护者，Ashcraft 推广了一种改良的 Thal 术式[9,10]，而 Boix-Ochoa 实施了一种相似的手术方式，并指出是用以重建胃食管的解剖学和生理学机制来阻止胃食管反流[27,29]。1991 年，Dallemagne 首先报道在成人施行腹腔镜胃底折叠术[64]。2 年后，Georgeson[88]和 Lobe[147]分别报道了在儿童中实施腹腔镜胃底折叠术的结果。今天，微创技术已经成为手术治疗儿童胃食管反流疾病新的标准手术途径[86,87,89,146,156,163,182,203,216,225,228,255]。

引言

呕吐和反流在儿童中经常发生，4 个月龄的婴儿有 70%每天都存在反流，而只有 25%的家长认为这是问题[165,246]。而医生要做的就是将能自然恢复的生理性症状从需要药物或手术治疗的病理性症状中区分开来。病理性胃食管反流的临床体征多变，需识别这些体征并进行诊断学评价和治疗，最重要的目的是阻止这一病理过程可能导致的严重后果。

胚胎学和解剖学

目前尚不清楚导致婴儿和儿童发生胃食管反流的确切胚胎学机制。许多对反流发生的胚胎学解释曾经被提出过[98,134,160,214,262,268]，其中比较有意思的一种解释是 Mansfield 提出的，他认为人类的胃食管反流根源在于从胚胎发生到宫外发育过程的改变[154]，以适应直
1121 立姿势和双足行走。为了适应直立姿势导致的许多体内脏器和系统的结构和相互关系发生改变，胃的旋转改变了从胃窦到胃底部的前后关系，使原来属于背侧的胃转移至左侧，而属于腹侧的胃体转移至右侧，这可能是反流发生病因学中的关键所在。这些改变造成了胃食管连接部内在钳闭功能的畸形以及重力因素对胃的牵拉，而位于腹侧的心脏在人类可以引起膈肌的紧张。Mansfield 认为上述改变存在限制性差异，并能够解释为何人类极易罹患胃食管反流及其后续并发症的潜在原因。

食管下端高压区在阻止胃食管反流中同样具有重要意义[214,267]。一定长度的腹腔内食管对阻止胃食管反流是必需的[267]，能够影响胃食管连接部高压区，而干扰对生理性胃食管反流之廓清功能的解剖畸形，如食管闭锁、膈疝和动力性疾病，都与反流发生的病理明显相关[14,23,49,70,78,104,111,115,124,137,222,223]。

定义

GERD 被定义为是偶尔发生的胃内容物反流至食管内的病理性结果[209,249]。在成人，GERD 首先是和消化性食管炎及其并发症同时考虑的，包括胃灼热感、食管狭窄和 Barrett 食管的形成[165,166,179,209,246,249]；在儿童，病理性胃食管反流的形成更加复杂。病理性胃食管反流最多见于神经系统功能障碍的患儿。神经功能受损而伴发胃食管反流的患儿常常存在吞咽困难、不发育、原发性误吸、全身僵直状态、腹腔压力升高以及中枢性原因导致的作呕、气哽和干呕。同时，他们往往伴有胃排空延迟、食管和胃肠道近段动力学功能障碍以及在仰卧位时往往主导反流发生的食管裂孔疝。神经系统功能正常的婴儿和儿童则多存在与反流相关的反复气道疾病，如误吸、吸入性肺炎、喉部症状和呼吸暂停。有时，这一呼吸暂停可以维持足够长的时间而威胁生命[177,186,209,245,256]。儿童也存在消化功能症状，包括频繁发作的反胃而导致不发育、易激惹、厌食、胃灼热感、呕血、黑便、吞咽困难以及与 Barrett 食管相关的食管上皮改变[96,100,101,183,209,210]。

病理生理学

GERD 由于胃内容物的反流引起临床症状并可导致组织病理学改变。GERD 导致的病理改变是复杂多因素的，其中主要的解剖学和生理学因素一旦失去功能将直接与胃食管反流的发生相关，讨论如下（图 71–1）[67,249]。

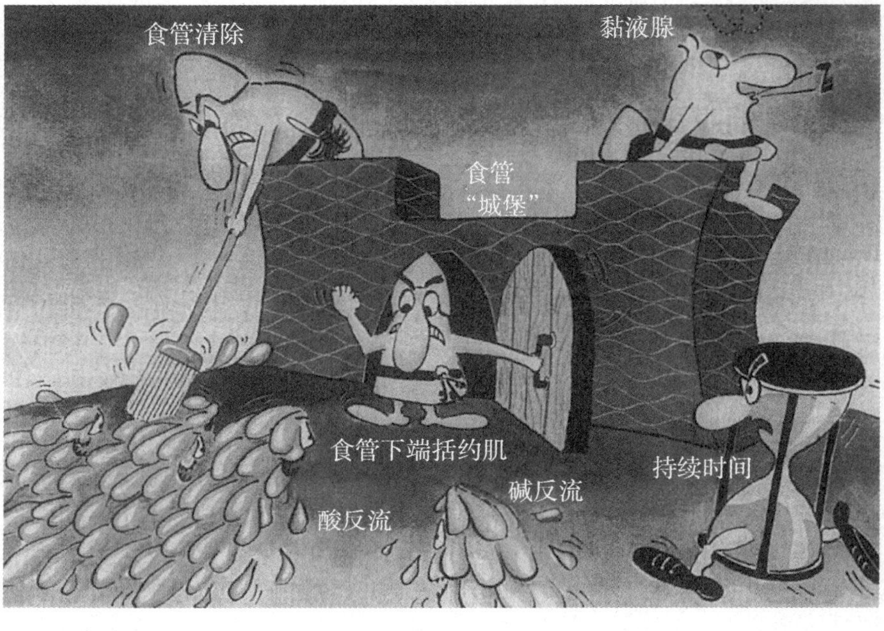

图 71–1 食管损伤的范围取决于反流物的攻击和食管黏膜防御功能之间的平衡。在对食管的冲击中，反流液的酸度和量以及与食管接触时间的长短由食管黏膜的清除功能和防御机制所抗衡。

唾液的分泌：唾液有助于食物的润滑而增强食管的转运，其碱性成分还有利于中和反流的胃液并刺激食管的蠕动。睡眠时唾液的分泌量及吞咽频率减少。咀嚼口香糖能增加唾液流，对某些 GERD 患者是一
1122 项非药物性的治疗方法[125,249]。

食管蠕动：食管的收缩被分成一期、二期和三期。吞咽运动导致了一期收缩波；二期蠕动是由食物进入食管腔内的反射运动所引发的，有助于食管的廓清[125,142]；三期收缩则是自发的协同性不能传播的收缩波，与吞咽或反射无关。吞咽引发的一期收缩起始于喉部并能通过横纹肌和平滑肌传导至贲门[58,73,121]。白天，反流次数及吞咽频率增加，这是对食管内酸性物质进行廓清的有效机制。

食管廓清：食管的廓清机制受三大主要因素影响：蠕动波、重力和唾液[102,122]。食管内酸性物质的廓清延迟是引起食管炎的首要因素[41,105]。吞咽的唾液有助于中和反流物的酸性，而 GERD 患者常常存在唾液分泌功能减退。体位治疗的效果可能部分源于重力因素[3,175,249,251]。食管壁内存在不同类型的外周神经元[15,67,249]，C 型无髓鞘神经纤维主导深部烧灼痛，A 型三角纤维能感觉锐痛。反复的不良刺激或强烈刺激能够同时使这两种神经纤维致敏，从而对非不良刺激同样产生应答。内脏的痛觉过敏能够导致动力学问题而引起反流[120,181]，因此，在某些患者中，GERD 首先可能由一些能够导致异常动力学问题的不良刺激引发。痛觉感受能够通过神经递质钙基因相关蛋白（cGRP）和 P 物质传送到大脑[8,266]，P 物质能引起平滑肌收缩和血管扩张，同时刺激黏膜通透性升高，它在组织损伤时释放。在食管炎患者中，P 物质释放越多，反流物质所引起的不良刺激越大，从而形成恶性循环。P 物质还能引起海马白质内肥大细胞释放组胺，从而导致气管痉挛。有人推测食管内 P 物质的释放有时可能与活动性呼吸道疾病发生有内在关联[190,224]。

食管下段括约肌：食管下段括约肌（LES）是引起病理性胃食管反流重要因素的概念是在 1971 年证实的[53]。LES 是一道功能性屏障，在成人中其长度介于 3～5cm，是食管远端一个静息压升高的区域，是抵御异常反流而避免胃内容物进入食管的屏障。在成人资料中发现，平均 LES 压小于 6mmHg 且总长度小于 2cm 时易产生病理性胃食管反流[198,269]。Boix-Ochoa 和 Canals 的研究表明，新生儿 LES 的长度只有 0.5～1.0cm，并随着年龄的增长而增长（图 71-2）[30]。

LES 在吞咽发生 2 秒后松弛，并维持开放状态 10～12 秒直到食团通过这一区域。Dodds 等人首先报道了由迷走反射所介导的食管下段括约肌的短暂松弛（TLESR）[71]，它最初是由于刺激了胃底的机械性刺激感受器或是胃底的牵张而发动[107]。LES 压在进餐后降低，而胃的收缩、胃内容物的碱化以及蛋白质则促使 LES 压力升高，胃泌素、促胃动素和 P 物质也能升高 LES 压；相反胆囊收缩素、胰高血糖素、血管活性肠肽、一氧化氮、多巴胺、胰泌素、雌激素、尼古丁、酒精、薄荷和巧克力则都能使 LES 压降低[249]。儿童中大部分的反流源于食管下段括约肌的交替松弛，是健康足月儿以及存在慢性肺部疾病患儿胃食管反流发生的主要机制[170,171]。大量进食能引起胃液分泌量的增加，从而引起更多的食管下段括约肌交替松弛，因此质子泵抑制剂（PPI）和组胺 H_2 受体竞争性抑制剂（H_2RA）的作用可能与减少胃液分泌量相关而不是影响 pH。而抗反流手术的效果可能是促使不完全性的 LES 松弛进一步完成，从而减少食管下段括约肌的短暂松弛发生的次数[128,129]。

腹腔段食管：腹腔段食管的长度是抗反流屏障的重要组成部分。腹腔段食管的直径大约是胃直径的 1/5。根据 Laplace 定律，如果腹腔段食管足够长，且其内径明显小于胃径，则能够阻止由于腹腔内压力升高所导致的胃食管反流是。如果腹腔段食管短，其长

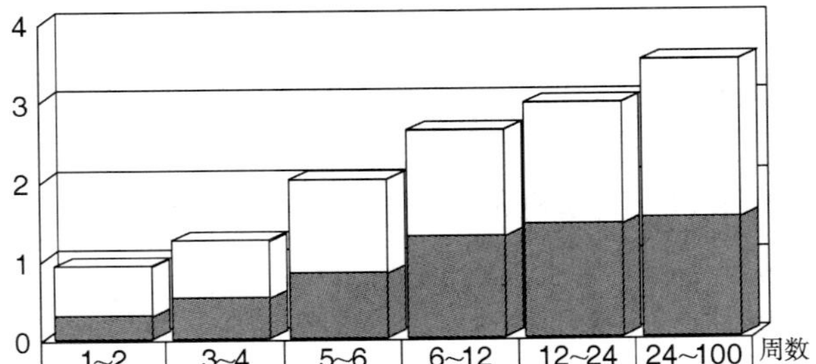

	1~2	3~4	5~6	6~12	12~24	24~100
胸段食管	0.65	0.75	1.2	1.35	1.55	2
腹腔段食管	0.27	0.5	0.8	1.25	1.4	1.48

图 71-2 新生儿和婴儿食管下端括约肌的平均水平。

度小于 2cm，或者是括约肌总长度小于 2cm，就容易引起胃食管反流[34,69,267]，出生后第 1 年，腹腔段食管存在生理性短小，从而导致反流在这一人群中发生率的升高。

His 角：His 是由食管和胃大弯所构成的，通常成锐角[11,28,144,189]。其抗反流作用体现在患儿试图呕吐时，胃内容物冲击胃底部，可以引起胃食管连接部的关闭。而一旦 His 成钝角，则胃的形态转变成漏斗型，腹内压突然升高将促使胃内容物直接反流入
1123 食管[18]。在胃食管连接部还存在有一簇卷曲的食管黏膜皱褶，随着胃内压的改变以及胸腔内食管内负压的作用，这些黏膜皱褶挤压在一起，能够形成一道有轻微作用的抗反流阀[144,189]。

弹簧夹作用：膈肌食管裂孔是由吊索状的右侧膈肌脚所构成的，深吸气时，这一吊索牵拉食管向右向下方移动，从而使食管远端腔径缩小[7,33,68,106,113,153,194,254]，膈肌的这一弹簧夹作用能在清醒状态下的内镜检查中看到[176]。

胃容量及其排空：存在明显 GERD 的儿童中，常发现其胃电活动异常以及胃排空延迟[59,201]，进食过程中胃存在两个重要反射，适应性舒张是指食物进入胃时胃底的舒张，而容受性舒张是指食物在食管内向下运动时胃底的舒张，在这两种反射途径中都有一氧化氮的参与，并引起胃底环形肌的松弛[196,229]。神经系统畸形的患儿常常患有胃动力学功能异常和（或）胃排空延迟[2,40,141,178,196]。

胃酸：大部分反流患者胃酸分泌正常，但是在几组 GERD 儿童病例中发现存在高胃酸分泌[55,123]，胃酸与胃蛋白酶相结合能够引起食管黏膜损伤[180,199]。大多数病例中，胃液分泌量增多比 pH 升高更重要，因此，无论是否存在夜间胃酸分泌过度，通过 PPI 减少胃液分泌是潜在的治疗食管炎的方法[36,45,90,93]。

幽门螺旋杆菌感染：过去的 30 年中，胃癌、胃溃疡和十二指肠溃疡的死亡率已经下降，而食管腺癌和 GERD 的死亡率却在上升[133]。部分研究表明，幽门螺旋杆菌的存在对严重的食管炎和 Barrett 食管有保护作用[52,265]。有人根据这一流行病学数据，提议在 GERD 患者中不应该完全消除幽门螺旋杆菌。然而幽门螺旋杆菌又是消化性溃疡和胃癌的高危因素，从而令医生进退两难，这一课题目前仍在研究中[92,140,151]。

胃蛋白酶、胰蛋白酶和胆盐：胃蛋白酶和胰蛋白酶属于蛋白溶解酶，对食管黏膜有损伤作用。胃蛋白酶在 pH介于 2～3 水平时破坏作用最大，而胰蛋白酶的作用区间为 pH介于 5～8 之间[200,243]。胆盐由于能够增加食管黏膜对酸的通透性，因此在酸性条件下对食管黏膜是有害的。结合性胆盐在 pH 酸性条件下对食管有害，而非结合性胆盐和胰蛋白酶在 pH 中性条件下对食管具有损伤性[193,234]。随着管腔内阻力和胆红素检测手段的进展，研究已经证实，在成人 GERD 患者反流成分中存在胆盐。混合成分的反流物可能较单一的酸性反流物对食管黏膜更具破坏力[240,241]。

腹腔内压：儿童腹腔内压力增高的机制尚未阐明，有些报道还存在矛盾[94]。在成人中，有 17%的胃食管反流与腹腔压力增高有关[72]。肥胖、腹水和腹膜透析均能因引起腹内压升高而诱发胃食管反流[17,162,164]。儿童腹壁缺损也存在较高的胃食管反流发病率，显然这与腹壁缺损关闭后升高的腹内压有关[19,136]。

胃食管反流引起的反流：胃食管反流通过触发正反馈弧而成为引发胃食管反流的重要因素。反流的胃酸刺激食管黏膜后能够通过增加局部血流而引起前列腺素 E_2 的分泌。前列腺素能在局部引起食管黏膜通透性增加，从而增进了食管黏膜炎性反应的易感性。炎症导致食管动力功能损伤并降低了 LES 的静息压，还能通过引起幽门痉挛而进一步产生更多的反流并引起食管炎[249]。胰蛋白酶、胃蛋白酶和胆盐的存在也具备潜在性的食管黏膜损伤作用。

呼吸因素：呼吸道问题导致深吸气运动和胸腔负压升高也能引起胃食管反流[127]。

药物和激素：药物和激素，如抗组胺药、黄嘌呤、茶碱、巧克力、咖啡因、钙通道阻滞剂、胃泌素、多巴胺、胰高血糖素和前列腺素，也与胃食管反流的发病率相关[139,192,226,230]。

潜在的先天性畸形：食管闭锁患儿存在病理性胃食管反流的高发倾向[23,70,137,145,219,223]。在这些患儿中，食管蠕动功能受损而 LES 也存在功能不全。虽然在这类患儿中，反流的发生率随着年龄的增长会逐步下降，但是 10%～30%的食管闭锁修复患儿仍将由于存在 GERD 的并发症而需要行抗反流手术[24,138,215]。在食管闭锁患儿并发 GERD 的病例中，最常见的现象是反复发作的吻合口狭窄。适当的预防性抗反流药物治疗能够减少这类患儿狭窄的形成。先天性膈疝患儿常常存在食管的功能性解剖学畸形而引起胃食管反流。病理性胃食管反流的发生率在这类存活的畸形患儿中高达 20%。大约 15%的先天性膈疝患儿需要同时行抗反流手术[78,115,124]。
1124 先天性腹壁缺损如腹裂和脐膨出也可能因为腹内压升高而导致胃食管反流发病率上升[19,136]。

神经系统受损患儿：神经系统受损的患儿也存在胃食管反流高发倾向。其潜在的原因可能与前肠动力学问题有关。在这类患儿中，食管动力受损和胃排空延迟是导致反流的主要因素。

诊断

很少有病例研究来比较各种诊断技术在诊断儿童胃食管反流中的价值。不同的胃食管反流检测方法仅在证明胃食管反流的各种表现时有用，而且仅在应用于适当的临床意义时有其价值。

病史和体格检查：对于可能存在 GERD 的婴儿和儿童，病史和体格检查是用于临床评价最重要的组成部分。记录生长曲线和原发症状，如瘦小、反复吸入性呛咳、活动性呼吸道疾病、喘鸣、呼吸暂停、反复肺炎发作、易激惹、胃灼热感、腹痛和吞咽困难，有助于引导该患儿后续诊治的进行[209,250]。

上消化道造影：上消化道造影检查对胃食管反流的诊断既无特异性，也无敏感性可言[1,47,187]。然而，它能够如实的反映患者的解剖学路径，从而排除其他可能引起呕吐的病因。需要排除的问题包括幽门狭窄、肠旋转不良、十二指肠出口不完全梗阻、食管裂孔疝和食管狭窄。

食管 pH 监测：食管 pH 监测记录了酸性反流发作的时程长短和频率。当与每日规律的活动相结合时，最能体现出其价值。患者症状的发生应当与 pH 探针的测定值平行记录。一次反流发作被定义为食管内 pH小于 4 的时程介于 15～30 秒之间。食管内 pH 小于 4 的总时程所占百分比则转换成反流指数，反映了食管被酸侵蚀的总时间[56]。应当记住的是，出生后 1 年内的婴儿酸性反流较为常见，成人的指标并不适用于这一年龄段。在儿童中，正常值的上限是 pH 小于 4 的总时程占 5.5%，而对小于 1 岁的婴儿来说，正常值高达 12%[31,75,209,221,248,266]。

内镜检查和病理组织学检查显示，食管炎与异常的 pH 呈很强的相关性。病理活检证实，存在食管炎的成人病例中，有 95%具有异常的 pH 监测结论[26,191,223]。然而在儿童中，食管炎并不是病理性胃食管反流的唯一显著症状[93,131,157]。pH 探针并不能够记录非酸性反流的发生。在一些研究中，十二指肠内容物反流的发生是通过记录胃食管反流物中是否存在胆汁来确认的[16,84,135,193,242]。Orel 和 Markovic 报道了一组 65 例有症状的 GERD 资料，发现其中十二指肠性胃食管反流发生率的升高与食管炎的严重程度相关。他们同时还指出，在具有食管炎和病理性十二指肠-胃食管反流的病例中，并不能够通过 pH 探针分析出病理性反流的存在。

近二十年来，能够探测所有反流类型（酸性、非酸性、液体和气体）能力的多导联腔内电阻技术发展起来，这一技术对检测非酸性反流十分有用[220,239,259]。Belaji 等人报道，59%的胃食管反流发生并非普通的酸性反流，所以不能够被 pH 电极所探测到[16]。在婴儿中，非酸性胃食管反流与呼吸道症状如呼吸暂停相关联。这一发现促使研究者提出假设，那就是婴儿期的呼吸暂停是为防止呼吸道反流所引起。需要进一步的研究探明阻抗以及其他新技术在确认婴儿和儿童病理性 GERD 中的重要性[188,260]。

内镜：内镜检查和病理活检有助于确认食管炎及其他疾病，如狭窄、索带和感染的存在及其严重程度。由于内镜下表现与病理间存在不一致，因此在内镜检查同时行病理活检是必需的[26,148,207]。上皮细胞间存在嗜酸性粒细胞或中性粒细胞，以及图像分析法测量基底细胞厚度和乳头层高度是反流性食管炎的可靠指标[26,46,209]。

核素闪烁成像：在核素闪烁成像法中，通过口服锝标记配方或食物，扫描寻找胃食管反流或气道吸入的证据，能够证实非酸性反流的存在并提供有关胃排空情况的信息[169,185,218,232]。由于缺乏相应的技术标准以及该检查持续时间短，限制了该检查的诊断价值[218]。

食管测压：食管测压技术能够评价食管上段及下段括约肌的活动并监测食管的整合性收缩运动。虽然这一检查并不用于诊断胃食管反流，但是有利于临床更好的认识其潜在的病理生理学改变。虽然该检查有助于鉴别原发性和继发性食管动力学改变，但是在儿童中诊断胃食管反流并不常用[91,110,114]。其他的一些新技术，如光纤内镜在感受器测试辅助下评价吞咽功能的检查，也有人评价过其对诊断儿童 GERD 的临床价值[143,233]。

对儿童疑似胃食管反流病的评价

婴儿和儿童 GERD 表现多样而复杂，对儿童疑似的胃食管反流适当的评价步骤目前仍存在争论。其中必须包括仔细的病史询问和体格检查，其他必须实
1125 施的部分检查包括：上消化道造影排除解剖畸形，24 小时 pH 监测或食管阻力监测，在一些病例中需行内镜检查并实施远段食管黏膜的病理活检。请参考 Box 71-1 由儿童胃肠和营养学会推荐的步骤[209]。

治疗

保守治疗

婴儿和儿童的胃食管反流症状可以通过改变生活方式来治疗。对婴儿应提倡少量多餐而不是无规律的大量进食。对于体重增长缓慢的病例，稠厚的饮食可能有益，有证据支持 1～2 周的低变应原配方对人工喂养呕吐的婴儿有用[97,209,235,246,249]。虽然体位治疗被广泛采用，但是争论仍然存在。即便食管 pH 监测证实婴儿在前倾位时胃食管反流的发生较仰卧位明显减少，但是前倾位却与较高的婴儿猝死（SIDS）发生率相关[76,161,184]。在从出生至 12 个月龄的婴儿中，前倾位睡眠所导致的 SIDS 危险度高于其所带来的优点。因此，美国儿科学会推荐非前倾位的睡眠姿势[126]。但是对于进食后清醒状态的儿童，前倾位还是能够接受的。在大儿童中，推荐的保守治疗包括减肥（如果患儿过重的话），并且避免暴饮暴食，回避咖啡因、巧 1126
克力和辛辣食物[159,209]。

药物治疗

抗反流药物治疗的目的是控制症状、预防并发症和促进食管炎的恢复。抑酸剂和促动力药物是两种主要的药物治疗方法，能用于防止由胃食管反流所引起的症状和损伤，制酸剂能中和胃酸，而抗分泌型药物，如 H_2RA 和 PPI 能减少胃酸的分泌。

组胺 H_2 受体拮抗剂

H_2RA 能通过抑制胃壁细胞的 H_2 受体而减少胃酸的分泌，口服 5.0mg/kg 剂量的雷尼替丁能够在婴儿中控制胃酸分泌 9～10 小时[152]。在成人病例中，不同的随机病例分析资料证实，西咪替丁、雷尼替丁和法莫替丁能有效地控制症状并治疗食管炎[48,236]。

质子泵抑制剂

PPI 穿过壁细胞膜并在分泌小管内累积，从而结合及灭活 H^+,K^+–ATP 酶[263]。这类药物在进食前半小时服用最为有效。一些研究证实，奥美拉唑对于其他一些药物，包括 H_2RA，难以治疗的食管炎十分有效[4,155]。最常见的奥美拉唑推荐剂量是 0.5～3.3mg/（kg·d）[57]。但是也有长期使用 PPI 可能导致高胃泌素血症的危险，病理学家发现，在长期服用 PPI 治疗的患儿胃底活检中存在壁细胞肥大和息肉[50]。此外，由于胃泌素是营养性激素，因此长期依赖 PPI 治疗的患者如果存在结肠癌遗传易感性，则将有潜在发生结肠癌的危险[36]。

制酸剂和表面制剂

由于制酸剂能中和胃酸，因此有利于短时间内缓解胃食管反流引起的症状，如胃灼热感和食管炎。研究发现，在婴儿中使用含铝制剂的抗酸剂会增加血浆

Box 71-1 儿童胃食管反流疾病的评价

1. 反复呕吐。存在反复呕吐症状的患儿需要进行详细的病史询问和体格检查进行评价，尤其需要注意存在评价意义的危险因素。这些因素包括：胆汁性或喷射样呕吐、生长受限、胃肠道（GI）出血、发热、肝脾肿大、颅内压增高症状、癫痫发作、腹肌紧张、腹泻或者是遗传性疾病。如果无上述症状存在，而患儿又能正常生长发育，就没有必要进入诊断程序。由于在这一阶段的患儿中，呕吐症状常常能在 12 个月后自愈，因此推荐采取保守治疗，包括对婴儿采取仰卧体位，短期内尝试性采用低变应原食物喂养或者给予较稠厚的食物。如果在 18～24 月龄时，呕吐症状仍无好转，就需要考虑进行进一步的上消化道造影检查进行评价。如果患有反复呕吐症状的患儿还存在其他症状，如生长发育受限或易激惹或者是年龄大于 2 岁，就应当进行上消化道造影检查、24 小时 pH 监测，必要时包括上消化道内镜活检以排除食管炎的存在。对于已经具备足够热量摄入而仍生长发育受限的婴儿，需要进行全套的血细胞计数检查、电解质、碳酸氢盐、尿素氮、肌酐、丙氨酸转氨酶、血氨、血糖、尿常规、尿酮体和降解物质检查，并回顾其新生儿筛查项目结论。
2. 胃灼热或胸痛。这部分患儿通常是大龄儿童或青少年，对于初次发病者，推荐采取改变生活方式、回避促发因素和实验性服用 2～4 周的组胺 H_2 受体拮抗剂（H_2RA）或质子泵抑制剂（PPI）治疗。如果症状没有缓解，建议采取上消化道造影检查排除食管动力学问题，如失弛缓症，上消化道内镜活检以确定是否存在食管炎，并评价其严重程度。
3. 食管炎。这一诊断能够通过上消化道内镜活检加以确认。对于初发患儿的治疗包括生活方式改变和 H_2RA 或 PPI 药物治疗。对疗效不佳的患儿，需要考虑是否存在诊断错误，如嗜酸性食管炎或者是治疗不当。食管 pH 检测有助于确认药物的疗效。
4. 吞咽困难或吞咽痛。对存在吞咽困难和吞咽疼痛的患儿建议采取上消化道造影检查，对可能食管炎存在的患儿需要进行上消化道内镜活检。
5. 窒息或明显的致命性因素（ALTE）。ALTE 被定义为婴儿的窒息发作或皮肤颜色和肌肉张力改变，是需要进行干预的情况。其初次发作通常在出生后 2 个月左右，而很少在 8 个月以后再出现。这类婴儿通常具有猝死的高危险率，60%～70%的患儿存在呕吐倾向，40%～80%的患儿需要行腹腔段食管的 pH 监测。即便有报道指出食管反流是导致窒息的潜在因素，在对随机选择的 ALTE 患儿进行的调查中并没有发现食管酸化与窒息或心动过缓之间存在必然的联系。如果在对婴儿的食管 pH 监测过程中发现 ALTE 发作时存在严重的呕吐或反胃，抗反流治疗通常对这类患儿有益。对于药物治疗无效的严重患儿，则需要考虑手术治疗。需要指出的是，有潜在可能导致 ALTE 的胃食管反流的诊断和处理需要十分小心。
6. 哮喘。儿童中同时患有哮喘和异常食管 pH 监测结果的发病率介于 25%～75%之间。有人指出，在哮喘患儿中，食管的酸化可能导致气道易激惹和不同程度的梗阻。因此在哮喘患儿中如果具有以下问题，需要采取食管 pH 监测和针对胃食管反流的试验性强化药物治疗。这些问题是：胃食管反流病，存在反流性肺炎的影像学依据，夜间哮喘发作的频率超过一周一次，需要大剂量或连续的激素治疗以及不能脱离药物治疗的状态。
7. 反复肺炎发作。临床研究证实，胃食管反流能够导致反复的肺炎发作并引起肺纤维化。纤维支气管镜结合肺灌洗液证实，存在大百分比的载脂巨噬细胞，而核素闪烁现象技术也能用于发现吸入现象，但两者的结论都缺乏特异性。神经系统损伤的患儿可能会因为不良的吞咽动作导致吸入，电视透视的吞咽功能检查或光纤内镜吞咽功能评价有助于对这部分病例的诊断。

铝浓度水平[264]，而由于有其他更安全的替代治疗，因此并不适合长期使用。硫糖铝作为表面制剂能够黏附于受损的食管黏膜，然而目前还没有足够的数据表明其在儿童中应用的安全性和有效性[209]。

促动力药物

在最近的研究中，食管下段括约肌的短暂松弛被认为是胃食管反流中最为重要的原因之一。促动力药物能提高 LES 压力，增进食管蠕动并加快胃排空。西沙比利是一种混合性 5-羟色胺能药物，能减轻胃酸对食管的侵蚀。研究表明，西沙比利能改善胃食管反流患者的症状评分，减轻食管炎，并促进肺功能[60,217,247]。然而，它同时存在导致严重心律失常的潜在危险，因而在许多国家已经禁止使用[13,63,74]。Meta 分析和随机病例分析表明，西沙比利在儿童病例中无明显临床优势[13,63]。甲氧氯普胺是抗多巴胺能制剂，虽然在一些研究中发现其存在部分模棱两可的作用[149,209]，然而其不良反应如运动障碍，则可能是不可逆的。总而言之，虽然促动力药物使用广泛，但是，目前已有的证据并不足以证明该类药物对胃食管反流存在治疗作用。

红霉素

有报告指出，红霉素在低于抗生素剂量水平应用时，存在对胃肠道的促动力作用，然而至今尚无随机对照临床研究[62]。

内镜治疗

内镜腔内治疗已经成为治疗成人 GERD 的新方向，并有取代手术治疗的趋势。目前正在研究的主要有两种方法。腔内胃折叠术是指通过内镜在食管胃交界处安置缝线的技术[150,204]。

另一种内镜腔内治疗技术则是应用射频能量刺激远段 LES 和胃贲门，这一方法被称为 Stretta 方法，能降低 LES 的顺应性，加强 LES 肌群，从而限制食管下段括约肌的短暂松弛对 GERD 的反应[238]。该技术在非盲前瞻性临床试验中已经显示出疗效[77,238]。Islam 及其同事报道了对 6 例存在反复 GERD 的儿童实施射频治疗，短期疗效似乎还令人满意[112]。

手术治疗适应证

在儿童中实施手术治疗主要针对以下情形[117,137,209,223,249]：

1. 药物治疗无效，持续存在下列症状的儿童需要考虑手术介入，包括持久的肺部症状、存在生命危险、呕吐而致生长发育困难、持续的胃灼热感或者是通过适当的药物治疗后不能脱离药物。
2. 存在解剖结构异常，如食管裂孔疝、肠旋转不良或腸疝。
3. GERD 继发食管狭窄。
4. 食管闭锁术后存在反复的食管狭窄而药物保守治疗无效。
5. 存在神经源性损害的儿童，并发存在喂养困难和严重的反流症状。

手术方式 1127

对胃食管反流手术治疗的目的是阻止反流的发生从而避免诸如吞咽困难、不能打嗝或呕吐等并发症的发生。有许多手术方式曾被应用于儿童，目前最为常用的包括：采用完全包裹的 Nissen 胃底折叠术、改良 Nissen-Rossetti 胃底折叠术和采取部分包裹的 Thal-Ashcraft 胃底折叠术、Toupet 胃底折叠术以及 Boix-Ochoa 胃底折叠术[32,82,216,223,250]。所有这些手术都试图通过制造一个食管远段生理性高压区而阻止反流。近 10 年来，上述方式都曾经由腹腔镜施行，虽然长期随访结果发现腹腔镜下手术和开腹手术相似，但是腹腔镜手术创伤更少，而且似乎并发症较少[158]。

上述手术方式都有其拥护者，而作者倾向于在任何情形下都采用松弛的 Nissen 胃底折叠术来纠正胃食管反流。有人指出通过完全包裹的胃底折叠术纠正存在神经源性损伤的儿童，而通过部分胃底折叠术纠正神经发育正常的胃食管反流患儿[54]。当然也有作者提出由部分胃底折叠术纠正所有类型的胃食管反流患者[44]。目前尚无高质量的随机病例研究来探讨何种手术更适合于何种情形。一位资深作者通过病例回顾指出，对神经系统发育正常的胃食管反流患儿，部分包裹的 Toupet 胃底折叠术与完全包裹的 Nissen 胃底折叠术相比，前者术后的复发率几乎是后者的 2 倍[51]。这一结果也与 Jobe 及其他一些作者报道的结果相一致。他们发现，在成人实施部分包裹的手术后存在较高的复发率。然而许多小儿外科医生们仍然认可部分包裹的术式在儿童中的疗效，而其复发率也能被接受[32,44,54]。

开放手术方式

Nissen 胃底折叠术

手术最好通过上腹部正中切口或左肋缘下切口施行，游离肝左叶，折叠后向右侧牵开，离断三组以上胃短血管以游离胃底部，横行切开覆盖于胃食管连接部前方的腹膜后，环形游离食管远端。如果需要的话，继续沿食管壁向胸腔内游离以确保腹腔段食管的 3cm 长度，迷走神经也随食管同时游离。游离食管远端时，通常可将一烟卷式引流管套住食管和迷走神经以作协助。以不可吸收线从后侧修补膈肌脚后，就可将胃底 360°包绕食管，在完成包裹时通常在胃底和食管上间断缝合 3～4 针。部分外科医生同时还在包裹上方用 4～6 针将食管和膈肌脚缝合一圈，用以防止胃底包裹或其他腹腔内容物疝入胸腔（图 71-3）。在缝合包裹时通常在食管内放置适当尺寸的探条以防止将包裹缝得太紧。此外，折叠部分需足够松弛，以能在胃底包裹和安置探条后的食管间可穿过钝头钳为准[81]。

Thal-Ashcraft 胃底折叠术

在这一手术中，远端需要环形游离至少 2cm 腹腔段食管，膈肌脚缺损用八字缝合方式关闭，缝合时缝线同时需要穿越食管后壁，在前方将胃底跨越腹腔段食管前壁后折叠并用不可吸收线间断或连续缝合固定。胃底与膈肌脚和食管相贴形成 270°的前侧折叠。虽然有一部分外科医生倾向于间断缝合完成上述折叠，但是大多数仍采用连续缝合方式。这样，腹腔段食管的前壁 270°被胃底包绕（图 71-4）[206]。

Toupet 折叠术

在 Toupet 术式中，食管的解剖与 Nissen 胃底折叠术相同，膈肌脚向后牵引靠拢以贴紧食管裂孔，游离胃底时可离断或不离断胃短血管，将胃底从食管后间隙牵引，并以间断缝合方式固定于左侧和右侧膈肌脚。大部分近端缝线均穿越三层结构：胃底、膈肌脚和食管。这一包裹在后壁用 2～3 针缝合固定于膈肌
脚。同时胃底被缝至食管的左右外侧壁形成后方 1128
270°的包裹，从而使食管前方 1/4 圈游离于包裹圈外（图 71-5）[258]。

Boix-Ochoa 术

这一手术方式需要重建 2～3cm 长度的腹腔段食管，膈肌脚的修补以及膈肌脚与食管壁的缝合在食管前壁及左右外侧壁完成。将胃底与食管裂孔的右侧边缘缝合以重建 His 角。在食管前壁和胃底间缝合数针。然后将胃底用缝线钉在膈肌上，从而使胃底像伞一样展开（图 71-6）[31]。

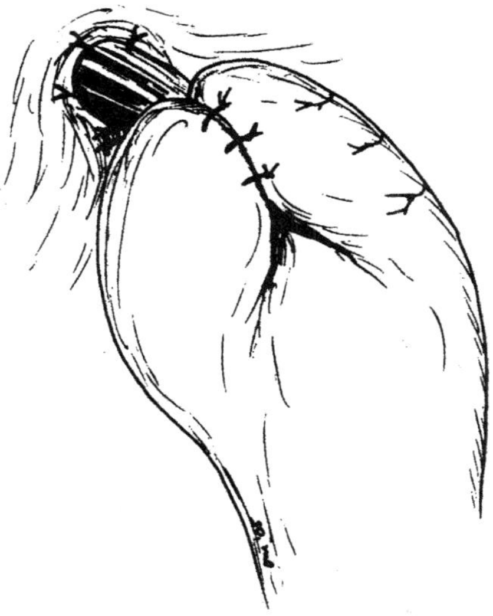

图 71-3 Nissen 胃底折叠术。

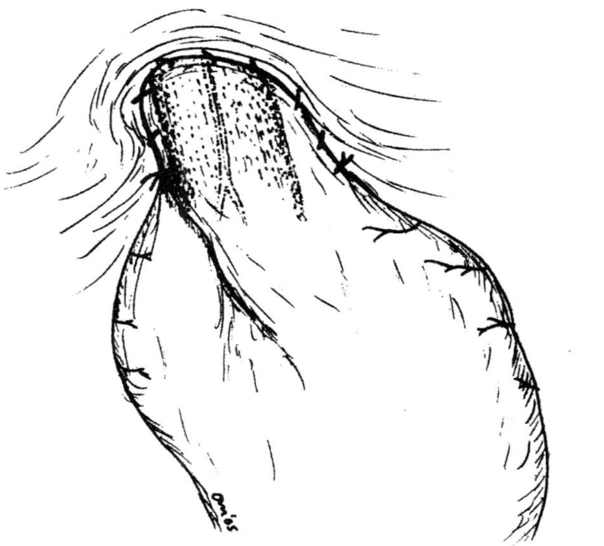

图 71-4 Thal-Ashcraft 胃底折叠术。

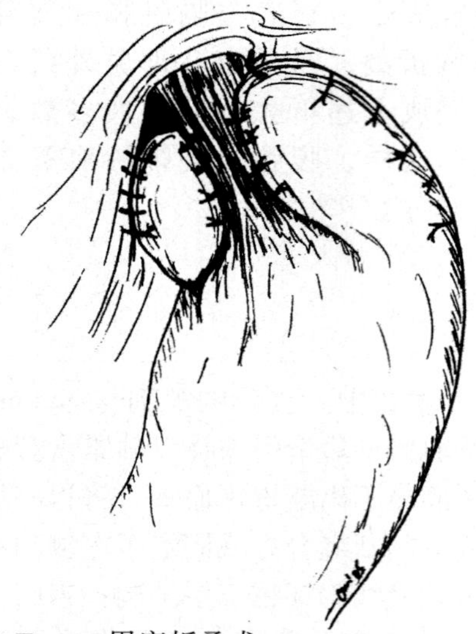

图 71-5 Toupet 胃底折叠术。

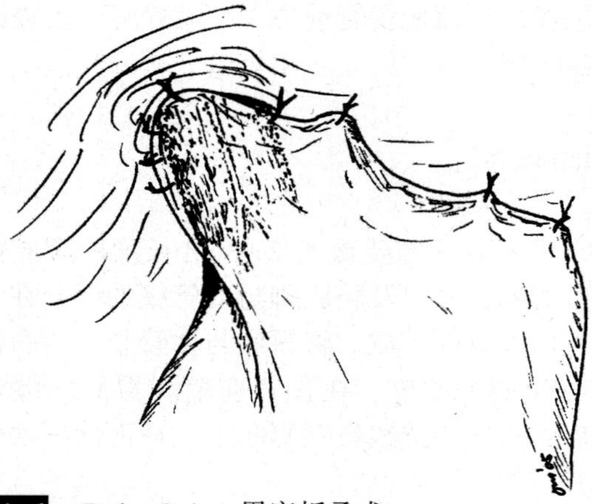

图 71-6 Boix-Ochoa 胃底折叠术。

腹腔镜下 Nissen 胃底折叠术

虽然上述的开放手术方式都曾经通过腹腔镜实施，但是最为普遍实施的是腹腔镜下 Nissen 胃底折叠术。腹腔镜手术存在提升手术视野和图像放大的技术优势，并能减轻术后疼痛。基于上述原因，近 10 年来，腹腔镜下胃底折叠术已经成为儿童病理性胃食管反流的治疗选择。在婴儿和儿童中实施安全和有效的腹腔镜手术治疗胃食管反流需要娴熟的腹腔镜技术，以及复杂的电子设备和特殊的腹腔镜器械。

手术体位和 Trocar 安置

将患儿安置在手术台尾端，并将下肢分叉固定，对于体重大于 30kg 的儿童可用脚蹬支撑固定。适当的棉垫支撑同样重要，能够防止受压酸痛或是外周神经损伤。在婴儿可以通过挤压耻骨联合上方的方法（Credé maneuver）将膀胱排空。而对于大龄儿童通常无需留置导尿管。在麻醉师完成气道保护后就可以安置适当尺寸的食管扩张器了。除非是术中认真对待并加以避免，不然吞咽困难将是最常见的术后早期问题，作者倾向于使用大尺寸的扩张器将食管完全扩开以避免造成包裹太紧。患儿成反向 Trendelenburg 体位，并轻度抬高左侧，以利用重力作用将小肠袢和横结肠从上腹部牵开，从而更好地暴露胃食管连接部。手术者站位于手术台末端，用开放方式安置第一枚套管针。作者倾向于用可扩张的 5mm 套管针经脐孔最低点进腹。可扩张的套管针能避免在操作过程中经套管针穿孔部位的气体外漏。气腹形成后就能够通过套管针置入 4mm 或 5mm 的 30°镜，余下的 4 枚套管针将在腹腔镜监视下放置，具体部位如图 71-7 所示。 1129
所有这些套管针都应当固定于腹壁，以防在手术操作过程中因器械的进出活动而致滑脱。3～4mm 的套管针均可适用于大多数儿童和青少年患者。用一把分

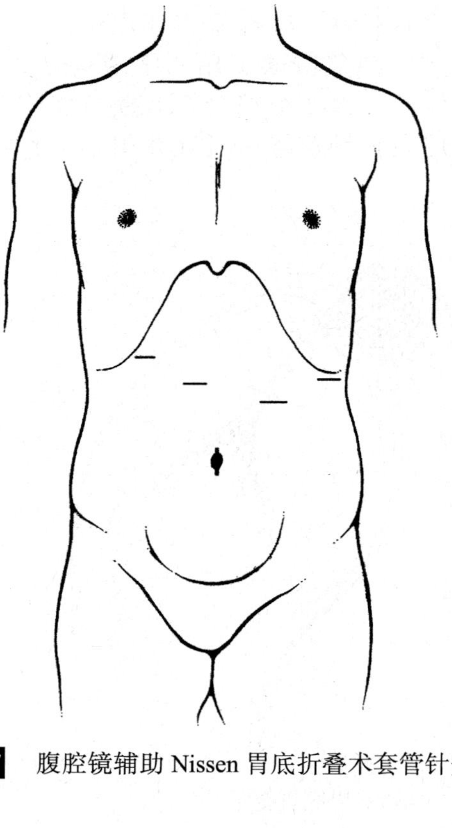

图 71-7 腹腔镜辅助 Nissen 胃底折叠术套管针安置部位示意。

叶、多关节拉钩牵引肝左叶离开食管裂孔。胃底折叠术由离断肝胃韧带开始。可以用电钩或剪刀来完成。需要一直解剖至右侧膈肌脚。肝胃韧带内的小血管和迷走神经的肝支均需要离断。如果肝胃韧带内存在有肝左动脉，则需要加以保留。仔细辨认右侧膈肌脚和食管间的空隙，并加以扩大直至跨过食管的顶部（图 71–8）。解剖过程需谨慎，勿伤及食管前侧的迷走神经，其通常黏附于食管基层。用电凝离断胃短血管，这一解剖沿胃底一直到食管（图 71–9），从而将左侧

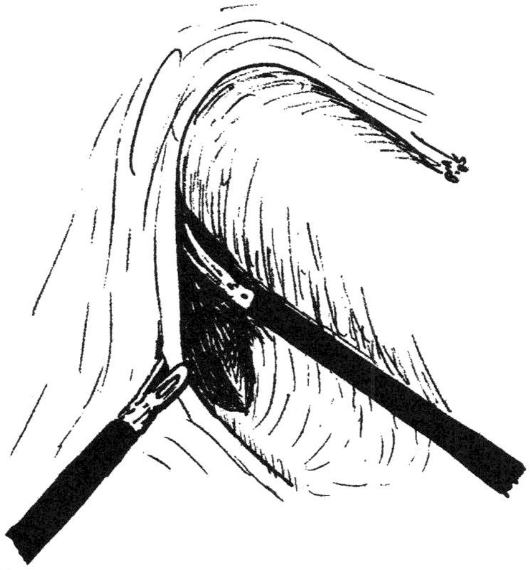

图 71–8　腹腔镜辅助 Nissen 胃底折叠术：在右侧膈肌脚和食管间形成一空隙。

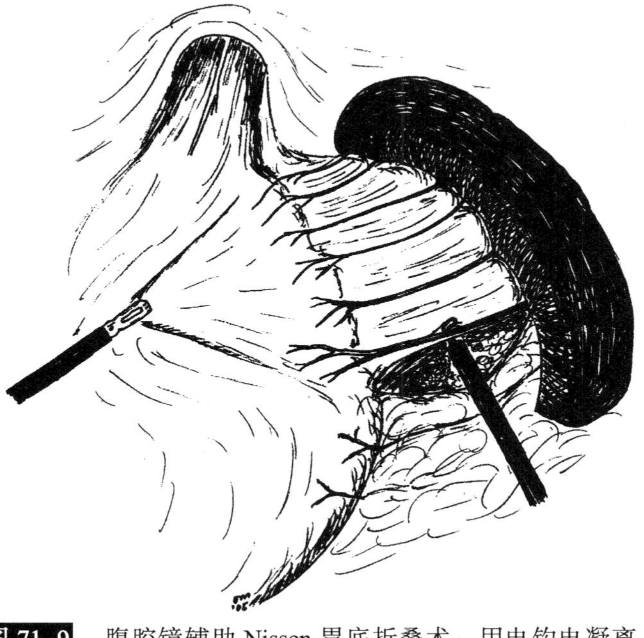

图 71–9　腹腔镜辅助 Nissen 胃底折叠术：用电钩电凝离断胃短血管。

食管从膈肌脚游离出来。继而沿食管一周解剖至食管完全从膈肌脚游离，并扩大食管后间隙。需要保证腹腔段食管有 3cm 的长度且无张力。膈肌脚在食管后方用不吸收线间断缝合，最头端的一针缝线需要同时穿过食管后壁，但要避免伤及迷走神经后支。食管和膈肌脚间需要缝合 3～5 针以防止胃底包裹存在疝入胸腔的风险（图 71–10）。此外还需要指出的是，腹腔段食管越长，患者胃底包裹滑入胸腔的可能性越低（图 71–11）。胃底由食管后间隙牵引包裹食管，并以不吸收线间断缝合固定（图 71–12）。包裹段长度在儿童大约为 2cm，在婴儿则是 1.5cm，更长的包裹段可能导致吞咽困难和打嗝及呕吐的功能障碍。检视伤口有无出血及内脏有无损伤后，退出操作器械和套管针，并根据手术医生的习惯关闭伤口。 1130

幽门成形术

在胃食管反流患儿中，前肠自主神经功能障碍的发生率较高[49,227]。大约有 50%存在胃排空延迟。胃底折叠术后由于胃排空延迟所引起的并发症包括：早期饱胀感和胃食管反流复发。小儿外科医生经常采用幽门成形术或改良的幽门手术来改善胃底折叠术后的胃排空状况，并且许多研究也证实了在胃底折叠和幽门成形术后，胃排空状况得以改善[170,212]。1997 年，Brown 等人报道了一组存在胃排空延迟的患儿，在仅行胃底折叠术后也得到了胃排空功能的改善[38]。

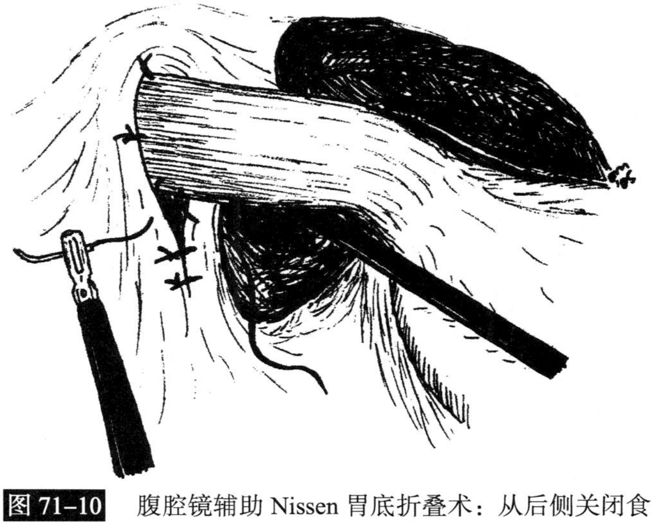

图 71–10　腹腔镜辅助 Nissen 胃底折叠术：从后侧关闭食管裂孔，用 4～6 针将食管固定在膈肌脚上。

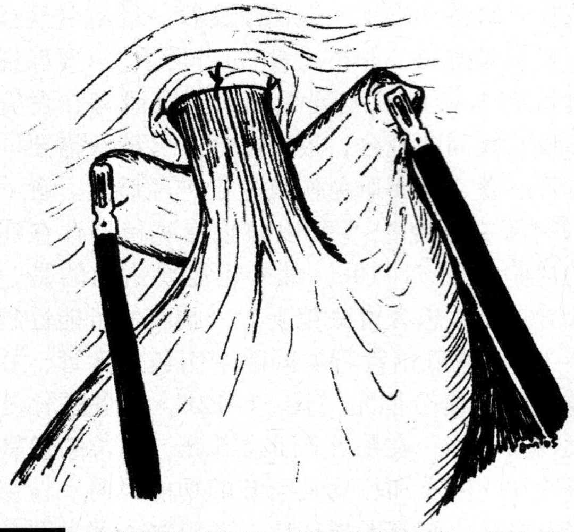

图 71-11　腹腔镜辅助 Nissen 胃底折叠术：从食管后方的间隙中牵拉出胃底，并通过“擦皮鞋”动作评价拟吻合部位的对称性。

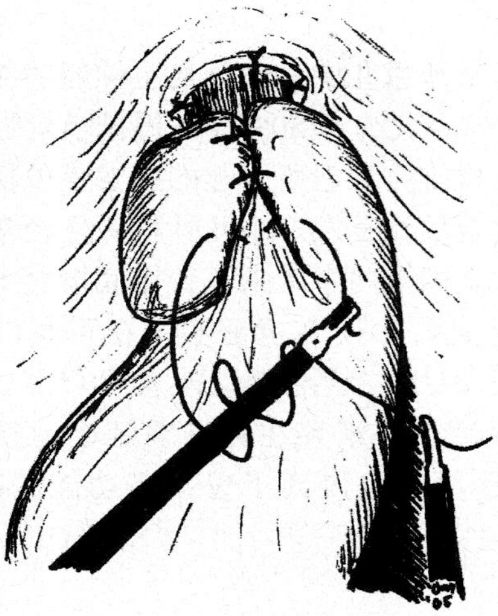

图 71-12　腹腔镜辅助 Nissen 胃底折叠术：滑动的折叠部位通过缝线被固定在 1.5～2.0cm 长度的食管上。

随后 Johnson 等人报道了一小组儿童前肠自主神经功能障碍的病例，在单独行幽门成形术后，胃排空功能未能得以改善[118]。因此，通过幽门成形术改善存在胃肠道自主神经功能障碍儿童的胃排空状况仍存在争议。而胃底折叠术所起的改善作用似乎较幽门成形术更大。

胃造口术

胃造口术通常施用于存在吞咽疾病、厌食症、慢性发育困难和吞咽吸入等问题的儿童。显然，对于需要短期胃肠营养的患儿，仅需要通过插鼻胃管或鼻肠管即可。然而对于需要长期进行胃肠营养支持的患儿，则适用胃造口术或空肠造口术。目前有多种肠饲器械可供外科使用，包括开放式胃造口术、经皮内镜胃造口术、经胃造口放置胃空肠造口管、腹腔镜胃造口术、小弯侧胃造口术、单纯空肠造口术和 Roux-en-Y 空肠造口术。

对于施行胃造口术的患儿是否需要同时实施针对胃食管反流的相应手术，目前仍存在争议。一部分学者认为无需上述操作[39,99]。其观点主要在于：胃造口术后患儿将不再呕吐，即便术后呕吐也能够通过经胃造口进食得以解决。然而这一观点并不为许多儿外科医生所认同，后者认为，在胃造口前必须就胃食管反流进行纠治[21,173]。如果存在明显的反流，抗反流手术必须与胃造口术同时施行。第三种观点认为，如果胃食管反流患儿需要肠道喂养，需要实施胃空肠吻合术或者安置空肠喂养管。这种观点的缺点在于：患儿必须通过持续滴注的方法喂养，而这恰恰是对需照料胃食管反流患儿的父母来说最没有吸引力的地方。胃空 1131
肠喂养管常常会滑脱，而患儿又居住在远离儿童诊疗中心的地区，因此管道的滑脱对他们来说是最难应付的后续顾虑。对于无抗反流手术保障的患儿，实施胃造口喂养也存在大量反流物被吸入的风险。就我们的经验来说，父母通常因患儿的反复呕吐和体重不升而操劳并精疲力竭。因此，笔者倾向于在实施胃造口术之前先解决大量反流的问题。对于存在明显反流的患儿或者存在术后反流预期风险的患儿，如大型的食管裂孔疝或者是与腹腔内压增高相关的食管痉挛，应同时实施胃造口术和胃底折叠术。

Richards 等人报道，2/3 的术后干呕反胃的患儿能通过详细的病史询问在术前得以确认。他们将其特征认定为呕吐而不是反流，并且倾向于在这部分患儿中避免实施胃底折叠术[197]。而另一方面，Owings 调查了 138 例接受了胃底折叠术的存在神经系统损伤的患儿。发现其中 33%的患儿在接受胃底折叠术后反胃和呕吐症状得以治愈，35%的患儿无论在术前还是在术后均无反胃症状，20%的患儿术前术后都存在反胃，而 12%的患儿是术后出现上述症状的（Owings E，私人交流经验）。由于 2/3 的神经系统损伤患儿术后无明显反胃症状发生，因此作者不会拒绝在这类患者身上施行胃底折叠术。

如果患儿需要缓慢的肠道喂养，有不少胃造口方案可供选择。通过开腹手术实施胃造口就有不同的方式。经典的方法是 Stamm 胃造口术，它通过一长约 4cm 的剑突与脐连线中点正中切口进腹。于胃前壁做 2 圈荷包缝线，然后于左上腹适当位置导入一个导管，将球形或伞形导管经荷包中央进胃（图 71–13）。适度收紧荷包，并将胃造口处通过可吸收线固定于腹壁（图 71–14），最后用缝线将胃造口管固定于皮肤。

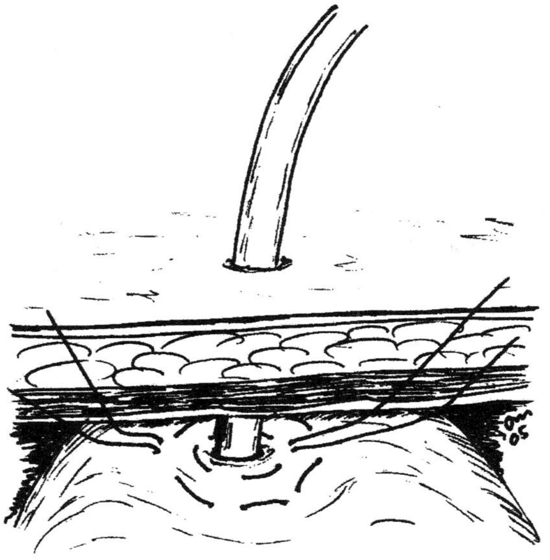

图 71–13　Stamm 胃造口术：在胃前壁安置 1～2 圈荷包缝线，并适当收紧固定胃造口管。

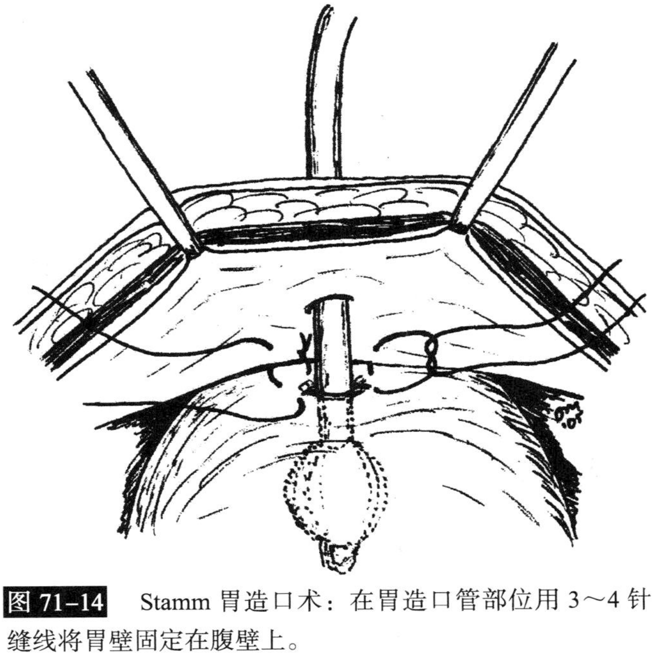

图 71–14　Stamm 胃造口术：在胃造口管部位用 3～4 针缝线将胃壁固定在腹壁上。

经皮内镜胃造口术（PEG）是由小儿外科医生 Michael Gauderer首先介绍的。详细的 PEG 操作过程在文献中均有介绍[79,85,195]。PEG 是微创技术，在儿童中通常需要全身麻醉。其缺点包括不能对造口的部位进行精确定位，盲目的操作容易造成结肠或者肝脏的穿透性损伤。另一项常用的安置胃造口管或造口扣的方法是腹腔镜胃造口术。作为微创手术，该方法同样需要全身麻醉。然而这一技术用途广泛，能够方便地通过其他腹腔镜技术来实施。它允许对安置胃造口装置的胃壁部位进行精确定位。对于初次安置造口扣的患儿，这一方法相对较为方便。

腹腔镜胃造口术通常有两种方法比较常用[213]。第一种是经套管针通道法，将左中上腹部的套管针通道扩大后，将拟安置造口装置部位的胃壁牵拉出腹壁，然后经筋膜、胃壁及对侧筋膜安置固定缝线 2 针，在
胃造口伤口远端再重复上述缝合 1 针。将胃壁经套管 1132
针通道牵拉出腹壁后，荷包固定 1 针。经荷包中心在胃壁上穿孔，再将造口管或造口扣安置在钻孔位置后回复胃壁至腹腔，然后适当收紧荷包缝线。造口管或造口扣能够根据医生的偏好在体外固定。经套管针通道法虽然简单但存在缺陷。经过扩大后的皮肤通道容易溃破从而导致胃壁外置于皮肤通道外，在腹壁较薄的婴儿中尤甚。这一技术最常见的问题是：难于完全回复胃壁至腹腔内，胃造口通道与胃黏膜平行，导致造口易于泄漏，而当移除造口管或造口扣后，容易反复产生难以关闭的胃皮肤窦道[213]。

另一项常用的腹腔镜胃造口术是 U 字缝线技术。它是将 U 字缝线于近中线邻近左上腹套管针通道部位进腹，穿过胃壁后回针出腹壁，第 2 针 U 字旁开 1cm 安置（图 71–15）。用穿刺针经套管针部位刺入已经由麻醉师通过 Levine 管注气扩张的胃腔内。穿刺部位位于两针 U 字缝线中间，经穿刺针置入导引钢丝（图 71–16）。沿导引钢丝置入扩张器并扩张通道至 20 号后，由钢丝引导 14 号球囊搭扣进入胃腔，用 8 号扩张器使进入胃腔后的球囊杆坚硬。将两 U 字缝线结扎固定胃造口搭扣的两个侧翼，如果是用造口管，则固定于套管（图 71–17）[213]。这一方法的主要缺点在于胃壁不是直接固定于腹壁。然而在应用这
种方法安置胃造口扣超过 1000 例后，这一固定问题 1133
似乎并不是主要问题，正如 PEG 导管通常并不会引起胃内容物漏入腹膜腔一样[255]。

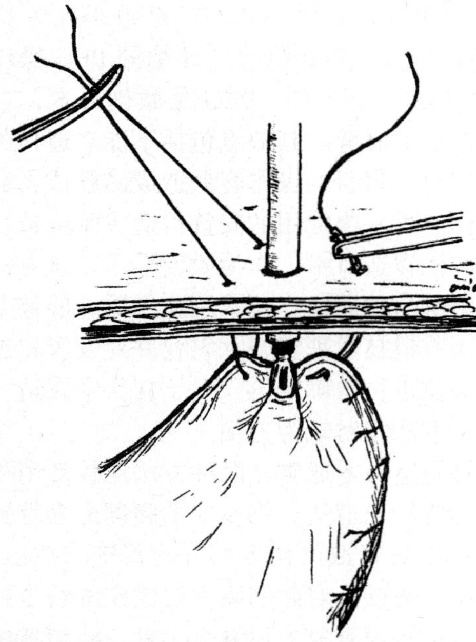

图 71-15 腹腔镜辅助 U 字缝线胃造口术：将胃壁钳夹并靠近腹壁，在胃前壁安置两针 U 字缝线对抗牵引。

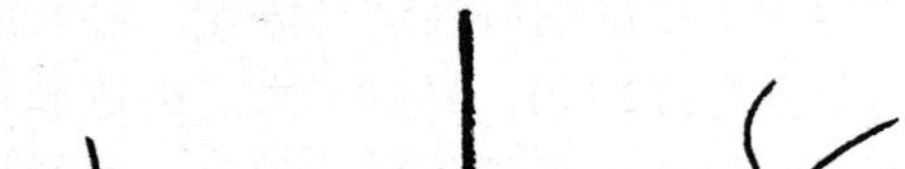

图 71-16 腹腔镜辅助 U 字缝线胃造口术：经由套管针安置部位将针头和导引钢丝穿入扩张的胃腔，沿导引钢丝置入扩张器至 20 号大小。

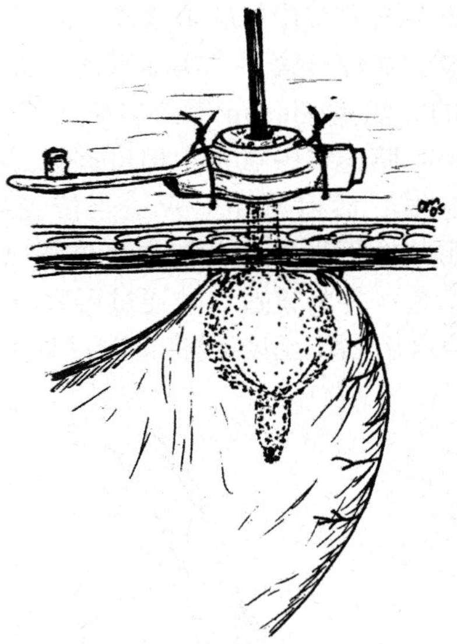

图 71-17 腹腔镜辅助 U 字缝线胃造口术：U 字缝线松松的扎在胃造口搭扣的两侧翼上，并在术后第 2 天除去。

抗反流手术的并发症

根据发生的时间，并发症可以分为术中、术后早期和术后晚期并发症。术中并发症包括胃短血管、脾或者游离的左肝动脉出血。在成人的腹腔镜手术病例中，报道有 1%的初次手术患者存在术中食管或胃穿孔[257]。而在我们所施行的 1000 多例初次腹腔镜胃底折叠术患儿中，仅有 1 例出现了胃穿孔，无食管穿孔发生。无论是腹腔镜手术，还是开腹手术，都可能发生气胸。气胸通常在试图延长腹腔段食管长度而解剖纵隔段食管时发生。气胸能够通过在同侧胸腔放置静脉导管，在手术结束关闭腹腔后拔出来缓解。腹腔镜操作对于初次接受手术的患儿，中转开腹的比例应该低于 3%。许多胃底折叠术患儿在术后几天由于胃底包绕水肿存在早期吞咽困难。这一症状能够通过胃底包绕完成得相对宽松、术中离断上端的胃短血管以及在术后 2～3 周进软食来加以避免[109]。食管裂孔太紧也可能是导致术后吞咽困难的原因而应当避免。另外还需要注意防止将胃底包绕做得太长。作者的经验是，3cm 长的胃底包绕比 2cm 长的宽松包绕更容易引起吞咽困难。存在严重食管动力学问题的患儿即便是具备了宽松的胃底包绕，仍会存在吞咽困难。对于这类患儿，促动力学药物通常有所帮助。

在儿童中，反流复发是常见的术后并发症[82]，通常与术后反胃呕吐相关。能够认识到胃底折叠术后反胃多由中枢神经系统异常引起而不是原发性的胃肠道症状非常重要。最常见的术后反胃原因是过度进食。表现积极的父母常常会因为患儿拥有了可以依赖的生理功能而非常兴奋，以至于看着他们半饥饿的患儿而给予过度的喂养。询问反胃发生的准确时间对明确其发作的根本原因非常重要。反胃能够通过以下途径来加以缓解：滴注式哺乳、开始哺乳前排空胃内气体、治疗便秘以及前面提到的避免对患儿过度喂养。然而反胃和呕吐仍然是胃底折叠术后的主要问题，尤其是在存在神经系统损伤的患儿。

其他胃底折叠术后并发症包括胃胀气综合征和呕吐无力。大多数具备宽松的胃底折叠包绕患儿能够在术后 6 个月内打嗝和呕吐（Owings E，个人交流）。真正意义上的胃胀气综合征在这些患儿中并不多见。其通常发生于存在神经系统损伤而又吞气的患儿。更为普遍的是，看上去胃胀气的患儿其实存在便秘，而其结肠内的积气要甚于胃。这类胃胀气综合征能够通过食用纤维类食物和适当的缓泻剂治疗便秘来得到缓解[35]。

倾倒综合征也常伴随着抗反流包绕的形成而发生。胃底折叠术精简了胃的结构，缩小了胃的尺寸，降低了其食物的储存功能。联合施行幽门成形术甚至增加了倾倒综合征的发生率。进食后出现发汗和腹泻的患儿应当予以限制进食，减少糖类的摄入，并采取滴注式喂养[132]。虽然小肠梗阻是腹腔镜辅助下胃底折叠术后相对罕见的并发症，但接受开腹方式做胃底折叠术的患儿中却并不罕见。有报道指出，开腹术后的发生率为 2.6%[82]。

结局和结果

开放式抗反流手术和腹腔镜抗反流手术的成功率均令人满意。一项多中心的 20 年回顾性研究调查了 7000 多名儿童病例，发现经由开腹手术施行胃底折叠后，在神经系统正常的儿童中，术后满意率达到 95%，而在神经系统有损伤的儿童中则是 84.6%。相同的满意率同样能够在腹腔镜手术后获得[82,159]。Chung 和 Georgeson 报道了他们施行腹腔镜 Nissen 和 Toupet胃底折叠术的成功经验，指出在实施腹腔镜 Nissen 胃底折叠术的患儿中，2 年后有 3.5%出现复发症状，相比较而言，Toupet 胃底折叠术后的复发率达 6.1%[51]。腹腔镜术后发生胃底折叠失败的最常见原因是胃底包绕向胸腔内滑脱（Ngerncham M，私人交流经验）。因此需要努力防止胃底包绕向胸腔内的滑动。最近有一篇报道评价了腹腔镜 Thal 抗反流术的效果，发现在无症状的儿童中，静息反流率达到 25%[108]。这也正如我们先前提到过的，部分胃底折叠术比完全胃底折叠术更容易引起胃食管反流的复发。

我们通常都会碰到如何去处理多次胃底折叠术后失败的问题。无论什么时候，只要可行，都可以通过药物控制反流复发的症状。正如 Islam 等人推荐的那样，射频消融是另一可行的方法。如果必需再次手术，Roux-en-Y 食管空肠吻合术被认为是有效的，但是这一方法容易引起严重的并发症[65]。另一种再次手术方式是施行 Collis-Nissen 术[108]或贲门成形术[40]，从而延长腹腔段食管长度。除此之外，已经没有其他可行的方法来处理儿童胃底折叠术后反流复发的问题。作者倾向于在第一次复发时再次行 Nissen胃底折叠术，而在第二次反流症状复发时则实施腹腔镜Collis-Nissen 术。 1134

小结

胃食管反流是儿童的常见病，通常需要手术纠治。婴儿和儿童的胃食管反流比成人的要复杂得多。药物治疗失败或应用抗反流药物后不能正常生长发育的患儿，是实施手术纠治反流的指征。虽然仍存在争论，但是完全性的胃底折叠术与部分胃底折叠术相比有着更好的效果。术后反胃和胃食管反流复发是抗反流术后最常见也是最让人苦恼的并发症。

（潘伟华译　吴晔明校）

参考文献

1. Aksglaede K, Funch-Jensen P, Thommesen P: Radiological demonstration of gastroesophageal reflux: Diagnostic value of barium and bread studies compared with 24-hour pH monitoring. Acta Radiol 1999;40:652.
2. Alexander F, Wyllie R, Jirousek K: Delayed gastric emptying affects outcome of Nissen fundoplication in neurologically impaired children. Surgery 1997;122:690.
3. Allen ML, Zamani S, Dimarino AJ Jr: The effect of gravity

on esophageal peristalsis in humans. Neurogastroenterol Motil 1997;9:71.
4. Alliet P, Raes M, Bruneel E, et al: Omeprazole in infants with cimetidine-resistant peptic esophagitis. J Pediatr 1998; 132:352.
5. Allison PR: Reflux esophagitis, sliding hiatus hernia and the anatomy of repair. Surg Gynecol Obstet 1951;92:419.
6. Allison PR, Johnston AS, Royce GB: Short esophagus with simple peptic ulceration. J Thorac Cardiovasc Surg 1943; 12:432.
7. Altorki NK, Skinner DB: Pathophysiology of gastroesophageal reflux. Am J Med 1989;86:685.
8. Andrews PL, Sanger GJ: Abdominal vagal afferent neurons: An important target for the treatment of gastrointestinal dysfunction. Curr Opin Pharmacol 2002;2:650.
9. Ashcraft KW, Goodwin CD, Amoury RW, et al: Thal fundoplication: A simple and safe operative treatment for gastroesophageal reflux. J Pediatr Surg 1978;13:643.
10. Ashcraft KW, Holder TM, Amoury RA: Treatment of gastroesophageal reflux in children by Thal fundoplication. J Thorac Cardiovasc Surg 1981;82:706.
11. Atkinson M, Summerling ME: The competence of the cardia after cardiomyotomy. Gastroenterologia 1959;92:123.
12. Au FC: The Stamm gastrostomy: A sound procedure. Am Surg 1993;59:674.
13. Augood C, MacLennan S, Gilbert R, et al: Cisapride treatment for gastro-oesophageal reflux in children. Cochrane Database Syst Rev (4):CD002300, 2003.
14. Axelrod FB, Schneider KM, Ament ME, et al: Gastroesophageal fundoplication and gastrostomy in familial dysautonomia. Ann Surg 1982;195:253.
15. Aziz Q, Thompson DG: Brain-gut axis in health and disease. Gastroenterology 1998;114:559.
16. Belaji NS, Blom D, DeMeester TR, et al: Redefining gastroesophageal reflux (GER). Surg Endosc 2003;17:1380.
17. Barak N, Ehrenpreis ED, Harrison JR, et al: Gastroesophageal reflux disease in obesity: Pathophysiological and therapeutic considerations. Obes Rev 2002;3:9.
18. Bardaji C, Boix-Ochoa J: Contribution of the His angle to the gastroesophageal antireflux mechanism. Pediatr Surg Int 1986;1:172.
19. Beaudoin S, Kieffer G, Sapin E, et al: Gastroesophageal reflux in neonates with congenital abdominal wall defect. Eur J Pediatr Surg 1995;5:323.
20. Belsey R: Diaphragmatic hernia. In Modern Trends in Gastroenterology. London, Butterworth, 1952, p 134.
21. Berezin S, Schwartz SM, Halata MS, Newman LJ: Gastroesophageal reflux secondary to gastrostomy placement. Am J Dis Child 1986;40:649.
22. Berger D, Bischof-Delaloye A, Reinberg O, et al: Esophageal and pulmonary scintiscanning in gastroesophageal reflux in children. Prog Pediatr Surg 1985; 18:68.
23. Bergmeijer JH, Hazebroek FW: Prospective medical and surgical treatment of gastroesophageal reflux in esophageal atresia. J Am Coll Surg 1998;187:153.
24. Bergmeijer JH, Tibboel D, Hazebroek FW: Nissen fundoplication in the management of gastroesophageal reflux occurring after repair of esophageal atresia. J Pediatr Surg 2000;35:573.
25. Billiard MC: Traite des maladies des enfans nouveaux-nes et a la mamelle. In Billiard M (ed): Atlas D'Anatomie Pathologique pour Servir A L'Historie des Maladies des Enfants. Paris, Imprimerie de H Balzac, 1828, p 271.
26. Black DD, Haggitt RC, Orenstein SR, et al: Esophagitis in infants. Morphometric histological diagnosis and correlation with measures of gastroesophageal reflux. Gastroenterology 1990;98:1408.
27. Boix-Ochoa J: Diagnosis and management of gastroesophageal reflux in children. Surg Ann 1981;13:123.
28. Boix-Ochoa J: Gastroesophageal reflux. In Welch K, Randolph JG, Rautch M, et al (eds): Pediatric Surgery. St Louis, Mosby–Year Book, 1986.
29. Boix-Ochoa J: Gastroesophageal reflux in children. In Jemieson G (ed): Surgery of the Esophagus. Edinburgh, Churchill Livingstone, 1988.
30. Boix-Ochoa J, Canals J: Maturation of the lower esophagus. J Pediatr Surg 1976;11:749.
31. Boix-Ochoa J, Lafuenta JM, Gil-Vernet JM: Twenty-four hour esophageal pH monitoring in gastroesophageal reflux. J Pediatr Surg 1980;15:74.
32. Boix-Ochoa J, Rowe MI: Gastroesophageal reflux. In O'Neill JA (ed): Pediatric Surgery, vol 2. St Louis, Mosby–Year Book, 1998, p 1007.
33. Bombeck CT, Dillard NH, Nyhus LM: Muscular anatomy of the gastroesophageal junction and role of phrenoesophageal competence. Ann Surg 1966;164:643.
34. Bonavina L, Evander A, DeMeester TR, et al: Length of the distal esophageal sphincter and competency of the cardia. Am J Surg 1986;151:25-34.
35. Borowitz SM, Satphen JL: Recurrent vomiting and persistent gastroesophageal reflux caused by unrecognized constipation. Clin Pediatr (Phila) 2004;43:461.
36. Boyle JT: Acid secretion from birth to adulthood. J Pediatr Gastroenterol Nutr 2003;37(Suppl):S12.
37. Bright R: Account of a remarkable misplacement of the stomach. Guys Hosp Rep 1836;1:598.
38. Brown RA, Wynehank S, Rode H: Is a gastric drainage procedure necessary at the time of antireflux surgery? J Pediatr Gastroenterol Nutr 1997;25:377.
39. Burd RS, Price MR, Whalen TV: The role of protective antireflux procedures in neurologically impaired children: A decision analysis. J Pediatr Surg 2002;37:500.
40. Bustorff-Silva J, Moreira AP, Cavalsco MA, et al: Extended hiatoplasty: Early experience with a simple technique increases the intraabdominal esophageal length in complicated gastroesophageal reflux. J Pediatr Surg 2001; 35:555.
41. Cadiot G, Bruhat A, Rigaud D, et al: Multivariate analysis of pathophysiological factors in reflux oesophagitis. Gut 1997;40:167.
42. Carré IJ: Natural history of partial thoracic stomach ("hiatal hernia") in children. Arch Dis Child 1959;34:344.
43. Carré IJ: Postural treatment of children with partial thoracic stomach ("hiatus hernia"). Arch Dis Child 1960;35:569.
44. Ceriati E, Guarino N, Zaccara A, et al: Gastroesophageal reflux in neurologically impaired children: Partial or total fundoplication? Arch Surg 1998;383:317.
45. Cezard JP: Managing gastro-oesophageal reflux disease in children. Digestion 2004;69:3.
46. Chadwick LM, Kurinczuk JJ, Hallam LA, et al: Clinical and endoscopic predictors of histological oesophagitis in infants. J Paediatr Child Health 1997;33:388.
47. Chen MY, Ott DJ, Sinclair JW, et al: Gastroesophageal reflux disease: Correlation of esophageal pH testing and radiographic findings. Radiology 1992;185:483.
48. Chiba N, Gara CJ De, Wilkinson JM, et al: Speed of healing and symptom relief in grade II to IV gastroesophageal reflux disease: A meta-analysis. Gastroenterology 1997;112:1798.
49. Chong SK: Gastrointestinal problems in the handicapped child. Curr Opin Pediatr 2001;13:441.
50. Choudhry U, Boyce HW Jr, Coppola D: Proton pump

inhibitor–associated gastric polyps: A retrospective analysis of their frequency, and endoscopic, histologic, and ultrastructural characteristics. Am J Clin Pathol 1998;110:615.
51. Chung DH, Georgeson KE: Fundoplication and gastrostomy. Semin Pediatr Surg 1998;7:213.
52. Clark GW: Effect of *Helicobacter pylori* infection in Barrett's esophagus and the genesis of esophageal adenocarcinoma. World J Surg 2003;27:994.
53. Cohen S, Harris LD: Does hiatus hernia affect competence of the gastroesophageal sphincter? N Engl J Med 1971; 284:1053.
54. Cohen Z, Fishman S, Yulevich A, et al: Nissen fundoplication and Boix-Ochoa antireflux procedure: Comparison between two surgical techniques in the treatment of gastroesophageal reflux disease in children. Eur J Pediatr Surg 1999;9:289.
55. Collen MJ, Ciarleglio CA, Stanczak VJ, et al: Basal gastric acid secretion in children with atypical epigastric pain. Am J Gastroenterol 1988;83:923.
56. Colletti RB, Christie DL, Orenstein SR: Statement of the North American Society for Pediatric Gastroenterology and Nutrition (NASPGN). Indications for pediatric esophageal pH monitoring. J Pediatr Gastroenterol Nutr 1995;21:253.
57. Colletti RB, Di Lorenzo C: Overview of pediatric gastroesophageal reflux disease and proton pump inhibitor therapy. J Pediatr Gastroenterol Nutr 2003;37(Suppl):S7.
58. Cook IJ, Dodds WJ, Dantos RO, et al: Opening mechanisms of the human upper esophageal sphincter. Am J Physiol 1989;257:G748.
59. Cucchiara S, Salvia G, Borrelli O, et al: Gastric electrical dysrhythmias and delayed gastric emptying in gastroesophageal reflux disease. Am J Gastroenterol 1997;92:1103.
60. Cucchiara S, Staiano A, Boccieri A, et al: Effects of cisapride on parameters of oesophageal motility and on the prolonged intraoesophageal pH test in infants with gastrooesophageal reflux disease. Gut 1990;31:21.
61. Cucchiara S, Staiano A, Di Lorenzo C, et al: Esophageal motor abnormalities in children with gastroesophageal reflux and peptic esophagitis. J Pediatr Gastroenterol Nurs 1986;108:907.
62. Curry JI, Lander TD, Stringer MD: Erythromycin as prokinetic agent in infants and children. Aliment Pharmacol Ther 2001;15:595.
63. Dalby-Payne JR, Morris AM, Craig JC: Meta-analysis of randomized controlled trials on the benefits and risks of using cisapride for the treatment of gastroesophageal reflux in children. J Gastroenterol Hepatol 2003;18:196.
64. Dallemagne B, Weerts JM, Jehaes C, et al: Laparoscopic Nissen fundoplication: Preliminary report. Surg Laparosc Endosc 1991;1:138.
65. Danielson PD, Emmers RW: Esophagogastric disconnection for gastroesophageal reflux in children with severe neurological impairment. J Pediatr Surg 1999;34:84.
66. Darling DB: Hiatal hernia and gastroesophageal reflux in infancy and childhood. AJR Am J Roentgenol 1975;123:724.
67. Davidson G: The role of lower esophageal sphincter function and dysmotility in gastroesophageal reflux in premature infants and in the first year of life. J Pediatr Gastroenterol Nutr 2003;37(Suppl):S17.
68. Delattre JF, Avisse C, Marcus C, et al: Functional anatomy of the gastroesophageal junction. Surg Clin North Am 2000;80:241.
69. DeMeester TR, Wernly JA, Bryant GH, et al: A clinical and in vitro analysis of determinants of gastroesophageal competence. A study of the principles of antireflux surgery. Am J Surg 1979;137(Suppl):39.
70. Deurloo JA, Ekkelkamp S, Bartelsman JF, et al: Gastroesophageal reflux: Prevalence in adults older than 28 years after correction of esophageal atresia. Ann Surg 2003;238:686.
71. Dodds WJ, Dent J, Hogan WJ, et al: Mechanisms of gastroesophageal reflux in patients with reflux esophagitis. N Engl J Med 1982;307:1547.
72. Dodds WJ, Stef JJ, Hogan WJ: Factors determining pressure measurement accuracy by intraluminal esophageal manometry. Gastroenterology 1976;70:117.
73. Duranceau A, Liebermann-Mefferret D: Physiology of the esophagus. In Zuidema G (ed): Shackelford's Surgery of the Alimentary Tract, 5th ed. Philadelphia, WB Saunders, 2002.
74. Enger C, Cali C, Walker AM: Serious ventricular arrhythmias among users of cisapride and other QT-prolonging agents in the United States. Pharmacoepidemiol Drug Saf 2002;11:477.
75. Euler AR, Byrne WJ: Twenty-four-hour esophageal intraluminal pH probe testing: A comparative analysis. Gastroenterology 1981;80:957.
76. Ewer AK, James ME, Tobin JM: Prone and left lateral positioning reduce gastro-oesophageal reflux in preterm infants. Arch Dis Child Fetal Neonatal Ed 1999;81:F201.
77. Fanelli RD, Gersin KS, Bakhsh A: The Stretta(r) procedure: Effective endoluminal therapy for GERD. Surg Technol Int 2003;11:129.
78. Fasching G, Huber A, Uray E, et al: Gastroesophageal reflux and diaphragmatic motility after repair of congenital diaphragmatic hernia. Eur J Pediatr Surg 2000;10:360.
79. Ferguson RD, Harig JM, Kozarek RA, et al: Placement of feeding button (One-Step Button) as the initial procedure. Am J Gastroenterol 1993;8:501.
80. Follette D, Fonkalsrud EW, Euler A, et al: Gastroesophageal fundoplication for reflux in infants and children. J Pediatr Surg 1976;11:757.
81. Fonkalsrud EW: Nissen fundoplication for pediatric gastroesophageal reflux disease. Semin Pediatr Surg 1998;7:110.
82. Fonkalsrud EW, Ashcraft KW, Coran AG, et al: Surgical treatment of gastroesophageal reflux in children: A combined hospital study of 7467 patients. Pediatrics 1998; 101:419.
83. Fonkalsrud EW, Foglia RP, Ament ME, et al: Operative treatment for the gastroesophageal reflux syndrome in children. J Pediatr Surg 1989;24:525.
84. Freedman J, Lindqvist M, Hellstrom PM, et al: Presence of bile in the oesophagus is associated with less effective oesophageal motility. Digestion 2002;66:42.
85. Gauderer MWL, Ponsky JL: A simplified technique for constructing a tube feeding gastrostomy. Surg Gynecol Obstet 1981;152:83.
86. Georgeson K: Results of laparoscopic antireflux procedures of neurologically normal infants and children. Semin Laparosc Surg 2002;9:172.
87. Georgeson K: Minimally invasive surgery in neonates. Semin Neonatal 2003;8:243.
88. Georgeson KE: Laparoscopic gastrostomy and fundoplication. Pediatr Ann 1993;92:675.
89. Georgeson KE: Laparoscopic fundoplication and gastrostomy. Semin Laparosc Surg 1998;5:25.
90. Gibbons TE, Gold BD: The use of proton pump inhibitors in children: A comprehensive review. Paediatr Drugs 2003;5:25.
91. Godoy J, Tovar JA, Vicente Y, et al: Esophageal motor dysfunction persists in children after surgical cure of reflux: An ambulatory manometric study. J Pediatr Surg 2001; 36:1405.

92. Gold BD: Outcomes of pediatric gastroesophageal reflux disease: In the first year of life, in childhood, and in adults. oh, and should we really leave *Helicobacter pylori* alone? J Pediatr Gastroenterol Nutr 2003;37(Suppl):S33.
93. Gold BD, Freston JW: Gastroesophageal reflux in children: Pathogenesis, prevalence, diagnosis, and role of proton pump inhibitors in treatment. Paediatr Drugs 2002;4:673.
94. Goldani HA, Fernandes MI, Vicente YA, et al: Lower esophageal sphincter reacts against intraabdominal pressure in children with symptoms of gastroesophageal reflux. Dig Dis Sci 2002;47:2544.
95. Gorenstein A, Levine A, Boaz M, et al: Severity of acid gastroesophageal reflux assessed by pH metry: Is it associated with respiratory disease? Pediatr Pulmonol 2003; 36:330.
96. Gorrotxategi P, Reguilon MJ, Arana J, et al: Gastroesophageal reflux in association with the Sandifer syndrome. Eur J Pediatr Surg 1995;5:203.
97. Gremse DA: Gastroesophageal reflux disease in children: An overview of pathophysiology, diagnosis, and treatment. J Pediatr Gastroenterol Nutr 2002;35(Suppl):S297.
98. Grosser O: The development of respiratory apparatus. In Keibel F, Mall F (eds): Manual of Human Embryology. Philadelphia, JB Lippincott, 1912, p 473.
99. Hamant JM, Bax NM, van der Zee DC, et al: Complications of percutaneous endoscopic gastrostomy with or without concomitant antireflux surgery in 96 children. J Pediatr Surg 2001;36:1412.
100. Hassall E: Co-morbidities in childhood Barrett's esophagus. J Pediatr Gastroenterol Nutr 1997;25:255.
101. Hassall E, Weinstein WM, Ament ME: Barrett's esophagus in childhood. Gastroenterology 1985;89:1331.
102. Helm JF: Esophageal acid clearance. J Clin Gastroenterol 1986;8:5.
103. Hill LD: An effective operation for hiatal hernia: An eight-year appraisal. Ann Surg 1967;166:681.
104. Hillemeier C, Buchin PJ, Gryboski J: Esophageal dysfunction in Down's syndrome. J Pediatr Gastroenterol Nutr 1982;1:101.
105. Ho SC, Chang CS, Wu CY, et al: Ineffective esophageal motility is a primary motility disorder in gastroesophageal reflux disease. Dig Dis Sci 2002;47:652.
106. Holloway RH: The anti-reflux barrier and mechanisms of gastro-oesophageal reflux. Baillieres Best Pract Res Clin Gastroenterol 2000;14:681.
107. Holloway RH, Hongo M, Berger K, et al: Gastric distention: A mechanism for postprandial gastroesophageal reflux. Gastroenterology 1985;89:779.
108. Hunter JG, Smith CD, Branum GD, et al: Laparoscopic fundoplication failures: Patterns of failure and response to fundoplication revision. Am Surg 1999;230:595.
109. Hunter JG, Swanstrom L, Waring JP: Dysphagia after laparoscopic antireflux surgery: The impact of operative technique. Ann Surg 1996;224:51.
110. Hussain SZ, Di Lorenzo C: Motility disorders. Diagnosis and treatment for the pediatric patient. Pediatr Clin North Am 2002;49:27.
111. Hyams JS: Functional gastrointestinal disorders. Curr Opin Pediatr 1999;11:375.
112. Islam S, Geiger JD, Coran AG, et al: Use of radiofrequency ablation of the lower esophageal sphincter to treat recurrent gastroesophageal reflux disease. J Pediatr Surg 2004; 39:282.
113. Jackson C: The diaphragmatic pinchcock. Laryngoscope 1922;32:139.
114. Jadcherla SR: Manometric evaluation of esophageal-protective reflexes in infants and children. Am J Med 2003;115(Suppl):157S.
115. Jaillard SM, Pierrat V, Dubois A, et al: Outcome at 2 years of infants with congenital diaphragmatic hernia: A population-based study. Ann Thorac Surg 2003;75:250.
116. Jobe BA, Wallace J, Hansen PD, et al: Evaluation of laparoscopic Toupet fundoplication as a primary repair for all patients with medically resistant gastroesophageal reflux. Surg Endosc 1997;11:1080.
117. Johnson DG: Current thinking on the role of surgery in gastroesophageal reflux. Pediatr Clin North Am 1985; 325:1165.
118. Johnson DG, Reid BS, Meyers RL, et al: Are scintiscans accurate in the selection of reflux patients for pyloroplasty? J Pediatr Surg 1998;33:573.
119. Johnson LF, DeMeester TH: Twenty-four hour pH monitoring of the distal esophagus: Quantitative measure of gastroesophageal reflux. Am J Gastroenterol 1974;63:325.
120. Kahrilas PJ: GERD pathogenesis, pathophysiology, and clinical manifestations. Cleve Clin J Med 2003;70(Suppl):S4.
121. Kahrilas PJ, Dodds WJ, Dent J, et al: Upper esophageal sphincter function during deglutition. Gastroenterology 1988;95:52.
122. Kahrilas PJ, Dodds WJ, Hogan WJ: Effect of peristaltic dysfunction on esophageal volume clearance. Gastroenterology 1988;94:73.
123. Kalach N, Badran AM, Jaffray P, et al: Correlation between gastric acid secretion and severity of acid reflux in children. Turk J Pediatr 2003;45:6.
124. Kamiyama M, Kawahara H, Okuyama H, et al: Gastroesophageal reflux after repair of congenital diaphragmatic hernia. J Pediatr Surg 2002;37:1681.
125. Kapila YV, Dodds WJ, Helm JF, et al: Relationship between swallow rate and salivary flow. Dig Dis Sci 1984;29:528.
126. Kattwinkel J, Brooks JG, Keenan ME, et al: Changing concepts of sudden infant death syndrome: Implications for infant sleeping environment and sleep position. Pediatrics 2000;105:650.
127. Kawahara H, Dent J, Davidson G, et al: Relationship between straining, transient lower esophageal sphincter relaxation, and gastroesophageal reflux in children. Am J Gastroenterol 2001;96:2019.
128. Kawahara H, Imura K, Nakajima K, et al: Motor function of the esophagus and the lower esophageal sphincter in children who undergo laparoscopic Nissen fundoplication. J Pediatr Surg 2000;35:1666.
174. Orel R, Markovic S: Bile in the esophagus: A factor in the pathogenesis of reflux esophagitis in children. J Pediatr Gastroenterol Nutr 2003;36:266.
175. Orenstein SR: Effects on behavior state of prone versus seated positioning for infants with gastroesophageal reflux. Pediatrics 1990;85:765.
176. Orenstein SR: Gastroesophageal reflux. Curr Probl Pediatr 1991;21:193.
177. Orenstein SR: An overview of reflux-associated disorders in infants: Apnea, laryngospasm, and aspiration. Am J Med 2001;111(Suppl):60S.
178. Orenstein SR, Di Lorenzo C: Postfundoplication complications in children. Curr Treat Options Gastroenterol 2001; 4:441.
179. Orenstein SR, Izadnia F, Khan S: Gastroesophageal reflux disease in children. Gastroenterol Clin North Am 1999; 28:947.
180. Orlando RC: Pathogenesis of gastroesophageal reflux disease. Gastroenterol Clin North Am 2002;31(Suppl):S35.
181. Orlando RC: Pathogenesis of gastroesophageal reflux

disease. Am J Med Sci 2003;326:274.
182. Ostlie D, Holcomb GW: Laparoscopic fundoplication and gastrostomy. Semin Pediatr Surg 2002;11:196.
183. Othersen HB Jr, Ocampo RJ, Parker EF, et al: Barrett's esophagus in children: Diagnosis and management. Ann Surg 1993;217:676.
184. Oyen N, Markestad T, Skaerven R, et al: Combined effects of sleeping position and prenatal risk factors in sudden infant death syndrome: The Nordic Epidemiological SIDS Study. Pediatrics 1997;100:613.
185. Ozcan Z, Ozcan C, Erinc R, et al: Scintigraphy in the detection of gastro-oesophageal reflux in children with caustic oesophageal burns. A comparative study with radiography and 24-h pH monitoring. Pediatr Radiol 2001; 31:737.
186. Page M, Jeffery H: The role of gastro-esophageal reflux in the aetiology of SIDS. Early Hum Dev 2000;59:127.
187. Pan JJ, Levine MS, Refern RO, et al: Gastroesophageal reflux: Comparison of barium studies with 24-h pH monitoring. Eur J Radiol 2003;47:149.
188. Pandolfino JE, Richter JE, Ours T, et al: Ambulatory esophageal pH monitoring using a wireless system. Am J Gastroenterol 2003;98:740.
189. Paterson WG: The normal antireflux mechanism. Chest Surg Clin North Am 2001;11:473.
190. Patterson PE, Harding SM: Gastroesophageal reflux disorders and asthma. Curr Opin Pulm Med 1999;5:63.
191. Patwari AK, Bajaj P, Kashyp R, et al: Diagnostic modalities for gastroesophageal reflux. Indian J Pediatr 2002;69:133.
192. Pehl C, Pfeiffer A, Wendl B, et al: The effect of decaffeination of coffee on gastro-oesophageal reflux in patients with reflux disease. Aliment Pharmacol Ther 1997;11:483.
193. Penagini R: Bile reflux and oesophagitis. Eur J Gastroenterol Hepatol 2001;13:1.
194. Pettersson GB, Bombeck CT, Nyhus LM: The lower esophageal sphincter: Mechanisms of opening and closure. Surgery 1980;88:307.
195. Ponsky JL: Percutaneous endoscopic gastrostomy: Techniques of removal and replacement. Gastrointest Endosc Clin North Am 1992;2:215.
196. Ravelli AM, Milla PJ: Vomiting and gastroesophageal motor activity in children with disorders of the central nervous system. J Pediatr Gastroenterol Nutr 1998; 26:56.
197. Richards CA, Milla PJ, Andrews PL, et al: Retching and vomiting in neurologically impaired children after fundoplication: Predictive preoperative factors. J Pediatr Surg 2001;36:1401.
198. Richter J: Do we know the cause of reflux disease? Eur J Gastroenterol Hepatol 1999;11(Suppl):S3.
199. Richter JE: Importance of bile reflux in Barrett's esophagus. Dig Dis Sci 2001;18:208.
200. Richter JE: Duodenogastric reflux–induced (alkaline) esophagitis. Curr Treat Options Gastroenterol 2004;7:53.
201. Riezzo G, Chiloiro M, Guerra V: Comparison of gastric electrical activity and gastric emptying in healthy and dyspeptic children. Dig Dis Sci 2000;45:517.
202. Rossetti M, Hell K: Fundoplication for the treatment of gastroesophageal reflux in hiatal hernia. World J Surg 1977;1:439.
203. Rothenberg SS: Laparoscopic Nissen procedure in children. Semin Laparosc Surg 2002;9:146.
204. Rothstein RI, Filipi CJ: Endoscopic suturing for gastroesophageal reflux disease: Clinical outcome with the Bard EndoCinch. Gastrointest Endosc Clin North Am 2003; 13:89.
205. Rowen SJ, Gyepes MT: 'The trumpeting elephant' sign of gastroesophageal reflux. Radiology 1978;167:188.
206. Roy-Choudhung S, Ashcraft KW: Thal fundoplication for pediatric gastroesophageal reflux disease. Semin Pediatr Surg 1998;7:115.
207. Ruchelli E, Wenner W, Voytek T, et al: Severity of esophageal eosinophilia predicts response to conventional gastroesophageal reflux therapy. Pediatr Dev Pathol 1999;2:15.
208. Rudolph CD: Supraesophageal complications of gastroesophageal reflux in children: Challenges in diagnosis and treatment. Am J Med 2003;115(Suppl):150S.
209. Rudolph CD, Mazur LJ, Liptak GS, et al: Guidelines for evaluation and treatment of gastroesophageal reflux in infants and children. Recommendations of the North American Society for Pediatric Gastroenterology and Nutrition. J Pediatr Gastroenterol Nutr 2001;32(Suppl):S1.
210. Sacher P, Stauffer UG: The Herbst triad: Report of two cases. J Pediatr Surg 1990;25:1238.
211. Sachs G: Improving on PPI-based therapy of GERD. Eur J Gastroenterol Hepatol 2001;13(Suppl):S35.
212. Sampson LK, Georgeson KE, Royal SA: Laparoscopic gastric antroplasty in children with delayed gastric emptying and gastroesophageal reflux. J Pediatr Surg 1998; 33:282.
213. Sampson LK, Georgeson KE, Winters DC: Laparoscopic gastrostomy as an adjunctive procedure to laparoscopic fundoplication in children. Surg Endosc 1996;10:1106.
214. Sanudo JR, Domenech-Mateu JM: The laryngeal primordium and epithelial lamina: A new interpretation. J Anat 1990;171:207.
215. Schalamon J, Lindahl H, Saarikoski H, et al: Endoscopic follow-up in esophageal atresia—for how long is it necessary? J Pediatr Surg 2003;38:702.
216. Schier F: Indications for laparoscopic antireflux procedures in children. Semin Laparosc Surg 2002;9:139.
217. Scott RB, Ferreira C, Smith L, et al: Cisapride in pediatric gastroesophageal reflux. J Pediatr Gastroenterol Nutr 1997; 25:499.
218. Seibert JJ, Byrne WJ, Euler AR, et al: Gastroesophageal reflux—the acid test: Scintigraphy or the pH probe. AJR Am J Roentgenol 2001;140:1087.
219. Somppi E, Tammela O, Ruuska T, et al: Outcome of patients operated on for esophageal atresia: 30 years' experience. J Pediatr Surg 1998;33:1341.
220. Sondheimer J: Expanding the definition of GE reflux. J Pediatr Gastroenterol Nutr 2002;34:511.
221. Sondheimer JM: Continuous monitoring of distal esophageal pH: A diagnostic test for gastroesophageal reflux in infants. J Pediatr 1980;96:804.
222. Sondheimer JM, Morris BA: Gastroesophageal reflux among severely retarded children. J Pediatr 1979;94:710.
223. Spitz L, McLeod E: Gastroesophageal reflux. Semin Pediatr Surg 2003;12:237.
224. Stein MR: Possible mechanisms of influence of esophageal acid on airway hyperresponsiveness. Am J Med 2003; 115(Suppl):55S.
225. Steyaert H, Al Mohaidly M, Lembo MA, et al: Long-term outcome of laparoscopic Nissen and Toupet fundoplication in normal and neurologically impaired children. Surg Endosc 2003;17:543.
226. Sturdivant RA: Is gastrin the major regulator of lower esophageal sphincter pressure? Gastroenterology 1974; 67:551.
227. Sullivan PB: Gastrointestinal problems in the neurologically impaired child. Baillieres Clin Gastroenterol 1997;

11:529.
228. Sydorak RM, Albanese CT: Laparoscopic antireflux procedures in children: Evaluating the evidence. Semin Laparosc Surg 2002;9:133.
229. Takahashi T: Pathophysiological significance of neuronal nitric oxide synthase in the gastrointestinal tract. J Gastroenterol 2003;38:421.
230. Terry P, Lagergren J, Wolk A, et al: Reflux-inducing dietary factors and risk of adenocarcinoma of the esophagus and gastric cardia. Nutr Cancer 2000;38:186.
231. Thal AP: A modified approach to surgical problems of the esophagogastric portion. Ann Surg 1968;168:542.
232. Thomas EJ, Kumar R, Dasan JB, et al: Gastroesophageal reflux in asthmatic children not responding to asthma medication: A scintigraphic study in 126 patients with correlation between scintigraphic and clinical findings of reflux. Clin Imaging 2003;27:333.
233. Thompson DM: Laryngopharyngeal sensory testing and assessment of airway protection in pediatric patients. Am J Med 2003;115(Suppl):166S.
234. Todd JA, de Caestecker J, Jankowski J: Gastro-esophageal reflux disease and bile acids. J Pediatr Gastroenterol Nutr 2003;36:172.
235. Tolia V, Wuerth A, Thomas R: Gastroesophageal reflux disease: Review of presenting symptoms, evaluation, management, and outcomes in infants. Dig Dis Sci 2003; 48:1723.
236. Tougas G, Armstrong D: Efficacy of H_2 receptor antagonists in the treatment of gastroesophageal reflux disease and its symptoms. Can J Gastroenterol 1997;11:51B.
237. Toupet A: Technic of esophago-gastroplasty with phrenogastropexy used in radical treatment of hiatal hernia as a supplement to Heller's operation in cardiospasms. Mem Acad Chir (Paris) 1963;89:384.
238. Triadafilopoulos G: Stretta: An effective, minimally invasive treatment for gastroesophageal reflux disease. Am J Med 2003;115(Suppl):192S.
239. Tutuian R, Castell DO: Use of multichannel intraluminal impedance to document proximal esophageal and pharyngeal nonacidic reflux episodes. Am J Med 2003; 115(Suppl):119S.
240. Tutuian R, Vela MF, Shay SS: Multichannel intraluminal impedance in esophageal function testing and gastroesophageal reflux monitoring. J Clin Gastroenterol 2003; 37:206.
241. Vaezi MF, Richter JE: Duodenogastro-oesophageal reflux. Baillieres Best Pract Res Clin Gastroenterol 2000;14:719.
242. Vaezi MF, Richter JE: Duodenogastroesophageal reflux and methods to monitor nonacidic reflux. Am J Med 2001; 111(Suppl):160S.
243. Vaezi MF, Singh S, Richter JE: Role of acid and duodenogastric reflux in esophageal mucosal injury: A review of animal and human studies. Gastroenterology 1995; 108:1897.
244. Vandenplas Y: Reflux esophagitis in infants and children: A report from the working group on gastro-esophageal reflux disease of the European Society of Paediatric Gastroenterology and Nutrition. J Pediatr Gastroenterol Nurs 1994;18:413.
245. Vandenplas Y: Invited review: Asthma and gastroesophageal reflux. J Pediatr Gastroenterol Nutr 1997; 24:89.
246. Vandenplas Y: Diagnosis and treatment of gastroesophageal reflux disease in infants and children. Can J Gastroenterol 2000;14:26D.
247. Vandenplas Y, de Roy C, Sacre L: Cisapride decreases prolonged episodes of reflux in infants. J Pediatr Gastroenterol Nutr 1991;12:44.
248. Vandenplas Y, Goyvaerts H, Helven R, et al: Gastroesophageal reflux, as measured by 24-hour pH monitoring, in 509 healthy infants screened for risk of sudden infant death syndrome. Pediatrics 1991;88:834.
249. Vandenplas Y, Hassall E: Mechanisms of gastroesophageal reflux and gastroesophageal reflux disease. J Pediatr Gastroenterol Nutr 2002;35:119.
250. Vandenplas Y, Hegar B: Diagnosis and treatment of gastro-oesophageal reflux disease in infants and children. J Gastroenterol Hepatol 2000;15:593.
251. Vandenplas Y, Sacre-Smits L: Seventeen-hour continuous esophageal pH monitoring in the newborn: Evaluation of the influence of position in asymptomatic and symptomatic babies. J Pediatr Gastroenterol Nutr 1985;4:356.
252. van der Zee DC, Arendo NJ, Bax NM: The value of 24-hour pH study in evaluating the results of laparoscopic antireflux surgery in children. Surg Endosc 1999;13:918.
253. van der Zee DC, Bax KN, Ure BM, et al: Long-term results after laparoscopic Thal procedure in children. Semin Laparosc Surg 2002;9:168.
254. Vantrappen G, Texter EC Jr, Barborka CJ, et al: The closing mechanism at the gastroesophageal junction. Am J Med 1960;28:564.
255. Wadre GM, Lobe TE: Gastroesophageal reflux disease in neurologically impaired children: The role of the gastrostomy tube. Semin Laparosc Surg 2002;9:180.
256. Waring JP, Lacayo L, Hunter J, et al: Chronic cough and hoarseness in patients with severe gastroesophageal reflux disease: Diagnosis and therapy. Dig Dis Sci 1995;40:1093.
257. Watson DI, de Beaux AC: Complications of laparoscopic antireflux surgery. Surg Endosc 2001;15:344.
258. Weber TR:. Toupet fundoplication for gastroesophageal reflux disease. Semin Pediatr Surg 1998;7:121.
259. Wenzl TG, Moroder C, Trachterna M, et al: Esophageal pH monitoring and impedance measurement: A comparison of two diagnostic tests for gastroesophageal reflux. J Pediatr Gastroenterol Nutr 2002;34:519.
260. Wenzl TG, Schenke S, Peschgens T, et al: Association of apnea and nonacid gastroesophageal reflux in infants: Investigations with the intraluminal impedance technique. Pediatr Pulmonol 2001;31:144.
261. Winkelstein A: Peptic esophagitis: A new clinical entity. JAMA 1935;104:906.
262. Winter HS: Disorders of the Oesophagus. Philadelphia, WB Saunders, 1984.
263. Wolfe MM, Sachs G: Acid suppression: Optimizing therapy for gastroduodenal ulcer healing, gastroesophageal reflux disease, and stress-related erosive syndrome. Gastroenterology 2000;118(Suppl):S9.
264. Woodard-Knight L, Fudge A, Teubner J, et al: Aluminium absorption and antacid therapy in infancy. J Pediatr Child Health 1992;28:257.
265. Wu JC, Chan FK, Ching JY, et al: Effect of *Helicobacter pylori* eradication on treatment of gastro-oesophageal reflux disease: A double blind, placebo controlled, randomised trial. Gut 2004;53:174.
266. Yoshida Y, Tanaka Y, Hirano M, et al: Sensory innervation of the pharynx and larynx. Am J Med 2000;108(Suppl):51S.
267. Zaninotto G, DeMeester TR, Schwizer W, et al: The lower esophageal sphincter in health and disease. Am J Surg 1988;155:104.

268. Zaw-Tun HA: The tracheo-esophageal septum: Fact or fantasy? Origin and development of the respiratory primordium and esophagus. Acta Anat (Basel) 1982; 114:1.

269. Zwischenberger JB, Alpard SK, Orringer MB: Esophagus. In Townsend CM (ed): Sabiston Textbook of Surgery, 16th ed. Philadelphia, WB Saunders, 2001.

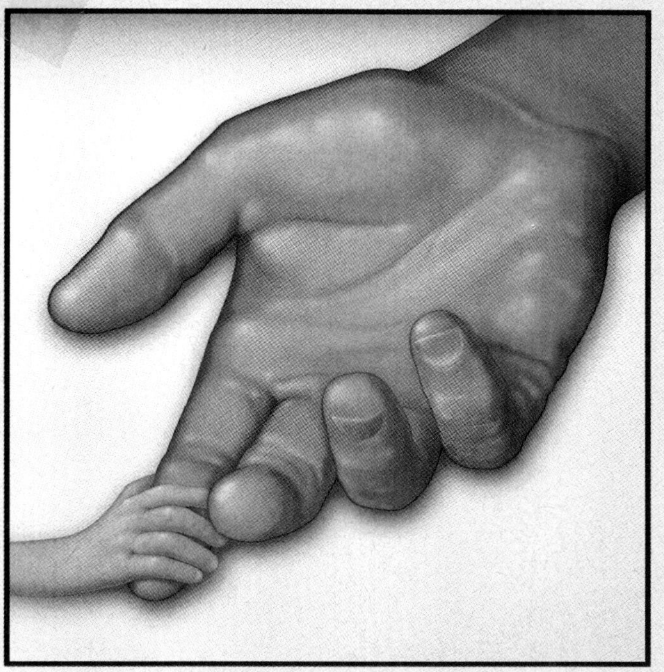

小儿外科学
Pediatric Surgery

（第6版·下卷）

注 意

在小儿外科领域中，医学相关知识和最佳实践都在不断进步。由于新的研究和临床经验在不断拓展我们的知识，在治疗和用药方面做出某种改变也许是必需或适宜的。建议读者核对本书所提供的：(1) 有关手术操作过程的最新信息；(2) 每种药品的生产厂商的最新产品信息，确认推荐剂量、服用方法与时间及相关的禁忌证。确定诊断、决定患者的最佳服药剂量和最佳治疗方式以及采取适当的安全预防措施是经治医师的责任，这有赖于他（她）们的个人经验和对每一位患者的了解。在法律允许的范围内，出版商和编著者对于因与本书所包含的资料相关而引起的任何人身损伤或财产损失，均不承担任何责任。

出版者

小儿外科学
Pediatric Surgery

（第 6 版·下卷）

主　　编　Jay L. Grosfeld
　　　　　James A. O'Neill, Jr.
　　　　　Eric W. Fonkalsrud
　　　　　Arnold G. Coran

主　　译　吴晔明

副 主 译　施诚仁　蔡　威　刘锦纷
　　　　　刘国华　董其刚

主译助理　顾　松

北京大学医学出版社
Peking University Medical Press

图书在版编目（CIP）数据

小儿外科学：第 6 版 /（美）格罗斯费尔德（Grosfeld，J. L.）等主编；吴晔明等译. — 北京：北京大学医学出版社，2008

书名原文：Pediatric Surgery: Sixth Edition

ISBN 978-7-81116-311-7

Ⅰ. 小… Ⅱ. ①格… ②吴… Ⅲ. 儿科学：外科学 Ⅳ. R726

中国版本图书馆 CIP 数据核字（2008）第 154800 号

北京市版权局著作权合同登记号：图字：01-2006-5583

Pediatric Surgery, 6th edition

Jay L. Grosfeld, James A. O'Neill, Jr., Eric W. Fonkalsrud and Arnold G. Coran

ISBN-13: 978-0-323-02842-4

ISBN-10: 0-323-02842-X

978-981-259-755-7

981-259-755-7

Elsevier (Singapore) Pte Ltd.

3 Killiney Road, #08-01 Winsland House I, Singapore 239519

Tel: (65) 6349-0200, Fax: (65) 6733-1817

First Published 2009

2009 年初版

小儿外科学

主　　译： 吴晔明

出版发行： 北京大学医学出版社（电话：010-82802230）

地　　址：（100191）北京市海淀区学院路 38 号 北京大学医学部院内

网　　址： http://www.pumpress.com.cn

E－mail： booksale@bjmu.edu.cn

印　　刷： 北京画中画印刷有限公司

经　　销： 新华书店

责任编辑： 马联华　李　娜　董彩萱　　**责任校对：** 杜　悦　　**责任印制：** 郭桂兰

开　　本： 889 mm × 1194 mm　1/16　**印张：** 75　**插页：** 2　**字数：** 2406 千字

版　　次： 2009 年 1 月第 1 版　2009 年 1 月第 1 次印刷

书　　号： ISBN 978-7-81116-311-7

定　　价： 760.00 元（上下卷）

编著者名单

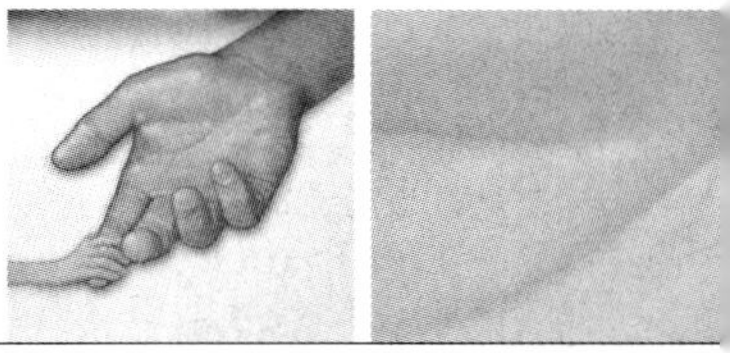

Mark C. Adams, MD, FAAP
Professor of Urology and Pediatrics, Vanderbilt University School of Medicine; Pediatric Urologist, Monroe Carell Jr. Children's Hospital at Vanderbilt, Nashville, Tennessee
Magaureter and Prune-Belly Syndrome

N. Scott Adzick, MD
C. Everett Koop Professor of Pediatric Surgery, University of Pennsylvania School of Medicine; Surgeon-in-Chief, The Children's Hospital of Philadelphia, Philadelphia, Pennsylvania
Cysts of the Lungs and Mediastinum

Craig T. Albanese, MD
Professor of Surgery, Pediatrics, and Obstetrics and Gynecology, and Chief, Division of Pediatric Surgery, Department of Surgery, Stanford Hospital & Clinics, Stanford; John A. and Cynthia Fry Gunn Director of Surgical Services, Lucile Packard Children's Hospital at Stanford, Palo Alto, California
Necrotizing Enterocolitis

Fred Alexander, MD
Associate Professor of Surgery, Cleveland Clinic Lerner School of Medicine of Case Western Reserve University; Staff Surgeon, Cleveland Clinic Foundation, Cleveland, Ohio
Crohn's Disease

R. Peter Altman, MD
Professor of Surgery, Columbia University College of Physicians and Surgeons; Surgeon-in-Chief, Morgan Stanley Children's Hospital of New York Presbyterian, New York, New York
The Jaundiced Infant: Biliary Atresia

Richard J. Andrassy, MD
Denton A. Cooley Professor and Chairman, Department of Surgery, University of Texas Medical School at Houston; Executive Vice President of Clinical Affairs and Associate Dean for Clinical Affairs, University of Texas at Houston, Houston, Texas
Rhabdomyosarcoma

Walter S. Andrews, MD
Professor of Surgery, University of Missouri–Kansas City School of Medicine; Director, Transplantation Program, Children's Mercy Hospital, Kansas City, Missouri
Gallbladder Disease and Hepatic Infections

Harry Applebaum, MD
Clinical Professor of Surgery, David Geffen School of Medicine at UCLA; Head, Division of Pediatric Surgery, Kaiser Permanente Medical Center, Los Angeles, California
Duodenal Atresia and Stenosis—Annular Pancreas

Marjorie J. Arca, MD
Assistant Professor of Surgery, Medical College of Wisconsin; Attending Surgeon, Children's Hospital of Wisconsin, Milwaukee, Wisconsin
Atresia, Stenosis, and Other Obstructions of the Colon

Robert M. Arensman, MD
Professor of Surgery, Louisiana State University School of Medicine; Attending Surgeon, Ochsner Clinic Foundation, New Orleans, Louisiana
Gastrointestinal Bleeding

James B. Atkinson, MD
Professor and Chief, Division of Pediatric Surgery, Department of Surgery, David Geffen School of Medicine at UCLA, Los Angeles, California
Liver Tumors

Richard G. Azizkhan, MD, PhD(Hon)
Professor of Surgery and Pediatrics, Lester Martin Chair of Pediatric Surgery, and Vice Chair, Department of Surgery, University of Cincinnati College of Medicine; Surgeon-in-Chief and Director, Division of Pediatric Surgery, Cincinnati Children's Hospital Medical Center, Cincinnati, Ohio
Teratomas and Other Germ Cell Tumors

Anwar Baban, MD
Laboratory of Molecular Genetics, Gaslini Children's Hospital, Genoa, Italy
Hirschsprung's Disease and Related Neuromuscular Disorders of the Intestine

Douglas C. Barnhart, MD, MSPH
Assistant Professor, Departments of Surgery and Pediatrics, University of Alabama at Birmingham School of Medicine; Attending Surgeon, The Children's Hospital of Alabama, Birmingham, Alabama
Biopsy Techniques for Children with Cancer

Robert H. Bartlett, MD
Professor of Surgery, University of Michigan Medical School, Ann Arbor, Michigan
Extracorporeal Life Support for Cardiopulmonary Failure

Laurence S. Baskin, MD
Professor of Urology, University of California, San Francisco, School of Medicine; Chief, Pediatric Urology, UCSF Children's Hospital at UCSF Medical Center, San Francisco, California
Hypospadias

Spencer W. Beasley, MB, ChB, MS
Clinical Professor of Pediatrics and Surgery, Christchurch School of Medicine and Health Sciences, University of Otago; Chief of Child Health Services, Division of Child Health, and Clinical Director, Paediatric Surgery, Christchurch Hospital, Christchurch, New Zealand
Torticollis

Michael L. Bentz, MD, FAAP, FACS
Professor of Surgery, Pediatrics, and Plastic Surgery, and Chairman, Division of Plastic Surgery, University of Wisconsin School of Medicine and Public Health; Chief of Plastic Surgery, University of Wisconsin Hospital and Clinics, Madison, Wisconsin
Hand, Soft Tissue, and Envenomation Injuries

Victor E. Boston, MD, FRCSI, FRCSEng, FRCSEd
Honorary Senior Lecturer, Department of Surgery, The Queen's University of Belfast Faculty of Medicine; The Royal Belfast Hospital for Sick Children, Belfast, Northern Ireland
Ureteral Duplication and Ureteroceles

Scott C. Boulanger, MD, PhD
Assistant Professor of Surgery, Division of Pediatric Surgery, University of Mississippi Medical Center School of Medicine, Jackson, Mississippi
Inguinal Hernias and Hydroceles

Edward L. Bove, MD
Professor of Surgery, University of Michigan Medical School; Head, Section of Cardiac Surgery, C.S. Mott Children's Hospital, Ann Arbor, Michigan
Congenital Heart Disease and Anomalies of the Great Vessels

Mary L. Brandt, MD
Professor and Vice Chair, Michael E. DeBakey Department of Surgery, Baylor College of Medicine, Texas Children's Hospital, Houston, Texas
Disorders of the Breast

John W. Brock III, MD
Professor of Urologic Surgery, Vanderbilt University School of Medicine; Director, Pediatric Urology, Vanderbilt Medical Center; Surgeon in Chief, Monroe Carell Jr. Children's Hospital at Vanderbilt, Nashville, Tennessee
Bladder Exstrophy

Rebeccah L. Brown, MD
Assistant Professor of Clinical Surgery and Pediatrics, University of Cincinnati College of Medicine; Associate Director of Trauma Services, Cincinnati Children's Hospital Medical Center, Cincinnati, Ohio
Genitourinary Tract Trauma

Marybeth Browne, MD
Surgical Resident, McGaw Medical Center of Northwestern University, Chicago, Illinois
Gastrointestinal Bleeding

Terry L. Buchmiller, MD
Formerly Assistant Professor of Surgery, Weill Medical College of Cornell University of New York, New York; Currently Assistant Professor of Surgery, Harvard Medical School; Assistant in Surgery, Children's Hospital Boston, Boston, Massachusetts
The Jaundiced Infant: Biliary Atresia

Ronald W. Busuttil, MD, PhD
Professor and Executive Chairman, Department of Surgery, David Geffen School of Medicine at UCLA; Chief, Division of Liver and Pancreas Transplantation, Dumont-UCLA Liver Cancer Center; Director, Pfleger Liver Institute, UCLA Medical Center, Los Angeles, California
Liver Transplantation

Michelle S. Caird, MD
Lecturer, Department of Orthopaedic Surgery, Alfred Taubman Health Care Center, University of Michigan, Ann Arbor, Michigan
Musculoskeletal Trauma

Anthony A. Caldamone, MD, FAAP
Professor of Surgery (Urology) and Pediatrics, Brown University School of Medicine; Chief of Pediatric Urology, Hasbro Children's Hospital, Providence, Rhode Island
Renal Infection, Abscess, Vesicoureteral Reflux, Urinary Lithiasis, and Renal Vein Thrombosis

Darrell A. Campbell, Jr., MD
Professor of Surgery, University of Michigan Medical School; Chief of Clinical Affairs, University of Michigan Health System, Ann Arbor, Michigan
Renal Transplantation

Donna A. Caniano, MD
Professor of Surgery and Pediatrics, The Ohio State University College of Medicine and Public Health; Surgeon-in-Chief, Children's Hospital, Columbus, Ohio
Ethical Considerations

Michael G. Caty, MD
Associate Professor of Surgery and Pediatrics, University at Buffalo School of Medicine and Biomedical Science; Surgeon-in-Chief, Women and Children's Hospital of Buffalo, Buffalo, New York
Adrenal Tumors

Dai H. Chung, MD
Associate Professor of Surgery and Pediatrics, The University of Texas Medical Branch School of Medicine at Galveston; Chief, Section of Pediatric Surgery, UTMB Children's Hospital, Galveston, Texas
Burns

Robert E. Cilley, MD
Professor of Surgery and Pediatrics, Penn State College of Medicine; Chief, Division of Pediatric Surgery, Milton S. Hershey Medical Center, Hershey, Pennsylvania
Disorders of the Umbilicus

Paul M. Colombani, MD
Professor of Surgery, Pediatrics, and Oncology, and Robert Garrett Professor of Surgery, Johns Hopkins University School of Medicine; Chief, Division of Pediatric Surgery, Johns Hopkins Medicine; Pediatric Surgeon-in-Charge, Johns Hopkins Hospital, Baltimore, Maryland
Surgical Implications Associated with Bone Marrow Transplantation

Joel D. Cooper, MD
Professor of Surgery, University of Pennsylvania School of Medicine; Chief, Division of Thoracic Surgery, Hospital of the University of Pennsylvania, Philadelphia, Pennsylvania
Lung Transplantation

Arnold G. Coran, MD
Professor of Pediatric Surgery, University of Michigan Medical School, Ann Arbor, Michigan
Nutritional Support; Congenital Anomalies of the Esophagus; Hirschsprung's Disease and Related Neuromuscular Disorders of the Intestine; Abnormalities of the Female Genital Tract

Robin T. Cotton, MD
Professor of Otolaryngology, University of Cincinnati School of Medicine; Director, Pediatric Otolaryngology–HNS, Cincinnati Children's Hospital Medical Center, Cincinnati, Ohio
Lesions of the Larynx, Trachea, and Upper Airway

Michael C. Dalsing, MD
Professor of Surgery and Director, Section of Vascular Surgery, Indiana University School of Medicine, Indianapolis, Indiana
Venous Disorders in Childhood

Alan Daneman, MBBCh, BSc, FRANZCR, FRCPC
Professor of Radiology, University of Toronto Faculty of Medicine; Staff Radiologist, Hospital for Sick Children, Toronto, Ontario, Canada
Intussusception

Andrew M. Davidoff, MD
Associate Professor, Department of Surgery and Pediatrics, University of Tennessee School of Medicine; Chief, Division of General Pediatric Surgery, St. Jude Children's Research Hospital, Memphis, Tennessee
Principles of Pediatric Oncology, Genetics of Cancer, and Radiation Therapy

Richard S. Davidson, MD
Associate Professor, University of Pennsylvania School of Medicine; Attending Surgeon, Children's Hospital of Philadelphia and Shrener's Hospital, Philadelphia
Musculoskeletal Trauma

Romano T. DeMarco, MD
Assistant Professor of Urologic Surgery, Division of Pediatric Urology, Vanderbilt University School of Medicine, Nashville, Tennessee
Bladder Exstrophy

Daniel A. DeUgarte, MD
Pediatric Surgery Fellow, University of Michigan Medical School and C.S. Mott Children's Hospital, Ann Arbor, Michigan
Liver Tumors

Eric Devaney, MD
Assistant Professor of Surgery, University of Michigan Medical School; Attending Surgeon, C.S. Mott Children's Hospital, Ann Arbor, Michigan
Congenital Heart Disease and Anomalies of the Great Vessels

William Didelot, MD
Professor of Pediatric Orthopaedics, Indiana University School of Medicine; Staff Surgeon, Riley Hospital for Children, Indianapolis, Indiana
Major Congenital Orthopedic Deformitites

John W. DiFiore, MD
Clinical Assistant Professor of Surgery, Case School of Medicine; Staff Pediatric Surgeon, Children's Hospital at Cleveland Clinic, Cleveland, Ohio
Respiratory Physiology and Care

Patrick A. Dillon, MD
Assistant Professor of Surgery, Washington University in St. Louis School of Medicine; Attending Surgeon, St. Louis Children's Hospital, St. Louis, Missouri
Gastrointestinal Tumors

Peter W. Dillon, MD
Professor of Surgery and Pediatrics, Penn State College of Medicine; Vice Chair, Department of Surgery, and Chief, Division of Pediatric Surgery, Penn State Children's Hospital, Hershey, Pennsylvania
Congenital Diaphragmatic Hernia and Eventration

Patricia K. Donahoe, MD
Marshall K. Bartlett Professor of Surgery, Harvard Medical School; Director, Pediatric Surgical Research Laboratories and Chief, Pediatric Surgical Services Emerita, Massachusetts General Hospital, Boston
Ambiguous Genitalia

James C. Y. Dunn, MD, PhD
Assistant Professor of Surgery, David Geffen School of Medicine at UCLA; Attending Surgeon, Mattel Children's Hospital at UCLA, Los Angeles, California
Appendicitis

Simon Eaton, BSc, PhD
Senior Lecturer in Pediatric Surgery and Metabolic Biochemistry, Department of Pediatric Surgery, Institute of Child Health, University College London, London, United Kingdom
Neonatal Physiology and Metabolic Considerations

Martin R. Eichelberger, MD
Professor of Surgery and Pediatrics, George Washington University School of Medicine and Health Sciences; Director, Emergency Trauma, Burn Service, and Senior Attending, Pediatric Surgery Service, Children's National Medical Center; President and CEO, Safe Kids Worldwide, Washington, DC
Accident Victims and Their Emergency Management

Sigmund H. Ein, MDCM, FRCSC, FAAP, FACS
Associate Professor of Surgery, Adjunct Clinical Faculty, Department of Surgery, University of Toronto Faculty of Medicine; Honorary Staff Surgeon, Division of General Surgery, The Hospital for Sick Children, Toronto; Courtesy Staff, Department of Surgery, Lakeridge Health Corporation, Oshawa, Ontario, Canada
Intussusception

Carolyn Ells, RTT, PhD
Assistant Professor of Medicine, McGill University Faculty of Medicine; Clinical Ethicist, Sir Mortimer B. Davis Jewish General Hospital, Montreal, Quebec, Canada
Ethical Considerations

Barry L. Eppley, MD, DMD
Professor of Plastic Surgery, Indiana University School of Medicine, Indianapolis, Indiana
Cleft Lip and Palate

Mary E. Fallat, MD
Professor of Surgery, and Director, Division of Pediatric Surgery, University of Louisville; Chief of Surgery, Kosdir Children's Hospital, Louisville, Kentucky
Ovarian Tumors

Diana L. Farmer, MD
Professor of Clinical Surgery, Pediatrics and Obstetrics, Gynecology, and Reproductive Medicine, University of California, San Francisco, School of Medicine; Surgeon-in-Chief, UCSF Children's Hospital, San Francisco, California
Cysts of the Lungs and Mediastinum

Douglas G. Farmer, MD
Associate Professor of Surgery, David Geffen School of Medicine at UCLA; Director, Intestinal Transplantation, Dumont-UCLA Transplant Center, Los Angeles, California
Liver Transplantation; Intestinal Transplantation

Steven J. Fishman, MD
Professor of Surgery, Harvard University Medical School; Senior Associate in Surgery, Children's Hospital Boston, Boston, Massachusetts
Vascular Anomalies: Hemangiomas and Malformations

Alan W. Flake, MD
Professor of Surgery and Obstetrics and Gynecology, University of Pennsylvania School of Medicine; Director, Children's Institute for Surgical Science, The Children's Hospital of Philadelphia, Philadelphia, Pennsylvania
Molecular Clinical Genetics and Gene Therapy

Robert P. Foglia, MD
Associate Professor of Surgery and Division Chief, Pediatric Surgery, Washington University in St. Louis School of Medicine; Surgeon-in-Chief, St. Louis Children's Hospital, St. Louis, Missouri
Gastrointestinal Tumors

Eric W. Fonkalsrud, MD
Professor of Surgery, David Geffen School of Medicine at UCLA; Emeritus Chief of Pediatric Surgery, UCLA Medical Center, Los Angeles, California
Ulcerative Colitis; Lymphatic Disorders

Henri R. Ford, MD
Vice-Chair and Visiting Professor of Surgery, Keck School of Medicine of USC; Surgeon-in-Chief and Vice President, Surgery, and Medical Director, Burtie Green Bettingen Surgery Center, Children's Hospital Los Angeles, Los Angeles, California
Sepsis and Related Considerations

Stephanie M. P. Fuller, MD
Clinical Fellow, Division of Cardiothoracic Surgery, The Children's Hospital of Philadelphia and Thomas Jefferson University Hospital, Philadelphia, Pennsylvania
Heart Transplantation

Victor F. Garcia, MD
Professor of Surgery, University of Cincinnati College of Medicine; Director of Trauma Services, Cincinnati Children's Hospital Medical Center, Cincinnati, Ohio
Genitourinary Tract Trauma; Bariatric Surgery in Adolescents

John M. Gatti, MD
Assistant Professor of Surgery and Urology, University of Missouri–Kansas City School of Medicine; Director of Minimally Invasive Urology, Children's Mercy Hospital of Kansas City, Kansas City, Missouri
Abnormalities of the Urethra, Penis, and Scrotum

Michael W. L. Gauderer, MD
Professor of Surgery and Pediatrics (Greenville), University of South Carolina School of Medicine, Columbia; Adjunct Professor of Bioengineering, Clemson University, Clemson; Chief, Division of Pediatric Surgery, Children's Hospital, Greenville Hospital System, Greenville, South Carolina
Stomas of the Small and Large Intestine

James D. Geiger, MD
Associate Professor of Surgery, University of Michigan Medical School; Staff Surgeon, C.S. Mott Children's Hospital, Ann Arbor, Michigan
Biopsy Techniques for Children with Cancer

Keith E. Georgeson, MD
Professor of Surgery, University of Alabama at Birmingham School of Medicine; Chief of Pediatric Surgery, The Children's Hospital of Alabama, Birmingham, Alabama
Gastroesophageal Reflux Disease

Cynthia A. Gingalewski, MD
Assistant Professor of Surgery and Pediatrics, George Washington University School of Medicine and Health Science; Pediatric Surgeon, Children's National Medical Center, Washington, DC
Other Causes of Intestinal Obstruction

Kenneth I. Glassberg, MD
Professor of Urology, Columbia University College of Physicians and Surgeons; Director, Division of Pediatric Urology, Morgan Stanley Children's Hospital of New York–Presbyterian, New York, New York
Renal Agenesis, Dysplasia, and Cystic Disease

Philip L. Glick, MD, MBA
Professor of Surgery, Pediatrics, and Obstetrics and Gynecology, University of Buffalo School of Medicine and Biomedical Sciences; Executive Director, Miniature Access Surgery Center (MASC), Women and Children's Hospital of Buffalo, Buffalo, New York
Inguinal Hernias and Hydroceles

Sherilyn A. Gordon, MD
Assistant Professor of Surgery, Division of Liver and Pancreas Transplantation, David Geffen School of Medicine at UCLA, Los Angeles, California
Intestinal Transplantation

Tracy C. Grikscheit, MD
Senior Fellow in Pediatric Surgery, Children's Hospital and Regional Medical Center and University of Washington School of Medicine, Seattle, Washington
The Impact of Tissue Engineering in Pediatric Surgery

Jay L. Grosfeld, MD
Lafayette Page Professor of Pediatric Surgery Emeritus, Indiana University School of Medicine; Surgeon-in-Chief Emeritus, Riley Hospital for Children, Indianapolis, Indiana
Neuroblastoma; Jejunoileal Atresia and Stenosis; Abnormalities of the Female Genital Tract

Angelika C. Gruessner, MS, PhD
Associate Professor of Surgical Science, University of Minnesota Medical School, Minneapolis, Minnesota
Pancreas and Islet Cell Transplantation

Rainer W. G. Gruessner
Professor of Surgery, University of Minnesota Medical School, Minneapolis, Minnesota
Pancreas and Islet Cell Transplantation

Philip C. Guzzetta, Jr., MD
Professor of Surgery and Pediatrics, George Washington University School of Medicine and Health Sciences; Interim Chief of Pediatric Surgery, Children's National Medical Center, Washington, DC
Nonmalignant Tumors of the Liver

Carroll M. Harmon, MD, PhD,
Associate Professor of Surgery, University of Alabama at Birmingham School of Medicine; Attending Surgeon, Children's Hospital, Birmingham, Alabama
Congenital Anomalies of the Esophagus

Michael R. Harrison, MD
Professor of Surgery, Pediatrics, and Obstetrics, Gynecology, and Reproductive Sciences, University of California, San Francisco, School of Medicine; Director, Fetal Treatment Center, UCSF Children's Hospital and Medical Center, San Francisco, California
The Fetus as a Patient

Andrea A. Hayes-Jordan, MD
Assistant Professor of Surgery and Pediatrics, University of Texas Medical School at Houston and M.D. Anderson Cancer Center; Pediatric Surgeon, Memorial Hermann Children's Hospital and M.D. Anderson Cancer Center, Houston, Texas
Lymph Node Disorders

Stephen R. Hays, MD, MS, FAAP
Assistant Professor of Anesthesiology and Pediatrics, Vanderbilt University School of Medicine; Director, Pediatric Pain Services, Vanderbilt Children's Hospital, Nashville, Tennessee
Pediatric Anesthesia

John H. Healey, MD
Professor of Orthopaedic Surgery, Weill Medical College of Cornell University; Chief of Orthopaedic Surgery, Memorial Sloan-Kettering Cancer Center, New York, New York
Bone Tumors

W. Hardy Hendren III, MD, FACS, FAAP, FRCS (Irel&Engl), FRCPS(Glasgow), DSc(Drexel), MD(HonCausa) Université Aix Marseilles
Robert E. Gross Distinguished Professor of Surgery, Harvard Medical School; Chief of Surgery Emeritus, Children's Hospital Boston; Honorary Surgeon, Massachusetts General Hospital, Boston, Massachusetts
Megaureter and Prune-Belly Syndrome

Bernhard J. Hering, MD
Assistant Professor of Surgery, University of Minnesota Medical School; Associate Director, Diabetes Institute for Immunology and Transplantation, University of Minnesota Medical Center, Fairview, Minneapolis, Minnesota
Pancreas and Islet Cell Tranplantation

David N. Herndon, MD
Professor of Surgery and Pediatrics and Jesse H. Jones Distinguished Chair in Burn Surgery, University of Texas Medical Branch School of Medicine at Galveston; Chief of Staff and Director of Research, Shriners Burns Hospital, Galveston, Texas
Burns

Ronald B. Hirschl, MD
Professor of Surgery, University of Michigan Medical School; Head, Section of Pediatric Surgery, and Surgeon-in-Chief, C.S. Mott Children's Hospital, Ann Arbor, Michigan
Extracorporeal Life Support for Cardiopulmonary Failure

George W. Holcomb III, MD, MBA
Katharine Berry Richardson Professor of Surgery, University of Missouri–Kansas City School of Medicine; Surgeon-in-Chief, Children's Mercy Hospital, Kansas City, Missouri
Gallbladder Disease amd Hepatic Infections

Charles B. Huddleston, MD
Professor of Surgery, Washington University in St. Louis School of Medicine; Chief, Pediatric Cardiothoracic Surgery, and Surgical Director, Lung Transplant Program, St. Louis Children's Hospital, St. Louis, Missouri
Lung Transplantation

Raymond J. Hutchinson, MS, MD
Professor of Pediatrics, University of Michigan Medical School; Director of Clinical Services, Pediatric Hematology/Oncology, C.S. Mott Children's Hospital, Ann Arbor, Michigan
Surgical Implications of Hematologic Disease

John M. Hutson, MD(Monash), MD(Melb), FRACS, FAAP(Hon)
Professor of Pediatric Surgery, Department of Pediatrics, University of Melbourne Faculty of Medicine, Melbourne; Director of General Surgery, Royal Children's Hospital, Parkville, Victoria, Australia
Undescended Testis, Torsion, and Varicocele

Thomas Inge, MD, PhD
Associate Professor of Surgery and Pediatrics, University of Cincinnati College of Medicine; Surgical Director, Comprehensive Weight Management Program, Cincinnati Children's Hospital Medical Center, Cincinnati
Bariatric Surgery in Adolescents

Vincenzo Jasonni, MD
Professor of Pediatric Surgery, University of Genoa Medical School; Surgeon-in-Chief and Chair of Pediatric Surgery, Gaslini Children's Hospital, Genoa, Italy
Hirschsprung's Disease and Related Neuromuscular Disorders of the Intestine

Nishwan Jibri, MD
Department of Pediatric Surgery, Gaslini Children's Hospital, Genoa, Italy
Hirschsprung's Disease and Related Neuromuscular Disorders of the Intestine

Byron D. Joyner, MD
Associate Professor of Urology, University of Washington School of Medicine; Residency Director, University of Washington Urology Program, and Faculty/Staff, Children's Hospital and Regional Medical Center, Seattle, Washington
Ureteropelvic Junction Obstruction

Martin Kaefer, MD
Associate Professor, Department of Urology, Indiana University School of Medicine; Pediatric Urologist, Riley Children's Hospital, Indianapolis, Indiana
Disorders of Bladder Function

Henry K. Kawamoto, Jr., MD, DDS
Clinical Professor of Surgery, Department of Surgery, Division of Plastic Surgery, David Geffen School of Medicine at UCLA; Director, Craniofacial Surgery, UCLA Medical Center, Los Angeles, California
Craniofacial Anomalies

Robert M. Kay, MD
Associate Professor of Orthopedic Surgery, Keck School of Medicine of USC; Orthopedic Surgeon, Children's Hospital Los Angeles, Los Angeles, California
Bone and Joint Infections

Kosmas Kayes, MD
Staff Surgeon, Riley Hospital for Children and St. Vincent Children's Hospital, Indianapolis, Indiana
Major Congenital Orthopedic Deformities

Mark L. Kayton, MD
Assistant Member, Memorial Sloan-Kettering Cancer Center; Assistant Attending Surgeon, Division of Pediatric Surgery, Memorial Hospital, New York, New York
Surgical Implications Associated with Bone Marrow Transplantation

Robert E. Kelly, Jr., MD, FACS, FAAP
Associate Professor of Clinical Surgery and Pediatrics, Eastern Virginia Medical School, Children's Hospital of the King's Daughters, Norfolk, Virginia
The Nuss Procedure for Pectus Excavatum [Chapter 59]

Stephen S. Kim, MD
Assistant Professor of Surgery, University of Washington School of Medicine; Attending, Division of Pediatric Surgery, Children's Hospital and Regional Medical Center, Seattle, Washington
Necrotizing Enterocolitis

Michael D. Klein, MD
Arvin I. Philippart Chair and Professor of Surgery, Wayne State University School of Medicine; Surgeon-in-Chief, Children's Hospital of Michigan, Detroit, Michigan
Congenital Defects of the Abdominal Wall

Giannoula Klement, MD
Instructor in Pediatrics (Hematology-Oncology), Harvard University Medical School; Assistant in Pediatrics, Children's Hospital Boston, Boston, Massachusetts
Vascular Anomalies: Hemangiomas and Malformations

Matthew J. Krasin, MD
Assistant Member and Radiation Oncologist, St. Jude Children's Research Hospital, Memphis, Tennessee
Principles of Pediatric Oncology, Genetics of Cancer, and Radiation Therapy

Thomas M. Krummel, MD, FACS
Professor in Surgery, Stanford University School of Medicine; Service Chief, Surgery, Stanford Hospital & Clinics, Stanford; Susan B. Ford Surgeon-in-Chief, Lucile Packard Children's Hospital at Stanford, Palo Alto, California
New and Emerging Surgical Technologies and the Process of Innovation

Jean-Martin Laberge, MD, FRCSC, FACS
Professor of Surgery, McGill University Faculty of Medicine; Director, Division of Pediatric General Surgery, The Montreal Children's Hospital, Montreal, Quebec, Canada
Infections and Diseases of the Lungs, Pleura, and Mediastinum

Ira S. Landsman, MD
Associate Professor of Anesthesiology and Pediatrics, Vanderbilt University School of Medicine; Director, Division of Pediatric Anesthesia, Vanderbilt Children's Hospital, Nashville, Tennessee
Pediatric Anesthesia

Michael P. La Quaglia, MD
Professor of Surgery, Weill Medical College of Cornell University; Chief, Pediatric Surgical Service, Memorial Sloan-Kettering Cancer Center, New York, New York
Hodgkin's Disease and Non-Hodgkin's Lymphoma

Stanley T. Lau, MD
Pediatric Surgery Fellow, Women and Children's Hospital of Buffalo, Buffalo, New York
Adrenal Tumors

Steven L. Lee, MD
Regional Pediatric Surgeon, Kaiser Permanente, Los Angeles Medical Center, Los Angeles, California
Duodenal Atresia and Stenosis—Annular Pancreas

Joseph L. Lelli, Jr., MD
Assistant Professor of Surgery, Wayne State Medical School; Pediatric Surgeon, The Children's Hospital of Michigan, Detroit, Michigan
Polypoid Diseases of the Gastrointestinal Tract

Marc A. Levitt, MD
Assistant Professor of Surgery and Pediatrics, University of Cincinnati College of Medicine; Associate Director, Colorectal Center for Children, Cincinnati Children's Hospital Medical Center, Cincinnati, Ohio
Anorectal Malformations

Harry Lindahl, MD, PhD
Lecturer in Pediatrics, University of Helsinki School of Medicine; Chief of Pediatric Surgery, Hospital for Children and Adolescents, Helsinki; University Central Hospital, Helsinki, Finland
Esophagoscopy and Diagnostic Techniques

Thom E. Lobe, MD
Professor of Surgery and Pediatrics, University of Tennessee School of Medicine, Memphis, Tennessee; Pediatric Surgeon, Blank Children's Hospital, Des Moines, Iowa
Other Soft Tissue Tumors

Randall T. Loder, MD
Garceau Professor of Orthopaedic Surgery, Indiana University School of Medicine; Director of Pediatric Orthopaedics, Riley Hospital for Children, Indianapolis, Indiana
Amputations in Children

Thomas G. Luerssen, MD
Professor of Neurological Surgery, Indiana University School of Medicine; Chief, Pediatric Neurosurgery Service, Riley Hospital for Children, Indianapolis, Indiana
Central Nervous System Injuries

Jeffrey R. Lukish, MD
Associate Professor of Surgery and Pediatrics, Uniformed Services University of the Health Sciences F. Edward Hébert School of Medicine, Bethesda, Maryland; Chief, Division of Pediatric Surgery, and Attending Pediatric Surgeon, The National Naval Medical Center and Walter Reed Army Medical Center, Washington, DC
Accident Victims and Their Emergency Management

Dennis P. Lund, MD
Chairman, Division of General Surgery, University of Wisconsin-Madison, and Surgeon-in-Chief, UW Children's Hospital, Madison, Wisconsin
Alimentary Tract Duplications

Mary Beth Madonna, MD
Assistant Professor of Surgery, Northwestern University Feinberg School of Medicine; Attending Surgeon, Children's Memorial Hospital and John H. Stroger, Jr. Hospital of Cook County, Chicago, Illinois
Gastrointestinal Bleeding

John C. Magee, MD
Associate Professor of Surgery, University of Michigan Medical School; Director, Adult and Pediatric Renal Transplantation, and Director, Pediatric Liver Transplantation, University of Michigan Health System, Ann Arbor, Michigan
Renal Transplantation

Giuseppe Martucciello, MD
Associate Professor of Pediatric Surgery, Faculty of Medicine, University of Genoa, Genoa, and University of Pavia, Pavia; Director, and Surgeon-in-Chief, Department of Pediatric Surgery, IRCCS Scientific Institute Policlinico San Matteo, Pavia, Italy
Hirschsprung's Disease and Related Neuromuscular Disorders of the Intestine

Stephen J. Mathes, MD
Professor of Surgery and Head, Division of Plastic and Reconstructive Surgery, University of California, San Francisco, School of Medicine, San Francisco, California
Congenital Defects of the Skin, Connective Tissues, Muscles, Tendons, and Hands

Eugene D. McGahren III, MD
Associate Professor of Surgery and Pediatrics, University of Virginia School of Medicine; Pediatric Surgeon, University of Virginia Health System, Charlottesville, Virginia
Laryngoscopy, Bronchoscopy, and Thoracoscopy; Ascites

Leslie T. McQuiston, MD, FAAP
Staff Pediatric Urologist, Urology Associates of North Texas, Cook Children's Hospital, Fort Worth, Texas
Renal Infection, Abscess, Vesicoureteral Reflux, Urinary Lithiasis, and Renal Vein Thrombosis

Peter Metcalfe, MD, FRCSC
Pediatric Urology Fellow, Indiana University School of Medicine and Riley Hospital for Children, Indianapolis, Indiana
Incontinent and Continent Urinary Diversion

Alastair J. W. Millar, MBChB(Cape Town), FRCS, FRACS, FCS(SA), DCh
Honorary Professor, Paediatric Transplantation and Hepatopancreaticobiliary Surgery, University of Birmingham; Consultant, Paediatric Liver and Intestinal Transplantation and Hepatopancreaticobiliary Surgery, Birmingham Children's Hospital, Birmingham, United Kingdom
Caustic Strictures of the Esophagus

Eugene Minevich, MD, FACS, FAAP
Assistant Professor of Surgery, Cincinnati Children's Hospital Medical Center, Cincinnati, Ohio
Structural Disorders of the Bladder, Augmentation

Edward P. Miranda, MD
Professor of Surgery, Division of Plastic Surgery, University of California, San Francisco, School of Medicine, San Francisco, California
Congenital Defects of the Skin, Connective Tissues, Muscles, Tendons, and Hands

Michael E. Mitchell, MD
Professor of Urology, University of Washington School of Medicine; Chief, Pediatric Urology, Children's Hospital and Regional Medical Center, Seattle, Washington
Ureteropelvic Junction Obstruction

Takeshi Miyano, MD, PhD
Professor, Department of Pediatric Surgery, Juntendo University School of Medicine; Director, Juntendo University Hospital, Tokyo, Japan
The Pancreas

Delora Mount, MD, FACS, FAAP
Assistant Professor of Surgery and Pediatrics, University of Wisconsin School of Medicine and Public Health; Chief of Pediatric Plastic Surgery, University of Wisconsin Hospital and Clinics; Director, Craniofacial Anomalies Clinic, American Family Children's Hospital, Madison, Wisconsin
Hand, Soft Tissue, and Envenomation Injuries

Pierre Mouriquand, MD
Professor of Pediatric Urology, Claude-Bernard University Medical School; Head, Department of Pediatric Urology, Debrousse Hospital, Lyon, France
Renal Fusions and Ectopia

Noriko Murase, MD
Associate Professor of Surgery, University of Pittsburgh School of Medicine, Pittsburgh, Pennsylvania
Principles of Transplantation

J. Patrick Murphy, MD
Professor of Surgery, University of Missouri–Kansas City School of Medicine; Chief, Urology Section, Children's Mercy Hospital of Kansas City, Kansas City, Missouri
Abnormalities of the Urethra, Penis, and Scrotum

Saminathan S. Nathan, MD
Director, Musculoskeletal Oncology Service, Department of Orthopaedics, National University Hospital, Singapore, Singapore
Bone Tumors

Kurt D. Newman, MD
Professor of Surgery and Pediatrics, George Washington University School of Medicine and Health Sciences; Surgeon-in-Chief, Children's National Medical Center; Executive Director, Joseph E. Robert, Jr. Center for Surgical Care, Washington, DC
Lymph Node Disorders

Alp Numanoglu, MD, FCS(SA)
Senior Lecturer in Paediatric Surgery, University of Cape Town School of Child and Adolescent Health; Senior Specialist, Department of Paediatric Surgery, Red Cross Children's Hospital, Institute of Child Health, Cape Town, South Africa
Caustic Strictures of the Esophagus

Donald Nuss, MB, ChB, FRCS(C), FACS, FAAP
Professor of Clinical Surgery and Pediatrics, Eastern Virginia Medical School; Children's Hospital of the King's Daughters, Norfolk, Virginia
The Nuss Procedure for Pectus Excavatum [Chapter 59]

Richard Ohye, MD
Assistant Professor of Surgery, University of Michigan Medical School; Surgical Director, Pediatric Cardiac Transplantation, and Director, Pediatric Cardiovascular Surgery Fellowship Program, C.S. Mott Children's Hospital, Ann Arbor, Michigan
Congenital Heart Disease and Anomalies of the Great Vessels

Keith T. Oldham, MD
Professor of Surgery, Medical College of Wisconsin; Surgeon-in-Chief, Children's Hospital of Wisconsin, Milwaukee, Wisconsin
Atresia, Stenosis, and Other Obstructions of the Colon

James A. O'Neill, Jr., MD, MA(Hon)
J.C. Foshee Professor and Chairman Emeritus, Section of Surgical Sciences, Vanderbilt University School of Medicine; Surgeon-in-Chief Emeritus, Vanderbilt University Medical Center, Nashville, Tennessee
Choledochal Cyst; Bladder and Cloacal Exstrophy; Conjoined Twins; Arterial Disorders

Evelyn Ong, MBBS, BSc, FRCS(Eng)
Joint Royal College of Surgeons of England/British Association of Paediatric Surgeons Research Fellow; Department of Paediatric Surgery, Institute of Child Health, University College London; Clinical Research Fellow, Great Ormond Street Hospital for Children NHS Trust, London, United Kingdom
Neonatal Physiology and Metabolic Considerations

William L. Oppenheim, MD
Professor of Orthopedic Surgery, David Geffen School of Medicine at UCLA; Director of Pediatric Orthopedics, UCLA Medical Center; Consultant, Shriners Hospital of Los Angeles, Los Angeles, California
Bone and Joint Infections

H. Biemann Othersen, Jr., MD
Professor of Surgery and Pediatrics and Emeritus Head, Division of Pediatric Surgery, Medical University of South Carolina College of Medicine; Attending Surgeon, MUSC Children's Hospital, Charleston, South Carolina
Wilms' Tumor

Mikki Pakarinen, MD, PhD
Consultant Pediatric Surgeon, Hospital for Children and Adolescents, University of Helsinki Medical Faculty, Helsinki, Finland
Other Disorders of the Anus and Rectum, Anorectal Function

Keshav Pandurangi, MD
Vascular Surgery Fellow, Indiana University School of Medicine, Indianapolis, Indiana
Venous Disorders in Childhood

Richard H. Pearl, MD, FACS, FAAP, FRCSC
Professor of Surgery and Pediatrics,University of Illinois College of Medicine at Peoria; Surgeon-in-Chief, Children's Hospital of Illinois, Peoria, Illinois
Abdominal Trauma

Alberto Peña, MD
Professor of Surgery and Pediatrics, University of Cincinnati College of Medicine; Director, Colorectal Center for Children, Cincinnati Children's Hospital Medical Center, Cincinnati, Ohio
Anorectal Malformations

Rafael V. Pieretti, MD
Chief, Section of Pediatric Urology, Department of Pediatric Surgery, Massachusetts General Hospital, Boston, Massachusetts
Ambiguous Genitalia

Agostino Pierro, MD, FRCS(Eng), FRCS(Ed), FAAP
Nuffield Professor of Paediatric Surgery and Head of Surgery Unit, Institute of Child Health, University College London; Consultant Paediatric Surgeon, Great Ormand Street Hospital for Children NHS Trust, London, United Kingdom
Neonatal Physiology and Metabolic Considerations

William P. Potsic, MD, MMM
Professor of Otorhinolaryngology–Head and Neck Surgery, University of Pennsylvania School of Medicine; Director, Division of Otolaryngology, and Vice Chair for Clinical Affairs, The Children's Hospital of Philadelphia, Philadelphia, Pennsylvania
Otolaryngologic Disorders

Pramod S. Puligandla, MD, MSc, FRCSC
Assistant Professor of Surgery and Pediatrics, McGill University Faculty of Medicine; Attending Staff, Division of Pediatric Surgery and Pediatric Critical Care Medicine, The Montreal Children's Hospital of the McGill University Health Center, Montreal, Quebec, Canada
Infections and Diseases of the Lungs, Pleura, and Medistinum

Devin P. Puapong, MD
Senior Surgical Resident, Kaiser Permanente Medical Center, Los Angeles,California
Duodenal Atresia and Stenosis—Annular Pancreas

Prem Puri, MS, FRCS, FRCS(Edin), FACS
Professor of Paediatrics, University College Dublin; Consultant Paediatric Surgeon and Director of Research, Children's Research Centre, Our Lady's Hospital for Sick Children, Crumlin, Dublin, Ireland
Intestinal Neuronal Dysplasia

Judson G. Randolph, MD
Professor of Surgery Emeritus, George Washington University School of Medicine and Health Sciences; Former Surgeon-in-Chief, Children's National Medical Center, Washington, DC
A Brief History of Pediatric Surgery

Frederick J. Rescorla, MD
Professor of Surgery, Indiana University School of Medicine; Surgeon-in-Chief, Riley Hospital for Children, Indianapolis, Indiana
The Spleen

Jorge Reyes, MD
Professor of Surgery, University of Washington School of Medicine; Chief, Division of Transplant Surgery, University of Washington Medical Center, Seattle, Washington
Principles of Transplantation

Richard R. Ricketts, MD
Professor of Surgery, Emory University School of Medicine; Chief, Division of Pediatric Surgery, Children's Health Care of Atlanta at Egleston, Atlanta, Georgia
Mesenteric and Omental Cysts

Richard C. Rink, MD
Robert A. Garrett Professor of Pediatric Urologic Research and Professor of Urology, Indiana University School of Medicine; Chief, Pediatric Urology, Riley Hospital for Children, Indianapolis, Indiana
Incontinent and Continent Urinary Diversion

Risto J. Rintala, MD
Professor of Pediatric Surgery, University of Helsinki Medical Faculty; Chief, General Pediatric Surgery, Hospital for Children and Adolescents, Helsinki, Finland
Other Disorders of the Anus and Rectum, Anorectal Function

Albert P. Rocchini, MD
Professor of Pediatrics and Director of Pediatrics Cardiology, University of Michigan Redical School; Director of Pediatric Cardiology, University of Michigan Hospital, Ann Arbor
Neonatal Cardiovascular Physiology and Care

Heinz Rode, M Med(Chir), FCS(SA), FRCS(Edin)
Professor of Paediatric Surgery, University of Cape Town School of Child and Adolescent Health; Head of Pediatric Surgery, Red Cross Children's Hospital, Institute of Child Health, Cape Town, South Africa
Caustic Strictures of the Esophagus

Bradley M. Rodgers, MD
Professor of Surgery and Pediatrics, University of Virginia School of Medicine; Chief, Division of Pediatric Surgery, Department of Surgery, University of Virginia Medical Center; Chief, Children's Surgery, UVA Children's Hospital, Charlottesville, Virginia
Laryngoscopy, Bronchoscopy, and Thoracoscopy

A. Michael Sadove MD, MS
James Harbaugh Professor of Surgery (Plastic), Indiana University School of Medicine; Chief of Plastic Surgery, Riley Hospital for Children, Indianapolis; Chairman of Surgery, Clarian North Medical Center, Carmel, Indiana
Cleft Lip and Palate

Bob H. Saggi, MD
Assistant Professor of Surgery, Department of Surgery, Division of Immunology and Organ Transplantation, University of Texas Medical School at Houston; Staff Surgeon, Memorial Hermann Hospital, Houston, Texas
Liver Transplantation

Arthur P. Sanford, MD
Assistant Professor of Surgery, The University of Texas Medical Branch School of Medicine at Galveston; Staff Physician, Shriners Burns Hospital, Galveston, Texas
Burns

L. R. Scherer III, MD
Associate Professor of Clinical Medicine, Indiana University School of Medicine; Director of Trauma, Riley Hospital for Children, Indianapolis, Indiana
Peptic Ulcer and Other Conditions of the Stomach

Jay J. Schnitzer, MD, PhD
Associate Professor of Surgery, Harvard Medical School; Associate Visiting Surgeon, Massachusetts General Hospital, Boston, Massachusetts
Ambiguous Genitalia

Marshall Z. Schwartz, MD
Professor of Surgery and Pediatrics, Drexel University College of Medicine; Director, Pediatric Surgery Research Laboratory, and Surgical Director, Pediatric Renal Transplantation, St. Christopher's Hospital for Children, Philadelphia, Pennsylvania
Hypertrophic Pyloric Stenosis

Robert C. Shamberger, MD
Robert E. Gross Professor of Surgery, Harvard Medical School; Chief, Department of Surgery, Children's Hospital Boston, Boston, Massachusetts
Congenital Chest Wall Deformities

Nina L. Shapiro, MD
Associate Professor of Surgery/Pediatric Otolaryngology, David Geffen School of Medicine at UCLA; Attending Surgeon, UCLA Medical Center, Los Angeles, California
Salivary Glands

Curtis A. Sheldon, MD
Professor, University of Cincinnati College of Medicine; Professor and Director (Pediatric Urology), Cincinnati Children's Hospital Medical Center, Cincinnati, Ohio
Structural Disorders of the Bladder, Augmentation

Stephen J. Shochat, MD
Professor of Surgery and Pediatrics, University of Tennessee School of Medicine; Surgeon-in-Chief and Chairman, Department of Surgery, St. Jude Children's Research Hospital, Memphis, Tennessee
Tumors of the Lung

Michael A. Skinner, MD
Associate Professor of Surgery and Pediatric Surgery, Duke University School of Medicine, Durham, North Carolina
Surgical Diseases of the Thyroid and Parathyroid Glands

C. D. Smith, MD, MS
Associate Professor of Surgery and Pediatrics, Medical University of South Carolina College of Medicine; Attending, Division of Pediatric Surgery, MUSC Medical Center, Charleston, South Carolina
Cysts and Sinuses of the Neck

Jodi L. Smith, MD, PhD
Assistant Professor of Neurological Surgery, Department of Neurological Surgery, Indiana University School of Medicine; Pediatric Neurosurgeon, Riley Hospital for Children, Indianapolis, Indiana
Management of Neural Tube Defects, Hydrocephalus, Refractory Epilepsy, and Central Nervous System Infections

Samuel D. Smith, MD
Professor of Surgery, University of Arkansas for Medical Sciences College of Medicine; Chief of Pediatric Surgery, Arkansas Children's Hospital, Little Rock, Arkansas
Disorders of Intestinal Rotation and Fixation

Charles L. Snyder, MD
Associate Professor of Surgery, University of Missouri–Kansas City School of Medicine, Kansas City, Missouri; Clinical Assistant Professor of Surgery, University of Kansas School of Medicine, Kansas City, Kansas; Director of Clinical Research, The Children's Mercy Hospital, Kansas City, Missouri
Meckel's Diverticulum

Lewis Spitz, MBChB, MD(Hon), PhD, FRCS, FRCPCH, FAAP(Hon), FCS(SA)(Hon)
Emeritus Nuffield Professor of Pediatric Surgery, Institute of Child Health, University College London; Consultant Paediatric Surgeon, Great Ormond Street Hospital, London, United Kingdom
Esophageal Replacement

Thomas L. Spray, MD
Professor of Surgery, University of Pennsylvania School of Medicine; Chief, Division of Cardiothoracic Surgery, and Alice Langdon Warner Endowed Chair in Pediatric Cardiothoracic Surgery, The Children's Hospital of Philadelphia, Philadelphia, Pennsylvania
Heart Transplantation

Thomas E. Starzl, MD, PhD
Distinguished Service Professor of Surgery, University of Pittsburgh School of Medicine; Director Emeritus, Thomas E. Starzl Transplantation Institute, Pittsburgh, Pennsylvania
Principles of Transplantation

Charles J. H. Stolar, MD
Professor of Surgery and Pediatrics, Columbia University College of Physicians and Surgeons; Chief, Pediatric Surgery, Morgan Stanley Children's Hospital of New York–Presbyterian, New York, New York
Congenital Diaphragmatic Hernia and Eventration

Phillip B. Storm, MD
Assistant Professor of Neurosurgery, University of Pennsylvania School of Medicine; Attending Neurosurgeon, Hospital of the University of Pennsylvania and The Children's Hospital of Philadelphia, Philadelphia, Pennsylvania
Brain Tumors

Steven Stylianos, MD
Professor of Surgery, University of Miami Leonard M. Miller School of Medicine; Chief, Department of Pediatric Surgery, Miami Children's Hospital, Miami, Florida
Abdominal Trauma

Wendy T. Su, MD
Fellow, Pediatric Surgical Service, Memorial Sloan-Kettering Cancer Center, New York, New York
Hodgkin's Disease and Non-Hodgkin's Lymphoma

Riccardo Superina, MD, CM, FRCSC, FACS
Professor of Surgery, Northwestern University, Director, Transplant Surgery, Children's Memoral Hospital, Chicago, Illinois
Portal Hypertension

David E. R. Sutherland, MD, PhD
Professor of Surgery, University of Minnesota Medical School; Head, Transplant Division, and Director, Diabetes Institute for Immunology and Transplantation, University of Minnesota Medical Center, Fairview, Minneapolis, Minnesota
Pancreas and Islet Cell Transplantation

Leslie N. Sutton, MD
Professor of Neurosurgery, University of Pennsylvania School of Medicine; Chairman, Division of Pediatric Neurosurgery, The Children's Hospital of Philadelphia, Philadelphia, Pennsylvania
Brain Tumors

Edward P. Tagge, MD
Professor of Surgery and Pediatrics, Division of Pediatric Surgery, Medical University of South Carolina College of Medicine; Attending Surgeon, MUSC Children's Hospital, Charleston, South Carolina
Wilms' Tumor

Daniel H. Teitelbaum, MD
Professor of Surgery, University of Michigan Medical School; Pediatric Surgeon, C.S. Mott Children's Hospital, Ann Arbor, Michigan
Nutritional Support; Hirschsprung's Disease and Related Neuromuscular Disorders of the Intestine

Claire L. Templeman, MD
Assistant Professor of Clinical Gynecology and Surgery, Keck School of Medicine at USC; Pediatric Surgeon, Children's Hospital Los Angeles, Los Angeles, California
Ovarian Tumors

Gonca Topuzlu Tekant, MD
Associate Professor of Pediatric Surgery, Istanbul University School of Medicine; Pediatric Surgeon, Cerrahpasa Medical Faculty, Istanbul, Turkey
Gastroesophageal Reflux Disease

Joseph J. Tepas III, MD
Professor of Surgery and Pediatrics, University of Florida College of Medicine; Staff Physician, Shands Jacksonville, Jacksonville, Florida
Vascular Injuries

Patrick B. Thomas, MD
Pediatric Surgery Fellow, Texas Children's Hospital, Baylor College of Medicine, Houston, Texas
Wilms' Tumor

Dana Mara Thompson, MD, MS
Associate Professor of Otorhinolaryngology, Mayo Graduate School of Medicine; Attending, Otorhinolaryngology Department, Mayo Clinic, Rochester, Minnesota
Lesions of the Larynx, Trachea, and Upper Airway

Juan A. Tovar, MD, PhD
Professor of Surgical Pediatrics, Department of Pediatrics, Universidad Autonoma de Madrid; Head, Department of Pediatric Surgery, Hospital Universitario LaPaz, Madrid, Spain
Disorders of Esophageal Function

Jeffrey S. Upperman, MD, MA
Assistant Professor of Surgery, Keck School of Medicine of USC; Attending Surgeon, Children's Hospital Los Angeles, Los Angeles, California
Sepsis and Related Considerations

Joseph P. Vacanti, MD
John Homans Professor of Surgery, Harvard Medical School; Chief, Pediatric Surgery, Massachusetts General Hospital, Boston, Massachusetts
The Impact of Tissue Engineering in Pediatric Surgery

Dennis W. Vane, MD, MS, MBA
Professor of Surgery, University of Vermont College of Medicine; Chair, Pediatric Surgery, and Vice-Chair, Clinical Affairs, Department of Surgery, Fletcher Allen Health Care, Burlington, Vermont
Child Abuse and Birth Injuries

Mirjana Vustar, MD
Assistant Professor of Anesthesiology and Pediatrics, Vanderbilt University School of Medicine; Director, Pediatric Anesthesia Education, Vanderbilt Children's Hospital, Nashville, Tennessee
Pediatric Anesthesia

Brad W. Warner, MD
Professor of Surgery and Pediatrics, University of Cincinnati College of Medicine; Attending Surgeon and Director of Surgical Research, Division of Pediatric General and Thoracic Surgery, Cincinnati Children's Hospital Medical Center, Cincinnati, Ohio
Short-Bowel Syndrome

Thomas R. Weber, MD
Professor of Surgery, Saint Louis University School of Medicine; Director, Pediatric Surgery, Cardinal Glennon Children's Hospital, St. Louis, Missouri
Esophageal Rupture and Perforation

David E. Wesson, MD
Professor of Surgery and Chief, Division of Pediatric Surgery, Baylor College of Medicine; Chief, Pediatric Surgery Service, Texas Children's Hospital, Houston, Texas
Thoracic Injuries

Karen W. West, MD
Professor of Surgery, Indiana University School of Medicine; Director of ECMO, Riley Hospital for Children, Indianapolis, Indiana
Primary Peritonitis

Ralph F. Wetmore, MD
Professor of Otorhinolaryngology–Head and Neck Surgery, University of Pennsylvania School of Medicine; Senior Surgeon, The Children's Hospital of Philadelphia, Philadelphia, Pennsylvania
Otolaryngologic Disorders

Eugene Wiener, MD
Professor, Department of Surgery (Pediatric), University of Pittsburgh School of Medicine; Executive Vice President and Chief Medical Officer, Children's Hospital of Pittsburgh, Pittsburgh, Pennsylvania
Testicular Tumors

Jay M. Wilson, MD
Associate Professor of Surgery, Harvard Medical School; Attending, Children's Hospital Boston, Boston, Massachusetts
Respiratory Physiology and Care

Russell K. Woo, MD
Instructor in Surgery, Department of Surgery, Stanford University School of Medicine; Staff Physician, Stanford Hospital and Clinic, Stanford, and Lucile Packard Children's Hospital at Stanford, Palo Alto, California
New and Emerging Surgical Technologies and the Process of Innovation

Hsi-Yang Wu, MD
Assistant Professor of Urology, University of Pittsburgh School of Medicine; Director of Pediatric Urology Research, Children's Hospital of Pittsburgh, Pittsburgh, Pennsylvania
Testicular Tumors

Elizabeth Yerkes, MD
Assistant Professor of Urology, Feinberg School of Medicine at Northwestern University; Attending Urologist, Children's Memorial Hospital, Chicago, Illinois
Incontinent and Continent Urinary Diversion

Daniel G. Young, MBChB, FRCS(Edin, Glasg), DTM&H
Honorary Senior Research Fellow, University of Glasgow; Former Head (Retired), Department of Surgical Pediatrics, Royal Hospital for Sick Children, Glasgow, United Kingdom
A Brief History of Pediatric Surgery

Moritz M. Ziegler, MD
Professor of Surgery, Division of Pediatric Surgery, University of Colorado School of Medicine; Surgeon-in-Chief, The Children's Hospital, Denver, Colorado
Meconium Ileus

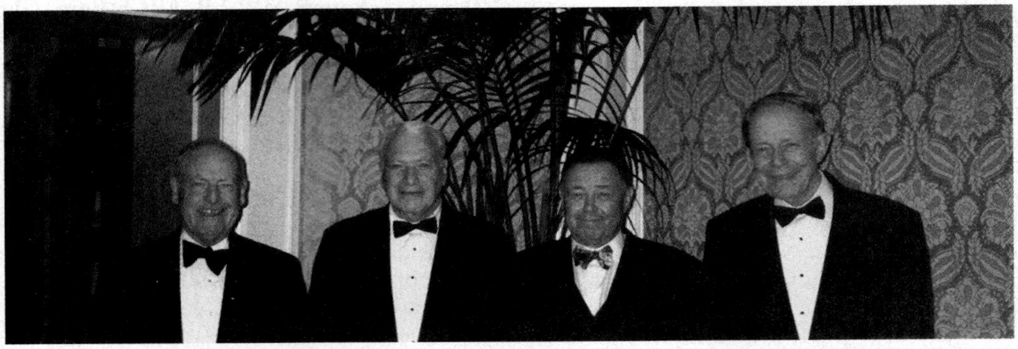

主编（从左到右）：James A. O’Neill, Jr.、Jay L. Grosfeld、Arnold G. Coran 和 Eric W. Fonkalsrud。

译校者名单

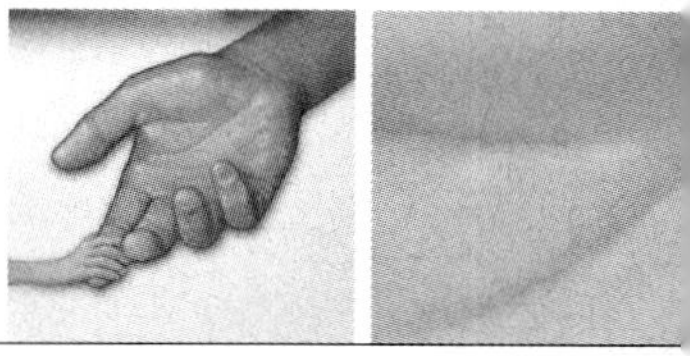

主　译

吴晔明　上海交通大学医学院附属上海儿童医学中心

副主译

施诚仁　上海交通大学医学院附属新华医院
蔡　威　上海交通大学医学院附属新华医院
刘锦纷　上海交通大学医学院附属上海儿童医学中心
刘国华　上海交通大学医学院附属上海第一人民医院
董其刚　上海交通大学医学院附属新华医院

主译助理

顾　松　上海交通大学医学院附属上海儿童医学中心

译校者（按姓氏笔画排序）

重庆医科大学附属儿童医院　王　珊
南京医科大学附属南京市儿童医院　王　浩
郑州大学第一附属医院　文建国
天津市儿童医院　叶祖萍
复旦大学附属儿科医院　吕志葆
苏州大学附属儿童医院　朱锦祥
上海交通大学医学院附属上海第一人民医院　刘国华
上海交通大学医学院附属瑞金医院　许　恩
宁夏医学院附属医院　杜　勇
北京首都儿科研究所　李　龙
浙江大学医学院附属儿童医院　李民驹
安徽省立医院　李巍松
苏州大学附属儿童医院　汪　健

首都医科大学附属北京儿童医院 陈永卫
湖南省儿童医院 周小渔
上海交通大学医学院附属上海第一人民医院 金惠明
广州市儿童医院 夏慧敏

上海交通大学医学院附属新华医院

沈涤华 陈锡民 周 莹 赵 黎 施诚仁 董其刚 蔡 威 潘伟华

上海交通大学医学院附属上海儿童医学中心

王 伟 王 俊 王宇鹏 王耀平 叶启东 刘锦纷 孙 杰 孙彦隽
严志龙 李 菁 吴晔明 何 蓉 张 震 张瑞冬 陈 盛 陈其民
胡 明 赵海腾 洪 莉 顾 松 顾 硕 徐 敏 徐建民 黄 萍
葛翼华 褚 珺 鲍 南

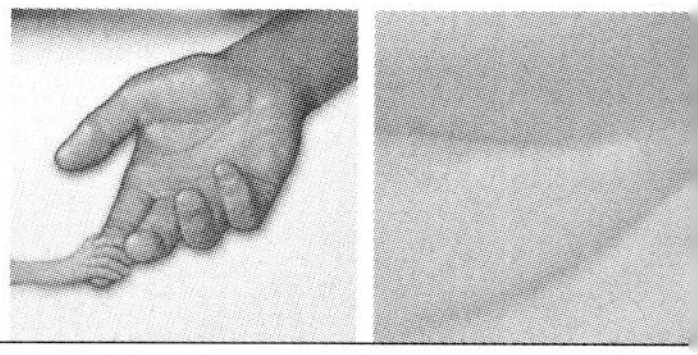

中文版序言

我国对应用科学的发展一向是主张“古为今用、洋为中用”，对医学的发展更是如此。国际上现代小儿外科学基本上是以 Ladd 和 Gross 的观点为主线的体系。小儿外科学在世界各国均有发展，而美国仍然是小儿外科学发展的前沿中心。我国小儿外科起步较晚，受时代背景的影响，创建了具有中国特色的小儿外科，并且在一个有 13 亿人口的发展中大国做出了令人瞩目的成绩。

回顾过去有利于未来。1950 年，我国始建小儿外科。其时正值西方国家对我国实行孤立与封锁。我国小儿外科的四位主要开创者从不同渠道间接引进了 Gross 观点：马安权毕业于圣约翰大学，使用英语渠道；佘亚雄毕业于震旦大学，用法语；童尔昌毕业于同济大学，用德语；我毕业于国立上海医学院，也用英语。四人分别在不同风格的医院通过实践开创了小儿外科。虽然基本观点仍是 Gross 体系，但是思路更宽。1960 年后又有李正等人留苏回国，带来了一些苏联的观点。难得的是，这一代人又都接受过系统的中医学补课教育。这样在多元化学术基础上，结合国情，融入自己的经验，形成了现时的中国小儿外科体系。

改革开放以后，我国小儿外科学书刊的出版空前繁荣，并且都反映了我国的特色。通过各种形式的国际交流，我国的小儿外科学在国际上也取得了一定地位。然而，作为占世界人口 1/4 的、有五千多年文明史的大国，在新的信息时代，随着经济发展，应该有责任也有能力为人类做出更大的贡献。我们小儿外科同道首先需要进一步提高我国小儿外科学水平，与国际先进学术接轨；还应该融入更多的中医精华，创立一个崭新的小儿外科学，作为 21 世纪对全世界儿童的献礼。因此当前需要的是充分、广泛、深入了解国际小儿外科学的体系和动态。

我国小儿外科队伍庞大，分布地域辽阔，水平参差不齐，对国际信息的获取很大程度上仍有语言和经济方面的障碍。上世纪 60 年代初，马安权曾组织翻译了 1953 年版《Gross 小儿外科学》。因为当时经济困难，只摘译出版了前半部。以后因国内十年动乱、盲目排外等等，再无一人出面问津。今天吴晔明教授主译本书正是填补空缺，将为我国小儿外科学界了解美国和国际学术体系提供很大便利。我国小儿外科能在贫困中以惊人的速度发展并壮大，这种精神已经闻名世界，有这本书出版，更将如虎添翼。

本书英文原版在国际上颇具盛名，已是第 6 次更新再版。本书译者校者都是我国当代小儿外科学界的精英，在小儿外科领域都有各自的专长造诣，并且都曾在国外学习，多次参加国际交流。相信本书译本质量必有保障，当为中国小儿外科一项时代硕果。我们国家提出“自主创新”，必先了解世界，了解历史。这部国际经典巨著正是一个理想的参考资料。我为本书的出版干杯。

张金哲

2008 年 2 月 23 日

中国工程院院士

小儿外科学教授

首都医科大学附属北京儿童医院

译者前言

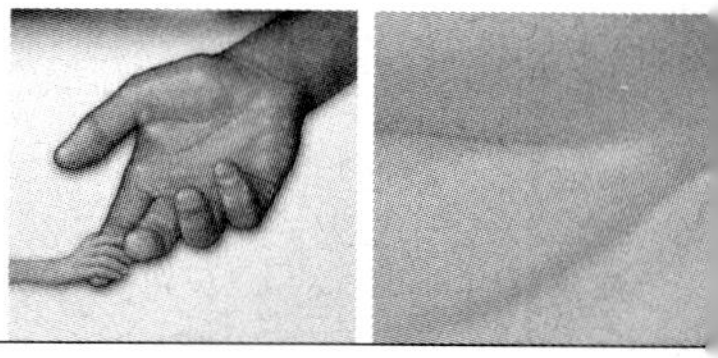

《小儿外科学》自1962年第1版出版以来，一直都是国际小儿外科界公认的最权威的经典教科书之一。该书因其为小儿外科领域内容最全面、与临床技术进步同步而深受小儿外科同行的推崇。四十多年来，该书先后出版了6版。在相隔8年后，这本最新的第6版在第5版的基础上，增加了大量的最新理论和临床新技术，极具参考价值。

由于《小儿外科学原则》一书的成功翻译和出版，我受北京大学医学出版社委托，翻译《小儿外科学》第6版。面对如此繁重和艰巨的任务，深感能力不足，一度动摇，后来在上海儿童医学中心全体小儿外科同仁的鼓励和支持下，我鼓起勇气承接了翻译任务。这一工作还得到了施诚仁老师、蔡威学兄的支持，也得到了我的同仁刘锦纷教授的支持，还获得了师长董其刚、刘国华教授的帮助；本书的翻译和校对工作也获得了来自全国各地的、近年来活跃于小儿外科领域的中青年专家的支持和协助，在此对他们表示衷心的感谢，他们是：浙江大学医学院附属儿童医院李民驹教授；天津市儿童医院叶祖萍教授；苏州大学附属儿童医院朱锦祥教授；复旦大学附属儿科医院吕志葆教授；苏州大学附属儿童医院汪健教授；首都医科大学附属北京儿童医院陈永卫教授；首都儿科研究所李龙教授；郑州大学第一附属医院文建国教授；广州市儿童医院夏慧敏教授；湖南省儿童医院周小渔教授；重庆医科大学附属儿童医院王珊教授。没有他们的帮助，本书的翻译和校对工作将更为困难。

我特别要感谢我的同事顾松博士，他为翻译稿的整理、校对、译校者的联系及出版事务做了大量工作。

希望本书的出版有助于我国小儿外科的普及和发展，并成为广大小儿外科专科医生的常用工具书之一。大多数译校者都是利用工作之余完成此项任务，由于时间较为仓促，在翻译和审校中难免存在错误之处，敬请批评指正，以便在再版中得以改正。

吴晔明

2008年1月21日

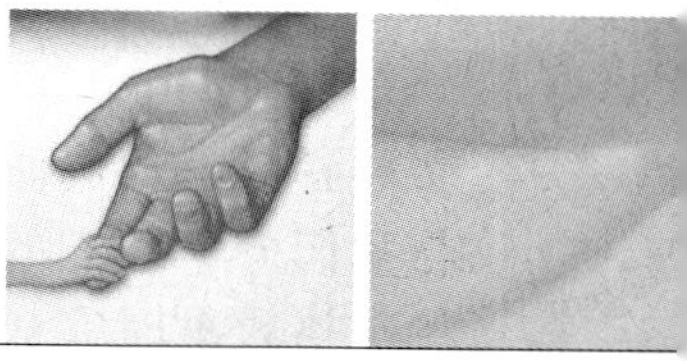

著者前言

《小儿外科学》第 1 版是 1962 年由医学年鉴出版社出版的，编委会由 Kenneth Welch、William Mustard、 Mark Ravitch、Clifford Benson 和 William Snyder 五位医生组成。其目的是为了满足小儿外科的总体工作需要，重点是放在普外、胸外和泌尿外科这些传统领域上。这本内容全面的教科书融入了众多著者的辛勤劳动，自第 1 版出版后，本书又先后出版了 4 版。44 年来各版一直是小儿外科领域中最好的世界闻名的综合性图书。

自 1998 年第 5 版出版以来又过去了 8 年。在这期间，我们经历了一场真正意义上的新的科学信息爆炸，其特征是人类基因组解读、组织工程发展和其他对诊断和如何处理病人已产生明确影响的新技术的引进。

本书第 6 版包含 133 章，拥有国际视角，著者来自美国、加拿大、欧洲、亚洲、澳大利亚、新西兰和非洲。主编者的目的是使本书融入各位专家各自感兴趣领域的重要或独特的经验，以便所有章节都遵循同一个目标：作为当代综合性和权威性教科书，提供可参考使用和实用的信息。本书第 6 版的写作还有很多新作者和共同作者参加。在新加的章节中有一章是小儿外科学简史，描述了英国、美国和亚洲小儿外科专业发展的简要背景。其他新的章节包括：临床分子遗传学和基因治疗、组织工程对小儿外科学的影响、先进而新兴的外科技术和创新历程、儿科肿瘤学 / 遗传学和放射治疗原理、小肠移植以及青春期肥胖治疗。

其他所有章节也都进行了大量修改和更新，并根据大量的最新参考文献进行了扩展。如胎儿作为患者的最新进展；先天性胸壁畸形，包括有关 Nuss 手术的最新信息；小儿麻醉；伦理学和法律问题；先天性巨结肠的遗传学；短肠综合征的新信息（即分期手术）；并且在适当的章节，将微创外科技术（腹腔镜、胸腔镜）融入其中。

第 6 版还包含其他重要修改和更新。第Ⅰ部分：新生儿生理学和代谢问题、呼吸生理学和监护、新生儿心血管生理学和护理、心肺衰竭的体外生命支持、脓毒症及相关问题、血液病和营养。第Ⅱ部分：创伤（包括烧伤护理）。第Ⅲ部分：儿童的主要肿瘤。第Ⅳ部分：器官移植（肝、肺、心脏、胰、肾和骨髓移植的外科含意），这部分也根据最新护理技术和结果的新指南和信息进行了重新组织和更新。第Ⅴ部分：累及头颈部的疾病。第Ⅵ部分：胸部疾病（包括食管闭锁和食管气管瘘以及其他各种食管病变、肺囊肿、先天性膈疝）；第Ⅶ部分：常见的先天性和获得性腹部疾病（包括疝、腹壁缺损、肠闭锁、胎粪性肠梗阻、先天性巨结肠、肛门直肠畸形、肠重复畸形、炎症性肠道疾病、胆道闭锁、胆总管囊肿、胰腺疾病、脾脏、门脉高压和其他）；第Ⅷ部分：泌尿生殖系统疾病；第Ⅸ部分：特殊的小儿外科疾病（联体儿、先天性心脏病、手和软组织、骨科、神经系统和血管疾病）。很多章节有很好的图解，并大量使用了图表、影像学、大体病理照片和组织学照片以及手术操作图示。

第 6 版的编委会由 Jay L. Grosfeld、James A. O'Neill Jr.、Eric W. Fonkalsrud 和 Arnold G. Coran 组成。这四位医生也是第 5 版编委会的成员。最初各章节的编写是由四位主编平均负责的。很高兴，Anthony A. Caldamone 医生作为第Ⅷ部分泌尿生殖系统疾病副主编，Grosfeld 医生作为编委会的主席和总编，成为整部手稿的最终审核者。《小儿外科学》第 6 版承袭的编辑标准承蒙我们之前的本书前 5 版的编辑所设立。

还要感谢我们的行政助理和秘书 Karen Jaeger、Donna Bock、Gale Fielding、Cheryl Peterson 和 Carol Simmons，他们除了完成日常工作外，还自愿帮助我们完成这一著作。没有他们的帮助，这一工作很难完成，非常感谢他们对本书的贡献。我们还要向来自世界各地的、在第 6 版的准备工作中做出重要贡献的众多著者表示我们诚挚的赞赏和感谢，感谢他们主动与我们分享他们的知识和经验，并能按照教科书的特殊格式准时完成写作，使我们能在限定时间内出版本书。

我们还要感谢 Elsevier/Mosby 的出版团队，感谢他们在第 6 版的准备和出版中保持高标准的支持和合作。我们感谢高级发展编辑 Janice Gaillard 女士和文字编辑 Faith Voit 为本书的编辑所做的贡献；感谢出版部主任 Judith Fletcher 和高级项目经理 Linda Grigg 女士为本书的整个出版过程所做的贡献。

本书主编者的照片摄于 2005 年 4 月，是在美国外科学会的一次会议期间。编者们将编写《小儿外科学》第 6 版视作他们钟爱的一项工作，我们希望这本教科书能成为从事小儿外科临床工作的医生、接受培训的医生以及其他对婴幼儿感兴趣的专业人员的专业参考书。我们希望这本教科书可成为有益于全世界遭受外科疾病困扰的儿童的一种知识资源。

主编

（吴晔明译）

目 录

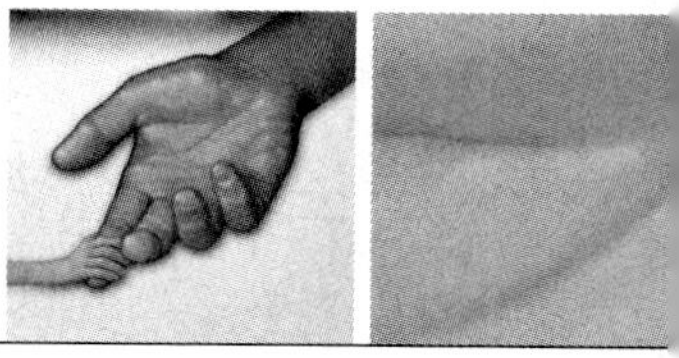

上 卷

下 卷

彩　图

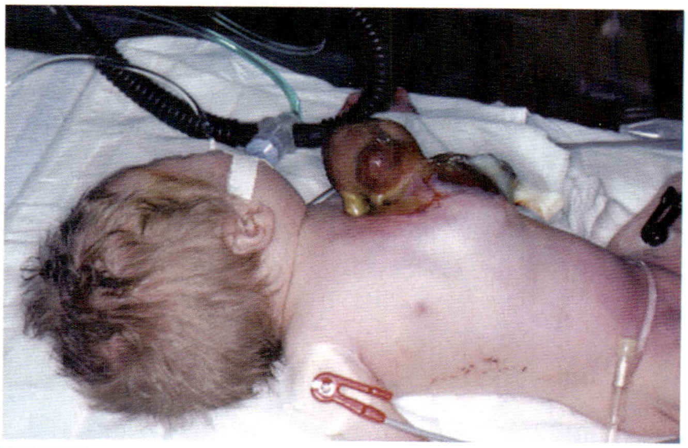

图 73-2 异位心。

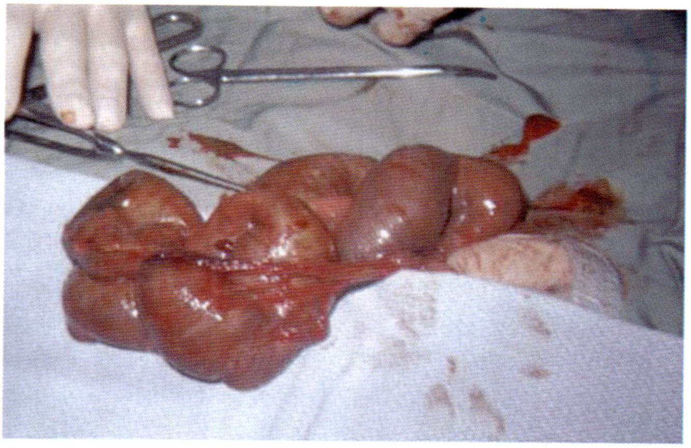

C

图 80-5 C. 剖腹手术中发现肠扭转及复杂性胎粪性肠梗阻引起的多发性肠闭锁。该婴儿患有囊性纤维化。

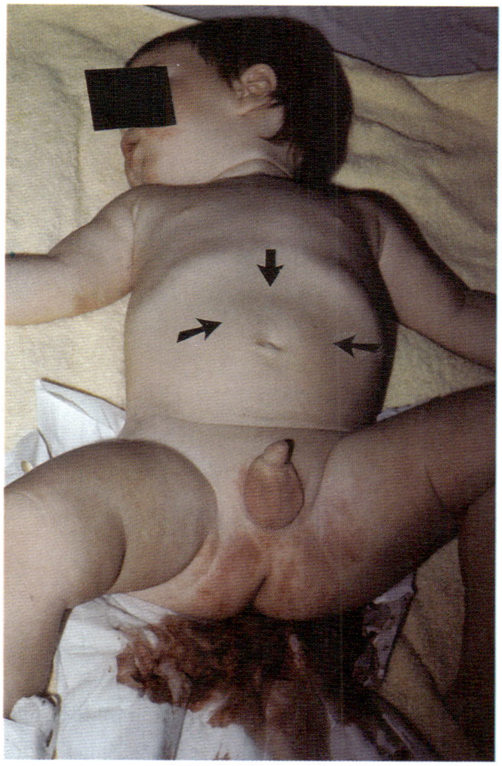

图 83-4 一名苍白、昏睡的肠套迭患儿以及典型的果酱样便。注意上腹部肿块（箭头）。

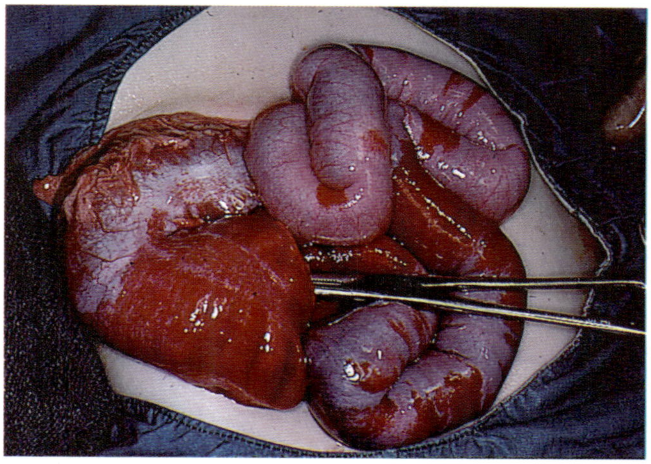

图 83-24 未完全复位的回结型肠套迭。盲肠和升结肠充血肿胀。注意部分复位、充血但有活力的末端回肠。

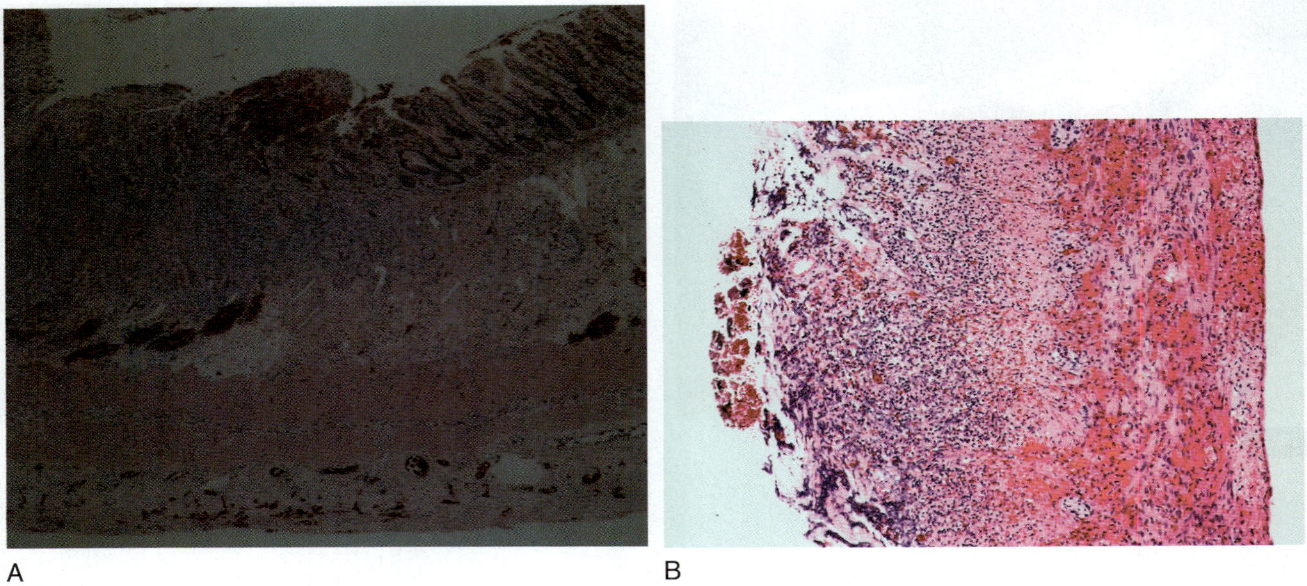

图 92–1 A. 组织切片显示早期坏死性小肠结肠炎有黏膜下炎症和肠壁囊样积气症（苏木精伊红染色 × 150）。B. 组织切片显示进展期坏死性小肠结肠炎有透壁性坏死以及绒毛和隐窝结构消失（苏木精伊红染色 × 150）。

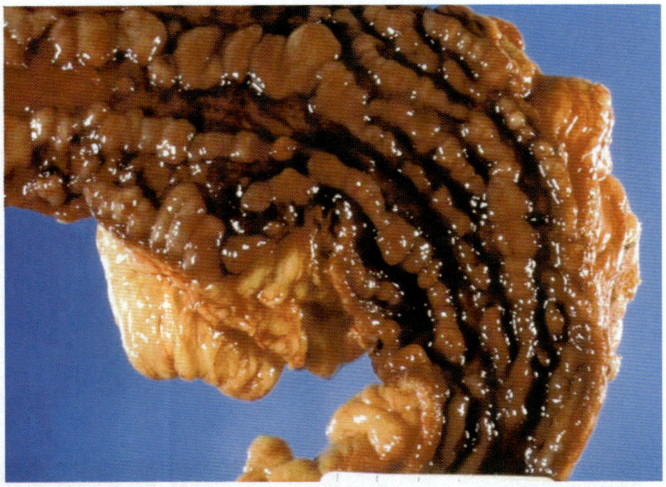

图 93–1 Crohn 病的熊掌样畸形。

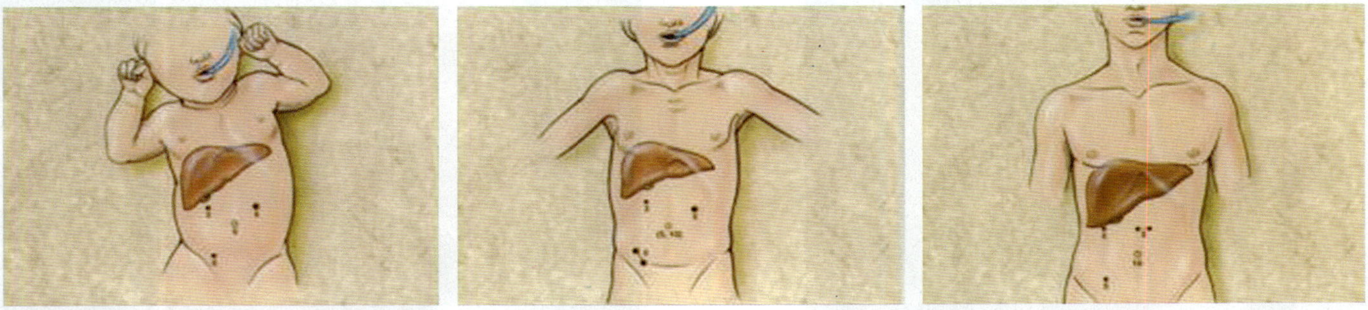

图 105–5 腹腔镜下胆囊切除手术时，插管和仪器位置的确定与患儿的年龄和体型有关。小婴儿用 3 mm 和 5 mm 的插管，并且插管之间的距离应尽可能大，以保证足够的操作空间（左图）。对于青春期前的儿童，插管之间的空间也要足够大。3 mm 的插管可以在外科医生的左手侧。对于此年龄段的患儿，可以用 5 mm 的脐部插管。但是许多患儿在取出胆囊时需要10 mm 脐部插管(中图)。青少年时期，插管的位置接近成年人（右图）。

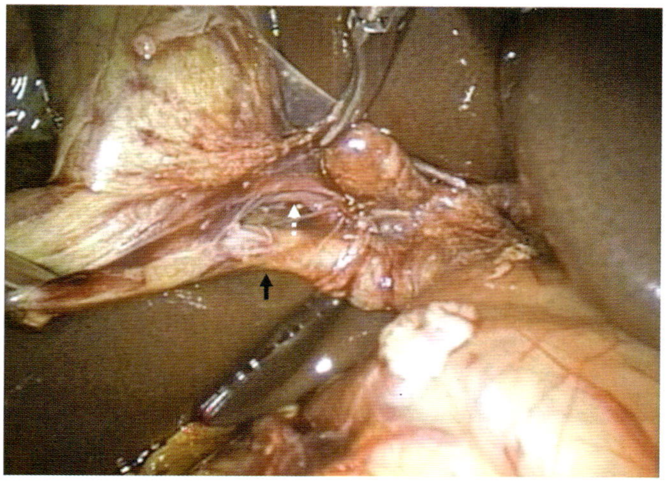

图 105-6 在腹腔镜下胆囊切除手术开始时，侧面牵拉漏斗部非常重要，这样可以在胆道（实心箭头）和共同通道间形成一个 90° 的角。注意胆囊管头侧的胆囊动脉（点状箭头）。

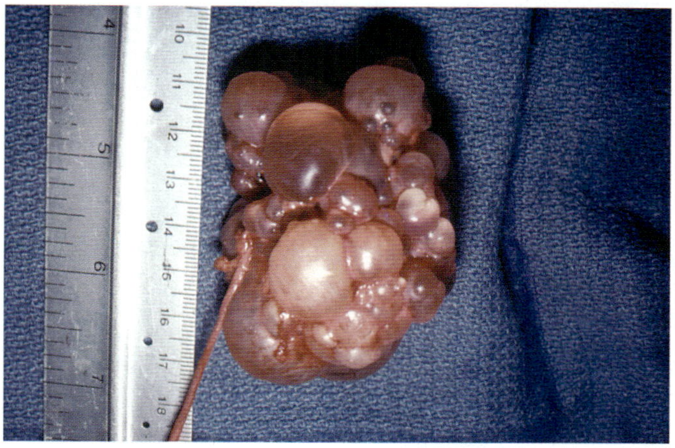

图 109-3 典型的多囊肾伴有输尿管闭锁。可见“葡萄串”外观。（From Shah SH, Glassberg KI: Multicystic dysplastic kidney disease. In Gearhart JP, Rink RC, Moriquand PDE [eds]: Pediatric Urology. Philadelphia, WB Saunders, 2001, p279.）

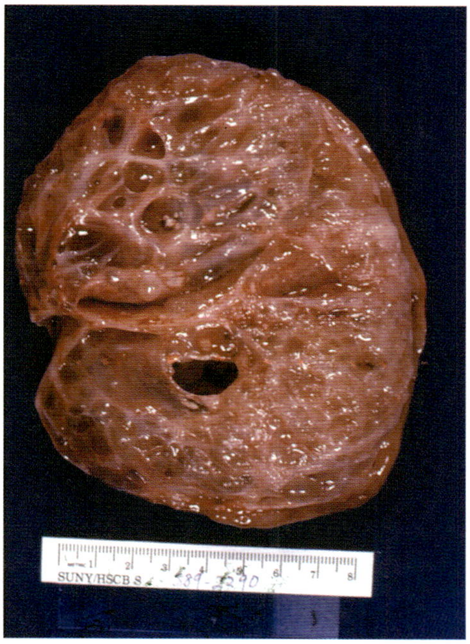

C

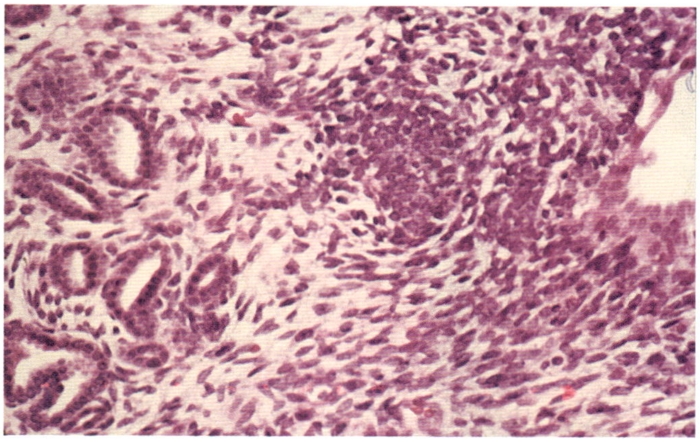

D

图 109-9 C. 肿块的大体标本可见有非交通性的小房。D. 显微镜下所见，可见胚芽细胞巢和小管系统，位于囊腔之间，为典型的多房性囊肿伴有部分分化的表现。

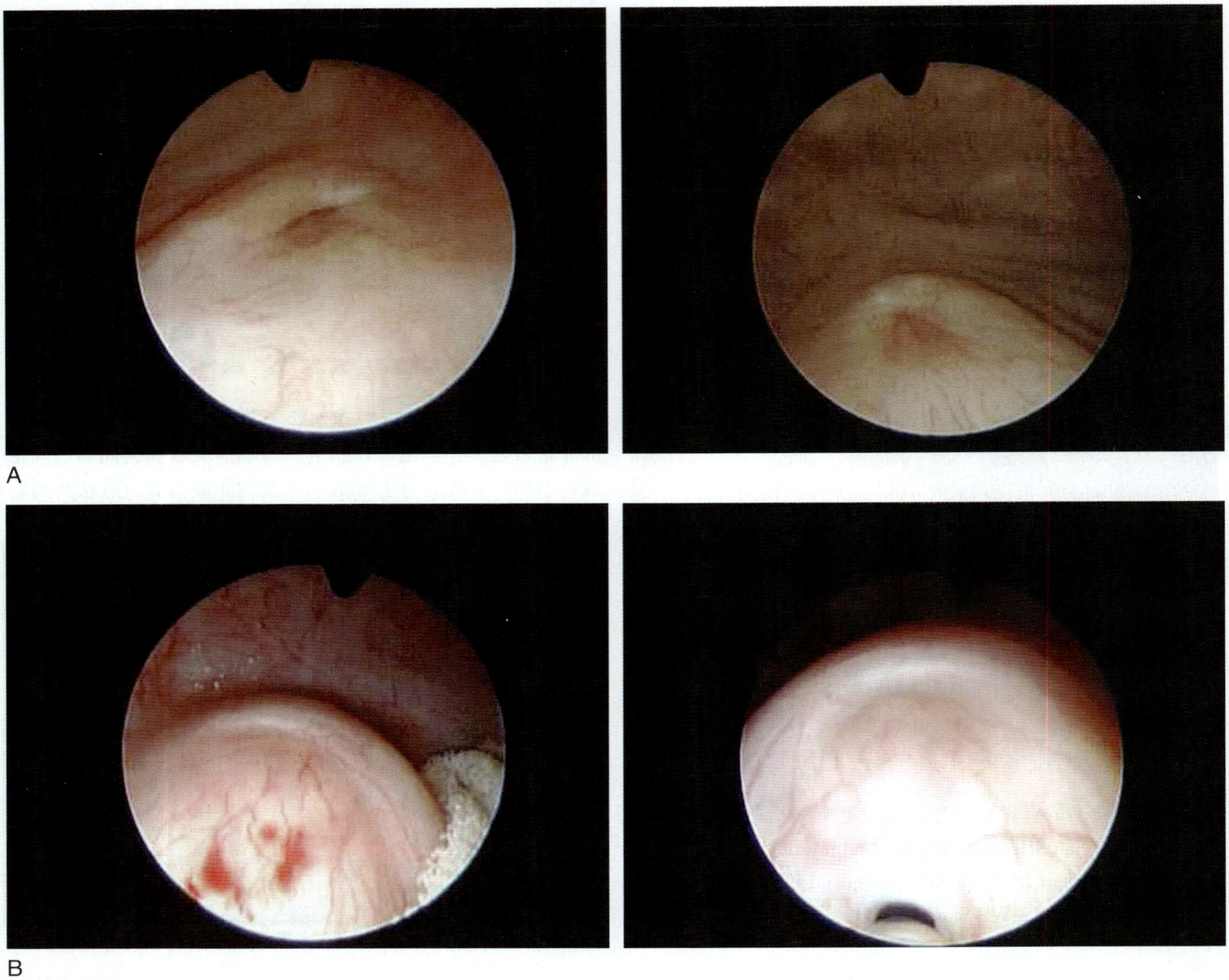

图 112-13 内镜注射。A. 注射前的左右输尿管开口。B. 注射后左右输尿管开口呈现半月形或火山口形外观。

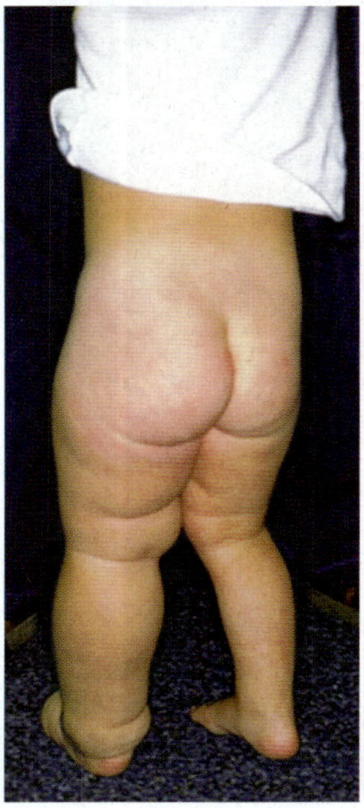

图 132-3 Klippel-Trenaunay 综合征。注意单侧下肢肥大、水肿，下肢长度有差异。

第七部分

腹部疾病

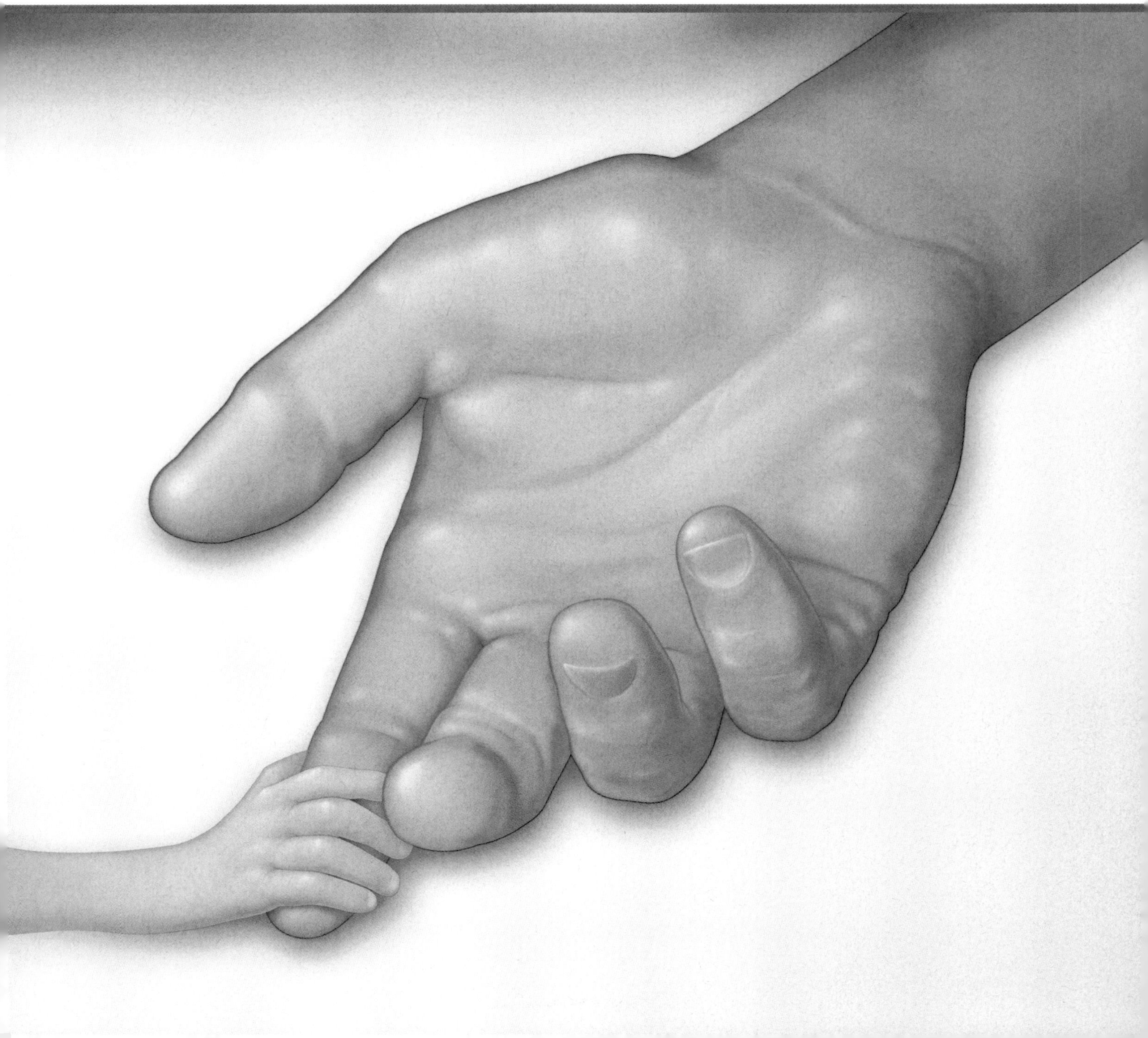

第 72 章

脐部疾病

Robert E. Cilley

历史回顾

1143 很早以前，艺术及雕塑作品已描绘过脐部畸形，但直到19世纪后期，人们才认识到这些畸形的发育基础。外科学教科书中，如 von Bergmann 在 1904 年清楚地描述了卵黄肠管的胚胎发育过程及瘘、窦道或囊肿的存在[105]。人们已知道脐部排出粪便（先天性脐位肛门）和肠管脱出的症状，提醒外科医生应避免的错误，如露出两个肠腔切除“脐部肿块”，这往往意味着切除卵黄肠残余物过多，以致切到了回肠。而作为卵黄管残留物的脐部息肉曾被称作“肠畸胎瘤”。

在过去的100年里，脐部畸形的外科治疗没有太多改变。有趣的是，直到今天仍然用硝酸银烧灼治疗脐部肉芽肿。很久之前人们对脐尿管发育畸形的胚胎基础及其手术治疗方法的认识就与今天一样。早在19世纪后期，人们就认识到大多数脐疝可自行消失。常推荐使用的方法是外部压迫，而且最重要的治疗方式是保留脐部形态而不是将其切除。对小婴儿实施脐部修补术是有风险的，因为那些尝试脐部矫形的外科先驱们对手术并发症准确的发生率和死亡率了解甚少。

1916 年，Cullen 撰写的一本经典著作对脐部作了完整描述[31]。这部百科全书式的著作仍是目前该学科最具权威性的著作。一个脐部恶性肿瘤的病例激发了 Cullen 的好奇心，驱使他去探索整个脐部疾病的病理。他写道：“对脐部的研究，刚开始时好像十分繁琐，但当猎奇了大多数的内容后，它变得如此迷人。[31]”

与出生后相比，胎儿在子宫时，脐的生理功能更为重要，胚胎通过它完成正常的发育。那些由于外科手术失去脐部的人，他们的感受证明了它同样具有心理方面的重要性。无论是新生儿还是大龄儿童，脐部有任何异常表现，应首先咨询小儿外科医生。脐疝修补术是儿童期经常实施的手术之一。此外，脐部是大多数腹腔镜手术的入口，而且它也可被用作尿道或肠道的造瘘口。脐部血管插管，无论是在原位，还是被手术移位，都为新生儿提供了一条血管通路。脐在审美中也很重要[28]，它可以是一个供展示或装饰的部位。露脐是很普遍的，人们常用珠宝和脐部穿刺来增加美感。

正常胚胎发育

脐部形成的经典描述显示，腹壁是在第 4 孕周时由圆盘样的三胚层胚胎的侧褶内翻和腹侧屈曲共同形成的。但胚胎的实际发育过程并不真正涉及机体结构“弯曲”和“折叠”，而是组织的分化生长。起初，羊膜在胚胎背侧，而卵黄囊占据了腹侧的位置。胚胎附着在胎盘的发源地——绒毛膜上，通过一个由胚外中胚层组织组成的体蒂相连，脐血管在这个体蒂中发育，尿囊也在其中生长（图 72-1A）。卵黄囊在腹侧，分为胚内体腔和胚外体腔两部分（图 72-1B）。胚内体腔从卵黄囊顶部发育起源，形成原始消化道，并通过卵黄管或脐肠系膜管与胚外体腔相连。正常情况下，这种连接在胚胎第 5～7 周消失[31,42]，如果连接管道持续存在，发育中的消化道或伴随的卵黄血管的残留物则形成一些畸形。该内容将在本章内详细描述。

早在胚胎第 3 周，一个被称作尿囊的腔隙，从卵
黄囊后壁起源并向胚胎的连接体蒂中延伸生长（图 1145
72-1A和1B）。在低级脊椎动物中，尿囊是发育中肾脏系统的储蓄池，但尚不清楚其在人胚胎发育中的作用。它本质上是短暂存在的脐尿管的胚外部分。当后肠末端或泄殖腔将腹侧的泌尿生殖窦和背侧的肛直肠管分隔开时，发育中的膀胱通过体蒂中脐尿管与尿囊

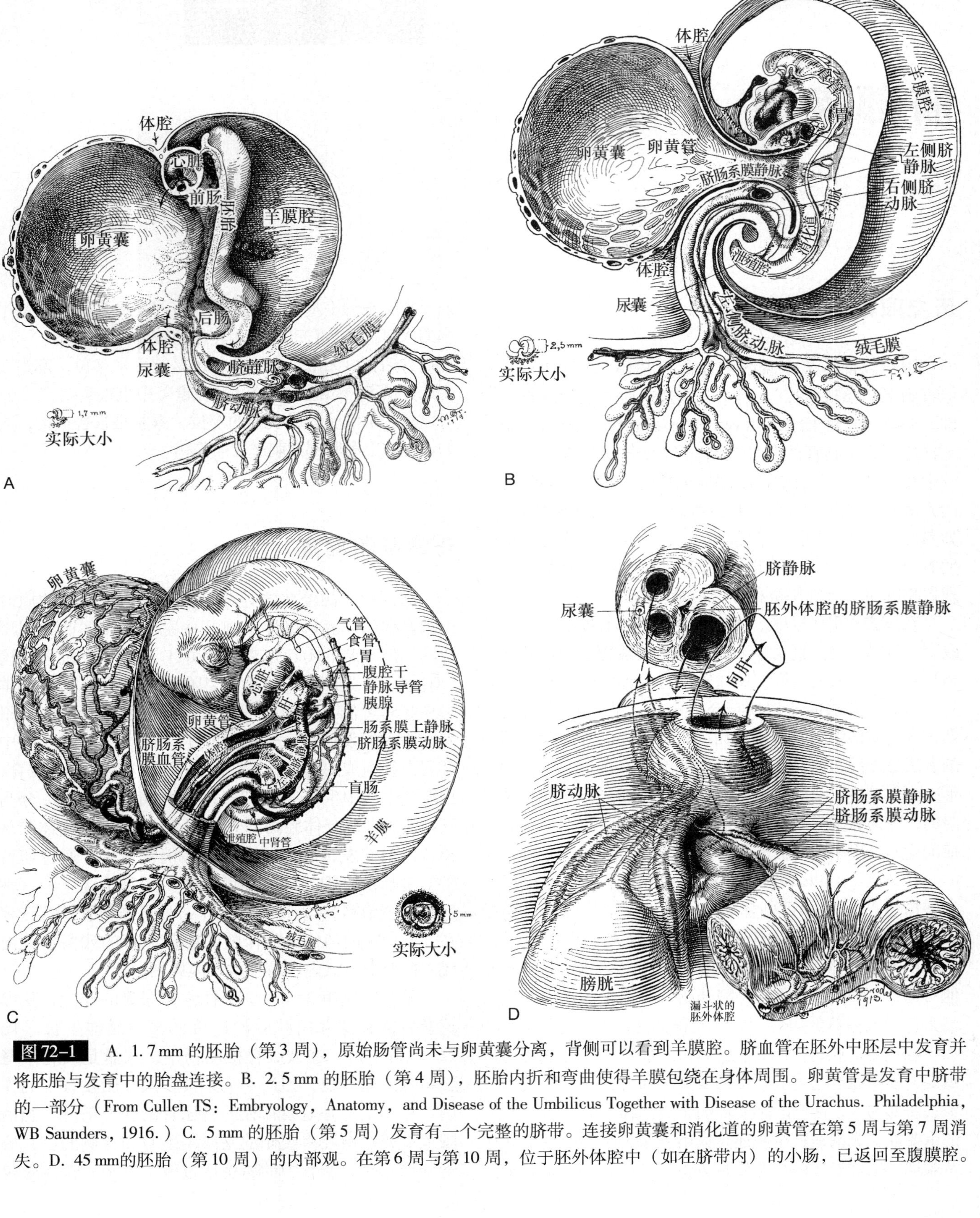

图 72–1　A. 1.7 mm 的胚胎（第 3 周），原始肠管尚未与卵黄囊分离，背侧可以看到羊膜腔。脐血管在胚外中胚层中发育并将胚胎与发育中的胎盘连接。B. 2.5 mm 的胚胎（第 4 周），胚胎内折和弯曲使得羊膜包绕在身体周围。卵黄管是发育中脐带的一部分（From Cullen TS：Embryology，Anatomy，and Disease of the Umbilicus Together with Disease of the Urachus. Philadelphia，WB Saunders，1916.）C. 5 mm 的胚胎（第 5 周）发育有一个完整的脐带。连接卵黄囊和消化道的卵黄管在第 5 周与第 7 周消失。D. 45 mm的胚胎（第 10 周）的内部观。在第 6 周与第 10 周，位于胚外体腔中（如在脐带内）的小肠，已返回至腹膜腔。

保持相通（图 72-1D）。脐尿管完全起源于发育中的膀胱，可以以各种方式存在，它的相关畸形将在随后讲述。

随着胚胎的发育，羊膜向四周延伸，包绕胚胎并覆盖发育中的脐带组织，包括尿囊、脐血管、卵黄管和原始间充质组织（脐带胶质）（图 72-1C）。在胚胎第 6～10 周，肠管快速生长，中肠的发育是在体腔外进行的。随着体腔壁的持续发育，肠管返回到体腔内并旋转和固定。脐环的肌纤维继续收缩，通常到出生时关闭（图72-1D）。筋膜的持续开放导致脐疝形成，通常见于早产儿。与其他腹壁缺损不同，由于出生后脐环组织的继续发育，脐疝有自愈的倾向，无特效疗法。该结构的发展结局与表 72-1 所示的脐的发育有关。

出生时的脐部

分娩时，现代的产科医生常在切断脐带的同时，在离脐部皮肤几厘米处放置一次性塑料脐带夹。出生后，常在脐带残端使用表面抗菌剂，如脐区消毒药、杆菌肽、磺胺嘧啶银、聚维酮碘、氯己定、六氯酚、酒精、水杨酸糖粉剂、绿黏土粉剂、过氧化-苯-银或 1% 碱性品红[89,90]。所有这些抗菌剂可有效降低细菌繁殖率，在不能保证适当的脐部护理时被推荐使用。这些物质可能会影响脐带脱落的时间，有些可能引起皮肤脱色，重复使用含抗菌剂的碘酒，可能导致机体碘吸收量过多而抑制甲状腺功能。在发达国家的做法是，尽量保持脐带干燥，局部不使用抗生素，而是常规每天用肥皂和清水清洗，并仔细洗手，与局部使用抗菌药物一样可以有效地减少感染[126]。

当存在不能识别的小的脐带疝（或小型脐膨出）时，错误放置脐带夹会导致肠管损伤。与脐相关的腹壁缺损（腹裂和脐膨出）将在第 73 章中阐述。

脐带脱落的正常时间范围是出生后 3 天～2 个月[120]。抗感染治疗因减少了白细胞浸润可能延长脐带脱落时间。脐带的延迟脱落也可能与遗传性中性粒细胞移动缺陷有关，此疾病可导致感染的迅速扩散并经常是致命的[51]。这种异常的中性粒细胞缺少一种膜表面糖蛋白，导致黏附、趋化及噬菌作用异常[120]。尽管出生后 3 周脐带附属物残留提示可能是免疫系统异常的表现，但最近对 600 余名新生儿的研究结果表明：正常新生儿的脐带脱落时间范围很大（3～67 天），平均 14～15 天[84,120]。在这些研究中，将近 10% 的正常新生儿脐带在出生 3 周后脱落，因此，脐带脱落延迟并不是免疫系统疾病的可靠指标。如果脐 1146
带脱落时间延长同时合并感染，则应考虑白细胞黏附缺陷，需进行免疫学评估[45,53,90]。

脐带脱落后，脐部外观不一。正常脐的特征是，下压脐部可以出现“乳头状物”（中央突出内含脐带残留物的坚硬部分）和“瘢痕”（厚实的瘢痕，胚内体腔与胚外体腔曾通过此处相连），“软垫”则是在

表 72-1　与脐发育相关结构的转归

结构	转归	残留物、病理状态
脐尿管（连接膀胱和尿囊）	消失	脐正中韧带、脐尿管开放、窦道、囊肿
脐肠系膜管（连接中肠和卵黄囊）	消失	Meckel 憩室、脐肠系膜管开放、窦道、囊肿、索带、息肉
脐肠系膜动脉	大部分退化，与腹腔、肠系膜上和脐下组织融合	优势动脉可伴随 Meckel 憩室和连接肠系膜动脉的纤维索带
脐肠系膜静脉	十二指肠周围的血管丛，形成肠系膜上和门静脉（可形成左和右静脉）	如果腹侧血管丛持续存在，则形成十二指肠前门静脉症
脐动脉	出生后消失	脐外侧韧带
脐静脉	右侧消失，左侧通过静脉导管引流胎盘的血液回流至下腔静脉	镰状韧带

下压脐部时周围轻微突起的皮肤边缘。Cullen 曾描绘过 60 种“正常”的脐部形态[31]。

脐部异常

获得性

脐部肉芽肿

脐带脱落以后，基底部可以长出小块状的肉芽组织。这些肉芽肿是由成纤维细胞及丰富的毛细血管组成的肉芽组织；肉芽肿的直径范围大约为 1 mm～1 cm 不等，表面常呈菌类植物形状。脐部肉芽肿可以用硝酸银一次或多次烧灼，直到表面上皮形成。脐部肉芽肿也可以切除，并用硝酸银或可吸收止血药物处理创面[80]。如果烧灼没有达到治疗效果，则应怀疑真性脐息肉或窦道存在的可能性（见下文）。

脐部感染

尽管现代的围生技术已大大降低了脐炎的发生率，但脐部感染的发病率和死亡率仍令人担忧，尤其在第三世界国家。严格无菌操作、洗手和脐部护理已使住院新生儿脐部感染的发生率低于 1%[72]。在这之前，脐炎的死亡率为 65%。导致感染的原发病原体为金黄色葡萄球菌和化脓性链球菌。目前，革兰阴性菌在脐部感染的发病机制中起重要作用。严重感染则常由多种微生物引起。脐炎可表现为脐部脓性分泌物或脐周蜂窝织炎。家中分娩、低出生体重、脐部插管及分娩败血症是脐炎发生的危险因素。少数情况下可以发生破伤风感染。静脉抗感染治疗可以治愈大多数感染。在发展中国家脐炎是常见疾病，可以超过入院新生儿人数的 1/4[4,101]。

蜂窝织炎可以发展为筋膜炎，且进展不易引起注意。坏死性筋膜炎的体征包括腹胀、心动过速、紫癜、疱疹、发热、体温过低、白细胞增多及抗生素治疗效果不佳的进展性蜂窝织炎。细菌培养显示为多种菌群生长[16]。坏死性筋膜炎或脐部坏疽可以是致死性的，需要快速而广泛的外科清创术以挽救患儿生命[63,66,72,79,94,95,106]。快速的手术切除应包括以下部分：所有感染的皮肤、脂肪和筋膜，直到显露有活力的组织及出血的腹壁肌肉组织，同时必须切除脐部。切除腹膜外的组织是至关重要的，包括脐部血管和脐尿管残余物，因为这些组织内可能会藏匿入侵的细菌，小范围的外科清创术可能会为感染扩散提供途径[63]。需要放置暂时的修复性补片以关闭留下的腹壁缺损，但最终的筋膜关闭和脐部重建需留下一个理想的外观。高压氧疗被推荐为辅助性治疗手段，但并未证明它的有效性。普遍报道，与坏死性筋膜炎相关的死亡率为 81%[63,66,72,79,94,95,106]。

已有报道显示脐部流液源于脐部残余物的慢性感染，如脐动脉残余[21]。通过切除残余物和清创术可以达到治愈效果。出生 2 个月内的脐炎可发生坏死和脐残端自行脱落，可能与门静脉血栓及继发的肝外门静脉高压有关。

先天性

脐肠系膜残余物

卵黄管或脐肠系膜管的残留可引起多种脐部畸形，往往脐部畸形需要外科手术矫治[76]。这些残余物包括瘘管、窦道、囊肿、黏膜残余和先天性索带。典型变异的病理类型图例见图 72-2A～F[31,60,77]。

从回肠末端至脐部的脐肠瘘，将见到粪便样排出物（图 72-3A）。尽管出现这样的状况对于患儿父母来说充满戏剧性，但这种畸形在体检时可以被立即识别并判断清楚，且可以告知患儿父母，迅速的外科矫治简单而有效，以消除他们的疑虑。近端和远端的回肠通过开放的卵黄管脱出是该病的一个特征表现。注射造影剂检查有助于诊断，但并不改变手术方法（图 72-3B）[29,125]。手术时要注意到可能存在的解剖异常，如卵黄管可能从较少见的阑尾处起源。除非有其他严重疾病存在，开放的卵黄管应迅速手术切除。不需要机械遵循术前肠道准备，尽管我们习惯上停止患儿的肠道喂养，并给予术前剂量的口服抗生素。围术期应给予静脉内抗生素。手术通常无需额外的腹部切口，经脐部或经脐下弧形切口进入，全面探查并确认脐部的所有结构，
包括一条静脉、两条动脉和脐尿管残余物。追踪卵黄管 1147
至回肠处并分离，关闭回肠，并注意处理主要的显露的卵黄血管。关闭筋膜后，应行脐成形术。

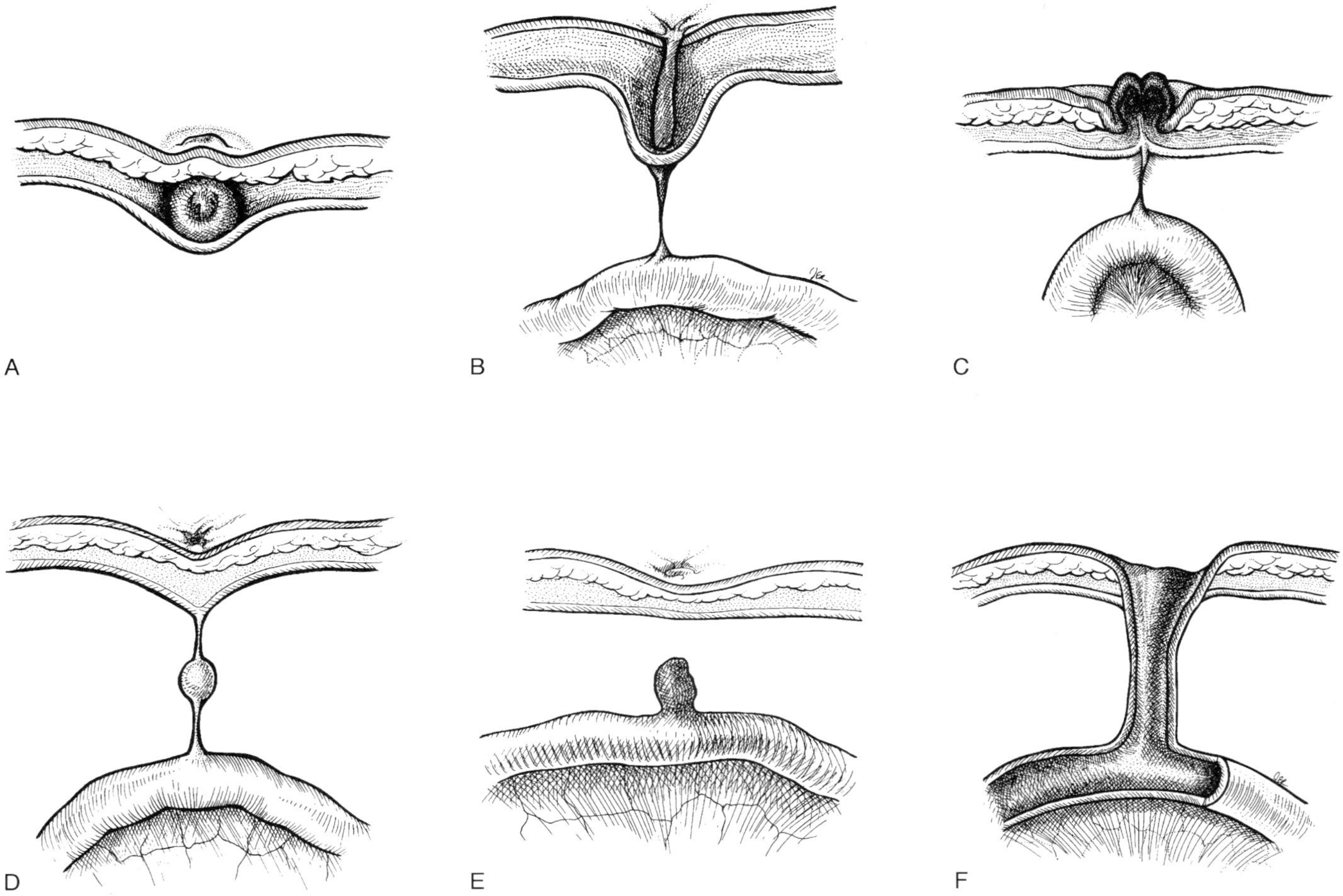

图 72-2　各种类型的卵黄管残留物。A. 包含肠组织的脐部囊肿。B. 伴随索带的脐窦。C. 包含肠黏膜的脐息肉。D. 包含囊肿的纤维索带。E. Meckel 憩室。F. 未闭的卵黄管。其他类型可合并存在。

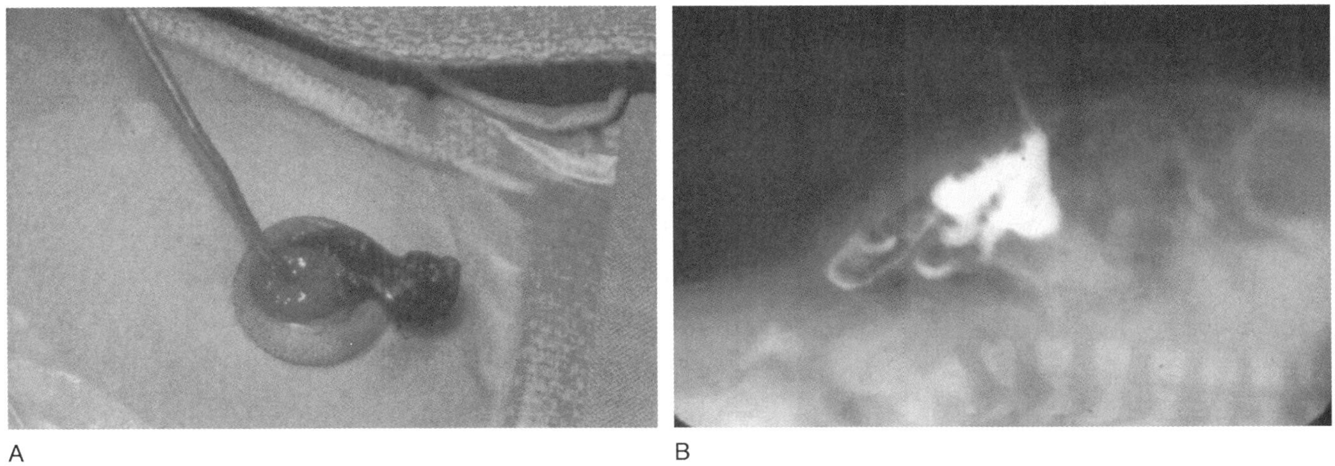

图 72-3　A. 一位新生儿的照片，显示探针可以通过开放的卵黄管到达回肠。B. 将造影剂注入开放的卵黄管的 X 光片，显示小肠内有造影剂充盈。这种诊断方式通常不是必需的。

小的卵黄管残余物和窦道很少有特征性的脐部流出物。在这些情况中，注射造影剂检查有助于发现问题的本质，但手术探查仍是确诊的手段。脐部全面探查非常重要，脐部所有结构，包括脐部腹膜内组织，都应予以肉眼鉴别，并去除任何附着在小肠表面的索
1148 带。如果探查时发现 Meckel 憩室与卵黄管索带相附着，则应予以切除。卵黄管的囊肿样残余物可以引起感染而出现急性症状，甚至是大龄患儿。如果形成脓肿，可能需要手术引流，并随后切除所有残余组织。卵黄管或任何附着在肠管与腹壁之间的残余物都可能引起肠管成角、扭转或肠管内疝而导致机械性肠梗阻，剖腹探查可以发现梗阻的原因。

少数情况下，开放的卵黄管可以自行退化[58,65]。1 例在出生后不久经瘘管造影发现脐肠瘘的患儿在其 3 个月大时实施了手术治疗，术中只发现 Meckel 憩室，但憩室并没有与脐部相连，由此提示在此期间可能存在着一些退化现象。

脐尿管残留

曾有多种脐尿管畸形被报道过[6,31,82]。典型的畸形如图 72-4 所示。开放的脐尿管伴有尿液从脐部排出。脐部有清亮的液体流出，尤其是出现尿液所致的皮疹时通常应怀疑存在脐尿管未闭。尽管在剖腹探查时可以明确解剖，但脐部单纯流出尿液时，需要进行泌尿系统检查，以判断是否存在膀胱出口梗阻，因为脐尿管在功能上可以作为缓解膀胱梗阻的阀门（图 72-5）[56]，但这种情况很少见。脐尿管未闭可以通过脐部或脐下切口手术。术中要确认脐部所有结构以明确诊断。将开放的脐尿管结扎并在膀胱水平离断，再用可吸收线双层关闭基底宽阔的连接部。

脐尿窦可以表现为脐部排液或在体检时被发现。
脐尿管囊肿常引起感染而表现为脐部和耻骨上的疼痛 1149
性包块。超声或 CT 有助于确诊。曾有报道显示其他一些少见的征象，如腹壁非正中区包块[14]。脐尿管曾被报道不在脐部下方正中线位置[30,86]。此外，脐尿管未闭可能是导致新生儿期巨脐的原因之一。当脐尿管囊肿感染形成脓肿时，需紧急行脓肿引流术。在脓肿引流后，脐尿管囊肿可完全治愈。随后是否必须行剖腹探查去除囊肿残留物还不确定。

脐尿管残余物可导致并发症。异常的上皮组织。包括结肠组织、小肠组织和鳞状上皮组织均可以出现在偶然移动的脐尿管残余物中[113]。这些组织的发展结局尚不清楚，但文献报道显示，有许多不同类型的恶性肿瘤起源于脐尿管。表 72-2 列出了部分起源于脐尿管的成人恶性肿瘤。儿童肿瘤，如横纹肌肉瘤和

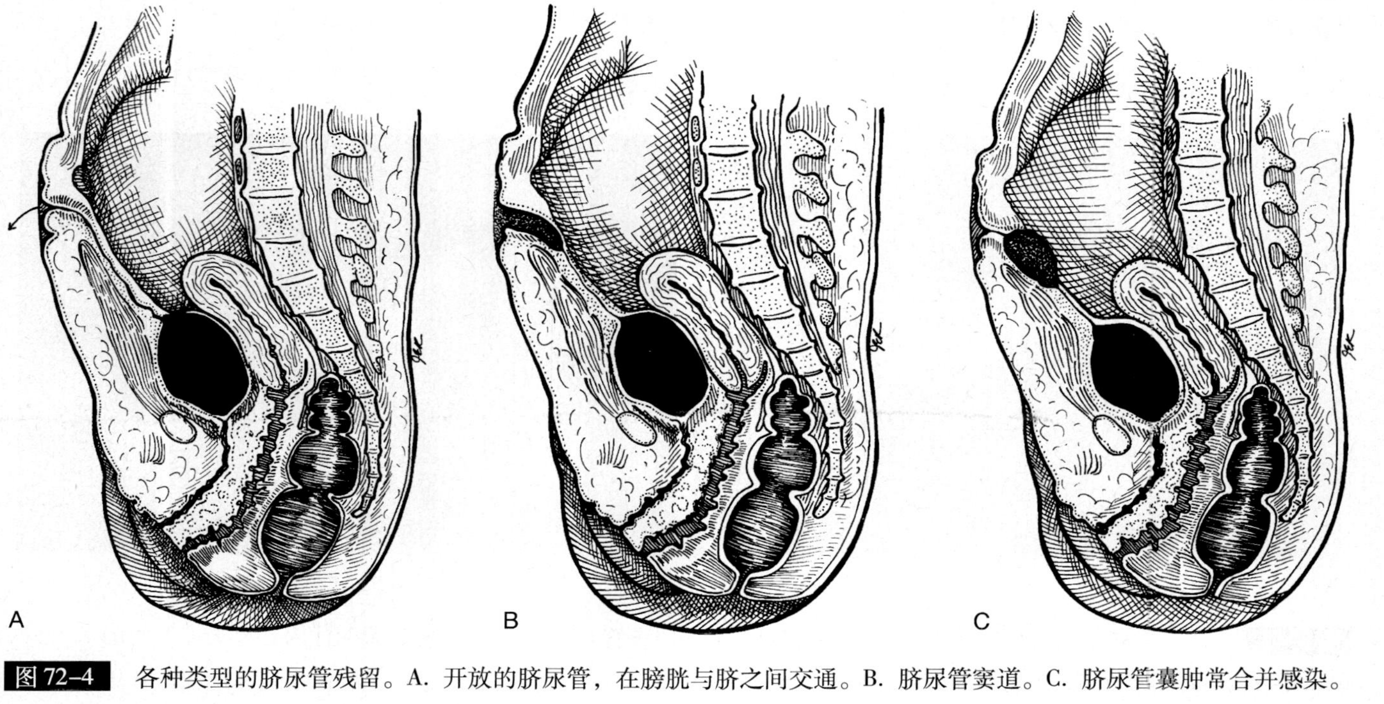

图 72-4　各种类型的脐尿管残留。A. 开放的脐尿管，在膀胱与脐之间交通。B. 脐尿管窦道。C. 脐尿管囊肿常合并感染。

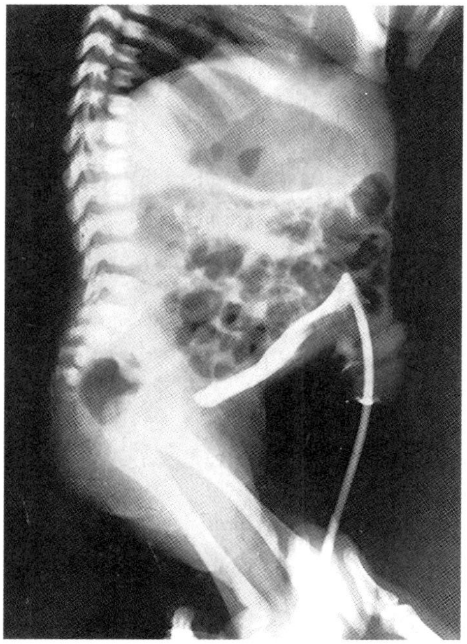

图 72-5　将造影剂注入开放的脐尿管的 X 光片，显示膀胱内有造影剂充盈。[From Jona JZ: Umbilical anomalies. In Raffensberger JG (ed): Swenson's Pediatric Surgery, 5th ed, Norwalk, Conn, Appleton & Lange, 1990. 经允许后使用。]

表 72-2　来源于脐尿管起源的肿瘤

腺癌
移行细胞癌
鳞状上皮细胞癌
黏液性（囊性）腺癌
恶性纤维组织细胞瘤
纤维肉瘤
多形细胞肉瘤
卵黄囊瘤
炎性假瘤
绒毛状腺瘤（癌前病变）

神经母细胞瘤也可能起源于脐尿管残余物[24,122]。

疼痛和排尿时脐部回缩是脐尿管异常的体征[61,93]。切除脐部残余物可以治愈。

诊断性影像学检查，如超声、造影、CT 和磁共振在脐部畸形的诊断和治疗中偶尔也有帮助[12]。曾报道一例患儿由于同时存在持久性脐尿管和脐肠瘘管表现为脐部排泄物[70]。

脐部畸形

单一的脐动脉可以出现在许多综合征中，并与 1/3 的先天性畸形病例有关。这些畸形包括 18 三体综合征和肾、心脏畸形。有畸形征象的儿童可能存在有助于诊断的特征性表现，而无医学意义的轻微畸形也可以为发育过程中畸形发生的本质和时间提供一些线索[41]。通常，皮纹、毛发分布、耳郭形状和生殖器外形是观察的内容之一。脐部结构的轻微异常可能对相关畸形的分类有帮助。以面部扁平、脐体短小及生殖器发育不全为特征的 Robinow 综合征的患儿为例，他们的脐部在腹壁的位置非常高，位于肋弓下缘且扁平，皮肤较少。如果脐部宽大且蒂比较长、脐周皮肤富赘，尤其当脐部异常合并前房角发育不良及牙齿发育不全时，则应怀疑为 Rieger 综合征。如脐部中央像纽扣一样，按压时呈纵向卵圆形深陷或扁平，周围皮纹呈放射状时，则应考虑为 Aarskog 综合征，其特征性表现为身材矮小、面部发育不良、并指（趾）和生殖器畸形[111]。

其他先天性或获得性脐部病变

脐下皮样窦道通常由耻骨上的皮肤延伸而来，沿着脐尿管，经过脐与膀胱之间的上表面区域[43,87]。这种窦道的胚胎来源尚不清楚，可能是背侧尿道重复畸形的一种变异。

膀胱和泄殖腔外翻畸形的患儿可以合并脐膨出或脐位置偏低，与开放的膀胱上段融合，常伴随下腹壁肌肉分离和耻骨联合分离[75]。外翻畸形还包括膀胱肠管瘘、外翻重复畸形以及膀胱完整而肌肉骨骼异常的假性外翻。

有许多脐部异常膨出的报道。卵黄管细胞具备多能造血干细胞的本质很好地解释了胰腺组织包括胰岛细胞的异位[19]。曾有与肝主要叶段有关的肝组织异常的报道，在关闭腹腔后，异常肝脏组织可能被脐环所压迫[97]。曾有一巨大的、直径 10 cm 未侵入腹腔的脐部错构瘤被完整切除且没有并发症的病例报道[23]。早期就有报道称在阑尾与脐之间存在瘘管（脐肠系膜残余物）的阑尾-脐。阑尾陷夹于脐部，如在小型脐膨出中，也可以解释一些脐至阑尾的瘘管[13,57]。分离脐带后可以看到瘢痕疙瘩形成[39]。巨大脐带常包含有脐尿

表 72-3 获得性脐部病变

病变	内容	出处
皮肤病	脂溢性皮炎、银屑病、妊娠疱疹、脂质贮积病	Powell 1988[91]
异物反应	淀粉、滑石粉、塞入的物体	Powell 1988
脐炎	角蛋白和皮脂物质凝结	Powell 1988
藏毛病	与毛发覆盖的窦道有关	Steck 1965[104]，Gupta 1990[46]
感染	细菌、真菌、病毒、寄生虫	Powell 1988
子宫内膜异位症	异位的子宫内膜组织	Powell 1988，Franklin 1990[40]
良性肿瘤	痣、化脓性肉芽肿、包涵囊肿、血管瘤、皮肤纤维瘤、神经纤维瘤、颗粒细胞肿瘤、畸胎瘤、硬纤维瘤、脂肪瘤	Powell 1988
恶性肿瘤（原发性）	恶性黑色素瘤、脐尿管腺癌、鳞状上皮癌、基底细胞癌、肉瘤	Shetty 1990[98]，Powell 1988，Cornil 1967[26]
恶性肿瘤（转移性）	胃、胰腺、子宫内膜、卵巢、子宫颈、结肠、小肠、胆囊、肺、前列腺、乳房、其他	Shetty 1990
肠瘘	继发于溃疡性结肠炎，穿孔性阑尾炎，其他的内脏穿孔如结肠、胆囊	Park 1991[88]，Veloso 1989[114]，Burchell 1989[18]
精神疾病	阴道幻想	Waltzer 1974[117]
各种疾病	脑室腹膜分流术穿孔、感染、皮肤病和穿刺后肉芽肿组织	Bryant 1988[17]，Lena 1994[69]

管残留物和扩张的血管，类似一个小型脐膨出。在有脐带异常表现时，可以在使用脐带夹时予以切除。

脐部可以发生一些与被覆毛发的皮肤相关的疾病，如皮样囊肿和感染。它也可以出现异位的组织，包括子宫内膜异位，除起源脐尿管的肿瘤以外，也是很多原发性和转移性肿瘤的好发部位（见表72-2）。
1150 表 72-3 总结了一些脐部获得性病变。

在治疗上脐部穿刺较常用，并可出现进退两难的局面。创伤外科医生应该熟悉人体穿刺的开放机制，以推进放射学研究及需要紧急手术救治的医疗程序[59]。如果已发生感染，不一定要去除穿刺装置[118]。局部感染应热敷和涂抹抗生素药膏。如果感染持续存在，则可以口服抗生素。感染处用含抗生素的肥皂清洗，去掉饰物，并留下空隙便于引流。需要行外科引流或清创术的脐部感染较少见。

脐棉绒屑

脐部棉绒屑聚集是脐部漩涡状毛发与衣物直接作用的结果，毛发围绕在脐周，毛发角蛋白鳞屑与朝向毛囊的基底部交错。这种情况受腹部与身体活动时衣物前后摩擦、棉绒布自由移动的影响。脐周的毛发起齿轮样的作用，使绒布头屑向脐深部移动。脐周没有毛发时，脐棉绒屑不会形成，棉绒屑的颜色就是所穿衣服的颜色。

脐疝

解剖

出生时，脐部被坚硬的筋膜环所包绕，并在腹白线处存在缺损。脐部开口被下方的脐尿管和脐动脉残留物紧密附着，并被上方的脐静脉较疏松地附着所加强。来源于腹横肌的筋膜（Richet 筋膜）支撑着脐的基底部。脐环下有完整的腹膜层，脐带离断后可见其上方覆盖的皮肤组织。当支持的筋膜缺损或薄弱时可形成直疝（图 72-6）[121]。脐疝患儿脐环周围有坚固的筋膜，中央有与外突的皮肤相附着的腹膜疝囊穿

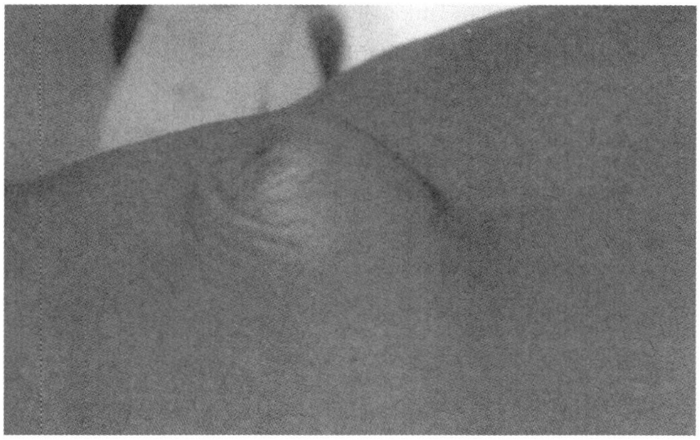

图 72-6 一位 5 岁女孩典型的脐疝相片。

过。脐环渐进性关闭和脐缺损的筋膜力量加强，使得大多数脐疝的患儿可以自愈。

曾有间接型脐疝的报道，腹膜内容物从脐环上方的位置疝入。疝沿着脐静脉从脐管突出，腹白线在其
1151 前方，薄薄的腹膜外筋膜在其后方[11]。这种疝的形成提示在儿童中可引起喙形疝（proboscoid hernias）。存在这种缺损，可因为疝的增大使得脐部残蒂向下方延伸。这种缺损也与一些成人脐疝有关。

儿童脐疝需与“脐带疝”鉴别，后者存在脐部腹膜及筋膜的开放性缺损，小肠疝入脐带中且只外被羊膜。脐带疝实际上是一种小型脐膨出。

发病率及自然病程

脐环关闭的分子学基础已不容置疑[109]。遗传因素决定一些儿童在出生时脐环开放，而在另一些儿童，脐环于脐带脱落后关闭。许多患儿的脐环在出生后数周、数月或数年中会逐渐闭合，而腹股沟疝及上腹壁疝与此不同，它们在出生后没有自行关闭的趋势。

脐疝在男孩与女孩中的发生率相同，很多文献报道非洲及非裔美国婴儿中脐疝的发生率较高[17,35,116]。脐环在孕期中的大部分时间是开放的，但随着孕龄的增加逐渐缩小。大多数婴儿的脐疝在脐带脱落后几周内被发现，几乎所有患儿在出生后 6 个月内发病。大多数患儿的脐疝在出生后 3 年内自行闭合。许多早产儿在脐带脱落后会发生脐部缺损。尽管脐疝在低体重儿中很常见（体重低于 1500 g 的新生儿中达 75%），但大多数可以自行愈合[115]。由于对脐部缺损儿童的纵向发展结局缺乏精确的研究，因此无法对其自然病程给出明确结论[96]。脐环直径较小的（脐疝小于 1.0 cm）更容易自行关闭，且比脐环较大（直径大于 1.5 cm）的脐疝关闭要早。脐部缺损的直径对预后很重要，而脐疝突出的长度与预后的关系不大。一些脐疝在 5 岁前无需手术治疗可自行关闭[47,52]。脐疝出现症状的时间与儿童期脐部缺损之间的关系尚不清楚。疝前突部分的大小常维持不变，直到筋膜环变小至疝囊不能容纳为止。因此，疝常表现为突然消失[52]。脐疝在 Down 综合征、18 三体、13 三体、黏多糖增多症和先天性甲状腺功能减退中较常见。脐部缺损（疝或脐膨出）也是 Beckwith-Wiedemann 综合征的部分表现。肠管或网膜的嵌顿、绞窄、穿孔、内脏脱出以及疼痛在儿童脐疝的自然病程中很少发生。对大多数小儿外科医生来说，较困难的是说服患儿家属，多数脐疝只需观察无需手术治疗，尤其是婴儿。教会父母用他们一个手指的尺寸来监测脐部缺损的大小有助于治疗。

未矫正的脐疝可以在任何年龄出现症状。疝囊破裂和内脏脱出很罕见但偶有发生[2,102]。嵌顿也很少见，但一旦发生，则常累及小肠。持续的腹腔压力升高增加了并发症的可能性。修补有腹水的患者的脐疝风险较大。脐疝可以在妊娠期出现症状，而且一旦嵌顿，应行手术治疗。较少见的疝内容物有子宫肌瘤和子宫内膜等组织[33,124]。

手术指征

尽管提倡儿童期疝修补术是为了避免成人后发生嵌顿疝的并发症，但这两者之间的关系尚不清楚[67,78]。一些少见的情况，如需要复位的嵌顿疝、绞窄性疝、穿孔和内脏脱出是手术的绝对指征。除了这些绝对指征外，在发达国家疝的持续存在及有临床症状是手术的相对指征。巨大喙形疝，且随访观察期间脐环未见缩小的婴儿也可在 2 岁前行手术治疗。典型的脐疝最少应观察至 2 岁，如果脐环的大小没有改变，可以考虑手术修补。有充分的证据支持可推迟修补。大的缺损（直径大于 1.5 cm）在 5 岁时仍然持续存在时需要手术修补。因为缺少证据支持的手术指征，是否手术治疗取决于个体情况，如家族史、双亲

意愿和当地的医疗习惯。疝的外部表现常使家属坚持要求行手术修补。在欠发达国家，积极观察脐疝情况，若出现并发症如嵌顿疝，再行手术治疗也是适当的[3,73]。

如果患儿脐部包块柔软，通过挤出嵌顿肠管中的气体并用坚实、持续的压力作用于嵌顿的包块上，可使疝减小。如果复位成功，由父母观察是否有腹膜炎体征并在第 2 天进行手术是恰当的。如果嵌顿疝复位不成功，则应进行急诊手术。对腹股沟疝合并脐疝的婴儿，通常不处理脐疝，因为它有自行闭合的可能。

手术技巧、结果和并发症

对腹膜囊内翻患儿的脐疝修补术可以采用打开腹膜，并逐层关闭腹腔的方式，或者像治疗腹股沟疝一样，用线结扎[7,10]。可吸收线和不吸收线均可使用。较大脐部缺损的多余皮肤可以保留在原处，随着时间的推移，脐外观可以自行改善。一些医生建议对巨大 1152
喙形疝可以切除多余皮肤并进行脐部重建（见下文）。但脐疝手术的基本原则在 1953 年 Gross 描述后改变不大[44]。关闭筋膜常采用横行方式，并保留脐部外观，是各种脐疝修补术中共同采用的技巧。脐部缺损采用胶布固定的方法已不被采用[100,121]。

脐疝修补也可以在基础麻醉下于门诊完成，在基础麻醉前或后可采用伤口浸润的方式行局部麻醉，但应避免因麻醉而导致脐周组织变形[27]。局部麻醉以切皮前无痛为原则。脐下的切口按皮肤皱褶的方向打开（图 72-7）。环绕疝囊进行皮下组织的解剖，横断疝囊并在脐部皮肤下方剥离出来。无需进行广泛而长时间的切割。注意在皮肤下方保留少量的疝囊残端以避免并发症的发生。疝囊可以修剪至坚固的筋膜边缘

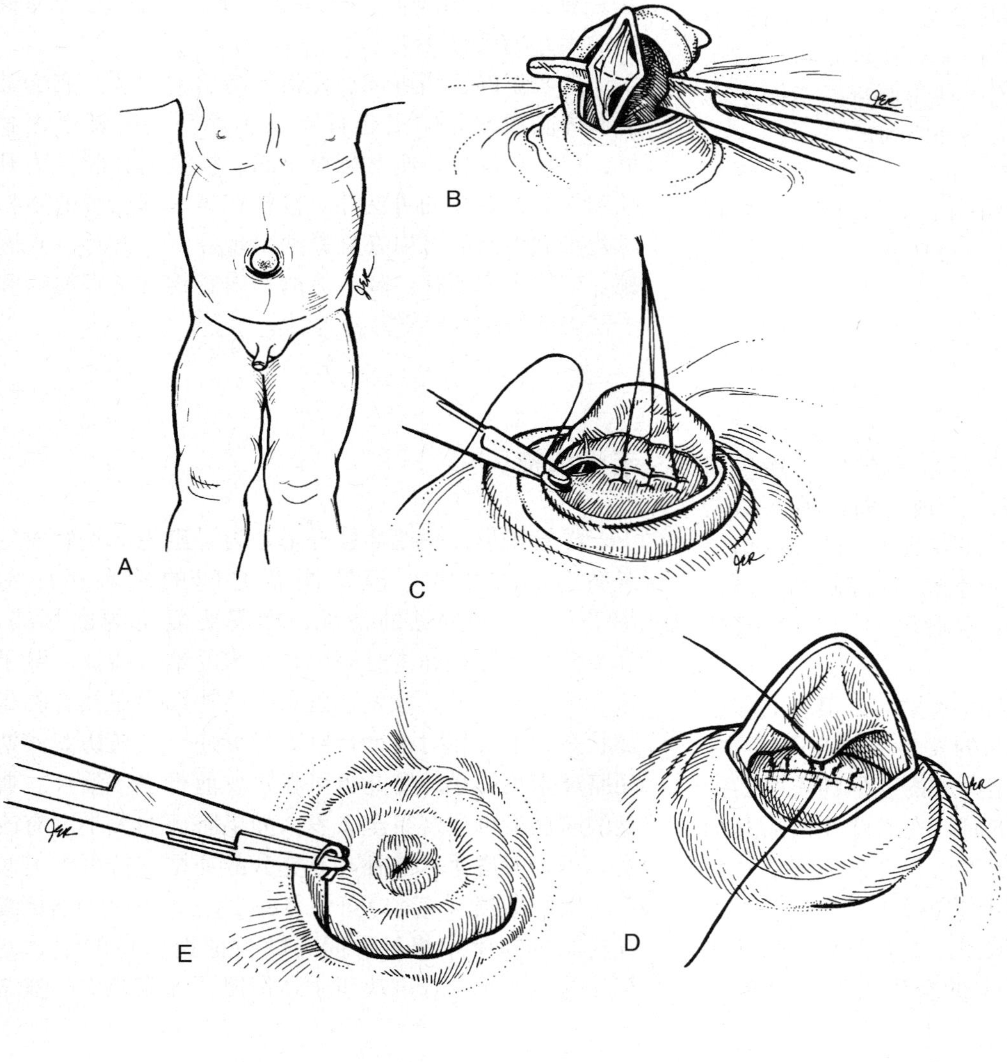

图 72-7 脐疝修补术。A. 脐下弧形切口。B. 环形打开疝囊。C. 横形关闭筋膜。D. 在脐部皮肤下方与筋膜间放置附加缝线。E. 最终效果。

或简单地向内翻折，以横向间断放置可吸收线。确保正确地放置缝线，缝线应全部放置完成后再进行打结，不需要关闭第 2 层。在脐部皮肤下方与筋膜中间部位放置精致的可吸收皮内缝线，以保持脐部皮肤内翻。皮肤采用可吸收线进行皮内缝合，并用可产生适当压力的小敷料覆盖伤口。

尽管感染可使疝复发，但很少见。可能会发生内脏损伤，但如果手术时筋膜的边缘暴露在视野内的话，损伤是可以避免的。

脐的用途

对于患病的新生儿，脐动脉或脐静脉插管是经常采用的方法，并为进行血管内采样和监测提供了便利。伴随的风险有感染、血栓和导管的直接损伤[22]。
1153 脐部常常是腹腔镜手术的入口。脐中央可能是开放的，在婴儿、低龄儿童和脐部较浅者，可探查筋膜环以提供快速的进腹途径。这种技术几乎不会留下易察觉的瘢痕，而脐较深的患者，最好采用脐下切口。脐孔常是腹腔镜手术的基本入口[38]，用于放置视镜。在手术结束，去掉套管后需关闭缺损的筋膜，以减少疝的发生。在肥厚性幽门狭窄的患儿，脐部常被用于环肌切开术的手术入口，这种入路几乎不留下可察觉的瘢痕。

脐部可以用做造口[20]。目前还没有研究比较脐部肠造口术及腹壁其他部位造口术的并发症情况，但常有脐造口术后并发症的单一研究的报道[37]。在关闭切口后，应进行脐部重建，并尽量使脐部的外观接近正常。我们曾应用脐部作为暂时的造口，取得了满意的效果。尽管这样做从生理角度来讲并没有太大的意义，但可以为患者留下一个不太明显的瘢痕。

脐部也可以用作尿流改道的出口，在早产儿，可以充分利用脐部的功能做暂时的脐部膀胱造口，取得了令人满意的结果。小肠也可以作为尿流改道的管道，并可从脐部引出[15]。

脐部重建与保留

脐部在审美上很重要，它的缺如会引起患者的不愉快感。脐部的外观应被患者及家属接受。对女性来说，从审美角度讲一个 T 形或卵圆形上方带帽样的脐部形态是最吸引人的[28]。很宽或突出的脐部却很难被人们所接受。脐部手术的目标之一是尽可能保持脐部的正常外观。标准的脐疝修补术可最低限度地减少脐部损伤，一般能形成令患者较为满意的外形。脐肠系膜和脐尿管残留物如前所述常被切除。在腹腔镜手术后，如果将脐部皮肤固定于关闭的筋膜上，则可以保留令人满意的凹陷形脐窝。

有多余皮肤的巨大疝的脐成形术

当进行巨大疝（巨大的喙形疝）的修补时，多余的皮肤使脐部外形异常，随着时间的推移虽然可有一些好转，但宽大、平坦、前突的形状可以永久存在，各种形式的重建手术可以立即和长期改善脐部的外观[8,9,25,54,92,110]。我们发现以 Reyna 等“三瓣脐成形术”为基础的手术技术对巨大疝的脐重建效果令人满意[92]。然而，这些方法均没有被广泛采用，但在长期随访上显示出其优越性。

腹壁缺损的脐成形术

腹壁畸形手术中常需要保留脐部或进行脐部重建。脐带结构也可以用于脐部的重建或用于形成新的脐部[50,64,68,81,85,112,119]。

在腹裂和脐膨出中，筋膜的修补可以通过脐结构切除后留下的环形皮肤缺损进行。这种情况需进行一期或分期关闭手术。环形的皮肤缺损可以采用荷包皮内缝合，与筋膜中央区域固定在一起（图 72-8）[64]。即使因为应用腹裂袋而扩大了筋膜缺损，缺损的部分也可以采用类似的环形方式重建脐部的外形[50]。一些医生建议在腹壁缺损修补术时保留脐部，并原位保留脐部残留物，直到皮肤切口关闭[81,112,119]。所有膀胱外翻的儿童都存在脐部位置的异常和小型脐膨出。在关闭外翻的膀胱时，常需将脐部向头侧移位，以维持脐部正常的外形[48]。梅干腹综合征的儿童脐部可能附着在血管蒂上，手术切除多余皮肤后，脐部可以放置在正常位置[34]。

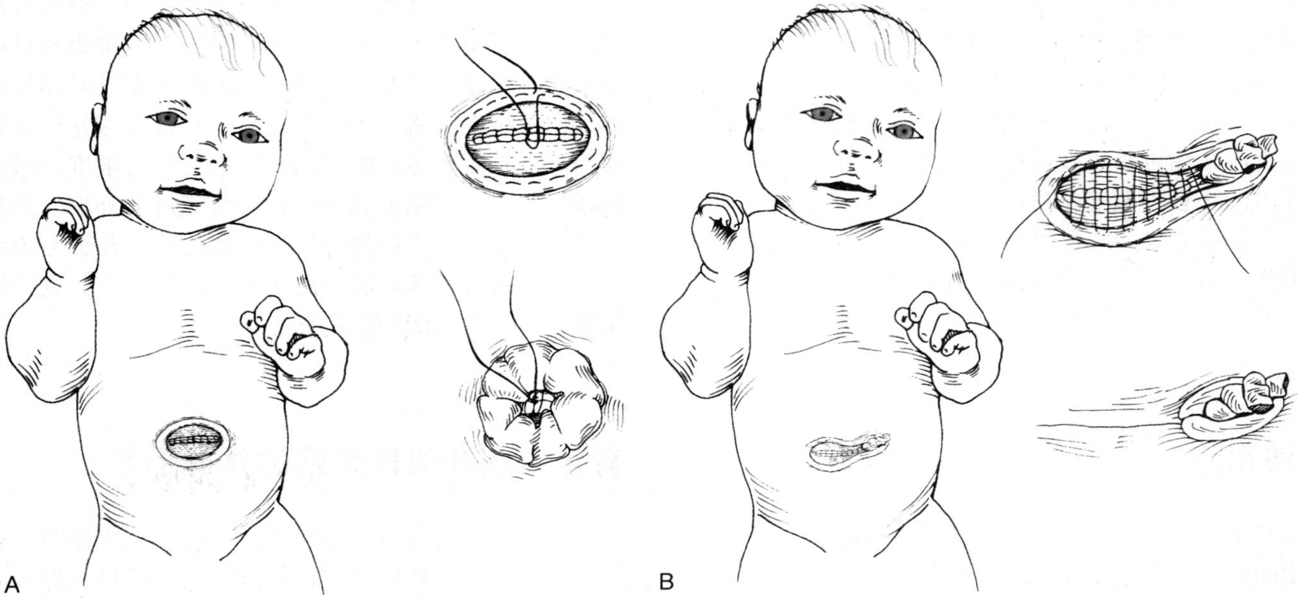

图 72-8　切除脐带组织或通过脐部进行的手术治疗（如腹裂或小型脐膨出的手术修补，通过脐环切除脐肠系膜残留物，通过脐切除脐尿管残留物）后的脐成形技术。A. 关闭筋膜后的腹裂患儿，在周围皮肤组织中放置荷包缝线，注意缝线应穿过筋膜。B. 腹裂修补术后保留脐带。

脐部缺如的重建

在一些情况下，因手术切除的脐部可以重建。脐部的正常位置是在髂嵴水平，第 3 或第 4 腰椎前方。脐部重建应形成一个圆形的或椭圆形的有陡壁的陷窝，以将脐部皮肤固定在腹壁中央筋膜上。随着时间推移，一些重建的脐部将变得扁平。管状皮肤重建维持的时间可能较长，也可能变得像软垫一样或脐窝周围的皮肤轻度升高。许多重建缺失脐部的手术技巧[5,32,55,62,64,71,74,85,99,107,123]各有各的复杂性，但长期随访均没有证实有优越性。有几种手术方法可特异性地用于外翻畸形手术修补后脐部缺失的重建[36,48,49,108]。

（杜　勇译　吴晔明校）

参考文献

1. Adzick NS, Harrison MR, Glick PL, et al: Temporary cutaneous umbilical vesicostomy in premature infants with urethral obstruction. J Pediatr Surg 1986;21:171-172.
2. Ahmed A, Ahmed M, Nmadu PT: Spontaneous rupture of infantile umbilical hernia: Report of three cases. Ann Trop Paediatr 1998;18:239-241.
3. Ameh EA, Chirdan LB, Nmadu PT, et al: Complicated umbilical hernias in children. Pediatr Surg Int 2003;19:280-282.
4. Ameh EA, Nmadu PT: Major complications of omphalitis in neonates and infants. Pediatr Surg Int 2002;18:413-416.
5. Bartsich SA, Schwartz MH: Purse-string method for immediate umbilical reconstruction. Plast Reconstr Surg 2003; 112:1652-1655.
6. Begg RD: The urachus: Its anatomy, histology and development. J Anat 1930;64:170-183.
7. Benjamin B, Vinocur CD, Wagner CW, et al: A closed technique for umbilical hernia repair. Surg Gynecol Obstet 1987;164:473-474.
8. Billmire DF: A technique for the repair of giant umbilical hernia in children. J Am Coll Surg 2002;194:677-680.
9. Blanchard H, St-Vil D, Carceller A, et al: Repair of the huge umbilical hernia in black children. J Pediatr Surg 2000; 35:696-698.
10. Blodgett JB: Transumbilical repair of congenital umbilical hernia. Surg Gynecol Obstet 1941;72:632-634.
11. Blumberg NA: Infantile umbilical hernia. Surg Gynecol Obstet 1980;150:187-192.
12. Boothroyd AE, Cudmore RE: Ultrasound of the discharging umbilicus. Pediatr Radiol 1996;26:362-364.
13. Borgna-Pignatti C, Andreis IA, Bettili G, Zamboni G: Delayed separation of an appendix-containing umbilical stump. J Pediatr Surg 1995;30:1717-1718.
14. Boyle G, Rosenberg HK, O'Neill JA: An unusual presentation of an infected urachal cyst. Review of urachal anomalies. Clin Pediatr (Phila) 1988;27:130-134.
15. Braren V, Workman CH, Johns OT, et al: Use of the umbilical area for placement of a urinary stoma. Surg Gynecol

Obstet 1979;148:543-546.
16. Brook I: Microbiology of necrotizing fasciitis associated with omphalitis in the newborn infant. J Perinatol 1998; 18:28-30.
17. Bryant MS, Bremer AM, Tepas JJ 3rd, et al: Abdominal complications of ventriculoperitoneal shunts. Case reports and review of the literature. Am Surg 1988;54:50-55.
18. Burchell MC: Spontaneous umbilical fistula in Crohn's disease. Report of a case. Dis Colon Rectum 1989;32: 621-623.
19. Caberwal D, Kogan SJ, Levitt SB: Ectopic pancreas presenting as an umbilical mass. J Pediatr Surg 1977;12: 593-599.
20. Cameron GS, Lau GY: The umbilicus as a site for temporary colostomy in infants. J Pediatr Surg 1982;17: 362-364.
21. Choi SO, Park WH, Kang JS: Purulent umbilical drainage from infection of left umbilical artery associated with open umbilocoperitoneal communication. J Pediatr Surg 1988; 23:382-383.
22. Cilley RE: Arterial access in infants and children. Semin Pediatr Surg 1992;1:174-180.
23. Cilley RE: Giant hamartoma protruding from the umbilicus in a newborn. Unpublished data.
24. Clapuyt P, Saint-Martin C, De Batselier P, et al: Urachal neuroblastoma: First case report. Pediatr Radiol 1999;29: 320-321.
25. Cone JB, Golladay ES: Purse-string skin closure of umbilical hernia repair. J Pediatr Surg 1983;18:297.
26. Cornil C, Reynolds CT, Kickham CJ: Carcinoma of the urachus. J Urol 1967;98:93-95.
27. Courreges P, Poddevin F, Lecoutre D: Para-umbilical block: A new concept for regional anaesthesia in children. Paediatr Anaesth 1997;7:211-214.
28. Craig SB, Faller MS, Puckett CL: In search of the ideal female umbilicus. Plast Reconstr Surg 2000;105:389-392.
29. Crankson SJ, Ahmed GS, Palkar V: Patent omphalomesenteric duct of the vermiform appendix in a neonate: Congenital appendicoumbilical fistula. Pediatr Surg Int 1998;14:229-230.
30. Crawford RA, Sethia KK, Fawcett DP: An unusual presentation of a urachal remnant. Br J Urol 1989;64:315-316.
31. Cullen TS: Embryology, Anatomy, and Diseases of the Umbilicus Together with Diseases of the Urachus. Philadelphia, WB Saunders, 1916.
32. de Lacerda DJ, Martins DM, Marques A, et al: Umbilicoplasty for the abdomen with a thin adipose layer. Br J Plast Surg 1994;47:386-387.
33. Ehigiegba AE, Selo-Ojeme DO: Myomectomy in pregnancy: Incarcerated pedunculated fibroid in an umbilical hernia sac. Int J Clin Pract 1999;53:80.
34. Ehrlich RM, Lesavoy MA: Umbilicus preservation with total abdominal wall reconstruction in prune-belly syndrome. Urology 1993;41:231-232.
35. Evans AG: The comparative incidence of umbilical hernias in colored and white infants. J Natl Med Assoc 1941;33: 158-160.
36. Feyaerts A, Mure PY, Jules JA, et al: Umbilical reconstruction in patients with exstrophy: The kangaroo pouch technique. J Urol 2001;165:2026-2027.
37. Fitzgerald PG, Lau GY, Cameron GS: Use of the umbilical site for temporary ostomy: Review of 47 cases. J Pediatr Surg 1989;24:973.
38. Fitzgerald PG, Lau GY, Langer JC, et al: Umbilical fold incision for pyloromyotomy. J Pediatr Surg 1990;25: 1117-1118.
39. Ford T, Widgerow AD: Umbilical keloid: An early start. Ann Plast Surg 1990;25:214-215.
40. Franklin RR, Navarro C: Extragenital endometriosis. Prog Clin Biol Res 1990;323:289-295.
41. Friedman JM: Umbilical dysmorphology. The importance of contemplating the belly button. Clin Genet 1985;28: 343-347.
42. Gray SW, Skandalakis JE: The bladder and urethra. In Gray SW, Skandalakis JE (eds): Embryology for Surgeons: The Embryological Basis for the Treatment of Congenital Defects. Philadelphia, WB Saunders, 1972, pp 519-552.
43. Groff DB: Suprapubic dermoid sinus. J Pediatr Surg 1993; 28:242-243.
44. Gross RE: The Surgery of Infancy and Childhood: Its Principles and Techniques. Philadelphia, WB Saunders, 1953, pp 423-427.
45. Guneser S, Altintas DU, Aksungur P, et al: An infant with severe leucocyte adhesion deficiency. Acta Paediatr 1996; 85:622-624.
46. Gupta S, Sikora S, Singh M, et al: Pilonidal disease of the umbilicus—a report of two cases. Jpn J Surg 1990;20: 590-592.
47. Hall DE, Roberts KB, Charney E: Umbilical hernia: What happens after age 5 years? J Pediatr 1981;98:415-417.
48. Hanna MK: Reconstruction of umbilicus during functional closure of bladder exstrophy. Urology 1986;27:340-342.
49. Hanna MK, Ansong K: Reconstruction of umbilicus in bladder exstrophy. Urology 1984;24:324-326.
50. Harmel RP Jr: Primary repair of gastroschisis with umbilicoplasty. Surg Gynecol Obstet 1985;160:464-465.
51. Hayward AR, Harvey BA, Leonard J, et al: Delayed separation of the umbilical cord, widespread infections, and defective neutrophil mobility. Lancet 1979;1:1099-1101.
52. Heifetz CJ, Bilsel ZT, Gaus WW: Observations on the disappearance of umbilical hernias in infancy and childhood. Surg Gynecol Obstet 1963;116:469-473.
53. Hung CH, Cheng SN, Hua YM, et al: Leukocyte adhesion deficiency disorder: Report of one case. Acta Paediatr Taiwan 1999;40:128-131.
54. Ikeda H, Yamamoto H, Fujino J, et al: Umbilicoplasty for large protruding umbilicus accompanying umbilical hernia: A simple and effective technique. Pediatr Surg Int 2004; 20:105-107.
55. Itoh Y, Arai K: Umbilical reconstruction using a cone-shaped flap. Ann Plast Surg 1992;28:335-338.
56. Jona JZ: Umbilical anomalies. In Raffensberger JG (ed): Swenson's Pediatric Surgery, 5th ed. Norwalk, CT, Appleton & Lange, 1990, pp 193-195.
57. Kadzombe E, Currie AB: Neonatal fistula from the appendix to the umbilicus. J Pediatr Surg 1988;23: 1059-1060.
58. Kamii Y, Zaki AM, Honna T, et al: Spontaneous regression of patient omphalomesenteric duct: From a fistula to Meckel's diverticulum. J Pediatr Surg 1992;27:115-116.
59. Khanna R, Kumar SS, Raju BS, et al: Body piercing in the accident and emergency department. J Accid Emerg Med 1999;16:418-421.
60. Kittle CF, Jenkins HP, Dragstedt LR: Patent omphalomesenteric duct and its relation to the diverticulum of Meckel. Arch Surg 1947;54:10-36.
61. Knoll LD, Pustka RA, Anderson JR, et al: Periumbilical pain secondary to persistent urachal band. Urology 1988; 32:526-528.
62. Korachi A, Oudit D, Ellabban M: A simplified technique for umbilical reconstruction. Plast Reconstr Surg 2004;114: 619-621.

63. Kosloske AM, Bartow SA: Debridement of periumbilical necrotizing fasciitis: Importance of excision of the umbilical vessels and urachal remnant. J Pediatr Surg 1991;26: 808-810.
64. Krummel TM, Sieber WK: Closure of congenital abdominal wall defects with umbilicoplasty. Surg Gynecol Obstet 1987;165:168-169.
65. Kurzbart E, Zeitlin M, Feigenbaum D, et al: Rare spontaneous regression of patent omphalomesenteric duct after birth. Arch Dis Child Fetal Neonatal Ed 2002;86:F63.
66. Lally KP, Atkinson JB, Woolley MM, et al: Necrotizing fasciitis. A serious sequela of omphalitis in the newborn. Ann Surg 1984;199:101-103.
67. Lassaletta L, Fonkalsrud EW, Tovar JA, et al: The management of umbilical hernias in infancy and childhood. J Pediatr Surg 1975;10:405-409.
68. Lee SL, DuBois JJ, Greenholz SK, et al: Advancement flap umbilicoplasty after abdominal wall closure: Postoperative results compared with normal umbilical anatomy. J Pediatr Surg 2001;36:1168-1170.
69. Lena SM: Pierced navels are troublesome. CMAJ 1994;150: 646-647.
70. Lizerbram EK, Mahour GH, Gilsanz V: Dual patency of the omphalomesenteric duct and urachus. Pediatr Radiol 1997;27:244-246.
71. Marconi F: Reconstruction of the umbilicus: A simple technique. Plast Reconstr Surg 1995;95:1115-1117.
72. Mason WH, Andrews R, Ross LA, et al: Omphalitis in the newborn infant. Pediatr Infect Dis J 1989;8:521-525.
73. Meier DE, OlaOlorun DA, Omodele RA, et al: Incidence of umbilical hernia in African children: Redefinition of "normal" and reevaluation of indications for repair. World J Surg 2001;25:645-648.
74. Miller MJ, Balch CM: "Iris" technique for immediate umbilical reconstruction. Plast Reconstr Surg 1993;92: 754-756.
75. Mitchell W, Venable D, Patel AJ: Pseudoexstrophy. Urology 1993;41:134-136.
76. Moore TC: Omphalomesenteric duct malformations. Semin Pediatr Surg 1996;5:116-123.
77. Moore TC: Omphalomesenteric duct anomalies. Surg Gynecol Obstet 1956;103:569-580.
78. Morgan WW, White JJ, Stumbaugh S, et al: Prophylactic umbilical hernia repair in childhood to prevent adult incarceration. Surg Clin North Am 1970;50:839-845.
79. Moss RL, Musemeche CA, Kosloske AM: Necrotizing fasciitis in children: Prompt recognition and aggressive therapy improve survival. J Pediatr Surg 1996;31:1142-1146.
80. Nagar H: Umbilical granuloma: A new approach to an old problem. Pediatr Surg Int 2001;17:513-514.
81. Nagaya M, Ando H, Tsudo M, et al: Preservation of the umbilical cord at the primary fascial closure in infants with gastroschisis. J Pediatr Surg 1993;28:1471-1472.
82. Nix JT, Menville JG, Albert M, et al: Congenital patent urachus. J Urol 1958;79:264-273.
83. Nobuhara KK, Lukish JR, Hartman GE, et al: The giant umbilical cord: An unusual presentation of a patent urachus. J Pediatr Surg 2004;39:128-129.
84. Novack AH, Mueller B, Ochs H: Umbilical cord separation in the normal newborn. Am J Dis Child 1988;142:220-223.
85. Park S, Hata Y, Ito O, et al: Umbilical reconstruction after repair of omphalocele and gastroschisis. Plast Reconstr Surg 1999;104:204-207.
86. Park WH, Choi SO: An unusual urachal sinus with external opening in the midline suprapubic area. J Pediatr Surg 2003;38:E18-E20.
87. Park WH, Choi SO, Park KK, et al: Prepubic dermoid sinus: Possible variant of dorsal urethral duplication (Stephens type 3). J Pediatr Surg 1993;28:1610-1611.
88. Park WH, Choi SO, Woo SK, et al: Appendicumbilical fistula as a sequela of perforated appendicitis. J Pediatr Surg 1991;26:1413-1415.
89. Pezzati M, Biagioli EC, Martelli E, et al: Umbilical cord care: The effect of eight different cord-care regimens on cord separation time and other outcomes. Biol Neonate 2002;81:38-44.
90. Pomeranz A: Anomalies, abnormalities, and care of the umbilicus. Pediatr Clin North Am 2004;51:819-827.
91. Powell FC, Su WP: Dermatoses of the umbilicus. Int J Dermatol 1988;27:150-156.
92. Reyna TM, Harris WH Jr, Smith SB: Surgical management of proboscoid herniae. J Pediatr Surg 1987;22:911-912.
93. Rowe PC, Gearhart JP: Retraction of the umbilicus during voiding as an initial sign of a urachal anomaly. Pediatrics 1993;91:153-154.
94. Samuel M, Freeman NV, Vaishnav A, et al: Necrotizing fasciitis: A serious complication of omphalitis in neonates. J Pediatr Surg 1994;29:1414-1416.
95. Sawin RS, Schaller RT, Tapper D, et al: Early recognition of neonatal abdominal wall necrotizing fasciitis. Am J Surg 1994;167:481-484.
96. Shaw A: Disorders of the umbilicus. In Welch KJ, Randolph JG, Ravitch MM, et al (eds): Pediatric Surgery. Chicago, Year Book, 1986, pp 731-739.
97. Shaw A, Pierog S: "Ectopic" liver in the umbilicus: An unusual focus of infection in a newborn infant. Pediatrics 1969;44:448-450.
98. Shetty MR: Metastatic tumors of the umbilicus: A review 1830-1989. J Surg Oncol 1990;45:212-215.
99. Shinohara H, Matsuo K, Kikuchi N: Umbilical reconstruction with an inverted C-V flap. Plast Reconstr Surg 2000; 105:703-705.
100. Sibley WL 3rd, Lynn HB, Harris LE: A twenty-five year study of infantile umbilical hernia. Surgery 1964;55:462-468.
101. Simiyu DE: Morbidity and mortality of neonates admitted in general paediatric wards at Kenyatta National Hospital. East Afr Med J 2003;80:611-616.
102. Singh UK, Singh S, Ojha P, et al: Spontaneous rupture of umbilical hernia in an infant. Indian Pediatr 2000;37: 341-342.
103. Sroujieh AS, Dawoud A: Umbilical sepsis. Br J Surg 1989;76:687-688.
104. Steck WD, Helwig EB: Umbilical granulomas, pilonidal disease and the urachus. Surg Gynecol Obstet 1965;120: 1043-1057.
105. Steinthal AJ: Malformations of the umbilicus and urachus: Faulty closure of the vitello-intestinal duct and its results. In von Bergmann E, von Bruns P, von Mikuliez J, et al (eds): A System of Practical Surgery. Philadelphia, Lea Brothers, 1904, pp 142-149, 593-606.
106. Stunden RJ, Brown RA, Rode H, et al: Umbilical gangrene in the newborn. J Pediatr Surg 1988;23:130-134.
107. Sugawara Y, Hirabayashi S, Asato H, et al: Reconstruction of the umbilicus using a single triangular flap. Ann Plast Surg 1995;34:78-80.
108. Sumfest JM, Mitchell ME: Reconstruction of the umbilicus in exstrophy. J Urol 1994;151:453-454.
109. Suzuki N, Labosky PA, Furuta Y, et al: Failure of ventral body wall closure in mouse embryos lacking a procollagen C-proteinase encoded by *Bmp1*, a mammalian gene related to *Drosophila tolloid*. Development 1996;122:3587-3595.
110. Tamir G, Kurzbart E: Umbilical reconstruction after repair

of large umbilical hernia: The "lazy-M" and omega flaps. J Pediatr Surg 2004;39:226-228.
111. Tsukahara M, Fernandez GI: Umbilical findings in Aarskog syndrome. Clin Genet 1994;45:260-265.
112. Uceda JE: Umbilical preservation in omphalocele repair. J Pediatr Surg 1994;29:1412-1413.
113. Upadhyay V, Kukkady A: Urachal remnants: An enigma. Eur J Pediatr Surg 2003;13:372-376.
114. Veloso FT, Cardoso V, Fraga J, et al: Spontaneous umbilical fistula in Crohn's disease. J Clin Gastroenterol 1989;11:197-200.
115. Vohr BR, Rosenfield AG, Oh W: Umbilical hernia in low birth weight infants (less than 1500 grams). J Pediatr 1977;90:807-808.
116. Walker SH: The natural history of umbilical hernia. A six-year follow up of 314 negro children with this defect. Clin Pediatr (Phila) 1967;6:29-32.
117. Waltzer H: The umbilicus as vagina substitute. A clinical note. Psychoanal Q 1974;43:493-496.
118. Weir E: Navel gazing: A clinical glimpse at body piercing. Can Med Assoc J 2001;164:864.
119. Wesson DE, Baesl TJ: Repair of gastroschisis with preservation of the umbilicus. J Pediatr Surg 1986;21;764-765.
120. Wilson CB, Ochs HD, Almquist J, et al: When is umbilical cord separation delayed? J Pediatr 1985;107:292-294.
121. Woods GE: Some observations on umbilical hernia in infants. Arch Dis Child 1953;28:450-462.
122. Yokoyama S, Hayashida Y, Nagahama J, et al: Rhabdomyosarcoma of the urachus. A case report. Acta Cytol 1997;41:1293-1298.
123. Yotsuyanagi T, Nihei Y, Sawada Y: A simple technique for reconstruction of the umbilicus, using two twisted flaps. Plast Reconstr Surg 1998;102:2444-2446.
124. Yuen JS, Chow PK, Koong HN, et al: Unusual sites (thorax and umbilical hernia sac) of endometriosis. J R Coll Surg Edinb 2001;46:313-315.
125. Zaidenstein L, Freud E, Schwartz M, et al: Clinical presentation of rare appendiculo-omphalic anomalies. J Pediatr Surg 1995;30:1702-1703.
126. Zupan J, Garner P, Omari AAA: Topical umbilical cord care at birth (Cochrane Review). Cochrane Database Syst Rev 2004;3:CD001057.

第 73 章

先天性腹壁缺损

Michael D. Klein

历史回顾

1157 公元1世纪，罗马医生 Aulus Cornelius Celsus 首先报道了新生儿腹部缺损。公元5世纪 Paulus Aegineta 也报道了相似内容[67]。16世纪 Ambrose Paré 在其著作中描述了脐膨出[123]，同一时期 Lycosthenes 首先对腹裂进行了描述[103]。1894 年 Taruffi 应用了“gastroschisis”这一术语[156]。许多年来腹裂与囊膜撕破的脐膨出相混淆[133]。Moore 和 Stokes 对这两种疾病的临床本质进行了明确界定，如我们今天所理解的一样[112]，不过他们将功劳归功于早期使用这些术语的作者如Bernstein等[19]，而不是最早收集了一些资料的 Massabuau 和 Guibal[107]。1802 年 Hey 首次报道一例成功的脐膨出修补术[60]。1873 年 Visick 报道了一例成功的腹裂修补术[166]。1899 年 Ahlfeld[1] 报道用酒精涂抹脐膨出患儿的外被囊膜，使其结痂挛缩和上皮化，而 Max Grob 普及了在囊膜涂抹红汞的治疗方法[52,53,122]，虽然随后有水银毒性的相关报道[32,46,150]。现代的治疗观念由 Ein 和 Shandling 引进，他们在治疗中使用了黏性的人造半透膜[45]。1887 年 Olshausen 首先报道去除囊膜后用皮瓣覆盖缺损处，而 Gross 进一步证实了这一技术的有效性并加以推广[56]。因为肠管脱出腹腔，腹腔没有得到发育并且肠管与皮瓣粘连，导致疝很难分阶段关闭。因此，有时要将皮肤覆盖在整个完整的囊膜上[55,105]。Schuter 发现只用皮肤关闭腹腔并不能促进腹腔的增大，他在 1967 年介绍了用聚炳乙烯材料分阶段缩减巨大脐膨出的方法[142]。新的技术不断涌现，皮肤移植[73,99]、造气腹扩大腹腔壁为以后关闭腹腔做准备[119,130]、肝部分切除[27,78]、筋膜的减压性侧切[14]和分离腹直肌等独创性方法的出现，使非手术治疗取得了普遍的成功或认可[85]。

先天性腹壁缺损的临床分类

临床上重要的先天性腹壁缺损都在脐部，并具有完整的腹直肌（表 73-1）。脐膨出是一种较大的缺损（直径超过 4 cm），并被羊膜所覆盖，内有中肠与其他腹部器官，如肝、脾和生殖腺（图 73-1）。一种罕见的脐膨出类型是头褶缺损或称 Cantrell 五联症，这种腹壁缺损是脐上缺损，心脏通过缺损的心包膜及隔膜中心腱突出到囊膜腔内[29]。异位心（心脏突出胸 1158
腔外，与脐膨出囊腔内的心脏相反，它没有心包膜覆盖）可以被认为是头褶缺损的另一种类型（图 73-2）。另一种罕见的脐膨出是尾褶缺损、泄殖腔外翻，这种畸形是脐下缺损，常合并膀胱外翻和肛门闭锁（见 118 章）。腹裂的腹肌缺损直径小于 4 cm，无囊膜覆盖，内容物通常为中肠和胃（图 73-3）。脐疝的缺损直径也小于 4 cm，内容物只是中肠，但有囊膜覆盖（图 73-4）。脐疝有两种特征与以上两种畸形相鉴别：它的缺损处外覆正常皮肤，并且在出生时很少

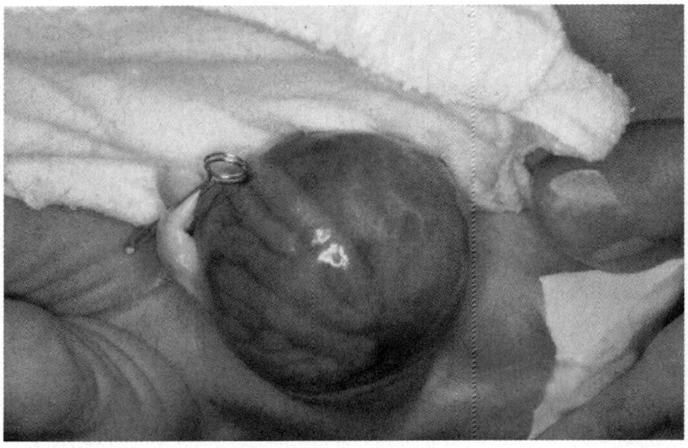

图 73-1 脐膨出。

表 73-1　先天性腹壁缺损的比较

缺损	位置	囊膜	内容物	发生频率	伴发畸形	预后
脐膨出——侧褶	脐部	有	肝、肠、脾、生殖腺	常见	染色体、心脏	好（取决于伴发畸形）
脐膨出——头褶（Cantrell 五联症）	脐上	有	肝、肠	罕见	心脏、胸骨裂、心包膜缺损、膈肌中心腱缺损	差
脐膨出——尾褶（泄殖腔外翻）	脐下	有	肠	罕见	膀胱外翻、无肛、尿道上裂	一般
脐疝	脐	有	肠	不常见	不常见	好
腹裂	脐右侧	无	肠	常见	肠闭锁	好
异位心	胸骨中线	无	心脏	罕见	心脏	差

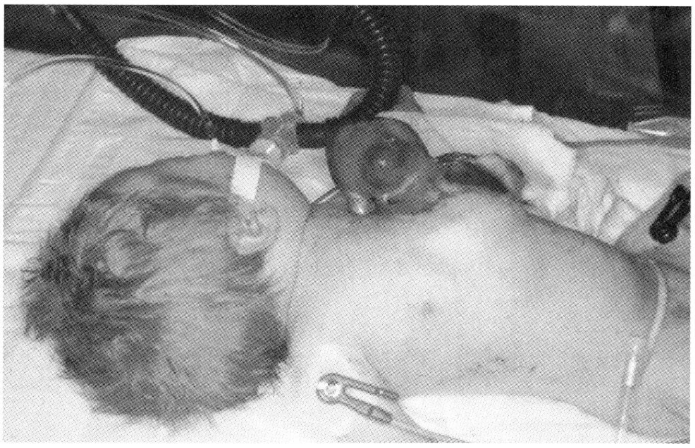

图 73-2　异位心（也见彩图）。

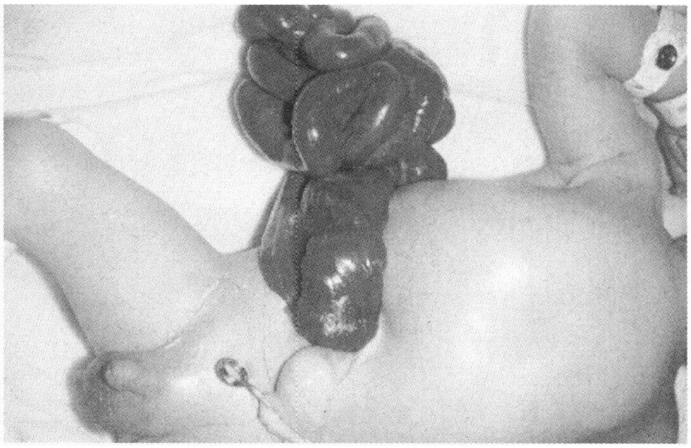

图 73-3　腹裂。

发生，而常出现在出生后头几周或数月内。1970 年以前的文献，甚至到今天的非小儿外科专业的文献中一直将这三种疾病混为一谈，尤其对腹裂和脐膨出，这使得一些相关的数据很难予以解释。

先天性腹壁缺损或梅干腹综合征的婴幼儿都有正常的腹壁层，但在疏松的蜂窝组织中肌肉很少。很多与此相似的肌肉缺陷畸形发生在泌尿生殖道和消化道（见 114 章）。

曾经报道的一些其他腹壁缺损常危及生命[97,127,154]，如肠切除术后的真性腹壁结构缺损[49,109]。

胚胎学

腹壁的胚胎发育

孕 3 周时胚胎的扁平细胞盘发育为 4 个褶，并将关闭形成体腔（图 73-5A 和 5B）。两个侧褶向前部中线处汇合形成胸腹膜管。起源于大脑远端的头褶逐渐被前胸壁所取代，向下发育为心脏。头褶中包含有原始横膈组织，向后延伸，将胸腹膜管分为胸腔和腹腔。尾褶（在平盘期）起始于肛门远端，将来发育为膀胱或尿囊。在这个时期，肠管沿着胚胎长轴生
长，并在脐部与卵黄囊相交通；卵黄囊最终将消失， 1159
有时只在远端回肠上留下卵黄管残余物。孕 5 周时，肠管在脐腔内即胚胎前表面体蒂中的腔内，开始延长并发育（图 73-5C）。孕 10 周时，肠管由脐腔中返回至腹腔，并旋转和固定。

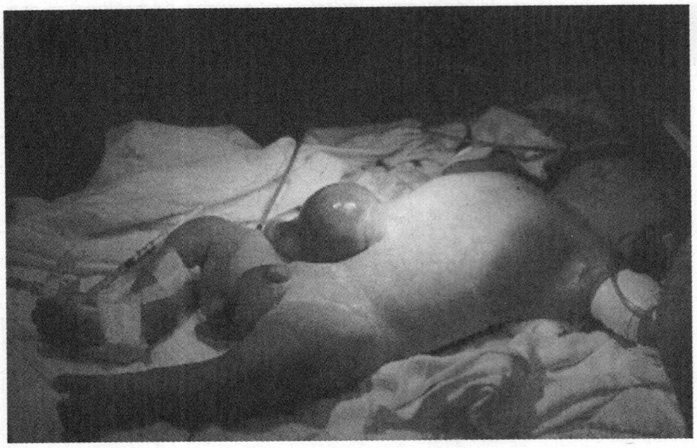

图 73-4 脐疝。

胚胎形成缺陷

脐膨出表现为体褶发育过程中的缺陷[43]。大多数脐膨出是侧褶缺损，且缺损总是在脐部。直肠肌起点常与肋缘处分开，因此修补时往往不能将两者缝合在一起。无论何种因素造成的损伤，该畸变总是发生在胚胎早期，因此也可能影响到其他器官系统发育， 1160
所以脐膨出的患儿常合并有其他畸形。头褶缺损导致心脏异位或 Cantrell 五联症，而尾褶缺损则引起膀胱和泄殖腔外翻。绒毛膜或卵黄囊破裂形成索带引起的机械性破坏可更好地解释异位心的发生，这些儿童常有其他索带损坏的特征，如颜面裂[70]。

腹裂即出生前内脏外露，可能与脐腔发育畸形有关[76]。随着肠管延长，体腔内没有空间，肠管扩张并正

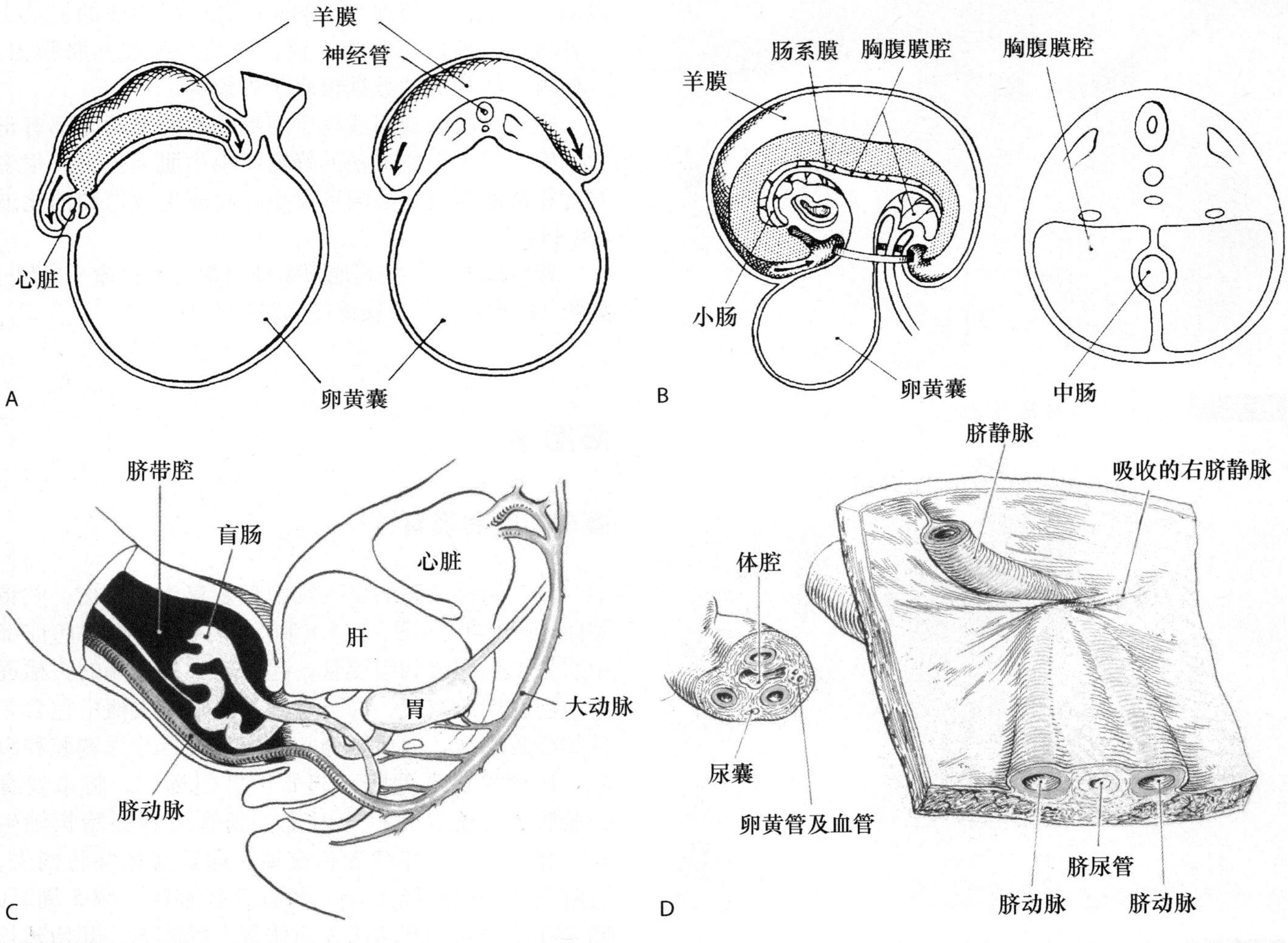

图 73-5 腹壁的胚胎发育。A. 2 周的胚胎，在体褶形成腹腔之前像一个扁平盘。B. 4 周时体褶完成，肠管从夹在卵黄囊中。C. 6 周时延长的中肠进入脐体腔。D. 从腹腔内侧看，因右脐静脉被吸收，脐右侧相对缺少支持物。

好在脐右侧破裂露出体壁，这可能是因为右脐静脉在孕4周时被吸收，脐右侧相对薄弱所致（图73-5D）[144]。因此，腹裂没有膜覆盖，肠管常常表现为壁厚、水肿、表面粗糙并被纤维素样膜状组织覆盖。有人根据胚胎肾发挥作用后，羊水的电解质成分发生改变，对后一种现象做出了解释[4,79,159,160]。动物实验显示膜状物既能在子宫内形成[34,102,138]，也能在出生后形成[38]。一些研究者认为肠管的这种情况与胎儿在羊水中形成胎粪有关[116,120]。最近的临床研究发现，羊水若被胎粪污染，则新生儿肠管会形成一种纤维素样膜，若未被污染则不会形成[116]。我们对50例新生儿的临床观察显示，腹裂肠管的变化最有可能发生在出生后（图73-6）。刚出生时，腹裂的肠管通常正常，20分钟后开始出现其特征性的变化。这些变化可能由于肠管暴露在空气中造成，但更可能与肠系膜血管在腹壁水平闭塞导致肠管水肿，以及蛋白质样液体渗出有关。

脐疝是中肠在第10～12孕周时返回腹腔时发生的缺陷引起的，因此这种缺损只包含有中肠并有被膜覆盖。疝比脐膨出要小得多，且外观相对较好。从胚胎学和临床角度区分脐疝和脐膨出对患者的治疗及预后均很重要。Margulies[106]首先将Pernkopf[124]、Politzer及Sternberg[126]的胚胎学著作翻译成英文，使得Benson、Penberty和Hill[18]将脐疝和脐膨出区分为不同本质的疾病。

对这些不同类型的缺损（尤其是腹裂）现有的解释并没有被广泛接受。一些人认为腹裂是腹壁组成部分缺损的“中胚层形成障碍”[66,68]。虽然这种畸形

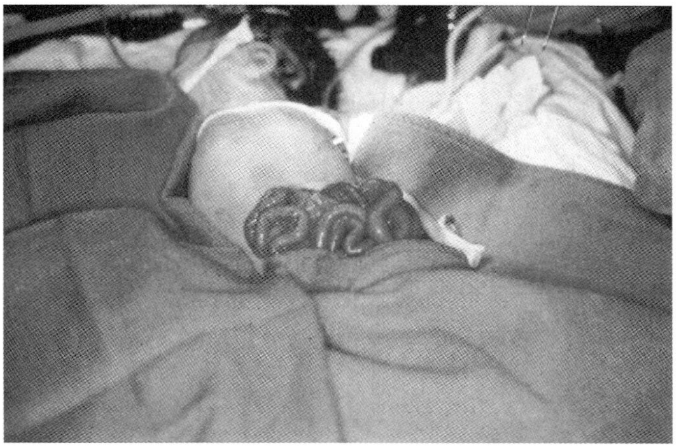

图 73-6　刚分娩的腹裂。肠管表面光滑、无水肿及覆盖剥脱的纤维素样渗出膜。

以前曾有报道，但通常是畸形死胎。几乎所有腹壁缺损的活产婴儿肌层结构均正常且腹壁层完整。其他的报道认为一些腹壁缺损不是发育性的而是获得性的，是脐部血流中断的结果[63]。这个解释无法说明一些缺损合并的畸形，也与缺损患儿腹壁正常，而脐部有一个巨大的且异常开口的事实不符。一项研究提示缺损的发生可能与吸烟，尤其是孕母还同时使用其他血管收缩剂相关[170]。许多早期的报道显示腹裂是一种破裂或囊膜撕裂的脐膨出[158]。腹裂没有如此多的囊膜残余物的事实否定了这种观点。

几种外源性物质能诱导形成腹壁缺损动物模型，尽管这些报道认为一些缺损是脐膨出，但它们更像腹裂、脊柱裂或少见的危及生命的体壁畸形。这些研究提出了这样一个问题，自1970年起，腹裂的发生率明显增加是否与新的环境致畸物的出现有关[42]。一位研究者发现致畸物与腹裂之间没有联系[95]，而一些人则认为避孕药、阿司匹林[83,169]及毒品可能与腹裂的发生有关[63]。

遗传和家族史

很少的几个报道显示腹壁缺损，尤其是脐膨出，在同一个家族里，甚至是在双胞胎中同时出现，但这种情况并不常见[129,134]。尚未发现与先天性腹壁缺损有关的特异性基因，但它们有些确实是一些综合征的表现之一，Beckwith-Wiedemann综合征（先天性腹壁缺损、巨舌和低血糖，日后可发展为腹部肿瘤）是最常见的综合征[17,172]。值得一提的是Beckwith-Wiedemann综合征中的腹壁缺损可以与以上提到的3个病变中的任何1个共同存在，然而我们推测它们可能有着不同的胚胎发生机制。其他一些存在这些缺损的综合征还有OEIS综合征（脐膨出、外翻、肛门闭锁和脊柱畸形）[144]；Gershoni-Baruch综合征（脐膨出、膈疝、心血管畸形和桡侧列缺损），可能是常染色体隐性遗传[48]；Donnai-Barrow综合征（膈疝、脐疝、胼胝体缺乏、器官距离过远、近视和感觉神经性耳聋），也是常染色体隐性遗传[31]；以及Fryns综合征（先天性膈疝、粗糙面容、肢端发育不全并常有脐膨 1161
出[8]）[13]。OEIS综合征与尾褶脐膨出有密切关系，可能与一个特定的基因有关[157]。脐膨出也似乎与一种染色体畸形有关[136,175]，尤其是13、18或21三体[28,131,148]。

很少有临床根据表明基因畸变与腹裂有关，但是一项研究显示，当仔细询问家族史时，6%的腹裂患者有一位亲属存在相似的疾病[161]。在小鼠动物模型的相关报道中，主动脉羧肽酶样蛋白（aortic-carboxypeptidase-like proterin）基因缺失与腹裂的发生有关[90]。

产前诊断

超声检查

目前，产前诊断常采用超声检查[150]。脐膨出可以通过存在囊膜及其缺损中有肝而分别与腹裂和脐疝区分。产前咨询时做出诊断一般预后较好。欧洲 11 个产前超声注册处的报道显示，超声发现脐膨出的敏感度是75%（范围 25%～100%），发现腹裂的敏感度为 83%（18%～100%）[15]。首次发现脐膨出的时间是(18±6）孕周，腹裂则是（20±7）孕周。仅有 41%的产前检查为脐膨出的胎儿出生时存活，22% 在胎儿期死亡，37% 中止妊娠；而 59% 的腹裂胎儿在出生时存活，12% 在胎儿期死亡，29% 中止妊娠。

产前超声检查也可以发现相关畸形[64]。腹裂常常伴发肠闭锁[10]，脐膨出常伴发心血管畸形，使得产前超声心动图检查很有意义[163]。

由于所有异位心脏预后不良，当超声证实心脏在胸腔外时，中止妊娠可能是合理的选择。一些超声医生试图通过产前超声发现腹裂患儿的肠道问题[11,86,127]，但包括我们目前的经验在内，所有的医疗中心都没有成功的报道[5,26]。

虽然常规产前超声检查对一些存在致命畸形的胎儿可能提高其存活率，但它的广泛应用并没有显示明显改善围生期发病率或母亲的预后。虽然这可能节省医疗费用，但多与母亲选择中止妊娠有关。脐膨出或腹裂病例不属此列[165]。

羊水和血清检测

所有不伴脊髓脊膜膨出的腹壁缺损胎儿的羊水及母亲血清中 α 甲胎蛋白（AFP）升高，其羊水中的乙酰胆碱酯酶（AChE）也增高[114]。一项对 23 例腹裂和 17 例脐膨出妊娠的研究发现，妊娠两三个月时，腹裂胎儿的血清 AFP 比正常高 9.42 倍，脐膨出比正常高 4.18 倍[137]。另一项研究报道发现 100% 的腹裂及仅 20% 的脐膨出胎儿羊水中 AFP 升高，80% 的腹裂及 27% 的脐膨出胎儿 AChE 升高[162]。

产科分娩

凭直觉，似乎剖宫产可以避免损伤肠管或撕裂囊膜，对患儿更适合。一些报道肯定剖宫产的益处[44,93,135]，但也有 2 例腹裂患儿在剖宫产时肠管被损伤的报道[40]。最近更多的产科文献显示剖宫产对腹壁缺损患儿不存在优势[58,62,94,143,147,153]。一些报道甚至认为腹壁缺损患儿的母亲在小儿外科医疗中心分娩没有好处[117,152]。它们认为分娩方式的选择应该由产科医生根据产科适应证决定，无需考虑有无腹壁缺损。

一些医生认为腹裂患儿的肠管状况与妊娠晚期（33周）时的宫内环境相关，因此建议腹裂患儿应在预产期前出生[111]。但我们认为腹裂患儿肠管表现发生在出生后，无需让患儿承担早产的风险。让患儿在预产期前出生的益处似乎表现在计划性剖宫产可以让患儿及时接受修补手术，以避免肠系膜静脉充血影响肠管的状态。其他医生则认为预产期前出生没有益处[44]。

产前介入治疗已被认为可用于治疗腹裂患儿，但还未得到验证。根据实验研究结果，腹裂患儿的肠管损伤与羊水有关[3]。一位土耳其的医生为 1 例患者更换了羊水，认为这样可使腹裂患儿出生时的肠管维持正常外观[2]。在法国有人用生理盐水对腹裂和羊水过少的患儿在妊娠期进行羊膜腔灌注，发现可以明显改善出生时肠管的性状[139,167]。

做好产前咨询并与产科医生协调很重要。因为腹裂的肠管状况和脐膨出的肠管扩张程度及肝大小常与分娩至手术修补的时间间隔相关，应尽快在患儿出生后即实施修补术。

临床表现

脐膨出

脐膨出是腹壁中心缺损，直径常大于 4 cm。它常被一个半透明膜所覆盖，脐带由其上伸出。囊膜在分

娩时可能被撕破，但很少发生。腹壁肌肉正常，但后
1162 来腹直肌嵌入肋缘，使得减压手术困难。囊内常包含肝、中肠和其他器官如脾或生殖腺。脐膨出患儿常常是足月产。

发生率

1970 年之前，脐膨出是腹壁缺损中最常见的类型，但现在退居第二位，排在腹裂之后。脐膨出的总发生率是每 5000 个活产婴儿中有 1 ~ 2.5 个[107]，男性占多数[28]。

伴发症

脐膨出伴发的畸形见表 73-2。据报道，多达 45% 的脐膨出患儿有心脏畸形，包括室间隔缺损、房间隔缺损、异位心脏、三尖瓣闭锁、主动脉缩窄和新生儿持续性肺动脉高压[51]。40% 的患儿存在染色体异常[118]，其与 Down 综合征之间的联系也有报道[131]。脐膨出患儿看起来常大于胎龄（巨大儿或出生体重大于 4 kg）[168]。据报道，肌骨骼及神经管畸形的发生率也比想象的高[7,98]。胃食管反流比较常见，在一项研究报道中，其发生率可达 43%[81]，且 33% 的患儿在 1 岁时存在隐睾症[71]。

脐膨出的头褶畸形（Cantrell 五联症）

这个五联症的基本表现是恒定的[29]，脐上脐膨出常仅包含肝或主要是肝。通过半透明膜常可以看到从膈肌缺损中挤出的心脏或左心室憩室。也可表现为

表 73-2　伴发情况

脐膨出	腹裂
心脏	肠闭锁
染色体异常	小于胎龄儿
Down 综合征	早产儿
巨大儿	胃食管反流
胃食管反流	隐睾症
隐睾症	
肌骨骼	
神经管缺损	

下胸骨裂、膈膜中心腱缺损、心包膜缺损和心脏内异常。

异位心

在这种罕见的畸形中，心脏没有包膜，从分离的两半胸骨之间突出，顶端朝向下颚。异位心常伴发心脏内畸形，偶尔也伴发其他畸形，如没有被列入 Cantrell 五联症的腹壁缺损。

脐膨出的尾褶畸形（泄殖腔外翻）

与头褶缺损不同，这种畸形的表现是变化多端的。通常为脐下脐膨出，很少包含肝、膀胱外翻合并尿道上裂、耻骨支分离和肛门闭锁。回肠在外翻的膀胱之间脱出。详细的临床情况将在第 118 章中讨论。

腹裂

与脐膨出相比，腹裂腹壁缺损较小，通常小于 4 cm。几乎在所有的病例中，腹裂紧邻脐部，位于脐带右侧，在脐带和缺损之间偶尔存在皮桥，但腹壁和肌层正常。没有囊膜和囊膜残余物。中肠，偶尔还有生殖腺从缺损中疝出。出生时，肠管表现十分正常，但出生 20 分钟以后，突出的肠管变厚并覆盖一层表面粗糙的纤维蛋白性渗出膜以至肠管很难辨认。有几个腹裂的病例报道显示在缺损上方有小的中肠残留物，该残留物的腔隙基本闭合，可能是出生前肠扭转所致[21,36]。

胎儿腹裂可能与宫内不良应激有关。腹裂的新生儿常为早产儿，并通常存在呼吸系统问题，甚至足月的腹裂新生儿也表现为小于胎龄儿[24,25,50]，并且可能其母亲较年幼[33]。

发生率

近 30 年来，腹裂成为最常见的腹壁缺损疾患[12,72,108,136]。这可能与早产儿增多及早产儿的存活

率增加有关，或与直到20世纪70年代才正式将腹裂和脐膨出区分的事实有关[76]。腹裂的发生率为每1万个活产婴儿中有2～4.9个[12,88,108,132]，男性占多数[28]。

伴发症

腹裂的伴发畸形常与中肠有关，最常见的是肠狭窄（见表73-2）[149]。腹裂患儿在1岁之前常出现胃食管反流（16%）[81]和隐睾（15%），但后者常可自愈[71,89]。

1163 脐疝

这种缺损通常很小且发生在脐部，脐部向外延伸，常外被囊膜，易与脐膨出混淆。区别在于它的包含物只有中肠，绝无肝，缺损处的腹壁正常，腹直肌向剑突中线处会合。很少报道这种缺损伴发其他畸形。与所有的腹壁缺损相同，中肠在胎儿期未能返回腹腔进行旋转和固定，脐疝患儿可存在肠旋转不良，虽然它通常并不是引起肠梗阻的原因。

治疗

脐膨出

早期治疗

虽然脐膨出肠管被囊膜保护，仍需要紧急手术以增加一期腹腔关闭的可能性。应早期放置鼻饲管（nasogastric，NG）以减轻肠道压力。直肠检查有助于排空胎粪。维持患儿体温尤为重要（见第6章）。必要时应给予机械通气和给氧。

因为常伴发心脏缺陷，应做心功能评估和超声心动图，检查的结果并不会延迟修补术的时间。最常见的心脏畸形是室间隔缺损，它在出生后1周内心室的顺应性变为左心室占优势之前，很少出现临床症状。

最好在上肢进行维持量的静脉输液。如果出生时未输液，应给予1 mg剂量的维生素K，并预防性应用抗生素。如果这种畸形在出生前被我们的医疗中心确诊，如同治疗腹裂一样，我们在产房里直接进行修补术。我们相信这个策略将增加筋膜及时关闭的可能性。

一期腹腔关闭的价值仍存在着争论。一些人认为，分期手术很成功，可以减少腹腔压力升高而导致的可能并发症，包括呼吸抑制、静脉回流受阻而导致的尿量和心输出量减少、肠血液供给减少和肝复位肝静脉扭曲导致的酸中毒。在无法实施手术时，初始的非手术治疗（抗菌剂涂抹囊膜）仍然有效[82]。

手术治疗

在手术室，消毒囊膜及腹部，并去除多余脐带，如果患儿缺氧或情况不稳定，可将脐动脉或静脉（或两者）置管后保留于侧腹壁以利于术后监测，但实际上这种情况很少[47]。我们常用黏性塑料切口保护膜，以保持患儿体温。像许多文献报道的一样，我们常首先试着在囊膜完整的情况下，将膨出物送回腹腔[59,74,178]。但因为腹腔太小或囊膜常与肝或镰状韧带粘连，这种复位很难成功。我们在缺损外沿囊膜四周切除几毫米皮肤，提起皮瓣直到显露腹直肌。在这个层次上切除囊膜并结扎脐血管及脐尿管。将肝与囊膜分离，一些小的残余物可以留在肝上，如果内脏复位困难，可以向后前方牵拉腹壁以扩大腹腔。首先放回肠管，然后放回肝。因为肝可以有效固定复位的肠管，而且，如果需要利用皮瓣关闭腹腔，这样可以使第2次手术更安全些。在一期手术中，除皮肤外所有腹壁层应褥式缝合，重要的是，应将缝线放置在腹直肌层，而不仅仅是在中线筋膜层，以避免手术后疝的发生。因为腹直肌大部分镶嵌入肋缘，故在让其合并贴近切口上部不太可能，且因为肝的存在，在这个区域也不需要分离腹直肌。曾有将腹直肌前筋膜翻转后覆盖在缺损上方的报道，但我们发现这样做没有必要。放置腹壁缝线最好不要打结，先相互向对侧牵拉，以观察患儿是否能耐受关闭筋膜。如果此时麻醉师给患儿的机械通气压力低于25 cmH_2O，则关闭是安全的。连续缝合关闭皮肤切口，在大多数患者，这样可以让手术瘢痕看上去像脐一样。此外，在初次手术时还有几种美化脐部的手术方法[57,84,92,173]。一般采用可吸收线荷包皮内缝合，需每间隔2～3针时同筋膜组织缝合在一起，并关闭切口。但大多数手术因皮肤不够用，使用的频率不高。在许多病例中，因腹壁皮肤的血供较差而显苍白。不要使用胶带敷贴包扎伤口。

其他一些方法可以判断关闭筋膜后张力是否太大：静脉输注的液体不再因重力而下滴，膀胱或胃管内的压力大于 20 cmH_2O 等[85,171]。如果关闭筋膜后腹腔张力太大，可以考虑只缝合皮肤。但以我们的经验，在此情况下，缝合皮肤张力也会很高。这时，可以利用 Silo 袋包裹内脏，使内脏在一个星期内缓慢复位于腹腔。其中最简单的装置是底部带弹簧圈的硅橡胶罩，可通过腹壁缺损放置在腹壁边缘的下方（图 73-7）[141]。应将弹簧圈缝合在腹壁上，防止内脏复位时压力增高使弹簧圈压出。在缺损边缘涂上含抗生素的药膏。如果没有该装置或合适的型号可以使用 0.007 英寸厚的 Dacro 增强硅橡胶袋（Dacro-reinforced
1164 Silastic）。我们将袋子一端与腹壁的每个侧边缝合，另一端放置在腹壁外并打结，使得腹壁筋膜边缘和硅橡胶袋都朝向腹腔外。然后在缺损顶部分上、下两层进行缝合（图 73-8）。

我们不行 Ladd 术或阑尾切除术。如果在囊膜内看到睾丸，可将睾丸放置入腹腔内，因为大多数病例在出生 1 年内睾丸可自行下降至阴囊内。如果存在明显的肠狭窄，我们只在正常腹壁处行单腔肠造口术，术后 3 周再行肠吻合术。

巨大脐膨出存在一个特殊的问题，即使在使用硅橡胶储袋分期将肠等内脏复位以后，因缺损太大，皮肤或筋膜都无法覆盖在缺损上面。有几种方法可以采用，如从其他剩余的比较开阔的区域移植皮瓣[177]，有人报道将可吸收的网塞固定在缺损上，然后在形成的肉芽组织上移植皮瓣或用皮肤移植物[16]。但这种技术有引起肠瘘的危险。有几例我们使用了 Gore-Tex（聚四氟乙烯），并在 Gore-Tex 表面上覆盖皮瓣或移植物，但每一例都发生了感染和败血症。然而，去除 Gore-Tex 后，在肉芽组织表面上使用皮瓣或植皮还是可行的，而且这个在下面的假包膜似乎稳定了腹壁。在较大婴儿，皮肤扩张器也可以使用[39]。

手术后治疗

在一期修补术后，大部分患者初期需要机械通气辅助呼吸，但几天以后，腹壁就可以容纳耐受腹腔内容物了。静脉液体可以大于等于 15 ml/(kg·h) 的速度输注以维持尿量在 1 ml/(kg·h)，可以中心静脉置管以输注静脉营养液。如果是行一期修补术，则在短期内使用抗生素。但在分期手术中，则需持续预防性使用抗生素。伤口上使用抗生素药膏，3 周后拆线。我们使用 10 号鼻饲管（NG）进行低压间断抽吸，直到患儿肠功能恢复，包括排便、腹胀缓解和鼻饲管引流量减少为止。去除鼻饲管 12 小时后可以逐渐开始喂养。肠功能恢复延迟并不少见。如果 3 周后肠功能仍未恢复，应行小肠造影检查。

如果使用了储袋，通常在手术后 1 天开始内脏复位，复位可以简单地由人工操作完成，可采用多种方式确保安全：用脐带线将长钳夹住的储袋悬吊在患儿头上温暖的地方，用 TIA90 吻合器、前后连续缝合或使用脐带夹（图 73-9）。一个特别有创意的方法是

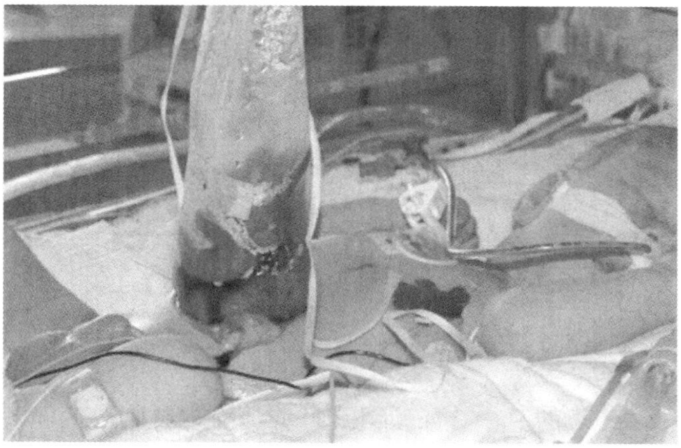

图 73-7　腹裂，肠管被放置于硅橡胶袋中。

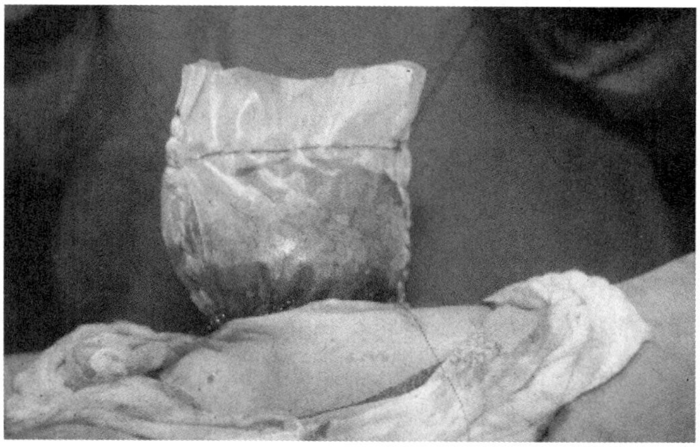

图 73-8　腹裂，肠管被放置于手缝制的硅橡胶袋中。

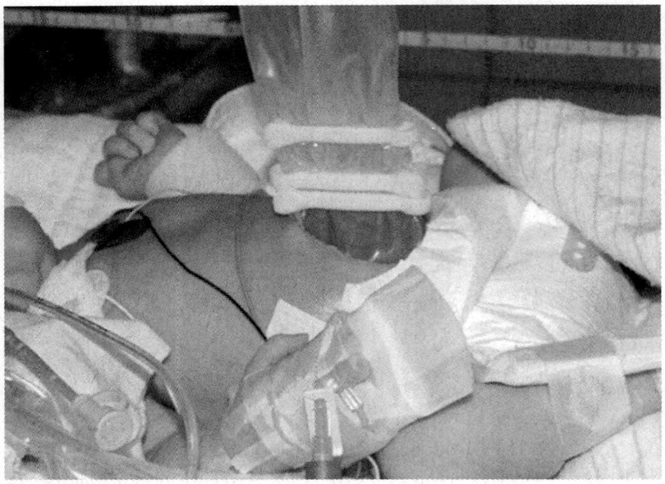

图 73-9 硅橡胶袋内肠管的复位。

Sawin 等[140]描述的套环装置，简单将储袋用脐带线打结，留下一个大的环形缺口，而不是两边靠拢关
1165 闭。但该装置没有被商业性使用。有医生认为应在储袋外面每侧都增加几针预置缝线，当储袋缩小变平更靠近底边时可以将缝线打结。

不管 Schuster 的最初设想如何，复位过程中腹腔容积未必增大[142]，更有可能是肠壁水肿消退以及肠内容物排空。

前文讨论过的在关闭腹壁时采用的几种检测腹腔内压力的方法在储袋内脏复位时仍可以采用。从这些研究中我们得到的最重要教训是，我们通常每隔一天为内脏复位的时间太慢，加快一些是很重要的。大部分储袋可以在 7 天内去除并关闭腹腔。如果 14 天时仍无法去除储袋，则储袋因为没能与周围组织长到一起，开始要同腹壁分离了。最近，Jona 的小宗病例报道认为主动去使内脏复位是不必要的[69]，他不对 silo 袋施加压力，储袋中的内容物可以在 8 天内自动复位至腹腔。

如果使用了皮瓣，则可以在任何时间进行根治手术，这主要依据患儿的一般情况。如果肠管开始向巨大的皮肤囊中生长，而不是向腹腔内复位，则需使用腹带以产生向腹腔内的直接压力。如果到了该关闭筋膜的时候，则应该将皮肤从肝上分割出来，虽然会产生小的创伤而不是轻微的压迫即止的出血。如果无法缝合双侧腹壁肌肉，只要能完全被健康皮肤所覆盖，可以使用修复性网塞补片。而如果有一部分补片不得不暴露在外，将无法愈合，会出现感染或将被排出。如果在初次手术时预测到皮瓣不能关闭腹腔，则不要对皮肤进行过多的解剖，如此这些组织在最后行修补术时会更健康。

如果手术后发生疝，一般可在 1 岁时修补，并不需要使用修复性补片。患者的疝偶尔可以自行消失。

异位心和头褶缺损

异位心和头褶缺损是很难处理的疾病。很难将心脏回纳入胸腔而不引起大血管或肺血管的扭曲。为赢得治疗时间而采用软组织填塞可能会导致心脏压塞，所以推荐在心脏和大血管周围广泛解剖，以增加胸腔的容积。头褶缺损（Cantrell 五联症）胸骨裂和心包膜缺损不需要特殊的外科治疗。可以立即关闭脐膨出的皮肤缺损，等待患者长大后再治疗心脏内缺损。因为中心腱缺损使得心脏很容易进入腹腔，可以用 Gore-Tex 补片关闭膈肌中心腱。随着患儿成长，补片被拉紧，心脏在胸腔里慢慢地被抬起，机体对此耐受。一旦循环呼吸系统稳定后，可以关闭腹部筋膜。在异位心，提供一个较硬的材料覆盖在心脏外是很重要的。曾报道将肋骨和修复材料放置在裂开的胸骨之间，修补这些复杂的临床缺损主要应强调创造性地利用可用的组织和个体解剖特征[61,91,113]。

尾褶缺损

第 118 章将详细讲述这些复杂疾病的处理方式。最初的治疗方式是关闭脐膨出和进行结肠造口。Lund 和其他医生已讨论了随后的治疗[100]。

腹裂

早期治疗

腹裂的两个特征使得其早期治疗与脐膨出不同。患者常是早产儿，关闭缺损时常要注意保温、呼吸支持及肠管大部分表面暴露在外的问题。后者常导致液体需要量增加和热量丧失。也许解决这个问题的最好办法是及时将患儿放置于有塑料拉带的肠袋中以控制热量散发和液体丢失[146]。因为大多数病例中，无论是自然分娩还是剖宫产，患儿的肠管未受到损伤。肠管复位越快，一期复位的可能性越大，肠管水肿和纤维素样渗出膜积聚得就越少。

我们选择在患儿出生后立即手术[35]，因为我们的产科医生对腹壁缺损的患儿均选择剖宫产，可以安排完整的小儿外科手术组人员在相邻的手术室为手术做准备。

手术技巧

首先小心去除掉胎儿皮脂以便以后的操作。如果没有急性呼吸抑制，则建立静脉通道，应用监护设备，并进行插管。在麻醉医生介入后手术医生将脐带提起，一段一段地将肠管复位。在大多数病例中，在术区皮肤准备完成之前，肠管已完全复位。扩张肛管以帮助胎粪排出是很重要的。其他的手术操作与术后监护和脐膨出大致相同。大多数腹裂患儿在初次手术后可保持脐部的完整（图 73-10）。在修整脐带后可
1166 以在腹膜水平分离脐血管和脐尿管。关闭皮下组织，将脐放置在切口中间或完整切口的左侧边缘，因为腹裂和脐带疝患儿的缺损常常很小。

在一些医疗中心，医生们常常在患者床边放置带弹簧圈的储袋[110,174]，也可以在床边进行肠管复位，只有最后的腹壁关闭手术在手术室里进行。Kidd 等发现采用这种技术行一期腹腔关闭的较少（34% 对 84%），而且住院时间延长（38 天对 30 天），但死亡率（约 3% 除外合并其他致死性畸形）和恢复肠道喂养的时间没有差异[75]。他们报道的还有机械通气时间、感染、狭窄、再次手术和坏死性小肠结肠炎发生减少。Bianchi 等报道，等待几个小时以后复位并没有想象中的有害[22,23]。

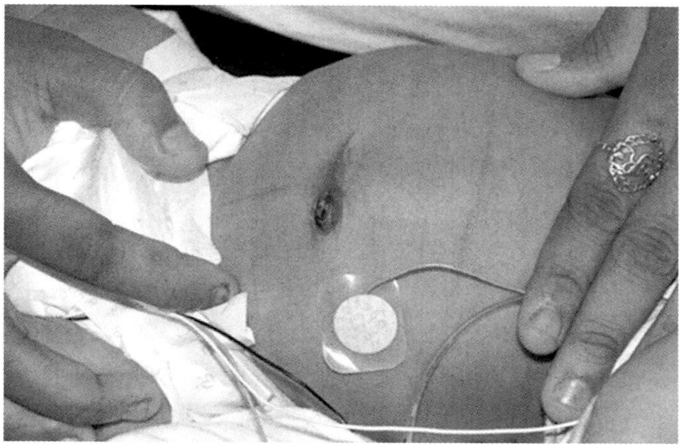

图 73-10　腹裂患儿经整形关闭并保留脐部。

脐疝

这种缺损在提高疝囊并轻柔按摩肠管后很容易将肠管复位，通常可以一期关闭筋膜，脐成形术通常也简单易行。

并发症

并发症的发生常与早产（腹裂）、伴发畸形（脐膨出）、消化道畸形（腹裂）和关闭腹壁后张力太大有关。前文已经提到了液体需要量增加和肠功能恢复延迟的可能性。此外，对早产儿相关问题的治疗准备非常重要，包括热量散失、呼吸衰竭、高胆红素血症、低血糖症、高血糖症和低血钙症。治疗呼吸抑制时从上肢采血进行毛细管血气分析很重要，因为下肢往往水肿，故血气分析结果要比实际代表的血氧值低而血碳酸值高。腹裂和囊膜破裂的脐膨出患儿常有血容量减少。Philippart 等将肌肉 pH 作为机体灌注充足和复苏的指标，以研究腹裂和脐膨出患儿液体复苏情况[125]。他们发现所有患儿在手术中至少需要 25% 的估计血容量（17 ~ 80 ml/kg，在 45 ~ 120 分钟内完成），在出生 24 小时内需要 82 ~ 312 ml/kg。在新生儿中，尿量是最好的监测指标，大多数消化道畸形的治疗可以延期，脐膨出中肠管可以是正常的足以承受吻合术，但随着手术时间的延长，所有的组织水肿将加剧，肝将向外膨大。在腹裂和脐膨出患儿，如果需要，狭窄的肠管甚至可以在不行造口的情况下放回腹腔，等待 3 ~ 6 周后腹壁缺损愈合时再做治疗。

关闭腹壁时张力太大会导致通气障碍、回心血量减少、心输出量减少和少尿。治疗措施是将患儿送回手术室拆除筋膜缝线，只关闭皮肤切口。也许需要一个假体，如果在治疗开始时就使用假体，则可以在床边再次开腹，重新关闭腹壁时就会松弛一些。在脐膨

出中，手术后代谢性酸中毒的出现常与肝复位时肝静脉扭曲有关。此时，去除并重新精加工假体很有必要。

无论肠管复位有多快或肠管看上去有多正常，所有患者都有肠功能恢复缓慢的倾向。脐膨出患儿的肠管功能恢复比腹裂患儿快[176]。我们应有耐心，但对手术后3周肠蠕动仍没有恢复的患儿应进行肠管造影检查。

结局

短期预后

在大多数系列报道中脐膨出和腹裂的存活率为90%[12,155]。在德克萨斯州的登记注册资料研究（registry study）中，1995—1997年腹裂患儿的存活率为93%[115]。曼彻斯特的一项研究中提到腹裂的存活率为94%[41]，其中7例患儿死亡，有5例死于不可逆转的败血症。80%的患儿进行了一期筋膜缝合，开始肠道喂养时间的中位数是30天（5～60天），住院时间的中位数是42天（11～183天）。需要储袋（silo）或合并有肠闭锁的患儿（91例患儿中有8例）开始肠道喂养的时间和住院时间更长，但死亡率没有增加。

脐膨出的存活率为70%～95%。大多数患儿的死亡与伴发的心脏或染色体异常有关[155]。Mabogunje和Mahour报道脐膨出患儿的死亡与其出生体重、缺损大小或一期关闭腹腔的方式无关[104]。他们也报道脐膨出患儿死亡率在1960—1970年间为23%，与1970—1980年间的19%相比，没有显著改变。死亡
1167 率主要与伴发畸形有关。腹裂患儿最近10年的存活率增加到了91%，死亡率主要与早产、肠道并发症和全静脉营养引起的念珠菌属败血症（*Candida* sepsis）有关。

任何类型的异位心脏存活者都很少[6,65]，但Groner报道了1例12岁儿童佩戴塑料护罩，可正常活动，至今未行骨骼缺损重建[54]。

底特律的密歇根儿童医院1990—2004年中期共治疗128例患儿，其中有78例腹裂（39例男性和39例女性）、47例脐膨出（28例男性和19例女性）和3例脐带疝患儿（均为女性）。腹裂患儿母亲的平均年龄是22岁，患儿的平均出生体重为2.5 kg，平均孕期为35.3孕周；脐膨出患儿母亲的平均年龄为29岁，患儿的平均出生体重为2.9 kg，平均孕期为36.6孕周。62%的腹裂患儿母亲和79%的脐膨出患儿母亲都进行了产前超声检查。

患儿普遍存活率为97%，其中腹裂为99%，脐膨出为94%，死亡常与伴发的心脏和染色体异常有关。腹裂的术后并发症为9%（伤口问题、肠扭转、败血症和粘连），脐膨出的术后并发症为17%（耐受肠道喂养的时间延迟、肠梗阻、少尿、血流动力学不稳定、代谢性酸中毒和心搏停止）。

长期预后

Lunzer等的一项澳大利亚的研究显示[101]，7例脐膨出存活者中的4例有严重的伴发畸形（2例Beckwith-Wiedemann综合征、1例脑穿通性囊肿和1例骨骼缺损），有这些畸形的孩子均有严重残疾，而另外3例发育正常。11例腹裂中1例智力迟钝，其他10例发育正常。

Davies和Stringer随访了1972—1984年间行腹裂手术的35例患儿中的12例，他们的存活时间均超过1年[37]，平均年龄为16岁。96%的患儿身体健康、生长发育正常，35%的患儿需要进一步手术治疗，其中2例有小肠梗阻，3例需要切口整形。据报道他们中57%的人因脐部缺失而导致儿童期情绪压抑。Swartz等报道了25例学龄期腹裂患儿，7例留级或进入了特殊班级，但都参加正常的体力活动[155]。84%的患儿有正常的肠功能。他们的腹部并发症常为非特异的或功能性的。22例在初始手术中需要进行肠管切除的患儿中10例有肠道并发症；而68例未行肠切除术的儿童中，只有2例出现肠道并发症。全部患儿的10%进行了更进一步的腹壁疝、伤口整形或隐睾的手术治疗。

在Tunell等脐膨出和腹裂的联合报道中，94例患儿的存活率为88%[164]，对其中61例患儿进行了平均14.2年的随访，19例进行了31次再手术，主要是因为腹壁疝和肠闭锁。80%的患者描述自己的生活质量较好，但40%的患者关心自己的身高，并感觉自己在体育运动和社会活动中存在不足。一些人表达了对脐部缺失的忧虑。

在瑞典 Lindham 进行的另一项患者平均随访年龄为 8.8 岁的研究中[96]观察到几例 1 岁之前偶发肠梗阻，并有无特殊畸形的再发性腹痛，其中一些女孩对伤疤及脐部缺失表示忧虑，但她们的生长发育正常。

Davies 和 Stringer 的研究中，腹裂患儿在 5 岁时体重比正常小儿低 32 个百分点，5 岁以后比正常小儿低 52 个百分点[37]。而复杂性腹裂的患儿（如腹裂合并肠闭锁）比正常小儿低 25 个百分点。斯坦福（Sanford）的 Berseth 等[20]发现腹裂和脐膨出患儿体重增加较慢，但根据放射学、粪便脂肪排泄（fecal fat excretion）和血清生化检查，在 3 岁时，没有人有胃肠道或代谢方面的问题。1/3 的患儿 IQ 低于 90，这与住院时间及非胃肠道畸形有关。

芬兰的 Koivusalo 等对 75 例（16 例脐膨出，11 例腹裂）17 岁以上的先天性腹壁缺损患者进行了详细的问卷调查，回收率 76%[80]。调查发现与正常人群相比，唯一一种发生频率较高的疾病是类风湿性关节炎，约 7%。37% 的患者具有与腹部瘢痕和脐部缺失相关的疾病，51% 具有功能性肠运动失调，12% 自尊低下。但 88% 的人认为自己身体健康，他们的生活质量和受教育程度与一般人群相比没有差异。

后期的心血管呼吸和肺部的负面效应在脐膨出或腹裂的患儿中很少见[176]。许多患儿在随后的生活中表达了对脐部缺失的忧虑。尽管应注意异位心脏、头褶和尾褶缺损的脐膨出患儿的近期和远期预后，但侧褶缺损的脐膨出、脐疝和腹裂患者的存活率和远期预后较好，多数问题与伴发疾病有关，而与腹壁缺损或它的修补术方式无关。

（杜 勇译 周小渔校）

参考文献

1. Ahlfeld F: Der Alkohol bei der Behandlung inoperabeler Bauchbrüche. Monatsschr Geburtsh Gynäkol 1899;10:124.
2. Aktug T, Demir N, Akgur FM, et al: Pretreatment of gastroschisis with transabdominal amniotic fluid exchange. Obstet Gynecol 1998;91:821.
3. Aktug T, Ucan B, Olguner M, et al: Amnio-allantoic fluid exchange for the prevention of intestinal damage in gastroschisis. III: Determination of the waste products removed by exchange. Eur J Pediatr Surg 1998;8:326.
4. Albert A, Margarit J, Julia V, et al: Morphology and mucosal biochemistry of gastroschisis intestine in urine-free amniotic fluid. J Pediatr Surg 2003;38:1217.
5. Alsulyman OM, Monteiro H, Ouzounian JG, et al: Clinical significance of prenatal ultrasonographic intestinal dilatation in fetuses with gastroschisis. Am J Obstet Gynecol 1996;175:982.
6. Amato JJ, Zelen J, Talwalkar NG: Single stage repair of thoracic ectopia cordis. Ann Thorac Surg 1995;59:518.
7. Ardinger HH, Williamson RA, Grant S: Association of neural tube defects with omphalocele in chromosomally normal fetuses. Am J Med Genet 1987;27:135.
8. Arnold SR, Debich-Spicer DD, Opitz JM, et al: Documentation of anomalies not previously described in Fryns syndrome. Am J Med Genet 2003;116A:179.
9. Arroyo Carrera I, Pitarch V, Garcia MJ, et al: Unusual congenital abdominal wall defect and review. Am J Med Genet 2003;119A:211.
10. Axt R, Quijano F, Boos R, et al: Omphalocele and gastroschisis: Prenatal diagnosis and peripartal management. A case analysis of the years 1989-1997 at the Department of Obstetrics and Gynecology, University of Homburg/Saar. Eur J Obstet Gynecol Reprod Biol 1999;87:47.
11. Babcook CJ, Hedrick MH, Goldstein RB, et al: Gastroschisis: Can sonography of the fetal bowel accurately predict postnatal outcome? J Ultrasound Med 1994;13:701.
12. Baerg J, Kaban G, Tonita J, et al: Gastroschisis: A sixteen-year review. J Pediatr Surg 2003;38:771.
13. Bamforth JS, Leonard CO, Chodirker BN, et al: Congenital diaphragmatic hernia, coarse facies, and acral hypoplasia: Fryns syndrome. Am J Med Genet 1989;32:93.
14. Banfield EE: Congenital omphalocele. Northwest Med 1955;54:258.
15. Barisic I, Clementi M, Hausler M, et al: Evaluation of prenatal ultrasound diagnosis of fetal abdominal wall defects by 19 European registries. Ultrasound Obstet Gynecol 2001; 8:309.
16. Bawazir OA, Wong A, Sigalet DL: Absorbable mesh and skin flaps or grafts in the management of ruptured giant omphalocele. J Pediatr Surg 2003;38:725.
17. Beckwith JB, Wang CI, Donnell GN, et al: Hyperplastic fetal visceromegaly with macroglossia, omphalocele, cytomegaly of adrenal fetal cortex, postnatal somatic gigantism, and other abnormalities: Newly recognized syndrome. Proc Am Pediatr Soc 1964;41:16.
18. Benson CD, Penberthy GC, Hill EJ: Hernia into umbilical cord and omphalocele. Arch Surg 1949;58:833.
19. Bernstein P: Gastroschisis, a rare teratological condition in the newborn. Arch Pediatr 1940;57:505.
20. Berseth CL, Malachowski N, Cohn RB, Sunshine P: Longitudinal growth and late morbidity of survivors of gastroschisis and omphalocele. J Pediatr Gastroenterol Nutr 1982;1:375.
21. Bhatia AM, Musemeche CA, Crino JP: Gastroschisis complicated by midgut atresia and closure of the defect in utero. J Pediatr Surg 1996;31:1288.
22. Bianchi A, Dickson AP: Elective delayed reduction and no anesthesia: 'Minimal intervention management' for gastroschisis. J Pediatr Surg 1998;33:1338.
23. Bianchi A, Dickson AP, Alizai NK: Elective delayed midgut reduction—no anesthesia for gastroschisis: Selection and conversion criteria. J Pediatr Surg 2002;37:1334.
24. Blakelock R, Upadhyay V, Kimble R, et al: Is a normally functioning gastrointestinal tract necessary for normal

growth in late gestation? Pediatr Surg Int 1998;13:17.
25. Blakelock RT, Upadhyay V, Pease PW, Harding JE: Are babies with gastroschisis small for gestational age? Pediatr Surg Int 1997;12:580.
26. Brun M, Grignon A, Guibaud L, et al: Gastroschisis: Are prenatal ultrasonographic findings useful for assessing the prognosis? Pediatr Radiol 1996;26:723.
27. Buchanan RW, Cain WL: A case of a complete omphalocele. Ann Surg 1965;143:552.
28. Calzolari E, Volpato S, Bianchi F, et al: Omphalocele and gastroschisis: A collaborative study of five Italian congenital malformation registries. Teratology 1993;47:47.
29. Cantrell JR, Haller JA, Ravitch MM: A syndrome of congenital defects involving the abdominal wall, sternum, diaphragm, pericardium, and heart. Surg Gynecol Obstet 1958; 107:602.
30. Castanon M, Guimaraes L, Tarrado X, et al: Congenital epigastric evisceration: A case report. J Pediatr Surg 2003; 38:1253.
31. Chassaing N, Lacombe D, Carles D, et al: Donnai-Barrow syndrome: Four additional patients. Am J Med Genet 2003;121A:258.
32. Clark JA, Kasselberg AG, Glick AD, O'Neill JA Jr: Mercury poisoning from merbromin (Mercurochrome) therapy of omphalocele: Correlation of toxicologic, histologic, and electron microscopic findings. Clin Pediatr (Phila) 1982; 21:445.
33. Colombani PM, Cunningham MD: Perinatal aspects of omphalocele and gastroschisis. Am J Dis Child 1977; 131:1386.
34. Correia-Pinto J, Tavares ML, Baptista MJ, et al: A new fetal rat model of gastroschisis: Development and early characterization. J Pediatr Surg 2001;36:213.
35. Coughlin JP, Drucker DE, Jewell MR, et al: Delivery room repair of gastroschisis. Surgery 1993;114:822.
36. Davenport M, Haugen S, Greenough A, Nicolaides K: Closed gastroschisis: Antenatal and postnatal features. J Pediatr Surg 2001;36:1834.
37. Davies BW, Stringer MD: The survivors of gastroschisis. Arch Dis Child 1997;77:158.
38. Deans KJ, Mooney DP, Meyer MM, et al: Prolonged intestinal exposure to amniotic fluid does not result in peel formation in gastroschisis. J Pediatr Surg 1999;34:975.
39. De Ugarte DA, Asch MJ, Hedrick MH, et al: The use of tissue expanders in the closure of a giant omphalocele. J Pediatr Surg 2004;39:613.
40. Dinatti LA, Meagher DP Jr, Martinez-Frontanilla LA: "Bucket handle" avulsion of intestine in gastroschisis. J Pediatr Surg 1993;28:840.
41. Driver CP, Bruce J, Bianchi A, et al: The contemporary outcome of gastroschisis. J Pediatr Surg 2000;35:1719.
42. Drongowski RA, Smith RK Jr, Coran AG, et al: Contribution of demographic and environmental factors to the etiology of gastroschisis: A hypothesis. Fetal Diagn Ther 1991;6:14.
43. Duhamel B: Embryology of exomphalos and allied malformations. Arch Dis Child 1963;38:142.
44. Dunn JC, Fonkalsrud EW, Atkinson JB: The influence of gestational age and mode of delivery on infants with gastroschisis. J Pediatr Surg 1999;34:1393.
45. Ein SH, Shandling B: A new nonoperative treatment of large omphaloceles with a polymer membrane. J Pediatr Surg 1978;13:255.
46. Fagan DG, Pritchard JS, Clark TW, Greenwood MR: Organ mercury levels in infants with omphaloceles treated with organic mercurial antiseptics. Arch Dis Child 1977;52:962.
47. Filston HC, Izant RJ: Translocation of the umbilical artery to the lower abdomen: An adjunct to the postoperative monitoring of arterial blood gases in major abdominal wall defects. J Pediatr Surg 1975;10:225.
48. Franceschini P, Guala A, Licata D, et al: Gershoni-Baruch syndrome: Report of a new family confirming autosomal recessive inheritance. Am J Med Genet 2003;122A:174.
49. Fraser N, Crabbe DC: An unusual left-sided abdominal-wall defect. Pediatr Surg Int 2002;18:66.
50. Fries MH, Filly RA, Callen PW, et al: Growth retardation in prenatally diagnosed cases of gastroschisis. J Ultrasound Med 1993;12:583.
51. Gibbin C, Touch S, Broth RE, Berghella V: Abdominal wall defects and congenital heart disease. Ultrasound Obstet Gynecol 2003;21:334.
52. Grob M: Lehrbuch der Kinderchirurgie. Stuttgart, Germany, Georg Thieme Verlag, 1957.
53. Grob M: Conservative treatment of exomphalos. Arch Dis Child 1963;38:148.
54. Groner JI: Ectopia cordis and sternal defects. In Ziegler MM, Azizkhan RG, Weber TR (eds): Operative Pediatric Surgery. New York, McGraw-Hill, 2003, p 279.
55. Gross RE: A new method for surgical treatment of omphaloceles. Surgery 1948;24:277.
56. Gross RE: Omphalocele (umbilical eventration). In Gross RE (ed): The Surgery of Infancy and Childhood. Philadelphia, WB Saunders, 1953, p 406.
57. Harmel RP Jr: Primary repair of gastroschisis with umbilicoplasty. Surg Gynecol Obstet 1985;160:464.
58. Heider AL, Strauss RA, Kuller JA: Omphalocele: Clinical outcomes in cases with normal karyotypes. Am J Obstet Gynecol 2004;190:135.
59. Hendrickson RJ, Partrick DA, Janik JS: Management of giant omphalocele in a premature low-birth-weight neonate utilizing a bedside sequential clamping technique without prosthesis. J Pediatr Surg 2003;38(10):E14.
60. Hey W: Practical Observation in Surgery. London, Cadell & Davis, 1802.
61. Hornberger LK, Colan SD, Lock JE, et al: Outcome of patients with ectopia cordis and significant intracardiac defects. Circulation 1996;94(9 Suppl):II32.
62. How HY, Harris BJ, Pietrantoni M, et al: Is vaginal delivery preferable to elective cesarean delivery in fetuses with a known ventral wall defect? Am J Obstet Gynecol 2000; 182:1527.
63. Hoyme HE, Higginbottom MC, Jones K: The vascular pathogenesis of gastroschisis: Intrauterine interruption of the omphalomesenteric artery. J Pediatr 1981;98:228.
64. Hughes MD, Nyberg DA, Mack LA, et al: Fetal omphalocele: Prenatal US detection of concurrent anomalies and other predictors of outcome. Radiology 1989;173:371.
65. Humpl T, Huggan P, Hornberger LK, McCrindle BW: Presentation and outcomes of ectopia cordis. Can J Cardiol 1999;15:1353.
66. Izant RJ Jr, Brown F, Rothmann BF: Current embryology and treatment of gastroschisis and omphalocele. Arch Surg 1966;93:49.
67. Jarcho J: Congenital umbilical hernia. Surg Gynecol Obstet 1937;65:593.
68. Johnson AH: Omphalocele and related defects. Am J Surg 1967;114:279.
69. Jona JZ: The 'gentle touch' technique in the treatment of gastroschisis. J Pediatr Surg 2003;38:1036.
70. Kaplan LC, Matsuoka R, Gilbert EF, et al: Ectopia cordis and cleft sternum: Evidence for mechanical teratogenesis following rupture of the chorion or yolk sac. Am J Med

Genet 1985;21:187.
71. Kaplan LM, Koyle MA, Kaplan GW, et al: Related association between abdominal wall defects and cryptorchidism. J Urol 1986;136:645.
72. Kazaura MR, Lie RT, Irgens LM, et al: Increasing risk of gastroschisis in Norway: An age-period-cohort analysis. Am J Epidemiol 2004;159:358.
73. Kearns JE, Clarke BG: One stage surgical repair of gastroschisis (omphalocele) by cutis graft technic. Plast Reconstr Surg 1950;6:41.
74. Kern HM: New and simplified procedure for repairing omphalocele. Am J Surg 1949;77:783.
75. Kidd JN Jr, Jackson RJ, Smith SD, Wagner CW: Evolution of staged versus primary closure of gastroschisis. Ann Surg 2003; 237:759.
76. Klein MD: Robot-enhanced fetoscopic surgery. J Pediatr Surg 2004;39:1463.
77. Klein MD, Hertzler JH: Congenital defects of the abdominal wall. Surg Gynecol Obstet 1981;152:805.
78. Kleinhaus S, Kauffer N, Boley SJ: Partial hepatectomy in omphalocele repair. Surgery 1968;64:484.
79. Kluck P, Tibboel D, van der Kamp AW, et al: The effect of fetal urine on the development of the bowel in gastroschisis. J Pediatr Surg 1983;18:47.
80. Koivusalo A, Lindahl H, Rintala RJ: Morbidity and quality of life in adult patients with a congenital abdominal wall defect: A questionnaire survey. J Pediatr Surg 2002; 37:1594.
81. Koivusalo A, Rintala R, Lindahl H: Gastroesophageal reflux in children with a congenital abdominal wall defect. J Pediatr Surg 1999;34:1127.
82. Kouame BD, Dick RK, Ouattara O, et al: Therapeutic approaches for omphalocele in developing countries: Experience of Central University Hospital of Yopougon, Abidjan, Cote d'Ivoire. Bull Soc Pathol Exot 2003;96:302.
83. Kozer E, Nikfar S, Costei A, et al: Aspirin consumption during the first trimester of pregnancy and congenital anomalies: A meta-analysis. Am J Obstet Gynecol 2002;187:1623.
84. Krummel TM, Sieber WK: Closure of congenital abdominal wall defects with umbilicoplasty. Surg Gynecol Obstet 1987;165:168.
85. Lacey SR, Carris LA, Beyer AJ 3rd, Azizkhan RG: Bladder pressure monitoring significantly enhances care of infants with abdominal wall defects: A prospective clinical study. J Pediatr Surg 1993;28:1370.
86. Lafer DJ: Rectus muscle transection for visceral replacement. Surgery 1968;63:988.
87. Langer JC, Khanna J, Caco C, et al: Prenatal diagnosis of gastroschisis: Development of objective sonographic criteria for predicting outcome. Obstet Gynecol 1993; 81:53.
88. Laughon M, Meyer R, Bose C, et al: Rising birth prevalence of gastroschisis. J Perinatol 2003;23:291.
89. Lawson A, de la Hunt MN: Gastroschisis and undescended testis. J Pediatr Surg 2001;36:366.
90. Layne MD, Yet SF, Maemura K, et al: Impaired abdominal wall development and deficient wound healing in mice lacking aortic carboxypeptidase-like protein. Mol Cell Biol 2001;21:5256.
91. Leca F, Thibert M, Khoury W, et al: Extrathoracic heart (ectopia cordis). Int J Cardiol 1989;22:221.
92. Lee SL, DuBois JJ, Greenholz SK, Huffman SG: Advancement flap umbilicoplasty after abdominal wall closure: Postoperative results compared with normal umbilical anatomy. J Pediatr Surg 2001;36:1168.
93. Lenke RR, Hatch EI Jr: Fetal gastroschisis: A preliminary report advocating the use of cesarean section. Obstet Gynecol 1986;67:395.
94. Lewis DF, Towers CV, Garite TJ, et al: Fetal gastroschisis and omphalocele: Is cesarean section the best mode of delivery? Am J Obstet Gynecol 1990;163:773.
95. Lindham S: Teratogenic aspects of abdominal wall defects. Z Kinderchir 1983;38:211.
96. Lindham S: Long-term results in children with omphalocele and gastroschisis—a follow-up study. Z Kinderchir 1984;39:164.
97. Lippman O: Ein seltener Fall von Spaltbildung der vorderen Leibenswand, nebst Beitrag zur Enstehung von Bauchspalten. Zentralb Gynakol 1937;61:516.
98. Loder RT, Guiboux JP: Musculoskeletal involvement in children with gastroschisis and omphalocele. J Pediatr Surg 1993;28:584.
99. Lore JM: Omphalocele treated with split-thickness skin graft. N Y State J Med 1963;63:3573.
100. Lund DP, Hendren WH: Cloacal exstrophy: Experience with 20 cases. J Pediatr Surg 1993;28:1360.
101. Lunzer H, Menardi G, Brezinka C: Long-term follow-up of children with prenatally diagnosed omphalocele and gastroschisis. J Matern Fetal Med 2001;10:385.
102. Luton D, de Lagausie P, Guibourdenche J, et al: Influence of amnioinfusion in a model of in utero created gastroschisis in the pregnant ewe. Fetal Diagn Ther 2000;15:224.
103. Lycosthenes C: Prodigiorum ac ostentorum chronicon. Henricum Petri, 1557.
104. Mabogunje OA, Mahour GH: Omphalocele and gastroschisis. Trends in survival across two decades. Am J Surg 1984;148:679.
105. Maguire CH: Surgical management of omphalocele. Arch Surg 1949;59:484.
106. Margulies I: Omphalocele (amniocele). Am J Obstet Gynecol 1945;49:695.
107. Massabuau G, Guibal A: L'éviscération ombilicale congénitale. Arch Mal l'App Difestif 1933;23:129.
108. McDonnell R, Delany V, Dack P, et al: Changing trend in congenital abdominal wall defects in eastern region of Ireland. Ir Med J 2002;95:236.
109. Melikoglu M, Karaguzel G, Ogus M, et al: A gastroschisis-like abdominal wall defect in the left hypochondrium. Case report and literature review. Eur J Pediatr Surg 1998;8:52.
110. Minkes RK, Langer JC, Mazziotti MV, et al: Routine insertion of a Silastic spring-loaded silo for infants with gastroschisis. J Pediatr Surg 2000;35:843.
111. Moore TC, Collins DL, Catanzarite V, et al: Pre-term and particularly pre-labor cesarean section to avoid complications of gastroschisis. Pediatr Surg Int 1999;15:97.
112. Moore TC, Stokes GE: Gastroschisis. Surgery 1953;33:112.
113. Morales JM, Patel SG, Duff JA, et al: Ectopia cordis and other midline defects. Ann Thorac Surg 2000;70:111.
114. Morrow RJ, Whittle MJ, McNay MB, et al: Prenatal diagnosis and management of anterior abdominal wall defects in the west of Scotland. Prenat Diagn 1993;13:111.
115. Nembhard WN, Waller DK, Sever LE, et al: Patterns of first-year survival among infants with selected congenital anomalies in Texas, 1995-1997. Teratology 2001;64:267.
116. Nichol PF, Hayman A, Pryde PG, et al: Meconium staining of amniotic fluid correlates with intestinal peel formation in gastroschisis. Pediatr Surg Int 2004;20:211.
117. Nicholls G, Upadhyaya V, Gornall P, et al: Is specialist centre delivery of gastroschisis beneficial? Arch Dis Child 1993;69:71.
118. Nicolaides KH, Snijders RJ, Cheng HH, et al: Fetal gastrointestinal and abdominal wall defects: Associated

malformations and chromosomal abnormalities. Fetal Diagn Ther 1992;7:102.
119. Nissan S: Pneumoperitoneum as aid for second stage repair of omphalocele. Arch Surg 1965;91:839.
120. Olguner M, Akgur FM, Api A, et al: The effects of intraamniotic human neonatal urine and meconium on the intestines of the chick embryo with gastroschisis. J Pediatr Surg 2000;35:458.
121. Olshausen RZ: Zur Therapie der Nabelschnurhernien. Arch Gynakol Berlin 1887;29:443.
122. Paltia V: Omphalocele. Acta Chir Scand 1960;30:119.
123. Paré A: The Workes of That Famous Chirugeon, Book 24, Chapter 66. Th Cotes and R Young, 1634, p 959.
124. Pernkopf E: Die Entwicklung der Form des Magendarmkanales beim Menschen. II Die weitere Auftretens der ersten Dunndarmschlingen. Z Anat Entwgesch 1925;77:1.
125. Philippart AI, Canty TG, Filler RM: Acute fluid volume requirements in infants with anterior abdominal wall defects. J Pediatr Surg 1972;7:553.
126. Politzer G, Sternberg H: Ueber die Entwicklung der ventralen Korperwand und des Nabelstranges beim Menschen. Z Anat Entwgesch 1930;92:279.
127. Pribram E: Anteromedian mero-crania (nosencephalos), combined with hypogastroschisis dextra and malformation of the fingers and toes. Arch Pathol Lab Med 1927; 3:400.
128. Pryde PG, Bardicef M, Treadwell MC, et al: Gastroschisis: Can antenatal ultrasound predict infant outcomes? Obstet Gynecol 1994;84:505.
129. Pryde PG, Greb A, Isada NB: Familial omphalocele: Considerations in genetic counseling. Am J Med Genet 1992;44:624.
130. Ravitch MM: Giant omphalocele: Second stage repair with the aid of pneumoperitoneum. JAMA 1963;185:42.
131. Reddy VN, Aughton DJ, DeWitte DB, Harper CE: Down syndrome and omphalocele: An underrecognized association. Pediatrics 1994;93:514.
132. Reid KP, Dickinson JE, Doherty DA: The epidemiologic incidence of congenital gastroschisis in Western Australia. Am J Obstet Gynecol 2003;189:764.
133. Remensnyder JP: Intrauterine rupture of omphalocele. Surgery 1963;54:681.
134. Rothenberg RE, Barnett T: Omphalocele in siblings. Arch Surg 1957;75:131.
135. Sakala EP, Erhard LN, White JJ: Elective cesarean section improves outcomes of neonates with gastroschisis. Am J Obstet Gynecol 1993;169:1050.
136. Salihu HM, Pierre-Louis BJ, Druschel CM, et al: Omphalocele and gastroschisis in the State of New York, 1992-1999. Birth Defects Res A Clin Mol Teratol 2003; 67:630.
137. Saller DN Jr, Canick JA, Palomaki GE, et al: Second-trimester maternal serum alpha-fetoprotein, unconjugated estriol, and hCG levels in pregnancies with ventral wall defects. Obstet Gynecol 1994;84:852.
138. Santos MM, Tannuri U, Maksoud JG: Alterations of enteric nerve plexus in experimental gastroschisis: Is there a delay in the maturation? J Pediatr Surg 2003;38:1506.
139. Sapin E, Mahieu D, Borgnon J, et al: Transabdominal amnioinfusion to avoid fetal demise and intestinal damage in fetuses with gastroschisis and severe oligohydramnios. J Pediatr Surg 2000;35:598.
140. Sawin R, Glick P, Schaller R, et al: Gastroschisis wringer clamp: A safe, simplified method for delayed primary closure. J Pediatr Surg 1992;27:1346.
141. Schlatter M, Norris K, Uitvlugt N, et al: Improved outcomes in the treatment of gastroschisis using a preformed silo and delayed repair approach. J Pediatr Surg 2003;38:459.
142. Schuster SR: A new method for the staged repair of large omphaloceles. Surg Gynecol Obstet 1967;125:837.
143. Segel SY, Marder SJ, Parry S, et al: Fetal abdominal wall defects and mode of delivery: A systematic review. Obstet Gynecol 2001;98:867.
144. Shanske AL, Pande S, Aref K, et al: Omphalocele-exstrophy-imperforate anus-spinal defects (OEIS) in triplet pregnancy after IVF and CVS. Birth Defects Res A Clin Mol Teratol 2003;67:467.
145. Shaw A: The myth of gastroschisis. J Pediatr Surg 1975; 10:235.
146. Sheldon RE: The bowel bag: A sterile, transportable method for warming infants with skin defects. Pediatrics 1974;53:267.
147. Singh SJ, Fraser A, Leditschke JF, et al: Gastroschisis: Determinants of neonatal outcome. Pediatr Surg Int 2003;19:260.
148. Snijders RJ, Brizot ML, Faria M, et al: Fetal exomphalos at 11 to 14 weeks of gestation. J Ultrasound Med 1995; 14:569.
149. Snyder CL, Miller KA, Sharp RJ, et al: Management of intestinal atresia in patients with gastroschisis. J Pediatr Surg 2001;36:1542.
150. Stanley-Brown EG, Frank JE: Mercury poisoning from application to omphalocele. JAMA 1971;216:2144.
151. Stoll C, Clementi M, Euroscan Study Group: Prenatal diagnosis of dysmorphic syndromes by routine fetal ultrasound examination across Europe. Ultrasound Obstet Gynecol 2003;21:543.
152. Stoodley N, Sharma A, Noblett H, et al: Influence of place of delivery on outcome in babies with gastroschisis. Arch Dis Child 1993;68:321.
153. Strauss RA, Balu R, Kuller JA, et al: Gastroschisis: The effect of labor and ruptured membranes on neonatal outcome. Am J Obstet Gynecol 2003;189:1672.
154. Stroer WFH: Zur Aetiologie der Bauchspalten. Beitr Pathol Anat Allg Pathol 1949;106:302.
155. Swartz KR, Harrison MW, Campbell JR, Campbell TJ: Long-term follow-up of patients with gastroschisis. Am J Surg 1986;151:546.
156. Taruffi G: Storia della Teratologia, vol VII. Bologna, Italy, Regia Tipografia, 1894.
157. Thauvin-Robinet C, Faivre L, Cusin V, et al: Cloacal exstrophy in an infant with 9q34.1-qter deletion resulting from a de novo unbalanced translocation between chromosome 9q and Yq. Am J Med Genet 2004;126A:303.
158. Thomas DF, Atwell JD: The embryology and surgical management of gastroschisis. Br J Surg 1976;63:893.
159. Tibboel D, Raine P, McNee M, et al: Developmental aspects of gastroschisis. J Pediatr Surg 1986;21:865.
160. Tibboel D, Vermey-Keers C, Kluck P, et al: The natural history of gastroschisis during fetal life: Development of the fibrous coating on the bowel loops. Teratology 1986; 33:267.
161. Torfs CP, Curry CJ: Familial cases of gastroschisis in a population-based registry. Am J Med Genet 1993;45:465.
162. Tucker JM, Brumfield CG, Davis RO, et al: Prenatal differentiation of ventral abdominal wall defects. Are amniotic fluid markers useful adjuncts? J Reprod Med 1992;37:445.
163. Tulloh RM, Tansey SP, Parashar K, et al: Echocardiographic screening in neonates undergoing surgery for selected gastrointestinal malformations. Arch Dis

Child Fetal Neonatal Ed 1994;70:F206.
164. Tunell WP, Puffinbarger NK, Tuggle DW, et al: Abdominal wall defects in infants. Survival and implications for adult life. Ann Surg 1995;221:525.
165. Vintzileos AM, Ananth CV, Smulian JC, et al: Routine second-trimester ultrasonography in the United States: A cost-benefit analysis. Am J Obstet Gynecol 2000;182:655.
166. Visick C: An umbilical hernia in a newly born child. Lancet 1873;1:829.
167. Volumenie JL, de Lagausie P, Guibourdenche J, et al: Improvement of mesenteric superior artery Doppler velocimetry by amnio-infusion in fetal gastroschisis. Prenat Diagn 2001;21:1171.
168. Waller DK, Keddie AM, Canfield MA, Scheuerle AE: Do infants with major congenital anomalies have an excess of macrosomia? Teratology 2001;64:311.
169. Werler MM, Sheehan JE, Mitchell AA: Maternal medication use and risks of gastroschisis and small intestinal atresia. Am J Epidemiol 2002;155:26.
170. Werler MM, Sheehan JE, Mitchell AA: Association of vasoconstrictive exposures with risks of gastroschisis and small intestinal atresia. Epidemiology 2003;14:349.
171. Wesley JR, Drongowski R, Coran AG: Intragastric pressure measurement: A guide for reduction and closure of the Silastic chimney in omphalocele and gastroschisis. J Pediatr Surg 1981;16:264.
172. Wiedemann HR: Complexe malformatif familial avec hernie ombilicale et macroglossie—un “syndrome nouveau”? J Genet Humaine 1964;13:223.
173. Williams AM, Brain JL: The normal position of the umbilicus in the newborn: An aid to improving the cosmetic results in exomphalos major. J Pediatr Surg 2001;36:546.
174. Wu Y, Vogel AM, Sailhamer EA, et al: Primary insertion of a Silastic spring-loaded silo for gastroschisis. Am Surg 2003;69:1083.
175. Yatsenko SA, Mendoza-Londono R, Belmont JW, et al: Omphalocele in trisomy 3q: Further delineation of phenotype. Clin Genet 2003;64:404.
176. Zaccara A, Iacobelli BD, Calzolari A, et al: Cardiopulmonary performances in young children and adolescents born with large abdominal wall defects. J Pediatr Surg 2003;38:478.
177. Zaccara A, Zama M, Trucchi A, et al: Bipedicled skin flaps for reconstruction of the abdominal wall in newborn omphalocele. J Pediatr Surg 2003;38:613.
178. Zaiem MM: Staged closure of omphalocele major using autogenous sac as supportive material. Saudi Med J 2003;24(5 Suppl):S57.

第 74 章

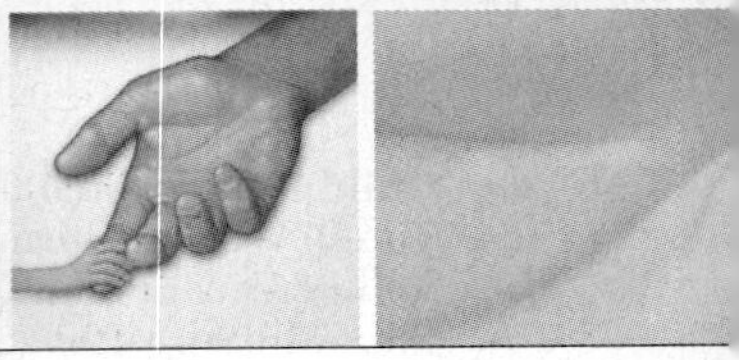

腹股沟疝和鞘膜积液

Philip L. Glick 和 Scott C. Boulanger

历史回顾

对腹股沟疝的认识至少可以追溯至公元前 1500 年，对腹股沟疝的描写出现在一个古老的希腊雕像上，埃及人的著作中也描述了由咳嗽引起的腹股沟区突出物（Ebers 的纸草书，约公元前 1552 年）[57]。有迹象显示，早在公元前 1200 年就已经用外科方法治疗疝。罗马医生 Celsus 被认为在公元 50 年左右实行了最早的疝手术[57]。与此同时，Galen 描述了腹股沟区的解剖，但他认为腹股沟疝是腹膜破裂并使其上方覆盖的肌肉和筋膜伸长的结果[57]。这可能是疝的俚语“rupture（破裂）”的起源。

现代疝外科学开始于 19 世纪，即当时人们对腹股沟管的解剖结构已有了准确了解[57]。这一时期，Richter、Camper 和 Scarpa 脱颖而出，为这一领域作出了贡献。1804 年 Cooper 描述了腹横筋膜和耻骨韧带或 Cooper 韧带。1811 年 Colles 描述了腹股沟韧带的反折。Cloque 在 1817 年观察到鞘状突在出生时很少关闭。在对腹股沟区解剖彻底了解之后，现代疝外科学只在等待无菌技术的发展。

1870 年 Lister 介绍了外科灭菌法的概念[57]。1896 年 Halsted 开始在外科手术时戴手套。1904 年，Von Mikulica 迈出了更大的一步，进行了无菌手术。这些发展使得疝外科学突飞猛进。1871 年 Marcy 实行的手术方法，今天的小儿外科医生依然沿用：经外环口高位结扎未打开的疝囊，并加强内环口。但这种术式在成人中复发率很高[87]。1887 年 Bassini 报道了一种手术方式：打开腹外斜肌，高位结扎疝囊，加强外环口并重建腹股沟后壁[87]。Bassini 和 Halsted 对现代疝修补术作出了巨大贡献。

疝外科学概况（北美的观点）

现代小儿疝修补术延续其标准原则：打开腹外斜肌，暴露内环口，高位结扎疝囊，修补腹股沟管前壁。这个看似简单的手术细节，不同外科医生实施起来差异很大。在美国，Ladd 和 Gross 被认为是小儿外科之父[38]。他们在“Abdominal Surgery of Infancy and Childhood”《婴儿和儿童腹部外科学》一书中，详细描述了疝修补术[56]，这同样也是 Ferguson 手术的本质[31]。手术步骤如下：暴露腹外斜肌和外环口，打开外环口并向近端延伸。钝性分离提睾肌，用镊子提出疝囊，将疝囊与周围组织锐性分离，打开疝囊，用外被纱布的手指继续钝性分离疝囊。用缝针刺穿疝囊颈并切除多余的疝囊。用双股线将疝囊颈缝在腹外斜肌和腹内斜肌下方并打结，并向后通过腹外斜肌和腹内斜肌将其提出。折叠方式关闭腹外斜肌，其上缘与腹股沟韧带缝合，下缘与腹外斜肌上部分缝合。关闭 Scarpa 筋膜，再关闭皮肤切口。

在最近一项北美小儿外科调查中，Levitt 等[61]回顾了近 60 年来疝修补术的变化。81% 的（640 名应答者）外科医生继承了 Ladd 和 Gross 的思想，很好地保留了他们有关疝修补术的要点。如在这些外科医生中，94% 的人关闭 Scarpa 筋膜，90% 的人钝性分离提睾肌，81% 的人识别髂腹股沟神经，79% 的人不探查睾丸，78% 的人除了引流外保留远端疝囊，65% 的人用剪刀打开 Scarpa 筋膜。有一些 Ladd 与 Gross 倡导的疝修补
方式已不再使用，如将一个手指放入疝囊，用纱布将其钝性分离，以及术后使用 Stiles 敷料等。作者认为手术方式的变化可以从手术训练、临床经验和文献分析中联合获得。疝手术是小儿外科医生最常做的手术，也是了解外科学如何演变发展的一个范例。

发生率

如上所述，腹股沟疝修补术是小儿外科医生最常做的手术。儿童腹股沟疝的发生率为 0.8%~4.4%[12]。

年龄

腹股沟疝常发生于 1 岁以内的幼儿，发病高峰在出生后数月内。大约 1/3 的患儿手术年龄在 6 个月以内[12]。腹股沟疝在早产儿中发病率最高，大约 16%~25%[79,105]。这与鞘状突未闭的发生相关；出生时，80% 的婴儿鞘状突未闭，这一比例在出生 6 个月内急剧下降[93]。不过无论其发病年龄，所有的腹股沟斜疝都继发于胎儿期和新生儿期的鞘状突发育障碍。

性别

男性更容易患腹股沟疝，报道显示男女发生率比例在 3∶1~10∶1[12]。早产儿的腹股沟疝发生率较高，患儿之间没有显著的性别差异[11,75,103]。

部位

不论男女，大约 60% 的腹股沟疝发生在右侧[83]。在男性，右侧睾丸下降较左侧晚可能导致了这一结果，但却无法解释女性中出现同样的现象。在腹股沟疝病例中，双侧疝的发生率约占 10%[83]。据推测，左侧腹股沟疝患儿发生右侧腹股沟疝比右侧腹股沟疝患儿发生左侧腹股沟疝更容易[22,64]，但最近更多的数据显示这可能不准确[9,37,100]。

家族史

大约 11.5% 的患者有腹股沟疝家族史[12]，双胞胎的疝发生率较高，男性双胞胎发生率为 10.6%，女性双胞胎则为 4.1%[3]。

胚胎学

腹股沟斜疝以鞘状突闭合障碍为发病基础（图 74-1），鞘状突是通过内环处的腹膜反折，在胚胎第 3 个月时出现[19]。有人认为腹腔内压力导致了鞘状突的形成[6]，也有人认为鞘状突形成是一个主动过程[1,2]。腹腔内睾丸在妊娠第 7~9 个月穿过鞘状突下降，与此同时，鞘状突得以延伸。随后，部分鞘状突在睾丸上方闭锁，并封闭了腹股沟内环口，而远端持续存在形成睾丸鞘膜。当这一过程出现障碍时，则引起鞘状突未闭，有可能形成腹股沟斜疝（如果肠管或其他脏器进入鞘膜腔）或鞘膜积液（仅为腹腔液体）。在女性，与鞘状突相对应的 Nuck 管与大阴唇（与男性的阴囊相对应）相连。正常情况下，Nuck 管大约在孕第 7 个月关闭，早于男性。

关闭的确切时间尚不清楚。研究显示约 80%~100% 的婴儿在出生时鞘状突未闭，并最可能在出生 6 个月内关闭（如果关闭的话）[82,93]。此后，鞘状突未闭的发生率逐渐下降，在 3~5 岁时趋于稳定。研究也显示左侧鞘状突关闭较右侧早。鞘状突关闭的起 1174

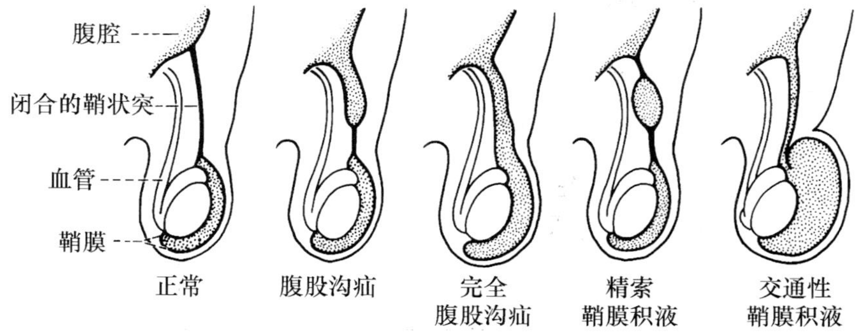

图 74-1 因鞘状突闭塞障碍引起的疝和鞘膜积液的常见类型。

始位置不清楚（如近端、中间和远端）。关闭后鞘状突变为索带，随后逐渐消失。较多的鞘状突未闭与睾丸未降相关联，提示鞘状突关闭发生在睾丸下降之后，且这两个过程有一定联系。

睾丸通过腹股沟管下降及鞘膜闭锁的大部分生物学信号和导向机制尚不清楚。雄性激素似乎起一定作用，因为鞘状突未闭常发生于雄激素不敏感综合征，但鞘膜本身并不存在雄激素受体。Clarnette 和 Hutson[19] 发现生殖股神经和钙基因相关肽（calcitonin gene-related peptide，GGRP）在睾丸下降及鞘状突闭锁中起作用。他们认为生殖股神经释放的钙基因相关肽在出生前减少可能导致睾丸未降，而在出生后的释放减少则导致疝和鞘膜积液的发生。

尽管已知鞘状突未闭是腹股沟疝发生的先决因素，但这一条件尚不充分，还涉及其他因素。表74-1列举了已明确的腹股沟疝发生的相关因素。

临床表现

一般情况下，腹股沟疝（除非特别指明，“腹股沟疝”指腹股沟斜疝）由患儿父母在为孩子洗澡时或由儿科医生在健康查体时发现，患儿有在腹腔压力增高（如哭闹或腹肌紧张时），腹股沟区、阴唇或阴囊内间断出现包块的典型病史。当询问病史时，鉴别腹股沟疝与交通性鞘膜积液、睾丸未降及腹股沟腺病很重要。斜疝可能在出生时被发现，或出生后数周、数月甚至数年出现，但这种缺陷在出生时已存在。有一点很重要，对于无症状疝，在其等待手术期间（如非急性期）应允许患儿参加一定的活动（如为无症状疝则不限制活动）。

表 74-1 先天性腹股沟疝形成的相关因素

泌尿生殖系统
睾丸未降
膀胱外翻
腹腔液体增加
腹水
脑室腹腔分流
腹膜透析
腹腔内压力增加
脐膨出或腹裂修补
急性腹水（乳糜腹）
胎粪性腹膜炎
慢性呼吸系统疾病
囊性纤维病
结缔组织疾病
Ehlers-Danlos 综合征
Hurrter-Hurler 综合征
Marfan 综合征
黏多糖病

腹股沟斜疝通常是无症状的。因为疝经常出现在婴儿不适时，父母亲常认为疝是引起不适的原因。这些能感觉到的症状可一直持续到修补术后。年长的孩子常主诉在运动时大腿根部或腹股沟区有不适感。

嵌顿疝是指疝囊内的肠管或其他内脏器官被卡住。嵌顿发生在内环口处还是在外环口处一直存在争论。尽管嵌顿在两处均可发生，但内环水平的嵌顿是主要因素。嵌顿可以引起间歇性疼痛和易激惹症状。随后产生肠梗阻的征象，如腹胀、呕吐和便秘。如果嵌顿未解除，可能会发生绞窄，嵌顿器官的血液供应减少而导致梗死，此时，患儿可以出现腹膜炎。这一过程短到可在 2 小时内完成。疝嵌顿一般在出生 6 个月内发生，并在 5 岁后相对减少。

值得注意的是尚无语言能力的患儿中，其监护人常不能及时认识嵌顿疝的症状和体征。我们指导患儿的家人在等待选择性疝手术时，对患儿的哭闹进行鉴别诊断：是饥饿、要换尿布、想睡觉，还是疝嵌顿需要手术。我们应指导患儿家长要留意什么（上级住院医生给 PLG 的忠告，Dr. Don Nakayama，1982）。

体格检查

患者应在温暖的房间，褪去衣物，取仰卧位进行检查。首先观察患儿在腹股沟区或阴部有无包块或不对称。用单指通过双侧阴囊顶部在阴囊内寻找睾丸，以区别真性腹股沟疝与回缩性睾丸。如果没有明显的包块，可以要求大一点的儿童站起来并做 Valsalva 动作；小婴儿则让其活动或哭闹以诱发腹股沟区包块的出现。如果包块依然没有出现，则仔细触诊精索有无增粗（丝弦征，silk string sign）[56]。让患儿仰卧，用一个手指在耻骨结节水平触摸精索，手指轻柔地从精索的一侧触摸到另一侧（图 74-2）。阳性体征是：与

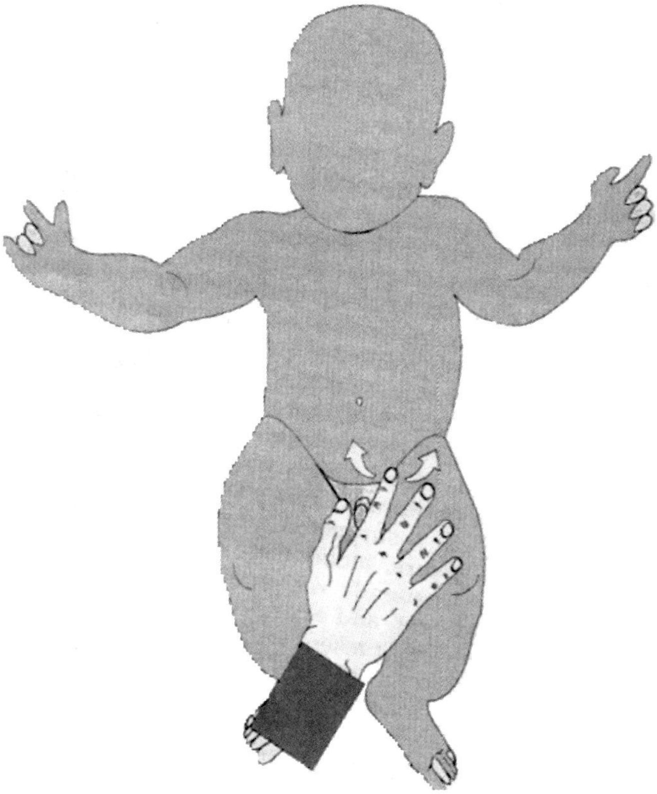

图 74-2　腹股沟疝的体格检查。一个手指放置在腹股沟区与腹股沟管平行，在耻骨结节水平，从一侧向另一侧横跨触摸精索。

正常侧精索相比，患侧腹股沟管内的精索增粗，检查者有触摸到两根丝线的感觉或触摸到内有少量液体的塑料包的感觉（plastic baggie sign），但只根据这些体征并不能完全确诊。

1175 如果在体格检查中未确诊有斜疝，但内科医生或家属能明确提供斜疝病史，外科医生往往仍选择手术[86]。然而，如果父母受到良好的教育、进行随访检查和借助现代放射学诊断技术，一些可疑病例可能会避免不必要的手术。

放射学研究

大多数情况下，腹股沟疝可以仅通过病史和体格检查确诊。但在一些患儿，放射学检查具有一定价值。如前所述，常用的技术是疝囊造影术（herniography），但现在已经被腹股沟区超声所取代。

疝囊造影术是经脐下荧光透视引导下将水溶性造影剂注入腹腔[47]。重力使造影剂在疝囊内逐渐积聚，分别在注射照影剂后 5 min、10 min、45 min 拍摄腹部平片。鞘膜积液可以通过这种方法鉴别，股疝也可以通过这种方法与腹股沟斜疝相鉴别。此方法在检查对侧斜疝或手术后同侧疝复发征象时有一定帮助。但在嵌顿疝，疝囊造影术无诊断价值，因为疝囊颈被封闭。该技术的并发症有肠穿孔、肠壁血肿及造影剂过敏反应等，但很少见[47,106]。尽管如此，疝囊造影术应用并不广泛。

作为体格检查的辅助手段，超声最近应用很广泛。它有迅速、非侵入性及无并发症等特点。Chen 等[17]对 224 例单侧或双侧斜疝男孩进行了双侧腹股沟区超声扫描。他们报道了正常腹股沟管直径的正常上限是 4 mm，并有 97% 的精确率。Erez 等[29]检查了 642 例患儿，在手术中发现正常腹股沟管手术前的直径范围是（3.6 ± 0.8）mm，而鞘状突未闭患儿腹股沟管直径为（4.9 ± 1.1）mm，斜疝患儿直径为（7.2 ± 2.0）mm 或更大。因此，随着仪器的正确应用，对有典型病史但体格检查未发现明显阳性体征的患儿，超声成为斜疝诊断值得信赖的工具。此外，在单侧斜疝患儿，超声也可用于术前评估对侧腹股沟区的情况（图 74-3）。然而，超声仍未得到广泛应用。

治疗

真性腹股沟疝不能自行愈合，一般需要手术治疗。因为嵌顿的几率较高，尤其在小婴儿，应迅速地行疝修补术。一些报道显示，如果在确诊 1 个月内行手术治疗，可以避免 90% 的并发症[85,107]。除早产儿、心脏或呼吸系统有问题的年长儿，大部分患儿可以在流动设施内（ambulatory setting）得到安全的治疗。

麻醉

患儿的麻醉方法各异，可以采用全身、区域或局

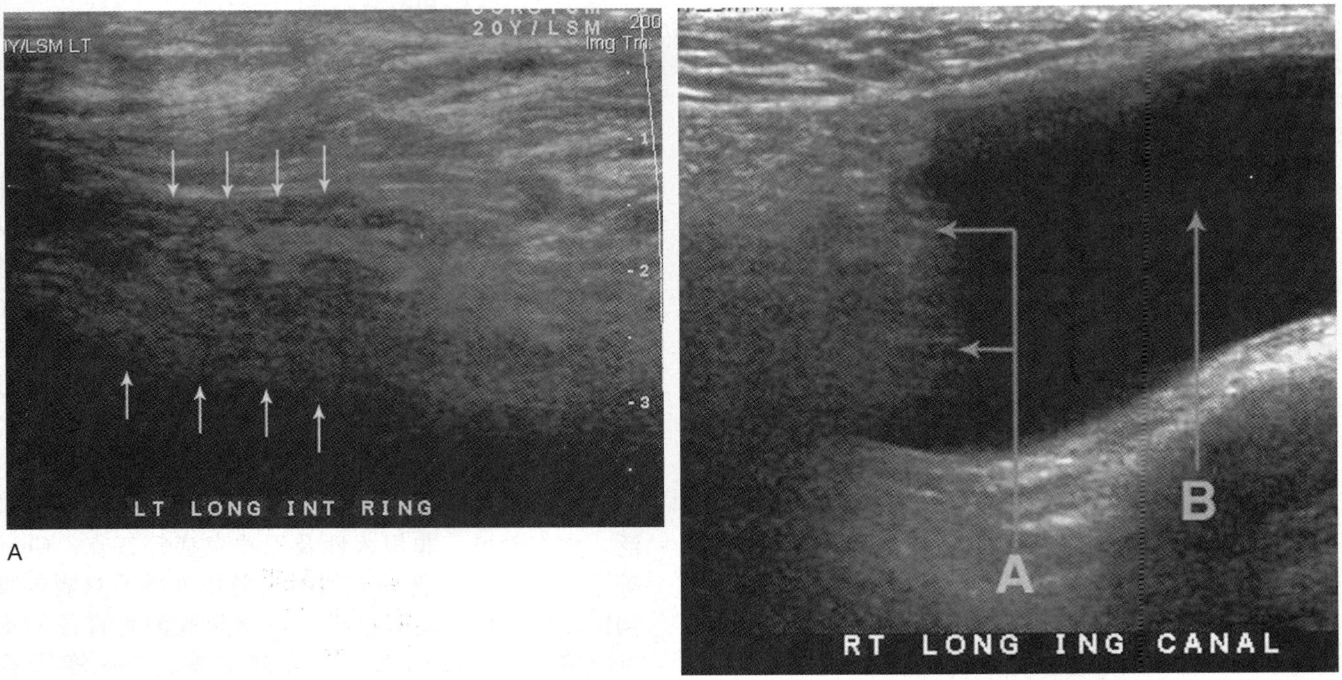

A　B

图 74-3　腹股沟管的超声检查。A. 没有疝。箭头所指的范围为腹股沟管，中间条索是输精管和精索结构。应用多普勒超声将看到阴囊内的动脉信号和下腔静脉的静脉信号。B. 腹股沟疝。双箭头指示嵌顿疝的前缘。如果嵌顿的是肠管，可以有蠕动；如果是网膜，则没有蠕动。单箭头所指为疝囊内液体。

部麻醉。可根据几个方面选择麻醉方式，包括患者的年龄或是否存在明显的合并症。大多数患者采用气管内插管或喉罩行全身麻醉。既往健康的足月患儿或年长患儿一般采用全身气管内麻醉，这种方法非常安全。其他患儿，特别是早产儿（早于孕 36 周出生和孕周加实足年龄小于 60 周）需要更适合的麻醉方法。在这种情况下，一般选择区域麻醉（脊麻、硬膜外或骶管麻醉等）效果较好[26]。最近一篇来自 Cochrane（循证医学数据库）的文章综述了几种区域麻醉方式与全麻的数据，显示其在术后呼吸暂停或心动过缓、呼吸频率及术后氧饱和度方面没有统计学差异，但整个实验组仅有 108 例患者。

1176 术后镇痛也是值得争论的问题。一些医疗机构常规采用骶管阻滞，而一些医院采用手术野局部滴注麻醉剂。一项随机的前瞻性研究对比了用无肾上腺素的 0.25% 丁哌卡因（2.5 mg/kg）局部浸润麻醉及骶管阻滞麻醉，发现它们在术后镇痛方面没有差异[23]。此外局部浸润麻醉（所谓的溅开技术）与伤口内注射麻醉药一样有效。

当天手术的年龄

大多数足月婴儿和年长儿童的腹股沟疝将接受当天（same-day）手术治疗，早产儿安全接受当天手术的年龄值得探讨。一项研究显示小于 41～46 孕周的早产儿和有新生儿窒息史的婴儿发生术后呼吸暂停的风险增加[62]。据另一项大型调查显示，应用先进的技术监测手术后呼吸紊乱情况，发现小于 44 孕周的婴儿术后发生临床上典型呼吸暂停的风险增加[63]。1995 年对 8 个前瞻性研究的联合分析显示，32 孕周出生而实际年龄为 56 孕周与 34 孕周出生而实际年龄为 54 孕周时，术后呼吸暂停的发生率不会低于 1%（可信度 95%）[25]。在我们的医疗中心，宁可失之过于谨慎，一般将 60 孕周作为单日住院手术的临界年龄。

手术时机

大多数医生推荐在确诊后不久即行疝手术[61]。

这可以大大减少疝手术的并发症，而且因现代麻醉的安全性，它也是可行的。对于早产儿，大多数外科医生推荐在患儿出院前，体重增加到 2 kg 时行手术治疗。1996 年之前，外科医生的观点则与之相反，当时只有 33% 的医生接受对早产儿进行手术[107]。对早产儿早期手术存在一个缺点即较小的患儿复发率比较高。在欧洲，正在对体重为 2. 5 kg 与 5 kg 的接受修补术的患儿进行一项随机的前瞻性研究[68]。

男性疝修补术

儿童腹股沟疝修补的基本原则是行疝囊高位结扎术。改良 Ferguson 修补术曾是 Ladd 和 Gross 的选择[56]。这与在英国很流行的 Mitchell-Bank 修补方式相比，他们首选该手术方式即不打开腹外斜肌，通过 1177
内环口简单地高位结扎疝囊[87]。在 Ferguson 修补术中，打开腹外斜肌，重建腹股沟管，但不改变精索与腹股沟管的关系。下面讲述一下我们采用的腹股沟斜疝修补术并强调主要的变化之处（图 74-4）。

患者仰卧位，寻找耻骨结节与髂前上棘连线中点。耻骨结节是很重要的解剖标志，因为外环口在其外侧下方。在耻骨结节外侧上方中点取皮肤切口，随儿童年龄增长，内环口更靠向外侧，而婴儿的外环口和内环口是重叠的。在较大的儿童，内环口与外环口之间距离增大，皮肤切口应更靠外侧一些。在任何年龄的儿童，过于靠中间的切口在找到腹股沟韧带之前会偏离外环口，增加损伤精索组织的危险。

切开皮肤，暴露皮下脂肪或 Camper 筋膜。剪开 Camper 筋膜，以暴露更重要的 Scarpa 筋膜，需小心

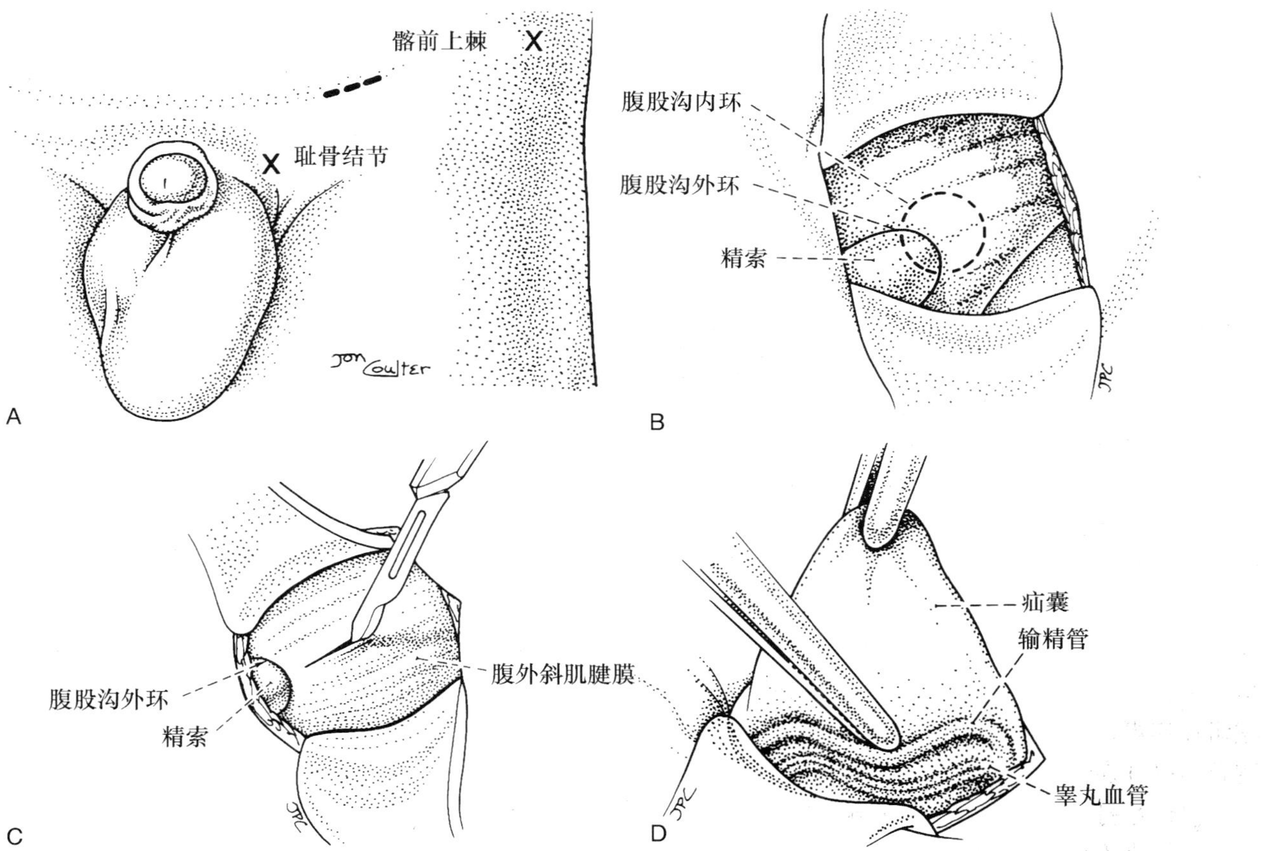

图 74-4　男性患儿腹股沟疝修补术技巧。A. 耻骨结节和髂前上棘是内环口前方腹股沟皮肤切口的标志物（阴影线）。B. 在1 岁以下的婴儿，内环口与外环口重叠，腹股沟较短。不需要经过常规的腹外斜肌切口到达内环。C. 年龄较大的患儿，越过内环口在外环口外侧打开腹外斜肌腱膜。腹外斜肌下面有清晰的提睾肌纤维。D. 切开提睾肌，用剪刀暴露精索，抓住并提起精索。从白色疝囊上轻柔分离输精管和精索血管，且不要碰触。

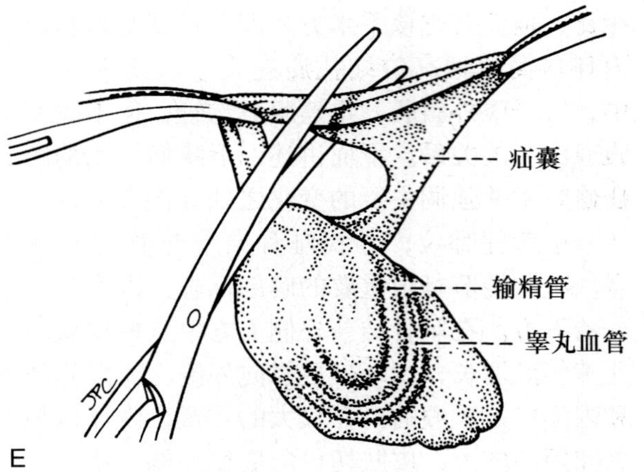

E

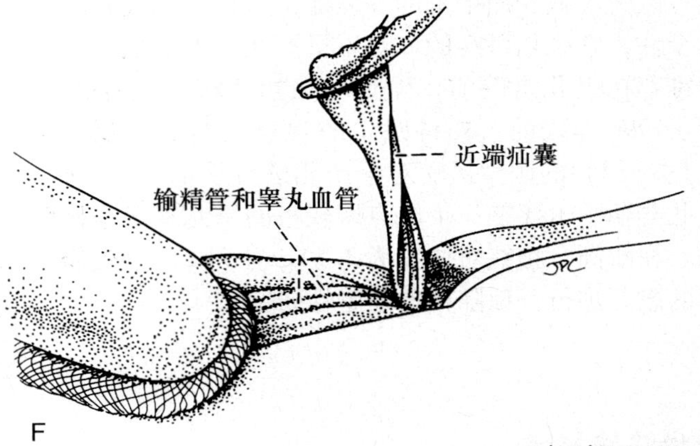

F

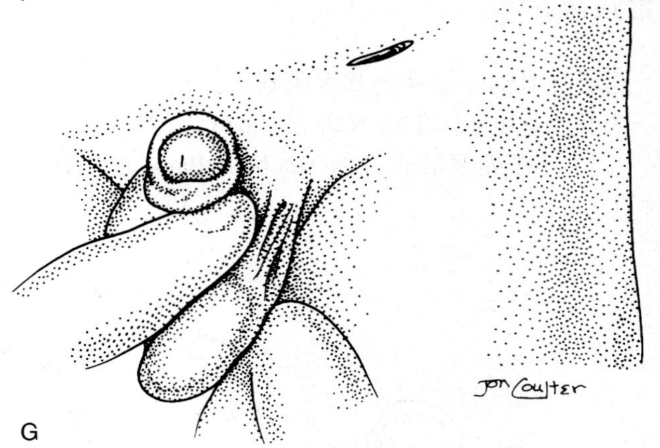

G

图 74-4 （续）E. 检查疝囊内容物，用钳子将空的疝囊直接分开。远端疝囊边缘电烙止血，并放回切口内。F. 轻柔地分离近端疝囊至内环口水平，此处可看到腹膜外脂肪。旋拧疝囊，注意不要夹入输精管和血管，并双层结扎疝囊。G. 将睾丸放回阴囊内，弄直精索，用可吸收线逐层关闭切口。

以避免损伤 Scarpa 筋膜上方的腹壁下血管。提起 Scarpa 筋膜并剪开以暴露腹外斜肌。在腹外斜肌显露以后，于外环口水平起轻柔分离，可以清楚看到从外到中线走向的腹股沟韧带。在腹股沟韧带上方解剖时需小心，以避免损伤股血管组织。用剪刀沿腹外斜肌肌纤维方向打开腹外斜肌，在近外环口处，用直的止血钳处理腹外斜肌边缘，以利于随后的层次分辨及关闭切口。在腹外斜肌底方、上方或下方，用镊子或一块医用纱布以利于辨认腹横肌筋膜、髂股神经、髂腹股沟神经及提睾肌纤维。在提睾肌上打开一个小切口，寻找疝囊。用一个较大的、口不太锐利的手术器械钳住疝囊，并将精索组织提出切口外，直到可以 V
1178 型翻转打开疝囊并清楚地显示疝囊内组织。将镊子由此切口钝性打开精索筋膜，并将输精管及血管与疝囊分离。检查有无疝内容物，并重新确认输精管和血管。两把止血钳靠近夹住疝囊，并离断疝囊。将近端疝囊向内环口处剥离干净，旋拧疝囊，在内环口处用单股可吸收线结扎疝囊。Ladd 和 Gross 用丝线结扎近端疝囊，但我们见到过疝修补术数年后线头从伤口中“冒出”的病例，用可吸收线可以避免这一现象。不必切开远端疝囊，因为可能会引起缺血性睾丸炎或术后血肿。同样非交通性鞘膜积液的远端鞘膜囊可以开窗，但不应完全剥除。无需一定进行睾丸探查。如果真的要探查，应避免损伤肉膜上的正常引带组织。探查结束后，牵拉阴囊皮肤及肉膜将睾丸放回阴囊内正常位置。逐层关闭切口，可吸收线间断缝合 Scarpa 筋膜。我们选择皮内缝合伤口，但间断缝合切口效果也不错。使用有塑料不渗水内膜的无菌敷料包扎伤口，以防治大小便的污染（在使用尿布的儿童）。因为安全性的问题，我们不使用医用胶封闭伤口。

女性疝修补术

因为不需要识别并保护精索，女性疝修补术比较简单。女性腹股沟管的手术途径与男性相同。确认疝囊后，应检查疝内容物，通常是卵巢、输卵管或输卵管系膜（图 74-5）。如果无内容物，在两把止血钳之

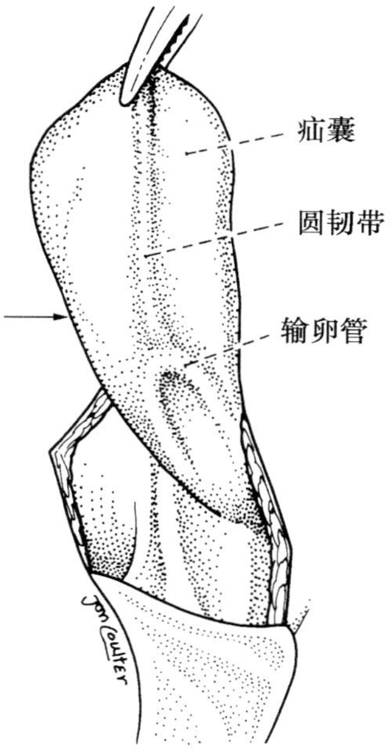

图 74-5　女性疝囊。常在疝囊壁上发现输卵管，形成滑疝，必须加以辨别。如果需要，打开疝囊，且圆韧带紧随输卵管。

间分开疝囊，远端疝囊止血后放回切口内，近端分离至内环口处，旋拧疝囊，双股可吸收线结扎。按标准程序用一或两针关闭外环口，并关闭切口。在旋拧并结扎疝囊之前，我们常规打开疝囊探查，因为多达40%的女性斜疝为滑疝。卵巢、输卵管或子宫是常见的疝内容物，也并非常常回缩至腹腔内。如果不容易看见输卵管，一些术者会牵拉圆韧带以在结扎疝囊前确认输卵管是否在疝囊内。我们并不常规地将疝囊与圆韧带缝合至联合肌腱重建子宫的正常支持物（Bastionelli 方法）。

如果是滑疝，输卵管作为疝囊壁的一部分，不将它从疝囊壁疝分离。相反，如 Bevan 描述的一样，我
1179 们在输卵管上方的疝囊外壁上缝一针荷包线，将疝囊内翻入内环口内，然后用一或两针关闭内环口[7]。作为选择，Goldstein 和 Potts[92] 介绍的皮瓣法也可以采用。

腹腔镜疝修补术

腹腔镜下腹股沟疝修补术在成人中已开展了多年。其优点是疼痛较轻，较早恢复工作，通过同一戳孔修补双侧腹股沟疝及更便利地修补复发疝。缺点有费用增加、手术时间延长与手术学习曲线延长等。此外，还有许多技术被提出，如经腹修补术和腹膜外修补术。因为儿童手术切口较小、手术较成人简单及儿童开放性手术的痛苦较轻，许多小儿外科医生认为没有必要对儿童的腹股沟疝行腹腔镜疝修补术。

El-Gohary[28] 报道了 28 例行腹腔镜疝修补术的女性病例，在这些病例中，疝囊被内翻至腹腔内，将腹腔镜圈套器放置在内翻疝囊基底部结扎。因为这种结扎方式不能将精索排除在外，该手术方法仅适用于女性。Schier[88] 报道了 14 例女性腹腔镜疝修补术，他在腹腔内放置 2～3 针 Z 型缝线以关闭鞘状突。

Montupet 和 Esposito[71] 首先成功地在男孩身上实施了腹腔镜疝修补术。荷包缝合疝囊颈部，小心地分离输尿管和精索血管。45 例行疝修补术的男性没有手术并发症，但有 2 例复发需要再次行腹腔镜疝修补术。2000 年 Schier[89] 报道包括男性在内的疝修补术，他改变手术方法，用几针间断缝合，而不是 Z 型关闭疝囊。129 例患儿（81 例男孩）采用了这种手术方法，有 1 例早期复发。最近，Schier 主张在腹腔内荷包缝合以减少疝复发。

一些手术者采用特殊的装置从腹膜外在疝囊颈放置缝线。Lee 和 Liang[60] 报道 450 例使用这种特殊手术治疗的患儿，与开放手术相比，前者复发率为 0.88%。Prasad 等发表了使用一种商品化的钢锥钻帮助缝合的小宗病例报道。

腹腔镜疝修补术仍在发展，但复发率较高。在男性患者中，因为有较高的复发率，且担心不能像开放手术那样很好地识别并保护精索组织，我们已经停止使用腹腔镜疝修补术。当然，技术上的重要革新仍将继续涌现。

男性腹腔镜疝修补术需要仰卧位全身麻醉，并需要放置胃管和 Foley 导尿管或直导尿管。脐部放置 5 mm套针，并造气腹进行腹腔镜探查。可以轻易鉴别双侧斜疝或不常见的股疝或直疝。分别在左下腹和右下腹造两个 3 mm 切口，放入 3 mm 操作器械，这种方式可以使双侧疝更容易处理。用腹腔镜 3 mm 缝针在疝囊颈放置荷包线。缝荷包线可以使精索很清楚地被识别和分开。应该避免形成血肿，因为随着手术进展它将使精索组织变得模糊不清，容易损伤。线放置好后，在体内打结，3 mm 的切口不需缝合，只需用可吸收线缝合脐部切口。

如前所述，也可以使用其他技术。其中，Prasad[77]等使用的技术最简单。他们通过脐下切口放置腹腔镜摄像头，这个切口是唯一放置套针的切口。内环口位置通过腹部触诊确定，并在此处用手术刀切开皮肤。在腹腔镜的直接导引下，利用一种腹腔外缝针传动器经过皮肤切口将荷包线缝于内环口半圈，将针暂时留在腹腔内，经过同一切口将一个弯曲的钢锥钻穿过另外半圈，注意不要损伤精索。用锥将针抓紧并拉出腹腔外，完成荷包缝合，于腹腔外打结，腹腔镜下关闭内环口。

1180 在女性患者，因为没有精索，我们使用腹腔镜内翻结扎技术（laparoscopic inversion ligation，LIL）[113]。选择与男性患者相同的位置放置套针，将肠钳或左弯钳（Malyland clamp）放入疝囊内（图 74-6），抓住疝囊顶端将其翻转放入腹腔，旋拧疝囊，将两个圈套器放在疝囊颈处结扎疝囊，要小心确保在拧紧疝囊颈时，疝囊内没有附件结构。我们手术的病例中没有复发者，手术并发症也很低。

对侧腹股沟区探查

1955 年 Rothenberg 和 Barnett[82]报道的腹股沟疝病例中，100% 的 1 岁以下患儿和 68.5% 的 1 岁以上患儿存在双侧腹股沟疝。从此，常规双侧腹股沟探查在小儿外科疝手术中成了争论最多的话题之一。最近，腹腔镜下双侧腹股沟探查术也被列入了争论之列。

因为双侧腹股沟疝的发生率较高，Rothenberg 和 Barnett 推荐常规进行对侧腹股沟区探查，但他们发现，一些患者存在的是未闭的鞘状突而不是真性疝囊。尽管一些医生支持常规探查，但另一些认为探查会产生较大的负面影响，因为并不是所有未闭的鞘状突都将发展成为腹股沟疝。此外，常规探查使睾丸和输精管是有危险的。即便如此，在 1981 年的小儿外科医生调查中，Rowe 和 Maichildon[86]发现，约 80% 的医生对 1 岁以下的男孩进行常规对侧探查，90% 的医生对女孩进行探查。最近，更多的调查显示了常规对侧腹股沟区探查术的趋势：40% 的医生主张对 2 岁以下患儿进行常规探查，13% 的医生常规探查 2～5 岁的男孩，39% 常规探查女孩，51% 常规探查早产儿[61]。这个调查也显现了另一个趋势：24% 的外科医生使用腹腔镜进行对侧探查。

我们认为常规对侧腹股沟区探查是不必要的，没必要使输精管和睾丸处于危险境地，也没必要增加费用。我们根据事实做出判断：虽然 60%～80% 1 岁以下婴儿和 40% 较大婴儿有未闭的鞘状突，但只有 20% 的单侧斜疝患儿对侧出现腹股沟疝[84,86,93]。也就是说，需要做 10 次手术来预防 2 例对侧疝的发生。一些医生认为，无症状者一侧发展为斜疝的发生率较低，仅为 7%。所以，许多医生根据患儿的性别、年龄及患侧部位实施选择性对侧腹股沟区探查。

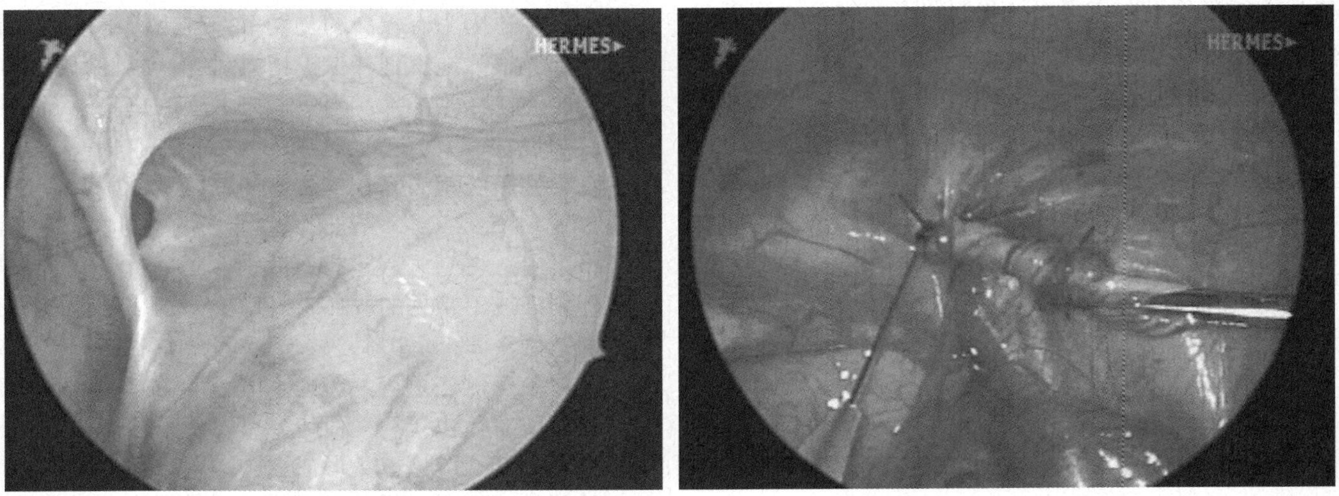

A B

图 74-6 鞘状突的腹腔镜征象。A. 开放的鞘状突。B. 鞘状突向腹腔内翻转并用套环结扎。

性别

过去，一些医生对女性行双侧探查术，主要因为在疝囊内较少发现生殖器官，损伤的危险很小。在1981 年的调查中，Rowe 和 Maichildon[86] 报道 90% 的医生对 1 岁以下女性患儿常规行对侧腹股沟区探查术。Wiener 等[107] 在 1996 年对小儿外科医生进行了一项调查，发现 84% 的人对 4 岁以下女性患儿行常规对侧探查术。现在看来这种趋势已在下降，因为 2002 年 Levitt 等[61] 发现只有 39% 的医生对 5 岁以下女性
1181 患儿进行双侧腹股沟区探查。尽管疝囊内很少发现生殖器官，但探查仍存在损伤腹股沟后壁、髂腹股沟神经和髂股神经的可能性。因为缺少有随访数据的文献，很难量化这些风险。然而，尽管我们知道仅有 20% 左右单侧腹股沟疝的女性患者将出现对侧疝，但为预防少数疝的发生，仍在大量进行对侧探查术。Chertin 等[18] 最近综述了 300 例单侧疝修补术的女孩，随访1 ~4年，只有 8% 发展为对侧斜疝，而且并不受手术年龄及患侧部位的影响。

年龄

基于 Rothenberg 和 Barnett[82] 的发现，100% 的 1 岁以下腹股沟疝婴儿存在双侧鞘状突未闭，许多医生选择常规对侧探查术。2002 年对外科医生的一项调查显示，51% 的被调查者对早产儿进行常规对侧探查，40% 探查 2 岁以下的男孩[61]。这与 1981 年的调查结果中 80% 的医生主张行对侧探查术相比大大下降[86]。对 1052 例患者随访 11 年的调查中显示，对侧疝在 1 岁以下男孩中的发生率为 13.1%，在 2 岁以下男孩中的发生率为 13.7%[49]。在女孩，约 9.6% 的 1 岁以下患儿出现对侧疝，5 岁以下患儿约 13.9% 出现对侧疝。最近，一项报道调查了 181 例 1 岁以下行单侧疝修补术的婴儿[4]，随访 5 ~ 10 年，7.7% 出现对侧疝。基于以上报道，单侧斜疝小婴儿将来是否有较高的风险出现对侧疝仍不清楚。

部位

人们推测，右侧疝比左侧更常见的原因是右侧鞘状突关闭较晚。所以，左侧斜疝患儿发生对侧疝的风险较右侧斜疝患儿发生对侧疝的几率要高。据此，一些医生推荐对左侧斜疝患儿常规进行对侧腹股沟区探查术。McGregor 等[64] 一项 20 年的回顾性调查显示，41% 原发为左侧斜疝的患儿日后出现右斜疝，而只有 14% 初发为右侧斜疝的患儿发生左侧疝。然而，其他一些报道显示在左侧疝修补术后出现对侧疝的几率要少。例如，Kemmotsu 等[50] 回顾了 1052 例行单侧疝修补术的儿童，发现原发疝修补的部位并不影响对侧疝的发生率。Miltenburg 等[67] 通过 Meta 分析发现行左侧疝修补术的儿童发生对侧疝的几率比右侧疝修补术高 11%。总体看来，原发疝的部位与对侧疝出现的概率无关。

其他探查术

为减少对侧疝探查手术的阴性结果，其他一些技术用于判断对侧鞘状突是否未闭。方法之一是诊断性气腹（Goldstein 实验），腹部经由对侧疝囊充气，如果对侧腹股沟区触诊到捻发音，则是鞘状突未闭的征象。在对 62 例患儿的研究中，7 例（11%）有阳性结果[49]，他们中每例探查均发现存在对侧斜疝。而其余 55 例患儿中，只有 3 例（5%）发生对侧疝。我们认为这项技术是安全而有效的。然而，一些医生认为该技术不可信，可能漏诊一些鞘状突未闭患儿。Bakes 扩张器可以用于探查对侧腹股沟区，但这项技术很难而且不可信。疝囊造影术前文已讨论过，现在已很少应用。超声检查很早已开始讨论，应用适合的诊断标准，超声对鞘状突未闭的检查具有相当的敏感性。

腹腔镜探查

20 世纪 90 年代早期，腹腔镜用来评估对侧腹股沟区。腹腔镜具有操作容易及可以直视下观察对侧内环口情况的优点，该技术目前已广泛应用。腹腔镜手术有多种方式，也许最常用的技术是放置套针通过患侧疝囊向腹腔内注气，使用有角度（如 70°）的镜子可以很容易评价对侧情况。一些医生通过脐部套管置腹腔镜或用腹腔镜通过腹壁置入一根血管造影用的套针给予同轴造影。软的或硬的镜子均可以使用[35]。

Yerkes 等[111]应用腹腔镜评价了 627 例 10 岁以下患单侧疝并在发病后 5 年出现对侧鞘状突未闭（contralateral patent processus vaginalis，CCPV）的患儿后发现，46%1 岁以下的患儿发生 CCPV，39%1 岁以上的患儿发生 CCPV。Geisler 等[36]评估了 358 例 1 月~13 岁的患儿，其总的 CCPV 发生率为 33%。按年龄分组，1 岁以下的发生率是 50%，2 岁以下为 45%，5 岁以下为 37%，5 岁以上为 15%。Pellegrin 等[76]研究了 50 例患者，发现 CCPV 发生率为 31%。Rescorla 等[81]报道的 CCPV 发生率为 48%。总的来讲，腹腔镜的 CCPV 发现率较一致，大约为 30%~45%。

问题是，这些 CCPV 中有哪些将发展为腹股沟疝？答案是不明确的，需要进行随机的、前瞻性的及终生的随访——这实际上是不可能的。Kieswetter 和 Parenzar[52]对 100 例 2 岁以下患儿进行了常规对侧腹股沟探查，发现 61% 为 CCPV；他们对 231 例行单侧疝修补术的患儿进行了密切随访，发现 31% 发生对
1182 侧疝，其中约一半是未预料到的。根据他们的以及 Rowe 与 Clatworthy[84]的调查数据，人们可以期待通过腹腔镜技术显著减少不必要的手术。持反对意见的人则指出超过一半的患者接受了不必要的手术（不包括腹腔镜检查为假阴性结果的患者），而且考虑到手术时间及所需手术设备，医疗费用大大提高。但是，腹腔镜手术中可多次重复使用的器械的出现已减少了费用及时间的消耗。

随着患儿年龄的增加，CCPV 的发生率明显下降。问题是到什么年龄将不需要腹腔镜进行诊断？Bhatia 等[8]调查了 101 例 2~8 岁的患儿及 171 例 2 岁以下患儿，后者中有 38% 发生 CCPV，年龄较大的儿童中有 20% 发生 CCPV，而在一组 12 例 8 岁以上的患儿中，只有 1 例发生 CCPV。作者认为腹腔镜技术对 2 岁以上患儿的作用可以做出结论，但因为研究的样本数较小，对 8 岁以上患儿的作用没有明确结论。Geisler 等[36]的研究中，有 15%5 岁以上的患儿发生 CCPV。似乎可以看出，5~8 岁的患儿应用腹腔镜诊断 CCPV 的效力显著下降。

难复性疝（嵌顿疝）

大多数腹股沟斜疝容易回缩至腹腔内，而嵌顿疝的疝内容物则很难复位。当内环口或外环口较紧，内脏血管受压血流减少，如果疝没有复位，大多数患儿会很快发展为绞窄性疝[101]。初期，由于疝环缩紧导致静脉和淋巴回流受阻及继发内脏肿胀。如继续发展，动脉血供的终止将导致肠或其他内脏器官坏死或穿孔。绞窄性疝也可阻止睾丸的血供而导致睾丸损伤。发生过嵌顿疝的患儿，在疝修补术后更容易发生睾丸萎缩。

各种研究显示，嵌顿疝在男孩和女孩中的发生率相似，均为 12%~17%[83,98]。1 岁以下的患儿更容易发生嵌顿疝，但此后，发生率逐渐下降（图 74-7）。在两个大型调查中，2~3 月龄以下的足月患儿，嵌顿疝发生率为 28%~31%[80,83]。在另一篇报道中，6 周以下的患儿发生率为 24%[69]。与足月儿相比，早产儿的嵌顿疝发生率较低（13% 对 18%）。这可能与环口较大及腹肌较薄弱有关。而且，很多这些婴儿在新生儿监护中心的持续监护下，嵌顿疝可以通过早期复位预防或干脆被漏报。

绞窄性疝诊断

如果肠管嵌顿入疝囊，患儿会变得易激惹并发展为剧痛，随之出现腹胀、呕吐、停止排气或排便等梗阻症状。在腹股沟区出现一个有张力、无波动的包块，可以向阴囊延伸。当内脏嵌顿时，包块会变得较

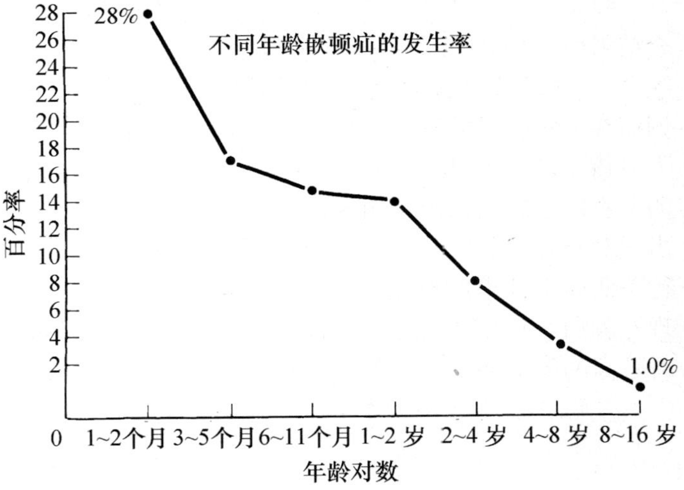

图 74-7 不同年龄嵌顿疝的发生率。嵌顿疝在出生 1 年内很常见，然后发生率明显下降。

柔软。包块偶尔透光试验阳性，容易同鞘膜积液混淆。不可对可疑的“鞘膜积液”肿块进行诊断性穿刺或抽液治疗。

绞窄性疝的后期症状是休克、便血和腹膜炎。通常可以触及睾丸，但它们往往大而硬，很难同睾丸扭转相鉴别。腹部平片显示不完全性或完全性肠梗阻，阴囊内也可见到肠管气体影。对可疑的病例，超声可以鉴别是肠管还是鞘膜积液或睾丸扭转。

非手术治疗

患者无明显休克和腹膜炎体征时，应首先尝试非手术治疗。在许多病例，嵌顿肠管突出于外环口并在此被卡压，所以我们采用以下的技术（图 74-8）：让患儿平躺并尽力让其平静，禁食，如果可能，可以将患儿的下肢抬高。站立在患儿的患侧，小婴儿的话站在其脚端，将左手示指和中指放在患侧髂前上棘前方，并沿腹股沟管向下，向同侧阴囊处滑动，将左手放在睾丸、腹股沟包块或阴囊皮肤上并保持一定压力。持续轻柔地牵拉阴囊，以保持疝囊长轴与腹股沟管长轴相一致。接下来，在同侧内环口水平，用右手 1183
的示指和拇指给疝囊颈的任一侧一个压力。同时牵拉阴囊，以利于外环口和内环口在一条线上并保持开放状态。而且，牵拉阴囊也可以防止疝囊过分重叠或成为疝内容物回缩入腹腔的障碍。最后，保持左手在包块顶部，右手示指和拇指在内环口处持续用力。左手在腹股沟上缓慢向内环口方向运动，并保持在疝内容物底部持续施压。这一过程可能需要数分钟，如果成功，疝内容物将缓慢消失，回缩至腹腔内。与对侧腹股沟区相比较，确保疝内容物完全消失。如果该方法没有成功或患儿难以忍受疼痛，可以使用镇静剂。但

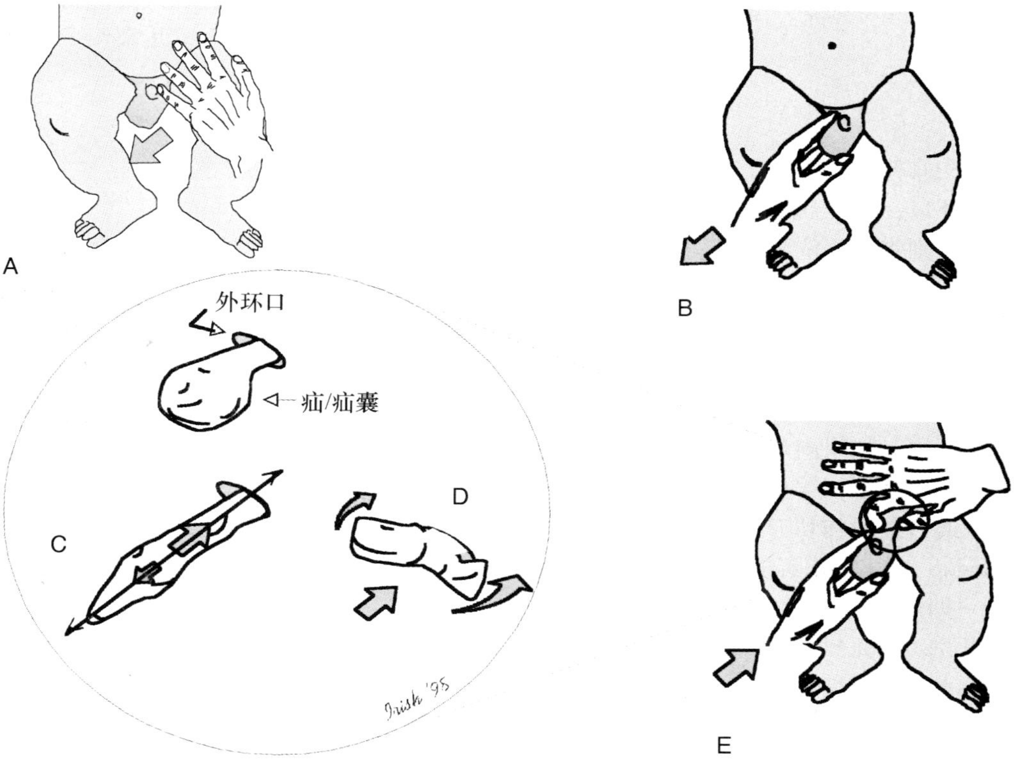

图 74-8　嵌顿疝复位示意图。A. 站在儿童患侧或婴儿的脚边，将左侧中指和示指放在患侧（图例为左侧）髂前上棘，并沿腹股沟管向同侧阴囊下滑。B. 用左手在睾丸、疝块或阴囊皮肤上施加压力。C. 持续轻柔地牵拉阴囊有助于疝囊长轴和腹股沟管长轴成一直线，然后，用右手的示指及拇指在疝囊颈任一侧施加压力。D. 牵拉阴囊，使内环口和外环口保持开放，并阻止疝囊重叠或成为复位时的潜在障碍。E. 最后，左手放在疝块顶端，用右手示指和拇指在腹股沟管上持续施压。向着内环口缓慢移动手指，并在疝内容物底部持续施压。

不主张使用全身麻醉，因为复位过程中有可能出现肠管损伤或复位肠管已有坏死，全麻下难以发现。通常单独使用镇静剂即可有助于疝内容物自行回缩。曾有坏死肠管回缩至腹腔的报道[99]，所以，对复位困难的患儿，我们建议在医院留观 24 小时。疝修补术至少推迟24～48小时进行，以使水肿消退。

手术治疗

当非手术治疗失败或患者出现休克或腹膜炎征象时，应行手术治疗。按标准流程完成术前准备，开放静脉，输注液体，留置尿管以利于监测。给予广谱抗生素，如果有肠梗阻症状应留置鼻胃管。在患者充分复苏后，将其送入手术室。如果疝内容物在全身麻醉后、手术之前复位至腹腔，仍继续进行手术治疗。有几种手术方式可用于治疗嵌顿疝，包括经腹股沟或腹膜外途径，腹腔镜也可用于嵌顿疝治疗。

腹股沟区途径

可采用腹股沟疝修补术的标准手术，只是该术式切口稍长。打开外环口，确认疝囊，如果疝内容物仍旧存在，如无坏死，则将其复位至腹腔，然后按标准
1184 方式实行疝修补术。如果无法将肠管复位至腹腔，结扎腹壁下血管，打开部分腹股沟管，扩大内环口，对这些病例应该行正规疝后壁修补术。

如果疝囊内的肠管怀疑有坏死，则用温纱布热敷肠管，几分钟后再观察。如果内环口仍狭小，可以再予以扩大，注意不要让肠管回缩至腹腔。如果确认肠管已坏死，则可以通过腹股沟切口或对口切开的腹横筋膜切口（La Roque 切口）或经另外的腹部切口切除坏死肠管，行一期肠吻合术[55]。如果肠管具有活力则将其复位至腹腔，并完成疝修补术。

如果肠管在检查前已回缩至腹腔，问题就变得复杂一些。如果没有发现肠坏死的迹象，如肠内容物或酸臭味或血性液体，许多医生选择直接行疝修补术。也可行腹腔镜手术，通过脐部切口或疝囊放置腹腔镜，再判断肠是否有活力。事实上，在手术开始即可使用腹腔镜监视疝内容物复位过程。如果内容物具有活力，则行标准的疝修补术[58]，如果怀疑肠管坏死，可以在疝修补术后再行观察，如果明确肠坏死，则将肠管从脐部切口拖出并切除。

腹腔外途径

一些医生选择腹腔外途径治疗嵌顿疝。1921 年 Cheatle[16]在成年患者中采用过的这种术式，也成功地应用于儿童。Kamalaedeen 和 Shanbhougue[48]报道 24 例，Turnock 等[102]报道 12 例，发现腹膜外途径在复位疝内容物和行疝切开术时更便利。如果需要，可以打开腹腔观察肠管活力。

腹膜外途径在髂前上棘水平沿皮纹切开皮肤，采用标准的支架（gridiron）途径到达腹膜外层。在腹壁下血管外侧确认内环口和疝囊。在疝囊底部打开腹膜，检查内容物活力，坏死的肠管经过此切口很容易被切除，否则，将有活力的肠管复位至腹腔，行疝切开术。如果外环口成为疝内容物复位的阻碍，则打开腹外斜肌浅层，扩大外环口。疝切开术完成后，按标准程序关闭切口。该切口如在右侧，与阑尾切除切口相似，应将这一点告之患儿家长。一些医生也经腹腔完成腹腔外途径手术。

Pfannenstiel 切口

Kaga 等[53]最近主张使用 Pfannenstiel 切口经腹腔途径治疗嵌顿疝。他们采用 Pfannenstiel 皮肤切口，随后打开中线筋膜，使肠管复位并检测其活力，如果需要切除肠管，该切口可以很好地暴露术野，疝囊也很容易修补。作者认为这个途径手术瘢痕较小。

作者选择的方式

我们选择经脐放置套针的腹腔镜手术方式，在腹腔镜监测下复位肠管，随后经腹股沟切口行标准的疝切开术。尚没有完全通过腹腔镜手术治疗儿童嵌顿疝的报道。

卵巢嵌顿

这里特别提及女性患者的无症状卵巢嵌顿疝。很久以来，许多人认为，这种嵌顿的、可移动的、无张

力的卵巢长期位于疝囊内，没有绞窄的危险。但随后的报道否认了这一看法[72]。现在一致认为，如果女性卵巢嵌顿应尽早行修补术[61]。

手术后并发症

阴囊肿胀

在疝修补术后，特别是交通性鞘膜积液手术后，液体可能积聚在远端疝囊内，形成积液。通常能自行吸收，少数需抽吸治疗。切除远端疝囊可引起阴囊血肿。

医源性隐睾

疝修补术后医源性隐睾不常见，但也有可能是被少报了的一种并发症。Kiesewetter 和 Oh[51] 报道的 248 例患者有 2 例发生医源性睾丸未降，Hecher 和 Ring-Mrozik[44] 报道 1957 例患者中有 5 例出现该并发症，发生率为 0.2%。除外先天性隐睾，这种异常与手术结束前未能成功将睾丸放置回阴囊或睾丸随后回缩有关。需要行睾丸固定术纠正这一问题。

复发

很难准确判定腹股沟斜疝修补术后复发率是多
185 少，因为一些因素，如性别和有无嵌顿，在报道的文献中并没有清楚说明。一般情况下，报道的不太复杂的疝修补术的复发率为 0～0.8%。早产儿复发率上升至 15%，嵌顿疝复发率则为 20%。在许多报道中，没有对患者进行长时间的随访，实际的复发率尚不清楚，可能比报道的要高。对腹股沟嵌顿疝患者的报道常不能明确原始治疗方案是手术还是非手术。

许多与疝发生相关的因素也与疝复发有关。例如，Grosfeld 等[41]报道的 25 例脑室腹膜分流术的患儿，3 例（12%）发生斜疝。嵌顿疝也是引起疝复发的主要因素，Steinau 等[97]报道 29 例（25 例男孩，4 例女孩）出现复发疝，其中患过嵌顿疝的为 24%。与此相反，2754 例未发生嵌顿疝的患者的疝复发率仅为 7.6%。其他危险因素有手术后并发症（9.4% 的复发率）及伴发疾病和畸形[96]。有趣的是，Harvey 等[43]发现尽管手术技术的不完善可引起疝复发，但手术医生的经验水平不是导致复发的因素。大部分腹股沟复发疝是斜疝，可能与疝囊撕裂、没有完整地解剖疝囊、疝囊颈线结滑脱或结扎疝囊位置不够高未达到内环口水平等有关。复发疝的另一个因素是早产，一些报道显示，早产儿的斜疝复发率增加，为 2%～15%。

虽然很少发生，但在首次手术中误诊的直疝或股疝也存在“疝复发”。Steinau 等[96]报道的 34 例复发疝中，4 例为直疝，1 例为股疝。Fonkalsrud 等[33]一组报道中发现，13 例直疝中有 4 例（31%）后来行斜疝修补术。斜疝修补术后出现直疝既可能是在首次手术中未被认识的伴发疾病，也可能是损伤腹股沟管后壁后的新发疾病。股疝的复发更多是因为首次手术中误诊，而不是真正的疝复发。

在几个大规模的腹腔镜疝修补术的报道中，Schier[89]报道的对 279 例患儿实施的 403 例腹腔镜疝修补术中，复发率为 2.3%。不同医生之间的腹腔镜手术技巧不同仍是疝复发的相关因素。而且，因存在腹腔镜学习中的认知曲线，复发更容易出现在医生的早期手术后。在我们施行的男性腹腔镜疝修补术中，复发率相当高，所以我们没有将这项技术用于男性。而在女性，使用上文提及的 LIL 术，没有疝复发。

输精管损伤

尽管输精管被离断后在手术中很容易看见，但直到成年才认识到术中输精管受到意外挤压损伤，即使如此，还必须是在双侧损伤的情况下。离断的输精管应立即用 2～3 针 8-0 单股可吸收线在放大镜的帮助下进行吻合。Sparkman[94]报道，经证实输精管损伤的发生率为 0.6%，他在 313 例行疝修补术的患儿中发现 5 例疝囊中存在输精管片断。但是这些病例的详细资料没有报道，也无法获得组织学和临床资料。Walker 和 Mills[104]发现约 6% 的青春期前的男孩疝囊里存在小腺体的包涵体，他们认为是苗勒管的残留物而非输精管片断。他们强调这些结构没有临床意义，Sparkman 报道中发现的可能是这种组织。也许

Steigman等[95]的估计更具有价值，他们综述了14.5年间7314例行疝修补术患者疝囊的组织学检查结果，发现17例（0.23%）有输精管组织，22例（0.3%）有附睾，30例（0.4%）有胚胎残余物，3例（0.04%）疝囊存在输精管和附睾。Partrick等[74]分析了1494例病例后发现输精管损伤的发生率为0.13%，并认为输精管损伤率如此之低，没有必要行常规的疝囊组织学检查。

Shangling和Janik等[91]证实输精管在疝囊修补术中很容易被损伤。他们在试验中使用手指、无齿镊、无创伤血管钳（bulldog vascular clamps）或蚊氏钳暴露和提抓大鼠的输精管。研究显示在手术后6个月，仍可在除手指操作外的所有操作中发现输精管存在损伤。Ceylan等[15]证实牵拉精索也可以造成输精管和睾丸的损伤，他们将不同力量的水平牵引力作用于大鼠精索，所有角度的牵拉都将明显导致输精管肌层变薄及睾丸的萎缩。

男性生育能力与疝修补术之间的关系还未得到证实，Homonnal等[46]报道了131例男性不育者曾在2~35岁之间进行腹股沟疝修补术，尽管其中14%的患者存在可能与疝修补术有关的睾丸萎缩或精子异常，但详细的临床资料，如嵌顿疝的发生率及手术医生的经验水平等没有被报道。Yavetz等[110]综述了有临床症状的8500例不育症患者，565例（6.65%）曾进行过腹股沟疝修补术，有或无睾丸萎缩。手术年龄与手术后精液质量之间无相关关系。

手术中输精管损伤可以导致输精管阻塞及睾丸淋巴液的精子抗原转向。血睾屏障的破坏引起抗原免疫反应，产生精子自身抗体。一篇综述报道了存在精子自身抗体的76例不育男性中，12例（16%）在儿童时期进行过单侧疝修补术[34]，其中10例行腹股沟区探
1186 查，有5例确认有输精管阻塞。作者认为在儿童疝修补术中误切或误扎输精管可能是男性不育症的原因之一。Parkhouse和Hendry等[73]报道了与此相似的发现。因此，尽管这些报道未指出腹股沟疝修补术后男性不育症的发生率，但他们认为两者之间是有关联的。

睾丸萎缩

睾丸血管在手术中易被损伤，尤其在小婴儿，但常规疝修补术后睾丸萎缩的报道很少。Fischer和Mumenthaler[32]以及Fahstrom等[30]各自报道睾丸萎缩的发生率为1%。在这些研究中，手术方式各异，嵌顿疝的数量也未报道，因此，它们并不能反映有经验的外科医生行单纯高位结扎术关闭疝囊时睾丸萎缩的真实发生率。

嵌顿疝有可能累及睾丸血供，腹股沟嵌顿疝睾丸血供损害的发生率约为2.6%~5%。嵌顿疝急诊手术中，大约11%~29%的患者可发现睾丸青紫。组织学检查确诊的睾丸萎缩或随访睾丸变小的实际发生率很低，约0~19%。但不幸的是，系列报道中的急诊手术的病例只是小部分患者，随访的时间长短及睾丸萎缩的诊断标准各异。Puri等[78]报道的87例非手术治疗的男性嵌顿疝患儿中发生单侧睾丸萎缩的为2例（2.3%）。根据这些数据，我们认为睾丸血管损伤很常见，但实际梗死的风险并不大，因此，除非睾丸明显梗死，不需要行睾丸切除术。

卵巢疝

卵巢、输卵管嵌顿或可能性更大的疝囊内卵巢扭转可能危及卵巢和输卵管血液供应。报道显示未复位的卵巢绞窄的发生率高达32%。Boley等[10]报道17例女性嵌顿疝中卵巢绞窄的发生率为27%。

肠管损伤

嵌顿疝中，肠管梗死的发生率很低。1960—1965年，Rowe和Clatworthy[83]报道了351例嵌顿疝中肠管切除率为1.4%。1978年以来发表的3篇系列报道中221例嵌顿疝患者没有一例行肠管切除。

腹腔容积损失

疝手术并发症中，尤其在早产儿，很少讨论腹腔容积（abdominal domain）损失而导致的术后呼吸衰竭。巨大腹股沟疝，特别是双侧疝，肠管主要在疝囊内、腹腔以外。如果这种状态持续时间过长，肠管则丢失了它的腹腔领域。行疝修补术时，肠管复位至腹腔易导致腹腔内压力过高和呼吸衰竭。Bascombe

等[5]报道 1 例患双侧巨大腹股沟疝的重度早产儿在疝修补术后需要机械通气辅助呼吸 41 天。

疝修补术后的呼吸衰竭比较常见。Gollin 等[39]发现 34% 的早产儿在疝修补术后需要机械通气辅助呼吸。由于腹腔容积丢失引起腹腔内压力增加，可能是尚未认识到的原因之一。我们的经验是对双侧巨大疝在选定的时间行分期手术，在现代技术的支持下，再次麻醉（机械通气辅助呼吸插管时需要）的风险很低。在急诊手术情况下，例如修补巨大嵌顿疝，可使用 silo 袋修补缺损的腹壁，以减少腹腔内压力，使得肠管缓慢复位至腹腔。

死亡率

腹股沟疝的死亡率与疝并发症或合并的危险因素如早产或心脏病等有关。1938 年，Thorndike 和 Ferguson[101]报道的 1927—1936 年的嵌顿疝死亡率大致为 2.8%。1954 年 Clatworthy 和 Thompson[21]报道的 135 例嵌顿疝患儿有 1 例死亡（0.7%）。1970 年，同一家医疗机构报道的 351 例嵌顿疝患儿中无死亡病例。从那时起，嵌顿疝的死亡率变得极低。但绞窄性疝的死亡率较高。1989 年，英国报道的因绞窄性疝而死亡的患儿有 5 例。危险因素包括：年龄小于 6 个月、手术医生和麻醉师缺少相关的儿科经验。

早产儿的手术死亡率现在很低，在最近的 2 篇早产儿行疝修补术的报道中，303 例患儿中无死亡病例[54,69]。

腹腔镜手术的并发症

腹腔镜手术最近被应用于儿童腹股沟疝的治疗，
1187 还未取得长期的研究结论，但有短期并发症的报道。Schier 等[90]联合发表了他们对 666 例患儿行 933 例腹腔镜疝修补术及随访 2 个月~7 年的经验，复发率为 3.4%。但作者没有按年龄或性别分析发生率的情况。他们也报道了 4 例术后鞘膜积液和 1 例男性患儿“睾丸位置和大小轻微改变”。Schier[89]个人报道了 279 例患儿实行了 403 例腹腔镜疝修补术，经过平均 23 月的随访，复发率为 2.7%。

如前文所述，对男性患者，因为复发率较高，我们不常规采用腹腔镜疝修补术。对女性患者行稍加变化的腹腔镜疝修补术。迄今为止，我们没有复发的病例，但手术的例数很少，随访也有限。

到目前为止，尚无腹腔镜手术致输精管损伤及睾丸萎缩的病例报道。支持者认为因为腹腔镜下输精管和精索容易被识别并避免被损伤，该技术可以更好地避免医源性损伤及使术后不育降到最低。因为病例数很少且随访时间有限，大部分开腹手术中的输精管损伤要到出现生育问题时才被认识到，故此结论尚待进一步观察。因此，我们推荐男性患儿的腹腔镜修补手术应限于特殊情况下使用，如最初经腹股沟区行腹股沟疝修补术的复发病例，或是因其他原因进行腹腔镜检查时偶然发现腹股沟斜疝的病例。

特殊病例

早产儿

已证实早产儿腹股沟疝的发生率更高，并更容易出现双侧疝。婴儿的未成熟度越大，越容易发生腹股沟疝。Walsh[105]的一篇 82 例体重低于 2000 g 的婴儿病例综述中，腹股沟疝的发生率为 13%；与 54 例体重大于 1500 g 的患儿中有 4 例（7%）发生腹股沟疝相比，28 例体重低于 1500 g 的患儿，7 例（25%）发生腹股沟疝。Rescorla 和 Grosfled[80]综述了 100 例小于 2 个月的需行腹股沟疝修补术的患儿，30% 为早产儿，44% 有双侧疝。Rajput 等[79]报道的 1391 例极低体重儿（体重小于 1500 g）中，222 例（16%）在 28 天龄~20 月龄（矫正后的）出现腹股沟疝。Peevy 等[15]研究了 397 例新生儿，发现体重 1000~1500 g 的婴儿腹股沟疝发生率为 9%，而体重 500~1000 g 的婴儿发生率为 30%。在 Harper 等[42]的一个小规模的病例报道中，体重低于 1000 g 的 37 例早产儿中，11 例（30%）发生腹股沟疝，其中 2 例（18%）发生嵌顿疝。尽管婴幼儿嵌顿疝的发生率高达 28%，但据报道，早产儿其发生率较低，为 13%~18%。

脑室腹腔分流术和腹膜透析

腹股沟疝的一个重要病因是腹腔内液体过多和压

力过大。在鞘状突未闭的患儿，将液体引导至腹腔可以导致疝或鞘膜积液的发生。疝的发生是液体的物理压力增高还是继发于腹腔压力增高尚不明确。神经肌肉功能异常可能也是原因之一。Moazam 等[70]综述了134 例行脑室腹腔分流术的病例，19.5% 的脑脊髓脊膜膨出患者和 47% 的脑室内出血患者出现疝，但后者全是早产儿。Grosfeld 等[41]报道，14% 的脑室腹腔分流术后患者出现腹股沟疝，其中 20% 发生嵌顿疝，复发疝为 16%。基于这些研究，作者推荐：（1）脑室腹腔分流术后的患儿应密切观察腹股沟疝的发生；（2）由于嵌顿疝发生率较高，疝明确诊断后应尽早手术；（3）单侧疝手术时应进行对侧腹股沟区探查。Clarnette 等[20]评价了 430 例行脑室腹腔分流术的患儿，15% 出现腹股沟疝，另外 6% 的男孩出现鞘膜积液，47% 的男孩及 27% 的女孩为双侧疝。腹股沟疝的发生率与患儿进行分流术的年龄密切相关。在出生后数月内行分流术的患儿，疝发生率为 30%，1 岁后行分流术的疝发生率下降为 10%。作者认为腹腔内压力增加可能与疝的发生有关。此外，他们发现出生数月内鞘状突未闭的发生率为 30%，并由此认为鞘状突有可能在出生 1 年内自行关闭。

已证实长期行腹膜透析的患者有发生腹股沟疝的危险，发生率为 7%～15%。在这些病例中，鞘状突未闭可以发展为直疝。建议在放置腹膜透析管时行疝囊造影术，通过导管注入水溶性造影剂，并让患者保持头高位 15 分钟。如果明确存在鞘状突未闭，应行修补术。此外，也可以在放置导管时通过腹腔镜直视下观察内环口情况，尤其在后者需要行腹腔镜手术时。可以采用开放式或腹腔镜途径行疝修补术。

滑疝

在女孩，输卵管或输卵管系膜常可以成为疝囊壁的一部分，并易被损伤。手术治疗前文已经探讨过。

1188 阑尾也可以成为滑疝的疝囊壁的一部分。如果条件允许，应按常规行疝囊高位结扎。对女孩滑疝也可以采用不同的方式，可结扎阑尾远端的疝囊，近端疝囊连同阑尾一起复位至腹腔，行或不行荷包关闭。婴儿的膀胱位于内环口下方中线处，可能在分离时与疝囊一起被下拖，如果辨认不清，高位结扎疝囊时可能会将膀胱壁结扎进去而引起血尿或膀胱壁坏死和尿外渗。在穿刺时仔细检查疝囊颈可避免该情况。当对此有疑问时，应打开疝囊壁并检查内容物。偶尔，膀胱可以延伸至疝囊内侧壁上，成为真性滑疝。Shaw 和 Santulli[92]推荐像 Goldstein－Potts 的女性疝修补术一样，行折叠手术。但我们只将膀胱由远端疝囊分离并结扎，翻转残端，并缩小内环口（Bevan 修补术）[7]。

直疝

直疝曾一度被认为在儿童中很少见，但随着腹腔镜手术的推广，发现直疝比以前认为的要多。过去，直疝常在腹股沟斜疝修补术后复发时发现，或许是因为在初次疝修补术时误诊或损伤了腹股沟管壁。Wright[108]在1600 多例腹股沟疝手术中，仅发现 19 例（1.2%）为直疝。然而，Gorsler 和 Schier[40]发现 403 例腹股沟疝中直疝的发生率为 3.9%。如果在斜疝手术中没有发现典型疝囊并且筋膜缺损位于腹壁下血管中下部，该诊断是有疑问的。治疗采用腹横筋膜修补术，例如 Bassini 修补术或 Cooper 韧带修补术。

股疝

股疝在儿童中也很少见，常在临床检查或行腹股沟斜疝修补术时误诊。Fonkalsrud[33]与 Burke[13]分别回顾了 5452 例与 5141 例共计 10593 例腹股沟疝患儿，年龄在 6 周～13 岁之间，21 例（0.2%）为股疝。男女比例为 1∶2。21 例患者中，术前诊断正确的为 8 例（38%），4 例为双侧股疝，5 例发生股疝嵌顿。

De Caluwe 等[27]描述了 20 年间的 38 例股疝，4 例为双侧股疝，术前的正确诊断率为 53%。18 例误诊的患儿中，7 例必须再次手术。当手术中遇到的情况（如未发现明显的斜疝）与术前诊断不一致时，应考虑到直疝或股疝的可能。这种情况下，在儿童腹腔镜应用以前，常打开腹股沟管后壁进行腹股沟管探查。但随着腹腔镜设备的广泛应用，Lee 和 DuBois[59]主张将诊断性腹腔镜检查作为疝修补术的辅助手段，尤其在复发病例中。他们对 4 例可疑斜疝复发的病例在第 2 次手术中应用了诊断性腹腔镜检查，3 例为股疝，也同时存在对侧股疝。

Wright[109]报道了 16 位股疝患者，并主张经股管

（infrainguinal，腹股沟下）途径，缝合腹股沟韧带与耻骨梳韧带和耻骨筋膜。Ceran 等[14]像 Lee 和 DuBois 一样，用网塞成功地治疗了 4 例股疝患儿[59]。对同侧股疝患者，我们在首次探查时选择标准的 Cooper 韧带修补术，并发现如前所述，网塞是有效的治疗方式。

遗传性结缔组织疾病

Hunter-Hurler 综合征（黏多糖增多症）、Ehlers-Danlos 综合征（皮肤过度干燥综合征）和 Marfan 综合征患者常发生腹股沟疝，并容易复发，除非在常规疝囊高位结扎同时行腹股沟管后壁修补术。Coran 和 Eraklis[24]发现 50 例 Hunter-Hurler 综合征患者中 36% 发生腹股沟疝。单纯疝囊高位结扎的复发率为 56%，所以推荐使用正规的疝修补术。在青少年患者，我们建议采用疝囊高位结扎并行无张力网塞疝修补术。

囊性纤维病

囊性纤维病患者的腹股沟疝发生率为 6%～15%[45]。基于输精管切除术的研究结果，该病的输精管缺失发生率为 0.5%～1%[65,112]。这些囊性纤维病患者的输精管异常类型各异，可以从阻塞到完全缺失，并经常是双侧的。所以输精管缺失患者应考虑到有囊性纤维病的可能。在非囊性纤维病的患儿，输精管发育不全与肾发育不良有一定联系，在这种情况下建议进行上尿路评估。

两性畸形

在女性表现型患者的大阴唇中触摸到男性生殖腺很少见，可能是基因型为男性的雄激素不敏感综合征
1189 或真两性畸形。如果在此类女性患者疝囊内发现卵巢，应仔细检查有无睾丸组织的迹象（卵睾体）。雄激素不敏感综合征的男性没有输卵管和子宫，但有小睾丸。两性体可以在疝囊内发现输卵管，但生殖腺的检查为不对称的卵睾体。在这两种情况中，如果存在畸形的生殖腺，不应该将其切除。生殖腺的每极均行部分楔形切除，并行生殖腺移位和疝修补。这种情况将在第 121 章和 122 章中进一步讨论。

脾生殖腺融合

脾组织可以和正常的睾丸组织融合生长（脾睾融合）。表现为阴囊内包块，并通常在手术前被诊断为睾丸肿瘤。不需要行睾丸切除，术中冰冻可以确诊，并允许保留睾丸。脾-卵巢融合也可以发生。另外，脾生殖腺融合可以表现为隐睾或腹腔内肿块。这种情况下，腹腔镜技术可以作为诊断和治疗的手段。

肾上腺残留

表现为小的浅黄色组织团块的异位肾上腺出现在疝囊顶部并不少见。385 例腹股沟疝手术中有 10 例（2.6%），均为偶尔发现[66]。在另一组调查中，1077 例疝囊中发现肾上腺残留的比率为 0.2%[74]。肾上腺组织出现在这个部位可能与胚胎发育中睾丸由后腹膜腔下降至阴囊内时，肾上腺组织附着在睾丸组织上有关。

先天性睾丸鞘膜积液

鞘膜积液是液体积聚在睾丸周围，位于两层睾丸鞘膜之间。鞘膜积液可以与腹腔交通（鞘状突未闭，液体自由流动），也可以不交通（通常位于男性阴囊内，腹股沟较薄弱）。鞘膜积液在婴儿和儿童中很常见，在许多病例中与斜疝有一定关联。鞘膜积液常常是双侧的，右侧的发生率较高。它们可以大小各异，并因重力作用，在白天患儿直立时增大，晚上患儿平卧时缩小。鞘膜积液偶尔可以由腹股沟管延伸至后腹膜，形成腹腔阴囊鞘膜积液，容易同斜疝发生混淆。患儿在阴囊上端或腹股沟区可以出现一个圆形、有张力的无痛性包块，这是精索鞘膜积液。每天包块大小发生改变的是交通性鞘膜积液。急性鞘膜积液可以继发于睾丸鞘膜内的急性病程或者在睾丸或其附件扭转时出现，常伴随疼痛和触痛。此外，急性鞘膜积液也可以在上呼吸道感染或腹泻同时或以后出现，这时咳

嗽或腹压增高压迫液体流入尚未发现的未闭合的鞘状突内。

通常，体格检查可以鉴别鞘膜积液与腹股沟疝。典型的表现是阴囊内无张力的囊性肿块包绕睾丸和透光试验阳性。单纯的透光试验并不能完全确诊鞘膜积液，因为嵌顿疝时充满气体的肠管也可以表现为透光试验阳性。因此，不要行穿刺抽吸以明确诊断。通常，在鞘膜积液上方可以触摸到细细的精索，但在较大的鞘膜积液或腹腔阴囊鞘膜积液中精索常较难触摸清楚。

在大多数先天性鞘膜积液的儿童，鞘状突在积液后方关闭（非交通性），积液在 2 岁以前可被吸收。因此，除非积液是交通性的或不能排除腹股沟疝，一般不建议在 2 岁内行手术治疗。大而张力较高的、引起不适感的鞘膜积液不在此列。2 岁以上或较大儿童出现的鞘膜积液应该行手术治疗。同成人鞘膜积液手术一样，手术步骤包括高位结扎鞘状突，打开远端鞘膜囊并放液，保留打开的鞘膜囊并引流，边缘不需要缝合。液体在囊膜内重新积聚很少发生，一般可以自行吸收。

（杜 勇译 周小渔校）

参考文献

1. Backhouse K: The gubernaculum testis Hunteri: Testicular descent and maldescent. Ann R Coll Surg Engl 1964; 35:15.
2. Backhouse K, Butler H: The gubernaculum testis of the pig. J Anat 1960;94:208.
3. Bakwin H: Indirect inguinal hernia in twins. J Pediatr Surg 1971;6:165-168.
4. Ballantyne A, Jawaheer G, Munro FD: Contralateral groin exploration is not justified in infants with a unilateral inguinal hernia. Br J Surg 2001;88:720-723.
5. Bascombe D, Caty M, Glick PL: Surgical Rounds 2004; 31:520-522.
6. Bergin WC, Gier HT, Marion GB, Coffman J R: A developmental concept of equine cryptorchism. Biol Reprod 1970;3:82-92.
7. Bevan A: Sliding hernias of the ascending colon and caecum, the descending colon, sigmoid, and the bladder. Ann Surg 1930;92:754.
8. Bhatia AM, Gow KW, Heiss KF, et al: Is the use of laparoscopy to determine presence of contralateral patent processus vaginalis justified in children greater than 2 years of age? J Pediatr Surg 2004;39:778-781.
9. Bock JE, Sobye JV: Frequency of contralateral inguinal hernia in children: A study of the indications for bilateral herniotomy in children with unilateral hernia. Acta Chir Scand 1970;136:707-709.
10. Boley SJ, Cahn D, Lauer T, et al: The irreducible ovary: A true emergency. J Pediatr Surg 1991;26:1035-1038.
11. Boocock GR, Todd PJ: Inguinal hernias are common in preterm infants. Arch Dis Child 1985;60:669-670.
12. Bronsther B, Abrams MW, Elboim C: Inguinal hernias in children—a study of 1000 cases and a review of the literature. J Am Med Womens Assoc 1972;27:522-525.
13. Burke J: Femoral hernia in childhood. Ann Surg 1967; 166:287-289.
14. Ceran C, Koyluoglu G, Sonmez K: Femoral hernia repair with mesh-plug in children. J Pediatr Surg 2002;37: 1456-1458.
15. Ceylan H, Karakok M, Guldur E, et al: Temporary stretch of the testicular pedicle may damage the vas deferens and the testis. J Pediatr Surg 2003;38:1530-1533.
16. Cheatle G: An operation for inguinal hernia. BMJ 1921; 2:1025.
17. Chen KC, Chu CC, Chou TY, Wu CJ: Ultrasonography for inguinal hernias in boys. J Pediatr Surg 1998;33:1784-1787.
18. Chertin B, De Caluwe D, Gajaharan M, et al: Is contralateral exploration necessary in girls with unilateral inguinal hernia? J Pediatr Surg 2003;38:756-757.
19. Clarnette TD, Hutson JM: The genitofemoral nerve may link testicular inguinoscrotal descent with congenital inguinal hernia. Aust N Z J Surg 1996;66:612-617.
20. Clarnette TD, Lam SK, Hutson JM: Ventriculo-peritoneal shunts in children reveal the natural history of closure of the processus vaginalis. J Pediatr Surg 1998;33:413-416.
21. Clatworthy HW, Thompson A: Incarcerated and strangulated inguinal hernia in infants: A preventable risk. JAMA 1954;154:123.
22. Clausen EG, Jake RJ, Binkley FM: Contralateral inguinal exploration of unilateral hernia in infants and children. Surgery 1958;44:735-740.
23. Conroy JM, Othersen HB Jr, Dorman BH, et al: A comparison of wound instillation and caudal block for analgesia following pediatric inguinal herniorrhaphy. J Pediatr Surg 1993;28:565-567.
24. Coran AG, Eraklis AJ: Inguinal hernia in the Hurler-Hunter syndrome. Surgery 1967;61:302-304.
25. Cote CJ, Zaslavsky A, Downes JJ, et al: Postoperative apnea in former preterm infants after inguinal herniorrhaphy: A combined analysis. Anesthesiology 1995;82:809-822.
26. Craven PD, Badawi N, Henderson-Smart DJ, O'Brien M: Regional (spinal, epidural, caudal) versus general anaesthesia in preterm infants undergoing inguinal herniorrhaphy in early infancy. Cochrane Database Syst Rev 2003;CD003669.
27. De Caluwe D, Chertin B, Puri P: Childhood femoral hernia: A commonly misdiagnosed condition. Pediatr Surg Int 2003; 19:608-609.
28. El-Gohary MA: Laparoscopic management of persistent mullerian duct syndrome. Pediatr Surg Int 2003;19: 533-536.
29. Erez I, Rathause V, Vacian I, et al: Preoperative ultrasound and intraoperative findings of inguinal hernias in children: A prospective study of 642 children. J Pediatr Surg 2002; 37:865-868.
30. Fahstrom C, Holmberg L, Johannson H: Atrophy of the testis following operations upon the inguinal region of

infants and children. Acta Chir Scand 1963;126:221.
31. Ferguson A: Oblique inguinal hernia: Typical operation for its radical cure. JAMA 1899;33:6.
32. Fischer V, Mumenthaler A: 1st bilaterale herniotomie bei sauglingen unde kleinkindern unit einseitiger Lesitenhernie angezeigt? Helv Chir Acta 1957;4:436.
33. Fonkalsrud E, deLorimier A, Clatworthy HW: Femoral and direct inguinal hernias in infants and children. JAMA 1965; 192:597.
34. Friberg J, Fritjofsson A: Inguinal herniorrhaphy and sperm-agglutinating antibodies in infertile men. Arch Androl 1979;2:317-322.
35. Gardner TA, Ostad M, Mininberg DT: Diagnostic flexible peritoneoscopy: Assessment of the contralateral internal inguinal ring during unilateral herniorrhaphy. J Pediatr Surg 1998;33:1486-1489.
36. Geisler DP, Jegathesan S, Parmley MC, et al: Laparoscopic exploration for the clinically undetected hernia in infancy and childhood. Am J Surg 2001;182:693-696.
37. Given JP, Rubin SZ: Occurrence of contralateral inguinal hernia following unilateral repair in a pediatric hospital. J Pediatr Surg 1989;24:963-965.
38. Glick PL, Azizkhan RG: A Genealogy of North American Pediatric Surgery: From Ladd until Now. St Louis, Quality Medical Publishing, 1997.
39. Gollin G, Bell C, Dubose R, et al: Predictors of postoperative respiratory complications in premature infants after inguinal herniorrhaphy. J Pediatr Surg 1993;28: 244-247.
40. Gorsler CM, Schier F: Laparoscopic herniorrhaphy in children. Surg Endosc 2003;17:571-573.
41. Grosfeld JL, Cooney DR, Smith J, Campbell RL: Intra-abdominal complications following ventriculoperitoneal shunt procedures. Pediatrics 1974;54:791-796.
42. Harper RG, Garcia A, Sia C: Inguinal hernia: A common problem of premature infants weighing 1000 grams or less at birth. Pediatrics 1975;56:112-115.
43. Harvey MH, Johnstone MJ, Fossard DP: Inguinal herniotomy in children: A five year survey. Br J Surg 1985; 72:485-487.
44. Hecker WC, Ring-Mrozik E: [Results of follow-up of operations in pediatric patients with indirect inguinal hernia]. Langenbecks Arch Chir 1987;371:115-121.
45. Holsclaw DS, Shwachman H: Increased incidence of inguinal hernia, hydrocele, and undescended testicle in males with cystic fibrosis. Pediatrics 1971;48:442-445.
46. Homonnai ZT, Fainman N, Paz GF, David MP: Testicular function after herniotomy: Herniotomy and fertility. Andrologia 1980;12:115-120.
47. Jewett TC Jr, Kuhn IN, Allen JE: Herniography in children. J Pediatr Surg 1976;11:451-454.
48. Kamaledeen SA, Shanbhogue LK: Preperitoneal approach for incarcerated inguinal hernia in children. J Pediatr Surg 1997;32:1715-1716.
49. Kapur P, Caty M, Glick P: Pediatric hernias and hydroceles. In Glick P, Irish M, Caty M (eds): The Pediatric Clinics of North America. Philadelphia, WB Saunders, 1998, pp 773-789.
50. Kemmotsu H, Oshima Y, Joe K, Mouri T: The features of contralateral manifestations after the repair of unilateral inguinal hernia. J Pediatr Surg 1998;33:1099-1102.
51. Kiesewetter WB, Oh KS: Unilateral inguinal hernias in children: What about the opposite side? Arch Surg 1980;115:1443-1445.
52. Kiesewetter WB, Parenzan L: When should hernia in the infant be treated bilaterally? JAMA 1959;171:287.
53. Koga H, Yamataka A, Ohshiro K, et al: Pfannenstiel incision for incarcerated inguinal hernia in neonates. J Pediatr Surg 2003;38:E16-E18.
54. Krieger NR, Shochat SJ, McGowan V, Hartman GE: Early hernia repair in the premature infant: Long-term follow-up. J Pediatr Surg 1994;29:978-981.
55. La Roque G: The permanent cure for inguinal and femoral hernia. Surg Gynecol Obstet 1919;29:507.
56. Ladd WE, Gross RE: Abdominal Surgery of Infancy and Childhood. Philadelphia, WB Saunders, 1941.
57. Lau WY: History of treatment of groin hernia. World J Surg 2002;26:748-759.
58. Lavonius MI, Ovaska J: Laparoscopy in the evaluation of the incarcerated mass in groin hernia. Surg Endosc 2000; 14:488-489.
59. Lee SL, DuBois JJ: Laparoscopic diagnosis and repair of pediatric femoral hernia: Initial experience of four cases. Surg Endosc 2000;14:1110-1113.
60. Lee Y, Liang J: Experience with 450 cases of micro-laparoscopic herniotomy in infants and children. Pediatr Endosurg Innov Techn 2002;6:25-28.
61. Levitt MA, Ferraraccio D, Arbesman MC, et al: Variability of inguinal hernia surgical technique: A survey of North American pediatric surgeons. J Pediatr Surg 2002;37: 745-751.
62. Liu L, Cote C, Goudsouzian N, et al: Life threatening apnea in infants recovering from anesthesia. Anesthesiology 1983;56:510.
63. Malviya S, Swartz J, Lerman J: Are all preterm infants younger than 60 weeks postconceptual age at risk for post-operative apnea? Anesthesiology 1993;78:1076.
64. McGregor DB, Halverson K, McVay CB: The unilateral pediatric inguinal hernia: Should the contralateral side be explored? J Pediatr Surg 1980;15:313-317.
65. Michelson L: Congenital anomalies of the vas deferens and epididymis. J Urol 1989;61:384.
66. Michowitz M, Schujman E, Solowiejczyk M: Aberrant adrenal tissue in the wall of a hernial sac. Am Surg 1979;45:67-69.
67. Miltenburg DM, Nuchtern JG, Jaksic T, et al: Meta-analysis of the risk of metachronous hernia in infants and children. Am J Surg 1997;174:741-744.
68. Miserez M: Inguinal hernia repair in a premature infant. J Pediatr Surg 2004;39:252.
69. Misra D, Hewitt G, Potts SR, et al: Inguinal herniotomy in young infants, with emphasis on premature neonates. J Pediatr Surg 1994;29:1496-1498.
70. Moazam F, Glenn JD, Kaplan BJ, et al: Inguinal hernias after ventriculoperitoneal shunt procedures in pediatric patients. Surg Gynecol Obstet 1984;159:570-572.
71. Montupet P, Esposito C: Laparoscopic treatment of congenital inguinal hernia in children. J Pediatr Surg 1999; 34:420-423.
72. Moss RL, Hatch EI Jr: Inguinal hernia repair in early infancy. Am J Surg 1991;161:596-599.
73. Parkhouse H, Hendry W: Vasal injuries during childhood and their effect on subsequent fertility. Br J Urol 1991; 67:91.
74. Partrick DA, Bensard DD, Karrer FM, Ruyle SZ: Is routine pathological evaluation of pediatric hernia sacs justified? J Pediatr Surg 1998;33:1090-1092.
75. Peevy KJ, Speed FA, Hoff CJ: Epidemiology of inguinal

hernia in preterm neonates. Pediatrics 1986;77:246-247.
76. Pellegrin K, Bensard DD, Karrer FM, Meagher DP Jr: Laparoscopic evaluation of contralateral patent processus vaginalis in children. Am J Surg 1996;172:602-605.
77. Prasad R, Lovvorn HN 3rd, Wadie GM, Lobe TE: Early experience with needleoscopic inguinal herniorrhaphy in children. J Pediatr Surg 2003;38:1055-1058.
78. Puri P, Guiney EJ, O'Donnell B: Inguinal hernia in infants: The fate of the testis following incarceration. J Pediatr Surg 1984;19:44-46.
79. Rajput A, Gauderer MW, Hack M: Inguinal hernias in very low birth weight infants: Incidence and timing of repair. J Pediatr Surg 1992;27:1322-1324.
80. Rescorla FJ, Grosfeld JL: Inguinal hernia repair in the perinatal period and early infancy: Clinical considerations. J Pediatr Surg 1984;19:832-837.
81. Rescorla FJ, West KW, Engum SA, et al: The "other side" of pediatric hernias: The role of laparoscopy. Am Surg 1997;63:690-693.
82. Rothenberg R, Barnett TM: Bilateral herniotomy in infants and children. Surgery 1955;37:949.
83. Rowe MI, Clatworthy HW: Incarcerated and strangulated hernias in children: A statistical study of high-risk factors. Arch Surg 1970;101:136-139.
84. Rowe MI, Clatworthy HW Jr: The other side of the pediatric inguinal hernia. Surg Clin North Am 1971;51:1371-1376.
85. Rowe MI, Copelson LW, Clatworthy HW: The patent processus vaginalis and the inguinal hernia. J Pediatr Surg 1969;4:102-107.
86. Rowe MI, Marchildon MB: Inguinal hernia and hydrocele in infants and children. Surg Clin North Am 1981;61:1137-1145.
87. Sachs M, Damm M, Encke A: Historical evolution of inguinal hernia repair. World J Surg 1997;21:218-223.
88. Schier F: Laparoscopic herniorrhaphy in girls. J Pediatr Surg 1998;33:1495-1497.
89. Schier F: Laparoscopic surgery of inguinal hernias in children—initial experience. J Pediatr Surg 2000;35:1331-1335.
90. Schier F, Montupet P, Esposito C: Laparoscopic inguinal herniorrhaphy in children: A three-center experience with 933 repairs. J Pediatr Surg 2002;37:395-397.
91. Shandling B, Janik J: The vulnerability of the vas deferens. J Pediatr Surg 1981;16:461.
92. Shaw A, Santulli TV: Management of sliding hernias of the urinary bladder in infants. Surg Gynecol Obstet 1967;124:1314-1316.
93. Snyder W Jr, Greaney E Jr: Inguinal hernia. In Benson C, Mustard W, Ravitch M, et al (eds): Pediatric Surgery. Chicago, Year Book Medical Publishers, 1962, pp 573-587.
94. Sparkman R: Bilateral exploration in inguinal hernia in juvenile patients. Surgery 1962;51:393.
95. Steigman CK, Sotelo-Avila C, Weber TR: The incidence of spermatic cord structures in inguinal hernia sacs from male children. Am J Surg Pathol 1999;23:880-885.
96. Steinau G, Schleef J, Lambertz M, Schumpelick V: [Incidence of contralateral inguinal hernias in infancy and childhood]. Langenbecks Arch Chir 1997;382:252-256.
97. Steinau G, Treutner KH, Feeken G, Schumpelick V: Recurrent inguinal hernias in infants and children. World J Surg 1995;19:303-306.
98. Stephens BJ, Rice WT, Koucky CJ, Gruenberg JC: Optimal timing of elective indirect inguinal hernia repair in healthy children: Clinical considerations for improved outcome. World J Surg 1992;16:952-956.
99. Strauch ED, Voigt RW, Hill JL: Gangrenous intestine in a hernia can be reduced. J Pediatr Surg 2002;37:919-920.
100. Tackett LD, Breuer CK, Luks FI, et al: Incidence of contralateral inguinal hernia: A prospective analysis. J Pediatr Surg 1999;34:684-687.
101. Thorndike AJ, Ferguson C: Incarcerated inguinal hernia in infancy and childhood. Am J Surg 1938;39:429.
102. Turnock RR, Jones MO, Lloyd DA: Preperitoneal approach to irreducible inguinal hernia in infants. Br J Surg 1994;81:251.
103. van Zeben-van der Aa TM, Verloove-Vanhorick SP: Inguinal hernias are common in preterm infants. Arch Dis Child 1986;61:99.
104. Walker AN, Mills SE: Glandular inclusions in inguinal hernial sacs and spermatic cords: Mullerian-like remnants confused with functional reproductive structures. Am J Clin Pathol 1984;82:85-89.
105. Walsh S: The incidence of external hernias in premature infants. Acta Paediatr 1962;51:161.
106. White JJ, Haller JA Jr, Dorst JP: Congenital inguinal hernia and inguinal herniography. Surg Clin North Am 1970;50:823-837.
107. Wiener ES, Touloukian RJ, Rodgers BM, et al: Hernia survey of the Section on Surgery of the American Academy of Pediatrics. J Pediatr Surg 1996;31:1166-1169.
108. Wright J: Direct inguinal hernia in infancy and childhood. Pediatr Surg Int 1994;9:161.
109. Wright JE: Femoral hernia in childhood. Pediatr Surg Int 1994;9:167.
110. Yavetz H, Harash B, Yogev L, et al: Fertility of men following inguinal hernia repair. Andrologia 1991;23:443-446.
111. Yerkes EB, Brock JW 3rd, Holcomb GW 3rd, Morgan WM 3rd: Laparoscopic evaluation for a contralateral patent processus vaginalis: Part III. Urology 1998;51:480-483.
112. Young D: Bilateral aplasia of the vas deferens. Br J Surg 1949;36:417.
113. Zallen, Glick PL: Laparoscopic inversion ligation hernia repair. J Laparoendosc Adv Surg Tech. Submitted for publication.

第 75 章

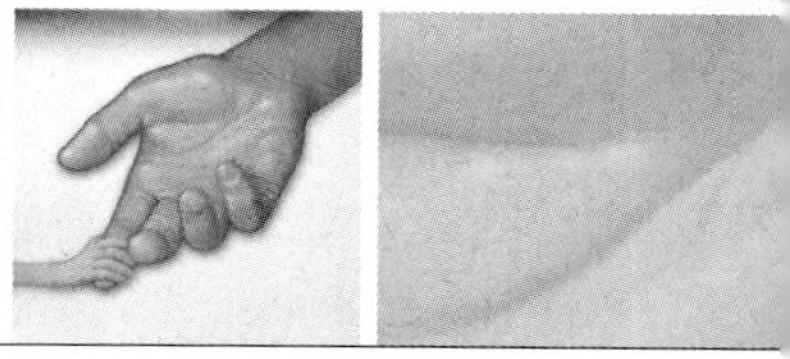

隐睾、睾丸扭转和精索静脉曲张

John M. Hutson

隐睾

历史回顾

1193 从古代起睾丸下降的重要意义就已被人们熟知，但造成其下降的真正机制却一直未能阐明。直到1786年，Hunter在对胎儿解剖时发现腹腔内的睾丸通过韧带连接到腹股沟腹壁上。这条韧带看似引导睾丸下降到阴囊，所以被命名为睾丸引带[79]。

胚胎学

在哺乳动物中，睾丸下降到温度较低的阴囊内是一个复杂的分期过程[190]。人类的性别分化开始于胎龄7～8周，起初胎儿睾丸和卵巢处于相同的位置。随着性别的分化，性腺位置发生不同的变化，睾丸逐渐靠近以后形成的腹股沟管，而卵巢逐渐向远离腹股沟的位置迁移。性腺同时被头端悬韧带（上极）和睾丸引带（下极）支持固定。

位于性腺头端的悬韧带在女孩体内持续存在，在男孩体内却随着睾丸引带的发育而退化，退化最明显的部位位于引带远端埋入腹股沟腹壁的部分。围绕于睾丸引带周围的间叶细胞浓缩形成腹股沟肌肉组织，进而再形成腹股沟管结构。睾丸引带的间叶细胞持续存在形成实质条索状结构，然后再被来自腹膜的憩室空化，形成鞘状突结构[5]。起初与性腺连接的近端睾丸引带随附睾尾的生长而膨大生长。鞘状突向睾丸引带的间质生长，使部分睾丸引带空化。睾丸引带的尾端保持实质结构，但近端分化成两部分，其中间的柱形结构与附睾连接，环状的壁层结构逐渐演化形成提睾肌。在妊娠晚期开始的时候，睾丸引带的尾端突出超过腹股沟腹壁（图75-1），同时经过耻骨水平向阴囊迁移[70]。鞘状突在睾丸引带内侧成比例延长，以保证离开腹腔的睾丸可以进入鞘状突并随之下降（见图75-1）。睾丸及其引带向阴囊迁移的过程在胚胎35周前完成[70,71]。迁移过程中，睾丸引带在腹股沟阴囊的间质中逐渐松解，提示其周围组织被酶解消化。迁移结束以后，鞘状突继发性地附着到阴囊底（见图75-1）。

睾丸下降的不同时期由激素调节[183]。激素控制睾丸下降，但对激素的作用机制尚存在争议[71]。睾丸从腹腔下降的早期过程与其在腹股沟阴囊内的迁移过程不同，各自受到不同的激素调控[80,88]。雄激素控制睾丸头端悬韧带的退化，但韧带的退化并不是睾丸下降所必需的[109]。睾丸引带的膨胀主要受到非雄激素调控，最近的研究发现该调控因子是类胰岛素因子-3（lnsulin-like factor 3，Insl3）[128]。

Insl3由两条被双硫键连接的肽链构成，与松弛素同源，目前公认其属于胰岛素家族，是众多生长因子中的一员[128]。研究发现，突变型Insl3敲除小鼠存在腹腔型隐睾和睾丸引带异常，该研究结果与Insl3能刺激睾丸引带发生“肿胀反应”和介导睾丸经腹腔下降的观点一致[42,105]。许多活体和离体的实验也证实，Insl3的主要作用之一是刺激睾丸引带的早期生长发育，除此以外，该因子还能继发性地刺激机体产生睾酮和苗勒氏管抑制因子[42,105]。

睾丸及其引带从腹股沟迁移至阴囊的过程由雄激素控制。在完全雄激素抵抗或垂体促性腺激素缺乏的情况下，这一迁移过程将缺失[59]。雄激素控制睾丸引带迁移的机制尚不清楚，但有部分证据认为其与生殖股神经的作用有关。有人提出，生殖股神经的感觉支能释放降钙素相关基因肽（CGRP），后者刺激睾

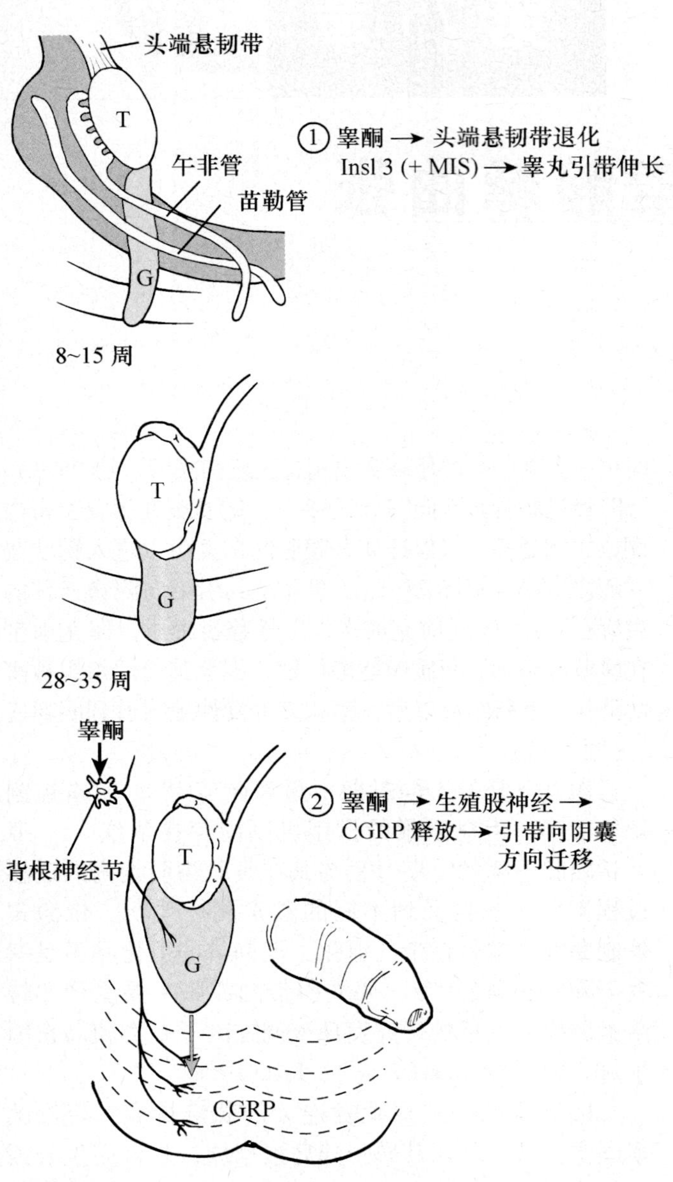

图 75-1　睾丸引带发育模式图。人类胚胎发育过程中，睾丸下降经过两个阶段。怀孕 8～15 周时，睾丸（T）下降处于第一（腹腔）阶段，睾丸引带（G）随胚胎发育而增大，睾丸逐渐靠近腹股沟内环。与卵巢比较，睾丸位置的相对变化受睾丸激素控制。Insl3 在 MIS/AMH 的作用下，参与睾丸发育。在睾酮的刺激下，睾丸头端引带退化。怀孕 28～35 周，睾丸下降处于第二（腹股沟阴囊）阶段，睾丸引带伸长向阴囊方向迁移。在睾酮的作用下，背根神经节处的生殖股神经分化为感觉纤维，释放降钙素基因相关蛋白（CGRP）。这一过程受 CGRP 调控。动物实验证明，CGRP 调控大鼠睾丸引带的生长和迁移方向。由此提出的假说认为人类睾丸的迁移机制与此相同。AMH，抗苗勒管激素；CSL，头端悬韧带；MIS，苗勒氏管抑制物质；GFN，生殖股神经。

丸引带发育，从而间接控制引带迁移，但这一观点尚未被完全证实[81]。腹腔内的压力通过开放的鞘状突传递，为睾丸下降提供了机械性动力。最近的研究还表明，睾丸引带壁上的提睾肌发育和交感神经刺激也为睾丸下降提供了协同作用[172]。 1194

任何抑制睾丸下降的因素都将造成临床上隐睾疾病的发生[84]。复杂的睾丸下降机制说明，隐睾的发生原因错综复杂。在绝大多数隐睾患者中，睾丸的位置多位于腹股沟管以外，或许提示腹股沟阴囊阶段的睾丸下降异常更为普遍。相反，在睾丸下降的腹腔阶段，睾丸引带的被动定位过程很少被干扰，所以相对而言，腹腔型隐睾的发病率很低，临床上只占到所有隐睾患者的 5%～10%[151]。大多数隐睾患者的睾丸位于腹股沟浅窝靠近阴囊入口处，正好位于腹股沟外环的外侧，或略偏于腹股沟外环外侧。睾丸引带迁移的异常可能与下降机制障碍或生殖股神经功能的丧失有关[31,88]。胚胎发育过程中，脑垂体与胎盘促性腺激素分泌不足使妊娠中晚期的雄激素分泌不足，这可能是造成与睾丸迁移有关的神经发育缺陷的原因。医学界目前认识到的内分泌功能紊乱同样会造成睾丸下降不全，其中包括苗勒管抑制因子不足、睾酮分泌低下以及激素受体功能不良，但这些原因相对次要。随着对 Insl3 基因及其功能的研究进展，一些学者试图证实 Insl3 基因突变是造成腹腔型隐睾的病因，但迄今为止只有极少量的研究结果被报道[7,51,176]。

下降不全的睾丸位于正常路径以外的位置较罕见，诸如会阴或大腿等部位，且发生的原因尚不完全清楚。Hutson 和他的助手[88]认为，这可能是因为异位的生殖股神经造成睾丸引带迁移异常所造成的。睾丸横向异位的原因同样未知，但在动物实验中，如果切除了附着在睾丸上的睾丸引带，使得睾丸不需要通过同侧腹股沟管离开腹腔，所以能够轻易诱导出睾丸横向异位的模型。性腺活动度的增大有时也能继发睾丸下降至对侧腹股沟管[87]。后一情况同样出现于患有永久性苗勒管综合征的儿童，由于这些患儿的睾丸引带异常增长，常造成睾丸意外迁移至对侧腹股沟管。

一些遗传综合征与隐睾发生有关。尽管这些患者常有小头畸形，提示其可能存在垂体激素或促性腺激素的不足，但其潜在原因尚不明确[63]。一些复杂的畸形综合征常与神经源性或器质性畸形相关，如先天性多关节挛缩症[45]。这些畸形引起胚胎受到外力挤压或内在的神经异常，可能导致隐睾的发生。实验证

1195 明，睾丸下降过程中压迫腹股沟阴囊可能造成隐睾[113]。腹腔型隐睾是梅干腹综合征的典型特征。造成隐睾的原因颇多且有争议，如中胚层缺损或产前暂时性尿路梗阻[9,122,132,138]、腹股沟管内鞘状突的缺如，以及睾丸位于膀胱后位的情况往往和梗阻有关。后尿道瓣膜的婴儿中 10% 存在隐睾[102]。

隐睾发生于腹壁缺损的婴儿中的现象很普遍，如腹裂（患者睾丸引带在此处发生断裂）、脐疝（脐膨出）和膀胱外翻[96]。其中隐睾在腹裂患者中的伴发比率超过 15%，在脐疝和脐膨出患者中至少有 1/3[63,69]。这是否与腹腔压力下降有关，或者是其他机械因素所造成尚不能肯定。而腹腔压力与隐睾发生的关系已经在一些动物实验中得到证实[3]。

神经管缺陷导致隐睾的发病率较高[103]。当脊髓脊膜膨出影响到上腰段脊索时，隐睾的发病率将超过 1/3。患者腹壁肌肉麻痹和腹腔压力低下或脊髓脊膜突出引起的生殖股神经运动核发育不良可能是造成隐睾的原因[85]。

睾丸与附睾体的分离常常出现在隐睾患者中[50,91,100]，而腹腔隐睾和高位腹股沟隐睾患者发生这种情况的可能性更大。这是否是造成隐睾的原因，或者仅仅是因为子宫内雄激素分泌减少所引起的伴随症状尚不清楚。实验研究发现，给啮齿动物喂养抵抗雄激素的饮食会造成子宫内胚胎的雄激素水平低下而导致附睾缺陷[19]。

输精管畸形在隐睾患者中很常见。极细的腹股沟管内的睾丸其输精管可形成长袢，从腹股沟管外环中突出。在对这些长袢输精管血供进行检查的基础上，Fowler 和 Stephens 认为在治疗高位隐睾时，可以利用输精管丰富的并行血管，切断睾丸原有的来自于精索的血供，从而达到既能完成睾丸下降，又能保证睾丸活力的目的[53]。由于该手术方法有引起睾丸萎缩的危险，所以开放手术中很少首选该术式，但目前常采用该术式在腹腔镜下行一期或二期手术。

隐睾的分类

由于睾丸在鞘膜内具有一定的活动度，根据性腺位置对隐睾进行分类较复杂。隐睾最恰当的定义是，在精索无张力的情况下，睾丸无法被牵拉进入阴囊底。正常下降的睾丸即使在首次体检时出现回缩，仍然会自动地降入阴囊。隐睾的位置可以分为停留在正常下降路线上的睾丸和异位的睾丸（图 75-2）。腹腔

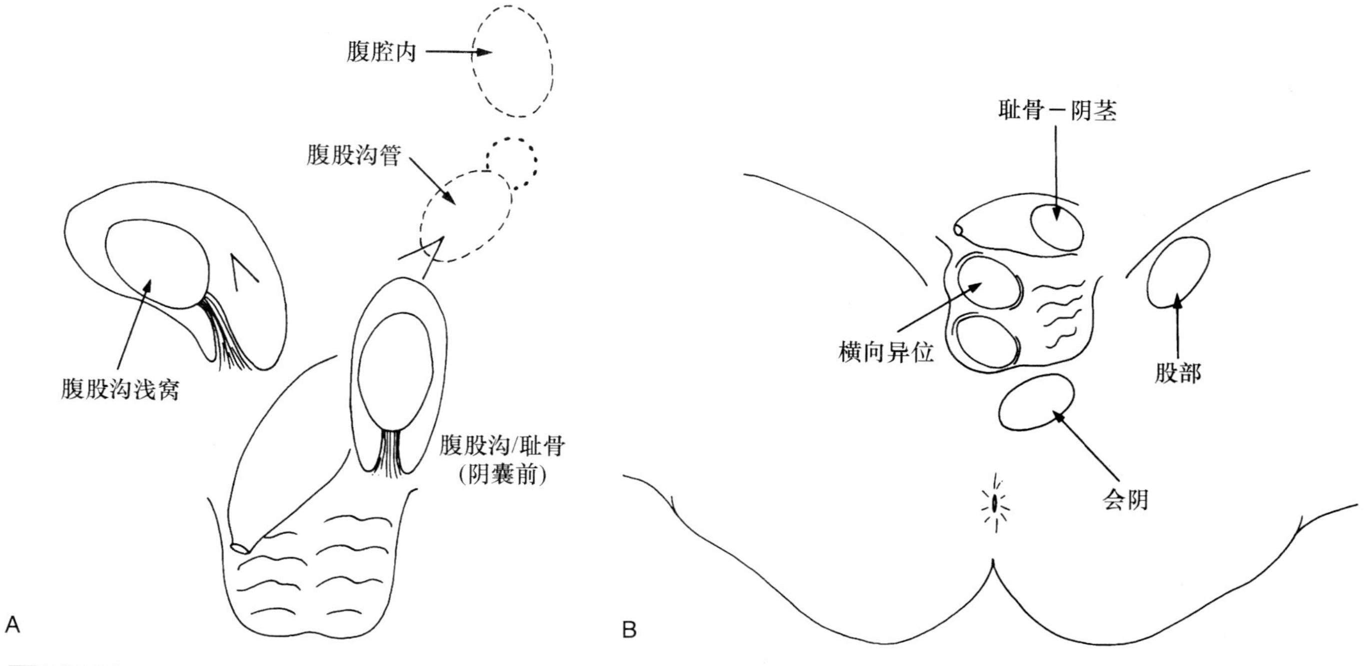

图 75-2 睾丸下降不全的可能位置。A. 正常下降线路（包括有争议的腹股沟浅筋膜，注意大多数病例的睾丸引带附着在阴囊颈附近）。B. 罕见的真性异位睾丸。

1196 内的睾丸常定位于距离腹股沟管内环数厘米处，其输精管和睾丸血管出腹腔以后通过短小的睾丸系膜进入睾丸。经腹股沟管的腹腔外探查术很难发现这些腹腔内的睾丸。但目前借助腹腔镜进行探查，手术已变得相对简单。

位于腹股沟管内的睾丸被肌肉组织覆盖，有时很难或不可能被触及，经挤压后则能出现于腹股沟外环以外，从而有利于触诊，因此这样的睾丸被称作“突现睾丸”。

根据 Browne 最早的描述，离开外环的睾丸通常位于靠近阴囊入口的位置，或是略高于或偏离外环，包裹于腹浅筋膜内（见图 75-2）[18]。后一种位置的睾丸在少数情况下预示着睾丸引带附着异常，这是因为手术中睾丸引带通常止于阴囊颈或是接近于这一区域[50,84]。从本质上来讲，位于腹股沟浅筋膜内的睾丸被自身的鞘膜包裹，其表面局限于腹壁浅筋膜的浅层，尾端潜行向腹股沟韧带，与阔筋膜相连。处于这一位置的睾丸是否该归类为异位睾丸仍有争议，但因为其引带通常向下止于或接近阴囊颈，所以一般还是认为位于腹股沟浅筋膜内的睾丸处于正常下降途径之中[69]。真正意义上的异位睾丸可以位于会阴、股部、耻骨上等，或是进入对侧半阴囊内形成睾丸横向异位。

回缩性睾丸

由于提睾肌的收缩，睾丸能够暂时性地回缩，这是正常的提睾反射。肌肉的这一功能可以调节睾丸的温度，也可以保护睾丸免受外伤[161]。睾丸回缩是由于低温或生殖股神经的皮支（腿内侧）受到刺激时的反应。

正常提睾反射在新生儿期很弱或缺如，阴囊经常呈悬垂状态。以后在儿童时期，当雄激素水平低下时，提睾肌的收缩明显加强，提睾反射也随之加强。10 岁以后，雄激素水平上升，青春期逐渐开始，反射再次变得不太显著。Farrington 的研究发现了提睾反射和正常的睾丸回缩，并发现在儿童阶段的中期睾丸回缩发病率很高[48]。

目前，对于回缩性睾丸发生的原因尚未达成共识[8]。多数临床医生认为，尽管回缩性睾丸不能始终保持下降状态而需要接受细致的随访，但依然属于下降的睾丸。或许回缩性睾丸反映的只是一个和年龄有关的提睾肌收缩效应，是正常的生理反应。Goh 和 Hutson 认为所谓的回缩性睾丸实际上是获得性的睾丸下降不良[57]。由于腹股沟管外环和阴囊底之间的距离随年龄的增加而增加（从婴儿时的 5 cm 增加到 10 岁左右的 10 cm），精索的长度也必须相应地增加，以保证睾丸能稳定地停留于阴囊内生长发育。回缩性睾丸或许反映的是精索不能随年龄增长，从而继发获得性睾丸下降不良。一些疾病如脑瘫和双侧肢体强直症等，会造成提睾肌过度收缩，这可能引起回缩性睾丸的出现[167]。

上升睾丸

上升睾丸是一个新名词，不同于回缩性睾丸[8,92]。在许多这类儿童中，长期的随访研究表明，儿童期继发性的睾丸上升常常与出生后前 3 个月内睾丸迟发性地下降到阴囊有关。目前，上升睾丸先后被证明[4,8]。上升睾丸和回缩性睾丸的差异尚不清楚，也许它们只是同一种疾病的不同命名而已。

研究表明，不是所有的隐睾在刚出生时就有临床表现的。尽管试图在婴儿期就进行筛查，但仍有许多孩子直到儿童阶段才被发现患有隐睾疾病[40]。而且，仔细询问这些患儿的病史后发现，在这些孩子中常常不存在出生后或早期儿童阶段的异常[60]。

获得性隐睾可能与精索不能随身体生长而增长有关。这些睾丸似乎是随着年龄的增长而逐渐移出阴囊外的，但实际上测量精索的长度后发现，睾丸上升的表面现象往往超过其真实情况。这一观察结果在脑瘫患者中得到了进一步印证，统计数据表明，严重的痉挛性瘫痪患者中，有近 50% 的青春期患者罹患获得性隐睾[167]。

Atwell 认为，上升睾丸或回缩性睾丸也许是由鞘状突持续开放所引起的，鞘状突的持续开放将影响到邻近输精管和睾丸血管的延长[4]。脑瘫患者中，已经证明其提睾肌处于痉挛状态，病因明确与异常的肌肉收缩有关。如果睾丸在出生以前就已经下降到阴囊，婴儿期保持停留在这一正常位置，而以后在儿童期再出现睾丸位置过高，那么一般通过阴囊切口就可以顺利地进行睾丸固定术[13,154]。

隐睾的发病率

1964 年 Scorer 报道婴儿隐睾的发病率是 4. 3%，这是一项划时代的研究[160]。1 岁左右，隐睾的发病率下降到 0. 96%。1986 年，有报道称 1 岁的英国儿童中，隐睾的发病率是 1. 58%。John Radcliffe 医院隐睾研究小组发现，出生以后 3 个月内睾丸可能出现自发性地下降，超过这一时限，睾丸自发下降的可能性很小[92,93]。近年来，在英格兰和威尔士的各大医院中，睾丸固定术的比例已经增加了 1 倍[143]。虽然隐
1197 睾的发病率和进行睾丸固定术的数量之间的差别提示部分睾丸固定术可能是没有必要的，但是我们也不能忽视这一事实，那就是隐睾的发病率的确在不断上升，而对于其中的原因尚留有许多争议[8]。有学者认为，睾丸固定术增加 1 倍的一个合理解释或许与获得性上升睾丸或回缩性睾丸有关[8]。因为先天性隐睾的手术推荐年龄已经下降至 1 岁甚至更小，所以那些获得性隐睾的患者更不容易与因先天性引带迁移异常而形成隐睾的患者区分开[40]。

早产儿中隐睾的发生率显著上升[125]。当出生体重小于 1500 g 时，隐睾的发病率接近 60%～70%[52]。造成隐睾高发的可能原因是，正常的睾丸下降过程直到胎龄 35 周的时候才能彻底完成。大多数早产儿的睾丸在出生以后能继续下降，所以对于这些儿童，如果随访至正常预产期以后 12 周，则可以发现隐睾的发病率已经明显下降到正常水平。

隐睾的并发症

隐睾和睾丸异常之间到底孰先孰后，是原发性的睾丸异常导致隐睾发生，还是未下降到正常位置的睾丸引起继发的睾丸发育异常，关于这一点的争论一直没有停止过。目前更多的证据似乎更倾向于下降不全的睾丸将造成睾丸继发性地异常。少数情况下，当下丘脑-垂体-性腺轴存在原发异常时，会造成性激素分泌缺乏、睾丸下降不全以及原发性的睾丸异常。

动物种群之间的差异造成有关隐睾并发症的研究结果之间难以比较。许多研究实验中选择了啮齿类动物，在这些动物中睾丸引带迁移的重要过程直至出生以后 10 天才完全结束。但是对于小鼠来讲，直到出生后的 2～3 周，睾丸才能进入阴囊。而大鼠的睾丸下降出现在动物进入青春期性成熟阶段，即出生以后的 3～4 周[46]。人类的睾丸引带迁移和睾丸下降同时发生，正常情况下在出生以前完成。因此，以青春期以后的大鼠作为模型研究隐睾的并发症，其结果将不会明显。

温度效应

阴囊中的睾丸处于一个特殊的低温环境中，机体为此特殊环境提供的保证包括蔓状血管丛、阴囊皮肤色素沉着、皮下脂肪缺如，以及随温度变化而能够敏感调节的肌肉，诸如提睾肌和肉膜的肌肉等，所有的上述结构都保证了性腺和附睾的温度能够有效地降低。人类阴囊内的温度保持在 33℃，而腹股沟的温度大约是 34～35℃，腹腔的温度在 37℃ 左右（图 75-3）[119,171]。睾丸的生理适应了低温的环境，因此周围环境温度的增加势必给下降不全睾丸造成持续性的损伤[190]。

内分泌效应

大鼠实验发现，糖皮质激素旁路途径使接受手术固定的隐睾患者在青春期以前不表现出明显异常，说明实验模型中的睾丸间质细胞仍然具有内分泌功能。测定结果表明，隐睾大鼠在刚出生的时候，体内睾酮含量与正常大鼠无明显差异。这一现象持续到出生以后的 2～3 周，此后大鼠进入青春期，睾酮产量明显低于对照组动物[47]。促性腺激素对睾丸间质细胞和支持细胞的调节同样处于异常情况。但是，睾丸支持细胞和间质细胞的数量相对正常[12]。隐睾患者睾丸

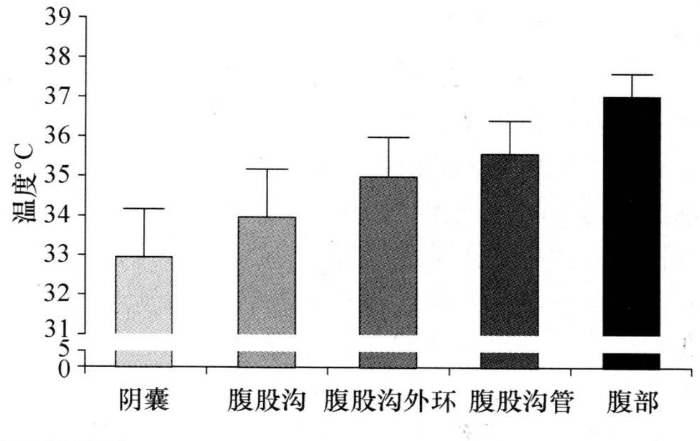

图 75-3　不同水平的睾丸温度（均值 ± 标准差）。

支持细胞的功能性紊乱最早由 Kretser 和 Risbridger 报道[35]。

测定隐睾婴儿血清的促性腺释放激素和睾酮水平，已经发现体内促黄体生成素（luteinizing hormone，LH）出生以后存在正常的上升，而睾酮含量明显低于正常[55,147]。很难判断出生后雄激素水平的缺乏属于原发异常还是继发于睾丸下降不全的结果。

在一项临床研究中，研究者随访调查了一些平均孕周为 30 周的早产儿，结果发现尽管其中有一些孩子的睾丸在出生以后下降，但在他们月龄满 18 个月的时候，隐睾的发病率仍高达 19%[6]。正常儿童出生后的第 2、3 个月时，体内睾酮水平有一个正常上升，但这一变化不存在于患有隐睾的早产儿之中。作者认为，由于缺乏子宫内人绒毛膜促性腺激素（human chorionic gonadotropin，hCG）的刺激，早产儿体内的睾酮含量低下，将影响到其隐睾疾病的预后。出生以后 1～4 个月中，隐睾婴儿的血清睾酮和 LH 浓度都降低[90]。尽管可能存在雄激素缺乏的病理情况，但研究双侧隐睾婴儿阴囊皮肤内的成纤维细胞，以及在行睾丸固定术时取睾丸标本活检，结果都证明这些细胞上的雄激素受体水平正常[17]。出生以后 4～12 个月期间，血清苗勒氏管抑制因子有个一正常上升过程，但在隐睾患者中这一上升过程被抑制[187]。

1198 生殖细胞发育

隐睾患者生殖细胞的缺乏被认为是先天性的[161]。但是据观察，刚出生时睾丸在组织学上的结构是正常的，随着年龄的增长，睾丸进行性地显现出异常。Mengle 和他的助手对 752 例 2 个月～15 岁的儿童行睾丸活检时首次发现，隐睾患者生精小管内的精原母细胞数在 3 岁时明显下降[118]。

凭借电子显微镜的帮助，Hadziselimovic 和他的同事们发现患儿 2 岁时睾丸间质细胞组织学上开始发生异常。更多深入的研究表明，隐睾患者中睾丸间质细胞损伤开始于出生后的 2～6 个月，而当时的睾丸支持细胞和生殖细胞仍然表现正常[64]。到年满 2 岁时，隐睾患者中有将近 40% 的患者丧失了生殖细胞。他们认为隐睾患者生殖细胞缺乏的现象是继发性的，因为在接近 100 名年龄小于 1 岁的患儿中只有 1 名被检测出缺乏生殖细胞，而这些小婴儿中 70% 的活检标本中有正常数量的生殖细胞[62]。在更新的研究报告中，Huff 和他的同事们研究了新生的精原细胞向 A 级精母细胞的转化，这是出生以后生殖细胞发育的一个早期阶段。通过研究，他们发现隐睾症患者缺少这一阶段[75-77]。

一些学者认为，这些早期的生殖细胞发育过程受雄激素调空，出生以后的雄激素缺乏会造成细胞发育缺如[75]。但是，也有一些学者对此持不同看法，他们认为苗勒氏管抑制因子控制了出生以后的生殖细胞发育[10,188]。当然，雄激素阻断或缺乏并不影响新生啮齿动物中精原细胞向 A 级精母细胞的转化[189]。

生育能力

有隐睾病史的男性生育能力相对低下。早先的观点认为，青春期以前的未降睾丸无明显异常，因此患者在 12 岁或者 15 岁以前无需外科干预[161]。自从研究明确隐睾的病损出现于出生后 6 个月以后，广大临床医生就认识到这一睾丸的退化过程不仅是严重的，而且急需早期干预以阻止病变加重。相对说来，采用动物实验很容易了解医源性或先天性隐睾引起的青春期后生殖细胞缺乏，是否会造成生育能力的降低[98]。单侧隐睾患者或动物的生育能力下降不明显，但双侧隐睾患者或动物的生育能力严重受损[107,108]。由于对早年接受睾丸固定术的患儿缺乏长期研究，目前还无法在患者生育率和接受手术的时间之间建立相关联系。有回缩性睾丸病史的男性生育能力尚存在争议，一些学者认为，这些患者精子数量的异常并不直接反映他们的生育能力[131,146,149]。

恶性变

过去认为，存在隐睾病史的男性患睾丸肿瘤的几率是正常人群的 35～50 倍[182]。通过使用不同的方法去计算相对风险，Woodhouse[185] 提出其癌变的实际风险是正常人群的 5～10 倍。综观所有睾丸肿瘤的患者，单侧隐睾患者的癌变风险是正常人的 15 倍，而双侧隐睾患者癌变风险是正常人的 33 倍，尤以腹腔型隐睾的癌变风险最高[11,23,170]。

隐睾患者生殖细胞进行性退化和发育不良被认为与癌变风险不断增加有关[67]。睾丸肿瘤在儿童中并不常见，正常下降睾丸癌变的发生多见于相同的年龄段（如 20～40 岁）。Giwercman 和他的同事推测，睾丸肿瘤的发生也许和组织内在的结构异常关系更密切，而不仅仅是简单地继发于睾丸发育不良[56]。他们认为，原位的睾丸生殖上皮癌实际上是恶性的精母细胞肿瘤，是侵袭性肿瘤的先兆。在不育或者两性畸形儿童的新生儿期间，这些表现出组织学特征的原位癌很容易被发现。Skakkabaek 和他的同事们描述了这些原位癌的组织学特征，并提供强有力的证据证明了这些异常细胞的出现预示了侵袭性睾丸肿瘤的发生[165]。他们建议有隐睾病史的年轻人能接受睾丸活检，以便于及早发现细胞恶性变。

腹股沟疝

正常情况下，鞘状突在腹腔内的睾丸下降以后闭合。睾丸下降不全与鞘状突开放或腹股沟斜疝高度相关，由于疾病增加了嵌顿疝的发病率，许多患者需要早期接受手术干预。临床证据表明，同时合并疝和隐睾的患者应该立即接受手术。绝大多数外科医生推崇在施行睾丸固定术的同时进行疝修补手术。

隐睾扭转

以前的外科教科书上提到，未经治疗的隐睾发生睾丸扭转的可能性高达 20%[161]。但在最近的 30 年中，由于隐睾的治疗倾向于早期干预，所以目前大多数儿外科医生几乎没有遇见过隐睾扭转病例。位于腹股沟浅筋膜内的睾丸活动度大，容易在睾丸鞘膜内发生扭转，但目前确切的扭转概率很难统计[157]。

外伤

一般认为，腹股沟睾丸遭遇直接外伤的风险略高于正常。但是，与睾丸扭转一样，早期的手术干预使这一问题发生的概率略微下降[52]。笔者所见的隐睾
1199 遭遇外伤的最常见情况发生于乘坐轮椅的脑瘫儿童。在这些儿童中，位于腹股沟的隐睾可能会被轮椅的皮带压伤。

心理影响

由于生殖器官的外观明显异常，患者的父母亲对孩子将来的生育问题非常焦虑，就诊心情急迫，这是隐睾涉及的一个重要的心理问题。

睾丸-附睾异常融合

隐睾中常见睾丸与附睾联结异常。睾丸-附睾异常融合的风险随睾丸位置的上升而增加，位于腹股沟管或腹腔内的睾丸发生上述异常的可能性大大超过了位于腹股沟外环附近或阴囊入口处的睾丸。出现该畸形的原因很大程度上与宫内雄激素缺乏有关，其结果足以影响日后的生育能力。

诊断

隐睾患者体检时，最重要的是需要明确未下降完全的睾丸是否可以被触及，以及了解在没有明显张力的情况下，睾丸可以被牵拉到的最低位置[86]。睾丸所能下降到的最低位置可能受到鞘状突尾端的限制。体检时要求环境温暖，并尽力使孩子放松。在患者躺下以后，要仔细在阴囊内触摸睾丸。当腹股沟区出现肿块时，应当考虑睾丸下降不全或者斜疝的可能。在耻骨上向头端方向牵拉皮肤常常使睾丸明显地回缩到阴囊上极。阴囊的外观随年龄的不同变化明显，新生儿时阴囊皮肤薄、下垂、松弛，学龄期儿童的阴囊相对较小易起皱折。当睾丸位于阴囊内时，通过薄弱的阴囊皮肤很容易被发现。单侧睾丸下降不全时，会出现半个阴囊发育不良的表现。如果两边阴囊发育相等而又出现隐睾疾病，常提示该患儿可能属于回缩性睾丸或是上升睾丸。

对阴囊上方的睾丸进行定位时，必须切记睾丸是被鞘状突包裹的器官，因此具有一定的活动度。另外，还需要注意腹股沟韧带的骨性标志。为了定位腹股沟浅筋膜内的睾丸，用伸开的手轻触诊就很有效。如果触摸时用力过度，往往会使手指下的睾丸移位而未被体检医生发现。至少有 80%~90% 的腹股沟区的睾丸可以被触诊到，或者可以被施力挤出腹股沟管，注意后者手法，必须在腹壁外环处施加稳定的压力，由侧面近髂前上棘向下、向中线阴囊方向按压。腹腔型隐睾或者腹股沟管内无法触摸到的睾丸并不常见。一旦睾丸在腹股沟区被触及时，检查者两手需要配合操作，一手在睾丸上方尝试把睾丸推向阴囊内，另一

手通过阴囊的皮肤试着抓住睾丸。这样做的目的是要明确在精索无明显张力时，睾丸最低能够到达的部位。正常情况下，回缩性睾丸应该可以被拉到阴囊底，并停留在该处。Scorer[160]曾阐述睾丸的位置可以通过体检时测量其与耻骨结节之间的距离来确定，虽然该定位通常并不必要。

最有价值的临床观察指标是睾丸是否能够自发地停留于阴囊内。阴囊内的睾丸很容易被发现和触摸到，所以对新生儿进行阴囊检查并不是一件困难的事情。如果体检发现睾丸位于阴囊以上水平时，应在3个月以后再次对患儿进行检查以排除睾丸延迟下降的可能。对于3个月后仍不能下降进入阴囊的睾丸，临床上可以确诊为先天性隐睾。一些患者的睾丸下降发生于出生以后12周内，由于这些患者睾丸有再次上升的可能性，所以临床上需要加强观察。

腹股沟疝嵌顿的时候很难正确判断睾丸的位置，而一旦嵌顿疝被复位，则睾丸的具体位置也可以明确。

临床上对正常的回缩性睾丸和先天性或获得性隐睾进行区分是困难的。一般认为正常的回缩性睾丸往往具有以下特征：

1. 在毫无困难的情况下，睾丸可以被完全拖到阴囊底。
2. 在被牵拉至阴囊以后，睾丸可以停留其中维持一定时间，而不表现为立即回缩。
3. 睾丸大小正常。
4. 有睾丸自发下降至阴囊的病史。

如果睾丸不能在腹股沟近外环的常见位置被触摸到，应当检查异位睾丸的存在部位，如股部或会阴区。真正意义上的不能触摸到的睾丸相对少见，据报道发病率大概为5%~28%[20,94,156,181]。如果睾丸不能被触诊到，则睾丸可能存在于腹腔内（45%）、腹股沟管内（25%）或睾丸不存在（45%）。最后一种情况被称为睾丸缺如，造成这一结果的原因大多是因为在睾丸引带迁移进入阴囊的时候，精索在宫腔内扭转所致[39,77,178]。精索扭转会造成患侧睾丸萎缩，而对侧睾丸通常增大，这是一个有价值的临床体征[76,99]。

盲目地对不能触摸到的睾丸进行腹股沟探查手术并不见得能成功。对此类睾丸，推荐使用多种影像学检查手段[74]。这些检查包括腹部和腹股沟超声、CT、MRI及精索动脉、静脉造影等。目前，腹腔镜检查已经成为一种主要的诊疗手段，借助这一技术，可以明确腹腔型隐睾的位置，排除睾丸继发性萎缩[14,123,142]。此外，在腹腔镜的协助下可以非常容易地对睾丸血管进行结扎，采用这一手段能提高分期Fowler-Stephens手术的疗效[14]。

治疗 1200

激素治疗

激素治疗隐睾的前提是该疾病的原因是由于下丘脑-垂体-性腺轴分泌激素缺乏引起，并且出生以后的治疗可以通过激素调节介导引带迁移从而使睾丸下降[61]。激素治疗包括使用睾酮、hCG和LHRH等。由于剂量过大会造成患者早熟，所以直接使用雄激素治疗的方法早已被淘汰。在过去的10~20年时间里，采用hCG治疗的方法在欧洲很普及，但在其他地区却比较少见。近年来，LHRH正逐渐得到应用。

对于激素治疗的结果报道不一，与许多因素有关，成功治愈的比例从10%~50%不等[38,73,148]。年龄大于4岁的儿童、双侧位于阴囊入口处的隐睾或回缩性睾丸对hCG的反应更好。而对于最常见的隐睾，即位于腹股沟浅筋膜内的睾丸，其治疗成功率相对较低。有人提出，前者疗效较好的原因是因为大多数疾病属于回缩性睾丸[148]。Christiansen和他的同事们报道[24]，有大约25%的隐睾患者在接受hCG治疗后睾丸完全下降，另有25%的患者睾丸位置表现为向下移动。回顾他们的论著发现，由于缺乏必要的参考要素，要从中排除隐睾的变异类型如回缩性睾丸或是上升睾丸几乎是不可能的。从统计学角度来讲，单侧隐睾更倾向属于先天性疾病，激素疗法的治疗成功率只有14%左右。

在一项随机双盲实验中，Rajfer和他的同事们比较了hCG和LHRH的疗效，发现接受hCG治疗的男童中有6%的患者痊愈，而接受LHRH治疗的男童中有19%的患者痊愈[148]。他们认为，无论是hCG还是LHRH，对于真正意义上的隐睾都没有肯定的疗效。在另一项双盲实验中，研究人员比较了安慰剂和LHRH鼻喷剂的治疗效果，发现鼻喷剂的疗效是9%，而安慰剂的疗效达到8%[37,38]。二期治疗使用 LHRH 时，疗效能上升到 18%。年幼儿对激素治疗的效果最差，LHRH 对临床上不能触及的睾丸是无效的。

一些临床医生建议在治疗回缩性睾丸的时候可以考虑使用激素，临床证实其确有一定疗效，能避免手术创伤。获得性隐睾，即严重回缩的睾丸或者继发性上升的睾丸对 hCG 有一定反应，推荐的使用方法是肌注 100 IU/kg，一周 2 次，连续使用 3～4 周，或使用 LHRH 鼻喷剂 100 mg，每侧鼻孔一天喷 6 次，连续使用 3～4 周。在笔者的外科部门，激素治疗很少被应用，几乎所有的先天性或获得性隐睾患者都接受睾丸固定术。

外科治疗

隐睾症的外科治疗是建立在早期干预可防止睾丸受高温影响而继发变性这一假设的基础上的[190]。阴囊内的温度比腹腔低 3～4℃，这对出生后睾丸的正常发育是至关重要的[19]。手术的时机问题仍然存在争议，一些学者认为在儿童期晚些时候行睾丸固定术的效果比较好，而另有些学者对此持反对意见。有研究表明生殖细胞在出生以后的 6～12 个月发生退化，显微镜下观察学龄期儿童的睾丸发现萎缩，所有这些结果都支持下降不完全的睾丸在出生以后进行性地发生变性[75,101]。尽管还没有证据表明早期手术能预防人类睾丸的退化变性，但动物实验的结果已经证实了这一点[129]。

许多年来，施行睾丸固定术推荐的年龄是 2 岁，但据笔者经验，手术时间应该选择在出生后 6 个月。这是因为睾丸最早表现出受损迹象的时间是在出生后 6 个月左右[75]。但是，对如此年幼的儿童实施睾丸固定术是一个挑战。在儿童外科中心，在患儿 6 个月以后实施睾丸固定术是非常合理的；但是对于一些在年幼儿手术方面经验不丰富的医疗中心而言，把手术时间定于 18 个月~2 岁会更安全些。笔者推荐家长选择儿童外科中心进行睾丸固定术，这样做的目的是在治疗的同时不增加并发症的风险[184]。

以笔者个人的临床经验，推荐对所有刚出生的男婴进行生殖器体检。对于那些刚出生时单侧或两侧睾丸未降的儿童，建议在 3 个月以后复查。如果那时睾丸仍然未完全下降到阴囊内，则需要考虑在患儿 6～12 个月或者出生后的第 2 年里进行睾丸固定术。如果患者的睾丸在出生以后 12 周内自行下降，则日后数年需要加强随访，以彻底排除睾丸在儿童晚期发生继发性上升的现象。隐睾伴发斜疝的患儿，在疝囊修补的同时进行睾丸固定术。如果在疝手术以后延期进行睾丸固定术的话，腹股沟管将遭遇二次探查，这样将大大提高输精管或精索血管损伤的机会。当年长儿表现为疑似获得性睾丸下降不良且不能自发下降至阴囊时，笔者推荐对这些孩子施行睾丸固定术。当然，这一意见仅代表个人观点，一些学者对此争议颇多。

睾丸固定术可以作为门诊手术，患儿在术前几小时进入医院或诊室，术后观察数小时后即可出院[82]。静脉注射前在患者的手背上涂擦局部麻醉药膏以减轻注射痛苦。手术过程在全身麻醉下进行，配合区域或局部麻醉以减少术后几个小时内产生的疼痛。

腹股沟隐睾手术选择经外环的皮肤切口，略向侧方延长（图 75－4A）。其余的手术细节描述如图75–4B～N。

隐睾症常伴发鞘状突开放（高达 70%），手术时需要将其从输精管和精索血管上分离出来（见图 75–4D）。精索前方的疝囊被血管环绕，输精管位于后中间位置，血管位于后外侧面。高位隐睾，尤其是 1203
处于腹股沟管内的隐睾，疝囊可以完全包裹睾丸，以致输精管和精索血管连同系膜一起居于疝囊内。常规行疝囊修补术时需要游离疝囊。具体操作时可以用示指钩住疝囊壁并保持张力，选择圆头的无齿镊把疝囊轻轻地从精索其他结构上剥离下来，剥离的时候注意不要损伤到输精管和睾丸血管。也可以分离输精管和血管以后再离断其余精索结构，相比之下，当疝囊完整的时候采用这一方法更为简便。如果鞘状突开口不明显，应该用镊子夹起腹膜的边缘，保持腹膜外翻开放。输精管粘在疝囊的后壁上，因此在游离疝囊时必须加以识别。

一旦精索结构被安全地分离出来，疝囊也就被游离了（见图 75–4E）。继续向内环方向游离疝囊，当腹膜外脂肪暴露以后，精索血管与输精管相互分开，血管向侧方行进，输精管向中线走行，见到这一特征性的结构即表明手术操作已经到达腹膜后区域（见图 75–4F）。紧接着，在内环水平贯穿缝扎鞘状突（见图 75–4G）。

在腹膜后区域离断精索周围的纤维组织粘连，可以进一步松解睾丸血管，轻柔地抓住睾丸将其下降到阴囊内（见图 75–4H）。在年长儿中，把睾丸血管行径路线上的弯曲捋直往往就可以有效地拉长精索（见

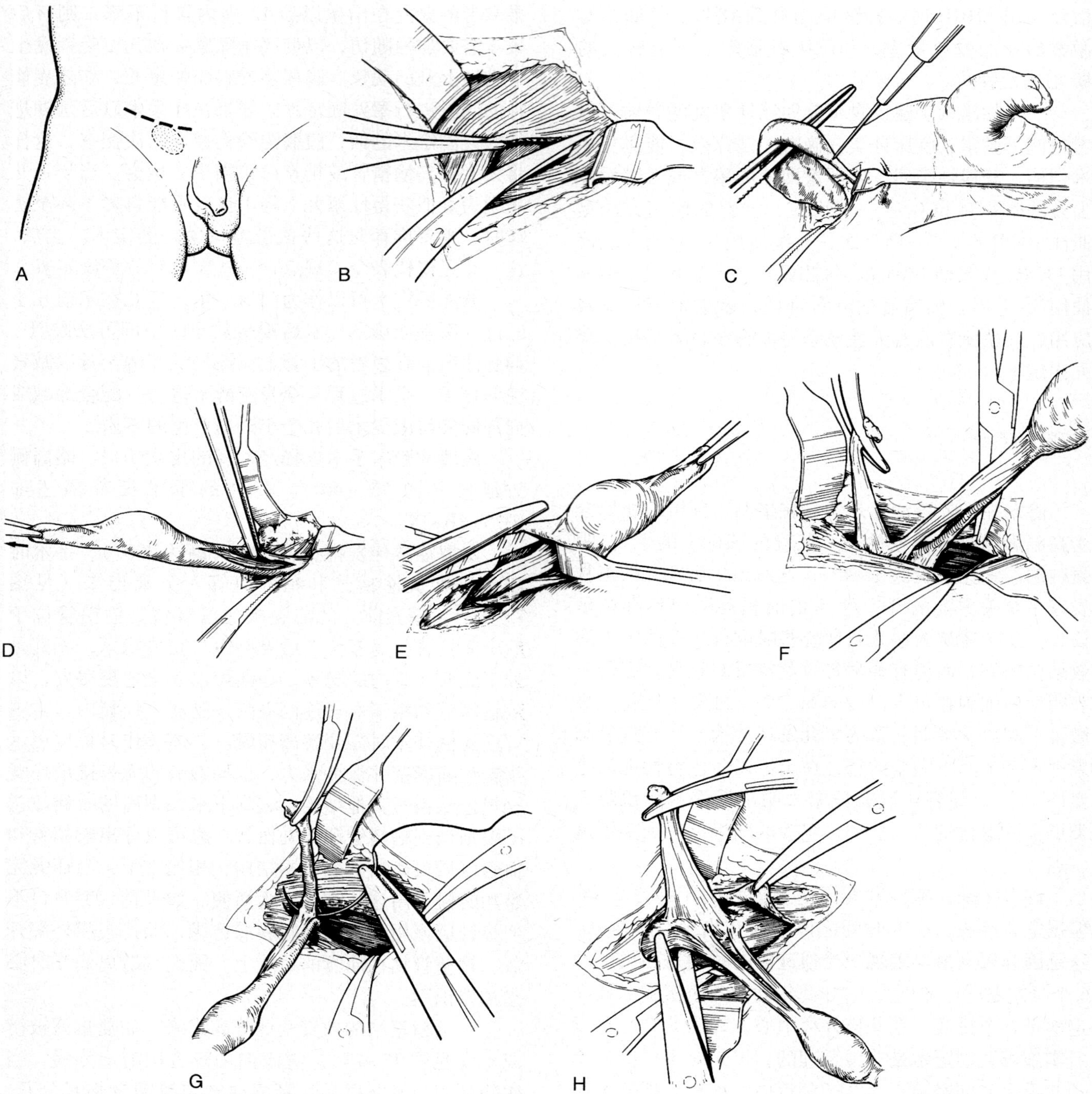

图 75-4　A. 皮纹切口，经腹股沟外环向外侧延伸。B. 分离 Scarpa 筋膜后，暴露腹外斜肌腱膜并用手术刀将其切开，以手术剪向腹股沟外环内侧延伸。应用蚊式血管钳探查，可协助辨认外环位置和术后关闭。C. 位于腹股沟浅筋膜内或耻骨区的睾丸易被发现，可将镊子穿过精索并加以牵拉，辨认睾丸引带后将其分离。大多数患者的睾丸引带位于阴囊颈上方或附着于旁边。D. 牵拉鞘膜，剥离提睾肌纤维，分离残留的鞘状突，保留输精管和精索血管。输精管和精索血管一般附着于疝囊的游离后壁上。E. 从疝囊上辨认分离输精管和精索血管，钳夹离断疝囊时以小型牵开器保护输精管和血管。F. 向腹股沟内环方向，由后外侧的性腺血管上分离出前内侧的鞘状突。在此位置，输精管走向内侧。G. 在腹股沟内环水平贯穿、缝扎鞘状突。操作以前，首先将疝囊扭转，以防缝针不小心钩带腹腔内容物。H. 在腹膜后范围内松解精索血管侧面粘连，可延长精索长度。

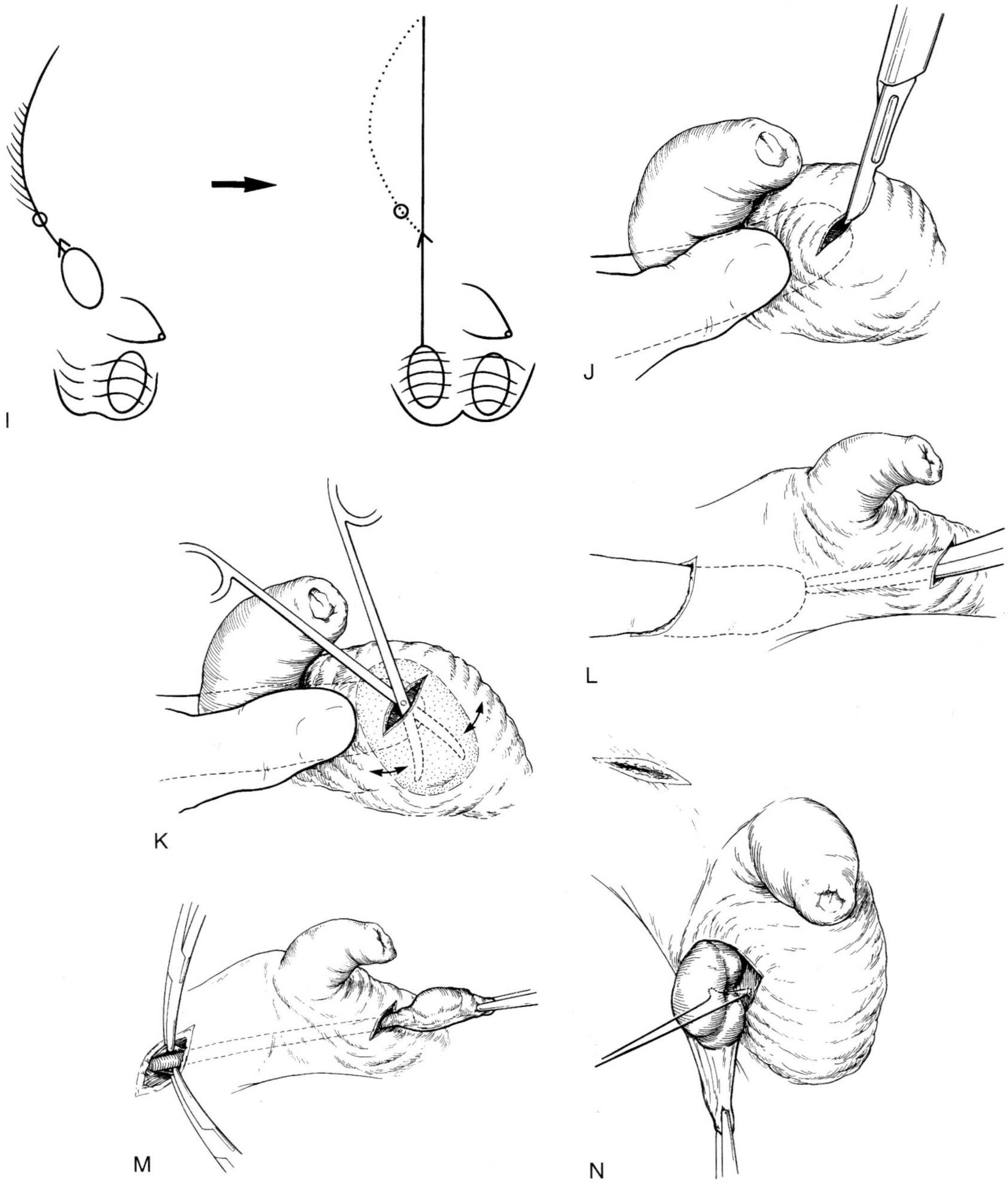

图 75-4　（续）I. 伸直精索血管，使睾丸下降到达阴囊。J. 从腹股沟切口探入手指，向阴囊方向钝性分离出一个空间供睾丸下降。然后，在阴囊皮肤上做一切口。经阴囊中线的切口或一侧阴囊的横切口都可以使睾丸下降到肉膜下。笔者选择后者，出血较少。K. 用剪刀或血管钳在阴囊皮下做一小囊。操作时注意止血，以免术后出现阴囊血肿。L. 在手指的引导下，经腹股沟阴囊筋膜将腹股沟切口和阴囊皮肤切口连通。M. 以血管钳夹住睾丸，小心勿造成精索扭转，将睾丸经腹股沟筋膜下降至肉膜下。N. 下降的睾丸可能不存在张力，可选择是否予以睾丸固定。为防止睾丸回缩，尤其在处理精索存在张力的患者时，可用细线将睾丸白膜固定到阴囊隔上，或者变化为缝线缩窄睾丸下降时通过的小孔。常规关闭阴囊和腹股沟切口。（From Spitz L，Coran AG：Pediatric surgery. In Rob and Smith's Operative Surgery，5th ed. London，Chapaman & Hall，1995.）

图 75-4I），但在年幼儿中，上述技巧却不起作用。通过腹腔镜可以看到，睾丸血管从腹主动脉走向腹股沟内环的路径几乎是笔直的，所以在腹膜后游离精索血管下降睾丸的动作实际上是对睾丸动脉的牵拉延长过程，而并非是把弯曲的血管伸直。

一般情况下，输精管有足够的长度可以下降到阴囊内，术中无须特别操作。但是，在一些手术困难的患者中，可以分离腹壁下血管，或者在腹壁下血管内侧切开腹股沟管后壁，睾丸经过腹壁下血管内侧下降。这样，输精管可以获得数厘米长的额外松解。阴囊内睾丸的固定方法见图 75-4J～N。

在 Bianchi 和 Squire[13]，以及 Russinko 和他的同事[154]们的报道中，都分别提到了选择阴囊切口的改良手术，这一改良手术尤其适用于获得性隐睾患者。手术选择经阴囊颈的横切口，暴露睾丸鞘膜，保持张力，把睾丸从伤口中拖出。分离与精索粘连的疏松结缔组织，充分暴露精索。通常，精索上会残留未完全闭锁的鞘状突纤维束。一旦这些纤维束被松解以后，输精管和血管都能毫不费力地下降到阴囊底部[25]。关闭阴囊颈伤口，将睾丸与之固定，或将睾丸缝合至阴囊中隔。

当睾丸位于腹股沟管或者腹腔内时，也许在经过前述努力以后，精索仍然不能被充分松解而到达阴囊。这种情况下，手术医生有下列一些选择。如果有足够的经验与设备保证，可以行微血管吻合术，横断睾丸血管，将它和腹壁下动静脉吻合。这一手术需要丰富的显微血管吻合经验，所以并不作为常规应用。通常情况下，在睾丸不能充分下降时，可以将其固定于腹股沟尽可能低的位置，作为一期手术，并在此之后 6～12 个月之间行二期手术再次尝试下降睾丸。据报道，分期睾丸固定术的成功率在 70%～90%[68]。

另一种可供选择的方法是 Fowler-Stephens 手术，将睾丸血管在腹腔外结扎，睾丸旋转到长环状血管内，该血管的血供由并行的动静脉供应，也可由一些精索、血管供应（见图 75-7A 和 B）[53]。在决定施实 Fowler-Stephens 手术前对腹股沟管进行基本的分离可能会损伤并行血管的血供使手术风险增加，可以通过最初先结扎睾丸血管并将 Fowler-Stephens 手术作为二期手术来克服这些并发症，避免影响并行血管的血供。二期手术可使睾丸及输精管在腹股沟管内获得较大的活动空间，从而下降到阴囊。在对二期手术患者随诊中发现 70%～90% 没有出现阴囊萎缩[15,41]。

表 75-1 睾丸固定术并发症
睾丸无法下降到阴囊
睾丸继发性萎缩
睾丸回缩
输精管梗阻
出血
伤口感染

现在，许多外科医生借助腹腔镜手段治疗位于腹股沟管内或者腹腔内的隐睾[94,142]。对于腹腔型隐睾，如果睾丸可以被顺利地拖至对侧内环，则睾丸固定术大多能够一次手术成功。分期的 Fowler-Stephens 手术同样受到推崇，其近期效果值得肯定。在一期手术中，腹腔镜下对发育弱小或发育不良的睾丸进行定位，可以对是选择睾丸固定手术还是睾丸切除手术做出决定。如果确定需实施睾丸固定术，则可以在腔镜下较容易地结扎或钳闭睾丸血管[14]。6 个月以后再行睾丸固定术，睾丸连带其周围伴行的腹膜血管通过腹股沟管内侧下降到阴囊底。目前，对分期的睾丸下降手术，笔者都能通过腹腔镜技术完成[157]。

手术并发症

一个经验丰富的外科医生，配合常规的手术放大技术，可以使睾丸固定术并发症出现的风险小于 5%（表 75-1）[84]。术中损伤睾丸血管会导致睾丸萎缩，这是手术造成的最严重的并发症，但相对少见。从理论上来讲，输精管损伤会造成管腔堵塞，继而影响到生育能力，这种损伤比较轻微，但它的确切发生率很难统计。凝血障碍造成伤口继发性出血也时有发生。

由于目前许多手术对象是婴儿，睾丸固定术后最常见的并发症是伤口感染。无论是腹股沟切口还是阴
囊切口，手术造成的伤口感染可以发生于任何年龄。1204
但据笔者的经验，婴儿更容易出现阴囊感染。通常，感染不会造成严重的后果，治疗上可以采用简单的抗生素或是伤口引流，效果良好。另一个出现几率不高但重要的并发症是睾丸固定术后回缩，造成该并发症的原因是术中对精索的游离不够充分或者睾丸位置固定不佳。睾丸手术以后常见阴囊水肿、血肿，一般无须处理，术后 1～2 个月后能自行吸收。

表 75-2 睾丸固定术后生育力情况

作者	病例数	平均手术年龄	生育力实验	生育力	
				单侧	双侧
Puri 等，1985	142	7～13	精液分析	74	30
Singer 等，1988	25	6.2	精液分析	70	40
Cendron 等，1989	40	7.0	已生育子女	87	33
Kumar 等，1989	56	7～18 +	已生育子女	84	60
Okuyama 等，1989	167	2～5	精液分析	95	24
Mandat 等，1994	135	8.9	精液分析	53	26
Lee 等，2001	51	7.1	已生育子女	90	—

手术以后 1～2 周，患儿应复查，稍后除去敷料，对手术近期效果进行评估。术后 6～12 个月需要对患儿做进一步的远期疗效随访，了解睾丸术后是否出现明显萎缩或者错位。值得肯定的是，在绝大多数患者中，睾丸最终的下降结果和外观是令人满意的。

已经通过腹股沟管外环的睾丸，其治疗成功率比较高。而位于腹股沟管内或者腹腔内的睾丸在下降手术以后结构仍然异常的发生率较高。腹腔型隐睾可能无法下降到阴囊，至少一次手术很难成功。即使手术能够成功，患者的性腺发育往往不正常，或者出现萎缩。术后睾丸坏死极其罕见，据报道术前睾丸无法触摸到的患者其发生的概率在 3% 左右。进一步随访发现术后出现部分萎缩的概率在 15%～20%。一些患者需要接受二期手术将睾丸下降到阴囊，这或许增加了术后发生萎缩的风险。但对这些情况，尚没有确切的数据统计。

在睾丸下降固定手术的同时进行嵌顿疝或绞窄疝复位会增加术后睾丸萎缩的风险。很难确定这是否同嵌顿疝压迫睾丸血供，或者是在广泛剥离疝囊时损伤睾丸的血管侧支循环有关。因此，睾丸固定术时间的选择需要综合多方面因素考虑。手术年龄越大，睾丸发育异常的可能性也越大；但是，手术年龄越小，术后继发睾丸萎缩的可能性又会增加。Wilson-Storey 和同事们[184]比较了 100 例年龄小于 2 岁的和 100 例年龄大于 2 岁的儿童的手术效果。研究结果表明，两组中睾丸萎缩的发生概率都在 5% 左右，说明在儿童外科中心，手术年龄与术后睾丸萎缩之间并不存在直接联系。

生育能力

研究统计的一些数据显示了睾丸固定术后男性的生育能力（表 75-2）[21,106,108,115,134,145,164]。尽管单侧隐睾的位置对疾病生育力的总体影响并不是很明显，但仍然可以看到，那些初始位置已经超过腹股沟管的睾丸的预后较好[107]。但是要想解释这些结果很难，因为就目前为止，参与调查的患者当年接受手术的时间大多在 6～13 岁，而处于这一年龄段的孩子所受到的客观干扰因素较多，诸如上升睾丸或回缩性睾丸等。由于婴儿期睾丸处于阴囊内，生殖细胞的早期发育正常，所以在这些患者中，睾丸所表现出的生育力异常远不同于真正意义上的隐睾。据报道，上升型睾丸在组织学上与先天性隐睾类似，而组织病理学形态与将来的生育力之间存在着潜在联系[152,153]。

一篇大型文献综述表明，在 4～14 岁早期手术对改善患者日后的生育力并没有明显的帮助[164]。尽管我们查阅了 27 篇文献，但近来只有 4 篇文献发表，而我们也无法推断上世纪五六十年代，处于青春期的患者手术以后的效果怎样。在过去的 25 年中，随着知识水平的提高和临床治疗的改变（如早期手术干预），比较历史的疾病疗效和现代疗效是不恰当的。婴儿期行睾丸固定术是否一定可以显著提高患者的生育力尚有待研究。

恶性变 1205

目前为止，尚无确切的数据表明早在婴儿期就施行睾丸固定术能减少继发睾丸癌的风险。但是据 Cortes 报道，获得性隐睾患者的恶变率非常低[30]。目前对隐睾的手术治疗时间倾向于婴儿期，这样的改变是否会造成先天性隐睾转归的变化，回答这一问题尚需时间观察。目前，临床医生所能做的全部事情就是明确所有可能影响疾病预后的因素。预后良好的指征包括睾丸靠近阴囊颈、疾病类型属于上升型睾丸或回缩型睾丸，也许还包括在婴儿期早期接受手术治疗。预后不良的指征包括原发性睾丸或附睾发育不良、腹腔型隐睾或腹股沟管内的隐睾、伴发腹股沟绞窄疝，或许还包括拖延手术时间直至儿童期或青春期。

睾丸扭转

Delasiauve 于 1840 年最早报道了睾丸扭转[36]。1897 年，Taylor 首先报道了新生儿睾丸扭转[173]。1922 年，Colt 第一个描述了睾丸附件扭转[27]。1913 年，Ombredanne记述了一个病损情况，就其叙述的内容分析，很可能是睾丸附件，但当时他对此并没有认识[136]。

睾丸扭曲或扭转导致血供障碍，如果不及时缓解，将引起睾丸坏死。虽然这不是儿童阴囊急症的最常见原因，但不容否认，它是所有阴囊急症中最重要的（图 75-5）。扭转通常发生于完全下降至正常位置的睾丸，由于极易导致睾丸坏死，该病属于外科急症。

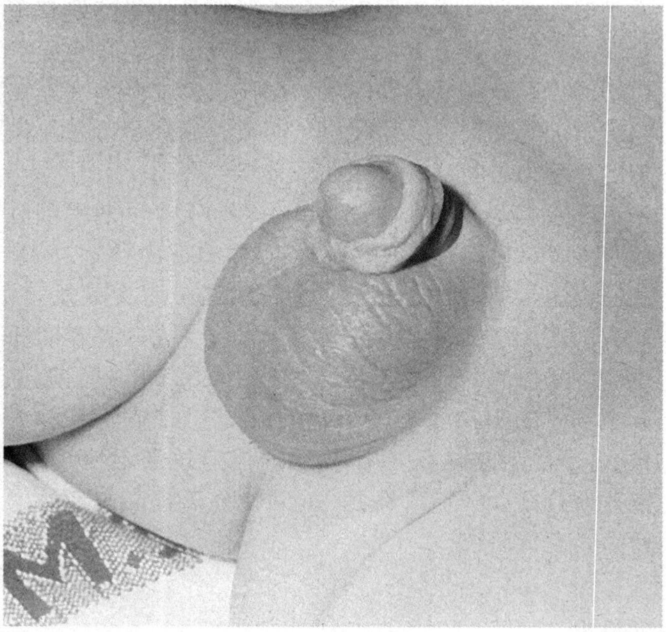

图 75-5 一例 1 岁婴儿器质性阴囊急症。由于一侧鞘膜对炎症的限制作用，疾病表现为半侧阴囊疼痛、水肿、发红。

被膜或鞘膜内的扭转是最常见的类型，精索在鞘膜内附着位置过高是疾病的易感因素。长而狭窄的睾丸系膜使睾丸无法正常垂直固定，睾丸在鞘膜内水平翻转导致发病。正常睾丸系膜较短，系膜附着于附睾全长，允许睾丸在鞘膜内小幅活动，但能防止完全扭转。悬垂于鞘膜内的睾丸在精索上的附着点较高，水平活动度大，随下肢的活动和提睾肌收缩，睾丸容易发生扭转。鞘内睾丸扭转的罕见类型出现于睾丸附睾之间，常由于睾丸附睾分离而造成扭转发生。这种情况多发生于隐睾患儿。

被膜或鞘膜外的扭转比较少见，局限于围生期。在睾丸引带迁移和睾丸下降至阴囊期间，局部结构周围组织疏松，可使得整个睾丸和精索发生扭转。

新生儿期以后，睾丸扭转几乎都伴发 bell-clapper 畸形。由于许多活动造成提睾肌运动，外伤和体育活动对睾丸扭转的意义重大[112]。提睾肌收缩既可以是睾丸扭转的原因，也可以是睾丸扭转的后果。青春期睾丸扭转高发的事实提示我们，睾丸的急剧增大和血清睾酮水平的突然增高或许是发病因素之一。

扭转并不总是引起睾丸坏死，前提是扭转的程度较小或扭转以后睾丸自行复位。在一次以犬为动物模型的研究中发现，精索完全扭转 4 圈以后的 2 小时内睾丸将完全坏死，而扭转 1 圈以后的 12 小时内睾丸都不会出现局部缺血[168]。对于青春期男孩，坏死通常发生于症状出现 24 小时后，但也可以短于 2 小时[95,162]。

1761 年，Morgagni 描述了睾丸附件的存在，因此，目前睾丸附件也被称作 Morgagni 附件[86]。该附件被认为属于胚胎期苗勒氏管头端或是中肾旁管的遗迹。多于 90% 的男性体内残留该附件，直径 1～10 mm不等。4 个睾丸附件之中，Morgagni 附件是扭转发生频率最高的。其他的睾丸附件包括属于午非管残留的附睾附件、旁睾及迷走小管。这些残留结构在组织学上有相似表现，均由呈胶态的结缔组织与血管构成，被覆柱状上皮细胞。Morgagni 附件通常基底狭小如蒂柄，这一结构是扭转的易发因素。睾丸附件扭转的好发年龄在 11 岁左右。这一发病高峰恰巧处于青春期开始阶段，疾病发生可能与青春期前雌激素刺激有关[26,155,166]。

阴囊的炎症表现常被称作睾丸附睾炎，即便通常

在青春期前只有附睾单独受累。青春期以后，附睾炎
1206 罕见，而睾丸附睾炎多发。腮腺炎病毒多影响青春期后的睾丸，而非青春期前。青春期前的附睾炎症通常由于细菌沿输精管经泌尿道逆行性感染所致。大肠埃希菌是常见的致病菌，泌尿道先天性畸形或尿道操作往往是造成感染的易发因素。目前儿童期罹患睾丸附睾炎的最常见人群是那些患有脊柱裂需要间歇性导尿的男孩，偶见于肛门闭锁及直肠尿道瘘的婴儿。

自发性阴囊水肿有时需要与睾丸扭转或睾丸附件扭转相鉴别。前者的症状是阴囊水肿迅速从腹股沟区、阴茎、会阴等处发展而来，或向上述区域扩散而去。阴囊水肿的原因并不总是很明显，但也许和细菌性蜂窝织炎或特异性变态反应有关。

阴囊脂肪坏死是一种罕见的疾病，需要与睾丸扭转鉴别。该病的特征性表现是突然出现的局部压痛，两侧阴囊皮肤上常常有小肿块出现。肥胖是疾病的易感因素，可能有在冷水里游泳的病史。

临床特点

睾丸扭转常见于青春期儿童，但在青春期开始以前，睾丸附件扭转更多见（表 75–3）。睾丸扭转的发病年龄有两个高峰：新生儿早期及 13～16 岁的青春期男孩。一项研究回顾了 771 例年龄 16 岁以下的阴囊急症儿童，发现其中 58% 属于睾丸附件扭转，29% 属于睾丸扭转，另有 13% 的儿童被诊断为附睾炎，但其中不少患者随后发现患有睾丸附件扭转，而在之前却被临床医生们忽略了[26]。

睾丸扭转的临床表现通常以突然出现的睾丸疼痛为前驱症状，疼痛可波及下腹部或腹股沟，伴有恶心和呕吐。发病偶尔表现为渐进过程，无严重疼痛，导致诊断延误。之前短时间持续的性质相似的疼痛往往提示睾丸不全扭转而后自行复位的发生。男童站立时睾丸呈水平方向提示其在精索的附着位置较高。除非睾丸和附睾已经坏死，否则在触碰阴囊局部时会感到异常疼痛。患侧阴囊迅速变红、水肿，如果不能得到及时治疗，睾丸梗死形成使半边阴囊皮肤将变成蓝紫色。由于腹膜和鞘膜的限制，这种炎症体征通常在患侧阴囊的边缘突然终止。水肿渗出液进入鞘膜，造成反应性鞘膜积液，这一现象使体征解释起来更困难（见图 75–5）。

表 75–3　阴囊急症原因

病理	频度	发病年龄
鞘膜外睾丸扭转	少见	围生期
鞘膜内睾丸扭转	常见	任何年龄，13～16 岁为发病高峰
睾丸附件扭转	非常多见	任何年龄，11 岁为发病高峰
附睾炎	罕见	0～6 个月
流行性腮腺炎并发睾丸炎	少见	只在青春期以后
自发性阴囊水肿	少见	0～5 岁
阴囊脂肪坏死	罕见	5～15 岁

睾丸附件扭转的临床表现几乎与睾丸扭转一样，但疼痛程度一般较轻。在阴囊皮肤相当于睾丸上极的位置可见紫黑斑（blue–dot 征），触摸局部时可引起患者剧烈疼痛，相反，对睾丸整体的触诊仅造成轻微不适。附件扭转导致附睾炎症程度不一。一旦疾病造成阴囊继发性地出现水肿和炎症时，再试图鉴别睾丸附件扭转和睾丸扭转几乎是不可能的。

辅助检查包括放射性同位素扫描和多普勒超声，以明确阴囊急症时睾丸的血液供应情况[133,186]。一般说来，上述方法只对青春期以后的患儿有意义，因为发育以后的睾丸已经有足够的体积供仪器探查，从而使结果具有高度准确性。相反，在青春期以前，睾丸体积只有 1～2 ml 左右，实验室检查准确度较低，临床实用性较小。笔者本人并不习惯对阴囊急症患者做这些检查，而倾向于急诊做阴囊探查手术，径路选择阴囊中线小切口。

治疗

阴囊急症怀疑睾丸扭转时需要立即行阴囊探查手术。选择阴囊中线切口，用电刀切开患侧阴囊。水肿的阴囊壁使鞘膜难以辨认，但是一旦其被打开，随着鞘膜内大量积液的涌出，鞘膜结构将会清晰地呈现在手术者面前。从鞘膜内托出睾丸，肉眼分辨睾丸是否存在扭转情况。如果睾丸外观血供良好，则可以把它放回阴囊，经切口切除扭转附件形成的囊泡样结构。

通常，在出血性梗死形成以后，睾丸附件形似黑豌豆。但是，有相当数量的睾丸附件在扭转后没有继发出血，手术可见其外观苍白。这些外观苍白的睾丸附件同样需要切除并送病理检查以明确是否存在坏死。

如果睾丸发生了扭转，手术复位的同时需要评价其活力。通常，这一方式对青春期前的儿童相对简单，复位后数分钟内，睾丸血循环即恢复。但对于青春期以后的儿童，尤其当病变继发出血时，判断睾丸的活力往往比较困难。在这种情况下，最好利用对侧阴囊探查的手术时间多观察几分钟，或许借助多普乐超声技术观察睾丸血流可以协助术中诊断。

1207 确诊睾丸扭转以后，一定要同时探查对侧阴囊，因为畸形往往同时存在于两侧睾丸上。仅仅用可吸收线在睾丸和阴囊壁之间固定数针是不够的。最好的方法是切除部分鞘膜，以不可吸收线将开窗鞘膜的边缘和阴囊壁进行固定[126]。这样，在睾丸表面和阴囊皮下结缔组织之间就建立了新的睾丸系膜，使之永久融合。固定不充分容易造成睾丸扭转复发[116,175]。

在一时无法判断睾丸活力时，对病变睾丸选择切除还是原位保留观察日后的内分泌功能，尚存在争议。目前充分的证据表明睾丸局部缺血会损伤血-睾屏障，对年龄大于 10 岁的儿童，将增加其精原细胞发生自身免疫反应的潜在风险[145]。一些缺血的睾丸在青春期时被手术固定，患者成年后的精子发生表现异常，这一潜在的严重并发症得到了临床医生们的关注。缺血引起的自身免疫应答在 10 岁以下的幼童中表现不明显，这是因为当时尚不存在血-睾屏障，精子发生也没有启动[120,180]。因此，根据笔者经验，对 10 岁以下的儿童，还是应该保留那些难以判断其活力的睾丸；而对于年龄超过 10 岁的儿童，笔者建议切除病变睾丸。

另一个引起争议的问题是，对于单侧睾丸因围生期扭转而明显表现为坏死的新生儿，对侧睾丸是否需要手术固定[34,121]。前文已经提到，围生期睾丸坏死的原因主要是在睾丸下降过程中出现了精索的扭转。然而，这些儿童中很大一部分对侧睾丸同样表现出固定不良或呈钟摆样，因而有潜在睾丸扭转的风险。很难对这些病例做出一个强有力的建议，但一些医生们仍然推崇早期行对侧阴囊的探查手术，尤其是对那些出生小于数周的婴儿。而出生 3 个月以后，睾丸引带将继发黏附于阴囊上，探查手术的作用会减小。

对间歇性出现睾丸疼痛的青春期儿童可以施行双侧睾丸固定手术，尤其对于那些临床体检时被发现睾丸横卧于阴囊内的儿童，手术的意义更为明显。差不多有 1/3 的青春期睾丸扭转患者曾出现过间歇性睾丸疼痛的病史。

精索静脉曲张

精索静脉丛中睾丸静脉扩张可引起精索静脉曲张[83]。由此造成精索静脉内热量交换的逆流倍增机制破坏，睾丸与阴囊的温度上升。异常增高的温度可以被温度计测量到，高温逐渐引起睾丸与附睾功能不良，继而可能导致睾丸萎缩和发育不育[29,190]。这一现象最早由 Tulloch 报道[177]。也许睾丸萎缩只有在患者成年以后才有明显表现，但有证据表明，早在青春期阶段，睾丸就有异常表现[144]。男性中，精索静脉曲张的总体发病率是 15%，在临床不育的患者中，20%～40% 的患者出现此病。10 岁以下的儿童中，精索静脉曲张的发生非常罕见，但在青春期末期儿童中，该病的发病率与成年人相似[137]。年幼儿中，精索静脉曲张可继发于肾母细胞瘤、神经母细胞瘤及肾积水，其发病机制是原发病造成了睾丸静脉回流障碍。精索静脉曲张好发于左侧，右侧精索静脉曲张很可能提示腹膜后存在肿瘤。

临床表现

精索静脉曲张表现为阴囊上部质软、扩张的团块（图 75-6）。左侧发病占总数的 80%～90%，双侧发病占 2%～20%，右侧发病占 1%～7%[159]。仰卧位时，可以观察到左半侧多余的阴囊皮肤，左侧睾丸横卧于阴囊内[32]。站立时，曲张的精索静脉内充满血液，造成典型的“蚯蚓团”状外观。通常，病损不会引起疼痛，但患儿可能会主诉阴囊坠胀感。

按照静脉扩张程度，精索静脉曲张可以分成Ⅰ～Ⅲ级，或轻度、中度和重度。轻度（Ⅰ级）精索静脉曲张可以在患者做 Valsalva 动作时观察到[127,169]，中度（Ⅱ级）精索静脉曲张无须做 Valsalva 动作就可以被触摸到，而重度精索静脉曲张时，静脉在阴囊内表现与占位性病变类似[174]。

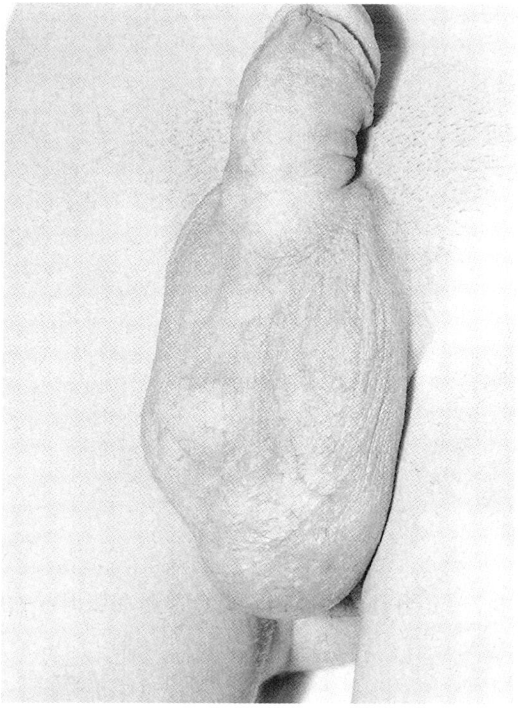

图 75-6　一名 14 岁男孩精索静脉曲张Ⅲ级，术前仰卧位时可见阴囊左半侧占位性病变。站立时，扩张的血管内血液充盈，形成“蚯蚓团”。

1208 病因学

左侧睾丸静脉缺少静脉瓣是精索静脉曲张的主要发病原因之一。尸检结果表明，40% 的左侧精索静脉内不存在静脉瓣，而相比之下，右侧精索静脉中只有 23% 无静脉瓣结构。同时，左侧精索静脉以几乎直角的形态注入左肾静脉，回流血管内的高压力状态是造成精索静脉曲张发病的另一个易感因素[2]。直立位时，静脉丛内的血液回流需克服阻力，回流路线较长，引起回流困难，静脉扩张。除此以外，还有一些其他的病因理论，包括静脉瓣被精索上的覆盖物损坏，左肾静脉压迫于肠系膜上动脉和主动脉之间，充盈的乙状结肠造成左睾丸静脉压迫以及左睾丸静脉起点处血管受到左肾上腺分泌的肾上腺素刺激而出现痉挛。在一项研究中，调查人员对 659 例患者进行了精索静脉造影，检查发现其中 484 例左侧睾丸静脉内没有静脉瓣结构[16]。另外 172 例患者虽然存在静脉瓣，但左肾静脉血流却能通过侧支循环注入睾丸静脉。103 例患者被发现肾静脉狭窄。精索外静脉（提睾肌静脉）也会出现皱褶，因 50% 的精索静脉曲张症中也可表现有精索外静脉扩张[22]。

由于睾丸血液受到 3 条独立的动脉供应，静脉回流路径同样不止 1 条。血液从腹主动脉经睾丸动脉（精索内动脉）到达睾丸，分支动脉供应输精管，而提睾肌动脉（精索外动脉）起源于髂外动脉和腹壁下动脉（图 75-7A）。上述 3 支血管在附睾尾部互相交通。睾丸与附睾的血液进入蔓状静脉丛，与睾丸动脉伴行。在超过腹股沟管内环水平处，精索静脉数量减少到 1 条或 2 条，最后融合成单一的睾丸静脉，右侧注入下腔静脉，左侧注入左肾静脉，后者成直角注入。静脉瓣可以阻止静脉血液倒流。静脉侧支沿输精管互相交汇至膀胱底，通过提睾肌静脉和阴囊静脉与大隐静脉汇合（见图 75-7B）。

精索静脉曲张的影响

精索静脉曲张可导致睾丸萎缩和成年后继发性不育，病因可能与局部温度过高有关[104]。但是，高温是如何造成睾丸功能低下的尚不清楚。在精索静脉曲张疾病中，许多激素功能和生理方面的参数异常都已经得到阐明，但是这些异常指标究竟属于原发性还是继发于疾病之后尚不能完全肯定。这一点在下丘脑-垂体-性腺轴缺陷中表现尤为突出[28]。尽管患者存在雄激素亚临床缺陷，但血清睾酮含量通常是正常的。成人睾丸萎缩时，大多数表现为睾丸间质细胞发育不良伴血清高浓度卵胞刺激素，这一情况已经得到临床认识[110,114,134]。青春期睾丸发育的抑制与其组织学改变有关，病变特征与精索静脉曲张造成成年不育时所见类同。睾丸萎缩时，促性腺激素释放激素刺激试验将造成垂体激素释放异常。

治疗指征 1209

治疗标准还存在争议，一般指征包括疾病造成患者长期疼痛或不适、青春期睾丸萎缩以及成年以后继发不育。Parrott 和 Hewatt[140] 主张在睾丸容积小于正常值 10% 以上时予以手术干预。Nagar 和 Levran[127] 建议对学龄儿童进行普检以便早期发现精索静脉曲张，而他们在对 800 名儿童调查以后，惊人地发现其

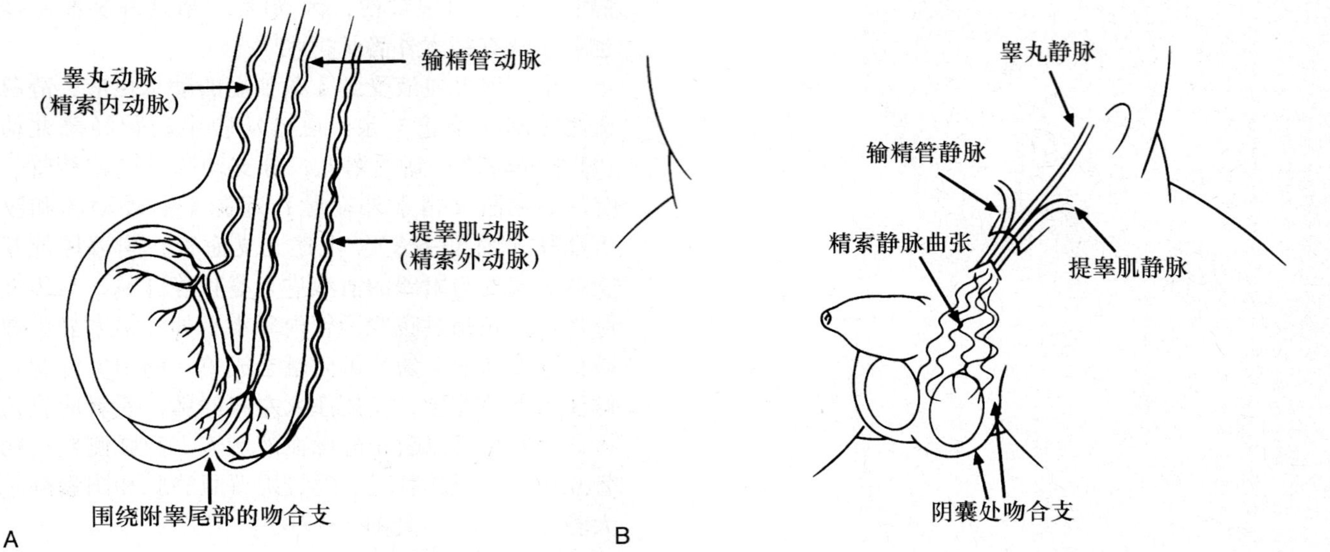

图 75-7　A. 睾丸、附睾和输精管动脉供应，血管网围绕于附睾尾。B. 睾丸静脉回流，图示精索静脉曲张时的血管网。（From Hutson JM：Varicocele and its treatment. Pediatr Surg Int 1995；10：509.）

中可确诊精索静脉曲张却没有明显临床表现的占到总数的近 10%。他们提出，筛查可以使疾病在较小年龄和早期阶段就得以诊断。他们推测，这样做应该可以改善患者成年以后的生育力，但最终结果尚需时间验证。对于成年不育患者，目前多采用多普勒超声排除亚临床型的精索静脉曲张[33]。但是，在青春期早期，由于患者睾丸容积和血流明显小于成年人，多普勒超声的可信度将明显下降。诊断或治疗性的静脉造影目前在男性精索静脉曲张中广泛应用[130,158]。对青春期患者，造影技术多在全身麻醉的基础上应用，虽然也有研究报道，在局部麻醉的条件下插入弹簧圈进行治疗性静脉造影治疗精索静脉曲张。

手术治疗

精索静脉曲张的众多发病学理论使其外科治疗有多种选择（图 75-8）。多年以来，腹股沟探查已经成为一个标准的手术方式，如同 Ivanissevich[89]、Sayfan 和他们的同事们[158] 所描述的一样，手术的主要技巧

图 75-8　精索静脉曲张不同手术方法。（From Hutson JM：Varicocele and its treatment. Pediatr Surg Int 1995；10：509.）

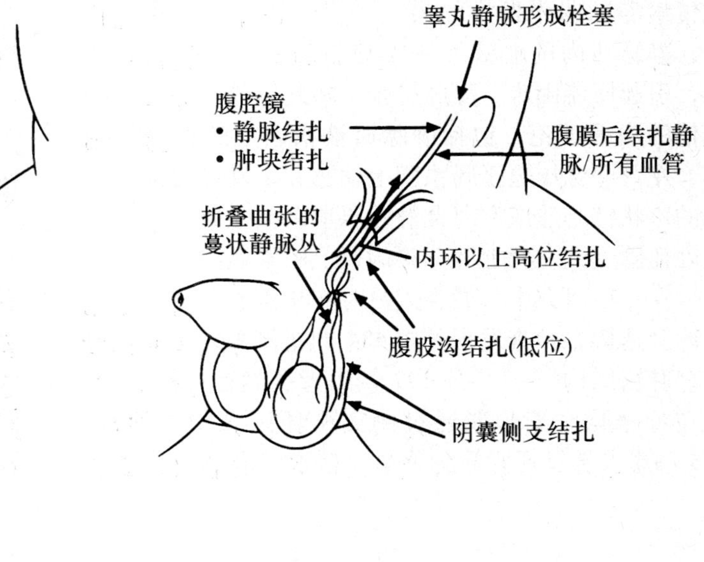

就是仔细结扎所有的精索静脉。过去，这一手术方式在实际应用中曾造成继发性的鞘膜积液高发病率，意外结扎睾丸动脉引起睾丸萎缩以及精索静脉曲张复发等问题[43,58]。这些不良的手术结果使人们对手术方式进行了不断研究改进，包括借助显微外科技术分离睾丸静脉、保留精索中的睾丸动脉和淋巴管结构。一些学者建议手术时注意区分动脉与静脉，以便保留动脉。为达到这一目的，医生们采用了多普勒超声和静脉造影手段，但它们在手术中的作用仍不能十分确定[58,66,111]。一些医疗机构还应用了顺行性注射硬化剂的治疗方式[117]。

Shafik 和同事们建议通过手术折叠精索外筋膜，以外力压迫蔓状血管丛的方法来治疗精索静脉曲张[163]。这一手术方法简单，但它不能彻底解决因肾静脉反流引起的精索静脉曲张。尽管目前还不十分明确，但如果术后静脉反流持续可能将导致疾病复发。

腹腔镜下手术可以在近腹股沟管内环处结扎睾丸静脉，这一方法目前非常流行[142]。一些作者建议在结扎血管时对静脉与动脉加以区分，以进一步保留睾丸动脉而仅结扎静脉。但另一些作者则认为这样做是完全没有必要的，手术时可以把动静脉作为一个整体予以结扎离断。许多文献不断证明了腹腔镜手术的简单易行，但不容否认，其长期随访情况尚不得而知[43,150]。

Palomo 是第一个提出在腹膜后范围，即腹股沟管内环水平以上结扎精索静脉时，无须区分动静脉而可以一并结扎离断的[139]。经观察，这一手术方式的成功率非常高，而术后睾丸萎缩的发生也很低，精索周围未遭损伤的并行血管为睾丸提供了充分的血液供应[72,97,140,150]。该手术方式的提出已经有很长时间了，但直到最近才得到广泛应用。许多临床医生担心睾丸丧失动脉后会继发萎缩，这一担心制约了该手术方式的推广。但是，如同 Palomo 所阐述的，只要保存了任何 2~3 支血管，睾丸的血液供应就可以得到维持。由于提睾肌和输精管保留完好，并行动脉可以为睾丸提供血液，而简单的手术步骤也避免了因误认精索动脉而意外结扎静脉。

Palomo 所采用的腹膜后结扎精索的手术方式也是笔者所采用的。笔者通常让患者家长选择是采用腹腔镜手术，还是以小切口行腹膜后的开放手术。腹腔镜手术方法与前文中介绍的相似，即采用的是一个
210 5-mm内镜窗口和两个 4-mm 窗口，其中 5-mm 窗口位于脐部，两个 4-mm 窗口，一个位于左侧脐水平，另一个在胃下水平。术者站在手术台右侧，助手站在左侧，显示屏置于患者左脚处。倾斜患者体位，使结肠倒向对侧。在距离内环数厘米处打开后腹膜，动脉和静脉一起，抓提整个血管蒂，以 3-0 的可吸收线缝扎。

开放手术同样简单，并可以建立在门诊手术的基础上。借助短暂的全身麻醉，于左侧髂窝内侧略低于髂前上棘处做皮肤切口，该切口通常距离腹股沟管内环几厘米处。沿肌纤维方向在靠近腹直肌处分离腹斜肌。一旦发现腹膜，则以剥离器将其向中线推开，钝性分离。在这一切口下，腹腔比较浅，向内侧略微推移腹膜即可立即暴露精索血管，通常位于入盆腔的输尿管水平以下。以直角钳从腹膜下游离出精索血管蒂，并用两根 3-0 的可吸收线连续缝扎血管。一般无须特别游离睾丸血管，但这样做也是一个选择。血管缝扎后移开拉钩，腹膜能立即回复原位。按常规方法，腹壁肌肉分层缝合，皮肤切口采用皮内缝合。由于这一方式不破坏腹股沟阴囊区的淋巴回流，而且精索与输精管和提睾肌之间的脉管交通都得到保留，所以术后并发急性鞘膜积液的风险低于一般手术。

结果

目前已知的精索静脉曲张术后并发症如表 75-4 所述。术后复发或精索静脉持续曲张的概率在 5%~45%[58]，发生鞘膜积液的风险在 7%~39%。最严重的并发症之一，即睾丸萎缩的发生与手术方式相关，由于报道罕见，所以不知道确切的发生概率。

根据报道，腹股沟径路手术可损伤髂腹股沟神经，腹腔镜手术可伤及生殖股神经与输精管。采用改良的 Ivanissevich 手术方式经腹股沟管手术的复发率是 16%。经腹膜后选择性地高位结扎精索静脉的复

表 75-4 静脉曲张术后并发症

疾病复发/持续	5%~45%
反应性鞘膜积液	7%~39%
睾丸萎缩	不详
髂腹股沟神经损伤	不详
输精管损伤	不详

发率是11%。有临床报道，采用 Palomo 手术方式成功治疗了 32 例儿童，术后随访无睾丸萎缩发生。据笔者经验，Palomo 手术方式为首选的术式。随着手术方式的不断改良，对精索静脉曲张的治疗方法也在不断变化，但就目前为止，无论是选择腹腔镜的手术方法还是选择采用开放手术，Palomo 手术方式都具有良好的预后。该术式在疾病治疗上成功率高、并发症少，与先前的众多手术方法比较，确实值得推广。

（孙 杰译 文建国校）

参考文献

1. Adamsen S, Bornesson B: Factors affecting the outcome of orchidopexy for undescended testis. Acta Chir Scand 1988;154:529.
2. Ahlberg NE, Bartley O, Chidekel N: Right and left gonadal veins: An anatomical and statistical study. Acta Radiol (Diagn) 1966;4:517.
3. Attah AA, Hutson JM: The role of intra-abdominal pressure in cryptorchidism. J Urol 1993;150:994.
4. Atwell JD: Ascent of the testis: fact or fiction. Br J Urol 1985;57:474.
5. Backhouse KM: Embryology of testicular descent and maldescent. Urol Clin North Am 1982;9:315.
6. Baker BA, Morley R, Lucas A: Plasma testosterone in preterm infants with cryptorchidism. Arch Dis Child 1988; 63:1198.
7. Baker LA, Nef S, Nguyen MT, et al: The insulin-3 gene: Lack of a genetic basis for human cryptorchidism. J Urol 2002;167:2534.
8. Barthold JS, Gonzalez R: The epidemiology of congenital cryptorchidism, testicular ascent and orchiopexy. J Urol 2003;170:2396.
9. Beasley SW, Bettenay F, Hutson JM: The anterior urethra provides clues to the aetiology of prune belly syndrome. Pediatr Surg Int 1988;3:169.
10. Behringer RR, Finegold MJ, Cate RL: Mullerian-inhibiting substance function during mammalian sexual development. Cell 1994;79:415.
11. Benson RC Jr, Beard CM, Kelalis PP, Kurland LT: Malignant potential of the cryptorchid testis. Mayo Clin Proc 1991;66:372.
12. Bergh A, Nikula H, Damber JE, et al: Altered concentrations of gonadotrophin, prolactin and GnRH receptors, and endogenous steroids in the abdominal testes of adult unilaterally cryptorchid rats. J Reprod Fertil 1985;74:279.
13. Bianchi A, Squire BR: Trans-scrotal orchidopexy: Orchidopexy revisited. Pediatr Surg Int 1989;4:189.
14. Bloom DA: Two-step orchiopexy with pelviscopic clip ligation of the spermatic vessels. J Urol 1991;145:1030.
15. Boddy S, Gordon AC, Thomas DF, Browning FS: Experience with the Fowler-Stephens and microvascular procedures in the management of intra-abdominal testes. Br J Urol 1991;68:199.
16. Braedel HU, et al: A possible ontogenic etiology for idiopathic left varicocele. J Urol 1994;151:62.
17. Brown TR, Berkovits GD, Gearheart JP: Androgen receptors in boys with isolated bilateral cryptorchidism. Am J Dis Child 1988;142:933.
18. Browne D: Some anatomical points in operation for undescended testicle. Lancet 1933;1:460.
19. Cain MP, Kramer SA, Tindall DK, Husmann DA: Expression of androgen receptor protein within the lumbar spinal cord during ontologic development and following antiandrogen induced cryptorchidism. J Urol 1994;152:766.
20. Canavese F, Lalla R, Linari A, et al: Surgical treatment of cryptorchidism. Eur J Pediatr 1993;152(Suppl 2):S43.
21. Cendron M, Keating MA, Huff DS, et al: Cryptorchidism, orchiopexy and infertility: A critical long-term retrospective analysis. J Urol 1989;142:559.
22. Chehval MJ, Purcell MH: Varicocelectomy: Incidence of external spermatic vein involvement in the clinical varicocele. Urology 1992;39:573.
23. Chilvers C, Pike MC: Epidemiology of undescended testis. In: Urological and Genital Cancer. Oxford, Blackwell Scientific, 1989.
24. Christiansen P, Muller J, Buhl S, et al: Treatment of cryptorchidism with human gonadotropin releasing hormone. Horm Res 1988;30:187.
25. Clarnette TD, Rowe D, Hasthorpe S, Hutson JM: Incomplete disappearance of the processus vaginalis as a cause of ascending testis. J Urol 1997;157:1889.
26. Clift VL, Hutson JM: The acute scrotum in childhood. Pediatr Surg Int 1989;4:185.
27. Colt GH: Torsion of the hydatid of Morgagni. Br J Surg 1922;9:464.
28. Comhaire F, Vermeulen A: Plasma testosterone in patients with varicocele and sexual inadequacy. J Clin Endocrinol Metab 1975;40:824.
29. Comhaire FH: Vasculature of the testis: Assessment and management of varicocele. In Burger H, de Kretser D (eds): The Testis, 2nd ed. New York, Raven Press, 1989.
30. Cortes D, Thorup J, Petersen BL: Testicular neoplasia in undescended testes of cryptorchid boys-does surgical strategy have an impact on the risk of invasive testicular neoplasia? Turk J Pediatr 2004;46(Suppl):35-42.
31. Costa WS, Sampaio FJ, Favorito LA, Cardoso LE: Testicular migration: Remodelling of connective tissue and muscle cells in human gubernaculum testis. J Urol 2000;167:2171.
32. Coveney EC, Fitzgerald RJ: Varicocele and the horizontal testis: A change in position? J Pediatr Surg 1994;29:452.
33. Cvitanic OA, Cronan JJ, Sigman M, et al: Varicoceles: Postoperative prevalence—a prospective study with color Doppler US. Radiology 1994;287:711.
34. Das S, Singer A: Controversies of perinatal torsion of the spermatic cord: A review, surgery and recommendations. J Urol 1990;143:231.
35. de Kretser DM, Risbridger GP: Changes in Sertoli cell structure and function. In Hutson JM, Beasley SW (eds): The Cryptorchid Testis. Boca Raton, FL, CRC Press, 1989.
36. Delasiauve LJF: Descente tardive du testicule gauche, prisé pour une hernie etranglée. Rev Med Fr Etrang 1840;1:363.
37. De Muinck Keizer-Schrama SMPF: Hormonal treatment of cryptorchidism. Horm Res 1988;30:178.
38. De Muinck Keizer-Schrama SMPF, Hazebroek FWJ, Drop SLS, et al: Double-blind, placebo-controlled study of luteinizing-hormone-releasing hormone nasal spray in treatment of undescended testes. Lancet 1986;1:876.
39. Diamond DA, Caldamone AA, Elder JS: Prevalence of the vanishing testis in boys with a unilateral impalpable testis: Is the side of presentation significant? J Urol 1994;152:502.
40. Donaldson KM, Tong SYC, Hutson JM: Prevalence of late

orchidopexy is consistent with some undescended testes being acquired. Indian J Pediatr 1996;63:725.
41. Elder JS: Two-stage Fowler-Stephens orchidopexy in the management of intra-abdominal testes. J Urol 1992; 148:1239.
42. Emmen JM, McLuskey A, Adham IM, et al: Hormonal control of gubernaculum development during testis descent: Gubernaculum outgrowth in vitro requires both insulin-like factor and androgens. Endocrinology 2000;141:4720.
43. Esposito C, Valla JS, Najmaldin A, et al: Incidence and management of hydrocele following varicocele surgery in children. J Urol 2004;171:1271.
44. Esposito C, Monguzzi GL, Gonzalez-Sabin MA, et al: Laparoscopic treatment of pediatric varicocele: A multicenter study of the Italian society of video surgery in infancy. J Urol 2000;163:1944.
45. Fallat ME, Hersh JH, Hutson JM: Theories on the relationship between cryptorchidism and arthrogryposis. Pediatr Surg Int 1992;7:271.
46. Fallat ME, Williams MPL, Farmer PJ, et al: Histologic evaluation of inguinoscrotal migration of the gubernaculum in rodents during testicular descent and its relationship to the genitofemoral nerve. Pediatr Surg Int 1992;7:265.
47. Farrer JH, et al: Impaired testosterone biosynthesis in cryptorchidism. Fertil Steril 1985;44:125.
48. Farrington GH: The position and retractability of the normal testis in childhood with reference to the diagnosis and treatment of cryptorchidism. J Pediatr Surg 1968; 3:53.
49. Favorito LA, Sampaio FJ, Javaroni V, et al: Proximal insertion of gubernaculum testis in normal human fetuses and in boys with cryptorchidism. J Urol 2000;164:792.
50. Favorito LA, Klojda CA, Costa WS, Sampaio FJ: Is there a relationship with anomalous insertions of the distal gubernaculum testis and testicular ectopia? Analysis in human fetuses and patients with cryptorchidism. J Urol 2003;170:554.
51. Ferlin A, Simonato M, Baroloni L, et al: The INSL3-LGR8/GREAT ligand-receptor pair in human cryptorchidism. J Clin Endocrinol Metab 2003;88:4273.
52. Fonkalsrud EW, Mengel W: The Undescended Testis. Chicago, Year Book Medical Publishers, 1981.
53. Fowler R, Stephens FD: The role of testicular vascular anatomy in the salvage of high undescended testes. Aust N Z J Surg 1959;29:92.
54. Frey P, Bianchi A: Microvascular autotransplantation of intra-abdominal testes. Progr Pediatr Surg 1989;23:115.
55. Gendrel D, Roger M, Job J-C: Plasma gonadotropin and testosterone values in infants with cryptorchidism. J Pediatr 1980;97:217.
56. Giwercman A, Muller J, Skakkebaek NE: Cryptorchidism and testicular neoplasia. Horm Res 1988;30:157.
57. Goh DW, Hutson JM: Can undescended testes be acquired? Lancet 1993;341:504.
58. Goldstein M, Gilbert BR, Dicker AP, et al: Microsurgical inguinal varicocelectomy with delivery of the testis: An artery and lymphatic sparing technique. J Urol 1992;148:1808.
59. Grocock CA, Charlton HM, Pike MC: Role of the fetal pituitary in cryptorchidism induced by exogenous maternal oestrogen during pregnancy in mice. J Reprod Fertil 1988; 83:295.
60. Hack WW, Meijer RW, van der Voort-Doedens LM, et al: Natural course of acquired undescended testis in boys. Br J Surg 2003;90:728.
61. Hadziselimovic F (ed): Cryptorchidism: Management and Implications. Berlin, Springer-Verlag, 1983.
62. Hadziselimovic F: Fertility and cryptorchidism. Am J Dis Child 1985;139:963.
63. Hadziselimovic F, Duckell JW, Snyder HM 3rd, et al: Omphalocele, cryptorchidism and brain malformations. J Pediatr Surg 1987;22:854.
64. Hadziselimovic F, Herzog B, Girard J, et al: Cryptorchidism—histology, fertility and treatment. Prog Reprod Biol Med 1984;10:1.
65. Hadziselimovic F, Herzog B, Seguchi H: Surgical correction of cryptorchidism at 2 years: Electron microscopic and morphometric investigations. J Pediatr Surg 1975;10:19.
66. Hart RR, Rushton HG, Belman AB: Intraoperative spermatic venography during varicocele surgery in adolescents. J Urol 1992;148:1514.
67. Haughey BP, Graham S, Brasure J, et al: The epidemiology of testicular cancer in upstate New York. Am J Epidemiol 1989;130:25.
68. Hazebroek FWJ, Molenaar JC: The management of the impalpable testis by surgery alone. J Urol 1992;148:629.
69. Herzog B, Steigert M, Hadziselimovic F: Is a testis located at the superficial inguinal pouch (Denis Browne pouch) comparable to a true cryptorchid testis? J Urol 1992; 148:622.
70. Heyns CF: The gubernaculum during testicular descent in the human fetus. J Anat 1987;153:93.
71. Heyns CF, Hutson JM: Historical review of theories on testicular descent. J Urol 1995;153:754.
72. Hirokawa M, Matsushita K, Iwamoto T, et al: Assessment of Palomo's operative method for fertile varicocele. Andrologia 1993;25:47.
73. Hoorweg-Nijman JJG, Havers HM, Delemarre-van de Waal HA: Effect of human chorionic gonadotrophin (hCG)/follicle-stimulating hormone treatment versus hCG treatment alone on testicular descent: A double-blind placebo-controlled study. Eur J Endocrinol 1994;130:60.
74. Hrebinko RL, Bellinger MF: The limited role of imaging techniques in managing children with undescended testes. J Urol 1993;150:458.
75. Huff DS, Hadziselimovic F, Snyder HM 3rd, et al: Early postnatal testicular maldevelopment in cryptorchidism. J Urol 1991;146:624.
76. Huff DS, Snyder HM, Hadziselimovic F: An absent testis is associated with contralateral testicular hypertrophy. J Urol 1992;148:627.
77. Huff DS, Wu HY, Snyder HM 3rd, et al: Evidence in favor of the mechanical (intrauterine torsion) theory over the endocrinopathy (cryptorchidism) theory in the pathogenesis of testicular agenesis. J Urol 1991;146:630.
78. Huhtaniemi I, Bergh A, Nikula H, Damber JE: Differences in the regulation of steroidogenesis and tropic hormone receptors between the scrotal and abdominal testes of unilaterally cryptorchid adult rats. Endocrinology 1984; 115:550.
79. Hunter J: A description of the situation of the testis in the foetus, with its descent into the scrotum. In Observations on Certain Parts of the Animal Oeconomy. London, Castle-Street Leicester Square, 1786.
80. Hutson JM: A biphasic model for the hormonal control of testicular descent. Lancet 1985;2:419.
81. Hutson JM, Sasaki Y, Huynh J, et al: The gubernaculum in testicular descent and cryptorchidism. Turk J Pediatr 2004; 46(Suppl):3-6.
82. Hutson JM: Orchidopexy. In Spitz L, Coran AG (eds): Operative Pediatric Surgery, Rob & Smith's Operative Surgery, 6th ed. London, Arnold Chapman, 2006.
83. Hutson JM: Varicocele and its treatment. Pediatr Surg Int 1995;10:509.

84. Hutson JM, Beasley SW: Descent of the Testis. Melbourne, Edward Arnold, 1992.
85. Hutson JM, Beasley SW, Bryan AD: Cryptorchidism in spina bifida and spinal cord transection: A clue to the mechanism of transinguinal descent of the testis. J Pediatr Surg 1988;23:275.
86. Hutson JM, Woodward AA, Beasley SW: Jones' Clinical Paediatric Surgery: Diagnosis and Management, 5th ed. Melbourne, Blackwell Scientific, 1999.
87. Hutson JM, Davidson PM, Reece LA, et al: Failure of gubernacular development in the persistent Mullerian duct syndrome allows herniation of the testes. Pediatr Surg Int 1994;9:544.
88. Hutson JM, Hasthorpe S, Heyns CF: Anatomical and functional aspects of testicular descent and cryptorchidism. Endocr Rev 1996;18:259.
89. Ivanissevich O: Left varicocele due to reflux: Experience with 4,470 operative cases in 42 years. J Int Coll Surg 1960; 34:742.
90. Job JC, Toublanc JE, Chaussain JL, et al: Endocrine and immunological findings in cryptorchid infants. Horm Res 1988;30:167.
91. Johansen TEB: Anatomy of the testis and epididymis in cryptorchidism. Andrologia 1987;19:565.
92. John Radcliffe Hospital Cryptorchidism Study Group: Cryptorchidism: An apparent substantial increase since 1960. BMJ 1986;293:1401.
93. John Radcliffe Hospital Cryptorchidism Study Group: Boys with late descending testes: The source of patients with "retractile" testes undergoing orchidopexy. BMJ 1986; 293:789.
94. Kanemoto K, Hayashi Y, Kojima Y, et al: The management of nonpalpable testis with combined groin exploration and subsequent transinguinal laparoscopy. J Urol 2002; 167:674.
95. Kaplan GW, King CR: Acute scrotal swelling in children. J Urol 1970;104:219.
96. Kaplan LM, Koyle MA, Kaplan GW, et al: Association between abdominal wall defects and cryptorchidism. J Urol 1986;136:645.
97. Kass EJ, Marcol B: Results of varicocele surgery in adolescents: A comparison of techniques. J Urol 1992;148:694.
98. Keel BA, Abney TO: Cryptorchidism-induced changes in spermatogenesis and fertility. In Abney TO, Keel BA (eds): The Cryptorchid Testis. Boca Raton, FL, CRC Press, 1989.
99. Koff S: Does compensatory testicular enlargement predict monorchism? J Urol 1991;146:632.
100. Koff WJ, Scaletscky R: Malformations of the epididymis in undescended testis. J Urol 1990;143:340.
101. Kogan SJ, Tennebaum S, Gill B, et al: Efficacy of orchiopexy at patient age 1 year for cryptorchidism. J Urol 1990;144:508.
102. Kreuger RP, Hardy BE, Churchill BM: Cryptorchidism in boys with posterior urethral valves. J Urol 1980;124:101.
103. Kropp KA, Voeller KKA: Cryptorchidism in meningomyelocele. J Pediatr 1981;99:110.
104. Ku JH, Son H, Kwak C, et al: Impact of varicocele on testicular volume in young men: Significance of compensatory hypertrophy of contralateral testis. J Urol 2002; 168:1541.
105. Kubota Y, Temelcos C, Bathgate RA, et al: The role of insulin 3, testosterone, Mullerian inhibiting substance and relaxin in rat gubernaculum growth. Mol Hum Reprod 2002;8:900.
106. Kumar K, Bremner DN, Brown PW: Fertility after orchiopexy for cryptorchidism: A new approach to assessment. Br J Urol 1989;64:516.
107. Lee PA, Coughlin MT, Bellinger MF: Paternity and hormone levels after unilateral cryptorchidism: Association with pretreatment testicular location. J Urol 2000; 164:1697.
108. Lee PA, Coughlin MT, Bellinger MF: No relationship of testicular size at orchiopexy with fertility in men who previously had unilateral cryptorchidism. J Urol 2001;166:236.
109. Lee SMY, Hutson JM: Effect of androgens on the cranial suspensory ligament and ovarian position. Anat Rec 1999; 225:306.
110. Lipshultz LI, Corriere JN Jr: Progressive testicular atrophy in the varicocele patient. J Urol 1977;117:175.
111. Loughlin KR, Brooks DC: The use of a Doppler probe to facilitate laparoscopic varicocele ligation. Surg Gynecol Obstet 1992;174:326.
112. Lrhorfi H, Manunta A, Rodriquez A, Lobel B: Trauma-induced testicular torsion. J Urol 2002;168:2548.
113. Luthra M, Hutson JM, Stephens FD: Effects of external inguinoscrotal compression on descent of the testis in rats. Pediatr Surg Int 1989;4:403.
114. Lyon RP, Marshall S, Scott MP: Varicocele in childhood and adolescence: Implication in adulthood fertility? Urology 1982;19:641.
115. Mandat KM, Wieczorkiewica B, Gubala-Kacala M, et al: Semen analysis of patients who had orchidopexy in childhood. Eur J Pediatr Surg 1994;4:94.
116. May RE, Thomas WEG: Recurrent torsion of the testis following previous surgical fixation. Br J Surg 1980;67:129.
117. Mazzoni G, Spagnoli A, Lucchetti MC, et al: Adolescent varicocele: Tauber antegrade sclerotherapy versus Palomo repair. J Urol 2001;166:1462.
118. Mengel W, Hienz HA, Sippe WG 2nd, Hecker WC: Studies on cryptorchidism: A comparison of histological findings in the germinative epithelium before and after the second year of life. J Pediatr Surg 1974;9:445.
119. Mieusset R, Fouda PJ, Vaysse P, et al: Increase in testicular temperature in case of cryptorchidism in boys. Fertil Steril 1993;59:1319.
120. Mininberg DT, Chen ME, Witkin SS: Antisperm antibodies in cryptorchid boys. Eur J Pediatr 1993;152(Suppl):S23.
121. Mishriki SF, Winkle DC, Frank JD: Fixation of a single testis: Always, sometimes or never. Br J Urol 1992;69:311.
122. Moerman P, Fryns JP, Goddeeris P, Lauweryns JM: Pathogenesis of the prune belly syndrome: A fractional urethral obstruction caused by prostatic hypoplasia. Pediatrics 1984;73:470.
123. Moore RG, Peters CA, Bauer SB, et al: Laparoscopic evaluation of the nonpalpable testis: A prospective assessment of accuracy. J Urol 1994;151:728.
124. Morgagni GB, cited in Jones PG: Torsion of the testis and its appendages during childhood. Arch Dis Child 1962; 37:214.
125. Morley R, Lucas A: Undescended testes in low birthweight infants. BMJ 1987;295:753.
126. Morse TS, Hollabaugh RS: The "window" orchidopexy for prevention of testicular torsion. J Pediatr Surg 1977; 12:237.
127. Nagar H, Levran R: Impact of active case-finding on the diagnosis and therapy of pediatric varicocele. Surg Gynecol Obstet 1993;177:38.
128. Nef S, Parada LF: Hormones in male sexual development. Genes Dev 2000;14:3075.
129. Nguyen MT, Showalter PR, Timmons CF, et al: Effects of orchiopexy on congenitally cryptorchid insulin-3 knockout mice. J Urol 2002;168:1779.

130. Nieschlag E, Behre HM, Schlingbeider A, et al: Surgical ligation vs. angiographic embolization of the vena spermatica: A prospective randomized study for the treatment of varicocele-related infertility. Andrologia 1993;25:233.
131. Nistal M, Paniagua R: Infertility in adult males with retractile testes. Fertil Steril 1984;41:395.
132. Nunn P, Stephens FD: The triad syndrome: A composite anomaly of the abdominal wall, urinary system and testes. J Urol 1961;86:782.
133. Nussbaum Blask AR, et al: Color Doppler sonography and scintigraphy of the testis: A prospective, comparative analysis in children with acute scrotal pain. Pediatr Emerg Care 2002;18:67.
134. Okuyama A, Koide T, Itatani H, et al: Pituitary-gonadal function in schoolboys with varicocele and indications for varicocelectomy. Eur Urol 1981;7:92.
135. Okuyama A, Nonomura N, Nakamura M, et al: Surgical management of undescended testis: Retrospective study of potential fertility in 274 cases. J Urol 1989;142:749.
136. Ombredanne L: Torsions testiculaires chez les enfants. Bull Mem Soc Chir Paris 1913;38:799.
137. Oster J: Varicocele in children and adolescents. Scand J Urol Nephrol 1971;5:27.
138. Pagon RA, Smith DW, Shephard TH: Urethral obstruction malformation complex: A cause of abdominal muscle deficiency and the "prune belly." J Pediatr 1979; 94:900.
139. Palomo A: Radical cure of varicocele by a new technique: Preliminary report. J Urol 1949;61:604.
140. Parrott TS, Hewatt L: Ligation of the testicular artery and vein in adolescent varicocele. J Urol 1994;152:791.
141. Patil KK, Duffy PG, Woodhouse CR, Ransley PG: Long-term outcome of Fowler-Stephens orchiopexy in boys with prune-belly syndrome. J Urol 2004;171:1666.
142. Peters CA: Laparoscopy in pediatric urology. Curr Opin Urol 2004;14:67.
143. Pike MC, Chilvers C, Peckham MJ: Effect of age at orchidopexy on risk of testicular cancer. Lancet 1986;1:1246.
144. Podesta ML, Gottlieb S, Medel R Jr, et al: Hormonal parameters and testicular volume in children and adolescents with unilateral varicocele: Preoperative and postoperative findings. J Urol 1994;152:794.
145. Puri P, Barton D, O'Donnell B: Prepubertal testicular torsion: Subsequent fertility. J Pediatr Surg 1985;20:598.
146. Puri P, Nixon HH: Bilateral retractile testes—subsequent effects on fertility. J Pediatr Surg 1977;12:563.
147. Raivio T, Toppari J, Kaleva M, et al: Serum androgen bioactivity in cryptorchid and noncryptorchid boys during the postnatal reproductive hormone surge. J Clin Endocrinol Metab 2003;88:2597.
148. Rajfer J, Handelsman DJ, Swerdloff RS, et al: Hormonal therapy of cryptorchidism: A randomised, double-blind study comparing human chorionic gonadotropin and gonadotropin-releasing hormone. N Engl J Med 1986; 314:466.
149. Rasmussen TB, Ingerslev HJ, Hostrup H: Natural history of the maldescended testis. Horm Res 1988;30:164.
150. Riccabona M, Oswald J, Koen M, et al: Optimizing the operative treatment of boys with varicocele: Sequential comparison of 4 techniques. J Urol 2003;169:666.
151. Rozanski TA, Bloom DA: The undescended testis. Urol Clin North Am 1995;22:107.
152. Rusnack SL, Wu HY, Huff DS, et al: The ascending testis and the testis undescended since birth share the same histopathology. J Urol 2002;168:2590.
153. Rusnack SL, Wu HY, Huff DS, et al: Testis histopathology in boys with cryptorchidism correlates with future fertility potential. J Urol 2003;169:659.
154. Russinko PJ, Siddiq FM, Tackett L, Caldomone AA: Prescrotal orchiopexy: An alternative surgical approach for the palpable undescended testis. J Urol 2003; 170:2436.
155. Samnakay N, Cohen RJ, Orford J, et al: Androgen and oestrogen receptor status of the human appendix testis. Pediatr Surg Int 2003;19:520.
156. Saw KC, Eardley I, Dennis MJ, Whitaker RH: Surgical outcomes of orchiopexy: I. Previously unoperated testes. Br J Urol 1992;70:90.
157. Sawchuk T, Costabile RA, Howards SS, Rodgers BM: Spermatic cord torsion in an infant receiving human chorionic gonadotropin. J Urol 1993;150:1212.
158. Sayfan J, Soffer V, Orda R: Varicocele treatment: Prospective randomized trial of 3 methods. J Urol 1992; 148:1447.
159. Saypol DC: Varicocele. Int J Androl 1981;2:61.
160. Scorer CG: The descent of the testis. Arch Dis Child 1964; 39:605.
161. Scorer CG, Farrington GH: Congenital Deformities of the Testis and Epididymis. London, Butterworths, 1971.
162. Sessions AE, Rabinowitz R, Hulbert WC, et al: Testicular torsion: Direction, degree, duration and disinformation. J Urol 2003;169:663.
163. Shafik A, Khalil AM, Saleh M: The fasciomuscular tube of the spermatic cord: A study of its surgical anatomy and relation to varicocele: A new concept for the pathogenesis of varicocele. Br J Urol 1972;44:147.
164. Singer R, Dickerman Z, Sagir M, et al: Endocrinological parameters and cell-mediated immunity post operation for cryptorchidism. Arch Androl 1988;20:153.
165. Skakkebaek NE, Berthelsen JG, Giwercman A, Muller J: Carcinoma in situ of the testis: Possible origin from gonocytes and precursor of all types of germ cell tumors except spermatocytomas. Int J Androl 1987;10:19.
166. Skoglund RW, McRoberts JN, Ragde H: Torsion of testicular appendages: Presentation of 43 new cases and a collective review. J Urol 1970;104:598.
167. Smith JA, Hutson JM, Beasley SW, Reddihough DS: The relationship between cerebral palsy and cryptorchidism. J Pediatr Surg 1989;23:275.
168. Sonda LP, Lapides J: Experimental torsion of the spermatic cord. Surg Forum 1961;12:502.
169. Steckel J, Dicker AP, Goldstein M: Relationship between varicocele size and response to varicocelectomy. J Urol 1993;149:769.
170. Stone JM, Cruickshank DG, Sandeman TF, Matthews JP: Laterality, maldescent, trauma and other clinical factors in the epidemiology of testis cancer in Victoria, Australia. Br J Cancer 1991;64:132.
171. Sutthoff-Lorey G, Waag KL: Die Pra und intraoperative Genebetemperaturmessung bei maldescensus Testis. In Schier F, Waldsschmidt J (eds): Maldescensus Testis. Munich, Zuckschwerdt Verlag, 1990.
172. Tanyel FC: The descent of testis and reason for failed descent. Turk J Pediatr 2004;46(Suppl):7-17.
173. Taylor MR: A case of testicle strangulated at birth: Castration: recovery. BMJ 1897;1:458.
174. Thomas JC, Elder JS: Testicular growth arrest and adolescent varicocele: Does varicocele size make a difference? J Urol 2002;168:1689.
175. Thurston A, Whitaker R: Torsion of testis after previous testicular surgery. Br J Surg 1983;70:217.
176. Tomboc M, Lee PA, Mitwally MF, et al: Insulin-like

3/relaxin like factor gene mutations are associated with cryptorchidism. J Clin Endocrinol Metab 2000;85:4013.
177. Tulloch WS: A consideration of sterility factors in the light of subsequent pregnancies: Subfertility in the male. Trans Edin Obstet Soc 1952;59:29.
178. Turek PJ, Ewalt DH, Snyder HM 3rd, et al: The absent cryptorchid testis: Surgical findings and their implications for diagnosis and etiology. J Urol 1994;151:718.
179. Uehling DT: Fertility in men with varicocele. Int J Fertil 1968;13:58.
180. Urry RL, Carrell DT, Starr NT, et al: The incidence of antisperm antibodies in infertility patients with a history of cryptorchidism. J Urol 1994;151:381.
181. Walker RD: Diagnosis and management of the nonpalpable undescended testicle. AUA Update Series 1992;11:153.
182. Whitaker RH: Neoplasia in cryptorchid men. Semin Urol 1988;6:107.
183. Wilson JD, George FW, Griffin JE: The hormonal control of sexual development. Science 1981;211:1278.
184. Wilson-Storey D, McGenity K, Dickson JAS: Orchidopexy: The younger the better? J R Coll Surg (Edinb) 1990; 35:362.
185. Woodhouse CRJ: Undescended testes. In Long-term Paediatric Urology. Oxford, Blackwell Scientific, 1991.
186. Wu HC, Sun SS, Kao A, et al: Comparison of radionuclide imaging and ultrasonography in the differentiation of acute testicular torsion and inflammatory testicular disease. Clin Nucl Med 2002;27:490.
187. Yamanaka J, Baker M, Metcalfe S, Hutson JM, et al: Serum levels of Mullerian inhibiting substance in boys with cryptorchidism. J Pediatr Surg 1991;26:621.
188. Zhou B, Watts LM, Hutson JM: The effect of Mullerian inhibiting substance (MIS) on germ cell development of the neonatal mouse in vitro. J Urol 1993;150:613.
189. Zhou B: Normal pre-pubertal development of spermatogonia in immature testicular feminized (TFM/y) mice with complete androgen resistance. J Pediatr Surg (in press).
190. Zorgniotti AW (ed): Temperature and environmental effects on the testis. Adv Exp Med Biol 1991;286:199.

第 76 章

肥厚性幽门狭窄

Marshall Z. Schwartz

历史回顾

1215 Blair[7]于1917年描述了一例死后尸解与肥厚性幽门狭窄相一致的婴儿。1888年Hirschsprung第一次完整地描述了肥厚性幽门狭窄[23]，他认为这是先天性的，与胎儿幽门内卷异常有关，并将其命名为"angeborener pylorusstenose"（先天性幽门狭窄）。Dufour和Fredet[12]于1908年提出，可通过分离肥大的幽门肌层至黏膜下层并横向缝合肌层以完成外科矫治。Ramstedt[46]于1912年提出不必缝合肌层，之后便建立了现在的标准术式。

婴儿肥厚性幽门狭窄（IHPS）是婴儿胃出口梗阻的常见原因之一。IHPS发病率在白种人中每1000名活产婴儿中有1.5～4人发病，但在非洲、美洲和亚洲儿童中发病率相对要低[35]。有报道称发病率还在上升[34,39]。众所周知男孩发病率比女孩要高，约为2∶1～5∶1[35]。IHPS由多种原因引起，包括环境和家族因素。

目前有观点认为IHPS是因机械性而非发育性缺陷引起。Wallgren[63]在对1000名男孩出生后立即行钡餐检查后未发现幽门解剖学异常，后来，其中有5例发生IHPS。类似的但更近期的研究连续对1400名新生儿行幽门超声检查也未发现异常[48]，但是其中9名婴儿之后发生IHPS。

解剖学与组织学

IHPS肉眼可见幽门呈增大苍白的肌肉团块，长约2～2.5 cm，直径约1～1.5 cm（图76-1）。组织学可见肌肉主要是环肌层明显肥大和增生[43]以及黏膜下层的增生[22]。肥大肌肉的免疫组化分析显示成纤维细胞、纤维连接蛋白、黏蛋白、软骨素、硫酸盐[45]、结合蛋白[19]、弹力蛋白[42]和胶原[36]增多。共聚焦显微镜可见异常扭曲增厚的神经纤维[29]。这些改变的直接结果就是幽门管的部分或完全性梗阻。

病因学

数十年来，IHPS的病因学已经引起学者们的极大兴趣。尽管大量的研究试图阐明IHPS的病因，但仍未确定起决定性的诱发因素。遗传与环境因素似乎都在病理生理学中起作用。遗传倾向的证据包括种族间的差异、明显的男性易患性、有家族史的头胎婴儿发病率增高以及某些ABO血型。Mitchell和Risch对

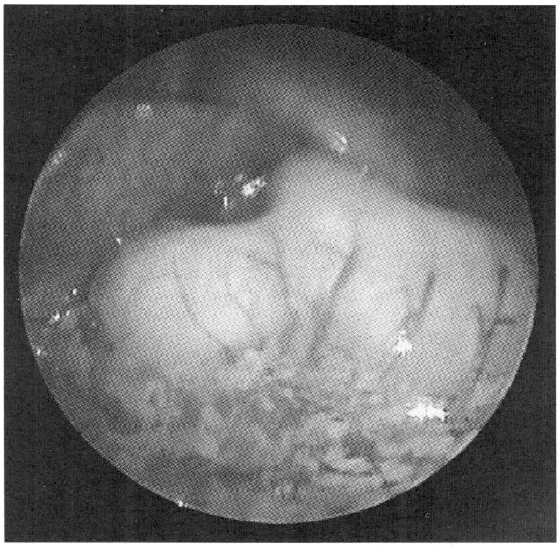

图 76-1　腹腔镜视野下肥厚的幽门。

1216 IHPS 的家族发病模式进行研究并提出，这与多因子遗传界限或多重相互干扰基因座的效应一致[35]。尽管幽门狭窄于男孩中更常见，但母亲患有幽门狭窄比父亲患有 IHPS 更容易引起子代患病。与 IHPS 相关的环境因素包括喂养方式（母乳喂养与人工喂养）、季节变换、琥乙红霉素接触史以及经幽门喂养的早产儿[25,35,47,58]。

另一个讨论焦点为幽门肌肉的松弛问题。一项研究指出幽门环肌神经节细胞减少[4]，但后续研究发现神经节细胞数量正常但发育不成熟[14]。Zuelzer[67]和 Jona[26]未发现神经节细胞有数量及超微结构的改变。随着新技术与新概念的发展，已有更多新的相关报道，包括 IHPS 与胃肠肽、生长因子、神经营养因子、神经发育的变化以及一氧化氮有关。

生长因子和胃肠肽

在过去的几十年中，通过直接或间接的方法已证明许多胃肠肽和生长因子与该病有因果关系，其中包括胃泌素、P 物质、表皮生长因子（EGF）、转化生长因子-α（TGF-α）、胰岛素样生长因子-I、生长抑素、胰泌素、肠高血糖素及神经降压素[10,56]。其他肽类也被证实可能与 IHPS 有潜在关系。P 物质是一种控制肠壁肌肉收缩的神经递质，可以引起慢性幽门痉挛导致肌肉肥厚[60]。此肽在 IHPS 患者幽门肌肉中浓度很高。Shima 等发现患者中 EGF、TGF-α 和胰岛素样生长因子-I 基因表达增高以及 EGF、TGF-α 免疫染色增强[40,53,54]。生长抑素、胰泌素、肠高血糖素和神经降压素也被提及[10,11,21]，但其作用仍未明确，也未证实明显与病因有关。

神经营养因子、神经发育和神经功能

神经营养因子对神经的分化及存活十分重要，已注意到在 IHPS 患者体内是减少的。进一步的研究表明，这些神经营养因子的特异性受体之一酪氨酸激酶 A 受体 c 试剂盒，在 IHPS 组织中不表达[20,61,65]。研究者们还发现 IHPS 的幽门缺乏神经胶质诱导生长因子，这也许暗示肠道神经系统发育不成熟[18]。

其他技术也被用来评估幽门的神经分布。Okazaki 等应用单克隆抗体标记神经末梢和神经微丝[41]，发现 IHPS 患者两种神经元素密度均降低。Kobavashi 等证实 IHPS 患儿环肌与纵肌层中神经支持细胞减少[30]。Piotrowska 等发现 IHPS 患者肌肉活检标本中胃肠道的起搏细胞即星形胶质细胞减少，以及在星形胶质细胞与平滑肌细胞间起联系作用的亚铁血红素加氧酶-2 缺乏[44]。

一氧化氮

一氧化氮可以诱导食管、胃和肠道平滑肌松弛。有理由相信幽门肌肉一氧化氮缺乏可导致肌肉无法松弛[1,57,59]。有人对 IHPS 患者肥大的幽门肌肉壁取活检，测量烟酰胺腺嘌呤二核苷酸磷酸（NADPH）黄递酶（本质上等同于一氧化氮合酶）后发现，肥大的幽门环肌未显示出任何 NADPH 黄递酶活性，但是幽门纵肌显示出正常活性。作者得出结论，幽门组织一氧化氮合酶缺乏可导致幽门痉挛并引起 IHPS[62]。

因此，目前 IHPS 的原因尚未明确定论。但不管其机制如何，必须认识到 IHPS 通常发生于出生后几周，幽门环肌肥大只是暂时性的甚至不需要肌切开术。但很明显，不管是什么机制触发了 IHPS，都可造成细胞结构和功能的巨大改变，该现象可能会引起更广泛的思考解决途径。

临床表现和鉴别诊断

IHPS 患儿典型临床表现为出生后 2～8 周出现非胆汁性的呕吐，高峰时间为 3～5 周。然而 IHPS 已可于出生时[66]甚至宫内诊断[27]。开始时呕吐可能并不频繁或剧烈，但经过几天时间可发展为几乎每次进食后就呕吐且变得剧烈（喷射性）。偶尔可因胃炎或食管炎而呕吐物呈血性，呈现出褐色或咖啡色。IHPS 患儿呕吐后有饥饿感，并且不显示出病态或发热。然而诊断的明显延误可引起严重脱水导致患儿嗜睡。一些患儿有腹泻（饥饿便）并被误诊为肠胃炎。大约有 2%～5% 的患儿因间接高胆红素血症而黄疸，可高达 15～20 mg/dL。我们认为这是继发于葡萄糖醛酰基转移酶缺乏[49]。早产儿 IHPS 诊断通常比足月产儿晚 2 周[58]，呕吐可能不呈喷射性且发展缓慢，易导致诊断延误。

如果没有进一步影像学评估，幽门痉挛及胃食管
217 反流很难与 IHPS 鉴别诊断。其他非胆汁性呕吐的内科原因包括胃肠炎、颅内压增高和代谢性疾病；外科原因包括胃窦蹼、幽门闭锁、胃窦幽门区重复囊肿和幽门肌内异位胰腺组织，发病率都低于 IHPS。

诊断

非胆汁性喷射性呕吐、左上腹肉眼可见蠕动波以及低氯低钾性碱中毒是 IHPS 的主要表现。75% 的 IHPS 患儿可通过上腹部详细体检明确诊断，但该方法已经很少被使用。内科医生经常首先要求影像学检查而非详细的体格检查。要成功触诊增大的幽门，患儿必须安静、注意保暖和合作。婴儿吸吮假乳头或少量喂食（5% 葡萄糖水溶液）可能会对触诊有帮助。如果胃扩张，经鼻胃管抽吸有助于成功触诊增大的幽门，通常描述为“橄榄样”。婴儿取仰卧位，腿屈曲以放松腹部肌肉，检查者手应放在上腹部。用指尖确定肝脏边缘后，轻轻深压肝脏并沿中线逐渐向尾侧移动，如果存在 IHPS，可在脐与剑突连线 1/3 处触及幽门。检查者必须耐心，必要时需要 5 ~ 15 分钟不间断触摸。检查者可在指尖下触及肥大的幽门以明确诊断。若未能触及幽门，则需要进一步确定呕吐的原因。IHPS 需与食物过敏、胃食管反流、胃窦蹼及幽门重复畸形鉴别，有时呕吐也可伴发肾上腺性腺综合征。

超声不但已经成为诊断 IHPS 最常用的影像学技术，也明显成为诊断 IHPS 的标准。在理想情况下，该技术准确度非常高，但这取决于超声检查医生的经验与专业知识。目前被普遍接受的超声检查阳性标准为幽门肌层厚度不少于 3.5 ~ 4 mm 以及幽门管长度不短于 16 mm（图 76–2）[28]。一些医学中心也测定幽门直径并认为超过 14 mm 为异常[28]。Lamki 等[32] 回顾其应用超声诊断的经验并得出结论，小于 30 天的儿童若肌层厚度达到 3 mm 应考虑为阳性。超声检查还可以免去 X 线检查的必要，避免射线照射。

如果超声检查不能诊断，上消化道（UGI）造影检查可有效诊断 IHPS。检查中可以发现延长的幽门管及胃窦轮廓处的凹陷，这是幽门肌肉增大的间接表现（图 76–3）。如果钡剂停留于胃中，就无法确诊 IHPS，因为幽门痉挛也可引起完全性胃出口梗阻。但

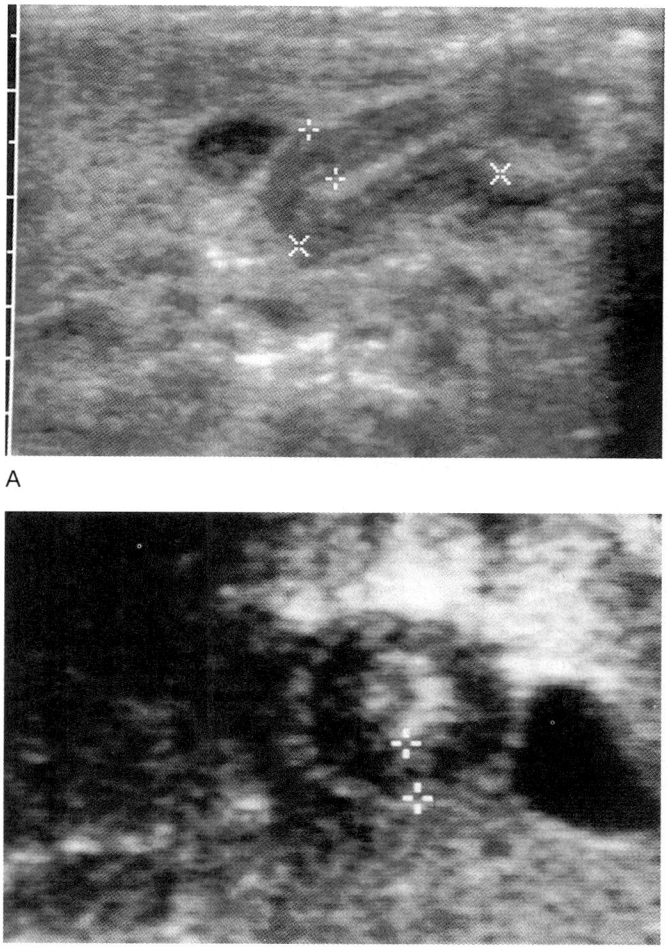

A

B

图 76–2　一名 5 周龄患儿肥厚幽门的超声图像。A. 纵向面显示幽门长（X–X）18 mm，幽门肌层厚（ + – + ）5.2 mm。（Courtesy of Dorothy Bulas，MD.）B. 横向面显示肌层厚度（ + – + ）。

如果花费足够长时间间断透视检查，应该可以鉴别两 1218
种疾病。建议放射科医生在放射检查结束后抽出胃中残留钡剂以避免术中倒吸。

1998 年我们团队对社区、大学及儿童医院的儿外科医生进行了一项有关 IHPS 诊断的实践模式的调查[3]。调查表被分发到 487 名符合标准的儿外科医生中，应答率 69%。91% 的被调查者表明他们在触摸到“橄榄样”幽门后不会行进一步诊断性检查。他们选择超声检查作为体检不明确时的诊断方法（约 86%）。最终有 82% 的儿外科医生在超声检查阳性时会进行手术，即使麻醉下体格检查结果为阴性。该调查结果表明选择超声检查可基本取代体格检查作为 IHPS 的诊断方法[3]。

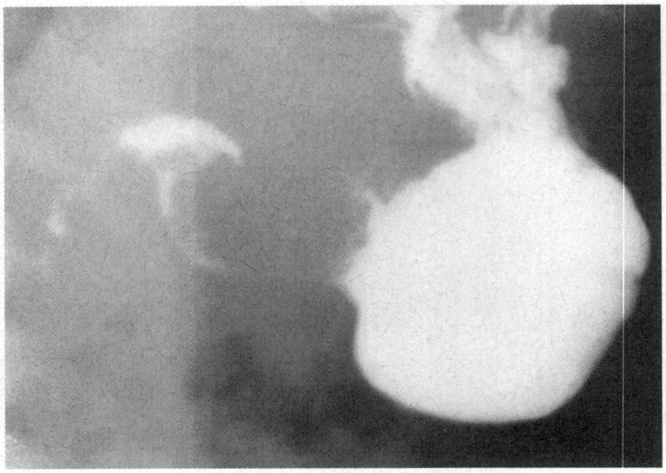

图 76-3　上消化道造影检查显示伸长的幽门管伴近端双角，间接证明幽门肌层肥厚。注意十二指肠球部的少量造影剂显示出肥厚幽门的长度。

治疗

术前准备

患儿充分适当的准备对于 IHPS 的麻醉与手术矫治是最重要的。术前准备的时间取决于水电解质紊乱的严重程度。Benson 和 Alpern[6] 主要根据血浆 CO_2 含量将严重程度分为三级（轻度，<25 mEq/L；中度，26~35 mEq/L；重度，>35 mEq/L）。除碳酸氢盐升高外，也会出现低钾血症、低氯血症、脱水和营养不良。

大多数 IHPS 患儿没有完全性胃出口梗阻，因此可以耐受胃分泌。术前应停止经口喂养，不必常规放置鼻胃管，因为这会从胃中吸走额外的液体及盐酸，可导致持续性电解质及酸碱失衡。

补液应基于脱水和电解质紊乱的程度。大多数 IHPS 患儿可给予 24 小时时段的补液。但在严重代谢体液紊乱的情况下，大量补液会引起体液和电解质快速转移，可能会导致癫痫发作及其他并发症。静脉内给予含有 20~40 mEq/L 氯化钾和 5% 葡萄糖的 0.45 生理盐水，这是补充水电解质的最佳补液方案。见尿补钾只会耽误治疗时机，原来有肾损害或有证据表明急性肾损害的患者是例外情况（很罕见）。低钠血症很容易处理。尽管如此，仍可以看到经常将生理盐水作为最初的补液，但没有理论证明生理盐水有用，因为它可通过稀释作用加重低钾血症并提供多余的钠。静脉补液疗法应根据脱水程度纠正。最初补液量应为正常需要量的 1.25~2 倍，直到体内达到足够的液体量为止。静脉补液中氯化钾的浓度应根据低钾血症的程度及输注量而定，同时要牢记氯化钾浓度不可超过 40 mEq/L，同时要检测尿量和血浆电解质情况，纠正血浆 CO_2 水平（目标为低于 30 mEq/dL）通常要晚于液体量补足和纠正血浆钾与氯水平。很少需要给予氯化铵或稀释盐酸。根据之前提到的，一小部分 IHPS 患儿会发生间接性高胆红素血症，临床表现为黄疸，但通常不用进一步监测高胆红素血症。在矫治术后，高胆红素血症会消退。

手术方法（开腹）

在手术室麻醉诱导前抽空胃很重要。如果之前进行过钡剂检查，建议通过胃灌洗和吸引抽出残留的造影剂以避免术中误吸。

选用的术式仍然为 Ramstedt 幽门肌切开术。该术式因其直观性、治愈性和极低的死亡率经受了时间的考验。标准途径为右上腹腹直肌上方或外侧、肝边缘正上方约 2.5~3 cm 横切口。在腹直肌上横向分离筋膜层，筋膜层向外侧牵开或从中纵向分开。除此之外还有其他几种切口[12]。另一种常见的可供选择的切口为脐上弧形皮肤切口，向上分离中线筋膜 1~2 cm。以非损伤抓钳抓住肝边缘并将其从切口牵出向上翻起以暴露胃大弯（近幽门），之后用湿纱布海绵抓住胃并向外下侧牵拉，幽门即可被拖出切口。用镊子直接抓住十二指肠或幽门会导致损伤或穿孔，因此应避免该操作。在肥厚幽门处用解剖刀沿胃窦幽门结合处至幽门静脉处切开肥大幽门前壁浆膜层（图76-4）。笔者和其他医生更倾向于使用解剖刀柄背侧钝性分离肥厚的肌层直至黏膜下层来完成手术（见图 76-4）。另一些外科医生倾向于使用幽门扩展钳如 Benson 描述的那种[5]。应在十二指肠端适当留一些完整的幽门肌纤维以减少十 121
二指肠穿孔的危险。大多数不完善的幽门肌层切开术是因为没有将切开处延伸至胃窦处。在将幽门放入腹腔前应仔细检查十二指肠与胃是否有漏。幽门肌层边缘或黏膜下层表面的出血通常是静脉血，几乎都会在幽门与胃纳入腹腔后止住。

幽门肌层切开术很少会穿破肠壁。一旦发生这种情况，应用好的吸收线间断缝合黏膜下层并在该点用

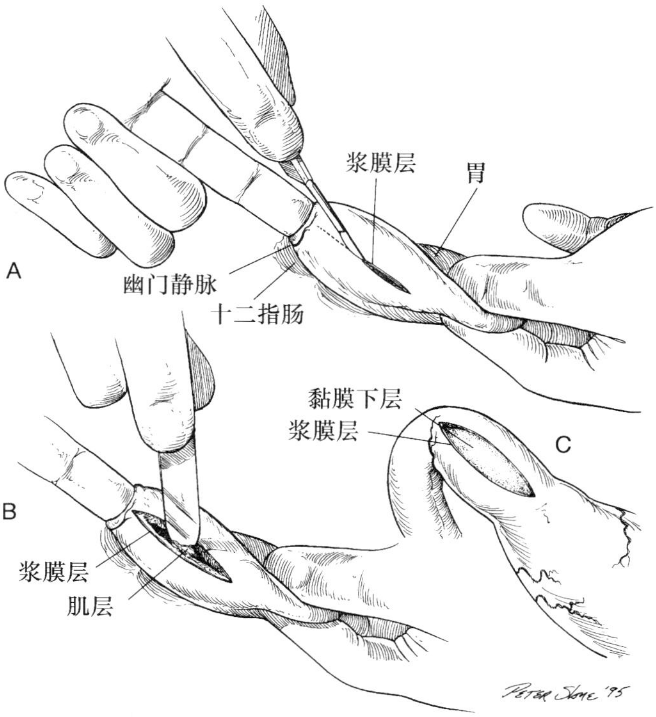

图 76-4　幽门狭窄手术操作。A. 从腹腔内取出幽门，术者食指顶住十二指肠端，助手抓住近胃端以固定。描出浆膜层切口然后开始操作。B. 用解剖刀柄背面劈开肥厚的肌层直至黏膜下层。C. 肌层完整切开可见黏膜下层经肌肉分开处膨出。

网膜覆盖。另一种可供选择但很少需要使用的方法是重新缝合切开点，180°旋转幽门，于幽门后壁行肌切开术，以可吸收线连续缝合腹壁筋膜层。皮肤可通过皮下缝合与免缝关闭并在表面贴 Op-Site 敷贴。

腹腔镜手术

1991 年 Alain 等首先报道了腹腔镜幽门肌层切开术[2]，后来有大量文献报道支持该术式，目前大多数医学中心都在采用。患儿取仰卧位置于手术台一端（图 76-5），于脐部置一 5 mm 的入孔并将 CO_2 注入腹腔，然后于左、右上腹（在镜头直视下）取两个辅助入口（图 76-6）。在局麻下用 11 号手术刀片做一个小的皮肤切口（3 mm），用关节切开刀穿透肌层，从左上腹切口置入一把抓钳，在幽门近端抓住胃窦部，用相同的方法将关节切开刀穿透右上腹切口，以抓钳固定

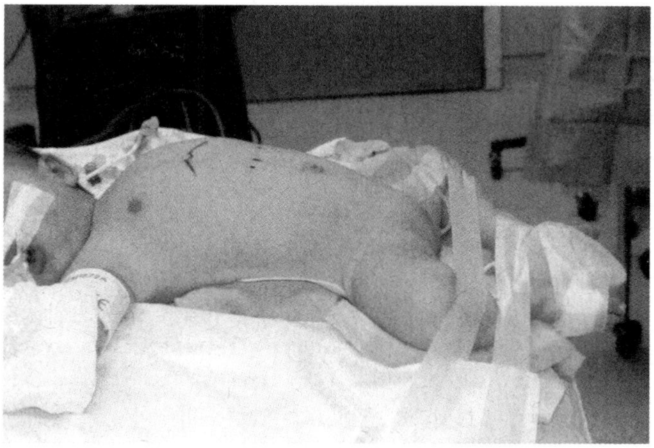

图 76-5　腹腔镜幽门肌层切开术患儿手术台上的体位。

幽门，用关节切开刀类似于开腹手术慢慢切开肥大幽门的浆膜层表面（图 76-7），收起刀刃，用关节切开刀刀鞘劈开肥厚的肌层，然后移去关节切开刀，将专门为腹腔镜手术设计的幽门扩展钳经右上腹切口置入。用该器械完成肌层切开（图 76-8）。手术完成后抓住被切开肌层的两侧向相反方向分离以确保肌层彻底切开。通过鼻胃管注入空气（通常为60 ml）以检查是否有漏。如果未发现，移去器械，抽去 CO_2 并移走脐部入孔，关闭脐部筋膜缺损并皮下缝合三处的皮肤。

开腹手术与腹腔镜手术的比较

虽然最初是麻醉的进步推动了腹腔镜手术的发展，但支持者们引证了许多腹腔镜手术的其他优点，包括术后恢复至正常喂养的时间较快、术后出院更早、术后呕吐发生减少及疼痛减轻[15]。然而主张开腹手术者认为两者恢复时间相近而腹腔镜手术并发症发生率更高，包括穿孔[9,13,15,55,63]、遗漏穿孔[13]、肌 1220
层切开不完全[13,64]、手术时间增加及费用增加[9]。他们对所有迄今已发表的研究进行回顾，得出的结论存在显著性差异。

已发表的文献中腹腔镜手术平均住院时间与开腹手术相近。4 组文献对住院时间进行了比较，只有一组发现有统计学意义，且差异仅有 4 个小时（表 76-1）[8,9,31,38,51,52,55]。

术后呕吐发生率差异较大。腹腔镜手术术后发生率为 1%～68%，而开腹手术则为 25%～65%，开腹

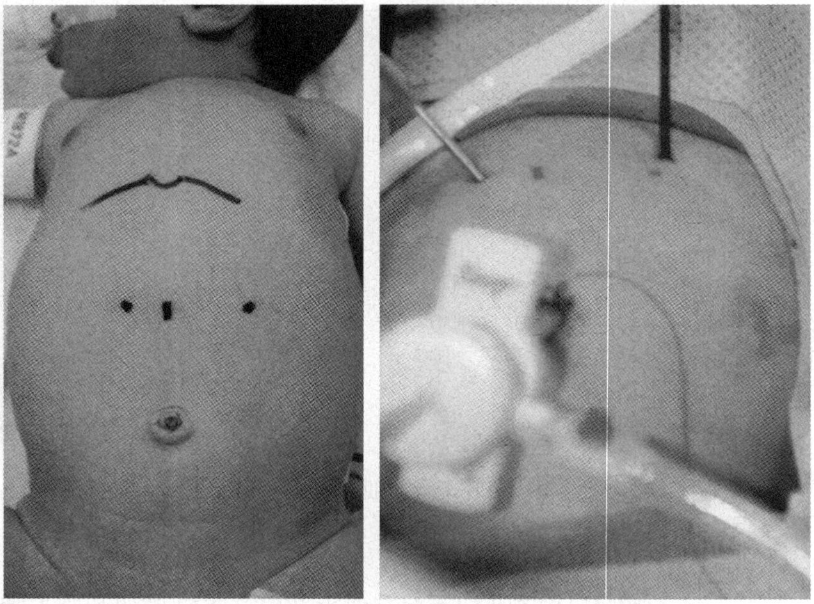

A B

图 76-6 入孔放置部位（A）及操作器械和内窥镜置入后（B）。

组与腹腔镜组之间差异无统计学意义[8,9,15,17,31]。

腹腔镜组恢复正常喂养的平均时间为 16～32 小时，而开腹组为 20～61 小时（表 76-2）[8,9,13,15,17]。如果排除 Fujimoto 无关项的研究，则结果无差异[15]。

两组伤口感染率相近，腹腔镜组为 0～6%，开腹组为 0～7%。没有研究表明两组间存在明显差异（表 76-3）[8,13,15,24,31,38,55]。

两组手术时间也相似，腹腔镜组为 24.3～41 分钟而开腹组为 18.9～32.5 分钟。Yagmurlu 等[64]（样本量最多的研究）指出腹腔镜手术比开腹组平均快4.7 分钟。 1221
而 Sitsen[55] 与 Scorpio[51] 等分别得出腹腔镜手术慢 14.3 分钟与 13 分钟的结论，但在各研究组中小样本量可能意味着研究时手术经验不足。另 5 组对照研究表明无统计学差异（表 76-4）[8,9,13,15,17,31,38,51,52,55,64]。

包括十二指肠和幽门损伤在内的穿孔率，腹腔镜组为 0.4%～10%，开腹组则为 0～6%。有 4 组对照研究发现腹腔镜组穿孔发生率稍高，但无统计学差异（表 76-5）[9,13,15,31,55,64]。

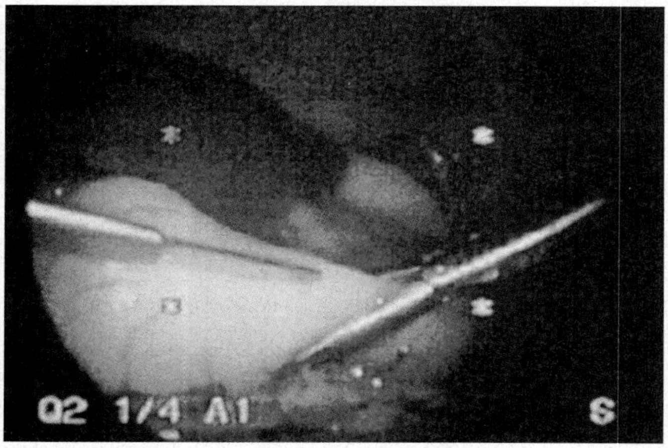

图 76-7 腹腔镜下使用关节切开刀切开肥大幽门浆膜层。

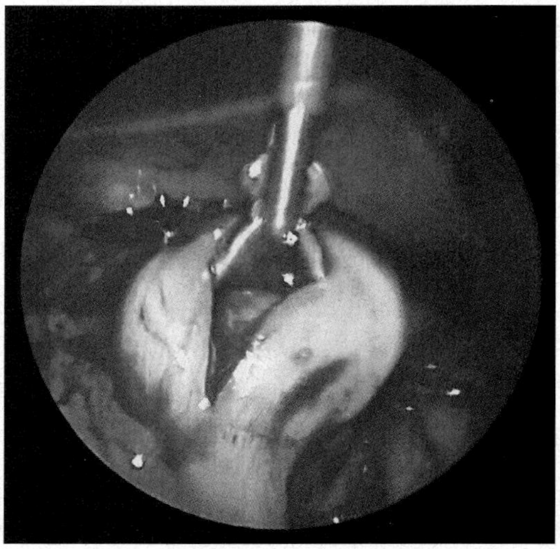

图 76-8 肥厚幽门肌层经幽门扩展钳分离后。

表 76-1　平均住院时间（小时）

作者	病例数	腹腔镜组	开腹组
Kramer WL 等	133	61.6	
Caceres M, Liu D	56	60	61.5
Campbell BT 等	117	31	28
Shankar KR 等*	86		58
Sitsen E, Bax NM, van der Zee DC	72	70	74†
Najmaldin A 等	37	28	
Scorpio RJ 等	63	44	63
范围		28～70	28～74

*仅为脐部入径。
†$P<.05$.

表 76-2　平均恢复正常喂养时间（小时）

作者	病例数	腹腔镜组	开腹组
Caceres M, Liu D	56	24.1	27
Campbell BT 等	117	19	20
Fujimoto T 等*	60	34.8	61.2†
Ford WD, Crameri JA, Holland AJ	84	32	41
Greason KL 等	25	19	23
范围		19～35	20～61

*仅为脐部入径。
†$P<.01$.

表 76-3　平均伤口感染率

作者	病例数	腹腔镜组	开腹组
Kramer WL 等	133	3%	
Caceres M, Liu D	56	0%	3%
Fujimoto T 等*	60	0%	7%
Sitsen E, Bax NM, van der Zee DC	72	6%	3%
Ford WD, Crameri JA, Holland AJ	84	3%	2%
Najmaldin A 等	37	0%	
Scorpio RJ 等	63	0%	5%
范围		0～6%	0～7%

*仅为脐部入径。

表 76-4　平均手术时间（分钟）

作者	病例数	腹腔镜组	开腹组
Yagmurlu A 等	457	24.3*	29
Kramer WL 等	133	29	
Caceres M, Liu D	56	36.1	32.5
Campbell BT 等	117	38	33
Shankar KR 等†	86		30
Fujimoto T 等†	60	27.4	31.9
Sitsen E, Bax NM, van der Zee DC	72	33.2	18.9*
Ford WD, Crameri JA, Holland AJ	84	41	28
Greason KL 等	25	25.4	26.1
Najmaldin A 等	37	29	
Scorpio RJ 等	63	40.2‡	27.3
范围		24～41	19～33

*$P<.01$.
†仅为脐部入径。
‡$P<.05$.

表 76-5　平均穿孔发生率

作者	病例数	腹腔镜组	开腹组
Yagmurlu A 等	457	0.40%	3.6%*
Kramer WL 等	133	3%	
Campbell BT 等	117	8%	4%
Fujimoto T 等†	60	3%	0%
Sitsen E, Bax NM, van der Zee DC	72	9%	6%
Ford WD, Crameri JA, Holland AJ	84	10%	6%
范围		0.4%～10%	0～6%

*$P<.05$
†仅为脐部入径。

表 76-6　幽门肌层切开术后喂养方案*

Pedialyte 溶液，30 ml 经口喂养每 3 小时一次
全能方案，30 ml 经口喂养每 3 小时一次
全能方案，45 ml 经口喂养每 3 小时两次
全能方案，60 ml 经口喂养每 3 小时一次
全能方案，75 ml 经口喂养每 3 小时一次
按需予以全能方案

*术后 4～6 小时开始喂养。对于特别小的婴儿，开始喂养量可减至 15 ml，并在达到 60～70 ml 时停止该治疗方案，因为这个量可提供足够热量。如果合适则可以此方案替代母乳喂养。

学者们还分析其他因素包括腹壁疝发生率（腹腔镜为4%~7%）[51,55]、白细胞介素-6 及热损失。Fujimoto 等发现腹腔镜组白细胞介素-6 峰值水平在术后24 小时内明显较低[15]。他们推测这可能表明患者应激水平降低。Holland 等发现腹腔镜较开腹手术可明显导致患儿体温降低，这可能会对生理有负面影响[24]。这些生物学指标显示了开腹手术与腹腔镜手术间的细微差别，但可能并无临床意义。

我们对迄今为止所有报道的文献进行回顾。随着腹腔镜手术经验的积累及外科医生学习曲线的缩短，该技术在不断发展，可能会成为常规操作。随着越来越大规模的腹腔镜手术研究指出了其与开腹手术之间在并发症发生率方面具有可比性，如疼痛或早期喂养之类的主观因素可能会减少，最终，两者之间的主要差异可能是腹腔镜手术费用的增加。但是对于由于客观条件限制无法很好掌握腹腔镜技术的外科医生，与其他方法相比，开腹 Ramstedt 手术仍然是治疗的金标准。

术后处理

大多数患儿可在术后 4 小时内开始喂养。因胃炎而呕血的患儿术后最好再过 6～12 小时进食。表76-6中列出了代表性的喂养方案。很明显，喂养方案越强力，术后初期呕吐发生率越高，但是该方法通常很有效且有助于更早出院[16]。表 76-6 所示喂养方案程度较温和，一般开始喂养后约 24 小时即可出院。将来患儿可在术后3～4小时即出院，并由家人在家中恢复喂养。

非手术治疗

该方法在北美地区从未被接受，过去只在几个欧洲国家应用过。虽然 IHPS 患儿可通过少量多次喂养来维持，但该方法需要的住院时间更长，同时需要周到的家属看护，并可能导致倒吸和营养不良。肥厚的幽门肌肉可能需要几个月才能缩小。偶发的死亡率导致该方法被废除。

1222 ## 并发症

如果由经验丰富的外科医生进行手术，术后并发症非常少。一般认为常于术后初期发生的呕吐继发于胃食管反流、胃蠕动失调和胃无力症，不应将其当作并发症。频繁呕吐持续超过 3～4 天可能说明幽门肌层切开不全或有未能预料的穿孔。术后造影检查可以确诊十二指肠漏但无助于诊断肌层切开不全。幽门影像学表现需数周才能改善[50]。幽门肌层切开术后持续频繁呕吐超过 1 周需重新探查。

预后

幽门肌层切开术后死亡率应很少发生，发病率也应该很低。在对一组大规模开腹手术患儿的研究中，穿孔发生率为 2. 3%，与切口有关的并发症发生率为 1%，只有 1 例死亡[5]。更近的研究报道的发病率与死亡率更低[37]。

随着腹腔镜幽门肌层切开术经验的增加，手术预后将会与开腹手术相近，再加上稍有力的术后喂养方案，患儿可在术后 24 小时内出院。

幽门肌层切开术后长期后遗症较少。Ludtke 等[33]评估了术后 17～27 年的 36 例成年人是否存在胃肠道症状，行胃排空闪烁成像并通过超声检查测量幽门。将他们的结论与年龄相匹配的对照组和性别相匹配的对照组进行比较，发现这些参数并无差异。

（王宇鹏译 董其刚校）

致谢

The author wishes to thank David Otterburn, MD, Pediatric Surgery Research Fellow, for his significant assistance in updating this chapter.

参考文献

1. Abel RM, Bishop AE, Dore CJ, et al: A quantitative study of the morphological and histochemical changes within the nerves and muscle in infantile hypertrophic pyloric stenosis. J Pediatr Surg 1998;33:682.
2. Alain JL, Grousseau D, Terrier G: Extramucosal pyloromyotomy by laparoscopy. Surg Endosc 1991;5:174.
3. Alavi K, Bauer TL, Wolfson PJ, Schwartz MZ: Pyloromyotomy without palpation: The new standard of care [abstract]? Paper presented at the Annual Meeting of the American Pediatric Surgical Association, Hilton Head, SC, 1998.

4. Belding HD, Kernohan JW: A morphologic study of the myenteric plexus and musculature of the pylorus with special reference to the changes in hypertrophic pyloric stenosis. Surg Gynecol Obstet 1953;97:322.
5. Benson CD: Infantile hypertrophic pyloric stenosis. In Welch KJ, Randolph JG, Ravitch MM, et al (eds): Pediatric Surgery, 4th ed. Chicago, Year Book, 1986.
6. Benson CD, Alpern EB: Preoperative and postoperative care of congenital pyloric stenosis. Arch Surg 1957;75:877.
7. Blair P: On the dissection of a child much emaciated. Phil Trans 1717;30:631.
8. Caceres M, Liu D: Laparoscopic pyloromyotomy: Redefining the advantages of a novel technique. J Soc Laparoendosc Surg 2003;7:123.
9. Campbell BT, McLean K, Barnhart DC, et al: A comparison of laparoscopic and open pyloromyotomy at a teaching hospital. J Pediatr Surg 2002;37:1068.
10. Christofides ND, Mallet E, Ghatei MA, et al: Plasma enteroglucagon and neurotensin in infantile pyloric stenosis. Arch Dis Child 1983;58:52.
11. Dick AC, Ardill J, Potts SR, Dodge JA: Gastrin, somatostatin and infantile hypertrophic pyloric stenosis. Acta Paediatr 2001;90:879.
12. Dufour H, Fredet P: La stenose hypertrophique du pylore chez le nourisson et son traitement chirurgical. Rev Chir 1908;37:208.
13. Ford WD, Crameri JA, Holland AJ: The learning curve for laparoscopic pyloromyotomy. J Pediatr Surg 1997;32:552.
14. Friesen SR, Boley JO, Miller DR: The myenteric plexus of the pylorus: Its early normal development and its changes in hypertrophic pyloric stenosis. Surgery 1956;39:21.
15. Fujimoto T, Lane GJ, Segawa O, et al: Laparoscopic extramucosal pyloromyotomy versus open pyloromyotomy for infantile hypertrophic pyloric stenosis: Which is better? J Pediatr Surg 1999;34:370.
16. Georgeson KE, Corbin TJ, Griffen JW, Breaux CW Jr: An analysis of feeding regimens after pyloromyotomy for hypertrophic pyloric stenosis. J Pediatr Surg 1993;28:1478.
17. Greason KL, Thompson WR, Downey EC, Lo Sasso B: Laparoscopic pyloromyotomy for infantile hypertrophic pyloric stenosis: Report of 11 cases. J Pediatr Surg 1995; 30:1571.
18. Guarino N, Shima H, Oue T, et al: Glial-derived growth factor signaling pathway in infantile hypertrophic pyloric stenosis. J Pediatr Surg 2000;35:835.
19. Guarino N, Shima H, Puri P: Structural immaturity of the pylorus muscle in infantile hypertrophic pyloric stenosis. Pediatr Surg Int 2000;16:282.
20. Guarino N, Yoneda A, Shima H, et al: Selective neurotrophin deficiency in infantile hypertrophic pyloric stenosis. J Pediatr Surg 2001;36:1280.
21. Heine W, Groger B, Litzenberger M, et al: Results of Lambling gastric juice analysis in infants with spastic hypertrophic pyloric stenosis (SHPS). Padiatr Padol 1986; 21:119.
22. Hernanz-Schulman M, Lowe LH, Johnson J, et al: In vivo visualization of pyloric mucosal hypertrophy in infants with hypertrophic pyloric stenosis: Is there an etiologic role? AJR Am J Roentgenol 2001;177:843.
23. Hirschsprung H: Falle von angeborener Pylorus Stenose. J Kinderheilk 1888;27:61.
24. Holland AJ, Ford WD: The influence of laparoscopic surgery on perioperative heat loss in infants. Pediatr Surg Int 1998;13:350.
25. Honein MA, Paulozzi LJ, Himelright IM, et al: Infantile hypertrophic pyloric stenosis after pertussis prophylaxis with erythromycin: A case review and cohort study. Lancet 1999;354:2101.
26. Jona JZ: Electron microscopic observation in infantile hypertrophic pyloric stenosis (IHPS). J Pediatr Surg 1978;13:17.
27. Katz S, Basel D, Brabski D: Prenatal gastric dilatation and infantile hypertrophic pyloric stenosis. J Pediatr Surg 1988; 23:1021.
28. Keller H, Waldermann D, Greiner P: Comparison of preoperative sonography with intraoperative findings in congenital hypertrophic pyloric stenosis. J Pediatr Surg 1987; 22:950.
29. Kobayashi H, Miyahara K, Yamataka A, et al: Pyloric stenosis: New histopathologic perspective using confocal laser scanning. J Pediatr Surg 2001;36:1277.
30. Kobayashi H, O'Briain DS, Puri P: Selective reduction of intramuscular nerve supporting cells in infantile hypertrophic pyloric stenosis. J Pediatr Surg 1994; 29:651.
31. Kramer WL, Van der Bilt JD, Bax NM, et al: Hypertrophic pyloric stenosis in infants: Laparoscopic pyloromyotomy. Ned Tijdschr Geneeskd 2003;147:1646.
32. Lamki N, Athay PA, Round ME, et al: Hypertrophic pyloric stenosis in the neonate—diagnosis criteria revisited. Can Assoc Radiol J 1993;44:21.
33. Ludtke FE, Bertus M, Michalski S, et al: Long-term analysis of ultrasonic features of the antropyloric region 17-27 years after treatment of infantile hypertrophic pyloric stenosis. J Clin Ultrasound 1994;22:299.
34. Mason PF: Increasing infantile hypertrophic pyloric stenosis? Experience in an overseas military hospital. J R Coll Surg Endinb 1991;36:293.
35. Mitchell LE, Risch N: The genetics of infantile hypertrophic pyloric stenosis. Am J Dis Child 1993;147:1203.
36. Miyazaki E, Yamataka T, Ohshiro K, et al: Active collagen synthesis in infantile hypertrophic pyloric stenosis. Pediatr Surg Int 1998;13:237.
37. Murtagh K, Perry P, Corlett M, Fraser I: Infantile hypertrophic pyloric stenosis. Dig Dis 1992;10:190.
38. Najmaldin A, Tan HL: Early experience with laparoscopic pyloromyotomy for infantile hypertrophic pyloric stenosis. J Pediatr Surg 1995;30:37.
39. O'Donoghue JM, Connolly KD, Gallagher MM, et al: The increasing incidence of infantile hypertrophic pyloric stenosis. Ir J Med Sci 1993;162:175.
40. Ohshiro K, Puri P: Increased insulin-like growth factor-I mRNA expression in pyloric muscle in infantile hypertrophic pyloric stenosis. Pediatr Surg Int 1998;13:253.
41. Okazaki T, Yamataka A, Fujiwara T, et al: Abnormal distribution of nerve terminals in infantile hypertrophic pyloric stenosis. J Pediatr Surg 1994;29:655.
42. Oue T, Puri P: Abnormalities of elastin and elastic fibers in infantile hypertrophic pyloric stenosis. Pediatr Surg Int 1999;15:540.
43. Oue T, Puri P: Smooth muscle cell hypertrophy versus hyperplasia in infantile hypertrophic pyloric stenosis. Pediatr Res 1999;45:853.
44. Piotrowska AP, Solari V, Puri P: Distribution of heme oxygenase-2 in nerves and interstitial cells of Cajal in the normal pylorus and in infantile hypertrophic pyloric stenosis. Arch Pathol Lab Med 2003;127:1182.
45. Pueyo Gil C, Oshiro K, Elias Pollina J, et al: Increase of the chondroitin-sulfate proteoglycan, fibronectin and fibroblasts in infantile hypertrophic pyloric stenosis. Cirugia Pediatr 2001;14:103.
46. Ramstedt C: Zur Operation der angeborenen Pylorus Stenose. Med Klin 1912;8:1702.

47. Rasmussen L, Green A, Hansen LP: The epidemiology of infantile hypertrophic pyloric stenosis in a Danish population. Int J Epidemol 1989;18:413.
48. Rollins MD, Shields MD, Quinn RJ, Woolridge MA: Pyloric stenosis: Congenital or acquired. Arch Dis Child 1989; 64:138.
49. Roth B, Statz A, Heinisch HM, Gladtke E: Elimination of indocyanine green by the liver of infants with hypertrophic pyloric stenosis and the icteropyloric syndrome. J Pediatr 1981;99:240.
50. Runstrom G: On the roentgen anatomical appearance of congenital pyloric stenosis during and after the manifest stage of the disease. Acta Pediatr Scand 1939;26:383.
51. Scorpio RJ, Tan HL, Hutson JM: Pyloromyotomy: Comparison between laparoscopic and open surgical techniques. J Laparoendosc Surg 1995;5:81.
52. Shankar KR, Losty PD, Jones MO, et al: Umbilical pyloromyotomy—an alternative to laparoscopy? Eur J Pediatr Surg 2001;11:8.
53. Shima H, Ohshiro K, Puri P: Increased local synthesis of epidermal growth factors in infantile hypertrophic pyloric stenosis. Pediatr Res 2000;47:201.
54. Shima H, Puri P: Increased expression of transforming growth factor-alpha in infantile hypertrophic pyloric stenosis. Pediatr Surg Int 1999;15:198.
55. Sitsen E, Bax NM, van der Zee DC: Is laparoscopic pyloromyotomy superior to open surgery? Surg Endosc 1998;12:813.
56. Spitz L, Zail SS: Serum gastrin levels in congenital hypertrophic pyloric stenosis. J Pediatr Surg 1976;11:33.
57. Subramaniam R, Doig CM, Moore L: Nitric oxide synthase is absent in only a subset of cases of pyloric stenosis. J Pediatr Surg 2001;36:616.
58. Tack ED, Perlman JM, Bower RJ, McAlister WH: Pyloric stenosis in the sick premature infant: Clinical and radiologic findings. Am J Dis Child 1988;142:68.
59. Takahashi T: Pathophysiological significance of neuronal nitric oxide synthase in the gastrointestinal tract. J Gastroenterol 2003;38:421.
60. Tam PK: Observation and perspectives of the pathology and possible aetiology of infantile hypertrophic pyloric stenosis: A histological, biochemical, histochemical and immunocytochemical study. Ann Acad Med Singapore 1985;14:523.
61. Vanderwinden JM, Liu H, DeLaet MH, et al: Study of the interstitial cells of Cajal in infantile hypertrophic pyloric stenosis. Gastroenterology 1996;111:1408.
62. Vanderwinden JM, Mailleux P, Schiffmann SN, et al: Nitric oxide synthase activity in infantile hypertrophic pyloric stenosis. N Engl J Med 1992;327:511.
63. Wallgren A: Preclinical stage of infantile hypertrophic pyloric stenosis. Am J Dis Child 1946;72:371.
64. Yagmurlu A, Barnhart DC, Vernon A, et al: Comparison of the incidence of complications in open and laparoscopic pyloromyotomy: A concurrent single institution series. J Pediatr Surg 2004;39:292.
65. Yamataka A, Fujiwara T, Kato Y, et al: Lack of intestinal pacemaker (c-kit positive) cells in infantile pyloric stenosis. J Pediatr Surg 1996;31:96.
66. Zenn MR, Redo SF: Hypertrophic pyloric stenosis in the newborn. J Pediatr Surg 1993;28:1577.
67. Zuelzer W: Infantile hypertrophic pyloric stenosis. In Welch KJ, Randolph JG, Ravitch MM, et al (eds): Pediatric Surgery, 4th ed. Chicago, Year Book, 1986.

第 77 章

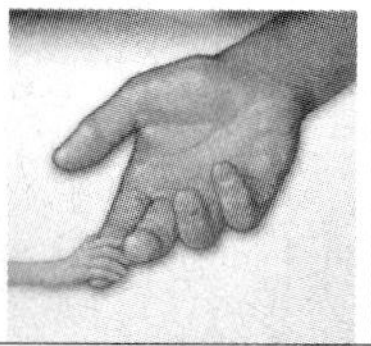

消化性溃疡及其他胃部疾病

L. R. Scherer III

急性和慢性消化性溃疡

1225 历史上消化性溃疡被认为是胃酸和胃蛋白酶联合作用于胃肠黏膜的结果。小儿消化性溃疡的历史可以追溯至 1826 年。1941 年 Bird 等对 243 例消化性溃疡病例进行了文献综述[16]，其中包括 119 例需要手术治疗的患儿。1～15 天患儿溃疡的特征性表现为无任何先兆或症状的急性出血或穿孔。而学龄前儿童通常在出血或穿孔前有前驱症状。消化性溃疡病因的多样性目前尚未公认，人们将这些差异归因于年龄。

消化性溃疡的学说及病因在以后的 45 年里保持一致。对具有溃疡样症状而无其他明确病因的患儿及由此引出消化性溃疡病家族史所做的详细组织学检验信息，在原发性胃十二指肠溃疡中很普遍[108,142]。Marshall 和 Warren[91] 于 1984 年报道原发性溃疡可能由细菌引起。继发性溃疡则证实由严重应激或危重疾病引起。本章沿用此分类法来讨论病因、诊断及治疗（表 77-1）。

流行病学

原发性消化性溃疡

儿童消化性溃疡发病率约为每年 5.4/10 万新发病例[97]。尽管男孩发病率比女孩高 2～3 倍，但在婴儿和小儿患者中，性别分布仍然相近。多种易感因素在各年龄层消化性溃疡患者发病过程中相互作用。

十二指肠和幽门前溃疡表现相似，常伴有高水平胃酸分泌。O 型血患儿更容易发病，与 A 型、B 型及 AB 型患儿相比其十二指肠溃疡发病率高 30%。成年十二指肠溃疡患者多为 ABH 血型物质的非分泌
型者，而消化性溃疡患儿中没有观察到这些物质的 1226
过度分泌[71]。胃溃疡（除位于幽门前位置外）主要发生于年轻患者，这些人通常胃酸分泌过少（但非无胃酸）且多为 A 型血。溃疡常发生于壁细胞和胃窦黏膜连接部[72]。

表 77-1　儿童胃炎和溃疡的病因及分类

分类/类别	病因
原发性	幽门螺杆菌
继发性	
胃酸分泌过多	Zollinger-Ellison 综合征 胃窦 G 细胞增生症 胃窦 G 细胞功能亢进 全身性肥大细胞增多症 肾衰竭，甲状旁腺功能亢进
应激	婴儿：产伤、新生儿败血症、窒息 儿童：休克、创伤、败血症、颅脑损伤、烧伤
其他情况	嗜酸细胞性胃肠炎 Ménétrier 病，肥厚性胃炎 淋巴细胞（天花样）胃炎 自身免疫性（萎缩性）胃炎 胃十二指肠 Crohn 病
药物有关	非甾体类抗炎药，不论有无幽门螺杆菌 阿司匹林 乙醇（酒精）

有人提出疑问，儿童消化性溃疡是否与成人发病情况相同，并已经注意到该病有明显的家族倾向。33%～56%的患儿一级亲属和二级亲属中有消化性溃疡患者[58,71,107,129]。同卵双胎消化性溃疡发病率也高于异卵双胎。儿童消化性溃疡遗传率经计算为每一级亲属0.91[71]，相对于成人0.37的遗传率要高。消化性溃疡阳性家族史对患儿而言是很重要的特征。在家庭个体成员感染幽门螺杆菌时，儿童原发性胃炎和消化性溃疡之间有一定联系[28,38]。幽门螺杆菌导致损伤的患者中胃黏膜炎症（胃炎）比溃疡多[39]。

目前证据显示，小于18岁表现出消化性溃疡而无其他明确病因者都为原发性胃十二指肠溃疡（见表77-1）。幽门螺杆菌于胃窦部种植，符合Koch法则成为人类病原体，引起儿童原发性溃疡和慢性活动型胃炎[159]。工业化国家幽门螺杆菌每年感染率估计为0.5%[52,90]，发展中国家则为3%～10%[121]。幽门螺杆菌传播途径为粪-口途径或口-口途径[4,51]。儿童幽门螺杆菌感染伴随的危险因素包括家族过密、地方病发源地、社会经济水平低下及种族特异性。幽门螺杆菌感染伴发的病变包括慢性浅表性胃炎、慢性活动性胃炎、原发性十二指肠溃疡、胃溃疡、Barrett食管、胃癌和MALT淋巴瘤[18,69,114,122]。

继发性消化性溃疡病

继发性溃疡（应激性溃疡）在儿童中常表现为继发于较大的身体或热创伤、败血症、休克或其他病重情况的急性溃疡（见表77-1）。应激性胃溃疡通常主要为发生于胃底部的多发性浅表黏膜糜烂。胃十二指肠溃疡的病因可为以下一种或三种因素的混合：(1) 黏膜血流量减少；(2)黏膜屏障的破坏；(3) 胃内酸性程度[1]。婴儿期和儿童早期消化性疾病80%为应激性溃疡[115]。药物和化学制品引起的溃疡在临床表现及分布上与应激性溃疡相似。但是因颅内疾病如脑肿瘤或头部损伤引起的溃疡通常为易于穿孔的单个深层溃疡（Cushing溃疡）。对成年患者的研究显示胃酸分泌过多与应激性溃疡或摄取药物引起的溃疡无关联[88,101]。相反，多数Cushing溃疡伴有胃酸分泌增加[90,116]。年长儿继发性溃疡通常具有单一性且深度较大（类似于Cushing溃疡），而非成人中常见多发性浅表性应激性溃疡。尚未有研究显示儿童应激性溃疡是否存在胃酸分泌过多。

过去通常认为儿童应激性溃疡与成人Cushing溃疡相似，因为两者都发生于十二指肠，具有单一性且侵蚀层次深；而成人应激性溃疡为多发性浅表性。随着儿童内镜技术的发展，发现儿童应激性溃疡的发病部位与成人相似，多发生于胃，但其他研究发现该病在胃与十二指肠的分布率相同[83]。Morden[103]等报道了10例患有严重内科疾病的病例，都有多发性胃溃疡。

Williams和同事[162]发表了1篇病例数最多的儿童应激性溃疡报道，194例主要由伴有严重烧伤的Cushing溃疡病例组成，其中100例由临床诊断，其余经尸检发现。63例明确发病部位的病例中有43例溃疡位于十二指肠。病例组中临床症状明显的胃溃疡在穿孔后才获得诊断。Grosfeld等报道29例病例中，胃与十二指肠损害分布几乎相同[56]。除1例外所有溃疡均为单发性；该患儿在尸解时发现多个溃疡。2例儿童溃疡继发于严重烧伤，但不伴颅内损伤。在另一组25例继发性溃疡中，损伤在十二指肠和胃的分布几乎相同[35]。这些研究中单个的胃溃疡通常位于幽门前区，临床表现与十二指肠溃疡相似。内镜技术优化了诊断手段，有助于更好地认识儿童溃疡病的表现和病程。最近，超过2/3接受过皮质激素或非甾体类抗炎药（NSAIDs）治疗的患儿发生继发性溃疡，表现为急性上腹痛[106]。

胃生理学和病理生理学

侵袭因子

早在妊娠19周胎儿胃已开始分泌胃酸，34周时出现胃蛋白酶分泌。足月儿可分泌胃酸和胃蛋白酶[19]。胃酸分泌不足发生于出生后5小时内，在之后的48小时内会增加直到pH稳定至3.0左右[61]。早产儿也能分泌胃酸和胃蛋白酶但少于足月产儿。33%的早产儿胃pH为碱性，20%的早产儿10天内无胃酸分泌。许多早产儿于4天时胃酸分泌量最大[106]。新生儿壁细胞总数每单位面积是成人的2～3倍[124]。婴儿在出生后1周～10天内胃酸分泌水平相对较高（表77-2）[61]。母体胃泌素分泌与壁细胞总数的增加和胃酸高分泌有关。胃酸分泌通常在出生10天后迅速下降[2]。在接下来的4个月内，胃酸和胃蛋白酶的分泌随着体重而非年龄增加，贯穿整个儿童期。 1227

表 77-2　胃十二指肠黏膜平衡的攻击和防御因素

攻击因素	黏膜防御因素
血管损伤：微循环减少	黏膜循环：足够的微循环
肿瘤化疗药物	上皮细胞更新因子
阿司匹林	碳酸氢盐分泌增加
非甾体类抗炎药	抑制胃酸分泌
传染因子：	维持血流/微循环
巨细胞巨化病毒，	
疱疹病毒	
系统应激：儿茶酚胺增加	修补上皮层表面
胃蛋白酶分泌增加	黏膜层：糖蛋白、多糖-蛋白质复合物
幽门螺杆菌	碳酸氢盐层：pH 梯度
	免疫球蛋白：IgG、IgA

有报道称消化性溃疡儿童体内胃酸分泌水平升高。与成人的研究相似，胃酸分泌增多对于诊断儿童消化性溃疡病并非必然有用。例如 Ghai[50] 应用加量组织胺试验对 18 名消化性溃疡病儿童及 16 名对照儿童进行研究，发现溃疡病患儿基础胃酸分泌并无明显增加，平均最大值和高峰酸排出量有增加，但两组结果有重叠；最大值和高峰值随患儿年龄和体重增加。Robb 等[129] 将 49 例十二指肠溃疡患儿与 30 例消化不良但无溃疡患儿进行比较，发现了年龄、体重和胃酸分泌量的相似关系，但未观察到两组之间胃酸分泌有任何不同。Nagita[112] 和助手测量了原发性消化性溃疡患儿和正常儿童胃内 pH 的昼夜变化，发现胃酸度随着年龄而增加并在 14 岁时达到成人水平。所有年龄段的胃溃疡组患儿平均 pH 高于同年龄对照组；十二指肠溃疡组患儿 pH 低于 2 的平均时间比已校正年龄的对照组患儿长[112]。

1984 年，Marshall 和 Warren[91] 报道在微需氧环境下成功地培养了人体胃窦黏膜处一种新型细菌（幽门螺杆菌）（见表 77-2）。成人复发的消化性溃疡可伴发主要涉及胃窦的胃炎。临床资料和实验室研究显示：幽门螺杆菌满足各项 Koch 法则，是人类慢性活动性胃炎的原因之一[159]。幽门螺杆菌是一种高自动力的 S 型革兰阴性杆菌，能够产生诸如尿素酶、过氧化氢酶和氧化酶之类的酶。以鞭毛支撑的幽门螺杆菌需微需氧环境培养，反映出它们因环境喜好穿过厚而黏稠的黏膜层至胃上皮层顶部[43]。所有感染幽门螺杆菌的患儿都逐渐患上慢性活动性胃炎。大多数为无症状感染，不会导致明显的临床症状。关于引起感染的机制的理论包括细菌产物尿素酶和空泡形成细胞毒素。尿素酶在胃黏膜表面将尿素水解为氨和碳酸氢盐。氨可直接对表皮细胞造成毒性作用，并伴发黏膜表面 pH 增加，影响胃上皮层功能，如分泌黏液[100]。最近，人们将注意力放到由特定幽门螺杆菌株分泌的空泡形成细胞毒素上。该细胞毒素于体外能在真核细胞细胞浆内产生空泡。这种毒素的基因（vac A）有两个等位基因并在隔离群内表达多样[127]。CagA，一种细胞毒素蛋白，在约 60% 幽门螺杆菌隔离群中被分离出来，且该蛋白的存在与空泡形成细胞毒素的表达有明显的关联[63]。分泌细胞毒素的菌株比细胞毒素阴性菌株有更强的毒力。目前一些研究者将菌株分类成 Ⅰ 型（细胞毒素阳性）和 Ⅱ 型（细胞毒素阴性）。Ⅰ 型菌株比 Ⅱ 型菌株伴发更严重的胃炎或十二指肠疾病[119]。

胃和十二指肠上皮细胞损伤开始于显著的免疫反应（见表 77-2）。炎症时胃黏膜层可有单核细胞、巨噬细胞、多形核白细胞和浆细胞[7,161] 浸润。在感染患儿炎症黏膜中可测得炎性细胞因子水平升高，包括干扰素-γ、白介素-1（IL-1）、IL-2、IL-6 和IL-8[143]。

防御因子

大量临床和实验室研究试图明确应激性消化性溃疡的发病机制。盐酸的存在是溃疡形成的必要条件，即使不存在分泌过多也如此，但 Cushing 溃疡除外。大多数促进应激性溃疡发展的因素减弱胃黏膜保护其不受胃酸损伤的能力，而非增加胃酸的分泌[147]。研究者普遍认为黏膜局部缺血也是消化性溃疡的发病机制之一（见表 77-2）[26]。通常少量氢离子会弥散入黏膜，但如果黏膜血流充足可迅速将其清除或中和。缺血会减少黏液分泌及中和胃酸进入组织的能力，导致氢离子的产生并继发溃疡[95]。缺血对能量代谢产生的不良作用可能是减弱黏膜防御损伤能力的额外因素。实验中出血性休克造成的黏膜损伤给予静脉输注碳酸氢钠有保护作用，这表明胃灌注动脉血的 pH 对 1228
于胃黏膜保护其不受胃酸损伤的能力也很重要[27]。这些发现说明缺血、能量不足和全身酸中毒在应激性溃疡发病机制中是重要因子。

在药物引起的溃疡中，药物可破坏黏膜通透屏障[102]。胃黏膜于胃腔内无法容纳氢离子，氢离子过度反扩散入黏膜细胞导致溃疡。上皮细胞和黏液细胞表层于胃的各处分泌稠厚的黏膜凝胶，黏液的分泌由胆碱能激动剂、前列腺素和炎性或免疫细胞因子激发。胃表面的黏液层约为上皮细胞表面的 20 倍且充满带电荷的蛋白质粒子。在生理情况下，这层黏膜可以提供有效屏障防止胃酸侵害。

前列腺素可以防止实验诱导的应激性溃疡的发展并起保护作用[98]。机制尚未明确但可能与前列腺素刺激氯离子转运出细胞外与碳酸氢根离子交换有关，这能阻断环磷酸腺苷（AMP）的生成。细胞内碳酸氢根的增加能增强细胞缓冲胃酸的能力。内源性前列腺素在维持胃黏膜足够血供、刺激黏液产生以及提高黏膜抵抗胃酸腐蚀方面也有作用[130]。皮质激素和 NSAIDs 已被认为是消化性溃疡病的致病因素。研究已证实前列腺素的细胞保护作用，并发现在 NSAIDs 和皮质激素治疗期间有溃疡发生以及胃内前列腺素水平降低。这些发现揭示了 NSAID 和皮质激素诱导的消化性溃疡发展的因果关系[106,144]。药物可损伤黏膜使其被胃酸消化导致继发性溃疡。阿司匹林是药物诱导的继发性溃疡的常见因素之一。另一种常用药物硫酸亚铁的过量使用也被认为是引起儿童溃疡的原因之一。关于皮质激素是应激性溃疡的促进因素的证据还存在矛盾[29]。虽然皮质激素和 NSAID 疗法与继发性溃疡发展之间的因果关系仍是争论的焦点，但越来越多的证据暗示了其因果关系[106,144]。一般来说，药物诱导的溃疡应该对停止用药和保守治疗有反应，除非发生并发症。

临床表现

儿童原发性溃疡病的临床表现易与许多疾病混淆，该相似性可夸大儿童溃疡病的实际发病率（表 77-3）。婴儿的临床表现包括拒食、持续哭闹以及呕吐[72]。阳性家族史儿童患病几率更高。多项研究证实双亲感染的特定人群中，特别是母亲在将幽门螺杆菌向儿童传播过程中起到关键作用[132]。通常不易诊断，直到发生穿孔或出血等并发症。呕吐在学龄前和学龄儿童中很常见。随着儿童年龄的增加，腹痛发生几率随之增大。疼痛通常为钝性且很难描述，可能由于饮食引起或者通过进食缓解，如同成人所见[35,137]。在年长儿和青少年中，消化性溃疡的临床表现和自然进程与成人更加接近。有消化性溃疡阳性家族的青少年溃疡表现为夜间上腹疼痛。这种情况下，不管急性溃疡治愈与否，该疾病的自然进程会导致溃疡复发。目前已明确这种溃疡与高胃蛋白酶遗传倾向无关，但会伴发幽门螺杆菌感染[141]。几乎所有原发性溃疡病患者都有腹痛。不幸的是，小儿最常见的胃肠疾病——儿童期精神性的反复腹痛的症状与溃疡病相同[25]。腹痛发作造成夜间惊醒可分为器质性的和心源性的。Gremse 和 Shakoor[55] 对胃镜下明确诊断消化性溃疡病的患儿进行症状体征预测值的评估，有 6 个症状明显与消化性溃疡病有关：上腹痛、夜间痛、进食后痛、返 1229
酸、体重减轻和消化性溃疡病家族史。与 60% 消化性溃疡病患儿相比，只有 7% 心理性反复腹痛儿童发生夜间腹痛。一项对 110 例十二指肠溃疡患儿的研究显示，平均获诊年龄为 11.3 岁；46% 的儿童于 10 岁前已表现出一些消化性溃疡病的症状[108]。

表 77-3　原发性和继发性胃炎及消化性溃疡病的临床表现

疾病本质	症状和体征
原发性胃炎	无症状（最常见） 反复腹痛（任何部位） 上腹痛 反酸，胃灼热（胃食管反流症状） 呕吐，恶心，食欲减退 缺铁性贫血 身材短小，生长停滞（？）
继发性胃炎	腹痛 上消化系统失血：呕血，便血 上腹疼痛部位（“痉挛性”） 易激性，随喂养方式改变 疲劳 缺铁性贫血
原发性消化性溃疡病	慢性、反复发作性腹痛 间断性上腹痛 呕吐，反复发作 夜间惊醒 贫血
继发性消化性溃疡病	危及生命的胃肠道出血 胃或十二指肠穿孔 休克 腹痛（少见）

继发性溃疡为急性发病。尽管继发性溃疡平均发病年龄为 1 天~18 岁，但大多数患儿小于 6 岁。继发性消化性溃疡常归因于有害因素（如皮质激素和 NSAIDs）的侵袭或发生于重大应激事件后（如烧伤、头部损伤、全身疾病）[141]。在这些情况下常发生上消化道出血、呕吐或穿孔，因此使诊断更加困难，常在如出血或穿孔等突发事件发生时才可作出诊断。约 92%6 岁以下的患儿可发生胃肠道出血，这是继发性溃疡最突出的症状[13]。若刺激因素或诱发黏膜溃疡形成的潜在疾病成功治愈，继发性溃疡在治愈后不会复发。

诊断

内镜诊断后给予组胺-2（H_2）受体拮抗剂治疗已经成功改善了儿童急性溃疡病的发病和转归。在儿童应用内镜前，消化性溃疡病患儿常表现为急腹症、大量出血或穿孔，在手术或尸检时才能作出诊断。目前早期诊断溃疡病的指征为胃肠道出血、吞咽困难、持续性呕吐以及上面提及的特征性腹痛[15]。胃液分析不是有效的诊断措施。过去继发性溃疡通过对比造影检查、血管造影术、开腹术和尸检来诊断。已知患有继发性溃疡伴生理应激时，应在症状体征出现前就做出诊断，以免病情加重造成不良后果。在消化道出血时影像学诊断会变得困难，因为血块可遮盖溃疡。因此内镜已经成为诊断急性出血性溃疡的标准。一份报告指出内镜可对 85% 上消化道出血患儿作出诊断，而放射学检查为 62%[153]。血管造影术有助于对出血速度大于 0.5 ml/min 的出血性溃疡进行定位[44,154]。

幽门螺杆菌

有创检查方法：内镜可准确诊断儿童消化性溃疡。胃窦处结节是儿童幽门螺杆菌感染活跃的一项特征（但不敏感）。应从胃内取组织活检并以多种技术测定幽门螺杆菌的存在，如活检切片染色（银染色、Giemsa 染色、Genta 染色、吖啶橙染色）和显微镜评估，进行细菌培养并测定尿素酶活性。对于同时接受质子泵抑制剂治疗的儿童和青少年，除胃窦处外，应在胃体、贲门（甚至移行区）取活检以减少假阴性结果[34]。在儿童人群中很少需要内镜随访，除非在消化性溃疡病有并发症的情况下（如大量出血或者穿孔）。

无创检查方法：幽门螺杆菌感染会引起强烈的免疫反应导致局部或全身抗体产生。幽门螺杆菌特异性 IgG 抗体可出现于血清、血浆、全血、唾液、胃液和尿液中。体液免疫反应在儿童中并不强烈，因此适用于成人的决定幽门螺杆菌感染与否的检测值并不适用于幼儿。对低患病率环境如发达国家儿童或青少年中抗体测定是否有实用性日益引发争议。尽管免疫测定法相对较便宜且技术上容易操作，但是这些应用于儿童的方法必须首先在各个国家或地区使用相关人群的血清样本加以验证[28]。应用稳定同位素 ^{13}C-或放射性标记的 ^{14}C-尿素作为底物的呼吸试验在成人无创诊断幽门螺杆菌感染方面表现出广阔的应用前景，但 ^{14}C 标记的底物不可用于儿童和育龄期妇女。尿素呼吸试验对大于 2 岁的儿童准确率高[23,75]。有报道称一种粪抗原试验作为成人的诊断性实验具有很高的准确率。血清学检测中抗体滴度在机体成功清除幽门螺杆菌后数月内持续升高，与此不同的是，粪抗原检测据称在幽门螺杆菌清除后一星期内即转阴性。粪抗原检测于各种临床环境下在儿童人群中的准确性验证了其有效性[75]。

治疗

儿童消化性溃疡病的治疗与成人相似。制酸剂和 H_2 受体拮抗剂（如西咪替丁）是药物治疗的主要手段。其他治疗方法包括选择性抗胆碱能药物、质子泵抑制剂、细胞保护药物和抗感染剂（表 77-4）。

质子泵抑制剂奥美拉唑和兰索拉唑抑制了刺激胃酸分泌的最后共同通路（AMP-腺苷酸环化酶循环，H^+-K^+ 三磷腺苷酶抑制），因此各种形式引起的胃酸分泌均被阻断（组胺神经能、胃酸神经能和胆碱神经能）。儿童奥美拉唑用量为 1 mg/(kg · d) 并逐渐增加到 20 mg/d；兰索拉唑为 30 kg 以下 0.5 mg/(kg · d)，30 kg 以上 30 mg/d，在 4 周内对 95% 的患儿有效[74]。虽然奥美拉唑耐受性很好，但副作用较多，包括头痛、恶心和腹痛。

对于确诊幽门螺杆菌胃炎或十二指肠溃疡的儿 1230
童，需使用标准抗微生物制剂和铋制剂才能根治（见表 7-4）。目前的标准疗法包括两种抗生素合用（选取以下任何两种）：阿莫西林［50 mg/(kg · d)］、克拉仙霉素［15 mg/(kg · d)］或甲硝唑［20 mg/(kg · d)］

表 77–4 对儿童合并幽门螺杆菌感染疾病的三种推荐联合根治方法

药物	剂量	治疗周期
阿莫西林	50 mg/(kg · d)	14 天 bid
克拉仙霉素	15 mg/(kg · d)	14 天 bid
质子泵抑制剂	1.0 mg/(kg · d)	1 月 bid
阿莫西林	50 mg/(kg · d)	14 天 bid
甲硝唑	20 mg/(kg · d)	14 天 bid
质子泵抑制剂	1.0 mg/(kg · d)	1 月 bid
克拉仙霉素	15 mg/(kg · d)	14 天 bid
甲硝唑	20 mg/(kg · d)	14 天 bid
质子泵抑制剂	1.0 mg/(kg · d)	1 月 bid

以及一种质子泵抑制剂。用法为连续 2 周，每天 2 次定量使用抗生素，连续 4 周应用质子泵抑制剂。该三联疗法可根治超过 80%~90% 的患者[34,74,75]。

与安慰剂相比，抗酸剂可有效中和胃酸分泌（分别为 75% 和 40%）。不幸的是，这些药物顺应性不太满意，且并发症如腹泻、便秘等让服药者不适。抗酸剂（0.5 ml/kg）需饭前 1 小时、饭后 3 小时及睡前服用。

组胺可刺激胃酸分泌。针对 H_2 的 H_2 受体分布于分泌胃酸的胃壁细胞，H_2 受体拮抗剂可抑制所有促分泌的信号，因此可有效抑制胃酸分泌。西咪替丁［20～40 mg/(kg · d)］是第一个商业用拮抗剂。其抗雄激素的副作用及作用于中枢神经系统的效应似乎与该复合物的咪唑环抑制肝细胞色素 P450 系统有关。雷尼替丁［2～4 mg/(kg · d)］是一种没有咪唑环的 H_2 受体拮抗剂，其效价为西咪替丁的 6～8 倍并在 8 周内可取得同样的疗效（85%～93%）。但有报道称复发率为 20%。法莫替丁和尼扎替丁也是在成人中使用的有效拮抗剂，但在儿童中的应用情况报道甚少。

硫糖铝的细胞保护作用来自于覆盖作用，通过硫酸化二糖铝盐的负电荷与损伤黏膜的蛋白质正电荷相吸附。该复合物似乎能刺激黏液分泌和前列腺素合成，结合胆盐并中和胃蛋白酶和胃酸。成人用量为每天 4 次，每次 1 g［1 g/10 ml 混悬剂］；儿童用量为 40～80 mg/(kg · d)。便秘是该药唯一明显的临床副作用。

E 族前列腺素如枸橼酸铋钾、恩前列腺素、甲基前列腺素 E_2 都具有细胞保护作用[106]。黏膜保护的作用机制与阻断 AMP 生成循环、刺激 HCO_3^- 分泌和增加黏膜血供有关。成人用量为每天 4 次，每次 200 μg，但是目前针对儿童的使用经验尚少。

外科治疗

从古至今，消化性溃疡病的手术治疗主要针对其并发症如穿孔、出血、梗阻和顽固性疼痛。对应用药物治疗原发性溃疡病患儿的随访提示：治疗中断后该病复发率很高，贯穿儿童期至成人期[108,125]。这些复发的患者数量越来越多，最终需要外科治疗。由于患者经药物治疗可造成发病率报告的延迟，因此有人推荐早期采取外科干预[128]。迷走神经切断术和幽门成形术而非胃切除术被推荐为有效治疗方法，对将来的生长发育影响最小[73]。过去 10 年间，高选择性或胃壁细胞迷走神经切断术已在数个中心广泛使用来治疗成人消化性溃疡病，但是尚无儿童方面的报道。该方法的高复发率（10%～15%）可能是个问题，但是有些学者认为该复发率在儿童中可以接受，因为该方法可能对生长发育造成的影响最小且长期预后相当好[62]。

出生后 1～2 周发生的出血或穿孔性溃疡（与其他疾病或应激无关）似乎是由母亲胃泌素导致胃酸过度分泌引起的一种急性溃疡。这种溃疡常伴发出血，可通过口胃管减压并给予盐水灌洗以保证从胃中抽出血凝块和适当补充容量。穿孔需迅速外科干预，应用最简单的方法（如 Graham 补片）安全修复缺损。如果因出血而手术，单纯缝扎溃疡底部就足够了。没有证据表明这些溃疡会复发。

尽管过去 20 年内出血和穿孔的发生率逐渐降低，消化性溃疡病引起的慢性梗阻并发症并未改变。在一篇对近 45 年研究的综述中，Azarow 和同事[8]发现需外科干预的胃出口梗阻发生率维持在很高的水平。迷走神经切断术和幽门成形术或胃肠切开术可缓解梗阻。继发于先天性疾病如十二指肠蹼[3,79]或肥厚性幽门狭窄的慢性、局部胃出口梗阻也可导致婴幼儿消化性溃疡。明确这些情况的发病原因尤为重要，因为溃疡可通过治疗远端梗阻完全缓解。

1231 Zollinger-Ellison 综合征

Zollinger-Ellison 综合征在儿童中相对少见[131]。可根据胃壁有较大的褶皱、十二指肠扩张和小肠黏膜水肿作出诊断，并通过升高的血清胃泌素确诊。钙负荷试验对于成人和儿童都很可靠，可用于明确诊断高胃泌素血症。除非原发胰腺肿瘤可完整切除，过去需常规行全胃切除术治疗 Zollinger-Ellison 综合征，一些报道称 H_2 受体拮抗剂或质子泵抑制剂可免除儿童胃切除的必要[37]。事实上许多内分泌肿瘤都为恶性，必须在得出疗效可靠的结论前，对使用 H_2 受体拮抗剂或质子泵抑制剂治疗的每个病例仔细评估以决定其转归并进行长期随访。此外，分泌胃泌素的肿瘤偶尔会发生在十二指肠壁并需要切除。多发性内分泌腺瘤综合征 1 型见于 25% 的病例。生长抑素受体闪烁显像有助于探测原发性或转移性胃泌素瘤。

应激性溃疡

预防是应激性溃疡的首选治疗目标。经实验证明在模拟临床环境下，应激性溃疡的进展需要很低的胃酸 pH 值。应用预防性抗酸剂维持胃内 pH 于 6.0 或更高是有效的方法。支持性疗法辅以改良通气支持、维持血容量、纠正酸碱平衡失调以及营养支持也有助于胃黏膜抵抗胃酸消化损伤作用。

H_2 受体拮抗剂或质子泵抑制剂对于预防应激性溃疡极其有效[30,74]。一种 H_2 受体拮抗剂可被用于预防和治疗 Cushing 溃疡，该溃疡伴有胃酸分泌过多。

当继发性溃疡表现为出血时，应用平衡盐溶液和输血作为紧急支持治疗通常已足够。经历上消化道大出血或反复出血的患儿需内镜治疗[164]。出血时的内镜治疗相比其他内镜操作需要更高的技巧和技能。内镜师不仅要明确出血部位还要有控制出血的知识及经验。可采取的干预措施包括治疗性注射（高渗 NaCl、肾上腺素、无水乙醇）、加热探针烧灼、双极电凝或激光（Nd：YAG 或氩）。如果内镜师不是外科医生，那么小儿外科医生应该在急诊内镜治疗前对患儿进行评估，之后外科医生可观察出血部位并在有需要时立即进行外科干预。

如果在药物和内镜治疗后大出血持续或复发，则是外科手术的指征。大出血的定义是小于 2 岁的婴儿 24 小时内失血量等于全身估计血容量，或年长儿 24 小时内失血量等于一半估计血容量（使用 80 ml/kg 作为估计全身血容量的指标）。该定义与 Williams 和同事的报道相关[162]，即所有 24 小时内丢失超过 60% 全身估计血容量的患儿在外科治疗下都得以康复。目前已有报道成功地选择性使用动脉内加压素治疗儿童出血性应激性溃疡[84]，但是其他研究尚未发现该方法有效[57,103]。尽管继发性溃疡出血通常在穿孔前发生，但穿孔可能是最初的临床表现并需立即手术治疗。

用于治疗应激性溃疡的外科手术包括单纯穿孔修补、出血性溃疡基底对缝缝合、胃切除等[24]。一般来说，这些溃疡患儿不伴有溃疡体质，因此应该用最简单有效的方法治疗现存的疾病。应激性溃疡由潜在的疾病导致，如果该疾病未解决，溃疡还是有复发的可能，在选择合适的手术方法时应考虑到这个因素。最简单的术式如折叠穿孔部位或对缝缝合出血点通常有效。另外，当明确潜在疾病在一段时期内无法根治时，采取进一步处理溃疡的手术是合适的。最常推荐的术式为迷走神经切断术和幽门成形术，因为这些术式不会影响患儿继续发育。有时对广泛烧伤和颅内疾病患者需采取迷走神经切断术和胃窦切除术以控制出血性溃疡[118]。对于幽门成形术无法解决的巨大穿孔需行胃窦切除术，尽管浆膜补片也有可能成功修补穿孔。成人中，即使是全胃切除术也很少被推荐用以治疗多发性溃疡引起的大出血，该术式在儿童中几乎没有应用指征。为消化性溃疡病患儿进行手术的外科医生必须注意患儿还要生长发育，因此应选择最简单、损伤最小的术式。有证据显示这些患儿术后确实会存在一些问题如血红蛋白水平低[157]。一项研究比较了胃切除术和迷走神经切断术、幽门成形术对小猪生长发育的影响，实验数据[120]显示迷走神经切断术加幽门成形术对生长发育的影响较小。随访数据表明迷走神经切断术加幽门成形术是有效的治疗手段，不会出现长期问题[73]。考虑到成人已有行各种消化性溃疡手术治疗骨质疏松症、铁缺乏和转储的报道[89,104]，长期随访是必须的。很少有胃次全切除术后残胃发生腺癌的报道[133]。但在 Billroth-Ⅱ式吻合术（胃空肠吻合术）后该风险会增加。我们有 1 例慢性梗阻性十二指肠溃疡的患者在迷走神经切断术和幽门成形术后 1232
12 年在 23 岁时残胃发生肿瘤。其他肿瘤也可发生于胃内并因侵蚀表现为出血。其中包括罕见的胃畸胎瘤、平滑肌肉瘤、胃肠道间质瘤（GIST）。这些疾病在第 31 章有详细介绍。

胃其他疾病

先天性胃出口梗阻

幽门闭锁

历史回顾

1937 年，一名出生 4 天的婴儿在“幽门狭窄术”后 36 小时死亡，尸检显示梗阻是由完全性幽门前瓣膜造成。1940—1959 年有外科成功治疗完全性幽门前瓣膜的报道，并有小于 1 周的早产儿和足月产儿发生双重隔膜的记录[14]。至少有 6 篇报道描述了家族性的发病情况[45]，并称该病为常染色体隐性遗传。

胚胎学和病理学

胃窦和十二指肠壶腹上部由前肠的尾端发育而成，该部位的闭锁以蹼、瓣膜或罕见的固体索带形式发生（表 77-5）。胃窦蹼或闭锁的原因尚未完全明确。有多种说法用来解释这种罕见畸形的发生。通常认为是宫内血管意外造成缺血坏死导致肠闭锁，但是对于胃来说这似乎不太可能，因为其血供非常丰富。同样将之前提出的血管再通失败作为胎儿肠梗阻的原因也很难解释，因为没有确切的证据表明胃也会发生此类梗阻。I 型梗阻在十二指肠或近端空肠多见[158]。Skandalakis 和 Gray[146]假设多余的移行上皮细胞会引起不完全隔膜的形成。Sharma 和同事[140]也对 1 小组后天性幽门黏膜梗阻病例的病因提出假设。尽管这些解释可能是瓣膜和蹼的病因，但仍有待推敲且目前尚无确实证据。在没有致畸因子的情况下，患者及发生该病的同胞和表亲间临床病理学特征的相似性，提示该病具有与家族遗传性幽门闭锁和表皮溶解性大疱患儿病理相似的遗传病因学[33,126]。胃出口梗阻的另一个具有相似胚胎学的病因为幽门十二指肠重复囊肿[60,177]。

表 77-5 胃窦和壶腹上闭锁分类

Ⅰ. 幽门
  A. 瓣膜
  B. 闭锁
Ⅱ. 胃窦（离幽门 1.0 cm 或更近）
  A. 瓣膜
  B. 闭锁

临床表现和病理生理学

幽门闭锁患儿的母亲通常有羊水过多史。随着产前超声检查应用增多，可在妊娠最后 3 个月内发现羊水过多及胎儿胃扩张[160]。患儿在出生后几天内表现为非胆汁性呕吐和完全性胃出口梗阻[40,134]。横膈可能会有穿孔，当孔径小于 10 mm 时内腔基本上还是完全梗阻的[13,158]。呼吸系统问题很常见，呼吸困难、呼吸急促、发绀以及过度流涎等临床表现可能会被误认为是食道闭锁的症状[20,81]。腹部体检可见上腹因胃扩张而膨隆。若诊断延误，胃过度扩张可导致穿孔。由于梗阻位于 Vater 壶腹的近端，胎粪通过可能会误导无经验的观察者。

诊断

腹部摄片可明确临床诊断（图 77-1）。可能需要抽出胃内液态内容物并注入同等量的空气，但通常无

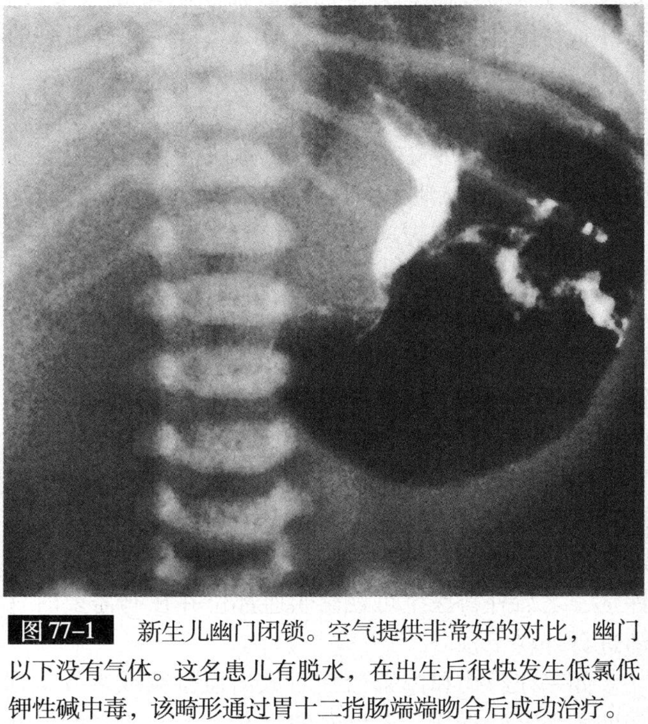

图 77-1 新生儿幽门闭锁。空气提供非常好的对比，幽门以下没有气体。这名患儿有脱水，在出生后很快发生低氯低钾性碱中毒，该畸形通过胃十二指肠端端吻合后成功治疗。

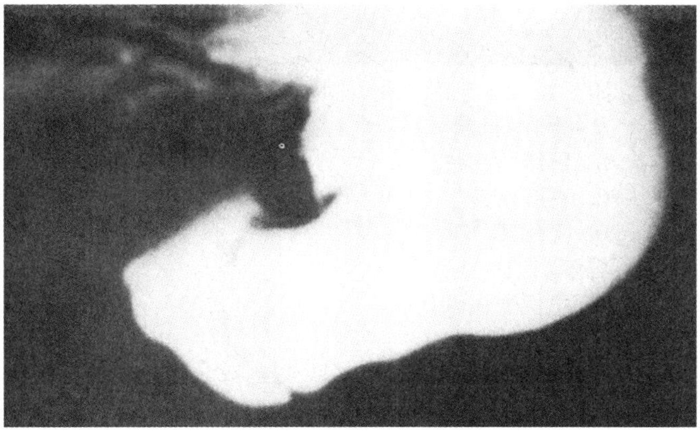

图 77-2　新生儿不全性胃窦横膈膜。该患儿于出生后不久出现非胆汁性呕吐，稀释吞钡造影检查诊断为不全性梗阻，经过 Heineke-Mikulicz 幽门成形术和蹼切除后成功治疗。

1233 需注射造影剂。抽出物通常不含胆汁。需要进行不同部位腹部摄片以建立正确诊断。可观察到单个胃泡且幽门后无空气。如果具有非胆汁性呕吐、胃扩张和胃远端有空气的特征，需使用稀释钡剂或可溶性造影剂来诊断不完全性幽门瓣膜（图 77-2）。

需要说明的是开腹手术难以鉴别幽门蹼，外科医生必须进行近端胃广泛切开术。Haller 和 Cahill[59] 提醒不要漏诊幽门蹼伴十二指肠闭锁，他们推荐胃广泛切开术并在切开幽门前隔膜后往远端置入导管以确定是否伴有十二指肠隔膜。

治疗

通常可在手术时发现幽门闭锁：一条纤维索带连接两个盲端（图 77-3），需行胃切开术及远端置管以检测膜状梗阻（图 77-4）。以 Heineke-Mikulicz 或

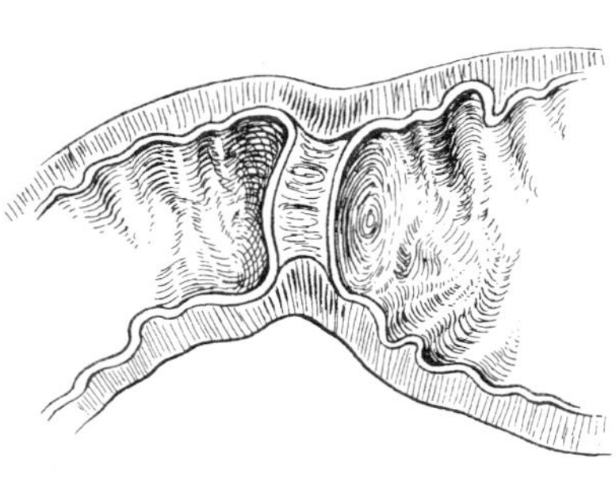

图 77-3　幽门闭锁。浆肌层连续。胃和十二指肠黏膜之间的组织有两种类型：纤维状和网状。

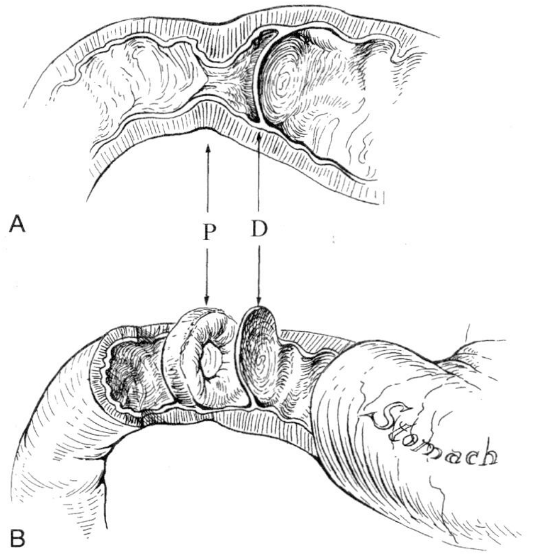

图 77-4　先天性幽门和幽门前梗阻。A. 幽门前瓣膜。B. 胃窦横膈膜。P. 幽门部。D. 横膈膜。

Finney 幽门切开术切开完全性或部分性隔膜是最直接的治疗方法。如果幽门闭锁其闭锁端被索带样结构或不连续结构分离，必须行胃十二指肠吻合术。Dessanti 和同事提出可利用闭锁的盲端穹窿行端端吻合以重建幽门括约肌[36]，该术式免除了因胃和十二指肠大小不一致而切除闭锁部分并行侧侧或端侧斜行吻合的情况。暂时胃切开减压术和经胃置饲管可能有帮助。近期内镜技术的进步促进了其他治疗策略的发展，包括球囊扩张、激光蹼切除和激光放射状切开 I 型瓣膜。这些技术的病例报道尚少且缺乏长期随访资料。

预后

如果能早期诊断和外科治疗及给予新生儿支持性监护，生存率是可以预见的。死亡常由于诊断延迟[10,79,117]或其他并发症[123]。59 例先天性幽门闭锁已被报道。6 个家庭 13 名患儿被发现有家族遗传性疾病，但无法解释在这些家族中的高死亡率。一些家族遗传性病例还伴有大疱性表皮松解。由于败血症、吸收不良、肾脏病和发育停滞，一些极端病例还会伴发结合性大疱性表皮松解/幽门闭锁综合征[81,117,150]。在医学文献报道的 70 名病例中，到 11 月龄时死亡 54 例。所有 16 例存活者都经受了表皮松解并发症的折磨，病程从 30 天~16 年不等[33]。幽门闭锁伴结合性大疱性表皮松解起因于 PLEC1 基因的变异，最致命

的形式是伴有细胞内 β-4 整联蛋白的降解。

1234 幽门重复畸形

胃和幽门重复畸形并不常见，约占消化道重复畸形的 3%。幽门重复畸形在女孩中稍多见。重复的部分与胃或幽门共壁但很少连通。患儿在出生后 2～3 周表现为非胆汁性呕吐和体重减轻[31,148]，易与肥厚性幽门狭窄相混淆。幽门重复畸形有时可触及包块，更易被误诊为肥厚性幽门狭窄，可通过超声检查显示腔外囊性包块压迫胃出口作出诊断。该病可能直到术中才被发现，手术方法为黏膜外切开，有时需行囊肿胃造瘘术。术后生存率很高且并发症少。影响胃的重复囊肿常于出生后出现，重复畸形在第 88 章有详细讨论。

胃扭转

历史回顾

胃扭转由 Berti 在 1886 年首次报道。1904 年，Borchardt 提出了经典的三联征：上腹部急性或局限性膨隆伴疼痛、无法置入鼻胃管以及反复干呕。成人和儿童中已有很多病例报道。儿童胃扭转比较少见，近期有一篇文献综述报道了 51 例婴幼儿胃扭转[22]。52% 小于 1 岁，26% 小于 1 月。Bautista-Casasnovas 及同事[12]报道了他们 25 年的经验，明确了早期诊断婴儿急性胃扭转的时机。更近期的一篇综述提出慢性胃扭转比急性胃扭转更常见；成人多并发食道旁裂孔疝[152]。另外，急性胃扭转是一个真正的外科急症。

胚胎学及分类

胃扭转比较少见，因为胃由胃膈韧带、食管裂孔、十二指肠后腹膜附着、胃短血管及胃结肠韧带牢牢固定在原位。只有当这些附着物松弛或缺失时才会发生胃扭转。有时胃扭转会伴发横膈突出、膈疝、先天性索带、胃附着物伸长或胃结肠韧带缺如。胃异常扭转的诱因可分为原发的固定物缺失、解剖结构异常和邻近脏器畸形[94,135]。详见表 77-6。

表 77-6　胃扭转的解剖学病因

Ⅰ. 附件缺如，无附着或胃固定物过长
- A. 胃脾韧带
- B. 胃结肠韧带
- C. 胃肝韧带
- D. 大网膜

Ⅱ. 胃解剖或功能异常
- A. 急性或慢性扩张
  1. 胃出口梗阻
  2. 胃动力不足
  3. 吞气过多
- B. 消化性溃疡病
- C. 胃新生物
- D. 沙漏胃
- E. 胃下垂

Ⅲ. 邻近器官畸形
- A. 横膈
  1. 裂孔疝、滑疝或食管旁疝
  2. Bochdalek 疝或其他先天性缺损
  3. 横膈破裂
  4. 横膈膨升
  5. 膈神经麻痹
- B. 巨脾、多脾
- C. 横结肠扭转
- D. 旋转不良和中肠扭转
- E. 肝左叶错位或发育不良

急性胃扭转在儿童中常见。大多数报道[11,94,110,139,149]和最大的单机构研究[12]证实，新生儿和小于 6 个月的婴儿是急性胃扭转最好发的年龄组。主要症状包括哭闹和急腹痛（90%）、恶心呕吐（67%）以及相对少见的腹胀、胃食管反流、生长发育停滞或者反复呼吸道感染。

胃扭转根据旋转的平面分类（图 77-5）。器官轴型扭转时胃沿其长轴旋转，胃大弯向前突出但向后移位。在不常见的系膜轴型扭转中，旋转沿胃大弯向胃小弯的方向进行（幽门或贲门常向前旋转）。反向扭转也可发生，扭转可以是完全性的，包括整个或部分胃，局限于幽门末端，扭转的部分通常向前突出。

X 线表现

X 线检查可确诊胃扭转，并且常常能发现伴发的潜在先天性畸形或缺损。急性胃扭转的 X 线表现包括

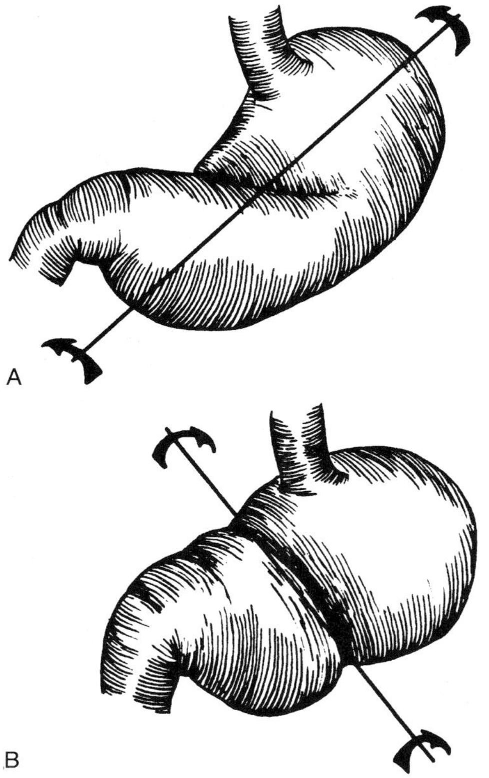

图 77-5 胃扭转。A. 器官轴型。胃大弯向前突出但向后旋转。B. 系膜轴型。幽门或贲门通常向前旋转，但相反方向也可发生。（From Cole BC，Dickinson SJ：Acute volvulus of the stomach in infants and children. Surgery 1971；70：707；with permission.）

（1）局限性上腹部巨大膨隆；（2）胃大弯上升（87%）；（3）胃大弯横跨胃体（83%）；（4）胃袢固定且不随体位改变；（5）咽入钡剂界限在食管远端逐渐变细，即所谓的“鸟嘴征”；（6）可能存在裂孔囊或其他形式的膈疝；（7）脾脏位置偏差。

治疗

胃扭转可急性发病，需要紧急手术干预以防止或
235 减少血管损伤。单纯鼻胃管减压可暂时缓解症状，但不宜做长期治疗。手术时胃减压有助于复位。一旦回复正常的解剖关系，应仔细探查以明确可能的穿孔或坏疽部位。之后的手术操作应集中预防扭转复发和纠正任何横膈缺陷（裂孔疝和 Bochdalek 裂孔疝）。婴幼儿应行胃造瘘术或胃前壁固定术。已有数篇报道应用这些技术开腹或内镜下修补，预后很好[11,12,149]，随访 1 ~ 10 年均无复发。固定后再次复发也有报道[152]。

新生儿胃穿孔

背景

新生儿期自发性胃穿孔常发生于需要复苏或出生不久即发生缺氧的婴儿。男孩比女孩更易患病，据报道发病率为 2900 名活产婴儿中有 1 名患病。导致胃穿孔的原因有两种理论。第一种认为缺血性创伤伴围生期应激导致黏膜缺氧损伤并在数天内发展为穿孔；第二种认为与胃过度膨胀有关，这可能是复苏过程中面罩过度加压、食管内插管意外和强力注气、口胃管通过时造成的损伤或幽门闭锁远端出口梗阻导致近端扩张穿孔的结果。胃局部缺血和穿孔也可见于广泛坏死性小肠结肠炎累及大部分胃肠道的早产儿。

历史回顾

1826 年首次报道了原因不明的新生儿胃肠道穿孔，即所谓的自发性穿孔。1943 年，成功关闭了一例新生儿胃肠道穿孔。1964 年，Lloyd 和同事[86]报道了 61 例新生儿自发性胃肠道穿孔，提出应注意无论部位如何，所有的病变都是缺血坏死的结果。由围生期应激、缺氧或休克激活的窒息防御机制的副作用即选择性循环缺血，被认为是造成这些病变的主要原因[9,42,155]。1969 年，Lloyd[87]回顾世界范围的研究，发现 315 例新生儿胃肠道穿孔符合缺血性损伤。此后，学者们提出了多种诱发因素和发病原因[5,46,145]。

胚胎学和病理学

尽管缺血可能是最常见的共同点，但也可能有多种病因，包括先天性胃壁肌层缺损[99]、致病菌在肠道内集群[82]、腔内存在高渗物质如碳水化合物、免疫系统不成熟[56]以及应用吲哚美辛引起的内皮损伤[145]。Gregory 等[54]报道 42 例肠道缺血坏死患儿中 39 例伴有围生期应激。

介导缺血性改变的确切机制目前尚不清楚，但学者们确信系因血液从周围循环、肾及肠系膜血管床分流注入心脏和脑所致。读者可参考 Elsner 及同事[42]关于哺乳动物和人类“潜水反射”理论的详细报道。出生时窒息且 Apgar 评分较低的婴儿尤其容易发生胃肠道穿孔。缺氧时血液重新分布、低血容量或其他应激状态[156]引起肠系膜血管床血液转流被认为是导致微血管损伤[64,65]及之后黏膜失去完整性的原因[68]。持续缺血性损伤可使微血管血栓扩散，导致肠穿孔中所见的透壁坏死。应激和潜在肠系膜缺血的时期可能暂时与穿孔关系不大。低体重出生儿吲哚美辛疗法也可引起消化道穿孔[53,111,145]。新生儿免疫系统也不完
1236 善，早产常伴发补体、调理机制、巨噬细胞功能、IgA 和 IgM 及 T 淋巴细胞功能缺乏[48,93]（胃肠穿孔在 92 章有详细介绍）。单纯性胃穿孔通常发生于胃大弯平滑肌层间，并且如之前提及的，可能与早产儿伴发胃结石、使用急救袋过度复苏造成的医源性损伤、食管插管不慎、胃管通过时造成的损伤、年长婴幼儿经皮内镜下放置胃造瘘管过程中不明原因的损伤有关[47,56]。

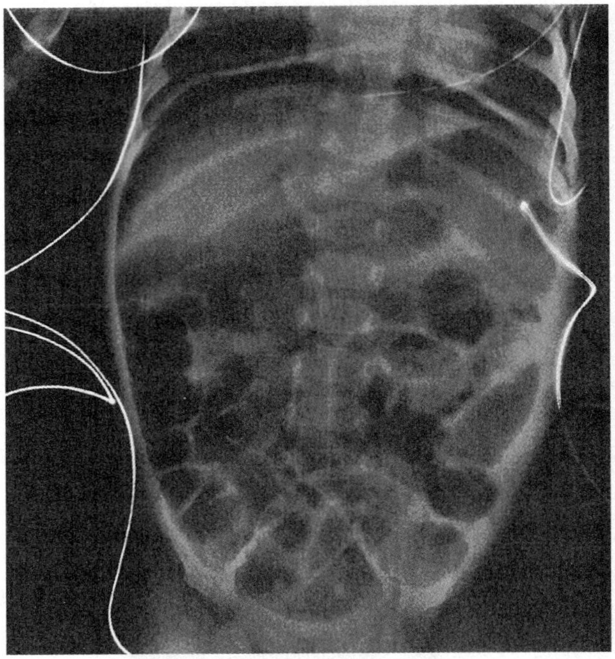

图 77-6　自发性胃穿孔患儿腹部 X 线片，显示出腹腔内游离气体。

症状、体征和诊断

肠穿孔的首要症状常发生于出生后 5～15 天，但自发性胃穿孔则常发生在出生后 3～5 天。腹胀常突然发生且进展迅速。常存在低血容量和灌注减少的征象，患儿表现为心动过速和嗜睡。巨大气腹导致呼吸困难可为首要症状。出生前合并胎盘早剥、前置胎盘和羊膜炎（严重的胎儿窘迫）以及经急诊剖宫产术出生的婴儿患病几率更大，需要仔细观察。

虽然许多有危险因素的早产儿没有开始喂养，但如果开始喂养，对于开始时喂养满意但突然拒绝进食或者无精打采、表情淡漠以及诊断为败血症的患儿应该停止喂养。应该进行连续腹部 X 线摄片直到明确问题原因。大多数胃穿孔患儿 X 线有腹腔游离气体的迹象（图 77-6）。进一步的诊断包括检测白细胞和血小板计数以及动脉血 pH 和血气分析。

治疗

胃穿孔婴儿的情况可迅速恶化，因此必须早期诊断及迅速治疗，包括快速补液复苏、输血、纠正酸中毒、应用抗生素、胃管抽吸、维持体温以及只进行必要的诊断性检查[85]。患儿通常需要立即插管和通气支持。使用钝性针头或塑料套管进行穿刺以抽出气腹，可缓解在复苏期间横膈抬高而危及生命的呼吸性窘迫。如果需要转送入特殊婴儿重症监护室，必须在转运前开始复苏。患儿必须由有经验的人员转运以便在途中维持复苏。

急诊剖腹术应用经脐上腹横切口。腹腔内容物必须做需氧菌、厌氧菌以及真菌培养。必须系统地探查腹腔，找到腹膜渗出液最多的部位。如果有明显的胃内容物或淡胆汁样液体常提示胃或者十二指肠穿孔，暗黑色或者粪汁样物质提示小肠或结肠穿孔。穿孔部位可以很隐蔽。在仔细检查食管裂孔至盆腔水平的肠道后，还必须检查小网膜区域。建议可在腹腔内充满温生理盐水后寻找气泡。大多数自发性胃穿孔发生在远离食管的胃大弯处。婴儿十二指肠溃疡的穿孔发生在十二指肠前壁或靠近幽门十二指肠结合部，而胃溃疡则沿胃小弯在近胃窦胃底结合处穿孔。胃穿孔通常可一期清创缝合。如果胃大弯广泛坏死，可切除并使用自动吻合器将残胃卷成管状。当胃窦有广泛坏死时，可行部分胃切除术和胃肠吻合术。首选 Billroth I 型手术（胃十二指肠吻合术）。如果合并个别的小肠

坏死穿孔但邻近肠管还是健康的，应一期修复穿孔。如果穿孔范围广泛，必须行肠切除术。行肠吻合术或外置残余肠管应取决于穿孔水平以及污染程度。由于婴儿无法很好耐受高位肠造瘘，所以如果局部缺血则倾向于行一期肠吻合术。但是，患儿最佳存活机会常
1237 依靠短期外置术。对于有肠穿孔的极低出生体重新生儿，经皮腹膜腔放置烟卷引流的腹腔引流法最早由 Ein 和同事在 25 年前报道[41]。最初，此法只推荐作为暂时性治疗措施，用于小而病情极为危重的坏死性小肠结肠炎患儿引流气体和粪便、减轻腹腔间隔综合征和败血症，以使其能更好地耐受接下来的剖腹手术。最近，临床医生发现早产儿肠穿孔中一种独立的亚群，其穿孔为自发性且不伴有坏死性小肠结肠炎。腹膜引流对这种被称作自发性、局灶性、特发性、吲哚美辛伴发的穿孔或单纯性小肠穿孔有很好的效果[5,21,145]。这种方法不能用于胃穿孔患儿，因为他们需要迅速手术修补。因此对于临床医生来说，提高警惕注意胃穿孔的发生以避免治疗时不必要的延误是很重要的。坏死性结肠小肠炎、特发性穿孔和腹膜引流的专题在第 92 章中有详细讨论。

单纯胃穿孔的患儿通常应用 7 天抗生素。在肠道休息以及应用抗生素一段时间后，当有迹象表明肠功能恢复、胃管内液体澄清且量少时可开始恢复肠道喂养。许多医生在开始喂养前先行造影检查。对于无法耐受肠道喂养的患儿常规行上、下消化道造影检查以评估是否存在胃漏或梗阻。

预后

目前单纯性胃穿孔的存活率为 75%~80%，患儿的死亡常因最初的损伤伴发腹膜炎、败血症以及免疫系统功能不完善，最后发生多脏器功能衰竭引起。胃坏死伴发广泛的坏死性小肠结肠炎的婴儿有很高的发病率和死亡率[56]。

先天性小胃

历史回顾

先天性小胃是一种罕见疾病，最早于 1800 年报道[17,32]。迄今只有 43 例报道。这种畸形常伴发其他先天性畸形，包括无脾、肠扭转不良、内脏反位、巨食管[66,151]和上肢畸形如桡骨、尺骨和鱼际发育不良（小胃–肢端缩小并发症）[17,32]。随着儿童医院婴幼儿护理区域化的增加，对该病的认识也逐渐增多[6,67,136]。目前报道的小胃疗法从对患者影响最小的保守食物疗法到外科小胃增大手术不等。

胚胎学和病理学

这是种罕见的先天性胚胎前肠尾部畸形，特征是小而管状的胃、巨食管和胃旋转不全，食管、胃、小肠和大肠的黏膜是正常的。胃肠道可伴发多种疾病如中肠不旋转伴十二指肠束带和无脾。内脏反位和无脾已有报道[80]。常见骨骼畸形包括小颌症、尺桡骨发育不良、脊柱畸形、少指（趾）畸形和指甲发育不良等，无眼也有报道[136]。

由于畸形伴发器官生长，因此认为器官生长发育停止发生在胚胎 4~8 周。胆囊缺如也已有报道[113]。可发生大量持续性胆管反流。患儿可有以单心房、单心室以及全肺静脉回流入门静脉异常为特征的先天性心脏病。

临床表现和病理生理学

随着产前超声检查应用的增多，羊水过多和小胃可在妊娠晚期发现。大多数患儿获得诊断的时间在新生儿期之后，多有扩张的食管及边界不清的胃食管结合部，因此易发生胃食管反流。最常见的临床表现为呕吐、误吸、肺炎以及生长停滞，可能会导致营养不良和发育迟缓，腹泻很常见。这些病例中都有食管下端括约肌不全。当伴有胃容量减少、食管扩张时，呕吐、食管腐蚀和误吸很常见。尽管研究不多，但我们设想营养不良和腹泻可能是胃容量过小、胃酸排空过快的结果。细菌过度生长和盲袢样综合征被用来解释腹泻和营养不良，但 Shilling 测试结果正常。

诊断

上消化道钡剂造影检查通常是首选检查手段，可提示上述特征性表现[138]。影像学检查可增加 X 线摄片。内镜检查经证实有难度且会产生混淆结果。特殊的发现需要进行适当的心脏检查，无脾可通过外周红

细胞 Howell-Jolly 小体以及核成像检查来诊断。如果临床上有胃食管反流的表现，食管测压和 pH 检测是恰当的做法。对于腹泻、营养不良和发育迟缓的患
1238 儿，应进行肠道吸收检查以明确病因。

治疗

最初应尝试药物治疗。持续性或夜间胃管喂养可以维持患儿生长，也能增大胃以耐受正常喂养。如果胃食管反流发展，可使用促动力药物或胃酸抑制疗法促进胃排空。胃食管反流的并发症需应用鼻空肠饲管或外科放置空肠造瘘管。空肠喂养补充口饲的不足，可让胃增大[109]。如果患儿的胃无法增大，一些专家建议通过双空肠贮袋结构增加胃容量[49,96,105]，早期随访结果令人满意。

（王宇鹏译　董其刚校）

参考文献

1. Acra SA, Nakagawa N, Ghishan FK: Peptic ulcer diseases in children. Comprehens Ther 1991;17:22-26.
2. Agunod M, Yamaguchi N, Lopez R, et al: Correlative study of hydrochloric acid, pepsin, and intrinsic factor secretion in newborns and infants. J Dig Dis 1969;14:400-414.
3. Airan B, Yadav K, Yadav RV: Congenital incomplete duodenal diaphragm with prediaphragmatic duodenal ulcer. Am J Gastroenterol 1979;72:426-427.
4. Allaker RP, Young KA, Hardie JM, et al: Prevalence of *Helicobacter pylori* at oral and gastrointestinal sites in children: Evidence for possible oral-to-oral transmission. J Med Microbiol 2002;51:312-317.
5. Alpan G, Eyal F, Vinograd I, et al: Localized intestinal perforation after enteral administration of indomethacin in premature infants. J Pediatr 1985;106:277-281.
6. Anderson KD, Guzzetta PC: Treatment of congenital microgastria and dumping syndrome. J Pediatr Surg 1983; 18:747-750.
7. Ashorn M: What are the specific features of *Helicobacter pylori* gastritis in children? Ann Med 1995;27:617-620.
8. Azarow K, Kim P, Shandling B, et al: A 45-year experience with surgical treatment of peptic ulcer disease in children. J Pediatr Surg 1996;31:750-753.
9. Barlow B, Santulli TV: Importance of multiple episodes of hypoxia or cold stress on the development of enterocolitis in an animal model. Surgery 1975;77:687-690.
10. Bar-Maor JA, Nissan S, Nevo S: Pyloric atresia: A hereditary congenital anomaly with autosomal recessive transmission. J Med Genet 1972;9:70-72.
11. Basaran UN, Inan M, Ayhan S, et al: Acute gastric volvulus due to deficiency of the gastrocolic ligament in a newborn. Eur J Pediatr 2002;161:288-290.
12. Bautista-Casasnovas A, Varela-Cives R, Fernandez-Bustillo JM, et al: Chronic gastric volvulus: Is it so rare? Eur J Pediatr Surg 2002;12:111-115.
13. Bell MJ, Keating JP, Ternberg JL, et al: Perforated stress ulcers in infants. J Pediatr Surg 1981;16:998-1002.
14. Bell MJ, Ternberg JL, McAlister W, et al: Antral diaphragm—a cause of gastric outlet obstruction in infants and children. J Pediatr 1977;90:196-202.
15. Benaroch LM, Rudolph CD: Pediatric endoscopy. Semin Gastrointest Dis 1994;5:32-46.
16. Bird C, Limper M, Mayer J: Surgery in peptic ulceration of the stomach and duodenum in infants and children. Ann Surg 1941;114:526.
17. Blank E, Chisolm AJ: Congenital microgastria, a case report with a 26-year follow-up. Pediatrics 1973;51:1037-1041.
18. Blaser MJ, Chyou PH, Nomura A: Age at establishment of *Helicobacter pylori* infection and gastric carcinoma, gastric ulcer, and duodenal ulcer risk. Cancer Res 1995;55:562-565.
19. Boyle JT: Acid secretion from birth to adulthood. J Pediatr Gastroenterol Nutr 2003;37(Suppl 1):S12-S16.
20. Bronsther B, Nadeau MR, Abrams MW: Congenital pyloric atresia: A report of three cases and a review of the literature. Surgery 1971;69:130-136.
21. Camberos A, Patel K, Applebaum H: Laparotomy in very small premature infants with necrotizing enterocolitis or focal intestinal perforation: Postoperative outcome. J Pediatr Surg 2002;37:1692-1695.
22. Cameron AE, Howard ER: Gastric volvulus in childhood. J Pediatr Surg 1987;22:944-947.
23. Canete A, Abunaji Y, Alvarez-Calatayud G, et al: Breath test using a single 50-mg dose of ^{13}C-urea to detect *Helicobacter pylori* infection in children. J Pediatr Gastroenterol Nutr 2003;36:105-111.
24. Chan KL, Tam PK, Saing H: Long-term follow-up of childhood duodenal ulcers. J Pediatr Surg 1997;32:1609-1611.
25. Chelimsky G, Czinn S: Peptic ulcer disease in children. Pediatr Rev 2001;22:349-355.
26. Cheung LY, Chang N: The role of gastric mucosal blood flow and H^+ back-diffusion in the pathogenesis of acute gastric erosions. J Surg Res 1977;22:357-361.
27. Cheung LY, Porterfield G: Protection of gastric mucosa against acute ulceration by intravenous infusion of sodium bicarbonate. Am J Surg 1979;137:106-110.
28. Chong SK, Lou Q, Zollinger TW, et al: The seroprevalence of *Helicobacter pylori* in a referral population of children in the United States. Am J Gastroenterol 2003;98:2162-2168.
29. Conn HO, Blitzer BL: Nonassociation of adrenocorticosteroid therapy and peptic ulcer. N Engl J Med 1976;294: 473-479.
30. Cook DJ, Reeve BK, Guyatt GH, et al: Stress ulcer prophylaxis in critically ill patients: Resolving discordant meta-analyses [see comment]. JAMA 1996;275:308-314.
31. Cooper S, Abrams RS, Carbaugh RA: Pyloric duplications: Review and case study. Am Surg 1995;61:1092-1094.
32. Cunniff C, Williamson-Kruse L, Olney A: Congenital microgastria and limb reduction defects. Pediatrics 1993;91: 1192-1194.
33. Dank JP, Kim S, Parisi MA, et al: Outcome after surgical repair of junctional epidermolysis bullosa-pyloric atresia syndrome: A report of 3 cases and review of the literature. Arch Dermatol 1999;135:1243-1247.
34. Das BK, Kakkar S, Dixit VK, et al: *Helicobacter pylori* infection and recurrent abdominal pain in children. J Trop Pediatr 2003;49:250-252.
35. Deckelbaum RJ, Roy CC, Lussier-Lazaroff J, et al: Peptic ulcer disease: A clinical study in 73 children. Can Med

Assoc J 1974;111:225-228.
36. Dessanti A, Iannuccelli M, Dore A, et al: Pyloric atresia: An attempt at anatomic pyloric sphincter reconstruction. J Pediatr Surg 2000;35:1372-1374.
37. Drake DP, Maciver AG, Atwell JD: Zollinger-Ellison syndrome in a child: Medical treatment with cimetidine. Arch Dis Child 1980;55:226-228.
38. Drumm B, Perez-Perez GI, Blaser MJ, et al: Intrafamilial clustering of *Helicobacter pylori* infection. N Engl J Med 1990;322:359-363.
39. Drumm B, Sherman P, Cutz E, et al: Association of *Campylobacter pylori* on the gastric mucosa with antral gastritis in children. N Engl J Med 1987;316:1557-1561.
40. Ducharme JC, Bensoussan AL: Pyloric atresia. J Pediatr Surg 1975;10:149-150.
41. Ein SH, Marshall DG, Girvan D: Peritoneal drainage under local anesthesia for perforations from necrotizing enterocolitis. J Pediatr Surg 1977;12:963-967.
42. Elsner R, Franklin DL, Van Citters RL, et al: Cardiovascular defense against asphyxia. Science 1966;153:941-949.
43. Figura N: Identifiable *Helicobacter pylori* strains or factors important in the development of duodenal ulcer disease. Helicobacter 1997;2(1).
44. Fliegel CP, Herzog B, Signer E, et al: Bleeding gastric ulcer in a newborn infant diagnosed by transumbilical aortography. J Pediatr Surg 1977;12:560-589.
45. Gahukamble DB: Familial occurrence of congenital incomplete prepyloric mucosal diaphragm. J Med Genet 1998; 35:1040-1042.
46. Garland J, Nelson D, Rice T, et al: Increased risk of gastrointestinal perforations in neonates mechanically ventilated with either face mask or nasal prongs. Pediatrics 1985;76:406-410.
47. Gauderer MW: Percutaneous endoscopic gastrostomy—20 years later: A historical perspective. J Pediatr Surg 2001; 36:217-219.
48. Gennari R, Alexander JW, Gianotti L, et al: Granulocyte-macrophage colony-stimulating factor improves survival in two models of gut-derived sepsis by improving gut barrier function and modulating bacterial clearance. Ann Surg 1994;220:68-76.
49. Gerbeaux J, Couvreur J, Vialas M, et al: Congenital absence of the stomach. Ann Pediatr 1971;18:349-356.
50. Ghai O: An assessment of gastric acid secretory response with "maximal" augmented histamine stimulation in children with peptic ulcer. Arch Dis Child 1965;40:77.
51. Goodman KJ, Correa P: The transmission of *Helicobacter pylori:* A critical review of the evidence. Int J Epidemiol 1995;24:875-887.
52. Granquist A, Bredberg A, Sveger T, et al: A longitudinal cohort study on the prevalence of *Helicobacter pylori* antibodies in Swedish children and adolescents. Acta Paediatr 2002;91:636-640.
53. Gray PH, Pemberton PJ: Gastric perforation associated with indomethacin therapy in a pre-term infant. Aust Pediatr J 1980;16:65-66.
54. Gregory JR, Campbell JR, Harrison MW, et al: Neonatal necrotizing enterocolitis: A 10 year experience. Am J Surg 1981;141:562-567.
55. Gremse DA, Shakoor S: Symptoms of acid-peptic disease in children. South Med J 1993;86:997-1000.
56. Grosfeld JL, Molinari F, Chaet M, et al: Gastrointestinal perforation and peritonitis in infants and children: Experience with 179 cases over ten years. Surgery 1996;120:650-655; discussion 655-656.
57. Grosfeld JL, Shipley F, Fitzgerald JF, et al: Acute peptic ulcer in infancy and childhood. Am Surg 1978;44:13-19.
58. Habbick BF, Melrose AG, Grant JC: Duodenal ulcer in childhood: A study of predisposing factors. Arch Dis Child 1968;43:23-27.
59. Haller JA Jr, Cahill JL: Combined congenital gastric and duodenal obstruction: Pitfalls in diagnosis and treatment. Surgery 1968;63:503-506.
60. Hamada Y, Inoue K, Hioki K: Pyloroduodenal duplication cyst: Case report. Pediatr Surg Int 1997;12:194-195.
61. Harada T, Hyman PE, Everett S, et al: Meal-stimulated gastric acid secretion in infants. J Pediatr 1984;104:534-538.
62. Harmon JW, Jordan PH Jr: Verdict on vagotomy. Gastroenterology 1981;81:809-810.
63. Harris PR, Godoy A, Arenillas S, et al: CagA antibodies as a marker of virulence in Chilean patients with *Helicobacter pylori* infection. J Pediatr Gastroenterol Nutr 2003;37:596-602.
64. Harrison MW, Connell RS, Campbell JR, et al: Microcirculatory changes in the gastrointestinal tract of the hypoxic puppy: An electron microscope study. J Pediatr Surg 1975;10:599-608.
65. Harrison MW, Connell RS, Campbell JR, et al: Fine structural changes in the gastro-intestinal tract of the hypoxic puppy: A study of natural history. J Pediatr Surg 1977;12:403-408.
66. Herman TE, Siegel MJ: Imaging casebook: Asplenia syndrome with congenital microgastria and malrotation. J Perinatal 2004;24:50-52.
67. Hochberger O, Swoboda W: Congenital microgastria: A follow-up observation over six years. Pediatr Radiol 1974; 2:207-208.
68. Hopkins GB, Gould VE, Stevenson JK, et al: Necrotizing enterocolitis in premature infants: A clinical and pathologic evaluation of autopsy material. Am J Dis Child 1970;120: 229-232.
69. Hussell T, Isaacson PG, Crabtree JE, et al: The response of cells from low-grade B-cell gastric lymphomas of mucosa-associated lymphoid tissue to *Helicobacter pylori*. Lancet 1993;342:571-574.
70. Idjadi F, Robbins R, Stahl WM, et al: Prospective study of gastric secretion in stressed patients with intracranial injury. J Trauma Inj Infect Crit Care 1971;11:681-688.
71. Jackson RH: Genetic factors in the development of duodenal ulcer in childhood. Gut 1971;12:856-857.
72. Johnson D, L'Heureux P, Thompson T: Peptic ulcer disease in early infancy: Clinical presentation and roentgenographic features. Acta Pediatr Scand 1980;69:753-760.
73. Johnston PW, Snyder WH: Survey of vagotomy and pyloroplasty in infants and children. Am J Surg 1970;120:173-181.
74. Kato S, Ebina K, Fujii K, et al: Effect of omeprazole in the treatment of refractory acid-related diseases in childhood: Endoscopic healing and twenty-four-hour intragastric acidity. J Pediatr 1996;128:415-421.
75. Kato S, Ozawa K, Okuda M, et al: Accuracy of the stool antigen test for the diagnosis of childhood *Helicobacter pylori* infection: A multicenter Japanese study. Am J Gastroenterol 2003;98:296-300.
76. Kato S, Takeyama J, Ebina K, et al: Omeprazole-based dual and triple regimens for *Helicobacter pylori* eradication in children. Pediatrics 1977;100:e3.
77. Kawashima H, Iwanaka T, Matsumoto M, et al: Pyloric stenosis caused by noncystic duodenal duplication and ectopic pancreas in a neonate. J Pediatr Gastroenterol Nutr 1998;27:228-229.
78. Keramidas DC, Voyatzis N: Pyloric atresia: Report of a second occurrence in the same family. J Pediatr Surg 1972; 7:445-446.
79. Keramidas DC, Voyatzis N: Duodenal ulcer associated with

incomplete duodenal diaphragm. J Pediatr Surg 1975;10: 837-838.
80. Kessler H, Smulewicz JJ: Microgastria associated with agenesis of the spleen. Radiology 1973;107:393-396.
81. Konvolinka CW, Steward RE Jr: Pyloric atresia. Am J Dis Child 1978;132:903-905.
82. Kosloske AM: Necrotizing enterocolitis in the neonate. Surg Gynecol Obstet 1979;148:259-269.
83. Kumar D, Spitz L: Peptic ulceration in children. Surg Gynecol Obstet 1984;159:63-66.
84. Lerner AG, Meng CH, Schneider KM: Selective intra-arterial vasopressin in the management of stress ulcers in childhood. Pediatrics 1973;51:126-128.
85. Linkner L, Benson C: Spontaneous perforation of the stomach in the newborn. Ann Surg 1959;149:525.
86. Lloyd J, Espiasse E, Bernstein J: Etiology of gastrointestinal perforations in the newborn. Harper Hosp Bull 1964;22:224.
87. Lloyd JR: The etiology of gastrointestinal perforations in the newborn. J Pediatr Surg 1969;4:77-84.
88. Lucas CE, Sugawa C, Riddle J, et al: Natural history and surgical dilemma of "stress" gastric bleeding. Arch Surg 1971;102:266-273.
89. Magnusson B, Hallberg L, Arvidsson B: Iron absorption from food and from ferrous ascorbate: A study in normal subjects, patients with peptic ulcer and patients after partial gastrectomy. Scand J Hematol 1976;26:69-85.
90. Malaty HM, Kim JG, Kim SD, et al: Prevalence of *Helicobacter pylori* infection in Korean children: Inverse relation to socioeconomic status despite a uniformly high prevalence in adults. Am J Epidemiol 1996;143:257-262.
91. Marshall BJ, Warren JR: Unidentified curved bacilli in the stomach of patients with gastritis and peptic ulceration. Lancet 1984;1:1311-1315.
92. Maton PN: Zollinger-Ellison syndrome. Recognition and management of acid hypersecretion. Drugs 1996;52:33-44.
93. Maxson RT, Jackson RJ, Smith SD: The protective role of enteral IgA supplementation in neonatal gut origin sepsis. J Pediatr Surg 1995;30:231-233; discussion 233.
94. McIntyre RC Jr, Bensard DD, Karrer FM, et al: The pediatric diaphragm in acute gastric volvulus. J Am Coll Surg 1994;178:234-238.
95. Menguy R: Role of gastric mucosal energy metabolism in the etiology of stress ulceration. World J Surg 1981; 5:175-180.
96. Menon P, Rao KL, Cutinha HP, et al: Gastric augmentation in isolated congenital microgastria. J Pediatr Surg 2003; 38:E4-E6.
97. Mezoff AG, Balistreri WF: Peptic ulcer disease in children. Pediatr Rev 1995;16:257-265.
98. Miller TA, Jacobson ED: Gastrointestinal cytoprotection by prostaglandins. Gut 1979;20:75-87.
99. Miserez M, Barten S, Geboes K, et al: Surgical therapy and histological abnormalities in functional isolated small bowel obstruction and idiopathic gastrointestinal perforation in the very low birth weight infant. World J Surg 2003;27: 350-355.
100. Mobley HL: The role of *Helicobacter pylori* urease in the pathogenesis of gastritis and peptic ulceration. Aliment Pharmacol Ther 1996;1:57-64.
101. Moody FG, Cheung LY: Stress ulcers: Their pathogenesis, diagnosis, and treatment. Surg Clin North Am 1976;56: 1469-1478.
102. Moody FG, Zalewsky CA, Larsen KR: Cytoprotection of the gastric epithelium. World J Surg 1981;5:153-163.
103. Morden RS, Schullinger JN, Mollitt DL, et al: Operative management of stress ulcers in children. Ann Surg 1982; 196:18-20.
104. Morgan DB, Hunt G, Paterson CR: The osteomalacia syndrome after stomach operations. Q J Med 1970;39:395-410.
105. Moulton SL, Bouvet M, Lynch FP: Congenital microgastria in a premature infant. J Pediatr Surg 1994;29:1594-1595.
106. Mulberg AE, Linz C, Bern E, et al: Identification of nonsteroidal antiinflammatory drug-induced gastroduodenal injury in children with juvenile rheumatoid arthritis. J Pediatr 1993;122:647-649.
107. Murphy MS, Eastham EJ: Peptic ulcer disease in childhood: Long-term prognosis. J Pediatr Gastroenterol Nutr 1987; 6:721-724.
108. Murphy MS, Eastham EJ, Jimenez M, et al: Duodenal ulceration: Review of 110 cases. Arch Dis Child 1987;62: 554-558.
109. Murray KF, Lillehei CW, Duggan C: Congenital microgastria: Treatment with transient jejunal feedings. J Pediatr Gastroenterol Nutr 1999;28:343-345.
110. Mutabagani KH, Teich S, Long FR: Primary intrathoracic gastric volvulus in a newborn. J Pediatr Surg 1999;34: 1869-1871.
111. Nagaraj HS, Sandhu AS, Cook LN, et al: Gastrointestinal perforation following indomethacin therapy in very low birth weight infants. J Pediatr Surg 1981;16:1003-1007.
112. Nagita A, Amemoto K, Yoden A, et al: Diurnal variation in intragastric pH in children with and without peptic ulcers. Pediatr Res 1996;40:528-532.
113. Neifeld JP, Berman WF, Lawrence W, et al: Management of congenital microgastria with a jejunal reservoir pouch. J Pediatr Surg 1980;15:882-885.
114. Newton M, Bryan R, Burnham WR, et al: Evaluation of *Helicobacter pylori* in reflux oesophagitis and Barrett's oesophagus. Gut 1997;40:9-13.
115. Nord KS, Lebenthal E: Peptic ulcer in children: A review. Am J Gastroenterol 1980;73:75-80.
116. Norton L, Greer J, Eiseman B: Gastric secretory response to head injury. Arch Surg 1970;101:200-204.
117. Olsen L, Grotte G: Congenital pyloric atresia: Report of a familial occurrence. J Pediatr Surg 1976;11:181-184.
118. O'Neill JA Jr, Pruitt BA Jr, Moncrief JA: Surgical treatment of Curling's ulcer. Surg Gynecol Obstet 1968;126: 40-44.
119. Orsini B, Ciancio G, Censini S, et al: *Helicobacter pylori* cag pathogenicity island is associated with enhanced interleukin-8 expression in human gastric mucosa. Dig Liver Dis 2000;32:458-467.
120. Othersen HB Jr, Garcia R, Doering EJ: The effect of gastric resections and denervation upon growth in miniature swine. J Pediatr Surg 1973;8:159-163.
121. Parsonnet J: The incidence of *Helicobacter pylori* infection. Aliment Pharmacol Ther 1995;2:45-51.
122. Parsonnet J: *Helicobacter pylori* in the stomach—a paradox unmasked [see comment]. N Engl J Med 1996;335: 278-280.
123. Peltier FA, Tschen EH, Raimer SS, et al: Epidermolysis bullosa letalis associated with congenital pyloric atresia. Arch Dermatol 1981;117:728-731.
124. Polacek MA, Ellison EH: Gastric acid secretion and parietal cell mass in the stomach of a newborn infant. Am J Surg 1966;111:777-781.
125. Puri P, Boyd E, Blake N, et al: Duodenal ulcer in childhood: A continuing disease in adult life. J Pediatr Surg 1978;13:525-526.
126. Puvabanditsin S, Garrow E, Kim DU, et al: Junctional epidermolysis bullosa associated with congenital localized absence of skin, and pyloric atresia in two newborn siblings.

J Am Acad Dermatol 2001;44(2 Suppl):330-335.
127. Qiao W, Hu JL, Xiao B, et al: cagA and vacA genotype of *Helicobacter pylori* associated with gastric diseases in Xi'an area. World J Gastroenterol 2003;9:1762-1766.
128. Ravitch MM, Duremides GD: Operative treatment of chronic duodenal ulcer in childhood. Ann Surg 1970;171: 641-646.
129. Robb JD, Thomas PS, Orszulok J, et al: Duodenal ulcer in children. Arch Dis Child 1972;47:688-696.
130. Robert A, Nezamis JE, Lancaster C, et al: Mild irritants prevent gastric necrosis through "adaptive cytoprotection" mediated by prostaglandins. Am J Physiol 1983;245: G113-G121.
131. Rosenlund ML: The Zollinger-Ellison syndrome in children: A review. Am J Med Sci 1967;254:884-892.
132. Rothenbacher D, Winkler M, Gonser T, et al: Role of infected parents in transmission of *Helicobacter pylori* to their children. Pediatr Infect Dis J 2002;21:674-679.
133. Sasaki H, Sasano H, Ohi R, et al: Adenocarcinoma at the esophageal gastric junction arising in an 11-year-old girl. Pathol Int 1999;49:1109-1113.
134. Saw EC, Arbegast NR, Comer TP: Pyloric atresia: A case report. Pediatrics 1973;51:574-577.
135. Scherer L, Haller J: Gastrostomy in infants and children: Gastric volvulus. In Scott HW, Sawyers JL (eds): Surgery of the Stomach, Duodenum, and Small Intestine. Boston, Blackwell Scientific, 1992.
136. Schulz RD, Niemann F: Congenital microgastria occurring in combination with skeletal malformations: New syndrome. Helv Pediatr Acta 1971;26:185-191.
137. Seagram CG, Stephens CA, Cumming WA: Peptic ulceration at the Hospital for Sick Children, Toronto, during the 20-year period 1949-1969. J Pediatr Surg 1973; 8:407-413.
138. Shackelford GD, McAlister WH, Brodeur AE, et al: Congenital microgastria. Am J Roentgenol Rad Ther Nucl Med 1973;118:72-76.
139. Shah A, Shah AV: Laparoscopic gastropexy in a neonate for acute gastric volvulus. Pediatr Surg Int 2003;19: 217-219.
140. Sharma KK, Agrawal P, Toshniwal H: Acquired gastric outlet obstruction during infancy and childhood: A report of five unusual cases. J Pediatr Surg 1997;32:928-930.
141. Sherman P, Czinn S, Drumm B, et al: *Helicobacter pylori* infection in children and adolescents: Working Group Report of the First World Congress of Pediatric Gastroenterology, Hepatology, and Nutrition. J Pediatr Gastroenterol Nutr 2002;35(Suppl 2):S128-S133.
142. Sherman PM: Peptic ulcer disease in children. Diagnosis, treatment, and the implication of Helicobacter pylori. Gastroenterol Clin North Am 1994;23:707-725.
143. Shimizu T, Haruna H, Ohtsuka Y, et al: Cytokines in the gastric mucosa of children with Helicobacter pylori infection. Acta Paediatr 2004;93:322-326.
144. Shimizu T, Yamashiro Y, Yabuta K: Impaired increase of prostaglandin E_2 in gastric juice during steroid therapy in children. J Pediatr Child Health 1994;30:169-172.
145. Shorter N, Liu J, Mooney D, et al: Indomethacin-associated bowel perforations: A study of possible risk factors. J Pediatr Surg 1999;34:442-444.
146. Skandalakis JE, Gray SW (eds): Embryology for Surgeons. Baltimore, Williams & Wilkins. 1994.
147. Skillman JJ, Silen W: Stress ulcers. Lancet 1972;2:1303-1306.
148. Stannard MW, Currarino G, Splawski JB: Congenital double pylorus with accessory pyloric channel communicating with an intraluminal duplication cyst of the duodenum. Pediatr Radiol 1993;23:48-50.
149. Stiefel D, Willi UV, Sacher P, et al: Pitfalls in therapy of upside-down stomach. Eur J Pediatr Surg 2000;10: 162-166.
150. Tan KL, Murugasu JJ: Congenital pyloric atresia in siblings. Arch Surg 1973;106:100-102.
151. Tanaka K, Tsuchida Y, Hashizume K, et al: Microgastria: Case report and a review of the literature. Eur J Pediatr Surg 1993;3:290-292.
152. Tanner NC: Chronic and recurrent volvulus of the stomach with late results of "colonic displacement." Am J Surg 1968;115:505-515.
153. Tedesco FJ, Goldstein PD, Gleason WA, et al: Upper gastrointestinal endoscopy in the pediatric patient. Gastroenterology 1976;70:492-494.
154. Ternberg JL, Koehler PR: The use of arteriography in the diagnosis of the origin of acute gastrointestinal hemorrhage in children. Surgery 1968;63:686-689.
155. Touloukian RJ: Gastric ischemia: The primary factor in neonatal perforation. Clin Pediatr 1973;12:219-225.
156. Touloukian RJ, Posch JN, Spencer R: The pathogenesis of ischemic gastroenterocolitis of the neonate: Selective gut mucosal ischemia in asphyxiated neonatal piglets. J Pediatr Surg 1972;7:194-205.
157. Tsuchida Y, Makino S, Ishida M: A follow-up study of subtotal gastrectomy in infancy and early childhood. J Pediatr Surg 1974;9:499-500.
158. Tunell WP, Smith EI: Antral web in infancy. J Pediatr Surg 1980;15:152-155.
159. Veldhuyzen van Zanten SJ, Sherman PM: Indications for treatment of *Helicobacter pylori* infection: A systematic overview. Can Med Assoc J 1994;150:189-198.
160. Weissman A, Achiron R, Kuint J, et al: Prenatal diagnosis of congenital gastric outlet obstruction. Prenat Diag 1994; 14:888-891.
161. Whitney AE, Emory TS, Marty AM, et al: Increased macrophage infiltration of gastric mucosa in *Helicobacter pylori*-infected children. Dig Dis Sci 2000;45:1337-1342.
162. Williams JW, Pannell WP, Sherman RT: Curling's ulcer in children. J Trauma Inf Infect Crit Care 1976;16:639-644.
163. Wilson SD: The role of surgery in children with the Zollinger-Ellison syndrome. Surgery 1982;92:682-692.
164. Wyllie R, Kay MH: Therapeutic intervention for nonvariceal gastrointestinal hemorrhage. J Pediatr Gastroenterol Nutr 1996;22:123-133.

第 78 章

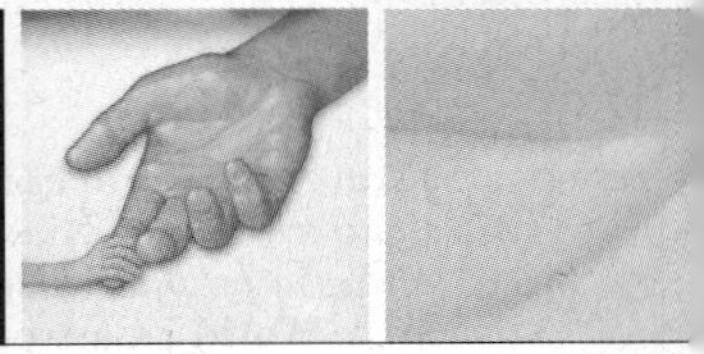

青春期肥胖症外科学

Victor F. Garcia 和 Thomas Inge

1242 美国以及世界范围内儿童肥胖发生率的增加已经成为公共健康危机的一个巨大组成部分[82,89,222,239]。肥胖是慢性进展性疾病，常不易治疗，且对目前的药物干预抵抗力强。在美国肥胖每年导致 40 万人死亡，仅次于吸烟这个可预防的早产儿的死亡原因[182]。近期的分析显示肥胖相关的预期寿命减少主要影响的年龄组比以前认识的要小，特别是在年轻的黑人男性中[101]。在美国，儿童在肥胖人群中增长最快[133]。但直到最近人们才广泛意识到儿童肥胖不只是社会问题，而且对目前和长远健康都有重大影响[70,268]。儿童和青少年肥胖对于成人发病率和早产儿死亡率是独立的危险因素[106,119]。此外，肥胖目前已经被当作儿童和青少年中最紧迫的营养性疾病[95,161,217]。最终，以至于最剧烈的常规减肥方法也无法治疗肥胖[87]。

目前，如果没有其他办法，肥胖手术是严重肥胖个体达到长期体重减轻和改善大多数肥胖相关并存病最有效的措施。它还可以降低病态肥胖患者的长期死亡率[54,100]。肥胖发病率在 5%~11%，死亡率估计在 0.05%~0.5%[49]。有经验的医疗中心已经显示肥胖手术后体重减轻是持久的[136,189,192,204,247]。成人最常见的肥胖手术营养问题已通过补给法得以良好解决。但在青少年中，还不知道该方法的预后是否同成人一致，会不会有难以接受的高复发率以及由于低顺应性或微量营养素吸收减少导致的长期营养后遗症[209,248]。尽管如此，对于极端肥胖青少年尚无有效的非手术治疗措施。随着严重肥胖儿童数量的增加以及严重健康问题的增多，外科手术减轻体重被公认为是治疗严重肥胖青少年的唯一有效方法。

本章中我们为青春期肥胖手术提供概念框架和临床指导。该手术很大程度上借鉴了成人最成功的肥胖手术以及治疗青少年囊性纤维化、哮喘和癌症等慢性疾病的“最佳实践经验”[131,199,211,215,253]。

基本前提是以家庭为中心处理青少年独特的生理、认知力、发展以及心理社会需求，并结合成功应用于其他长期模型中的行为矫正技术。考虑到肥胖手术的困难性、患者术后处理的复杂性以及青少年长期预后的不确定性，为了获得与成人研究最相近的结果，有必要对前瞻性临床资料收集进行集中区域化管理。此外，这也可以增加我们对于青少年肥胖手术短期和长期预后的认识。

青少年肥胖手术的历史回顾

儿童肥胖手术最早报道是 Randolph 和 Weintraub 介绍的空肠回肠旁路术的经验[206]，预后与成人相似。更特别的是，体重减轻非常明显且持久，生活质量显著提高。但代谢性并发症也很明显[231]且按照今天的标准难以承受。Greenstein 和 Rabner[126]报道了大量垂直捆绑胃成形术的成功经验，并得出结论：接受充分饮食指导的青少年可获得与进行完全局限性胃手术的成人相同的手术效果。后继报道的儿童肥胖手术包括一些青少年小宗病例，大多数为开腹以及最近的腹腔镜下 Roux-en-Y 胃旁路术（RYGBP）[1,10,45,142,205,234,238,243,248]或腹腔镜下可调式胃捆绑手术（LAGB）[1,77]，术后预后良好，并发症少
且无手术相关性死亡。如同儿童腹腔镜胆囊切除术、漏 1243
斗胸微创修复术以及腹腔镜抗反流手术一样，青少年肥胖手术尚无前瞻性和对照研究。目前仍未有行可调式胃捆绑手术的青少年术后随访时间超过 4 年的相关报道。一项青少年可调式胃捆绑手术短期研究显示患者 2 年内平均体重减轻 35 kg，表明捆绑术安全且有效[77]。

Sugerman和同事[248]发表了病例最多且随访时间最长的报道，包括33名行肥胖手术——一期胃旁路术的青少年[平均术前体重指数BMI（公斤体重/身高平方米）= $52\ kg/m^2$]。术后5年63%的患者体重明显减轻（平均 $BMI=33\ kg/m^2$），10年为56%（平均 $BMI=34\ kg/m^2$）。14年前行手术治疗的9名患者目前只随访到6名，这6名患者中33%保持体重减轻（平均 $BMI=38\ kg/m^2$）[248]，15%体重回复到以前的部分或全部超重状态，说明术后青少年和成人复发率相同。这些数据提出几个问题——青少年的手术选择标准或术后处理措施是否与成人不同，以及幼年时手术和不手术的肥胖青少年长期营养和代谢状况孰优孰劣？

2001年，Garcia和Inge在辛辛那提儿童医学中心建立了首个以医院为基础的儿童肥胖手术方案[114,142]。该方案被并入到现有的儿童和青少年以行为为基础的减重方案中。这种综合性减重方案为临床顽固性严重肥胖青少年提供减肥服务。候选人先经过评估，然后由2名儿童肥胖手术医生、1名有儿童肥胖专门经验的儿童心脏病专家、经验丰富的护士、营养师、心理学家和运动生理学家对其进行治疗。

肥胖科学

肥胖研究是目前科学研究中最热门的领域之一，融合了生理学、遗传学、神经生物学、内分泌学、分子生物学以及胃肠外科的内容。近几年我们对于肥胖的某些病因认识及其科学基础的难处理性有了相当大的进步。我们对进食行为的神经解剖学基础[127,145,223]、调控摄取食物和能量消耗的分子生物学机制[108,109]、影响能量平衡的基因[56,121,228]以及过剩脂肪组织的炎性成分[272]等作了一些初步的观察。这些系统与环境、发育、情感、心理因素之间复杂相互作用的研究无疑消除了过于简单的观念，即少吃以及多锻炼可控制体重的“决定”性观点，同样也为肥胖伴发一系列代谢疾病如胰岛素抵抗综合征、多囊卵巢综合征和心血管疾病提供了研究基础[109]。简单说来，有确切科学依据指出机体存在一个精确且强大的生物系统维持体重于一个狭窄范围内[109,221]，这说明严重肥胖不是某一个人的选择问题而是慢性、高度顽固且具有连续性风险的疾病。

能量消耗

人体遵循热力学第一定律。因此如果摄入的能量与消耗的能量不相等就会引起体重增加。长期过量摄入能量后，能量在体内以三酰甘油形式贮存，但通常体重会维持相对稳定，证明潜意识中神经系统扮演了调整能量摄入和消耗的波动以维持平衡的角色。数项研究表明能量消耗的高遗传性调节对体重有显著影响。严重肥胖患者减肥时会碰到以下问题：遗传介导的代偿性能量消耗降低、代谢活性以及食欲增加抵抗体重改变[157]。一名青少年如果需要将体重从300磅减到250磅，与体重稳定在250磅的人相比必须消耗更少的日常卡路里以维持新减去的体重。因此对于减肥的人来说，维持体重减轻是非常困难的事。

遗传学

基因通过平衡卡路里摄入和能量消耗来控制体重。家族聚集性和孪生子的研究证明基因对肥胖发生的遗传指数达到0.7~0.8，与基因影响身高的遗传指数相近[6,214]。只有5%的儿童期病态性肥胖是单基因缺损的结果，通常表现为黑皮质素受体亚型即α-促黑激素受体[180]。在其余人群中，肥胖是多基因与环境因素相互作用的结果。有证据表明诱发肥胖的基因和代谢过程为我们祖先在食物紧缺的时候提供生存优势[99,151]。这也许可以解释曾经生活在逆境中的不同群体（非裔美国人、美国本土人群和西班牙人）之间肥胖发生率的高差别性。

肥胖诱导的炎症

肥胖及伴随的病理代谢可伴发以细胞因子生成异常、急性期反应物增多和炎症标志性途径激活为特征的慢性炎症反应[156,265]。超重以及肥胖的儿童和成人
血清C反应蛋白、白介素-6、肿瘤坏死因子-α和瘦 1244
素水平升高，这些都是炎症标记物，并且与心血管危险因素以及心血管性、非心血管性死因密切相关。这可以解释为什么肥胖人群患糖尿病、心脏病以及其他慢性疾病的危险性高。有人推测肥胖伴发的炎症与2型糖尿病、多囊卵巢综合征、非酒精源性肝脂肪化以

及心血管病有关系[31,47,65,137]。随着肥胖的进展，伴随的炎症应答被触发并主要发生于脂肪组织内[137]。

这些炎症改变的细胞来源不只有脂肪细胞，还有巨噬细胞或脂肪细胞前体。巨噬细胞渗入脂肪组织是人类肥胖的特征[263,265]。BMI 和脂肪细胞平均体积是脂肪组织内巨噬细胞积聚的灵敏指标[263]。基因表达分析显示：渗入脂肪的巨噬细胞是脂肪组织内炎症的重要来源[272]。脂肪细胞同时也可生成细胞因子并能激活补体级联反应[139]。过去 10 年的研究有力证明了炎症途径在胰岛素抵抗和 2 型糖尿病中起关键作用[137]。肥胖症中炎症应答如何触发并维持以及如何导致代谢性疾病目前仍然不清楚[265]。对炎症和代谢结果关系的进一步研究可能会取得更深的认知以及治疗学进展，但目前手术减肥仍然是改善严重肥胖代谢状况最有效的方法[5,75,76,148,191,192,204]。

定义

理想情况下，以健康为主导的超重和肥胖的定义应建立在增加健康风险的过剩体脂量上。伴随超重和肥胖的健康风险是连续体的一部分，在一定肥胖水平上可根据特定观察到的人群发生变化[141]。事实上肥胖的健康风险因人种而异。因此极难精确定义什么样的肥胖水平与特定个体健康风险的增加有关。

虽然如此，成人引起发病风险增加的肥胖水平可根据 BMI 精确得出[44,257]。BMI 是被广泛接受的与脂肪负荷相关的体重身高指数。尽管 BMI 与理想的肥胖测量手段相差很大，但大多数临床和流行病学研究仍依据 BMI 检测肥胖。例如，众所周知许多运动员体重超过理想指标且 BMI 偏高。但他们不属于肥胖，因为他们的超重是由于肌肉量的增加。成人 BMI 最常用的域值超重为 25 kg/m^2，肥胖为 30 kg/m^2。成人肥胖的标准通常不适用于尚未完全发育的儿童和青少年，因为脂肪量的生理学变化在发育成熟期间是变化的[97]。例如，出生时平均 BMI 为 13 kg/m^2，1 岁时增至 17 kg/m^2，6 岁时又降回 15 kg/m^2，20 岁时再次升至 21 kg/m^2。在各种测量儿童肥胖的方法中，如果年龄和性别使用百分位数来说明生长发育时 BMI 的正常变化，那么 BMI 是合理的方法。同年龄段的 85% 和 95% 的 BMI 被用来定义超重和肥胖（图 78-1）[16,17,73]。

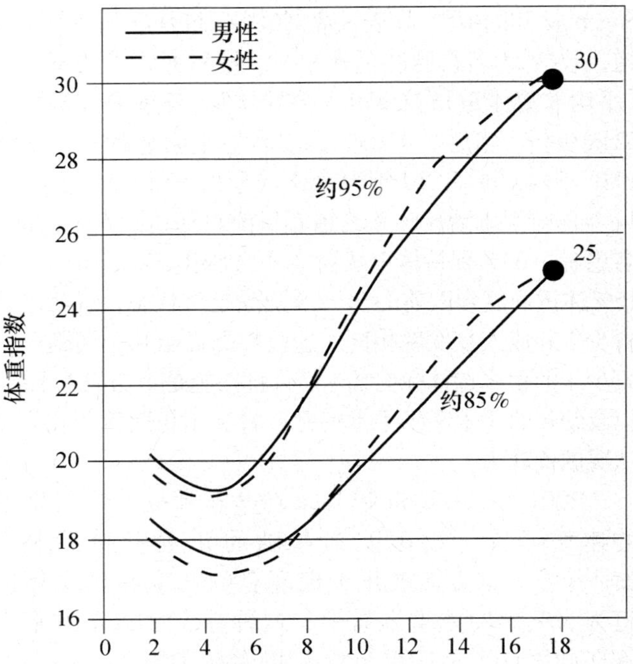

图 78-1 肥胖和超重年龄的体重指数曲线。

儿童肥胖的“95% 可信区间”是一种统计学设计，而不是一种以健康风险为基础的标准。可能肥胖健康风险与向心性肥胖的关系比与 BMI 的关系更直接。事实上一些脂肪库（如腹内）比其他脂肪库（如皮下）更危险，BMI 也不能给出局部脂肪分布的信息，这对于使用 BMI 为标准定义肥胖来说是另一个内在缺陷。

青少年肥胖

流行病学

肥胖是美国最普遍的严重营养疾病。约有 60% 的成年人超重或者肥胖。在过去 14 年中，成人肥胖发病率增加了 2 倍（BMI > 30 kg/m^2），而 BMI 超过 40 kg/m^2 的则增加了 4 倍，超过 50 kg/m^2 的增加了 5 倍[245]。过去 20 年中美国儿童超重和肥胖的发生 1245
率也有上升[194]。在过去 30 年里儿童和青少年肥胖的比例翻了三番[193,194]。儿童是美国超重与肥胖人口增长最快的人群[98]。儿童肥胖的显著增长在其他国家也有发生[78,110,115,153,169,174,274]。与成人肥胖趋势相似，儿童极端肥胖发生率比一般肥胖发生率高[73]。

男孩和女孩的肥胖发生率存在显著的种族差异。男孩中肥胖百分比最高的是墨西哥裔美国人，而女孩中则是非西班牙裔黑人，其次为墨西哥裔美国人。女孩肥胖百分比最低的是非西班牙裔白人[80,123,244]。黑人女孩超重（85%可信区间）的发生率比白人女孩高约 1/3：分别为 31% 和 22%[150]。黑人女孩肥胖（95%可信区间）的发生率为白人女孩的 2 倍：分别为 18% 和 8%。该研究中令人担心的是超重和肥胖发生率几乎翻倍。到 19 岁时超过一半的黑人女孩和 1/3 的白人女孩发生超重，而超过 1/3 的黑人女孩和 1/5 的白人女孩发生肥胖[150]。黑人中逐渐增高的肥胖易感性可能与能量平衡的种族差异有关，因为非裔美国人静息时能量消耗比白人低[113,152]。

危险因素

肥胖的危险随着年龄增长而累积，并受到基因、生物学因素、心理学因素、社会文化以及贯穿一生的环境因素的影响。近期对于胎儿、新生儿和肥胖发展起源的深入了解[195]与肥胖手术青少年候选者的临床评估有很大关联。青少年肥胖的发展在孕前和青春期之间存在临界期[18,22,103,154,179,259]。有流行病学证据显示出生体重与儿童期[21]和成年期[235]BMI[198]有关联。低出生体重可增加向心性肥胖[21,43]和胰岛素抵抗[43]的危险。这种关联的机制目前尚不明确，可能与“节约遗传型或表型”[195]有关。糖尿病母亲下一代患有儿童肥胖的危险性更高[232]。出生后，更长时间的母乳喂养[117,118]和迟发的脂肪反弹[267]可降低青少年超重的危险性。在前面提到的所有危险因素中，低出生体重和青春期高 BMI 对于慢性肥胖来说危险性最高。

家庭成员的肥胖是青春期肥胖的另一项危险因素。如果家庭中双亲有一人肥胖，那么从儿童期到成人期持续肥胖发生的优势比为 3，如果双亲均肥胖，则优势比为 10[268]。这种情况在 10 岁以下的儿童中尤其显著。青春期也是肥胖发生的临界时期[132]。肥胖儿童中可见月经初潮早发。BMI 超过 85%可信区间的女孩月经初潮早发的几率要增大 2 倍[164,262]。青少年肥胖持续至成年的危险比超重幼儿高。最后，发生肥胖的危险性还有事先存在的种族差异[244]。由于饮食匮乏和体力活动机会有限，社会经济较差的人群可能特别易发生肥胖[123]。

健康影响

表 78-1 列出了青春期肥胖对健康的重要影响。随着美国儿童肥胖普遍性和严重性的增高，已经出现了全新的或重新定义的儿童健康问题[71]，其发病

表 78-1 青春期肥胖的健康影响

社会心理方面
自尊心低下[107,243]
抑郁[71,120]
饮食紊乱[3,42]
神经系统
脑假瘤[14,55]
呼吸系统
睡眠呼吸暂停[8,34,160,270]
哮喘和无法耐受运动[128,259]
心血管系统
血脂障碍[10,152,257-260]
高血压[19,20,24-26,41,188,237]
凝血障碍
慢性炎症[64]
内皮机能紊乱[5,111,138,255]
胃肠道系统
胆结石
脂肪肝炎[183,197,219-221]
泌尿系统
肾小球硬化症[4]
内分泌系统
2 型糖尿病[12,13,79,83,84,89,140]
胰岛素抵抗[21,26,46,60,81,149]
代谢综合征[60,61,144,265,275]
性早熟[155,262]
多囊卵巢综合征[104,163]
肌肉骨骼系统
股骨骺脱位
Blount 病
前臂骨折
扁平足

年龄更低[185,186]，成年发病和死亡的风险更高[185]。儿
1246 童肥胖同样还存在负面的社会及经济影响[124,241,260]。约70%~80%的超重儿童成年后发展为肥胖[70]，这种肥胖的持续性[129]与特定并发症有特殊关联。

高血压、血脂异常、慢性炎症、血液高凝状态、内皮功能不全、高胰岛素血症的综合发病，即所知的胰岛素抵抗综合征或代谢综合征[116]，已在5岁的儿童中发现[275]。Bogalusa心脏研究所指出心血管疾病的危险因素与非典型性冠状动脉粥样硬化有关。个体肥胖程度越严重，损伤越大[176,177]。最近一项研究表明代谢综合征在儿童和青少年中的发生远比之前报道的普遍，并且其发病率正好随着肥胖程度增加而增加[264]。该综合征的每个方面都随着肥胖加重而恶化，与年龄、性别和青春期体质无关。

糖尿病前期的一些表现如葡萄糖耐受不良和胰岛素抵抗，在严重肥胖儿童中发病率很高，甚至在临床诊断糖尿病前就可发病[233]。即便以往认为成年发病的2型糖尿病，目前也有将近一半新诊断的儿童糖尿病为该型[90,202]，多半可能是儿童肥胖流行的结果。目前特别值得关注的是从疾病预防控制中心得出的数据，指出于2001年出生的美国人33%会患糖尿病[187]。对于黑人和西班牙人，该数字上升至近50%[187]。英国糖尿病前瞻性研究的发现令人震惊并使人清楚地认识到，虽然目前我们能进行强化治疗并能良好控制血糖，但2型糖尿病仍会自然进展。该资料表明糖尿病伴β细胞功能异常发生于高血糖之前，可在疾病诊断前数年出现[77,146,162,256]。其他研究明确指出儿童期或成人早期发生的2型糖尿病比成年期发病的进展更快[7]，可能比成人后期发生的糖尿病更严重[67]。这可能有宿主依赖性（如年龄小因此更易受到伤害的宿主）或者与儿童多余中心脂肪组织比成人更快积聚有关。

非酒精性脂肪肝炎被认为是儿童慢性肝病的一种常见原因[219]，常伴有肥胖。一项报告称超过25%的超重儿童肝功能检测异常升高[105]。有人指出儿童肥胖源性非酒精性脂肪肝炎[212]可能会成为肝衰竭的主要病因并在未来数十年内成为肝移植的首要指征[52,53,219,220]。

无法耐受运动、睡眠障碍性呼吸和哮喘是青春期肥胖的呼吸系统并发症[94,216]。哮喘和无法耐受运动还会限制体力活动从而进一步增加体重[82]。阻塞性睡眠呼吸暂停（OSA）是睡眠障碍性呼吸中最严重的表现，可明显损害肥胖青少年的与健康相关的生活质量[229]，导致左心室形态异常[9]，并增加他们过度兴奋、学习困难的风险[51]。一些文献还证明阻塞性睡眠呼吸暂停儿童可患有躯体发育减慢和系统性高血压[227]。有一些研究指出肥胖儿童患OSA的危险性是非肥胖儿童的4~5倍[216]。虽然OSA是与BMI直接相关的严重临床问题，但已出版的文献中尚未有对肥胖儿童OSA发病率和生长发育及心血管问题的绝对危险进行定量分析的文章[227]。另外在肥胖引起OSA的青少年患者中，我们发现通过外科手术减重可使他们免受气管造口术之苦。术后6个月内，多睡眠图显示无睡眠呼吸暂停或阻塞性睡眠呼吸暂停。

青春期肥胖对患者最大的影响在于社会心理方面[71,242]。社会言论施加于肥胖儿童身上所产生的心理应激可能与医学疾病一样对他们造成伤害[57]。许多肥胖青少年感到自卑和悲伤并且容易作出高危举动[242]。最近一项健康相关生活质量指数指出，肥胖儿童生活质量评分比苗条儿童明显要低，与小儿肿瘤患者评分相近[229]。超重还和低社会经济水平有关。超重的青春期女性可能更不想结婚，而且更早地结束学校生涯[124]。

儿童肥胖对健康造成的影响比以前认识的范围更广、发病率更高、特定时间点的疾病进展更严重[12,26,60,83,168,175,237,252,264]。肥胖的BMI域值并不能解释疾病负担的人种差异，也无法解释特定人群中肥胖青少年的加速发病[84,188,196]。随着成人疾病在儿童中发病越来越年轻化[70-72,275]，糖耐量降低、胰岛素抵抗、代谢综合征以及2型糖尿病在年幼儿童中发病率逐渐增高[23,50,90,233,237,275]，以及研究显示2型糖尿病儿童期发病比成人期发病更严重[67]，证实了目前儿童肥胖定义的临床关联性，以及疾病负担会随时间而影响控制并发症的能力[167,170,225]。

青少年认知发育：青少年肥胖手术的相关概念和原则

认知发育与思考推断能力的发育有关。在6~12岁时儿童具体思考的能力开始发育。青春期标志着更加复杂思维的开始。在任何年龄，青少年都处于不同的认知和社会心理发育阶段，相比实际年龄，这种情况和处于青春期状态的关系更为密切[251]。

此外，形式运演的成就和个性的形成存在性别差
247 异，这使得达到新的智力水平、进行抽象思维[201]以及认知能力成为可能，而这些对于治疗方案的适用性和针对性都至关重要。形式运演的实例包括思考事物可能性、运用假设进行逻辑推理、预测尚未发生的事件、考虑一些传统的限制以及退一步审视自己的思维过程。在形式运演形成前，青少年运用具体运演分析和推理。在这个阶段的发育过程中，青少年解决问题仅局限于可直接感知或想象的具体事物，只有当心理活动运用于从直接经验中获得的信息时，才有可能发展成心理运演。通过形式运演，青少年可获得推理能力、逻辑抽象思维、进行假设并考虑各种行为的后果。有这种能力的儿童能更好地思考并理解采取营养补充与否的后果，以及之后坚持规定的蛋白质节约食谱。通常青春期也被当作社会实践、挑战传统限制、冒险以及自我中心主义的时期，这些无疑增加了青少年依从保健行为的挑战。

青少年肥胖手术患者术后治疗需进行认识发育水平评估以及对青少年冒险倾向的了解[85]。需要注意的是认知成熟度水平因人而异，与实际年龄无关[58]。获得新的心理能力后并不能立即熟练应用，单单教育也无法增进认知成熟度。增强儿童对于丰富营养及生活方式疗法的依从性需要运用认知发育理论进行有效教育，还需要通过同龄人和家庭帮助其对自身弱点有更现实的了解。

依从性

肥胖手术长期治疗成功的前提是遵守规定的食谱、生活方式以及营养补充疗法。通常认为青春期是一个不断尝试以及会做出各种影响健康的行为如饮食和锻炼的阶段。为加强预防性健康实践和治疗方法的依从性，专业指导至关重要。以往，青少年人群中能遵从健康指导的比率非常低，大约只有40%～50%患有慢性疾病如囊性纤维化病、糖尿病和哮喘的青少年能够遵从[32,220]。Rand 和 McGregor 发现肥胖手术后只有不超过20%的青少年能够非常严格地遵守维生素和微量元素补充疗法[205]。对于患有慢性疾病的青少年，坚持严格的药物和食物疗法实际上是行为疗法应用的进步[69,93,158,208,271]。不幸的是对于服从治疗的患者，目前尚无长期社会心理因素方面的详细资料，因此事先排除“食谱”能够帮助已行肥胖手术但依从性较差的青少年解决预防和治疗问题。为了促使青少年遵从术后终身的食谱和营养补充疗法，青少年肥胖手术方案应该聘请专业人士负责评估认知发育程度、人格特征比如自尊心和自控能力，以及家庭差异如凝聚力和有效沟通能力[58,59]。对这些因素的事先了解有助于增强肥胖手术团队和初级护理医生在术后提供有效的先期辅导的能力，比如有助于知道何时及和谁消耗的非营养性卡路里最多，这样工作团队就可以意识到哪个时期或哪个人会使青少年不易适应术后饮食习惯。

青少年依从性可通过以下几方面提高：（1）视觉辅助；（2）关注治疗立即获得的效果；（3）参加自我管理；（4）自我监督；（5）自我巩固加强[207]。青少年自我管理和相关策略鼓励独立于家庭外，这是青少年发展过程中很重要的一步。随着肥胖手术后饮食模式的改变，需要不断自我巩固加强以形成有利于健康的长期习惯。患者及其家庭需要不断辅导并密切随访以促进其生理和心理稳定。

青春期肥胖手术方案应建立在其他青春期疾病管理方案的最佳实践经验上[210,240]，因此需基于一个前提，即青少年长期体重控制能够获得有组织的家庭参与以及不断的支持。

为了增加青少年依从性，可采取特殊策略，包括教育、根据患者社会文化背景调整治疗方案，以及获得家庭和同龄人的支持（表 78-2）[58]。一些青
少年乐于遵从形式化的自我加强模式，如立约。 1248

表 78-2　改善术后依从性的策略

- 在术前预先采用饮食疗法以在手术干预前明确问题并予解决。
- 使用量杯、食物量表以及建议摄入的特定食物图片以促进青少年遵从饮食计划。
- 为青少年提供一本饮食日记和一本锻炼日记，以表格形式填写并在术前练习。
- 列出患者术后每个恢复阶段可摄取的食物（第 1 周，第 2～4 周，第 2～3 月等）包括该食物的卡路里、蛋白质、碳水化合物和脂肪含量以供参考。
- 详细列出术后所需补充的微量元素以及为什么要补充和如果不补充的后果。

肥胖手术

肥胖手术应被视为一门手术学科而非操作程序。肥胖手术患者是一个有诸多问题的特殊人群，常伴有多种严重并发症。他们有着特殊的术后需求，且术后并发症并不能通过常规诊断方法解决。他们需要长期严密随访，使进行肥胖手术的患者在从青春期到成年的过渡中注意临床护理计划中的主要部分。

目前肥胖手术的大多数步骤在腹腔镜下完成。微创肥胖手术相比开腹手术有明显优点，但也是技术上难度最大的手术之一[226]，手术学习曲线比较陡峭[100]。Schauer 和同事提出学习曲线在 100 例手术时开始呈平稳走向[224]。前肠手术的腹腔镜技术并不能直接转用于肥胖手术，微创手术的熟练度也不能与微创肥胖手术的熟练度画等号。随着肥胖手术数量的攀升，相比早期经常引用的文献而言，并发症发病率和术后死亡率都有所上升[100,165]。因此，一些协会和机构制定了肥胖手术的标准条例和指导方针，最近美国肥胖手术协会提出了肥胖手术优化中心的标准。希望从事肥胖手术的儿外科医生应至少参加一门肥胖手术课程，并在经验丰富的腹腔镜肥胖手术外科医生指导下获得初期手术经验。此外他们必须在选择患者的时候认识并考虑到可引起术中并发症和死亡危险的特征[49,91,92,125,166,203]。

手术选择

目前肥胖手术常用术式有四种：Roux-en-Y 胃旁路术（RYGBP；分为标准、长臂、超长臂 Roux）；腹腔镜可调胃束带术（LAGB）；胃垂直捆扎成形术；以及胆胰转道伴或不伴十二指肠翻转。每种术式均有其特殊潜在并发症或营养问题[40]。所有这些术式均可改善或逆转肥胖并发症，达到明显减轻体重的效果。每种术式均可在腹腔镜下完成，这样住院时间更短、恢复更快[92,168,190]、伤口并发症也更少。但与开腹手术相比，腹腔镜肥胖手术腹腔内并发症发生率较高[189]。目前有学者试图根据患者特点决定哪种术式可能最适合个体需求，但尚无任何前瞻性评估[39]。在大部分地区，胃垂直捆扎成形术已成为历史，不再被应用。表 78-3 列出了各种术式体重减轻的百分比、并发症发生率和死亡率以及手术是否能改进或转换。

Roux-en-Y 胃旁路术

胃旁路术主要是一种调整正常食欲并保持适度吸收不良的限制性手术。在美国这是最早也是最常用的一种肥胖手术。发挥限制作用的主体是小胃袋（15～20 ml）以及缩小的胃出口（1～2 cm），这样能早期且持续保持饱腹感。根据不同肠段通过胃肠旁路重建肠的连续性：标准为 75 cm；长臂为150 cm；超长臂或远端胃旁路为 250 cm[226]。旁路可置于结肠前或结肠后，胃空肠吻合可用端端吻合器或线性吻合器完成或通过手工缝合[226]。我们使用的是 Higa 和同事报道的技术（图 78-2）[135]。这种技术胃空肠吻合口漏的发生率报道最低，而吻合口漏是与手术所致死亡率相关的独立危险因素[91,92,226]。

对于 BMI 达到 50 kg/m^2 的患者而言，旁路越长，减轻的体重才能与采取标准胃旁路术的相对较瘦的患者相比较。术后体重持续减轻（术前体重的 30%～40%）1～2 年，之后趋于平稳。术后并发症包括倾倒综合征、胃空肠吻合口狭窄、吻合口溃疡以及内疝。对这项术式的研究已超过 14 年，在此期间可获得持久的体重减轻[204]。

表 78-3　各种肥胖手术的比较

术式	体重减轻（%EBW）	死亡率（%）	发病率（%）	能逆转	能改进	体重减轻的持久性
RYGBP	65～70	0.5	5	Yes	Yes	＋＋＋＋
LAGB	47	0.1	5	Yes	Yes	?
VGB	60～65	0.1	5	Yes	Yes	＋
BPD ± DS	70	1.5	5	Yes	Yes	＋＋＋＋

RYGBP = Roux-en-Y 胃旁路术；LAGB = 腹腔镜可调胃束带术；VGB = 胃垂直捆扎成形术；BPD ± DS = 胆胰转道伴或不伴十二指肠翻转；EBW = 超重体重

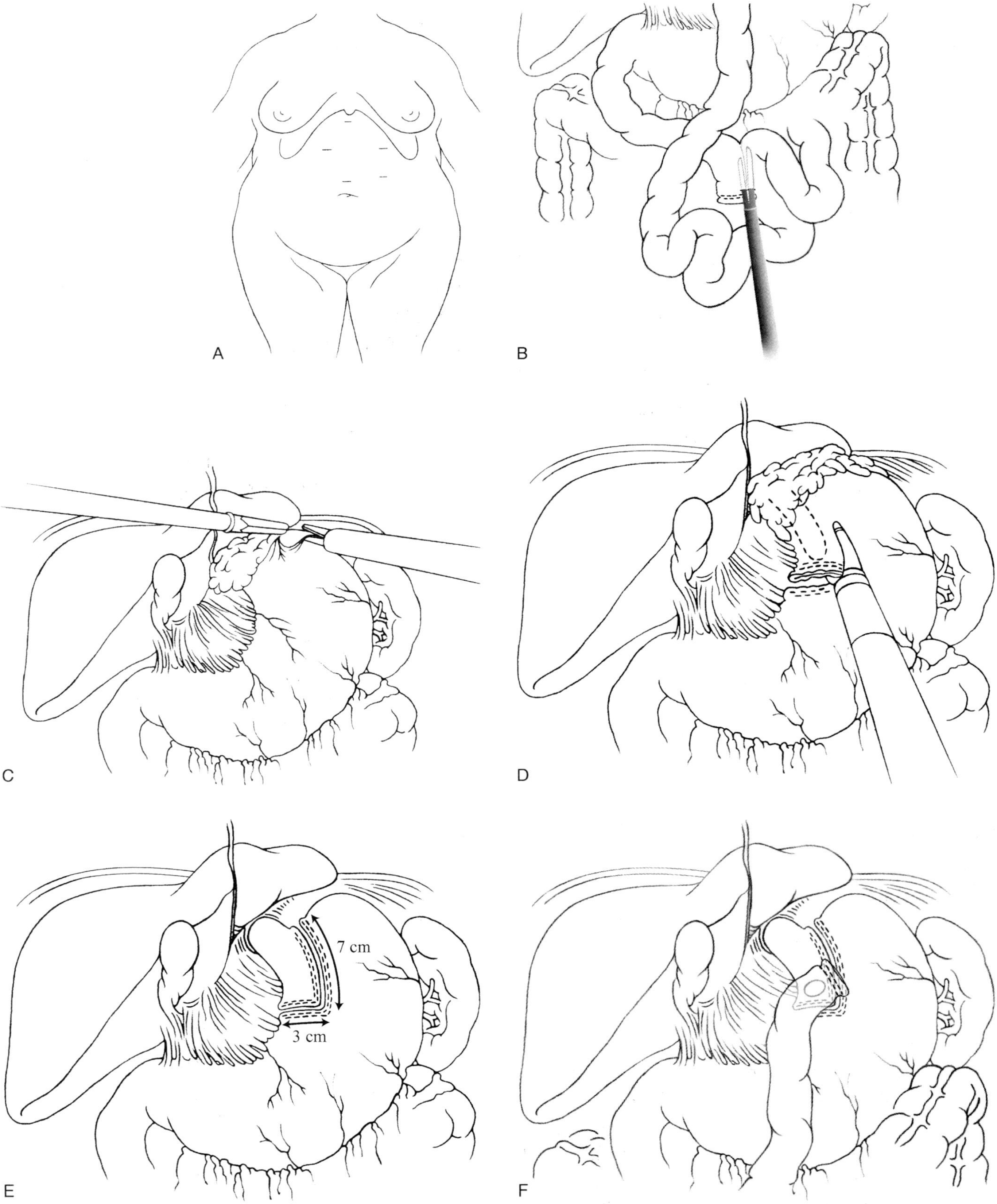

图 78-2　Roux-en-Y 胃旁路手术。A. 各种腹腔镜入径部位。B. 准备进行 Roux 支的吻合。C. 松解胃。D. 准备形成旁路袋。E. 旁路袋宽 3.0 cm，长 7.0 cm。F. 胃空肠吻合。

腹腔镜可调胃束带术

腹腔镜可调胃束带术是创伤最小的肥胖手术，在欧洲、拉丁美洲和澳大利亚开展最广泛。美国食品与药品管理局已于2001年批准使用胃箍。接受和使用该技术的美国医院正不断增加。通过腹腔镜放置的束带在胃较高位置处形成一个小口袋和吻合口。于前腹壁处打孔以调节束带。定期调节束带对取得良好预后非常关键。使用胃箍的并发症包括胃脱垂、吻合口狭窄、束带侵蚀胃壁和进入孔问题。松弛部技术显著降低了胃脱垂的危险[184,218]。最近一篇文献综述显示：尽管胃束带术短期发病率和死亡率风险比胃旁路术低，但可调式胃束带术长期效果尚无定论。建议通过随机对照试验比较胃箍和胃旁路术以明确其优点[49]。

胆胰转道伴或不伴十二指肠翻转术

胆胰转道术[230]在欧洲使用广泛。十二指肠翻转术由Hess和同事一起改进[134]。两种术式都主要是保持吸收不良，包括建立100～150 ml的胃袋。通过将小肠在回盲瓣处分成的肠支和胆胰支吻合，建立一条50～150 cm长的共同通道，并可避免空肠回肠旁路术中碰到的中毒问题。相比胆胰转道加其他减肥术式，胆胰转道加十二指肠翻转术体重减轻更加明显。但这些术式造成的维生素、营养和蛋白质缺乏也比之前提及的减肥手术更加常见[11]。

营养代谢问题

肥胖手术后的营养代谢问题已经详细叙述过了[35,38,74,243,246]。所有在胃下部和近端小肠处做旁路手术的术后患儿都会发生铁、叶酸、钙以及维生素B_{12}吸收障碍。即使术后增补，铁、维生素、叶酸和钙缺乏也会发生。考虑到青少年术后依从性较差[205]，某些特定营养素如维生素B_1、叶酸和钙等需要特别考虑。

叶酸对于DNA和RNA的合成以及氨基酸循环非常重要，尤其是甲硫氨酸-半胱氨酸循环中的甲基化，对于生长发育、细胞分化、基因调节、修复以及宿主防御均必不可少[37,130]。一般人群中叶酸缺乏发生率比之前文献提到的更普遍。孕期中器官形成阶段如果母体叶酸充足，可降低神经管缺损、室间隔缺损、泌尿道梗阻畸形、肢体缺损、面裂和先天肥厚性幽门狭窄的发生率。神经管闭合发生于受孕后26～28天（如在意识到怀孕前第一次月经未来后的1～2周）。因此在此期间后开始补充叶酸不太可能预防神经管缺损。

母体叶酸缺乏还可伴发围生期并发症如低出生体重、早产、胎盘早剥、梗死形成以及儿童发生神经外胚层瘤。叶酸缺乏表现为血清半胱氨酸水平升高，还可伴发心血管疾病、发育不良危险增加以及肿瘤形成。考虑到叶酸缺乏的蛋白表现，通常建议所有适龄妇女都应补充叶酸。对于经历肥胖手术的青少年，仅靠食补（如谷类食物）还不够，因此富含多种维生素的额外补给治疗至关重要。检测血清叶酸和半胱氨酸浓度有助于诊断是否存在叶酸缺乏[33,74,112,181]。

青少年是骨骼成长的飞速阶段，也是增加骨骼矿物质的高峰时机，对于终生骨健康的影响可正可负。青春期个人钙营养的不同可导致绝经后髋骨骨折发生率高达50%的差异[172,173]。尽管普遍认为肥胖青少年骨量超过正常标准[159]，而且由于钙吸收、骨折危险或将来骨质疏松等这些因素不利于手术，但目前已有人对这个观点提出不同看法[86]。目前尚不清楚减肥手术后骨密度降低以及服用维生素D和钙剂依从性较差，是否会增加青少年肥胖手术患者将来骨折的风险。因此我们认为，有必要对行肥胖手术特别是胃旁路术和胆胰转道术的青少年，严密检测其骨矿物质密度。

青少年肥胖手术指导方针

对非手术减肥疗法无效且有多种严重并发症的严重肥胖，应将其考虑为肥胖手术的适应证。其他适应证包括极端肥胖严重影响日常生活的，以及肯定会导致健康问题的肥胖。图78-3列出了由儿童肥胖专家组制定的治疗计划[143]。对于在专家指导下6个月未能减重的青少年，可以考虑选择肥胖手术（表78-4）。

日益增多的术前超重及男性都是导致手术相关并发症和死亡率的危险因素[91,92]。考虑到这些因素以及参照指导方针，选择进行减肥手术的青少年平均体

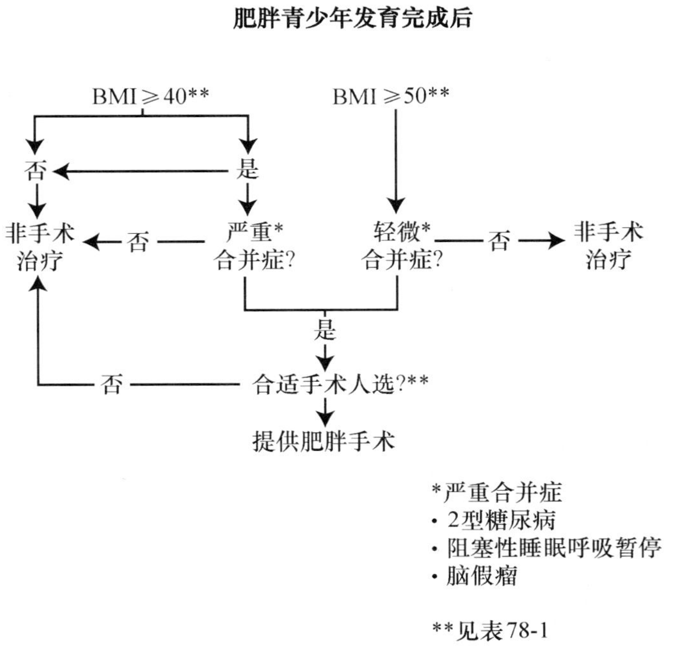

图 78-3 肥胖青少年治疗流程图。（From Inge TH, Krebs NF, Garcia VF, et al: Bariatric surgery for severely overweight adolescents: Concerns and recommendations. Pediatrics 2004; 114; 217-223）

重比成年患者更重。对于手术医生来说，考虑患者体形可能会增加手术的潜在风险是很重要的。一些专家建议处于学习曲线早期的医生应该避免治疗高风险患者以降低术后并发症[91]。

青少年肥胖手术应在具备多学科综合小组的医疗中心进行，并能提供长期随访和处理青春期年龄组独特的行为学问题。根据美国肥胖手术协会和美国外科医师学会制定的标准[249]，综合小组应包括具有专业知识的青春期肥胖评估治疗专家、心理学家、营养师、行为指导专家以及肥胖手术医生。根据个体需要，治疗小组还需具备青春期用药、内分泌学、肺病学、胃肠病学、心脏病学、整形外科学和伦理学等方面的专业知识。同时还应包括类似于多学科儿童肿瘤学和移植方案中使用的评估程序。这个评估程序应能为患者及其家庭提供特别制定的治疗建议。

对于超重青少年并没有实行肥胖手术特定的最佳时间，多数取决于患者迫切的健康需求。需要考虑的还有生长发育和成熟因素。生理成熟通常在性成熟（Tanner）第三阶段或第四阶段完成。女孩达到骨骼成熟（达到成人身高）为 13 ~ 14 岁，男孩则为 15 ~ 16岁。超重儿童通常青春期提早开始。因此，与同年龄非超重儿童相比，他们可能长得更高或者骨龄更长。如果无法确定是否已达到成人身高水平，可通过手和手腕 X 线片来客观评价骨骼成熟度（骨龄）。如果个体已达到成人身高水平的 95%，肥胖手术可能无法明显影响其线性生长的完成。

因此决定患者合适与否，所有的候选人都应进行广泛的心理学评估。评估的目的在于（1）确定心理应激原或家庭内冲突，以及过去和现在的精神、情感、行为或饮食异常；（2）明确患儿依从性潜在的促进和阻碍因素，以及其家庭是否准备好进行手术和改变生活方式（特别是家长中一方或双方肥胖的家庭）；（3）最重要的是评估能否达到合理的期望结果；（4）评估青少年患者认知力和社会心理发育水平。在变更肥胖手术后饮食模式的同时，需反复强化以帮助形成促进健康的终生习惯。这个年龄段的肥胖手术应基于一个前提，即有强大的和规律的术后心理支持以保持体重控制。行为治疗学家的作用取决于青少年智力功能水平，包括术前视觉-运动行为演练疗法，运用行为合约描述治疗要求并获得患者同意坚持该行为合约，制定患儿及家长坚持监督和意外强化的计划。治疗学家在建立家长-青少年之间的沟通、化解家庭冲突、改变行为习惯和进行家庭干预中起到关键作用，这有助于家
庭疗法帮助患者建立新的生活方式。稳定的家庭环 1252
境以及家庭成员无条件的全力支持是青少年肥胖手术的必要条件。

表 78-4　青少年肥胖手术候选人标准

- 患儿有动力和良好的洞察力
- 患儿期望值符合现实
- 家庭能支持和实行治疗计划
- 患儿能遵从健康康复计划
- 患儿及其家属明白需要长期改变生活习惯
- 患儿同意长期随访
- 患儿具有决断力
- 明确患儿有减重愿望
- 无证据表明患儿存在影响术后治疗依从性的严重精神疾病
- 没有较严重的指导/行为问题
- 之前无精神性药物滥用
- 患儿在未来 2 年内无怀孕计划

青少年肥胖手术的临床处理路径

肥胖手术可减少进食并降低富含必须脂肪酸、维生素和其他特殊营养物质的食物的吸收，这项手术的长期结果目前正受到质问和立法关注[15,68,88,102,178,213,273]。肥胖手术后体重急剧减轻能改善严重肥胖妇女的生育能力，还能使妊娠增加的体重正常化，减少巨大儿发生率以及使胎儿出生体重正常化[171,270]。然而，正如荷兰饥荒[213]时所反应的那样，胎儿发育期间营养不良可导致成年肥胖。因此青少年肥胖手术的成功需要更广泛的定义，不仅要维持体重减轻，还必须在日后的青春期、成年期发育正常并最终顺利地生出正常的后代。

肥胖手术对于青少年的长期影响目前尚无前瞻性评估。青少年肥胖手术中心以及治疗方案的目标不应局限于获得显著持续的体重减轻，还应致力于研究最有效的手术方法、复发的危险因素以及长期预后。实施青少年肥胖手术的医疗中心应高度关注患儿骨密度以及终生维生素和营养吸收减少方面的细节，尤其是育龄期妇女及其后代。为了取得这方面的进展，这些医学中心必须进行广泛的临床和基础研究工作。部分地区选择的复杂手术如青少年肥胖手术的潜在优势已被证实[27-30,48,96,122]。为了达到这个目标，青少年肥胖手术应集中在愿意且能够提供综合的术前、术后研究包括实验室检查和诊断评估的医学中心开展。因此位于辛辛那提儿童医学中心的综合体重治疗中心设计出临床路径，用于更好地了解行肥胖手术的青少年中肥胖相关并发症的发生和处理，以及对在更小年纪中广泛开展的肥胖手术已知和未知的影响进行监督。

我们的术前常规包括完整的化学指标、肝功能检测、尿酸、转铁蛋白、铁离子、叶酸、脂类指标、尿液分析、心电图、血常规、血红蛋白 A_{1C}、空腹血糖、空腹胰岛素、促甲状腺激素，女性还需进行妊娠试验。非糖尿病患儿进行 2 小时葡萄糖耐量试验。除葡萄糖耐量试验外，之前提及的实验室和诊断学常规检查在术后 3、6、9、12 个月必须复查，之后每年复查即可。对于体重超过 300 磅的患儿可通过生物电阻抗评估身体成分，对于体重小于 300 磅的患儿则通过双能 X 线吸收仪（DEXA）进行分析，分析需在术前和术后 3、6、12 个月时进行。DEXA 不仅可以测量脂肪和瘦肌肉的减少率和相对量，还能为骨密度变化提供定量分析。身体成分分析可在减肥期间用于调整饮食计划以保存瘦肌肉。有证据表明青少年骨矿物质含量即使只有 2 个标准差的改变，也能明显增加将来骨质疏松和骨折的风险，这强调了严密广泛监测营养、维生素和矿物质吸收的重要性[147]。由于与非肥胖青少年相比，肥胖者心脏形态畸形[62,63,66]和睡眠障碍发生率[9]更高，准备肥胖手术的患儿应进行超声心动图和儿童特异性多导睡眠描记检查。

我们的肥胖手术经验

第一个儿童医院综合性肥胖治疗方案在 2001 年于美国辛辛那提市制定[114,142]。迄今为止已有 66 例患儿进行了 Roux-en-Y 胃旁路术（4 例开放手术，62 例腹腔镜下完成）。在随访为 1 年或 1 年以上的患儿中，术前平均体重为 361 磅（164 kg），BMI 范围为 44～85 kg/m²，平均 57 kg/m²。术后 1 年，平均体重为 222 磅（101 kg），BMI 范围为 26～58 kg/m²，平均 35 kg/m²。这表示 1 年中 BMI 降低了 39%，过剩体重减轻则为 63%。BMI 为 85 kg/m²的这名患者在 1 年中减掉 71 kg，但术后第 2 年底体重恢复了 6 kg。没有因手术而死亡的病例，尽管有两例发生术后吻合口漏，但手工缝合的胃空肠吻合口无 1 例发生这种情况。2 例术后漏均通过微创修补，没有造成患儿生理创伤。胃旁路术明显逆转了肥胖术前并存疾病。3 例 2 型糖尿病患儿和 7 例 OSA 患儿术后症状完全缓解，不再需要降血糖药物和连续气道正压通气。在这最初的一组患儿中发生的并发症与成人组中相似。有一个例外需要注意即 2 例青少年胃旁路术后发生脚气病[255]，提示我们在治疗中加入复合维生素 B。只有一些极度肥胖患儿需要预先注意，并在术后短期住在监护室内。

青少年肥胖代表着一类比成人更加严重[101]和难治的疾病[205,248]。但是目前我们还缺乏对该人群肥胖手术长期预后（肯定和否定的）的了解。因此提供肥胖手术治疗的医学中心有义务准确评价手术结果，确保建立适当机制以详细收集所有行肥胖手术青少年的术后并发症变化以及有害事件的资料。这能够帮助我们更好地明确肥胖手术在这些患儿治疗过程中的作用。

总结

在美国，肥胖流行已使一部分青少年过早患上成人疾病。临床和流行病学研究已阐明一些儿童和青少年肥胖发展过程中的危险因素。目前肥胖手术是维持体重减轻以及解决或改善肥胖主要并发症的最有效手段。青少年肥胖手术成功的定义不仅应包括体重减轻以及死亡率减少，还应包括患者在儿童和成人阶段的正常发育。为实现这个目标，青少年肥胖手术小组应由专业成员组成，这样能增加患儿复合营养和生活方式疗法终生的依从性，也就是说专家可以评估和满足青少年特殊的医疗、认知、生理和社会心理方面的需求。肥胖手术的指导方针应以保守治疗为主，易于察觉对青少年生长潜能可能造成的影响，并能在手术相关并发症风险最小时进行手术并确保尽可能治疗肥胖相关并发症。青少年肥胖手术后对于严格的营养和生活方式疗法的依从性最佳的维持方式是家庭-医学中心小组模式，即结合行为策略以尽可能保证术后饮食、体力活动指导的依从性。肥胖手术是极其复杂和高难度的手术。手术导致的死亡率和预后体现出医院和医生开展该手术的能力，其相对效果与该医院能否开展治疗有直接关系。考虑到目前青少年肥胖手术长期预后的不确定性，区域化治疗和建立全国患儿数据库刻不容缓，我们必须达到和成人最佳结果相同的水平，并提高对青少年肥胖手术短期和长期影响的认识。

（王宇鹏译　董其刚校）

参考文献

1. Abu-Abeid S, Gavert N, Klausner JM, Szold A: Bariatric surgery in adolescence. J Pediatr Surg 2003;38:1379-1382.
2. Adami GF, Meneghelli A, Scopinaro N: Night eating and binge eating disorder in obese patients. Int J Eat Disord 1999;25:335-338.
3. Adelman RD, Restaino IG, Alon US, Blowey DL: Proteinuria and focal segmental glomerulosclerosis in severely obese adolescents. J Pediatr 2001;138:481-485.
4. Aggoun Y, Tounian P, Dabbas-Tyan M, et al: [Arterial rigidity and endothelial dysfunction in obese children]. Arch Mal Coeur Vaiss 2002;95:631-635.
5. Albrecht RJ, Pories WJ: Surgical intervention for the severely obese. Baillieres Best Pract Res Clin Endocrinol Metab 1999;13:149-172.
6. Allison DB, Miller RA, Austad SN, et al: Genetic variability in responses to caloric restriction in animals and in regulation of metabolism and obesity in humans. J Gerontol A Biol Sci Med Sci 2001;56(Spec No 1):55-65, 2001.
7. American Diabetes Association: Type 2 diabetes in children and adolescents. Pediatrics 2000;105:671-680.
8. Amin R, Daniels S: Relationship between obesity and sleep-disordered breathing in children: Is it a closed loop? J Pediatr 2002;140:641-643.
9. Amin RS, Kimball TR, Bean JA, et al: Left ventricular hypertrophy and abnormal ventricular geometry in children and adolescents with obstructive sleep apnea. Am J Respir Crit Care Med 2002;165:1395-1399.
10. Anderson AE, Soper RT, Scott DH: Gastric bypass for morbid obesity in children and adolescents. J Pediatr Surg 1980;15:876-881.
11. Anthone GJ, Lord RV, DeMeester TR, Crookes PF: The duodenal switch operation for the treatment of morbid obesity. Ann Surg 2003;238:618-627; discussion 627-628.
12. Arslanian S: Type 2 diabetes in children: Clinical aspects and risk factors. Horm Res 2002;57(Suppl 1):19-28.
13. Aye T, Levitsky LL: Type 2 diabetes: An epidemic disease in childhood. Curr Opin Pediatr 2003;15:411-415.
14. Balcer LJ, Liu GT, Forman S, et al: Idiopathic intracranial hypertension: Relation of age and obesity in children. Neurology 1999;52:870-872.
15. Barker DJ, Eriksson JG, Forsen T, Osmond C: Fetal origins of adult disease: Strength of effects and biological basis. Int J Epidemiol 2002;31:1235-1239.
16. Barlow SE, Dietz WH: Obesity evaluation and treatment: Expert Committee recommendations. The Maternal and Child Health Bureau, Health Resources and Services Administration and the Department of Health and Human Services. Pediatrics 1998;102:E29.
17. Barlow SE, Dietz WH, Klish WJ, Trowbridge FL: Medical evaluation of overweight children and adolescents: Reports from pediatricians, pediatric nurse practitioners, and registered dietitians. Pediatrics 2002;110:222-228.
18. Bartley M, Blane D, Montgomery S: Health and the life course: Why safety nets matter. BMJ 1997;314:1194-1196.
19. Barton M, Furrer J: Cardiovascular consequences of the obesity pandemic: Need for action. Expert Opin Invest Drugs 2003;12:1757-1759.
20. Bartosh SM, Aronson AJ: Childhood hypertension: An update on etiology, diagnosis, and treatment. Pediatr Clin North Am 1990;46:235-252.
21. Bavdekar A, Yajnik CS, Fall CH, et al: Insulin resistance syndrome in 8-year-old Indian children: Small at birth, big at 8 years, or both? Diabetes 1999;48:2422-2429.
22. Ben-Shlomo Y, Kuh D: A life course approach to chronic disease epidemiology: Conceptual models, empirical challenges and interdisciplinary perspectives. Int J Epidemiol 2002;31:285-293.
23. Berenson GS: Bogalusa Heart Study: A long-term community study of a rural biracial (black/white) population. Am J Med Sci 2001;322:293-300. 1253
24. Berenson GS, Srinivasan SR: Emergence of obesity and cardiovascular risk for coronary artery disease: The Bogalusa Heart Study. Prev Cardiol 2001;4:116-121.
25. Berenson GS, Wattigney WA, Webber LS: Epidemiology of hypertension from childhood to young adulthood in black, white, and Hispanic population samples. Pub Health Rep 1996;111(Suppl 2):3-6.
26. Bhatia V: IAP National Task Force for Childhood Prevention of Adult Diseases: Insulin resistance and type 2 diabetes mellitus in childhood. Indian Pediatr 2004;41:443-457.
27. Birkmeyer JD, Dimick JB: Potential benefits of the new

Leapfrog standards: Effect of process and outcomes measures. Surgery 2004;135:569-575.
28. Birkmeyer JD, Dimick JB, Birkmeyer NJ: Measuring the quality of surgical care: Structure, process, or outcomes? J Am Coll Surg 2004;198:626-632.
29. Birkmeyer JD, Finlayson EV, Birkmeyer CM: Volume standards for high-risk surgical procedures: Potential benefits of the Leapfrog initiative. Surgery 2001;130:415-422.
30. Birkmeyer JD, Siewers AE, Finlayson EV, et al: Hospital volume and surgical mortality in the United States. N Engl J Med 2002;346:1128-1137.
31. Black PH: The inflammatory response is an integral part of the stress response: Implications for atherosclerosis, insulin resistance, type II diabetes and metabolic syndrome X. Brain Behav Immun 2003;17:350-364.
32. Borowitz D, Wegman T, Harris M: Preventive care for patients with chronic illness: Multivitamin use in patients with cystic fibrosis. Clin Pediatr 1994;33:720-725.
33. Borson-Chazot F, Harthe C, Teboul F, et al: Occurrence of hyperhomocysteinemia 1 year after gastroplasty for severe obesity. J Clin Endocrinol Metab 1999;84:541-545.
34. Bower CM, Gungor A: Pediatric obstructive sleep apnea syndrome. Otolaryngol Clin North Am 2000;33:49-75.
35. Boylan LM, Sugerman HJ, Driskell JA: Vitamin E, vitamin B-6, vitamin B-12, and folate status of gastric bypass surgery patients. J Am Diet Assoc 1988;88:579-585.
36. Brolin RE, Gorman JH, Gorman RC, et al: Prophylactic iron supplementation after Roux-en-Y gastric bypass: A prospective, double-blind, randomized study. Arch Surg 1998;133: 740-744.
37. Brolin RE, Gorman JH, Gorman RC, et al: Are vitamin B_{12} and folate deficiency clinically important after Roux-en-Y gastric bypass? J Gastrointest Surg 1998;2:436-442.
38. Brolin RE, Gorman RC, Milgrim LM, Kenler HA: Multivitamin prophylaxis in prevention of post-gastric bypass vitamin and mineral deficiencies. Int J Obes 1991;15:661-667.
39. Buchwald H: A bariatric surgery algorithm. Obes Surg 2002;12:733-746; discussion 747-750.
40. Buchwald H: Overview of bariatric surgery. J Am Coll Surg 2002;194:367-375.
41. Buiten C, Metzger B: Childhood obesity and risk of cardiovascular disease: A review of the science. Pediatr Nurs 2000;26:13-18.
42. Burrows A, Cooper M: Possible risk factors in the development of eating disorders in overweight pre-adolescent girls. Int J Obes Relat Metab Disord 2002;26:1268-1273.
43. Byberg L, McKeigue PM, Zethelius B, Lithell HO: Birth weight and the insulin resistance syndrome: Association of low birth weight with truncal obesity and raised plasminogen activator inhibitor-1 but not with abdominal obesity or plasma lipid disturbances. Diabetologia 2000;43:54-60.
44. Calle EE, Thun MJ, Petrelli JM, et al: Body-mass index and mortality in a prospective cohort of U.S. adults. N Engl J Med 1999;341:1097-1105.
45. Capella JF, Capella RF: Bariatric surgery in adolescence: Is this the best age to operate? Obes Surg 2003;13:826-832.
46. Caprio S: Insulin resistance in childhood obesity. J Pediatr Endocrinol Metab 2002;15(Suppl 1):487-492.
47. Chan JC, Cheung JC, Stehouwer CD, et al: The central roles of obesity-associated dyslipidaemia, endothelial activation and cytokines in the Metabolic Syndrome—an analysis by structural equation modelling. Int J Obes Relat Metab Disord 2002;26:994-1008.
48. Chang RK, Klitzner TS: Can regionalization decrease the number of deaths for children who undergo cardiac surgery? A theoretical analysis. Pediatrics 2002;109:173-181.
49. Chapman AE, Kiroff G, Game P, et al: Laparoscopic adjustable gastric banding in the treatment of obesity: A systematic literature review. Surgery 2004;135:326-351.
50. Chen W, Bao W, Begum S, et al: Age-related patterns of the clustering of cardiovascular risk variables of syndrome X from childhood to young adulthood in a population made up of black and white subjects: The Bogalusa Heart Study. Diabetes 2000;49:1042-1048.
51. Chervin RD, Dillon JE, Archbold KH, Ruzicka DL: Conduct problems and symptoms of sleep disorders in children. J Am Acad Child Adolesc Psychiatry 2003;42:201-208.
52. Chitturi S, Farrell GC: Etiopathogenesis of nonalcoholic steatohepatitis. Semin Liver Dis 2001;21:27-41.
53. Chitturi S, Farrell GC, George J: Non-alcoholic steatohepatitis in the Asia-Pacific region: Future shock? J Gastroenterol Hepatol 2004;19:368-374.
54. Christou NV, Sampalis JS, Liberman M, et al: Surgery decreases long-term mortality, morbidity, and health care use in morbidly obese patients. Ann Surg 2004;240:416-423; discussion 423-424.
55. Cinciripini GS, Donahue S, Borchert MS: Idiopathic intracranial hypertension in prepubertal pediatric patients: Characteristics, treatment, and outcome. Am J Ophthalmol 1999;127:178-182.
56. Clement K, Boutin P, Froguel P: Genetics of obesity. Am J Pharmacogenomics 2002;2:177-187.
57. Committee on Nutrition of the American Academy of Pediatrics: Prevention of pediatric overweight and obesity. Pediatrics 2003;112:424-430.
58. Cromer B: Compliance with health recommendations. In Stanford Friedman MF, Schonberg SK, Alderman E (eds): Comprehensive Adolescent Health Care, 2nd ed. New York, Mosby-Year Book, 1998, pp 104-108.
59. Cromer BA, Tarnowski KJ: Noncompliance in adolescents: A review. J Dev Behav Pediatr 1989;10:207-215.
60. Cruz ML, Goran MI: The metabolic syndrome in children and adolescents. Curr Diab Rep 2004;4:53-62.
61. Csabi G, Torok K, Jeges S, Molnar D: Presence of metabolic cardiovascular syndrome in obese children. Eur J Pediatr 2000;159:91-94.
62. Daniels SR, Kimball TR, Morrison JA, et al: Effect of lean body mass, fat mass, blood pressure, and sexual maturation on left ventricular mass in children and adolescents. Statistical, biological, and clinical significance. Circulation 1995;92:3249-3254.
63. Daniels SR, Witt SA, Glascock B, et al: Left atrial size in children with hypertension: The influence of obesity, blood pressure, and left ventricular mass. J Pediatr 2002;141: 186-190.
64. Das UN: Is obesity an inflammatory condition? Nutrition 2001;17:953-966.
65. Das UN: Obesity, metabolic syndrome X, and inflammation. Nutrition 2002;18:430-432.
66. de Simone G, Devereux RB, Daniels SR, et al: Stroke volume and cardiac output in normotensive children and adults: Assessment of relations with body size and impact of overweight. Circulation 1997;95:1837-1843.
67. Dean H, Flett B: Natural history of type 2 diabetes mellitus diagnosed in childhood: Long term follow-up in young adults. Diabetes 2002;51:A24.
68. Delisle H: [Foetal programming of nutrition-related chronic diseases]. Sante 2002;12:56-63.

69. Denzer C, Reithofer E, Wabitsch M, Widhalm K: The outcome of childhood obesity management depends highly upon patient compliance. Eur J Pediatr 2004;163:99-104.
70. Dietz WH: Childhood weight affects adult morbidity and mortality. J Nutr 1998;128(Suppl):411S-414S.
71. Dietz WH: Health consequences of obesity in youth: Childhood predictors of adult disease. Pediatrics 1998; 101:518-525.
72. Dietz WH: Overweight and precursors of type 2 diabetes mellitus in children and adolescents. J Pediatr 2001;138:453-454.
73. Dietz WH: Overweight in childhood and adolescence. N Engl J Med 2004;350:855-857.
74. Dixon JB, Dixon ME, O'Brien PE: Elevated homocysteine levels with weight loss after Lap-Band surgery: Higher folate and vitamin B_{12} levels required to maintain homocysteine level. Int J Obes Relat Metab Disord 2001;25:219-227.
75. Dixon JB, O'Brien PE: Health outcomes of severely obese type 2 diabetic subjects 1 year after laparoscopic adjustable gastric banding. Diabetes Care 2002;25:358-363.
76. Dixon JB, O'Brien PE: Lipid profile in the severely obese: Changes with weight loss after lap-band surgery. Obes Res 2002;10:903-910.
77. Dolan K, Creighton L, Hopkins G, Fielding G: Laparoscopic gastric banding in morbidly obese adolescents. Obes Surg 2003;13:101-104.
78. Dorosty AR, Siassi F, Reilly JJ: Obesity in Iranian children. Arch Dis Child 2002;87:388-391; discussion 388-391.
79. Drake AJ, Smith A, Betts PR, et al: Type 2 diabetes in obese white children. Arch Dis Child 2002;86:207-208.
80. Dwyer JT, Stone EJ, Yang M, et al: Prevalence of marked overweight and obesity in a multiethnic pediatric population: Findings from the Child and Adolescent Trial for Cardiovascular Health (CATCH) study. J Am Diet Assoc 2000;100:1149-1156.
81. Dwyer T, Blizzard L, Venn A, et al: Syndrome X in 8-year-old Australian children: Stronger associations with current body fatness than with infant size or growth. Int J Obes Relat Metab Disord 2002;26:1301-1309.
82. Ebbeling CB, Pawlak DB, Ludwig DS: Childhood obesity: Public-health crisis, common sense cure. Lancet 2002;360: 473-482.
83. Ehtisham S, Barrett TG: The emergence of type 2 diabetes in childhood. Ann Clin Biochem 2004;41:10-16.
84. Ehtisham S, Hattersley AT, Dunger DB, Barrett TG: First UK survey of paediatric type 2 diabetes and MODY. Arch Dis Child 2004;89:526-529.
85. Elkind D: Cognitive development. In Stanford Friedman MF, Schonberg SK, Alderman E (eds): Comprehensive Adolescent Health Care, 2nd ed. St. Louis, Mosby-Year Book, 1998, pp 34-37.
86. Ellis KJ, Shypailo RJ, Wong WW, Abrams SA: Bone mineral mass in overweight and obese children: Diminished or enhanced? Acta Diabetol 2003;40(Suppl 1):S274-277.
87. Epstein LH, Myers MD, Raynor HA, Saelens BE: Treatment of pediatric obesity. Pediatrics 1998;101:554-570.
88. Eriksson J, Forsen T, Osmond C, Barker D: Obesity from cradle to grave. Int J Obes Relat Metab Disord 2003;27:722-727.
89. Fagot-Campagna A: Emergence of type 2 diabetes mellitus in children: Epidemiological evidence. J Pediatr Endocrinol Metab 2000;13(Suppl 6):1395-1402.
90. Fagot-Campagna A, Pettitt DJ, Engelgau MM, et al: Type 2 diabetes among North American children and adolescents: An epidemiologic review and a public health perspective. J Pediatr 2000;136:664-672.
91. Fernandez AZ Jr, DeMaria EJ, Tichansky DS, et al: Experience with over 3,000 open and laparoscopic bariatric procedures: Multivariate analysis of factors related to leak and resultant mortality. Surg Endosc 2004;18:193-197.
92. Fernandez AZ Jr, DeMaria EJ, Tichansky DS, et al: Multivariate analysis of risk factors for death following gastric bypass for treatment of morbid obesity. Ann Surg 2004;239:698-702; discussion 702-703.
93. Fielding D, Duff A: Compliance with treatment protocols: Interventions for children with chronic illness. Arch Dis Child 1999;80:196-200.
94. Figueroa-Munoz JI, Chinn S, Rona RJ: Association between obesity and asthma in 4- to 11-year old children in the UK. Thorax 2001;56:133-137.
95. Filozof C, Gonzalez C, Sereday M, et al: Obesity prevalence and trends in Latin-American countries. Obes Rev 2001;2:99-106.
96. Finlayson EV, Goodney PP, Birkmeyer JD: Hospital volume and operative mortality in cancer surgery: A national study. Arch Surg 2003;138:721-725; discussion 726.
97. Flegal KM: Defining obesity in children and adolescents: Epidemiologic approaches. Crit Rev Food Sci Nutr 1993; 33:307-312.
98. Flegal KM, Troiano RP: Changes in the distribution of body mass index of adults and children in the US population. Int J Obes Relat Metab Disord 2000;24: 807-818.
99. Flodmark CE: Thrifty genotypes and phenotypes in the pathogenesis of early-onset obesity. Acta Paediatr 2002; 91:737-738.
100. Flum DR, Dellinger EP: Impact of gastric bypass operation on survival: A population-based analysis. J Am Coll Surg 2004;199:543-551.
101. Fontaine KR, Redden DT, Wang C, et al: Years of life lost due to obesity. JAMA 2003;289:187-193.
102. Forsen T, Eriksson J, Tuomilehto J, et al: The fetal and childhood growth of persons who develop type 2 diabetes. Ann Intern Med 2000;133:176-182.
103. Fox J: A life course approach to chronic disease epidemiology. BMJ 1998;317:421.
104. Franks S: Adult polycystic ovary syndrome begins in childhood. Best Pract Res Clin Endocrinol Metab 2002;16: 263-272.
105. Franzese A, Vajro P, Argenziano A, et al: Liver involvement in obese children: Ultrasonography and liver enzyme levels at diagnosis and during follow-up in an Italian population. Dig Dis Sci 1997;42:1428-1432.
106. Freedman DS, Dietz WH, Srinivasan SR, Berenson GS: The relation of overweight to cardiovascular risk factors among children and adolescents: The Bogalusa Heart Study. Pediatrics 1999;103:1175-1182.
107. French SA, Story M, Perry CL: Self-esteem and obesity in children and adolescents: A literature review. Obes Res 1995;3:479-490.
108. Friedman JM: The function of leptin in nutrition, weight, and physiology. Nutr Rev 2002;60(Suppl):S1-S14; discussion S68-S84.
109. Friedman JM: A war on obesity, not the obese. Science 2003;299:856-858.
110. Galal OM: The nutrition transition in Egypt: Obesity, undernutrition and the food consumption context. Public Health Nutr 2002;5:141-148.
111. Gallistl S, Sudi KM, Borkenstein M, et al: Correlation between cholesterol, soluble P-selectin, and D-dimer in obese children and adolescents. Blood Coagul Fibrinolysis 2000;11:755-760.
112. Gallistl S, Sudi KM, Erwa W, et al: Determinants of homocysteine during weight reduction in obese children and

adolescents. Metabolism 2001;50:1220-1223.
113. Gannon B, DiPietro L, Poehlman ET: Do African Americans have lower energy expenditure than Caucasians? Int J Obes Relat Metab Disord 2000;24:4-13.
114. Garcia VF, Langford L, Inge TH: Application of laparoscopy for bariatric surgery in adolescents. Curr Opin Pediatr 2003;15:248-255.
115. Ghannem H, Darioli R, Limam K, et al: Epidemiology of cardiovascular risk factors among schoolchildren in Sousse, Tunisia. J Cardiovasc Risk 2001;8:87-91.
116. Gidding SS, Bao W, Srinivasan SR, Berenson GS: Effects of secular trends in obesity on coronary risk factors in children: The Bogalusa Heart Study. J Pediatr 1995;127:868-874.
117. Gillman MW: Breast-feeding and obesity. J Pediatr 2002; 141:749-757.
118. Gillman MW, Rifas-Shiman SL, Camargo CA Jr, et al: Risk of overweight among adolescents who were breastfed as infants. JAMA 2001;285:2461-2467.
119. Glanz K, Croyle RT, Chollette VY, Pinn VW: Cancer-related health disparities in women. Am J Public Health 2003;93:292-298.
120. Goodman E, Whitaker RC: A prospective study of the role of depression in the development and persistence of adolescent obesity. Pediatrics 2002;110:497-504.
121. Goran MI: Genetic influences on human energy expenditure and substrate utilization. Behav Genet 1997;27:389-399.
122. Gordon TA, Bowman HM, Tielsch JM, et al: Statewide regionalization of pancreaticoduodenectomy and its effect on in-hospital mortality. Ann Surg 1998;228:71-78.
123. Gordon-Larsen P, Adair LS, Popkin BM: Ethnic differences in physical activity and inactivity patterns and overweight status. Obes Res 2002;10:141-149.
124. Gortmaker SL, Must A, Perrin JM, et al: Social and economic consequences of overweight in adolescence and young adulthood. N Engl J Med 1993;329:1008-1012.
125. Gould JC, Garren MJ, Starling JR: Lessons learned from the first 100 cases in a new minimally invasive bariatric surgery program. Obes Surg 2004;14:618-625.
126. Greenstein RJ, Rabner JG: Is adolescent gastric-restrictive antiobesity surgery warranted? Obes Surg 1995;5:138-144.
127. Grill HJ, Kaplan JM: The neuroanatomical axis for control of energy balance. Front Neuroendocrinol 2002; 23:2-40.
128. Guerra S, Wright AL, Morgan WJ, et al: Persistence of asthma symptoms during adolescence: Role of obesity and age at onset of puberty. Am J Respir Crit Care Med 2004;170:78-85.
129. Guo SS, Wu W, Chumlea WC, Roche AF: Predicting overweight and obesity in adulthood from body mass index values in childhood and adolescence. Am J Clin Nutr 2002;76:653-658.
130. Hall J, Solehdin F: Folic acid for the prevention of congenital anomalies. Eur J Pediatr 1998;157:445-450.
131. Hazzard A, Hutchinson SJ, Krawiecki N: Factors related to adherence to medication regimens in pediatric seizure patients. J Pediatr Psychol 1990;15:543-555.
132. Heald FP, Khan MA: Teenage obesity. Pediatr Clin North Am 1973;20:807-817.
133. Hedley AA, Ogden CL, Johnson CL, et al: Prevalence of overweight and obesity among US children, adolescents, and adults, 1999-2002. JAMA 2004;291:2847-2850.
134. Hess DS, Hess DW: Biliopancreatic diversion with a duodenal switch. Obes Surg 1998;8:267-282.
135. Higa KD, Boone KB, Ho T, Davies OG: Laparoscopic Roux-en-Y gastric bypass for morbid obesity: Technique and preliminary results of our first 400 patients. Arch Surg 2000;135:1029-1033; discussion 1033-1034.
136. Higa KD, Ho T, Boone KB: Laparoscopic Roux-en-Y gastric bypass: Technique and 3-year follow-up. J Laparoendosc Adv Surg Tech A 2001;11:377-382.
137. Hirosumi J, Tuncman G, Chang L, et al: A central role for JNK in obesity and insulin resistance. Nature 2002;420: 333-336.
138. Hirsch S, Pia De la Maza M, Yanez P, et al: Hyperhomocysteinemia and endothelial function in young subjects: Effects of vitamin supplementation. Clin Cardiol 2002;25:495-501.
139. Hotamisligil GS, Shargill NS, Spiegelman BM: Adipose expression of tumor necrosis factor-alpha: Direct role in obesity-linked insulin resistance. Science 1993;259: 87-91.
140. Hotu S, Carter B, Watson PD, et al: Increasing prevalence of type 2 diabetes in adolescents. J Paediatr Child Health 2004;40:201-204.
141. Hubbard VS: Defining overweight and obesity: What are the issues? Am J Clin Nutr 2000;72:1067-1068.
142. Inge TH, Garcia V, Daniels S, et al: A multidisciplinary approach to the adolescent bariatric surgical patient. J Pediatr Surg 2004;39:442-447; discussion 446-447.
143. Inge TH, Krebs NF, Garcia VF, et al: Bariatric surgery for severely overweight adolescents: Concerns and recommendations. Pediatrics 2004;114:217-223.
144. James PT, Rigby N, Leach R: The obesity epidemic, metabolic syndrome and future prevention strategies. Eur J Cardiovasc Prev Rehabil 2004;11:3-8.
145. Jequier E: Leptin signaling, adiposity, and energy balance. Ann NY Acad Sci 2002;967:379-388.
146. Kahn SE: Clinical review 135: The importance of beta-cell failure in the development and progression of type 2 diabetes. J Clin Endocrinol Metab 2001;86:4047-4058.
147. Kalkwarf HJ, Khoury JC, Lanphear BP: Milk intake during childhood and adolescence, adult bone density, and osteoporotic fractures in US women. Am J Clin Nutr 2003; 77:257-265.
148. Karason K, Lindroos AK, Stenlof K, Sjostrom L: Relief of cardiorespiratory symptoms and increased physical activity after surgically induced weight loss: Results from the Swedish Obese Subjects study. Arch Intern Med 2000; 160:1797-1802.
149. Keller KB, Lemberg L: Obesity and the metabolic syndrome. Am J Crit Care 2003;12:167-170.
150. Kimm SY, Barton BA, Obarzanek E, et al: Obesity development during adolescence in a biracial cohort: The NHLBI Growth and Health Study. Pediatrics 2002;110:e54.
151. Kimm SY, Glynn NW, Aston CE, et al: Racial differences in the relation between uncoupling protein genes and resting energy expenditure. Am J Clin Nutr 2002;75: 714-719.
152. Kimm SY, Glynn NW, Aston CE, et al: Effects of race, cigarette smoking, and use of contraceptive medications on resting energy expenditure in young women. Am J Epidemiol 2001;154:718-724.
153. Krassas GE, Tzotzas T, Tsametis C, Konstantinidis T: Prevalence and trends in overweight and obesity among children and adolescents in Thessaloniki, Greece. J Pediatr Endocrinol Metab 2001;14(Suppl 5):1319-1326; discussion 1365.
154. Lacour M, Zunder T, Dettenkofer M, et al: An interdisciplinary therapeutic approach for dealing with patients attributing chronic fatigue and functional memory disorders to environmental poisoning—a pilot study. Int J Hyg Environ Health 2002;204:339-346.
155. Lazar L, Kauli R, Bruchis C, et al: Early polycystic ovary–like

syndrome in girls with central precocious puberty and exaggerated adrenal response. Eur J Endocrinol 1995; 133:403-406.
156. Lehrke M, Lazar MA: Inflamed about obesity. Nat Med 2004;10:126-127.
157. Leibel RL, Rosenbaum M, Hirsch J: Changes in energy expenditure resulting from altered body weight. N Engl J Med 1995;332:621-628.
158. Lemanek KL, Kamps J, Chung NB: Empirically supported treatments in pediatric psychology: Regimen adherence. J Pediatr Psychol 2001;26:253-275.
159. Leonard MB, Shults J, Wilson BA, et al: Obesity during childhood and adolescence augments bone mass and bone dimensions. Am J Clin Nutr 2004;80:514-523.
160. Lessell S: Pediatric pseudotumor cerebri (idiopathic intracranial hypertension). Surv Ophthalmol 1992;37:155-166.
161. Levine J, Melanson EL, Westerterp KR, Hill JO: Measurement of the components of nonexercise activity thermogenesis. Am J Physiol Endocrinol Metab 2001; 281:E670-E675.
162. Levy J, Atkinson AB, Bell PM, et al: Beta-cell deterioration determines the onset and rate of progression of secondary dietary failure in type 2 diabetes mellitus: The 10-year follow-up of the Belfast Diet Study. Diabet Med 1998; 15:290-296.
163. Lewy VD, Danadian K, Witchel SF, Arslanian S: Early metabolic abnormalities in adolescent girls with polycystic ovarian syndrome. J Pediatr 2001;138:38-44.
164. Lin-Su K, Vogiatzi MG, New MI: Body mass index and age at menarche in an adolescent clinic population. Clin Pediatr 2002;41:501-507.
165. Livingston EH: Procedure incidence and in-hospital complication rates of bariatric surgery in the United States. Am J Surg 2004;188:105-110.
166. Livingston EH, Huerta S, Arthur D, et al: Male gender is a predictor of morbidity and age a predictor of mortality for patients undergoing gastric bypass surgery. Ann Surg 2002;236:576-582.
167. Long SD, O'Brien K, MacDonald KG Jr, et al: Weight loss in severely obese subjects prevents the progression of impaired glucose tolerance to type II diabetes: A longitudinal interventional study. Diabetes Care 1994;17:372-375.
168. Lujan JA, Frutos MD, Hernandez Q, et al: Laparoscopic versus open gastric bypass in the treatment of morbid obesity: A randomized prospective study. Ann Surg 2004; 239:433-437.
169. Luo J, Hu FB: Time trends of obesity in pre-school children in China from 1989 to 1997. Int J Obes Relat Metab Disord 2002;26:553-558.
170. MacDonald KG Jr, Long SD, Swanson MS, et al: The gastric bypass operation reduces the progression and mortality of non-insulin-dependent diabetes mellitus. J Gastrointest Surg 1997;1:213-220.
171. Marceau P, Kaufman D, Biron S, et al: Outcome of pregnancies after biliopancreatic diversion. Obes Surg 2004; 14:318-324.
172. Matkovic V: Osteoporosis as a pediatric disease: Role of calcium and heredity. J Rheumatol Suppl 1992;33:54-59.
173. Matkovic V, Ilich JZ, Andon MB, et al: Urinary calcium, sodium, and bone mass of young females. Am J Clin Nutr 1995;62:417-425.
174. Matsushita Y, Yoshiike N, Kaneda F, et al: Trends in childhood obesity in Japan over the last 25 years from the national nutrition survey. Obes Res 2004;12:205-214.
175. Matthews DR, Wallace TM: Children with type 2 diabetes: The risks of complications. Horm Res 2002;57(Suppl 1): 34-39.
176. McGill HC Jr, Herderick EE, McMahan CA, et al: Atherosclerosis in youth. Minerva Pediatr 2002;54: 437-447.
177. McGill HC Jr, McMahan CA, Herderick EE, et al: Obesity accelerates the progression of coronary atherosclerosis in young men. Circulation 2002;105:2712-2718.
178. Mi J, Law C, Zhang KL, et al: Effects of infant birthweight and maternal body mass index in pregnancy on components of the insulin resistance syndrome in China. Ann Intern Med 2000;132:253-260.
179. Michels KB: Early life predictors of chronic disease. J Womens Health 2003;12:157-161.
180. Miraglia Del Giudice E, Cirillo G, Nigro V, et al: Low frequency of melanocortin-4 receptor (MC4R) mutations in a Mediterranean population with early-onset obesity. Int J Obes Relat Metab Disord 2002;26:647-651.
181. Misra A: Risk factors for atherosclerosis in young individuals. J Cardiovasc Risk 2000;7:215-229.
182. Mokdad AH, Marks JS, Stroup DF, Gerberding JL: Actual causes of death in the United States, 2000. JAMA 2004; 291:1238-1245.
183. Molleston JP, White F, Teckman J, Fitzgerald JF: Obese children with steatohepatitis can develop cirrhosis in childhood. Am J Gastroenterol 2002;97:2460-2462.
184. Msika S: [Surgery for morbid obesity: 2. Complications. Results of a Technologic Evaluation by the ANAES]. J Chir 2003;140:4-21.
185. Must A, Jacques PF, Dallal GE, et al: Long-term morbidity and mortality of overweight adolescents: A follow-up of the Harvard Growth Study of 1922 to 1935. N Engl J Med 1992;327:1350-1355.
186. Must A, Spadano J, Coakley EH, et al: The disease burden associated with overweight and obesity. JAMA 1999;282: 1523-1529.
187. Narayan KM, Boyle JP, Thompson TJ, et al: Lifetime risk for diabetes mellitus in the United States. JAMA 2003;290: 1884-1890.
188. Nesbitt SD, Ashaye MO, Stettler N, et al: Overweight as a risk factor in children: A focus on ethnicity. Ethn Dis 2004;14:94-110.
189. Nguyen NT, Goldman C, Rosenquist CJ, et al: Laparoscopic versus open gastric bypass: A randomized study of outcomes, quality of life, and costs. Ann Surg 2001; 234:279-289; discussion 289-291.
190. Nguyen NT, Wolfe BM: Laparoscopic versus open gastric bypass. Semin Laparosc Surg 2002;9:86-93.
191. O'Brien PE, Dixon JB: Lap-band: outcomes and results. J Laparoendosc Adv Surg Tech A 2003;13:265-270.
192. O'Brien PE, Dixon JB, Brown W, et al: The laparoscopic adjustable gastric band (Lap-Band): A prospective study of medium-term effects on weight, health and quality of life. Obes Surg 2002;12:652-660.
193. Ogden CL, Carroll MD, Flegal KM: Epidemiologic trends in overweight and obesity. Endocrinol Metab Clin North Am 2003;32:741-760.
194. Ogden CL, Flegal KM, Carroll MD, Johnson CL: Prevalence and trends in overweight among US children and adolescents, 1999-2000. JAMA 2002;288:1728-1732.
195. Oken E, Gillman MW: Fetal origins of obesity. Obes Res 2003;11:496-506.
196. Palaniappan LP, Carnethon MR, Fortmann SP: Heterogeneity in the relationship between ethnicity, BMI, and fasting insulin. Diabetes Care 2002;25: 1351-1357.
197. Palasciano G, Portincasa P, Vinciguerra V, et al: Gallstone prevalence and gallbladder volume in children and ado-

lescents: An epidemiological ultrasonographic survey and relationship to body mass index. Am J Gastroenterol 1989;84:1378-1382.
198. Parsons TJ, Power C, Logan S, Summerbell CD: Childhood predictors of adult obesity: A systematic review. Int J Obes Relat Metab Disord 1999;23(Suppl 8):S1-S107.
199. Partridge AH, Avorn J, Wang PS, Winer EP: Adherence to therapy with oral antineoplastic agents. J Natl Cancer Inst 2002;94:652-661.
200. Phipps S, DeCuir-Whalley S: Adherence issues in pediatric bone marrow transplantation. J Pediatr Psychol 1990; 15:459-475.
201. Piaget J: The Growth of Logical Thinking From Childhood to Adolescence. New York, Basic Books, 1958.
202. Pinhas-Hamiel O, Dolan LM, Daniels SR, et al: Increased incidence of non-insulin-dependent diabetes mellitus among adolescents. J Pediatr 1996;128:608-615.
203. Podnos YD, Jimenez JC, Wilson SE, et al: Complications after laparoscopic gastric bypass: A review of 3464 cases. Arch Surg 2003;138:957-961.
204. Pories WJ, Swanson MS, MacDonald KG, et al: Who would have thought it? An operation proves to be the most effective therapy for adult-onset diabetes mellitus. Ann Surg 1995;222:339-350; discussion 350-352.
205. Rand CS, McGregor AM: Adolescents having obesity surgery: A 6-year follow-up. South Med J 1994;87:1208-1213.
206. Randolph JG, Weintraub WH, Rigg A: Jejunoileal bypass for morbid obesity in adolescents. J Pediatr Surg 1974;9: 341-345.
207. Rapoff M, Barnard MU: Compliance with pediatric medical regimens. In Cramer JA (ed): Patient Compliance in Medical Practice and Clinical Trials. New York, Raven Press, 1991, pp 73-98.
208. Rapoff MA: Assessing and enhancing adherence to medical regimens for juvenile rheumatoid arthritis. Pediatr Ann 2002;31:373-379.
209. Rapoff MA: Commentary: Pushing the envelope: Furthering research on improving adherence to chronic pediatric disease regimens. J Pediatr Psychol 2001;26: 277-278.
210. Rapoff MA, Belmont J, Lindsley C, et al: Prevention of nonadherence to nonsteroidal anti-inflammatory medications for newly diagnosed patients with juvenile rheumatoid arthritis. Health Psychol 2002;21:620-623.
211. Rapoff MA, Purviance MR, Lindsley CB: Educational and behavioral strategies for improving medication compliance in juvenile rheumatoid arthritis. Arch Phys Med Rehabil 1988;69:439-441.
212. Rashid M, Roberts EA: Nonalcoholic steatohepatitis in children. J Pediatr Gastroenterol Nutr 2000;30:48-53.
213. Ravelli AC, van der Meulen JH, Osmond C, et al: Obesity at the age of 50 y in men and women exposed to famine prenatally. Am J Clin Nutr 1999;70:811-816.
214. Ravussin E, Lillioja S, Knowler WC, et al: Reduced rate of energy expenditure as a risk factor for body-weight gain. N Engl J Med 1988;318:467-472.
215. Reddington C, Cohen J, Baldillo A, et al: Adherence to medication regimens among children with human immunodeficiency virus infection. Pediatr Infect Dis J 2000;19:1148-1153.
216. Redline S, Tishler PV, Schluchter M, et al: Risk factors for sleep-disordered breathing in children: Associations with obesity, race, and respiratory problems. Am J Respir Crit Care Med 1999;159:1527-1532.
217. Reitman A, Friedrich I, Ben-Amotz A, Levy Y: Low plasma antioxidants and normal plasma B vitamins and homocysteine in patients with severe obesity. Isr Med Assoc J 2002; 4:590-593.
218. Ren CJ: Controversies in bariatric surgery: Evidence-based discussions on laparoscopic adjustable gastric banding. J Gastrointest Surg 2004;8:396-397; discussion 404-405.
219. Roberts EA: Nonalcoholic steatohepatitis in children. Curr Gastroenterol Rep 2003;5:253-259.
220. Roberts EA: Steatohepatitis in children. Best Pract Res Clin Gastroenterol 16:749-765, 2002.
221. Rosenbaum M, Leibel RL, Hirsch J: Obesity. N Engl J Med 1997;337:396-407.
222. Rosenbloom AL, Joe JR, Young RS, Winter WE: Emerging epidemic of type 2 diabetes in youth. Diabetes Care 1999; 22:345-354.
223. Sainsbury A, Cooney GJ, Herzog H: Hypothalamic regulation of energy homeostasis. Best Pract Res Clin Endocrinol Metab 2002;16:623-637.
224. Schauer P, Ikramuddin S, Hamad G, Gourash W: The learning curve for laparoscopic Roux-en-Y gastric bypass is 100 cases. Surg Endosc 2003;17:212-215.
225. Schauer PR, Burguera B, Ikramuddin S, et al: Effect of laparoscopic Roux-en Y gastric bypass on type 2 diabetes mellitus. Ann Surg 2003;238:467-484; discussion 484-485.
226. Schauer PR, Ikramuddin S: Laparoscopic surgery for morbid obesity. Surg Clin North Am 2001;81:1145-1179.
227. Schechter MS: Technical report: Diagnosis and management of childhood obstructive sleep apnea syndrome. Pediatrics 2002;109:e69.
228. Schonfeld-Warden NA, Warden CH: Uncoupling proteins: A molecular basis for racial differences in energy expenditure (and obesity?). Am J Clin Nutr 2002;75:607-608.
229. Schwimmer JB, Burwinkle TM, Varni JW: Health-related quality of life of severely obese children and adolescents. JAMA 2003;289:1813-1819.
230. Scopinaro N, Adami GF, Marinari GM, et al: Biliopancreatic diversion. World J Surg 1998;22:936-946.
231. Silber T, Randolph J, Robbins S: Long-term morbidity and mortality in morbidly obese adolescents after jejunoileal bypass. J Pediatr 1986;108:318-322.
232. Silverman BL, Rizzo TA, Cho NH, Metzger BE: Long-term effects of the intrauterine environment. The Northwestern University Diabetes in Pregnancy Center. Diabetes Care 1998;21(Suppl 2):B142-B149.
233. Sinha R, Fisch G, Teague B, et al: Prevalence of impaired glucose tolerance among children and adolescents with marked obesity. N Engl J Med 2002;346:802-810.
234. Soper RT, Mason EE, Printen KJ, Zellweger H: Gastric bypass for morbid obesity in children and adolescents. J Pediatr Surg 1975;10:51-58.
235. Sorensen HT, Sabroe S, Rothman KJ, et al: Relation between weight and length at birth and body mass index in young adulthood: Cohort study. BMJ 1997;315:1137.
236. Sorof J, Daniels S: Obesity hypertension in children: A problem of epidemic proportions. Hypertension 2002; 40:441-447.
237. Srinivasan SR, Frontini MG, Berenson GS: Longitudinal changes in risk variables of insulin resistance syndrome from childhood to young adulthood in offspring of parents with type 2 diabetes: The Bogalusa Heart Study. Metabolism 2003;52:443-450; discussion 451-453.
238. Stanford A, Glascock JM, Eid GM, et al: Laparoscopic Roux-en-Y gastric bypass in morbidly obese adolescents. J Pediatr Surg 2003;38:430-433.
239. Steinberger J, Moran A, Hong CP, et al: Adiposity in childhood predicts obesity and insulin resistance in young adulthood. J Pediatr 2001;138:469-473.

240. Stewart KS, Dearmun AK: Adherence to health advice amongst young people with chronic illness. J Child Health Care 2001;5:155-162.
241. Strauss RS: Childhood obesity. Pediatr Clin North Am 2002;49:175-201.
242. Strauss RS: Childhood obesity and self-esteem. Pediatrics 2000;105:e15.
243. Strauss RS, Bradley LJ, Brolin RE: Gastric bypass surgery in adolescents with morbid obesity. J Pediatr 2001;138:499-504.
244. Strauss RS, Pollack HA: Epidemic increase in childhood overweight, 1986-1998. JAMA 2001;286:2845-2848.
245. Sturm R: Increases in clinically severe obesity in the United States, 1986-2000. Arch Intern Med 2003;163:2146-2148.
246. Sugerman HJ: Bariatric surgery for severe obesity. J Assoc Acad Minor Phys 2001;12:129-136.
247. Sugerman HJ: Gastric bypass surgery for severe obesity. Semin Laparosc Surg 2002;9:79-85.
248. Sugerman HJ, Sugerman EL, DeMaria EJ, et al: Bariatric surgery for severely obese adolescents. J Gastrointest Surg 2003;7:102-108.
249. Surgeons, American College of: Recommendations for Facilities Performing Bariatric Surgery. Bulletin of the American College of Surgeons, No. 85, 2000.
250. Surgery, American Society for Bariatric: Guidelines for Bariatric Surgery. Bulletin of the American College of Surgeons, No. 85, 2000.
251. Taranger J, Engstrom I, Lichenstein H, Svennberg-Redegren I: Somatic pubertal development. Acta Paediatr Scand Suppl 1976;258(Suppl):121-135.
252. Ten S, Maclaren N: Insulin resistance syndrome in children. J Clin Endocrinol Metab 2004;89:2526-2539.
253. Thompson SM, Dahlquist LM, Koenning GM, Bartholomew LK: Brief report: Adherence-facilitating behaviors of a multidisciplinary pediatric rheumatology staff. J Pediatr Psychol 1995;20:291-297.
254. Tounian P, Aggoun Y, Dubern B, et al: Presence of increased stiffness of the common carotid artery and endothelial dysfunction in severely obese children: A prospective study. Lancet 2001;358:1400-1404.
255. Towbin A, Inge TH, Garcia VF, et al: Beriberi after gastric bypass surgery in adolescence. J Pediatr 2004;145:263-267.
256. Turner RC, Cull CA, Frighi V, Holman RR, and for the UK Prospective Diabetes Study Group: Glycemic control with diet, sulfonylurea, metformin, or insulin in patients with type 2 diabetes mellitus: Progressive requirement for multiple therapies (UKPDS 49). JAMA 1999;281:2005-2012.
257. Van Itallie TB: Health implications of overweight and obesity in the United States. Ann Intern Med 1985;103:983-988.
258. von Mutius E, Schwartz J, Neas LM, et al: Relation of body mass index to asthma and atopy in children: The National Health and Nutrition Examination Study III. Thorax 2001;56:835-838.
259. Wahlqvist ML: Chronic disease prevention: A life-cycle approach which takes account of the environmental impact and opportunities of food, nutrition and public health policies—the rationale for an eco-nutritional disease nomenclature. Asia Pac J Clin Nutr 2002;11(Suppl 9):S759-S762.
260. Wang G, Dietz WH: Economic burden of obesity in youths aged 6 to 17 years: 1979-1999. Pediatrics 2002;109:E81.
261. Wang Y: Is obesity associated with early sexual maturation? A comparison of the association in American boys versus girls. Pediatrics 2002;110:903-910.
262. Wattigney WA, Srinivasan SR, Chen W, et al: Secular trend of earlier onset of menarche with increasing obesity in black and white girls: The Bogalusa Heart Study. Ethn Dis 1999;9:181-189.
263. Weisberg SP, McCann D, Desai M, et al: Obesity is associated with macrophage accumulation in adipose tissue. J Clin Invest 2003;112:1796-1808.
264. Weiss R, Dziura J, Burgert TS, et al: Obesity and the metabolic syndrome in children and adolescents. N Engl J Med 2004;350:2362-2374.
265. Wellen KE, Hotamisligil GS: Obesity-induced inflammatory changes in adipose tissue. J Clin Invest 2003;112:1785-1788.
266. Whitaker RC: Understanding the complex journey to obesity in early adulthood. Ann Intern Med 2002;136:923-925.
267. Whitaker RC, Deeks CM, Baughcum AE, Specker BL: The relationship of childhood adiposity to parent body mass index and eating behavior. Obes Res 2000;8:234-240.
268. Whitaker RC, Wright JA, Pepe MS, et al: Predicting obesity in young adulthood from childhood and parental obesity. N Engl J Med 1997;337:869-873.
269. Wing YK, Hui SH, Pak WM, et al: A controlled study of sleep related disordered breathing in obese children. Arch Dis Child 2003;88:1043-1047.
270. Wittgrove AC, Jester L, Wittgrove P, Clark GW: Pregnancy following gastric bypass for morbid obesity. Obes Surg 1998;8:461-464; discussion 465-466.
271. Wysocki T, Greco P, Harris MA, et al: Behavior therapy for families of adolescents with diabetes: Maintenance of treatment effects. Diabetes Care 2001;24:441-446.
272. Xu H, Barnes GT, Yang Q, et al: Chronic inflammation in fat plays a crucial role in the development of obesity-related insulin resistance. J Clin Invest 2003;112:1821-1830.
273. Yajnik C: Interactions of perturbations in intrauterine growth and growth during childhood on the risk of adult-onset disease. Proc Nutr Soc 2000;59:257-265.
274. Yarnell JW, McCrum EE, Patterson CC, et al: Prevalence and awareness of excess weight in 13- and 14-year-olds in Northern Ireland using recent international guidelines. Acta Paediatr 2001;90:1435-1439.
275. Young-Hyman D, Schlundt DG, Herman L, et al: Evaluation of the insulin resistance syndrome in 5- to 10-year-old overweight/obese African-American children. Diabetes Care 2001;24:1359-1364.

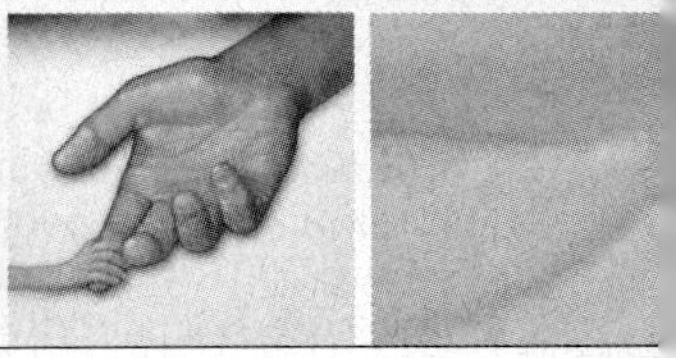

第 79 章

十二指肠闭锁和狭窄——环状胰腺

Harry Applebaum、Steven L. Lee 和 Devin P. Puapong

1260 十二指肠是新生儿肠梗阻最好发的部位，约有一半病例发生于此[16]。尽管早在 18 世纪就已认识到十二指肠闭锁、狭窄和环状胰腺，但是直到 20 世纪，先天性高位肠梗阻都很少有治疗成功的病例。Calder 在 1733 年第一次报道了十二指肠闭锁[12]。Cordes[15] 于 1901 年描述了该先天性缺损的典型临床表现，而法国的 Vidal 和荷兰的 Ernst 分别于 1905 年和 1914 年成功进行了外科手术修复[24,84]。到 1929 年，Kaldor 确认文献报道的十二指肠闭锁病例有 250 例，但是 1931 年 Webb 和 Wangensteen 的综述中提到只有 9 名存活者[41,85]。与此形成鲜明对比的是，现代外科技术已使存活率超过 95%，偶尔在伴有其他器官畸形的情况下才发生死亡[33]。

过去，当十二指肠闭锁伴发 21 三体（Down 综合征）时，近 1/3 的新生儿梗阻往往不进行治疗。直到 20 世纪 70 年代，社会学和医学伦理学的改变才促使医生对这些患儿进行手术治疗[58,69,82]。随着妊娠早期围生期医生对染色体异常的诊断能力的提高，多数孕妇可选择中止妊娠，使新生儿十二指肠梗阻发病率逐渐降低[14,67,76,83]。

十二指肠闭锁的发病率估计为 6000～10 000 名活产儿中有 1 名[28]。最近一个大型综述对欧洲登记的 18 种先天性畸形进行了统计，在 670 093 名活产儿中发现 64 例患有十二指肠闭锁，即 10 500 名活产儿中有 1 名[35]。尽管至今仍未明确有特定基因缺陷可导致十二指肠闭锁，但有一些报道显示畸形发生于同胞和同一家庭多代人，并常伴有 21 三体，提示可能存在特定基因缺陷[13,29,37,53,57,59,71,83,90]。

胚胎学

在胚胎发育第 3 周，原肠胚形成。面向卵黄囊的胚胎细胞表层发育成内胚层，面向羊膜囊的细胞层发育为外胚层，而中间层则发育为中胚层。内胚层在胚胎发育第 4 周起开始形成消化管道。第 6 周开始，消化道上皮细胞迅速增殖，导致肠腔闭塞。肠道在接下来的几周后逐渐再通。再通过程中发生的错误被认为是十二指肠闭锁和狭窄的主要原因。再通完全失败导致闭锁，而部分失败导致膜状狭窄[6,66,74]。这种发病机制与其他肠段的肠闭锁和狭窄的发病机制不同，后者通常认为是由妊娠后期血管意外引起[52]。

胰腺从妊娠第 4 周开始由十二指肠内胚层内层发育而成。先形成两个囊状结构，之后一个变成较大的背侧胰腺原始胚基，另一个变成较小的腹侧胰腺原始胚基。在第 8 周时腹侧胰腺芽向背侧旋转并与背侧胰腺芽融合。如果腹侧胰腺芽未能完全旋转，则停留在十二指肠前面并与腹侧胰腺原始胚基融合形成环绕十二指肠的环状胰腺[6,42,62,66,74]。

约有半数以上十二指肠闭锁或狭窄患儿伴有其他器官的先天性畸形[5,7,44,65,70,80,87,91]。Sweed 对照统计了大量十二指肠梗阻伴发畸形的病例，发现 Down 综合征、环状胰腺、先天性心脏病和肠旋转不良是最常见的畸形（表 79-1）[81]。

相关疾病谱

多种内源性和外源性先天性病变可造成完全性
（81%）或部分性（19%）十二指肠梗阻[16]。造成 12
内源性梗阻的畸形包括闭锁或连续肠管内厚度不一的

表 79-1　伴发畸形（收集病例统计）

畸形	%
Down 综合征	28.2
环状胰腺	23.1
先天性心脏病	22.6
旋转不良	19.7
食管闭锁/食管气管瘘	8.5
泌尿生殖系统	8.0
肛门直肠	4.4
其他肠道闭锁	3.5
其他畸形	10.9
无畸形	45.0

Data from Sweed Y: Duodenal obstruction. In Puri P (ed): Newborn Surgery, 2nd ed, London, Arnold, 2003, p 423.

膜状狭窄以及完全性或近完全性肠道中断。造成外源性梗阻的畸形包括环状胰腺、十二指肠前门静脉、Ladd 束带以及肠扭转[37,39,43,50,51,54,55,60]。

Gray 和 Skandalakis 将各种十二指肠闭锁归为 3 种类型[32]：

Ⅰ型（92%）[25]：由黏膜和黏膜下层形成的，且肌层无缺损的梗阻性隔膜（蹼）。肠系膜完整。如果隔膜很薄且可伸长，则称之为Ⅰ型十二指肠闭锁的变异体——“风向袋样畸形”（图 79-1A）。隔膜的基底通常位于十二指肠第二部分，但向远端膨胀如气球，延伸至十二指肠第三、第四部分。因此表面上看起来闭锁部位要比实际位置更远[73]。

Ⅱ型（1%）：一条短纤维索带连接十二指肠的两个盲端。肠系膜完整（见图 79-1B）。

Ⅲ型（7%）：十二指肠两个盲端间无任何联系。肠系膜存在 V 型缺损（见图 79-1C）。

Ⅰ型闭锁中梗阻性隔膜厚度可从 1 毫米至数毫米不等。闭锁间隔导致完全性梗阻，而当中有孔的隔膜则导致不完全性梗阻。在隔膜有孔的情况下，孔径直接决定了梗阻的程度并与症状轻重呈反比关系（图79-2）[73]。

虽然内源性梗阻可发生于十二指肠任何部位，但85%的病例发生于第一、第二段结合部周围。胆总管的远端常越过隔膜的中部，而壶腹部常位于梗阻近端面。少数病例胆总管远侧部出现分叉即有近端和远端开口，使之第一眼看起来似乎是难以想象的，即同时有空气和胆汁出现在先天性完全性梗阻的十二指肠远端[9,10]。

环状胰腺中胰腺环绕十二指肠可造成外源性不全性梗阻。然而更为常见的是十二指肠闭锁或狭窄的隔膜在环状胰腺的下面，才是造成梗阻的真正原因[22]。胰管的解剖学构造改变，主胰管横越环状部分（图 79-3）。远端胰管通常位于下方内源性梗阻组织内，壶腹部开口于其表面。如果没有内源性梗阻，远端胰管解剖结构正常，则很有可能在日后行不相关的开腹手术中才能发现并诊断环状胰腺[39]。

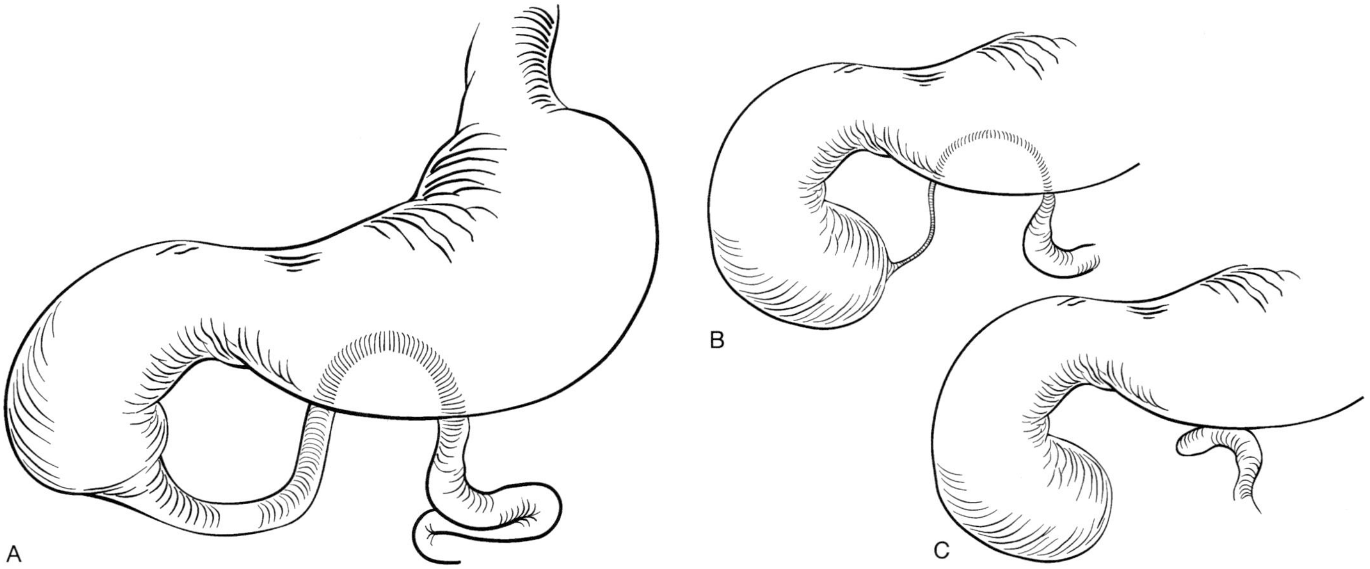

图 79-1　A. Ⅰ型十二指肠闭锁。B. Ⅱ型十二指肠闭锁。C. Ⅲ型十二指肠闭锁。

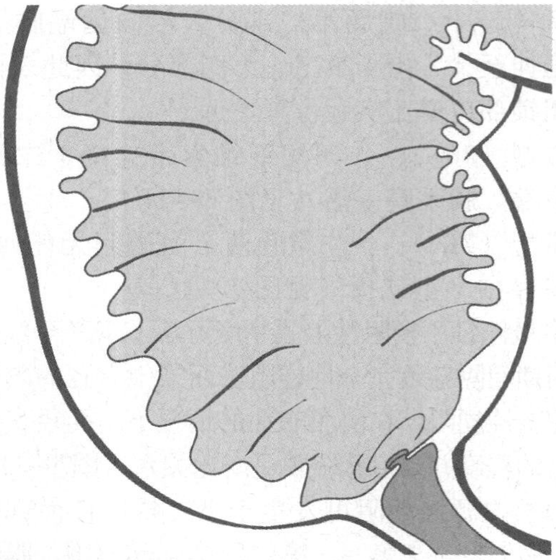

图 79-2　典型十二指肠隔膜伴中央孔。

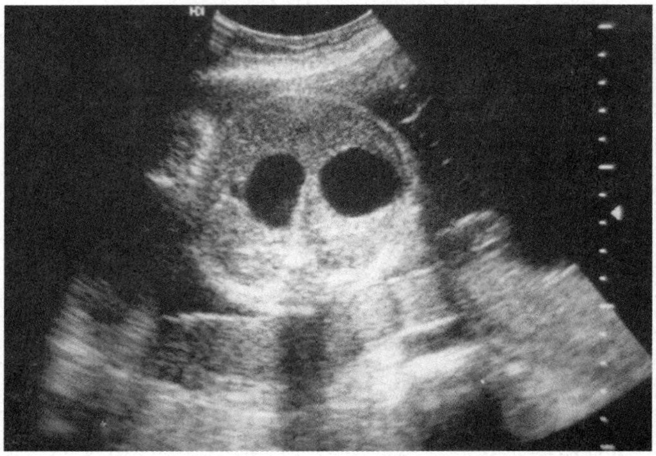

图 79-4　胎儿超声显示“双泡征”。

1262 十二指肠前门静脉于十二指肠第二段前方而非后方越过，可能会因压迫造成十二指肠不完全性梗阻。这种少见的外源性十二指肠压迫常见于复杂性先天性心脏病患儿[33,60]。

肠旋转不良形成 Ladd 束带通常会引起十二指肠第二至第三段外源性不完全性梗阻。这些患儿可发生不同程度的中肠扭转（急性、间断性或慢性），也可引起梗阻[75]。

临床表现

产前保健的进步使大部分十二指肠梗阻（包括完全性和不完全性）可在产前检测出[36]。30%～65% 的

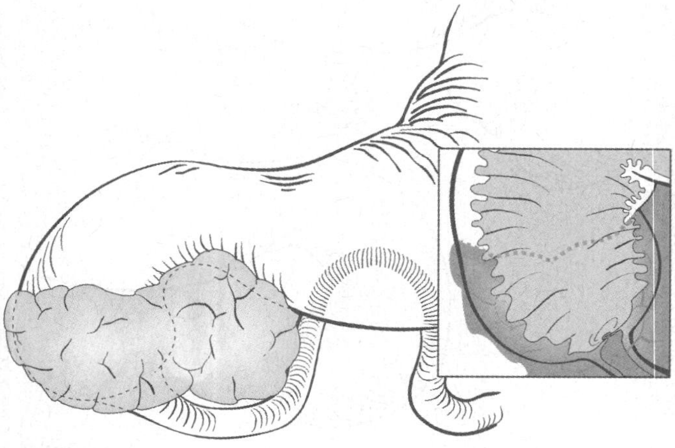

图 79-3　环状胰腺伴下方隔膜造成不完全性梗阻。

患儿母亲有羊水过多，这是需要进一步检查的早期线索[16,55]。由于羊水过多常导致早产，因此约有一半患儿是早产儿。在早期胎儿超声中很容易辨认出典型的“双泡征”梗阻图像。位于胎儿腹腔内并排的双泡中较大的那个是扩张且充满液体的胃，而另一个是扩张的近端十二指肠（图 79-4）。环状胰腺有时也可有这种表现[63,88]。

反复胆汁性呕吐是几乎所有十二指肠梗阻新生儿的特征性临床表现。由于肠梗阻的水平较高，患儿可能不会表现出腹胀，有时可出现轻微上腹饱满感。放置鼻胃管后抽出超过多于 30 ml 液体即提示有肠梗阻。如果缺乏产前诊断，很容易作出胎粪吸入的错误诊断。在分娩后吸痰清理气道时，气管导管可能会不小心进入食管，导致将胆汁性胃液误认为是气管内抽吸物。

对于完全性或严重十二指肠梗阻患儿，可通过腹部平片看到“双泡征”帮助确诊。远端肠道内无气体是完全性梗阻的特征，而存在气体则表明是不完全性梗阻。当高度怀疑但是“双泡征”看不清楚时，通过鼻胃管注入 30～60 ml 空气可使“双泡征”更加明显（图 79-5）。

如果梗阻程度相对较轻，那么不完全性梗阻的诊断可能会有延误[28]。这种情况下当婴儿进食由奶改为固体食物后或婴儿晚期、儿童期甚至罕见的成人期才首次出现症状也很常见，此时肠动力减弱、食物阻塞或异物可造成更明显的症状[27,56,68]。

当腹部平片有十二指肠梗阻的特征性表现时，可以直接进行手术干预而无需行造影检查。有时上消化

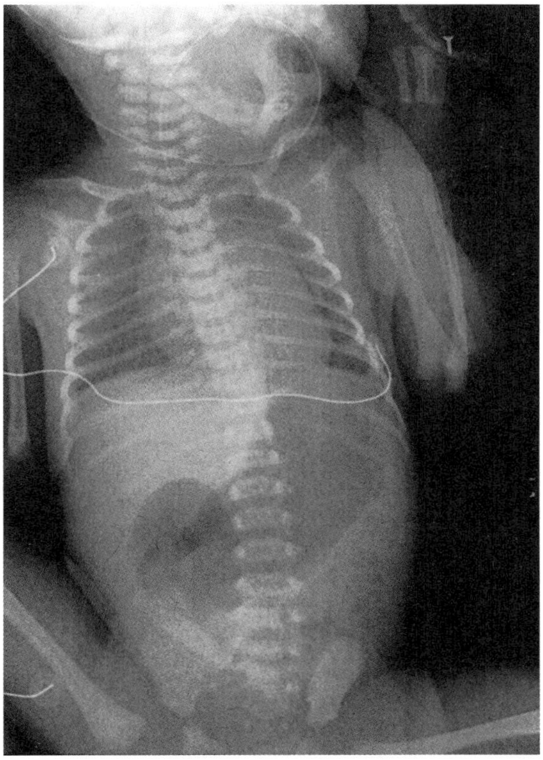

图 79-5　新生儿十二指肠梗阻腹部平片（孔型隔膜）。注意“双泡”远端有少量空气。相同征象但无远端积气提示十二指肠闭锁。

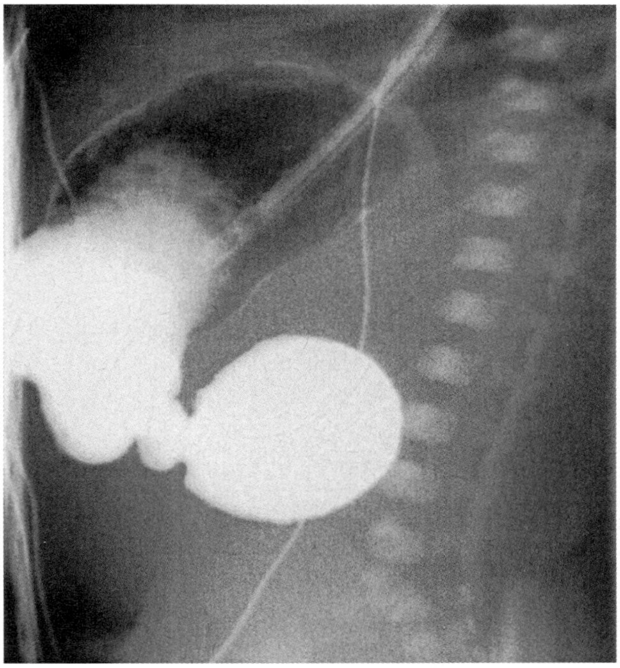

图 79-6　上消化道造影检查显示十二指肠闭锁。

1263 道造影检查有助于鉴别内源性十二指肠梗阻和中肠扭转。内源性梗阻时可在十二指肠第二段梗阻水平看到光滑、圆形末端，如果梗阻不完全，则可看到十二指肠悬韧带（图 79-6）。十二指肠第三段远端“鸟喙”样结构应考虑肠扭转并需要急诊手术。然而如果患者准备在短时间内进行探查手术，完全不必在术前鉴别这两种疾病[26]。

上消化道造影检查有助于评估具有慢性不完全性梗阻症状的婴儿和儿童[11]。胃十二指肠镜检查有助于诊断，有时也是治疗方法之一[49,64]。

治疗

十二指肠梗阻新生儿最初治疗包括鼻胃管或口胃管减压及静脉补液。需适当补足胃肠损失量，并推荐在周围静脉插入中心导管给予肠外营养，因为喂养通常要延迟至修补术后数周。假如中肠扭转已被排除，则十二指肠梗阻不需要急诊手术。可在患儿血液动力学调整到最佳状态和了解其伴发的畸形后再进行手术[44]。对于非常小的早产儿，其肺功能状态和肺容量可妨碍早期手术干预，可能在手术前需要进行数周的胃肠减压和肠外营养。

手术最好取右上象限肝下缘和脐当中横切口，稍微越过腹中线。在探查腹腔之后游离右结肠和肝曲并推移结肠至中腹部以完全暴露近端十二指肠。将小肠和结肠拖出腹腔，放在切口左侧以更好暴露十二指肠第三、第四段。这个操作可以充分暴露肠系膜根部和十二指肠悬韧带。尽管许多十二指肠严重梗阻患儿同时可伴有旋转不良，但仔细检查的话会发现一部分是假性扭转不良，这是因为明显扩张的十二指肠可造成右结肠和肝曲向左侧异常异位。十二指肠悬韧带缺失见于真性扭转不良患儿。

检查整个十二指肠及可能发生梗阻的部位及梗阻类型。对于完全性或几乎完全性梗阻，近端十二指肠呈巨大、沼泽样、增厚的球状。Ⅰ型中，梗阻远端细小无气体的小肠表明梗阻为完全性。Ⅱ型和Ⅲ型中不 1264
连续的肠段在分离过程中清晰可见。在环状胰腺患儿中可见到胰腺组织环形包绕十二指肠第二段。

当近端肠段扩张明显时，将十二指肠尾状成形术

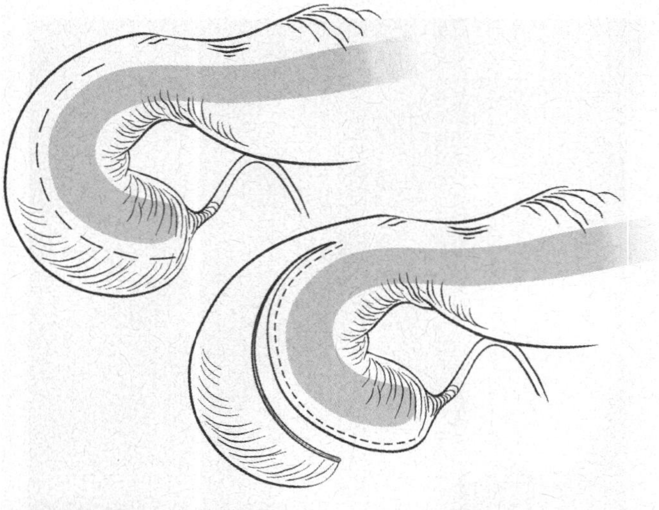

图 79-7 锥形裁剪成形扩张的近端十二指肠。

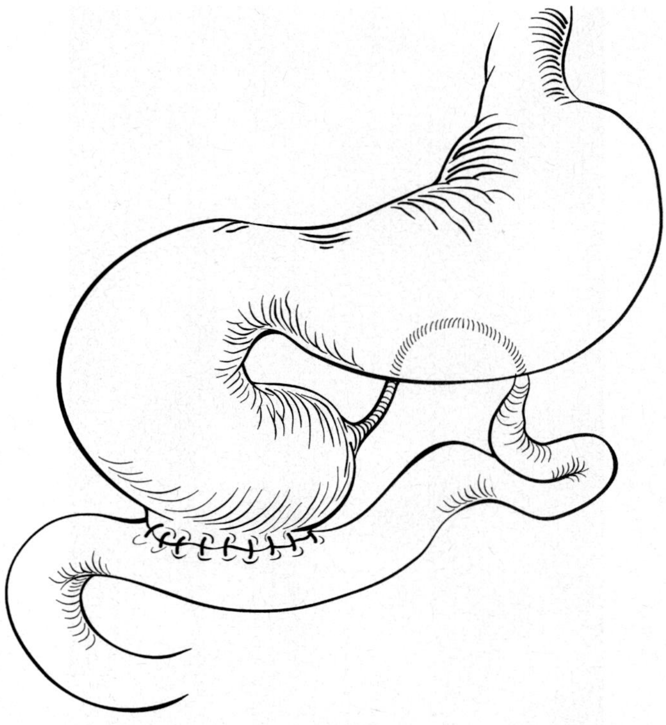

图 79-8 十二指肠空肠吻合术。

作为初期手术可加速术后蠕动功能恢复[1,3,19,38,46,77,92]。成形术可通过缝扎折叠完成，亦或使用 GIA 吻合器或针式电刀切除部分扩张肠管加缝合关闭。在肠管前面或前外侧面进行尾状成形术以避免损伤胆总管、胰腺以及壶腹部（图 79-7）[40]。此外，游离十二指肠悬韧带以帮助移动远端肠段可以使吻合口无张力且不会扭曲。

如果近端和远端十二指肠连续，最好在肉眼可见梗阻部位附近打开远端肠管，打开部位和打开方向应适合将来可能进行的旁路手术。如果明确隔膜是梗阻原因，有时可进行切除而非进行旁路手术。这种情况下延长切口越过隔膜至近端肠腔，切除并烧灼隔膜。如果壶腹位于隔膜的中部或辨认不清楚，只切除隔膜外侧部分。同成形术一样横向关闭十二指肠以缩短和增宽隔膜处的肠腔，这样可以降低狭窄的风险。只有在隔膜很薄且是引起梗阻的唯一原因时才可行隔膜切除术。

大多数情况下，十二指肠与十二指肠吻合术即将梗阻近端和远端肠管吻合是最好的矫治术。这是最直接最符合生理学的修复方法，并且在可供选择的方法中日后发生并发症的可能性最小。如果由于患儿解剖结构特别是小的早产儿而较难实施该方法时，可考虑选择十二指肠空肠吻合术。选择一段可充分提至近端十二指肠的近端空肠肠袢，并将其从右横结肠肠系膜中穿过置于结肠后位置。十二指肠空肠吻合术术后效果和十二指肠与十二指肠吻合术基本相同（图 79-8）。胃空肠吻合术术后可频繁发生吻合口溃疡和盲袢综合征等晚期并发症，因此应避免采取该术式。

在最近报道的一组十二指肠梗阻患儿中，十二指肠与十二指肠吻合术已成为大多数患儿选择的术式（>80%），而十二指肠空肠吻合术大约为 10%，隔膜切除术则为 5%～10%，很少选择胃空肠吻合术[8,16,25,34]。

在进行旁路吻合时，首选“菱形吻合”（近端横行切开，远端纵行切开）（图 79-9A）而非“单纯吻合”（近端和远端均纵行切开）（图 79-9B），这最早由 Kimura 提出[45,47,86]。有证据表明这种不对称吻合可维持吻合口宽大张开的形状并更早允许十二指肠内容物通过。

每个肠段系膜对侧缘的切口应有 1～2 cm 长，这取决于患儿体型，以保证足够宽的吻合口。对于Ⅲ型闭锁，适当将远端肠段末端修剪。在切开远端肠段前，向肠腔内注射生理盐水有助于远端封闭的肠壁轻微伸展，在技术上使吻合更加容易。此外，可放置 10 号法式 Foley 导管，近端通过胃，远端达到空肠，气囊充气后往回拉，这样可以确保没有遗漏其他隔膜

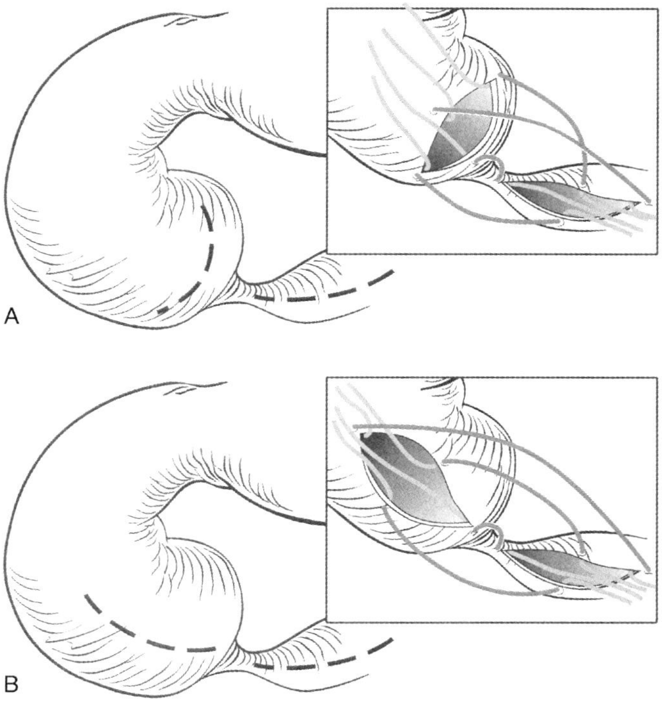

图 79-9　A.“菱形吻合”。B.“单纯”吻合。

1265 或风向袋样畸形。在开始吻合前，可在近端扩张肠段内放置小型带状牵引器以检查梗阻部位和确定 Vater 壶腹的位置。该解剖标志甚至是早产小婴儿通常也很容易看见。大多数患儿的 Vater 壶腹位于十二指肠近端，靠近或位于狭窄或隔膜的前内侧面。其余患儿的 Vater 壶腹可位于靠近或位于梗阻部位的十二指肠远端。

菱形吻合是通过先置缝线将各切口的中点与另一个切口的终点相对合完成的。置缝线时应预先在后壁打结于腔内，前壁打结于腔外。通过二分法吻合后壁以保证缝线之间距离相等和吻合口接合良好。之后以相同方式完成吻合口前面部分。仔细检查吻合口的通畅性后将肠管回纳腹腔至原位。如果右结肠移动性很大且十二指肠悬韧带被游离，或者如果存在旋转不良，将肠管重置即小肠置于右侧而结肠置于左侧，如 Ladd 术式那样。放置一根鼻胃管于胃中。尽管过去经常使用胃造瘘管，但现在认为这个方法只对那些近期无法经口喂养的患儿有用。虽然目前尚未明确其好处，一些外科医生常规将饲管放至吻合口以下[4,86]。

位于十二指肠悬韧带处或其附近的先天性远端十二指肠梗阻是一个特别棘手的问题。失去张力的扩张的十二指肠段很难做尾状修剪，因此重建的肠道和吻合可能在很长时间内功能很差甚至无功能。这种情况下建议行保留壶腹部的十二指肠扩张部的次全切除术(图 79-10A)[23,48]。打开十二指肠第二段前壁并找到 Vater 壶腹。游离十二指肠悬韧带，从胰腺向近端逆行分离扩张的十二指肠至壶腹部远端。然后在近壶腹

图 79-10　A. 分离十二指肠悬韧带后移动远端扩张的十二指肠。B. 切除远端十二指肠后与正常空肠相嵌合（注意：斜形切除以保留壶腹部）。

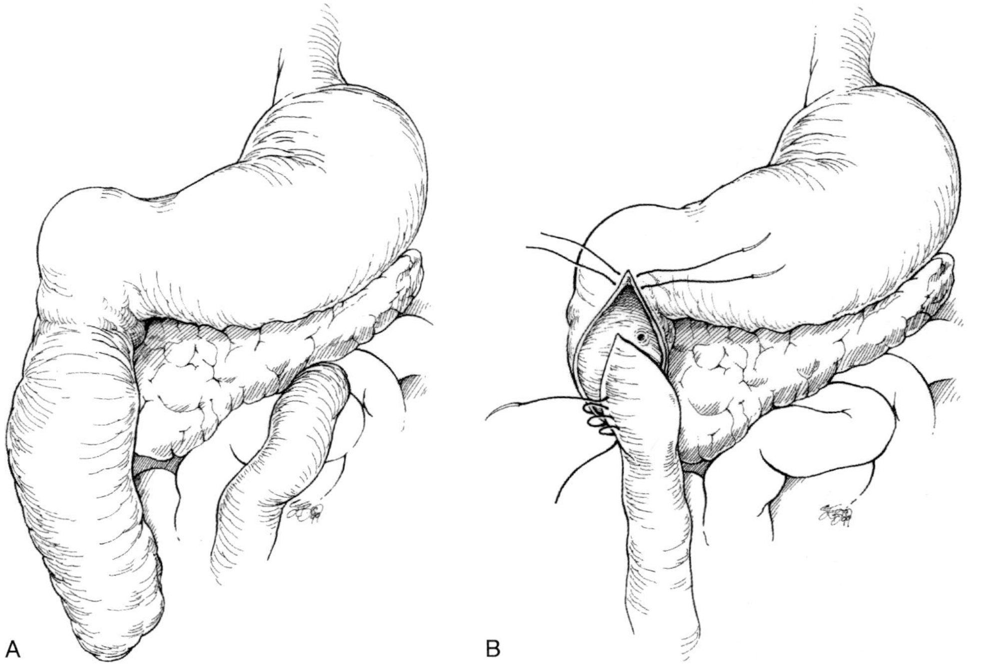

1266 部水平尾状修剪十二指肠第一和第二段，将离断的近端十二指肠连同远端十二指肠一起切除。修剪梗阻远端的正常空肠并与锥形成形后的近端肠段吻合（见图79-10B）。

当发现十二指肠梗阻伴有环状胰腺时，常选择旁路手术。不要横断胰腺环因为主胰管结构横穿其中。这些结构的损伤可导致胰液漏和/或胰腺炎。十二指肠前门静脉梗阻也可采取相同的术式。

最近有数例腹腔镜下旁路手术成功矫治新生儿十二指肠梗阻的病例报道[8,31,79]。由于受到患儿病例数的限制，目前还无法比较该技术与经典开腹手术之间长期预后的差异。

术后持续给予全肠外营养并监测鼻胃管排出量。和其他新生儿肠道手术一样，喂养要在鼻胃管排出量减少且颜色变浅变清时才开始。这个阶段通常需要术后几天至一周，也有可能延长。开始时少量喂养，当耐受后再增加量和浓度。对于大多数婴儿这个过程非常快，绝大多数可在一周至几周内出院。

并发症

术中并发症

有几种术中判断和技术上的缺陷会引起术后的问题[17]。很长且松软的隔膜（风向袋样畸形）最易引起梗阻部位判断失误。基底位于近端的隔膜充满了胃肠道分泌物并向远端十二指肠球形膨出，使远端十二指肠扩张并使梗阻部位看似比实际所在的位置远得多。没有认识到隔膜真正位置的粗心的外科医生可能会在完全远离隔膜实际位置的部位进行旁路吻合术。另外，在罕见情况下，梗阻不止一处。由于临近肠管无明显扩张，远端隔膜很容易遗漏。因此在开始吻合前小心地将近端置入胃、远端置入空肠的球囊导管往回拉可预防上述情况出现[2,11,72]。

术后并发症

恢复进食的时间延长是十二指肠梗阻术后最常见的并发症。对于需要进行旁路吻合术或隔膜切除术的患儿来说，恢复功能的时间变异性很大。尽管有人提出多种促动力药物可缩短这个过程，但至今没有发现任何一种药物有连贯的疗效。总之，如果初期手术中没有发生特别问题，而术后2～3周功能尚未恢复相对正常的患儿应予以关注。此时，上消化道系列检查有助于发现残留吻合口梗阻、吻合口狭窄、之前未发现的其他部位梗阻以及肠蠕动差。初期手术时在吻合口放置小夹子可以帮助确定吻合部位以及引起残留问题的原因。任何进一步手术治疗的决定应基于影像学检查和临床胃肠道功能评估的基础上。在旁路吻合术后完全恢复功能之前，可在X片上看到扩张的近端十二指肠长达数月之久[78]。

与持续性蠕动功能减弱相比，如果肠功能较差的时间延长，则更不容易发现吻合口梗阻。近端十二指肠单纯尾状锥形修剪可提供足够的额外动力，而如果最初梗阻位于十二指肠远端则可选择十二指肠次全切除加近端锥形成形[48]。一旦胃肠道功能得以恢复，可能会发生更多问题，但这种情况不常见。

十二指肠后期梗阻偶尔可在年长婴儿和儿童中发生。这种情况发生于看似成功的新生儿旁路手术或隔膜切除术后，也可以是最初不完全性十二指肠梗阻诊断遗漏后新形成的。前者可由于一片纤维性食物或异物在部分切除的隔膜或相对较窄的吻合口处嵌塞，吻合口狭窄可能是由于吻合口不够大，随时间推移变得狭窄或没有随着儿童一起生长引起的。后一种情况，梗阻可发生于因近端肠管扩张以及无效蠕动加重，逐渐引起症状的狭窄程度相对轻的部位。在其他情况中，最初手术纠治后不会出现持续的解剖性梗阻，但某些持续扩张或进行性扩张的肠管可能会出现蠕动功能减弱[18]。

这时无论是在原来未充分矫治的连接部还是在自身没有明显的解剖性狭窄的情况下，近端尾状修剪均很有帮助[20,21]。

大多数年长婴儿和儿童已适合进行上消化道内镜全功能检查，这有助于诊断，也可进行吻合口狭窄扩张或隔膜切除等治疗[49,64]。

预后

十二指肠梗阻患儿存活率在过去半个世纪内已由45%上升至95%[30,32,61,89]。虽然选择性终止妊娠起到一定作用，但这个显著的进步主要与诊断、外科手术

1267 以及术后处理的进展有关。几乎所有死亡都与其他器官系统的伴发畸形有关，主要是心、肺和脑的伴发疾病。

（王宇鹏译　陈永卫校）

参考文献

1. Adzick NS, Harrison MR, deLorimier AA: Tapering duodenoplasty for megaduodenum associated with duodenal atresia. J Pediatr Surg 1986;21:311.
2. Akhtar J, Guiney EJ: Congenital duodenal obstruction. Br J Surg 1992;79:133.
3. Alexander F, DiFiore J, Stallion A: Triangular tapered duodenoplasty for the treatment of congenital duodenal obstruction. J Pediatr Surg 2002;37:862.
4. Arnbjornsson E, Larsson M, Finkel Y, Karpe B: Transanastomotic feeding tube after an operation for duodenal atresia. Eur J Pediatr Surg 2002;12:159.
5. Andrassy RJ, Mahour GH: Gastrointestinal anomalies associated with esophageal atresia or tracheoesophageal fistula. Arch Surg 1979;114:1125.
6. Arey LB: Developmental Anatomy: A Textbook and Laboratory Manual of Embryology, 7th ed. Philadelphia, WB Saunders, 1974.
7. Bailey PV, Tracy TFJ, Connors RH, et al: Congenital duodenal obstruction: A 32-year review. J Pediatr Surg 1993;28:92.
8. Bax NM, Ure BM, van der Zee DC, van Tuijl I: Laparoscopic duodenoduodenostomy for duodenal atresia. Surg Endosc 2001;15:217.
9. Bickler SW, Harrison MW, Blank E, Campbell JR: Microperforation of a duodenal diaphragm as a cause of paradoxical gas in congenital duodenal obstruction. J Pediatr Surg 1992;27:747.
10. Boyden EA, Cope JG, Bill AHJ: Anatomy and embryology of congenital intrinsic obstruction of the duodenum. Am J Surg 1967;114:190.
11. Brown RA, Millar AJ, Linegar A, et al: Fenestrated duodenal membranes: An analysis of symptoms, signs, diagnosis, and treatment. J Pediatr Surg 1994;29:429.
12. Calder E: Two examples of children born with preternatural conformation of the guts. Med Essays (Edinburgh) 1733;1:203.
13. Celli J, van Bokhoven H, Brunner HG: Feingold syndrome: Clinical review and genetic mapping. Am J Med Genet 2003;122A:294.
14. Chasen ST, Sharma G, Kalish RB, Chervenak FA: First-trimester screening for aneuploidy with fetal nuchal translucency in a United States population. Ultrasound Obstet Gynecol 2003;22:149.
15. Cordes L: Congenital occlusion of the duodenum. Arch Pediatr 1901;18:401.
16. Dalla Vecchia LK, Grosfeld JL, West KW, et al: Intestinal atresia and stenosis: A 25-year experience with 277 cases. Arch Surg 1998;133:490.
17. Danismend EN, Brown N: Morbidity and mortality in duodenal atresia. Z Kinderchir 1986;41:86.
18. de Lorimier AA: Bowel motility in infants and children born with duodenal atresia and stenosis. J Pediatr Surg 1998;33:950.
19. Dewan LA, Guiney EJ: Duodenoplasty in the management of duodenal atresia. Pediatr Surg Int 1990;5:253.
20. Ein SH, Shandling B: The late nonfunctioning duodenal atresia repair. J Pediatr Surg 1986;21:798.
21. Ein SH, Kim PC, Miller HA: The late nonfunctioning duodenal atresia repair—a second look. J Pediatr Surg 2000;35:690.
22. Elliot GB, Kliman MR, Elliot KA: Pancreatic annulus: A sign or cause of duodenal obstruction. Can J Surg 1968;11:357.
23. Endo M, Ukiyama E, Yokoyama JMK: Subtotal duodenectomy with jejunal patch for megaduodenum secondary to congenital duodenal malformation. J Pediatr Surg 1998;33:1636.
24. Ernst NP: A case of congenital atresia of the duodenum treated successfully by operation. BMJ 1916;1:1644.
25. Escobar MA, Ladd AP, Grosfeld JL, et al: Duodenal atresia and stenosis: Long-term follow-up over 30 years. J Pediatr Surg 2004;39:867.
26. Eustace S, Connolly B, Blake N: Congenital duodenal obstruction: An approach to diagnosis. Eur J Pediatr Surg 1993;3:267.
27. Ferraris VA, McPhail JF: Adult duodenal web associated with peptic ulcer disease. Surg Gynecol Obstet 1984;158:461.
28. Fonkalsrud EW, DeLorimier AA, Hays DM: Congenital atresia and stenosis of the duodenum: A review compiled from the members of the Surgical Section of the American Academy of Pediatrics. Pediatrics 1969;43:79.
29. Gahukamble DB, Khamage AS, Shaheen AQ: Duodenal atresia: Its occurrence in siblings. J Pediatr Surg 1994;29:1599.
30. Girvan DP, Stephens CA: Congenital intrinsic duodenal obstruction: A twenty-year review of its surgical management and consequences. J Pediatr Surg 1974;9:833.
31. Gluer S, Petersen C, Ure BM: Simultaneous correction of duodenal atresia due to annular pancreas and malrotation by laparoscopy. Eur J Pediatr Surg 2002;12:423.
32. Gray SW, Skandalakis JE: Embryology for Surgeons: The Embryological Basis for the Treatment of Congenital Defects. Philadelphia, WB Saunders, 1986.
33. Grosfeld JL, Rescorla FJ: Duodenal atresia and stenosis: Reassessment of treatment and outcome based on antenatal diagnosis, pathologic variance, and long-term follow-up. World J Surg 1993;17:301.
34. Grosfeld JL, Ballantine TV, Shoemaker R: Operative management of intestinal atresia and stenosis based upon pathologic findings. J Pediatr Surg 1979;14:368.
35. Haeusler MC, Befghold A, Stoll C, et al: EUROSCAN Study Group: Prenatal ultrasonographic detection of gastrointestinal obstruction: Results from 18 European congenital anomaly registries. Prenat Diagn 2002;22:616.
36. Hancock BJ, Wiseman NE: Congenital duodenal obstruction: The impact of an antenatal diagnosis. J Pediatr Surg 1989;24:1027.
37. Hendricks SK, Sybert VP: Association of annular pancreas and duodenal obstruction—evidence for Mendelian inheritance? Clin Genet 1991;39:383.
38. Hutton KA, Thomas DF: Tapering duodenoplasty. Pediatr Surg Int 1988;3:132.
39. Irving IM: Duodenal atresia and stenosis: Annular pancreas. In Lister J, Irving IM (eds): Neonatal Surgery, London, Butterworths, 1990, p 424.
40. Jona JZ, Belin RP: Duodenal anomalies and the ampulla of Vater. Surg Gynecol Obstet 1976;143:565.
41. Kaldor J: Atresia of the duodenum and duodenal diverticula. Ann Surg 1929;89:6.
42. Kamisawa T, Yuyang T, Egawa N, et al: A new embryologic

hypothesis of annular pancreas. Hepatogastroenterology 2001;48:277.
43. Kiernan PD, ReMine SG, Kiernan PC, et al: Annular pancreas: Mayo Clinic experience from 1957 to 1976 with review of the literature. Arch Surg 1980;115:46.
44. Kimble RM, Harding J, Kolbe A: Additional congenital anomalies in babies with gut atresia or stenosis: When to investigate and which investigation. Pediatr Surg Int 1997;12:565.
45. Kimura K, Tsugawa C, Ogawa K, et al: Diamond-shaped anastomosis for congenital duodenal obstruction. Arch Surg 1977;112:1262.
46. Kimura K, Perdzynski W, Soper RT: Elliptical seromuscular resection for tapering the proximal dilated bowel in duodenal or jejunal atresia. J Pediatr Surg 1996;31:1405.
47. Kimura K, Mukohara N, Nishijima E, et al: Diamond-shaped anastomosis for duodenal atresia: An experience with 44 patients over 15 years. J Pediatr Surg 1990;25:977.
48. Kling K, Applebaum H, Dunn J, et al: A novel technique for correction of intestinal atresia at the ligament of Treitz. J Pediatr Surg 2000;35:353.
49. Kokkonen ML, Kalima T, Jaaskelainen J, Louhimo I: Duodenal atresia: Late follow-up. J Pediatr Surg 1988;23:216.
50. Komuro H, Makino S, Tahara K: Choledochal cyst associated with duodenal obstruction. J Pediatr Surg 2000;35:1259.
51. Knechtle SJ, Filston HC: Anomalous biliary ducts associated with duodenal atresia. J Pediatr Surg 1990;25:1266.
52. Lambrecht W, Kluth D: Hereditary multiple atresias of the gastrointestinal tract: Report of a case and review of the literature. J Pediatr Surg 1998;33:794.
53. Lemire EG, Evans JA, Giddins NG, et al: A familial disorder with duodenal atresia and tetralogy of Fallot. Am J Med Genet 1996;66:39.
54. McCollum MO, Jamieson DH, Webber EM: Annular pancreas and duodenal stenosis. J Pediatr Surg 2002;37:1776.
55. Merrill JR, Raffensperger JG: Pediatric annular pancreas: Twenty years' experience. J Pediatr Surg 1976;11:921.
56. Mikaelsson C, Arnbjornsson E, Kullendorff CM: Membranous duodenal stenosis. Acta Paediatr 1997;86:953.
57. Mitchell CE, Marshall DG, Reid WD: Preampullary congenital duodenal obstruction in a father and son. J Pediatr Surg 1993;28:1582.
58. Molenaar JC: The legal investigation of a decision not to operate on an infant with Down's syndrome and a duodenal atresia: A report from the Netherlands. Bioethics 1992;6:35.
59. Moore SW, de Jongh G, Bouic P, et al: Immune deficiency in familial duodenal atresia. J Pediatr Surg 1996;31:1733.
60. Mordehai J, Cohen Z, Kurzbart E, Mares AJ: Preduodenal portal vein causing duodenal obstruction associated with situs inversus, intestinal malrotation, and polysplenia: A case report. J Pediatr Surg 2002;37:E5.
61. Nixon HH, Tawes R: Etiology and treatment of small intestinal atresia: Analysis of a series of 127 jejunoileal atresias and comparison with 82 duodenal atresias. Surgery 1971;69:41.
62. Nobukawa B, Otaka M, Suda K, et al: An annular pancreas derived from paired ventral pancreata, supporting Baldwin's hypothesis. Pancreas 2000;20:408.
63. Norton KI, Tenreiro R, Rabinowitz JG: Sonographic demonstration of annular pancreas and a distal duodenal diaphragm in a newborn. Pediatr Radiol 1992;22:66.
64. Okamatsu T, Arai K, Yatsuzuka M, et al: Endoscopic membranectomy for congenital duodenal stenosis in an infant. J Pediatr Surg 1989;24:367.
65. Pameijer CR, Hubbard AM, Coleman B, Flake AW: Combined pure esophageal atresia, duodenal atresia, biliary atresia, and pancreatic ductal atresia: Prenatal diagnostic features and review of the literature. J Pediatr Surg 2000;35:745.
66. Patten BM: Human Embryology, 3rd ed. New York, McGraw-Hill, 1968.
67. Pinette MG, Egan JF, Wax JR, et al: Combined sonographic and biochemical markers for Down syndrome screening. J Ultrasound Med 2003;22:1185.
68. Pittschieler K, Gentili L: Endoscopic diagnosis of duodenal stenosis. J Pediatr Gastroenterol Nutr 1997;24:359.
69. Randolph JG: The doctor's dilemma in Down's syndrome and duodenal atresia. Hosp Physician 1974;10:23.
70. Ried IS: Biliary tract anomalies associated with duodenal atresia. Arch Dis Child 1973;48:852.
71. Rogers JC, Harris DJ, Holder T: Annular pancreas in a mother and daughter. Am J Med Genet 1993;45:116.
72. Rossello PJ: Congenital duodenal atresia associated with a separate duodenal diaphragm. J Pediatr Surg 1978;13:441.
73. Rowe MI, Buckner D, Clatworthy HW Jr: Wind sock web of the duodenum. Am J Surg 1968;116:444.
74. Sadler T: Langman's Medical Embryology, 9th ed. Philadelphia, Lippincott Williams and Wilkins, 2003.
75. Samuel M, Wheeler RA, Mami AG: Does duodenal atresia and stenosis prevent midgut volvulus in malrotation? Eur J Pediatr Surg 1997;7:11.
76. Schuchter K, Hafner E, Stangl G, et al: The first trimester "combined test" for the detection of Down syndrome pregnancies in 4939 unselected pregnancies. Prenat Diagn 2002;22:211.
77. Sherman JO, Schulten M: Operative correction of duodenomegaly. J Pediatr Surg 1974;9:461.
78. Spigland N, Yazbeck S: Complications associated with surgical treatment of congenital intrinsic duodenal obstruction. J Pediatr Surg 1990;25:1127.
79. Steyaert H, Valla JS, Van Hoorde E: Diaphragmatic duodenal atresia: Laparoscopic repair. Eur J Pediatr Surg 2003; 13:414.
80. Sumner TE, Auringer ST, Cox TD: A complex communicating bronchopulmonary foregut malformation: Diagnostic imaging and pathogenesis. Pediatr Radiol 1997;27:799.
81. Sweed Y: Duodenal obstruction. In Puri P (ed): Newborn Surgery, 2nd ed, London, Arnold, 2003, p 423.
82. Todres ID, Krane D, Howell MC, Shannon DC: Pediatricians' attitudes affecting decision-making in defective newborns. Pediatrics 1977;60:197.
83. Torfs CP, Christianson RE: Anomalies in Down syndrome. Am J Med Genet 1998;77:431.
84. Vidal E: 18e Congrès de chirurgie, Paris: Procès verbaux mémoires et discussion. Assoc Fr Chir 1905;18:739.
85. Webb CH, Wangensteen OH: Congenital intestinal atresia. Am J Dis Child 1931;41:262.
86. Weber TR, Lewis JE, Mooney D, Connors R: Duodenal atresia: A comparison of techniques of repair. J Pediatr Surg 1986;21:1133.
87. Wei JL, Rodeberg D, Thompson DM: Tracheal agenesis with anomalies found in both VACTERL and TACRD associations. Int J Pediatr Otorhinolaryngol 2003;67:1013.
88. Weiss H, Sherer DM, Manning FA: Ultrasonography of fetal annular pancreas. Obstet Gynecol 1999;94:852.
89. Wesley JR, Mahour GH: Congenital intrinsic duodenal obstruction: A twenty-five year review. Surgery 1977; 82:716.
90. Yokoyama T, Ishizone S, Momose Y, et al: Duodenal atresia in dizygotic twins. J Pediatr Surg 1997;32:1806.
91. Young DG, Wilkinson AW: Abnormalities associated with neonatal duodenal obstruction. Surgery 1968;63:832.
92. Young JS, Goco I, Pennell T: Duodenoplasty and reimplantation of the ampulla of Vater for megaduodenum. Am J Surg 1993;59:685.

第 80 章

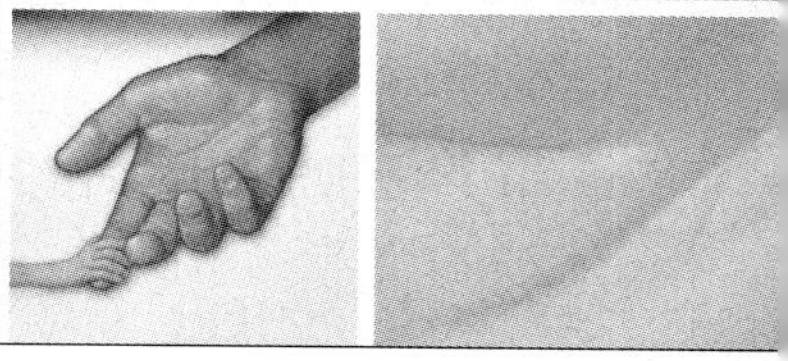

空回肠闭锁及狭窄

Jay L. Grosfeld

历史回顾

1269 Goeller 于 1684 年首先描述了回肠闭锁[37]。Calder（1773）[153]和 Osiander（1779）[47]记录了其他有关肠闭锁的早期观察。Voisin 于 1804 年对肠闭锁施行了肠造瘘手术。Meckel 于 1812 年发表了关于这个疾病的综述并对病因进行了推测。1889 年，Bland-Sutton[15]提出肠闭锁的分型，并推测肠闭锁发生于“闭塞性胚胎事件”的位置，如卵黄管萎缩。1894 年，Wanitschek 首次尝试对肠闭锁行肠切除和吻合术，但未成功[47]。1900 年，Tandler[137]提出肠闭锁与肠发育中实心索带阶段的再通（空泡化）失败相关的学说。1910 年，Johnson 证实了此结论[64]。1911 年，Fockens[39]首先成功地对肠闭锁实施肠吻合术。1912 年，Spriggs[132]提出机械性意外（包括血管闭塞）可能与肠闭锁的发生有关。Davis 和 Poynter（1922）[31]，以及 Webb 和 Wangensteen（1931）[153]通过对肠闭锁的临床观察支持这个观点。Evans 对 1498 例消化道闭锁病例的广泛回顾（1951）[37]显示仅有 139 例婴儿治疗取得成功。Louw 和 Barnard 经典的实验观察（1955）[80]证实子宫内晚期肠系膜血管意外是大多数空肠回肠闭锁的原因，这为现代对这些畸形的理解和治疗奠定了基础。

发生率

空肠回肠闭锁及狭窄是新生儿肠梗阻的主要原因。肠闭锁是肠腔完全闭塞引起的先天性梗阻，占新生儿肠梗阻的 95%。肠狭窄定义为肠腔部分闭塞，从而引起不完全肠梗阻，占空回肠梗阻的 5%。在过去的 20 年中，人们对病因及受损的肠功能有了更好的了解，并且在儿科麻醉、手术技术、术前术后护理（特别在营养支持领域）上有了改进，这使患儿存活率有了明显的提高。

空肠回肠闭锁的发生率据报道为 1/1500 活产儿至 1/400（丹麦）或 1/330（美国）活产儿[37]。Cragan 及其同事[28,29]和 Harris 及其同事[55]的流行病学研究发现非裔美国儿童和双胞胎中小肠闭锁的发生率更高。在荷兰，异性的双胞胎中空肠闭锁的发生率也有相似的增加[92]。夏威夷的一项人群普查研究显示，与白人相比，空肠回肠闭锁在远东的亚洲人中更常见[41]。在怀孕期间，母亲单独使用伪麻黄碱或与对乙酰氨基酚联合使用，或母亲有偏头痛而使用麦角胺和咖啡因（咖啡角）后，胎儿发生小肠闭锁的危险性增加[46,156]。

1972～2004 年间在印第安纳州印第安纳波利斯 Riley 儿童医院治疗的 387 例肠闭锁及肠狭窄病例中，194 例为空肠回肠病变，169 例为十二指肠病变，24 例为结肠病变。Nixon 和 Tawes[99]注意到空肠回肠闭锁与十二指肠闭锁的发生率之比为 2∶1。在美国儿科学会外科组成员做的 619 例空肠回肠闭锁及狭窄病例的回顾研究中，de Lorimier 及其同事[32]发现男孩和女孩的发病率相等。尽管在此相对大样本的人群中，婴儿的平均出生体重为 2.7 kg（范围：0.9～4.8 kg），但有1/3的婴儿为空肠闭锁，1/4 为回肠闭锁，一半以上的多发性闭锁患儿为低出生体重儿[32]。产前超声检查发现肠闭锁的患儿常为低出生体重儿[4]。十二指肠闭锁或狭窄患儿中有 30% 为 Down 综合征，而空肠回肠闭锁患儿中 21 三体相对少见。Nixon 和 Tawes[99]在 127 例空肠回肠闭锁病例中仅观察到 2 例 21 三体，de Lorimier 及其同事[32]在 619 例中仅观察到 5 例。Riley 儿童医院的 194

例空肠回肠闭锁病例中仅有的1例Down综合征患儿合并十二指肠闭锁。

1270 **病因学**

追溯历史，有关空肠回肠闭锁原因的早期概念曾被简单思考过。1900年，Tandler[137]提出肠闭锁与肠发育中实心索带阶段的再通失败相关的理论。1959年，Lynn和Espinas[82]证实了Tandler的一些有关上皮堵塞肠腔的观察。虽然黏膜闭锁常见于十二指肠闭锁病例，但上皮堵塞引起的空肠回肠闭锁少见。大多数空肠回肠闭锁被索带样节段或V形肠系膜缺损分隔开。Louw和Barnard[80]、Santulli和Blanc[121]以及Nixon[98]的临床观察发现闭锁段远端常可见胆汁色素、鳞状物和胎毛，这强烈提示除了上皮堵塞之外还有其他原因。胎儿分泌胆汁和吞咽羊水开始于妊娠11~12周，即在实心索带再通之后。尸体解剖观察发现有血管畸形如肠系膜动脉弓缺乏，更增加了存在其他病因学因素的怀疑。

1955年，Louw和Barnard[80]为妊娠晚期的胎狗结扎肠系膜血管，形成绞窄性肠梗阻。10~14天之后，检查受影响的肠管后发现其闭锁症状与临床上观察到的人类新生儿肠闭锁相似。这些发现强烈提示大多数空肠回肠闭锁是子宫内晚期肠系膜血管病变的结果。Courtois[26]证实胎兔手术后，宫内肠穿孔可愈合且无任何痕迹（有或无胎粪性腹膜炎的迹象），或导致肠狭窄或肠闭锁。他进一步发现如果肠袢孤立，在血供不好的情况下可发生肠袢的再吸收。Santulli和Blanc[121]、Abrams[1]、Koga及其同事[72]以及Tovar及其同事[144]在对胎兔、胎羊、胎狗和鸡胚中进行的各种实验性研究也证实了这些发现。2001年，Sweeney及其同事注意到空肠闭锁（42%）患儿比回肠闭锁（2%）患儿有更高的畸形发生率，提示一些空肠闭锁可能来源于一种畸变过程[135]。Glǔ er报道在羊膜内注射染料后4对双胞胎发生空肠回肠闭锁，由此提出了一种畸形形成的机制[44]。Gillich及其同事给大鼠模型使用多柔比星（阿霉素）后，证实在发育中的中肠区域异常地形成脊索，并伴有多发性肠闭锁[43]。

临床上常可见到宫内晚期肠系膜血管损伤，如肠扭转、肠套迭、内疝以及紧张的腹裂或脐膨出缺损压迫肠系膜引起的肠闭锁病例[14,50,51,62,74,151]。de Lorimier及其同事[32]发现619例空肠回肠闭锁病例中42%有肠梗死的迹象。Nixon和Tawes[99]在127例肠闭锁病例中观察到61例有肉眼或显微镜下可见的宫内腹膜炎，44例有明显的肠扭转。Murphy[95]注意到5%的肠闭锁与胎儿内疝有关。Santulli和Blanc[121]、Nixon和Tawes[99]、Okmian和Kovamees[101]报道肠闭锁病例与脐膨出时肠管嵌顿有关。Vassy和Boles[146]、Landor及其同事[76]报道隐性脐膨出脐带钳夹后可引起医源性产后回肠闭锁。Grosfeld和Clatworthy[51]观察到空肠闭锁伴紧张的腹裂缺损内整个中肠梗死的病例。在美国儿科学会的调查中，2%的患儿为空肠回肠闭锁伴腹裂[32]。但近期调查发现腹裂并发肠闭锁的发生率更高，为10%~25%[45,91,129]。在我院，194例空肠回肠闭锁病例中，28例（14.4%）伴有腹裂。据报道，宫内肠套迭不是肠闭锁的常见病因。Evans[37]回顾1498例肠闭锁病例中仅9例伴有肠套迭。然而，据Komuro描述，在48例肠闭锁病例中，12例（25%）的病因为宫内肠套迭，并常伴发单纯性中小肠闭锁[73]。在高位空肠闭锁、苹果皮样肠闭锁或多发性闭锁病例中，未发现肠套迭是肠闭锁的病因。与出生后肠套迭相似，宫内肠套迭的原因不明[62,151]。这些患儿大多为没有合并畸形的足月儿，有条索型或裂隙型肠闭锁，不伴有囊性纤维化[52,103,113,131,140]。据报道，早产儿出生后肠套迭也是空肠闭锁的病因之一[109]。在Riley儿童医院治疗的194例空肠回肠闭锁或狭窄的患儿中，64例伴肠扭转，32例伴肠旋转不良，5例伴肠套迭，2例伴内疝，28例伴腹裂，24例有胎粪性腹膜炎的迹象。这些迟发事件解释了为什么肠外合并畸形的发生率相对较低（7%）[32]。少数情况下，在同卵双生的双胞胎中可发现空肠回肠闭锁与胆道闭锁、十二指肠闭锁、结肠闭锁、胃闭锁、先天性巨结肠和关节挛缩共存[24,49,52,75,77,89,159]。所幸的是，大多数空肠回肠闭锁的婴儿仅此单纯畸形，而在其他方面是正常的。Gross及其同事报道并发十二指肠和空肠闭锁的家族性病例[53]。Guttman及其同事[54]、Aigrain及其同事[2]、Kimble及其同事[69]、Puri和Fujimoto[108]、Fourcade及其同事[42]报道了无血管损伤迹象或胆汁色素、胎毛或闭锁远端鳞状物的遗传性多发性肠闭锁病例，指出畸形发生可能与常染色体隐性遗传有关。Kilani及其同事描述了可能为常染色体显性遗传的空肠闭锁伴肾发育不良的家族系谱图[66]。Walker及其同事[150]报道了1例多发性肠闭锁伴移植物抗宿主病及免疫抑制的病例。Rothenberg 及其同事发现 1 例多发性肠闭锁伴有以无丙球蛋白血症、B 细胞缺乏和 T 细胞功能受损为特征的严重免疫缺陷病例[119]。

1271 诊断

临床表现

空肠回肠闭锁的相关表现包括母亲羊水过多、胆汁性呕吐、腹胀、黄疸，以及出生后第 1 天不能排出胎粪（表 80-1）[32,48,79,95,114,148]。24% 的病例出现母亲羊水过多，多见于近端空肠闭锁的病例（38%）[32]。胆汁性呕吐稍多见于空肠闭锁（84%），而腹胀更多见于回肠闭锁（98%）[48]。黄疸发生于 32% 的空肠闭锁患儿及 20% 的回肠闭锁患儿[32]。这些小肠梗阻病例的黄疸特征性地伴有间接胆红素升高[17,100]。尽管大多数患儿无法在出生后 24 小时内排出胎粪，但偶尔可经直肠排出胎粪及坏死组织[48,51,99,114,140]。腹胀是空肠回肠闭锁病例的常见临床特征。近端空肠闭锁可伴有上腹胀。更加广泛性的腹胀常表示有低位梗阻（如远端小肠或结肠梗阻），梗阻水平近端大量肠袢充满气体。严重的腹胀可伴发横膈抬高引起的呼吸窘迫，腹壁静脉显露，体检时在腹壁上发现以可见的肠袢为特征的肠型（有时有蠕动波）。虽然腹胀常在出生后 12～24 小时发生，但在出生时即发现腹胀则提示有巨大的囊性胎粪性腹膜炎[19,48]。

产前超声

羊水过多的孕妇行产前超声检查可确认有无小肠梗阻伴发肠闭锁、肠扭转及胎粪性腹膜炎[3,4,78,83]。

表 80-1　空肠回肠闭锁的临床表现

临床表现	空肠闭锁（%）	回肠闭锁（%）
羊水过多	38	15
胆汁性呕吐	84	81
腹胀	78	98
胎粪不能排出	65	71
黄疸	32	20

产前超声探测十二指肠闭锁比更远端的病变更可靠。有多处扩张肠袢伴强烈肠蠕动应怀疑是否有产前小肠闭锁[116]。产前超声检查发现胎儿有腹裂伴肠管扩张时，也应怀疑是否有肠闭锁[3,91]。Phelps 及其同事[105]报道，产前诊断为消化道畸形的只有 42% 在婴儿出生后被证实患有该病，220 例出生后发现有消化道畸形的病例在产前被超声检测出的仅有 35 例（16%），虽然产前超声表现为有回声的肠管常说明有消化道畸形，但 44 例中仅有 12 例（27%）在出生后被证实[105]。Basu 和 Burge 报道经产前超声诊断为小肠闭锁的患儿有 31%[4]，他们发现在妊娠较晚期时做超声扫描更易检测出消化道畸形，如果孕妇仅在孕 16 周时接受 1 次超声检查，就可能漏诊。Dalla Vecchia 及其同事、Tam 和 Nicholls 均发现肠闭锁的产前诊断相对较少，只有不到 1/3 的病例可被超声识别[30,136]。如果被识别，闭锁常位于近端，患儿需延长生后的治疗时间。这些观察结果提示产前超声对肠道畸形的预测价值相对较差，在检测或排除胎儿消化道畸形方面仍然是一种不太可靠的方法。有关胎儿磁共振的早期研究显示该方法可识别消化道畸形，并且在肠闭锁的产前诊断上可能比超声更准确[120,147]。

放射学检查

腹部放射学检查常可确诊空肠回肠闭锁。应为每位患儿做直立位及卧位的腹部摄片。拇指大小的肠袢（拇指法则）及气液平强烈提示有新生儿肠梗阻[50]。高位空肠闭锁可呈现少许气液平，除此以外没有任何气体（图 80-1）。闭锁越靠近远端，腹胀越明显，腹部平片上扩张的肠袢及气液平越多。闭锁处可为一个有明显气液平的大肠袢（图 80-2）。12% 的病例在腹部平片上可见到腹膜内钙化，说明有胎粪性腹膜炎，此为宫内肠穿孔的征象（图 80-3）。此外，可观察到肠腔内钙化（木乃伊化）的病例，说明出生前有肠扭转[9,60]。巨大囊性胎粪性腹膜炎病例的腹部平片可见胎粪性假囊肿处有一大的气液平[19]。这与晚期宫内穿孔有关，导致穿孔肠管处形成包裹性肿块（假囊肿），并含有胎粪[48,114]。

新生儿在腹部平片上很少见到结肠袋，可能只单纯显示扩张的肠袢，无法在小肠和结肠之间准确

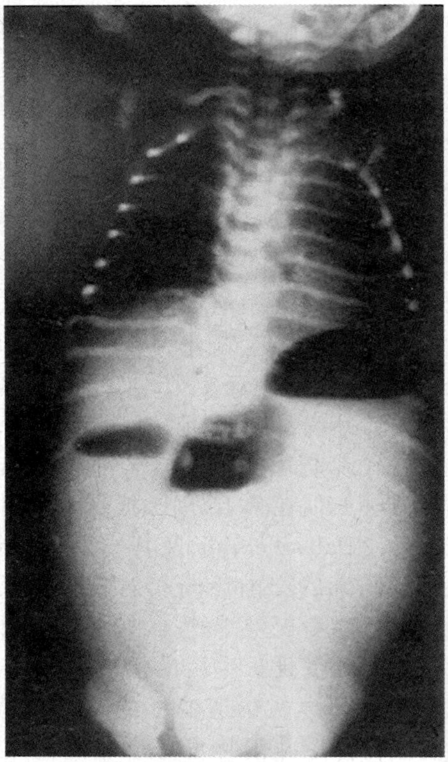

A

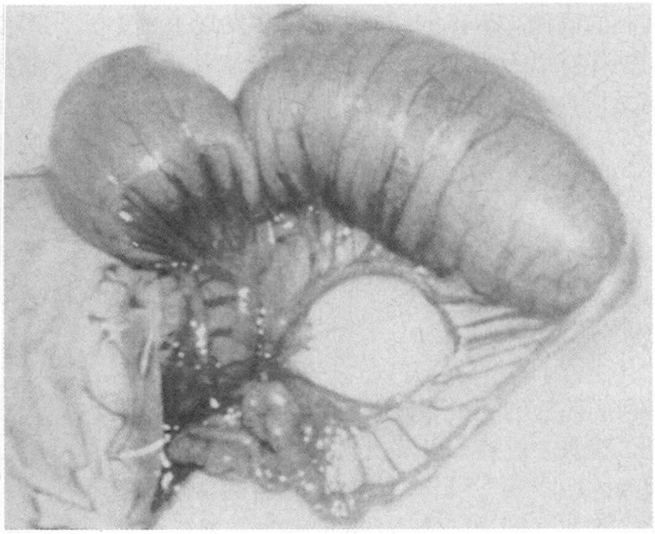

B

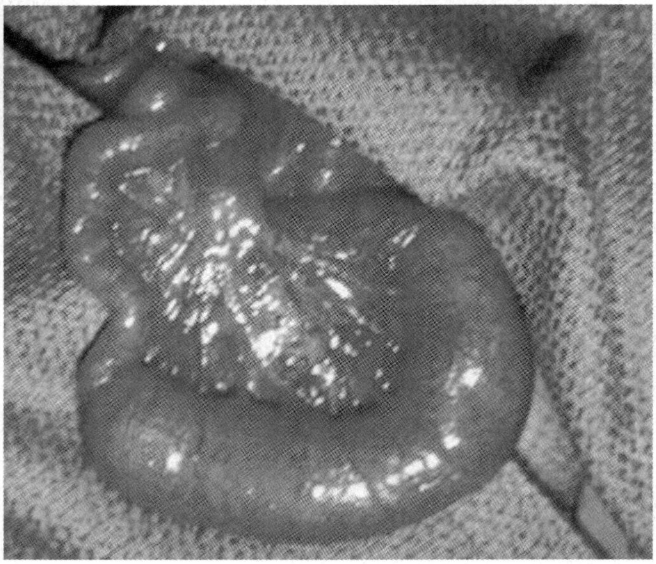

C

图 80-1　高位空肠闭锁。A. 腹部平片。3 个气泡说明梗阻仅在十二指肠远处。B. 在剖腹手术中发现近端空肠 I 型黏膜闭锁。C. 另一例 I 型空肠闭锁患儿的照片，在黏膜闭锁处移行带不太明显。（A 和 B 引自 Grosfeld JL：Alimentary tract obstruction in the newborn. Curr Probl Pediatr 1975；5:3.）

地区分。应给每个疑为新生儿肠梗阻的病例做钡剂
1272 灌肠检查。患儿接受的第一次灌肠应该是对比灌肠，由对新生儿及婴儿肠梗阻有经验的放射科医生执行以使风险降至最低。对比灌肠检查有 3 个目的：（1）鉴别小肠与结肠扩张；（2）确定使用或不使用结肠（小结肠）；（3）确定盲肠的位置，因为可能存在肠旋转和固定的异常[48]。绝大多数空肠回肠闭锁的婴儿存在小结肠，这就把梗阻限制于远端小肠（见图80-3）。小结肠的形成与肠液不能通过胎儿远端小肠梗阻的区域有直接的关系，且未使用的结肠并不扩张[8]。然而，在少数情况下，如果导致肠闭锁的宫内血管病变发生于孕晚期，结肠可有正常的管径。特别在与宫内肠套迭有关的肠闭锁病例中常有这种情况发生（图 80-4）[51,111,140]。肠旋转不良可见于约 10% 的空肠回肠闭锁患儿[32,99]，我们儿童医院 194 例空肠回肠闭锁患儿中有 32 例肠旋转不良（16.5%）。

完全性肠梗阻病例常无行上消化道造影的指征。然而对于不完全梗阻的肠狭窄病例，这项检查非常有用。小肠对比灌注造影法比常规的小肠系列检查有更高的诊断率。

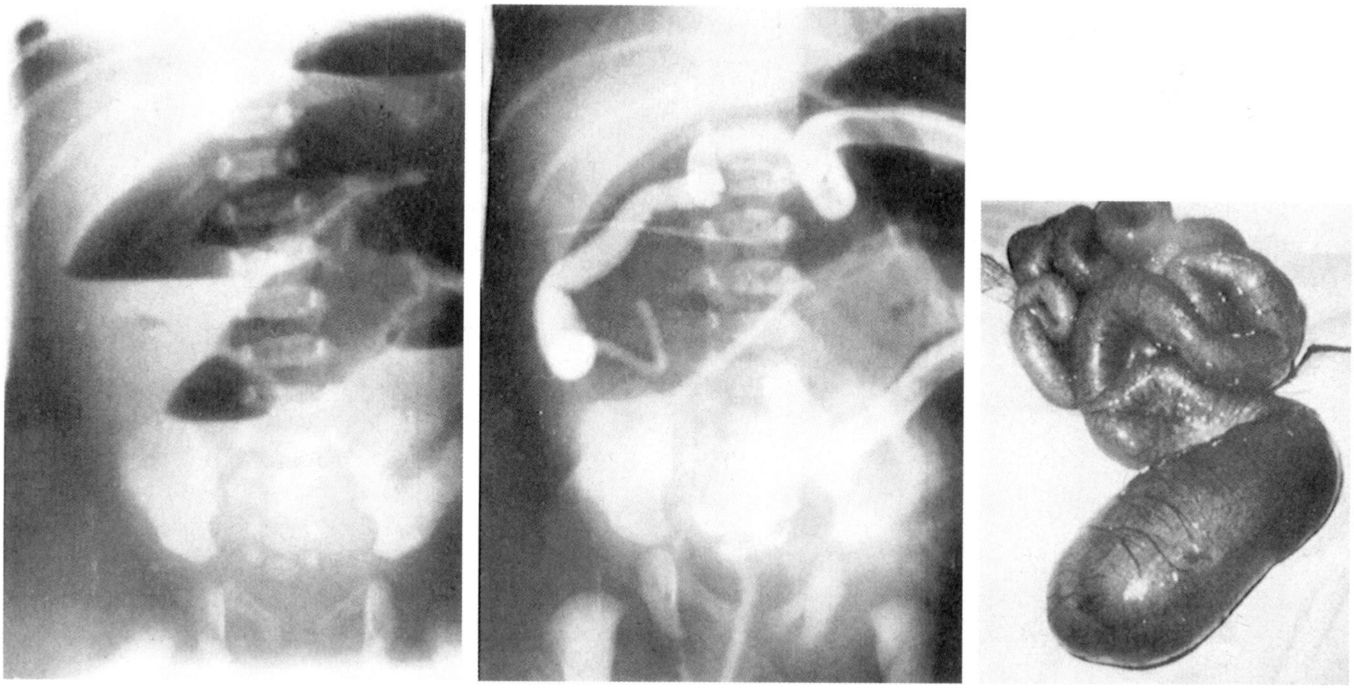

A　B　C

图 80-2 回肠闭锁。A. 腹部直立位平片显示肠袢扩张伴有气液平。B. 对比灌肠证实为小结肠（未使用的），说明有小肠梗阻。C. 剖腹手术中发现（Ⅲ型）回肠闭锁。（From Grosfeld JL：Alimentary tract obstruction in the newborn. Curr Probl Pediatr 1975；5:3.）

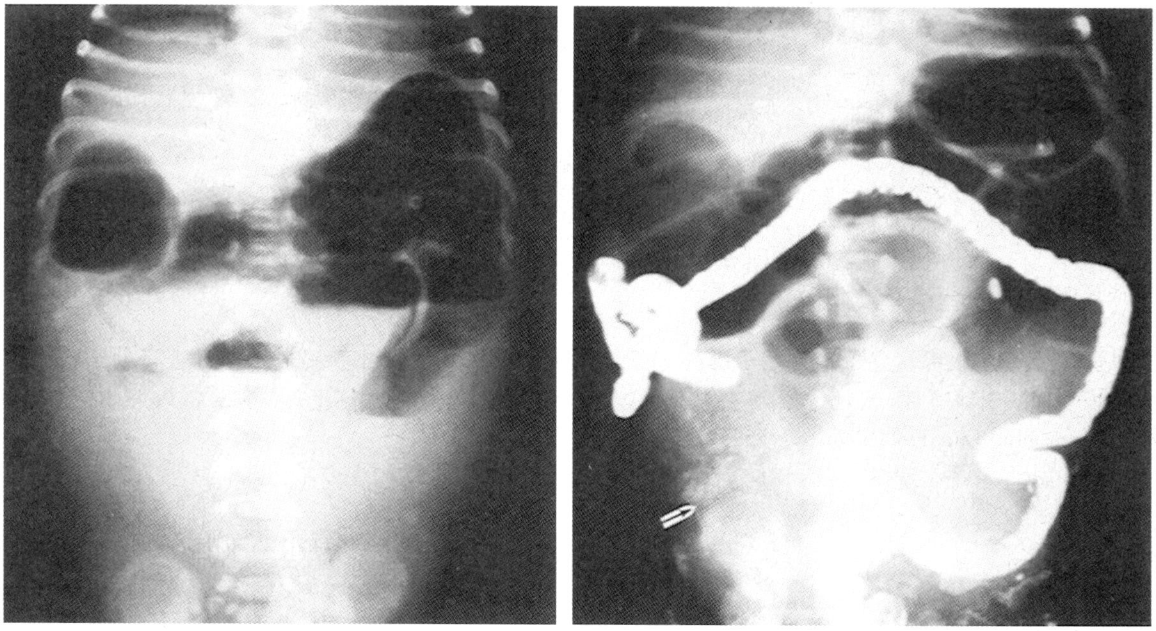

A　B

图 80-3 胎粪性腹膜炎。A. 腹部直立位平片发现有大于拇指大小的肠袢，伴有多个气液平。B. 钡剂灌肠证实有未使用的结肠（小结肠），伴不完全性肠旋转不良（盲肠位于右上腹）。右下腹有钙化（箭头）说明有胎粪性腹膜炎。（From Grosfeld JL：Alimentary tract obstruction in the newborn. Curr Probl Pediatr 1975；5:3.）

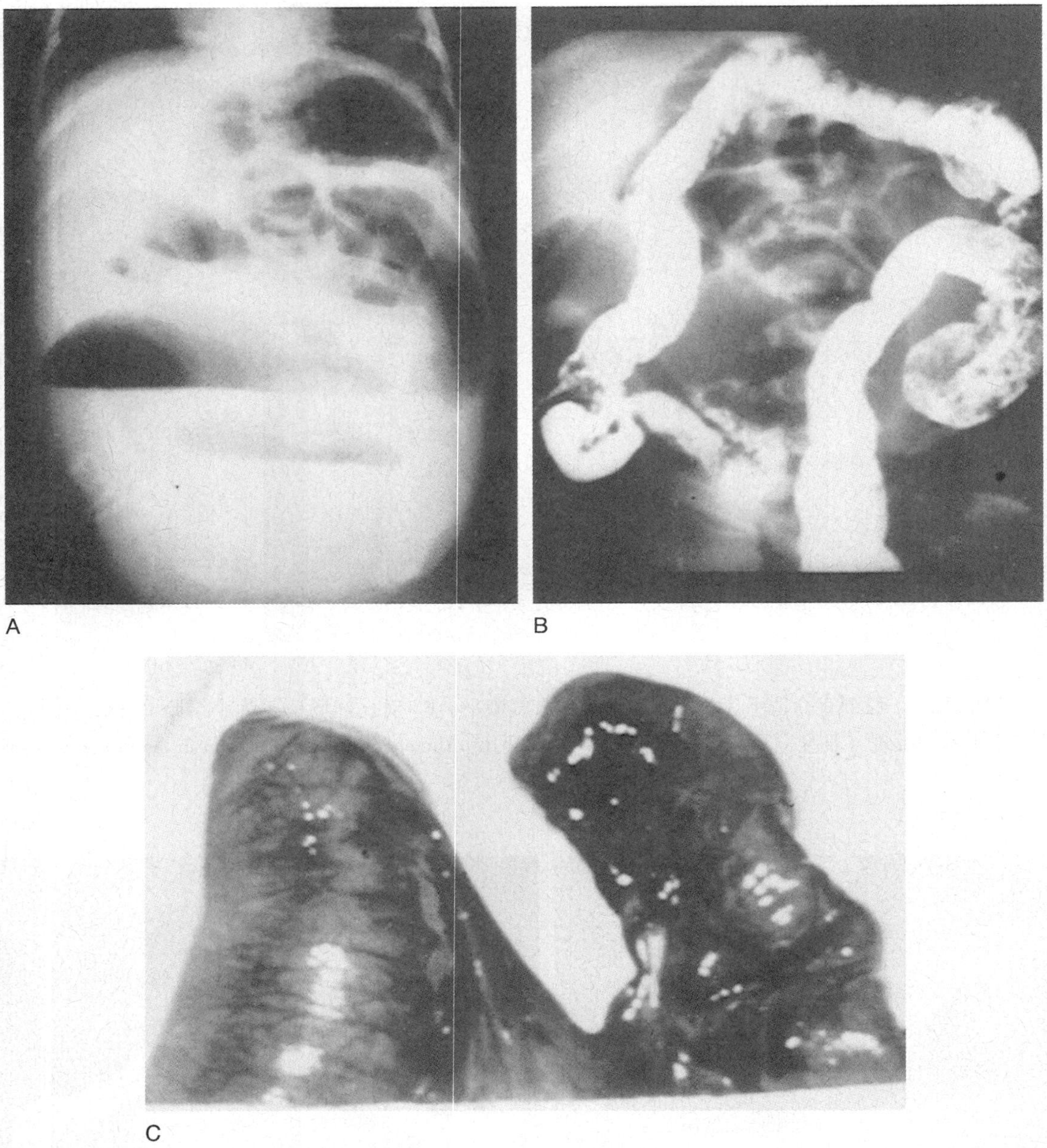

图 80-4 回肠闭锁。A. 腹部直立位平片显示肠袢扩张，伴有气液平。B. 对比灌肠显示正常管径的结肠内充满碎屑。C. 剖腹手术中发现回肠闭锁（Ⅲa 型），肠系膜有 V 形缺损，并发现宫内肠套迭的证据。（From Grosfeld JL：Alimentary tract obstruction in the newborn. Curr Probl Pediatr 1975；5:3.）

鉴别诊断

其他原因引起的新生儿肠梗阻的临床表现可能与
1274 空肠回肠闭锁很相似。其他原因包括肠旋转不良伴或不伴肠扭转、胎粪性肠梗阻、肠重复畸形、内疝、结肠闭锁、与败血症有关的麻痹性肠梗阻以及全结肠无神经节细胞症[20,75,80]。钡剂灌肠常可获得有价值的信息，并排除某些肠梗阻的原因，特别是结肠闭锁和低肠段的神经节细胞缺失症。空肠回肠闭锁可与肠旋转不良（10%～18%）、胎粪性腹膜炎（12%）、胎粪性肠梗阻（9%～12%）、全结肠无神经节细胞症共存，偶尔与肠神经元发育不良共存，故有时不能清楚地区分[13,48,63,75,80,86,99,102]。仔细询问囊性纤维化的家族史可在手术前鉴别胎粪性肠梗阻[30,48,49,114]。

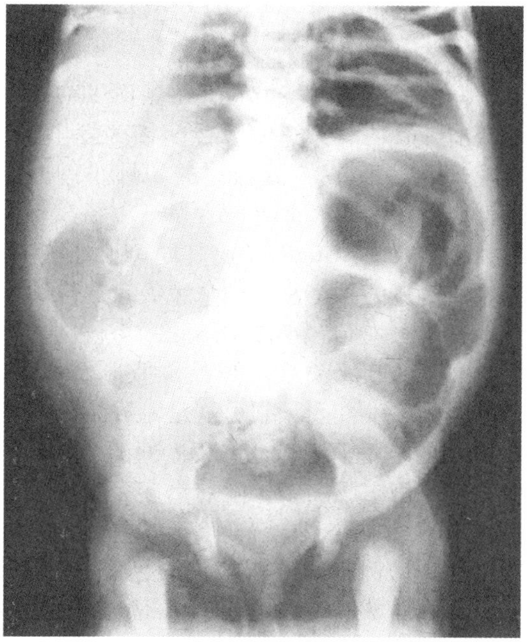
A

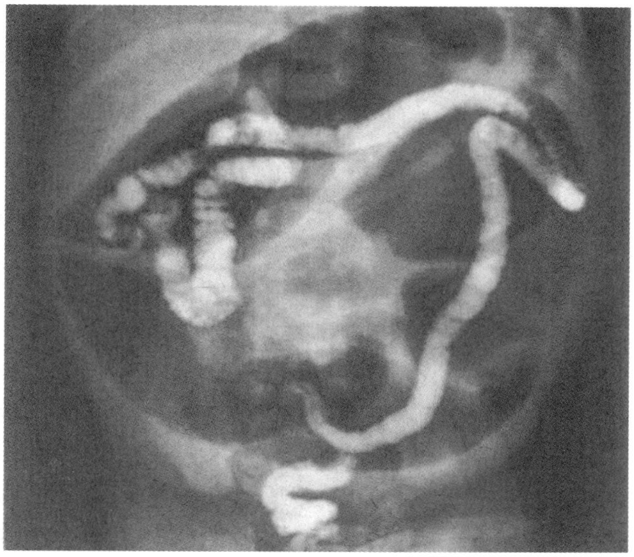
B

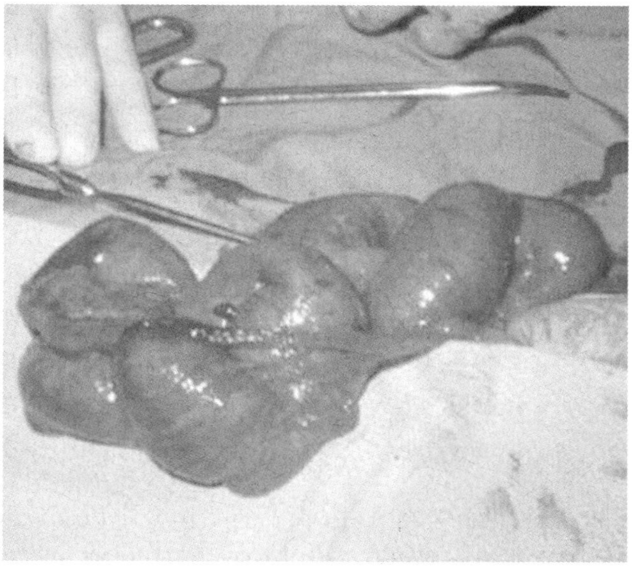
C

图 80–5　A. 一个新生儿的腹部平片显示有多个扩张肠袢。B. 钡剂灌肠显示有未使用的小结肠，说明扩张的肠段为小肠。C. 剖腹手术中发现肠扭转及复杂性胎粪性肠梗阻引起的多发性肠闭锁（也见彩图）。该婴儿患有囊性纤维化。

非复杂性胎粪性肠梗阻患儿常有明显扩张、大小相似的肠袢，有时无气液平。后一种情况见于胎粪非常粘滞，不能分层成气液交界面[48]。可在右下腹观察到毛玻璃样外观（Neuhauser 征）[96] 或
275 Singleton皂泡征[127]，表明黏滞的胎粪与空气混合。对这些患儿进行仔细评估可避免不必要的手术，因为用泛影葡胺（Gastrografin）灌肠的非手术治疗对至少一半的非复杂性胎粪性肠梗阻病例有效（见 81 章）。胎粪性肠梗阻并发肠闭锁、肠扭转或肠坏疽需要手术干预，给这些肠梗阻患儿行剖腹手术可明确诊断（图 80–5）。结肠闭锁的闭锁肠段在腹部平片上偶尔也可有肥皂泡样外观[30]。

病理学表现

小肠闭锁的病变平均分布于空肠（51%）和回肠（49%）。31% 的病例闭锁处位于近端空肠，20% 位于远端空肠，13% 位于近端回肠，36% 位于远端回肠[27]。闭锁常为单发性（>90%），但 6%~20% 的病例为多发[31,32,49]。多发性闭锁常累及近端

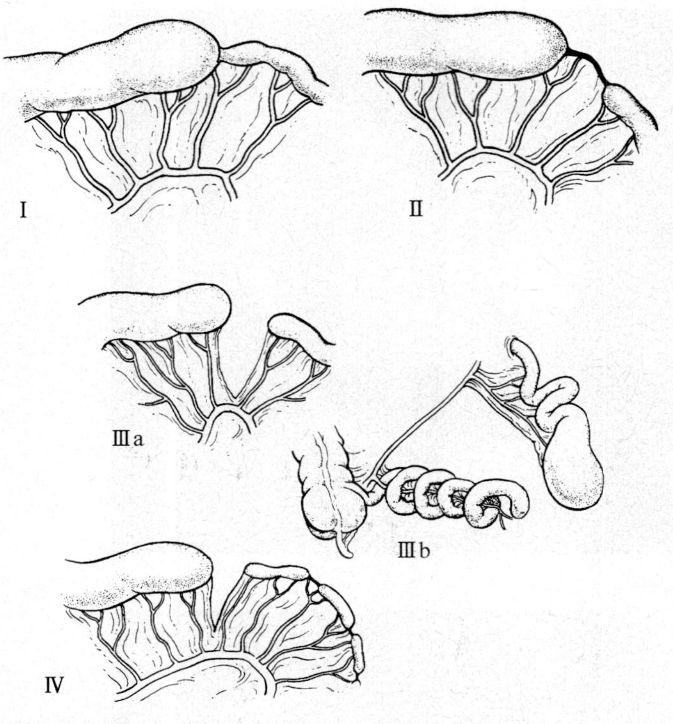

图 80-6 肠闭锁的分类。Ⅰ型，黏膜（膜状）闭锁，肠壁及肠系膜完整。Ⅱ型，闭锁盲端被纤维索带隔开。Ⅲa型，闭锁盲端被V形（裂隙）肠系膜缺损隔开。Ⅲb型，苹果皮样闭锁。Ⅳ型，多发性闭锁（像一串香肠）。（From Grosfeld JL，Ballantine TVN，Shoemaker R：Operative management of intestinal atresia and stenosis based on pathologic findings. J Pediatr Surg 1979；14:368.）

空肠[5,57,107,108]。

自从 Bland-Sutton[15] 和 Spriggs[132] 的早期发现以来，空肠回肠闭锁的分型稍有变化。Louw[81] 认为空肠回肠闭锁有3种类型。Ⅰ型为黏膜（间隔）闭锁，肠壁及肠系膜完整；Ⅱ型有两个闭锁盲端由纤维组织（索带）连接，肠系膜完整；Ⅲ型闭锁肠管的两端被肠系膜裂隙（V形缺损）分开（图80-6）。这种分型在肠闭锁的早期文献特别是大型综述中使用最广泛[32,99,141,142]。de Lorimier 及其同事[32] 对559例空肠
1276 回肠闭锁进行评估后，发现19%为Ⅰ型，31%为Ⅱ型，46%为Ⅲ型。Nixon 和 Tawes[99] 也发现Ⅲ型是最常见的类型。很多Ⅲ型闭锁由于血管损伤造成胎儿肠管在宫内被吸收，故肠管长度较短，但大多数Ⅰ型和Ⅱ型闭锁剩余的肠管长度正常。Foglia 及其同事[40] 报道1例罕见的Ⅰ型闭锁患者有40 cm长的一段肠管闭锁。

到目前为止，对多发性闭锁及伴有早产及高死亡率的肠管短缩病例的关注仍然很少，手术中可发现其有串珠样或香肠串样的外观（见图80-6）。Rittenhouse 及其同事[115] 报道多发性闭锁的发生率为14%，并发现一个婴儿有25处独立的闭锁。宫内炎症被认为是可能的发病原因。有学者发现小肠憩室病与多发性闭锁相关[126]。Guttman 及其同事[54] 报道了魁北克圣约翰河附近的一个法裔加拿大人家族性多发性闭锁累及胃、十二指肠、小肠和结肠的系谱图。由于该组成员有高度的亲缘关系，作者和 Teja 及其同事[138] 均提出广泛的多发性闭锁很可能是一种罕见的常染色体隐性基因的表达。Mishalany 和 Najjar[90] 报道一个家庭中发生3例空肠闭锁。随后更多多发性闭锁的病例被报道[2,24,69,107,108,150]。已观察到家族性空肠闭锁伴肾发育不良的病例，这可能为常染色体显性遗传[58,66]。Bilodeau 及其同事[11] 报道了16例多发性肠闭锁伴 IgM 缺乏（最初由 Guttman[54] 于1974年报道此病种）病例为常染色体隐性遗传方式，并随访30余年。所有的患者均已死亡，其病因学仍不清楚，并未能找到可靠的产前诊断或有效的手术治疗方法。作者认为该致命的疾病可能由一种特定的、未被阐明的基因突变所致[11]。

另一组少见的病例为苹果皮样（apple-peal）闭锁或圣诞树样（Christmas-tree）畸形。这些患儿表现为空肠闭锁接近十二指肠悬韧带、肠管短缩、肠系膜有大的裂隙、闭锁远端肠管的血供不稳定——来源于回结肠动脉、右结肠动脉或肠系膜下动脉的吻合弓以逆行的方式供血[36,47,124,155,160,161]。Ros Mar 及其同事[118] 在37例空肠回肠闭锁患者中观察到12例（32.4%）苹果皮样畸形。然而，Zerella 和 Martin[160] 在59例空肠回肠闭锁患者中仅发现7例（11%）苹果皮样闭锁的变异体。有此种特殊的闭锁变异的患儿常有家族遗传性，常为低出生体重（70%）或早产（70%），有肠旋转不良（54%），并多数伴发畸形[16,129]。苹果皮样闭锁也见于有眼部畸形和小头畸形的同胞中[133]。

1976年，Martin 和 Zerella[85] 提出一种包括多发性闭锁和苹果皮样闭锁的新分型方法。笔者于1979年修改了这种分型，保留了先前 Louw 的命名，增加苹果皮样闭锁作为Ⅲ型中的一种特殊类型（Ⅲb），将多发性闭锁命名为Ⅳ型（见图80-6）[49]。在过去的25年中，这种分型方法已被广泛接受用以描述肠闭锁[49]。

治疗

起初评估时，婴儿应被置于温暖湿润的环境（婴儿保温箱或头顶放置取暖器）以避免体温过低。置入口胃管（10F）。抽出胃内容物，注意有无胆汁。留置胃管使胃减压，并防止呕吐及吞入空气后梗阻肠道进一步充气扩张。如果要将婴儿从社区医院或综合性医院转运至三级新生儿重症监护室，这是关键的先决条件。在放射科检查婴儿前这些预防措施也是有效的，因为误吸是转运过程中严重的并发症，应注意避免。在转运过程中，婴儿应由有经验的人员照看。

应确定婴儿的体重，应用微量技术采集血样本用
277 于基本实验室检查（例如全血细胞和血小板计数、血尿素氮、血清胆红素、血糖、血钙、pH、血气分析、血清电解质）以及确定血型和交叉配血。同时要测定尿量、尿比重和渗透压。术前准备的程度主要取决于是否有诊断延迟、体液和电解质失衡的程度、有无严重的伴随畸形和腹膜炎。在手背或足背经皮穿刺置入 22 或 24 号短的硅管，建立足够的静脉通路。笔者通常避免静脉切开，因为很少需要。可从外周经皮置入中心静脉导管及传统的中心静脉锁骨下导管用于全肠外营养（total parenteral nutrition，TPN）。同时也应避免常规脐静脉插管，因为可增加败血症的风险；然而，对于间接胆红素过高的患儿，脐静脉插管偶尔可用于短期交换输血。如果患儿合并与误吸呕吐物或严重腹胀有关的呼吸窘迫，需经皮将动脉导管插入右侧桡动脉，经开放的动脉导管和卵圆孔，在右向左分流水平以上更准确地监测新生儿动脉血氧分压。对于病情稳定的患儿，脉搏血氧定量法足以监测血氧饱和度。

评估患儿的液体不足，并开始补液治疗。用等量的乳酸林格液补充口胃管引流出的含胆汁的液体。对于有腹膜炎和/或严重腹胀的患儿，将乳酸林格液以 20 ml/kg 的速度在 30 多分钟内输入体内，对于没有穿孔的肠梗阻患儿，10 ml/kg 的经验性输液可用于纠正隔离于腹腔或梗阻的近端肠管内的第三间隙体液丧失引起的血容量不足。需要额外的液体（低盐血清白蛋白或乳酸林格液）使患儿血压维持在 50 mm Hg 以上，并有一定的尿量［1～2 ml/(kg · h)］。内含 10% 的葡萄糖的 0.25% 或 0.33% 的生理盐水用于维持机体所需。

常规给予氧化维生素 K_1［phytonadione（Aqua-MEPHYTON），1 mg 肌注］和静脉注射抗生素［氨苄西林 125 mg/(kg · d)，以及庆大霉素 5 mg/(kg · d)］。术前准备需要 1～4 小时，取决于患儿病情及低血容量的严重程度。

手术室准备

适当的准备后，将患儿送至手术室，采取相应的预防措施，包括转运及保持合适的环境温度。手术室温度保持在 75～80℉。将患儿置于加热毯上，或用取暖灯照射，四肢用柔软的棉花卷包裹。给患儿头部盖上小块布或戴上衬铝的帽子，防止辐射热损失。用温热的碘伏溶液清洗脐带，钳夹切断后用缝线结扎。肠梗阻患儿应在清醒时进行插管以避免误吸，气管内导管的位置应通过仔细听诊来评估。使用脉搏血氧计监测氧饱和度。每位患者都常规监测血压（多普勒）、心电图、脉搏和体温（皮肤或腋窝探针）。必要时测定动脉血 pH 和血气分析。麻醉气体需加热并增湿，以防止热量损失及呼吸道干燥。干燥的麻醉气体可引起纤毛破坏、细胞脱落进入气管支气管腔以及黏液产生减少[22,84]。这些变化可导致与支气管内清除延迟及堵塞有关的术后肺部并发症发生率增高。用温热的碘伏溶液［聚维酮碘（Betadine）］轻柔地消毒准备腹部皮肤（涂抹而不是擦洗）。用手术巾覆盖腹部，并用无菌透明的含碘塑料薄膜粘贴于手术野并固定手术巾。用儿科剖腹手术孔巾覆盖塑料薄膜，手术在开孔处进行。大的塑料贴膜可帮助保持体温。

右侧脐上横切口使新生儿腹腔的所有区域都能很好地暴露。笔者通常使用带有铅笔样指尖控制器的婴儿精细电凝器来止血。这种方法可减少进腹过程中失血及术中费时的钳夹、结扎。术中以 5～10 ml/(kg · h) 的补液量给予含 5% 葡萄糖的乳酸林格液，用以补充切开造成的隐性组织液丢失。用等量的乳酸林格液补充术中经口胃管丢失的液体及吸出的肠内容物。如果损失量多于估计血容量（80 ml/kg）的 10%～15%，需输入温热的浓缩红细胞。使用小容量的吸引收集系统并密切观察海绵纱布重量便于评估液体的损失。血液损失达估计血容量的 10%～15% 时，可输入含 5% 葡萄糖的乳酸林格液纠正。

手术方法

空肠回肠闭锁及狭窄的手术选择与病理学表现及每个个体的具体情况有关[48]。最合适的手术方式取决于梗阻的病理学类型（例如狭窄或Ⅰ型、Ⅱ型、Ⅲa型、Ⅲb型及Ⅳ型闭锁），有无肠旋转不良、肠扭转、胎粪性肠梗阻或胎粪性腹膜炎，以及婴儿一般状况（图80-7）。其他的复杂情况可见于伴发腹裂或脐膨出的肠闭锁或狭窄患儿，这时一期关闭腹壁可能产生问题[45,91,114,125,129,145]。

任何吻合方式中，保留及使用扩张的闭锁近端肠
1278 段常常引起功能性梗阻。虽然在手术纠治空肠回肠闭锁的早期尝试中常使用侧侧吻合，但是该方法常并发功能性吻合口梗阻及随后出现的盲袢综合征[8,80,98,99]。Nixon[98,99]注意到扩张的闭锁近端肠段出现平滑肌肥大及肠管直径变大。他认为该肠段的蠕动为无效蠕动，在手术后肠管压力降低的情况下不能起作用。de Lorimier及其同事[34]以及Cloutier[23]认为增生是慢性梗阻发生后肠平滑肌发生的主要变化。在慢性完全性梗阻的病例中，如空肠闭锁，增生非常严重达到失代偿状态，即使强烈收缩也不能充分关闭肠腔，也不能在正常的入口压力下增加压力或有效地推进[23]。Schoenberg和Kluth[123]描述了实验诱导的小肠闭锁小鸡的肠神经系统结构变化，他们把这些异常归因于近端肠管的扩张。Masumoto及其同事描述了切取自新生儿闭锁近端肠段的肠壁内神经及C-kit阳性的起搏细胞的发育不全[87]。

在临床上，经验已经证明对于大多数近端空肠闭锁的病例（肠道长度足够），在十二指肠悬韧带处切除扩张的闭锁肠段，然后做端-斜侧吻合常可避免这些并发症，并且预后良好。当剩下的肠管长度有限时（例如短肠），Thomas[139]提出的系膜对侧空肠锥形成形术是有用的。Howard和Othersen[61]、Weber及其同事[154]以及其他人[65,104,152]均证实了肠锥形成形术在部分病例中的适用性。de Lorimier和Harrison[33]报道肠覆瓦状重叠可有效缩小扩张肠管的管径并恢复功能。虽然肠覆瓦状重叠技术保留了黏膜表面的区域，但它有损坏的倾向，使扩张复发。Kimura及其同事[70]改进了这种方法，椭圆形切除肠管浆肌层使得扩张的近端肠管变细，保留黏膜层。Kling及其同事介绍了对发生于十二指肠悬韧带的空肠闭锁病例行十二指肠侧面切开及十二指肠空肠造口吻合术，肠管锥形成形术对这种病例效果欠佳[71]。

近端广泛切除并吻合也用于肠道长度足够、中段小肠或远端回肠有单处或多处闭锁的病例。对于远端回肠闭锁的病例，回肠-升结肠端侧吻合是合理的选

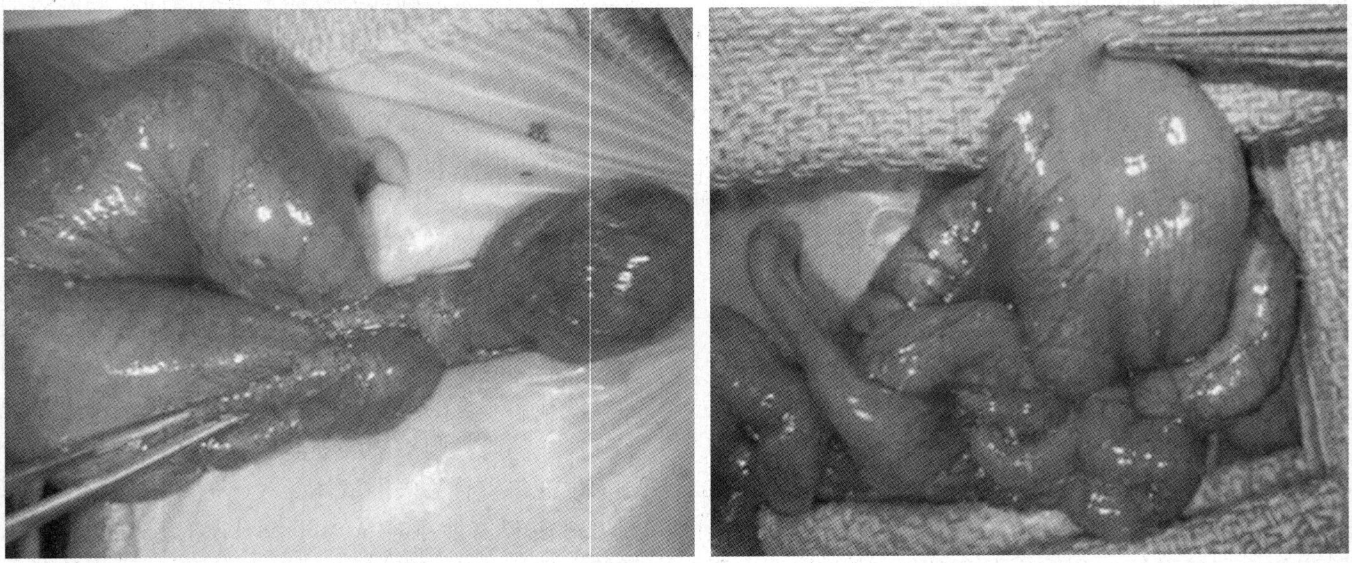

A　　B

图80-7 A. 照片显示围绕腹膜带的宫内肠扭转引起的回肠闭锁。B. 肠旋转不良引起的宫内中肠扭转造成空肠闭锁。注意阑尾位于中上腹的扭转处。

择[8]。这种术式的主要缺点是绕过了回盲瓣。

手术中要仔细检查肠管，辨别闭锁肠管的近端和远端。轻柔地将内脏外置常可便于检查。可见到肠旋转不良、肠扭转或宫内肠扭转后部分再吸收胎肠的肠段。仔细地将扭曲的肠管复位，以便能够完整地评估病理解剖。在肠管的远端闭锁端做荷包缝合，用 24 号静脉导管注入盐水（或空气）以排除潜在的闭锁远端肠管的黏膜隔膜或蹼。如果肠管长度足够，将闭锁近端扩张的肠段切除至肠管直径为 1.0～1.5 cm 处（回肠闭锁的病例）或近端空肠闭锁病例的十二指肠 1279
悬韧带附近。将 Bainbridge 婴儿肠钳呈 90°角钳夹近端肠管，将另一把 Bainbridge 肠钳，呈 45°角在系膜缘对侧较远处切除远端闭锁肠段（图80-8A）。如果两端肠腔大小仍不相称，在闭锁远端肠管的系膜缘对侧做一个小切口即可解决这个问题。用 5-0 丝线做双层间断端-斜吻合（见图 80-8B）。先在肠管后方的浆

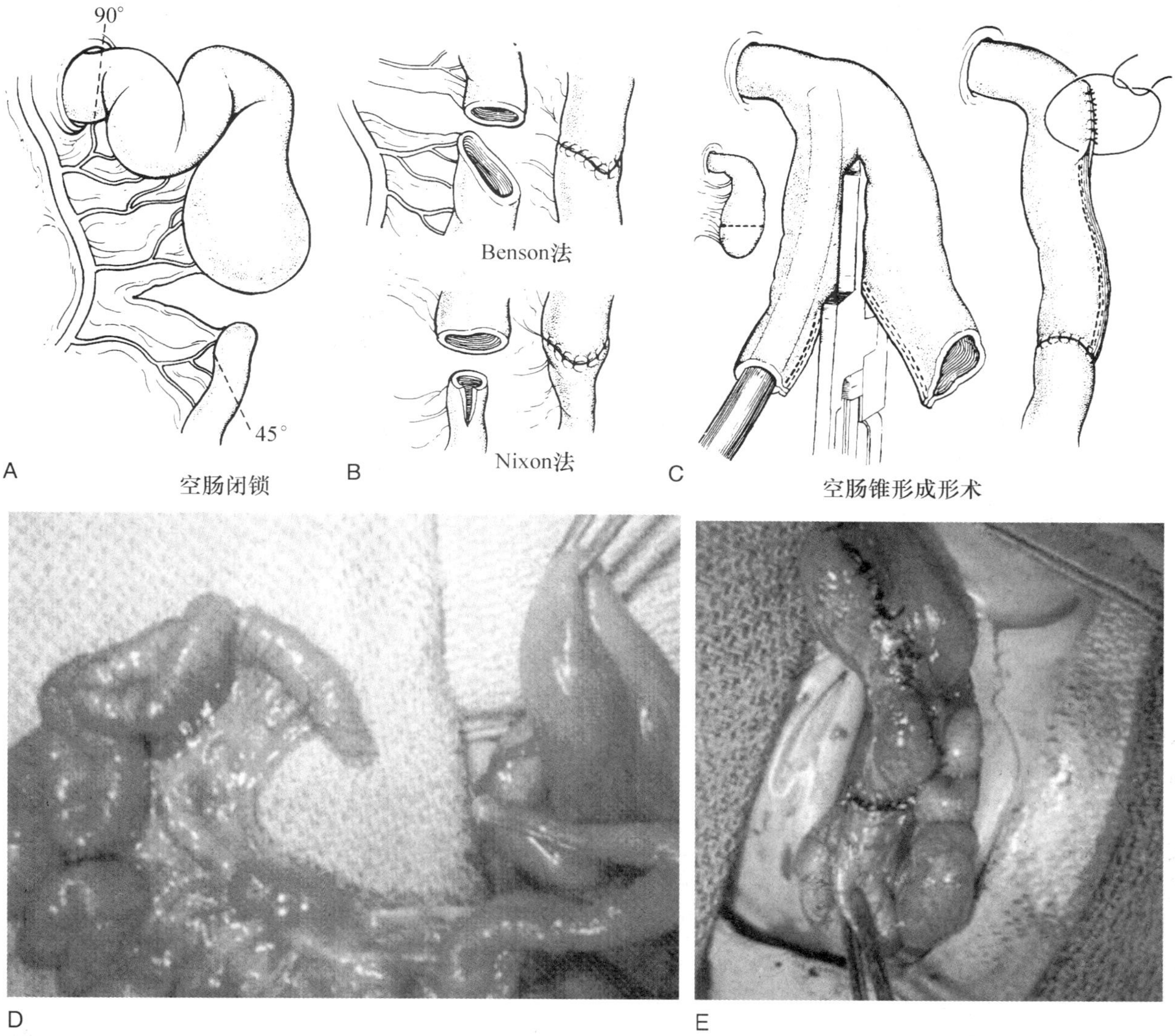

图 80-8　空肠闭锁：吻合技术。A. 在十二指肠悬韧带处以 90°角切断空肠闭锁近端肠管，以 45°角切断闭锁远端肠管。B. 按Benson 法（单层）或 Nixon 法（双层）用丝线做精细的间断端-斜吻合。C. 近端空肠锥形成形术：切除球状的闭锁远端肠段，将导管置于肠腔的肠系膜侧，用自动 U 形钉吻合装置切除系膜缘对侧肠管直至十二指肠悬韧带，做端端吻合完成手术。注意用 5-0 丝线间断缝合吻合钉缘。D. 空肠闭锁近端，伴有Ⅲb 型裂隙和苹果皮样外观的远端闭锁的照片。E. 完成空肠锥形成形术及吻合。

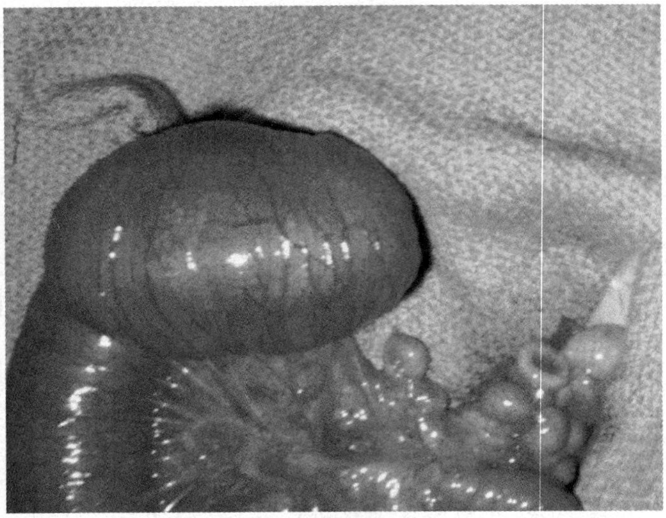

A

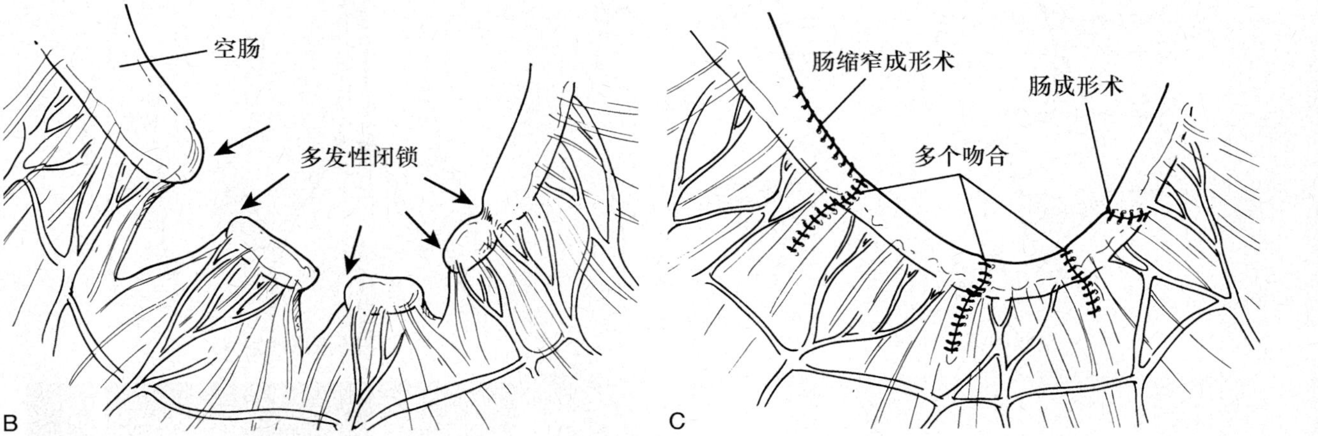

图 80-9 A. 一个婴儿的手术照片，其空肠闭锁近端肠管扩张，有各种类型的多个远端闭锁（Ⅰ型、Ⅱ型和Ⅲa 型）。B. 图例示多发性闭锁，闭锁远端不扩张。C. 近端空肠锥形成形术，Ⅱ型和Ⅲa 型闭锁做多个吻合，Ⅰ型闭锁做横向肠成形术以保留肠管长度。

肌层外层留置缝线（一般不超过 5 根），然后打结。除去肠钳，修剪被挤压的组织。将肠管后方内层的缝线向前拉，做间断的反向 Connell 缝合（内-外，外-内），结打在里面。在肠管前方外层浆肌层用 5-0 丝线做 Lembert 缝合完成吻合。也可用5-0 Vicryl 或 PDS 缝线缝合内层，PDS 缝线缝合外层。一些小儿外科医生较喜欢做单层吻合。但我们发现单层吻合发生漏的机会稍微大一些，且双层间断修补后很少发生狭窄。仔细修补肠系膜缺损，褶起较长的近端肠系膜以避免
1280 吻合处扭结[99]。对于多发性闭锁的病例，尤其是肠管长度有问题者，需保留尽可能多的肠管。可能需做多次吻合以达到这个目的[56,122]。减压的闭锁远端肠段常不扩张，如果肠腔完全通畅，不必切除肠管，对于Ⅱ型或Ⅲ型闭锁可将其直接与下一肠段吻合，对于Ⅰ型黏膜闭锁可做横向肠成形术（图 80-9）。Dinsmore 及其同事[35]、Chaet 及其同事[21]介绍了肠腔内支架术来处理多发性闭锁或穿孔，但笔者没有关于该技术的经验。

对于肠管明显短缩的空肠闭锁病例，可用自动 U 形钉吻合装置（U. S. Surgical Corporation，Norwalk，CT）来完成系膜缘对侧空肠锥形成形术（见图 80-8C）。切除闭锁近端肠段呈球形扩张的远侧部分，沿肠系膜侧将 24～26F 的导管插入肠腔。在两排自动吻合钉之间切除系膜缘对侧的肠管边缘直至十二指肠悬韧带。用 5-0 丝线或 PDS 缝线缝合覆盖剩余的吻合钉，手术最后做如前介绍的端-斜吻合术（见图 80-8D和图 80-8E）。现在可借助 2.5～3 倍的放大镜进行解剖和吻合。放大镜使得吻合处缝线的位置更加精确，极大地方便了手术操作，特别是早产儿的手术。虽然首选一期吻合（80-10A 和图 80-10B），但

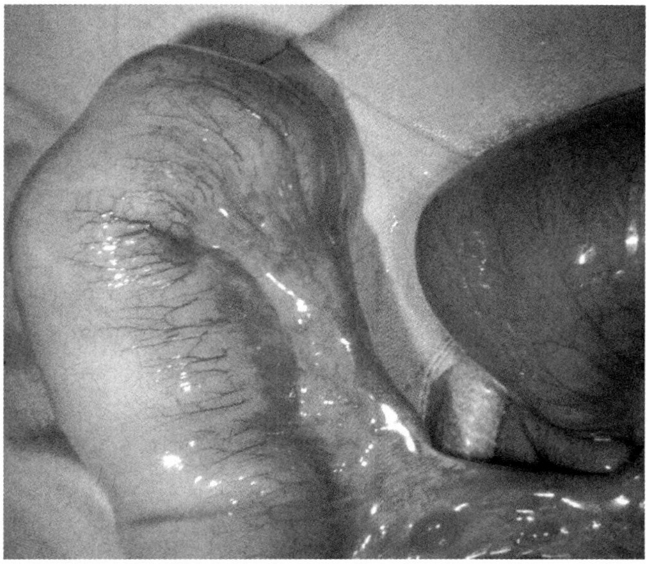

A

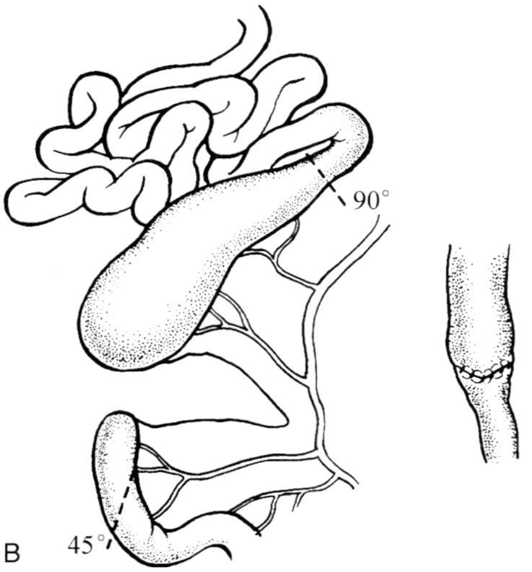

B

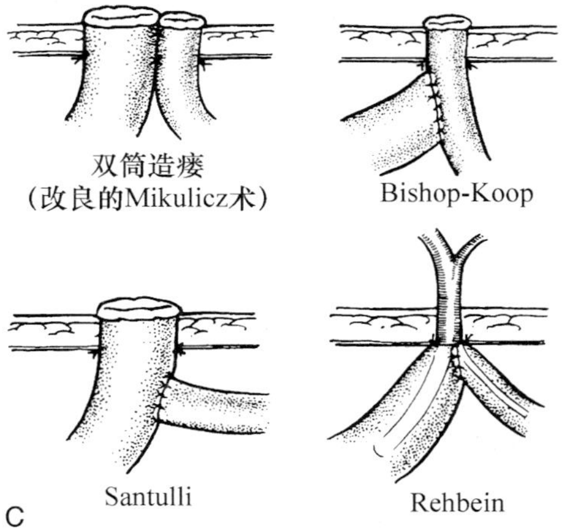

C

图 80-10　回肠闭锁的手术方式。A. 回肠闭锁近端肠管扩张（Ⅲa型）。B. 向后切除回肠闭锁近端肠管直至肠管直径为 1.0~1.5 cm，做端-斜吻合。C. 用于严重腹膜炎、肠管活力可疑及胎粪性肠梗阻病例的肠外置手术的类型。首选双筒并列肠造瘘术（改良的 Mikulicz 术）。

对于肠道血管完整性有问题的回肠闭锁伴肠扭转、严重胎粪性腹膜炎，以及复杂性胎粪性肠梗阻病例，一期吻合是不可取的。对于这些病例，需切除闭锁的回肠并做肠管外置术。最快速的术式是将肠管经切口拖出，做并列双筒肠造瘘（改良的 Mikulicz 手术）[6,12,112,117]，用5-0 丝线将造瘘肠管间断缝合固定于腹壁（见图 80-10C）。Bishop-Koop（远端造瘘）[13]、Santulli（近端造瘘）[121]以及 Rehbein（置管造瘘）[113]肠吻合肠造瘘可能在这种情况下都是同样可取的。笔者偏向于做双筒肠造瘘，因为可快速完成，避免初期腹腔内吻合，并在术后易于评估造瘘口的肠管活力。虽然这形成了回肠造瘘末端，但适当的
81 造瘘口和皮肤护理，以及通过中心静脉或外周静脉给予肠外营养常可避免其他问题的发生。以后再次手术需做局限的有目的的剖腹手术，通过端端吻合恢复肠道连续性。笔者在近端空肠吻合处不使用经吻合口的硅胶减压导管[60]，在做远端回肠吻合的病例中也不使用阑尾造瘘导管（Suruga 及其同事建议使用[134]）。分层关闭腹壁，用4-0 羟乙酸乳酸聚酯 910（Vicryl）缝线或聚葡糖酸酯（Maxon）缝线连续缝合腹膜，用4-0 Vicryl 或 Maxon 缝线间断内翻缝合筋膜层。PDS 缝线也是一种合理的选择。Scarpa 筋膜用 5-0 Vicryl 缝线连续缝合，皮缘用 5-0 的皮内缝线缝合，并贴以 Steri-Strips 免缝胶带。在手术伤口处覆以干燥无菌敷料，再贴上敷贴。

在 Riley 儿童医院，194 例行手术治疗的空肠回

肠闭锁及狭窄患儿中，38%行闭锁肠段一期肠切除及肠吻合，18%行肠切除及肠锥形成形和肠吻合术，23%行肠切除及暂时性肠造瘘，19%行肠造瘘而未行肠切除，4例患儿行肠造瘘及肠蹼切除术（2%）。6例腹裂患儿在关腹时首先将闭锁肠管放回腹腔，延迟至3周时吻合。其他22例腹裂患儿中，2例行一期肠切除和肠吻合，其余20例行暂时性肠造瘘。这些病例包含在前面提到的数据中。肠切除和肠吻合组中的6例在转到我们医院之前在别处已经用闭锁肠段行空肠吻合术。其中每例都发生了功能性梗阻，最终需切除闭锁肠段并重新吻合或锥形成形。在5例短肠患儿中放置胃造瘘管，但并不列为常规。

1282 手术后治疗

在恢复室里作短暂的密切观察后，将患儿送回新生儿重症监护室，置于温暖、湿润、有良好的中性温度监测的环境中。婴儿保温箱的头端上抬30°。以80～100 ml/(kg · d) 的量给予维持补液，补液为含有10%葡萄糖的0.25%或0.33%的生理盐水。同时补充氯化钾［2～3 mEq/(kg · d)］，不要超过40 mEq/L。如果口胃管引流液清亮（胃液），用含0.45%生理盐水的5%葡萄糖等量补充口胃管引流丢失的液体量；如果引流液为绿色（肠液），则用含5%葡萄糖的乳酸林格液等量补充。静脉输注需含有维生素B和维生素C，这是伤口愈合所必需的。偶尔需额外快速输注液体来对抗过量的第三间隙液体丢失。排尿量为40～50 ml/(kg · d)、尿比重为1.005～1.015、体重稳定常表示水合作用适当。密切监测婴儿的葡萄糖水平、酸碱平衡及血清胆红素水平，以避免低血糖、酸中毒及核黄疸。术后最初几天内需每日监测血清电解质水平。

当患儿有自发的肠蠕动，并且胃引流液变清、量变少后，可将口胃管往上拔作为刺激打嗝的导管。如果没有过度胃反流或肠反流发生，可拔除口胃管并以0.5盎司/3小时的量开始进食清澈的液体（Pedialyte），逐渐增加液体量，然后给予半浓度低渗小凝块配方奶（Isomil），最后给予全浓度配方奶。新生儿需要120 kcal/(kg · d) 的热卡以满足生长需要。乳糖不耐受是大量肠切除后常见的问题，如果起初就喂以大凝块配方奶（Similac或Enfamil），则小肠吻合口处可发生奶块梗阻[25]。吸收不良和腹泻常见于短肠、回盲瓣切除，以及多发性闭锁或苹果皮样闭锁的患儿[48,49,85,114,124]。应避免给这些患儿喂含有长链脂肪的配方奶，而应给予含中链三酰甘油或酪蛋白水解物的食物（Pregestimil）。有时也可给予不含碳水化合物或易于吸收的要素饮食，如婴儿Vivonex。

如果不能耐受上述配方奶，可经留置于中心静脉的硅胶（Broviac）导管给予高热量的TPN（18%葡萄糖，2.5%氨基酸），导管经胸壁插入切开的颈外或颈内静脉或头静脉进入上腔静脉。这种溶液每毫升可提供1卡热量。此外，应静脉输入10%的脂肪溶液（Intralipid）。这种溶液是等渗的，含游离脂肪酸，每毫升可额外提供1.1卡热量。对于长时间消化道功能障碍的病例，这些重要的辅助治疗方法可预防蛋白质-热量营养不良，并为肠道适应提供了时间。Riley儿童医院194例空肠回肠闭锁患儿中有94例（49%）接受了TPN（49%）。为了排除囊性纤维化，术后所有空肠回肠闭锁患儿都接受了检测氯离子浓度的汗液检查和检测DF508基因突变的细胞遗传学检查，有24例（12.5%）发现囊性纤维化（见81章）。

发病率和死亡率

空肠回肠闭锁婴儿最常见的早期死亡原因是与肺炎、腹膜炎或败血症有关的感染[32]。最重要的术后并发症包括吻合口处的功能性肠梗阻及吻合口漏[32,99]。其他影响发病率和死亡率的因素包括伴发畸形、呼吸窘迫、早产、短肠综合征及肠扭转、肠梗死引起的术后肠梗阻[32]。Nixon和Tawes[99]发现死亡最常见最重要的原因是吻合口漏或功能障碍，发生率为15%。

过去，空肠闭锁的存活率相对较低（58%）[32]。远端梗阻的预后相对较好，回肠闭锁的存活率为75%。同时发现多发性闭锁（57%）、苹果皮样闭锁（71%）、肠闭锁合并胎粪性肠梗阻（65%）、胎粪性腹膜炎（50%）以及腹裂（66%）的死亡率较高[32,48,85,108,114,124,128,145]。

1971年，Nixon和Tawes[99]建议使用风险分组和治疗分组对肠闭锁患儿的存活率做临界评价。患儿被分至3个风险组：A组患儿体重超过5.5磅，无其他严重畸形；B组患儿体重在4.0～5.5磅或有中度严重的伴发畸形；C组患儿体重低于4.0磅或伴发严重畸形。结果C组患儿存活率最低（32%），而A组或B组患儿的存活率为81%。治疗组分为高位空肠闭锁组、中段小肠闭锁组和末端回肠闭锁组。结果A组或B组高位空肠闭锁患儿的存活率为60%，而C组所有8例高位空肠闭锁患儿死亡。A组或B组中段小肠闭锁患儿的存活率为82%，而C组中段小肠闭锁患儿的存活率仅为32%。A组或B组末端回肠闭锁患儿的存活率为100%，但C组末端回肠闭锁患儿的存活率降至50%。

de Lorimier及其同事[32]评估了近端肠管广泛切除和端端吻合的存活率。肠切除将空肠闭锁的存活率从39%提高至66%，但对回肠闭锁总体存活率的改善没有效果。Louw[80]报道33例空肠回肠闭锁患儿行近端肠管广泛切除和端-斜单层吻合术后的存活率为94%，其中2例发生吻合口漏，该研究中仅有的2例死亡发生于被分至C组的患儿。据Martin和Zerella[85]报道，自1968年以来，23例空肠回肠闭锁患儿的存活率为100%。

近年来，大多数研究报道空肠回肠闭锁的总体存
283 活率为80%~90%或更高（表80-2）[30,114,135,143]。随着新生儿重症监护室治疗的进步，与先前几十年相比，早产已不是一个很不利的因素。1971年Nixon介绍的按出生体重分型的风险预测方式已不太适用[98,99]。Smith和Glasson[128]报道的存活率为78%，将肠旋转不良、伴发畸形及使用造瘘作为风险因素。Riley儿童医院的手术死亡率（术后30天内）为1.5%，194例中死亡3例，其中2例伴胎粪性腹膜炎患儿的死亡与败血症及多器官功能衰竭有关，另1例早产儿的死亡与败血症及呼吸衰竭有关。然而，有21例在初次治疗后的3个月~8年内发生迟发性死亡（总死亡率为12.5%），10例死于败血症及多器官系统衰竭，其中5例有短肠综合征，3例肠闭锁伴腹裂。3例短肠综合征患儿在长期使用TPN后发生肝衰竭，1例腹裂并有支气管肺发育不良死于进行性呼吸衰竭，1例苹果皮样闭锁患儿死于败血症，1例吻合口漏发生于回肠闭锁及肠扭转的患儿。只有1例多发性闭锁病例存活，11例苹果皮样闭锁患儿中9例存活，28例伴发腹裂的患儿中有24例存活。对于伴发腹裂的患儿，如果需用人工假体装置（silo）来关闭腹壁缺损，应避免一开始就做肠造瘘[91,129]。将闭锁肠段放回腹腔，再延迟行一期吻合效果较好。有多发性闭锁伴不明原因的免疫缺陷综合征的家族遗传性病例的死亡率更高[11]。

表80-2 空肠回肠闭锁的存活率

作者/年份	存活率（%）
de lorimier 等，1969[32]	68
Nixon 和 Tawes，1971[99]	62
Louw，1967[81]	94
Martin 和 Zerella，1976[85]	100
Rescorla 和 Grosfeld，1983[114]	90
Smith 和 Glasson，1989[128]	78
Touloukian，1993[142]	91
Dalla Vecchia 等，1998[30]	84
Hou 和 Zhang，1999[59]	82
Sweeney 等，2001[135]	80
Grosfeld，2004（最近的数据）	87

空肠结肠闭锁患儿存活率的提高与对部分病例行恰当的肠切除术或肠锥形成形术，以及端-斜吻合术或延迟吻合的肠外置术有关。积极使用TPN作为辅助疗法明显改善了这些患儿的总体治疗效果[110]。北京儿童医院对449例肠闭锁患儿的回顾分析显示，使用TPN及纵向斜吻合后，近期该病的死亡率从64.7%降低至18.6%[59]。即使是苹果皮样闭锁的患儿也获得了很好的远期效果（存活率为80%）[30,38,149]。TPN避免了蛋白质-热量营养不良的发生，有助于建立正氮平衡，并使伴有吻合口功能障碍或腹裂的空肠回肠闭锁患儿有相对安全的等待时间。TPN对短肠综合征及做肠造瘘后功能障碍行暂时性肠外置的病例也非常有用。对于小肠闭锁合并腹裂的患儿，Molik及其同事发现27例中有7例发生短肠综合征，其住院时间延长并需要长期TPN支持[91]。肠管大量切除后，TPN维持患儿的营养需求，使患儿能很好地恢复并有了适应的时间[110]。肠道适应以绒毛肥大、黏膜细胞增生、肠壁厚度及周径增加为特征。短肠综合征这一主题将在本书的其他章节进行重点介绍（见86章）。不幸的是，TPN可并发严重的胆汁淤积，偶尔可引起进行性肝病，继发肝衰竭。我们医院2例患儿的死亡与TPN引起肝衰竭有关。

中段小肠切除的患儿的预后优于回盲瓣切除的患儿。Wilmore[158]回顾了50例切除较多小肠的病例，结果显示大多数中段小肠切除后肠管长度大于35 cm、回盲瓣完整的患儿存活下来。如果剩余肠管长度仅为

15～25 cm，存活率降至 50%；如果剩余肠管长度短于 15 cm、回盲瓣完整，或近端肠管短于 40 cm、回盲瓣切除，存活率则为 0。笔者认为 TPN 和特殊要素饮食可在一定程度上改善这种情况，因为笔者治疗了 2 例剩余肠管长度分别为 20 cm 和 30 cm 且回盲瓣切除的患儿，最终适应并存活。一个有力的证据是早产儿的肠道可在第一年内增长，在这些情况下可起到一定作用[143,157]。对于部分病例，给予生长激素、谷氨酰胺以及其他生长因子可能是有益的[74,88,158]。对于非常严重的短肠综合征病例，Bianchi 纵向延长术和 Kim 及其同事发明的连续横向肠成形术（serial transverse enteroplasty，STEP）是试图增加肠管长度的方法（详见 86 章）[10,67,68]。对不能适应的患儿，同种异体肠移植可能是另一种治疗选择（见 46 章）。除短肠综合征以外，机体不能适应并发生 TPN 相关性肝衰竭的患儿，多脏器移植或许可挽救生命（见 46 章）。肠延长术对手术时有严重肝功能障碍的患儿一般无益，常需要进行移植[18]。

虽然大多数接受 50% 中段小肠切除术的患儿能
1284 够正常生长发育，但接受更广泛肠管切除的患儿则不能。较远端肠管切除，特别是切除回盲瓣的患儿，更易发生吸收不良（脂肪、胆盐、维生素 B_{12}、钙、镁）、腹泻（脂肪泻）及小肠细菌增生[7,157,158]。虽然很多短肠综合征的婴儿能够存活，但他们会继发很多问题，需要密切监测，包括肾结石、胆结石及吸收不良。我院的 1 例患儿发生缺铁性贫血，并有粪便中带血的迹象，11 岁时内镜下发现吻合口溃疡，予以切除。Sondheimer 及其同事[130]、Couper 及其同事[26]也报道了相似的迟发性吻合口溃疡引起出血的情况。故强烈建议对新生儿期接受空肠回肠闭锁治疗的患儿进行长期随访。

（陈　盛译　董其刚校）

参考文献

1. Abrams JS: Experimental intestinal atresia. Surgery 1968; 64:185-191.
2. Aigrain Y, Enezian G, Sonsino E, et al: Multiple intestinal atresias: Report of 2 cases. Chir Pediatr 1989;30:61-64.
3. Alyulymon OM, Monteiro H, Ouzounian JG, et al: Clinical significance of prenatal ultrasonographic intestinal dilatation in fetuses with gastroschisis. Am J Ostet Gynecol 1996; 175:982-984.
4. Basu R, Burge DM: The effect of antenatal diagnosis on the management of small bowel atresia. Pediatr Surg Int 2004;20:177-179.
5. Baxi LV, Yeh MN, Blanc WA, Schullinger JN: Antepartum diagnosis and management of in-utero intestinal volvulus with perforation. N Engl J Med 1983;308:1519-1521.
6. Bell RH, Johnson FE, Lilly JR: Intestinal anastomosis in neonatal surgery. Ann Surg 1976;83:276-281.
7. Benson CD, Lloyd JR: Surgical lesions of the small intestine in the newborn. Dis Colon Rectum 1962:5:89-104.
8. Benson CD, Lloyd JR, Smith JD: Resection and primary anastomosis in the management of stenosis and atresia of the jejunum and ileum. Pediatrics 1960;26:265-272.
9. Berdon WE, Baker DH, Santulli TV, et al: Microcolon in newborn infants with intestinal obstruction: Its correlation with the level and time of onset of obstruction. Radiology 1968;90:878-885.
10. Bianchi A: Experience with intestinal lengthening and tailoring. Eur J Pediatr Surg 1999;9:256-259.
11. Bilodeau A, Prasil O, Cloutier R, et al: Hereditary multiple intestinal atresia: 30 years later. J Pediatr Surg 2004;39: 726-730.
12. Birtch AG, Coran AG, Gross RE: Neonatal peritonitis. Surgery 1967;61:305-313.
13. Bishop HC, Koop CE: Management of meconium ileus: Resection, Roux-en-Y anastomosis and ileostomy irrigation with pancreatic enzymes. Ann Surg 1957;145:410-414.
14. Black PR, Meuller D, Chow J, et al: Mesenteric defect as a cause of intestinal volvulus after malrotation and as the possible primary etiology of intestinal atresia. J Pediatr Surg 1994;29:1339-1343.
15. Bland-Sutton J: Imperforate ileum. Ann J Med Sci 1889; 98:457.
16. Blyth H, Dickson JAS: Apple-peel syndrome (congenital intestinal atresia): A family study of 7 index patients. J Med Genet 1969;6:275-277.
17. Boggs TR Jr, Bishop H: Neonatal hyperbilirubinemia associated with high obstruction of the small bowel. J Pediatr 1965;66:349-356.
18. Bueno J, Guiterrez J, Mazariegos GV, et al: Analysis of patients with longitudinal lengthening procedure referred for intestinal transplantation. J Pediatr Surg 2001;36:178-183.
19. Careskey JM, Grosfeld JL, Weber TR, Malangoni MA: Giant cystic meconium peritonitis (GCMP): Improved survival based on clinical and laboratory observations. J Pediatr Surg 1982;17:482-489.
20. Careskey JM, Weber TR, Grosfeld JL: Total colonic aganglionosis: Analysis of 16 cases. Am J Surg 1982;143:160-168.
21. Chaet MS, Warner BW, Sheldon CA: Management of multiple jejunoileal atresias with an intraluminal Silastic stent. J Pediatr Surg 1994;29:1604-1606.
22. Chalon J, Loew DA, Malebranche J: Effects of dry anesthetic gases on tracheobronchial ciliated epithelium. Anesthesiology 1972;37:338-343.
23. Cloutier R: Intestinal smooth muscle response to chronic obstruction: Possible application in jejunal atresia. J Pediatr Surg 1975;10:3-8.
24. Collins DL, Kimura K, Morgan A: Multiple intestinal atresia and amyoplasia congenita in four unrelated infants. J Pediatr Surg 1986;21:331-333.
25. Cook RCM, Rickham PP: Neonatal intestinal obstruction due to milk curds. J Pediatr Surg 1969;4:599-605.
26. Couper RT, Durie PR, Stafford SE, et al: Late gastrointestinal bleeding and protein loss after distal small-bowel resection in infancy. J Pediatr Gastroenterol Nutr 1989;9:454-460.
27. Courtois B: Des origines foetales des occlusions congeni-

tales due grele dites par atresia. J Chir 1959;78:405.
28. Cragan JD, Martin ML, Moore CA, Khoury MJ: Descriptive epidemiology of small intestinal atresia, Atlanta, Georgia. Teratology 1993;48:441-450.
29. Cragan JD, Martin ML, Waters GD, Khoury MJ: Increased risk of small intestinal atresia among twins in the United States. Arch Pediatr Adolesc Med 1994;148:733-739.
30. Dalla Vecchia L, Grosfeld JL, West KW, et al: Intestinal atresia and stenosis: A 25 year experience with 277 cases. Arch Surg 1998;133:490-496.
31. Davis DL, Poynter CWM: Congenital occlusions of intestine with report of a case of multiple atresias of jejunum. Surg Gynecol Obstet 1922;34:35.
32. de Lorimier AA, Fonkalsrud EW, Hays DM: Congenital atresia and stenosis of the jejunum and ileum. Surgery 1969;65:819-827.
33. de Lorimier AA, Harrison MR: Intestinal imbrication in the treatment of atresia. J Pediatr Surg 1983;18:734-737.
34. de Lorimier AA, Norman DA, Goodling CA, Preger L: A model for the cinefluoroscopic and manometric study of chronic intestinal obstruction. J Pediatr Surg 1973;8:785-791.
35. Dinsmore JE, Jackson RJ, Wagner CW: Management of multiple atresias and perforation with intraluminal stenting. Pediatr Surg Int 1998;13:226-228.
36. Dickson JA: Apple-peel small bowel: An uncommon variant of duodenal and jejunal atresia. J Pediatr Surg 1970;5:595-600.
37. Evans CH: Atresias of the gastrointestinal tract. Surg Gynecol Obstet 1951;92:1-8.
38. Festen S, Brevoord JC, Goldhoorn GA, et al: Excellent long-term outcome for survivors of apple peel atresia. J Pediatr Surg 2002;37:61-65.
39. Fockens P: Ein operativ geheilter Fall von Kongenitaler Duenndarm Atresie. Zentrlbl Chir 1911;38:532.
40. Foglia RP, Jobst S, Fonkalsrud EW, Ament ME: An unusual variant of a jejuno-ileal atresia. J Pediatr Surg 1983;18:182-184.
41. Forrester MB, Merz RD: Population-based study of small intestinal atresia and stenosis, Hawaii, 1986-2000. Public Health 2004;118:434-438.
42. Fourcade L, Shima H, Miyazaki E, Puri P: Multiple gastrointestinal atresias result from disturbed morphogenesis. Pediatr Surg Int 2001;17:361-364.
43. Gillick J, Giles S, Bannigan S, Puri P: Midgut atresias result from abnormal development of the notochord in an Adriamycin rat model. J Pediatr Surg 2002;37:719-722.
44. Gluer S: Intestinal atresia following intraamniotic use of dyes. Eur J Pediatr Surg 1995;5:240-242.
45. Gornall P: Management of intestinal atresia complicated by gastroschisis. J Pediatr Surg 1989;24:522-524.
46. Graham JN, Marin-Padilla M, Hoefnagel D: Jejunal atresia associated with Cafergot ingestion during pregnancy. Clin Pediatr 1983;22:226.
47. Gray SW, Skandalakis JE: Embryology for Surgeons. Philadelphia, WB Saunders, 1994.
48. Grosfeld JL: Alimentary tract obstruction in the newborn. Curr Probl Pediatr 1975;5:3-47.
49. Grosfeld JL, Ballantine TVN, Shoemaker R: Operative management of intestinal atresia and stenosis based on pathologic findings. J Pediatr Surg 1979;14:368-375.
50. Grosfeld JL, Clatworthy HW Jr: Intrauterine midgut strangulation in a gastroschisis defect. Surgery 1970;67:519-520.
51. Grosfeld JL, Clatworthy HW Jr: The nature of ileal atresia due to intrauterine intussusception. Arch Surg 1970;100:714-717.
52. Grosfeld JL, Dawes L, Weber TR: Current management of abdominal wall defects: Gastroschisis and omphalocele. Surg Clin North Am 1981;61:1037-1049.
53. Gross E, Armon Y, Abu-Dalu K, et al: Familial combined duodenal and jejunal atresia. J Pediatr Surg 1996;31:1573.
54. Guttman FN, Braun P, Garance PH, et al: Multiple atresias and a new syndrome of hereditary multiple atresias involving the gastrointestinal tract from stomach to rectum. J Pediatr Surg 1973;8:633-640.
55. Harris J, Kallen B, Robert E: Descriptive epidemiology of alimentary tract atresia. Teratology 1995;52:15-29.
56. Hasegawa T, Sumimura J, Nose K, et al: Congenital multiple intestinal atresia successfully treated with multiple anastomoses in a premature infant: Report of a case. Surg Today 1996;26:849-851.
57. Heij HA, Moorman-Voestermans CG, Vos A: Atresia of the jejunum and ileum: Is it the same disease? J Pediatr Surg 1990;25:635-637.
58. Herman TE, McAlister WH: Familial type I jejunal atresia and renal dysplasia. Pediatr Radiol 1995;25:272-274.
59. Hou D, Zhang J: 40 years' review of intestinal atresia. China Med J (Engl) 1999;112:583-585.
60. Houston CS, Wittenborg MH: Roentgen evaluation of anomalies of rotation and fixation of the bowel in children. Radiology 1965;84:1-18.
61. Howard ER, Othersen HB: Proximal jejunoplasty in the treatment of jejunal atresia. J Pediatr Surg 1973;8:685-690.
62. Imai Y, Nishijima E, Muraji T, et al: Fusion of intussusceptum and intussuscipiens in intrauterine intussusception: A rare type of intestinal atresia. Pathol Int 1999;9:962-967.
63. Janik JP, Wayne ER, Janik JS, Price MR: Ileal atresia with total colonic aganglionosis. J Pediatr Surg 1997;32:1502-1503.
64. Johnson FP: The development of the mucous membrane of the esophagus, stomach, and small intestine in the human embryo. Am J Anat 1910;10:521.
65. Kazandjian V, Aigrain Y, Enezian G, et al: Upper jejunal atresia: Treatment using jejunal resection, duodenal modeling, and duodenal jejunal or ileal anastomosis. Chir Pediatr 1989;30:191-195.
66. Kilani RA, Hmiel P, Garver MK, et al: Familial jejunal atresia with renal dysplasia. J Pediatr Surg 1996;31:1427-1429.
67. Kim HB, Fauza D, Garza J, et al: Serial transverse enteroplasty (STEP): A novel bowel lengthening procedure. J Pediatr Surg 2003;38:425-429.
68. Kim HB, Lee PW, Garza J, et al: Serial transverse enteroplasty for short bowel syndrome: A case report. J Pediatr Surg 2003;38:881-885.
69. Kimble RM, Harding JE, Kolbe A: Jejuno-ileal atresia, an inherited condition? Pediatr Surg Int 1995;10:5.
70. Kimura K, Perdzynski W, Soper RT: Elliptical seromuscular resection for tapering the proximal dilated bowel in duodenal or jejunal atresia. J Pediatr Surg 1996;31:1405-1406.
71. Kling K, Applebaum H, Dunn J, et al: A novel technique for correction of intestinal atresia at the ligament of Treitz. J Pediatr Surg 2001;36:353-355.
72. Koga Y, Hayashida Y, Ikeda K, et al: Intestinal atresia in fetal dogs produced by localized ligation of mesenteric vessels. J Pediatr Surg 1975;10:949-953.
73. Komuro H, Hori T, Amagai T, et al: The etiologic role of intrauterine volvulus and intussusception in jejunoileal atresia. J Pediatr Surg 2004;39:1812-1814.
74. Ladd AP, Grosfeld JL, Pescovitz OH, Johnson NB: The effect of growth hormone supplementation on late nutritional independence in pediatric patients with short bowel syndrome. J Pediatr Surg 2005;40:442-445.

75. Lally KP, Chwals WJ, Weitzman JJ, et al: Hirschsprung's disease: A possible cause of anastomotic failure following repair of intestinal atresia. J Pediatr Surg 1992;27:469-470.
76. Landor JH, Armstrong JH, Dickerson OB, Westerfeld RA: Neonatal obstruction of bowel caused by accidental clamping of small omphalocele: Report of two cases. South Med J 1963;56:1236-1238.
77. LeCoultre C, et al: An unusual association of small bowel atresia and biliary atresia: A case report. J Pediatr Surg 1983;18:136.
78. Lituania M, Cordone MS: Prenatal diagnosis of jejunal atresia by ultrasound (apple-peel syndrome). Gaslini 1980;12:197.
79. Lloyd JR, Clatworthy HW Jr: Hydramnios as an aid to the early diagnosis of congenital obstruction of the alimentary tract: A study of maternal and fetal factor. Pediatrics 1958;21:903-909.
80. Louw JH, Barnard CN: Congenital intestinal atresia: Observations on its origin. Lancet 1955;2:1065-1067.
81. Louw JH: Resection and end-to-end anastomosis in the management of atresia and stenosis of the small bowel. Surgery 1967;62:940-950.
82. Lynn HB, Espinas EE: Intestinal atresia: An attempt to relate location to embryologic processes. Arch Surg 1959; 79:357-361.
83. Mogliner BM, Appelman Z, Lancet M, Casif R: Antenatal diagnosis of fetal intestinal obstruction by ultrasonography. Harefuah 1981;101:5.
84. Marfatia S, Donahoe PK, Hendren WH: Effect of dry and humidified gases on the respiratory epithelium in rabbits. J Pediatr Surg 1975;10:583-592.
85. Martin LW, Zerella JT: Jejunoileal atresia: Proposed classification. J Pediatr Surg 1976;11:399-404.
86. Martucciello G, Torre M, Pini Prato A, et al: Associated anomalies. I: intestinal neuronal dysplasia. J Pediatr Surg 2002;37:219-223.
87. Masumoto K, Suita S, Nada O, et al: Abnormalities of enteric neurons, intestinal pacemaker cells, and smooth muscle in human intestinal atresia. J Pediatr Surg 1999; 34:1463-1468.
88. Matarese LE, Seidner DL, Steiger E: Growth hormone, glutamine and modified diet for intestinal adaptation. Am J Diet Assoc 2004;104:1265-1272.
89. Matsumoto Y, Komatsu K, Tabata T: Jejuno-ileal atresia in identical twins: Report of a case. Surg Today 2000;30:438-440.
90. Mishalany HG, Najjar FB: Familial jejunal atresia: Three cases in one family. J Pediatr Surg 1968;73:753-755.
91. Molik KA, Gingalewski CA, West KW, et al: Gastroschisis: A plea for risk categorization. J Pediatr Surg 2001;36:51-55.
92. Moorman-Voestermans CG, Heij HA, Vos A: Jejunal atresia in twins. J Pediatr Surg 1990;25:638-639.
93. Moreno LA, Gottrand F, Tvack D, et al: Severe combined immunodeficiency syndrome associated with autosomal recessive familial multiple gastrointestinal atresia: Study of a family. Am J Med Genet 1990;37:143-146.
94. Moya F, Apgar V, James LS, Berrien C: Hydramnios and congenital anomalies: Study of a series of 74 patients. JAMA 1960;173:1552-1556.
95. Murphy DA: Internal hernias in infancy and childhood. Surgery 1964;55:311-316.
96. Neuhauser EB: Roentgen changes associated with pancreatic insufficiency in early life. Radiology 1946;46:319.
97. Nixon HH: Intestinal obstruction in the newborn. Arch Dis Child 1955;30:13-22.
98. Nixon HH: An experimental study of propulsion in isolated small intestine and applications to surgery in the newborn. Ann R Coll Surg Engl 1960;24:105-124.
99. Nixon HH, Tawes R: Etiology and treatment of small intestinal atresia: Analysis of a series of 127 jejunoileal atresias and comparison with 62 duodenal atresias. Surgery 1971;69:41-51.
100. Odell GB: Physiologic hyperbilirubinemia in the neonatal period. N Engl J Med 1967;277:193-195.
101. Okmian LG, Kovamees A: Jejunal atresia with intestinal aplasia: Strangulation of the intestine in the extraembryonic coelom of the belly stalk. Acta Paediatr Scand 1964; 53:65-69.
102. Olsen MM, Luck SR, Lloyd-Still J, Raffensperger JG: The spectrum of meconium disease in infancy. J Pediatr Surg 1982;17:479-481.
103. Parkkulainen KV: Intrauterine intussusception as a cause of intestinal atresia: A contribution to the etiology of intestinal atresia. Surgery 1958;44:1106-1111.
104 Paterson-Brown S, Stalewski H, Brereton RJ: Neonatal small bowel atresia, stenosis and segmental dilatation. Br J Surg 1991;78:83-86.
105. Phelps S, Fisher R, Partington A, Dykes E: Prenatal ultrasound diagnosis of gastrointestinal malformations. J Pediatr Surg 1997;32:438-440.
106. Pokorny WJ, Harberg FJ, McGill CW: Gastroschisis complicated by intestinal atresia. J Pediatr Surg 1981;16:261-263.
107. Prasad SR, Mitra DK, Bhatnagar V, Mathur M: Multiple atresias of the bowel with reference to Tandler's theory of embryogenesis. Ind Pediatr 1993;30:1036-1039.
108. Puri P, Fujimoto T: New observations in the pathogenesis of multiple intestinal atresias. J Pediatr Surg 1988;23: 221-225.
109. Puvabandisin S, Garrow E, Sanransamraujkit R, Lopez LA: Postnatal intussusception in a premature infant causing intestinal atresia. J Pediatr Surg 1996;31:711-712.
110. Quiros-Tejeira RE, Ament ME, Reyen L, et al: Long-term parenteral nutritional support and intestinal adaptation in children with short bowel syndrome: A 25-year experience. J Pediatr 2004:145:157-163.
111. Rachelson MH, Jernigan JR, Jackson WF: Intussusceptum in the newborn infant with spontaneous expulsion of the intussusception: Case report and review of the literature. J Pediatr 1955;47:87-94.
112. Randolph JG, Zollinger RM Jr, Gros RE: Mikulicz resection in infants and children: A 20-year survey of 196 patients. Ann Surg 1963;158:481-491.
113. Rehbein F, Halsband H: A double tube technique for the treatment of meconium ileus and small bowel atresia. J Pediatr Surg 1968;3:723.
114. Rescorla FJ, Grosfeld JL: Intestinal atresia and stenosis: Analysis of survival in 120 cases. Surgery 1983;98:668-676.
115. Rittenhouse EA, Beckwith JB, Chappell JS, Bill AH: Multiple septa of the small bowel: Description of an unusual case with review of the literature and consideration of etiology. Surgery 1972;71:371-379.
116. Romero R, Shidini A, et al: Gastrointestinal tract and abdominal wall defects. In Brock DJH, Rodeck CH, Ferguson-Smith MA (eds): Prenatal Diagnosis and Screening. Edinburgh, Churchill Livingstone, 1992, p 237.
117. Rosenman JE, Kosloske AM: A reappraisal of the Mikulicz enterostomy in infants and children. Surgery 1982;91:34-37.
118. Ros Mar Z, Diez Pardo JA, Ros Miquel M, Benavent I: Apple-peel small bowel: A review of 12 cases. Z Kinderchir Grenzgeb 1980;29:313-317.
119. Rothenberg ME, White FV, Chilmonczyk B, Chatila T: A syndrome involving immunodeficiency and multiple intestinal atresias. Immunodeficiency 1995;5:171-178.
120. Saguintaah M, Couture A, Veyrac C, Baud C: MRI of the

fetal intestinal tract. Pediatr Radiol 2002;32:395-404.
121. Santulli TV, Blanc WA: Congenital atresia of the intestine: Pathogenesis and treatment. Ann Surg 1961;154:939-948.
122. Sapin E, Carricaburu E, De Boissieu D, et al: Conservative intestinal surgery to avoid short-bowel syndrome in multiple intestinal atresias and necrotizing enterocolitis: 6 cases treated by multiple anastomoses and Santulli-type enterostomy. Eur J Pediatr Surg 1999;9:24-28.
123. Schoenberg RA, Kluth D: Experimental small bowel obstruction in chick embryos: Effects on the developing enteric nervous system. J Pediatr Surg 2002;37:735-740.
124. Seashore JH, Collins FS, Markowitz RI, Seashore MR: Familial apple-peel atresia: Surgical, genetic and radiographic aspects. Pediatrics 1987;80:540-544.
125. Shah R, Wooley MM: Gastroschisis and intestinal atresia. J Pediatr Surg 1991;26:788-790.
126. Shenoy MU, Robson K, Broderick N, Kapila L: Congenital small bowel diverticulosis and intestinal atresia: A rare association. J Pediatr Surg 2000;35:636-637.
127. Singleton EB: Congenital abnormalities of the small bowel: Meconium ileus. In Singleton EB (ed): X-Ray Diagnosis of the Alimentary Tract in Infants and Children. Chicago, Year Book , 1959, pp 199-205.
128. Smith GH, Glasson M: Intestinal atresia: Factors affecting survival. Aust N Z J Surg 1989;59:151-156.
129. Snyder CL, Miller KA, Sharp RJ, et al: Management of intestinal atresia in patients with gastroschisis. J Pediatr Surg 2001;36:1542-1544.
130. Sondheimer JM, Sokol RJ, Narkewicz MR, Tyson RW: Anastomotic ulceration: A late complication of ileocolonic anastomosis. J Pediatr 1995;127:225-230.
131. Spencer R: The various patterns of intestinal atresia. Surgery 1968;64:661-668.
132. Spriggs NL: Congenital intestinal occlusion. Guys Hosp Rep 1912;66:143.
133. Stromme P, Dahl E, Flage T, Sten-Johansen H: Apple peel intestinal atresia in siblings with ocular anomalies and microcephaly. Clin Genet 1993;44:208-210.
134. Suruga K, Hirai Y, Nagashima K, et al: Congenital intestinal atresia. Shujutsu 1968:22:726-733.
135. Sweeney B, Surana R, Puri P: Jejunoileal atresia and associated malformations: Correlation with timing of in-utero insult. J Pediatr Surg 2001;36:774-776.
136. Tam PK, Nicholls G: Implications of antenatal diagnosis of small-intestinal atresia in the 1990s. Pediatr Surg Int 1999;15:486-487.
137. Tandler J: Zur Entwicklungsgeschichte des menschlichen Duodenum in fruhen Embryonalstadien. Morphol Jahrb 1900;29:187.
138. Teja K, Schnatterly P, Shaw A: Multiple intestinal atresia: Pathology and pathogenesis. J Pediatr Surg 1981;16:194-199.
139. Thomas CG Jr: Jejunoplasty for correction of jejunal atresia. Surg Gynecol Obstet 1969;129:545-546.
140. Todani T, Tabuchi K, Tanaka S: Intestinal atresia due to intrauterine intussusception: Analysis of 24 cases in Japan. J Pediatr Surg 1975;10:445-451.
141. Touloukian RJ: Intestinal atresia and stenosis. In Holder TM, Ashcraft KW (eds): Pediatric Surgery. Philadelphia, WB Saunders, 1980.
142. Touloukian RJ: Diagnosis and treatment of jejunoileal atresia. World J Surg 1993;17:310-317.
143. Touloukian RJ, Smith GJ: Normal intestinal length in preterm infants: An autopsy study. J Pediatr Surg 1983; 18:720-723.
144. Tovar JA, Sunol M, Lopez de Torre B, et al: Mucosal morphology in experimental intestinal atresia: Studies in the chick embryo. J Pediatr Surg 1991;26:184-189.
145. Van Hoorn WA, Hazebrook FW, Molenaar JC: Gastroschisis with atresia—a plea for delay in resection. Z Kinderchir 1985;40:368-370.
146. Vassy LE, Boles ET: Iatrogenic ileal atresia secondary to clamping of an occult omphalocele. J Pediatr Surg 1975; 10:797-800.
147. Veyrac C, Coutre A, Saguintaah M, Baud C: MRI of fetal GI tract abnormalities. Abdom Imaging 2004;29:411-420.
148. Wagner ML, Rudolph AJ, Singleton EB: Neonatal defects associated with abnormalities of the amnion and amniotic fluid. Radiol Clin North Am 1968;6:279-294.
149. Waldhausen JH, Sawin RS: Improved long-term outcomes for patients with jejunoileal apple peel atresia. J Pediatr Surg 1997;32:1307-1309.
150. Walker MW, Lovell MA, Kelly TC, et al: Multiple areas of intestinal atresia associated with immunodeficiency and post-transfusion graft-versus-host disease. J Pediatr 1993;123:93-95.
151. Wang NL, Yeh ML, Chang PY, et al: Prenatal and neonatal intussusception. Pediatr Surg Int 1998;13:232-236.
152. Ward HC, Leake J, Milla PJ, Spitz L: Brown bowel syndrome: A late complication of intestinal atresia. J Pediatr Surg 1992;27:1593-1595.
153. Webb CH, Wangensteen OH: Congenital intestinal atresia. Am J Dis Child 1931;41:262.
154. Weber TR, Vane DW, Grosfeld JL: Tapering enteroplasty in infants with bowel atresia and short gut. Arch Surg 1982;117:684-688.
155. Weitzman JJ, Vanderhoof RS: Jejunal atresia with agenesis of the dorsal mesentery with "Christmas tree" deformity of the small intestine. Am J Surg 1966;111:443-449.
156. Werler MM, Sheehan JE, Mitchell AA: Maternal medication use and risks of gastroschisis and small intestinal atresia. Am J Epidemiol 2002;155:26-31.
157. Wilkinson AW: Some effects of extensive intestinal resection in childhood: Symposium on resection in the newborn infant. Bibl Pediatr 1968;87:191-207.
158. Wilmore DW: Factors correlating with a successful outcome following extensive intestinal resection, intestinal absorption and malabsorption, Zurich 1967. Mod Probl Paediatr 1968;11:191.
159. Yanagihara J, Nakamura K, Shimotake D, et al: An association of multiple intestinal atresia and biliary atresia. Eur J Pediatr Surg 1995;5:372-374.
160. Zerella JT, Martin LW: Jejunal atresia with absent mesentery and a helical ileum. Surgery 1976;80:550-553.
161. Zwiren GT, Andrews HG, Ahmann P: Jejunal atresia with agenesis of the dorsal mesentery ("apple-peel small bowel"). J Pediatr Surg 1972;7:414-419.

第 81 章

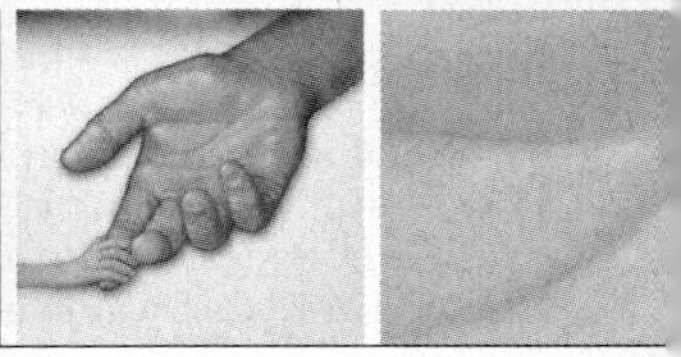

胎粪性肠梗阻

Moritz M. Ziegler

历史回顾

1289 Landsteiner 于 1905 年首次描述了胎粪性肠梗阻，将胎粪阻塞小肠的发现与胰腺的病理学改变联系起来，并推测后者是由于一种酶缺乏引起的。之后的学者们也认识到了黏稠的胎粪与胰管机械性梗阻或狭窄间存在相似的联系[4,31,54,64]。“胰腺囊性纤维化”这个名词于 1936 年由 Fanconi 首先提出，用以描述婴儿慢性肺病与胰腺功能不全之间的关系[124]。然而，Anderson 于 1938 年提出胎粪性肠梗阻和囊性纤维化（cystic fibrosis，CF）均有类似的胰腺异常的组织学表现，并描述胎粪性肠梗阻是全肺及胰腺功能不全的早期且更严重的表现[2,3]。之后的学者确定了胎粪浓缩的本质，发现其与胰腺功能不全和 CF 患儿肠道分泌的异常黏液有关[38,94,102,103,104,125]。

随着遗传学的进步，人们已经认识到 CF 是白种人中最常见的潜在致命性常染色体隐性遗传疾病。在上世纪 40 年代后期[]，胎粪性肠梗阻的预后几乎都是患儿死亡[39,48,125]，那时发明出很多干预方法，包括去除或旁路分流肠腔内阻塞的浓缩胎粪，将术中肠道操作减到最少，甚至使用全身麻醉药以对婴儿生理方面的损伤降到最低。1969 年，一种新的治疗方法是使用高渗性泛影葡胺（Gastrografin）经直肠灌肠，其对干燥黏滞的胎粪具有增溶作用，使得非复杂性胎粪性肠梗阻无需接受手术治疗，并在 2/3 以上的患儿中取得成功[81]。直到上世纪 70 年代早期，这些进步加上对 CF 的电解质、营养和肺部畸形治疗方面的进步，使得患儿的存活率提高到约 75%[20,99。]

在过去的 20 年中，我们不断看到进步。首先，CF 跨膜调节蛋白（CF transmembrane regulator，CFTR）变异的遗传学损害被确定为 CF 的发病原因[60,61]，现在认识到胎粪性肠梗阻患儿可能是一种症状更早、肺功能恶化的特殊表型[69,78]。其次，临床诊断标准基本保持不变，生化检测结合目前的遗传学检测可确诊。有趣的是，当灌肠无法治疗胎粪性肠梗阻或减轻其梗阻症状时，首选的手术干预方式是 1948 年首次描述的肠切开冲洗，典型的是使用胎粪溶解剂。这些策略的应用以及对患儿肺部情况和营养状况的密切监测，使胎粪性肠梗阻患儿的存活率持续上升，现已达到 95%~100%。

病理生理学

遗传学

囊性纤维化是一种常染色体隐性遗传疾病，白种人中杂合子的发生率为每 29 名新生儿中有 1 名。在黑色人种中罕见（1/17 000 活产儿），在亚洲人（1/90 000活产儿）和非洲人中几乎未听说过这种病。5%~6% 的异常基因携带率使得 CF 在白种人中的发生率达到每 1150~2500 名活产儿中有 1 名。父母均为杂合子时，其后代患病的概率为 1/4[1]。胎粪性肠梗阻是 CF 特有的，是以肠腔内累积浓缩干燥的胎粪引起肠梗阻为特征的新生儿疾病。因为这些患儿在新生儿期会及时得到诊断和治疗，故胎粪性肠梗阻是 CF 最早的临床表现[23]。据报道，在美国 CF 人群中 20. 8% 的患儿，胎粪性肠梗阻是其主要特征。10%~40% 的胎粪性肠梗阻患儿中有 CF 家族史，这对宫内诊断来说尤为重要。由于存在胎粪性肠梗阻合并 CF 的标准病例，报道已经提示 CF 随后发生胎粪性肠梗阻的发生率为 30%~40%。

290 1989 年，Francis Collins 确定了编码被称为 CF 跨膜调节蛋白的细胞膜蛋白的基因突变，该位点和 CF 的诊断有关[91,92]。它位于 7 号染色体的长臂上的 q31 带[63]。这种蛋白质被确定为一种环磷腺苷诱导的、能够调节离子通过上皮细胞顶端表面的氯通道[113]。CFTR 的变异（已有 400 多种变异被确认）引起上皮细胞膜顶端外环境的电解质含量异常。受影响的上皮管状结构排列的特点是干燥及分泌物清除降低，受影响的系统包括呼吸道、胃肠道、胆道、胰腺和生殖道的上皮细胞。其病理生理学的临床表现包括胰腺功能不全（90%）、胎粪性肠梗阻（10%~20%）、糖尿病（20%）、阻塞性胆道疾病（15%～20%）和无精症（几乎 100%）。上皮腺体异常和产生高黏度的黏蛋白的确切机制尚未明确。当然，黏稠的胎粪蛋白、含水量以及增加的黏度都在前面有所描述。

ΔF508 突变是许多 CFTR 基因位点中最常见的，约 50% 的 CF 患儿为纯合子，另外 25%～30% 的患儿只有单个突变。纯合子个体几乎总是在表型上表现为胰腺外分泌功能不足，且胎粪性肠梗阻的发生率更高。相似地，同时表达 ΔF508 和 G542X 的患儿发生胎粪性肠梗阻的概率也更高。然而，不是所有这种基因型的患儿都发生胎粪性肠梗阻，所以该病的病因学仍不是很明确。阻塞性肺疾病和胎粪性肠梗阻的同时出现说明存在其他 CFTR 修饰基因，甚至环境因素也可能在其中发挥作用。此外，大宗病例组未能确定 CF 并发症的预测因子，包括胎粪性肠梗阻的发病率。

发病机制

CF 的缺陷是外分泌腺功能障碍，特别是黏液分泌腺和汗腺功能障碍[15]。由于对先天性胰管狭窄的患儿伴发胎粪性肠梗阻很早就有报道，所以胰腺消化液缺乏被认为是胎粪性肠梗阻的发病机制。然而，上世纪 40 年代以来的数据显示 CF 患儿的胰腺病变具有变异性，在大于 1 岁的患儿中最复杂。相比之下，CF 伴胎粪性肠梗阻患儿亚组中的肠黏膜腺体异常更加突出，说明这些腺体病变更可能是引起胎粪性肠梗阻患儿肠腔内梗阻的黏性物质产生的原因[30]。其他的病理学资料显示在胎粪性肠梗阻的发病机制中肠道腺体病变起主要作用，而胰腺病变起次要作用[50,111]。

关于腺体异常是否能解释或引起这些改变，尚不很确定。各种解释包括钙离子介导的腺体分泌高渗黏液使得黏液的理化性质变得黏滞并有渗透性导致水分流失，促进管腔内的分泌物浓缩。这种腺体阻塞性黏液可引起先前提到的病理学损害。第二种假说是液体通过分泌细胞出入血管外的空间减少，这可能阻止了细胞腔的正常稀释[23,24]。高度浓缩的物质可对那些充满分泌物的细胞产生毒性。

通过限制性片段长度多态性分析知道 CFTR 基因定位于 7 号染色体后，不久人们认识到 CFTR 其本身是一个细胞膜氯通道，它可通过其他途径进一步调节氯化物转导[27]。这个机制可能是 CF 患儿特征性的外泌汗腺分泌物中钠离子和氯离子水平升高的原因。小管细胞再吸收水钠电解质障碍以及这些细胞对氯离子的不可渗透性导致排泄产物含大量的钠和氯。该理论符合已知的 CFTR 膜蛋白的特征，它是一种氯通道，起调节盐和水转运至上皮表面的作用。其功能被扰乱后可改变外分泌电解质含量并导致分泌物的干燥及清除减少。

胎粪自身具有可变的成分，这可以从不同胎龄正常婴儿的不同肠道部位的胎粪和 CF 患儿（有或无胎粪性肠梗阻）的胎粪比较中看出来[65]。正常婴儿或正常同胞胎粪中钠、钾、镁的浓度几乎是 CF 患儿（有或无胎粪性肠梗阻）的两倍。同样，对照组婴儿和正常同胞胎粪中酶催化重金属的水平也比 CF 患儿（有或无胎粪性肠梗阻）高。胎粪性肠梗阻患儿的胎粪标本蛋白氮含量较高，而碳水化合物含量较低，这也区别于正常胎粪。分析异常胎粪的蛋白含量可进一步发现异常的黏蛋白。这些产物 2/3 为蛋白质，1/3 为碳水化合物，成分类似于 CF 患儿的十二指肠液。这些蛋白质的来源不确定，可能来自腺体分泌或胎儿在子宫内吞咽的羊水。由于这种蛋白质大部分为白蛋白，故推测肠腔内的蛋白质来源于血浆。它们与黏多糖反应，在没有降解酶的情况下，它们使相关的分泌物具有高黏性的橡皮样特征。这些黏蛋白的黏度可进一步受周围电解质环境的影响。最后，由于 CF 患儿 1291
胎粪中白蛋白含量升高，因此出现了胎粪筛查试验用以诊断该病。

总之，胎粪性肠梗阻两个同时存在的发病机制似乎开始于子宫内，并导致患儿肠腔内积聚高度黏稠的胎粪：胰腺外分泌酶缺乏和病理学上异常的肠道腺体分泌高黏度的黏液。增厚的胎粪逐渐累积，在子宫内就开始阻塞肠道。胎粪的累积解释了胎粪性肠梗阻并发症的发生机制（即巨大的肠袢扭转后发生穿孔、腹膜炎、囊肿或闭锁）和新生儿腹部膨隆和肠梗阻的形态。近端回肠内充满柏油样黏滞的胎粪后变得扩张、肠壁增厚。同时，狭窄的远端小肠（有时还有结肠）内含有呈灰白色、油灰样的串珠状或车厢状的浓缩胎粪结石。更远端结肠细小或废用，呈细小结肠。

临床特征

疾病谱

新生儿的胎粪性肠梗阻表现可分为非复杂性、单纯性以及复杂性。在大龄儿童或年轻人表现为胎粪性肠梗阻等位症或远端回肠梗阻综合征。

非复杂性的胎粪性肠梗阻在出生后即有典型的表现，可发现患儿腹部膨隆，这是浓缩的胎粪充满并阻塞远端小肠的独特表现。可通过 CF 的宫内遗传学诊断及超声提示有回声的肠梗阻来预测。除了腹部膨隆，胆汁性呕吐及无法排便也预示将发生肠梗阻。

与之相反，复杂性胎粪性肠梗阻可表现为宫内或出生后有肠梗阻，同时之前有并发肠穿孔和/或肠坏死的迹象：即腹腔内出现新月形或斑点状的钙化，或临床评估可能有腹膜炎的迹象，包括腹壁红斑或水肿，和/或明确的腹部触痛[21]。

临床病史

10%~33% 胎粪性肠梗阻患儿有 CF 的家族史[25]。该病史再结合宫内羊膜穿刺液及限制性片段长度多态性分析，可为 CF 胎儿做出准确诊断。将这一结果与一系列宫内超声结果结合后，就可准确预测哪些患儿有发生胎粪性肠梗阻的危险（约占 CF 人群的 20%），以及有无并发胎粪囊肿的可能。母亲羊水过多可能是宫内胎粪性肠梗阻的特征之一，推测这是由高位肠梗阻引起的。羊水的过度累积可发生在 20% 胎粪性肠梗阻患儿的母亲，对于并发复杂性胎粪性肠梗阻的患儿这一比例更高。虽然宫内生长发育迟缓常见，但早产和其他伴随畸形较罕见。

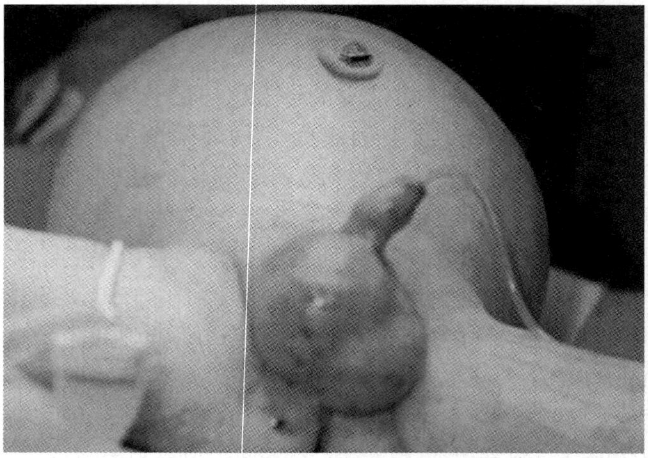

图 81-1 新生儿出生后腹部膨隆。有囊性纤维化的家族史，且新生儿在宫内时就作出囊性纤维化的细胞学诊断。胎儿超声检查证实有肠壁高回声，与胎粪性肠梗阻的诊断相符。

体格检查

胎粪性肠梗阻新生儿出生后常有腹部膨隆（图 81-1）。事实上，胎粪性肠梗阻是可引起刚出生的新生儿在吞咽空气前就发生腹部膨隆的新生儿肠梗阻的唯一类型。常可见蠕动波，并触及面团样肠袢。指压坚实的肠袢可留下压痕，这就是所谓的油灰征。对于单纯性或非复杂性胎粪性肠梗阻，无腹膜刺激征的表现。直肠检查通常无明显发现，但将检查者手指抽出后，患儿典型地表现为不能自发排出胎粪。宫内发生穿孔伴胎粪性腹膜炎及“囊肿”形成后，常可触及腹部肿块，出现腹壁变色和腹膜刺激征。有腹膜炎的患儿很快就出现血容量不足的体征。置入鼻胃管后，抽出的含胆汁的胃液常超过 20 ml。

影像学检查

在子宫内，胎粪性肠梗阻患儿的肠管不仅可表现为膨胀，而且在妊娠末 3 个月时超声可见具有回声的胎儿肠壁，这是具有诊断价值的[5,56,79]。出生后非复杂性胎粪性肠梗阻患儿在腹部平片上有典型的梗阻表现（图 81-2）[47,59]。除了仰卧位和直立位平片明显相似外，其特征性的表现包括以下几点：（1）不同肠

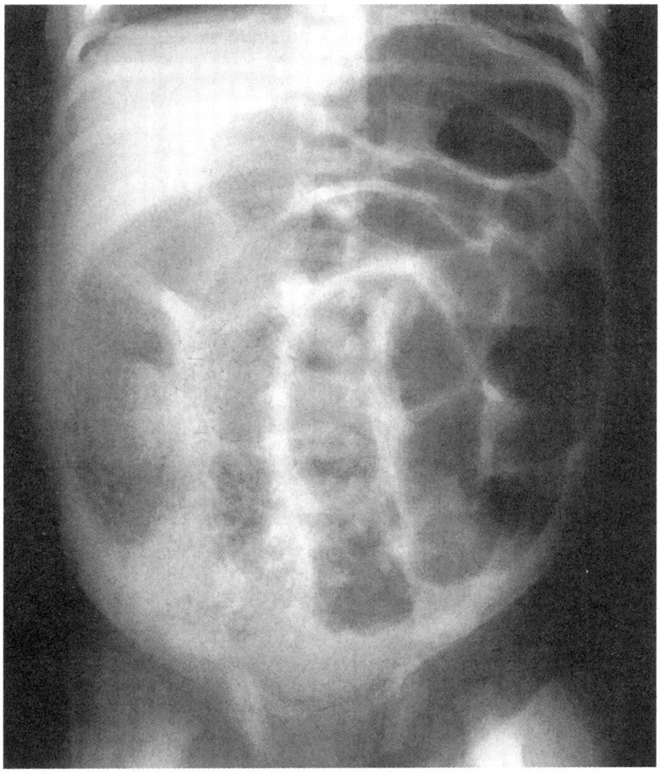

图 81-2 腹部直立位平片符合胎粪性肠梗阻的诊断。小肠袢扩张、大小不等、少量气液平、右下腹呈“毛玻璃”或“肥皂泡”样外观。(From Rescorla FJ, Grosfeld JL: Contemporary management of meconium ileus. World J Surg 1993; 17:381.)

段的外形不同，肠袢的大小有很大差异；（2）因为吞咽下去的空气不能浮在增厚浓缩的胎粪之上，故直立位片上没有或极少有气液平；（3）右半腹常可见颗粒状、“肥皂泡样”或“毛玻璃样”外观，这是由吞咽下的气泡与黏性的胎粪混合而形成的（图 81-3）[121]。这些特征中的每一个都不能单独特异性地诊断胎粪性肠梗阻，因为它们也可见于其他原因引起的肠梗阻。然而，将它们集中在一起就可有力地提示有胎粪性肠梗阻。如果将平片用于鉴别诊断，将包含所有远端小肠梗阻的原因，包括回肠闭锁、先天性巨结肠或胎粪栓塞综合征。可支持平片诊断胎粪性肠梗阻的确诊性检查是对比灌肠。对比灌肠（无论使用钡剂、泛影葡胺或任何水溶性造影剂）将显示出位置正常、长度适当的结肠，但肠管管径偏小（见图 81-3）[70]。结肠内可能是空的，或含有小块的浓缩胎粪。结肠可能为典型的“失用性”结肠或“小结肠”。如果造影剂反流入末端回肠，将显示出小块的浓缩胎粪[12,59]。如果造影剂反流入更近端的回肠，可发现小肠袢变得扩张。如造影剂未能反流入近端扩张的小肠，就无法诊断胎粪性肠梗阻，也不能明确肠梗阻的确切水平。在造影剂无法反流入扩张肠段的情况下，需行手术干预进行诊断和治疗。

实验室检查

能够确诊 CF 的检查为发汗试验。通过毛果芸香碱电离子导入法，收集患儿前臂、腿部或背部的汗液并定量，然后测定汗液样本中钠和氯的浓度[36,87]。最少需收集 100 mg 的汗液，如果汗液中氯浓度超过 60 mEq/L 就可诊断 CF。因为需要收集足够的汗液，所以这项检查常常不能应用于新生儿，但是也有相反的报道。个别汗液中的氯含量升高，但没有 CF 的其他特征。由于这些问题，再加上正常新生儿汗液中钠和氯的水平也可能升高，故需将这项试验延迟至婴儿出生几周后再进行。

通过分析 CFTR 的细胞 DNA 可进行 CF 的遗传检测，从而可确定有胎粪性肠梗阻特征的可疑 CF 患儿父母的基因携带状态。然而，由于这些商业性分析能检测出的基因突变很少，得出的阴性结果意义不大。如果知道其家族有 CFTR 突变，通过羊膜穿刺进行胎儿 DNA 限制性片段长度多态性分析可预测胎儿有无 CF。

胎粪中白蛋白浓度升高这一病理生理改变可能是一项有用的、针对胎粪性肠梗阻的诊断性筛查方法[43,44]。这项试验用四溴苯酚乙酯蓝作为指示剂，能够检测每克粪便浓度在 20 mg 以上的胎粪白蛋白；然而，假阳性结果可见于早产、黑粪症、腹裂及宫内感染等情况。假阴性率也有报道。这个简单且相对便宜的方法直接、快速，其比色指示剂简明易懂[52,107]。正常新生儿胎粪中的白蛋白浓度为每克粪便低于 5.0 mg，而 CF 患儿胎粪的白蛋白浓度有时超过80 mg/g[9,10]。

过去，粪便的胰蛋白酶和糜蛋白酶分析是筛查胎粪性肠梗阻的常用试验[9,10,46]。每克粪便中胰蛋白酶
水平低于 80 mg，并结合手术探查的结果，可支持胎 1293
粪性肠梗阻的诊断。某些医疗中心提倡在人群中通过检测血液中的免疫反应性胰蛋白酶原来筛查 CF。

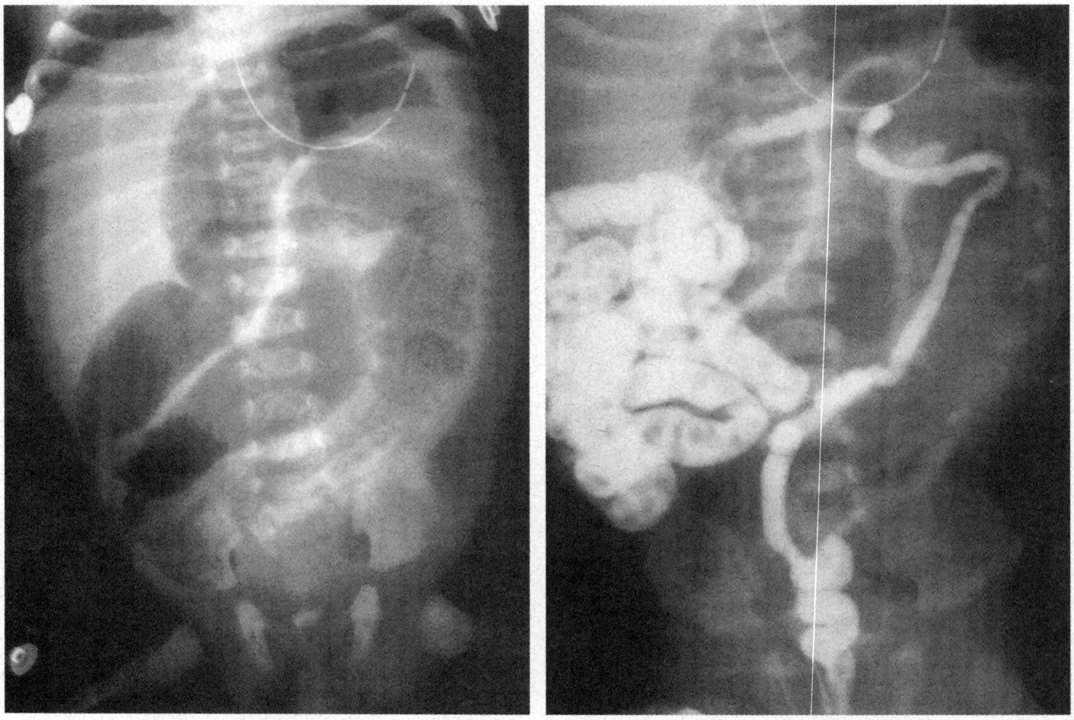

A B

图 81-3 A. 腹部平片符合胎粪性肠梗阻的诊断。肠袢扩张、大小不等、少量气液平、右下腹呈“肥皂泡”样外观。B. A 图中的同一位患儿进一步接受对比灌肠检查，证实有小结肠或失用性结肠，造影剂反流入更近端扩张的小肠，可见肠腔内有小块状的浓缩胎粪。这些发现强烈提示胎粪性肠梗阻的诊断。

手术取得的组织标本若有肠道（直肠）或阑尾的特异病理性改变，包括杯状细胞增生、隐窝或管腔内分泌物积聚，则有助于诊断 CF[84]。如果给疑为胎粪性肠梗阻的患儿施行手术，阑尾造口可用作肠腔灌洗的入口，为了获得诊断性的病理标本，需做阑尾切除术。

鉴别诊断

新生儿的家族史、体格检查和影像学评估是 3 个高灵敏度的诊断标准，可准确作出胎粪性肠梗阻的临床诊断。加上母亲羊膜穿刺标本或婴儿发汗试验的连锁分析可确诊 CF。最终诊断取决于肠梗阻原因的确定。胎粪性肠梗阻占新生儿肠梗阻病例的 10%～25%。因此，主要鉴别诊断的是各种新生儿肠梗阻的原因，包括回肠闭锁、先天性巨结肠、新生儿小左结肠和胎粪栓塞综合征[73]。

回肠闭锁在平片上常显示为远端肠梗阻伴气液平[19,97]。如果对比灌肠证实为小结肠，造影剂不会反流至近端扩张的“闭锁”肠段，而胎粪性肠梗阻和先天性巨结肠则有这种现象（图 81-4）。一旦疑为回肠闭锁，最终确诊需手术探查。胎粪性肠梗阻可伴有回肠闭锁，手术时若发现胎粪性肠梗阻特征性的黏性胎粪，则回肠闭锁的可能性大（图 81-5）。先天性巨结肠，特别是全结肠神经节细胞缺失和扩展至小肠的神经节细胞缺失，可与胎粪性肠梗阻类似[62,109,122]。事实上，几乎所有全肠型神经节细胞缺失症起初都被误诊为胎粪性肠梗阻[55]。确诊先天性巨结肠可通过 X 线和肛门直肠测压，但最终取决于组织化学检查结果示乙酰胆碱酯酶含量升高，或直肠活检的组织病理学检查结果示神经节细胞缺失。结肠型先天性巨结肠的 X 线特征可能包括一个移行区。对于全结肠型的先天性巨结肠患儿，典型的表现是造影剂反流至末端回 129 肠，不显示为胎粪性肠梗阻的充盈缺损，而表现为气液平和近端扩张的肠管。

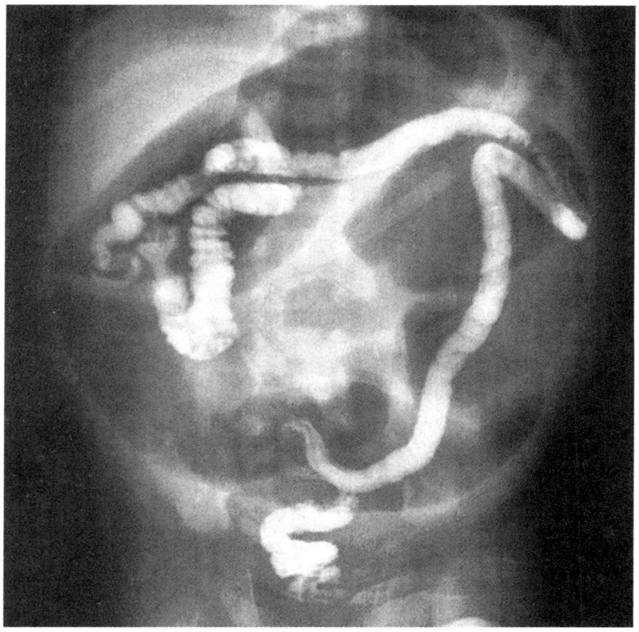

图 81-4　平片上明显有远端肠梗阻迹象的新生儿做对比灌肠检查。发现小结肠通往小管径的远端回肠，造影剂未反流至扩张的肠管，完全符合远端肠闭锁的诊断。(From Rescorla FJ, Grosfeld JL: Contemporary management of meconium ileus. World J Surg 1993; 17:381.)

新生儿小左结肠综合征也要与胎粪性肠梗阻相区别[18,86,108]。这种病变局限于左结肠，对比灌肠显示肠管变细呈漏斗样，并常与母亲的糖尿病、甲亢、药物滥用或子痫有关（图 81-6）。需行直肠活检以排除先天性巨结肠。一般没有胎粪性肠梗阻的其他特征。

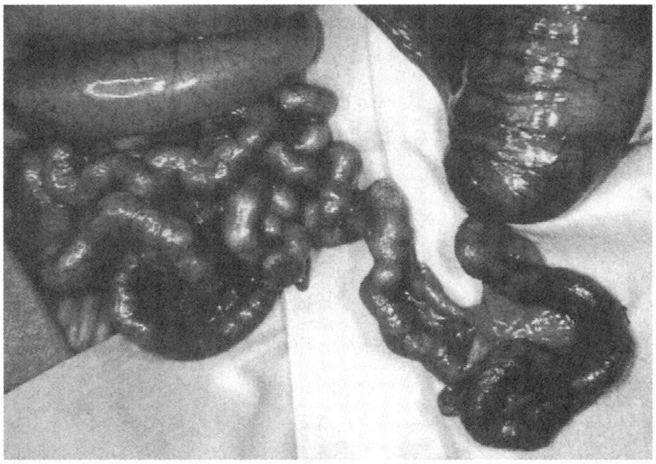

图 81-5　一例胎粪性肠梗阻合并获得性回肠闭锁患儿的手术所见。闭锁近端的小肠扩张，远端回肠和结肠有小块的浓缩胎粪。

胎粪栓塞综合征通常可通过对比灌肠摄片显示乙状结肠或降结肠内的栓状或模具状胎粪来确诊（见图 81-6）[14,29,93,110]。胎粪栓常可在灌肠管抽出、灌肠剂排出后自行排出。胎粪栓塞综合征和其他胃肠道畸形之间有明显联系，多达 14% 的 CF 新生儿有胎粪栓塞综合征[112]。胎粪栓的发病机制尚未明确，可能和肠管运动不足有关。胎粪栓塞综合征也与早产、肌张力减退、高镁血症、呼吸窘迫、败血症、甲状腺功能减退、糖尿病和先天性巨结肠有关[16,106]。这些联系说明在肠梗阻症状缓解后，需对胎粪栓塞综合征患儿进行发汗试验和直肠活检以分别排除 CF 和先天性巨结肠[37,115]。

胎粪性肠梗阻可发生于多种原因引起的胰腺或肠道功能不全但无 CF 的足月儿或早产儿[25,89,101]。肠腔梗阻是由于浓缩的黏性胎粪在末端回肠或右结肠内积聚引起的，但胎粪既不呈柏油样，也不耐受常规的清洁灌肠，后者通常具有治疗作用。至于病因是肠分泌功能不全还是胰液缺乏尚不确定，但很少有胰腺功能不全的报道。要确切排除 CF，临床上需做汗液氯含量分析和/或 DNA 分析。

非手术治疗

胎粪性肠梗阻的非手术治疗取决于通畅的、未受损害的回结肠肠腔内浓缩胎粪的溶解度[8,11,82]。尽管历史上曾通过口服、手术中或经直肠使用各种增溶剂，但胎粪性肠梗阻的主要治疗方法仍是手术[82]。1969 年，另外儿篇报道提出溶剂是有效的，并且在临床和试验中都提出了使用溶剂的非手术治疗价值[98]。Noblett 报道了高渗性对比灌肠成功应用于 4 例非复杂性胎粪性肠梗阻的新生儿。她介绍使用这种疗法前需要遵循以下标准：（1）首先需行诊断性对比灌肠排除其他原因引起的远端肠梗阻；（2）必须排除肠旋转不良、肠闭锁、肠穿孔或腹膜炎等并发症；（3）必须在小心的透视控制下进行灌肠；（4）应给予静脉内抗生素；（5）操作过程中患儿应该由一位小儿外科医生照看；（6）在操作过程中应给患儿积极补充液体（1～3 倍的维持量），以保证充分的液体复苏；（7）如果发生 1295

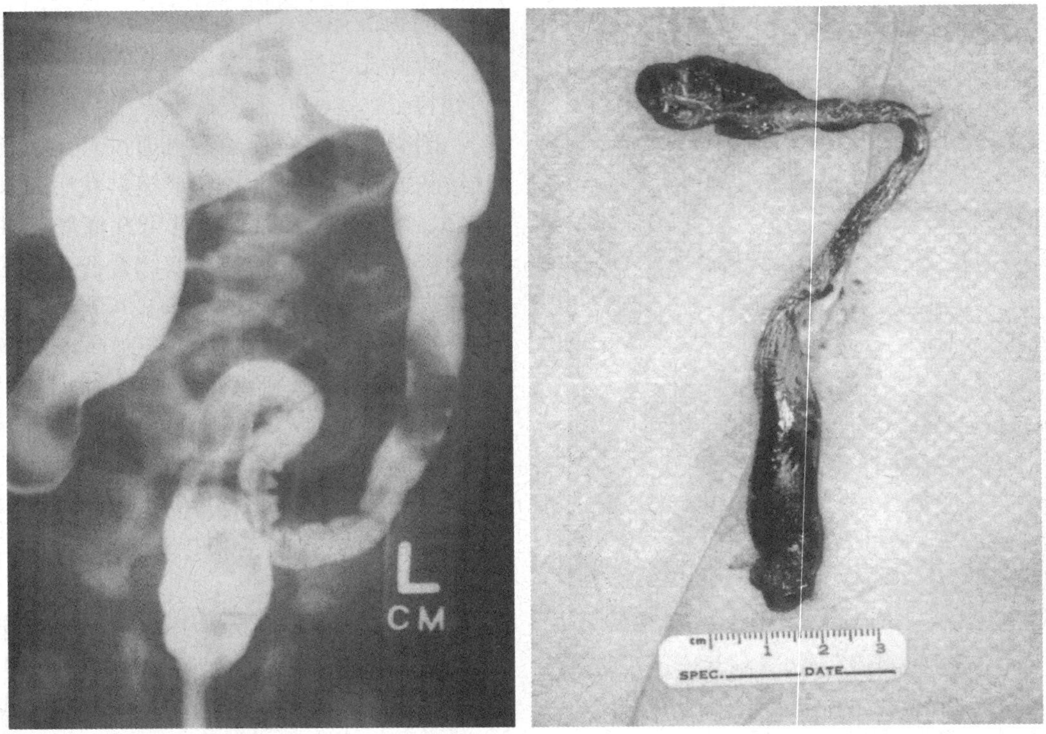

A B

图 81-6 胎粪性肠梗阻的鉴别诊断包括一些以左结肠病变为特征的疾病。A. 平片示远端肠管梗阻的新生儿，其对比灌肠显示脾曲下的结肠逐渐变细，直肠乙状结肠内有充盈缺损。这些发现提示可能存在先天性巨结肠、新生儿小左结肠综合征或胎粪栓塞综合征。B. 拔除灌肠导管后，患儿自行排出一条胎粪栓，梗阻解除。发汗试验和直肠活检可分别用以排除囊性纤维化及先天性巨结肠。

并发症，准备紧急手术[95,96]。自这篇报道之后，泛影葡胺灌肠成为非手术治疗的标准方法。泛影葡胺是一种高渗的、水溶性、辐射不能透过的溶液，含 0.1% 的聚山梨酯 80（Tween 80）（一种增溶剂或湿润剂）和 37% 的有机结合碘。葡甲胺是 n1n1-二乙酰-3，5-二氨基-2，4，6-三碘苯甲酸钠-甲基葡胺盐的 76% 含水溶液，此高渗溶液的渗透压浓度为 1900 mOsm/L，其特性是可使液体流向肠腔并帮助浓缩的胎粪排出。使用泛影葡胺后，可发生暂时性的渗透性腹泻及可能的渗透性利尿，故强调积极液体复苏的重要性。此外，这种物质是辐射透不过的，从而能够安全地在 X 线透视监测下给药。聚山梨酯 80（Tween 80）是一种非离子型表面活性乳化剂，不仅能在 X 线下更好地确定肠黏膜纹，也有助于高渗的泛影葡胺在梗阻处的黏膜和粘连的胎粪之间通过。10% 的聚山梨酯 80 溶液可在手术中经肠造瘘给药，以使得胎粪液化。其他不含聚山梨酯 80 的水溶性物质［如 40% 的泛影酸钠（40% Hypaque）］也可有效地解除梗阻，并可避免泛影葡胺对结肠黏膜造成的不良影响[11,34]。

使用胎粪性肠梗阻增溶性灌肠治疗技术也要遵守上述 Noblett 提到的指导方针。在液体复苏、鼻胃管减压、体检评估及腹部平片排除腹膜炎或肠穿孔后，用钡剂或水溶性造影剂进行诊断性对比灌肠。预先的诊断性检查完成后，将无球囊灌肠导管的头端插入肛门，围绕导管用胶带固定在臀部。将泛影葡胺配成 50% 的水溶液，在 X 线透视引导下，通过导管顶端的注射器缓缓注入造影剂。当造影剂通过结肠进入扩张的被胎粪阻塞的回肠时停止检查，送患儿返回病床接受监护、补液（两倍的维持量），并使体温恢复正常。随后浓缩的胎粪可自行经直肠排出。8～12 小时后复查腹部平片以确定梗阻是否减轻。如果胎粪未完 129
全排出，梗阻仍然存在，可用相同浓度的泛影葡胺重复灌肠。如果在成功的反流性灌肠后没有排便，或造影剂不能反流至扩张的肠段，应放弃这种方法而准备行手术干预。同样，如果有梗阻加重、腹胀、X 线片上肠袢扩张加重或有可能的穿孔引起腹膜炎的征象，均应行手术干预。Noblett 建议在灌肠成功之后，经鼻胃管每 6 小时给予 5 ml 10% N-乙酰半胱氨酸溶液以使上消化道分泌物液化[76]。此外，开始用配方奶喂养，每餐必须补充胰酶[85,105]。

非手术治疗的成功率各不相同[58,118]。Noblett 最初报道用这种方法成功治疗 2/3 的患儿。非手术治疗的优势包括肺部发病率降低、住院时间减少。弊端包括延误了灌肠治疗不成功患儿的手术干预时机、有即刻或延迟性肠损伤或穿孔的危险，以及引起血容量减少。肠管损伤后有穿孔的危险，这是由于重复灌肠、灌肠导管球囊扩张不当或造影剂直接致黏膜损伤导致的[33,42,68,71,123]。损伤的机制可能和肠管扩张或聚山梨酯 80 的含量有关。后一种损伤可通过使用将等张的泛影葡胺用水稀释至 320～340 mOsm/L、含 1%～2% 聚山梨酯 80 的增溶灌肠剂或替代的等张造影剂来预防。

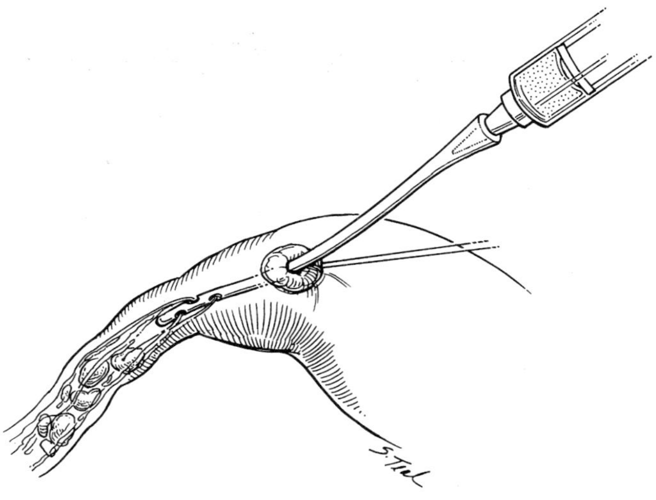

图 81-7　图中所示为胎粪性肠梗阻最常见的、首选的现代手术处理方法。在有浓缩胎粪的肠段近端切开扩张的小肠，置入冲洗导管。注入增溶剂后拔除导管、关闭肠切开处；或者将导管留在原处或替换成 T 管，以便于术后继续注入增溶剂。（From Rescorla FJ, Grosfeld JL: Contemporary management of meconium ileus. World J Surg 1993; 17: 381.）

手术治疗

胎粪性肠梗阻的手术治疗指征有多种[22,26,41]。1/3～1/2 接受手术治疗的患儿为增溶灌肠剂治疗失败的单纯或非复杂性的胎粪性肠梗阻。其余 1/2～2/3 为有并发症的病例，包括肠闭锁、肠旋转、肠穿孔、伴腹膜炎的胎粪性囊肿形成、肠坏疽或这些并发症的结合。对于单纯的胎粪性肠梗阻，手术的目的是解除回结肠的肠腔内梗阻，排出肠腔内黏附的胎粪或切除充满浓缩胎粪的肠段[83]。

单纯性胎粪性肠梗阻

对于胎粪性肠梗阻患儿有多种手术方式（图 81-7和图 81-8）[83]。起初该病的存活者接受肠切开灌洗及局限性肠管切除。这种手术技术是目前最常应用的。灌洗液包括温盐水、50% 泛影葡胺溶液、1% 胰酶溶液（Viokase; A. H. Robbins Co., Richmond, VA）、过氧化氢以及最常见的 2% 或 4% 的 N-乙酰半胱氨酸溶液（Mucomyst; Apothecon, Princeton, NJ）[76,100]。更高浓度的 N-乙酰半胱氨酸或泛影葡胺，或过氧化氢及其伴随的空气栓塞可能带来的危险大于益处。从肠切开导管注入增溶剂后，将胎粪轻轻地挤向远端的结肠，或从肠切开处排出（见图81-7）。关闭肠切开处及腹腔并做肠造瘘或在肠切开处置入 T 管[45,74,80,116]。T 管应置于近端扩张回肠与远端（较萎陷的）回肠的连接处，此处可发现肠腔内浓缩的胎粪团。将导管留于原位，使肠切开处紧贴前腹壁，从而保证有一可控的瘘管以及可供术后第一天起滴注胰酶溶液的胃肠道通路。术后 7～14 天冲洗液可畅通地进入结肠，说明梗阻解除，此后可拔除导管。这避免了再次手术及关闭造瘘。另一种方法是行阑尾切除及阑
尾造口术，通过此途径抽出胎粪或灌洗[32]。也可暂 1297
时留置盲肠造瘘管。为了保证此灌洗技术的成功，必须轻柔地操作肠管，肠管不可过度扩张，也不可为了使浓缩的胎粪排出而过度按摩或挤压肠管。

肠切开灌洗的一个替代手术是做暂时性解除梗阻的造瘘，可做或不做部分肠切除。Gross 首先提倡做 Mikulicz 双筒肠造瘘，此手术可快速完成且不需要术中抽空胎粪（见图 81-8）。可在关闭腹部切口后打开外置的肠管，如此可使腹腔内污染降至最低。当梗阻解除、婴儿康复后，可在造瘘处体外使用带刺的 Mikulicz 夹完成侧侧吻合。不必返回手术室关闭造瘘，

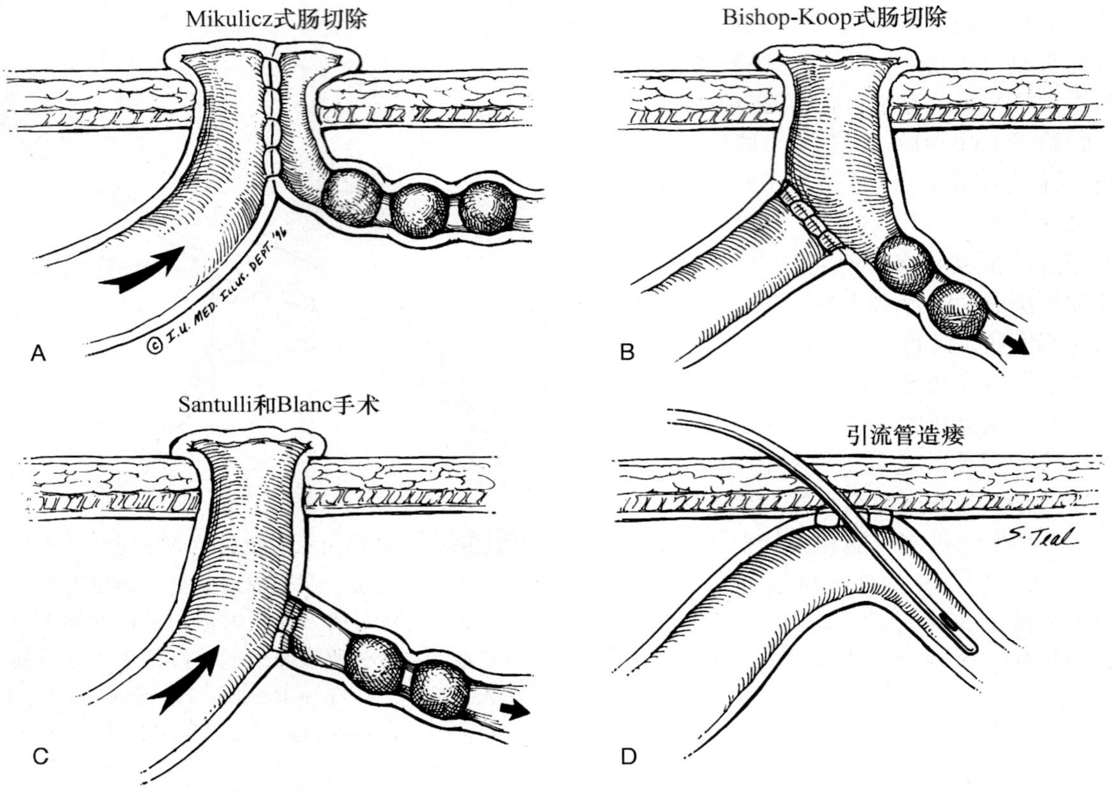

图 81-8　单纯性胎粪性肠梗阻的手术方式。A. Mikulicz 式肠切除及造瘘。B. Bishop-Koop 式肠切除及造瘘。C. Santulli 式造瘘。D. 引流管造瘘。（From Rescorla FJ, Grosfeld JL: Contemporary management of meconium ileus. World J Surg 1993; 17:381.）

因为在钳夹吻合后残余的肠外瘘可自行关闭。此腹腔外肠切除、延迟关闭造瘘的一种替代方法是 10 年后由 Swenson 和 Noblett 介绍的一期肠切除和吻合术。排出胎粪后，可行一期腹腔内吻合，或在患儿完全康复后做端端吻合、延迟关闭造瘘。

另一种替代的手术是做肠切除及远端烟囱状肠造瘘，即所谓的 Bishop-Koop 手术（见图 81-8）[67]。该技术可满足以下标准：（1）减少新生儿期术中肠损伤；（2）切除异常扩大的、充满浓缩增厚胎粪的回肠袢；（3）近端回肠口径合适并与远端回肠侧面吻合，吻合口靠近腹壁，远端回肠外置，当远端梗阻存在时作为能够为肠管减压的“近端造瘘口”；（4）为导管置入远端含有浓缩胎粪块的肠管提供了通路，便于手术后滴注增溶的胰酶；（5）最终可在床边通过结扎烟囱状造瘘口来关闭肠造瘘，使 CF 患儿避免再一次麻醉的风险。术中将 8F 的橡胶导管经烟囱状造瘘口插入远端回肠。术后 12～24 小时后经导管注入胰酶溶液（1 茶匙胰酶加 1 盎司水）进行灌洗，每 4～6小时重复一次直至远端肠腔梗阻解除，梗阻解除后拔除导管。起初肠造瘘排出量很多，当远端梗阻解除后会逐渐减少。随后粪便经结肠排出。此后造瘘口 1298
就停止排泄。最终有两种方式处理烟囱状造瘘口。可在床边结扎造瘘口。如果经这种非侵袭性的方法处理后有持续的肠外瘘，可在全麻下行正规的腹腔内或腹腔外造瘘关闭术，大约 75% 的患儿需用后一种方法处理[20]。

Santulli 描述了近端烟囱状造瘘术，本质上与切除肠管后远端做烟囱状造瘘相反（见图 81-8）。将远端回肠末端与近端回肠在紧贴筋膜下的平面做端侧吻合，近端回肠外置作为造瘘末端。通过这种造瘘，可加强对近端回肠的灌洗和减压。和 Bishop-Koop 手术一样，术中将导管经造瘘口插到远端回肠用于术后滴注增溶剂。由于建立了高排出量的功能性末端造瘘，需早期关闭造瘘口以避免液体和电解质过度丢失引起并发症。

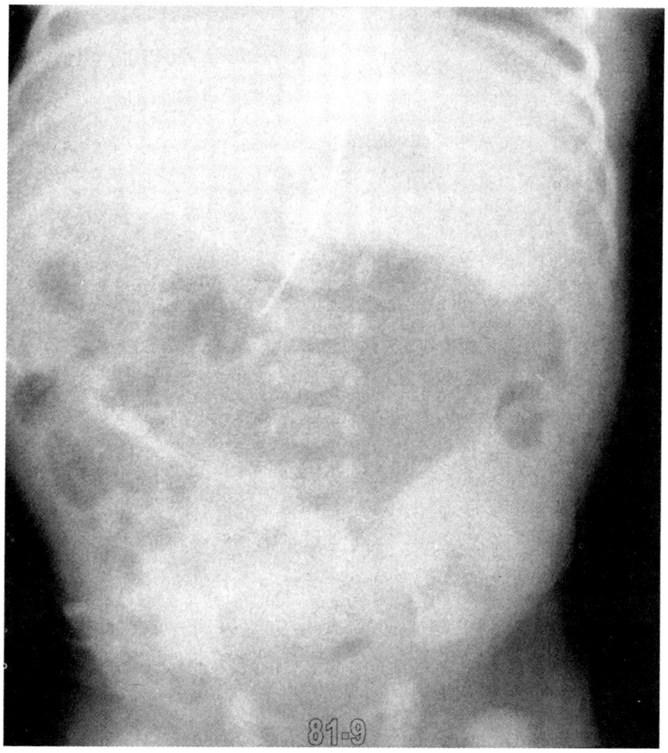

图 81-9　腹部平片符合复杂性胎粪性肠梗阻的诊断。中央巨大的被空气充盈的肿块提示有肠穿孔及巨大的胎粪性囊肿形成。如果穿孔时间更长，可出现腹腔内钙化。（From Rescorla FJ, Grosfeld JL: Contemporary management of meconium ileus. World J Surg 1993; 17:381.）

复杂性胎粪性肠梗阻

复杂性胎粪性肠梗阻一般需要手术治疗，罕见的例外是子宫内肠穿孔后钙化胎粪残留于肠腔外、腹膜内，穿孔处自行关闭，并且肠道保持连续性而无需手术[67]。而后者的另一种情况是疝手术时在开放的鞘状突内，或在以后腹部摄片时见到钙化的胎粪。相反，手术的指征则包括持续性肠梗阻、增大的腹部肿块、有腹膜炎征象，包括腹壁水肿、变色、体检时有压痛，以及有进行性败血症的临床及实验室征象（图 81-9）。

胎粪性腹膜炎是其中一种情况。胎粪性假囊肿是胎粪在腹腔内积聚数周或数月后形成的。胎粪被钙化的假囊肿的纤维囊壁包裹，多余的肠袢在假囊肿的周围（见图 81-9）。在出生前的几周或几月，胎粪污染腹腔后形成粘连的胎粪性腹膜炎。密集的肠管粘连及血管粘连使手术难以解除粘连性肠梗阻。腹腔内可有散在的钙化。如果肠穿孔发生在出生前几天，则腹腔内充满胎粪性腹水而没有钙化。胎粪性腹膜炎的第 4 种情况是细菌感染性腹水，当定殖于肠道的细菌经穿孔的肠管进入腹腔后就会发生这种情况。

手术中必须评估剩余肠管的长度，保守性切除是很关键的。需有效的手术医疗设备，从而使可能遇到的胎粪性腹膜炎、肠扭转、肠闭锁或肠缺血得到最佳治疗。只有出现弥漫性细菌性腹膜炎时才不能做一期吻合。治疗复杂性胎粪性肠梗阻患儿时，Bishop-Koop 手术、Mikulicz 手术及 Santlli 手术都有其各自的适用性。

术后处理

胎粪性肠梗阻行手术治疗后，需关注患儿全身的生理性支持以及近端或远端胃肠道内残余的浓缩胎粪的排出情况。一般可经鼻胃管注入 2% 或 4% 乙酰半胱氨酸（痰易净）以溶解残余的胎粪。当临床或 X 线摄片证实肠道通畅后，可从要素配方奶开始肠内营养，如哺力美（Mead-Johnson, Evansville, IN）。当肠内营养开始后，必须添加补充的胰酶［可供选择的有 Viokase，Pancrease（McNeil Pharmaceuticals, Spring Hill, PA）和 Cotazym-S（Organon Inc., West Orange, NJ）］。如果手术后肠梗阻时间延长或手术治疗后发 1299
生短肠综合征，则全肠外营养成为重要的术后早期营养治疗，并且其使用时间可延长。早期的肠内或肠外营养治疗必须保持盐分和矿物质平衡；适当补充维生素，如维生素 K；以及积极治疗短肠综合征引起的任何营养缺乏。CF 固有的吸收不良如伴发复杂性胎粪性肠梗阻引起的严重短肠综合征将给治疗带来很大困难[114,120]。

单纯性或复杂性胎粪性肠梗阻术后可短期使用静脉内抗生素，而有针对性的、较长时间的抗感染治疗可使潜在的肺部并发症降至最低。有力的肺部物理治疗应在手术后及早开始并无限制地持续应用。教会患儿家长进行包括体位引流在内的肺部物理治疗是出院前计划中的一个必需部分。对于做造瘘的患儿，教会家长正确地护理造瘘口也很重要。只有对于做 Bishop-Koop 或 Mikulicz 回肠造瘘的患儿，才可在出院前考虑为其在床边结扎烟囱状造瘘口或使用 Mikulicz 钳。

术后处理中最重要的一点可能是确定 CF 为胎粪性肠梗阻的原因。一些文章报道新生儿肠腔内浓缩的胎粪是小肠梗阻的原因，并应用了以上概括的相同的治疗方案。然而，这些患儿术后未被发现汗液电解质异常。由于胎粪栓塞局限于小肠，故这些病例已经与结肠性胎粪栓塞综合征清楚地区别开来。据报道这种情况见于早产儿、无 CF 的同胞、胰腺部分发育不良及胰管狭窄的患儿[117]。这些发现也是与伴 CF 的胎粪性肠梗阻的重要区别。

并发症

胃肠道并发症

胎粪性肠梗阻有许多胃肠道并发症，如肠套迭及直肠脱垂，其发生率均较高。然而，对于患有 CF 的儿童和青少年，最常见的胃肠道问题是远端肠梗阻，称为胎粪性肠梗阻等位症或远端肠梗阻综合征[40]。肠腔内物质所致的部分肠梗阻可能是由于脂肪泻或不耐受口服酶治疗引起的。痉挛性腹痛、腹胀和可触及的右下腹肿块等症状和体征提示该疾病的发生，高位肠梗阻可伴有顽固性便秘、腹胀、呕吐。需考虑其他多种疾病，包括便秘、肠套迭甚至阑尾炎，腹部平片结合对比躯体显像具有诊断价值。一旦确立诊断，首选的治疗是增溶剂，比如乙酰半胱氨酸和泛影葡胺，口服及经直肠同时给药。很少需手术治疗。调整口服酶疗法辅以更好的水合作用以及使用粪便软化剂可预防复发。组胺 H_2 受体阻滞剂和质子泵抑制剂均可通过提高肠道 pH 而起效，也可应用促运动剂。

阑尾腔梗阻产生的症状、体征可与急性或慢性阑尾炎相似[17]。阑尾病理学诊断取决于临床评估及造影剂的应用——增强 CT。这些并发症，以及最常见的胃肠道并发症吸收不良，通过适当的酶替代治疗可以得到改善。碳水化合物、蛋白质、脂肪吸收不良都可发生，腹腔内炎症的范围和短肠综合征的严重程度都可促使病情恶化。后者可能为功能性或解剖性的，解剖学上的短缩是由肠闭锁或肠切除造成的。双糖酶缺乏或胆汁浓缩加重了吸收不良，也可引起黄疸及脂肪吸收障碍。相同的病理生理学过程可造成 1/4 的 CF 患儿患胆结石，也可引发有症状的慢性结石性胆囊炎或胆道运动障碍，这也是 CF 患儿特征性的表现。如果出现反复或慢性肺部感染使得能量需求增加时，营养吸收不良的问题就显得更为严重。完全肠外营养证明能有效补充肠内营养物，在长时间的手术后肠梗阻期间提供适当的热卡，并使得肠道休息，特别在吻合口愈合或需要关闭肠外瘘时更有益。此外，有证据显示，与无胎粪性肠梗阻的同龄 CF 患儿相比，胎粪性肠梗阻的营养吸收不良明显不同甚至更严重。

年龄较大的 CF 患儿中，肠套迭的发生率约为 1%，肠腔内浓缩的粪便可能是诱发点。典型的发病部位是回结肠结合部，但小肠或结肠套迭也可发生。通常难以作出诊断，并且很难和 CF 的其他右下腹疾病鉴别，手术整复和/或肠管切除是常用的治疗方式。

直肠脱垂可能是发汗试验证实为 CF 后患儿的首个临床表现。1/5～1/3 的 CF 患儿可在 1～3 岁特征性地发生直肠脱垂。CF 确诊后首选的治疗方法为口服酶，很少需要进行经肛门直肠黏膜下硬化治疗或行直肠固定术。

据报道 CF 患儿发生的结肠狭窄[33,85,105,123]可能 1300
继发于大剂量口服酶治疗，其中一半患儿之前有胎粪性肠梗阻。这种疾病最常局限于右结肠，也有节段性结肠炎甚至全结肠病变的报道。梗阻和疼痛的局部征象需与胎粪性肠梗阻的症状相鉴别，对比灌肠具有诊断价值。可尝试调整酶疗法，但顽固性狭窄需行最常用的肠管切除术。

肺部并发症

胎粪性肠梗阻的早期发病和死亡的原因主要是肺源性的，包括细菌性败血症和支气管肺炎。一些学者认为胎粪性肠梗阻治疗 6 个月后，其预后和发病率与无胎粪性肠梗阻的 CF 患儿相似。但是其他研究显示胎粪性肠梗阻患儿在 8～12 岁时比无胎粪性肠梗阻的 CF 患儿肺功能差，更易患阻塞性肺疾病。这些改变的发生可相对减少肺容量。当确定有假单胞菌、大肠杆菌或其他特定的定殖或致病微生物时，早期积极使用（即使是预防性地使用）氨基糖苷类和半合成青霉素已证实能提高存活率、改善预后。最后，使用物理治疗和体位引流可进一步使肺部并发症降至最低。

腹股沟阴囊疾病

据报道，CF 患儿腹股沟疝、鞘膜积液和隐睾的发生率增加[53,119]。腹股沟疝修补术中的两个发现能够提示潜在的 CF，即在疝囊内出现钙化的胎粪和输精管缺如[90]。在先前未作出 CF 诊断的情况下，这两个发现提示需要做诊断性发汗试验。此外，输精管缺如的不育男性可能是无症状的携带 CF 基因的杂合子。

治疗效果

无论是复杂性或是单纯性的胎粪性肠梗阻，在过去的 30 年中其治疗效果有了稳步提高，根据最新报道，其存活率接近 100% （图 81-10）[13,20]。在一组接受非手术和手术治疗的患儿中，其 5 年和 10 年存活率从上世纪 60 年代（分别为 30% 和 10%）到 70 年代（分别为 80% 和 70%）和 80 年代（随访 5 年为 100%）在稳步提高[35,57,75,77]。过去，存活率的提高归功于非手术治疗，但在过去的 10 年中，手术和非手术治疗的存活率均达到 100%。自从上世纪 60 年代以来（6 个月存活率仅为 33%），手术存活率有了显著提高[72]。在 1979 年之前，手术后 6 个月存活率为 60%，1979—1989 年间达到 100%[88]。不论患儿的性别、是否有胎粪性肠梗阻的并发症，以及手术类型（回肠造瘘、一期肠切除加肠吻合、肠切除后做 Mikulicz 回肠造瘘，以及 Bishop-Koop 肠造瘘），治疗结果总体上没有显著差异。此外，用 Bishop-Koop 手术治疗的长期存活率（6 年为 62%）与接受其他手术治疗的患儿没有区别，并且所有大于 6 个月的患儿均死于和 CF 有关的心肺疾病或肺炎，而和手术并发症无关。有趣的是，单纯性和复杂性胎粪性肠梗阻病例的 10 年存活率均为 72%。

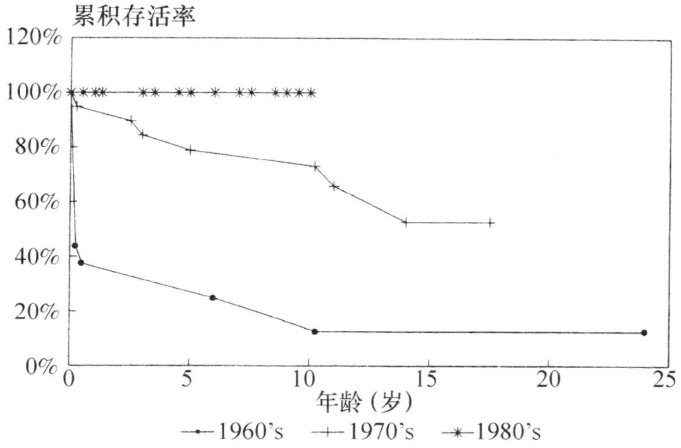

图 81-10 以 10 年分界描述的胎粪性肠梗阻患儿的长期存活率。通过比较上世纪 60 年代、70 年代、80 年代的存活率数据，可以发现存活率在统计学上有明显提高（$P < 0.0001$）。（From Del Pin CA, Czyrko C, Ziegler MM, et al: Management and survival of meconium ileus: A 30-year review. Ann Surg 1992; 215: 179-185.）

死亡的原因很多，包括未发现的漏引起的腹腔内脓毒症、肺部脓毒症、支气管肺炎或短肠综合征并发肝衰竭。

（陈 盛译 董其刚校）

参考文献

1. Allan DL, Robbie M, Phelan PD, et al: Familial occurrence of meconium ileus. Eur J Pediatr 1981;135:291-292.
2. Anderson DH: Cystic fibrosis of the pancreas and its relation to celiac disease. Am J Dis Child 1938;56:344-399.
3. Anderson DH: Cystic fibrosis of the pancreas. J Chron Dis 1958;7:58-90.
4. Auburn RP, Feldman SA, Gadacz TR, et al: Meconium ileus secondary to partial aplasia of the pancreas: Report of a case. Surgery 1969;65:689-693.
5. Benacerraf BR, Chaudhury AK: Echogenic fetal bowel in the third trimester associated with meconium ileus secondary to cystic fibrosis: A case report. J Reprod Med 2001; 46:697-698.
6. Bishop HC, Koop CE: Management of meconium ileus: Resection, Roux-en-Y anastomosis and ileostomy irrigation with pancreatic enzymes. Ann Surg 1957;145:410.
7. Bishop HC, Ziegler MM: Meconium ileus. In Spitz L, Nixon HH (eds): Rob and Smith's Operative Surgery, 4th ed. Boston, Butterworth, 1988, vol 10, pp 300-310.
8. Bowring AC, Jones RFC, Kern IB: The use of solvents in the intestinal manifestations of mucoviscidosis. J Pediatr Surg 1970;5:338-343.
9. Bruns WT, Connell TR, Lacey JA, et al: Test strip meconium screening for cystic fibrosis. Am J Dis Child 1977;131:71-73.
10. Buchanan DJ, Rapoport S: Chemical comparison of normal meconium and meconium from a patient with meconium ileus. Pediatrics 1952;9:304-310.
11. Burke MS, Rag JM, Karamanoukian HL, et al: New strategies in nonoperative management of meconium ileus. J Pediatr Surg 2002;37:760-764.
12. Byrk D: Meconium ileus: Demonstration of the meconium mass on barium enema study. AJR Am J Roentgenol 1965;95:214-216.
13. Caniano DA, Beaver BL: Meconium ileus: A fifteen year experience with forty-two neonates. Surgery 1987;102: 699-703.

14. Clatworthy HW Jr, Howard WHR, Lloyd J: The meconium plug syndrome. Surgery 1956;39:131-142.
15. Colin AA, Wohl MEB: Cystic fibrosis. Pediatr Rev 1994; 15:192-200.
16. Cooney DR, Rosevear W, Grosfeld JL: Maternal and postnatal hypermagnesemia and the meconium plug syndrome. J Pediatr Surg 1976;11:167-172.
17. Coughlin JP, Gauderer MWI, Stern RC, et al: The spectrum of appendiceal disease in cystic fibrosis. J Pediatr Surg 1990;25:835-839.
18. Davis WS, Allen RP, Favara BE, et al: Neonatal small left colon syndrome. AJR Am J Roentgenol 1974;120:322-329.
19. Delorimier AA, Fonkalsrud EW, Hays DM: Congenital atresia and stenosis of the jejunum and ileum. Surgery 1969;65:819-827.
20. Del Pin CA, Czyrko C, Ziegler MM, et al: Management and survival of meconium ileus, a 30 year review. Ann Surg 1992;215:179-185.
21. Dirkes K, Crombleholme TM, Craigo SD, et al: The natural history of meconium peritonitis diagnosed in utero. J Pediatr Surg 1995;30:979-982.
22. Dey DL: The surgical treatment of meconium ileus. Med J Aust 1963;50:179-180.
23. di Sant'Agnese PA, Davis PB: Research in cystic fibrosis. N Engl J Med 1976;295:481-485.
24. di Sant'Agnese PA, Dische Z, Danilczenko A: Physiochemical differences of mucoproteins in duodenal fluid of patients with cystic fibrosis of the pancreas and controls. Pediatrics 1957;19:252-260.
25. Dolan TF Jr, Touloukian RJ: Familial meconium ileus not associated with cystic fibrosis. J Pediatr Surg 1974;9: 821-824.
26. Donnison AB, Shwachman H, Gross RE: A review of 164 children with meconium ileus seen at the Children's Hospital Medical Center, Boston. Pediatrics 1966;37:1-18.
27. Egan M, Flotte T, Alfone S, et al: Defective regulation of outwardly rectifying Cl channels by protein kinase A corrected by insertion of CFTR. Nature 1992;358:581-584.
28. Ein S, Shandling B, Reilly B, et al: Bowel perforation with nonoperative treatment of meconium ileus. J Pediatr Surg 1987;22:146-147.
29. Ellis DG, Clatworthy HW Jr: The meconium plug syndrome revisited. J Pediatr Surg 1966;1:54-61.
30. Emery JL: Laboratory observations of the viscidity of meconium. Arch Dis Child 1954;29:34-37.
31. Farber SJ: The relation of pancreatic achylia to meconium ileus. J Pediatr 1944;24:387-392.
32. Fitzgerald R, Conlan K: Use of the appendix stump in the treatment of meconium ileus. J Pediatr Surg 1989;24: 899-900.
33. Fitzsimmons SC, Burkhart GA, Borowitz D, et al: High dose pancreatic enzyme supplements and fibrosing colonopathy in children with cystic fibrosis. N Engl J Med 1997;336: 1283-1289.
34. French RS, McAlister WH, Ternberg J, et al: Meconium ileus relieved by 40% water-soluble contrast enemas. Radiology 1970;94:341-342.
35. George L, Norman AP: Life tables for cystic fibrosis. Arch Dis Child 1971;46:139-143.
36. Gibson LE, Cooke RE: A test for concentration of electrolytes in sweat in cystic fibrosis of the pancreas utilizing pilocarpine by iontophoresis. Pediatrics 1959;23:545-549.
37. Gilis DA, Grantmyre EB: The meconium plug syndrome and Hirschsprung's disease. Can Med Assoc J 1965;92: 225-227.
38. Glanzmann E: Dysporia entero-broncho-pancreatica congenita familiaris. Ann Paediat 1946;166:289.
39. Glanzmann E, Berger H: Uber mekoniumileus. Ann Pediatr 1950;175:33.
40. Goldschmidt Z, Cohen H, Issacsohn M, et al: Meconium ileus equivalent in an infant, aggravated by soybean formula. Clin Pediatr 1977;16:284-286.
41. Graham WP, Halden A, Jaffe BF: Surgical treatment of patients with cystic fibrosis. Surg Gynecol Obstet 1966;122:373.
42. Grantmyre EB, Butler GJ, Gillis DA: Necrotizing enterocolitis after Renografin-76 treatment of meconium ileus. Am J Radiol 1981;136:990.
43. Green MN, Clarke JT, Shwachman H: Studies in cystic fibrosis of the pancreas: Protein pattern in meconium ileus. Pediatrics 1958;21:635-641.
44. Green MA, Shwachman H: Presumptive tests for cystic fibrosis based on serum protein in meconium. Pediatrics 1968;41:989-992.
45. Harberg FJ, Senekjian EK, Pokorny WJ: Treatment of uncomplicated meconium ileus via T-tube ileostomy. J Pediatr Surg 1981;16:61-63.
46. Hauerback BJ, Dyce BJ, Gutentag PJ, et al: Measurement of trypsin and chymotrypsin in stool. Gastroenterology 1963;44:588-597.
47. Henson RE: Meconium ileus. Radiology 1957;68:568-571.
48. Hiatt RB, Wilson PE: Celiac syndrome: Therapy of meconium ileus: Report of eight eases with a review of the literature. Surg Gynecol Obstet 1948;87:317-327.
49. Hill JT, Snyder WH, Pollock WF: Management of complicated meconium ileus. Am J Surg 1964;108:233-238.
50. Hinden E: Meconium ileus with no pancreatic abnormality. Arch Dis Child 1950;25:99-100.
51. Holsclaw DS, Eckstein HB, Nixon HH: Meconium ileus: A 20 year review of 109 cases. Am J Dis Child 1965;109: 101-113.
52. Holsclaw DS Jr, Keith HH, Palmer J: Meconium screening for cystic fibrosis. Pediatr Ann 1978;7:29-40.
53. Holsclaw DS, Schwachman H: Increased incidence of hydrocele and undescended testicles in males with cystic fibrosis. Pediatrics 1971;3:442.
54. Hurwill ES, Arnheim EE: Meconium ileus associated with stenosis of the pancreatic ducts. Am J Dis Child 1942;64:443-454.
55. Ikeda K, Goto S: Total colonic aganglionosis with or without small bowel involvement: An analysis of 137 patients. J Pediatr Surg 1986;21:319-322.
56. Irish MS, Ragi JM, Karamanoukian H, et al: Prenatal diagnosis of the fetus with cystic fibrosis and meconium ileus. Pediatr Surg Int 1997;12:434-436.
57. Kalayoglu M, Sieber WK, Rodnan JB, et al: Meconium ileus: A critical review of treatment and eventual prognosis. J Pediatr Surg 1971;6:290-300.
58. Kao SCS, Franken EA Jr: Non-operative treatment of simple meconium ileus: A survey of the Society for Pediatric Radiology. Pediatr Radiol 1995;25:97-100.
59. Keats TE, Smith TH: Meconium ileus: A demonstration of the ileal meconium mass by barium enema examination. Radiology 1967;89:1073-1074.
60. Kerem BS, Rommens JM, Buchanan JA, et al: Identification of the cystic fibrosis gene: Genetic analysis. Science 1989;245:1073-1080.
61. Kerem E, Corey M, Kerem B, et al: Clinical and genetic comparisons of patients with cystic fibrosis, with or without meconium ileus. J Pediatr 1989;114:767-773.
62. Kleinhaus S, Boley SJ, Sheran M, et al: Hirschsprung's disease: A survey of the members of the surgical section of the

American Academy of Pediatrics. J Pediatr Surg 1979;14:588-597.
63. Knowlton RG, Cohen-Haguenauer O, VanCong N, et al: A polymorphic DNA marker linked to cystic fibrosis is located on chromosome 7. Nature 1985;318:380-382.
64. Kornblith BA, Otani S: Meconium ileus with congenital stenosis of the main pancreatic duct. Am J Pathol 1929;5:249-262.
65. Kopito L, Shwachman H: Mineral composition of meconium. J Pediatr 1966;68:313-314.
66. Lansteiner K: Darmverschlus durch eingedictes meconium pankreatitis. Zentralbl Allg Pathol 1905;16:903-907.
67. Leonidas JC, Berdon WE, Baker DH, et al: Meconium ileus and its complications: A reappraisal of plain film roentgen diagnostic criteria. AJR Am J Roentgenol 1970;108:598.
68. Leonidas JC, Burry VF, Fellows RA, et al: Possible adverse effect of methylglucamine diatrizoate compounds on the bowel of newborn infants with meconium ileus. Radiology 1976;121:693-696.
69. Li Z, Lai HC, Kosorok MR, et al: Longitudinal pulmonary status of cystic fibrosis children with meconium ileus. Pediatr Pulmonol 2004;38:277-284.
70. Lillie JG, Chrispin AR: Investigation and management of neonatal obstruction by Gastrografin enema. Ann Radiol 1972;15:237.
71. Lutzger LG, Factor SM: Effects of some water-soluble contrast media on the colonic mucosa. Radiology 1976; 118:545-548.
72. MacDonald JA, Trusler GA: Meconium ileus: An eleven-year review at the Hospital for Sick Children, Toronto. Can Med Assoc J 1960;83:881-885.
73. Manchaurin C: Functional ileus of the newborn. Aust NZ J Surg 1964;34:196.
74. Mak GZ, Harberg FJ, Hiatt P, et al: T-tube ileostomy for meconium ileus: Four decades of experience. J Pediatr Surg 2000;35:349-352.
75. McPartlin JF, Dickson JAS, Swain VAJ: Meconium ileus immediate and long-term survival. Arch Dis Child 1972;47:207-210.
76. Meeker IA, Kincannon WN: Acetylcysteine used to liquefy inspissated meconium causing intestinal obstruction in the newborn. Surgery 1964;56:419-425.
77. Mabogunje OA, Wang CI, Mahour GH: Improved survival of neonates with meconium ileus. Arch Surg 1982;117: 37-40.
78. Mornet E, Serre JL, Farrell M, et al: Genetic differences between cystic fibrosis with or without meconium ileus. Lancet 1988;1:376-378.
79. Neuhauser EBD: Roentgen changes associated with pancreatic insufficiency in early life. Radiology 1946;46: 319-328.
80. Nguyen LT, Youssef S, Guttman FM, et al: Meconium ileus: Is a stoma necessary? J Pediatr Surg 1986;21:766-768.
81. Noblett HR: Treatment of uncomplicated meconium ileus by Gastrografin enema: A preliminary report. J Pediatr Surg 1969;4:190-197.
82. Olim CB, Ciuti A: Meconium ileus: A new method of relieving obstruction. Ann Surg 1954;140:736-740.
83. O'Neill JA, Grosfeld JL, Boles ET Jr, et al: Surgical treatment of meconium ileus. Am J Surg 1970;119:99-105.
84. Oppenheimer EH, Easterly JR: Pathological evidence of cystic fibrosis patients with meconium ileus. Pediatr Res 1973;7:339.
85. Pettei MJ, Leonidas JC, Levine JJ, Garvoy JD: Pancolonic disease in cystic fibrosis and high dose pancreatic enzyme therapy. J Pediatr 1994;125:587-589.
86. Philipart AI, Reed JO, Georgenson KE: Neonatal small left colon syndrome: Intramural not intraluminal obstruction. J Pediatr Surg 1975;10:733-740.
87. Quinton PM, Bijman J: Higher bioelectric potentials due to decreased chloride absorption in the sweat glands of patients with cystic fibrosis. N Engl J Med 1983;308: 1185-1189.
88. Rescorla FJ, Grosfeld J, West KJ, et al: Changing patterns of treatment and survival in neonates with meconium ileus. Arch Surg 1989;124:837-840.
89. Rickham DP, Boeckman CR: Neonatal meconium obstruction in the absence of mucoviscidosis. Am J Surg 1965;109:173-177.
90. Rigot JM, Lafitte JJ, Dumur V, et al: Cystic fibrosis and congenital absence of the vas deferens. N Engl J Med 1991; 325:64-65.
91. Riordan JR, Rommens JM, Kerem BS, et al: Identification of the cystic fibrosis gene: Cloning and characterization of complementary DNA. Science 1989;245:1066-1073.
92. Rommens JM, Iannazzi MC, Kerem B, et al: Identification of cystic fibrosis gene: Chromosome walking and jumping. Science 1989;245:1059-1065.
93. Rosenstein BJ: Cystic fibrosis presenting with the meconium plug syndrome. Am J Dis Child 1978;132:167-169.
94. Rosenstein BJ, Langbaum TS: Incidence of meconium abnormalities in newborn infants with cystic fibrosis. Am J Dis Child 1980;134:72-73.
95. Rowe MI, Furst AJ, Altman DH, et al: The neonatal response to Gastrografin enema. Pediatrics 1971;48:28-35.
96. Rowe MI, Seagram G, Weinberger M: Gastrografin-induced hypertonicity. Am J Surg 1973;125:185-188.
97. Santulli TV, Blanc WA: Congenital atresia of the intestine: Pathogenesis and treatment. Ann Surg 1961;154: 939-948.
98. Schiller M, Grosfeld JL, Morse TS: Nonoperative treatment of meconium ileus: An experimental study in rats. Am J Surg 1971;122:22-26.
99. Shariatzadeh AN, Enderle FJ, Fitzgerald JF, et al: Meconium ileus. Surg Gynecol Obstet 1973;136:234-236.
100. Shaw A: Safety of *N*-acetylcysteine in treatment of meconium obstruction of the newborn. J Pediatr Surg 1969;4:119-125.
101. Shigemoto H, Endo S, Isomoto T, et al: Neonatal meconium obstruction in the ileum without mucoviscidosis. J Pediatr Surg 1978;13:475-479.
102. Shwachman H: Gastrointestinal manifestations of cystic fibrosis. Pediatr Clin North Am 1975;22:787-805.
103. Shwachman H, Dooley RR, Guilmette R, et al: Cystic fibrosis of the pancreas with varying degrees of pancreatic insufficiency. Am J Dis Child 1956;92:347-368.
104. Shwachman H, Lebenthal E, Khaw KT: Recurrent acute pancreatitis in patients with cystic fibrosis with normal pancreatic enzymes. Pediatrics 1975;55:86-95.
105. Smyth RH, Van Velzen D, Smyth AR, et al: Stricture of ascending colon in cystic fibrosis and high-strength pancreatic enzymes. Lancet 1994;343:85-86.
106. Sokol MM, Koenigsberger MR, Rose JS, et al: Neonatal hypermagnesemia and the meconium plug syndrome. N Engl J Med 1972;286:823-825.
107. Stephan U, Busch EW, Kollberg H, et al: Cystic fibrosis detection by means of a test strip. Pediatrics 1975;55:35-38.
108. Stewart DR, Nixon GW, Johnson DG, et al: Neonatal small left colon syndrome. Ann Surg 1977;186:741-745.
109. Stringer MD, Brereton RJ, Drake DP, et al: Meconium ileus due to extensive intestinal aganglionosis. J Pediatr Surg 1994;29:501-503.

110. Swischuk LE: Meconium plug syndrome: a cause of neonatal intestinal obstruction. Am J Roentgenol Radiat Ther Nucl Med 1968;103:339-346.
111. Thomaidis TS, Arey JB: The intestinal lesions in cystic fibrosis of the pancreas. J Pediatr 1963;63:444-453.
112. Townes PL, Kopelman AE: Meconium plug syndrome, cystic fibrosis, and exocrine pancreatic deficiency. Am J Dis Child 1978;132:1043-1044.
113. Tsui LC, Buchwald M: Biochemical and molecular genetics of cystic fibrosis. Adv Human Genet 1991;202:153.
114. Vaisman N, Pencharz P, Corey M, et al: Energy expenditure of patients with cystic fibrosis. J Pediatr 1987;111: 496-500.
115. VanLeeuwen G, Riley WC, Glenn L, et al: Meconium plug syndrome with aganglionosis. Pediatrics 1967;40: 665-666.
116. Venugopal S, Shandling B: Meconium ileus: Laparotomy without resection, anastomosis or enterostomy. J Pediatr Surg 1979;14:715-718.
117. Vinograd I, Mogle P, Peleg O, et al: Meconium disease in premature infants with very low birth weight. J Pediatr 1983;103:963-966.
118. Wagget J, Bishop HC, Koop CE: Experience with Gastrografin enema in the treatment of meconium ileus. J Pediatr Surg 1970;5:649-654.
119. Wang CI, Kwok S, Edelbrock H: Inguinal hernia, hydrocele, and other genitourinary abnormalities in boys with cystic fibrosis and their male siblings. Am J Dis Child 1970;119:236-237.
120. Warner BW, Ziegler MM: Management of the short bowel syndrome in the pediatric population. Pediatr Clin North Am 1993;40:1335-1350.
121. White H: Meconium ileus: A new roentgen sign. Radiology 1956;66:567.
122. Wildhaben J, Seelentag WKF, Spiegel R, Schoni MH: Cystic fibrosis associated with neuronal intestinal dysplasia type B: A case report. J Pediatr Surg 1996;31:951-954.
123. Wood BP, Katzberg RW, Ryan DH, et al: Diatrizoate enemas: Facts and fallacies of colonic toxicity. Radiology 1978;126:441-444.
124. Ziegler MM: Meconium ileus. Curr Probl Surg 1994;31:736-777.
125. Zuelzer WW, Newton WA: Pathogenesis of fibrocystic disease of the pancreas. Pediatrics 1949;4:53-69.

第 82 章

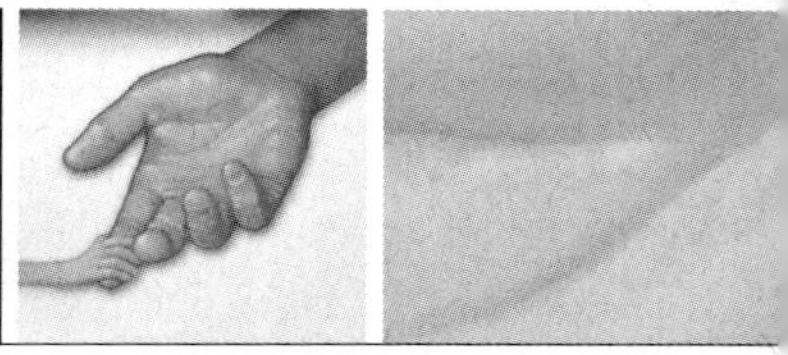

Meckel 憩室

Charles L. Snyder

历史回顾

1304 Hildanus 于 1598 年首次描述了 Meckel 憩室[23,32]。Lavater 和荷兰解剖学家 Ruysch 也分别于 1672 年和 1701 年描述了此病[50]。在同一时代，Littre 报道在疝中发现憩室[33]。1809 年，解剖学家及医生 Meckel（小 Meckel）确定脐肠系膜管是憩室的来源[38,39]，并提出是该病的潜在病因。1861 年，Zenker[67] 发现憩室内有异位的胰腺黏膜。1904 年，Salzer[51] 发现憩室内有胃黏膜。19 世纪末 20 世纪初，有学者对 Meckel 憩室的炎症及梗阻并发症进行了首次描述[17,30,56,63]。

胚胎学和解剖学

在胎儿发育的早期，胚盘与卵黄囊相连。随着胚胎生长，胚盘向内合拢，卵黄囊变窄变长。体腔内的卵黄囊形成肠道。胎儿的中肠通过脐肠系膜管与卵黄囊相连（也称为卵黄管或卵黄蒂；图 82-1）。卵黄管常在妊娠 5~7 周时发生退化，此时有功能的胎盘取代卵黄囊成为发育中胎儿的主要营养来源[59]。近端卵黄管未能闭塞则导致 Meckel 憩室的发生。卵黄管的异常退化也可引起另一种畸形——卵黄管囊肿，有纤维索带连接肠道及腹壁、脐窦，如卵黄管完全存留（卵黄管未闭）则形成脐回肠瘘[42]。这些畸形如图 82-2 所示。左右卵黄动脉在卵黄蒂内起源于主动脉：左卵黄动脉退化，右卵黄动脉则保留成为肠系膜上动脉，末端给 Meckel 憩室供血。卵黄动脉远端残留部分可成为憩室系膜带，延伸至憩室的顶端，偶尔与腹壁连接。

Meckel 憩室是最常见的卵黄管畸形。它位于小肠的系膜对侧缘，为真性肠道憩室（含有肠壁所有正常层次）[56]。25% 的患儿憩室与腹壁相连[59]。Meckel 憩室的位置多变，虽然大多数位于距回盲瓣 90 cm（约 3 英尺）以内，但还有 1/3 位于更近端的肠道。对于年长的儿童，至少需检查 5 英尺的小肠以充分排除 Meckel憩室[26,59]。发现异位黏膜（正常组织位于异常位置）的频率取决于临床表现。约 15% 切除的憩室偶尔有异常黏膜。然而，约 67% 有症状的患儿有异位组织[65,66]，主要是胃组织和胰腺组织。据报道，出现的概率分别为 60%~85% 及 5%~16%[12,35,62,42]。其他类型的黏膜（结肠、子宫内膜、胰岛）非常罕见。

“2 规则” 常用来记忆 Meckel 憩室。Meckel 憩室位于小肠末端 2 英尺内，长度为 2 英寸，人群中发生率为 2%，男性为女性的 2 倍，常在 2 岁时出现症状，含有两种异位黏膜——胃黏膜和胰腺黏膜。

发病率

Meckel 憩室是最常见的先天性消化道畸形，大量尸检和外科手术中的检出率大约为 1%~2%[2,20,21,36,60]。尚未明确引起 Meckel 憩室的潜在基因缺陷。在无症状患儿中，男女比例几乎相等；然而，在有症状的患儿中，男性发病更多（3:1~4:1）[4]。许多有 Meckel 憩室的个体未出现症状，但超过 3/4 的有症状患者在 20 岁以内发病，且常在 2 岁以内[59]。

伴发疾病 1305

虽然大多数病例是单发的，但据报道 Meckel 憩室伴发的很多其他先天性畸形的发生率在增加，包括

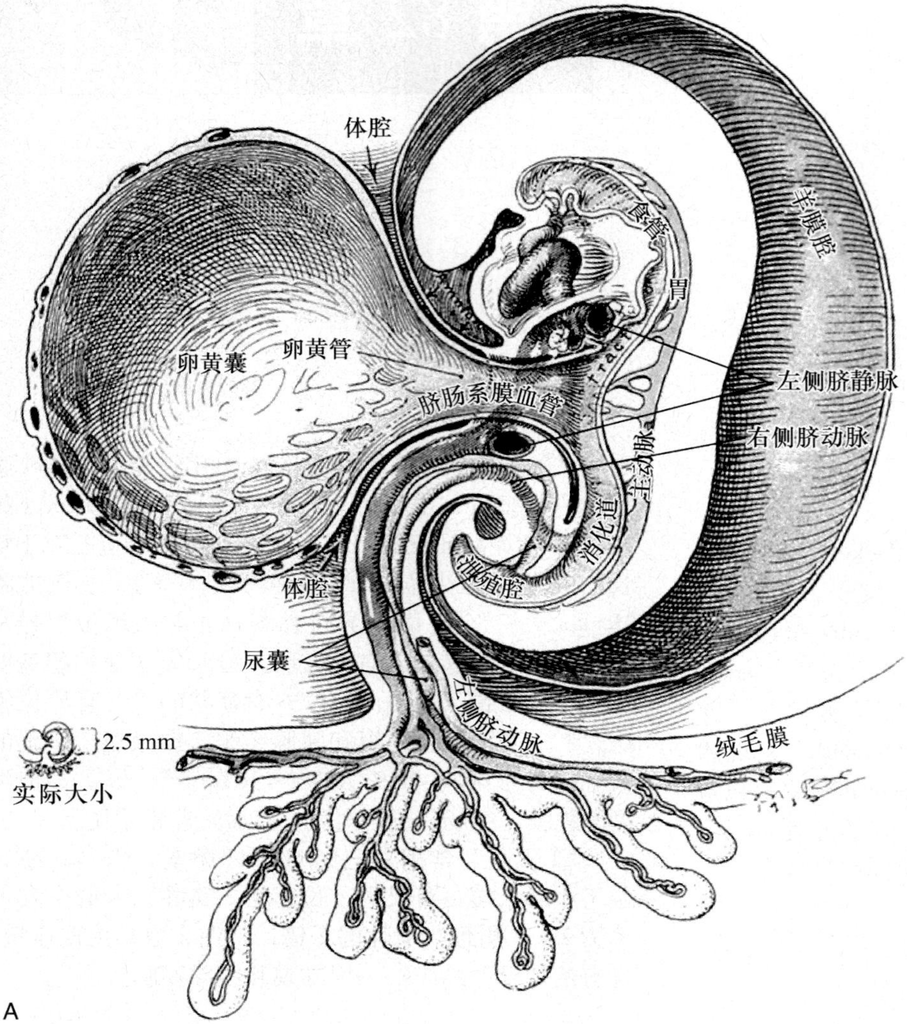

A

图 82-1 脐肠系膜结构未完全退化的胚胎。A. 在较早期阶段，膨大的卵黄囊通过卵黄管或脐肠系膜管向胎儿中肠排空。可见通向胎盘的体蒂及脐血管与卵黄管相邻。

食管闭锁、十二指肠闭锁、肛门闭锁、脐膨出、肠旋转不良、先天性巨结肠、Down 综合征、先天性膈疝和各种先天性神经系统及心血管畸形[44,58,60,62]。尸检发现伴随畸形的发生率远高于临床数据[10,59]。在一项大型尸检报道中，Meckel 憩室伴发食管闭锁或肛门闭锁的发生率超过 10%，约 5% 患有神经系统或心血管畸形的患儿有 Meckel 憩室。有 Meckel 憩室的患儿一般不需检查有无其他畸形，因为少于 5% 的患儿有伴发畸形[58]。有趣的是，Meckel 憩室很少伴有脐尿管和脐肠系膜畸形。

连续 294 例因 Crohn 病行右半结肠切除术的患儿中，约 6% 发现有 Meckel 憩室，比预期的普通人群发病率要高得多[3]。据另一个小样本的 Crohn 病患儿的报道显示，该组患儿中无一例有异位黏膜[14]。

流行病学

很难准确地评估偶然发现的 Meckel 憩室患者一生中发生并发症的可能性。两个大型研究估计此可能性为 4.2% 和 6.4%[11,61]。随着年龄增加，并发症的发生率可能会下降，但有报道得出相反的结果[5,11,65]。据报道，Meckel 憩室发生并发症的可能性增加的相关因素包括年龄小于 40 岁、男性、有异位黏膜以及憩室长度超过 2 cm[6,18,34-36]。

对于可扪及憩室增厚（说明有异位的黏膜）的非复杂性、有无法解释的腹痛史，以及憩室与腹壁附着的偶然发现的病例，需行选择性切除术。对于免疫缺陷、植入人工材料及腹裂（由于浆膜皮增厚或有人工补片）的患儿，一般禁忌选择性切除偶然发现的憩室。

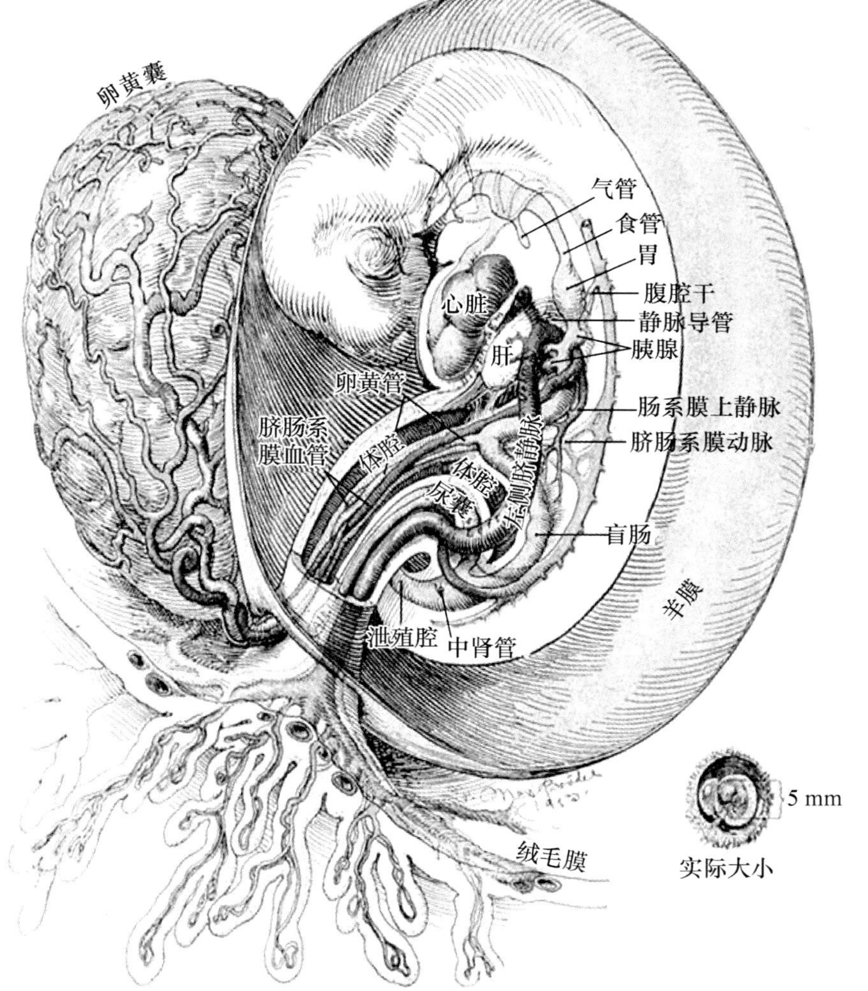

B

图 82-1 （续）B. 在稍晚阶段，卵黄管与体蒂融合形成脐带。注意卵黄血管覆盖在卵黄囊上。卵黄囊最初是胎儿营养的主要来源，最终胎盘承担这种功能。（From Cullen TS：Embryology, Anatomy and Diseases of the Urachus. Philadelphia, WB Saunders, 1916. Drawings by Max Brödel）

Meckel 憩室选择性切除后最常见的并发症是粘连性肠梗阻，发生率可高达 5%～10%[31]。对无症状患儿行 Meckel 憩室选择性切除术的死亡率应接近 0[36,64]。据报道，Meckel 憩室并发症的死亡率为 0～10%[5,11,13,34,35,40,66]。近来报道 Meckel 憩室选择性切除术并发症的发生率和死亡率极低，这反映出外科护理及外科技术（特别是使用吻合钉的腹腔镜下切除）的进步，从而倾向于切除偶然发现的憩室[65]。然而，还缺乏长期观察的数据。

临床表现

Meckel 憩室最常见的症状和体征是出血、梗阻和炎症。Meckel 憩室被称为“伟大的模仿者”，因为其相对少见、表现各异。大多数有症状的患儿年龄小于 10 岁[59]。临床表现的类型也与年龄有关（图 82-3）。

出血

出血是 Meckel 憩室最常见的症状。常可在憩室的回肠和异位胃黏膜交界处发现溃疡，但溃疡也可位于异位黏膜内或邻近憩室对侧的肠系膜侧的正常回肠上。这些溃疡通常较小，只有通过组织病理学检查才能发现。

Meckel 憩室将近占所有儿童低位消化道出血病例 1307
的 50%，常发生于婴儿和幼儿。有症状的成人患者

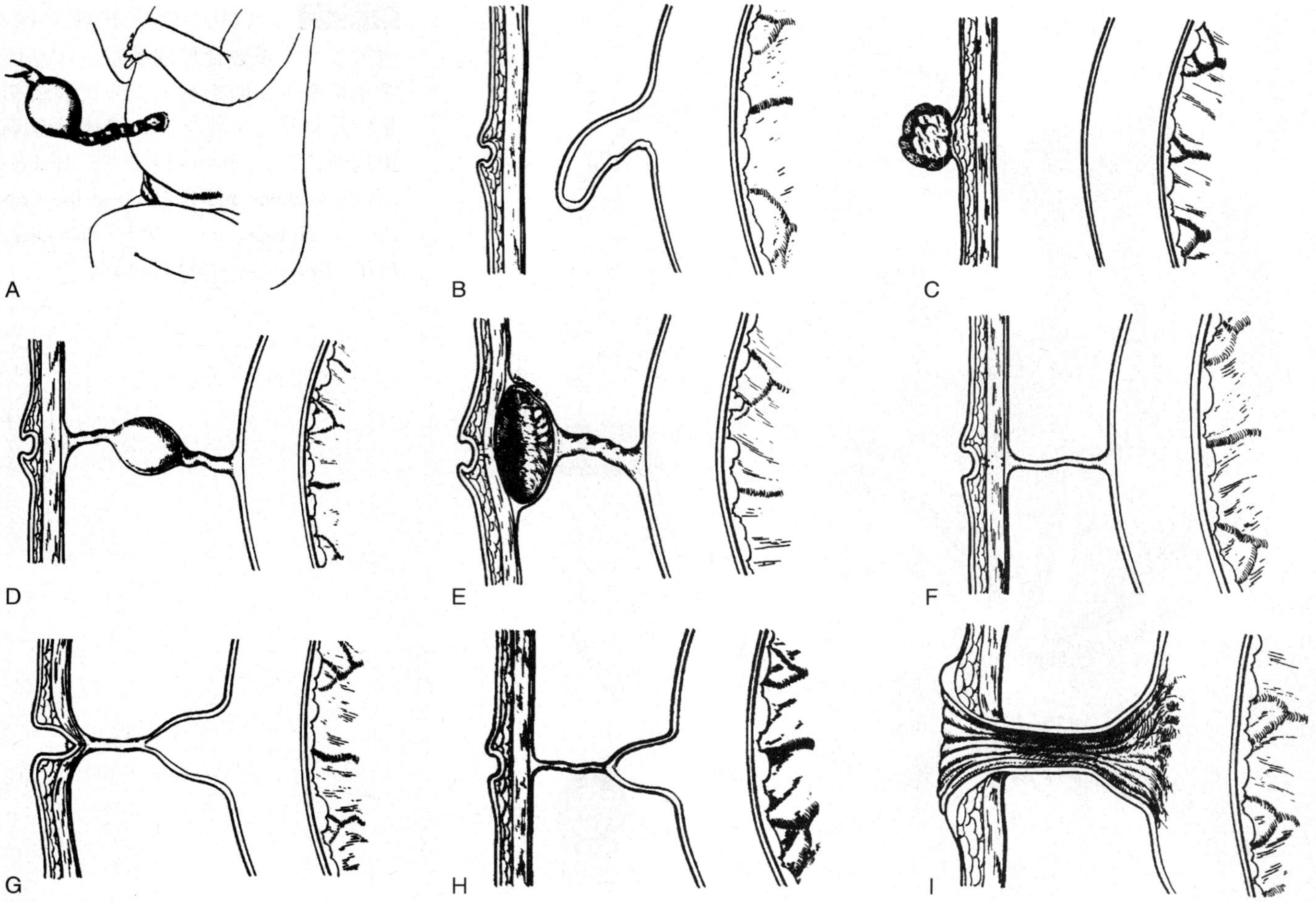

图 82-2 Meckel 憩室及脐部畸形。A. 脐带上含有黏膜的囊肿，囊肿远离脐部。这没有临床意义，因为出生时囊肿连同脐带将一起被切除。B. Meckel 憩室。大约 3/4 的 Meckel 憩室不与腹壁相连。C. 脐息肉为脐凹内淡红色肠黏膜的突出部分。虽然通常为单独畸形，但息肉也可透过腹壁与深部结构相连。黏膜息肉可被误认为是更常见的脐部肉芽肿。D. 有黏膜内衬及肌肉覆盖的卵黄管囊肿，在卵黄管近端及远端闭合后持续存在。E. 前腹膜内有肌壁及黏膜的囊肿，位于脐下，有时经脐向皮肤延伸。F. 憩室完全退化后，卵黄（脐肠系膜）血管成为与腹壁相连的纤维索带。G. 持续存在的脐窦为外露的卵黄管残迹，可能成为有脓液排出的感染的来源。图示脐窦通过闭合的卵黄管体内部分或开放连续的卵黄管与 Meckel 憩室连接。少数情况下，瘘道直接与卵黄管相连，不插入 Meckel 憩室。H. 卵黄管远端退化后 Meckel 憩室通过纤维索带与腹壁相连，可围绕索带发生肠扭转。I. 卵黄管持续开放与胎肠相通引起脐回肠（脐肠）瘘。注意肠皱襞从回肠肠腔延伸至皮肤。在有些病例中，这层黏膜含有胃黏膜。治疗方式为沿脐的开口切开，将瘘管剥离至回肠，然后切断并关闭回肠。

更易出现炎症或梗阻症状（见图 82-3）[13,35]。一般为多次发作的无痛性出血，有时可大量出血。粪便可为鲜红、砖红或红褐色[37,49]。柏油样便不常见。常可发现血红蛋白水平明显降低。隐匿性出血伴贫血的情况罕见。

儿童低位消化道出血的鉴别诊断包括炎性肠病、肠息肉、肠重复畸形、血管瘤或动静脉畸形。消化性溃疡及静脉曲张破裂出血可能与 Meckel 憩室的出血方式相似，但可通过血性鼻胃管吸引物或上消化道内镜检查来鉴别。即使仔细寻找也很少能在出血的 Meckel 憩室异位胃黏膜中发现幽门螺旋杆菌[1,8,16,24,28,41]。这种细菌在其他部位溃疡的发病机制中起主要作用，但在 Meckel 憩室异位胃黏膜引起的炎症或出血中不是重要因素。胆盐毒性对幽门螺旋杆菌的影响可能与之缺失有关。

自上世纪 70 年代起 Tc99m 扫描就已用于检测异

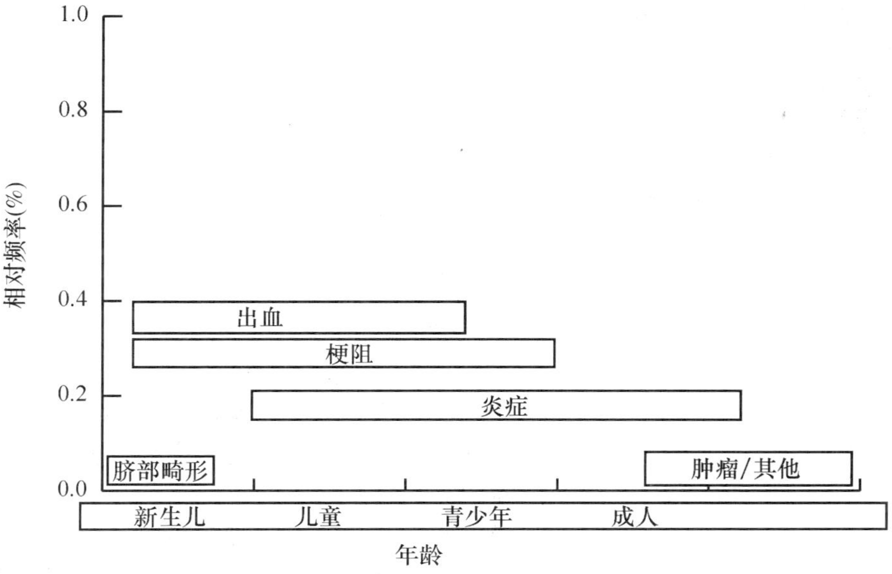

图 82-3 Meckel 憩室各种临床表现的近似发生率（相对和绝对）和出现症状的常见年龄。脐部畸形出现于新生儿期，肿瘤主要见于成人。出血、梗阻及炎症可出现于更广的年龄范围。

位胃黏膜[27]。运送 Tc99m 同位素的高锝酸盐离子被胃黏膜细胞贮存并分泌至肠腔[55]。少量同样的细胞分散至整个肠道，但与胃黏膜相比，肠黏膜的排泄率较低。图 82-4 显示了阳性的 Meckel 憩室同位素扫描图像。对 10 年内 954 例 Meckel 憩室 Tc99m 扫描的回顾发现假阴性率为 1.7%，假阳性率为 0.05%，敏感性为 85%，特异性为 95%，准确率为 90%[54]。对于成人，闪烁显像的准确率明显降低[13,53]。

五肽胃泌素、组胺阻滞剂及胰高血糖素可增加扫描的准确性[55]。五肽胃泌素促进胃对高锝酸盐的摄取，当高锝酸盐被摄取后，组胺阻滞剂可抑制其分泌。胰高血糖素可抑制蠕动，减少胃将高锝酸盐排入小肠，并增加其在憩室中停留的时间。禁食、鼻胃管吸引及留置导尿可增加扫描的效率。如果第一次同位素扫描结果为阴性，但诊断结果仍然可疑，有时可重复检查。有异位胃黏膜的肠重复畸形引起的出血 Tc99m 扫描结果为阳性。其他情况在鉴别诊断时行 Meckel 憩室同位素扫描为阴性结果，例如幼年性息肉或错构瘤性息肉、炎性肠病、溃疡、肠道血管畸形。虽然血管造影为侵袭性检查，但有时可发现 Meckel 憩室，甚至在没有出血的情况下[46]。如果同位素扫描及内镜检查结果为阴性，但仍强烈怀疑 Meckel 憩室的诊断，腹腔镜（或剖腹手术）是合理的选择[15,25,52]。危及生命的严重出血少见，如果一旦出现，不需明确术前诊断即可手术探查。

择期手术常可推迟到患儿情况稳定之后，因为 Meckel 憩室的出血一般为阵发性，常可自行停止。常

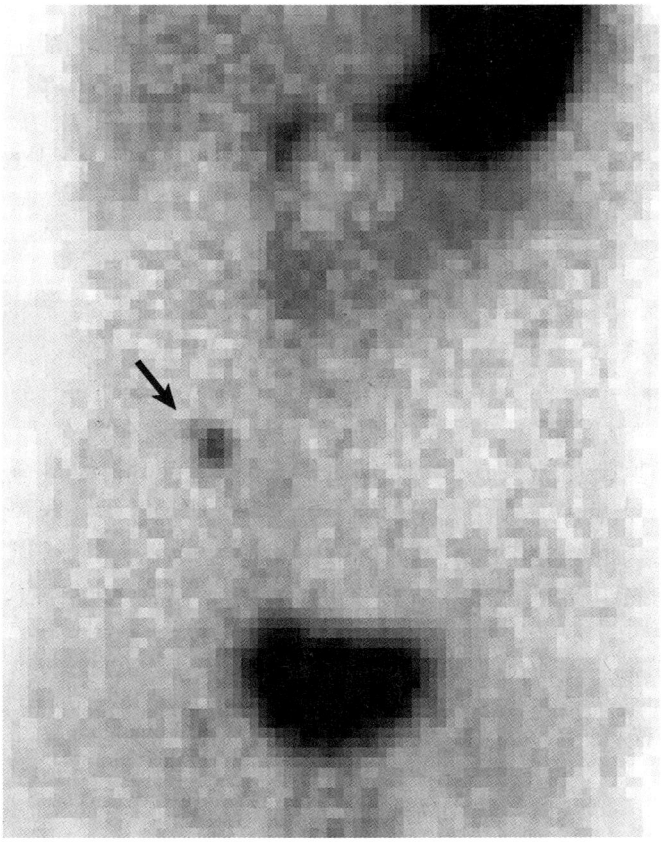

图 82-4 Meckel 憩室同位素扫描。Tc99m 高碍酸盐在有胃黏膜的胃部或 Meckel 憩室处选择性聚集，它由胃向十二指肠及近端小肠排泄。在尿中被排泄的同位素被膀胱收集。同位素聚集处扫描时为黑色区域。在该病例中，同位素显示出胃、近端小肠、Meckel 憩室（箭头）和膀胱的轮廓。

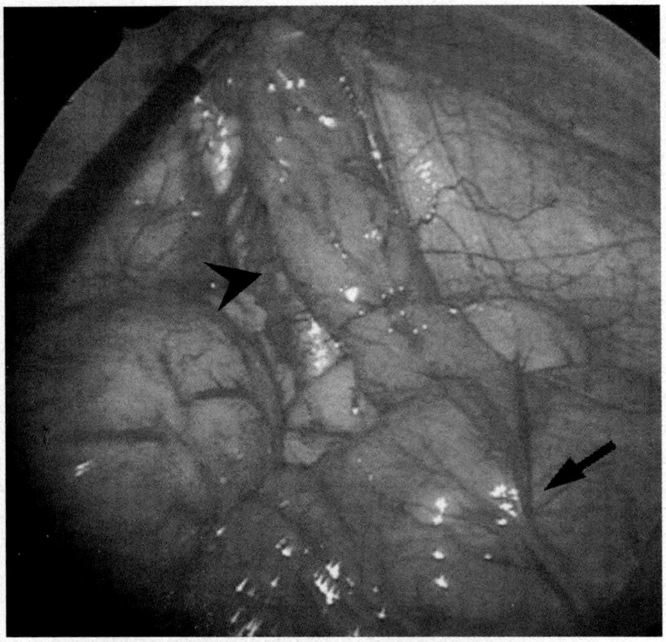

图 82-5　腹腔镜下切除出血的 Meckel 憩室。肠腔内的血液使憩室蒂部变色（箭头的头部）。动脉血供来自持续存在的右侧卵黄动脉（箭头），通常可辨认并将其结扎。可能无法见到溃疡，溃疡常位于异位胃黏膜和回肠黏膜的交界处，或在憩室底部的正常回肠内。

需要输血及补液。治疗可采取腹腔镜或开放性手术（图 82-5）。

Meckel 憩室切除可采用单纯性憩室切除和横向关闭基底部或切除一小段含憩室的回肠后行再吻合术。溃疡可能位于憩室对侧的肠系膜边缘，故切除一段含憩室的回肠是最安全的手术方式。应明确并结扎回肠表面的滋养动脉（憩室的）（见图 82-5），通常顺带切除阑尾。总的说来，憩室切除术治疗出血的效果很好。

梗阻

Meckel 憩室可通过以下几种机制的其中之一引起肠梗阻：肠套迭（最常见）、肠扭转、内疝、炎症性过程（见后）、经开放的卵黄管脱出（罕见）。在 1000 例以上的联合研究中，肠套迭占肠梗阻的 46%，肠扭转占 24%[21,29,35,40,49,62,64]。

当 Meckel 憩室翻转并成为病理性诱发点时可发生肠套迭。大于 5 岁的肠套迭患儿更有可能伴有潜在病理性因素，其中 Meckel 憩室的可能性较大。总的说来，小于 3% 的肠套迭由 Meckel 憩室引起（图 82-6A）[21]。一项对发生肠套迭的 160 例 Meckel 憩室患儿的经典回顾性研究显示，将近一半的患儿小于 10 岁[21]。

儿童肠套迭的临床表现包括呕吐、间歇性腹痛、血便、下腹部有可触及的肿块，最终发展为脱水及嗜睡。超声或空气灌肠常可证实肠套迭的诊断，但很少能确定潜在的病因。如果空气灌肠或对比灌肠后肠套迭完全复位，可行选择性憩室切除术。但通常不能完全复位，常在手术中或检查切下的标本时意外发现憩室。Meckel 憩室引起肠梗阻的外科治疗包括切除梗阻肠段并做端端吻合。

与 Meckel 憩室有关的肠扭转的发生可由几种机制造成。肠管上有血管或卵黄管的持续残留物，或憩室与腹壁相连可引起肠管扭转、纽结或形成疝（见图 82-2D～I，图 82-6B 和 C）。长的憩室甚至可自己打结，引起梗阻（图 82-6E）。从憩室顶部至肠系膜的憩室系膜索带可使肠袢在下方形成疝，引起梗阻、缺血和坏疽。这些索带是胎儿卵黄循环的胚胎残留物，可给憩室供血（图 82-6F）。巨大的 Meckel 憩室或卵黄管囊肿可引起新生儿肠扭转[7,19]。

术前准备包括静脉补液、纠正电解质紊乱、鼻胃管减压及使用抗生素（特别在怀疑肠绞窄时）。复苏后的治疗为切除憩室及受累的肠段（如果有不可逆的损伤），常可行端端吻合。

炎症

Meckel 憩室的炎症表现一般出现较晚，常被误认为阑尾炎。怀疑为阑尾炎但术中发现阑尾正常时，要探查有无 Meckel 憩室（图 82-7）。在一组 8000 多例疑为阑尾炎的病例中，0.76% 的患儿被发现有 Meckel 憩室[2]。虽然严重的炎症可能掩盖切下的标本中的异位黏膜，但一般总是存在的（通常为胃黏膜，偶尔为胰腺黏膜）。Meckel 憩室可能会与消化性溃疡病、胃肠炎、胆绞痛、炎性肠病及其他疾病混淆。肠穿孔可导致局部或弥散性污染。可单纯切除憩室或切除憩室及受累肠段来治疗炎症性并发症。常可行一期吻合。少数情况下，由于患儿病情严重需行肠外置或暂时性肠造瘘。

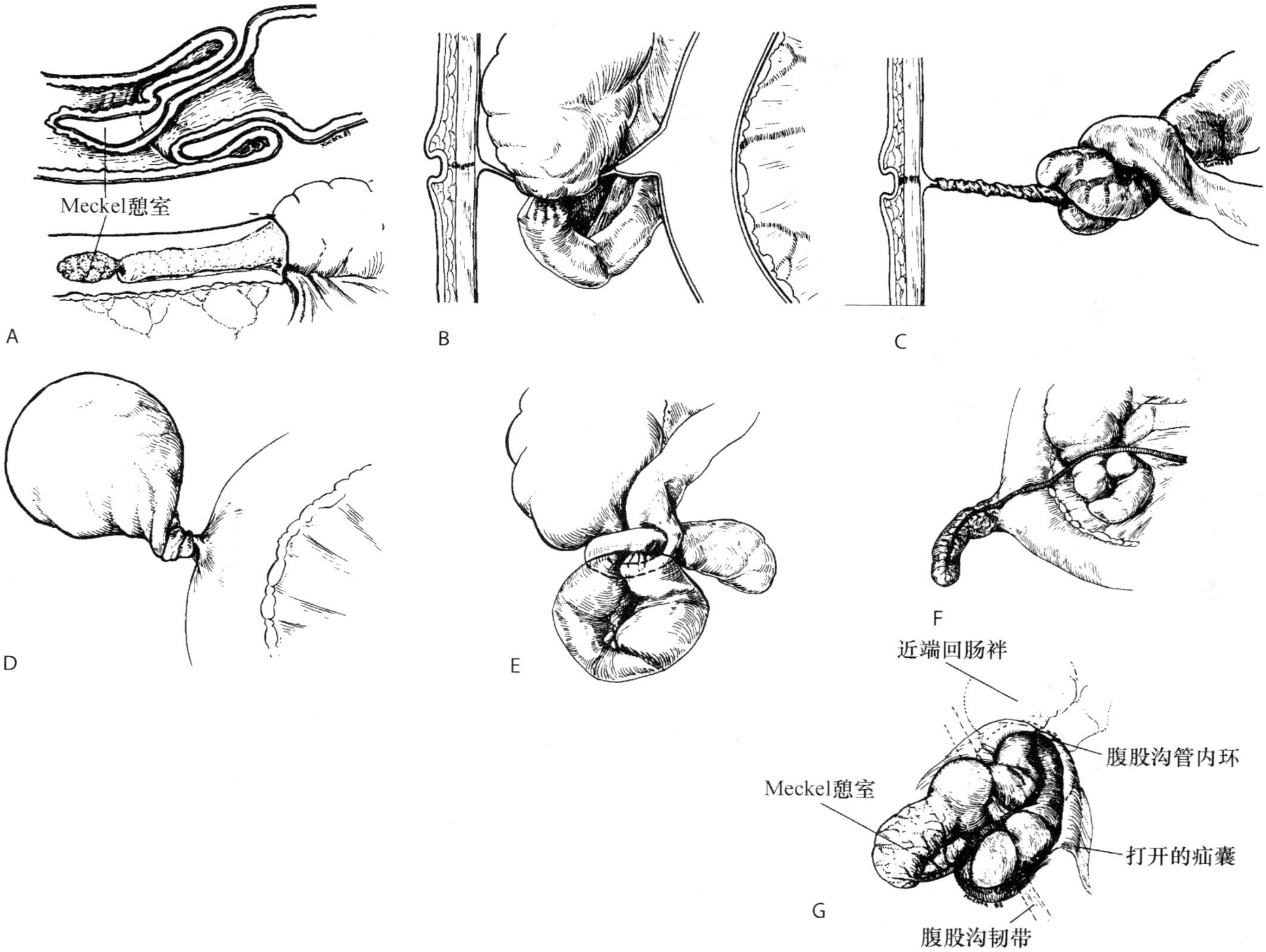

图 82-6 Meckel 憩室及肠梗阻形成的可能机制。与卵黄管索带样残留物（B 和 C）有关的肠套迭（A）和肠梗阻是最常见的机制，很少涉及其他机制（D～G）。A. 肠套迭。上一幅图，Meckel 憩室翻转入回肠成为回肠-回肠型肠套迭的诱发点。憩室的内面可能不会翻向外。下一幅图，憩室套入更远，可进入升结肠形成回肠-回肠结肠型肠套迭。B. 一段小肠在 Meckel憩室和脐之间的卵黄管索带样残留部分上扭结。C. 小肠袢围绕卵黄管纤维索带残留部分的固定点发生扭转。D. Meckel憩室基底部扭转，引起憩室梗阻并可能发生梗死。E. 长的 Meckel 憩室自身打结后引起回肠梗阻，可引起回肠及憩室本身梗阻。F. 含有卵黄血管的憩室系膜索带跨过回肠到达憩室，它从肠系膜分出并可形成索带使一段小肠疝入而发生梗阻。G. Littre 疝有一段含 Meckel 憩室的回肠在腹股沟疝囊内。图示为含有肠管和憩室的斜疝。在疝内容物回纳及腹股沟疝修补之前已打开疝囊。腹股沟管内环收缩引起肠梗阻，故近端肠管扩张。远端肠管在梗阻处之外，已经排空。

10 **其他表现**

约有 5% 有症状的 Meckel 憩室患儿存在脐部畸形（见图 82-2C、G 和 I）[60-62]。外露的、有黏膜的脐带囊肿是出生时罕见的病变。这些为典型的单独畸形，与肠道无关（见图 82-2A）。

脐部持续的息肉组织或肉芽组织残留是新生儿的常见问题。大多数脐息肉不伴有腹腔内畸形，局部治疗（结扎或用硝酸银涂于脐部肉芽肿）就足够了。如果结扎后息肉未消退，或 1～2 次治疗后脐部肉芽肿仍然存在，或患儿有脐部流液的病史，或脐部可见瘘道，则需进一步治疗。“息肉”或瘘道内可有肠黏膜（见图 82-2C）。有时可通过小心地插入小口径的导管来确认脐部瘘道，或通过腔窦 X 线摄片也可证实。

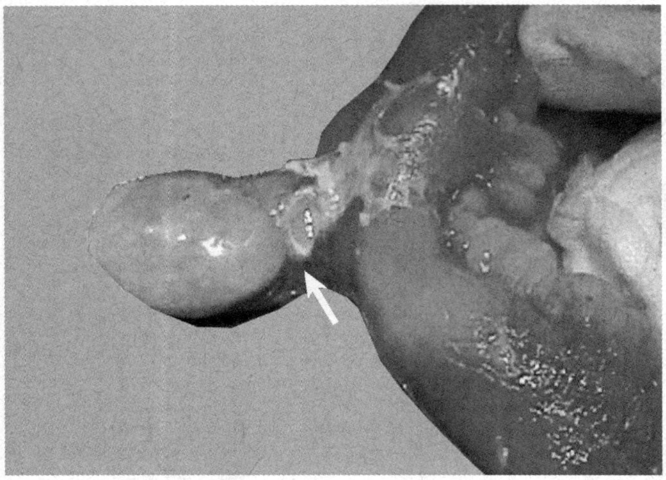

图 82-7　伴有炎症的 Meckel 憩室，底部穿孔（箭头）。憩室尖端由于异位胃黏膜及炎症性改变而明显增厚。可行节段性肠切除或单纯性憩室切除，这取决于临床情况及邻近肠管的特征，以及炎症反应的严重程度。

由于持续存在的卵黄管黏膜向外脱垂，脐部可有回肠造瘘样外观（见图 82-2I；图 82-8）。严重脱垂
1311 可引起肠梗阻，甚至可影响肠管血供。做脐下或经脐切口最易处理脐部窦道或瘘管。在瘘道内放置导管有助于分离。将瘘道的脐端横断或沿周围切开、分离，并与其他持续存在的异常结构一起完整切除。一般切除与肠道的附属物，并横行关闭肠管。

有异物或结石位于 Meckel 憩室内的报道，憩室内也可有寄生虫感染如血吸虫病、蛔虫病[22,47,48,65]。

很少有 Meckel 憩室患儿患有原发性消化道癌（类癌、肉瘤、淋巴瘤、腺癌、平滑肌瘤）的报道[9,43,57]。这些肿瘤一般见于成人，其中类癌最常见。在一篇回顾 104 例类癌瘤的文献中，患者的平均年龄为 57 岁，其中男性患者是女性患者的 2.5 倍[45]。这些是具有相对侵袭性的肿瘤（3/4 在诊断时有转移），免疫表型及生物学上它们类似于空肠回肠类癌而不像阑尾类癌[43]。大于 5 mm 的肿瘤发生转移的风险明显增加。也可发生类癌综合征。治疗方法是切除含憩室及其肠系膜的回肠肠段。对于同时患有类癌和 Meckel 憩室的患儿，有发生第二种原发性恶性肿瘤的报道[57]。

（陈　盛译　董其刚校）

参考文献

1. Ackerman Z, et al: Role of *Helicobacter pylori* infection in complications from Meckel's diverticulum. Dig Dis Sci 2003;48:1068.
2. Albu I, et al: The ileal diverticulum: Morpho-clinical and epidemiological study. Rom J Morphol Embryol 1993;39:37.
3. Andreyev HJ, et al: Association between Meckel's diverticulum and Crohn's disease: A retrospective review. Gut 1994;35:788.
4. Androulakis JA, et al: The sex ratio of Meckel's diverticulum. Am Surg 1969;35:455.
5. Arnold JF, Pellicane JV: Meckel's diverticulum: A ten-year experience. Am Surg 1997;63:354.

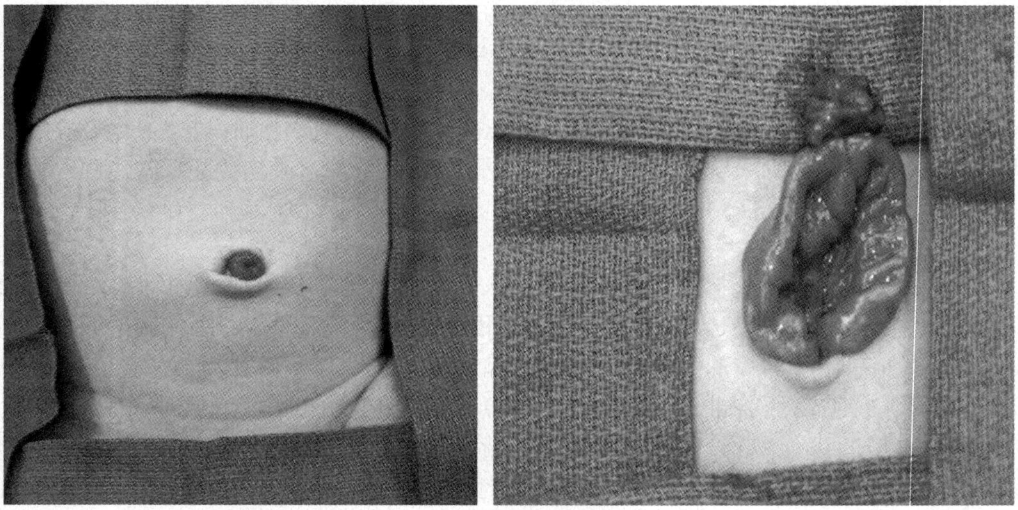

A　B

图 82-8　脐回肠瘘。A. 脐部有回肠造瘘样的外观。B. 瘘管宽而短。分开与瘘管粘连的皮肤及腹壁，经脐部缺损提出回肠并横形关闭。这种缺损相对罕见。

6. Artigas V, et al: Meckel's diverticulum: Value of ectopic tissue. Am J Surg 1986;151:631.
7. Bell MJ, et al: Ileal dysgenesis in infants and children. J Pediatr Surg 1982;17:395.
8. Bemelman WA, et al: Role of *Helicobacter pylori* in the pathogenesis of complications of Meckel's diverticula. Eur J Surg 1993;159:171.
9. Chatterjee CR: Sarcomas of Meckel's diverticulum. Can J Surg 1970;13:163.
10. Christie A: Meckel's diverticulum: A pathologic study of 63 cases. Am J Dis Child 1931;42:544.
11. Cullen JJ, et al: Surgical management of Meckel's diverticulum: An epidemiologic, population-based study. Ann Surg 1994;220:564.
12. DeBartolo HM Jr, van Heerden JA: Meckel's diverticulum. Ann Surg 1976;183:30.
13. Diamond T, Russell CF: Meckel's diverticulum in the adult. Br J Surg 1985;72:480.
14. Eckman CN: Regional enteritis associated with Meckel's diverticulum: A report of five cases. Gastroenterology 1958;34:130.
15. Fansler RF: Laparoscopy in the management of Meckel's diverticulum. Surg Laparosc Endosc 1996;6:231.
16. Fich A, et al: Does *Helicobacter pylori* colonize the gastric mucosa of Meckel's diverticulum? Mayo Clin Proc 1990;65:187.
17. Gramen K: Chronischen ulcus in einem Meckelshen Divertikel mit perforation and diffuser peritonitis. Nord Med Ark Kirkurgi 1915;48:1.
18. Groebli Y, et al: Meckel's diverticulum in adults: Retrospective analysis of 119 cases and historical review. Eur J Surg 2001;167:518.
19. Grosfeld JL, Franken EA: Intestinal obstruction in the neonate due to vitelline duct cysts. Surg Gynecol Obstet 1974;138:527.
20. Haber J: Meckel's diverticulum. Am J Surg 1947;73:468.
21. Harkins H: Intussusception due to invaginated Meckel's diverticulum. Ann Surg 1933;98:1070.
22. Haynes S, Reid HA: Meckel's diverticulitis due to *Schistosomiasis mansoni.* Am J Gastroenterol 1976;66:559.
23. Hildanus F: Opera observationum et curationum medico—chururgicarum, quae extant omnia, etc. Francof, J Beyeri, 1646.
24. Hill P, Rode J: *Helicobacter pylori* in ectopic gastric mucosa in Meckel's diverticulum. Pathology 1998;30:7.
25. Huang CS, Lin LH: Laparoscopic Meckel's diverticulectomy in infants: Report of three cases. J Pediatr Surg 1993;28:1486.
26. Jay GD III, et al: Meckel's diverticulum: A survey of one hundred and three cases. Arch Surg 1950;61:158.
27. Jewett TC, et al: The visualization of Meckel's diverticulum with 99m Tc-pertechnetate. Surgery 1970;68:567.
28. Kumar S, et al: *Helicobacter pylori* and Meckel's diverticulum. J R Coll Surg Edinb 1991;36:225.
29. Kusumoto H, et al: Complications and diagnosis of Meckel's diverticulum in 776 patients. Am J Surg 1992;164:382.
30. Kuttner H: Ileus durch intussusception eines Meckelschen divertikel. Beitr Klin Chir 1898;21:289.
31. Leijonmarck CE, et al: Meckel's diverticulum in the adult. Br J Surg 1986;73:146.
32. Lichtenstein ME: Meckel's diverticulum. Q Bull Northwest Univ Med 1941;15:296.
33. Littre A: Observation sur une nouvelle espece de hernia. Hist Acad Roy Sci 1719;300.
34. Ludtke FE, et al: Incidence and frequency of complications and management of Meckel's diverticulum. Surg Gynecol Obstet 1989;169:537.
35. Mackey WC, Dineen P: A fifty year experience with Meckel's diverticulum. Surg Gynecol Obstet 1983;156:56.
36. Matsagas MI, et al: Incidence, complications, and management of Meckel's diverticulum. Arch Surg 1995;130:143.
37. Mayo CW: Meckel's diverticulum. Proc Mayo Clin 1933;8:230.
38. Meckel J: Uber die Divertikel am Darmkanal. Arch Physiol 1809;9:421.
39. Meckel J: Handbuch der pathologischen Anatomie. Leipzig, CH Reclam, 1812, p 533.
40. Meguid M, et al: Complications of Meckel's diverticulum in infants. Surg Gynecol Obstet 1974;139:541.
41. Morris A, et al: *Campylobacter pylori* infection in Meckel's diverticula containing gastric mucosa. Gut 1989;30:1233.
42. Moses WR: Meckel's diverticulum: A report of two unusual cases. N Engl J Med 1947;237:118.
43. Moyana TN: Carcinoid tumors arising from Meckel's diverticulum: A clinical, morphologic, and immunohistochemical study. Am J Clin Pathol 1989;91:52.
44. Nicol JW, MacKinlay GA: Meckel's diverticulum in exomphalos minor. J R Coll Surg Edinb 1994;39:6.
45. Nies C, et al: Carcinoid tumors of Meckel's diverticula. Dis Colon Rectum 1992;35:589.
46. Okazaki M, et al: Angiographic findings of Meckel's diverticulum: The characteristic appearance of the vitelline artery. Abdom Imaging 1993;18:15.
47. Pujari BD, Deodhare SG: Ascarideal penetration of Meckel's diverticulum. Int Surg 1978;63:113.
48. Roessel CW: Perforation of Meckel's diverticulum by foreign body: Case report and review of the literature. Ann Surg 1962;156:972.
49. Rutherford RB, Akers DR: Meckel's diverticulum: A review of 148 pediatric patients, with special reference to the pattern of bleeding and to mesodiverticular vascular bands. Surgery 1966;59:618.
50. Ruysch F: Thesaurus Anatomicus. 2nd ed. Amsterdam, 1701.
51. Salzer H: Uber das Offerene Meckelesche Divertikel. Wien Klin Wochenschr 1904;17:614.
52. Schier F, et al: Laparoscopic removal of Meckel's diverticula in children. Eur J Pediatr Surg 1996;6:38.
53. Schwartz MJ, Lewis JH: Meckel's diverticulum: Pitfalls in scintigraphic detection in the adult. Am J Gastroenterol 1984;79:611.
54. Sfakianakis GN, Conway JJ: Detection of ectopic gastric mucosa in Meckel's diverticulum and in other aberrations by scintigraphy. I. Pathophysiology and 10-year clinical experience. J Nucl Med 1981;22:647.
55. Sfakianakis GN, Conway JJ: Detection of ectopic gastric mucosa in Meckel's diverticulum and in other aberrations by scintigraphy. II. Indications and methods—a 10-year experience. J Nucl Med 1981;22:732.
56. Sibley WL: Meckel's diverticulum: Dyspepsia meckeli from heterotopic gastric mucosa. Arch Surg 1944; 49:156.
57. Silk YN, et al: Carcinoid tumor in Meckel's diverticulum. Am Surg 1988;54:664.
58. Simms MH, Corkery JJ: Meckel's diverticulum: Its association with congenital malformation and the significance of atypical morphology. Br J Surg 1980;67:216.
59. Skandalakis JE, et al: The small intestines. In Skandalakis JE, Gray SW (eds): Embryology for Surgeons, 2nd ed. Baltimore, Williams & Wilkins, 1994, p 184.
60. Soderlund S: Meckel's diverticulum, a clinical and histologic study. Acta Chir Scand Suppl 1959;248:213.
61. Soltero MJ, Bill AH: The natural history of Meckel's diverticulum and its relation to incidental removal: A study of 202 cases of diseased Meckel's diverticulum found in

King County, Washington, over a fifteen year period. Am J Surg 1976;132:168.
62. St-Vil D, et al: Meckel's diverticulum in children: A 20-year review. J Pediatr Surg 1991;26:1289.
63. Thompson JE: Perforated peptic ulcer in Meckel's diverticulum. Ann Surg 1937;105:44.
64. Vane DW, et al: Vitelline duct anomalies: Experience with 217 childhood cases. Arch Surg 1987;122:542.
65. Yahchouchy EK, et al: Meckel's diverticulum. J Am Coll Surg 2001;192:658.
66. Yamaguchi M, et al: Meckel's diverticulum: Investigation of 600 patients in Japanese literature. Am J Surg 1978; 136:247.
67. Zenker FA: Nebenpancreas in des Darmwand. Virchow Arch Pathol Anat 1861;21:369.

第 83 章

肠套迭

Sigmund H. Ein、Alan Daneman

历史回顾

313 我们能通过回顾过去学到知识，这同样适用于肠套迭（intussusception）[111,144,145,183]。早在 17 世纪晚期，人们就认识了肠套迭（Barbette、Peyer），但直到 1793 年才由 Hunter 第一次对其作了详细的描述[93,167]。Raffensperger[142] 写到远在希波克拉底（Hippocrates）时代就有向直肠内灌入空气或液体以使肠套迭复位的典故。然而，Ravitch[144] 提到在 Littré 的译文中，希波克拉底只提到肠梗阻，因此像人们预期的一样，对于历史记录及报告存在一些疑问。那时建议对肠套迭进行放血及汞治疗，Hunter 在此基础上作了补充，如前者无效，可采用先催吐后导泻的方法进行治疗。随后，Hunter 的肠套迭复位方法得到改进，用手动鼓风机向肛门内用力鼓风，以试图使套迭的肠管回复至正常的位置。显然，希波克拉底时代人们已尝试过这种治疗方式[110]，但直到 19 世纪早期，医学文献上才第一次有了肠套迭空气灌肠复位的记载（Blacklock，1818；Mitchell，1836；Gorham，1838）[111]。这些病例没能被很好地记录下来，其中包括一些成人病例，和希波克拉底时代一样，其中很多病例被怀疑是否为真正的肠套迭。1864 年，外科医生 Greig[68,111] 首次对肠套迭的临床诊断制定了严格的标准。他试图让他人相信他应用手动鼓风机使 5 个真正肠套迭患儿中的 4 个复位成功，他说："出乎我们的意料，空气很容易地就通过了肠管，看上去患儿的病情也得到了很大缓解。"然而，这种技术只是当时很多种治疗方法（泡腾剂粉、冷水、高渗盐水、长的直肠探条、电流、颠茄、鸦片）中的一种，正如人们所料，它并未获得很大成功。因此，肠套迭对于大多数婴幼儿来说仍是致命的。

1831 年，Wilson[183] 手术整复 1 例成人肠套迭，但直到 40 年后（1871 年），Hutchinson[94,183] 才首次对 1 名婴儿成功实施肠套迭复位手术。但在当时，手术干预是非常危险的。1885 年，Treves[167,171] 提出了一种治疗方案，与现今的治疗方法差别不大，尽管如此，他报道首次手术治疗的 33 例肠套迭病例中死亡率仍高达 73%。1876 年，Hirschsprung[84] 首次报道液体静压复位（死亡率为 23%）效果优于手术治疗，直到 20 世纪中期仍是如此。19 世纪晚期，人们开始了解液体静压或空气灌肠能否使肠管成功复位取决于施加的压力大小。由于采用该治疗方法的患者日益增多，故研制出了各种设备以满足治疗需要。一些学者（Forest，1886 年[61]）甚至怀疑液体和/或空气是否为最好的灌肠物质，后来 Forest 计算出肠套迭复位合适的压力为 6 磅每平方英寸。1891 年，Mortimer[123] 也表示对这些新方法带来的风险感到担忧。

20 世纪初时，液体静压复位的方法被广泛接受，但这并不妨碍一些有进取心和大胆的外科医生尝试用手术方法来治疗肠套迭。1900 年左右，Clubbe[22] 和 Peterson[145] 均首次成功地为患儿行肠套迭切除术。虽然 Hirschsprung 于 1905 年报道液体静压复位的死亡率（23%，共 84 名患者）远低于外科手术，但随着手术方法的逐步改进以及术后疗效的提高，特别是在美国、英国和澳大利亚，手术治疗已开展起来[85,111]。

大概在 1913 年，肠套迭的诊断和治疗有了很大改进。Ladd[144] 首先报道使用铋剂灌肠进行诊断性成像，并首次公布了肠套迭 X 线照片。尽管 Lehman[144] 在 3 年前就进行了同样的观察，但直到 1914 年才报道了和 Ladd 相同的发现。Ladd 认为铋剂灌肠是一个较好的诊断方法，但没有任何治疗价值[144]。又过了 14 年（1927 年），Olsson 和 Pallin[131]、Poulquien[137]、Retan[147] 等成功在 X 线透视下，通过钡剂灌肠液体静压复

位的方法来治疗肠套迭。此时，澳大利亚仍热衷于使
1314 用非手术方法治疗小儿肠套迭。1926 年，Hipsley[83] 报道了 100 例肠套迭患者中 62 例采用盐水灌肠，只有 1 例死亡。同时，钡剂灌肠的方法开始在斯堪的纳维亚和南美流行开来[111]。尽管最近报道放射科医生可诊断及复位肠套迭，但在美国，外科手术仍是首选的治疗方法，然而这种治疗方法的选择并不是以循证为基础。

直到 Ravitch 和 McCune[146]（1948 年）报道肠套迭的手术死亡率达 32%，人们又开始关注非手术治疗。在这篇报道之后，X 线透视下钡剂灌肠（barium enema，BE）的方法又逐渐引起大家的重视。Ravitch 和 McCune[146] 先后于 1948 年、1952 年、1954 年和 1958 年通过实验室研究及临床证据最先支持这种方法，他们报道其复位率达 75% 而死亡率为 0。即便如此，1953 年 Gross[69]（像他的前辈 Ladd 一样）虽然承认该非手术治疗方法的有效性，但仍然对其表示强烈反对，他认为手术治疗具有决定性作用。但液体静压的复位方法还是保留了下来，并成为肠套迭首选的、最安全、最成功的治疗方法。

从那以后，放射科医生开始参予肠套迭的临床治疗，并对肠套迭的非手术治疗作了进一步改进，用空气（空气灌肠复位）作为对比剂（1959 年 Fiorito 等[59]；1986 年 Guo 等[73]）；超声（ultrasonography，US）被用于筛查、诊断和监测复位情况（1977 年 Burke 和 Clarke[16]）；也有医生尝试采用延时重复灌肠的复位方式（1986 年 Guo 等）。目前，手术治疗已成为放射学引导下行肠套迭复位的替代方案。

引言

“肠套迭”一词来源于拉丁语“intus”（在里面）和“suscipere”（容纳）[74]。肠套迭是一部分肠管陷入另一部分肠管内（图 83-1）。Swenson[169] 对其做了清晰的描述：肠套迭是一个包括 3 个肠壁的圆柱体，内层和中间的圆柱体为内陷的肠管（肠套迭套入部），外层的圆柱体则容纳内陷的肠管（肠套迭鞘 1315
部）。肠套迭可能是除了便秘以外，婴儿及学龄前儿童急性腹痛的第二类最常见的病因。此外，肠套迭也是该年龄组患儿急性小肠梗阻（small bowel obstruc-

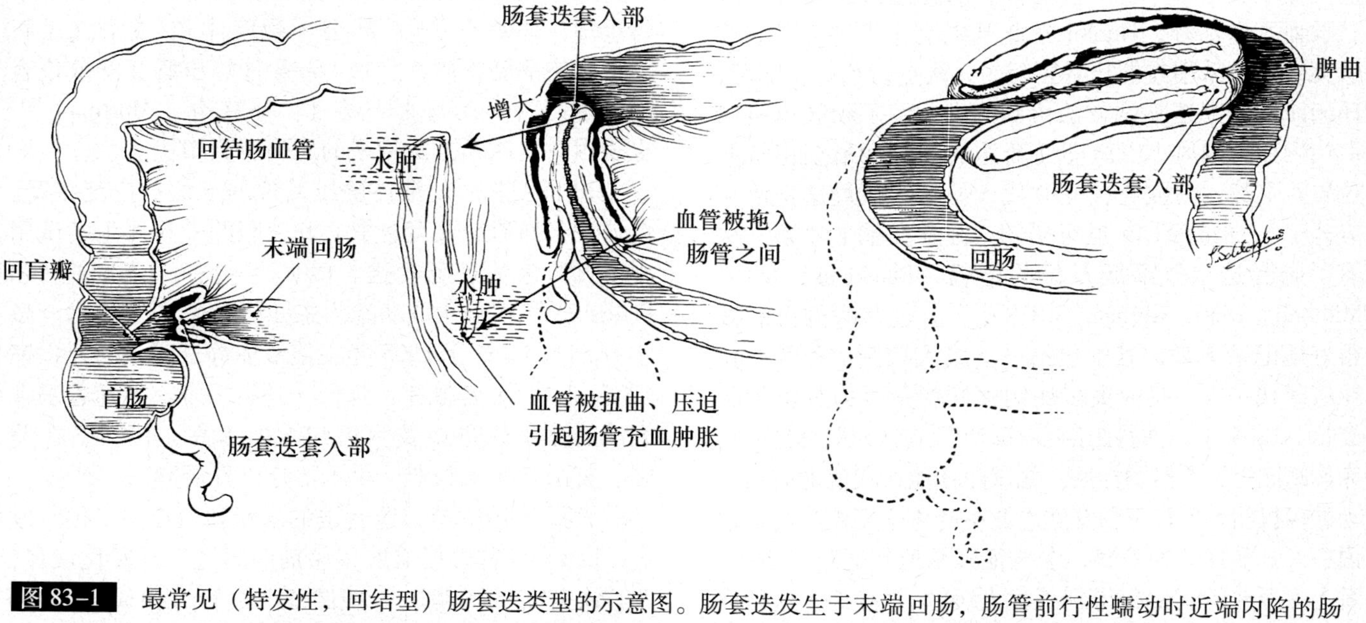

图 83-1 最常见（特发性，回结型）肠套迭类型的示意图。肠套迭发生于末端回肠，肠管前行性蠕动时近端内陷的肠管（肠套迭套入部）携带肠系膜进入容纳肠管（肠套迭鞘部），肠系膜血管在套入部的肠管之间被扭曲成角、挤压和压迫，导致套入部局部严重水肿，引起静脉压迫、充血及血液淤滞，进而使肿胀的套入部排出黏液和血液，常形成果酱样外观的粪便。若此恶性循环持续下去，肠管充血加剧、压力增高，随后肠管发生缺血性改变并导致肠坏死（坏疽）。套入部的最外层肠管最先失活，最内层肠管较晚才发生坏疽，最外层肠管（肠套迭鞘部）最晚失活[144]。然而，对液体静压灌肠复位时发生肠穿孔的回顾性研究显示，穿孔处位于靠近套入部的结肠（肠套迭鞘部）[48,92,113]。

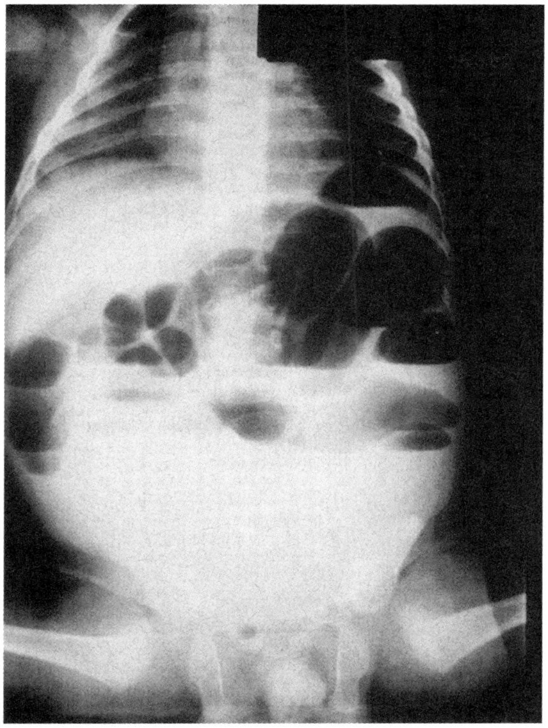

图 83-2　小肠梗阻的放射学图像。小肠梗阻可发生于婴儿或学龄前儿童，最常由特发性肠套迭（通常为回回结型）或手术后肠套迭引起。

tion，SBO）的常见原因（图 83-2）。因此，对于儿科医务人员来说，了解肠套迭，特别是对其所有的变化和变异类型都能作出诊断是非常必要的。一些作者提出肠套迭难以诊断，但只要儿科医生了解、思考过该病，并且知道少数患儿（15%）没有典型的绞痛症状，这些困难便可迎刃而解[52]。50 年前，Gross[69] 就明确声称："很少有疾病其临床病史和体征能很好地提示医生作出正确的诊断。"

小儿放射科医生在诊断和治疗肠套迭方面做出的许多改进和创新，包括超声的使用、从液体静压复位向空气复位的转变以及延时重复灌肠的采用，都超出了地方及非权威儿科中心的关注、兴趣或专业知识的范围[8]。一些小型医疗机构遇到及治疗的肠套迭病例较少，故对这种常见的儿科疾病不够熟悉并缺乏经验，因此也不愿尝试一些新方法[14]。与预期的一样，这种情况导致无法改变的、难以被大家接受的高手术率，而正常情况下这是不应发生的。如果儿科中心（三级及四级医疗中心）能够构建一个持续支持的交流、教育及合作的网络来提高整体医疗水平，即使所有肠套迭的婴儿或儿童获得相似的治疗效果，这个问题就能得以解决[18]。

本章的资料和数据引自多伦多儿童医院（The hospital for Sick Children，HSC）治疗肠套迭的丰富经验，自 1952 年来已经发表了 40 多篇文章。在头 53 年中（1915—1968），有 1000 多例肠套迭病例（25 例/年），1968 年后又有 1300 例肠套迭（35 例/年）患儿被诊断及治疗[51]。这些病例均包括在他们发表的许多文章里。

本章的许多内容是 Ravitch[146] 和 Young[183] 的经典著作中智慧和经验的集合，之前他们也是这本分上下册的教科书中肠套迭相关章节的作者。本版在 1998 出版的《小儿外科学》（第五版）的基础上，增加了其他资料、数据和观点，以及临床研究的最新成果（表 83-1 和 83-2）（超过 500 种摘要和出版物）。

目前，肠套迭的诊断和治疗需要小儿放射科医生和小儿外科医生的共同努力，目前小儿放射科医生能成功治疗大多数肠套迭病例。然而不应忘记 Zachary 的箴言，他在 1954 年于伦敦举行的首届英国小儿外科医生年会上指出："……手术医生应对患儿负责，并亲自监测患儿的情况。[40,179,184]"

表 83-1　1998—2004 年病例报道中的病理性诱发点

阑尾-28	囊性纤维化-2
脂肪瘤-22	错构瘤-2
息肉-17	白血病-2
Peutz-Jeghers 综合征-13	淋巴样增生-2
十二指肠胃套迭-11	Meckel 憩室-2
腺瘤-10	纤维平滑肌瘤-2
淋巴瘤-7	骨肉瘤-2
导管-6	血管神经性水肿-1
癌-5	类癌瘤-1
小肠结肠炎-5	绒毛膜癌-1
乳糜泻-4	异位胃黏膜-1
Crohn 病-4	异位胰腺-1
过敏性紫癜-4	异物-1
积气症-4	内疝-1
外伤-4	淋巴管瘤-1
重复畸形-3	淋巴组织增生-1
子宫内膜异位-3	神经鞘瘤-1
组织细胞瘤-3	肾细胞癌-1
黑素瘤-3	结节病-1
血管瘤-2	脾组织植入-1
粪石-2	蠕虫-1

表 83-2 1998—2004 年文献中以肠套迭为主题的文献
病例报告-200
临床观察-102
影像学-77
病毒-39
上消化道逆行套迭-24
产前及新生儿肠套迭-18
腹腔镜-14
手术-7
家族性肠套迭-6
肠旋转不良-4
病史-4
死亡率-4
总计-499

1316 发病率及人口统计学

只要有需要治疗的儿童，就可见到肠套迭的发生，但各儿科中心报道的肠套迭病例数有明显的差异[51,144,145,183]。回顾这些报道后给人一个直接的印象，即迄今为止，中国是肠套迭发病率最高的国家(5000 例/年)[73]，但这也许是人口因素所致。斯堪的纳维亚位居第二（50～60 例/年），其次是多伦多、格拉斯哥和墨尔本（35 例/年），英格兰（伯明翰，泰恩河旁的纽卡斯尔）和波士顿（20～30 例/年）。美国其他儿童医院（巴尔的摩、芝加哥、辛辛那提、丹佛、洛杉矶、密尔沃基、纽奥尔良、纽约、圣路易斯）报道的肠套迭病例数为 5～14 例/年。

Young[183]从资料回顾中得出一些结论。他注意到澳大利亚、加拿大、新西兰报道的肠套迭发病率与欧洲和美国相似，而埃及、罗得西亚和南非报道的发病率与苏格兰相似。但奇怪的是，在尼日利亚肠套迭更常见于 5 岁以上的儿童，且有成为亚急性或慢性肠套迭的趋势。Ravitch[145]认为在中国大陆及台湾同样如此。

婴儿和儿童的肠套迭发生率约为 1/2000。据两份英国和苏格兰的研究报道显示，肠套迭的发生率为每 1000 例活产儿中有 1.5～4 例[145,183]。相比之下，患儿腹股沟疝的发生率为 1/50，阑尾炎的发生率为 6/100。

大多数报道显示，肠套迭患儿中男孩多于女孩，

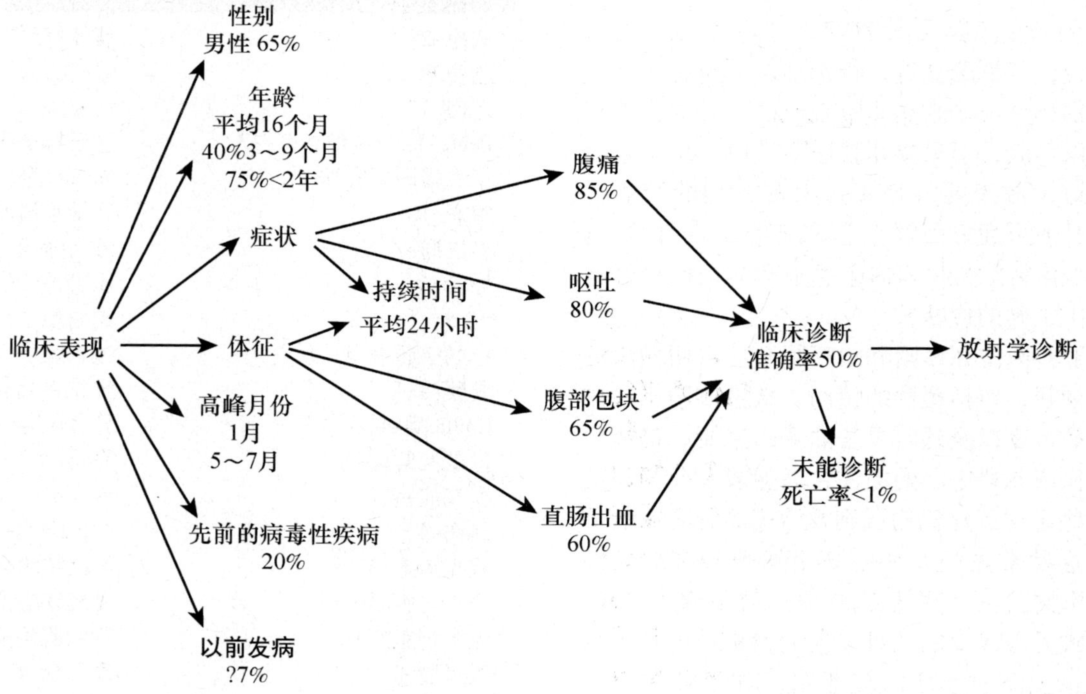

图 83-3 肠套迭临床特征及诊断规则系统的详细描述（注意其他规则系统都能按顺序加入此规则系统）。

通常为 2∶1 或 3∶2（图 83-3）。Ravitch[145] 宣称对此还没有令人满意的解释，而 Macmahon183 报道，这种情况在 9 个月以上的婴儿中（男性占 78%）比 9 个月以下的婴儿（男性占 55%）更加明显。据报道，白人婴儿和儿童中患肠套迭的更多，而具体发生率则取决于研究的地区。

尽管肠套迭可发生于从产前胎儿到大龄青少年的所有年龄组（成人甚至动物也会发生肠套迭），但在多伦多 75% 的肠套迭发生于 2 岁前，超过 40% 的肠套迭见于 3～9 个月的婴儿[51]。大多数研究倾向支持多伦多的结果，因为差异较小。肠套迭可发生于子宫内[136]，并可导致肠闭锁（通常是回肠闭锁）[54,154,170]。有些病例可在远端肠管找到肠套迭头部[141,183]，但至
317 今未能解释为什么会发生这种情况。肠套迭也可发生于新生儿（出生 30 天以内）[120]，但对于年龄较大的患儿，有病理性诱发点（pathologic lead point，PLP）的可能性较大[174]。大多数有 PLP 的肠套迭患儿（占所有肠套迭患儿的 0.3%）在其他方面均是正常的[183]。

据报道，肠套迭患儿的家属[165] 及亲属也可能患该病［根据特拉维夫、特内里费（加那利群岛）、美国等 4 个不同地区的报道显示，肠套迭可发生于同卵双胎、同胞及父子］，但他们的病史似乎都提示有病毒感染的原因，而不是遗传因素[144,145]。没有证据表明肠套迭和幽门狭窄一样，一旦家族中的一个孩子患病，其同胞也可能患病。

从不同的研究可以看出，肠套迭的发生率有随季节变化的趋势，即使在不同年代的同一个中心也是如此[46,51]。大多数而不是所有作者确实注意到肠套迭发病的季节性常和病毒感染（呼吸道和/或胃肠道病毒）有关[145,183]。多伦多儿童医院回顾其 25 年间的肠套迭病例后，发现实际上只有季节性发病高峰月份发生了明显变化，即从一个发病高峰（1959—1968 年的 5 月和 6 月[51]）变化至两个高峰（1985—1990 年的 1 月和 7 月[46]）。在这两组病例资料中，约 20% 的患儿之前有过病毒感染。除了病毒性疾病在多伦多的寒冷月份更常见这个原因之外，对于这种发病高峰月份的分离现象还没有明确的解释。在大多数报道中，肠套迭最好发于 5 月、6 月和 7 月[144,145,183]。

1905 年，Hirschsprung[85] 宣称他从未见到营养不良的小儿患肠套迭。从那以后，人们认为只有健康、结实、发育及营养状况良好的儿童才会患肠套迭[95]。虽然我们无法得知 Hirschsprung 的经典论述试图传达的确切含意，但 Ravitch[144,145] 和 Mayell[109a] 的回顾性研究表明这种观点并不一定正确。Janik 和 Firor[97] 指出芝加哥的肠套迭患儿表现为低体重率，且与社会经济状况无关。Hirschsprung 所说的“营养良好”指大部分肠套迭患儿有高体重率或高体重/身高率，这同样未被多伦多的研究所证实[95]。

尽管难以证实，但据 Ravitch[145] 报道，有 7% 的患儿在明显的肠套迭症状出现之前的 10 天至 6 个月内有过相似的腹痛发作。他认为这可能说明在这些患儿中有 PLP，并暗示肠套迭可自行复位，但这是值得探讨的。

发病机制

病理解剖

每例肠套迭患儿都有以下的病理解剖学（见图 83-1）：发病时肠管向前蠕动，近端内陷的肠管（肠套迭套入部）携带肠系膜进入远端容纳肠管（肠套迭鞘部），肠系膜血管在套入部的肠管之间被扭曲成角、挤压、压迫，如此导致套入部局部严重水肿，这又反过来引起静脉压迫、充血及血液淤滞，进而使肿胀的套入部排出黏液和血液，常（但不总是）形成典型的红色果酱样便（图 83-4）。如果这个过程不能缓解，肠管充血加剧、压力增高，最终肠管发生缺血性改变并导致套入部肠管坏死（坏疽）。这种解剖学发现也已被 Ravitch 的实验证明[144]，他注意到套入部的最外层肠管最先失活，最内层肠管要晚很久才发生坏疽，而肠套迭鞘部的最外层肠管很少失活。然而，1981 年多伦多和渥太华的一项联合研究回顾了 25 年间因液体静压复位而发生肠穿孔的 7 例病例[48,92,113]，研究显示在套入部附近坏死的结肠上（肠套迭鞘部）有一处或多处穿孔，从针尖大小到 2 cm 的裂口不等，穿孔处常有数英寸的间隔，其中 3 例结肠有多处穿孔[48]。在肠套迭病例的末端回肠（套入部）有一缺
血区域。显微镜检查发现穿孔区域的肠管全层缺血。 1318
7 例病例的套入部肠管都有水肿，有的有坏死，这些病例均为回结肠型肠套迭，均无 PLP。1995 年，多伦多又对 7 例因灌肠所致的肠穿孔病例（这次是空气灌肠）作了回顾，穿孔仍位于肠套迭鞘部（结肠）[33]。

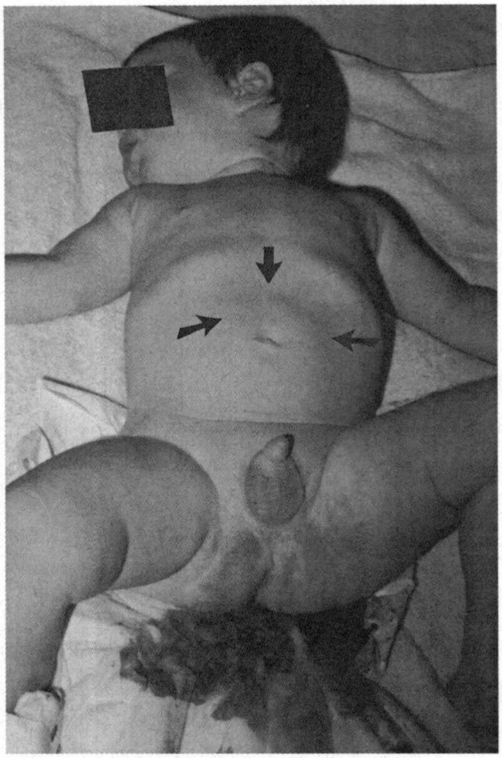

图 83-4　一名苍白、昏睡的肠套迭患儿以及典型的果酱样便。注意上腹部肿块（箭头）（也见彩图）。

1999 年 Karnak 等[98]在 5 例行套迭肠段切除术的患儿中发现了一个纵型病理性薄弱区域。该处肠管明显变薄，沿这个带状区域几乎不能扪及肠壁。该区域就像一条白线，显微镜检查发现该处肠黏膜坏死、黏膜肌层破裂、一部分肌肉组织缺失。据说这条线是由位于套入部肠管和无顺应性的外层结肠带之间的肠套迭鞘部肠管壁内层受压迫而形成的。这条压痕位于肠系膜对侧缘独立带下的部分可解释为局部血管受损所致，因为此处有结肠终动脉分布。因此需仔细检查肠管的肠系膜对侧缘（以及肠系膜侧）有无薄弱的纵型压痕。在肠壁上发现这种具有潜在危险性的薄弱压痕是切除肠管的指征。多伦多和渥太华儿童医院的研究[48]进一步计算出当肠管发生缺血性坏死时，肠套迭鞘部（通常是结肠）已经容纳肿胀的套入部超过 72 小时。此外，由于之前已经提到的机制，完全性小肠梗阻说明肠套迭套入部在鞘部受到压迫。

当肠缺血的过程持续而未被诊断时，会发生两种情况，这是 Ravitch[145] 所认为的“忽视的证据”。Ravitch 推测（如果未得到治疗）在 2～5 天内这将是致命的。尽管很少见，人们很早就知道只要患儿没有死于肠梗阻或败血症，肠套迭可发生坏疽及肠脱落，肠管可发生融合，分离坏死的套入部脱落并从直肠排出。肠脱落在肠套迭历史中很早就发生过，并且几乎是存活的唯一希望。早期的出版物[145]介绍需 10～20 天才发生肠脱落，且大多发生于年长的儿童。儿童肠套迭的这两种严重并发症现在已很罕见。

类型

根据不同的特征，肠套迭可分为 4 种类型（普通型、特殊型、解剖型、其他型）：（1）两种普通型为永久性（肠套迭固定，占 80%）和暂时性（可自行复位，占 20%）；（2）特殊型可分为特发性肠套迭（无 PLP，占 95%）、PLP（占 4%）和术后肠套迭（占 1%）；（3）解剖型分为回结型（占 85%）、回回结型（占 10%）、阑尾结肠型、盲肠结肠型、结肠结肠型（共占 2. 5%）、空肠空肠型、回肠回肠型（共占 2. 5%），以及管周肠套迭；（4）第 4 种是其他型，其中包括复发性肠套迭（5%）。以下将按照发病机制规则系统的表现对列出的肠套迭类型进行讨论（图 83-5）。

普通型

永久性肠套迭（固定性）

大部分（80%）肠套迭为永久性（固定性），大多有症状（85%），并且全都需要治疗。

暂时性肠套迭（可自行复位） 131

自行复位的肠套迭并不少见，据报道约 20% 的肠套迭（暂时性肠套迭）病例可自行复位（见图 83-5）[126]。这可能涉及患病前的经历，7% 的患儿家长称他们的婴儿或儿童有过类似的发作（未经证实的肠套迭?），如果是这样则肯定发生过肠套迭完全自行复位[145]。当然这仍值得推敲。根据 1968 年多伦多的研究[51]，当时肠套迭的复位成功率不如现在，钡剂灌肠后仍有 10% 的患儿不能复位，而在随后的剖腹手术中中发现肠套迭已自行复位，诱发点区域的挫伤

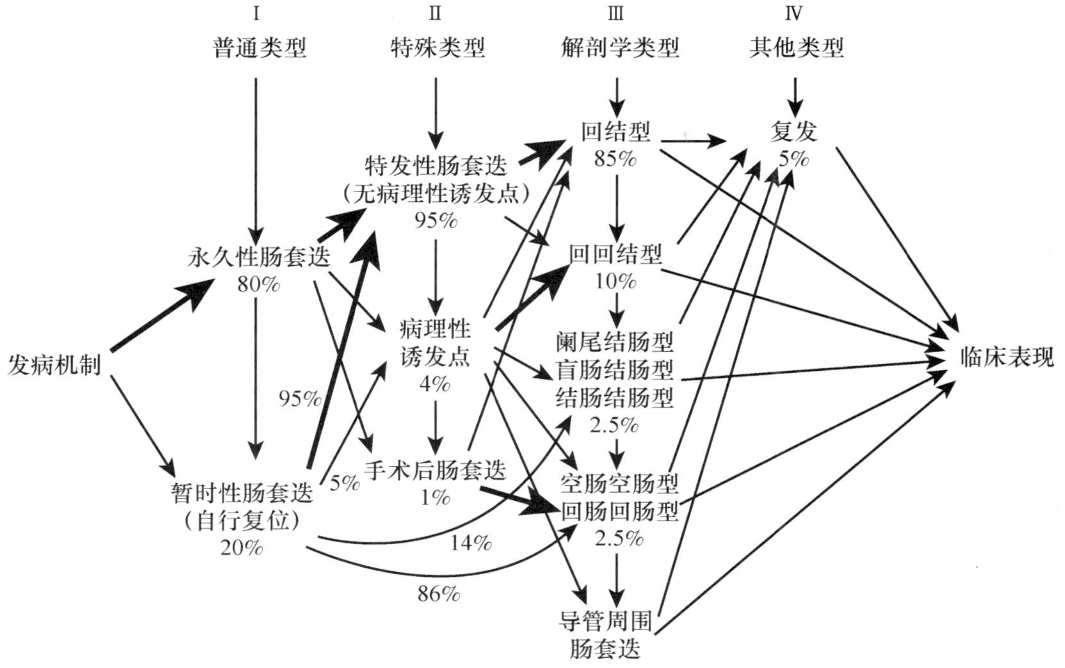

图 83-5　肠套迭发病机制的规则系统。

及水肿说明此处发生过肠套迭。另外一个公认的发现，即剖腹手术（术中需清除或切除后腹膜，很多肠管经过处理会发生回缩）时偶尔（有时为多次）也可发现不同位置的小肠套迭几厘米（ <2 cm）后自行复位。最近有大量自行复位的婴幼儿肠套迭的病例报道，这可能和腹部超声的频繁使用[121]，以及小肠钡剂检查和 CT 等影像学检查能更好地识别肠套迭有关[126]。这些自行复位的肠套迭中有 86% 仅累及小肠[168]，并位于中腹部及左侧腹部[126]。其中一半以上的患儿没有症状，而是由于其他疾病或异常时接受上述检查才偶然发现。由于其中一些疾病可能会引起肠壁增厚及肠管活动异常，从而诱发暂时性肠套迭。由于有炎症的肠管过度活动，暂时性肠套迭也可与胃肠炎症状同时出现。有趣的是小肠发生暂时性套迭时并不常伴有腹部绞痛。此外，Kornecki 等[104] 和 Siaplaouras 等[158]报道只有 5%~6% 的有症状的患者消化道存在某些病理情况，可能会成为 PLP[126]。而其他有报道称 PLP 的比例更高[126]。可自行复位的暂时性肠套迭例数较少说明可能存在抽样差异，因为一些小儿放射科医生未给无症状的患儿常规行肠道超声检查[126]。另外对于正常的、无症状的儿童，小肠套迭（以及伴有急性胃肠炎的婴儿或儿童）估计可自行复位，只需临床观察，只要肠套迭无症状就无需额外行影像学检查。

特殊型

特发性肠套迭（无 PLP）

大多数（95%）特发性肠套迭发生于回结肠区（回结型占 85%，回回结型占 10%），并且无 PLP（见图 83-5）。实际上，所有肠套迭都有某种诱发点，但绝大多数（超过 90%）的诱发点是增厚的肠壁淋巴组织（Peyer 斑）[129,144,145,183]。婴幼儿有大量的淋巴组织（扁桃体、腺样体、淋巴结），当病毒感染（呼吸道病毒、胃肠道病毒）累及淋巴组织时，远端回肠壁的淋巴组织可能会增大（肥大），即淋巴样增生。Peyer 斑通常位于肠壁的肠系膜对侧，但是一旦靠近远端回肠，Peyer 斑可累及肠管的四周使肠腔狭窄，肠蠕动时就可能发生梗阻性回结肠套迭。此外，病毒性疾病和/或肠套迭后邻近的肠系膜淋巴结也可能增大。病毒性疾病先于肠套迭发生或引起小儿肠套迭的情况见于 20% 的病例（Dennison[41]、Strang[163]，多伦多[51]）。腺病毒[119,176]和轮状病毒[124,185]感染（及其疫苗）可引起淋巴样增生，因此和小儿肠套迭有关。事实上，这使得美国食品药品管理局于1999年7月停止使用四价的轮状病毒疫苗，因为该疫苗可能和20例肠套迭有关。文献对该问题仍有激烈的争论[159]，对该领域仍在进行大量研究（见表83-2）。毫无疑问，当一年中的某个时候病毒感染出现一个高峰（暴发）时，肠套迭发生最为频繁[46,51]。

病理性诱发点

Blakelock和Beasley[11]在回顾文献后发现可引发肠套迭的PLP在婴儿或儿童中的发生率为1.5%～12%（见图83-5），平均为8%。根据多伦多的经验，PLP的发生率为4%[34,36,44-46,50,51,53,126,128]。PLP的发生率随着年龄增长而增加：出生后第1年为5%，5～14岁年龄组中为60%。据Turner[183]报道，PLP在大于2岁的患儿中发生率为22%。Navarro和Daneman[126]报道，44%的PLP发生在5岁以前。有过1次肠套迭复发的婴儿或儿童中，PLP的发生率为4%，而多次复发的患儿中为14%。

可发生两种类型的PLP：胃肠道局部（单个）或弥漫性病变。事实上，所有关于这个问题的文章都证实翻转的Meckel憩室是PLP最常见的原因[36,134]，其次是息肉6（多数为回肠息肉）（图83-6）和重复畸形（多数为回肠和盲肠的重复畸形）[1,7,45]。据报道，

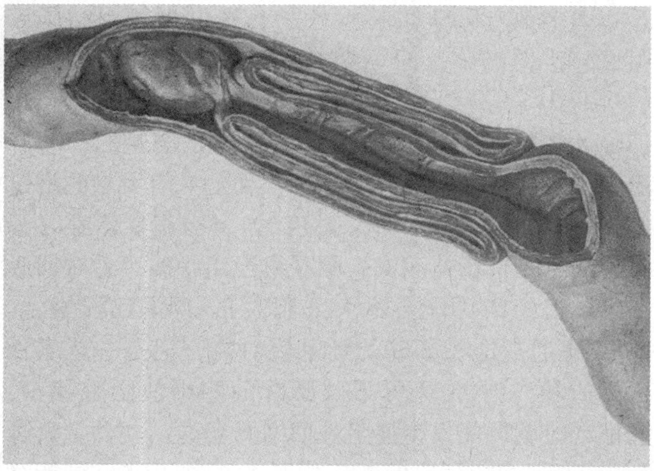

图83-6 由第二常见的局部（单个）病理性诱发点（息肉，大都位于远端回肠）引起的小肠套迭。

其他不太常见的局部PLP有阑尾周围炎、阑尾残端、阑尾黏液囊肿、局部缝线、局部淋巴组织大量增生、异位胰腺、腹部外伤、良性肿瘤（腺瘤、平滑肌瘤、类癌瘤、神经纤维瘤、血管瘤）及恶性肿瘤（淋巴 132
瘤、肉瘤、白血病）[126]。可广泛累及肠道、引起肠壁增厚和/或影响肠管活力，从而导致肠套迭[126]的疾病包括过敏性紫癜（henoch-Schönlein purpura，HSP）[89]、囊性纤维化[87]、腹部疾病、凝血功能障碍、血友病、中性粒细胞减少性结肠炎、巨结肠小肠结肠炎、Peutz-Jeghers综合征及家族性息肉。1992年，Stringer等[166]的报道列出了更多不太常见的PLP，从1998—2004年这份列表中的病例报告一直在持续更新（见表83-1）。

由于临床表现各异且常为非特异性，并且病变类型广泛、肠道异常为弥漫性[126,128]，故诊断PLP引起的肠套迭仍具有挑战性[32,37]。PLP引起的肠套迭和常见的回结型肠套迭（因为没有PLP，故为特发性）的差异是有关联的，因为两者的处理方法可能不同。因为局部病变引起的肠套迭常无特定的始发症状或体征，所以有可能诱发肠套迭的潜在病变是最重要的临床线索[126]。肠套迭的发生是由于肠壁增厚、肠管活动异常、分泌受阻或有多发性息肉。这些疾病可导致肠壁及身体其他部分的广泛异常。Navarro和Daneman[126]报道，35%有PLP的患儿有这些诱发情况中的一种（潜在疾病）。和PLP有关的另外4个重要因素是回回结型肠套迭、较年长的儿童、慢性症状伴发体重减轻及复发性肠套迭。

大多数PLP在解剖学上表现为回回结型肠套迭，一小部分为空肠空肠型、回肠回肠型、回结肠型、阑尾结肠型、盲肠结肠和结肠结肠型肠套迭。尽管回回结型肠套迭可在没有PLP的情况下发生，但40%还是有明确的PLP[45]。

虽然PLP相关性肠套迭发生于较年长的儿童（或者较年长的儿童肠套迭一般由PLP引起），但Ong和Beasley[132]文献指出PLP相关性肠套迭最好发于1岁以内。Blakelock和Beasley[11]认为PLP引起的肠套迭的比例随年龄增长，从1岁以内的5%到5～14岁的60%。因此，虽然年龄可能是PLP的预测因素（特别是肠套迭发生于新生儿或大于5岁的儿童时），但是必须注意到PLP也可见于婴儿和儿童，他们是回结肠型（特发性）肠套迭最好发的年龄段。

大多数PLP相关性肠套迭和常见的特发性回结型肠套迭有相同的症状和体征。遗漏小肠恶性肿瘤（淋

巴瘤）的顾虑在文献中被过于夸大了[114,174]。一项对40年内多伦多1200名婴儿和儿童的研究发现11例淋巴瘤表现为PLP引起的肠套迭[53]。大多数患儿年龄大于4岁半，长期患病，有时迁延数月，有体重减轻及腹部肿块，这些都指向恶性肿瘤的过程。11例回结型淋巴瘤肠套迭中有10例采用钡剂灌肠复位，但均有残余的充盈缺损。在超声下，淋巴瘤在肠套迭套入部中呈小叶状的低回声肿块[126]。然而据报道，极少数情况下，良性反应性淋巴增生明显突出，外观如同淋巴瘤，需手术切除做组织学检查[128]。因此，各方面综合考虑后便很难遗漏罕见的、可引起小儿肠套迭的淋巴瘤。

报道的婴儿及儿童的PLP总体发生率差异很大，可达12%，但多伦多的经验表明复发性肠套迭的PLP发生率更高，可高达33%[34]。Navarro等[127]注意到肠套迭复发或临床表现都不能预测PLP。因此，影像学检查在确定有无PLP时起到主要作用[117]。据他们介绍，在肠套迭仅复发一次的患儿中，仅4%~5%有PLP，而多次复发的患儿中，14%~19%（在几个研究中）有PLP。虽然多次复发表明存在PLP，但大多数有PLP的患儿仅复发一次，因为根据影像学表现（肠套迭第一次发作时所做的检查）或由于肠套迭无法复位行手术治疗，就可诊断PLP。必须记住大多数肠套迭复发的患儿没有PLP。在多伦多的研究中[126]，对肠套迭复发患儿（有多达8例成功复位的患儿复发）的长期随访显示在最后一次肠套迭发生后没有进一步的临床问题或发现PLP，由此提示复发不太可能由PLP造成。

肠套迭不能复位（经一次或多次灌肠后）并不一定表示有PLP，但这个问题并不重要，因为无法复位是手术的绝对指征。一份早期的文章称所有PLP引起的肠套
321 迭都不能通过液体静压灌肠复位，必须手术治疗[45]。这种观点已经被证明是不正确的（多伦多，1986）[50]，随后的研究（多伦多，2000）[128]显示对于PLP引起的肠套迭，BE的复位成功率为50%，空气灌肠（air enema，AE）的复位成功率高达60%[42]。PLP相关性肠套迭用BE复位时，在回结肠或结肠常常（40%）可见持续性的钡柱充盈缺损（图83-7），然而用AE复位时这种情况并不多见（11%）。在这个研究中，超声被证明是最基本的诊断方式，它可诊断2/3的PLP[35]。

超声检查在很大程度上取决于操作人员的技术。多伦多的研究人员可诊断出64%的PLP，其中局灶性PLP的诊断率为74%，弥漫性PLP的诊断率为40%，并且为32%的PLP的明确分型提供了特异性诊断[126]。

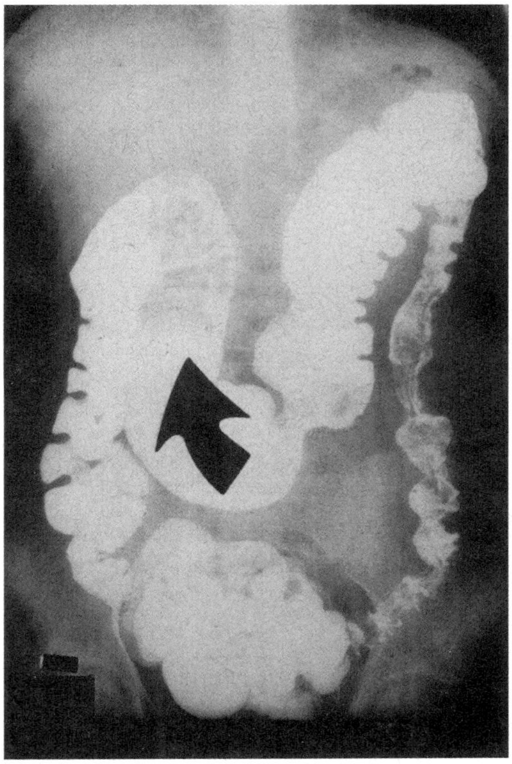

图 83-7 罕见的、由右侧横结肠巨大的Peutz-Jeghers息肉引起的肠套迭行液体静压对比灌肠复位。成功复位后病理性诱发点仍为一处充盈缺损。

他们总结出超声对诊断重复性囊肿和淋巴瘤构成的PLP特别有效，但对Meckel憩室[35]和息肉的诊断则较差，并且对广泛影响肠道的PLP的诊断特异性较差。

如果超声常规用于肠套迭的诊断，放射科医生就有机会发现PLP。对于高度怀疑有PLP但超声检查结果为阴性的患儿，没有科学的数据指导我们该如何处理[126]。如何应用其他影像学方法寻找超声无法辨别的PLP的文献资料很少。而CT的价值是有限的，疑有息肉而超声检查结果为阴性时，小肠、结肠造影[39]以及结肠镜检查可有一定的诊断价值。对于疑似病例，如果起初超声检查结果为阴性，应重复行超声检查。

术后肠套迭

第三种常见的肠套迭类型为术后肠套迭[3,10,47,86,118,177]（1%）（见图83-5），表现为SBO

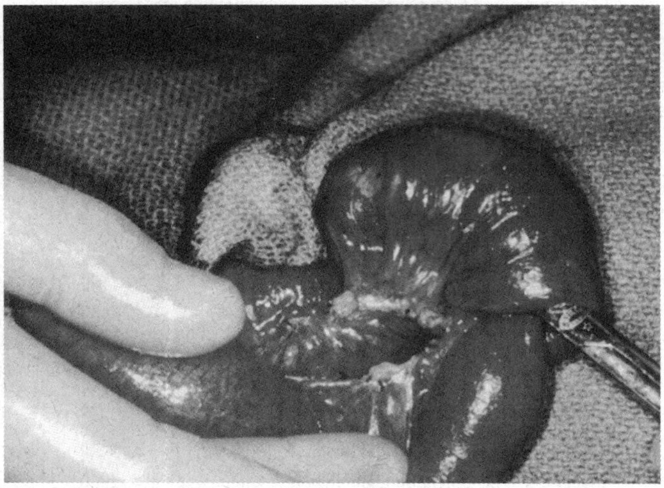

图 83-8　小肠套迭常由 PLP 引起。它是最常见的手术后肠套迭类型，但后一种情况几乎不伴有 PLP。

（见图 83-2）。这种肠套迭常发生于有明显肠管收缩及肠管操作的长时间开腹手术之后，一般只累及小肠，偶尔会累及回结肠。小肠套迭（回回结型肠套迭的第一部分）常因 PLP 发病（40%）[51]，但典型的术后小肠套迭并非如此（图 83-8）[20]。小儿因各种原因行剖腹手术后发生粘连性肠梗阻的比例为 5%（80% 发生于术后 2 年内），据估计在儿科患者中此型肠套迭约占所有术后 SBO 的 5%～10%[96]。大多数 SBO 似乎发生于腹膜后清除术后（肾母细胞瘤、神经母细胞瘤）或广泛的肠道手术（腹会阴拖出手术，即 Ladd 手术）后[126]。在开腹手术时，发生累及小肠的一处或几处小的（<2 cm）肠套迭并不少见，并可自行复位，一般不是病理性的，故很少有临床意义，也不能预示手术后会发生肠套迭。

另一方面，很多作者[11,100,177]已经报道对腹部以外的结构进行手术后也会发生肠套迭。异常的肠蠕动
1322 有很多原因，已发现的有血清电解质异常、化疗、放疗、麻醉、药物和神经源性因素等。这似乎很具有偶然性，可能是推测的，这和某位住院患者在术后恢复过程中得急性阑尾炎一样。诊断真正的术后肠套迭的要点是术后确实发生了肠套迭，特别是发生于一个大型剖腹手术后。早期表现为术后 SBO，并且因术后发生的无力性肠梗阻而难以察觉。超声具有诊断性，如果为罕见的回结型肠套迭，可尝试灌肠复位。否则需手术复位，可最终治愈，且术后复发很少见[55]。

解剖型

回结型

回结型是最常见的肠套迭类型，已在之前的“特发性肠套迭（无 PLP）”部分中作了讨论（见图 83-5）。

回回结型

回回结型（见图 83-5）是第二常见的肠套迭类型（4%）[51]，它有两个解剖部分：第一个是回肠回肠部分，该部分套入盲肠和结肠后即为回回结型肠套迭（图 83-9）。其他研究中此类型肠套迭的发生率高达 5%～12%[69,169]。此型肠套迭的特征性表现为更完全的 SBO，且难以复位（BE 的复位成功率为 25%[48]，AE 的复位成功率可能高一些）。虽然回回结型肠套迭可发生在无 PLP 的特发性肠套迭患儿，但其中 40% 的潜在病因为 PLP[51]。

阑尾结肠型、盲肠结肠型和结肠结肠型

这些类型的肠套迭较少见（2.5%），并且常伴有 PLP（见图 83-5）。

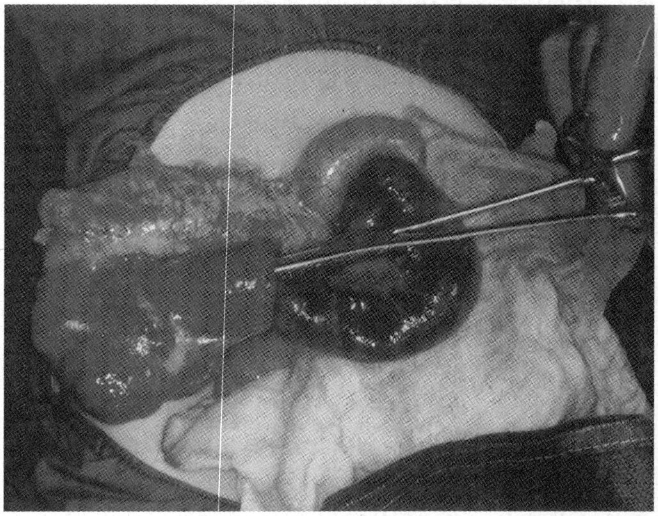

图 83-9　回回结型肠套迭的回结部复位（注意盲肠及升结肠充血但空虚）及回回部部分复位，末端回肠明显坏死。

空肠空肠型和回肠回肠型

空肠空肠型和回肠回肠型肠套迭不常见（2.5%），除非是术后肠套迭（见图 83-8），否则通常伴有 PLP（见图 83-5）。

导管周围肠套迭

在过去 10 年中，由于导管在胃肠减压或喂养中的普遍使用，肠道导管周围肠套迭已日益引起人们的关注。（见图 83-5）。据报道（Hughes 和 Connolly[90]）放置胃空肠造瘘管后有 16% 的患儿发生肠套迭[91]。所有放入空肠的各型导管（不论放置的途径）都有发生该并发症的风险，其中以猪尾形导管最为常见。这种肠套迭是顺行（前行）的，常发生于空肠，并且沿着胃空肠造瘘管[25]或鼻肠管[90]的末端，可引起高位 SBO 伴胆汁性呕吐，但无痉挛或疼痛，通过超声检查即可确诊。拔除、置换、回拉导管，或将导管更换为胃造瘘管或鼻胃管可解决问题。这种肠套迭很少需要手术复位，但可能复发，并且可以是暂时性的，可自行复位，提示其实际发生率可能被低估了。这种导管引起的肠套迭并不少见，常偶发且无症状，唯一的治疗方法是保守性的临床监测。当胃造瘘管随着胃蠕动通过幽门进入十二指肠和/或空肠时，可发生逆行性空肠十二指肠胃套迭[60,63,175]。此外，这种肠套迭发生时患儿无疼痛，喂养导管仍有功能（食物从导管远端流出），可发生高位 SBO 伴胆汁性呕吐，而呕吐物中无食物。此病的诱发因素是当移位的胃造瘘管在球囊（如果存在的话）仍然膨胀时，将造瘘管往外拉拽造成的。尽管超声可诊断，但仍需手术治疗。偶有研究报道，一种更罕见的肠套迭是经胃肠吻合处的顺行性或逆行性空肠胃套迭，常表现为胃出口梗阻，此时常需手术复位。

其他类型

复发性肠套迭

在 1968 年多伦多的研究中[51]，肠套迭总复发率为 5%；BE 复位的复发率为 11%；手术复位的复发率为 3%；有趣的是，肠套迭切除术后的复发率为 0%（见图 83-5），其他报道中肠套迭的总复发率为 8%～15%[38]。1998 年，多伦多的一项 17 年回顾性研究[34]（与 1968 年的回顾性研究相比[51]）显示，不管之前用 BE 或是 AE 复位，肠套迭复发患儿的人口社会学资料相似。因为资料中用 AE 复位的信息较少，所以以前的报道认为复发率主要和 BE 有关。 1323

复发的模式显示 68% 的肠套迭复发病例只复发过一次，且大多发生于首次肠套迭之后的最初几天内（图 83-10）[34]。一些病例复发于成功复位后的几小时内，甚至超声记录到一个病例刚从放射台上被移下就复发。复发离首次复位（时间上）越近，首次复位不完全或未复位的可能性越大。剩下 32% 的病例有多次复发，在几天、几周、几月甚至几年内独立发作，或在首次住院过程中连续复发甚至达 8 次之多[34]。2000 年，Lin 等[107]在 AE 前给患儿肌肉注射地塞米松，试图把淋巴增生降到最低，从而减少早期复发率。经过 6 个月的随访，在 122 例接受激素治疗的病例中只有一例复发，其治疗效果在统计学上优于对照组。尽管这种方法表面上有效，但其效果还需进一步证实。

几个研究[34,44,57]显示肠套迭复发病例的首次及复发性套迭都有很高的复位率（分别为 90% 及 95%），且一组研究中无肠穿孔发生[34]。这种高复位率是由几个因素造成的：（1）对于之前有过肠套迭的患儿，其家长的警惕性增高，故从出现症状及体征至到达医院的时间缩短（平均为 8 小时）[44]。越早诊断，成功复位的机会就越大。（2）复发性肠套迭被认为套迭较松（血流灌注可能更好），因此更容易复位，但复发的机会也更大[34]。近期的研究显示复位率更高（95%）[34]，这反映出复位技术更具持续性（但受控制）。

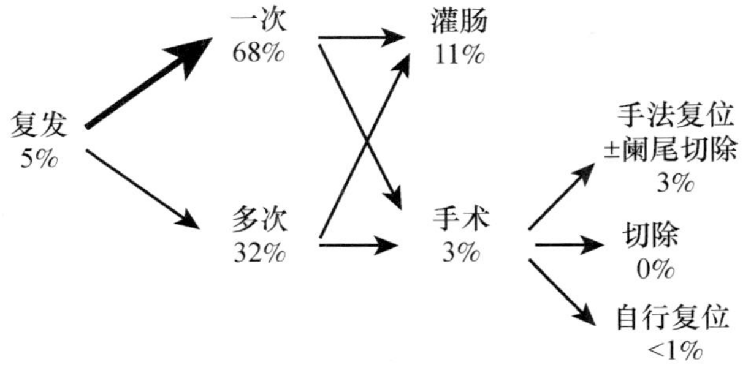

图 83-10　复发性肠套迭的规则系统。

有过一次肠套迭复发的患儿的 PLP 发生率为 4%，多次复发的则为 14%[126]。因此对于所有肠套迭复发的婴儿及儿童，有必要考虑 PLP 存在的可能性，特别是多次复发的患儿。尽管如此，我们必须记住大多数的小儿复发性肠套迭与 PLP 无关。除了一些弥漫性的肠道问题能够提示 PLP 是复发性肠套迭的原因，一般没有临床迹象也没有任何复发的方式能提示有 PLP。对于肠套迭复发几次后再寻找 PLP，没有绝对原则，需尽早并经常行超声检查，可能的话再辅以肠道造影。治疗取决于个体对于治疗方式的适应水平，以及考虑手术治疗前是否接受有经验的放射科和外科治疗。之前报道[57]建议对一次或两次复发的患儿行手术复位，其理由包括可寻找 PLP（特别是远端回肠淋巴瘤），以及试图减少以后复发的可能性。然而，大多数复发的婴儿和儿童（即使多次复发）没有 PLP，虽然手术复位使复发的风险从 11% 降至 3%，但并不能保证不复发[51]。由于复发性肠套迭的复位率高（95%），穿孔率低（<1%），长期随访的效果满意，故一般建议给所有复发性肠套迭的患儿行影像学引导下的复位（首选 AE）。手术只用于反复尝试仍无法复位、灌肠时发生穿孔或影像学检查发现 PLP 的患儿。

临床发现及诊断

两种典型的症状（腹痛、呕吐）及体征（腹部包块、直肠出血）有助于诊断婴儿或儿童肠套迭（见图 83-3）[51]。结合这四种症状和体征，做出诊断的平均时间约为 24 小时（42% 在 12 小时内，70% 在 24 小时内）[51]。奇怪的是，多伦多有研究者回顾
1324 1985—1990 年间的 300 多例肠套迭（在之前 1959—1968 年间的 300 多例肠套迭的研究后 25 年[51]）后发现，平均诊断时间延长至 36 小时却无法解释[46]。然而并无意外的是，由于家长的敏锐性，诊断复发性肠套迭仅需 8 小时[44]。

只要了解肠套迭的症状和体征，就不难加以识别并做出诊断[69,145]。但诊断所需的是腹部绞痛史，特别是对于婴儿。其他典型症状或体征中的一个、两个或三个（呕吐、直肠出血、腹部肿块）通常有助于确诊。如果等到所有的四个典型症状、体征都出现后（只见于 30% 的病例）再诊断，会延误病情[51]。同样，四个症状、体征中出现三个的概率仅为 40%，而出现两个的概率为 20%，出现一个的概率为 10%[52]。此外，在约 20% 的肠套迭患儿中，（病毒性）腹泻[51]先于肠套迭的症状、体征出现，这也是诊断延迟的原因之一。将这些有腹泻症状的婴儿和儿童误诊为胃肠炎而让其回家或收入传染病病房的例子并不少见[51]。像这样延误病情会带来潜在的严重后果[145]。体温和实验室检查一般与临床情况有关，休克和血容量过低常较晚才会出现。

症状

小儿肠套迭最常见的（85%）典型症状是突发的、剧烈的、间歇性腹部绞痛，可使大腿抬起（在婴儿）并持续几分钟[51]。腹痛过后，婴儿通常安静、皮肤苍白、出汗，并可暂时恢复正常活动。较年长的患儿常诉腹痛，并可指出腹痛的部位。很重要的一点是 15% 的肠套迭婴儿及儿童无明显的腹痛。这在 1976 年一份多伦多的报告中有过介绍[52]，其中一位作者（已故的 Clint Stephens）主张这种观点。事实上，《小儿外科杂志》的第一位编辑（C. Everett Koop）曾询问作者无腹痛史的肠套迭的真实性。无腹痛的肠套迭患儿（无法解释其原因）首次就诊时（较一般晚）皮肤苍白、神志淡漠，呈重病面容。无腹痛症状（即使呕吐、腹部肿块、直肠出血等症状都出现）确实使诊断时间加倍，延长到 51 小时[52]。Ravitch[145]注意到腹痛更多见于 2 岁以上的患儿。更不用说，无腹痛也不能排除肠套迭。

Ravitch[145]和 Young[183]指出不但大多数国家对于肠套迭的临床描述相似，而且令人惊奇的是，他们还发现呕吐是最常见的首发症状（44%），先于典型的腹痛出现。多伦多两项相隔 25 年的研究均发现呕吐是继腹痛后第二个最常见的症状，1959—1968 年间为 80%[51]，1985—1990 年间为 48%[46]。婴儿较年长的儿童更易发生呕吐，SBO 引起的胆汁性呕吐更多见于诊断延迟的肠套迭患儿[48]。但没有呕吐也不能排除肠套迭。

体征

两个典型体征（腹部肿块和直肠出血）出现的

频率基本相同[51]。

所谓的腊肠样腹部肿块常可在右上腹触及，并可沿着横结肠向左（上腹）延伸。在大多数研究中，65% 的病例可出现腹部肿块，但在 1997 年多伦多的研究中[46]，该比例无明显原因地降至 22%。肿块可能稍有触痛，只有在腹痛发作的间歇、患儿安静平卧时才能被触及。因此不难理解无腹痛的肠套迭患儿的诊断可能会被拖延较长时间。其中许多患儿在初次就诊时即有休克、皮肤苍白、神志淡漠，呈重病面容，常在此时才首次发现腹部肿块，有时未触摸就能看到肿块（见图 83-4）。最不易引起注意的是右下腹不能触及肠管，称为“Dance 征”[69]。肠套迭偶尔可达远端肠管，5% 可在直肠指检时触及。在 2 个病例中，肠套迭脱出直肠，被误诊为“直肠脱垂”[51]。Ravitch[145] 报道，这种所谓的直肠脱垂的发生率为 3%。这些发现提示无可触及的腹部肿块并不能排除肠套迭。

第二个体征是直肠出血。根据 Ravitch[145] 的研究，直肠出血比腹部肿块更多见（婴儿为 95%，较年长的儿童为 65%）。在 1968 年多伦多的研究中[51]，直肠出血的发生率为 60%，而在 1997 年的研究中，该比例无明显原因地下降至 43%[46]。当发生肠套迭并且结肠自行清除粪便后，经直肠流出的血液量较多，并有黏液样组织，呈典型的果酱样外观（见图 83-4）。这对家长最具有提醒性，如果之前有延误，但出现这样的情况后，家长会迅速将患儿送至医院就诊。虽然不能找到一个能促使家长为他们的婴儿或儿童寻求治疗的特异性症状或体征，但在我们的印象中，除腹痛以外，直肠出血无疑是重要的体征[46,51]。大多数对肠套迭有所了解的医生对于腹部绞痛及果酱样便均有警惕性，但通常是由于后者未出现而延误了诊断。由于出血的最初证据一般只有做直肠检查后才能发现，或者因为出血较隐蔽，故怀疑肠套迭时一定不能遗漏做粪便隐血试验。直肠出血通常是最后出现的体征[51]。很明显，无直肠出血不能排除肠套迭。

Wansbrough 介绍的肠套迭诊断的 5 个原则 1325
（1953 年一项研究回顾了多伦多 1915—1950 年这 35 年内约 600 例病例[51]）仍然适用：“为拒食或呕吐长达几小时的婴儿排除肠套迭是内科医生的责任；应在这些患儿中寻找有无直肠出血或腹部肿块；有腹泻时不能排除肠套迭；较年长的儿童有肠梗阻体征时可能患肠套迭；任何直肠出血的婴儿都应考虑肠套迭的可能性。”此外还应加上一点：不要忘记腹部绞痛。

放射学诊断

腹部平片

临床病史和体检毫无疑问可提示肠套迭的诊断。然而，临床诊断的准确率只有约 50%[9]，因此需要依靠小儿放射科医生及影像学检查来确认或做出正确诊断[75]（图 83-11）。这仅是他们共同参与的开始，随后他们还要参与治疗（见后）。

腹部 X 线在诊断可疑的小儿肠套迭方面仍有争议[32]。1999 年一项对儿科放射学欧洲协会成员的调查发现[153]，73% 的放射科医生常规使用腹部 X 线。这反映出如果患儿存在任何提示腹部问题的症状和体征时，腹部 X 线为常规检查。通常有两种腹部 X 线表现可明确排除典型的特发性回结型肠套迭：（1）腹部平片可见肠道充满气体；（2）结肠内充满粪便。有趣的是虽然可在复位前知道肠道内气体和液体的容量和分布情况，但这些特征可在开始灌肠时通过超声或 X 线透视很容易确定。文献资料显示，由于可出现假阴性（远多于假阳性），且 X 片的解读也不尽相同，故腹部摄片（仰卧位、直立位、水平线侧

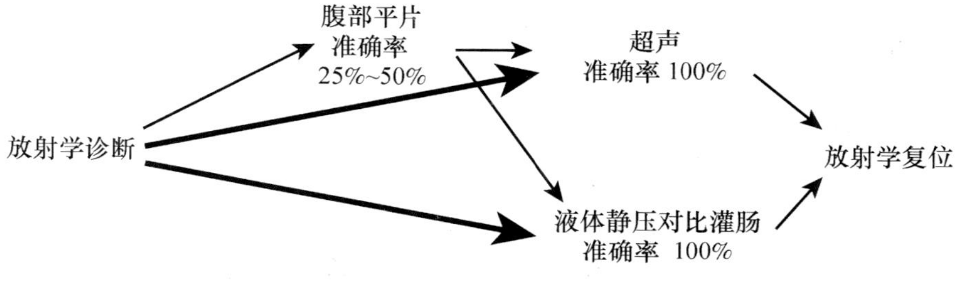

图 83-11　肠套迭放射学诊断的规则系统。

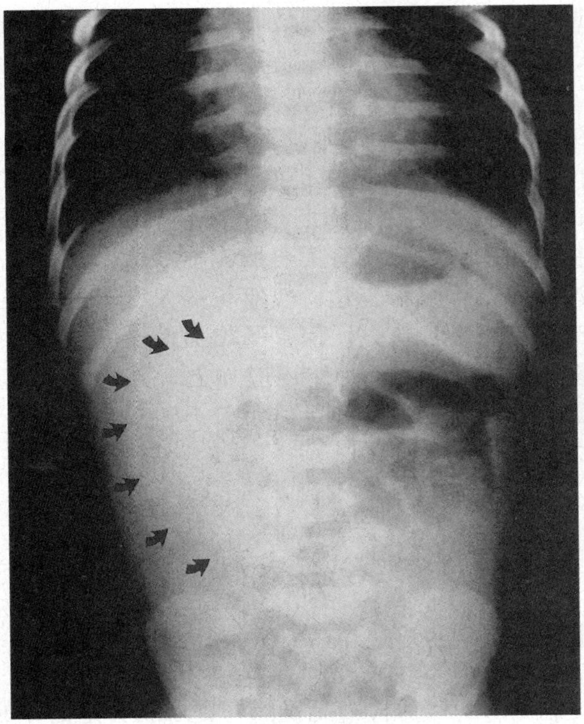

图 83-12　腹部平片的非特异性发现，提示右侧软组织肿块（箭头）伴盲肠气体消失。

位）常不能协助诊断[143]。但有些肠套迭征象在腹部平片上具有特征性（如半月征和靶征）[37]。较易引起注意的是右侧软组织肿块影伴盲肠内气体缺如这一非特异性 X 线表现（图 83-12）。然而，在 45% 的 5 岁或 5 岁以下的患儿中，乙状结肠（充满气体和粪便）常位于右下腹，可被误认为是盲肠[58]。一些医疗机构仍依靠腹部平片来诊断或排除肠套迭，但很少有研究对目前的临床环境下腹部平片的准确性进行评估。两项研究显示，腹部平片诊断肠套迭的准确率仅为 45%（Sargent 等[151]）和 50%（Bolin[12]）。因此，这些作者得出这样的结论，即腹部平片常不能提供帮助，并且对 X 片的解读也经常不一致[178]。Eklöf 和 Hartelius[56] 发现即使 3 次摄片后也只有 25% 的患儿可
1326 排除肠套迭。额外的摄片主要用于确定气液平和腹腔内游离气体。气液平在肠套迭或非肠套迭患儿中出现的频率几乎相同。文献记载，一名未经治疗的肠套迭患儿在灌肠复位前发现有肠穿孔，腹部平片上可见游离气体[32]。

目前普遍认为对于大多数疑似肠套迭的婴儿和儿童，如使用超声辅助诊断（见后），就可安全地省去

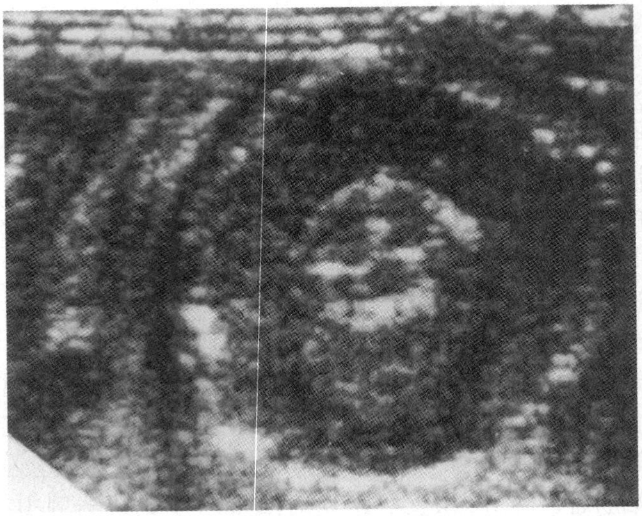

图 83-13　超声图在横截面上显示肠套迭位于右下腹前腹壁正下方。这被称为环形征或靶征。

腹部 X 线检查。这适用于发达国家的情况，因为通常患儿会被更及时地送往医院就诊。而在发展中国家用于诊断的时间较长，患儿肠管失活的发生率更高，故发生腹膜炎和肠穿孔的可能性更大，因此更需要做腹部 X 线检查[112,172]。

超声检查

1987 年，Pracros 等[140] 报道超声诊断肠套迭的准确率为 100%。之后，其他作者也证实了超声检查的高准确性（见图 83-11）。

肠套迭的特征性超声表现使诊断非常容易：常可在前腹壁正下方发现一个 3～5 cm（直径）的肿块（环形或靶征），一般位于右侧（图 83-13）[37]。很明显，检查的质量、准确性和对图像的解释取决于操作人员，因此如果放射科医生对这项技术缺乏经验和自信，其操作就值得担心。经过适当的训练，并配备有高频率、高分辨率的探头，放射科医生就可使用超声诊断肠套迭，并和其他情况作鉴别。此外，非侵入性是超声的一个主要优势。然而和预料的一样，超声诊断肠套迭的准确率在世界各地各不相同，主要有以下原因：缺乏经验、费用问题以及设备的可用性[37,153]。

对于怀疑为肠套迭的患儿，超声检查的作用不仅是单纯诊断或排除这种疾病，还可有效证实有无

PLP。Navarro 等[128]的研究发现，超声能够诊断出 66% 的 PLP，比 BE 高 26%，比 AE 高 55%。Pracros 等[140]报道，当疑似为肠套迭的病例行超声检查未发现患有该病时，却对其他腹部疾病（尿道异常、卵巢囊肿扭转、小肠扭转）有 4% 的检出率。

为了预测灌肠治疗肠套迭的复位率及有无肠坏死，已有学者对超声的特征进行了评估[36]。这些征象包括肠套迭增厚的外周低回声边缘、腹腔内游离液体、肠套迭套入部的液体、与肠系膜一同套入的增大的淋巴结和 PLP，最重要的是多普勒检查发现肠套迭区域的血流消失。许多研究显示，这些超声征象并不能 100% 地预测是否能够成功复位[36]。因此，在实践中仅根据超声特征很难预测哪个肠套迭病例不可复位或可能发生坏死。然而，观察到以上提到的任何超声特征后可对肠套迭不可复位和/或坏死的可能性有所警惕，但不应该放弃尝试灌肠复位。

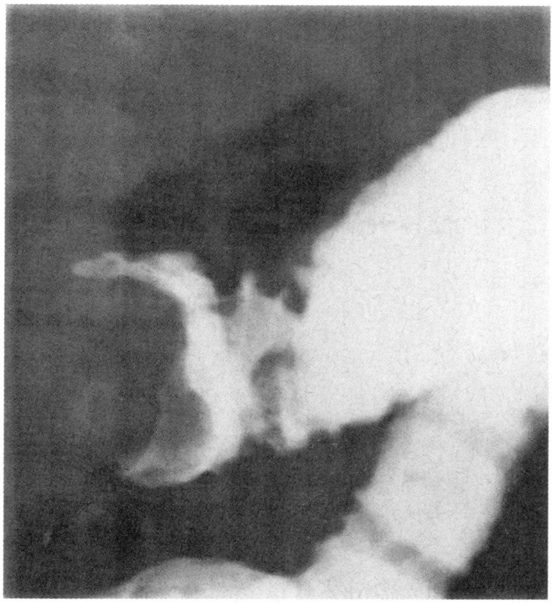

图 83-14　液体静压钡剂对比灌肠显示肠套迭位于左侧横结肠。注意钡剂在肠套迭头部（套入部）形成的新月形凹面。

对比灌肠

20 世纪 80 年代中期超声的价值被人们公认之前，结肠的钡剂检查（BE）在世界各地被认为是诊断或排除肠套迭的金标准[36]。然而，目前一些医疗机构仍然认为对比灌肠（用钡剂）是最快速、成本效率最高的方法[181]。1999 年对欧洲儿科放射科医生的调查显示[153]，34% 的被调查者使用对比灌肠诊断肠套（图 83-14）。主要理由包括：很少遗漏肠套迭的诊断、放射科医生都了解这项检查方式、诊断过程（如果为阳性）也是治疗过程。毫无疑问，对比灌肠在世界各地是诊断肠套迭的首选方法，其诊断准确率达 100%（见图 83-11）[139,181]。

对比灌肠的缺点在于它是一项侵入性操作，并有少量的放射线[36]。如果只用以诊断肠套迭，决定用对比灌肠代替超声时需考虑这些因素。一些作者认为，怀疑为肠套迭的婴儿和儿童行诊断性对比灌肠检查时，50% 以上为阴性结果[36]。这说明有其他急性腹部病变的临床表现常类似于肠套迭。最后，对比灌
327 肠（钡剂，40%）不能像超声（66%）那样很好地描述其他腹腔内病变（如果无肠套迭）或 PLP（如果有肠套迭）[128]。

尽管其他诊断方法（小肠追踪检查[39]、CT[28]、磁共振成像[173]）能够描述肠套迭，但用于诊断最常见的回结型和回回结型肠套迭，临床很少使用。但可用于临床表现更复杂或超声表现不典型的肠套迭患者做进一步的检查，或用于更好地描述可疑的 PLP[36,128]。

治疗

对肠套迭婴儿或儿童的治疗必须从第一个接诊患儿的急诊科开始，并且外科医生必须从一开始就参与其中[179]。如果患儿有呕吐，必须经过适当的液体复苏，并放置鼻胃管用于吸引，这是非常重要的。如果病史较短、患儿无呕吐，可省略后一步骤。如果肠管血供受损并可行肠道手术，应给予抗生素（包括抗厌氧菌）。如需输血，则患儿应行交叉配型。这些都完成之后，应准备行放射学检查以确诊（见图 83-11），接着是其他必要的治疗。应通知手术室，以便于在非手术治疗失败后，患儿可直接从放射科转到手术室行手术治疗。

治疗方法非常简单：包括药物治疗（在偶然及特殊情况下）、放射学复位（图 83-15）（液体或空气）、手术复位、切除肠管、关闭灌肠引起的穿孔及

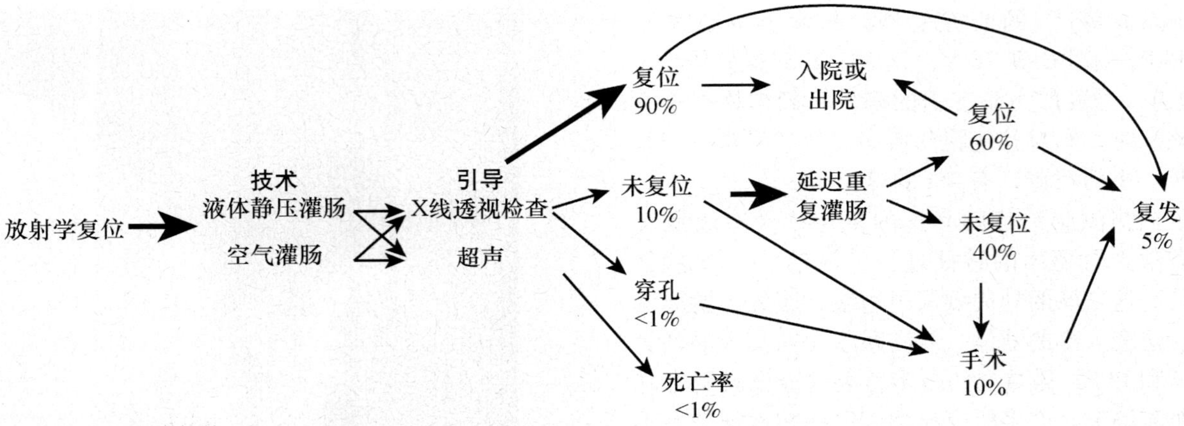

图 83-15　肠套迭放射学复位的规则系统。

开腹手术或腹腔镜切除 PLP（图 83-16）。毫无疑问，过去 25 年间肠套迭治疗的最大改变（进步）是更多地尝试放射学复位[102]。在 1968 年多伦多的研究中[51]，只有 75% 的肠套迭患儿接受 BE 复位。但是目前不论患儿病史长短，事实上，所有的婴儿和儿童均会尝试钡剂或水溶性造影剂的液体静压复位或空气灌肠复位。

药物治疗

在非常特殊的情况下，一些由 PLP 引起的弥漫性肠壁增厚的肠套迭可在尝试放射学复位（成功或不成功）之前、之中和/或之后用类固醇激素治疗。已报道至少有两种疾病［淋巴样增生、过敏性紫癜（HSP）］用这种方法治疗后取得了一定的成功（淋巴样增生 2 例，成功率 100%[157]；HSP 7 例，成功率 50%[161]）。

类固醇激素治疗影响淋巴样增生的机制仍不清 1328
楚。Kokkonen 和 Karttunen[103] 推测淋巴样增生“可能作为对肠腔内食物抗原的反应，代表了长期上调的肠道免疫反应。如果真是如此，类固醇激素治疗的淋巴细胞减少效应可能是减轻淋巴样增生的原因。”

大多数 HSP 患儿有胃肠道症状[64]，起初采用保守治疗[26,27]。然而，由于可能发生致命的并发症，

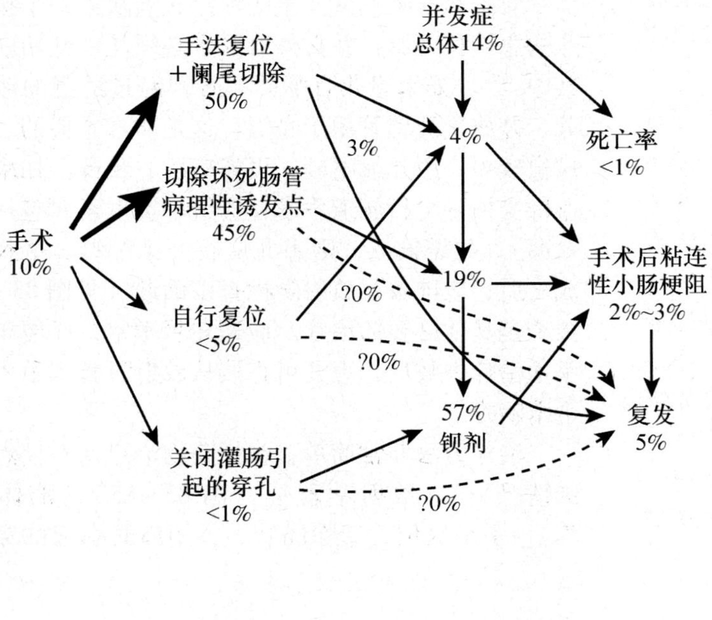

图 83-16　肠套迭外科干预的规则系统。

其中 5%~22% 的患儿需行开腹手术[30,76,161]。这些并发症中最常见的是肠套迭，发生于 3% 的 HSP 患儿[21]。据报道，虽然回回型和回结型肠套迭的发生率相等，但在前面提到的 7 例中有 6 例为回回型。灌肠复位只对回结型肠套迭有效。

总的来说，用激素治疗 HSP 患儿是有争议的[161]。一项研究（比较使用激素和不用激素的患儿）表明，激素治疗组的患儿胃肠疼痛可在更短时间内消失（一般为 24~48 小时）。从文献中可得知激素有助于缓解、但无法治愈 HSP 引起的症状。激素对于胃肠道症状的作用可归因于其可消除肠壁水肿。尚未明确激素是否可有效预防 HSP 过程中的肠套迭。

如果在肠套迭还未复位时就开始激素治疗，必须对患儿进行密切观察。正如 Sönmez 等[161]所说的："只要知道起病时间，超声及 X 线检查已确诊，有急诊手术设备，并有经验丰富的小儿外科医生对患儿进行随访，伴有小肠套迭的 HSP 患儿进行保守治疗是可行的。"

放射学复位

仔细挑选适于尝试液体静压或空气灌肠复位的婴儿和儿童是很重要的，只有少数患儿需直接行手术治疗（见图 83-15）。应在液体复苏开始后，并且患儿情况已经稳定、适于接受任何检查或治疗时再进行选择。一些研究者提出，灌肠复位的禁忌证是有腹膜炎或腹腔内游离气体的迹象，前者非常少见，后者在多伦多的研究中还没有遇到，也没有一例起初就穿孔的肠套迭的病例报道[32,37]。几个因素提示 BE 后可能会发生穿孔：年龄小于 6 个月、出现症状达 72 小时和完全性 SBO。出现这些症状和体征甚至可禁止行诊断性灌肠[48]。一般来说，很少有理由禁止尝试灌肠复位[38,130]。医疗中心之间以及世界各地对此看法迥异。在发达国家，绝大多数肠套迭患儿可经诊断发现，并给予及时治疗。相比之下，在很多发展中国家，正如近来尼日利亚[112]和印度尼西亚[172]的报道显示，手术治疗仍然是常用的、基本的和必要的治疗方法。在这些地方，婴儿和儿童患者的症状和体征明显持续时间更长，肠管失活的发生率也更高，死亡率达 18%~20%[38]。对这种病例，Meier 等[112]认为使用非手术的 BE 复位并不能明显降低高死亡率。

目前被经常使用的四种非手术的放射学复位技术包括[38]：X 线透视引导下的空气灌肠复位、超声引导下的空气灌肠复位、超声引导下的液体静压复位以及 X 线透视引导下的液体静压复位（见图 83-15）。评估这四种复位技术时，需谨慎比较不同的研究结果，即使有些放射科医生表面使用了相似的技术[116]。来自北美小儿放射科[115]和欧洲儿科放射学协会成员[153]的两份调查显示，即使在前几年，他 1329
们对肠套迭的处理也是不同的，但趋势是从液体静压复位转向空气灌肠复位，并且更多地使用超声检查[150]。超声的明显优势是避免暴露于放射线中，相比 X 线透视能提供更多的信息，监测复位过程时有更高的准确性和可靠性，能看到肠套迭的各部分，包括复位后水肿的回盲瓣，并能更容易地辨认 PLP[38]。主要缺点是需要一名能够熟练使用超声引导复位的放射科医生。超声引导下空气灌肠复位的经验较少，特别是液体静压或空气灌肠复位时辨认肠穿孔的经验很少[38]。

液体静压钡剂灌肠

液体静压 BE 复位的主要优点是大多数（即使不是全部）放射科医生对这项技术有丰富的经验，并且熟悉这种造影剂和荧光屏透视检查的使用方法[18,19,38,133]。这是一项简单、安全、有效的技术。钡剂（及任何液体介质）的缺点是使用时会弄脏身体，如发生穿孔，结肠撕裂会更大，尤其是钡剂会（永久性）增加腹腔内污染，并且因为有高渗的水溶性物质而发生快速的体液转移[33,48,92]。

过去，多伦多使用 Ravitch[145]改进的液体静压 BE 复位技术。钡柱高度从 3 英尺开始，如果需要可缓慢上升至更高的水平。如果 10 分钟内钡柱无改变，他们仍不放弃 BE，但不会像 Ravitch 建议的那样持续 45 分钟[145]。肠管复位的速度差异很大，时快时慢。当钡柱碰到肠套迭部分时，常有一个停顿。典型的情况是，圆形的钡柱突然下凹，在肠套迭头部周围变成新月形（见图 83-14）。当肠套迭被钡柱充盈时，则新月形的凹面变平（图 83-17）。因为肠套迭套入部在管径较大的鞘部内显得较松动，故钡剂可渗入两者之间，产生特征性的像卷曲弹簧般的放射学外观（图 83-18）。盲肠充盈常较慢，在钡剂突然灌入远端回肠，即复位之前，盲肠可短时间内极度膨胀（图

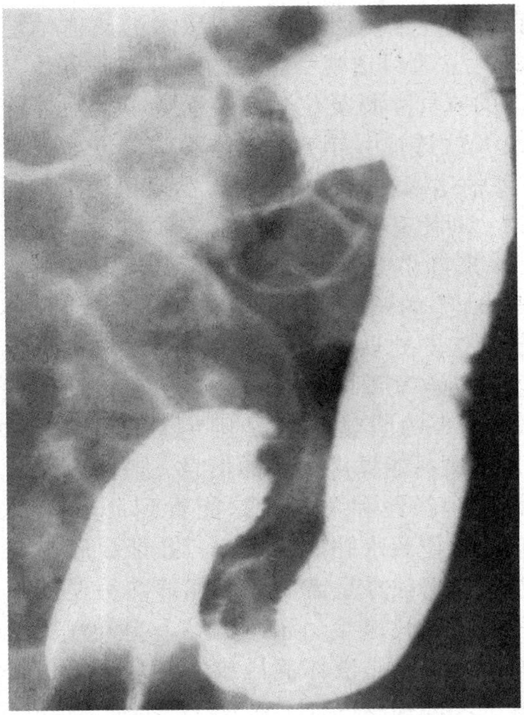

图 83-17　液体静压对比灌肠显示当肠套迭被充满时，新月形凹面（图 83-14）就变平。

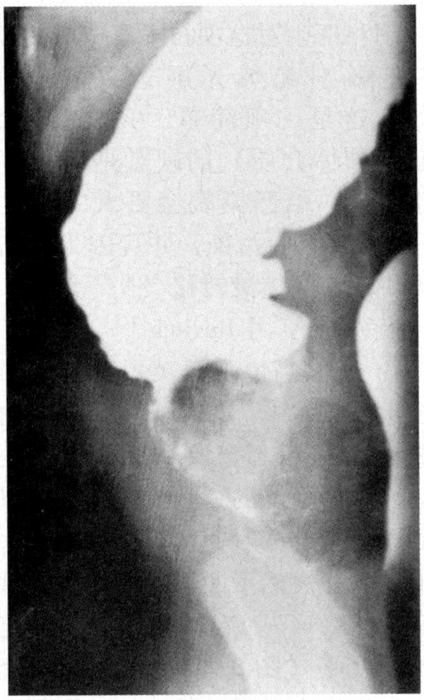

图 83-19　液体静压对比灌肠显示盲肠充盈常较慢，在钡剂突然灌入远端回肠（表示复位）之前，盲肠可在一段时间内变得极度膨胀。

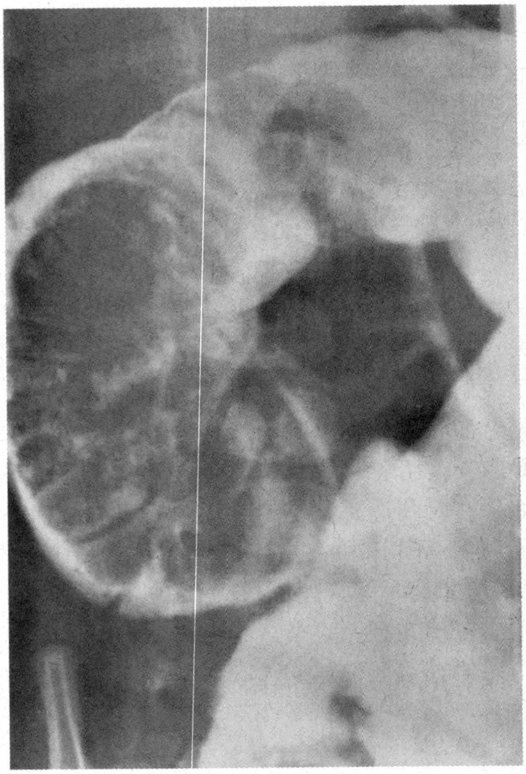

图 83-18　液体静压对比灌肠显示当肠套迭套入部在管径较大的鞘部内较松弛时，渗入两者间的造影剂产生特征性的卷曲弹簧样的外观。

83-19）。如果回肠没有通畅地被钡剂充盈数英尺（不是英寸），就不能（绝对不能）认为已经完全复位（图 83-20）。如果钡剂从直肠漏出或导管滑出和/或堵塞，就必须重复 BE 的过程。一旦复位成功，婴儿或儿童即可解除疼痛，并常可入睡。

空气灌肠

由于 X 线透视下空气灌肠复位具备一些优点，故已被广泛接受：它容易操作、可快速施行、无腹腔污染、释放的放射线较少、更舒适，及造成的穿孔更小、腹腔污染较轻（图 83-21）[164]。这项技术的缺点是在回结型肠套迭没有完全复位时，空气进入末端回肠后可能产生张力性气腹[79,125]，并偶尔可发生肠穿孔[164]。自从 Gu 等[70] 将空气灌肠技术介绍给多伦多的小儿放射科医生后，他们经常发表这方面的著作[32,35-38,46,133]。他们从 50 mmHg 的低气压（经常成功复位）开始缓慢加压，但不超过 110～120 mmHg[156]。

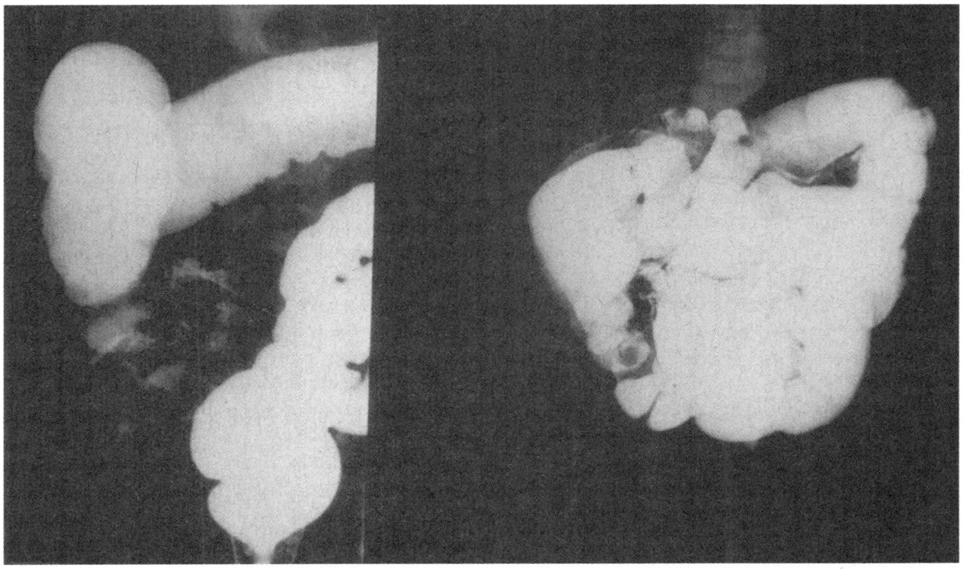

图 83-20　液体静压对比灌肠显示肠套迭不完全复位，左图中只有一条很细的造影剂进入末端回肠。右图可见造影剂充满末端回肠，说明完全复位。

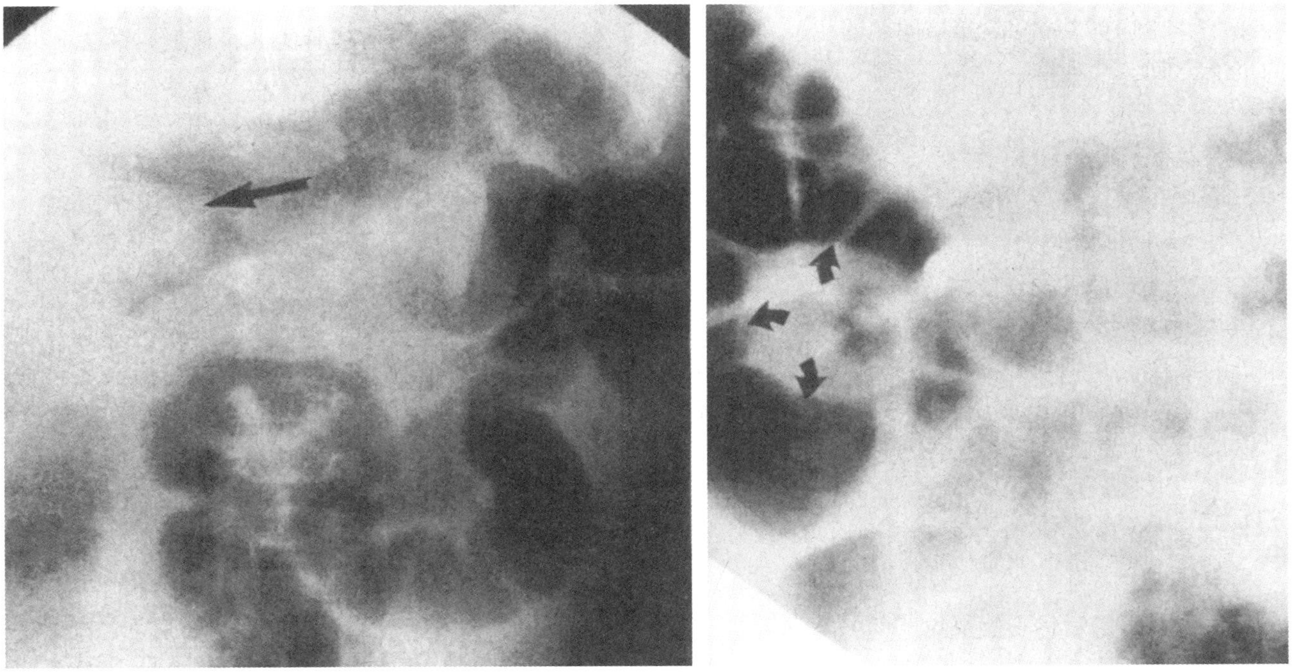

图 83-21　左图为空气灌肠显示位于右侧横结肠的肠套迭新月形凹面（箭头）。右图显示空气倒灌入末端回肠，说明肠套迭复位成功。注意回盲瓣的残余水肿（箭头）。

改善复位率的方法

一些作者提倡用一些他们认为能够改善灌肠复位率的方法。

药物

关于激素的使用，见之前的“药物治疗”部分。平滑肌松弛剂（特别是胰高血糖素[62,88]）及镇静剂被用以帮助肠套迭复位，但结果不确定且有差别[2,62,108,122]。近来小儿放射科医生小心、持续地尝试复位，提高了需手术治疗的不可复位型肠套迭的复位率，其中 10% 在手术室内已经复位，可能是自行复位，但全身麻醉的镇静、肌松作用使之复位的可能性更大。1992 年 Meyer[115] 调查发现，北美多数小儿放射科不使用胰高血糖素和镇静剂。同样，1999 年一项对欧洲小儿放射科医生的调查显示，常规使用镇静剂的只占 35%[153]。总之，既不支持也不反对在肠套迭复位时使用镇静剂的临床证据很少。这些结论与 Ravitch[145] 回顾 1977—1986 年该问题的相关文献后所作的报道类似。

经腹操作法

尽管 Ravitch[145] 反对用手施压的经腹操作法，但 Grasso 等[67] 发现这种操作能将 AE 的复位率从 58% 提高至 76%。虽然一些学者认为该技术的使用要比文
1331 献报道的更广泛，但难以评估其真正的益处[38]。此外，其他医疗机构在不使用辅助性手法操作的情况下，已取得了更高的 AE 复位率。

延迟重复灌肠

过去，对灌肠后仍不能复位的肠套迭立即行手术治疗被认为是标准的治疗方法[145]。然而，术中发现 10% 的肠套迭已经复位，另有 40% 的病例可简单通过手法使其复位[51]。故推测如果放射科医生采取不同的灌肠方式，一半的病例有可能无需手术治疗。根据这种理论，手法难以复位，或有坏死、灌肠后穿孔，或有 PLP 的肠套迭才需要手术。Guo 等[73] 和 Collins 等[23] 早先报道介绍了在进手术室前使用延迟重复灌肠的方法。然而这些研究以及其他一些研究[65,66,152] 并未清楚地规定灌肠的时间间隔。虽然非麻醉下延迟重复灌肠近来才在文献上引起学者较多的关注，但在多伦多及其他医疗机构已成功应用多年[24,32,38,49,127,149,152]。鉴于目前的放射学灌肠技术的初次复位成功率已达到 90%，延迟重复灌肠只适用于少数（必要的）儿科肠套迭病例（多伦多，12%）[127]（见图 83-15）。据说，肠套迭的部分复位及延迟重复灌肠的时间间隔可减轻静脉充血和肠壁水肿，因此使余下的水肿较轻的肠套迭在重复灌肠过程中易于复位。多伦多的一项研究[149] 根据他们的经验制定出延迟重复灌肠的指南如下：（1）肠套迭症状、体征的持续时间少于 36 小时；（2）患儿体温低于 38℃；（3）脉率小于 150 次/分；（4）肠套迭有移动（越靠近回盲瓣越好）；（5）患儿转为无症状；（6）重复灌肠的间隔为 2～4 小时似乎是合适和安全的（如果患儿情况稳定，可尝试更长的间隔）。第一次重复灌肠的成功率为 60%，10 例患儿中有 9 例成功复位。Collins 等[23] 第 2 次重复灌肠的成功率为 84%，但这是在手术室中于全麻下完成的。

这种方法需要有经验的儿科放射科医生和儿外科医生的密切合作。除非严格遵守上述原则，在延迟重复灌肠间隙中仔细监测患儿的情况，否则风险可能超过益处。

复位后治疗

灌肠复位后，根据患儿的一般情况及是否成功复位，至少需密切观察患儿几小时。有时，如果肠套迭发现较早、患儿无呕吐、灌肠复位成功并且过程顺利、家长可以信赖、患儿住处与医院的距离适当，并
且患儿无症状、在复位后短时间内可耐受流质饮食， 133
可回家而不需要住院[106]。大多数患儿（即使是那些成功复位的）需收入小儿普外科病房进行观察并进一步治疗。

如果灌肠复位成功，患儿可开始进流食，如果能耐受可进一步过渡到普食。可减少静脉补液，直至停止补液。如果患儿一开始有 SBO，需放置鼻胃管（即使肠套迭复位后 SBO 解除），梗阻的小肠需数小后才能减压。因此，最好将鼻胃管留置过夜（如果未使用鼻胃管，保持禁食）并维持静脉补液。除非患儿在复

位前后有发热，以及复位困难（紧张的肠套迭），否则无需术前使用抑制革兰阴性菌和厌氧菌的抗生素。出现发热通常表明有菌血症、内毒素血症、细胞因子（肿瘤坏死因子、白介素）和溶菌酶的释放，甚至产生反应性淋巴细胞。在这种情况下，至少需持续抗菌治疗 48 小时[145,160,176,180,182]。动物研究显示，即使肠管有活力的肠套迭在无菌条件下进行手术复位，并且做细菌培养的组织取自外观完整的肠管浆膜表面，通常仍有致病菌生长[144]。除了上述提到的因素，细菌异位（细菌透壁迁移的旧理论）也可能是常见的、伴发复位的高热的原因之一[138]。Somekh 等[160]在 AE 复位之前、AE 后即刻，以及 1 小时后做了一系列的血培养以评估与 AE 复位相关的菌血症的风险。结果显示，虽然在 AE 复位后可能有发热，但临床上发生严重菌血症和败血症的风险非常低。

虽然 Ravitch 坚持给患儿口服或经鼻胃管给予碳片以证明 SBO 已解除（见患儿排出含有炭末的粪便）[145]，但只要患儿不发热、无腹痛，并且胃肠道功能正常，大多数小儿外科医生就感到满意。通常无需随访性的预约就诊，但患儿家长应意识到灌肠复位后有 10% 的复发率［钡剂灌肠（10%），高于空气灌肠（4%）］[108,133]。

如果对灌肠复位是否成功仍有疑问和/或腹痛复发，可行重复超声检查[43]。如果肠套迭复发，可重复灌肠复位。灌肠复位成功后，回盲瓣常在 1 天或更长时间内水肿、增厚（见图 83-21）[38]。其表现易与肠套迭复发进行区别，因为它没有典型的同心圆外观和内陷的肠系膜、比肠套迭典型的靶征小，并且会随着时间而消失[78,148]。如进行对比灌肠检查，回盲部增厚处亦可见有充盈缺损或狭窄（图 83-22）。当试图证实肠套迭已完全复位，以及区分复位后水肿的肠管与 PLP 或复发性肠套迭时，认识这些征象很重要。复位后行超声检查对以下复杂情况是必要的[43]：当用 AE 复位后肠套迭消失但远端小肠气体较少或无气体时，用以确定肠套迭是否复位；当回回结型肠套迭结肠小肠里均有大量气体时，描述其未复位的回结部或回回部[125]；排除 PLP。如果超声只显示增大的肠系膜淋巴结、肠壁明显增厚且充血（多普勒检查），则可能是进行性的炎症过程（艰难梭菌、小肠结肠炎耶尔森氏菌）引起的肠套迭[15,82]。超声在尝试延迟重复灌肠复位前再评估先前部分复位的肠套迭，以排除自发性复位时也很重要。

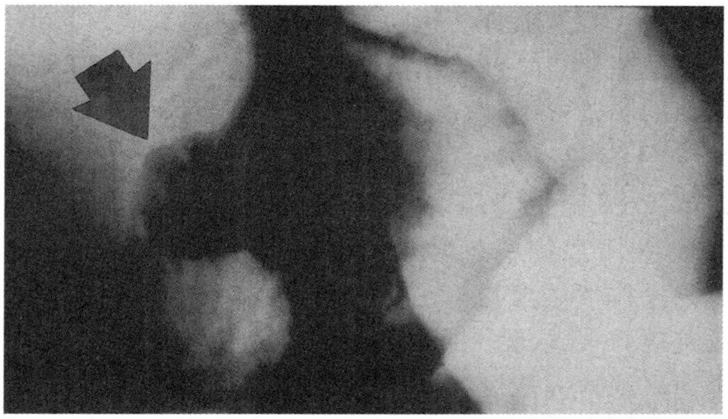

图 83-22　回结型肠套迭在行液体静压对比灌肠成功复位后回盲瓣水肿（箭头）。

手术治疗

剖腹手术

如果上述所有的复位尝试都失败了（10%），则需行手术治疗（见图 83-16）。此时患儿需放置静脉导管和鼻胃管。需逐步进行液体复苏，并给予患儿 3 倍量的静脉抗生素，并为可能的输血进行交叉配型。气管内全身麻醉后，为开腹手术做腹部准备并铺巾。通常做小的右侧腹部横切口（脐上或脐下）。麻醉下常可触及肠套迭肿块，这有助于外科医生选择切口。另一种选择是做上方的中线切口，可经过（或绕过）脐在中线上向下或下方延长切口（这取决于术中所见及需要做什么操作）。切口的大小和位置必须保证能接近肠套迭处，肠套迭通常位于右侧，有时位于上腹部中央，位于结肠左侧较少见。肠套迭的位置越远，1333
复位的难度越大。婴儿的盲肠一般较难固定，所以大多数位于右面的肠套迭能很容易地从上述切口提出。这看起来似乎比将肠套迭在腹腔内复位更明智，正如 Ravitch[144]和 Gross[69]一开始提出的。多数右下腹横切口（因为像阑尾切除术的切口）需切除阑尾。另一方面，很多（不是所有的）外科医生手法复位肠套迭后切除阑尾，并声称分离明显的腹腔粘连（Jackson 帆）和局部手术粘连可减少复发的机会，但这仍有待证实[183]。

进腹后，若看到浆液血性的（红色而非澄清的黄色）腹腔内液体，一般就可诊断肠坏死。一旦吸出所有的液体，多数为漏出液，常可经切口不费力地提出肠套迭部分。手法复位成功的关键是缓慢并持续地捏、挤（就像挤牙膏一样）或逆行经肠套迭鞘部的肠壁向后（向近端）挤肠套迭套入部的最远端（图 83-23）。助手可轻柔地、缓慢地将肠套迭套入部拉出肠套迭鞘部。Ravitch 建议不可如此拉，但 Gross 说可以用“最轻柔的方式”拉[69,145]。这一系列的操作（主要是捏、挤或向近端挤）是手法复位的绝对必要步骤，必须在没有干扰的情况下缓慢地、平稳地完成。事实上，这种技术如灌肠一样增加了肠管内压力。Ravitch[145]建议在肠套迭套入部和鞘部之间轻柔地注入无菌矿物油，可能有助于复位。另一方面，他反对在这个空隙内轻轻伸入手指或用 Kelly 钳排出一些水肿液（图 83-24）。同样，可将示指轻柔地插入肠套迭套入部和鞘部从而在两者之间产生一个更大的空间（改良的 Hutchinson 手法）。Gross[69]说：“只有凭经验，术者才能知道复位需持续多久。有时花 20 分钟复位比急于切除肠管更好。另一方面，长时间的复位不成功可能会使患儿筋疲力尽。”一些外科医生提出，在尝试手法复位时发生浆膜撕裂是不可复位的肠管发生坏疽（坏死）并需切除的指征。然而，事实并不总是如此。

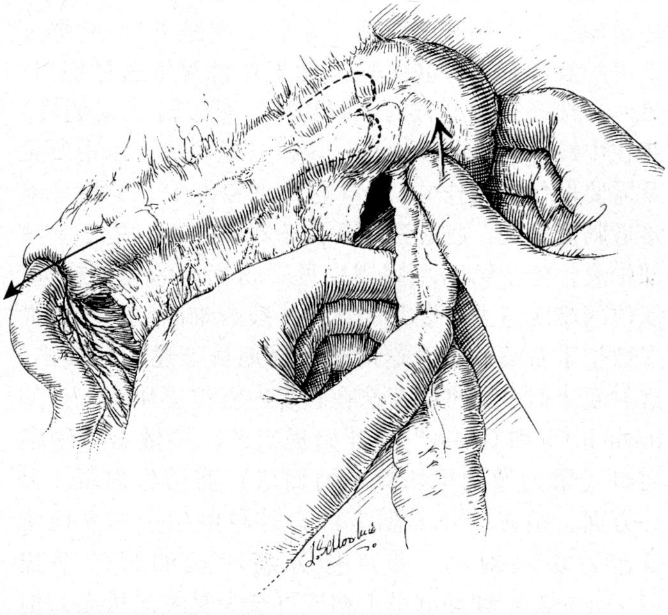

图 83-23 成功手法复位的关键是缓慢并持续地捏、挤（就像挤牙膏一样）或用逆行的方式经肠套迭鞘部的肠壁向后（向近端）挤肠套迭套入部的最远端。助手可轻柔地、缓慢地将肠套迭套入部拉出肠套迭鞘部。

Gross[69]写道：“肠管浆膜层小的撕裂并不十分危险，但这是对术者的一个警告，提示如果向肠管施加的压力不当则可能很快会使肌层或黏膜层撕裂。如果浆膜撕裂口长或深（延伸至肌层），快速缝合几针就足以修补裂口。”因此，如果复位有进展，无论浆膜（腹膜）有无撕裂，而应小心地挤压。如果浆膜（腹膜）有撕裂而复位无进展，就应切除不可复位的肠套迭部（通常是右半结肠切除术）。如果是回回结型肠套迭，常分两个步骤复位：首先是回结部，通过回盲瓣后再是回回部的复位（见图 83-9）。复位后肠管（尤其是套入部的头端）可能发蓝、充血、有淤伤，并可影响其活力（见图 83-24）。然而，耐心等待一段时间（5～10 分钟），
经温盐水湿敷后肠管常会恢复变为粉红色。儿科患 1334
者的坏死肠管不可能复位的观点并不总是正确的。Ein 和 Stephens 称 50% 无活力的肠管可在切除前手法复位（见图 83-9）[51]。在尝试复位时必须权衡其益处和穿孔的风险（随后伴有污染），成功复位后仅需切除一小段坏死的肠管，该手术较不可复位的肠套迭的回结肠切除术或右半结肠切除术小。

如果已复位的肠套迭（通常是远端回肠）的肠管活力较差，应将其切除。少数情况下，如果疑为一块很小的区域坏死，同样可切除或用一层不可吸收缝线将其倒置。

灌肠时发生穿孔的病例（$<1\%$[38]）行手术治

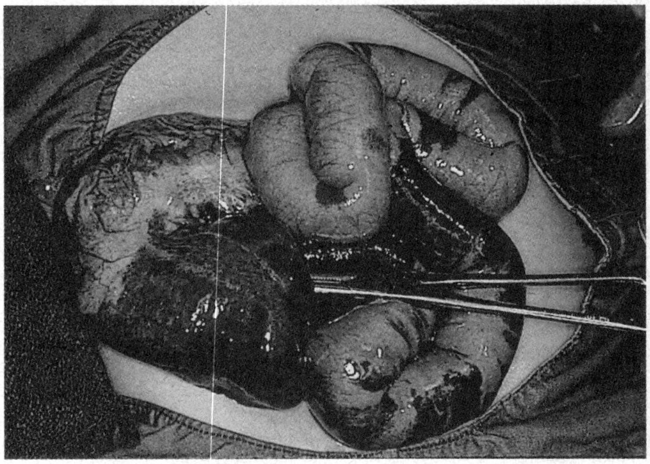

图 83-24 未完全复位的回结型肠套迭。盲肠和升结肠充血肿胀。注意部分复位、充血但有活力的末端回肠（也见彩图）。

疗存在一些问题[33,48,92]。穿孔通常发生于肠套迭复位前，并且出现比预计的要早。虽然这些穿孔的肠套迭大多（但不是全部）有肠管坏死，50% 仍可手法复位（用肠钳关闭穿孔后），因此可减少需要切除的肠管长度[51]。如果不可能复位，则需一同切除整个肠套迭部分及附近的结肠穿孔处。液体静压灌肠引起的穿孔常导致大的结肠撕裂，如使用钡剂，腹腔内会留下不可除去的钡剂和粪便的混合物（图 83-25），并且留下永久的暴风雪状的放射学影像（图 83-26）。Daneman 等认为，与空气灌肠穿孔的患儿相比，钡剂灌肠穿孔者的麻醉时间更长，行肠切除术的可能性更大，且发病率更高、住院时间更长[33]。除了这些重要的、令人忧虑的观察结果，已对豚鼠模型进行实验研究以评估腹腔内粪便和各种造影剂的有害效应[80]。Hernanz-Schulman 等[81]提出与含水溶性造影剂、生理盐水及空气相比，含钡剂的粪便溢出造成的有害作用更大。钡剂是吞噬细胞的重要激活剂，可使吞噬细胞激发后的应答反应变得迟钝，并且对所有受试细菌的应答反应造成不利影响。这解释了为什么上述的钡剂粪便污染增强及不良临床效应延长。

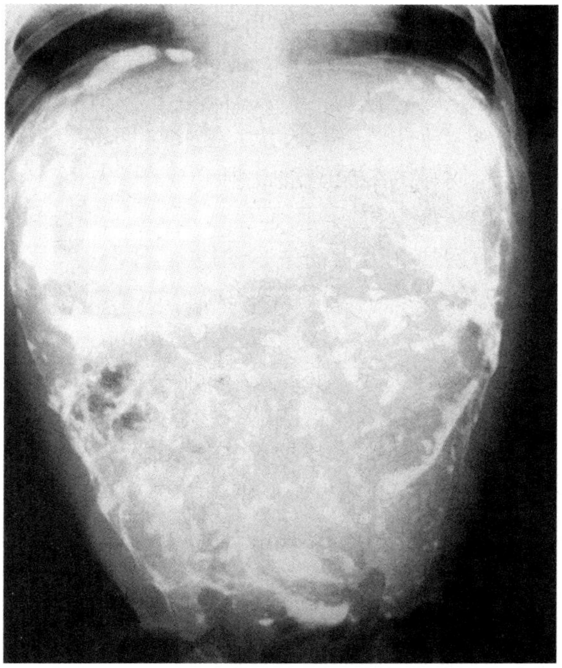

图 83-26　钡剂灌肠穿孔手术后的 X 线片。注意整个腹腔内被污染。这种暴风雪样的影像将终身存在。

水溶性造影剂（如果不是等张的）可迅速吸引大量液体进入腹腔，故增加了粪便污染。相比之下，空气灌肠穿孔后结肠的破孔较小，腹腔内污染的程度较轻并且更容易清除[33,71]。在新式的荧光检查设备的协助下可很容易地发现游离气体。

少数情况下，当发生穿孔时，患儿仍在放射台上，此时患儿可能会表现为张力性气腹，症状明显并需紧急穿刺抽气（最好用 18 号针在脐上的腹中线穿刺）[70]。然而，一旦发现游离气体，立即停止灌肠并开放直肠灌肠导管使结肠减压可避免穿刺抽气。如果无需切除肠管，常可一期关闭破口，最多对创缘进行局部修剪。

如果需切除不可复位或坏死的肠管（见图 83-9），应按照术者最喜欢的方式进行手术。大多数 1335
病例可行一期端端吻合。如果婴儿（可能性更大）或儿童病情危急，肠管切除后（紧急切除肠管而不结扎标本侧的血管）肠的两端应外置作为临时造瘘[69,144,145]。现在这种情况很少见。

如果手法复位得以成功实施，特别对于回回结型肠套迭（见图 83-9）必须仔细检查有无 PLP[128]，最常见的是翻转的 Meckel 憩室[101]或远端回肠息肉（见图 83-6）[127,128]，如果发现，应予切除。回回结型肠

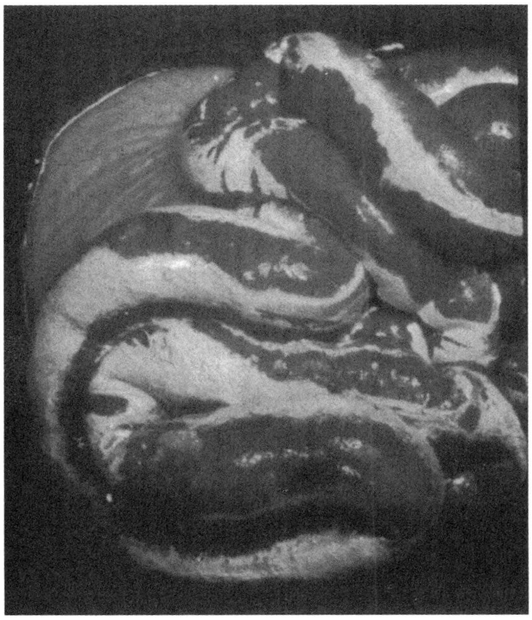

图 83-25　液体静压钡剂灌肠肠穿孔后的腹腔。注意腹腔内的钡剂和粪便混合造成严重污染，这是难以除去的。

套迭常表现为完全性（紧密的）SBO（见图 83-2），常（40%[51]）由 PLP 引起，很少（25%[48]）能通过灌肠复位。BE 的成功率为 50%，AE 则高达 60%[48,51,128]。如果复位成功，在末端回肠、盲肠或结肠将会有明显的残余充盈缺损（见图 83-7）（不论用钡剂还是空气复位），而不是很常见的水肿回盲瓣，后者常在随后的几天内消失，灌肠（图 83-22）或超声检查均不能发现（见图 83-21）。如果充盈缺损残留，应切除 PLP。因为是择期手术，故病变的部位常决定切口的选择。不幸的是，有时会给所谓的 PLP，通常是末端回肠系膜缘对侧的一小块皱褶，而被误认为是 PLP 淋巴肉瘤行不必要的手术切除，但实际上是最常见的非 PLP，即硬的 Peyer 斑。大多数远端回肠的淋巴肉瘤是比上述浆膜皱褶（小凹）大得多的肿块[126]。

腹腔镜

近来腹腔镜已应用于前述的外科领域，同样效果良好。自从这本两册的教科书的上一版（第五版）于 1998 年出版以来（里面未提到腹腔镜）[183]，已有 6 篇有关腹腔镜应用于小儿肠套迭的文章发表，其中一篇仅涉及用腹腔镜确认（取代了剖腹手术）放射学复位[78]。在没有超声或超声证据不足的情况下，用腹腔镜证实是否充分复位是适当的[29]。其他文章则涉及对灌肠复位失败的肠套迭进行成功复位，效果良好（50%~65%）[40]。虽然有争议，但剖腹手术的切口常比那些倾向于在腹腔镜辅助下行肠切除术的外科医生所做的切口小[105]。腹腔镜也可辅助切除 PLP[31]。近来大多数报道（来自 Ann Arbor，Michigan99）显示，腹腔镜手术均只能将住院时间缩短几天。尚需观察腹腔镜下是否能和开腹手法复位一样，对难以复位的肠套迭在技术上易于操作。可以推测，由于腹腔镜可能对肠道的操作更少、肠管收缩更少，所以术后肠套迭、肠粘连及肠梗阻的可能性更小。2003 年 Davis 等[40]提出，腹腔镜的作用在肠套迭讨论会上仍未确定，其未来运用将取决于当地医生的腹腔镜技术和热情。

术后处理取决于手术操作的程度。需注意患儿有无发热，如果有发热，需使用抗生素 48 小时，如果行肠切除（未做肠道准备）或关闭穿孔（无论有无粪便漏出），至少需使用抗生素 5 天。

并发症

放射学并发症

灌肠复位的主要并发症是肠穿孔（见图 83-15）[38]。有经验的医生在行各种灌肠操作时穿孔率很低（低于 1%），只有一些报道高于 1%[33,48,92,155]。应运用各种技术识别穿孔。1989 年一篇来自北美 40 所儿童医院的综述中，Campbell[19]发现在 14 000 例接受液体静压灌肠复位的患儿中，只有 55 例发生穿孔（0.39% = 1/250）。然而，1992 年 Stein 等[162]报道了相对高的 AE 穿孔率（2.8%）。这引发了对空气灌肠技术安全性的争议。相比之下，Guo 等[73]于 1986 年报道了在 6000 多例肠套迭中 AE 穿孔率为 0.14%；1993 年，Gu 等[71]报道在 9000 例患儿中穿孔率为 0.16%；此外，Gu 等[72]报道从 1988 年起他们使用一种新的、能限制压力的气泵后，在大约 3000 次 AE 中未发生穿孔。估计一些医院的穿孔率更低，在那里一些患儿被认为有高的穿孔风险，故不进行灌肠而直接被送到手术室。

Bramson 和 Blickman[13]提出穿孔仅和肠壁坏死有关，因此可推测穿孔位于肠套迭套入部的内部。然而，Daneman 等介绍的 14 例穿孔均发生于肠套迭鞘部的外部[33]。此外，该 14 例中的 8 例无肠坏死，这就说明在一些患儿中技术因素起到一定作用。这些因素包括在灌肠中过度持续使用过高或变化过快的压力。新技术的掌握必定会有一条学习曲线，应强调在低至 60 mm Hg 的压力下也会发生穿孔[33,71]，这说明可能在灌肠复位之前就已经发生了穿孔。肠套迭套入部（有可疑的穿孔）和鞘部的对合可能会阻止肠管内的气体进入腹腔[13]。这解释了为什么这类患儿在灌肠复位前腹部平片上未见腹腔内游离气体。灌肠后部分复位可能会使已经存在的穿孔暴露，从而使造影剂或空气进入腹腔。Daneman 等将 7 例 BE 后肠穿孔和另外 7 例 AE 后肠穿孔患儿的临床状况做了比较[33]，结果显示两组临床状况相似：穿孔发生于小于 6 个月、症状及体征持续时间更长（>36 小时）的婴儿。其他有关患儿肠穿孔的报道也证实了这一点（Bramson 和 Blickman[13]，Maoate 和 Beasley[109]）。无论采用何种技术，应谨慎对待，对症状、体征持续时间较长的小婴儿进行灌肠复位时需给予特别的关心[48]。对于这种特殊的临床情况如何区别对待，尚未建立特别的指导方针。较缓慢地进行灌肠并尽量保持低的压力可能会在一些患儿中降低穿孔风险[156]。

外科并发症

开腹及腹腔镜术后的常见并发症是可以预料到的（见图 83-16）。术前应使用抗生素，如果患儿有发热、败血症，或行肠切除术（未做肠道准备）或关闭穿孔后，术后应继续使用。在一项对 336 名婴儿和儿童，其中包括 354 例肠套迭患儿的研究中，Ein 和 Stephens 报道 251 例手术病例的总体术后并发症发生率为 14%，其中仅接受手法复位（切除或不切除阑尾）的患儿为 4%，行肠切开术或切除术的患儿则为 19%[51]。如果行肠道手术，发生伤口感染的比例为 26%，伤口裂开及突出的比例为 8%。相比之下，未行肠道手术的则分别为 2% 和 0%。两组发生术后粘连性 SBO 的比例相等（2%～3%）。虽然有作者报道肠套迭术后会发生 SBO，但多伦多一项对 SBO 的大型回顾性研究显示[96]，术后肠套迭是第三个最常见的原因（7%）。任何儿科剖腹手术后（特别是阑尾切除术和结肠次全切除术）发生粘连性 SBO 的的风险为 5%，80% 的 SBO 发生于初次手术后的 2 年内，并且不论之前 SBO 的发生次数多少，其复发率相同[96]。1981 年多伦多的报道显示[48]，BE 穿孔的术后并发症发生率为 57%。

结果及预后

临床结果

目前（2004 年中期），诊断小儿肠套迭的总体结果很好。目前小儿肠套迭临床诊断的准确率为 50%（见图 83-3）[9]，而超声及液体静压或空气灌肠的准确率均为 100%（见图 83-11）[37]。治疗小儿肠套迭的结果也同样很好。过去 25 年中（基于 1968[51] 年和 1997[46] 年多伦多的两项大型研究）的主要进步是提高了非手术治疗的效果，液体静压和/或空气灌肠复位的成功率接近 90%。通过更持续的放射学方法，包括谨慎使用延迟重复灌肠复位（成功率为 60%）（见图 83-12）[127]，进入手术室的肠套迭患儿（10%）仅是那些需接受长时间并艰难的手法复位（50%）、需切除坏死肠管或去除 PLP（45%）、自行复位（<5%）或需关闭灌肠后穿孔（<1%）的病例（见图 83-16）[149]。8%～15% 的病例会发生复发性肠套迭[37]。液体静压或空气灌肠复位后约 10% 的病例复发，手法复位（切除或不切除阑尾）后有 3% 复发，事实上肠切除后不复发（见图 83-10）。此复发率在 25 年内未有变化[46]。在所有肠套迭复发的婴儿和儿童中，68% 的病例只有一次复发（大多发生于首次肠套迭的最初几天内）；32% 多次复发，可在几天、几周、几月甚至几年内独立发作，或在最初的住院过程中集中发作（可多达 8 次）[38]。由于患儿家长能较早地诊断肠套迭，因此复发性肠套迭的复位率较高（95%）。据说复发性肠套迭较松（血液灌注更好），因此更容易复发，但也更容易复位[34]。另外肠套迭婴儿和儿童一旦恢复，其远期效果通常是正常的。

死亡率

小儿肠套迭的死亡率在 100 年里已逐步下降[183]。Gross[69] 报道波士顿的肠套迭死亡率从 1922 年的 59% 下降至 1947 年的 2.7%。其他报道也显示了相似的趋势。Gross[69] 在 1948 年的发现直至今日仍是准确的："症状出现与开始治疗之间的时间间隔是最重要的，如果有更多的治疗在症状出现后的 24 小时内进行，则肠套迭的死亡率将更接近 0。"但死亡仍偶有报道。Stringer 等[166] 注意到在他们的研究中 61% 的死亡是可以避免的。可避免的因素包括诊断延迟、静脉液体复苏和抗生素治疗不足、非手术复位后对复发性肠套迭或残余肠套迭的诊断延迟，以及外科并发症。自从本书的上一版（第五版）于 1998 年出版后，已有四篇有关儿童肠套迭死亡率的文章发表（美国，2000 年；澳大利亚，2001 年；另外两篇来自尼日利亚，2002 年）。Parashar 等[135]（美国疾病预防控制中心）报道，婴儿肠套迭的死亡率从 1979—1981 年间的每 100 万名活产儿中死亡 6.4 名降至 1985—1997 年间的每 100 万名活产儿中死亡 2.3 名。这些作者从他们的回顾中得出结论：若肠套迭患儿的母亲小于 20 岁、非白种人、未婚、教育程度程度低于 12 年级，则患儿的死

亡风险增加。澳大利亚的 Byard 和 Simpson[17] 对
1337 1961—1995 年间两例死于肠套迭的病例（5 个月和 6 个月的婴儿）进行了报道，患儿的表面症状较轻，呈非特异的，但随后症状迅速恶化。从中可以得出结论，虽然意外死亡更可能发生于年龄较大的完全小肠套迭的儿童，但这两个病例证明意外死亡可在任何时间发生于任何级别的肠套迭。两篇来自 Ameh（尼日利亚）[4,5] 的文章报道手法复位后的死亡率为 8%，肠套迭切除术后的死亡率为 67%。目前在发达国家，小儿肠套迭总死亡率非常低（<1%），未诊断的肠套迭的死亡率低于 1%（见图 83-3），放射学复位的死亡率低于 1%（见图 83-15），外科干预的死亡率低于 1%（见图 83-16）[32,46,51,183]。2000 年一项美国研究[135] 对死亡率风险进行了最恰当的概括：“虽然在过去的二十年里和肠套迭有关的婴儿死亡率在美国已明显下降，但一些死亡似乎与复位的方法，或诊断及卫生保健的延迟有关，这些都是可以避免的。”

最新研究及未来

自从本书的上一版出版以后，已经有超过 500 篇有关小儿肠套迭的出版物发表[183]。在这段时间内，作者们专门为小儿外科杂志、小儿放射学杂志及儿科杂志撰写了 40 多篇和肠套迭有关的综述性文章。所有这些送检及发表的文章都满足了读者的兴趣。几乎一半（200 篇）的文章为病例报告，介绍了超过 40 种特定的引起肠套迭的病变（PLPs）（见表 83-1）。最常见的 PLP 为阑尾、脂肪瘤、息肉、Peutz-Jeghers 错构瘤性息肉和十二指肠胃套迭。除了这些病例报告，6 个最常见的肠套迭主题是临床观察、影像学、病毒（特别是轮状病毒）、十二指肠胃逆行套迭、产前及新生儿肠套迭以及腹腔镜（见表 83-2）。

进入 21 世纪后，小儿肠套迭仍会继续发生，除非病毒性疾病及表 83-1 中列出的所有 PLP 被消灭。现实中我们可以期待的是运用空气灌肠复位技术治疗肠套迭的比例增加至 90% 以上，只有 10% 或更少的病例接受外科治疗（见图 83-16）[149]。理想的情况是在这 10% 的病例中没有已经自行复位的；手术治疗的肠套迭病例应行艰难的手法复位，切除缺血、坏疽及坏死的肠管，修补 AE 引起的穿孔，或切除 PLP。

总结

肠套迭是腹痛及胃肠道梗阻相对常见的原因，发生率为每 2000 名婴儿或儿童中有 1 名。仔细询问病史是诊断的主要依据，85% 的病例有典型的病史。对于不典型的病例必须保持高度怀疑，比如 15% 无腹痛的肠套迭[52]。腹部平片，尤其超声是临床诊断的主要辅助检查。采用液体静压或空气灌肠复位治疗肠套迭（通常为回结型，占 95%）效果较好。如果这些非手术方法失败，应行手术修复（手法复位和/或切除）。诊断延迟与发病率及死亡率有关，该原因是最主要的并可避免[51]。在过去的一个世纪里，工业化（发达）国家的肠套迭死亡率已逐步下降至 1% 以下[183]。

（陈　盛译　董其刚校）

参考文献

1. Adamsbaum C, Sellier N, Helardot P: Ileocolic intussusception with enterogenous cyst: Ultrasonic diagnosis. Pediatr Radiol 1989;19:325.
2. Allan RA, Heenan S, Given-Wilson R, Adam EJ: Re: K. Rosenfeld, K. McHugh. Survey of intussusception reduction in England, Scotland and Wales: How and why we could be better. Clin Radiol 2000;55:895.
3. Allbery SM, Swischuk LE, John SD, et al: Post-operative intussusception: Often an elusive diagnosis. Pediatr Radiol 1998;28:271.
4. Ameh EA: The morbidity and mortality of laparotomy for uncomplicated intussusception in children. West Afr J Med 2002;21:115.
5. Ameh EA: The morbidity and mortality of right hemicolectomy for complicated intussusception in infants. Niger Postgrad Med J 2002;9:123.
6. Baldisserotto M, Spolidoro JVN, Bahu MGS: Graded compression sonography of the colon in the diagnosis of polyps in pediatric patients. AJR Am J Roentgenol 2002;179:201.
7. Barr LL, Hayden CK Jr, Stansberry SD, et al: Enteric duplication cysts in children: Are their ultrasonographic wall characteristics diagnostic? Pediatr Radiol 1990;20:326.
8. Beasley S: Intussusception. Pediatr Radiol 2004;34:302.
9. Beasley SW, Auldist AW, Stokes KB: The diagnostically difficult intussusception: Its characteristics and consequences. Pediatr Surg Int 1988;3:135.

10. Beek FJ, Rövekamp MH, Bax NM, et al: Ultrasound findings in post-operative jejunojejunal intussusception. Pediatr Radiol 1990;20:601.
11. Blakelock RT, Beasley SW: The clinical implications of non-idiopathic intussusception. Pediatr Surg Int 1998;14:163.
12. Bolin H: Conventional roentgenography in diagnosis of intussusception in children. Acta Radiol Diagn 1964;2:32.
13. Bramson RT, Blickman JG: Perforation during hydrostatic reduction of intussusception: Proposed mechanism and review of the literature. J Pediatr Surg 1992;27:589.
14. Bratton SL, Haberkern CM, Waldhausen JH, et al: Intussusception: Hospital size and risk of surgery. Pediatrics 2001;107:299.
15. Burchfield DJ, Rawlings D, Hamrick HJ: Intussusception associated with *Yersinia enterocolitica* gastroenteritis. Am J Dis Child 1983;137:803.
16. Burke LF, Clarke E: Ileocolic intussusception—a case report. J Clin Ultrasound 1977;5:346.
17. Byard RW, Simpson A: Sudden death and intussusception in infancy and childhood—autopsy considerations. Med Sci Law 2001;41:41.
18. Calder FR, Tan S, Kitteringham L, et al: Patterns of management of intussusception outside tertiary centres. J Pediatr Surg 2001;36:312.
19. Campbell J: Contrast media in intussusception. Pediatr Radiol 1989;19:293.
20. Carnevale E, Graziani M, Fasanelli S: Post-operative ileo-ileal intussusception: Sonographic approach. Pediatr Radiol 1994;24:161.
21. Choong CK, Kimble RM, Pease P, et al: Colo-colic intussusception in Henoch-Schönlein purpura. Pediatr Surg Int 1988; 14:173.
22. Clubbe CPB: The Diagnosis and Treatment of Intussusception, 2nd ed. London, Hodder & Stoughton, 1921.
23. Collins DL, Pinckney LE, Miller KE, et al: Hydrostatic reduction of ileocolic intussusception: A second attempt in the operating room with general anesthesia. J Pediatr 1989;115:204.
24. Connolly BL, Alton DJ, Ein SH, et al: Partially reduced intussusception: When are repeated delayed reduction attempts appropriate? Pediatr Radiol 1995;25:104.
25. Connolly BL, Chait PG, Siva-Nandan R, et al: Recognition of intussusception around gastrojejunostomy tubes in children. AJR Am J Roentgenol 1998;170:467.
26. Connolly BL, O'Halpin D: Sonographic evaluation of the abdomen in Henoch-Schönlein purpura. Clin Radiol 1994; 49:320.
27. Courture A, Veyrac C, Baud C, et al: Evaluation of abdominal pain in Henoch-Schönlein syndrome by high frequency ultrasound. Pediatr Radiol 1992;22:12.
28. Cox TD, Winters WD, Weinberger E: CT of intussusception in the pediatric patient: Diagnosis and pitfalls. Pediatr Radiol 1996;26:26.
29. Cuckow PM, Slater RD, Najmaldin AS: Intussusception treated laparoscopically after failed air enema reduction. Surg Endosc 1996;10:671.
30. Cull DL, Rosario V, Lally K, et al: Surgical implications of Henoch-Schönlein purpura. J Pediatr Surg 1990;23:741.
31. Cunningham JD, Vine AJ, Karch L, et al: The role of laparoscopy in the management of intussusception in the Peutz-Jeghers syndrome: Case report and review of the literature. Laparosc Endosc Percutan Techn 1998;8:17.
32. Daneman A, Alton DJ: Intussusception: Issues & controversies related to diagnosis and reduction. Radiol Clin North Am 1996;34:743.
33. Daneman A, Alton DJ, Ein S, et al: Perforation during attempted intussusception reduction in children—a comparison of perforation with barium and air. Pediatr Radiol 1995;25:81.
34. Daneman A, Alton DJ, Lobo E, et al: Patterns of recurrence of intussusception in children: A 17-year review. Pediatr Radiol 1998;28:913.
35. Daneman A, Lobo E, Alton DJ, et al: The value of sonography, CT and air enema for detection of complicated Meckel diverticulum in children with nonspecific clinical presentation. Pediatr Radiol 1998;28:928.
36. Daneman A, Myers M, Shuckett B, et al: Sonographic appearances of inverted Meckel diverticulum with intussusception. Pediatr Radiol 1997;27:295.
37. Daneman A, Navarro O: Intussusception Part 1: A review of diagnostic approaches. Pediatr Radiol 2003;33:79.
38. Daneman A, Navarro O: Intussusception Part 2: An update on the evolution of management. Pediatr Radiol 2004;34:97.
39. Daneman A, Reilly BJ, De Silva M, et al: Intussusception on small bowel examination in children. AJR Am J Roentgenol 1982;139:299.
40. Davis CF, McCabe AJ, Raine PAM: The ins and outs of intussusception: History and management over the past fifty years. J Pediatr Surg 2003;38:60.
41. Dennison WM: Acute intussusception in infancy and childhood. Glasgow Med J 1948;29:71.
42. Don S, Cohen MD, Wells LJ, et al: Air reduction of an intussusception caused by a pathologic lead point in an infant. Pediatr Radiol 1992;22:326.
43. Dugougeat F, Navarro O, Daneman A: The role of sonography in children with abdominal pain after recent successful reduction of intussusception. Pediatr Radiol 2000;30:654.
44. Ein SH: Recurrent intussusception in children. J Pediatr Surg 1975;10:751.
45. Ein SH: Leading points in childhood intussusception. J Pediatr Surg 1976;11:209.
46. Ein SH, Alton D, Palder SB, et al: Intussusception in the 1990s: Has 25 years made a difference? Pediatr Surg Int 1997;12:374.
47. Ein SH, Ferguson JM: Intussusception—the forgotten post-operative obstruction. Arch Dis Child 1982;57:788.
48. Ein SH, Mercer S, Humphry A, et al: Colon perforation during attempted barium enema reduction of intussusception. J Pediatr Surg 1981;16:313.
49. Ein SH, Palder SB, Alton DJ, et al: Intussusception: Toward less surgery? J Pediatr Surg 1994;29:433.
50. Ein SH, Shandling B, Reilly BJ, et al: Hydrostatic reduction of intussusceptions caused by lead points. J Pediatr Surg 1986;21:883.
51. Ein SH, Stephens CA: Intussusception: 354 cases in 10 years. J Pediatr Surg 1971;6:16.
52. Ein SH, Stephens CA, Minor A: The painless intussusception. J Pediatr Surg 1976;11:563.
53. Ein SH, Stephens CA, Shandling B, et al: Intussusception due to lymphoma. J Pediatr Surg 1986;21:786.
54. Ein SH, Venogopal S, Mancer K: Ileocaecal atresia. J Pediatr Surg 1985;20:525.
55. Eke N, Adotey JM: Postoperative intussusception, causal or casual relationships? Int Surg 2000;85:303.
56. Eklöf O, Hartelius H: Reliability of the abdominal plain film diagnosis in pediatric patient with suspected intussusception. Pediatr Radiol 1980;9:199.
57. Fecteau A, Flageole H, Nguyen LT, et al: Recurrent intussusception: Safe use of hydrostatic enema. J Pediatr Surg 1996; 31:859.
58. Fiorella DJ, Donnelly LF: Frequency of right lower quadrant position of the sigmoid colon in infants and young

children. Radiology 2001;219:91.

59. Fiorito ES, Recalde Cuestas LA: Diagnosis and treatment of acute intestinal intussusception with controlled insufflation of air. Pediatrics 1959;24:241.
60. Fisher D, Hadas-Halpern I: Jejunoduodenogastric intussusception—A rare complication of gastrostomy tube migration. Pediatr Radiol 2001;31:455.
61. Forest WE: Intussusception in children. Am J Obstet 1886; 19:673.
62. Franken EA Jr, Smith WL, Chernish SM, et al: The use of glucagon in hydrostatic reduction of intussusception: A double-blind study of 30 patients. Radiology 1983; 146:687.
63. Gasparri MG, Pipinos II, Kralovich KA: Retrograde jejunogastric intussusception. South Med J 2000;93:499.
64. Glasier CM, Siegel MJ, McAlister WH, et al: Henoch-Schönlein syndrome in children: Gastrointestinal manifestations. AJR Am J Roentgenol 1998;136:1081.
65. González-Spínola J, Del Pozo G, Tejedor D, et al: Intussusception: The accuracy of ultrasound-guided saline enema and the usefulness of a delayed attempt at reduction. J Pediatr Surg 1999;34:1016.
66. Gorenstein A, Raucher A, Serour F, et al: Intussusception in children: Reduction with repeated, delayed air enema. Radiology 1998;206:721.
67. Grasso SN, Katz ME, Presberg HJ, et al: Transabdominal manually assisted reduction of pediatric intussusception: Reappraisal of this historical technique. Radiology 1994; 191:777.
68. Greig D: On insufflation as a remedy in intussusception. Edinb Med J 1864;10:306.
69. Gross RE: Intussusception. In The Surgery of Infancy and Childhood. Philadelphia, WB Saunders, 1953, p 281.
70. Gu L, Alton DJ, Daneman A, et al: Intussusception reduction in children by rectal insufflation of air. AJR Am J Roentgenol 1988;150:1345.
71. Gu L, Wong S, Gu A: Perforations during attempted intussusception reduction: 14 patients from 9,028 examinations over a 20 year period. J Intervent Radiol (China) 1993;2:36.
72. Gu L, Zhu HY, Wang S, et al: Sonographic guidance of air enema for intussusception reduction in children. Pediatr Radiol 2000;30:339.
73. Guo JZ, Ma XY, Zhou QH: Results of air pressure enema reduction of intussusception: 6396 cases in 13 years. J Pediatr Surg 1986;21:1201.
74. Hamby LS, Fowler CL, Pokorny WJ: Intussusception. In Donnellan WL (ed): Abdominal Surgery of Infancy and Childhood. Australia, Harwood, 1996, p 1.
75. Harrington L, Connolly BL, Hu X, et al: Ultrasonographic and clinical predictors of intussusception. J Pediatr 1998; 132:836.
76. Harvey JG, Colditz PB: Henoch-Schönlein purpura—A surgical review. Aust Pediatr J 1994;20:13.
77. Hase T, Kodama M, Mizukuro T, et al: Manual reduction with the index finger for infantile intussusception. A modification of Hutchinson's maneuver. Pediatr Surg Int 1998;13:223.
78. Hay SA, Kabesh AA, Soliman HA, et al: Idiopathic intussusception: The role of laparoscopy. J Pediatr Surg 1999; 34:577.
79. Hedlund GL, Johnson JF, Strife JL: Ileocolic intussusception: Extensive reflux of air preceding pneumatic reduction. Radiology 1990;174:187.
80. Hernanz-Schulman M, Foster C, Maxa R, et al: Experimental study of mortality and morbidity of contrast media and standardized fecal dose in the peritoneal cavity. Pediatr Radiol 2000;30:369.
81. Hernanz-Schulman M, Vanholder R, Waterloos MA, et al: Effect of radiographic contrast agents on leukocyte metabolic response. Pediatr Radiol 2000;30:361.
82. Hervás JA, Alberti P, Bregante JI, et al: Chronic intussusception associates with *Yersinia enterocolitica* mesenteric adenitis. J Pediatr Surg 1992;27:1591.
83. Hipsley PL: Intussusception and its treatment by hydrostatic pressure: Based on an analysis of one hundred consecutive cases so treated. Med J Aust 1926;2:201.
84. Hirschsprung H: Tilfaelde af subakut tarminvagination. Hospitals-Tilende 1876;3:321.
85. Hirschsprung H: 107 Falle von Darminvagination bei Kindern, behandelt in Konigen Louis-en-Kinderhospital in Kopenhagen vahrend der Jahre 1871-1904. Mitt Grenzgeb Med Chir 1905;14:555.
86. Holcomb GW 3rd, Ross AJ 3rd, O'Neill JA Jr: Postoperative intussusception: Increasing frequency or increasing awareness? South Med J 1991;84:1334.
87. Holsclaw DS, Rocmans C, Shwachman H: Intussusception in patients with cystic fibrosis. Pediatrics 1971;48:51.
88. Hsiao JY, Kao HA, Shih SL: Intravenous glucagon in hydrostatic reduction of intussusception: A controlled study of 63 patients. Acta Paediatr Sinensis 1988;29:242.
89. Hu SC, Feeney M, McNicholas M, et al: Ultrasonography to diagnose and exclude intussusception in Henoch-Schönlein purpura. Arch Dis Child 1991;66:1065.
90. Hughes UM, Connolly BL: Small-bowel intussusceptions occurring around nasojejunal enteral tubes—Three cases occurring in children. Pediatr Radiol 2001;31:456.
91. Hughes UM, Connolly BL, Chait PG, et al: Further report of small-bowel intussusceptions related to gastrojejunostomy tubes. Pediatr Radiol 2000;30:614.
92. Humphry A, Ein SH, Mok PM: Perforation of the intussuscepted colon. AJR Am J Roentgenol 1981;137:1135.
93. Hunter J: On introsusception. Trans Soc Improv Med Surg Knowledge 1793;1:103.
94. Hutchinson J: A successful case of abdominal section for intussusception. Proc R Med Chir Soc 1873;7:195.
95. Janik JS, Cranford J, Ein SH: The well-nourished infant with intussusception. Am J Dis Child 1981;135:600.
96. Janik JS, Ein SH, Mancer K: An assessment of the surgical treatment of adhesive small bowel obstruction in infants and children. J Pediatr Surg 1981;16:225.
97. Janik JS, Firor HV: Intussusception and nutritional status. J Pediatr 1976;99:358.
98. Karnak I, Senocak ME, Kale G, et al: A previously unmentioned surgical observation in the treatment of intussusception. Surg Today 1999;29:979.
99. Kia K, Mony V, Eustace S, et al: Laparoscopic versus open surgical approach for intussusception requiring operative intervention. Paper presented at a meeting of the American Pediatric Surgical Association, May 2004, Ponte Vedra Beach, Florida.
100. Kidd J, Jackson R, Wagner CW, et al: Intussusception following the Ladd procedure. Arch Surg 2000;135:713.
101. Kim G, Daneman A, Alton DJ, et al: The appearance of inverted Meckel diverticulum with intussusception on air enema. Pediatr Radiol 1997;27:647.
102. Kirks DR: Diagnosis and treatment of pediatric intussusception: How far should we push our radiologic techniques? Radiology 1994;191:622.
103. Kokkonen J, Karttunen JK: Lymphonodular hyperplasia on the mucosa of the lower gastrointestinal tract in children: An indication of enhanced immune response? J Pediatr Gastroenteral Nutr 2002;34:42.

104. Kornecki A, Daneman A, Navarro O, et al: Spontaneous reduction of intussusception: Clinical spectrum, management and outcome. Pediatr Radiol 2000;30:58.
105. Lai IR, Huang MT, Lee WJ: Mini-laparoscopic reduction of intussusception for children. J Formos Med Assoc 2000;99:510.
106. Le Masne A, Lortat-Jacob S, Sayegh N, et al: Intussusception in infants and children: Feasibility of ambulatory management. Eur J Pediatr 1999;158:707.
107. Lin SL, Kong MS, Houng DS: Decreasing early recurrence rate of acute intussusception by the use of dexamethasone. Eur J Pediatr 2000;159:551.
108. Liu KW, MacCarthy J, Guiney EJ, et al: Intussusception—current trends in management. Arch Dis Child 1986;61:75.
109. Maoate KM, Beasley SW: Perforation during gas reduction of intussusception. Pediatr Surg Int 1998;14:168.
109a. Mayell MJ: Intussusception in infancy and childhood in South Africa. Arch Dis Child 1972;47:20.
110. McAlister WH: Intussusception: Even Hippocrates did not standardize his technique of enema reduction. Radiology 1998;206:595.
111. McDermott VG: Childhood intussusception and approaches to treatment: A historical review. Pediatr Radiol 1994; 24:153.
112. Meier DE, Coln CD, Rescorla FJ, et al: Intussusception in children: International perspective. World J Surg 1996; 20:1035.
113. Mercer S, Carpenter B: Mechanism of perforation occurring in the intussusception. Can J Surg 1982;25:481.
114. Mestel AL: Lymphosarcoma of the small intestine in infancy and childhood. Ann Surg 1959;149:87.
115. Meyer JS: The current radiologic management of intussusception: A survey and review. Pediatr Radiol 1992;22:323.
116. Meyer JS, Dangman BC, Buonomo C, et al: Air and liquid contrast agents in the management of intussusception: A controlled, randomized trial. Radiology 1993;188:507.
117. Miller SF, Landes AB, Dautenhahn LW, et al: Intussusception: Ability of fluoroscopic images obtained during air enemas to depict lead points and other abnormalities. Radiology 1995;197:493.
118. Mollitt DL, Ballantine TVN, Grosfeld JL: Postoperative intussusception in infancy and childhood: Analysis of 119 cases. Surgery 1979;86:402.
119. Montgomery EA, Pokek EJ: Intussusception, adenovirus, and children: A brief reaffirmation. Hum Pathol 1994; 25:169.
120. Mooney DP, Steinthorsson G, Shorter NA: Perinatal intussusception in premature infants. J Pediatr Surg 1996;31:695.
121. Morrison SC, Stork E: Documentation of spontaneous reduction of childhood intussusception by ultrasound. Pediatr Radiol 1990;20:358.
122. Mortensson W, Eklöf O, Laurin S: Hydrostatic reduction of childhood intussusception: The role of adjuvant glucagon medication. Acta Radiol Diagn 1984;25:261.
123. Mortimer JD: On the treatment of intussusception by injection or inflation and its dangers. Lancet 1891;1:1144.
124. Mulcahy DL, Kamath KR, deSilva LM, et al: A two part study of the aetiological role of rotavirus in intussusception. J Med Virol 1982;9:51.
125. Murakami JW, Winters WD, Weinberger E, et al: Extensive reflux of air during enema for intussusception without reduction: Case report. Can Assoc Radiol J 1998;49:334.
126. Navarro O, Daneman A: Intussusception Part 3: Diagnosis and management of those with an identifiable or predisposing cause and those that reduce spontaneously. Pediatr Radiol 2004;34:305.
127. Navarro O, Daneman A, Chae A: Intussusception: The use of delayed repeat reduction attempts and the management of intussusceptions due to pathologic lead points in pediatric patients. AJR Am J Roentgenol 2004;182:1169.
128. Navarro O, Dugougeat F, Kornecki A, et al: The impact of imaging in the management of intussusceptions owing to pathologic lead points in children: A review of 43 cases. Pediatr Radiol 2000;30:594.
129. Nissan S, Levy E: Intussusception in infancy caused by hypertrophic Peyer's patches. Surgery 1966;59:1108.
130. Okuyama H, Nakai H, Okada A: Is barium enema reduction safe and effective in patients with a long duration of intussusception? Pediatr Surg Int 1999;15:105.
131. Olsson G, Pallin G: Uber das Bild der akuten Darminvagination mit Hilfe von Kontrastlavements. Acta Chir Scand 1927;61:371.
132. Ong NT, Beasley SW: The leadpoint in intussusception. J Pediatr Surg 1990;25:640.
133. Palder SB, Ein SH, Stringer DA, et al: Intussusception: Barium or air? J Pediatr Surg 1991;26:271.
134. Pantongrag-Brown L, Levine MS, Elsayed AM, et al: Inverted Meckel diverticulum: Clinical, radiologic, and pathologic findings. Radiology 1996;199:693.
135. Parashar UD, Holman RC, Cummings KC, et al: Trends in intussusception-associated hospitalizations and deaths among US infants. Pediatrics 2000;106:1413.
136. Parkkulainen KV: Intrauterine intussusception as a cause of intestinal atresia. Surgery 1958;44:1106.
137. Poulquien M: Indication du lavement bismuthe dans certaines formes d'invaginations intestinales. Bull Mem Soc Nat Chir 1927;53:1016.
514-516.
139. Poznanski AK: Why I still use barium for intussusception. Pediatr Radiol 1995;25:92.
140. Pracros JP, Tran-Minh VA, Morin DE, et al: Acute intestinal intussusception in children: Contribution of ultrasonography (145 cases). Ann Radiol 1987;30: 525-530.
141. Rachelson MH, Jernigan JP, Jackson WF: Intussusception in the newborn infant with spontaneous expulsion of the intussusception: A case report and review of the literature. J Pediatr 1955;47:87.
142. Raffensperger JG: The Acute Abdomen in Infancy and Childhood. Philadelphia, JB Lippincott, 1970, p 52.
143. Ratcliffe JF, Fong S, Cheong I, et al: The plain abdominal film in intussusception: The accuracy and incidence of radiographic signs. Pediatr Radiol 1984;22:110.
144. Ravitch MM: Intussusception in Infants and Children. Springfield, IL, Charles C Thomas, 1959.
145. Ravitch MM: Intussusception. In Welch KJ, Randolph JG, Ravitch MM, et al (eds): Pediatric Surgery, 4th ed. Chicago, Year Book, 1986, p 868.
146. Ravitch MM, McCune RM Jr: Reduction of intussusception by hydrostatic pressure: An experimental study. Bull Johns Hopkins Hosp 1948;82:550.
147. Retan GM: Nonoperative treatment of intussusception. Am J Dis Child 1927;33:765.
148. Rohrschneider W, Tröger J, Betsch B: The post reduction donut sign. Pediatr Radiol 1994;24:156.
149. Sandler AD, Ein SH, Connolly BL, et al: Unsuccessful air-enema reduction of intussusception: Is a second attempt worthwhile? Pediatr Surg Int 1999;15:214.
150. Sanz N, Sánchez M, García Aroca J, et al: Intussusception: Barium vs. pneumatic reduction. Cir Pediatr 1996;9:21.
151. Sargent MA, Babyn P, Alton DJ: Plain abdominal radiography in suspected intussusception: A reassessment.

Pediatr Radiol 1994;24:17.
152. Saxton V, Katz M, Phelan E, et al: Intussusception: A repeat delayed gas enema increases the nonoperative reduction rate. J Pediatr Surg 1994;29:588.
153. Schmit P, Rohrschneider WK, Christmann D: Intestinal intussusception survey about diagnostic and nonsurgical therapeutic procedures. Pediatr Radiol 1999;29:752.
154. Senocak ME, Büyükpamakcu N, Hicsönmez A: Ileal atresia due to intrauterine intussusception caused by Meckel's diverticulum. Pediatr Surg Int 1990;5:64.
155. Shiels WE 2nd, Kirks DR, Keller GL, et al: Colonic perforation by air and liquid enemas: Comparison study in young pigs. AJR Am J Roentgenol 1993;160:931.
156. Shiels WE 2nd, Maves CK, Hedlund GL, et al: Air enema for diagnosis and reduction of intussusception: Clinical experiences and pressure correlates. Radiology 1991; 181:169.
157. Shteyer E, Koplewitz BZ, Gross E, et al: Medical treatment of recurrent intussusception associated with intestinal lymphoid hyperplasia. Pediatrics 2003;111:682.
158. Siaplaouras J, Moritz JD, Gortner L, et al: Dünndarminvaginationen im Kindesalter: Diagnostik und Bedeutung (Small bowel intussusception in childhood). Klin Padiatr 2003;215:53.
159. Simonsen L, Morens D, Elixhauser A, et al: Effect of rotavirus vaccination programme on trends in admission of infants to hospital for intussusception. Lancet 2001; 358:1224.
160. Somekh E, Serour F, Gonçalves D, et al: Air enema reduction of intussusception in children: Risk of bacteremia. Radiology 1996;200:217.
161. Sönmez K, Turkyilmaz Z, Demirogullari B, et al: Conservative treatment for small intestinal intussusception associated with Henoch-Schönlein's purpura. Surg Today 2002;32:1031.
162. Stein M, Alton DJ, Daneman A: Pneumatic reduction of intussusception: 5-year experience. Radiology 1992;183:681.
163. Strang RP: Intussusception in infancy and childhood: A review of 400 cases. Br J Surg 1959;46:484.
164. Stringer DA, Ein SH: Pneumatic reduction: Advantages, risks and indications. Pediatr Radiol 1990;20:475.
165. Stringer MD, Homes SJK: Familial intussusception. J Pediatr Surg 1992;27:1436.
166. Stringer MD, Pablot SM, Brereton RJ: Paediatric intussusception. Br J Surg 1992;79:867.
167. Stringer MD, Willetts IE: John Hunter, Frederick Treves and intussusception. Ann R Coll Surg Engl 2000;82:18.
168. Strouse PJ, DiPietro MA, Sáez F: Transient small bowel intussusception in children on CT. Pediatr Radiol 2003; 33:316.
169. Swenson O: Pediatric Surgery, 2nd ed. New York, Appleton-Century-Crofts, 1962, p 328.
170. Todani T, Tabuchi K, Tanake S: Intestinal atresia due to intrauterine intussusception: Analysis of 24 cases in Japan. J Pediatr Surg 1975;10:445.
171. Treves F: The treatment of intussusception. Proc Med Soc London 1885;8:83.
172. van Heek NT, Aronson DC, Halimun EM, et al: Intussusception in a tropical country: Comparison among patient populations in Jakarta, Jogyakarta, and Amsterdam. J Pediatr Gastroenterol Nutr 1999;29:402.
173. Warshauer DM, Lee JKT: Adult intussusception detected at CT or MR imaging: Clinical-imaging correlation. Radiology 1999;212:853.
174. Wayne ER, Campbell JB, Kosloske AM, et al: Intussusception in the older child—suspect lymphosarcoma. J Pediatr Surg 1976;11:789.
175. Weber A, Nadel S: CT appearance of retrograde jejunoduodenogastric intussusception: A rare complication of gastrostomy tubes. AJR Am J Roentgenol 1991; 156:957.
176. West KW, Grosfeld JL: Intussusception in infants and children. In Wyllie R, Hyams JS (eds): Pediatric Gastrointestinal Disease. Philadelphia, WB Saunders, 1993, p 472.
177. West KW, Stephens B, Rescorla FJ, et al: Postoperative intussusception: Experience with 36 cases in children. Surgery 1988;104:781.
178. White SJ, Blane CE: Intussusception: Additional observations on the plain radiograph. AJR Am J Roentgenol 1982; 139:511.
179. Wilson-Storey D, MacKinlay GA, Prescott S, et al: Intussusception: A surgical condition. J R Coll Surg Edinb 1988;33:270.
180. Willetts IE, Kite P, Barclay GR, et al: Endotoxin, cytokines and lipid peroxides in children with intussusception. Br J Surg 2001;88:878.
181. Winstanley JHR, Doig CM, Brydon H: Intussusception: The case for barium reduction. J R Coll Surg Edinb 1987; 32:285.
182. Yeung CP, Ip SM, Lee KH, et al: The significance of bacteraemia, endotoxaemia and cytokine release in the production of fever in childhood intussusception. Paper presented at the 42nd Meeting of the British Association of Paediatric Surgeons, 1995, Sheffield, England.
183. Young DG: Intussusception. In O'Neill JA Jr, Rowe MI, Grosfeld JL, et al (eds): Pediatric Surgery, 3rd ed. Chicago, Year Book, 1998, p 1185.
184. Zachary RB: Acute intussusception in children. Arch Dis Child 1955;30:32.
185. Zanardi LR, Haber P, Mootrey GT, et al: Intussusception among recipients of rotavirus vaccine: Reports to the vaccine adverse event reporting system. Pediatrics 2001; 107:E97.

第 84 章

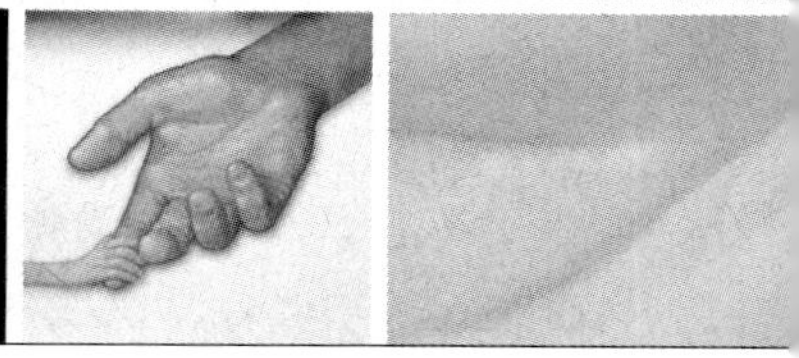

肠旋转和固定的异常

Samuel D. Smith

342 ## 历史回顾

有关肠道发育过程中的旋转和固定异常的研究进展一直比较缓慢，在 1900 年之前只有在外科手术和尸体解剖中发现个案性描述，在该现象从胚胎学上得到解释前，这些报告间并无关联。

在胚胎学上第一次有意义的描述是 1898 年由约翰霍普金斯大学解剖学教授 Mall 提出的[36]，在自己有关重构胚的研究基础上，他在德国与著名的胚胎学家 His 共同研究，Mall 描述了肠旋转和固定的过程。Fraser 和 Robbins[19] 通过大规模的胚胎学研究扩展了 Mall 的发现。

1923 年，Dott[15] 发表了关于肠旋转异常胚胎学和外科表现的经典文章，首次阐明了临床和胚胎表现之间的关系。Dott 在他的 2 例和其他文献中收集的 40 例病例不同的发育异常中找出这两者之间的相关性。其后多数文章中报道的临床病例均与 Dott 报道的胚胎期发育异常的分析有关。1928 年 Waugh[55] 描述了 2 例由于肠不旋转造成的肠扭转；1931 年 Haymond 和 Dragstedt[24] 描述了一种内疝的临床表现和胚胎学；在 20 世纪 30 年代 Gardner 和 Hart[21] 报告了 2 例并将其他报告中的 104 例进行分类；Wakefield 和 Mayo[53] 描述了 13 例；McIntosh 和 Donovan[39] 描述了 20 例；1932 年 Ladd[32] 描述了 10 例合并肠扭转的肠旋转不良，同时建议通过逆时针扭转纠正进行治疗；在 1936 年 Ladd[33] 发表了经典的肠旋转不良治疗的文章，描述了 21 例患者，他强调了十二指肠上束带的分离和将回盲部放置在左上腹的重要性。这篇文章表明 Ladd 关注了以前很少有人注意的延伸到十二指肠右侧的束带，他没有辨别包裹十二指肠和回盲部的经常出现的束带。Ladd 的手术步骤是游离十二指肠然后把回盲部放置在左上腹，这仍然是外科治疗肠不旋转合并中肠扭转的基石。以前有报道通过缝合将回盲部固定在左上腹部，但现在不再提倡，因为这并没有什么效果[9,10]。在 1953 年 Gross[23] 首次详细回顾性报道了有关这个主题的 156 例病例；波士顿儿童医院的相关经验一直在改进[24,51]。

在 1954 年 Snyder 和 Chaffin[48] 清晰和深入地描述了肠旋转异常，在该报告中通过一个中央有带子（用来表示肠系膜上血管）的绳圈的扭转来展示肠旋转不良胚胎学上的变化。

正常的旋转和固定

在肠旋转的描述中可能主要是针对肠道的两端，即近端的十二指肠空肠袢和远端的盲结肠袢，以及这两者间持续旋转的变化。大多数作者仅提及中肠，但最好是包括整个肠道[23,34]。

十二指肠空肠袢

正常成人的胃、十二指肠以及空肠起始部的位置是众所周知的。从成人肠道的起始部开始观察它的固定与肠系膜上动脉之间的关系，可以清楚地看见胃在该动脉的上部或前面，十二指肠第二部在动脉的右侧，第三部在动脉的下方，第四部（十二指肠末端和空肠一端）位于动脉的左侧。胚胎期十二指肠空肠袢也是从与成人胃相同的部位起始（图 84-1）。如果肠袢的其他部分最终定位于前面描述的位置，即十二指肠空肠袢围绕着肠系膜上动脉从上（见图 84-1）向

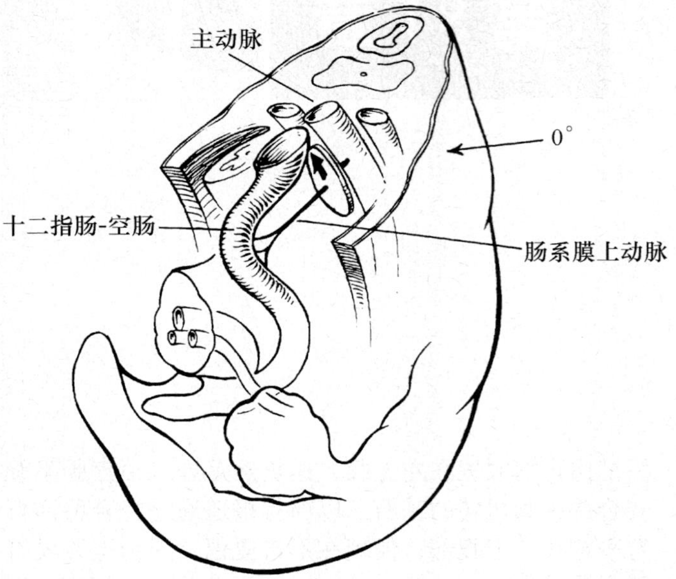

图 84-1 5 mm 胚胎的腹侧简图。肠道形成一个轻微向前的弯曲，肠系膜上动脉（SMA）呈直角从主动脉到肠管的弯曲，围绕肠系膜动脉根部画了一个圆盘；箭头上方指向点是十二指肠空肠袢起始点或者是 0°旋转，以动脉为轴心发生旋转。

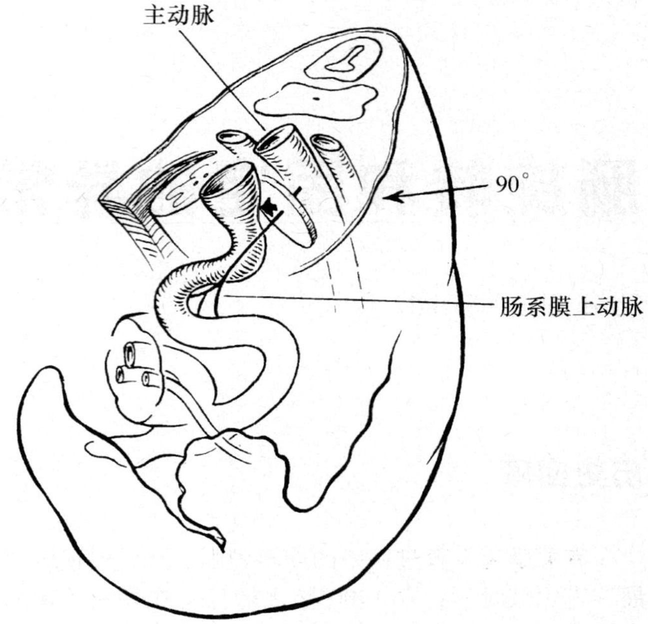

图 84-2 10 mm 胚胎的腹侧简图。十二指肠空肠袢从肠系膜上动脉（SMA）上方到动脉的右侧，从其原始的位置旋转了 90°的弧度，如图中箭头所示。

右侧旋转 90°（图 84-2），同时向下旋转 90°，总共为 90°（图 84-3），然后再旋转 90°最终到达动脉的左侧，则总共的弧度为 270°（图 84-4）。旋转的方向取决于正常胃和十二指肠 4 个部分的最后位置。

向侧面的旋转及旋转方向

在前面的描述中，右侧是指患者的右侧，并不是面对患者的观察者的右侧。然而通常描述旋转方向的是用时钟方向，是从观察者的方向而来。如果一个想象中的时钟放置在胚胎或患者后面墙上，指针的轴点（即旋转的中轴）即是肠系膜上动脉，十二指肠空肠袢沿逆时针方向旋转。

盲肠袢

在成人，末端回肠、盲肠和右半结肠位于右侧腹部，肠系膜上动脉的右侧。在胚胎期，它们位于该动

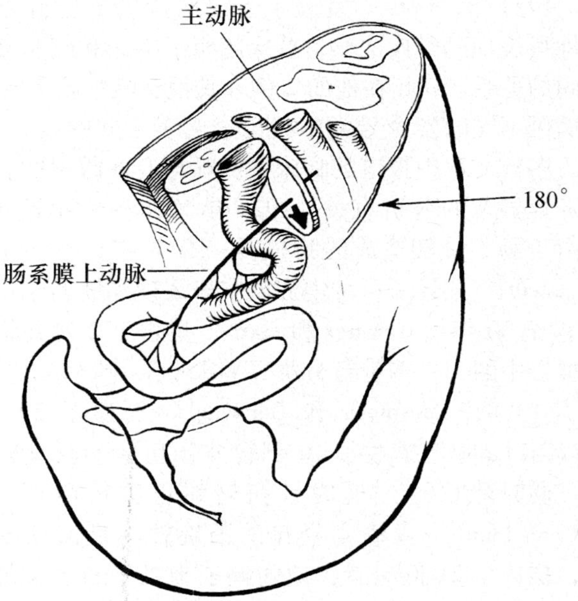

图 84-3 25 mm 胚胎的腹侧简图。显示十二指肠空肠袢进一步旋转到肠系膜上动脉（SMA）下方，其旋转弧度为 180°，肠道向脐带内延伸的部分在此图中没有显示。

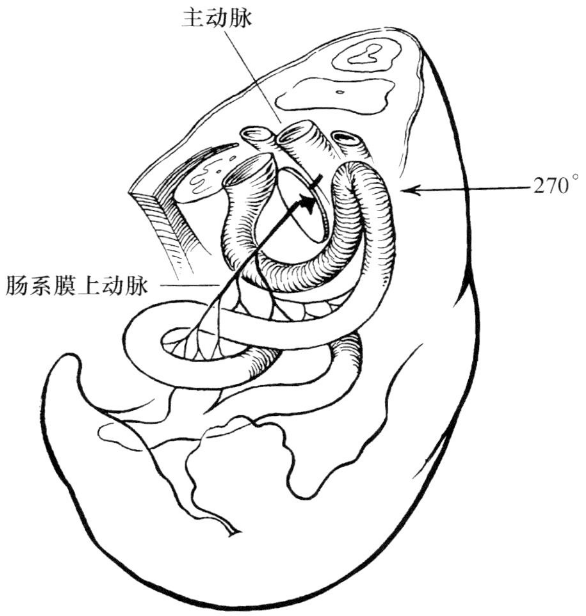

图 84-4　40 mm 胚胎的腹侧简图。显示十二指肠空肠袢最后旋转至肠系膜上动脉（SMA）的左侧，此袢先从上面的位置旋转到右下然后到达左侧，总共逆时针旋转了 270°，十二指肠空肠袢最终旋转使肠道沿着脐带退回腹腔内。

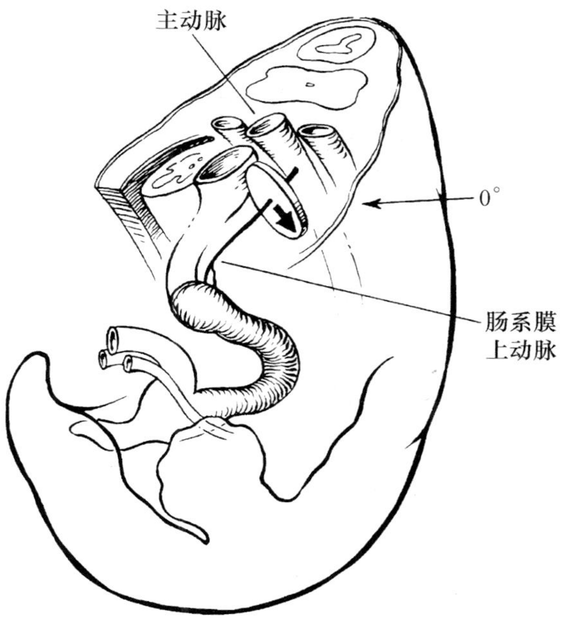

图 84-5　5 mm 胚胎的腹侧简图。显示肠道向前弯曲，强调回盲袢在肠系膜上动脉（SMA）的下方，或从围绕 SMA 根部的圆盘状显示图所示在 0°旋转的位置，此袢 0°位时正好在 SMA 的下方，而十二指肠空肠袢则在其上方。

脉的下方。回盲袢从其在该动脉下方的起始部起，和十二指肠空肠袢一样逆时针旋转（图 84-5），到动脉的左侧 90°（图 84-6），向上 180°转向动脉右侧（图 84-7），总共 270°（图 84-8）。回盲袢以此方式到达如同成人的位置。

345 **在两端和整个肠道同时发生的旋转**

旋转过程好比在一块木板上的一根金属轮辐（铁丝）上下附着的一段绳圈的变化（图 84-9）。用左手抓住绳圈向左旋转 3/4 圈，注意绳圈上臂的近端部分，这部分从最初在铁丝的上方位置，转到铁丝的右侧然后到其下方到达左侧。与此同时，下半段从铁丝的下方开始旋转，到达左侧、上方，最终到达铁丝的右侧。如果将上半段的绳子比作十二指肠空肠袢、下半段绳子比作回盲袢、中间的铁丝比作肠系膜上动脉，这些结构在旋转中位置的变化就很清楚了。这整个过程可以通过在立体显微镜下对一系列 4～12 周大的胚胎研究了解其细节，在胚胎的第 4 周或者胚胎只

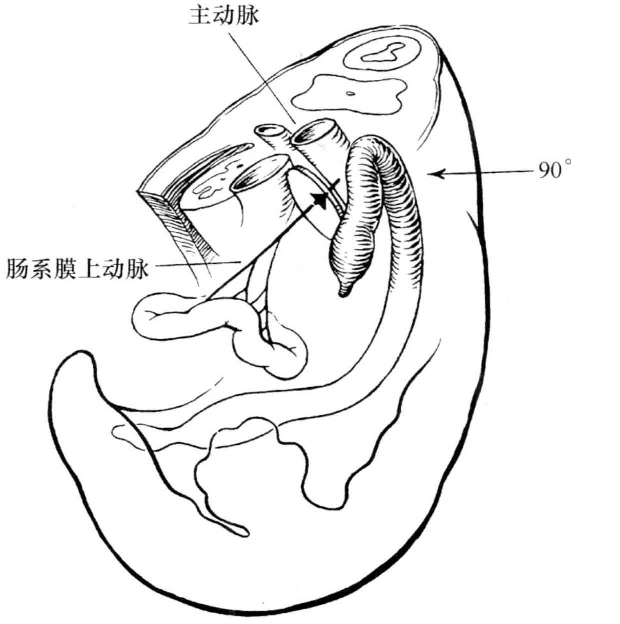

图 84-6　40 mm 胚胎的腹侧简图。显示回盲袢在肠系膜上动脉（SMA）的左侧，该袢已经从起始部位旋转 90°至肠系膜上动脉的下方（见 SMA 根部的圆盘示意图），这个时期的旋转过程一直位于脐带内，并在此过程中肠管回纳到腹腔内。

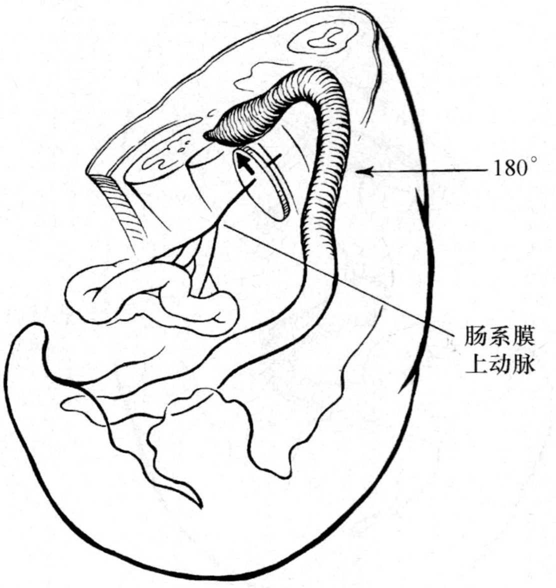

图 84-7　40 mm 胚胎的腹侧简图。显示回盲肠袢旋转到肠系膜上动脉（SMA）上方的位置，或从起始部位起旋转 180°到 SMA 下方，这一过程在肠管从脐带回纳到腹腔内时立即发生。

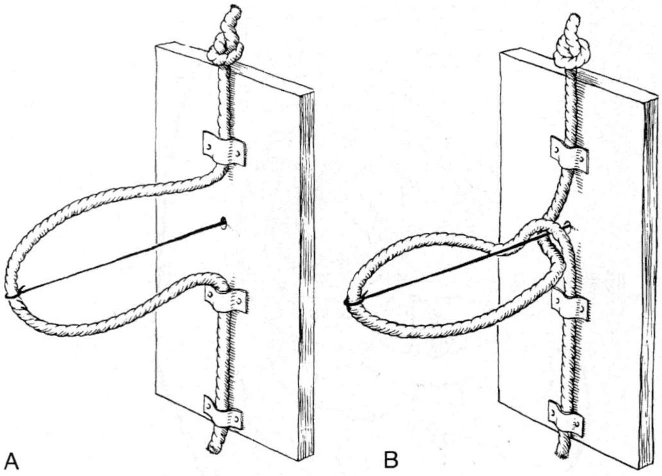

图 84-9　肠道旋转的摸拟演示。一根绳索两端固定在一块板上，中央有根线成直角从板拉到绳圈的基底。A. 绳圈的上半部分代表十二指肠空肠袢，那根线代表肠系膜上动脉，底部代表回盲部分。B. 绳圈被手抓住然后以那根线为轴逆时针旋转 270°，或者 3/4 圈。这样上面的部分到下面去了，下面的部分到上面去了。通过这样的运动，绳子的两部分离后面的板更近了，可以在胚胎中观察到肠道旋转的过程。

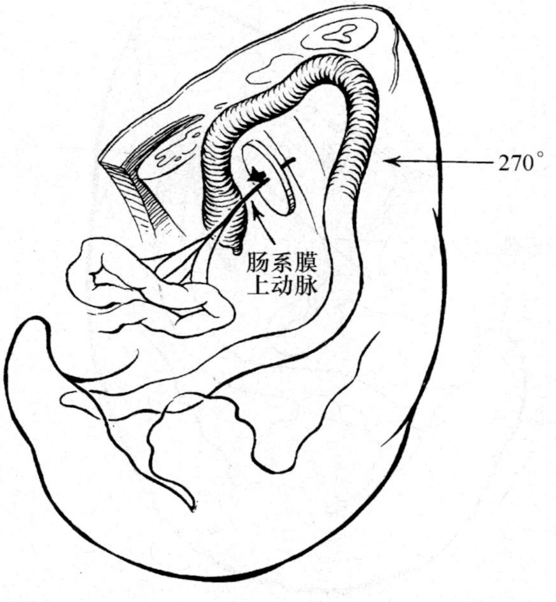

图 84-8　40 mm 胚胎的腹侧简图。显示回盲袢的最终位置是在肠系膜上动脉（SMA）的右侧，该袢从下面穿到左侧，然后到上方，最后到 SMA 的右侧，总共在逆时针方向旋转了 270°。

有 5 mm 大小时，肠道几乎是直的管道，中间稍稍向前膨出，肠系膜上动脉从后壁向前到达膨出部分的中点（见图 84-1 到 84-5）。当肠的形态在扩张的腹腔和脐索中时就开始迅速地变化，胃还是处于原始位置，肠系膜上动脉的上方和前面，十二指肠开始向下弯曲并到达动脉的右侧，空肠和小肠延伸进入脐索，伴随着盲肠、升结肠和部分横结肠。所有的肠袢均从动脉前面的位置到达动脉的一边（见图 84-2 和图 84-6）。

以前认为所有的肠袢在脐索中没有回纳到腹腔之前时位置保持不变[15,19]，但 Mall[36] 证明在肠道回到体腔之前十二指肠空肠袢也在持续旋转，这同时也被 Snyder 和 Chaffin[48] 证明，到第 8 周时十二指肠第三部到达肠系膜上动脉的下方（见图 84-3），这部分的旋转增加了 180°，最后大约在第 10 周（或者胚胎有 40 mm 长时）肠道回到腹腔，这是一个非常快的过程，因为几乎没有描述这个时期的标本。小肠最先进入腹腔，然后推动十二指肠第四部和空肠到肠系膜上动脉的左侧，完成这段小肠的完全旋转（见图 84-4）。盲肠和升结肠最后进入腹腔，位于左侧腹（见图 84-6），并最终从前方或上方跨于肠系膜上动脉（见图 84-7）定位于动脉的右侧（见图 84-8）。

可以用另外一种模拟来表示，把手放置在一个想象中的汽车方向盘的上面，向左侧旋转 3/4 圈，如同十二指肠空肠袢围绕着中轴（肠系膜上动脉）旋转，把手放在方向盘的下方向左转动 3/4 圈，如同回盲袢的旋转。

346 上述过程为正常旋转过程，这种旋转顺序过程的假设来源于很多人观察到的少量证据，这一过程中并没有明显 Ⅰ 期、Ⅱ 期、Ⅲ 期的分界线，因为这是个连续的过程，可以通过摆动一根扭动的绳索或者转动方向盘来理解[19]。这种描述有点过于简单化，但是能够帮助手术医生记忆和理解。

Kluth 和 Lambrecht[31] 提出了一个基于老鼠胚胎研究的与此稍有不同的肠旋转异常的解释，他们强调十二指肠快速的生长和延伸使十二指肠空肠袢顶端向肠系膜根部的下方生长。远端的中肠同样也迅速生长延长推动盲肠从尾端向头端移位，这看上去像旋转但是其余部分的结肠直肠并不参与这个过程。这些作者认为肠道的固定和定位是一个不同的生长过程而并非旋转，因为在他们的胚胎学研究中没有发现直肠和中肠的明显变化。在涉及中肠发育畸形的发病机制上，他们推测胚胎期十二指肠袢发育异常是一个主要问题。十二指肠袢长度的减少或者异常插入系膜根部造成十二指肠袢的生长障碍，可以解释十二指肠和 Treitz 韧带定位异常。他们认为盲肠和结肠移动在肠道定位和固定异常中起到的作用较为被动或者甚微。

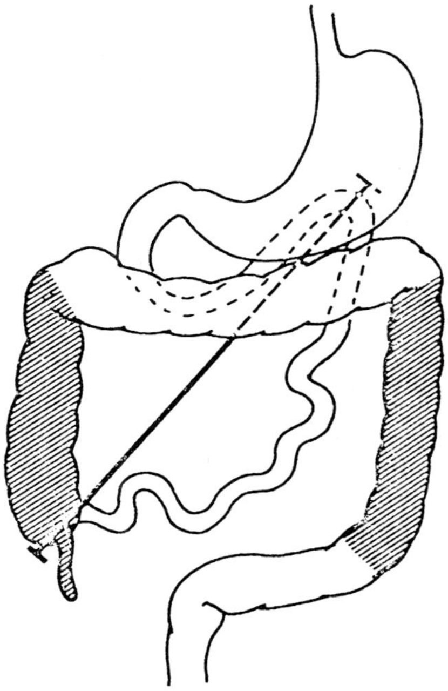

图 84-10 正常中肠系膜的固定。正常情况下有宽广的基底从 Treitz 韧带延伸到回盲肠交界处，以防止肠道扭转。升结肠和降结肠固定于后腹膜。（From Fliston HG，Kirks DR：Malrotation—the ubiquitous anomaly. J Pediatr Surg 1981；16:614.）

肠旋转异常的分类

十二指肠和结肠的正常固定见图 84-10。正常的肠系膜附着从 Treitz 韧带部位也就是胃出口的水平延伸到盲肠，升结肠和降结肠一同固定在后腹膜。肠旋转不良可有多种不同表现，如何对这些异常造成的外科问题进行恰当的分类，取决于如何理解发育、旋转、十二指肠和 Treitz 韧带位置异常，任何分期都是任意的，但都是参考了图 84-11，该图显示了正常旋转过程，有助于确定每个病例所出现的发育异常[4]。

肠旋转不良这个术语是指所有的肠道位置和固定异常[16]，包括近期提出的不典型旋转不良的概念和肠旋转不良的变异类型。非典型的肠旋转不良是指当 Treitz 韧带在中线的左侧（通过和椎体的关系来明确），或者是通过上消化道对比造影发现其位于胃出口的下方。肠不旋转这个术语是指第一期的异常（见图 84-10），而不完全性的旋转和混合性旋转是指第二期的异常。

反向旋转很少见，在这种类型中十二指肠和结肠以肠系膜上动静脉为中心顺时针方向旋转，这时候横结肠不可避免地位于血管下方，可造成急性或慢性结肠梗阻。

肠旋转和固定异常也被认为与内脏异位同时存在，但很少伴有内脏反位。内脏异位是指内脏位置异常排列或者完全反位，内脏异位常常伴有主要的心血管异常，消化道异常包括中位肝、胃异位、肠旋转和固定的异常、腹腔内胰腺以及无脾或多脾[11]。

肠旋转不良是先天性膈疝和腹部缺损这两类畸形的一部分表现，在腹裂中，肠不旋转且悬挂于胎儿腹腔外，这会导致缺血性损害而不伴有肠扭转。而脐膨出和膈疝的婴儿往往有不同程度的肠旋转和固定异常，这取决于肠道异位的程度。

大约有 30%～60% 的肠旋转不良患儿有合并畸形[17,30,41,53]，可以发现十二指肠闭锁合并肠旋转不良

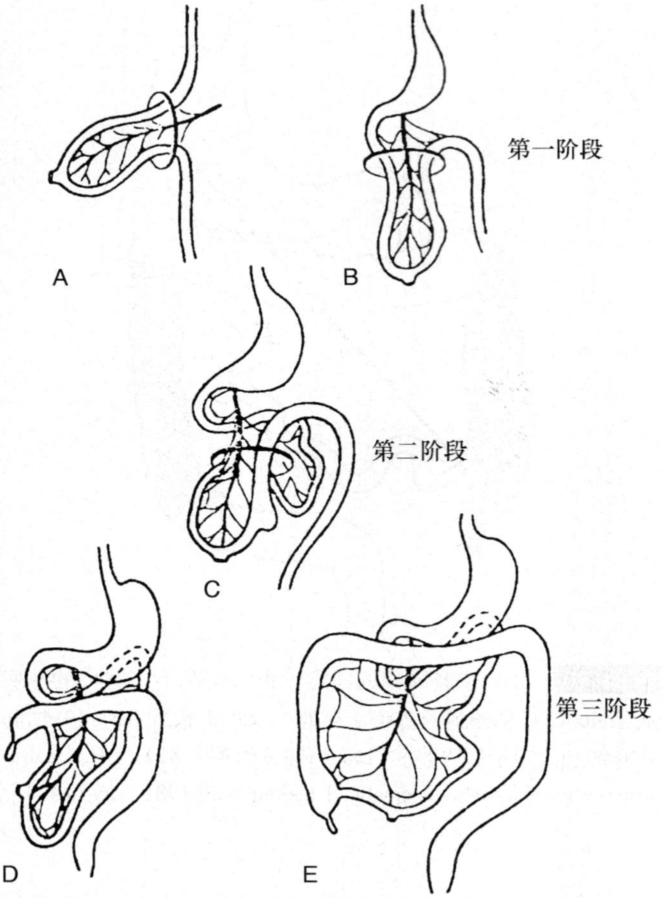

图 84-11 正常肠道的旋转。A. 妊娠 6 周：没有旋转。B. 妊娠 8 周：不完全旋转。C. 妊娠 9 周：不完全旋转。D. 妊娠 11 周。E. 妊娠 12 周。（From Fliston HG，Kirks DR：Malrotation—the ubiquitous anomaly. J Pediatr Surg 1981；16:614.）

和围生期肠扭转，在肠旋转不良患儿中不能忽视十二指肠腔内膜状闭锁造成的梗阻。Filston 和 Kirks[17] 发现中肠扭转常常合并存在于半数的空肠闭锁和 1/3 的十二指肠闭锁病例中。肠旋转不良在 Hirschsprung 病和肛门直肠畸形中很罕见[36]。肠系膜囊肿可以伴有肠旋转不良，但囊肿是由于先天性原因还是由于慢性
1347 扭转引起淋巴梗阻造成的尚不清楚[7]。

临床表现

肠旋转和固定异常可有多种临床表现从慢性腹痛到急性中肠扭转伴有缺血性肠损伤。一般情况下可以

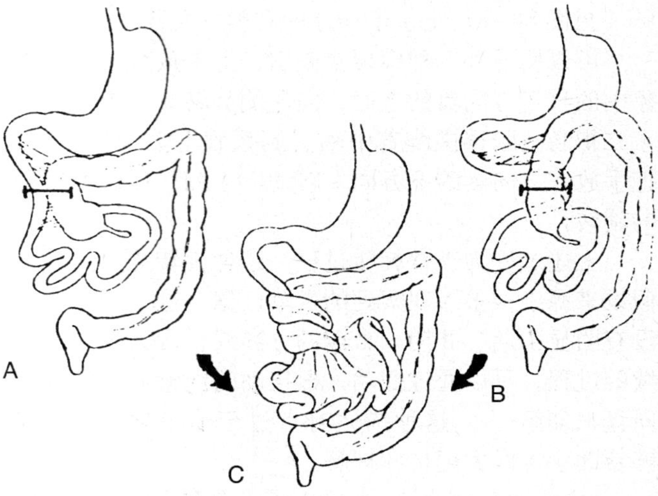

图 84-12 中肠扭转合并有肠旋转不良的病理生理学。A. 在无旋转情况下狭窄的肠系膜附属物。B. 不完全的旋转。C. 容易使患儿发生中肠扭转。（From Fliston HG，Kirks DR：Malrotation—the ubiquitous anomaly. J Pediatr Surg 1981；16:614.）

把临床上各种表现和解剖学上的发现相联系，但也有些例外。

急性中肠扭转

肠旋转不良造成肠系膜根部狭窄所形成的蒂易使中肠从十二指肠到横结肠顺时针方向扭转（图84-12）[15]，肠系膜过长或者在肠袢间点状粘连都可以成为扭转的中轴，其机制不明，原因可能有多种，包括躯干非正常运动、肠道异常蠕动或者是节段性肠管扩张[13]。

大多数中肠扭转在出生后 1 个月内出现[46]，在对一组 74 例患儿的研究中发现 23 例出现在出生后的 7 天，16 例在 7～30 天，24 例是 1～12 月，仅 11 例超过 1 岁[3]。Torres 和 Ziegler[52] 描述的 22 例患儿中有 14 例在出生后第 1 个月就发病。

最初的临床表现是健康的婴儿突然发作的胆汁性呕吐[43]。在呕吐发生后迅速出现近端小肠梗阻，远端结肠空虚，呕吐开始后不久下腹部可能呈舟状。随着血管受压的加重，可能发生肠腔内出血，出现便血，常见痉挛性腹痛。胆汁性呕吐可排除肥厚性幽门狭窄痉挛性肠绞痛或良性“急腹痛”。

婴儿完全性梗阻可迅速出现肠壁缺血并出现腹部

紧张和腹胀、低血容量、休克。腹部肌紧张和血管受压的程度有关，不可避免地常出现腹膜炎体征。

高度怀疑中肠扭转应建立于病史、体格检查、代谢性酸中毒的表现的基础上。通过多普勒超声检查和上消化道造影可进一步诊断，应根据患儿的临床表现和延迟诊断易致血管受压的危险性行直接剖腹探查或腹腔镜探查。

慢性中肠扭转

间歇性和部分中肠扭转会导致淋巴管和静脉的梗
348 阻、肠系膜淋巴结肿大，这种情况在 2 岁以上的儿童中常见[18,26,27,43,49]。基于 2 岁以上肠旋转不良儿童的临床资料回顾，最常见的临床症状是慢性呕吐（68%）、间断性腹痛（55%）、腹泻（9%）、呕血（5%）和便秘（5%）[37]。手术前平均症状持续时间为 28 个月，在长期肠道不完全扭转并伴有部分梗阻的严重病例中，可能因为淋巴管和静脉血管淤滞造成吸收和营养物质传送障碍，最后导致蛋白-热卡性营养不良[26,49]，可增加感染的易感性[26]。

在一些患者中，对此诊断的忽视可能导致医生对患者进行饮食治疗，甚至怀疑有精神疾病。伴有腹痛的胆汁性呕吐需考虑外科性疾病[14]，需排除胃十二指肠扩张的神经源性反应，该反应也能引起非胆汁性呕吐。

无症状或轻微症状的典型肠旋转不良

在影像学检查或术中偶然发现肠旋转不良的一些无症状的患儿中，值得思考的是它们最终会不会引起并发症。在通过对 50 例成人肠旋转不良的研究中，Wang 和 Welch[54] 发现 26 例症状与该异常有关。普遍的观点是在任何年龄发现该病均需要手术纠正[17,20,46]。

Chang 等[11]注意到无症状性肠旋转不良，他们报道了 34 例内脏异位和和复杂先天性心脏病的患儿合并有肠旋转不良，28 例中的 4 例发生了急性和慢性中肠扭转，进行了急诊 Ladd 术，还有 6 例合并有内脏转位的患儿行上消化道造影发现肠固定和旋转异常，这些患儿均在心血管系统稳定情况下进行了选择性 Ladd 术。

在急腹症的探查术中首先要注意是否存在肠旋转不良的问题，肠旋转不良的患儿有炎症的阑尾可能不在右下腹，需要进一步的影像学检查来确定。在 Collin[12] 的研究中观察了 71 000 例阑尾标本，2849 例出现因为结肠旋转不完全造成阑尾位置异常，当患儿急诊外科治愈出院后，应行上消化道造影检查以进一步评估。

继发于先天性束带的急性十二指肠梗阻

急性十二指肠梗阻是由于来源于腹膜的束带（Ladd 束）延伸跨过十二指肠第三部，外源性压迫引起肠腔狭窄，或者是肠管在固定的位置发生扭结。十二指肠梗阻常见于新生儿和婴儿，但可在年龄稍大时延迟发病，且肠扭转也并非主要症状。

婴儿和新生儿通常会出现剧烈的胆汁性呕吐，间或存在腹胀，这取决于呕吐后胃排空的程度，可见胃蠕动波[40]。梗阻可以是完全性或不完全性，因此胎粪或粪便有时可以排出，可有黄疸[42]。在新生儿中，有症状的肠旋转不良通常表现为十二指肠梗阻症状，腹部平片通常可见因十二指肠梗阻造成的“双泡征”，上消化道十二指肠造影可以明确诊断。

继发于先天性束带的慢性十二指肠梗阻

慢性、复发性或者亚急性十二指肠梗阻是因为血管周围的肠袢没有完成其正常的旋转，粘连和腹膜束带会造成十二指肠扭转、成角、纠结[35]，一定程度的肠扭转会牵拉束带造成纠结加剧，梗阻的位置通常在十二指肠第三部。

最主要的临床表现是胆汁性呕吐，体重不增和间断性腹部绞痛是常见症状。确诊的年龄从婴儿到学龄前儿童不等。不伴有反流的暂时性十二指肠扩张可刺激胃的反流，在胃肠道造影时候观察需要非常仔细，因为这种扩张可能非常轻微。

反向旋转伴有结肠梗阻

这种情况很罕见，十二指肠和空肠位于肠系膜上动脉的前方（图 84-13），导致其后方的横结肠梗阻，横结肠从肠系膜下方通过，造成了慢性完全性或不完全性结肠梗阻，这可以在成人见到，很少见于儿童[54]。

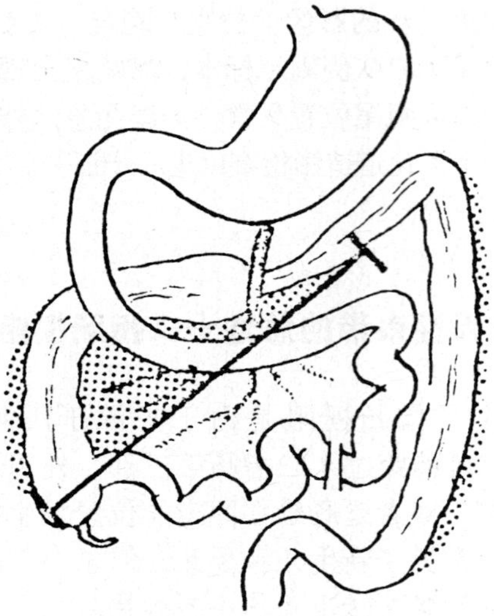

图 84-13　十二指肠和结肠反向旋转，当结肠在肠系膜上动脉下方旋转时，横结肠中段可能出现部分梗阻，这是由血管和从系膜到小肠形成的束带压迫造成。

内疝

右半结肠、左半结肠或者十二指肠系膜缺乏固定可能会导致腹腔内形成潜在的疝的腔隙。内疝与反复发生的不全性肠梗阻有关，并可最后导致完全性肠梗阻和绞窄。最常见的内疝为 Willwerth 等[56]描述的右侧或者左侧的结肠系膜疝，还有一种说法称为十二指肠旁疝。右侧结肠系膜疝是因为动脉周围的肠管没有 134
围绕肠系膜上动脉根部旋转，而导致肠袢被盲肠和结肠系膜包裹（图 84-14A）。左侧结肠系膜疝是因为在肠系膜下静脉和结肠后侧壁部分附着处之间的降结肠系膜区域无支持，小肠在此区域像气球样突出，占据左上腹腔。通常盲肠完全旋转并定位于右下腹位置，回肠从囊中穿出，但是和回盲瓣间距离变化较大（图

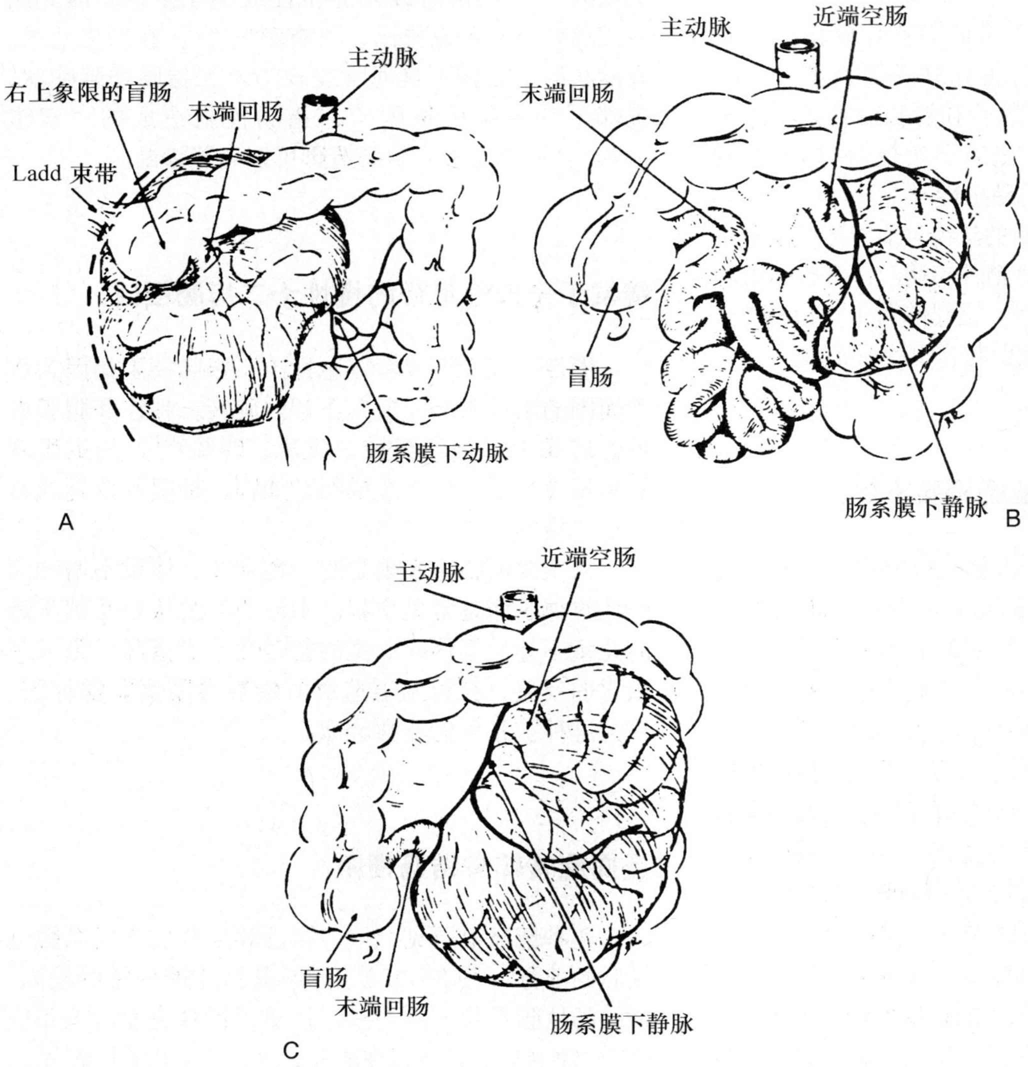

图 84-14　结肠系膜疝。A. 右侧系膜疝。中肠动脉前部分未能旋转，动脉后部分不发生旋转，同时大量的小肠被结肠系膜束缚在右系膜后方，阴影线表示外科切口使内疝复位。B. 左侧结肠系膜疝。最初小肠的旋转是正常的，在移行到左上腹的过程中，肠管陷入左侧结肠系膜无血管区，位于肠系膜下静脉后面。C. 左侧结肠系膜疝。小肠除了末端回肠被包裹于左侧结肠系膜之下，值得注意的是肠系膜下静脉勾勒出囊袋右侧边缘处，构成了疝囊的颈部。［From：Willwerth BM，Zollinger RM，Izant RJ：Congenital mesocolic （paraduodenal） hernia：Embryologic basis of repair. Am J Surg 1974；128：358，1974. B and C，Based on Callander CL，et al：Surg Gynecol Obstet 1935；60：1052.］

84-14B 和 C)。

内疝的临床表现为反复、间断发作性的小肠梗阻伴有复发性肠绞痛，后期则导致持续性腹痛、呕吐，有时会有便秘，这些症状有可能比较轻微，有时会被认为是精神症状，在发作时候行放射性检查可提示小肠梗阻。

50 盲肠扭转

盲肠扭转通常见于 60 岁以上的患者，这是因为盲肠、末端回肠和升结肠近端缺乏固定造成的，主要症状是急性剧烈腹痛、恶心，伴有右侧腹部胀满，经常出现完全性梗阻，腹部平片的典型表现为一个巨大充满气体的肠袢占据着左上腹部（凸面朝向左下腹)，伴有小肠梗阻[2]。

肠旋转和固定异常的放射学诊断

放射学造影检查对于临床诊断和评估肠旋转和固定异常是最基本的，胃、十二指肠、Treitz 韧带以及回盲部的正常位置关系见图 84-11，放射学结果见图 84-15。正常肠系膜附着的长度在放射学上对诊断有很大的预见性[4,8,25,45]。

腹部平片往往不能作出诊断，因为在新生儿和小婴儿中充气的小肠和大肠很难区分[28]，然而可以见到有些有价值的征象，包括急性十二指肠梗阻时可以见到“双泡征”（图 84-16A)，或者在老年患者中缺乏正常的结肠气体显示图像伴有盲肠异位，中肠扭转特点是腹部往往没有气体，但有时是远端小肠梗阻的表现[28]。在这些情况下肠壁往往增厚水肿（图84-16B)。

超声检查对于研究腹腔内病变已经成为一个有用的手段，当怀疑婴儿患有中肠扭转时是个很好的筛查手段，可以监测肠系膜上血管的血流情况。Pracros 等[44]报告了 18 例肠扭转中有 15 例在超声下看到肠系膜上静脉呈现涡流型态，同时发现肠系膜围绕着肠系膜上动脉，这种情况使用多普勒彩超显示最清楚（图 84-17)。其他的超声检查结果还有十二指肠积液、扩张，大部分扩张增厚的小肠袢位于脊柱的右侧。口服和静脉增强造影 CT 检查亦可发现肠系膜上

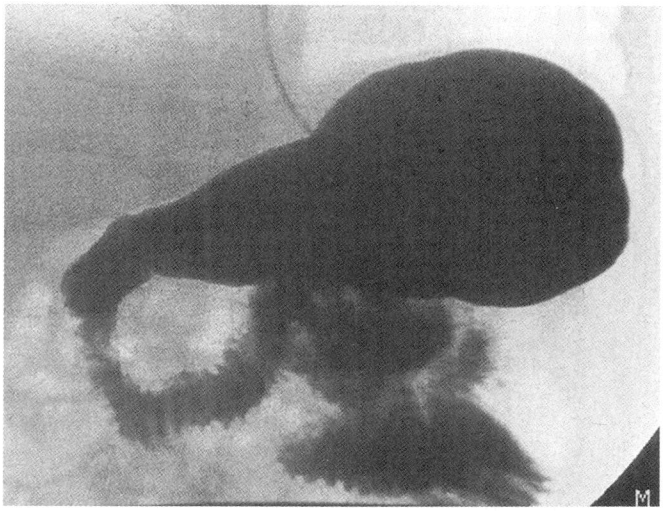

图 84-15　正常十二指肠的旋转和十二指肠空肠的固定。在超过十二指肠和空肠连接部的部分成为腹膜内器官之前，十二指肠从中线右侧下降，然后转向左侧，然后上升到中线的左侧到十二指肠球部水平。(Courtesy of Marc S. Keller, MD, Yale University School of Medicine.)

静脉的涡流征象（图 84-18)。

当患者可能存在肠旋转不良时应行上消化道造影，对十二指肠空肠轮廓进行仔细观察是目前首选的检查。Treitz 韧带位于中线或者椎体中央附近以及胃出口水平，正常情况下 Treitz 韧带位于椎体左侧和胃出口水平（图 84-19)。许多儿科放射学医生认为 Treitz 韧带位于中线右侧或者缺失是典型的旋转不良的表现，而位于中线或者位于左侧和胃出口水平的下方被认为是非典型性肠旋转不良的表现（图 84-20)。盲肠位置在右下腹为正常，位于右下腹之外均为异常。非典型性肠旋转异常的外科处理难点将在后面讨论。

在放射片上中肠扭转还是束带压迫造成的肠梗阻差异非常细微。Ablow 等[1]描述了在间歇性腹痛和呕吐的大龄儿童中的 Z 形十二指肠空肠袢，上消化道造影显示远端十二指肠到空肠呈锐角往返的过程，可能穿到中线的左侧，而不是正常情况下在 Treitz 韧带部位的平滑的十二指肠袢（图 84-21B)。Z 形征象是不完全肠旋转的诊断性标志，同时腹膜形成宽阔的束带延伸横过小肠并固定小肠，并不发生肠扭转，这些 Z 形征象和中肠扭转的螺丝锥征象有明显的区别。

内脏异位的婴儿放射片检查是非常具有挑战性

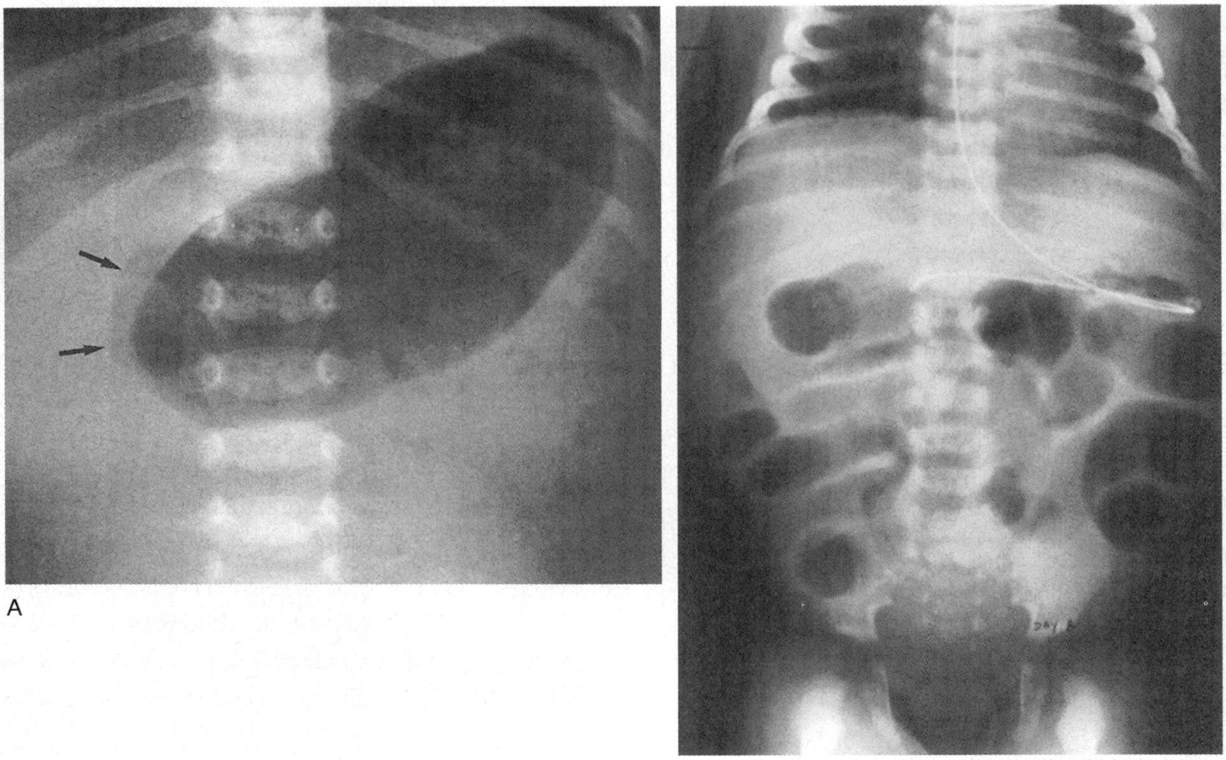

A

B

图 84-16 A. 婴儿中肠扭转的腹部平片。十二指肠降部梗阻会导致胃和十二指肠胀气（箭头所示），而远端无气。B. 伴有中肠扭转的 8 天的婴儿。远端小肠梗阻伴有肠壁增厚比近端的十二指肠梗阻少见，但它常常引起更严重的血管受压和临床后果。（Courtesy of Marc S. Keller，MD，Yale University School of Medicine.）

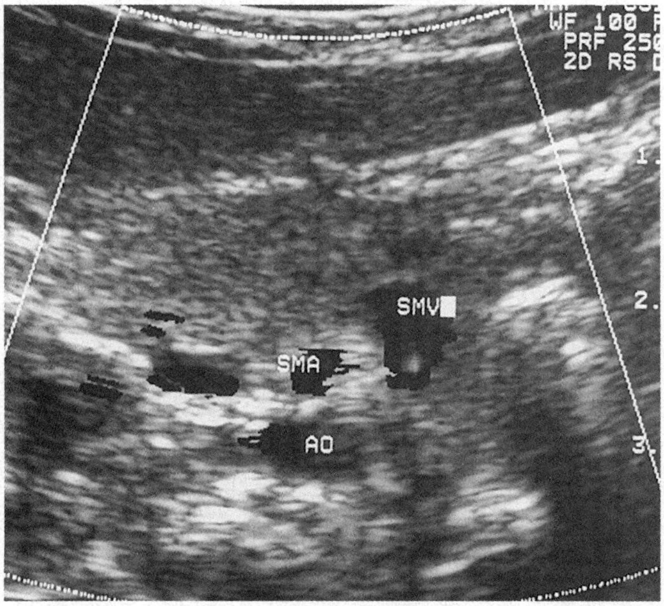

图 84-17 肠旋转不良的上腹部横向彩超图像。肠系膜上静脉（SMA）的位置异常，位于肠系膜上动脉（SMA）左侧，并可看见位于腹主动脉（AO）正前方。（Courtesy of Marc S. Keller，MD，Yale University School of Medicine.）

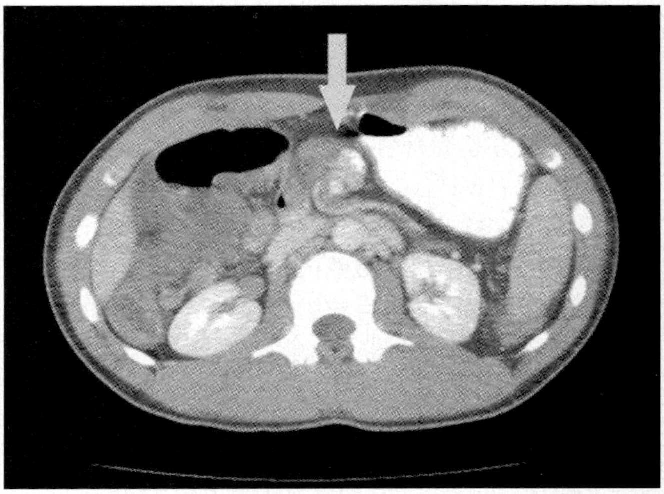

图 84-18 肠旋转不良伴有肠扭转 CT 扫描［注意肠系膜血管的螺旋结构（箭头所示）］。

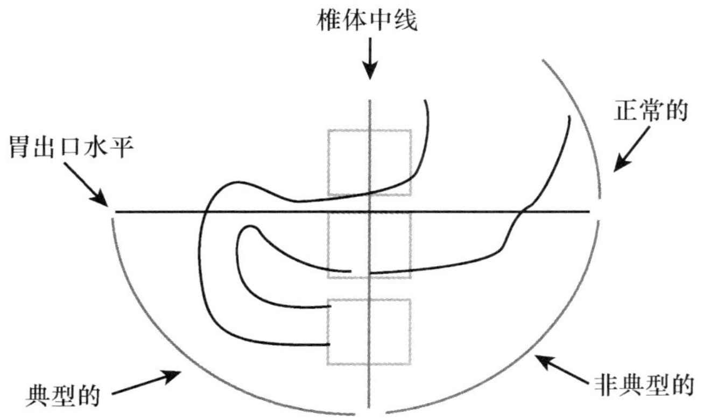

图 84-19　基于椎体中线位置和胃出口水平与 Treitz 韧带位置关系比较的肠旋转不良的分级。

的，因为胃、肝和脾的位置是不确定的。以我们的经验[11]，大多数患儿都存在十二指肠和空肠的固定异常，且均有可能通过造影被发现，无论胃是在左侧还是右侧（图 84-22）。

在吸收不良综合征中常常可以见到小肠黏膜增厚，这是慢性梗阻和扭转的另一个征象[16]。在右侧结肠系膜疝的患儿，升结肠和横结肠的相互关系一般是异常的，造影检查可见小肠被包裹。

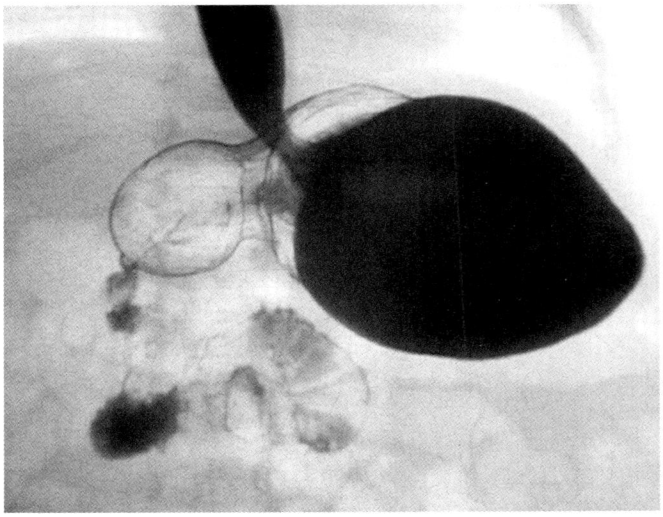

图 84-20　非典型性肠旋转不良或肠旋转不良变异的造影检查。Treitz 韧带不能到达正常的位于中线左侧和位于胃出口水平的位置。

治疗 1352

术前处理

当怀疑婴儿有中肠扭转和呕吐时会存在脱水、低血容量和低氯血症的表现，需要快速使用生理盐水进行静脉复苏。但不要延长复苏过程，因为迅速施行剖腹探查术对于患儿存活是非常必要的。其他需尽快实施的治疗包括放置鼻胃管，建立良好的静脉通道和胃肠道外应用抗生素。

手术技巧

Ladd 术可纠正伴有或不伴有中肠扭转的与旋转不良相关的基本病理异常。该操作包括以下重要步骤，且需要按正确的顺序进行：（1）托出小肠并探查肠系膜根部；（2）逆时针方向旋转以矫正中肠扭转；（3）松解 Ladd 束带，并沿着腹腔右侧沟伸直十二指肠；（4）切除阑尾；（5）把盲肠放置在左下腹。

肠旋转和固定异常的辨认

手术入路应取通过右侧脐上横切口，从中线延伸到对侧，切口要足够长能够暴露整个中肠，全部小肠要移出切口，以便完整地检查肠腔定位和固定。

在腹部两个重要的解剖学标志是幽门和脾曲，它们的位置在肠旋转不良的患儿中没有变化，表面上盲肠位于右中腹或下腹部以及部分十二指肠在左侧并不表示旋转正常，也不能排除肠旋转不良。

有几个征象提示有旋转异常：（1）异常的腹膜束带从回肠或右半结肠延伸到腹腔侧壁处十二指肠或者覆盖十二指肠；（2）十二指肠或空肠上段与盲肠或右半结肠相固定；（3）可以看见整个十二指肠、部分第三段和第四段位于横结肠系膜根部；（4）盲肠位置异常或游离度大，或十二指肠位于右侧腹腔旁沟。

确定回盲区域和定位回肠系膜有助于术者将肠系膜在手中展平。正常情况下盲肠位于回肠的右侧，在许多病例中肠系膜的位置不确定，但是通常可以见到系膜根部附着处狭窄，有时候只有在盲肠和右半结肠从十二指肠结肠峡部处分离后才能确诊肠旋转不良。

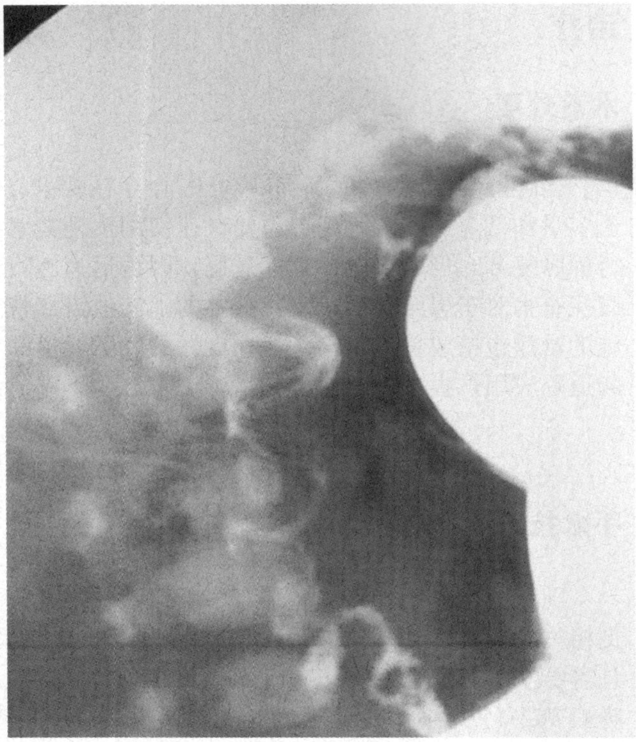

A

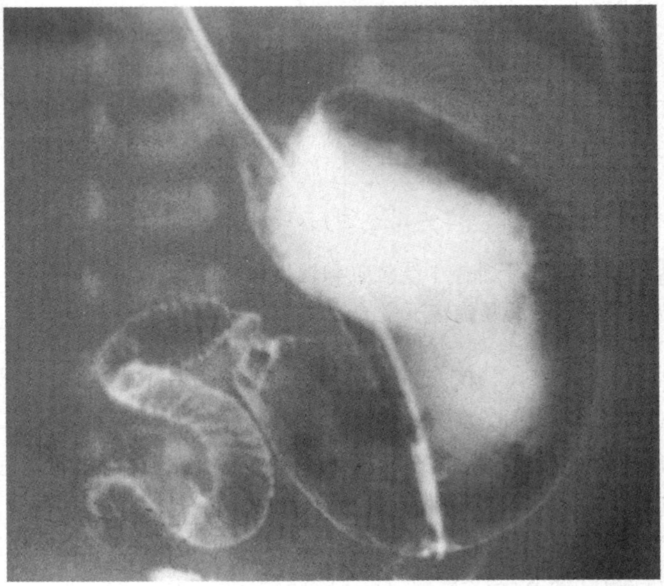

B

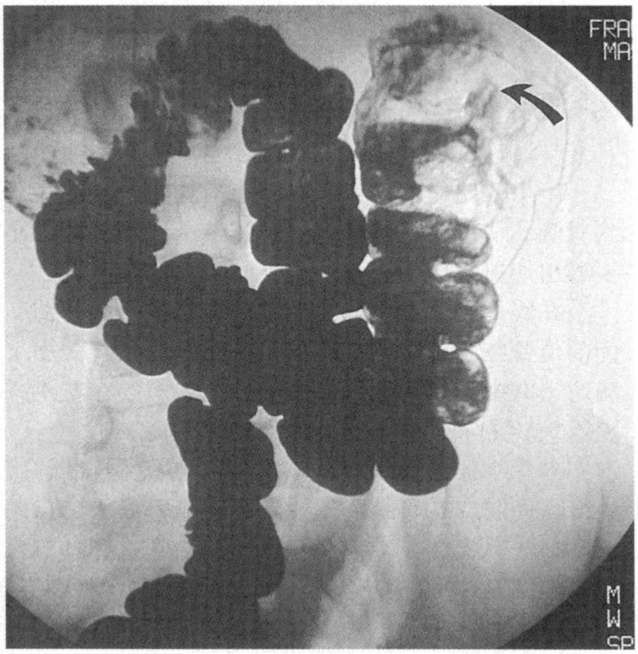

C

图 84-21 A. 肠旋转不良伴有中肠扭转。整个十二指肠和空肠近端非固定状态位于中线左侧并螺旋形向下呈螺丝锥结构。B. 十二指肠呈 Z 型带状结构的肠旋转不良。这例肠旋转不良婴儿异常的十二指肠被先天性的束带固定。C. 结肠的位置异常。上消化道造影的延迟摄片显示，回盲部（箭头所示）和未固定的结肠位于左上腹部。（Courtesy of Marc S. Keller，MD，Yale University School of Medicine.）

解除扭转

伴有中肠扭转时，当手术打开腹腔后，小肠充血呈紫色，伴有肠系膜静脉扩张。此时，因为结肠位于后方所以无法立刻看到回盲部异位（图 84-23A）。

整个小肠和大肠需从腹腔内托出，以避免肠系膜牵拉，这样可以看到系膜根部的扭曲（图 84-23B）。术者把肠管托在手中，逆时针方向解除扭转（图 84-23C）。作者较喜欢把肠管按 180°复位，直到看到横结肠和盲肠位于系膜带前面（图 84-23D）。当梗阻

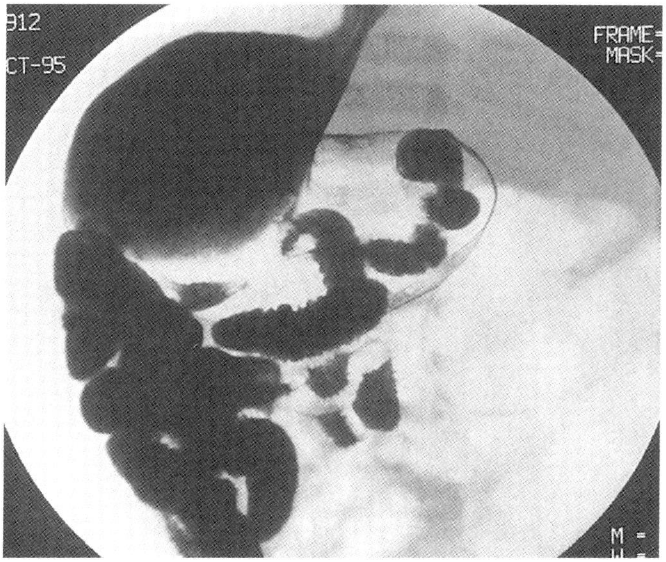

图 84-22　肠旋转不良伴有内脏异位。这例先天性心脏病的新生儿可见肝边缘的阴影和胃位于右上腹，十二指肠从中线左侧下降然后转向右侧但并不上升到十二指肠空肠交界处的固定点。(Courtesy of Marc S. Keller, MD, Yale University School of Medicine.)

解除后肠管的颜色会明显好转，除非肠管严重受压或坏死。一般来说需要旋转 2～3 圈才能完全解除扭转。

53 解除十二指肠梗阻并分离 Ladd 束带

当解除扭转之后需辨别引起梗阻的十二指肠束带，需从幽门或十二指肠空肠末端分离束带（见图 84-23D）。该束带通常附着在十二指肠到盲肠或者邻近肠系膜上血管的右半结肠，即所谓的十二指肠峡部。切断束带需靠近十二指肠浆膜层和肝十二指肠韧带中间和上部（接近肠系膜上血管时要小心），梗阻性的束带可能累及回肠或向下延伸累及空肠。Hous-
54 ton 和 Wittenborg[25] 指出这些束带可以向上延伸到胆囊和肝。在大多情况下使用锐性分离，在慢性十二指肠梗阻的年长儿童中可以清晰见到束带中的血管附着。

在所有的患儿必须探明没有内源性的梗阻存在，可以通过放置适当直径的鼻胃管或者经胃造瘘放置导管通过十二指肠进入空肠来检查（图 84-23E）。气体通过十二指肠不能排除有十二指肠隔膜或者“风帽样”蹼存在，这种情况在新生儿可能完全被忽视。

一旦 ladd 束带被分离，十二指肠可以相对较直地向下置入腹腔右侧旁沟（图 84-23E），如果不能完全解除束带则会导致十二指肠梗阻或肠扭转复发。任何试图通过固定十二指肠或者结肠以稳定肠系膜的方法都不能采用，因为这些方法都会增加由于粘连和内疝造成肠梗阻复发的危险[3,30,50,51]。

Ladd 术中最后一步是阑尾切除术。有些作者[52]推荐使用内翻结扎阑尾切除术避免可能出现的粪便污染，最后把盲肠放在左下腹部使肠系膜最大限度地增宽。

腹腔镜和开放手术

关于应用腹腔镜诊断和纠正肠旋转不良目前已有一些小规模的或者个案报道[5,6,38]，所有的研究报道中成功通过腹腔镜诊断和治疗的病例数均在 12 例或以下，由于缺乏大规模或前瞻性的随机研究来比较开放手术和腹腔镜手术，因此哪种方法是最好的外科治疗方式尚不明确。

肠切除和二次手术探查

当肠管状态良好，简单的肠粘连松解和 Ladd 术就足够了。局部的阶段性肠坏死但剩余的肠管状态良好时，可进行坏死肠管切除和一期吻合。缺血损伤造成的肠切除几率和症状持续的时间不同，Torres 和 Ziegler 的患儿中 30% 出现肠坏死[52]，而在 Seashore 和 Touloukian 的 40 例患儿中只有 3 例（7.5%）出现肠坏死需要肠切除[46]。

当出现多段肠管有状态不良或整个中肠看上去无法存活以及临床症状和体征表明有进行性肠管病变加重时，可行二次探查术。在 12～24 小时之后，或有问题的肠管得到恢复，或坏死的肠管界限明显，则通常需要行切除术。

对于肠管坏死或坏死边缘明显的患儿需根据其具体情况作出个体化处理，但应该遵循 3 个原则：（1）保留肠管长度至少要满足患儿的生存，这一点至关重要，二次手术中在肠管保留方面易犯错误，尤其在末端回肠和回盲瓣处理方面；（2）应该避免对血运有问题的肠管进行吻合；（3）整个小肠的切除

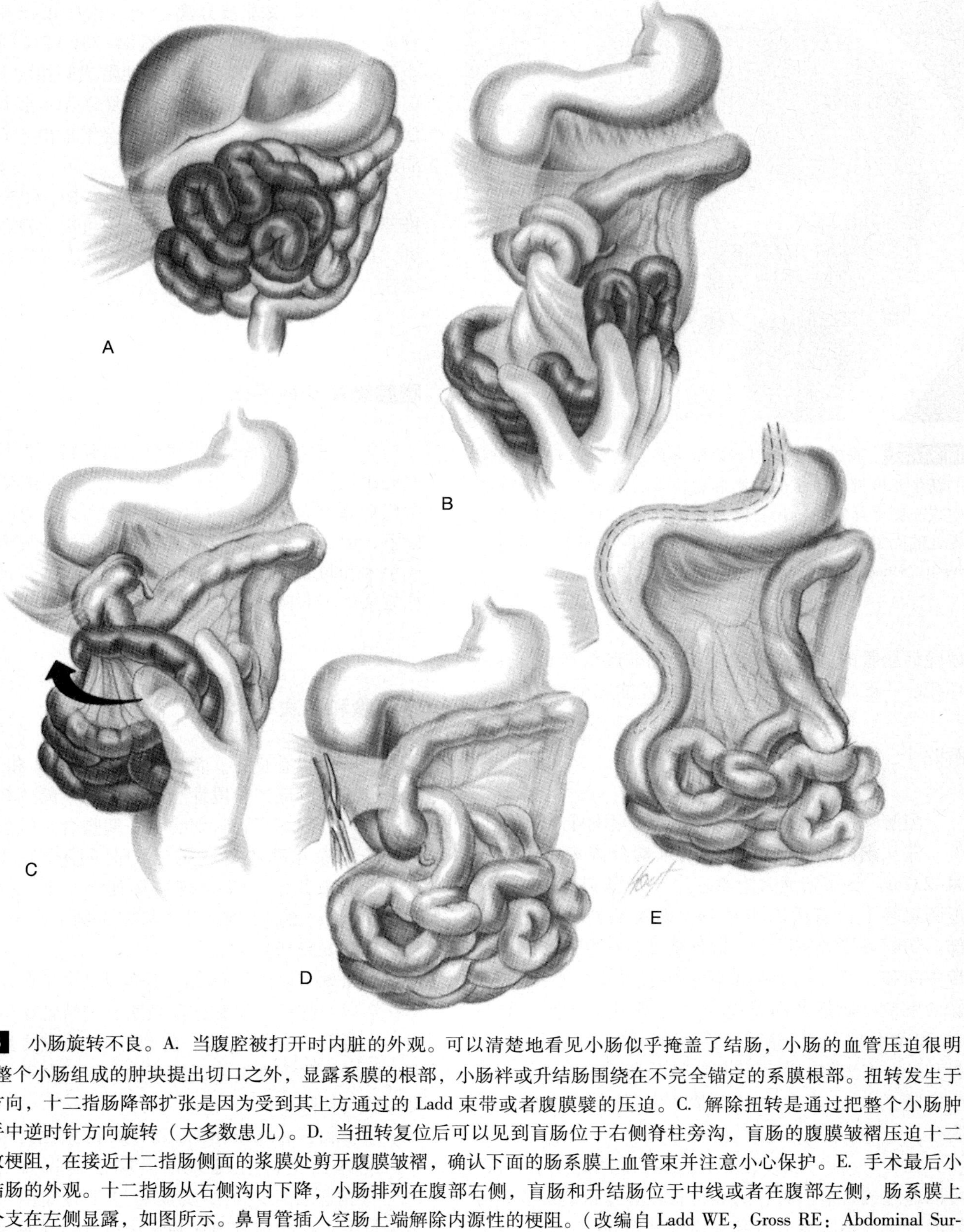

图 84-23　小肠旋转不良。A. 当腹腔被打开时内脏的外观。可以清楚地看见小肠似乎掩盖了结肠，小肠的血管压迫很明显。B. 整个小肠组成的肿块提出切口之外，显露系膜的根部，小肠袢或升结肠围绕在不完全锚定的系膜根部。扭转发生于顺时针方向，十二指肠降部扩张是因为受到其上方通过的 Ladd 束带或者腹膜襞的压迫。C. 解除扭转是通过把整个小肠肿块握在手中逆时针方向旋转（大多数患儿）。D. 当扭转复位后可以见到盲肠位于右侧脊柱旁沟，盲肠的腹膜皱褶压迫十二指肠导致梗阻，在接近十二指肠侧面的浆膜处剪开腹膜皱褶，确认下面的肠系膜上血管束并注意小心保护。E. 手术最后小肠和升结肠的外观。十二指肠从右侧沟内下降，小肠排列在腹部右侧，盲肠和升结肠位于中线或者在腹部左侧，肠系膜上动脉及分支在左侧显露，如图所示。鼻胃管插入空肠上端解除内源性的梗阻。（改编自 Ladd WE，Gross RE：Abdominal Surgery of Infancy and Childhood. Philadelphia，WB Saunders，1941.）

会导致患儿需要终生肠外营养或小肠移植。

非典型的肠旋转不良和肠旋转不良变异

通过上消化道造影越来越多的非典型肠旋转不良得以诊断，这些患儿被介绍给儿外科医生以评价和进行可能的外科治疗。儿外科医生对这些患儿往往是进退两难，因为手术风险和非手术治疗风险两者间优劣尚不清楚。许多患儿常常在进行胃食管反流的系列检查中被确诊。笔者和同事回顾了 5 年间不同类型肠旋转不良的外科治疗[40]，在 201 例肠旋转不良患儿（不包括脐疝、腹壁缺损的婴儿）的外科治疗中，典型的肠旋转不良为 75 例，其他类型肠旋转不良 101 例，在典型肠旋转不良患儿中肠扭转和内疝较为常见（分别为 16% 对 2% 和 21% 对 7%）。在变异型肠旋转不良患儿中症状持续存在和出现术后肠梗阻等并发症则更为常见（分别为 21% 对 12% 和 12% 对 0%），只有在典型肠旋转不良才会出现缺血性肠扭转。这些资
1356 料再次证实了典型肠旋转不良手术治疗的重要性。然而，在不典型患儿中因为发生扭转和内疝的可能性小且有较多的术后并发症，因此我们对无症状的非典型肠旋转不良或仅仅有胃食管反流症状的患儿行手术纠正的必要性提出疑问。

继发于反向旋转的结肠梗阻

在过去分离结肠和十二指肠前面相连之处是推荐的治疗方式，现在认识到这种梗阻可以通过游离十二指肠并将肠系膜血管放在前面同时把横结肠放在侧面来解决[54]。

肠系膜疝

右侧结肠系膜疝最好的处理方式是切开右结肠腹膜并返折，将结肠转向左侧，然后游离小肠[56]。左侧结肠系膜疝的治疗更有技术上的挑战性，有时小肠可以通过疝囊颈部复位，修补和复位的关键是移动肠系膜下静脉，该静脉沿疝囊颈前部边缘走向，要注意保留（见图 84-14B 和 C）。在静脉的右侧切开可以使肠管复位，腹膜和静脉的连接处要和后腹膜缝合以闭合疝囊颈部。

盲肠扭转

盲肠扭转的治疗在盲肠血运好时可以采用盲肠固定或者盲肠造瘘术，当肠管无法保留时可切除盲肠。

术后处理和并发症

肠功能恢复的时间取决于梗阻的持续时间和肠管损害的程度。在不复杂的十二指肠束带造成的十二指肠外源性梗阻，肠蠕动会在 1～5 天恢复，此时可以恢复喂养[30]。在没有扭转或梗阻的病例中，不常规使用鼻胃管进行胃肠减压。大龄患儿伴有慢性旋转不良或者反复发生的慢性肠梗阻往往长时间存在梗阻而需要鼻胃管引流和肠外营养支持。

当患儿的肠管处于存活边缘伴有黏膜损伤或短肠综合征时会引发特殊问题，完全胃肠外营养支持对于切除大段小肠的患儿是必要的，直到残留肠道适应生长所需和发生代偿性的生长[22]。少量的肠内营养推荐使用以促进肠道的适应过程同时提供肠黏膜的营养，是否需要胃造瘘来进行营养支持要根据具体情况。

Coombs 等[13]描述了一组 1 岁以上的肠旋转不良患儿反复出现长时间的肠动力不足的症状，这些患儿看上去没有从 Ladd 术中受益，这些假性肠梗阻的表现可能是偶发的或者是因为长期不完全性梗阻造成的神经性肠损伤。

并发症（除了短肠综合征导致的营养不良、腹泻、脱水）和其他腹部手术的并发症相类似，值得注意的是术后肠套迭，其发生率是 3.1%，而其他腹部手术的发生率为 0.05%[29]，典型表现是术后 5～8 天出现腹胀和胆汁性呕吐。术后粘连性肠梗阻的发生率为 4%。

复发性肠扭转的比例很低，在 Boston 的系列研究里，441 例中只有 2 例出现复发性肠梗阻；在 Los Angeles 的系列研究中没有病例出现复发[3]，159 例施行 Ladd 术的患儿中只有 2 例出现复发性中肠扭转[40]。

死亡原因主要和中肠扭转造成大面积肠坏死引起

的腹膜炎、后期营养相关性并发症或插管所致败血症等有关，特别是在1岁以下的患儿中。当超过75%的肠管出现坏死时其死亡率至少为65%[40]。

（李巍松译 王 俊校）

参考文献

1. Ablow RC, et al: Z-shaped duodenojejunal loop: Sign of mesenteric fixation anomaly and congenital bands. Am J Radiol 1983;141:461.
2. Anderson A, Bergdahl L, Van der Linden W: Volvulus of the cecum. Ann Surg 1975;181:876.
3. Andrassy RJ, Mahour GH: Malrotation of the midgut in infants and children. Arch Surg 1981;116:158.
4. Balthazar EJ: Intestinal malrotation in adults: Roentgenographic assessment with emphasis on isolated complete and partial nonrotations. AJR Am J Roentgenol 1976;126:358.
5. Bass KD, Rothenberg SS, Chang JH: Laparoscopic Ladd's procedure in infants with malrotation. J Pediatr Surg 1998; 33:279.
6. Bax NM, ven der Zee DC: Laparoscopic treatment of intestinal malrotation in children. Surg Endosc 1988;12:1314.
7. Bentley JFR: Mesenteric cysts with malrotated intestine. BMJ 1959;2:223.
8. Berdon WE, et al: Midgut malrotation and volvulus. Radiology 1970;96:365.
9. Bill AH, Grauman D: Rationale and technic for stabilization of the mesentery in cases of nonrotation of the midgut. J Pediatr Surg 1966;1:127.
10. Brennom WS, Bill AH: Prophylactic fixation of the intestine for midgut nonrotation. Surg Gynecol Obstet 1974;138:181.
11. Chang J, Brueckner M, Touloukian RJ: Intestinal rotation and fixation abnormalities in heterotaxia: Early detection and management. J Pediatr Surg 1993;28:1281.
12. Collins DC: 71,000 Human appendix specimens: A final report, summarizing forty years' study. Am J Proctol 1963; 14:365.
13. Coombs RC, Burch RG, Gornall PG: Intestinal malrotation: The role of small intestinal dysmotility in the cause of persistent symptoms. J Pediatr Surg 1991;26:553.
14. Devlin HB: Midgut malrotation causing intestinal obstruction in adult patients. Ann R Coll Surg Engl 1971;48:227.
15. Dott NM: Anomalies of intestinal rotation: Their embryology and surgical aspects with report of five cases. Br J Surg 1923;11:251.
16. Estrada RL: Anomalies of Intestinal Rotation and Fixation. Springfield, Ill, Charles C Thomas, 1958.
17. Filston HC, Kirks DR: Malrotation—the ubiquitous anomaly. J Pediatr Surg 1981;16:614.
18. Firor HV, Steiger E: Morbidity of rotational abnormalities of the gut beyond infancy. Cleve Clin Q 1983;50:303.
19. Fraser JE, Robbins RH: On the factors concerned in causing rotation of the intestine in man. J Anat Physiol 1915;50:75.
20. Fukuya T, Brown BP, Lu CC: Midgut volvulus as a complication of intestinal malrotation in adults. Dig Dis Sci 1993; 38:438.
21. Gardner CE, Hart D: Anomalies of intestinal rotation as a cause of intestinal obstruction. Arch Surg 1934;29:942.
22. Georgeson KE, Breaux CW Jr: Outcome and intestinal adaptation in neonatal short-bowel syndrome. J Pediatr Surg 1992;27:344.
23. Gross RE: The Surgery of Infancy and Childhood. Philadelphia, WB Saunders, 1953.
24. Haymond HE, Dragstedt LR: Anomalies of intestinal rotation. Surg Gynecol Obstet 1931;53:316.
25. Houston CS, Wittenborg MH: Roentgen evaluation of anomalies of rotation and fixation of the bowel in children. Radiology 1965;84:1.
26. Howell CG, et al: Malrotation, malnutrition and ischemic bowel disease. J Pediatr Surg 1982;17:469.
27. Janik JS, Ein SH: Normal intestinal rotation with nonfixation: A cause of chronic abdominal pain. J Pediatr Surg 1979;14:670.
28. Kassner EG, Kottmeier PK: Absence and retention of small bowel gas in infants with midgut volvulus: Mechanisms and significance. Pediatr Radiol 1975;4:28.
29. Kidd J, Jackson R, Wagner C, Smith S: Intussusception following the Ladd's procedure. Arch Surg 2000;135:713.
30. Kiesewetter WB, Smith JW: Malrotation of the midgut in infancy and childhood. Arch Surg 1958;77:483.
31. Kluth D, Lambrecht W: Disorders of intestinal rotation. In Freeman NV, Burge DM, Griffiths DM, Malone PSJ (eds): Surgery of the Newborn. New York, Churchill Livingstone, 1994.
32. Ladd WE: Congenital obstruction of the duodenum in children. N Engl J Med 1932;206:277.
33. Ladd WE: Surgical diseases of the alimentary tract in infants. N Engl J Med 1936;215:705.
34. Ladd WE, Gross RE: Abdominal Surgery of Infancy and Childhood. Philadelphia, WB Saunders, 1941.
35. Lewis JE Jr: Partial duodenal obstruction with incomplete duodenal rotation. J Pediatr Surg 1966;1:47.
36. Mall FP: Development of the human intestine and its position in the adult. Bull Johns Hopkins Hosp 1898;9:197.
37. Maxson RT, Franklin PA, Wagner CW: Malrotation in the older child: Surgical management, treatment, and outcome. Am Surg 1995;61:135.
38. Mazziotti MV, Strasberg SM, Langer JC: Intestinal rotational anomalies without volvulus: The role of laparoscopy. J Am Coll Surg 1997;185:172.
39. McIntosh R, Donovan EJ: Disturbances of rotation of the intestinal tract. Am J Dis Child 1939;57:116.
40. Mehall JR, et al: Management of typical and atypical intestinal malrotation. J Pediatr Surg 2002;37:1169.
41. Messineo A, et al: Clinical factors affecting mortality in children with malrotation of the intestine. J Pediatr Surg 1992;27:1343.
42. Porto SO: Jaundice in congenital malrotation of the intestine. Am J Dis Child 1969;117:684.
43. Powell DM, Othersen HB, Smith CD: Malrotation of the intestines in children: The effect of age on presentation and therapy. J Pediatr Surg 1989;24:777.
44. Pracros JP, et al: Ultrasound diagnosis of midgut volvulus: The "whirlpool" sign. Pediatr Radiol 1992;22:18.
45. Schey WL, Donaldson JS, Sty JR: Malrotation of bowel: Variable patterns with different surgical considerations. J Pediatr Surg 1993;28:96.
46. Seashore JH, Touloukian RJ: Midgut volvulus: An ever present threat. Arch Pediatr Adolesc Med 1994;148:43.
47. Simpson AJ, et al: Roentgen diagnosis of midgut malrotation: Value of upper gastrointestinal radiographic study. J Pediatr Surg 1972;7:243.
48. Snyder WH, Chaffin L: Embryology and pathology of the intestinal tract: Presentation of 48 cases of malrotation.

Ann Surg 1954;140:368.
49. Spigland N, Brandt ML, Yazbeck S: Malrotation presenting beyond the neonatal period. J Pediatr Surg 1990;25:1139.
50. Stauffer UG, Herrmann P: Comparison of late results in patients with corrected intestinal malrotation with and without fixation of the mesentery. J Pediatr Surg 1980;15:9.
51. Stewart DR, Colodny AL, Daggett WC: Malrotation of the bowel in infants and children: A 15-year review. Surgery 1976;79:716.
52. Torres AM, Ziegler MM: Malrotation of the intestine. World J Surg 1993;17:326.
53. Wakefield EG, Mayo CW: Intestinal obstruction produced by mesenteric bands. Arch Surg 1936;33:47.
54. Wang CA, Welch CE: Anomalies of intestinal rotation in adolescents and adults. Surgery 1963;54:839.
55. Waugh GE: Congenital malformation of the mesentery: A clinical entity. Br J Surg 1928;15:438.
56. Willwerth BM, Zollinger RM, Izant RJ: Congenital mesocolic (paraduodenal) hernia: Embryologic basis of repair. Am J Surg 1974;128:358.

第 85 章

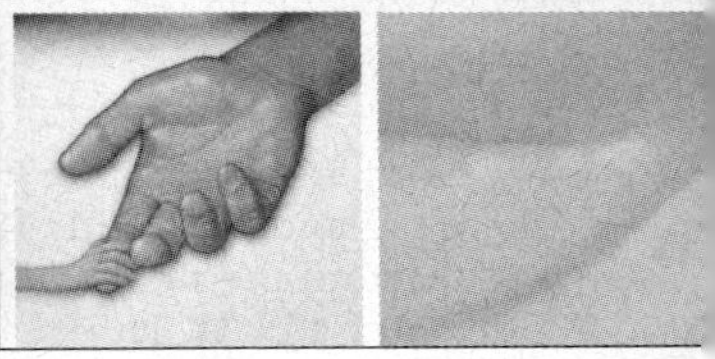

肠梗阻的其他原因

Cynthia A. Gingalewski

1358 肠梗阻可以发生在从新生儿到成人的任何年龄，根据患者发病的年龄以及以往的外科手术史，其病因学有很大的不同。常见的先天性肠梗阻原因包括肠闭锁/狭窄、旋转不良、巨结肠、肛门闭锁以及新生儿胎粪导致的疾病。在其他章节将详细讨论上述这些疾病，而本章主要回顾其他引起小肠和结肠梗阻的常见和不常见的病因。

早期诊断有赖于对梗阻症状（胆汁性呕吐、腹胀和腹部触痛）的识别和对 X 线片的解释。多数情况下，婴幼儿肠梗阻需要进行儿外科治疗。

胚胎学

除少数病例外，在大多数婴儿和儿童的肠梗阻均为胚胎性原因所致，尤其是在 1 岁以下的患儿中，在其他章节已经讨论过此类问题，本章中将探讨与其相关的胚胎学基础。

疾病谱

在婴儿和儿童中小肠梗阻较结肠梗阻更为常见，多数病因均为先天性或者获得性的，包括小肠粘连性梗阻、疝（先天性疝和后天性疝）、肠内和肠外的病变。其中粘连性小肠梗阻最常见，约占各类小肠梗阻的 60%。肿瘤（20%）、疝（10%）、肠道炎症性疾病（5%）、肠扭转（3%）以及其他各种原因引起的肠梗阻可导致粘连[4]。

术后肠粘连

区分术后肠麻痹和术后肠梗阻较为困难，两者在 X 线片上均显示出肠袢扩张，因此很难区别。粘连性小肠梗阻多见于盆腔手术后包括阑尾切除、妇科手术和结直肠手术。通常认为是由于盆腔内粘连产生束带导致继发性梗阻，在这个部位小肠游离度大并容易扭转从而在粘连周围发生梗阻。

儿童腹部手术后小肠梗阻的发生率约为 2%～30%，在新生儿更多见。Festen[22] 的资料显示在 1476 例腹部手术的患儿中小肠粘连性梗阻的发生率为 2.2%，80% 的梗阻发生在初次术后 3 个月内，70% 为单纯粘连束带所造成。在新生儿术后肠梗阻发生率要比婴儿和儿童高 57%，且常见于腹裂和肠闭锁术后。在儿童中阑尾切除术是引起术后粘连性肠梗阻最常见的原因，但发生率在阑尾有无穿孔或单纯性阑尾炎中无明显差别。多伦多儿童医院也得出类似的结果，在儿童肠梗阻中，术后粘连性肠梗阻排第七位[28]，最常见于阑尾术后（16%），且大多数发生在术后 2 年（82%）。

诊断

粘连性肠梗阻的诊断要点是：有腹部手术史的患儿出现腹胀和胆汁性呕吐，在疾病初期很难与胃肠炎相区分。最初呕吐物可能不含胆汁，但随着疾病的进展出现胆汁性或粪汁样呕吐，患儿主诉腹部
绞痛、食欲减退。在不完全性肠梗阻时会有持续性 1359
排气排便，但在完全性肠梗阻时排气排便均消失。随着梗阻病情进展患儿出现嗜睡，发热提示有肠坏

死的可能。

疾病初期可能无明显的体征，但随着疾病进展会出现腹胀及肠鸣音亢进或减弱，最后导致局部持续性腹痛，通过胃肠减压不能缓解，这是肠管出现血运障碍的不良预兆。持续性的局限性腹痛是肠缺血的唯一可靠的征象，Janik[28]等在一组 131 例患儿的报告中指出，如胃肠减压之后仍然存在持续性腹痛则 100% 发生肠坏死。

放射学检查有助于区分炎症性梗阻，所有患儿都需要进行腹部平片检查，至少包括腹部平卧位和直立位两项检查（图 85-1）。肠袢扩张和液气平面征象表明梗阻的存在，结肠和直肠出现气体表明是不完全性肠梗阻，腹腔游离气体表明有肠穿孔，需要急诊手术。肠梗阻还可以通过 CT 检查和上消化道肠对比造影（UGISBFT）进一步明确诊断，CT 的优点是可以排除其他诊断，发现梗阻的部位，而且与 UGISBFT 检查相比较，水溶性造影剂不容易被稀释。

治疗

目前对于小肠梗阻的患儿是采取急诊手术还是采用保守的减压治疗仍然有争论，所有怀疑存在肠梗阻的患儿均需接受积极的静脉补液和补充电解质，同时放置胃管进行胃肠减压，行血常规检查，当出现白细胞总数上升，且中性粒细胞上升明显要考虑有肠缺血坏死的可能，是否手术需取决于患儿的临床表现，如果为完全性肠梗阻没有排气或排便则应该立即行剖腹探查术。当部分肠梗阻的时候，同时不伴有发热、白细胞上升和局限性腹部压痛，则可先观察，观察过程中要经常对患儿进行腹部体检、动态腹部平片检查，测量血电解质。在一项 230 例粘连性肠梗阻患儿的回顾性调查中，保守治疗的成功率为 74%[1]，但保守治疗患儿中肠梗阻复发率为 36%，而行粘连松解术后复发率为 19%。粘连松解术后肠梗阻复发的比率为 5%~19% 不等。

在存在扩张肠袢时也能施行腹腔镜下的粘连松解术，梗阻的部位越靠近近端，施行腹腔镜粘连松解术就越容易。在开放性肠粘连松解术中肠道损伤的比率为 11%[28]。一项有关成人的肠梗阻剖腹手术或腹腔镜手术的回顾性研究中表明，腹腔镜手术成功的比率为 32%，原因主要为不能发现梗阻部位、不能建立 1360
气腹、严重的肠粘连和小肠坏死[16]。术中肠损伤在开放手术是腹腔镜手术的 4 倍，开放手术术后并发症的比率较高，包括肺炎、肠麻痹时间延长、切口感染，死亡和梗阻未解除只发生在腹腔镜组。在另一项关于成人的回顾性研究中[52]，腹腔镜治疗中转开腹手术的比例超过 50%，在腹腔镜组有较高的并发症发生率，包括肠道损伤和吻合口漏。在儿童没有类似的对比研究。

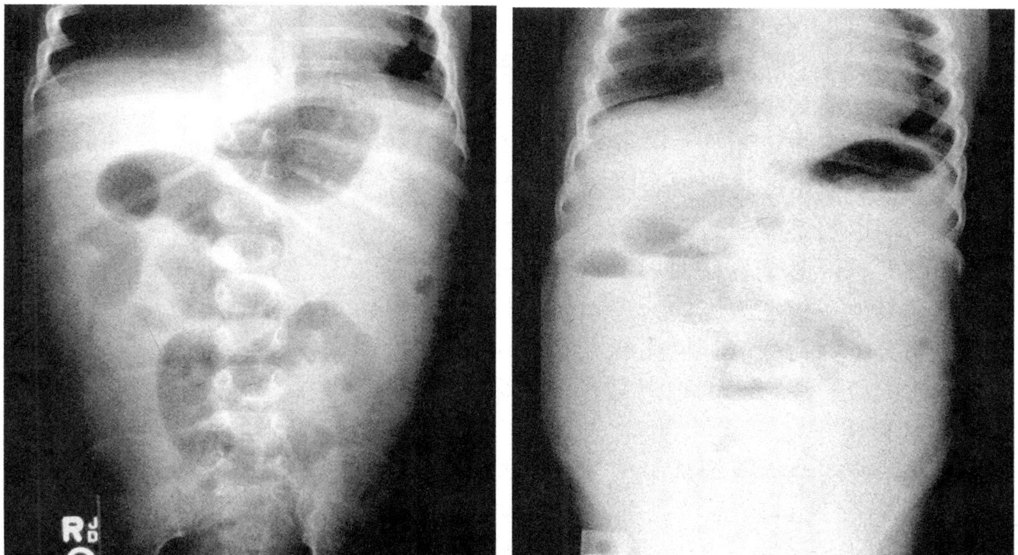

A　　B

图 85-1　完全性小肠梗阻。A. 一名肠旋转不良儿童行 Ladd 术后腹部仰卧位平片显示小肠肠管扩张，结肠无气体。B. 该患儿的腹部立位平片显示扩张的小肠内液气平面同时结肠没有气体。

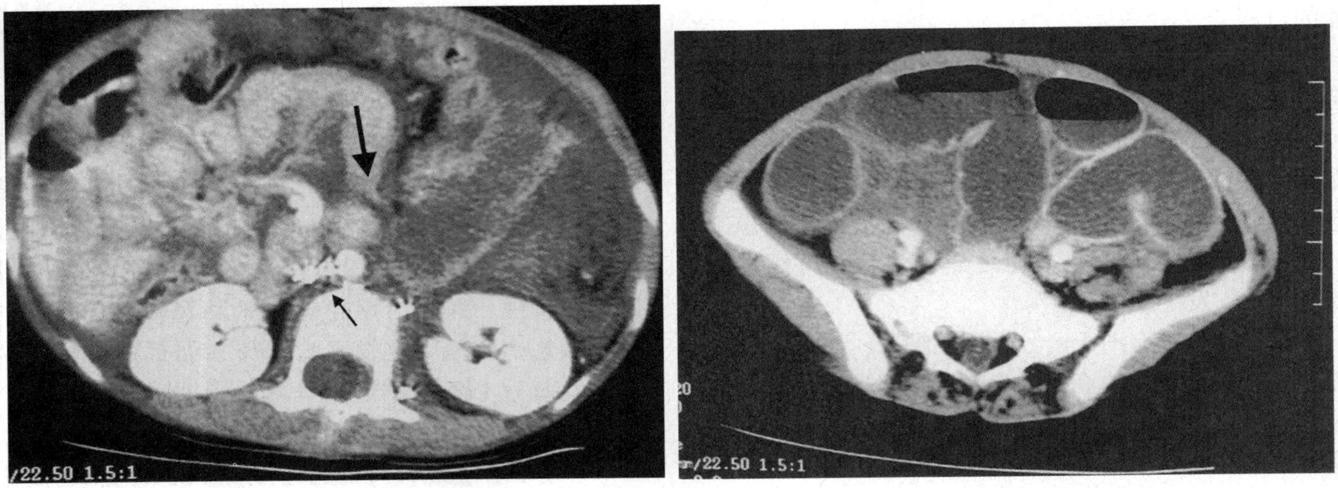
A　B

图 85-2　不全性小肠梗阻。A. CT 腹部增强造影，对神经节细胞瘤切除术后不全性肠梗阻的患儿进行腹部扫描，小箭头指向前次手术修剪的部位，大箭头表示梗阻的移行部位。注意到在扩张的肠管可以见到造影剂被稀释，部分性梗阻的特点是可以见到造影剂从移行部位通过。B. 同样的病例显示近端肠管扩张充满液体，在盆腔可以见到液气平面。

预防

很多报道介绍了预防腹腔内粘连的方法，然而还没有发现有效防止粘连形成的“魔力子弹”。一般性的措施包括：轻柔的操作、彻底的止血、冲洗腹腔、减少肠管暴露在空气中的时间，但这些并不能消除粘连的发生。有些商品化抗粘连介质如透明质酸为主的生物可吸收膜、透明质酸、羧甲基纤维素膜都已经被广泛使用和报道。透明质酸为主的生物可吸收膜在 24 小时形成胶体，然后在 7 天内逐渐缓慢被吸收。几个临床使用透明质酸为主的生物可吸收膜试验表明其能减少术后肠粘连[7,8,50]，然而应该避免使用该膜包裹吻合口，因为这会增加吻合口漏的可能性。使用该膜的困难主要是它黏度大，很难操作使用以及不能通过腹腔镜使用，它的改进品透明质酸Ⅱ，因为很容易使用所以很快在市场上流行开来。其他一些在腹腔内使用预防肠粘连发生的物质有高分子葡萄糖酐、氧化纤维素、纤维蛋白封闭剂和水凝胶。在临床试验中只有氧化纤维素显示了抗粘连的效果[6]。

在肠粘连的动物模型试验中，Springhall 和 Spitz 在大鼠术后使用口服西沙比利，粘连发生率降低 50%[48]。由于该药品已经从市场上被剔除，因此没有人体临床试验来证实其效果。

术后肠麻痹

有时很难区分术后肠麻痹和肠梗阻，X 线片上出现扩张的肠袢无法区分这两种情况，因此胃肠道对比增强造影可能是必须的。大多数术后肠麻痹在术后 5～7天消失，肛门排气提示结肠功能的恢复，表明肠麻痹消失。术后肠麻痹时间的延长与麻醉药使用呈剂量相关性。麻醉剂、严重的肠道创伤、腹腔内出血、术前肠梗阻的存在均导致肠功能恢复时间延长。

鸦片制剂有抑制胃肠动力、增加胃窦和十二指肠第一段张力的作用，对小肠的运动具有双向性[11]。
吗啡最初刺激肌移动复合波（MMC）的第Ⅱ相，但 1361
这种刺激伴随着胃肠传输时间的迟缓而减慢[24]。使用吗啡对抗剂盐酸钠洛酮并未发现其在缩短术后肠麻痹时间上的益处[24,33]。

因为缺乏细胞间的缝隙连接，麻醉剂对结肠运动的抑制作用最大[33]，麻醉药氟烷和安氟醚均能减少胃排空，局麻药物胸部的硬膜外麻醉还会导致内脏血流增加，阻碍传入和传出神经抑制反射，在胸段应用时可明显减少术后肠麻痹时间[12,29]，有趣的是腰段的硬膜外麻醉并没有类似的效果[32,41]。

人们试图通过腹腔镜手术、早期进食和应用各种药物以缩短术后肠麻痹的时间。早期进食并不能缩短肠麻痹时间[35]，而在动物试验和临床试验中均表明经腹腔镜手术可以明显减少术后肠麻痹时间[10,30]。在很多药物试验中，唯一证明对人有效的是西沙比利（目前一般不使用，除非特殊情况下酌情使用）。生长抑素类似物奥曲肽具有抑制多种胃肠激素的作用，可以减少狗术后肠麻痹的时间[13,18,31]。非甾体类抗炎药物（NSAIDs）对减少肠麻痹时间有帮助，这是因为它可以减少麻醉止痛药物的应用；盐酸甲氧氯普胺作为动力促进剂具有促胆碱能和抗多巴胺作用，刺激肌移动复合波（MMC）的第Ⅱ相，但反复试验研究均表明其不能减少术后肠麻痹时间。在前瞻性随机化试验中，胃动素受体刺激物琥乙红霉素也不能缩短术后肠麻痹时间[47]。

术后肠套迭

儿童更容易发生术后肠套迭，特别是后腹膜肿瘤术后以及巨结肠和其他神经嵴细胞病变。在术后肠功能恢复后突然出现大量的胆汁性呕吐应怀疑小肠套迭发生的可能，可以通过上消化道增强造影作出诊断。大多数的术后肠套迭发生在小肠，因此需要手术纠正。

炎症性粘连

腹腔内炎症性疾病均可导致粘连形成，继而在没有手术史的患儿中引起粘连性肠梗阻，这类疾病包括卵巢扭转、脑室腹腔分流感染、Crohn 病、艾滋病和盆腔炎症性疾病等等。

疝

尽管疝只占小肠梗阻病因的 10%，但更容易造成肠绞窄，这些疝包括腹股沟疝、直疝和内疝。内疝是因为腹腔内的束带和肠切除后肠系膜缺损造成的，很容易造成“闭袢性”肠梗阻，这种情况很容易在短时间内导致肠缺血，其特点是与腹部体征不相符的腹痛。

先天性疝包括十二指肠旁疝、腹股沟疝、继发于脐肠管残留所引起的内疝、非胚胎源性的先天性束带、镰状韧带未固定造成的内疝，外科术后造成的内疝包括肠系膜关闭不全和造瘘口周围疝。

十二指肠旁疝

十二指肠旁疝（结肠系膜疝）是较少见的先天性病变，是由于肠旋转不良造成的，十二指肠旁疝的命名不甚确切，但是提示小肠会在结肠系膜的后方疝出。右侧结肠系膜疝是因为中肠袢未能围绕肠系膜上动脉正常旋转造成的，大多数的小肠在此动脉的右侧（图 85-3A）。左侧结肠系膜疝的病因尚不明确，因为此时肠道的旋转往往正常，小肠从 Treitz 韧带和横结肠之间的无血管区进入，位于肠系膜下静脉的下方（图 85-3B），十二指肠系膜和结肠系膜融合不完全[15]，结果导致疝的发生，同时可能引起空肠嵌顿和左上腹回肠长度的变化。尽管这种变化是先天性的，但大多在成人中被发现。左侧系膜疝发生率是右侧的 3 倍，是内疝中最多见的类型，占 50%。

当高度怀疑内疝的时候需要进行进一步诊断，这些内疝症状往往不典型，包括阵发性剧烈腹痛、呕吐、腹胀和黑便[39]。影像学检查包括上消化道造影或 CT 检查，是唯一能进行术前准确诊断的方法。

十二指肠旁疝的外科处理包括打开疝囊、小肠复位和修补缺损，不要试图去切除疝囊。腹腔镜下十二指肠旁疝的修补也有报道[49]。

脐肠管残留 1362

脐肠管（卵黄管）是胚胎发育中的正常结构，连接胎儿的肠管和卵黄囊，当该结构在婴儿出生后还存在则成为脐肠管残留物，可以表现为通向脐部的瘘管、回肠和脐部间的纤维束带以及 Meckel 憩室。这是最常见的先天异常之一（占人口的 2%），但有症状的只占 2%。在一个 46 例的回顾性调查中，脐肠管残留患儿中 28% 伴有肠梗阻（肠套迭、内疝、肠扭转）[38]，需外科治疗，目前也有腹腔镜治疗的报道[14]，在第 82 章中已深入讨论。

先天性非胚胎性和炎性来源束带

有关先天性束带造成肠梗阻有散在文献报道，病因学尚不清楚，但它们不是胚胎源性如脐肠管或者卵黄管残留所致。在一篇回顾中 8 例有异常束带的患

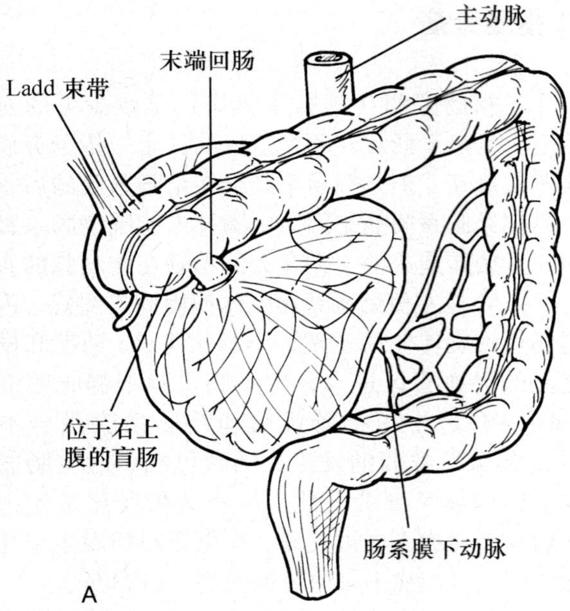

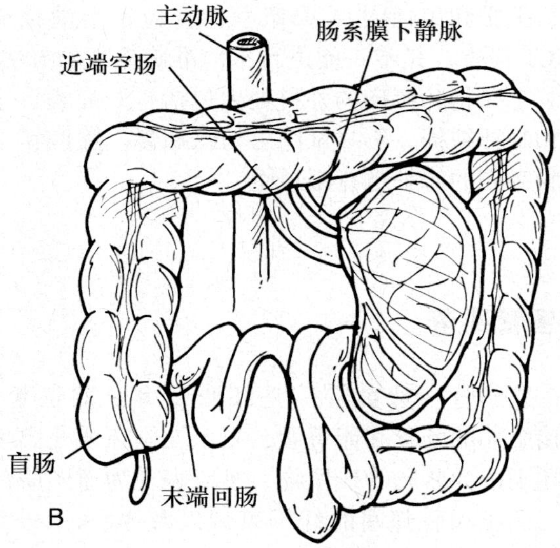

图 85-3 十二指肠旁疝（结肠系膜疝）。A. 右十二指肠旁疝。肠管异常旋转，盲肠位于右上腹，可以看见 Ladd 带。大部分小肠被包裹于右侧结肠系膜后。B. 左侧十二指肠旁疝。小肠旋转正常，包裹于左侧结肠系膜后，位于肠系膜下静脉后。［改编自 Willwerth BM, Zollinger RM Jr, Izant RJ Jr, et al: Congenital mesocolic (paraduodental) hernia. Embryologic basis of repair. Am J Surg 1974; 128:358-361.］

儿，50%发生在升结肠和末端回肠之间，Treitz 韧带和末端回肠占 25%，肝右叶和末端回肠占 12.5%，肝右叶和升结肠占 12.5%[2]。

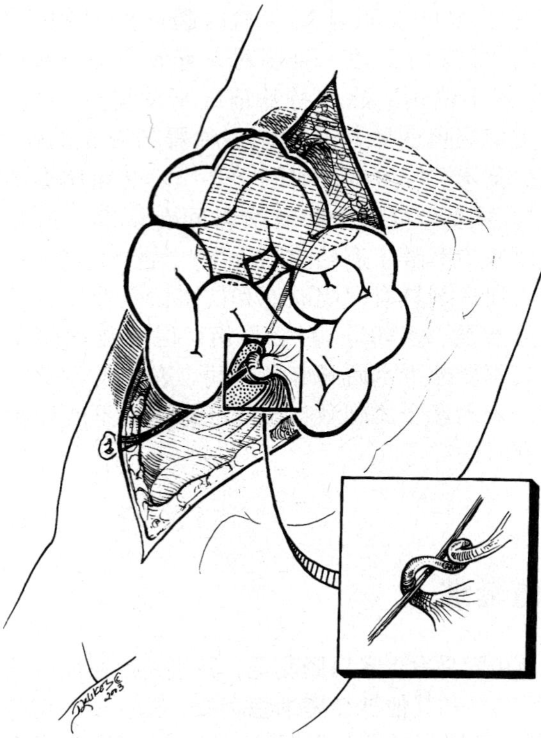

图 85-4 继发于镰状韧带未完全腹膜化的内疝。镰状韧带没有和前腹壁通过双层腹膜固定，如同先天性索带，使小肠疝入其周围，导致内疝发生。

患儿可能有慢性腹痛或者急性肠梗阻，需及时诊断，分离束带即可治愈。

镰状韧带未固定

镰状韧带通常由两层腹膜构成，将肝和前腹壁固定，它有 3 个边界：膈肌、前腹壁到脐的水平、肝下缘游离部分，其中有闭锁的脐静脉。如果腹膜不能沿着脐静脉融合，会导致这种罕见的镰状韧带未固定，引起小肠进入形成疝，如同先天性束带（图85-4），在新生儿中曾有这种情况发生的报道[9,19,45]。

自从 1937 年首次报道该疾病之后，在世界文献中报道该病不超过 10 例，这些病例中只有 2 例在新生儿期被发现，其余发现于成人，没有儿童期发病的报道。镰状韧带的缺陷包括从游离的镰状韧带到韧带腹膜叶上的孔，通常这种疝内容物为小肠，也可以是大网膜或大肠[27]。

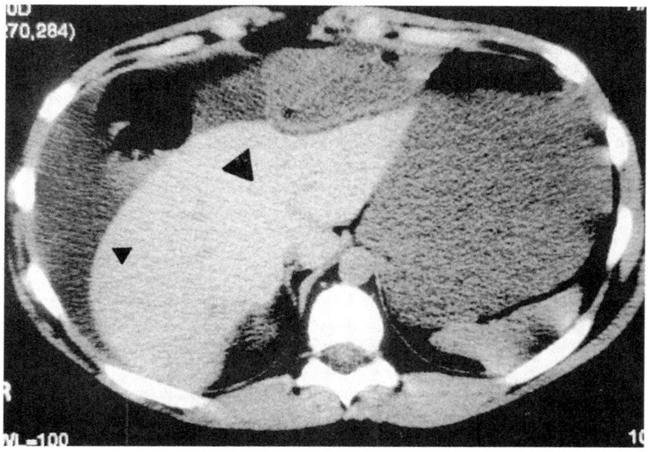

图 85-5　镰状韧带周围内疝患儿术前 CT 增强造影。患儿出现粪便样呕吐，无既往手术史。大箭头表示小肠袢位于肝缘之上，镰状韧带周围，右侧结肠可以见到位于右上腹肝之上，小箭头表明有腹水存在。术中发现小肠坏疽，行镰状韧带分离，切除坏死小肠并行一期吻合。

通常是在无手术史和无外疝的急性小肠梗阻急诊手术探查当中发现并作出该病的诊断，术前 CT 检查
363 中发现小肠围绕镰状韧带位于肝之上提示该病（图 85-5），当出现腹水的时候提示有肠管血运障碍，通过分离镰状韧带解除梗阻可以治愈该病。

系膜缺损

在所有涉及小肠切除的手术操作中必须注意关闭所有的缺损系膜，可以使用可吸收或者不可吸收缝线，连续缝合或间断缝合。间断缝合的好处在于拆散一针不会形成大的缺损而导致内疝形成。

造瘘口周围疝

造瘘口周围疝是结肠造口术后常见的问题。造瘘口旁疝的发生率为 2%～35%，大多数出现在术后 2 年内，肥胖或营养不良的患儿中更为常见，使用皮质激素和术后切口感染同样会增加该病的风险。为了减少其发生的可能性，结肠应该从腹直肌中穿出，应保留皮下脂肪，筋膜的缺损不要太大，缝合肠管浆膜和造瘘口周围的皮肤可以减少婴儿疝发生的风险。

永久性造瘘的患儿如果有小的无症状的造瘘口周围疝，修补时造瘘口必须去除。当出现较大的疝，妨碍造瘘袋具的放置、出现疼痛或者出现嵌顿时需要外科手术修补，处理方法包括造瘘重新换位、筋膜关闭、补片修补，成人的手术修补效果不佳，造瘘口重新换位复发率为 33%～50%，筋膜修补复发率为 50%～100%，补片修补复发率为 50%，复发后再修补其效果更差，复发率为 90%～100%。

结肠梗阻

肠扭转

在成人中结肠扭转是引起结肠梗阻的常见病因，但在儿童中非常罕见，曾经有些个案报道儿童盲肠、乙状结肠、横结肠扭转[5,36,43,46]，常伴有精神发育迟缓、Hirschsprung 病、肠动力缺乏和慢性便秘。当儿童出现突发性腹痛和梗阻时，腹部平片提示梗阻近端
肠袢扩张，钡剂灌肠显示在病变的肠管部位出现特征 1364
性的“鸟嘴征”。

治疗包括通过结肠镜非手术复位或者直接剖腹探查手术矫正扭转，盲肠扭转应行一期切除吻合或者盲肠固定术[25]，横结肠扭转是唯一逆时针方向扭转的肠管，切除加端端吻合是横结肠、结肠脾曲、乙状结肠扭转的治疗方式。在所有患儿中，不主张行单纯非手术复位，因为其复发率高。

肿瘤

结肠癌是最常见的癌症之一，然而只有大约 1% 的结肠恶性肿瘤发生在 30 岁以下，10 岁以下的儿童更为罕见。男性发病率稍高，病变可以发生在结肠的任何部位，48% 的肿瘤为黏液腺癌和印戒细胞癌。儿童结肠癌往往病情发展迅速，预后差，总体 5 年生存率为 2.5%[3]。

儿童结肠癌的症状和体征与成人相似，不易诊断。腹痛、贫血、腹胀、大便习惯改变和直肠出血为最常见的表现，此外儿童还可能有急性或隐匿性肠梗阻表现。

诊断和分期的方法包括结肠镜检查加活检和腹部及盆腔 CT 扫描，癌胚抗原的诊断价值在儿童中尚不确定，通过手术切除治疗可获得治愈或缓解，与成人不同的是化疗和放疗无缓解或治愈的价值[42]。

结肠狭窄

获得性结肠狭窄可以引起不完全性肠梗阻。狭窄可能继发于坏死性小肠结肠炎、炎性肠病、外伤或囊性纤维化（囊性纤维性结肠病变），对该疾病的治疗均可采用病变肠管切除和肠吻合。

多种原因的小肠和结肠梗阻

肠内和肠外的疾病

在整个胃肠道中有很多肠内和肠外病变可引起肠梗阻，梗阻可以由病变本身造成，也可能是病变的继发性改变如肠套迭，或肠管围绕病变形成扭转造成。

很多恶性肿瘤可发生于肠腔内和肠腔外，包括淋巴瘤（特别是 Burkitt 淋巴瘤）和平滑肌肉瘤，任何一个超过 3 岁的患儿的肠套迭需考虑有无此类疾病，此时需专门的儿科放射科医生进行细致的小肠检查来发现病变，尤其要注意右下腹部。

非肿瘤性因素包括幼年型结肠息肉、炎性息肉、黏膜下出血、血管瘤和消化道异物。幼年型息肉在小儿中最多见，在儿童中的发病率为 1%～2%[26]，高峰期在 2～5 岁。该病的表现是无痛性直肠出血，最初的症状可能包括直肠肿块脱出、黏液便、腹痛、结肠肠套迭。该病病因学不明，属错构瘤。结肠镜可以明确诊断同时切除息肉。

炎性息肉是一种非肿瘤性的疾病，常位于胃和小肠，结肠少见，由慢性炎性细胞如嗜酸性细胞组成，它们可以导致小肠任何部位的套迭和梗阻，通常表现为腹部疼痛，治疗方法为手术切除，因为病变位于小肠因此诊断非常困难，胶囊式内镜和术中肠镜检查有助于息肉的定位[37]。

黏膜下血肿可以发生在消化道的任何部位，病因包括过敏性紫癜、血小板病变、抗凝治疗和化疗并发症，同样可以导致小肠套迭的发生。

各种不同的消化道异物包括花生、植物粪石、毛粪石以及精神异常造成的异食癖均可导致部分或者完全性肠梗阻，通常发生梗阻的位置为胃的出口、末端回肠，胃出口梗阻可通过内镜治疗，回肠梗阻则需要手术探查去除异物。

炎性假瘤

炎性假瘤（IPT）和炎症性纤维母细胞瘤（IMT）或者浆细胞性肉芽肿是同一疾病。IPTs 是发生在消化道任何部位，还有胸部、头部和颈部的一组肿瘤，病因尚不清楚。从组织学上来说，肿瘤由浆细胞、组织细胞和分布于成纤维细胞构成间质的淋巴细胞组成，尽管它们有局部侵犯的特性，但总体上是良性的。

消化道的 IMTs 可以导致梗阻症状出现、体重减 136
轻和腹痛。实验室检查提示贫血、血沉增快。典型的病变位于阑尾和胃，但是也有报道病变来源于小肠、结肠和 Meckel 憩室。

治疗方式主要是手术完全切除。该肿瘤复发率约 18%～40%[44]，如肿瘤未完整切除则复发率会增高，肿瘤多次复发会导致恶变。有报道术前和术后应用非甾体类药物治疗取得了一定疗效。

乳凝块综合征

1969 年 Cook 和 Richman[17] 首次报道了因为乳凝块造成的新生儿肠梗阻，主要由于脂肪酸和钙浓缩形成的凝块引起远端小肠的梗阻，易发生于出生后 6 周的新生儿中。确切的发病率尚不清楚，似乎好发于男婴和极低体重儿，有时也可见于足月儿。

主要症状为胎粪已排出的婴儿出现远端小肠梗阻，如胆汁性呕吐、腹胀。放射学检查可提供诊断依据，因为形成的凝块和肠壁不粘连，腹部平片上可以见到肠腔内肿块周围有气体的光晕或者其中有气体影。所有患儿均配方奶喂养，有些是完全配方奶，有些为母乳混合喂养。可以通过非手术方法治疗。

治疗与胎粪栓塞的治疗类似，使用泛影葡胺灌肠，但在患儿不能排除存在坏死性肠炎时应慎用。在保守治疗无效的情况下手术治疗，最常见的乳栓部位是末端回肠，通常 2～3 cm 长，可以挤过回盲瓣。如果该方法失败，则需切开肠管使用生理盐水或 N-乙酰半胱氨酸灌洗。

该病病因学尚不明确，直肠活检可以见到正常的神经节细胞，梗阻可能与越来越多的极低体重儿摄入高脂肪和高钙有关。

腹茧症

腹茧症是引起肠梗阻的罕见病因，主要见于来自热带或亚热带的青少年女孩[23]。该病的特点是小肠被厚壁、纤维化囊覆盖，病因不明确，临床上均表现为慢性小肠梗阻、体重下降或是急性梗阻伴有疼痛和可触及的腹部包块。术前通过应用对比造影 CT 检查显示“菜花征”有助于诊断，但大多术中明确诊断[40]。小肠呈蛇样盘绕成圈，包裹肠管的长度从若干英尺到整个小肠，外科手术仍然是标准的治疗方式，主要是切除厚壁纤维囊并分离小肠。

蛔虫病

最常见的寄生虫感染就是线虫属的人蛔虫感染，据估计全世界范围内的蛔虫感染超过 10 亿例。肠梗阻是引起死亡的主要原因。通过手口传染，感染通常无症状，然而严重感染（虫体超过 60 个）会导致部分或完全性的肠梗阻或胆道梗阻[20]。通过 B 超可以发现虫体位于胆道、胰管或肠道，主要使用驱虫药治疗，如甲苯达唑、阿苯达唑（肠虫清）、左旋咪唑或噻嘧啶。如果药物治疗无效，可使用 ERCP（内镜下胰胆管造影）去除胆道内的虫体，亦可外科施行肠切开术去除肠道内的虫体。

外伤后肠狭窄

车祸伤最常见的消化道损伤就是胃肠道穿孔[34]，是继发于安全带造成的损伤，症状通常在外伤后迅速出现，安全带损伤造成的迟发性后遗症为肠管狭窄导致肠梗阻。

钝性损伤 10 天~3 周后出现腹痛和胆汁性呕吐应怀疑存在外伤性肠管狭窄。腹部放射学检查提示有部分小肠狭窄，造影检查提示梗阻近端肠管扩张，病灶部位肠管狭窄或者造影剂通过延迟，也可有多种征象合并出现。

其病因为小肠受到座位带和脊柱的直接挤压造成损伤，当损伤足够严重会导致病变部位缺血、血肿以及继发性纤维化导致肠腔狭窄，有时不止一段肠管受损，这一进行性过程导致症状在损伤后 1～3 周延迟出现。

淋巴管畸形

腹部囊性淋巴管畸形形成腹部肿块在婴幼儿中少见，一般为肠系膜囊肿或者大网膜囊肿，表现为无症状的腹部包块，伴或不伴腹痛和肠梗阻以及肠扭转。它们均为真性囊肿，内衬内皮细胞，其发病 1366
机理为淋巴结构异常增生且与正常淋巴管系统缺乏交通[21]。肠系膜囊肿可以发生在胃肠道的任何部位，最常见的部位是回肠。B 超检查是最佳的诊断方法，表现为圆形的囊性结构，壁很薄伴有分隔。通过 CT 扫描也可以明确诊断，可显示病变程度，排除肾囊肿、胰腺囊肿和卵巢囊肿。治疗原则是囊肿完整切除，有时需同时进行肠切除术，如不能完整切除时可行造袋术，最近有报道在儿童进行腹腔镜囊肿切除[51]。

重复畸形囊肿

消化道重复畸形是罕见的先天性异常，位于肠壁内或肠系膜，其病理诊断是囊肿壁内见平滑肌细胞，可以存在于消化道的任何部位。通常在出生后早期出现症状，症状包括腹部包块、疼痛、肠扭转或者肠套迭造成的肠梗阻，穿孔后会出现腹腔游离气体。术前通过 CT 和 B 超可以明确诊断，治疗采用手术切除。

假性梗阻

假性肠梗阻是一种综合征，表现为肠梗阻症状或体征，但是却没有机械性因素造成肠腔梗阻。尽管通常见于老年患者，但假性肠梗阻也可在新生儿出现，

表 85-1 假性肠梗阻的辅因
内分泌疾病
糖尿病
嗜铬细胞瘤
甲状旁腺功能减退
甲状腺功能减退
神经系统疾病
先天性巨结肠
南美洲锥虫病
家族性自主神经系统功能障碍
多发性神经纤维瘤
肠道平滑肌异常疾病
肌营养不良
非热带性口炎性腹泻
系统性红斑狼疮
药物引起
麻醉药
三环类抗抑郁药物
酚噻嗪类药物
可乐定
蘑菇中毒

青少年患者往往是由其他疾病引起的（表 85-1），病变并不局限于小肠。一般认为是肠道的运动功能发生异常，病因可以是肌源性或者是神经源性的。

患儿反复出现不同时间长度和频率的症状发作，包括恶性、呕吐、腹部扩张、腹泻或者是便秘。因为小肠传输时间过长和细菌过度繁殖，可频繁发生脂肪泻。放射学检查显示胃肠传输时间延长伴有小肠和结肠袢扩张。

该病的治疗效果不佳，钡剂造影排除机械性因素后主要靠药物治疗。红霉素（50～100 mg）刺激胃动素受体，促进胃排空，低剂量的时候刺激肠道收缩，并非越多越好，在大剂量时候反而抑制肠蠕动。奥曲肽（50 μg）皮下注射可以刺激小肠节律性收缩。新的治疗药物主要针对肠道 5-羟色胺受体（阿洛司琼，1 mg 口服），目前证实有效，同时也在临床试验中。外科治疗仅限于短段型无动力肠段的患儿。弥漫性肠动力低下的患儿不宜施行外科手术，因为症状复发时很难与术后肠粘连造成的梗阻相鉴别。

（李巍松译 王 俊校）

参考文献

1. Akgur FM, Tanyel FC, Buyukpamukcu N, et al: Adhesive small bowel obstruction in children: The place and predictors of success for conservative treatment. J Pediatr Surg 1991;26:37-41.
2. Akgur FM, Tanyel FC, Buyukpamukcu N, et al: Anomalous congenital bands causing intestinal obstruction in children. J Pediatr Surg 1992;27:471-473.
3. Andersson A, Bergdahl L: Carcinoma of the colon in children: A report of six new cases and a review of the literature. J Pediatr Surg 1976;11:967-971.
4. Angood PB, Gingalewski CA, Andersen DK: Surgical complications. In Townsend C (ed): Sabiston's Textbook of Surgery, 16th ed. Philadelphia, WB Saunders, 2001, pp 189-225.
5. Asabe K, Ushijima H, Bepu R, et al: A case of transverse colon volvulus in a child and a review of the literature in Japan. J Pediatr Surg 2002;37:1626-1628.
6. Azziz R: The INTERCEED (TC7) adhesion barrier study group II. Microsurgery alone or with Interceed absorbable adhesion barrier for pelvic sidewall adhesion re-formation. Surg Gynecol Obstet 1993;77:135-139.
7. Beck DE, Cohen Z, Fleshman JW, et al: Prospective, randomized, multicenter, controlled study of the safety of Seprafilm adhesion barrier in abdominopelvic surgery of the intestine. Dis Colon Rectum 2003;46:1305-1309.
8. Belluco C, Meggiolaro F, Pressato D, et al: Prevention of postsurgical adhesions with an autocrosslinked hyaluronan derivative gel. J Surg Res 2001;100:217-221.
9. Blunt A, Rich GF: Intestinal strangulation through an aperture in the falciform ligament. Aust N Z J Surg 1968; 37:310.
10. Bohm B, Milsom JW, Fazio VW: Postoperative intestinal motility following conventional and laparoscopic intestinal surgery. Arch Surg 1995;130:415-419.
11. Borody TJ, Quigley EM, Phillips SF, et al: Effects of morphine and atropine on motility and transit in the human ileum. Gastroenterology 1985;89:790-796.
12. Bredtmann RD, Herden HN, Teichmann W, et al: Epidural analgesia in colonic surgery: Results of a randomized prospective study. Br J Surg 1990;77:638-642.
13. Brown TA, McDonald J, Williard W: A prospective randomized, double-blinded, placebo controlled trial of cisapride after colorectal surgery. Am J Surg 1999;177: 399-401.
14. Bueno LJ, Serralta SA, Planeeis RM, et al: Intestinal obstruction caused by omphalomesenteric duct remnant: Usefulness of laparoscopy. Rev Esp Enferm Dig 2003;95: 736-738.
15. Callander CL, Rusk GH, Nemir A: Mechanism, symptoms and treatment of hernia into the descending mesocolon (left duodenal hernia). A plea for a change in nomenclature. Surg Gynecol Obstet 1935;60:1052-1064.
16. Chopra R, McVay C, Phillips E, et al: Laparoscopic lysis of adhesions. Am Surg 2003;69:966-968.
17. Cook RC, Richman PP: Neonatal intestinal obstruction due to milk curds. J Pediatr Surg 1969;4:599-605.
18. Cullen JJ, Eagon JC, Kelly KA: Gastrointestinal peptide hormones during postoperative ileus: Effect of octreotide. Dig Dis Sci 1994;39:1179-1184.
19. Davies CJ, Franks RE: Herniation through a defect in the falciform ligament. Guys Hosp Rep 1974;123:171-175.
20. De Silva NR, Guyatt HL, Bundy DA: Worm burden in intestinal obstruction caused by *Ascaris lumbricoides*. Trop Med

Int Health 1997;2:189-190.
21. Egozi EI, Ricketts RR: Mesenteric and omental cysts in children. Am Surg 1997;63:287-290.
22. Festen C: Postoperative small bowel obstruction in infants and children. Ann Surg 1982;196:580-583.
23. Foo KY, Ng KC, Rauff A, et al: Unusual small intestinal obstruction in adolescent girls: The abdominal cocoon. Br J Surg 1978;65:427-430.
24. Foss JF: A review of the potential role of methylnaltrexone in opioid bowel dysfunction. Am J Surg 2001;182(Suppl 5A): 19S-26S.
25. Gupta S, Gupta SK: Acute caecal volvulus: Report of 22 cases and review of the literature. Ital J Gastroenterol 1993;25: 380-384.
26. Horrileno EG, Eckert C, Ackerman LV: Polyps of the rectum and colon in children. Cancer 1957;10: 1210-1220.
27. Jamieson NV: The 'falciform ligament window': An unusual site for an internal hernia causing small bowel obstruction. J R Coll Surg Edinb 1987;32:374-375.
28. Janik JS, Ein SH, Filler RM, et al: An assessment of the surgical treatment of adhesive small bowel obstruction
29. Jorgensen H, Fomsgaard JS, Dirks J, et al: Effect of epidural bupivacaine vs. combined bupivacaine and morphine on gastrointestinal function and pain after major gynaecological surgery. Br J Anaesth 2001;87: 727-732.
30. Lacy AM, Garcia-Valdecasas JC, Pique JM, et al: Short-term outcome analysis of a randomized study comparing laparoscopic vs. open colectomy for colon cancer. Surg Endosc 1995;9:1101-1105.
31. Lander, B, Redkar R, Nicholls G, et al: Cisapride reduces neonatal postoperative ileus: Randomized placebo controlled trial. Arch Dis Child Fetal Neonatal Ed 1997;77: F119-F122.
32. Liu SS, Carpenter RL, Mackey DC, et al: Effects of perioperative analgesic technique on rate of recovery after colon surgery. Anesthesiology 1995;83:757-765.
33. Livingston EH, Passaro EP: Postoperative ileus. Dig Dis Sci 1990;35:121-131.
34. Lynch JM, Albanese CT, Meza MP, et al: Intestinal stricture following seat belt injury in children. J Pediatr Surg 1996; 31:1354-1357.
35. Macmillan SLM, Kammer-Doak D, Rogers RG, et al: Early feeding and the incidence of gastrointestinal symptoms after major gynecologic surgery. Obstet Gynecol 2000; 96:604-608.
36. Mercado-Deane MG, Burton EM, Howell CG: Transverse colon volvulus in pediatric patients. Pediatr Radiol 1995;25: 111-112.
37. Miyata T, Yamamoto H, Kita H, et al: A case of inflammatory fibroid polyp causing small bowel intussusception in which retrograde double-balloon enteroscopy was useful for the preoperative diagnosis. Endoscopy 2004;36: 344-347.
38. Moore TC: Omphalomesenteric duct anomalies. Surg Gynecol Obstet 1956;103:569-580.
39. Moran JM, Salas J, Sanjuan S, et al: Paramesocolic hernias: Consequences of delayed diagnosis. Report of three new cases. J Pediatr Surg 2004;39:112-116.
40. Navani S, Shah P, Pandya S, Doctor N: Abdominal cocoon—the cauliflower sign of barium small bowel series. Indian J Gastroenterol 14:19, 1995.
41. Neudecker J, Schwenk W, Junghans T, et al: Randomized controlled trial to examine the influence of thoracic epidural analgesia on postoperative ileus after laparoscopic sigmoid resection. Br J Surg 1999;98:1292-1295.
42. Pratt CB, Rivera G, Shanks E, et al: Colorectal carcinoma in adolescents: Implications regarding etiology. Cancer 1977; 40(5 Suppl):2464-2472.
43. Salas S, Angel CA, Salas N, et al: Sigmoid volvulus in children and adolescents. J Am Coll Surg 2000;190: 717-723.
44. Sanders BM, West KW, Gingalewski C, et al: Inflammatory pseudotumor of the alimentary tract: Clinical and surgical experience. J Pediatr Surg 2001;36:169-173.
45. Schutz RB, Zeigler AM: Persistent fetal tachycardia and neonatal intestinal obstruction due to internal hernia beneath the umbilical vein. Am J Obstet Gynecol 1937;33: 692-694.
46. Shah SS, Louie JP, Fein JA: Cecal volvulus in childhood. Pediatr Emerg Care 2002;18:300-302.
47. Smith AJ, Nissan A, Lanouette NM, et al: Prokinetic effect of erythromycin after colorectal surgery: Randomized, placebo-controlled, double-blind study. Dis Colon Rectum 2000;43:333-337.
48. Springhall RG, Spitz L: The prevention of post-operative adhesions using a gastrointestinal prokinetic agent. J Pediatr Surg 1989;24:530-533.
49. Uematsu T, Kitamura H, Iwase M, et al: Laparoscopic repair of a paraduodenal hernia. Surg Endosc 1998;12:50-52.
50. Vrijland WW, Tseng LNL, Eijkman HJM, et al: Fewer intraperitoneal adhesions with the use of hyaluronic acid–carboxymethylcellulose membrane: A randomized clinical trial. Ann Surg 2002;235:193-199.
51. Vu JH, Thomas EL, Spencer DD: Laparoscopic management of a mesenteric cyst. Am Surg 1999;65:264-265.
52. Wullstein C, Gross E: Laparoscopic compared with conventional treatment of acute adhesive small bowel obstruction. Br J Surg 2003;90:1147-1151.

第 86 章

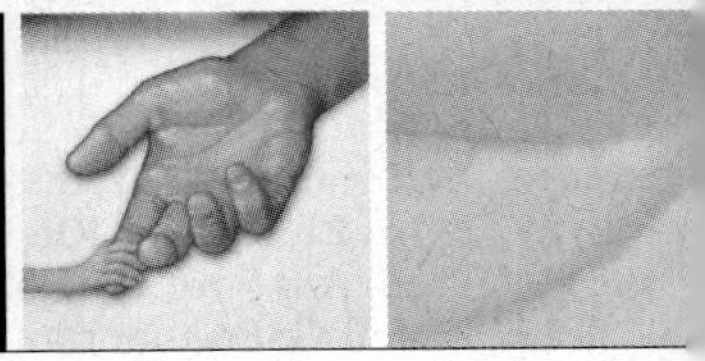

短肠综合征

Brad W. Warner

1369 短肠综合征（SBS）是一组由于小肠黏膜表面吸收和消化不良而发生的病理生理紊乱。SBS 的临床特征大体包括进行性营养不良、体重下降和腹泻。虽然这些问题通常是由于肠黏膜解剖学上的缺陷造成的，但由于肠的吸收、动力紊乱，或者是二者兼具，在肠黏膜表面积正常的情况下也可发生。由于大多数儿童的 SBS 发生于手术切除病变的肠管后和先天性短肠，因此讨论大部分集中于肠管变短后引起的病变。

病因学

SBS 在儿童群体中的特殊病因这些年来已得到认识和发展。在早期的报道中，最常见的病因是中肠扭转和肠闭锁[87]。在最近的报道中，SBS 最常见的病因是新生儿坏死性小肠结肠炎（图 86-1）[80,81]。儿童 SBS 其他常见病因包括肠闭锁和继发于中肠扭转的肠坏死。少见的病因包括由于侵入性主动脉监视装置而造成的肠系膜血管闭塞、新生儿主动脉栓塞或者心源性栓子。继发于心源性、低血容量性或败血症性休克的血流灌注不足和影响血管收缩药物的应用也会导致肠管的缺血坏死。胎粪性肠梗阻或胎粪栓塞可能会促进扭转的发生，导致肠管坏死。

肠的实际长度正常，但是肠的动力和提供肠内营养的能力削弱的功能性疾病包括长段型的神经节细胞缺如、特发性假性肠梗阻综合征。由于合并肠管长度缩短和增厚的肠袢蠕动功能失调，腹裂与 SBS 相关。由于多次和广泛的肠管切除、瘘管造成的旁路吸收黏膜或黏膜吸收能力的减弱，Crohn 病也可能与 SBS 有关。

肠适应

大量的肠切除后在剩余肠段中有一种代偿反应，术语称为肠适应。肠切除诱发的肠适应引起的变化影响肠细胞形态学、细胞更新动力和整体的功能[51]。肠的长度和管径增加以及肠的所有组织层均以形态变化的方式增生和肥大。随着肠管径和长度的增加，由于绒毛的增高和隐窝的加深其表面积也会增加。除了形态学的改变，肠上皮细胞的转化率也在增加，表现为肠细胞内的增生变强和程序性细胞死亡（凋亡）

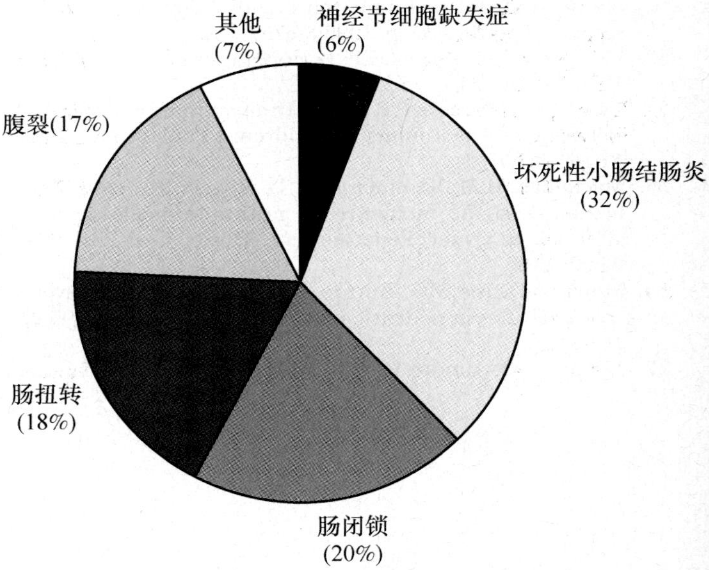

图 86-1 466 例患儿的短肠综合征病因。神经节细胞缺失症（6%）、坏死性小肠结肠炎（32%）、闭锁（20%）、扭转（18%）、腹裂（17%）、其他（7%）。（数据来自参考文献 3，13，40，78 和 81）

率增加[29]。通过估算每单位面积消化和吸收酶的活性，肠的功能性适应也增强。

370 临床观察很好地显示了适应反应的重要性，随着时间进展，那些当时不能耐受肠道喂养的患儿最后能够完全脱离补充的肠外营养。另一方面，如果适应不完全，患儿必须终生伴随肠外营养和与其相关的疾病。因此，深入地理解适应的病理生理学和提升这一过程的能力是一个热点研究领域。

现已经提出了很多引发和维持肠切除后适应的机制和介质。有 3 个主要的机制，涉及体液因素、肠内营养和胰胆管的分泌。肠大量切除后发现血浆中多肽、激素和生长因子水平升高。个别病例中肠大量切除后应用这些因子可诱导适应反应的增强。更加引人注目的证实激素对适应贡献的实验之一是联体模型。两个动物共用一个循环，一个动物的肠切除后会引发另一个未手术动物出现适应性变化[86]。另外，来自于大量肠切除动物的血清可以刺激一种原型的肠上皮细胞株的生长[37]。尚未确定血清中某种单一的因子能充分解释所有的肠形态和功能的适应性变化。

肠内营养通过与肠上皮细胞的直接接触和刺激与营养有关的胃肠道激素和胰胆的分泌等几种机制来刺激肠道的适应[84]。由于肠黏膜萎缩与饥饿有关，再喂食会逆转肠黏膜萎缩的观察证实了肠道营养对肠适应反应的作用。此外，手术将一部分回肠移位到更近端的肠道会导致移位的回肠结构和功能“空肠化”，不但肠内营养的存在对于适应很重要，而且营养成分也很重要[2,22]。肠道注入非营养物质对于适应作用不大。越复杂的营养需要更多的代谢能量去消化和吸收，似乎能诱发最大的适应反应，显示出所谓的功能负荷假说[80]。肠道中的脂肪是诱导适应反应的最有效的营养素[11]。更特别的是，长链和多不饱和的脂肪会提供一个更大的适应刺激[76]。

许多实验观察认为内源性的胃肠道分泌对适应很重要。手术将 Vater 壶腹移位到胃肠道更远区域的实验模型显示绒毛的增生超过了移位的肠管[1,85]。胆汁单独递送到中段小肠会刺激肠道 DNA 和 RNA 含量增加，但与胰腺分泌结合时这种影响效应更加明显[1]。在其他研究中，与胆汁相比较，胰腺的分泌对肠黏膜更有营养[85]。胰胆管分泌对切除后的适应很重要的进一步证据是生长抑素，一种能够极大地减少内源性胃肠道分泌量的介质，也与抑制适应反应有关[5]。

其他对适应发生有作用的因素还有宿主的营养状态。肠切除后限制热卡的摄入与迟钝的适应反应有关[20]。这种情况的出现是否是由于肠道营养含量的减少或热卡缺乏造成的尚不清楚。在适应的产生和维持中，其他的考虑因素还有机械因素。猪部分肠梗阻的实验显示其能诱导近段小肠的适应性变化[18]。这一观察已被临床延伸至在同一组患者施行肠管延长术前先使其肠管扩张[25]。沿着这些思路，肠动力可能对适应也很重要。大量肠切除后已经观察到了许多肠动力的异常[56,57]。现在还不清楚这种反应是原发于适应的发生还是继发于几种之前提到的因素。药物阻滞紊乱的肠动力对适应反应的影响尚不清楚。

影响短肠综合征的因素

大量肠丢失的临床反应依赖于几个关键特征，包括肠切除的部位、长度以及回盲瓣存在与否。可能其中最根本的因素是肠管切除的长度。正常足月新生儿的肠管长度是 200～250 cm。在胎儿，胃肠道总的生长率随胎龄而增加，生长最快速的时期出现在妊娠的最后 3 个月。实际上，在胎龄的 19～27 周和 35 周，小肠长度可能会增加 1 倍[73]。单就生长而言，婴幼儿期的小肠仍保持快速增长，直到头足长达到约 60 cm。然后，在头足长 60～100 cm 时，肠生长较缓慢，在头足长 100～140 cm 时肠的变化很小。因此，新生儿大量肠切除后，需要根据小肠增长情况估计最终的小肠长度。

对于长期全肠外营养（TPN）需求能力的预测还很困难，因为许多 SBS 的系列研究是由伴有不同基础疾病的多种患者群体构成。同样地，一个因坏死性小肠结肠炎需大量肠切除的新生儿显示的适应反应与有相同的肠长度但患有腹裂的新生儿明显不 1371
同。尽管有这些局限，Sondheimer 和助手在一组婴幼儿的研究中发现，最初切除时的肠长度和 12 周龄时肠道热卡耐受的百分数能独立地预测长期 TPN 依赖[62]。在这个报道中，Cox 比例风险方程可用来推算这两种参数预测的 TPN 依赖。例如，如果最初肠切除后留下25 cm，但到 3 个月时肠道途径能耐受 50% 的热卡，预测大约 20% 的婴幼儿将永久依赖 TPN。如果有75 cm肠管剩余，即使他们在相同的年龄能够耐受类似的肠道营养，但几乎所有的患儿都可以脱离 TPN。另一方面，如果剩余 25 cm 的肠管而3个月后他们仅能够耐受25%的营养，预测接近40%的患儿会永久依赖TPN。

法国一项对成年人的重要研究中，Messing和同事主要通过依据最初的肠长度来计算存活概率[48]。这一研究由连续的124个患者组成，区别暂时还是永久TPN依赖的小肠长度截断值在远端肠造口术的患儿为100 cm，空肠结肠吻合的为65 cm，30 cm也是可能的。影响TPN依赖的概率的变量如图86-2所示。

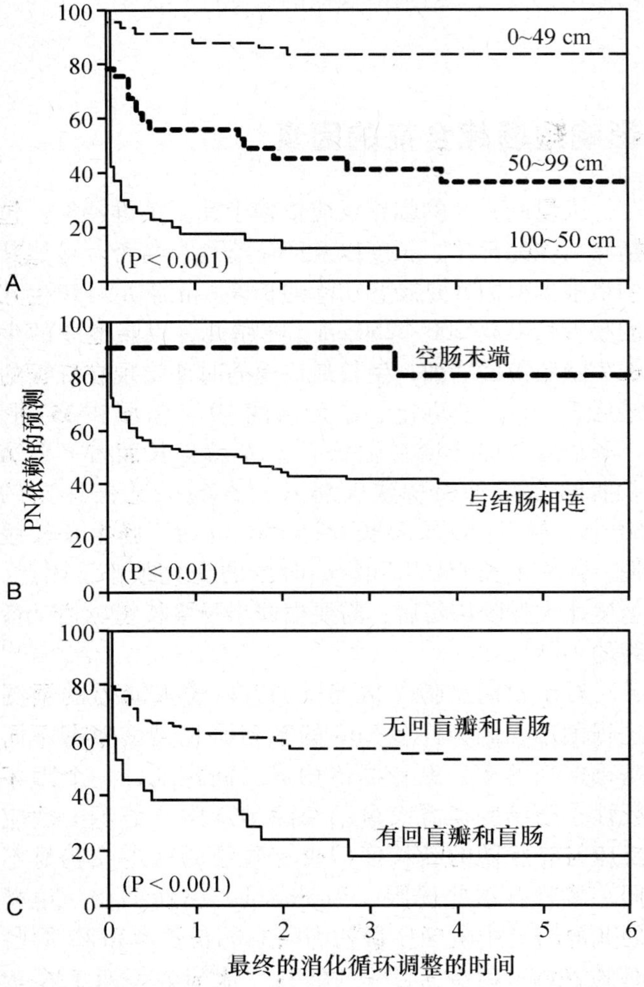

图86-2 对124例短肠综合征成年患者的肠外营养（PN）依赖的预测。预测肠外营养（PN）依赖的3个主要因素包括：（A）残留肠的长度，（B）有或没有与结肠相接，（C）有或没有回盲瓣。（From Messing B，Crenn P，Beau P，et al：Long-term survival and parenteral nutrition dependence in adult patients with the short bowel syndrome. Gastroenterology 1999；117：1043.）

虽然肠管的长度作为主要的预后因素很重要，但实际测量肠的长度量是很主观和多变的。而且，在进行广泛肠切除的过程中，花费时间去测量剩余肠的长度经常被忽视，尤其是在身体薄弱的患儿。因此，应寻找其他更客观和更有重复性的肠衰竭的指标来预测是否需要长期TPN。除了提升肠内营养的临床能力外，Grenn和他的同事报道在一组成人SBS患者中，血浆瓜氨酸与TPN的依赖之间有强烈的相关性[19]。这一几乎唯一在肠黏膜产生的低水平的氨基酸，将可能在儿科人群中作为预测TPN依赖的一个有用的指标。

TPN的应用已使SBS患儿的存活率显著改善。不幸的是，这种患儿最常见的死亡原因是TPN导致的肝功能紊乱[67]。尽管存在这个问题，剩余小肠的长度不足40 cm的患儿存活较常见，剩余小肠长度不足20～30 cm的婴儿长期存活也是有可能的。的确有报道，一个仅剩余11 cm小肠和没有回盲瓣的新生儿在没有TPN支持下存活下来[34]。总体上，至少有70%的SBS患儿出院，几乎所有人1年后还活着。

肠造瘘的位置也是影响肠切除临床反应的一个重要因素。切除空肠会产生大量营养素和电解质吸收的永久缺陷，因为回肠有较强的适应能力并能够取代这些吸收功能。几种抑制胃酸分泌的肠激素主要由空肠分泌，因此空肠切除可能会导致胃酸分泌过多[61]。

相反，回肠在减慢肠转运中有显著的效应。因此，回肠切除通常会导致转运增加。回肠也是胆盐吸收和再循环的一个重要部位。同样地，广泛的回肠切除与胆盐池的耗损有关，导致胆石病发生增多和脂肪吸收不良。由于该原因可行预防性胆囊切除[68]。脂肪吸收不良导致脂溶性维生素A、D、E、K缺乏，回 13
肠切除超过60 cm后将出现维生素B_{12}吸收不良。肠管似乎在很大程度上不能在残存的回肠或空肠适应性地补充新的维生素B_{12}受体。

如需大量切除小肠时，应尽可能地保留结肠，因为这将减轻SBS的严重程度。结肠不仅能提供吸收的表面积，而且对早期的胃排空有制动作用，还可被动地吸收碳水化合物、蛋白质和脂肪。

回盲瓣减慢肠的转运，进而增加肠道营养物质与肠黏膜表面的接触时间。在一个新生儿SBS的研究中，回盲瓣的存在与成功脱离TPN之间无明显的相关性，但是，的确降低了TPN依赖的持续时间[16,26]。

另外，回盲瓣作为一个屏障可防止结肠腔内的微生物迁移进入远端小肠。

广泛肠切除的宿主效应

SBS 患儿的临床过程包括几个期，包括最初的水和电解质极度丢失的围术期，继而开始肠道营养和不断变化的适应期，最后，在 1～2 年后达到一个慢性或平台期。因此，在最后的阶段，如果肠适应不完全则会出现吸收不良、腹泻、肠外营养和慢性营养缺乏等问题。

最初的术后处理应直接针对水和电解质的补充。大量的液体会从造瘘口丢失，需要补充含有类似电解质浓度的溶液，以防止水和电解质失衡。由于腹腔内感染和（或）瘘需要再次手术探查，使术后早期的处理会变得更复杂。

广泛的肠切除后腹泻不可避免，它是由多种因素造成的：吸收表面积减少，肠运转增加，胃、小肠和结肠分泌过多，结肠内容物的渗透压增加，小肠内细菌过度增长。另外，胆汁酸溢出和脂肪进入结肠增加，在那里它们被腔内的细菌转化为促分泌的刺激物而使结肠分泌过多。

肠切除后高胃泌素血症和胃酸过多症几乎在肠切除后立即发生，可导致大量的水和电解质丢失，潜在地形成消化道溃疡和肠吸收障碍。在较酸的十二指肠环境中，胰脂肪酶活性下降，导致微团的形成减少和脂肪吸收下降。胃酸分泌过多对组胺受体拮抗剂和质子泵抑制剂反应良好，通常自行缓解。

没有吸收的碳水化合物进入结肠被细菌代谢分解成短链脂肪酸，通过直接渗透作用也可以直接刺激结肠分泌水分和电解质，进一步加重腹泻。广泛肠切除的患儿很少出现 D-乳酸酸中毒，这继发于结肠内 pH 的改变和拟杆菌属的生长抑制，因此，有利于抗酸性厌氧菌的生长产生 D-乳酸[10]。由于肠腔内游离脂肪酸的含量很大，结合并妨碍了钙的吸收，食物中草酸盐的生物利用度提高，导致高草酸尿和肾石病。

矿物质不足很常见，需要积极的补充。钠和钾的丢失常见，需要迅速补充。吸收不良的脂肪酸与钙镁形成皂化复合物。尽管维生素 D 和钙的补充通常对于防止钙缺乏有帮助，但镁缺乏的处理更加复杂，因为肠道输入大量的镁盐通常与腹泻有关。

内科和营养治疗

SBS 最重要的治疗目标是维持患儿的营养状况，并支持其继续生长发育。TPN 应该早期使用以防止严重的体重丢失，并建立正氮平衡。尽可能早地开始肠道营养非常重要，对患儿来讲最大目标是尽可能恢复正常的饮食[81]。第一个需要作出的决定是采取哪种喂养方式。小于 1 岁的婴儿，增加食物的渗透性可能会产生抗原，导致对配方的蛋白质过敏。因此，低过敏原的配方理论上有优势，包括 Nutramigen、Pregestimil（Mead Johnson Laboratories，Evansville，IN）和 Alimentum（Ross Laboratories，Columbus，OH）。为了进一步降低高危易感患儿的过敏风险，可以用一种叫 Neocate（SHS，Liverpool，英国）的氨基酸配方。这些配方的另一大优势是它们主要为脂肪形式，热卡百分率高，比碳水化合物更容易耐受。如果可以的话，对新生儿而言母乳是最好的营养来源。众所周知，母乳对于细胞的增殖和剩余肠管的适应性变化有积极的影响。对于这些好处的可能解释是存在一种尚未完全明确的营养生长因子的过剩。大龄的孩子能耐受更复杂但花费少的肠道喂养。在大龄孩子中很少有蛋白质的吸收问题。

在这些患儿的治疗中，胃造瘘管是一个重要的辅助，因为它可以允许连续的肠道营养。由于小肠中吸收转运蛋白持续饱和，总的热卡吸收百分数最高，持续喂养优于快速推注的方式。肠内输注应该保持等渗并以缓慢的速率增加。最后，根据患者的耐受力，肠道喂养的容量可以随肠外营养的减少而逐渐增加。粪
便丢失的增加在 24 小时内超过 50% 时，禁忌补液。 1373
粪便丢失超过 40～50 ml/(kg·d)，强烈提示应减少喂养，表明肠道喂养不应该再增加。在这种情况下，喂养率已经达到患儿吸收能力的极限[74]。

一旦结合肠内和肠外营养的患儿情况稳定，TPN 应该从日夜不停的持续输注过渡到夜间循环输注。这一输注方案对于患儿和家长而言是安全的并且能允许患儿白天自由活动。

喂养行为是 SBS 患儿管理中的一个很重要的成分。幼婴应该鼓励持续的吸吮和吞咽，同时鼓励间断的少量配方奶的奶瓶喂养。因为较大孩子是很难完全

禁食的，他们可允许尝试口感好的但不会产生大量粪便的食物。

减少胃酸分泌过多的药物包括 H_2 受体拮抗剂和质子泵抑制剂，可用于 SBS 患儿的早期治疗。因为胃酸分泌过多通常在广泛肠切除后的 6～12 月减少，过了这段时间就很少需要治疗了。

也可以应用抑制肠转运的药物，这样可以改善营养的吸收，可能使患儿摆脱肠外营养。减慢肠运转的药物主要是阿片类物质。阿片制剂通常用来治疗腹泻，包括可待因、地芬诺酯和络派丁胺。在几个临床试验中络派丁胺比地芬诺酯控制腹泻更有效[23,52]。可待因虽然控制腹泻十分有效，但有显著的中枢神经系统副作用和明显的成瘾性。

生长抑素和它的长效类似物奥曲肽已被用于治疗严重顽固性腹泻的研究，但得出的结论尚不明确。奥曲肽本质上抑制所有内分泌和外分泌的胃肠道和胰腺分泌。在成人 SBS 的一些临床试验中，需要补充的电解质和营养物质减少、水分泌和电解质的丢失减少以及生活质量得到改善[50,55]。在更近的一个试验中，奥曲肽导致肠转运减慢，但对于大营养物质的吸收和体重的增加却没有显著的效应[49]。在一个 SBS 动物模型中，给予奥曲肽导致黏膜主动转运营养物质下降[59]。在一些研究中，奥曲肽也显示抑制肠道适应，可能是通过降低外分泌的胃肠道分泌物明显的适应增强效应而发挥作用[5,65]。另一方面，奥曲肽对肠适应的抑制效应还没有普遍观察到[75]。儿童人群中奥曲肽的应用受到某些限制，一个理论上的问题是这一制剂对生长潜在的长期影响。由于上述这些原因，奥曲肽在儿童 SBS 患儿中尚未被认可得到常规应用。

考来烯胺可治疗 SBS 患儿的腹泻。但是仅针对由于胆盐到达结肠发生导泻作用所引起的腹泻有效。在广泛回肠切除的患儿应该考虑用它治疗[69]。另一方面，一部分 SBS 患儿脂肪吸收不良也可能由于胆汁分泌不足所致。外源性合成结合胆汁酸无导泻作用可以抵抗细菌降解，通过促进脂肪的吸收对 SBS 患儿可能有效[31]。

SBS 患儿除了有大量的水、电解质和营养障碍，其他并发症也应预料到，包括中心静脉导管并发症、TPN 诱导的肝病和肠道细菌过度生长。TPN 诱导的肝病经常发生在婴幼儿 SBS 中并且脓毒血症是他们死亡的主要原因，表现为多因素的过程，该过程经常可逆转但是也可导致严重的胆汁淤积、脂肪变性甚至肝硬化。儿童比成人多见并且长期接受 TPN 的患儿中有 1/3 死于该病。TPN 诱导的肝病依然是肝/小肠移植的主要适应证之一。

避免过量的肠道外营养并且通过肠道给予尽可能多的热量将可能有助于预防这些并发症[69]。外源性胆囊收缩素对 SBS 患儿 TPN 诱导的肝病可能会改善其肝功能[66]，另外，脱氧胆汁酸盐通过刺激胆汁的流动可能减轻这些患儿的肝功能异常程度[6]。最近发现了一种相关的胆汁酸盐牛黄脱氧胆汁酸盐，并发现其无显著的效应[30]。这可能因为在 SBS 患儿中胆盐是通过口服的且吸收受限。避免中央静脉脓毒血症和严格管理小肠内细菌过度生长可能会减少 TPN 相关胆汁淤积的进展。

在功能失调的肠段检出过度生长的细菌值得高度怀疑。小肠增殖导致结合胆汁酸的浓缩功能降低同时会导致脂肪吸收不良。由于脂肪吸收不良会出现分泌性腹泻，增加了短链脂肪酸的形成同时伴有渗透梯度、气体增加和维生素 B_{12} 的吸收减少[45]，另外，细菌过度生长导致黏膜发炎，因此加重了所有营养素的吸收不良。没有回盲瓣的患儿，由于潜在的细菌从结肠内反流可能使这种并发症的风险增加。当患儿的吸收能力和腹泻急剧改变时应考虑结肠化，并且扩张的肠袢是影像学证据。要使用针对厌氧菌和革兰阴性和阳性需氧菌的抗生素，主要有头孢氨苄-甲硝唑联合 137
或者单用甲硝唑、甲氧苄叮-磺胺甲基异噁唑或口服庆大霉素。需进一步研究通过抑制细菌的过度生长是否能阻止其发生和在治疗中起作用[33]。

肠功能的药物治疗

像以前提到的一样，在各种 SBS 动物模型中生长因子、肽和激素治疗结果出现肠适应增强。在临床中，通过生长激素（GH）、谷酰胺（GLN）和高血糖多肽-2（GLP-2）的联合使用，大部分数据已经获得。虽然这里列出的几个临床研究显示对这些因子的反应仅仅是适度的改善，结果还是令人鼓舞的。不幸的是，许多这些研究的 SBS 患者具有多个诊断，而且经常是超过切除后适应阶段好多年。有实验证据表明，为了最大限度地支持适应和肠道功能，切除后的时间、给药途径和剂量都是应该考虑的关键变量[63]。

在第一个主要的研究中，Byrne 和合作者报道了一组 47 个主要依靠 TPN 的成年 SBS 患者，接受 GLN

（首选的肠上皮细胞能量来源）、GH 和配方饮食（高碳水化合物、低脂肪）治疗[14]。治疗 28 天后，57% 的患者不再需要 TPN，而另外 30% 的患者降低了每天的 TPN 需要量。研究结束后，他们出院回家，只需依靠节食和单独的 GLN 治疗，GH 治疗已停止。随访 5 月~5年，TPN 依赖已降到 40% 而 TPN 减少的患者已增加到 40%。

与这个报道相反，Scalopio 和同事在 8 例成年 SBS 患者中做了一个随机、6 周、双盲、安慰剂对照、交叉的 GLN/GH/配方饮食（高碳水化合物、低脂肪）的研究[58]。这种联合治疗仅观察到细微的好处。用这种相同的研究设计，Seguy 和同事最近的报道发现 GLN/GH 在西方饮食过量的背景下导致肠道内营养素的显著吸收，同时增加体重和肌肉组织[60]。GLN/GH 的应用经验在儿童中非常有限。目前，用这种激素和特殊肠细胞营养素联合一个选定的饮食用于治疗 SBS 患儿仍有争议。

胰高血糖素原衍生肽类 GLP-2 与肠道营养有关[15]，营养摄取后由远端肠 L 细胞分泌。因此，远端肠广泛切除的患儿血清中 GLP-2 的水平显著降低并不奇怪[35]。在一个回结肠切除和 SBS 患者的研究中发现，给予 GLP-2 可导致体重增加和肠道吸收能量的改善[36]。目前，GLP-2 还没有商品化；然而，用这种多肽的特定类似物治疗 SBS 的研究正在进行中。

提高肠功能的外科治疗

预防 SBS 是最早和最好的方法。坏死性小肠结肠炎和（或）肠扭转患儿及时对肠管手术切除行保守治疗对于避免 SBS 非常重要。一旦患儿超过了最初设想的手术期，最大的目标就是尽可能地通过肠道途径提供所有的热卡和停止 TPN。患儿经常会出现 TPN 相关的并发症，或出现排便和（或）电解质的丢失，故限制了进一步的肠道营养。另外，有些患儿情况更糟，需要增加而不是减少 TPN 的量。这类患儿（如出现 TPN 并发症，不能进一步的肠道营养且肠道营养耐受力恶化）应该考虑手术干预。

外科干预最佳时机的选择很重要。如果手术太早，可能没有必要，由于正常肠切除后适应或随正常生长发育的肠增长可能会避免 TPN 的应用。如果手术太迟，患儿可能会出现并发症，也会增加 TPN 支持的费用。至少 1 年是一个使适应完成的较合理的最短间隔时间。即使过了这个时期，如果患儿正在逐渐耐受肠道营养而 TPN 的支持只是个小问题，手术干预应该推迟。然而，这一策略在有明显 TPN 并发症的情况下需要重新考虑。

手术干预的最大目标是提高肠道的吸收和消化能力。沿着这一思路，作为早期治疗计划的一部分，如果可行的话有造瘘口的患儿应尽可能恢复肠的连续性。许多手术步骤是针对 SBS 患儿的特殊的肠道解剖和生理异常而产生的。这些异常包括肠转运增快、黏膜表面积减少、无效蠕动和肠的长度减少。各种各样的手术步骤选择取决于它们的最初异常分类。

决定每一个步骤的适应证需要一个仔细的术前诊断检查和一个精心的手术计划。第一步，应对患儿肠道的解剖和功能有一个详细的了解。这些可以通过腹部平片和上消化道对比造影检查获得。应寻找部分梗阻的区域和转运的效率。解除部分肠梗阻的简单干预如松解粘连或切除局部的缩窄，对于患儿病情的显
著改善是必要的。为减慢肠转运而设计的手术步骤对 1375
于明显转运延迟的患儿显然不是适应证。尽管并不完全准确，可以通过上消化道造影来推算小肠的长度和直径。对于近端有瘘口的患儿，行灌肠造影也应谨慎，它将提供一些信息，如远端肠管有多少可以用于接下来的再吻合以及确定缩窄的潜在区域。

肠瓣膜

通过对 SBS 患儿的治疗已经认识到回盲瓣的重要性。1972 年，Wilmore 证明有回盲瓣的婴儿生存需要的最小肠长度是 15 cm[87]。然而，没有回盲瓣的婴儿，生存所需的最小肠长度要明显增长（40 cm）。更最近的报道显示，89% 没有回盲瓣并且小肠少于 40 cm的患儿可以存活[16]。同一报道也显示没有回盲瓣的患儿 TPN 持续期更长。因此，保存回盲瓣应该是任何手术干预的主要目标。

基于观察到的回盲瓣的重要性，多种构建类似回盲瓣的技术已经有报道。最简单的技术包括在肠的周围放置缝线或放置一个外置的聚四氟乙烯树脂垫圈[64]。一个更有技术含量的方法是外翻一段肠管产生一个小的套入部来减慢转运（图 86-3）。这些方法

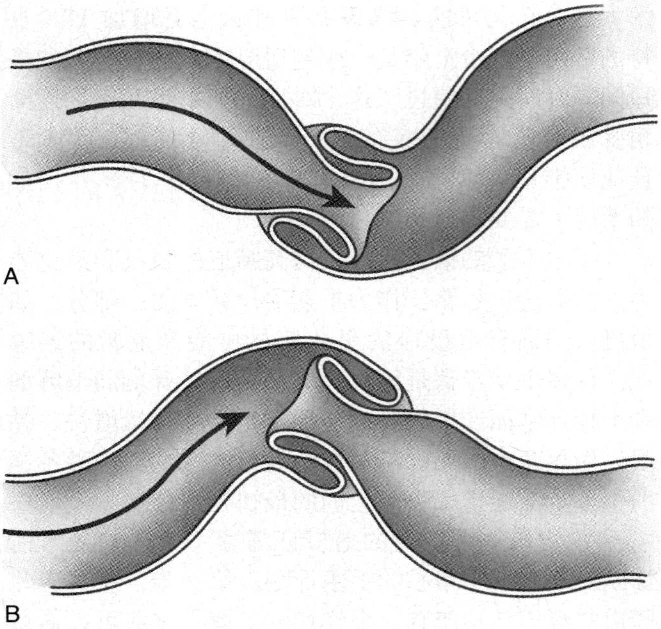

图 86–3　减慢肠转运的肠瓣膜的构建。瓣膜可以同向（A）或对抗（B）蠕动支构建，然后套入另一支中。

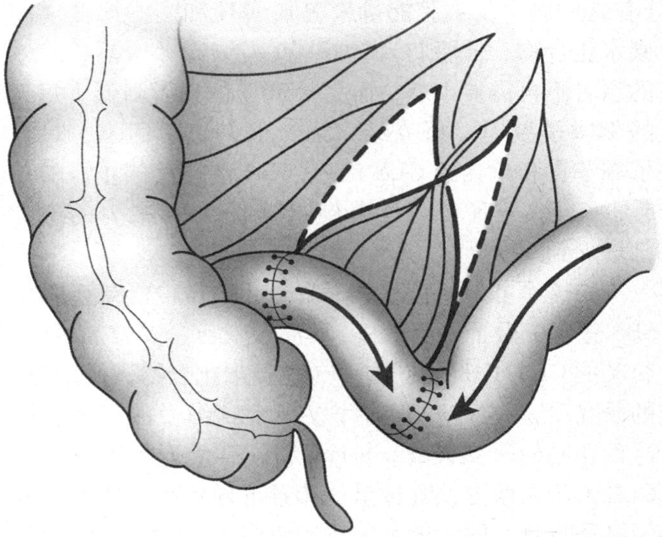

图 86–4　减慢肠转运的反转肠段。切除肠系膜血供完整的一小段远端肠管，然后翻转 180°，与留下的胃肠道吻合恢复连续性。理论上，反转肠段的蠕动方向将与本身的肠管蠕动波相对抗，其作用为一生理瓣，因此减慢转运。

的多变性和不易理解的地方集中在外翻肠管的最佳长度和套迭的方向，如果被套迭的一段肠管太大，则会造成功能性肠梗阻。

肠瓣膜的临床经验很少，仅局限于小规模的病例报告。构建一个部分梗阻瓣膜已显示可以诱导肠扩张和黏膜适应[18]。利用这一观察结果，Gerogeson 和同事报道了一组 SBS 儿童，这些患儿最初构建套迭瓣，紧接着后期实施一个肠延长手术[25]。这些患儿中的几例由于延长了以前未扩张的肠管而使病情得到改善。

逆转肠段

在迷走神经切除后腹泻或倾倒综合征的患儿用肠段逆转来减慢肠蠕动已积累了许多经验。用部分肠段产生一个“生理性”瓣，在瓣内肠的蠕动是反方向的（图 86–4）。逆转肠段的实际长度很重要，因为太短对减慢肠蠕动无效，而太长则会产生功能性肠梗阻。各种逆转肠管的长度在许多实验和临床研究中会产生不一样的结果。虽然在成年患者中 10 cm 是最常用的肠长度，在婴儿有逆转长度短至 3 cm 却同样有效的报道[79]。从技术上讲，逆转的肠段应该放在肠的最远端部分，以便在减慢转运和增加黏膜吸收方面收效最大。逆转肠段在肠管极其短的患儿中应用性有限，因为逆转肠段的构建可能会损害已经脆弱的肠黏膜团块。

已有 30 多例 SBS 成年患者用逆转肠段取得了良好效果的报道[4,53]。逆转肠段的长期效果目前尚不清楚。在儿童，逆转的肠段可能继续生长，可能导致肠梗阻。另外，逆转肠段可能不发挥正常功能，因此应有效地缩短残留肠的长度，尤其是有并发症如梗阻和缺血出现时。逆转肠段的应用在适应出现之前的短时间内有帮助[61]。大多数逆转肠段的报道是作为一件趣事，很少和其他的手术方法进行比较。当肠的直径正常和运转加快时，这一逆转肠段也许和肠瓣膜的作用一样。

再循环袢

理论上，如果构建一个营养在进入远端前可被循环几次的肠袢，营养物质与肠黏膜的暴露时间就会延长。此外，全部的肠转运会减慢。不幸的是，这些理论的优点很少变成现实。几个实验研究没有显示出这些方法的任何益处。总的发病率和死亡率升高，与袢的复杂性直接相关。另一个有趣的发现是虽然肠的内容物再循环已得到影像学的证明，但吸收并没有改善。

再循环袢已在少数患儿实施但是效果并不理想。目前，在 SBS 患儿的治疗中再循环袢的应用相对有限。较高的死亡率抑制了该手术的实施，而且效果没有得到证实。再循环肠袢可能不应实施，提及它只是为了完整性。

结肠间置

在快转运的患儿中用一段结肠插入到两支小肠中已被实验研究和应用于临床（图 86–5）。尽管应用这种有效方法的具体机制尚不清楚，间置的结肠一般放在肠的近端，依靠它缓慢的、部分的蠕动性收缩来减慢营养素转运到远端肠管的速度。间置的结肠也有吸收营养素、水和电解质的能力。包括黏膜[47]和纵向平滑肌的间置结肠似乎会出现适应性改变[46]。

首次报道同向蠕动的结肠间置治疗 SBS 是在切除 90% 小肠的小猎犬中实施的[32]。与单独肠切除比较，间置结肠的犬肠转运时间延长、体重增加、大便排出

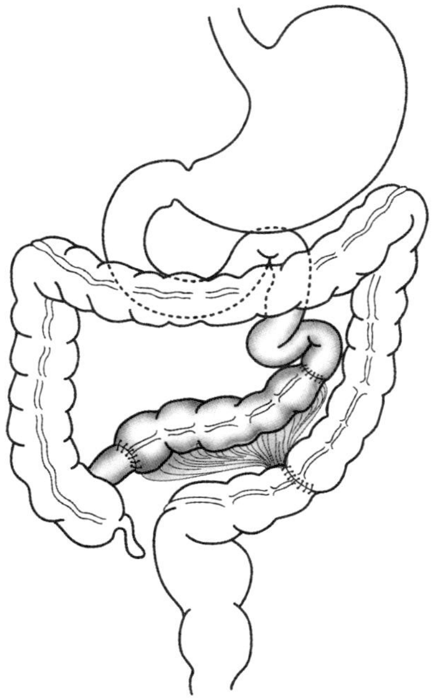

图 86–5　结肠间置。一段有完整血供的乙状结肠被间置在小肠间，作为一个生理的闸门，因此可减慢转运。

减少和粪便中脂肪排泄减少。临床上结肠间置在儿童和成人都有效。在一项大宗的儿童 SBS 研究中，同向蠕动结肠间置使 6 个患儿中的 3 个摆脱了 TPN[27]，另外 3 个死于继发的 TPN 并发症，与结肠间置有关的发病率和病死率尚未报道。

用于间置的结肠的理想长度尚不明确。在上面提到的研究中，结肠长度在 8～15 cm 不等，其他报道最长可达 24 cm。患儿数量太少无法确定用于间置的结肠的最合适长度。这似乎是一个增加肠转运的有用技术，有 50% 的成功率，对小肠的发育能力没有损害。该技术可考虑用于那些有完整结肠且小肠尚未扩张的患儿。

肠裁剪（变细）成形术

肠段扩张是功能性肠梗阻的一个公认的原因，收
缩时肠壁的对合失败导致无效蠕动。扩张的小肠收缩 1377
压低，导致肠内容物往复运动，这种情况会形成淤积、细菌过度生长及毒素产生和营养不良。如果患儿受累的肠段较短并且有足够长的剩余肠，切除扩张的肠段被认为是一个最佳的治疗。遗憾的是，SBS 患儿大多数肠管已经显著扩张并且总的长度很短。因此，切除通常并不是一个可行的选择。

变细成形术减小了肠管的直径同时保留了肠的长度。该手术切除肠系膜对侧的肠管，并保留系膜部分的肠管完整（图 86–6）。变细的肠直径显著减小，因此蠕动变得更有效[82]。

这一技术的一个改变是系膜对侧肠管的折叠术。替代切除肠系膜对侧的部分肠管，肠管被折叠到肠腔内形成褶皱。这在理论上保留了肠黏膜以便于吸收，同时又减小了肠管总的直径[21]。遗憾的是，随着时间推移，缝线可能会损坏，肠管扩张，且功能性梗阻再发。

在一个 160 例儿童和成年 SBS 的大规模研究中[70]，11 例年龄 6 月~9 岁的儿童肠段扩张，剩余肠管大于 30 cm。所有这些儿童都有细菌过度生长和营养不良。肠成形术分别在十二指肠（n＝3）、空肠（n＝3）或回肠（n＝5）进行，11 例中的 7 例成形的肠长度超过 15 cm，9 例完全摆脱 TPN，另外 2 例 TPN 需要量减少。由于再发的吸收不良，这 2 个患儿随后进行了肠延长术。肠变细术较肠延长术死亡率低，只

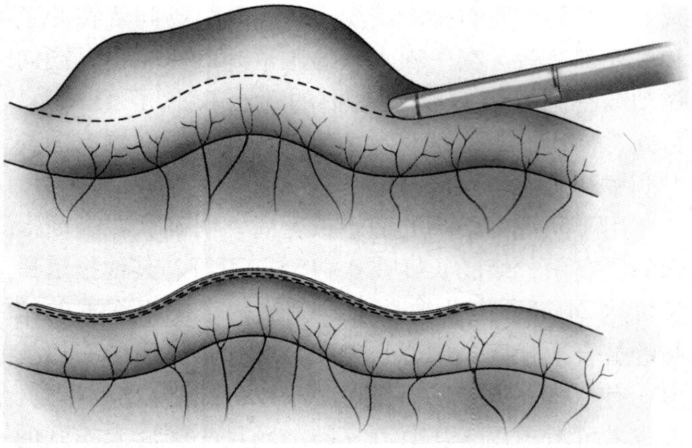

图 86-6　肠裁剪（变细）成形术。利用吻合器沿纵轴切除系膜对侧的部分小肠。留下的肠管管径因此变小，显示动力改善。

要患儿有足够的小肠就可选择此手术。

肠延长术

1980 年 Bianchi 首次描述了一个重要的真正意义上的肠延长手术方法[7]。像其他切除后的手术方法一样，这一方法对最初肠切除后已经历了一段时期正常肠适应的患者最为成功[8]。该方法利用了提供肠管血运的肠系膜的解剖特点。正好在到达肠壁边缘前，肠系膜内的血管分叉供应肠管圆周的一半。这种节段性供血形式使肠管沿着纵轴被分成两个管，其管径为原来肠管的一半。用胃肠道吻合器（GLA）会容易些但也可以用手缝合。一旦肠沿着纵轴被一分为二，两段新建的肠管可以按照同向的蠕动方式缝合在一起（图
1378 86-7）。总的结果就是肠的长度增加了一倍而周径减到一半。因此，这一手术不但增加了肠管的长度以增加吸收，而且通过减小肠管的直径改善了蠕动。该技术的一个改进是在最初肠延长时进入肠支的一侧，一旦延长完成后从另一侧出来[17]。这可允许仅仅单层吻合，是一个非常有用的技术改进。

由于 GLA 吻合器的应用，扩张的肠段一般很容易延长。由于以前手术的广泛腹膜内粘连在实施肠延长术时经常碰到，应小心避免伤到肠系膜血供。另外，可能会出现供应肠壁的血管变异而使该技术失败[72]。在没有显著的自发性肠管扩张的患儿，Bianchi 手术是可行的，可以实施 Georgeson 和同事所描述的阶段性连续的肠延长术[25]。

Thompson 和同事报道了一项研究，该研究中 6 例患儿接受了 Bianchi 手术[71]。其中，1 例患儿死于脓毒血症，4 例完全摆脱了 TPN，最后 1 例患儿减少了 TPN 的需要量。在另一研究中，Figueroa-Colon 和合作者报道 7 例患儿接受了肠延长术，9 个月时显示肠道耐受的热卡显著增加[24]。他们也发现患儿所有的生长参数或者维持原状或者改善，并且肠延长术后的第 2 年里住院天数减少。Bianchi 的一项大宗病例报道中，实施这一肠延长手术的 20 例儿童[9]，16 年

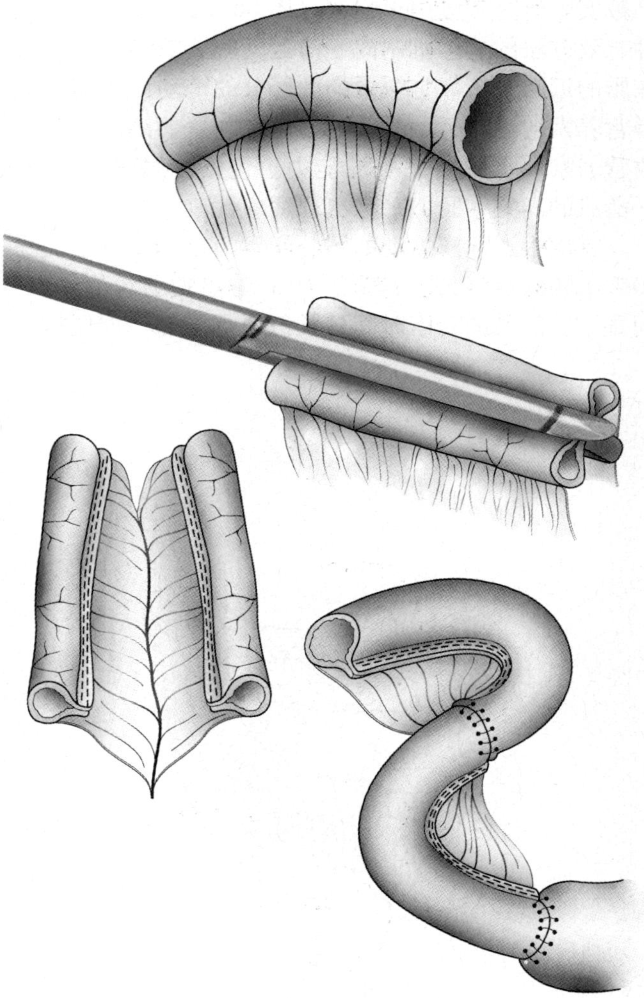

图 86-7　Bianchi 肠延长术步骤。肠管在纵向剖面分离产生 2 个管，再吻合后肠壁周径变为原来的一半，但肠长度增加 1 倍。

后长期生存率是45%。生存者一般肠长度大于40 cm，在肠道重建时有无明显的肝病迹象通过有无黄疸来判断。匹斯堡的一项研究认为如实施这一手术的患儿肠长度极短（小于 50　cm）、有黄疸或处在新生儿期，肠成形失败的患儿都被推荐行小肠移植[77]。最后，Waag 和助手阐明了接受这一手术的患儿的持续发病率。在这一研究中，18 例接受了 Bianchi 手术存活者的远期发病包括摄食过量、低血钠、低血氯、代谢性酸中毒、D-乳酸酸中毒、胆石症及尿石症、胃食管反流和延长的肠袢继发扩张引起的症状。因此，有理由要继续对这些病情复杂的患儿进行长期随访。

对那些不是 Bianchi 手术候选者或者是肠系膜有限且肠很短的 SBS 患儿，Iowa（Kimura）手术可作为一种治疗的手段[44]。这个手术有两个阶段，第一步是对肠系膜对侧表面肠管与机体的血供进行初始接合。首先做一个纵形的浆肌层切开，顺着肠系膜的对侧缘延伸，暴露黏膜下层。然后，肝前缘的包膜和腹壁肌层下面的壁腹膜被除去产生一个裸露的组织表面。黏膜下层和肝以及腹壁肌层的裸露组织面用两个连续缝合形成一个肝肌层肠固定。大约 8 周后实施第二步手术，这涉及纵向劈开肠管以提供两个肠袢。然后，这两个肠袢依次排列短短吻合使肠管长度增加 1 倍（图 86-8）。迄今为止，只有一个运用该技术的报
道[25,44]，特别适合于剩余肠仅限于十二指肠而不能 1379
行 Bianchi 手术的儿童。有人提出一个类似的方法用大网膜作为寄生的血供来源。在对犬的初步研究中显示新生的血管形成改善了吸收和适应[77]。

最近，一个新颖的称为连续横向肠成形术的肠延长手术被报道[41]。在一个猪模型中，通过 GIA 吻合器连续横向分别从对侧方向，构建一个锯齿形的通道，使扩张的小肠延长（图 86-9）。肠管的长度几乎

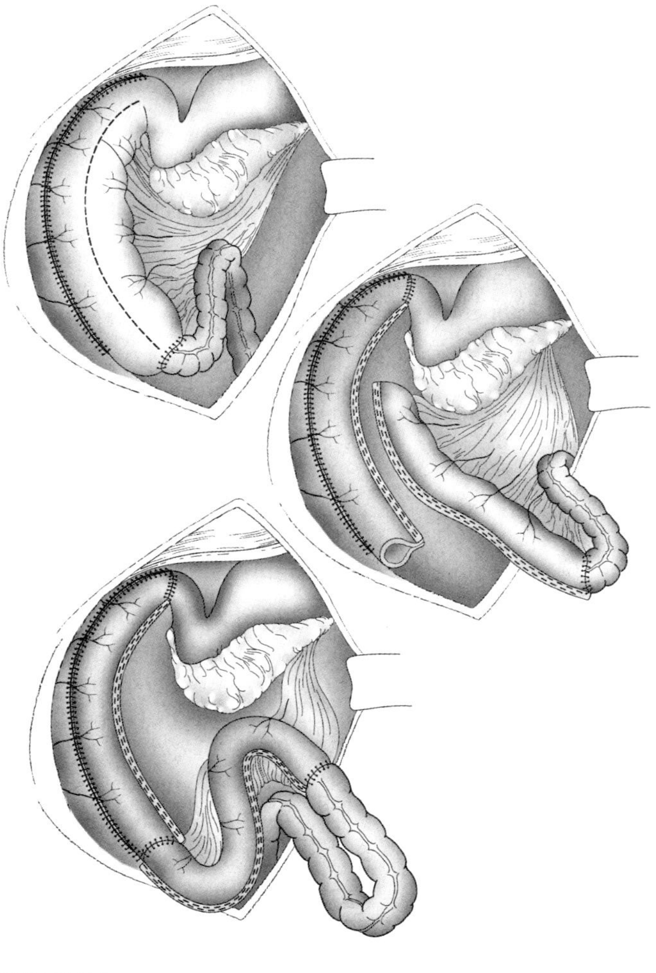

图 86-8　Iowa（Kimura）肠延长术步骤。肠系膜对侧的肠壁被固定于腹壁下面。依靠系统衍生的腹壁在固定前，沿着肠壁浆肌层切开和腹壁机械性摩擦促进肠系膜对侧的肠管新血管形成。几个月后，肠管可沿着纵轴分成两支，第一支依靠系统血供，而另一支依靠肠系膜血供。这两支大约可使肠长度延长 1 倍。

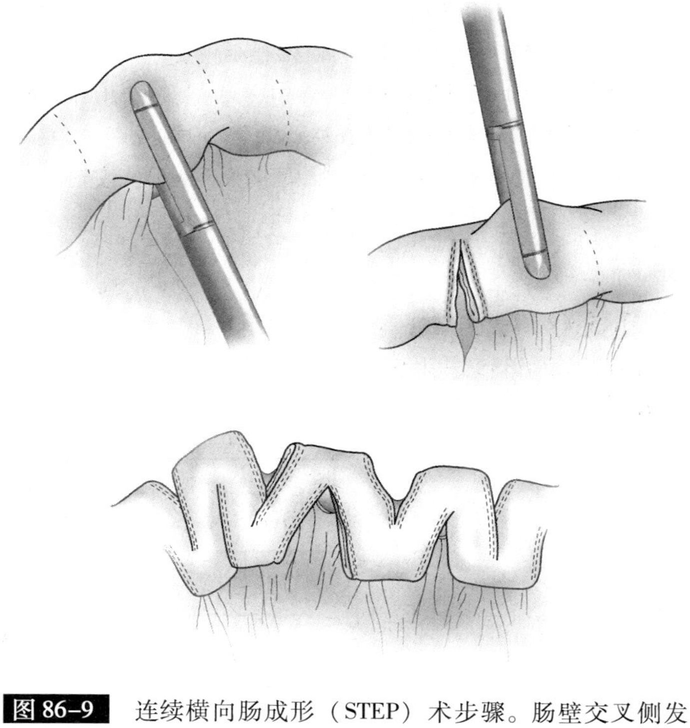

图 86-9　连续横向肠成形（STEP）术步骤。肠壁交叉侧发射吻合器使管径减小伴肠内营养转运长度增加。

增加 1 倍。这一手术随后被用于临床，结果令人鼓舞[42]。但还需要进一步研究，并与传统的 Bianchi 手术比较，作出详细的临床评价。

图 86-10 为在有或无肠管直径的情况下 SBS 患儿治疗的路线图。

组织工程

组织工程是一个令人激动的新领域，目前处在研究的早期。这些模型利用管状多微孔的生物可降解聚合体，用肠上皮类器官单位种植。血液供应来自于肠系膜。注意到会有新生的肠管形成，然后再被吻合到原始的小肠上[38,39,43]。在人体尚未有应用新生肠的报道，但是组织工程领域在将来 SBS 患儿的治疗中将发挥重要的作用[28]。

肠移植

肠移植是 SBS 患儿治疗的一个重要的也是最后的选择，在本书的其他地方也有阐述。小肠移植是一个可行的成形治疗方法，但是发病率和死亡率很高。最近的结果显示，患儿和移植物的 1 年存活率分别为 70% 和 65%。然而，移植 3 年后，患儿和移植物的存活率分别降到 40%～55% 和 50%[42,56]。复杂的免疫抑制和各种感染并发症仍然是治疗这些复杂患儿的障碍。

结论

总体上，SBS 患儿的治疗进展显著。然而，针对大量 SBS 所致的肠异常设计了很多手术方法，但都没有足够病例数来进行临床试验以进行有效结果的比较。所有手术的最终目标就是让患儿进展到肠道营养以避免 TPN 并发症和让患儿能够尽量回归正常的生活。也许，SBS 患儿治疗最重要的是理解黏膜生长的内源性调节和切除后适应反应的遗传调控。

（汪　健译　朱锦祥校）

参考文献

1. Altmann GG: Influence of bile and pancreatic secretions on the size of the intestinal villi in the rat. Am J Anat 1971; 132:167.
2. Altmann GG, Leblond CP: Factors influencing villus size in the small intestine of adult rats as revealed by transposition of intestinal segments. Am J Anat 1970;127:15.
3. Andorsky DJ, Lund DP, Lillehei CW, et al: Nutritional and other postoperative management of neonates with short bowel syndrome correlates with clinical outcomes. J Pediatr 2001;139:27.
4. Barros D'sa AB: An experimental evaluation of segmental reversal after massive small bowel resection. Br J Surg 1979; 66:493.
5. Bass BL, Fischer BA, Richardson C, et al: Somatostatin analogue treatment inhibits post-resectional adaptation of the small bowel in rats. Am J Surg 1991;161:107.
6. Beau P, Labat-Labourdette J, Ingrand P, et al: Is ursodeoxycholic acid an effective therapy for total parenteral nutritrion related liver disease? J Hepatol 1994;20:240.
7. Bianchi A: Intestinal loop lengthening—a technique for increasing small intestinal length. J Pediatr Surg 1980;

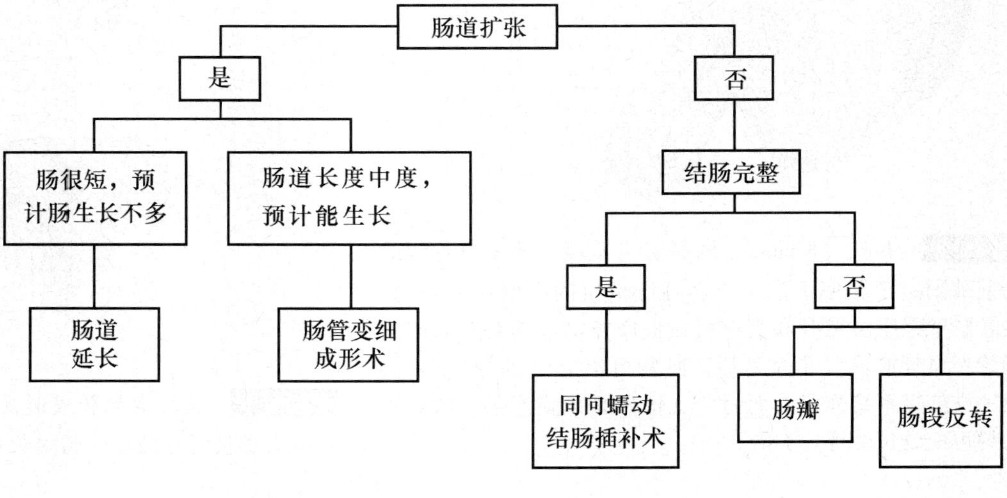

图 86-10　有或无肠管直径的情况下 SBS 患儿治疗路线图。

15:145.
8. Bianchi A: Autologous gastrointestinal reconstruction. Semin Pediatr Surg 1995;4:54.
9. Bianchi A: Experience with longitudinal intestinal lengthening and tailoring. Eur J Pediatr Surg 1999;9:256.
10. Bongaerts G, Bakkeren J, Severijnen R, et al: Lactobacilli and acidosis in children with short small bowel. J Pediatr Gastroenterol Nutr 2000;30:288.
11. Booth IW: Enteral nutrition as primary therapy in short bowel syndrome. Gut 1994;35(Suppl):S69-S72.
12. Bueno J, Guiterrez J, Mazariegos GV, et al: Analysis of patients with longitudinal intestinal lengthening procedure referred for intestinal transplantation. J Pediatr Surg 2001;36:178.
13. Bueno J, Ohwada S, Kocoshis S, et al: Factors impacting the survival of children with intestinal failure referred for intestinal transplantation. J Pediatr Surg 1999;34:27.
14. Byrne TA, Persinger RL, Young LS, et al: A new treatment for patients with short-bowel syndrome: Growth hormone, glutamine, and a modified diet. Ann Surg 1995; 222:243.
15. Chance WT, Foley-Nelson T, Thomas I, et al: Prevention of parenteral nutrition-induced gut hypoplasia by co-infusion of glucagon-like peptide-2. Am J Physiol 1997;273(2 pt 1): G559-G563.
16. Chaet MS, Farrell MK, Ziegler MM, et al: Intensive nutritional support and remedial surgical intervention for extreme short bowel syndrome. J Pediatr Gastroenterol Nutr 1994;19:295.
17. Chahine AA, Ricketts RR: A modification of the Bianchi intestinal lengthening procedure with a single anastomosis. J Pediatr Surg 1998;33:1292.
18. Collins J III, Vicente Y, Georgeson K, et al: Partial intestinal obstruction induces substantial mucosal proliferation in the pig. J Pediatr Surg 1996;31:415.
19. Crenn P, Coudray-Lucas C, Thuillier F, et al: Postabsorptive plasma citrulline concentration is a marker of absorptive enterocyte mass and intestinal failure in humans. Gastroenterology 2000;119:1496.
20. Cronk DR, Ferguson DC, Thompson JS: Malnutrition impairs postresection intestinal adaptation. J Parenter Enteral Nutr 2000;24:76.
21. de Lorimier AA, Harrison MR: Intestinal plication in the treatment of atresia. J Pediatr Surg 1983;18:734.
22. Dowling RH, Booth CC: Structural and functional changes following small intestinal resection in the rat. Clin Sci 1967; 32:139.
23. Ericsson CD, Johnson PC: Safety and efficacy of loperamide. Am J Med 1990;88(Suppl):10S.
24. Figueroa-Colon R, Harris PR, Birdsong E, et al: Impact of intestinal lengthening on the nutritional outcome for children with short bowel syndrome. J Pediatr Surg 1996; 31:912.
25. Georgeson K, Halpin D, Figueroa R, et al: Sequential intestinal lengthening procedures for refractory short bowel syndrome. J Pediatr Surg 1994;29:316.
26. Georgeson KE, Breaux CW Jr: Outcome and intestinal adaptation in neonatal short-bowel syndrome. J Pediatr Surg 1992;27:344.
27. Glick PL, de Lorimier AA, Adzick NS, et al: Colon interposition for the short bowel syndrome. J Pediatr Surg 1984; 19:719.
28. Grikscheit TC: Tissue engineering of the gastrointestinal tract for surgical replacement: A nutrition tool of the future? Proc Nutr Soc 2003;62:739.
29. Helmrath MA, Erwin CR, Shin CE, et al: Enterocyte apoptosis is increased following small bowel resection. J Gastrointest Surg 1998;2:44.
30. Heubi JE, Wiechmann DA, Creutzinger V, et al: Tauroursodeoxycholic acid (TUDCA) in the prevention of total parenteral nutrition-associated liver disease. J Pediatr 2002;141:237.
31. Heydorn S, Jeppesen PB, Mortensen PB: Bile acid replacement therapy with cholylsarcosine for short-bowel syndrome. Scand J Gastroenterol 1999;34:818.
32. Hutcher NE, Mendez-Picon G, Salzberg AM: Prejejunal transposition of colon to prevent the development of short bowel syndrome in puppies with 90 per cent small intestine resection. J Pediatr Surg 1973;8:771.
33. Hwang ST, Shulman RJ: Update on management and treatment of short gut. Clin Perinatol 2002;29:181.
34. Iacono G, Carroccio A, Montalto G, et al: Extreme short bowel syndrome: A case for reviewing the guidelines for predicting survival. J Pediatr Gastroenterol Nutr 1993;16:216.
35. Jeppesen PB, Hartmann B, Hansen BS, et al: Impaired meal stimulated glucagon-like peptide 2 response in ileal resected short bowel patients with intestinal failure. Gut 1999;45:559.
36. Jeppesen PB, Hartmann B, Thulesen J, et al: Glucagon-like peptide 2 improves nutrient absorption and nutritional status in short-bowel patients with no colon. Gastroenterology 2001;120:806.
37. Juno RJ, Knott AW, Erwin CR, et al: A serum factor(s) after small bowel resection induces intestinal epithelial cell proliferation: Effects of timing, site, and extent of resection. J Pediatr Surg 2003;38:868.
38. Kaihara S, Kim SS, Benvenuto M, et al: Successful anastomosis between tissue-engineered intestine and native small bowel. Transplantation 1999;67:241.
39. Kaihara S, Kim SS, Kim BS, et al: Long-term follow-up of tissue-engineered intestine after anastomosis to native small bowel. Transplantation 2000;69:1927.
40. Kato T, Mittal N, Nishida S, et al: The role of intestinal transplantation in the management of babies with extensive gut resections. J Pediatr Surg 2003;38:145.
41. Kim HB, Fauza D, Garza J, et al: Serial transverse enteroplasty (STEP): A novel bowel lengthening procedure. J Pediatr Surg 2003;38:425.
42. Kim HB, Lee PW, Garza J, et al: Serial transverse enteroplasty for short bowel syndrome: A case report. J Pediatr Surg 2003;38:881.
43. Kim SS, Kaihara S, Benvenuto MS, et al: Effects of anastomosis of tissue-engineered neointestine to native small bowel. J Surg Res 1999;87:6.
44. Kimura K, Soper RT: A new bowel elongation technique for the short-bowel syndrome using the isolated bowel segment Iowa models. J Pediatr Surg 1993;28:792.
45. King CE, Toskes PP: Small intestine bacterial overgrowth. Gastroenterology 1979;76:1035.
46. King DR, Anvari M, Jamieson GG, et al: Does the colon adopt small bowel features in a small bowel environment? Aust NZ J Surg 1996;66:543.
47. Kono K, Sekikawa T, Iizuka H, et al: Interposed colon between remnants of the small intestine exhibits small bowel features in a patient with short bowel syndrome. Dig Surg 2001;18:237.
48. Messing B, Crenn P, Beau P, et al: Long-term survival and parenteral nutrition dependence in adult patients with the short bowel syndrome. Gastroenterology 1999;117:1043.
49. Nehra V, Camilleri M, Burton D, et al: An open trial of octreotide long-acting release in the management of short bowel syndrome. Am J Gastroenterol 2001;96:1494.

50. Nightingale JMD, Walker ER, Burnham WR: Octreotide (a somatostatin analogue) improves the quality of life in some patients with a short intestine. Aliment Pharmacol Ther 1989;3:367.
51. O'Brien DP, Nelson LA, Huang FS, et al: Intestinal adaptation: Structure, function, and regulation. Semin Pediatr Surg 2001;10:56.
52. O'Brien JD, Thompson DG, McIntyre A: Effect of codeine and loperamide on upper intestinal transit and absorption in normal subjects and patients with postvagotomy diarrhoea. Gut 1988;29:312.
53. Panis Y, Messing B, Rivet P, et al: Segmental reversal of the small bowel as an alternative to intestinal transplantation in patients with short bowel syndrome. Ann Surg 1997; 225:401.
54. Reyes J: Intestinal transplantation for children with short bowel syndrome. Semin Pediatr Surg 2001;10:99.
55. Rodrigues CA, Lennard-Jones JE, Thompson DG: The effects of octreotide, soy polysaccharide, codeine and loperamide on nutrient, fluid and electrolyte absorption in the short-bowel syndrome. Aliment Pharmacol Ther 1989;3:159.
56. Schmidt T, Pfeiffer A, Hackelsberger N, et al: Effect of intestinal resection on human small bowel motility. Gut 1996;38:859.
57. Scolapio JS, Camilleri M, Fleming CR: Gastrointestinal motility considerations in patients with short-bowel syndrome. Dig Dis 1997;15:253.
58. Scolapio JS, Camilleri M, Fleming CR, et al: Effect of growth hormone, glutamine, and diet on adaptation in short-bowel syndrome: A randomized, controlled study. Gastroenterology 1997;113:1074.
59. Seydel AS, Miller JH, Sarac TP, et al: Octreotide diminishes luminal nutrient transport activity, which is reversed by epidermal growth factor. Am J Surg 1996;172:267.
60. Seguy D, Vahedi K, Kapel N, et al: Low-dose growth hormone in adult home parenteral nutrition-dependent short bowel syndrome patients: A positive study. Gastroenterology 2003;124:293.
61. Shanbhogue LKR, Molenaar JC: Short bowel syndrome: Metabolic and surgical management. Br J Surg 1994; 81:486.
62. Sondheimer JM, Cadnapaphornchai M, Sontag M, et al: Predicting the duration of dependence on parenteral nutrition after neonatal intestinal resection. J Pediatr 1998; 132:80.
63. Shin CE, Helmrath MA, Falcone R Jr, et al: Epidermal growth factor augments adaptation following small bowel resection: Optimal dosage, route, and timing of administration. J Surg Res 1998;77:11.
64. Stahlgren LH, Roy RH, Umana G: A mechanical impediment to intestinal flow: Physiological effects on intestinal absorption. JAMA 1964;187:41.
65. Sukhotnik I, Khateeb K, Krausz MM, et al: Sandostatin impairs postresection intestinal adaptation in a rat model of short bowel syndrome. Dig Dis Sci 2002;47:2095.
66. Teitelbaum DH, Han-Markey T, Drongowski RA, et al: Use of cholecystokinin to prevent the development of parenteral nutrition-associated cholestasis. J Parenter Enteral Nutr 1997;21:100.
67. Teitelbaum DH, Tracy T: Parenteral nutrition-associated cholestasis. Semin Pediatr Surg 2001;10:72.
68. Thompson JS: The role of prophylactic cholecystectomy in the short-bowel syndrome. Arch Surg 1996;131:556.
69. Thompson JS: Management of the short bowel syndrome. Gastroenterol Clin North Am 1994;23:403.
70. Thompson JS, Langnas AN, Pinch LW, et al: Surgical approach to short-bowel syndrome: Experience in a population of 160 patients. Ann Surg 1995;222:600.
71. Thompson JS, Pinch LW, Murray N, et al: Experience with intestinal lengthening for the short-bowel syndrome. J Pediatr Surg 1991;26:721.
72. Thompson JS, Vanderhoof JA, Antonson DL: Intestinal tapering and lengthening for short bowel syndrome. J Pediatr Gastroenterol Nutr 1985;4:495.
73. Touloukian RJ, Walker Smith GJ: Normal intestinal length in preterm infants. J Pediatr Surg 1983;18:720.
74. Vanderhoof JA: Short bowel syndrome. Clin Perinatol 1996; 23:377.
75. Vanderhoof JA, Kollman KA: Lack of inhibitory effect of octreotide on intestinal adaptation in short bowel syndrome in the rat. J Pediatr Gastroenterol Nutr 1998; 26:241.
76. Vanderhoof JA, Park JH, Herrington MK, et al: Effects of dietary menhaden oil on mucosal adaptation after small bowel resection in rats. Gastroenterology 1994;106:94.
77. Waag KL, Hosie S, Wessel L: What do children look like after longitudinal intestinal lengthening. Eur J Pediatr Surg 1999;9:260.
78. Wales PW, de Silva N, Kim J, et al: Neonatal short bowel syndrome: Population-based estimates of incidence and mortality rates. J Pediatr Surg 2004;39:690.
79. Warden MJ, Wesley JR: Small bowel reversal procedure for treatment of the "short gut" baby. J Pediatr Surg 1978; 13:321.
80. Warner BW, Vanderhoof JA, Reyes JD: What's new in the management of short gut syndrome in children? J Am Coll Surg 2000;190:725.
81. Warner BW, Ziegler MM: Management of the short bowel syndrome in the pediatric population. Pediatr Clin North Am 1993;40:1335.
82. Warner BW, Chaet MS: Nontransplant surgical options for management of the short bowel syndrome. J Pediatr Gastroenterol Nutr 1993;17:1.
83. Williams JK, Carlson GW, Austin GE, et al: Short gut syndrome: Treatment by neovascularization of the small intestine. Ann Plast Surg 1996;37:84.
84. Williamson RC: Intestinal adaptation. Structural, functional and cytokinetic changes. N Engl J Med 1978; 298:1393.
85. Williamson RC, Bauer FL, Ross JS, et al: Proximal enterectomy stimulates distal hyperplasia more than bypass or pancreaticobiliary diversion. Gastroenterology 1978;74:16.
86. Williamson RC, Buchholtz TW, Malt RA: Humoral stimulation of cell proliferation in small bowel after transection and resection in rats. Gastroenterology 1978;75:249.
87. Wilmore DW: Factors correlating with a successful outcome following extensive intestinal resection in newborn infants. J Pediatr 1972;80:88.

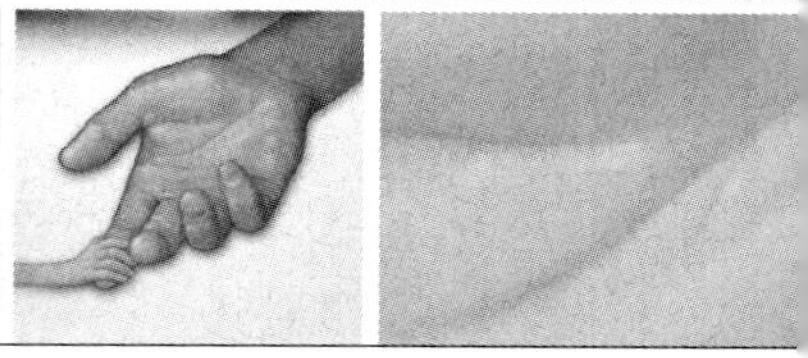

第 87 章

胃肠道出血

Robert M. Arensman、Marybeth Browne 和 Mary Beth Madonna

383 胃肠道（GI）出血中 10%～15% 的病例需要转诊至儿科胃肠病学专家。当与大便或呕吐物混合后即使是很少量的血都会感觉很多，它可能引起家长及医生的警觉。在儿童中，这样的出血通常是自限性的，出血的原因可以通过仔细地询问病史和体格检查来确定（图 87–1 和图 87–2）。

经验表明，大多数患儿自发地或在住院早期即停止出血；然而，因为儿童的血容量小，尽可能早地开

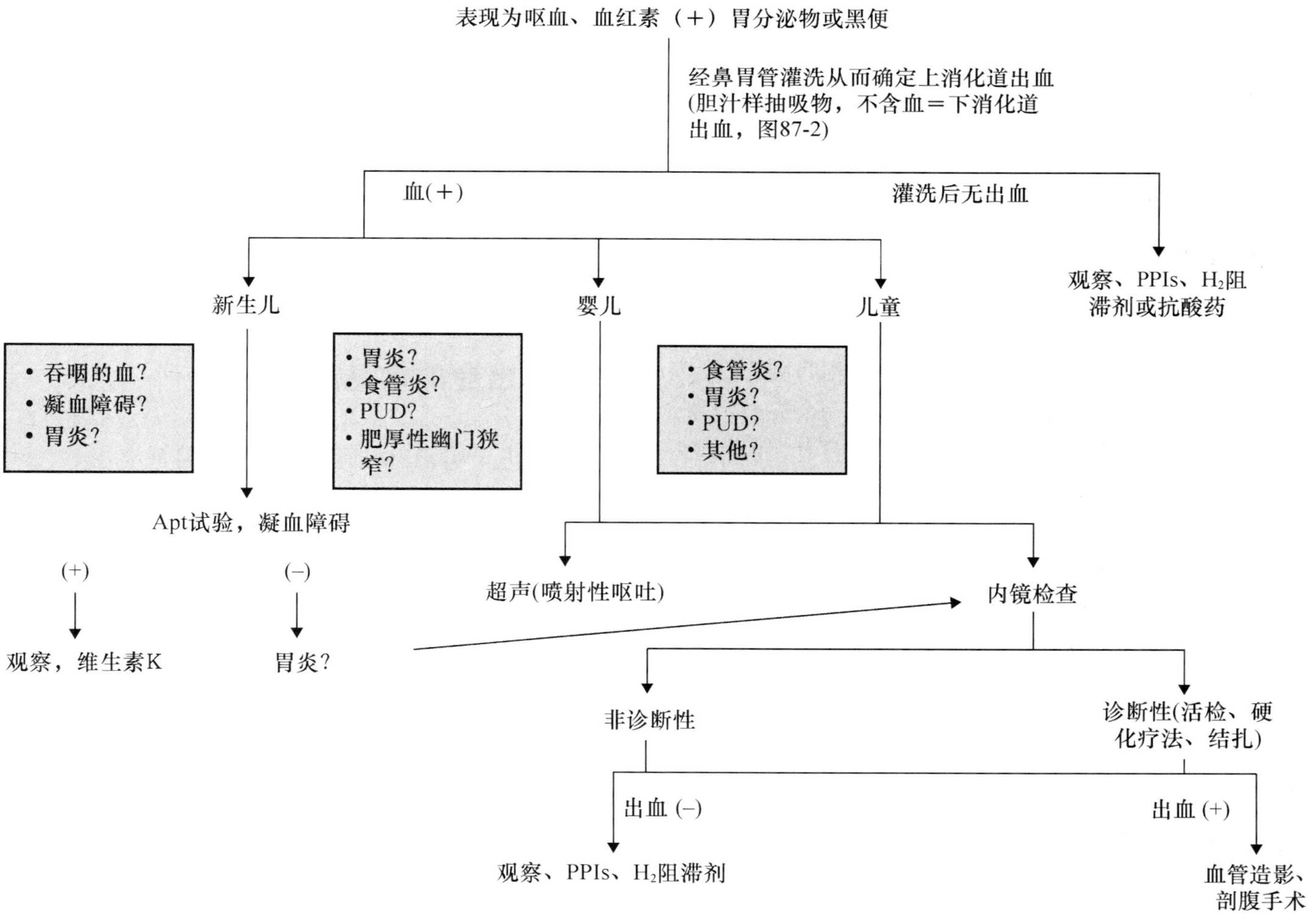

图 87–1 上消化道出血的诊断示意图。PPI，质子泵阻滞剂；PUD，消化性溃疡病。

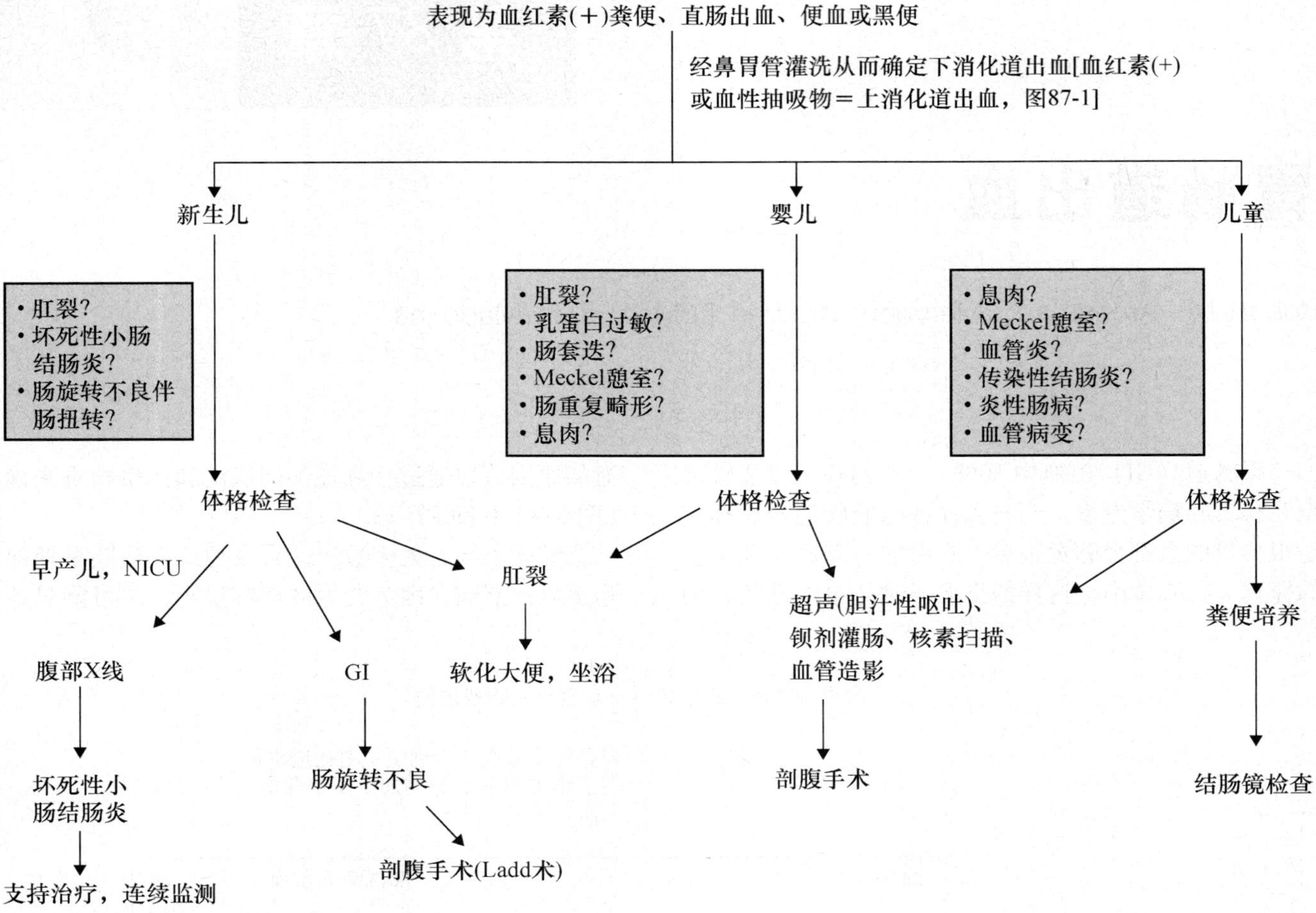

图 87–2 下消化道出血的诊断示意图。NICU，新生儿重症监护病房。

始液体复苏很重要。在患儿中，与年龄相当的心动过速是急性失血的一个最敏感指标，任何一个失血量超过 10% 的患儿都应该在重症监护室监护[7]。记住绝
1384 大多数的患儿尽管大量丢失血液但仍可以维持血压，这一点非常重要[1,10]。出血的量决定液体复苏的程度。当采集完病史时，应放置鼻胃管估计上消化道出血情况，同时开始静脉输液。开始液体复苏时，最初给予 20 ml/kg 生理盐水或林格液。血制品只有在输入晶体液无效、持续出血或先前存在心肺疾病时才考虑使用。

在儿童中，胃肠道出血可以出现在所有的年龄组，每个都有与其年龄相对应的诊断（表 87–1）。本章节讨论各个年龄组最常见的出血原因的评估与处理，同时也讨论一些较少见的原因。

新生儿出血的常见原因

新生儿上消化道出血最常见的原因是：

新生儿出血性疾病
吞下了母亲的血液
应激性胃炎

新生儿下消化道出血最常见的原因是：

肛裂
坏死性小肠结肠炎
肠旋转不良伴扭转

表 87-1　消化道出血的原因

年龄	上消化道出血	下消化道出血
新生儿	新生儿出血性疾病	肛裂
	吞咽母血	坏死性小肠结肠炎
	应激性胃炎	肠旋转不良伴扭转
	凝血病	先天性巨结肠合并小肠结肠炎
	败血症	
	血管畸形	
婴儿（1 月~2 岁）	胃炎	肛裂
	食管炎	乳蛋白过敏症（过敏性直肠结肠炎）
	肥厚性幽门狭窄	肠套迭
	继发于胃造口管的损伤	淋巴结节状增生
	异物	肠重复畸形
	非甾体抗炎病	肠管坏疽
		感染性腹泻
		嗜酸细胞性胃肠病
		获得性血小板减少（症）
儿童（2 岁以上）	消化性溃疡	息肉
	食管静脉曲张	淋巴结节状增生
	胃静脉曲张	Meckel 憩室
	胃炎	溶血性尿毒性综合征
	食管炎	过敏性紫癜
	Mallory-Weiss 裂伤	感染性结肠炎
	胃造口管继发损伤	肛裂
	嗜酸细胞性胃肠病	嗜酸细胞性胃肠病
	Munchausen 综合征	炎性肠病
	非甾体抗炎病	血管病变
	异物	
	化学治疗	

NSAIDS，非甾体抗炎药物。

健康新生儿大多数胃肠道出血是良性的和自限性的。早产儿或是经历了生理性应激的婴儿经常会有“咖啡样”胃吸出物或黑便。即使出血很少，也应考虑维生素 K 缺乏的可能，并做凝血试验。新生儿出血性疾病是一种自限性的出血性疾病，是由于维生素 K 依赖的凝血因子缺乏所致。维生素 K 依赖的凝血因子出生后迅速下降，生后 48 ~ 72 小时达到最低点。自新生儿生后不久常规应用维生素 K 以来，这种疾病几乎消失。然而，随着维生素 K 治疗失败、抗生素治疗导致的肠道菌群改变、囊性纤维化导致的脂肪吸收不良、新生儿病毒或细菌性败血症和母乳喂养的增多，使得发生出血性疾病的危险增加[7]。

呕血或在胃吸出物中有大量的出血很可能来自分
娩时吞咽了母亲的血液所致[4]，Apt 试验可确诊。具 1385
体做法是将新生儿胃中鲜红的血液放在有 1% NaOH 的滤纸上，母亲的血会减少和变成深棕色，如果是胎儿自身的血，那么就不会减少，颜色仍保持粉红或红色。

出生时窘迫、需要液体复苏的新生儿、早产儿或是正进行机械通气的新生儿由于应激性胃炎，更容易出现“咖啡样”的胃吸出物。在新生儿重症监护病房中，高达20%的患儿出现这种情况。如Apt试验阴性和排除凝血障碍，这些新生儿应该经口腔插入胃管洗胃和静脉输注 H_2 阻断剂。如果出血持续或恶化，可推迟进一步的评估。

当在婴儿的大便外面发现鲜红色血或是在尿布中有几滴鲜血时，在那些看起来正常的婴儿中最常见的诊断是肛裂或是直肠黏膜撕裂，大多数是由于坚硬的大便损伤所致。后正中线评估和简单肛检通常能确诊[12]。治疗是给予粪便软化剂和温水坐浴，很少需要切除。如果在较大的婴儿中或是直肠黏膜前方有裂隙应该考虑炎性肠病的可能。

早产儿如果经直肠排出血液应该考虑坏死性结肠炎，这种情况下的死亡率可高达40%，在新生儿加强监护病房中1%~7.7%的婴儿被诊断为坏死性结肠炎[12]。这些婴儿可以表现为麻痹性肠梗阻、腹胀、胆汁性呕吐、腹壁红斑或包块和消化道出血。腹部X线平片显示肠壁增厚、肠壁积气症、门静脉积气或是气腹[13]。造影检查既不被推荐也不是适应证。这些患儿的处理包括置胃管、应用广谱抗生素、静脉液体复苏、肠道休息、全静脉营养和连续的检查。在临床症状恶化或有肠坏死或穿孔证据时应考虑手术治疗，包括剖腹探查、引流、切除或减压。经过初次治疗后的再发性出血提示坏死性结肠炎的再次发生或是坏死性结肠炎后的肠狭窄（见92章）。

伴中肠扭转的肠旋转不良是新生儿期一个最危急的外科急症，表现为先前正常的婴儿突发黑粪和胆汁性呕吐。在病程的初期，临床检查无异常，随后出现
1386 进行性的腹胀和触痛。紧急的上消化道造影是必要的，可以显示一个异常的十二指肠空肠连接部和近端小肠“螺丝锥征”或是“鸟喙状中断征”（如果肠梗阻是完全性的）[13]。对反旋的肠管应迅速实施剖腹探查术，判断肠管的活力，松解Ladd束带，同时行阑尾切除术（Ladd手术）（见84章）。

1月~2岁婴儿最常见的出血原因

婴儿上消化道出血最常见的原因：

食管炎
胃炎
肥厚性幽门狭窄
消化性溃疡病

婴儿下消化道出血最常见的原因：

肛裂
乳蛋白过敏（过敏性直肠结肠炎）
肠套迭
肠重复畸形
Meckel 憩室

1月~2岁婴儿上消化道出血最常见的两个原因是食管炎和胃炎。消化性食管炎是由于胃食管反流所致，这些患儿表现为反胃、吞咽时疼痛（吞咽痛）、吞咽困难导致的厌食症或是生长停滞[1]。由单纯性疱疹病毒、巨细胞病毒或带状疱疹病毒引起的病毒性食管炎在免疫受损的儿童中更常见但是有类似的症状。食管摄片、食管腔内pH探针、带活组织检查的食管镜检、食管测压和99Tc乳剂扫描有助于区别是病毒性还是消化性的食管炎，并可以评估反流的程度。对消化性的食管炎，质子泵抑制剂（PPIs）和推动剂是第一线的治疗[8]。阿昔洛韦和更昔洛韦被分别用来治疗单纯性疱疹病毒和巨细胞病毒感染。抗反流的方法很少用来控制出血，但是当药物治疗无效、有狭窄形成的危险以及由误吸引起肺部并发症的患儿可考虑使用。

儿童中胃炎最常见的原因是原发性胃炎和消化性溃疡病（PUD），两者都与幽门螺旋杆菌感染有关[1]。感染最多见于胃窦，但也可发生在全胃[6]。继发性胃炎及PUD的发生与严重的全身性疾病如烧伤、头外伤或Crohn病、来自异物或胃造口管的机械性损伤或是使用非皮质激素抗炎药相关。胃炎是一个组织学诊断，需要上消化道内镜和活组织检查。幽门螺旋杆菌感染需联合用质子泵抑制剂、抗生素和铋剂。随着质子泵抑制剂的出现，消化性溃疡或胃炎只有在持续性的出血、慢性溃疡或穿孔时才需要手术[12]（见77章）。

肥厚性幽门狭窄由于胃炎偶尔出现微带血性或“咖啡样”的呕吐[14]。在适当的年龄和性别并伴有非胆汁性的喷射性呕吐时，应怀疑此诊断。幽门括约肌切开术可纠正并可抑制出血（见76章）。

婴儿直肠出血最常见的原因是乳蛋白过敏症或过敏性结肠炎[15]，这些过敏症可以产生隐性失血或肉

眼可见的出血，与易怒、饮食不佳、腹泻、呕吐和生长停滞有关[1]。通常可根据临床表现作出诊断，但是血及大便中有嗜酸性粒细胞显著增多和结肠活检可支持此诊断。大豆不耐受仅仅被发现存在于 14% 的患儿中，如果配方已改变而症状持续存在时应考虑大豆蛋白质或肽敏感[16]。另外，如果症状严重，母乳喂养的母亲应该避免饮用奶制品。

肠套迭是引起 6～18 个月婴幼儿便血的常见原因，90% 的肠套迭是回结肠型，可能是因为在婴儿回肠末段 peyer 斑处有丰富的淋巴组织。60% 的病例表现为阵发性的腹部绞痛、非胆汁性或胆汁性呕吐和血黏液样或果酱样大便[2]。超声有 97%～100% 的诊断准确率和 100% 的阴性预测价值。然而许多放射科医生仍喜欢钡灌肠，因为它既可以用于诊断，也可以用于治疗[5]。超声下或荧光透视指导下的空气整复也是有效的。如果空气整复不成功，标准的治疗依然是立即外科手术，但一些报道已经强调重复的空气灌肠可以将整复率从 71% 提高到 90%[9]。在手术的整复过程中，肠管要从远段向近段小心地挤压，如果有明显的浆膜撕裂或肠管看上去缺血则需要切除此段肠管，许多外科医生同时行阑尾切除术来避免将来因为右下象限切口的存在引起混淆。肠套迭在非手术整复后有 5%～10% 的复发率，在手术整复后有 1%～4% 的复发率[5]（见 83 章）。

1 月～2 岁儿童血液大量丢失的两个可能原因是胃肠道重复畸形和 Meckel 憩室。Meckel 憩室是儿童中严重直肠出血最常见的原因[3]，憩室中的异位胃黏膜引起邻近的回肠黏膜消化性溃疡，导致无痛性、间断或大量的直肠出血[3]。如果高度怀疑是 Meckel 憩室引起的出血，99Tc 扫描应是最初选择的一项检查。这项检查在局部有异位胃黏膜的病例中有 85% 的敏感性和 95% 的特异性。如果出血严重而扫描结果是阴性的，应实施血管造影来定位和栓塞。有出血症状

时，Meckel 憩室诊断可成立，则行憩室切除并同时施行阑尾切除术（见 82 章）。

像 Meckel 憩室一样，由于异位胃黏膜的存在胃肠道重复畸形也可以引起直肠出血。重复畸形可发生在消化道的任何地方，这些患儿通常表现为直肠出血或痛性及增大的腹部肿块。如果存在异位胃黏膜，则 99Tc 扫描是有用的，然而，肠道重复畸形经常在手术前没有得到诊断，当剖腹探查中发现病变的话，必需切除。

2 岁以上患儿最常见的出血原因

2 岁以上儿童上消化道出血最常见的原因：

食管静脉曲张
消化性溃疡病
胃炎
食管炎

2 岁以上患儿下消化道出血最常见的原因：

息肉
Meckel 憩室
炎性肠病
外伤
血管病变
感染性结肠炎

食管静脉曲张的发生是由于肝前、肝内、肝后阻塞引起门静脉高压的结果。患儿通常表现为突然的大量呕血。如果是肝前阻塞引起的，因为肝功能正常，出血经常会自行停止或是经轻微干预即停止。在这些患儿中，治疗的方法主要是长期消除门静脉高压。肝内、肝后阻塞伴有肝硬化的患儿通常采取姑息治疗直至肝移植成为可能[10]。尽管过量输液可能会增加门静脉压和导致血液继续丢失，食管静脉曲张引起的出血应立即开始液体复苏[10]。一旦患儿病情稳定，应用食道胃十二指肠镜检查来证实食管静脉曲张的诊断和评估胃和十二指肠的情况。硬化疗法和结扎静脉曲张处在检查中也可以运用。血管收缩药物如垂体后叶加压素、生长抑素、奥曲肽已成功用于控制儿童静脉曲张破裂出血，明确诊断后应着手应用此类药物。对于那些应用内镜不成功的肝硬化患儿，可以考虑经颈静脉的肝内门体循环分流。不得已时可以考虑紧急的外科手术分流（见 106 章）。

间断少量或持续的直肠出血可由消化道息肉引起。幼稚的炎症性息肉是 2 岁以上儿童直肠出血最常见的原因。出血通常与肠管暂时的位置变动相关，而且很少有大量的出血。可以用钡剂灌肠造影或是结肠镜检做出诊断，可采用简单的内镜息肉切除术做保守处理。这些息肉经常会自行脱落并排出。在儿童期，易形成幼稚性息肉，而到青春期该趋势会逐渐减少（见 91 章）。

15%~20%的炎性肠病通常在儿童期被诊断[11]。溃疡性结肠炎和 Crohn 病两者都可以表现为血样腹泻。尽管病因可以通过钡剂灌肠的特异性表现来推断，最终确诊仍需要带活组织检查的结肠镜检。该疾病通过药物治疗出血通常可自发停止（见 93 章和 94 章）。

患儿表现为腹泻和下消化道出血时应该考虑感染性结肠炎。也许从症状上很难和炎性肠病区别，但是通过大便培养可以很容易地排除该病。在任何先前经抗生素治疗的患儿，都应该考虑有艰难梭状芽胞杆菌感染的可能。然而，这个诊断不大可能出现在新生儿和婴幼儿中，因为该年龄段的儿童肠上皮缺乏毒素受体[1]。口服 10 天甲硝唑或是万古霉素对 95% 的患儿有效。其他细菌如大肠杆菌（0157:H7）、沙门菌、志贺菌属和弯曲杆菌是侵袭性的，可以引起血样腹泻。这些感染通常是自限性的，仅仅只需要支持治疗，除非那些有严重疾病的患儿。

在儿科人群中，影响消化道的血管病变相对罕见，但是可以引起急性的或慢性的血液丢失。这些病变包括血管瘤、静脉畸形、动静脉畸形和血管炎。如果血量丢失较少，上或下消化道内镜检查通常是第一线的治疗，它不仅可以诊断，而且可以治疗。如果内镜检查不能确诊或是肉眼出血量大，则要考虑核素扫描或血管造影。只有已局部准确定位或经过上述其他治疗无效的持续出血才考虑手术治疗。

（汪 健译 朱锦祥校）

参考文献

1. Arain Z, Rossi TM: Gastrointestinal bleeding in children: An overview of conditions requiring nonoperative management. Semin Pediatr Surg 1999;8:172-180.
2. Bisset GS III, Kirks DR: Intussception in infants and children: Diagnosis and therapy. Radiology 1988;168:141-145.
3. Brown RL, Azizkhan RG: Gastrointesinal bleeding in infants and children: Meckel's diverticulum and intestinal duplication. Semin Pediatr Surg 1999;8:202-209.
4. Bulstrode NW, Cuckow PM, Spitz LS: Neonatal gastrointestinal pseudohaemorrhage. J R Coll Surg Edinb 1998;43:355-356.
5. DiFiore JW: Intussusception. Semin Pediatr Surg 1999;8:214-220.
6. Drumm B: *Helicobacter pylori* in the pediatric patient. Gastroenterol Clin North Am 1993;22:169.
7. Fox VL: Gastrointestinal bleeding in infancy and childhood. Gastroenterol Clin North Am 2000;29:37-66.
8. Glassman M, George D, Grill B: Gastrointestinal reflux in children. Gastroenterol Clin North Am 1995;24:71-98.
9. Gorenstein A, Raucher A, Serour F: Intussusception in children: Reduction with repeated delayed air enema. Radiology 1998;206:721-724.
10. Karrer FM, Narkewicz MR: Esophageal varices: Current management in children. Semin Pediatr Surg 1999;8:193-201.
11. O'Hara SM: Acute gastrointestinal bleeding. Radiol Clin North Am 1997;35:879-895.
12. Pearl RH, Irish MS, Caty MG, Glick PL: The approach to common abdominal diagnoses in infants and children: Part II. Pediatr Clin North Am 1998;45:1287-1326.
13. Racadio JM, Agha A, Johnson ND, Warner BW: Imaging and radiological interventional techniques for gastrointestinal bleeding in children. Semin Pediatr Surg 1999;8:181-192.
14. Spitz L, Batcup G: Haematemesis in infantile hypertrophic pyloric stenosis: The source of the bleeding. Br J Surg 1979;66:827.
15. Teach SJ, Fleicher GR: Rectal bleeding in pediatric emergency department. Ann Emerg Med 1994;23:1252-1258.
16. Zeiger RS, Sampson HA, Bock SA, et al: Soy allergy in IgE-associated cow's milk allergy. J Pediatr 1999;134:614-622.

第 88 章

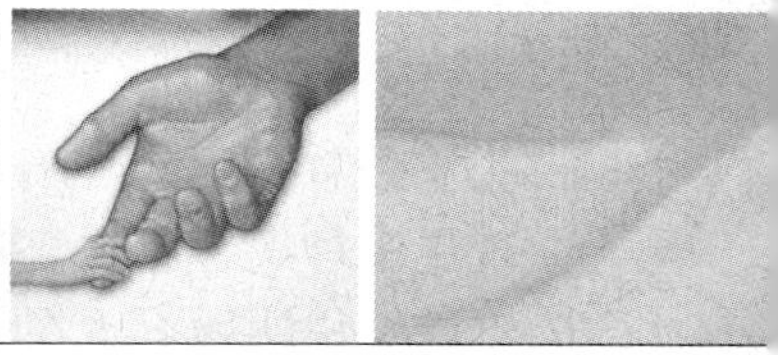

消化道重复畸形

Dennis P. Lund

1389 术语“消化道重复畸形”包括贯穿整个胃肠道的各种包块性病变，或是管状的或是囊性的。由Calder在1733年首次报道，被提及的这些病变大多是依据位置和相关组织结构来描述的[6]。现在通常指的消化道或肠道重复畸形已经被冠以不同的名称如巨大憩室、肠囊肿、回肠或结肠重复、巨大胸腔囊肿重复和再重复及不常用的 Meckel 憩室。没有单一的分类系统可以合理地解释所有这些病变的胚胎学、部位和临床表现。

1937 年，William Ladd 建议用消化道重复这一术语试图简化命名[26]，我们将这个名词的广泛应用归功于他的影响。Ladd 把这个词用于具有 3 个特征的先天性病变：（1）有发育良好的平滑肌层；（2）内衬的上皮代表某一部分肠道黏膜；（3）与胃肠道某些部分有密切的解剖联系。Ladd 和 Gross 在 1941 年的教科书《婴幼儿腹部外科学》中报道了 18 例这样的病例[27]。Gross 在 1953 年的教科书《婴幼儿外科学》中报道了 68 例[16]。1958 年 Swenson 在《小儿外科学》中对这个主题引入了一个章节[50]，但是 Potts 在 1959 年的短篇著作《外科医生和孩子》中并未提及重复畸形[39]。

消化道重复畸形的发生率在一个尸解系列报道中为 1/4500[38]，从口咽部到肛门的任何部位都可以发生，男性稍多[20]。Heiss 用 Meta 分析法分析了 12 个大的系列包含 580 名患者，见表 88-1，显示大约 20% 的病变发生在胸腔，其余的位于腹腔，小部分位于胸腹腔[17]。虽然胚胎的起源部位并不明确，但根据它们的位置，通常所说的重复畸形为前肠、中肠及后肠衍生的。肠重复畸形经常含有与相邻的胃肠道类似的黏膜，但也不总是这样。例如，有些重复畸形含有胃黏膜，会表现与位置无关的消化道溃疡或出血症状，有报道在颈部重复畸形中出现直肠黏膜。有 10%~20% 的患者肠重复是多发的，出现一个病变时应寻找其他部位的病变[20]。

最后，肠重复畸形的儿童并发其他异常疾病的发病率似乎也很高。在一些病例里已发现脊柱异常，尤其是胸腔或是胸腹部病变者。肠旋转不良和肠闭锁已发现伴腹部重复畸形。有报道泌尿道异常合并中肠和后肠重复畸形。在所有患者都是多发的重复畸形的一个系列中，发现有骨骼或泌尿道畸形[20]。

胚胎学

Ladd 采用消化道重复畸形这一术语是由于他认

表 88-1　580 例肠重复畸形的位置

部位	数量	%
颈部	6	1
纵隔	95	18
胸腹部	13	2
胃	35	7
十二指肠	30	6
空、回肠	282	53
结肠	68	13
直肠	19	4
其他	3	0.5
总计	580	100

来自 Heiss K 的 Meta 分析：肠重复畸形。

摘自 Oldham KT, Colombani PM, Foglia RP (eds): Surgery of Infants and Children: Scientific Principles and Practice. Philadelphia, Lippincott-Raven, 1997。

1390 为它们有相同的胚胎学机制。随着胚胎学的发展，出现了多种解释肠重复畸形的理论，但是没有哪一种理论能够说明所有现在知道的变异体。有 4 种主要的理论可以解释大多数目前看到的变异体。

部分或中断的孪生作用

重复畸形的第一个可能机制是由于部分或者中断的孪生作用。已有头、口腔、上消化道、后肠和下泌尿生殖道双倍畸形的报道，该机制似乎最能够说明这些情况。多个病例报道描述了完全双倍的结肠、膀胱、尿道和外生殖器[2]，这些孩子中有些还有严重的骨骼异常。孪生畸形的时间可以用来解释孪生的程度，例如，妊娠早期原条的分裂，紧接着尾端的生长会导致胎儿尾端完全的孪生，然而，晚期的分裂可能只导致结肠的重复畸形。

分裂的脊索理论和异常附着

1960 年，Bentey 和 Smith 提出了脊索分裂综合征的理论来描述涉及脊柱、胃肠道、胸部皮肤的多种畸形[3]。根据该理论，在妊娠的第 3 周（第 8 期），脊索似乎向头侧生长。脊索开始与内胚层紧密联系，与内胚层细胞正常分离。在分离中，有时会出现一个沟，经过这个沟，来自前肠（内胚层）的一个憩室以不完全分离的方式突出。然后这些来自于发育中的前肠的内胚层细胞附着在外胚层上并形成一个囊，或者，如果它们继续附着在脊索上，可以作为以后脊柱中胚层前部融合的一个屏障，导致在神经肠源性囊肿中看到的脊柱前裂。因此，这种机制可以解释许多胸部消化道重复畸形背侧的位置，也可以解释那些与其有联系的脊柱异常情况。它是否能解释所有的前肠重复畸形尚不明确。一个类似的异常附着机制可以解释发生在腹腔，但似乎在胸腔高位束缚于脊柱的少见的长段重复畸形。这种附着可能早期发生，甚至可能早于脊索出现，因此解释了这种重复畸形为何跨越如此长的距离[48]。

憩室和腔化不全

胎儿胃肠道经过胚胎学家称作的“实心期”之后，肠道会逐渐按从头部到尾部方向形成一个腔道。多年来，已认识到在哺乳动物胚胎中存在一些憩室[30]。这些憩室最常位于回肠，这是许多肠重复畸形的位置。因此，推测这种理论对肠重复畸形的形成有作用的假设似乎是合理的。然而，这种理论不能解释有异位黏膜尤其是胃的情况，也不能解释大部分重复畸形位于背侧，而许多憩室位于肠系膜的对侧面。Bremer 推测一些少见的重复畸形是由于肠道腔化异常引起的[5]。通过检查许多胚胎后，Moutsouris 认为这可能在闭锁段的形成上起作用[35]。已经明确肠腔完全恢复出现在 18 mm期。Bremer 提出肠重复畸形是由于肠道腔化不完全或缺陷的结果。该理论解释了重复畸形而不伴有其他相关畸形出现的原因，但是也存在一些与憩室理论相同的缺点，尤其是不能够解释重复畸形或黏膜的异位为何大多数位于肠系膜。

环境因素

众所周知，不同时期的胎儿存在明显的环境应激。Mellish 和 Koop 提出缺氧和创伤会诱导重复畸形和孪生[34]。一些资料支持这一理论，即其他的畸形尤其是肠闭锁，可能是由宫腔内血管意外诱导的[32]。这些胚胎理论在肠重复畸形中发挥的作用尚不清楚。很明显，在胚胎发育过程中，会有许多组织的生长、分化、迁移、程序性细胞死亡和组织粘连。这些发育机制的任何一个环节障碍都可能涉及肠重复畸形的形成。最可能的是，如同有多种形式的肠重复畸形一样，也会有许多因素导致它们的形成。

临床表现

肠重复畸形通常是囊状或者管状肿块。根据大小、位置、毗邻和它们是否有异位黏膜会有不同的表现。大多数重复畸形在 2 岁前诊断。通常，肠重复畸形表现的症状可以和其他胃肠道疾病相混淆，例如急性阑尾炎。许多重复畸形仅有少量或者是没有症状，而是在检查其他症状例如咳嗽、腹痛、胃食管反流时意外发现的。肠重复畸形可以通过产前超声就得到诊断。囊性肿块在超声下表现为黑洞，如果足够大很容易看到[11]。

1391 如果肿块在胸部，可以表现为哮喘、肺炎或者吞咽困难，促使患者行 X 线检查。其他潜在症状包括发育停滞、呼吸困难和呕吐。除非出血或感染使肿块突然增大，胸痛是很罕见的症状。

腹痛、呕吐和腹部肿块是腹腔肠重复畸形最常见的症状和体征[21]。由于重复畸形是一个囊性肿块，因此肿块感染或分泌突然增多会导致急性腹痛。如果重复畸形有异位黏膜，可导致溃疡、出血甚至穿孔。急性增大的囊肿会引起邻近肠管的梗阻，导致恶心、呕吐和绞痛。巨大囊肿可能引起邻近肠管的局部扭转。50% 的患者可以触到移动性肿块[14]。胃和十二指肠重复畸形可引起呕吐、腹胀、黑便和穿孔。胃重复畸形可以特别大。有报道胃重复畸形表现类似幽门肥厚性狭窄并伴有胃出口的梗阻[15]。十二指肠重复可能是复发性胰腺炎的一个原因，可导致很高的死亡率[54]。

中肠和后肠的重复畸形更容易引起腹痛、腹胀、黑便或穿孔。那些发生在回肠的重复畸形容易与急性阑尾炎相混淆，很难在术前作出诊断。小肠重复畸形也可以表现为肠套迭，其作用是作为套迭的头部。

结肠和后肠的重复畸形可以简单地表现为在会阴部的第二个开口。在女性，这个开口可能在阴道的后壁，提示有直肠阴道瘘的可能[43]。后肠的重复畸形也可引起由肿块所致的症状，特别是肿块位于盆腔时，可压迫尿道或者导致严重便秘。骶骨前的重复畸形可以类似于骶尾部肿瘤如畸胎瘤和皮样囊肿。

诊断

由于产前超声的应用，消化道重复畸形的产前诊断变得更加普遍。早在 1984 年文献中就有了产前诊断的经验[51]，但是报道很少。随后的几十年随着经验的积累，大部分确诊的病例位于胸腔或者是上腹部，这些地方比较容易被超声发现。由于纵隔移位，胸部的病变可偶尔引起胎儿水肿，可采用宫内胸腔羊膜腔分流进行治疗[10]。到 2000 年为止，14 例腹部重复畸形病例被产前诊断[7]。

产前超声检查的经验迅速增加，2003 年，Montreal 小组报道了他们 22 年肠重复畸形的经验，18 名患儿得到产前诊断[40]。有趣的是，在他们的新生儿肠重复畸形组中，肠扭转的发生率是 23.8%，这就引发了当产前诊断出肠重复畸形后是早期手术干预还是密切观察的争议。

病史和体格检查在诊断中非常重要，这在肠重复畸形中也不例外。病史包括上面提到的症状，以及体格检查时腹部可以触到肿块。典型肿块似“沼泽状”（boggy）并可活动，根据患儿的症状可有或没有触痛。如果胸部肿块巨大可以伴有局部呼吸音减弱。除非患儿由于异位胃黏膜导致肿块出血而出现贫血，实验室检查几乎对诊断无帮助。如果患儿重复囊肿位于胰腺头部时，会有血淀粉酶和脂肪酶升高，同时伴有其他胰腺炎的表现。

超声检查也可有助于产后的诊断，因为这些病变通常很容易看到。除非有溃疡和出血，囊肿在超声上显示典型的无回声。由于是由平滑肌和黏膜组成，囊壁常有 2～3 mm 厚，这与其他囊肿如肠系膜、大网膜囊肿或卵巢囊肿不同，这些典型的囊肿更大，只含有简单的壁。肠重复囊肿的黏膜内衬在囊肿内产生特征性的有回波的信号（图 88-1）[51]。其他形式的超声如内镜超声检查[12]，已经可准确诊断肠重复畸形特别是前肠重复畸形。

其他放射学检查如平片、胃肠道造影和 CT 或 MRI 可能也有助于肿块的诊断和定位（图88-2）。由于囊性重复畸形并不与肠管相通，胃肠道成像本身并不能显示病变。然而，胃肠道成像可以反映肿块对肠
道的压迫，在诊断中很有帮助（图88-3）。肠重复畸 1392

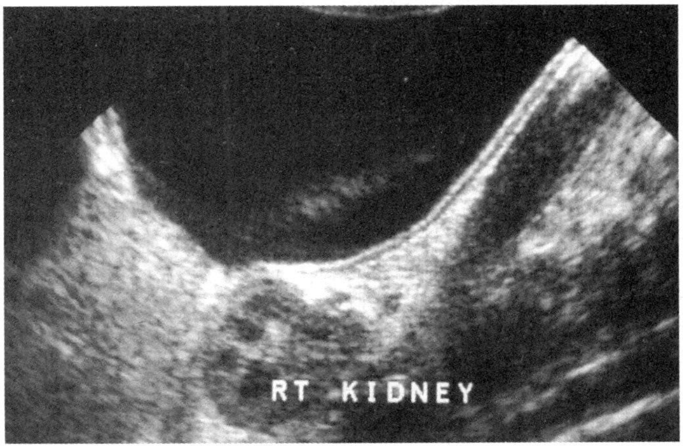

图 88-1 回肠重复畸形的超声检查显示黏膜内衬特征性的回声信号。

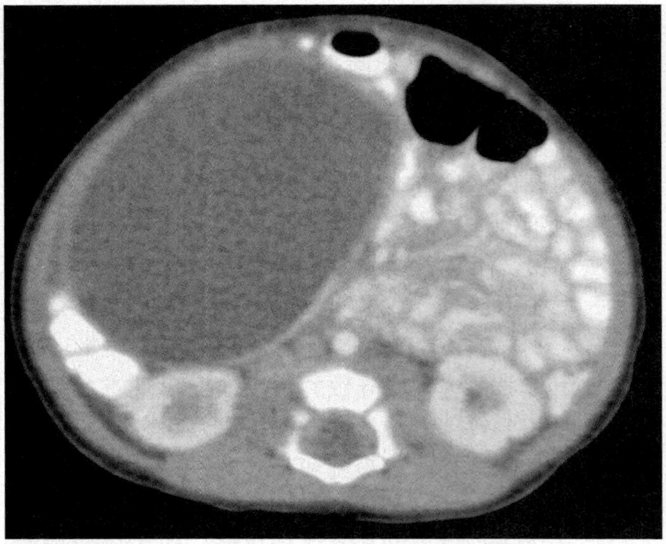

图 88-2　CT 扫描显示胰腺头部有一个巨大的囊性肿块，诊断为十二指肠重复畸形。（Courtesy of Dr. Aimen Shaaban）

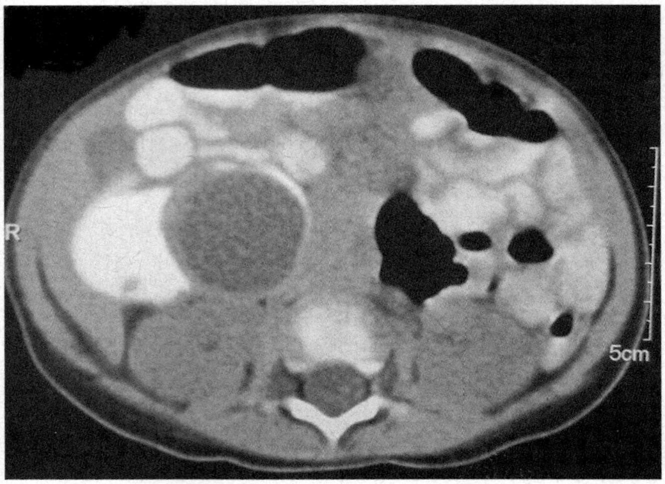

图 88-4　一个婴儿的 CT 扫描显示存在一个边缘增强的回肠囊性重复畸形。

形的 CT 扫描表现为典型的囊性肿块并有增强的边缘，因此容易和脓肿相混淆（图88-4）。然而，在缺乏脓毒血症的临床征象（例如发热和白细胞计数升高）时，这样的 CT 影像应该提示重复畸形而不是脓肿。需要对包括尿道的其他结构进行术前检查，了解重复畸形的范围和对周围结构的影响，这些检查可能会影响病变的安全处理。

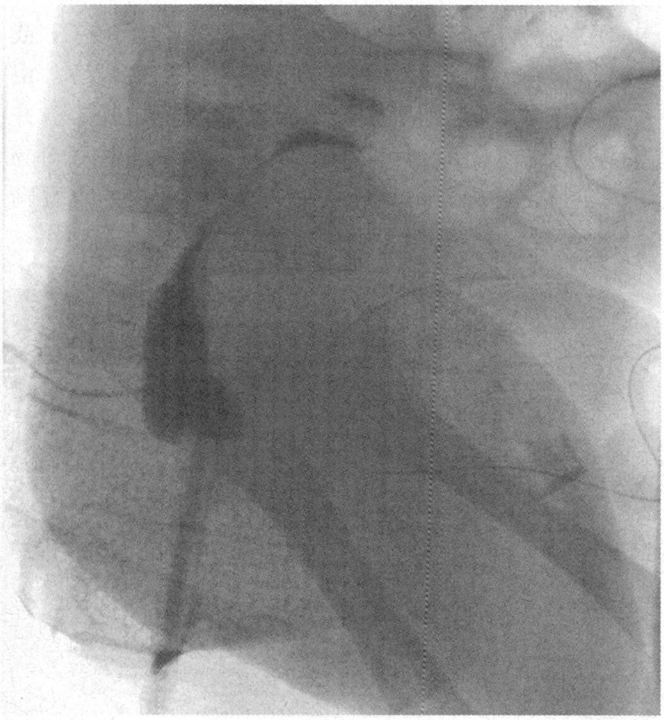

图 88-3　钡灌肠检查显示一个少见的前方直肠重复畸形压迫直肠。

中肠和后肠重复畸形可能更难诊断，经常在手术时才作出诊断。这些病变可以表现为肠扭转或肠套迭，有时只在手术时才发现。正如先前提到的，许多重复畸形含有异位胃黏膜。有合适的临床环境下，例如，在一个有贫血和腹痛的患儿，就像诊断 Meckel 憩室一样，Tc99m 扫描可能会有帮助[52]。实际上，由于两者都位于回肠，肠重复畸形常与 Meckel 憩室相混淆。因此，谨慎的外科医生在鉴别诊断时应考虑这两种情况。

颈食管重复畸形

颈食管重复囊肿极其罕见。在本书的上一版中提到，文献报道少于 10 例。从那以后，仅有 1 例报道[55]。几乎所有这些病例都在出生后早期发病，并伴有威及生命的呼吸困难。症状通常在出现肿块前表现出来。通常需要插管、快速诊断和干预。肿块可以在体格检查时鉴别，但是 CT 是最好的诊断方式。鉴别诊断包括其他的颈部囊性肿块，例如淋巴管畸形和气道囊肿、鳃器或甲状舌管囊肿。可能的话，治疗包括手术切除。如果不能完全切除，应该去掉重复畸形的黏膜以闭塞囊腔。

393 ## 胸腔和胸腹部重复畸形

大约有 20% 的消化道重复畸形发生于胸腔或位于胸腹部。在婴幼儿纵隔肿块的鉴别诊断时，重复畸形仅次于神经源性肿瘤排在第二位[42]。大多数病变位于后纵隔的下部，并可以突入到两侧胸廓。许多这类病变被列入神经管原肠囊肿的分类中，因为它们与重复畸形和椎管连接有关，同时伴脊柱异常。也有一类非常少见的囊性病变位于中枢神经系统如小脑和视神经，与胃肠道没有联系，但含有异位胃肠道黏膜，局部压迫神经结构而引起症状[33,34]。虽然神经管与原肠囊肿最常见于胸部，但可发生于其他部位，组成位于膈以下肠重复畸形的一小部分[1]。当发现脊柱异常时应该怀疑胸部的病变。几乎所有的神经管与原肠囊肿会有脊柱异常，但不是所有位于胸腔的囊肿都是神经管与原肠的。在 Holcomb 和他的助手报道的一个系列研究中，21 个胸腔重复畸形患者中 5 个有脊柱异常[19]。

正如前面提到的，胸腔病变已经被产前超声确诊，并尝试在胎儿呼吸困难时进行宫内治疗[10]。虽然胸腔重复畸形通常没有症状并可由于其他原因行常规影像学检查时发现，但是最常见的症状是呼吸困难[19,20]。重复畸形偶尔与其他畸形有关如食管闭锁或膈疝。胸腔重复畸形与其他畸形包括脊柱异常同时发生，提示应寻找多发的重复畸形，因为它可出现在多达 1/3 的病例中。一旦胸部有可疑的囊性肿块，评估的最佳手段是 CT，应该包括腹部，因为 1/4 的胸腔重复畸形会伴有腹部的第 2 处重复畸形。钡餐检查对于描述重复畸形与食管的关系和制定手术计划有帮助（图 88-5）。如果怀疑为心包的囊肿，超声心动图也可能有帮助；尽管大多数肠重复畸形位于后纵隔，心包囊肿可能位于前或中纵隔。最后，如果囊肿是神经管与原肠的，脊柱 MRI 对于了解囊肿与脊柱和椎管的密切关系会有帮助。在这点上，MRI 在很大程度上取代了脊柱造影。

胸腔和胸腹部消化道畸形的治疗主要为切除，只要有可能就要实施。可以通过胸腔镜切除，尽管并不总是可行。囊肿减压可能有助于切除，但如果囊肿小的话，尽可能保留囊肿完整有利于切除。位于食管壁内的囊肿，可以打开食管平滑肌进行囊肿黏膜外切除术，保留黏膜的完整。囊肿切除后，特别是通过胸腔镜切除的，外科医生必须确保液体或空气没有进入食管腔，未识别的食管漏将导致纵隔炎和严重的死亡率。

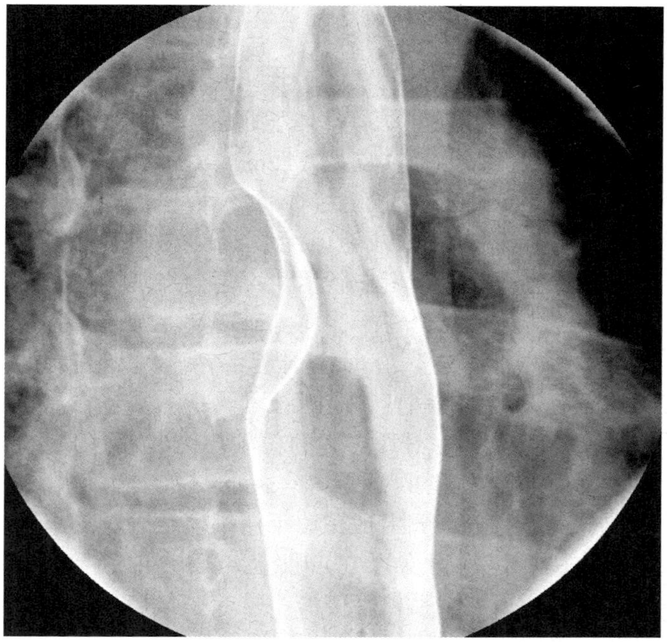

图 88-5　吞钡造影显示一个食管重复畸形对中段食管形成压迫。这个男孩表现为胸痛，通过胸腔镜切除重复畸形。

如果有脊柱内成分进入神经管与原肠囊肿，应该寻求与神经外科医生协作，并且脊柱内部分应尽可能先切除。这样将减少可能的脑膜炎发病率和减少囊肿切除后的水肿。

胸腹部巨大囊肿可以分阶段切除，以减少大型胸腹部切开术的死亡率。当分阶段实施手术时，囊肿的剩余部分应采用一种减压机制（例如引流入肠腔），避免术后由于囊肿阻塞而致泄漏，引起脓毒血症。万一囊肿不能完全切除，去除全部黏膜非常重要，这样囊肿就不会再复发，并且也切除了异位的胃黏膜。不提倡刮除术和纱布填塞囊腔以促进硬化，因为这种治疗形式比完全切除或正规的黏膜剥离有较高的并发症发生率。

腹部的前肠重复畸形

1394 胃和十二指肠重复通常体积很大（图 88-6）并且常有症状。大部分重复是囊性的。由于肿块的影响和对周围组织的压迫引起症状，导致胃出口梗阻、胰腺炎[54]，或伴有食欲减退但无缓冲胃酸过多的溃疡型的症状和腹痛，或者在新生儿可能会出现类似肥厚性幽门狭窄的症状[41]。

术语“胃重复”有时会引起混淆，因为它有时指的是与胃有关的病变，有时该术语指的是包含异位胃黏膜的病变，而不管它们的位置。为此经过讨论，术语“胃重复”指的是与胃有关的那些病变，最常出现在胃大弯。一般出现在幼年期，通常表现为可触及的肿块。这些病变可在产前超声检查时看到[13]。症状和体征可能包括发育停滞、呕吐、贫血、胃食管反流和腹痛。如此病变也可以导致伴气性腹膜炎的穿孔[24]或自发性腹腔积血[22]。超声评估对于上腹部的巨大囊肿是有诊断性的，并可与肥厚性幽门狭窄鉴别。如果肿块位于右上象限，可与胆总管囊肿相混淆，除非它们阻塞胆总管，前肠重复畸形通常不会伴有黄疸。上消化道造影可有助于描述病变的内容物及

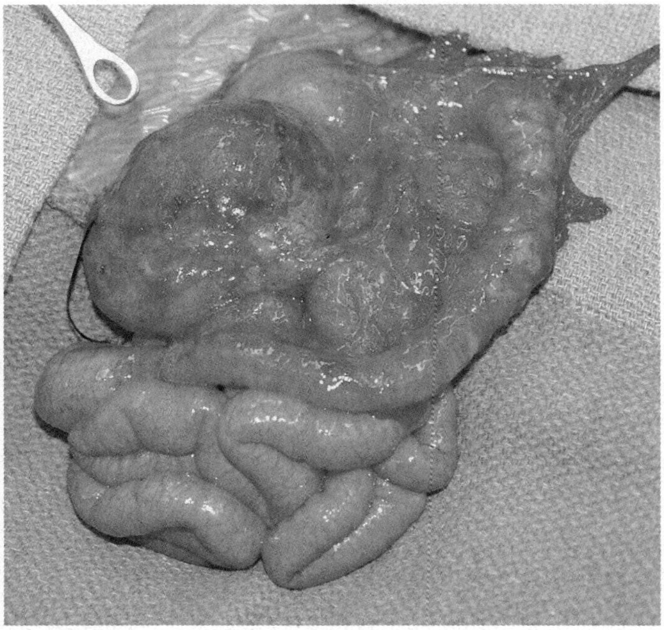

图 88-6 这一囊性肿块发生在一个有呕吐和胃出口梗阻症状的婴儿，肿块被完全切除。这一巨大十二指肠重复的 CT 扫描结果见图 88-2。（Courtesy of Dr. Aimen Shaaban）

与胃、十二指肠和胰腺的关系。

胃重复畸形的治疗方法是切除。通常，这些病变非常大并且与胃食管连接部或者幽门有密切关系。切除但不侵犯胃腔是最理想的，但是通常不可能做到。可能需要做部分胃切除或者部分囊肿切除加黏膜剥离。如果术后有胃排空延迟的话，胃造口术甚至营养性空肠造瘘术是有益的。最后，外科医生应该意识到胃重复囊肿与胰管系统相通的少见情况，尽管这更可能发生于十二指肠的重复畸形[18]。

十二指肠重复可以表现为胆道或胰腺的症状如黄疸和胰腺炎。典型的是症状表现较模糊，包括右上腹痛、早期饱胀感或生长停滞。病变最常位于十二指肠第 2、3 段的中后部。这些囊肿可能被混淆为胆总管囊肿，尤其是以黄疸为主要症状的胆总管囊肿。复发性胰腺炎也有报道。这些病变通常累及十二指肠或小肠黏膜，偶尔会与十二指肠腔相通。在检查模糊的腹部症状时，行上消化道造影检查或超声检查可注意到有一个压迫十二指肠的肿块。好的术前影像对十二指肠重复畸形特别重要，CT、内镜逆行胰胆管造影术（ERCP）和核磁共振胆管造影术对确定囊肿与胰腺和胆道系统的关系都有帮助。

虽然内镜或者经皮穿刺引流十二指肠重复畸形的治疗手段是可行的，最佳的治疗仍是切除。在那些切除了有潜在的高发病率的病例中，内引流是安全和有效的。因为这些病例很有挑战性，手术医生必须掌握多种技术来实施这样的手术。例如，局部的十二指肠切除和重建可能足够了[47]，但是囊肿与十二指肠的造袋术或者是囊肿与小肠袢的 Roux-en-Y 造袋术哪种更可取则要根据病变的解剖位置。最后，胰十二指肠切除术（Whipple 术式）对于充分地处理囊肿几乎没有必要[54]。无论选择哪种手术方式，术中胆道造影对确保囊肿切除后胆道完整和没有阻塞是最安全的。在囊肿含有胃黏膜的病例中，明智的方法是通过囊肿切除或者是黏膜剥离去除所有的异位胃黏膜。

小肠重复畸形

小肠近端的重复畸形是最常见的肠重复畸形，大多数位于回肠。它们可能是囊性或者是管状的，并且大多数位于小肠的系膜侧。这与 Meckel 憩室是相反的，Meckel 憩室位于肠系膜的对侧。通常，重复畸形

与相邻的肠管有共同的平滑肌壁和血供，以致于重复
395 畸形就位于肠系膜上。这提示在重复畸形的治疗中，切除重复畸形可能需要切除相邻的肠管，因其与肠腔交通可能是变异的。肠重复畸形通过产前超声诊断为肠畸形的日益增多。

小肠重复畸形的症状和体征多样，但是腹痛和（或）肿块是最常见的。小的囊性重复畸形可以作为小肠套迭的头部或导致局部的扭转。如果重复畸形增大或者肿胀，可以导致邻近肠管受压和引起梗阻症状。如果重复畸形为管状或者与相邻肠管交通，这种可能性更大。有远端交通的重复畸形很少变得充盈或引起梗阻型的症状。一些含有异位胃黏膜的重复畸形能够引起消化性溃疡、出血或穿孔。有异位黏膜的可以用 Tc99m 扫描诊断（Meckel 憩室扫描），便血的患者也可应用这个试验来评价。通常，很难在术前作出重复畸形这一准确的诊断。

1998 年来自北京儿童医院的一个报道中，李和他的同事研究了 80 例小肠重复畸形的血供[31]。基于它们的血供不同将重复畸形分为两种类型。在Ⅰ型病变（平行型）中，有动脉供应的重复畸形位于肠系膜的一侧，而相对的静脉供应的直接进入原来的肠管。Ⅱ型（肠系膜内型）重复正好位于肠系膜并且静脉来自于肠系膜的两侧，横过肠系膜进入原来的肠管。有趣的是，李和他的同事发现Ⅱ型占整个病变的少数（24.6%），但是超过 90% 与胸部脊柱畸形有关，而Ⅰ型病变中仅有 5% 有脊柱畸形。李和他的同事根据这些发现提出这两种类型的肠重复畸形必然有不同的胚胎学原因。他们也提出了解肠重复畸形的血管解剖使得可以只切除病变部位而不需切除邻近的肠管[31]。

小肠重复畸形理想的治疗是切除。囊性重复畸形通常切除重复畸形和邻近的肠管，行再吻合术（图 88-7）。这可以通过开腹或者是腹腔镜技术实施[29,45,46]。腹腔镜对于开腹手术也是有辅助作用的，它可以诊断病变和减压，便于通过一个小的切口来做开腹切除手术。限制性切除对患者应该没有害处。如果不能切除，可以将病变引流入小肠的 Roux-en-Y 肠袢或者与邻近肠管构建一个很大的窗。手术时，彻底探查全部的肠管是明智的，因为这些患者常有较多的多发性病变。也有报道在新生儿期肠重复畸形与肠闭锁联合出现。除非表现为肠梗阻，产前超声诊断为肠重复的新生儿不必在新生儿期行切除手术[19]。然而，应该在几个月内实施切除以避免发生并发症例如梗阻

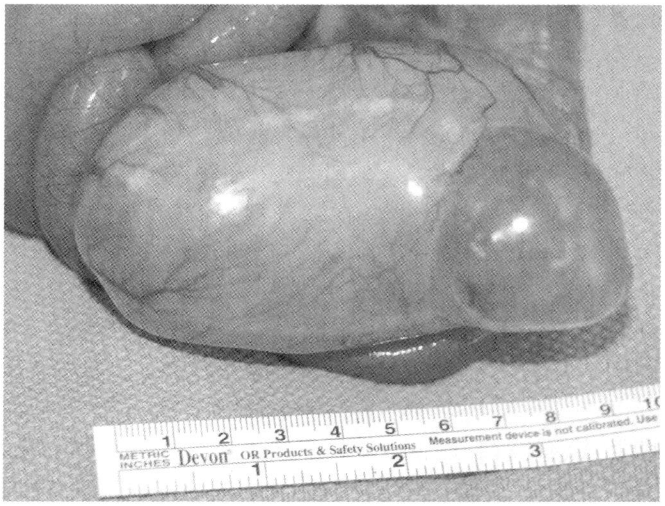

图 88-7　这个回肠囊性重复连同相邻的 5.0 cm 肠管从一 2 个月的女婴身上切除。肠的连续性通过一期吻合重建。这个肿块由产前超声诊断。

和（或）扭转。至少有 6 例腺癌出现在小肠重复畸形的报道，常较晚出现。所以如果能够切除就没有如此高的死亡率，应尽快切除这些病变[25]。

小肠长的管状重复畸形给手术治疗带来极大挑战，特别是如果切除邻近肠管会导致短肠综合征时。如果有异位胃黏膜出现，应该通过限制性切除或者是黏膜剥脱而去除，因为这可导致出血或者穿孔。重复畸形应该仔细检查，打开肠系膜以确定是否可以只切除重复畸形同时保留邻近肠管完整。由 Bianchi 提出的纵形肠延长技术可用于肠系膜的解剖[4]。另外，无论是近端还是远端在重复畸形与邻近肠管之间构建的大窗（造袋术），都应满足要求，以使重复畸形充分引流。这用线性胃肠吻合器很容易完成。如果选择造袋术治疗，这些病例必须随访以防日后由于保留的胃黏膜而出现症状。

后肠重复畸形

结肠和直肠重复畸形占所有肠重复畸形的 17%。它们可以是结肠壁或系膜上简单的囊性病变，或者十分广泛，延续结肠全长和作为一个单独的开口出现在
会阴部，有时在阴道的后壁。它们也可能与流产的孪 1396
生异常有关，在联体儿中亦有报道[36]，与尿道和生

殖器的重复或其他畸形有关。在这些病例中，这些复杂的畸形也可能与下半部的脊柱畸形有关。重复结肠通常只含有结肠黏膜而很少含有异位的胃黏膜。Kottra和 Dodds[23]描述了一种后肠重复畸形的分类系统，分为短的重复（Ⅰ型）和长管状重复（Ⅱ型）。然而，这种分类法在临床很少应用。尽管偶尔可见到位于前面的肿块，直肠重复畸形的典型表现为位于直肠后骶前间隙的大小各异的囊性肿块（见图88-3），可以出现在新生儿期或者是儿童后期的任何时间，甚至偶尔出现在青少年（图88-8）。

后肠重复畸形似乎有三种大体的分类。第一种是囊性或短柱状肿块，位于结肠系膜上，与许多中肠重复畸形相似，这一类型较少见。第二种是肿块位于中线，通常位于骶骨和尾骨的前方和直肠的后面。有时可能与直肠血供紧密联系，特别是病变向上延伸进入腹腔，需要广泛切除和重建。其他时候，它们可能更像囊性肿块，可以被切除而不影响直肠的血供。最后一种，结肠和直肠边对边的重复，在重复长度和位置上变异很大。该型女性更多见，可能与其他下腹部和尾部的畸形如泌尿生殖道畸形或脊柱裂相关。这些病变的治疗可能非常复杂，通常包括部分切除和（或）额外腔的开窗术。

很多重复畸形出现在后肠，与它们相联系的症状多种多样，这并不奇怪。可以表现为囊性肿块，或者

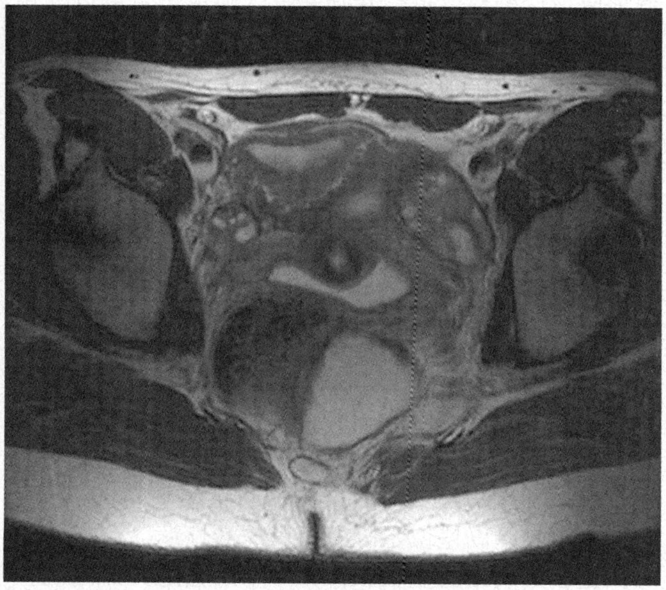

图88-8 一个17岁女孩直肠重复畸形合并感染的MRI影像。初期做了经皮外引流，然后通过后矢状途径切除。

出现腹胀和梗阻症状。还有许多表现为轻微症状或者伴有模糊的腹痛、便秘或生长停滞。开口在阴道处的重复畸形可以出现直肠阴道瘘的症状和体征（图88-9），如阴道排出气体或粪便。极少数病例也可伴有泌尿系统的梗阻或者潴溜。如果感染的话可与直肠周围脓肿或瘘相混淆。其他表现有直肠出血或者脱垂[28]。

后肠重复的诊断可能很困难。利用CT、MRI和钡灌肠准确地成像和术前评估对于确定治疗方法是非常重要的。会阴部的第2个开口可以逆行注入造影剂进行评估。直肠重复应该借助CT和MRI进行评估，这样可以显示病变的范围以及和直肠、脊柱和尿道的关系。一个三联征——骶前肿块、直肠狭窄和骶骨畸形——被称为Currarino三联征，是以常染色体显性方式遗传的[8]。正如有些小肠重复、短的或者囊性的后肠重复有时仅在手术中得以诊断。由于后肠重复很少含有胃黏膜，Tc99m扫描用处不大。

与大多数肠重复畸形一样，手术切除（如果可能）是最理想的治疗。对于短的结肠囊性重复可以行局限性的结肠切除或简单地从肠系膜将病变剥离。

如果骶前重复表现为脓肿，理想的方法是向外引流而不是通过直肠引流。经直肠引流会因为粪便菌群污染，导致脓肿复发。中线骶前的直肠重复可以通过后矢状路径切除[9]，有时可合并局限性的直肠壁切除，但是大多数不采用。神经刺激仪可能在解剖和重建过程中描绘盆部肌肉和括约肌有帮助。万一需要做肠切除术的病例，有可能的话，术前应做肠道准备。同样，在手术室里为患者做术前准备时应考虑到有时需要经腹部和会阴的联合途径。幸运的是，直肠前中线处的重复畸形非常少，但是它是一个艰难的手术挑战。切除病变是非常困难和危险的，因为需要移开直肠，并且可能损伤膀胱颈和括约肌。在一些病例中，手术可通过从上面去除病变的黏膜而把肌壁留于原位。为避免盆部脓毒血症的发生，当切除和重建变得困难或复杂时，外科医生应该准备利用临时转向的结肠造瘘术。如果重复畸形的所有黏膜没有去除，则会导致直肠重复切除最常见的并发症即复发。

长管状的后肠重复畸形需要创造性的手术方式。由于原始肠管与重复畸形有共同的血供，通常需要全部或者次全结肠切除术。在儿童中这并不是一个理想的选择。同样，在回盲瓣区域的重复畸形也经常会有变异，例如，在回肠远端可能有一个囊性的部分，邻

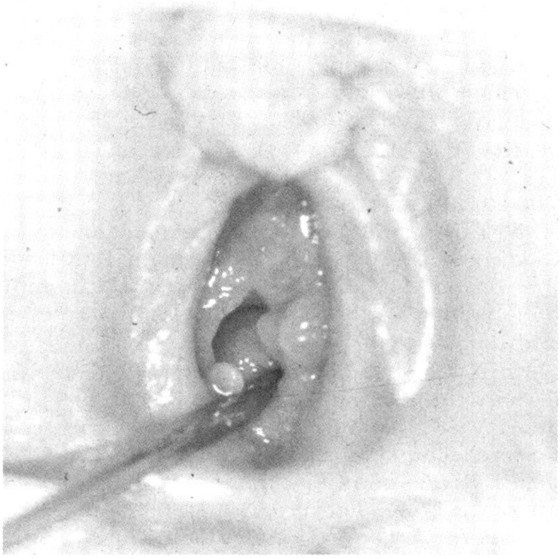

A

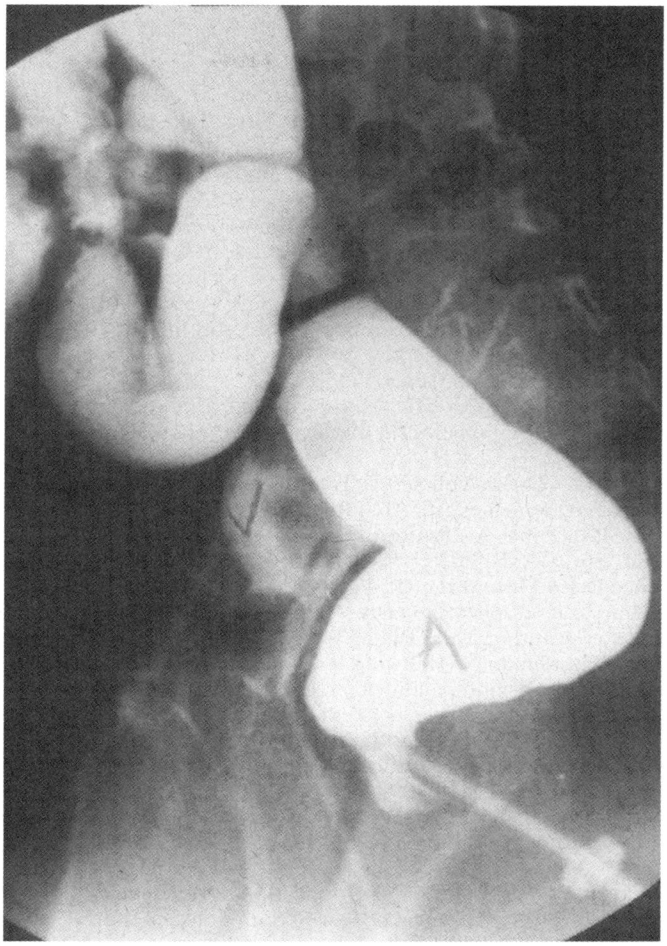

B

图 88-9　A. 这个女婴的父母发现她的大便从阴道排出。探针显示在阴道后壁上有第 2 个孔。B. 钡灌肠显示远端有 2 个腔，证明是一个完全的结肠重复畸形。

近结肠处伴有一个长的管状部分[43]。另外，如果重复的部分开口于会阴部或者进入泌尿生殖道，交通的部分也必须做处理。长的边对边的结肠重复可通过两个管腔的近段和远端广泛的开窗来治疗，也可以通过线性吻合器或者是手工侧侧吻合的方式做结肠切开术。如果开口于会阴，重复的远端不会通过括约机制（例如有一个通到阴道后壁的通道），应该很容易被切除。黏膜应该去除或者只有一小部分剩余以便可以将引流和粪便通道分开。为了适当地治疗这种重复畸形，外科医生需切除直肠或者切除后重建括约肌复合体。

结论

肠重复畸形可以多种多样的方式出现，可包括从颈部到肛门的多种病变。可以是单纯、囊性、复杂、多发或者是柱状的，也可以伴有其他畸形包括脊柱和泌尿生殖道畸形。最佳的治疗方式是手术切除，但是对于复杂的病例需要采用多种方法，包括开窗或黏膜剥离。通过合适的治疗，先天有肠重复畸形的患儿可以治愈，并且有良好的长期预后和生活质量。

（汪　健译　朱锦祥校）

参考文献

1. Alrabeeah A, Gillis DA, Giacomantonio M, Lau H: Neurenteric cysts—a spectrum. J Pediatr Surg 1988;23:752.
2. Beach PD, Brascho DJ, Hein WR, et al: Duplication of the primitive hindgut of the human with double colon, anus, bladder, uterus, vagina and vulva. Surgery 1961;49:794.
3. Bentley JFR, Smith JR: Developmental posterior enteric remnants and spinal malformations. Arch Dis Child 1960;35:76.
4. Bianchi A: Intestinal loop lengthening—a technique for increasing small intestine length. J Pediatr Surg 1980;15:145.
5. Bremer JL: Diverticula and duplications of the intestinal tract. Arch Pathol 1952;38:132.
6. Calder J: Medical Essays Obser 1733;1:205.
7. Correia-Pinto J, Tavares ML, Monteiro J, et al: Prenatal diagnosis of abdominal enteric duplications. Prenat Diagn 2000;20:163.
8. Currarino G, Coln D, Votteler T: Triad of anorectal, sacral, and presacral anomalies. AJR Am J Roentgenol 1981;137:395.
9. deVries PA, Pena A: Posterior sagittal anorectoplasty. J Pediatr Surg 1982;17:638.
10. Martinez-Ferro MM, Milner R, Voto L, et al: Intrathoracic alimentary tract duplication cysts treated in utero by thoracoamniotic shunting. Fetal Diagn Ther 1998;13:343.
11. Foley PT, Sithasanan N, McEwing R, et al: Enteric duplications presenting as antenatally detected abdominal cysts: Is delayed resection appropriate? J Pediatr Surg 2003;38:1810.
12. Geller A, Wang KK, DiMagno EP: Diagnosis of foregut duplication cysts by endoscopic ultrasonography. Gastroenterology 1996;109:838.
13. Granata C, Dell'Acqua A, Lituania M, et al: Gastric duplication cyst: Appearance on prenatal US and MRI. Pediatr Radiol 2003;33:148.
14. Grosfeld JL, Boles ET, Reiner C: Duplication of the pylorus in the newborn: A rare cause of gastric outlet obstruction. J Pediatr Surg 1970;5:365.
15. Grosfeld JL, O'Neill JA, Clatworth HW: Enteric duplications in infancy and childhood: An 18-year review. Ann Surg 1970;172:83.
16. Gross RE: Surgery of Infancy and Childhood. Philadelphia, WB Saunders, 1953.
17. Heiss K: Intestinal duplications. In Oldham KT, Colombani PM, Foglia RP (eds): Surgery of Infants and Children: Scientific Principles and Practice. Philadelphia, Lippincott-Raven, 1997.
18. Hoffman M, Sugerman HJ, Herman D: Gastric duplication cyst communicating with aberrant pancreatic duct: A rare cause of recurrent acute pancreatitis. Surgery 1987; 101:369.
19. Holcomb GW 3rd, Gheissari A, O'Neill JA Jr, et al: Surgical management of alimentary tract duplications. Ann Surg 1989;209:167.
20. Ildstad ST, Tollerud DJ, Weiss RG, et al: Duplications of the alimentary tract: Clinical characteristics, preferred treatment, and associated malformations. Ann Surg 1988;208:184.
21. Iyer CP, Mahour GH: Duplications of the alimentary tract in infants and children. J Pediatr Surg 1995;30:1267.
22. Kleinhaus S, Boley SJ, Winslow P: Occult bleeding from a perforated gastric duplication in an infant. Arch Surg 1981; 116:122.
23. Kottra JJ, Dodds WJ: Duplication of the large bowel. AJR Am J Roentgenol 1971;113:310.
24. Kremer RM, Kepoff RB, Izant RJ Jr: Duplication of the stomach. J Pediatr Surg 1970;5:360.
25. Kusunoki N, Shimada Y, Fukumoto S, et al: Adenocarcinoma arising in a tubular duplication of the jejunum. J Gastroenterol 2003;38:781.
26. Ladd WE: Duplications of the alimentary tract. South Med J 1937;30:363.
27. Ladd WE, Gross RE: Abdominal Surgery of Infancy and Childhood. Philadelphia, WB Saunders, 1941.
28. LaQuaglia MP, Feins N, Eraklis A, et al: Rectal duplications. J Pediatr Surg 1990;25:980.
29. Lee KH, Tam YH, Yeung CK: Laparoscopy in the management of intestinal duplication in childhood. Aust N Z J Surg 2000;70:542.
30. Lewis FT, Thyng FW: Regular occurrence of intestinal diverticula in embryos of pig, rabbit and man. Am J Anat 1908;7:505.
31. Li L, Zhang JZ, Wang YX: Vascular classification for small intestinal duplications: Experience with 80 cases. J Pediatr Surg 1998;33:1243.
32. Louw JH: Congenital intestinal atresia and stenosis in the newborn. Ann R Coll Surg Engl 1959;25:209.
33. Mehta VS, Chowdhury C, Bhatia R: Neuroenteric cyst of the cerebellum. Postgrad Med J 1984;60:287.
34. Mellish RWP, Koop CE: Clinical manifestations of duplication of the bowel. Pediatrics 1961;27:397.
35. Moutsouris C: The "solid stage" and congenital intestinal atresia. J Pediatr Surg 1966;1:446.
36. O'Neill JA Jr, Holcomb GW 3rd, Schnaufer L, et al: Surgical experience with thirteen conjoined twins. Am Surg 1988;208:299.
37. Pokorny WJ, Golstein IR: Enteric thoracoabdominal duplications in children. J Thorac Cardiovasc Surg 1984;87:821.
38. Potter EL: Pathology of the Fetus and Newborn. Chicago, Year Book Medical Publishers, 1961.
39. Potts W: The Surgeon and the Child. Philadelphia, WB Saunders, 1959.
40. Puligandla PS, Nguyen LT, St-Vil D, et al: Gastrointestinal duplications. J Pediatr Surg 2003;38:740.
41. Ramsey GS: Enterogenous cyst of the stomach simulating hypertrophic pyloric stenosis. Br J Surg 1957;44:632.
42. Ravitch MM: Duplications of the alimentary tract. In Ravitch MM, et al (eds): Pediatric Surgery, 3rd ed. Chicago, Year Book Medical Publishers, 1982.
43. Sarpel U, Le MN, Morotti RA, Dolgin SE: Complete colorectal duplication. J Am Coll Surg 2005;200:304.
44. Scaravilli F, Lidov H, Spalton DJ, Symon L: Neuroenteric cyst of the optic nerve: Case report with immunohistochemical study. J Neurol Neurosurg Psychiatry 1992;55:1197.
45. Schalamon J, Schleef J, Hollwarth ME: Experience with gastro-intestinal duplications in childhood. Langenbeck Arch Surg 2000;385:402.
46. Schleef J, Schalamon J: The role of laparoscopy in the diagnosis and treatment of intestinal duplication: A report of two cases. Surg Endosc 2000;14:865.
47. Siddiqui AM, Shamberger RC, Filler RM, et al: Enteric duplications of the pancreatic head: Definitive management by local resection. J Pediatr Surg 1998;33:1117.
48. Skandalakis JE, Gray SW (eds): Embryology for Surgeons: The Embryologic Basis for the Treatment of Congenital Anomalies, 2nd ed. Baltimore, Williams & Wilkins, 1994.
49. Smith ED, Stephens FD: Duplication and vesicointestinal fissure. Birth Defects Orig Article Series 1988;24:551.
50. Swenson O: Pediatric Surgery. New York, Appleton-Century-Crofts, 1958.
51. Teele RL, Share JC: Ultrasonography of Infants and Children. Philadelphia, WB Saunders, 1991.
52. Torgerson CL, Young DW, Vaid YN, et al: Intestinal duplication: Imaging with Tc-99m sodium pertechnetate. Clin Nucl Med 1996;21:968.
53. Van Dam LJ, de Groot CJ, Hazebroek FW, Wladimiroff JW:

Case report: Intrauterine demonstration of bowel duplication by ultrasound. Eur J Obstet Gynecol Reprod Biol 1984;18:229.
54. Williams WH, Hendren WH: Intrapancreatic duodenal duplication causing pancreatitis in a child. Surgery 1971; 69:708.
55. Wootton-Gorges SL, Eckel GM, Poulos ND, et al: Duplication of the cervical esophagus: A case report and review of the literature. Pediatr Radiol 2002;32:533.

第 89 章

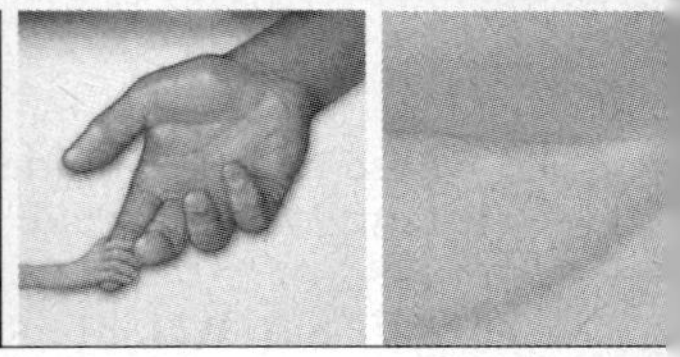

肠系膜和大网膜囊肿

Richard R. Ricketts

历史回顾

1399 1507 年，弗拉伦萨解剖学家 Benevieni 首次记录了一名 8 岁男孩尸检时发现肠系膜囊肿[2]。1842 年 Vonrokitansky 首先描述了 1 例乳糜肠系膜囊肿[41]；1852 年 Gairdener 报道了 1 例大网膜囊肿[12]。1880 年法国外科大夫 Tillaux 首次成功切除了 1 例肠系膜上的囊性肿块[38]。1883 年 Pean 第一个成功地开展了囊肿造口术[40]。1890 年 Carson 发表了美国第 1 例肠系膜乳糜样囊肿的报告[2]。截止到 1950 年，文献记载大约有 600 例肠系膜囊肿[40]。到 1994 年数量增加到了约 820 例[9,72]。Beahrs 等将肠系膜囊肿分为 4 类：胚胎和发育性的囊肿、创伤或获得性囊肿、肿瘤性囊肿、感染或退变性囊肿[2]。本章只讨论第一类。

引言

肠系膜和大网膜囊肿非常少见。发病率在综合性医院的入院病例中接近 1/105 000，而儿童医院的发病率则为 1/20 000[7,20,40]。本章节报道的是来自于 Egleston 的亚特兰大儿童医院 30 多年来的 16 例病例。现代研究资料显示近 1/3 的肠系膜囊肿患儿小于 15 岁，1/4 为小于 10 岁的患儿[3,5,27]。据报道显示，女性和白种人比男性和非白种人更易患该病[4,5,34,39,40,42]。然而，在儿童组，年龄范围从出生至 18 岁（平均 4. 35 岁），并且囊肿在男孩中稍多见（60%）。表 89–1 中列出了亚特兰大 16 例患儿的年龄和性别分布；注意有一例患儿是宫内诊断，所有患儿除了 2 例都小于 10 岁。

有些作者对囊性淋巴管瘤和肠系膜大网膜囊肿进行了区分[3,18,24,37]。囊性淋巴管瘤是单纯囊肿，囊壁含上皮细胞、泡沫细胞、小的淋巴腔隙、淋巴组织和平滑肌。肠系膜囊肿的壁缺少平滑肌和淋巴腔隙，内衬细胞是立方或柱状细胞[37]。淋巴管瘤出现在肠系膜或后腹膜，易在生后早期发病且伴有急腹症症状，而肠系膜囊肿局限于肠系膜，常在成年期发病且表现为无症状肿块[18,37]。由于肠系膜、大网膜囊肿和腹膜后囊肿的评价和治疗目标相同，并且它们都是胚胎期腹膜后组织的向前伸展[14]，因此具有相同的特点。在本章，肠系膜囊肿被定义为任何位于肠系膜的囊肿，它可以延伸或不延伸到后腹膜，有一个可识别的上皮内衬或间皮细胞[3]。大网膜囊肿有相同的组织特点但是主要局限在大网膜或者是小网膜。

胚胎学

已经提出的一些肠系膜或大网膜囊肿形成的机制包括胚胎淋巴腔隙和静脉系统连接障碍、结旁组织正常的淋巴管静脉分流不足、淋巴结离开肠系膜融合、

表 89–1　肠系膜囊肿患儿年龄性别分布

年龄	男	女	总数
0 ~ 1	1	1	2*
1 月~ 1 岁	2	1	3
1 ~ 5 岁	4	3	7
5 ~ 10 岁	1	1	2
>10 岁	2	0	2
总数	10（62. 5%）	6（37. 5%）	16

*其中一名患儿囊肿在宫内被诊断。

表 89-2　肠系膜和大网膜囊肿的位置

作者	日期	病例数	肠系膜	大网膜	后腹膜
Mollitt[27]	1978	11	8	0	3
Molander[26]	1982	6	3	3	0
Radhakrishma[31]	1989	8	5	3	0
Adejuyigbe[1]	1990	5	3	2	0
Kosir[18]	1991	13	9	0	4
Chung[7]	1991	15	9	2	4
Hebra[14]	1993	22	13	6	3
Bliss[3]	1994	10	10	0	0
Senocak[35]	1994	19	14	5	0
Okur[29]	1997	10	7	1	2
Egozi[10]	1997	14	10	2	2
总数		133	91 (68%)	24 (18%)	18 (14%)

400 隐蔽的创伤、肿瘤形成和淋巴结的局部变性[2,37]。通常被接受的理论是由 Gross 提出的[13]，即位于肠系膜的异位淋巴系统良性增生，缺乏与其他剩余的淋巴系统的交通。他认为这些囊肿来自于与胚胎腹膜后淋巴囊有关联的淋巴腔隙，类似于颈部水囊状淋巴管瘤，与颈静脉淋巴囊有关联[36]。淋巴梗阻这一机制是有争议的。由于淋巴系统内存在丰富的脉络，因此动物体内试验性的淋巴隙梗阻不能产生这些囊肿[2,36,37]。除此之外，淋巴管造影也不能表明存在淋巴系统梗阻[40]。

疾病谱和鉴别诊断

肠系膜囊肿可出现在从十二指肠到直肠的胃肠道肠系膜的任何部位[2]；它们可以从肠系膜根部延伸进入后腹膜。大网膜囊肿则位于大、小网膜。肠系膜囊肿通常是大网膜囊肿的 4.5 倍[42]。在一个 1950—1985 年 162 个病例的综述中，Kurtz 等发现[20]，肠系膜囊肿 60% 位于小肠系膜，24% 位于大肠系膜，14.5% 位于后腹膜。最常见的部位是回肠系膜。在结肠系膜，囊肿常位于乙状结肠[5,40]。几个有关儿童囊肿的系列报道的位置如表 89-2 所示。

肠系膜囊肿和大网膜囊肿的鉴别诊断见表 89-3。现代影像学检查通常可以确定囊性病变在腹腔中起源的器官。肠重复畸形和肠系膜囊肿的鉴别很难，因为它们都与肠壁密切相关。前者与邻近的肠管享有共同的血液供应和肌肉层，并且有界限清楚的黏膜层，而肠系膜囊肿则没有[3,6,7,26,27]。手术时，肠重复畸形需切除病变的肠管，而肠系膜囊肿通常能够从肠系膜上剜除[11]。

这些囊肿的病理特征各异。可以单个或多个，也可单房或多房；可以是浆液性、乳糜性、血性或者是混合内容物；其壁可以从单层扁平内皮细胞到立方或柱状上皮细胞到杂乱的纤维组织[5,8,14,24,42]。囊壁钙化极少见[4,8,40]。与肠重复畸形不同，肠系膜或大网膜囊肿没有产生黏液的细胞[5]。肠系膜囊肿通常是单房和多房，当涉及远端小肠或结肠系膜时，囊肿液体通常是浆液性的；而位于近端小肠系膜时则为乳糜性[27,40]。大网膜囊肿总是浆液性的[8]。表 89-4 为该组囊肿的病理特征。

表 89-3　肠系膜和大网膜囊肿的鉴别诊断

肠重复畸形囊肿
卵巢囊肿
胆总管囊肿
胰腺、脾、肾囊肿
肾积水
畸胎瘤、皮样囊肿
包虫囊肿
腹水

表 89-4　肠系膜和大网膜囊肿的病理特征

特点	数量（%）
数量	
单个	11（69）
多个	5（31）
类型	
多房	14（88）
单房	2（12）
液体内容物	
血性	7（44）
浆液性	3（19）
乳糜性	2（12）
感染性	1（6）
非特异性	3（19）
大小（cm）	
最小 4×4.5×1.7	
最大 30×40×10	

数据来自于参考文献 2，6，7，11，12，15，16。

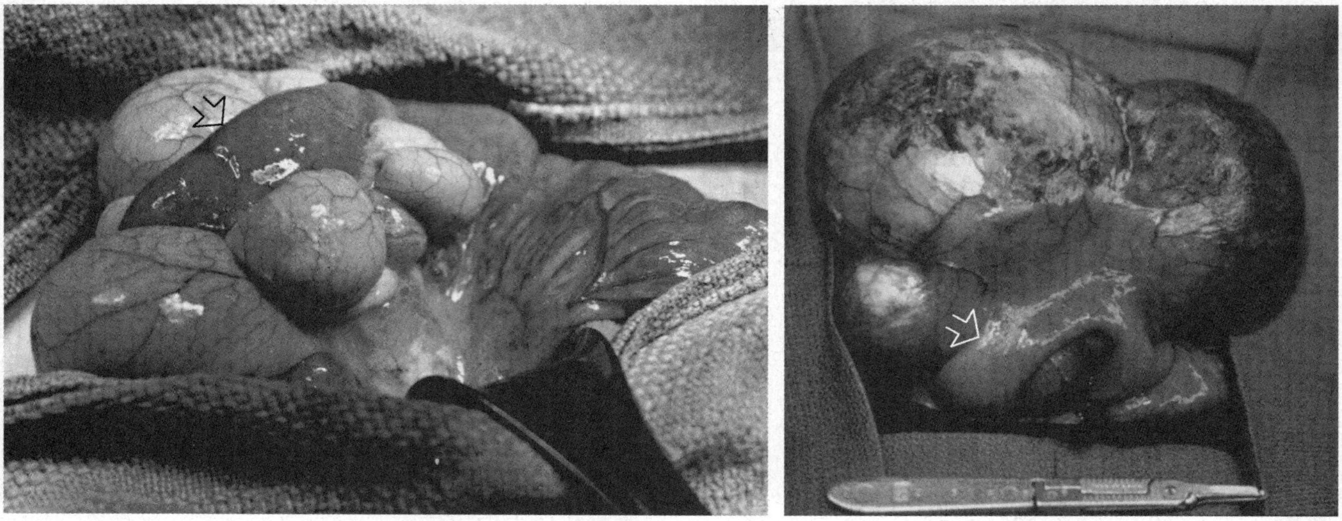

A B

图 89-1 A. 充满乳糜液的多发性肠系膜囊肿围绕近端小肠（箭头）。B. 巨大的多房性肠系膜囊肿压迫下面的小肠（箭头），引起一个慢性局部梗阻。为了完整切除囊肿，2 例患者均需要行肠切除。

临床表现

肠系膜和大网膜囊肿的临床表现各异，可以由于其他原因实施剖腹探查时偶然发现，也可是急性的、威胁生命的腹腔内疾病。在成年人，偶然发现的囊肿大约占患者的 40%[34,40,42]，大于 60% 的患者表现为
1401 急腹症。典型的症状是低位不全性肠梗阻伴有一可触及的腹部活动性肿块[4]。儿童最常见的急性表现是小肠梗阻，有时伴有肠扭转和肠梗死[8,18,27]。小肠梗阻可以是继发于出血而造成的肿块突然增大或者是由于附着在肿块上方的肠管受到肿块的压迫造成的（图 89-1）。

表 89-5 肠系膜囊肿和大网膜囊肿的症状和体征

症状	数量	体征	数量
腹痛	8	腹胀	10
呕吐	7	肿块	8
食欲减退	6	发热	3
腹泻	3	蠕动波	3
便秘	1	触痛	1
腹壁红斑	1		
无症状	4		

数据自参考文献 2，6，7，11，12，15，16。

表 89-5 为 16 个患儿的症状和体征，一般的临床表现形式见表 89-6。尽管 4 个患儿无症状，但无一例患儿的囊肿是偶然发现的。4 个中的一个在产前超声检查时发现有一个囊性腹腔肿块。在本组中，75% 的患儿有腹部症状，并且所有的患儿均在腹部检查时发现有囊肿。只有 2 个患儿（12.5%）表现为急腹症。

下面是 5 个患儿的病例摘要，显示肠系膜和大网膜囊肿的表现多样化：

1. 一个 7 天的女婴呕吐和腹泻 48 小时，并有发热、腹胀和腹壁红斑。证实有大肠杆菌性败血症。该患儿有多个累及大网膜和横结肠的感染的大网膜和肠系膜囊肿，所有的病变被切除，该患儿痊愈。

2. 一个出生 3 天的男婴，症状和体征与小肠梗 1402
阻的表现一致。发现回肠有一个多房性的肠系膜囊肿并有扭转，需要切除小肠并行 I 期肠吻合。

3. 一个 2 岁男孩表现为无症状的腹部包块，发现有一个累及横结肠系膜和胰腺的多房性肠系膜囊肿。给予了囊肿和远端胰腺切除治疗。

4. 一个 2 岁女孩表现为无症状腹胀 2 周。发现有一个 30 cm × 40 cm × 10 cm 多房性肠系膜囊肿，肿块延着肠系膜根部从 Treitz 韧带延伸到横结肠。采用造袋术将残留的囊肿引入腹腔，切除几乎全部的囊肿并袋装缝合剩余的囊于附壁，并且用碘酒硬化其壁以

作长期治疗。

5. 一个女性胎儿在产前常规检查时发现有一个腹腔囊性肿块。出生后，同时存在的婴儿黄疸提示是胆总管囊肿，用标准放射性核素扫描可以排除。光疗后，无症状的可触的无痛性腹部活动肿块仍然存在。在6个月时进行了选择性大网膜囊肿切除（图89–2）。

肠系膜和大网膜囊肿有多种并发症，包括肠梗阻（最常见）、肠扭转、囊内出血、感染[16]、破裂、囊肿扭转[42]、输尿管或胆管梗阻[21]和恶性肿瘤[2,20,27,39,40]。报道恶化（肉瘤、淋巴管内皮瘤或罕见的腺癌）的几率为3%[20]；在儿童还没有恶性肠系膜或者大网膜囊肿的报道。

诊断

体检时大多数肠系膜和大网膜囊肿的患儿有腹胀，可触及或者触不到肿块。由于肿块巨大、柔软和液体黏度及活动度大，可能不容易触到明显的肿块。肿块可以很大，充满整个腹腔并导致腹水[15-17,32,33,35]，不容易叩诊。通过腹壁视诊可以区分大网膜囊肿和腹水，腹水可以导致腹壁外突而囊肿则不会。如果没有其他原因所致的腹水（例如肝、肾脏疾病）应考虑肠系膜囊肿或大网膜囊肿[11]。如果明确触到肿块，肠系膜囊肿常在横断面上活动，而大网膜囊肿则在横断面和前后方向移动[3,40]。

现代影像学检查常可以确诊（或至少在很大程度上）肠系膜和大网膜囊肿。腹部平片可见一个无气、同质、透明的肿块取代周围的肠袢[8]。大网膜囊肿可以压迫后面的肠管而肠系膜囊肿常被周围的肠袢环绕（图 89–3）[6]，有时可以看到少量的钙化[48]。腹部超声和计算机断层成像（CT）可以排除造影检查的必要，例如上消化道造影、钡灌肠、静脉肾盂造影。腹部超声是常用的影像学方法[6,18,26]。该检查可显示一个局限、薄壁、充满液体的囊性组织，常会有薄的内隔和由于出血、感染或碎屑产生的内部回声（图 89–4）[3,6,26]。肠重复畸形的肠壁组织和相邻的肠管有共同的肌壁[6]。超声可见明显的黏膜层。CT 可提供的其他信息很少，然而，使用胃肠道对比剂可以显示囊肿与肠管的关系（图 89–5），表明囊肿不是来自于其他组织例如肾、胰腺或卵巢[40]。胆道放射性核素扫描可以排除胆总管囊肿。

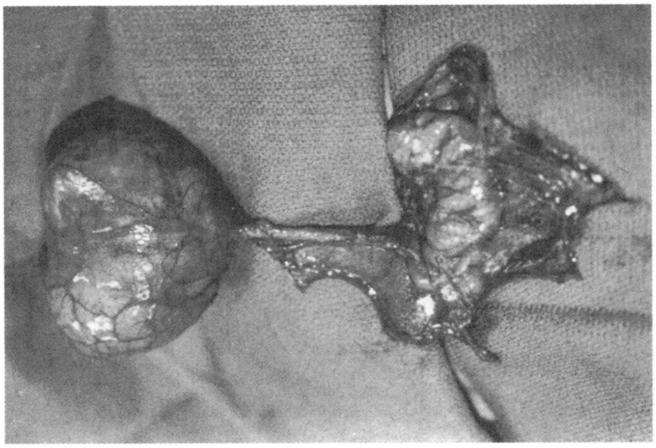

图 89–2　无症状但可以触及的可活动的大网膜囊肿，可在产前超声首次发现，6 个月时可择期切除。

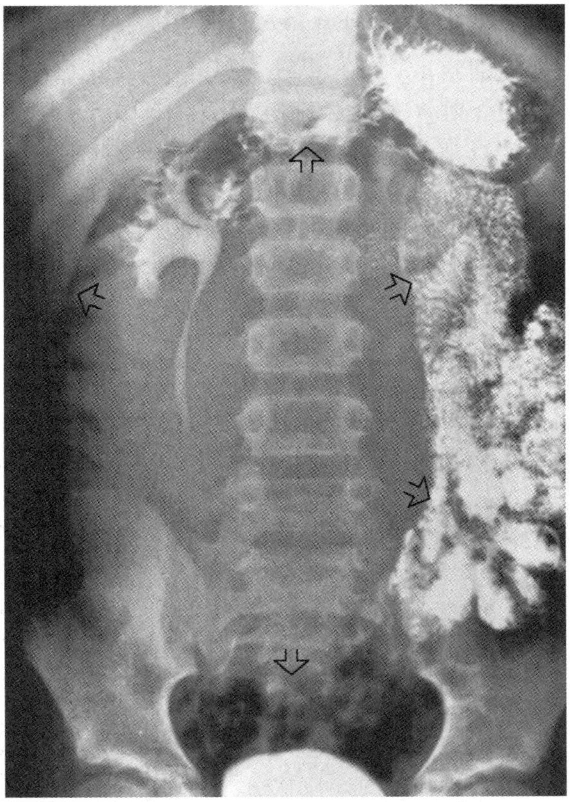

图 89–3　给予胃肠道和静脉注射造影剂后拍摄的腹部 X 线片，可见被肠袢围绕的一巨大肿块（箭头），肿块没有使腹膜后组织移位，这些是肠系膜囊肿典型的特征。

1403 ## 治疗

外科治疗的目标是完整切除肿块。大网膜囊肿比较容易切除并且不用切除肠管[8,14]。大网膜囊肿也可以采用腹腔镜切除[15,19,44]。囊肿部分引流对确定囊肿的原始位置并通过脐部切除是有必要的[28]。肠系膜囊肿最好的治疗方法是囊肿切除术[11,14,20,40]。在成人，肿块可以从剩余的肠系膜上完整地剥离[11]；然而在儿童，要完整切除肿块常需要切除肠段来保证正常的血供不受影响。成人肠系膜囊肿大约仅有 33% 需要肠切除而儿童则达到 50%～60%[3,8,18,20,23,27,29]。由于这一原因，如果时间允许的话，术前需要做肠道
1404 准备[7]。如果需要做肠切除的话，最初应该重建肠的连续性。有记载用腹腔镜切除肠系膜囊肿[9,25,28,30]。因为这些病例需伴有肠切除，所以无论是体内技术还是腹腔镜辅助的体外技术都可以采用。

如果不能剥离或是切除，第三个选择是部分切除，剩余部分在腹腔内造袋。约 10% 的患者需要采用这样的治疗[20]。如果部分切除，囊的内面可以用 10% 葡萄糖溶液[5]、电灼或碘酊使其硬化以防止复发。经皮注射 A 型化脓性链球菌 OK432 低压冷冻卵胚混合液已成功治疗儿童不可切除的淋巴管瘤[24]。OK432 的作用机制可能是激活白细胞（增加自然杀伤细胞和 T 细胞的数量），提高细胞因子介导的内皮渗透性（提高肿瘤坏死因子和白介素-6 活性），导致囊肿缩小[24]。这一试剂可以用来作为后腹膜囊肿手术的辅助治疗。由于部分切除和引流与高复发率有关，所以这些方法并不常用[20]。

最近，针对各种不同的肠系膜囊肿，提出了一种简单并通用的病理分类体系（图 89-6）[24]。1 型和 2 型用切除或剜出法很容易治疗，伴或者不伴有肠切除。3 型和 4 型延伸至后腹膜，手术步骤复杂，常需硬化治疗。3 型和 4 型较 1 型和 2 型更容易复发。

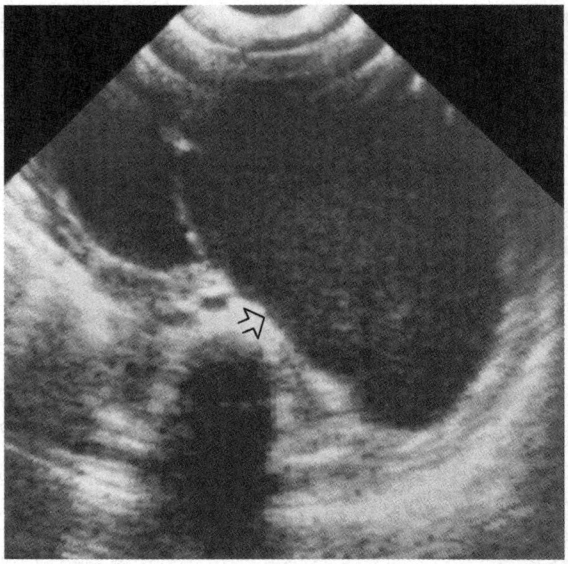

图 89-4 超声显示前腹部有一个巨大、多房的囊性肿块，与肠系膜囊肿的诊断一致。细小的内部回声代表囊内出血（箭头）。

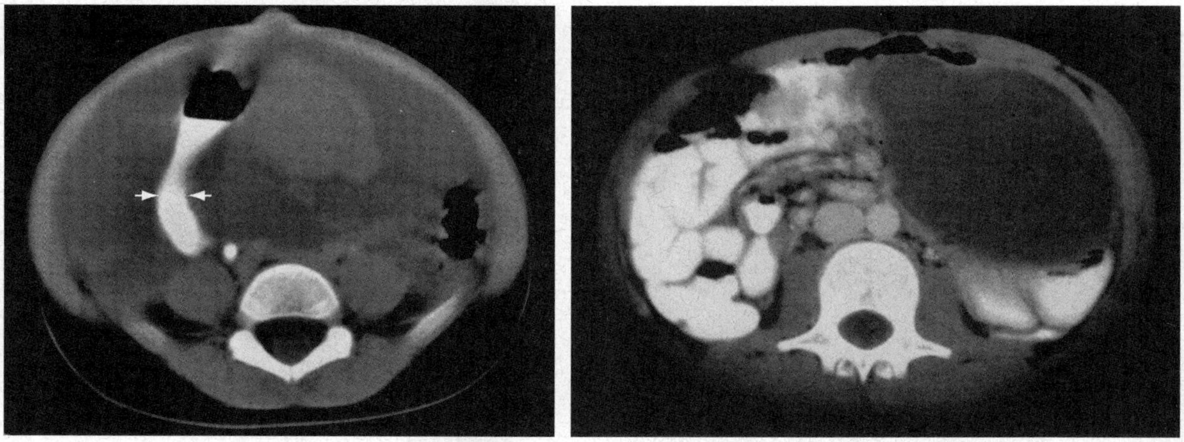

A B

图 89-5 A. 胃肠道造影和 CT 扫描可见围绕小肠袢的一个巨大的囊性肿块（箭头）。B. CT 扫描可见一个巨大的单房性囊肿，肠袢向侧后方移位。

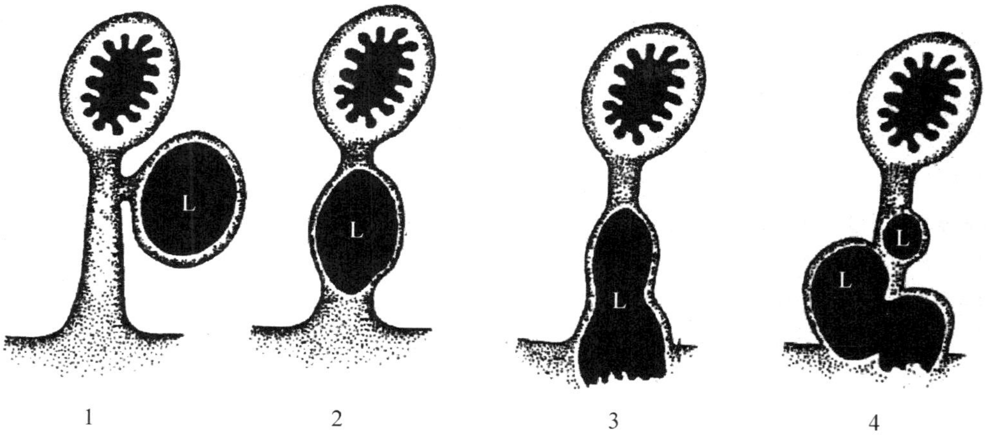

图 89-6　肠系膜囊肿分类。1 型-有蒂型；较易切除。2 型-固定的肠系膜；需做肠切除。3 型-延伸到腹膜后；常不能完全被切除。4 型-多中心型，可能需要复杂的手术、硬化治疗或二者兼用。（From Losanoff JE，Richman BW，El-Sherif A，et al：Mesenteric cystic lymphangioma. J Am Coll Surg 2003；196：598.）

表 89-6　肠系膜囊肿和大网膜囊肿的首发症状

首发症状	数量
慢性腹部症状（<2 月）	5
亚急性腹部症状（<2 月）	5
腹痛、呕吐、腹围增大	3
腹痛、呕吐、食欲不振	1
腹痛、食欲不振	1
无症状腹部肿块、腹胀	4
急腹症（<48 小时）	2
呕吐、腹胀	1
呕吐	1

数据来自参考文献 2，6，7，11，12，15。

表 89-7 列出了目前手术治疗的病例。3 例大网膜囊肿被完整切除。13 例中 11 例（85%）肠系膜囊肿被全部切除；2 例（15%）在腹腔行囊袋缝合并用电灼（1）或者碘酊硬化囊壁（1）。全部切除的囊肿中 5 例（45%）需同时行肠切除，1 例需远端胰腺切除，没有一例行单纯囊肿引流。在该组中没有长期或短期并发症、死亡或复发病例。

预后

所有的患者尤其是儿童肠系膜或者大网膜囊肿均预后良好。报道的复发率为 0～13.6%，在一组有 162 例儿童和成人病例的报道中平均为 6.1%[20]。大部分复发出现在后腹膜囊肿或部分切除的病例。在所有成人和儿童中死亡率为 2%[20]。从 1950 年以来只报道过一例患儿死亡，是一个 26 月大的女婴，表现为肠系膜囊肿伴肠扭转导致肠梗死[43]。

总结

肠系膜囊肿和大网膜囊肿发病率低，在儿童医院
较普通成人医院多见。大部分囊肿是原发的，并与先 1405
天性淋巴系统异常有关。这些异常导致了淋巴在异位
淋巴组织中生成和流动，而这些淋巴又不能回流到中
心管。囊肿可以位于大网膜或肠系膜的任何位

表 89-7　肠系膜囊肿和大网膜囊肿的手术治疗

治疗	肠系膜囊肿（N=13）NO.（%）	大网膜囊肿（N=3）NO.（%）
剥离、切除	5（38.5）	3（100）
肠切除 *	5（38.5）	0
切除、远端胰腺切除	1（8）	0
囊袋缝合、电灼	2（15）	0
引流	0	0

* 一个患者有肠扭转。数据来自参考文献 2，4，6，11，12，24，没有死亡和复发病例。

置甚至可延伸到后腹膜。随着现代影像学研究的发展，囊肿通常能够与腹腔内其他脏器的病变相鉴别。可以偶然发病，或呈隐匿性或者表现为威及生命的急症。在儿童，来自肠梗阻伴或不伴肠扭转的急性表现相对常见。在成人，常为亚急性表现。治疗目标是通过切除或者是剥离完全去除囊肿，在儿童常需肠切除。有时，必须留下部分囊壁于原位，并袋形缝合于腹腔和硬化。儿童肠系膜或大网膜囊肿的长期或短期预后良好，复发率很低，与治疗相关的并发症较少，基本上没有死亡。

（汪　健译　朱锦祥校）

参考文献

1. Adejuyigbe O, Lawal OO, Akinula DO, et al: Omental and mesenteric cysts in Nigerian children. J R Coll Surg Edinb 1990;35:181.
2. Beahrs OH, Judd ES, Docherty MB: Chylous cysts of the abdomen. Surg Clin North Am 1950;30:1081.
3. Bliss DP Jr, Coffin CM, Bower RJ, et al: Mesenteric cysts in children. Surgery 1994;115:571.
4. Burnett WE, Rosemand GP, Bucher RM: Mesenteric cysts: Report of three cases, in one of which a calcified cyst was present. Arch Surg 1950;60:699.
5. Chirathivat S, Shermeta D: Recurrent retroperitoneal mesenteric cyst. Gastroenterol Radiol 1979;4:191.
6. Chou YH, Tiu CM, Lui WY, et al: Mesenteric and omental cysts: An ultrasonographic and clinical study in 15 patients. Gastrointest Radiol 1991;16:311.
7. Chung MA, Brandt ML, St-Vil D, et al: Mesenteric cysts in children. J Pediatr Surg 1991;26:1306.
8. Colodny A: Mesenteric and omental cysts. In Welch KJ (ed): Pediatric Surgery, 4th ed. Chicago, Year Book Medical Publishers, 1986.
9. Dequanter D, Lefebvre JC, Belva P, et al: Mesenteric cysts: A case treated by laparoscopy and a review of the literature. Surg Endosc 2002;16:1493.
10. Egozi EI, Ricketts RR: Mesenteric and omental cysts in children. Am Surg 1997;63:287.
11. Feins NR, Raffensperger JG: Cystic hygroma, lymphangioma, and lymphedema. In Raffensperger JG (ed): Swenson's Pediatric Surgery, 5th ed. Norwalk, Conn, Appleton & Lange, 1990.
12. Gairdner WT: A remarkable cyst in the omentum. Trans Pathol Soc Lond 1852;3:1851.
13. Gross RE: Omental cysts and mesenteric cysts. In Gross RE (ed): The Surgery of Infancy and Childhood. Philadelphia, WB Saunders, 1953.
14. Hebra A, Brown MF, McGeehin KM, et al: Mesenteric, omental, and retroperitoneal cysts in children: A clinical study of 22 cases. South Med J 1993;86:173.
15. Horiuchi T, Shimomatsuya T: Laparoscopic excision of an omental cyst. J Laparoendosc Adv Surg Tech A 1999; 9:411.
16. Iuchtman M, Soimu U, Amar M: Peritonitis caused by a ruptured infected mesenteric cyst. J Clin Gastroenterol 2001; 32:452.
17. Klin B, Lotan G, Efrati Y, et al: Giant omental cyst in children presenting as pseudoascites. Surg Laparosc Endosc 1997;7:291.
18. Kosir MA, Sonnino RE, Gauderer MWL: Pediatric abdominal lymphangiomas: A plea for early recognition. J Pediatr Surg 1991;26:1309.
19. Kuriansky J, Bar-Dayan A, Shabtai M, et al: Laparoscopic resection of huge omental cyst. J Laparoendosc Adv Surg Tech A 2000;10:283.
20. Kurtz RJ, Heimann TM, Beck AR, et al: Mesenteric and retroperitoneal cysts. Ann Surg 1986;203:109.
21. Lawrence RA, Putnam TC, Webb SR: Omental cyst: Presentation in an infant with jaundice and increasing abdominal girth. J Pediatr Gastroenterol Nutr 1992;15:97.
22. Liew SCC, Glenn DC, Storey DW: Mesenteric cyst. Aust N Z J Surg 1994;64:741.
23. Lin JI, Fisher J, Caty MG: Newborn intraabdominal cystic lymphatic malformations. Semin Pediatr Surg 2000;9:141.
24. Losanoff JE, Richman BW, El-Sherif A, et al: Mesenteric cystic lymphangioma. J Am Coll Surg 2003;196:598.
25. Mason JE, Soper NJ, Brunt LM: Laparoscopic excision of mesenteric cysts: A report of two cases. Surg Laparosc Endosc Percutan Tech 2001;11:382.
26. Molander ML, Mortenssen W, Uden R: Omental and mesenteric cysts in children, Acta Pediatr Scand 1982; 71:227.
27. Mollitt DL, Ballantine TVN, Grosfeld JL: Mesenteric cysts in infancy and childhood. Surg Gynecol Obstet 1978; 147:182.
28. Morrison CP, Wemyss-Holden SA, Maddern GJ: A novel technique for laparoscopic resection of mesenteric cysts. Surg Endosc 2002;16:219.
29. Okur H, Kucukaydin M, Ozokutan BH, et al: Mesenteric, omental, and retroperitoneal cysts in children. Eur J Surg 1997;163:673.
30. Polat C, Ozacmak ID, Yucel T, et al: Laparoscopic resection of giant mesenteric cyst. J Laparoendosc Adv Surg Tech A 2000;10:337.
31. Radhakrishma K, Rao PLNG: Intraabdominal lymphatic cysts in children. Indian Pediatr 1989;26:1214.
32. Rahman GA, Johnson AW: Giant omental cyst simulating ascites in a Nigerian child: Case report and critique of clinical parameters and investigative modalities. Ann Trop Paediatr 2001;21:81.
33. Rattan KN, Budhiraja S, Pandit SK, et al: Huge omental cyst mimicking ascites. Indian J Pediatr 1996;63:707.
34. Sardi A, Parikh KJ, Singer JA, et al: Mesenteric cysts. Am Surg 1987;53:58.
35. Senocak ME, Gundogdu H, Buyukpamukcu N, et al: Mesenteric and omental cysts in children: Analysis of nineteen cases. Turk J Pediatr 1994;36:295.
36. Skandalakis JE, Gray SW, Ricketts RR: The lymphatic system. In Skandalakis JE, Gray SW (eds): Embryology for Surgeons, 2nd ed. Baltimore, Williams & Wilkins, 1994.
37. Takiff H, Calabria R, Yin L, et al: Mesenteric cysts and intraabdominal cystic lymphangiomas. Arch Surg 1985;120:1266.
38. Tillaux PJ: Cyste du mesentere un homme: Ablation par la gastromie: Quersion. Rev Ther Med Chir Paris 1880; 47:479.
39. Tykka H, Koivuniemi A: Carcinoma arising in a mesenteric cyst. Am J Surg 1975;129:709.

40. Vanek VW, Phillips AK: Retroperitoneal, mesenteric, and omental cysts. Arch Surg 1984;119:838.
41. vonRokitansky CF: Handbuch der pathologischen anatomie, bd2. Handbuch der Speciellen Pathologischen Anatomie. Wien, Braumuller & Seidel, 1842.
42. Walker AR, Putnam TC: Omental, mesenteric, and retroperitoneal cysts. Ann Surg 1973;178:13.
43. Wong SW, Gardner V: Sudden death in children due to mesenteric defect and mesenteric cyst. Am J Forensic Med Pathol 1992;13:214.
44. Yao CC, Wu TL, Wong HH, et al: Laparoscopic resection of an omental cyst with pedicle torsion. Surg Laparosc Endosc Percutan Tech 1999;9:372.

第 90 章

腹水

Eugene D. McGahren III

1407 腹水是指过多的液体在腹膜腔内的病理性积聚。单词“ascites”来自于希腊语“askos”和“askites”，意思是“囊”、“（气）囊”或“凸部”[18]。自希波格拉底时代（公元前 400）以来，腹水就已经得到认识，然而现代对胎儿和婴儿腹水的描述可追溯至 17 世纪[9,14,17,67]。有很多情况，无论是先天性的还是获得性的，均可引起婴儿和儿童腹水（表 90-1）。本章节将介绍腹水的常见原因。

解剖和病理生理学

腹腔淋巴液有两大主要来源，一是来自肝的血流。来自肝动脉和门静脉的血流灌注肝血窦，然后经肝静脉流出。由于毛细血管前阻力要高于毛细血管后阻力，肝血窦里的压力非常低。Disse 腔的界定为肝细胞在一侧，窦状的内皮细胞在另一侧。肝的淋巴液是由血窦内血浆滤过进入 Disse 腔内而形成的。这些淋巴液通过横膈淋巴从肝引流至胸导管，然后注入锁骨下静脉。静脉窦上皮对清蛋白有很高的通透性，并且肝淋巴中蛋白的浓度接近血浆。因此，正常情况下通过静脉窦膜没有明显的渗透梯度[18]。

腹腔淋巴液的第二大来源是来自于肠系膜静脉系统的淋巴液。来自肠系膜毛细血管的血液通过肠系膜静脉流入门静脉。肠系膜毛细血管的平均压力大约是 20 mmHg。肠系膜淋巴液从局部淋巴系统引流入胸导管。肠系膜毛细血管膜相对不易透过清蛋白。由于肠系膜淋巴液的蛋白质浓度仅为血浆的 20%，在正常状态下有一个明显的渗透梯度，促进淋巴液回流到毛细血管。一个成年患者腹腔里的游离液体不超过 150 ml，正常流入胸导管的淋巴量为 800～1000 ml/d[18]。

表 90-1　腹水的原因

肝细胞性

糖原累积病，溶酶体累积病，半乳糖血症，α_1-抗胰蛋白酶缺乏，病毒性肝炎，新生儿肝炎，先天性肝纤维化，肝硬化，肝静脉或门静脉栓塞，Budd-Chiari 综合征，恶性肿瘤，静脉闭塞性疾病，胆道闭锁

胆汁性

胆道穿孔，胆道外伤

染色体

21-三体，Turner 综合征

心脏

先天性心衰，心律失常

感染

阑尾炎，结核和非典型抗酸杆菌，巨细胞病毒，细小病毒组，梅毒，水痘带状疱疹，肠道病毒，李斯特菌病，弓形体病，甲型肝炎，*衣原体*，真菌

肾/泌尿道

后尿道瓣膜，输尿管囊肿，输尿管狭窄，输尿管狭窄或闭锁，神经源性膀胱，膀胱穿孔，肾病综合征，泌尿生殖窦，泄殖腔畸形

胃肠道

闭锁，旋转不良，扭转，肠穿孔，肠病，胎粪性腹膜炎，淋巴管扩张，创伤（包括虐待儿童），腹膜带引起的先天性梗阻，腹裂，心脏手术，肿瘤的腹部手术，其他腹部手术，淋巴管瘤，肠套迭

胰腺

各种原因的胰腺炎，假性囊肿，创伤

妇科

卵巢囊肿破裂，子宫阴道积水

混杂

脑室腹膜分流术，腹膜透析，腹膜假黏液瘤，肉芽肿性腹膜炎，黏液水肿，肿瘤（如淋巴瘤、神经母细胞瘤、卵巢肿瘤），代谢累积疾病

当正常流体静力学的、渗透性的以及电化学性的力等决定液体平衡的因素发生改变时就会出现腹水，如肝和肠系膜毛细血管流体静力和渗透压引起液体从血管到淋巴管的净转运超过了淋巴系统的引流能力的时候，腹水就会产生。要注意的是，静水压的改变可
408 能来自于心脏的功能不全或通过腔静脉或门静脉系统的血流减少。胶体渗透压的改变可能来自继发于肝损害的低蛋白血症或者是由于各种感染、代谢、遗传或是肿瘤等所致的毛细血管膜的通透性紊乱。淋巴液引流异常可能来自于包括外科和虐童的创伤、先天畸形或者是其他导致淋巴系统阻塞的畸形。最后，腹水也可以由尿道和腹腔直接相通而引起[18,65,69]。

临床特点

腹胀是与腹水有关联的最常见的体征[66,67]。其他体征有胁腹膨胀、腹壁静脉显露、脐外翻（假如伴有脐疝）或者脐内翻（假如没有脐疝）、腹股沟斜疝、阴囊或大阴唇水肿、液波震颤、全身水肿和叩诊呈移动性浊音[1,59,65,66,69]。其他与腹水有关的一些体征还包括如心脏杂音、肝肾脾大或腹部肿块等情况。由于血管内衰竭、腹内压增加或尿液漏出使得尿量减少[6]。腹膜刺激征提示有原发性炎症、感染等原因引起腹水和腹水继发感染[67]，可出现恶心和呕吐。如果腹水积聚引起膈肌抬高，可能会出现呼吸困难[5,14]。

诊断

腹部平片的特征性表现为肠管向中间移位腹腔弥漫性浑浊呈毛玻璃样外观（图 90–1）。腹膜外脂肪条纹与结肠的分离和充气肠袢的分离是另外两个非特异性表现。肝可以呈圆形并被推至中央。如果腹水伴有穿孔或者是腹膜炎时可出现钙化[20,65,69]。

超声（US）对探测腹腔内的游离液体是很敏感的。根据其位置，腹腔内的游离液体可以表现为不同位置的游离无回声区。在肝区、肾区还有盆腔可以探测到少量的液体。在 US 中，少量甚至 50 ~ 100 ml 的液体都可有助于（见图 90–1）[65]。变动患者的体位可以区分是游离液体还是原位聚集的液体。US 可有助于鉴别腹水的诱发因素，尤其是诊断与腹水有关的尿道畸形，例如后尿道瓣膜[66]。然而，超声检查不能区别腹水的类型。产前 US 常规探测胎儿腹水，有助于医生考虑对婴儿产前或产后的对策[20,24]。CT 可

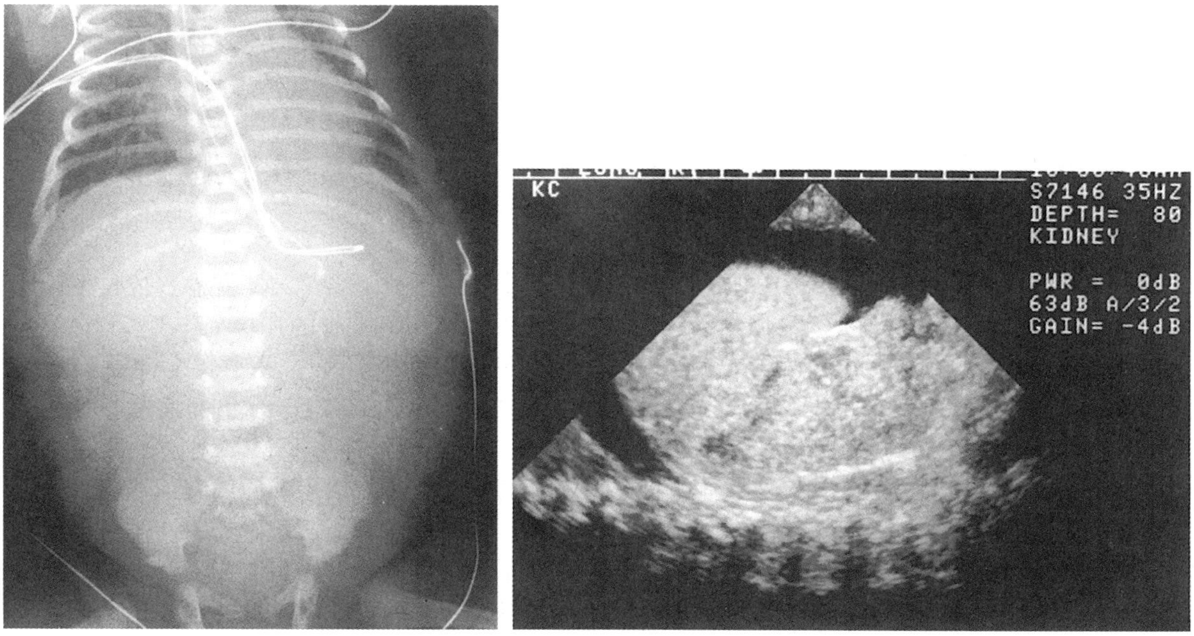

图 90–1　一例有肝性腹水的新生儿。平片显示大片的浑浊伴极少的肠道积气；超声显示肝肾隐窝积液。

表 90-2　腹水的实验室分析

腹水的类型	清蛋白水平	胆红素水平	三酰甘油水平	pH	肌酐水平
肝细胞性	2～3 g/dl	≈血清水平	<50 mg/dl	7.35	<1 mg/dl
胆汁性	≈3 g/dl	血清水平的2～3 倍	<50 mg/dl	>7.4	<1 mg/dl
乳糜性	<3 g/dl	<1 mg/dl	1000～1500 mg/dl	7.5	<1 mg/dl
尿性	<1 g/dl	<1 mg/dl	<50 mg/dl	<7.0	<5～10 mg/dl

以帮助诊断腹水的原因，但提供的信息通常并不会比超声所提供的更多。

腹水的液体应通过穿刺术获得并根据临床可能的诊断进行分析（表 90-2）。US 在穿刺定位上很有帮助，特别是存在以前手术瘢痕影响的时候[18]。抽吸
1409 10～20 ml 腹水对于完整的分析已经足够。应评估大体外观，液体可能是淡黄色、浑浊的、血性的或者乳糜性的。腹水液体的实验室评估应该包括细胞计数和分类、革兰氏染色和培养和细胞学的评估，有指征的话，作包括 pH、乳酸脱氢酶、清蛋白、蛋白质、淀粉酶、胆红素、肌酐、三酰甘油水平在内的化学分析[60,65,69]。

肝细胞性腹水

新生儿肝炎、胆道闭锁、先天性代谢缺陷、先天性肝纤维化、α_1-抗胰蛋白酶缺乏通常导致肝硬化、门静脉高压，紧接着出现腹水。腹水液体是渗透性的，由于门静脉压增加、肠系膜毛细血管内压增加和液体丢失而进入腹腔。清蛋白丢失加剧了这种损失和激发肾脏重吸收钠和水[60]。诊断这种情况要依据不同的测试结果，包括先天性异常的特殊生化分析、病毒培养、病毒抗体滴度试验和肝组织学测定。腹水液体分析应包括血清-腹水清蛋白梯度。梯度大于 1.1 g/dl 时预测门静脉高压的准确性达 97%[55]。细胞计数应该是低的，不应该看到细菌，尽管原发腹膜炎能使已经形成的腹水复杂化。

肝源性腹水的最初治疗包括限制水和钠。钠的摄入应该限制在 1～2 mEq/（kg·d），水的摄入不超过每日维持量的 75%，除非出现明显的低钠血症（<125 mg/dl）[60,66]，严格的限水并无必要。在限制钠和水的同时通常给予温和的利尿剂，为了防止钾的丢失，利尿的目标是为了排泄细胞外水和钠。在治疗的初期常服用螺内酯[60,69]。对于那些限制水盐失败尤其是有呼吸功能不全症状的患者，需要反复的大容量穿刺术。用低盐清蛋白或右旋糖酐代替穿刺移去的腹水液体被证明是安全和有效的，特别是与利尿治疗和限钠结合使用时[6,35,62,64]。

已有报道腹腔静脉分流术对一些婴儿和儿童的肝源性或其他原因所致的顽固性腹水疗效很好[27,52,56]。但由于大尺寸的机械装置和静脉管道的限制，使得这种装置在儿科患者中很少使用。制造商已作出改良以帮助定制用于新生儿的 Denver 型分流装置[52]。腹膜内的血管通道已成功用于姑息性缓解由肝细胞癌所致的张力性恶性腹水[12]。用新生儿腹膜透析导管控制腹水引流也是有效的。经颈静脉肝内门体静脉分流术（TIPS）已经成功地治疗了 1 例青少年腹水，故可用于治疗某些患儿[36]。

胆汁性腹水

胆汁性腹水通常来自于胆总管的自发性穿孔，最常见的是在和胆囊管的连接处[25,37,38,40,61]。胆囊穿孔的实例很少有报道[29]。胆道自发性穿孔是一种相对少见的情况，到 2003 年为止的文献报道大约有 150 例[20]。虽然已经提出了很多理论，胆道穿孔的原因尚不确定。已提出的可能原因有远端胆管梗阻、胰液向上反流至胆总管、胆总管先天性薄弱、胆总管局部管壁的畸形和胰胆管连接异常[22,30,38,48]。有人提出胆管壁缺陷可能会促使胆道易发生穿孔，包括一些先天性畸形，如胆总管囊肿。值得一提的是胆道系统的穿孔也可能来自于外伤[49,61]。

由于胆管穿孔所致的典型的胆汁性腹水常出现在从刚出生到 2 岁的婴幼儿和学步的孩子，但是也可以发生在大龄儿童[7,15,28,30,32,61]。胆汁性腹水也可能发生在胎儿期。大多数患儿在其他方面是健康的，没有与该病有关联的易感因素。典型的表现是进行性无痛性腹胀伴黄疸超过 1～4 周，也可以出现呕吐、腹痛和白色陶土样大便。尽管胆汁性腹膜炎是最初的表现，但也可以看到中毒症状，患儿通常无腹痛。然而，大多数患儿可以耐受腹腔内有大量胆汁却没有感染或腹膜炎的迹象[61]。体格检查会有明显的腹胀、腹腔内有液体，也可能在腹股沟斜疝内出现液体和胆汁样的鞘膜积液[7,15,28,30,32,61,70]。

当没有任何肝病而出现这些明显的症状时应该怀疑胆汁性腹水。超声可以证实腹腔内有液体，核闪烁描记法可以辅助诊断和胆汁泄漏定位[23,32,70]。通过穿刺可以明确诊断。尽管伴有慢性疾病的患儿胆红素水平可以很低，但当胆红素水平为 100～400 mg/dl 时，液体可被胆汁染色[7]。

胆源性腹水治疗的主要手段是外引流[7,15,31,32,61,70]。手术行右上腹部剖腹探查，同时切除胆囊和采用胆囊造影术确定穿孔的大小和位置。如果有远端梗阻的证据，有些人提倡胆－肠吻合术；否则，很少有必要[7,31]。此外，其他的内引流手术，如胆囊空肠吻合术或伴有括约肌成形术的十二指肠切开术通常没有必要而且较复杂，因为并不存在内在的梗阻并且炎症会使得解剖困难[38,53]。这些区域会有严重的瘢痕，并且充满胆汁的囊可能被误以为是胆总管囊肿[70]。外引流术可以通过在肝门放置一个 Penrose 或者闭合的吸引引流管来实施。胆囊造口术对于减压和以后进一步评估胆道系统有帮助[7]。外引流术也可以经皮实施，这样就避免了剖腹术[32]。腹腔镜检查提供了这一选择，它可以确定穿孔位置和精确地放置引流管[7]。胆道狭窄是外引流最常见的并发症，门静脉栓塞、胆漏和胆管炎也有报道[32,70]。

采用合适的外引流，大部分患儿可以存活并且不需要另外的手术干预。80% 的穿孔在 3 周内痊愈[7,25,32,38,40,53,61]。抗生素和全静脉营养（TPN）使肠道彻底休息，对这些患者是重要的辅助治疗。无脂的婴儿肠道营养配方也被采用，但对胆源性腹水患儿没有这两种营养选择的比较研究。胆囊造瘘术和腹膜引流应该保留在原位，直到胆囊造影术显示胆道的解剖结构正常。

乳糜性腹水

乳糜性腹水是淋巴液在腹腔内的过多聚集。在婴儿或儿童大多都是特发性的（45%～60%），推测可能是淋巴管的先天性畸形[17,41,57,66,67]。已知的导致乳糜性腹水的先天性畸形包括肠系膜根部或乳糜池的主乳糜管狭窄或闭锁、肠系膜囊肿、全身性淋巴管瘤病和淋巴管瘤[13,19,34,66,67]。乳糜性腹水的其他常见原因包括肠套迭、肠旋转不良、嵌顿疝、原发或转移性癌症、结核病、腹裂、感染性疾病所致的淋巴结增大等情况造成的淋巴管阻塞[13,19,30,41,59,66,67]。最后，还有 15%～20% 的乳糜性腹水是淋巴系统的外伤所致。这些外伤的类型包括创伤、各种情况下手术损伤和虐童。腹水可能直到应激事件发生后数天或数周后才出现[8,9,17,23,39,68]。

尽管大多数患者为婴儿或者学步的孩子[41,66,67]，但乳糜性腹水可以发生在任何年龄段的儿童，最常见的初发症状是腹胀。它可以是进展性的或者急性发病，也可伴有腹痛或呼吸困难[4,9,17,39,41,46,66,67]。其他症状和体征包括呕吐、腹泻、腹股沟斜疝和水肿[43,67]。

主要的诊断手段是腹腔穿刺，如果患儿接受的是含脂肪的饮食，穿刺可以得到白色乳样液体。液体的特点是三酰甘油的浓度升高（通常大于 1000 mg/dl）、细胞分类以淋巴细胞为主（70%～90%）、总蛋白和胆固醇升高[17,41,55,65-67]。

确定乳糜性腹水的原因很难，特别是在患儿没有通常易造成淋巴泄漏的明显疾病时。US、CT 和胃肠道造影检查可能有助于确定诱发疾病如肠旋转不良、淋巴管瘤、肿瘤或肠系膜囊肿。新生儿腹水原因不明，先天性淋巴管畸形是最可能的诊断。淋巴管造影术在大龄的患儿中有报道，但是在儿童中很难实施。通过足部的径路不总是能显示肠系膜淋巴系统，行淋巴管造影术的患儿中只有一小部分对直接治疗有帮助[55,66]。此外，在缺乏明显的诱发原因以及非手术干预作为首选治疗时，淋巴管造影术对治疗策略的制定作用不大。

手术能治疗的病变例如肠旋转不良、肠系膜囊肿、肠套迭或嵌顿疝应该给予纠治。对于手术不能矫治的患儿，最初治疗的目的就是减少通过受损或者阻塞淋巴管的淋巴液。这可以通过暂停肠内进食和开始 TPN 而实现。一些患儿对这种干预的反应比较快，腹水2周内即可消退。如果患儿的营养和水合状况可以维持的话，TPN的时间可以考虑延长到10周[4,68]。由于中链三酰甘油（MCTs）可以直接吸收入门脉系统，因此，不会刺激淋巴液产生，一直被推荐用于治疗乳糜性腹水。目前尚缺乏MCT方案优点的确切数据。然而，有低脂、MCT增强配方如Portagen在多个非手术治疗的过程中应用成功的报道，应考虑将其作为TPN的辅助或者是作为对TPN有效的患儿肠道营养的初始配方[4,8,23,59,68]。长期应用低脂配方的婴幼儿可有神经系统发育不良，可能与脂肪酸缺乏有关[57]，因此低脂配方治疗应该限制在3～6个月。对于有呼吸障碍的患儿可行腹腔穿刺同时使肠道休息。

如果非手术治疗6～10周还没有治愈或者是患儿
1411 出现其他方面的症状，有必要行外科干预[41,57,66,68]。如同早前所述，术前淋巴管造影的作用并不确定，因为这种检查不能清楚地显示肠系膜和肝门淋巴系统[46,51]。较常用的是在手术探查前6小时给予患儿高脂肪饮食（经常是牛奶），大量奶油色的淋巴液为确定泄漏的部位提供了良好的机会。另外，对牛奶苏丹染色会更有助于确定泄漏的位置[46,51]。虽然也累及腹膜后和肠系膜淋巴管，最常见的淋巴泄漏出现在肠系膜上血管的基底部[5,41,46,51,57,66]。应完全松解十二指肠和胰腺头部，彻底探查整个后腹膜[13]。结扎泄漏部位明确的淋巴管可以治愈85%的患儿[46,66]。最近也有报道腹腔镜有助于确定泄漏的位置以及用纤维蛋白胶来控制淋巴液泄漏[5,46]。腹腔静脉分流术可能是一种有用的治疗策略，可作为主要的手术治疗方案或者用于治疗那些手术探查治疗失败的孩子。在一些大龄患儿，乳糜性腹水死亡率可高达24%～30%[66,67]。然而，随着最近营养支持和手术干预能力的提高，预后将越来越好。

尿性腹水

尽管尿性腹水是新生儿腹水的常见原因，但却不多见，占孤立性腹水病例的1/3[14,65]。男性多于女性，比例为7∶1[21]。下尿道梗阻，特别是来自后尿道瓣膜的梗阻，约占尿性腹水病例的70%。尿性腹水的其他原因包括输尿管囊肿、尿道狭窄、神经源性膀胱或闭锁[14,21,26,44,65]。约65%有梗阻原因的患儿的尿外渗来自于不连续的穿孔。后穹窿是泌尿系统最薄弱的地方。因此，尽管膀胱穿孔也很常见，但穿孔部位最常见于肾盂[14,44]。其他尿性腹水在性质上为非梗性的，包括试图脐动脉插管时造成的脐尿管残余物的损伤、婴儿结缔组织疾患引起的膀胱自发破裂和女性尿生殖窦开放或者泄殖腔的畸形，尿液可通过子宫和输卵管直接漏入腹腔[2,14,21,26,44,45,54,58,63,65]。

大多数尿性腹水的患儿在出生后不久即被发现[3,10,11,32,42]。然而，产前超声也可以探测到腹水。体格检查时，腹胀及通常可触到的侧腹部包块是最常见的表现。可以出现呼吸窘迫和酸中毒（从腹腔吸收尿液），可出现Potter综合征（母体羊水过少和肾、肺和胸壁发育不良）[14,42,50]，也可以在体格检查时发现Prune-belly综合征。低钠血症、高钾血症、血清尿素氮水平升高和肌酐水平升高也很常见[14,16,21]。

诊断检查应该从腹部超声开始，它可以显示腹水，还可以确定与尿性腹水有关的常见的泌尿道畸形，例如肾积水、输尿管扩张以及扩张或增厚的膀胱[65]。排泄性膀胱尿道造影术（VCUG）可以显示任何部位的阻塞性病变并且也可以显示外渗点[26,44,63]。静脉肾盂造影（IVP）或用二乙烯三胺五乙酸（DTPA）或者是硫醇醋酸三甘油（MAG3）的肾扫描可以提供由于长期阻塞肾实质受损程度的信息和显示外渗点[22]。

治疗主要集中在解除潜在的泌尿道梗阻。患儿的最初治疗包括液体复苏、抗生素、远端泌尿道引流[26,44,63]。对于明显的泌尿道梗阻可考虑产前干预[47]。可以用Foley导管插入术来使泌尿道减压，尤其是有后尿道瓣膜的患儿[47]。如果Foley插管引流成功的话，可择期用膀胱镜除去瓣膜。根据所侵犯的病变和患儿的情况，其他减压的方法有经皮肾造瘘术、膀胱造口术或肾盂造口术[26,44]。虽然一些人主张常规引流腹水，但引流腹水或修补穿孔通常并不需要，因为一旦尿引流成功，穿孔很快愈合，尿性腹水随之被吸收[14,21,44]。但如存在呼吸障碍或者感染时，腹水引流是必要的[14]。一旦成功完成上述措施，可以实施针对受侵犯病变的手术。由于慢性梗阻，会有长期肾功能损害的危险。然而，由于导致腹水的梗阻自发性减压对肾功能有保护作用，因此，虽然要长期监测，但有很多患儿仍维持了良好的肾功能[3,14,21,33,65]。随着对新生儿护理和对这些情况的早期认识，尿性腹水的死亡率已从70%降到0%[44]。

（汪　健译　朱锦祥校）

参考文献

1. Ackerman Z: Ascites in nephrotic syndrome: Incidence, patients' characteristics, and complications. J Clin Gastroenterol 1996;22:31.
2. Adams MC, Ludlow J, Brock JW 3rd, Rink RC: Prenatal urinary ascites and persistent cloaca: Risk factors for poor drainage of urine or meconium. J Urol 1998;160:2179.
3. Adzick NS, Harrison MR, Flake AW, deLorimier AA: Urinary extravasation in the fetus with obstructive uropathy. J Pediatr Surg 1985;20:608.
4. Alliet P, Young C, Lebenthal E: Chylous ascites: Total parenteral nutrition as primary therapeutic modality. Eur J Pediatr 1992;151:213.
5. Antao B, Croaker D, Squire R: Successful management of congenital chyloperitoneum with fibrin glue. J Pediatr Surg 2003;38:7.
6. Baden HB, Morray JP: Drainage of tense ascites in children after cardiac surgery. J Cardiothorac Vasc Anesth 1995; 9:720.
7. Banani SA, Bahador A, Nezakatgoo N: Idiopathic perforation of the extrahepatic bile duct in infancy: Pathogenesis, diagnosis, and management. J Pediatr Surg 1993;28:950.
8. Beshay VE, Beshay JE, Rosenberg AJ: Chylous ascites: A case of child abuse and an overview of a rare condition. J Pediatr Gastroenterol Nutr 2001;32:487.
9. Besson R, Gottrand F, Saulnier P, et al: Traumatic chylous ascites: Conservative management. J Pediatr Surg 1992; 27:1543.
10. Bettelheim D, Pumberger W, Deutinger J, Bernaschek G: Prenatal diagnosis of fetal urinary ascites. Ultrasound Obstet Gynecol 2000;16:473.
11. Blessed WB, Sepulveda W, Romero R, et al: Prenatal diagnosis of spontaneous rupture of the fetal bladder with color Doppler ultrasonography. Am J Obstet Gynecol 1993; 169:1629.
12. Borger JA, Pitel P, Crump G: Management of malignant ascites with a vascular port. J Pediatr Surg 1993;28:1606.
13. Chang JHT, Newkirk J, Carlton G, et al: Generalized lymphangiomatosis with chylous ascites—treatment by peritoneo-venous shunting. J Pediatr Surg 1980;15:748.
14. Checkley AM, Sabharwal AJ, MacKinlay GA, et al: Urinary ascites in infancy: Varied etiologies. Pediatr Surg Int 2003; 19:443.
15. Chilukuri S, Bonet V, Cobb M: Antenatal spontaneous perforation of the extrahepatic biliary tree. Am J Obstet Gynecol 1990;163:1201.
16. Clarke HS, Mills ME, Parres JA, Kropp KA: The hyponatremia of neonatal urinary ascites: Clinical observations, experimental confirmation and proposed mechanisms. J Urol 1993;150:778.
17. Cochran WJ, Klish WJ, Brown MR, et al: Chylous ascites in infants and children: A case report and literature review. J Pediatr Gastroenterol Nutr 1985;4:668.
18. Colletti RB, Krawitt EL: Ascites. In Wyllie R, Hyams JS (eds): Pediatric Gastrointestinal Disease, 2nd ed. Philadelphia, WB Saunders, 1999.
19. Craven CE, Goldman AS, Larson DL, et al: Congenital chylous ascites: Lymphangiographic demonstration of obstruction of the cisterna chyli and chylous reflux into the peritoneal space and small intestine. J Pediatr 1967;70:340.
20. DeRusso PA, Benson J, Lau H: Intestinal malrotation and omental cyst presenting as fetal ascites. J Pediatr Gastroenterol Nutr 2003;36:283.
21. De Vries SH, Klijn AJ, Lilien MR, De Jong TP: Development of renal function after neonatal urinary ascites due to obstructive uropathy. J Urol 2002;168:675.
22. Donahoe PK, Hendren WH: Bile duct perforation in a newborn with stenosis of the ampulla of Vater. J Pediatr Surg 1976;11:823.
23. Drinnen D, Filston HC: An unusual case of gastroschisis with gallbladder evisceration and late postrepair chylous ascites. J Pediatr Surg 1997;12:1804.
24. Favre R, Dreux S, Dommergues M, et al: Nonimmune fetal ascites: A series of 79 cases. Am J Obstet Gynecol 2004; 190:407.
25. Fitzgerald RJ, Parbhoo I, Guiney EJ: Spontaneous perforation of bile ducts in neonates. Surgery 1978;83:303.
26. Greenfield SP, Hensle TW, Berdon WE, Geringer AM: Urinary extravasation in the newborn male with posterior urethral valves. J Pediatr Surg 1982;17:751.
27. Guttman FM, Montupet P, Bloss RS: Experience with peritoneovenous shunting for congenital chylous ascites in infants and children. J Pediatr Surg 1982;17:368.
28. Haller JO, Condon VR, Berdon WE, et al: Spontaneous perforation of the common bile duct in children. Radiology 1989;172:621.
29. Hammar B, Sanders E: Spontaneous biliary peritonitis in infancy. J Pediatr Surg 1968;3:84.
30. Hasegawa T, Udatsu Y, Kamiyama M, et al: Does pancreaticobiliary maljunction play a role in spontaneous perforation of the bile duct in children? Pediatr Surg Int 2000; 16:550.
31. Ibanez DV, Vila JJ, Fernandez MS, et al: Spontaneous biliary perforation and necrotizing enterocolitis. Pediatr Surg Int 1999;15:401.
32. Kasat LS, Borwankar SS, Jain M, Naregal A: Spontaneous perforation of the extrahepatic bile duct in an infant. Pediatr Surg Int 2001;17:463.
33. Kobata R, Isukahara H, Takeuchi M, et al: Early detection of prune belly syndrome in utero by ultrasonography. Acta Paediatr Jpn 1997;39:705.
34. Konen O, Rathous V, Dlugy E, et al: Childhood abdominal cystic lymphangioma. Pediatr Radiol 2002;32:88.
35. Kramer RE, Sokol RJ, Yerushalmi B, et al: Large-volume paracentesis in the management of ascites in children. J Pediatr Gastroenterol Nutr 2001;33:245.
36. Lee WS, McKiernan PJ, de Ville de Goyet JV, et al: Successful treatment of refractory ascites in a child with transjugular intrahepatic portosystemic shunt. Acta Paediatr 2001;90:1352.
37. Lees W, Mitchell JE: Bile peritonitis in infancy. Arch Dis Child 1966;48:188.
38. Lilly JR, Weintraub WH, Altman RP: Spontaneous perforation of the extrahepatic bile ducts and bile peritonitis in infancy. Surgery 1974;75:664.
39. Lloyd D: Gastroschisis, malrotation, and chylous ascites. J Pediatr Surg 1991;26:106.
40. Lloyd DA, Mickel RE: Spontaneous perforation of the extra-hepatic bile ducts in neonates and infants. Br J Surg 1980;67:621.
41. Loiterman DL, Bleicher MA: Chylous ascites: An etiology of peritonitis in infancy. J Pediatr Surg 1985;5:538.
42. Lowenstein L, Solt I, Talmon R, et al: In utero diagnosis of bladder perforation with urinary ascites. A case report. Fetal Diagn Ther 2003;18:179.
43. Man DWK, Spitz L: The management of chylous ascites in children. J Pediatr Surg 1985;20:72.
44. Mann CM, Leape LL, Holder TM: Neonatal urinary ascites: A report of 2 cases of unusual etiology and a review of the literature. J Urol 1974;111:124.

45. Mata JA, Livne PM, Gibbons MD: Urinary ascites: Complication of umbilical artery catheterization. Urology 1987;30:375.
46. Mitsunaga T, Yoshida H, Iwai J, et al: Successful surgical treatment of two cases of congenital chylous ascites. J Pediatr Surg 2001;36:1717.
47. Nakayama DK, Harrison MR, de Lorimier AA: Prognosis of posterior urethral valves presenting at birth. J Pediatr Surg 1986;21:43.
48. Ohkawa H, Takahashi H, Maie M: A malformation of the pancreaticobiliary system as a cause of perforation of the biliary tract in childhood. J Pediatr Surg 1977; 12:541.
49. Pandit SK, Budhiraja S, Rattan KN: Post traumatic bile ascites. Indian J Pediatr 2000;67:72.
50. Patil KK, Wilcox DT, Samuel M, et al: Management of urinary extravasation in 18 boys with posterior urethral valves. J Urol 2003;169:1508, discussion 1511.
51. Pearl J, Joyner J, Collins DL: Chylous ascites: The first reported surgical cure by direct ligation. J Pediatr Surg 1977;12:687.
52. Pettitt BJ: Use of a modified Denver peritoneovenous shunt in a newborn with intractable ascites. J Pediatr Surg 1992;27:108.
53. Prevot J, Babist M: Spontaneous perforation of the biliary tract. In Rickham PP, Hecker WC, Prevot J (eds): Progress in Pediatric Surgery. Baltimore, University Park Press, 1971.
54. Redman JF, Seibert JJ, Arnold W: Urinary ascites in children owing to extravasation of urine from the bladder. J Urol 1979;122:411.
55. Runyon BA, Montano AA, Akriviadis EA, et al: The serum-ascites albumin gradient in the differential diagnosis of ascites is superior to the exudate/transexudate concept. Ann Intern Med 1992;117:215.
56. Ryan JA, Smith MD, Page CP: Treatment of chylous ascites with peritoneovenous shunt. Am Surg 1981;47:384.
57. Sanchez RE, Mahour GH, Brennan LP, Woolley MM: Chylous ascites in children. Surgery 1971;69:183.
58. Sayan A, Demircan M, Erikci VS, et al: Neonatal bladder rupture and unusual complication of umbilical catheterization. Eur J Pediatr Surg 1996;6:378.
59. Solans CV, Sockolow RE: Chylous ascites associated with gastroschisis. Clin Pediatr (Phila) 1996;35:415.
60. Squires R: Complications of end-stage liver disease. In Rudolph CD, Rudolph AM (eds): Rudolph's Pediatrics, 21st ed. New York, McGraw-Hill, 2003.
61. Stringel G, Mercer S: Idiopathic perforation of the biliary tract in infancy. J Pediatr Surg 1983;18:546.
62. Terg R, Berreta J, Abecasis R, et al: Dextran administration avoids hemodynamic changes following paracentesis in cirrhotic patients: A safe and inexpensive option. Dig Dis Sci 1992;37:79.
63. Thompson IM, Bruns TNC: Neonatal ascites: A reflection of obstructive disease. J Urol 1972;107:509.
64. Tito L, Gines P, Arroyo V, et al: Total paracentesis associated with intravenous albumin management of patients with cirrhosis and ascites. Gastroenterology 1990;98:146.
65. Towers H: Neonatal ascites. In Burg FD (ed): Gellis & Kagan's Current Pediatric Therapy 17. Philadelphia, WB Saunders, 2002.
66. Unger SW, Chandler JG: Chylous ascites in infants and children. Surgery 1983;93:455.
67. Vasko JS, Tapper RI: The surgical significance of chylous ascites. Arch Surg 1967;95:355.
68. Weiser AC, Lindgren BW, Ritchey ML, Franco I: Chylous ascites following surgical treatment for Wilms tumor. J Urol 2003;170:1667, discussion 1669.
69. Wyllie R, Arasu TS, Fitzgerald JF: Ascites: Pathophysiology and management. J Pediatr 1980;97:167.
70. Xanthakos SA, Yazigi NA, Rychman FC, Arkovitz MS: Spontaneous perforation of the bile duct in infancy: A rare but important cause of irritability and abdominal distension. J Pediatr Gastroenterol Nutr 2003;36:28.

第 91 章

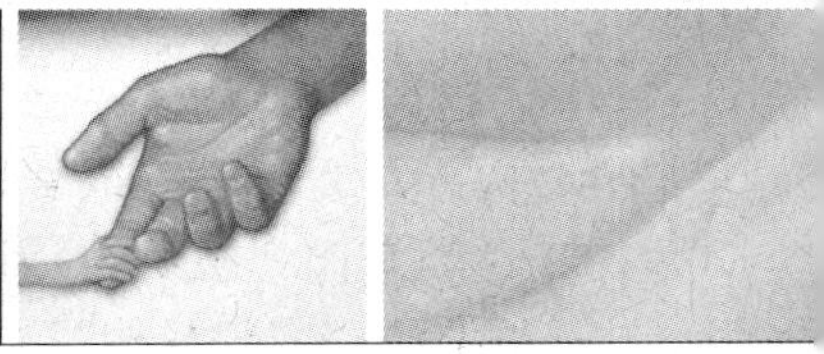

胃肠道息肉性疾病

Joseph L. Lelli, Jr.

14 胃肠道息肉性疾病包括孤立于肠道的病变（幼年型、淋巴型和腺瘤型）、一些少见的综合征及身体其他部位疾病（Peutz-Jeghers 综合征、Gardner 综合征和 Turcot 综合征）。大多数胃肠道息肉是良性的，由黏膜下淋巴组织增生或黏膜错构瘤引起。但腺瘤样息肉是黏膜发生紊乱改变的表现，有潜在的恶变倾向。

儿童息肉很常见，学龄前和学龄期儿童息肉的发生率为 1%[173]。由于其发病率高，胃肠道息肉是 2~5岁的幼儿及学龄前儿童直肠出血最常见的原因。幼年型息肉最常见（80%），其次是淋巴样息肉（15%）[106]，腺瘤型息肉在所有息肉患儿中比例小于 3%。

幼年型息肉

历史回顾

1908 年，Verse 首先描述了幼年型息肉[177]。许多年来所有儿童的息肉都被认为是腺瘤[66]，通常用放疗来治疗。1957 年，Horrileno[75] 第一个用“幼年型息肉”这个词来描述主要发生在儿童期的、有组织学特点的结直肠息肉。1962 年，Morson[116] 做了一个很重要的贡献，证明幼年型息肉是良性的错构瘤，因此，完全区别于有潜在恶性变的腺瘤样息肉。然而减少放疗以后，息肉增长缓慢。1964 年，McColl 和他的同事[109]第一次将孤立性幼年型息肉与幼年型息肉病区别开来。三种不同形式的幼年型息肉病在 1972 年被 Sachatello 进一步确认[146]。1971 年 Kaschula 及其后的 1976 年 Enterline[39] 报道了同时患有幼年型和腺瘤型息肉的儿童病例。1982 年 Billingham 及其合作者[12]报道发现有幼年型息肉的儿童同时患有单独的腺瘤。这些早期关于幼年型息肉和腺瘤型息肉并存的报道，使得人们认识到幼年型息肉具有腺瘤样变和恶性变的可能[60,114,131]。然而，只有伴有幼年型息肉病的儿童，息肉才具有恶变倾向[25,55,147]。区分常见的孤立性良性幼年型息肉和较少见的可能是恶性的幼年型息肉综合征，已经变得非常重要了[25,55,83,119]。

Jass[81] 建议在有息肉的儿童中具备以下标准就有恶性变的风险：（1）结肠内超过 5 个幼年型息肉；（2）息肉累及整个胃肠道；（3）任何数目的息肉伴有家族性幼年型息肉病病史。Jass 标准将 Sachatello 于 1972 年报道的 3 种不同的幼年型息肉病综合征区分开来[146]。基于 Jass 和 Sachatello 的研究，以下是最常用的幼年型息肉的分类：

Ⅰ. 孤立性幼年型息肉（非恶性）：结肠内少于 5 个息肉，无家族性幼年型息肉病的病史。

Ⅱ. 幼年型息肉病综合征（恶性倾向）：

A. 婴儿广泛幼年型息肉病：小于 6 个月的婴儿整个胃肠道布满幼年型息肉。

B. 广泛幼年型息肉病：多发性息肉分布整个胃肠道，但大多数在胃内、远端结肠和直肠，通常发生在 6 月~5 岁的儿童。

C. 幼年型结肠息肉：5 ~ 15 岁儿童远端结肠和直肠有多发性幼年型息肉。

孤立性幼年型息肉

病理

幼年型息肉亦被认为是固定的、炎症性或囊性息

1415 肉，是胃肠道中最常见的息肉，占儿童息肉的 80%。这类息肉常被认为是正常结肠黏膜组织偶然重组产生的错构瘤[116]或构成异常[81]。

大体上，典型的息肉有一个具有光泽、光滑、圆形、红色的头部，直径在 2 毫米至几厘米之间（图 91–1），息肉表面通常溃疡，故易引起直肠出血。横切面显示囊腔内充满黏液（图 91–2）。典型的幼年型息肉有一个表面覆有结肠黏膜的细长蒂部，该蒂部易使息肉扭转，导致静脉淤血，表面发生溃疡、出血并可自行脱落。

显微镜下，息肉表面覆有单层结肠上皮，这层上皮通常有溃疡或被肉芽组织所替代。当有炎症时，上皮出现增生，形成轻度发育不良或腺瘤样改变[10]。息肉的主体主要由内衬正常结肠上皮的扩张的或囊状上皮样管构成。这些管状和囊状湖位于黏膜固有层大量疏松的具有血管和纤维的间质中（图 91–3）。这种间质内充满大量中性粒细胞、嗜酸性粒细胞、单核细胞和淋巴细胞，有丝分裂现象少见。在文献中，有 2 例实质性幼年型息肉有恶性改变的报道[103,149]。根据 Jass 的观点[81]，只有 1 例是属于真正的恶性表现，在对有单个息肉患儿的长期随访中，没有发现其能增加结直肠癌的风险[130]。

病因学

幼年型息肉的病因不明，但有几个作者认为基因[96]、遗传[58]、错构瘤样畸形[116]以及炎症[143]是其发病的因素。近年的资料表明，幼年型息肉是由继发于炎症后黏膜结构的重新排列引起的[49]。最初可能表现为溃疡，接着黏膜发生炎症，导致局部小的结肠黏膜腺体发生梗阻，进而梗阻的腺体增生、分裂以及扩张，形成一个囊状结构，囊状结构挤压黏膜，导致进一步溃疡、炎症和肉芽组织形成。当这个循环继续时，形成越来越大的团块突出于肠腔，大便的通过和肠管的蠕动推挤团块突落于肠腔，使蒂柄更长，最终形成了幼年型息肉典型的肉茎样表现。

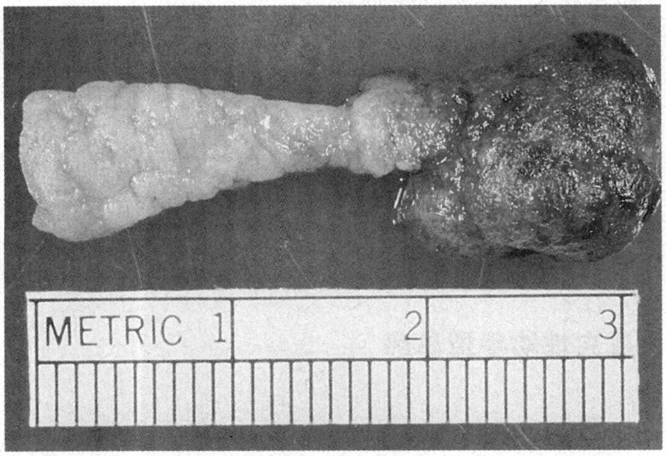

图 91–1　与柄附在一起的典型幼年型息肉。

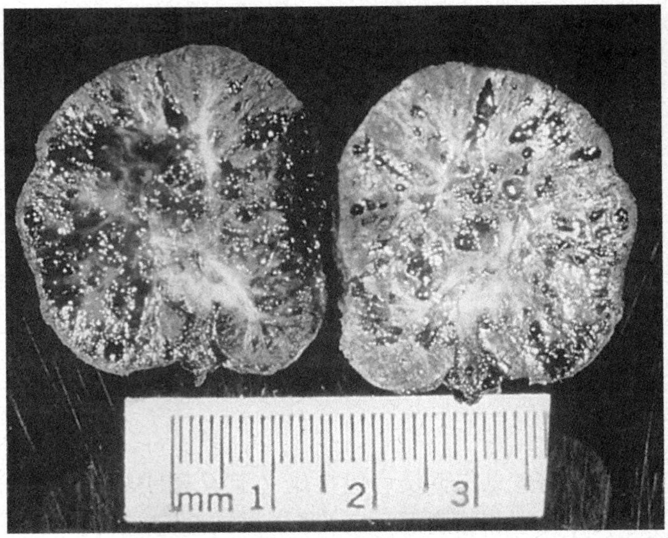

图 91–2　幼年型息肉冠状切面上有典型的囊状湖，其间充满了黏液。

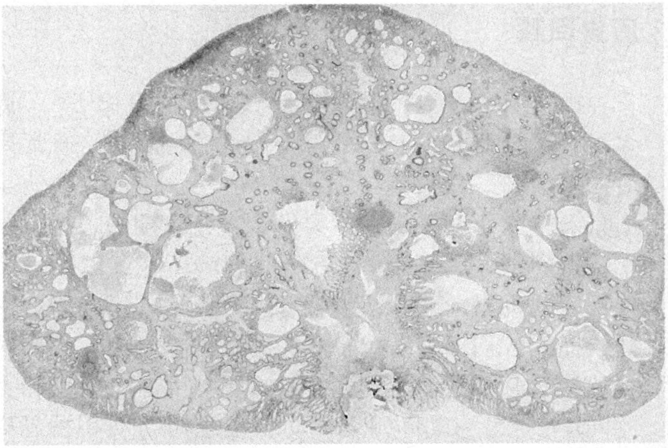

图 91–3　典型幼年型息肉显微镜下的照片。表面光滑、平坦、覆盖结肠上皮，有大的管状和囊状湖，嵌入多量稀疏的基质内。

发病率

尽管幼年型息肉的发病率尚不清楚，但在所有学龄前儿童中的发病率约为 1%[113]。大多数幼年型息肉发生在 10 岁前的儿童，发病率高峰为 3～5 岁[113]。
16 50% 病例的息肉是单发的，其余的病例有 2～10 个息肉不等。这些息肉的位置在过去 10 年中已发生了变化，以前 70% 的息肉发生在直肠，目前，只有 40% 发生在直肠或乙状结肠，而 60% 发生在近端结肠，在青春期后，幼年型息肉较少见。

临床表现

幼年型息肉最常见的表现是由息肉表面的溃疡引起的出血（93%）。失血常很少表现为大便表面有鲜红的血丝。腹痛（10%）被认为是由于肠管蠕动牵拉息肉引起的。息肉脱垂（4%）是另一个少见的症状，直肠脱垂和大便失禁亦有报道[113]。许多幼年型息肉会自行脱落，直肠出血随之自行停止[122]。

幼年型息肉的鉴别诊断要考虑引起幼儿和 6 岁前儿童直肠出血的所有原因。肛裂和直肠脱垂引起的直肠出血通过体检较容易区别开来。Meckel 憩室或肠重复畸形引起的出血比息肉的失血量多，血与大便混在一起而不是覆盖于大便表面。肠套迭引起的出血同时伴有腹痛，这种腹痛比息肉的腹痛更严重。肠道炎症性疾病通常伴有腹泻，而息肉不伴有腹泻。血恶瘤质、肠壁血管瘤和自身免疫性疾病如过敏性紫癜在鉴别诊断亦要考虑。

治疗

幼年型息肉的诊断和治疗要通过确切的病史、直肠指检和结肠镜检查结合起来考虑。幼年型息肉可移行至近端结肠[122]以及要考虑有幼年型息肉病的存在（超过 5 个息肉），它增加了恶变的风险，有必要行整个结肠的检查。疑有息肉的儿童应首先做直肠指检，直肠内的息肉很容易通过肛门镜切除。直肠幼年型息肉去除后，在肠道准备充分的前提下，应进行全结肠镜检查来发现近端结肠有无另外的息肉存在[64]。幼年型息肉病和腺瘤样息肉的儿童，息肉通常在右半结肠[73]。因此，应去除所有息肉并进行组织学检查。结肠镜下去除息肉的并发症较少见。

幼年型息肉病综合征

幼年型息肉病综合征较少见，这些综合征被分成 3 种不同的临床类型：婴儿弥漫性幼年型息肉病、弥漫性幼年型息肉病和幼年型结肠息肉病[146]。

类型

婴儿弥漫性幼年型息肉病

婴儿弥漫性幼年型息肉病常发生在出生后几个月[25]，通常无家族史[81]，出现的症状包括腹泻、直肠出血、肠套迭、肠源性蛋白丢失、巨颅、杵状指（趾）以及肌张力减退[62,140,148,158]、腹泻、直肠出血、肠源性蛋白丢失的程度与息肉的数量直接相关，整个胃肠道通常受累及。这种综合征通常采用不保守治疗，首先是全静脉营养使肠道休息，接下来是减少蛋白和血液的丢失，降低肠套迭的发生率[157]。当患儿的营养状况稳定后，切除息肉较多的肠管。尽管采取了适当的治疗，该病儿乎都导致死亡。有报道，12 例患儿中只有 2 例活过 2 岁[3,18,62,98,109,140,145,147,148,158,175]。

弥漫性幼年型息肉病

患弥漫性幼年型息肉病的儿童常见的发病年龄为 6 个月～5 岁，表现为轻度直肠出血和脱垂，但亦可以出现肠源性蛋白丢失、肠套迭和营养不良[25]。在这个年龄段中，重要的是要把幼年型息肉病同家族性腺瘤样息肉病区分开来。弥漫性息肉病的息肉累及整个肠管，最常见的病变位于胃、远端结肠和直肠[25]。肠镜下息肉摘除和节段性肠管切除可治疗该病，尽管通常需要反复治疗，但患儿通常恢复较好。

幼年型结肠息肉病

结肠幼年型息肉病发生在 5～15 岁的儿童。该病有典型的特征，包括直肠流出鲜红色血液、贫血、直肠脱垂或这些症状均有。息肉通常局限于远端结肠和直肠内[25]，约 50% 的患儿有家族史，提示是常染色体显性遗传[147]。已有报道其可能伴随的先天缺陷有腭裂和肠旋转不良，多指（趾）以及心脏和头颅畸形[81]。

病理

有5个或更多息肉的儿童，甚至息肉布满胃肠道，或即使只有一个息肉的家族性幼年型息肉病儿童，都被认为是幼年型息肉病综合征[81]，大多数患该综合征的儿童有50～100个结肠息肉，有弥漫性幼年型息肉病的婴儿和儿童在胃和小肠内或二者兼有息肉。由于该病有癌变可能（17%），且癌变年龄早
1417 （平均诊断年龄为35.5岁）[25]，确诊息肉病综合征很重要，需进行长期随访。

幼年型息肉病的息肉大体外观与孤立性幼年型息肉相似，大约20%表现为多叶性的团块，组成一串息肉连在一个蒂上（图91-4）[83]。组织学上，这些息肉有许多绒毛或乳头状上皮，幼年型息肉[53,58,60,63,65,79,83,89,102,114,131,142,176]及其共存的腺瘤中[5,6,23,55,83,89,131,139,142,176]可能发生上皮异常增生。被认为是原位癌的严重上皮发育不良可在伴有幼年型息肉病综合征的幼年型息肉患儿身上发现[87]。分叶息肉发生严重发育不良的几率（47%）较不分叶的息肉（10%）高[83]。已有几例报道发现幼年型息肉病患儿结直肠中有浸润性腺癌[57,60,79,142,146,156,162]，根据St. Mark在伦敦的息肉病登记资料显示，在60岁时，幼年型息肉病综合征患儿的癌变累积风险为68%[65,119]。

治疗

常染色体显性遗传和60岁时癌变的累积风险为68%，意味着治疗必须包括对患有息肉的患儿和他的家庭成员进行长期随访。一些人建议可行预防性结肠切除和直肠黏膜切除，并在直肠内作回肠肛管拖出吻合作为最初的治疗[79]，还有人建议定期（每2年）结肠镜检查并随机活检[77]，接下来如果有严重发育不良、息肉生长迅速或出血要作结肠切除[55]。一个患儿4岁时作了结肠切除和回肠乙状结肠吻合术，但在27岁时乙状结肠发展成无法手术的癌症[83]。因该病具有家族性特点，应对直系亲属进行筛查。幼年型息肉病儿童的治疗方法与家族性腺瘤样息肉病相似。

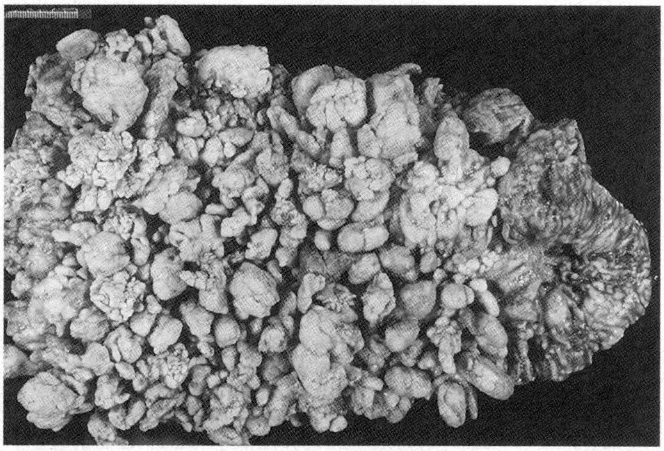

图91-4　幼年型息肉病综合征的患儿结肠大体标本，可见小的腺瘤与多叶状息肉群附着在柄上。

PEUTZ-JEGHERS 综合征

历史回顾

在1921年Peutz[135]首先报道肠息肉同时伴有口、手和足的皮肤黏膜色素沉着斑；1944年，Jeghers[84]报道2例；1949年，他和同事[85]又报道了8例以及本人收集来的其他12例病例；接着，Jeghers和同事[85]定义了该综合征的两个主要特点：（1）颊黏膜和口唇上的黑色素斑，同时，睑和手指数目不定的黑色素斑；（2）肠道息肉病。1954年，Bruwer和同事[15]首先使用Peutz-Jeghers综合征这个词。近来，有肠道和肠道外癌症患者的报道引起了对这些患者治疗的重新评估[136]。

病理

Peutz-Jeghers综合征的特征是黑色素斑，颜色从棕色到黑色，常发生在口唇的周围和颊黏膜上，在手、足、鼻黏膜、结膜和直肠内亦可出现这些斑点[136]，这种黑色素斑常见于婴儿，通常在青春期消退。

尽管Peutz-Jeghers综合征的息肉分布从胃到直肠，但最常见于小肠（55%），大约30%的息肉位于胃和十二指肠，15%位于结肠和直肠[169]，息肉大体观为大小从几毫米到几厘米，光滑、坚实带蒂并有分叶，而幼年型息肉不分叶。Peutz-Jeghers综合征组织学上为肌黏膜错构瘤[136]并有平滑肌纤维丝将息肉分成几个部分（图91-5）[82,117,118]。Peutz-Jeghers息肉可同时伴有腺瘤。

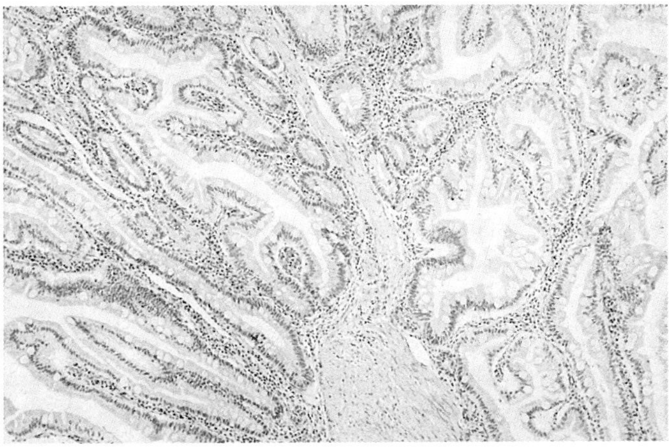

图 91-5　Peutz-Jeghers 息肉的显微镜照片显示肌性黏膜的错构瘤样改变，平滑肌纤维将息肉分成几个部分。

病因和发病率

Peutz-Jeghers 综合征较少见，男女发病相似，在所有年龄组中均有报道。大多数 Peutz-Jeghers 综合征的病例是常染色显性遗传，但一些是新发病例，大多数表现为新的自发性变异。近来，2 个研究小组发现 Peutz-Jeghers 综合征与基因变异有关，在 Peutz-Jeghers 综合征受累的个体中，许多（不是全部）患儿发生了一种异常的丝氨酸/苏氨酸酶（LKB1 或 STK11）的变异，使激酶失去活力[67,86]。常规基因检测和基因治疗还在研究中，目前还未应用[110]。

临床表现

因 Peutz-Jeghers 综合征与家族遗传相关，常可通过筛查发现该病，如果无家族史，患者通常有腹痛，往往是由息肉引起暂时性肠套迭。腹部平片通常发现扩张或部分梗阻的小肠，但很少完全梗阻。贫血由隐匿的失血引起，可有恶病质样症状。在前 10 年中，30% 的患儿出现症状和体征，在 20 岁时，达到 50%[35,169]。

有报道 Peutz-Jeghers 综合征伴有小肠肿瘤[16,45,56,74,159,171]。在 Peutz-Jeghers 综合征错构瘤样息肉中常有恶变的报道[26,76,94,108,126,134,152,154,159]。独立的腺瘤和癌症样改变在错构瘤中也有报道，认为在 Peutz-Jeghers 综合征患儿的小肠中会发生腺瘤样癌变[26]。回顾 72 例该综合征的患儿，显示 22% 的患儿发展为癌症，9 例发生在胃肠道或胰腺，7 例发生在肠道外。与年龄相似的一般人群相比，Peutz-Jeghers 综合征患儿发生胃肠道癌症的死亡风险高出 13 倍多，发生各类癌症的死亡风险要高出 9 倍多，Peutz-Jeghers 综合征患者在 60 岁时，发生癌症导致死亡的机会大约为 50%[136]。

Peutz-Jeghers 综合征肠道外肿瘤包括卵巢、宫颈和睾丸肿瘤。报道的卵巢肿瘤包括囊腺瘤[35,78,107]、生殖细胞肿瘤[23] 和性索肿瘤[9,70,150,190]，宫颈腺癌的发生往往与卵巢肿瘤相关[189]，已发现有睾丸 Sertoli 细胞肿瘤以及 50% 的病例出现男性乳房女性化。这些肿瘤通常是良性的，但有恶变可能，因此需要作睾丸切除。Peutz-Jeghers 综合征患者亦有乳腺、甲状腺、胆道、胰腺和胆囊癌的报道[136]。

治疗

任何儿童出现绞窄性腹痛或隐匿性贫血以及黑色素斑时要怀疑 Peutz-Jeghers 综合征。由于对恶变的认识增加，近 10 年对于该病的治疗建议有所改变。Phillips 和 Spigelman[136] 推荐的治疗方案包括每年评价以下情况：（1）息肉相关症状；（2）血液丢失引起血细胞计数下降的贫血；（3）女孩宫颈涂片和盆腔超声来检查盆腔和乳腺；（4）男孩行超声检查睾丸；（5）胰腺超声检查以及至少两年 1 次的食管、胃十二指肠镜和结肠镜检查，同时小肠造影检查。近来，核磁共振（MRI）作为对小肠筛查的一种监测方式[95]，在 25、30、35 和 38 岁时，要进行乳腺 X 线检查，两年 1 次，直到 50 岁，以后每年 1 次。

内镜下发现大于 0.5 mm 的息肉均要切除，可在剖腹时结合术中肠镜去除所有直径大于 15 mm 的小肠息肉。由于息肉有复发的特点以及会导致短肠综合征，所以之前的根治性小肠切除方法应避免。任何肠道内或肠道外的肿瘤应积极治疗。历史资料显示 Peutz-Jeghers 综合征患者 60 岁前死亡率接近 60%，而一般人群此年龄段为 25%[136]。

淋巴样息肉

历史回顾

Marina-Fid 和 Rof-Carballo 在 1941 年报道第一例回肠末端淋巴样增生的病例，同年 Patel 和 Awen 也有报道[133]；Fieber 和 Schaefer[43] 在 1966 年回顾以前文献报道的 8 例以及他们自己收集的 4 例病例；Byrne 和同事[20] 报道了世界范围内仅有的 44 例该病病例；然而，Franker 发现放射性腹痛的患儿中 60% 有淋巴样息肉[48]。因此，淋巴样息肉的发生率远高于所报道的，但他们中大多数是没有症状的，因此从未被发现。

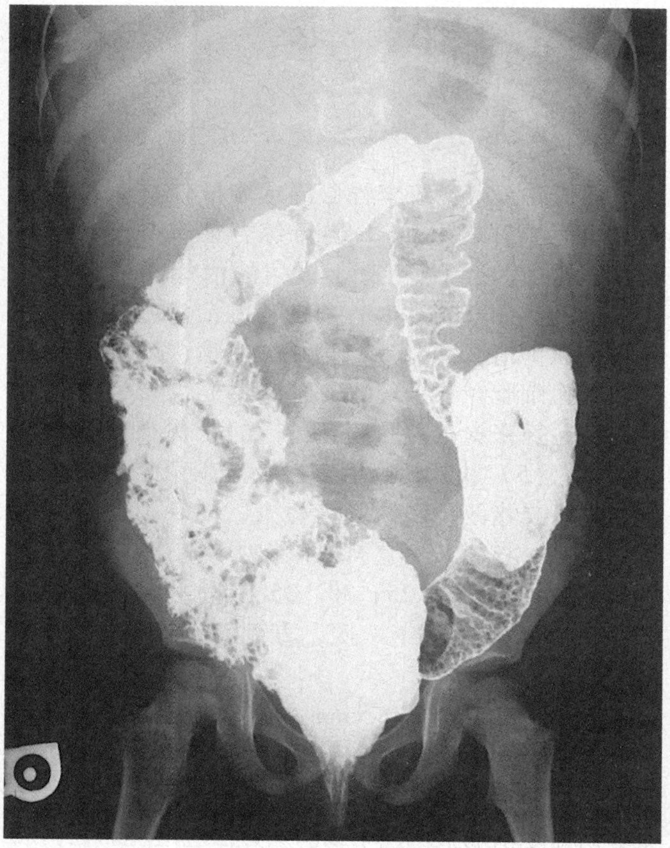

图 91-6　钡灌肠显示多发性、小的 1～2 mm 黏膜样小瘤，分布于整个结肠和末端回肠，在这张排空后的 X 线片上，可以看到这些小瘤中央凹陷，可诊断为弥漫性淋巴增生。

病理

淋巴样息肉直径大小从几毫米到 3. 0 cm，通常无蒂。息肉是由黏膜下集合淋巴结增生突起引起的，被
覆的黏膜通常出现溃疡，使息肉出现火山口样表现， 141
黏膜溃疡导致隐匿性失血。黏膜下淋巴组织的增生被认为是由于儿童非特异性感染引起的[1,2,4,106]。

发病率

淋巴样息肉多发生于婴幼儿生后几年内，是因其暴露于新的病毒和细菌所致[157]，发病高峰期在 4 岁，5 岁时明显减少。

临床表现

失血引起贫血以及偶尔大量直肠出血是淋巴样息肉的常见表现。结肠镜、气钡灌肠造影或两者均为结肠淋巴样息肉的诊断性检查。气钡灌肠造影显示小的、均匀的、中央凹陷的息肉状充盈缺损（图 91-6 和 91-7）[20,48]，有别于幼年型和腺瘤样息肉内镜下看到的小的异常黏膜突起，活检可明确诊断，组织学检

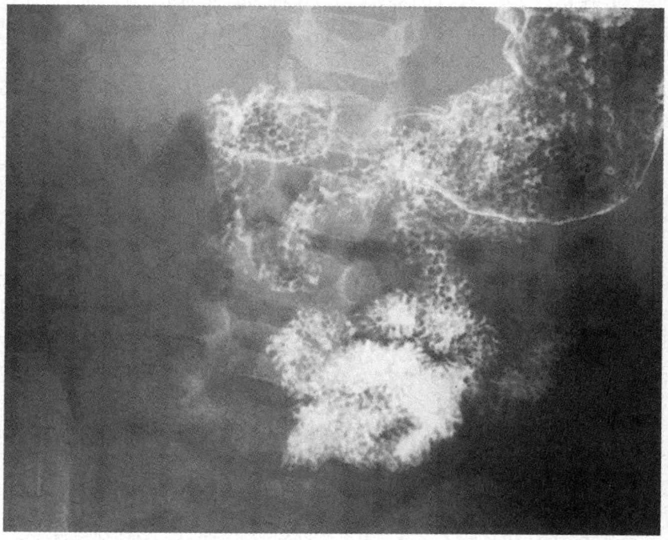

图 91-7　上消化道造影显示整个胃和小肠弥漫性淋巴增生。

查可发现大量生发滤泡的淋巴样聚集[157]。

治疗

淋巴样息肉是良性自限性疾病，倾向于自行消退[21,106]，一旦组织学诊断成立，在病灶消退前常需进行监测，不能控制的大量出血和肠套迭可能需要作进一步外科处理。

家族性腺瘤样息肉病

历史回顾

1847 年 Covisart 记录了第一例腺瘤样息肉病[28]，但在 12 年后，Chargelaigue[22] 在患有该病的 16 岁女孩和 21 岁男孩中首次对该病进行了明确说明。1867 年 Virchow[178] 第一个报道这些结肠息肉的病理改变。1881 年，Woodward[188] 第一个区别了新生性和炎症性息肉。1882 年，Cripps[32] 第一次在一名 9 岁男童及其 17 岁姐姐间描述了该息肉病的家族相关性，然而直到 1890 年，Handford 才认识到这些息肉有恶变的可能[66]。

正如 Thomson 和 Watne 报道的[168,185]，第一例有记载的息肉病手术要归功于北美的 Lilienthal[10] 及其后伦敦 St. Mark 医院的 Lockhart-Mummery。1925 年，Lockhart-Mummery[104] 得出：（1）多发性腺瘤样息肉可以传代；（2）受累的个体可在早期发展成癌症；（3）腺瘤是一种癌前病变。1927 年，Cockayne[27] 描
20 述该病遗传模式为孟德尔显性遗传，在 1930 年被 Dukes[37] 所证实，在 1939 年，亦被 Lockhart-Mummery 和 Dukes 证实[105]。从那时起，家族性腺瘤样息肉病（FAP）已成为了解腺癌顺序的一种模型[36]。

Gardner 综合征的患者 5 号染色体 q69 位点的缺失是 FAP 的基因基础，即 APC 基因[13,61,71,88,92,93,100,111,115,127]，在 APC 基因中 5q 的缺失或改变产生了一种截短的蛋白基因产物，该产物使 APC 基因充当肿瘤抑制剂。FAP 的小鼠模型已经建立[164]，并将为基因治疗研究提供便利。

病理

在结肠内至少有 100 个可见的腺瘤样息肉才能定义为家族性腺瘤样息肉病[17]，然而较少息肉的患者亦能诊断为 FAP，如一个患儿早期有结直肠癌和 5q 基因缺失，而结肠镜下只发现一个息肉也可诊断为 FAP[99]。

结直肠息肉是 FAP 的标志，尽管通常需要发现 100 个息肉才可诊断该病，但在青少年期结肠切除的患儿中，可发现典型的上千个息肉（图 91-8），似乎有两种类型的 FAP 存在：以数百个息肉为特征的稀疏型和以几千个息肉为特征的密集型。Utsunomiya 及其同事[174] 发现两种类型的病情发展不同——密集型息肉患儿更易于在早年发生腺癌。

在 FAP 中，息肉典型地分布在整个结肠，通过乙结肠镜可诊断。息肉的直径从 1.0～2.0 mm 不等，有时出现带蒂柄的直径 1 cm 或更大的息肉（图 91-9）。在十二指肠镜检时，看似正常的十二指肠黏膜活检可发现肉眼见不到的微腺瘤，这些微腺瘤由 3 或 4 个发育不良的隐窝构成，并且通常有管状腺瘤样结构[185]。

腺瘤样息肉是由至少一种上皮细胞在隐窝处增生导致的一种瘤性转化[121]，这种转化克隆被出芽分隔，并占据了隐窝的上半部分[121]，隐窝融合促进了腺瘤的生长。这种瘤性转化称作发育不良，具有非典型形态学特征，伴有核增大和分层。腺瘤似乎通过逐渐的

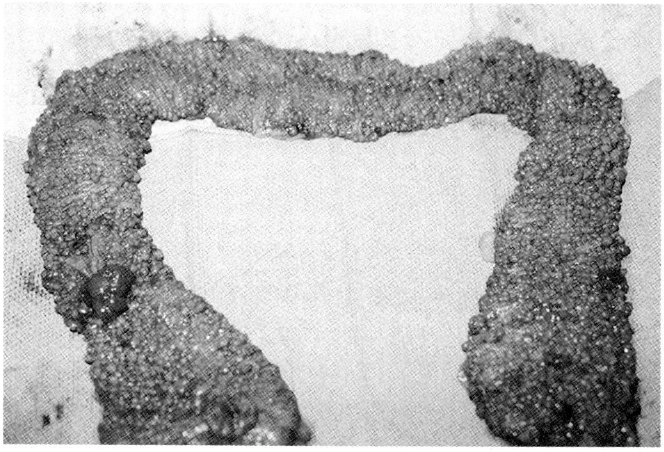

图 91-8 家族性腺瘤样息肉病患者的全结肠大体标本，可见几千个腺瘤样息肉，并在升结肠部位有一个大的腺瘤。

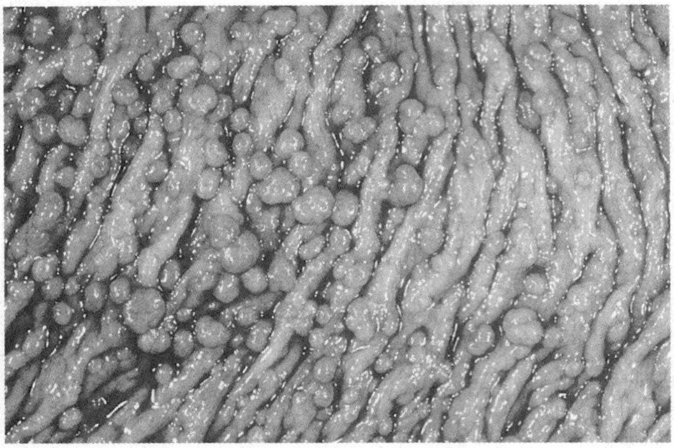

图 91-9　结肠黏膜的特写镜头。在这例家族性腺瘤样息肉病的患者中可以看到一条小的 1～2 mm 腺瘤“地毯”。

发育不良发展成浸润性腺癌[120]。肿瘤细胞侵入结肠上皮基底膜即为原位癌，当肿瘤细胞侵入超过基底膜时，肿瘤在显微镜下即变成浸润的。由于结肠黏膜不包含淋巴组织，通常不发生转移，直到肿瘤侵入肌黏膜到达黏膜下层。

小肠黏膜亦能被腺瘤样息肉所累及，小肠息肉通常位于胆总管开口周围的十二指肠内[160]。这个部位的息肉大小不一，通常是微腺瘤，仅累及一部分隐窝，十二指肠乳头和壶腹部周围地区腺癌发生率为所有 FAP 患儿的 2.9%[160]，在这些患儿中亦可发生胆总管腺癌[161]。

FAP 的患儿亦有胃息肉发生，但它们通常是有基底腺的良性息肉[34]。这些息肉是由于特殊胃壁腺体囊状扩张导致，而不是发育不良引起，没有证据显示在基底腺的息肉中有瘤性转化的发生[165]。

病因学

FAP 的发病率从新生儿中 1/6000～1/12 000 不
1421 等[80,141,184]。FAP 是以一种中度（10%）突变的常染色体显性遗传病[72]。FAP 的表现各不相同，可能是 APC 基因突变的多样化所致。尽管息肉的发生与基因密切相关，但是在 1988 年发现结肠切除和乙状结肠、回肠吻合后有直肠息肉退化的现象[42,125]，同时指出肠腔环境在息肉的发展上亦起着一定的作用。

FAP 是由于第 5 号染色体长臂上的 APC 基因突变引起的，5 号染色体上基因的各种缺失或改变与该病有关。APC 基因编码一种蛋白产物，该产物可作为一种肿瘤抑制剂[72]。由于该基因的缺失，到 25 岁患癌症（乙状结肠镜活检诊断）的可能性为 90%[66]。在结直肠癌细胞系中引入完整的 5 号染色体，小鼠发生肿瘤的倾向大大减弱[59,166]。相同的结果亦出现在其他肿瘤抑制基因中，它们是 17p 上的 TP53 基因和 18q 上缺失的结直肠癌基因（DCC 基因）[72]，在 FAP 中，存在明显的基因异质性，APC 基因某个基因种系的突变易减弱疾病的表达[31,112]，进一步的证据显示附加的改良基因可影响 FAP 的严重程度[30]。

临床表现

尽管 FAP 在婴儿和低龄儿童中发病，但最常见于青少年早期，大多数患儿无症状，但有些表现为大便次数增多、直肠出血、贫血和腹痛。因为这些患儿有腺瘤样息肉病的家族史，大多数（90%）通过常规监测能被发现。

FAP 可通过乙状结肠镜诊断，有时也可通过气钡灌肠诊断。乙状结肠镜常发现整个结肠表面均覆盖有息肉，至少需活检 10 个息肉才能确诊。在一些 FAP 患儿中，大多数息肉集中在近端结肠。如果一个患儿 FAP 诊断成立，且表现为一种新的突变（不知道其他家庭成员患该病），则需要仔细检查所有家庭成员。

胃内发现息肉占 FAP 患儿的 50%，但只有 6% 是腺瘤样息肉[34]，其余的为基底腺息肉（错构瘤）。十二指肠内的息肉较胃内少见，但十二指肠内多见腺瘤样息肉。有几组报道显示，多达 98% 的 FAP 患儿有可见的十二指肠息肉，或者至少是一种组织学上的异常，伴有发育不良的单隐窝腺瘤或十二指肠黏膜异常增生[34,160,173]。十二指肠乳头或壶腹部周围区域最终发展为腺瘤占 FAP 患儿的 2.9%[160]，因此，患该病的所有患儿均有必要进行上消化道内镜检查。

治疗

所有 FAP 患儿如果不治疗都会发生结肠恶变，

发展为癌的平均年龄是 39 岁，其中 7% 为 20 岁，15% 为 25 岁[128]。外科切除整个结肠黏膜将阻止结直肠癌的发生。大多数有症状的息肉患儿已经发生了癌变[128]，因此，如果患儿出现症状，在任何年龄均要切除结肠。

外科治疗有多种方法，全直肠与结肠切除同时做永久性回肠造瘘可阻止癌变发生。但在年龄较小的婴儿会在腹壁留下一个永久性的造瘘口。在青少年期，永久性造瘘对患儿的生理和精神影响是巨大的，这种手术能引起很多并发症，因为广泛的盆腔分离破坏了神经而发生膀胱无力，在男性可引起阳痿。由于这些原因，全结肠切除不作为治疗儿童 FAP 的方法。

在过去，腹部全结肠切除同时作回直肠吻合，并连续监测剩余的直肠，已成为治疗 FAP 患儿最常用的手术方式。伦敦的 St. Mark 医院报道了接受该手术的 215 例患儿的结果，术后早期并发症包括长段性肠梗阻（7%）、吻合口漏（2%）和出血（小于 1%），全部并发症发生率为 10%。后期随访（6.5 年）大便次数为每天 3 次。报道有晚间污粪的小于 10%，72% 的患儿大便控制完全正常，44% 的患儿仍需要继续治疗直肠息肉。根据直肠息肉的密度，每 3～6 个月进行一次评估，直径大于 5.0 mm 的任何息肉可采用乙状结肠镜进行电切，在直肠残端 10% 发展成癌症。到 50 岁时直肠癌的累积风险率为 10%，到 60 岁时为 29%[128]。如果一开始直肠就没有息肉，则其风险就会低一些。

近来，直肠黏膜剥除的全结肠切除加上回肠肛管的储袋方法已成为治疗儿童 FAP 的首选手术方式[155]。J-储袋是首选的方法，因为其构成简单，并发症较少[47]。Geiger 和同事[54]报道一种新颖的双分隔、回肠肛管 J-储袋吻合技术，获得很好的效果。储袋大小与排便次数存在反比关系[11,68,94,124]。其他影响大便次数的因素包括炎症、括约肌功能以及小肠的肠管动力。大的储袋使排便次数减少，但易引起储袋器的炎症（“储袋炎”）。这是由大便滞留引起的。近来有报道 450 例有储袋的患儿大便次数在 3.3～7.2 次/天，平均每天大便次数 5.8 次[7,44,46,123,132,172]。大样本研究发现有储袋的患儿储
422 袋炎的发生率平均为 23%，盆腔脓毒症发生率为 8%。FAP 患儿储袋炎的发生率要小于那些做同样手术的溃疡性结肠炎患儿。

随访

所有 FAP 患儿应每年进行上消化道内镜和乙状结肠镜检查。十二指肠内的息肉可通过内镜或切开十二指肠来切除。直径大于 1.0 cm、生长迅速、息肉变硬、严重发育不良或有绒毛状改变的，需要行进一步的干预。近年资料显示，直径大于 1.0 cm 的 Vater 壶腹部腺瘤，42% 包含癌症病灶，而直径小于 1.0 cm 的只有 13%[151]。在做过回肠肛管拖出术的患儿中，很容易行乙状结肠镜检查。肛管和任何片段的直肠黏膜残留都必须仔细加以评估。

其他治疗

药物和饮食添加物亦用于治疗息肉，包括维生素 C[19,179]、舒林酸[179]、膳食纤维[33]和钙剂[163,167]。在使用舒林酸的随机双盲研究中，可看到十二指肠和直肠的息肉生长受到抑制[129]，并且其他研究亦得到证实[96,187]。但在有安慰剂对照的随机双盲研究中，标准剂量的舒林酸在 FAP 患儿中不能阻止腺瘤的发展。

Gardner 综合征

在 1951—1955 年，Gardner 和同事[50-53]确立了结肠 FAP 和多发性骨瘤、纤维瘤和表皮样囊肿结肠外表现的相关性，亦证明了该病是常染色体显性遗传[50,52]。结肠息肉的演变史和治疗与 FAP 患儿相似。骨肉瘤最常发生在颅骨和面部骨骼，可以发现异常嵌塞的牙列和早期牙齿腐烂以及多生牙[40]。在腿部经常可以看到皮脂囊肿，在脸、头皮、手臂上亦经常可以看到，亦可发现脂肪瘤和纤维瘤。

壶腹周围癌在综合征中比在 FAP 患儿中更普遍，但对 FAP 患儿的十二指肠监测显示，所有患儿十二指肠异常的发生率较高。对所有家族性息肉病患儿的详细监测，发现了许多微妙的结肠外表现。Gardner 综合征和 FAP 之间的区别正变得日益模糊了。FAP 涉及面更广，可根据受累情况不同而有不同的临床表现[14]。

Gardner 综合征患儿的腹壁和小肠系膜韧带样纤

维瘤的发生率为 20%。这些肿瘤亦可发生在只有结肠症状的 FAP 患儿，并且是已经做过预防性结肠切除患儿死亡的主要原因。韧带样纤维瘤是一种质地硬、纤维样增生的肿瘤，它可以位于局部亦可以广泛播散于整个肠系膜、腹壁，偶尔位于后腹膜。可以发现纤维发育不良的各个时期，包括纤维肉瘤。大多数韧带样纤维瘤出现在外科手术后，通常是 6～30 个月[41]。最先看到的是体表的纤维瘤，因为它们中的许多保持静止，或几年后消退[41]。由于这些原因，所以当纤维瘤继续生长或直径达到 10 cm，有可能的话建议完全切除肿瘤，它的复发率小于 10%，相当令人满意。大多数腹腔内纤维瘤无症状，直到长成手术无法切除的尺寸时才有表现。由于腹腔内纤维瘤切除的困难性，所以，试用几种药物有不同的成功率。这些药物包括皮质激素、抗雌激素药物（黄体酮、他莫昔芬和托瑞米芬）和非甾体类抗炎药物[8,38,91,180-182,186]。

Turcot 综合征

Turcot 和同事[170]报道了两个兄弟起病初期表现为家族性腺瘤样息肉，最后死于颅内肿瘤（成胶质细胞瘤和髓母细胞瘤）。Turcot 认为颅脑肿瘤是 FAP 的结肠外表现。室管膜瘤和甲状腺癌（通常是乳头状）[14]在 Turcot 综合征中亦有报道。

（严志龙译　叶祖萍校）

参考文献

1. Ackerman LV: Malignant potential of polypoid lesions of the large intestine. S Afr Cancer Bull 1965;9:5.
2. Alvear DT: Localized lymphoid hyperplasia: An unusual cause of rectal bleeding. Contemp Surg 1984;25:29-33.
3. Arbeter AM, Courtney RA, Gaymor AF: Diffuse gastrointestinal polyposis associated with chronic blood loss, hypoproteinemia, and anasarca in an infant. J Pediatr 1970;76:609-611.
4. Atwell JD, Burge D, Wright D: Nodular lymphoid hyperplasia of the intestinal tract in infancy and childhood. J Pediatr Surg 1985;20:25-29.
5. Baptist SJ, Sabatini MT: Coexisting juvenile polyps and tubulovillous adenoma of colon with carcinoma in-situ: Report of a case. Hum Pathol 1985;16:1061-1063.
6. Barge J, Desvignes G, Maillard J-N, et al: Polypose colique associant des aspects juveniles et adenomataux. Gastroenterol Clin Biol 1977;1:159-164.
7. Beart RW, Metcalf AM, Dozois RR, et al: The J ileal pouch-anal anastomosis: The Mayo Clinic experience. In Dozois RR (ed): Alternatives to Conventional Ileostomy. Chicago, Year Book Medical Publishers, 1985.
8. Belliveau P, Graham AM: Mesenteric desmoid tumor in Gardner's syndrome treated by sulindac. Dis Colon Rectum 1984;27:53-54.
9. Benagiano G, Bigotti G, Buzzi M, et al: Endocrine and morphological study of a case of ovarian sex-cord tumor with annular tubules in a woman with Peutz-Jeghers syndrome. Int J Gynaecol Obstet 1988;26:441-452.
10. Berg HK, Herrera L, Petrelli NG, et al: Mixed juvenile-adenomatous polyp of the rectum in an elderly patient. J Surg Oncol 1985;29:40-42.
11. Berger A, Tiret E, Parc R, et al: Excision of the rectum with colonic J pouch anal anastomosis for adenocarcinoma of the low and mid-rectum. World J Surg 1992;16:470-477.
12. Billingham RP, Bowman HE, MacKeigan J: Solitary adenomas in juvenile patients. Dis Colon Rectum 1980;23:26-30.
13. Bodmer WF, Bailey CJ, Bodmer J, et al: Localization of the gene for familial adenomatous polyposis on chromosome 5. Nature 1987;328:614-616.
14. Brett MCA, Hershman MJ, Glazer G: Other manifestations of familial adenomatous polyposis. In Phillips RKS, Spigelman AD, Thomson JPS, et al (eds): Familial Adenomatous Polyposis and Other Polyposis Syndromes. Boston, Little, Brown, 1994.
15. Bruwer A, Bargen JA, Kierland RR: Surface pigmentation and generalized intestinal polyposis (Peutz-Jeghers syndrome). Mayo Clin Proc 1954;29:168-171.
16. Burdick D, Prior JT, Scanlon GT: Peutz-Jeghers syndrome: A clinical-pathological study of a large family with a 10-year follow-up. Cancer 1963;16:854-867.
17. Bussey HJ: Familial Polyposis Coli Family Studies: Histopathology, Differential Diagnosis, and Results of Treatment. Baltimore, Johns Hopkins University Press, 1975.
18. Bussey HJ: Gastrointestinal polyposis. Gut 1970;11:970-978.
19. Bussey HJ, DeCosse JJ, Deschner EE, et al: A randomized trial of ascorbic acid in polyposis coli. Cancer 1982;50:1434-1439.
20. Byrne WJ, Jimenez JF, Euler AR, Golladay ES: Lymphoid polyps (focal lymphoid hyperplasia) of the colon in children. Pediatrics 1982;69:598-600.
21. Capitanio MA, Kirkpatrick JA: Lymphoid hyperplasia of the colon in children: Roentgen observations. Radiology 1970;94:323-327.
22. Chargelaigue A: Des polypes du rectum. Thesis. Paris, 1859.
23. Chevrel JP, Amouroux J, Guerad JP: La polypose juvenile—apropos des 3 familial cases. Med Chir Dig 1976;5:47-54.
24. Christian CD, McCloughlin TG, Cathcart CR, Eisenberg MM: Peutz-Jeghers syndrome associated with functioning ovarian tumor. JAMA 1964;190:935-938.
25. Cobum MC, Pricolo VE, DeLuca FG, Bland KI: Malignant potential in intestinal juvenile polyposis syndromes. Ann Surg Oncol 1995;2:386-391.
26. Cochet B, Carrel J, Desbaillets L, Widgren S: Peutz-Jeghers syndrome associated with gastrointestinal carcinoma: Report of two cases in a family. Gut 1979;20:169-175.
27. Cockayne EA: Heredity in relation to cancer. Cancer Rev 1927;2:337.
28. Covisart L: Hypertrophie partielle de la muquese intestinale. Bull Soc Anat 1847;22:400.
29. Cottrell S, Bicknell D, Kaklamanis L, Bodmer WF: Molecular analysis of APC mutations in familial adenomatous polyposis and sporadic colon carcinomas. Lancet 1992;340:626-630.

30. Crabtree MD, Tomlinson IP, Hodgson SV, et al: Explaining variation in familial adenomatous polyposis: Relationships between genotype and phenotypes and evidence for modifier genes. Gut 2002;51:420-423.
31. Crabtree MD, Tomlinson IP, Talbot IC et al: Variability in the severity of colonic disease in familial adenomatous polyposis results from differences in tumor initiation rather than progression and depends relatively little on patient age. Gut 2001;49:540-543.
32. Cripps WH: Two cases of disseminated polypus of the rectum. Trans Pathol Soc Lond 1882;33:165.
33. DeCosse JJ, Miller HH, Lesser ML: Effect of wheat fiber and vitamins C and E on rectal polyps in patients with familial adenomatous polyposis. J Natl Cancer Inst 1989;81:1290-1297.
34. Domizio P, Talbot IC, Spigelman AD, et al: Upper gastrointestinal pathology in familial adenomatous polyposis: Results from a prospective study of 102 patients. J Clin Pathol 1990; 43:738-743.
35. Dorrnandy TL: Gastrointestinal polyps with mucocutaneous pigmentation (Peutz-Jeghers syndrome). N Engl J Med 1957; 236:1093, 1141-1186.
36. Dukes C: Simple tumors of the large intestine and their relation to cancer. Br J Surg 1925;13:720.
37. Dukes CE: The hereditary factor in polyposis intestine or multiple adenomata. Cancer Rev 1930;5:241.
38. Eagel BA, Zentler-Munro P, Smith IE: Mesenteric desmoid tumors in Gardner's syndrome—review of medical treatments. Postgrad Med J 1989;65:497-501.
39. Enterline HT: Polyps and cancer of the large bowel. In Morson C (ed): Current Topics in Pathology, Vol 63, Pathology of the Gastro-intestinal Tract. Berlin, Springer Verlag, 1976.
40. Fader M, Kline SM, Spatz SS, Zobrow HG: Gardner's syndrome (intestinal polyposis, osteomas, sebaceous cysts) and a new dental discovery. Oral Surg 1962;15:153-172.
41. Farmer KCR, Hawley PR, Phillips RKS: Desmoid disease. In Phillips RKS, Spigelman AD, Thomson JPS, et al (eds): Familial Adenomatous Polyposis and Other Polyposis Syndromes. Boston, Little, Brown, 1994.
42. Feinberg SM, Jagelman DG, Sarre RG, et al: Spontaneous resolution of rectal polyps in patients with familial polyposis following abdominal colectomy and ileorectal anastomosis. Dis Colon Rectum 1988;31:169-175.
43. Fieber SS, Schaefer HJ: Lymphoid hyperplasia of terminal ileum—clinical entity. Gastroenterology 1966;50:83-98.
44. Fleshman JW, Cohen Z, McLeod RS, et al: The ileal reservoir and ileoanal anastomosis procedure: Factors affecting technical and functional outcomes. Dis Colon Rectum 1988;31:10-16.
45. Foley TR, McGarrity TJ, Abt AB: Peutz-Jeghers syndrome: A clinicopathologic survey of the Harrisburg family with a 49-year follow-up. Gastroenterology 1988;95:1535-1540.
46. Fonkalsrud EW, Stelzner M, McDonald N: Experience with the endorectal ileal pull-through with lateral reservoir for ulcerative colitis and polyposis. Arch Surg 1988;123: 1053-1058.
47. Fonkalsrud EW, Thakur A, Beanes S: Ileoanal pouch procedures in children. J Pediatr Surg 2001;36:1689-1692.
48. Franken EA: Lymphoid hyperplasia of the colon. Radiology 1970;94:323-334.
49. Franzin G, Zamboni G, Dina R, et al: Juvenile and inflammatory polyps of the colon: A histological and histochemical study. Histopathology 1983;7:719-728.
50. Gardner EJ: A genetic and clinical study of intestinal polyposis: A predisposing factor for carcinoma of the colon and rectum. Am J Hum Genet 1951;3:167-176.
51. Gardner EJ: Mendelian pattern of dominant inheritance for a syndrome including intestinal polyposis, osteomas, fibromas, and sebaceous cysts in a human family group. In Gedda L (ed): Novant'anni delle Leggi Mendelione, Milan, Italy, 1995, pp 321-329.
52. Gardner EJ, Plenk HP: Hereditary pattern for multiple osteomas in a family group. Am J Hum Genet 1952;4:31-36.
53. Gardner EJ, Richards RC: Multiple cutaneous and subcutaneous lesions occurring simultaneously with hereditary polyposis and osteomatosis. Am J Hum Genet 1953;5:139-147.
54. Geiger JD, Teitelbaum DH, Hirschl RB, et al: A new operative technique for restorative proctocolectomy: The endorectal pull-thru combined with a double-stapled ileo-anal anastomosis. Surgery 2003;134:492-495.
55. Giardiello FM, Hamilton SR, Kern SE, et al: Colorectal neoplasia in juvenile polyposis or juvenile polyps. Arch Dis Child 1991;66:971-975.
56. Giardiello FM, Welsh FB, Hamilton SR, et al: Increased risk of cancer in Peutz-Jeghers syndrome. N Engl J Med 1987;316:1511-1514.
57. Goodman ZD, Yardley JH, Milligan FD: Pathogenesis of colonic polyps in multiple juvenile polyposis: Report of a case associated with gastric polyps and carcinoma of the rectum. Cancer 1979;43:1906-1913.
58. Gowin TS: Polyps of colon and rectum in children. South Med J 1961;54:526-529.
59. Goyette MC, Cho K, Fasching CL, et al: Progression of colorectal cancer is associated with multiple tumor suppressor gene defects but inhibition of tumorigenicity is accomplished by correction of any single defect via chromosome transfer. Mol Cell Biol 1992;12:1387-1395.
60. Grigioni WF, Alampi G, Martinelli G, Piccaluga A: Atypical juvenile polyposis. Histopathology 1981;5:361-376.
61. Groden J, Thliveris A, Samowitz W, et al: Identification and characterization of the familial adenomatous polyposis coli gene. Cell 1991;66:589-600.
62. Grosfeld JL, West KW: Generalized juvenile polyposis coli: Clinical management based on long-term observations. Arch Surg 1986;121:530-534.
63. Grotsky HW, Rickert RR, Smith WD, Newsome JF: Familial juvenile polyposis coli. Gastroenterology 1982;82:494-501.
64. Gupta SK, Fitzgerald JF, Croffie JM, et al: Experience with juvenile polyps in North American children: The need for pancolonoscopy. Am J Gastroenterol 2001;96: 1695-1697.
65. Haggitt RC, Pitcock JA: Familial juvenile polyposis of the colon. Cancer 1970;26:1232-1238.
66. Handford H: Disseminated polypi of the large intestine becoming malignant; strictures (malignant adenoma) of the rectum and of the splenic flexure of the colon; secondary growths of the liver. Trans Pathol Soc Lond 1890;41: 133-137.
67. Hemminki A, Markie D, Tomlinson I, et al: A serine/threonine kinase gene defective in Peutz-Jeghers syndrome. Nature 1998;391:184-187.
68. Heppell J, Kelly KA, Phillips SF: Physiologic aspects of continence after colectomy, mucosal proctocolectomy, and endorectal ileoanal anastomosis. Ann Surg 1982;195: 435-443.
69. Herrera L, Kakati S, Gibas L, et al: A brief clinical report: Gardner syndrome in a man with an interstitial deletion of 5q. Am J Med Genet 1986;25:473-476.
70. Herruzo AJ, Redondo E, Perez de Avila I, et al: Ovarian sexcord tumour with annular tubules and Peutz-Jeghers syndrome. Eur J Gynaecol Oncol 1990;11:141-144.
71. Hockey KA, Mulcahy MT, Montgomery P, Levitt S: Deletion of chromosome 5q and familial adenomatous polyposis.

J Med Genet 1989;26:61-62.
72. Hodgson SV, Spigelman AD: Genetics. In Phillips RKS, Thomson JPS, et al (eds): Familial Adenomatous Polyposis and Other Polyposis Syndromes. Boston, Little, Brown, 1994.
73. Hoffenberg EJ, Sauaia A, Maltzanos T, et al: Symptomatic colonic polyps in childhood: Not so benign. J Pediatr Gastroenterol Nutr 1999;28:175-181.
74. Hood AB, Krush AJ: Clinical and dermatologic aspects of the hereditary intestinal polyposes. Dis Colon Rectum 1983;26:546-548.
75. Horrileno E, Eckert C, Ackerman L: Polyps of the rectum and colon in children. Cancer 1957;10:1210-1220.
76. Hsu SD, Zaharopoulos M, May JT, Costanzi JJ: Peutz-Jeghers syndrome with intestinal carcinoma: Report of the association in one family. Cancer 1979;44:1527-1532.
77. Huer W, Beveridge I, Domizio P, et al: Clinical management and genetics of gastrointestinal polyps in children. J Pediatr Gastroenterol Nutr 2000;31:469-479.
78. Humphries AL, Shepherd MH, Peters HJ: Peutz-Jeghers syndrome with colonic adenocarcinoma and ovarian tumor. JAMA 1966;197:138-140.
79. Jarvinen H, Fransilla KO: Familial juvenile polyposis coli: Increased risk of colorectal cancer. Gut 1984;25:792-800.
80. Jarvinen HJ, Peltokallio P, Landtman M, Wolf J: Gardner's stigma in patients with familial adenomatosis coli. Br J Surg 1982;69:718.
81. Jass JR: Juvenile polyposis. In Phillips RKS, et al (eds): Familial Adenomatous Polyposis and Other Polyposis Syndromes. Boston, Little, Brown, 1994.
82. Jass JR: The large intestine: Epithelial polyps. In Morson BC (ed): Systemic Pathology, Vol 3, Alimentary Tract. London, Churchill Livingstone, 1987.
83. Jass JR, Williams CB, Bussey HJ, Morson BC: Juvenile polyposis: A precancerous condition. Histopathology 1988;13: 619-630.
84. Jeghers H: Pigmentation of the skin. N Engl J Med 1944; 231:122.
85. Jeghers H, McCusick VA, Katz KH: Generalized intestinal polyposis and melanin spots of the oral mucosa, lips, and digits: A syndrome of diagnostic significance. N Engl J Med 1949;241:1031-1036.
86. Jenne DE, Reimann H, Nezu J, et al: Peutz-Jeghers syndrome is caused by mutations in a novel serine threonine kinase. Nat Genet 1998;18:38-43.
87. Jones MA, Herbert JC, Trainer TD: Juvenile polyp with intramucosal carcinoma. Arch Pathol Lab Med 1987; 111:200-201.
88. Joslyn G, Carlson M, Thliveris A, et al: Identification of genetic mutations and three new genes at the familial polyposis locus. Cell 1991;66:601-613.
89. Kaschula ROC: Mixed juvenile, adenomatous and intermediate polyposis coli: Report of a case. Dis Colon Rectum 1971;14:368-374.
90. Kennedy RLJ: Polyps of rectum and colon in infants and in children. Am J Dis Child 1941;62:481.
91. Kinzbrunner B, Ritter S, Domingo J, Rosenthal CJ: Remission of rapidly growing desmoid tumors after tamoxifen therapy. Cancer 1983;52:2201-2204.
92. Kinzler KW, Nilbert NC, Su LK, et al: Identification of FAP locus gene from chromosome 5q 21. Science 1991;253: 661-665.
93. Kinzler KW, Nilbert NC, Vogelstein B, et al: Identification of a gene located at chromosome 5q 21 that is mutated in colorectal cancers. Science 1991;251:1366-1370.
94. Konishi F, Wyse NE, Muto T, et al: Peutz-Jeghers polyposis associated with carcinoma of the digestive organs: Report of three cases and review of the literature. Dis Colon Rectum 1987;30:790-799.
95. Kurugoglu S, Aksoy H, Kantarci F, et al: Radiological work-up in Peutz-Jeghers syndrome. Pediatr Radiol 2003;33:766-771.
96. Labayle D, Fischer D, Vielh P, et al: Sulindac causes regression of rectal polyps in familial adenomatous polyposis. Gastroenterology 1991;101:635-639.
97. Lazorthes F, Fages P, Chiotassol P, et al: Resection of the rectum with construction of colonic reservoir and coloanal anastomosis for carcinoma of the rectum. Br J Surg 1986; 73:136-138.
98. LeFevre HWJ, Jacques TF: Multiple polyposis in an infant of four months. Am J Surg 1951;81:90.
99. Leppert M, Burt R, Hughes JP, et al: Genetic analysis of an inherited predisposition to colon cancer in a family with a variable number of adenomatous polyps. N Engl J Med 1990;332:904-908.
100. Leppert M, Dobbs M, Scambler P, et al: The gene for familial polyposis maps to the long arm of chromosome 5. Science 1987;238:1411-1413.
101. Lindegaard-Madsen E, Morck-Hultberg B: Metastasizing Sertoli cell tumors of the testis: A report of two cases and a review of the literature [letter]. Acta Oncol 1990;129: 946-949.
102. Lipper S, Kahn LB, Sandler RS, Varma V: Multiple juvenile polyposis: A study of the pathogenesis of juvenile polyps and their relationship to colonic adenomas. Hum Pathol 1981;12:804-813.
103. Liu T-H, Chen MC, Tseng HC, et al: Malignant change of juvenile polyp of colon: A case report. Chin Med J 1978; 4:434-439.
104. Lockhart-Mummery JP: Cancer and heredity. Lancet 1925; 1:427-429.
105. Lockhart-Mummery JP, Dukes CE: Familial adenomatosis of the colon and rectum: Its relationship to cancer. Lancet 1939;2:586-589.
106. Louw JH: Polypoid lesions of the large bowel in children with particular reference to benign lymphoid polyposis. J Pediatr Surg 1968;3:195-209.
107. Lucidarme P, Dribda M, elKhoury S, et al: Ovarian tumour and Peutz-Jeghers syndrome: A case report. Gastroenterol Clin Biol 1990;14:1015-1018.
108. Matuchansky C, Babin P, Coutrot S, et al: Peutz-Jeghers syndrome with metastasizing carcinoma arising from a jejunal hamartoma. Gastroenterology 1979;77:1311-1315.
109. McColl I, Bussey HJ, Veale AM, Morson BC: Juvenile polyposis coli. Proc R Soc Med 1964;57:896-897.
110. McGarrity TJ, Kulin HE, Zaino RJ: Peutz-Jeghers syndrome. Am J Gastroenterol 2000;95:596-604.
111. Meera Khan P, Tops CM, vd Broek M, et al: Close linkage of a polymorphic marker (DSS37) to familial polyposis (FAP) and confirmation of FAP localization on chromosome 5q21-q22. Hum Genet 1988;79:183-185.
112. Meldrum RJ, Croaks R, Spigelmen AD, et al: Familial adenomatous polyposis: More evidence for disease diversity and genetic heterogeneity. Gut 2001;48:508-514.
113. Mestre JR: The changing pattern of juvenile polyps. Am J Gastroenterol 1986;81:312-314.
114. Mills SE, Fechner RE: Unusual adenomatous polyps in juvenile polyposis coli. Am J Surg Pathol 1982;6:177-183.
115. Miyoshi Y, Ando H, Nagase H, et al: Germ-line mutations of the *APC* gene in 53 familial adenomatous polyposis patients. Proc Natl Acad Sci U S A 1992;89:4452-4456.
116. Morson BC: Some peculiarities in the histology of intestinal polyps. Dis Colon Rectum 1962;5:337-344.
117. Morson BC, Dawson IMP: Developmental abnormalities. In

Gastrointestinal Pathology, 2nd ed. Oxford, Blackwell, 1979.
118. Morson BC, Jass JR: Histological classification of precancerous lesions of the gastrointestinal tract. In Gastrointestinal Pathology, 2nd ed. Oxford, Blackwell, 1979.
119. Murday V, Slack J: Inherited disorders associated with colorectal cancer. Cancer Surveys 1989;8:138-157.
120. Muto T, Bussey HJR, Morson BCM: The evolution of cancer of the colon and rectum. Cancer 1975;36:2251-2270.
121. Nakamura S, Kino I: Morphogenesis of minute adenomas in familial polyposis coli. J Natl Cancer Inst 1984;3:41-49.
122. Nelson EW, Rodgers BM, Zawatsky L: Endoscopic appearance of auto amputated polyps in juvenile polyposis coli. J Pediatr Surg 1977;12:773-776.
123. Nicholls RJ, Lubowski DZ: Restorative proctocolectomy: The four loop (W) reservoir. Br J Surg 1987;74:564-566.
124. Nicholls RJ, Pezim ME: Restorative proctocolectomy with ileal reservoir for ulcerative colitis and familial adenomatous polyposis: A comparison of three reservoir designs. Br J Surg 1985;72:470-474.
125. Nicholls RJ, Springall RG, Gallagher P: Regression of rectal adenomas after colectomy and ileorectal anastomosis for familial adenomatous polyposis. BMJ 1988;296: 1707-1708.
126. Niimi K, Tomoda H, Furusawa M, et al: Peutz-Jeghers syndrome associated with adenocarcinoma of the cecum and focal carcinomas in hamartomatous polyps of the colon: A case report. Jpn J Surg 1991;21:220-223.
127. Nishisho I, Nakamura Y, Miyoshi Y, et al: Mutations of chromosome 5q21 genes in FAP and colorectal cancer patients. Science 1991;253:665-669.
128. Nugent KP, Northover J: Total colectomy and ileorectal anastomosis. In Phillips RKS, Spigelman AD, Thomson JPS, et al (eds): Familial Adenomatous Polyposis and Other Polypoid Syndromes. Boston, Little, Brown, 1994.
129. Nugent KP, Farmer KC, Spigelman AD, et al: Randomized controlled trial of the effect of sulindac on duodenal and rectal polyposis and cell proliferation in familial adenomatous polyposis. Br J Surg 1993;80:1618-1619.
130. Nugent KP, Talbot IC, Hodgson SV, Phillips RK: Solitary juvenile polyps: Not a marker for subsequent malignancy. Gastroenterology 1993;105:698-700.
131. O'Riordain DS, O'Dwyer PJ, Cullen AF, et al: Familial juvenile polyposis coli and colorectal cancer. Cancer 1991;68:889-892.
132. Oresland T, Fasth S, Nordgren S, Hulten L: The clinical and functional outcome after restorative proctocolectomy: A prospective study in 100 patients. Int J Colorect Dis 1989;4:50-56.
133. Patel VK, Awen CF: Benign lymphoid polyposis of ileum: Three cases and a review of the literature. Can J Surg 1971;14:402-405.
134. Pesta J, Orlowska J: Small intestine carcinoma in the Peutz-Jeghers syndrome. Materia Med Polona 1989;21:43-47.
135. Peutz JLA: On a very remarkable case of familial polyposis of the mucous membrane of the intestinal tract and nasopharynx accompanied by peculiar pigmentations of the skin and mucous membrane. Ned Tijdschr Geneesk 1921;10:136-146.
136. Phillips RKS, Spigelman AD: Peutz-Jeghers syndrome. In Phillips RKS, Spigelman AD, Thomson JPS, et al (eds): Familial Adenomatous Polyposis and Other Polypoid Syndromes. Boston, Little, Brown, 1994.
137. Powell SM, Zilz SN, Beazer-Barclay Y, et al: APC mutations occur early during colorectal carcinogenesis. Nature 1992;359:235-237.
138. Proppe KH, Scully RE: Large-cell calcifying Sertoli cell tumor of the testis. Am J Clin Pathol 1980;74:607-619.
139. Rabin ER, Patel T, Chen FH, et al: Juvenile colonic polyposis coli with villous adenoma and retroperitoneal fibrosis: Report of a case. Dis Colon Rectum 1979;22:63-67.
140. Ravitch MM: Polypoid adenomatosis of the entire gastrointestinal tract. Ann Surg 1948;128:283.
141. Reed TE, Neal JV: A genetic study of multiple polyposis of the colon. Am J Hum Genet 1955;7:236-263.
142. Restrepo C, Moreno J, Duque E, et al: Juvenile colonic polyposis in Colombia. Dis Colon Rectum 1978;21: 600-612.
143. Roth SI, Helwig EB: Juvenile polyps of the colon and rectum. Cancer 1963;16:468-479.
144. Rozen P, Baratz M: Familial juvenile polyposis with associated colon cancer. Cancer 1982;49:1500-1503.
145. Ruymann FB: Juvenile polyps with cachexia. Gastroenterology 1969;57:431-438.
146. Sachatello CR: Gastrointestinal polypoid diseases. J Ky Med Assoc 1972;70:540-544.
147. Sachatello CR, Hahn IS, Carrington CB: Juvenile gastrointestinal polyposis in a female infant: Report of a case and review of the literature of a recently recognized syndrome. Surgery 1974;75:107-113.
148. Scharf GM, Becker JHR, Laage NJ: Juvenile gastrointestinal polyposis or the infantile Cronkite-Canada syndrome. J Pediatr Surg 1986;21:953-954.
149. Schilla FW: Carcinoma in a rectal polyp. Am J Surg Pathol 1954;4:434-439.
150. Scully RE: Sex-cord tumor with annular tubules: A distinctive ovarian tumor of the Peutz- Jeghers syndrome. Cancer 1970;25:1107-1121.
151. Sellner F: Investigations on the significance of the adenoma-carcinoma sequence in the small bowel. Cancer 1990; 66:702-715.
152. Settaf A, Mansori F, Bargach C, et al: Peutz-Jeghers syndrome with carcinomatous degeneration of a duodenal hamartomatous polyp. Ann Gastroenterol Hepatol 1990;26:285-288.
153. Sharma S, Seam RK, Kapoor HL: Malignant Sertoli cell tumor of the testis in a child. J Surg Oncol 1990;44:129-131.
154. Shibata HR, Phillips MJ: Peutz-Jeghers syndrome with jejunal and colonic adenocarcinomas. Can Med Assoc 1970;103:285-287.
155. Shilyansky J, Lelli JL, Drongowski RA, Coran AG: The efficacy of the straight endorectal pull-through in the management of familial adenomatous polyposis: A 16 year experience. J Pediatr Surg 1997;32:1139-1143.
156. Smilow PC, Pryor CA, Swinton NW: Juvenile polyposis coli: A report of three patients in three generations. Dis Colon Rectum 1966;9:248-254.
157. Soper RT: Gastrointestinal neoplasms. In Ashcraft KW, Holder TM (eds): Pediatric Surgery. Philadelphia, WB Saunders, 1993.
158. Soper RT: Intestinal polyps. In Holder T, Ashcraft K (eds): Pediatric Surgery, 2nd ed, Philadelphia, WB Saunders, 1980.
159. Spigelman AD, Murday V, Phillips RKS: Cancer and the Peutz-Jeghers syndrome. Gut 1989;30:1588-1590.
160. Spigelman AD, Williams CB, Talbot IC, et al: Upper gastrointestinal cancer in patients with familial adenomatous polyposis. Lancet 1989;2:783-785.
161. Spigelman AD, Farmer KC, James M, et al: Tumors of the liver, bile ducts, pancreas, and duodenum in a single patient with familial adenomatous polyposis. Br J Surg 1991;78:979-980.
162. Stemper TJ, Kent TH, Summers RW: Juvenile polyposis and gastrointestinal carcinoma. Ann Intern Med 1975;83:

639-646.
163. Stern HS, Gregoire RC, Kashtan H, et al: Long-term effects of dietary calcium on risk markers for colon cancer in patients with familial polyposis. Gut 1990;108:528-533.
164. Su LK, Kinzler KW, Vogelstein B, et al: Multiple intestinal neoplasia caused by a mutation in the murine homolog of the *APC* gene. Science 1992;256:668-670.
165. Talbot IC: Pathology. In Phillips RKS, Spigelman AD, Thomson JPS, et al (eds): Familial Adenomatous Polyposis and other Polypoid Syndromes. Boston, Little, Brown, 1994.
166. Tanaka K, Oshimura M, Kikuchi R, et al: Suppression of tumorigenicity in human colon carcinoma cells by introduction of normal chromosome 5 or 18. Nature 1991;349: 340-342.
167. Thomas MG, Thomson IPS, Williamson RCN: Oral calcium inhibits rectal epithelial proliferation in familial adenomatous polyposis. Br J Surg 1993;80:499-501.
168. Thomson JPS: Familial adenomatous polyposis: The large bowel. Ann R Coll Surg Engl 1990;72:177-180.
169. Tovar JA, Eizaguirre AA, Jimenez J: Peutz-Jeghers syndrome in children: Report of two cases and review of the literature. J Pediatr Surg 1983;18:1-6.
170. Turcot J, Despres J-P, St. Pierre F: Malignant tumors of the central nervous system associated with familial polyposis of the colon: Report of two cases. Dis Colon Rectum 1959;2:465-468.
171. Utsunomiya J, Gocho H, Miyanaga T, et al: Peutz-Jeghers syndrome: Its natural course and management. Johns Hopkins Med J 1975;136:71-82.
172. Utsunomiya J, Iwama T: The J ileal pouch-anal anastomosis: The Japanese experience. In Dozois RR (ed): Alternatives to Conventional Ileostomy. Chicago, Year Book Medical Publishers, 1985.
173. Utsunomiya J, Maki T, Iwama T, et al: Gastric lesion of familial polyposis coli. Cancer 1974;34:745-754.
174. Utsunomiya J, et al: Phenotypic expressions of Japanese patients with familial adenomatous polyposis. In Herrera L (ed): Familial Adenomatous Polyposis. New York, Alan R. Liss, 1990.
175. Veale AM, McColl I, Bussey HJ, Morson BC: Juvenile polyposis coli. J Med Genet 1966;3:5-16.
176. Velcek FT, Coopersmith IS, Chen CK, et al: Familial juvenile adenomatous polyposis. J Pediatr Surg 1976;11:781-787.
177. Verse M: Ueber die Histogenese der Schleirnhautcarcinome. Verh Dtsch Ges Pathol 1908;2:95.
178. Virchow RL: Die Frankhaften Geschwulste. Berlin, A. Hirshwald, 1863, p 243.
179. Waddell WR, Ganser GF, Cerise EJ, Loughry RW: Sulindac for polyposis of the colon. Am J Surg 1989;57:175-179.
180. Waddell WR, Gerner RE: Indomethacin and ascorbic acid inhibit desmoid tumors. J Surg Oncol 1980;5:85-90.
181. Waddell WR, Gerner RE, Reich MP: Nonsteroidal anti-inflammatory drugs and tamoxifen for desmoid tumors and carcinoma of the stomach. J Surg Oncol 1983;2:197-211.
182. Waddell WR, Kirsch WM: Testolactone, sulindac, warfarin, and vitamin K for unresectable desmoid tumors. Am J Surg 1991;61:416-421.
183. Watne AL: The syndromes of intestinal polyposis. Curr Probl Surg 1987;24:269-340.
184. Watne AL: In Syndromes of Polyposis Coli and Cancer. Chicago, Year Book Medical Publishers, 1982.
185. Williams CB: Imaging: Endoscopy. In Phillips RKS, Spigelman AD, Thomson JPS, et al (eds): Familial Adenomatous Polyposis and Other Polypoid Syndromes. Boston, Little, Brown, 1994.
186. Wilson AJ, Baum M, Singh L, Kangas L: Anti-estrogen therapy of pure mesenchymal tumor. Lancet 1987;1:508.
187. Winde G, Gumbinger HG, Osswald H, et al: The NSAID sulindac reverses rectal adenomas in colectomized patients with familial adenomatous polyposis: Clinical results of a dose-finding study on rectal sulindac administration. Int J Colorect Dis 1993;8:13-17.
188. Woodward JJ: Pseudo-polypi of the colon: An anomalous result of follicular ulceration. Am J Med Sci 1881;81:142-155.
189. Young RH, Scu1ly RE: Mucinous ovarian tumors associated with mucinous adenocarcinomas of the cervix: A clinicopathological analysis of 16 cases. Int J Gynecol Pathol 1988;7:99-111.
190. Young RH, Welch WR, Dickersin GR, Scully RE: Ovarian sex-cord tumor with annular tubules: Review of 74 cases including 27 with Peutz-Jeghers syndrome and four with adenoma malignum of the cervix. Cancer 1982;50: 1384-1402.

第 92 章

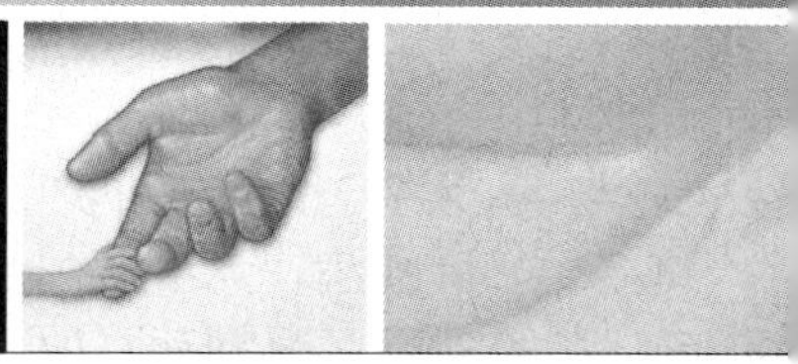

坏死性小肠结肠炎

Stephen S. Kim 和 Craig T. Albanese

427 在世界范围内，坏死性小肠结肠炎（NEC）是新生儿重症监护室中导致发病和死亡最主要的原因。对早产儿和新生儿监护的研究进展发现，早产儿有发生NEC的风险，目前为新生儿最常见的外科急症，与其他需要手术的胃肠道疾病相比有较高的死亡率，尽管对其已进行了广泛的研究，但是确切的病因和发病机制尚不清楚。

在20世纪60年代，NEC的治疗是早期手术，到70年代，人们通过早期诊断认识该病，大多数患儿通过非手术治疗而痊愈。1978年Bell等[21]出版了一个以严重程度为基础的分类方案，有助于选择治疗方案和结果的比较。1979年，国际疾病分类制定了一个由NEC引起死亡的编码，因此可进行更精确的流行病学和预后的分析。

历史回顾

1888年，Paltauf[223]描述了5位死于暴发性腹膜炎的患儿，其中有3位由NEC引起。除此之外，1891年Generisch[88]发表了第一篇有关NEC的报道，但对所描述的内容进行仔细回顾，可以确定其是一例胎粪性腹膜炎而不是NEC。

1939年，Thelander[289]报道了16例胃穿孔、30例十二指肠穿孔、39例小肠和结肠穿孔病例，许多肠穿孔的患儿同时有NEC。1943年，Agerty等[2]首次报道成功治疗因NEC导致局限性回肠穿孔的患儿。1953年，Schmid和Quaiser[264]首次使用“坏死性小肠结肠炎”这个名词。1959年，Rossier与其同事[249]报道了15例患儿，有14例死于“早产儿溃疡性坏死性小肠结肠炎”。

1964年，Berdon等[22]报道了21例NEC患儿的临床表现和放射学检查结果。1年后Mizrahi等[195]报道了18例早产儿的NEC。1953—1963年，纽约儿童医院婴儿室NEC的发生率为0.9%，但该病的病死率占婴儿室总死亡数的2.3%。1975年，Santulli等[257]推测，该病的发展需要有3个必要条件：肠黏膜损伤、细菌存在及代谢底物的获得。

发病率

NEC确切的发病率还不清楚，在美国和世界范围有明显的差别，NEC在美国NICU入院的患儿中占1%～7%，即每1000个活产儿中有1～3例[100,102,131,152]，极低体重婴儿（<1500 g）该病的发病率为10%～12%，但也有报道在2%～22%，这取决于每个调查中心的调查结果不同而不同[44,51,131,174,291]。在日本，极低体重婴儿NEC的发病率为1%～2%，澳大利亚为7%，希腊为10%，阿根廷为14%，香港为28%[44,76,101,131,271]。

几个混淆因素可能导致这种差异，包括极低体重婴儿的数量和存活者、患儿相关的病因（出生时或出生后）和诊断标准的使用。一个相对大型的多中心调查显示极低体重婴儿中确诊NEC的为10.1%，可疑NEC的为17.2%，虽然各个中心之间存在一定差异[291]。另一个研究显示，确诊NEC与可疑NEC的发生率分别为8.6%和18.6%[152]。在Pokorny等[234]的报道中，超过18 000例新生儿NEC的发生率为3‰，其中包括1735例极低体重婴儿，这和许多其他的研究一样低估了NEC的发病率，因为其发病率代表的是全部NEC的病例占整个NICU患者的比例，这些数字包括许多早产儿，这些患儿在生后3天内死于心肺疾病，无法活到足够长时间而发生NEC。一项研究排除了早期死亡的新生儿，只包括已经开始喂养的患儿，其得出NEC发病率为15%[146]。

大多数近来的报道证实NEC与早产密切相关，低孕龄和低体重的早产儿是主要的危险人群。据估
1428 计，足月新生儿发生的NEC只占所有患儿的7%～13%[27,221,311]，早期表面活性物质的运用和改良的机械通气方法已明显改善了低和极低体重婴儿的存活率[57,113]。因此，较小婴儿数量增多是目前NEC发生的一个危险因素，将来NEC可能取代呼吸窘迫综合征成为早产儿死亡的主要原因[141]。

流行病学和发病机制

流行病学

年龄和成熟度

NEC成为早产低体重婴儿的一个主要疾病，比小样儿多见。Kliegman 和 Fanaroff[142] 报道123例NEC患儿的平均孕龄是31周（平均出生体重1460 g），足月儿只占7.3%而小样儿占10.5%。极低体重婴儿（＜1000 g）和那些孕期28周或少于28周的婴儿发病风险最大[115,254]。一个大的多中心前瞻性研究报道了4438例体重在501～1500 g的婴儿，Lemons等[174]证实出生体重和NEC发病率之间存在反比的关系，NEC的发病率在体重501～750 g的婴儿中是最高的（14%），随着体重增加发病率下降，751～1000 g为9%、1001～1250 g为5%、1251～1500 g为3%。

Tesdale等[288]报道NEC的发病年龄与孕龄间存在反比的关系，生后第1周发生NEC的患儿（平均孕龄为36.1周），比那些出生1周后发生NEC的患儿（平均孕龄为33.4周）发育更成熟，发病较早的患儿其并发症和死亡率更高。Ostcie等[221]同样证实孕龄和NEC的发生存在反相关，足月（≥38周）婴儿平均于生后4.9天发病，比那些早产（＜38周）婴儿平均于生后13天发生NEC明显提早。Martinez-Tallo等[187]亦证实出生体重超过2000 g的婴儿较早出现NEC（3.3天）。

Wilson等[310]计算出在NEC的患儿中特殊的出生体重与每周发作的比例，随着出生体重增加，NEC的危险期亦缩短。他们发现孕期35～36周的发病风险明显下降这个固定的形式，因此推测胃肠道功能的成熟度可能在决定NEC的风险上起重要作用。早产儿胃肠道胃酸分泌下降以及低浓度水平的保护性黏液[19,213]，可增加黏膜的通透性[292]，缺乏正常协调的蠕动能力，直至孕期34～35周才恢复[19,213]。

喂养

90%的NEC发生于开始喂养后的婴儿，只有10%或更少发生在喂养之前[144,147,157,185,281]。1978年，Brown和Sweet[33]认为快速喂养方式是导致NEC发病的原因。他们发现在1974年7月，在改成缓慢递增的喂养方式之前，1745例低出生体重的婴儿有14例发生NEC。1974年7月—1978年6月，当采用谨慎的喂养方法后，在收入NICU的2557例患儿和932例低体重婴儿中只有1例发生NEC。一个纵向队列研究回顾了体重在1250～2500 g，孕龄小于35周的婴儿，在“执行标准喂养方案”之前和之后的3年期间NEC的发病率，Kamitsuka等[132]报道NEC的风险下降84%，其他研究亦认为，NEC的发病率增加与配方奶喂养的热卡超过20 kcal/(kg · d)有关[9,165,291,313]。但是，随机试验并没有证实快对慢、早期对延期，或者连续性对间断性的食团喂养之间NEC的发病率有任何不同[136,137,238,243]。一项随机研究对185例分别给予慢喂养［15 ml/(kg · d)；10天全量喂养］和快喂养［35 ml/(kg · d)；5天全量喂养］的极低体重儿进行了比较。Rayyis等[243]证实在两组中NEC的发生率（13%对9%）穿孔率（4%对2%）和死亡率（2%对3%）没有明显的不同。在一项对体重低于1500 g的早产婴儿比较连续和间断性食团喂养的随机性研究中，Premji和Chessell[238]发现在两组中NEC发病率没有明显不同。

在最近的一个随机研究中，极低体重婴儿被分成在接受全奶量喂养之前最少剂量喂养组［20 ml/(kg · d)］或者标准的喂养方式组［开始时20 ml/(kg · d)逐渐增加到全量］。Berseth等[24]报道，最小剂量喂养组NEC的发生率明显低于标准组（1.4%对10%）。NEC的发病风险存在如此大的差别以致该项研究早期就停止了。延长使用“营养喂养量”被认为可促进胃肠功能的成熟，这项研究再次证实了先前的研究有

关肠道刺激方式对极低体重的婴儿是有用的[71]，以及开始最少剂量喂养，7～11 天后再进行适度的添加喂养可最大限度减少 NEC 的发病率[258]。

高渗性配方奶和药物

渗透压和肠内喂养的内容物与 NEC 的发病率增加有关。高渗透压的配方奶可增加婴儿 NEC 的发病率，并且在动物模型中可引起肠黏膜损伤。Delem-
429 os[65]等证实给予新生山羊高渗透奶粉，可出现类似于 NEC 的肠管损伤。Book 等[293]在一项前瞻性研究中对 16 例早产儿喂养 650 mOsm/kg 的要素饮食或 350 mOsm/kg的牛奶，发现喂养要素饮食的婴儿 NEC 发生率为 85%，而牛奶喂养婴儿的发生率为 25%。Grantmyre 及其同事[96]报道一个患儿因胎粪性肠梗阻而使用 Renografin-76（渗透压为 1900 mOsm/kg）进行灌肠后而导致了致命性的 NEC 发生。

许多口服药，如一些维生素制剂，其中的高渗成份可导致肠内黏膜潜在性损伤。Willis 等[309]报道，服用未稀释乳酸钙（1700 mOsm/kg）的婴儿 NEC 发生率要比非钙剂喂养或用水或奶粉稀释的乳酸钙喂养的婴儿高。White 和 Harkavy 报道[306]，即便是与奶粉相混合，许多新生儿监护室常用的口服药仍有很高的渗透压浓度。通常药物的辅料比药物本身更易引起高渗透压。Finer 等[82]报道，口服高渗维生素 E 的早产儿 NEC 的发生率为 13.4%，那些给予肠外维生素 E 的婴儿 NEC 的发生率为 5.7%。高渗溶液进入胃肠道内造成损伤的机制，尽管在临床上未被证实，但是已证明由于血管腔内的液体快速转移到肠腔而引起肠黏膜血供减少[108,252,255]。目前临床对 NEC 的发展过程中相关的肠损伤机制尚不明确。

药物

黄嘌呤衍化物（如胆茶碱、氨茶碱）可以降低肠道活性并在代谢为尿酸时会产生氧自由基，这被认为与 NEC 有关。1980 年，Williams[307]和 Robinson 等[248]描述了 3 个患儿因早产呼吸困难而口服和静脉使用黄嘌呤类药物，导致 NEC 的发生。在动物试验中，Cronin 等[59]证实给予新生小羊氨茶碱，使胃肠道血流和氧的释放发生改变并导致胃肠道氧储备耗尽和黏膜损伤。尽管有这些早期报道，但是在后来的大样本的病例研究中未证实存在这种相关性[63,112]。

早产儿给予大剂量的维生素 E 与 NEC 的发生增加有关[124]，给予早产儿维生素 E 可减少视网膜病不良后遗症的发生率，已证实其通过干扰白细胞在胞内杀灭细菌。NEC 的高发生率，只有在口服高渗药物后才会发生，而肌肉注射给药后不会发生[82]。

吲哚美辛阻断前列腺素合成酶并引起血管收缩，该作用可关闭充血性心衰的早产儿未闭的动脉导管（PDA）。低体重儿用大剂量吲哚美辛治疗时可以发生胃肠道穿孔和 NEC[7,98,162]。已经证实，吲哚美辛可增加肠系膜血管阻力，并减少 16%～20% 的肠系膜血流[99]。Norton 等[215]证实吲哚美辛用作抑制分娩的药物时，可增加 30 周前分娩的婴儿 NEC 的发病率（平均分娩年龄为 27.6 周），但吲哚美辛并不能增加 32 周后分娩的婴儿 NEC 发病率。一项对 252 例静脉给予吲哚美辛治疗有症状的 PDA 患儿的回顾性研究中，Grosfeld 等[97]发现 NEC 的发病率为 35%。相反，一项超过 500 例的低体重早产儿的随机对照研究中，一组早期给予小剂量吲哚美辛，另一组给予安慰剂来治疗 PDA，结果发现随后两组在 NEC 的发病率上无差别[89,183]。吲哚美辛本身可能不足以引起 NEC，但是低氧、心衰或败血症、不良的胃肠道反应可导致极低体重患儿发生 NEC[156]。

可卡因

可卡因有较强的血管收缩作用，自从 20 世纪 80 年代以来由于其大量滥用，被认为是发生 NEC 的一个危险因素[235,265,286]，加上其血管收缩作用，可卡因亦能阻止神经末梢的儿茶酚胺再摄取，从而增加孕妇体内儿茶酚胺的血药浓度[312]。产前可卡因的使用与许多围生期疾病相关，包括死产、胎盘早剥、宫内发育迟缓、早产、婴儿猝死综合征和母体高血压[16,70,125]，可能的机制包括增加了子宫血管阻力，降低子宫血流以及慢性胎盘不成熟伴有胎儿缺氧、高血压和心动过速[37,110,202]。

除这些论述外，还有少数研究调查了可卡因对新生儿胃肠道的血管和炎症作用。对怀孕鼠的研究发现可卡因的应用可使胚胎的胃肠道、子宫和胎盘发生严重的炎症改变[37]；新生小猪服用高剂量的可卡因可使肠系膜血管阻力增加，并通过多普勒超声检查发现肠系膜血流下降[110]；在用放射标记技术比较孕鼠和非孕鼠的研究中，接受可卡因的孕鼠组发生以剂量为基础的子宫、胎盘和胎儿的灌注明显下降，而在非孕鼠组中子宫的灌注没有改变[138]。

一项确诊为 NEC 的患儿的回顾性研究中，在产前接受以及不接受可卡因的两组患儿中，出现几种不同的报道。Czyrko 等[61]注意到在产前接受可卡因的比未接受可卡因的患儿更需要外科干预（72.7%对 38%），并有较高的肠坏疽（54%对 12%）和死亡率
1430 （54.5%对 18%）。对种族、性别和出生体重进行匹配的病例对照分析得出，可卡因组比非可卡因组 NEC 发生的风险增加 2.5 倍。Lopez 等[178]报道，接受可卡因组 NEC 的发生率为 12%，而未接受可卡因组为 3%；另外，在可卡因组生后头 7 天内的患儿 NEC 发生率明显增多。在一项对出生体重在 750～1500 g 的患儿的回顾性研究中，Hand 等[106]比较了 48 例产前接受可卡因与 101 例产前未接受可卡因的 NEC 的发生率，结果两组没有明显差异。

尽管已知可卡因的不良反应，但很难与 NEC 建立起一个确切的因果关系。孕妇滥用可卡因时常叙述不清服用的时间和剂量，可能在产前已服用了很长时间，并且没有足够的产前保健。另外，母亲服用可卡因时同时还服用其他药物、饮酒和吸烟，这些母亲生出的孩子发生早产或小于胎龄，或两者均有的风险就增高了。

细胞因子和生长因子

细胞因子和生长因子在介导增殖、成熟、趋化性、造血细胞和免疫细胞的活化上扮演重要角色。人们已经认识到，细胞因子和生长因子对各种组织的许多细胞有重要作用，包括胃肠道内的细胞（表 92-1）。肠内细胞可接触到肠内皮细胞、黏膜成纤维细胞和肠细胞本身分泌的细胞因子[172,214,224,226,316]。

上皮生长因子（EGF）是胃肠道发育的一个重要的促进因子。EGF 受体普遍存在于整个胎儿和新生儿的肠道内[50,57,126,184]。EGF 最初由唾液腺和十二指肠的 Brunner 腺体分泌入肠腔的，在母乳中的浓度较高[233,244]。已证实与年龄相匹配的对照组相比，早产的 NEC 患儿唾液和血清中 EGF 明显降低。这些 NEC 患儿的对照组设定是与年龄相匹配的[111,267]。已证实灭活敲除小鼠 EGF 受体可导致在组织学上与 NEC 相似的出血性肠炎[191]。在新生大鼠 NEC 模型的研究中，使鼠窒息和接受冷刺激，肠内给予 EGF 可以明显降低鼠群中 NEC 的发生率和严重度[72]，故提示这种保护性的作用可能通过介导致炎细胞因子白介素-18（IL-18）的下调和增加抗炎细胞因子 IL-10 的生成来实现的[103]。Fagbemi 等[80]研究了因严重的 NEC 而行肠切除的早产儿小肠黏膜EGF受体与NEC的相

表 92-1 细胞因子和生长因子在胃肠道中的重要作用

细胞因子	血细胞生成作用	促炎	抑炎	肠道保护作用	肠上皮细胞营养作用
EGF		无	有	有	有
Epo	红细胞增殖	无	无	有	有
IL-1	急性期反应	有	无	不清楚	有
IL-2	T、B 细胞和自然杀伤细胞生长和活化	有	无	有	不清楚
IL-3	早期亚铁血红素细胞的增殖和分化	有	无	不清楚	有
IL-4	T、B 细胞和巨噬细胞的调节	有	有	有	不清楚
IL-10	降低巨噬细胞活化	无	有	有	不清楚
IL-11	增加巨核细胞和巨噬细胞生成	无	有	有	有
IL-15	T、B 细胞和自然杀伤细胞活化	有	不清楚	不清楚	有
NO	调节血小板聚集和黏附，调节内皮白细胞相互作用	有	有	有	无

EGF，表皮生长因子；EPO，促红细胞生长素；IL，白介素；NK，自然杀伤；NO，一氧化氮。

数据改编自 Ledbetter DJ，Juul SE：Necrotizing enterocolitis and hematopoietic cytokines. Clin Perinatol 2000；27：697.

关性，并证实完整的 EGF 受体存在于肠上皮细胞的基底外侧膜上。

促红细胞生成素（Epo）是由肾产生的一种生长因子，在贫血时促进红细胞生成。随着重组蛋白的发展，重组红细胞生成素（rEpo）广泛应用于 NICU[127,218]。人母乳中有 Epo，在胎儿和新生儿小肠内发现有功能性的 EPO 受体，故提示在胃肠道发育中起到一定的作用[128,130,149]。在一项 260 例服用 rEpo 的极低体重婴儿与 233 例对照组的回顾性对照研究中，Ledbetter 和 Juul[171] 证实 rEpo 组 NEC 发生率
431 （4.6%）比对照组（10.8%）明显降低。肠内给予新生大鼠 rEpo 的研究结果表明，肠黏膜的绒毛表面积表现与剂量相关的增长，且细胞增生加快，故提示 rEpo 是小肠发育的一种促进因素[129]。之前腹腔内注射 rEpo，在涉及低氧和再氧合的 NEC 的新生鼠模型中，可明显降低黏膜炎症和坏死，这被认为是通过减少一氧化氮（NO）生成来介导的[163]。

细胞因子是引发一连串炎症反应的内源性介质，促炎和抑炎细胞因子产物通过复杂的反馈机制来调整并维持内环境稳定[285,297]，它们中任何一种生成过多都会产生明显的不良反应。致炎细胞因子［IL-1、IL-2、IL-6、IL-8、IL-12；肿瘤坏死因子-α（TNF-α）、干扰素-γ、血小板活化因子（PAF）］过多可导致休克、多器官衰竭和死亡[188,232]。抑炎细胞因子（IL-4、IL-10、IL-11）过多会引起严重的免疫抑制[28,83]。NEC 的发病机制涉及许多不同的炎症介质[47,107]，通过比较成熟肠内皮细胞系与胎儿肠内皮细胞系对 TNF-α、IL-1β 或脂多糖（LPS）炎症刺激的反应，证实了胎儿细胞可分泌过多的 IL-8[56,210]，之前用 Epo 治疗的细胞可抑制 TNF-α 介导的 IL-8 分泌并控制其水平。在一项评价两种促炎细胞因子（IL-1β、IL-β）和两种抑炎细胞因子（IL-1 受体拮抗剂、IL-10）在 NEC 婴儿中的血清浓度的研究中，Edelson 等[73] 证实在发病的 24 小时内，严重 NEC 患儿的IL-8、IL-10 的水平比轻度 NEC 的患儿明显高出许多，他们注意到阻止调控的介质的释放在早产儿中是以合适浓度分泌的。发病后才释放，可作为严重病变的一种标记。Nadler 等[209] 评估了因严重 NEC 作肠切除的患儿和在其他炎症情况下作肠切除患儿的细胞因子的表达形式，与对照组相比，NEC 患儿的样本中可以看到 IL-8 的 mRNA 明显上调，另外，他们注意到 NEC 患儿的 IL-11 的 mRNA 明显上调，并发现 IL-11的表达与全坏死样改变之间存在一种负相关，故认为 IL-11 分泌是对限制肠损伤扩大的一种适应性反应。几种白介素（IL-4、IL-10、IL-11）在胃肠道中扮演保护或营养的角色，IL-4 被证实通过减少细菌易位，增加细胞超氧化物产物并减少促进蜕变的因子，来保护宿主免受自身补体激活的攻击，而在人肠道上皮细胞内起细胞保护作用[10,268]。IL-10 是一个潜在的抗炎细胞因子，抑制了促炎细胞因子的生成[168]。在低氧-再氧合的新生大鼠 NEC 模型中，重组 IL-10 通过皮下注射与对照组相比可以发现肠损伤的程度明显减轻，因此被认为是在抗炎过程中起保护作用[222]。IL-11 被认为是一种多效的细胞因子，能促进上皮再生，增强肠切除后的适应性[177]。在放置无功能肠袢或大部小肠切除的老鼠皮下注射重组 IL-11，可以防止去功能肠袢的黏膜萎缩并促进切除后残留肠管的黏膜适应和吸收功能[4,68]。

为确定 NO 在许多不同炎症过程的发病机制中的作用，人们进行了大量的研究，有证据显示，NO 有两种功能，既有益又有害，尤其对消化道[159,161]。NO 通过一氧化氮合成酶（NOS）的 3 种亚型作用于精氨酸而形成，NOS-1（神经元型，nNOS）和 NOS-3（内皮型，eNOS）在小肠中的浓度较低，NOS-2（诱导型，iNOS）是通过对炎症细胞因子的反应而产生的[5,211]。NOS 的基本形式和 NO 基本水平已被证实可有改善胃肠道的许多重要功能，包括维持黏膜完整性，调节黏膜渗透性和血流，调节肠管活力以及抑制细胞因子的黏附力和活力[6,18,90,198,279]。

多种肠损伤的动物模型可通过缺血再灌注、LPS 或 PAF 诱导抑制 NO 的合成，这将会明显加剧黏膜损伤[41,117,158,181,193,239]。给予外源性的 NO，包括 L-精氨酸、硝普钠以及硝酸甘油，可以很大程度上减轻这些有害效应[3,69,95,228]。在一项 53 例早产儿的前瞻性研究中，Zamora 等[317] 证实 NEC 患儿血浆精氨酸水平要比对照组明显降低。在一项极低体重婴儿的前瞻性随机安慰剂对照研究中，每天口服或肠外给予 L-精氨酸（261 mg/kg）或在胎儿的第 28 天给予安慰剂，Amin 等[8] 发现 NEC 的发生率在精氨酸组（6.7%）要明显低于对照组（27.3%），该研究中，精氨酸组患儿其血浆精氨酸浓度明显高于对照组。有意思的是，两组 NEC 患儿诊断时的精氨酸浓度明显低于各自的同龄婴儿，是否精氨酸水平的下降可促进 NO 产物利用，消耗其他蛋白合成物，或者降低肠内吸收尚不清楚。该研究认为，给予精氨酸和其他潜在的 NO 供体对预防 NEC 的发生可能有益。

NOS 的诱导形式（NOS-2、iNOS）被认为可上调对炎症性细胞因子的反应。在刺激后的几小时内，在肠上皮内 NOS-2 的表达和活力增加了 15 倍，并导
1432 致大量 NO 生成[287]，尽管由 NOS 组成的亚型产生的 NO 水平较低，但可保持胃肠道的内环境稳定。已有学者提出由于 NOS-2 的上调引发了 NO 持续释放的有害效应，可造成细胞损伤和黏膜屏障衰竭[53,60,287]。这被认为是由于超氧化物（O_2^-）和过量 NO 发生反应产生了过亚硝酸盐（$ONOO^-$），这是一个有效的活性氮中间物，可触发细胞毒性过程，包括脂质过氧化反应和 DNA 破坏[60,242,256]。在一项因 NEC 而行肠切除患儿的 NOS-2 表达的前瞻性研究中，Ford 等[84]证实在肠上皮中有标记的 NOS-2 的基因表达上调，并促进绒毛顶端肠内细胞的凋亡。另外，在绒毛顶端发现残余的硝基酪氨酸水平增高，故提示黏膜损伤和凋亡增加是通过 NO 和过亚硝酸盐的形成介导的。在新生鼠 NEC 低氧模型中，Nadler 等[208]证实了 NEC 的发生率、NOS-2 的表达、肠上及细胞的凋亡以及 IL-12mRNA降低，在配方喂养组的发生率要明显高于母乳喂养组。IL-12 表达下降被认为是通过 NO 介导的，并且理论上是通过减少细菌清除率导致肠管损伤。

PAF，一种内源性磷脂炎症介质，在人和动物的肠损伤研究的病理生理学中起重要作用[44]。PAF 有多种生物学功能，包括肠系膜血管收缩、毛细血管漏、肠黏膜渗透性增加和中性粒细胞和血小板活化[105,160,274]。临床上，配方奶喂养的早产儿 PAF 水平增高，这与 NEC 的发生一样[107,182]。在新生鼠 NEC 的模型中，Caplan 等[39]发现肠 PAF 浓度、肠磷脂酶-A2（PAF 合成酶）RNA 表达和肠 PAF 受体表达增强。在其他动物实验中，给予外源性 PAF 可导致严重肠管坏死[94]。内源性肠 PAF 的产生是对多种刺激的反应上调的结果，包括 LPS、缺氧和肿瘤坏死因子-α[48,79,116,284]，给予 PAF 受体拮抗剂或者 PAF 乙酰水化酶（PAF 降解酶）可减少发生 NEC 的风险[40,45,79]。在人类研究中，PAF 乙酰水化酶活性被证实存在于母乳中，在新生儿期减少，在生后 6 周左右酶活性达到成人的水平，并发现在 NEC 患儿中是缺乏的[42,47,206]。在一项 164 例患儿有关 NEC 风险的前瞻性研究中，Rabinowitz 等[241]监测了一系列血浆 PAF 和与脂有关的 PAF（PAF-LL）水平以评估发生 NEC 时的改变。在 NEC 组，其 PAF-LL 与对照组相比有一个明显高的峰值。另外，升高的 PAF-LL水平与 NEC 的严重度呈正相关，疾病痊愈时，其水平恢复至基线水平。

TNF-α 有多种促炎作用，包括中性粒细胞活化，诱导白细胞和内皮黏附分子及其他细胞因子如 PAF[121,300]。已证实 TNF-α 可使 NEC 动物发生严重的高血压和肠管坏死，且该作用是通过 PAF 介导的，PAF 受体拮抗剂可减弱其作用[284]。

LPS（内毒素）是一种细菌产物，可通过诱导多种促炎细胞因子，如 PAF 和 TNF 而产生较强的炎症反应。注射内毒素可引起低血压、休克以及严重的肠坏死[115]，它已用于 NEC 的动物模型中，产生与 NEC 相似的肠管损伤。LPS 引起的肠管损伤被证实是由 PAF 和 TNF-α 介导的，并能通过 PAF 拮抗剂来预防[116]。

环氧合酶（COX）催化花生四烯酸代谢产生前列腺素、白三烯和血栓烷[212]。已发现两种环氧合酶的亚型。COX-1 出现在许多组织中，包括胃肠道[308]。COX-2 在胃肠道炎症状况下如炎性肠病时表达[11,270]。促炎细胞因子（IL-1、IL-6、TNF-α），与促炎转录因子核因子-κB（NF-κB）一样，可促进 COX-2 的表达[266]。NF-κB 在许多炎症介质和细胞因子的活化作用中是一个重要蛋白[189]。在严重 NEC 而行肠切除的患儿中已证实 COX-2 的表达明显增强[55]。为阐明 NEC 有关的 COX-2 表达的机制，Chung 等[55]在 NEC 的新生大鼠模型中，证实在损伤早期存在NF-κB活化和 COX-2 表达上调的协同诱导。

发病机制

尽管多年的广泛研究并发现了一些危险因子，NEC 的发病机制至今未明。病因可能是多因素的并且涉及黏膜受损、病原菌和喂养的协同作用，导致易感宿主发生肠管损伤和一连串炎症。早产是最重要的危险因子，其他危险因素包括配方奶肠道喂养。商品用配方奶粉缺乏母乳中许多有益的成分。这些保护性物质包括肠生长激素、诱导肠成熟的因子、增强非致病性细菌集落形成的因子、抗炎介质、维生素和其他抗氧化物质以及参与细胞免疫和体液免疫的物质[34,38,92,104]。

受损肠屏障的证据

早产儿的胃肠道特征是细胞和机体免疫还未成熟[32,278]。通透性增高[294]、胃酸分泌减少[12]、消化酶
434 浓度较低、不完全去神经化和动力下降[19,23]以及肠上皮和微绒毛未成熟[225]。屏障功能下降在健康早产儿中亦存在，但它们有能力系统地吸收和释放未消化的大分子、完整的细菌和 LPS[91,247,303]。肠上皮黏膜屏障的损害作为最初症状出现，导致一连串炎症反应的激活。

黏膜血流减少导致细胞缺氧和损伤，是发生 NEC 最常见的病因之一。Touloukian[290]强调围生期较频繁的生理应激，可能是引起肠缺血的原发或继发性的原因。这些因素主要是低氧和低血压、脐静脉换血、脐动脉插管、心血管损伤和血清黏滞性过高。一种隔代遗传的“潜水反射”学说认为在这些情况下，内脏的血液灌注减少，以保证脑和心脏的血液供应[216]。在低血流量和再灌注的时期，Parks 等[227]发现黄嘌呤氧化酶、次黄嘌呤和氧分子之间发生反应，产生大量的超氧自由基，这些自由基可引起细胞和体线粒膜的损伤，并改变肠黏膜屏障的通透性。尽管动物实验支持这种理论，但缺乏相关临床研究以及前瞻性临床研究来证实在低氧和 NEC 的发生上存在一种持久的相关性[145]。

大量研究已经得出，多种炎症介质在 NEC 的发病机制上扮演重要的角色。对动物模型和人类标本的研究中已确定 PAF、LPS、NO 和 TNF-α 是疾病发生的潜在介质[48,84,94]。LPS 和 TNF-α 的作用是通过 PAF 所介导的。黏膜通透性和易感性的增加使细菌发生易位，或者细菌毒素和一连串炎症反应激活被认为是导致肠上皮完整性最终发生塌陷的关键步骤[154,167]。

一直以来对于发生组织损害早期的情况了解得很少。近来研究认为，凋亡加速导致了肠黏膜屏障的破坏。在 NEC 中所有关键的介质已经明确（PAF、NO、LPS、TNF-α），可引起肠上皮细胞的凋亡[58,84,119,314]。在 NEC 新生大鼠模型中，配方奶喂养组动物接受缺氧和冷刺激，对照组接受母乳喂养，Jilling 等[123]证实在 NEC 组，肠上皮层的凋亡比对照组明显增多，但发生的机制尚未明确。在肠上皮中可看见凋亡加速位于肉眼形态改变之前，给予一种 caspase 家族抑制剂可以抑制肠细胞凋亡并明显降低上皮凋亡率，同时 NEC 发生率也下降。故提示凋亡是随后发生黏膜损伤并最终导致 NEC 的根本原因。

胃肠道对炎症刺激的反应导致 NOS-2 的高表达，并使 NO 产量过多，可引起细胞损伤，并且强氧化剂过亚硝酸盐生成能破坏肠上皮屏障[53]。Ford 等[84]证实，NEC 患儿的肠壁中 NOS-2 和 NO 有高表达，并通过过亚硝酸盐介导加速肠上皮细胞的凋亡。这种凋亡的加速导致了在绒毛顶端出现一个“裸区”，表示肠黏膜屏障已被破坏，在这个部位可发生细菌黏附、易位并开始一连串的炎症反应[236]。另外，过亚硝酸盐在 NEC 的大鼠模型中可抑制肠上皮细胞的增殖[237]。结果提示这与 NO 或过亚硝酸盐生成过多相关（如 NEC）。上皮损伤加速和钝性组织修复机制引起的失衡，可导致肠上皮屏障功能不良。

感染性病菌的作用

喂养的方式和肠细菌集落的形式可决定发生 NEC 的风险。母乳喂养的婴儿肠道以双叉杆菌定殖为主（革兰阳性菌），它可抑制革兰阴性菌生长[139,315]。相比之下，配方奶喂养的婴儿肠道主要以大肠杆菌、肠球菌和假菌体定殖为主[140]。

以下几点可证明细菌在 NEC 的发病机制中的重要性：（1）NEC 的发生是突发性的，有发作曲线，患儿与地点、时间或有相同的感染源相关，实行感染控制措施则可阻止疾病的流行[26,31]；（2）在群体发生时，可在患儿和他们的照顾者中分离出相同的病原菌[109]；（3）NEC 可发生在没有危险因素的婴儿中；（4）NEC 在新生儿期发生时可发展几周或几月[148,154]，此时胃肠道全层修复并有足够的时间恢复；（5）给予早产儿大剂量的维生素 E（干扰白细胞对细菌的胞内杀伤作用）与 NEC 的发生率增加相关连[124]；（6）一种 NEC 样的疾病可发生在梭状芽孢杆菌感染的易感宿主中[169]；（7）NEC 样损害可通过实验给予 LPS 来再现[47]；（8）80% 的 NEC 患儿有内毒素血症，并且革兰阴性菌的血培养呈阳性[263]；（9）肠壁积气是一个常见的放射学表现，表明细菌发酵使黏膜下气体积聚[33,78]。

坏死性小肠结肠炎的统一假说

以下常见的临床方案为 NEC 的发病机制提供了一个一致的假说。一个收入 NICU 的早产儿，通常由于对呼吸窘迫的治疗，并且暴露在潜在性的致病性院内菌 1434

落中，婴儿可能有间歇性呼吸暂停和心动过缓发作。常规给予广谱抗生素来消灭厌氧菌群，这潜在地破坏了防止致病的革兰阴性菌过度生长和繁殖的屏障。替代母乳而给予人工喂养，而配方奶提供了细菌生长的基质，并且缺乏母乳中所含有的保护性因子。胃肠道蠕动减少，使得致病菌过度生长，基于微生物的数量与毒力以及黏膜损伤与否，细菌可突破黏膜屏障。由于特异性和非特异性免疫防御不足，不能杀灭细菌。灌注和再灌注减少或轻度感染，使得黏膜屏障破坏，促炎细胞因子产生并导致发生一连串的炎症反应。这个串联反应增加了黏膜通透性，反过来进一步破坏了肠黏膜和肠壁，更多的细菌和细菌产物通过黏膜破口侵入并进一步加重肠管损伤导致全层坏死以及穿孔。

病理

NEC累及单段（50%）或多段（不连续）肠管，最常累及末端回肠，其次是结肠[15]。44%的病例，大小肠均受累。全肠累及（全坏死、NEC全炎症）是NEC的一种暴发性的形式，特征是至少有55%的肠管坏死，占所有手术治疗病例的19%，并且大多数死亡[254]。

在术中，NEC的肉眼外观相当多变，肠管显著扩张，局部变薄，浆膜层典型的从红变为苍白色，可有纤维素样渗出物覆盖。有坏死时，浆膜层是黑的，通常可看到浆膜下有气体积聚，黏膜表面呈广泛上皮脱落样的溃疡。当肠管坏死时可见血性腹水，穿孔时可见褐色的浑浊液体。

在NEC中，肠管炎症普遍存在（图92-1A）。但炎症的程度和性质各个部位不同。在60%的病例中同时存在急慢性炎症。最常见的镜下改变是颜色变淡或浅表黏膜凝固样坏死（89%）[133]。发展至完全黏膜坏死时，黏膜下出现水肿和出血。起初在黏膜下层可见肠壁囊样积气症，随后在肌层和浆膜下层。40%的病例在肠腔以及肠壁内可检测到细菌，偶尔在气性囊肿内可发现。全层坏死时，特征性的改变是嗜酸性玻璃样变。在疾病进展期，在肌层内可出现细胞核的缺失，并常出现上皮再生，肉芽形成和早期纤维化，这提示化脓性过程至少要持续几天。在黏膜和黏膜下坏死的区域附近可见肉芽组织黏膜和黏膜下纤维化，导致一部分在后期形成狭窄。肠系膜小血管以及黏膜下小动脉有时可出现血管栓塞。在坏死组织内小血管

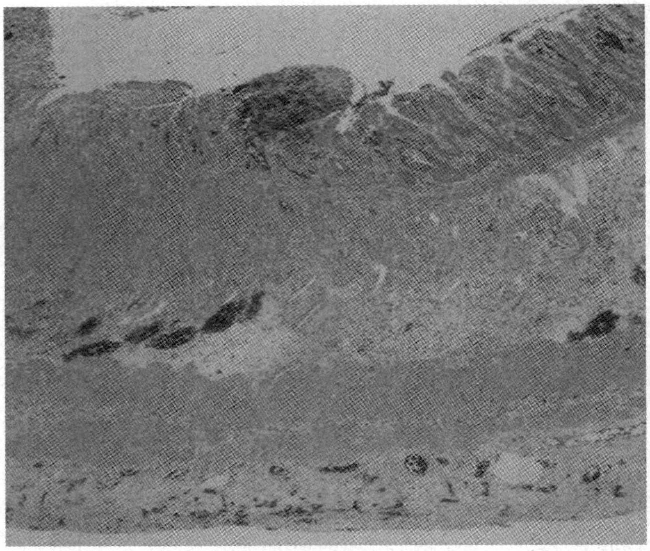

A

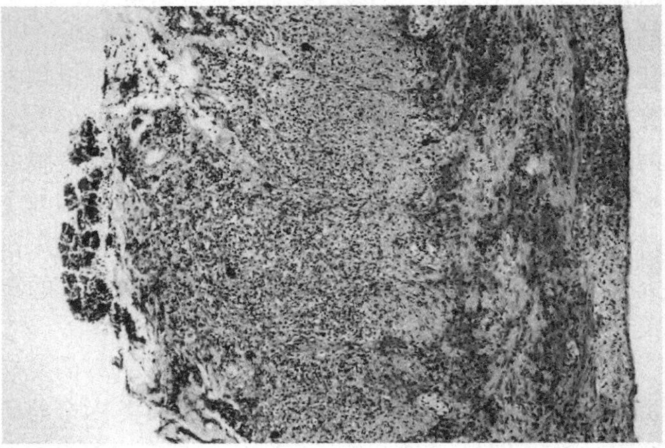

B

图92-1　A. 组织切片显示早期坏死性小肠结肠炎有黏膜下炎症和肠壁囊样积气症（苏木精伊红染色×150）。B. 组织切片显示进展期坏死性小肠结肠炎有透壁性坏死以及绒毛和隐窝结构消失（苏木精伊红染色×150）（也见彩图）。

栓塞被认为是一种继发性改变。大血管栓塞在尸检时相对少见。

诊断

临床表现

NEC开始时常有非特异性临床表现，并只表现为

35 生理紊乱[52,133]，包括嗜睡、体温不稳、反复呼吸暂停、心动过缓、低血糖和休克。许多与胃肠道相关的特异性症状，包括腹胀（70%~98%）、便血（79%~86%）、喂食后胃内食物大量滞留（>70%）、呕吐（>70%）和腹泻（4%~20%）。25%~63% 的病例大便带血，22%~59% 大便隐血阳性，直肠出血量很少。

因为疾病严重程度不同，最初体检可只有轻微的腹胀和轻微触痛。当疾病发展时，腹部触诊有疼痛，并可触及肠袢，为一个固定或移动的团块，或者腹壁有捻发音。约 4% 的病例出现早期腹膜炎，表现为腹壁水肿、红斑，但在疾病后期较常见。在男性，可有阴囊脱色，提示有穿孔。少部分病例，疾病进展迅速，通常较早出现典型临床表现，患儿可在 24 小时内死亡。

实验室检查

NEC 的患儿通常有中性粒细胞减少、血小板减少以及代谢性酸中毒。白细胞计数可能升高，但大多是下降的。在一项研究中，37% 的患儿中性粒细胞绝对计数小于 1500/mm^3[118]，其中白细胞计数最低的预后最差，中性粒细胞计数小于 6000/mm^3 的常伴发革兰阴性菌败血症。

血小板减少几乎都存在，似乎与革兰阴性细菌脓毒症以及血小板被内毒素结合有关。NEC 中血小板减少的发生率为 65%~90%，本质上讲，从 20 世纪 70 年代最早报道起一直没有变化[118,275]。O'Neill[219] 在一组 40 例患儿的研究中发现，接受手术的 NEC 患儿中，95% 血小板计数小于 150 000/mm^3。Rowe 等[251,253] 发现血小板计数小于15 000/mm^3 的患儿，革兰阴性细菌培养阳性。在患病的过程中，血小板计数越低的患儿，往往病情越严重，并且这些患儿通常会死亡[299]。血小板计数小于 10^9/L，或者快速下降，往往是预后差的一个指征。

代谢性酸中毒较常见（40%~85% 的 NEC 患儿），被认为与低血容量和败血症有关，它不是肠坏死的特异性指征。大便隐血试验常阳性，并且有还原性物质。Book 等[30] 认为，NEC 的肠黏膜损伤导致了糖类吸收不良，未消化的碳水化合物进入结肠内发酵，并随大便排出。笔者用 Clinitest 片来检测人工喂养患儿的大便还原性物质，发现人工喂养的 NEC 患儿中，70% 大便还原性物质超过 + +。结肠内细菌发酵，引起局部 D-乳酸盐生成增多，该乳酸盐通过肾脏吸收和分泌。Garcia 等[86] 发现在 NEC 组的患儿中，D-乳酸盐水平增高，但在对照组中不增高，随着患儿的康复或给予口服抗生素，D-乳酸分泌减少。同样当发酵增加时，呼吸时氢的排出亦增加。这项试验有助于排除 NEC。氢呼吸试验阴性准确率达 99%，可用来排除 NEC[54]。

C-反应蛋白（CRP）是一种急性期反应物。该物质水平的测量与疾病的发生、消失或缓解有关[120]。CRP 可作为 NEC 早期的一个指标。在 48 小时内，其水平超过 10 mg/L 要怀疑其诊断（报道其敏感性为 92%，特异性为 81%）。CRP 在 10 天内没有恢复至正常水平，则提示有脓肿、狭窄或败血症。

微生物学

已证实要确认常见的感染性病原菌是相当困难的。在 NEC 患儿血液和大便中找出病原菌取决于胃肠道菌落、院内菌落、局部培养和先前的抗生素治疗时间，且无法证实培养出的细菌是否为引起 NEC 的病原菌，或者由于抗感染治疗而继发的机会性致病菌。由于在相似环境下的其他患儿中缺乏完全匹配的对照组和完整的细菌学资料，使得 NEC 微生物学的研究变得很困难。

细菌学

NEC 的细菌学资料主要从对血液、大便和腹膜腔采集的标本培养获得的。30%~50% 的患儿血培养阳性[140]，通常有大肠杆菌、肺炎克雷白杆菌、奇异变形杆菌、金黄色葡萄球菌、表皮葡萄球菌、肠球菌和产气荚膜梭状芽孢杆菌，并且血培养多数为阳性。从大便样本中培养的细菌有大肠杆菌、肺炎克雷伯杆菌、肠球菌、铜绿假单胞菌、沙门杆菌、凝固酶阴性葡萄球菌（表皮葡萄球菌）、产气荚膜梭状芽孢杆菌、艰难梭状芽孢杆菌和酪酸梭状芽孢杆菌[25,304]。腹腔培养常见的为克雷白菌属、大肠杆菌、凝固酶阴性葡萄球菌、肠内菌属和酵母菌[197]。

真菌培养

与细菌相反，没有数据显示真菌是引起 NEC 病理机制的最初生物体。真菌是一种继发性的感染菌。在 1991 年，儿童健康国立学院和人类发育新生儿研
1436 究协作网关于 NEC 的研究中报道，5%～17% 的真菌血培养为阳性[293]。1993 年，Karlowicz[135] 报道在同一机构中真菌性腹膜炎在增加，从 1980—1989 年的 7% 上升到 1989—1991 年的 35%。在后期死亡的 NEC 病例中发现有念珠菌性真菌性败血症[272]。Smith 等对 30 例死于 NEC 的患儿的体液和组织培养结果进行了一项回顾性和前瞻性研究发现，47% 的病例有真菌存在[272]，20% 的病例发现有真菌集落，第一个阳性结果在术后平均（22 ±8.9）天获得。8 个患儿（27%）有真菌性败血症，7 个有念珠菌性败血症和球拟酵母菌属败血症。第一个阳性真菌培养结果在术后（16.5 ±7.0）天获得，8 个患儿中有 4 个在死亡前被诊断为真菌性败血症。

细菌毒素

在一些 NEC 的病例中，黏膜损伤可通过细菌毒素介导[259]。在 NEC 发作时，艰难梭状芽孢杆菌、酪酸梭状芽孢杆菌和大肠杆菌产生的毒素可从大便样本中被分离出来。Scheifele 等[260,261]研究认为，ε-毒素可以从凝固酶阴性葡萄球菌中分离出，56% 凝固酶阴性葡萄球菌 NEC 患儿的大便中存在毒素。这种毒素很少被发现存在于无 NEC 的凝固酶阴性葡萄球菌感染的患儿中。

群集性流行

在大多数大样本中，散发的病例出现在相对大量病例的突然发作之后。在多次发作中，没有发现特异性病原菌。作为院内感染监督方案的一部分，Book 等[31]在 1972—1977 年对 74 例 NEC 患儿作了一项前瞻性研究，发生 6 例暂时性以及地域相关的 NEC 群发病例，没有分离出特异性的病原菌。在研究中，个别护理人员伴发急性胃肠道疾病，感染控制措施得力使 NEC 的发生率明显降低。在 1972 年、1973 年、1974 年、1975 年和 1978 年[140]，发生于彩虹婴儿和儿童医院的 NEC 有相似的流行，但无特异的病原。在费城儿童医院[199]，有 11 例散发 NEC 病例，但在监护室婴儿的大便中没有发现病原菌。Van Acker 等[295]报道 12 例婴儿在超过 2 个月的时间内暴发 NEC 与 Sakazakii 肠杆菌有关，这个病原菌的出现是 NICU 使用的配方奶污染所导致的。其他暴发流行的病原菌包括大肠杆菌、沙门杆菌、艰难梭状芽孢杆菌、轮状病毒和冠状病毒样病原体[26,259]。

影像学检查

NEC 诊断的重要方法是前后位和左外侧位平片，以下任何一个或全部的表现与 NEC 有关：肠梗阻表现（非特异性肠管扩张）、肠壁囊样积气症（线状或囊状）（图 92-2）、门静脉积气、气腹、腹腔游离液体和持续性扩张、固定的肠袢[204]。肠壁积气和门静脉积气通常是短暂的症状。

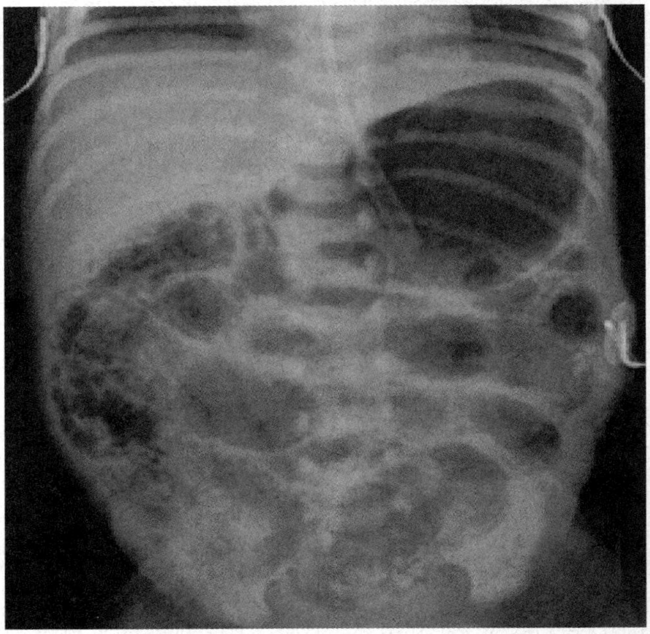

图 92-2　腹部平片显示广泛的肠壁囊样积气（囊状和线状）以及在肝脏阴影的上方有分叉样气体影提示在门静脉系统分支内有气体扩散。

肠管扩张

大多 NEC 患儿早期在放射学检查时有多发性肠袢积气表现（55%～100%）[62]。由于气体和液体积聚，在卧位片上可看见气液平面。肠袢的分布与扩张程度与疾病的临床严重程度和进展有关。在一些病例中，非特异性肠管扩张先于临床症状出现，提示几小时内可出现 NEC。

肠壁囊样积气症

在适当的临床环境中，肠壁囊样积气症（肠内积气）的出现对 NEC 的诊断来说是一个典型的临床表现。气体主要成分是氢，它是细菌代谢的副产物。尽管肠壁囊样积气症的发生率为 19%～98%，但多达 14% 的 NEC 患儿缺乏该表现（即使是严重的病变）[143]，反过来，广泛积气的表现可能非常轻微，通常对药物治疗起效迅速。

积气是暂时的，在临床症状出现前出现，通常为
37 早期表现。与未喂养的患儿（14%）相比[185]，在已经喂养的患儿中最常见（84%）。肠壁囊样积气症对 NEC 是非特异性的。在巨结肠的小肠结肠炎、浓缩牛奶综合征、幽门狭窄、严重的腹泻、糖不耐受以及其他疾病中亦有出现。

肠壁囊样积气症在放射学上有两种表现：囊状和线状。囊状积气有一种颗粒状或泡状表现，并在黏膜下出现，易与大肠内的大便相混淆；线状积气由肌层和浆膜下小水泡积聚形成，构成一条细小线状或绒毛样的气体形态，分布在一段肠管肠壁的周围。

门静脉积气

门静脉积气是以分支样放射线状覆盖在肝脏表面，并通常扩展至肝脏周围。气体通过放射状门静脉系统扩散。门静脉积气是短暂的，其发生率约为 10%～30%[35]。在大多数病例，门静脉积气预后较差[143]。全肠管累及的病例，61% 有气体存在。门静脉积气的机制可能是细菌侵入引起肠壁气体积聚并扩散至静脉系统，再移行至放射状的门静脉中，另外它可能是门静脉系统内产气细菌所致。

气腹

腹腔内游离气体与肠管穿孔有关，约占 12%～30% 的患儿，左侧卧位或横向侧卧位片可清楚地观察到，不必要做直立位片。腹部平卧片显示镰状韧带（“足球征”）、脐动脉或脐尿管残留物周围有游离气体或有双壁征。这种征象代表的是肠壁两侧的气体（肠腔和腹腔）影像，在手术中证实有肠穿孔的病例，放射学上显示有游离气体的只占 63%。因此，放射学诊断无游离气体的患儿穿孔发生率相当高。

必须牢记气腹可能出现在没有肠管穿孔，但因严重肺部疾患行机械性通气的患儿。在这种临床情况下，气压伤引起肺泡破裂，气体通过纵隔扩散到腹部。患儿的症状、体征和实验室检查结果通常能鉴别气体的来源。如果不确定，可进行腹腔穿刺，抽吸液体进行分析。如果没有腹水，通过胃管注入一种水溶性的造影剂可排除胃穿孔。

腹腔内液体

若平片显示腹腔内有游离液体要进行穿刺：（1）严重的非气体性扩张；（2）充满气体的肠管被包围在腹部中央，远离腹壁轮廓；（3）腹腔内模糊影增多；（4）肠袢分离。据报道 11% 的病例出现这些表现。腹水和门静脉积气是与高死亡率相关的放射学表现。手术证实 21% 的肠穿孔患儿有腹水。然而，所有被证实穿孔的患儿，其中 16% 在平片上既没有腹水亦没有游离气体。

持续性扩张的肠袢

持续性扩张肠袢征是一个放射学平片表现，曾由 Wexler[305] 描述，他在一项 5 例 NEC 患儿的研究中发现，有单个或几个扩张的肠袢，24～36 小时内在位置和外形上没有发生改变，这些患儿随后发生肠管全层坏死。但这种表现不总是提示有肠坏死。Leonard 等[175] 发现，21 例患儿中 33% 发现有持续性肠袢，57% 的持续性肠袢患儿在手术或尸检时发现有肠管坏死，但 43% 的患儿没有发生坏死，并且通过非手术治疗康复。

造影

对那些通过临床表现和放射学检查怀疑为NEC的患者，上消化道造影检查偶尔有助于提高其诊断的精确性。然而，过度依靠放射造影检查来诊断有时可导致不必要的治疗。仔细检查造影剂的使用类型是有必要的[305]。钡剂从不被使用，因为钡剂和大便混合，通过穿孔处渗入到腹腔可加重腹膜炎。而水溶性造影剂可被肠管或腹膜腔吸收。这种吸收可一过性地（6～12小时）增加尿液比重。过去，水溶性造影剂是高渗的，有引起大量腹腔内液体转移的危险，尤其是在早产儿。目前，水溶性造影剂是非离子性的，有较低的渗透压，可产生较好的胃肠道造影。当肠道造影增强显示肠管壁袢被水肿的肠壁分开，有边界不清的不规则黏膜、黏膜溃疡、肠壁针刺样或肠壁囊样积气，要怀疑NEC。该检查可在床旁进行。

尽管有人[134]提到因为有直肠乙状结肠穿孔的风险而不应做肠道造影检查，除非有结肠疾病或造影剂反流入病变的回肠末端，造影检查不能诊断NEC。实际上，由于造影剂灌肠可引起积气以及暂时性门静脉积气，所以，可能引起不恰当的NEC诊断。不像床旁的上消化道造影，灌肠造影需同时进行X线透视检查，需要将重病的新生儿转移到放射室。对近期已完成治疗但有部分小肠梗阻或大便出血的NEC患儿，采用造影检查对鉴别肠管狭窄非常有用。

表92-2　坏死性小肠结肠炎分期系统

Ⅰ期（怀疑期）
任何一个或更多的既往因素导致的围生期应激
全身表现——体温不稳、嗜睡、呼吸暂停、心动过缓
胃肠道表现——进食差、鼻饲前胃残留物增加、呕吐（可能是胆汁样或OB试验阳性）、轻度腹胀、大便隐血（无肛裂）
腹部平片显示肠管扩张伴有轻度肠梗阻
Ⅱ期（确定期）
一个或更多既往因素
以上症状和体征加上持续性隐性或肉眼有胃肠道出血，明显腹胀
腹部平片显示肠管显著扩张合并肠梗阻、小肠分开（肠壁水肿或腹腔积液）
不变或持久存在的“僵硬的”肠袢，肠壁囊样积气、门静脉积气
Ⅲ期（进展期）
一个或更多的既往因素
以上症状和体征加上生命体征恶化，有败血症休克表现或者明显的胃肠道出血
腹部平片显示气腹加上Ⅱ期所列举的表现

From Bell MJ, Temberg JL, Feigin RD, et al: Neonatal necrotizing enterocolitis: Therapeutic decisions based upon clinical staging. Ann Surg 1978; 187: 1.

超声

超声被用来发现坏死肠管、腹腔内液体和门静脉积气。理论上，如果超声能发现需要手术的患儿，比其他方便的临床和影像方法更敏感和及时的话，那么则有其重要的价值。

异常肠袢超声的特点是低回声边缘伴中央回声聚焦（“目标体征”）[150]。Avni等[13]发现，胆囊周围高回声表示胆囊周围血管内有气体或者有泡状的炎症浸润扩展至胆囊周围。

超声主要用于诊断临床上可疑的并且影像学检查或穿刺有局限性腹腔内液体的患儿。

核磁共振

核磁共振（MRI）是一种非侵袭性方法，近来用于鉴别继发于NEC的肠缺血患儿：尽管MRI能证实NEC的基本表现，但大多数情况下，这种技术的应用是有限的[180]。

分类

为了选择合适的治疗方法（非手术和手术），以及为了决定该疗法对存活率和远期结果的影响，研究者用可比较的标准对NEC的各阶段进行分类是很有必要的。现已提出几种分类方法。1978年，Bell等[21]提出了目前最常见的分类方法，一种三期分类（怀疑、确定和进展），以患儿的病史因素、胃肠道症状、影像学检查和全身症状（表92-2）进行分类。目前Bell的分期方法已经得到改良[148]，三阶段仍被使用，但加入亚型以辨别特殊的预后因素。Ⅰ期患儿有可疑的 NEC 表现，Ⅱ期患儿有明显的 NEC 表现，但没有进行外科干预的指征，Ⅲ期患儿为进展性 NEC 伴有肠管坏死或穿孔表现。

治疗

非手术治疗

在没有肠坏死或穿孔的情况下，NEC 患儿治疗的主要措施为支持性的。停止喂养，通过胃管进行胃肠道减压，经静脉液体复苏治疗，测定全血细胞计数、血小板计数、血气分析以及 CRP 和 血清电解质，进行血和尿标本培养，通过静脉给予广谱抗生素。直到现在，常用抗生素有青霉素、氨基糖苷类以及有效抑制厌氧菌的药物。因为这些患儿通常为 1～2 周大，抗生素应用包括抗厌氧菌的药物似乎是合乎逻辑的，但在仔细研究时，厌氧菌较少见。到目前为止，没有对照研究显示这种治疗的有效性。抗生素的选择最好不仅要针对 NEC 中最常见的病原体，而且也要针对院内监护室内的菌落。因为近来报道，患儿的大便和血培养凝固酶阴性金葡菌呈阳性。目前一些小组经验性地联合应用万古霉素和庆大霉素或者万古霉素加上三代头孢菌素来治疗这些患儿[262]。NEC 患儿死于真菌性败血症的发生率很高，因此，如果患儿连续有症状出现，但没有明确的细菌感染，则是进行经验性的抗真菌治疗的有力指征。

39 密切的临床观察包括：经常体检、每隔 6～8 小时进行二维的腹部影像学检查、血小板和白细胞计数以及血气分析。

一旦喂养重新开始就要进行大便还原性物的测试和隐血试验。如果其中一个结果阳性，就要停止喂养。确定为严重程度为中度的患儿（Bell 分期Ⅱ期）至少要治疗 7～14 天，给予肠道休息和胃肠减压，放置中心静脉导管进行静脉营养。如果患儿临床状况较好，可重新开始给予小剂量稀释配方奶。患儿要对腹胀、呕吐或 NEC 的非特异性症状和体征进行连续仔细的监测。喂养量逐渐加大同时避免浓缩配方奶或大剂量喂养。接受手术的患儿，术后进行 1～2 周的静脉抗感染治疗，一旦临床症状较好以及肠功能恢复，就可以开始喂养。

手术指征

在 NEC 中，外科干预的目标是切除坏死肠管以及保留肠管的长度[81,229]。比较理想的情况是直到发生坏死但未穿孔时才进行手术。不幸的是，没有临床检查或与辅助检查联合应用能显示出对肠坏死有较高的敏感性[153,155]。因此，对外科手术指征、最佳手术时间以及最佳手术治疗方法仍存在争议。最广泛接受的手术指征是有气腹存在。有人尝试确定某种特征来作为肠坏死的预兆，Kosloske[153] 回顾了 12 条用于 147 例 NEC 患儿的手术标准，根据敏感性、特异性、阳性/阴性预示值和患病率将这些标准进行分层。“最佳的”手术指征［特异性和阳性预示值（PPV）约 100%，患病率大于 10%］为气腹、腹腔穿刺阳性（抽吸量超过 0.5 ml 棕色或黄色液体，细菌革兰染色为阳性）、门静脉积气。“优良的”指征（特异性和 PPV 约 100%，患病率小于 10%）为肠袢固定、腹壁红斑以及可触及的腹部包块。“较好的”指征（特异性 91%、PPV 94%、患病率 20%）为通过影像系统进行分级的“严重的”肠壁囊样积气。“较差的”指征为临床症状恶化（PPV78%）、血小板计数小于 10 万/mm^3（PPV50%）、腹部触痛（PPV58%）、严重胃肠道出血（PPV50%）以及腹腔有腹水但无游离气体（0%）。不幸的是，没有一个指征的敏感性超过 48%。目前，只有气腹是手术的绝对指征，相对指征包括腹腔穿刺阳性、可触及的腹部肿块、腹壁红斑、门静脉积气、肠袢固定以及虽进行最大剂量药物治疗，但临床症状进一步恶化。

气腹

在非手术治疗过程中，出现气腹的患儿要进行剖腹手术或者放置腹腔引流。不幸的是，气腹在新生儿中不总是能证实有消化道穿孔，一项研究显示穿孔患儿证实有游离气体的只占 63%[85]。

腹腔穿刺

腹腔穿刺抽吸超过 0.5 ml 棕色或黄色液体，内含革兰染色的细菌，则定义为穿刺阳性，该结果对诊断肠坏死是特异的[53]。肠坏死时腹腔穿刺结果阴性很少，但在局限性肠壁穿孔或者某段肠管受损但没有穿孔的情况下也能发生[246]。没有绝对的腹腔穿刺指征。Kosloske[153]推荐对广泛积气性肠炎或经非手术治疗后没有改善的患儿需要做腹腔穿刺。如果未抽吸到腹腔液体，要将 30 ml/kg 生理盐水注入腹腔内进行灌洗，翻动患儿从一侧到另一侧，再抽出这些液体。Ricketts 和 Jerles[246]报道腹腔穿刺阳性作为 51% 的患儿的手术指征，其存活率超过 70%，有 3 个假阳性发生。当出现腹壁红斑和水肿、门静脉积气，连续腹部影像检查显示固定并扩张的肠袢、固定伴有触痛的腹部肿块或临床症状持续恶化要进行腹腔穿刺。在这个报道中，腹腔穿刺的指征被许多外科医生认为是手术的指征。

门静脉积气

为确定门静脉积气与肠管坏死的出现和程度以及死亡率的关系的意义，Kurkchubasche 等[164]回顾了匹兹堡儿童医院的经验，与各国文献报道相同，在 616 例患儿中，118 例（19%）腹部平片显示有门静脉积气，通常 X 线显示有门静脉积气 24 小时后，在这 118 例患儿中有 102 例进行了手术。102 例患儿均有全层肠壁坏死，52% 的患儿病变肠段超过整个小肠的 75%。门静脉积气患儿的总体死亡率为 52%，并且全肠累及的患儿死亡率为 90%。在 15 例门静脉积气但没有进行手术的患儿中，肠坏死需要进一步手术的有 6 例（40%），其中 5 例死亡。在另一项研究中，Rowe 等[254]认为超过 90% 门静脉积气的患儿将会发生肠管坏死，52% 发展为全肠受累。最近，在对一项 40 例 NEC 及门静脉积气患儿的回顾性研究中，Molik 等[196]报道手术总体死亡率为 54% 并且 25% 的患儿全肠受累。

1440 持续固定的肠袢

肠袢固定扩张即肠袢位置、形态持续不变超过 24 小时，约一半的患儿通过非手术治疗可治愈[230]。腹腔镜已用来评估 2 例有扩张肠袢的患儿[231]，其中一例确诊为 NEC，另一例被排除。

临床症状恶化

尽管有足够的支持措施，但病情仍持续恶化的儿童有需要进行手术的指征[245]，但没有一个为绝对的指征。这些指征包括腹壁红斑、体检发现有腹膜炎、持续性/进行性酸中毒以及持续性/进展性血小板减少。

腹水

如前所述，气腹不总是肠穿孔的证据。一个无游离气体、充满液体的腹腔可能是穿孔的唯一体征。Frey 等[85]报道，21% 的肠穿孔患儿，唯一的影像学证据即腹水，他们认为影像学检查是不精确的，腹水的证据需在恰当的情况下通过穿刺来获得，并做进一步的评估。

手术处理

疾病进展并需要手术干预的占所有 NEC 患儿的 50%[36,151]。因为缺乏严谨的前瞻性随机试验，NEC 的最佳手术方法仍有争议。手术目的是去除坏死肠管、保留肠管的长度。在这方面观点各异，但大多数人同意，手术途径的选择应依据肠管受累的程度。

在手术前患儿的一般情况应为最佳状态，包括较好的通气支持、休克治疗、给予广谱抗生素以及贫血、凝血异常的纠治。理想情况下，尿量至少为 1 ml/（kg · h），要有与年龄相适应的平均动脉压，手术过程可在 NICU 合适的条件下进行，并且不增加并发症发生的风险[87]。

初期腹腔引流

极低体重婴儿肠穿孔的治疗仍有争议。1977 年，Ein 等[77]报道将腹腔引流（PD）作为肠穿孔早产儿在剖腹术前稳定和改善全身状况的一种方法。从那时起，PD 作为初期治疗用于多种状况，并且有一些研究者建议可作为一种关键性的治疗[14,66,93,176,203]。在一项 44 例进展期 NEC 患儿的前瞻性研究中，PD 作为一项主要治疗方法，Demestre 等[66]报道，28 例患儿（63.3%）只做了 PD，有 16 例患儿（36.4%）在 PD 后需要做剖腹手术。只做 PD 的生存率为 64%，但引流后 86% 有症状改善。在 PD 后，54% 的患儿需要做进一步的手术。Morgan 等[203]报道将 PD 作为体重小于 1500 g，以及体重大于 1500 g 的不稳定 NEC 患儿的主要治疗手段，他们报道 PD 后存活率为 79%，23 例中的 17 例（73.9%）存活者不需要手术干预。Moss 等[205]近来对接受 PD 与剖腹手术的穿孔的 NEC 患儿比较做了一个 Meta 分析，并回顾了 10 项已发表的该类研究。因为在治疗手段上有显著的偏倚，同时小婴儿进行 PD 的比例比剖腹术大，作者亦未能确定 PD 的相对优点。目前，大多数外科医生建议把 PD 作为极低体重伴 NEC 穿孔患儿在进行最终的手术前复苏和维持稳定的最初治疗手段。为了强调这个观点，近来两组多中心前瞻性随机对照试验正在进行中，对 PD 和剖腹手术在体重小于 1000 g（A. Pierro：NET trial）或小于 1500 g（R. L. Moss：NECSTEPS trial）的早产儿中进行比较。

剖腹手术

在手术中，NEC 的病变范围分为局限性、多发性或全肠性（活力肠管 <25%）。基于疾病和患儿手术的特征，可采取不同的手术方式，包括切除并肠造瘘、切除并吻合、近端肠造瘘、“修剪和下降（clip and drop）”技术以及“补片、引流和等待（patch, drain and wait）”技术。腹部做一个右脐上横切口，注意不要损伤肝。腹水标本作需氧菌、厌氧菌和真菌培养。要系统地检查整个胃肠道来评估病变的范围以及肠管的活力。在手术结束时，必须记录剩余的有活力的肠管长度并注意有无回盲瓣。

NEC 手术时罕见的并发症之一为被牵开器或手指分离引起损伤，导致自发性腹腔内肝出血。Vanderkolk 等[296]报道这种并发症在超过 5 年的时间里占 NEC 手术者的 11.8%。有肝出血患儿的平均孕龄为 28 周（平均体重 1262 g），在这些患儿中只有一例存活。笔者认为术前较低的动脉血压和术前过量液体补充超过 24 小时，是导致其发生的主要因素。这种并发症在腹部打开和肠管切除后很短时间内发生。肝充血后接着发生包膜下血肿和破裂。

1 ## 局限性病变

当单个肠管区域出现坏死或穿孔，只需作局灶切除，行近端肠管造瘘并作造瘘口护理。笔者倾向于造瘘口经切口（可并列或分开）外置是因为：（1）肠系膜通常厚且短，因此阻碍了通过造瘘口以及腹壁的血供；（2）造瘘口关闭方便；（3）切口并发症相比较远处造瘘口的发生率没有增加，小肠造瘘口通过用间断缝线将肠管缝到筋膜上。预留肠管超过腹壁皮肤约 2 cm，而不用缝线将肠管末端加以固定。如果在手术后造瘘口的活力有问题，可在床旁切断一小段全层肠管，并观察切口末端的出血情况。

切除并作一期吻合必须在经过仔细选择的患儿，在孤立性病变的情况下进行。一期吻合相对于有较高死亡率的肠造瘘患儿来讲有优势，并无需进行第二次手术[1]。为安全执行该技术，必须遵循以下标准：（1）精确定位，通常是近段病变肠管；（2）不损伤剩余肠管外观；（3）患儿全身情况较好，没有快速进展的败血症或凝血异常发生。

多发性病变（有活力的肠管 >50%）

如果患儿有多发性肠管坏死，并被有活力的肠管隔开，有以下方法可供选择。以前，外科医生切除每一处病变的肠管，并做多个造瘘，而不做一个大段的肠管切除。相反，可做单个高位造瘘（靠近空肠），同时和远端肠管拼接在一起，避免多个造瘘。近端空肠造瘘可引起大量的液体和电解质丢失，以及造瘘口周围皮肤的并发症，尽管有了较好的皮肤护理以及造瘘口装置的置换技术能避免这些潜在的并发症。吻合口狭窄较多见，并且可发生在空肠造瘘口关闭时。切除多余的吻合口目前已获得广泛认可，为严重 NEC 和多发性病变提供了一个有效的治疗方法[229]。在一项 46 例多发性病变的 NEC 患儿的研究中，Fasoli 等[81]报道，切除加上一期吻合（85%）比肠造瘘（50%）有较高的存活率。

1989 年 Moore 等[200]描述了一个有争议的途径，术语为“补片、引流和等待”（patch, drain and wait）的过程。保留潜在肠管长度的原则是在穿孔近处做横行单层缝合（补片），下腹部放两根 Penrose 引流管行低位引流（引流），并给予长期的肠外营养（等待）。烟卷式引流可产生粪瘘，并且功能上相当于肠造瘘，因为腹腔粘连会很快闭合[201]。这个过程不会导制败血症的发生，因为坏死肠管未被切除，腹腔整体很难引流，并且薄壁穿孔肠管通常不能做缝合。

Vaugham 等[298]描述了一项新颖的技术来避免多发性肠造瘘、高位空肠造瘘的并发症并保留肠管的长度。作者在 3 例 NEC 患儿中运用了“修剪和下降”

(clip and drop）技术。在这个过程中，切除明显坏死的肠管，切缘末端用钛夹或切割器关闭。在 48～72 小时之后再次探查，去除夹子，所有的肠段进行再吻合不做造瘘。3 个患儿中有 1 个在第 2 次探查时，再次切除坏死肠管，肠管断端再上夹子，在第 3 次手术时，成功进行一期吻合。随访了小部分病例 6 个月～7 年，无吻合口并发症或者后来再行手术。

全肠管受累（NEC 全肠炎，有活力的肠管 <25%）

19% 的患儿为全肠管受累[164]。该情况面临许多治疗难题，并且是一个存在许多争议的问题。最重要的需考虑的问题是尽可能多地保留肠管。主要的治疗方法包括切除所有坏死的肠段并做近端或多个造瘘，或者近端改道不做肠切除，并计划作第 2 次手术。在许多研究中证实了全肠累及的患儿的死亡率高达 42%～100%，存活下来的所有患儿几乎都有短肠综合征，体重不足 1000 g 的患儿其死亡率接近 100%，因此有学者认为应放弃任何治疗。

通过高位近端空肠造瘘（不做肠切除）而使肠管改道，通过远端肠管的减压可能有利于受损肠管愈合，代谢产物、细菌及其可能的产物数量减少。这项技术由 Martin 和 Neblett[186] 首先报道，他们做了一个不切肠管的高位空肠造瘘，计划在术后 6～8 周，再进行第 2 次探查。在 10 例全肠管受累的患儿中，Sugarman 和 Kiely[283] 报道 8 例存活者进行了二次探查，切除坏死肠段并成功进行肠管吻合，但长期存活率只有 50%。

造瘘口关闭和并发症

目前对重建肠管连续性既没有一个理想的体重和年龄要求，亦没有一个公认的时间。原则上关瘘手术时间根据上次手术以来的时间、体重增加和造瘘口排出情况而定。一般来讲，小肠造瘘关闭在最后一次手术即狭窄的风险期后 4 周进行是安全的。由于血管相连和正在吸收的炎症，手术后不到 4 周进行关闭可能
1442 会造成腹腔闭塞。在小肠造瘘口关闭前，必须确认肠管远端的通畅性，可通过逆行或顺行造影检查判断。Musemeche 等[20] 研究发现，术后小于 3 个月、3～5 个月以及超过 5 个月的并发症发生率三者之间没有明显不同，他们亦注意到体重小于 2.5 kg、2.5～5.0 kg 以及大于 5.0 kg 的患儿进行造瘘口关闭后，在并发症上没有区别。

尽管，在新生儿行小肠造瘘是可以挽救患儿生命的，但它亦是导致患病的一个主要因素。在近来的研究中报道，新生儿小肠造瘘有关的并发症发生率从 34%～68% 不等[217,302]，并发症包括伤口感染、伤口裂开、造瘘口狭窄需要再手术、切口疝、造瘘口旁疝、造瘘口脱垂或套迭以及小肠梗阻。

存活率

过去十年，NEC 患儿的存活率已经有了显著的提高（表 92-3）[250]。这归功于对早产儿 NEC 的早期诊断和更加有效的支持性治疗。有效的支持性治疗包括改善通气、表面活性物质疗法、全静脉营养以及对患病新生儿的处理和病理生理的进一步了解，以及小儿麻醉的改进。最值得注意的是出生体重小于 1000 g、胎龄小于 28 周的患儿成活率有所提高。在近来一项 754 例胎龄为 22～25 周早产儿的回顾性研究中，总体存活率为 63%，范围为从胎龄 22 周 14% 的存活率到胎龄 25 周 76% 的存活率[51]。极低体重患儿的死亡率仍显著高于体重较重的患儿。一项研究通过调查极低体重患儿与有全肠累及的 NEC 标准早产儿（大于 1000 g）两者预后间的差异，Snyder 等[273] 发现体重小于 1000 g 的患儿更需要手术治疗（51% 对 34%），以及最后发展为全肠受累要比体重大于 1000 g 的患儿多（10% 对 4%）。在两组中，全肠受累的患儿 100% 死亡。在一项 70 例体重小于 1000 g 有穿孔的 NEC 患儿的回顾性研究中，Erhlich[75] 证实存活率并不取决于外科手术的方式（是引流还是剖腹），而与患儿伴发的疾病数量有关。

笔者不认为死亡率的不同是由于所使用的措施的有效性不同。在不同的患儿组中，病变从局限性病变到广泛性坏死，各种情况的患儿数量亦不同，其死亡率亦大不相同，取决于出生体重、伴发疾病、病变的严重性和该患儿是当地出生的还是转运来的。状态不稳定的患儿有发生 NEC 的风险，必须强调这样一个事实，那就是 NEC 的患儿与对照组相比，对照组中的死亡率是 33%[280]。

表 92-3 药物和手术治疗坏死性小肠结肠炎的存活率

作者	年份	病例数（N）	存活率（%）	
			药物治疗	手术治疗
Touloukian[290]	1955—1966	25	20	27
Wilson 等[310]	1958—1968	16	14	13
Dudgeon 等[250]	1970—1972	63	59	26
O'Neill[219]	1970—1974	52	69	60
Philippart 和 Rector[250]	1974—1976	73	73	81
Grosfeld 等[98]	1972—1982	176	68	51
Ricketts 和 Jerles[246]	1980—1988	100	–	70
Grosfeld 等[98]	1983—1990	126	95	75
Lemelle 等[173]	1985—1990	331	82	65
Snyder 等[273]	1971—1996	226	–	68
Ehrlich 等[75]	1991—1998	70	–	75
Guthrie 等[100]	1998—2000	390	95	77

摘自 Rowe MI：Necrotizing enterocolitis. In Welch KJ, Randolph JG, Ravitch MM, et al（eds）: Pediatric Surgery, 4th ed. Chicago, Year Book, 1986.

并发症

胃肠道

肠狭窄

1968 年，Rabinowitz 等[240]首先报道了在急性 NEC 恢复后出现的肠狭窄的临床和放射学表现，所报道的总体发病率从 9%~36% 不等[114,269]，并且在非手术治疗后，更易发生肠管狭窄。随着疾病死亡率的下降，NEC 后肠狭窄的发生率在增高。肠狭窄是由于严重缺血损伤部位的纤维化愈合所导致的。不管狭窄是发生在手术后或者非手术治疗后，最常见的受累部位是结肠（80%），其次是末端回肠（15%）。60% 的结肠狭窄位于左半结肠，最常见的结肠狭窄位于脾曲（21%）。大多数患儿有单个狭窄，但亦有多个狭窄产生（15%）[122]。NEC 非手术治疗后，患儿出现生长发育迟缓、直肠出血或者肠梗阻，要怀疑有肠管狭窄发生。50% 肠狭窄的患儿会出现这些症状和体征，应用造影剂灌肠来进行评估，如果有症状的患儿造影发现有狭窄，通常建议做选择性的狭窄切除并吻合。

肠吸收不良和短肠综合征

吸收不良可由许多因素引起，包括肠管长度缩短、可吸收黏膜面积下降、酶缺乏、肠管蠕动功能亢进、胃酸分泌过多、细菌过度生长、肠管传输时间减少、维生素 B_{12} 缺乏和胆盐缺乏。短肠综合征（见第 86 章）是外科手术治疗 NEC 后最严重的长期胃肠道并发症。行肠切除的 NEC 存活患儿，短肠综合征的发生率高达 23%[245]。

胆汁淤积性肝病

胆汁淤积性肝病由多种因素引起，但主要是由于长期全静脉营养引起的。它是以直接高胆红素血症、肝肿大和转氨酶水平增高为特征。尽管是多因素的，但最重要的因素可能是长期的禁食。目前已证实最有效的治疗方法是早期的、小剂量的肠内喂养，同时给予全静脉营养，通过对肠黏膜施加一个营养作用并刺激胆流，帮助肠管适应。

复发的坏死性小肠结肠炎

NEC 可在手术以及非手术治疗后复发，其复发率为 4%~6%[246,282]，目前还未注意到在复发的 NEC 与肠内喂养的类型或时间、解剖位点或者初始治疗的方法之间存在稳固的联系。Stringer 等报道，超过 70% 复发的 NEC 患儿可通过非手术成功治愈[282]。

吻合口溃疡

NEC 肠切除多年后可出现一个较晚的并发症，即吻合口溃疡。Sondheimer 等[276]报道，6 例患儿在新生儿期行回结肠切除并吻合，这些患儿在 5～13 岁时有低位胃肠道出血。6 例患儿中有 5 例通过结肠镜检诊断出有吻合口溃疡，需要作溃疡切除。在行切除的 5 例患儿中，有 4 例患儿发生边缘溃疡复发，组织学检查发现浅表溃疡只穿透至肌层。引起溃疡的原因尚未明确。

神经发育并发症

患儿住院时间与患儿 1～2 岁时的生长发育密切相关[269]。这反映出医疗和社会因素对患儿大脑发育的不良影响。推荐在第 1 年时每 4 个月以及第 2 年时每 6 个月进行生长发育的评估，因为长期随访的数据表明，正常早产儿和严重 NEC 存活者有较高的神经发育异常的风险。

约 50% 的 NEC 患儿的神经发育正常[246,280]。在过去，认为接受治疗的 NEC 患儿神经发育异常与早产及其相关的状况，而不是 NEC 本身有关。但近来对存活婴儿的评估，对这种假设提出质疑。Vohr 等[301]研究了 1151 例极低体重（401～1000 g）存活儿，在 18～22 月这个可纠治的年龄段的神经发育、神经感觉和功能结果，发现神经发育有明显缺陷（25%），Bayley Ⅱ精神发育指数小于 70（37%），精神运动发育指数小于 70（29%），视觉障碍（9%）和听力障碍（11%）。NEC 作为异常神经性检查和低 Bayley 精神运动发育指数的一个危险因素而呈特异性相关。在一项评估 NEC 对神经发育影响的研究中，Sonntag 等[277]在 12 和 20 个月这个可纠治年龄段，对极低体重 NEC 患儿和没有 NEC 的对照组进行比较。虽然正常生长的 NEC 患儿不伴发短肠综合征，但作者证实了在 12 和 20 个月这两个年龄段均有明显的神经发育迟缓。55% 的 NEC 患儿有严重的智力迟钝，而没有 NEC 的患儿只有 22.5%。

预防

要减少 NEC 的发病率或预防 NEC 的发生，必须考虑到该病可能的发病机制以及一些被公认的围生期危险因素。预防 NEC 的方法包括：限制院内微生物传播、增强宿主防御、减少胃肠道内细菌繁殖和过度生长、给予促进肠管成熟的因子以及减少炎症串联反应可能是有效的。感染控制方法、母乳喂养、谨慎喂养患病的早产儿、喂养中添加免疫球蛋白、激素治疗、补充生长因子以及使用炎症介质拮抗剂，这些是已经被研究的部分预防措施。

感染控制措施

在婴儿室内采取感染控制措施可减少感染发生并限制感染的传播，因此，可潜在性地减少 NEC 的流行。传统的院内流行的预防措施包括：严格使用杀菌剂洗手、长袖衣服和手套、分开每个患儿的尿片和洗衣袋、隔离确诊的患儿以及对确诊的患儿安排独立的房间和护理人员（不要交叉）。已经证实，采取的感染控制措施可以阻止 NEC 的流行[31,109]。在群体发病时，相同的微生物能从患病的新生儿以及护理人员中分离出来。

加强宿主防御

口服免疫球蛋白制剂

预防性的免疫球蛋白，主要是 IgA，在早产儿的消化道中是缺乏的。如缺乏母乳喂养，则只有极少量的分泌型 IgA 以及肠道相关的 IgM 和 IgG。分泌型 IgA

通过黏附细菌和防止细菌黏附于肠黏膜而起到“抗体护层”的作用。Eibl 等证实肠内给予一种 IgG-IgA 制剂可降低 NEC 的发生率。他们随机分析了 179 例体重在 800~2000 g 的婴儿，在他们的奶粉中加入了一种人 IgG-IgA 制剂，对照组只给奶粉，两组均不给母乳，在免疫球蛋白组没有发生 NEC，但 91 例对照组中有 6 例发生 NEC。近来在兔子的实验研究中，Dickinson 等[67]证实在喂养中添加 IgA，通过加强黏膜屏障功能可预防细菌易位，这种作用在 IgG 和乳铁蛋白中是没有的。在一组随机双盲对照试验中，肠内给予婴儿 IgG 并不能减少 NEC 的发生[170]。

母体给予糖皮质激素

糖皮质激素可促进黏膜细胞成熟和改善肠道屏障功能，这种功能是通过肠表面的糖基化所介导的，它能影响细菌的黏附。糖皮质激素通过刺激血小板黏附因子的酶降解来下调炎症反应[274]。这些现象已通过临床和实验获得。Bauer 等[20]通过回顾性分析注意到母体产前使用糖皮质激素可促进胎儿肺成熟，而出生的婴儿与对照组相比其 NEC 的发生率显著下降(2% 对 7%)。这个大型的、多中心安慰剂对照试验很好地控制了许多潜在的混杂因素。Halac 等[101]进行了一项对早产儿母亲给予糖皮质激素的随机对照试验，对照组母亲给予安慰剂，但她们的婴儿出生后，立即给予 7 天的大剂量的地塞米松，NEC 的发生率在产前和产后激素治疗的两组中均显著下降。尽管产后治疗不如产前治疗在降低发生率上一样有效，但它改善了 NEC 的临床预后。然而，在这项研究中，许多潜在的混杂因素没有被评估，确定的预期的数据以及生后潜在毒性的评估是必须的。

母乳

母乳可降低许多新生儿感染的风险，包括下呼吸道病变、中耳炎、菌血症、脑膜炎和 NEC[34]。人乳提供一类体液和细胞抗感染因子、生长因子、益生菌以及必须的维生素和营养素。母乳因子包括 IgA、巨噬细胞、淋巴细胞、补体成分、溶菌酶、乳铁蛋白、运铁蛋白、干扰素、表皮生长因子、α-甲胎蛋白、促红细胞生成素、前生物因子、益生菌婴儿双歧杆菌和噬酸乳杆菌、血小板黏附因子乙酰水解酶和几种炎症介质。有力的证据显示分泌型 IgA 有保护作用，是构成肠-乳腺轴的主要免疫成分。母乳通过提供一个酸性环境抑制大肠杆菌的生长，促进双歧乳杆菌以及结合铁（一种大肠杆菌生长的必须元素）[17]的竞争性生长。

因为感染性病原菌的侵入似乎是 NEC 发病的主要因素，所以母乳对婴儿抵抗疾病来说是最理想的。母乳喂养可预防实验性的 NEC[17,65]。配方奶喂养的婴儿 NEC 的发生率比母乳喂养的婴儿高出 4~6 倍[179]。

喂养

有关 NEC 多见于奶粉喂养的婴儿中，以及奶粉所提供的底物为细菌过度生长提供了便利，很少有不同意见。尽管仔细的、有规律的喂养可防止 NEC 发生的潜在益处已被广泛接受，但是随机对照试验没有证实，在慢与快、早期与晚期，或者连续与间断喂养之间 NEC 发生率有任何不同[136,137,166,220,238,243]。

低出生体重婴儿和患儿或者产前有异常的婴儿要禁食 7~10 天，并给予静脉营养。如果没有任何症状表明 NEC 发生，可开始小心喂养。尽管许多临床医生以一个低比例的、低热卡配方开始喂养，但喂养的类型、浓度和增加的比例是没有统一的。如果胃内残留物增加或者任何潜在的与 NEC 有关的临床表现出现，则要停止喂养并对婴儿进行评估。

减少肠道细菌定殖和过度生长的方法

给予益生菌

益生菌被定义为“能在肠道内生长并对宿主有帮助的活的微生物”[43,192]。在治疗和预防胃肠道疾病中利用厌氧菌已有报道，对使用益生菌来预防 1445
NEC 已越来越引起人们的兴趣。双歧杆菌是革兰阳性的厌氧菌，是母乳喂养的婴儿肠道内主要的菌落，但是在有较高 NEC 风险的早产儿肠道内很少。在新生大鼠 NEC 模型中使用益生菌已证实可明显减少 NEC 的发病率[43,46]，未来亦需要进行人的临床试验。

肠内抗生素

非吸收性的广谱抗生素可抑制细菌生长以阻止NEC的发生。肠道内使用氨基糖苷类（如庆大霉素或卡那霉素），已作为一种方法来降低保守治疗中穿孔的发生率。然而，随机对照试验发现，在接受抗生素和未接受抗生素的两组婴儿中，在临床过程、并发症或死亡率上没有区别[74,194]。另外，口服氨基糖苷类药物可通过受损的肠道吸收，使其血清水平增加，并且有潜在的药物毒性。在肠内卡那霉素治疗后可发生细菌耐药[74]，并普遍存在促进真菌生长的风险。在近来一组早产儿口服万古霉素预防NEC的随机安慰剂对照研究中，Sin等[271]报道，与对照组相比，万古霉素组NEC的发生率下降了50%。

这些可行的研究并不支持对所有高风险早产儿常规使用肠内抗生素，早产儿中有许多肠管活力差，其有效性亦未被证实，并可能发生细菌耐药。在婴儿室给予特殊的抗生素是有指征的，NEC的暴发与某一特殊的生物体相关。

配方奶的酸化作用

Carrion和Egan[49]做了一项小型的前瞻性双盲研究，在这研究中，早产儿给予用盐酸酸化的pH值在2.5~5.5的食物，发现喂养物酸化可明显降低胃pH值小于4.0的婴儿的胃内细菌定殖率，他们亦发现，给予酸化食物婴儿的NEC发生率要比对照组明显降低。

炎症介质拮抗剂

有报道显示血小板黏附因子（PAF）的作用是通过受体介导的，许多混合物其功能为受体拮抗剂或者酶来降解这些蛋白，动物实验中运用PAF拮抗剂（WEB2086、WEB2170、SRI63-441）或者PAF降解酶（PAF乙酰水解酶）已经证实，它具有防止大鼠因给予内毒素或缺氧而导致肠管损伤的能力[47,115]。PAF乙酰水解酶也存在于母乳中，尽管在动物模型中得到了预期的结果，但是有关运用PAF拮抗剂或者降解酶治疗NEC的人体实验尚没有报道。

（严志龙译 叶祖萍校）

参考文献

1. Ade-Ajayi N, Kiely E, Drake D, et al: Resection and primary anastomosis in necrotizing enterocolitis. J R Soc Med 1996; 89:385.
2. Agerty HA, Ziserman AJ, Shollenberger CL: A case of perforation of the ileum in a newborn infant with operation and recovery. J Pediatr 1943;22:233.
3. Akisu M, Ozmen D, Baka M, et al: Protective effect of dietary supplementation with L-arginine and L-carnitine on hypoxia/reoxygenation-induced necrotizing enterocolitis in young mice. Biol Neonate 2002;81:260.
4. Alavi K, Prasad R, Lundgren K, et al: Interleukin-11 enhances small intestine absorptive function and mucosal mass after intestinal adaptation. J Pediatr Surg 2000; 35:371.
5. Alderton WK, Cooper CE, Knowles RG: Nitric oxide synthases: Structure, function and inhibition. Biochem J 2001; 357:593.
6. Alican I, Kubes P: A critical role for nitric oxide in intestinal barrier function and dysfunction. Am J Physiol 1996; 33:G225.
7. Alpan G, Eyal F, Vinograd I, et al: Localized intestinal perforation after enteral administration of indomethacin in premature infants. J Pediatr 1985;106:277.
8. Amin HJ, Zamora SA, McMillan DD, et al: Arginine supplementation prevents necrotizing enterocolitis in premature infants. J Pediatr 2002;140:425.
9. Anderson DM, Kliegman RM: The relationship of neonatal alimentation practices to the occurrence of endemic necrotizing enterocolitis. Am J Perinatol 1991;8:62.
10. Andoh A, Fujiyama Y, Sumiyoshi K, et al: Interleukin-4 acts as an inducer of decay-accelerating factor gene expression in human intestinal epithelial cells. Gastroenterology 1996;111:911.
11. Appleby SB, Ristimaki A, Neilson K, et al: Structure of the human cyclooxygenase-2 gene. Biochem J 1994;302: 723.
12. Auricchio S, Rabino A, Murset G: Intestinal glycosidase activities in the human embryo, fetus, and newborn. J Pediatr 1965;35:944.
13. Avni EF, Rypens F, Cohen E, Pardou A: Peri-cholecystic hyper-echogenicity in necrotizing enterocolitis: A specific sonographic sign? Pediatr Radiol 1991;21:179.
14. Azarow KS, Ein SH, Shandling B, et al: Laparotomy or drain for perforated necrotizing enterocolitis: Who gets what and why. Pediatr Surg Int 1997;12:137.
15. Ballance WA, Dahms BB, Shenker N, et al: Pathology of neonatal necrotizing enterocolitis: A ten-year experience, J Pediatr 1990;117:56.
16. Bandstra ES, Bukett G: Maternal-fetal and neonatal effects of in utero cocaine exposure. Semin Perinatol 1991;15:288.
17. Barlow B, Santulli TV, Heird WC, et al: An experimental study of neonatal enterocolitis—the importance of breast milk. J Pediatr Surg 1984;9:587.
18. Barry MK, Aloisi JD, Pickering SP, et al: Nitric oxide modulates water and electrolyte transport in the ileum. Ann Surg 1994;219:382.
19. Bates MD: Development of the enteric nervous system. Clin Perinatol 2002;29:97.
20. Bauer CR, Morrison JC, Poole WK, et al: A decreased incidence of necrotizing enterocolitis after prenatal glucocorticoid therapy. Pediatrics 1984;73:682.
21. Bell MJ, Temberg JL, Feigin RD, et al: Neonatal necrotizing

enterocolitis: Therapeutic decisions based upon clinical staging. Ann Surg 1978;187:1.
22. Berdon WE, Grossman H, Baker DH, et al: Necrotizing enterocolitis in the premature infant. Radiology 1964;83:879.
23. Berseth CL: Gestational evolution of small intestine motility in preterm and term infants. J Pediatr 1989;115:646.
24. Berseth CL, Bisquera JA, Paje VU: Prolonging small feeding volumes early in life decreases the incidence of necrotizing enterocolitis in very low birth weight infants. Pediatrics 2003;111:529.
25. Blakey JL, Lubitz L, Campbell NT, et al: Enteric colonization in sporadic neonatal necrotizing enterocolitis. J Pediatr Gastroenterol Nutr 1985;4:591.
26. Boccia D, Stolfi I, Lana S, et al: Nosocomial necrotising enterocolitis outbreaks: Epidemiology and control measures. Eur J Pediatr 2001;160:385.
27. Bolisetty S, Lui K: Necrotizing enterocolitis in full-term neonates. J Paediatr Child Health 2001;37:413.
28. Bone RC: Immunologic dissonance: A continuing evolution in our understanding of the systemic inflammatory response syndrome and the multiple organ dysfunction syndrome. Ann Intern Med 1996;125:690.
29. Book LS, Herbst JJ, Atherton SO, et al: Necrotizing enterocolitis in low birth weight infants fed elemental formula. J Pediatr 1975;87:602.
30. Book LS, Herbst JJ, Jung AL: Carbohydrate malabsorption in necrotizing enterocolitis. Pediatrics 1976;57:201.
31. Book LS, Overall JC, Herbst JJ: Clustering of necrotizing enterocolitis: Interruption by infection-control methods. N Engl J Med 1977;297:984.
32. Bousvaros A, Walker WA: Development and function of the intestinal mucosal barrier. In McDonald TT (ed): Ontogeny of the Immune System of the Gut. Boca Raton, FL, CRC Press, 1990, p 2.
33. Brown EG, Sweet AY: Preventing necrotizing enterocolitis in neonates. JAMA 1978;240:2452.
34. Buescher ES: Host defense mechanisms of human milk and their relations to enteric infections and necrotizing enterocolitis. Clin Perinatol 1994;21:247.
35. Buonomo C: Neonatal imaging: The radiology of necrotizing enterocolitis. Radiol Clin North Am 1999;37:1187.
36. Butter A, Glageole H, Laberge J: The changing face of surgical indications for necrotizing enterocolitis. J Pediatr Surg 2002;37:496.
37. Buyukunal C, Kilic N, Dervisoglu S, et al: Maternal cocaine abuse resulting in necrotizing enterocolitis—an experimental study in a rat model. Acta Paediatr Suppl 1994;396:91.
38. Caplan MS, Amer M, Jilling T: The role of human milk in necrotizing enterocolitis. Adv Exp Med Biol 2002;503:83.
39. Caplan MS, Hedlund E, Adler L, et al: Role of asphyxia and feeding in a neonatal rat model of necrotizing enterocolitis. Pediatr Pathol 1994;14:1017.
40. Caplan MS, Hedlund E, Adler L, et al: The platelet-activating factor receptor antagonist WEB 2170 prevents necrotizing enterocolitis in rats. J Pediatr Gastroenterol Nutr 1997;24:296.
41. Caplan MS, Hedlund E, Hill N, et al: The role of endogenous nitric oxide and platelet-activating factor in hypoxia-induced intestinal injury in rats. Gastroenterology 1994;106:346.
42. Caplan MS, Hsueh W, Kelly A, et al: Serum PAF acetylhydrolase increases during neonatal maturation. Prostaglandins 1990;39:705.
43. Caplan MS, Jilling T: Neonatal necrotizing enterocolitis: Possible role of probiotic supplementation. J Pediatr Gastroenterol Nutr 2000;30:S18.
44. Caplan MS, Jilling T: New concepts in necrotizing enterocolitis. Curr Opin Pediatr 2001;13:111.
45. Caplan MS, Lickerman M, Adler L, et al: The role of recombinant platelet-activating factor acetylhydrolase in a neonatal rat model of necrotizing enterocolitis. Pediatr Res 1997;42:779.
46. Caplan MS, Miller-Catchpole, R, Kaup S, et al: Bifidobacterial supplementation reduces the incidence of necrotizing enterocolitis in a neonatal rat model. Gastroenterology 1999;117:577.
47. Caplan MS, Sun XM, Hsueh W, et al: Role of platelet activating factor and tumor necrosis factor-alpha in neonatal necrotizing enterocolitis. J Pediatr 1990;116:960.
48. Caplan MS, Sun XM, Hsueh W: Hypoxia causes ischemic bowel necrosis in rats: The role of platelet-activating factor. Gastroenterology 1990;99:979.
49. Carrion V, Egan E: Prevention of neonatal necrotizing enterocolitis. J Pediatr Gastroenterol Nutr 1990;11:317.
50. Chailler P, Menard D: Ontogeny of EGF receptors in the human gut. Font Biosci 1999;4:D87.
51. Chan K, Ohlsson A, Synnes A, et al: Survival, morbidity, and resource use in infants of 25 weeks' gestational age or less. Am J Obstet Gynecol 2001;185:220.
52. Chandler JC, Hebra A: Necrotizing enterocolitis in infants with very low birth weight. Semin Pediatr Surg 2000;9:63.
53. Chen K, Inoue M, Okada A: Expression of inducible nitric oxide synthase mRNA in rat digestive tissues after endotoxin and its role in intestinal mucosal injury. Biochem Biophys Res Commun 1996;224:703.
54. Cheu HW, Brown DR, Rowe MI: Breath hydrogen excretion as a screening for the early diagnosis of necrotizing enterocolitis. Am J Dis Child 1989;143:156.
55. Chung DH, Ethridge RT, Kim S, et al: Molecular mechanisms contributing to necrotizing enterocolitis. Ann Surg 2001;233:835.
56. Claud EC, Savidge T, Walker WA: Modulation of human intestinal epithelial cell IL-8 secretion by human milk factors. Pediatr Res 2003;53:419.
57. Cohen S: The epidermal growth factor (EGF). Cancer 1983;51:1787.
58. Coopersmith CM, O'Donnell D, Gordon JI: Bcl-2 inhibits ischemia-reperfusion–induced apoptosis in the intestinal epithelium of transgenic mice. Am J Physiol 1999;276:G677.
59. Cronin CM, Canose J, Buchanan D, et al: The effect of aminophylline on gastrointestinal blood flow and oxygen metabolism in the conscious newborn lamb. J Pediatr Gastroenterol Nutr 1989;8:371.
60. Crow JP, Beckman JS: Reactions between nitric oxide, superoxide, and peroxynitrite: Footprints of peroxynitrite in vivo. Adv Pharmacol 1995;34:17.
61. Czyrko C, Del Pin CA, O'Neill JA Jr, et al: Maternal cocaine abuse and necrotizing enterocolitis: Outcome and survival. J Pediatr Surg 1991;26:414.
62. Daneman A, Woodward S, deSilva M: The radiology of neonatal necrotizing enterocolitis: A review of 47 cases and the literature. Pediatr Radiol 1978;7:70.
63. Davis JM, Abbasi S, Spitzer AR, et al: Role of theophylline in pathogenesis of necrotizing enterocolitis. J Pediatr 1986;109:344.
64. Deitch EA: Role of bacterial translocation in necrotizing enterocolitis. Acta Paediatr Suppl 1994;396:33.
65. de Lemos RA, Rogers JR Jr, McLaughlin GW: Experimental production of necrotizing enterocolitis in newborn goats [abstract]. Pediatr Res 1974;8:830.

66. Demestre X, Ginovart G, Figueras-Aloy J, et al: Peritoneal drainage as primary management in necrotizing enterocolitis: A prospective study. J Pediatr Surg 2002;37:1534.
67. Dickinson EC, Gorga JC, Garrett M, et al: Immunoglobulin A supplementation abrogates bacterial translocation and preserves the architecture of the intestinal epithelium. Surgery 1998;124:284.
68. Dickinson EC, Tuncer R, Nadler EP, et al: Recombinant human interleukin-11 prevents mucosal atrophy and bowel shortening in the defunctionalized intestine. J Pediatr Surg 2000;35:1079.
69. Di Lorenzo M, Bass J, Krantis A: Use of L-arginine in the treatment of experimental necrotizing enterocolitis. J Pediatr Surg 1995;30:235.
70. Downing GJ, Horner SR, Kilbride HW: Characteristics of perinatal cocaine exposed infants with necrotizing enterocolitis. Am J Dis Child 1991;145:26.
71. Dunn L, Hulman S, Weiner J, et al: Beneficial effects of early hypocaloric enteral feeding on neonatal gastrointestinal function: Preliminary report of a randomized trial. J Pediatr 1988;112:622.
72. Dvorak B, Hallpern MD, Holubec H, et al: Epidermal growth factor reduces the development of necrotizing enterocolitis in a neonatal rat model. Am J Physiol Gastrointest Liver Physiol 2002;282:G156.
73. Edelson MB, Bagwell CE, Rozycki HJ: Circulating pro- and counterinflammatory cytokine levels and severity in necrotizing enterocolitis. Pediatrics 1999;103:766.
74. Egan EA, Nelson RM, Mantilla G, Eitzman DV: Additional experience with routine use of oral kanamycin prophylaxis for necrotizing enterocolitis in infants under 1,500 grams. J Pediatr 1977;90:331.
75. Ehrlich PF, Sato TT, Short BL, et al: Outcome of perforated necrotizing enterocolitis in the very low birth weight neonate may be independent of the type of surgical treatment. Am Surg 2001;67:752.
76. Eibl MM, Wolf HM, Furnkranz H, et al: Prevention of necrotizing enterocolitis in low-birth-weight infants by IgA-IgG feeding. N Engl J Med 1988;319:1.
77. Ein SH, Marshall DG, Girvan D: Peritoneal drainage under local anesthesia for necrotizing enterocolitis. J Pediatr Surg 1977;12:963.
78. Engel RR, Virning NL, Hunt CE, et al: Origin of mural gas in necrotizing enterocolitis. Pediatr Res 1973;7:292.
79. Ewer AK, Al-Salti W, Coney AM, et al: The role of platelet-activating factor in a neonatal piglet model of necrotising enterocolitis. Gut 2004;53:207.
80. Fagbemi AO, Wright N, Lakhoo K, et al: Immunoreactive epidermal growth factor receptors are present in gastrointestinal epithelial cells of preterm infants with necrotising enterocolitis. Early Hum Dev 2001;65:1.
81. Fasoli L, Turi RA, Spitz L, et al: Necrotizing enterocolitis: Extent of disease and surgical treatment. J Pediatr Surg 1999;34:1096.
82. Finer NN, Peters KL, Hayek Z, et al: Vitamin E and necrotizing enterocolitis. Pediatrics 1984;73:387.
83. Fisher CJ, Agosti JM, Opal SM, et al: Treatment of septic shock with the tumour necrosis factor: Fc fusion protein. N Engl J Med 1996;334:1697.
84. Ford H, Watkins S, Reblock K, et al: The role of inflammatory cytokine and nitric oxide in the pathogenesis of necrotizing enterocolitis. J Pediatr Surg 1997;32:275.
85. Frey EE, Smith W, Franken EA, et al: Analysis of bowel perforation in necrotizing enterocolitis. Pediatr Radiol 1987; 17:380.
86. Garcia J, Smith FR, Cucinell SA: Urinary D-lactate excretion in infants with necrotizing enterocolitis. J Pediatr 1984; 104:268.
87. Gavilanes A, Heineman E, Herpers M, et al: Use of neonatal intensive care unit as a safe place for neonatal surgery. Arch Dis Child 1997;76:F51.
88. Generisch A: Bauchfellentzündung beim Neugeborenen in folge von Perforation des Ileums. Virchows Arch Pathol Anat 1891;126:485.
89. Gersony WM, Peckham GJ, Ellison RC, et al: Effects of indomethacin in premature infants with patent ductus arteriosus: Results of a national collaborative study. J Pediatr 1983;102:895.
90. Gianotti L, Alexander JW, Pyles T, et al: Arginine-supplemented diets improve survival in gut-derived sepsis and peritonitis by modulating bacterial clearance. The role of nitric oxide. Ann Surg 1993;217:644.
91. Glode MP, Sutton A, Moxon ER, et al: Pathogenesis of neonatal *Escherichia coli* meningitis: Induction of bacteremia and meningitis in infant rats fed *E coli* K1. Infect Immunol 1977;16:75.
92. Goldman AS, Thorpe LW, Goldblum RM, et al: Anti-inflammatory properties of human milk. Acta Paediatr Scand 1986;75:689.
93. Gollin G, Abarbanell A, Baerg J: Peritoneal drainage as definitive management of intestinal perforation in extremely low-birth-weight infants. J Pediatr Surg 2003; 38:1814.
94. Gonzalez-Crussi F, Hsueh W: Experimental model of ischemic bowel necrosis: The role of platelet-activating factor and endotoxin. Am J Pathol 1983;112:127.
95. Graf JL, Vanderwall KJ, Adzick NS, et al: Nitroglycerin attenuates the bowel damage of necrotizing enterocolitis in a rabbit model. J Pediatr Surg 1997;32:283.
96. Grantmyre EB, Butler GJ, Gillis DA: Necrotizing enterocolitis after Renografin-76 treatments of meconium ileus. AJR Am J Roentgenol 1981;136:990.
97. Grosfeld JL, Chaet M, Molinari F, et al: Increased risk of necrotizing enterocolitis in premature infants with patent ductus arteriosus treated with indomethacin. Ann Surg 1996;224:350.
98. Grosfeld JL, Cheu H, Schlatter M: Changing trends in necrotizing enterocolitis: Experience with 302 cases in two decades. Ann Surg 1991;214:300.
99. Grosfeld JL, Kamman K, Gross K, et al: Comparative effects of indomethacin, prostaglandin E, and ibuprofen on bowel ischemia. J Pediatr Surg 1983;18:738.
100. Guthrie SO, Gordon PV, Thomas V, et al: Necrotizing enterocolitis among neonates in the United States. J Perinatol 2003;23:278.
101. Halac E, Halac J, Begue EF, et al: Prenatal and postnatal corticosteroid therapy to prevent neonatal necrotizing enterocolitis: A controlled trial. J Pediatr 1990;117:132.
102. Hallstrom M, Koivisto AM, Janas M, et al: Frequency of and risk factors for necrotizing enterocolitis in infants born before 33 weeks of gestation. Acta Paediatr 2003; 92:111.
103. Halpern MD, Dominguiz JA, Dvorakova K, et al: Ileal cytokine dysregulation in experimental necrotizing enterocolitis is reduced by epidermal growth factor. J Pediatr Gastroenterol Nutr 2003;36:126.
104. Hamosh M: Bioactive factors in human milk. Pediatr Clin North Am 2001;48:69.
105. Hanahan DJ: Platelet activating factor: A biologically active phosphoglyceride. Annu Rev Biochem 1986;55:483.
106. Hand IL, Noble L, McVeigh, et al: The effects of intrauterine cocaine exposure on the respiratory status of the very

low birth weight infant. J Perinatol 2001;21:372.

107. Harris MC, Costarino AT Jr, Sullivan JS, et al: Cytokine elevations in critically ill infants with sepsis and necrotizing enterocolitis. J Pediatr 1994;124:105.

108. Harris PD, Neuhauser EBD, Gerth R: The osmotic effect of water soluble contrast media on circulating plasma volume. Am J Roentgenol Radium Ther Nucl Med 1964;91:694.

109. Healthy People 2000: National Health Promotion and Disease Prevention Objective (DHHS Publication [PHS] No. 21-59212:365). Washington, DC, Department of Health and Human Services, 1991.

110. Hebra A, Brown MF, McGeehin K, et al: Systemic and mesenteric vascular effects of platelet-activating factor and cocaine. In vivo effects on a neonatal swine model. Am Surg 1993;59:50.

111. Helmrath MA, Shin CE, Fox JW, et al: Epidermal growth factor in saliva and serum of infants with necrotising enterocolitis. Lancet 1998;351:266.

112. Henderson-Smart DJ, Subramaniam P, Davis P: Continuous positive airway pressure versus theophylline for apnea in preterm infants. Cochrane Database Syst Rev 2001;4: CD001072.

113. Horbar JD, Wright EC, Onstad L: NICHD Neonatal Research Network: Decreasing mortality associated with the introduction of surfactant therapy: An observational study of neonates weighing 601 to 1300 grams at birth. Pediatrics 1993;92:191.

114. Horwitz JR, Lally KP, Cheu HW, et al: Complications after surgical intervention for necrotizing enterocolitis: A multicenter review. J Pediatr Surg 1995;30:994.

115. Hsueh W, Caplan MS, Qu XW, et al: Neonatal necrotizing enterocolitis: Clinical considerations and pathogenetic concepts. Pediatr Dev Pathol 2002;6:6.

116. Hsueh W, Gonzalez-Crussi F, Arroyave JL: Platelet activating factor is an endogenous mediator for bowel necrosis in endotoxemia. FASEB J 1987;1:403.

117. Hutcheson IR, Whittle BJR, Boughton-Smith NK: Role of nitric oxide in maintaining vascular integrity in endotoxin-induced acute intestinal damage in the rat. Br J Pharmacol 1990;101:815.

118. Hutter JJ, Hathaway WE, Wayne ER: Hematologic abnormalities in severe neonatal necrotizing enterocolitis. J Pediatr 1976;88:1026.

119. Inagaki-Ohara K, Yada S, Takamura N, et al: P53-dependent radiation-induced crypt intestinal epithelial cell apoptosis is mediated in part through TNF-TNFR1 system. Oncogene 2001;20:812.

120. Isaacs D, North J, Lindsell D, Wilkinson AR: Serum acute phase reactants in necrotizing enterocolitis. Acta Paediatr Scand 1987;76:923.

121. Jaattela M: Biologic activities and mechanisms of action of tumor necrosis factor-alpha/cachectin. Lab Invest 1991; 64:724.

122. Janik JS, Ein SH, Mancer K: Intestinal strictures after necrotizing enterocolitis. J Pediatr Surg 1981;16:438.

123. Jilling T, Lu J, Jackson M, et al: Intestinal epithelial apoptosis initiates gross bowel necrosis in an experimental rat model of neonatal necrotizing enterocolitis. Pediatr Res 2004;55:622.

124. Johnson L, Bowen FW Jr, Abbasi S, et al: Relationship of prolonged pharmacologic serum levels of vitamin E to incidence of sepsis and necrotizing enterocolitis in infants with birth weight 1500 grams or less. Pediatrics 1985; 75:619.

125. Jones KL: Developmental pathogenesis of defects associated with prenatal cocaine exposure: Fetal vascular disruption. Clin Perinatol 1991;18:139.

126. Jones MK, Tomikawa M, Mohajer B, et al: Gastrointestinal mucosal regeneration: Role of growth factors. Front Biosci 1999;4:D303.

127. Juul SE: Erythropoietin in the neonate. Curr Probl Pediatr 1999;29:129.

128. Juul SE, Joyce AE, Zhao Y, et al: Why is erythropoietin present in human milk? Studies of erythropoietin receptors on enterocytes of human and rat neonates. Pediatr Res 1999;46:263.

129. Juul SE, Ledbetter DJ, Joyce AE, et al: Erythropoietin acts as a trophic factor in neonatal rat intestine. Gut 2001;49:182.

130. Juul SE, Yachnis AT, Christensen RD: Tissue distribution of erythropoietin and erythropoietin receptor in the developing human fetus. Early Hum Dev 1998;52:235.

131. Kafetzis DA, Skevaki C, Costalos C: Neonatal necrotizing enterocolitis: An overview. Curr Opin Infect Dis 2003; 16:349.

132. Kamitsuka MD, Horton MK, Williams MA: The incidence of necrotizing enterocolitis after introducing standardized feeding schedules for infants between 1250 and 2500 grams and less than 35 weeks of gestation. Pediatrics 2000;105:379.

133. Kanto WP Jr, Hunter JE, Stoll BJ: Recognition and medical management of necrotizing enterocolitis. Clin Perinatol 1994;21:335.

134. Kao SCS, Smith KWL, Franklin EA Jr, et al: Contrast enema diagnosis of necrotizing enterocolitis. Pediatr Radiol 1992; 22:115.

135. Karlowicz MG: Risk factors associated with fungal peritonitis in very low birth weight neonates with severe necrotizing enterocolitis: A case-control study. Pediatr Infect Dis J 1993;12:574.

136. Kennedy KA, Tyson JE, Chamnanvanakij S: Rapid versus slow rate of advancement of feedings for promoting growth and preventing necrotizing enterocolitis in parenterally fed low-birth-weight infants. Cochrane Database Syst Rev 2000;(2):CD001241.

137. Kennedy KA, Tyson JE, Chamnanvanakij S: Early versus delayed initiation of progressive enteral feedings for parenterally fed low birth weight or preterm infants. Cochrane Database Syst Rev 2000;(2):CD001970.

138. Kilic N, Buyukunal C, Dervisoglu S, et al: Maternal cocaine abuse resulting in necrotizing enterocolitis. An experimental study in a rat model. II. Results of perfusion studies. Pediatr Surg Int 2000;16:176.

139. Kleessen B, Bunke H, Tovar K, et al: Influence of two infant formulas and human milk on the development of faecal flora in newborn infants. Acta Paediatr 1995;84: 1347.

140. Kliegman RM: Neonatal necrotizing enterocolitis: Implications for an infectious disease. Paediatr Clin North Am 1979;26:327.

141. Kliegman RM: Neonatal necrotizing enterocolitis: Bridging the basic science with the clinical disease. J Pediatr 1990;117:833.

142. Kliegman RM, Fanaroff AA: Neonatal necrotizing enterocolitis: A nine-year experience. Am J Dis Child 1981; 135:608.

143. Kliegman RM, Fanaroff AA: Neonatal necrotizing enterocolitis in the absence of pneumatosis. Am J Dis Child 1982;136:608.

144. Kliegman RM, Fanaroff AA: Neonatal necrotizing enterocolitis. N Engl J Med 1984;310:1093.

145. Kliegman RM, Hack M, Jones P, et al: Epidemiologic study

of necrotizing enterocolitis among low-birth-weight infants. J Pediatr 1982;100:440.
146. Kliegman RM, Pittard WB, Fanaroff AA: Necrotizing enterocolitis in neonates fed human milk. J Pediatr 1979; 95:450.
147. Kliegman RM, Walker WA, Yolken RH: Necrotizing enterocolitis: Research agenda for a disease of unknown etiology and pathogenesis. Pediatr Res 1993;34:701.
148. Kliegman RM, Walsh MC: Neonatal necrotizing enterocolitis: Pathogenesis, classification, and spectrum of illness. Cur Probl Pediatr 1987;17:213.
149. Kling PJ, Sullivan TM, Roberts RA, et al: Human milk as a potential enteral source of erythropoietin. Pediatr Res 1998;43:216.
150. Kodroff MB, Hartenberg MA, Goldschmidt RA: Ultrasonographic diagnosis of gangrenous bowel in neonatal necrotizing enterocolitis. Pediatr Radiol 1984; 14:168.
151. Kosloske AM: Surgery for necrotizing enterocolitis. World J Surg 1985;9:277.
152. Kosloske AM: Epidemiology of necrotizing enterocolitis. Acta Paediatr Suppl 1994;396:2.
153. Kosloske AM: Indications for operation in necrotizing enterocolitis revisited. J Pediatr Surg 1994;29:663.
154. Kosloske AM, Musemeche CA: Necrotizing enterocolitis of the neonate. Clin Perinatol 1989;16:97.
155. Kosloske AM, Papile LA, Burstein J: Indications for operation in acute necrotizing enterocolitis of the neonate. Surgery 1980;87:502.
156. Krasna IH, Kim H: Indomethacin administration after temporary ischemia causes bowel necrosis in mice. J Pediatr Surg 1992;27:805.
157. Krouskop RW, Brown EG, Sweet AY: The relationship of feeding to necrotizing enterocolitis. Pediatr Res 1974; 8:383.
158. Kubes P: Ischemia-reperfusion in feline small intestine: A role for nitric oxide. Am J Physiol 1993;264:G143.
159. Kubes P: Inducible nitric oxide synthase: A little bit of good in all of us. Gut 2000;47:6.
160. Kubes P, Arfors KE, Granger DE: Platelet-activating factor–induced mucosal dysfunction: Role of oxidants and granulocytes. Am J Physiol 1991;260:G965.
161. Kubes P, McCafferty DM: Nitric oxide and intestinal inflammation. Am J Med 2000;109:150.
162. Kuhl G, Wille L, Bolkenius M, et al: Intestinal perforation associated with indomethacin treatment in premature infants. Eur J Pediatr 1985;143:213.
163. Kumral A, Baskin H, Duman N, et al: Erythropoietin protects against necrotizing enterocolitis of newborn rats by the inhibiting nitric oxide formation. Biol Neonate 2003;84:325.
164. Kurkchubasche AG, Smith SD, Rowe MI: Portal venous air—an old sign and new operative indication for necrotizing enterocolitis [abstract]. Paper presented at the 38th BAPS Annual International Congress, July 1991, Budapest.
165. La Gamma EF, Browne LE: Feeding practices for infants weighing less than 1500 g at birth and the pathogenesis of necrotizing enterocolitis. Clin Perinatol 1994;21:271.
166. La Gamma EF, Ostertag SG, Birenbaum H: Failure of delayed oral feedings to prevent necrotizing enterocolitis. Results of study in very-low-birth-weight neonates. Am J Dis Child 1985;139:385.
167. Langer JC, Sohal SS, Mumford DA: Mucosal permeability in the immature rat intestine: Effects of ischemia-reperfusion, cold stress, hypoxia, and drugs. J Pediatr Surg 1993;28:1380.
168. Lauw FN, Pajkrt D, Hack CE, et al: Proinflammatory effects of IL-10 during human endotoxemia. J Immunol 2000;165:2783.
169. Lawrence G, Bates J, Gaul A: Pathogenesis of neonatal necrotizing enterocolitis. Lancet 1982;72:317.
170. Lawrence G, Tudehope D, Baumann K, et al: Enteral human IgG for prevention of necrotising enterocolitis: A placebo-controlled, randomized trial. Lancet 2001;357: 2090.
171. Ledbetter DJ, Juul SE: Erythropoietin and the incidence of necrotizing enterocolitis in infants with very low birth weights. J Pediatr Surg 2000;35:178.
172. Ledbetter DJ, Juul SE: Necrotizing enterocolitis and hematopoietic cytokines. Clin Perinatol 2000;27:697.
173. Lemelle JL, Schmitt M, de Miscault G, et al: Neonatal necrotizing enterocolitis: A retrospective and multicentric review of 331 cases. Acta Paediatr Suppl 1994;396:70.
174. Lemons JA, Bauer CR, Oh W, et al: Very low birth weight outcomes of the National Institute of Child Health and Human Development Neonatal Research Network, January 1995 through December 1996. Pediatrics 2001; 107:e1.
175. Leonard T Jr, Johnson F, Pettett PG: Critical evaluation of the persistent loop sign in necrotizing enterocolitis. Radiology 1982;142:385.
176. Lessin MS, Luks FI, Wesselhoeft CW Jr, et al: Peritoneal drainage as definitive treatment for intestinal perforation in infants with extremely low birth weight (less than 750 grams). J Pediatr Surg 1998;33:370.
177. Liu Q, Du XX, Schindel DT, et al: Trophic effects of interleukin-11 in rats with experimental short bowel syndrome. J Pediatr Surg 1996;31:1047.
178. Lopez SL, Taeusch HW, Findlay RD, et al: Time of onset of necrotizing enterocolitis in newborn infants with known prenatal cocaine exposure. Clin Pediatr (Phila) 1995;34:424.
179. Lucas A, Cole TJ: Breast milk and neonatal necrotizing enterocolitis. Lancet 1990;336:1519.
180. Maalouf EF, Fagbemi A, Duggan PJ, et al: Magnetic resonance imaging of intestinal necrosis in preterm infants. Pediatrics 2000;105:510.
181. MacKendrick W, Caplan M, Hsueh W: Endogenous nitric oxide protects against platelet-activating factor–induced bowel injury in the rat. Pediatr Res 1993;34:222.
182. MacKendrick W, Hill N, Hsueh W, et al: Increase in plasma platelet-activating factor levels in enterally fed preterm infants. Biol Neonate 1993;64:89.
183. Mahony L, Caldwell RL, Girod DA, et al: Indomethacin therapy on the first day of life in infants with very low birth weight. J Pediatr 1985;106:801.
184. Malo C, Menard D: Influence of epidermal growth factor on the development of sucking mouse intestinal mucosa. Gastroenterology 1982;83:28.
185. Marchildon MB, Buck BE, Abdenour G: Necrotizing enterocolitis in the unfed infant. J Pediatr Surg 1982;17:620.
186. Martin LW, Neblett WW: Early operation with intestinal diversion for necrotizing enterocolitis. J Pediatr Surg 1981; 16:252.
187. Martinez-Tallo E, Claure N, Bancalari E: Necrotizing enterocolitis in full-term or near-term infants: Risk factors. Biol Neonate 1997;71:292.
188. Marty C, Misset B, Tamian F, et al: Circulating interleukin-8 concentrations in patients with multiple organ failure of septic and nonseptic origin. Crit Care Med 1994;22:673.
189. Mercurio F, Manning AM: NF-κB as a primary regulator of

the stress response. Oncogene 1999;42:477.
190. Merritt CRB, Goldsmith JP, Sharp MJ: Sonographic detection of portal venous gas in infants with necrotizing enterocolitis. AJR Am J Roentgenol 1984;143:1059.
191. Miettinen PJ, Berger JE, Meneses J, et al: Epithelial immaturity and multiorgan failure in mice lacking epidermal growth factor receptor. Nature 1995;376:337.
192. Millar M, Wilks M, Costeloe K: Probiotics for preterm infants? Arch Dis Child 2003;88:F354.
193. Miller MJS, Zhang XJ, Sadowska-Krowicka H, et al: Nitric oxide release in response to gut injury. Scand J Gastroenterol 1993;28:149.
194. Miranda JC, Schimmel MS, Mimms GM, et al: Gentamicin absorption during prophylactic use for necrotizing enterocolitis. Dev Pharmacol Ther 1984;7:303.
195. Mizrahi A, Barlow O, Berdon W, et al: Necrotizing enterocolitis in premature infants. J Pediatr 1965;66:697.
196. Molik KA, West KW, Rescorla FJ, et al: Portal venous air: The poor prognosis persists. J Pediatr Surg 2001;36:1143.
197. Mollit DL, Tepas JJ, String DL, et al: Does patient age or intestinal pathology influence the bacteria found in cases of necrotizing enterocolitis? South Med J 1990;84:879.
198. Moncada S, Palmer RM, Higgs EA: Nitric oxide: Physiology, pathophysiology, and pharmacology. Pharmacol Rev 1991; 43:109.
199. Moomjian AS, Sokal MM, Vijayan S: Necrotizing enterocolitis—endemic vs epidemic form. Pediatr Res 1978; 12:530.
200. Moore TC: Management of necrotizing enterocolitis by "patch, drain, and wait." Pediatr Surg Int 1989;4:110.
201. Moore TC: Successful use of the "patch, drain, and wait" laparotomy approach to perforated necrotizing enterocolitis: Is hypoxia-triggered "good angiogenesis" involved? Pediatr Surg Int 2000;16:356.
202. Moore TR, Sorg J, Miller L, et al: Hemodynamic effects of intravenous cocaine on the pregnant ewe and fetus. Am J Obstet Gynecol 1986;157:686.
203. Morgan JL, Shochat SJ, Hartman GE: Peritoneal drainage as primary management of perforated NEC in the very low birth weight infant. J Pediatr Surg 1994;29:310.
204. Morrison SC, Jacobson JM: The radiology of necrotizing enterocolitis. Clin Perinatol 1994;21:347.
205. Moss RL, Dimmitt RA, Henry MCW, et al: A meta-analysis of peritoneal drainage versus laparotomy for perforated necrotizing enterocolitis. J Pediatr Surg 2001;36:1210.
206. Moya FR, Eguchi H, Zhao B, et al: Platelet-activating factor acetylhydrolase in term and preterm human milk: A preliminary report. J Pediatr Gastroenterol Nutr 1994; 19:236.
207. Musemeche CA, Kosloske AM, Ricketts RR: Enterostomy in necrotizing enterocolitis: An analysis of techniques and timing of closure. J Pediatr Surg 1987;22:479.
208. Nadler EP, Dickinson E, Knisely A, et al: Expression of inducible nitric oxide synthase and interleukin-12 in experimental necrotizing enterocolitis. J Surg Res 2000; 92:71.
209. Nadler EP, Stanford A, Zhang XR, et al: Intestinal cytokine gene expression in infants with acute necrotizing enterocolitis: Interleukin-11 mRNA expression inversely correlates with extent of disease. J Pediatr Surg 2001;36:1122.
210. Nanthakumar NN, Fusunyan RD, Sanderson I, et al: Inflammation in the developing human intestine: A possible pathophysiologic contribution to necrotizing enterocolitis. Proc Natl Acad Sci U S A 2000;97:6043.
211. Nathan C, Xie Q: Nitric oxide synthases: Roles, tolls, and controls. Cell 1994;78:915.
212. Needleman P, Turk J, Jakschik BA, et al: Arachidonic acid metabolism. Annu Rev Biochem 1986;55:69.
213. Neu J, Bernstein H: Update on host defense and immunonutrients. Clin Perinatol 2002;29:41.
214. Nilsen EM, Johansen FE, Jahnsen FL, et al: Cytokine profiles of cultured microvascular endothelial cells from the human intestine. Gut 1998;42:635.
215. Norton ME, Merrill J, Cooper BA, et al: Neonatal complications after administration of indomethacin for preterm labor. N Engl J Med 1993;329:1602.
216. Nowicki P: Intestinal ischemia and necrotizing enterocolitis. J Pediatr 1990;117:S14.
217. O'Connor A, Sawin RS: High morbidity of enterostomy and its closure in premature infants with necrotizing enterocolitis. Arch Surg 1998;133:875.
218. Ohls RK: Erythropoietin to prevent and treat the anemia of prematurity. Curr Opin Pediatr 1999;11:108.
219. O'Neill JA Jr: Neonatal necrotizing enterocolitis. Surg Clin North Am 1981;61:1013.
220. Ostertag SG, LaGamma EF, Reisen CE, Ferrentino FL: Early enteral feeding does not affect the incidence of necrotizing enterocolitis. Pediatrics 1986;77:275.
221. Ostlie DJ, Spilde TL, St Peter SD, et al: Necrotizing enterocolitis in full-term infants. J Pediatr Surg 2003;38:1039.
222. Ozturk H, Dokucu A, Ogun C, et al: Protective effects of recombinant human interleukin-10 on intestines of hypoxia-induced necrotizing enterocolitis in immature rats. J Pediatr Surg 2002;37:1330.
223. Paltauf A: Die spontane dickdarm Rupture der Neugeborenen. Virchows Arch Pathol Anat 1888;111:461.
224. Pang G, Couch L, Batey R, et al: GM-CSF, IL-1 alpha, IL-1 beta, IL-6, IL-8, IL-10, ICAM-1, and VCAM-1 gene expression and cytokine production in human duodenal fibroblasts stimulated with lipopolysaccharide, IL-1 alpha and TNF-alpha. Clin Exp Immunol 1994;96:437.
225. Pang KY, Bresson JL, Walker WA: Development of the gastrointestinal mucosal barrier. III. Evidence for structural differences in microvillus membranes from newborn and adult rabbits. Biochem Biophys Acta 1983;727:201.
226. Parikh AA, Salzman AL, Kane CD, et al: IL-6 production in human intestinal epithelial cells following stimulation with IL-1 beta is associated with activation of the transcription factor NF-kappa B. J Surg Res 1997;69:139.
227. Parks DA, Bulkley GB, Granger DN: Role of oxygen-derived free radicals in digestive tract diseases. Surgery 1983;94:415.
228. Payne D, Kubes P: Nitric oxide donors reduce the rise in reperfusion-induced intestinal mucosal permeability. Am J Physiol 1993;265:G189.
229. Pierro A: Necrotizing enterocolitis: Pathogenesis and treatment. Br J Hosp Med 1997;58:126.
230. Pierro A, Hall N: Surgical treatment of infants with necrotizing enterocolitis. Semin Neonatol 2003;8:223.
231. Pierro A, Hall N, Ade-Ajayi A, et al: Laparoscopy assists surgical decision making in infants with necrotizing enterocolitis. J Pediatr Surg 2004;39:902.
232. Pinsky MR, Vincent JL, Deviere J, et al: Serum cytokine levels in human septic shock: Relation to multiple-system organ failure and mortality. Chest 1993;103:565.
233. Playford RJ, Wright NA: Why is epidermal growth factor present in the gut lumen? Gut 1996;38:303.
234. Pokorny WJ, Garcia-Prats JA, Barry YN: Necrotizing enterocolitis: Incidence, operative care, and outcome. J Pediatr Surg 1986;21:1149.
235. Porat R, Brodsky N: Cocaine: A risk factor for necrotizing enterocolitis. J Perinatol 1991;11:30.
236. Potoka DA, Nadler EP, Upperman JS, et al: Role of nitric

oxide and peroxynitrite in gut barrier failure. World J Surg 2002;26:806.
237. Potoka DA, Upperman JS, Zhang XR, et al: Peroxynitrite inhibits enterocytes' proliferation and modulates Src kinase activity in vitro. Am J Physiol Gastrointest Liver Physiol 2003;285:G861.
238. Premji S, Chessell L: Continuous nasogastric milk feeding versus intermittent bolus milk feeding for premature infants less than 1500 grams. Cochrane Database Syst Rev 2003;(1):CD001819.
239. Qu XW, Rozenfeld RA, Huang W, et al: Roles of nitric oxide synthases in platelet-activating factor–induced intestinal necrosis in rats. Crit Care Med 1999;27:356.
240. Rabinowitz JG, Wolf BS, Feller MR, et al: Colonic changes following necrotizing enterocolitis in the newborn. Am J Roentgenol Radium Ther Nucl Med 1968;103:359.
241. Rabinowitz SS, Dzakpasu P, Piecuch S, et al: Platelet-activating factor in infants at risk for necrotizing enterocolitis. J Pediatr 2001;138:81.
242. Radi R, Beckman JS, Bush KM, et al: Peroxynitrite-induced membrane lipid peroxidation: The cytotoxic potential of superoxide and nitric oxide. Arch Biochem Biophys 1991;288:481.
243. Rayyis SF, Ambalavanan N, Wright L, et al: Randomized trial of "slow" versus "fast" feed advancements on the incidence of necrotizing enterocolitis in very low birth weight infants. J Pediatr 1999;134:293.
244. Read LC, Francis GL, Wallace JC, et al: Growth factor concentrations and growth-promoting activity in human milk following premature birth. J Dev Physiol 1985;7:135.
245. Ricketts RR: Surgical treatment of necrotizing enterocolitis and the short bowel syndrome. Clin Perinatol 1994;21:365.
246. Ricketts RR, Jerles ML: Neonatal necrotizing enterocolitis: Experience with 100 consecutive surgical patients. World J Surg 1990;14:600.
247. Robertson DM, Paganilli R, Dinwiddie R, et al: Milk antigen absorption in the preterm and term neonate. Arch Dis Child 1982;57:369.
248. Robinson MJ, Clayden GS, Smith MF: Xanthines and necrotizing enterocolitis. Arch Dis Child 1980;55:494.
249. Rossier A, Sarrot S, Deplanque J: L'entcolite ulceronecrotique du premature. Semin Hop Paris 1959;35:1428.
250. Rowe MI: Necrotizing enterocolitis. In Welch KJ, Randolph JG, Ravitch MM, et al (eds): Pediatric Surgery, 4th ed. Chicago, Year Book, 1986.
251. Rowe MI, Buckner DM, Newmark S: The early diagnosis of gram negative septicemia in the pediatric surgical patient. Ann Surg 1975;182:280.
252. Rowe MI, Furst AJ, Poole CA: The neonatal response to Gastrografin enema. Pediatrics 1971;48:29.
253. Rowe MI, Marchildon MB, Arango A, et al: The mechanisms of thrombocytopenia in experimental gram-negative septicemia. Surgery 1978;84:87.
254. Rowe MI, Reblock KK, Kurkchubasche AG, et al: Necrotizing enterocolitis in the extremely low birthweight infant. J Pediatr Surg 1994;29:987.
255. Rowe MI, Seagram G, Weinberger M: Gastrografin-induced hypertonicity. Am J Surg 1973;125:185.
256. Rubbo H, Radi R, Trujillo M, et al: Nitric oxide regulation of superoxide and peroxynitrite-dependent lipid peroxidation. Formation of novel nitrogen-containing oxidized lipid derivatives. J Biol Chem 1994;269:26066.
257. Santulli TV, Schullinger JN, Heird WC, et al: Acute necrotizing enterocolitis in infancy: A review of 64 cases. Pediatrics 1975;55:376.
258. Schanler RJ, Shulman RJ, Lau C, et al: Feeding strategies for premature infants: Randomized trial of gastrointestinal priming and tube-feeding method. Pediatrics 1999; 103:434.
259. Scheifele DW: Role of bacterial toxins in neonatal necrotizing enterocolitis. J Pediatr 1990;117:S44.
260. Scheifele DW, Bjornson GL: Delta toxin activity in coagulase-negative staphylococci from the bowels of neonates. J Clin Microbiol 1988;26:279.
261. Scheifele DW, Bjornson GL, Dyer RA, Dimmick JE: Delta-like toxin produced by coagulase-negative staphylococci is associated with necrotizing enterocolitis. Infect Immun 1983;55:2268.
262. Scheifele DW, Ginter GL, Olsen E, et al: Comparison of two antibiotic regimens for neonatal necrotizing enterocolitis. J Antimicrobial Chemother 1987;30:421.
263. Scheifele DW, Melton PW: Endotoxinemia in neonates with necrotizing enterocolitis [abstract]. Clin Res 1981; 29:127.
264. Schmid O, Quaiser K: Uer eine besondere schwere Verlaufende form von Enteritis beim Saugling. Oesterr Z Kinderh 1953;8:114.
265. Sehgal S, Ewing C, Waring P, et al: Morbidity of low-birthweight infants with intrauterine cocaine exposure. J Natl Med Assoc 1993;85:20.
266. Serou MJ, DeCoster MA, Bazan NG: Interleukin-1 beta activates expression of cyclooxygenase-2 and inducible nitric oxide synthase in primary hippocampal neuronal culture: Platelet-activating factor as a preferential mediator of cyclooxygenase-2 expression. J Neurosci Res 1999;58:593.
267. Shin CE, Falcone RA Jr, Stuart L, et al: Diminished epidermal growth factor levels in infants with necrotizing enterocolitis. J Pediatr Surg 2000;35:173.
268. Shou J, Motyka LE, Daly JM: Intestinal microbial translocation: Immunologic consequences and effects of interleukin-4. Surgery 1994;116:868.
269. Simon NP: Follow-up for infants with necrotizing enterocolitis. Clin Perinatol 1994;21:411.
270. Singer II, Kawka DW, Schloemann S, et al: Cyclooxygenase 2 is induced in colonic epithelial cells in inflammatory bowel disease. Gastroenterology 1998;115:297.
271. Siu YK, Ng PC, Jung SC, et al: Double blind, randomized, placebo controlled study of oral vancomycin in prevention of necrotizing enterocolitis in preterm, very low birth weight infants. Arch Dis Child Fetal Neonatal Ed 1998; 79:F105.
272. Smith SD, Tagge ED, Miller J, et al: The hidden mortality in surgically-treated necrotizing enterocolitis: Fungal sepsis. J Pediatr Surg 1990;25:1030.
273. Snyder CL, Gittes GK, Murphy JP, et al: Survival after necrotizing enterocolitis in infants weighing less than 1,000 grams: 25 years' experience at a single institution. J Pediatr Surg 1997;32:434.
274. Snyder F: Platelet-activating factor and related acetylated lipids as potent biologically active cellular mediators. Am J Physiol 1990;259:C697.
275. Sola M, Vecchio A, Rimsza L: Evaluation and treatment of thrombocytopenia in the neonatal intensive care unit. Neonatal Hematol 2000;27:655.
276. Sondheimer JM, Sokol RJ, Narkewicz MR, et al: Anastomotic ulceration: A late complication of ileocolonic anastomosis. J Pediatr 1995;127:225.
277. Sonntag J, Grimmer I, Scholz T, et al: Growth and neurodevelopmental outcome of very low birthweight infants with necrotizing enterocolitis. Acta Paediatr 2000;89:528.
278. Spencer T, McDonald TT: The ontogeny of human mucosal barrier immunity. In McDonald TT (ed): Ontogeny of the

Immune System of the Gut. Boca Raton, FL, CRC Press, 1990, p 23.
279. Stark ME, Szurszeski JH: Role of nitric oxide in gastrointestinal and hepatic function and diseases. Gastroenterology 1992;103:1928.
280. Stevenson DK, Kerner JA, Malachowski N, et al: Late morbidity among survivors of necrotizing enterocolitis. Pediatrics 1980;66:925.
281. Stoll BJ: Epidemiology of necrotizing enterocolitis. Clin Perinatol 1994;21:205.
282. Stringer MD, Brereton RJ, Drake DP, et al: Recurrent necrotizing enterocolitis. J Pediatr Surg 1993;28:979.
283. Sugarman ID, Kiely EM: Is there a role for high jejunostomy in the management of severe necrotising enterocolitis? Pediatr Surg Int 2001;17:122.
284. Sun XM, Hsueh W: Bowel necrosis induced by tumor necrosis factor in rats is mediated by platelet-activating factor. J Clin Invest 1988;81:1328.
285. Taniguchi T, Koido Y, Aiboshi J, et al: Change in the ratio of interleukin-6 to interleukin-10 predicts a poor outcome in patients with systemic inflammatory response syndrome. Crit Care Med 1999;27:1262.
286. Telsey AM, Merrit TA, Dixon SD: Cocaine exposure in a term neonate. Necrotizing enterocolitis as a complication. Clin Pediatr (Phila) 1988;27:547.
287. Tepperman BL, Brown JF, Whittle BJR, et al: Nitric oxide synthase induction and intestinal cell viability in rats. Am J Physiol 1993;265:G214.
288. Tesdale F, Le Guennec JC, Bard H, et al: Neonatal necrotizing enterocolitis: The relationship of age at the time of onset and prognosis. Can Med Assoc J 1980;123:387.
289. Thelander HE: Perforation of the gastro-intestinal tract of the newborn infant. Am J Dis Child 1939;58:371.
290. Touloukian RJ: Neonatal necrotizing enterocolitis: An update on etiology, diagnosis and treatment. Surg Clin North Am 1976;56:281.
291. Uauy RD, Fanaroff AA, Korones SB, et al: Necrotizing enterocolitis in very low birth weight infants: Biodemographic and clinical correlates. J Pediatr 1991; 119:630.
292. Udall JN Jr: Gastrointestinal host defense and necrotizing enterocolitis. J Pediatr 1990;117:S33.
293. Uauy RD, Fanaroff AA, Korones SB, et al: Necrotizing enterocolitis in very low birth weight infants: Biodemographic and clinical correlates. National Institute of Child Health and Human Development Neonatal Research Network. J Pediatr 1991;119:630.
294. Udall JN, Pang K, Fritze L, et al: Development of gastrointestinal mucosal barrier. I. The effect of age of intestinal permeability to macromolecules. Pediatr Res 1981; 15:241.
295. Van Acker J, De Smet F, Muyldermans G, et al: Outbreak of necrotizing enterocolitis associated with *Enterobacter sakazakii* in powdered milk formula. J Clin Microbiol 2001;39:293.
296. VanderKolk WE, Kurz P, Daniels J, et al: Liver hemorrhage during laparotomy in patients with necrotizing enterocolitis. J Pediatr Surg 1996;31:1063.
297. van Dissel JT, van Langevelde P, Westendorp RGJ, et al: Anti-inflammatory cytokine profile and mortality in febrile patients. Lancet 1998;351:950.
298. Vaughan WG, Grosfeld JL, West K, et al: Avoidance of stomas and delayed anastomosis for bowel necrosis: The 'clip and drop-back' technique. J Pediatr Surg 1996; 31:542.
299. Ververidis M, Kiely EM, Spitz L, et al: The clinical significance of thrombocytopenia in neonates with necrotizing enterocolitis. J Pediatr Surg 2001;36:799.
300. Vilcek J, Lee TH: Tumor necrosis factor. New insights into the molecular mechanisms of its multiple actions. J Biol Chem 1991;266:7313.
301. Vohr BR, Wright LL, Dusick AM, et al: Neurodevelopmental and functional outcomes of extremely low-birth-weight infants in the National Institute of Child Health and Human Development Neonatal Research Network, 1993-1994. Pediatrics 2000;105:1216.
302. Weber TR, Tracy TF Jr, Silen ML, et al: Enterostomy and its closure in newborns. Arch Surg 1995;130:534.
303. Wells CL, Maddaus MA, Simmons RL: Proposed mechanism for the translocation of intestinal bacteria. Rev Infect Dis 1988;10:958.
304. Westra-Meijer CMM, Degener JE, Dzoljic-Danilovic G, et al: Quantitative study of the aerobic and anaerobic fecal flora in neonatal enterocolitis. Arch Dis Child 1983; 58:523.
305. Wexler HA: The persistent loop sign in neonatal necrotizing enterocolitis: A new indication for surgical intervention? Radiology 1978;126:201.
306. White KC, Harkavy KL: Hypertonic formula resulting from added oral medications. Am J Dis Child 1982; 136:931.
307. Williams AJ: Xanthines and necrotizing enterocolitis. Arch Dis Child 1980;55:973.
308. Williams CS, Dubois RN: Prostaglandin endoperoxide synthase: Why two isoforms? Am J Physiol 1996;270:G393.
309. Willis DM, Chabot J, Radde IC, et al: Unsuspected hyperosmolarity of oral solutions contributing to necrotizing enterocolitis in very low birth weight infants. Pediatrics 1977;60:535.
310. Wilson R, Kanto WP Jr, McCarthy BJ, et al: Age at onset of necrotizing enterocolitis: An epidemiologic analysis. Pediatr Res 1982;16:82.
311. Wiswell TE, Robertson CF, Jones TA, et al: Necrotizing enterocolitis in full-term infants. A case-control study. Am J Dis Child 1988;142:532.
312. Woods JR, Plessinger MA, Clark KE: Effect of cocaine on uterine blood flow and fetal oxygenation. JAMA 1987;257:957.
313. Wright LL, Uauy RD, Younes N, et al: Rapid advances in feeding increase the risk of necrotizing enterocolitis in very low birth weight infants [abstract]. Pediatr Res 1993; 33:313.
314. Xu DZ, Lu Q, Swank GM, et al: Effect of heat shock and endotoxin stress on enterocytes viability apoptosis and function varies based on whether the cells are exposed to heat shock or endotoxin first. Arch Surg 1996;131:1222.
315. Yoshioka H, Iseki K, Fujita K: Development and differences of intestinal flora in the neonatal period in breast-fed and bottle-fed infants. Pediatrics 1983;72:317.
316. Yu Y, Chadee K: *Entamoeba histolytica* stimulates interleukin-8 from human colonic epithelial cells without parasite-enterocyte contact. Gastroenterology 1997;112:1536.
317. Zamora SA, Amin HJ, McMillan DD, et al: Plasma L-arginine concentrations in premature infants with necrotizing enterocolitis. J Pediatr 1997;131:226.

第 93 章

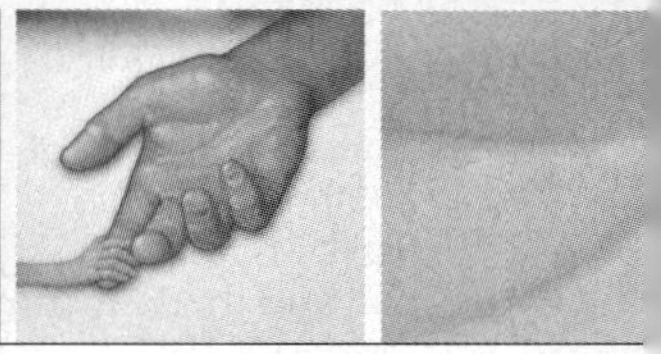

Crohn 病

Fred Alexander

1453 Crohn 病是一种胃肠道慢性炎症，目前，它已成为影响青少年身体健康并且治疗费用最高的慢性疾病之一。尽管在 19 世纪末和 20 世纪早期就有散在的“慢性小肠结肠炎”的报道[11,25]，但直到 1932 年 Crohn、Oppenheimer 和 Ginsberg 才第一次将 Crohn 病作为一种临床疾病来报道[10]，他们描述该疾病的特征为末端回肠亚急性或慢性坏死性炎症导致肠腔狭窄和肠瘘。

Crohn 病的病因尚不清楚。然而，有许多重要的影响因素，包括基因、感染和免疫。同样重要的是，事实上第三世界国家还不知道该病。典型的 Crohn 病的炎症是以全肠管炎、肠壁全层增厚以及口疮样溃疡和直肠内少量鹅卵石样溃疡为特征。在结肠内，Crohn 病可能与溃疡性结肠炎相混淆，两者有时在临床表现和组织学上很难区别开来。事实上，10% 的慢性结肠炎患儿，其组织学是不明确的。Crohn 病和溃疡性结肠炎两者有相似的肠道外表现。两者均有结直肠癌高发的风险。尽管存在这些明显相同点，但是两种疾病的外科治疗和预后有很大的不同。因此，有必要对每一个患儿进行完整的评估，所有的治疗措施需经儿科胃肠医生、外科医生和病理科医生组成的多学科团队进行充分权衡和讨论。

流行病学

Crohn 病较溃疡性结肠炎更常见。在儿童中，Crohn 病的发病率为每年 11 例/10 万人，而溃疡性结肠炎的发病率为 2.3 例/10 万人[17]。Crohn 病的发病率有年龄特点，年龄小于 15 岁的儿童，其发病率为每年 2.5 例/10 万人，年龄在 15～19 岁的患者，其发病率为每年 16 例/10 万人[36]。男女发病率相似。Crohn 病好发于白种人和犹太人。另外，青少年 Crohn 病的发病率在西方国家呈现出增长趋势，在 1968—1983 年间，苏格兰发现其发病率呈 3 倍增长[16]。

病因学

Crohn 病的病因尚不清楚，然而，许多危险因素显示与该病的形成有关。例如，具有 Crohn 病遗传倾向的患儿与肠道炎症性疾病存在 5%～25% 的低度相关性[35]。Crohn 病在同胞间的发病率是 7%，而在后代子女中的发病率为 9%，在单合子双胎中也表现为相当高的一致性。另外，某些感染性病原菌，如副结核分枝杆菌和麻疹病毒，两者可引起肉芽肿性炎症、败血症和瘘的形成。

在 Crohn 病患儿组织破坏的区域被大量淋巴细胞浸润，表现为失去对抗原刺激的常见自限性反应，并伴有细胞因子释放、花生四烯酸代谢和活泼氧中间体的失控。近年来研究显示[29]细胞因子，包括白介素-1（IL-1）、IL-4、IL-8、IL-12、肿瘤坏死因子（TNF）和干扰素-γ 的共同作用补充炎症细胞，促进胶原沉积和诱发嗜酸性细胞脱颗粒，从而刺激氯化物的分泌引起腹泻。其步骤从免疫活化到组织损伤这个过程仍不清楚。但是，可能涉及异常的辅助 T 细胞反应或者氧代谢物释放的可能，可有潜在的细胞毒性作用（或两者都有）[30]。最后，尽管没有直接的证据显示 Crohn 病可能是由食物过敏原引起，但是已经证实，牛奶蛋白的血清抗体在许多 Crohn 病患儿体内是升高的。

54

病理

在 Cleveland 临床中心治疗的 361 例 Crohn 病患儿中，60% 的患儿病变累及末端回肠和结肠，小肠受累仅 30%，而大肠受累只有 10%[31]。受累肠管和肠系膜因胶原沉积和水肿而增厚，并有脂肪沿浆膜层浸润（脂肪环绕）。组织学上，黏膜有大量的口疮样溃疡。在大体上，由于黏膜溃疡附近区域再生形成鹅卵石样变，亦称熊掌样变（图 93-1）。通常这种炎症间隔有正常的肠道组织而呈跳跃式出现。炎症通常穿过黏膜并且侵入邻近的结构中，形成肠管与其他结构之间的瘘管，包括肠道、膀胱、腹壁、阴道或会阴部。瘘管通常一端是盲端，并且形成局部炎症或蜂窝织炎。受损小肠中 40% 有组织学上的肉芽肿改变。60%～80% 的内镜活检样本取自胃内以及 25% 的内镜样本取自结肠[38]。

临床特征

Crohn 病在大年龄组中的发病率日益增加。4% 的新病例发生在 6～10 岁，31% 发生在 11～15 岁，以及 65% 发生在 15～20 岁[11]。大多数年龄较小的患儿在诊断 Crohn 病时，已有 2 年的临床症状。诊断依据为有慢性病史、间歇性痉挛性腹痛伴腹泻、体重减轻、直肠出血以及家族性肠道炎症病史。临床体征包括腹部压痛或肿块，并有肛周病变、杵状指、口炎或皮疹，身高和体重的连续测量可证明体重减轻或生长障碍。

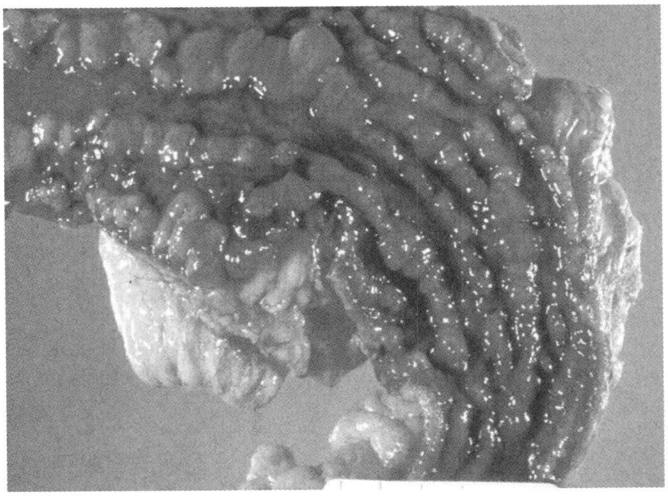

图 93-1 Crohn 病的熊掌样畸形（也见彩图）。

生长障碍表现为青春期延迟、幼稚型性征以及由于厌食、营养不良、腹泻和胰岛素样 1 型生长因子及胶原代谢的激素抑制导致的身材矮小。在这些表现中，最重要的影响因素是厌食导致低蛋白和热卡的摄入减少，在该病的其他症状和体征出现前，40% 的患儿出现生长障碍、体重减轻或两者均有发生。以下是单独或联合随访观察的情况：体重增加在国家健康状况统计中心制定的相对年龄体重的 5% 以下，低于正常的身高增长速度，为每年 5 cm 以下，另外根据 Tanner 生长速度曲线，身高增长小于前年的 2 cm 以下。总之，85% 的 Crohn 病患儿出现身高和（或）体重增长障碍。

另外，肠道外的症状也发生在许多 Crohn 病患儿中，关节痛和关节炎发生率为 10%，并且在肠道疾病出现前几年就已出现。皮肤表现如红斑性结节，坏疽性脓皮症的发生率为 1%～4%，眼睛表现如虹膜炎，葡萄膜炎发生率小于 10%（表 93-1）[23]。在 Crohn 病的患儿中，5% 患有草酸钙和尿酸构成的肾结石，同样，2%～5% 的患儿有胆囊结石[30]。

诊断

实验室检查对 Crohn 病患儿无特异性，但有时可有帮助。70% 的患儿有贫血，60% 有血小板增加以及 80% 有红细胞沉降率增加。营养标志物包括清蛋白和

表 93-1 有关 Crohn 病的临床和内镜特点

临床	肛周病变（肛裂/肛瘘/脓肿/赘生物）
	肛门手术史
	腹部肿块
	口腔溃疡
	肠道外症状
内镜影像	小肠病变
	直肠病变
	黏膜鹅卵石样改变
	匍行溃疡
	结肠狭窄
	跳跃式病变

前清蛋白，转铁蛋白和维生素结合蛋白在多于一半的 Crohn 病患儿中有异常降低。I 型胶原 C-端前肽或Ⅲ型胶原 N-端前肽的测定与生长速度相关。在 1/3 的患儿中大便愈创木脂试验阳性，并且所有大便均需作彻底的内源性病原菌评价，如艰难梭状芽孢杆菌、轮状病毒以及弯曲杆菌属。

1455 影像学检查在 Crohn 病患儿中是一个有用的筛查工具。超过 80% 的患儿有小肠受累。因此，在大多数病例中要进行上消化道造影以及整个小肠显影。阳性发现包括末端回肠结节化和狭窄，并与肠袢分离（图 93-2）。静脉胃肠道增强的 CT 检查可发现增厚的肠袢以及对发现蜂窝织炎和脓肿形成有帮助。

最后，上、下消化道内镜检查可直接观察和组织学取样。结肠镜检直肠病变可排除溃疡性结肠炎的可能性，如回肠受累或肉芽肿形成可确诊 Crohn 病。

药物治疗

目前，Crohn 病的药物治疗是各种药物的混合治疗。包括糖皮质激素、5-氨基水杨酸（ASA）制剂、甲硝唑、6-巯基嘌呤或硫唑嘌呤、氨甲蝶呤、环孢霉素 A、单克隆抗体［如英夫利昔单抗（抗类风湿药）］

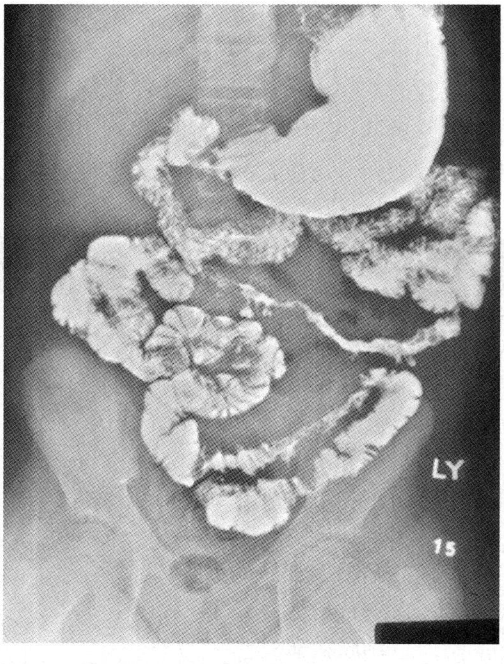

图 93-2 全肠道 Crohn 病。

以及肠内营养支持。糖皮质激素仍是治疗小肠以及大肠病变的一线药物。泼尼松口服剂量 1～2 mg/（kg・d）（最大 40～60 mg），直至缓解，然后剂量每 1～2 周减少 5 mg。对于住院患儿相同剂量的泼尼松龙（美卓乐）可通过静脉给药。糖皮质激素的抗炎作用主要通过阻止 IL-1 的表达，刺激辅助 T 细胞吸引并且激活自然杀伤细胞和巨噬细胞。激素的不连贯使用可导致在 1 年内有 70% 的高复发率。另一方面，重复或连续使用糖皮质激素亦导致一系列不良反应，包括库欣综合征、生长抑制、白内障、青光眼以及骨质疏松症椎体塌陷、肌无力以及情绪压抑。维持治疗的替换疗法包括隔日糖皮质激素来降低对全身的影响或应用激素类似物加强受体结合特性，以及加快代谢。布地奈德有比可的松高 100 倍的受体结合能力[23]，并且首次以失活的形式通过肝，更多的临床试验表明[18,46]，该药在缓解 Crohn 病病情上略逊于泼尼松龙，但其副作用明显减少。

其他达到缓解的治疗方法是口服 5-ASA 的替代物[47]，柳氮磺胺吡啶（杨柳磺胺吡啶）在结肠内代谢为磺胺吡啶，是一种磺胺类抗生素，可以用来充当载体或代替 5-ASA，是一种有效的抗炎药。临床试验已证实柳氮磺胺吡啶治疗较轻疾病是有作用的，亦能缓解回结肠 Crohn 病和 Crohn 病结肠炎的患儿[34,50]。柳氮磺胺吡啶的副作用基于其剂量并与其剂量相关联，包括头痛、恶心、疲劳、氮质血症以及超敏反应如皮疹、发热、肝炎、溶血性贫血以及骨髓抑制。丙烯酸树脂（美沙拉秦片）或乙基纤维素中心体（皮质得斯安）包裹的 5-ASA 能在炎症部位最大限度释放并且减少吸收[20]，两者均能缓解激素和外科治疗后的 Crohn 病。5-ASA 亦能做成栓剂形式，在肛周 Crohn 病的患儿通过灌肠直肠给药。

免疫调节药物如硫唑嘌呤和 6-巯基嘌呤与 5-ASA合用可逐渐减少激素应用以及防止 Crohn 病的复发。硫唑嘌呤在红细胞内转变为 6-巯基嘌呤，在肝再转换成活性代谢物，抑制 DNA 的合成[22]。两种药物在 2/3 激素依赖或难治性 Crohn 病的患儿中均能耐受并且有效[27]，其作用机制是抑制淋巴细胞、原始 T 细胞和自然杀伤细胞。这些药物起效较晚（通常 3～6 个月），其副作用包括胰腺炎、骨髓抑制和肝损害[43]。这些药物亦能引起与剂量相关的中性粒细胞减少，必须密切监护。不过，它们潜在的致癌作用在儿童中是比较弱的[9]。甲氨蝶呤是另一种免疫抑制剂，对 Crohn 病相当有效，尤其在伴有关节炎和关节

痛的患儿。甲氨蝶呤每周注射 25 mg 时有显著的作用[15]。临床研究显示[33]，在 3～4 周内，64% 的儿童
456 有反应，像其他免疫抑制药物一样，甲氨蝶呤亦能引起骨髓抑制和肝病。环孢霉素 A 很少用于未实施其他疗法的难治性、重症 Crohn 病和不适宜外科治疗的患儿。环孢霉素 A 选择性阻断辅助性和细胞毒性淋巴细胞活性，并相对于其他免疫药物产生较短的作用。最有效的是通过连续静脉给药，给予小剂量的口服药不能有效维持缓解[6,48]。环孢霉素 A 是一种有效的免疫抑制剂，它可引起肾功能不全、神经毒性以及癫痫发作，同时亦有机会性感染的可能，最后，英夫利昔单抗是一种新的免疫调节剂，在治疗 Crohn 病上显示出巨大的作用，尤其是结肠或肛周受累的患儿（或两者兼有）。它是一种针对肿瘤坏死因子的单克隆抗体，通过静脉给药，与肿瘤坏死因子结合，在几天至几周内产生较高的应答率[24]。许多 Crohn 结肠炎的患儿取得了较好的疗效，但需要多次静脉给药，因为其复发率较高。

抗生素尤其是环丙沙星和甲硝唑（灭滴灵制剂），在治疗 Crohn 病时有辅助作用。大剂量的抗生素对治疗肛周疾病有效。甲硝唑与柳氮磺胺吡啶对治疗轻度或中度活跃期病例有效[52]。甲硝唑可推迟手术后吻合口复发[45]，但必须长期服用以避免复发。长期应用甲硝唑，尤其是剂量超过 40 mg/(kg · d) 可引起恶心、口中有金属味以及周围神经损害。

最后，以要素饮食和全肠外营养构成的营养疗法，不仅可成功改善生长障碍，同时亦改善症状和减少激素应用[4,44]。除此之外，肠衣包裹的鱼油在维持 Crohn 病的缓解上也有作用[5]。据推测，黏膜内充满 Ω-3 脂肪酸可转变花生四烯酸代谢，针对白三烯 C 或 D 类的弱活性产物[21]，使其远离白三烯 B_4 炎症前体[21]。大多数临床试验证实，再生长和症状减轻是对连续应用鼻胃管或胃造瘘喂养的肠内支持的反应[4,39,42,44]。许多青少年反对该种治疗方法，还有患儿不喜欢口服大量鱼油，因呼吸时有鱼味，一旦停止肠内支持，症状很快复发。目前，还不清楚是否液体聚合物饮食更便宜和可口，并在促进生长和缓解症状方面与要素饮食同样有效。最后，严重的且不能忍受任何类型的肠内饮食的 Crohn 病患儿，让肠道休息的全肠外营养将改善症状并作为外科治疗的一个桥梁。如患儿治疗不能获得一个满意的生活质量或者发生有害的副作用时，要考虑进行外科治疗。

手术指征和外科治疗

外科不能治愈 Crohn 病，而用于处理药物治疗无效的 Crohn 病和（或）Crohn 病的并发症。另外，由于 Crohn 病的复发不可避免，所以总体上要求保守的外科治疗。特殊的外科处理方式依据每个病例受损的部位以及并发症的类型来实施（表 93-2）。Crohn 病最常见的并发症包括肠梗阻、肠穿孔、腹腔内和肛周脓肿、瘘管以及巨结肠。在许多病例，这些并发症呈现出暴发的症状和体征，并通过外科治疗能完全消除。

由于病变局限在末端回肠和盲肠，故 50%～60% 的儿童和青少年的 Crohn 病有右下腹疼痛。该区域的肠管病变经常并发机械性肠梗阻、脓肿、蜂窝织炎、瘘管形成或同时有几种症状出现。许多有这些并发症和相关症状的患儿，可通过静脉抗生素和激素成功治疗。如果症状通过药物治疗未完全消除或者同时有生长障碍（或两者兼有），就有必要进行外科干预。这种状况下可进行回盲部切除并一期吻合，同时切除瘘管和蜂窝织炎，受累小肠的切除边缘可含该病的大体病变。因为该病的镜下切除并不能预防复发，可安全切除瘘管而不需要广泛切除终末器官，无论是小肠、大肠、膀胱或阴道的壁层组织。在这些患儿中，瘘管可横断并冲洗末端器官，缺损处用两层缝线关闭。

约 20%～30% 的儿童和青少年的 Crohn 病患者，常有多发性小肠狭窄所导致的急性或慢性小肠梗阻（或两者兼有）。另外，这些患儿一开始对抗炎和免疫药物治疗有反应。但是，大多数慢性肠梗阻患儿有长期间歇性腹痛和生长障碍。在过去，外科治疗局限于切除每一段狭窄的小肠，有时由于多处小肠切除而

表 93-2　Crohn 病外科保守治疗原则（伯明翰，英国）
Crohn 病变累及全肠道
外科不能治愈该病
外科应尽可能安全
外科医生只要求处理并发症
复发是（几乎）不可避免的，所以尽可能保留肠管
不切除肠管的情况下，可安全治疗肠管狭窄的并发症

导致短肠综合征。目前，小肠切除的指征是有小肠穿
1457 孔、瘘管形成或肠壁极度肥厚需防止狭窄者，另外，肠管狭窄临近受累超过 30 cm 或者回盲部病变需要尽早作肠切除的。事实上，狭窄整形是外科治疗的选择（图 93-3）。短段狭窄 7～10 cm 以上者，可通过 Heineke-Mikulicz 狭窄整形进行治疗。这种方法通过做一个经过狭窄的纵向切口，并且达到狭窄任一端正常肠管 1～2 cm。肠管使用不可吸收线（通常为慢吸收）做单层间断横行缝合。长段狭窄达到 25～30 cm，可运用 Finney 侧侧吻合来治疗，通过肠管前后壁用可吸收线全层缝合，并后壁浆肌层加强。狭窄整形适用于通过 Folley 导管球囊测量的内径小于或等于 2 cm 的所有狭窄。然而，由于疾病的进行性特征，建议治疗所有的狭窄，除了肠管管径受影响的病例。狭窄整形能使梗阻症状消失，在保持小肠长度的同时，85% 的患儿不需要连续服用激素[40]。狭窄整形的并发症包括吻合口漏和出血，与肠切除术相近，其发生率为 5%～10%。该病的复发率在之前做过狭窄整形和切除后的部位无差别。然而有人报道，早期实施狭窄整形的肠管可完全治愈。因此，病变肠管的保留不一定会诱发狭窄部位的早期复发。

10%～20% 较早出现疾病表现的 Crohn 病患儿，病变局限于结肠和直肠。Crohn 结肠炎如片状或呈弥漫性病变，通常有直肠受累。而在溃疡性结肠炎中从未发生过。Crohn 结肠炎伴有肛周病变，然而，肛周病变不是 Crohn 结肠炎必然出现的症状。并发症如穿孔、脓肿以及瘘管形成较少见，尽管偶尔亦出现乙状结肠和降结肠狭窄，大多数 Crohn 结肠炎患儿需要手术治疗难治性腹痛和腹泻。当 Crohn 结肠炎药物治疗不起作用时，可实施的外科治疗包括部分结肠切除、全结肠切除并回肠造瘘或者回肠直肠吻合以及全结直肠切除并末端回肠造瘘。由于 5 年内有近 60% 的高复发率[51]，应避免部分结肠切除。全结肠切除是一个较好的方法，使大便能正常排出。当直肠病变严重或者有严重的肛周病变时，要作全结肠切除同时做末端回肠造瘘，以及 Hartmann 储袋作为一期手术。当直肠受累较轻并有正常的括约肌和直肠张力时，就可以安全进行一期回肠直肠吻合。回肠直肠吻合亦可作为直肠病变消失后的二期手术（图 93-4）。全结直肠切除并做永久性回肠造瘘可治疗严重直肠和肛周病变。因为 Crohn 病复发而导致回肠直肠吻合失败或者肠道活检证实有原位癌的患儿可选择该治疗，做该手术时保留直肠壁肌层外的所有组织，包括括约肌是很重要的，以避免术后会阴部窦道问题。

尽管回肠储袋肛管吻合（IPAA）已成为溃疡性结肠炎的治疗方法，但对 Crohn 病患儿不合适，因为该病在储袋内的高复发风险，使得储袋要进一步切除，并失去宝贵的小肠。未确诊的结肠炎不是回肠储袋肛管吻合的禁忌证[1]。然而，如果由于直肠或肛周病变而怀疑 Crohn 病，全结肠切除加上末端回肠造瘘以及 Hartmann 储袋是其指征。接下来可基于标本病理结果进行回肠储袋肛管吻合加回肠直肠吻合。

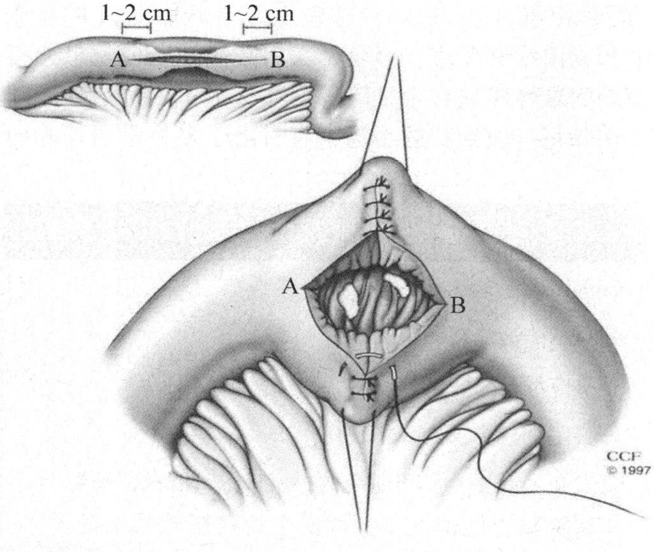

图 93-3　Heineke-Mikulicz 狭窄整形。（Courtesy of Cleveland Clinic Foundation，1997.）

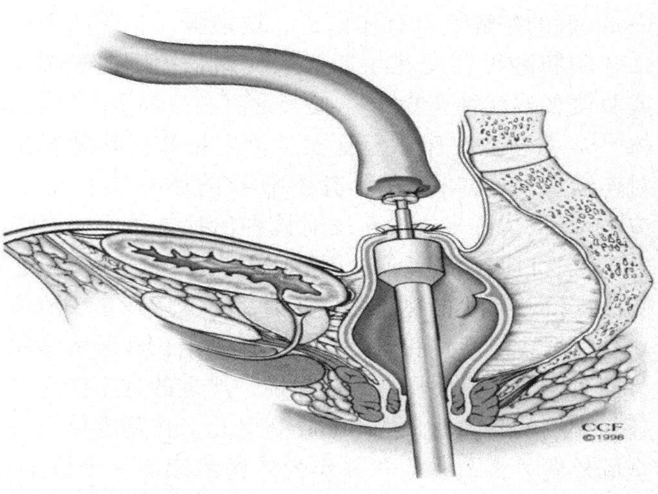

图 93-4　严重 Crohn 结肠炎的回直肠吻合术。（Courtesy of Cleveland Clinic Foundation，1998.）

458 青少年 Crohn 病严重肛周病变的发生率为 5%～10%，通常伴有回肠或远端结肠病变。在溃疡性结肠炎中肛周病变非常少见。像肠道 Crohn 病一样，肛周 Crohn 病对药物治疗亦有反应。外科手术用作处理并发症，最常见的手术指征是肛周脓肿需要切开、引流以及清创。小的脓肿可疏松地填塞纱布，24～48 小时后清除。大的脓肿累及直肠周围间隙，具体根据受累的范围，要放置蘑菇头引流管引流。可在手术室应用荧光透视使用水溶性造影剂来确定需要二次引流的马蹄形脓肿，引流管放置 4～8 周，以构建一个可控制的瘘管。患儿可用甲硝唑或用环丙沙星进行治疗，并每天擦洗，直至随访造影检查证实脓腔已完全愈合，此时可拔除引流管。引流管可用硝酸银以及注射纤维胶进行治疗[7]。肛瘘是肛周 Crohn 病的另一个并发症，它对抗生素（甲硝唑或环丙沙星）或免疫抑制剂治疗（糖皮质激素和英夫利昔单抗）敏感。对括约肌下瘘管宜采用瘘管切开或瘘管切除术，与该药在肠道其他部位的药物治疗效果相同。括约肌上的瘘管治疗较困难，瘘管的切开或切除会引起大便失禁，最好通过放置 Seton 缝线，或通过清创并注入硝酸银以及纤维胶来治疗[40]。近端改道（如末端结肠造瘘术）用于先前的药物或外科治疗无效的患儿，根据病变部位和疾病累及的范围，该手术可同时结合局限性肠管切除或部分结肠次全切除。许多病例在肠管改道后，瘘管将在 6～12 月愈合。在这时，患儿可做一个Ⅱ期尿流复道加结肠造瘘术或回肠直肠吻合术。肛裂在 Crohn 病患儿中最好是通过药物治疗。在 Crohn 病患儿中不主张做肛裂切除，因为伤口愈合较差，并且复发相当常见。严重的肛裂要根据患儿的实际情况治疗，可通过饮食控制以及全肠外营养或者通过近端改道治疗。

手术预后

Crohn 病手术后复发需再次手术的累积风险在 5 年内达到 20%，10 年达到 35%，15 年内接近 45%（图 93-5）[35]，而且这种风险在第 2 次手术后仍存在[49]。包括 Cleveland 临床基金会在内的几个研究显示，外科手术后的复发风险与患儿的临床特征无关（表 93-3）[31]。复发不受性别、发病年龄、出现症状到手术的时间或者手术指征，包括梗阻、肿块、瘘管或难处理性的影响。而且，肠切除术后复发的风险在并发末端回肠与大肠疾病，以及小肠与大肠疾病的患儿中类似[35]。另外，组织学研究显示，切除边缘距病变组织距离不影响复发。切缘超过正常组织 3～5 cm，对预防复发是没有必要的。唯一减少复发的外科方法是做永久性的造瘘，这种方法被用来补救约 25% 具有 10 年病史的 Crohn 病幼年患儿[1]。

由于病变累及全肠管的特点以及高复发率，1459
Crohn 病有面临短肠综合征的风险。Douglas Wilmone 医生[53]的儿组成年人大样本回顾性研究显示，空回肠长度少于 200 cm 的患儿中 24% 是由于 Crohn 病造成的，而空回肠长度少于 50 cm 的患儿中 90% 是由 Crohn 病造成。为了减少 Crohn 病患者的短肠风险，伯明翰大学治疗组推荐常规使用狭窄整形来治疗小肠狭窄而不是切除狭窄的肠段[14]。狭窄整形是安全有效的，出血以及狭窄复发的并发症小于 5%，并且漏、瘘管、脓肿形成小于 10%[3]，狭窄整形可 100% 解除梗阻，并且 75% 的年轻患儿身高、体重增加[38]。狭窄整形后 Crohn 病复发与肠切除的形式一样，10 年内约 50%（图 93-6）[49]。然而，在许多病例中，当再次手术时，狭窄整形部位并没有病变发生。

表 93-3　Crohn 病：复发的临床特征

临床特征	无复发的患者数	复发患者数	*P* 值
Crohn 病的病变部位			
空-回肠	5	2	无意义
末端回肠	20	23	无意义
结肠和回肠	25	25	无意义
手术指征			
梗阻	20	20	无意义
肿块	1	18	无意义
瘘管	14	16	无意义
难治性	8	9	无意义

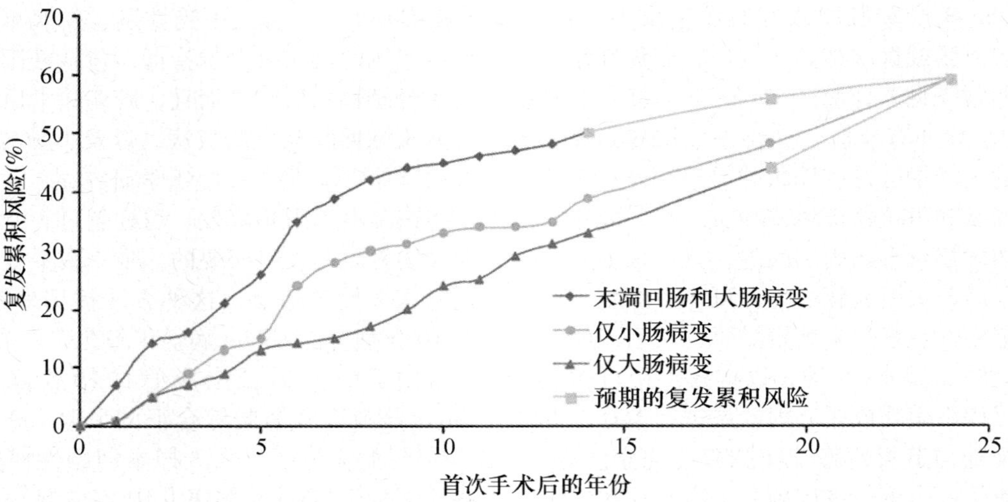

图 93-5 病变开始部位复发积累风险的影响。(From Lock MR, Farmer RG, Fazio VW, et al: Recurrence and reoperation for Crohn's disease: The role of disease location in prognosis. N Engl J Med 1981; 304: 1586-1588.)

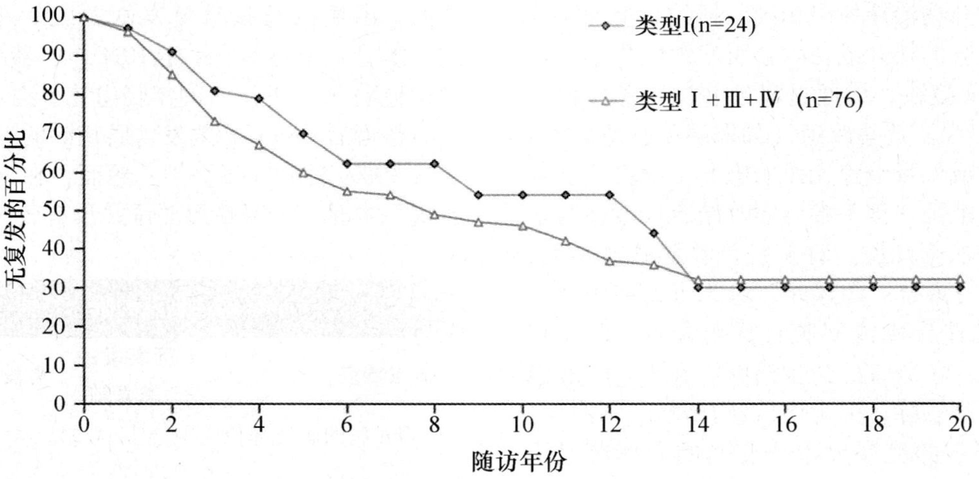

图 93-6 切缘正常组织学与异常组织学的累积复发比例。两组曲线无差异(From Kotanagi H, Kramer K, Fazio VW, Petras RE: Do microscopic abnormalities at resection margins correlate with increased anastomotic recurrence in Crohn's disease? Dis Colon Rectum 1991; 34: 909-916.)

Crohn 结肠炎不同于小肠疾病，在青少年的 Crohn 病中，外科手术的主要指征是难治性疾病以及药物治疗反应较差，而不是小肠梗阻。外科治疗方法包括部分结肠切除、全结肠切除并做回直肠吻合或回肠造瘘以及 Hartmann 储袋，以及直结肠切除并做回肠造瘘。大多数临床研究显示，直结肠切除复发率较低，5 年约 15%，10 年约 20%[13]。全结肠切除的复发率 5 年为 30%，10 年为 50%。而部分结肠切除复发率最高，5 年接近 50%，10 年为 65%[49]。

在目前最常用的 I 期或 Ⅱ 期手术为全结肠切除及回肠直肠吻合，整个并发症发生率为 15%，包括 3% 的吻合口漏、4% 的败血症、2% 的肠梗阻以及 6% 的其他并发症[32]。回肠直肠吻合与储袋功能相似，白天和夜晚排便，每天约 4 次大便。在一组 131 例行回肠直肠吻合术患儿的报道中，术后 72 例有功能，36 例没有功能，平均随访 7.5 年[53]。36 例行直肠切除或大便改道的患儿指征包括排便功能差、超量的激素依赖以及出血，在这些患儿中，会阴部直肠切除提供了良好的补救治疗。

严重的肛周 Crohn 病治疗起来相当困难，约 20%～30% 的患儿可通过近端肠管切除或大肠或小肠改道来治疗[41]。如果这些治疗措施仍不能治疗肛周疾病，那么直肠切除或直结肠切除可用作补救，在 5 年内有 10% 的再次手术的风险，在 10 年内有 30% 的风险[40]。

癌变

评估 Crohn 病或溃疡性结肠炎患儿癌变风险最重要的因素是疾病的持续时间。据估计，溃疡性结肠炎
60 患儿癌变的风险在疾病的第一个 10 年以每年 1% 的比率递增[12]，全结肠病变的患儿风险最高。但是，部分溃疡性结肠炎的患儿要比正常人群有较高的癌变风险[3,8]。另外，Crohn 病亦有较高的癌变风险[19]。在 Cleveland 临床基金会 20 年回顾研究中发现，454 例青少年溃疡性结肠炎患者中，有 10 例发生结直肠癌，834 例青少年 Crohn 病患儿中有 2 例发生癌变[37]。因此，溃疡性结肠炎诊断后的 8～10 年内，不管有无症状的青少年患者要每年进行检查[26]。另外，严重肛周或直肠病变的 Crohn 病患儿应定期检查，以及对任何可疑的肛直肠肿物要进行活检。

（严志龙译　叶祖萍校）

参考文献

1. Alexander F, Sarigol S, DiFiore J, et al: Fate of the pouch in 151 pediatric patients after ileal pouch anal anastomosis. J Pediatr Surg 2003;38:78-82.
2. Alexander-Williams J, Haynes IG: Conservative operations for Crohn's disease of the small bowel. World J Surg 1985; 9:945-951.
3. Bansai P, Sonnenberg A: Risk factors of colorectal cancer in inflammatory bowel disease. Am J Gastroenterol 1996; 91:44-48.
4. Belli DC, Seidman E, Bouthillier L, et al: Chronic intermittent elemental diet improves growth failure in children with Crohn's disease. Gastroenterology 1988;94:503-510.
5. Belluzzi A, Brignola C, Campieri M, et al: Effect of an enteric-coated fish-oil preparation on relapses in Crohn's disease. N Engl J Med 1996;334:1551-1560.
6. Benkov KJ, Rosh JR, Schwersenz A, et al: Cyclosporine as an alternative to surgery in children with inflammatory bowel disease. J Pediatr Gastroenterol Nutr 1994;19:290-294.
7. Cintron JR, Park JJ, Orsay CP, et al: Repair of fistulas-in-ano using fibrin adhesive. Dis Colon Rectum 2000;43:944-950.
8. Collins RH, Feldman M, Fordtran JS: Colon cancer, dysplasia, and surveillance in patients with ulcerative colitis. A critical review. N Engl J Med 1987;316:1654-1658.
9. Connell WR, Kamm MA, Dickson M, et al: Long-term neoplasia risk after azathioprine treatment in inflammatory bowel disease. Lancet 1994;343:1249-1252.
10. Crohn BB, Ginsberg L, Oppenheimer GD: Regional enteritis: A pathologic and clinical entity. JAMA 1932;99:1323-1329.
11. Dalziel TK: Chronic intestinal enteritis. BMJ 1913;2: 1068-1069.
12. Devroede GJ, Taylor WT, Sauer WG, et al: Cancer risk and life expectancy of children with ulcerative colitis. N Engl J Med 1971;285:17-21.
13. Dietz DW, Lauret S, Strong SA, et al: Safety and long term efficacy of strictureplasty in 314 patients with obstructing small bowel Crohn's disease. J Am Coll Surg 2001;192:333-337.
14. Fazio VW, Galandiuk S, Jagelman DG, Lavery IC: Strictureplasty in Crohn's disease. Ann Surg 1989;210: 621-625.
15. Feagan BG, Rochon J, Fedorak RN, et al: Methotrexate for the treatment of Crohn's disease. N Engl J Med 1995;332: 292-297.
16. Gilat T: Incidence of inflammatory bowel disease: Going up or down? Gastroenterology 1983;85:196-197.
17. Grand RJ, Ramakrishna J, Calenda KA: Inflammatory bowel disease in the pediatric patient. Gastoenterol Clin North Am 1995;24:613-632.
18. Greenberg GR, Feagan BG, Martin F, et al: Oral budesonide for active Crohn's disease. N Engl J Med 1994;331:36-41.
19. Greenstern AJ, Sachar DB, Smith H, et al: A comparison of cancer risk in Crohn's disease and ulcerative colitis. Cancer 1981;12:2742-2745.
20. Hanauer SB: Drug therapy: Inflammatory bowel disease. N Engl J Med 1996;334:841-848.
21. Hawthorne AB, Daneshmend TK, Hawkeg CJ, et al: Treatment of ulcerative colitis with fish oil supplementation: A prospective 12 month randomized controlled trial. Gut 1992;33:922-928.
22. Hawthorne AB, Hawkey CJ: Immunosuppressive drugs in inflammatory bowel disease: A review of efficacy and place in therapy. Drugs 1989;38:267-288.
23. Hyams JS: Extraintestinal manifestations of inflammatory bowel disease. J Pediatr Gastroenterol Nutr 1994;19:7-21.
24. Hyams JS, Markowitz J, Wyllie R: Use of infliximab in the treatment of Crohn's disease in children and adolescents. J Pediatr 2000;137:192-196.
25. Janowitz HD: Inflammatory Bowel Disease, New York, Field, Rich & Associates, 1985.
26. Jonsson B, Ahsgren L, Anderson LO, et al: Colorectal cancer surveillance in patients with ulcerative colitis. Br J Surg 1994;81:689-691.
27. Kirschner BS: Safety of azathioprine and 6-mercaptopurine in pediatric patients with inflammatory bowel disease. Gastroenterology 1998;115:813-821.
28. Kotanagi H, Kramer K, Fazio VW, Petras RE: Do microscopic abnormalities at resection margins correlate with increased anastomotic recurrence in Crohn's disease? Dis Colon Rectum 1991;34:909-916.
29. Lawrance IC, Wu F, Leite AZ, et al: A murine model of chronic inflammation-induced intestinal fibrosis down-regulated by antisense NF-Kappa B. Gastroenterology

2003;125:1750-1761.
30. Levin KE, Pemberton JH, Phillips SF, et al: Role of oxygen free radicals in the etiology of pouchitis. Dis Colon Rectum 1992;35:452-456.
31. Lock MR, Farmer RG, Fazio VW, et al: Recurrence and reoperation for Crohn's disease: The role of disease location in prognosis. N Engl J Med 1981;304:1586-1588.
32. Longo WE, Oakley JR, Lavery K, et al: Outcome of ileorectal anastomosis for Crohn's colitis. Dis Colon Rectum 1992; 35:1066-1070.
33. Mack DR, Young R, Kaufman SS, et al: Methotrexate in patients with Crohn's disease after 6-mercaptopurine. J Pediatr 1998;132:830-835.
34. Malchaw H, Ewe K, Brandes JW, et al: European Cooperative Crohn's Disease Study (ECCDS): Results of drug treatment. Gastroenterology 1984;86:249-266.
35. Michener WM, Caufield M, Farmer RG, et al: Genetic counseling and family history in IBD: 30 years experience at The Cleveland Clinic. Can J Gastroenterol 1990;4:350-354.
36. Michener WM, Caulfield M, Wyllie R, Farmer RG: Management of inflammatory bowel disease: 30 years of observation. Cleve Clin J Med 1990;57:685-691.
37. Michener WM, Farmer RG, Mortimer EA: Long-term prognosis of ulcerative colitis with onset in childhood or adolescence. J Clin Gastroenterol 1979;1:301-305.
38. Michener WM, Wyllie R: Management of children and adolescents with inflammatory bowel disease. Med Clin North Am 1990;74:103-117.
39. Morin CL, Roulet M, Roy CC, Weber A: Continuous elemental enteral alimentation in children with Crohn's disease and growth failure. Gastroenterology 1980;79:1205-1210.
40. Oliva RT, Wyllie R, Alexander F, et al: The results of strictureplasty in pediatric patients with multifocal Crohn disease. J Pediatr Gastroenterol Nutr 1994;18:307-311.
41. Orkin BA, Telander RL: The effect of intra-abdominal resection or fecal diversion on perianal disease in pediatric Crohn's disease. J Pediatr Surg 1985;20:343-347.
42. Polk DB, Hattner JA, Kerner JA Jr: Improved growth and disease activity after intermittent administration of a defined formula diet in children with Crohn's disease. J Parenter Enteral Nutr 1992;16:499-504.
43. Present DH, Korelitz BL, Wisch N, et al: Treatment of Crohn's disease with 6-mercaptopurine: A long-term randomized double-blind study. N Engl J Med 1981;302:981-987.
44. Russka T, Vaajalahti P, Arajarvi P, Maki M: Prospective evaluation of upper gastrointestinal mucosal lesions in children with ulcerative colitis and Crohn's disease. J Pediatr Gastroenterol Nutr 1994;19:181-186.
45. Rutgeerts P, Hiele M, Geboes K, et al: Controlled trial of metronidazole treatment for prevention of Crohn's recurrence after ileal resection. Gastroenterology 1995;108: 1617-1621.
46. Rutgeerts P, Lofgerg R, Malchaw H, et al: A comparison of budesonide with prednisolone for active Crohn's disease. N Engl J Med 1994;331:842-845.
47. Sachar DB: Maintenance therapy in ulcerative colitis and Crohn's disease. J Clin Gastroenterol 1995;20:117-122.
48. Sandborn WJ: A critical review of cyclosporin therapy in inflammatory bowel disease. Inflamm Bowel Dis 1995;1: 48-63.
49. Sedgwick DM, Barton JR, Hamer-Hodges DW, et al: Population-based study of surgery in juvenile onset Crohn's disease. Br J Surg 1991;78:171-175.
50. Summer RW, Switz DM, Sessions JT Jr, et al: National Cooperative Crohn's Disease Study: Results of drug treatment. Gastroenterology 1979;77:847-869.
51. Tjandra JJ, Fazio VW: Surgery for Crohn's colitis. Int Surg 1992;77:9-14.
52. Ursing B, Alm T, Barany F, et al: A comparison study of metronidazole and sulfasalazine for Crohn's disease: The Cooperative Crohn's Disease Study in Sweden II. Gastroenterology 1982;83:550-562.
53. Wilmore D: Short bowel syndrome. World J Surg 2000;24: 1487-1493.

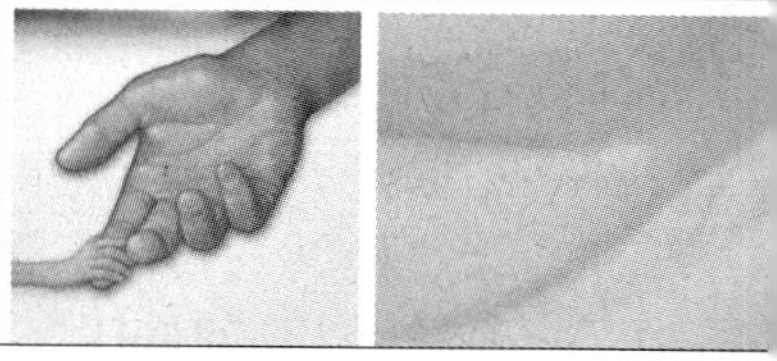

第 94 章

溃疡性结肠炎

Eric W. Fonkalsrud

1859 年，Wilks 和 Moxon[91]首次描述了溃疡性结肠炎（ulcerative colitis，UC）。19 世纪末，对于严重的病例，大便改道是常规方法，尽管症状改善是暂时的。20 世纪早期，管状阑尾造瘘和碳酸氢盐溶液反复结肠灌洗为主要的治疗方法[89]。1913 年，Browne[8]通过回肠造瘘使大便完全改道，尽管有较高的发病率和死亡率，但仍被广泛应用。直到 20 世纪 40 年代中期，回肠造瘘装置还较原始，并常伴有大便污染及皮肤刺激，往往直至患者病情较重，才行外科手术进行干预。造瘘口关闭后常出现疾病复发。

直到 1944 年，Strauss[81]采取直肠结肠切除和回肠造瘘来治疗严重的 UC。它分三期：（1）回肠造瘘术；（2）结肠次全切除术和乙型结肠造瘘术；（3）经腹直肠切除（1948 年由 Cattell[9]推荐）。不久以后，在 1951 年，回肠造瘘并同时行结肠次全切除所组成的二期手术方法开展起来，这种手术方法死亡率仅为 4.4%[35]。Ripstein[67]在 1952 年和 Goligher[88]在 1954 年采用回肠造瘘并 I 期直肠结肠切除术，直到 20 年前，一直被认为是治疗 UC 的标准术式。

尽管回肠造瘘加直肠结肠切除为 UC 的治疗方法，但许多患者不愿意接受永久性的回肠造瘘，所以手术被拖延，直至患者的病情加重、出现营养不良以及大量药物治疗后发生并发症时才接受手术。改善回肠造瘘患者生活质量的器械因素包括 1952 年由 Brooke[7]倡导的回肠造瘘的外翻技术以及黏附性回肠造口肛门袋的发展。随后，Turnbull[86]和其他人改进了造瘘口周围皮肤护理，及对护士进行专门培训，使大多数患者可使肛门袋保持黏附于皮肤达 4～6 天。1969 年，Kock[48]发明了在回肠造瘘时做一个在腹腔内乳头样瓣膜装置，使患者达到无需使用肛门袋自我控制排便和随时随地灌肠的目的。

60 年前医生们开始为 UC 患者寻找一个保存括约肌的手术，墨尔本的 Devine[15]医生采用了分期的回肠乙状结肠吻合术，伦敦的 Avlett[3]医生是结肠切除并回肠直肠吻合术的倡导者。1966 年，他报道的 300 例患者都取得良好的效果，死亡率仅为 5.7%。Parc[59]等人回顾了 17 项研究总共 1206 例患者，因为 UC 做结肠切除并回肠直肠吻合术的患者平均每天大便 4.5 次，大多数可自我控制。由于持久的直肠病变，15%以上的患者最终需行直肠切除，保留直肠发生癌变的风险为 2%～20%。目前，回肠直肠吻合术很少使用，只用于轻度直肠病变的患者。

1947 年，Ravitch 和 Sabiston[65]改良了之前不成功的回肠肛管吻合术，加入了直肠黏膜切除的术式，大多数患者行该手术后，大便次数异常增多，大便急迫。随后 30 年中该手术很少运用[64]。1964 年 Soave[74]描述了远端直肠黏膜切除后直肠内结肠拖出术治疗先天性巨结肠病，并报道取得良好的临床效果。1973 年，Safaie 和 Soper[70]在 4 例年轻家族性结肠息肉病的患者中运用远端直肠黏膜切除加全结肠切除，并直接在直肠内行回肠肛管吻合术。1977 年，Martin[54]等人报道运用该技术，在年轻 UC 患者中取得了满意的效果。

回肠肛管拖出术，在过去的几年中进行了多种改良，最重要的是增加了远端回肠构成的储袋并与肛管行吻合术以减少大便次数以及大便急迫感。回肠储袋的发展建立于 1955 年 Valente 和 Bacon[88]对犬的研究基础上，他们使用一个三袢的回肠储袋。Karlan[44]等人使用一个双排的同蠕动储袋。Ferrari 和 Fonkalsrud[23]采用了 S 形储袋以及回肠肛管吻合术。1978 年，Parks 和 Nicholls[60]联合使用 S 形的回肠储袋切除直肠黏膜同时，行储袋与肛管吻合术，在成人

1463 中取得了较好的效果。全结肠切除并作回肠肛管储袋法（IAPP）已被广泛接受认为是目前外科处理所有年龄组 UC 的最佳方法[14,19,29,58,66]。

病因

UC 的病因仍未明确。许多人认为细菌或病毒感染是其病因，然而，研究发现致病微生物不相一致[39]。还有人认为细菌或病毒是继发性侵入的而非原发性病原菌，饮食因素起了重要作用[4]。目前，认为 UC 的病因是对自身细菌或化学性抗原引起的自身免疫性反应是最有吸引力的理论。约 15% 的 UC 患者有一个或多个炎症性肠道疾病的家庭成员。对特发性强直性脊椎炎及虹膜炎和 UC 患者进行HLA-W27测试，结果表明存在遗传倾向，然而没有发现确切的相关性。尽管在 UC 患者中没有确定存在特异性的基因位点，但是在一些研究中发现与染色体 3、5、7 和 12 上的基因有相关性。尽管精神因素对 UC 亦有作用，但目前不认为它作为一个单独的病前个体存在，精神因素和应激可能导致复发以及对疾病的慢性病程有作用，但不能引起原发病变。

病理

UC 是一个直肠和结肠黏膜及黏膜下的慢性炎症性疾病，超过 95% 的病例直肠受累，炎症以接连的方式向邻近扩展[73]。如果回肠末端受累，必须考虑患者可能为 Crohn 病。“回流性回肠炎”的概念可能用词不当，因为没有科学证据显示有结肠内容物反流入回肠，引起回肠末端炎症。当结肠受累时（全结肠炎），最严重的改变通常发生在直肠和乙状结肠，儿童比成人更易发生全结肠炎。

UC 显微镜下特征性改变为腺窝脓肿。该脓肿导致黏膜溃疡，并影响相邻黏膜，假息肉形成并黏膜桥样改变，通常以环状面的形式出现，相反，肉芽肿性结肠炎的溃疡通常为线形的并位于结肠的肠系膜侧（图 94-1）。急性期，随着病情进展，结肠扩张、蠕动减慢、结肠肌层变薄和弥漫性出血，如果治疗不充分，疾病最终发展为结肠急性扩张、菌血症、腹膜炎以及少见的继发性中毒性巨结肠穿孔。慢性 UC 患者

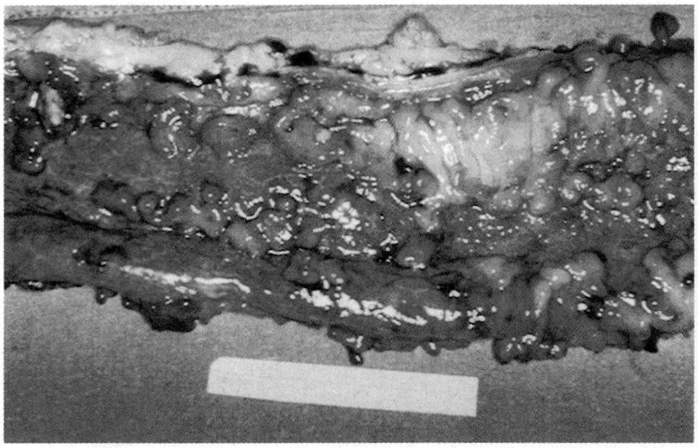

图 94-1 一个 16 岁的慢性 UC 患者左半结肠剖面样本，可以看到巨大的假息肉，并且正常的黏膜皱折消失。

黏膜肌层变厚、纤维化、结肠袋变平坦及蠕动收缩减少；长期病变中黏膜出现萎缩以及发育不良、结肠系膜变短、结肠表面浆膜层血管增生，并有大量脂肪组织覆盖；缓解期，黏膜可恢复接近显微镜下的正常外观。黏膜活检对确诊以及评估疾病活动度有帮助。

从免疫角度出发，UC 的黏膜内主要由 T 淋巴细胞的 $CD4^+$ 群构成[43]。这些 T 细胞有一个不典型的表型即转化生长因子-β 和白介素（IL）-5 的产物增加。T 细胞可被邻件上皮细胞的抗原激活。加上活化巨噬细胞产生的炎症介质，分泌许多炎症细胞因子包括肿瘤坏死因子、IL-1 和 IL-6，这些炎症因子形成了一些治疗 UC 的新疗法的基础。

临床表现

10 岁前，不足 4% 的患者出现症状，约 18% 的患者症状出现在 10～20 岁。UC 最常发生于 20 岁以后的患者，男和女发生比例相同。白种人的发病率是黑种人、拉丁美洲人以及亚洲人的 4 倍，犹太人是非犹太人的 3 倍。典型的症状始于腹泻，并伴有大便带血、黏液和脓液、间歇性下腹部绞痛和里急后重，贫血较常见。慢性炎症可引起厌食、体重下降、生长发育迟缓以及胃口差。当疾病变为慢性时，需长期使用激素，导致许多儿童感到乏力和不愿参加社会实践及体育锻炼。大多数儿童发展为迁延性结肠炎，并经常由于情绪紧张或间断性感染而引起复发。患儿偶尔获

464 得永久性的缓解，然而许多慢性结肠炎患儿的改善是短暂的，并且很少缓解，完全缓解的单个发作患者少于 10%。

约 15% 的儿童，UC 的发作是暴发性的，伴有大量血性腹泻、严重的腹部绞痛、发热以及偶尔出现的败血症，需要紧急处理[29]。虽然一些患儿（5%）可发展为中毒性巨结肠，需要外科急诊处理[1]，大多患儿通过药物治疗有所改善。我们的经验是，超过 50% 的 UC 儿童最终需要做结肠切除。

据报道在头 10 年中有 3% 的儿童患结肠或直肠癌，在随后的每 10 年中约以 10%~15% 的速度递增，恶变甚至可以发生在结肠炎缓解的患儿中[16]。癌变更常见于全结肠炎的患者，多在 17 岁前出现症状，这类患者常突发原发性硬化性胆管炎[17,76]。活检发现结肠黏膜发育不良提示继发癌变的可能性较大。

UC 外在表现包括生长发育迟缓、关节痛、性成熟延迟、皮肤病变、贫血、骨质疏松症、原发性硬化性胆管炎、肾石病、眼葡萄膜炎以及口炎（图 94-2），青少年慢性 UC 患者常伴有生长发育迟缓及骨生长延迟。尿促性腺激素水平降低常引起性成熟延迟[55]。生长激素水平在各年龄段患者通常是正常的。

约 25% 的 UC 患者有关节痛，通常与疾病的严重性和病程有关。膝、踝、腕、手指以及髋关节最常受累。关节症状有时先于肠道症状出现，可与青少年类风湿性关节炎相混淆。1%~6% 发生强硬性脊柱炎。4%~18% 的患者有骶髂关节炎。患者接受激素治疗后症状可改善，但当停止使用激素时，又会复发。无论 UC 的严重程度如何，患者最终都可能会留下永久性的功能障碍。

最常见的皮肤病变为躯干部红斑结节，偶见于四肢。少于 5% 的 UC 患儿发生坏疽性脓皮病（慢性皮肤溃疡），通常位于下肢。这些病变通常对局部或全身治疗无反应，并且迁延不愈，直到患者病情缓解或通过外科治愈。

15% 的患者肝功能异常，可由各种肝功能紊乱导致。几乎 80% 的 UC 患者肝活检有异常。超过 50% 的患者有不同程度的脂肪浸润。尽管在成人 UC 患者中有 15% 发生硬化性胆管炎[45]，但在儿童中不常见。贫血较常见，通常由于大便显性或隐性失血所导致。

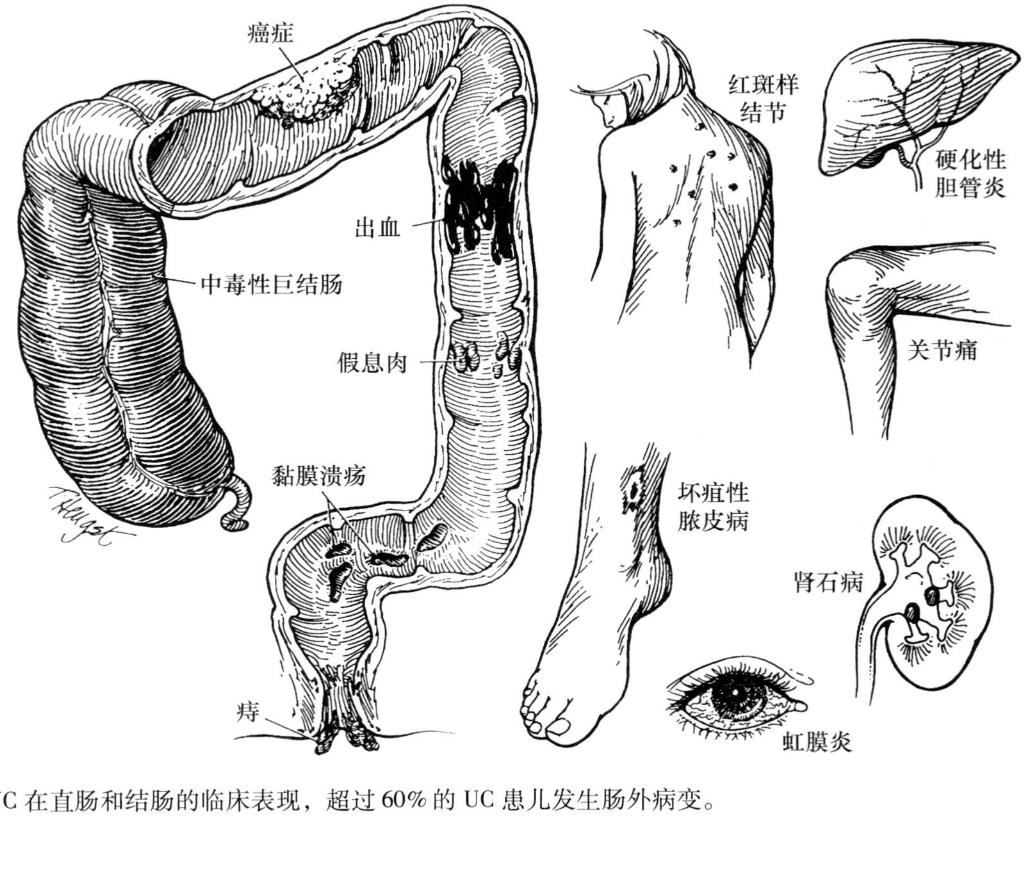

图 94-2 UC 在直肠和结肠的临床表现，超过 60% 的 UC 患儿发生肠外病变。

1465 骨质疏松症和骨软化症是由于钙吸收下降，伴有脂溶性维生素摄入减少以及激素治疗后尿钙丢失增加所致。患者由于没有摄入足够的水以补充腹泻所引起的液体丢失，约8%的UC发生肾结石[80]。葡萄膜炎（虹膜炎）发生率小于2%。溃疡性口炎在UC的患者中常见，尤其在疾病的突发期。

临床检查

尽管内镜检查可发现易碎以及水肿的黏膜伴薄的脓性分泌物，但是，轻度UC患儿或者缓解期患儿，体检时很少有阳性表现。慢性UC的患儿通常有身高发育延迟、性成熟延迟、贫血、苍白以及存在长期激素治疗后的库欣样特征。急性期，有发热、脱水以及全身中毒症状。乙状结肠部位通常有触痛，大便次数增多及腹泻常导致外痔。然而，肛裂、肛瘘以及脓肿少见。如果出现，则要考虑Crohn病。乙状结肠或结肠镜检常发现黏膜水肿和出血，并且黏膜表面有溃疡以及覆盖脓性、血性分泌物（图94-3）。

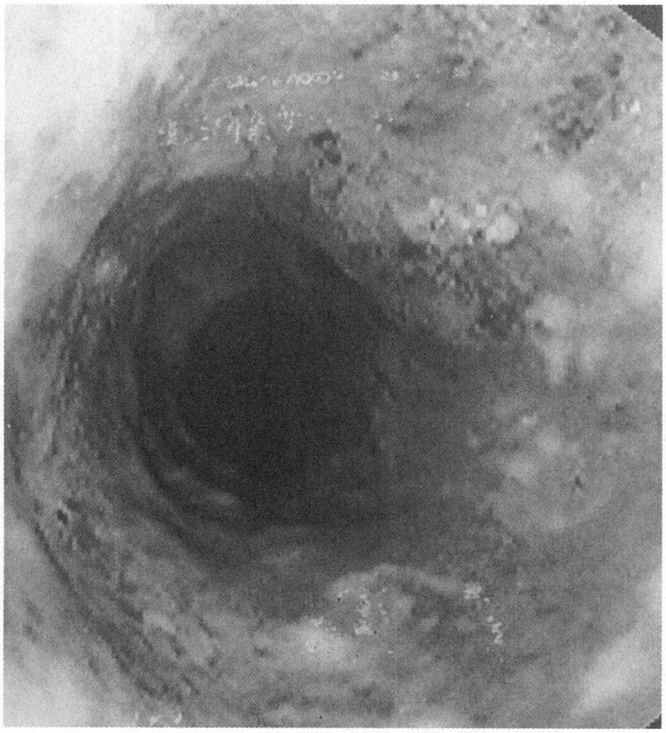

图94-3 一个18岁严重UC患者通过结肠镜镜所看到的横结肠外观，可发现黏膜溃疡和黏膜皱折消失。

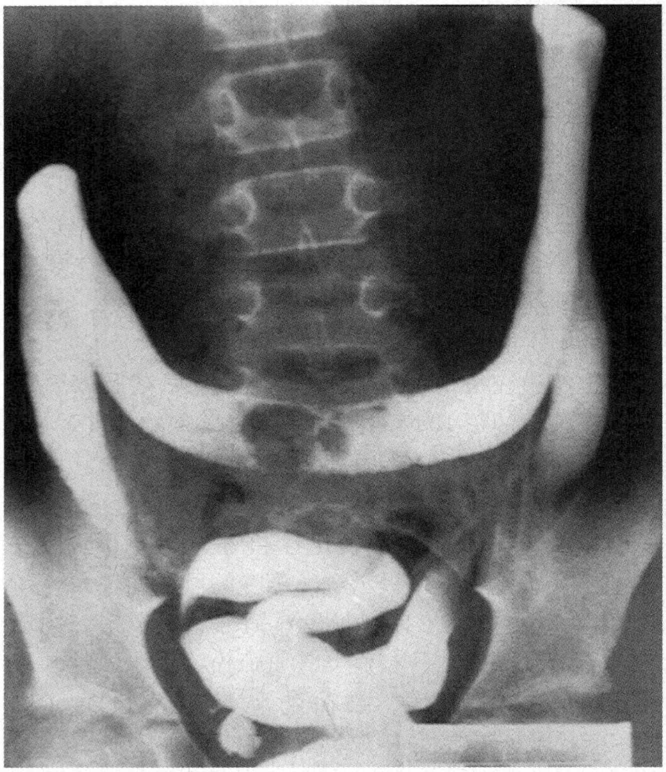

图94-4 1个患有慢性UC的17女孩钡剂灌肠片，可看到结肠变短且储袋标志消失使结肠表现为特征性的“铅管”样外观。

2/3的患儿因便血而出现贫血、红细胞沉降率升高、凝血酶原时间延长和血清白蛋白水平下降。因迁延性腹泻而出现低钠和低钾血症。大便培养细菌和寄生虫持续阴性。

慢性UC患儿钡剂灌肠造影显示结肠短、狭窄、坚硬、结肠袋消失（铅管状外观）以及广泛的假息肉形成（图94-4）。急性结肠炎时，肠管外形不规则，黏膜溃疡导致锯齿状边缘。溃疡区之间的黏膜水肿外观看上去像假息肉，由于钡剂灌肠能刺激产生结肠炎的急性表现，而且更多有意义的发现可通过结肠镜获得，故钡剂灌肠现在很少使用。

药物处理

药物治疗严重的UC没有特异性，主要基于症状的改善。然而，最终病程可能将改变或通过非手术治疗来治愈。许多儿童轻度UC的病变位于直肠和乙状

结肠。这些患儿长期服用 5-氨基水杨酸盐化合物如柳氮磺胺吡啶或 5-氨基水杨酸后症状可缓解[62]。抗
66 炎复合物被认为是通过阻止前列腺素和白三烯的产物而发生作用。同时亦阻止细菌肽诱导的分泌作用以及清除激活的氧代谢产物。慢性患者发展为急性发作型，2~3 个月的皮质醇激素（泼尼松）的治疗可达到缓解。逐步快速减少激素剂量，或尽可能快地开始使用隔日疗法。幼小儿童长期应用激素的相关副作用，包括生长障碍、骨质疏松症、高血压、高血糖症以及库欣样特征如在女孩躯干和大腿上有皮纹的表现。直肠内给激素（氢化可的松）或 5-氨基水杨酸复合物如彼得斯安、美沙拉秦片或 Rowasa 灌肠剂，对局限于直肠和低位左结肠的结肠炎有帮助。激素与 H_2 受体阻滞剂合用加上口服抗酸药可以减少消化性溃疡或胃炎的发生率。接受激素治疗的患者应摄入钙剂、维生素 D 和双磷酸盐。

止泻剂如盐酸地芬诺酯加硫酸阿托品（止泻宁）或者盐酸氯苯呱酰胺（盐酸洛哌丁胺）可减少肠蠕动及直肠痉挛，但使用时需注意，因为这些药物同阿片类药物，可偶尔引起中毒性巨结肠[36]。其他有效的药物包括镇静剂和抗菌药如甲硝唑。饮食要求改良以减少肠道刺激如减少巧克力、醋及辣的食物、新鲜蔬菜和硬果的摄入。严重贫血和低蛋白血症需要输血、输白蛋白或两者都输。

免疫抑制药包括硫唑嘌呤、6-巯基嘌呤（6-MP）以及环孢霉素 A，常用于治疗慢性 UC 的患儿。然而，其有效性未得到统一的认识，而且其副作用也较明显[34]。硫唑嘌呤和 6-巯基嘌呤可影响 T 细胞亚群，并且需要长期服用才有效。这些药物有一定的毒性可能引起胰腺炎或肝炎。其可使激素治疗减量和维持病情缓解。环孢霉素 A 比硫唑嘌呤起效快，与激素一样对治疗严重的 UC 有效。环孢霉素 A 有较强的免疫抑制作用，能阻止 T 细胞活化以及抑制 IL-2 和 IL-2 受体的表达。前炎症细胞因子——肿瘤坏死因子-α 的单克隆抗体（英夫利昔单抗）对治疗 UC 尚存在争议[18]。

精神治疗有助于慢性 UC 患者正确对待该病以及它的并发症和副作用。更重要的是获得医生的同情和关心，以及家庭的支持和理解。

在 UC 急性发作期，大多数患者需要住院治疗，静脉补液、禁食、增加激素剂量以及肠外营养。这些措施通常能纠正代谢紊乱以及减轻临床症状，但不能改变结肠炎的病程。肠外营养的主要作用在于通过改善患者的氮平衡来减少外科手术的风险。结肠炎进一步发展或对药物治疗无反应是进行急诊手术的指征。

UC 儿童外科手术后的并发症随着病程以及药物剂量和服用时间的增加而增加[24,58]。我们的经验是，接受过大剂量皮质类固醇激素和免疫抑制剂治疗的患儿，进行外科治疗后，其并发症发生率相当高[29]。虽然有报道指出，静脉应用环胞霉素 A 对严重激素抵抗的患儿能迅速起效，但激素治疗中断后 6 个月内，超过 60% 的患儿需行结肠切除，所以认为药物治疗仅仅是延迟结肠切除的手段[51]。

激素被证明在对结肠吻合口的愈合有不良影响[23]。过量的药物治疗 UC 可能增加急诊分期结肠切除的发生率。结果它增加了患者的发病率、住院时间和花费，而且不能获得最理想的功能[24]。修复性直肠结肠吻合术，在因严重急性 UC 而需急诊手术的患者中进行可能是安全的。对于许多病例，如果不能快速控制结肠炎，那么药物治疗应减少[40]。

有报道指出，吸烟可能减少 UC 的发生率，阑尾切除术也是预防 UC 的一个保护因素[69]。初步研究认为，在传统的维持治疗基础上加上经皮尼古丁治疗可改善 UC 的症状[63]。

外科处理

尽管药物治疗能缓解各时期的 UC，但是不将病变的结肠和直肠切除是很难治愈的。因为 IAPP 的长期效果较好，所以在严重残疾和并发症出现前外科治疗对 UC 患者是很有必要的。药物治疗后，溃疡性结肠炎患者仍持续出现症状、生长发育迟缓、严重活动受限以及生活质量差，可选择外科治疗。当患儿影响上学，以及由于严重的症状而不能参加社会活动和体育锻炼时，这常使患者和家人感到痛苦和烦恼。暴发性且药物治疗效果差的直肠大量出血或中毒性巨结肠（约 20%），是进行急诊手术的指征。儿童 UC 相对成人更易急性发病和出现更严重的症状。在儿童，当骨骺仍开放处于生长和发育的最佳时期时，病变严重的结肠应被切除。儿童的状况在治疗过程中应由外科和胃肠病医生定期评估，并考虑除长期药物治疗外的其他疗法。约 8% 的慢性结肠炎患者，无论高级的诊断测试还是组织样本

的病理检查，都很难清楚地区分 UC 和 Crohn 病，这
1467 些病例通常称为“不确定结肠炎”[2]。尽管约 1/4 的患者最终需要切除储袋，但笔者倾向对这些患儿按 UC 来治疗[13]。对不确定结肠炎而做 IAPP 的患者，要告知有因急性 Crohn 病而导致储袋失败的风险，那么必须要做永久性回肠造瘘。

手术方法的选择应与患儿及其父母详细讨论。与做过手术的患儿交谈有助于减少手术患儿的恐惧，以及对回肠造瘘的担心并有助于他们做出行外科治疗的决定。术前与肠造口专家讨论，有助于为患儿和家长对暂时性回肠造瘘做准备。尽管，对于儿童较容易掌握造瘘口的护理，但是造瘘口器具通常会给患儿参加锻炼和社会活动带来尴尬。在儿童中，直肠结肠吻合术后发生阳痿和膀胱功能障碍少见，但是，这些问题已引起许多患儿、父母，以及医生抵制手术治疗，直到结肠炎患儿身体虚弱并且激素和免疫抑制治疗引起全身并发症。

贫血、低蛋白血症以及电解质紊乱在术前必须纠正，但很少需要短期肠外高营养。激素治疗仍需维持直到手术，以避免急性发作。术前 48 小时禁止口服液体、泻药和高渗溶液如 GOLYTELY，避免清洁灌肠，因为这样做会引起结肠炎的急性发作。术前 1 天口服抗生素（琥乙红霉素和新霉素），静脉抗生素（庆大霉素和克林霉素）在术前 2 小时开始使用。

60 年以来，对药物难治性的 UC，全直肠切除加永久性回肠造瘘已成为标准外科治疗方式。此方式可治愈该病，并发症率相对低，长期预后较好。但是，所有年龄段的患儿发现清洗回肠造瘘肛门袋使日常生活增加了很多麻烦。约 30% 的患儿有回肠造瘘肛门袋相关的问题，包括皮肤不适、皮肤过敏、漏以及异味。在美国，估计每年用于回肠造瘘术后护理的费用约每人 1500 美元以上。目前，当有好的替代手术出现时，很少有患者选择带永久性回肠造瘘的直肠结肠切除术。

带有乳头样瓣膜的 Kock 可控性回肠贮器，省略了造瘘袋的冲洗——贮器内放入 1 根硅橡胶管，1 天引流几次，是最初报道为较好的永久性回肠造瘘术的替代术[49]。然而，许多患者需要多次手术，并且由于乳头样瓣膜相关并发症和伴发储袋炎的停滞袢综合征而要进行储袋切除[5]。Kock 储袋的改良目前主要用于少数患者如有括约肌损伤、肛周脓肿或窦道阻碍 IAPP 使用者。

结肠次全切除并做回肠直肠吻合术目前只应用于诊断不明的患儿，这些患儿中很少是 UC 和有相关的直肠受累。如果直肠内结肠炎继续活跃，那么几乎所有患儿最终需要行全结肠切除手术。

回肠储袋肛管吻合术

因为 UC 是原发于黏膜的一种疾病。结肠并直肠黏膜切除和 IAPP 已成为药物难治性 UC 最常用的治疗方法。切除整个直肠下至齿状线的黏膜，不影响肛门括约肌的功能或者辨别气体、液体及固体内容物的能力[61]。该方法避免了一个永久性回肠造瘘口，不需要反复插管排便（是 Kock 储袋法所必需的）并且有一个接近正常的排便方式[41]。

早期手术方式直接行直肠内回肠拖出术，大多数患者术后大便次数增多、大便急，并有不同程度的大便失禁。偶尔报道在儿童中预后较好[11,56]。直接直肠内回肠拖出术保留了肠管蠕动收缩功能，并且产生的波峰下降至肛管吻合口。近来，有报道当外科医生行直接拖出术时，同时在接近肛管吻合口远端12～15 cm 处行多个垂直肌切开术取得了较好的结果[26]。几乎所有的外科医生目前做拖出术后再在回肠肛门吻合口上做一个回肠储袋或储存装置，以减少远端回肠的蠕动，达到储存粪便的作用[19]。不管使用何种储存装置，只要不破坏远端 4 cm 长的直肠肌层，肛管括约肌的收缩和松弛压可在 3 个月内恢复正常值[77]。IAPP 后长期生活质量通常与肠功能是一致的[47]。

尽管在儿童中提倡进行 I 期 IAPP 手术，但经验显示，约 3 个月的回肠造瘘可最大限度减少储袋漏或盆腔感染的风险[27]。注意手术的许多细节对减少潜在的并发症是很有必要的。如不做回肠造瘘，漏的发生超过 2 倍并且恢复时间通常要延长[10]。I 期 IAPP 后要考虑的是，患儿应有好的营养，给予最小剂量的免疫抑制药物或激素治疗，避免直肠感染以及肥胖[20]。同时应避免有害的手术意外情况发生，吻合应在最适宜并且没有张力的条件下进行。尽管，笔者倾向于在所有 UC 患者中采用暂时性的回肠造瘘术，但是，任何未经过仔细评估的患者，在行 I 期 IAPP 后，没有并发症发生。当回肠造瘘省略后，患者应被告知恢复期将延长。

4 种形态的储袋用于临床，包括侧面、S、J 和 W 形的储袋（图 94-5）。S 和 W 储袋为人工缝合，较吻

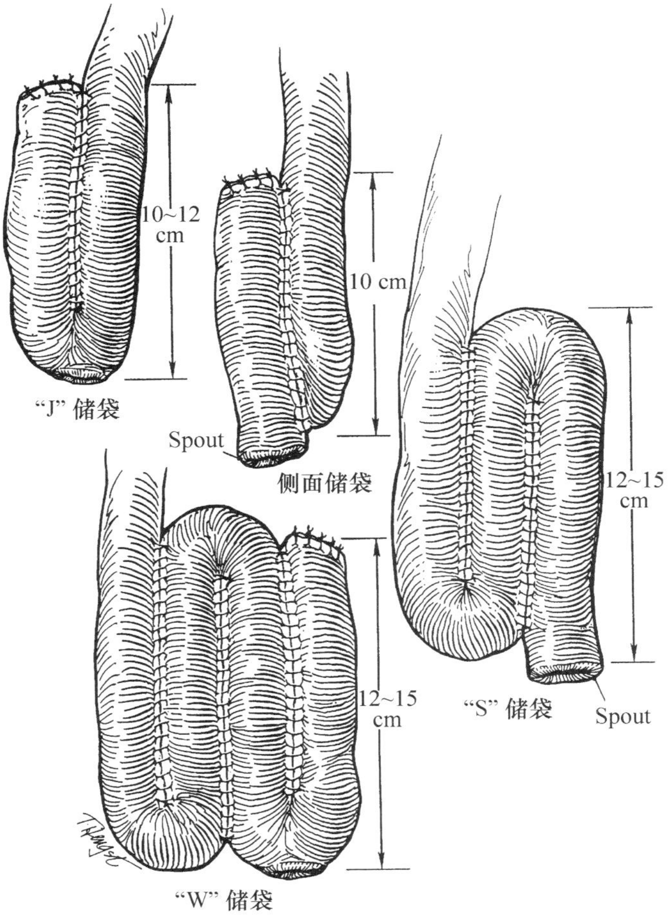

图 94-5 4 种回肠储袋的构型已用于临床，侧面和“S”形储袋有一个较短的出口，J 形储袋使用最频繁。

合器吻合的 J 形和侧面储袋的手术时间要长。大的储袋通常会发生粪便滞留，有时为了排空需要用导管冲洗[78]。几个月后，许多有回肠出口的储袋变大且发生粪便滞留。

468 J 形储袋的结构由 Utsunomiya[87] 等人第一个描述，目前广泛被应用，结构最简单，在成人和儿童中长期并发症最少。侧面回肠储袋曾经应用于儿童，并获得了较好的长期效果，在储袋最低点和肛管之间的回肠出口较短[29]。目前，侧面储袋仅用于回肠系膜较短以及不能有足够长度做 J 形储袋的患者（如在无张力下不能到达肛管）。只要储袋保持较短长度（＜12 cm），袋形态相对不重要，考虑到要有足够的功能，如果有可能可避免出口。如果出口存在，不要超过 1.5 cm。腹腔镜辅助下结肠切除并行 IAPP 的方法使用逐渐在增加。但手术时间较长，储袋结构更复杂，住院时间与开放手术相比没有缩短。

Ⅱ期回肠肛管储袋构建

大多数患者，IAPP 通过Ⅱ期手术形成。在第 1 次手术时，患者予以全身麻醉，并以截石位置于手术台上，留置鼻胃管和导尿管。正中切口，从耻骨上到脐上，切除整个结肠及网膜。如果末端回肠有炎症出现，那么有可能是 Crohn 病，这时不要做 IAPP，直到明确诊断。近来研究显示，IAPP 的患者切除超过 15 cm 的远端回肠可促进胃排空并且增加大便次数[84]。直肠用抗生素溶液彻底冲洗。腹膜返折环形切开，直肠用电凝分离游离至齿状线下 4 cm，然后再断开（图 94-6）。由病理医生检查标本来排除 Crohn 病的可能，扩张肛管，直肠黏膜用剪刀和电凝分离，从直肠肌层下将其剥离。注射稀释的肾上腺素溶液于黏膜与肌层之间，有利于创造分离的空间。所有黏膜剥离到齿状线，仔细止血。有些医生自骨盆行直肠内分离而不从会阴部分离。

回肠系膜游离要贴近上腹部肠系膜上血管，使远端回肠获得足够的长度，使其无张力到达肛门。远端回肠 10～12 cm 自行折返，系膜对侧面互相靠在一起（图 94-7A）。在袢的顶部做一个小切口。GIA 从这个切口伸入切割吻合，就构成了储袋（图 94-7B）。储袋的上端开口内翻缝合关闭，用可吸收线加强由吻合器吻合的储袋吻合线，将储袋拖至盆腔，通过直肠肌鞘，顶端开口与肛管直肠肌层在齿状线水平用可吸收线间断缝合（图 94-8）。通过充分游离回肠系膜以避免吻合口张力过大。在回肠储袋靠近上端约 15 cm 处横断回肠。近端回肠拖出构成末端回肠造瘘（图 94-9）。在儿童，不必做外翻的造瘘口，因为回肠浆肌层与临近皮肤做吻合，在 2 周内会产生一个外翻的造瘘口，不会引起造瘘口水肿或梗阻，远端回肠关闭，松弛地贴附在邻近造瘘口的腹内壁，当关闭造瘘口时方便进入。儿童也不需要做回肠袢造瘘，因为肠系膜血管张力增加，并延伸至盆腔的储袋，给安装一个功能良好的回肠造瘘器械带来困难[32]。经腹腔的盆腔引流管放置大约 4 天。

静脉用激素在手术后应快速减量，口服泼尼松 3 周内停止。大多数患儿手术后 6 天出院。在 2 个月内行泛影葡胺灌肠造影确认回肠储袋有无漏或者窦道形 1469
成（图 94-10）。大多数患儿 3 周内能进行体育活动。

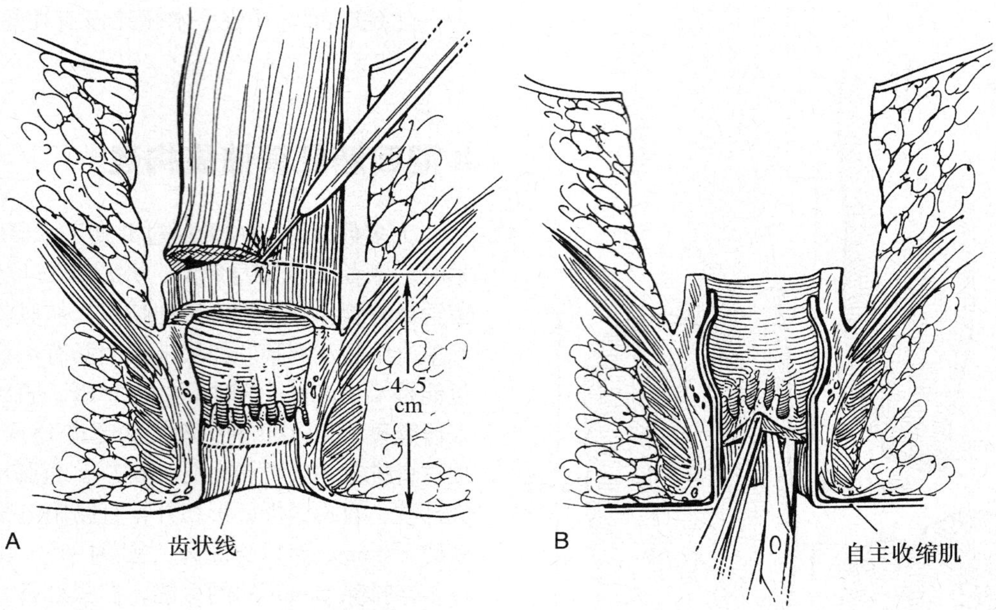

图 94-6　A. 直肠用电刀游离至齿状线 4 cm 以内，进行切断。B. 在齿状线水平用电凝环形切开直肠黏膜，黏膜用剪刀或电刀分离，从肌层提起。

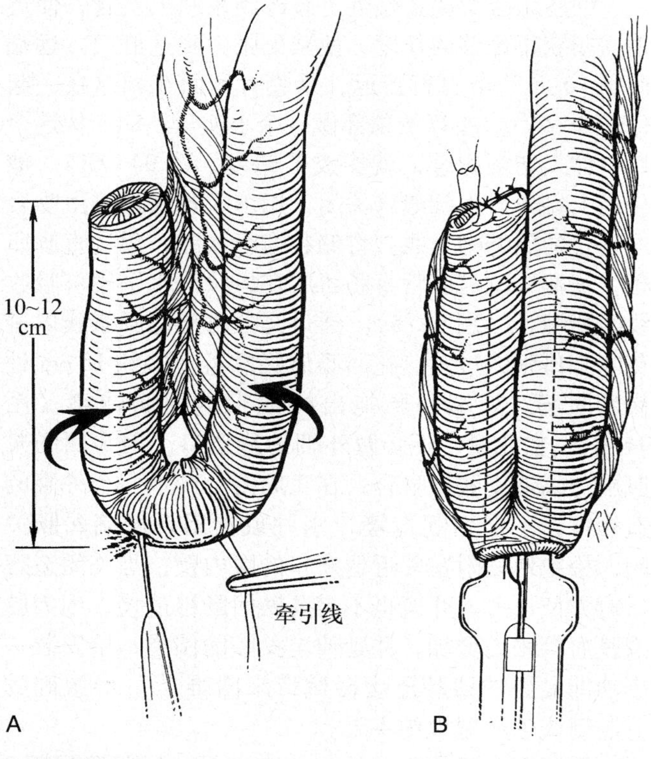

图 94-7　A. 回肠远端 10～12 cm 向回返折，对系膜侧肠管靠在一起，在袢的顶端做一个小切口，可放入 GIA 肠吻合器。B. 把 GIA 肠吻合器通过 J 袢顶端的小切口放置后，并切割吻合，储袋上端开口采用内翻缝合关闭。

大约第 1 次手术 3 个月后，患儿再次入院作剖腹手术和乙状结肠镜检及造瘘口关闭。回肠肛管吻合口在麻醉下进行扩张。当能经口进食后，调味料应避免辛辣食物、巧克力和加醋色拉，以减少腹泻。服用约 6 周小剂量的甲硝唑，以减少储袋内粪便滞留引起的回肠黏膜炎症。减少蠕动的药物（如地芬诺酯、盐酸洛哌丁胺）可抵消引起储袋收缩的正常刺激，促进粪便滞留，因此应少用。除了在手术后短短几周内减少频繁的夜间排便次数外，膨胀剂很少有帮助。术后第 4 天，做过回肠肛管吻合术的患者如出现吻合口狭窄，需要每天用大号的黑加尔扩张器进行扩张。至少每周扩张 2 次，持续 3～6 个月，以预防远期直肠狭窄而导致储袋扩张以及粪便滞留。

临床经验

过去的 20 年，在 UCLA 医疗中心，184 例小于 19 岁的儿童（141 例 UC、29 例息肉病、12 例巨结肠和 2 例特发性结肠无力）进行了结肠切除、直肠黏膜切除以及直肠内回肠拖出术，19 例患儿小于 10 岁。同期，另外 604 例患有 UC 或结肠息肉病的年龄在 19

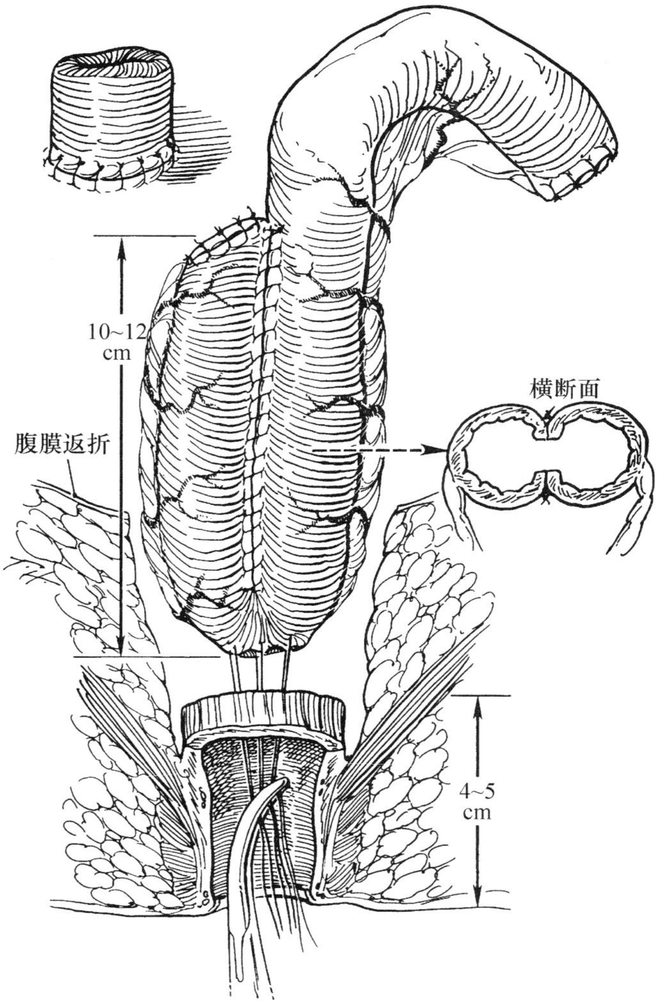

图 94-8　用牵引缝线将完成好的储袋通过盆腔拖至直肠肌鞘内，回肠储袋的开口在齿状线水平用可吸收线与肛管上皮及直肠肌层作间断缝合。

470 岁或 19 岁以上的患儿施行了 IAPP。

对 J 形和侧面储袋的患者进行长期随访显示，3 个月内平均每天的大便次数为 6.1 次，在 6 个月时下降为 4.2 次[26]。在 3 个月内有 17% 的患者出现夜间大便或污染超过每周 2 次，尤其是年轻的 UC 患者；在 6 个月时，发生率下降至 6%。在另外一组成人的大样本中，90% 的患者无夜间失禁症状[6]。在 IAPP 后，68 例女性患者中有 19 例生下了健康的宝宝，其中 10 例是经阴道分娩的。因 UC 而行 IAPP 的女性患者中，卵巢囊肿较常见，并且生育能力轻度降低[57,82]。没有出现膀胱功能障碍。尽管有 1 例出现逆行射精，73 例男性患者中没有 1 例发生阳

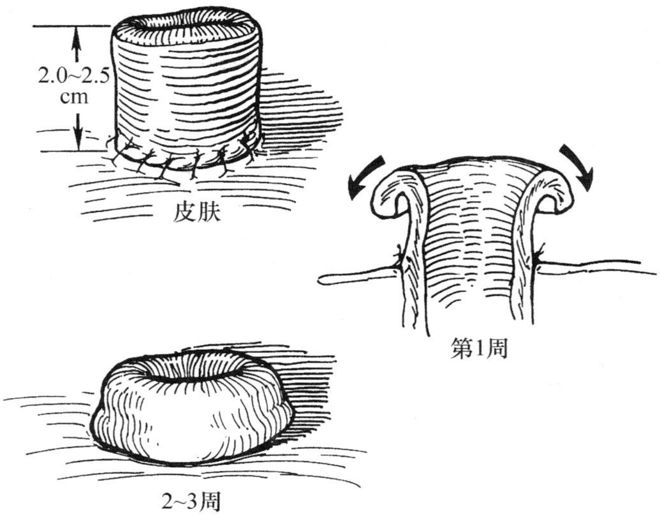

图 94-9　儿童单腔回肠造瘘术技术，肠系膜从回肠远端 3 cm 游离，约 2.0～2.5 cm 长的回肠高出皮肤表面，回肠肌层用细的单丝可吸收线与皮肤做间断缝合，不需要做深部缝针。2～3 周内，回肠末端将外翻并附着于皮肤。

痿，许多患者能参加剧烈的体育运动，包括足球、游泳以及马拉松赛跑。

19 例患儿大便胆盐和血清 B_{12} 水平的测量值在正常范围内[46]。几个月内，回肠储袋的黏膜开始与正常大肠黏膜一样起作用[79]。一篇综述详细回顾了最近 85 例患儿，显示除 2 例外其余目前功能均较好，并提示并发症的下降与临床经验的提高有关。95% 的患儿的功能和生活质量是相当好的，这与其他年长患儿的大样本资料相似[14,21,75]。

排便后残余大便量与患儿的临床功能密切相关，这与残余尿量和膀胱功能的关系相似。在最近一组 150 例儿童和成人的病例综述中，术后 6 个多月进行检查时发现，当残余大便量小于 10 ml 时，每天大便的次数为 4.6 次，污粪发作的次数是每周 0.4 次；相对应，当残留大便量超过 30 ml 时，其每天大便次数为 9.4 次，污粪为每周 4.8 次；当残余大便量小于 10 ml时，在第一次大便后能维持 2 小时以上的时间，78% 的患者残留少量大便，但放屁时不带出大便，并且 82% 的患者排尿时无粪便排出。

IAPP 的并发症发生率报道为 35% ～ 65%[21,22,25-27,33,72,75,90]（141 例 UC 患儿中为 41%），死亡率小于 1%。在长期随访中，储袋炎是最常见的并发症，发生率为 10%～50%。小肠梗阻发生率为

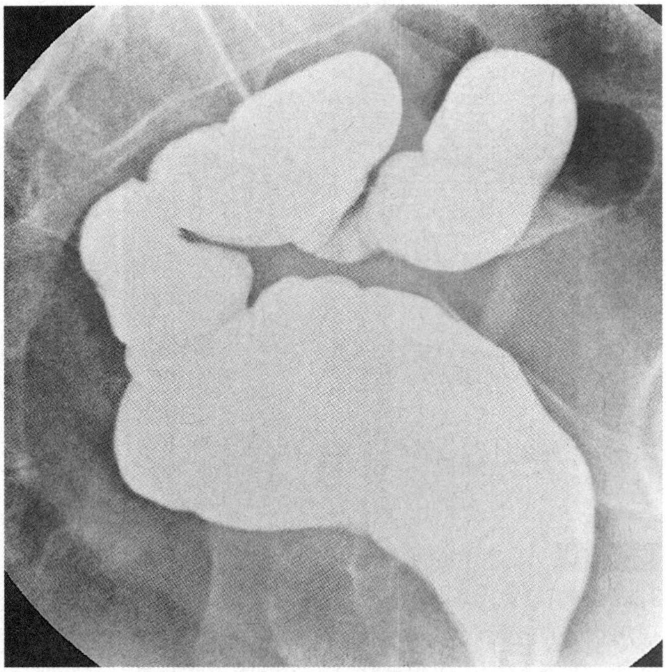

图 94-10 一个患 UC 的 16 岁儿童在完成结肠切除以及回肠肛管 J 形储袋手术后 8 周所做的泛影葡胺灌肠侧位片。

10%～25%；盆腔脓肿、瘘或败血症发生率为
1471 3%～10%；回肠造瘘口梗阻或功能不良占 1%～6%；伤口感染为 5%～15%；切口疝为 3%～8%；肛管狭窄为 2%～15%；直肠阴道瘘为 1%～6%；储袋出血为1%～5%；严重的失禁为 2%～6%。约 15%～45% 的患者需要再次手术[42,85]，3%～15% 患者需要切除储袋以及做一个永久性的回肠造口[6]。由于被诊断为 Crohn 病而不是 UC，近 1/4 患者需要切除储袋。

储袋炎是一个持续储袋感染的临床综合征。患者常有水样腹泻、发热、不适，偶尔有关节痛和其他肠道外症状[53,71]。储袋炎在 IAPP 术后头 2 年最常见，在儿童中发作更频繁更严重[68]。引起储袋炎的原因不明，但通常腔内发现需氧菌数增多。血清标记物 PANCA 阳性的患者发生储袋炎的风险最大。全结肠炎的患者，尤其是“倒灌性回肠炎”患者易发生储袋炎。随着回肠储袋的建立，远端回肠的主要功能由吸收转为储存，粪便在储袋内保留时间过长常导致细菌过度繁殖，这可能引起黏膜炎症[6,50]。有效的储袋排空、最小的残留大便量与储袋炎的低发生率相关[26]。常规 IAPP 术后直肠扩张并且进一步外科纠治出口梗阻，使 UC 患者储袋炎的发生率小于 10%。IAPP 术后头几年常规乙状结肠镜检，通常能早期发现储袋炎，这时的储袋炎对治疗有反应。患者因息肉病或巨结肠而行 IAPP 术后很少发生储袋炎。抗生素（甲硝唑或环丙沙星）治疗储袋炎效果较好。每天用清水或 5-氨基水杨酸冲洗储袋也有效。对于慢性的病例，可口服 5-氨基水杨酸并且加上氢化可的松保留灌肠。储袋炎的治疗应连续进行，直至完全治愈；有时即便症状消失，对于顽固性储袋炎的患者，要进行黏膜活检和评估以发现 Crohn 病。对引起生长发育迟缓的慢性储袋炎的 UC 患者，要考虑做回肠造瘘口改道。近来研究提示，活的微生物（如乳酸杆菌和链球菌和益生菌制剂）可改变储袋细菌群落，并减少储袋炎的发生率[37]。

做过 IAPP 的患者在回肠造瘘关闭后头几个月内会发生许多并发症；在以后 1 年内或更长时间里，储袋功能不良可逐渐加重，储袋的有效收缩因储袋扩张、变大或慢性炎症而减少。任何原因的出口不畅将影响储袋的完全排空，包括出口狭窄、出口延长或者因皮肤刺激或肛周瘘管及肛裂引起的括约肌痉挛。储袋内大便滞留时间过长及不完全排空常导致滞留性储袋炎和腹泻、大便急及次数增多、短链脂肪酸增加、经口摄入减少，偶尔出现失禁并有全身症状如关节痛。回肠造瘘口关闭后，有回肠肛管吻合口狭窄的患者，可常规做直肠扩张，可大大减少因储袋出口梗阻所产生的症状发作的频率。

成人 IAPP 后 24 小时内，大便排出量很少超过 750 ml，然而，这几乎是正常结肠排便 3 倍还多。储袋接近排空同时每次肠管运动每日能产生大约 3～5 次总共 150～200 ml 的大便，不完全储袋排空将导致大便量少且次数频繁。在过去的 20 年中，回肠储袋被大多数外科医生逐渐缩短到约 10～15 cm，使临床结果得到改善，并且并发症发生率降低。

有症状的儿童和成人储袋功能不良是由于机械因素引起的，对大多数患者我们已行重建手术，并取得了良好的效果[30,33]。17 例患者做了直接的直肠内回肠拖出术，因出现症状而要求再次手术，每个患者均成功从盆腔游离回肠并做 J 形储袋[31]。尽管在术前很难识别这些患者，但偶然有一个没有储袋的患者亦取得较好的结果。因此我们在所有儿童中运用储袋，83 例患者做了腹腔腹膜储袋重建，并且 95% 的患者获得较好的结果；58 例有侧面储袋的患者缩短出口，97% 获得良好的结果；7 例患者去除原有储袋而构建

一个新的储袋；暂时性的回肠造瘘只用于做过第 2 次重建手术的 5% 的患者中。

争议围绕在手法缝合的回肠储袋与肛管吻合，与保留肛管移行区而做的吻合器吻合之间的优点比
72 较上[52,83]。一方面，吻合器吻合技术要求较低，可最大限度减少对直肠肌肉复合体的损伤，而且回肠与直肠的吻合可以在无张力下进行；另一方面，UC 患者通常直肠病变较重，它会干扰回肠肛管或直肠吻合口的愈合，并且引起瘘或者储袋出口梗阻。Coull[12] 等人对 105 例患者的研究显示，吻合器做储袋肛管吻合后平均 5.5 年，黏膜活检发现有活跃的非典型以及严重的急慢性炎症。肛管移行区保留并做吻合器吻合可能最适用于将回肠储袋拖至肛管有一定张力的患者，严重的直肠 UC，同时有结肠癌或者黏膜发育不良是保留直肠黏膜的禁忌证。16 岁之前发生 UC 的儿童，发生直肠或结肠癌的风险比大年龄患儿更高。已行吻合器吻合的患者，需每年行乙状结肠镜检查。

结论

UC 是一个严重的疾病，儿童比成人有更多的急性症状，可能是由于长期激素和免疫抑制剂的使用所致。儿童的生长发育延迟，直到青少年后期，如果外科医生未治愈该病，则患儿的生长发育无法赶上同龄者，并将终生受到儿童期药物治疗的影响。因为大多数有严重 UC 的儿童症状持续到成年并最终需要做直肠结肠切除，要考虑在儿童期骨骺关闭前做结肠切除以及治愈该病。

目前患者普遍能接受直肠内 IAPP 是一个安全且可行的治疗，对 UC 和家族性结肠息肉病的患者来说是直肠结肠切除并永久性回肠造瘘术的替代方法。事实上所有患者宁可选择该方法而不愿做一个永久性的回肠造瘘。术后主要并发症可被纠治，许多功能不良的储袋可进行重建，减少了储袋切除和永久性回肠造瘘的必要性。J 形储袋使用最广泛，约 95% 的儿童和 96% 的成人在术后 5 年余仍有良好的功能。

（严志龙译　叶祖萍校）

参考文献

1. Adams JT: Toxic dilatation of the colon: A surgical disease. Arch Surg 1973;106:678.
2. Atkinson KG, et al: Restorative proctocolectomy and indeterminate colitis. Am J Surg 1994;167:516.
3. Aylett SO: Three hundred cases of diffuse ulcerative colitis treated by total colectomy and ileo-rectal anastomosis. BMJ 1966;1:1001.
4. Bacon HE: Ulcerative Colitis. Philadelphia, JB Lippincott, 1958.
5. Beahrs OH: Use of ileal reservoir following proctocolectomy. Surg Gynecol Obstet 1975;141:363.
6. Becker JM: Surgical management of inflammatory bowel disease. Curr Opin Gastroenterol 1993;9:600.
7. Brooke BN: The management of an ileostomy including its complications. Lancet 1952;2:102.
8. Browne JY: Value of complete physiological rest of large bowel in ulcerative and obstructive lesions. Surg Gynecol Obstet 1913;16:610.
9. Cattell RB: The surgical treatment of ulcerative colitis. Gastroenterology 1948;10:63.
10. Cohen Z, et al: Continuing evolution of the pelvic pouch procedure. Ann Surg 1992;216:506.
11. Coran A: A personal experience with 100 consecutive total colectomies and straight ileoanal endorectal pull-throughs for benign disease of the colon and rectum in children and adults. Ann Surg 1990;212:242.
12. Coull DB, et al: Risk of dysplasia in the columnar cuff after stapled restorative proctocolectomy. Br J Surg 2003;90:72.
13. Delaney CP, et al: Equivalent function, quality of life and pouch survival rates after ileal pouch-anal anastomosis for indeterminate and ulcerative colitis. Ann Surg 2002;236:43.
14. Delaney CP, et al: Prospective age-related analysis of surgical results, functional outcome, and quality of life after ileal pouch-anal anastomosis. Ann Surg 2003;238:221.
15. Devine H: Method of colectomy for desperate cases of ulcerative colitis. Surg Gynecol Obstet 1943;76:136.
16. Devroede GJ, et al: Cancer risk and life expectancy of children with ulcerative colitis. N Engl J Med 1971;185:17.
17. Ekborn A, et al: Ulcerative colitis and colorectal cancer, a population-based study. N Engl J Med 1990;323:1228.
18. Escher JC, et al: Treatment of inflammatory bowel disease in childhood: Best available evidence. Inflam Bowel Dis 2003;9:34.
19. Farouk F, et al: Functional outcomes after ileal pouch-anal anastomosis for chronic ulcerative colitis. Ann Surg 2000;231:919.
20. Fazio VW: Surgery of the colon and rectum. Am J Gastroenterol 1994;89:S106.
21. Fazio VW, et al: Ileal pouch-anal anastomoses complications and function in 1005 patients. Ann Surg 1995;222:120.
22. Fazio VW, et al: Quantification of risk for pouch failure after ileal pouch anal anastomosis surgery. Ann Surg 2003;238:605.
23. Ferrari BT, Fonkalsrud EW: Endorectal ileal pullthrough operation with ileal reservoir after total colectomy. Am J Surg 1978;136:113.
24. Ferzoco SJ, Becker JM: Does aggressive medical therapy for acute ulcerative colitis result in a higher incidence of staged colectomy? Arch Surg 1994;129:420.
25. Fleshman JW, et al: The ileal reservoir and ileoanal anastomosis procedure: Factors affecting technical and functional outcome. Dis Colon Rectum 1988;31:10.

26. Fonkalsrud EW: Clinical and physiologic studies with restorative proctocolectomy. In Deutsche Gesellsch: Langenbeck's archiv chirurg suppl kongressbericht. Berlin, Springer Verlag, 1994.
27. Fonkalsrud EW: Long-term results after colectomy and ileoanal pullthrough procedure in children. Arch Surg 1996;131:881.
28. Fonkalsrud EW: In Bayless TM, Hanauer SB (eds): Ileoanal pouch surgery in childhood. Advanced Therapy of Inflammatory Bowel Disease. Hamilton, Ontario, BC Decker, 2001, p 215.
29. Fonkalsrud EW, Loar N: Long-term results after colectomy and endorectal ileal pullthrough procedure in children. Ann Surg 1992;215:57.
30. Fonkalsrud EW, Phillips JD: Reconstruction of malfunctioning ileoanal pouch procedures as an alternative to permanent ileostomy. Am J Surg 1990;160:245.
31. Fonkalsrud EW, Stelzner M, McDonald N: Construction of an ileal reservoir in patients with a previous straight endorectal ileal pullthrough. Ann Surg 1988;208:50.
32. Fonkalsrud EW, Thakur A, Roof L: Comparison of loop versus end ileostomy for fecal diversion after restorative proctocolectomy for ulcerative colitis. J Am Coll Surg 2000; 190:418.
33. Fonkalsrud EW, et al: Reconstruction for chronic dysfunction of ileoanal pouches. Ann Surg 1999;229:1.
34. Furst MB, et al: Colonic anastomoses: Bursting strength after corticosteroid treatment. Dis Colon Rectum 1994; 37:12.
35. Gardner C, Miller CG: Total colectomy for ulcerative colitis. Arch Surg 1951;63:370.
36. Garrett JM, Sauer WG, Moertel CG: Colonic motility in ulcerative colitis after opiate administration. Gastroenterology 1967;53:93.
37. Gionchetti P, et al: Prophylaxis of pouchitis onset with probiotic therapy: A double-blind, placebo-controlled trial. Gastroenterology 2003;124:1202.
38. Goligher JC: Primary excisional surgery in the treatment of ulcerative colitis. Ann R Coll Surg Engl 1954;15:316.
39. Hanauer SB: Medical therapy of ulcerative colitis. Lancet 1993;342:412.
40. Harms BA, et al: Management of fulminant ulcerative colitis by primary restorative proctocolectomy. Dis Colon Rectum 1994;39:971.
41. Heppell J, et al: Physiologic aspects of continence after colectomy, mucosal proctectomy, and endorectal ileoanal anastomosis. Ann Surg 1982;195:435.
42. Heuschen UA, et al: Risk factors for ileoanal J pouch-related septic complications in ulcerative colitis and familial adenomatous polyposis. Ann Surg 2002;235:207.
43. Joossens S, et al: The value of serologic markers in indeterminate colitis: A prospective follow-up study. Gastroenterology 2002;122:1240.
44. Karlan M, McPherson RC, Watman RN: An experimental evaluation of fecal continence, sphincter and reservoir in the dog. Surg Gynecol Obstet 1959;108:469.
45. Kartheuser AH, et al: Complications and risk factors after ileal pouch-anal anastomosis for ulcerative colitis associated with primary sclerosing cholangitis. Ann Surg 1993;217:314.
46. Kelly RE Jr, et al: Early and long-term effects of colectomy and endorectal ileal pullthrough on bile salt profile. Ann Surg 1993;217:321.
47. Ko CY, et al: Long-term outcomes of the ileal pouch anal anastomosis: The association of bowel function and quality of life 5 years after surgery. J Surg Res 2001;98:102.
48. Kock NG: Intra-abdominal reservoir in patients with permanent ileostomy: Preliminary observations on a procedure resulting in fecal continence in five ileostomy patients. Arch Surg 1969;99:223.
49. Kock NG, et al: The quality of life after proctocolectomy and ileostomy: A study of patients with conventional ileostomies converted to continent ileostomies. Dis Colon Rectum 1974;17:287.
50. Levitt MD, Kuan M: The physiology of ileo-anal pouch function. Am J Surg 1998;176:384.
51. Lichtiger S, et al: Cyclosporine in severe ulcerative colitis refractory to steroid therapy. N Engl J Med 1994;330:1841.
52. Luukkonen P, Jarvinen H: Stapled vs hand-sutured ileoanal anastomosis in restorative proctocolectomy: A prospective randomized study. Arch Surg 1994;128:437.
53. Mahadevan U, Sanborn WJ: Diagnosis and management of pouchitis. Gastroenterology 2003;124:1636.
54. Martin LW, Le Coultre C, Schubert WK: Total colectomy and mucosal proctectomy with preservation of continence in ulcerative colitis. Ann Surg 1977;186:477.
55. McCaffery TD, et al: Severe growth retardation in children with inflammatory bowel disease. Pediatrics 1970;45:386.
56. Morgan RA, Manning PB, Coran AG: Experience with the straight endorectal pullthrough for management of ulcerative colitis and familial polyposis in children and adults. Ann Surg 1987;206:595.
57. Olsen KO, et al: Female fecundity before and after operation for familial adenomatous polyposis. Br J Surg 2003; 90:227.
58. Orkin BA, et al: The surgical management of children with ulcerative colitis: The old vs the new. Dis Colon Rectum 1990;33:947.
59. Parc R, et al: Current results: Ileorectal anastomosis after total abdominal colectomy for ulcerative colitis. In Dozois RR (ed): Alternatives to Conventional Ileostomy. Chicago, Year Book Medical Publishers, 1985.
60. Parks AG, Nicholls RJ: Proctocolectomy without ileostomy for ulcerative colitis. BMJ 1978;2:85.
61. Pescatori M, Parks AG: The sphincteric and sensory components of preserved continence after ileoanal reservoir. Surg Gynecol Obstet 1984;158:517.
62. Podolsky DK: Inflammatory bowel disease. N Engl J Med 2002;347:417.
63. Pullan RD, et al: Transdermal nicotine for active ulcerative colitis. N Engl J Med 1994;330:811.
64. Ravitch MM: Anal ileostomy with sphincter preservation in patients requiring total colectomy for benign conditions. Surgery 1948;24:170.
65. Ravitch MM, Sabiston DC: Anal ileostomy with preservation of the sphincter: A proposed operation in patients requiring total colectomy for benign lesions. Surg Gynecol Obstet 1947;84:1095.
66. Rintala RJ, Lindahl HG: Proctocolectomy and J-pouch ileoanal anastomosis in children. J Pediatr Surg 2002;37:66.
67. Ripstein CB: Results of the surgical treatment of ulcerative colitis. Ann Surg 1952;135:14.
68. Robb BW, et al: Restorative proctocolectomy with ileal pouch-anal anastomosis in very young patients with refractory ulcerative colitis. J Pediatr Surg 2003;38:863.
69. Rutgeerts P, et al: Appendectomy protects against ulcerative colitis. Gastroenterology 1994;106:1251.
70. Safaie S, Soper RT: Endorectal pullthrough procedure in the surgical treatment of familial polyposis coli. J Pediatr Surg 1973;8:711.
71. Sanborn WJ: Pouchitis following ileal pouch-anal anastomosis: Definition, pathogenesis, and treatment.

Gastroenterology 1994;107:1856.
72. Sarigol S, et al: Ileal pouch-anal anastomosis in children with ulcerative colitis. Inflam Bowel Dis 1996;2:82.
73. Sloan WP, Bargen JA, Gage RP: Life histories of patients with chronic ulcerative colitis: A review of 2000 cases. Gastroenterology 1950;16:25.
74. Soave F: A new surgical technique for treatment of Hirschsprung's disease. Surgery 1964;56:1007.
75. Stavio P, et al: Pediatric pouch-anal anastomosis: Functional outcomes and quality of life. J Pediatr Surg 2003;28:935.
76. Stelzner M, Fonkalsrud EW: The endorectal ileal pullthrough procedure in patients with ulcerative colitis and familial polyposis with carcinoma. Surg Gynecol Obstet 1989;169:187.
77. Stelzner M, Fonkalsrud EW: Assessment of anorectal function after mucosal proctectomy and endorectal ileal pullthrough for ulcerative colitis. Surgery 1990;107:201.
78. Stelzner M, et al: Significance of the reservoir length in the endorectal ileal pullthrough with ileal reservoir. Arch Surg 1988;123:1265.
79. Stelzner M, et al: Adaptive changes in ileal mucosal nutrient transport following colectomy and endorectal ileal pullthrough with ileal reservoir. Arch Surg 1990; 125:586.
80. Stelzner M, et al: Nephrolithiasis and urine ion composition in ulcerative colitis patients undergoing colectomy and endorectal ileal pullthrough. J Surg Res 1990; 48:552.
81. Strauss AA, Strauss SF: Surgical treatment of ulcerative colitis. Surg Clin North Am 1994;24:211.
82. Thakur A, et al: Management of ovarian cysts in women undergoing restorative proctocolectomy for ulcerative colitis. Am Surg 2003;69:339.
83. Thompson-Fawcett MW, et al: "Cuffitis" and inflammatory changes in the columnar cuff, anal transition zone, and ileal reservoir after stapled pouch-anal anastomosis. Dis Colon Rectum 1999;42:348.
84. Tomita R, et al: Gastric emptying function after ileal J-pouch anal anastomosis for ulcerative colitis. Surgery 2004;135:81.
85. Tulchinsky J, et al: Long-term failure after restorative proctocolectomy for ulcerative colitis. Ann Surg 2003;238:229.
86. Turnbull RP: Management of an ileostomy. Am J Surg 1953;86:617.
87. Utsunomiya AJ, et al: Total colectomy, mucosal proctectomy and ileoanal anastomosis. Dis Colon Rectum 1980; 23:459.
88. Valente MA, Bacon HE: Construction of pouch using "pantaloon" technique for pull-through following total colectomy. Am J Surg 1955;90:6621.
89. Weir RF (1902): Quoted by Corbet RS: A review of the surgical treatment of chronic ulcerative colitis. Proc R Soc Med Lond 1945;38:277.
90. Wexner SD, et al: Long-term functional analysis of the ileoanal reservoir. Dis Colon Rectum 1989;32:275.
91. Wilks S, Moxon DW: Lectures on Pathologic Anatomy. London, Longmans, Green, 1875.

第 95 章

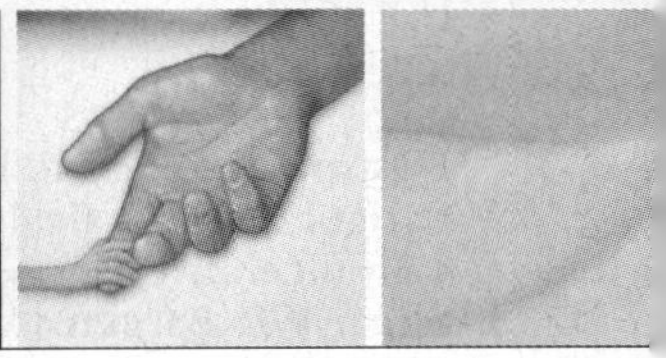

原发性腹膜炎

Karen W. West

1475 原发性腹膜炎（primary peritonitis，PP）（亦指特发性或自发性腹膜炎）被定义为非腹腔内因素引起的腹膜腔感染的过程[7,10,11]。这种感染是通过血液或淋巴途径或直接通过阴道扩散至腹腔的。除了输卵管的末端，腹膜腔是完全封闭的，这个腔能被异物如脑室腹膜分流术和腹膜透析导管所穿透。在青春期前和青少年期的女孩中，液体通过输卵管进行的逆行播散是上行性外阴阴道炎或“游泳池腹膜炎”发生的原因[5,13,25,51]。

1581 年报道了第一例致死性自发性细菌性腹膜炎（spontaneous bacterial peritonitis，SBP）的病例，患者是一名女孩，经历一段时间无痛性腹泻后死亡[21]。在 20 世纪早期，多达 10% 的儿童腹部手术都归到 PP 的范畴中，相关死亡率上升到 50%[10]。今天，这种状况的发生率在所有儿童剖腹手术中小于 1%，这是由于诊断明确而且最初的治疗无需手术干预[11]。在大多数儿童组中的患儿中，PP 患儿伴有肾病综合征（nephrotic syndrome，NS）或慢性肝病。在这些患者中，通常存在腹水或肝硬化。这一组中包括患有胆道闭锁、囊性纤维病、肝纤维化以及红斑狼疮的儿童和婴儿（表 95-1）[9,24,26]。在不同的相关情况下，从腹膜腔分离出的病原菌也不同（表 95-2）。例如革兰阳性菌，包括肺炎链球菌以及 A 族链球菌。在 NS 的患儿中，各种革兰阴性菌最常见[1,17,22]。相同的革兰阳性菌在肝病的患儿中亦能培养出。分离出的革兰阴性菌谱包括大肠杆菌、肺炎克雷白杆菌以及假单胞菌属。

在早期报道的病例中，大多数患儿是女孩，而且阴道通常被认为是引起感染的根源，然而，阴道炎不常见，感染的最终原因仍不清楚[21]。青春期前，子宫颈缺乏可潜伏细菌的颈内腺体，所以，这一年龄段发生的上行性感染很可能与推动细菌从阴道进入腹腔的外力有关，如性虐待或跳水时足先入游泳池或水中[13]。近来文献报道，男女童发生 PP 的发病率相同[31,35,50]，在一些病例中，引起腹膜感染的相同病菌也可从呼吸道、泌尿道和口腔中培养出来[7]。

表 95-1　儿童原发性腹膜炎伴发症
肾病综合征
肝功能不全
肾上腺性腺综合征
囊性纤维病
慢性肾衰竭需要长期不卧床腹膜透析
脾切除术后并发症
需要长期激素治疗的疾病（系统性红斑狼疮、皮肌炎）

表 95-2　与原发性腹膜炎相关的病原菌
链球菌标本（肺炎链球菌、A 族链球菌）
大肠杆菌
淋球菌
流感嗜血杆菌
肺炎克雷白杆菌
单核细胞增多性李司忒菌
副流感
伤寒沙门杆菌
黏质沙雷菌
小肠结肠炎耶尔森菌

临床病史、实验室指标和诊断性检查

PP 患儿有急性腹痛并伴有发热、恶心、呕吐、腹
76 泻或其他病毒感染症状。原发性腹膜炎比继发性腹膜炎的病程长，常常出现弥漫性肌反跳痛，没有局限性疼痛的出现可能是因为腹腔脏器表面受到了刺激[31,37]。

出现腹水时，做诊断性腹腔穿刺可能会有帮助，如在肾衰竭患儿中进行的移动性腹膜透析。当腹腔液体白细胞计数超过 500/mm^3 同时以中性粒细胞为主时（正常腹膜腔液体以淋巴细胞为主），就可诊断为 PP。液体的 pH 小于 7.35 且乳酸水平升高（大于 25 mg/dl）。送至少 10 ml 液体标本做革兰染色和培养分析将提高阳性的检出率，但在所报道的病例中，60% 的病例培养可能为阴性[15]。如果革兰染色中有一种以上细菌存在，要怀疑有脏器穿孔的可能。特殊细菌的分离缩小了所需抗生素的抗菌谱，并且潜在地排除对肾功能受损患儿肾毒性药物的使用[17]。血和尿标本送去做培养，同时还要拍摄胸腹部的平片，这对排除脏器穿孔或肺炎引起的腹腔感染有帮助。血清蛋白降低以及伴随的调理素下降可能促进了 PP 的进展[36]。

在临床平片有混淆时，腹部超声和 CT 检查有助于鉴别原发和继发性腹膜炎（通常由常见的儿科疾病引起如阑尾炎）。在 SBP 中，双重增强 CT 扫描可发现阑尾腔未闭，广泛的腹腔内液体以及肠壁的继发性增厚。

肾病综合征

NS 的儿童 PP 的发生率为 17%，这个发生率在过去的 30 年中都没有发生改变[1,3,19,39,48,49]。在使用抗生素治疗前，PP 是引起这一组患儿死亡的主要原因。在这些患儿中，由于细胞免疫受损、发生趋化现象、调理作用下降以及循环中的免疫球蛋白水平下降，发生感染的可能性将增加。在患有腹膜炎和 NS 的患儿中，血清中补体蛋白 I 和 B 的水平是下降的，但在尿中含量升高[29]。腹膜炎的复发率为 26% 并且伴有循环中的 IgG 水平下降[19]。

大量儿童病例报道显示，在 6%～30% 患有 NS 综合征和腹膜炎的患儿中，能分离出革兰阴性菌，4%～38% 的患儿能培养出肺炎链球菌[1,19,47]。即使腹腔液体没有分离出细菌，患儿静脉内滴注青霉素也能使症状有所改善。不论是用激素治疗，还是 NS 综合征复发，80% NS 的患儿会发展为 SBP[1,19,49]。

在诊断时，最常见的症状是弥漫性腹痛、发热、反跳痛、恶心和呕吐。多达 29% 的病例胸片显示有渗出，15%～27% 的患儿会发生不止一次的腹膜炎。在这组患儿中建议接种肺炎球菌疫苗，尽管进行了预防性免疫，但腹膜炎仍会发生[33,47]。另外有报道指出，预防性的口服青霉素治疗可能会引起细菌耐药[33]。PP 的最初治疗应选择兼顾革兰阳性和阴性细菌的抗生素，应对那些在最初治疗开始后 24 小时内临床症状没有改善的病例进行进一步的诊断性检查，如腹部 CT 或诊断性腹腔镜探查以排除腹膜炎的其他原因。在临床状况没有改善的情况下，运用腹腔镜和腹腔灌洗并联合药物治疗的方法在临床上已取得成功，然而，腹部 CT 扫描不能鉴别是原发性还是继发性腹膜炎。

肝功能不全

伴有肝功能受损、肝硬化和腹水的 SBP 患儿，通常 SBP 与在肠道内正常生长的革兰阴性菌，如大肠杆菌和肺炎克雷白杆菌，以及革兰阳性菌包括肺炎链球菌和金黄色葡萄球菌有关[32,35]。富含网状内皮组织的肝正常情况下能过滤门脉循环中的细菌。随着肝硬化的发展，门静脉血流部分从肝分流，所以降低了对血液和淋巴系统中的细菌和真菌的清除率。这种清除水平的下降可能使腹水中的细菌持续存在[26,40,41~43]。50% 的 SBP 的儿童出现发热和腹痛。穿刺液体的白细胞数大于 500/mm^3，细菌的革兰染色阳性，同时 pH 小于 7.35，穿刺对活跃期的 SBP 检验有 100% 的敏感性和 96% 的特异性[17]。肝硬化或综合功能受损导致的囊性纤维化和肝功能不良的患儿，也有发生 PP 的风险[9]。

原发性腹膜炎及腹膜透析

在两个独立的多中心研究中，持续性不卧床腹膜透析（continuous ambulatory peritoneal dialysis，CAPD）的患儿发生（细菌或真菌性）腹膜炎的概率为每

11.1～13.2 名患儿一日中发生 1 次[14,22,34,38]。革兰阳性菌的检出率为 48.7%，革兰阴性菌为 21.6%，真菌为 1.8%，21.6% 有症状的患儿没有阳性的培养结果[14]。在这组患儿中，导致腹膜炎的危险因素包括透析液体交换的接头处污染、出口处或管道的感染、管道处的局部损伤和鼻腔葡萄球菌的生长[14]。因为有局部或管道感染的患儿发生腹膜炎的机会将
1477 增加 1 倍，所以解决这些问题就能降低感染的发生。临床表现包括腹痛、发热和浑浊的透析液中中性粒细胞计数升高。进行液体培养，联合应用静脉和腹腔内抗生素，密切监测抗生素的浓度水平。目前治疗的准则包括，联合应用一代和三代头孢菌素治疗非复杂性腹膜炎，同时应用糖肽类和三代头孢菌素治疗复发感染和近期有耐甲氧西林腹膜炎病史的年幼儿童[46]。开始治疗后，24～36 小时内症状有改善[44]。正常皮肤菌落，包括金黄色葡萄球菌和表皮葡萄球菌，仍是从腹膜液体中培养出的最常见的病原菌，但还培养出一些其他细菌（表 95-3）。有性生活活跃的进行腹透的青少年发生淋球菌腹膜炎的病例[51]。长期多中心纵向研究表明，当假单胞菌属、念珠菌属、非典型分枝杆菌属的菌体标本出现时，应去除腹膜透析导管以杜绝感染[2,14,23,25]。感染这些病原菌有发生腹膜功能衰竭的危险，故不能继续进行腹膜透析。使用双套囊系统及将出口朝下，可降低腹膜炎的发病率[14,50]。CAPD 相关腹膜炎的其他危险因素包括，CAPD 持续的时间（超过 1 年）、年龄小于 2 岁和血清 IgG 水平下降[25]。

表 95-3 在长期不卧床腹膜透析（CAPD）的腹膜炎患儿中存在的细菌

病原菌	百分比
金黄色葡萄球菌	38.9
表皮葡萄球菌	13.2
A 族链球菌	9.7
假单胞菌属	9.0
其他细菌或真菌	13.9
培养没有发现病原菌	13.9

* Data from 144 episodes of peritonitis in 66 children at J. W. Riley Hospital for Children, Indianapolis, IN.

健康儿童中的自发性细菌性腹膜炎

1950 年 Gross 报道了 58 例 PP 病例，58 例均为有过上呼吸道感染的既往体健的婴幼儿（平均年龄 2 岁），开始的症状包括呕吐、发热、易激惹、腹胀和触痛，肺炎球菌是主要的致病菌。在接下来的 30 年中，该机构报道了 33 例 SBP 患儿（平均年龄 5 岁）接受了治疗[21,28]。口服抗生素变得更加普遍被认为是腹膜炎患儿数目下降的原因。尽管存在多种潜在感染源，包括血源性的（拔牙过程、菌血症）、淋巴的、肠道菌群移位和多发的妇科疾病，但在大多数的病例中病因仍未明确。在 1985 年，有报道两个曾经健康的儿童发生脱水、腹胀，以及 A 族链球菌感染的腹膜炎。尽管其中一名患儿有右侧膈疝，但剖腹探查时，并没有发现感染源[45]。文献确定了一组发生特发性腹膜炎的健康儿童，同时从气管、咽喉、扁桃体处培养出了 A 族链球菌[4,12,18,20]。有淋球菌阴道炎的青春期前的女孩，6% 可能有腹膜炎症状。可使用非肠道途径的头孢菌素进行治疗，同时检查其他相关的可通过性传播的细菌[23]。原先腹腔探查没有发现肠道病原菌存在，近来分离出副流感嗜血杆菌[30]。

如果使用了静脉抗生素临床症状仍没有改善，应进行诊断性腹腔镜或剖腹探查。即使有浑浊的渗出液，亦可以安全地进行阑尾切除手术，以及检查肠管表面，以期发现引起感染的继发性原因。在外科干预后，应继续使用抗生素直至白细胞计数正常、肠梗阻症状消失为止[10,37]。

少见情况下的原发性腹膜炎

家族性地中海热（反复性浆膜炎、周期性发作）是常染色体隐性遗传性疾病，主要发生于从地中海地区移民来的美国人、土耳其人和犹太人，经常发生腹膜炎（85%）、关节炎（50%）和胸膜炎（38%）并伴有高热、腹部触痛。腹部症状在 12 小时内开始减轻，在 24～48 小时内消失。如果进行外科干预，术中特征性的表现为肠管上覆盖着含纤维素的无菌渗出物。远期并发症包括小肠粘连性肠梗阻，其发生率为 3%。秋水仙素的运用能减轻疼痛的发作程度，以及减少远期小肠粘连性疾病的发生[6,27]。

SBP，亦可发生在没有脑脊液感染的行脑室腹腔分流术的儿童中，这些患儿的腹膜液培养中可获得多种革兰阳性的细菌。一旦把转流管从腹内取出后，腹膜刺激症状即可以得到改善[16]。

（严志龙译 叶祖萍校）

参考文献

1. Alwadhi RK, Mathew JL, Roth B: Clinical profile of children with nephrotic syndrome not on glucocorticoid therapy but presenting with infection. J Pediatr Child Health 2004;40:28.
2. Andreoli SP, Langefield CD, Stadler S: Risks of peritoneal membrane failure in children undergoing long-term peritoneal dialysis. Pediatr Nephrol 1993;7:543.
3. Barness LA, Moll GH, Janeway CA: Nephrotic syndrome I. Natural history of the disease. Pediatrics 1950;5:486.
4. Brase R, Kuckelt W, Manhold C, et al: Spontaneous bacterial peritonitis without ascites. Anasthesiol Intensivmed Notfallmed Schmerzther 1992;27:325.
5. Burry VF: Gonococcal vulvovaginitis and possible peritonitis in prepubertal girls. Am J Dis Child 1971;121:536.
6. Ciftci AO, Tanyel FC, Buyukpamukcu N, et al: Adhesive small bowel obstruction caused by familial Mediterranean fever: The incidence and outcome. J Pediatr Surg 1995;30:1319.
7. Clark JH, Fitzgerald JF, Kleiman MB: Spontaneous bacterial peritonitis. J Pediatr 1984;104:495.
8. Dann PH, Amodio JB, Rivera R, et al: Primary bacterial peritonitis in otherwise healthy children: Imaging findings. Pediatr Radiol 2005;35:198.
9. Doershuk CF, Stern RC: Spontaneous bacterial peritonitis in cystic fibrosis. Gut 1994;35:709.
10. Ein SH: Primary peritonitis. In Welch KJ, Randolph JG (eds): Pediatric Surgery, 4th ed. Chicago, Year Book, 1986, p 976.
11. Fowler R: Primary peritonitis: Changing aspects 1956-1970. Aust Paediatr J 1971;7:73.
12. Freij BJ, Votteler TP, McCracken GH: Primary peritonitis in previously healthy children. Am J Dis Child 1984;138:1058.
13. Fuld GL: Gonococcal peritonitis in a prepubertal child. Am J Dis Child 1968;115:621.
14. Furth SL, Donaldson LA, Sullivan EK, et al: Peritoneal dialysis catheter infections and peritonitis in children: A report of the North American Pediatric Renal Transplant Cooperative Study. Pediatr Nephrol 2000;15:179.
15. Garcia-Tsao G, Conn HO, Lerner E: The diagnosis of bacterial peritonitis: Comparison of pH lactate concentration and leukocyte count. Hepatology 1985;5:91.
16. Gaskill SJ, Marlin AE: Spontaneous bacterial peritonitis in patients with ventriculoperitoneal shunts. Pediatr Neurosurg 1997;36:115.
17. Gilbert JA, Karnath PS: Spontaneous bacterial peritonitis, an update. Mayo Clin Proc 1995;70:365.
18. Gillespie RS, Hauger SB, Holt RM: Primary group A streptococcal peritonitis in a previously healthy child. Scand J Infect Dis 2002;34:847.
19. Gorensek MJ, Lebel MH, Nelson JD: Peritonitis in children with nephrotic syndrome. Pediatrics 1988;81:849.
20. Graham JC, Moss PJ, McKendrick MW: Primary group A streptococcal peritonitis. Scand J Infect Dis 1995;27:171.
21. Harken AH, Shochat SJ: Gram-positive peritonitis in children. Am J Surg 1973;125:769.
22. Holitta TM, Ronnholm KA, Jalanko J, et al: Peritoneal dialysis in children under 5 years of age. Perit Dial Int 1997;17:573.
23. Ingram DL: *Neisseria gonorrhoeae* in children. Pediatr Ann 1994;23:341.
24. Krensky AM, Ingelfinger JR, Grupe WE: Peritonitis in childhood nephrotic syndrome. Am J Dis Child 1982;136:732.
25. Kuizon B, Melocoton TL, Holloway M, et al: Infections and catheter related complications in pediatric patients treated with peritoneal dialysis at a single institution. Pediatr Nephrol 1995;9(Suppl):S12.
26. Larcher VF, Manolaki N, Vegnente A, et al: Spontaneous bacterial peritonitis in children with chronic liver disease: Clinical features and etiologic factors. J Pediatr 1985;106:907.
27. Majeed HA, Barakat M: Familial Mediterranean fever (recurrent hereditary polyserositis) in children: Analysis of 88 cases. Eur J Pediatr 1989;148:636.
28. Marshall R, Teele DW, Klein JO: Unsuspected bacteremia due to *Haemophilus influenzae*: Outcome in children not initially admitted to hospital. J Pediatr 1979;95:690.
29. Matsell DG, Wyatt RJ: The role of I and B in peritonitis associated with the nephrotic syndrome of childhood. Pediatr Res 1993;34:84.
30. Mayer MP, Schweizer P: Primary peritonitis in a child caused by *Haemophilus parainfluenzae*. Pediatr Surg Int 2002;18:728.
31. McDougal WS, Izant RJ Jr, Zollinger RM Jr: Primary peritonitis in infancy and childhood. Ann Surg 1974; 181:310.
32. Mihas AA, Toussaint J, Hsu HS, et al: Spontaneous bacterial peritonitis in cirrhosis: Clinical and laboratory features, survival and prognostic indicators. Hepatogastroenterology 1992;39:520.
33. Milner LS, Berkowitz FE, Ngwenya E, et al: Penicillin resistant pneumococcal peritonitis in nephrotic syndrome. Arch Dis Child 1987;62:964.
34. Mocan H, Murphy AV, Beattie TJ, et al: Peritonitis in children on continuous ambulatory peritoneal dialysis. J Infect 1988;16:243.
35. Moskovitz M, Ehrenberg E, Grieco R, et al: Primary peritonitis due to group A streptococcus. J Clin Gastroenterol 2000;30:332.
36. Nguyen MH, Yu VL: *Listeria monocytogenes* peritonitis in cirrhotic patients: Value of ascitic fluid gram stain and a review of the literature. Dig Dis Sci 1994;39:215.
37. Nohr CW, Marshall DA: Primary peritonitis in children. Can J Surg 1984;27:179.
38. Orkin BA, Fonkalsrud EW, Saluksy IB, et al: Continuous ambulatory peritoneal dialysis catheters in children. Arch Surg 1983;118:1398.
39. Pahmer M: *Pneumococcus* peritonitis in nephrotic and nonnephrotic children. J Pediatr 1940;17:90.
40. Rimola A, Soto R, Bory F, et al: Reticuloendothelial system phagocytic activity in cirrhosis and its relation to bacterial infections and prognosis. Hepatology 1984;4:53.
41. Runyon BA: Patients with deficient ascitic fluid opsonic activity are predisposed to spontaneous bacterial peritonitis. Hepatology 1980;8:632.
42. Runyon BA: Low-protein-concentration ascitic fluid is predisposed to spontaneous bacterial peritonitis. Gastroenterology 1986;91:1343.
43. Runyon BA, Umland ET, Merlin T: Inoculation of blood culture bottles with ascitic fluid: Improved detection of spontaneous bacterial peritonitis. Arch Intern Med 1987; 147:73.

44. Schaefer F: Management of peritonitis in children receiving chronic peritoneal dialysis. Paediatr Drugs 2003;5:315.
45. Serlo W, Heikkinen E, Kouvalainen K: Group A streptococcal peritonitis in infancy. Ann Chir Gynaecol 1985; 74:183.
46. Silva MM, Pecoits-Filho R, Rocha CS, et al: The recommendations from the International Society for Peritoneal Dialysis for Peritonitis Treatment: A single-center historical comparison. Adv Perit Dial 2004;20:74.
47. Speck WT, Dresdal SS, McMillan RW: Primary peritonitis and the nephrotic syndrome. Am J Surg 1974;127:267.
48. Tapaneya-Olarn C, Tapaneya-Olarn W: Primary peritonitis in childhood nephrotic syndrome: A changing trend in causative organisms. J Med Assoc Thailand 1991;74:502.
49. Tsau YK, Cxhen CH, Tsai WS, et al: Complications of nephrotic syndrome in children. J Formosan Med Assoc 1991;90:555.
50. Warady BA, Sullivan EK, Alexander SR: Lesson from the peritoneal dialysis patient database: A report of the North American Pediatric Renal Transplant Cooperative Study. Kidney Int Suppl 1996;53:568.
51. Wolfson AB, Naehamkin I, Singer I, et al: Gonococcal peritonitis in a patient treated with CAPD. Am J Kidney Dis 1985;6:257.

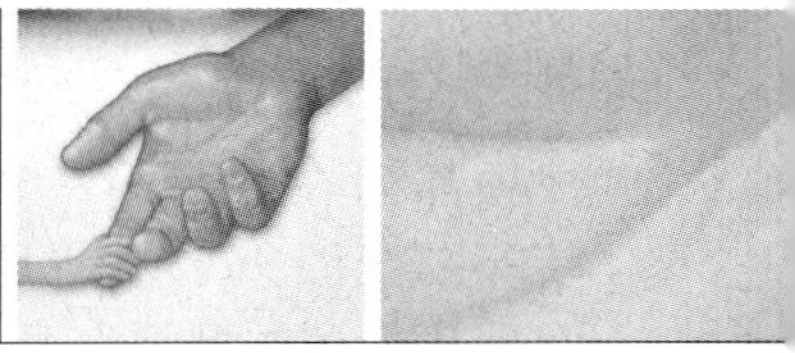

第 96 章

小肠和大肠造瘘

Michael W. L. Gauderer

历史回顾

479 肠造瘘，被认为是基本的外科手术，有着悠久而多彩的历史。作为治疗肠梗阻的一种方法，结肠造瘘可追溯到18世纪后期，第一批接受该术式并存活下来的人中有一部分是肛门闭锁的患儿[52,77,90,95,97]。尽管早期有个别手术成功的病例，但儿童中小肠后半段和大肠造瘘手术发展却很慢，有的外科医生勉强理解，有的甚至强烈反对实施这些合并有重大并发症的手术[77,95]。然而，随着外科医生经验的积累，在19世纪末和20世纪初，结肠造瘘和偶然的空肠造瘘被用来治疗一些儿童疾病。随着现代小儿外科的进展以及患有致命疾病的患儿的存活，造瘘的需要在不断增加。肠造瘘技术最初只在成人中实施[10,54,55,98]，经过不断改良后应用于儿童，尤其是在有先天性肠梗阻的新生儿中运用[5,6,11,53,63,69,76]。接下来将介绍近端减压加上远端喂养治疗新生儿十二指肠或高位空肠闭锁的新技术[16,35,71]。为前肠功能障碍的患儿实施幽门后喂养途径的手术方法需要进一步的发展和评估[3,20,62,74,80,88]，并且不断发展的微创外科为新的喂养途径、造口、减压、灌洗以及特殊目的的造瘘方式的发明，提供了新的和令人振奋的机会[34,36,37,57,62,81]。

在过去的几十年中，肠造瘘治疗已逐渐发展成一门独立的专业[7,91,97]，并且儿童造瘘护理方面也取得很大的进步，包括特殊的儿童造瘘装置、耐受性较好的生物材料以及非药物支持系统的发明[19,46,60]。另外，同人们对耐受力的认识一样，肠造瘘正在得到更广泛的认识和接受[7,9,60,97]。对肠造瘘生理的理解以及对肠内外营养的各项研究改善了肠造瘘的护理和预后。肠造瘘的构建、护理和关闭，现在已成为现代小儿外科的重要组成部分[56]。

儿童造瘘

儿童造瘘会严重地扰乱其正常生活状态，并且会使患儿和其父母遭受很大的精神创伤。然而，大多数儿童时期的小肠造瘘是暂时的，待根本问题解决后，常常要关闭改道的开口。尽管儿童外科医生一直在寻找替代肠管外露的治疗方法[84,89]，但适当提示的、准确进行的暂时性的肠造瘘常常是不可避免并且是救命的。在一些远端大肠存在不能纠正的情况以及病理缺陷的病例中，一个永久性的功能良好的肠造瘘可以提高生活质量[9,93,99]。尽管认为肠造瘘机制简单，但是肠造瘘有许多种基本类型、技术和护理方法，并且其早晚期并发症的发生率高得惊人。这些是外科医生、肠造瘘专家、护士、父母和患儿面临的主要挑战*。因此，当需要做一个造瘘时必须通过评估患儿的病理状况和健康状态，衡量改道的利弊，尽可能地事前计划以及考虑构建和拆除作为主要的干预手段才能获得最佳的结果。除了有成人较好的造瘘口部位选择作为治疗指导外，以下因素如解剖和生理不同点、具体结构、生长以及身体和情感成熟度都需要被考 1480
虑。外科医生和外科团队的成员必须牢记造瘘患儿的生活质量与造瘘口的质量密切相关。

肠造瘘的类型

肠造瘘的4种基本类型，其主要目的和技术选

---

* 见参考文献2，4，6，8，11，13～15，17，23，27，30，32，33，38，40，49，50，53，56，58，64～66，68，70，72，78，82，83，87，96和97。

项都列在表 96-1 中，这些方法的图示举例在图 96-1至图 96-3，将近端造瘘口置于腹壁上以及远端造瘘处理的列举在表 96-2 中，举例在图 96-3 至图 96-5中。

儿童肠造瘘的指征

在新生儿、婴幼儿以及儿童中，暂时性的和偶然的永久性小肠、大肠造瘘被广泛地用来治疗外科和非外科的病理状况。除了提供喂养途径之外，超过一半的造瘘发生在新生儿时期而另外 1/4 进行该手术的儿童年龄小于 1 岁[56]。

空肠造瘘主要用于有神经系统损伤且伴有前肠动力不良引起的状况复杂的儿童的肠内喂养[20,21,62,74,100]，以及一些能够通过早期肠内喂养获益的存在急诊外科问
1481 题的患儿中，如大的创伤[3,74]。也运用于需要长期提供喂养的儿童，如囊性纤维病的儿童（图 96-6）[82]。

表 96-1 肠造瘘的应用和考虑因素

喂养、给药或两者

- 不进入空肠壁：胃空肠管、胃造瘘-空肠造瘘管[34,74]
- 直接进入空肠壁：隧道样导管[98]、针式导管[3]、T 管[41]、纽扣[88]、其他
- 独立的空肠袢直接提出腹壁：R-Y 术[20,100]

近端减压和远端喂养

- 胃造瘘和远端营养管、同一个造瘘或单独的[16,34]
- 双腔管放入扩张的近端空肠且营养管末端通过吻合口[71]；或者两根单腔管分开放入，关闭小肠袢[35]
- 分开的肠段直接拉至皮肤水平，造瘘袋黏附在近端造瘘口处，并将营养导管放入远端肠管

逆行灌肠的通路

- 阑尾或者其他肠道的导管拖至腹壁作间歇性导入[5,52,85]
- 导管、T 管，皮肤水平装置放入肠腔内[37,41,81,88]

减压、改道或排空

- 单腔造瘘、单个开口[10]
- 双腔造瘘[55,69,73]
- 单腔造瘘伴腹壁下一个吻合口[5,76]
- 小棒或者皮桥上的肠袢[6,54,63]
- 有导管的关闭的肠袢[35]或者开放式肠袢并有瓣膜样装置[28,67]，可控制出口
- 特殊的造瘘，如一个导管样造瘘袋[36,47]

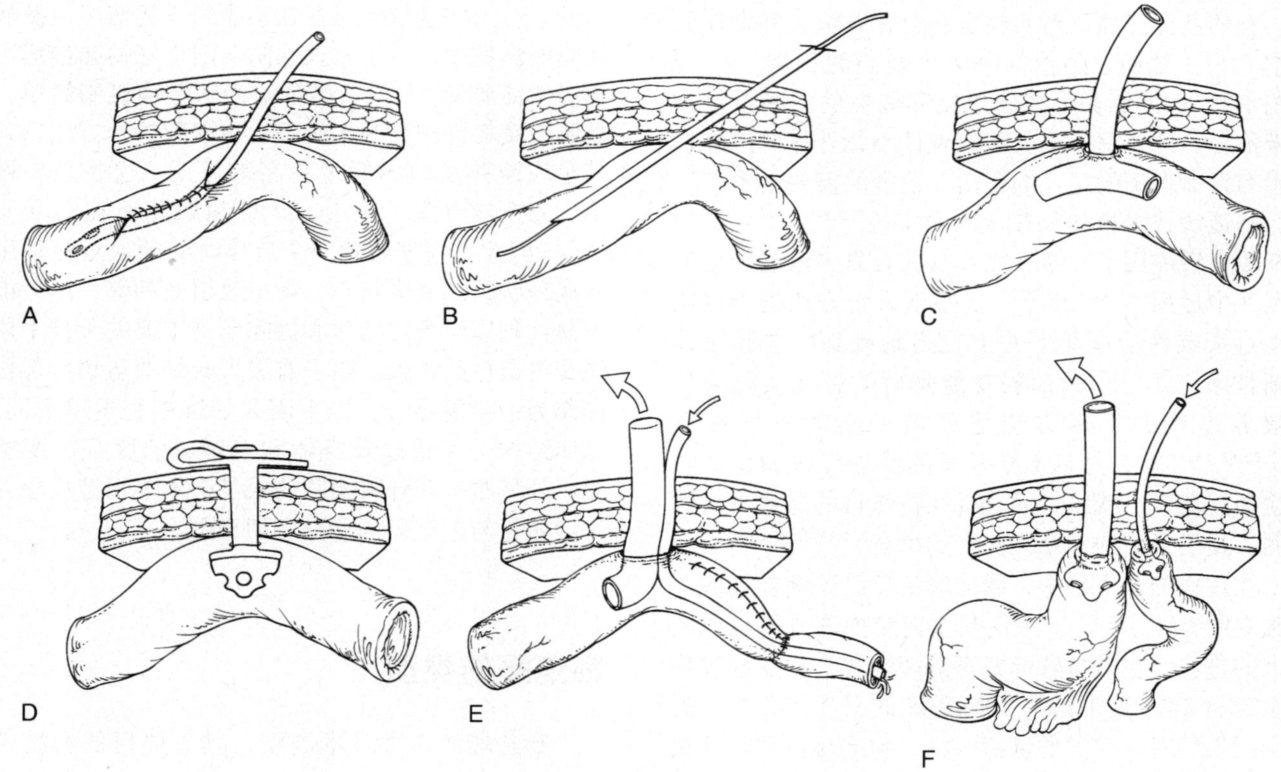

图 96-1 选择性营养以及减压-营养空肠造瘘的图示。A. 隧道样导管[98]。B. 针式导管[3]。C. T 管[41]。D. 纽扣[88]。E. 近端减压和远端营养管通过吻合口[71]。F. 当初期吻合不安全并且不能做肠外露时暂时性的减压营养用导管[35]。

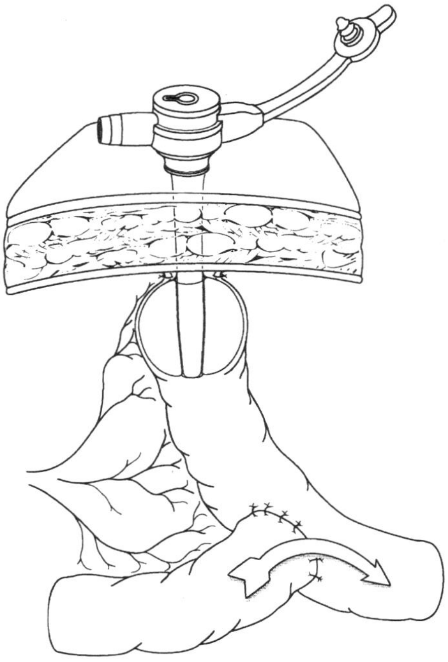

图 96-2 Roux-en-Y 营养性空肠造瘘并有一个球囊样皮肤通路装置[20]。

表 96-2 肠造瘘出口

近端造瘘
- 通过盲肠切口
- 通过分开的开口
- 远近端肠管靠在一起
- 远近端分开的开口
- 多个造瘘
- 以上多种结合

远端造瘘
- 黏膜瘘管外翻接近或远离近端肠管
- 部分关闭并靠近近端造瘘口
- 关闭并放在腹腔内
- 放置导管后关闭，并作为接下来灌洗或造影检查的通路

胃管减压结合经空肠吻合口喂养对于选择性十二指肠或高位空肠闭锁的患儿来说是一种古老而有效的疗法[16,34]。多种外露空肠类型被应用于胆道闭锁的患

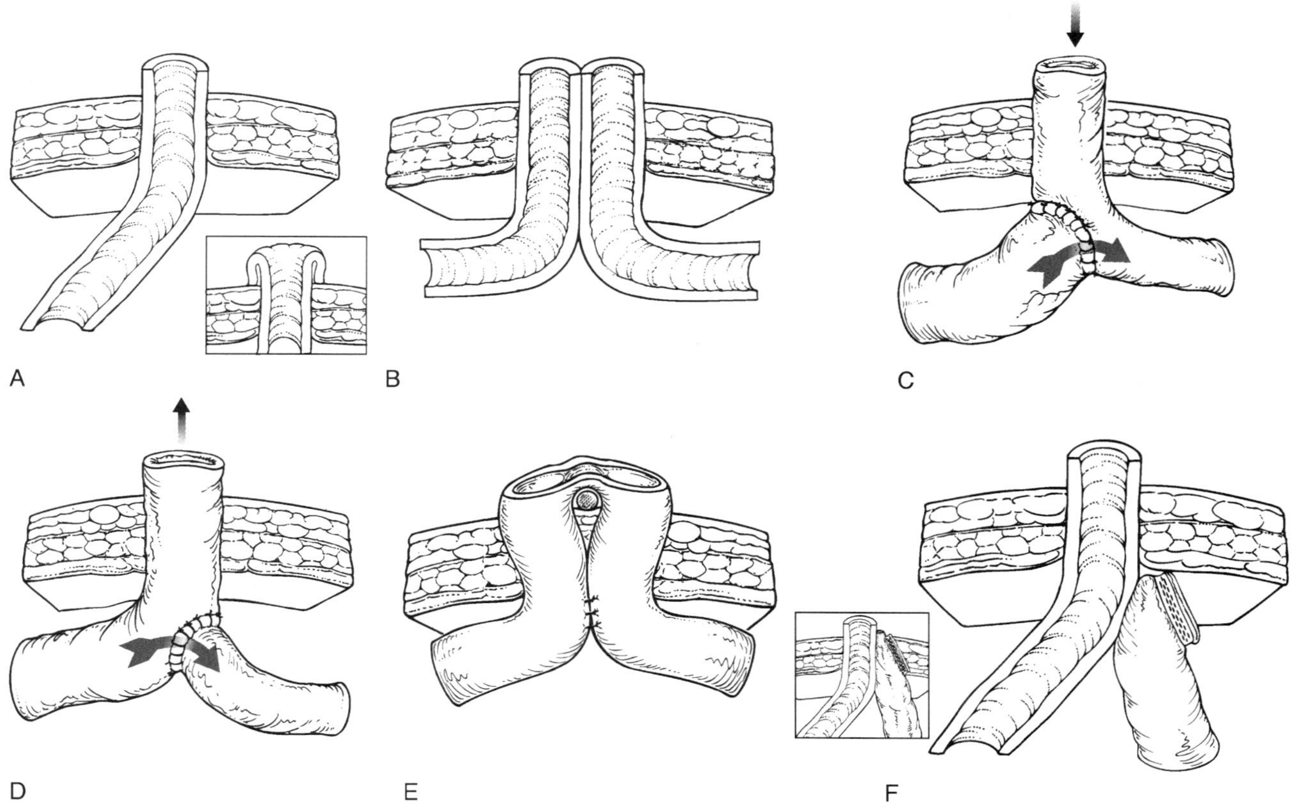

图 96-3 减压、改道或排空造瘘图示。A. 单腔造瘘（小图显示典型的样式）[10]。B. 双腔造瘘[55]。C. 端侧吻合并远端作灌洗[5]。D. 侧端吻合并近端排出[76]。E. 肠袢式造瘘[54]。F. 单腔造瘘并筋膜下远端肠管一端关闭（小图显示无棒的单袢式造瘘[92]）。

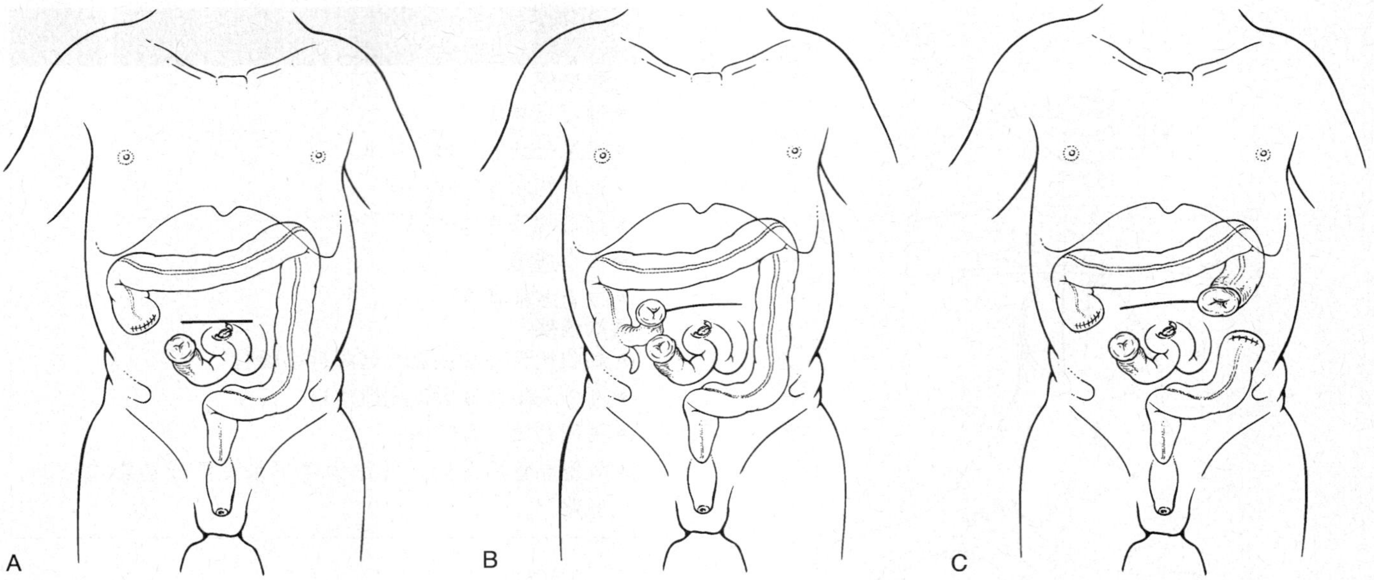

图 96-4　婴儿肠切除后造瘘部位选择图示。A. 近端肠管通过一个对缝切口拖出外露并远端肠管关闭放在腹壁下。B. 步骤同 A. 远端肠管通过切口边缘外露。C. 两段肠管切除后的排列。

儿[42]。然而，因为有继发性的问题出现如与门脉高
1482 压相关的造瘘口出血，运用该手术方式的积极性有所下降[83]。另一方面，介于膀胱和腹壁的一段肠管可以用于胆汁淤积症的儿童，作为部分胆汁外引流通道[24,36]。当有腹膜炎或肠缺血存在时，空肠切除后，应做肠造褛或肠管减压[1,40,61,73]。

当初级吻合术不能做或不安全时，回肠造瘘被广泛地应用。典型的指征包括坏死性小肠结肠炎（图 96-7和 96-8）或其他严重的腹腔内病变[1,40,52,56,61,73]。远端小肠造瘘对处理新生儿的肠梗阻是必不可少的，如长段型巨结肠、复杂的胎粪性肠梗阻和腹裂伴有肠闭锁[5,41,56,69]。回肠造瘘亦广泛应用于溃疡性结肠炎

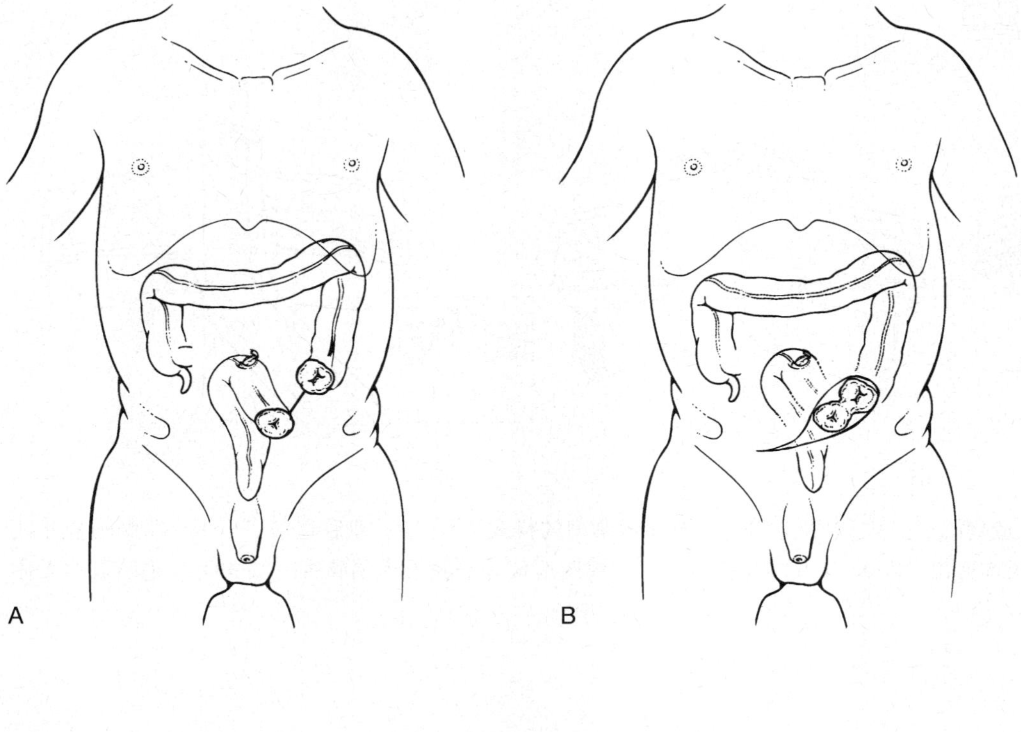

图 96-5　乙状结肠造瘘。A. 分开的造瘘口。近端肠管在切口的上端，下面为黏膜瘘管。B. 袢式结肠造瘘。外露肠管在一根棒或皮桥上，或者通过缝线的帮助完成。造瘘卸除和拖出时使用菱形切口。

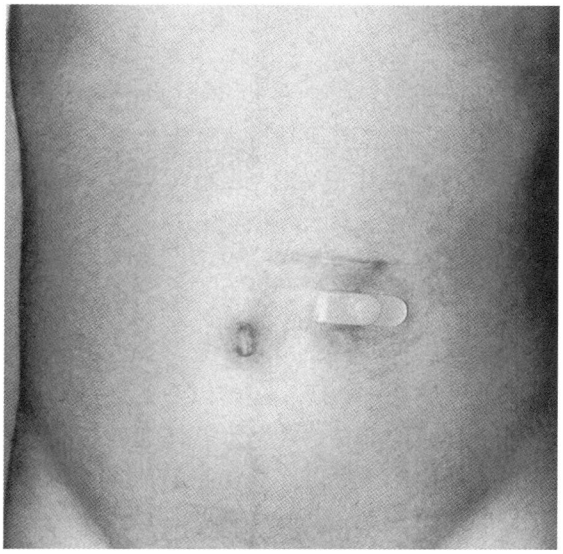

图 96-6　囊性纤维病患儿使用空肠纽扣式造瘘提供营养，通过一个对缝切口安置皮肤水平装置。

483 和家族性息肉病，作为暂时性、预防性或者永久性的造瘘[10,30,31,47,52,67,91,97]。

盲肠造瘘、阑尾造瘘以及乙状结肠造瘘（图 96-9）被用作有复杂的肛门括约肌和后肠问题或脊髓发育不良的儿童冲洗肠管的进入点[22,37,81,85]。

结肠造瘘的历史最长[77]，多种状况的处理，包

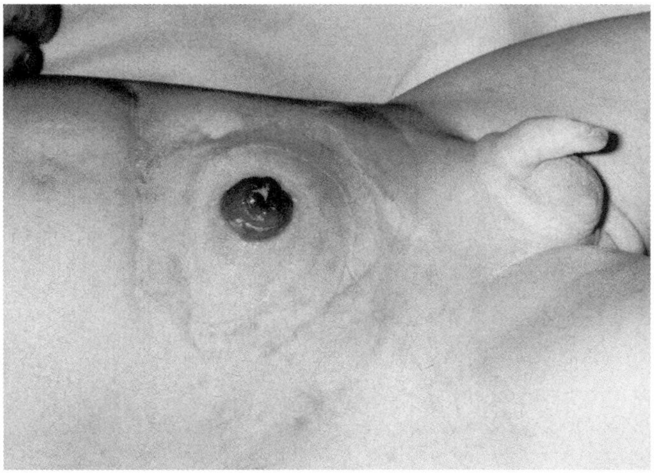

图 96-7　一个没有远端回肠的严重坏死性小肠结肠炎的男孩，其结肠在再吻合前下降至腹膜返折处。液体状大便妨碍了患儿早期肠连续性的重建。注意装置标记和与切口、脐部、腹股沟腹壁褶皱以及右髂前上棘的合适距离。

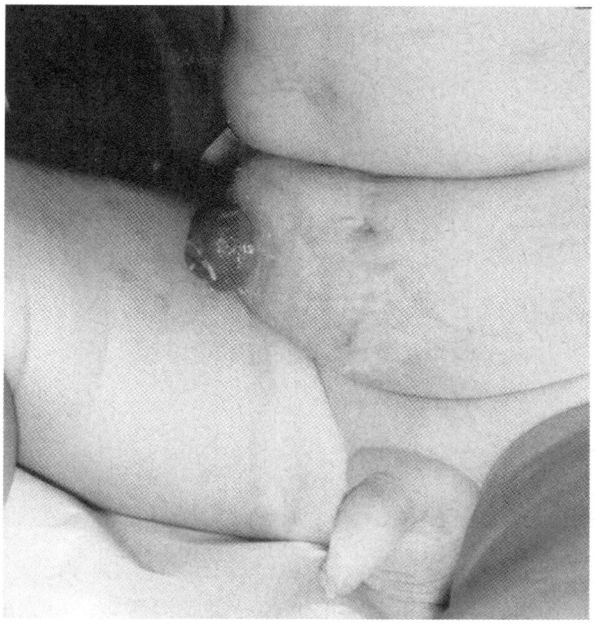

图 96-8　图 96-7 中的同一男孩的坐姿，注意到脐上横切口所产生的较深的皱痕，一个通过这样的切口拖出的造瘘口将不能很好地使用造瘘袋，有必要进行修正。

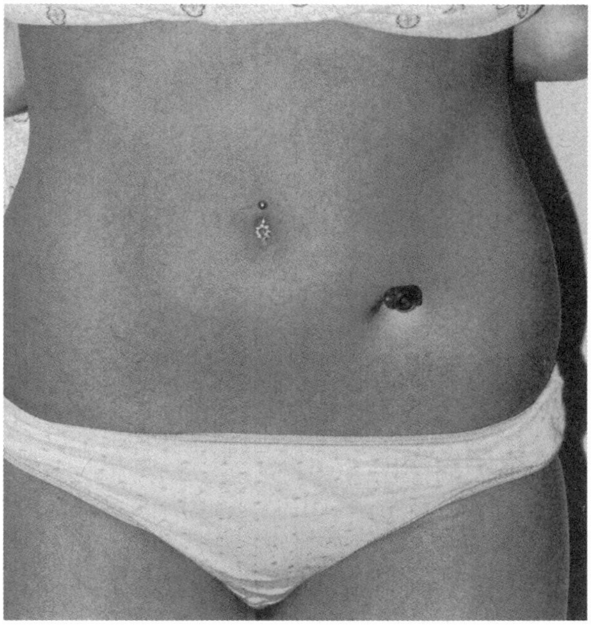

图 96-9　一个 16 岁患者乙状结肠冲洗管放置后 7 年。她从婴儿期在没有灌肠情况下就不能排空大便。直肠活检是正常的。结肠不透光标志物传输试验和肛门检测确定了盆底功能不良的诊断，同时伴发获得性巨直肠症并且出现直肠敏感性阈值提高，她对松弛反应、生物反馈治疗已经没有反应了。她自己每 2～3 天用 600～900 ml 清水冲洗，没有排便相关的并发症。皮肤装置已经换了两套。

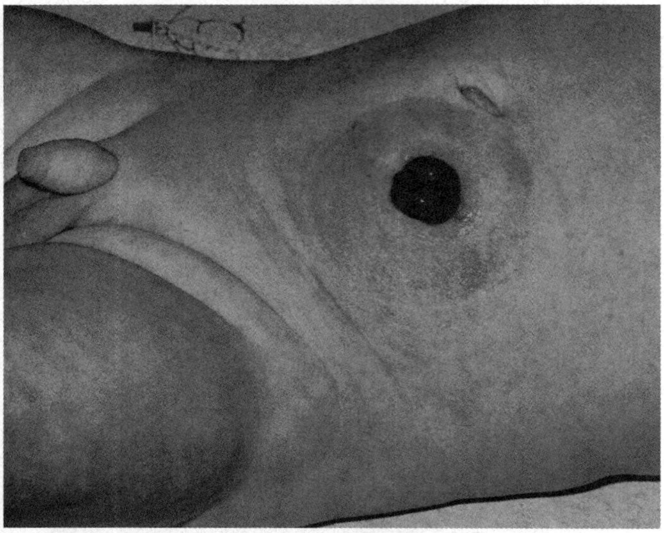

图 96-10 一个 5 个月大的高位肛门闭锁患儿。高位乙状结肠袢式造瘘与脐部、髂前上棘和腹股沟褶皱是等距的，原始的切口比造瘘口稍长些，注意在两肠腔间开起的“骨刺”，对适当的大便改道很有必要。

1484 括高位肛门闭锁（图 96-10）以及复杂的骨盆畸形、巨结肠、结肠闭锁、结肠或肛门直肠外伤和恶性病变为造瘘积累了大量的经验。回肠或结肠的外翻段曾被用作尿路构建。然而，随着现代尿道再建技术的发展，这种方法很少应用于儿童[43]。另一方面，游离的阑尾被用作通向膀胱的管道[57,86]。

肠造瘘的选择

喂养性空肠造瘘

留置鼻空肠和胃空肠管仅适用于短时或间歇性的应用（几天到几周）[34,74]，因为它们易于阻塞、移位以及引起肠穿孔。由于一般的直、长的导管[98]（见图96-1A 和 B）固定和替换较困难，我们倾向于在婴儿和年龄较小的儿童中用 T 管[88]（见图 96-1C）。在年长儿中用纽扣样造瘘（见图 96-1D 和 96-6）做空肠长期通路。在这些空肠造瘘中，通过使用传统的腹腔切开术、经皮内镜或腹腔镜技术使肠管直接附着于腹壁上，如同胃造瘘一样[12,62,74]。在管理过程中 T 管和纽扣造瘘管两者皆是可更换的，方法是使用带线引导的可替换的直管[80]。因为有发生造瘘口漏的可能，所以一些外科医生倾向于做 R-Y 空肠造瘘，或者是在原始部位做可插入导管的黏膜通道或者是改良方法，改良方法使用一根导管或一个皮肤水平装置进入附着在壁腹膜上的肠袢内（见图 96-2）[20,100]。

回肠造瘘

了解儿童的病理状况、年龄以及估计造瘘口的长度有助于造瘘口的选择。在新生儿坏死性小肠结肠炎或其他主要的腹内病变需要肠切除的情况下，我倾向于（见图 96-3A）通过另一个戳孔切口将一个单腔造瘘口拖出（见图 96-4A～C 和 96-7）。一个更方便的方法是将近端肠管从切口末端拖出。然而，以我的经验，该方法更易发生伤口并发症；并且如果造瘘口需放置较长时间加上儿童的生长，通过回盲部切口产生的褶皱可能会干扰造瘘口装置的服帖（见图96-7 和 96-8）。预期到一个有活力的远端肠管有回缩可能，我先关闭远端肠管口，并且把它放在接近近端造瘘口的腹腔内（图 96-11）。另外，一个黏膜瘘的外置术需要慎重对待（见图 96-4B）。应用肠袢代替单腔造瘘口可为肠管系膜提供最充分的血供。双腔造瘘是另

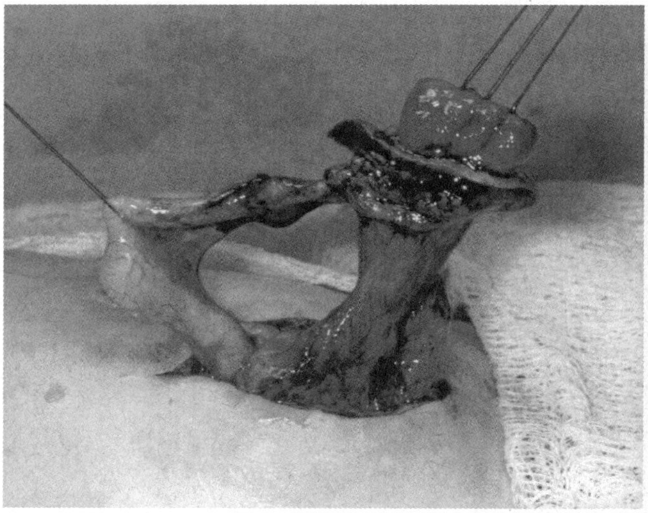

图 96-11 一个 4 个月大的患有腹裂和小肠闭锁患儿在进行肠道连续性的重建。通过脐孔将扩张和水肿的回肠作为单腔造口拖出，近端关闭的结肠端附着在回肠一侧的腹壁下，这种方式可快速识别远端肠管，减少切口和分离的范围。

一个选择（见图 96–3B）。为了保住尽可能多的肠管，可能有必要做多个造瘘口（见图96–4C）。在溃疡性结肠炎或家族性息肉病的患儿中，进行肠造瘘遵循的
485 原则与成人的相似（见图 96–3A；96–12B 和 96–13）。一个暂时性保护性回肠改道的造瘘的选择包括一个单纯肠袢（见图 96–3E）、一个末端肠袢（见图 96–3F）以及在筋膜下的一个末端关闭的单腔造瘘（见图 96–3F）。

阑尾造瘘、管状盲肠造瘘、管状乙状结肠造瘘

有几种途径，无论是从左或右半结肠进入，均可进行逆行灌肠。如果阑尾存在，可通过一个开口外置阑尾[22,85]，瓣膜的功能可有可无，也可以运用腹腔镜辅助技术完成；如果没有阑尾，盲肠壁可以被卷成管状拖至皮肤上。另外，导管[81]或皮肤上装置，如纽扣样结构[88]，可通过开腹或腹腔镜手术放置。对于结肠动力正常的患儿，灌肠液直接进入乙状结肠可能具有生理上的优势（见图 96–9）[37]。

结肠造瘘

大多数结肠造瘘口位于三种部位：右侧横结肠、左侧横结肠和乙状结肠。无肛患儿做大便改道与肠造瘘的主要不同点在表 96–3 已列出。我们倾向于做一个高位乙状结肠袢式造瘘（见图 96–5B 和96–10）。然而分开结肠断端，尤其在男孩中（见图 96–5A）[32]，已经成为一种强烈推荐的替代方法[14,96]。分开的优势是可以减少尿道感染以及减少造瘘口脱垂，在远端肠管最为明显。缺点包括一个较长的切口，伤口存在更多潜在的危险，并且在新生儿中放置造瘘口装置较困难，或者体重增长时产生褶皱。

巨结肠患儿最好的造瘘口位于移行段近端扩张的结肠，因为该段结肠有正常的神经节细胞。通常选择袢式造瘘，因为其结构简单并且容易拆除。由于大多数移行区位于乙状结肠，正确手术时，将造瘘口定

表 96–3　肛门闭锁的结肠造瘘

乙状结肠造瘘	
优点	**缺点**
直肠乙结肠腹膜返折可正确识别肠袢	如果低位或中间位乙状结肠造瘘，拖出的肠管长度可能不够
大便较硬，不是总需要造瘘袋，较少发生表皮脱落或脱水	可能干扰血供
在使用袢式造瘘时，由于大便较硬，很少进入远端肠管	有远端梗阻、乙状结肠可能大于横结肠
造瘘口脱垂发生率低	
尿液吸收的表面积较少	
远端结肠较易清洗	
结肠造影较易进行	
上腹部没有瘢痕	
横结肠造瘘	
优点	**缺点**
肠管长度足够	大便松，尤其在右半结肠，必须要有造瘘袋，皮肤反应和脱水较常见
较易游离	脱垂发生率高
直径较小，并且胎粪较少	
	在远端肠管，尿液的吸收面积较大
	远端肠管的清洗较困难或不可能
	上腹部瘢痕更明显

于左下腹（见图 96-5B）。然而，有时更倾向于做一个单腔造瘘，因为大量的肠管扩张会使袢式造瘘难以构建以及术后较难管理。如果选择分开式造瘘，远端肠管较短时，远端肠管只做对缝。由于黏膜不能被合理地排空或清洗掉，因此在所有其他病例中，不宜采用这个方法。尽管在儿童中没有获得相似的统计资料，但在成人中已全部采用袢式结肠造瘘[59]。

技术方面

通过“开放”技术造瘘放置喂养管时，通过左上腹的小切口到达近端空肠（见图 96-6）。确认 Treitz韧带，在距 Treitz 韧带 10～20 cm 的空肠前系膜侧放置导管或皮肤水平装置。用多丝可吸收合成线在
1486 造瘘口周围做荷包样路线缝合并打结。导管通过另外一个切口取出。第二个荷包样线路缝合，用可吸收单丝合成线进行缝合，缝线在导管拖出处的腹壁与肠管间交替。固定后第二肠浆膜层在不透水的情况下接近体壁腹膜[34,88]。这种方式的替代方法为经皮内镜下空肠造瘘术和腹腔镜辅助的空肠造瘘术[74]。

减压回肠造瘘通常位于右下腹（见图 96-4 和 96-7）。图 96-12A 列举了新生儿、婴幼儿和小年龄儿童中（如患有坏死性小肠结肠炎的儿童）合适的和不合适的造瘘口部位，图 96-12B 展示了大年龄儿童或青少年的理想造瘘口部位（如溃疡性结肠炎或家族性息肉病患儿）。在需长期或永久造瘘的患儿中应避免下腹部切口，因为这样的切口产生的不平坦表面会干扰造瘘装置的依附。脐孔是一个造瘘可取的部位[29]，尤其对近端肠管扩张、同时有腹裂和小肠闭锁的新生儿尤为适合（见图 96-11）。在儿童中，在做腹壁切口前，尽可能将选择好的造瘘口位置或候选位置在腹壁上进行标记，这对患儿是有帮助的。该计划既适宜于选择性病人又适合于急诊状况，对于选择性病人的长期造瘘口最好在手术前 1 天做好定位标记（图 96-13）。造瘘口的位置应定位于腹直肌中线的凸面上，远离切口、脐部、骨头突出以及皮肤折叠处。要特别留意超重的患儿因为其有腹壁较深的皱痕产生。当在婴幼儿小肠造瘘使用一个对缝切口时，我有几次用眼科环锯，因为这种有不同直径的环形切割装置，可以在腹壁腹直肌前形成一个直径几厘米、边缘锐利的圆形切口。用电刀或单纯分离做腹直肌横行切口。腹直肌后壁作横行或环形切开。在年长儿中，我倾向于在做中线垂直的腹腔切口之前为计划好的回肠造口术选择开放方式的切口，该切口可获得直接的进入途径，并可避免在切口边缘拖曳引起肌层扭转。切

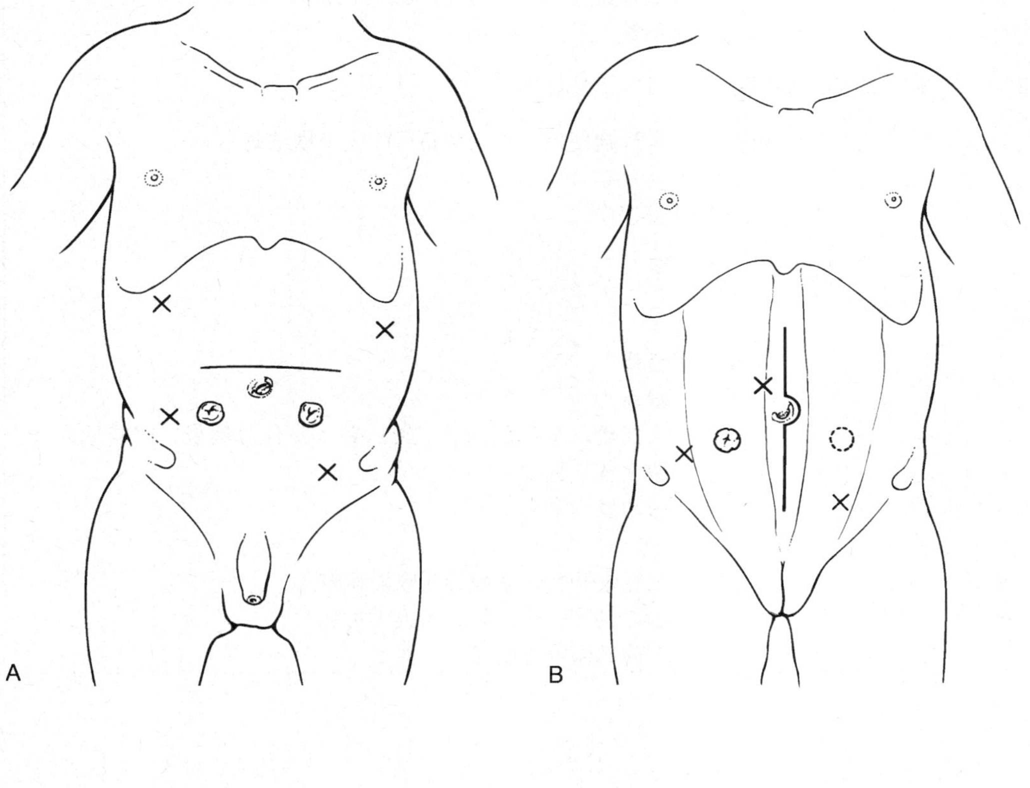

图 96-12　理想的造瘘点：A. 婴儿，单腔造瘘可通过对缝切口在右下腹或左下腹拖出，“X”标记处不适合做造瘘，因为太靠近肋缘、髂前上棘、胸廓或腹膜沟。B. 大年龄儿童或青少年，最好的造瘘点位于右下腹腹直肌中段，对侧点亦可选择，标记“X”区域不适宜做造瘘。

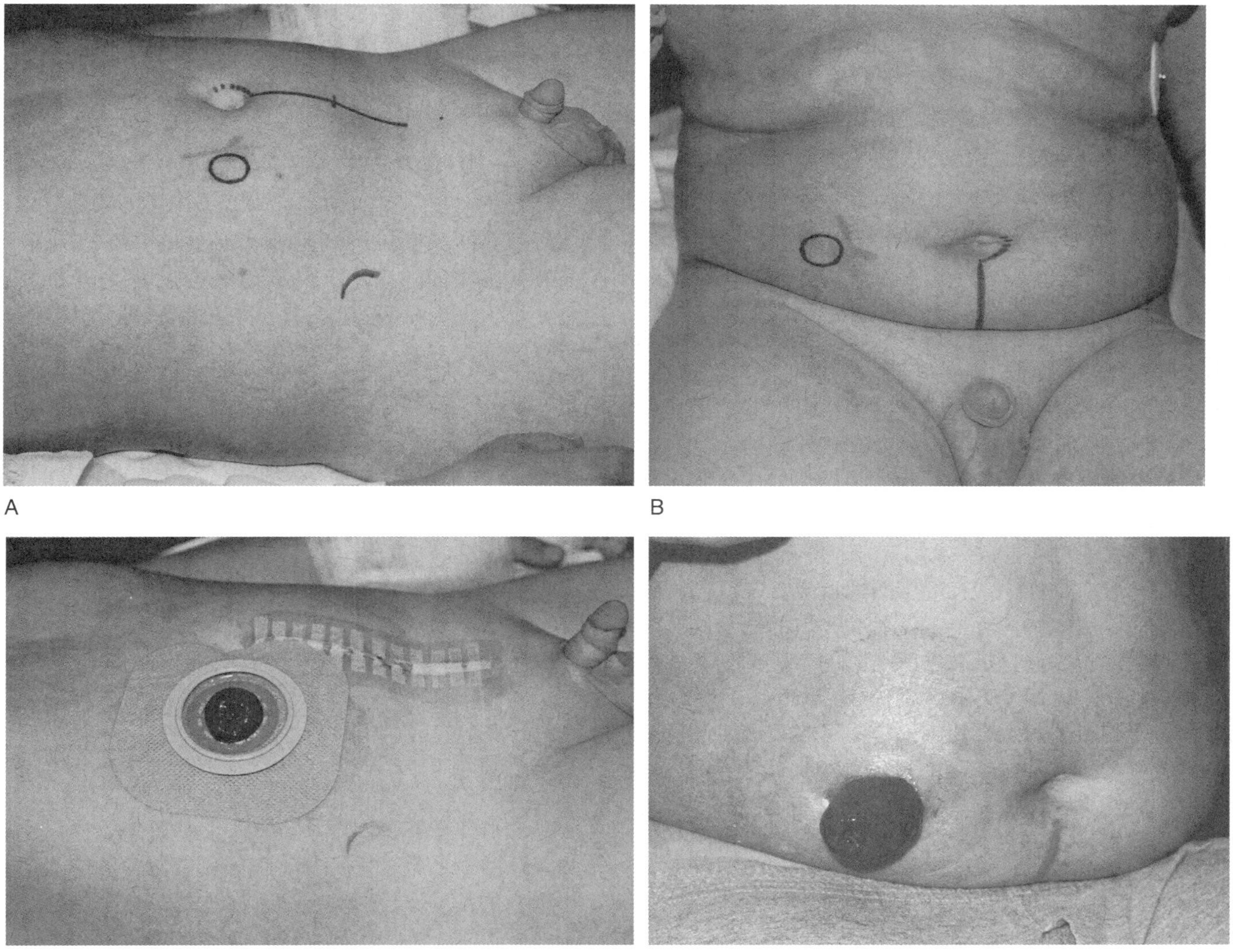

A　B　C　D

图 96-13　一个患有难治性溃疡性结炎的 8 岁男孩，进一步的药物治疗失败，包括皮质类固醇激素、硫唑嘌呤和 Inffiximab，他做了一个全结肠切除和回肠造瘘，作为回肠肛管吻合的过渡期。A. 患儿平卧位，造瘘点几天前就决定好了，男孩被要求戴上双件套的造瘘袋，用选好的位点作为引导。B. 将麻醉好的患儿改为坐姿，确认造瘘口部位远离腹壁的主要褶皱。C. 在结肠切除完成后，用法兰作皮肤屏障（二件套装置）粘贴于回肠造瘘口。D. 6 周后，造瘘口愈合很好，只有轻度残余水肿。E. 该男孩戴上一个附有透明造瘘袋的二件套装置，他白天排空集粪袋 3～4 次，晚上排空 2～3 次。他能参加体育运动，包括打篮球，他不需要使用造瘘绷带，并且每 3 天更换一次皮肤屏障和造瘘袋。

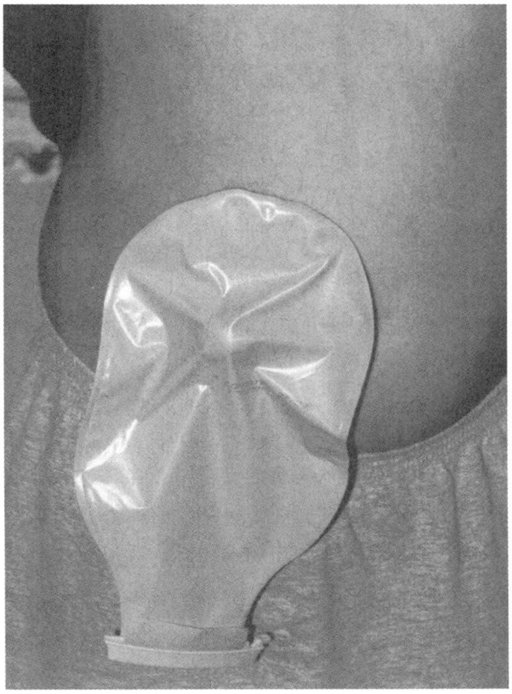

E

口应大小刚好使回肠顺利拖出，而且不影响其血液供应。基于患儿的体形，皮肤上回肠造瘘口的大小可以从1厘米到几厘米，以便固定合适的造瘘袋。

新生儿造瘘，尤其是为那些坏死性小肠结肠炎患儿造瘘，应避免缝合固定，因为它将影响已经脆弱的血液供应。外露的造瘘口末端用合成的可吸收线与皮肤做四针单纯的缝合，并涂抹抗生素软膏，且不要覆盖敷料，大便排出后用集粪袋黏附于造瘘口。婴幼儿黏膜生长速度要快于外露的浆膜层。大年龄儿童的瘘口应直接缝于腹壁组织上，并且该技术一开始就已成熟了（见图96-2A）。应避免深的全层缝合，因为这会产生从肠管到腹膜组织的瘘管。一些医生不论患儿的年龄如何都不固定造瘘口，因为直立外翻的肠管在没有额外缝线时能自动翻转。在大年龄患儿中，我将回肠袢从腹腔内移至腹壁，这样可以预防扭转和内疝，也可减少脱垂的可能。手术结束时，再黏附上造瘘袋。

1488 左下腹应是优先选择的结肠造瘘点。在肛门闭锁的患儿中，腹腔打开后要辨认胎粪充填的乙状结肠和盆腔腹膜返折，选择近端乙状结肠的合适部位，并且使肠管外露。使用断开技术时（见图96-5A），使造瘘口位于切口的两端，用细的合成可吸收线将肠管缝合至腹壁的所有层次。两个开口之间要有足够的空间使造瘘袋能覆盖在近端造瘘口上（或者远端造瘘口皮肤必须清洗）。为避免造瘘口过分狭窄，在关闭伤口时，应将一个大小合适的黑加宫颈扩张器或导管放入肠腔内。单腔造瘘口应只轻度脱出皮面，做一个袢式造瘘（见图96-5B和96-10），切口长度为肠袢的长度或轻度延长。要通过所选择肠段的系膜放置导管，然后将这段肠管提出皮面。靠近两个造瘘口的每一边固定三针，并且每一边与腹膜固定，以防止内疝发生。整圈肠壁固定在腹膜和筋膜上，缝线将肠管后壁提起高出皮面。我已经不再放置黑加宫颈扩张器或导管，因为它们会影响装置的适配[79]。纵向切开肠管并使其边缘外翻。所有肛门闭锁患儿其远端充填胎粪的肠管，在结肠造瘘时都要被冲洗干净，这对避免粪块的形成很重要。巨结肠患儿，袢式造瘘时也必须非常细致，包括将已扩张的肠管绷紧以降低肠管脱垂的可能（见图96-10）。

为方便以后小肠或大肠造瘘的拆卸，肠管的两端应靠近；然而，必须避免干扰造瘘袋。如果远端肠袢被放在腹壁下，用不可吸收缝线或一个金属夹（或两者）做标记并使其尽可能靠近造瘘口以便能方便地确认并做再吻合。放置一个金属夹有助于用X片显示远端肠管的近端。这对患有坏死性小肠结肠炎的患儿在重建肠管的连续性前进行钡剂灌肠时尤其有帮助。

造瘘口护理

适当的造瘘口护理是相当必要的。在离开医院前和接下来的随访中，必须要教会患儿父母和大龄患儿本人如何护理造瘘口。回肠造瘘和近端结肠造瘘总需要集粪袋。对于乙状结肠造瘘后形成的成形粪便，一些父母用一个皮肤屏障、卫生纸以及尿布代替集粪袋。大多数造瘘装置可以购买到，包括适合所有年龄和尺寸的一次性的和反复使用的集粪袋，甚至适合最小的早产儿尺寸的产品都可以购买到。产品中有皮肤屏障、黏合剂、粉剂、有开口的集粪袋以及清除异味的溶液，这都为今天的人工造瘘者提供了方便[7,17,19,52,60,91,97]。

合适恰当的装置可以放置几天，3天是过得去的。有两个小儿基本类型装置：一片集粪袋装置，其中皮肤黏合屏障已经黏附于集粪袋上，两片装置其皮肤黏合屏障与集粪袋是分开的。在后者中，这两片装置通过一个法兰胶合在一起（看图96-13C和E）。由于现在的皮肤黏合屏障具有较强的结合力，所以不必另外用纱带或带来固定它。在集粪袋附带的造瘘口大小模板的帮助下，可剪出合适的造瘘口皮肤屏障。除了医生、护士，以及肠造瘘治疗专家提供的用法说明外，我们还鼓励父母与肠造瘘社团工作者取得联系并利用更多的教育材料[46,52,60,97]。尽管已经尝试使用特殊的腹腔内肠道集粪袋[26,47]、磁性帽子[28]、短球囊导管的“自制的肠造瘘”[67]以及其他腔内闭合形式[52,97]，但在儿童中进行这种手术或使用这种装置的经验仍有限[26]。

在造瘘口周围皮肤上的念珠菌感染仍是一个难题，局部抗真菌药应在炎症出现早期就开始使用。感染一般伴有表皮脱落，所以该区域应暴露在空气中，并且同时使用一个人造屏障，吹风机对此是非常有帮助的。轻度造瘘口出血通常自行止住，硝酸银可以用来控制早期皮肤黏膜交界处周围肉芽组织的增生。残留的缝线可能成为感染源，所以应该去除。我不常规地扩张造瘘口，偶尔才冲洗远端肠管。在更严重的并发症出现前，功能不良的造瘘口通常需要早期进行手术卸除或修正。饮食和选择性药物的运用对形成成形大便有帮助，高位回肠造瘘的患儿必须仔细监护以防电解质失衡和营养吸收不充分[8,27,38,44]。

肠道连续性的再建

肠造瘘口关闭的时间很大程度上依赖于以下状况，儿童的健康状况和肠造瘘相关并发症的发生情况[45,61,94]。不必要地延迟肠连续性的再建易增加并发症的发生率，应尽量避免[4,14]。越近端的造瘘口，应越早关闭，以减少并发症[14,27,38]。进行造瘘并需切除缺血性肠管的患儿必须在术前做远端肠管造影，以排除肠管狭窄或完全性肠腔闭锁。小肠肠管连续性的再建一般不需要肠道准备。结肠造瘘关闭时要在传统灌肠器的辅助下进行逆行灌肠。尽管，我常规在围术期静脉给予抗生素，但我不用肠腔内抗生素溶液。当肠
489 道连续性再建涉及左半结肠或乙状结肠时，我在直肠内放置一根软的导管，以便在术中辨认肠袢。良好的暴露和充分游离的肠管盲端是非常重要的。尽管，腹膜外关闭亦已用于儿童，但是不推荐常规使用[18]。进行肠道吻合时，我用细的可吸收合成线单层缝合伤口。

表 96-4　肠造瘘常见并发症
脱垂
狭窄
回缩
伤口分开、开裂
伤口感染、术后败血症
造瘘口旁疝
换导管后肠壁分开或穿孔
错误的肠管或断端外露
肠梗阻（粘连、内疝）
肠扭转缺血
瘘管形成
营养或冲洗管穿孔
造瘘袋不匹配或漏
精神创伤
皮肤表皮脱落、念珠菌感染、皮炎
黏膜脱落和出血
黏膜皮肤交界处肉芽组织
门脉高压的静脉曲张出血
电解质失衡
酸中毒（远端肠管吸收尿液引起）
大便嵌塞（远端肠袢）

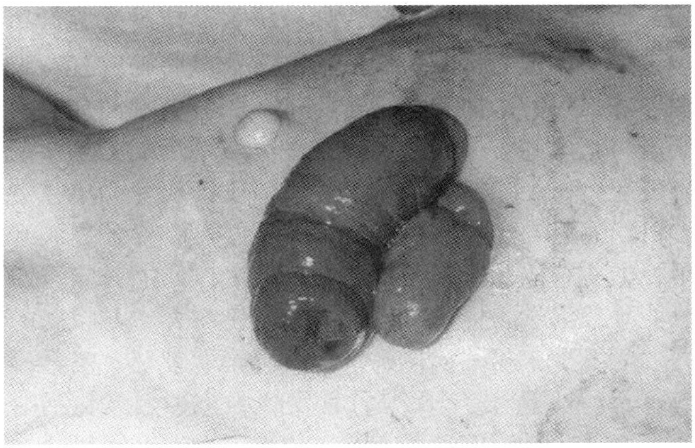

图 96-14　一个患有 Down 综合征和巨结肠病的 6 个月大的患儿，左半结构袢式造瘘后出现远端结肠脱垂，可以看到在大的翻转肠袢的末端有 3 个开口，包括盲端腔、回盲瓣开口以及阑尾腔。

造瘘口并发症

涉及小肠和大肠造瘘口的构建、护理和造瘘口关闭的并发症数量众多而且非常常见，并可导致较高的患病率并偶有死亡（表 96-4）。对儿童的系列分析表明并发症率通常达到有时甚至超过 50% *。此外造瘘口的修正或早期卸除通常是必要的[45,56,58,94]。基础疾病会加重用作喂养的肠造瘘的并发症，尤其是营养不良、神经系统受损的患儿[12,82,100]。用于小肠排空的造瘘的相关发病率要比结肠的高，因为这些造瘘伴有液体、电解质和吸收物质丢失[8,27,38]。横结肠造瘘比乙状结肠造瘘更易发生并发症[2,14,15,32,58]，在几个造瘘方式中，分开的结肠造瘘要优于袢式结肠造瘘[14,32,96]（图 96-14）。

较常见的严重并发症是脱垂、狭窄和回缩†。儿童造瘘口脱垂的发生率高达 21.7%[11]，如果远端肠袢外露的话其发生率更高‡，大的脱垂需要立即干预，通常需要在全麻下进行肠管回纳。暂时性控制脱垂的方法包括改良的荷包缝线技术[39,49,50]或从回纳肠管的肠腔放置一个 U 形缝线，在通过腹壁时，内外都放置小拭子，小拭子使肠管背对腹壁并且防止缝线切割。造瘘口狭窄如果较轻，扩张有效[11,58]。然而，如果

* 见参考文献 2，11，14，23，40，53，56，58，64~66，70，72，78，87，94.

† 见参考文献 2，4，11，14，40，56，58，64~66，78.

‡ 见参考文献 2，5，11，14，15，32，56，58，70，78.

排大便减少，并且近端肠管开始扩张，建议修改造瘘口。这个方法通常需要切除狭窄造瘘口周围所有的腹壁层并拖出健康的肠管，有时是扩张的肠管。开口不必过大，因为它可能会导致脱垂。如果问题更复杂或出现造瘘口旁疝时，通过对缝切口进行治疗。单腔造瘘口回缩可导致造瘘装置黏附困难并可能导致皮肤水平处的狭窄以及梗阻。如果袢式造瘘口回缩影响排便可能导致远端肠袢充满大便。肠道再吻合亦与较高的并发症发生率相关，特别是伤口感染、裂开、瘘管形成以及肠梗阻[14,45,58,64,94]。其发病的多种因素包括时间不合适、肠道准备不充分、技术错误和缝线材料选择不当以及电烙术的过分使用等。营养不良、虚弱、贫血和激素治疗的患儿发生并发症的风险最大，这些致病因素在进行肠道连续性建立之前应纠正。

1490 任何造瘘口的安装和卸除应仔细计划，应被考虑为主要程序，其要求包括理想的手术条件、一个教育环境和合适的监管。儿童肠造瘘与成人造瘘大不相同，对细节保持谨慎的重要性不容忽视。

（严志龙译 叶祖萍校）

参考文献

1. Alaish SM, Krummel TM, Bagwell CE, et al: Loop enterostomy in newborns with necrotizing enterocolitis. J Am Coll Surg 1996;182:457-458.
2. Al-Salem AH, Grant C, Khawaja S: Colostomy complications in infants and children. Int Surg 1992;77:164-166.
3. Andrassy RJ, Page CP, Feldtman RW, et al: Continual catheter administration of an elemental diet in infants and children. Surgery 1977;82:205-210.
4. Bakx R, Busch OR, Benelman WA, et al: Morbidity of temporary loop ileostomies. Dig Surg 2004;21:277-281.
5. Bishop HC, Koop CE: Management of meconium ileus: Resection, Roux-en-Y anastomosis and ileostomy irrigation with pancreatic enzymes. Ann Surg 1957;145:410-414.
6. Bishop HC: Colostomy in the newborn: Indications, techniques, complications and care. Am J Surg 1961;101:642-648.
7. Borkowski S: Pediatric stomas, tubes, and appliances. Pediatr Clin North Am 1998;45:1419-1435.
8. Bower TR, Pringle KC, Soper RT: Sodium deficit causing decreased weight gain and metabolic acidosis in infants with ileostomy. J Pediatr Surg 1988;23:567-572.
9. Branagan G, Tromans A, Finnis D: Effect of stoma formation on bowel care and quality of life in patients with spinal cord injury. Spinal Cord 2003;41:680-683.
10. Brooke BN: Historical perspectives. In Dozois RR (ed): Alternatives to Conventional Ileostomy. Chicago, Year Book Medical Publishers, 1985, pp 19-28.
11. Cain WS, Kieswetter WB: Infant colostomy. Arch Surg 1965;91:314-320.
12. Campos AC, Marchesini JB: Recent advances in the placement of tubes for enteral nutrition. Curr Opin Clin Nutr Metab Care 1999;2:265-269.
13. Caldamone AA, Emmens RW, Rabinowitz R: Hyperchloremic acidosis and imperforate anus. J Urol 1979;122:817-818.
14. Chandramouli B, Srinivasan K, Jagdish S, et al: Morbidity and mortality of colostomy and its closure in children. J Pediatr Surg 2004;39:596-599.
15. Chowdhary SK, Chalapathi G, Narasimhan KL, et al: An audit of neonatal colostomy for high anorectal malformations: The developing world perspective. Pediatr Surg Int 2004;20:111-113.
16. Coln D, Cywes S: Simultaneous drainage gastrostomy and feeding jejunostomy in the newborn. Surg Gynecol Obstet 1977;145:594-595.
17. Cooney DE, Grosfeld JL: Care of the child with a colostomy. Pediatrics 1977;59:469-472.
18. Das S: Extraperitoneal closure of colostomy in children. J Indian Med Assoc 1991;89:253-255.
19. Davies A: Children with ostomies: Parents helping parents. JET Nurs 1992;19:207-212.
20. DeCou JM, Shorter NA, Karl SR: Feeding Roux-en-Y jejunostomy in the management of severely neurologically impaired children. J Pediatr Surg 1993;28:1276-1279.
21. Di Lorenzo C, Flores AF, Buie T, et al: Intestinal motility and jejunal feeding in children with chronic intestinal pseudo-obstruction. Gastroenterology 1995;108:1379-1385.
22. Driver CP, Barrow C, Fishwick J, et al: The Malone antegrade colonic enema procedure: Outcome and lessons of six years' experience. Pediatr Surg Int 1998;13:370-372.
23. Duchesne JC, Wang YZ, Weintraub SL, et al: Stoma complications: A multivariated analysis. Am Surg 2002;68:961-966.
24. Emond JC, Whitington PF: Selective surgical management of progressive familial intrahepatic cholestasis (Byler's disease). J Pediatr Surg 1995;30:1635-1641.
25. Ein SH: Divided loop colostomy that does not prolapse. Am J Surg 1984;147:250-252.
26. Ein SH: A ten-year experience with the pediatric Kock pouch. J Pediatr Surg 1987;22:764-766.
27. Festen C, Severijnen RSVM, vd Staak FHJ: Early closure of enterostomy after exteriorization of the small intestine for abdominal catastrophes. J Pediatr Surg 1987;22:144-145.
28. Feustel H, Henning G: Kontinente Kolostomie durch Magnetverschluss. Dtsch Med Wochenschr 1975;100:1063-1064.
29. Fitzgerald PG, Lau GY, Cameron GJ: Use of the umbilical site for temporary ostomy: Review of 47 cases. J Pediatr Surg 1989;24:973.
30. Fonkalsrud EW: Special aspects of ostomies in infancy and childhood. In Barker WF, et al (eds): The Creation and Care of Enterocutaneous Stomas. Curr Probl Surg 1975;12:54-62.
31. Fonkalsrud EW, Thakur A, Roof L: Comparison of loop versus end ileostomy for fecal diversion after restorative proctocolectomy for ulcerative colitis. J Am Coll Surg 2000;190:418-422.
32. Gauderer MWL: Colostomy for anorectal malformations—problems related to technique and management. In Hofmann V, Kap-herr S (eds): Anorektale Fehlbildungen. Stuttgart, Gustav Fisher, 1983, pp 99-104.
33. Gauderer MWL, Izant RJ Jr: A technique for temporary control of colostomy prolapse in children. J Pediatr Surg 1985;20:653-655.
34. Gauderer MWL, Stellato TA: Gastrostomies: Evolution,

techniques, indications and complications. Curr Probl Surg 1986;23:657-719.
35. Gauderer MWL: Double-tube enterostomy for temporary small bowel decompression. Pediatr Surg Int 1986;1:60-62.
36. Gauderer MWL, Boyle JT: Cholecystoappendicostomy in a child with Alagille syndrome. J Pediatr Surg 1997;32: 166-167.
37. Gauderer MWL, DeCou JM, Boyle JT: Sigmoid irrigation tube for the management of chronic evacuation disorders. J Pediatr Surg 2002;37:348-351.
38. Gertler JP, Seashore JH, Touloukian RJ: Early ileostomy closure in necrotizing enterocolitis. J Pediatr Surg 1987;22: 140-143.
39. Golladay ES, Bernay F, Wagner CW: Prevention of prolapse in pediatric enterostomies with purse string technique. J Pediatr Surg 1990;25:990-991.
40. Haberlik A, Hollworth ME, Windhager U, Schober PH: Problems of ileostomy in necrotizing enterocolitis. Acta Paediatr Suppl 1994;396:74-76.
41. Harberg FJ, Senekjian EK, Pokorny WJ: Treatment of uncomplicated meconium ileus via T-tube ileostomy. J Pediatr Surg 1981;16:61-63.
42. Hays DM, Kimura K: Biliary atresia: New concepts of management. Curr Probl Surg 1981;18:541-608.
43. Hendren WH: Diversion and undiversion. In O'Neill JA Jr, et al (eds): Pediatric Surgery, 5th ed. St. Louis, Mosby, 1998, pp 1653-1670.
44. Hill GL: Physiology of conventional ileostomy. In Dozois RR (ed): Alternatives to Conventional Ileostomy. Chicago, Year Book Medical Publishers, 1985, pp 129-139.
45. Kiely EM, Sparnon AL: Stoma closure in infants and children. Pediatr Surg Int 1987;2:95-97.
46. Kirkland S: Ostomy dolls for pediatric patients. J Enterostomal Ther 1985;12:104-105.
47. Kock NG, Dare N, Hulten L, et al: Ileostomy. Curr Probl Surg 1977;14:6-52.
48. Koga H, Yamataka A, Yoshida, et al: Laparoscopic-assisted repair for prolapsed colostomy in an infant. Pediatr Endosurg Innov Tech 2004;8:275-278.
49. Krasna IH: A simple pursestring suture technique for treatment of colostomy prolapse and intussusception. J Pediatr Surg 1979;14:801-802.
50. Lau JTK, Saing H, Ong GB: Double pursestring suture technique for loop colostomy prolapse in infants. Aust Paediatr J 1982;18:58-59.
51. Lyerly HK, Mault JR: Laparoscopic ileostomy and colostomy. Ann Surg 1994;219:317-322.
52. MacKiegan JM, Cataldo PA: Intestinal Stomas: Principles, Techniques and Management. St. Louis, Quality Medical Publishing, 1993.
53. MacMahon RA, Cohen SJ, Eckstein HB: Colostomies in infancy and childhood. Arch Dis Child 1963;38:114-117.
54. Maydl K: Zur Technik der Kolostomie. Zentalbl Chir 1888; 15:433-436.
55. Mikulicz J: Chirurgische Erfahrungen über das Darmkarzinom. Arch Klin Chir 1903;69:28-47.
56. Millar AJ, Lakhoo K, Rode M, et al: Bowel stomas in infants and children: A five-year audit of 203 patients. S Afr J Surg 1993;31:110-113.
57. Mitrofanoff P: Cystostomie continente trans-appendiculaire dans le traitement des vessies neurologiques. Chir Pediatr 1980;21:297-305.
58. Mollitt DL, Malangoni MA, Ballantine TV, et al: Colostomy complications in children: An analysis of 146 cases. Arch Surg 1980;115:455-458.
59. Morris DM, Rayburn D: Loop colostomies are totally diverting in adults. Am J Surg 1991;161:668-671.
60. Mullen BD, McGinn KA: The ostomy book: Living comfortably with colostomies, ileostomies and urostomies. Palo Alto, CA, Bull Publishing, 1992.
61. Musemeche CA, Kosloske AM, Ricketts RR: Enterostomy in necrotizing enterocolitis: An analysis of techniques and timing of closure. J Pediatr Surg 1987;22:479-483.
62. Nagle AP, Murayama KM: Laparoscopic gastrostomy and jejunostomy. J Long Term Eff Med Implants 2004; 14:1-11.
63. Nixon HH: Colostomy: A simple technique, and observations on indications. Z Kinderchir 1966;3:98-103.
64. Nour S, Beck J, Stringer MD: Colostomy complications in infants and children. Ann R Coll Surg Engl 1996;78: 526-530.
65. Park JJ, Del Pindo A, Orsay CP, et al: Stoma complications: The Cook County Hospital experience. Dis Colon Rectum 1999;42:1575-1580.
66. Pearl RK, Prasad ML, Orsay CP, et al: Early local complications from intestinal stomas. Arch Surg 1985;120: 1145-1147.
67. Pemberton JH, Kelly KA, Phillips SA: The continent ostomy valve: Concept and experience. In Dozois RR (ed): Alternatives to Conventional Ileostomies. Chicago, Year Book Medical Publishers, 1985, pp 211-225.
68. Quarmby CJ, Millar AJ, Rode H: The use of diverting colostomies in paediatric peri-anal burns. Burns 1999;25: 645-650.
69. Randolph JG, Zolinger RM Jr, Gross RE: Mikulicz resection in infants and children: A 20 year survey of 196 patients. Ann Surg 1963;158:481-485.
70. Rees BI, Thomas DF, Negam M: Colostomies in infancy and childhood. Z Kinderchir 1982;36:100-102.
71. Rehbein F, Halsband M: A double-tube technique for the treatment of meconium ileus and small bowel atresia. J Pediatr Surg 1968;3:723-726.
72. Rokhsar S, Harrison EA, Shaul DB, et al: Intestinal stoma complications in immunocompromised children. J Pediatr Surg 1999;34:1757-1761.
73. Rosenman JE, Kosloske AM: A reappraisal of the Mikulicz enterostomy in infants and children. Surgery 1982;91:34-37.
74. Ryan JA Jr, Page CP: Intrajejunal feedings: Development and current status. J Parenter Enteral Nutr 1984;8:187-198.
75. Sangkhathat S, Patrapinyokul S, Tadyathikom K: Early enteral feeding after closure of colostomy in pediatric patients. J Pediatr Surg 2003;38:1516-1519.
76. Santulli TV, Blanc WA: Congenital atresia of the intestine, pathogenesis and treatment. Ann Surg 1961;154:939-948.
77. Schärli WF: The history of colostomy in childhood. Prog Pediatr Surg 1986;20:188-198.
78. Schier F, Antoniu D, Waldschhmidt J: Komplikationen der Kolostomie im Kindesalter. Zentralbl Chir 1990;115: 1435-1440.
79. Simson JNL, Brereton RJ: Temporary antimesenteric stomas without a skin bridge in infants. Ann R Coll Surg Engl 1985;67:363-365.
80. Schimpl G, Mayr J, Gauderer MWL: Jejunostomy with replaceable feeding tube: A new technique. J Am Coll Surg 1997;184:652-654.
81. Shandling B, Chait PG, Richards HF: Percutaneous cecostomy: A new technique in the management of fecal incontinence. J Pediatr Surg 1996;31;534-537.
82. Smith D, Soucy P: Complications of long-term jejunostomy in children. J Pediatr Surg 1996;31:787-790.
83. Smith S, Wiener ES, Starzl TE, et al: Stoma-related variceal bleeding: An under-recognized complication of biliary

atresia. J Pediatr Surg 1988;23:243-245.
84. So HB, Becker JM, Schwartz DL, et al: Eighteen years' experience with neonatal Hirschsprung's disease treated by endorectal pull through without colostomy. J Pediatr Surg 1998;33:673-675.
85. Squire R, Kiely EM, Carr B, et al: The clinical application of the Malone antegrade colonic enema. J Pediatr Surg 1993;28:1012-1015.
86. Stein JP, Daneshmand S, Dunn M, et al: Continent right colon reservoir using a cutaneous appendicostomy. Urology 2004;63:577-580.
87. Steinau G, Ruhl KM, Hornchen H, et al: Enterostomy complications in infancy and childhood. Langenbecks Arch Surg 2001;386:346-349.
88. Stellato TA, Gauderer MWL: Jejunostomy button as a new method for long-term jejunostomy feedings. Surg Gynecol Obstet 1989;168:552-554.
89. Teitelbaum DH, Cilley RE, Sherman NJ, et al: A decade of experience with the primary pull-through for Hirschsprung's disease in the newborn period: A multicenter analysis of outcomes. Ann Surg 2000;232:372-380.
90. Turnbull RB Jr, Weakley FL: Atlas of Intestinal Stomas. St. Louis, CV Mosby, 1967.
91. Turnbull RW, Turnbull GB: The history and current status of paramedical support for the ostomy patient. J ET Nurs 1993;20:102-104.
92. Unti JA, Abcarian H, Pearl RK, et al: Rodless end-loop stomas: A seven-year experience. Dis Colon Rectum 1991; 34:999-1004.
93. Villarreal J, Sood M, Zangen T, et al: Colonic diversion for intractable constipation in children: Colonic manometry helps guide clinical decision. J Pediatr Gastroenterol Nutr 2001;33:588-591.
94. Weber TR, Tracy TF Jr, Silen ML, Powell MA: Enterostomy and its closure in newborns. Arch Surg 1995;130:534-537.
95. Webster R: Historical review. In Stephens FD, Smith ED (eds): Ano-rectal Malformations in Children. Chicago, Year Book Medical Publishers, 1971, pp 1-13.
96. Wilkins S, Peña A: The role of colostomy in the management of anorectal malformations. Pediatr Surg Int 1988; 3:105-109.
97. Winkler R: Stoma Therapy: An Atlas and Guide for Intestinal Stomas. New York, Thieme, 1986, pp 2-104.
98. Witzel O: Zur Technik der Magenfistelanlegung. Zentralbl Chir 1891;18:601-618.
99. Woodward MN, Foley P, Cusick EL: Colostomy for treatment of functional constipation in children: A preliminary report. J Pediatr Gastroenterol Nutr 2004;38:75-78.
100. Yoshida NR, Webber EM, Gillis DA, et al: Roux-en-Y jejunostomy in the pediatric population. J Pediatr Surg 1966;31:791-793.

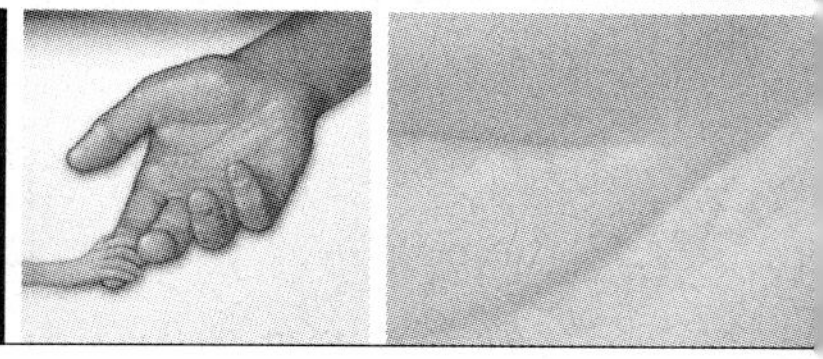

第 97 章

结肠闭锁、狭窄和其他梗阻性疾病

Keith T. Oldham 和 Marjorie J. Arca

先天性结肠闭锁和狭窄

历史回顾

93
1673 年 Binniger[22] 首先描述结肠闭锁。一直到 1922 年，Gaub[27] 采用近端结肠造口术成功治疗一名乙状结肠闭锁的儿童后，才有了此病存活者的相关报道。1947 年 Potts[48] 对一名新生儿进行了一期横结肠吻合术，该患儿成功存活。先天性结肠狭窄文献报道较少，从 1966 年起只有 8 例报道[1,9,21,55,56]。大部分患儿采用了病变肠段切除和端端吻合术，但个别病例采用了近端扩张肠管造口的分期手术方式。所有被报道的先天性结肠狭窄的患儿都存活了下来。

引言

结肠闭锁是引起新生儿期肠梗阻的罕见原因。报道的发生率差异很大，从 1∶1498[22] 到 1∶40 000[25] 活产婴儿不等。最常被引用的数据是约 20 000 个活产婴儿中有 1 例结肠闭锁患儿[9,69]，比较与事实相接近。在美国主要的儿童医院，每年有 1 或 2 例结肠闭锁的患儿。肠闭锁中约 1.8%[26] 至 15% 发生在结肠，这一估计值不包括一直以来被认为属于肛门闭锁范畴的直肠畸形[9,49,56]。结肠闭锁或狭窄没有性别和种族间的差异。尽管在霍斯坦牛[64] 中存在与此类似的常染色体隐性遗传的畸形，但在人类未见到相关报道。

结肠闭锁常伴随一些重要的肌肉骨骼系统（如并趾、多趾、畸形足和桡骨缺损）[46]、眼[49]、心脏[49]、胃肠道和腹壁[46]（如腹裂、脐膨出、膀胱或泄殖腔外翻）[12,58] 畸形等，也有颜面部发育不全、无眼等合并泄殖腔外翻的报道[65]。在一个大样本病例报道中，36 例先天性结肠闭锁的患儿中 22 例没有合并其他畸形[46]，其余 14 例婴儿中 9 例合并腹壁中线缺损，5 例合并空肠狭窄。

约 15%～20% 的结肠闭锁患儿合并近端小肠闭锁[46,49]，所以患中、远端小肠闭锁的新生儿应常规在术中探查结肠或术前行结肠造影检查。

至少有 2% 的结肠闭锁儿童合并先天性巨结肠[3,23,33,35,70]，一些学者推测是胚胎第 11 周结肠后腹膜固定之前发生血管损伤，影响了肠神经系统向后端的迁移[23]。所以为结肠闭锁的患儿重建连续肠管通道之前，必须先排除先天性巨结肠。

胚胎学

现代多数分析认为器官形成阶段宫内供血不足可导致肠闭锁的发生[37,44,54]。血管损伤的原因可能是结肠扭转、套迭、栓子或血栓形成，或结肠因为疝或腹壁缺损导致嵌顿或绞窄。缺血坏死后损伤肠管病灶被重吸收。Louw[37]、Barnard 和 Louw[6] 的实验研究发现结肠闭锁畸形的类型与小肠闭锁相似，证实了宫内血管梗死是导致结肠闭锁的病因。Barnard-Sutton[11] 和 Louw[37] 对小肠闭锁的分类方法同样也适用于结肠。简而言之，Ⅰ型闭锁为肠腔内隔膜样闭锁；Ⅱ型闭锁为近远闭锁端之间有纤维索带相连；Ⅲ型闭锁为肠完
全分离，系膜呈 V 型缺损。Ⅲ型闭锁是最常见的类 1494
型[12,49]。也可见完全的系膜分离和多发性肠闭锁。这种分类方式的临床价值有限，因为手术治疗原则及预后与闭锁的类型无关。

先天性结肠狭窄比结肠闭锁少见。有报道称 8 例结肠狭窄中有 7 例狭窄肠段的长度为 3～16.5 cm[1,9,21,55,56]，导致狭窄的原因认为是发育中的结肠血液供应受到了影响。最近，肠腔内瓣膜部分梗阻认为是引起结肠狭窄的原因[42]。

临床表现

现代超声技术使远端小肠闭锁的产前诊断成为可能。B 超可以显示小肠袢或结肠扩张，超过该孕周应有的肠管大小[5,25]。羊水过多不太明显，因为羊水可以在梗阻的小肠近端被吸收。

结肠闭锁或狭窄的患儿在出生时一般无明显异常，但在出生后 24～48 小时出现腹胀。因为梗阻的部位在远端肠管并通常是完全性梗阻，腹胀一般比较明显并逐渐加重，如果不治疗，在出生第 2 或第 3 天腹胀会非常明显。因为极度的肠扩张和腹胀，常需机械通气辅助呼吸。因为梗阻的位置在远端，呕吐可以出现较晚或相对较轻。粪汁样呕吐常较晚出现。结肠闭锁的患儿只能排出很少的胎粪或不排出胎粪。直肠指检也只能见到白色粪便而不是胎粪。在患儿查体时可能会发现合并运动系统畸形或腹壁缺损。

诊断

任何疑为肠梗阻的新生儿均应拍摄腹部平片。肠闭锁患儿的腹部平片可以出现多发性胀气肠袢和气液平面，也可以出现远端肠管梗阻征象（图 97-1）。尽管在新生儿期小肠和结肠很难分辨，但在结肠，其梗阻近端肠管的扩张程度比小肠梗阻更为明显（见图 97-1）。气腹征是近端结肠穿孔的表现，约 10% 的结肠闭锁患儿在诊断时存在气腹征[46]。回盲瓣的存在造成结肠近、远端节段性闭袢梗阻，理论上增大了肠穿孔的危险性。

诊断结肠闭锁或狭窄的标准检查方法是使用等渗性造影剂进行对比灌肠的放射学检查。完全梗阻的特征是远端的“细小结肠”因废用而狭小，但一般情况下本质上为正常的肠管。造影剂充填了远端结肠，而在梗阻的位置中断，并与近端扩张肠管内的气体影（梗阻点）相连接。先天性肠狭窄的特征是肠腔狭窄，近端肠管造影剂充盈受限，并常可见近端肠管扩张。

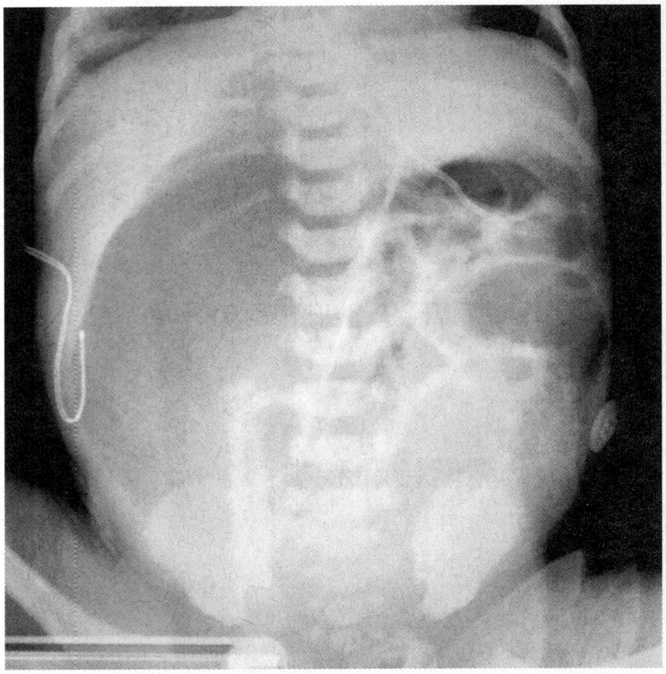

图 97-1 结肠闭锁。24 小时患儿腹部平片显示近端肠管显著扩张，直肠或左下腹无气体影。剖腹探查发现闭锁位于结肠肝区水平。（Courtesy of J. Sty，MD.）

对所有疑为远端肠闭锁的新生儿进行对比灌肠放射学检查是十分必要的，因为手术医生在手术前需要确认远端肠管是否存在梗阻。此外，这项检查对诊断其他原因，如胎粪性栓塞综合征、先天性巨结肠及新生儿左小结肠综合征[5]等引起的远端肠管梗阻具有决定性意义。结肠闭锁或狭窄的患儿，不需要其他的影像学检查明确肠道的解剖结构。如果患儿合并心血管系统的畸形应进行心脏的扫描。

治疗

肠梗阻的患儿应置鼻胃管减压并静脉补液以利于患儿复苏。手术前应给予广谱抗生素。肠闭锁的常见类型是两个盲端之间没有肠系膜附连的类型（Ⅲ型）。因为存在肠穿孔和局部扭转的风险，手术治疗不应该拖延。以往强调根据闭锁或狭窄的位置决定手术方式[49]，认为右半结肠闭锁应行一期肠吻合术；

左半或乙状结肠闭锁应先行近端结肠造口术；二期重建肠管连续性以降低感染的风险及肠瘘的发生率。现代的实践中，只要患儿医学情况能稳定，无论肠闭锁的位置如何，均应行一期肠吻合术。但是，如果涉及肠管血供、两端肠管的直径相差过大或大量的粪便污染等因素，也不能盲目行一期肠吻合术。

手术治疗的原则如下：采用损伤比较小的切口，通常是横行，在脐上位置，进行剖腹探查，切除极端膨胀的近端肠管（通常是右结肠）和梗阻部位，以利于肠功能的恢复，需保留一定长度的肠管和回盲瓣。术前和术中都应注意远端结肠的情况。采用单层端端斜形吻合重建肠管的连续性。

因为可能合并先天性巨结肠，行一期肠吻合术时应在手术中行直肠黏膜抽吸活检以评价肠神经节的情况。同样，如果决定行结肠造口术，术中应检查造口处的肠肌丛并在肠管重新吻合前行直肠黏膜抽吸活检。

已知切除肠管并吻合的预后很好，不推荐行结肠成形术，因为局部结肠成形术的经验较少。合并中线腹壁缺损的复杂结肠闭锁应采取另外的手术方案，如近端造口成形及分期结肠修补术。

预后

结肠闭锁和狭窄修补术的并发症与其他类型的结肠手术类似，最常见的并发症是吻合口狭窄、吻合口漏和近端肠管功能失调。粘连性小肠梗阻、伤口感染及肠造口相关的问题也常有报道[4,46,49]。Powell 和 Raffensperger 报道[49]，1946—1978 年治疗的 19 例结肠闭锁或狭窄患儿有 15 例出现并发症，结肠闭锁的死亡率为 10.5%。DellaVecchia[19] 等报道 1972—1997 年治疗的 21 例结肠闭锁和狭窄患儿，12 例出现并发症，包括伤口感染（1 例）、造口回缩（1 例）、肠蠕动不良性肠梗阻（2 例）、后期粘连性肠梗阻（8 例）。这些患者中手术死亡率为 0，长期存活率为 100%。

获得性结肠狭窄

不同类型的炎症、感染、创伤和肿瘤可导致婴儿和儿童发生获得性肠狭窄[59]。其中，新生儿坏死性小肠结肠炎是最常见的原因。多达 10%～25% 的新生儿坏死性小肠结肠炎患儿将发展为结肠狭窄[7,8,51]。病变局部过度分泌的肿瘤坏死因子是引起狭窄病变的原因。Gobet[29] 等报道了 47 例进行手术治疗的坏死性小肠结肠炎患儿，22 例（47%）发展为结肠狭窄，需要手术切除。狭窄通常在原发病发生后 3 个月内发生。狭窄通常发生在乙状结肠，也可以发生在腹腔内结肠和小肠的任何部位。可以发生几处狭窄，但通常为不全性肠梗阻（图 97-2）。典型的症状是拒食、胆汁性呕吐和腹胀。对比灌肠的放射学检查可以明确诊断。治疗采用病变肠管手术切除。在高危患儿中，则采用近端肠管分流和分期肠管连续性重建。曾经有球囊扩张狭窄结肠的成功报道，但经验很少，现代治疗中很少使用这种技术[45]。

还有一些感染性疾病与获得性结肠狭窄的发生相关，曾报道的有：溶血性尿毒症综合征[67]和甲氧苯青霉素耐药的金黄色葡萄球菌小肠结肠炎[39]。在

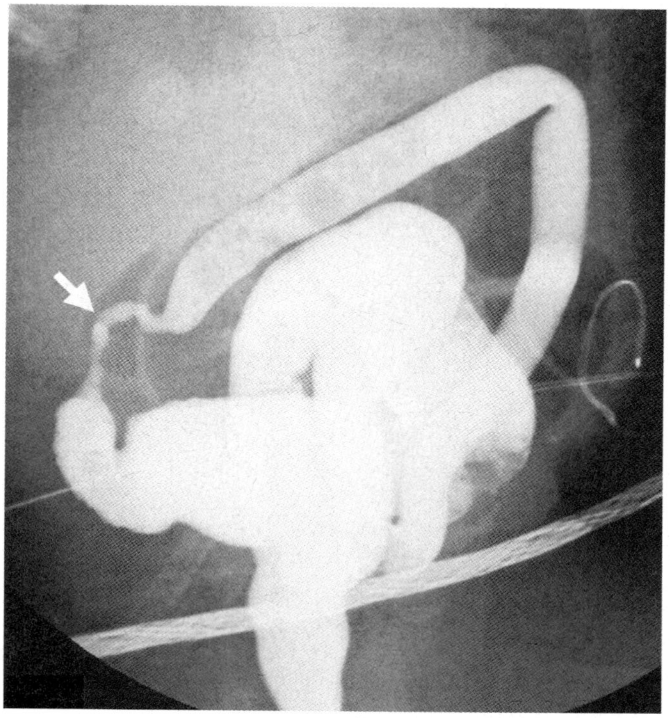

图 97-2　一例有坏死性小肠结肠炎病史，未行手术治疗的 3 个月婴儿的灌肠对比造影的放射学摄片。患儿表现为厌食、呕吐和腹胀。升结肠可见一处狭窄（箭头）。患儿行病变肠管阶段性切除并一期肠吻合术获治愈。（Courtesy of J. Sty，MD.）

人类免疫缺陷性病毒感染的儿童，曾有侵入血管壁的念珠菌感染引起急性结肠梗阻和死亡的报道[38]。慢性非甾体抗炎药物的使用可以导致成人结肠狭窄
1496 的发生[34]，但至今为止在儿童人群中尚无此类疾病的报道。

肿瘤样物质可以由于腔内生长（息肉、神经纤维瘤[31,53]和腺癌[13,16,22]）和外在压迫（淋巴瘤、腹膜后肉瘤或畸胎瘤）或腹腔内浸润（结节性硬化和神经纤维瘤病）[61]引起结肠梗阻，这些情况都不常见。在所有的病例中，如果可能，原发病因均应加以控制。一般情况下，良性病变应予以切除，并行一期结肠吻合。恶性和复杂性病变需要粪便引流、分期手术或更为复杂的结肠连续性重建。

结肠腺癌很少发生于年轻患者，21 岁以下的 97% 腺癌患者最常见的主述是梗阻性疼痛[29]。儿童腺癌的总体生存率约为 25%，成人的生存率约为 50%[62]。诊断延误[52,68]、晚期[67]和不好的病理分型[40]是儿童生存率较低的原因。LaQuaglia[36]等综述了 29 例儿童腺癌患者，结论是与成人中等分化或原位腺癌（31%）相比，儿童腺癌更倾向于预后不良，如“印戒细胞”或未分化癌（69%）。手术患儿的病理类型及淋巴结转移情况是切除术后患儿死亡率的主要预测指标。高危类型患儿及区域性淋巴结转移者，除手术外还要进行其他辅助治疗[36]。

功能性结肠梗阻

许多疾病的过程与功能性结肠梗阻有关，这些类型的结肠梗阻在第 99 章和第 100 章已经进行了详细的讨论，这里主要讲述婴儿和儿童结肠梗阻的鉴别诊断。

肠神经发育不良是一种肌间肠神经系统异常的疾病，其临床表现与先天性巨结肠类似（参见第 99 章和 100 章）[41]。A 型肠神经发育不良的特征是肠交感神经减少，而副交感神经纤维中度增多；B 型肠神经发育不良有巨大或不成熟的神经节细胞和神经纤维粗大。这些组织病理学改变可见于结肠的一段或整个消化道。

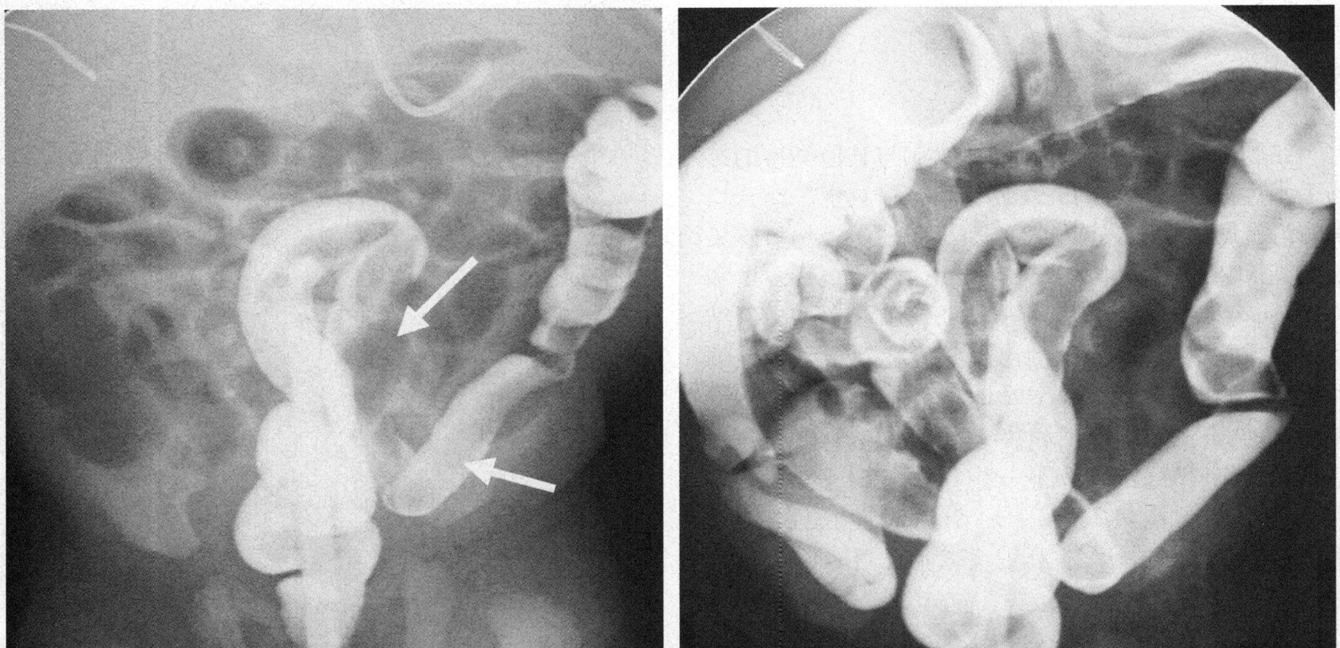

A B

图 97-3 一例正常的早产合并胎粪性栓塞综合征的婴儿放射学摄片。A. 造影剂灌肠最初摄片显示结肠肠腔内充盈缺损（胎粪塞）（箭头）可以确诊。B. 造影剂灌肠最终摄片显示结肠完全被充盈。（Courtesy of J. Sty，MD.）

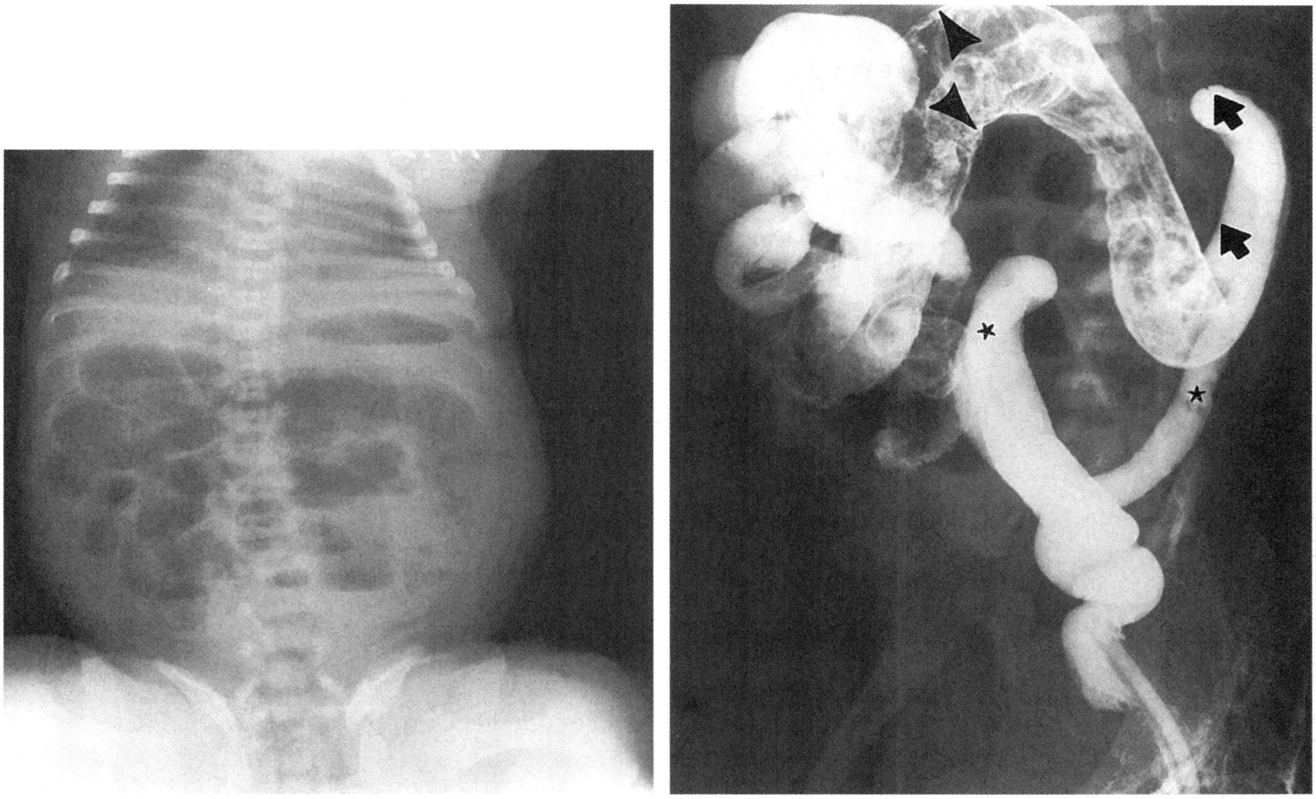

A　　B

图 97-4　A. 一例母亲为糖尿病的婴儿的腹部平片显示远端肠梗阻。　B. 钡剂灌肠造影显示典型的左小结肠综合征。标记处为细小结肠（星形），脾区移行段（箭头）和梗阻处近端扩张的横结肠（箭头）（Courtesy of D. Frush，MD.）

Ogilvie 综合征（假性结肠肠梗阻）是缺少任何明确机械性原因而发生的急性结肠扩张。通常见于成人，偶尔也见于儿童和青少年，主要累及盲肠和右半结肠。发展成为 Ogilvie 综合征的高危因素包括电解质紊乱和某些药物，特别是麻醉药物的使用，它能减弱肠道动力。盲肠的扩张抑制了结肠的自主推动性活动，也可引起缺血性坏死。胃肠减压、停用相关的药物和结肠镜减压是主要的治疗措施。最近，儿科文献上报道了乙酰胆碱酯酶抑制剂新斯的明（0.007～0.75 mg/kg）的治疗效果[28]。新斯的明的确切作用机制尚不清楚，推测是由于其类胆碱作用纠正了结肠自主神经系统的获得性功能失调。

慢性特发性假性肠梗阻可以发生在儿童和成人[15,57]。肠平滑肌（肌病）与肠肌间神经丛（神经病变）的异常，或两种病变合并均可发生。

在新生儿，一种内脏肌病被称为巨膀胱-小结肠-肠蠕动迟缓综合征，特征是解剖上肠道未闭，肠神经节细胞正常，临床上表现为继发于无效蠕动的肠梗阻。因为无有效的药物和手术治疗方法，这种疾病常常是致命的[4,10,50,59]。

胎粪性栓塞综合征与左小结肠综合征看起来比较特殊，但它们从本质上来说是一种新生儿期的结肠功能性梗阻，为充分阐明，以下将分节讨论。

胎粪性栓塞综合征

胎粪性栓塞综合征是引起新生儿功能性肠梗阻相对常见的原因（参见第 99 章）[17,20]。患儿可能是早产儿，且大体情况正常。推测该综合征是由于未成熟的肌间神经系统导致肠无效蠕动[14]，以及肠内水分过度吸收，形成胎粪性便秘阻塞结肠。这一发病机制尚未得到证实，但确定其与肠的暂时失动力有关。其临床表现与远端肠梗阻相似，直肠指检有

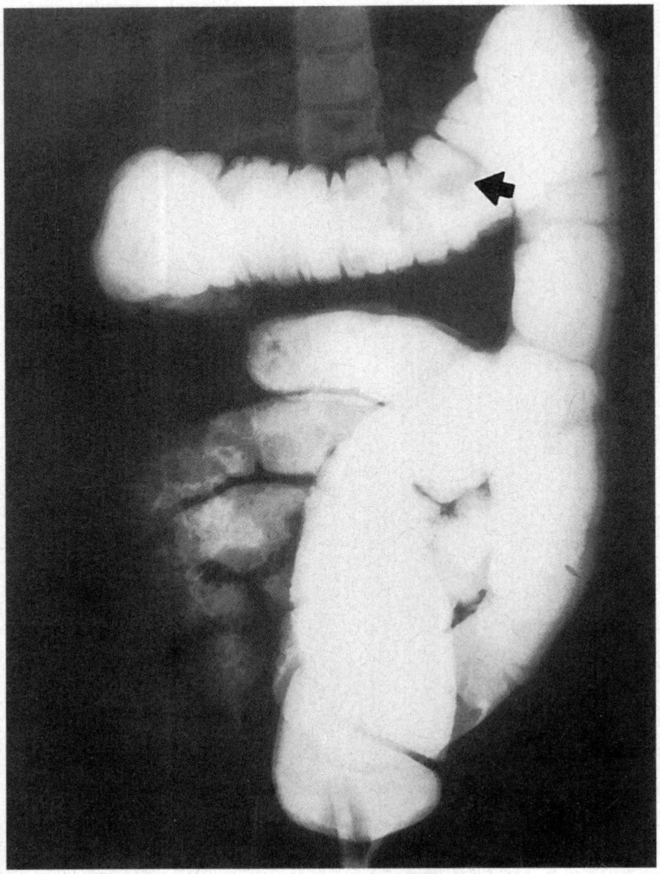

图 97-5 钡剂灌肠摄片显示横结肠浓缩的粪便影（箭头）。此为一名有胎粪性肠梗阻及复发性肠梗阻病史的囊性纤维病患儿。

助于诊断，可以刺激排出稠厚的胎粪而缓解临床症状。水溶性造影剂灌肠检查常常用于诊断及治疗，但往往需要多次灌肠（图 97-3）。很少需要手术介入。推荐使用直肠抽吸活检，与个别先天性巨结肠症患儿相鉴别，但这一检查常用于胎粪排出后依旧存在便秘症状的儿童。同样地，该综合征可与结肠胎粪性肠梗阻混淆。另外，诊断性汗水试验是排除囊性纤维病的常用方法。

左小结肠综合征

左小结肠综合征是一种动力失调、左结肠细小引起暂时性结肠梗阻的综合征，偶尔可导致穿孔的发生[18,47]。约 40%~50% 患儿的母亲患糖尿病，且几乎均为胰岛素依赖型。Davis 和 Campbell[18] 报道，患糖尿病的母亲所产婴儿中约 50% 无症状的婴儿存在左小结肠的放射学征象。梗阻常是不完全的，病变常累及降结肠远端直到结肠脾区（图 97-4）。梗阻的程度各不相同，有很多近端肠管穿孔的报道，尤其是盲肠。低血糖诱导的胰高血糖素释放被认为与此病有关，病因尚不清楚[45]，但新生儿左半结肠似乎对胰高血糖素及其他物质所致的结肠肌肉收缩敏感[47]。其临床症状是暂时的，随着婴儿自身产生的胰岛素含量正常，常在出生后 24 ~ 48 小时得以缓解。可采用灌肠造影检查以明确诊断，也可以作为治疗方法促进缓解功能性肠梗阻。因为脾曲存在移行区，左小结肠的放射学征象与先天性巨结肠相似，所以应常规采用直肠抽吸活检以排除先天性巨结肠的可能性。也应谨慎地排除囊性纤维病。

胎粪性肠梗阻

胎粪性肠梗阻的本质是与囊性纤维病相关的肠梗阻，相关内容已在第 81 章讨论过。囊性纤维病的特征是胰腺的外分泌不足及肠分泌物中水分缺乏，导致粪便稠厚坚硬难以排出而阻塞小肠或结肠。这一疾病常见于新生儿，也见于囊性纤维病的青少年患儿，他们与外源性酶替代疗法的依从性较难保持。病史和腹部平片有助于诊断，但确诊依靠对比灌肠造影检查（图 97-5）。顺向或逆向的结肠灌洗及胰酶替代治疗是首选的治疗手段。慢性梗阻常采用胃造口术或规范的盲肠造口，以定期灌洗肠道。

结肠梗阻的其他原因

这里主要讲述几种少见的结肠梗阻，包括盲肠或乙状结肠扭转、各种肿瘤侵害、先天性腹膜异常索带[2]、后肠重复畸形[62] 或先天性节段性结肠扩张（膨胀）[30]。节段性结肠扩张是婴儿或儿童先天性疾病，临床表现为不全性结肠梗阻。它是一种肠管局限性及功能性疾病，病变的结肠肠管缺少蠕动能力及结肠带。因为其近远端结肠的结构及功能均正常，手术切除病变肠管可治愈[24]。

结肠的节段性扭转可以出现在乙状结肠或盲肠

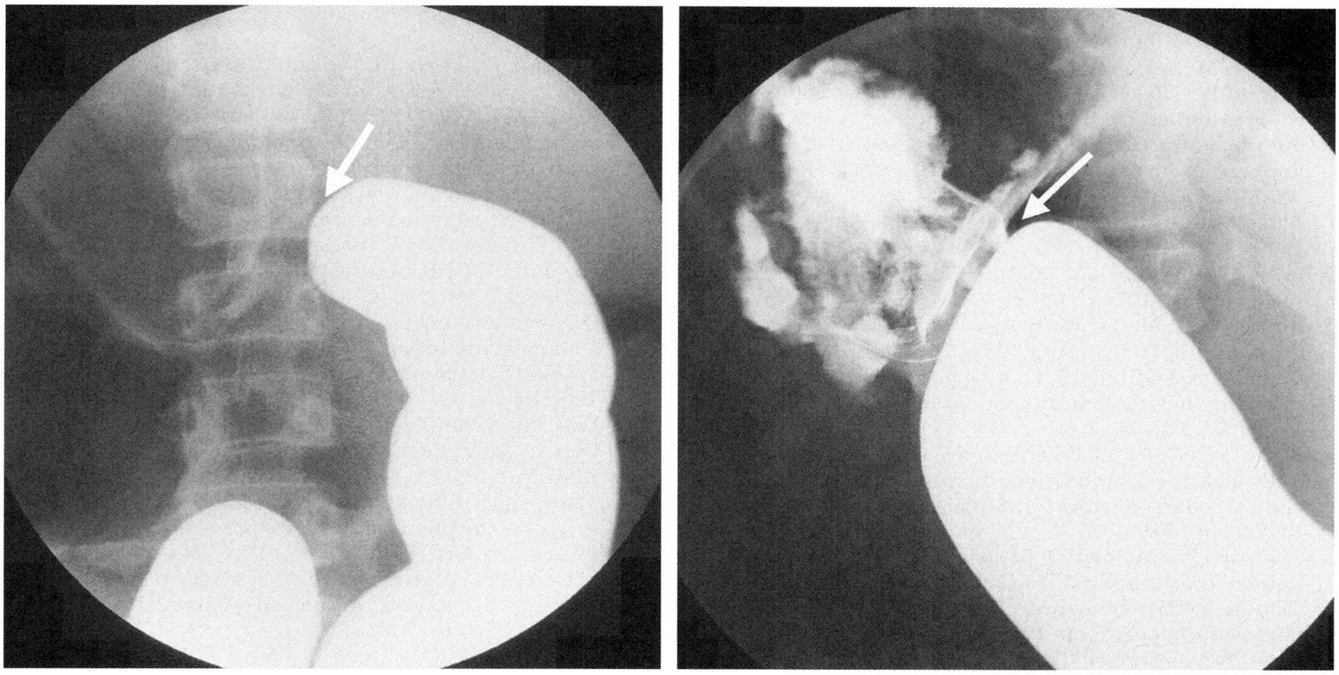

A　　B

图 97–6　A. 一例乙状结肠扭转患儿的造影剂灌肠检查。箭头显示梗阻部位。B. 造影剂最低限度地充盈梗阻近端结肠。（Courtesy of J. Sty，MD.）

（图 97–6），典型的表现为儿童或青少年患者有较长时间的便秘或假性肠梗阻病史，临床表现为腹胀、恶心和呕吐。一些患儿，结肠的节段性扭转与恶化的假性肠梗阻很难鉴别。据报道，有两例 Cornelia de Lange 综合征的患儿出现盲肠扭转[32]。诊断依靠造影剂灌肠检查。治疗则常规需要手术切除病变肠管。

20 世纪 90 年代中期，有报道囊性纤维病患儿出现长段的结肠纤维化，认为是摄入大剂量的胰酶（每日 >19 000 U/kg）导致结肠损伤[24]。许多此类患儿需要切除病变肠管。近年来，改变胰酶的剂量降低了这种并发症的发生。

小结

婴儿和儿童结肠梗阻的病因各异。一般情况下，解剖因素导致的梗阻采用病变肠管切除和一期肠吻合较易达到治疗目的。功能性肠梗阻的发病机制各不相同，一般首选非手术方法治疗。在现代小儿外科手术实践中，解剖因素导致的梗阻的临床预后较好，除非有其他并发疾病或腹膜炎败血症。

（杜　勇译　周小渔校）

参考文献

1. Abu-Jedeh HH, Methratta S, Ybasco A, et al: Congenital colonic stenosis. South Med J 2001;94:344-346.
2. Akgur FM, Tanyel FC, Buyukpamukcu N, et al: Anomalous congenital bands causing intestinal obstruction in children. J Pediatr Surg 1992;27:471-473.
3. Akgur FM, Tanyel FC, Buyukpamukcu N, et al: Colonic atresia and Hirschsprung's disease association shows further evidence for migration of enteric neurons. J Pediatr Surg 1993;28:635-636.
4. Al-Rayess M, Ambler MW: Axonal dystrophy presenting as the megacystis-microcolon-intestinal hypoperistalsis syndrome. Pediatr Pathol 1992;12:743-750.
5. Anderson N, Malpas T, Robertson R: Prenatal diagnosis of colon atresia. Pediatr Radiol 1993;23:63-64.
6. Barnard CN, Louw JF: The genesis of intestinal atresia. Minn Med 1956;39:745-753.
7. Beardmore HE, Rodgers BM, Outerbridge E: Necrotizing enterocolitis (ischemic enteropathy with the sequel of colonic atresia). Gastroenterology 1978;74:914-917.
8. Bell MJ, Ternberg JL, Askin FB, et al: Intestinal stricture in

necrotizing enterocolitis. J Pediatr Surg 1976;11:319-327.
9. Benson CD, Lotfi MW, Brough AJ: Congenital atresia and stenosis of the colon. J Pediatr Surg 1968;3:253-257.
10. Berdon WE, Baker DH, Blanc WA, et al: Megacystis-microcolon-intestinal hypoperistalsis syndrome: A new cause of intestinal obstruction in the newborn. Report of radiologic findings in five newborn girls. AJR Am J Roentgenol 1976;126:957-964.
11. Bland-Sutton JD: Imperforate ileum. Am J Med Sci 1889;98:457-462.
12. Boles ET Jr, Vassy LE, Ralston M: Atresia of the colon. J Pediatr Surg 1976;11:69-75.
13. Brown RA, Rode H, Millar AJ, et al: Colorectal carcinoma in children. J Pediatr Surg 1992;27:919-921.
14. Bughaighis AG, Emery JL: Functional obstruction of the intestine due to neurological immaturity. Prog Pediatr Surg 1971;3:37-52.
15. Byrne WJ, Cipel L, Euler AR, et al: Chronic idiopathic intestinal pseudo-obstruction syndrome in children—clinical characteristics and prognosis. J Pediatr Surg 1977;90:585-589.
16. Chabalko JJ, Fraumeni JF Jr: Colorectal cancer in children: Epidemiologic aspects. Dis Colon Rectum 1975;18:1-3.
17. Clatworthy HW Jr, Howard WHR, Lloyd JR: The meconium plug syndrome. Surgery 1956;39:131-142.
18. Davis WS, Campbell JB: Neonatal small left colon syndrome: Occurrence in asymptomatic infants of diabetic mothers. Am J Dis Child 1975;129:1024-1027.
19. DellaVecchia LK, Grosfeld JL, West KW, et al: Intestinal atresia and stenosis: A 25-year experience with 277 cases. Arch Surg 1998;133:490-496.
20. Ellis DG, Clatworthy HW Jr: The meconium plug syndrome revisited. J Pediatr Surg 1966;1:54-61.
21. Erskine JM: Colonic stenosis in the newborn: The possible thromboembolic etiology of intestinal stenosis and atresia. J Pediatr Surg 1970;5:321-333.
22. Evans CW: Atresias of the gastrointestinal tract. Surg Gynecol Obstet 1951;92:1-8.
23. Fishman SJ, Islam S, Buonoma C, et al: Nonfixation of an atretic colon predicts Hirschsprung's disease. J Pediatr Surg 2003;36:202-204.
24. FitzSimmons SC, Burkhart GA, Borowitz D, et al: High-dose pancreatic-enzyme supplements and fibrosing colonopathy in children with cystic fibrosis. N Engl J Med 1997;336:1283-1289.
25. Franken EA Jr (ed): Gastrointestinal Imaging in Pediatrics, 2nd ed. New York, Harper & Row, 1982.
26. Freeman NV: Congenital atresia and stenosis of the colon. Br J Surg 1966;53:595-599.
27. Gaub OC: Congenital stenosis and atresia of the intestinal tract above the rectum, with a report of an operated case of atresia of the sigmoid in an infant. Trans Am Surg Assoc 1922;40:582.
28. Gmora S, Poenau, D, Tsai E: Neostigmine for the treatment of pediatric acute colonic pseudoobstruction. J Pediatr Surg 2002;37:E28.
29. Gobet R, Sacher P, Schwobel MG: Surgical procedures in colonic strictures after necrotizing enterocolitis. Acta Paediatr Suppl 1994;396:77-79.
30. Helikson MA, Shapiro MB, Garfinkel DJ, et al: Congenital segmental dilatation of the colon. J Pediatr Surg 1982;17:201-202.
31. Hochberg FH, Dasilva AB, Galdabini J, et al: Gastrointestinal involvement in von Recklinghausen's neurofibromatosis. Neurology 1974;24:1144-1151.
32. Husain K, Fitzgerald P, Lau G: Cecal volvulus in the Cornelia de Lange syndrome. J Pediatr Surg 1994;29:1245-1247.
33. Johnson JF, Dean BL: Hirschsprung's disease coexisting with colonic atresia. Pediatr Radiol 1981;11:97-98.
34. Khan AZ, George K, Defriend DJ: Non-steroidal anti-inflammatory drug-induced colonic stenosis: An unusual cause of a right-sided colonic mass: Report of a case. Dis Colon Rectum 2003;46:403-405.
35. Kim PCW, Superina RA, Ein S: Colonic atresia combined with Hirschsprung's disease: A diagnostic and therapeutic challenge. J Pediatr Surg 1995;30:1216-1217.
36. LaQuaglia MP, Heller G, Filippa DA, et al: Prognostic factors and outcome in patients 21 years and under with colorectal carcinoma. J Pediatr Surg 1992;27:1085-1089.
37. Louw JH: Jejunoileal atresia and stenosis. J Pediatr Surg 1966;1:8-23.
38. Loveland J, Bowley DMG, Beavon IR, et al: Bowel obstruction in an infant with AIDS. Arch Dis Child 2003;88: 825-826.
39. Masunaga K, Masaki R, Endo A, et al: Colonic stenosis after severe methicillin-resistant *Staphylococcus aureus* enterocolitis in a newborn. Pediatr Infect Dis J 1999;18:169-171.
40. Mayo CW, Pagtalunan RJG: Malignancy of the colon and rectum in patients under 30 years of age. Surgery 1963;53:711-718.
41. Meier-Ruge WA, Schmidt PC, Stoss F: Intestinal neuronal dysplasia and its morphometric evidences. Pediatr Surg Int 1995;10:447-450.
42. Mizuno M, Kato T, Hebiguchi T, et al: Congenital membranous colonic stenosis—case report of an extremely rare anomaly. J Pediatr Surg 2003;38:E13-E15.
43. Nixon GW, Condon VR, Stewart DR: Intestinal perforation as a complication of the neonatal small left colon syndrome. Am J Roentgenol Rad Ther Nuclear Med 1975;125:75-80.
44. Peck DA, Lynn HB, Harris LE: Congenital atresia and stenosis of the colon. Arch Surg 1963;87:428-439.
45. Peer A, Klin B, Vinograd I: Balloon catheter dilatation of focal colonic strictures following necrotizing enterocolitis. Cardiovasc Intervent Radiol 1993;16:248-250.
46. Philippart AI: Atresia, stenosis, and other obstructions of the colon. In Welch KJ, et al (eds): Pediatric Surgery, 4th ed. Chicago, Year Book Medical Publishers, 1986.
47. Philippart AI, Reed JO, Georgeson KE: Neonatal small left colon syndrome: Intramural not intraluminal obstruction. J Pediatr Surg 1975;10:733-740.
48. Potts WJ: Congenital atresia of intestine and colon. Surg Gynecol Obstet 1947;85:14-18.
49. Powell RW, Raffensperger JG: Congenital colonic atresia. J Pediatr Surg 1982;17:166-170.
50. Puri P, Lake BD, Gorman F, et al: Megacystis-microcolon-intestinal hypoperistalsis syndrome: A visceral myopathy. J Pediatr Surg 1983;8:64-69.
51. Rabinowitz JG, Wolf BS, Feller MR, et al: Colonic changes following necrotizing enterocolitis in the newborn. AJR Am J Roentgenol 1968;103:359-364.
52. Rao BN, Pratt CB, Fleming ID, et al: Colon carcinoma in children and adolescents: A review of 30 cases. Cancer 1985;55:1322-1326.
53. Riccardi VM: Von Recklinghausen neurofibromatosis. N Engl J Med 1981;305:1617-1627.
54. Santulli TV, Blanc WA: Congenital atresia of the intestine: Pathogenesis and treatment. Ann Surg 1961;154:939-948.
55. Sax EJ: Pediatric case of the day: Congenital colonic stenosis. AJR Am J Roentgenol 1991;156:1315-1317.
56. Schiller M, Aviad I, Freund H: Congenital colonic atresia

and stenosis. Am J Surg 1979;138:721-724.
57. Schuffler MD, Deitch EA: Chronic idiopathic intestinal pseudo-obstruction: A surgical approach. Ann Surg 1980;192:752-761.
58. Shah R, Woolley M: Gastroschisis and intestinal atresia. J Pediatr Surg 1991;26:788-790.
59. Shono T, Suita S, Taguchi T, Nagasaki A: Manometric evaluation of gastrointestinal motility in a case of megacystis-microcolon-intestinal hypoperistalsis syndrome (MMIHS). Eur J Pediatr Surg 1992;1:52-54.
60. Srikanth MS, Ford EG, Isaacs H Jr, et al: Megacystis microcolon intestinal hypoperistalsis syndrome: Late sequelae and possible pathogenesis. J Pediatr Surg 1993;28:957-959.
61. Staple TW, McAlister WH, Anderson MS: Plexiform neurofibromatosis of the colon simulating Hirschsprung's disease. Am J Roentgenol Rad Ther Nuclear Med 1964; 91:840-845.
62. Stringer MD, Spitz L, Abel R, et al: Management of alimentary tract duplication in children. Br J Surg 1995;82:74-78.
63. Sugarbaker PH, Gunderson LL, Wittes RE: Colorectal cancer. In DeVita VT Jr, Hellman S, Rosenberg S (eds): Cancer: Principles and Practice of Oncology. Philadelphia, JB Lippincott, 1985.
64. Syed M, Shanks RD: Atresia coli inherited in Holstein cattle. J Dairy Sci 1992;75:1105-1111.
65. Szavay PO, Schiephake H, Hubert O, Gluer S: Colon atresia, facial hemiaplasia and anophthalmia: A case report. J Pediatr Surg 2002;37:1498-1500.
66. Tan X, Hsueh W, Gonzalez-Crussi F: Cellular localization of tumor necrosis factor (TNF)-α transcripts in normal bowel and in necrotizing enterocolitis. Am J Pathol 1993;142:1858-1865.
67. Tapper D, Tarr P, Avener E, et al: Lessons learned in the management of hemolytic uremic syndrome in children. J Pediatr Surg 1995;30:158-163.
68. Umpleby HC, Williamson RCN: Carcinoma of the large bowel in the first four decades. Br J Surg 1984;71:272-277.
69. Webb CH, Wangensteen OH: Congenital intestinal atresia. Am J Dis Child 1932;14:262-284.
70. Williams MD, Burrington JD: Hirschsprung's disease complicating colon atresia. J Pediatr Surg 1993;28:637-639.

第 98 章

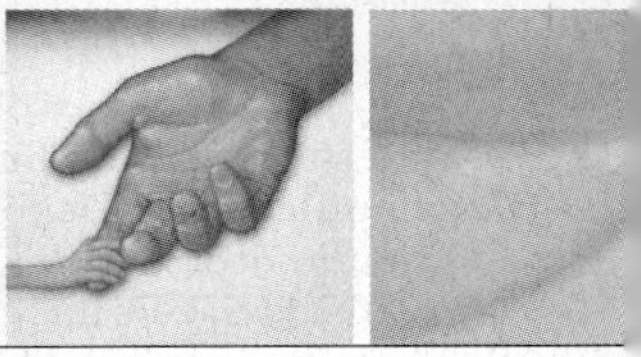

阑尾炎

James C. Y. Dunn

阑尾炎是外科最常见的急腹症及最容易误诊的疾病。对它的治疗仍有许多争议，激起小儿外科医生无穷的兴趣并有许多相关的文献报道。阑尾炎的发病率存在很大的地域差异。在美国，1997 年对 25.4 万个住院日及 6.8 亿美元的住院费用的调查显示，每年有 70000 个儿童诊断为阑尾炎，每年 1000 个儿童中约有 1 个儿童发病[65]。阑尾炎在第三世界国家的发病率较低[96]，在过去的几十年中，阑尾炎的发病率已稳步降低[9,75,96,160]。

历史回顾

首次报道与阑尾炎相似的疾病的医学文献大约出现在 500 年之前[99]，疾病的病理改变描述为盲肠周围炎。盲肠曾一度被认为是该疾病的原发病灶，直到 1827 年 Melier 声称阑尾的炎症才是该病的发生原因。1886 年 Fitz[54] 最终证明盲肠周围炎起源于阑尾的炎症，并提出了“阑尾炎”这一术语。

Amyand 首次成功施行了阑尾切除术，1735 年他通过阴囊切口成功切除了穿孔的阑尾并引流阴囊脓肿。1887 年 Morton 在美国第一次演示了阑尾切除术[99,132]。1889 年 McBurney[95] 在他的手术切除治疗阑尾炎的文章中描述到：“疼痛最显著的位置准确位于髂前上棘与脐连线上，距髂前上棘 1～2.5 英寸。”从此，这一位置就称为麦氏点。虽然现代外科治疗与抗生素应用使得这一曾经的不治之症罕有死亡病例，阑尾炎仍然是儿童及青少年的常见疾病[122]。

胚胎与解剖

在胚胎发育中，阑尾作为盲肠前尖部的一个延续器官出现于胚胎第 8 周[28,148]。在儿童后期，阑尾最终旋转到盲肠中后位，回盲瓣下方 2 cm 的位置。这一旋转过程存在许多变异，导致阑尾最终位置的多样性。95% 的病例阑尾位于腹膜内，但确切位置存在很多变异[172]。30% 的病例中阑尾尖位于盆腔，65% 位于盲肠后，5% 位于腹膜外结肠后或盲肠后。在旋转不良或内脏转位的病例中，异位阑尾导致炎症的体征出现在异常位置。

阑尾的长度为 0.3～33 cm，平均 8 cm。阑尾的直径为 5～10 mm。阑尾动脉来自回结肠动脉，从末段回肠后穿过。阑尾起源于三根结肠带的交汇处，这是定位异位阑尾时一个很有用的标志。阑尾的上皮层、环肌和纵肌层均为盲肠的延续。在出生时，阑尾黏膜下有很少的淋巴结，12 岁时数量增加 200 倍，30 岁时急剧下降，60 岁消失，只留下痕迹。

盲肠发育的突然停止导致阑尾的发育不良或发育不全。每 10 万人中有 4 例存在阑尾重复畸形[20,23]。阑尾重复畸形可以是部分（双阑尾）或全部，它们可以有共同的或分离的盲肠开口，而阑尾开口也可以存在重复畸形。

阑尾的功能尚不明确。灵长类有阑尾，但多数哺乳动物没有。奇怪的是兔子有阑尾，而且兔子的阑尾是 B 细胞发育的很重要的免疫器官[153]。

疾病谱

人一生阑尾炎的发生率在女性为 7%，男性为

9%[1]。约 1/3 的阑尾炎发生于 18 岁以下人群。在美
02 国，阑尾炎更容易发生于白种人，并常于夏季发病。发病的高峰年龄在 11～12 岁。尽管阑尾炎不常见于婴幼儿，但一旦延误诊断，该年龄组的患者出现并发症的比例很高。阑尾穿孔也可能是其他疾病的后果，比如新生儿期的先天性巨结肠[90]。即使不去讨论阑尾炎如何起病以及它的发病率，它依然是个谜团——一种普通的疾病，尽管我们尽了最大努力但依然是误诊最多的外科急腹症。尽管诊断和治疗都得到改善，阑尾炎仍然是不容忽视的疾病，并且依然有死亡病例，虽然已很少见[111,125]。

有许多描述阑尾炎不同发病阶段的术语，包括“急性阑尾炎、化脓性阑尾炎、坏疽性阑尾炎和穿孔性阑尾炎”。它们之间的界限很模糊，只是在单纯性和复杂性阑尾炎之间存在着较清晰的区别。因为坏疽性阑尾炎的病理特征是肠坏死，而在功能上则表现为肠穿孔，我们用复杂性阑尾炎来描述坏疽性和穿孔性阑尾炎。

慢性或复发性阑尾炎是否存在，几十年来一直存在争议。最近的文献认为它确实存在，并应在复发性下腹部疼痛的鉴别诊断中予以重视[93,150]。阑尾的炎症并不都发展为穿孔，因为自发性炎症消散确实存在[36,68]。认识这一点有助于减少阑尾切除术[75,160]。

临床表现

传统学说认为阑尾炎的病程包括单纯炎症直至阑尾穿孔各个阶段。典型穿孔发生在起病后 24～36 小时，2～3 天后继发性脓肿形成[24,143]。然而阑尾炎的临床表现各异，使得剖腹术并不都能反映出阑尾炎症，临床经验增加及影像学检查的发展提高了诊断的准确性，但并不意味着 100% 确诊。从阑尾炎的病理生理学角度出发可理解它的临床表现。

炎症发生后的管腔梗阻容易导致阑尾炎的发生，这一过程在 1905 年由 van Zwalenberg[169] 首先描述，1939 年由 Wangensteen[173] 实验证实。Wangensteen 发现阑尾腔的压力超过 93 mmHg 时，人类的阑尾黏膜仍可以持续分泌黏液。尽管已经证实管腔阻塞可导致阑尾炎，但阻塞产生的原因尚不明确。粪便浓缩和有时钙化的粪便物质称为粪石，常在发病中起一定作用[114]。外科手术时，在 20% 急性阑尾炎和 30%～40% 穿孔性阑尾炎患儿中可以发现粪石的存在[40,159]。文献报道，放射学检查中也经常发现阑尾粪石的存在。阑尾淋巴滤泡的异常增生常造成阑尾管腔的阻塞，阑尾炎发生率高低与淋巴滤泡数量的多少成正比[27]。可以引起淋巴组织对局部或全身反应的细菌如 耶尔森鼠疫杆菌、沙门杆菌和志贺杆菌等感染可以导致阑尾管腔的阻塞，同时还有寄生虫感染如内 阿米巴属、类圆线虫属、蛲虫和血吸虫或蛔虫[2,108,146]等。肠病毒和全身病毒感染如麻疹、水痘和巨细胞病毒等也可导致阑尾炎的发生[81,167]。囊性纤维化的患儿由于黏膜分泌腺体的病变也可能导致阑尾炎的发生[38,115]。类癌也可造成管腔阻塞，特别是其位于近 1/3 段时。近 200 年来，各种异物，如大头针、蔬菜种子和樱桃核等被提及可导致阑尾炎发生。创伤、心理压力[39]及遗传[8]也是相关报道中提及的原因[69]。

病初腹痛之前，患儿出现轻微胃肠道症状，如食欲减退、消化不良及排便习惯的改变。食欲减退是一个对诊断有帮助的表现，尤其在儿童，因为儿童有饥饿感时很少是阑尾炎。但疼痛开始前任何严重的胃肠道症状提示也可存在其他疾病。阑尾腔的扩张刺激内脏疼痛纤维，典型的内脏疼痛是非特异性的脐周疼痛。最初的局限的深钝痛由脊髓的第 10 胸节神经传导。阑尾管壁的持续扩张引起恶心和呕吐，并典型地在数小时后开始腹痛。恶心很常见，呕吐往往并不严重。腹痛前的这些表现常提示阑尾炎。

梗阻的阑尾是定殖细菌很好的繁殖地。随着腔内压力的增高，淋巴回流受阻，进一步加剧水肿和肿胀。最终，压力的升高造成阑尾静脉的阻塞，导致组织缺血、梗死及坏疽，细菌侵入阑尾壁。缺血组织、白细胞和细菌释放的炎症介质导致发热、心动过速和白细胞升高。当阑尾壁的炎性渗出物接触到壁腹膜，刺激体神经纤维，在临近阑尾的位置，通常是麦氏点产生固定疼痛。疼痛偶尔仅出现于右下腹而无早期内脏疼痛。当有盲肠后位或盆腔位阑尾时，因为炎性渗出物在阑尾穿孔和炎症扩散之前无法接触到壁腹膜，固定疼痛常出现较晚。盲肠后位阑尾疼痛常出现在肋腹部或后背处，盆腔位阑尾因靠近输尿管和睾丸组织，可引起尿频和（或）睾丸疼痛。发炎的阑尾可以导致输尿管和膀胱炎症而产生排尿疼痛和继发于尿潴留的膀胱胀痛。

进一步阑尾壁破裂穿孔，腔内炎性内容物外流形
成局限性脓肿或弥漫性腹膜炎。这一病理过程的发展 1503
取决于穿孔的速度和患儿对流出的炎性肠内容物的反

应能力。阑尾穿孔的体征包括：体温升高超过38.6℃（101.5℉）、白细胞计数高于4000/mm^3[137]和其他弥漫性腹膜炎的表现。一些报道指出穿孔阑尾炎的高危因素还包括男性、小婴儿、老年人以及解剖因素如盲肠后位阑尾[119,143]。但是，穿孔性阑尾炎和非穿孔性阑尾炎是完全不同的[9]。某些阑尾炎症的自发消散确实存在。阑尾穿孔前可没有任何症状，也可以在症状出现48小时后仍未穿孔。但一般情况下，症状的长时间持续存在提高了穿孔的危险性。便秘不常出现，但常会出现直肠的充盈感或里急后重感。儿童比成人更容易出现腹泻，而误诊为胃肠炎。腹泻在短时间内持续存在并经常发生末端回肠或回盲部的激惹症状提示有盆腔脓肿的发生。

对于小婴儿，因为不能提供准确的病史和医生的警觉性低，更容易发生误诊而导致复杂性阑尾炎[64,67,84]。学龄前儿童的典型症状是呕吐和随后的发热和腹痛[5]。阑尾穿孔几乎都在剖腹探查时才发现，患儿可继发广泛的末端回肠和回盲部炎症而导致小肠梗阻。

诊断

体格检查

与大多数疾病进展类似，患儿查体前就已经基本明确。阑尾炎的患儿通常卧床不愿意活动，乱动尖叫的孩子很少是阑尾炎患者。比较特殊的是盲肠后位阑尾炎常因输尿管刺激表现为类似肾绞痛的疼痛。年长儿常跛行或卷曲着身体，而小婴儿常将右腿向腹部屈曲。如果有在来院就诊途中因颠簸而加剧疼痛的情况，将有助于阑尾炎的诊断。

询问病史后，常常让患儿用单个手指指出腹部最疼痛的部位。屈膝放松腹肌，从不疼痛的区域开始轻柔触诊腹部。远离疼痛部位的触诊如引起右下腹压痛（牵涉痛引起的Rovsing征），则提示腹膜激惹征。用小婴儿自己的手或听诊器触诊腹部，患儿将会更为配合。听诊器在阑尾炎诊断中作用很多，其中最不重要的是可用于听诊。尽管一些患儿会出现肠鸣音减弱或消失，但不具有普遍性，腹部听诊意义不大。然而胸部听诊对下呼吸道炎症的诊断有帮助，因为右下肺叶炎症可以产生和阑尾炎相类似的症状。T10至L1神经根传导的感觉神经异常所引起的皮肤感觉过敏征，是一种早期即出现但与阑尾炎不相符合的体征，听诊器的轻触诊可诱使患儿产生这种不舒适的感觉。

在触诊或叩诊时要注意局部压痛情况，这是阑尾炎的诊断要点。局部压痛可以十分轻微，甚至可被更泛化的腹痛所掩盖，尤其在发病初期。压痛通常固定于麦氏点，盲肠后位的阑尾炎在髂后上棘和第十二后肋之间有固定压痛，盆腔位阑尾产生直肠内触痛。肠旋转不良的患儿的压痛点取决于发炎阑尾渗出物的流向区域。

随着病程进展，阑尾穿孔，发生腹膜炎。疼痛的类型同样与阑尾的位置有关。穿孔后随着内脏胀痛的缓解，症状可以暂时减轻。开始，腹膜炎可以表现为局部腹肌紧张。随着单纯的不自主的自我防护，腹肌紧张可以泛化。其他的体征包括腰大肌征（右髋后伸或上抬伸直的下肢对抗阻力时可以引出）或闭孔内肌征（被动向内侧旋转右大腿时可以引出）均可引出时，提示为盲肠后位阑尾炎。其他一些腹膜炎体征的检查如反跳痛因可引起不舒适感很少被使用。

常规的直肠触诊在阑尾炎诊断中的使用仍存在争议[23,43,47]。该检查所产生的疼痛不是阑尾炎所特异的。如果已有的体征可以诊断阑尾炎，则不需要进行直肠检查。然而，它对可疑病例的诊断，如盆腔位阑尾炎、怀疑有脓肿形成或需要排除输卵管、子宫病变时还是有帮助的。

如果阑尾炎进一步发展，可引起弥漫性腹膜炎和休克；或炎症局限，脓肿形成。可能是因为缺少网膜脂肪，婴幼儿更容易发生弥漫性腹膜炎，年长儿或青少年则更容易形成脓肿。一些病例可以在脓肿部位触及沼泽状的柔软的团块。

经常有由同一人进行的一系列有确诊意义的体格检查却不报道的情况。1975年White和同事[16]首先报道了安全而有效的系列检查方式，后有其他研究进一步对其补充。Surana和同事们[161]的一项前瞻性研究显示，在同一医院，严密观察后行阑尾切除术与立即行阑尾切除术的病例相比死亡率没有增多。诊断不明确时，进行一系列的腹部检查，可减少不必要的腹部手术，也并不增加患儿的风险。

实验室检查

许多与阑尾炎相关的实验室检查已有很多讨论。

全白细胞计数和中性粒细胞计数得到广泛研究[21,45,72]，白细胞升高的灵敏度为 52%~96%，中性粒细胞核左移的灵敏度为 39%~96%。后者诊断价值更高，但常存在对其诊断价值的错误解释。5% 的阑尾炎患儿白细胞计数可以正常。中性粒细胞与淋巴细胞的比值超过 3.5 时特异性和灵敏性更大[61]。

C-反应蛋白和红细胞沉降率阳性值对诊断有帮助[123]，但阴性结果不能排除阑尾炎，因此限制了这些检查的临床应用。这些检查的联合应用对诊断最有帮助。Dueholm[46] 发现白细胞计数、中性粒细胞百分比和 C-反应蛋白水平正常对排除阑尾炎的准确率是 100%。然而，这些数值的异常并不是诊断阑尾炎所必需的。

大多数儿童阑尾炎的可疑病例，结合病史、体格检查和实验室检查可以为诊断提供充分的证据。然而据报道，误诊导致的阴性阑尾切除的发生率为 10%~30%[138]。基于 8 个临床因素的阑尾炎评分（右下腹固定压痛、白细胞增多、转移性腹痛、核左移、发热、恶心或呕吐、厌食和腹膜刺激征）有助于提高诊断的准确性[6,76]。对急性腹痛儿童的前瞻性研究，评分系统的敏感度为 76%~100%，特异性为 79%~87%[88,138]。对可疑病例有必要连续观察并进一步行影像学检查。

放射学检查

放射成像和放射性药物学检查均能提高诊断的准确性。腹部平片有一定意义，10%~20% 的患儿可见粪石影，这对症状轻微的患儿是手术指征。右下腹异常的气体分布，腰椎偏离右下腹，右侧腰大肌阴影或腹脂线消失有助于诊断。有必要行胸片检查排除肺炎。

钡剂灌肠造影检查可显示阑尾充盈缺失或不完全、不规则的阑尾腔以及盲肠或末端回肠的壁外包块。该项检查的敏感度与特异性均很低[140]，最好用于非特异性腹痛的诊断。

白细胞标记扫描的灵敏度为 87%，特异度为 92%，但需要 3~5 小时完成检查[51]。一项在儿童中进行的研究证明，怀疑为阑尾炎的早期病例，Tc99m 四氮六甲环胺肟白细胞标记扫描对儿童患者诊断的准确度和可信度均较差[74]。

对有经验的医生，B 超检查对阑尾炎的诊断有帮助。在一项前瞻性研究中，B 超检查比外科医生的最初临床印象更具有准确性[171]。大多数研究证实，B 超有高于 85% 的灵敏度和高于 90% 的特异度[178]。阑尾管腔直径≥7 mm 有早期诊断意义。粪石的存在对诊断有帮助。这一技术需要压力阶梯以及自我定位[32]，经阴道或经直肠 B 超检查[103]或许能提高诊断准确性。

在过去几十年中，计算机 X 线断层扫描（CT）被广泛用于阑尾炎的诊断[19,29,89,157]。发现阑尾增粗（>6 mm）、阑尾壁增厚（>1 mm）、阑尾周围脂肪线和阑尾壁信号增强对诊断有意义[34,66]。CT 扫描的灵敏度高于 90%，特异度高于 80%[14]。比较 B 超和 CT 检查，后者有更高的灵敏度，而前者有更高的特异度[19,73,178]。这两种影像学检查只在诊断不明确时应用。在一项记录中，盆腔 B 超与局限性 CT 直肠对比的扫描联合应用有 94% 的灵敏度和 94% 的特异度[59]。这一记录显示，研究期间在同一研究机构阴性阑尾切除术发生率由 12% 下降为 6%，而 80% 儿童阑尾炎可疑病例进行了影像学检查。尽管没有确切证据证明常规行 CT 检查有助于阑尾炎的诊断，但可以认为在儿童患者中 CT 扫描增多可使诊断准确性提高[25,60,124]。另一方面，要考虑 CT 检查对医院医疗资源的利用是否得当及是否延误了外科治疗，以及 CT 电离辐射致癌的潜在危险[25]。

这些诊断方法只在诊断不明确时应用。常规的钡剂对比灌肠检查、B 超及 CT 扫描并没有对急性阑尾炎患儿的诊断和临床病程产生本质的影响[140]。尽管一些研究报道，与单一外科体格检查的诊断结果相比，由同一检查者采用更安全和更准确的系列辅助诊断手段更具有优越性[12]。最近的一项回顾性研究报道显示，小儿外科医生的评估联合选择性的有意义的影像学检查结果（<40% 为阑尾炎可疑儿童）的诊断具有更高的灵敏度（99%）和特异度（92%）以及较低的阴性阑尾切除率（5%）[79]。 1505

鉴别诊断

急性阑尾炎可以有一些与腹腔内其他疾病相类似的表现[37]，阑尾炎的鉴别诊断见表 98-1。手术前考虑到这些疾病及在术中和麻醉状态下发现阑尾正常时认真探查均十分重要。

阑尾炎的临床诊断具有一定的挑战性，因为阑尾炎的许多临床症状是非特异性的，且存在着很多变异。急性胃肠炎是引起儿童腹痛的常见病因。它常由病毒性感染性疾病引起，并具有自限性。常表现为水样泻、痉挛性腹痛、发热、恶心和呕吐。便秘是儿童腹痛、恶心和呕吐的另一种常见原因。腹痛常是持续性的，但无渐进性加重，病史和腹部平片对诊断有提示作用。泌尿系感染也可以引起发热、恶心和呕吐，如果存在泌尿系症状应进行尿液分析检查。

尽管影像学诊断有新进展，手术有时却发现阑尾并无炎症。以前，术中发现不存在阑尾炎的发生率为15%~40%[143]。最近的文献报道，这一比率在阴性阑尾切除术中要低于10%[22,49,110,123]。当手术中发现阑尾正常时，大多数手术者选择切除阑尾进行病理检查，以避免患儿将来出现右下腹疼痛而混淆诊断。同时应进行右下腹器官的探查以寻找引起“阑尾炎”症状的病因，验证回肠末端是否有肠系膜淋巴结炎——回肠肠系膜上是否有继发于上呼吸道感染而增大的淋巴结。患儿可以有腹痛、发热和恶心，但腹部压痛点与阑尾压痛点位置不同。淋巴细胞增多也可见于白细胞分类计数中。Meckel 憩室也应排除，但它很少引起腹痛，无痛性出血及肠梗阻是其常见的症状。如果是 Crohn 病，阑尾或盲肠受累也不应切除阑尾，因为切除阑尾后肠瘘的发生率较高[177]。

表 98-1　急性阑尾炎的鉴别诊断

阑尾	**泌尿系统**
阑尾肿瘤、类癌瘤	肾盂积水
阑尾黏液囊肿	肾盂肾炎
Crohn 病	输尿管或肾脏结石
	肾母细胞瘤
盲肠和结肠	
盲肠癌	**子宫、卵巢**
憩室炎	异位妊娠
Crohn 病	卵巢扭转
肠梗阻	卵巢囊肿破裂
粪性溃疡	输卵管炎
盲肠炎（白血病性、阿米巴性）	输卵管-卵巢脓肿
肝胆管	**其他**
胆囊炎	巨细胞病毒感染
肝炎	糖尿病酮症酸中毒
胆管炎	过敏性紫癜
	川崎病
小肠	Burkitt 淋巴瘤
淋巴结炎	网膜扭转
十二指肠溃疡	腹直肌鞘血肿
胃肠炎	胰腺炎
肠梗阻	寄生虫感染
套迭	胸膜炎
Meckel 憩室	卟啉病
结核	肺炎
伤寒（溃疡穿孔）	腰大肌脓肿
	镰状红细胞贫血症
	肠脂垂扭转

阑尾炎在年轻女性中诊断准确率最低，因为许多妇科疾病可以引起下腹部疼痛。有下腹部疼痛的青少年女性应考虑到异位妊娠的可能，可以出现阴道流血、停经、眩晕、恶心或呕吐。卵巢囊肿破裂和卵巢扭转也可出现下腹部疼痛。对于性生活活跃的女性，盆腔炎症也可以引起下腹部疼痛、阴道流液及附件增大。大多数有宫颈活动性触痛，抗生素治疗有效。抗生素治疗无效或脓肿持续存在时需手术介入治疗。

阑尾切除术时发现为阑尾类癌的发生率低于1%[63]。与其他肠类癌相比，大多数的阑尾类癌瘤缺少含5-羟色胺的内分泌细胞，该细胞为中肠类癌瘤特有的，因而没有相应症状，常在行阑尾切除术时偶尔发现[135]。此病大多为良性，单纯行阑尾切除术即可治愈[102,121]。对潜在恶性的阑尾类癌瘤，正确的治疗方法一直有争议。一般认为如果癌肿直径超过2 cm，且有明显的转移，并位于阑尾基底部时则应行右半结肠切除术。如果直径小于1 cm，在诊断时没有转移的征象，则仅行阑尾切除术[118,135]。对直径在1～2 cm肿瘤的治疗仍存在争议。Moertel 和他的同事[102]认为，如果肿瘤没有转移，可以采用相对保守的外科治疗，而无须考虑肿瘤的大小和位置。

治疗

尽管所有外科医生都认为阑尾炎的治疗方法是手术切除，但围术期管理的细节仍各有不同[107]，很多治疗细节的最佳方案仍不清楚。例如，引流物的应用、是否需要腹腔冲洗、阑尾残端的处理方法和切口的缝合方法等仍存在争论。阑尾脓肿时 B 超和 CT 诊断并在其引导下放置引流物正对是否需要早期手术产生影响。在非手术治疗阑尾蜂窝组织炎后是否需要手术介入仍存在争议。对于抗生素的选择和应用时间，不同外科医生的观点也不尽相同。

抗生素

抗生素的应用对治疗阑尾炎有显而易见的好处[97,104]。目前尚无数据证明术中细菌培养对治疗结果有影响[97,104]。抗生素的最佳疗法和疗程仍存在着争议。最近对一项小儿外科医生的调查显示对抗生素的应用存在很大分歧[107]。静脉内连续 10 天应用氨苄西林、庆大霉素和克林霉素或甲硝唑是治疗复杂性阑尾炎的金标准[149]，而其他抗生素的联合使用的有效性常常挑战着这一经验法则。根据细菌谱不同包括大肠杆菌、肠球菌、克雷白杆菌属、类杆菌属等而采用不同的抗生素联合应用。因为新一代抗生素的广泛应用，一些其他联合疗法也是有效的，例如：头孢噻肟合用克林霉素[14]、单独用头孢噻吩[101]、克林霉素合用阿米卡星[15]、克林霉素合用氨曲腩[15]、头孢吡肟合用甲硝唑[18]、替卡西林合用克拉维酸钾及哌拉西林合用三唑巴坦[109]。

目前有减少抗生素使用疗程的趋势[142]。早期阑尾炎只在围术期使用抗生素，推荐单一药物应用 48 小时[16,83]。一项前瞻性双盲研究显示，使用单一剂量的头孢噻吩（半衰期为 0.8 小时）不如单一剂量的头孢双硫唑甲氧（半衰期为 3.5 小时）或 24 小时维持使用头孢噻吩有效[83]。因此药物使用时间取决于选择何种药物。对于复杂性阑尾炎，最近的研究报道显示仅用 48 小时的抗生素治疗已足够[103]。一些研究认为，抗生素需连续使用 5 天，并根据患儿的白细胞计数、是否发热而决定增加的天数[18,35,154]。另一种倾向是在胃肠道功能恢复后改为使用口服抗生素。一项前瞻性随机研究显示治疗复杂性阑尾炎时，静脉内使用 10 天抗生素与静脉内使用 10 天抗生素后改为口服的疗效是等同的[133]。我们所在医疗机构内抗生素的使用标准是：手术前，对怀疑为单纯性阑尾炎的患儿使用头孢噻吩，而对复杂性阑尾炎的患儿使用氨苄西林、庆大霉素和克林霉素。如果临床上出现发热、白细胞计数升高则继续使用抗生素。

阑尾切除术

急性阑尾炎普遍接受的治疗方法是迅速手术。但有证据显示，一些急性阑尾炎可以自发消退[36]，但无报道显示早期不进行手术治疗，会使发展为复杂性阑尾炎的风险增加。目前并不认为放射学检查、实验室检查或临床体征对判断单纯性阑尾炎症是消退还是导致并发症发生有帮助，而且采用非手术方法治疗急性阑尾炎的病例很少。一种趋势是对急性阑尾炎不进行急诊手术治疗，包括半夜手术[162,179]。根据美国小儿外科协会的一份调查显示，只有约半数的外科医生在半夜里行阑尾切除术[107]。对单纯性阑尾炎，在入院后 6 小时内手术与 6～18 小时内手术相比，后者并没有增加阑尾穿孔或并发症的风险[161,176]。然而，对大多数确诊为急性阑尾炎的患儿还是采取了急诊手术治疗，大部分小儿外科医生选择在 8 小时内行阑尾切除术[107]。

开腹手术时，选择右下腹经麦氏点的横形或斜形手术切口（图 98-1）。常规分离腹壁肌肉，进入腹腔后，牵动盲肠和阑尾，将阑尾提出腹壁切口。分离阑尾系膜，结扎阑尾基底部，基底部残端短一些以避免残株炎的发生[52]。残株在简单结扎后用袋式的或 Z 型抽线法内翻缝合，或不结扎直接内翻缝合[158]。简单结扎很快就可完成并可减少粘连发生。理论上内翻缝合可以较好地控制出血、双重可靠地关闭以及减少污染，但它在将来的造影检查中会产生一个假象并能引起套迭[70]。一篇关于单纯结扎与结扎后内翻缝合对比的综述中提到，单纯结扎和结扎后内翻缝合同样有效，而且可以减少肠粘连的形成[158]。对单纯性阑尾炎不需要进行伤口冲洗。逐层关闭伤口，无需放置引流物。手术后不久就可以正常进食，术后 1～2 天可以出院。如果发现阑尾正常，则应探查腹腔，以排除感染性肠疾病、肠系膜淋巴结炎、Meckel 憩室炎或女性卵巢方面的疾患。

1983 年首次报道“内镜”下阑尾切除术[151]。腹腔镜下阑尾切除术借助腹腔镜辅助技术，通过腹壁上小切口，使用 1～2 把腹腔镜钳拖出阑尾，并采用标准的开腹阑尾切除方式切除阑尾[50,168]。另外，阑尾切除也可以完全在腹腔镜下完成，通常用 3 个套管
针：一个放置在脐下用于置入腹腔镜，一个放置在右 1508
上腹，一个放置在左下腹用于牵开组织并解剖（图 98-2）。沿着盲肠寻找阑尾，将阑尾头部向腹壁方向牵开，靠近阑尾尖处抓住阑尾系膜。在靠近阑尾基底

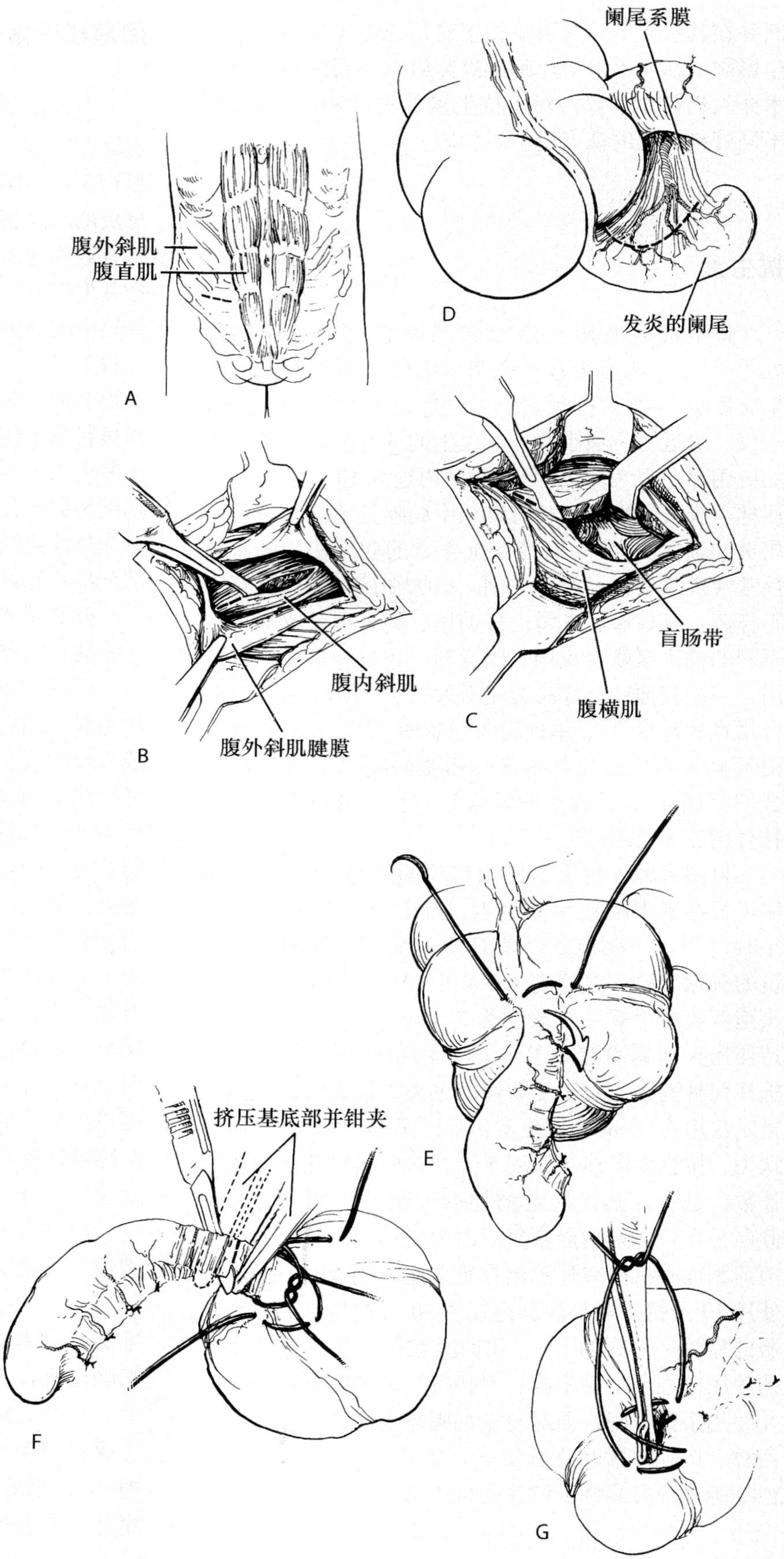

图 98-1 A. 右下腹横切口。B. 分离腹外斜肌腱膜，显露腹内斜肌腱膜和肌肉。C. 打开腹横肌和腹膜，暴露盲肠。D. 确认发炎的阑尾，游离阑尾系膜，钳夹、分离并打结。E. 在盲肠壁上放置袋式缝合线。F. 挤压阑尾基底部并打结，切除阑尾。G. 内翻阑尾残端，袋式缝合线打结。（From Rowe M，O'Neill J，Grosfeld J，et al：Essentials of Pediatric Surgery. Philadelphia，CV Mosby，1995.）

部的系膜上开窗，以利于被血管钳、抓手或止血钳等分离，结扎和切除阑尾的方法有许多种[49,152]，最简单的是用内镜吻合器抓紧阑尾基底部，将阑尾从脐部的套管针中拖出。

尽管前瞻性的随机研究对开腹及腹腔镜手术进行了比较，但腹腔镜手术的优缺点一直仍存在争议*。其优势集中在：缩短住院时间、减轻了手术后疼痛、减少伤口并发症、提高对未确诊病例的诊断能力、使肥胖患儿的手术更加容易以及加快了手术后的恢复[22,42,49,57,58,80,87]。劣势在于：因手术设备的需要及手术时间的延长增加了住院费用、增加了对手术医生训练及经验的培养、增加了不必要的阑尾手术的比率及增加了腹腔内感染的发生率等[10,22,97,144,165]。尽管对于腹腔镜手术相比开腹手术的优势评价不一，但对儿童，腹腔镜下阑尾切除术似乎更为安全有效，随机的前瞻性研究支持了这一点。

关于复杂性阑尾炎治疗的争论比单纯性阑尾炎多。因为社会、文化、经济及医疗状况对诊断和治疗的影响，在不同情况下阑尾炎穿孔率为 16%～57% 不等。不存在公认的复杂性阑尾炎的最佳治疗方案。各种治疗意见都有：非手术治疗、积极手术治疗并抗生素冲洗、腹腔引流和延迟关闭切口[17,31,53,94,101]。Weiner 和同事[175]报道对复杂性阑尾炎先采用非手术 1509
治疗，8 周后进行阑尾切除术，其住院时间、治疗费用及并发症的发生率并没有显著差异。在另一项研究中，对经影像学检查确诊的复杂性阑尾炎开始采用非手术治疗，其中 22% 的患儿因继发的小肠梗阻而行

* 见参考文献 30，82，85，86，92，116，120，130，134，141。

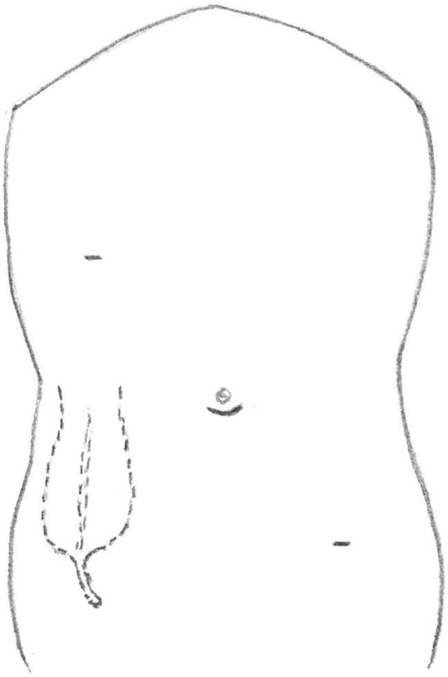
A

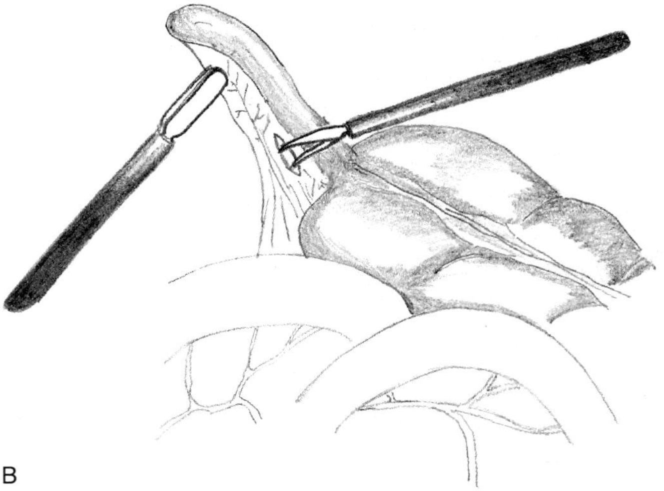
B

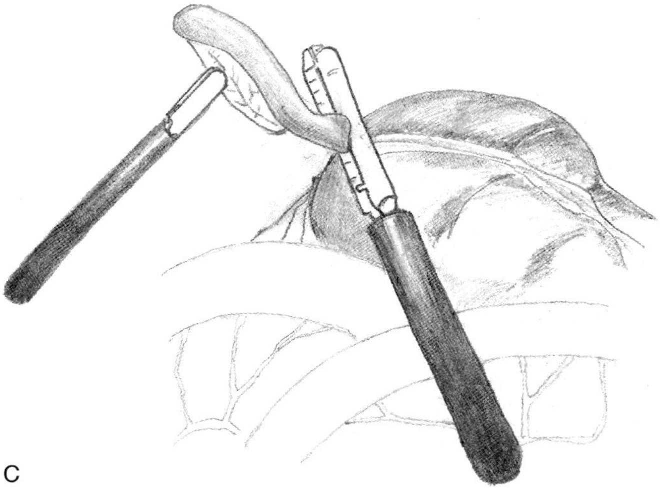
C

图 98-2　A. 腹腔镜下阑尾切除术中放置 3 把手柄。脐部放置 12 mm 套管以放入内镜切割器，另外两个分别为 3 mm和 5 mm 套管以放入解剖器械。B. 朝上提起阑尾头端，在阑尾系膜上放置抓钳，用分离器在阑尾根部系膜上开窗，止血电凝分离阑尾系膜。C. 将内镜移到右下腹，以利于内镜切割器穿过脐部切口分离阑尾，烧灼阑尾残端，从脐部切口将阑尾提出。

阑尾切除术[77]。Bandemia 报道约超过 15% 的患儿非手术治疗失败。因为手术前很难判定阑尾是否穿孔，手术治疗仍然是复杂性阑尾炎的标准治疗方案。

复杂性阑尾炎手术方式是阑尾切除术，手术细节仍存在争议：是否行腹腔引流、是关闭切口还是先开放再进行延迟缝合、是否进行腹腔冲洗及如果冲洗是否使用抗生素溶液等。腹腔引流被认为既可能增加发生感染性并发症的几率也可能减少感染性并发症[40,41,137,145,159,164]。大多数医生不支持放置引流物，因为盲肠后的脓肿可能不能被正常清除。文献不支持切口延迟关闭[49,110,137,149]，并认为它似乎没有起到保护作用，因为阑尾炎的切口感染率仅为 3%。是否进行腹腔冲洗仍存在争议。Putnam 及同事[128]认为冲洗回肠将增加小肠梗阻发生的几率，并报道不进行腹腔冲洗仍有很好的治疗效果。最近一些报道支持生理盐水冲洗腹膜腔，可以加或不加抗生素[40,49,110,139,149]。我们对复杂性阑尾炎的标准治疗是：阑尾切除、排尽脓液、生理盐水冲洗、不放置引流及一期关闭切口。

对能触摸到腹部包块的患儿的治疗方案是另一个争议的主题。它出现在少数但很严重的复杂性阑尾炎患儿，尤其是在穿孔后的年幼患儿。一些医生主张行急诊阑尾切除术[166]，一些医生认为应在麻醉下确诊阑尾包块的存在再行手术治疗。如果手术，应小心操作，避免损伤邻近器官而受到感染，如小肠、卵巢、输卵管和输尿管等。Surana[163]和 Nitecki[113]认为应静脉应用抗生素直到白细胞计数正常和患儿体温正常 24 小时。如果患儿情况恶化或 B 超随访检查中发现包块增大，应经皮引流包块，并进行延迟性阑尾切除术。延迟性阑尾切除可以避免阑尾炎症复发，并增加手术医生正确评价其他类似阑尾包块的机会。是否进行延迟性阑尾切除也存在着争议[13,26,48,71,105,113,131]。Nitecki 及同事[113]认为不需要进行延迟性阑尾切除术，因为仅有 14% 的患儿在初次诊断为阑尾炎后两年内出现复发症状。目前标准治疗方案是行保守治疗，8～12 周后行延迟性阑尾切除术。

并发症

随着阑尾炎严重程度的增加，并发症的发生率也增加，但最近几年阑尾炎的并发症持续减少。并发症包括伤口感染、腹腔内脓肿形成、手术后肠梗阻、慢性肠梗阻以及比较少见的肠外瘘。伤口感染是最常见的并发症，但其发生率已由 50% 降低为 5%，即使是在复杂性阑尾炎患者[40,49,110,119,128,159]。腹腔内脓肿也是复杂性阑尾炎较常见的并发症，其发病率低于 2%，脓肿可以在 CT 导引下经皮引流或在手术室经直肠进行引流，更保守的治疗方法也有报道[44,62,117]。约 1% 复杂性阑尾炎患儿并发术后肠梗阻，并往往需行粘连松解术[3]。肠外瘘是较少见的并发症，通常需要非手术治疗。化脓性门静脉炎是很严重但更为少见的并发症[170]。确诊前病程较长的患儿可能会发生败血症和多器官衰竭。目前阑尾炎的主要并发症，如术后肠梗阻和腹腔脓肿等的发生率已下降至 5% 以下。

一个未解决的问题是复杂性阑尾炎对女性生育能力的影响，现有的研究结果之间存在着矛盾。Puri 及同事[127]报道青春期前复杂性阑尾炎对女性生殖功能影响很小，不会引起输卵管性不孕。而 Mueller 及同事报道[106]，复发性阑尾炎女性发生输卵管性不孕症的风险比普通阑尾炎大 4 倍。随着公众及医疗教育力度的加大，使阑尾炎在穿孔前即得到迅速治疗，复杂性阑尾炎的预后也将会有大的改观。

预后

复杂性阑尾炎的死亡率已接近 0，抗生素的使用使感染性并发症也大大减少。尽管复杂性阑尾炎的住院时间和死亡率远远超过单纯性阑尾炎，整个儿童复杂性阑尾炎的发生率仍低于 10%。

方法各异的阑尾炎手术后管理开始集中于以循证为基础的临床路径[156,174]，经济状况的转变改善了患儿治疗和预后[55,56,112]。早期预后的相关研究显示每周行阑尾切除术少于 1 例的医院，阑尾炎的误诊率也较高[155]。也有报道显示，由小儿外科医生主治的阑尾炎儿童预后较好[4,78]。联合手术评估、在诊断清楚时予以急诊手术、诊断有疑问时观察一段时间再辅助以影像学检查，由有经验的医疗机构和临床医生进行治疗将使儿童阑尾炎的预后越来越好。

（杜 勇译 周小渔校）

参考文献

1. Addiss DG, Shaffer J, Fowler BS, Tauxe RV: The epidemiology of appendicitis and appendectomy in the United States. Am J Epidemiol 1990;132:910.
2. Adebamowo CA, Akang EE, Ladipo JK, Ajao OG: Schistosomiasis of the appendix. Br J Surg 1991;78:1219.
3. Ahlberg G, Bergdahl S, Rutqvist J, et al: Mechanical small-bowel obstruction after conventional appendectomy in children. Eur J Pediatr Surg 1997;7:13.
4. Alexander F, Magnuson D, DiFiore J, et al: Specialty versus generalist care of children with appendicitis: An outcome comparison. J Pediatr Surg 2001;36:1510.
5. Alloo J, Gerstle T, Shilyansky J, Ein SH: Appendicitis in children less than 3 years of age: A 28-year review. Pediatr Surg Int 2004;19:777.
6. Alvarado A: A practical score for the early diagnosis of acute appendicitis. Ann Emerg Med 1986;15:557.
7. Andersen BR, Kallehave FL, Andersen HK: Antibiotics versus placebo for prevention of postoperative infection after appendicectomy. Cochrane Database Syst Rev 2003; CD001439.
8. Andersson N, Griffiths H, Murphy J, et al: Is appendicitis familial? BMJ 1979;2:697.
9. Andersson R, Hugander A, Thulin A, et al: Indications for operation in suspected appendicitis and incidence of perforation. BMJ 1994;308:107.
10. Apelgren KN, Molnar RG, Kisala JM: Laparoscopic is not better than open appendectomy. Am Surg 1995;61:240.
11. Attwood SE, Mealy K, Cafferkey MT, et al: *Yersinia* infection and acute abdominal pain. Lancet 1987;1:529.
12. Bachoo P, Mahomed AA, Ninan GK, Youngson GG: Acute appendicitis: The continuing role for active observation. Pediatr Surg Int 2001;17:125.
13. Bagi P, Dueholm S: Nonoperative management of the ultrasonically evaluated appendiceal mass. Surgery 1987; 101:602.
14. Balthazar EJ, Megibow AJ, Siegel SE, Birnbaum BA: Appendicitis: Prospective evaluation with high-resolution CT. Radiology 1991;180:21.
15. Barboza E, del Castillo M, Yi A, Gotuzzo E: Clindamycin plus amikacin versus clindamycin plus aztreonam in established intraabdominal infections. Surgery 1994;116:28.
16. Bauer T, Vennits B, Holm B, et al: Antibiotic prophylaxis in acute non-perforated appendicitis. Ann Surg 1989;209:307.
17. Bennion RS, Thompson JE: Early appendectomy for perforated appendicitis in children should not be abandoned. Surg Gynecol Obstet 1987;165:95.
18. Berne TV, Yellin AE, Appleman MD, et al: A clinical comparison of cefepime and metronidazole versus gentamicin and clindamycin in the antibiotic management of surgically treated advanced appendicitis. Surg Gynecol Obstet 1993;177(Suppl):18.
19. Birnbaum BA, Balthazar EJ: CT of appendicitis and diverticulitis. Radiol Clin North Am 1994;32:885.
20. Bluett MK, Halter SA, Salhany KE, O'Leary JP: Duplication of the appendix mimicking adenocarcinoma of the colon. Arch Surg 1987;122:817.
21. Bolton JP, Craven ER, Croft RJ, Menzies-Gow N: An assessment of the value of the white-cell count in the management of suspected acute appendicitis. Br J Surg 1975;62:906.
22. Bonanni F, Reed J 3rd, Hartzell G, et al: Laparoscopic versus conventional appendectomy. J Am Coll Surg 1994;179:273.
23. Bonello JC, Abrams JS: The significance of "positive" rectal examination in acute appendicitis. Dis Colon Rectum 1979; 22:97.
24. Brender JD, Marcuse EK, Keopsell TD, Hatch EI: Childhood appendicitis: Factors associated with perforation. Pediatrics 1985;76:301.
25. Brenner DJ: Estimating cancer risks from pediatric CT: Going from the qualitative to the quantitative. Pediatr Radiol 2002;32:228.
26. Bufo AJ, Shah RS, Li MH, et al: Interval appendectomy for perforated appendicitis in children. J Laparoendosc Adv Surg Tech A 1998;8:209.
27. Burkitt DP: The aetiology of appendicitis. Br J Surg 1971; 58:695.
28. Buschard K, Kjaeldgaard A: Investigation and analysis of the position, fixation, length and embryology of the vermiform appendix. Acta Chir Scand 1973;139:293.
29. Callahan MJ, Rodriguez DP, Taylor GA: CT of appendicitis in children. Radiology 2002;224:325.
30. Canty TG Sr, Collins D, Losasso B, et al: Laparoscopic appendectomy for simple and perforated appendicitis in children: The procedure of choice? J Pediatr Surg 2000; 35:1582-1585.
31. Chen C, Botelho C, Cooper A, et al: Current practice patterns in the treatment of perforated appendicitis in children. J Am Coll Surg 2003;196:212.
32. Chesbrough RM, Burkhard TK, Balsara ZN, et al: Self-localization in US of appendicitis: An addition to graded compression. Radiology 1993;187:349.
33. Chew DK, Borromeo JR, Gabriel YA, Holgersen LO: Duplication of the vermiform appendix. J Pediatr Surg 2000; 35:617.
34. Choi D, Park H, Lee YR, et al: The most useful findings for diagnosing acute appendicitis on contrast-enhanced helical CT. Acta Radiol 2003;44:574.
35. Ciftci AO, Tanyel FC, Buyukpamukcu N, Hicsonmez A: Comparative trial of four antibiotic combinations for perforated appendicitis in children. Eur J Surg 1997; 163:591.
36. Cobben LP, de Van Otterloo AM, Puylaert JB: Spontaneously resolving appendicitis: Frequency and natural history in 60 patients. Radiology 2000;215:349.
37. Cope Z: Appendicitis and the differential diagnosis of acute appendicitis. In Silen W (ed): Cope's Early Diagnosis of the Acute Abdomen. New York, Oxford University Press, 1991.
38. Coughlin JP, Gauderer MW, Stern RC, et al: The spectrum of appendiceal disease in cystic fibrosis. J Pediatr Surg 1990;25:835.
39. Creed F: Life events and appendectomy. Lancet 1981; 1:1381.
40. Curran TJ, Meunchow SK: The treatment of complicated appendicitis in children using peritoneal drainage: Results from a public hospital. J Pediatr Surg 1993;28:404.
41. David IB, Buck JR, Filler RM: Rational use of antibiotics for perforated appendicitis in childhood. J Pediatr Surg 1982; 17:494.
42. DeWilde RL: Goodbye to late bowel obstruction after appendicectomy [Letter]. Lancet 1991;338:1012.
43. Dixon JM, Elton RA, Rainey JB, Macleod DA: Rectal examination in patients with pain in the right lower quadrant of the abdomen. BMJ 1991;302:368.
44. Dobremez E, Lavrand F, Lefevre Y, et al: Treatment of post-appendectomy intra-abdominal deep abscesses. Eur J Pediatr Surg 2003;13:393.
45. Doraiswany NV: Leucocyte counts in the diagnosis and prognosis of acute appendicitis in children. Br J Surg 1979;66:72.
46. Dueholm S, Bagi P, Bud M: Laboratory aid in the diagnosis of acute appendicitis: A blinded, prospective trial concerning diagnostic value of leukocyte count, neutrophil differential

count and C-reactive protein. Dis Colon Rectum 1989; 32:855.
47. Dunning PG, Goldman MD: The incidence and value of rectal examination in children with suspected appendicitis. Ann R Coll Surg Engl 1991;73:233.
48. Ein SH, Shandling B: Is interval appendectomy necessary after rupture of an appendiceal mass? J Pediatr Surg 1996; 31:849.
49. El Ghoneimi A, Valla JS, Limonne B, et al: Laparoscopic appendectomy in children: Report of 1379 cases. J Pediatr Surg 1994;29:786.
50. Esposito C: One-trocar appendectomy in pediatric surgery. Surg Endosc 1998;12:177.
51. Evetts BK, Foley CR, Latimer RG, Rimkus DS: Tc-99 hexamethylpropyleneamineoxide scanning for the detection of acute appendicitis. J Am Coll Surg 1994;179:197.
52. Feigin E, Carmon M, Szold A, Seror D: Acute stump appendicitis. Lancet 1993;341:757.
53. Fishman SJ, Pelosi L, Klavon SL, O'Rourke EJ: Perforated appendicitis: Prospective outcome analysis for 150 children. J Pediatr Surg 2000;35:923.
54. Fitz RH: Perforating inflammation of the vermiform appendix, with special reference to its early diagnosis and treatment. Trans Assoc Am Phys 1886;1:107.
55. Flum DR, Morris A, Koepsell T, Dellinger EP: Has misdiagnosis of appendicitis decreased over time? A population-based analysis. JAMA 2001;286:1748.
56. Flum DR, Koepsell T: The clinical and economic correlates of misdiagnosed appendicitis: Nationwide analysis. Arch Surg 2002;137:799.
57. Frazee RC, Roberts JW, Symmonds RE, et al: A prospective randomized trial comparing open versus laparoscopic appendectomy. Ann Surg 1994;219:725.
58. Fritts LL, Orlando R: Laparoscopic appendectomy. Arch Surg 1993;128:521.
59. Garcia Pena BM, Mandl KD, Kraus SJ, et al: Ultrasonography and limited computed tomography in the diagnosis and management of appendicitis in children. JAMA 1999;282:1041.
60. Garcia Pena BM, Cook EF, Mandl KD: Selective imaging strategies for the diagnosis of appendicitis in children. Pediatrics 2004;113:24.
61. Goodman DA, Goodman CB, Monk JS: Use of the neutrophil: Lymphocyte ratio in the diagnosis of appendicitis. Am Surg 1995;61:257.
62. Gorenstein A, Gewurtz G, Serour F, Somekh E: Postappendectomy intra-abdominal abscess: A therapeutic approach. Arch Dis Child 1994;70:400.
63. Gouzi JL, Laigneau P, Delalande JP, et al: Indications for right hemicolectomy in carcinoid tumors of the appendix. Surg Gynecol Obstet 1993;176:543.
64. Grosfeld JL, Weinberger M, Clatworthy HW Jr, et al: Acute appendicitis in the first two years of life. J Pediatr Surg 1973;8:285.
65. Guthery SL, Hutchings C, Dean JM, Hoff C: National estimates of hospital utilization by children with gastrointestinal disorders: Analysis of the 1997 kids' inpatient database. J Pediatr 2004;144:589.
66. Gwynn LK: Appendiceal enlargement as a criterion for clinical diagnosis of acute appendicitis: Is it reliable and valid? J Emerg Med 2002;23:9.
67. Huang CB, Yu HR, Hung GC, et al: Clinical features and outcome of appendicitis in children younger than three years of age. Chang Gung Med J 2001;24:27.
68. Heller MB, Skolnick LM: Ultrasound documentation of spontaneously resolving appendicitis. Am J Emerg Med 1993;11:51.
69. Hennington MH, Tinsley EA Jr, Proctor HJ, Baker CC: Acute appendicitis following blunt abdominal trauma: Incidence or coincidence? Ann Surg 1991;214:61.
70. Hoehner JC, Kimura K, Soper RT: Intussusception as a complication of inversion appendectomy. Pediatr Surg Int 1995;10:51.
71. Hoffman J, Lindhard A, Jensen HE: Appendix mass: Conservative management without interval appendectomy. Am J Surg 1984;148:379.
72. Hoffman J, Rasmussen OO: Aids in the diagnosis of acute appendicitis. Br J Surg 1989;76:774.
73. Kaiser S, Frenckner B, Jorulf HK: Suspected appendicitis in children: US and CT—a prospective randomized study. Radiology 2002;223:633.
74. Kanegaye JT, Vance CW, Parisi M, et al: Failure of technetium-99m hexamethylpropylene amine oxime leukocyte scintigraphy in the evaluation of children with suspected appendicitis. Pediatr Emerg Care 1995;11:285.
75. Kang JY, Hoare J, Majeed A, et al: Decline in admission rates for acute appendicitis in England. Br J Surg 2003;90:1586.
76. Klein MD, Rabbani AB, Rood KD, et al: Three quantitative approaches to the diagnosis of abdominal pain in children: Practical applications of decision theory. J Pediatr Surg 2001;36:1375.
77. Kogut KA, Blakely ML, Schropp KP, et al: The association of elevated percent bands on admission with failure and complications of interval appendectomy. J Pediatr Surg 2001;36:165.
78. Kokoska ER, Minkes RK, Silen ML, et al: Effect of pediatric surgical practice on the treatment of children with appendicitis. Pediatrics 2001;107:1298.
79. Kosloske AM, Love CL, Rohrer JE, et al: The diagnosis of appendicitis in children: Outcomes of a strategy based on pediatric surgical evaluation. Pediatrics 2004;113:29.
80. Kum CK, Ngoi SS, Goi PM, et al: Randomized controlled trial comparing laparoscopic and open appendectomy. Br J Surg 1993;80:1599.
81. Kwong MS, Dinner M: Neonatal appendicitis masquerading as necrotizing enterocolitis. J Pediatr 1980;96:918.
82. Lavonius MI, Liesjarvi S, Ovaska J, et al: Laparoscopic versus open appendectomy in children: A prospective randomised study. Eur J Pediatr Surg 2001;11:235.
83. Liberman MA, Greason KL, Frame S, Ragland JJ: Single-dose cefotetan or cefoxitin versus multiple-dose cefoxitin as prophylaxis in patients undergoing appendectomy for acute appendicitis. J Am Coll Surg 1995;180:77.
84. Lin YL, Lee CH: Appendicitis in infancy. Pediatr Surg Int 2003;19:1.
85. Lintula H, Kokki H, Vanamo K: Single-blind randomized clinical trial of laparoscopic versus open appendicectomy in children. Br J Surg 2001;88:510.
86. Little DC, Custer MD, May BH, et al: Laparoscopic appendectomy: An unnecessary and expensive procedure in children? J Pediatr Surg 2002;37:310.
87. Lujan Mompean JA, Robles Campos R, Parrilla Paricio P, et al: Laparoscopic versus open appendectomy: A prospective assessment. Br J Surg 1994;81:133.
88. Macklin CP, Radcliffe GS, Merei JM, Stringer MD: A prospective evaluation of the modified Alvarado score for acute appendicitis in children. Ann R Coll Surg Engl 1997; 79:203.
89. Malone AJ Jr, Wolf CR, Malmed AS, Melliere BF: Diagnosis of acute appendicitis: Value of unenhanced CT. AJR Am J Roentgenol 1993;160:763.
90. Martin LW, Perrin EV: Neonatal perforation of the appendix in association with Hirschsprung's disease. Ann Surg 1967;166:799.

91. Martin AE, Vollman D, Adler B, Caniano DA: CT scans may not reduce the negative appendectomy rate in children. J Pediatr Surg 2004;39:886.
92. Marzouk M, Khater M, Elsadek M, Abdelmoghny A: Laparoscopic versus open appendectomy: A prospective comparative study of 227 patients. Surg Endosc 2003; 17:721.
93. Mattei P, Sola JE, Yeo CJ, et al: Chronic and recurrent appendicitis are uncommon entities often misdiagnosed. J Am Coll Surg 1994;178:385.
94. Mazziotti MV, Marley EF, Winthrop AL, et al: Histopathologic analysis of interval appendectomy specimens: Support for the role of interval appendectomy. J Pediatr Surg 1997;32:806.
95. McBurney C: Experience with early operative interference in cases of disease of the vermiform appendix. NY Med J 1889;50:676.
96. McCahy P: Continuing fall in the incidence of acute appendicitis. Ann R Coll Surg Engl 1994;76:282.
97. McKinlay R, Neeleman S, Klein R, et al: Intraabdominal abscess following open and laparoscopic appendectomy in the pediatric population. Surg Endosc 2003;17:730.
98. McNamara MJ, Pasquale MD, Evans SRT: Acute appendicitis and the use of intraperitoneal cultures. Surg Gynecol Obstet 1993;177:393.
99. Meade RH: The evolution of surgery for appendicitis. Surgery 1964;55:741.
100. Meier DE, Guzzetta PC, Barber RG, et al: Perforated appendicitis in children: Is there a best treatment? J Pediatr Surg 2003;38:1520.
101. Meller JL. Reyes HM, Loeff DS, et al: One-drug versus two-drug antibiotic therapy in pediatric perforated appendicitis: A prospective randomized study. Surgery 1991;110:764.
102. Moertel CL, Weiland LH, Telander RL: Carcinoid tumor of the appendix in the first two decades of life. J Pediatr Surg 1990;25:1073.
103. Moore L, Wilson SR: Ultrasonography in obstetric and gynecologic emergencies. Radiol Clin North Am 1994; 32:1005.
104. Mosdell DM, Morris DM, Fry DE: Peritoneal cultures and antibiotic therapy in pediatric perforated appendicitis. Am J Surg 1994;167:313.
105. Mosegaard A, Nielson OS: Interval appendectomy. Acta Chir Scand 1979;145:109.
106. Mueller BA, Daling JR, Moore DE, et al: Appendectomy and the risk of tubal infertility. N Engl J Med 1986; 315:1506.
107. Muehlstedt SG, Pham TQ, Schmeling DJ: The management of pediatric appendicitis: A survey of North American Pediatric Surgeons. J Pediatr Surg 2004;39:875.
108. Nadler S, Coppell MS, Bhatt B, et al: Appendiceal infection by *Entamoeba histolytica* and *Strongyloides stercoralis* presenting like acute appendicitis. Dig Dis Sci 1990; 35:603.
109. Nadler EP, Reblock KK, Ford HR, Gaines BA: Monotherapy versus multi-drug therapy for the treatment of perforated appendicitis in children. Surg Infect 2003; 4:327.
110. Neilson IR, Laberge JM, Nguyen LT, et al: Appendicitis in children: Current therapeutic recommendations. J Pediatr Surg 1990;25:1113.
111. Neuspiel DR, Kuller LH: Fatalities from undetected appendicitis in early childhood. Clin Pediatr 1987;26:573.
112. Newman K, Ponsky T, Kittle K, et al: Appendicitis 2000: Variability in practice, outcomes, and resource utilization at thirty pediatric hospitals. J Pediatr Surg 2003;38:372.
113. Nitecki S, Assalia A, Schein M: Contemporary management of the appendiceal mass. Br J Surg 1993;80:18.
114. Nitecki S, Karmeli R, Sarr MG: Appendiceal calculi and fecaliths as indications for appendectomy. Surg Gynecol Obstet 1990;171:185.
115. Oestreich AE, Adelstein EH: Appendicitis as the presenting complaint in cystic fibrosis. J Pediatr Surg 1982; 17:191.
116. Oka T, Kurkchubasche AG, Bussey JG, et al: Open and laparoscopic appendectomy are equally safe and acceptable in children. Surg Endosc 2004;18:242.
117. Okoye BO, Rampersad B, Marantos A, et al: Abscess after appendicectomy in children: The role of conservative management. Br J Surg 1998;85:1111.
118. Parkes SE et al: Carcinoid tumours of the appendix in children 1957-1986: Incidence, treatment and outcome. Br J Surg 1993;80:502.
119. Pearl RH, Hale DA, Molloy M, et al: Pediatric appendectomy. J Pediatr Surg 1995;30:173.
120. Pedersen AG, Petersen OB, Wara P, et al: Randomized clinical trial of laparoscopic versus open appendicectomy. Br J Surg 2001;88:200.
121. Pelizzo G, La Riccia A, Bouvier R, et al: Carcinoid tumors of the appendix in children. Pediatr Surg Int 2001;17:399.
122. Peltokallio P, Tykka H: Evolution of the age distribution and mortality of acute appendicitis. Arch Surg 1981; 116:153.
123. Peltola H, Ahlqvist J, Rapola J, et al: C-reactive protein compared with white blood cell count and erythrocyte sedimentation rate in the diagnosis of acute appendicitis in children. Acta Chir Scand 1986;152:55.
124. Pena BM, Taylor GA, Fishman SJ, Mandl KD: Effect of an imaging protocol on clinical outcomes among pediatric patients with appendicitis. Pediatrics 2002;110:1088.
125. Pledger HG, Fahy LT: Deaths in children with a diagnosis of acute appendicitis. BMJ Clin Res 1987;295:1233.
126. Pokorny WJ, Kaplan SL, Mason EO: A preliminary report of ticarcillin and clavulanate versus triple antibiotic therapy in children with ruptured appendicitis. Surg Gynecol Obstet 1991;172(Suppl):54.
127. Puri P, McGuinness EPJ, Guiney EJ: Fertility following perforated appendicitis in girls. J Pediatr Surg 1989;24:547.
128. Putnam TC, Gagliano NG, Emmons RW: Appendicitis in children. Surg Gynecol Obstet 1990;170:527.
129. Rabau MY, Avigad I, Wolfstein I: Rubella in acute appendicitis. Pediatrics 1980;66:813.
130. Rangel SJ, Henry MC, Brindle M, Moss RL: Small evidence for small incisions: Pediatric laparoscopy and the need for more rigorous evaluation of novel surgical therapies. J Pediatr Surg 2003;38:1429.
131. Ranson JHC: Nonoperative treatment of the appendiceal mass: Progress of regression? Gastroenterology 1987; 93:1439.
132. Ravitch MM: Appendicitis. In Welch KJ, et al (eds): Pediatric Surgery. Chicago, Year Book Medical Publishers, 1986.
133. Rice HE, Brown RL, Gollin G, et al: Results of a pilot trial comparing prolonged intravenous antibiotics with sequential intravenous/oral antibiotics for children with perforated appendicitis. Arch Surg 2001;136:1391.
134. Richards W, Watson D, Lynch G, et al: A review of the results of laparoscopic versus open appendectomy. Surg Gynecol Obstet 1993;177:473.
135. Roggo A, Wood WC, Ottinger LW: Carcinoid tumors of the appendix. Ann Surg 1993;217:385.
136. Rodgers B, Karn G: *Yersinia* enterocolitis. J Pediatr Surg 1975;10:497.

137. Samelson SL, Reyes HM: Management of perforated appendicitis in children revisited. Arch Surg 1987;122:691.
138. Samuel M: Pediatric appendicitis score. J Pediatr Surg 2002;37:877.
139. Sanders DY, Cort CR, Stubbs AJ, et al: Shigellosis associated with appendicitis. J Pediatr Surg 1972;7:315.
140. Sarfati MR, Hunter GC, Witzke DB, et al: Impact of adjunctive testing on the diagnosis and clinical course of patients with acute appendicitis. Am J Surg 1993; 166:660.
141. Sauerland S, Lefering R, Neugebauer EA: Laparoscopic versus open surgery for suspected appendicitis. Cochrane Database Syst Rev 2002;CD001546.
142. Schein M, Assalia A, Bachus H: Minimal antibiotic therapy after emergency abdominal surgery: A prospective study. Br J Surg 1994;81:989.
143. Scher KS, Coil JA Jr: Appendicitis: Factors that influence the frequency of perforation, South Med J 1980;73:1561.
144. Schirmer BD, Schmieg RE Jr, Dix J, et al: Laparoscopic versus traditional appendectomy for suspected appendicitis. Am J Surg 1993;165:670.
145. Schmit PJ, Hiyama DT, Swisher SG, et al: Analysis of risk factors of postappendectomy intraabdominal abscess. Surg Gynecol Obstet 1994;179:721.
146. Schnell VL, Yandell R, Van Zandt S, Dinh TV: *Enterobius vermicularis* salpingitis: A distant episode from precipitating appendicitis. Obstet Gynecol 1992;80:553.
147. Schropp KP, Kaplan S, Golladay ES, et al: A randomized clinical trial of ampicillin, gentamicin and clindamycin versus cefotaxime and clindamycin in children with ruptured appendicitis. Surg Gynecol Obstet 1991;172:351.
148. Schumpelick V, Dreuw B, Ophoff K, Prescher A: Appendix and cecum: Embryology, anatomy, and surgical applications. Surg Clin North Am 2000;80:295.
149. Schwartz MZ, Tapper D, Solenberger RI: Management of perforated appendicitis in children. Ann Surg 1983;197:407.
150. Seidman JD, Andersen DK, Ulrich S, et al: Recurrent abdominal pain due to chronic appendiceal disease. South Med J 1991;84:913.
151. Semm K: Endoscopic appendectomy. Endoscopy 1983; 15:5.
152. Shalaby R, Arnos A, Desoky A, Samaha AH: Laparoscopic appendectomy in children: Evaluation of different techniques. Surg Laparosc Endosc Percutan Tech 2001; 11:22.
153. Sinha RK, Mage RG: Developing neonatal rabbit appendix, a primary lymphoid organ, is seeded by immature blood-borne B cells: Evidence for roles for CD62L/PNAd, CCR7/CCL21, alpha4beta1 and LFA-1. Dev Comp Immunol 2004;28:829.
154. Sirinek KR, Levine BA: A randomized trial of ticarcillin and clavulanate versus gentamicin and clindamycin in patients with complicated appendicitis. Surg Gynecol Obstet 1991;172(Suppl):30.
155. Smink DS, Finkelstein JA, Kleinman K, Fishman SJ: The effect of hospital volume of pediatric appendectomies on the misdiagnosis of appendicitis in children. Pediatrics 2004;113:18.
156. Smink DS, Finkelstein JA, Garcia Pena BM, et al: Diagnosis of acute appendicitis in children using a clinical practice guideline. J Pediatr Surg 2004;39:458.
157. Stephen AE, Segev DL, Ryan DP, et al: The diagnosis of acute appendicitis in a pediatric population: To CT or not to CT. J Pediatr Surg 2003;38:367.
158. Street D, Bodai BI, Owens LJ, et al: Simple ligation vs stump inversion in appendectomy. Arch Surg 1988;123:689.
159. Stringel G: Appendicitis in children: A systematic approach for a low incidence of complications. Am J Surg 1987;154:631.
160. Stringer MD, Pledger G: Childhood appendicitis in the United Kingdom: Fifty years of progress. J Pediatr Surg 2003;38(7 Suppl):65.
161. Surana R, O'Donnell B, Puri P: Appendicitis diagnosed following active observation does not increase morbidity in children. Pediatr Surg Int 1995;10:76.
162. Surana R, Quinn F, Puri P: Is it necessary to perform appendicectomy in the middle of the night in children? BMJ 1993;306:1168.
163. Surana R, Puri P: Appendiceal mass in children. Pediatr Surg Int 1995;10:79.
164. Tander B, Pektas O, Bulut M: The utility of peritoneal drains in children with uncomplicated perforated appendicitis. Pediatr Surg Int 2003;19:548.
165. Tate JJ, Dawson JW, Chung SC, et al: Laparoscopic versus open appendectomy: Prospective randomised trial. Lancet 1993;342:633.
166. Vakili C: Operative treatment of appendix mass. Am J Surg 1976;131:312.
167. Valerdiz-Casasola S, Pardo-Mindan FJ: Cytomegalovirus infection of the appendix in patient with the acquired immunodeficiency syndrome. Gastroenterology 1991; 101:247.
168. Valioulis I, Hameury F, Dahmani L, Levard G: Laparoscope-assisted appendectomy in children: The two-trocar technique. Eur J Pediatr Surg 2001;11:391.
169. van Zwalenburg C: The relation of mechanical distention to the etiology of appendicitis. Ann Surg 1905;41:437.
170. Vanamo K, Kiekara O: Pylephlebitis after appendicitis in a child. J Pediatr Surg 2001;36:1574.
171. Wade DS, Marrow SE, Balsara ZN, et al: Accuracy of ultrasound in the diagnosis of acute appendicitis compared with the surgeon's clinical impression. Arch Surg 1993; 128:1039.
172. Wakeley CPG: Position of vermiform appendix as ascertained by analysis of 10,000 cases. J Anat 1933;67:277.
173. Wangensteen OH, Dennis C: Experimental proof of obstructive origin of appendicitis. Ann Surg 1939;110:629.
174. Warner BW, Rich KA, Atherton H, et al: The sustained impact of an evidenced-based clinical pathway for acute appendicitis. Semin Pediatr Surg 2002;11:29.
175. Weiner DJ, Katz A, Hirschl RB, et al: Interval appendectomy in perforated appendicitis. Pediatr Surg Int 1995;10:82.
176. White JJ, Santillana M, Haller JA: Intensive in-hospital observation. a safe way to decrease unnecessary appendectomy. Am Surg 1975;41:793.
177. Wolff BG: Current status of incidental surgery. Dis Colon Rectum 1995;38:435.
178. Yacoe ME, Jeffrey RB: Sonography of appendicitis and diverticulitis. Radiol Clin North Am 1994;32:899.
179. Yardeni D, Hirschl RB, Drongowski RA, et al: Delayed versus immediate surgery in acute appendicitis: Do we need to operate during the night? J Pediatr Surg 2004;39:464.

第 99 章

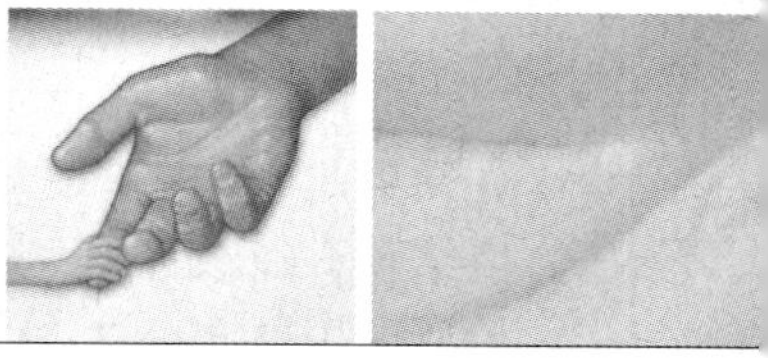

先天性巨结肠和相关的肠神经肌肉疾病

Daniel H. Teitelbaum 和 Arnold G. Coran

历史回顾

514 Harald Hirschsprung 是哥本哈根路易斯女王儿童医院的一名高级儿科医生。在 1886 年柏林儿科大会上，他第一次报告了先天性巨结肠的临床情况，故后人用他的名字来命名这个疾病[131,213]。他描述了两个这类疾病患儿的典型临床症状和解剖特征。这两个患儿分别在 7 个月和 11 个月时死于反复发生的小肠结肠炎。对儿童巨结肠的描述可以追溯到 17 世纪，一位荷兰解剖学家 Frederick Ruysch 于 1691 年报道了一个 5 岁女孩死于肠梗阻的病例。尽管当时也有其他人报告了一系列与 Hirschsprung 描述相类似的病例，但是在 Hirschsprung 报告之前人们对这个疾病没有一个正确的评价。后来也有几个病例报告，其中包括 Hirschsprung 在 1904 年的 10 例患儿的报道，他称这个疾病为先天性结肠扩张症。

又经过了几十年对先天性巨结肠发病机制的研究，人们提出了三个基本的学说。第一个是“功能紊乱学说”，是指结肠肥大起源于最初的先天性缺陷[233]。第二个是“梗阻学说”，是指结肠或者直肠瓣的冗长引起机械性梗阻而造成的结肠扩张[339]。第三个是“痉挛学说”，这个学说是由 Fenwick 在 1900 年最先提出，是指远端结肠痉挛性收缩而引起功能性的梗阻[339]。1901 年，Tittel[333] 证实了一位先天性巨结肠儿童的远端结肠缺少神经节细胞，从而做出了远端结肠异常才是疾病发生根源的正确评价。由于起初一些原发性便秘的患儿也被诊断为先天性巨结肠，所以直到 20 世纪 40 年代晚期先天性巨结肠的发病原因依旧很混乱。1946 年，Ehrenpreis[75] 报告了扩张的结肠继发于远端结肠梗阻的结论。1948 年 Whitehouse 和 Kernohan[361] 以及 Zuelzer 和 Wilson[383] 证明了先天性巨结肠患儿的肠肌间神经丛神经节细胞的缺如。1948 年 Swenson 和 Bill[311] 第一次进行了先天性巨结肠纠正手术。Swenson[309,310] 最近还发表了关于这个疾病的病因和治疗的历史上的观点。这些标志性的进展引出了先天性巨结肠临床治疗的基本原则。近期关于肠神经系统的分子遗传学和病理生理学上的进展使得对于这个疾病的理解有了明显的突破。在过去十年内有将近一半关于发病机制的文章发表。

发病率

成活儿先天性巨结肠的发病率为 1/4400 ~ 1/7000[245,304]。典型的先天性巨结肠其男女比例为4:1，男性多见[278,296]。而长段型的先天性巨结肠，其男女比例接近 1:1，女性多见[245]。在大多数调查中，此病在人种中的分布与总人口中的分布是相似的。家族中有先天性巨结肠的患儿，其发病率可上升接近至 6%，范围在 2%~18% 之间[250,305]。Badner[21] 等致力于先天性巨结肠遗传学上的研究，他们发现短段型患者的兄弟患病的几率（4%）明显高于姐妹俩（1%）。在长段型的女性患者中其兄弟和儿子患此病的危险最高（分别为 24% 和 29%）。

诊断 1515

临床表现

先天性巨结肠的诊断目前在临床上仍是一种挑战。

在新生儿时期就有便秘病史的患儿要考虑是否有先天性巨结肠。确诊的平均年龄经过几十年发展逐步提前，从1920—1930年的2～3岁，提前到1950—1970年的3～6个月[314]。最近的文献报道在新生儿期就能明确诊断的先天性巨结肠超过90%以上[127,183,260]。新生儿先天性巨结肠常见的临床表现包括出生后48小时内胎粪排出延迟[57]。95%的足月新生儿在出生24小时内排出胎粪，剩余的在48小时内首次排便。要注意的是也有6%~42%的患儿缺乏这一个病史[162,314]。其他的体征和症状还包括便秘、腹胀、食欲缺乏、呕吐。除了新生儿期的体征外，先天性巨结肠的临床体征还表现为便秘、腹胀、生长发育不良[37,86,325]。在年长的儿童中鉴别先天性巨结肠与其他表现如便秘或大便失禁的一些疾病是十分困难的(以后讨论)。先天性巨结肠的患儿也可表现为先是便秘紧接着出现暴发性的腹泻，这提示有小肠结肠炎的发生。在所有患儿中都应该询问有无家族史。当从新生儿期过渡到年长儿，此病的诊断率也逐渐减少，对于这类患儿的合理处理是非常重要的[155,219]。

体格检查经常表现为腹胀，但在出生时不明显。会阴部肛门位置的评估很重要。轻微闭锁的肛门位置前移也可引起便秘。先天性巨结肠患儿如有肛门收缩在直肠指检中可以被误诊为肛门狭窄。

放射学检查

造影检查首先做腹部的平片和各种体位的摄片(包括侧位水平摄片、直立位片、俯卧位片)。通常这些检查显示扩张的肠袢和直肠位置少量的气体。这些影像学上的发现与其他原因引起的新生儿远端肠梗阻的表现相似。肠管的移行路径被肠管内的气体完整显示很少见，尽管新生儿腹部的游离气体是极其少见的，但是这可能是先天性巨结肠近端肠管穿孔的最初表现[15,238]。对于外科医生来说从这点上就应该考虑并排除先天性巨结肠是引起这一表现的病因。在新生儿时期先天性巨结肠的漏诊和误诊都可能导致小肠或者大肠的自发性穿孔，这是跟它的高发病率和死亡率相关的。穿孔在婴儿长段型巨结肠中最常见。

对比造影可以帮助先天性巨结肠的诊断。在新生儿期，钡灌肠可以将先天性巨结肠与其他原因引起的远端肠管梗阻相鉴别。在对疑似先天性巨结肠进行钡灌肠时有几个相关的技术要点。首先，在新生儿不可预计有无自发性穿孔时采用水溶性的造影剂优于钡剂灌肠，可以防止钡剂引起的腹膜炎，而且可更有效地缓解胎粪性肠梗阻。在诊断新生儿先天性巨结肠时水溶性的造影剂与钡剂一样准确[241]。应该避免采用高渗透性的溶液，这样可以避免水电解质紊乱的发生。新生儿期以后，此时自发性穿孔不再是关注的重点，在怀疑先天性巨结肠时优先选择钡剂灌肠，因为它的清晰度更强。在发生小肠结肠炎时不推荐使用造影灌肠。

在钡灌肠前应该避免直肠检查和清洁灌肠，因为这些操作可能掩盖病变的移行段。灌肠管插入肛门，气囊不要充盈。早期灌注钡剂时需要非常仔细，造影初期要缓慢灌注，而且开始的时候患儿最好采取俯卧位，这样可以在侧位上使直肠显影。偶尔仅在造影初期可以看到病变段，再注入钡剂后就变得模糊不清，最后表现为明显的扩张。直到病变段显示或者整个结肠显影时，才可以逐渐将造影剂抽出。这时可以去除肛管，允许患儿排便，从而获得排泄后的造影显像。

先天性巨结肠典型的X线表现为痉挛性狭窄的远端肠管伴有扩张的近端肠管。钡剂灌肠诊断先天性巨结肠时，关键在于发现肠管管径的改变或者病变段(图99-1)。病变段可以发生在结肠的任何部位，但最常见的位于乙状结肠。造影剂的潴留是存在畸形的有力证据[277]。24小时延迟摄片已经不再作为常规检查，但是可以用来评估造影剂的潴留情况。即使没有显示病变段，但是只要有钡剂潴留就应该怀疑为先天性巨结肠并做进一步的检查。

不幸的是钡剂灌肠不能诊断所有的先天性巨结肠。一些学者已经报道了诊断的准确率：Swenson 等[314]报道为76%，Lister[193]为87%，Klein 等[162,163]为92%。也有学者认为钡剂灌肠的帮助不大。Taxman等[322]认为用钡剂潴留诊断先天性巨结肠依据不足，因为其假阳性率可达29%，假阴性率可达20%。在那些病变段不明确的患儿中，钡灌肠的诊断作用也是有限的。在新生儿和短段型的巨结肠以及全结肠神经节细胞缺乏症的患儿中要明确病变段是非常困难的。

进行钡灌肠可以明确病变段，这样有利于手术方案及手术方式的选择。虽然放射科的医生认为90%的钡灌肠可以显示出病变段的区域[299]，然而一群学者认为在决定病变区域的时候近53%的钡灌肠是误诊的。放射显像上的病变区域与肠无神经节细胞的病理范围相一致的仅达62.5%。而在长段型的巨结肠中，仅有25%是一致的[147]。因此在制定手术方案时用钡灌肠明确病变段是要非常仔细的。

15

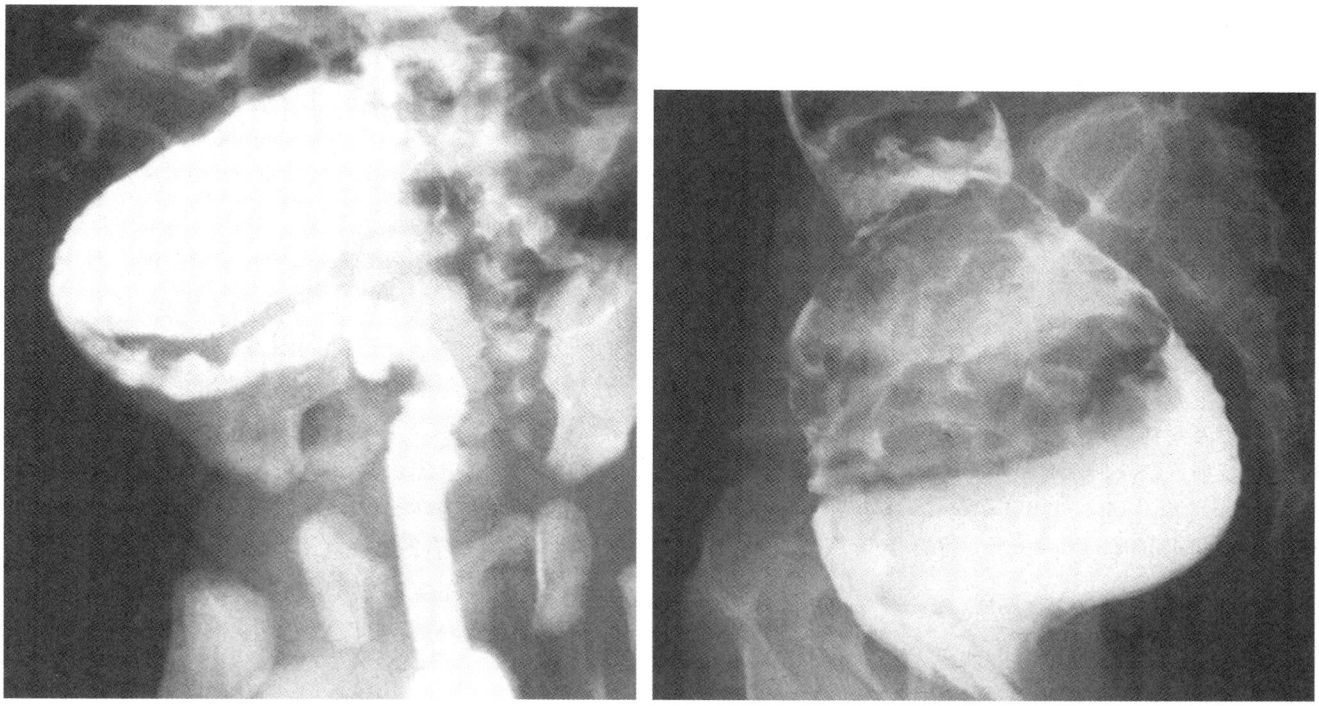

A　B

图 99-1　先天性巨结肠患儿的造影对比（A）和便秘患儿的造影对比（B）。注意先天性巨结肠患儿的狭窄段和便秘患儿扩张的直肠壶腹部。

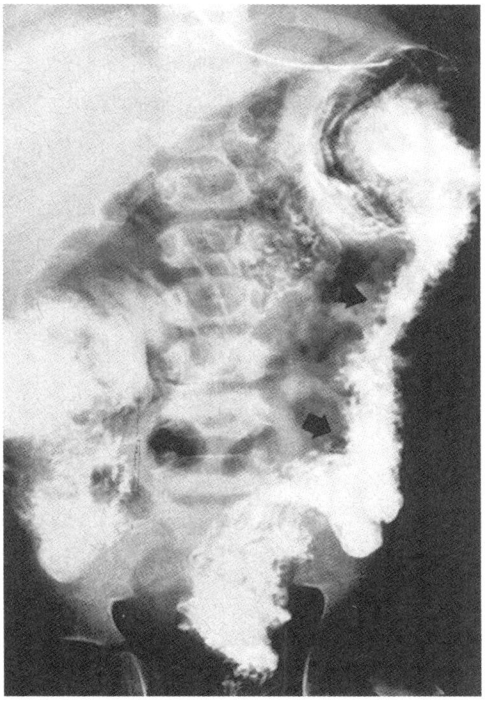

图 99-2　小肠结肠炎患儿的钡灌肠显示明显的不规则的肠黏膜一直向下延伸到无神经节细胞的直肠。

钡灌肠有时也可以显示出反复发作的小肠结肠炎、肠壁的水肿及痉挛，甚至肠黏膜的溃疡（图 99-2）。远端无神经节细胞痉挛的肠管经常可见锯齿样的改变，但这并不是结肠炎的指征。应该注意到如果患儿在临床上怀疑有小肠结肠炎，那么钡灌肠是禁忌疗法，因为其可以增加穿孔及败血症的危险。

直肠肛管测压法

直肠肛管测压是诊断先天性巨结肠的另一种方法。该技术的生理学基础将在以后的病理生理学部分
进行讨论。在这里要分析 3 个参数，第一个典型的测 1517
量指标就是直肠腔扩张后内括约肌松弛反射的缺如（图 99-3）。通过这个检查还可以获得静息时肛门括约肌的压力（先天性巨结肠时有升高），此外还可以了解年长儿球囊扩张时的整个感觉。这个操作在住院病房或在门诊都可进行，事实上没有任何的并发症。Swenson[308,311,313]最先提出将这个技术作为诊断该疾

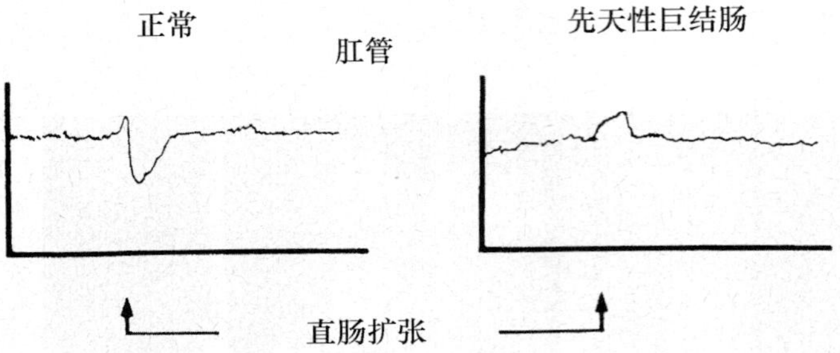

图 99-3 正常儿童的直肠肛管测压（左图）和先天性巨结肠患儿的直肠肛管测压（右图）。可以注意到先天性巨结肠患儿肛管上方有异常收缩的增加（箭头所示）并伴有直肠的扩张以及内括约肌松弛反射的缺如。正常儿童有一适当的松弛反射（箭头所示）。（From Walker AW, et al: Pediatric Gastrointestinal Disease: Pathophysiology, Diagnosis, Management. Philadelphia, BC Decker, 1990.）

病的首要方法，1964 年 Callaghan 和 Nixon[47] 又进一步改善了这个操作。直肠肛管测压的局限性为测试结果与测试时的正常生理状态相关。假如患儿在检查时处于非正常生理状态下（例如败血症、甲状腺机能减退），那么检查结果不准确是可能的[377]。另一些局限性包括年幼儿还需要使用镇静剂避免活动或者哭吵产生的众多人为因素。

关于直肠肛管测压准确率的一系列报道差别很大。一些学者认为这个检查的诊断率很高[319,377]，而其他学者则报告了许多不准确的结果[64]。假阴性率（也就是指有些确诊为先天性巨结肠的患儿该检查结果却提示是正常）0[319]～24%[217]不等。假阳性率（也就是指有些正常儿童进行这个检查却不能引出内括约肌松弛反射）0[195,319]～62%[222,223]不等。Holschneider[135]等不建议对早产儿或者年龄小于 12 天的足月儿进行肛直肠反射检查。Ito[143]等认为这种检测手段对于孕期加出生后年龄小于 39 周，体重低于 2.7 kg的患儿是不可靠的。Loening-Baucke[196]等报道由于反应装置敏感性这个局限性，在新生儿期进行直肠肛管测压存在很大难度。有经验的医生实施检查可以明显提高准确率。

该技术也可用于评估进行肛门直肠拖出术后的患儿的异常排便功能[218,344,380]。对于长期存在排便功能问题的患儿进行全结肠测压可以获得非常有用的信息。有趣的是在实施典型的肛门直肠拖出术后，患儿虽然不能恢复内括约肌松弛反射，但是这不影响他们对排便的控制能力[344,380]。

直肠活检

直肠活检是诊断先天性巨结肠的金标准（图 99-4）。1959 年，Swenson[312]等首次描述了直肠全层活检的方法，它的缺点有出血、瘢痕、需要全身麻醉。通过对远端直肠病理学的了解，经过一系列的改 15

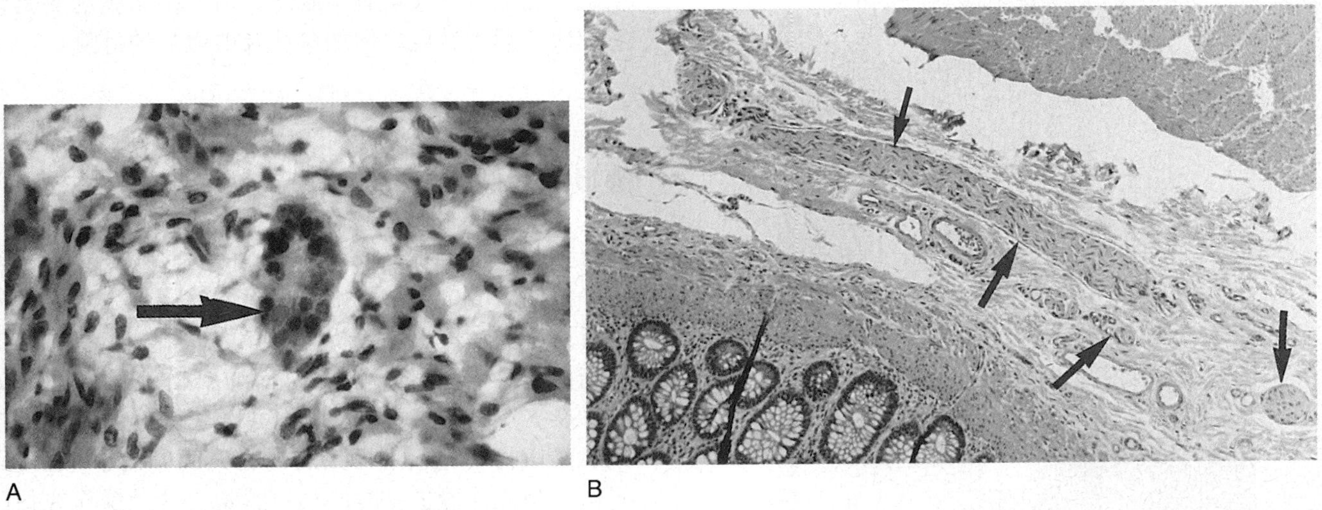

图 99-4 先天性巨结肠的组织病理学。A. 近端（有神经节细胞的）肠管典型的神经节细胞团（箭头所示）。B. 无神经节细胞部分神经节细胞的缺如和明显粗大的神经（箭头所示）。

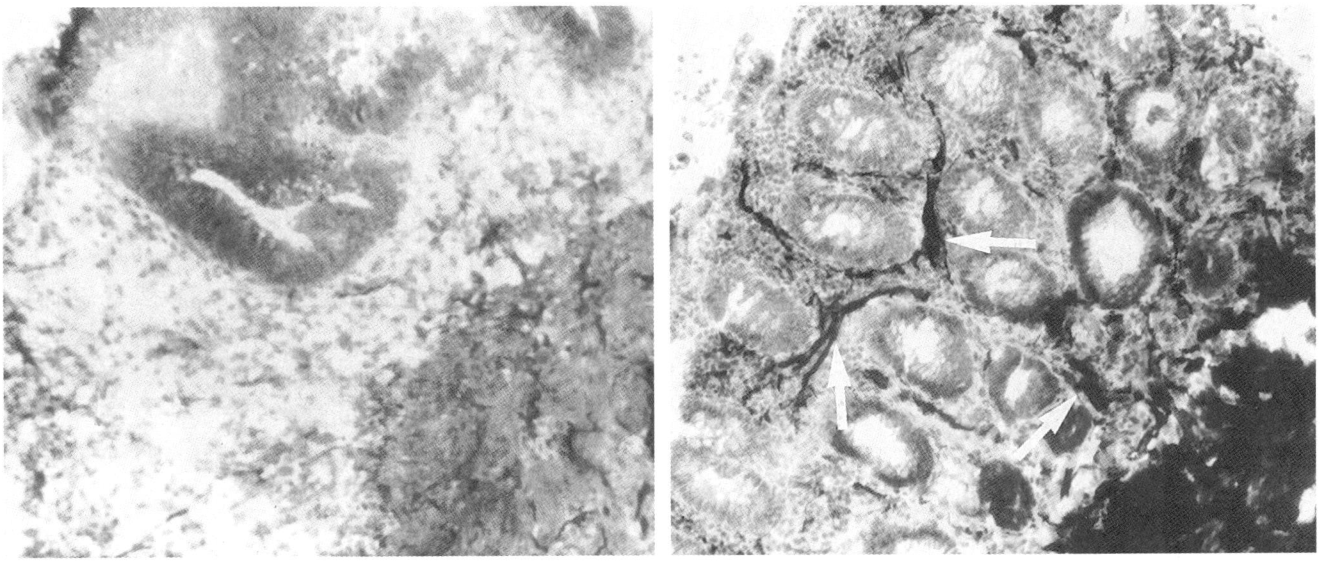

A　B

图 99-5　A. 肠壁神经节细胞乙酰胆碱酯酶染色。B. 肠壁无神经节细胞乙酰胆碱酯酶染色。在无神经节细胞的肠管（白色箭头所指的黑色神经纤维）中的黏膜固有层和肌固有层（右下方）显示出乙酰胆碱酯酶的强染色反应。（Stephen Qualman，MD 提供）

进后发明了直肠黏膜吸吮活检的方法。Shandling 认[293]为更浅表的活检对于先天性巨结肠的诊断已经足够了。1960 年 Gherardi[106]证明了在肠管的黏膜下和肌间神经丛中同样存在神经节细胞。同年，这个发现使得 Bodian[34]最先进行了黏膜下活检。随着这个技术的改进和吸吮活检手段的发展，1965 年 Dobbins 和 Bill[69]将直肠黏膜活检做了进一步的改进，使得先天性巨结肠的诊断更加容易。

吸吮活检可以在床旁和门诊进行。虽然据报道该诊断的准确性可高达 99.7%，但也有错误发生。最常见的问题就是所取的黏膜下组织较少造成标本不够，从而无法对神经节细胞进行评估。另一个问题就是活检部位太接近肛门括约肌。正常的肛管在内括约肌水平都缺少或者含有极少量的神经节细胞。Aldridge 和 Campbell[6]通过对早产儿、足月儿、年长儿的尸解进行详细的分析后发现在肛管中正常的神经节细胞减少区在黏膜下神经丛比肌间神经丛更长。此外，在所有年龄组中正常的神经节细胞减少区的长度相似，平均 9～10 mm 位于齿状线上（范围3～17 mm）。这使得医生通常在肛管 2 cm 以上进行吸吮活检。肌间神经丛中正常的神经节细胞减少区平均长度为齿状线上 2～6 mm，因此在进行全层活检时要选取更远的部位。

虽然有直肠吸吮活检并发症的报道，但是这项技术还是十分安全的。一所研究机构对 1340 例连续性活检病例进行的回顾性研究发现，3 例穿孔（占 0.2%），3 例直肠出血需要输血治疗[267]。其中 1 例穿孔的患儿因为继发臀部的坏疽而死亡。这个检查的准确率已被很好地证明了。在关于直肠吸吮活检应用的大型综述文章中，Andrassy[11]等发现 444 例患儿中仅 1 例出现假阴性结果。

对于先天性巨结肠的诊断而言，直肠吸吮活检的病理学评估比全层活检更困难。最近关于先天性巨结肠诊断方法的多中心分析结果显示，诊断策略存在很大差异，且强调需要一位很有经验的病理学家[266]。乙酰胆碱酯酶染色可以使诊断更容易。Meier-Ruge[215]等最先介绍了这项技术用于诊断先天性巨结肠，这项技术起源于 Karnovsky 和 Roots 的染色方法。这个方法是从暗斑的生长上进行改进而成的[179]。在先天性巨结肠中整个固有层和黏膜肌层都可以看到强染色的肥大的神经纤维（图 99-5）。一些学者检测了这种染色的诊断准确率，获得了满意的结果[137,178]。Schofield[288]等回顾了 497 例直肠吸吮活检的病例，8 例为先天性巨结肠的患儿，9 例不需要进行乙酰胆碱酯酶染色，因为只采用伊红-苏木精染色不能获得明确诊断。然而另有一篇综述显示 96 例先天性巨结肠病例中5例在乙酰胆碱酯酶染色时缺乏典型的表现，而需要通过标准的伊红-苏木精染色明确诊断[55]。假阴性率很少见，但有报道[18]。

当直肠吸吮活检不能明确诊断时，应该在手术室
1519 进行直肠后壁的全层活检。在那些年龄较大的儿童吸吮活检不能获得足够的黏膜下组织时全层的活检是有用的。在以后的病例中通常不需要进行黏膜肌层的完整活检。

鉴别诊断

在诊断先天性巨结肠时应该考虑还有其他的疾病。表99-1列出了最常见的鉴别诊断。在出生后的最初几天，胎粪性肠梗阻的临床表现与先天性巨结肠相似。腹部平片显示腹部呈现毛玻璃状，特别是在右下腹，钡灌肠可提示细小结肠。全结肠闭锁或者远端小肠闭锁的患儿也可表现为低位的肠梗阻，与初期的先天性巨结肠相仿。钡灌肠显示完全性肠梗阻例如肠闭锁也可导致细小结肠。在发生胎粪塞综合征时，钡灌肠既是诊断方法又是治疗方法[81]。钡灌肠后患儿经常排出胎粪，梗阻的症状也就缓解了。在左小结肠综合征患儿中，钡灌肠显示左侧有明显的结肠狭窄，且婴儿的母亲可能是糖尿病患者。然而此时钡灌肠的表现与先天性巨结肠非常相似。需要对胎粪塞综合征或者是左小结肠综合征的患儿进行直肠吸吮活检排除先天性巨结肠，因为后者可以伴有这两种综合征中的任何一种[253,268]。功能性肠梗阻可由多种全身性的和胃肠道的疾病引起。早产儿的大肠功能较差，许多这样的婴儿在出生后的最初几天内没有大便排出。功能性肠梗阻或者大肠功能减退的患儿可以表现为细小结肠[9]。在婴儿期，败血症、电解质紊乱和甲状腺机能减退也可与胃肠道梗阻表现相似。最后，年长儿童的良性功能性便秘的症状可能类似于先天性巨结肠的症状。这两类疾病的鉴别要点将在《先天性便秘和大便失禁》这一节讨论。

表99-1　先天性巨结肠的鉴别诊断
其他的机械性梗阻
胎粪性肠梗阻
远端回肠或者结肠闭锁
小肠狭窄
低位肛门闭锁
功能性肠梗阻
早产儿
左小结肠综合征
胎粪塞综合征
败血症和电解质紊乱
克汀病和黏液性水肿
功能性便秘
肠神经发育不良

病因

对先天性巨结肠的病理生理学的了解可以提出合理的诊断和治疗方法，但是其确切的病因仍在探索中。该部分总结了目前对这一发病过程的认识，首先介绍已知的与先天性巨结肠发生相关的基因突变，然后将这些变化与该过程中发现的病理生理学的失调相联系。

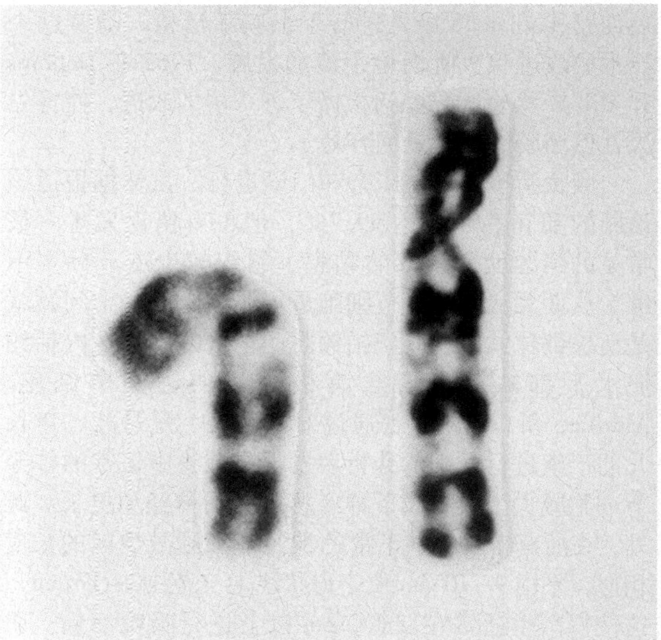

图99-6　1例全结肠型的无神经节细胞症在10号染色体的长臂上（10qll-21）存在中间缺失。

表 99-2　神经嵴病的分类

简单的神经嵴病
无瘤形成的
先天性巨结肠
白化病
下颌面骨发育障碍
无下颌并耳畸形
先天性中央性肺换气不足综合征（CCHS）
有瘤形成的
神经母细胞瘤
嗜铬细胞瘤
甲状腺髓样癌
非嗜铬细胞副神经节瘤
类癌瘤
复杂的神经嵴病（有瘤形成的和无瘤形成的）
神经纤维瘤病（von Recklinghausen 病）
多发性内分泌瘤（MEN）1 型
MEN2A
MEN2B
神经皮肤黑素沉着病
家族性神经母细胞瘤伴有先天性巨结肠
Haddad 综合征（先天性中央性肺换气不足综合征 + 先天性巨结肠）
Shan-Waardenburg 综合征（Waardenburg 综合征 + 先天性巨结肠）

先天性巨结肠遗传分子学基础

G. Martucciello、A. Baban、N. Jibri 和 V. Jasonni

散发性先天性巨结肠占先天性巨结肠总病例数的 80%~90%。可以观察到不同的表现度（患儿无神经节细胞段的长度不同）和不完全的伴性外显率（是否这个个体显示出他或她的基因型）。经过多年的研究，先天性巨结肠的多种特征表明其是多因素遗传、涉及多种基因变异的一种疾病。意大利热那亚 Gaslini 研究中心率先致力于确定先天性巨结肠主要遗传基因的研究。其报道了 1 例全结肠型的无神经节细胞症的女孩 10 号染色体的长臂上存在基因的中间缺失（46XX，缺失位点 10qll. 21–q21. 2）（图 99–6）[207]。
通过对缺失区域的绘图，进一步将这个区域缩小到 1520
RET 原癌基因所在的一个 200 kb 的区域之间[53]。这个发现引发了对这个基因的特定方面以及其他与先天性巨结肠有关的基因缺失的进一步研究。最初大量的遗传信息是通过无神经节细胞症的动物模型获得的，这样有助于对人类无神经节细胞症基因缺陷的了解。对不同组患儿及其家庭成员的分离分析表明有不同形式的遗传，这取决于无神经节细胞节段的长度。通过检查基因突变如何与神经嵴病相关联，可以了解与先天性巨结肠相关的基因突变，因为它们有许多相似的

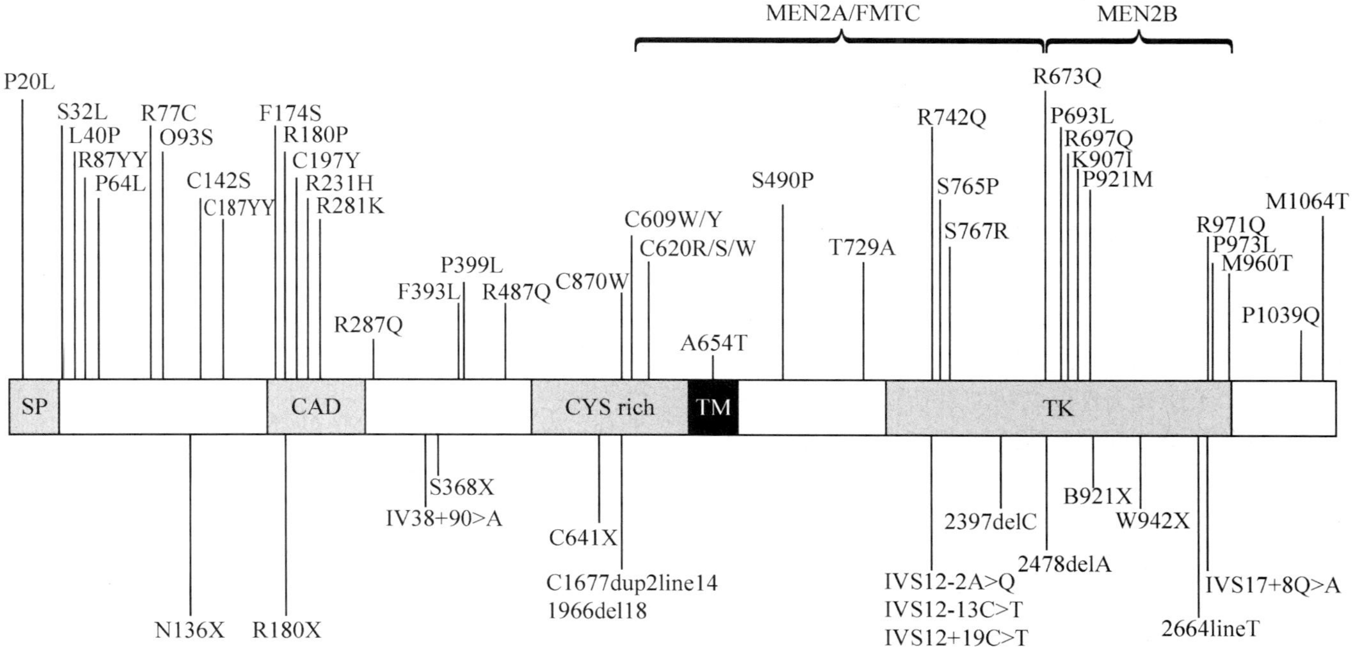

图 99-7　导致先天性巨结肠的 *RET* 基因突变在该基因的 21 个外显子中都有发生。

遗传模式。运用 Bolande 分类法可将神经嵴病分成两个基本类型。第一种单一类型是指涉及单一的病理过程即单病灶和局部化，更进一步可分为非遗传无瘤形成型（例如先天性巨结肠）和有瘤形成型（例如甲状腺髓样癌和其他）。第二种神经嵴病更加复杂，甚至包括综合征的形式，这与多病灶疾病和单一的神经嵴病相关（表 99-2）[35]。

RET 蛋白的表达

RET 是一个原癌基因，在胚胎期最初表达于神经嵴、泌尿生殖器的前身、肾上腺髓质、甲状腺，出生后贯穿中枢和周围神经系统及内分泌系统[216]。*RET* 基因突变近 35% 发生于散发的先天性巨结肠，49% 发生于家族性先天性巨结肠，长段型的比率（占 76%）高于短段型（占 32%）[54,231]。导致先天性巨结肠的 *RET* 突变可以通过基因的 21 个外显子发生[216]，已经证实至少有 89 种突变，包括无义突变、错义突变、细小的
1521 删除和插入（图 99-7）[54]。相反，导致多发性内分泌瘤 2A 型（MEN2A）或者家庭性甲状腺髓样癌（FMTC）的突变位点在细胞外 5 个半胱氨酸之一上，与那些引起先天性巨结肠的不同，它们的突变非常活跃[41,89,143]。先天性巨结肠 *RET* 基因的突变导致功能性的等位基因的缺失和自然的杂合，提示单功能不全。虽然先天性巨结肠和 MEN2 经常单独地出现在一些病例中，这可能是因为不同的分子细胞机制导致不同类型突变的结果，但是在既有先天性巨结肠又有 MEN2（FMTC 和 MEN2A）的家庭中确定的 *RET* 突变（C618 和 C620）是令人惊讶的。导致这两种疾病的根本机制还不清楚[232]，一些先天性巨结肠的家庭携带有可导致 MEN2 的基因突变。这个关系可能提示在每个疾病中有一种特殊的分子机制。为了解释相同的突变怎样产生不同的表现形式，我们可以假设那是由于突变发生在不同的胚胎时期和出生后的时间内的缘故。

另一个关于先天性巨结肠的复杂遗传模式和 *RET* 基因突变的低检测率的解释就是存在几种常见的 *RET* 基因的多形变态，这与引起先天性巨结肠的危险因素相关。特殊的 *RET* 单模标本既可作为保护因子又可作为诱病因素，也可用于调节疾病的严重程度[40,41,52,88,89,111,112]。一个少见的外显子 2（A45A）单核苷多形态（SNP）的等位基因的特殊单模标本与先天性巨结肠密切相关，反之，外显子 14 的 SNP（S836s）的等位基因的单模标本好像是与此病相关的

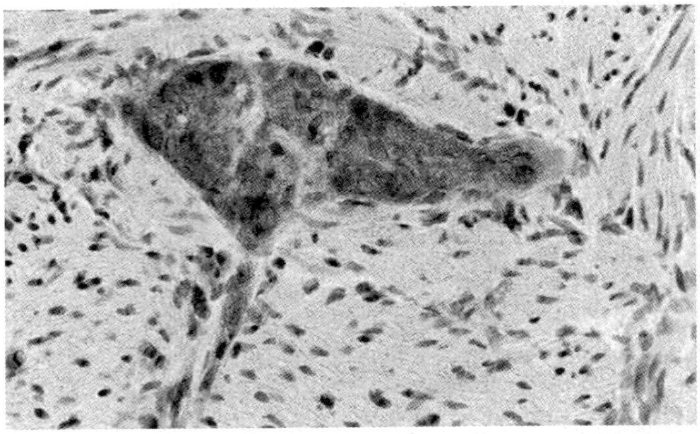

A

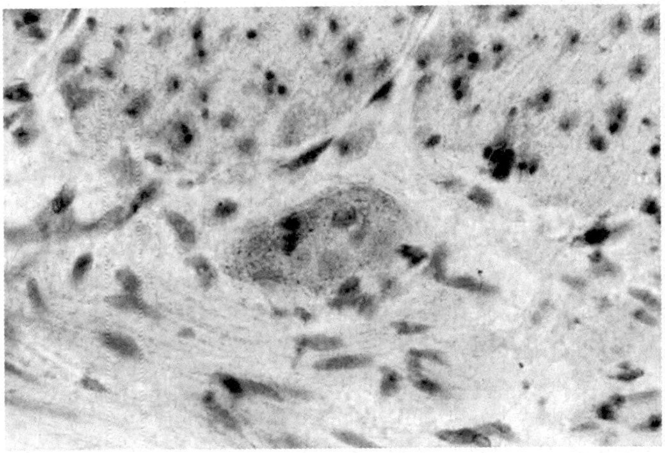

B

图 99-8　A. RET 蛋白在正常神经节中的免疫染色。B. 先天性巨结肠患儿 RET 蛋白免疫反应减少并伴有密码突变的停顿。

低渗透性的保护因素[88,111]。

RET 原癌基因的表达最初是在许多与神经嵴病相关的肿瘤中发现的。这种关系是在神经母细胞瘤的细胞系、嗜铬细胞瘤、甲状腺髓样癌中被发现的[286]。这些在人类肿瘤中的发现暗示 RET 蛋白可能与神经嵴细胞的分化相关，它们的过度表达和激活可能导致恶变。这些研究提示 RET 的受体在分化的特定阶段或者在世系中都可以有正常的功能，但是其所在细胞的类型并不多，它的表达仅局限于有限的局部组织[340]。关于免疫组化方面，1995 年首先在肠神经系统中开始 RET 蛋白定位的研究，神经节细胞显示出强阳性的染色[208]。有 *RET* 基因的完整缺失和密码子突变的先天性巨结肠的病例中可以看到染色明显减少（图99-8）。这个发现可支持由于 RET 蛋白数量的减

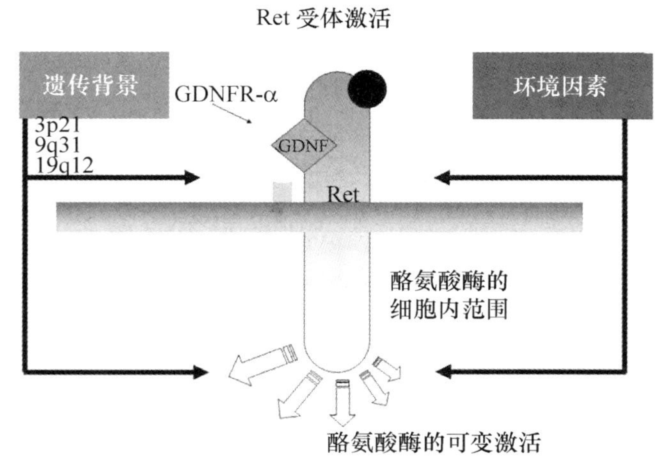

图 99-9　GDNF-RET 受体信号系统。

少导致功能降低的假说。

很多学者试图解释 *RET* 突变是不存在的，尤其在那些无规则的孟德尔遗传的家庭中的病例。在对家族几代中有超过 3 个患者的研究表明，其易感性集中在人染色体 9q31 上有密码顺序缺失的 *RET* 突变[38]。另外，对短段型先天性巨结肠家庭的连锁分析研究表明，除 *RET* 等位基因外还有另外两个染色体位点（3p21 和 19q12）[19]。

与先天性巨结肠有关的其他基因

约 5%～10% 的患儿还有其他基因的突变，例如神经胶质细胞源性的神经营养因子（GDNF）、neuturin 基因（NTN）、内皮素-3 基因（EDN3）、内皮素 B 受体（EDNRB）、内皮素转化酶-1（ECE1）、转录因子 SOX10、Smad 作用蛋白-1（SIP1）以及成对的同源异形盒 2B（PHOX2B）。在少部分的已知基因突变的患儿中（少于半数）要高度怀疑有其他修饰基因或另外一些危险因子受累，它们中的一些已经被定位[38,52,100]。这个领域的研究仍然在继续，基于我们目前的知识，以下的基因突变可能与先天性巨结肠的表现型相关。

神经胶质细胞源性的神经营养因子

GDNF（染色体 5p13）是 RET 受体的一种配体（图 99-9）。合成的糖基磷脂酰肌醇联结蛋白GDNFR-α
提供 RET 蛋白与 GDNF 之间的配体连接。GDNF 和 1522
GDNFR-α 中的任何一个缺失都会导致 RET 信号的减少或者缺失（见图 99-9）。已经证实有 2 种 GDNF 外显子 2 的杂合突变。约在 0.9%～5.5% 先天性巨结肠患儿中可以发现这些突变，且在大多数发现 RET 突变的患儿中发现，所以猜想单独存在的 GDNF 突变是不足以引起先天性巨结肠的[13,145]。事实上即使没有基因突变，与正常对照组相比 GDNF 蛋白的表达在一部分先天性巨结肠患者中也是减少的[209]。在无神经节细胞段的 GDNF 表达缺乏可能是先天性巨结肠发病机制中的一个重要辅助因子，可以导致在无 *RET* 原癌基因突变的情况下 RET 受体激活的减少和缺失，从而引起肠神经母细胞迁移停止和先天性巨结肠。

Neurturin 基因

除 GDNF 外，RET 还有另一个配体 NTN（位于染色体 19p13.3 上），它是一个联合受体（NTNR-α）。这个多亚单位配体可以作用于 RET 的激活[23,285]。还证实有其他的联合受体，包括 GDNF-β、GDNFR-α2、GDNFR-α3 等（见图 99-7）[150,371]。Doray[70] 等首次报道了在一个无血缘关系的大家庭中杂合的 NTN

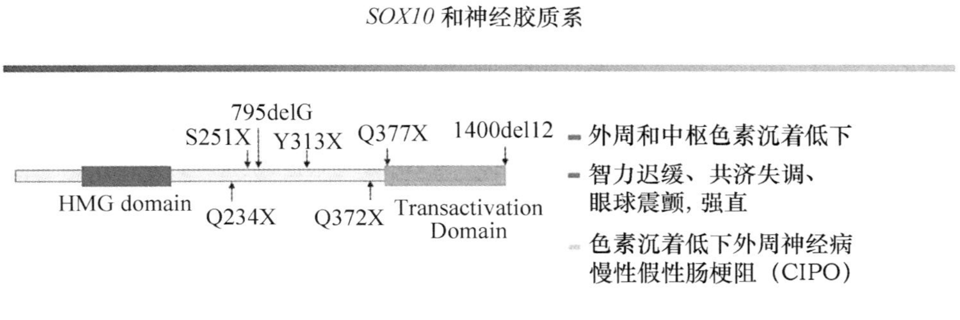

图 99-10　*SOX10* 基因的结构。*SOX10* 的不同突变可以导致不同的表现型（Gossens et al., personal communication, 2004）。

的错义突变，其中有四个长段型先天性巨结肠的患儿。他们也证实了在这个家庭中有 *RET* 基因的错义突变，其遗传来源于未受明显影响的父亲。除此之外，还有两个未受影响的儿童伴有单个杂合的 NTN 突变，还有一个儿童有单个的 *RET* 突变。总的来说，NTN 可以在先天性巨结肠的发生中起一定的作用，但是单独的 NTN 突变不足以引起先天性巨结肠；还需要 *RET* 突变的相互作用，还有一些其他的易感位点未被证实[70]。这也可能说明了在多途径的神经嵴细胞迁移和分化中 *RET* 仅是一个普通的传感器。

内皮素-3 基因和内皮素-B 受体

内皮素属于 21 氨基酸血管活性异构肽家族的，包括 EDN1、EDN2 和 EDN3。这 3 个异构肽的变化不超过 6 个氨基酸。它们每一个都是作为已知的“大内皮素”未活化的多肽而产生的。EDN3 是内皮素 B 受体（EDNRB）的一个配体；这个配体-受体系统在肠神经系统的发生过程中起重要的作用。

在肠神经系统发育早期，EDN3 和 EDNRB 在神经嵴迁移和分化中起一定的作用。EDNRB 缺失可以导致两个神经嵴亚群的激活受影响——成黑素细胞（色素细胞）和肠神经系统的神经母细胞前体。因为黑素细胞和肠神经系统都有共同的信号路径，导致皮肤、头发和眼睛着色异常，总称为 Waardenburg 综合征。这个复杂的神经嵴综合征包括色素沉着异常（多位于中线上的前额白发以及皮肤浅色斑）、感觉神经丧失、异色症或淡蓝色虹膜（蓝宝石色）伴基底色素低下和远端肠管不同长短的肠神经系统的缺如。伴有先天性巨结肠的 Waardenburg 综合征又称 Shah-Waardenburg 综合征或 Waardenburg 四型[70]，该病有
1523 复杂的遗传背景是因为它是由 *EDN3*、*EDNRB* 突变和 *SOX10* 引起的。*EDNRB* 或者 *EDN3* 纯合子的患者显示了这个疾病包括先天性巨结肠的所有特征[173,347]，然而杂合子的患者显示了 Waardenburg 综合征、先天性巨结肠或者两者共同的特征。带有 *EDNRB* 或 *EDN3* 突变的患者的父母经常是无症状的，属于常染色体隐性遗传，发病率为 25%；*SOX10* 是常染色体的显性遗传，在受影响的同胞中的发病率为 50%[347]。单独的先天性巨结肠伴有 EDNRB 突变在其散发的病例中是少见的病因[8,20,133,142,176,281,307,320]。

表 99-3 先天性巨结肠相关的基因突变

人类基因	位点	发病率
RET	10q11	散发 35%
		家族性 49%
		长段型 76%
GDNF	5p13	0.9%~5.5%
NTN	1qp13.3	少见（1 个已知突变）
EDNRB	13q22	少见（15 个已知突变）
EDN3	20q13	少见（2 个已知突变）
ECE1	1p36	少见（1 个已知突变）
SOX10	22q12-13	少见
ZFHX1B (*SIP1*)	2q22-23	少见
PHOX2B	4p12	少见

转录因子 *SOX10*

人类 *SOX10*（染色体 22q12-q13）是转录调节因子 *SOX* 基因家族成员中的一员。它在神经嵴细胞早期发育过程中以及胚胎期和成人期的外周和中枢神经系统的神经胶质细胞中选择性地表达[174]。先前已经提及 *SOX10* 突变以及 *EDN3* 和 *EDNRB* 突变可以引起神经嵴病（Shah-Waardenburg 综合征）[271]。在 Shah-Waardenburg 综合征中无神经节细胞段的长度不一，但是与单纯的先天性巨结肠患者不同的是，大多数 Shah-Waardenburg 综合征患者有长段型或者全结肠型的无神经节细胞症。

最近的资料显示，与 *EDN3* 和 *EDNRB* 不同，*SOX10* 突变也可通过其他一些已知或者未知因素的相互作用而引起一系列影响中枢神经系统、外周神经系统、肠神经系统和黑素细胞的综合征。包括（1）Waardenburg 综合征，外周神经脱鞘病和中枢脱髓鞘脑白质营养不良症[234,255]；（2）慢性假性肠梗阻，可以发生在有正常肠神经节细胞存在时，这说明无神经节细胞症不只是 *SOX10* 突变患者肠功能低下的唯一根本机制[256]；（3）在也门聋哑色素沉着减低综合征，该病的患者皮肤色素沉着低下或者亢进，角膜微小，眼组织残缺，耳聋并有其他症状，但没有先天性巨结肠[39]。*SOX10* 基因的不同突变可以导致不同的显型，如图 99-10 上所示。

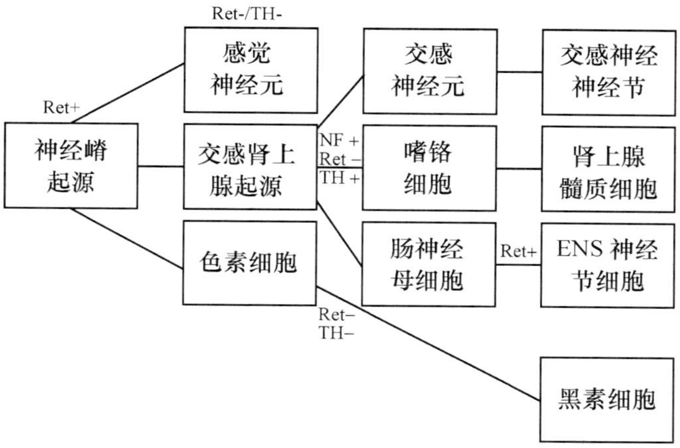

图 99-11　神经嵴细胞的发育。神经嵴前身可分化成不同的类型。

其他基因突变

还证实有一些其他基因的突变（表 99-3），但不在本章节对它们进行讨论。这些突变包括 PHOX2B，伴有 Ondine 呼吸困扰[152]或者中枢肺换气不足综合征；SIP1，伴有 Mowat-Wilson 综合征和 ECE1，伴有一些其他先天性畸形。

遗传咨询

先天性巨结肠是一个受多基因或者多因素影响的疾病，所以有关遗传咨询方面的问题正逐渐受到关注。先天性巨结肠被定义为受性别影响的多因子疾病，在先证者同胞和直系亲属中发病率为 4%。在一些孤立的病例中很难估计其发病风险，但是也可通过考虑一些数据包括先证者和其他家庭成员的性别以及

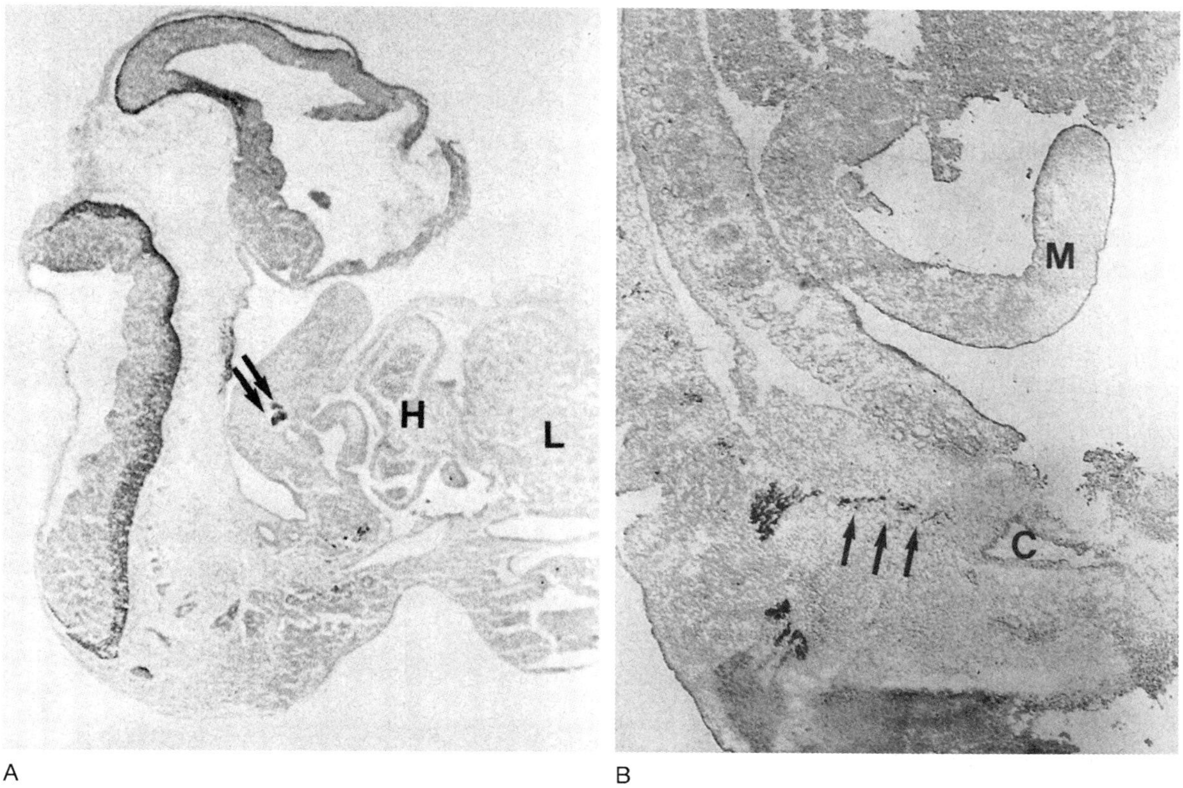

图 99-12　胚胎第 4 周的神经丝蛋白。A. 神经嵴起源的细胞首次出现在食管上部（双箭头）。B. 同时在神经嵴细胞出现前免疫反应束（纤维）移向泄殖腔（箭头）。C. 泄殖腔。H. 心脏。L. 肺。M. 口。（From Fujimoto T，HataJ，Yokoyama S，Mitomi T：A study of the extracellular matrix protein as the migration pathway of neural crest cells in the gut：Analysis in human embryos with special reference to the pathogenesis of Hirschsprung's disease. J Pediatr Surg 1989；24：550-556.）

无神经节细胞段的长度来估计发病风险[21]。对已知家庭中有 *RET* 突变常染色体显性遗传的病例进行遗传咨询比较容易，其儿女有 50% 的突变率，但是还未能预知它的外显率和表达率。对 17 个先天性巨结肠的家庭进行的研究发现 *RET* 的外显率是伴性遗传的（72% 为男性，51% 为女性）[19]。因此我们能够假定先天性巨结肠呈现出明显的性别差别，这取决于无神经节细胞段的长度和性别；男性发病率几乎比女性高出 2～4 倍[54]。所有这些因素使基因咨询变得非常困难，同时也使先天性巨结肠的产前诊断不能实行。另外，遗传咨询必须考虑最近几十年先天性巨结肠外科治疗的进展。特别要注意那些携带细胞外 *RET* 基因外显子 10 和 11 的一个半胱氨酸残基上的突变的患儿，该突变有发生 MEN2A 的倾向[12,230,292]。对这些患者和其他的易感家庭成员应该进行仔细随访、实施合理的监控和生物学测试，因为他们有发生神经内分泌瘤的危险。

胚胎学

正常肠神经系统的胚胎形成

了解正常肠神经系统的胚胎发育对于正确认识先天性巨结肠的发生是必需的。正常神经节细胞的发育由几个特定的阶段组成。首先是诱导期，主要是指受空间和时间需要的影响，这取决于多种因素和不同的分子信号[186]。第二步就是神经嵴细胞迁移到远端遍及整个胚胎[185,186]。第三步是神经嵴细胞前体分化为
1524 多种细胞类型。这个分化机制还有很多地方不清楚（图 99-11）。在正常的胚胎发育中，肠神经母细胞从神经嵴由消化道的上端向尾端迁移[187]。第一批神经细胞在胚胎第 5 周到达食管[242]，第 7 周出现在中肠，第 12 周迁移到远端结肠（图 99-12）。迁移首先发生在 Auerbach 神经丛（肌间神经丛）；随后这些细胞移至黏膜下神经丛。在这个迁移过程中神经嵴细胞被一些糖蛋白例如纤维结合素和透明质酸（薄片蛋白）[95]和一些神经生长因子所引导。

关于先天性巨结肠胚胎发育缺失有两个基本理论："迁移失败"理论和"敌对环境"理论。很明显因为确定了与先天性巨结肠相关的其他基因突变的因素，我们能够更好地认识一些临界蛋白，这些临界蛋白在正常神经节细胞发育过程中必须在适当的时间和空间下进行表达[146]。在发现 RET 与其他信号蛋白（GDNF和 NTN）相互作用的基础上，多因素的结合对于无神经节细胞症全部表现型的发生是必需的。图 99-13 给出了先天性巨结肠发生不同机制的概述图。

异常的肠神经元迁移

组成肠神经系统的所有神经元和神经胶质细胞都起源于神经嵴[186]。正常的迁移过程是复杂的，取决
于许多因素。原先认为肠道接受迷走神经和骶部起源 152
的神经嵴细胞。现在认为迷走神经嵴细胞是神经节细胞的主要来源，它们比其他来源的细胞更早地迁移至内脏[46]。骶部的神经嵴细胞是肠神经系统组成的一小部分，主要作用于后肠。一些学者假定先天性巨结肠发生时神经嵴细胞迁移出现异常，神经母细胞不能迁移到更远端的位置引起先天性巨结肠。Okamoto 和 Ueda[242] 首先提出了这样的假设：神经节细胞的缺如是因为正常的神经嵴迁移无法进行所导致的。实验证实了切除全部迷走神经嵴细胞会导致从肛门到中肠的完全无神经节细胞症；切除邻近 3～5 个体节仅会导致后肠的无神经节细胞症，只要不切除这个节段就不会影响肠神经系统的发育[251,252]。学者们还证实了远端结肠无神经节细胞症可能与后肠水平的鸡胚横断有关。将鸽子的神经节细胞移植于横断处的远端，远端肠壁就会有正常的神经节细胞结合了。因此先天性巨结肠的病因之一就是正常的神经嵴细胞迁移障碍。

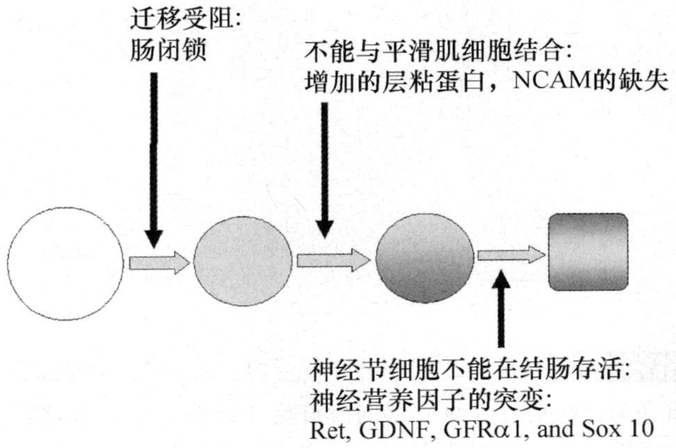

图 99-13 先天性巨结肠潜在的发病机制。

细胞外基质的改变

引导神经嵴细胞迁移机制之一是通过一系列在神经嵴迁移过程发生前产生的糖蛋白和纤维进行的[95,248,249]。这些糖蛋白包括纤维结合素和透明质酸，它们的出现为神经嵴细胞的迁移创造了路径途径。这些支持纤维从消化道移至整个结肠，开始于基膜层终止于肌层。随后神经嵴细胞利用这些结构迁移至肠壁。迁移到肠壁后可能这些神经母细胞处在一个“敌对”的或者不利的环境中，从而导致神经节细胞发育停顿[101,247~249,330]。许多学者指出在无神经节细胞症的肠壁内纤维结合素和层粘蛋白分布异常。这些学者还指出大量的层粘蛋白在细胞外异常堆积，推测这些堆积可能阻止神经节细胞迁移至新的环境。

神经营养因子的缺失

阻止神经嵴细胞迁移和结合的确切原因还不为人知。一个可能对先天性巨结肠发病有重要影响的关键因素就是神经营养因子的表达。RET 信号通路就是这样一个因子。RET 和它的结合受体 GFR-α 在迁移的迷走神经嵴细胞中被表达，同时也对肠神经系统的发育起至关重要的作用[46]。RET-GFR-α1 的联合体配体是 GDNFR。GDNF 在消化道壁内被表达，作为肠神经元的化学引诱剂。最大的 GDNF 反应发生在神经嵴细胞将要迁移进去的地方，因此可以作为向导引导正常迁移，且似乎被内皮素-3（EDN3）反向调节[123]。正如上文所指出的，所有这些因素在先天性巨结肠患者中都有基因突变从而阻止正常迁移。引导神经嵴细胞迁移的其他重要因素还包括 NTN 和 END3[144]。一旦神经嵴细胞成功地迁移至消化道壁中，就可以发生一系列细胞的成熟变化。神经嵴细胞功能的缺失也可能在先天性巨结肠的发生中起重要的作用[146]。在胚胎学上，在神经嵴细胞首先探测到的可表达的因子是氧化亚氮，随后是其他的许多神经传递介质。已经证实在肠道无神经节细胞的区域有氧化亚氮表达的缺失（见后）。另外两个作用于神经嵴突变的亲神经因子是转录因子 Mash1 和 SOX10；*SOX10* 的突变已经在先天性巨结肠的一些病例中被证实了（前面已述）[246]。

细胞内粘连分子表达的缺失

为了支持“敌对”环境因素理论，Langer 等[181]证实了从无神经节的结肠的平滑肌组织中培养出神经节细胞，其黏合平滑肌细胞的能力明显减低，说明缺乏细胞-细胞粘连。这个发现由先天性巨结肠中神经细胞黏合分子（NCAM）活性缺失这一现象所证实。Kobayashi 等[147]研究了先天性巨结肠患者的结肠标本中 NCAM 的反应力，并将它们与年龄和性别相匹配的正常对照组进行对照。含有神经节细 1526
胞的肠管 NCAM 的反应力很强（无论在对照组的患者还是在先天性巨结肠的患者中），而在无神经节细胞的节段的肌间神经丛中缺乏 NCAM 阳性反应的神经纤维。NCAM 被认为在胚胎形成时对神经细胞的迁移和神经细胞定位于特殊部位是很重要的。还发现另有其他一些黏合分子在无神经节细胞的区域表达减少，包括 L1CAM 和 N-钙粘连素[378]。可能为了弥补神经迁移的缺失，细胞间黏合分子 1（ICAM-1）在无神经节细胞区域有明显的增加[166]。

免疫因素

主要的组织相容性Ⅱ级抗原在无神经节细胞区域有明显的增加[175]。其他一些学者[130,166]还发现神经

表 99-4　先天性巨结肠无神经节细胞症的范围

过渡区	一些研究的范围（%）					
	Polley[260]	Kleinhaus[164]	Klein[163]	Teitelbaum[327]	Ikeda[140]	Swenson[314]
直肠乙状结肠	74	74	58	71	79	73
长段型	11	18	26	13	13	24
全结肠	12	8	12	10	5	3
小肠	3	*	0	0	3	0.4

*小肠包含在全结肠中。

节细胞缺如的另一个机制就是在神经节细胞上对抗自身抗原的免疫反应加剧。正如早期发现的，ICAM-1表达的增加，可能是对已察觉的异质组织炎症反应的结果。另一个神经节细胞缺如的潜在机制就是因为细胞凋亡的增加。虽然这个研究领域还较新，但是已经有证据显示在无神经节细胞的区域有一个阻止凋亡的主要因子 Bcl-2 的缺失，从而潜在地允许有更大范围的神经节细胞缺如[302]。

基因和病理生理信息未来的应用

通过基因控制，可以在小鼠和大鼠中建立无神经节细胞症的模型。这些模型有两个种类组成，致死花斑株（S^LS^L-纯合子）和致死位点株（L^S-杂合子）。这些老鼠发展为巨结肠，并通常在出生后的头几个月内死于腹泻和假性小肠结肠炎[50,94]。虽然这与人类疾病的描述不完全一样，但是这些模型和发现可以帮助我们确定其他潜在的基因突变，引导我们研究治疗先天性巨结肠的新方式。随着对干细胞研究的进展，治疗方法可能有进一步发展，包括在肠道的无神经节细胞部分移植入神经节细胞。最近研究显示神经细胞的干细胞可以从啮齿动物中分离出来[172,297]。最近通过 *EDNRB* 基因胎内转染成功地治疗了 EDNRB 被破坏或者 S^L（致死位点）突变的大鼠[102]。这使得在这些大鼠中 EDNRB 得到完整表达并且结肠内也有了神经节细胞，从而阻止了巨结肠的发生。这个令人兴奋的新探索领域提出了是否应该在人类中应用这个治疗手段的问题，对与先天性巨结肠相关的突变有更好的理解并且在胎内就发现这些疾病可能是至关重要的。另一个挑战就是该方法应用的时机。这表明该治疗方法应该应用于胚胎期从而使得神经节细胞得到足够的表达。在早期发现这个遗传性疾病，并将遗传物质转染到胚胎将是一个严峻的挑战。

病理学

先天性巨结肠的大体表现随着疾病未治疗时期的变化而变化。在新生儿早期，肠管可以接近正常。随着婴儿的年龄增长，近端神经节细胞的肠管过度生长，比正常的肠管更粗更长。没有清晰的软组织带，但可以看见肥厚的纵肌层完全地围绕在结肠的周围。肠管有神经节细胞的区域到无神经节细胞的过渡区呈漏斗形，长度不一，远端大肠正常或者狭窄。

组织学上，这个疾病的特点就是远端肠管神经节细胞的缺如。在黏膜下神经丛（Meissner's）和肌间神经丛（Auerbach's）中都有神经节细胞的缺如（见图 99-4A）。与这个发现相关的是明显增粗的神经纤维延伸至黏膜下（见图 99-4B）。这些纤维可以通过常规的苏木精-伊红染色被看见，但是用乙酰胆碱酯酶染色更容易发现（见“诊断”一节，图 99-5A 和 B）。无神经节细胞症最典型的病变区域就是乙状结肠，发病率占 80%[195,222,223,238]。几大系的无神经节细胞症的病变段在表 99-4 中列出。无神经节细胞症在本质上是连续的、无间断的直至到达近端有神经节的节段。也有例外情况的报道，但这种病例非常少见，在无神经节细胞段发现神经节细胞，提示已经到达移行区了。虽然外科医生使用拖出手术时的冰冻切片确认移行区，但是仍有错误发生。在一篇有冰冻切 152
片的 80 例先天性巨结肠患者的综述中，固定标本和冰冻切片的符合率仅达 80%。此外，有两名患者因为冰冻切片报告不准确而导致手术效果不佳。这些都说明了需要一个有经验的病理科医生来协助外科医生。新技术乙酰胆碱酯酶或 NADPH-心肌黄酶染色的应用，可帮助我们避免这类错误的发生[168,237]。

移行段的长度不一，可以延伸至几厘米。虽然神经节细胞可能在移行区出现，但是结肠的动力可能不正常。这个区域出现过度生长的神经纤维，说明过渡区还是存在的。这些过度生长的神经纤维的出现和在移行区中可能发现的肠神经元发育不良，都可能是在明确拖出肠段后引起肠功能低下的原因[217]。此外，虽然在肠壁的一侧可以出现神经节细胞，但在过渡区可能存在于周边其他地方，这样就支持了拖出肠管的长度选择应比冰冻切片所建议的高出几个厘米的想法[107]。

多种神经元和肽的标志物的发现有助于明确先天性巨结肠中神经和神经节分布的改变。在无神经节细胞段中可以发现肠管血管活性多肽、P 物质、胃泌素释放多肽和 met-脑啡肽浅染[114,341,342]。在无神经节细胞段中其他固有的神经纤维既可以没有变化（甘丙肽或降钙素基因有关的多肽）也可以有所增加（神经肽 Y）[184]。这些变化的病理生理学重要性还未被阐明。

已经确定许多其他组织学标志物在先天性巨结肠患儿的消化道中呈现特定的形式。其中包括神经元特异的烯醇酶、神经丝蛋白和 S-100 蛋白数量的减少[165,316,353,373]。在无神经节细胞组织中 Schwann 细胞的单克隆抗体，D_7 完全缺如，这可能是无神经节细胞症最好的标志物之一[96]。此外，NADPH－心肌黄酶染色缺如可能对明确先天性巨结肠有帮助[225]。最后在先天性巨结肠患者中有 Cajal 肠神经细胞的改变，包括在肛门括约肌中这些细胞缺如[258]以及在先天性巨结肠患儿结肠无神经节细胞段的染色完全缺如[346]。虽然这些标志物没有被普遍地使用，但是最终有一些可能成为该疾病诊断的有效指标。

病理生理学

肠管包含三个神经丛：黏膜下神经丛或称 Meissner 神经丛、肌间神经丛或称 Auerbach 神经丛和许多小的黏膜神经丛[291,370]。每一个丛都有相当完整的神经网络，用来控制肠管的许多功能（吸收、分泌、血流、运动），同时它们也较少受到身体中枢神经的控制。事实上，肠管包含与脊髓相等数量的神经元[370]。正常的肠管运动最初是受每个神经节细胞内固有的神经元控制。即使外部控制缺失，肠管也能发挥足够的功能[326]。这些神经节可以使平滑肌收缩或松弛；然而正常情况下松弛占优势。肠管外来的控制是通过神经节前的胆碱能纤维和神经节后的肾上腺素能纤维来进行的。胆碱能纤维通过乙酰胆碱神经传递素控制收缩。肾上腺素能纤维主要控制抑制反应，但也包含一些产生兴奋的路径，它们用去甲肾上腺素来调节其功能。肠管也包含了一个有神经传递素的固有的神经系统，起到自发的抑制作用；这个系统就是先前所指的非胆碱能、非肾上腺素能神经系统。直到 1990 年才确定了对这级神经起作用的神经传递素，Bult[45]等指出一氧化氮（NO）是这个抑制反应的介质。在正常肠管中收缩力和舒张力的平衡可以有效地控制平滑肌（图 99-14）。

除了神经节细胞的异常迁移之外，肠管的起搏细胞-肠道 Cajal 细胞（ICCs）——也被认为在先天性巨结肠的病变段是减少的。已经发表的文章指出先天性巨结肠中有正常和减少的 ICC 分布[239,301]。有趣的是 ICCs 使用 NO 作为神经传递介质。ICCs 的缺失可能对先天性巨结肠的病理生理学改变有明显的作用[257]。

远端直肠可以存在正常的运动反射。这个机制最初在 1877 年由 Gowers[110]提出。远端直肠适度的扩张使该点上端的肠管收缩，而下端的肠管舒张。这个反射纯粹是肠管本身固有的。这个反射的消失表示肠管壁内的神经节细胞异常或缺如。

当神经节细胞缺如时，外部的神经系统对肠管的控制明显增加。在无神经节细胞的肠管中胆碱能和肾 1528
上腺素能系统的神经分布增加 2～3 倍[26,138,335,337]。这样可以推测在无神经节细胞的节段中肾上腺素能的兴奋作用超过其抑制功能，因此平滑肌的紧张性增加。在无神经节细胞的组织中胆碱能神经也明显增加且主要产生兴奋。解释无神经节细胞节段收缩功能机制的另一个成分就是正常神经节细胞表达的 NO 缺如[317]。一些学者已经证实了在无神经节细胞肠管的肌间神经丛中缺乏 NO 合成酶（NO 形成需要这个酶）[27,167,243]，然而在有神经节细胞的节段中 NO 合成酶的数量正常[317]。NO 的缺如伴有肾上腺能和起兴奋作用的胆碱能纤维的增加可以导致平滑肌的过度收缩。这些研究中难以解决的问题就是 NO 合成酶在无神经节区的黏膜下神经丛有很强的反应力，但是在肌间神经丛中却没有。这可能是这些区域的 NO 源于外部神经的向内生长，且肌间神经丛 NO 合成酶的缺乏足以解释结肠的痉挛状态。

相关畸形

先天性巨结肠通常在足月健康的婴儿中是散在发病的。然而还有几个与之相关的先天性畸形。最常见的相关畸形就是 21－三体（Down 综合征），据报道在先天性巨结肠儿童中其发病率为 4.5%～16%[49,109]。在

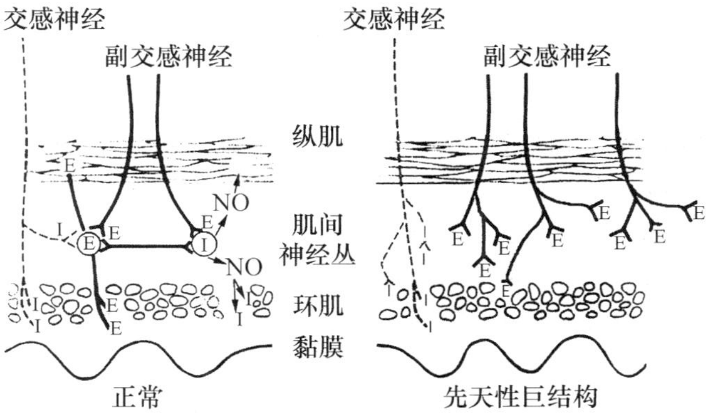

图 99-14　有神经节细胞肠管（左侧）和无神经节细胞肠管（右侧）的神经分布示意图。E：兴奋性纤维。I：抑制纤维。NO：一氧化氮。

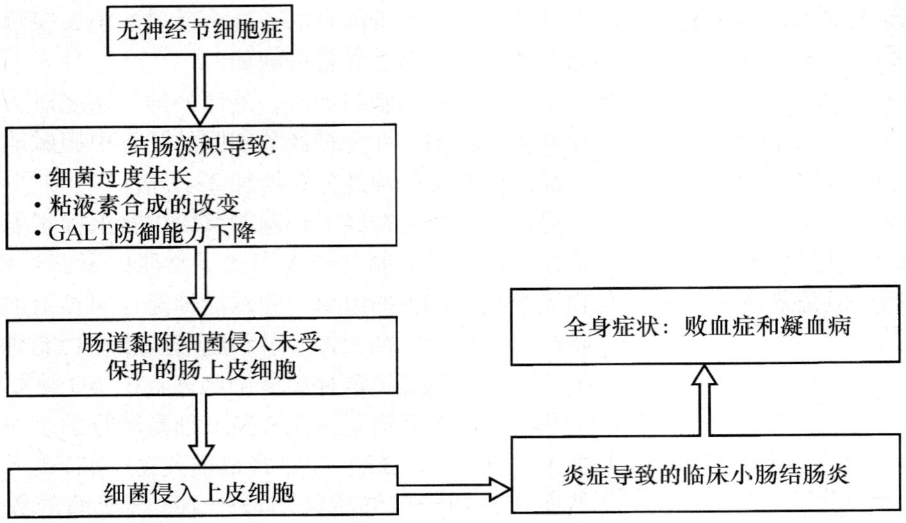

图 99-15 先天性巨结肠伴小肠结肠炎可能的病理生理学基础。

Quinn[267]等的研究中，13%的先天性巨结肠患儿伴有21-三体。这些患儿的预后较差。尽管17例患儿中13例进行了最终的巨结肠拖出术，但是只有1例有正常的肠道功能。也有其他人报告了较好的临床效果。在Caniano[49]等的文章中13例21-三体中的6例需进行拖出术。尽管婴儿夜晚排便失禁，但是白天有较好的排便控制力。最近有更多的报道相似的结果，而且建议对高功能21-三体患儿像其他先天性巨结肠患儿一样进行治疗[116]。重要的是，曾有报道[323]伴有21-三体的先天性巨结肠患儿小肠结肠炎的发病率增高，可能是由这些患者中T和B淋巴细胞功能减低引起的[189]。

在先天性巨结肠患儿中曾有小肠和大肠闭锁的报道。也有几篇病例报告指出结肠闭锁与先天性巨结肠有关[3,136,368]。其发病的原因还不知道，可能是晚期血管事件的结果[3]。虽然少见，儿外科医生应该坚持对无神经节细胞症远端结肠做仔细的病理学检查[3]和直肠吸吮活检。发现有连续的肠管后会经常错过先天性巨结肠的诊断，从而发展成肠梗阻[227,365]。先天性巨结肠伴有小肠闭锁比伴有结肠闭锁更常见，大约占所有先天性巨结肠患者的0.25%~0.8%[140,227]。Gauderer等[103]建议在小肠闭锁的病例中应常规检查远端肠管有无先天性巨结肠。伴有肛直肠闭锁的先天性巨结肠也曾有报道，Kiesewetter等[156]报道了在296例先天性巨结肠患者中发病率达3.4%，Watanatittan等[354]在321例中发现了9例（占2.8%）。一些关于超短段型巨结肠的报道可能仅说明了有瘘管的无肛患儿缺乏神经节细胞而已。

先天性巨结肠伴有的其他畸形为18-三体、Ondine病[77]和先前已经讨论过的许多神经嵴病[58,157,244]。Currarino三联征也与先天性巨结肠相关[24]，又称Smith-Lemli-Opitz综合征。曾经认为与先天性巨结肠相关的其他畸形如尿道畸形已经被否定了。

小肠结肠炎

小肠结肠炎仍是先天性巨结肠主要的发病和死亡原因。其临床主要表现为暴发性的腹泻、腹胀和发热[32,77]。先天性巨结肠的小肠结肠炎的病理生理机制尚未完全明确，然而基于临床和实验室的研究，已经证实的几个因素可能对解释其发展有帮助。图99-15阐明了与先天性巨结肠相关的小肠结肠炎发生的理论。因为无神经节细胞，所以小肠和结肠发生淤积。如果这种淤积未得到治疗，那么就可以观察到小肠结肠炎的发病率明显增高[48,108]。许多学者认为肠内容物的淤积可以导致细菌的过度生长以及黏膜血流状态的改变。由于肠防御机制减弱，具有肠黏附性和侵袭性的细菌就可以进入肠壁的上皮细胞[323]。在先天性巨结肠中至少有两个防御机制减弱。第一是黏液素合成物的明显异常[4,16,17,212]。黏液素基因表达和翻译后特性的变化可以干扰黏液素的正常保护功能。特别是小肠结肠炎的婴幼儿实际上缺乏MUC2，它是人类结肠黏液素的主要形式[212]。第二是先天性巨结肠的婴幼儿存在局部的免疫异常，包括肠道中免疫球蛋白A数量的缺乏[50,94,366,367]。另外在人类小肠结肠炎和大鼠模型

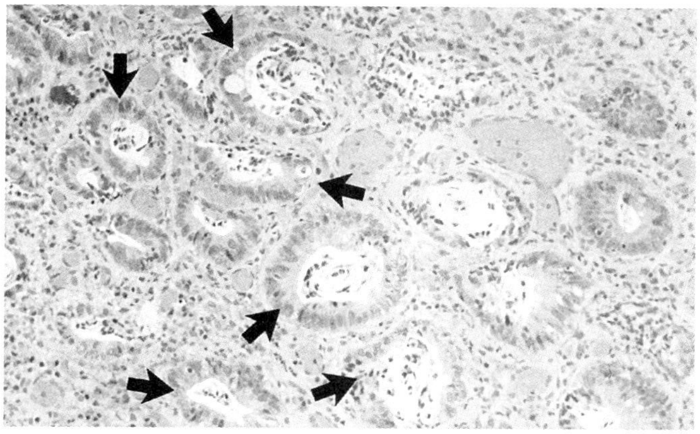

图 99-16 小肠结肠炎患儿的组织病理学表现。箭头所示的是大量的腺管脓肿。

中都证实有 T 淋巴细胞功能的缺失。先天性巨结肠伴
29 有 21-三体患者中小肠结肠炎发病率增高这一现象可支持这一观点[325]。现在也证实了在 21-三体患者中缺少体液免疫和细胞免疫系统[189]。一旦细菌进入到肠上皮细胞，具有肠黏附特性的细菌就可以黏附然后侵入肠壁从而导致临床上小肠结肠炎的发生[323]。

小肠结肠炎在病理学上是指浸润结肠和小肠上皮黏膜和腺管的急性炎症（图 99-16）。组织学上可以看到进行性的改变。早期结肠腺管内可见大量浓缩的黏液素，具有这个特征性表现的只有两种疾病——先天性巨结肠和囊性纤维化[80,323]。随后可以出现腺管脓肿、黏膜溃疡，最后是肠壁完全穿孔。也可发生假膜性结肠炎，这是致命的[61,323]。这个过程在有神经节细胞的肠管中与无神经节细胞的肠管是一样的[80,323]。有报道初次发生先天性巨结肠和小肠结肠炎的患儿实施拖出术后小肠结肠炎复发的危险性增高[19,323]。虽然有不同的观点[115]，但是早期的小肠结肠炎组织学活检证实了这些患儿进行拖出术后有小肠结肠炎复发的危险[80]。也有人认为拖出术后严重的小肠结肠炎可能与直肠内局部肠神经发育不良有关[169]。严重的小肠结肠炎患儿小肠内可发生与吸收障碍有关的变化[44]。

作为先天性巨结肠初期表现的小肠结肠炎在过去 50 年中发生率有了明显的下降，那是因为现在先天性巨结肠在早期就可以得到诊断。目前小肠结肠炎最经常发生于拖出术后。拖出术后小肠结肠炎的发病率可以是 5%～46% 不等，但是通常在 20%～30%，这取决于诊断标准的制定[48,80,85,115,183,226,262,323,327]。拖出术后小肠结肠炎可能是因为拖出太紧或者是由肛门内括约肌痉挛所引起[120,327]。解剖上的狭窄和吻合口的狭窄都与小肠结肠炎密切相关[115,323,327]。虽然还未被所有的专家证实，但是与小肠结肠炎发生率增加有关的另一个危险因素就是长段型的病变[48,272,325]。

小肠结肠炎可依据腹泻（69%）、呕吐（51%）、发热（34%）和昏睡（27%）[78] 的临床表现来诊断。体检可以发现患儿腹胀，直肠指检后可有暴发性的腹泻[32,48]。除了这些病史和体征外，腹部 X 线出现“结肠中断征（cut-off sign）”对诊断有较高的敏感性（74%）和特异性（86%）（图 99-17）[78]。由于有穿孔的危险，应尽量避免做造影灌肠，然而钡灌肠肠黏膜可以呈现典型的“锯齿样”不规则外观（见图 99-2）。先天性巨结肠小肠结肠炎的死亡率为 0～30% 不等[32,115,140,164,325]。

治疗先天性巨结肠相关的小肠结肠炎首先将肛管插入直肠内括约肌上方进行主动清洗，以使结肠减 1530
压。单纯的灌肠因不能使结肠充分减压而效果不佳。在进行连续灌肠的同时，应根据临床表现的严重程度静脉给予抗生素或口服甲硝唑。在长段型的先天性巨

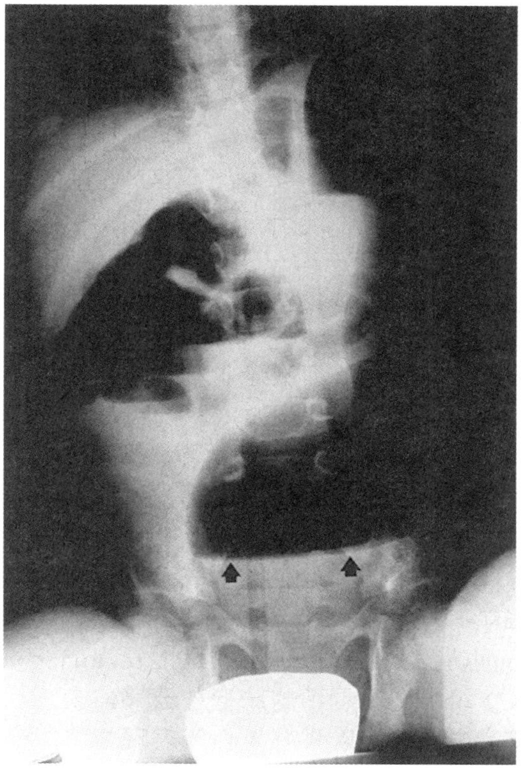

图 99-17 小肠结肠炎患儿的腹部 X 片。箭头所示的是盆腔上缘的“中断征”现象。

结肠中灌肠常常是无效的，可能需要使用结肠造瘘术进行减压[220]。有些患者通过注射内毒素可以使直肠扩张或者肛门内括约肌松弛。色甘酸钠（一种不被吸收的大细胞稳定剂，用于治疗炎症性的肠道疾病）的应用有利于防止小肠结肠炎的复发[275]。大多数的小肠结肠炎患者有过度生长的表现。实施肠管拖出术后小肠结肠炎反复发作的患者可以进行肌层后切术或者肌条部分切除术[364]。曾经有人提倡用拖出术后灌肠来减少小肠结肠炎的发病率[211]。

阑尾

通常在新生儿期，先天性巨结肠最初表现为阑尾炎穿孔[15,201,287]。有这种表现的婴幼儿需要进行连续的结肠活检。一般来说，这些穿孔表示无神经节细胞症区域的长度较长。关于使用阑尾诊断全结肠型巨结肠存在大量的争论，但是阑尾的组织学检查通常是明确诊断最好的方法[10]。阑尾的神经支配与其他小肠有轻微的不同；在全结肠无神经节细胞症中，阑尾缺乏神经纤维和神经内分泌细胞[295]。早期对先天性巨结肠患儿进行手术探查时对阑尾进行评估可以快速明确诊断。有一个病例，推测患儿是全结肠及阑尾无神经节细胞症，随后在其横结肠发现有神经节细胞[10]。这个极少见的病例提示有节段性的先天性巨结肠。

节段性和获得性疾病

节段性无神经节细胞症非常少见，是指单独的一个节段无神经节细胞而远端结肠有神经节细胞。跳跃式的病变就是这样一个例子。曾经报道过一些区域性的无神经节细胞症的病例[69,153,379]，在成人中也有描述[93]。它们的胚胎学发生仍未明确，但是Okamoo 和 Ueda[242]猜测可能是由于神经母细胞从颅端至尾端有序迁移的过程中遭到干扰所致。同样地，Kapur 等[153]从死亡的花斑鼠上发现跳跃的病变是继发于结肠神经母细胞肠壁外迁移的表现。这种情况非常少见，所以只有当临床表现与组织病理学描述不同时才需要考虑。

获得性的先天性巨结肠是指先天性巨结肠患儿最初在肠管的特定区域有神经节细胞，但是后来此处的神经节细胞缺如。该情况不常见，但是对于临床是个挑战[67,366,338]。获得性病变的原因尚未明确，但在一些病例中发现组织学上有缺血的改变，所以认为是由选择性缺血导致的[59,336]。相关实验包括将氯化汞注入直肠的网膜血管，这可以模拟出先天性巨结肠无神经节细胞的节段[242]。在婴儿中可见获得性先天性巨结肠的变种，这些患儿在进行结肠造口术后发生造瘘口功能减退，这是因为术后缺血造成了神经节细胞的缺如。同样，获得性无神经节细胞症可发生于肛门闭锁肠管拖出术后。另一种潜在的原因就是在拖出术后远端直肠残留的无神经节细胞节段增长。

青少年和成年人先天性巨结肠

在青春期少年和成年人中先天性巨结肠的临床表现不典型。十年间我们所里诊断 32 例青少年和 3 例成人先天性巨结肠，约占我们诊断的全部先天性巨结肠患者的 3%[260]。有一篇综述提到大约有 200 例成人先天性巨结肠[359]。一般来讲，这些患者通过近端肠管的代偿性扩张及规律性地使用泻药和灌肠，已基本适应了他们的病症[14]。Swenson 等[313]报道了成人先天性巨结肠的治疗经验；282 名患者进行了 Swenson 拖出术，其中 71 例是成人，占 25%。但是未比较成人与儿童的预后[315]。一般来说，多数手术后成人和青少年各种并发症的发生率比儿童高。因此在青春期少年和成人中要采取比较保守的方法。因为结肠扩张明显，所以不可以直接行无肠造瘘的巨结肠拖出术。如果是超短段型先天性巨结肠（<5 cm）可以考虑行直肠后壁括约肌切除术[199]。然而在 Wu 等[372]报道的 5 例成人先天性巨结肠中有 2 例只行括约肌切除术的仍然存在排便问题。对于成人无神经节细胞组织采用后壁括约肌切除术加低位的前壁切除术可以取得较好的结果[87]。

超短段型先天性巨结肠

超短段型先天性巨结肠（又称肛直肠失弛缓症）关于其诊断、治疗及疾病自身的发病引发了许多疑惑。主要的问题在于如果对超短段型先天性巨结肠患者取的标本太靠近近端，那么作为巨结肠诊断的金标

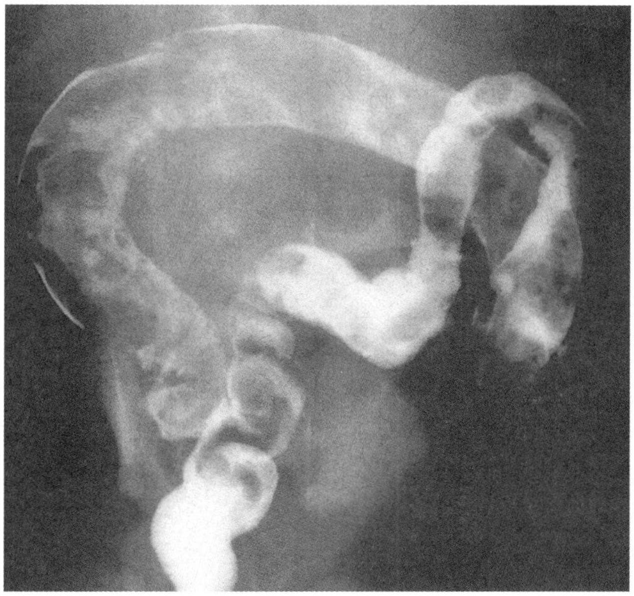

图 99-18　全结肠型无神经节细胞症患者的钡灌肠。注意问号形的结肠以及变圆的肝曲和脾曲。

准——直肠活检可能显示神经节细胞。许多患儿不仅有长时间的便秘史，而且有漏粪，使得很难同污粪相鉴别[236,290]。几篇关于该疾病的详细综述明确了一些普遍的特征，包括有慢性便秘病史、3 cm 和 5 cm 处吸吮活检发现神经节细胞以及钡灌肠造影未发现移行段。肛管直肠测压十分有用，可以显示内括约肌松弛反射缺乏[236]。这就造成在没有常规开展肛管直肠测压的医疗中心内，一些超短段型先天性巨结肠可能会被漏诊。同样，如果直肠活检时取样位置太低，刚好在正常肛管无神经节细胞处时，那么特发性便秘的患儿可能被误诊为超短段型巨结肠。对明确诊断的超短段型巨结肠推荐使用肛直肠肌条切除术[199]。

全结肠型无神经节细胞症

全结肠型无神经节细胞症约占婴幼儿先天性巨结肠患儿的 3%~12%（见表 99-4）。这些患儿是发病率和死亡率都有所升高的一类具有挑战性的群体。诊断全结肠型无神经节细胞症可能比较困难。放射学检查显示扩张的肠袢，结肠造影显示脾曲和肝曲不常见的圆形边缘导致的空的或问号形的结肠（图 99-18）。只有 20%~30% 的全结肠型无神经节细胞症根据放射性检查可以得到明确诊断[30]。全结肠型无神经节细胞症一般是在对疑似肠梗阻或穿孔患儿进行剖腹探查或对先天性巨结肠患儿行结肠造口术时确诊的。阑尾冰冻切片检查会有助于诊断，而且明显缩短了手术时间[10,240]。在先天性巨结肠家族史中，全结肠型的无神经节细胞症比乙结肠型的发病率高，约为 12.4%~33%[10,240]。另外，男女比例更低，大约为1.3∶1[261]；在广泛的无神经节细胞症中（包括广泛的小肠无神经细胞症），此比例降至0.8∶1[141]。无神经节细胞肠管近端在回肠末段的占 75%，回肠中段的占 20%，空肠段的占 5%[148,240]。全结肠型的无神经节细胞症并发症较多，且比普通型的先天性巨结肠更常出现并发症。许多全结肠型先天性巨结肠患儿可能因为体液的过度丢失、制造导管引起的败血症、生长障碍、造瘘口机能不良、电解质失衡、脱水等常见并发症需要肠外营养。全结肠型无神经节细胞症的死亡率为 0[151]~44%[141,363]，这更突出了这种先天性巨结肠的变种疾病的严重程度。

全结肠型无神经节细胞症的治疗方法始于合理的肠造口术的发明。应严密监测水电解质的摄入情况。
起初常给予肠外营养，以后逐渐过渡到肠内营养。生 1532
长发育弛缓较常见，但是注意钠和碳酸盐的替代可以预防此类并发症[280,290]。虽然有在新生儿期进行最基础的直肠内拖出式根治术的成功案例[80]，但是这个手术最好在较大的年龄进行，因为无结肠时会阴部表皮脱落可能非常严重。根据心理学的评估和肛门括约肌腔内的超声检查，全结肠型与普通型无神经节细胞症患儿的长期预后是相似的[198]。全结肠型无神经节细胞症患儿理想的拖出术仍被热烈地争论着。详细的外科手术方法将在下一节叙述。

早产儿的先天性巨结肠

先天性巨结肠常发生在足月儿中，但是也有一些早产儿先天性巨结肠的报道。对在我们医院治疗的 172 例患儿进行的回顾性研究发现，有确切孕龄的 142 例，其中孕龄小于或者等于 36 周的有 14 例，占 9.5%。其他的文献报道的范围在4%~8%。这个发病率与美国报道的早产儿的发病率 6.5%~10% 非常相似[161]。先天性巨结肠在更小的早产儿中极其少见，但也有报道[288]。

外科手术

先天性巨结肠的治疗方法经过反复实践正逐步趋于成熟。最初是通过采用改道的结肠造瘘术缓解患儿的症状，然而当造瘘口关闭后症状又出现了[213]。企图通过旁路或者切除多余的结肠治疗先天性巨结肠均未获得成功。最令人感兴趣的方法之一就是采用腰部交感神经切断术或者脊髓麻醉[2,122,349]。理论上切断直肠末端交感神经的输入可以导致副交感或者松弛冲动占优势。通过这种方法有几名患者的症状得到改善，但是 Ladd 最终还是认为不适用。图 99-19 总结了几种在先天性巨结肠外科治疗发展史上最常见的治疗方法。Swenson 和 Bill[311]第一次成功创立了先天性巨结肠的外科手术方法。该方法包括直肠乙结肠切除术和接近或含肛门括约肌拖出段的端-端吻合术。一些作者报告了较好的结果，其他学者发现大便失禁和吻合口狭窄的发生率较高。以后 Swenson 对这个手术进行了改良，包括进行一个更斜形的吻合而不涉及内括约肌。

以下是治疗先天性巨结肠的几个常见术式的讨论。虽然过去十年经肛门的直肠内拖出术占主要地位，但是对于儿外科医生来说熟悉其他几种手术方法也是非常重要的。假如经肛门直肠内拖出术不能进行或者需要重做，那么这些手术方式就会派上用场。

直肠全层活检

因为直肠吸引活检相对容易，并发症少，所以成为诊断先天性巨结肠的推荐方法。然而有时需要进行 153
直肠全层活检。对于多次直肠吸引活检不能明确诊断的患儿，最常见的是进行直肠全层活检。

术前准备

不需要进行正规的肠道准备。只要在手术时用生理盐水进行直肠灌洗，在近端直肠瓣处放置一块纱布防止大便进入手术区域就可以了。

体位、切口和标本的收集

患儿取截石位，臀部应置于手术床的末端用折叠的毛巾支撑。双足用纱布卷绕放在一起（脚底相对），两腿分开，悬在两侧，在髋部弯曲。

置入两个牵开器扩张狭窄的肛直肠。确定齿状线的后缘将 Vicryl（多乙醇酸）缝线（3-0）置于其上方用作牵引。在距齿状线 1 cm 和 2 cm 处的直肠后壁另外缝合两针（图 99-20A）。外科医生用非优势手拉住中间的缝线，用尖的弯头剪刀在齿状线和中间那根牵引线之间沿着直肠壁下半部做全层的切口。切开

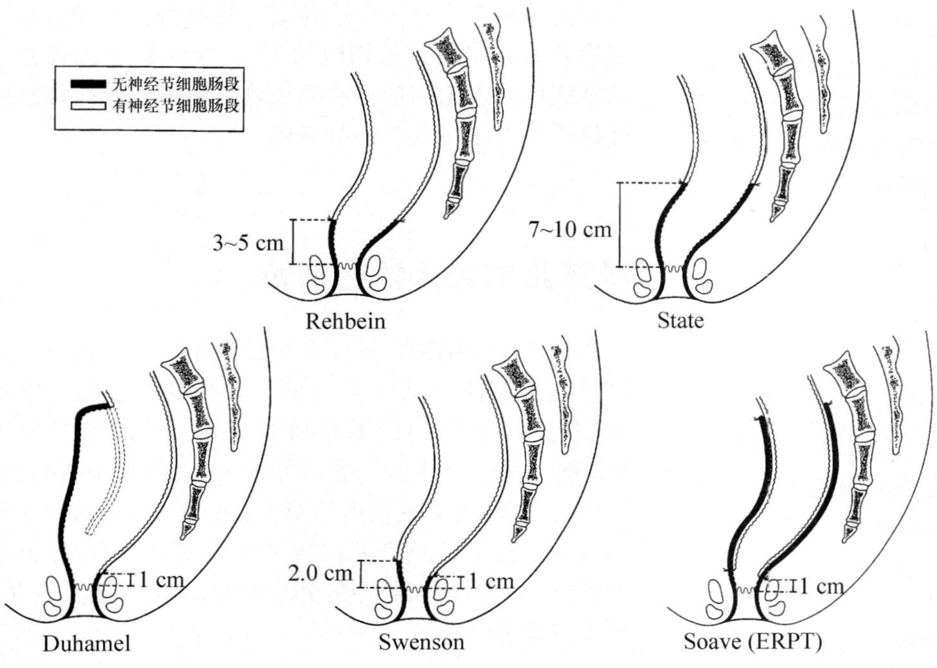

图 99-19　上半世纪常见的几种先天性巨结肠的手术方法。State 手术只因历史关系而列出。ERPT：直肠内拖出术。［From Spitz L，Coran A（eds）：Rob & Smith's Operative Surgery：Pediatric Surgery. London，Chapman HallMedical，1995.］

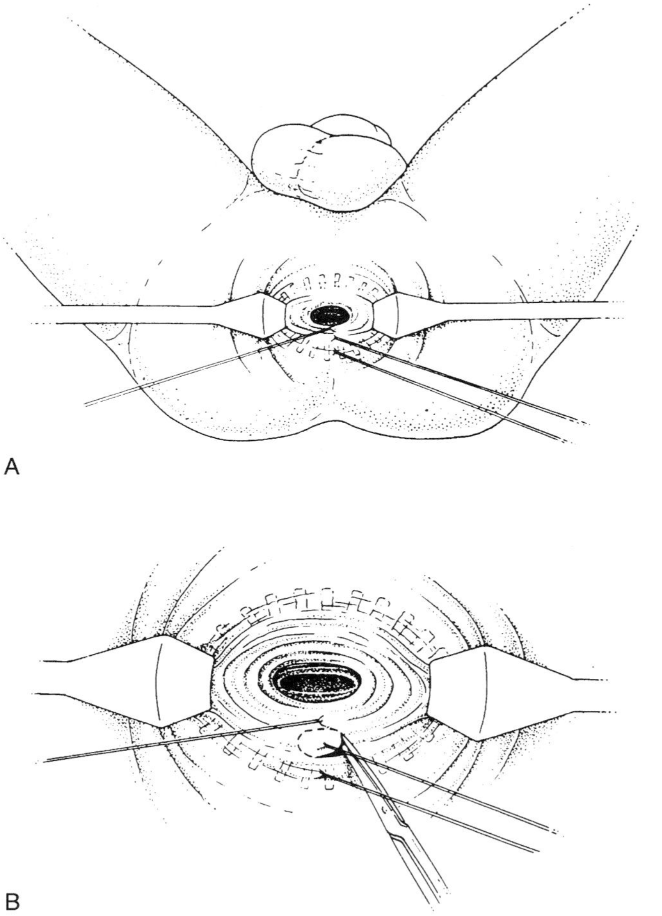

图 99-20　直肠全层活检。A. 活检时放置的牵引线。B. 在近远端牵引线之间取中间处做活检的标本。［From Spitz L，Coran A（eds）：Rob & Smith's Operative Surgery：Pediatric Surgery. London，Chapman Hall Medical，1995.］

后，可将剪刀置于前骶骨处，然后缓慢地剪。此时，出血可能影响手术视野，然而通过保持中间缝线的牵引，可以用剪刀平滑地切入直肠的上半部。每一次切开应取中间缝线吊起的组织的一半。假如所取的标本满意可送病理检查（图 99-20B）。用可吸收线单层或间断关闭切口。一旦缝合后可迅速止血。

标准的结肠造瘘术

虽然先天性巨结肠患儿的推荐手术是基础的拖出根治术，但是对有些患儿进行早期结肠造瘘术是有益的。结肠造瘘术的适应证是有严重小肠结肠炎的患儿或者因为有明显的近端结肠扩张不能进行基础的拖出根治术的患儿。

一般来说，做左下腹部斜切口可以暴露总的移行区。近端有神经节细胞的肠管通常有过度生长的纵向肌层，这层缺乏清晰可见的软组织带，在肠系膜对侧缘上用细尖的剪刀切入平滑肌组织取活检，切开的深度达黏膜下层。重要的是移行段可以延伸至几个厘米。顺着移行区向上，一部分周围的肠管出现神经节细胞，因此将造瘘处选择在更近端的肠管处是最安全的[360]。先天性巨结肠的肌层是相当厚的，所以容易切开。取 0.5 cm 大小的组织送去做冰冻切片，用间断的可吸收线缝合关闭肌层。在近端结肠移行段上方选择合适的位置做活检是非常重要的。用于造瘘的结肠要有许多神经节细胞，但没有肥大的神经。在此处附近行肠袢结肠造瘘术。因为初期肠管管径较大，所以造瘘口的回缩是常见的问题。因此在这个部位要将结肠与筋膜多处缝合以保证安全。为了保证以后肠管的安全，筋膜缝合的每一针都要避开肠系膜血管与筋膜缝合。

直肠内拖出术 1534

历史

虽然 1964 年 Soave 提出了直肠内的手术方式，但是该手术方式是 1952 年由 Yancey 首次使用，治疗了 2 例成人先天性巨结肠[374]。这个方法与目前开放的直肠内拖出术很相似，但是最初小儿外科协会并没有对这个术式完全认可。这个手术要剥除直肠的黏膜和黏膜下层，从无神经节细胞的肌鞘中拖出正常的有神经节细胞的肠管。Boley 改良了该手术[36]，在肛门处进行基础吻合。Coran 和 Weintraub[60] 又进一步改良了手术，将黏膜-黏膜下层管腔外翻至会阴部，使吻合更容易进行。由于保留了无神经节细胞直肠的肌鞘，重要的感觉神经纤维和内括约肌的完整性得以保存。尽管理论上在正常肠管周围保留无神经节细胞直肠的肌肉将导致术后较高的便秘发生率，但在临床上还没有这样的案例发生。

在新生儿中不进行最初的标准结肠造瘘而直接行基础直肠内拖出术是常见的手术方式[51,56,300]。将一期修补术与标准的两期手术进行全面的比较发现，两者并发症发生率相同[117,254,327]，技术上直肠内拖出术在新生儿期比年长儿期更易进行。

过去十年间直肠内拖出术由腹部的横切口改为经肛门的切口。这个显著的改变是由许多外科手术方式的革新引发的。Rintala 和 Lindahl[274]最先报道采用经肛门切口进行儿童先天性巨结肠手术，同时联合剖腹探查切口完成无神经节细胞肠管的移动。随后，Georgeson 等[105]提出了经肛门切口到达黏膜和黏膜下层的同时使用腹腔镜辅助无神经细胞结肠的移动。在无神经节细胞肠管的长度受直肠限制的病例，de la Torre-Mondragon 和 Ortega-Salgado[66]通过肛门入路进行完整的切除和移动。有报道指出采用经肛门术式的早期结果与腹部横切口的相似[5,79,118,134,183]。因为许多文章是最近发表的，所以还没有评估排便功能的长期研究。然而通过压力测定，经肛门手术和经腹部横切口手术术后肛门括约肌的压力是相似的[344]。

术前准备

即使在新生儿期，直肠内拖出术前也都要进行连续的生理盐水（10 ml/kg）灌肠和远端直肠扩张。在最后一次灌肠时加用 1% 的新霉素溶液。术前 1 小时静脉应用抗生素，术后继续给予 2 倍剂量的抗生素。

外科手术

经腹开放手术

存在许多直肠内拖出术的方式，该章节中不做详细的描述。图 99-21 显示了经腹开放的直肠内拖出术的主要步骤。成功进行拖出术的关键是儿童的体位，良好的体位有助于腹部和会阴部切口的进入。儿童的臀部通常放置于手术台的一端，将腿垫起放置于手术台边的木板或者支架上。取左下腹的斜切口，（如果之前没有进行的话）通过肉眼和一系列仔细标记的浆肌层冰冻活检决定无神经节细胞病变的范围。因为接近移行区进行拖出术可能预后欠佳，所以最好在距离首次发现正常神经节细胞的区域至少 5 cm 处行切断。直肠内切除通常在腹膜返折下 2 cm 处进行，用锐性或电切打开浆肌层。新生儿是在齿状线上 0.5 cm 内开始切除，所有的患儿都采用经腹切口（见图 99-21A 和 B）。一个确定有神经节细胞的结肠长度是否足够的简单方法就是将肠管伸展后观察其是否超过耻骨到达肛缘水平。可能需要近端移动至或跨过脾结肠韧带。当需要更长的肠管时，那么从其源头结扎肠系膜下动脉和保护好接近肠壁的边缘血管弓是有益的。

然后将注意力集中在会阴部。主刀医生将黏膜-黏膜下管腔外翻，管腔在齿状线上 0.5 cm 处被切开（见图 99-21C）。将 Kelly 钳放进开口处，通过先前放置的牵引线将正常有神经节细胞的肠管拖下来（见图 99-21D）。将肠管从肌鞘中拖出时应十分小心不要扭转肠管。在肠管两边用不同颜色（未染色的和染色的）的缝线对保持方向感十分有用。然后用可吸收线间断缝合进行吻合（见图 99-21E 和 F）。

内括约肌可以引起持续的梗阻症状[334]，因此许多外科医生在进行标准的拖出术时选择更远的接近尾端内括约肌的切口[224,350]。这可能是有益的，不会出现大便失禁的危险。

腹腔镜手术

腹腔镜手术与经腹开放手术的基本原则是一样的。套针放置如图 99-22A 所示，主要的一个放置在 153
右上腹，其余的放置在上腹部、左上腹和耻骨区。与开放手术一样进行无神经节细胞肠管的切除和拉平。用外科钳结扎血管或者电烙小血管（图 99-22B）。当完成肠管移动后，将其拖至会阴部，进行经肛门切除和吻合术（详见以后的章节）。

经肛门手术

手术开始的关键在于放置肛门牵开器（如：Lone Star Medical Products，Houston，Tex.）或者做多根牵引线可以使肛缘回缩（图 99-23A）。在齿状线上 0.5 cm 处电切一个环形的切口（图 99-23B）。在黏膜-黏膜下管腔处做多根牵引线，然后钝性切开。分离至近端腹膜返折处进入肌层，做全层切开（图 99-23C）。重要的是切开肌层直到直肠后壁中线的内括约肌，同时避免肌鞘的回缩以防引起相应的梗阻（图 99-23D 和 E）。对于直肠型先天性巨结肠而言，虽然在腹腔镜手术中系膜血管的结扎很容易，但是在经肛门手术中也会被切断。活检可以明确有神经节细胞肠管的水平，然后再行吻合术。

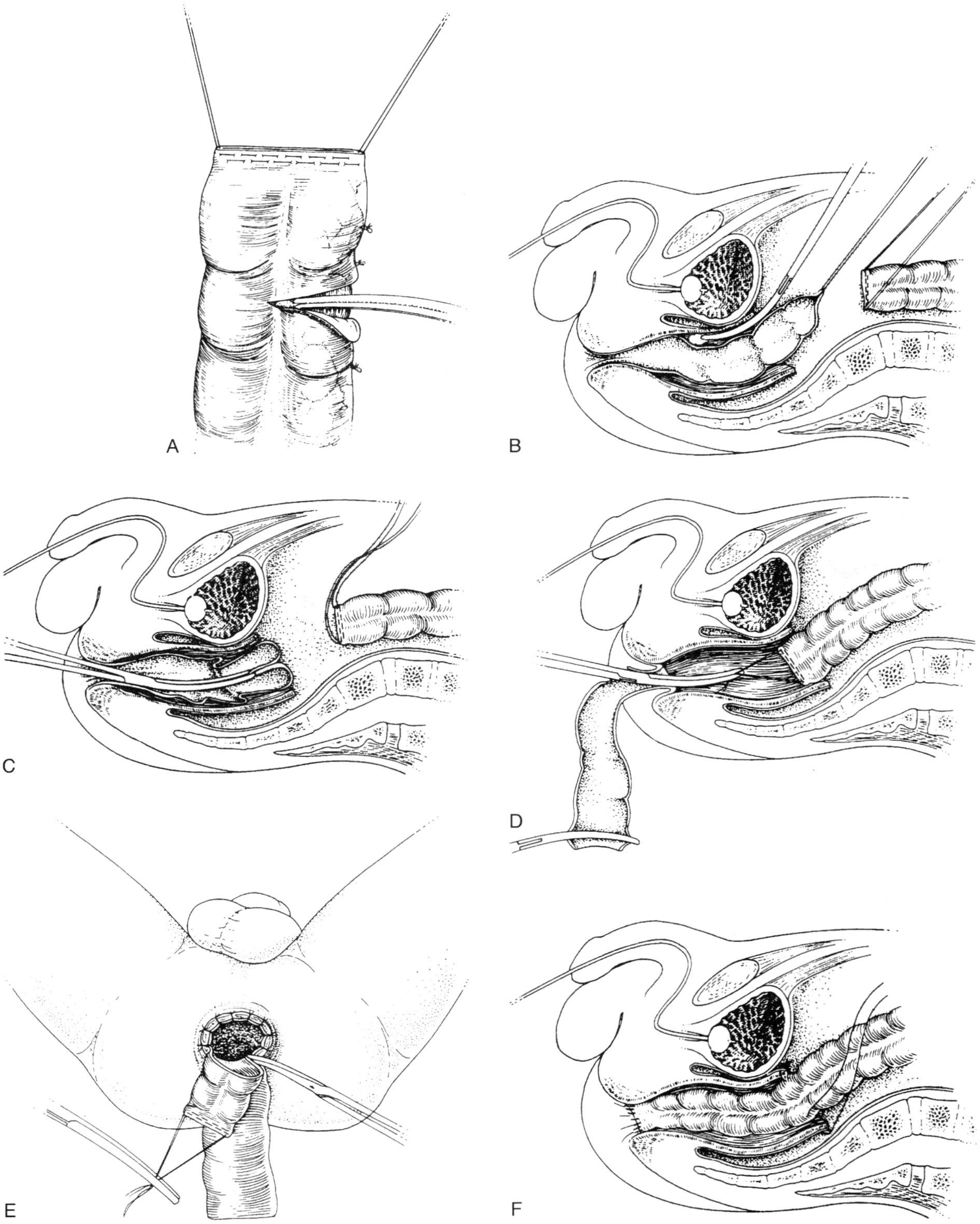

图 99-21　开放手术步骤。A. 直肠内切除首先在黏膜下肌层做环形切开。B. 下一步的切除在距肛门口 1.5 cm 的组织内进行。C. 将黏膜下-黏膜管腔外翻至会阴。D. 在接近齿状线 1 cm 处前方切开外翻的黏膜下-黏膜管腔后，将有神经节细胞的肠管从肌鞘拖出。E. 吻合黏膜下-黏膜管腔与有神经节细胞的肠管。F. 吻合口的最后形状。[From Spitz L, Coran A (eds): Rob & Smith's Operative Surgery: Pediatric Surgery. London, Chapman Hall Medical, 1995.]

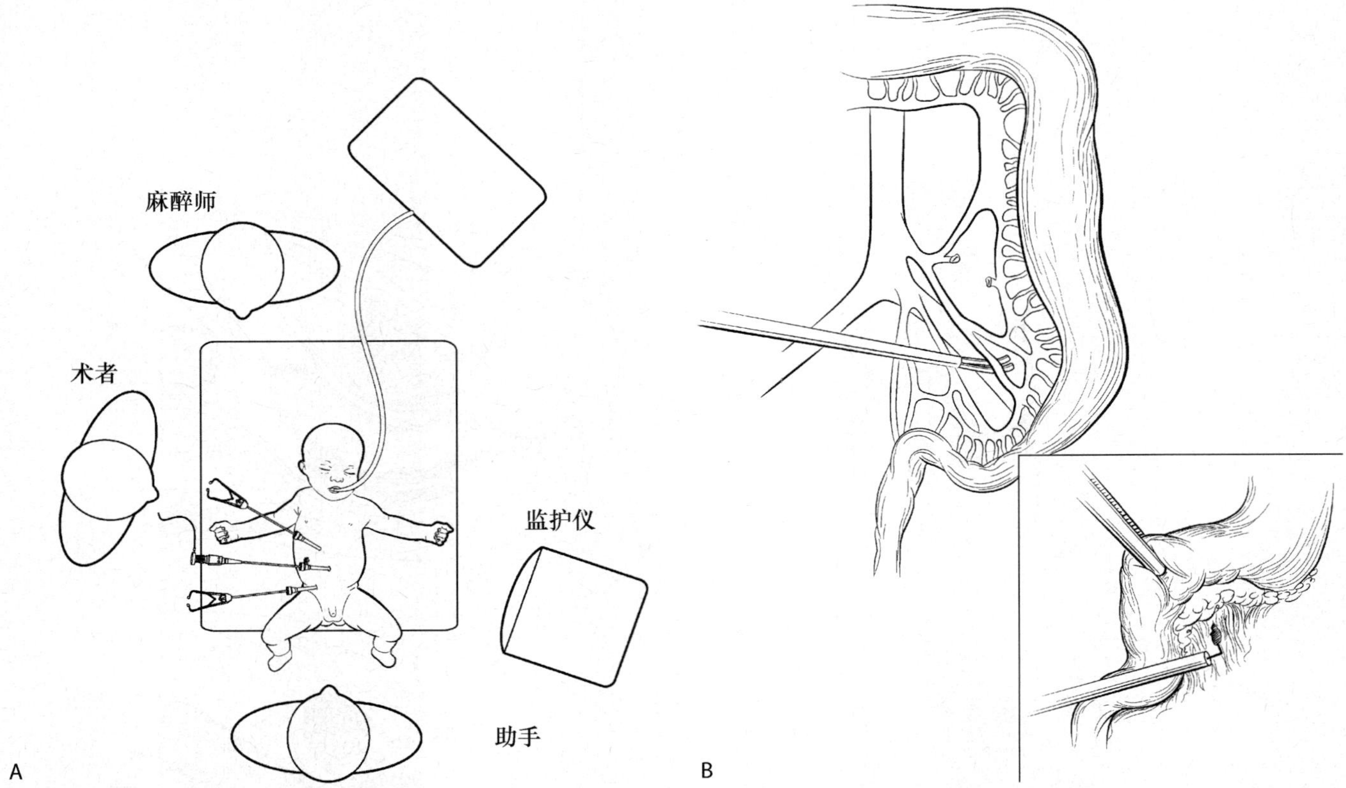

图 99-22 腹腔镜手术。A. 腹腔镜辅助的拖出术套针放置的位置。B. 腹腔镜辅助的拖出术。切除结肠血管的示意图。

Duhamel 手术

历史

1956 年 Duhamel 首次描述了他的先天性巨结肠的手术方法[71,72]。这个术式包含了直肠后的切除，保留部分无神经节细胞的直肠前壁与有神经节细胞的近端结肠进行吻合。这个手术的优点在于操作容易，减少了吻合口漏及狭窄的发生，保护了肛门的感觉受体和神经。实际上最初这个术式避免了肠管的吻合，用压钳将有神经细胞节替代无神经节细胞的肠管[73,74]。Duhamel 设计的这个手术是 Swenson 直肠乙结肠切除术的简化变体，适用于婴幼儿早期实施[73,74]。与 Swenson 手术的报道的相比，他早期的文章指出该手术的死亡率、功能性失禁、便秘或者腹泻、吻合口漏的发生率都有明显的减少[73,74]。

改良的 Duhamel 手术很多，包括将吻合口置于内括约肌的上方以避免大便失禁的发生[113]。其他的改良术包括用一个机械性的装置进行吻合等[139,303,318]。另一个改良是围绕消除无神经节细胞的直肠内的近端直 15
肠盲袋的刺激而产生的，那里可以潴留大便。Martin 和 Altemeier[203] 以及 Martin 和 Caudill[204] 阐述了运用钳挟装置完全去除直肠盲袋刺激的方法。最近 Duhamel 手术采用了腹腔镜技术，获得了满意的效果[62]。

经典的拖出术

虽然有几组关于 Duhamel 拖出术用于更年幼患儿的报道，但是这个手术主要适用于 9～12 个月的婴儿[194,221,343]。如用于更年幼的患儿，则需应用更小的内置 GIA 吻合器进行吻合。

肠管灌洗干净后，先做结肠造瘘口处理（假如存在），从左侧结肠造瘘处结肠做一个斜形至中线的切口打开腹膜。假如先前未行标准的结肠造瘘术，则需要使用冰冻切片决定有正常神经节细胞肠管的水平。然后移动近端结肠从而确保无张力的拖出。

远端将无神经节细胞的肠管移至腹膜返折下方，同时小心地保护输尿管。然后轻轻地钝性分离骶骨前

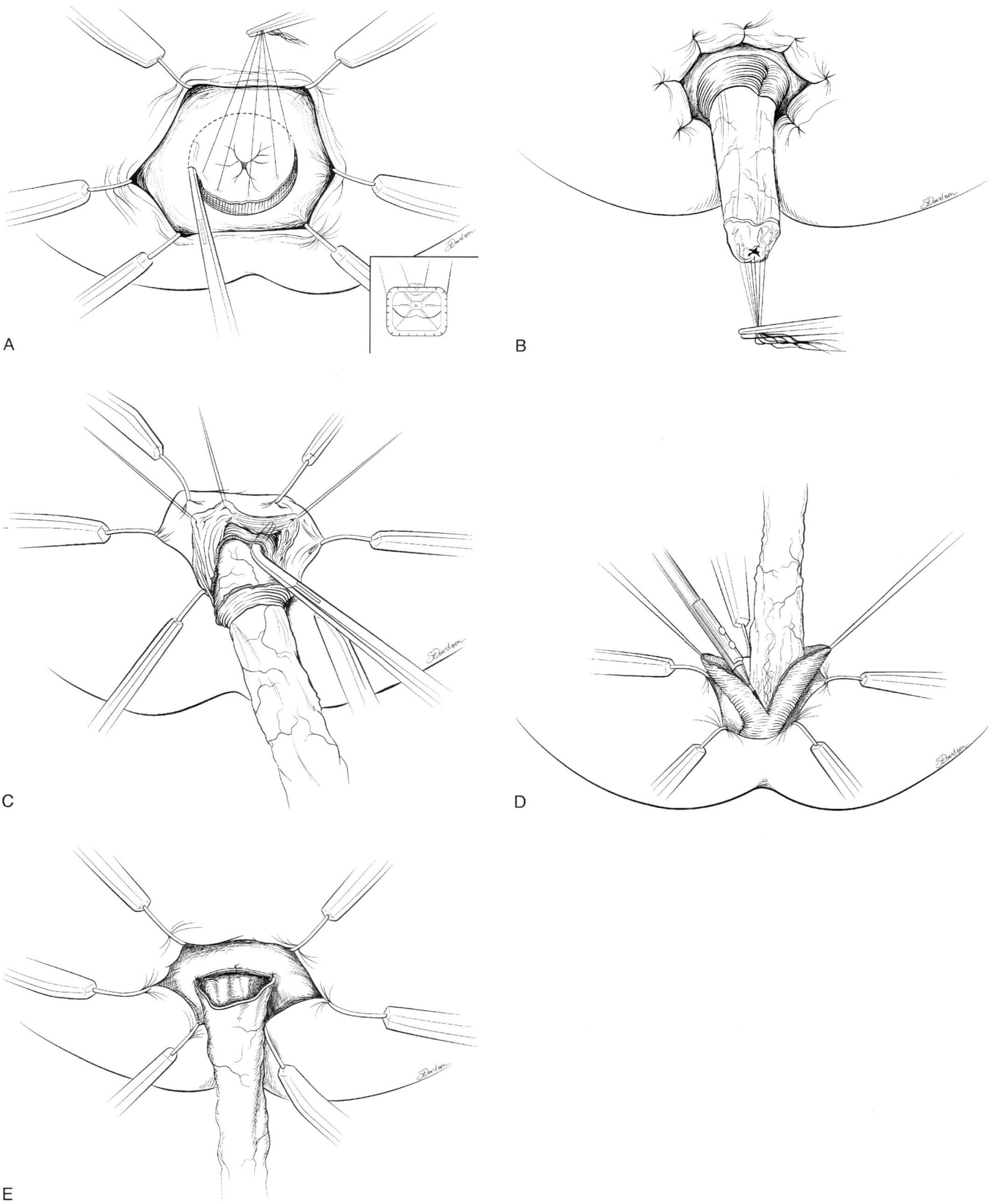

图 99-23 经肛门拖出术。A. 经肛门直肠内切除术的实施。使用了一个肛门牵开器（小图）。（Lone Star Medical Products，Houston，Tex）。B. 用一把细的电刀尖开始直肠内切除。这里还需要用多根缝线在肛门口作牵引。C. 切至腹膜水平全层打开直肠。D. 在拖出更近端的结肠以前，用电灼将直肠肌鞘从后劈开。E. 用间断的可吸收缝合进行吻合。

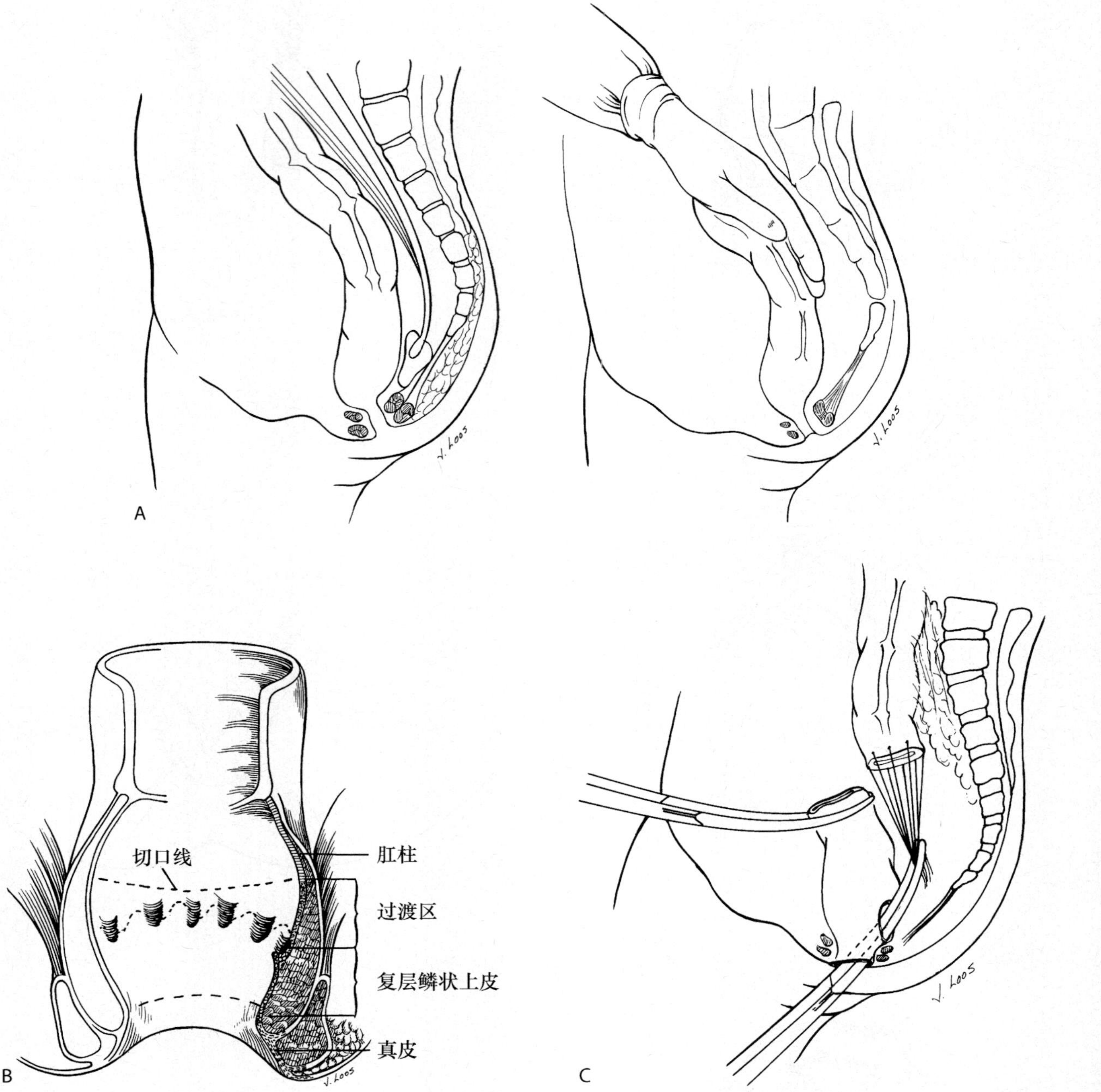

图 99–24 A. 通过钝性切割制造一条直肠后骶骨前的通道。B. 在接近齿状线 1～2 cm 处从 3 点到 9 点的位置作合层的直肠后壁切口。C. 将近端有神经节细胞的肠管，其肠系膜位于后侧，通过直肠后间隙拖至原直肠后壁切口的水平。

直肠后区域。通常为手术医生用手指或者小的纱条进行分离（图 99–24A）。近端有神经节细胞的肠管左右两侧留置牵引线（两边用不同的颜色），可以防止拖出时的扭转。

然后外科医生移向会阴部。轻轻地扩张肛门括约肌，可用狭窄的牵引器。暴露直肠后壁 3 点到 9 点的位置，确定齿状线的标志和 Morgagni 柱。术者用电切在齿状线上 1 cm 处从 3 点到 9 点的直肠后壁做全层的弧形切口（图 99–24B）。这个操作连接了上面分离的直肠后区域和无神经节细胞直肠的肠管。用可吸收线在切缘两侧做全层牵引线。当骶骨前的通道足够大时，将有神经节细胞的直肠在保证正常方向的前提下

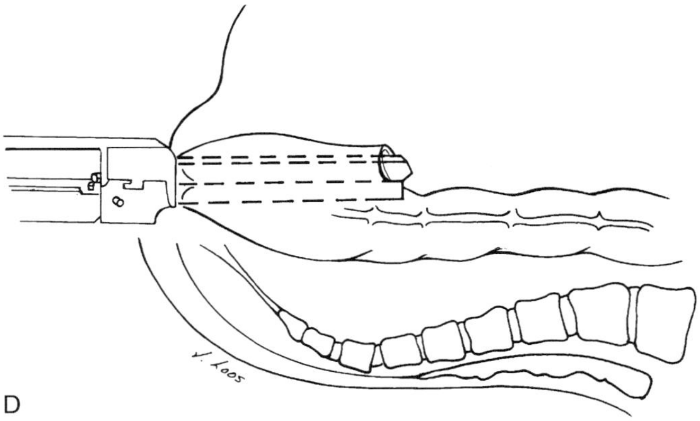

D

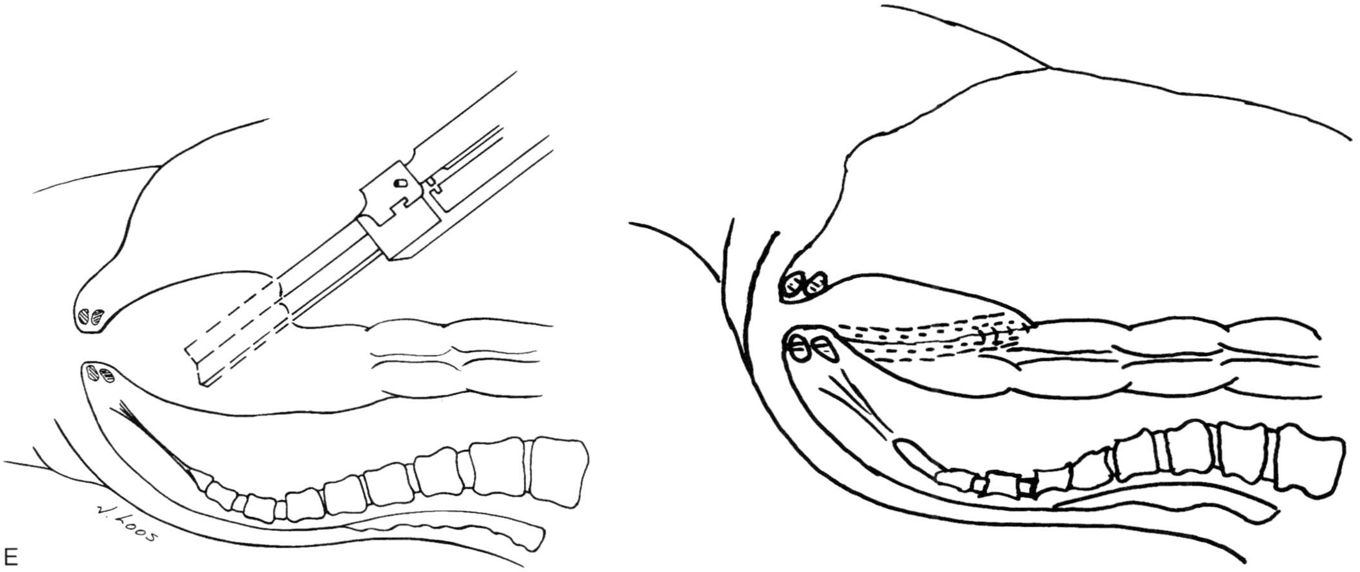

E

图 99-24　D. 从 3 点到 9 点的位置缝合新的直肠后壁和肛缘的皮肤以后，GIA 吻合器的一支插入原来的直肠腔，另一支进入新的肠腔。通过盆腔触诊明确吻合器的位置后闭合吻合器并发射，肠管的端-边吻合也就完成了。E. 回到下腹部盆腔区，将 GIA 吻合器从近端到远端重新插入，去除残留的共壁。关闭造瘘口。

从上面拖出，拖至肛门位置，此时管腔是开放的（图 99-24C）。用可吸收线吻合开放近端的结肠。外科吻合器通常采用 GIA80 mm 型，在小婴儿中用内置的 GIA 吻合器。重要的是，由于吻合口的厚度增加所以还需要 4. 8 mm 吻合钉。在发射这个装置前要确认会阴部和腹部肠管的方向（图 99-24D）。延着原先直肠及上吻合钉线，做结肠切除的切口。外侧的可吸收牵引线放在靠近两层肠壁处。重新装钉的 GIA 指向每个肠腔的远端在医生手指的引导下插入直肠（图 99-24E）。射出钉子后通过指检确定直肠壁完全消失。盆腔内多余的近端原始直肠被切除，进行两层的结肠-结肠吻合术。

Swenson 手术

图 99-25 为 Swenson 手术的示意图。虽然此术式还在应用，但这几年已经不流行了。优点即该手术的预后可能比 Duhamel 手术和直肠内拖出术更好，然而该手术技术要求非常高，还可能损伤邻近的神经血管组织。因此在这里不叙述 Swenson 手术的详细步骤了。读者可以参考关于此手术的其他书籍[324,357,358]。

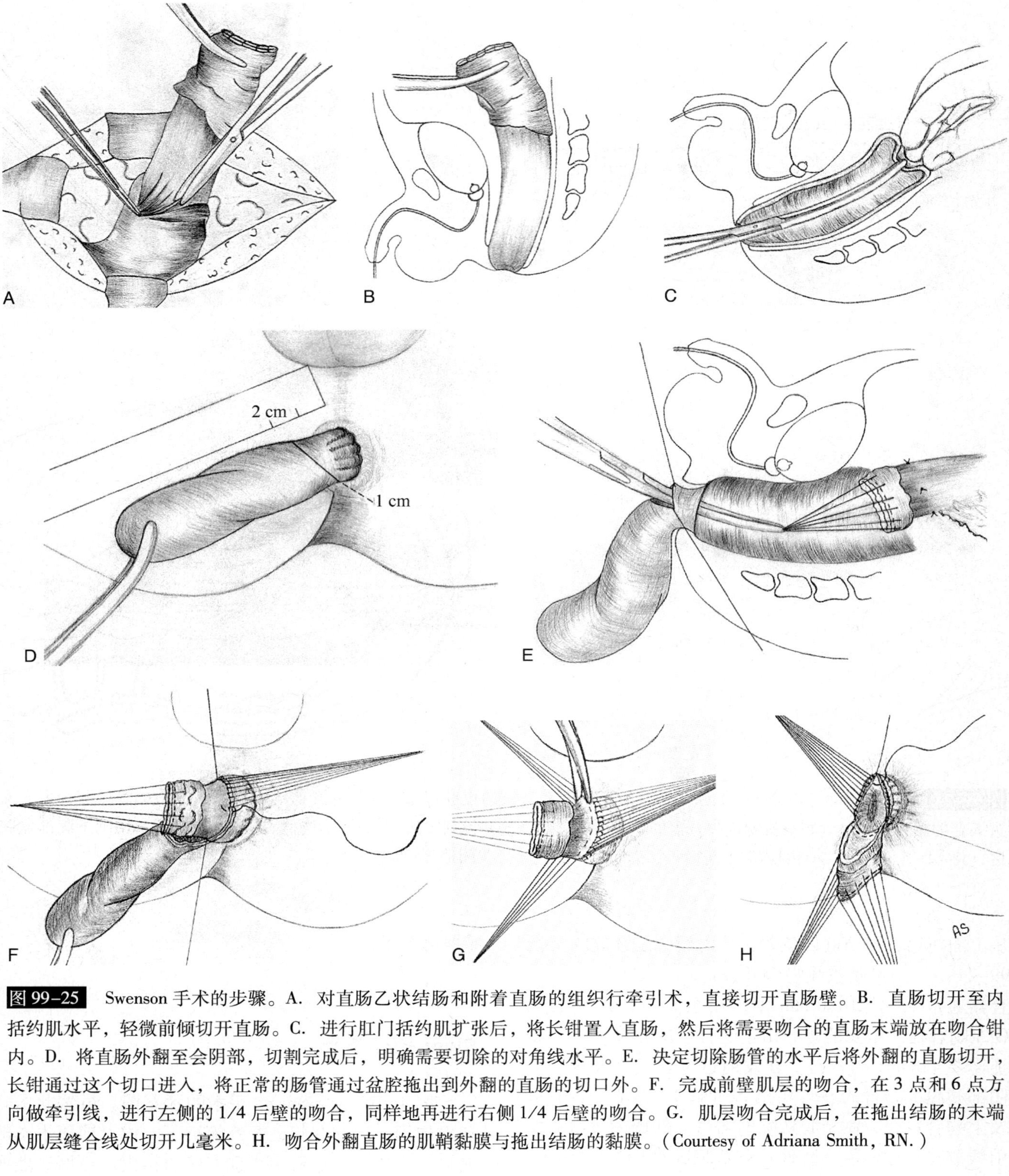

图 99-25 Swenson 手术的步骤。A. 对直肠乙状结肠和附着直肠的组织行牵引术，直接切开直肠壁。B. 直肠切开至内括约肌水平，轻微前倾切开直肠。C. 进行肛门括约肌扩张后，将长钳置入直肠，然后将需要吻合的直肠末端放在吻合钳内。D. 将直肠外翻至会阴部，切割完成后，明确需要切除的对角线水平。E. 决定切除肠管的水平后将外翻的直肠切开，长钳通过这个切口进入，将正常的肠管通过盆腔拖出到外翻的直肠的切口外。F. 完成前壁肌层的吻合，在 3 点和 6 点方向做牵引线，进行左侧的 1/4 后壁的吻合，同样地再进行右侧 1/4 后壁的吻合。G. 肌层吻合完成后，在拖出结肠的末端从肌层缝合线处切开几毫米。H. 吻合外翻直肠的肌鞘黏膜与拖出结肠的黏膜。（Courtesy of Adriana Smith，RN.）

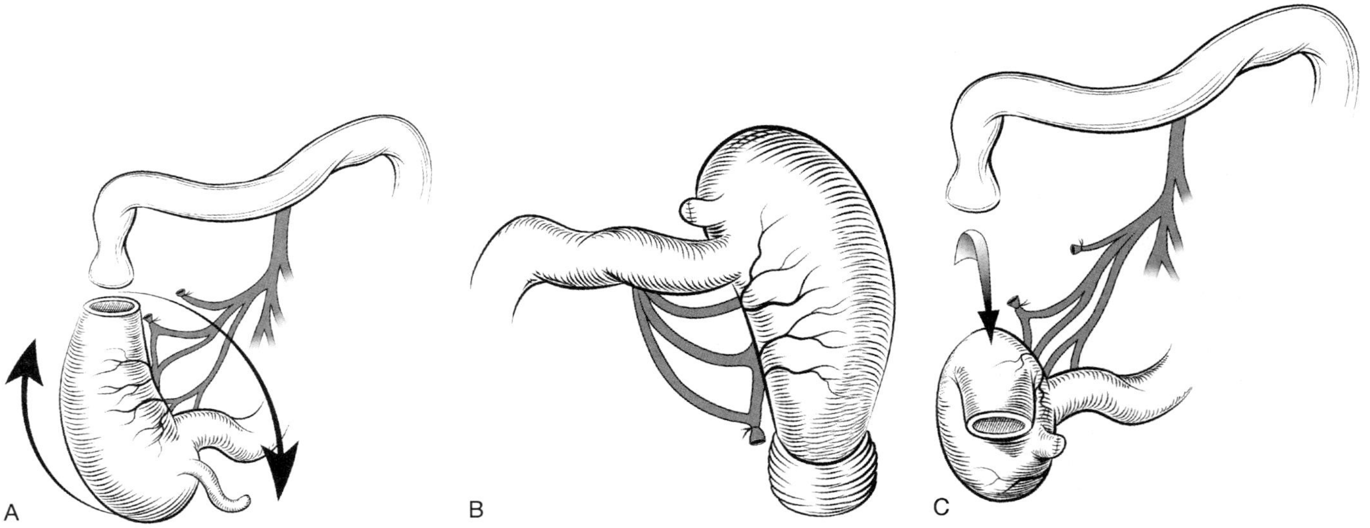

图 99-26 近结肠中动脉结肠无神经节细胞症患儿的手术方法。A. 肠管顺时针方向旋转。B. 结果导致患儿的回肠进入右侧的盲肠，这可能需要松解 Treitz 韧带。C. 另一个选择是向前旋转结肠。

先天性巨结肠罕见问题的手术治疗

右半结肠疾病

当对患有广泛的结肠疾病（至结肠中部血管右侧）的患儿进行拖出术时，要保证结肠正确的方向是很困难的，拖出的肠管发生扭转的危险性很高。这个问题 Duhamel 很早就认识到了，最好的解决方法就是将右半结肠逆时针旋转拖出（图 99-26A 所示）。因为小的肠管从患儿左侧离开结肠，所以有时需要完全地松解 Treitz 韧带（也就是肠旋转不良，图 99-26B）。也可以选择向前翻转结肠，可获得良好的效果（图 99-26C）。

全结肠型先天性巨结肠

已经有一些全结肠型巨结肠的手术方式被提出了。1953 年 Sandegard[282] 首先报道了用拖出术成功地治疗了此类患者。Martin[202] 在 Duhamel 拖出术式上做了进一步改良，即保留较长的无神经节细胞的直肠和左结肠以辅助水电解质的吸收。这个技术现在仍然被一些外科医生运用[76]。然而另有许多学者发现结肠保留过长会反向地影响患儿的排便能力，增加术后小肠结肠炎的发生率[63,132]。Kimura 等[160] 提出了一种手术方式把带有血供的盲肠补片缝合到有神经节细胞的小肠上。这个盲肠补片具有与无神经节细胞的直肠一样的吸收能力，临床效果很好[160,164,190]。然而大部分的医生选 1539
择标准长度的直肠内拖出术或者 Duhamel 手术治疗这类疾病，获得了良好的结果[30,151]。直肠内拖出术的预后与 Duhamel 手术的预后十分相似，然而进行 Duhamel 手术改良的 Martin 术（无神经节细胞的结肠与有神经节细胞的回肠延长的吻合）效果都不好[132]。尽管这些患者自我感觉生活质量比同龄差[129]，但大多数患者的长期预后是相当好的[129,198]。

广泛的小肠疾病

累及小肠病变的患者极少见。所有这些患儿需要长期的肠外营养支持，死亡率非常高（可达 50%）[159,160]。对于更广泛的累及小肠的先天性巨结肠的外科治疗较为复杂，因为必须考虑剩余的有神经节细胞的小肠的长度及功能，同时外科手术医生必须估 1540
计短肠综合征的程度。对于空回肠的疾病，许多人采用回肠补片[170] 或者更常见的右半结肠补片的方法进行治疗[159,306]。对这类患者应采用分期手术的方法，首先做造瘘术。即右半结肠吻合到有功能的近端造瘘口（Kimura-Stringel 术）。几周后保留这两段肠管的血供，通过 Soave 术或者 Swenson 术将这个端-端吻合的肠管拖出（图 99-27）。无神经节细胞的肠管应予以切除，因为这通常被视为败血症发生的潜在根源。

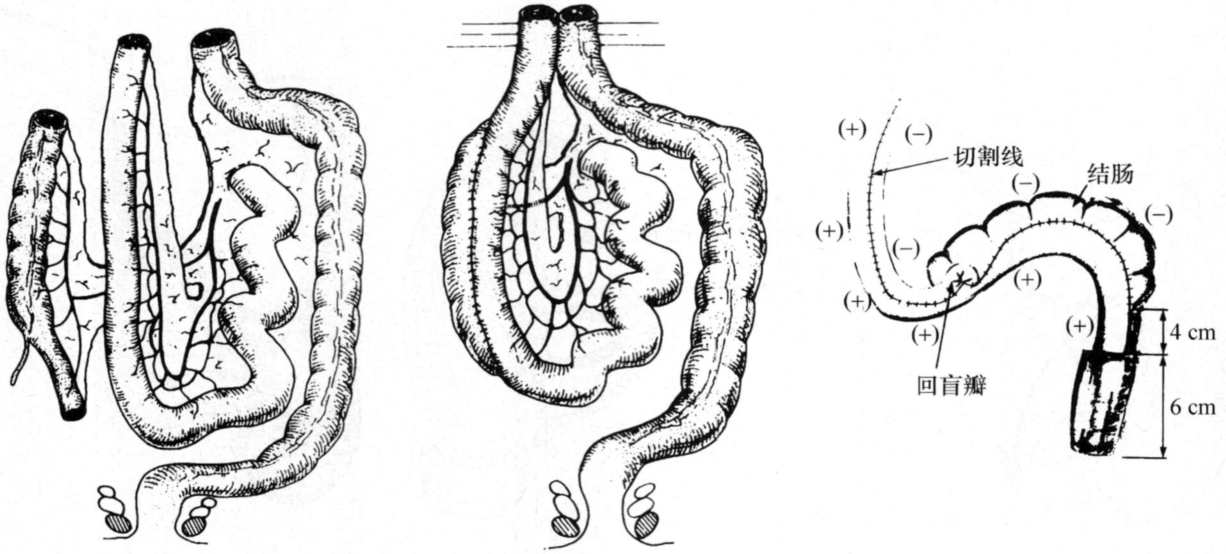

图 99-27 进行 Kimura-Stringel 手术是指将有神经节细胞的小肠作补片贴在无神经节细胞的回肠末端和右半结肠。在第二阶段，分离右半结肠的系膜，准备拖出有小肠系膜血管供应的合成肠管。

对于有神经节细胞的小肠少于 40 cm 的患儿，最好的方法是进行延长的肌层或肌切开术（图 99-28）。Ziegler 等[381,382]认为肌层切除术最好在有神经节细胞和无神经节细胞小肠的移行区进行。平行于小肠纵轴的对系膜缘做两个切口，切口的深度至表面的黏膜下层，使得浆肌层有宽度约 1 cm 的开口可以切除多余的肠管（其下的黏膜管腔要完好无损）。正常有神经节细胞肠管的延伸应该受限制，这样近端肠管的蠕动

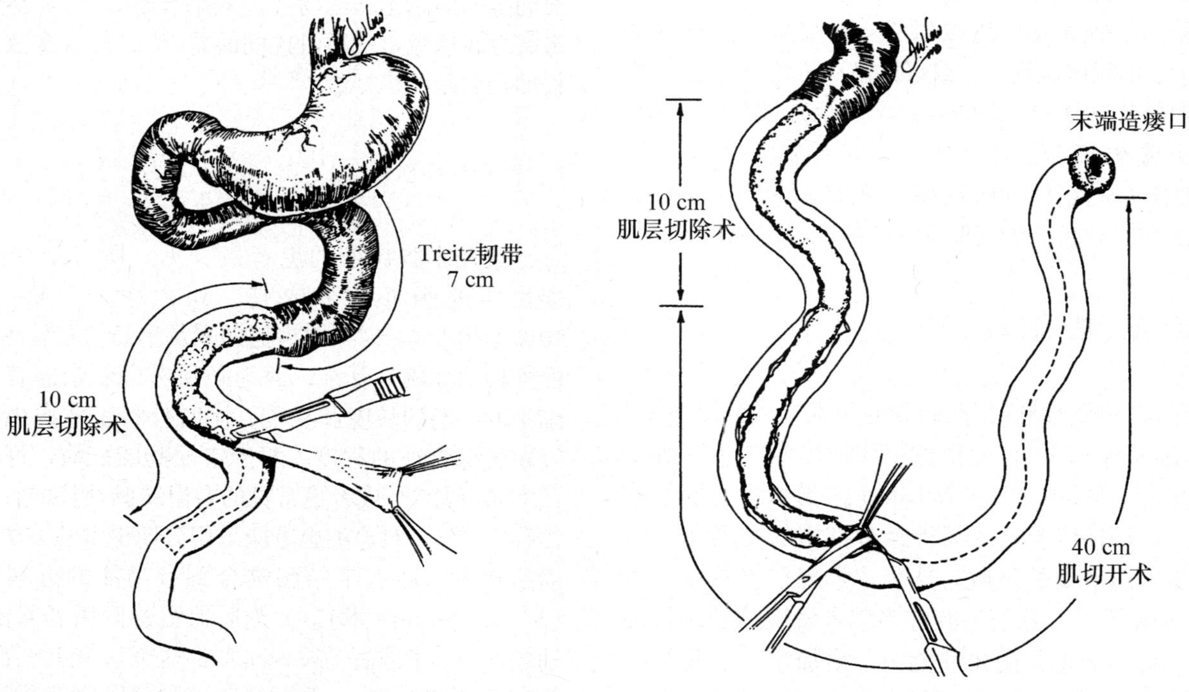

图 99-28 延长的肠管的肌切开术-肌层切除术从移行段的近端开始，延伸的范围取决于患者存活需要的小肠长度。

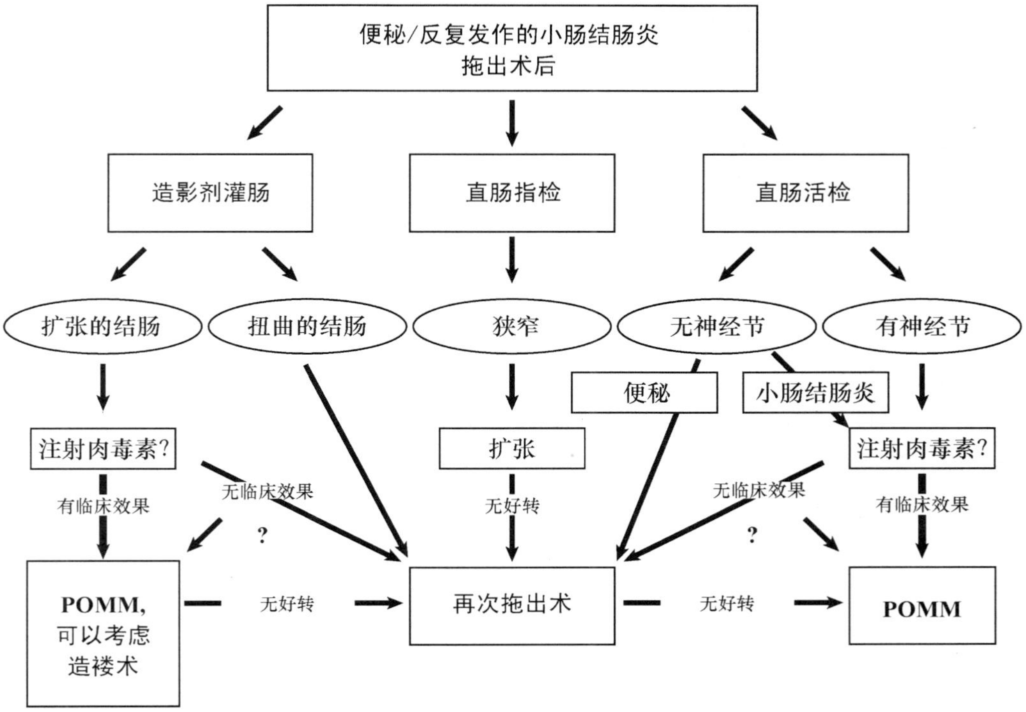

图 99-29 先天性巨结肠拖出术后慢性便秘或反复发作的小肠结肠炎（EC）患儿检查和治疗的流程图。在进行肌层切除术之前要注射肉毒素（Botox）。假如患儿接受 Botox 治疗长期获益的话，那么不需要进一步的治疗。假如 Botox 治疗只有短暂的效果，应考虑使用肌层切除术。POMM 是指后壁肌切除术或肌层切开术。

就不能推动肠内容物进入远端了。在这个节段的末端，最好是位于 Treitz 韧带下 50～70 cm 处，肠管末端造瘘口末端离开。假如存在任何的无神经节细胞远端的肠管残余，那么必须给它一个出口。

最后，当任何肠管的处理都失败了，则可能需要进行小肠移植或者肝肠移植。有两组关于小肠移植成功治疗全结肠型无神经节细胞症患者的报道[294,376]。

41 顽固性排便困难

对明显成功的拖出术后患儿的便秘和反复发作的小肠结肠炎进行评估需要完整的病史、体检和诊断性检查的结果。排便困难可能由保留的有神经节细胞肠管的神经系统异常引起，这不能归咎于手术[284]。通常症状持续的时间较短，且随着时间的推移而改善。
42 体检可以排除术后吻合口狭窄的可能性（见以后的章节）。内镜或者钡灌肠检查可以显示由于 Duhamel 手术操作不当导致的扭曲的拖出肠管和突起的形成。在没有机械性梗阻时，需要进行全面的诊断性评估。一篇关于这个问题的综述指出能提供最多信息的检查为直肠活检[229]。在一系列的文章中，作者在 178 例先天性巨结肠患儿中检出 16 例年龄在 4 岁以上仍有便秘或者梗阻症状的儿童。进一步检查发现这 16 例患儿中 13 例有异常的病变，其中 4 例保留有无神经节细胞的肠管，9 例有肠神经发育不良（见第 100 章）。直肠测压检查不能提示预后不良，也对患儿的全面评估没有帮助；然而肛管测压可为内括约肌的持续痉挛提供有用的信息以及预测便秘或失禁的原因[154]。根据最近两篇关于排便问题的综述，已经制定了详细的合理的检查方案（见 99-29）[180,364]。

肛直肠肌层切除术 1543

肛直肠肌层切除术是治疗短段型先天性巨结肠患者的标准手术。这个手术有经肛门[199]或者骶骨后[331,332]两种径路。该手术的优点在于避免了腹部的手术。这个手术只适用于治疗极短段的先天性巨结肠患者（一般≤5 cm）。外科医生必须确定肌层切除延伸到有正常神经
节细胞的肠管的水平。肌层切除不充分可能影响后续的 1544
拖出术的预后。假如不能确定病变的水平，则不能进行肌条切除术。患者的术前准备与其他拖出术的相同。

肌层切除术是治疗术后排便困难较常用的一种治疗方法（见图 99-29）。研究表明用这种方法对治疗先天性巨结肠拖出术后持续的排便困难或者反复发作的小肠结肠炎有良好的效果[25,33,158]。尽管进行了正常的

拖出术，但是据推测肌层切开术的作用可能是使持续痉挛的内括约肌被切开[224]。进行了后侧肌切除术或者肌层切除术的患者一般术后有明显改善[158]。Wildhaber 等[364]最近发表了关于这个手术效果的大量文章，文章中指出反复发作的小肠结肠炎患者的手术效果非常好；然而在那些存在无神经节细胞肠管的患者中，肌层切除术几乎均不成功，需要再次行拖出术。

患儿被置于行直肠全层活检术相同的位置。进行食指扩张肛门后由助手放入并抓住两个狭窄的牵开器。确认齿状线的后壁，在其上方 1 cm 处做 2 cm 的横切口，切开黏膜和黏膜下层。接着向上几个厘米进行黏膜下层的剥离。用丝线提起黏膜瓣，在两侧纵向地向近端延伸切口（图 99-30A）。

肌层切除术是指锐利地切开整个肌层，随后用 Bovie 电切在中线处切除一条宽 0. 5～1 cm 的肌条。最初切下的肌条应该至少长 5 cm（图 99-30B）。在横断肌条前，在靠近横断处放置两根牵引线。这样可以防止仍需进一步切除时近端肌肉的回缩超出外科医生的视野。应该用针或者缝线将这个肌条装在舌形的压板上，必须清楚地标明近远端。在手术完成之前，必须获得证实近端边缘有神经节细胞的冰冻切片。用这种方法切割约 7～8 cm。切除足够长的肌肉，然后电灼止血。冲洗伤口，用细的可吸收线间断缝合关闭黏膜和黏膜下层。

经过几次手术的患者要保存完整的黏膜下层是非常困难的，只进行纵向的椭圆形的全层切除比较简单（图 99-31A）。留下肌层的缺口，用连续的可吸收缝线缝合黏膜和黏膜下层（图 99-31B）。

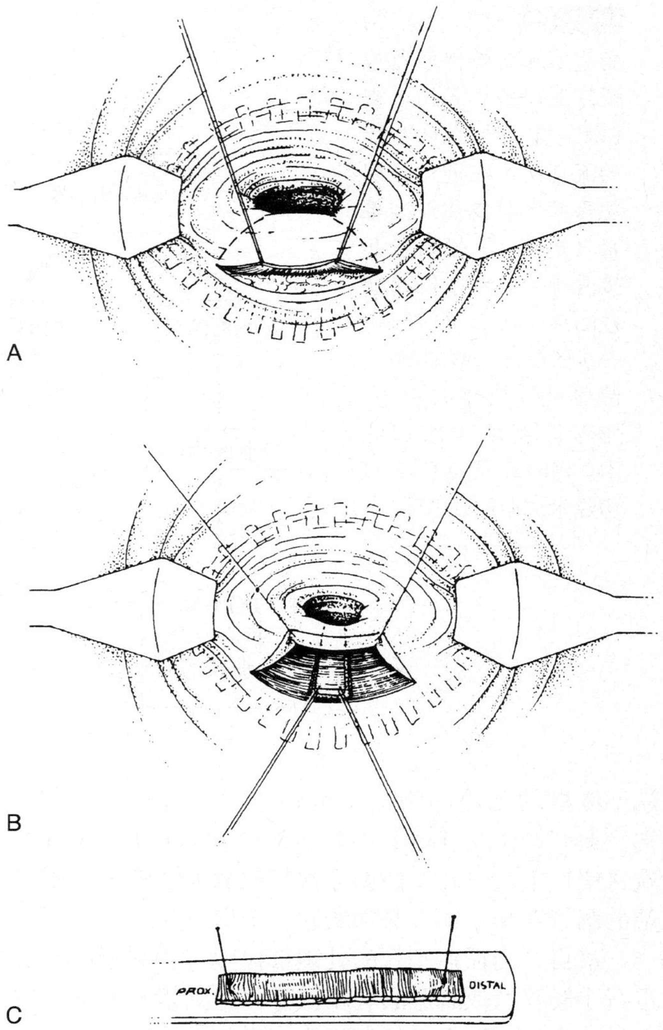

图 99-30 经肛门肌层切除术。A. 切开黏膜下-黏膜皮瓣暴露出肌固有层。做牵引缝合，辅助向上切开。B 和 C. 对于病理科医生来说标明标本的近远端是很重要的。［From Spitz L, Coran A (eds): Rob & Smith's Operative Surgery: Pediatric Surgery. London, Chapman Hall Medical, 1995.］

再次拖出术

虽然绝大多数患儿采用了拖出术后预后良好，但是约有 5% 的患儿预后差，其中一小部分患儿可能需要再次手术。再次拖出术的适应证包括残留的或者获得性的无神经节细胞症、严重的狭窄、肠功能不良和肠神经元发育不良。另外还有继发于多年便秘的直肠乙状结肠明显扩张和不能恢复肌肉节律的患儿。这类患儿手术步骤的示意图如图 99-32 所示。需要再次行拖出术的患者的预后不如首次行拖出术的好。然而有学者指出 70%～80% 的患儿再次行拖出术后排便功能有一定程度的改善[182,345,356,362]。但是在这些患儿中肛门失禁的发生率相当高。

并发症和预后 15

先天性巨结肠婴幼儿的预后评估一般分为早期和晚期并发症以及总体的生活质量。在过去的半个世纪中，先天性巨结肠患儿的预后有了明显的改善。然而其发病较普遍，据报道只有 1 例意外死亡[327,357]。

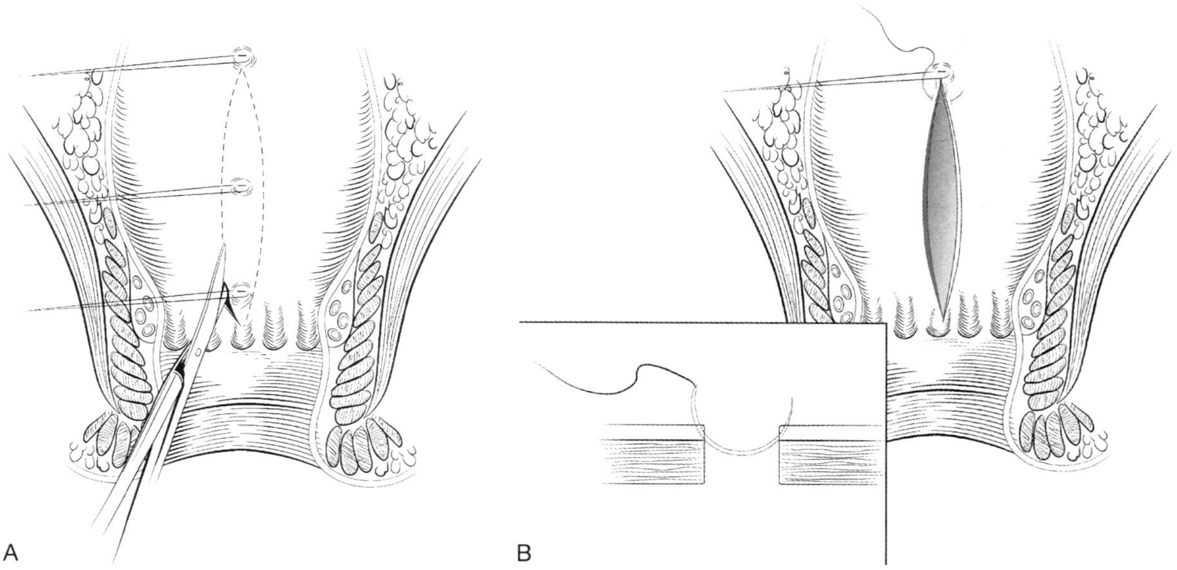

图 99-31　经肛门肌层切开术的另一种方法。A. 纵向地设置一系列的牵引线。用剪刀做全层的切口。最前端的缝线留作牵引。出血会影响手术视野，采用电凝止血。B. 从前端边缘开始连续缝合关闭黏膜和黏膜下层。

早期的拖出术后并发症

早期的拖出术后的并发症包括需要进行剖腹探查的肠梗阻，发病率约 8%～13%。与其他许多直肠结肠手术一样，伤口感染发生率约为 10%～15%。早期肛直肠狭窄约 10%～20%，对大多数的患儿可以使用肛门扩张在医院或在家进行治疗。吻合口破裂和吻合口漏的发生率约为 2%。可以将已拖出肠管进一步拖出治疗大的吻合口破裂，这样可以防止盆腔感染。二次行吻合术，与 Soave 使用的原始方法相似[117]。

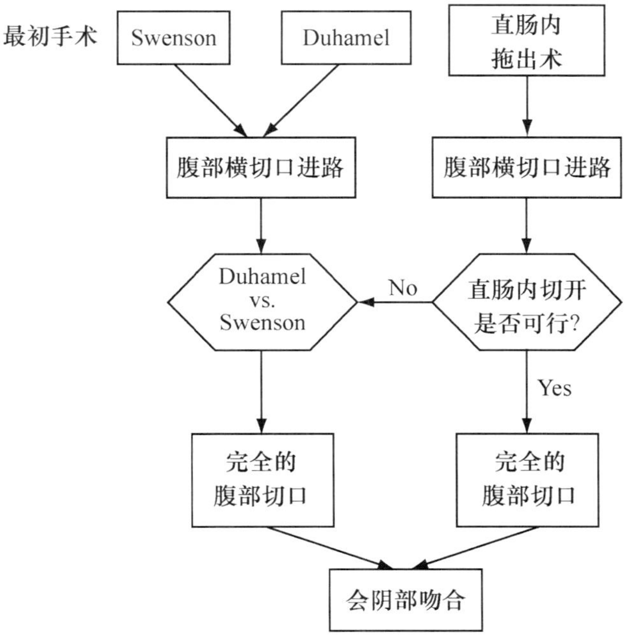

图 99-32　各种先天性巨结肠拖出术后再次行拖出术需要遵守的步骤。

晚期的拖出术后并发症

先天性巨结肠患儿的晚期随访为评估任何一种特定手术的有效性和预后提供了最好的机会。一般来说，最常遇见的问题是肛门失禁、便秘和小肠结肠炎，以及该疾病对生活方式的总体影响。其他的并发症如瘘管的形成、梗阻和阳痿是很少见的。

肛门失禁

可能没有比肛门失禁对生活质量影响更大的并发症了，但肛门失禁的发生率未见有文献报道。总的说来，关于排便控制率有一些一般性原则。首先，一些
学者发现在 21-三体或者与智力障碍相关的其他综合 1546
征的患者中肛门失禁的发病率较高[49,117,267]。通常肛

门失禁的发病率为3%～8%，但是还有文献报道比这更高的发病率。新生儿期以后，神经学上正常的患者预后较好，排便控制率不随年龄的增长而改变[125,329]。关于经肛门手术是否会增加肛门失禁发生率的问题还在争论中。虽然许多研究中随访的时间较短，但是一些文献指出该手术预后良好[105,118,183]。此外肛门括约肌张力测压的结果与那些进行开腹术的患者相似[344]。但是括约肌的张力与年龄匹配的对照组相比有所减少[126]。一般来说肛门失禁随年龄增长而改善[126,273]。这些结果有力地说明了在对肛门失禁的患儿进行任何形式的外科治疗前，儿外科医生应该进行积极的内科治疗、调整饮食并运用缓泻剂。

排便次数增多和便秘

先天性巨结肠排便次数增多在多数文献中很少有报道，但是大多数患者有正常排便次数增多[191,321]。在拖出术后的头3个月排便次数增多相当明显，到6个月时下降至正常（每天2～3次）[329,352]。

先天性巨结肠拖出术后便秘是常见的并发症。大多数便秘没有组织病理学的改变，无需进行全面的评估就可以进行治疗。大多数文章指出便秘的发生率为6%～30%。Puri 和 Nixon[264] 发现 Swenson 术后34.5%的患儿有便秘。Rescorla 等[273] 指出 Duhamel 术后27%的患儿有便秘，需要药物治疗，但是这个比率随年龄增长进行性地降低。

小肠结肠炎

小肠结肠炎的病理生理学机制已经讨论过了。文献中拖出术后小肠结肠炎的发病率有很大的不同，范围在2%～40%；这可能与作者对于小肠结肠炎和内括约肌痉挛的定义不同有关。术后小肠结肠炎的发病率中等，偶有死亡。当考察先天性巨结肠引起的死亡时，很多文献注意到近50%的死亡是由与小肠结肠炎直接相关的并发症引起的[48,328]。所有的小肠结肠炎都发生在拖出术后的头2年内。对这些患者的适当治疗可以避免小肠结肠炎。许多医院的常规做法是嘱患者口服甲硝唑1～2个月。Marty 等[211] 提倡在拖出术后对所有出院患儿进行预防性的直肠灌洗，这使总的临床预后有了明显的改善。假如小肠结肠炎持续发作，患儿需要进行后壁的肌层切除术[364]。然而首先应该进行较长时间的保守治疗，因为绝大多数拖出术后并发小肠结肠炎的患者的情况随时间延长而有所改善。

狭窄形成

根据狭窄形成的定义不同，文献报道的发生率不等，从0[84,191]～20%[321]。大多数狭窄可以经过传统的直肠扩张治疗好转。Heikkinen 等[25] 认为在术后早期出现吻合口漏的患者中狭窄的发生率最高。然而 Swenson 等[315] 指出23例术后早期有吻合口漏史的患者中只有3例出现晚期狭窄，而且没有发现明显的易感因素。拖出术后早期狭窄的患者小肠结肠炎的发生率较高[183,327]。

阳痿和排尿功能障碍

盆腔内进行任何手术操作都可能导致神经的损伤。先天性巨结肠的许多手术方式都是特别为避开这些组织结构而设计的。总的来说，阳痿和排尿功能不良的发生率很低，直觉上 Swenson 手术因其设计发生神经损伤的危险最高。然而对282例患者进行的回顾性研究表明101名已经度过青春期的男性患者没有1人出现阳痿；80名患者已经结婚，并有146个孩子出生[314]。Puri 和 Nixon[264] 发现在 Swenson 手术后84例患者中有2例尽管可以正常勃起但无射精。晚期泌尿系统障碍是极少见的并发症。可以认为最少量的盆腔操作与排尿障碍发病率的降低密切相关。1977年 Puri 和 Nixon[264] 回顾了52例进行 Duhamel 手术的患者，其中有7例出现夜间遗尿，2例出现白天滴尿。最近的文献未报道有阳痿或排尿问题的发生[105,183,327]。

全结肠型无神经节细胞症的预后

全结肠型无神经节细胞症患者的长期预后需要另行评估，因为此类型的患者比普通型或者长段型的先天性巨结肠患者的总体预后要差。然而其总体生活质量大多数还是好的[121]。

由于在许多研究中未将此类型患者进行区分，同时由于一个特定的研究机构见到的全结肠型无神经节细胞症患者数量较少，所以预后分析受到了限制。在 Ikeda 和 Goto[140] 的研究中有67例全结肠型的患者（占

4%）。在这篇报道中主要施行的是 Duhamel 手术，总体死亡率达 13%。美国儿科协会的回顾性研究发现，大多数外科医生采用 Duhamel 手术或者 Swenson 手术，相关的并发症发病率分别为 62% 和 70%；死亡率分别是 25% 和 30%[164]。在前面提到的两个报道中直肠内
1547 拖出术有较好的预后，且没有并发症和死亡发生，然而只有 9 例是此类型的患者。在这些文献中未提及排便次数增多，但 Marty 等[210]的研究发现排便次数较多且失禁的发生率非常高，他们发现将近 40% 的全结肠型无神经节细胞症患者有严重的污粪存在。Heij 等[124]注意到 7 例全结肠型无神经节细胞症患者中有 6 例出现便失禁。在后面的研究中大多数患者进行了 Duhamel 手术或者 Martin 手术。这与 Endo 等[83]的研究形成了对比，Endo 等发现尽管所有 9 例患者都有排不成形便的病史（每天 1～5 次），但随着时间的推移肠蠕动的次数明显增多，通常到 2～3 岁时降低至每天排便 2～5 次。所有全结肠型无神经节细胞症的患者都在接近回肠肛门吻合处进行 Kimura 补片手术。同时这些作者也注意到在更近端和广泛的无神经节细胞症患者中排便次数有明显增高。

生活质量

关于先天性巨结肠患者总体生活质量的研究相对较少。但是存在一些普遍性的规则。首先，总体生活质量是相当好的[125]，而且比其他肛直肠畸形患者的更好[121]。Bai 等[22]将 45 例先天性巨结肠患者与 44 例同年龄正常对照组的生活质量进行了比较研究。他们发现 87% 的先天性巨结肠患者的生活质量评分是较好或者一般，但明显比对照组低。其次，有任何程度污粪存在的患者生活质量的评分明显较低；其他一些研究也发现有相似的趋势[121,125,228,375]。随着时间的推移，大多数生活质量的问题有所改善，特别是当患者进入青春期后[375]。随着患者生活质量问题研究新方法的出现，将得到更多其他的信息[119]。

其他肠动力不良疾病

随着有关胃肠道动力的生理知识的不断增加，除先天性巨结肠以外还发现其他胃肠道动力性疾病的存在。胃肠道的运动受不同的机制控制，包括内在的神经系统和中枢神经系统的控制，同时胃肠道运动也受不同的胃肠道多肽的调节[98,99,219]。已知有几种疾病，一般表现为慢性（特发性）的假性肠梗阻。尽管提出了几种分类法[171]，但是肠动力不良性疾病可分为两个基本类型：胃肠道的原发性疾病和累及两个或多个部位的全身性疾病。最终，这些病变可以是家族性的，但更常见的是散发性的。大多数患者有腹胀的表现，并伴有间断性的腹痛、梗阻或者便秘的症状以及营养不良。常有肠道细菌的过度生长。

肠神经发育不良

1971 年 Meier-Ruge[214]首先描述了肠神经发育不良。虽然这个疾病可以累及胃肠道的任何部位，但是被划分为结肠发育不良。关于这个疾病将在第 100 章中作进一步的讨论。

慢性肠道假性梗阻综合征

慢性肠道假性梗阻综合征（CIP）是以肠道异常蠕动为特征的临床病理综合征[128]。这个综合征可以分为三种基本的疾病：继发于平滑肌畸形的疾病（肌病）、肠肌间神经丛疾病（神经病）和间质病，或者是肠 Cajal 间质细胞网（ICC）的改变。CIP 可以由原发的疾病引起，或者继发于系列的病理性疾病[65]。大多数这类患者有极其明显的腹胀（图 99-33）和肠营养摄入不足。有家族性发病的报道，特别是在神经 1548
病的患儿中[128]，但是大多数还是散发的。典型的临床表现有反复发作的腹痛、腹胀、恶心和呕吐。体重减轻很常见，大多数患者需要延长全肠外营养的疗程[128]。一些患者还可能伴有相关的泌尿系统综合征。

这类疾病常常在出生头几个月（3/4 的患儿在出生第一年内）就能确诊，有些在胎内就能诊断[128]。关于药物滥用、累及泌尿系统和家族史的病史尤为重要。实验室的检查不能明确诊断。检查应包括直肠吸引活检，直肠吸引活检可以排除不典型或者迟发的先天性巨结肠同时可以对肠神经发育不良进行评估。虽然造影检查不总是有帮助，但是可以排除机械性的梗阻。另外，在大量患者中已发现肠旋转不良、短肠综

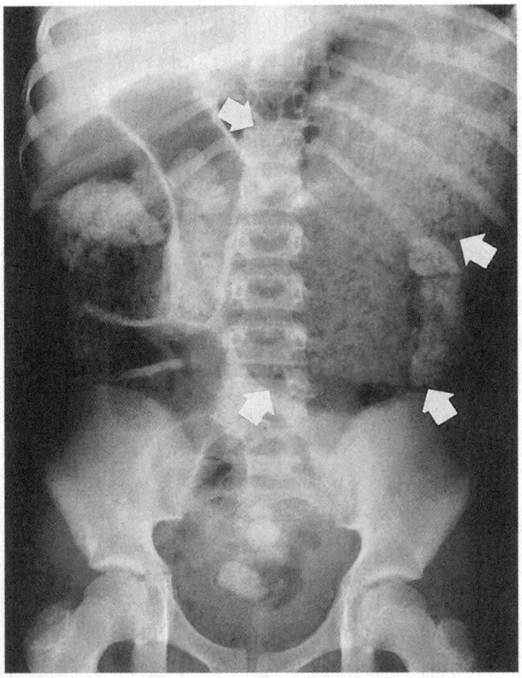

图 99-33　患有内脏肌病的患儿腹部 X 线表现。患儿胃（箭头所示“肥皂泡样”表现）和其他肠袢极度扩张。患儿有婴儿期膀胱和结肠功能不良的病史。（Courtesy of Robert Murrray，MD）

合征以及痉挛的左半结肠和小结肠[128]。然而在一些神经性疾病中，在上消化道中可以存在正常的胃和近端小肠的排空，但是肠内容物的排空却是异常的。一般来说，在肌肉性的病变中可见肠收缩力减弱、肠直径增加，而在肌间神经丛疾病中可见增强但不协调收缩的较小的肠腔。泌尿生殖系统的评估也是很重要的，因为一些研究显示多达有 1/3 的 CIP 患者存在膀胱和输尿管的扩张[92]。

虽然不是一个有效的方法，但在一些病例中也有应用胃电图进行诊断的[42]。一些报告支持使用连续的全层活检，不幸的是不熟悉这些疾病的病理科医生可能误诊[65]。此外，胃肠道的手术操作可以加重动力性疾病。Krishnamurthy 和 Schuffer[171]对 CIP 的病理学分类进行了全面的回顾。

另外普遍认为 CIP 的每个分类都有一些特点。

内脏肌病

内脏肌病是很少见的，其特点是胃肠道平滑肌退化，随后肌肉组织被纤维组织所替代。内脏肌病可以家族性发病，也可以散发。家族性的内脏肌病有 3 种基本类型[171]。Ⅰ型是常染色体显性遗传，伴有食管、十二指肠和结肠的扩张以及巨膀胱症。Ⅱ型是常染色体隐性遗传，伴有上睑下垂和眼肌麻痹，近端的肠管常常扩张。Ⅲ型可能是常染色体隐性遗传不伴有任何肠管外的症状。散发的原发性的内脏肌病可以累及整个消化道，偶有膀胱受累。巨膀胱-小结肠-肠蠕动迟缓综合征与该疾病有关，将在以后讨论。

内脏神经病

家族性的内脏神经病至少有两种类型[279,289]。一种类型是全身性的神经异常和胃肠道动力的紊乱，属于常染色体隐性遗传。尸体解剖显示肌间神经丛有退化变性。第二种类型是常染色体显性遗传，仅累及消化道。神经病也可以被分为炎性的或退行性的神经病。炎症改变可以使淋巴细胞和浆细胞在两个主要的有神经节细胞的神经丛中和肠神经系统的轴突上发生浸润。这类疾病也伴有肠外的疾病，包括 Chagas 病（由克鲁氏锥虫引起）、类癌瘤、神经母细胞瘤、胸腺瘤和结缔组织疾病。组织通常对抗细胞核神经元抗体和抗-Hu 抗体起反应。退行性变可能是由内源性和外源性因素造成的神经元损伤引起的。其他患者有 CIP 同时伴有 MEN2[235]。

间质性疾病

这类疾病包括 ICCs 的改变。用 cKIT 抗体进行免疫组化染色显示 ICCs 数量明显减少。另外，还存在其他结构上的异常，包括神经元结构的缺失。

巨膀胱-小结肠-肠蠕动迟缓综合征

1976 年 Berdon 等[29]率先描述了巨膀胱-小结肠-肠蠕动迟缓综合征。虽然与其他假性肠梗阻不同，但是这个疾病是功能性肠梗阻中最严重的类型之一，应该属于内脏肌病的一种。该疾病常见于新生儿期，被 Puri[262]命名为新生儿饥饿内脏肌病综合征。据 Puri 和 Tsuji[265]的文章报道，女性多见，男女比例为 1∶4，且被认为是常染色体隐性遗传。该疾病中最严重的是累及小肠的动力，这可以导致结肠的排便功能丧失。巨膀胱和相关的肾盂积水与胃肠道病变有关，常常需要进行引流。另外，这些患者有腹壁肌肉系统松弛、肠管旋转不全和细小结肠。进行外科旁路手术常常是无效的。病理学上，该综合征的特征性表现为神经节细胞数量的增多，但是当疾病进一步恶化时可以出现神经节细胞数量的减少。电镜下可显示一层薄的纵形肌膜及丰富的结缔组织[263]。这些患者的长期
549 预后并不乐观，死亡率达 87%，且长期存活者依赖全肠外营养。

治疗

在一些研究中运用促进肠动力的药物进行治疗，但是反应通常是短暂的或者是缺失的[65]。虽然反应常常不完全，但是 Cisapride 是最有效的药物[128,298]。最近因为这个药物可以引起心律失常，因而该药物的使用受到严格的限制。据一个研究报告显示，15 例成人患者中 6 例对大剂量的红霉素有中等程度的反应[82]。对于内科治疗无效的患者，最好的方法是进行胃肠减压造瘘。一般来说，肠造瘘口减压并给予肠内营养（通常是空肠造瘘术）是有效的。结肠造瘘术仅在一半的患者中有效，回肠末端造瘘术相对略好些[128]。造瘘口并发症较常见，如胃下垂，且几乎一半的婴儿至少有一处造瘘口需要修改。采用多种保守治疗无效的患者可以选择小肠移植。最近发表的文献显示 CIP 的肠移植取得了良好的效果，但在尿道膀胱异常的患者中仍存在问题[197]。

因为胃肠道内容物淤积时间延长，所以需要周期性地评估细菌滋生和维生素 B_{12} 的缺乏情况。细菌过度滋生的诊断可以通过呼气试验和大量小肠内容物的培养明确（$>10^5/mm^3$）。大便 pH 小于或等于 5.0 也提示细菌过度滋生[91]。

原发性的便秘和大便失禁

在儿童中便秘是常见的一个问题。在教学医院和诊所中慢性便秘伴有污粪的患儿多达 3%[188]。尽管这个问题频繁发生，但是便秘的定义还是模糊的。母乳喂养或者牛乳喂养的婴儿在生后第 1 个月中平均每天排便 2.7 次，1 岁时下降到 1.7 次[369]，4 岁时下降到 1.2 次[355]。为了制定统一的诊断标准，各国签订了

表 99-5　功能性排便障碍的 ROMEⅡ分类法

婴儿大便困难：年龄小于 6 个月的其他都正常的儿童，在排出柔软的大便之前有至少 10 分钟的扭动和哭闹

功能性便秘：婴儿或者学龄前儿童，持续至少 2 周；大多数大便为坚硬的颗粒石头样或者每周排 2 或 2 次以下坚硬的大便；没有其他结构、内分泌或者代谢性疾病

功能性大便潴留：从婴儿期到 16 岁的儿童，每周排出少于 2 次直径较粗的大便，持续 12 周；有目的的盆底收缩仍无排便，存在大便潴留；当盆底肌肉疲劳时，儿童用臀部的肌肉挤压臀部

无大便潴留性污粪：年龄大于 4 岁的儿童每周排便至少 1 次以上，持续 12 周；在与社会环境不符的时间、地点排便；没有结构性和炎症性病变；没有大便潴留的表现

《关于功能性胃肠道疾病 Rome Ⅱ 多国协定》。虽然有些诊断并未落入这个标准中[348]，但是协定将排便异常分为 4 种主要类型：婴儿大便困难、功能性便秘、功能性大便潴留和无大便潴留性污粪（表 99-5）。

引起便秘的原因很多，包括解剖结构的、生理性的和遗传性的因素。最常见的便秘为原发性原因。多达 65% 的便秘儿童在 6 个月时就表现出这种疾病的倾向，所以这种类型的便秘可能具有遗传易感性[322]。此外，该类型常常有家族史。当孩子意识到可以自行控制排便时（例如进行排便训练），便秘可能更加明显或者进一步加重。当便秘进一步加重时肛直肠壶腹部进行性扩张，容纳更多的大便。当大便更加坚硬时，排便时的疼痛可以引起肛瘘，从而加重症状。假如便秘症状持续，直肠将扩张至不能再容纳大便的最大容积。液性的大便从梗阻的粪块周围流出，从而引起污粪（也就是大便失禁）。

功能性无大便潴留的污粪或者大便失禁被定义为没有明显器官病变的粪便污染[90]。虽然大便失禁与心理情感问题有关，但是一个更加详细的分析表明只有 20% 大便失禁的患儿有严重的心理问题，而且许多这些问题是发生在大便失禁以后的[1]。大便失禁常开始于 3 岁以后。Levin[188] 的研究发现平均年龄为 7 岁。这类疾病可以并发尿路感染。

鉴别先天性巨结肠与慢性便秘是儿外科医生经常遇见的问题。一些症状、体征和检查有助于鉴别这两种类型的疾病。原发性便秘患者的典型特征有污粪

表 99-6 原发性便秘和先天性巨结肠的临床比较

症状、体征、诊断检查	原发性便秘	先天性巨结肠
污粪	常见	不常见
壶腹部的大便	常见	不常见
梗阻症状	少见	常见
大便潴留	常见	少见
小肠结肠炎	无	可能
肛直肠检查	壶腹扩张	狭窄
钡灌肠	壶腹扩张	远端肠管狭窄

（常常由液性大便溢出导致）和充满粪便的扩张的直肠壶腹。这两种表现在典型的先天性巨结肠患者中不常见。事实上，先天性巨结肠患者的壶腹部常常是狭窄的，直肠指检时可能是空的。钡灌肠造影显示在慢性便秘中壶腹扩张直到肛缘，而在先天性巨结肠中显示为狭窄收缩的直肠或者直肠乙状结肠（见图99-1）。表
1550 99-6 比较和对比了两种疾病的症状与体征。

便秘的治疗包括饮食调整、药物治疗、灌肠治疗和年轻儿童的行为治疗。在婴幼儿中简单地给予有通便作用的水果（例如杏子、洋李）就可能有效地治疗便秘。另外药物治疗也是有帮助的。虽然有多种推

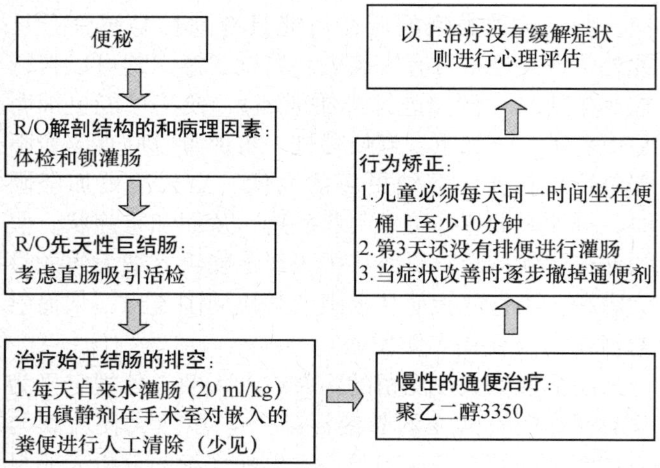

图 99-34 原发性便秘的治疗方案。在治疗之前，通过体检，钡灌肠和直肠吸吮活检排除（R/O）解剖结构和病理方面的病因。因为大多数患者有与便秘有关的大便嵌塞，所以需要排空结肠以打破大量粪便潴留的扩张的结肠周期。这需要每天进行灌肠 1～2 周。假如患者 3 天内未排便，则需要继续灌肠。通过这些治疗没有缓解症状，则需要进行心理评估。

荐药物，但是只有聚乙二醇 3350 在儿童中长期应用是安全的。在诊断功能性原发性便秘之前，必须排除其他解剖结构的和生理性的病因，常常需要进行直肠吸引活检。肛门前移位（可能是微小的）类似于良性便秘，可能需要外科治疗。对于慢性严重便秘或大便失禁的儿童，需要进行一系列的手术破除慢性损害的周期，从而改变以及增加排便的次数。图 99-34 为对这种类型患儿的推荐治疗方案。注意应根据症状的持续时间和严重程度以及父母和儿童的依从性对每个患儿进行个性化的治疗是非常重要的。

（褚 珺译 施诚仁校）

参考文献

1. Abrahamian F, Lloyd-Still J: Chronic constipation in childhood: A longitudinal study of 186 patients. J Pediatr Gastroenterol Nutr 1984;3:460-467.
2. Adson A: Hirschsprung's disease: Indications for and results obtained by sympathectomy. Surgery 1937;1:859.
3. Akgur F, Tanyel F, Buyukpamukcu N, Hicsonmez A: Colonic atresia and Hirschsprung's disease association shows further evidence for migration of enteric neurons. J Pediatr Surg 1993;28:635-636.
4. Akkary S, Sahwy E, Kandil W, Hamdy M: A histochemical study of the mucosubstances of the colon in cases of Hirschsprung's disease with and without enterocolitis. J Pediatr Surg 1981;16:664-668.
5. Albanese CT, Jennings RW, Smith B, et al: Perineal one-stage pull-through for Hirschsprung's disease. J Pediatr Surg 1999; 34:377-380.
6. Aldridge R, Campbell P: Ganglion cell distribution in the normal rectum and anal canal: A basis for the diagnosis of Hirschsprung's disease by anorectal biopsy. J Pediatr Surg 1968;3:475-490.
7. Amiel J, Attie T, Jan D, et al: Heterozygous endothelin receptor B (EDNRB) mutations in isolated Hirschsprung disease. Hum Mol Genet 1996;5:355-357.
8. Amiel J, Lyonnet S: Hirschsprung disease, associated syndromes, and genetics: A review. J Med Genet 2001;38:729-739.
9. Amodio J, Berdon W, Abramson S, Stolar C: Microcolon of prematurity: A form of functional obstruction. AJR Am J Roentgenol 1986;146:239-244.
10. Anderson K, Chandra R: Segmental aganglionosis of the appendix. J Pediatr Surg 1986;21:852-854.
11. Andrassy R, Isaacs H, Weitzman J: Rectal suction biopsy for the diagnosis of Hirschsprung's disease. Ann Surg 1981; 193:419-424.
12. Angrist M, Bolk S, Halushka M, et al: Germline mutations in glial cell line-derived neurotrophic factor (GDNF) and RET in a Hirschsprung disease patient. Nat Genet 1996; 14:341-344.
13. Angrist M, Bolk S, Thiel B, et al: Mutation analysis of the RET receptor tyrosine kinase in Hirschsprung disease. Hum Mol

Genet 1995;4:821-830.
14. Anuras S, Hade J, Soffer E, et al: Natural history of adult Hirschsprung's disease. J Clin Gastroenterol 1984;6:205-210.
15. Arliss J, Holgersen L: Neonatal appendiceal perforation and Hirschsprung's disease. J Pediatr Surg 1990;25:694-695.
16. Aslam A, Spicer RD, Corfield AP: Turnover of radioactive mucin precursors in the colon of patients with Hirschsprung's disease correlates with the development of enterocolitis. J Pediatr Surg 1998;33:103-105.
17. Aslam A, Spicer RD, Corfield AP: Histochemical and genetic analysis of colonic mucin glycoproteins in Hirschsprung's disease. J Pediatr Surg 1999;34:330-333.
18. Athow A, Filipe M, Drake D: Problems and advantages of acetylcholinesterase histochemistry of rectal suction biopsies in the diagnosis of Hirschsprung's disease. J Pediatr Surg 1990;25:520-526.
19. Attie T, Pelet A, Edery P, et al: Diversity of RET protooncogene mutations in familial and sporadic Hirschsprung disease. Hum Mol Genet 1995;4:1381-1386.
20. Auricchio A, Casari G, Staiano A, Ballabio A: Endothelin-B receptor mutations in patients with isolated Hirschsprung disease from a non-inbred population. Hum Mol Genet 1996;5:351-354.
21. Badner J, Sieber W, Garver K, Chakravarti A: A genetic study of Hirschsprung disease. Am J Hum Genet 1990;46: 568-580.
22. Bai Y, Chen H, Hao J, et al: Long-term outcome and quality of life after the Swenson procedure for Hirschsprung's disease. J Pediatr Surg 2002;37:639-642.
23. Baloh R, Tansey M, Golden J, et al: TrnR2, a novel receptor that mediates neurturin and GDNF signaling through RET. Neuron 1997;18:793-802.
24. Baltogiannis N, Mavridis G, Soutis M, Keramidas D: Currarino triad associated with Hirschsprung's disease. J Pediatr Surg 2003;38:1086-1089.
25. Banani SA, Forootan H: Role of anorectal myectomy after failed endorectal pull-through in Hirschsprung's disease. J Pediatr Surg 1994;29:1307-1309.
26. Baumgarten H, Holstein A, Stelzner F: Nervous elements in the human colon of Hirschsprung's disease (with comparative remarks on neuronal profiles in the normal human and monkey colon and sphincter ani internus). Virchows Arch A Pathol Anat 1973;358:113-136.
27. Bealer J, Natuzzi E, Flake A, et al: Effect of nitric oxide on the colonic smooth muscle of patients with Hirschsprung's disease. J Pediatr Surg 1994;29:1025-1029.
28. Bell E, Wall G: Pediatric constipation therapy using guidelines and polyethylene glycol 3350. Ann Pharmacother 2004;38:686-693.
29. Berdon W, Baker D, Bland W: Megacystis-microcolon intestinal hypoperistalsis syndrome: A new cause of intestinal obstruction in the newborn. Report of radiologic findings in five newborn girls. Ann Roentgenol 1976;126:957-964.
30. Bickler S, Harrison M, Campbell T, Campbell J: Long-segment Hirschsprung's disease. Arch Surg 1992;127: 1047-1050.
31. Bielschowsky M, Scholfield G: Studies on the inheritance and neurohistology of megacolon in mice. Proc Univ Otago Med Sch 1960;38:14-15.
32. Bill AH Jr, Chapman N: The enterocolitis of Hirschsprung's disease: Its natural history and treatment. Am J Surg 1962; 103:70-74.
33. Blair GK, Murphy JJ, Fraser GC: Internal sphincterotomy in post-pull-through Hirschsprung's disease. J Pediatr Surg 1996;31:843-845.
34. Bodian M: Pathological aids in the diagnosis and management of Hirschsprung's disease. In Recent Advances in Clinical Pathology. London, Churchill, 1960.
35. Bolande R: The neurocristopathies: A unifying concept of disease arising in neural crest maldevelopment. Hum Pathol 1974;5:409-429.
36. Boley S: An endorectal pull-through operation with primary anastomosis for Hirschsprung's disease. Surg Gynecol Obstet 1968;127:353-357.
37. Boley S, Dinari G, Cohen M: Hirschsprung's disease in the newborn. Clin Perinatol 1978;5:45-60.
38. Bolk S, Pelet A, Hofstra R, et al: A human model for multigenic inheritance: Phenotypic expression in Hirschsprung disease requires both the RET gene and a new 9q31 locus. Proc Natl Acad Sci U S A 2000;97:268-273.
39. Bondurand N, Kuhlbrodt K, Pingault V, et al: A molecular analysis of the Yemenite deaf-blind hypopigmentation syndrome: SOX10 dysfunction causes different neurocristopathies. Hum Mol Genet 1999;8:1785-1789.
40. Borrego S, Ruiz A, Saez M, et al: RET genotypes comprising specific haplotypes of polymorphic variants predispose to isolated Hirschsprung disease. J Med Genet 2000;37:572-578.
41. Borrego S, Saez M, Ruiz A, et al: Specific polymorphisms in the RET proto-oncogene are over-represented in patients with Hirschsprung disease and may represent loci modifying phenotypic expression. J Med Genet 1999;36:771-774.
42. Bracci F, Iacobelli B, Papadatou B, et al: Role of electrogastrography in detecting motility disorders in children affected by chronic intestinal pseudo-obstruction and Crohn's disease. Eur J Pediatr Surg 2003;13:31-34.
43. Brandborg L, Rubin G, Quinton W: Multipurpose instrument for suction biopsy of esophagus, stomach, small bowel and colon. Gastroenterology 1959;37:1-16.
44. Branski D, Lebenthal E: Small intestinal changes in enterocolitis complicating Hirschsprung's disease. J Clin Gastroenterol 1979;1:237-240.
45. Bult H, Boeckxstaens G, Pelckmans P: Nitric oxide as an inhibitory non-adrenergic non-cholinergic neurotransmitter. Nature 1990;345:346-347.
46. Burns A, Pasricha P, Young H: Enteric neural crest-derived cells and neural stem cells: Biology and therapeutic potential. Neurogastroenterol Motil Suppl 2004;1:3-7.
47. Callaghan R, Nixon H: Megarectum: Physiological observation. Arch Dis Child 1964;39:153.
48. Caneiro P, Brereton R, Drake D, et al: Enterocolitis in Hirschsprung's disease. Pediatr Surg Int 1992;7:356-360.
49. Caniano D, Teitelbaum D, Qualman S: Management of Hirschsprung's disease in children with trisomy 21. Am J Surg 1990;159:402-404.
50. Caniano D, Teitelbaum D, Qualman S, Shannon B: The piebald-lethal murine strain: Investigation of the cause of early death. J Pediatr Surg 1989;24:906-910.
51. Carcassonne M, Morisson-Lacombe G, Letourneau JN: Primary corrective operation without decompression in infants less than three months of age with Hirschsprung's disease. J Pediatr Surg 1982;17:241-243.
52. Carrasquillo M, McCallion A, Puffenberger E, et al: Genome-wide association study and mouse model identify interaction between RET and EDNRB pathways in Hirschsprung disease. Nat Genet 2002;32:237-244.
53. Ceccheini I, Yin L, Pasini B, et al: Close linkage with RET protooncogene and deletion mutation in autosomal dominant Hirschsprung disease. Hum Mol Genet 1993;2:1803-1808.
54. Chakravarti A, Lyonnet S: Hirschsprung disease. In Scriver C, Beaudet A, Valle D, Sly W (eds): The Metabolic and Molecular Bases of Inherited Disease, 8th ed. New York, McGraw-Hill, 2000.

55. Challa V, Moran J, Turner C, Lyerly A: Histologic diagnosis of Hirschsprung's disease: The value of concurrent hematoxylin and eosin and cholinesterase staining of rectal biopsies. Am J Clin Pathol 1987;88:324-328.
56. Cilley R, Statter M, Hirschl R, Coran A: Definitive treatment of Hirschsprung's disease in the newborn with a one-stage procedure. Surgery 1994;115:551-556.
57. Clark D: Times of first void and first stool in 500 newborns. Pediatrics 1977;60:457-459.
58. Clausen N, Andersson P, Tommerup N: Familial occurrence of neuroblastoma, von Recklinghausen's neurofibromatosis, Hirschsprung's aganglionosis and jaw-winking syndrome. Acta Paediatr Scand 1989;78:736-741.
59. Cohen MC, Moore SW, Neveling U, Kaschula RO: Acquired aganglionosis following surgery for Hirschsprung's disease: A report of five cases during a 33-year experience with pull-through procedures. Histopathology 1993;22:163-168.
60. Coran A, Weintraub W: Modification of the endorectal procedure for Hirschsprung's disease. Surg Gynecol Obstet 1976;143:277-282.
61. Corkery JJ: Hirschsprung's disease. Clin Gastroenterol 1975;4:531-544.
62. Curran TJ, Raffensperger JG: Laparoscopic Swenson pull-through: A comparison with the open procedure. J Pediatr Surg 1996;31:1155-1156.
63. Davies M, Cywes S: Inadequate pouch emptying following Martin's pull-through procedure for intestinal aganglionosis. J Pediatr Surg 1983;18:14-20.
64. Davies M, Cywes S, Rode H: The manometric evaluation of the rectosphincteric reflex in total colonic aganglionosis. J Pediatr Surg 1981;16:300-303.
65. De Giorgio R, Sarnelli G, Corinaldesi R, Stanghellini V: Advances in our understanding of the pathology of chronic intestinal pseudo-obstruction. Gut 2004;53:1549-1552.
66. de la Torre-Mondragon L, Ortega-Salgado JA: Transanal endorectal pull-through for Hirschsprung's disease. J Pediatr Surg 1998;33:1283-1286.
67. Dimler M: "Acquired" Hirschsprung's disease. J Pediatr Surg 1981;16:844-845.
68. Diseth TH, Bjornland K, Novik TS, Emblem R: Bowel function, mental health, and psychosocial function in adolescents with Hirschsprung's disease. Arch Dis Child 1997;76:100-106.
69. Dobbins W, Bill A: Diagnosis of Hirschsprung's disease excluded by rectal suction biopsy. N Engl J Med 1965;272:990.
70. Doray B, Salomon R, Amiel J, et al: Mutation of the RET ligand, neurturin, supports multigenic inheritance in Hirschsprung disease. Hum Mol Genet 1998;7:1449-1452.
71. Duhamel B: Une nouvelle operation pour le megacolon congenital: L'abaissement retrorectal et trans-anal du colon, et son application possible au traitement de quelques autres malformations. Presse Med 1956;64:2249.
72. Duhamel B: Therapies Chirurgicale Infantile. Paris, 1957.
73. Duhamel B: A new operation for the treatment of Hirschsprung's disease. Arch Dis Child 1960;35:38-40.
74. Duhamel B: Retrorectal and transanal pull-through procedure for the treatment of Hirschsprung's disease. Dis Colon Rectum 1964;7:455.
75. Ehrenpreis T: Megacolon in the newborn. Acta Chir Scand Suppl 1946;94:7-113.
76. Ein SH, Shandling B, So H: A new look at an old operation for aganglionosis. J Pediatr Surg 1994;29:1228-1230.
77. Elhalaby E, Coran A: Hirschsprung's disease associated with Ondine's curse: Report of three cases and review of the literature. J Pediatr Surg 1994;29:530-535.
78. Elhalaby E, Coran A, Blane C, et al: Enterocolitis associated with Hirschsprung's disease: A clinical-radiological characterization based on 168 patients. J Pediatr Surg 1995;30:76-83.
79. Elhalaby EA, Hashish A, Elbarbary MM, et al: Transanal one-stage endorectal pull-through for Hirschsprung's disease: A multicenter study. J Pediatr Surg 2004;39:345-351.
80. Elhalaby EA, Teitelbaum DH, Coran AG, Heidelberger KP: Enterocolitis associated with Hirschsprung's disease: A clinical histopathological correlative study. J Pediatr Surg 1995;30:1023-1026.
81. Ellis D, Clatworth H: The meconium plug revisited. J Pediatr Surg 1966;1:54-61.
82. Emmanuel A, Shand A, Kamm M: Erythromycin for the treatment of chronic intestinal pseudo-obstruction: Description of six cases with a positive response. Aliment Pharmacol Ther 2004;19:687-694.
83. Endo M, Watanabe K, Fuchimoto Y, et al: Long-term results of surgical treatment in infants with total colonic aganglionosis. J Pediatr Surg 1994;29:1310-1314.
84. Erdek M, Wilt E: Hirschsprung's disease: One institution's ten year experience and long-term follow-up. Am Surg 1994;60:625-628.
85. Estevao-Costa J, Carvalho JL, Soares-Oliveira M: Risk factors for the development of enterocolitis after pull-through for Hirschsprung's disease. J Pediatr Surg 1999;34:1581-1582.
86. Felman A, Talbert J: Failure to thrive. How about Hirschsprung's disease? Clin Pediatr 1971;10:125-126.
87. Fishbein R, Handelsman J, Schuster M: Surgical treatment of Hirschsprung's disease in adults. Surg Gynecol Obstet 1986;163:458-464.
88. Fitze G, Cramer J, Ziegler A, et al: Association between c135G/A genotype and RET protooncogene germline mutations and phenotype of Hirschsprung's disease. Lancet 2002;359:1200-1205.
89. Fitze G, Schreiber M, Kuhlisch E, et al: Association of RET protooncogene codon 45 polymorphism with Hirschsprung disease. Am J Hum Genet 1999;65:1469-1473.
90. Fitzgerald J: Encopresis, soiling, constipation. What's to be done? Pediatrics 1975;56:348-349.
91. Forstner G, Sherman P, Lichtman S: Bacterial overgrowth. In Walker W, Durie P, Hamilton J, et al (eds): Pediatric Gastrointestinal Disease, vol 1. Philadelphia, BC Decker, 1991, pp 689-700.
92. Framken E, Smith W, Frey E, et al: Intestinal motility disorders of infants and children: Classification, clinical manifestations, and roentgenology. CRC Crit Rev Diagn Imaging 1987;27:203-237.
93. Fu CG, Muto T, Masaki T, Nagawa H: Zonal adult Hirschsprung's disease. Gut 1996;39:765-767.
94. Fujimoto T, Reen DJ, Puri P: Inflammatory response in enterocolitis in the piebald lethal mouse model of Hirschsprung's disease. Pediatr Res 1988;24:152-155.
95. Fujimoto T, Hata J, Yokoyama S, Mitomi T: A study of the extracellular matrix protein as the migration pathway of neural crest cells in the gut: Analysis in human embryos with special reference to the pathogenesis of Hirschsprung's disease. J Pediatr Surg 1989;24:550-556.
96. Fujimoto T, Reen D, Puri P: Immunohistochemical characterization of abnormal innervation of colon in Hirschsprung's disease using D7 monoclonal antibody. J Pediatr Surg 1987;22:246-251.
97. Fujimoto T, Reen DJ, Puri P: Inflammatory response in enterocolitis in the piebald lethal mouse model of Hirschsprung's disease. Pediatr Res 1988;24:152-155.
98. Furness J, Costa M: The adrenergic innervation of the gastrointestinal tract. Erg Physiol 1974;69:1.

99. Furness J, Costa M: Types of nerves in the enteric nervous system. Neuroscience 1980;5:1-20.
100. Gabriel S, Salomon R, Pelet A, et al: Segregation at three loci explains familial and population risk in Hirschsprung disease. Nat Genet 2002;31:89-93.
101. Gaillard D, Birembaut P, Ploton D, et al: Colonic nerve network demonstrated by quinacrine. Bull Assoc Anat 1982;66:63-70.
102. Gariepy CE, Williams SC, Richardson JA, et al: Transgenic expression of the endothelin-B receptor prevents congenital intestinal aganglionosis in a rat model of Hirschsprung disease. J Clin Invest 1998;102:1092-1101.
103. Gauderer M, Rothstein F, Izant R Jr: Ileal atresia with long-segment Hirschsprung's disease in a neonate. J Pediatr Surg 1984;19:15-17.
104. Georgeson K, Fuefner M, Hardin W: Primary laparoscopic pull-through for Hirschsprung's disease in infants and children. J Pediatr Surg 1995;30:1017-1022.
105. Georgeson KE, Cohen RD, Hebra A, et al: Primary laparoscopic-assisted endorectal colon pull-through for Hirschsprung's disease: A new gold standard. Ann Surg 1999;229:678-682.
106. Gherardi G: Pathology of the ganglionic-aganglionic junction in congenital megacolon. Arch Pathol (Chicago) 1960;69:520.
107. Ghose SI, Squire BR, Stringer MD, et al: Hirschsprung's disease: Problems with transition-zone pull-through. J Pediatr Surg 2000;35:1805-1809.
108. Glotzer D, Gpihl B: Experimental obstructive colitis. Arch Surg 1966;92:1-8.
109. Goldberg E: An epidemiological study of Hirschsprung's disease. Int J Epidemiol 1984;13:479-485.
110. Gowers W: The automatic action of the sphincter ani. Proc R Soc Med 1877;26:77.
111. Griseri P, Pesce B, Patrone G, et al: A rare haplotype of the RET proto-oncogene is a risk-modifying allele in Hirschsprung disease. Am J Hum Genet 2002;71:969-974.
112. Griseri P, Sancandi M, Patrone G, et al: A single-nucleotide polymorphic variant of the RET proto-oncogene is under-represented in sporadic Hirschsprung disease. Eur J Hum Genet 2000;8:721-724.
113. Grob M: Intestinal obstruction in the new born infant. Arch Dis Child 1960;35:40.
114. Guo R, Nada O, Suita S, et al: The distribution and co-localization of nitric oxide synthase and vasoactive intestinal polypeptide in nerves of the colon with Hirschsprung's disease. Virchows Arch 1997;430:53-61.
115. Hackam DJ, Filler RM, Pearl RH: Enterocolitis after the surgical treatment of Hirschsprung's disease: Risk factors and financial impact. J Pediatr Surg 1998;33:830-833.
116. Hackam DJ, Reblock K, Barksdale EM, et al: The influence of Down's syndrome on the management and outcome of children with Hirschsprung's disease. J Pediatr Surg 2003;38:946-949.
117. Hackam DJ, Superina RA, Pearl RH: Single-stage repair of Hirschsprung's disease: A comparison of 109 patients over 5 years. J Pediatr Surg 1997;32:1028-1031.
118. Hadidi A: Transanal endorectal pull-through for Hirschsprung's disease: Experience with 68 patients. J Pediatr Surg 2003;38:1337-1340.
119. Hanneman MJ, Sprangers MA, De Mik EL, et al: Quality of life in patients with anorectal malformation or Hirschsprung's disease: Development of a disease-specific questionnaire. Dis Colon Rectum 2001;44:1650-1660.
120. Harrison M, Deitz D, Campbell J, Campbell T: Diagnosis and management of Hirschsprung's disease: A 25 year perspective. Am J Surg 1986;152:49-56.
121. Hartman EE, Oort FJ, Aronson DC, et al: Critical factors affecting quality of life of adult patients with anorectal malformations or Hirschsprung's disease. Am J Gastroenterol 2004;99:907-913.
122. Hawksley M: Spinal anaesthsia in the treatment of Hirschsprung's disease. Br J Surg 1943-1944;31:245-252.
123. Hearn C, Murphy M, Newgreen D: GDNF and ET-3 differentially modulate the numbers of avian enteric neural crest cells and enteric neurons in vitro. Dev Biol 1998;197:93-105.
124. Heij HA, de Vries X, Bremer I, et al: Long-term anorectal function after Duhamel operation for Hirschsprung's disease. J Pediatr Surg 1995;30:430-432.
125. Heikkinen M, Rintala R, Louhimo I: Bowel function and quality of life in adult patients with operated Hirschsprung's disease. Pediatr Surg Int 1995;10:342-344.
126. Heikkinen M, Rintala R, Luukkonen P: Long-term anal sphincter performance after surgery for Hirschsprung's disease. J Pediatr Surg 1997;32:1443-1446.
127. Helbig D: Hirschsprung's disease in infancy and childhood. In Holschneider A (ed): Hirschsprung's Disease. New York and Stuttgart, Hippokarates Verlag, Thieme-Stratton, 1982, pp 93-102.
128. Heneyke S, Smith V, Spitz L, Milla P: Chronic intestinal pseudo-obstruction: Treatment and long term follow up of 44 patients. Arch Dis Child 1999;81:21-27.
129. Hengster P, Pernthaler H, Gassner I, Menardi G: Twenty-three years of follow-up in patients with total colonic aganglionosis. Klin Padiatr 1996;208:3-7.
130. Hirobe S, Doody DP, Ryan DP, et al: Ectopic class II major histocompatibility antigens in Hirschsprung's disease and neuronal intestinal dysplasia. J Pediatr Surg 1992;27:357-362.
131. Hirschsprung H: Stuhltragheit neugeborner in folge von dilatation and hypertrophie des colons. Jaharb Kinderch 1887;27:1-7.
132. Hoehner JC, Ein SH, Shandling B, Kim PC: Long-term morbidity in total colonic aganglionosis. J Pediatr Surg 1998;33:961-965.
133. Hofstra R, Osinga J, Tan-Sindhunata G, et al: A homozygous mutation in the endothelin-3 gene associated with a combined Waardenburg type 2 and Hirschsprung phenotype (Shah-Waardenburg syndrome). Nat Genet 1996;12:445-447.
134. Hollwarth ME, Rivosecchi M, Schleef J, et al: The role of transanal endorectal pull-through in the treatment of Hirschsprung's disease: A multicenter experience. Pediatr Surg Int 2002;18:344-348.
135. Holschneider A, Kellner E, Streibl P, Sippell W: The development of anorectal continence and its significance in the diagnosis of Hirschsprung's disease. J Pediatr Surg 1976;11:151-156.
136. Hyde G Jr, De Lorimier A: Colon atresia and Hirschsprung's disease. Surgery 1968;64:976-978.
137. Ikawa H, Kim S, Hendren W, Donahoe P: Acetylcholinesterase and manometry in the diagnosis of the constipated child. Arch Surg 1986;121:435-438.
138. Ikawa H, Yokoyama J, Morikawa Y, et al: A quantitative study of acetylcholine in Hirschsprung's disease. J Pediatr Surg 1980;15:48-52.
139. Ikeda K: New techniques in the surgical treatment of Hirschsprung's disease. Surgery 1967;61:503-508.
140. Ikeda K, Goto S: Diagnosis and treatment of Hirschsprung's disease in Japan: An analysis of 1628 patients. Ann Surg 1984;199:400-405.

141. Ikeda K, Goto S: Total colonic aganglionosis with or without small bowel involvement: An analysis of 137 patients. J Pediatr Surg 1986;21:319-322.
142. Inoue M, Hosoda K, Imura K, et al: Mutational analysis of the endothelin-B receptor gene in Japanese Hirschsprung's disease. J Pediatr Surg 1998;33:1206-1208.
143. Ito S, Iwashita T, Asai N, et al: Biological properties of RET with cysteine mutations correlate with multiple endocrine neoplasia type 2A, familial medullary thyroid carcinoma, and Hirschsprung's disease phenotype. Cancer Res 1997; 57:2870-2872.
144. Ito Y, Donahoe P, Hendren W: Maturation of the rectoanal response in premature and perinatal infants. J Pediatr Surg 1977;12:477-481.
145. Ivanchuk SM, Myers SM, Eng C, Mulligan LM: De novo mutation of GDNF, ligand for the RET/GDNFR-alpha receptor complex, in Hirschsprung disease. Hum Mol Genet 1996;5:2023-2026.
146. Iwashita T, Kruger G, Pardal R, et al: Hirschsprung disease is linked to defects in neural crest stem cell function. Science 2003;301:972-976.
147. Jamieson D, Dundas S, Belushi S, et al: Does the transition zone reliably delineate aganglionic bowel in Hirschsprung's disease? Pediatr Radiol 2004;34:811-815.
developing bowel and pancreas. Dev Biol 2003;258: 364-384.
148. Jasonni V, Martucciello G: Total colonic aganglionosis. Semin Pediatr Surg 1998;7:174-180.
149. Jiang Y, Liu M, Gershon M: Netrins and DCC in the guidance of migrating neural crest-derived cells in the developing bowel and pancreas. Dev Biol 2003;258: 364-384.
150. Jing S, Yu Y, Fang M, et al: GFRalpha-2 and GFRalpha-3 are two new receptors for ligands of the GDNF family. J Biol Chem 1997;272:33111-33117.
151. Jordan F, Coran A, Weintraub W, Wesley J: An evaluation of the modified endorectal procedure for Hirschsprung's disease. J Pediatr Surg 1979;14:681-685.
152. Kanai M, Numakura C, Sasaki A, et al: Congenital central hypoventilation syndrome: A novel mutation of the RET gene in an isolated case. Tohoku J Exp Med 2002;196: 241-246.
153. Kapur RP, deSa DJ, Luquette M, Jaffe R: Hypothesis: Pathogenesis of skip areas in long-segment Hirschsprung's disease. Pediatr Pathol Lab Med 1995;15:23-37.
154. Keshtgar AS, Ward HC, Clayden GS, de Sousa NM: Investigations for incontinence and constipation after surgery for Hirschsprung's disease in children. Pediatr Surg Int 2003;19:4-8.
155. Khan AR, Vujanic GM, Huddart S: The constipated child: How likely is Hirschsprung's disease? Pediatr Surg Int 2003;19:439-442.
156. Kiesewetter W, Sukarochana K, Sieber W: The frequency of aganglionosis associated with imperforate anus. Surgery 1965;58:877-880.
157. Kim E, Boutwell W: Smith-Lemli-Opitz syndrome associated with Hirschsprung disease, 46,XY female karyotype, and total anomalous pulmonary venous drainage [letter]. J Pediatr 1985;106:861.
158. Kimura K, Inomata Y, Soper RT: Posterior sagittal rectal myectomy for persistent rectal achalasia after the Soave procedure for Hirschsprung's disease. J Pediatr Surg 1993;28:1200-1201.
159. Kimura K, Nishijima E, Muraji T: A new surgical approach to extensive aganglionosis. J Pediatr Surg 1981;16: 840-843.
160. Kimura K, Nishijima E, Muraji T, et al: Extensive aganglionosis: Further experience with the colonic patch graft procedure and long-term results. J Pediatr Surg 1988;23: 52-56.
161. Klaus M, Fanaroff A: Care of the High-Risk Neonate, 4th ed. Philadelphia, WB Saunders, 1993.
162. Klein M, Coran A, Wesley J, Drongowski R: Hirschsprung's disease in the newborn. J Pediatr Surg 1984;19: 370-374.
163. Klein M, Philippart A: Hirschsprung's disease: Three decades' experience at a single institution. J Pediatr Surg 1993;28:1291-1293.
164. Kleinhaus S, Boley S, Sheran M, Sieber W: Hirschsprung's disease—a survey of the members of the Surgical Section of the American Academy of Pediatrics. J Pediatr Surg 1979;14:588-597.
165. Kluck P, van Muijen G, van der Kamp A, et al: Hirschsprung's disease studied with monoclonal antineurofilament antibodies on tissue sections. Lancet 1984;1:652-654.
166. Kobayashi H, Hirakawa H, Puri P: Overexpression of intercellular adhesion molecule-1 (ICAM-1) and MHC class II antigen on hypertrophic nerve trunks suggests an immunopathologic response in Hirschsprung's disease. J Pediatr Surg 1995;30:1680-1683.
167. Kobayashi H, O'Briain D, Puri P: Lack of expression of NADPH-diaphorase and neural cell adhesion molecule (NCAM) in colonic muscle of patients with Hirschsprung's disease. J Pediatr Surg 1994;29:301-304.
168. Kobayashi H, O'Briain DS, Hirakawa H, et al: A rapid technique of acetylcholinesterase staining. Arch Pathol Lab Med 1994;118:1127-1129.
169. Kobayashi H, Yamataka A, Lane GJ, Miyano T: Inflammatory changes secondary to postoperative complications of Hirschsprung's disease as a cause of histopathologic changes typical of intestinal neuronal dysplasia. J Pediatr Surg 2004;39:152-156.
170. Kottmeier P, Jongco B, Velcek F: Absorptive function of the aganglionic ileum. J Pediatr Surg 1981;16:275-278.
171. Krishnamurthy S, Schuffler M: Pathology of neuromuscular disorders of the small intestine. Gastroenterology 1987; 93:610-639.
172. Kruger G, Mosher J, Bixby S, et al: Neural crest stem cells persist in the adult gut but undergo changes in self-renewal, neuronal subtype potential, and factor responsiveness. Neuron 2002;35:657-669.
173. Kruger GM, Mosher JT, Tsai YH, et al: Temporally distinct requirements for endothelin receptor B in the generation and migration of gut neural crest stem cells. Neuron 2003;40:917-929.
174. Kuhlbrodt K, Herbarth B, Sock E, et al: SOX10, a novel transcriptional modulator in glial cells. J Neurosci 1998; 18:237-250.
175. Kuroda T, Doody D, Donahoe P: Aberrant colonic expression of MHC class II antigens in Hirschsprung's disease. Aust N Z J Surg 1991;61:373-379.
176. Kusafuka T, Wang Y, Puri P: Novel mutations of the endothelin-B receptor gene in isolated patients with Hirschsprung's disease. Hum Mol Genet 1996;5:347-349.
177. Laberge JM, Adolph VR, Flageole H, Guttman FM: Salvage of Soave-Boley endorectal pull-through by conversion to a classical Soave procedure. Eur J Pediatr Surg 1996;6: 362-363.
178. Lake B, Malone M, Risdon R: The use of acetylcholinesterase (AChE) in the diagnosis of Hirschsprung's disease and intestinal neuronal dysplasia. Pediatr Pathol 1989;9:351-354.

179. Lake B, Puri P, Nixon H, Claireaux A: Hirschsprung's disease: An appraisal of histochemically demonstrated acetylcholinesterase activity in suction rectal biopsy specimens as an aid to diagnosis. Arch Pathol Lab Med 1978;102:244-247.
180. Langer J: Persistent obstructive symptoms after surgery for Hirschsprung's disease: Development of a diagnostic and therapeutic algorithm. J Pediat Surg 2004;39:1458-1462.
181. Langer J, Betti P, Blennerhassett M: Smooth muscle from aganglionic bowel in Hirschsprung's disease impairs neuronal development in vitro. Cell Tissue Res 1994;276: 181-186.
182. Langer JC: Repeat pull-through surgery for complicated Hirschsprung's disease: Indications, techniques, and results. J Pediatr Surg 1999;34:1136-1141.
183. Langer JC, Durrant AC, de la Torre ML, et al: One-stage transanal Soave pullthrough for Hirschsprung disease: A multicenter experience with 141 children. Ann Surg 2003;238:569-576.
184. Larsson L, Malmfors G, Sundler F: Neuropeptide Y, calcitonin gene-related peptide, and galanin in Hirschsprung's disease: An immunocytochemical study. J Pediatr Surg 1988;23:342-345.
185. Le Douarin N: Cell migrations in embryos. Cell 1984;38: 353-360.
186. Le Douarin N, Kalcheim C: The Neural Crest. Cambridge, UK, Cambridge University Press, 1999.
187. Le Dourin F, Teillet M: The migration of neural crest cells to the wall of the digestive tract in avian embryo. J Embryol Exp Morphol 1973;30:31-48.
188. Levin M: Children with encopresis: A descriptive analysis. Pediatrics 1975;56:412-416.
189. Levin S: The immune system and susceptibility to infections in Down's syndrome. In McCoy E, Epstein C (eds): Oncology and Immunology in Down's Syndrome. New York, Alan R Liss, 1987, pp 143-162.
190. Levy M, Reynolds M: Morbidity associated with total colon Hirschsprung's disease. J Pediatr Surg 1992;27:364-366.
191. Liem NT, Hau BD, Thu NX: The long-term follow-up result of Swenson's operation in the treatment of Hirschsprung's disease in Vietnamese children. Eur J Pediatr Surg 1995; 5:110-112.
192. Lifschitz C, Bloss R: Persistence of colitis in Hirschsprung's disease. J Pediatr Gastroenterol Nutr 1985;4:291-293.
193. Lister J: Hirschsprung: The man and the disease. J R Coll Surg Edinb 1977;22:378-384.
194. Liu CS, Chin TW, Wei CF: Neonatal Duhamel's pull-through for Hirschsprung's disease. Chung Hua I Hsueh Tsa Chih 2002;65:398-402.
195. Loening-Baucke V: Anorectal manometry: Experience with strain gauge pressure transducers for the diagnosis of Hirschsprung's disease. J Pediatr Surg 1983;18:595-600.
196. Loening-Baucke V, Pringle K, Ekwo E: Anorectal manometry for the exclusion of Hirschsprung's disease in neonates. J Pediatr Gastroenterol Nutr 1985;4:596-603.
197. Loinaz C, Mittal N, Kato T, et al: Multivisceral transplantation for pediatric intestinal pseudo-obstruction: Single center's experience of 16 cases. Transplant Proc 2004;36: 312-313.
198. Ludman L, Spitz L, Tsuji H, Pierro A: Hirschsprung's disease: Functional and psychological follow up comparing total colonic and rectosigmoid aganglionosis. Arch Dis Child 2002;86:348-351.
199. Lynn H, van Heerden J: Rectal myectomy in Hirschsprung disease: A decade of experience. Arch Surg 1975;110: 991-994.
200. Maia DM: The reliability of frozen-section diagnosis in the pathologic evaluation of Hirschsprung's disease. Am J Surg Pathol 2000;24:1675-1677.
201. Managoli S, Chaturvedi P, Vilhekar KY, et al: Perforated acute appendicitis in a term neonate. Indian J Pediatr 2004;71:357-358.
202. Martin L: Surgical management of Hirschsprung's disease involving the small intestine. Arch Surg 1968;97:183-189.
203. Martin L, Altemeier W: Clinical experience with a new operation (modified Duhamel procedure) for Hirschsprung's disease. Ann Surg 1962;156:678.
204. Martin L, Caudill D: A method for elimination of the blind rectal pouch in the Duhamel operation for Hirschsprung's disease. Surgery 1967;62:951-953.
205. Martin L, Perrin E: Neonatal perforation of the appendix in association with Hirschsprung's disease. Ann Surg 1967; 166:799-802.
206. Martin MJ, Steele SR, Mullenix PS, et al: A pilot study using total colonic manometry in the surgical evaluation of pediatric functional colonic obstruction. J Pediatr Surg 2004;39:352-359.
207. Martucciello G, Biocchi M, Dodero P, et al: Total colonic aganglionosis associated with interstitial deletion of the long arm of chromosome 10. Pediatr Surg Int 1992;7: 308-310.
208. Martucciello G, Favre A, Takahashi M, et al: Immunohistochemical localization of RET protein in Hirschsprung's disease. J Pediatr Surg 1995;30:433-436.
209. Martucciello G, Thompson H, Mazzola C, et al: GDNF deficit in Hirschsprung's disease. J Pediatr Surg 1998;33:99-102.
210. Marty T, Seo T, Matlak M, et al: Gastrointestinal function after surgical correction of Hirschsprung's disease: Long-term follow-up in 135 patients. J Pediatr Surg 1995;30:655-658.
211. Marty TL, Seo T, Sullivan JJ, et al: Rectal irrigations for the prevention of postoperative enterocolitis in Hirschsprung's disease. J Pediatr Surg 1995;30:652-654.
212. Mattar A, Drongowski R, Coran AG, Teitelbaum DH: MUC-2 mucin production in Hirschsprung's disease: Possible association with enterocolitis development. J Pediatr Surg 2003;38:417-421.
213. McCready R, Beart R Jr: Classic articles in colonic and rectal surgery: Constipation in the newborn as a result of dilation and hypertrophy of the colon: Harald Hirschsprung, Jahrbuch fur Kinderheilkunde, 1888 adult Hirschsprung's disease: Results of surgical treatment at Mayo Clinic. Dis Colon Rectum 1981;24:408-410.
214. Meier-Ruge W: [Casuistic of colon disorder with symptoms of Hirschsprung's disease.] Verh Dtsch Ges Pathol 1971;55:506-510.
215. Meier-Ruge W, Lutterbeck P, Herzog B, et al: Acetylcholinesterase activity in suction biopsies of the rectum in the diagnosis of Hirschsprung's disease. J Pediatr Surg 1972;7:11-17.
216. Meijers JH, van der Sanden MP, Tibboel D, et al: Colonization characteristics of enteric neural crest cells: Embryological aspects of Hirschsprung's disease. J Pediatr Surg 1992;27:811-814.
217. Meunier P, Marechal J, Mollard P: Accuracy of the manometric diagnosis of Hirschsprung's disease. J Pediatr Surg 1978;13:411-415.
218. Miele E, Tozzi A, Staiano A, et al: Persistence of abnormal gastrointestinal motility after operation for Hirschsprung's disease. Am J Gastroenterol 2000;95:1226-1230.
219. Milla P, Cucchiara S, DiLorenzo C, et al: Motility disorders in childhood: Working group report of the First World

Congress of Pediatric Gastroenterology, Hepatology, and Nutrition. J Pediatr Gastroenterol Nutr 2002;35 (Suppl 2):S187-S195.
220. Minkes RK, Langer JC: A prospective study of botulinum toxin for internal anal sphincter hypertonicity in children with Hirschsprung's disease. J Pediatr Surg 2000;35: 1733-1736.
221. Mir E, Karaca I, Gunsar C, et al: Primary Duhamel-Martin operations in neonates and infants. Pediatr Int 2001;43: 405-408.
222. Mishalany H, Woolley M: Chronic constipation: Manometric patterns and surgical considerations. Arch Surg 1984;119: 1257-1259.
223. Mishalany H, Woolley M: Postoperative functional and manometric evaluation of patients with Hirschsprung's disease. J Pediatr Surg 1987;22:443-446.
224. Miyano T, Yamataka A, Urao M, et al: Modified Soave pull-through for Hirschsprung's disease: Intraoperative internal sphincterotomy. J Pediatr Surg 1999;34:1599-1602.
225. Miyazaki E, Ohshiro K, Puri P: NADPH-diaphorase histochemical staining of suction rectal biopsies in the diagnosis of Hirschsprung's disease and allied disorders. Pediatr Surg Int 1998;13:464-467.
226. Moore S, Albertyn R, Cywes S: Clinical outcome and long-term quality of life after surgical correction of Hirschsprung's disease. J Pediatr Surg 1996;31:1496-1502.
227. Moore S, Rode H, Miller A, et al: Intestinal atresia and Hirschsprung's disease. Pediatr Surg Int 1990;5:182-184.
228. Moore SW, Albertyn R, Cywes S: Clinical outcome and long-term quality of life after surgical correction of Hirschsprung's disease. J Pediatr Surg 1996;31: 1496-1502.
229. Moore SW, Millar AJ, Cywes S: Long-term clinical, manometric, and histological evaluation of obstructive symptoms in the postoperative Hirschsprung's patient. J Pediatr Surg 1994;29:106-111.
230. Mulligan L, Eng C, Attie T, et al: Diverse phenotypes associated with exon 10 mutations of the RET proto-oncogene. Hum Mol Genet 1994;3:2163-2167.
231. Mulligan L, Ponder B: Genetic basis of endocrine disease: Multiple endocrine neoplasia type 2. J Clin Endocrinol Metab 1995;80:1989-1995.
232. Murthi GV, Raine PA: Preoperative enterocolitis is associated with poorer long-term bowel function after Soave-Boley endorectal pull-through for Hirschsprung's disease. J Pediatr Surg 2003;38:69-72.
233. Mya G: Due asservazioni di dilatazione ed impertrofia congenita del colon. Sperimentale 1894;48:215.
234. Nakagawa M, Takashima H: Molecular mechanisms of hereditary neuropathy: Genotype-phenotype correlation. Rinsho Byori 2003;51:536-543.
235. Navarro J, Sonsino E, Boige N, et al: Visceral neuropathies responsible for chronic intestinal pseudo-obstruction syndrome in pediatric practice: Analysis of 26 cases. J Pediatr Gastroenterol Nutr 1990;11:179-195.
236. Neilson I, Yazbeck S: Ultrashort Hirschsprung's disease: Myth or reality. J Pediatr Surg 1990;25:1135-1138.
237. Nemeth L, O'Briain S, Puri P: Whole-mount NADPH-diaphorase histochemistry is a reliable technique for the intraoperative evaluation of extent of aganglionosis. Pediatr Surg Int 1999;15:195-197.
238. Newman B, Nussbaum A, Kirkpatrick J Jr, Colodny A: Appendiceal perforation, pneumoperitoneum, and Hirschsprung's disease. J Pediatr Surg 1988;23: 854-856.
239. Newman C, Laurini R, Lesbros Y, et al: Interstitial cells of Cajal are normally distributed in both ganglionated and aganglionic bowel in Hirschsprung's disease. Pediatr Surg Int 2003;19:662-668.
240. N-Fekete C, Ricour C, Martelli H, et al: Total colonic aganglionosis (with or without ileal involvement): A review of 27 cases. J Pediatr Surg 1986;21:251-254.
241. O'Donovan A, Habra G, Somers S, et al: Diagnosis of Hirschsprung's disease. AJR Am J Roentgenol 1996;167: 517-520.
242. Okamoto E, Ueda T: Embryogenesis of intramural ganglia of the gut and its relation to Hirschsprung's disease. J Pediatr Surg 1967;2:437-443.
243. O'Kelly T, Davies J, Tam P, et al: Abnormalities of nitric-oxide-producing neurons in Hirschsprung's disease: Morphology and implications. J Pediatr Surg 1994;29: 294-299.
244. Omenn G, McKusick V: The association of Waardenburg syndrome and Hirschsprung megacolon. Am J Med Genet 1979;3:217-223.
245. Orr J, Scobie W: Presentation and incidence of Hirschsprung's disease. BMJ 1983;287:1671.
246. Paratore C, Goerich D, Suter U, et al: Survival and glial fate acquisition of neural crest cells are regulated by an interplay between the transcription factor SOX10 and extrinsic combinatorial signaling. Development 2001;128: 3949-3961.
247. Parikh DH, Tam PK, Lloyd DA, et al: Quantitative and qualitative analysis of the extracellular matrix protein, laminin, in Hirschsprung's disease. J Pediatr Surg 1992; 27:991-995.
248. Parikh DH, Tam PK, Van Velzen D, Edgar D: Abnormalities in the distribution of laminin and collagen type IV in Hirschsprung's disease. Gastroenterology 1992;102: 1236-1241.
249. Parikh DH, Tam PK, Van Velzen D, Edgar D: The extracellular matrix components, tenascin and fibronectin, in Hirschsprung's disease: An immunohistochemical study. J Pediatr Surg 1994;29:1302-1306.
250. Passarge E: The genetics of Hirschsprung's disease: Evidence for heterogeneous etiology and a study of sixty-three families. N Engl J Med 1967;276:138-143.
251. Peters van der Sanden M: The Hindbrain Neural Crest and the Development of the Enteric Nervous System. Rotterdam, Erasmus University, 1994.
252. Peters van der Sanden M, Kirby M, Gittenberger-de Groot A, et al: Ablation of various regions within the avian vagal crest has differential effects on ganglion formation in the fore, mid and hindgut. Dev Dyn 1993;196:183-194.
253. Philippart A, Reed J, Georgeson K: Neonatal small left colon syndrome: Intramural not intraluminal obstruction. J Pediatr Surg 1975;10:733-740.
254. Pierro A, Fasoli L, Kiely EM, et al: Staged pull-through for rectosigmoid Hirschsprung's disease is not safer than primary pull-through. J Pediatr Surg 1997;32:505-509.
255. Pingault V, Bondurand N, Le Caignec C, et al: The SOX10 transcription factor: Evaluation as a candidate gene for central and peripheral hereditary myelin disorders. J Neurol 2001;248:496-499.
256. Pingault V, Girard M, Bondurand N, et al: SOX10 mutations in chronic intestinal pseudo-obstruction suggest a complex physiopathological mechanism. Hum Genet 2002;111: 198-206.
257. Piotrowska A, Solari V, de Caluwe D, Puri P: Immunocolocalization of the heme oxygenase-2 and interstitial cells of Cajal in normal and aganglionic colon. J Pediatr Surg 2003;38:73-77.

258. Piotrowska AP, Solari V, Puri P: Distribution of interstitial cells of Cajal in the internal anal sphincter of patients with internal anal sphincter achalasia and Hirschsprung disease. Arch Pathol Lab Med 2003;127:1192-1195.
259. Polley T, Coran A: Hirschsprung's disease in the newborn. Pediatr Surg Int 1986;1:80-83.
260. Polley T Jr, Coran A, Wesley J: A ten-year experience with ninety-two cases of Hirschsprung's disease: Including sixty-seven consecutive endorectal pull-through procedures. Ann Surg 1985;202:349-355.
261. Prevot J, Bodart N, Babut J, Mourot M: Hirschsprung's disease with total colonic involvement: Therapeutic problems. Prog Pediatr Surg 1972;4:63-89.
262. Puri P: Hirschsprung's disease: Clinical and experimental observations. World J Surg 1993;17:374-384.
263. Puri P, Lake D, Gorman F, et al: Megacystis-microcolon-intestinal hypoperistalsis syndrome: A visceral myopathy. J Pediatr Surg 1983;18:64-69.
264. Puri P, Nixon HH: Long-term results of Swenson's operation for Hirschsprung's disease. Prog Pediatr Surg 1977;10:87-96.
265. Puri P, Tsuji M: Megacystis-microcolon-intestinal hypoperistalsis syndrome (neonatal hollow visceral myopathy). Pediatr Surg Int 1992;7:18-22.
266. Qualman SJ, Jaffe R, Bove KE, Monforte-Munoz H: Diagnosis of Hirschsprung disease using the rectal biopsy: Multi-institutional survey. Pediatr Dev Pathol 1999;2:588-596.
267. Quinn F, Surana R, Puri P: The influence of trisomy 21 on outcome in children with Hirschsprung's disease. J Pediatr Surg 1994;29:781-783.
268. Rangecroft L: Neonatal small left colon syndrome. Arch Dis Child 1979;54:635-637.
269. Rantis PC Jr, Vernava AM 3rd, Daniel GL, Longo WE: Chronic constipation—is the work-up worth the cost? Dis Colon Rectum 1997;40:280-286.
270. Rasquin-Weber A, Hyman P, Cucchiara S, et al: Childhood functional gastrointestinal disorders. Gut 1999;45:II60-II68.
271. Read A, Newton V: Waardenburg syndrome. J Med Genet 1997;34:656-665.
272. Reding R, de Ville de Goyet J, Gosseye S, et al: Hirschsprung's disease: A 20-year experience. J Pediatr Surg 1997;32:1221-1225.
273. Rescorla F, Morrison A, Engles D, et al: Hirschsprung's disease: Evaluation of mortality and long-term function in 260 cases. Arch Surg 1992;127:934-941.
274. Rintala R, Lindahl H: Transanal endorectal coloanal anastomosis for Hirschsprung's disease. Pediatr Surg Int 1993;8:128-131.
275. Rintala RJ, Lindahl H: Sodium cromoglycate in the management of chronic or recurrent enterocolitis in patients with Hirschsprung's disease. J Pediatr Surg 2001;36:1032-1035.
276. Romeo G, Ronchetto P, Luo Y, et al: Point mutations affecting the tyrosine kinase domain of the RET proto-oncogene in Hirschsprung's disease. Nature 1994;367:377-378.
277. Rosenfield N, Ablow R, Markowitz R, et al: Hirschsprung disease: Accuracy of the barium enema examination. Radiology 1984;150:393-400.
278. Ross M, Chang J, Burrington J, et al: Complications of the Martin procedure for total colonic aganglionosis. J Pediatr Surg 1988;23:725-727.
279. Roy A, Bharucha H, Nevin N, et al: Idiopathic intestinal pseudo-obstruction: A familial visceral neuropathy. Clin Genet 1980;18:290-297.
280. Sacher P, Hirsig J, Gresser J, Spitz L: The importance of oral sodium replacement in ileostomy patients. Prog Pediatr Surg 1989;24:226-231.
281. Sakai T, Nirasawa Y, Itoh Y, et al: Japanese patients with sporadic Hirschsprung: Mutation analysis of the receptor tyrosine kinase proto-oncogene, endothelin-B receptor, endothelin-3, glial cell line-derived neurotrophic factor and neurturin genes: A comparison with similar studies. Eur J Pediatr 2000;159:160-167.
282. Sandegard E: Hirschsprung's disease with ganglion cell aplasia of the colon and terminal ileum: Report of a case treated with total colectomy and ileo-anostomy. Acta Chir Scand 1953;106:367-376.
283. Sanders K, Ordog T, Ward S: Physiology and pathophysiology of the interstitial cells of Cajal: From bench to bedside. IV. Genetic and animal models of GI motility disorders caused by loss of interstitial cells of Cajal. Am J Physiol Gastrointest Liver Physiol 2002;282:G747-G756.
284. Sandgren K, Larsson L, Ekblad E: Widespread changes in neurotransmitter expression and number of enteric neurons and interstitial cells of Cajal in lethal spotted mice: An explanation for persisting dysmotility after operation for Hirschsprung's disease? Dig Dis Sci 2002;47:1049-1064.
285. Sanicola M, Hession C, Worley D, et al: Glial cell line-derived neurotrophic factor-dependent RET activation can be mediated by two different cell-surface accessory proteins. Proc Natl Acad Sci U S A 1997;94:6238-6243.
286. Santoro M, Rosati R, Greco M, et al: The RET proto-oncogene is consistently expressed in human pheochromocytoma and medullary thyroid carcinoma. Oncogene 1990;5:1595-1598.
287. Sarioglu A, Tanyel FC, Buyukpamukcu N, Hicsonmez A: Appendiceal perforation: A potentially lethal initial mode of presentation of Hirschsprung's disease. J Pediatr Surg 1997;32:123-124.
288. Schofield D, Devine W, Yunis E: Acetylcholinesterase-stained suction rectal biopsies in the diagnosis of Hirschsprung's disease. J Pediatr Gastroenterol Nutr 1990;11:221-228.
289. Schuffler M, Bird T, Sumi S, Cook A: A familial neuronal disease presenting as intestinal pseudo-obstruction. Gastroenterology 1978;75:889-898.
290. Schwarz K, Ternberg J, Bell M, Keating J: Sodium needs of infants and children with ileostomy. J Pediatr 1983;102:509-513.
291. Scott B: Motility disorders. In Walker W, Durie P, Hamilton J, et al (eds): Pediatric Gastrointestinal Disease, vol 1. Philadelphia, BC Decker, 1991, pp 784-799.
292. Seri M, Yin L, Barone V, et al: Detection of RET mutation is higher among long segment than short segment Hirschsprung patients. Hum Mutat 1996;9:243-249.
293. Shandling B: New technique in diagnosis of Hirschsprung's disease. Can J Surg 1961;4:298-305.
294. Sharif K, Beath SV, Kelly DA, et al: New perspective for the management of near-total or total intestinal aganglionosis in infants. J Pediatr Surg 2003;38:25-28.
295. Shaw P: The innervation and neuroendocrine cell population of the appendix in total colonic aganglionosis. Histopathology 1990;17:117-121.
296. Sherman J, Snyder M, Weitzman J, et al: A 40-year multinational retrospective study of 880 Swenson procedures. J Pediatr Surg 1989;24:833-838.
297. Sidebotham EL, Kenny SE, Lloyd DA, et al: Location of stem cells for the enteric nervous system. Pediatr Surg Int 2002;18:581-585.
298. Sinha SK, Kochhar R, Rana S, et al: Intestinal pseudo-obstruction due to neurofibromatosis responding to cisapride. Indian J Gastroenterol 2000;19:83-84.

299. Smith G, Cass D: Infantile Hirschsprung disease: Is a barium enema useful? Pediatr Surg Int 1991;6:318-321.
300. So HB, Schwartz DL, Becker JM, et al: Endorectal "pull-through" without preliminary colostomy in neonates with Hirschsprung's disease. J Pediatr Surg 1980;15:470-471.
301. Solari V, Piotrowska A, Puri P: Histopathological differences between recto-sigmoid Hirschsprung's disease and total colonic aganglionosis. Pediatr Surg Int 2003;19:349-354.
302. Song Y, Li J, Li M: Bcl-2 expression in enteric neurons of Hirschsprung's disease and its significance. Shi Yan Sheng Wu Xue Bao 2002;35:155-158.
303. Soper R: Surgery for Hirschsprung's disease. AORN J 1968;8:69-81.
304. Spouge D, Baird P: Hirschsprung disease in a large birth cohort. Teratology 1985;32:171-177.
305. Stannard V, Fowler C, Robinson L, et al: Familial Hirschsprung's disease: Report of autosomal dominant and probable recessive X-linked kindreds. J Pediatr Surg 1991;26:591-594.
306. Stringel G: Extensive intestinal aganglionosis including the ileum: A new surgical technique. J Pediatr Surg 1986; 21:667-670.
307. Svensson PJ, Tapper-Persson M, Anvret M, et al: Mutations in the endothelin-receptor B gene in Hirschsprung disease in Sweden [letter]. Clin Genet 1999;55:215-217.
308. Swenson O: My early experience with Hirschsprung's disease. J Pediatr Surg 1989;24:839-844.
309. Swenson O: How the cause and cure of Hirschsprung's disease were discovered. J Pediatr Surg 1999;34:1580-1581.
310. Swenson O: Hirschsprung's disease: A review. Pediatrics 2002;109:914-918.
311. Swenson O, Bill A: Resection of rectum and rectosigmoid with preservation of the sphincter for benign spastic lesions producing megacolon. Surgery 1948;24:212-220.
312. Swenson O, Fisher J, Gherardi G: Rectal biopsy in the diagnosis of Hirschsprung's disease. Surgery 1959;45:690-695.
313. Swenson O, Rheinlander H, Diamond I: Hirschsprung's disease: A new concept of the etiology—operative results in thirty-four patients. N Engl J Med 1949;241:551-556.
314. Swenson O, Sherman J, Fisher J: Diagnosis of congenital megacolon: An analysis of 501 patients. J Pediatr Surg 1973;8:587-594.
315. Swenson O, Sherman J, Fisher J, Cohen E: The treatment and postoperative complications of congenital megacolon: A 25 year follow-up. Ann Surg 1975;182:266-273.
316. Taguchi T, Tanaka K, Ikeda K: Immunohistochemical study of neuron specific enolase and S-100 protein in Hirschsprung's disease. Virchows Arch A Pathol Anat Histopathol 1985;405:399-409.
317. Takahashi T: Pathophysiological significance of neuronal nitric oxide synthase in the gastrointestinal tract. J Gastroenterol 2003;38:421-430.
318. Talbert J, Seashore J, Ravitch M: Evaluation of a modified Duhamel operation for correction of Hirschsprung's disease. Ann Surg 1974;179:671-675.
319. Tamate S, Shiokawa C, Yamada C, et al: Manometric diagnosis of Hirschsprung's disease in the neonatal period. J Pediatr Surg 1984;19:285-288.
320. Tanaka H, Moroi K, Iwai J, et al: Novel mutations in the endothelin-B receptor gene in patients with Hirschsprung's disease and their characterization. J Biol Chem 1998; 273:11378-11383.
321. Tariq GM, Brereton RJ, Wright VM: Complications of endorectal pull-through for Hirschsprung's disease. J Pediatr Surg 1991;26:1202-1206.
322. Taxman T, Yulish B, Rothstein F: How useful is the barium enema in the diagnosis of infantile Hirschsprung's disease? Am J Dis Child 1986;140:881-884.
323. Teitelbaum D, Caniano D, Qualman S: The pathophysiology of Hirschsprung's-associated enterocolitis: Importance of histologic correlates. J Pediatr Surg 1989;24:1271-1277.
324. Teitelbaum D, Langer J: Hirschsprung's disease. In Ziegler M, Weber TR, Azizkhan RG (eds): Operative Pediatric Surgery. New York, McGraw-Hill, 2002.
325. Teitelbaum D, Qualman S, Caniano D: Hirschsprung's disease: Identification of risk factors for enterocolitis. Ann Surg 1988;207:240-244.
326. Teitelbaum D, Sonnino R, Dunaway D, et al: Rat jejunal absorptive function after intestinal transplantation: Effects of extrinsic denervation. Dig Dis Sci 1993;38: 1099-1104.
327. Teitelbaum DH, Cilley RE, Sherman NJ, et al: A decade of experience with the primary pull-through for Hirschsprung disease in the newborn period: A multicenter analysis of outcomes. Ann Surg 2000;232:372-380.
328. Teitelbaum DH, Coran AG: Enterocolitis. Semin Pediatr Surg 1998;7:162-169.
329. Teitelbaum DH, Drongowski RA, Chamberlain JN, Coran AG: Long-term stooling patterns in infants undergoing primary endorectal pull-through for Hirschsprung's disease. J Pediatr Surg 1997;32:1049-1052.
330. Tennyson V, Pham T, Toth T, Gershon M: Abnormalities of smooth muscle, basal laminae, and nerves in the aganglionic segments of the bowel of the lethal spotted mutant mouse. Anat Rec 1986;215:267-281.
331. Thomas C Jr: Posterior sphincterotomy in Hirschsprung's disease. Surg Gynecol Obstet 1967;124:365-366.
332. Thomas C Jr, Bream CA, DeConnick P: Posterior sphincterotomy and rectal myotomy in the management of Hirschsprung's disease. Ann Surg 1970;171:796-810.
333. Tittel K: Uber eine angeborene Missbildung des Dickdrmes. Wien Klin Wochenschr 1901;14:903.
334. Tomita R: Regulation of the enteric nervous system in the internal anal sphincter in Hirschsprung's disease. Hepatogastroenterology 1999;46:215-219.
335. Touloukian R, Aghajanian G, Roth R: Adrenergic hyperactivity of the aganglionic colon. J Pediatr Surg 1973;8:191-195.
336. Touloukian R, Duncan R: Acquired aganglionic megacolon in a premature infant: Report of a case. Pediatrics 1975;56:459-462.
337. Touloukian R, Morgenroth V, Roth R: Sympathetic neurotransmitter metabolism in Hirschsprung's disease. J Pediatr Surg 1975;10:593-598.
338. Towne G, Stocker J, Thompson H: Acquired aganglionosis. J Pediatr Surg 1979;14:688-690.
339. Treeves F: Idiopathic dilatation of the colon. Lancet 1898;1:276.
340. Trupp M, Arenas E, Fainzilber M, et al: Functional receptor for GDNF encoded by the c-ret proto-oncogene. Nature 1996;381:785-789.
341. Tsuto T, Obata-Tsuto HL, Iwai N, et al: Fine structure of neurons synthesizing vasoactive intestinal peptide in the human colon from patients with Hirschsprung's disease. Histochemistry 1989;93:1-8.
342. Tsuto T, Okamura H, Fukui K, et al: An immunohistochemical investigation of vasoactive intestinal polypeptide in the colon of patients with Hirschsprung's disease. Neurosci Lett 1982;34:57-62.
343. van der Zee DC, Bax KN: One-stage Duhamel-Martin procedure for Hirschsprung's disease: A 5-year follow-up study.

J Pediatr Surg 2000;35:1434-1436.
344. van Leeuwen K, Geiger JD, Barnett JL, et al: Stooling and manometric findings after primary pull-throughs in Hirschsprung's disease: Perineal versus abdominal approaches. J Pediatr Surg 2002;37:1321-1325.
345. van Leeuwen K, Teitelbaum DH, Elhalaby EA, Coran AG: The long-term follow-up of redo-pullthrough procedures for Hirschsprung's disease. J Pediatr Surg 2000;35:829-834.
346. Vanderwinden JM, Rumessen JJ, Liu H, et al: Interstitial cells of Cajal in human colon and in Hirschsprung's disease. Gastroenterology 1996;111:901-910.
347. Verheij J, Hofstra R: EDNRB, EDN3 and SOX10 and the Shah-Waardenburg syndrome. In Epstein C, Erickson R, Wynshaw-Boris A (eds): Inborn Errors of Development. New York, Oxford University Press, 2004.
348. Voskuijl W, Heijmans J, Heijmans H, et al: Use of Rome II criteria in childhood defecation disorders: Applicability in clinical and research practice. J Pediatr 2004;145:213-217.
349. Wade R, Royle N: The operative treatment of Hirschsprung's disease: A new method. Med J Aust 1927;14:137.
350. Wang G, Sun X, Wei M, Weng Y: Heart-shaped anastomosis for Hirschsprung's disease: Operative technique and long-term follow-up. World J Gastroenterol 2005;11:296-298.
351. Wang J, Lee JC, Huang F, et al: Unexpected mortality in pediatric patients with postoperative Hirschsprung's disease. Pediatr Surg Int 2004;20:525-528.
352. Wang NL, Lee HC, Yeh ML, et al: Experience with primary laparoscopy-assisted endorectal pull-through for Hirschsprung's disease. Pediatr Surg Int 2004;20:118-122.
353. Watanabe Y, Ito F, Ando H, et al: Morphological investigation of the enteric nervous system in Hirschsprung's disease and hypoganglionosis using whole-mount colon preparation. J Pediatr Surg 1999;34:445-449.
354. Watanatittan S, Suwatanaviroj A, Limprutithum T, Rattanasuwan T: Association of Hirschsprung's disease and anorectal malformation. J Pediatr Surg 1991;26:192-195.
355. Weaver L, Steiner H: The bowel habits of young children. Arch Dis Child 1984;59:649-652.
356. Weber TR, Fortuna RS, Silen ML, Dillon PA: Reoperation for Hirschsprung's disease. J Pediatr Surg 1999;34:153-156.
357. Weitzman J: Management of Hirschsprung's disease with the Swenson procedure with emphasis on long-term follow-up. Pediatr Surg Int 1986;1:100-104.
358. Weitzman J, Hanson B, Brennan L: Management of Hirschsprung's disease with the Swenson procedure. J Pediatr Surg 1972;7:157-162.
359. Wheatley M, Wesley J, Coran A, Polley T Jr: Hirschsprung's disease in adolescents and adults. Dis Colon Rectum 1990;33:622-629.
360. White F, Langer J: Circumferential distribution of ganglion cells in the transition zone of children with Hirschsprung disease. Pediatr Dev Pathol 2000;3:216-222.
361. Whitehouse E, Kernohan J: Myenteric plexus in congenital megacolon. Arch Intern Med 1948;82:75-111.
362. Wilcox DT, Kiely EM: Repeat pull-through for Hirschsprung's disease. J Pediatr Surg 1998;33:1507-1509.
363. Wildhaber B, Coran A, Teitelbaum D: Total colonic Hirschsprung's disease: A 28-year experience. J Pediatr Surg 2005;40:203-206.
364. Wildhaber B, Pakarinen M, Rintala R, et al: Posterior myotomy/myectomy for persistent stooling problems in Hirschsprung's disease. J Pediatr Surg 2004;39:920-926.
365. Williams M, Burrington J: Hirschsprung's disease complicating colon atresia. J Pediatr Surg 1993;28:637-639.
366. Wilson-Storey D, Scobie W: Impaired gastrointestinal mucosal defense in Hirschsprung's disease: A clue to the pathogenesis of enterocolitis? J Pediatr Surg 1989;24:462-464.
367. Wilson-Storey D, Scobie W, Raeburn J: Defective white blood cell function in Hirschsprung's disease: A possible predisposing factor to enterocolitis. J R Coll Surg Edinb 1988;33:185-188.
368. Wolloch Y, Dintsman M: Colonic atresia associated with Hirschsprung's disease. Isr J Med Sci 1976;12:202-207.
369. Wolman I: Intestinal motility in infancy and childhood. In Wolman I (ed): Laboratory Applications in Clinical Pediatrics. New York, McGraw-Hill, 1957, p 696.
370. Wood J: Physiology of the enteric nervous system. In Johnson L (ed): Physiology of the Gastrointestinal Tract, 2nd ed. New York, Raven Press, 1987, p 67.
371. Worby C, Vega Q, Chao H, et al: Identification and characterization of GFRalpha-3, a novel co-receptor belonging to the glial cell line-derived neurotrophic receptor family. J Biol Chem 1998;273:3502-3508.
372. Wu JS, Schoetz DJ Jr, Coller JA, Veidenheimer MC: Treatment of Hirschsprung's disease in the adult: Report of five cases. Dis Colon Rectum 1995;38:655-659.
373. Yamataka A, Nagaoka I, Miyano T, et al: Quantitative analysis of neuronal innervation in the aganglionic bowel of patients with Hirschsprung's disease. J Pediatr Surg 1995;30:260-263.
374. Yancey AG, Cromartie JE, Ford JR, et al: A modification of the Swenson technique for congenital megacolon. J Nat Med Assoc 1952;44:356-363.
375. Yanchar NL, Soucy P: Long-term outcome after Hirschsprung's disease: Patients' perspectives. J Pediatr Surg 1999;34:1152-1160.
376. Yann R, Yves A, Dominique J, et al: Improved quality of life by combined transplantation in Hirschsprung's disease with a very long aganglionic segment. J Pediatr Surg 2003;38:422-424.
377. Yokoyama J, Namba S, Ihara N, et al: Studies on the rectoanal reflex in children and in experimental animals: An evaluation of neuronal control of the rectoanal reflex. Prog Pediatr Surg 1989;24:5-20.
378. Yoneda A, Wang Y, O'Briain DS, Puri P: Cell-adhesion molecules and fibroblast growth factor signalling in Hirschsprung's disease. Pediatr Surg Int 2001;17:299-303.
379. Yunis E, Sieber W, Akers D: Does zonal aganglionosis really exist? Report of a rare variety of Hirschsprung's disease and review of the literature. Pediatr Pathol 1983;1:33-49.
380. Zaslavsky C, Loening-Baucke V: Anorectal manometric evaluation of children and adolescents postsurgery for Hirschsprung's disease. J Pediatr Surg 2003;38:191-195.
381. Ziegler H, Heitz P, Kasper M, et al: Aganglionosis of the colon: Morphologic investigations in 524 patients. Pathol Res Pract 1984;178:543-547.
382. Ziegler M, Ross AI, Bishop H: Total intestinal aganglionosis: A new technique for prolonged survival. J Pediatr Surg 1987;22:82-83.
383. Zuelzer W, Wilson J: Functional intestinal obstruction on a congenital neurogenic basis in infancy. Am J Dis Child 1948;75:40-64.

第 100 章

肠神经元发育不良（IND）

Prem Puri

历史回顾

1971 年 Meier-Ruge 首次将肠神经元发育不良描述为肠神经丛异常[21]。Puri 和他的同事第一个报道了一个阿拉伯 5 岁男孩患有直肠乙状结肠无神经节症，并且合并有降结肠和横结肠处肠神经元发育异常(IND)[33]。1983 年，Fadda 和他的同事[4] 将 IND 按临床和组织学分为两类：A 型，发病率小于 5%，特点是先天性交感神经减少或者发育不良，新生儿期出现肠道急性梗阻、腹泻和血便；B 型，占 95%，临床难以和巨结肠相鉴别，特点是黏膜下和肌间神经丛内副交感神经分布异常[41,15]。IND 伴巨结肠的是 B 型。由于 IND A 型很少有资料描述，所以一般说的 IND 是指 IND B 型。

发病机制

肠道神经系统是最大最复杂的外周神经系统[31,32]。它含有比脊髓更多的神经元细胞，调节肠道运动功能，同时维持肠道的分泌功能[5]。随着对肠神经系统认识的提高，我们意识到单纯测定肠神经节细胞是否存在还不够，重要的是要了解这些神经节细胞的数量和类型。肠肌间神经丛的形态随着年龄增大而变化，同时出现的位置也随着年龄而变化[48]。多年以来，神经管嵴发育问题主要在鸟类胚胎的分子水平上进行研究。近年研究发现，神经管嵴的发育受到基因调控[36]。目前有些基因已经明确，它们控制了肠道神经系统的形态和分化。这些基因通过突变或者缺失，影响肠道神经系统发育[5,31,32,36,48]。

很多研究者怀疑 IND 是否作为一种特殊的组织病理形态存在[16,40]。IND 的病理形态改变可以出现在正常肠管发育过程中，也可以是先天性梗阻和炎症性疾病引起的继发性改变[16,26]。另一方面，有资料表明 IND 可具有家族性，提示 IND 可能受到基因调控。Martuccielo 等[19] 曾报告过三个多发 IND 病例的家族。Moore[29] 及 Kobayashi 等[13] 发现 IND 可以发生在同卵双胞胎中。其中最有力的证据来自 IND 的动物模型。Hox11L1 是一个同源基因，为与外周神经系统发育相关基因，它与神经管嵴增殖和分化密切相关。两只不同的 Hox11L1 基因敲除老鼠 3～5 周后都出现了巨结肠。组织和免疫组织化学显示了肌间神经节细胞增生，类似于人类 IND B 型改变[8,44]。但是，对 48 例 IND 患者进行 Hox11L1 基因筛查并没有发现该基因的异常[3]。

2002 年，Von Boyen 等[47] 报道杂合子 EDNRB 缺失老鼠的肠道神经元异常，类似人类 IND 的表现。它们发现 EDNRB 基因中 301 号碱基对缺失导致肠神经元发育异常。肠神经元发育异常包括神经节增多、神经节巨大和黏膜下神经纤维过度肥大，类似人类的 IND B 型。这些发现都支持 IND 可能伴随有基因缺陷。但是 EDNRB 基因突变没有在小样本 IND 患者中检查出来[6]。

发病率

IND 可以发生在各种类型的巨结肠中。各个临床中心报告，吸引活检中局限型 IND 发病率为 0.3%～40%[2,18,22,34]。在不同国家，IND 发病率各不相同。IND 出现在无神经节肠管的近端，通常在巨结肠手术后出现持续性梗阻症状[12]。有研究者发现巨结肠患者中 25%～35% 合并 IND[4,41]。但是，其他学者认为巨结肠很少伴有IND。IND发病率不明确的主要原因是IND没有明确的诊断标准。诊断困难是因为文献报道各不相同[23,24,35]，不仅是患者的年龄，诊断样本、染色方法和所用的诊断标准也各不相同[35]。

临床表现

典型的IND临床表现是：小于1岁的婴幼儿出现便秘和腹胀病史，类似巨结肠表现。Montedonico和他的同事[28]根据直肠活检的免疫组化严重程度将IND分类。诊断标准：黏膜下神经丛增生、固有层或黏膜下血管周围出现巨大神经节、异位神经节及乙酰胆碱酯酶（acetylcholinesterase，AChE）活性增加。任何活检显示黏膜下神经丛巨大神经节和其他诊断标准中任意一条，则被认为是轻度。Montedonico和他的同事还报告严重IND患儿出现症状的年龄比轻度IND早（5.2±112个月比17.5±23个月）。在Meier-Ruge和他同事的研究中[23]发现所有局限型IND的患儿，半数年龄大于2周岁，其余半数患儿的平均年龄是18个月。

IND伴发畸形的发生率为25%～30%[19,28]。常见的伴发畸形有：肠旋转不良、巨膀胱、小结肠、肠蠕动减弱症、先天性短肠、肥厚性幽门狭窄、坏死性小肠结肠炎和Down综合征。

诊断标准

自从1971年首次描述IND以来，关于IND的诊断存在很多争议。争议的关键问题是使用哪一种组织学诊断作为确认诊断的标准。目前的诊断标准是神经节细胞增多和巨大的神经节，此外直肠黏膜活检至少满足以下一条：固有层内异位的神经节及固有层内和黏膜下血管周围AChE阳性神经纤维增多[1,2,11,15,34,36,41]。但是，Lumb和Moore[17]认为巨大神经节是正常的，因为成人结肠和直肠肿瘤病理中也可以见到巨大的神经节。Borchard等人[1]为直肠黏膜活检设立了IND诊断标准，包括两个必要条件（黏膜下神经丛增生和黏膜下血管周围AChE染色阳性神经纤维增多）和两个附加条件（肠神经元异位和固有层AChE活性增加）。我们认为神经丛增生和巨大神经节是直肠黏膜活检诊断IND的重要指标。但新生儿例外，新生儿神经丛增生属正常现象[36]。

另一个围绕IND争论的观点是组织学结果是否与年龄相关。最新的有关神经节增多的描述被认为是IND最重要的诊断标准之一，并且与年龄相关，因而引起了更多的争议。近来研究证实，整个肠道神经系统发育在出生后是一个持续的过程。Wester和他同事[48]研究了单个神经节的细胞数目和正常远端结肠黏膜下神经丛中神经节细胞的密度，发现随着年龄增长神经节细胞的密度显著下降，但是单个神经节的细胞数目保持不变。关于正常肠神经系统中神经节细胞密度的资料很少，因为有关正常肌间神经丛中神经元密度的报告差异很大，在不同的研究中有关神经元密度的报告可以相差200倍以上[9,20,46]。这一结果对诊断某些疾病如神经节细胞增多症造成了困难。Schofield和Yunis[43]报道的456例病例研究中以出现固有层中AChE染色阳性增多和神经节细胞增多（定义为每个高倍视野下黏膜下层中神经节>5个）为诊断标准，有8.3%符合此IND特征性表现。其中大多是早产未成熟儿，这提示IND和年龄以及发育情况相关。Smith[45]进一步研究了肠道神经节与年龄的相关性，发现年龄小于4周的新生儿中黏膜下神经节细胞数量明显比大年龄儿童多，这对于更好地认识肠道神经系统和区别正常变异还是病态的IND量化诊断标准都是必需的。Moore和同事[30]介绍了一种建立在神经节增多、巨大神经节、神经元成熟、异位神经元细胞和固有层内黏膜肌层或黏膜下血管外膜AChE活性增加基础上的形态学评分系统。神经节细胞增多和固有层内神经纤维AChE活性增加是评分系统的关键因素。

诊断

直肠吸引活检是诊断肠神经元分布异常的主要方法。样本必须含有足够量的黏膜下层。直肠吸引活检标本的HE染色和AChE组织化学染色（图100-1和图100-2）为诊断性评价IND提供基础。但是AChE组织化学是否足以准确诊断IND仍有争议，有人已经 1562
提出其他染色方法。Meier-Ruge和他的同事提出乳酸脱氢酶组织化学染色法[23~25]。在我们实验室里，正在采用新的神经元标志物，如还原型烟酰胺腺嘌呤二核苷酸磷酸（nicotinamide-adenine dinucleotide phos-

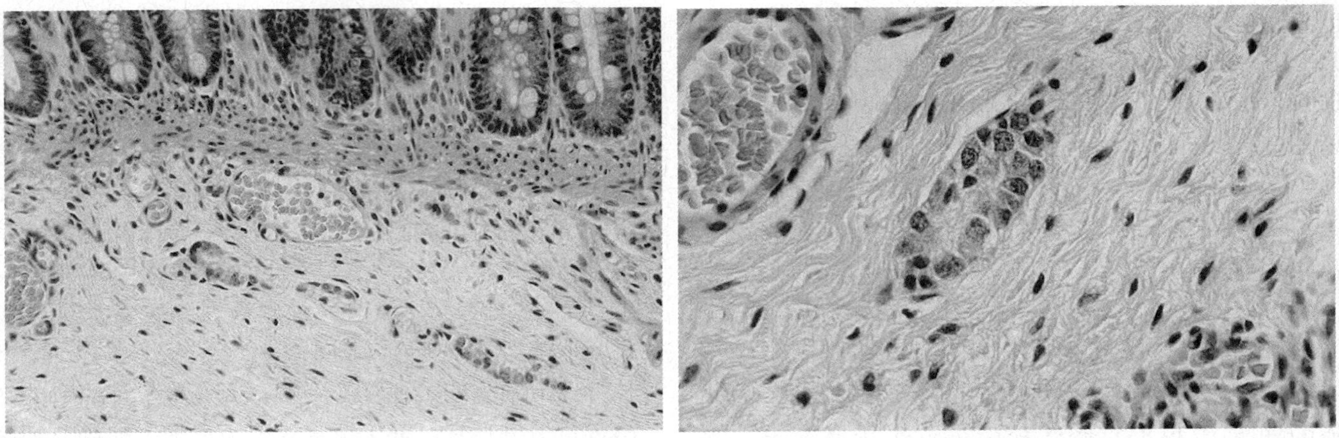

A　B

图 100-1　1 例 IND 患者直肠吸引活检 HE 染色。A. 神经节细胞增多。B. 巨大的神经节。

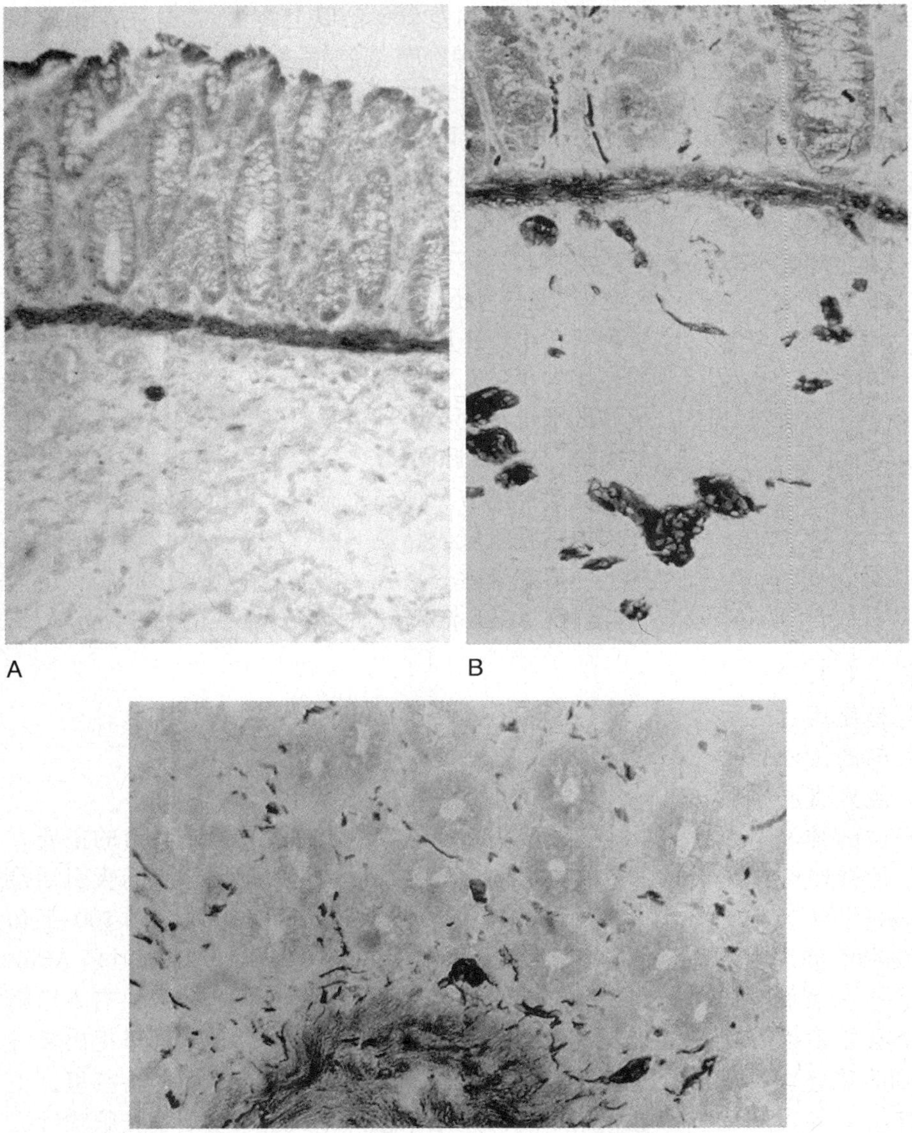

A　B　C

图 100-2　直肠吸引活检乙酰胆碱酯酶染色。A. 正常活检显示黏膜下神经丛。B. IND 患者的神经节细胞增多和巨大的神经节。C. IND患者活检标本中固有层内异位的神经节和固有层内 AChE 活性增加。

phate，NADPH）组织化学以及神经细胞黏附分子、蛋白基因产物 9.5（Protein Gene Product 9.5，PGP 9.5）、S-100、外周蛋白和突触素的抗体的免疫组化。神经节细胞计数有困难。标准的免疫组织化学技术使用的神经特异性烯醇化酶或者 PGP 9.5 也不适于肠神经系统计数，主要是因为它们不仅染色细胞体而且还能染色轴突[48]。近年来，核酸铜蓝染色可以仅染色神经元细胞体不染色轴突，可以作为用于细胞计数的染色方法。

除了直肠乙状结肠部扩张外，IND 患者进行钡剂灌肠不能显示任何特异性放射学特征。同样，肛门直肠测压可以显示直肠括约肌反射存在、消失或者不典型。

组织学发现与临床症状间的相关性

有些研究还对 IND 是否作为一个独立的组织病理学类型存在提出质疑[16,40]。其中一个原因是临床症状的严重程度与组织学异常之间相关性不强[14]。IND 的一些组织学发现可以提示是正常发育的一部分或者继发于便秘。近来，Montedonico 等[28]就 20 年内 44 例 IND 患者的临床特异性、放射结果和测压结果同组织病理学结果进行比较分析。他们将 IND 按照组织化学变化的严重程度分为两组：轻度 IND 和重度 IND。重度 IND 诊断标准：黏膜下神经丛增生、巨大神经节（大于 7 个神经节细胞）、固有层或黏膜下血管旁 AChE 活性增高和固有层内异位的神经元细胞。任何活检标本显示黏膜下神经丛内巨大神经节，再加上其他任意一条就可诊断为轻度 IND。按照他们的结果，临床诊断的重度 IND 可以在小于 1 岁的便秘和腹胀的婴幼儿中发现，肛门直肠测压缺少内括约肌松弛反射，类似于巨结肠，但是钡剂灌肠是正常的。发生重度 IND 的平均年龄为 5 个月，此结果在其他研究中也得到了证实。他们发现组织学严重性和临床表现间有某种相关性，提示 IND 是独立存在的疾病。虽然很多 IND 患者在临床上与巨结肠患者很难区分，但是 IND 患者的钡剂灌肠通常正常或者直肠乙状结肠轻度到中度扩张，但是缺少无神经节细胞症的典型狭窄段。

处理

IND B 型的治疗首先是保守治疗，可以用缓泻剂和灌肠。大多数患者临床症状可以缓解甚至消失。如果治疗 6 个月后肠症状仍持续，可以考虑行内括约肌部分切除术。病变肠管切除和拖出手术很少对 IND 患者使用。手术指征不能仅仅依靠组织病理学检查结果，而必须建立在每个患者的临床症状基础上。

预后 1563

近来，Gillick 等[7]报告了 33 例 IND 患者的治疗结果，随访 1～8 年，平均 2.4 年。21 例（64%）患者保守治疗后，效果很好，目前有正常的大便习惯。12 例（36%）患者保守治疗失败，行内括约肌部分切除术。其中 7 例患者有正常的大便习惯，2 例需要灌肠排空大便，3 例患者经过部分肌切除术后出现持续性便秘，在切除扩张的乙状结肠后大便正常。Scharli 等[41]报告 22 例 IND 患者中 13 例需行内括约肌部分切除术，90% 患者术后 3 个月取得满意的效果。

（沈涤华译　李　龙校）

参考文献

1. Borchard F, Meier-Ruge W, Wiebecke B, et al: [Disorders of the innervation of the large intestines—classification and diagnosis.] Pathologe 1991;12:171-174. German.
2. Cord-Udy CL, Smith VV, Ahmed S, et al: An evaluation of the role of suction rectal biopsy in the diagnosis of intestinal neuronal dysplasia. J Pediatr Gastroenterol Nutr 1997: 24:1-6.
3. Costa M, Fava M, Seri M, et al: Evaluation of the *HOX11L1* gene as a candidate for congenital disorders of intestinal innervation. J Med Genet 2000;37:Eq (Electronic letters).
4. Fadda B, Maier WA, Meier-Ruge W, et al: [Neuronal intestinal dysplasia: Critical 10-years' analysis of clinical and biopsy diagnosis.] Z Kinderchir 1983;38:302-312. German.
5. Gariepy CE: Intestinal motility disorders and development of the enteric nervous system. Pediatr Res 2000;49: 605-613.
6. Gath R, Goessling A, Keller KM, et al: Analysis of the *RET, GDNF, EDN3* and *EDNRB* genes in patients with intestinal neuronal dysplasia and Hirschsprung's disease. Gut 2001; 48:671-675.
7. Gillick J, Tazawa H, Puri P: Intestinal neuronal dysplasia: Results of treatment in 33 patients. J Pediatr Surg 2001: 36:777-779.
8. Hatano M, Aoki T, Dezawa M, et al: A novel pathogenesis of megacolon in *Ncx/Hox11L1* deficient mice. J Clin Invest 1997;100:795-801.

9. Ikeda K, Goto S, Nagasaki A, Taguchi T: Hypogenesis of intestinal ganglion cells: A rare cause of intestinal obstruction simulating aganglionosis. Z Kinderchir 1988;43: 52-53.
10. Kapur RP: Neuronal dysplasia: A controversial pathological correlate of intestinal pseudo-obstruction. Am J Med Genet 2003;122:287-293.
11. Kobayashi H, Hirakawa H, Puri P: What are the diagnostic criteria for intestinal neuronal dysplasia? Pediatr Surg Int 1995;10:459-464.
12. Kobayashi H, Hirakawa H, Surana R, et al: Intestinal neuronal dysplasia is a possible cause of persistent bowel symptoms after pull-through operation for Hirschsprung's disease. J Pediatr Surg 1995;30:253-259.
13. Kobayashi H, Mohamed A, Puri P: Intestinal neuronal dysplasia in twins. J Pediatr Gastroenterol Nutr 1996;22: 398-401.
14. Koletzko S, Ballauff A, Hadziselimovic F, Enck P: Is histological diagnosis of neuronal intestinal dysplasia related to clinical and manometric findings in constipated children? Results of a pilot study. J Pediatr Gastroenterol Nutr 1993; 17:59-65.
15. Koletzko S, Jesch I, Faus-Kebetaler T, et al: Rectal biopsy for diagnosis of intestinal dysplasia in children: A prospective multicentre study on inter-observer variation and clinical outcome. Gut 1999;44:853-861.
16. Lake BD: Intestinal neuronal dysplasia: Why does it only occur in parts of Europe? Virchows Arch 1995;426:537-539.
17. Lumb PD, Moore L: Are giant ganglia a reliable marker of intestinal neuronal dysplasia type B (IND B). Virchow's Arch 1998;432:103-106.
18. Martucciello G, Caffarena PE, Lerone M, et al: Neuronal intestinal dysplasia: Clinical experience in Italian patients. Eur J Pediatr Surg 1994;4:287-292.
19. Martucciello G, Torre M, Pini Prato A, et al: Associated anomalies in intestinal neuronal dysplasia. J Pediatr Surg 2002;37:219-223.
20. Meier-Ruge W, Morger R, Rehbein F: Das hypoganglionare Megakolon als Begleitkrankheit bei Morbus Hirschsprung. Z Kinderchir 1970;8:254-264.
21. Meier-Ruge W: Uber ein Ekrankungsbild des colon mit Hirschsprung-Symptomatik. Vehr Dtsch Ges Pathol 1971; 55:506-510.
22. Meier-Ruge W: Epidemiology of congenital innervation defects of the distal colon. Virchows Arch A Pathol Anat 1992;420:171-177.
23. Meier-Ruge W, Gambazzi F, Kaufeler RE, et al: The neuropathological diagnosis of neuronal intestinal dysplasia (NID B). Eur J Pediatr Surg 1994;4:267-273.
24. Meier-Ruge W, Bronnimann PB, Gambazzi F, et al: Histopathological criteria for intestinal neuronal dysplasia of the submucous plexus (type B). Virchows Arch 1995; 426:549-556.
25. Meier-Ruge W: Is intestinal neuronal dysplasia really a myth or an invented disease? Pediatr Surg Int 1995;10:439.
26. Milla PJ, Smith VV: Intestinal neuronal dysplasia. J Pediatr Gastroenterol Nutr 1993;17:356-357.
27. Miyazaki E, Ohshiro K, Puri P: NADPH-diaphorase histochemical staining of suction rectal biopsies in the diagnosis of Hirschsprung's disease and allied disorders. Pediatr Surg Int 1998;13:464-467.
28. Montedonico S, Acevedo S, Fadda B: Clinical aspects of intestinal neuronal dysplasia. J Pediatr Surg 2002;37:1772-1774.
29. Moore SW, Kaschula ROC, Cywes S: Familial and genetic aspects of intestinal neuronal dysplasia and Hirschsprung's disease. Pediatr Surg Int 1993;8:406-409.
30. Moore SW, Laing D, Kaschula RD, Cywes S: A histological grading system for the evaluation of co-existing NID with Hirschsprung's disease. Eur J Pediatr Surg 1994;4: 293-297.
31. Newgreen D, Young HM: Enteric nervous system: Development and developmental disturbances: I. Pediatr Dev Pathol 2002;5:224-247.
32. Newgreen D, Young HM: Enteric nervous system: Development and developmental disturbances: II. Pediatr Dev Pathol 2002;5:329-349.
33. Puri P, Lake BD, Nixon HH, et al: Neuronal colonic dysplasia: An unusual association of Hirschsprung's disease. J Pediatr Surg 1977;12:681-685.
34. Puri P: Variant Hirschsprung's disease. J Pediatr Surg 1997; 32:149-157.
35. Puri P, Wester T: Intestinal neuronal dysplasia. Semin Pediatr Surg 1998;7:181-186.
36. Puri P, Shinkai T: Pathogenesis of Hirschsprung's disease and variants: Recent progress. Semin Pediatr Surg 2004; 13:18-24.
37. Puri P, Rolle U: Variant Hirschsprung's disease. Semin Pediatr Surg 2004;13:293-299.
38. Rolle U, Nemeth L, Puri P: Nitrergic innervation of the normal gut and in motility disorders of childhood. J Pediatr Surg 2002;37:551-567.
39. Rolle U, Piotrowska AP, Puri P: Abnormal vasculature in intestinal neuronal dysplasia. Pediatr Surg Int 2003;19: 345-348.
40. Sacher P, Briner J, Hanimann B: Is neuronal intestinal dysplasia (NID) a primary disease or a secondary phenomenon? Eur J Pediatr Surg 1993;3:228-230.
41. Scharli AF: Neuronal intestinal dysplasia. Pediatr Surg Int 1992;7:2-7.
42. Schimpl G, Uray E, Ratschek M, et al: Constipation and intestinal neuronal dysplasia type B: A clinical follow-up study. J Pediatr Gastroenterol Nutr 2004;38:308-311.
43. Schofield DE, Yunis EJ: Intestinal neuronal dysplasia. J Pediatr Gastroenterol Nutr 1991;12:182-189.
44. Shirasawa S, Yunker AM, Roth KA, et al: *Enx (Hox11L1)*-deficient mice develop myenteric neuronal hyperplasia and megacolon. Nat Med 1997;3:646-650.
45. Smith VV: Isolated intestinal neuronal dysplasia: A descriptive pattern or a distinct clinicopathological entity. In Hadziselimovic F, Herzog B (eds): Inflammatory bowel disease and morbus Hirschsprung. Dordrecht, The Netherlands, Kluwer Academic, 1992, pp 203-214.
46. Smith VV: Intestinal neuronal density in childhood: A baseline for the objective assessment of hypo- and hyperganglionosis. Pediatr Pathol 1993;13:225-237.
47. Von Boyen GBT, et al: Abnormalities of the enteric nervous system in heterozygous endothelin B receptor deficient (spotting lethal) rats resembling intestinal neuronal dysplasia. Gut 2002;51:414-419.
48. Wester T, O'Briain DS, Puri P: Notable postnatal alterations in the myenteric plexus of normal human bowel. Gut 1999; 44:666-674.

第 101 章

肛门直肠畸形

Alberto Peña 和 Marc A. Levitt

历史

566 历史上，外科医生们一直在尝试治疗患有肛门直肠畸形的婴儿和儿童，但描述这类患者的文字记载非常少，这可能是因为大多数患者未经治疗就已经死亡了[45,58]。成功的治疗方法包括用手指或刀尖[17]戳破阻塞的膜，并进而在会阴部[4]或骶骨窝做一切口寻找肠管。1783 年进行了首例腹股沟结肠造口术[21,36]，但大多数婴儿死亡，结肠造口术被认为是最后的处理手段。1835 年 Amussat 将肠管通过会阴部切口拖出与皮肤缝合[3]，因而能避免早期手术常见的狭窄。18 世纪和 19 世纪，一些作者建议如果在下面没有见到肠管则行开腹手术[26,31,38,62]。在 20 世纪中叶，一期的腹部会阴手术变得非常流行[42,54]，并常常包括直肠乙状结肠切除。这些报告出现后不久，Stephens 描述了一种术式，强调直肠应从耻骨直肠肌之间通过[60]。直到 20 世纪 80 年代早期，这一术式加上其改良术式一直是标准手术方式，但这种术式在接近后尿道部位的切割是盲切的。为了增加会阴部切口的长度以获得更好的暴露，最终促使后矢状肛门直肠成形术的形成[20]，由于可以完全暴露括约肌的复合肌群并能清晰显示直肠和尿道系统以及周围重要结构的关系，这一手术方式被迅速地推广开来。

发病率

发生肛门直肠畸形的原因仍不清楚。尽管在某些地区可能更为常见，但大多数作者报道世界范围内的平均发病率是每 5000 个活产儿中有 1 例[11]。一些家庭有遗传易感性，肛门直肠畸形可以在连续几代人中都有发生。另外，肛门闭锁可发生在一些综合征中[51,66]。男性略多发[60]。

女性患儿中最常见的畸形是直肠前庭瘘，而男性患儿中最常见的畸形是直肠尿道瘘。泄殖腔畸形要比原先认为的更多见，可能因为其中许多以前被误诊为直肠阴道瘘[53]。不伴瘘管的肛门闭锁约占肛门直肠畸形的 5%，有趣的是，其中一半同时有 Down 综合征。在同时患有 Down 综合征和肛门直肠畸形的患者中，95% 有这种缺陷[66]。

分类

表 101-1 为一个纯描述性的分类系统，对治疗和预后有一定指导意义。

胚胎学

胚胎中的泄殖腔是一腔隙，后肠、原肠、尿囊和

表 101-1 肛门直肠畸形分类

男性	女性
会阴瘘	会阴瘘
直肠尿道瘘	前庭瘘
球部	泄殖腔存留
前列腺部	共同通道 <3 cm
直肠膀胱瘘（膀胱颈）	共同通道 >3 cm
不伴瘘的肛门闭锁	不伴瘘的肛门闭锁
直肠闭锁	直肠闭锁
复杂畸形	复杂畸形

后来的中肾管均开口于此。泄殖腔最初在妊娠21天左右形成，呈“U”形，尿囊位于前部，后肠居后。中间的隔膜向下生长，并与侧壁皱褶融合（Rathke皱襞）直至融入泄殖腔膜。在为时6周的过程中，前
1567 方形成了泌尿生殖腔，后方形成了肛门直肠腔。生殖结节的快速发育改变了泄殖腔的形态和泄殖腔膜的方向，使泄殖腔膜向后转移。在妊娠第7周，泄殖腔膜分裂产生两个开口：泌尿生殖开口和肛门开口[19,61,68]。同时围绕直肠的肌肉也在发育，妊娠6~7周时已可看到[32]；到第9周，所有相关的结构都已成形。在这一阶段，男女性外生殖器的分化还没有开始。

伴发畸形

多数肛门闭锁患儿伴有影响其他系统的一个或多个畸形[9,57]，发生率为50%~60%。发生畸形的位置越高则伴发畸形的种类越多。许多畸形是偶然被发现的，但有些，如心血管缺陷，可以是致命的。

心血管异常

接近1/3的肛门闭锁患儿可出现心血管异常[9,24,64,65]，但仅10%的患儿需要治疗。最常见的病变是房间隔缺损和动脉导管未闭，其次是Fallot四联症和室间隔缺损。大动脉转位和左心发育不全综合征少见。

胃肠道畸形

多种并发的胃肠道畸形已有描述，约10%的患者可有食管气管异常[24,57]，由闭锁或旋转不良引起的十二指肠梗阻的发生率为1%~2%[24,44]。在作者研究的1710例病例中发现3例先天性巨结肠，这一伴发症的过度诊断可能是由于在肛门直肠畸形患者中有较高的便秘发生率。

脊髓和脊椎畸形

常见的腰骶椎异常有半椎体、脊柱侧凸、蝶样脊柱和半骶骨畸形。最常见的脊髓问题是脊髓栓系[30,35]，但脊髓脂肪瘤、脊髓空洞症和脊髓脊膜膨出也很常见。越复杂的肛门直肠畸形，越容易伴发相关的脊髓脊椎异常。肛门直肠畸形患者中约1/3~1/2可发现（通过超声或磁共振）这些问题[4,12,55,63]。这些病变中多少具有临床意义和哪些需要预防仍不清楚[33,67]。骶骨缺陷，尤其是半骶椎畸形，伴肛门闭锁和骶前肿块称为Currarino三联症[18]，具有明显的家族性遗传倾向[1,5,15]。骶骨比例是一个有价值的预后评估工具（图101-1），因为它量化了骶骨发育不良的程度。骶骨比例小于0.3的患者，排便不能自制，骶骨比例接近1.0通常预后良好。

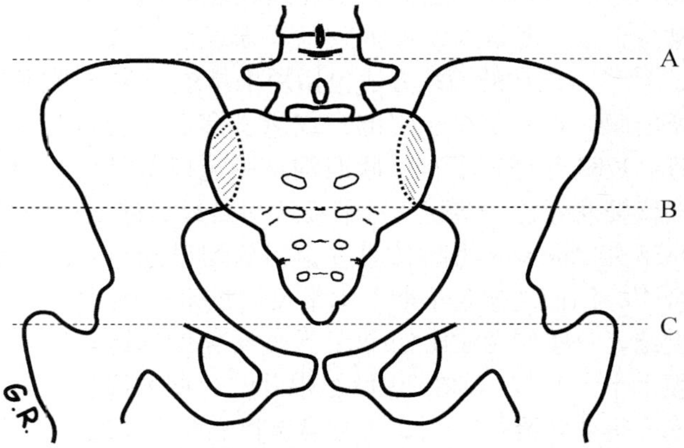

A 正常比例：BC/AB=0.74

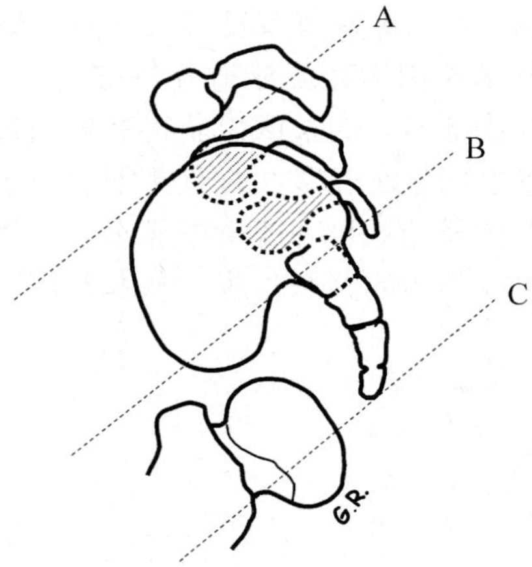

B 正常比例：BC/AB=0.77

图101-1 前后位（A）和侧位（B）的骶骨比例

泌尿生殖系统异常

泌尿生殖系统异常以泌尿系统异常为主。改进的成像方法使其显示上、下尿路异常的范围有所增加。一些研究表明其在肛门直肠畸形患者中的发病率为 1/3～1/2，并随着肛门直肠畸形复杂程度的增加而增加[39,44]。膀胱输尿管反流是最常见的畸形，肾发育不全或发育不良是第二常见的异常情况[16,39]。男性肛门闭锁患者中隐睾的发生率为 3%～19%[16,28]，尿道下裂的发生率约为 5%[28]。

68

女性生殖系统异常

肛门直肠畸形患者中相关的妇科畸形已经引起极大的关注。在新生儿期，阴道积液能导致尿道梗阻或阴道积脓。青春期月经排出受阻时可证实苗勒氏管畸形存在。苗勒氏管结构的缺失，可以导致大量的腹腔积液、腹膜炎或闭经。不对称的月经排出梗阻可由任何水平的解剖结构异常引起，如阴道梗阻、宫颈闭锁或有一盲端的半阴道[35,69]。约 1/3 的患者会出现子宫畸形（主要是双角子宫和双子宫）和阴道畸形（尤其是阴道隔膜[35]）。为了预防近期和远期的后遗症，在新生儿期、定型修复时以及造瘘口关闭时需要对存在阴道积液的患儿做生殖系统的检查。这些畸形对产科方面的影响仍不清楚。

肛门直肠的解剖和病理生理学

排便控制指察觉和保留胃肠气及粪便直到适当的时候排出的能力。这是括约肌功能、肛门直肠感觉和结肠运动之间复杂的相互作用的结果，在肛门直肠畸形的患儿中所有这些因素均会被影响。

括约肌机制

传统意义上的括约肌肌群包括：外括约肌的自主横纹肌、肛提肌和非自主的平滑肌（内括约肌）。这些肌肉受阴部神经支配，包括支配外括约肌的运动和肛周皮肤的感觉。阴部神经源自于 S2 至 S4 的骶神经丛根；同时，经过勃起神经的自主神经系统也起源于脊髓的 S2 至 S4 段。后矢状径路已证明外括约肌为旁正中方向走向。另外，外括约肌肌肉之间的边界是融合的，因此 ，外括约肌之间的成分无法被区别。在后矢状解剖时，通过一组被称为复合肌的垂直横纹肌纤维可辨认肛提肌和外括约肌的接合点。电刺激肛提肌组的上端可向前牵拉直肠，刺激复合肌（垂直纤维）可提升肛门，刺激外括约肌的正中旁纤维可关闭肛门。肛门直肠畸形患儿的横纹肌发育程度千差万别，从几乎完全正常的肌肉到完全没有肌肉。在非常高位的畸形中，直肠可位于漏斗状肌肉结构的上部；在较低的畸形中，直肠可穿过肌性隧道的基底。

在正常的个体中，内括约肌的特征和准确的界限还没有被精确地描述过。在肛门直肠畸形患者中，这一结构还没有被重视，也很少有人试图对其做出科学的评估[27]。

感觉和本体感受

在正常情况下，肛管是一个精敏的感觉区域，它使人能将固体与液体，甚至是与气体区分开。绝大多数肛门直肠畸形的患儿出生时没有肛管，因此他们不能像正常人那样进行区分。然而，有另一种感觉被称为本体感受，其被描述为一种模糊的感觉，当直肠扩张时被感觉到，并可能与围绕直肠的自主肌的伸展同时发生。似乎本体感受在多数肛门直肠畸形患者中出现的程度不同，其临床意义是显著的。患腹泻时这些患者无法控制排便。当他们能形成固体大便并能学习去感知大便时，就有能力做排便训练。

结肠和直肠乙状结肠的运动

正常情况下，胃内容物全部通过小肠需要 3～6 小时。小肠内容物以液体的形式进入盲肠。排泄物进入直肠并成形（固体）大约需要 20～24 小时。直肠乙状结肠作为粪便的储存袋，可以储留粪便的时间不同。肛管（齿状线以下）因周围括约肌机制的作用通常是排空的。然而，偶尔有蠕动波将排泄物推向肛门。直肠内容物向远端运动并触及肛管精敏的感觉组织，从而为机体提供关于直肠内容物的性质（气体、固体或液体）的有价值的信息。根据周围的社会情境，人体可让直肠内容物排泄，或收缩括约肌将粪便或气体推回到直肠内。直肠的扩张产生一种模糊的充盈感或甚至可产生痉挛性疼痛（本体感受），但并不提供有关内容物物理特征的具体信息。我们对于触发直肠乙状结肠蠕动以排空内容物的机制了解甚少，但已清楚直肠充盈的程度起非常重要的作用。因此，当到了一定时间，直肠乙状结肠为了排空肠腔产生蠕动波。机体能运用自主括约肌暂时地制止这一过程。当
1569 个人意愿允许粪便排出时，括约肌松弛，机体等待下一次的蠕动波。正常的排泄使得直肠乙状结肠大量排空，随之是另一次大约 24 小时的静息期，期间直肠乙状结肠再次作为一个储存袋。然而，直肠乙状结肠动力的重要性及其与排便关联性常被大大低估。

肛门直肠畸形患儿存在许多直肠乙状结肠动力紊乱。外科手术使患儿保留了直肠乙状结肠，但也导致一部分患儿便秘。便秘是最主要的功能性后遗症之一，可能是由直肠乙状结肠动力不足所致。如果不治疗，动力不足是终身存在并可逐渐加重的，最后形成巨乙状结肠。在极端的例子中，可以产生粪便嵌塞和大便失禁或溢出性假性失禁。低位肛门直肠畸形的患儿便秘更加严重。已知动力不足是导致巨乙状结肠恶性循环的开始，避免动力不足-便秘-巨乙状结肠的循环是小儿外科医生的职责。对患者进行密切随访加上饮食、物理和药物治疗可以预防这一循环。

不管什么原因，丧失直肠乙状结肠的肛门直肠畸形患儿会遭受完全相反的情况（也就是腹泻倾向）。这些儿童没有储存能力，对水果、蔬菜高度敏感，最糟的是形成失禁。

临床表现和初期治疗

图 101-2 显示了制定男性患儿初期治疗决策的流程。

当一位临床医生诊治患有肛门直肠畸形的新生男婴时必须做彻底的会阴部检查，这通常能提供有关患儿畸形类型的最重要的线索（图 101-3）。不要在胎儿出生后 24 小时内做进行结肠造口术或一期手术的决定，这一点很重要。推迟的理由是胎粪通过瘘孔排出需要很大的腔内压力。在这些婴儿中，胎粪通过瘘管排出是瘘管定位最有价值的指征。如果在会阴部看到胎粪，则是直肠会阴瘘的证据。如果尿中有胎粪，则显然可诊断为直肠尿道瘘（见图 101-3）。

因出生后 24 小时内直肠是萎瘪的，所以影像学检查还不能显示其真正的解剖结构。克服围绕直肠下部的括约肌的肌张力需要很大的腔内压力，因此，影像学检查做得过早（24 小时内）很容易出现“非常高位直肠”的表现，并做出错误的诊断。

在最初 24 小时，应给予婴儿静脉补液、抗生素，并使用鼻胃管减压以防止气道吸入。临床医生应利用这些时间排除伴发畸形的存在，如心脏畸形、食管闭锁和尿道问题。应做超声心动图检查，还应检查是否存在食管闭锁。应摄腰骶椎平片以排除半椎体和骶骨畸形。脊髓超声有助于筛查脊髓栓系和其他的脊髓问题。腹部超声检查可排除肾盂积水。

如果婴儿有会阴部瘘，则可施行肛门成形术而无需在 48 小时内做保护性的结肠造口术。

如果 24 小时后，在会阴部或尿中没有见到胎粪，我们建议婴儿取俯卧位做水平侧位 X 线投照[40]。如果直肠内的气体位于尾骨下方，患儿情况良好且没有

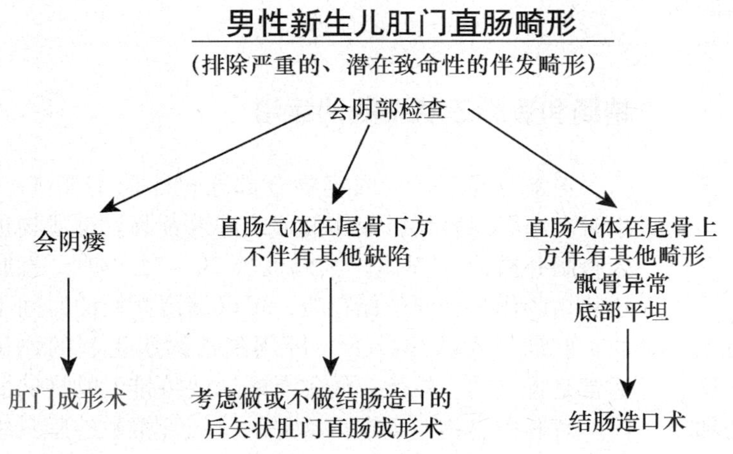

图 101-2　男性新生儿肛门直肠畸形的治疗流程图。

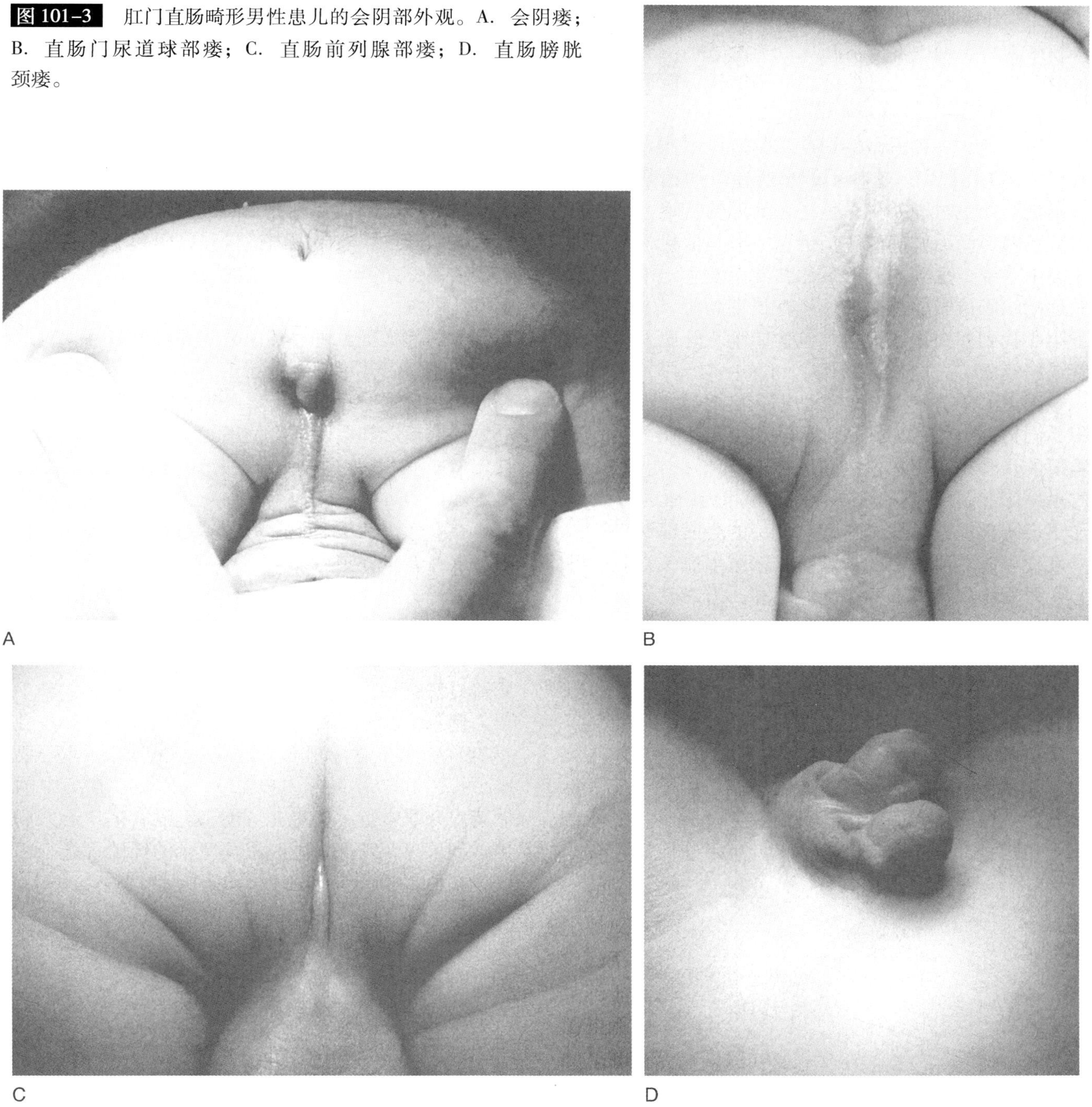

图 101-3　肛门直肠畸形男性患儿的会阴部外观。A. 会阴瘘；B. 直肠门尿道球部瘘；C. 直肠前列腺部瘘；D. 直肠膀胱颈瘘。

严重的伴发畸形，则根据外科医生的经验，可考虑在不做保护性结肠造口术的情况下进行后矢状径路手术。更保守的治疗方法是结肠造口术加二期的成形修复手术。

如果在尾骨上方看到直肠内气体，患儿尿中出现胎粪，有严重的伴发畸形，并且有骶骨异常或平坦的底部，则推荐做结肠造口术，主要的修复手术推迟为二期手术。如果患儿体重增加正常，二期手术可在 4 1570
周后进行。

在患儿一个月时做成形修复手术有很多优点，包括缩短腹部造口时间、减少结肠造口术关闭时远近端肠管大小的差别、肛门扩张更容易，并且会阴部操作所引起的疼痛不会留下明显的心理性后遗症。另外，至少在理论上，早期将直肠放在正确的部位可能有益于在生长中获得局部感觉的潜能。

必须将早期手术的潜在优点与经验不足的外科医生由于不熟悉小婴儿盆腔微细解剖结构可能造成的缺点进行权衡。

现在存在一种不做保护性结肠造口术而直接修复畸形的倾向[2,23,37]。这种不做结肠造口的修复手术令人担忧之处是对于外科医生正在处理的特定类型的肛门直肠畸形尚无精确的解剖信息。在其他机构进行的这类手术中，见到的最严重的并发症发生于术前没有
1571 做远端结肠造影的患儿中。当查找直肠时，术者可能不小心找到并损伤尿道、异位输尿管、膀胱颈、输精管或精囊腺[29]。

图 101–4 显示了制定女性患儿初期治疗决策的流程。同男性患儿一样，做出诊断和决定治疗方案时最重要的步骤是会阴部检查（图 101–5）。最初的 24 小时也用来排除重要的、严重的、可能致命的伴发畸形。会阴部检查可显示仅存在单一的会阴部开口，这一发现可确立泄殖腔的诊断。临床医生应该知晓这种患儿并发泌尿道畸形的可能性很高，需对其做泌尿系统评估，并应通过超声排除阴道积液。

这类患儿需要结肠造瘘。尽量在近端结肠做造口非常重要，这使得畸形纠治手术不受结肠造口的影响。也就是说，外科医生必须留出足够长的远端直肠乙状结肠，使拖出手术能顺利进行。在结肠造口术中，如存在阴道积液，则需要做引流。如果阴道积液没有达到膀胱上方的腹壁，可用橡胶管引流。这些患儿中相当一部分有双半阴道，术者必须确认插入阴道积液的引流管，使两个半阴道都得到引流。偶尔，术者必须在阴道隔膜上开窗，用一根管引流两侧的阴道。阴道积液过多时甚至可以引起呼吸窘迫；可以通过将阴道壁直接向腹壁开放引流这些巨大的阴道，这如同没有引流管的阴道造口术。罕见的一些有泄殖腔的患儿由于其共同通道几乎闭锁，导致膀胱不能排空。这种情况下，婴儿可能需要做膀胱造瘘术或耻骨上膀胱切开术。建议做内镜检查以明确泄殖腔婴儿的解剖结构，尤其是共同通道的长度，这将有助于制定手术计划。

会阴部检查也可以发现会阴部瘘的存在，对这种类型的畸形患儿不需要做结肠造口，而是直接施行一期肛门成形术。有时，外科医生可能面对早产儿或有严重伴发畸形和会阴部瘘的患儿。对于这种病例，可行瘘口扩张以便于结肠排空，同时延迟进行修复成形术。

在女性患儿中，最常见的畸形是前庭瘘，这种畸形可以在新生儿期纠治而无需保护性的结肠造口术。遗憾的是，在这类患儿中，这些手术是并发症的最常见的来源。应该根据将要施行该手术的外科医生的经验来决定是直接纠治这种畸形还是进行结肠造口。结肠造口术仍是保护这些患儿最有效的方法。

偶尔（少于 10% 的病例）看不到瘘口，并且观察 24 小时后仍没有出现胎粪。这一小组患儿需要做水平投影侧位 X 线片。如果 X 线片显示直肠中的气体离皮肤非常近，则患儿可能患有没有瘘口的肛门闭锁。如果患儿情况良好，根据医生的经验可施行一期

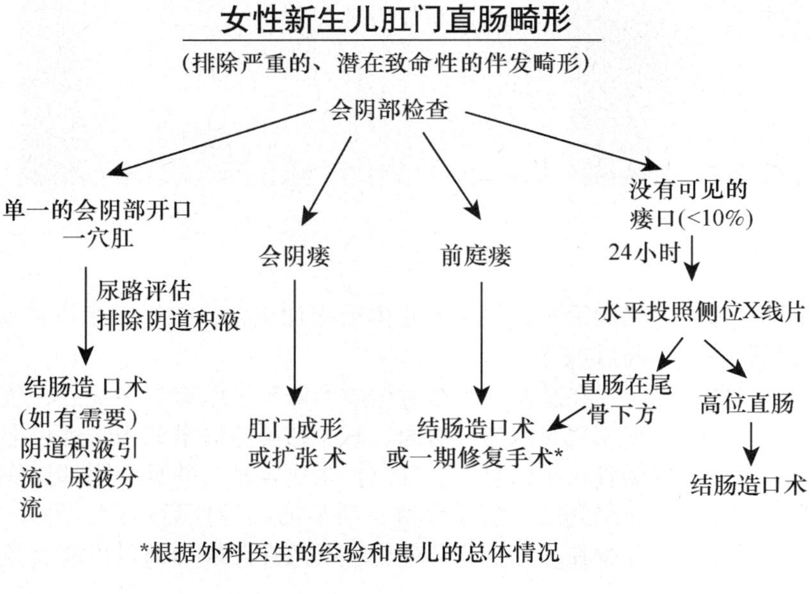

图 101–4 女性新生儿肛门直肠畸形的治疗流程图。

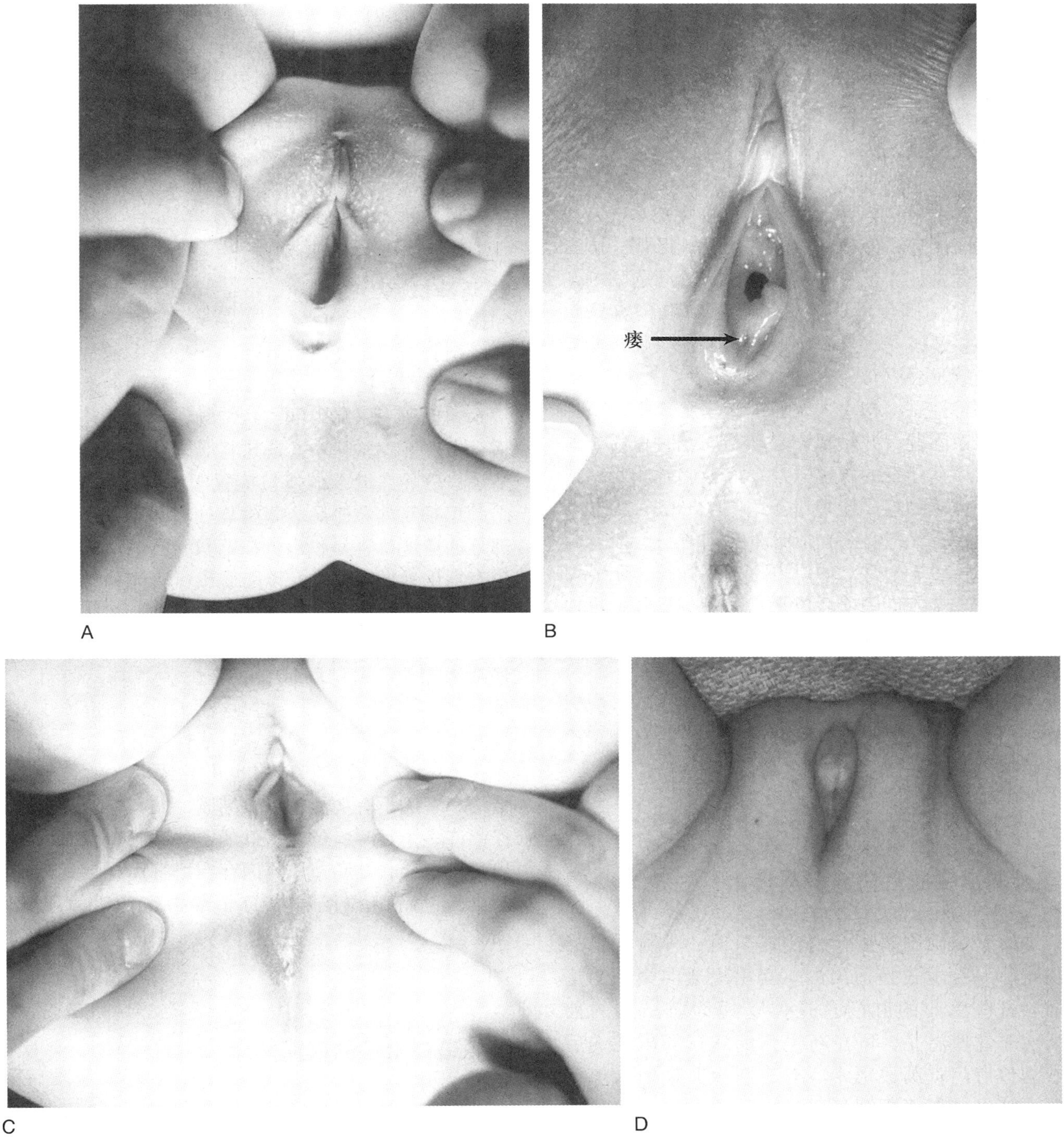

图 101-5　肛门直肠畸形女性患儿的会阴部外观。A. 会阴瘘；B. 前庭瘘；C. 一穴肛；D. 非常高位的一穴肛，平坦的底部。

手术，无需结肠造口。许多这些没有瘘口的患儿也可有 Down 综合征[66]。

有时，伴有会阴瘘或前庭瘘的患儿由于其他医学原因而非常虚弱，可以仅做瘘口的扩张使结肠减压。这些患儿可以晚些时候做纠治手术。是做保护性结肠造口的同时做纠治术，还是以一期的方式进行修补也

是根据术者的经验决定的。当患儿晚些时候接受一期
1572 前庭或会阴瘘修复手术时，应该提前24小时进行严格的术前肠道灌洗。术中应做中心静脉插管，术后禁食7天，并给予肠外营养。在我们的研究中，这种类型的患儿没有感染发生。

随着围生医学的进步和产前超声技术的发展，肛门直肠畸形在产前更容易被发现。超声检查发现诸如扩张的直肠或阴道积液，或显示有伴发畸形如一侧肾缺失、脊椎异常如半骶骨畸形或其他矫形问题如一侧桡骨缺失，会使围生学医生怀疑胎儿有肛门直肠畸形。随着科技的发展，这一领域的诊断甚至是对胎儿的干预将继续发展[13,56]。

1573 无论哪种性别，初次入院后应该用腹部超声评估伴发的泌尿系问题，并做超声心动图。此时也便于做脊髓超声以评估伴发的脊髓异常，如脊髓脊膜膨出或脊髓栓系。这样的超声检查对于这些畸形是一种非常好的筛查性检查，但必须在骶骨骨化前进行，骶骨骨化出现在出生后3个月。如果更迟进行筛查，则需要磁共振检查。从骶骨的前后位平片和侧位平片，可以计算出骶骨比例，骶骨比例有助于预测排便控制的预后（见图101-1）。

在进行肛门成形或结肠造口的术前评估时，应保留静脉内补液，并放置鼻胃管使胃减压，禁食。手术时给予抗生素。

局限性的后矢状肛门直肠成形术

当诊断为低位畸形（会阴瘘）时，外科医生必须决定哪一种术式是适当的。当出现通向会阴的瘘管时，这些患儿的肛门总是位于括约肌结构的前部。对于这些患儿，可在新生儿期施行局限性的后矢状切口肛门直肠成形术。对于新生儿期因为疾病和明显伴发畸形而无法经受这一手术的婴儿，应当先做瘘口扩张并制定将来的修复计划。在出生48小时内做这一手术是有利的，因为此时胎粪是无菌的。当这一手术被延迟到几个月后施行时，为避免会阴部感染，建议做完善的肠道准备，包括术后禁食和肠外营养。

对于局限性的后矢状肛门成形术而言，应将患儿置于俯卧位。对于男性患者，插入导尿管。直肠的远端紧贴后尿道，必须避免尿道损伤。沿着瘘管开口在黏膜皮肤交界处用6-0丝线缝数针。在正中切开分离后方括约肌，沿瘘口继续切开，当牵引瘘口向上暴露肠管时，沿肠管周围切开分离肠管，并重新将其放置在外括约肌的界限内，用细的可吸收线在有轻微张力的情况下缝合黏膜与皮肤，重建会阴体。

结肠造口术

结肠造口术在高位畸形的新生儿中常常作为第一期手术进行。降结肠造口术是相对容易的造口术。这一术式也留下了完整的乙状结肠以用于重建术。手术适合做左下腹斜切口。通过将肠管开口于切口两端使造瘘口分隔。近端的造口应置于乙状结肠的起始部，结肠正好从其左侧后腹膜附着处离开。置于结肠活动部分的造瘘口容易脱出。在乙状结肠上部的远端造口应有意识地做得偏小，以防脱出。应充分地灌洗远端肠段，清除所有胎粪。

结肠造口能导致严重的并发症，所以必须非常仔细地操作。横结肠造口经常发生脱垂，使得清洁远端结肠困难，也使通过远端加压结肠造影了解远端的直肠尿道解剖情况具有挑战性，并可能引起结肠穿孔[25]。这样的结肠造口也可导致巨大的直肠乙状结肠和左侧没有功能的细小结肠，尤其是当结肠造口保留许多个月时。位置太低的乙状结肠造口可限制拖出手术。袢状结肠造口可因存在瘘管而导致远端尿流污染，也可因粪便溢出而导致扩张的巨直肠乙状结肠。

结肠造口术后的后期处理

在重建前，通过远端结肠高压造瘘口造影（肠袢造影）了解肛门直肠畸形的解剖结构[25]。还没有做膀胱尿道造影的患儿，必要的信息可通过远端造瘘口
造影获得（图101-6和101-7）。当进行造瘘肠袢造 15
影时，需要耐心等远端直肠慢慢扩张。盆腔肌肉通常是收缩的，并因此压迫远端直肠，使远端直肠最初在耻骨尾骨线呈扁平状。轻微地加压，这一扁平线开始膨胀，并且在这一部位，检查者能观察到直肠真正的范围和直肠尿道瘘的存在情况。

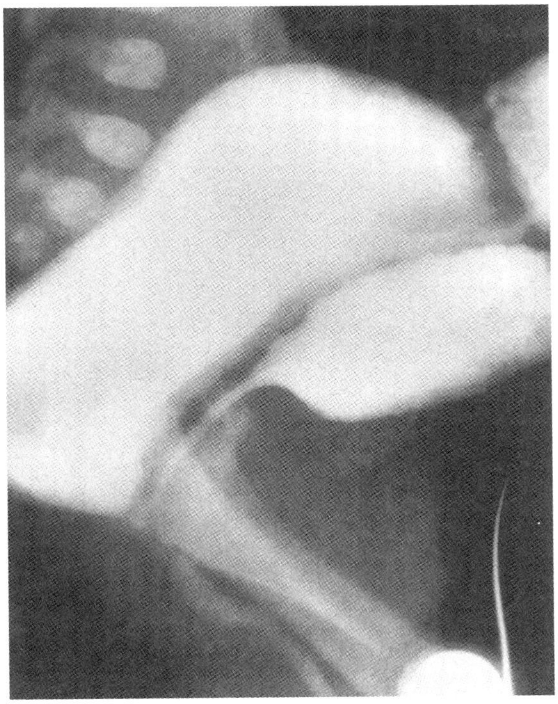

图 101-6　远端结肠造影显示直肠尿道球部瘘。

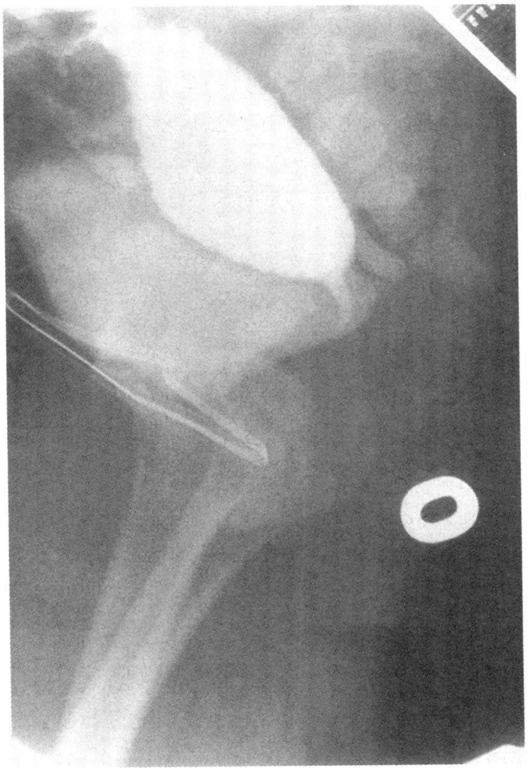

图 101-7　远端结肠造影显示直肠膀胱颈瘘。

肛门直肠重建术

基本原则

所有缺陷都能通过后矢状手术被纠治。接近10% 的男性患儿（直肠膀胱颈瘘）和约 40% 存在一穴肛畸形的女性患儿可能另外需要进行经腹的手术，可通过腹腔镜或开腹游离高位直肠或阴道。因为存在不同的畸形，术者必须准备探查解剖区域，并根据具体的解剖特点应用不同的技术。

将患儿置于俯卧位，骨盆抬高。必须特别注意在所有患儿身体受压部位加衬软垫。在两侧胸三角凹前必须用二个小的垫子，以防颈部和肩部过度伸展。在患儿置体位前插入 Foley 导管，导管有时经瘘管进入直肠而没有进入膀胱，为了避免放错，术者可在 Foley 导管的顶部插入起引导作用的泪腺探针以引导导管。有时，导管必须在术中瘘管暴露后放置。会阴部电刺激可以评估括约肌收缩的强度。做正中线切口，准确地在正中线处分开括约肌结构，使两侧的肌肉相等。这一方法的基本原理是基于正中线没有重要的神经、血管经过，似乎所有组织都在中线处终结，甚至有正中缝帮助术者确认开口确实在正中线上。用尖 Weitlaner 牵开器以获得良好的暴露，牵开器应放在表面以避免压迫周围的神经。

男性患儿后矢状径路肛门直肠成形术

直肠尿道瘘（球部和前列腺部）

切口的大小必须与患儿具体的解剖结构相适应（图 101-8）。在正中线上延长切口不会导致不良后果。切口通常从骶骨下部开始延伸，经过肛门凹中央；有时切口需要延伸到会阴体，尤其是在伴有直肠尿道球部瘘的男孩中。矢状旁肌纤维在皮下与中线平行走向。其他与上述肌肉垂直走向的肌肉结构延伸至中间并终止于肛门凹陷周围。这些结构从皮肤延伸到肛提肌，并被称为肌肉复合体。矢状旁纤维的深部有明显的直肠坐骨脂肪，在这个部位正中线缝变得非常细，因此切口容易偏离中线。肛提肌位于直肠坐骨脂肪的深部，也在正中线被分割。电刺激肛提肌可将直肠推向前，刺激肌肉复合体可以使肛门凹陷更明显，

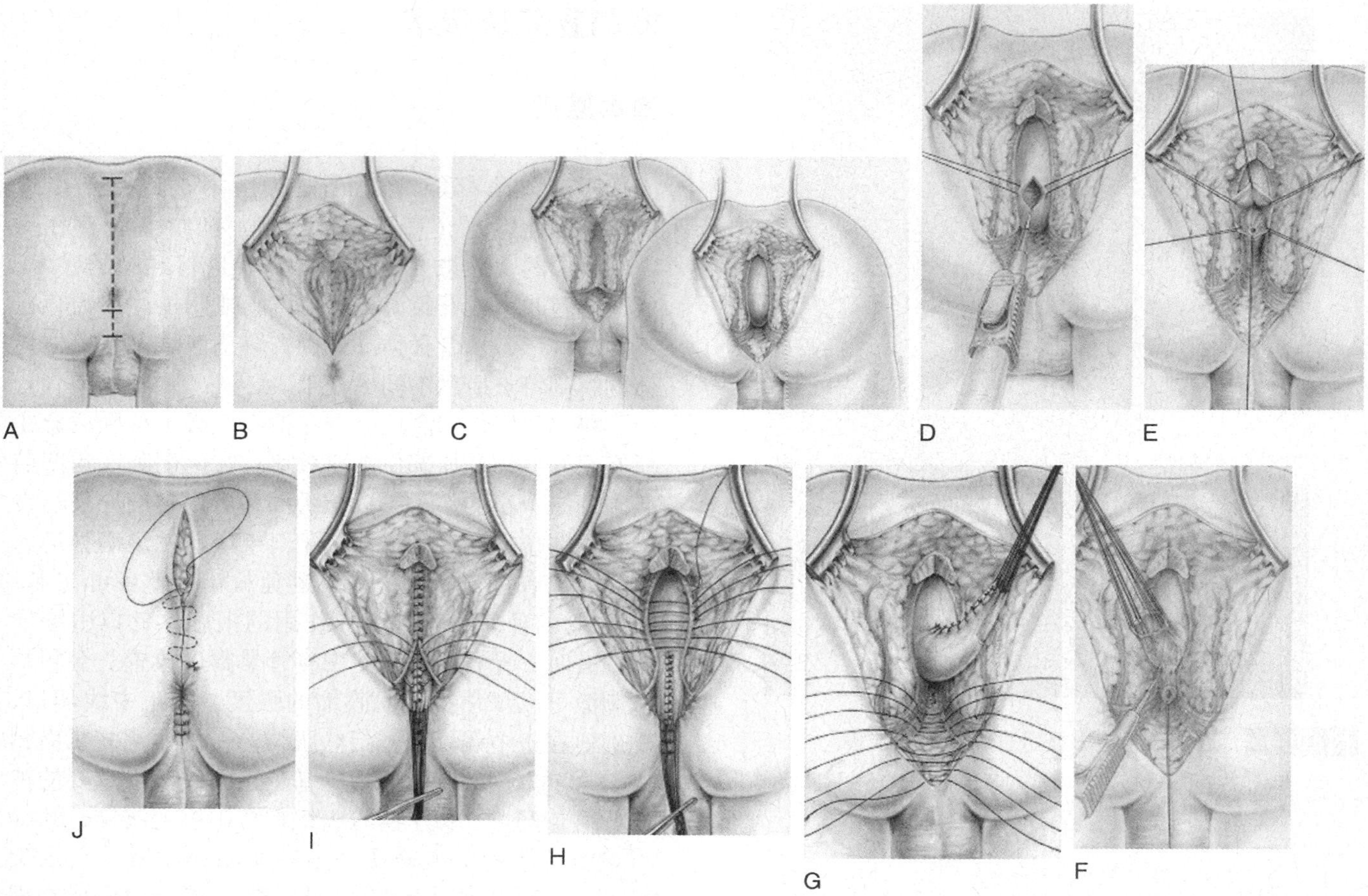

图 101-8　男性患者后矢状肛门直肠成形术的主要步骤。A. 计划好的后矢状切口。B. 通过后矢状径路在正中线处分离矢状旁纤维和坐骨直肠脂肪。C. 暴露直肠后壁。D. 在正中线处打开直肠后壁。E. 打开直肠后壁直至明确直肠尿道瘘的位置。F. 在瘘口上方分离后尿道和直肠。G. 直肠完全游离并被修剪，在前方缝合关闭会阴体。H. 将直肠置于括约肌结构的前后缘间拖出。I. 关闭肛提肌，并将直肠后壁与复合肌后缘缝合固定。J. 关闭后矢状切口，完成肛门成形术。

并将皮肤向骨盆上方提升。肌肉复合体和矢状旁肌肉结构的交叉处作为新肛门的前后界。使用电刺激器可最清晰地确定这些界限。

在直肠—尿道球部瘘的男孩中，肠管非常明显突出且向切口下部延伸。在直肠前列腺瘘的男孩中，直肠要小得多，并位于切口较高的位置。远端结肠造影提供的信息对于确定直肠的位置是有价值的。在直肠-膀胱颈瘘的病例中，经后矢状径路找不到直肠，不应该在这一途径寻找直肠。

在直肠后壁用丝线临时做牵引后在正中线打开直
1575 肠。向远端延长直肠壁的切口。当直肠被打开时，缝更多针牵拉直肠壁的边缘且能更好地暴露直肠腔。切口一直向远处延伸直到发现瘘管的位置（图 101-9）。

由于在直肠和尿道之间没有间隙，所以术者必须极其小心地将直肠与尿道分离。用 6-0 丝线在瘘口上方半圈缝数针（图 101-10）。这些缝线使外科医生在切割、分离直肠与尿道时能够尽量均衡地牵拉直肠。切割在直肠黏膜下层进行，尤其是在正中线部位，约 5～7 mm；两个结构，直肠和尿道逐渐分离最终变得各自独立。在瘘管位置缝一针使其以后能被容易地辨认出和关闭。一旦直肠与尿道完全地分离开，沿着直肠一周向上游离，延长直肠使其足以到达会阴部。为了达到这一目的，必须分离直肠周围的筋膜，包括附在直肠上的血管和神经。术者一边用先前放置的缝线牵拉直肠，一边沿直肠一周向上切割。电灼对直肠有牵拉的血管并分离直肠与血管，直到获得足够长的直肠。直肠有非常好的肠壁内血供；甚至在非常高位的前列腺瘘中，也可游离足够长度的直肠而不发生直肠缺血。然而，当直肠壁被损伤时，血供可能被破坏，并可发生缺血。因此，必须努力做到尽可能地靠近直肠壁切割但又不损伤到肠壁内的血供。一旦获得足够长的直肠，就进行无张力的直肠皮肤吻合。判断直肠的大小并与可用的空间作比较，如有需要可通过切除部分直肠后壁来剪裁。然后，通过用长期可吸收线双层间断缝合关闭直肠后切口，重建直肠。对于曾经附着于后尿道的一部分直肠前壁，缝合数针使浆肌层靠拢，以加强肠壁。尿道瘘管用可吸收线间断缝合关闭。

通过将先前用丝线做临时标记的外括约肌前缘缝 1576
合在一起重建会阴体。肛提肌必须在直肠后缝合（图 101–11，并且见图 101–8），复合肌的后缘必须在中线位置与部分直肠后壁缝合在一起以固定直肠，防止脱出（图 101–12）。坐骨直肠窝脂肪和皮下组织必须重新靠拢以免留下无效腔。皮肤通常用皮下缝合关 1577
闭。将直肠置于外括约肌前后缘之间，用长期可吸收线间断缝合，重建肛门。

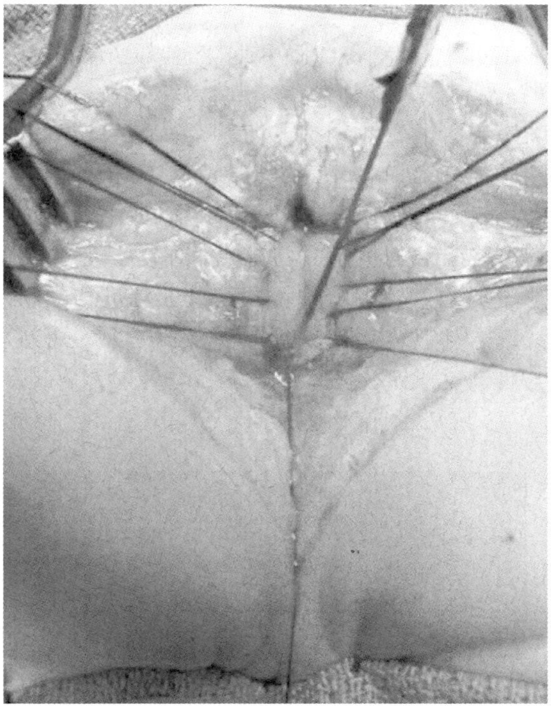

图 101–9　手术图示，可见直肠尿道瘘；一根金属探针插入其中。

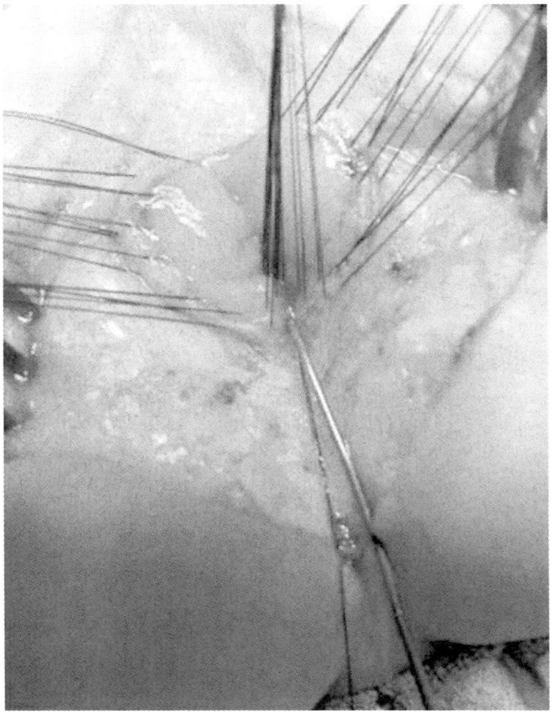

图 101–10　手术图示，细丝线经黏膜穿过瘘管上端（头侧）半圈。

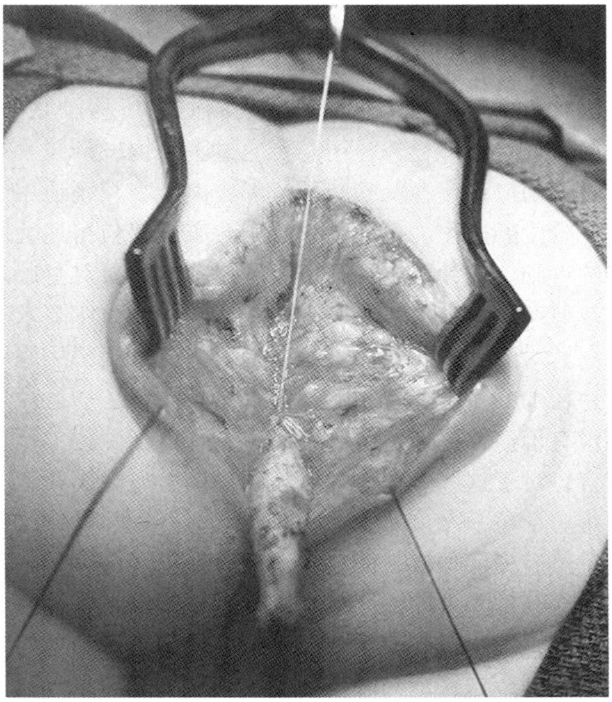

图 101–11　在直肠后缝合肛提肌。

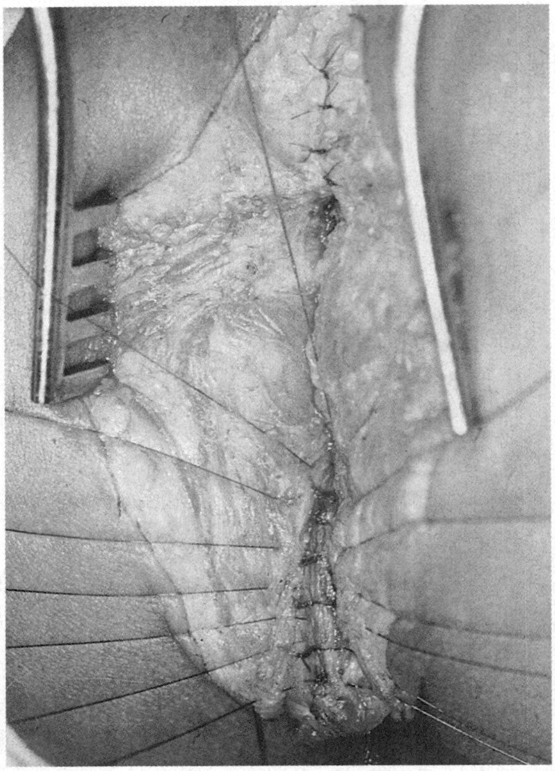

图 101-12 在复合肌后缘缝针固定直肠。

直肠膀胱颈瘘

对于直肠膀胱颈瘘的患儿而言，为了移动直肠，除了后矢状切口之外，还需要通过腹腔镜或剖腹手术做腹部切口将瘘管从膀胱颈背部分离。腹腔镜适用于这一阶段的操作。挑战常来自于游离足够长可达会阴部的直肠。这种游离加上这一畸形常常需要对直肠进行裁剪缩小这个事实，对腹腔镜下的操作技术要求非常高。对于其他病变如直肠尿道瘘，有人提倡用腹腔镜途径加一个非常小的会阴部切口[22]。这一途径可能很有价值，尤其是对于有高位直肠前列腺瘘的病例而言，对于这些患儿单经后矢状切口游离直肠常较为困难。低位病变如直肠尿道球部瘘，无需腹腔镜帮助，经后矢状切口就能安全地完成修复。

在开始手术前，从胸到脚趾做皮肤准备，使医生在同时进行腹部和会阴部手术时可以毫不费力地将患儿从俯卧位翻转到仰卧位。在正中线处分离括约肌结构。在骶骨间隙尿道之后肛提肌之前放置一根橡皮管。这根橡皮管放在复合肌的前后缘之间、骶骨前方，以模拟直肠。围着橡皮管重建整个括约肌结构。翻转患儿为仰卧，可经腹腔镜或剖腹进入腹腔（图101-13B）。找到乙状结肠并向下游离到膀胱颈（图101-13A）。膀胱颈通常位于腹膜底下方约 2 cm 处，因此需要很少的盆腔切割，无需做直肠内切割。必须牢记输精管和输尿管非常接近直肠，因此，切割必须尽可能地靠近直肠壁。直肠迅速变窄，并 T 形进入膀胱颈。分离直肠与尿道非常容易，因为越是高位的畸形，形成的共壁越少。直肠在其最远端被切断，用可吸收线缝合瘘管。将橡皮管置于后腹膜上，将直肠的大小与橡皮管比较，以确定是否需要对直肠进行裁

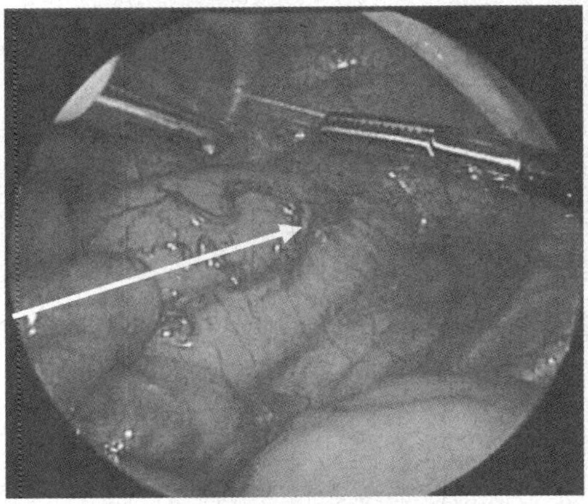

A

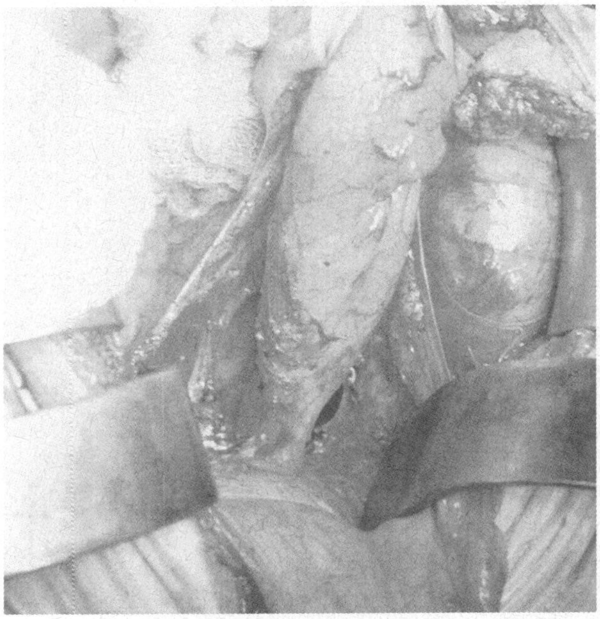

B

图 101-13 术中显示直肠乙状结肠终止于膀胱颈。A. 腹腔镜图示；B. 开腹探查图示。

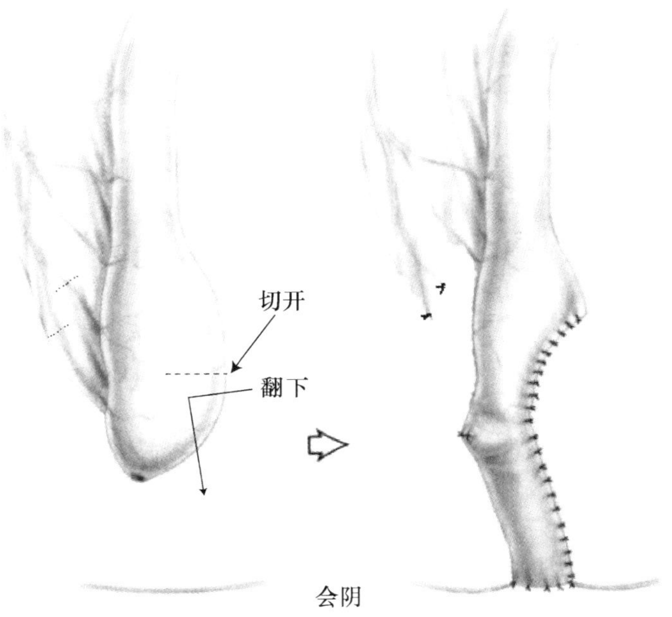

图 101-14 为了保护主干结扎肠系膜下血管的外周分支。做直肠成形术以获取额外的长度。

剪。然后将肠管与橡皮管连接固定，并向下拖出，延着直肠达到会阴部。

在这种非常高位的畸形中，有时直肠的拖出由于肠系膜下血管的分支受到限制。传统上建议外科医生将肠系膜下动脉在从腹主动脉发出的源头结扎切断。对于那些肠系膜下血管是直肠乙状结肠唯一血供的患儿，切断肠系膜下血管是禁忌的，因为这些患儿常常在结肠造口时已将中结肠血管与肠系膜下血管连接的血管弓阻断。因此，直肠远端的血供可能仅依靠肠系膜下血管。主干的保护对于保护直肠的壁内血供至关重要（图 101-14）。在特别高位的畸形，可通过直肠成形来延长直肠。肛门成形应按前面叙述的进行。将直肠与复合肌粘合在一起尤其重要，因为这些患儿的盆腔肌肉发育差，特别容易引起脱垂。

不伴瘘的肛门闭锁

不伴瘘的肛门闭锁患儿的直肠盲端与伴有尿道球部瘘患儿处于相同水平。然而，因为不伴瘘的肛门闭锁患儿的直肠仍与后尿道紧密相连，所以需将其与尿道仔细分离。接下去的纠治手术同直肠尿道瘘的病例。

直肠闭锁和狭窄

直肠闭锁和狭窄的纠治比较简单。这一手术的目的是将近端扩张的直肠盲端与远端的肛管相连接。二者常常被数毫米的纤维组织隔开。直肠必须被充分地游离这样才可以与肛管作端端吻合。然后如前面描述，通过重建所有肌肉结构关闭切口。

女性畸形的后矢状肛门直肠成形术

前庭瘘

这种畸形的复杂性常常被低估。前庭瘘的患儿具有控制排便的潜能，因此应努力为这些患儿提供最好的机会，以通过一次简单手术而得到成功重建。伤口裂开和感染可危及最终的功能效果，而保护性结肠造口大大减少了这些并发症的发生。

如果外科医生对这一畸形有相当的经验，可在新生儿期进行一期修复。偶尔，这类患儿在新生儿期没有被发现，而在几个月后做手术。这种情况下也能不做结肠造口而直接进行一期纠治。然而，为了避免会阴部感染，小心的操作、很好的肠道准备、禁食一周和术后肠外营养是至关重要的。

患儿取俯卧位，做中线切口，但通常不必将切口向上延伸至骶骨中部。中线切口继续围绕瘘管切割达到前庭，用多根 5-0 缝线沿瘘口缝一周。牵拉这些缝线，环形地分离直肠。直肠后壁很容易辨认，切割必须从后侧开始，然后再向外延伸。最后的步骤，即将直肠与阴道分离，是手术中最精细的部分。这种类型的畸形，直肠和阴道之间的共壁长且薄。常在直肠侧面发现痔血管的分支，分离这些血管，直肠可像之前描述的那样被游离并获得足够长度进行无张力的直肠—皮肤吻合。用电刺激确认括约肌结构的边缘，并缝丝线作为临时标记。然后，通过将外括约肌前缘缝合重建会阴部。将复合肌前缘如之前在男性患儿中叙述的一样重新靠拢。肛提肌通常不暴露，因此无需重建。然而，必须在直肠后重建复合肌，并与直肠后壁缝几针固定。肛门成形和切口关闭的操作与在男性患儿中的相同。

阴道瘘的病例极其少见，除了需要更长的游离直肠使其能拖至会阴部之外，其他技术操作都是相同的。

泄殖腔存留

通过后矢状肛门直肠成形术的变体手术处理这类女性畸形。由于它的复杂性，常被单独考虑。纠治泄殖腔存留存在一系列的挑战。它的治疗需要一位精细、技术高明，同时又具有创造性和想象力，并且足智多谋、经验丰富的外科医生。纠治这一畸形有三个目的：控制排便、控制排尿和保持性功能。因为存在一系列的缺陷，所以这些目标在一些病例中可以实现，而在另一些病例中，虽然在解剖结构上修复了缺陷，但患儿留有功能上的后遗症，需要更多的医疗帮助来提供良好的生活质量。在手术探查中，医生必须对直肠、阴道和尿道的异常解剖排列有足够的心理准备（图101-15A至C)。做一个长的正中矢状切口，切口从骶骨中部经外括约肌延伸到会阴部的单一开口。

在进行一穴肛的修复手术前，外科医生应先进行内镜检查，以确定共同通道的长度。一穴肛患儿可根据特点分为两个组[50]，这两组患儿代表了不同的技术性挑战，需要在术前就被认识到。第一组由共同通道短于3 cm的患儿组成。幸运的是这一组占据一穴肛病例的大多数。这些患儿通常能够仅通过后矢状途径手术纠治，而无需经腹手术。

1580 第二组由长共同通道的患儿组成。这些患儿常常需要开腹探查，随后需要泌尿科有经验并受过特殊训练的医生作出手术决策。这组患儿应在有治疗这些畸形专门经验的中心治疗。

共同通道短于3 cm的一穴肛

切口从骶骨中部向下延伸至单一的会阴部开口。所有的括约肌结构在正中线被分开。在括约肌组织被分开后外科医生最先发现的结构是直肠。沿正中线将直肠打开，并沿直肠后壁边缘缝丝线做牵拉。切口沿共同通道后壁向远端延长。整个共同通道被暴露出来，因此可以直接确认共同通道的长度（图101-16A）。然后，将直肠从阴道上分离出来（图101-16B）。这一操作与直肠膀胱瘘的纠治手术相同，因为如前所述直肠和阴道共壁。在有阴道隔膜的患儿中，必须在这一隔膜的后方探查直肠。

1581 一旦直肠与阴道完全分离，使用一种称为泌尿生殖整体移位的方法进行手术[47]。在过去，将阴道与尿道分离，这是一种技术上要求非常高的方法，伴有严重的并发症。泌尿生殖整体移位将阴道和尿道作为一个整体而不做分离地整体移动。直肠被分离后，在阴道和共同通道边缘缝多根丝线对泌尿生殖道做均匀的牵拉（图101-16C）。另外，跨过泌尿生殖道在距阴蒂5 mm处缝数针。在上一排缝线和阴蒂之间将共同通道横向切断。这一切割利用了泌尿生殖道与耻骨之间的自然平面。通过这一平面，术者能很快地并在出血很少的情况下到达耻骨上缘。在那儿可以看到支持阴道和膀胱的纤维性无血管结构，这一结构被称为尿道膀胱悬韧带。切开这一韧带，立即能使泌尿生殖复合体明显移动（2～3 cm）（图101-16D）。然后切割阴道外侧和背侧可另外得到5～10 mm。这一操作足以修复60%的一穴肛患儿，而且是一种可重复的方法。另外的优点是这一方法保留了尿道和阴道的良好血供，并将尿道开口置于可见位置，以便在需要时做 158
间断插管导尿。这也提供了一个平滑的便于插管的尿道。将共同通道在中线处劈开形成二侧瓣，与皮肤缝合构建新的阴唇（图101-16E）。然后将阴道边缘拉至皮肤，缝合建立一个良好的入口。用电刺激确认括约肌的边缘。将括约肌的前缘缝合重建会阴体。如前所述，将直肠置于括约肌的前后缘之间（图101-16F）。患儿可在手术当天进食，疼痛常容易控制。术后48小时患儿可出院。

共同通道长于3 cm的一穴肛

当内镜显示患儿有一个长的共同通道时，术者必须准备面对一项很有意义的技术性挑战。如果术者经验有限或缺乏专业泌尿外科的训练，应该请求在这方面有经验的医生帮助。小儿泌尿科医生并不意味着一定熟悉泄殖腔手术技术上的挑战，熟悉这一问题需要专业的训练。

具有长的共同通道的患儿术前应做全身的准备，因为可能需要进行腹部探查。经后矢状切口将直肠与阴道和尿道分离，如位置非常高则需经腹分离。存在非常长的共同通道（长于5 cm），表明无法用泌尿生殖整体移位法来修复畸形，建议将共同通道留在原位，可被用作间断插管导尿的尿道。在这种情况下通过用6-0丝线牵引阴道壁，在阴道和尿道之间建立一个解剖平面，将阴道部分地从尿道上分离出来。这是

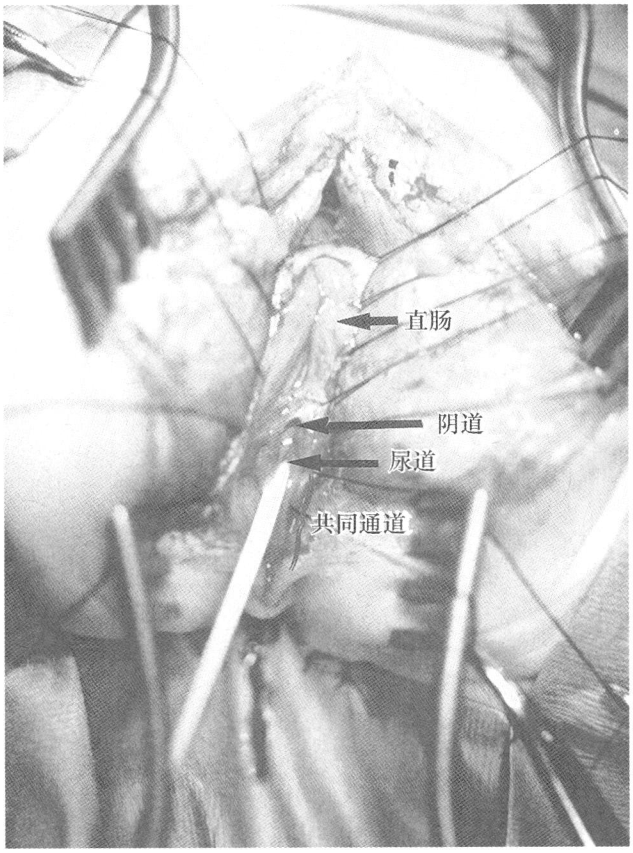

A

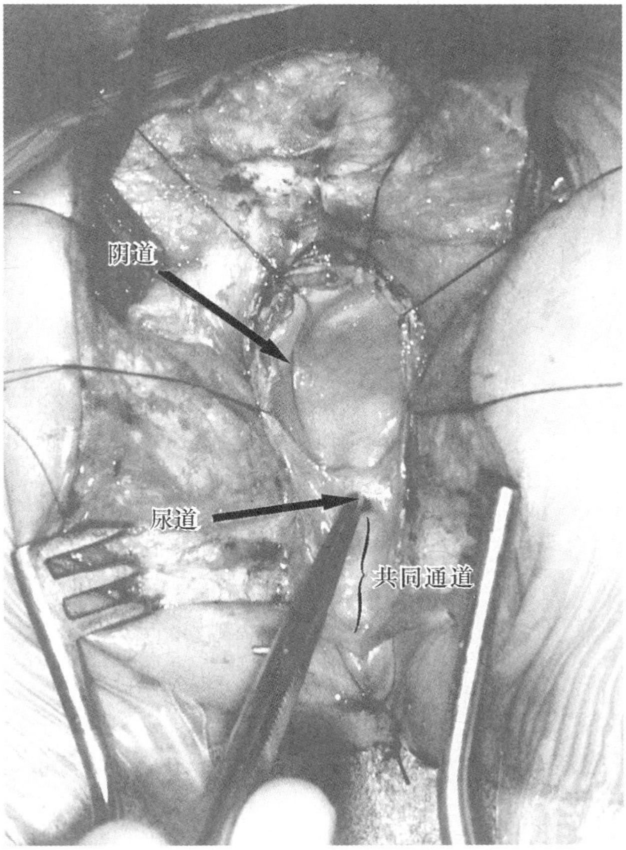

B

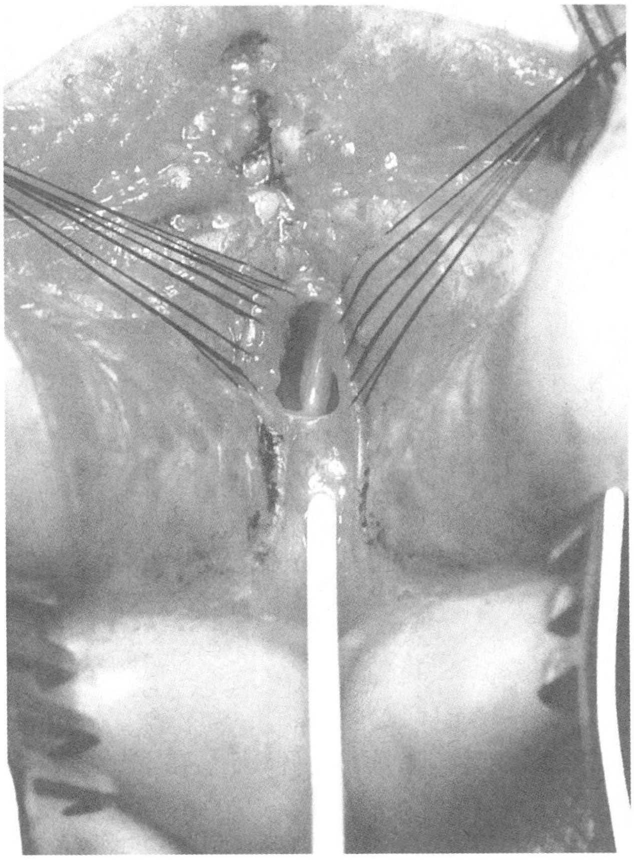

C

图 101-15 A. 典型的一穴肛，共同通道约为 2.5 cm。B. 一穴肛，伴有巨大阴道（阴道积液），直肠在阴道的开口位置较高，此处看不见。C. 伴有阴道隔膜的一穴肛，直肠开口于阴道隔膜的后面。

一项非常精细、谨慎而冗长的操作。这一切割能将阴道与尿道分离约 2 cm，剩下的分离必须通过腹部切口来完成。

建议采用腹部中线切口，在正中线处打开膀胱，将饲管插入两侧输尿管以保护输尿管。在这些类型的畸形中，阴道和膀胱间有大面积的共壁，两侧输尿管都穿过共壁。因此，在分离阴道与尿道时，有时需将支架插入输尿管，并需要保护输尿管。手术医生必须熟悉不同的输尿管再植技术，因为这些患儿在同一手术中常常需做这类手术。

一旦进入腹腔，通过插入一根经输卵管伞部的 3 号饲管和注入生理盐水来确认苗勒氏结构是否开放。如

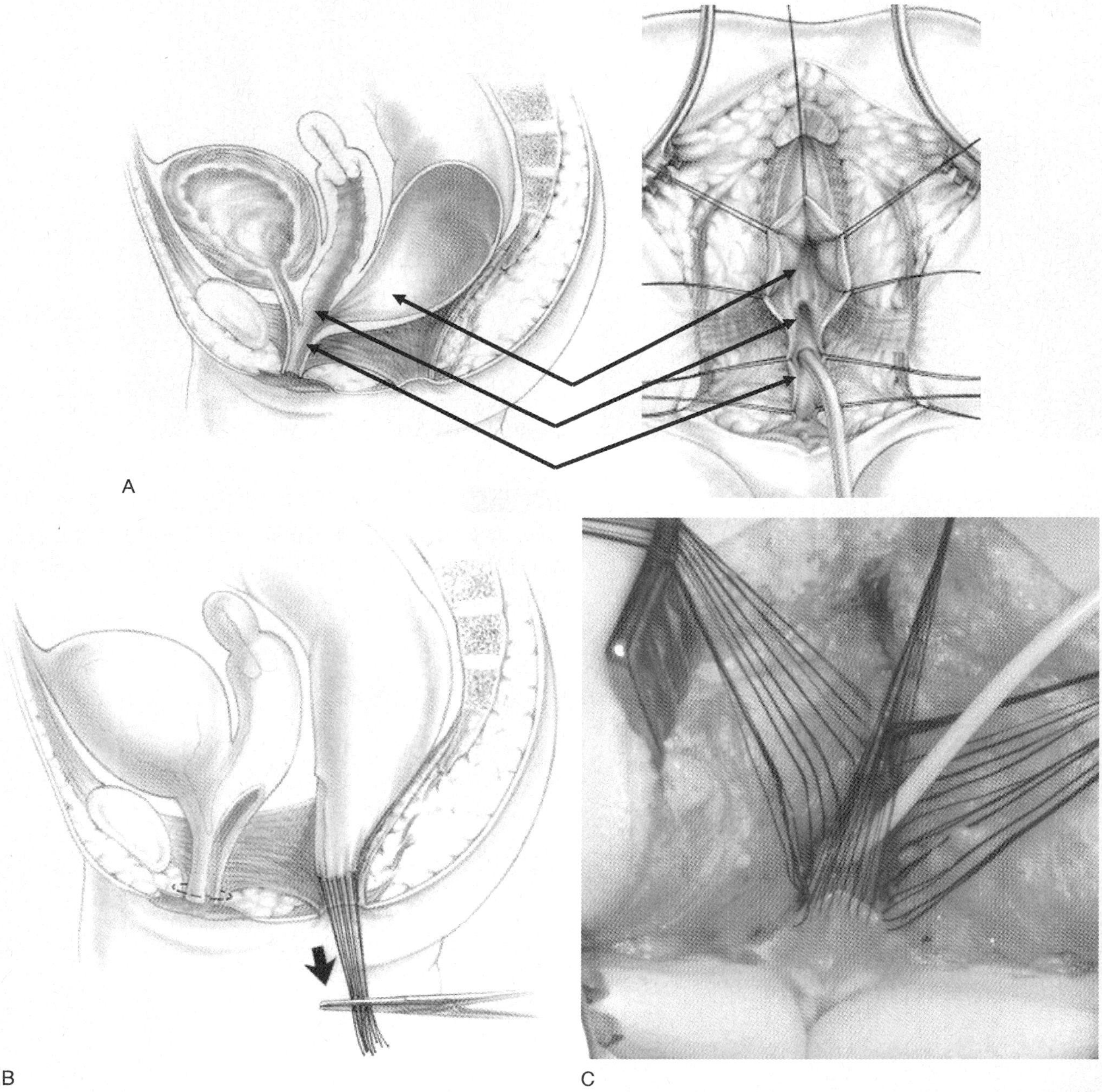

图 101-16　泌尿生殖道整体移位（共同通道 <3 cm 的泄殖腔）。A. 切口向下延长到会阴部的单一开口。B. 将直肠从泌尿生殖窦上分离。C. 沿泌尿生殖窦放置缝线用于牵拉。

图 101-16　（续）D. 移动泌尿生殖窦。E. 缝合泌尿生殖窦与阴蒂。F. 手术完成。

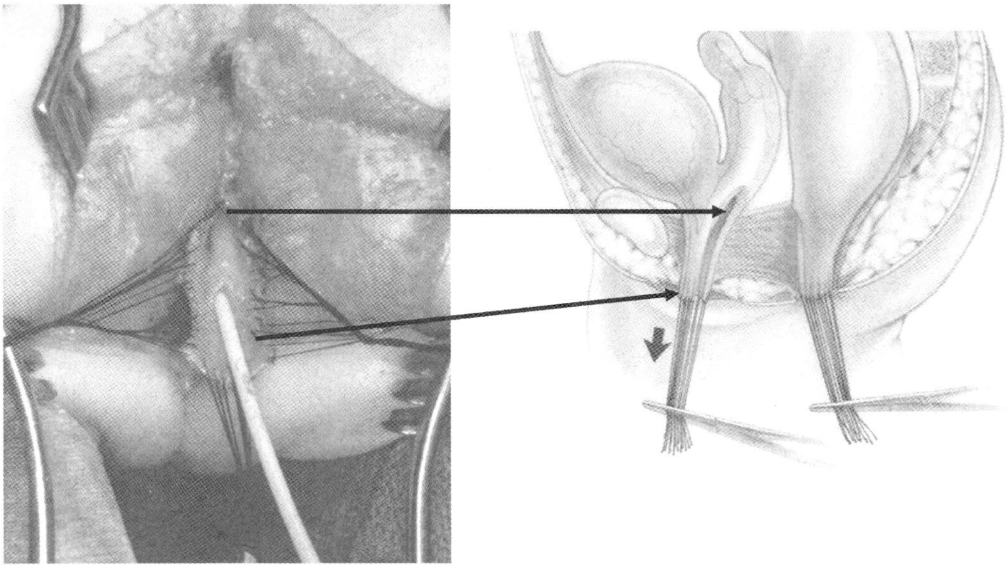

D

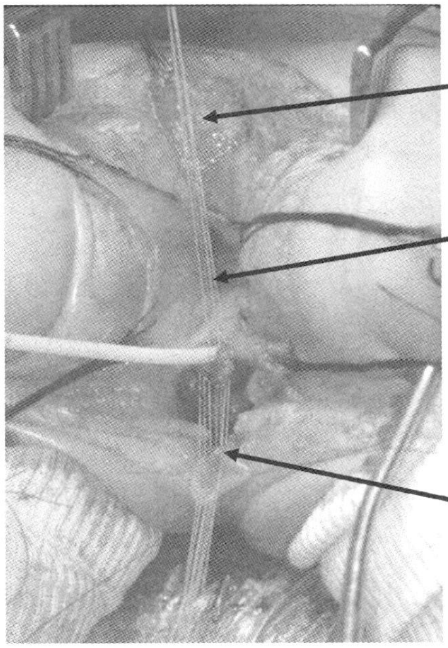

E

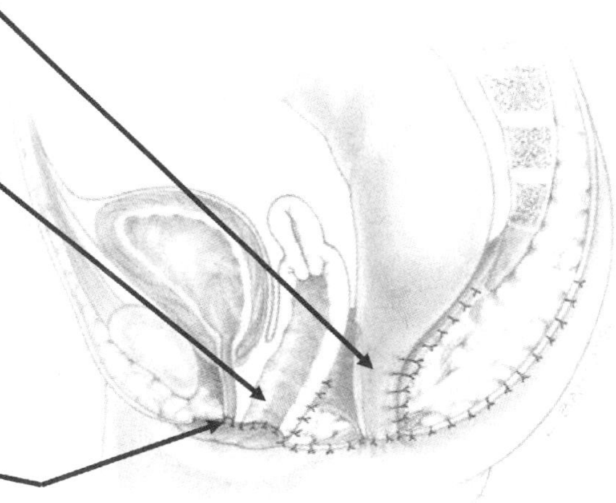

F

果系统中的一部分不开放，应切除闭锁的苗勒氏结构，需特别小心避免损伤卵巢血供。当双侧苗勒氏管闭锁时，我们建议将其留在原位，同时必须密切地监测患儿，当其接近青春期时，进一步做超声检查。

阴道和尿道的分离是最烦琐、最具有技术要求的手术步骤；通常阴道和尿道共享一条非常长的共同通道，所处的部位不容易到达。将膀胱打开并将导管插入两侧输尿管后进行分离，一旦分离完成，术者必须根据具体的解剖发现做出决定。

阴道转变手术

一组特殊类型的患儿，在出生时即伴有阴道积水和双侧半阴道（双阴道畸形）。双侧半阴道都非常大，并且两侧子宫可完全分离，子宫间的距离长于两个阴道的垂直长度。对于这些病例，理想的手术方式是“阴道转变”手术（图 101-17）。

切除一侧子宫和同侧输卵管，特别注意保存卵巢

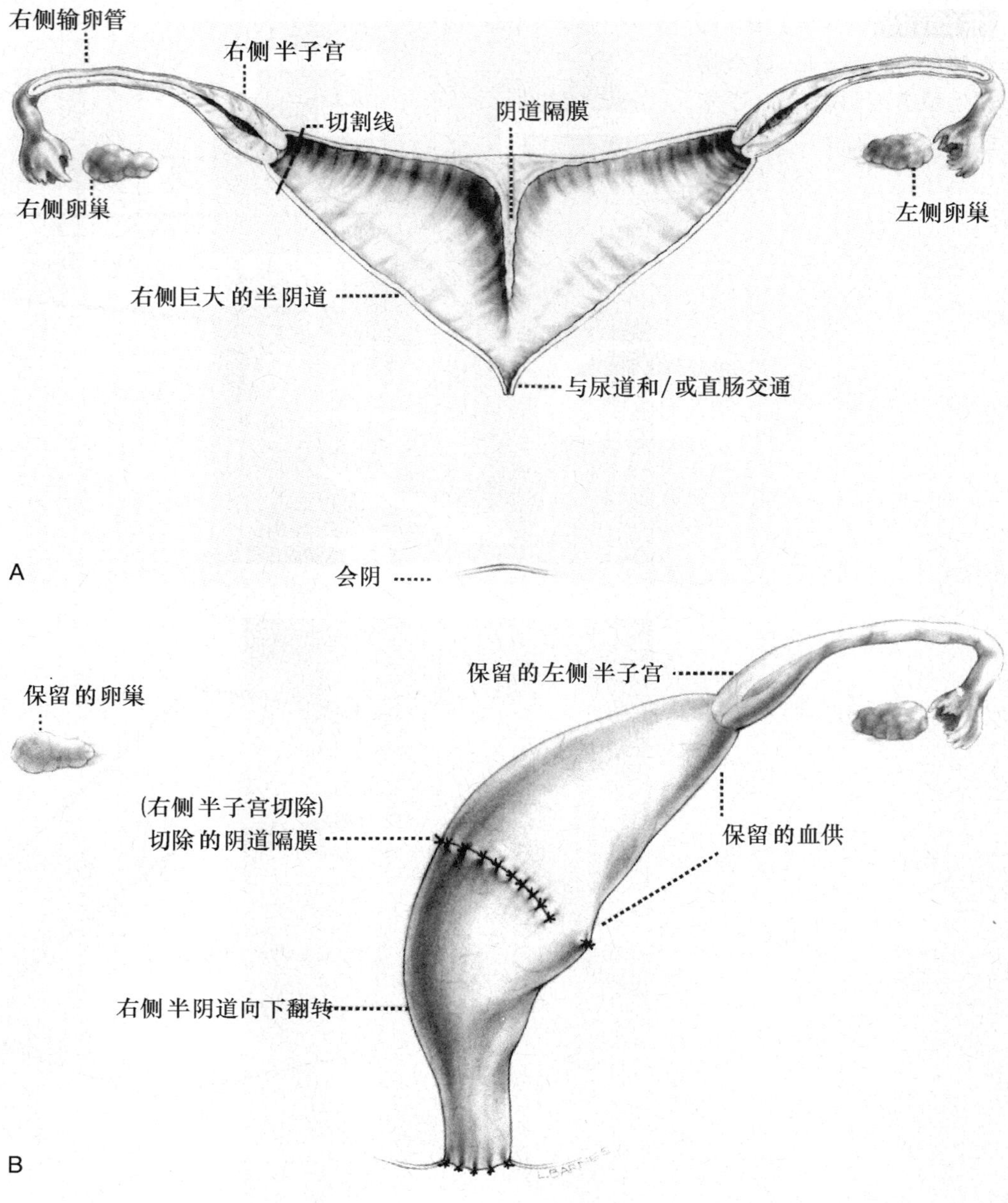

图 101-17　A．有阴道隔膜的巨大半阴道和长共同通道。B．阴道转变手术。

的血供。牺牲同侧半阴道的血供而保存对侧半阴道的血供，但多数时候两侧半阴道都可保留很好的血供。切除阴道分隔，将两侧半阴道切除分隔的侧面吻合，使阴道形成单一的管状阴道。然后，将切除子宫的一侧半阴道穹窿向下降至会阴。这是一种有用的办法，仅当解剖特征符合这里描述的要求时才可以施行。

阴道替代

当患儿的阴道很短或极少数的患儿有阴道缺失时，必须做替代手术。在这些病例中，可选择直肠、结肠或小肠作为替代。当患儿具有内生殖器或阴道鞘或子宫颈时，需要将替代的肠管上端与短小的阴道鞘吻合。当患儿不具备内生殖器（没有阴道和子宫）时，建立一个其上端是盲端的阴道，其仅用于性生活目的，没有生殖功能。

直肠：这一形式的阴道替代术仅适用于有巨大直肠的患儿，直肠大到足以能纵向地劈成两部分，一部分带有血供的肠壁将被重建为新的阴道，其余部分有足够的周径用于重建一个适当大小的直肠（图 101-18）。直肠的血供将由肠系膜下血管的分支通过肠壁

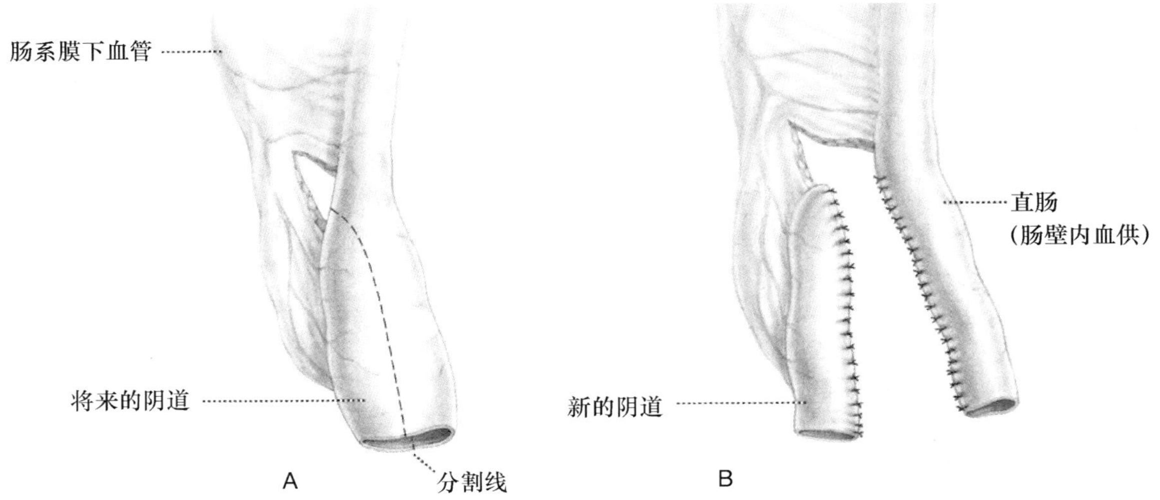

图 101-18　A 和 B，直肠阴道替代手术。

提供。在直肠乙状结肠足够长的患儿中也可以施行该手术，可用带有血供的远端肠管重建新的阴道，而将近端肠管拖下重建新的直肠。

583 **结肠：**结肠似乎是阴道替代的理想材料。然而，有时结肠造口的位置会影响这种类型的重建术。当条件允许时，乙状结肠替代更为可取。为了获得足够长的带有系膜的肠管，应取乙状结肠活动度最大的部分（图 101-19）。

小肠：当无法利用结肠时，小肠活动度最大的部分可用于阴道重建。在近回盲瓣约 15 cm 处的小肠系膜较长，是小肠用于阴道替代的最佳部分。分离这段回肠的一部分并保留血供，将其拖下用于替代阴道（图 101-20）。

在很高位的泄殖腔中，可以发现两个半阴道附着于膀胱颈，甚至附着于膀胱三角。在这些病例中，直肠也开口于膀胱三角（图 101-21）。分离这些结构要开腹进行。不幸的是，当分离完全后，常常已没有了膀胱颈或已将其严重损伤。这时，外科医生必须要有足够的经验决定要重建膀胱颈还是永久性将其关闭。在前一种情况下，多数患儿将需要间断性导尿以排空膀胱，并且不能保证重建的膀胱有正常的功能。在后一种情况下（永久地关闭膀胱颈），需进行膀胱造瘘，并且患儿将需要可控性转流手术，
84 有时为膀胱扩大术。这些手术到患儿能自控小便的年龄进行（3～4 岁）。在这种特殊类型的畸形中，患儿通常也需要做阴道替代术。术式可取前述几种术式中的一种。

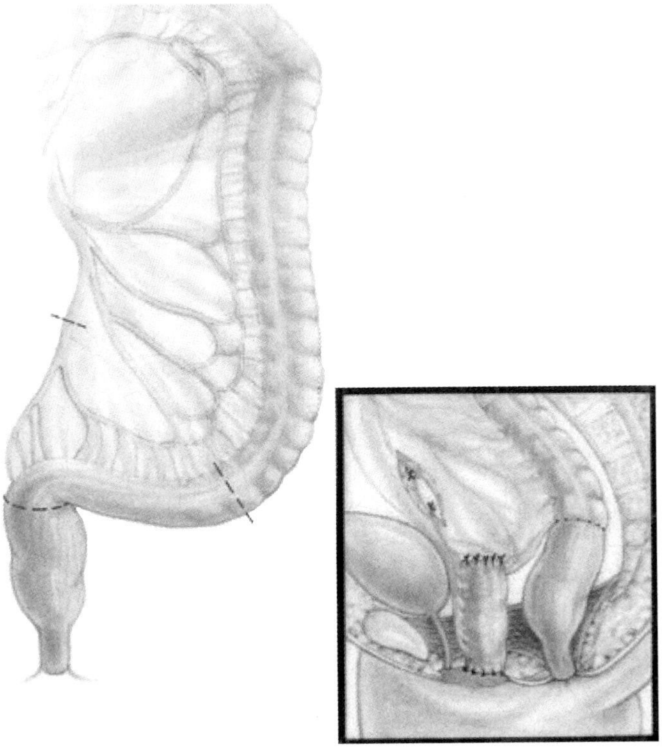

图 101-19　乙状结肠阴道替代手术。

在结肠造口关闭时，应做内镜检查来确定畸形已被完全地纠治。如果泄殖腔纠治术没有经腹，则关闭结肠造瘘是探查苗勒氏结构是否开放的好机会。

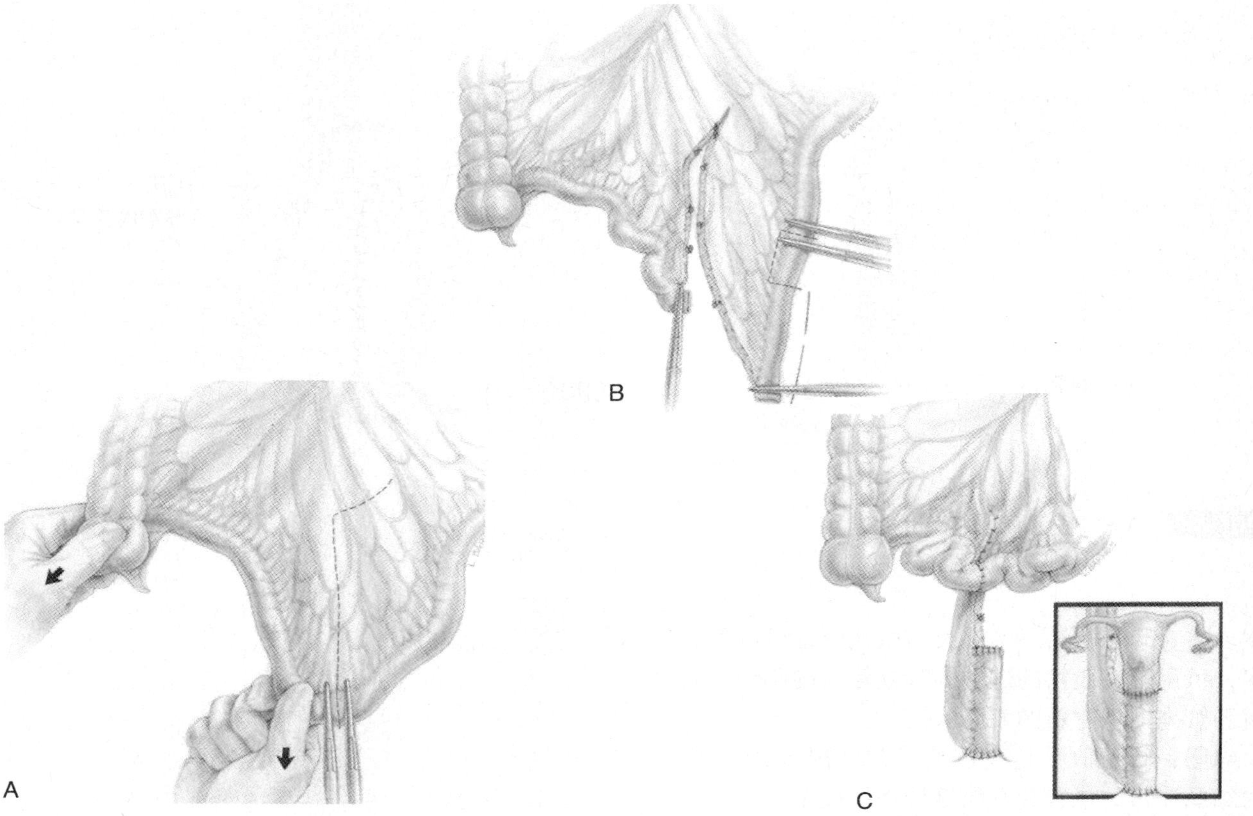

图 101-20　小肠阴道替代手术。A 和 B，使用肠系膜最长的回肠部分。C. 将小肠拖下作为新的阴道（插入的小图显示与阴道上半部分的吻合）。

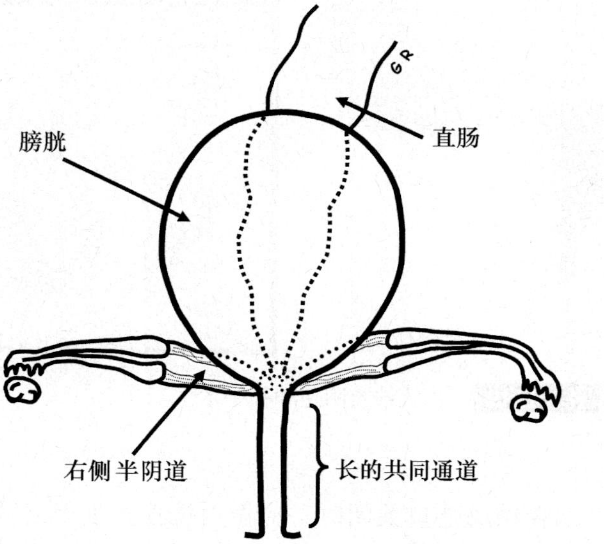

图 101-21　特别长的共同通道——半阴道和直肠开口于膀胱颈。

术后护理的一般原则

在没有开腹的病例中，术后几小时内就可开始经口进食。抗生素一般使用 48 小时。在有直肠尿道瘘的男孩中，导尿管应留置 7 天；在做过泄殖腔纠治手术的患儿中，导尿管至少要留置 3 周。如果纠治术需要开腹，有时应用耻骨上膀胱造瘘，在一些患儿中则需要运用膀胱切开术。

术后 2 周开始扩肛。测定肛门的口径，最开始用大小刚好合适的扩张器每天扩张肛门 2 次。扩张器的尺寸每周增加 1 号直至达到所设定的尺寸。扩张器的最佳尺寸在表 101-2 中列出。一旦达到合适的尺寸就关闭结肠造瘘。在关瘘后必须继续扩肛。一旦扩张器能被轻松地插入，则扩肛次数应调整为每天 1 次，连续 1 个月，然后每周 2 次 1 个月、每周 1 次 1 个月，再每周 1 次 3 个月。

在结肠造瘘口关闭后，患儿可能会频繁地排便，

表 101-2　肛门扩张程序

患儿年龄	Hegar 扩张器
1～4 个月	12 号
4～8 个月	13 号
8～12 个月	14 号
1～3 岁	15 号
3～12 岁	16 号
>12 岁	17 号

并可形成会阴部瘢痕。便秘饮食可能会对治疗这类问题有帮助。几周后，排便的次数会减少，多数患儿会
585 出现便秘。6 个月后，会形成更加规则的排便形式。患儿每天排便 1～3 次，在两次排便间保持清洁，并在排便过程中有推挤的感觉都说明排便形式好，而且通常预后好。可对这类患儿进行训练。如果患儿大便次数多或持续排便，且没有任何有感觉或有推挤的迹象，则通常提示预后功能差。

一穴肛纠治术后，患儿常常要留置 Foley 导管 2～3周。如果尿道开口因水肿而不能看得很清楚，我们选择保留 Foley 导管。一旦能看清楚尿道开口，就可拔除 Foley 导管。观察患儿是否能够排空膀胱。如果不能排出尿液，可以教会看护者间断地插入导尿管。在有非常长的共同通道的患儿中，要留置耻骨上膀胱造瘘管，并在术后 1 个月进行耻骨膀胱造影；然后患儿开始夹管并测量剩余尿，剩余尿是膀胱功能有效性的指标。保留耻骨上膀胱造瘘管直至有证据表明膀胱功能良好或护理者已学会在有指征时应如何插管导尿。

结果

并发症

这类外科手术术后，患儿可发生各类常见的术后并发症。另外，一些特殊问题也可在术后早期和晚期形成。

86 已知的并发症例如伤口感染和拖出结构的回缩。当感染仅影响到伤口的表层时，被拖出的结构不会伴发开裂，而且及时治愈则不会导致功能上的后遗症。相反，感染伴发拖出组织开裂可导致严重后果，并留下后遗症，包括失禁（原本预后良好）、狭窄、继发性闭锁、复发性瘘管和严重的骨盆纤维化。在我们的研究中心，我们已为超过 200 例患有这类并发症并被转到这里的患儿施行了第二次手术。在我们的研究中，小的没有后遗症形成的感染 23 例，发生直肠回缩的 6 例，发生阴道回缩的 8 例。

严重感染和开裂主要发生在没有做结肠造瘘而直接进行一期手术的患儿中。因此，虽然我们认识到不进行结肠造口而早期施行一期手术的好处，但也坚持结肠造口术在处理这些畸形中是非常有辅助价值的。每一个手术医生必须根据个人的经验做出有关决定。

确定这些并发症的确切病因非常困难，然而我们已知的起主要作用的因素有明显的粪便污染、缺血和缝合张力。

直肠或阴道（或两者）的狭窄常常由前面提到的并发症引起，尽管它们也可单独发生。推荐进行肛门扩张从而避免狭窄，但是这些方法仅预防小的环状狭窄。肛门扩张困难常反映与缺血相关的主要问题，缺血可导致细长的狭窄，甚至是继发性闭锁。我们仍推荐应用肛门扩张术，尤其是对于具有可在术后维持肛门关闭的良好的括约肌的患儿。

直肠黏膜脱垂在重建术后也很常见。在笔者的研究中，后矢状肛门直肠成形术后直肠黏膜脱垂的发生率是 3.8%[6]。后矢状肛门直肠整形术后的黏膜脱垂并不常见，这可能与下列关键技术步骤有关：(1) 直肠后壁与复合肌后缘的缝合固定；(2) 必要时裁剪扩张的直肠；(3) 在有张力的情况下进行肛门成形术，切断缝线后，直肠略回缩，黏膜不可见。当黏膜脱垂引起过多的黏液分泌或溃疡或影响肛门感觉时，可施行手术，切除脱垂黏膜后缝合。

对一组在其他研究机构进行手术的患儿的回顾研究显示，在经过试图纠治肛门直肠畸形手术的男性患儿中，泌尿道损伤的发生率较高。术前没有做良好的远端结肠造影而直接施行后矢状手术是引起这些并发症的最重要的原因。可发生尿道、输尿管、输精管和精索血管损伤。在经过正确手术治疗的肛门直肠畸形的男性患儿中，术后神经性膀胱极少见，因为它仅发生在有明显骶骨畸形的患儿中[8]。另一方面，在修复术中去除了膀胱和膀胱颈的神经支配也可导致神经性膀胱[29]。

肛门直肠畸形手术纠治后，便秘是最常见的后遗症，但在一定程度上可以预防。畸形越低位，便秘越

容易发生。巨大的直肠乙状结肠可导致便秘，便秘没有得到适当处理也能导致巨大的直肠乙状结肠。这样的恶性循环会导致充盈性的假性肛门失禁。对这些出现失禁的患儿，如果适当地处理便秘，他们的排便将会恢复节制。偶尔，这些患儿因乙状结肠的切除改善了便秘的症状[14,48,52]。

我们有证据表明术前扩张的直肠乙状结肠会导致严重的便秘。因此，应尽一切努力使婴儿从出生那刻起就保持肠道的萎瘪和清洁。横结肠造口保留较长时间后可导致严重的巨直肠乙状结肠。袢状结肠造口也可导致远端粪便嵌塞、肠管扩张和继发性的便秘。

排便控制

不清楚有多少出生时有肛门闭锁的患者具有正常的控制排便的能力。如果不知道患儿原来的潜在功能，很难对各种手术类型的结果进行评估[41]。长期的研究表明，约75%的患者可获得良好的排便控制能力。

表 101-3 至 101-6 中列出了作者根据畸形的类型分类获得的结果。低位畸形和直肠闭锁的患者效果较好，那些高位畸形的患者效果较差。

在造瘘口关闭后的数月中可以预测将来的排便控
1587 制能力。每天排便 1～3 次，两次排便之间没有粪污提示预后良好，并可以认为这是一种良好的排便方式。婴儿排便前的特殊行为和排便时用力说明排便感觉完整，这些都与好的预后有关。尽可能早地确定预后对于避免家长的错误期待至关重要。

所有肛门直肠畸形的患儿，不论畸形的复杂性如何，3 岁后必须完全无漏尿和溢粪，因为到了这个年龄他们已经能控制排尿和排便，又或因为我们进行的治疗能够使他们人为地保持干燥和清洁。

表 101-3　畸形的类型和便秘

	畸形患儿	便秘患儿	
畸形	数量	数量	%
前庭瘘	101	64	60.3
尿道球部瘘	91	53	58.3
会阴瘘	53	30	56.6
不伴瘘的肛门闭锁	40	22	55
直肠闭锁或狭窄	8	4	50
前列腺部瘘	94	42	44.7
共同通道 <3 cm 的一穴肛	87	33	37.9
共同通道 >3 cm 的一穴肛	45	17	37.7
膀胱颈部瘘	45	7	15.5
阴道瘘	45	0	
总计	568	269	47.4

表 101-4　畸形的类型和自主排便

畸形类型	患儿数量	自主排便的患儿	
		数量	%
直肠闭锁或狭窄	8	8	100
会阴瘘	41	41	100
前庭瘘	98	90	91.8
不伴瘘的肛门闭锁	35	30	86.7
尿道球部瘘	83	68	81.9
阴道瘘	4	3	75
前列腺部瘘	72	53	73.6
共同通道 <3 cm 的一穴肛	73	53	72.6
共同通道 >3 cm 的一穴肛	41	17	41.5
膀胱颈瘘	29	9	31.0
总计	484	372	76.9

表 101-5　畸形的类型与粪污

畸形	患儿数量	有粪污的患儿	
		数量	%
会阴瘘	45	4	8.9
直肠闭锁或狭窄	8	2	25
前庭瘘	101	37	36.6
不伴瘘的肛门闭锁	37	18	48.6
尿道球部瘘	89	48	53.9
共同通道 <3 cm 的一穴肛	77	47	61.0
前列腺部瘘	88	68	77.3
阴道瘘	5	4	80
共同通道 >3 cm 的一穴肛	40	35	87.5
膀胱颈部瘘	41	36	87.8
总计	531	299	56.3

表 101-6　畸形的类型与完全能节制排便的患儿

畸形	患儿数量	完全能控制排便的患儿	
		数量	%
会阴瘘	41	36	87.8
直肠闭锁或狭窄	8	6	75
前庭瘘	98	63	64.3
不伴瘘的肛门闭锁	35	18	51.4
尿道球部瘘	83	34	41.0
共同通道 <3 cm 的一穴肛	73	28	38.4
阴道瘘	4	1	25
前列腺部瘘	72	16	22.2
共同通道 >3 cm 的一穴肛	41	4	9.8
膀胱颈部瘘	29	2	6.9
总计	484	208	43.0

肠道处理使用灌肠剂来保证肠道排空后 24 小时的清洁期。通过合理地应用肠道灌洗、饮食和药物，大多数患儿，包括那些大便严重失禁的患儿，都能保持清洁长达 24 小时[49]。只有继发于短结肠或结肠缺失的严重腹泻患儿才是永久性结肠造瘘术的适用人群。

对患有大便失禁的患儿进行评估，将其分为便秘型和肠蠕动增加型（常有腹泻倾向）。在第一组中，必须彻底灌洗肠道。橡胶管通常要插入到高达乙状结肠的位置去清洁肠道。这种方法利用了便秘患儿肠蠕动性差的特点，使肠道在 24 小时内保持清洁。轻泻剂和饮食安排不是这个方案的一部分。第二组患儿因直肠储存功能的丧失，肠蠕动增加，需要依靠减少大便的饮食和药物来减少肠蠕动，并给予结肠灌洗。

经过一个星期的试验和调整治疗，95% 的患儿能够保持清洁，并有可接受的社会生活。当患儿必须上学以及所有同学都已经穿上常规内衣裤时，肠道管理可以开始进行。大多数患儿和家长非常乐意进行这一项目。然而，当患儿到 7 岁至 12 岁时，有时甚至更小，他们通常已经开始谋求更多的独立性。

这时，建议进行有排便节制的阑尾造口术（Malone 手术）[35,59]。这一手术通过患儿的阑尾在腹壁盲肠间建立一个通道，瓣膜的机制使盲肠能进行插管但防止了粪漏。患儿坐在马桶上能自行灌肠。手术包括用盲肠包绕阑尾，再将阑尾外置于脐深部，使其不引人注意。很多患儿没有阑尾，我们用部分盲肠壁制成管状的阑尾样结构，然后再用盲肠包绕这个结构。造口仍从脐部拖出。大多数接受过这一手术的患儿表示非常满意。

我们的生物反馈经验不如其他作者所报告的那样令人鼓舞[43]。

在首次手术中直肠被放在错误位置的患儿需要再 1588
次进行手术。仅在那些出生时有正常骶骨、良好括约肌和良好预后的畸形患儿中推荐再次手术。这个手术的结果不一，15%～46% 的患儿能获得有价值的排便控制能力[10,46]。

非一穴肛的男性和女性患儿中泌尿外科方面的问题少见[8]。在一穴肛患儿中，28% 共同通道短于 3 cm 的患儿需要间断插管或可控性的分流来排空膀胱；共同通道长于 3 cm 的患儿 70%～80% 需要间断插管导尿或进行可控性的分流排尿（表 101-7）。

（吴晔明译　施诚仁校）

表 101-7　一穴肛患儿的排尿节制

	共同通道 <3 cm		共同通道 >3 cm		总计	
	数量	%	数量	%	数量	%
正常	59	72.0	11	20.4	70	51.5
间断插管导尿后保持干燥	16	19.5	20	37.0	36	26.5
可控性转流后保持干燥	7	8.5	23	42.6	30	22.0
总计	82		54		136	

参考文献

1. Aaronson I: Anterior sacral meningocele, anal canal duplication and covered anus occurring in one family. J Pediatr Surg 1970;5:559-563.
2. Albanese CT, Jennings RW, Lopoo JB, et al: One-stage correction of high imperforate anus in the male neonate. J Pediatr Surg 1999;34:834-836.
3. Amussat JZ: Histoire d'une operation d'anus artificial practique avec success par un nouveau procede. Gaz Med Paris 1835;3:753.
4. Appignani BA, Jaramillo D, Barnes PD, Poussaint TY: Dysraphic myelodysplasias associated with urogenital and anorectal anomalies: Prevalence and types seen with MR imaging. AJR Am J Roentgenol 1994;163:1199-1203.
5. Ashcraft KW, Holder TM: Hereditary presacral teratoma. J Pediatr Surg 1974;9:691-697.
6. Belizon A, Levitt MA, Shoshany G, et al: Rectal prolapse following posterior sagittal anorectoplasty for anorectal malformations. J Pediatr Surg 2005;40:192-196, discussion 196.
7. Bell B: A System of Surgery, vol 2, 3rd ed. Edinburgh, 1787.
8. Boemers TM, van Gool JD, de Jong TP, Bax KM: Urodynamic evaluation of children with caudal regression syndrome (caudal dysplasia sequence). J Urol 1994;151: 1038-1040.
9. Boocock GR, Donnai D: Anorectal malformation: Familial aspects and associated anomalies. Arch Dis Child 1987;62:576-579.
10. Brain AJL, Kiley EM: Posterior sagittal anorectoplasty for reoperation in children with anorectal malformations. Br J Surg 1989;76:57-59.
11. Brenner EC: Congenital defects of the anus and rectum. Surg Gynecol Obstet 1975;20:579-588.
12. Carson JA, Barnes PD, Tunell WP, et al: Imperforate anus: The neurological implication of sacral abnormalities. J Pediatr Surg 1984;19:838-842.
13. Cilento BG Jr, Benacerraef BR, Mandell J: Prenatal diagnosis of cloacal malformation. Urology 1994;43:386-388.
14. Cloutier R, Archambault H, D'Amours C, et al: Focal ectasia of the terminal bowel accompanying low anal deformities. J Pediatr Surg 1987;22:758-760.
15. Cohn J, Bay-Nielsen E: Hereditary defect of the sacrum and coccyx with anterior sacral meningocele. Acta Paediatr Scand 1969;58:268-274.
16. Cortes D, Thorup JM, Nielsen OH, Beck BL: Cryptorchidism in boys with imperforate anus. J Pediatr Surg 1995;30:631-635.
17. Cule JH: John Pugh, 1814-1874. A scholar surgeon's operation on the imperforate anus in 1854. Ann R Coll Surg Engl 1965;37:247-257.
18. Currarino G, Coln D, Votteler T: Triad of anorectal, sacral and presacral anomalies. AJR Am J Roentgenol 1981;137: 395-398.
19. de Vries PA, Friedland GW: The staged sequential development of the anus and rectum in human embryos and fetuses. J Pediatr Surg 1974;9:755-769.
20. de Vries PA, Pena A: Posterior sagittal anorectoplasty. J Pediatr Surg 1982;17:638-643.
21. Dubois A: Recueil Periodique de la Societe de Medecine de Paris 1783;3:125.
22. Georgeson KE, Inge TH, Albanese CT: Laparoscopically assisted anorectal pullthrough for high imperforate anus: A new technique. J Pediatr Surg 2000;35:927-931.
23. Goon HK: Repair of anorectal anomalies in the neonatal period. Pediatr Surg Int 1990;5:246-249.
24. Greenwood RD, Rosenthal A, Nadas AS: Cardiovascular malformations associated with imperforate anus. J Pediatr 1975;86:576-579.
25. Gross GW, Wolfson PJ, Peña A: Augmented-pressure colostogram in imperforate anus with fistula. Radiology 1991;21:560-562.
26. Hadra R: Demonstration zweier Fälle von Atresie ani vulvalis. Berlin Klin Wochenschr 1885;22:340.
27. Hedlund H, Peña A: Does the distal rectal muscle in anorectal malformations have the functional properties of a sphincter. J Pediatr Surg 1990;25:985-989.
28. Hoekstra WJ, Scholtmeijer RJ, Molenoar JC, et al: Urogenital tract abnormalities associated with congenital anorectal anomalies. J Urol 1983;130:962-963.
29. Hong AR, Rosen N, Acuña MF, et al: Urological injuries associated with the repair of anorectal malformations in male patients. J Pediatr Surg 2002;37:339-344.
30. Karrer FM, Flannery AM, Nelson MD Jr, et al: Anorectal malformations: Evaluation of associated spinal dysraphic syndromes. J Pediatr Surg 1988;23:45-48.
31. Leisrink H: Atresia Ani, Fehlen des Rectum: Operation nach der Methode von Stromeyer. Dtsch Z Chir 1872;1:494.
32. Levi AC, Borghi F, Garavoglia M: Development of the anal canal muscles. Dis Colon Rectum 1991;34:262-266.
33. Levitt MA, Patel M, Rodriguez G, et al: The tethered spinal cord in patients with anorectal malformations. J Pediatr Surg 1997;32:462-468.
34. Levitt MA, Soffer SZ, Peña A: Continent appendicostomy in the bowel management of fecal incontinent children. J Pediatr Surg 1997;32:1630-1633.
35. Levitt MA, Stein DM, Peña A: Gynecological concerns in the treatment of teenagers with cloaca. J Pediatr Surg 1998;33:188-193.
36. Littre A: Diverses observations anatomiques, histoire de l'acadamemie royale de Science. Paris, 1710.
37. Moore TC: Advantages of performing the sagittal anoplasty operation for imperforate anus at birth. J Pediatr Surg 1990;25:276-277.
38. McLeod N: Case of imperforate rectum, with a suggestion for a new method of treatment. BMJ 1880;2:657.
39. McLorie GA, Sheldon CA, Fleisher M, Churchill BM: The genitourinary system in patients with imperforate anus. J Pediatr Surg 1987;22:1100-1104.
40. Narasimharao KL, Prasad GR, Katariya S, et al: Prone cross-table lateral view: An alternative to the invertogram in imperforate anus. AJR Am J Roentgenol 1983;140:227-229.
41. Nixon HH, Puri P: The results of treatment of anorectal anomalies: A thirteen to twenty year follow up. J Pediatr Surg 1977;12:27-37.
42. Norris WJ, Brophy TW III, Brayton D: Imperforate anus: A case series and preliminary report of one-stage abdomino-perineal operation. Surg Gynecol Obstet 1949;88:623-625.
43. Olness K, McParland FA, Piper J: Biofeedback: A new modality in the management of children with fecal soiling. J Pediatr 1980;96:505-509.
44. Partridge JP, Gough MH: Congenital abnormalities of the anus and rectum. Br J Surg 1961;49:37-50.
45. Paulus A: On the imperforate anus. In The Seven Books, Book VI, Section LXXXI; translated by Adams F for the Sydenham Society, London, 1844.
46. Peña A: Advances in the management of fecal incontinence secondary to anorectal malformations. Surg Annu 1990; 22:143-167.
47. Peña A: Total urogenital mobilization—an easier way to repair cloacas. J Pediatr Surg 1997;32:263-268.

48. Peña A, El-Behery M: Megasigmoid—a source of pseudo-incontinence in children with repaired anorectal malformations. J Pediatr Surg 1993;28:1-5.
49. Peña A, Guardino K, Tovilla JM, et al: Bowel management for fecal incontinence in patients with anorectal malformations. J Pediatr Surg 1998;33:133-137.
50. Peña A, Levitt MA, Hong AR, Midulla PS: Surgical management of cloacal malformations: A review of 339 patients. J Pediatr Surg 2004;39:470-479.
51. Pinsky L: The syndromology of anorectal malformation (atresia, stenosis, ectopia). Am J Med Genet 1978;1:461-474.
52. Powell RW, Sherman JO, Raffensperger JG: Megarectum: A rare complication of imperforate anus repair and its surgical correction by endorectal pullthrough. J Pediatr Surg 1982;17:786-795.
53. Rosen NG, Hong AR, Soffer SZ, et al: Recto-vaginal fistula: A common diagnostic error with significant consequences in female patients with anorectal malformations. J Pediatr Surg 2002;37:961-965.
54. Rhoads JE, Pipes RL, Randall JP: A simultaneous abdominal and perineal approach in operations for imperforate anus with atresia of the rectum and rectosigmoid. Ann Surg 1948;127:552.
55. Rivosecchi M, Lucchetti MC, Zaccara A, et al: Spinal dysraphism detected by magnetic resonance imaging in patients with anorectal anomalies: Incidence and clinical significance. J Pediatr Surg 1995;30:488-490.
56. Shimada K, Hosokawa S, Matsumoto F, et al: Urological management of cloacal anomalies. Int J Urol 2001;8:282-289.
57. Smith ED, Saeki M: Associated anomalies in anorectal malformations in children: Update 1988. Birth Defects 1988; 24:501.
58. Soranus E: On the care of the newborn. In Soranus' Gynecology Book II; translated by Temkin O. Baltimore, Johns Hopkins University Press, 1956.
59. Squire R, Kiely EM, Carr B, et al: The clinical application of the Malone antegrade colonic enema. J Pediatr Surg 1993;28:1012-1015.
60. Stephens FD: Malformations of the anus. Aust N Z J Surg 1953;23:9-24.
61. Stephens FD: Embryology of the cloaca and embryogenesis of anorectal malformations. Birth Defects Orig Artic Ser 1988;24:177-209.
62. Stromeyer H: Handbuch der Chirurgie, vols 1 and 2. Freiburg, Germany, 1844-1848.
63. Tasakyannis DE, Shamberger RC: Association of imperforate anus with occult spinal dysraphism. J Pediatr Surg 1995; 30:1010-1012.
64. Teixera OHP, Malhotra K, Sellers J, Mercer S: Cardiovascular anomalies with imperforate anus. Arch Dis Child 1983;58:747-749.
65. Templeton JM, Ditesheim JA: High imperforate anus—quantitive results of long-term fecal continence. J Pediatr Surg 1985;20:645-652.
66. Torres P, Levitt MA, Tovilla JM, et al: Anorectal malformations and Down's syndrome. J Pediatr Surg 1998;33:1-5.
67. Tuuha SE, Aziz D, Drake J, et al: Is surgery necessary for asymptomatic tethered cord in anorectal malformation patients? J Pediatr Surg 2004;39:773-777.
68. von de Putte SCJ, Neeteson FA: The pathogenesis of hereditary congenital malformations of the anorectum in the pig. Acta Morphol Neerl Scand 1984;22:17-40.
69. Warne SA, Wilcox DT, Creighton S, Ransley PG: Long-term gynecologic outcome of patients with persistent cloaca. J Urol 2003;170:1493-1496.

第 102 章

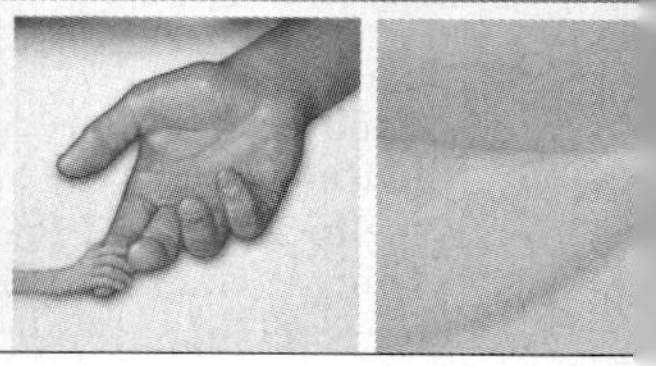

肛门直肠其他畸形和肛门直肠功能异常

Risto J. Rintala 和 Mikko Pakarinen

解剖学（图 102-1）

1590 肛管长 2.5~4.0 厘米[10]。直肠肛管连接处是立方上皮和柱状上皮移行区（齿线处）[61]。肛管的起始部被覆鳞状上皮，此处有皮脂腺和毛囊，向上被柱状和立方上皮所替代。上皮内和肛管黏膜内的感受器可以感受各种刺激，它们可以清楚分辨固体、液体和气体的刺激。直肠黏膜在齿状线处和肛管上皮相连，肛管黏膜形成 4~6 个纵形皱襞。

内括约肌的平滑肌部分是直肠内环肌的延续，主要位于肛管的底部。大约长 3 厘米，厚 5 毫米[45]。内括约肌被外括约肌和肛门周围的肌肉束包绕，形成一个强大收缩环，提供了至少 85% 的静止期肛管压力，使肛管处于闭合状态[23]。内括约肌可以轻度收缩，但是它可以通过直肠扩张反射完全放松[105]。这个反射是由肠肌间神经丛调节的，是一个内源性过程。这个反射持续存在不依赖于外在神经。

交感和副交感神经分布于内括约肌[36]。交感神经是主要的兴奋性神经，收缩内括约肌，来自于腰 2~4神经节段和肠系膜下神经节的腹下神经。α-肾上腺素刺激引起兴奋性传导，但是 β-肾上腺素刺激后引起抑制性传导。内括约肌持续性收缩状态受控于胆
碱能和肾上腺素能兴奋性刺激。副交感神经来自于骶 15
2~4神经节段，通常引起抑制性反应，导致内括约肌松弛[3,12]。

内括约肌本身也是内在神经分布的重要区域，直肠扩张时出现反射性松弛。这些内在神经包括位于肌间和肠壁内的神经丛（Auerbach）、深部的黏膜下神经丛（Henke）、黏膜下神经丛（Meissner）和非胆碱能非肾上腺素能神经丛[3,36]。

外括约肌可以随意控制。在齿状线以下的外括约肌环绕肛门，前面附着于会阴体部，后面附着于肛门

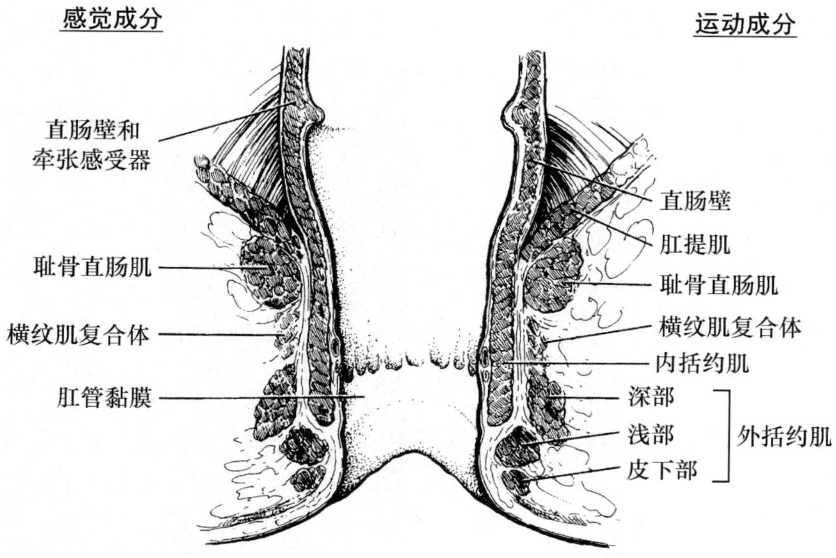

图 102-1 直肠和肛管的解剖。

尾骨处。外括约肌通常分为三部分：皮下部、浅部和深部。它们由来源于骶部 2～4 的阴部神经和会阴神经支配[64]。

外括约肌虽然是节段性收缩，但是它也可以出现强直收缩[17]。和内括约肌不同，外括约肌的强直收缩受外在输出神经支配。这个阶段的收缩包含主动和被动的过程，外括约肌维持 10%～15% 的肛管内压力[77]。

盆底肌肉是由肛提肌组构成的，其中耻骨直肠肌形成一个连接肛门直肠的索带。虽然是条索状的肌肉，但是耻骨直肠肌有保持强直性收缩的能力[48]。这造成了肛门和直肠在静息时有 80～90 度的角度，在排便时角度增大为 100～105 度的钝角[42]。大笑、用力或者其他突然间用力造成腹压升高时，耻骨直肠肌自动增加它的收缩压力。因此保持肛门直肠角为锐角，在控制排便中起重要作用[48]。肛提肌是围绕直肠、托起肛管的肌肉，它是肛管随意肌的一部分。肛提肌前部组成阴道和尿道括约肌，除了耻骨直肠肌以外，肛提肌是收缩和附着在骨盆后方的肌肉。

排便控制的生理

适当的结肠顺应性和肛门直肠处的储存机制对于排便控制来说是必需的。由于消化道远端不是一个简单的直线形管道，所以可以阻止大便直线性下降。直肠瓣和乙状结肠形成的角度可以阻碍大便向下移动。80 度的肛门直肠角度也可以控制排便[91]。除了排便反射，这些角度在平时腹部内压力突然增高（如喷嚏、大笑或姿势改变）的时候可以控制大便不至于从肛门排出。即使在内括约肌部分松弛的情况下，肛管的纵形黏膜折叠对于控制半固体或液体粪便也是有帮助的。

肛门内括约肌在控制排便中起到重要作用。自主性的外括约肌和不随意的内括约肌共同作用以维持肛管的静息压力。排便控制需要正常功能的内括约肌、外括约肌复合体和肛提肌，以及肛管直肠内正常的感觉器[10,38]。肛管有舒张功能的感受器越在远端，它的灵敏度越高。肛管内有丰富的感受器[88]，可以感觉是气体、液体，还是固体大便。

排便控制粗调节——控制体积较大的固体或者液体大便的能力——是由完善的肛门直肠角和内外括约肌系统控制的紧张性收缩完成的。排便控制细调节——控制体积较小的大便或者气体排出——是由括约肌协同完成的。远端直肠齿状线到齿状线以上 2 厘米是控制排便的重要区域[113]。这个区域是所谓的“简单反射区”，是控制固体、液体大便和气体的基础[30]。

排便生理

排便过程是一个随意肌和不随意肌协同作用的复杂过程，受比较高级的中枢系统的控制。通过结肠的运动，直肠渐渐充满大便，直肠扩张刺激直肠壁压力感受器和肛提肌，同时刺激引起括约肌复合体初步收缩，逆行排空远端直肠并使得内括约肌松弛，产生便意。粪便可以暂时性刺激肛管壁感受器，并被肛管黏膜内的精确感受器感知，分辨粪便的密度及识别是否为气体。便意产生，但此时便意可以受意志控制。肛门外括约肌和耻骨直肠肌可以自发收缩，抑制排便。直肠和肛管顺应性伸展可以降低直肠内压力和抑制便意。

当更多的大便进入直肠，感受度明显增加，直肠蠕动波明显加强，排便欲望增加。括约肌抑制性反射增加，抑制外括约肌和耻骨直肠肌强直性收缩；如果时间和地点允许，自主排便开始。

个体采用坐位或者蹲位的方式排便时，紧闭声门，使腹内压力增加。蹲位时，肛门直肠角被拉直，肛提肌收缩，这些运动可以防止骨盆下垂，结肠出现
大量的非蠕动性收缩，大段结肠顺应性排空[98]。在 1592
大便排出后，外括约肌系统收缩，内括约肌出现关闭肛管的活动，肛门直肠角重新建立。

*排便控制*可以被定义为能够控制到达肠管终末端的肠内容物，并可以无意识或有意识地控制潴留大便或者排便。排便生理机制的重点过程是储存大便、排便的连贯性和功能性内括约肌系统[125]。

幼儿的肠道转运时间短于大龄儿童。这和肠道蠕动频率密切相关[27]。婴幼儿由母乳或者牛乳喂养，造成每天 1～7 次肠运动[127]。1～4 岁儿童，85% 每天排便 1～2 次[128]。正常英国学龄儿童平均转运时间是 26 小时，便秘儿童转运时间是 80 小时。健康的成年人转运时间是 30～48 小时[117]。

便秘

儿童中便秘现象非常常见，尤其在西方。无法解决的便秘可以导致大便潴留和便秘恶性循环的发生。大多数人发生便秘的主要原因仍然不清楚，这种情况被称为*功能性便秘*。

定义

功能性便秘 不是由先天性异常、获得性疾病或药物所引起的便秘。便秘被定义为每周排便少于三次，如果同时伴有症状，如腹痛、溢粪，伴或不伴有污粪的大便潴留，即使大便超过每周三次[66,121]，也属于功能性便秘。便秘和污粪常见于小于 7 岁的儿童，据报道污粪在约 3% 的小于 4 岁的儿童中发生。临床上便秘发生率至少为 3%，儿童胃肠道门诊中便秘的发生率是 25%[29,35,62,67]。50% 以上的便秘儿童有家族史。很多研究提示其具有男性倾向，男女性比例为 1.5∶1～3∶1[1,63]。

Clayden 提出排便功能异常的分类如下[19]：

便秘 排便困难或延迟。

污粪 内裤上频繁有半固体的大便。

功能性大便失禁 正常排便但是出现在不合适的环境和地点。

因为新生儿期的便秘多伴有腹胀和呕吐，所以便秘是非功能性的，需要考虑解剖异常或机械性梗阻。94%～98% 的足月儿和 76% 的早产儿在生后 24 小时内排出胎粪。几乎所有的婴儿（100% 的足月儿和 99% 的早产儿）在出生后 48 小时排出胎粪。在出生后第一年，对于有便秘症状的患儿需要进行评价并且排除器质性病变。

在婴儿期，便秘通常出现在饮食结构发生变化的时候，如母乳转到人工喂养，或者开始食用固体食物[109]。尤其在儿童期，由于肛裂或 A 型*链球菌*引起的肛周皮炎可以导致排便疼痛，患儿因此不愿意排便，大便积聚，造成恶性循环，慢性便秘形成。A 型*链球菌* 感染提示患儿对于牛奶中蛋白物质不能耐受[50]。除大年龄儿童外，食物中的纤维素和便秘发生的相关性很小[99]。父母便秘的儿童常常也会发生便秘[55]。传输慢与成年人便秘密切相关，也是部分儿童便秘的主要原因[11,49]。心理问题在儿童便秘患儿中很常见，但多继发于便秘[1,68]。

急性便秘

急性便秘可以继发于活动少、饮食改变或肛裂。常见症状是腹部急性疼痛。当腹痛作为急性便秘首发症状时，可以通过简单的灌肠缓解。急性便秘的治疗通常是直接的，尤其是对婴幼儿和学龄前儿童。饮食中加入更多的水或者限制牛奶的摄入可以缓解症状。大年龄儿童和有急性肛裂的患儿需要用缓泻剂治疗一定时间。

慢性便秘

不能对饮食改变产生反应或者通过简单的缓泻剂治疗无效的持续性便秘可以定义为慢性便秘。慢性便秘的儿童可以出现污粪。功能性大便失禁（在不合适的时间和地点排便）和心理因素密切相关[20]。在慢性便秘的诊断中应该考虑一些器质性病变，详细见表 102-1。

儿童便秘和溢粪的研究显示，40% 的患者是因为没有足够的排便训练，30% 以上的患者发生过遗尿[62]。慢性便秘和污粪一般在 2～4 岁发生[24]，然而 1/4 的儿童在出生后第一年内便发生便秘。当 1 岁左右儿童开始进行排便训练时，便秘和污粪发生率明显增高。

慢性便秘的诊断有赖于病史和临床检查。详细的排便情况应该包括便秘第一次发生时的年龄、排便的频率和排便的性状以及以往的干预，包括药物治疗。抗惊厥剂、利尿剂、制酸剂及补充的铁剂都可以导致便秘发生。家族病史非常重要，尤其是巨结肠病史、囊性纤维病或家族性便秘。慢性便秘患者某些临床特点的发生率总结见表 102-2。

临床检查时儿童腹部通常没有触痛，很少有腹胀。在耻骨联合上方和左下腹常常可以摸到粪块。会阴和肛门的结构必须仔细检查，同时注意肛门周围皮肤是否有大便。因为肛门位置异常容易引起便秘，所以必须明确肛门位置是否正常[8,119]。Reisner 和他的同事[95]对定义男女孩正常肛门位置的测定标准做了具体规定。女孩为肛门中心到阴唇系带的距离比阴唇系带到尾骨的距离，男孩为肛门中心到阴囊后方的距

表 102-1 慢性便秘的鉴别诊断：器质性或获得性原因

巨结肠类缘病
内括约肌失弛缓症
肠神经元发育异常（肠神经元增多症）
神经元减少症
先天性异常
肛门狭窄
肛门前移位
获得性疾病
慢性肛裂
慢性肛瘘
Crohn 病
伴系统性疾病
低钾
高钙血症
脑瘫和神经损伤
尿毒症
心理性疾病
抑郁症
神经性厌食症
原发性功能性大便失禁
药物
抗抑郁药物
精神性药物
抗胆碱能药物

表 102-2 严重功能性便秘的临床特点

发病年龄	
0～1 岁	20%～25%
1～5 岁	70%
>5 岁	10%～15%
男女性比	1～3∶1
以往治疗	80%～90%
污粪	70%～75%
不成功的排便训练	70%～80%
排便时疼痛	70%～80%
腹部疼痛	50%～60%
偶发大便带血	25%～30%
食欲差	20%～30%
尿失禁	20%～30%
原发性心理疾病	15%～20%
直肠脱垂	3%

离比阴囊后方到尾骨的距离。女孩此比例小于 0.34（一般比例：新生儿为 0.44，4～18 个月为 0.40）和男孩此比例小于 0.46（一般比例：新生儿为 0.58，4～18个月为 0.56）时，需要引起重视，特别是伴有便秘的患儿。鉴别肛门前移位和会阴部异位肛门常很困难，尤其是肛门前移位伴有肛门狭窄时。最终诊断需要麻醉下行肌肉刺激，才能明确。

对于肛门周围感觉的检查可以用棉签棒在肛周皮肤上进行刺激，观察肛门周围组织是否会皱缩及会阴是否出现收缩。同时还需要注意检查患儿的内裤是否有污粪存在。

肛门指检可以提示肛管缩短。括约肌紧张性可能消失，尤其是直肠壶腹部充满大便时。大便堆积在直肠内可形成坚硬粪块。溢粪可以伴随粪块的出现而出现。外括约肌通常是完整的，肛门指检时患儿可以随意收缩外括约肌。必须检查直肠后间隙，在骶骨窝内可以触及粪块。手指拔出后，括约肌出现收缩反射。缺少会阴部皮肤反射或者括约肌收缩反射提示存在神经系统异常。

如果临床病史和体检没有提示器质性病变，可以进行实验性药物治疗。新生儿期即出现症状并早期出现便秘的患儿，需要行钡剂灌肠检查，检查前不需要进行肠道准备。若钡剂灌肠出现异常，应该行直肠黏膜活检和直肠测压以排除巨结肠类缘病。对新生儿期或婴儿期没有便秘史的大年龄患儿，没有必要在药物治疗以前进行钡剂灌肠或直肠活检[39,56]。对于药物治疗效果欠佳或者临床有异常表现如神经系统异常的儿童，可以进行钡剂灌肠和其他影像学检查，如腹部平片、传输时间分析或者核磁共振检查。对于合理药物治疗效果差的患儿才需要做直肠黏膜活检或直肠测压，以排除神经元发育不良如肠神经元发育不良和内括约肌失弛缓症（见第 99 章和 100 章）。

钡剂灌肠显示直肠乙状结肠到肛管部扩张，则可以排除巨结肠，但是不能排除内括约肌失弛缓症。腹 1594
部平片可以提示临床上有神经源性异常的患者是否存在椎管异常。如果有椎管异常，需要做核磁共振以排除脊髓内病变，如脊髓栓塞或者脊髓内脂肪瘤[100]。传输时间分析是依靠辐射不能穿透的标志[11,96]或放射性同位素[49]来估计药物治疗效果差的患儿的结肠运动情况。此分析方法显示难治性便秘患者中有相当一部分存在慢性便秘。该方法目前应用的主要问题是缺少健康儿童的正常值和诊断标准。

肛门直肠测压是诊断巨结肠和内括约肌失弛缓

症的有效手段。这两类疾病，患儿肛门直肠松弛反射消失。对于功能性便秘患儿，直肠肛管测压不能提高诊断和治疗的准确性[121]。对其他神经节细胞异常症，如神经节细胞减少症和肠神经元发育不良症，肛门直肠测压可以提示各种异常，但是不能作为诊断的依据[58]。另一方面，对于肠神经元发育异常或神经节细胞减少症，肛门直肠测压可以对治疗有帮助。按照我们的经验，如果患者肛管静息压力很高（>100 cm H_2O），则需要行内括约肌切除或部分切除术。有些患者组织病理学检查显示正常，但是直肠测压提示肛门出口梗阻和与之矛盾的内括约肌复合体收缩，临床上称为肛门直肠协调不良[5,54,69,76]。

处理

便秘儿童的常规治疗包括对父母提供咨询和教育。首先判断是否有粪块堵塞情况，如果有，先清除粪块，然后口服药物治疗[20,68]。

家庭咨询和教育是治疗的第一步。便秘的病因应该向患儿父母解释清楚。如果患儿有污粪，需要和家长商量，并鼓励家长在漫长的治疗过程中保持积极的心态。对患儿和家长进行宣教、情感支持，并对该家庭保持关注直到患儿正常排便，这都是康复计划的重要组成部分[20,51,54]。父母和患儿必须知道建立正常的排便需要 6~12 个月，甚至更长时间。

如果患儿出现大便干结成团或者粪块，在药物治疗以前需要去除干结的大便或粪块。体检发现下腹部较硬的肿块、直肠指检或者放射学检查可以提示粪块的存在。粪便嵌塞的典型症状是滞留性失禁。对于粪块治疗首选灌肠。口服药物也是有效的[32,116]。

口服的泻剂可以含有高剂量刺激性缓泻药、多库酯（阴离子表面活性物质）、矿物油和甘露醇。等渗性缓泻剂如乳果糖或山梨醇可以和其他药物联合应用。口服泻剂可以引起腹部疼痛或绞痛，也会增加污粪的机会。

灌肠的效果较口服泻剂快，但这种方法对肛门异常患儿具有侵袭性，并可引起疼痛，因此，灌肠对肛裂的患者是禁止使用的。许多研究人员提出可用生理盐水、多库酯（阴离子表面活性物质）、矿物油或磷酸盐灌肠[20,85,103]。当清除直肠内粪块时，灌肠次数应减少到最低，通常 1~3 次灌肠可以完全清除直肠内粪块。对于依从性差的患儿，可考虑全麻下行粪块清除。

维持治疗的目的是保证每天有 1~2 次的松软大便，防止粪块再次形成。这样可以阻断大便干结成团的恶性循环和减少排便时的剧烈疼痛。

治疗还包括饮食调节、心理放松和日常行为习惯的改变。饮食调节是必须强调的，尤其是增加水分和纤维素的摄入。纤维素的作用在儿童中并不十分明显[99]，不提倡过多的牛奶摄入[87]，尚无证据证明何种药物治疗效果更好。在粪块清除后的早期，需要有效的药物治疗。刺激性泻药番泻叶及吡啶甲叉双苯氧磺酸钠应在尽可能短的时间内应用，以后用毒性小的药物替代。等渗性泻药，如乳果糖或山梨醇，可以安全使用数月或数年。肠蠕动规则后，药物需要继续使用一段时间，通常几个月或者几年。一般推荐的原则是只要患儿还存在治疗前的症状就维持治疗。药物治疗剂量逐渐减少，以最小剂量达到治疗效果为宜。

不同年龄段有不同的行为治疗。对于婴幼儿，行为治疗不起作用。太早或者激进的排便训练都不提倡。小于 2~3 岁的儿童不进行排便训练，可以使用尿布。可以在白天饭后对大于 2~3 岁的儿童进行排便训练。应该给予奖赏与鼓励，并且持之以恒以取得满意的效果[32]。

长期预后

很少有关于长期慢性自发性便秘患儿的研究[55,73,110]。有报道称随访 5 年后，最终仅有 50% 的治愈率。有家族史的患儿预后差。但是值得欣慰的是，症状性便秘和溢出性便失禁在青春期并不常见[1,9]。有家族史和早期出现排便异常的患儿以后仍可能有持续性排便异常[116]。

外科选择

绝大多数慢性便秘患儿的症状由于选择了正确的治疗时机和使用合适的药物治疗而得到改善。很多患儿可以遵守医嘱进行治疗，但是有一些患儿尽管有理想的药物治疗还是持续出现便秘、腹部症状和污粪。没有对照研究说明外科方法对儿童原发性便秘有治疗作用。

对于药物治疗无效的病例有些可行外科治疗，但是器质性因素必须排除。Malone 顺行节制性灌肠（MACE）[75]最早用于神经性失禁或者肛门直肠畸形治疗后的失禁，现在也用于原发性便秘的治疗[57,130]。MACE 可逆性强，是灌肠和缓泻剂的替代方法，尤其受到青少年患者和成年患者的喜爱[129]。结肠造瘘也可以选择性用于患者，并取得良好效果。结肠测压可以给外科医生提供依据，但是此类研究仍处于初级阶段[49,137]。

无便秘的功能性污粪

有很小一部分患者不存在便秘或者器质或心理疾病，但是出现污粪[28,41,122]。出现的年龄是 4～8 岁。主要症状是每天不自主地排大便 1 次以上。污粪主要发生在白天。至少 1/3 的患者可出现白天或夜间遗尿。在过去 10 年中我们遇到约 20 例患者。

这种污粪一直被认为是心因性的。但是，在这些儿童中没有发现严重的心理异常，单纯心理治疗的效果往往令人失望[14]。我们对 20 例患者进行了广泛研究，没有发现心理异常，核磁共振显示脊髓无病变，钡剂灌肠和脊柱 X 线检查都正常；白天或夜间遗尿的发生率是 40%。仅肛门直肠测压提示直肠敏感性下降，内括约肌功能和正常人一样。治疗主要是对父母的宣教、排便训练和日常行为规范及饮食调整。大多数患者可以降低污粪次数。所有患者在青春期后污粪消失。

直肠脱垂

直肠脱垂是相对常见的疾病，在儿童期为自限性疾病。发病高峰是 1～3 岁。可以分为部分或完全脱垂。在部分脱垂的患者中，直肠黏膜距肛门缘处脱出 1～3 厘米。完全脱垂时，整个直肠全层脱出，一般有 5 厘米以上的直肠脱出（图 102-2）。对于儿童直肠脱垂中完全脱垂与部分脱垂的定义仍存在较大争议。

病理和诊断

下述解剖特点对儿童直肠脱垂提供了重要的病因学依据：

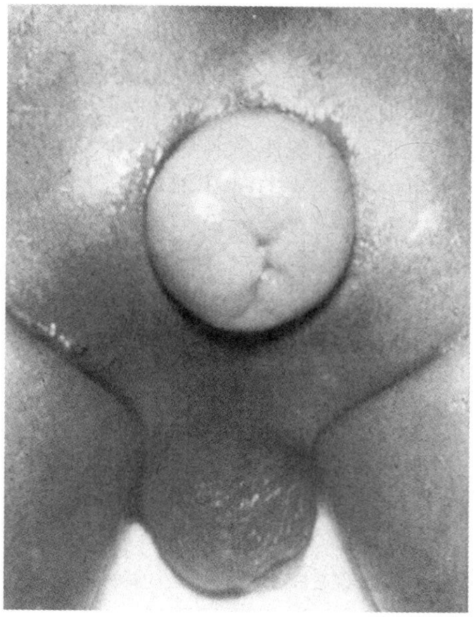

图 102-2　2 岁直肠脱垂男孩。

- 直肠呈垂直方向
- 侧向及前后部到直肠曲线不明显
- 较平坦的尾椎骨平面和骶骨平面
- 直肠和其他骨盆器官的位置相对较低
- 缺乏肛提肌的支撑

大多数直肠脱垂患者不存在易患因素。自发性直肠脱垂儿童通常其他方面都健康。便秘作为直肠脱垂的病因存在争议：仅有 3% 的严重慢性便秘患儿有直肠脱垂[1]。

其他器质性病变可以造成直肠脱垂，如囊性纤维病变伴有直肠脱垂[132]。大于 1/5 的囊性纤维病变伴 1596
有直肠脱垂[59,108]。神经性病变如脊髓脊膜膨出可以造成完全性直肠脱垂，但是很少见。另外，肛提肌麻痹引起腹内压增高可导致脱垂。膀胱外翻时广泛的耻骨联合和耻骨直肠肌分离，易于导致盆腔内脏器脱垂，包括直肠脱垂。

医源性的直肠全层脱垂发生于高位肛门直肠畸形经肛门手术后，常见的是黏膜脱垂[97]。直肠脱垂或者黏膜异位在经后矢状进路手术后患者中常见[90]。直肠息肉也可以导致直肠脱垂。严重的营养不良也是导致直肠脱垂的原因之一。

直肠脱垂的诊断通常依据病史。最常见症状的是排便后直肠黏膜呈现花瓣状。有时候患儿主诉肛门脱出。通常，肛门脱垂可以自发性复位，但是有时候需要手法复位。轻度的直肠脱垂可以由于用力或者腹泻，直肠偶尔脱出。如果每次排便都出现直肠脱垂，父母和患儿对此会出现焦虑和担心。

直肠脱垂在门诊咨询时并不发生。直肠指检可以排除直肠息肉。即使有直肠出血病史，也很少需要进行结肠镜检查以排除高位的结肠息肉或者其他位点的出血。通常不需要其他检查方法。

治疗

对于急性脱垂，站位时多可以自然复位。如果脱垂未能自行复位，应设法尽早复位。第一次发生脱垂时，父母通常会马上送患儿到医院。将脱垂的肠管头端缓慢地推入肛门内。如果肠壁有水肿，复位时挤压手法要轻柔。同时要将肛门脱垂的复位方法教给父母。

大部分复发性脱垂可以自愈[2]，很多情况下肛门脱垂会自行缓解。如果没有自行缓解，患儿父母获得正确的指导后，也可以对脱垂进行手法复位。保守治疗如臀部包扎、排便时用坐便器改变体位或侧卧位排便对于减少脱垂都无帮助。软化大便可以治疗脱垂。局部经肛门治疗如脱垂处注射、多处电灼黏膜、切除多余的黏膜或者肛门周围皮下缝合（Thiersch 线）都被证实无效。我们的经验也证实这一点。但是很多小儿外科医生认为以上方法是有效的，尤其是肛门周围皮下缝合，因为他们发现对于很多患儿来说都是有效的。

手术治疗用于极少的难治性脱垂患者，如经治疗后随访 12～18 个月仍不能痊愈的患儿。大于 4 岁的患者比小于 4 岁患者更需要外科治疗。有一些外科手术治疗方法可以治疗难治性脱垂。后矢状进路肌肉修补和直肠悬吊至骶骨[6,7,89,104]、直肠后折叠术[118]和 Ekehorn 直肠耻骨固定术[102]都可以治疗难治性脱垂。我们倾向于用腹腔镜进行直肠和前耻骨的悬吊。该手术方式术后疼痛最小，住院时间短。

经肛门拖出术后出现医源性脱垂且有症状的患儿需要进行二次手术治疗。典型的症状包括黏膜出血和黏液漏。对于黏膜脱出的患者，治疗包括切除异位黏膜和肛门局部皮瓣整形。完全脱垂需要肛提肌和外括约肌的重建及直肠悬吊术。

肛裂

肛裂是远端肛管沿纵轴裂开或溃疡裂开至肛门缘。绝大多数肛门裂开数周后可以自行愈合，但是有一部分可以转变为慢性。肛裂是儿童期便血的常见原因，也是肛门疼痛时需要鉴别诊断的疾病之一。肛裂是常见疾病，但是儿童肛裂的发生率还不明确。

发病机制

自发性肛裂的发病机制目前尚未明确，成人和儿童的发病机制可能不同[20]。儿童期肛裂由于排便时疼痛，多继发有便秘。认为发生肛裂的首要原因是由坚硬的粪块造成的机械性撕裂的经典理论可能过于简单和陈旧了。但是，有意识地减少排便的确可以造成直肠扩张、直肠敏感性下降，继而大便干结，影响肛裂愈合。害怕排便时的疼痛将导致大便潴留和恶性循环。

关于成人肛裂的发病理论，现在已经被广泛接受[80,120]。按照这个理论，增加内括约肌压力及肌肉痉挛可以导致组织灌注受损伤并且最终形成上皮溃疡。内括约肌痉挛可以导致严重的缺血和肛裂形成。最常见的部位是后正中位，这个部位的血管明显少于其他部位。肛裂患者的肛管静息压力明显增加。手术或药物治疗使肛管压力下降，进而增加肛 1
膜的灌注和促进慢性肛裂的愈合。目前，这个理论是否适用于儿童患者仍未可知。在儿童期，有很多未接受正规治疗的肛裂自发愈合。这是由于儿童期肛管组织具有相对良好的灌注和更好的再生能力。由于细菌的入侵和化学性或机械性因素，肛裂发生感染。长期肛裂慢性感染导致肛乳头肥大和前哨痔。儿童期慢性肛裂很少见，如果发生慢性肛裂需要考虑 Crohn 病的存在[112]。

诊断

肛裂可发生于任何年龄。发生肛裂的典型年龄是 2 岁左右。大多数肛裂有鲜红色血便和排便时疼痛。表现为大便时婴儿出现哭闹，大便表面有鲜红色血液。肛裂多伴有便秘，这是由于患儿畏惧排便时的疼痛，不敢排便，导致大便在直肠内滞留。

肛门视诊可以明确诊断。检查时发现典型的纵形至齿状线的远端开裂，即可明确诊断。肛裂的位置最常见于后正中线，还可以发生在肛门的其他部位，尤其是婴儿。女婴常见部位是前正中线。慢性或亚急性肛裂可以伴有前哨痔或者皮赘。不典型的肛裂可以多发，大多远离中线，常为巨大和不规则形。不典型肛裂出现时需要进一步检查，包括直肠活检、培养和直肠镜检查，以排除 Crohn 病、免疫低下、结核病、性病和恶性疾病。

治疗

绝大多数肛裂在儿童期可不进行治疗，数月内可自行愈合[53,115]，只有有症状的肛裂需要治疗。如果肛裂伴有便秘和（或）排便疼痛，可以进行饮食调整使大便软化，也可以使用容积性泻药。润滑油可以减轻排便时的疼痛，目的是阻断由大便秘结、粪便滞留及抑制肛裂愈合等因素引起的恶性循环[53]。软化大便后大多数肛裂可以愈合，便血也停止。除非无临床症状和便血，一般患者都愿意治疗。

成人肛裂治疗获得令人满意的效果。近年来又通过安慰剂对比试验评价了局部应用硝酸甘油治疗儿童肛裂的效果[53,81,114,115]。两项研究报道了使用硝酸甘油药膏治疗后肛裂快速愈合和症状缓解的情况，其中一项研究报告无明显改善[53]，另一项研究显示使用硝酸甘油药膏可以降低肛管最大静息压力[115]。使用硝酸甘油治疗时，很少有儿童出现一过性失禁，也没有头痛的报道[53,114,115]。近来一项包含成人和儿童患者的 meta 分析发现，硝酸甘油治疗肛裂与安慰剂对比可以取得满意的效果[81]。当润滑剂治疗无效时，硝酸甘油药膏可以选择性应用。每天使用膏药，持续至少 6～8 周才会有效[114,115]。

儿童期肛裂外科治疗包括：肛裂切除、麻醉下肛门扩张和内括约肌侧切术。肛裂切除手术结合使用润滑剂与单纯润滑剂治疗比较，二者治愈率相当（80%）[53,60]。侧面皮下括约肌切开对儿童有效[22]。肛门扩张可以导致不同程度的内括约肌损伤，应该避免。成年患者括约肌侧切术后约有 10% 的患者出现失禁[82]。肛门扩张与括约肌切开术相比，危险性明显增高[82]。不同的外科治疗方法对控制儿童排便效果无特殊性，所以对于局部使用硝酸甘油治疗无效的慢性肛裂患者，可考虑使用括约肌侧切术。对于这些患者需要做直肠活检以排除 Crohn 病。

肛周脓肿和肛瘘

肛周脓毒血症常见于小婴儿[86]。绝大多数患者为男性[34,106]。婴幼儿肛瘘有先天性因素存在。男性婴儿由于雄性激素导致上皮隐窝深，所以易于发生肛周脓肿[4,106]。典型的临床表现是小于 12 个月的婴儿出现肛周脓肿（图 102-3），主要发生于 6 个月以前。早期切开可以导致复发和瘘管形成。肛周脓肿转变为肛瘘的发生率是 10%～20%[73,84]。肛瘘可以不伴有肛周脓肿而独立存在。典型瘘管位于皮下，直形。瘘管起源于感染的隐窝，经过外括约肌皮下部直达肛周皮肤。瘘管常均匀分布于肛门周围。多发病变的发生率为 15%～20%（图 102-4）[84,126]。

肛周脓肿的传统治疗是切开和引流。传统治疗可有很高的复发率[79,126]。但是，大多数脓肿可以通过 1598
治疗而治愈[101,126]。肛瘘可以考虑手术治疗，传统方法是确定感染隐窝后行瘘管切开术。瘘管复发率是 10%～20%。近来报告提示无症状的肛瘘可以在 12～

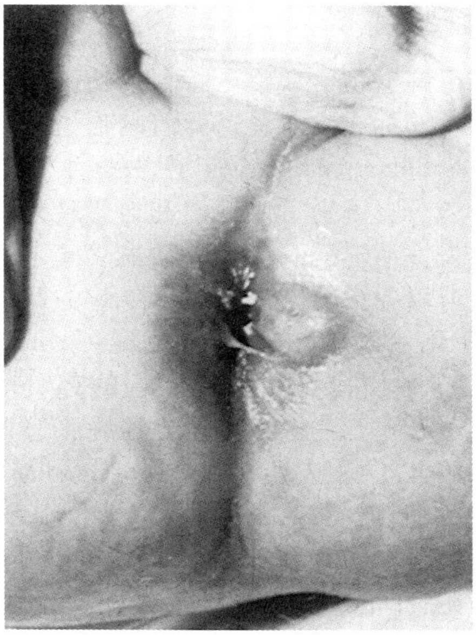

图 102-3　男婴典型肛周脓肿。

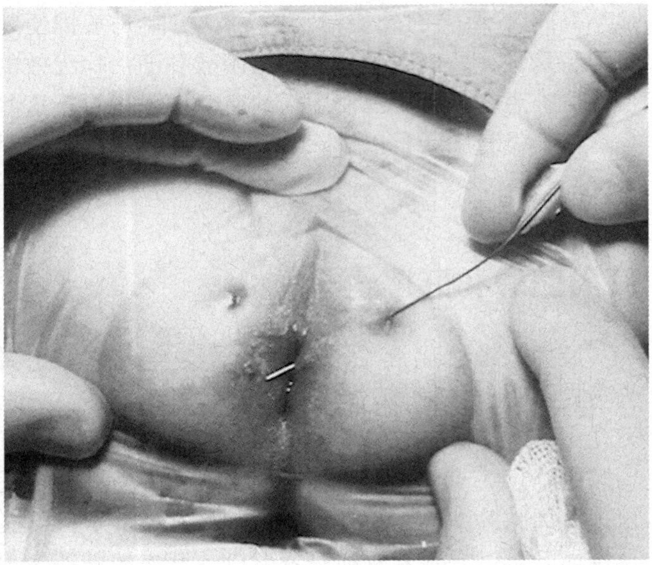

图 102-4 两侧肛瘘。探针从皮肤开口直达肛管隐窝。

24 个月内自行愈合[101,126]。

大龄儿童或青少年时期肛瘘是隐窝腺瘤病或伴有炎症性肠炎，主要是 Crohn 病。除了典型年龄的患儿，一般不考虑 Crohn 病。青少年期肛瘘的治疗方法与成年人的治疗相同。瘘管一旦明确，需要切除或者切开已经闭合的肉芽组织。

脉管性畸形

在不了解生物学和临床特性的情况下，根据相似病变的不同标志物对肠道脉管畸形进行分类易产生混淆。Mulliken 和 Glowacki[78] 根据生物学特性对其分类，该分类区别了血管瘤和血管畸形。血管瘤是可以自发性消退的新生物，而血管畸形是无法自行消退、非增生性的。血管畸形导致的肠道出血在儿童中少见，远端结肠和直肠是常见的出血部位[26]。有少数出血为系统性疾病的部分表现，如 Klippel-Trenaunay 综合征（先天性肿胀静脉、皮肤血管瘤和下肢扩张肥大）和 Osler-Rendu-Weber 综合征（毛细血管扩张综合征）。

血管畸形的诊断比较困难。内镜可以发现远端肠管的局部炎症，但很少看到扩张的静脉。近段尤其是小肠病变可以通过胶囊内镜观察[123]。MRI 和血管造影仍然是诊断学上定位肠道血管病变的最好方法。非手术方法可以控制出血，但要获得永久性治疗效果则需行病灶完全切除术。如病灶延伸至低位直肠和肛管，最好的治疗方法是经内镜拖出，行直肠肛管吻合术[33,71]。这种括约肌保留手术即使不能根治病灶，也能在较长时间段内保证无肠道出血。

痔疮

除门脉高压，儿童期痔疮不常见。1/3 的门脉高压患儿有痔疮。肝外型门脉高压患儿痔疮发生率高于肝内型门脉高压患儿[43]。但是有症状的痔疮仍很少见。

痔疮也可以发生在健康儿童，但是少见（图 102-5）。我们在过去的 15 年中，每年仅看到 1 例正常儿童的痔疮，而且通常是无症状的，但是患儿和家长可以发现有东西从肛门口脱出。这种情况常见于便秘儿童，肛门口有静脉丛形成，是便秘儿童出血的主要来源。不典型的痔疮开始于青春期，可以并发痔疮外部血栓形成。

健康儿童痔疮不需要外科治疗，有症状的门脉高压患儿需要治疗。大多数患儿病情可以通过捆扎或硬 15
化治疗控制[44]。

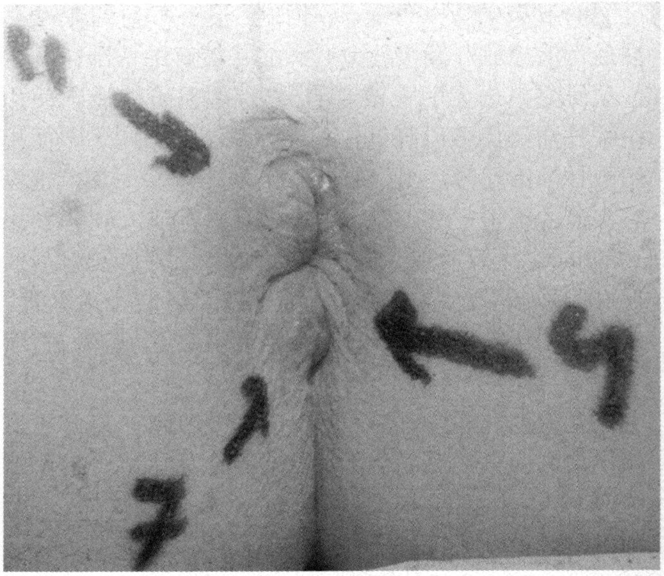

图 102-5 5 岁男孩痔疮。注意成人常见部位为 4、7 及 11 点。

单独的直肠溃疡

单独的直肠溃疡是一个慢性、良性的病变，以血便、黏液便、里急后重和局部肛周疼痛为主要表现。儿童时期少见，但可存在轻度的局部肛门症状[31]。内镜检查发现肠壁增厚和水肿，距肛门口 2～5 厘米的直肠前壁有溃疡或息肉存在。在过去 10 年中我们发现 6 例患者。有的患者表现为里急后重。直肠脱垂在大多数病例中发生[40]。按照我们的经验，软化大便的保守治疗和局部应用糖皮质激素栓剂可以治疗很多患者。直肠固定手术可以纠正单独直肠溃疡伴发的直肠脱垂。

婴儿期直肠结肠炎

除肛裂外，婴儿期直肠结肠炎也是导致小于 3 个月婴儿便血的常见原因。婴儿期直肠结肠炎典型表现是 3～4 周婴儿出现与大便混合的新鲜血丝。大便常是软的，无其他症状，婴儿的生长和发育正常[59a]。结肠镜检查显示斑片状结肠炎，很少超出左半结肠。组织学检查显示明显增多的嗜酸性粒细胞浸润。有些患者显示外周血中嗜酸性粒细胞计数增多。这些现象提示了过敏性因素的存在[74]。该疾病具有自限性，症状持续数周，饮食调节可以缓解直肠结肠炎[16]。

性虐待

性虐待是一个普遍存在的世界性问题。在欧洲小于 16 岁儿童中，女孩中发生率是 6%～36%，男孩中发生率是 1%～15%[52]。性虐待很少导致死亡，但是结果是严重的，可以影响人的一生。鉴定儿童时期性虐待时，阴道和处女膜具有重要意义，但是对肛交的鉴定存在争议而且难以证实。

Hobbs 和 Wynne[46] 提出“肛门扩张和反射性肛门扩张”在正常儿童中不常见，可以作为肛交的证据。社会健康机构、出院儿童门诊部、社区医院和直肠门诊对 200 名儿童的常规检查发现，28 名有反射性肛门扩张[111]。没有遭受性虐待的儿童，由于便秘或者粪块积聚在直肠也可以造成肛门扩张[21]。Hobbs 和 Wynne[47] 还提出肛裂是性虐待的特征，因为 143 例遭受性虐待的儿童中 53% 存在肛裂。Pierce[92] 发现儿童中有肛交的大多数出现肛裂或瘢痕。但是肛裂在临床上太常见了，不能作为肛交的直接证据，只能作为怀疑的证据[37]。

明显撕裂、肛门周围或者内侧大腿淤青和抓痕，尤其是有疑似或明确受虐待史的，需要更多确凿的证据。由于体检和暴力相隔太长时间，法庭证据明显减少。

如果体检时孩子出现完全被动和冷淡的反应，而且直肠指检横纹肌没有出现收缩或紧张的反应，临床医生应该警惕可能有性虐待存在。

发现由人乳头瘤病毒引起的肛周疣时可以怀疑有性虐待存在，因为这是性传播疾病[25,72]。很多研究（60%～90% 的研究）表明它与性虐待有关，但是近年来又对此提出质疑。父母患有非生殖系统的湿疣，有可能通过母亲垂直传播给婴儿。所以小于 1 岁的婴儿可能由母婴垂直传播获得，但是对于大年龄儿童则有可能存在性虐待。

（沈涤华译　李　龙校）

参考文献 1600

1. Abrahamian FP, Lloyd-Still JD: Chronic constipation in children: A longitudinal study of 186 patients. J Pediatr Gastroenterol Nutr 1984;3:460.
2. Adeyemi SD: Childhood rectal prolapse: A prospective clinical study including trial of a rationalized conservative treatment modality. Int J Pediatr Surg 1991;5:21.
3. Aldridge RT, Campbell PE: Ganglion cell distribution in the normal rectum and anal canal. J Pediatr Surg 1968;3:475.
4. Al-Salem AH, Laing W, Talwalker V: Fistula-in-ano in infancy and childhood. J Pediatr Surg 1994;29:436.
5. Arhan P, Devroede G, Jehannin B, et al: Idiopathic disorders of fecal continence in children. Pediatrics 1983;71:774.
6. Ashcraft KW, Amoury RA, Holder TM: Levator repair and posterior suspension for rectal prolapse. J Pediatr Surg 1977;12:241.
7. Ashcraft KW, Garred JL, Holder TM: Rectal prolapse—17-year experience with the posterior repair and suspension. J Pediatr Surg 1990;25:992.
8. Bar-Maor JA, Eitan A: Determination of the normal position of the anus. J Pediatr Gastroenterol Nutr 1987;6:559.
9. Bellman M: Studies on encopresis. Acta Paediatr Scand 1966;1(Suppl):170.
10. Bennett DL, Duthie HL: The functional importance of the internal anal sphincter. Br J Surg 1964;51:355.
11. Benninga MA, Buller HA, Tytgat GN, et al: Colonic transit time in constipated children: Does pediatric slow-transit constipation exist? J Pediatr Gastroenterol Nutr 1996;

23:241.
12. Bitar KN, Makhlour GM: Purinergic receptors on isolated smooth muscle cells. Gastroenterology 1982;82:1018.
13. Bonnard A, Mougenot JP, Ferkdadji L, et al: Laparoscopic rectopexy for solitary ulcer of the rectum syndrome in a child. Surg Endosc 2003;17:1156.
14. Brazzelli M, Griffiths P: Behavioural and cognitive interventions with or without other treatments for defaecation disorders in children. Cochrane Database Syst Rev 2001;4: CD002240.
15. Burkitt D, Morley D, Walker A: Dietary fibre in under- and overnutrition in childhood. Arch Dis Child 1980; 55:803.
16. Chang JW, Wu TC, Wang KS, et al: Colon mucosal pathology in infants under three months of age with diarrhea disorders. J Pediatr Gastroenterol Nutr 2002;35:387.
17. Christensen J: Motility of the colon. In Johnson LR (ed): Physiology of the Gastrointestinal Tract, 2nd ed. New York, Raven Press, 1987.
18. Clark DA: Times of first void and first stool in 500 newborns. Pediatrics 1977;60:457.
19. Clayden GS: Constipation and soiling in childhood. BMJ 1976;1:515.
20. Clayden G, Agnarsson U: Constipation in Childhood. Oxford, Oxford Medical Publications, 1991.
21. Clayden GS: Reflex anal dilatation associated with severe chronic constipation in children. Arch Dis Child 1988;63:832.
22. Cohen A, Dehn TCB: Lateral subcutaneous sphincterotomy for treatment of anal fissure in children. Br J Surg 1995;82:1341.
23. Culver PS, Rattan S: Genesis of anal canal pressures in the opossum. Am J Physiol 1986;251:765.
24. Davidson M, Kugler MM, Bauer CH: Diagnosis and management in children with severe and protracted constipation and obstipation. J Pediatr 1964;62:261.
25. de Jesus LE, Cirne Neto OL, Monteiro do Nascimento LM, et al: Anogenital warts in children: Sexual abuse or unintentional contamination? Cad Saude Publica 2001; 17:1383.
26. de la Torre L, Carrasco D, Mora MA, et al: Vascular malformations of the colon in children. J Pediatr Surg 2002; 37:1754.
27. Di Lorenzo C, Flores AF, Hyman PE: Age-related changes in colon motility. J Pediatr 1995;127:593.
28. Di Lorenzo C, Benninga MA: Pathophysiology of pediatric fecal incontinence. Gastroenterology 2004;126:S33.
29. Doyles DM: Enuresis and encopresis. In Ollendick TH, Hersen M (eds): Handbook of Child Psychopathology. New York, Plenum Press, 1983.
30. Duthie HL: Dynamics of the rectum and anus. Clin Gastroenterol 1975;4:467.
31. Ertem D, Acar Y, Karaa EK, et al: A rare and often unrecognized cause of hematochezia and tenesmus in childhood: Solitary rectal ulcer syndrome. Pediatrics 2002; 110:E79.
32. Felt B, Wise CG, Olson A, et al: Guideline for the management of pediatric idiopathic constipation and soiling. Multidisciplinary team from the University of Michigan Medical Center in Ann Arbor. Arch Pediatr Adolesc Med 1999;153:380.
33. Fishman SJ, Shamberger RC, Fox VL, et al: Endorectal pull-through abates gastrointestinal hemorrhage from colorectal venous malformations. J Pediatr Surg 2000; 35:982.
34. Fitzgerald R, Harding B, Ryan W: Fistula-in-ano in childhood, a congenital etiology. J Pediatr Surg 1985; 20:80.
35. Fleisher DR: Diagnosis and treatment of disorders of defecation in children. Pediatr Ann 1986;5:71.
36. Freckner B, Ihre T: Influence of autonomic nerves on the internal anal sphincter in man. Gut 1976;17:306.
37. Freeman NV: Anorectal problems in childhood. In Taylor I (ed): Progress in Surgery. Edinburgh, Churchill Livingstone, 1989, p 92.
38. Gaston EA: The physiology of fecal continence. Surg Gynecol Obstet 1948;87:280.
39. Ghosh A, Griffiths DM: Rectal biopsy in the investigation of constipation. Arch Dis Child 1998;79:266.
40. Godbole P, Botterill I, Newell S, et al: Solitary rectal ulcer syndrome in children. J R Coll Surg Edinb 2000; 45:411.
41. Griffiths DM: The physiology of fecal continence: Idiopathic fecal constipation and soiling. Semin Pediatr Surg 2002;11:67.
42. Hardcastle JD, Parks AG: A study of anal incontinence and some principles of surgical treatment. Proc R Soc Med 1970;63:116.
43. Heaton ND, Davenport M, Howard ER: Incidence of haemorrhoids and anorectal varices in children with portal hypertension. Br J Surg 1993;80:616.
44. Heaton ND, Davenport M, Howard ER: Symptomatic hemorrhoids and anorectal varices in children with portal hypertension. J Pediatr Surg 1992;27:833.
45. Henry MM: Anorectal neuromuscular physiology. In Decosse JJ, Todd IP (eds): Anorectal Surgery. Edinburgh, Churchill Livingstone, 1988.
46. Hobbs CJ, Wynne JM: Buggery in childhood: A common syndrome of child abuse. Lancet 1986;2:792.
47. Hobbs CJ, Wynne JM: Child sexual abuse: An increasing rate of diagnosis. Lancet 1987;2:837.
48. Holschneider AM: The problem of anorectal continence. Prog Pediatr Surg 1976;9:85.
49. Hutson JM, Catto-Smith T, Gibb S, et al: Chronic constipation: No longer stuck! Characterization of colonic dysmotility as a new disorder in children. J Pediatr Surg 2004;39:795.
50. Iacono G, Cavataio F, Montalto G, et al: Intolerance of cow's milk and chronic constipation in children. N Engl J Med 1998;339:1100.
51. Ingebo KB, Heyman MB: Polyethylene glycol-electrolyte solution for intestinal clearance in children with refractory encopresis. Am J Dis Child 1988;142:340.
52. Johnson CF: Child sexual abuse. Lancet 2004;364:462.
53. Kenny SE, Irvine T, Driver CP, et al: Double blind randomized controlled trial of topical glyceryl trinitrate in anal fissure. Arch Dis Child 2001;85:404.
54. Keren S, Wagner Y, Heldenberg D, Golan M: Studies of manometric abnormalities of the rectoanal region during defecation in constipated and soiling children: Modification through biofeedback therapy. Am J Gastroenterol 1988;83:827.
55. Keuzenkamp-Jansen CW, Fijnvandraat CJ, Kneepkens CM, Douwes AC: Diagnostic dilemmas and results of treatment for chronic constipation. Arch Dis Child 1996; 75:36.
56. Khan AR, Vujanic GM, Huddart S: The constipated child: How likely is Hirschsprung's disease? Pediatr Surg Int 2003; 19:439.
57. Kokoska ER, Keller MS, Weber TR: Outcome of the antegrade colonic enema procedure in children with chronic constipation. Am J Surg 2001;182:625.

58. Koletzko S, Ballauff A, Hadziselimovic F, Enck P: Is histological diagnosis of neuronal intestinal dysplasia related to clinical and manometric findings in constipated children? Results of a pilot study. Pediatr Gastroenterol Nutr 1993;17:59.
59. Kopel FB: Gastrointestinal manifestations of cystic fibrosis. Gastroenterology 1972;62:483.
59a. Lake AM: Food-induced eosinophilic proctocolitis. J Pediatr Gastroenterol Nutr 2000;30(Suppl):S58.
60. Lambe GF, Driver CP, Morton S, Turnock RR: Fissurectomy as a treatment for anal fissures in children. Ann R Coll Surg Engl 2000;82:254.
61. Lawson JO: Pelvic anatomy II: Anal canal and associated sphincters. Ann R Coll Surg Engl 1974;54:288.
62. Levine MD: The school child with encopresis. Pediatr Rev 1981;2:285.
63. Levine MD: Children with encopresis: A descriptive analysis. Pediatrics 1975;56:412.
64. Lockhart RD, Hamilton GF, Fyfe FW: Anatomy of the Human Body. London, Faber and Faber, 1969.
65. Lockhart-Mummery JP: Surgical procedures in general practice: Rectal prolapse. BMJ 1939;1:345.
66. Loening-Baucke V: Encopresis. Curr Opin Pediatr 2002; 14:570.
67. Loening-Baucke VA: Sensitivity of the sigmoid colon and rectum in children treated for chronic constipation. J Pediatr Gastroenterol Nutr 1984;3:454.
68. Loening-Baucke V: Encopresis and soiling. Pediatr Clin North Am 1996;43:279.
69. Loening-Baucke V: Persistence of chronic constipation in children after biofeedback treatment. Dig Dis Sci 1991; 36:153.
70. Loening-Baucke V: Constipation in early childhood: Patient characteristics, treatment, and long-term follow up. Gut 1993;34:1400.
71. Luukkonen P, Jarvinen HJ, Rintala R: Colo-anal sleeve resection for rectal hemangioma: Case report. Acta Chir Scand 1989;155:613.
72. McCoy CR, Appelbaum H, Besser AS: Condylomata acuminata: An unusual presentation of child abuse. J Pediatr Surg 1982;17:505.
73. Macdonald A, Wilson-Storey D, Munro F: Treatment of perianal abscess and fistula-in-ano in children. Br J Surg 2003;90:220.
74. Machida HM, Catto Smith AG, Gall DG, et al: Allergic colitis in infancy: Clinical and pathologic aspects. J Pediatr Gastroenterol Nutr 1994;19:22.
75. Malone PS, Ransley PG, Kiely EM: Preliminary report: The antegrade continence enema. Lancet 1990;336: 1217.
76. Meunier P, Louis D, Jaubert de Beaujeu M: Physiologic investigation of primary chronic constipation in children: Comparison with the barium enema study. Gastroenterology 1984;87:1351.
77. Monges H, Salducci V, Nardy F, et al: Electrical activity of internal anal sphincter. In Christensen J (ed): Gastrointestinal Motility. New York, Raven Press, 1980 p 495.
78. Mulliken JB, Glowacki J: Classification of pediatric vascular lesions. Plast Reconstr Surg 1982;70:120.
79. Murthi GV, Okoye BO, Spicer RD, et al: Perianal abscess in childhood. Pediatr Surg Int 2002;18:689.
80. Nelson R: Nonsurgical therapy for anal fissure (Cochrane review). In The Cochrane Library, Issue 2. Chichester, UK, John Wiley & Sons, 2004.
81. Nelson R: A systematic review of medical therapy for anal fissure. Dis Colon Rectum 2004;47:422.
82. Nelson R: Operative procedures for fissure in ano (Cochrane review). In The Cochrane Library, Issue 2. Chichester, UK, John Wiley & Sons, 2004.
83. Nigro ND: Restoration of the levator sling in the treatment of rectal procidentia. Dis Colon Rectum 1958;1:123.
84. Nix P, Stringer MD: Perianal sepsis in children. Br J Surg 1997;84:819.
85. Nurko S, Garcia-Aranda JA, Guerrero VY, Worona LB: Treatment of intractable constipation in children: Experience with cisapride. J Pediatr Gastroenterol Nutr 1996;22:38.
86. Oh JT, Han A, Han SJ, et al: Fistula-in-ano in infants: Is nonoperative management effective? J Pediatr Surg 2001;36:1367.
87. Olness K, Tobin J: Chronic constipation in children: Can it be managed by diet alone? Postgrad Med J 1982; 72:149.
88. Ottaviani G: Histologische-anatomische untersuchungen uber die innervation des mesdarmes. A Microscop-Anat Forsch 1940;47:151.
89. Pearl RH, Ein SH, Churchill B: Posterior sagittal anorectoplasty for paediatric recurrent rectal prolapse. J Pediatr Surg 1989;24:1100.
90. Peña A: Anorectal malformations: Experience with the posterior sagittal approach. In Stringer MD, Oldham KT, Mouriquand PDE, Howard ER (eds): Pediatric Surgery and Urology: Long Term Outcomes. Philadelphia, WB Saunders, 1998, p 375.
91. Phillips SE, Edwards DAW: Some aspects of anal continence and defaecation. Gut 1965;6:396.
92. Pierce AM: Anal fissures and anal scars in anal abuse—are they significant? Pediatr Surg Int 2004;20:334.
93. Potter NH: A physiological study of the pelvic floor in rectal prolapse. Ann R Coll Surg Engl 1962;31:379.
94. Puri P: Variant Hirschsprung's disease. J Pediatr Surg 1997;32:149.
95. Reisner SH, Sivan Y, Nitzan M, Merlob P: Determination of anterior displacement of the 1 anus in newborn infants and children. Pediatrics 1984;73:216.
96. Rintala RJ, Marttinen E, Virkola K, et al: Segmental colonic motility in patients with anorectal malformations. J Pediatr Surg 1997;32:453.
97. Rintala R, Lindahl H, Louhimo I: Anorectal malformations: Results of treatment and long-term follow-up in 208 patients. Pediatr Surg Int 1991;6:36.
98. Ritchie JA: Mass peristalsis in the human colon after contact with oxyphenisatin. Gut 1972;13:211.
99. Roma E, Adamidis D, Nikolara R, et al: Diet and chronic constipation in children: The role of fiber. J Pediatr Gastroenterol Nutr 1999;28:169.
100. Rosen R, Buonomo C, Andrade R, Nurko S: Incidence of spinal cord lesions in patients with intractable constipation. J Pediatr 2004;145:409.
101. Rosen NG, Gibbs DL, Soffer SZ, et al: The nonoperative management of fistula-in-ano. J Pediatr Surg 2000;35:938.
102. Sander S, Vural O, Unal M: Management of rectal prolapse in children: Ekehorn's rectosacropexy. Pediatr Surg Int 1999;15:111.
103. Sarahan T, Weintraub WH, Coran AG, Wesley JR: The successful management of chronic constipation in infants and children. J Pediatr Surg 1982;17:171.
104. Sarin YK, Sharma AK: Posterior sagittal rectoplasty for rectal prolapse. Indian Pediatr 1993;30:541.
105. Schuster MM, Hendrix TR, Mendeloff AI: The internal anal sphincter response: Manometric studies on its normal physiology, neural pathways and alteration in bowel disor-

ders. J Clin Invest 1963;42:196.
106. Shafer AD, McGlone TP, Flanagan RA: Abnormal crypts of Morgagni: The cause of perianal abscess and fistula-in-ano. J Pediatr Surg 1987;22:203.
107. Shapiro O: Applied anatomy of infants and children: Proctology. Rev Gastroenterol 1948;15:307.
108. Shwachman H, Redmond A, Khaw K-T: Studies in cystic fibrosis: Report of 130 patients diagnosed under 3 months of age over a 20-year period. Pediatrics 1970;46:335.
109. Silverberg M: Constipation in infants and children. Pract Gastroenterol 1987;11:43.
110. Staiano A, Andreotti MR, Greco L, et al: Long-term follow-up of children with chronic idiopathic constipation. Dig Dis Sci 1994;39:561.
111. Stanton A, Sutherland R: Prevalence of reflex anal dilatation in 200 children. BMJ 1989;298:802.
112. Sweeney JL, Ritchie JK, Nichols RJ: Anal fissure in Crohn's disease. Br J Surg 1988;75:57.
113. Swenson O, Bill AH: Resection of the rectum and rectosigmoid with preservation of the sphincter. Surgery 1948;24:212.
114. Sönmez K, Demirogullari B, Ekingen G, et al: Randomized, placebo-controlled treatment of anal fissure by lidocaine, EMLA, and GTN in children. J Pediatr Surg 2002;37:1313.
115. Tander B, Güven A, Demirbag S, et al: A prospective, randomized, double-blind, placebo-controlled trial of glyceryl-trinitrate ointment in the treatment of children with anal fissure. J Pediatr Surg 1999;34:1810.
116. Tolia V, Lin CH, Elitsur Y: A prospective randomized study with mineral oil and oral lavage solution for treatment of faecal impaction in children. Aliment Pharmacol Ther 1993;7:523.
117. Triboulet H: Durée de la traverse chez l'enfant modale épreuve du carmin. Bull Soc Pediatr Paris 1909; 11:512.
118. Tsugawa C, Matsumoto E, Muraji T, et al: Posterior plication of the rectum for rectal prolapse in children. J Pediatr Surg 1995;30:692.
119. Upadhyaya P: Mid-anal sphincteric malformation, cause of constipation in anterior perianal anus. J Pediatr Surg 1984;19:183.
120. Utzig MJ, Kroesen AJ, Buhr HJ: Concepts in pathogenesis and treatment of chronic anal fissure—a review of the literature. Am J Gastroenterol 2003;98:968.
121. van Ginkel R, Buller HA, Boeckxstaens GE, et al: The effect of anorectal manometry on the outcome of treatment in severe childhood constipation: A randomized, controlled trial. Pediatrics 2001;108:E9.
122. van Ginkel R, Benninga MA, Blommaart PJ, et al: Lack of benefit of laxatives as adjunctive therapy for functional nonretentive fecal soiling in children. J Pediatr 2000; 137:808.
123. Van Gossum A, Hittelet A, Schmit A, et al: A prospective comparative study of push and wireless-capsule enteroscopy in patients with obscure digestive bleeding. Acta Gastroenterol Belg 2003;66:199.
124. Wald A: Diagnosis of constipation in primary and secondary care. Rev Gastroenterol Disord 2004;4:S28.
125. Wald A: Disorders of defecation and fecal continence. Cleve Clin J Med 1989;56:491.
126. Watanabe Y, Todani T, Yamamoto S: Conservative management of fistula in ano in infants. Pediatr Surg Int 1998; 13:274.
127. Weaver LT, Ewing G, Taylor LC: The bowel habits of milkfed infants. J Pediatr Gastroenterol Nutr 1988;7:568.
128. Weaver LT, Steiner H: The bowel habit of young children. Arch Dis Child 1984;59:649.
129. Woodward MN, Foley P, Cusick EL: Colostomy for treatment of functional constipation in children: A preliminary report. J Pediatr Gastroenterol Nutr 2004;38:75.
130. Youssef NN, Barksdale E Jr, Griffiths JM, et al: Management of intractable constipation with antegrade enemas in neurologically intact children. J Pediatr Gastroenterol Nutr 2002;34:402.
131. Youssef NN, Pensabene L, Barksdale E Jr, Di Lorenzo C: Is there a role for surgery beyond colonic aganglionosis and anorectal malformations in children with intractable constipation? J Pediatr Surg 2004;39:73.
132. Zempsky WT, Rosenstein BJ: Cause of prolapse in children. Am J Dis Child 1988;142:338.

第 103 章

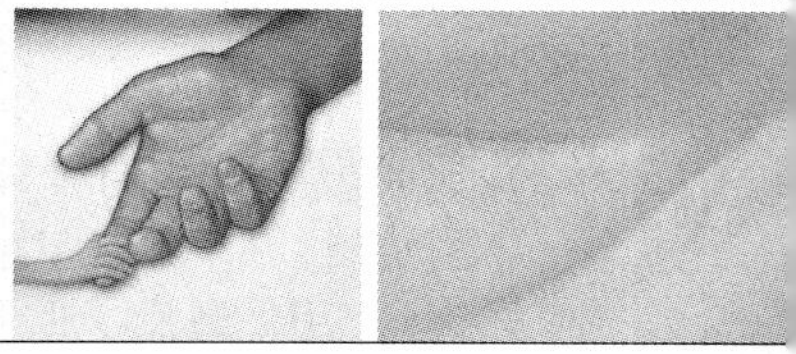

婴儿黄疸：胆道闭锁

R. Peter Altman 和 Terry L. Buchmiller

历史回顾

603 1892 年，Thomson[177] 在《爱丁堡医学杂志》发表文章，其中将胆道闭锁界定为一种特有的疾病。Holmes 回顾了所有已经报道的病例，于 1916 年提出了可纠治型和不可纠治型的疾病分类。目前该术语已经很少应用。Ladd[108] 于 1928 年报道了首例可纠治型胆道闭锁手术成功。1953 年，Gross[63] 注意到胆道闭锁是引起新生儿梗阻性黄疸最常见的原因，但是大多数患儿属于不可纠治型。Bill 等[24] 随后报告在 1927—1970 年间，仅 52 例胆道闭锁手术成功。在 20 世纪 50 年代及 60 年代早期，有几种新颖的但不成功的手术方法曾被报道，包括部分肝脏切除伴肝内胆管空肠吻合术[119]、人工胆管替代[166] 以及通过肝门[55] 和胸导管[2,141] 建立淋巴引流术。

20 世纪 60 年代，由于大部分胆道闭锁不能与新生儿肝炎或胆汁淤积综合征鉴别，因此对持续性黄疸的早期手术存在争议。1968 年，Thaler 和 Gellis[176] 对胆道闭锁的处理提出不同意见，他们认为由于手术干预使得新生儿肝炎病情恶化，因此建议手术应推迟至出生后 4 个月。胆道闭锁自愈的报道[93,106] 进一步动摇了早期手术的地位。二次探查手术偶尔被推荐用于纤维化的肝外胆管可能最终开放的病例中[34,50]。那些被诊断为不可纠治型胆道闭锁的患儿最终会死亡。

1957 年，通过引入肝门肠吻合术，Kasai 等[96,99] 迎来了可治疗传统认为不可纠治的胆道闭锁的新时代。尽管该主张最初遭到怀疑[32,105]，但包括 Bill[24] 等和 Lilly 及 Altman[115] 等在内的日本和美国小儿外科医生的报告逐渐证实了 Kasai 的结果。Kasai 的肝门肠吻合术包括 Roux-en-Y 重建，目前改良摒弃了肠造瘘术，保留了标准的胆道闭锁手术方法。尽管将近一半的患儿最终进展为肝功能衰竭，但超过 2/3 的患儿得到了基本的胆汁引流。

1963 年，Starzl[165] 首先介绍了肝移植术，它成为最初肝门肠吻合术治疗失败和那些进展为终末期肝病的患儿补救治疗的最终手段。随着减体积的活体器官的提供，胆道闭锁患儿的治疗前景变得更加乐观。

背景介绍

新生儿高胆红素血症通常是生理性的未结合胆红素增高，病程具有自限性。仅 2%～15% 的新生儿在出生后 2 周仍表现黄疸，而仅有 0.2%～0.4% 为肝内胆汁淤积或结构异常造成的胆道梗阻引起的胆汁淤积性黄疸[41]。肝内胆汁淤积可以由许多感染性或炎症性疾病以及遗传代谢性的缺陷引起。主要的结构异常疾病包括胆道闭锁和胆总管囊肿（第 104 章）。多种形式的肝细胞功能障碍对上述所有疾病来说均常见，这造成最初对内科和外科性胆汁淤积性疾病进行鉴别时较为困难。

胆道闭锁的发病率在活产儿中为 1/10 000～1/16 700，在过去的几十年中发病率稳定[95,126,139,143]。患者中女性占优势，男女比例为 1∶1.4～1.7。胆道闭锁中肝外胆管并没有完全缺如。它们通常是作为闭塞的纤维索带的结合物存留。胆道闭锁多种分类系统的产生均是以这些纤维胆管残余物的解剖学作为基础。

图 103-1 描述了胆道闭锁的常见类型。最常见的类型是肝外胆道系统完全闭塞，第二常见的类型发病率接近 20%，特点为远端胆囊及胆囊管、胆总管开放。

日本小儿外科学会已经提出了其他分类系统，其

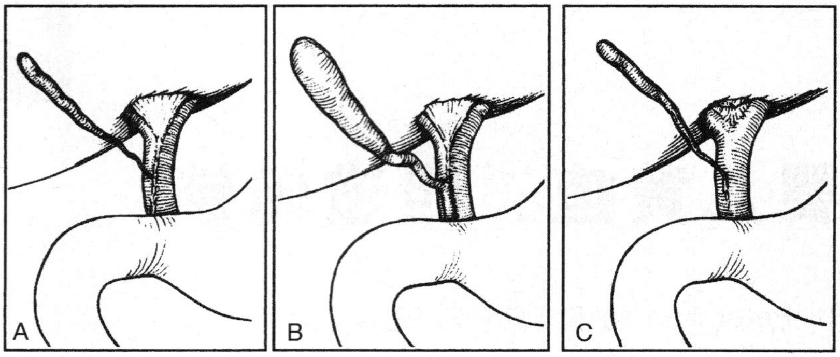

图 103-1 探查时发现肝外胆道纤维闭塞的不同类型。A. 最常见的类型为肝外胆道整体纤维化。B. 胆囊、胆囊管、胆总管开放伴有肝门区纤维闭塞。C. 胆囊表现为纤维索样，残留的胆管树从稀疏至缺如。（From Altman RP, Lilly JR, Greenfeld J, et al: A multivariable risk factor analysis of the portoenterostomy [Kasai] procedure for biliary atresia: Twenty-five years of experience from two centers. Ann Surg 1997; 226: 348, discussion 353. Courtesy of Lippincott Williams & Wilkins.）

1604 中将胆道闭锁分为三种主要类型：Ⅰ型，闭锁位于胆总管（相对频率为 11.9%）；Ⅱ型，闭锁位于肝管（2.5%）；Ⅲ型，闭锁位于肝门（84.1%）[139]。亚型也被描述，但由于超出本章范围，故在此不做完整回顾。

目前尚未发现种族差异或遗传因素与疾病的发生相关。伴发的先天性畸形发生率为 11%～20%[139]。多脾是最常见的伴发畸形，占总病例数的 7.5%。多脾综合征被定义为多脾伴有不同类型的畸形，包括十二指肠前门静脉、肠旋转不良和腹腔内脏转位。如多脾综合征患儿的母亲患糖尿病，则预后可能不好[44]。其他先天性畸形如无脾、心脏病、下腔静脉畸形、环状胰腺、肠闭锁和泌尿生殖系统畸形偶尔合并胆道闭锁[35,49,126]。

胆道闭锁的迅速诊断评估至关重要，大多数病例需结合血清学、超声、放射性核扫描检查和肝活检。必须强调高效率的诊断性检查和早期手术治疗对胆道闭锁治疗获得更高成功率是必要的。

胚胎学和病因学

胆道系统起源于胚胎第四周前肠的肝憩室，并分化成头尾两部分。头端产生近端肝外胆道和大部分肝内胆道系统，而尾端产生胆囊、胆囊管和胆总管。

胆道闭锁的发病机制涉及遗传、免疫介导和感染因素，但仍然没有被证明。先天性起源学说认为胆道闭锁是胆管胚胎形成期间肝外胆道系统再通障碍所致，然而胚胎胆管闭塞和随后再通至今仍然没有被证明[171]。有人认为发育期间肝内外胆管的汇合障碍可能导致胆管系统部分开放的特定类型胆道闭锁发生。

Desmet[46]最先提出了胆管原基（ductal plate）畸形理论。Tan 等[171]认为肝门处胆管重构障碍导致了胆道闭锁。他们假设这些畸形的胎儿胆管很少被间充质细胞支持，之后在围生期胆汁流量增加，出现胆汁渗漏。胆汁的渗漏触发强烈的局部炎性反应，引起胆管树闭塞。

许多学说认为胆道闭锁是获得性的而不是先天性的畸形[26]。该假说被一些临床观察所支持，大约 40% 的患儿可以在出生时排出正常胎粪，多达 60% 的患儿最初及出生后短期内排出含有胆汁的粪便[38]。

尽管胆道闭锁偶然发生于孪生儿[81,135]，但遗传病因仍未得到证实。其他推测的胆道闭锁病因包括血供丧失[104]、异常的胆汁酸代谢[92]、胰胆管连接异常[131]和 Landing 的“婴儿梗阻性胆管病”理论[109]。有人提出包括轮状病毒[156]和呼肠病毒 3 型[180]在内的病毒也是致病原因，但因果关系尚未被证实。已经建立了呼肠病毒感染导致胆道闭锁的动物模型[150]。

对胆道闭锁实验模型的积极研究正在进行，包括新生儿病毒感染的诱导。尽管存在前面所述的理论，但胆道闭锁病因仍然不明。它可能被证明是由多种因素结合导致发病的，比如病原体在具有遗传易感性的宿主中触发免疫反应。

病理特征

纤维化胆道残余物的组织病理学检查显示了不同阶段的炎症，这被认为是胆管系统进行性的破坏过程[36,56,101,116]。标本中偶尔可见变形胆管的管腔。不同改变的出现表明胆道系统整体开放的丧失是一个逐渐的过程。最终，胆管残余物完全闭塞，形成伴有慢性炎症的瘢痕肉芽组织（图 103-2）。在切除的肝门

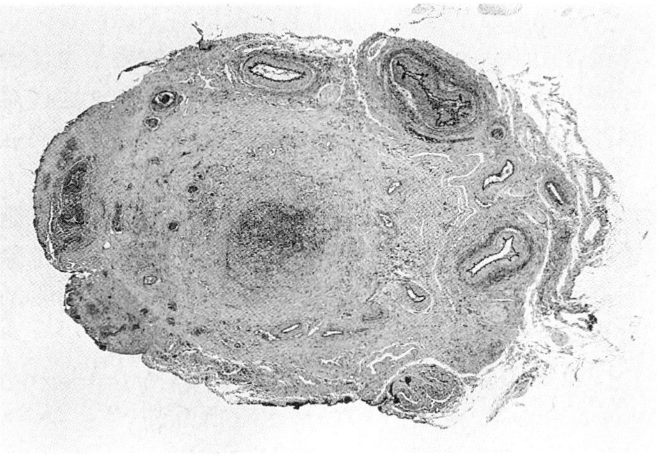

图 103-2 胆道闭锁中胆总管完全闭塞的组织病理学显示瘢痕样肉芽组织并伴有慢性炎症反应（苏木素伊红染色，40X）。

纤维板中胆管残余物的类型及大小有重要的预后意义（见后）。

605 显微镜下，肝门纤维残余物的横断面上可见三种特殊类型的胆管结构：已经存在的胆管、集合小管和胆汁腺[147]。仅胆小管与肝内胆道系统相连，它是肝门肠吻合术后引流胆汁的潜在管道。如果胆汁流持续存在，几个月内这些胆小管会在肝门处形成内部胆瘘（图 103-3）。

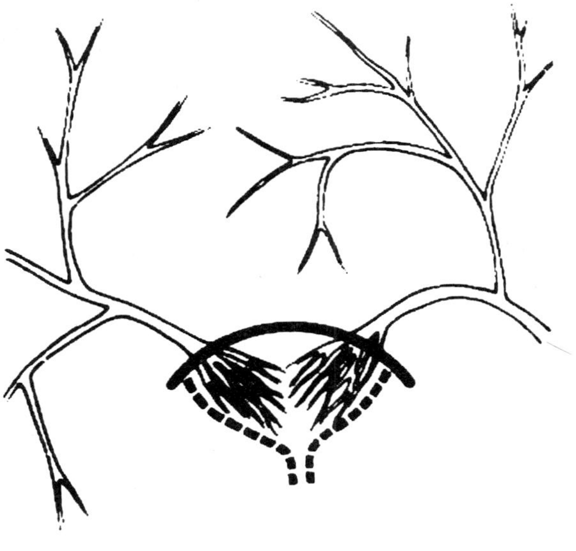

图 103-3 模式图显示开放增生的胆小管被纤维束锥包被。成功实施 Kasai 手术后肝门区通过这些内部胆瘘建立胆汁引流。（M. Kasai，MD. 惠赠）

胆道闭锁患儿的肝脏组织学检测显示标志性的胆小管增生表现。其他重要的诊断特征是胆汁淤积、肝细胞索扭曲、巨细胞转化、局部坏死和小叶内汇管区纤维化[26,97,134,144]。小叶间区域可见汇管区增宽、肝纤维化、门脉周围水肿、细胞浸润和不同程度的胆汁淤积。汇管区肝动脉分支过度增生和肥厚是特征性的表现，但其意义仍然不清楚[75]。当经皮肝活检标本含有足够的汇管区组织时，可以可靠地用于诊断胆道闭锁。

胆道系统的病理学改变首先影响了肝内和肝外胆管结构的理论逐渐被人们所接受[64,87,153]。肝内胆管结构狭窄扭曲，形状不规则[115]。然而一些作者认为肝内胆道系统的损害继发于肝脏发育期间肝外肝管闭塞[144]。后一个理论被手术纠治越早预后越好的临床观察结果所支持。肝内胆管受累对病理学和临床都有非常重要的意义，因为肝内胆管的损害程度与肝门肠吻合术后发生的许多疾病有关。肝门肠吻合术后肝内胆管受累的预后仍然存在争论。

临床表现

症状和体征

当有黄疸的婴儿伴有无胆汁性大便、深色尿、肝脏增大变硬时，应该高度怀疑胆道闭锁。胆道闭锁的病理性黄疸典型地出现于出生后数周，但是该种情况也可见于某些良性的新生儿黄疸。大多数患儿首次胎便是正常的，超过 50% 的病例一段时期内有不同程度的胆汁性大便[38]。黄疸持续存在，大便变成无胆汁样。患儿最初很活跃，在出生后几周到数月其生长发育可表现正常。

由于胆道梗阻持续存在，肝脏体积逐渐增大变硬，最终发展成肝硬化，继而出现脾大。脂溶性维生素吸收障碍可以引起贫血、营养不良及生长停滞。如果不进行治疗，大多数患儿在 19 个月内会死于肝失代偿、食管静脉曲张出血或感染。Karrer 等[95]报告未行胆汁引流手术的患儿 3 年生存率小于 10%。

诊断

当结合胆红素的比例超过总血清胆红素的 20% 时，

表 103-1 胆道闭锁的诊断
体检着重于：
粪便颜色
肝脏质地
肝功能检测
超声
肝胆管闪烁扫描［二异丙基亚氨基二乙酸（DISIDA）］
采用苯巴比妥预处理
经皮肝脏活检

应考虑为病理性黄疸，需要对此进行迅速评估[20]。由于有多种病因，血清学检查可以有助于将胆道闭锁与感染、血液学疾病、代谢性疾病和遗传异常（如 α_1-抗胰蛋白酶缺乏）鉴别开来。新生儿肝炎和
1606 胆道发育不良（小叶内胆管缺乏）最易与胆道闭锁混淆。由于没有任何一项检查是绝对可靠的，所以将血清学评估、超声、肝胆管闪烁扫描和经皮肝脏活检相结合，用于疑似胆道闭锁的迅速诊断（表 103-1）。通过审慎地结合这些检查结果，术前诊断胆道闭锁的准确率预计超过 90%。明确诊断需要外科手术探查。

血清学评估

常规血清学肝功能检测经常是没有特异性的，但是通常可以鉴别肝实质和肝外胆管疾病。继发于肝内胆汁淤积或胆道梗阻的高胆红素血症以间接和直接胆红素比例升高为特征。患有胆道闭锁时，血清胆红素轻微波动是典型特征。除非有严重的肝细胞疾病，否则胆汁淤积与胆道闭锁的转氨酶水平升高程度类似。肝脏合成功能通过凝血酶原时间、部分凝血活酶时间、总蛋白及血清白蛋白测定进行评估，在胆道闭锁早期很少受到损害。

由于子宫内感染可能表现为出生后黄疸，因此应常规监测 TORCH（弓形虫、其他病毒、风疹病毒、巨细胞病毒和单纯疱疹病毒）抗体滴度。同样，由于婴儿代谢性异常，α_1-抗胰蛋白酶缺乏也可以表现为出生后黄疸，建议进行筛查。受累患儿在编码 α_1-抗胰蛋白酶的蛋白酶抑制位点（Pi）表现为纯合子，具有 PiZZ 基因型[152]。目前对 α_1-抗胰蛋白酶缺乏症的治疗仅限于对肝功能衰竭者进行器官移植[186]。

其他血清学检查在此提及，但目前不建议作为常规检查用于疾病评估。胆汁淤积性黄疸的婴儿血清胆汁酸升高。日本新生儿群体筛查计划[124]发现通过总胆汁酸水平或鹅去氧胆酸与胆酸的比例鉴别胆道闭锁和其他胆汁淤积性疾病具有挑战性。

血清脂蛋白 X（lipoprotein X，Lp-X）在所有胆道闭锁患儿中均为阳性[151,174]，Lp-X 缺乏可以排除胆道闭锁。然而，阳性诊断与新生儿肝炎有 40% 的重叠，因此限制了其特异性。

胆道闭锁患儿 γ-谷氨酰转肽酶（γ-Glutamyl transpeptidase，γ-GPT）水平也有所升高[192]。Lp-X 和 γ-GPT 的检测相结合仍在研究中[175]。

超声

腹部超声是一种简单的无创性检查，有时对评估胆汁淤积和疑似胆道闭锁的婴儿很有帮助[1,161]。为了检测到正常的胆囊（长度 >1.5 cm），检查前婴儿必须禁食 4 小时[11]。发现胆囊或肝内胆管扩张可以有效地排除胆道闭锁的诊断[11]。如果胆囊萎瘪或不能找到，应怀疑胆道闭锁。进食后胆囊尺寸缩小，排除胆道闭锁的可能。熟练的超声技术有时可以检测到胆道闭锁时出现的纤维索残留和肝门纤维板[39]。十二指肠前门静脉、无脾、多脾的表现进一步支持了胆道闭锁的诊断[1]。注意勿将并行的肝动脉管道误诊为开放的胆管结构。多普勒超声的应用有助于提高诊断的准确性[11]。

肝胆管闪烁扫描

肝胆管闪烁扫描常用同位素锝 99m［如 Tc 标记的二异丙基亚氨基二乙酸（DISIDA）］。DISIDA 扫描广泛地用于确定胆管开放并帮助鉴别胆道闭锁和其他原因导致的婴儿胆汁淤积[47,120,145]。由于肝功能不良，严重的肝内胆汁淤积可能会影响示踪物的摄取。检查前预先给苯巴比妥［5 mg/(kg·d)］3~5天可以增强分泌功能，提高鉴别胆道闭锁和非梗阻性胆汁淤积疾病的能力[120]，因而该方法一直被推荐使用。肠道内可见放射性核素可以确定胆管开放，排除胆道闭锁。由于肝功能不良可以导致同位素分泌延迟，因此如果早期影像不能确定肠道内有放射性核素，则注射后 24 小时再次照相是必要

的。24 小时后同位素没有出现在肠道内，尤其是在苯巴比妥预处理之后，应该高度怀疑是由于胆道闭锁导致的胆道梗阻。

肝脏活检

有经验的肝脏病理学家根据经皮肝脏活检结果所做的诊断对黄疸婴儿的评估具有高度的准确性。笔者认为肝脏组织学是诊断胆道闭锁最可靠的方法[20,113]。应检测多处肝门束以获得最大的诊断准确率。胆道闭锁中具有鉴别作用的主要特征是胆管增生，这在非梗阻性症候群中不会见到。此外支持闭锁的诊断还包括汇管区内胆管栓，胆管及细胞胆汁淤积，肝门束水肿和纤维化，肿胀、空泡形成和胆管上皮脱落入胆管腔，炎症细胞浸润，以及肝细胞巨细胞化。胆道闭锁与胆道发育不良综合征易于鉴别[113]。

607 ### 辅助检查

经鼻十二指肠置管抽吸十二指肠液作为一种廉价无创且迅速的检查方法被推荐使用[54,60]。假如通过 24 小时收集引流液或连续十二指肠置管探测到典型的胆红素染色的黄色液体，则胆道闭锁的诊断可以被排除。但是由于主观性限制了该方法的广泛应用。通过近红外反射光谱分析技术评估粪便染色已经被介绍用于婴儿胆汁淤积性黄疸的鉴别[4]。

随着小型侧视内镜的发展，婴儿内镜逆行胆胰管造影（ERCP）的应用也得到了发展，甚至用于小婴儿的诊断[111,169]。但是 ERCP 在评估婴儿黄疸时具有局限性，不能作为常规检测开展。

当标准的诊断检查不能得出结论时，一些人主张采用超声引导的经皮胆管造影。经皮穿刺要求胆囊必须是扩张的，因此在大多数常见类型的胆道闭锁中的应用受到了限制。Meyers 及其同事[128]提出这种方法可以作为 ERCP 的一种替代方法使用，并且当诊断结果明确时可以避免手术探查。

在一个对胆道闭锁患儿进行的小型研究中，磁共振胆胰管造影对胆道和胰腺疾病的诊断具有 100% 的准确率[132]，然而在普遍推荐使用前仍需要进一步评估。

腹腔镜探查胆管造影评估新生儿胆汁淤积性黄疸仍然没有被广泛地接受。

没有任何一项检查或联合检查绝对可靠。对于高度怀疑胆道闭锁的婴儿或通过诊断评估仍不能明确病因者，推荐迅速行手术探查。

治疗

术前处理

除了常规的婴幼儿腹部手术术前处理外，还要每日给一次维生素 K（1～2 mg/kg 肌肉注射），术前给药数天。我们不进行常规的肠道准备。婴儿通常在手术当天早晨收住院，皮肤切开前在手术室内应用广谱抗生素。

手术技术

肝门肠吻合术（Kasai 手术）是治疗胆道闭锁的标准术式，已经成为基本的治疗方法近 30 年。完全整体切除肝外胆道结构，在肝门水平横向切断纤维束锥，并与空肠支行 Roux-en-Y 吻合[96]。横断的纤维组织中包含的细微胆管结构将胆汁引流进入肠道。随着时间推移，肠管和胆管上皮间自行发生吻合，胆汁引流通道得以建立（见图 103-3）。Kasai 肝门肠吻合术的细节将在下面描述。

婴儿取仰卧位，确保充分暴露，应该行胆道造影，它不是常规检查但有必要。取以右侧为中心的上腹横切口开始手术探查。如果需要进行胆道重建，切口可以延伸跨越中线。笔者首先探查左上腹了解脾脏的解剖结构。多脾提示患儿可能有十二指肠前门静脉和内脏反位。

下一步观察肝脏的坚硬度和检查肝门。一些外科医生在分离左右三角韧带后将肝脏托出腹腔[13,45]。此操作既没必要也不建议用于常规的病例。胆道闭锁的肝脏质地粗糙，纤维化且呈绿色。在新生儿肝炎和 Alagille 综合征（见后）的患儿中，肝脏平滑，呈巧克力棕色。

大多数拟诊断胆道闭锁行探查术的患儿有一个纤维化的未发育的胆囊。当胆囊作为残余物持续存在时，胆道闭锁的诊断成立，应行肝门切开术。假如不能确定胆囊是否正常，应做一个可吸收荷包缝合，从胆囊底部抽吸，“白色胆汁”通常可以确定胆道闭锁的诊断。在这种情况下应该继续切开肝门，无需进行胆道造影。但是有一些婴儿胆囊大小可以接近正常或者有胆汁存留。胆道造影可以在鉴别不同的亚型时起到一定作用。

如果胆囊有腔隙，注入稀释的造影剂［泛影葡胺（泛影钠）］来判断肝脏和十二指肠之间胆管树的连续性。当造影剂在远端十二指肠和近端肝脏根部显影，提示肝外胆道完全开放。通过胆管造影评估胆管的尺寸，确定是否存在胆管发育不良或由于胆汁浓缩造成的梗阻。如果造影剂仅进入远端十二指肠而没有进入肝脏，则再次注入造影剂时轻柔地挤压远端胆总管可能会使近端胆道充盈，然而这种方法很少奏效。如果证实肝外胆道开放，不管胆管管径正常还是变小（图 103-4），都需进行肝脏活检，并关闭切口。我们发现保留胆囊造口导管不是很有用，相反，我们将导管拔出，收紧荷包打结，将胆囊保留在原位。如果不能确定胆管是开放的，应该进行肝门切开和胆道重建（Kasai 手术）。

尽管对于 20% 远端胆道开放的病例可以行肝
1608 门胆囊吻合术，但历史上此种术式与吻合口并发症的高发生率相关。许多患儿需要重新改行肝门肠吻合术[9]。因此，即使胆囊、胆囊管和胆总管是开放的，目前的胆道重建仍然采用最初的肝门肠吻合术。

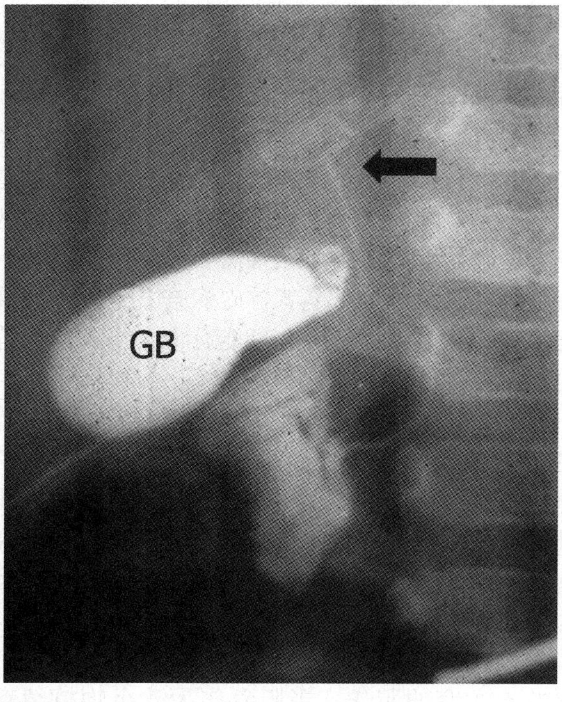

图 103-4 胆管发育不全：术中胆管造影显示胆道开放，但肝外胆道结构明显细小（箭头）。GB，胆囊。

肝门探查从先游离胆囊残迹开始，这样易于辨认纤维化的肝管。切开肝十二指肠韧带表面的腹膜。应用电凝可减少术后淋巴液的渗漏。注意胆管及肝动脉的解剖结构。

用不可吸收缝线结扎并横向切断远端纤维化的胆总管。轻柔地牵引残留物便于解剖肝门区，可见到门静脉分叉前方的纤维组织束锥。偶尔，需要用血管牵引带小心地环绕右侧肝动脉将其轻轻牵开。

必须强调门静脉分为左右支处是横向切断纤维束锥的唯一可靠标志[15,103]。必须识别几个小的但经常存在的进入纤维组织的门静脉“中间”分支，以免引起出血。虽然也可以仔细地结扎，但笔者倾向于用电凝分离这些小的分支。肝门处缺乏纤维束锥的情况极少见，应进行进一步的细致探查。

当胆管树不连续时，探查门静脉分支上方几乎均可见到纤维束锥。在该纤维组织中置缝线有助于在门静脉上方建立一个平面。

一旦完成解剖分离，在纤维束锥的两侧外缘缝上精细的固定线。在维持适中张力的情况下将纤维束锥锐性地横向切断，这样就切除了肝外胆道结构。没有必要也不应该切开肝实质，因为 Glisson 被膜瘢痕化可能会潜在地妨碍胆汁引流。手术的成功取决于纤维束锥中开放的显微胆管通道的存在。冲洗后将温盐水纱垫放置在肝门处，肝门处手术完成。

切除的胆道及附属的胆囊残余物送检行永久性切片，要求测量胆小管的尺寸用于预后评估。尽管一些作者[12,115]通过冰冻切片确定吻合处有开放的显微胆管存在，但我们不认为这种方法很有用，因为确切的横断面水平不能随意选取。最终，一些日本的小儿外科医生建议使用更宽的横断面、更宽的缝合面延伸超过肝门处血管。读者可以参考这些出版物以便了解更多的技术细节[52,88,148,178]。

在距屈氏韧带约 10 cm 处横向切断空肠作为 Roux-en-Y 支。内翻缝合远端空肠断面。在空肠断面以下 40 cm 处行空肠空肠端侧吻合以恢复小肠的连续性。日本医生倾向于选择长 50 cm 的 Roux-en-Y 支[90]。在横结肠系膜无血管处打一个孔，将 Roux-en-Y支穿过该孔提到先前横向切断的纤维组织近端。管道开口于距关闭的空肠末端远端数厘米的对系膜缘。

用预先缝在纤维束锥两侧的缝线作为标志，沿着纤维组织断面下缘在后壁置 6 根左右双臂缝针，开始肝门肠吻合。随后肠管并列时，需小心放置以确保潜在的胆管引流完全汇入吻合处的肠腔。术中常常需要轻柔地向下牵拉门静脉以使门平面得到充分暴露。

每一针的第二根针需缝在开放的空肠后壁上，缝线打结使得空肠与纤维组织切缘并列，然后进行前排的间断缝合。完成缝合后，整个纤维组织切面完全被包在空肠腔内。单层重建基本上是我们的手术唯一区别于最初报道的 Kasai 手术的地方。

最后，仔细地修补 Roux 支的系膜缺损，将 Roux 支固定至肠系膜开窗处以防系膜过度紧张或内疝的发生。于肝门肠吻合口附近放置一根引流管，在右下腹切口引出引流管。分层关闭腹部创面。图 103-5 显示手术完成后的示意图。

Lee 及其同事[112]最先报道了腹腔镜下进行 Kasai 肝门肠吻合手术的情况。极少数患有终末期肝功能衰竭（Child 分级 C 级）没有诊断胆道闭锁的婴儿，应慎重考虑最初就采用肝移植进行治疗。

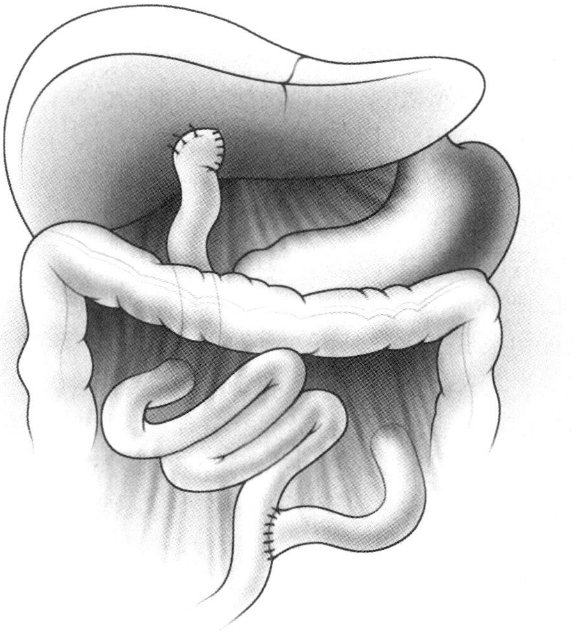

图 103-5　Kasai 手术：肝门肠吻合术完成后的模式图。Roux-en-Y 支长 40 cm，穿过横结肠系膜。

手术的改良 1609

日本儿外科医生最先设计了许多改良方法以降低术后胆管炎的发生率[38]。历史上曾经将重建的胆道作为造口外置以监测胆汁引流，理论上胆汁与肠内容物的分离减少了术后胆管炎的发生[10,117]。一旦胆汁引流得以建立，造瘘口在 3～6 个月后关闭以恢复管道的连续性。虽然造口可以降低最初胆管炎发生的严重程度[38]，但是经验表明重建胆道的外置造口不但不能降低胆管炎的发生率，还可能加重肝功能损害[17]、引起造瘘口并发症[112]以及使未来的肝移植手术更加复杂[147]。目前不推荐使用重建胆道造瘘术。

同样地，用肠套迭瓣理论上可以防止肠内容物的反流[38,52,138,172]，但是目前并不被推荐使用[110,121]。仅一个前瞻性的非随机对照研究显示肠套迭抗反流瓣的应用既不能降低胆管炎的发病率，也不能缩短发病的病程[142]。

用阑尾代胆道行肝门阑尾十二指肠吻合术有不同的结果被报道。在 Tsao 及其同事[179]最近发表的一篇综述中显示，患儿行该手术的最初总生存率相似于 Kasai 手术，但仅 31% 的患儿成功建立胆汁引流，88% 最终需行肝移植手术。目前不支持应用这种手术。

几乎没有人提倡将肝移植作为胆道闭锁婴儿最初的治疗方法[158]。这将使 1/3 通过肝门肠吻合手术可以得到明显纠治的患儿面对由于肝移植而导致的长期风险。另一些人提出将肝移植作为一种可选择的方法，并首选用于诊断时年龄超过 120 天或者那些具有预后不良的组织学表现的患儿[19,98,191]。我们认为肝门肠吻合术和肝移植应作为序列的、互补的手术方法用于治疗胆道闭锁[16]。

术后处理

持续鼻胃管减压直至肠功能恢复，肠功能通常在 48 小时内恢复。持续静脉应用抗生素直到开始饮食，并开始长期口服抗生素。引流管通常在出院之前拔除。平均住院时间为 5 天。事实上大多数人认为应延长抗生素的使用时间，同时应用促胆汁分泌药物来预防术后胆管炎的发生。类固醇的应用存在争议，将在下一节讨论。我们目前的术后用药在表 103-2 中列

表 103-2 胆道闭锁术后药物治疗
熊去氧胆酸（Actigall），10～15 mg/(kg·d)
SMZ 混悬剂；甲氧苄啶成分，2 mg/(kg·d)
维生素 ADEK 滴剂，1 ml/d
泼尼松，2 mg/(kg·d)，分 2 次口服；超过 2～3 周后逐渐减量。

出，其中包括类固醇的使用。

类固醇的使用

类固醇被公认有抗炎和免疫抑制的效应。类固醇还可以减轻水肿和胶原沉积，抑制单核细胞和淋巴细胞的迁移，抑制瘢痕的形成。据推测它有促胆汁分泌的作用，通过 Na^+，K^+-ATP 酶活性诱导产生不依赖胆盐的部分胆汁分泌，进而刺激胆流产生胆汁效应。有人尝试通过一个外置的管道测量胆汁排出量，记录增加的胆汁引流，但没有成功[14]。由于许多潜在混杂变异的存在，类固醇治疗胆道闭锁的优点很难被证明。此外，许多研究不能有力地得出有统计学意义的结论[136]。

但是，许多作者已经报道术后应用类固醇治疗可以改善预后。1985 年，Karrer 和 Lilly 报道了持续约一周的冲击性类固醇治疗（高剂量/短期）成功地治疗 Kasai 术后胆管炎或胆流减少的病例。Dillon 等[48]首先倡导长期应用类固醇（最少 6 周），并报道术后
1610 依靠自体肝脏的患儿随访 4 年后 76% 无黄疸。Muraji 等[137]报道了肝门肠吻合后继发胆管狭窄一周后应用类固醇治疗。假如粪便不含胆汁，则重复给药。Meyers和其同事[127]对静脉应用甲泼尼龙（Solu－Medrol）减量后继续 8～12 周口服泼尼松结合熊去氧胆酸的治疗组和不用类固醇的治疗组进行了对比研究。结果显示接受类固醇治疗的患儿术后 3～4 个月直接胆红素的水平比未用类固醇组明显降低，1 年内需要肝移植治疗或死亡的人数也相对较少[127]。

与类固醇相关的副作用包括水潴留和食欲增加。没有感染、切口疝及腹水发病增加的报道。尽管类固醇使用的最佳剂量、常规给药方式和应用疗程仍然存在争论，但越来越多的报道证明了类固醇应用的疗效。过去几年，我们已经将 2～3 周逐渐减量的类固醇应用纳入到术后处理中。

预后

Kasai 肝门肠吻合术明显提高了 40 年前被认为是患有绝症的患儿的生存率。死亡率在出生后头 30 天内极低，约 0～0.5%[16,137,179]。胆汁引流的最初建立表现为大便胆汁染色和黄疸减轻，通常出现在 10～14 天内。超过 2/3 的患儿有胆汁引流的建立（25%～86%[16,121,179]），但是并不能保证治愈。当然那些最初建立胆汁引流的患儿约一半（占总数的 25%～35%）将获得“治愈”，维持胆汁流量并且黄疸消退，不存在长期的后遗症。这些患儿生长发育达到正常标准，不需要进行肝移植治疗。

另一半建立胆汁引流的患儿（约占总数的 35%）逐渐出现进行性的肝功能衰竭，21% 伴有门脉高压及其后遗症的患儿再次出现黄疸。14% 伴有胆汁流量减少的患儿黄疸在术后有所消退，但是不能达到正常水平。他们可能出现生长停滞。虽然起初术后病情有所缓解，但是平均 5.4 年后需要进行肝移植治疗[16]。

剩余 15%～30% 的患儿行肝门肠吻合术后仍然没有胆汁引流，黄疸也没有改变，并且出现进行性的肝功能衰竭，只能通过肝移植挽救生命。婴儿供体肝短缺曾经严重限制了移植治疗，目前活体减体积肝移植手术的应用使得肝移植的数量大大增加。这样可以挽救肝门肠吻合术失败的患儿，使其在终末期肝衰竭之前得到治疗[27]。

肝门肠吻合术后的 10 年生存率已经稳步提高，目前在 40%～67% 之间。美国和加拿大胆道闭锁登记处最初报道 1976—1989 年 670 例患儿的 5 年和 10 年准确生存率大约为 48% 和 30%。英国的经验表明 64% 的患儿在最初进行肝门肠吻合术后可依靠自体肝生存 3.6 年[126]。香港大学报道 68% 的患儿行肝门肠吻合术后 10 年可以避免肝移植[184]。尽管最初效果喜人，但是仅有 20%～30% 未行肝移植的患儿存活年龄超过 20 岁[140,162]。Tsao 及其同事报道 50% 最终需要肝移植治疗[179]。我们已经报道了未行肝移植的患儿生存时间中位数为 15 年，20 年生存率达 49%[16]。

日本胆道闭锁登记处提供了自 1989 年以来 1400 例患儿的健康随访情况[139]。无肝移植的 5 年生存率

在 53%～64% 之间，行移植手术后增加到 78%[138]。他们报道依靠自体肝的 10 年生存率为 67%，非自体肝的 10 年生存率为 53%[139]。总体 5 年和 10 年生存率分别为 75% 和 67%[139]。

预测结果

我们[16]和其他作者[74,185,187]曾尝试预报肝门肠吻合术后的临床结果（1/3 治愈，1/3 进行性肝功能不良，1/3 无效）。每一类患儿的相对百分比取决于许多因素，如手术时的年龄、准确的切割和横向切断肝门、肝脏疾病的严重程度、初次术后的恢复过程以及术后并发症尤其是胆管炎的发生。

在多变量分析中，有意义的自变量包括手术时年龄[16]。患儿被分为 3 组进行分层分析（0～49 天，50～70 天，＞70 天）。前两个较小年龄组之间没有显示出差异，但是大于 70 天的婴儿比其他两个年龄较小组失败的风险更高。长期存活率亦随婴儿手术时年龄的增长而降低。在 60 天前进行手术治疗的患儿 10 年生存率为 68%，61～70 天为 39%，71～90 天为 33%，大于 91 天者 10 年生存率仅为 15%。

另有许多其他报道[33,62,74,129,159]亦确证了婴儿在 8～12周时手术预后有所改善。日本胆道闭锁登记处目前报道了 90 天日龄的婴儿也有类似的治疗成功率，但是此后的胆汁流量会变差。虽然日龄超过 70 天手术被广泛认为是一个危险因素，但最近一些报告提出了不一致的看法[42,121,127,184]。

Davenport 等最近研究了在较大日龄行肝门肠吻合术的婴儿（＞100 天）的预后情况[43]。尽管 37% 显示存在肝硬化，但 5 年和 10 年依靠自身肝脏的精确生存率分别为 45% 和 40%。1/3 的患儿有自体肝，28% 经过肝移植手术。没有发现有差异的因素。由于具有合理的中间生存期，因此 Kasai 手术，甚至是作为较大婴儿最初的手术治疗方法也得到了广泛认可。

另一个自变量与残余胆管的肉眼和显微镜下表现有关。当检测三种类型的胆道解剖结构时（见图
11 103-1），具有开放胆囊的患儿（B 型）比那些胆道完全纤维化闭塞（A 型）或缺乏肝门纤维块束锥的患儿（罕见的 C 型）预后好[105]。

肝门平面微小的胆管病理改变也与预后有关。许多研究检测了肝门处胆管结构的数量和大小与肝门肠吻合术成功率之间的关系。我们认为肝门平面管状残余物的组织学特征对预测临床结果具有重大意义[16]。三种不同类型的胆管被鉴定并依据管腔大小进行了归类：Ⅰ型，管腔大于 150 μm；Ⅱ型，管腔小于 150 μm并被大量结缔组织包绕；Ⅲ型，同心样纤维组织不能见到胆管腔[36]。所有Ⅰ型胆管患儿都可以建立胆汁引流，86% 的Ⅱ型胆管患儿具有胆汁引流，仅 12% 的Ⅲ型胆管患儿获得引流。我们断言胆管大小是很重要的预测临床结果的独立因素[16]。其他研究者[16,64,87,101,147,153,168]也支持上述的高度相关性，但是另有一些研究者不支持[56,111,127,171]。

肝脏组织学在行成形手术时被认为是评估预后的决定因素[160,170]。虽然与直觉相违背，但我们[16]和其他[8]一些研究者发现肝纤维化的程度与患儿的年龄、胆管的组织学类型或临床结果没有相关性。

最终，早年（20 世纪 70 年代）开展的手术治疗比近期的失败率高。这种差异可能很好地反映了手术的“学习曲线”以及在处理如胆管炎、门脉高压和营养缺乏并发症方面的成熟。

其他反映肝功能和临床结果的标志物也在研究中，尽管它们对于预后评估的意义仍属推测。下面将讨论几个较有前景的研究。^{99m}Tc－二亚乙基三胺五乙酸（DTPA）－半乳糖基标记的人血清白蛋白直接与肝细胞受体结合并允许闪烁扫描直接测量功能性的肝脏储备，借此显示与预后的相关性[85]。连续评估方法用于肝脏的预后分析并且在预测没有被认知的病情恶化或未来肝移植的需要方面有一定作用。

Ⅰ型胰岛素样生长因子（IGF－Ⅰ）已经作为肝脏储备功能的血清学标志物被研究[194]。在胆道闭锁患儿中即使没有生长迟缓并且生长激素水平正常，IGF－Ⅰ水平也较低。

对 35 例无黄疸（胆红素＜1.0 mg/dl）长期存活（＞5 年）的患儿进行的研究表明，术后 1 年时血清谷草转氨酶（AST）作为一个独立的预测指标与生活质量和肝功能不全的预后密切相关[182]。在胆道闭锁中血清透明质酸水平是肝纤维化的敏感指标[70]。可溶性细胞间黏附分子－1（ICAM－1）是一个有前景的标志物，可以用于显示胆道闭锁肝脏疾病的活动性[130]。肝动脉的多普勒超声检测用于计算“抵抗指数”。“抵抗指数”在预测 Kasai 手术后病情迅速恶化方面有一定的价值[28]。

试图预测肝门肠吻合术后结果的数学模型已经被

应用 30 年[74]。用于预测最初手术后结果的由多因素线性回归模型得出的胆道闭锁预后指数已经被确立[53]，变量包括按年龄分层的（<1 岁）血清学和体格参数。进行性肝纤维化的发病风险被量化，可用于早期考虑肝移植治疗。

儿童终末期肝病危险评分系统[189]已经作为胆道闭锁严重程度的指标被评估[163]，在区别未行移植的生存者与未生存者方面有很好的相关性。但是在小于 1 岁的婴儿和伴有严重并发症的年龄较大患儿中要谨慎应用，这就限制了该评分系统的整体适用性[163]。

并发症

营养并发症

如果肝功能不良持续存在，将会延缓术后体重的增长。另外，由于肝肠循环已经减退数月，可能发生涉及脂肪和蛋白代谢、维生素和微量元素吸收的各种代谢紊乱[18,61]。多达 32% 的患儿出现必需脂肪酸缺乏和佝偻病[22]。需要长期监测临床状态和补充营养。当胆汁流很少或缺乏时，推荐使用含有中链三酰甘油的配方。

胆管炎

胆管炎是肝门肠吻合术后最常见、最严重的并发症，发病率为 33%～60%[77,90,143,184]。胆管炎更多见于术后前几年，会导致肝脏进行性的功能衰竭和肝硬化。预防胆管炎发生最重要的是在肝门肠吻合术后维持胆汁的引流。

胆管炎的病因仍然不明，理论上包括 Roux 支肠内容物反流引起的直接污染、门静脉感染[40]、肝门处淋巴引流障碍[73]和全身细菌的移位。易感因素可能包括由于肝内胆管部分梗阻导致的胆汁淤积和肠道内细菌的过度生长。

发热、胆汁流减少和进行性黄疸提示胆管炎的发生。患儿出现嗜睡、烦躁并可能出现败血症。血清学评估出现血清胆红素水平增高、白细胞核左移和 C 反应蛋白增多证实有胆管炎。碱性磷酸酶、转氨酶和 γ-GGT升高超过正常值上限。肝脏活检不推荐作为常规检查，但是如果进行了肝活检，在肝门及其周围区域包括胆管上皮处可见急性炎症细胞浸润。在更严重 1612 的病例中可见微小脓肿的形成。经常可以分离到肠道革兰阴性菌和厌氧菌[29]。

术后早期胆管炎（3 个月内）经常伴有暂时性的胆汁流停止，其反复发作导致进行性的肝功能恶化。术后 6～9 个月胆汁淤积消除，胆流通畅，胆管炎的发生率降低。

胆管炎的治疗包括液体治疗、静脉应用广谱抗生素（抗厌氧菌）并使用促胆汁分泌的药物。在减少水肿和抗炎方面，类固醇的应用是经验性的方法。短期大剂量应用已经取得成功并被推荐[94]。大鼠胆道闭锁和胆管炎模型的实验研究目前正在测定类固醇抗炎效应的调节因子[80]。

研究者已经尝试预防胆管炎的复发。预防性应用口服抗生素的有效性仍然被肯定，但是存在争议[51,133]。历史对照分析表明患儿首次胆管炎发作后应用复方磺胺甲唑（TMP-SMZ）或新霉素在延迟和减少未来发作次数上是有效的［4 mg/(kg·d) TMP，20 mg/(kg·d) SMZ 分两次服用；或新霉素25 mg/(kg·d) 分 4 次应用，每周四天］[31]。术后类固醇药物的应用降低了胆管炎的发生率（28% 比 43%）[127]。新的治疗方法包括草药[84]，在有限的试验中显示有效。

当患儿在最初行 Kasai 手术成功后再次出现胆流停止[9]或顽固性胆管炎[12]时，有人提出尝试再行改进的肝门肠吻合手术重建胆汁引流。但是，值得注意的是二次手术有可能严重影响未来的肝移植。尽管二次手术最初较为流行，但是逐渐增多的经验表明当打算再次手术治疗时需要极度慎重。

Hasegawa 等回顾了 25 例由于胆道闭锁胆汁引流不足经历再次肝门肠吻合手术的病例[69]。仅 20% 的患儿在 3 个月内黄疸消退，生存时间是 6 个月到 11 年。剩余的 20 例中，8 人死亡，10 人进行了肝移植。此外，如果再次手术探查时肝组织学显示进一步的纤维化或肝硬化，则预后不良。我们也得出了相似的结论，7 例中仅有 2 例获得持续的胆汁流[9]。只有那些首次手术后有活跃的胆汁分泌的患儿晚期预后良好[83]。

Muraji 和同事[137]报告了再手术治疗 11 例严重顽固性胆管炎患儿的情况。在 Roux 肠支上创建一个长约 3 cm 的抗反流肠套迭瓣，如果肠支短于 50 cm 则将其延长。胆管炎在术后几次短期发作之后痊愈。2 例最终需要肝移植，但是过渡期的生活质量得到了改善。日本胆道闭锁登记处认为创建瓣膜与否结果没有差异[139]。

最近报道了一项用于治疗 2 例晚期发作的肝功能衰竭患儿的新技术[86]：一例肝内胆管扩张，另一例肝内胆湖形成。通过经皮减压及支撑架放置相结合，扩张的胆管最终通过手术与 Roux 肠支相连。在短期（<2 年）随访中黄疸消退。

即使再次手术偶有成功，但是由于现代肝移植时代的到来，我们不鼓励对 Kasai 手术失败的患儿进行二次手术。

门脉高压

胆道闭锁患儿初次手术后不可避免地会出现不同程度的肝纤维化，肝纤维化可以根据组织学特征进行分级。尽管成功地实行了肝门肠吻合术，但肝内疾病仍可能进展[8]。门脉高压是最严重的晚期并发症，发生率为 34%~76%，甚至在术后黄疸消退的患儿中也可以发生[3,118,167]。术后胆管炎是与门脉高压进展相关的一个很有意义的预测因素[146]。门脉高压自发性的缓解尽管很罕见，但与肝门压力降低和肝组织学改善有关[102,141]。

门脉高压出现腹水表现的占 63%。在长期存活者（>3 岁）中发生食管静脉曲张的比例为 49%，20%~60% 并发出血。有患病危险的患儿应该通过上消化道内镜进行监测，每年 1~2 次[53]。在一个随机对照试验中，预防性硬化疗法大大地降低了食管静脉曲张出血的发生率[58]。

严重的食管静脉曲张或静脉曲张出血最初通过内镜注射硬化疗法进行治疗。通常需要多次注射（平均每个患儿 6.3 次）[84]。奥曲肽或 β-阻滞剂以及曲张静脉结扎治疗已经得到了应用[66,78,79]。静脉曲张出血并非肝移植的绝对适应证，也并非一定是反映终末期肝衰竭预后的因素[184]。

肝门肠吻合术后脾功能亢进在长期生存者中的发生率为 16%~35%。血小板严重减少增加了胃肠道出血的危险[157]。应该考虑对伴有显著血小板减少（血小板计数 <5000 个/立方毫米）的有症状的脾功能亢进进行治疗。干预门脉高压和脾功能亢进的早期手术包括脾切除和脾肾分流手术。部分脾栓塞也已有成功的报道[71]。然而，在现代肝移植的时代，笔者不推荐行干预手术，如门体分流手术、食管离断手术和脾栓塞手术。相反，应该加快与肝移植有关的治疗安排。

长期生存者的心理社会随访已经得到了评估。65% 的患儿生长发育迟缓[22]。Kuroda 和同事[107]报告了 44 例随访超过 15 年的患者的情况，大多数患者（93%）被雇佣或具有高等学历，或者二者兼有。心理问题的发生率约为 18%[107]。

胆道闭锁手术治疗后成人期的长期随访目前已经 1613
开展。月经紊乱如月经初潮推迟、闭经与青春期的肝功能密切相关。青春期的紊乱被人认为是进行性肝功能障碍的预示指征，也是肝移植的一个预示因素。肝移植成功后月经将恢复正常[107]。

对怀孕妇女产生影响的报道开始出现。怀孕期间母亲门脉高压均逐渐加重，在所有依赖自身肝脏生存的患者中均发生食管静脉曲张[107]。新生儿为小孕龄儿，但不伴有先天性畸形的新生儿生长发育良好。产后问题包括 37.5% 肝功能恶化、25% 上行性胆管炎以及由于喂养导致的肝功能严重衰弱，所有这些最终均导致肝移植[162]。

即使患者最初的术后过程良好，在怀孕期间未能预料的并发症仍可能会发生。怀孕期间细致的监护是必要的，包括增加内镜监测静脉曲张的次数。可以建议对希望怀孕的妇女采用预防性的硬化疗法。

肝移植

肝移植在第 45 章有详细的讨论，它用于终末期肝病的治疗。胆道闭锁患儿约占所有肝移植儿童的近一半。考虑对胆道闭锁患儿行肝移植术的指征有：（1）首次肝门肠吻合术后不能建立胆汁引流；（2）胆流不足导致慢性肝功能衰竭、发育迟缓；（3）慢性肝脏疾病的后遗症得不到有效控制。

在等待移植的过程中患者的死亡率约为 4%[126]。为了解决婴儿和儿童供体肝脏不足的问题，另外两种移植技术目前已经开始得到运用。第一种方法是 Bismuth 和 Houssin 在 1984 年介绍的应用减体积或劈开的供体肝脏进行移植[25]。第二种方法涉及活体肝移植[27]。移植计划已经将这些技术推广至全球，用于治疗儿童患者[59,173]。综合的综述介绍已经超出了本章的范围，读者可以参考几个多中心的综述来进一步了解详情[57,59,154,155]。

随着免疫抑制剂的发展，肝移植生存率显著提高，人们提出了对胆道闭锁进行直接肝移植的问题[89,164]。尽管存在争论[191]，但小儿外科医生一致认为Kasai肝门肠吻合手术是胆道闭锁最初治疗的首选方法。理由包括将近一半的患儿在Kasai手术后获得足够的肝功能，以及肝门肠吻合手术延迟了许多患儿肝移植的需要[183]。儿童组供体短缺是主要的问题，而且肝移植与相关疾病（包括严重感染和肿瘤形成）的发病和死亡有关。然而肝移植仍是胆道闭锁救治的一个完整部分，最近的5年生存率接近85%[125]。

其他引起婴儿黄疸的外科疾病

除了胆道闭锁外，在婴儿和儿童期可以引起黄疸的其他外科疾病包括胆总管囊肿（第104章）、小叶间胆管发育不全、浓缩胆汁综合征、胆结石、自发性胆道穿孔、硬化性胆管炎、化脓性胆管炎、创伤性狭窄、胆囊炎、肝外胆道良性或恶性肿瘤以及胆管壁外压迫。三种最常见的疾病将在下面介绍。

胆管发育不全

胆管发育不全在胆汁淤积疾病中是一种独特的类型，常常被错误地诊断为“肝内胆道闭锁”。肝组织学以缺乏肝内胆管为特征，不像胆道闭锁那样肝内胆管增生。小叶间胆管缺乏被定义为小叶间胆管数量的减少（也就是说小叶间胆管数量与门脉管道之比显著下降）[65]。胆管发育不全最应被看做是继发于肝脏胆汁流减少的疾病而不是原发的胆管结构异常[72]。

婴儿和儿童中可见两种类型的胆管发育不全[7]，分为综合征型（Alagille）或非综合征型。非综合征型患儿最初可能与那些胆道闭锁的患儿相混淆。鉴别是很关键的，因为对于胆管发育不全引起的终末期肝病而言，肝移植是唯一适当的治疗方法。

来自患病婴儿经皮肝脏活检的标本显示，胆管发育不全缺乏胆道闭锁特征性的肝纤维化和胆管增生。如果行诊断性探查手术，肝脏是光滑的，并且经常呈“巧克力棕色”。胆管造影证实胆树细小，不需要进行胆道重建（见图103-4）。广泛的肝门探查可能危及这些精细管道的完整性，因此不推荐使用[114]。取而代之，要获得大量的肝活检标本。我们不推荐放置胆囊造口管用于术后研究。预后从胆汁淤积消退的临床症状改善到进行性肝纤维化的终末期肝病不等。

小叶间胆管缺乏综合征（Alagille综合征）

Alagille及同事最早描述了婴儿胆管缺乏综合征，其具有5个主要的临床特点：特殊面容、慢性胆汁淤积引起的黄疸、后部角膜胚胎环、蝴蝶样椎弓缺损、肺动脉分支发育不全或狭窄[5,6]。不常见的特征还包括生长停滞、智力障碍、肾功能紊乱、骨骼异常、声音音调高和青春期延迟[6]。这种被明确定义的综合征 161
型较非综合征型更常见。

患有Alagille综合征的婴儿1岁前表现为胆汁淤积和瘙痒。所有患儿均有肝大，但仅25%的患儿发展为肝硬化和门脉高压。血清学证实胆汁淤积会伴有总胆汁酸、胆固醇及三酰甘油水平的明显升高。Alagille综合征的诊断是以组织学上的小叶间胆管缺乏和特征性的临床特点为基础做出的。它以常染色体显性遗传的方式家族发病。由于大多数患有该病的患者可以活到成人期，所以这个综合征可以伴有长期慢性肝病的表现。

非综合征性小叶间胆管缺乏

在胆管发育不全非综合征性类型中，患儿胆汁淤积引起的不全梗阻出现在出生后1个月，瘙痒随之发生。实验室检查与在综合征型患儿中所见一致，为非特异性。诊断通过胆管造影和肝活检确定，显示小叶间胆管减少或缺乏，并伴有不同程度的肝门纤维化。

非综合征型胆管发育不全可以由胆管活动性的破坏或已成形的胆管萎缩引起。它也可以发生在其他临床情况中，包括并存的肝脏疾病如巨细胞病毒感染、风疹病毒感染、α_1-抗胰蛋白酶缺乏、囊性纤维化、移植物抗宿主疾病、Down综合征和垂体机能减退。可以见到三羟基粪甾烷酸水平增加。胆管发育不全非综合征型患儿比综合征型患儿预后差。半数患儿发展为肝硬化伴门脉高压，他们可能在1岁内死于肝功能衰竭。曾经有临床和组织病理学症状消退的个案报道[23]。

治疗

除了肝移植外，胆管发育不全不能通过其他手术治愈。药物治疗是支持性的，包括中链三酰甘油的喂养、脂溶性维生素的添加，以及对于有症状的严重瘙痒服用苯巴比妥和考来烯胺治疗。对具有终末期肝病或严重瘙痒并发症的患儿需要进行肝移植治疗[181]。

胆汁浓缩综合征

胆汁浓缩综合征被定义为新生儿期胆总管远端被稠厚的胆汁或泥沙阻塞引起的肝外胆道系统部分或完全的梗阻。据推测易感因素是引起胆汁黏滞性增加或溶解度降低的疾病。胆汁浓缩综合征可以发生在患有脱水、溶血、肝脏分泌胆汁功能受损、囊性纤维化和接受利尿剂[188]或全肠外营养治疗的婴儿中[123]。由于浓缩胆汁综合征和胆道闭锁二者均表现为黄疸和无胆汁性粪便，因此最初很难将其与胆道闭锁鉴别。胆汁的浓缩可以先于胆石症发生。

腹部超声显示轻度到中度的近端胆管扩张，泥沙或结石存在于远端胆总管中。放射核素扫描显示肝脏同位素浓度不能分泌进入肠道。

浓缩胆汁综合征通常在潜在的疾病被治愈或易感因素被消除后自限性地消退[100]。持续梗阻需要进行评估，手术探查中通过胆囊底部进行胆管造影可以确定诊断和排除胆道闭锁（图 103-6）。胆道造影经常是治疗性的，可以通过术中盐水冲洗胆道增强效果，很少需要十二指肠切开或胆总管切开。

胆总管自发性穿孔

肝外胆道系统自发性穿孔很罕见，是婴儿时期发生的重要临床疾病，需要迅速诊断并进行手术治疗。大多数患儿的穿孔发生在胆囊和胆总管的连接处。自发性穿孔的病因仍然基于推测。普遍接受的理论假说认为是胆道先天性薄弱所致[37,149]，其他原因有胆汁浓缩、病毒感染、胰腺炎和伴有胆管压力升高的 Va-

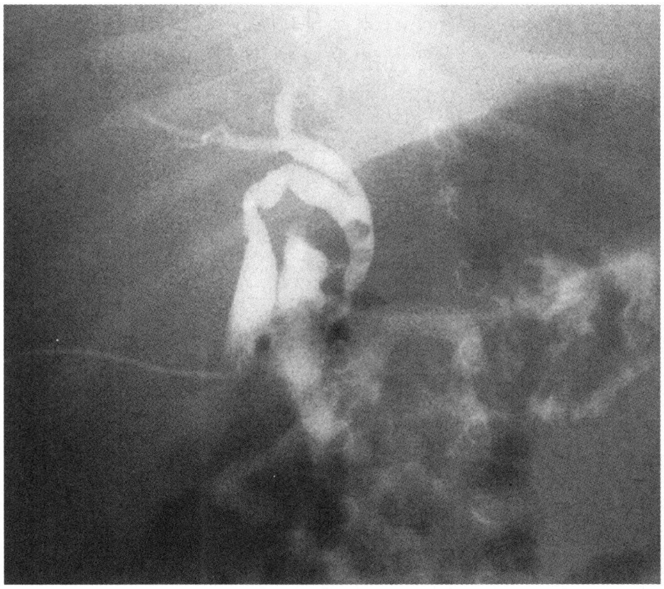

图 103-6　2 个月婴儿术中胆道造影显示浓缩胆汁位于胆总管远端。通过胆囊进行治疗性的冲洗。

ter 壶腹乳头狭窄。一些作者[149,193]已经证实在许多患
儿中存在胰胆管连接异常，并认为胆道自发穿孔和胆 1615
总管囊肿可能是先天性胆道畸形中同一疾病谱的不同表现形式。

临床特征和诊断

大多数婴儿有黄疸、无痛性腹胀伴腹水、陶土样大便和生长停滞[21]。腹水引起的腹内压增加可以引起腹股沟疝和脐疝。胆道穿孔经常很微小，胆汁缓慢流出。偶尔，漏液被包裹形成假性囊肿[111]。婴儿暴发性胆汁性腹膜炎的急性发作很少见[82]。

典型的血清胆红素水平不超过 8 mg/dl，伴有转氨酶的轻度升高。腹部超声显示广泛的腹水或右上腹局限性积液，但未见胆管扩张[67]。放射性核素扫描（DISIDA）证实同位素存在于腹水中或积聚在少见的假性囊肿内[122]。

治疗和预后

胆总管自发穿孔的患儿可以出现营养不良和脱水，术前积极开展急救至关重要。手术探查可以确定治疗方案。通过胆囊的术中胆管造影术可以排除胰胆

管连接异常、远端梗阻或其他的病理性疾病。当确诊胆道穿孔后，最有帮助的是原位保留胆囊造口管，这样既可以为胆道减压，又可以在术后开展胆道造影，评估愈合情况[68]。不建议缝合修补微小的穿孔，相反，推荐在穿孔区肝门处单纯引流而不予缝合修补穿孔的方法。大多数完全康复、不伴有长期肝胆管后遗症的患儿预后良好。

（周 莹译 吴晔明校）

参考文献

1. Abramson SJ, Berdon WE, Altman RP, et al: Biliary atresia and noncardiac polysplenic syndrome: US and surgical considerations. Radiology 1987;1632:377.
2. Absolon KB, Rikkers H, Aust JB: Thoracic duct lymph drainage in congenital biliary atresia. Surg Gynecol Obstet 1965:120:123.
3. Akiyama H, Saeki M, Ogata T: Portal hypertension after successful surgery for biliary atresia. In Kasai M (ed): Biliary Atresia and Its Related Disorders. Amsterdam, Excerpta Medica, 1983.
4. Akiyama T, Yamauchi Y: Use of near infrared reflectance spectroscopy in the screening for biliary atresia. J Pediatr Surg 1994:29:645.
5. Alagille D: Cholestasis in the first three months of life. Prog Liver Dis 1979:6:471.
6. Alagille D, Estrada A, Hadchouel M, et al: Syndromic paucity of interlobular bile ducts (Alagille syndrome or arteriohepatic dysplasia): Review of 80 cases. J Pediatr 1987;110:195.
7. Alagille D, Odievre M, Gautier M, Dommergues JP: Hepatic ductular hypoplasia associated with characteristic facies, vertebral malformations, retarded physical, mental, and sexual development, and cardiac murmur. J Pediatr 1975;86:63.
8. Altman RP: The portoenterostomy procedure for biliary atresia: A five year experience. Ann Surg 1978;188:351.
9. Altman RP: Results of re-operations for correction of extrahepatic biliary atresia. J Pediatr Surg 1979;14:305.
10. Altman RP: Long term results after the Kasai procedure. In Daum F (ed): Extrahepatic Biliary Atresia. New York, Marcel Dekker, 1983.
11. Altman RP, Abramson S: Potential errors in the diagnosis and surgical management of neonatal jaundice. J Pediatr Surg 1985;20:529.
12. Altman RP, Anderson KD: Surgical management of intractable cholangitis following successful Kasai procedure. J Pediatr Surg 1982;176:894.
13. Altman RP, Chandra R, Lilly JR: Ongoing cirrhosis after successful porticoenterostomy in infants with biliary atresia. J Pediatr Surg 1975;10:685.
14. Altman RP, Levy J: Biliary atresia. Pediatr Ann 1985;14:481.
15. Altman RP, Lilly JR: Technical details in the surgical correction of extrahepatic biliary atresia. Surg Gynecol Obstet 1975;140:952.
16. Altman RP, Lilly JR, Greenfeld J, et al: A multivariable risk factor analysis of the portoenterostomy (Kasai) procedure for biliary atresia: Twenty-five years of experience from two centers. Ann Surg 1997;226:348, discussion 353.
17. Ando H, Ito T, Nagaya M: Use of external conduit impairs liver function in patients with biliary atresia. J Pediatr Surg 1996;311:1509.
18. Andrews WS, Pau CM, Chase HP, et al: Fat soluble vitamin deficiency in biliary atresia. J Pediatr Surg 1981;16:284.
19. Azarow KS, Phillips MJ, Sandler AD, et al: Biliary atresia: Should all patients undergo a portoenterostomy? J Pediatr Surg 1997;32:168, discussion 172.
20. Balistreri WF: Neonatal cholestasis. J Pediatr 1985;106:171.
21. Banani SA, Bahador A, Nezakatgoo N: Idiopathic perforation of the extrahepatic bile duct in infancy: Pathogenesis, diagnosis, and management. J Pediatr Surg 1993;28:950.
22. Barkin RM, Lilly JR: Biliary atresia and the Kasai operation: Continuing care. J Pediatr 1980;96:1015.
23. Berezin S, Beneck D, Altman RP, Schwarz SM: Resolution of nonsyndromic paucity of intrahepatic bile ducts in infancy. Dig Dis Sci 1995;40:82.
24. Bill AH, Brennom WS, Huseby TL: Biliary atresia. New concepts of pathology, diagnosis, and management. Arch Surg 1974;109:367.
25. Bismuth H, Houssin D: Reduced-sized orthotopic liver graft in hepatic transplantation in children. Surgery 1984;95:367.
26. Brent RL: Persistent jaundice in infancy. J Pediatr 1962;61:111.
27. Broelsch CE, Whitington PF, Emond JC, et al: Liver transplantation in children from living related donors. Surgical techniques and results. Ann Surg 1991;214:428, discussion 437.
28. Broide E, Farrant P, Reid F, et al: Hepatic artery resistance index can predict early death in children with biliary atresia. Liver Transpl Surg 1997;36:604.
29. Brook I, Altman RP: The significance of anaerobic bacteria in biliary tract infection after hepatic portoenterostomy for biliary atresia. Surgery 1984;95:281.
30. Brown WR, Sokol RJ, Levin MJ, et al: Lack of correlation between infection with reovirus 3 and extrahepatic biliary atresia or neonatal hepatitis. J Pediatr 1988;113:670.
31. Bu LN, Chen HL, Chang CJ, et al: Prophylactic oral antibiotics in prevention of recurrent cholangitis after the Kasai portoenterostomy. J Pediatr Surg 2003;38:590.
32. Campbell DP, Poley JR, Alaupovic P, Smith EI: The differential diagnosis of neonatal hepatitis and biliary atresia. J Pediatr Surg 1974;9:699.
33. Canty TG Sr: Encouraging results with a modified Sawaguchi hepatoportoenterostomy for biliary atresia. Am J Surg 1987;154:19.
34. Carlson E: Salvage of the "noncorrectable" case of congenital extrahepatic biliary atresia. Arch Surg 1960;81:893.
35. Chandra RS: Biliary atresia and other structural anomalies in the congenital polysplenia syndrome. J Pediatr 1974; 85:649.
36. Chandra RS, Altman RP: Ductal remnants in extrahepatic biliary atresia: A histopathologic study with clinical correlation. J Pediatr 1978;93:196.
37. Chen W, Chang C, Hung W: Congenital choledochal cyst: With observations on rupture of the cyst and intrahepatic ductal dilatation. J Pediatr Surg 1973;8:529.
38. Chiba T: Japanese Biliary Atresia Registry. In Ohi R (ed): Biliary Atresia. Tokyo, Icom Associates, 1991.
39. Choi SO, Park WH, Lee HJ, Woo SK: 'Triangular cord': A sonographic finding applicable in the diagnosis of biliary atresia. J Pediatr Surg 1996;31:363.
40. Danks DM, Campbell PE, Clarke AM, et al: Extrahepatic biliary atresia: The frequency of potentially operable cases. Am J Dis Child 1974;128:684.
41. Davenport M, Betalli P, D'Antiga L, et al: The spectrum of

surgical jaundice in infancy. J Pediatr Surg 2003;38:1471.
42. Davenport M, Kerkar N, Mieli-Vergani G, et al: Biliary atresia: The King's College Hospital experience (1974-1995). J Pediatr Surg 1997;32:479.
43. Davenport M, Puricelli V, Farrant P, et al: The outcome of the older (> or =100 days) infant with biliary atresia. J Pediatr Surg 2004;39:575.
44. Davenport M, Savage M, Mowat AP, Howard ER: Biliary atresia splenic malformation syndrome: An etiologic and prognostic subgroup. Surgery 1993;113:662.
45. Davies MR: Facilitating the operative exposure of the portal plate in cases of biliary atresia by dislocating the whole liver onto the abdominal wall. J Pediatr Surg 1992;27:1391.
46. Desmet VJ: Intrahepatic bile ducts under the lens. J Hepatol 1985;15:545.
47. Dick MC, Mowat AP: Biliary scintigraphy with DISIDA. A simpler way of showing bile duct patency in suspected biliary atresia. Arch Dis Child 1986;61:191.
48. Dillon PW, Owings E, Cilley R, et al: Immunosuppression as adjuvant therapy for biliary atresia. J Pediatr Surg 2001;361:80.
49. Dimmick JE, Bove KE, McAdams AJ: Extrahepatic biliary atresia and the polysplenia syndrome [letter]. J Pediatr 1975;86:644.
50. Donovan EJ: Congenital atresia of the bile ducts. Ann Surg 1937;106:737.
51. Ecoffey C, Rothman E, Bernard O, et al: Bacterial cholangitis after surgery for biliary atresia. J Pediatr 1987;111:824.
52. Endo M, Katsumata K, Yokoyama J, et al: Extended dissection of the portahepatis and creation of an intussuscepted ileocolic conduit for biliary atresia. J Pediatr Surg 1983;18:784.
53. Endo M, Masuyama H, Watanabe K, et al: Calculation of biliary atresia prognostic index using a multivariate linear model. J Pediatr Surg 1995;30:1575.
54. Faweya AG, Akinyinka OO, Sodeinde O: Duodenal intubation and aspiration test: Utility in the differential diagnosis of infantile cholestasis. J Pediatr Gastroenterol Nutr 1991;13:290.
55. Fonkalsrud EW, Kitagawa S, Longmire WP Jr: Hepatic lymphatic drainage to the jejunum for congenital biliary atresia. Am J Surg 1966;112:188.
56. Gautier M, Jehan P, Odievre M: Histologic study of biliary fibrous remnants in 48 cases of extrahepatic biliary atresia: Correlation with postoperative bile flow restoration. J Pediatr 1976;89:704.
57. Goldstein MJ, Salame E, Kapur S, et al: Analysis of failure in living donor liver transplantation: Differential outcomes in children and adults. World J Surg 2003;27:356.
58. Goncalves ME, Cardoso SR, Maksoud JG: Prophylactic sclerotherapy in children with esophageal varices: Long-term results of a controlled prospective randomized trial. J Pediatr Surg 2000;35:401.
59. Goss JA, Shackleton CR, Swenson K, et al: Orthotopic liver transplantation for congenital biliary atresia. An 11-year, single-center experience. Ann Surg 1996;224:276, discussion 284.
60. Greene H: Nutritional aspects in the management of biliary atresia. In Daum F (ed): Extrahepatic Biliary Atresia. New York, Marcel Dekker, 1983.
61. Greene HL, Helinek GL, Moran R, O'Neill J: A diagnostic approach to prolonged obstructive jaundice by 24-hour collection of duodenal fluid. J Pediatr 1979;95:412.
62. Grosfeld JL, Fitzgerald JF, Predaina R, et al: The efficacy of hepatoportoenterostomy in biliary atresia. Surgery 1989;106:692, discussion 700.
63. Gross R: Obstructive jaundice in infancy. In Gross R (ed): The Surgery of Infancy and Childhood. Philadelphia, WB Saunders, 1953.
64. Haas JE: Bile duct and liver pathology in biliary atresia. World J Surg 1978;2:561.
65. Hadchouel M, Hugon RN, Gautier M: Reduced ratio of portal tracts to paucity of intrahepatic bile ducts. Arch Pathol Lab Med 1978;102:402.
66. Hall RJ, Lilly JR, Stiegmann GV: Endoscopic esophageal varix ligation: Technique and preliminary results in children. J Pediatr Surg 1988;23:1222.
67. Haller JO, Condon VR, Berdon WE, et al: Spontaneous perforation of the common bile duct in children. Radiology 1989;172:621.
68. Hammoudi SM, Alauddin A: Idiopathic perforation of the biliary tract in infancy and childhood. J Pediatr Surg 1988;23:185.
69. Hasegawa T, Kimura T, Sasaki T, et al: Indication for redo hepatic portoenterostomy for insufficient bile drainage in biliary atresia: Re-evaluation in the era of liver transplantation. Pediatr Surg Int 2003;19:256.
70. Hasegawa T, Sasaki T, Kimura T, et al: Measurement of serum hyaluronic acid as a sensitive marker of liver fibrosis in biliary atresia. J Pediatr Surg 2000;35:1643.
71. Hayashi Y: Effect of partial splenic embolization on hypersplenism in patients with biliary atresia. In Ohi R (ed): Biliary Atresia. Tokyo, Professional Postgraduate Services, 1987.
72. Hays DM, Woolley MM, Snyder WH Jr, et al: Diagnosis of biliary atresia: Relative accuracy of percutaneous liver biopsy, open liver biopsy, and operative cholangiography. J Pediatr 1967;71:598.
73. Hirsig J, Kara O, Rickham PP: Experimental investigations into the etiology of cholangitis following operation for biliary atresia. J Pediatr Surg 1978;13:55.
74. Hitch DC, Shikes RH, Lilly JR: Determinants of survival after Kasai's operation for biliary atresia using actuarial analysis. J Pediatr Surg 1979;14:310.
75. Ho CW, Shioda K, Shirasaki K, et al: The pathogenesis of biliary atresia: A morphological study of the hepatobiliary system and the hepatic artery. J Pediatr Gastroenterol Nutr 1993;16:53.
76. Holmes JB: Congenital obliteration of the bile ducts: Diagnosis and suggestions for treatment. Am J Dis Child 1916;11:405.
77. Howard ER: Extrahepatic biliary atresia: A review of current management. Br J Surg 1983;70:193.
78. Howard ER, Stamatakis JD, Mowat AP: Management of esophageal varices in children by injection sclerotherapy. J Pediatr Surg 1984;19:2.
79. Howard ER, Stringer MD, Mowat AP: Assessment of injection sclerotherapy in the management of 152 children with oesophageal varices. Br J Surg 1988;75:404.
80. Hsieh CS, Huang CC, Huang LT, et al: Glucocorticoid treatment down-regulates chemokine expression of bacterial cholangitis in cholestatic rats. J Pediatr Surg 2004;39:10.
81. Hyams JS, Glaser JH, Leichtner AM, Morecki R: Discordance for biliary atresia in two sets of monozygotic twins. J Pediatr 1985;1073:420.
82. Hyde GA Jr: Spontaneous perforation of bile ducts in early infancy. Pediatrics 1965;35:453.
83. Ibrahim M: Indications and results of reoperation for biliary atresia. In Ohi R (ed): Biliary Atresia. Tokyo, Icom Associates, 1991.
84. Iinuma Y, Kubota M, Yagi M, et al: Effects of the herbal medicine Inchinko-to on liver function in postoperative patients with biliary atresia—a pilot study. J Pediatr Surg 2003;38:1607.

85. Ishii T, Nio M, Shimaoka S, et al: Clinical significance of 99mTc-DTPA-galactosyl human serum albumin liver scintigraphy in follow-up patients with biliary atresia. J Pediatr Surg 2003;38:1486.
86. Islam S, Dasika N, Hirschl RB, Coran AG: A novel approach to the management of late-onset liver failure in biliary atresia. J Pediatr Surg 2004;39:371.
87. Ito T, Horisawa M, Ando H: Intrahepatic bile ducts in biliary atresia—a possible factor determining the prognosis. J Pediatr Surg 1983;18:124.
88. Ito T, Nagaya M, Ando H, et al: Modified hepatic portal enterostomy for biliary atresia. Z Kinderchir 1984;39:242.
89. Iwatsuki S, Shaw BW Jr, Starzl TE: Liver transplantation for biliary atresia. World J Surg 1984;8:51.
90. Japanese Biliary Atresia Society: Nationwide Registry of Biliary Atresia, 1998. Jpn J Pediatr Surg 2000;36:311.
91. Javitt NB, Keating JP, Grand RJ, Harris RC: Serum bile acid patterns in neonatal hepatitis and extrahepatic biliary atresia. J Pediatr 1977;90:736.
92. Jenner RE, Howard ER: Unsaturated monohydroxy bile acids as a cause of idiopathic obstructive cholangiopathy. Lancet 1975;2:1073.
93. Kanof A, Donovan EJ, Berner H: Congenital atresia of the biliary system;delayed development of correctibility. Am J Dis Child 1953;86:780.
94. Karrer FM, Lilly JR: Corticosteroid therapy in biliary atresia. J Pediatr Surg 1985;20:693.
95. Karrer FM, Lilly JR, Stewart BA, Hall RJ: Biliary atresia registry, 1976 to 1989. J Pediatr Surg 1990;25:1076, discussion 1081.
96. Kasai M: Treatment of biliary atresia with special reference to hepatic porto-enterostomy and its modifications. Prog Pediatr Surg 1974;6:5.
97. Kasai M, Kimura S, Asakura Y, et al: Surgical treatment of biliary atresia. J Pediatr Surg 1968;3:665.
98. Kasai M, Mochizuki I, Ohkochi N, et al: Surgical limitation for biliary atresia: Indication for liver transplantation. J Pediatr Surg 1989;24:851.
99. Kasai M, Okamoto A, Ohi R, et al: Changes of portal vein pressure and intrahepatic blood vessels after surgery for biliary atresia. J Pediatr Surg 1981;16:152.
100. Kasai M, Suzuki S: A new operation for "non-correctable" biliary atresia: Hepatic portoenterostomy. Shujyutsu 1959;13:733.
101. Kasai M, Yakovac WC, Koop CE: Liver in congenital biliary atresia and neonatal hepatitis. A histopathologic study. Arch Pathol 1962;74:152.
102. Keller MS, Markle BM, Laffey PA, et al: Spontaneous resolution of cholelithiasis in infants. Radiology 1985;157:345.
103. Kimura K, Tsugawa C, Kubo M, et al: Technical aspects of hepatic portal dissection in biliary atresia. J Pediatr Surg 1979;14:27.
104. Klippel CH: A new theory of biliary atresia. J Pediatr Surg 1972;7:651.
105. Koop CE: Biliary atresia and the Kasai operation. Pediatrics 1975;55:9.
106. Krovetz LJ: Congenital biliary atresia. Surgery 1960;47:453.
107. Kuroda T, Saeki M, Nakano M, Morikawa N: Biliary atresia, the next generation: A review of liver function, social activity, and sexual development in the late postoperative period. J Pediatr Surg 2002;37:1709.
108. Ladd WE: Congenital atresia and stenosis of the bile ducts. JAMA 1928;91:1082.
109. Landing BH: Considerations of the pathogenesis of neonatal hepatitis, biliary atresia and choledochal cyst—the concept of infantile obstructive cholangiopathy. Prog Pediatr Surg 1974;6:113.
110. Lazar EL, Altman RP: Surgical disease of the biliary tract. In Oxford Textbook of Surgery. Oxford, Oxford University Press, 1999.
111. Lebwohl O, Waye JD: Endoscopic retrograde cholangiopancreatography in the diagnosis of extrahepatic biliary atresia. Am J Dis Child 1979;133:647.
112. Lee H, Hirose S, Bratton B, Farmer D: Initial experience with complex laparoscopic biliary surgery in children: Biliary atresia and choledochal cyst. J Pediatr Surg 2004;39:804, discussion 807.
113. Lefkowitch JH: Biliary atresia. Mayo Clin Proc 1998;73:90.
114. Lilly JR: The surgery of biliary hypoplasia. J Pediatr Surg 1976;11:815.
115. Lilly JR, Altman RP: Hepatic portoenterostomy (the Kasai operation) for biliary atresia. Surgery 1975;78:76.
116. Lilly JR, Hitch DC: Postoperative ascending cholangitis following portoenterostomy for biliary atresia: Measures for control. World J Surg 1978;2:581.
117. Lilly JR, Stellin G: Variceal hemorrhage in biliary atresia. J Pediatr Surg 1984;19:476.
118. Lilly JR, Weintraub WH, Altman RP: Spontaneous perforation of the extrahepatic bile ducts and bile peritonitis in infancy. Surgery 1974;75:664.
119. Longmire WP Jr, Sanford MC: Intrahepatic-cholangiojejunostomy with partial hepatectomy for biliary obstruction. Surgery 1948;24:264.
120. Majd M, Reba RC, Altman RP: Hepatobiliary scintigraphy with ^{99m}Tc-PIPIDA in the evaluation of neonatal jaundice. Pediatrics 1981;67:140.
121. Maksoud JG, Fauza DO, Silva MM, et al: Management of biliary atresia in the liver transplantation era: A 15-year, single-center experience. J Pediatr Surg 1998;33:115.
122. Marshall DG, Brabyn DG, Vezina WC: Spontaneous perforation of the common bile duct in infancy detected by ^{99m}Tc HIDA scanning. Can J Surg 1984;27:590.
123. Matos C, Avni EF, Van Gansbeke D, et al: Total parenteral nutrition (TPN) and gallbladder diseases in neonates. Sonographic assessment. J Ultrasound Med 1987;6:243.
124. Matsui A, Ishikawa T: Identification of infants with biliary atresia in Japan. Lancet 1994;343:925.
125. McDiarmid SV: Current status of liver transplantation in children. Pediatr Clin North Am 2003;50:1335.
126. McKiernan PJ, Baker AJ, Kelly DA: The frequency and outcome of biliary atresia in the UK and Ireland. Lancet 2000;355:25.
127. Meyers RL, Book LS, O'Gorman MA, et al: High-dose steroids, ursodeoxycholic acid, and chronic intravenous antibiotics improve bile flow after Kasai procedure in infants with biliary atresia. J Pediatr Surg 2003;38:406.
128. Meyers RL, Book LS, O'Gorman MA, et al: Percutaneous cholecysto-cholangiography in the diagnosis of obstructive jaundice in infants. J Pediatr Surg 2004;39:16.
129. Middlesworth W, Altman RP: Biliary atresia. Curr Opin Pediatr 1997;9:265.
130. Minnick KE, Kreisberg R, Dillon PW: Soluble ICAM-1 (sICAM-1) in biliary atresia and its relationship to disease activity. J Surg Res 1998;76:53.
131. Miyano T, Suruga K, Suda K: Abnormal choledochopancreatico ductal junction related to the etiology of infantile obstructive jaundice diseases. J Pediatr Surg 1979;14:16.
132. Miyazaki T, Yamshita Y, Tang Y, et al: Single-shot MR cholangiopancreatography of neonates, infants, and young

children. AJR Am J Roentgenol 1998;170:33.
133. Mones RL, DeFelice AR, Preud'Homme D: Use of neomycin as the prophylaxis against recurrent cholangitis after Kasai portoenterostomy. J Pediatr Surg 1994; 29:422.
134. Moore TC: Congenital atresia of the extrahepatic bile ducts; report of 31 proved cases. Surg Gynecol Obstet 1953;96:215.
135. Moore TC, Hyman PE: Extrahepatic biliary atresia in one human leukocyte antigen identical twin. Pediatrics 1985; 76:604.
136. Muraji T, Higashimoto Y: The improved outlook for biliary atresia with corticosteroid therapy. J Pediatr Surg 1997;32:1103, discussion 1106.
137. Muraji T, Tsugawa C, Nishijima E, et al: Surgical management for intractable cholangitis in biliary atresia. J Pediatr Surg 2002;37:1713.
138. Nakajo T, Hashizume K, Saeki M, Tsuchida Y: Intussusception-type antireflux valve in the Roux-en-Y loop to prevent ascending cholangitis after hepatic portojejunostomy. J Pediatr Surg 1990;25:311.
139. Nio M, Ohi R, Miyano T, et al: Five- and 10-year survival rates after surgery for biliary atresia: A report from the Japanese Biliary Atresia Registry. J Pediatr Surg 2003;38:997.
140. Nio M, Ohi R, Shimaoka S, et al: [Long-term outcome of surgery for biliary atresia.] Nippon Geka Gakkai Zasshi 1996;97:637.
141. Odièvre M: Long-term results of surgical treatment of biliary atresia. World J Surg 1978;2:589.
142. Ogasawara Y, Yamataka A, Tsukamoto K, et al: The intussusception antireflux valve is ineffective for preventing cholangitis in biliary atresia: A prospective study. J Pediatr Surg 2003;38:1826.
143. Ohi R: The present status of surgical treatment for biliary atresia: Report of the questionnaire for the main institutions in Japan. In Ohi R (ed): Biliary Atresia. Tokyo, Professional Postgraduate Services, 1987.
144. Ohi R, Chiba T, Endo N: Morphologic studies of the liver and bile ducts in biliary atresia. Acta Paediatr Jpn 1987;29:584.
145. Ohi R, Klingensmith WC 3rd, Lilly JR: Diagnosis of hepatobiliary disease in infants and children with Tc-99m-diethyl-IDA imaging. Clin Nucl Med 1981;6:297.
146. Ohi R, Mochizuki I, Komatsu K, Kasai M: Portal hypertension after successful hepatic portoenterostomy in biliary atresia. J Pediatr Surg 1986;21:271.
147. Ohi R, Shikes RH, Stellin GP, Lilly JR: In biliary atresia duct histology correlates with bile flow. J Pediatr Surg 1984;19:467.
148. Ohi R, Takahashi T, Kasai M: Intrahepatic biliary obstruction in congenital bile duct atresia. Tohoku J Exp Med 1969;99:129.
149. Ohkawa H, Takahashi H, Maie M: A malformation of the pancreatico-biliary system as a cause of perforation of the biliary tract in childhood. J Pediatr Surg 1977;12:541.
150. Petersen C, Biermanns D, Kuske M, et al: New aspects in a murine model for extrahepatic biliary atresia. J Pediatr Surg 1997;32:1190.
151. Poley JR, Smith EI, Boon DJ, et al: Lipoprotein-X and the double 131 I-rose bengal test in the diagnosis of prolonged infantile jaundice. J Pediatr Surg 1972;7:660.
152. Povey S: Genetics of alpha 1-antitrypsin deficiency in relation to neonatal liver disease. Mol Biol Med 1990;7:161.
153. Raweily EA, Gibson AA, Burt AD: Abnormalities of intrahepatic bile ducts in extrahepatic biliary atresia. Histopathology 1990;17:521.
154. Renz JF, Emond JC, Yersiz H, et al: Split-liver transplantation in the United States: Outcomes of a national survey. Ann Surg 2004;239:172.
155. Renz JF, Yersiz H, Reichert PR, et al: Split-liver transplantation: A review. Am J Transplant 2003;3:1323.
156. Riepenhoff-Talty M, Gouvea V, Evans MJ, et al: Detection of group C rotavirus in infants with extrahepatic biliary atresia. J Infect Dis 1996;174:8.
157. Saeki M, Ogata T, Nakano M: Problems in long-term survivors of biliary atresia. In Ohi R (ed): Biliary Atresia. Tokyo, Professional Postgraduate Services, 1987.
158. Sandler AD, Azarow KS, Superina RA: The impact of a previous Kasai procedure on liver transplantation for biliary atresia. J Pediatr Surg 1997;323:416.
159. Schweizer P: Treatment of extrahepatic bile duct atresia: Results and long-term prognosis after hepatic portoenterostomy. Pediatr Surg Int 1986;1:30.
160. Segawa O, Miyano T, Fujimoto T, et al: Actin and myosin deposition around bile canaliculi: A predictor of clinical outcome in biliary atresia. J Pediatr Surg 1993;28:851.
161. Sera Y, Ikeda S, Akagi M: Ultrasonographic studies for the diagnosis of infantile cholestatic disease. In Ohi R (ed): Biliary Atresia. Tokyo, Professional Postgraduate Services, 1987.
162. Shimaoka S, Ohi R, Saeki M, et al: Problems during and after pregnancy of former biliary atresia patients treated successfully by the Kasai procedure. J Pediatr Surg 2001;36:349.
163. Shinkai M, Ohhama Y, Take H, et al: Evaluation of the PELD risk score as a severity index of biliary atresia. J Pediatr Surg 2003;38:1001.
164. Starzl TE, Iwatsuki S, Van Thiel DH, et al: Evolution of liver transplantation. Hepatology 1982;2:614.
165. Starzl TE, Marchioro TL, VonKaulla KN, et al: Homotransplantation of the liver in humans. Surg Gynecol Obstet 1963;117:659.
166. Sterling JA: Artificial bile ducts in the management of congenital biliary atresia: A clinical report. J Int Coll Surg 1961;36:293.
167. Stringer MD, Howard ER, Mowat AP: Endoscopic sclerotherapy in the management of esophageal varices in 61 children with biliary atresia. J Pediatr Surg 1989;24:438.
168. Suruga K, Miyano T, Kitahara T, et al: Treatment of biliary atresia: A study of our operative results. J Pediatr Surg 1981;16(4 Suppl 1):621.
169. Takahashi H: ERCP in jaundiced infants. In Ohi R (ed): Biliary Atresia. Tokyo, Professional Postgraduate Services, 1987.
170. Tan CE, Davenport M, Driver M, Howard ER: Does the morphology of the extrahepatic biliary remnants in biliary atresia influence survival? A review of 205 cases. J Pediatr Surg 1994;29:1459.
171. Tan CE, Driver M, Howard ER, Moscoso GJ: Extrahepatic biliary atresia: A first-trimester event? Clues from light microscopy and immunohistochemistry. J Pediatr Surg 1994;29:808.
172. Tanaka K, Shirahase I, Utsunomiya H, et al: A valved hepatic portoduodenal intestinal conduit for biliary atresia. Ann Surg 1991;213:230.
173. Tanaka K, Uemoto S, Tokunaga Y, et al: Surgical techniques and innovations in living related liver transplantation. Ann Surg 1993;217:82.
174. Tazawa Y, Konno T: Semiquantitative assay of serum lipoprotein-X in differential diagnosis of neonatal hepatitis and congenital biliary atresia. Tohoku J Exp Med

1980;130:209.
175. Tazawa Y, Yamada M, Nakagawa M, et al: Significance of serum lipoprotein-X and gammaglutamyltranspeptidase in the diagnosis of biliary atresia. A preliminary study in 27 cholestatic young infants. Eur J Pediatr 1986;145:54.
176. Thaler MM, Gellis SS: Studies in neonatal hepatitis and biliary atresia. I. Long-term prognosis of neonatal hepatitis. Am J Dis Child 1968;1163:257.
177. Thomson J: On congenital obliteration of the bile ducts. Edinb Med J 1892;37:724.
178. Toyosaka A, Okamoto E, Okasora T, et al: Extensive dissection at the porta hepatis for biliary atresia. J Pediatr Surg 1994;29:896.
179. Tsao K, Rosenthal P, Dhawan K, et al: Comparison of drainage techniques for biliary atresia. J Pediatr Surg 2003;38:1005.
180. Tyler KL, Sokol RJ, Oberhaus SM, et al: Detection of reovirus RNA in hepatobiliary tissues from patients with extrahepatic biliary atresia and choledochal cysts. Hepatology 1998;27:1475.
181. Tzakis AG, Reyes J, Tepetes K, et al: Liver transplantation for Alagille's syndrome. Arch Surg 1993;128:337.
182. Uchida K, Urata H, Suzuki H, et al: Predicting factor of quality of life in long-term jaundice-free survivors after the Kasai operation. J Pediatr Surg 2004;39:1040.
183. Vacanti JP, Shamberger RC, Eraklis A, Lillehei CW: The therapy of biliary atresia combining the Kasai portoenterostomy with liver transplantation: A single center experience. J Pediatr Surg 1990;25:149.
184. van Heurn LW, Saing H, Tam PK: Portoenterostomy for biliary atresia: Long-term survival and prognosis after esophageal variceal bleeding. J Pediatr Surg 2004;39:6.
185. Vazquez-Estevez J, Stewart B, Shikes RH, et al: Biliary atresia: Early determination of prognosis. J Pediatr Surg 1989;24:48, discussion 50.
186. Vennarecci G, Gunson BK, Ismail T, et al: Transplantation for end stage liver disease related to alpha 1 antitrypsin. Transplantation 1996;61:1488.
187. Weber TR, Grosfeld JL, Fitzgerald JF: Prognostic determinants after hepatoportoenterostomy for biliary atresia. Am J Surg 1981;141:57.
188. Whitington PF, Black DD: Cholelithiasis in premature infants treated with parenteral nutrition and furosemide. J Pediatr 1980;97:647.
189. Wiesner RH, McDiarmid SV, Kamath PS, et al: MELD and PELD: Application of survival models to liver allocation. Liver Transpl 2001;7:567.
190. Williams LF, Dooling JA: Thoracic duct–esophagus anastomosis for relief of congenital biliary atresia. Surg Forum 1963;14:189.
191. Wood RP, Langnas AN, Stratta RJ, et al: Optimal therapy for patients with biliary atresia: Portoenterostomy ("Kasai" procedures) versus primary transplantation. J Pediatr Surg 1990;25:153, discussion 160.
192. Wright K, Christie DL: Use of gamma-glutamyl transpeptidase in the diagnosis of biliary atresia. Am J Dis Child 1981;135:134.
193. Yano H, Matsumoto H: Choledochal cyst following operation for idiopathic perforation of the biliary tract in childhood. Jpn J Surg 1983;13:441.
194. Yoshida S, Nio M, Hayashi Y, et al: Serum insulinlike growth factor-I in biliary atresia. J Pediatr Surg 2003;38:211.

第 104 章

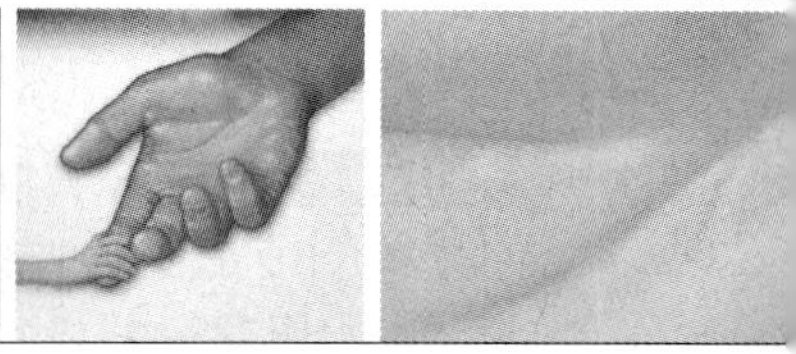

胆总管囊肿

James A. O'Neill, Jr.

620 1723 年 Vater 出版了一本专著，书中阐述了关于胆道系统正常和异常解剖的一系列研究成果，包括首次描述了 1 例胆总管梭形扩张的病例[91]。1852 年，Douglas 发表文章首次在临床上描述了一例胆总管扩张的患儿，他提出胆总管扩张可能是先天性的[14]。之后，胆总管囊肿偶有报道，直到 1959 年 Alonso-Lej 及其同事首次发表了对胆总管囊肿患儿进行回顾的成果，他们报道了自己的 2 例病例并回顾了 94 例之前文献中报道的病例[1]。该篇标志性的论文首次描述了胆总管囊肿的分类，包括 3 种常见类型及它们不同的手术处理方式。这篇文章的发表使得随后对该种畸形的病理生理学有了更好的理解，最终导致了新的治疗方法的产生。

解剖学分类

Alonso-Lej 及其同事首次将胆总管囊肿分为Ⅰ、Ⅱ和Ⅲ型[1]。之后，Todani 和其同事及其他研究者进一步根据胆道造影的分析将该种畸形分成 5 个主要类型及其他亚型[83,85]。常见类型如下（图 104-1）：

Ⅰ型——肝外胆道囊性或弥漫性梭形扩张
Ⅱ型——肝外胆道憩室
Ⅲ型——胆总管囊肿（十二指肠壁内型）
Ⅳ型——肝内或肝外胆道多发囊肿（或肝内外均有）
Ⅴ型——单发或多发肝内胆道囊肿

我们及其他研究者均发现Ⅲ型和Ⅳ型有时并存。Ⅰ型的不常见变异型也已经被观察到（参见 104-1b 和 c），如孤立的胆囊管或单一的肝管扩张，以及胆囊管汇入胆总管囊肿或汇入肝外胆总管囊肿水平以上的正常肝管处。比如，White 和 Becker[95] 报道了一例成人患孤立的左肝管囊肿的病例，我和我的同事们遇到了一例儿童患孤立的右肝管囊肿的病例。单发或多发的肝内胆管囊肿被归为Ⅴ型，当伴有肝纤维化时也称为 Caroli 病，有时可以见到这种类型的囊肿在许多年以后相继产生[7]。90%～95% 的胆总管囊肿属于Ⅰ型，梭形或囊状，梭形更为常见[57]。在最常见的类型中，胆囊汇入胆总管囊肿，左右肝管及肝内胆管大小正常。在Ⅱ型憩室型中，整个肝内及肝外胆道有别于正常胆道。Ⅲ型胆总管囊肿常发生在十二指肠壁内，有时发生在胆道胰腺段。另外，胆管系统是正常的，胆总管通常在十二指肠壁内与囊肿交汇。在胆总管囊肿的病例中，胆总管和主胰管可以共同或独立地汇入囊肿，但是开口通常因为慢性炎症而狭窄。胆总管囊肿本身通过狭窄的开口与十二指肠肠腔相通（图 104-2）。Manning 及其同事回顾了 40 例胆总管囊肿的病例，描述了两种主要的解剖学变异类型[47]。其中胆总管和胰管分别汇入十二指肠内的胆总管囊肿更常见。在第二种类型中，胆总管囊肿呈憩室样在 Vater 乳头水平从胆总管壁突出，胰管在通常的部位汇入胆总管末端。我曾经全面地回顾了胆总管囊肿的其他变异类型[55]。

病理学

在我治疗的患儿中，肝外胆总管囊肿的组织学切片显示了一个致密结缔组织与平滑肌纤维交错排列的 1621
厚壁结构。在大多数病例中，可以见到一定程度的炎

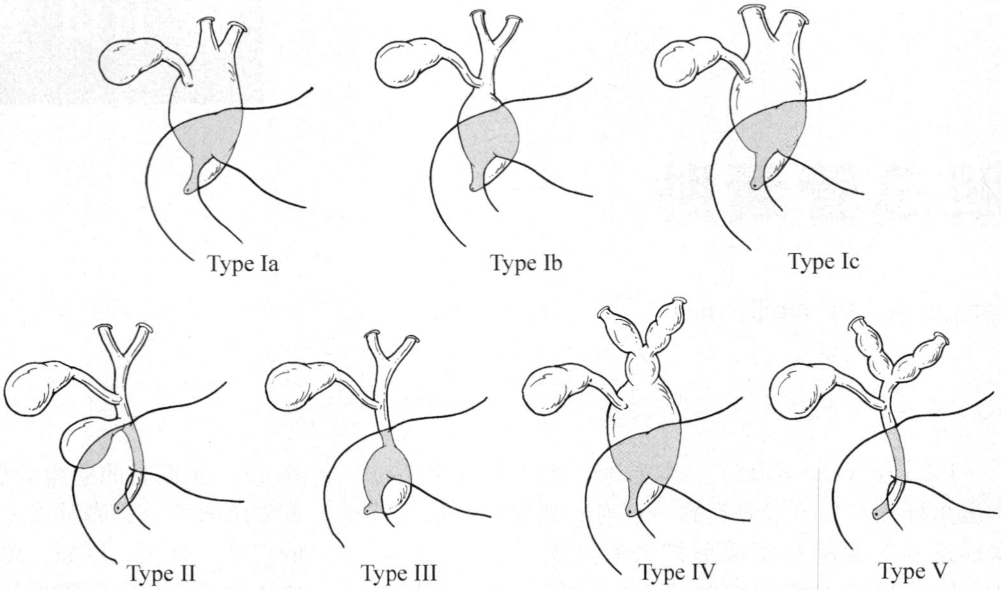

图 104-1　通过胆管造影显示 5 类主要的胆总管囊肿。通过术中胆管造影对解剖结构的细致描绘给外科治疗提供了方法。参见文中对解剖亚型的描述。

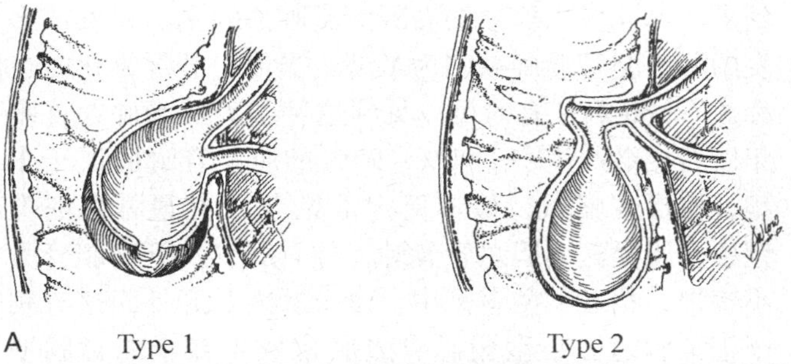

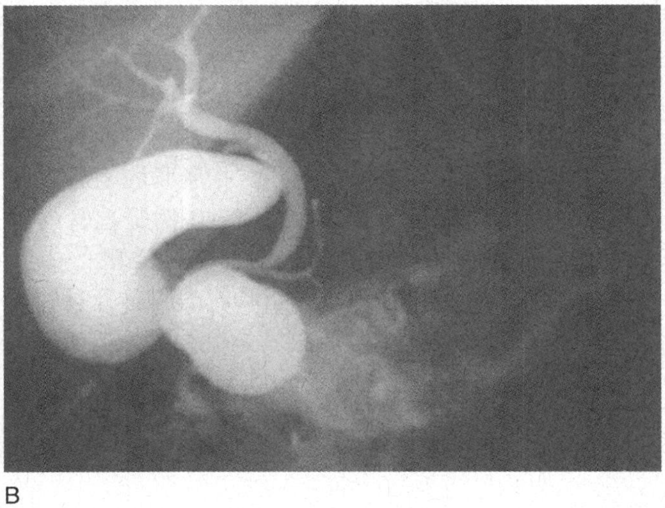

图 104-2　A. 两类经常遇到的十二指肠壁内型胆总管囊肿类型：Ⅰ型更常见。这些畸形最常见于十二指肠段，罕见情况下可见于胰腺头部。B. 6 岁男孩，术中通过胆囊行胆管造影显示十二指肠内的胆总管囊肿，囊肿部分梗阻，胰胆管连接异常，并可见正常的胆管系统。（A 引自 O'Neill JA：Curr Probl Surg 1992；29：374. 经作者允许）

症反应，尽管在婴儿中炎症反应最小，但随着年龄增长炎症反应会逐渐变得明显。此外，在超过 10 岁的患儿中，囊肿周围的炎症反应变得更加严重，与周围结构的粘连也变得更加明显；典型时仅仅可见到一个相对无细胞的囊肿内壁，而不是典型的胆道黏膜。在年龄小的患儿中，偶尔在囊肿壁可见柱状上皮岛及显微镜下胆管。当看到壁内腺体和管样结构，包括黏液分泌细胞、免疫反应性胃泌素及含生长激素抑制素的细胞时，说明胃肠道黏膜曾经遭到破坏并已再生[63]。患儿年龄越大，囊肿内壁越没有可能残留黏膜层。在肝内囊肿病例中，炎症反应通常更加显著。

除了Ⅲ型胆总管囊肿，其他类型胆总管囊肿的组织学表现相似。在这些病例中，囊肿内壁通常为十二指肠黏膜，偶尔内壁类似胆管黏膜。虽然胆道的组织学切片通常表现正常，但胆总管可见炎症反应、结石及泥沙，在年龄大的患儿中肝内胆管偶尔也可见到类似情况。

在远端，胆总管通常可见两种情况。大多数患病婴儿的胆道在十二指肠水平完全梗阻，这是胆道闭锁的一种类型。年龄较大患儿远端胆总管通常是开放的，Suda 及其同事曾经提出这些胆总管的狭窄段来自腹侧胰管[77]。在病因学部分中，将会提到胆总管和胰管的异常连接，表现为共同通道位于乳头外。在大多数胆总管囊肿患儿中存在异常的胰胆管连接。

肝活检结果随患儿年龄不同而不同。新生儿期肝的组织学表现通常为正常或有轻度胆管增生，伴有慢性胆道梗阻。在年龄较大患儿中，偶尔可以见到轻度的肝门周围纤维化。虽然我治疗的患儿在最初发现疾病时没有肝硬化，但 Ramirez 及其同事[65]和其他研究者曾经报道过先天性肝纤维化和胆总管囊肿并存。Landing 曾经提出了一个将胆总管囊肿、新生儿肝炎和胆道闭锁联系起来的新生儿梗阻性胆道疾病的概念。他指出在后来表现为胆总管囊肿的患儿中偶尔可以见到肝细胞巨细胞化[38]。此外，Landing 及其他研究者亦曾报道过胆总管囊肿可以发生在患有胆道闭锁的婴儿中[56]。除非患儿术后长期持续存在的胆管炎进展为胆汁性肝硬化，否则在我们治疗的胆总管囊肿患儿中，门脉高压不是一个重要的伴随特征，这种患儿也很少见。胆总管囊肿囊壁癌变已经得到了充分的认识，它是慢性炎症的结果。胆管癌也可发生在无胆总管囊肿但胰胆管连接异常的患者中[2,35,63]。胆总管囊肿壁癌变很少发生在儿童期，它是成人的一个主要问题。癌变的类型主要是腺鳞癌，偶尔为小细胞癌。尽管癌变大多数发生在胆总管囊肿壁，但其他发生部位包括胆囊和胰胆管连接的胰头处。由于这些病变进展似乎需要很长的间隔期，所以癌变被推测是由于胆管炎引起的慢性炎症所致。虽然慢性的轻微炎症可能导致胆总管和胰管狭窄，但炎症在Ⅲ型胆总管囊肿的患儿中似乎不是一个显著的特征。

病因学和胚胎学

由于多年来不断增加的认识，关于胆总管囊肿病因的理论已经发生了改变。最近准确的影像诊断技术的发展已经肯定了这些新增加的病因学理论。1852年，Douglas 推断常见的梭形畸形可能是胆总管的某些先天性缺陷[14]。1936 年，Yotsuyanagi 报道了采用当时已知的实验胚胎学知识分析 3 例患有胆总管囊肿患儿的情况。他提出缺陷的形成可能与原始胚胎发育期不适当的胆管形成有关[96]。他认为在胆总管区域发育实变期，上皮细胞的过度增殖可能导致再通过程后产生一个异常扩张的结构。而相似的理论已经被提出用于解释肠管特定区域的孤立性扩张，大多数研究者不接受 Yotsuyanagi 的假说。Alonso-Lej 及其同事们将病变归因于 Douglas 提出的先天性胆道发育缺陷理论。1973 年，Glenn 和 McSherry 对胆总管囊肿的病因学进行了回顾，并推断病因是先天性的[1,14,18]。他们推测先天性的缺陷可能是一种原发性缺陷或者是由胆总管内在结构畸形和胆管梗阻并存所致。从此，远端梗阻被认为至少是与胆总管囊肿病因相关的一个因素。1984 年，Todani 及其同事通过对内镜逆行胰胆管造影（ERCP）和其他胆管造影的研究，提出大多数患者具有胰胆管系统的排列异常，胰管汇入胆总管的部位恰好位于 Vater 壶腹环肌外，这样在胚胎发育期就使得含有胰蛋白酶的胰液向上反流进入胆总管，引起管壁破坏，进而出现扩张[81]。事实上我也在我们所有有胆道造影检查结果的患儿中注意到了这种异常的解剖排列（图 104-3）[55]。这种与胆总管囊肿病因

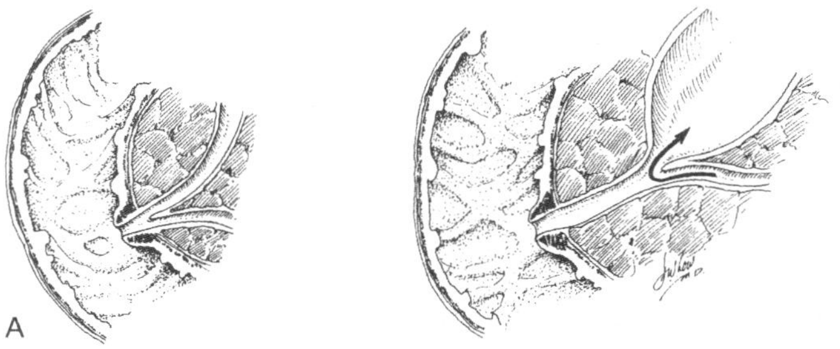

A

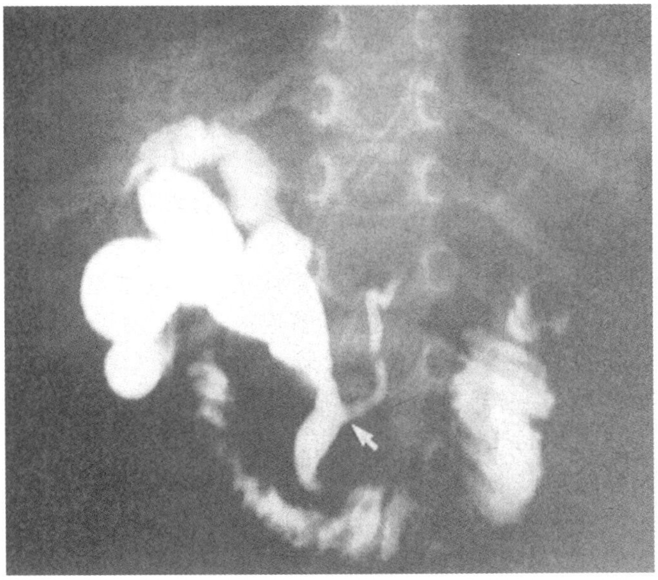

B

图 104-3　A. 正常解剖（左）与异常共同通道的解剖相对比（右，箭头），认为后者导致胰酶反流，引起宫内胆总管囊肿形成。B. 3 岁女孩术中胆管造影证实为典型的Ⅰ型梭形胆总管囊肿。可以看到胰管与胆总管连接部位较高（箭头），括约肌外的共同通道长，胰液容易反流入胆管系统。（引自 O' Neill JA：Choledochal cyst. Curr Probl Surg 1992；29：279. 经许可引用）

相关的“共同通道”理论在1969年首先被Babbitt提出[5]。Ito、Miyano、Spitz和其他研究者提出在十二指肠水平的胆道梗阻是疾病形成过程的一个附加因素，导致胆总管囊性扩张，这在多种实验准备中已经得到了证实[28,50,51,75]。如果将所有可供参考的研究考虑在内，那么有足够的证据支持胚胎时期的远端梗阻与胰胆管反流相结合引起了肝外胆道系统的变性扩张。Ito和其同事[28]以及其他研究者提出远端胆总管狭窄可能与胆总管异常插入十二指肠、先天性胆总管远端狭窄、上皮膜持续存在、瓣膜本身的畸形或括约肌神经肌肉运动失调有关。Ando及同事回顾了124例病例，他们注意到发生在胰胆管共同通道处的胆道连接异常在非胆总管囊肿的患者中偶尔可以见到[2]。在他们的研究中，有117例胆总管囊肿和7例不伴有胆总管扩张的胰胆管连接异常。因为这种连接异常可能发生于慢性反流和炎症的基础上，而且我们也已经注意到它与成人期胆道系统的癌变有很高的相关性，所以它可能不是一个良性状况。有趣的是，在Ando和其同事的研究中，所有患儿的症状均与黏膜栓引起的间歇性梗阻有关[3]。Rustad和Lilly[69]提出胰胆管连接异常仅仅是一种伴胆总管囊肿的结构畸形。但在我的经验中大量证据表明二者之间存在相关性。

显然这种常见的胆道结构畸形是先天性的，以下
1623 事实可以支持这个学说：胆总管囊肿在女性中占优势，表明这是与性别相关的畸形；亚洲人群比其他人群发病率更高。Jaunin-Stalder及其合作者报道了一对同卵双生双胞胎均患有胰胆管连接异常，然而也有同卵双生双胞胎之一患胰胆管连接异常的报道[30,54]。Wong和Lister曾经提出胰胆管连接异常是由于孕8周前胰胆管汇合进入十二指肠壁的迁移出现停顿所致[95]。在一篇高质量的胚胎学综述中，Li及其同事注意到Vater乳头远端异位有很高的发病率，它在先天性胆道扩张中作为一种梗阻因素起作用[40]。

关于其他类型的胆总管囊肿，如Ⅲ型胆总管囊肿和Caroli病，没有证据显示它们与常见的Ⅰ型病因相同。此外，Ⅱ型憩室型可能代表胆总管在产前破裂愈合后的终末期改变。已被提出的Ⅲ型胆总管囊肿的病因表明，它可能是由壶腹低位插入和壶腹梗阻导致的壶腹部和胆总管括约肌成分之间发生的一种单纯憩室，或者是在该区域发生的一种先天性十二指肠重复畸形。总而言之，两个最广为接受的病因是：(1)由于胰管先天性异常汇入胆总管，引起胰蛋白酶和其他胰酶反流进入近端胆管系统。该理论被Davenport和同事以及我和我同事的研究所支持。我们的研究显示先天性胆总管囊肿患者的胆汁中含有高水平的淀粉酶和其他胰酶。(2)完全或不完全的远端胆道梗阻[13,55,57]。任何程度的远端梗阻都会使胰酶反流进入近端胆道的机会增加。

产前诊断

产前超声诊断胎儿胆总管囊肿已经被许多研究者报道[25,44,45,48,57]。我的其中一位患者，母亲在孕17、18和27周采用超声随访，没有发现任何胎儿畸形，但是在孕31.5周，母亲超声显示胎儿肝脏下方有一个囊性包块，在孕37.5周观察到包块与轻微扩张的
肝内胆管相连（图104-4）。在其他作者发表的文章 16
中，有在孕15、19、20、25和37周通过母亲产前超声检查诊断出胆总管囊肿的报道[25,44,45,48,55]。在至少20个观察研究中发现胆总管囊肿在妊娠中期发生，这可能是由于时间的延长对于胰酶破坏胆道来说是必要的，尽管可能不是每个胎儿都对胰胆管反流敏感。

当产前发现胎儿患有胆总管囊肿时，关键问题是

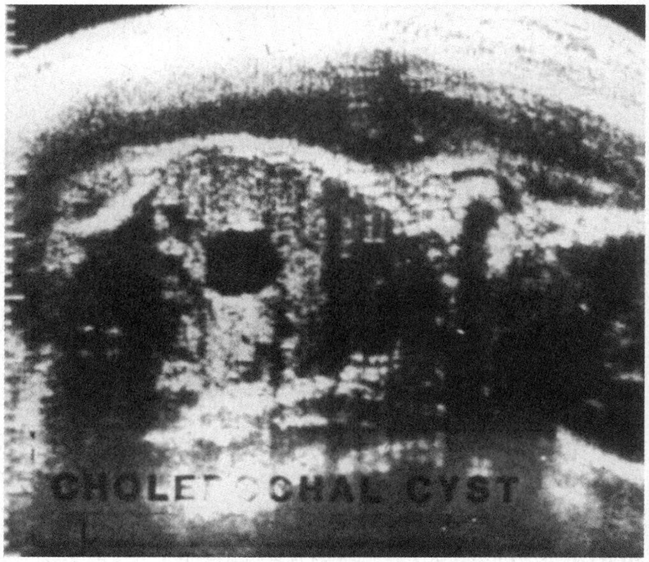

图104-4 孕31周母亲产前超声检查怀疑胆总管囊肿，之后得到证实。但是，产前超声应该作为一种筛查手段，因为它经常是不可靠的。该患者在出生后2周行囊肿切除术和内引流手术。

产前诊断后如何选择合适的手术干预时机。首先，应该意识到母亲超声检查仅仅是一种筛查研究，并不是非常可靠。Redkar 和其同事[66]以及 MacKenzie 和其同事[45]的研究显示母亲超声检查尽管很有帮助，但并不准确，也无法可靠地鉴别胎儿胆总管囊肿和其他胆道畸形。然而，当怀疑胆总管囊肿时，进行产后超声检查是必要的。一旦先前怀疑的胆总管囊肿在产后确诊，应当制订治疗方案。

Redkar 及其同事建议无症状的患儿最好在大约3个月时进行手术[66]。Suita 及其同事提出在出生后1个月内手术比1个月后手术的患儿肝纤维化发生率低，他们认为在出生后3个月内手术可能是理想的[79]。在一系列产前诊断胆总管囊肿的病例中，我和我的同事注意到除非是胆道完全梗阻，否则患有胆总管囊肿的新生儿大约在2周左右出现泥沙样结石，与黄疸出现的时间相对应。因此，我们倾向选择出生后2周内或2周左右进行纠治手术。Burnweit 和同事报道了6例出生前诊断的患儿，没有症状，平均在出生后6周左右进行手术，所有患儿均顺利康复[6]。Ohama 及同事报道了4例胆总管囊肿穿孔，并提出早期治疗可能会避免此类问题[58]。Lugo-Vicenti 提出对无症状无黄疸的患儿采用超声和血生化检查进行系列随访，在出生后大约6周行选择性的囊肿切除手术是比较合理的[44]。其他研究者亦同意此观点[60]。正如先前提到的，我不同意产前已做出诊断的患儿延迟手术时间是因为肝纤维化发生率高，有时甚至在出生时即可观察到肝纤维化，而采用手术是可以逆转的。此外还因为有囊肿增大及发生炎症、近端肝管狭窄形成、肝功能不全和穿孔等潜在并发症发生的可能。因此我和同事选择在大约2周时手术，此时婴儿通常病情稳定。

临床表现

胆总管囊肿患者的临床表现通常分为两种：婴儿型和成人型。除产前检查发现的患儿外，婴儿型的患儿在生后1~3个月通常表现为梗阻性黄疸、无胆汁粪便及肝大，临床表现与胆道闭锁很难鉴别[12]。有时，甚至在年龄小的患儿中也可以出现肝纤维化的表现，对于它的早期处理存在激烈的争论。婴儿型患儿不易发现腹痛及腹部包块。与胆道闭锁一样可能会有低热，但并没有胆管炎。产前检查已经诊断为胆总管囊肿的患儿通常在出生后1~3周出现黄疸。囊状和梭形胆总管囊肿通常在婴儿期都会出现黄疸，尽管梭形囊肿中黄疸可能是暂时性的。虽然一些人提倡如果检查胆汁分泌正常则在婴儿期保守治疗，仅在出现持续性或间歇性黄疸时，手术治疗是唯一的对策。我们不同意这种处理方式，因为以这种方式处理的患儿发生进行性肝纤维化的可能性很大。偶尔也可以发生囊肿穿孔[4]。目前，婴儿型和成人型胆总管囊肿发生率被认为是相等的。腹腔镜胆总管囊肿切除时代的到来为处理婴儿型胆总管囊肿提供了新的信息。

所谓成人型胆总管囊肿通常在2岁以后才出现明显症状，此类患儿通常有梭形胆总管囊性畸形，不伴有严重或完全的梗阻。偶尔可见成人型胆总管囊肿的典型三联征，即腹痛、触痛性肿块、黄疸，最先被 Alonso-Lej 和其同事所描述[1]。由于仅仅是部分胆道梗阻，所以症状通常是间歇性的。黏液栓和胆汁泥沙的形成伴有间歇性黄疸和右上腹偶尔是背部的非固定性疼痛。虽然肝大可以在成人型患儿中观察到，但与婴儿型胆总管囊肿相比不显著，因为婴儿型的胆道梗阻通常是完全性的。疼痛通常类似复发性胰腺炎的疼痛，经常可以检测到血清淀粉酶水平升高，尽管大多数人认为这种发作不是胰腺炎，但是具有异常的淀粉酶清除率。在许多患有胆总管囊肿的病例中，该病直到成年才被发现，可以表现为胆道症状和胆结石症状。这样导致了相当数量的此类患者行腹腔镜胆囊切除术，术中胆管造影摄片后发现存在胆总管囊肿（图104-5）。这样显得成人型胆总管囊肿的发生率高于婴儿型。我们已经见到很多在腹腔镜胆囊切除术和胆管造影摄片后发现胆总管囊肿而进行治疗的患者。复发性胆管炎可能是年龄较大患者的一个特征性的临床过程。但是，必须强调较大年龄患者的症状非常轻微并且是间断的，因此通常不容易做出诊断。肝损害是进行性的，所以有时此类患者发病最初表现为肝硬化 1625
和门脉高压。许多对这一课题感兴趣的研究者观察到年龄较大患者的临床症状几乎与胆道结石患者的症状一致。

胆总管囊肿并发胰腺炎问题应该特别提及。正如先前提到的，大多数血清淀粉酶浓度升高的患者清除率降低，但不是临床胰腺炎。另外，有一小部分患者表现为真正的胰腺炎，正像 Narasimhan[53]、Ando[3]、Sugiyama[78]及其同事阐述的，大多可能是蛋白栓堆积

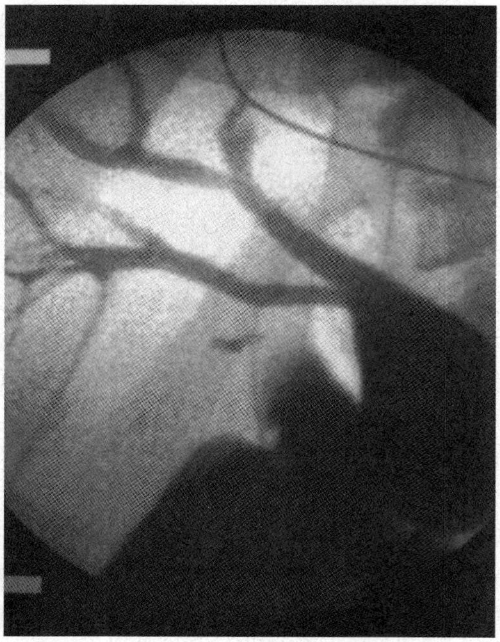

图 104-5　该图片显示一名 30 岁妇女因胆石症在术中进行胆管造影证实胆总管囊肿，行腹腔镜胆总管囊肿切除术。自从腹腔镜被应用以来，发现了更多类似的胆总管囊肿。

阻塞异常的胰胆管系统所致。在这些患者中胰胆管连接异常可能是首要的易感因素。胰腺分裂也偶尔会在一些患有胆总管囊肿的患者中观察到。这些患者仅很少一部分是病理性的，伴有可能与胰腺炎发生相关的区域梗阻。

诊断

实验室研究

实验室检查不可能确诊胆总管囊肿，但可以提示患者的临床状况。由于胆总管囊肿最常见的表现是黄疸，因此主要的实验室发现是结合胆红素升高，血清碱性磷酸酶及其他梗阻性黄疸的血清学标志物水平升高。尽管在年龄大的患者中黄疸是间歇性的和轻微的，但婴儿血清结合胆红素显著增高是一个规律。假如胆道梗阻表现已经持续了相当一段时间，患者甚至可能出现凝血异常。

影像学研究

无论是何种类型的解剖异常，一些影像学技术是确定诊断的关键。上消化道对比造影可以确诊十二指肠内的胆总管囊肿（壁内囊肿），但对其他类型的诊断不是很有用。CT 胆管造影曾经在确诊胆总管囊肿方面很有用，但现在已经被更准确的影像技术所取代。对于大多数胰胆管异常的患者而言，超声是最好的筛查手段，而所有婴儿均需要行超声检查。如果超声筛查怀疑胆总管囊肿，锝 99-DISIDA 闪烁扫描显像可以确诊，并可以提供胆汁引流、胆道梗阻和肝功能的一些信息。所有的 IDA 衍生物扫描中 DISIDA 可能是最好的，因为该试剂是亲脂性的，与其他同位素相比，与胆红素的结合更少，而且在新生儿期也容易开展[94]。超声作为筛查研究的其他好处在于它可以显示胰胆管口径的变化，也可以提供一些关于肝脏密度及肝纤维化状态的信息。

有创性影像学研究，如经皮肝穿刺胆管造影，被认为是年龄较大患者怀疑胆总管囊肿和肝内胆管囊肿时最好的诊断方法。年龄较大患者怀疑胰胆管畸形时，其他技术如 ERCP 有时很有帮助，它可以提供胰胆管连接异常发生率的信息[55,94]。它也可以提供数据，通过这些数据可以推动定义胰胆管畸形的构成标准[80]。ERCP 也可以确诊胰腺分裂畸形。最近几年，因为是无创性检查，磁共振胰胆管造影（MRCP）作为 ERCP 的替代检查已经较为普及[34,53]。现在行 MRCP 检查已经不需要屏气，该技术同样也已经在婴儿中得到应用[9]。其他同等的技术包括精细重建和仿真内镜 CT，该技术对于不伴有完全性胆道梗阻的大年龄患儿可能有帮助[70]。我们已经发现不需屏气的 MRCP 作为一种诊断胰胆管畸形的技术很有发展前景。无论是否用于术前诊断，都应该在术中行胆管造影，因为它可以提供最准确的解剖学信息。术中胆管造影可以通过胆囊或直接通过扩张的胆管进行，造影剂反流入肝内胆管系统对于诊断可能的胆管畸形或是否伴有近端胆管梗阻或肝内胆管囊肿很重要。

在随访期，腹部超声、DISIDA 闪烁扫描和 MRCP 都很有帮助，因为它们可以对比术前和术后胆管管径大小的变化，了解胆汁分泌率、胆汁淤积程度以及是否有胆结石或泥沙样结石存在。

尽管肝活检作为术前的诊断缺乏有效性，但术中肝活检对于确定是否存在肝硬化和达到何种程度很有帮助，并可以根据活检情况开展适当的随访。

在怀疑有胆总管囊肿的大年龄患儿中，鉴别诊断包括先天性肝纤维化、伴有肝纤维化的 Caroli 病、原发性硬化性胆管炎、先天性肝硬化、先天性肝总管或胆总管狭窄，所有这些疾病都可以通过结合前面提及的影像学检查来鉴别。

手术处理

多种手术治疗Ⅰ、Ⅱ和Ⅳ型胆总管囊肿的方法已经应用多年。过去，许多患者在出现症状时病情已相当严重，因此仅仅可采用有限的手术方式如抽吸术、开窗术和外引流术。Alonso-Lej 和其同事在 1959 年的报告中分析了当时采用的不同方法，他们指出单纯的外引流是不成功的，因为早已患病的患者在长期胆外瘘存在的情况下不能生存[1]。此外，其他形式的胆道外引流如胆囊造口、囊肿置管引流或切除囊肿后肝管引流的方法被尝试，但是由于高死亡率而被禁止使用。因此更多可靠的手术方法被提出。

1924 年，McWhorter 发表了通过肝总管十二指肠吻合术切除胆总管囊肿的第一篇报告[46]。在当时这种手术被认为是有技术难度的，确实，在 1960 年以前报道的与囊肿切除相关的死亡率为 30%。1933 年，Gross 发表了一篇文献综述，并加入了自己治疗的两个病例，他断定胆总管囊肿十二指肠吻合是一种安全有效的手术方法，并且死亡率低，所以许多年来他都继续倡导这种方法（图 104-6）。1965 年，Fonkalsrud 和 Boles 证实了囊肿十二指肠吻合的技术优点和低死亡率，因此不切除囊肿的内引流技术变成了首选的手术方法[16]。不幸的是在行囊肿十二指肠吻合术患者的长期随访中发现，15 年随访期间并发症的患病率为 30%~50%，这与远期死亡率有关[1,56]。行该手术的患者随访期越长，并发症发生的数量越多[56]。其中尤为重要的是观察到慢性复发性胆管炎，这可能与十二指肠液反流入胆道引起慢性炎症和吻合口狭窄有关，它的特点是症状轻微以至于没有诊断证据，导致隐匿性地发展为严重的胆汁性肝硬化和门脉高压。在大多数行此类手术的病例中，肝硬化的临床症状直到术后 5 年才表现出来。

上述原因最终导致 Roux-en-Y 囊肿空肠吻合术作为一种避免囊肿十二指肠吻合术后十二指肠内容物反流入胆道的替代术而产生（见图 104-6）。在 20 世纪 70 年代，许多报告表明倾向于选择 Roux-en-Y 囊

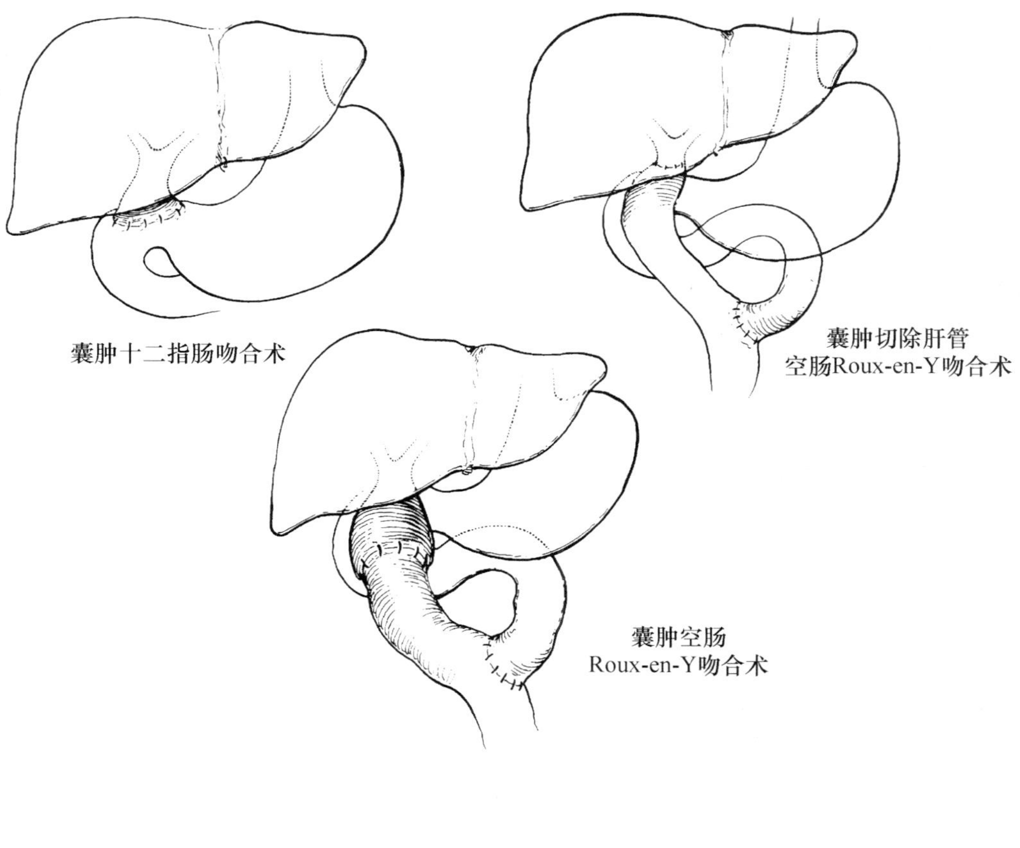

图 104-6 术中胆总管囊肿的不同处理方式。囊肿切除肝管空肠 Roux-en-Y 吻合术式为首选。

肿空肠吻合术[72]。尽管并发症发生率明显减少，但行囊肿空肠吻合的患儿仍然偶尔可以发生胆管炎，并出现与囊肿十二指肠吻合术患者相似的问题。Spitz 和 O' Neill 报道超过三分之二的行此类手术患者具有良好的远期随访结果[57,74]。然而这种手术的一个主要缺点是保留囊肿的患者有癌变的远期危险。尽管全囊肿切除被认为是理想的手术，但由于相关的死亡率过高，所以先前提及的早期死亡率和发病率低的引流手术被推荐为首选。

由于 20 世纪 70 年代早期术前术后监护水平开始提高，所以囊肿切除术开始被重新考虑。1970 年，Kasai 和其同事[32]及 Ishida 和其同事[27]报道了囊肿切除和 Roux-en-Y 空肠吻合术具有良好的结果，这使得世界其他医疗中心再次引入这种手术。根据我的经验，在所有婴儿型胆总管囊肿的患者和几乎所有成人型患者中都可以进行全囊肿切除（图 104-7）。对于许多患者，尤其是较大年龄患有反复发作的胆管炎的患者及伴有囊肿周围炎症和周围血管结构粘连的患者，采用最初被 Lilly 报道的手术方法很有用[41,42]。该手术在囊肿壁内外层之间进行平面解剖完成囊肿切除，内外层囊肿壁分离起始于胆总管与胆囊管汇合处，以胆囊管作为正确解剖层次的指导（图 104-8）。此外，在解剖前外侧囊肿壁时可以在中部打开囊肿，在直视下决定解剖平面。与门静脉和肝动脉粘连的部分囊肿壁被保留，如图 104-8D 所示。囊肿切除后，应该探查肝内胆管并用盐水冲洗去除泥沙及可能的胆道结石。此外，偶尔可以发现近端胆道梗阻，近端胆道系统可以是扩张的。我甚至遇到过主肝管中的一支为膜状完全性梗阻的病例。因此我倾向于选择 Roux-en-Y 肝管空肠吻合术，在大年龄患儿中采用 40 cm 的 Roux 肠袢，婴儿采用 30 cm 的肠袢，这是因为考虑到肠袢会随时间而增长。这样的长度似乎对预防反流很有效。Todani 和其同事倾向于在囊肿切除术后进行 Roux-en-Y 肝门十二指肠吻合术[82]。Gonzalez 和其同事[19]曾经提出将 30 cm 长的单独的近端空肠肠管置 162
于肝管汇合处和十二指肠第二段之间，而 Raffensperger[64]建议采用带瓣的空肠间置肝管十二指肠吻合术。随访研究表明 Roux-en-Y 肝管空肠吻合术是首选的手术方式，但没有足够的关于其他手术方式的随访研究。有证据显示，被 Raffensperger 及其他人推荐的乳头瓣手术方式随时间推移而被淘汰[51]。我和其他作者认为乳头瓣的构建使手术更加复杂，对Ⅰ、Ⅱ、Ⅳ型胆总管囊肿患者而言，这种手术方式并没有显示出比标准的 Roux-en-Y 肝管空肠吻合术更好的结果[51,55]。

对Ⅰ型和Ⅳ型胆总管囊肿患者行囊肿切除和 Roux-en-Y 空肠吻合术时，术中胆管造影偶尔会发现 162
有副胆管存在。Narasimhan 和其同事曾经报告了与单纯结扎副胆管相关的不良结果，因此他们提出将副胆管和胆管一同与肠管吻合[53]。Ming 及其同事报道了一项有 234 例患者的研究，在研究中他们采用了囊肿切除术，并将一短段带有裂隙样瓣的空肠间置，与十二指肠降部端侧吻合，或将阑尾作为间置物与十二指肠降部端侧吻合[49]。他们指出这两种手术方法都出现了我们不希望发生的较高的胆道狭窄发病率以及其他复杂问题。Hay 和其同事[23]、Li 等人[40]及 Liu 和其同事[43]曾经报告并讨论了腹腔镜技术在处理黄疸和胆总管囊肿患者时所起的作用。Liu 和其同事描述

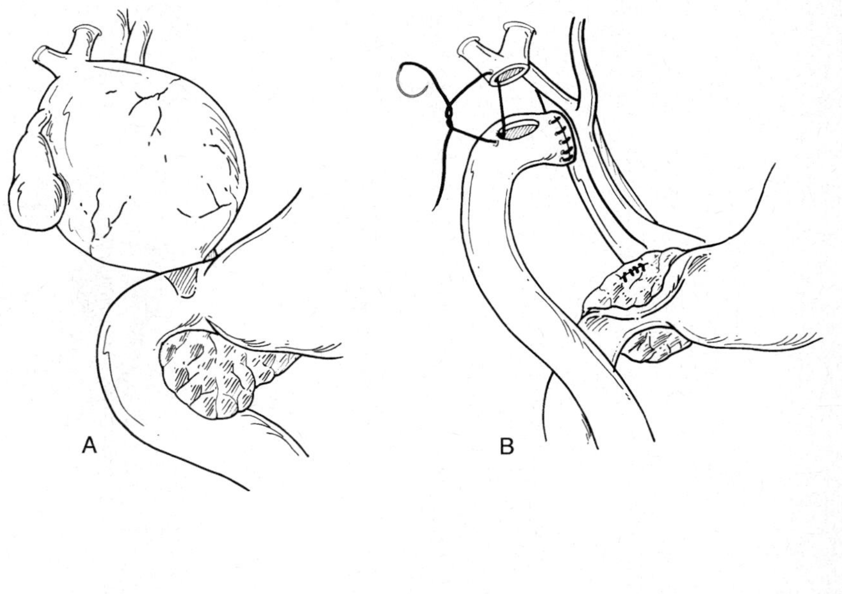

图 104-7 囊肿完全切除。A. 囊肿完全切除 Roux-en-Y 胆道重建术（B）。解剖图例显示 Roux 肠袢端或侧壁用于吻合。

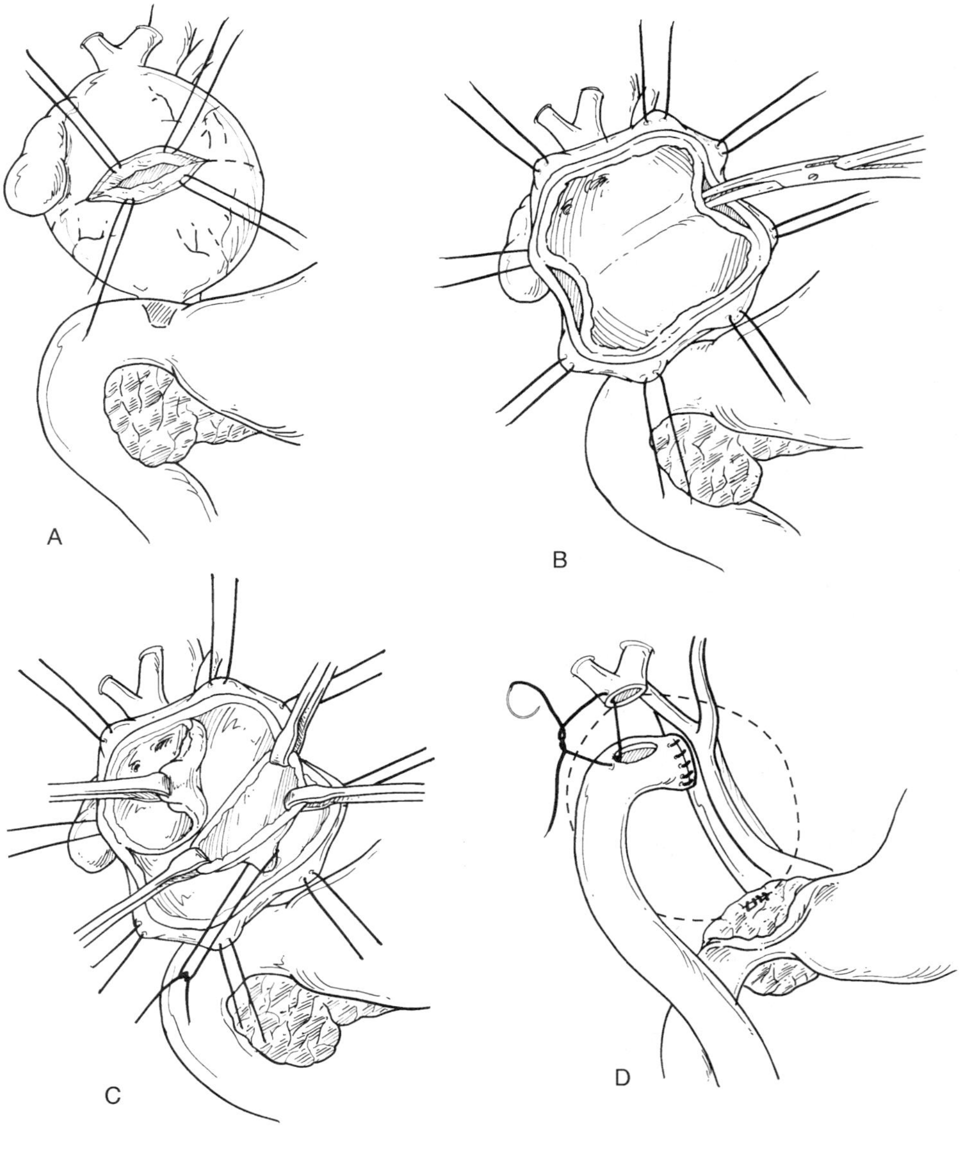

图 104-8 胆总管囊肿壁内切除 Lilly 术式步骤。A. 做横切口延至囊肿整个前壁中部和侧壁。B. 囊肿的后壁外层被完整地保留。在前壁切口一端剩余的后方囊肿壁任意选择一个解剖平面，切开后将囊肿壁分离为薄外层和厚内层。利用小弯止血钳在此平面解剖分离直至到达另一端切缘。横断完成后，后壁内层被完全分离。C. 通过钝性切割游离胆总管囊肿。断面继续向近端和远端游离，该处胆总管与门静脉和肝动脉粘连。D. Roux-en-Y 胆总管空肠端侧吻合完成手术。远端胆总管被尽可能切开至十二指肠下方胰腺段水平，然后缝合结扎关闭。虚线表示原先胆总管囊肿的位置。（修改后引自 O'Neill JA：Choledochal cyst. Curr Probl Surg 1992；29：398. 经许可引用）

了一例通过腹腔镜切除和胆管关闭治疗Ⅱ型憩室型囊肿的病例。但微创技术是否可以应用于范围更广的胆总管囊肿畸形患者仍然有待观察。至少目前标准的开放手术是首选。另外，我们有理由相信机器人技术提供了微创外科的其他途径，也许对治疗是有用的。

因为Ⅲ型胆总管囊肿（壁内囊肿）临床症状的特点是间歇性腹痛，不具有特异性，所以胆总管囊肿（壁内囊肿）的患者通常在至少 5 岁时才被确诊。通过上腹部横切口进行标准的胆道探查同样适用于胆总管囊肿的患者。一旦打开十二指肠侧腹膜，我选择纵向切开十二指肠，这样可以完整地暴露十二指肠内的胆总管囊肿。一旦胆总管囊肿完整地显露出来，很容易看到囊肿表面一引流胆汁的小孔。胆管造影应该通过胆囊或在囊肿开口处置一个小导管进行（见图 104-2B）。应该从囊肿的小孔处开始将囊腔去顶，然后用可吸收线间断地重新缝合黏膜。重要的是鉴别和标定胆总管和胰管的汇入点，以便决定是否需要进行胆总管和胰管的括约肌成形术。通常由于轻微的慢性炎症，胆总管开口处狭窄，所以许多病例都需要进行胆总管开口括约肌成形术。罕见胆总管囊肿位于胰头部，有时伴有胰腺炎，部分病例不能通畅引流进入十二指肠。如果没有替代的内引流手术，对于这些罕见病例通常需要进行胰管十二指肠切除术。

患有肝内胆管囊肿或 Caroli 病的患者很难处理，因为他们趋向于发展成严重的复发性胆管炎，之后发展为胆汁性肝硬化和进行性的节段性胆管扩张。因此，这些患者经常需要通过超声随访许多年。许多手术方法可以用于治疗肝内胆管囊肿。当病变是局部的并可以切除时，行部分肝叶切除术，但当近端胆管梗阻时可能需要行囊肿去顶，然后将胆汁引流至空肠 Roux 支[52]。

进行囊肿切除内引流的患者比胆道闭锁进行相似引流手术的患者术后胆管炎的发病率低。虽然胆道闭锁患者通常持续应用大剂量抗生素一段时间，但胆总管囊肿患者没有必要这样做。连续 6 周保护性地应用低剂量的氨苄西林或复方磺胺甲唑抗胆管炎是我的常规做法，这样可降低胆管炎并发症的发生率。

术后第一年应该每 3 个月随访一次，之后对于无症状的患者每年随访一次。每次随访都应该检测肝功能和血清淀粉酶水平，每年一次或当患者出现症状时做肝脏和胰腺超声检查。对于术前发现肝内胆管扩张的患者，肝脏超声检查相当重要。由于患者有时会出现晚期吻合口狭窄或结石，所以超声检查也有助于对 Roux-en-Y 吻合手术进行长期评估。

手术效果、随访和并发症

我和同事的研究中包含 46 例患者的随访数据，其中 37 例为女性。约一半左右的患者在新生儿期到 9 个月时出现症状，另一半在 2～32 岁出现症状。婴儿型患者临床表现的特点是接近完全或完全性的胆道梗阻，而成人型患者有多种不同的表现，包括腹痛、腹部触痛性包块和黄疸。2 例患者行囊肿十二指肠吻合术后，均重新行囊肿切除术和肝管空肠 Roux-en-Y 吻合术，平均随访 18 年，效果良好。6 例行囊肿空肠吻合术，其中 3 例再次手术，1 例是由于吻合口狭窄和胆管炎重新手术，而另外 2 例是由于囊肿恶变的远期风险再次手术。所有 6 例患者包括未行再次手术的患者目前状况均良好，平均随访 15 年。我们目前建议对所有这些患者都应行二期囊肿切除术。33 例患者行一期囊肿切除，5 例患者行二期手术囊肿切除，平均随访 10 年，所有患者情况都良好。3 例行单纯囊肿肠吻合术的患者有不同程度的胆汁性肝硬化和轻度门脉高压，需要仔细关注，但目前为止尚没有人需要肝移植治疗。1 例患 Caroli 病的肝内胆管囊肿的患者 15 年前行左肝叶切除术，另 1 例 12 年前行右肝囊肿空肠 Roux 支吻合内引流术，目前健康状况均良好。对这两名患者进行了预期肝内胆管囊肿再发的随访。3 名患者为胆总管囊肿（壁内囊肿）：2 例行十二指肠内胆总管囊肿切除及括约肌成形术，另 1 例将胰腺内胆总管囊肿内引流入十二指肠。所有 3 名患者平均随访 8 年，情况均良好。迄今为止，我们的患者中有 1 例行囊肿切除和内引流术后因吻合口狭窄和肝内胆管结石而再次进行治疗。自从再次吻合手术之后，该患者的状况良好。没有一个患者因保留囊肿壁或囊肿切除后的少量囊肿残余而发生恶变，但是长期的潜在风险可能存在，尤其是那些保留囊肿的患者。文献中的证据不仅支持行一期囊肿切除，而且支持对先前行单纯囊肿肠吻合的患者行二期囊肿切除术[76,84,89]。内引流术的类型可能对结果并不产生实质性的影响，但单纯的 Roux-en-Y 肝管空肠吻合手术与其他更复杂的手术一样有效，这就是为什么它应该被首先选用。

许多其他研究者的长期随访研究被发表。Saing 及其同事发表了他们 20 多年对大量病例进行随访研究的结果，由于有时甚至是在术后 17 年会发生晚期并发症，所以他们强调了长期随访的重要性[71]。研究中的主要问题是吻合口狭窄、胆管炎和肝内结石的形成。他们也承认有癌变的风险，但通过囊肿切除可以明显减少。此外，他们提出在最初的手术中可能出现膜样狭窄，这表明胆管造影和胆道探查冲洗残渣的重要性，尤其是对肝内胆管扩张的患者。我和我的同事也做了同样的观察，认为如果没有胆管或肝管空肠吻合口狭窄，即使将来有结石发生，这些结石也可以通过胆道排出。Tsuchida 和同事对 103 例患者平均随访了 12.5 年，观察到结石产生在术后 3～22 年的任何时间段[88]。他们观察到以下有趣的现象：（1）在 50 例最初没有肝内胆管扩张的患者中，仅有 1 例术后发生肝内结石；（2）在 43 例被诊断为肝内胆管扩张但没有下游胆管狭窄的患者中，1 例患者术后发生肝内结石；（3）在 10 例有肝内胆管扩张同时下游胆管有不同程度梗阻的患者中，4 例术后发生肝内结石。所有患者在最初均未观察到结石。术后结石形成的现象首先被 Tsuchida 等提出。Uno 和同事在对一期囊肿切除术后远期发生肝内结石的研究中注意到，每一例远期结石形成的患者总是之前存在胆管狭窄；他们也观察到结石容易产生在患 Caroli 病的患者中，这些患者通常有不同程度的相关胆管梗阻[90]。Cetta 提供的数据显示了同样的结果，由于胆管狭窄引起胆汁淤积，导致肝内结石的形成，这在发病机制中起重要作用[8]。Miyano 领导的小组报告了 180 例胆总管囊肿 30 年的治疗经验，他们的数据得出了同样的结论[51]。Okada 研究组中的 Hasegawa 测量了胆总管囊肿术后长期随访患者的血清总胆汁酸水平，显示总胆酸水平升高，这提示有不同程度的胆汁淤积，胆汁酸在半数以上的患者中持续升高，尤其容易发生在小年龄最初有严重胆汁淤积和肝纤维化的患者中[22]。他们得出结论认为一旦出现这些情况就容易发生肝内胆管结石。Okada 做了其他观察，他选择 Roux-en-Y 肝管空肠吻合术而不是空肠间置肝管十二指肠吻合术，因为即使后一种手术方式理论上很有吸引力，但在他的病例研究中显示该手术后经常发生胆汁反流性胃炎，以致他放弃了后一种手术方式[62]。Chijiiwa 和 Tanaka 回顾了 28 例长期随访 1～18 年行囊肿切除和肝管空肠吻合术的患者[11]。所有患者均存活，没有发生恶变。其中 3 例发生肝内胆管结石，但被认为与胆管炎而非吻合口狭窄相关。建议长期随访以避免并发症的发生。对于保留囊肿的患者，在 Rush 及同事、Katyal 和 Lees 以及 Chijiiwa 和 Koga 各自的报道中，并发症的发生率均超过 90%，包括胆管炎、胆总管结石和肝内结石[10,33,68]。大多数患者需要再次手术，而行囊肿切除术和内引流手术的患者长期预后都很好。远期肝内结石形成的可能机制目前已得到认可，大量证据表明结石发生的基础是肝管空肠吻合口或近端胆管水平的狭窄引起的胆汁淤积。在一项历时 25 年、对切除治疗胆总管囊肿进行的回顾性研究中，Todani 和其同事报道了 10 例由于复发性胆管炎伴有肝内结石再次手术的病例[86]。10 例中的 9 例吻合口在胆总管水平，1 例在肝管分叉水平，但 10 例中都存在胆管狭窄，这导致了结石的产生。这个研究表明胆道并发症可能发生在囊肿切除后吻合口狭窄的患者或原发性胆管狭窄的患者中，因此他们提出在肝门水平创建宽大的吻合口。

Miyano 和其助手有 30 年的临床经验，他们对 30 年间通过囊肿切除和肝管空肠吻合治疗的 180 例病例进行了回顾，这些数据提供了关于并发症发生率的信息[51]。他们对 171 例患者平均观察了 11 年，对其均行常规肝管肠吻合术，其中 4 例发生了胆管炎和肝内结石。这些并发症并没有发生在手术时年龄小于 5 岁的患儿中。由于这些患者中一些人存在肝内胆管狭窄，所以他们也提倡在切除囊肿时行术中囊肿内镜检查。他们认为大多数患者可以通过传统的肝总管引流得到治疗，仅有很少一部分患者需要更高水平的吻合。但 Todani 和他的小组不同意该观点，他们认为在左右肝管分叉水平做一个宽敞的吻合口很重要，因为这样可以在囊肿切除后使胆汁引流通畅无阻[86]。

Okada 和其同事根据他们丰富的经验对治疗胆总管囊肿的技术细节[61]提出了建议[62]。他们强调假如没有发生左右肝管狭窄，则胆总管水平的吻合是足够的，我同意此观点。我也同意仔细探查及胆管造影以避免遗留胆管狭窄就足够了。Okada 和同事也强调在十二指肠下方进入胰腺头部处彻底切除远端胆总管囊肿，但是我认为在胰腺头部广泛解剖是没有必要的。

到目前为止，已经有许多保留囊肿壁的病例发生恶变的报道[11,15,35,67,83]。理论上，假如慢性炎症减轻[92]，那么完全或囊肿壁内的切除就可以预防囊肿壁的恶变。否则，可能由于不同程度甚至是广泛的囊 1631
肿切除后遗留小的囊壁残留导致恶变发生。Kobayashi 和同事讨论了胰胆管连接异常包括胆总管囊肿患者行肝外胆道切除后胆管癌发生的风险。他们提出存在任何程度的慢性炎症和胆汁淤积，都有相当高的胆囊和近端胆道癌变的风险，且比正常人群发病年龄早。然而毫无疑问，先前已行囊肿肠吻合术同时保留囊肿的患者具有最大的癌变风险。Tsuchiya 及其同事报道了 13 例之前行囊肿肠吻合的病例，3 例囊肿发生腺癌，另有 1 例胆囊发生腺癌[89]。20% 的癌变率与 Rossi 及其同事报道的相同[67]。这些病例报告提出了对之前行囊肿内引流手术的患者是否应该行选择性囊肿切除的问题。我选择采用实用性的方法，如果能够证明行囊肿内引流术的患者没有慢性复发性胆管炎或其他慢性炎症的表现，那么可以对他们继续观察而不采取干预措施。我曾经建议仅将选择性的囊肿切除用于复发性胆管炎的患者，在这些情况下可以采用壁内切除的技术。随着保留囊肿晚期发生癌变病例报告的积累[31]和对病因学更好的认识，我开始对无症状的保留囊肿切除采取更积极的态度。但是二期囊肿切除可能更复杂。尽管我曾经仅遇到过一例囊肿完全切除术后发生复发性胆管炎的病例，但长期随访表明应该如 Ohi 和其同事建议的那样[59]仔细检查，以便发现肝管空肠吻合术后吻合口的狭窄或肝内囊肿感染。迄今，我们的患者中没有一例发生恶变，但可能与他们的年龄仍不够大有关。

据推测，慢性炎症是胆总管囊肿壁或胆管系统发生癌变的基本原因，但在囊肿完全切除的患者中则不同。Imazu 和其同事最近报道了关于胆总管囊肿癌变的相关因素[26]。他们报道患有梭形囊肿的患者胆囊黏膜过度增生，胆汁淀粉酶水平较高，并且与淀粉酶水平低的患者相比其 Oddi 括约肌和十二指肠之间具有更大的压力差。他们报道了一例 12 岁患囊状胆总管囊肿的儿童发生腺癌的病例。该患者胆汁淀粉酶水平高，这表明胰胆管连接部畸形伴有胰液慢性反流入胆管系统是癌变的基础病因。Iwai 和同事[29]报道了由于 Oddi 括约肌功能缺乏导致的胰液反流引起胆管壁多种组织学损害，这可能导致胆管恶变的发生。Todani 和其同事提出了同样的观点。Tokiwa 和 Iwai 也报道了胰胆管排列异常患者胆囊的早期黏膜改变[87]。Shimotake 和同事提供的数据显示，胰胆管连接异常的患者的癌变与伴随多基因逐级突变事件的慢性炎症所导致的 DNA 改变有关[73]。他们研究胰胆管连接异常儿童胆管上皮的基因突变，发现 *KRAS* 基因突变发生在早期上皮过度增生或化生时，而 *DPC4* 基因失活发生在胆道癌变进展晚期。Pushiparani 和 Redkar 及其同事进行了相似的研究[63,66]。Hahn 和同事也报道了 *DPC4/SMAD4* 基因在胆道腺癌中发生突变[21]。Fumino 和同事[17]、Hayashi 和同事[24]报道环氧合酶–2 表达的增强与胰胆管连接异常患者的胆囊黏膜过度增生有关，此外，与正常胆管上皮细胞相比，胆管肿瘤的环氧合酶–2 表达上调。因此提示采用环氧合酶–2 抑制剂可能是在易感个体中防止晚期胆管癌发生的一种方法。

最后，很少的患者在囊肿切除术和 Roux–en–Y 空肠吻合术后可能发生胰腺炎，尽管我没有遇到过这种并发症。Komuro 和其同事对 62 名胆总管囊肿患者随访观察多年，患者包括了所有年龄组[36]。由蛋白栓形成引起的急性胰腺炎在超过 20% 的随访患者中被观察到。他们的研究表明，术前有胰腺问题的患者术后胰腺方面的并发症得不到解决，括约肌成形术在预防残余胆管出现复发性蛋白栓方面无效。但是他们认为早期诊断和完整切除降低了复发性胰腺炎的发生率。Koshinaga 和 Fukuzawa 提出胰液长期滞留可能导致胰管形态学改变和胰管扩张，这些可能与胆总管囊肿患者术后胰腺炎的发生有关[37]。总之，胰腺炎是囊肿切除和内引流术后的一个少见并发症。

（周　莹译　吴晔明校）

参考文献

1. Alonso-Lej F, Revor WB, Pessagno DJ: Congenital choledochal cyst, with a report of 2, and an analysis of 94 cases. Surg Gynecol Obstet Int Abstr Surg 1959;108:1-30.
2. Ando H, Ito T, Nagaya M, et al: Pancreaticobiliary maljunction without choledochal cyst in infants and children: Clinical features and surgical therapy. J Pediatr Surg 1995;30:1658-1662.
3. Ando H, Kaneko K, Ito F, et al: Surgical removal of protein plugs complicating choledochal cysts: Primary repair after adequate opening of the pancreatic duct. J Pediatr Surg 1998;33:1265-1267.
4. Ando K, Miyano T, Kohno S, et al: Spontaneous perforation of choledochal cyst: A study of thirteen cases. Eur J Pediatr Surg 1998;8:23-25.
5. Babbitt DP: Congenital choledochal cyst: New etiological concept based on anomalous relationships of common bile duct and pancreatic bulb. Ann Radiol 1969;12: 231-240.
6. Burnweit CA, Birken JA, Heiss K: The management of choledochal cyst in the newborn. Pediatr Surg Int 1996; 11:130-133.
7. Caroli J, Soupalt R, Kossakowski J, et al: La dilatation polykystique congenitale des voies biliaires intrahepatiques: Essai de classification. Semin Hop Paris 1958;34:488-495.
8. Cetta F: Biostasis due to bile duct stricture precedes, not follows, the formation of primary intrahepatic stones and plays a basic role in their pathogenesis. Am J Gastroenterol 1996;91:2451-2452.
9. Chen JH, Chai JW, Chu WC, et al: Free breathing cholangiopancreatography (MRCP) at end expiration: A new technique to expand clinical application. Hepatogastroenterology 2002;49:593-596.
10. Chijiiwa K, Koga A: Surgical management and long-term follow-up of patients with choledochal cyst. Am J Surg 1993:165:238-242.
11. Chijiiwa K, Tanaka M: Late complications after excisional operation in patients with choledochal cyst. J Am Coll Surg 1994;179:139-144.
12. Davenport M, Betalli P, D'Antiga L, et al: The spectrum of surgical jaundice in infancy. J Pediatr Surg 2003;38: 1471-1479.
13. Davenport M, Stringer MD, Howard ER: Biliary amylase and congenital choledochal dilatation. J Pediatr Surg 1995;30:474-477.
14. Douglas AH: Case of dilatation of the common bile duct. Monthly J Med Sci (Lond) 1852;14:97.
15. Fieber SS, Nance FC: Choledochal cyst and neoplasm: A comprehensive review of 106 cases and presentation of two original cases. Am Surg 1997;63:982-987.
16. Fonkalsrud EW, Boles ET: Choledochal cysts in infancy and childhood. Surg Gynecol Obstet 1965;121:733-742.
17. Fumino S, Takewa K, Ono S, Iwai N: Cyclooxygenase-2 expression in the gallbladder of patients with anomalous arrangement of the pancreaticobiliary duct. J Pediatr Surg 2003;38:585-589.
18. Glenn F, McSherry CK: Congenital segmental cystic dilatation of the biliary ductal system. Ann Surg 1973;177:705-713.
19. Gonzalez EM, Garcia IG, Pascual H, et al: Choledochal cyst resection and reconstruction by biliary-jejuno-duodenal diversion. World J Surg 1989;13:232-237.
20. Gross RE: Idiopathic dilatation of the common bile duct in children. J Pediatr 1933;3:370-375.

21. Hahn SA, Bartsch D, Schroers A, et al: Mutations of the *DPC-4/Smad-4* gene in biliary tract carcinoma. Cancer Res 1998;58:1124-1126.
22. Hasegawa T, Shukri N, Sasaki T, et al: Measurement of serum total bile acid levels in long-term postoperative follow-up of patients with congenital bile-duct dilatation. Pediatr Surg Int 2002;18:227-230.
23. Hay SA, Soliman HE, Sherif HM, et al: Neonatal jaundice: The role of laparoscopy. J Pediatr Surg 2000;35:1706-1709.
24. Hayashi N, Yawamoto H, Hiraoka N: Differential expression of cyclooxygenase-2 (COX-2) in human bile duct epithelial cell and bile duct neoplasm. Hepatology 2001;34:638-650.
25. Howell CG, Templeton JM, Weiner S, et al: Antenatal diagnosis and early surgery for choledochal cyst. J Pediatr Surg 1983;18:387-393.
26. Imazu M, Iwai N, Tokiwa K, et al: Factors of biliary carcinogenesis in choledochal cyst. Eur J Pediatr Surg 2001;11:24-27.
27. Ishida M, Tsuchida Y, Saito S, et al: Primary excision of choledochal cysts. Surgery 1970;68:884-888.
28. Ito T, Ando H, Nagaya M, et al: Congenital dilatation of the common bile duct in children—the etiologic significance of the narrow segment distal to the dilated common bile duct. Z Kinderchir 1984;39:40-45.
29. Iwai N, Yanagihira J, Tokiwa K, et al: Congenital choledochal dilatation with emphasis on pathophysiology of the biliary tract. Ann Surg 1992;215:27-30.
30. Jaunin-Stalder N, Stahelin-Massik J, Knuchel J, Gnehm HE: A pair of monozygotic twins with anomalous pancreaticobiliary junction and pancreatitis. J Pediatr Surg 2002;37:1485-1487.
31. Kaneko K, Ando H, Watanabe Y, et al: Secondary excision of choledochal cyst after previous cyst-enterostomies. Hepatogastroenterology 1999;46:2772-2775.
32. Kasai M, Asakura Y, Taira Y: Surgical treatment of choledochal cyst. Ann Surg 1970;172:844-851.
33. Katyal D, Lees GM: Choledochal cyst: A retrospective review of 28 patients and a review of the literature. Can J Surg 1992;35:584-588.
34. Kim MJ, Han SJ, Yoon CS, et al: Using MR cholangiopancreatography to reveal anomalous pancreaticobiliary ductal union in infants and children with choledochal cysts. AJR Am J Roentgenol 2002;179:209-214.
35. Kobayashi S, Asano T, Yamasaki M, et al: Risk of bile duct carcinogenesis after excision of extrahepatic ducts in pancreaticobiliary maljunction. Surgery 1999;126:939-944.
36. Komuro H, Makino SI, Yasuda Y, et al: Pancreatic complications in choledochal cyst and their surgical outcomes. World J Surg 2001;25:1519-1523.
37. Koshinaga T, Fukuzawa M: Pancreatic ductal morphological pattern and dilatation in postoperative abdominal pain in patients with congenital choledochal cyst: An analysis of postoperative pancreatograms. Scand J Gastroenterol 2000;35:1324-1329.
38. Landing BH: Considerations of the pathogenesis of neonatal hepatitis, biliary atresia and choledochal cyst—the concept of infantile obstructive cholangiopathy. Prog Pediatr Surg 1974;6:113-139.
39. Levy AD, Rohrmann CA, Murakata LA, Lonergan GJ: Caroli's disease: Radiologic spectrum with pathologic correlation. AJR Am J Roentgenol 2002;179:1053-1057.
40. Li L, Yamataka A, Wang Y-X, et al: Ectopic distal location of the papilla of Vater in congenital biliary dilatation: Implications for pathogenesis. J Pediatr Surg 2001;36:1617-1622.
41. Lilly JR: The surgical treatment of choledochal cyst. Surg Gynecol Obstet 1979;149:36-42.
42. Lilly JR: Total excision of choledochal cyst. Surg Gynecol Obstet 1978;146:254-258.
43. Liu DC, Rodriguez JA, Merick F, Geiger JO: Laparoscopic excision of a rare type II choledochal cyst: Case report and review of the literature. J Pediatr Surg 2000;35:1117-1119.
44. Lugo-Vicente HL: Prenatally diagnosed choledochal cysts: Observation or early surgery? J Pediatr Surg 1995;30:1288-1290.
45. MacKenzie TC, Howell LJ, Flake AW, Adzick NS: The management of prenatally diagnosed choledochal cysts. J Pediatr Surg 2001;36:1241-1243.
46. McWhorter GL: Congenital cystic dilatation of the common bile duct: Report of a case with cure. Arch Surg 1924;8:604-626.
47. Manning PB, Polley TZ, Oldham KT: Choledochocele: An unusual form of choledochal cyst. Pediatr Surg Int 1990;5:22-26.
48. Marchildon MB: Antenatal diagnosis of choledochal cyst: The first four cases. Pediatr Surg Int 1988;3:431-436.
49. Ming F, Wang Y-X, Zhang J-Z: Evolution in the treatment of choledochus cyst. J Pediatr Surg 2000;35:1344-1347.
50. Miyano T, Suruga K, Suda K: Anomalous pancreatocholedochal ductal junction syndrome: A proposal of a new classification. J Jpn Soc Pediatr Surg 1985;21:75-81.
51. Miyano T, Yamataka A, Kato Y, et al: Hepaticoenterostomy after excision of choledochal cyst in children: A thirty-year experience with 180 cases. J Pediatr Surg 1996;31:1417-1421.
52. Nakayama H, Masuda H, Ugajin W, et al: Left hepatic lobectomy for type IV-A choledochal cyst. Am Surg 2000;66:1020-1022.
53. Narasimhan KL, Chowdhry SK, Rao KLN: Management of accessory hepatic ducts in choledochal cysts. J Pediatr Surg 2001;36:1092-1093.
54. Narita H, Tsuruga N, Hashimoto T, et al: Congenital choledochal dilatation in one of monozygotic twins. J Jpn Soc Pediatr Surg 1990;26:89-95.
55. O'Neill JA: Choledochal cyst. Curr Probl Surg 1992;29:365.
56. O'Neill JA, Clatworthy HW: Management of choledochal cysts: A 14-year followup. Am Surg 1971;37:230-237.
57. O'Neill JA, Templeton JM, Schnaufer L, et al: Recent experience with choledochal cyst. Ann Surg 1987;205:533-540.
58. Ohama K, Tsuchida K, Yazaki U, et al: Perforated choledochal cyst in childhood: Four cases and a review of Japanese literature. J Jpn Soc Pediatr Surg 1996:32:776-780.
59. Ohi R, Yaoita S, Kamiyama T, et al: Surgical treatment of congenital dilatation of the bile duct with special reference to late complications after total excisional operation. J Pediatr Surg 1990;25:613-617.
60. Ohtsuka Y, Yoshida H, Matsunaga T, et al: Strategy of management for congenital biliary dilatation in early infancy. J Pediatr Surg 2002;37:1173-1176.
61. Okada A, Hasegawa T, Oguchi Y, Nakamura T: Recent advances in pathophysiology and surgical treatment of congenital dilatation of the bile duct. J Hepatobiliary Pancreat Surg 2002;9:342-351.
62. Okada A, Nakamura T, Okumura K, et al: Surgical treatment of congenital dilatation of bile duct (choledochal cyst) with technical considerations. Surgery 1987;101:238-243.
63. Pushparani P, Redkar RG, Howard ER: Progressive biliary pathology associated with common pancreatico-biliary channel. J Pediatr Surg 2000;35:649-651.
64. Raffensperger J (ed): Choledochal cyst. In Swenson's Pediatric Surgery. New York, Appleton-Century-Crofts, 1980, pp 614-619.
65. Ramirez MJ, Nieto J, Valencia P: Fibrosis hepatica con-

genita asociada a quiste de coledoco. Bol Med Hosp Infant Mex 1989;46:803-807.
66. Redkar R, Davenport M, Howard ER: Antenatal diagnosis of congenital anomalies of the biliary tract. J Pediatr Surg 1998;33:700-704.
67. Rossi RL, Silverman ML, Braasch JW, et al: Carcinomas arising in cystic conditions of the bile ducts: A clinical and pathologic study. Ann Surg 1987;205:377-384.
68. Rush E, Podesta L, Norris M, et al: Late surgical complications of choledochal cystoenterostomy. J Am Surg 1994;60: 620-624.
69. Rustad DG, Lilly JR: Letter to the editor. Surgery 1987; 101:240-251.
70. Saing T, Chan JKF, Lam WWM, Chan K-L: Virtual intraluminal endoscopy: A new method for evaluation and management of choledochal cyst. J Pediatr Surg 1998;33: 1686-1689.
71. Saing T, Han H, Chan KL, et al: Early and late results of excision of choledochal cyst. J Pediatr Surg 1997;32:1563-1566.
72. Scharli A, Bettex M: Congenital choledochal cyst: Reconstruction of the normal anatomy. J Pediatr Surg 1968;3:604-607.
73. Shimotake T, Aoi S, Tomiyama H, Iwai N: *DPC-4 (Smad-4)* and *K-ras* gene mutations in biliary tract epithelium in children with anomalous pancreaticobiliary ductal union. J Pediatr Surg 2003;38:694-697.
74. Spitz L: Choledochal cyst. Surg Gynecol Obstet 1978; 146:444-452.
75. Spitz L: Experimental production of cystic dilatation of the common bile duct in neonatal lambs. J Pediatr Surg 1977; 12:39-42.
76. Stringer MD, Dhawan A, Davenport M, et al: Choledochal cyst: Lessons learned from twenty year experience. Arch Dis Child 1995;73:528-531.
77. Suda K, Matsumoto Y, Miyano T: Narrow duct segment distal to choledochal cyst. Am J Gastroenterol 1991;86:1259-1263.
78. Sugiyama M, Atomi Y, Kuroda A: Pancreatic disorders associated with anomalous pancreaticobiliary junction. Surgery 1999;126:492-497.
79. Suita S, Shono K, Kinugasa Y, et al: Influence of age in the presentation and outcome of choledochal cyst. J Pediatr Surg 1999;34:1765-1768.
80. Todani T, Akita E, Ito T: (The Japanese Study Group on Pancreaticobiliary Maljunction) Diagnostic criteria of pancreaticobiliary maljunction. J Hep Bil Pancr Surg 1994; 1:219-221.
81. Todani T, Watanabe Y, Fujii T, et al: Anomalous arrangement of the pancreaticobiliary ductal system in patients with a choledochal cyst. Am J Surg 1984;147:672-676.
82. Todani T, Watanabe Y, Mizuguchi T, et al: Hepaticoduodenostomy at the hepatic hilum after excision of choledochal cyst. Am J Surg 1981;142:584-587.
83. Todani T, Watanabe Y, Narusue M, et al: Congenital bile duct cyst: Classification, operative procedures, and review of 37 cases including cancer arising from choledochal cyst. Am J Surg 1977;134:263-269.
84. Todani T, Watanabe Y, Toki A, et al: Carcinoma related to choledochal cyst with internal drainage operations. Surg Gynecol Obstet 1987;164:61-64.
85. Todani T, Watanabe Y, Toki A, et al: Co-existing biliary anomalies and anatomical variants in choledochal cyst. Br J Surg 1998;85:760-763.
86. Todani T, Watanabe Y, Urushishra N, et al: Biliary complications after excision procedure for choledochal cyst. J Pediatr Surg 1995;30:478-481.
87. Tokiwa K, Iwai N: Early mucosal changes of the gallbladder in patients with anomalous arrangement of the pancreaticobiliary duct. Gastroenterology 1996;110:614-618.
88. Tsuchida Y, Takahashi A, Suzuki N, et al: Development of intrahepatic biliary stones after excision of choledochal cyst. J Pediatr Surg 2002;37:165-167.
89. Tsuchiya R, Harada N, Ito T, et al: Malignant tumors in choledochal cyst. Ann Surg 1977;186:22-28.
90. Uno K, Isuchida Y, Kawarasaki H, et al: Development of intrahepatic cholelithiasis long after primary excision of choledochal cyst. J Am Coll Surg 1996;183:583-588.
91. Vater A: Dissertation in Auguralis Medica, Poes Diss.qua Scirris Biscerum Dissert, c.c. Ezlerus, vol 70. Edinburgh, University Library, 1723, p 19.
92. Watanabe Y, Toki A, Todani T: Bile duct cancer developed after cyst excision for choledochal cyst. J Hepatobiliarypancreat Surg 1999;6:207-212.
93. White JB, Becker JM: Left hepatic choledochal cyst. Surgery 1996;125:567-569.
94. Wilkinson M: The art of diagnostic imaging: The biliary tree. J Hepatol 1996;25(Suppl 1):5-19.
95. Wong KC, Lister J: Human foetal development of the hepato-pancreatic duct junction—a possible explanation of congenital dilatation of the biliary tract. J Pediatr Surg 1981;16:139-145.
96. Yotsuyanagi S: Contribution to aetiology and pathology of idiopathic cystic dilatation of the common bile duct with report of three cases. Gann 1936;30:601-752.

第 105 章

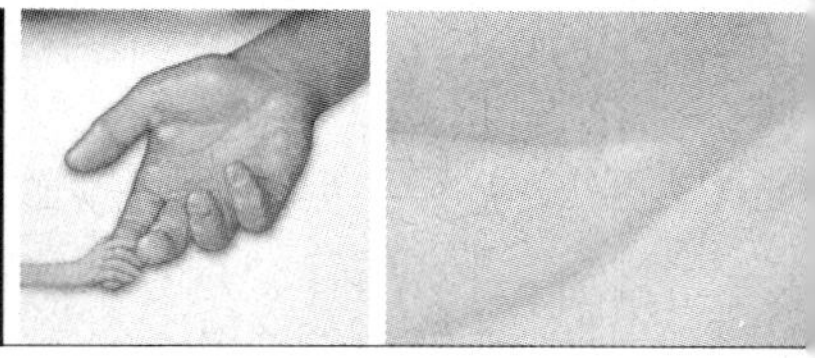

胆囊疾病和肝脏感染

George W. Holcomb III 和 Walter S. Andrews

胆囊疾病

35 在最近30年，儿童胆结石病例不断增加。究其原因，是发病率增高还是超声诊断技术的精确度增加，现在不得而知。但是，溶血性疾病不再是胆石症发生的前提条件[48,49,61]。此外，胆囊运动障碍和非结石性胆囊炎在儿童中比较常见。

非溶血性胆石症

目前已经知道可能引起儿童胆石症的几个因素，其中全肠道外营养（TPN）与儿童尤其是新生儿、婴幼儿非溶血性胆石形成有密切关系[60,78,98]。长期使用全肠外营养的患儿胆石症发生率可达43%[63]。关于全肠外营养引起胆石症的原因还不明确，但是与氨基酸输入、缺乏肠内摄入导致的胆汁成分改变有关。肠内摄入缺乏可导致胆囊无效收缩和胆汁肠肝循环减少。全肠外营养中的脂肪可以减轻全肠外营养中氨基酸的毒性。

由于很多婴幼儿进行全肠外营养治疗，只有很少一部分发展成胆石症，所以胆石症发生还和其他因素有关。败血症、脱水、长期应用利尿药物、囊性纤维病、短肠综合征和坏死性小肠结肠炎以及回肠切除都是发生胆石症的相关因素[37,74,93,98]。胆石症是多因素作用下产生的。胆石症的形成过程中，胆汁淤积、败血症、胆汁肠肝循环过程的变化都是重要因素。而且，新生儿尤其是早产儿由于胆盐的肠肝循环不完善而更易发生胆石症。儿童胆结石的组成成分和成人不同。成人结石的成分是胆固醇；而在胆石症患儿中胆结石的成分以碳酸钙和黑色素为主，特别是在10岁以下患儿[115]。

使用口服避孕药、囊性纤维病、妊娠、肥胖和回肠切除都是大龄儿童胆结石的病因[67,108,112]。有报道，心脏移植患者、使用环孢霉素和在新生儿期使用体外膜肺氧合的患者也可以出现胆石症[3,47,82,127]。

溶血性胆石症

虽然非溶血性胆石症发病率增加，但是溶血性胆石症（通常继发于镰状细胞贫血病）仍然是儿童胆石形成的常见原因，尤其在镰状细胞贫血病好发的边远乡村。镰状细胞贫血病合并胆色素结石与年龄有关。50%的镰状细胞贫血患者在20岁左右发生胆囊结石[30,65,102]。有趣的是，患镰状细胞贫血合并胆石症的患者胆红素生成率、清除率以及血浆胆红素水平与未合并胆石症的镰状细胞贫血患者相似[36]。研究提示过高的血非结合型胆红素并不是胆囊结石形成的主要原因。有实验发现胆囊结石者在禁食和餐后胆囊体积都增大，这提示胆囊静止时期未完全排空，胆汁滞留，泥沙形成，最终形成胆石。由于镰状细胞贫血患者经常有胆泥形成，所以不论有无结石，当胆囊有泥沙形成时应该考虑行选择性胆囊切除术[129]。有研究表明，35例镰状细胞贫血病合并有胆道泥沙的患者中，23例（65.7%）发展为胆囊结石[4]。

镰状细胞贫血患者在胆囊切除术后出现较多的并发症。在364例镰状细胞贫血患者中，术后并发症总 1636
发生率是39%，与镰状细胞相关的并发症占19%，围术期并发症占11%，输血并发症占10%，手术后遗症占4%，死亡占1%[43]。58%的患者接受开腹手术，42%的患者用腹腔镜手术。两组术后并发症没有差异。但是术前输血患者的并发症明显多于未输血患者。而且，推荐使用腹腔镜治疗。20%的患者出现急性胸腔综合征。此外，腹腔镜并不减少并发症的发生率[124]。围术期仔细处理、严格控制输血指征和加强呼吸道管理都可以减少胸腔综合征的发生。

其他两个常见并发胆石症的溶血性疾病是遗传性球形红细胞增多症和地中海贫血。遗传性球形红细胞增多症患者合并胆石症的发生率是43%~63%，女孩略多于男孩[6,68]。由于有合并胆石症的可能，所以行脾切除术前应行超声检查，明确是否要同时行胆囊切除术。以前，地中海贫血患儿合并胆石症的几率很高[25]。但是，由于高灌注治疗可以阻断骨髓产生脆性细胞[13]，目前地中海贫血患者很少出现胆石症。

临床表现

婴幼儿期的胆石症主要发生在患有系统性疾病和使用TPN的患者中。有些患者由于某些获得性疾病如坏死性肠炎或者先天性异常需要行回肠切除术。黄疸发生于超声可以检测到结石以前。大部分结石是含胆红素钙结石。

2~12岁间发生的胆结石是由胆红素钙、碳酸钙、胆固醇3种成分以不同比例混合构成的。有时X线平片可以看到不透光的结石，但是诊断还需依靠超声检查。虽然出现腹部疼痛、恶心、呕吐和偶尔出现发热，但是在年龄偏低的儿童中胆石症的诊断可能会延迟。腹痛表现可不同，可以在典型的右上腹，也可能无法定位，尤其是低年龄儿童。大龄儿童大多可以明确告知疼痛位于右侧肋下区域。

青少年患者表现和成年人类似。疼痛位于右侧肋下，放射到右侧肩胛下区域。常伴有恶心呕吐，不能耐受脂肪类食物。

胆囊水肿、非结石性胆囊炎、胆囊运动障碍和胆囊息肉常常发生。胆囊积水是胆囊无结石、炎症或先天性异常时发生的胆囊广泛扩张。胆囊积水常见于Kawasaki病，是由于胆囊管暂时性阻塞或者胆囊黏液分泌增多导致排空障碍[10,22,26,33]。随着胆囊扩张，胆囊管角度增大，也可促进梗阻的发生[105]。在疾病早期提倡保守治疗。败血症患者选用正确的抗生素和早期肠道内喂养能促进胆道排空，有利于治疗。如果一系列的超声检查显示进行性胆囊扩张，同时伴有明显腹痛或者胆囊坏疽，建议行胆囊切除术。

无胆石症的胆囊炎通常继发于严重的疾病，如败血症、烧伤、外伤导致的脱水、低血压和肠梗阻。在这些疾病中，常用TPN进行治疗。如果TPN治疗时间延长，随后胆囊收缩力下降并进行性扩张、胆汁淤积和胆道感染的发生率增加。近来有报道对12例患者进行研究，每天行超声检查作为是否行胆囊切除术的依据。其中3例患者由于胆囊壁增厚、胆囊扩张、胆囊周围积液而实施手术治疗。其他患者每天行超声检查，发现病情有不同程度改善，继续保守治疗。最终所有患者都治愈[53]。

胆囊运动障碍在儿童中的发病率不断增加[2,20,21,41,44,70,81,130]。据报道，腹腔镜行胆囊切除术是治疗这种疾病的有效手段，可以治愈80%以上的患者[2,20,21,41,70,81]。胆囊运动障碍以胆囊收缩力差、出现胆固醇结晶为特征。在出现典型的胆囊性疼痛且超声检查未发现明显异常时，应考虑该病。对胆囊收缩运动能力的评估可用注射胆囊收缩素后进行同位素扫描的方法。近年来，脂肪乳剂也可以产生相同的效果[44]。在胆囊运动障碍患者中，收缩分数小于35%[16]。组织病理学可以证实慢性胆囊炎[83]。回顾51例腹腔镜辅助下行胆囊切除术的胆囊收缩障碍患者，发现对于恶心、腹痛和胆囊收缩分数小于15%的患儿，胆囊切除术治疗有效。该报道也发现患儿的胆囊收缩分数大于15%时，胆囊切除术的效果不理想[20]。

最后，胆囊息肉在儿童中非常常见。如果有症状或者息肉大于1 cm，需要行胆囊切除术[113,114]。

在胆石症患儿中行选择性胆囊切除术的根本目的是减少并发症的发生。四个主要并发症是胆囊炎、黄疸、胆管炎和胆源性胰腺炎。急性胆囊炎的发生率在不断增加。有报道100例行腹腔镜胆囊切除术的患者，22%早期出现与结石有关的并发症[47]。7例出现急性胆囊炎表现，6例出现黄疸和腹痛，5例发展成为胆源性胰腺炎，4例出现急性胆源性非炎性绞痛。还有很多研究报道患者出现胆道梗阻症状[64,123]。对这些患者的治疗首先是控制局部感染，经过几天治疗后，可以在腹腔镜下行胆囊切除术。

放射学评价

虽然儿童时期腹部疼痛多采用腹部平片检查，但这对诊断胆石症的帮助不大，除非是胆囊结石钙化。溶血性疾病患者发生结石时，50% 以上是透光性结石。而成人中约有 15% 为胆固醇结石[111]。由于超声诊断的正确性很高，目前口服胆道造影很少应用。实时超声诊断对胆囊疾病诊断的正确率约为 96%，对于诊断肝脏和胆总管疾病也同样有效，同时也能发现增厚的胆囊壁及肝和胰头的任何异常表现[29]。胆囊炎最有效的诊断方法是用锝-99 标记的亚氨二醋酸胆管闪烁照相术。在这项检查中，急性胆囊炎患者的胆囊是不显影的。在危急患者中，尤其是禁食、病变严重或接受 TPN 治疗的患儿，可以存在假阳性结果。静脉给予吗啡是有帮助的，因为吗啡可以使 Oddi 括约肌收缩，胆道压力增加。后者可以使胆囊显影，减少假阳性率[38]。胆囊收缩素辅助或者脂肪乳剂改良的胆管闪烁照相术可以准确发现慢性无结石的胆囊疾病，也可提示可能需要胆囊切除术来缓解症状[2,20,41,44,71,94]。

非手术治疗

对儿童或者成人胆石症的非手术治疗已成为历史。以前对于成人患者曾用口服药物溶石或体外震波碎石治疗，但疗效甚微[99,103,104]。有文献报道，碎石治疗时间长、费用高，且 5 年内复发率高（50%）[99]。以上研究中未将儿童患者包括在内，其原因众多，包括这些治疗方法对色素结石无明显效果。目前，不主张对 2～3岁左右的结石患儿采用保守治疗。但是也有报道指出长期使用 TPN 的患儿，结石有自行消退的可能[17,50,54,116]。对于这个年龄阶段的患儿，在停止完全肠外营养并改为胃肠内营养后保守观察 6～12 个月比较合理。

外科治疗

外科治疗有症状的胆石症患者可以采用胆囊切除或胆囊碎石术。有报道曾经对在青春期前发生胆结石的患者在腹腔镜辅助下行胆囊碎石[121]，但是缺少长期随访资料。另一个报道称 10 例患者行胆道碎石术，经过 25 年随访，平均随访期限是 5 年，30% 的患者再次出现右上腹疼痛和结石复发[31]。由于碎石治疗有较高的复发率，所以这些学者认为对胆石症患者应行胆囊切除术。

过去 10 年中认为腹腔镜辅助下行胆囊切除术是治疗儿童胆石症的标准手术方式。手术的优点是减少不适和减少住院天数，手术伤口更符合美观的要求，并且很快可以恢复正常的生活，如工作、学习、玩耍和参加体育锻炼。这些优点是由于切口小造成的肌肉损伤较轻和对组织的创伤较小，比开腹手术造成的肠粘连和不适感更少。又有报道称没有并发症的腹腔镜手术患者术后 1～2 天就可以出院[35,47,71,95,117]。

虽然大多数患儿可以在 48 小时内出院，但是镰状红细胞症患者术前需要特别护理，以减少术后并发症。有些学者报道镰状红细胞症患者预后良好，而且强调术前输血的必要性[7,43,101,124,126]。近年来报道，腹腔镜对于镰状红细胞症患儿的治疗风险不大，可以首选此方法[43,47,101,124]。

一些特殊情况值得关注。首先是遗传性球形红细胞增多症患者，拟行脾切除术。脾切除术前必须行超声检查。如果胆石症存在，在脾切除的同时需行胆囊切除术。脾切除是否可以防止遗传性球形红细胞症患者胆石症形成不得而知。但是有研究报告，17 例只行脾切除的患者术前未发现胆石，术后平均随访 15 年，没有发现胆石形成[100]。因此，对于行脾切除术的没有胆石症的遗传性球形红细胞症患儿，预防性行胆囊切除是不必要的。

第二个值得关注的问题是胆石症患者出现或者怀
疑有胆总管结石症。治疗方法多种多样[73,86,106,131]， 1638
包括术前内镜逆行胰胆管造影（ERCP）下内括约肌切开术和取石术，在腹腔镜辅助下行胆囊切除术时腹腔镜或者开腹手术探查胆总管，或内窥镜下内括约肌切开取石术。选择哪种手术方法取决于两个因素：外科医生腹腔镜探查胆总管的经验以及在这所治疗机构中 ERCP 和括约肌成形术的效果如何。熟悉腹腔镜辅助下行胆总管探查的儿外科医生可以对手术效果不满意的患儿进行术后内镜下内括约肌切开术。但是大多数儿外科医生很少能够做内括约肌手术，这是由于病例较少而没有足够的经验。所以如果发现结石，最好术前在 ERCP 下行内括约肌切开取石术。如果成功，数天后行腹腔镜下胆囊切除术。但是如果没有成功，外科医生需要知道是否有必要行开腹或者腹腔镜辅助下胆总管探查手术。我院具体流程图见 105-1。

最后需要关心的问题是是否需要术中做胆道造影。上世纪 90 年代早中期，没有对儿童实施腹腔镜

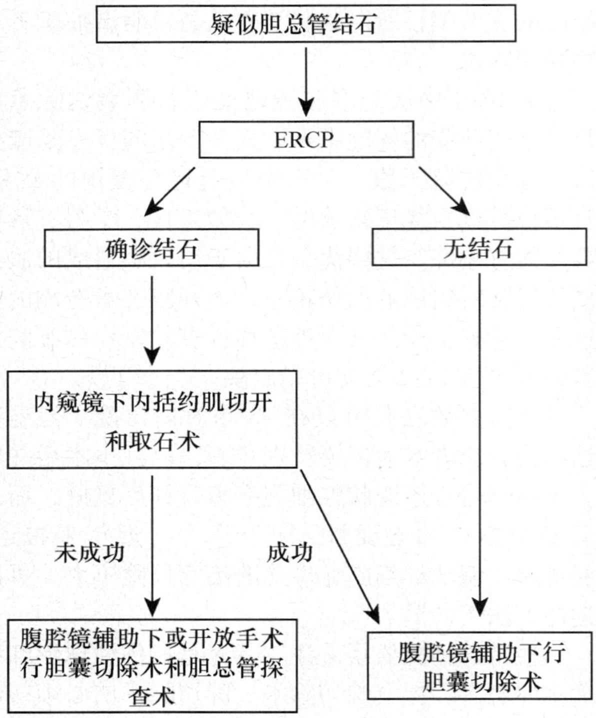

图 105-1 作者处理拟诊胆总管结石患者首选诊疗决策流程。必要时，可以在腹腔镜手术前 ERCP 下进行取石和内括约肌切开。如果 ERCP 不能够显示胆总管结石，再行腹腔镜胆囊切除术。术前运用 ERCP 检查的目的是让医生知道是否有必要进行腹腔镜或开腹胆总管探查。

手术的经验，为了达到培训外科医生和通过造影了解胆道系统解剖关系的目的，主张对大多数患儿实施术中胆道造影。还有一个原因是术中胆道造影可以明确共同通道中是否有结石，虽然术前症状、超声和术中腹腔镜检查也可以对这些加以明确。当外科医生对腹腔镜辅助下胆囊切除手术熟悉后，就无需胆道造影了。因此，我们的观点是，术中胆道造影可以确认胆道系统的解剖关系及了解是否有胆总管结石。我们在使用腹腔镜胆囊切除术前常规用超声证实胆囊结石和评价胆总管梗阻。上述方法可以减少手术时间和费用（表 105-1）。依据这个诊疗模式，我们研究所没有误诊一例胆总管结石。因此，手术时行胆管造影的目的是确保胆道正确的解剖。如果腹腔镜下解剖结构清楚，则可以不做常规的胆道造影。虽然有其他方法来
确保造影管进入腔内，但是如果做胆道造影，我们仍 163
喜欢用 Kumar 夹技术[48,51]。由于透视正确性比静止的 X 线高，所以能更好地动态评价胆管（图 105-2）。

另外，过去几年中作者改进的一项技术值得一提。在很多腹腔镜手术包括胆囊切除手术中，作者采用“刺入切口”方式，使得手术器械不再是持续停留在腹腔内，而是可以反复多次进入腹腔。511 例患者能经受各种腹腔镜手术，该手术只用 1～2 个 Innerdyne 插管（US. Swgical，Norwalk，CT），节省 187 180 美金[88]。如果用 Ethicon（Ethicon Endosurgery，Cincinnati，OH）插管，能节省 123 000 美金。胆囊切除时，右侧腹部的两个切口没有改变。这两个切口是理想的切口（图 105-3）。内镜可以通过脐部切口伸入，主操作孔在左上腹，所以 2 个 Innerdyne 插管可以用在这两个地方。

机器人手臂（Aesop）也可用来行胆囊切除[107]。这个设备的优点是提供了稳定的视野。而且，外科医生可以声控移动内镜和摄像头。我们发现放置 Aesop 的最佳位置是手术台的右侧，患者右侧股骨头水平。Aesop 不能倾斜，依患者体型调整机器臂可以到-1 位置，有时候可到 0 位（中间位）（图 105-4）[107]。

腹腔镜胆囊切除术 16

患者仰卧于手术台上，两台监视器置于患者头侧。

表 105-1 Mercy 儿童医院术前超声和术中胆道造影检测胆管结石的效价比

术前超声	费用	术中胆道造影	费用
超声检查（包括放射医生费用）：	$307. 67	15 分钟手术室时间	$734. 25
		C-arm 机放射科医生的费用	$365. 41
		C-arm 机无菌单	$20. 00
		胆道造影管	$83. 50
		胆道造影剂	$40. 00
总计	$307. 67	总计	$1243. 16

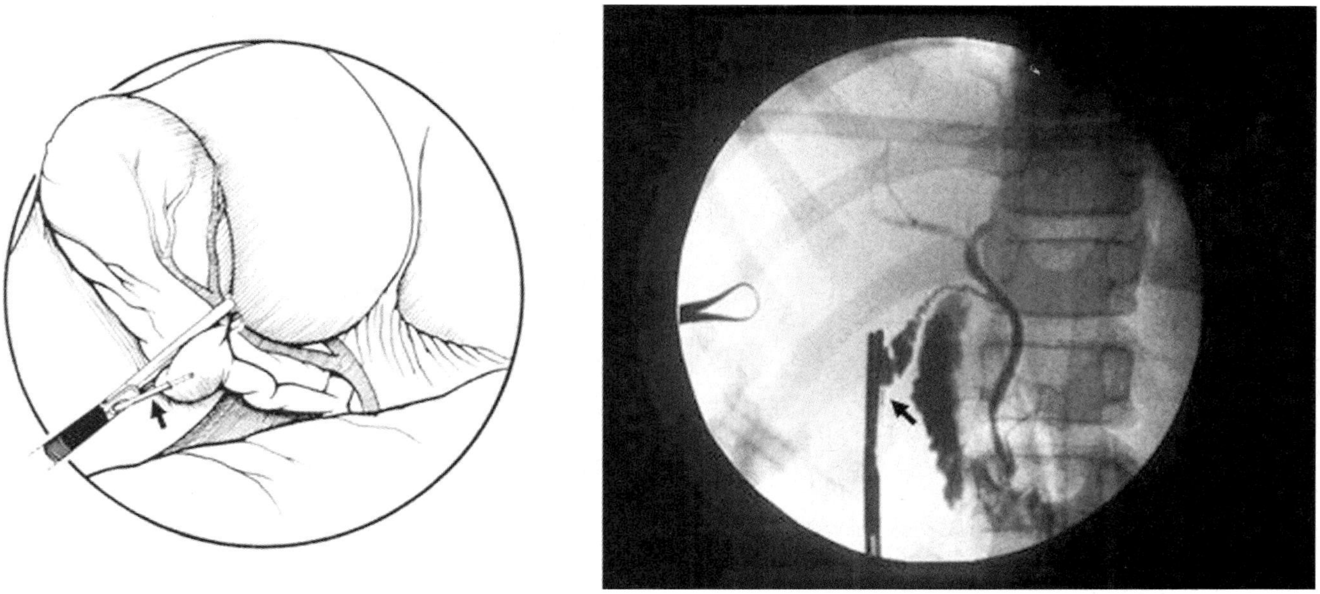

图 105-2　Kumar 夹技术在婴幼儿胆道造影中的应用。注意胆囊颈周围的夹子和夹子侧臂进入近端漏斗部的硬化治疗针头（箭头所示）。这个技术的优点是侧面切开，不需要对细小的胆囊管进行插管。

麻醉诱导后，经鼻插入胃管进行胃肠减压，插导尿管。采用两个插管和两个“穿刺切口”，但是具体位置取决于患者的年龄和体型（图 105-5）。对于婴幼儿，右侧下腹部切口应位于腹股沟皱褶区，上腹部套管应位于患者的左侧，以便在手术器械间提供足够的手术空间。

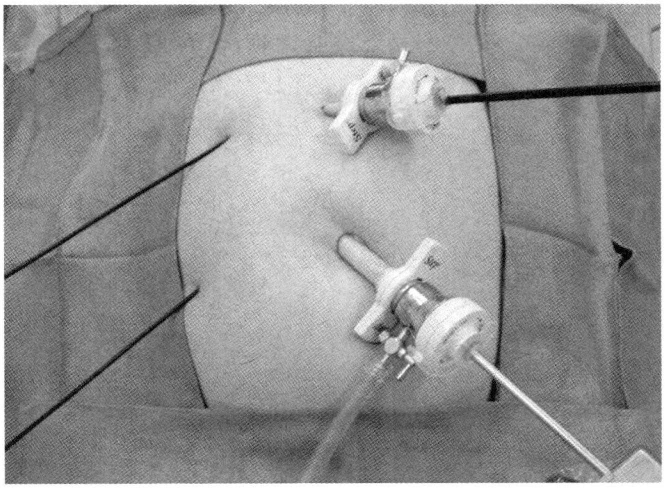

图 105-3　该操作图显示采用穿刺插入技术对 5 岁儿童行腹腔镜下胆囊切除术。患者右侧的 2 个 3 mm 的器械经穿刺插入技术导入，而没有用插管。1 个 5 mm 的插管位于右上腹。10 mm 的插管位于脐周，这是胆囊取出部位。穿刺插入技术的优点是花费小，不需要 2 个插管。

脐部做一个 10 mm 的切口，10 mm 的套管插入腹腔后充气。建立良好气腹后，将 0°或 45°内镜通过脐部套管插入腹腔，然后和摄像机相连。图像显示在监视器上。用 11 号刀片在右下腹做穿刺切口，将一把锁闭抓钳经该切口插入，助手用抓钳在肝脏上方牵拉胆囊。通常采用 5 mm 的套管，小婴儿可以用 3 mm 的。在右上腹的穿刺切口中插入未锁定的抓取钳，抓住胆囊漏斗部并向侧方牵拉。上腹部的通道多为 5 mm，是主要的操作通道。对于年龄大的青少年，如果需要 10 mm 的内镜夹来完全夹闭胆囊管，则需要 10 mm 的操作通道，手术原则和成人操作一样。这时内镜连接在 Aesop 上。

为了提高暴露的程度，患者和床通常旋转到头低 1641
脚高位和左侧倾斜位，可以使得其他内脏不至于挡住手术视野。此外，漏斗部的侧方牵拉也很重要，因为此时胆囊管和胆总管的角度大于 90°，而不牵拉时是倾斜或者平行的（图 105-6）。这个特点可以导致胆囊管和胆总管混淆，造成共同通道的损伤。

首先是暴露胆囊管和明确胆囊动脉。为了显露漏斗部和 Calot 三角，需要松解十二指肠和胃之间的粘连。一旦胆囊管明确，有两个选择。一个是行胆囊造影，前面我们已经讨论了。如果解剖很清楚，术前超

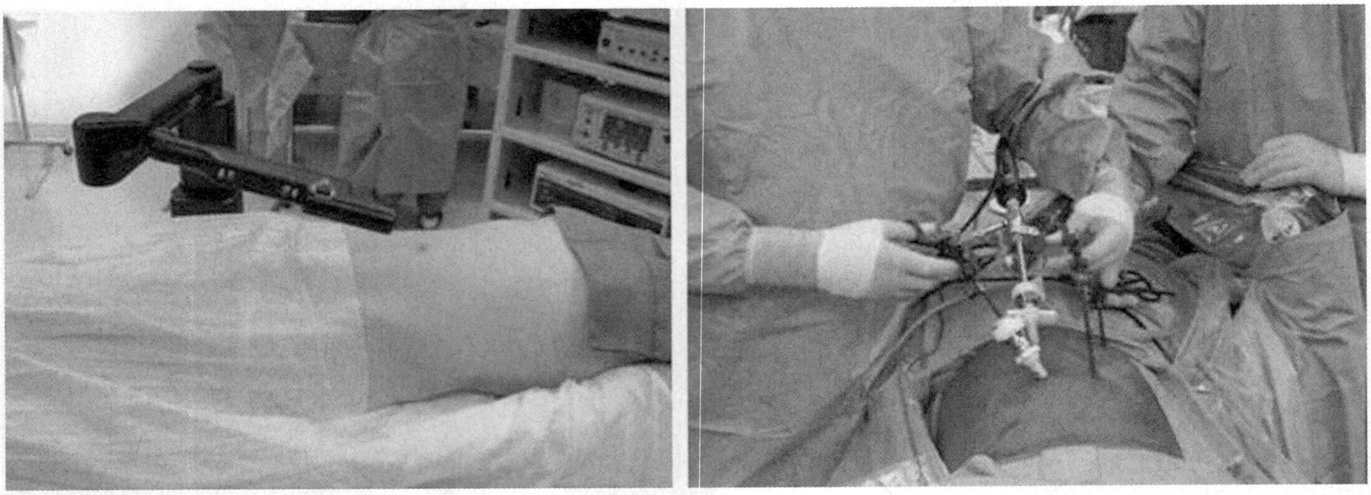

图 105-4　作者使用 Aesop 行腹腔镜下胃底折术和腹腔镜下胆囊切除术。腹腔镜下胆囊切除术时，Aesop 放置在手术台的右侧，相当于患者右侧股骨头水平。Aesop 通常位于-1 度水平（左侧）。为了使 Aesop 有效操作，外科医生通常在臂侧（右侧）操作。注意右侧的仪器都没有用插管。

声没有胆道狭窄存在，就分离和结扎胆囊管。虽然大龄儿童需要 10 mm 的夹子，但是通常使用 5 mm 的夹子已足够了。放在胆囊管上的两个夹子距离胆总管 5 mm（图 105-7）。另外一个或两个夹子夹住近漏斗部的胆囊管，防止胆囊内石头漏出。然后切断胆囊管和结扎断离胆囊动脉。一旦这两个结构分离了，胆囊就可以用器械（电钩、电刀和内镜剪）逆行分离。

在胆囊完全从胆囊床上分离下来以前，仔细检查 Calot 三角区，以便确保所有的夹子都夹紧，没有出血迹象。胆囊分离完全以后，镜子从脐部转到上腹部。如果上腹部通道是5 mm，那么采用5 mm 镜。抓钳通过脐部切口进入腹腔。胆囊从脐部切口取出。大龄患儿由于胆囊较大，需要切开脐部筋膜。脐部切口应该扩大，这样可以防止胆囊破裂，胆石和胆汁渗漏到胆囊外。一旦渗漏，必须清除渗漏物，因为有报道成人由于胆石滞留造成并发症[9,19,108]。胆囊取出后，分离的部位需要仔细检查，确保完全止血。所有的冲洗必须吸干净，丁哌卡因注射到切口上以确保术后止痛。对于低年龄的患儿，5 mm 切口周围的筋膜需要关闭。对于高年龄患儿，5 mm 切口或者刺入切口不需要关闭，但是 10 mm 切口需要仔细关闭以防止疝形成。对于刺入切口，通常需要关闭皮肤切口。患者术后第二天早

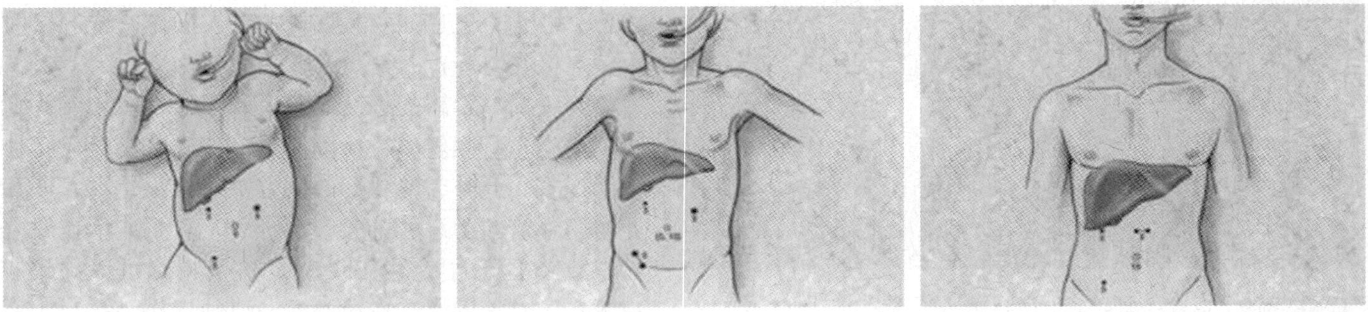

图 105-5　腹腔镜下胆囊切除手术时，插管和仪器位置的确定与患儿的年龄和体型有关。小婴儿用 3 mm 和 5 mm 的插管，并且插管之间的距离应尽可能大，以保证足够的操作空间（左图）。对于青春期前的儿童，插管之间的空间也要足够大。3 mm的插管可以在外科医生的左手侧。对于此年龄段的患儿，可以用 5 mm 的脐部插管。但是许多患儿在取出胆囊时需要 10 mm脐部插管（中图）。青少年时期，插管的位置接近成年人（右图）（也见彩图）。

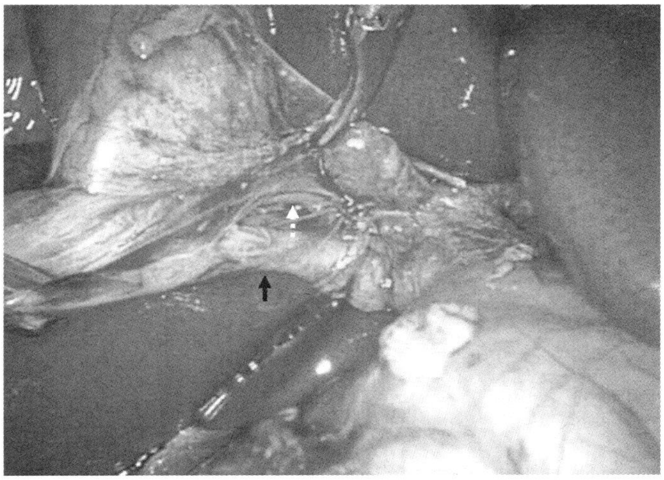

图 105-6　在腹腔镜下胆囊切除手术开始时，侧面牵拉漏斗部非常重要，这样可以在胆道（实心箭头）和共同通道间形成一个 90°的角。注意胆囊管头侧的胆囊动脉（点状箭头）（也见彩图）。

上出院，但是成人门诊腹腔镜胆囊切除增多。

Mercy 儿童医院的经验

尽管目前在儿童中广泛使用腹腔镜胆囊切除术，但是很少有文献报道，只有 3 篇报道病例数达 100 人[47,73,123]。1999 年对 Vanderbilt 大学医学中心 100 例腹腔镜胆囊切除手术进行回顾，其中 78 例为选择性手术，22 例为胆石症出现并发症需要急诊手术[47]。其中 19 例为溶血性疾病，2 例为胆囊运动障碍。6 例出现黄疸的患者在腹腔镜胆囊切除术前行 ERCP 检查。2 例患者的胆道结石取出，2 例行腹腔镜下胆总 1642
管探查。有并发症组的手术时间和术后住院天数都明显比选择性手术者长。均未发生严重的手术并发症，如再次手术、胆总管或其他内脏损伤、胆汁漏和持续胆总管结石。

2000—2003 年，Mercy 儿童医院有 93 例患儿进行腹腔镜下胆囊切除术（表 105-2）。1 例为遗传性球形红细胞增多症，腹腔镜脾切除术同时进行胆囊切除。62 例为女性，平均年龄 12. 3 岁，平均体重 55. 3 公斤。17% 有血液性疾病。2 例因为白血病行骨髓移植，另外 1 例视网膜母细胞瘤需要化疗，这 3 例都存在胆道运动障碍。胆囊切除后其中 2 例有症状改善。

在这四年中，6 例因为急性胆绞痛急诊入院。2 例发展为胆石性胰腺炎，1 例出现明显黄疸。2 例经过术前 ERCP 检查发现胆总管结石症，但是没有证据证明有共同通道内结石。2 例患者都接受了腹腔镜胆囊切除术。另外 2 例怀疑胆总管结石的患者在术中行胆道造影证实结石存在，行腹腔镜下胆囊切除术，术后行 ERCP 检查。此 2 例患者在术后第五天和第十一天分别进行 ERCP 检查和内括约肌切开术。共同通道

表 105-2　在 Mercy 儿童医院需要腹腔镜辅助下行胆囊切除术的患者（2000—2003 年）

患者总例数	93
男性	31
女性	62
平均年龄（岁）	12. 3（2～20）
平均体重（公斤）	55. 3（11～126）
血液疾病	
镰状红细胞增多症	9
遗传性球形红细胞症	6
丙酮酸激酶缺乏症	1
胆道运动障碍	3
急性胆绞痛	6
胆源性胰腺炎	2
黄疸	1

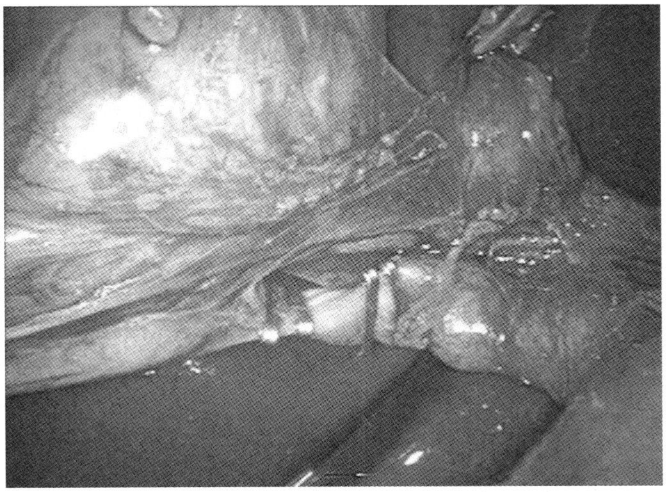

图 105-7　在明确和游离胆囊管后，各用两个夹子双重结扎胆囊管的近端和远端。胆囊管在两个中型内镜夹中间被分成两段。

内的结石移除，第二天 2 例患者都出院。

11 例患者行术中胆道造影，其他 82 例没有。手术中没有胆道和其他组织结构损伤，也没有患者需要二次手术（除了前面提到的 ERCP）。平均手术时间为 108 分钟。

除了上文提到的 2 例术后行 ERCP 的患者，只有 3 例术后住院时间超过 2 天。1 例有神经系统损伤，另外 1 例患有镰状红细胞增多症，恢复缓慢。1 例球形红细胞增多症的患者出现术后肠梗阻。这 3 名患者在术后第三天都出院。

过去的 10 年里，在腹腔镜辅助下行胆囊切除术成为儿童和成年人胆囊切除的标准术式。其并发症较少，并且尚无报道发生胆总管损伤，虽然此种损伤在所难免。此外，外科医生可以利用术中超声检查诊断胆总管结石，了解胆道解剖关系。

肝脏感染

不同的肝脏感染发生在婴幼儿不同时期（表 105–3）。本章讨论的重点是需要进行外科诊断或治疗的肝脏感染，包括肝脓肿和非病毒原因造成的肝脏感染。儿童时期肝脓肿大多继发于阑尾穿孔。肝脏感染的发生是由于门静脉炎和细菌由门静脉系统迁移到肝脏所致。儿童时期的肝脓肿发生于严重的疾病、粒细胞功能异常、镰状红细胞和先天性或获得性免疫功能抑制性疾病。约有一半以上的肝脓肿患者年龄小于 5 岁，25% 以上发生在 1 岁以内，而且多发脓肿较单发脓肿更多见[5,14,56]。 1643

表 105–3　儿童肝脏感染

细菌	**寄生虫**
化脓性肝脓肿	溶组织阿米巴
胆管炎	包虫病
猫抓病	肝吸虫
肝周炎	
布氏杆菌病	**真菌**
结核病	念珠菌病
放线菌病	曲霉病
伤寒性肝炎	组织胞浆菌病
兔热病	隐球菌病
梅毒	球孢子菌病
Lyme 病	放线菌病
钩端螺旋体病	
	立克次体
病毒	落基山斑疹热
肝炎	Q 热
巨细胞病毒感染	
疱疹	
单核细胞增多症	

病理生理学

细菌和其他微生物可以通过多种途径进入肝脏。最常见的是胆道系统、门静脉和肝动脉。微生物也可以在开放性外伤时直接进入。有报道称，16 例外伤后肝被膜下血肿的患者中 4 例发生肝脓肿[40]。此外，一小部分的肝脓肿原因不明。

肝脓肿的临床症状和体征通常无特异性。往往是发热、腹部疼痛和肝大，还有白细胞计数异常、肝酶异常或者胆红素水平异常。症状可以持续数天或数月。肝脏超声和 CT 的检查可以诊断肝脓肿（图 105–8 和 105–9）[5,14]。

化脓性肝脓肿

化脓性肝脓肿在儿童中不常见，有报告其比例可

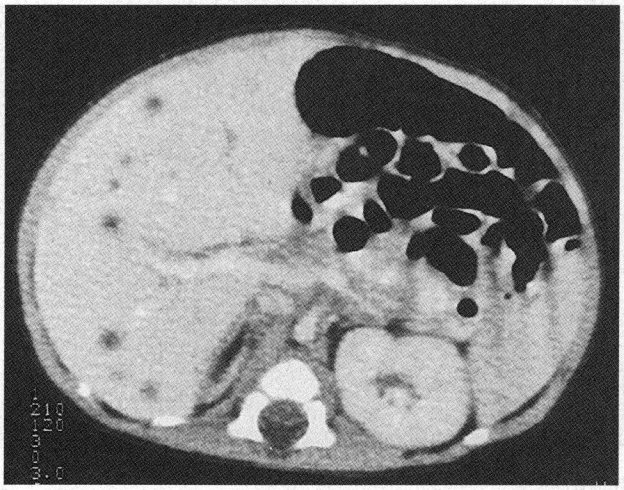

图 105–8　CT 扫描显示儿童葡萄球菌感染相关慢性肉芽肿性疾病的肝脓肿（缺损部位）。

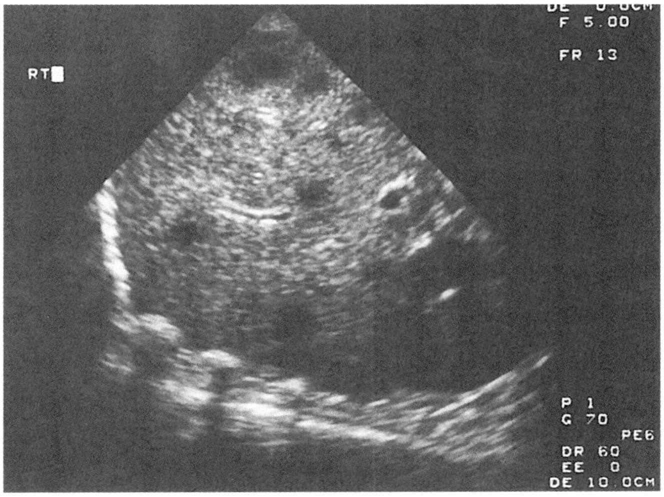

图 105-9　超声显示图 105-6 所示患者的肝脓肿（回声区域）。

占儿科住院患者的 3～25/10 万[92]。由于抗生素的应用，其发病率下降。与成人不同，儿童的化脓性肝脓肿主要见于免疫缺陷的患者。儿童时期的慢性肉芽肿病是常见的免疫缺陷。化疗或者移植后用免疫抑制剂造成免疫损伤，患者易于发生肝脓肿。继发于胆道疾病的肝脓肿常见于胆道闭锁、胆总管囊肿或肝移植术后。腹部钝性或锐性外伤所致的肝损伤可使肝脓肿发生率增加。以上原因造成的脓肿继发于坏死的肝组织和血肿。但是值得注意的是，肝脓肿患儿仅表现为原因不明的发热，而其他方面表现正常[8,45]。

在免疫力正常的儿童中，化脓性肝脓肿发生的其他原因有肠道感染（阑尾炎）、胆道闭锁患者具有慢性胆管炎伴肝内脓肿、新生儿期脐静脉插管，其他原因造成的全身性菌血症也是化脓性肝脓肿的原因[59]。此外，20% 的患者病因未明确[27]。

化脓性肝脓肿的诊断通常依靠鉴别诊断。在儿童时期肝脓肿的发生率很低，所以经常漏诊，有时直到几周或几个月时才被发现。如果患儿同时有发热、腹痛、黄疸和肝脏增大，一般很少漏诊。但是这些症状往往出现缓慢，而且常伴有体重减轻，容易使医生向肿瘤方面考虑。症状往往是不典型的，最主要的症状是腹痛[8,92]。症状持续的时间各不相同，通常在病后 1 周~1 个月。大多数患者出现发热，只有大约 2/3 的患者有肝脏增大。一项报告指出只有 40% 的患者出现右上腹触痛[59]。血液学检查帮助不大，一般只能发现轻微的白细胞增多。大约有一半的患者会出现肝功能亢进。

儿童化脓性肝脓肿的细菌学检查发现，37%～50% 的脓肿是由金黄色葡萄球菌引起的[8,15,27,92]。然而，大多数肝脓肿含有多种病原菌，包括 G^+ 球菌和 G^- 杆菌，如大肠杆菌、克雷白杆菌、肠道细菌和假单胞菌。最近，至少在 20% 的脓肿细菌培养中发现了厌氧菌[15,23,39]。大约 50% 的患者血培养阳性，然而血培养获得的细菌类型要少于直接脓液培养获得的细菌类型。需要注意的是，有 1/3 的血培养获得的细菌与脓液直接培养获得的细菌不同。肝脓肿穿刺抽液后对脓液进行革兰染色，对 G^+ 球菌具有高度敏感性，然而对 G^- 细菌只有 50% 的敏感性。真菌性肝脓肿在一些急性白血病的患儿中逐渐增多，表现为在治疗过程中出现发热、中性粒细胞下降[42]。一项前瞻性研究报道在这一群体中，真菌性肝和（或）脾脓肿的发生率为 29%。有报道描述了肝和脾念珠菌病的特殊超声表现[90]。

新生儿是肝脓肿的另一个特殊亚群体。在围生期，细菌有可能直接经胎盘侵入肝脏，这一播散过程可能伴有胎膜早破。不管有没有脐静脉置管，脐炎都很少会造成细菌性肝炎或肝脓肿。大多数新生儿肝脓肿是粟粒性的，具有高比例的 G^- 细菌。因为通常是粟粒性的，所以不适合做经皮引流，而需要长期大剂量的抗生素治疗。

一些新生儿肝脓肿表现为单个孤立的脓肿，通常为金黄色葡萄球菌感染造成。这些患儿表现为逐渐增大的右上腹包块，很难和肿瘤相鉴别。而就是因为很难鉴别脓肿和实性肿瘤，对这些孤立的肝脓肿一般行手术切除[118]。

放射学评价

诊断肝囊肿或脓肿最好的放射学诊断方法是腹部超声和 CT。由于超声不需要镇静剂和没有辐射，可作为初步筛查的首选方法。但是，CT 敏感性高，可以发现超声遗漏的问题。此外，CT 通常作为经皮穿刺引流时脓肿定位的首选方法[92]。

治疗

化脓性肝脓肿的初步治疗应该首先用针对革兰阴

性、阳性和厌氧菌的广谱抗生素，而且还应将假单胞菌考虑在内。穿刺引流应该在 CT 或者超声引导下进行。在脓肿引流和特异性细菌感染明确后，应该调整抗生素。静脉使用抗生素 4～6 周后，改口服抗生素 4～8周[56]。

近年来，经皮穿刺引流成为肝脓肿引流的首选方法。穿刺引流并发症的发生率为 4% 左右，失败率为 15% 左右[122]。但是，如果患者对于外引流没有反应或者外引流无法进行，则需要行手术治疗[8,62]。近来有报道腹腔镜下行化脓性肝脓肿外引流术[125]，可以缩短手术时间，减少出血和止疼剂的应用。应用这种强有力的治疗方法，化脓性肝脓肿的死亡率从 1970 年的 36% 下降到 1980 年的 15% 和现在的 10%。

成人化脓性肝脓肿的并发症是眼内炎，报道该病的发生率是 3.5%，可以导致各种眼科疾病，甚至失明[119]。治疗的最佳时机是发生该病的 24 小时以内。所以对于儿童的化脓性肝脓肿，一旦发现视力改变都需要行眼科检查。

猫抓病

猫抓病是接触感染的猫后发生的亚急性疾病，以局部淋巴结炎为特征，可以累及多个系统，如肝脏、脑和骨骼。该病 1889 年首次被描述为眼和腺体的异常。1950 年，Debre 报道该病伴有猫的抓痕[18]。从那时起，曾有多种感染性微生物被作为引起该病的病原体。目前，猫抓病被认为是由汉赛巴尔通体引起的。这个疾病主要发生于儿童和青少年（占 75%～80%）。多数病例首发病变主要位于感染部位，一般在 1～2 周内发生。典型病变是直径 2～5 mm 的单个丘疹。局部淋巴结病变发生于 3 周后，主要在腋窝、腹股沟和颈部淋巴结。当腺体发生病变时，最初的皮肤病变常已消退。其他相关症状有发热、食欲减退、不适、乏力和头痛等。

约有 5%～10% 的患者出现多系统症状或者症状
1645 不典型。这些患者缺乏典型的局部腺体病表现[77]，肝脏变化可以通过 CT 检查明确。CT 检查可以发现的典型表现是左右两叶多个病灶，有时候脾也受累[18,97]。通过开放手术或腹腔镜辅助下手术进行肝活检可以明确诊断。组织学检查显示肉芽肿性反应伴有坏死。细菌和真菌培养都是阴性。在 1 例患者的脓液和组织的 PCR 检查中都发现对汉赛巴尔通体的敏感性和特异性均很高。目前正在开发一种酶联反应。猫抓病的治疗一直是有争议的，因为很多患者可以自行缓解。但是有明显症状或内脏受累时，需要用抗生素治疗（如庆大霉素、环丙沙星、利福平或者复方磺胺甲唑）[79]。

肝周炎

在儿童时期，肝脏细菌性感染在青少年女性中常为奈瑟氏菌或者沙眼衣原体感染。起源于盆腔感染，由腹部向头侧发展，导致肝周炎发生。如果肝周炎不经治疗，典型的“小提琴弦”状粘连出现于肝和腹膜腔之间，伴有 Fitz-Hugh-Curtis 综合征。

除了痛经、阴道溢液和下腹部疼痛等典型的盆腔感染症状，还会出现严重的右上腹部疼痛，向右肩放射。也有患者诉左上腹疼痛。患者肝区常有触痛，同时在肋区可以听见摩擦音。常常合并有急性输卵管炎。实验室检查表现包括白细胞增多、转氨酶升高，偶尔有高胆红素血症。

肝周炎可以出现类似于患其他疾病如胆石症、肝炎、消化性溃疡穿孔、阑尾炎和胰腺炎时的腹痛。在青春期女性中，若有盆腔感染病史，当出现右上腹疼痛时，肝周炎必须作为鉴别诊断之一。

除非直接看到肝周炎，否则诊断很难明确。无法明确诊断或者有持续症状的患者需要进行诊断性的腹腔镜检查，直接观察肝周情况。如果发现有粘连，需要在腹腔镜下行松解手术，术后腹痛会明显改善[89]。

近年来有报道显示奈瑟氏菌和沙眼衣原体是本病的病因[96]。治疗的重点是控制奈瑟氏菌和沙眼衣原体感染。抗生素包括四环素、多西环素，当四环素无法使用时改用红霉素[96]。

阿米巴脓肿

阿米巴肝脓肿在美国的发病率在逐渐上升。溶组织内阿米巴不仅是引起成人阿米巴肝脓肿的病因，也是儿童阿米巴肝脓肿的病因[84]。卫生条件差和人口密集度高是阿米巴病发生和传播的条件。阿米巴肠炎患者的滋养体从结肠溃疡处进入，通过门静脉移行入肝脏，起初在肝脏中形成坏死性变化，然后是脓肿形成。在成人中，肝脏受累的阿米巴脓肿的发生率为 10%~50%，其中 90% 为男性。在儿童中，肝脏受累的阿米巴脓肿的发生率为 1%~7%，无性别差异[52,91,120]。使用皮质激素和免疫抑制剂容易形成脓肿。

超过 80% 的阿米巴肝脓肿发生在肝右叶。症状包括发热、寒战、恶心、体重下降和腹部膨隆。体格检查时，可见肝大，但是腹部疼痛和肝区压痛相对不明显。右下肺部的呼吸音减弱，常有右侧胸腔积液。黄疸少见。接触史和曾去过疫区（墨西哥、南美和东南亚）是一个重要的指征，比影像学检查更有利于诊断[28]。

实验室检查包括除嗜酸性粒细胞以外的白细胞增多、轻度贫血和肝功能正常或轻度异常。腹部超声和 CT 可用来确定脓肿部位和数量。典型的超声检测发现低回声的薄壁脓肿，有时可以含有气体。CT 显示非特异性低密度缺损，大多为实质性，主要位于肝右叶。现代影像学技术可将肝脏多发的阿米巴脓肿显示得非常清楚[110]。

阿米巴肝脓肿的诊断依赖于肝脏占位性病变和阿米巴阳性血清学结果。诊断阿米巴肝脓肿时，血清学（间接血红蛋白或者免疫扩散琼脂凝胶沉淀）有较高敏感度（>94%）和特异度（>95%）。如果临床区分肝脓肿和阿米巴肝脓肿困难，或者脓肿对于药物治疗无效，或阿米巴血清学检查无法确诊，可以抽吸脓液送培养。

目前，阿米巴脓肿治疗时用口服甲硝唑［30～50 mg/(kg·d)连续用药 7～10 天］。大多数患者治疗有效，发热和腹痛缓解。目前，没有并发症的阿米巴
46 肝脓肿不需要进行抽吸，主要是因为脓肿可以在药物治疗后自行消退[1,12,55,110]。如果在药物治疗后 4 天没有效果，或者肝脓肿直径大于 10 cm，或者局限于肝左叶，或者有破裂的危险，才行抽吸或经皮穿刺引流。此外，脓肿破入右侧胸膜腔也是穿刺引流的指征。脓肿完全吸收需要数月到数年，期间可以进行超声随访。

阿米巴肝脓肿最常见的并发症是膈肌的腐蚀后破裂，脓液流入右侧胸腔。临床上约有 10% 发生自发性破裂。脓肿破入心包很少见，但是可以引起心脏压塞。脓肿在腹腔内破裂可以导致腹膜炎和休克。如果发生脓肿破裂，需要补液、运用抗生素、抗阿米巴治疗和外科手术探查。

曾经想研制一种针对溶组织内阿米巴的疫苗，但是溶组织内阿米巴的感染不是终生免疫的。在溶组织内阿米巴流行地区，复发性阿米巴肝脓肿是个棘手的问题[11,85,87]。

包虫囊肿

包虫病是由来源于狗的棘球绦虫的幼虫感染引起的。被咽下的虫卵经过肠道黏膜再经过肠系膜静脉进入肝脏。少部分虫卵经过肝脏停留于肺部。报道包虫感染的高峰时期是 5～15 岁的儿童[69,128]。常见症状包括右上腹疼痛或约一半患者出现右侧下肋部疼痛或肿块[32]。有趣的是，约有 1/4 的患者没有症状[110]。囊肿不治疗可以不断长大，直到突出于肝脏表面，发生自发性破裂，导致寄生虫进入腹腔，造成过敏。约有 1/4 的患者囊肿可以继发细菌感染。包虫性肝脓肿最好的诊断是血清学诊断。间接血细胞凝集反应是特异性试验，但对于包虫病敏感性差。实验滴度 1∶512 为阳性，1∶128 为可疑，1∶32 为阴性。相比而言，补体结合试验中 80% 的包虫病患者为阳性。免疫电泳分析的敏感性和特异性较高。两个血清学试验结合起来诊断有效率可达 94% 以上[66]。如果考虑到囊肿为炎性或者为阿米巴性脓肿，可以行诊断性抽吸，但是不能诊断包虫病。腹部平片或者 CT 中包虫囊或子囊显示为钙化影，在阿米巴脓肿时没有钙化影（图 105-10）。

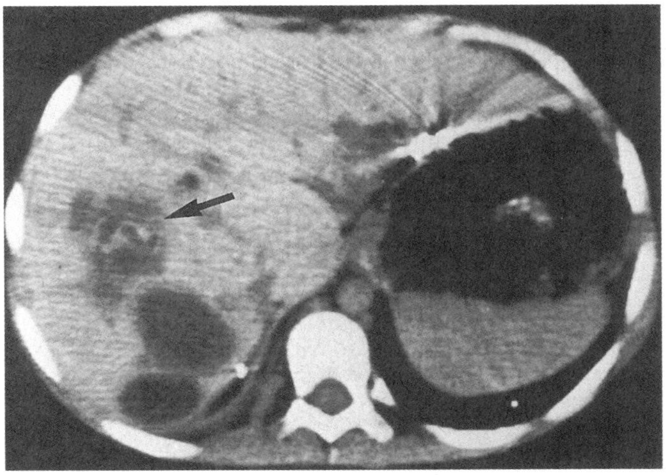

图 105-10 CT 扫描显示一些肝脓肿，其中一个（箭头）含有包虫病特征性的子囊肿。

包虫囊肿的药物治疗包括第二代驱虫药阿苯达唑。尽管有些资料提示阿苯达唑不降低术前肝脏包虫囊生存能力，但可以减少术后复发率[57,75]。

外科治疗成功依赖于肝脏隔离，应用高渗盐水或聚维酮碘海绵处理，防止囊内液渗出。囊液吸出后，用高渗盐水（20%）或者聚维酮碘灌洗囊肿来杀死所有子囊。但是，这些方法值得讨论[72]。然后将囊肿去顶，所有的子囊也被去除。有些学者建议不仅仅去除囊肿的复层膜，还应去除整个囊周壁[72,75]。标准切除囊周复发率为10%~20%，而根治性切除囊周壁后复发率小于2%[72,75]。

（沈涤华译 李 龙校）

参考文献

1. Ahsan T, Jehangir MU, Mahmood T, et al: Amoebic versus pyogenic liver abscess. J Pak Med Assoc 2002;52:497-501.
2. Al-Homaidhi HS, Sukerek H, Klein M, et al: Biliary dyskinesia in children. Pediatr Surg Int 2002;18:357-360.
3. Almond PS, Adolph VR, Steiner R, et al: Calculous disease of the biliary tract in infants after neonatal extracorporeal membrane oxygenation. J Perinatol 1992;12:18-20.
4. Al-Salem AH, Qaisruddin S: The significance of biliary sludge in children with sickle cell disease. Pediatr Surg Int 1998;13:14-16.
5. Baetz-Greenwalt B, Goske M: Intra-abdominal infection. In Wylie R, Hyams JS (eds): Pediatric Gastrointestinal Disease: Pathophysiology, Diagnosis, Management. Philadelphia, WB Saunders, 1993.
6. Bates GC, Brown CH: Incidence of gallbladder disease in chronic hemolytic anemia (spherocytosis). Gastroenterology 1952;21:104-109.
7. Bhattacharyya N, Wayne AS, Kevy SV, Shamberger RC: Perioperative management for cholecystectomy in sickle cell disease. J Pediatr Surg 1993;28:72-75.
8. Bilfinger TV, Hayden CK, Oldham KT, et al: Pyogenic liver abscesses in nonimmunocompromised children. South Med J 1986;79:37-40.
9. Birkett DH: Spilled cells, spilled clips, spilled stones. Surg Endosc 1995;9:269-271.
10. Bishop WP, Kao SCS: Prolonged postprandial abdominal pain following Kawasaki syndrome with acute gallbladder hydrops: Association with impaired gallbladder emptying. J Pediatr Gastroenterol Nutr 1991;13:307-311.
11. Blessmann J, Pham L Van, Nu Pat, et al: Epidemiology of amebiasis in a region of high incidence of amebic liver abscess in Central Vietnam. Am J Trop Med Hyg 2002;66:578-583.
12. Blessmann J, Binh HD, Hung DM, et al: Treatment of amoebic liver abscess with metronidazole alone or in combination with ultrasound-guided needle aspiration: A comparative, prospective and randomized study. Trop Med Int Health 2003;8:1030-1034.
13. Borgna-Pignatti C, DeStefano P, Pajno D, et al: Cholelithiasis in children with thalassemia major: An ultrasonographic study. J Pediatr 1981;99:243-244.
14. Branum GD, Tyson GS, Branum MA, et al: Hepatic abscess: Changes in etiology, diagnosis and management. Ann Surg 1990;212:655-662.
15. Brook I, Fraizer EH: Role of anaerobic bacteria in liver abscesses in children. Pediatr Infect Dis J 1993;12:743-747.
16. Brugge WR, Brand DL, Atkins HL, et al: Gallbladder dyskinesia in chronic acalculous cholecystitis. Dig Dis Sci 1986;31:461-467.
17. Carbajo Ferreira AJ, Urbaez Romero M, Medina Benitez W, et al: Biliary lithiasis in childhood. An Esp Pediatr 1992;36:281-284.
18. Carithers HA: Cat-scratch disease: Notes on its history. Am J Dis Child 1990;119:200-203.
19. Carlin CB, Kent RB Jr, Laws HL: Spilled gallstones—complications of abdominal-wall abscesses. Surg Endosc 1995;9:341-343.
20. Carney DE, Evan R, Kokoska ER, et al: Predictors of successful outcome after cholecystectomy for biliary dyskinesia. J Pediatr Surg 2004;39:813-816.
21. Cay A, Imamoglu M, Kosucu P, et al: Gallbladder dyskinesia: A cause of chronic abdominal pain in children. Eur J Pediatr Surg 2003;13:302-306.
22. Chamberlain JW, Hight DW: Acute hydrops of the gallbladder in childhood. Surgery 1970;68:899-905.
23. Charara AI, Rockey DC: Pyogenic liver abscess. Curr Treat Op Gastroenterol 2002;5:437.
24. Chemaly RF, Hall GS, Keys TF, et al: Microbiology of liver abscesses and the predictive value of abscess Gram stain and associated blood cultures. Diagn Microbiol Infect Dis 2003;46:245-248.
25. Chittmittrapap S, Buachum V, Dharmklong-at A: Cholelithiasis in thalassemic children. Pediatr Surg Int 1990;5:114-117.
26. Choi YS, Sharma B: Gallbladder hydrops in mucocutaneous lymph node syndrome. South Med J 1989;82:397-398.
27. Chusid MJ: Pyogenic hepatic abscesses in infancy and childhood. Pediatrics 1978;62:554-555.
28. Conter RL, Tomkins RK, Longmire WP Jr, et al: Differentiation of pyogenic from amebic hepatic abscesses. Surg Gynecol Obstet 1986;162:114-120.
29. Cooperberg PL, Burhenne HJ: Real-time ultrasonography: Diagnostic treatment of choice in calculous gallbladder disease. N Engl J Med 1980;302:1277-1279.
30. Cunningham JJ, Houlihan SM, Altay C: Cholecystosonography in children with sickle cell disease: Technical approach and clinical results. J Clin Ultrasound 1981;9:231-235.
31. DeCaluwe D, Akl U, Corbally M: Cholecystectomy versus cholecystolithotomy for cholelithiasis in childhood: Long-term outcome. J Pediatr Surg 2001;36:1518-1521.
32. deRosa F, Teggi A: Treatment of *Echinococcus granulosus* hydatid disease with albendazole. Ann Trop Med Parasital 1990;84:467-472.
33. Edwards KM, Glick AD, Greene HL: Intrahepatic cholangitis associated with mucocutaneous lymph node syndrome. J Pediatr Gastroenterol Nutr 1985;4:140-142.
34. El-Shafie M, Mah CL: Transient gallbladder distention in sick premature infants: The value of ultrasonography and radionuclide scintigraphy. Pediatr Radiol 1986;16:468-471.
35. Esposito C, Gonzalez Sabin MA, Corcione F, et al: Results and complications of laparoscopic cholecystectomy in childhood. Surg Endosc 2001;15:890-892.
36. Everson GT, Nemeth A, Kourourian S, et al: Gallbladder

function is altered in sickle hemoglobinopathy. Gastroenterology 1989;96:1307-1316.
37. Fabian TC, Croce, MA, Stanford GG, et al: Factors affecting morbidity following hepatic trauma: A prospective analysis of 482 injuries. Ann Surg 1991;213:540-547.
38. Flancbaum L, Alden SM: Morphine cholescintigraphy. Surg Gynecol Obstet 1990;171:227-232.
39. Garrison RN, Polk HC: Liver abscess and subphrenic abscess. In Blumgart LH (ed): Surgery of the Liver and Biliary Tract. New York, Churchill Livingstone, 1998.
40. Geis WP, Schultz KA, Giacchino JL, et al: The fate of unruptured intrahepatic hematomas. Surgery 1981;90: 689-697.
41. Gollin G, Raschbaum GR, Moorthy C, et al: Cholecystectomy for suspected biliary dyskinesia in children with chronic abdominal pain. J Pediatr Surg 1999;34:854-857.
42. Grois N, Mostbeck G, Scherrer R, et al: Hepatic and splenic abscesses—a common complication of intensive chemotherapy of acute myeloid leukemia (AML): A prospective study. Ann Hematol 1991;63:33-38.
43. Haberkern CM, Neumayr LD, Orringer EP, et al: Cholecystectomy in sickle cell anemia patients: perioperative outcome of 364 cases from the National Preoperative Transfusion Study. Preoperative Transfusion in Sickle Cell Disease Study Group. Blood 1997;89:1533-1542.
44. Hadigan C, Fishman SJ, Connolly LP, et al: Stimulation with fatty meal (Lipomul) to assess gallbladder emptying in children with chronic acalculous cholecystitis. J Pediatr Gastroenterol Nutr 2003;37:178-182.
45. Harrington E, Bleicher MA: Cryptogenic hepatic abscess in two uncompromised children. J Pediatr Surg 1980;15: 660-662.
46. Holcomb GW III: Pediatric laparoscopic cholecystectomy: An initial five-year experience. Pediatr Ann 1993;22: 657-662.
47. Holcomb GW III, Morgan WM III, Neblett WW III, et al: Laparoscopic cholecystectomy in children: Lessons learned from the first 100 patients. J Pediatr Surg 1999;34:1236-1240.
48. Holcomb GW III, Sharp KW, Neblett WW III, et al: Laparoscopic cholecystectomy in infants and children: Modifications and cost analysis. J Pediatr Surg 1994;29: 900-904.
49. Holcomb GW Jr, O'Neill JA Jr, Holcomb GW III: Cholecystitis, cholelithiasis and common duct stenosis in children and adolescents. Ann Surg 1980;191:626-635.
50. Holgersen LO, Stolar C, Berdon WE, et al: Therapeutic and diagnostic implications of acquired choledochal obstruction in infancy; spontaneous resolution in three infants. J Pediatr Surg 1990;25:1027-1029.
51. Holzman MD, Sharp K, Holcomb GW III: An alternative technique for laparoscopic cholangiography. Surg Endosc 1994;8:927-930.
52. Hotez PJ, Strickland AD: Amebiasis. In Feigin RD, Cherry JD (eds): Textbook of Pediatric Infectious Diseases, 4th ed. Philadelphia, WB Saunders 1998;2389.
53. Imamoglu M, Sarihan H, Sari A, et al: Acute acalculous cholecystitis in children: Diagnosis and treatment. J Pediatr Surg 2002;37:36-39.
54. Jacir NN, Anderson KD, Eichelberger M, et al: Cholelithiasis in infancy: Resolution of gallstones in three or four infants. J Pediatr Surg 1986;21:567-569.
55. Jamil B, Hamid SS: Abscesses in the liver: Amoebic or pyogenic? J Pak Med Assoc 2002;52:495-496.
56. Kaplan SL: Pyogenic liver abscess. In Feigin RD, Cherry JD (eds): Textbook of Pediatric Infectious Disease. Philadelphia, WB Saunders, 1987.
57. Karpathios T, Syriopoulou V, Nicolaidou P, et al: Mebendazole and the treatment of hydatid cysts. Am J Dis Child 1984;59:894-896.
58. Katzenstein D, Rickerson V, Braude A: New concepts of amebic liver abscess derived from hepatic imaging, serodiagnosis, and hepatic enzymes in 67 consecutive cases in San Diego. Medicine (Baltimore) 1982;61:237-246.
59. Kays DW: Pediatric liver cysts and abscesses. Semin Pediatr Surg 1992;1:107-114.
60. King DR, Ginn-Pease ME, Lloyd TV, et al: Parenteral nutrition with associated cholelithiasis: Another iatrogenic disease of infants and children. J Pediatr Surg 1987;22: 593-596.
61. Kirtley JA Jr, Holcomb GW Jr: Surgical management of diseases of the gallbladder and common duct in children and adolescents. Am J Surg 1966;111:39-46.
62. Klatchko BA, Schwartz SI: Diagnostic and therapeutic approaches to pyogenic abscess of the liver. Surg Gynecol Obstet 1989;168:332-336.
63. Komura J, Yano H, Tanaka Y, et al: Increased incidence of cholestasis during total parenteral nutrition in children—factors affecting stone formation. Kurume Med J 1993; 40:7-11.
64. Kumar R, Nguyen K, Shun A: Gallstones and common bile duct calculi in infancy and childhood. Aust N Z J Surg 2000; 70:188-191.
65. Lachman BS, Lazerson J, Starshak RJ, et al: The prevalence of cholelithiasis in sickle cell disease as diagnosed by ultrasound and cholecystography. Pediatrics 1979;64:601-603.
66. Lewis RT, Barkun J: Infection in the upper abdomen: Biliary tract, pancreas, liver, and spleen. In Meakins JL (ed): Surgical Infections. New York, Scientific American, 1994.
67. Lindberg MC: Hepatobiliary complications of oral contraceptives. J Gen Intern Med 1992;7:199-209.
68. Lobe TE: Cholelithiasis and cholecystitis in children. Semin Pediatr Surg 2000;9:170.
69. Lofi M, Hashemian H: Hydatid disease of the liver and its treatment. Int Surg 1973;3:166-168.
70. Lugo-Vicente HL: Gallbladder dyskinesia in children. JSLS 1997;1:61-64.
71. Lugo-Vicente HL: Trends in management of gallbladder disorders in children. Pediatr Surg Int 1997;12:348-352
72. Magistrelli P, Masetti R, Coppola R, et al: Surgical treatment of hydatid disease of the liver. Arch Surg 1991;126:518-522.
73. Mah D, Wales P, Njere I, et al: Management of suspected common bile duct stones in children: Role of selective intraoperative cholangiogram and endoscopic retrograde cholangiopancreatography. J Pediatr Surg 2004;39: 808-812.
74. Manji N, Bistrian BR, Mascioli EA, et al: Gallstone disease in patients with severe short bowel syndrome dependent on parenteral nutrition. J Parent Enter Nutr 1989;13:461-464.
75. Manterola C, Barroso M, Vial M, et al: Liver abscess of hydatid origin: Clinical features and results of aggressive treatment. ANZ J Surg 2003;73:220-224.
76. Marglieth AM: Antibiotic therapy for cat scratch disease: Clinical study of therapeutic outcome in 268 patients and a review of the literature. Pediatr Infect Dis 1992;11:474-478.
77. Matalack JJ, Jaffe R: Granulomatous hepatitis in three children due to cat-scratch disease without peripheral adenopathy: An unrecognized cause of fever of unknown origin. Am J Dis Child 1993;147:949-953.
78. Matos C, Avni EF, VanGansbeke D, et al: Total parenteral nutrition (TPN) and gallbladder diseases in neonates. J Ultrasound Med 1987;6:243-248.
79. Maxwell AJ, Mamtora A: Fungal liver abscesses in acute

leukemia: A report of two cases. Clin Radiol 1988;39:197-202.
80. McDermott EWM, Alkhalifa K, Murphy JJ: Laparoscopic cholecystectomy without exchange transfusion in sickle cell disease. Lancet 1993;342:1181.
81. Michail S, Preud'Homme D, Christian J, et al: Laparoscopic cholecystectomy: Effective treatment for chronic abdominal pain in children with acalculous biliary pain. J Pediatr Surg 2001;36:1394-1396.
82. Milas M, Ricketts RR, Amerson JR, et al: Management of biliary tract stones in heart transplant patients. Ann Surg 1996;223:747-753.
83. Misra DC, Blossom GB, Fink-Bennett D, et al: Results of surgical therapy for biliary dyskinesia. Arch Surg 1991; 126:957-960.
84. Mount AP: Liver Disorders in Childhood, 3rd ed. Oxford, Butterworth-Heinemann, 1994.
85. Nazir Z, Moazam F: Amebic liver abscess in children. Pediatr Infect Dis J 1993;12:929-932.
86. Newman KD, Powell DM, Holcomb GW III: The management of choledocholithiasis in children in the era of laparoscopic cholecystectomy. J Pediatr Surg 1997;32: 1116-1119.
87. Nordestgaard AG, Stapelford L, Worthen N: Contemporary management of amebic liver abscess. Am Surg 1992;58: 315-320.
88. Ostlie DJ, Holcomb GW III: The use of stab incisions for instrument access in laparoscopic operations. J Pediatr Surg 2003;38:1837-1840.
89. Owens S, Yeko TR, Bloy R, et al: Laparoscopic treatment of painful perihepatic adhesions in Fitz-Hugh-Curtis syndrome. Obstet Gynecol 1991;78:542-543.
90. Pastakia B, Shawker TH, Thaler M, et al: Hepatosplenic candidiasis: Wheels within wheels. Radiology 1988;166: 417-421.
91. Petri WA Jr, Sing U: Diagnosis and management of amebiasis. Clin Infect Dis 1999;29:1117-1125.
92. Pineiro-Carrerro VM, Andres JM: Morbidity and mortality in children with pyogenic liver abscess. Am J Dis Child 1989; 143:1424-1427.
93. Quigley EM, Marsh MN, Shaffer JL, et al: Hepatobiliary complications of total parenteral nutrition. Gastroenterology 1993;104:286-301.
94. Reed DN Jr, Fernandez M, Hicks RD: Kinevac-assisted cholescintigraphy as an accurate predictor of chronic acalculous gallbladder disease and the likelihood of symptom relief with cholecystectomy. Am Surg 1993;59:273-277.
95. Rescorla FJ: Cholelithiasis, cholecystitis, and common bile duct stones. Curr Opin Pediatr 1997;9:276-282.
96. Ris HW: Perihepatitis (Fitz-Hugh–Curtis syndrome): A review and case presentation. J Adolesc Health Care 1984;5:272-276.
97. Rizkallah MF, Meyer L, Nayoub EM: Hepatic and splenic abscesses in cat-scratch disease. Pediatr Infect Dis J 1988; 7:191-195.
98. Roy CC, Belli DC: Hepatobiliary complications associated with TPN: An enigma. J Am Coll Nutr 1985;4:651-660.
99. Sackmann M, Delius M, Sauerbruch T, et al: Shock-wave lithotripsy of gallbladder stones: The first 175 patients. N Engl J Med 1988;318:393-397.
100. Sandler A, Winkel G, Kimura K, et al: The role of prophylactic cholecystectomy during splenectomy in children with hereditary spherocytosis. J Pediatr Surg 1999;34: 1077-1078.
101. Sandoval C, Stringel G, Ozkaynak MF, et al: Perioperative management of children with sickle cell disease undergoing laparoscopic surgery. JSLS 2002;6:29-33.
102. Sarnaik S, Slovis TL, Corbett DP, et al: Incidence of cholelithiasis in sickle cell anemia using the ultrasonic gray-scale technique. J Pediatr 1980;96:1005-1008.
103. Schoenfield LJ, Berci G, Carnovale RL, et al: The effect of ursodiol on the efficacy and safety of extracorporeal shock-wave lithotripsy of gallstones: The Dornier National Biliary Lithotripsy study. N Engl J Med 1990;323:1239-1245.
104. Schoenfield LJ, Lachin JM, Steering Committee, National Cooperative Gallstone Study Group: Chenodiol (chenodeoxycholic acid) for dissolution of gallstones; The National Cooperative Gallstone Study: A controlled trial of efficacy and safety. Ann Intern Med 1981;95:257-282.
105. Scobie WB, Bentley JF: Hydrops of the gallbladder in a newborn infant. J Pediatr Surg 1969;4:457-459.
106. Shah RS, Blakely ML, Lobe TE: The role of laparoscopy in the management of common bile duct obstruction in children. Surg Endosc 2001;15:1353-1355.
107. Shew SB, Ostlie DJ, Holcomb GW III: Robotic telescopic assistance in pediatric laparoscopic surgery. Pediatr Endosurg Innovative Tech 2003;7:371-376.
108. Shocket E: Abdominal abscess from gallstones spilled at laparoscopic cholecystectomy. Surg Endosc 1995;9: 344-347.
109. Snyder CL, Ferrell KL, Saltzman DA, et al: Operative therapy of gallbladder disease in patients with cystic fibrosis. Am J Surg 1989;157:557-561.
110. Stanley SL Jr: Amoebiasis. Lancet 2003;361:1025-1034.
111. Stephens CG, Scott RB: Cholelithiasis in sickle cell anemia. Arch Intern Med 1980;140:648-651.
112. Stern RC, Rothstein FC, Doershuk CF: Treatment and prognosis of symptomatic gallbladder disease in patients with cystic fibrosis. J Pediatr Gastroenterol Nutr 1986;5: 35-40.
113. Stringel G, Beneck D, Bostwick HE: Polypoid lesions of the gallbladder in children. JSLS 1997;1:247-249.
114. Stringer MD, Ceylan H, Ward K, et al: Gallbladder polyps in children—classification and management. J Pediatr Surg 2003;38:1680-1684.
115. Stringer MD, Taylor DR, Soloway RD: Gallstone composition: Are children different? J Pediatr 2003;142: 435-440.
116. St-Vil D, Yazbeck S, Luks FL, et al: Cholelithiasis in newborns and infants. J Pediatr Surg 1992;27:1305-1307.
117. Tagge EP, Hebra A, Goldberg A, et al: Pediatric laparoscopic biliary tract surgery. Semin Pediatr Surg 1998;7: 202-206.
118. Tai YT, Shieh CC, Wang SM, et al: Neonatal solitary liver abscess: Report of one case. Acta Paediatr Taiwan 2002;43: 50-52.
119. Tan YM, Chee SP, Soo KC, et al: Ocular manifestations and complications of pyogenic liver abscess. World J Surg 2004;28:38-42.
120. The American Academy of Pediatrics: Amebiasis. In Pickering LK (ed): 2000 Redbook: Report of the Committee on Infectious Diseases, 25th ed. Elk Grove Village, IL, American Academy of Pediatrics, 2000.
121 Ure BM, deJong MM, Bax KN, et al: Outcome after laparoscopic cholecystectomy and cholecystectomy in children with symptomatic cholecystolithiasis: A preliminary report. Pediatr Surg 2001;17:396-398.
122. Vachon L, Diament MJ, Stanley P: Percutaneous drainage of hepatic abscesses in children. J Pediatr Surg 1986;21: 366-368.
123. Waldhausen JHT, Graham DD, Tapper D: Routine intraoperative cholangiography during laparoscopic cholecystectomy minimizes unnecessary endoscopic retrograde

cholangiopancreatography in children. J Pediatr Surg 2001;36:881-884.
124. Wales PW, Carver E, Crawford MW, et al: Acute chest syndrome after abdominal surgery in children with sickle cell disease: Is a laparoscopic approach better? J Pediatr Surg 2001;36:718-721.
125. Wang W, Lee WJ, Wei PL, et al: Laparoscopic drainage of pyogenic liver abscesses. Surg Today 2004;34:323-325.
126. Ware R, Filston HC, Schultz WH, et al: Elective cholecystectomy in children with sickle hemoglobinopathies. Ann Surg 1988;208:17-22.
127. Weinstein S, Lipsitz EC, Addonizio L, Stolar CJ: Cholelithiasis in pediatric cardiac transplant patients on cyclosporine. J Pediatr Surg 1995;30:61-64.
128. Weirich W: Hydatid disease of the liver. Am J Surg 1979; 138:805-808.
129. Winter SS, Kinney TR, Ware RE: Gallbladder sludge in children with sickle cell disease. J Pediatr 1994;125: 747-749.
130. Wood J, Holland AJ, Shun A, et al: Biliary dyskinesia: Is the problem with Oddi? Pediatr Surg 2004;20:83-86.
131. Zargar SA, Javod G, Khan BA, et al: Endoscopic sphincterotomy in the management of bile duct stones in children. Am J Gastroenterol 2003;98:586-589.

第 106 章

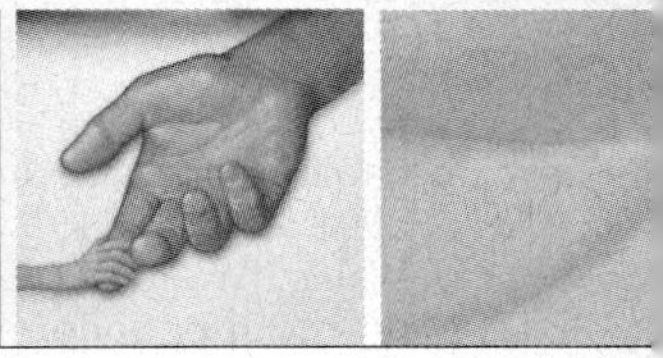

门脉高压症

Riccardo Superina

一个认为科学是无所不能或自然可以完成非自然事情的人是无知的，比缺乏学习更疯狂。我们的经验被由自然或艺术创造出来的仪器所限制。如果一个人感染了无药可医的疾病，不要期望药物能战胜病魔。

——希波克拉底

1651 门脉高压症的治疗在近数十年来取得了令人瞩目的改变，这一改变在儿童中更有意义。新的影像学技术以及药物和药物治疗的改善，使得已经存在的新的外科技术以精确的方式寻找潜在的导致门脉压力升高的疾病。

历史回顾

意大利内科医生和病理学家 Guido Banti 最早描述了脾大、贫血及肝硬化之间的关系。1903 年，由 Florence 施行了第一例用于治疗脾功能亢进的脾切除术。这个症候群后来被称作 Banti 综合征（Banti's syndrome）[168]。

更早期，德国解剖学家 Nikolai Eck 在狗的门静脉与下腔静脉之间建立了一个通道。稍后的研究说明门静脉与体静脉的合流与门体静脉性脑病的高血氨症发生有关[71,125]。

第一例门体静脉分流术报道于 20 世纪 50 年代与 60 年代之间[30,31,106,168]。当发现肠系膜静脉血流入体静脉可以减轻脑病后，出现了更多类型的选择性门体静脉分流术[77,127,228,229]。而报道的非分流性手术则主要用于阻断胃和食管的血流[206]。

最后，随着肝移植术的出现，替换患病器官以治疗由进展性和未治愈的肝病引起的门脉高压症，比有较高并发症、只能在短时间内改善症状的姑息性手术治疗要好[26,78,137,202]。

胚胎学和解剖学

门静脉的发育经过一个涉及原始血管形成和退化的复杂过程，并随后影响出生时已成熟的门脉循环系统的循环改变。

左、右脐肠系膜静脉在胚胎 4～6 周引流从卵黄囊发育而来的肠管血流。同时，脐静脉从胚胎胎盘传输血液。来自脐和脐肠系膜静脉的血液通过发育中的肝窦间隙进入肝血管，回流至发育中的心脏。一些血液从脐静脉经肝旁途径通过静脉导管进入静脉窦。尽管在胚胎早期脐肠系膜静脉与许多中间血管交通，但右侧的血管在第六周时退化并消失。左侧的血管发育为永久的门静脉，通过肠系膜上静脉及其分支引流肠系膜静脉床。右脐静脉也退化，左脐静脉直到出生后不久因栓塞而关闭，成为圆韧带。

门静脉的形成也受胰头后方的脾静脉及肠系膜上静脉的影响。冠状静脉引流胃静脉床，在脾肠系膜静脉汇合处或稍远端的位置汇入门静脉，肠系膜下静脉在胰后方、沿脾静脉长轴的任一位置汇入脾静脉。

肝动脉解剖存在相对多的变异，但门静脉的变异较少。肝外静脉主干分为左右两支。左支位于肝第Ⅳ段表面供应肝左叶，再向前转向Ⅱ、Ⅲ、Ⅳ段之间的 16
Rex 隐窝，最后供应这些肝段。肝右支正位于肝床被膜之前，分为前、后扇形分支。

很容易想象从原始的胚胎期脐肠系膜静脉发育形成单一的门静脉过程中，一系列的静脉交汇分支间复杂的相互连接、退化关闭等作用可能会出错。生物步骤序列的失调可能导致静脉空洞的形成。出生后脐静脉形成的血栓也可以进入肝门静脉并阻塞肝外静脉血流。这些过程导致了肝外或肝内门脉高压综合征的发生。

定义

肠系膜血管床包括来自小肠、胃、脾和胰腺的血流，流动受影响时发生门脉压力增高。门脉高压最常见病因是这些血管自然阻塞[210]。也就是说，来自脐肠系膜血管床经肝流向心脏的肝前血流出现阻碍。但回流至肝脏的血量增加或供应肝的静脉与动脉之间血管的直接交通使得血管床暴露于异常的高压下，也可以导致门静脉高压症。

当门静脉血管床的压力超过 5～8 cmH_2O 或肝静脉与体循环之间的压力梯度超过 5 cmH_2O 时，称为门脉高压症。无论是什么病因，当体循环的压力超过这些数值时，一系列的物理改变就会导致门脉高压症所有症状的出现。

侧支循环

正常情况下，随着门静脉压力的增加，从肠系膜上静脉及其属支进入肝脏的血流将改变其返回心脏的途径。门体静脉网之间侧支形成最容易的三条途径位于直肠、脐固及胃食管区域。在直肠，直肠上静脉与直肠下、中静脉的分支之间存在的丰富的直肠血管丛是一个通路。在肝圆韧带与脐中韧带之间，小的静脉（脐周部）在前腹壁、脐孔、下腹壁和髂部形成一个吻合支。最后，胃静脉通过引流肝血液进入半奇静脉的黏膜下静脉丛与食管静脉交通。

一些因门脉高压而自发分流的区域还有：结肠、十二指肠静脉和左肾静脉之间；Sappey 附属门脉系统，其分支穿过圆韧带和镰状韧带（尤其是后者），与上腹部和乳内静脉交汇，通过膈肌静脉与奇静脉连接；脐周血管通过圆韧带从肝门到脐部，形成被称为“海蛇头”的极其迂曲的血管团；肠壁静脉丛（Retzius 静脉）联系肠血管与下腔静脉及其腹腔后分支的血管网；肠系膜下静脉和开放汇入下腹壁的直肠静脉；以及少见的未闭的静脉导管提供了门静脉和下腔静脉间的直接通路。

表 106-1 门静脉高压症的分类

类型	病因
肝细胞	肝纤维化增加的肝内在疾病（见表 106-2）
血管	
肝前性	肝外门静脉栓塞
	门静脉海绵样变性
	门静脉外在性狭窄
肝后性	Budd-Chiari 综合征
	内在瓣膜
	肝静脉管径狭窄
高分流性（高动力性）	动静脉交通——肝内或肝外型
	先天性
	获得性

病因：疾病分类

门静脉高压症分为两类：（1）肝细胞损伤和肝纤维化而引起的门静脉高压症，（2）原发性血管因素引起的门静脉高压症（表 106-1）。

肝细胞损伤

表 106-2 列举了导致儿童门静脉高压的常见原因。各种毒性物质引起肝细胞损伤，肝纤维化启动并进展，最终导致肝硬化。肝组织进展性损害以及正常肝组织被纤维组织取代，导致流经肝脏的血流阻力增高。肝细胞损伤引起的胶原沉积是炎性因子如骨桥蛋

表 106-2 导致门脉高压症的肝细胞疾病

胆道闭锁
感染后肝硬化
先天性肝纤维化
先天性胆汁酸代谢异常
硬化性胆管炎
自身免疫性肝炎
药物毒性
代谢性疾病（如 α_1-抗胰蛋白酶缺乏）

白转录和星形细胞等介导的复杂过程[40]。星形细胞是肝窦细胞的正常组成成分，是肝纤维化时细胞外基质过度增生的最初来源[44,75]。它能改变自身的表型，由正常肝动脉平衡时的静止表型转变为在肝细胞损伤
1653 期经历成纤维细胞分化或激活的表型。凋亡错误或损伤的持续存在引起星形细胞活力和数量的失调，从而导致细胞外基质蛋白进行性沉积。最终，肝窦内胶原的过度沉积导致门静脉高压。

血管因素

肝前性门静脉高压

肝外水平的血管阻塞引起肝前性门静脉高压。儿童和成人中均可见到肝外门静脉栓塞，它可能是一种先天性或年长儿的获得性损害。即使这些症状有一定损害性，但因肝功能相对正常，患者能很好地耐受血管曲张出血[11,84]。门静脉主干闭塞将导致血管重建并形成一系列小的侧支血管，在超声检查中表现为静脉海绵样变性（图 106-1）。在大多数病例中，肝结构中的门静脉是完好的。门静脉血栓形成与脐炎、出生时脐部血管进行过仪器检查或插管、婴儿期败血症、脱

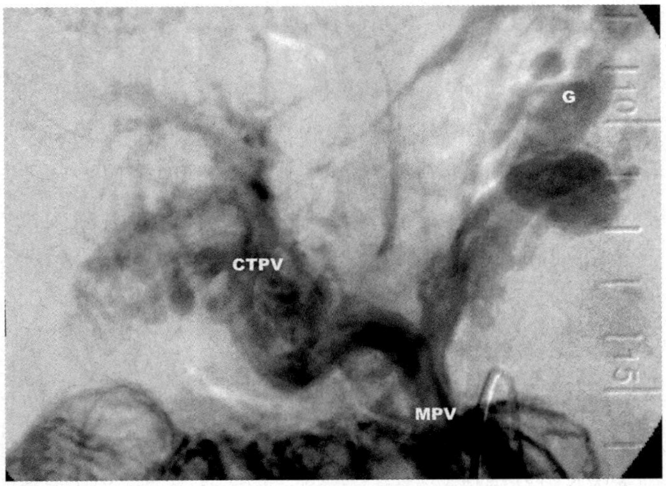

图 106-1 1 例肝外型门静脉梗阻和食管静脉曲张出血儿童的数字造影检查。这是经肠系膜上动脉注射造影剂的静脉影像。造影显示门静脉主干近端（MPV），门静脉内海绵样变（CTPV），正常肝内门静脉解剖结构缺失，以及从肝脏分流血液进入胃食管连接处和食管曲张静脉的大冠状静脉（G）。

水、肿块引起的血管外压迫等有关。这些损伤可以是炎症性的或恶性的。例如，肝门组织胞浆菌病引起的淋巴结反应性增多或肝门非 Hodgkin 淋巴瘤的压迫等。

与存在肝脏疾病的患儿不同，肝外静脉栓塞的儿童可以状态良好而突然发病。以作者的经验，约 50% 的患儿可出现无先兆的出血或胃底血管破裂便血。其他病例可能被诊断为原因不明的脾大和怀疑为血液系统恶性肿瘤。

脾功能亢进通常很明显，血小板计数少于 50 000、白细胞计数低于 1000 的并不少见。一些儿童需要造血生长因子，以降低血小板减少症或严重的白细胞减少症导致细菌感染引起的自发出血[160]。

过去，治疗被两种原则引导：患儿能很好地耐受出血和手术治疗非常困难且很少成功。因此，这些儿童以经常住院、多次输血和因肝硬化或食管静脉曲张重复进行内镜检查为特征。这种情况一直没有改变，直到儿童的探索性手术治疗越来越多，可信而有效的手术方法出现为止。手术以减轻肠系膜循环压力为主，包括选择性和非选择性门体静脉分流。因非选择性分流手术在门脉高压症并发出血的儿童中存在潜在的分流后脑病的危险，所以选择性分流手术如 Warren 手术在儿童中很受欢迎。一个大规模手术系列报道显示，在 50 例肝外型门脉栓塞的儿童中，选择性分流手术有很好的疗效，死亡率为零[25]。一些报道显示，随着治疗小婴儿肝病的手术专家的经验积累和儿童肝移植的出现及小血管吻合技术的提高，手术治疗取得了相当好的效果[69,137,159,194,195]。最近有报道，对肝移植后门静脉栓塞的儿童采用一种将肠系膜血液转流回肝脏的手术方式，该手术方式对先天性门静脉栓塞也有效[19,59,61,62]。

肝后性门静脉高压症

肝后性门静脉高压由引流肝脏血液进入下腔静脉的大或小血管阻塞而引起。这些血管的阻塞导致肝被动充血和肝叶中心区的肝细胞坏死。除非有紧急的救
治方法，急性静脉梗阻将导致大片肝坏死和细胞死 16
亡。Budd-Chiari 综合征，有时也称为 Chiari 综合征，在 1854 年首次被报道[40,50]，它在儿童中不常见[9]。肝静脉内先天性静脉瓣膜[219]、包虫病[110]、骨髓组织增生性疾病[17,47]、血液高凝状态[22,49,102,107,111,153,174]和因经常口服避孕药而致雌激素水平增高等可引起肝

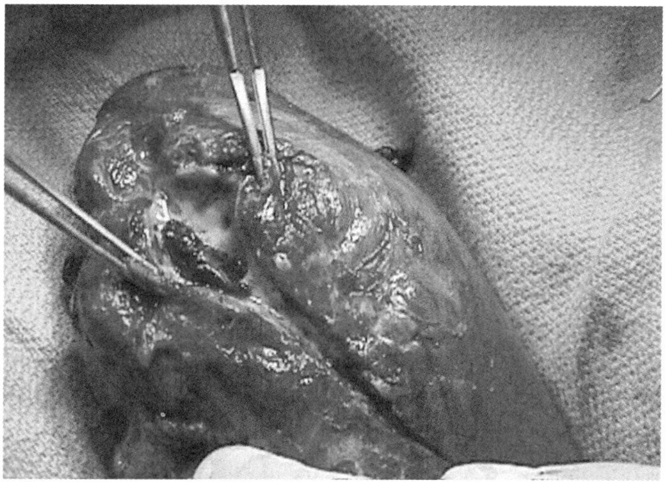

图 106-2 劈离式肝移植后因左肝Ⅱ、Ⅲ段内静脉凝血块引起的急性肝静脉阻塞。该患儿重新进行了肝移植。

内血液流出受阻[118,124,133]。静脉梗阻也可以发生在肝移植后（图 106-2）。

非血栓性肝微血管阻塞也可称为静脉闭塞性疾病，常发生于骨髓移植的患者[126,170,226,230]。白消安和环磷酰胺能引起肝内小血管的闭塞性静脉炎，并引起细胞内源性谷胱甘肽 S 转移酶储备衰竭而损伤内皮细胞[199]。另外，引起血管闭塞的还有食用含有双吡咯烷类生物碱的草药茶[117,156,197]。其他包括造影剂、雌激素和硫鸟嘌呤等也被报道与静脉闭塞性疾病有关[4,15,16,38,148,155,169,205,220]。这种疾病的死亡率较高，而且治疗只限于消除致病因素。如果可能，可联合溶栓治疗和经颈静脉肝内门体分流术[16,18,134]。

高分流状态

肠系膜循环中先天性或获得性动静脉交通很少见，但也是引起门静脉高压的已知原因。因门静脉循环的动静脉之间异常交通而引起门脉高压症也被称为高动力性门脉高压[94]，因为是高动力性循环导致了门静脉压力的增高。患者肝功能良好，表现为胃肠道出血、腹水或脾大。动静脉交通的位置变异很大，有报道脾、胃动脉为交通位点，肝实质内的肝动脉是更常见的交通位点。各年龄组均有动静脉瘘引起门脉高压的报道[6,23,73,93]，大多数是先天性的，但也有一些是获得性的，可因致病性病原体或医源性行为引起[87,99,109,113,157,167,204,233,237]。因动静脉交通的位置不同，其临床表现各异。曲张的血管出血可以很严重，而且因暴露于动脉压力，常规的治疗方法常不容易控制病情[68]。

治疗高流量的动静瘘需要阻断动静脉之间的异常交通。虽然手术，包括半肝切除术[23]和手术结扎肝外瘘管[20,68]，在某种意义上能去除瘘管，但是在这种情况下，通过放射学方法并采用经导管选择性栓塞阻断血流也是治疗的一种选择[6,46]。

临床表现

胃肠道出血

胃肠道出血是最常见的症状，也是门脉高压的危险征象。食管远端和胃贲门是常见的出血位点。尽管成人非曲张性血管出血的发生率为 25%[39]，但没有证据表明儿童中有类似情况[232]。在一项儿童临床表现为上消化道出血的研究中，大多数患者的出血继发于门脉高压的曲张静脉而非其他原因[203]。在世界的不同地区，门脉高压作为引起儿童上消化道出血的重要因素，其发生率各不相同。在西半球，消化性溃疡病仍旧是经内镜发现的经常引起儿童上消化道出血的病因。在任何原因引起门脉高压症的儿童中，虽然少数急性出血由门脉高压敏感性胃病所引起，但上消化道出血几乎普遍是由曲张静脉引起的[114]。所以，曲张静脉出血通常是门脉高压症儿童上消化道出血的唯一原因，也是 2 岁以上非住院患者上消化道出血最常见的原因。

曲张静脉出血可以表现为呕血、黑便或慢性贫血，出血常来源于下段食管和胃贲门。薄壁的曲张血管在升高的静脉压力下充满血液，可被胃酸或药物如阿司匹林或非类固醇类抗炎药物所腐蚀，血液流入胃内。在非进展性肝病中，出血会凝结，并积聚在胃内，引起胃扩张，最终达到动态平衡。出血可以是突发的，且常不伴随腹痛。平素健康的儿童可以呕吐大量变色或新鲜的血液。尽管这可能会令患儿及其家长极度恐慌，但出血往往会自发停止。静脉曲张也可以存在于下消化道。直肠出血很少见，常因直肠和乙状结肠静脉曲张而引起；表现为没有呕血，但会出现黑便或肉眼血便或排便次数增加。 1655

尽管大多数门脉高压患者都存在静脉曲张，但并不是所有的曲张静脉都出血。可以通过 Laplace 定律（Laplace's law）预测曲张静脉的出血危险度，即血管的透壁压与血管内的压力直接相关，与血管壁的厚度负相关[161]。然而血管内的压力并不容易测定。因此，对于成人，出血的危险度与曲张静脉的大小、肝病的严重程度和可提示上皮厚度的血管壁上红色凸纹等有关系[196]。

预测哪个患者容易出血对治疗方案的选择是很重要的，尤其是对任何类型的拟行预防性治疗的患者。据估计，约30%~50%的患者确诊时即发生静脉曲张出血[32]，且每年有10%~50%的肝病患者在第一次出血后死亡[234]。该比例在行门体静脉分流的Child A级患者和需肝移植的进展性肝病患者有所不同。非侵袭性或侵袭性手术治疗对出血风险高但未出血的患者有一定作用，可以使与出血相关的疾病的发病率与死亡率降低，并且手术并发症的危险在一个可以接受的较低范围内。

在肝外栓塞型门脉高压症儿童中，其出血所致的死亡率比肝病性门脉高压症儿童要低，而且患者常对出血耐受。然而，治疗原则相同，即早期医疗介入和落实长期治疗计划，以减少患者住院和侵袭性治疗次数。因为这些儿童门脉高压的原因是血管问题而不是肝脏本身的问题。对他们多采用手术治疗，一般能取得良好的远期效果。

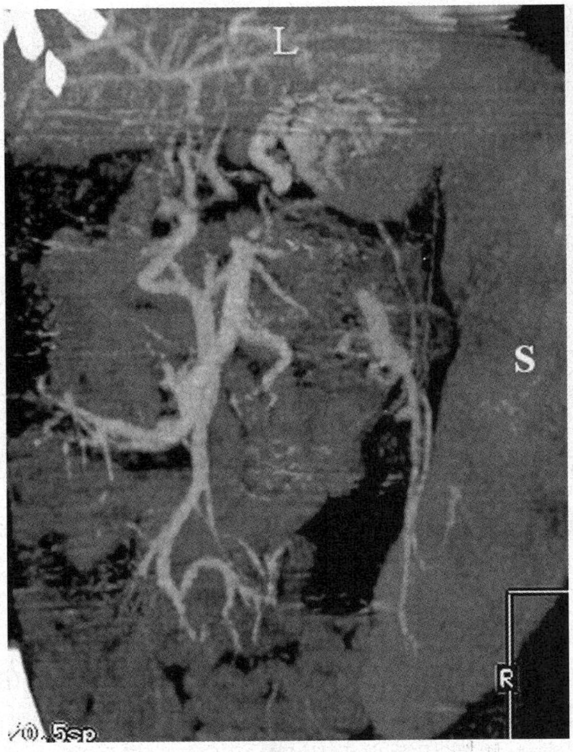

图106-3 1例有巨大脾大、严重血小板减少及粒细胞减少症的3岁女孩。CT血管成像显示延伸至盆腔的脾（S）及缩小的肝（L）。造影清楚地显示肝外门静脉栓塞和明显的肝内门静脉树。

脾功能亢进

没有其他门脉高压症状的静息脾大常是门脉高压症的第一个严重征象（图106-3）。发生于婴儿或儿童早期的脾大常被认为是血液系统恶性病变，尤其是在肝外门静脉栓塞而没有其他肝病征象的患者。随着腹部多普勒超声检查的出现，门静脉栓塞更易发现并可采取适当监测。此外，脾增大时，因脾隔离了血小板和白细胞，患者可表现为严重的血小板减少和粒细胞减少。应阻止这些患儿参加体育运动，因为即使轻微的腹部损伤也能导致脾破裂和因静脉内压力增高和血小板计数减少而引起的严重腹腔内出血。

脑病

在没有进展性肝病征象如黄疸、肝依赖性凝血因子和蛋白水平较低等患者中，脑病是极其少见的。与常在成人中出现的传统方向知觉丧失、记忆丧失和昏睡征象相比，学习障碍和行为异常是儿童脑病的症状。儿童也常伴随高血氨症[3]。

胃肠道外器官出血

严重的血小板减少可以引起血尿、月经过多、鼻出血和便血。严重病例也可以自发颅内出血，引起严重的神经系统后果。肝依赖性凝血因子缺乏也可导致出血，典型的症状发生于生殖道或鼻腔。在进展性肝病患者中，肺出血的并发症可以引起严重的呼吸系统损害。

腹水

进展性肝病儿童因合成障碍可出现腹水。腹水可伴随低蛋白血症和胶体渗透压降低。门静脉各支流的静水压增加时，毛细血管渗透性增加，导致腹腔内液体增多积聚。其他因素有毛细血管内氧化亚氮产物增加，引起血管扩张，以及代谢失调性肝硬化患者肾小管钠吸收增多[120,146,200]。Budd-Chiari 综合征及流出道梗阻也导致腹水产生。一般说来，腹水的出现是肝功能失调一个值得警惕的先兆。

肺部疾病

肺动脉高压可以发生于硬化性或非硬化性门静脉高压症患者。肺动脉高压继发于血管活性物质的增加对肺血管产生血管收缩作用或其直接的毒性作用[214]。肺动脉和门静脉高压患者血液中前列腺素 $F_{2\alpha}$、血栓素和血管紧张素 I 升高，提示这些经肝脏进入肺循环的物质在疾病中起一定的介导作用。在动物实验研究中，与对照组相比，通过结扎肝门血管导致的门脉高压伴有肺内诱导性氧化亚氮合酶升高和血红素氧合酶-1 的 mRNA 及其蛋白产物升高[186]，由此提示门静脉高压中的肺部病变与肺内的氧化亚氮及一氧化碳产物有关。

门静脉高压伴有肺动脉高压的患者在门静脉高压引起的出血发生前即出现肺部症状。这些症状包括呼吸困难或胸痛，无先兆的假死或突然死亡[189,214]。对具有进展性肺动脉高压的门脉高压患儿来说，治疗是一个问题，对这两种情况采取有效的药物治疗在应用范围及应用时间上受到限制[64,173]。

肝肺综合征的患者因肺内存在动静脉分流而引起持续低氧血症，除了门静脉高压症，还可能出现肝硬化，这也是肝肺综合征的临床征象。肝内皮素-1 产物、循环内皮素-1 及肺内内源性氧化亚氮合酶产物增加，导致这些症状的发生[88,131]。

因为肝前性门静脉高压症导致的肺动脉高压在门体静脉分流后依然存在[76]，所以肝肺综合征需要肝移植治疗[88]。门体静脉分流术将加重两者的病情[89,189]。

诊断

门静脉高压的诊断依靠父母和患儿提供的临床信息、影像学及实验室检查的综合结果。

临床资料

肝大

肝大通常是肝细胞性疾病的征象，但肝硬化的患者因肝脏缩小常触摸不到。如果肝脏触诊质地变硬或有结节，则更进一步证明肝脏病变是引起门静脉高压的原因。先天性肝纤维化的儿童常可触诊到延伸至髂嵴的巨大肝脏。静脉流出道梗阻的儿童也易触诊到增大的肝脏。

脾大

在门静脉高压症儿童中常可发现增大的脾脏，而且经常是患儿出血前常规体检时首先被发现的异常体征。脾大可出现于所有类型的门静脉高压症，对病因诊断没有帮助。

黄疸

除了进展性肝病，黄疸通常不和门静脉高压同时出现。肝外门静脉梗阻的儿童血总胆红素水平有轻微增高，但黄疸不是一个临床特征。如果门静脉高压症的患儿临床出现明显的黄疸症状，则意味着即将发生肝功能衰竭。

脑病

临床上症状明显的脑病是进展性肝病的一个征象。脑病可能因肠道蛋白负荷升高引起的急性出血而加剧，通常是进展性肝细胞疾病的征象，需要对患者进行肝移植评估。

实验室检查

对门静脉高压症病因的正确评估通常需要全面的实验室检查。在紧急情况下，出血患者常需要进行全血细胞计数和电解质水平的监测。 1657

长期存在门静脉高压的儿童常仅仅表现为血小板减少和粒细胞减少。血清直接胆红素增高、白蛋白水平降低和凝血酶原时间延长等均明显提示肝细胞疾病和肝硬化可能是引起门脉高压的根本原因。血氨水平显著升高提示门体静脉分流的出现，这在所有类型的门脉高压症中均可能发生。

肝外门静脉栓塞儿童的实验室检查特征是促凝血和纤溶途径中的肝依赖性凝血因子合成失调，但在未经详细检查时，一般不存明显的临床征象[132]。

内镜检查

在重症监护病房稳定病情以后，内镜检查可以提供上消化道出血来源的直接证据。如果存在静脉曲张，常在食管远端第三段和胃贲门处最明显。只有经过良好训练及熟悉仪器操作的医生才能对患者进行内镜检查。内镜可以提供介入治疗的机会并排除其他来源的出血，如消化性溃疡、食管 Mallory-Weiss 撕裂（胃食管撕裂综合征）或胃出血。

如果对怀疑为门静脉高压症的患者在出血之间进行内镜检查，曲张血管的征象为即将发生的出血提供了有价值的线索[92]。静脉曲张直径超过 5 mm、黏膜皱褶上的红色凸形条纹和肝功能 Child-Pugh 分级显示为进展性肝病则预示出血的风险很大，并证明医疗机构进行预防性治疗是正确的。

影像学检查

任何呕血的患儿首先应进行的影像学检查是腹部超声[116]。门静脉的情况是诊断时最重要的指标之一。肝血管的多普勒超声检查中发现门静脉多腔和栓塞是最好的诊断依据。对腹腔内主要的静脉血管包括肝静脉、脾静脉、肠系膜上静脉和下腔静脉进行评估是可能的。此外，脾的大小有助于确定临床检查的结果。也可以观察到肝实质异常，如结节、形态不一或囊肿。肾的形态也能提供有用的诊断线索，因为先天性肝纤维化的儿童常患有常染色体显性遗传的多囊肾和其他一些肾脏异常[149,127]。

CT 和磁共振血管成像检查是很好的诊断工具，在大多数情况下可以代替传统的数字化血管造影。大多数检查可以清晰地提供所有腹腔内血管信息及肝脏、胆管解剖的详细信息。CT 血管成像检查具有一些优点：检查更为迅速；与磁共振血管造影相比，可以减少影像的运动伪影等，除非磁共振检查在较长时间抑制呼吸的全身麻醉状态下进行。

传统的血管造影是一种侵袭性检查，在儿童门静脉高压中很少作为诊断工具。少数具有罕见血管畸形的病例，如腹部或肝脏的动静脉交通，可以在血管造影中得到最好的显示。而且，血管造影的可视性是进行血管造影栓塞或在畸形血管内放置支架的基础。

脾门静脉造影术在过去曾应用广泛，但以诊断为目的的脾门静脉造影术目前几乎不再使用[150,151]。

经颈静脉肝血管造影能有效地检测肝静脉压力，而且能提供肝静脉及其与腔静脉交汇处的确切影像[231]。这种技术也可以用于治疗，如放置经颈静脉肝内门体静脉分流（TIPS）或扩张先天性或获得性静脉流出道梗阻的狭窄。

肝活检

几乎所有的门静脉高压症儿童都需要进行肝活检，在大多数病例中可以经皮穿刺进行。在轻微凝血异常的儿童中，可以用维生素 K、新鲜冰冻血浆和血小板来纠正。该检查可以在重症监护病房内进行，任何肝活检的出血均能得到快速治疗。多数患凝血疾病的儿童，当凝血酶原时间明显超过 20 秒时，需要在介入性影像学器械下进行经颈静脉肝活检或在手术室经开放手术肝活检。一般情况下，限制放射科医生进行经颈静脉肝活检的因素是患者的年龄以及该技术的难度。在幼儿和小婴儿中该技术受限制最大。肝活检结果从肝外静脉栓塞病例的轻微异常到儿童慢性肝脏疾病的进展性肝纤维化和肝硬化不等。

治疗

儿童门脉高压症的治疗首先是针对疾病病理生理学本质的治疗，然后是针对症状的严重程度。

肝脏病变型门静脉高压症和那些肝脏正常、由血管畸形引起门静脉高压的儿童均不能耐受出血。急性出血会对可能已经异常的肝脏功能产生不利影响。肝脏病变和门静脉高压症患儿的预后完全依赖于肝储备能力。与存在低蛋白血症、生长障碍和凝血性疾病的患儿相比，肝硬化和合成能力储备相对稳定的儿童治疗方法完全不同。Child-Pugh 积分[51]根据患者肝储备等级分类，并依此来判断如果未治疗或采用手术治疗的预后[10,135,192,193]。最近，一种儿童终末期肝疾病评分（pediatric end-stage liver disease，PELD）可以将等待肝移植的患儿进行分级，能较准确地反映肝脏病变的严重程度[57,144]。生长发育程度与年龄符合、凝血功能正常且没有黄疸的儿童 PELD 积分较低。其门静脉高压并发症的治疗与高积分儿童有很大差异，这些患儿肝移植的效果良好。

Child-Pugh 积分为 5 或 6 分，或 PELD 积分低于 10 分的儿童 1 年的预期生存率在 90% 以上，该结果可以被认为是复杂的手术治疗缓解了门静脉高压症状。这些患儿的长期预后良好，在手术后能很好地存活，并在短期内不需要肝移植。曲张静脉出血、腹水或进展性凝血疾病的儿童 PELD 积分较高，在他们等待肝移植的过程中需要对门静脉高压采取积极的药物治疗。因为不能很好地耐受手术及较差的肝储备能力，进展性肝脏疾病的患儿不能进行其他手术治疗。

儿科医生和儿童胃肠病专家应密切随访所有门静脉高压和肝脏疾病儿童。这样，当门静脉高压进展为综合征时，患儿的父母将不会很惊讶，并通常能在医院内熟练应对。理想的情况下，在将要发生出血或将要复发时，一般采取选择性分流，这将在后面予以论述。

相反，非肝硬化的门脉高压也可能在毫无预料之中出现症状，并且首发症状即处于严重状态之下。

静脉曲张出血的药物治疗

急性曲张静脉出血的患儿需要血液及晶体液快速复苏，应用冰冻新鲜血浆替代缺乏的凝血因子并控制出血。广泛的血管内凝血、纤溶激活和循环血小板计数下降会加剧曲张静脉的出血。应用外源性凝血因子Ⅶ治疗肝合成功能损害的儿童能加强对这些患者的保护。尽管凝血因子Ⅶ替代物的昂贵价格限制了它的应用范围，但凝血因子Ⅶ的应用减少了纠正肝依赖性因子缺乏所必需的钠盐和液体量[7,41]。患儿最好安置于重症监护病房内，可以监测包括中心静脉压、动脉血压、每小时尿量和氧饱和度在内的生命体征。对肝硬化患者，监测神志情况也很重要，因为血液流入胃肠道内可以加剧或激发脑病。

制止出血及补充细胞外液体和血液是最重要的治疗目标。以往，三腔管（Sengstaken-Blakemore tube）压迫曲张静脉是能短期控制出血最有效的方法[70]。在成人中药物治疗有效，使球囊压迫止血法几乎被摈弃[14,103]。静脉内应用生长抑素的八肽类似物奥曲肽，大大改善了对曲张静脉出血的控制。它的半衰期比生长抑素长，且副作用少。奥曲肽在治疗曲张静脉出血中代替了血管加压素，因后者具有严重的血管副作用。

奥曲肽和其他生长抑素的类似物，如伐普肽（vapreotide），能降低肝血流量和肝静脉楔压，并通过对动脉平滑肌的直接作用使得脾动脉收缩。生长抑素类似物对降低和暂时中止门静脉高压症的出血很有效，并可以在等待对曲张静脉进行直接内镜治疗的开始 24～72 小时内使用[1,2,42,82,172]。将奥曲肽以 1.0～2.0 μg/（kg·h）的初始剂量连续输注，最大剂量为 100 μg/h，并持续到出血症状停止。

门脉高压症儿童的长期用药还包括单独使用非选择性 β 受体阻断药例如普萘洛尔或纳多洛尔，或与亚硝胺血管扩张剂如 5-单硝酸异山梨醇酯（isosorbide-5-mononitrate）联合使用。然而，一些作者认为局部套扎曲张静脉与长期药物治疗作用相同。对于大多数患儿，内镜监测及间歇性曲张静脉套扎治疗可能已足够[32]，与内镜及长期药物治疗有相同的存活率和再出血率。β 受体阻断药在减少脾血流和肝静脉楔压中的作用已有文献报道。它们的使用可以降低再出血发生率的 50%，并减少了肝病儿童对肝移植的需要[224,225]。对肝静脉楔压下降的评估将决定对降低门静脉压力有效的药物的用量，并指导及精确药物治疗的最佳方案[2,212]，但这些研究均以成人为基础，在儿童中的实际用途还很小。

静脉曲张的预防性治疗

在任何类型门静脉高压症曲张静脉出血之前均进行干预性治疗仍存在着争议，但应阻止患者的第一次
出血，且进行早期的预防性治疗。对成人及儿童的研 1659
究均显示，通过药物[86,130]和内镜套扎[48]预防性治疗静脉曲张可以降低出血的频率。但如果没有明确的指征，如严重的脾功能亢进，则是否手术防止初次出血仍存在争议。

内镜下硬化或套扎静脉曲张

外科医生很早就试图通过在血管周围或直接在血管中注射硬化剂溶液来治疗曲张静脉出血[104,105,211]。该技术在儿童曲张静脉出血的治疗中安全且有效[29,97,138,158,180,181]。硬化剂包括鱼肝油酸钠、氨基乙醇、十四烷硫酸钠和聚乙二醇单十二醚（polidocanol）。长期随访结果显示，硬化剂治疗在约90%的患者中获得成功。开始的硬化剂治疗应在规律的间隔时间中在内镜下重复应用，直到消除所有的静脉曲张或静脉曲张太小难以注射治疗为止，然后延长观测间隔时间至少4年，以监测静脉曲张的再次出现。一般情况下，每个曲张的静脉需注射2～3次，每次注射1 ml，最大总注射量为每次10～15 ml。在食管胃连接处，内镜医生应从远端食管环周起向近端食管靠近。

硬化治疗并发症的发生率比较高，包括主要和次要并发症，约发生在1/3的患者中。急性并发症有胸痛、食管溃疡和纵隔炎，慢性并发症有在多次注射后纤维化导致的食管狭窄。

在静脉曲张的治疗中，食管套扎是使用较广泛的方法。在一项肝外静脉栓塞型门静脉高压患儿的前瞻性研究中，套扎是较有效、迅速和安全的减少静脉曲张出血的方法[235]。套扎的并发症及长期再出血的发生率较低。另一项小的调查显示，与其他方法相比，套扎具有相同的有效性和安全性，甚至对具有内在肝病的门脉高压患儿同样有效[108,166]。新技术如多道式套扎内镜（multiband ligator scope），使得治疗多发性静脉曲张成为可能。这项技术在成人中首先使用，最近延伸至儿童中使用[145]。该技术提高了操作的速度和安全性，可以在3个月大小的婴儿中进行套扎；在1～2次治疗后，几乎可以100%地消除静脉曲张。

与药物治疗一样，食管曲张静脉套扎成为早期治疗曲张静脉出血的方法之一。接下来的治疗是结扎残余的曲张血管或在大血管套扎后出现的新的曲张血管。对大多数儿童来说，结扎是有效的，且没有硬化治疗的并发症多。

注射治疗胃静脉曲张

随着更多治疗食管静脉曲张的有效方法出现，食管以下消化道的曲张静脉出血成了问题所在。注射N-丁基-氰基丙烯酸盐粘合剂（N-butyl-cyanoacrylate）在胃静脉出血的成人患者中取得一定疗效[181]，但在儿童中没有相关报道。约15%～20%的患者胃静脉曲张与食管静脉曲张并存，两者也可以单独存在[182～184]。胃静脉曲张可以在消除了食管静脉曲张后出现，或在食管曲张静脉结扎后存留[8]。成人患者的治疗经验显示，胃静脉曲张、肝硬化和进展性肝病患者的出血可以被有效控制，但1年后再出血的发生率较高。在成人中，胃静脉曲张注射治疗对肝外静脉栓塞型门静脉高压患者出血的控制情况（35%）与肝病型门脉高压患者（75%）相比相对较低[112]。鉴于与成人相比，儿童中肝外门静脉栓塞是引起胃静脉曲张出血的更重要的因素，所以对于胃静脉曲张的儿童，注射治疗不适用，除非在正式的研究中证实其与手术或其他药物相比是安全和有效的。

经颈静脉肝内门体静脉分流术

经皮穿刺血管在肝实质内、门静脉与体静脉之间放置支架、创建通道为治疗进展性肝病和门脉高压患者提供了新的治疗途径[55]。经颈静脉肝内门体静脉分流术（transjugular intrahepatic portosystemic shunts，TIPS）的主要治疗指征是经内镜及奥曲肽等保守治疗后胃曲张静脉仍出血。它也是肝病性门脉高压症患者的保留治疗方法，并为肝移植搭桥[91,143]。其他一些应用指征包括：顽固性腹水、移植或未移植患者肝静脉流出道梗阻和肝肾综合征。

在儿童中，治疗经验有限。TIPS是门静脉高压性胃病或用其他方法难以控制的曲张静脉出血儿童实行肝移植的桥梁。TIPS用于囊性纤维病（图106-4）[163]、胆道狭窄[98]和先天性肝纤维化[21]，甚至用于小至1岁左右的儿童[45]，并取得成功。

TIPS主要的限制是分流后栓塞的高发生率，需要提高警惕监测分流是否明显，栓塞时要去除血凝块。其他不足是激发约20%的患者出现门体分流性脑病和加快已在衰竭边缘的肝功能衰竭。TIPS利于在那些肝功能差的极其虚弱的患者中进行血液分流[201]。

儿童在TIPS术后发生肝性脑病的几率比成人低，但因分流直径较小，分流后再闭塞的发生率较高。

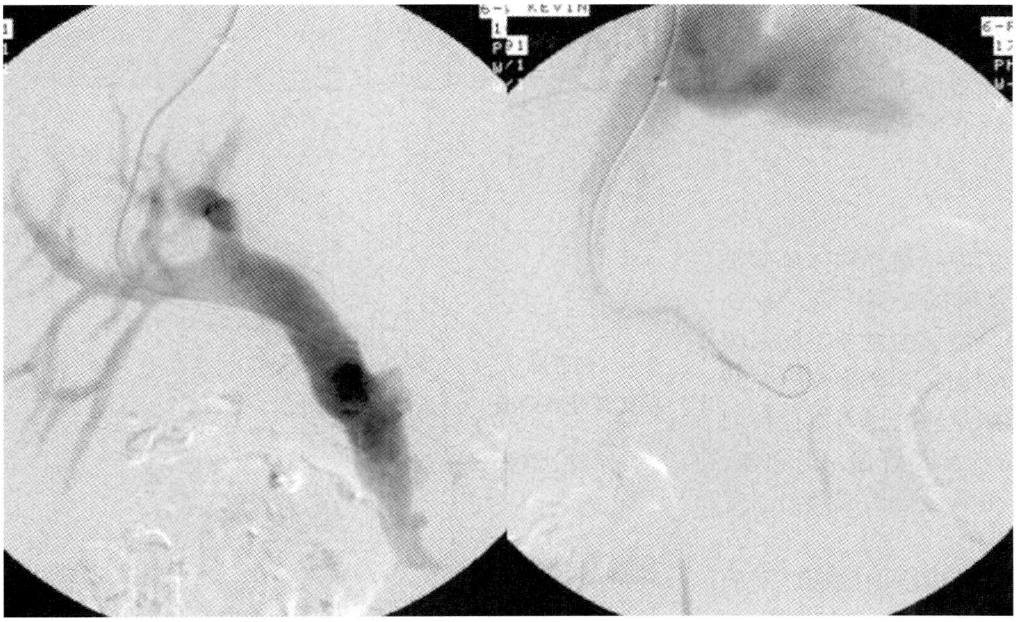

图 106-4　患囊性纤维病的男孩发生食管胃静脉曲张出血。为了使其在等待肝移植过程中病情平稳，采用经颈静脉肝内门体静脉分流术（TIPS）。一根经皮导管由颈静脉放置入右肝静脉。导管正向右门静脉前进（左图），然后放置支架，使得近端在门静脉主干内，远端在肝静脉远心端内。

60

分流手术

正如 Eck 首先描述的那样[65]，早期的分流手术将所有的肠系膜血流转向体循环。以后的作者报道，对具有严重出血的门静脉高压症的进展性肝病成人[27,28,118,119,141,162,165]及肝前型和肝内型门静脉高压症儿童[24,25,52-54]使用门腔静脉分流术。

分流可以是选择性的或非选择性的。选择性分流是在将血液从高压力的胃食管曲张静脉分流进入低压力的体静脉循环时保存流向肝的重要门静脉或肠系膜血流。实质上，选择性分流将门静脉循环分为两个独立的部分，虽然完全分离所有的交通是不可能的。相反的，非选择性分流将大部分的肠系膜血流从肝脏分流，从而使整个消化道包括脾和胰腺得到减压。非选择性分流可以进一步细分为完全和部分门静脉转流。

非选择性分流

完全转流

Eck[65]首先描述的端侧门腔分流术是完全门静脉转流的经典例子。门静脉血流完全在肝下转流入下腔静脉，缝合门静脉的肝侧静脉末端。

完全性转流分流术的另一个例子是近端脾肾静脉分流术。在靠近脾的位置分离脾静脉，将肠系膜静脉末端与左肾静脉缝合，这样所有肠系膜上静脉和下静脉的血液通过肾静脉进入体循环。该术式包括脾切除并有时直接缝扎食管胃曲张静脉[35,67,95,147,187,209]。

大直径的肠系膜腔静脉分流几乎能完全将肠系膜的血液从肝脏中分流。该方法可以在两根静脉之间进行侧侧吻合或使用短的自体血管移植或假体移植物移植[63,80,175]。自体血管移植更常用。需要在肠系膜根部暴露肠系膜上静脉，在十二指肠下暴露下腔静脉。

在儿童中，肠系膜腔静脉分流广泛应用于各种疾病，并有统一的较好的效果[12,24,85,142]。一些医生选择这种方式是因为它可以在两个直径较大的静脉之间进行吻合，也因为它能延伸应用范围，使建立大静脉瘘更为便利。该手术方法比脾肾分流更容易。此外，与近端脾肾分流相比，该方法更容易保留脾脏，这对于预防脾切除后败血症很重要[92,213]。

门腔静脉侧侧分流让肠和脾的血液更容易流入腔静脉。此外，与门腔静脉端端吻合术不同，门静脉的肝支末端被改为一个流出道。对于肝后型门静脉高压的 Budd-Chiari 综合征，肝脏也可以通过该手术方式减压，它可能会使疾病得以长期缓解，并可以阻止或延缓肝纤维化及最终肝功能衰竭的进展[5,9,43,118]。治疗 Budd-Chiari 综合征的另一个有效的手术方式是肠系膜腔静脉和中央性脾肾分流，通过开放的门静脉将肝内的门静脉血液以逆行性的方式排空。

1661 部分分流

部分转流分流术依赖于在门静脉循环和体静脉循环血管之间建立一个固定、狭窄的交通[177]。Sarfeh 分流可以从门静脉循环中转流出足够的血液将肠系膜压力降低至 12 cmH_2O，并因此使曲张静脉减压并减少出血机会，同时维持门静脉床足够的压力以保留回肝血流及肝血流[179]。Sarfeh 分流术尽管保留肝血流，减少门体分流性脑病的发生，但其血栓形成及出血复发的发生率较高[56]。

门腔静脉分流术后门静脉血流减少与脑病之间的相关关系已经报道了很长时间[71,122]。Sarfeh 术[179]可以控制分流的直径以保留流向肝脏的门静脉血流，降低门静脉循环的压力，也因此减少了曲张静脉的出血，并使门体静脉分流性脑病的发生率降为最低。

选择性分流

为了减少门腔分流后脑病的发生，Warren 等[228]描述了一种在脾静脉的门静脉端和肾静脉侧之间分流的手术方式（图 106-5）。在脾静脉与肠系膜上静脉汇合处缝扎脾静脉，并离断胃冠状静脉。这种方式中，胃食管曲张静脉血流通过胃短静脉引流，经左肾静脉进入腔静脉而获得减压。长期研究显示低压力的脾循环与高压力的肝循环的不连接不总是维持，一段时间后可能重新连通。流向肝的血流减少，并被再次引入胃周围的冠状静脉循环，如此一来，就像大多数的中央分流一样可以减少肝血流[90,185,198]。这个例子中，血管成像及内镜检查显示，随着时间的推移，选择性分流量逐渐减少。更完全的胰脾离断术避免了脾肾循环之间交通侧支的重建。在成人中，选择性分流与非选择性分流的远期死亡率和再出血率相似[83]，但选择性分流的门体分流性脑病发生率较低[36,77]。

对于儿童，由 Warren 等[228]描述了选择性分流术或稍加改良后成功治疗静脉曲张出血[25,34,66,69,90,121,137-139,142,194,218,222]和脾功能亢进[194]的手术方式。多数的系列报道显示该手术的长期有效率超过 90%，在所有分流保持通畅的患儿中没有出血。

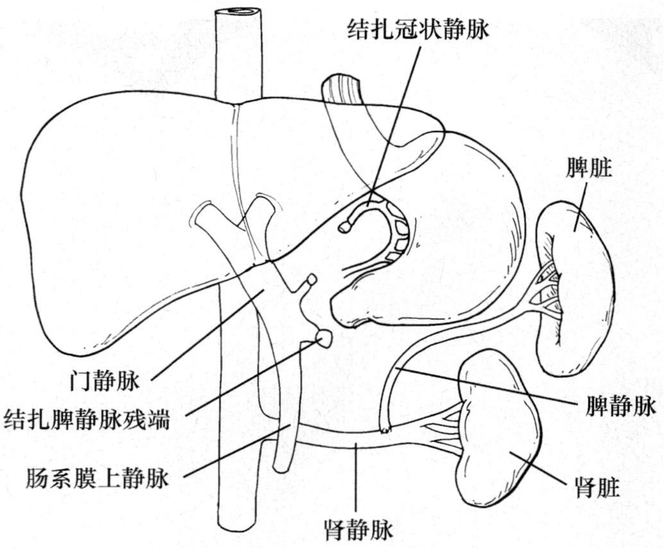

图 106-5 远端脾肾静脉分流术。已进入网膜囊，在胰下缘离断脾静脉，结扎并分离小的胰腺分支血管。寻找并分离左肾静脉，保留生殖腺和肾上腺属支，在与肠系膜上静脉汇合处离断脾静脉，并与左肾静脉端侧吻合。血管应沿平滑肌弧形放置以避免扭结。分离并结扎冠状静脉和胃网膜静脉。血流从胃和食管曲张的静脉经由胃短静脉，穿过脾并进入脾静脉。这种方式使得脾脏减压，并保留回肝脏的门脉血流。

远端脾肾分流术用于肝外门静脉栓塞[194]、稳定的 Child 分级 A 或 B 肝硬化[34,137,171]或较少见类型的肝内型门脉高压，如肝功能储备良好但存在静脉曲张出血症状的先天性肝纤维化的患儿。

在儿童中，保留神经识别功能很重要，因此应避免任何形式的非选择性分流手术。儿童脑病明显的认知失调或行为异常并不完全由门体分流术所引起[227]。尽管没有远端脾肾分流术后长期随访神经认知功能的研究报道，但也没有稳定性肝硬化或肝外型门静脉高压患儿脑病临床证据的系列报道。

在门脉高压症儿童中，脾功能亢进是一个特别的问题，一些儿童需行脾切除术或脾栓塞术[101,178,190,215,223]。远端脾肾分流对进展期脾功能亢进的儿童有帮助。术后脾脏消退，血小板、白细胞计数回归正常。分流术使得脾脏减压，凝血性疾病可以在该手术后得到改善并维持很长时间。

过去，对脾功能亢进患者主张行脾切除术和脾栓塞术。然而这些方法并不是没有并发症，在很长时间内患儿可以出现胃食管曲张静脉出血恶化和脾切除后败血症倾向[89]。此外，脾切除术后，仍存在曲张静脉出血的患儿将不能再行远端脾肾分流术。儿外科医生应该在任何可能的情况下保留脾脏，让脾切除成为
662 患儿没有其他手术方式可供选择时的最后选择。

肠系膜-左门静脉旁路术

1992 年，肠系膜-左门静脉旁路手术（mesenteric-to-left portal vein bypass）的出现推动了肝外型门静脉高压栓塞的治疗（图 106-6）。最初认为该手术是一种肝移植后门静脉栓塞时移植肝脏血管再成形的手术方法[58,61]，但后来延伸为儿童自发性门静脉栓塞的治疗途径。一个世界范围的小型研究团队报道了近 30～50 例接受该治疗的患儿[13,19,59,60,62,76]。

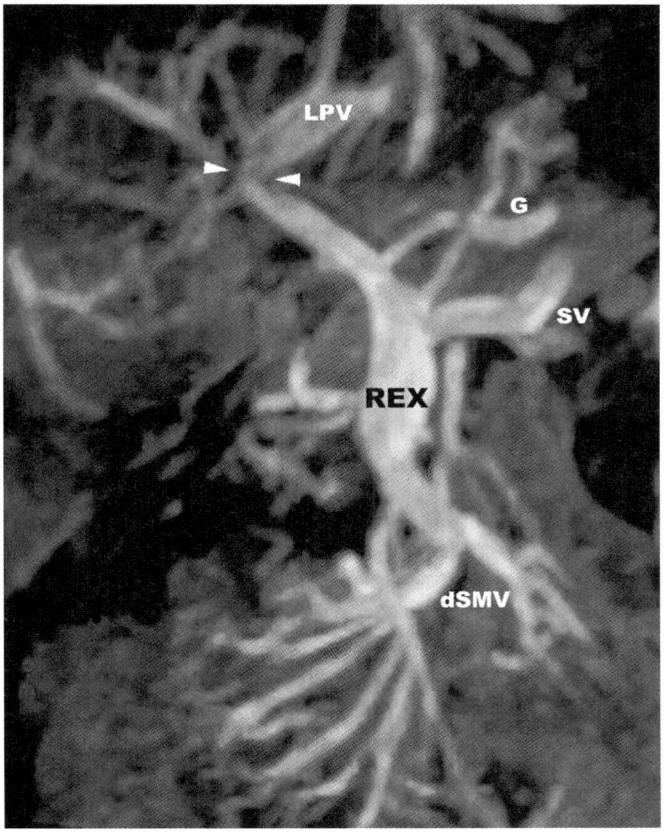

图 106-6　CT 血管成像图显示肝外型门静脉栓塞患者成功行肠系膜-左门静脉旁路移植 1 周后的征象。增强造影剂从肠系膜上静脉（dSMV），通过移植的静脉（REX），最终进入肝内门静脉（LPV）。血液从脾静脉（PV）和冠状静脉（G）流入移植的静脉和肝脏。

实质上，该手术是通过将阻塞的肠系膜血流转向肝内门静脉，从而缓解门静脉高压。该旁路手术的成功需要三个先决条件：（1）肝脏没有内在疾病；（2）肝内门静脉分支良好；（3）肠系膜循环中存在一条合适的静脉，功能上可以作为引流肠系膜血流的合适通道。

在门静脉栓塞中，肝外门静脉被一些小的侧支网所替代，该侧支网中的少量肠系膜血流供应肝脏并保持了肝内门脉循环。这些儿童的肝内门脉分支明显但发育不全。

术前的准备工作包括 CT 血管成像以评估静脉的直径和肝内门静脉的明显度，肝活检以排除肝脏内在疾患，凝血试验排除遗传性高凝血状态。过去认为遗传性高凝血状态导致了门静脉栓塞的形成[96,128,136,154]。然而，也有报道纤溶系统缺陷可能继发于肝内门脉血流缺失并可随门静脉血流再充盈而逆转。

手术以将肝内门静脉从肝第Ⅲ和Ⅳ段之间圆韧带中的 Rex 隐窝中解剖出来开始，去除部分Ⅲ和Ⅳ段肝组织。控制Ⅱ、Ⅲ、Ⅳ肝段的所有属支。如果合适，可在肠系膜根部解剖肠系膜上静脉。旁路术的血液来源已在前描述，包括肠系膜下静脉和胃冠状静脉。

当流入静脉被游离后，切取颈静脉（右颈静脉或左颈静脉），先与肝内门静脉缝合，然后与肠系膜上静脉缝合。移植的静脉通常穿过结肠系膜和小网膜囊（the lesser sac），在胃后向上穿过网膜囊，到达肝脏。对于旋转不良和其他先天性疾病患儿，根据患儿的自身条件，移植血管的穿行途径各异。

与门体静脉分流不同，肠系膜-左门静脉旁路或 Rex 分流恢复了向肝的门脉血流并缓解了门脉高压症状。正确选择患者使得该手术的有效率大于 90%。有效率依赖于肝内静脉的质量以及允许通过足够的维持血流的侧支数量。手术前的影像学检查很难完全辨别肝内门静脉情况，最后的评估只能在手术中完成。

非分流手术

门静脉高压的非分流手术一般只限于手术阻断或结扎出血的曲张静脉，以及横断食管以阻断食管腔内的曲张静脉[121,191,216]。因为存在较高的死亡率及复发

率，食管横断及再缝合或纤维包扎术的使用受到很大限制。

Sugiura 等[206,207]提出了在下肺静脉水平从胃切迹到中段食管处分离胃周围和食管周围血管的手术方式。此外，离断并重置食管。这种彻底的门脉高压治
1663 疗途径与分流手术不同，但也有并发疾病。改良的 Sugiura 术对儿童患者用吻合器设备进行食管横断再吻合，并保留脾脏[208]。在儿童中，随着分流及其他血管手术经验的增加及有效的应用，切除性和非生理性手术的应用减少。

手术并发症

分流后血栓症

任何血管手术都有血栓的潜在危险。可以在手术后立即使用低剂量的肝素和抗血小板药物如阿司匹林或双嘧达莫来预防血栓，并持续应用 3～6 个月。当分流后血栓症发生时，不需要急救，但如果出血再发生，则必须寻求其他解决办法，如血行阻断等。幸运的是，在相关专家的报道中手术后的血栓症发生率低于 5%。

腹水

腹膜后淋巴管道破裂常导致腹水的发生。大多数病例中腹水能自行消失，但在短时间内需要口服利尿剂。因为所有腹水的本质是乳糜，所以低脂饮食对改善腹水也有帮助。腹水张力很大或持续存在的情况很少，需行腹部穿刺。这种情况下，短时间内使用静脉营养可以减少乳糜的产生，直到淋巴漏闭合。如果这些方法不能消除腹水，常提示肝储备能力很低，可能需要行肝移植术。

食管狭窄

在食管横断并采取伴行血管阻断术后，横断部位的食管狭窄并非不常见。瘘少见但却是很严重的并发症，需要胸腔引流、延长抗生素使用时间及再手术。幸运的是，大部分食管狭窄可以通过扩张治疗，尽管一些病例需要重复进行扩张才能获得满意效果。

预后

门静脉高压症患儿的治疗结果依赖于门静脉高压形成的原因及治疗时肝脏的状态。过去 10 年里，因为药物和手术方式的改进及可以对肝贮备能力低的患儿行肝移植术，门静脉高压患者的状况得到很大改善。

曲张静脉紧急出血

门脉高压的药物控制使得不再常规对儿童行紧急分流术。内镜结扎曲张的食管静脉有较好的效果。必要时，紧急分流术对控制出血非常有效，据报道有较好的远期效果[69]。但也有报道，紧急分流术的显效率低于 90%，而选择性手术的显效率较高。因为药物和内镜控制急性曲张静脉出血有相似的效果，故紧急肠系膜腔静脉分流术已很少有报道。

间歇性食管和胃曲张静脉出血

现在由于内镜和药物治疗的有效性，肝外门静脉血栓导致的急性曲张静脉出血患者很少需要手术治疗。患者较多地表现为进展性脾功能亢进和控制良好的静脉曲张。但控制曲张静脉出血需要多次的内镜治疗，偶尔静脉输注 β 受体阻断药和血管扩张剂。

因为手术治疗变得更有效及其结果的可预见性更强，所以针对肝外性门脉高压的根治手术应提早进行，而不是等到其他治疗方法均失败后才进行。这点尤其与 Rex 分流手术的出现有关，因为 Rex 手术保留了正常的门脉压力，并通过改变肠系膜静脉向肝的血流以缓解脾功能亢进。恢复门脉血流向肝脏的效果还不明显，但可能在儿童早期发育过程中的代谢方面产生深远影响。保留门脉血流后，相关的凝血参数恢复正常，这可能只是众多肝功能改善的指标之一。患有门静脉血栓和门静脉高压的儿童具有“正常”肝功

能的看法可能是不正确的。

选择性分流如远端脾肾分流或胃冠状静脉-腔静脉移植，可以纠正门静脉血栓导致的门静脉高压，并已成为一种死亡率最低的手术方式，特别是当有经验的外科医生实施手术时，其死亡率可为零。其显效率高于95%，住院时间通常少于 1 周。在长期的病程中，与反复入院进行内镜下套扎和长期药物治疗以控制出血相比较，选择性分流对儿童更适合。此外，许多门静脉血栓患儿在确定性手术治疗延迟时，常出现进展性脾功能亢进。许多患儿在预防性套扎曲张静脉时，出血甚至由食管转移至胃。手术治疗（Rex 分流或远端脾肾分流）以符合生理的方式控制出血，减少了住院时间，降低了药物使用，缓解脾功能亢进，并且避免使患儿暴露在脾切除后致死性败血症的远期风险下。

因为要考虑到肝脏的健康状况，故由内在性肝病 1664
引起的门脉高压症的分流术更为复杂。对于低 Child-pugh 或 PELD 积分的患儿，选择性分流能很好地对门静脉树进行减压。尽管远端脾肾分流术理论上将脾和胃的静脉引流从肠和肠系膜静脉血流中分离出来，但研究显示两个系统的分离并不完全，并且可能在一定时间后，随着机体形成侧支循环替代被离断的血管，

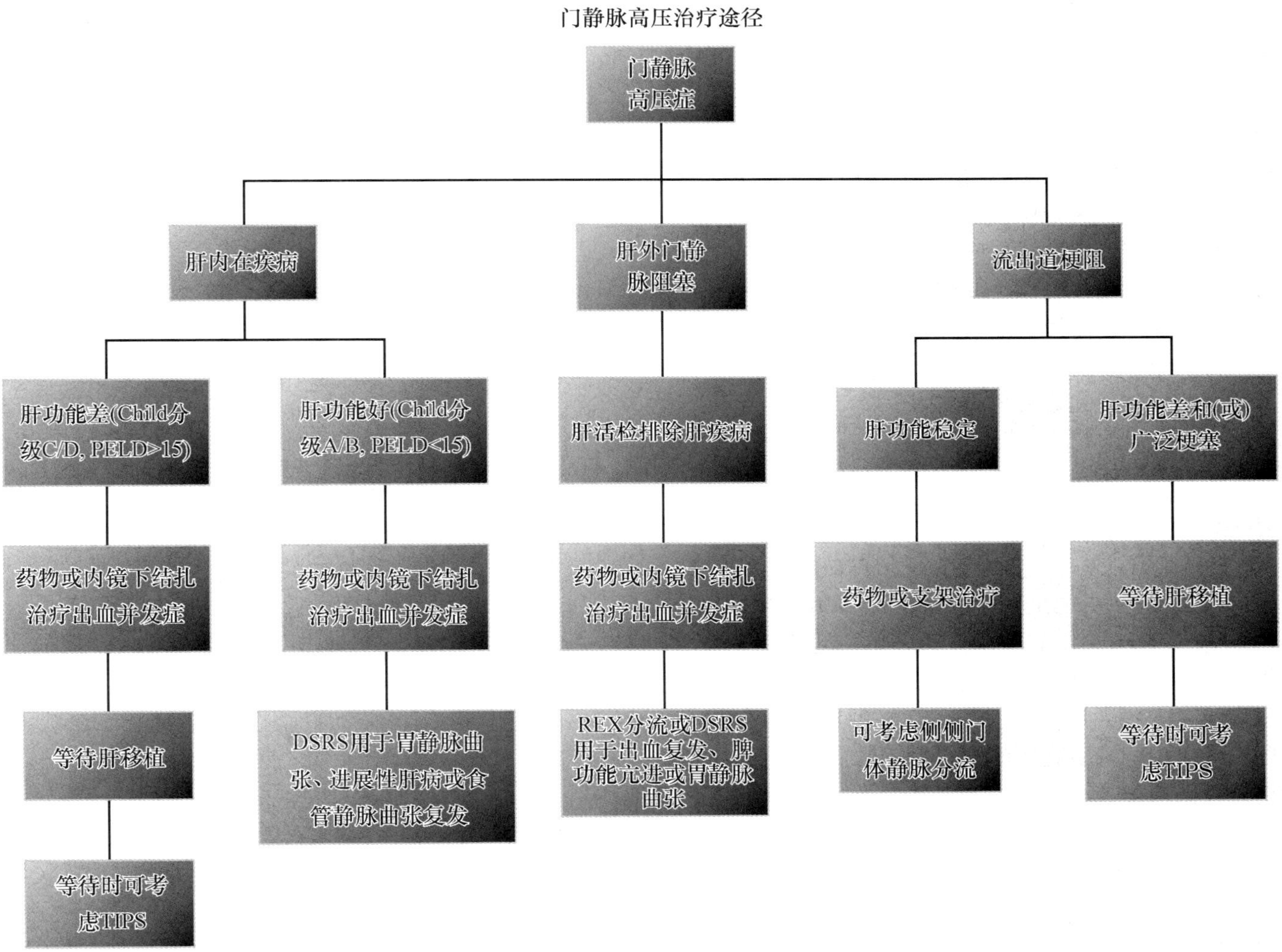

图 106-7 治疗法则根据门脉高压症的病因制定。由静脉流出道梗阻或内在性肝病导致进展性肝功能失调的门脉高压症患者，无论行或不行经皮肝内门体静脉分流术（TIPS），其最终的治疗方法是行肝移植治疗。如果肝功能失调不严重并没有迅速进展，分流术可能具有良好的远期效果。具有门静脉高压症状的肝外型门静脉高压患者可以选择肠系膜-左门静脉旁路术，随后进行远端脾肾分流术（DSRS）。PELD：儿童终末期肝病分级。

这种分离消失[79,199]。但在儿童和成人患者中，与非选择性分流相比，选择性分流试图保留向肝血流，从而减少门体分流性脑病，并使肝功能恢复较好[81]。

如果患儿的肝储备较好，并因以往手术失败或解剖状况不理想不能采用选择性分流术时，最好考虑实行血行中断以减少潜在的门体静脉分流性脑病。儿童非选择性分流的唯一作用是在少数肝储备功能良好及不能行血管移植或传统的放射性介入治疗的梗阻性血管病变患者中应用[176]。

脾功能亢进

随着食管曲张静脉出血治疗的改善，更多儿童表现为胃曲张静脉出血、门脉高压性胃病[81]或进展性的使人虚弱的脾功能亢进的并发症[194]。除了刺激骨髓的粒细胞集落刺激因子，没有药物能够治疗脾功能亢进[100]。手术是唯一可以替代上述药物的治疗方法。

在症状性曲张静脉出血初始治疗中，几乎所有的分流都显示能减轻脾功能亢进的严重程度。脾功能亢
1665 进的手术治疗需遵循两个原则：保留脾脏和避免门体分流性脑病。据报道，远端脾肾分流术能改善儿童的脾功能亢进。在肝外型门静脉栓塞的儿童中，Rex 分流是解决脾功能亢进的较好方式[19]。

小结

儿童门静脉高压对外科医生而言是个挑战。近10 年来，出现了许多治疗方式，包括减少肠系膜血管树及门静脉循环血流的更广泛而有效的药物治疗。这些治疗方法大大减少了门脉高压患者的急诊手术。图 106-7 以门静脉高压的原因为依据，总结了本章内讨论过的治疗方法。

辅助的介入治疗，如内镜下结扎曲张静脉和放射线引导下放置肝内支架，也可减少手术依赖，控制进展性肝病患儿的出血。这些介入治疗增加了患者存活以接受肝移植的机会。

尽管手术的需求减少，但手术结果得以改善，分流和非分流方法可以为肝前型、肝后型门静脉高压症和代偿良好的肝硬化患者的出血及脾功能亢进提供永久性的解决方法。随着门脉高压手术相关疾病发生率的下降，有报道甚至在婴儿和小年龄儿童中手术都有良好的远期效果。适合儿童的手术方式增加，甚至使我们在治疗的早期就可以在门静脉高压症手术与药物治疗之间进行更好的选择。

（杜 勇译 吴晔明校）

参考文献

1. Abraldes JG, Bosch J: Somatostatin and analogues in portal hypertension. Hepatology 2002;35:1305-1312.
2. Abraldes JG, et al: Hemodynamic response to pharmacological treatment of portal hypertension and long-term prognosis of cirrhosis. Hepatology 2003;37:902-908.
3. Abramowsky C, Romero R, Heffron T: Pathology of noncirrhotic portal hypertension: Clinicopathologic study in pediatric patients. Pediatr Dev Pathol 2003;6:421-426.
4. Adler M, et al: Hepatic vascular disease after kidney transplantation: Report of two cases and review of the literature. Nephrol Dial Transplant 1987;2:183-188.
5. Ahn SS, et al: Selective surgical therapy of the Budd-Chiari syndrome provides superior survivor rates than conservative medical management. J Vasc Surg 1987;5:28-37.
6. Aithal GP, et al: Portal hypertension secondary to arterio-portal fistulae: Two unusual cases. Liver 1999;19:343-347.
7. Aitken MG: Recombinant factor VIIa. Emerg Med Australas 2004;16:446-455.
8. Akahoshi T, et al: Long-term results of endoscopic Histoacryl injection sclerotherapy for gastric variceal bleeding: A 10-year experience. Surgery 2002;131(1 Suppl):S176-S181.
9. Alagille D, Le Tan V, Odievre M: [Budd-Chiari syndrome and veno-occlusive disease in children (apropos of 3 cases)]. Arch Fr Pediatr 1968;25:1039-1058.
10. Albers I, et al: Superiority of the Child-Pugh classification to quantitative liver function tests for assessing prognosis of liver cirrhosis. Scand J Gastroenterol 1989;24:269-276.
11. Aldrete JS, Slaughter RL, Han SY: Portal vein thrombosis resulting in portal hypertension in adults. Am J Gastroenterol 1976;65:236-243.
12. Altman RP: Portal decompression by interposition mesocaval shunt in patients with biliary atresia. J Pediatr Surg 1976;11:809-814.
13. Ates O, et al: Extrahepatic portal hypertension treated by anastomosing inferior mesenteric vein to left portal vein at Rex recessus. J Pediatr Surg 2003;38:E10-E11.
14. Avgerinos A, et al: A prospective randomized trial comparing somatostatin, balloon tamponade and the combination of both methods in the management of acute variceal haemorrhage. J Hepatol 1991;13:78-83.
15. Avner ED, Ellis D, Jaffe R: Veno-occlusive disease of the liver associated with cysteamine treatment of nephropathic cystinosis. J Pediatr 1983;102:793-796.
16. Azoulay D, et al: Successful treatment of severe azathioprine-induced hepatic veno-occlusive disease in a kidney-transplanted patient with transjugular intrahepatic portosystemic shunt. Clin Nephrol 1998;50:118-122.
17. Bachleitner-Hofmann T, Grumbeck E, Gisslinger H: Oral anticoagulants as secondary prophylaxis of thrombosis in patients with polycythemia vera: A retrospective analysis of

15 patients. Thromb Res 2003;112:229-232.
18. Bajwa RP, et al: Recombinant tissue plasminogen activator for treatment of hepatic veno-occlusive disease following bone marrow transplantation in children: Effectiveness and a scoring system for initiating treatment. Bone Marrow Transplant 2003;31:591-597.
19. Bambini DA, et al: Experience with the Rex shunt (mesenterico-left portal bypass) in children with extrahepatic portal hypertension. J Pediatr Surg 2000;35:13-18.
20. Baranda J, et al: Mesenteric arteriovenous fistula causing portal hypertension and bleeding duodenal varices. Eur J Gastroenterol Hepatol 1996;8:1223-1225.
21. Benador N, et al: Transjugular intrahepatic portosystemic shunt prior to renal transplantation in a child with autosomal-recessive polycystic kidney disease and portal hypertension: A case report. Pediatr Transplant 2001;5: 210-214.
22. Bhattacharyya M, et al: Inherited prothrombotic defects in Budd-Chiari syndrome and portal vein thrombosis: A study from north India. Am J Clin Pathol 2004;121:844-847.
23. Billing JS, Jamieson NV: Hepatic arterioportal fistula: A curable cause of portal hypertension in infancy. HPB Surg 1997;10:311-314.
24. Bismuth H, Franco D: Portal diversion for portal hypertension in early childhood. Ann Surg 1976;183:439-446.
25. Bismuth H, Franco D, Alagille D: Portal diversion for portal hypertension in children: The first ninety patients. Ann Surg 1980;192:18-24.
26. Bismuth H, Houssin D: Reduced-sized orthotopic liver graft in hepatic transplantation in children. Surgery 1984; 95:367-370.
27. Blakemore AH: Portacaval shunt for portal hypertension: Follow-up results in cases of cirrhosis of the liver. JAMA 1951;145:1335-1339.
28. Blakemore AH: The portacaval shunt for portal hypertension with special reference to cirrhosis of the liver. Bull N Y Acad Med 1951;27:477-494.
29. Blanchard H, et al: [Portal hypertension of extra-hepatic origin in children]. Chir Pediatr 1982;23:221-225.
30. Bolton GC: Portal vena caval shunt surgery Eck fistula. Med Arts Sci 1951;5:131-134.
31. Bono RF, et al: Studies on portal hypertension. V. A comparison between the experimentally induced state of portal hypertension and that observed in human beings. Surgery 1960;48:119-141.
32. Bosch J, Garcia-Pagan JC: Complications of cirrhosis. I. Portal hypertension. J Hepatol 2000;32(1 Suppl):141-156.
33. Bosch J, Garcia-Pagan JC: Prevention of variceal rebleeding. Lancet 2003;361:952-954.
34. Botha JF, et al: Portosystemic shunts in children: A 15-year experience. J Am Coll Surg 2004;199:179-185.
35. Boyd DP: Portal hypertension following stricture of the common duct: A report of 2 cases in which splenectomy and splenorenal shunt were carried out. Lahey Clin Bull 1954;8:217-220.
36. Britton RC: The clinical effectiveness of selective portal shunts. Am J Surg 1977;133:506-511.
37. Broelsch CE, et al: Liver transplantation in children from living related donors: Surgical techniques and results. Ann Surg 1991;214:428-437.
38. Broxson EH, et al: Portal hypertension develops in a subset of children with standard risk acute lymphoblastic leukemia treated with oral 6-thioguanine during maintenance therapy. Pediatr Blood Cancer 2005;44:226-231.
39. Buccino RV, et al: Endoscopic approach to patients with portal hypertension: A complex diagnosis. A retrospective study based on 10 years' experience. Surg Endosc 1990;4:76-79.
40. Budd G: On Diseases of the Liver. London, John Churchill, 1845, p 146.
41. Caldwell SH, Chang C, Macik BG: Recombinant activated factor VII (rFVIIa) as a hemostatic agent in liver disease: A break from convention in need of controlled trials. Hepatology 2004;39:592-598.
42. Cales P, et al: Early administration of vapreotide for variceal bleeding in patients with cirrhosis. French Club for the Study of Portal Hypertension. N Engl J Med 2001;344:23-28.
43. Cameron JL, et al: The Budd-Chiari syndrome: Treatment by mesenteric-systemic venous shunts. Ann Surg 1983;198: 335-346.
44. Canbay A, Friedman S, Gores GJ: Apoptosis: The nexus of liver injury and fibrosis. Hepatology 2004;39:273-278.
45. Cao S, et al: Emergency transjugular intrahepatic portosystemic shunt (TIPS) in an infant: A case report. J Pediatr Surg 1997;32:125-127.
46. Capron JP, et al: Inferior mesenteric arteriovenous fistula associated with portal hypertension and acute ischemic colitis: Successful occlusion by intraarterial embolization with steel coils. Gastroenterology 1984;86:351-355.
47. Cario H, et al: Familial polycythemia vera with Budd-Chiari syndrome in childhood. Br J Haematol 2003;123:346-352.
48. Celinska-Cedro D, et al: Endoscopic ligation of esophageal varices for prophylaxis of first bleeding in children and adolescents with portal hypertension: Preliminary results of a prospective study. J Pediatr Surg 2003;38:1008-1011.
49. Chen LH, et al: Antiphospholipid syndrome: A survey of clinical characters in ten cases. J Zhejiang Univ Sci 2003;4: 616-619.
50. Chiari H: Über die selbstandige phlebitis obliterans der hauptstamme der venae hepaticae als todesursache. Beitr Z Pathol Anat 1899;26:1-18.
51. Child CG, Turcotte JG: Surgery and portal hypertension. In Child CG (ed): Major Problems in Clinical Surgery, vol 1, The Liver and Portal Hypertension. Philadelphia: WB Saunders, 1964.
52. Clatworthy HW Jr, Boles ET Jr: Extrahepatic portal bed block in children: Pathogenesis and treatment. Ann Surg 1959;150:371-383.
53. Clatworthy HW Jr, Delorimer AA: Portal decompression procedures in children. Am J Surg 1964;107:447-451.
54. Clatworthy HW Jr, Nahmad M, Hollabaugh RS: Presinusoidal extrahepatic portal hypertension: A review of thirty-five cases variously treated. Prog Pediatr Surg 1978;11:125-139.
55. Colapinto RF, et al: Formation of intrahepatic portosystemic shunts using a balloon dilatation catheter: Preliminary clinical experience. AJR Am J Roentgenol 1983;140:709-714.
56. Collins JC, Rypins EB, Sarfeh IJ: Narrow-diameter portacaval shunts for management of variceal bleeding. World J Surg 1994;18:211-215.
57. Davies DB: The impact of PELD on OPTN liver allocation: Preliminary results. Clin Transpl 2003:13-20.
58. de Ville de Goyet J, Clapuyt P, Otte JB: Extrahilar mesenterico-left portal shunt to relieve extrahepatic portal hypertension after partial liver transplant. Transplantation 1992;53:231-232.
59. de Ville de Goyet J, et al: Original extrahilar approach for hepatic portal revascularization and relief of extrahepatic portal hypertension related to later portal vein thrombosis after pediatric liver transplantation: Long term results. Transplantation 1996;62:71-75.
60. de Ville de Goyet J, et al: Direct bypassing of extrahepatic portal venous obstruction in children: A new technique for

combined hepatic portal revascularization and treatment of extrahepatic portal hypertension. J Pediatr Surg 1998; 33:597-601.
61. de Ville de Goyet J, et al: Mesenterico-left intrahepatic portal vein shunt: Original technique to treat symptomatic extrahepatic portal hypertension. Acta Gastroenterol Belg 1998;61:13-16.
62. de Ville de Goyet J, et al: Treatment of extrahepatic portal hypertension in children by mesenteric-to-left portal vein bypass: A new physiological procedure. Eur J Surg 1999; 165:777-781.
63. Drapanas T: Interposition mesocaval shunt for treatment of portal hypertension. Ann Surg 1972;176:435-448.
64. D'Souza R, et al: Lessons to be learned: A case study of the temporal onset of pulmonary hypertension with pre-existent cirrhotic portal hypertension. J R Soc Health 2001; 121:257-261.
65. Eck N: On the question of ligature of the portal vein. Voyenno Med 1973;130:1.
66. Eizaguirre I, et al: [Warren's shunt in the treatment of portal hypertension in children]. Cir Pediatr 1991;4:134-139.
67. Ellis EE, Holman E: Portal hypertension accompanying cholangitis due to stricture of the common bile duct: Correction by splenorenal shunt; a case report. Surgery 1955;37:463-468.
68. Estrada O, et al: Posttraumatic intrapancreatic aortosplenic fistula causing portal hypertension. Asian Cardiovasc Thorac Ann 2003;11:272-274.
69. Evans S, et al: Selective distal splenorenal shunts for intractable variceal bleeding in pediatric portal hypertension. J Pediatr Surg 1995;30:1115-1118.
70. Feneyrou B, et al: Initial control of bleeding from esophageal varices with the Sengstaken-Blakemore tube: Experience in 82 patients. Am J Surg 1988;155:509-11.
71. Fischer JE: Hepatic coma in cirrhosis, portal hypertension, and following portacaval shunt: Its etiologies and the current status of its treatment. Arch Surg 1974;108:325-336.
72. Fonkalsrud EW, Longmire WP Jr: Reassessment of operative procedures for portal hypertension in infants and children. Am J Surg 1969;118:148-157.
73. Foster JH, Sandblom P: Portal hypertension secondary to an hepato-portal arteriovenous fistula. Ann Surg 1961;154: 300-304.
74. Freeman RB Jr: MELD/PELD: One year later. Transplant Proc 2003;35:2425-2427.
75. Friedman SL: Seminars in medicine of the Beth Israel Hospital, Boston. The cellular basis of hepatic fibrosis: Mechanisms and treatment strategies. N Engl J Med 1993;328:1828-1835.
76. Fuchs J, et al: Mesenterico-left portal vein bypass in children with congenital extrahepatic portal vein thrombosis: A unique curative approach. J Pediatr Gastroenterol Nutr 2003;36:213-216.
77. Galambos JT, et al: Selective and total shunts in the treatment of bleeding varices: A randomized controlled trial. N Engl J Med 1976;295:1089-1095.
78. Gartner JCJ, et al: Orthotopic liver transplantation in children: Two-year experience with 47 patients. Pediatrics 1984;74:140-145.
79. Gawish Y, et al: Devascularization procedure and DSRS: A controlled randomized trial on selected haemodynamic portal flow pattern in schistosomal portal hypertension with variceal bleeding. Int Surg 2000;85:325-330.
80. Gliedman ML: The mesocaval shunt for portal hypertension. Am J Gastroenterol 1971;56:323-333.
81. Goncalves ME, Cardoso SR, Maksoud JG: Prophylactic sclerotherapy in children with esophageal varices: Long-term results of a controlled prospective randomized trial. J Pediatr Surg 2000;35:401-405.
82. Gonzalez-Abraldes J, Bosch J, Garcia-Pagan JC: Pharmacological treatment of portal hypertension. Curr Opin Investig Drugs 2001;2:1407-1413.
83. Grace ND, et al: Distal splenorenal vs portal-systemic shunts after hemorrhage from varices: A randomized controlled trial. Hepatology 1988;8:1475-1481.
84. Grauer SE, Schwartz SI: Extrahepatic portal hypertension: A retrospective analysis. Ann Surg 1979;189:566-574.
85. Grosfeld JL, et al: Portal hypertension in infants and children with histiocytosis X. Am J Surg 1976;131:108-113.
86. Groszmann RJ, et al: Hemodynamic events in a prospective randomized trial of propranolol versus placebo in the prevention of a first variceal hemorrhage. Gastroenterology 1990;99:1401-1407.
87. Handa M, et al: [Portosystemic A-V fistula and portal hypertension associated with islet-cell tumor of the pancreas]. Nippon Geka Gakkai Zasshi 1985;86:953-958.
88. Hannam PD, et al: Post-surgical shunt hepatopulmonary syndrome in a case of non-cirrhotic portal hypertension: Lack of efficacy of shunt reversal. Eur J Gastroenterol Hepatol 1999;11:1425-1427.
89. Hansen K, Singer DB: Asplenic-hyposplenic overwhelming sepsis: Postsplenectomy sepsis revisited. Pediatr Dev Pathol 2001;4:105-121.
90. Hasegawa T, et al: Distal splenorenal shunt with splenopancreatic disconnection for portal hypertension in biliary atresia. Pediatr Surg Int 1999;15:92-96.
91. Hassoun Z, Pomier-Layrargues G: The transjugular intrahepatic portosystemic shunt in the treatment of portal hypertension. Eur J Gastroenterol Hepatol 2004;16:1-4.
92. Hay JM, Valayer J, Maillard JN: [Experience with mesocaval shunt with jugular vein interposition for treatment of portal hypertension in children]. Chir Pediatr 1982;23:211-213.
93. Helikson MA, Shapiro DL, Seashore JH: Hepatoportal arteriovenous fistula and portal hypertension in an infant. Pediatrics 1977;60:920-924.
94. Hirner A, et al: [Hyperkinetic portal hypertension. Arterioportal fistula: problems—case reports—review of the literature]. Chirurg 1978;49:303-310.
95. Holliday RW: Splenorenal shunt combined with ligation of esophageal varices through left thoracotomy. N Y State J Med 1961;61:4088-4090.
96. Horing E, et al: [Portal hypertension due to thromboses of the portal, splenic and mesenteric veins in congenital protein C deficiency]. Dtsch Med Wochenschr 1988; 113:1847-1849.
97. Howard ER, Stringer MD, Mowat AP: Assessment of injection sclerotherapy in the management of 152 children with oesophageal varices. Br J Surg 1988;75:404-408.
98. Huppert PE, et al: Transjugular intrahepatic portosystemic shunts in children with biliary atresia. Cardiovasc Intervent Radiol 2002;25:484-493.
99. Hyde GL: Postsplenectomy arteriovenous fistula causing portal hypertension. J Ky Med Assoc 1979;77:113-115.
100. Ishizone S, et al: Effect of granulocyte colony-stimulating factor on neutropenia in liver transplant recipients with hypersplenism. J Pediatr Surg 1994;29:510-513.
101. Israel DM, et al: Partial splenic embolization in children with hypersplenism. J Pediatr 1994;124:95-100.
102. Jagtap A, Shanbag P, Vaidya M: Budd-Chiari syndrome due to antithrombin III deficiency. Indian J Pediatr 2003;70:1003-1005.
103. Jaramillo JL, et al: Somatostatin versus Sengstaken balloon

tamponade for primary haemostasia of bleeding esophageal varices: A randomized pilot study. J Hepatol 1991;12: 100-105.
104. Johnston GW: Bleeding oesophageal varices in the absence of intrahepatic or extrahepatic obstruction of the portal system and without portal hypertension. Ulster Med J 1965;34:23-26.
105. Johnston GW, Rodgers HW: Management of bleeding oesophageal varices when portal systemic shunt is inadvisable, with particular reference to the use of balloon tamponade and sclerosing injections. Ulster Med J 1964; 33:110-115.
106. Jones JD: The results of treatment of portal hypertension. Br J Surg 1961;49:168-173.
107. Karasu Z, et al: Liver transplantation in a patient with Budd-Chiari syndrome secondary to factor V Leiden mutation. Transplant Proc 2003;35:3008-3010.
108. Karrer FM, et al: Portal vein thrombosis: Treatment of variceal hemorrhage by endoscopic variceal ligation. J Pediatr Surg 1994;29:1149-1151.
109. Kayser S, et al: Rapidly progressive portal hypertension 23 years after post-traumatic arterioportal fistula of the liver. Am J Gastroenterol 1996;91:1442-1446.
110. Khaldi F, et al: [Hepatic hydatidosis and portal hypertension in children: Is it the Budd-Chiari syndrome?]. Ann Pediatr (Paris) 1993;40:631-634.
111. Khubchandani RP, D'Souza S: Antiphospholipid antibody syndrome as a cause of Budd-Chiari syndrome. Indian Pediatr 2003;40:907-908.
112. Kind R, et al: Bucrylate treatment of bleeding gastric varices: 12 years' experience. Endoscopy 2000;32:512-519.
113. Kirchgatterer A, et al: Portal hypertension due to traumatic hepatic arterioportal fistula: Report of successful embolization. Eur J Gastroenterol Hepatol 1998;10:1057-1059.
114. Kitano S, Dolgor B: Does portal hypertension contribute to the pathogenesis of gastric ulcer associated with liver cirrhosis? J Gastroenterol 2000;35:79-86.
115. Klempnaue J, Schrem H: Review: Surgical shunts and encephalopathy. Metab Brain Dis 2001;16:21-25.
116. Koslin DB, Mulligan SA, Berland LL: Duplex assessment of the portal venous system. Semin Ultrasound CT MR 1992;13:22-33.
117. Kumana CR, et al: Hepatic veno-occlusive disease due to toxic alkaloid herbal tea. Lancet 1983;2:1360-1361.
118. Lang H, et al: The Budd-Chiari syndrome: Clinical presentation and diagnostic findings in 45 patients treated by surgery. Bildgebung 1994;61:173-181.
119. Large A, Johnston CG, Preshaw DE: The portacaval venous shunt, with special reference to side-to-side portacaval anastomosis. Ann Surg 1952;135:22-33.
120. Lauler DP: An overview of the pathophysiology and management of portal hypertension and ascites. J Hepatol 1993;17(Suppl 2):S1-S3.
121. Le Tourneau JN, Carcassonne M: [Portal hypertension: Choice of therapy for children under 10 years: Shunt or palliative surgery?]. Chir Pediatr 1983;24:34-36.
122. Leffman H, Payne JT: Episodic coma due to meat intoxication as a fatal complication of portacaval shunt in the human being. Am Surg 1955;21:488-498.
123. Levine OR, et al: Progressive pulmonary hypertension in children with portal hypertension. J Pediatr 1973;83: 964-972.
124. Lewis JH, Tice HL, Zimmerman HJ: Budd-Chiari syndrome associated with oral contraceptive steroids: Review of treatment of 47 cases. Dig Dis Sci 1983;28:673-683.
125. Lichtenheld FR: [Eck fistula coma and hepatic coma: An experimental study]. Z Gesamte Exp Med 1959;132:42-50.
126. Litzow MR, et al: Veno-occlusive disease of the liver after blood and marrow transplantation: Analysis of pre- and post-transplant risk factors associated with severity and results of therapy with tissue plasminogen activator. Leuk Lymphoma 2002;43:2099-2107.
127. Longmire WP Jr: Personal reflections on the surgical treatment of portal hypertension. Jpn J Surg 1985;15:243-248.
128. Lopez Serrano P, et al: [Extrahepatic portal hypertension: Spleno-portal thrombosis secondary to protein C deficiency]. An Med Interna 2003;20:473-476.
129. Lowe RC, Grace ND: Pharmacologic therapy for portal hypertension. Curr Gastroenterol Rep 2001;3:24-29.
130. Lui HF, et al: Primary prophylaxis of variceal hemorrhage: A randomized controlled trial comparing band ligation, propranolol, and isosorbide mononitrate. Gastroenterology 2002;123:735-744.
131. Luo B, et al: ET-1 and TNF-alpha in HPS: Analysis in prehepatic portal hypertension and biliary and nonbiliary cirrhosis in rats. Am J Physiol Gastrointest Liver Physiol 2004;286:G294-G303.
132. Mack CL, Superina RA, Whitington PF: Surgical restoration of portal flow corrects procoagulant and anticoagulant deficiencies associated with extrahepatic portal vein thrombosis. J Pediatr 2003;142:197-199.
133. Maddrey WC: Hepatic vein thrombosis (Budd Chiari syndrome): Possible association with the use of oral contraceptives. Semin Liver Dis 1987;7:32-39.
134. Maedler U, et al: Restoration of liver function and portosystemic pressure gradient after TIPSS and late TIPSS occlusion. Cardiovasc Intervent Radiol 2002;25:148-151.
135. Maggi U, et al: Child-Pugh score and liver transplantation. Transplant Proc 1993;25:1769-1770.
136. Majluf-Cruz A, et al: The incidence of protein C deficiency in thrombosis-related portal hypertension. Am J Gastroenterol 1996;91:976-980.
137. Maksoud JG, Goncalves ME: Treatment of portal hypertension in children. World J Surg 1994;18:251-258.
138. Maksoud JG, et al: The endoscopic and surgical management of portal hypertension in children: Analysis of 123 cases. J Pediatr Surg 1991;26:178-181.
139. Malec Z: [Two cases of Warren's distal splenorenal anastomosis in children with portal hypertension]. Wiad Lek 1984;37:677-683.
140. Mann DA, Smart DE: Transcriptional regulation of hepatic stellate cell activation. Gut 2002;50:891-896.
141. Mantz FA Jr, Craige E: Portal axis thrombosis with spontaneous portacaval shunt and resultant cor pulmonale. AMA Arch Pathol 1951;52:91-97.
142. Martelli H, et al: [Surgical treatment of portal hypertension in children: Retrospective study of 157 cases]. Chir Pediatr 1982;23:171-178.
143. McCashland TM: Current use of transjugular intrahepatic portosystemic shunts. Curr Gastroenterol Rep 2003;5: 31-38.
144. McDiarmid SV, et al: Selection of pediatric candidates under the PELD system. Liver Transpl 2004;10(10 Suppl 2):S23-S30.
145. McKiernan PJ, Beath SV, Davison SM: A prospective study of endoscopic esophageal variceal ligation using a multiband ligator. J Pediatr Gastroenterol Nutr 2002;34: 207-211.
146. Michielsen PP: Physiopathology of ascites in portal hypertension. Acta Gastroenterol Belg 1996;59:191-197.
147. Mino RA, Murphy AI Jr, Livingstone RG: Sarcoidosis producing portal hypertension: Treatment by splenectomy

and splenorenal shunt. Ann Surg 1949;130:951-957.
148. Mion F, et al: Azathioprine induced liver disease: Nodular regenerative hyperplasia of the liver and perivenous fibrosis in a patient treated for multiple sclerosis. Gut 1991;32:715-717.
149. Misra A, Loyalka P, Alva F: Portal hypertension due to extensive hepatic cysts in autosomal dominant polycystic kidney disease. South Med J 1999;92:626-627.
150. Misra S, et al: Splenoportovenography: Safety, success rate and hemodynamic changes, and incidence and natural history of splenic hematoma. Indian J Gastroenterol 1991;10:49-50.
151. Nagabhusan G, et al: Ultrasonography in portal hypertension: A sensitive noninvasive test to demonstrate portal-vascular anatomy. Gastroenterol Jpn 1989;24:442-445.
152. Nakatani Y, et al: Pulmonary hypertension associated with portal hypertension in childhood: Case report of a 6-year-old child and review of the literature. Acta Pathol Jpn 1988;38:897-907.
153. Nezakatgoo N, et al: Liver transplantation for acute Budd-Chiari syndrome in identical twin sisters with factor V Leiden mutation. Transplantation 2003;76:195-198.
154. Okuda K: Idiopathic portal hypertension and protein C deficiency. Hepatology 1989;10:903.
155. Olsen TS, Fjeldborg O, Hansen HE: Portal hypertension without liver cirrhosis in renal transplant recipients. APMIS Suppl 1991;23:13-20.
156. Ortiz Cansado A, et al: [Veno-occlusive liver disease due to intake of *Senecio vulgaris* tea]. Gastroenterol Hepatol 1995;18:413-416.
157. Osborne DR: Porto-biliary fistula and portal hypertension due to gallstones: A case report. Acta Chir Scand 1980;146:363-365.
158. Pasqualini M, et al: [Role of sclerotherapy in bleeding esophageal varices in children with portal hypertension]. Minerva Chir 1988;43:1027-1030.
159. Paulus H, et al: [Diagnosis and therapy of portal hypertension caused by portal vein thrombosis]. Med Klin (Munich) 1987;82:860-864.
160. Peck-Radosavljevic M: Hypersplenism. Eur J Gastroenterol Hepatol 2001;13:317-323.
161. Polio J, Groszmann RJ: Hemodynamic factors involved in the development and rupture of esophageal varices: A pathophysiologic approach to treatment. Semin Liver Dis 1986;6:318-331.
162. Postlethwait RW, Moseley V: Esophageal varices: The treatment of portal hypertension by portacaval shunt. J S C Med Assoc 1950;46:305-308.
163. Pozler O, et al: Transjugular intrahepatic portosystemic shunt in five children with cystic fibrosis: Long-term results. Hepatogastroenterology 2003;50:1111-1114.
164. Prediction of the first variceal hemorrhage in patients with cirrhosis of the liver and esophageal varices: A prospective multicenter study. The North Italian Endoscopic Club for the Study and Treatment of Esophageal Varices. N Engl J Med 1988;319:983-989.
165. Preshaw DE, Large A, Johnson AF: Effect of portacaval venous shunt on sulfobromophthalein (bromsulphalein) retention. AMA Arch Surg 1951;62:801-805.
166. Price MR, et al: Management of esophageal varices in children by endoscopic variceal ligation. J Pediatr Surg 1996;31:1056-1059.
167. Rajiv M, et al: Splenic artery aneurysm with arteriovenous fistula as a cause of portal hypertension. Indian J Gastroenterol 2004;23:36-37.
168. Ratnoff OD, Conley CL, Berthrong M: The differentiation between extrahepatic and intrahepatic obstruction of the portal circulation: A clinical study of the Banti syndrome. Bull Johns Hopkins Hosp 1950;87:305-327.
169. Read AE, et al: Hepatic veno-occlusive disease associated with renal transplantation and azathioprine therapy. Ann Intern Med 1986;104:651-655.
170. Reiss U, et al: Hepatic venoocclusive disease in blood and bone marrow transplantation in children and young adults: Incidence, risk factors, and outcome in a cohort of 241 patients. J Pediatr Hematol Oncol 2002;24:746-750.
171. Renard TH, et al: Use of distal splenorenal shunt in children referred for liver transplant evaluation. J Pediatr Surg 1994;29:403-406.
172. Reynaert H, Geerts A: Pharmacological rationale for the use of somatostatin and analogues in portal hypertension. Aliment Pharmacol Ther 2003;18:375-386.
173. Ribas J, et al: Isosorbide-5-mononitrate in the treatment of pulmonary hypertension associated with portal hypertension. Eur Respir J 1999;13:210-212.
174. Rizzati R, et al: Budd-Chiari syndrome associated with systemic lupus erythematosus: Diagnostic imaging and percutaneous treatment. Radiol Med (Torino) 2003;105: 519-523.
175. Rosenberg N, Konigsberg SF, Noronha J: Mesocaval and portacaval shunts using panelled bovine arterial H grafts. Arch Surg 1974;109:754-758.
176. Rossle M, et al: The Budd-Chiari syndrome: Outcome after treatment with the transjugular intrahepatic portosystemic shunt. Surgery 2004;135:394-403.
177. Rypins EB, Sarfeh IJ: Partial portal decompression: Two approaches to the management of portal hypertension. Hepatology 1990;12:370-372.
178. Santambrogio R, et al: [Role of splenectomy in the therapy of hypersplenism associated with intrahepatic portal hypertension]. Minerva Chir 1984;39:953-956.
179. Sarfeh IJ, et al: Portacaval H-graft: Relationships of shunt diameter, portal flow patterns and encephalopathy. Ann Surg 1983;197:422-426.
180. Sarin SK, et al: Endoscopic sclerotherapy for varices in children. J Pediatr Gastroenterol Nutr 1988;7:662-666.
181. Sarin SK, et al: Endoscopic sclerotherapy in the treatment of gastric varices. Br J Surg 1988;75:747-750.
182. Sarin SK, et al: The natural history of portal hypertensive gastropathy: Influence of variceal eradication. Am J Gastroenterol 2000;95:2888-2893.
183. Sarin SK, et al: A randomized controlled trial of cyanoacrylate versus alcohol injection in patients with isolated fundic varices. Am J Gastroenterol 2002;97:1010-1015.
184. Sarin SK, et al: Isolated gastric varices: Prevalence, clinical relevance and natural history. Dig Surg 2003;20:42-47.
185. Saubier EC, et al: [Warren's operation for portal hypertension: Evaluation of results by early angiography in 23 cases]. J Chir (Paris) 1980;117:147-153.
186. Schroeder RA, et al: Pulmonary expression of iNOS and HO-1 protein is upregulated in a rat model of prehepatic portal hypertension. Dig Dis Sci 2000;45:2405-2410.
187. Sedgwick CE, Poulantzas JK, Kune GA: Management of portal hypertension secondary to bile duct strictures: Review of 18 cases with splenorenal shunt. Ann Surg 1966;163:949-953.
188. Selzner M, et al: Current indication of a modified Sugiura procedure in the management of variceal bleeding. J Am Coll Surg 2001;193:166-173.
189. Shah HA, Piris J, Finlayson ND: Primary pulmonary hypertension developing 11 years after a splenorenal shunt for portal hypertension in hepatic cirrhosis. Eur J

Gastroenterol Hepatol 1995;7:283-286.

190. Shah R, et al: Partial splenic embolization: An effective alternative to splenectomy for hypersplenism. Am Surg 1990;56:774-777.

191. Sharma D, et al: A modified technique of devascularization for surgical management of portal hypertension in children. Trop Doct 2001;31:93-95.

192. Shetty K, Rybicki L, Carey WD: The Child-Pugh classification as a prognostic indicator for survival in primary sclerosing cholangitis. Hepatology 1997;25:1049-1053.

193. Shibata M: [Clinical course and prognostic value of Child-Turcotte criteria and Child-Pugh score in medically treated cirrhosis positive for HCV antibody—in comparison with cirrhosis positive for HBs Ag]. Nippon Rinsho 1995;53(Suppl):711-719.

194. Shilyansky J, Roberts EA, Superina RA: Distal splenorenal shunts for the treatment of severe thrombocytopenia from portal hypertension in children. J Gastrointest Surg 1999;3:167-172.

195. Shun A, et al: Portosystemic shunting for paediatric portal hypertension. J Pediatr Surg 1997;32:489-493.

196. Snady H, Feinman L: Prediction of variceal hemorrhage: A prospective study. Am J Gastroenterol 1988;83: 519-525.

197. Sperl W, et al: Reversible hepatic veno-occlusive disease in an infant after consumption of pyrrolizidine-containing herbal tea. Eur J Pediatr 1995;154:112-116.

198. Spina GP, et al: Early hemodynamic changes following selective distal splenorenal shunt for portal hypertension: Comparison of surgical techniques. World J Surg 1990;14:115-121.

199. Srivastava A, et al: Glutathione S-transferase M1 polymorphism: A risk factor for hepatic venoocclusive disease in bone marrow transplantation. Blood 2004;104: 1574-1577.

200. Stanley AJ, Bouchier IA, Hayes PC: Pathophysiology and management of portal hypertension. 2. Cirrhotic ascites. Br J Hosp Med 1997;58:74-78.

201. Stanley AJ, et al: Longterm follow up of transjugular intrahepatic portosystemic stent shunt (TIPSS) for the treatment of portal hypertension: Results in 130 patients. Gut 1996;39:479-485.

202. Starzl TE, et al: Extended survival in 3 cases of orthotopic homotransplantation of the human liver. Surgery 1968;63: 549-563.

203. Stav K, Reif S: [Gastrointestinal bleeding in children—etiology and diagnosis: Survey of patients in a Tel Aviv medical center, in the years 1990 to 1997]. Harefuah 2000;138: 534-538, 615.

204. Steffani KD, et al: [Recurrent intestinal bleeding in a patient with arterio-venous fistulas in the small bowel, limited mesenteric varicosis without portal hypertension and malrotation type I]. Z Gastroenterol 2003;41:587-590.

205. Stickel F, Seitz HK: The efficacy and safety of comfrey. Public Health Nutr 2000;3:501-508.

206. Sugiura M, Futagawa S: A new technique for treating esophageal varices. J Thorac Cardiovasc Surg 1973;66: 677-685.

207. Sugiura M, Futagawa S, Hidai K: A new technique for the treatment of esophageal varices. Bull Soc Int Chir 1975; 34:175-177.

208. Superina RA, Weber JL, Shandling B: A modified Sugiura operation for bleeding varices in children. J Pediatr Surg 1983;18:794-799.

209. Szecseny A: [Results of splenectomy and splenorenal shunt in a case of splenomegalic cirrhosis]. Orv Hetil 1954;95:218-219.

210. Tahan V, et al: Adrenomedullin in cirrhotic and non-cirrhotic portal hypertension. World J Gastroenterol 2003; 9:2325-2327.

211. Terblanche J, et al: A prospective controlled trial of sclerotherapy in the long term management of patients after esophageal variceal bleeding. Surg Gynecol Obstet 1979;148:323-333.

212. Thalheimer U, et al: Monitoring target reduction in hepatic venous pressure gradient during pharmacological therapy of portal hypertension: A close look at the evidence. Gut 2004;53:143-148.

213. Tocornal J, Cruz F: Portosystemic shunts for extrahepatic portal hypertension in children. Surg Gynecol Obstet 1981;153:53-56.

214. Tokiwa K, et al: Pulmonary hypertension as a fatal complication of extrahepatic portal hypertension. Eur J Pediatr Surg 1993;3:373-375.

215. Trobs RB, Bennek J: Partial splenectomy, transposition of the spleen to the abdominal wall or splenohepatoplasty in portal hypertensive rats: Effects on portal venous pressure and homeostasis—microscopical appearance of the transposed spleen. Eur J Pediatr Surg 1998;8:155-162.

216. Uchiyama M, et al: Long-term results after nonshunt operations for esophageal varices in children. J Pediatr Surg 1994;29:1429-1433.

217. Uno A, et al: Portal hypertension in children and young adults: Sonographic and color Doppler findings. Abdom Imaging 1997;22:72-78.

218. Valayer J: [The choice of an operation for correction of portal hypertension in children]. Chir Pediatr 1982;23:214-217.

219. Vallat G, et al: [Portal hypertension by membranous occlusion of the inferior vena cava at its termination. Budd-Chiari-type syndrome]. Med Chir Dig 1980;9: 717-719.

220. van Erpecum KJ, et al: Generalized peliosis hepatis and cirrhosis after long-term use of oral contraceptives. Am J Gastroenterol 1988;83:572-575.

221. van Hoek B: The spectrum of liver disease in systemic lupus erythematosus. Neth J Med 1996;48:244-253.

222. van Vroonhoven TJ, Molenaar JC: Distal splenorenal shunt for decompression of portal hypertension in children with cystic fibrosis. Surg Gynecol Obstet 1979; 149:559-560.

223. Vazquez-Estevez J, et al: [Partial splenic embolization in hypersplenism]. An Esp Pediatr 1984;21:798-802.

224. Villanueva C, et al: Nadolol plus isosorbide mononitrate compared with sclerotherapy for the prevention of variceal rebleeding. N Engl J Med 1996;334:1624-1629.

225. Villanueva C, et al: Maintenance of hemodynamic response to treatment for portal hypertension and influence on complications of cirrhosis. J Hepatol 2004;40: 757-765.

226. Vogelsang GB, Dalal J: Hepatic venoocclusive disease in blood and bone marrow transplantation in children: Incidence, risk factors, and outcome. J Pediatr Hematol Oncol 2002;24:706-709.

227. Voorhees AB Jr, et al: Portal-systemic encephalopathy in the noncirrhotic patient: Effect of portal-systemic shunting. Arch Surg 1973;107:659-663.

228. Warren WD, Zeppa R, Fomon JJ: Selective trans-splenic decompression of gastroesophageal varices by distal splenorenal shunt. Ann Surg 1967;166:437-455.

229. Warren WD, et al: Preoperative assessment of portal hypertension. Ann Surg 1967;165:999-1012.

230. Willner IR: Veno-occlusive disease. Curr Treat Options Gastroenterol 2002;5:465-469.
231. Wilson MW, et al: Percutaneous transhepatic hepatic venography in the delineation and treatment of Budd-Chiari syndrome. J Vasc Interv Radiol 1996;7:133-138.
232. Yachha SK, et al: Gastrointestinal bleeding in children. J Gastroenterol Hepatol 1996;11:903-907.
233. Yamamoto S, et al: Case report of a pancreatic pseudocyst ruptured into the splenic vein causing extrahepatic portal hypertension. Jpn J Surg 1982;12:387-390.
234. Zaman A: Current management of esophageal varices. Curr Treat Options Gastroenterol 2003;6:499-507.
235. Zargar SA, et al: Endoscopic ligation compared with sclerotherapy for bleeding esophageal varices in children with extrahepatic portal venous obstruction. Hepatology 2002;36:666-672.
236. Zargar SA, et al: Fifteen-year follow up of endoscopic injection sclerotherapy in children with extrahepatic portal venous obstruction. J Gastroenterol Hepatol 2004;19:139-145.
237. Zheng RQ, Chung H, Kudo M: Hepatobiliary and pancreatic arterioportal fistula causing portal hypertension. J Gastroenterol Hepatol 2003;18:873.

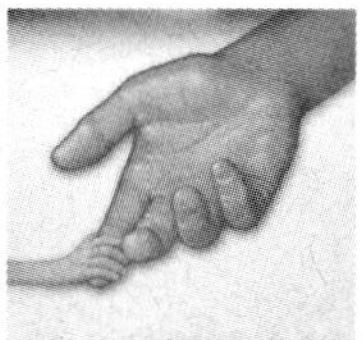

第 107 章

胰腺

Takeshi Miyano

胚胎学

671 胰腺起源于由前肠尾部发育而来的两个内胚层芽。其中一个是腹侧芽，起源于肝憩室的基底部，与胆道密切相关；另一个起源于十二指肠背部的表面，与十二指肠正对，并呈一个轻微的嘴形突向肝憩室[142]。两个内胚层芽大约在妊娠第六或者第七周时发生融合。

背侧芽先于腹侧芽出现，生长速度较快，因此体积较大[129,137]。在妊娠第六周初期形成轴向管道开口并进入肠管，随后很快便出现短的分支[73,128]。

胰腺的腹侧芽短时间内是由两个小叶组成的[105]；在这些小叶中形成小胰管，并开口进入到靠近胆囊的肝憩室中。近端部分从起始处开始延长肝憩室，并从十二指肠上发出腹侧芽。这个近端部分就是所谓的胆总管。左边的腹侧芽小叶后期完全退化。由于十二指肠的快速生长，限制了十二指肠本身环状面的左半部分形成[63]。右边的腹侧芽和发育中的胆总管向后旋转，位置靠近背侧胰腺芽表面的后下方。这种旋转的结果使胆总管的开口位于背侧芽相同方位，这样胆总管就位于开口的腹侧，并低于开口。右边腹侧芽小叶的头部最终位于肠系膜上动脉的后方。

在妊娠第七周，较小的腹侧芽与背侧的胰腺近端部分融合。

分泌型腺泡出现在妊娠第三个月，分泌型细胞簇起源于导管的末端，并聚集在其周围[109]。即使从妊娠第五个月开始就出现了酶原颗粒，也尚无证据表明胎儿腺泡有分泌活性[24]。胰蛋白酶可能早在妊娠第二十二周时就已经出现，但是在接近足月时才出现脂肪酶分泌[197]。腺泡细胞和胰岛细胞都起源并分化自胰腺的导管细胞。这种分化是否是永久性的，或者腺泡细胞是否可能通过以后的分化变成胰岛细胞还不清楚[1,11,88]。

胰腺的异常有许多种，都列在表 107–1 中。

环状胰腺

在妊娠的第六周，总导管和右边的腹侧芽小叶都位于背侧，环绕在十二指肠周围。较长的背侧胰腺导管与腹侧胰腺导管汇合，形成主胰腺导管。这个阶段的发育异常可导致环状胰腺。这种异常的发生率为每 20 000 例新生儿中有 1 例，男性比女性更为常见，男女比例为 2∶1[55]。在一名妇女及其孩子中出现了环状胰腺[155]，同样在连续两代成员中出现了环状胰腺[74]，提示环状胰腺可能与遗传有关，然而还没有得到证实。环状胰腺可表现为刚出生几天就出现十二指肠狭窄或者梗阻症状[119]。

表 107–1　胰腺发育中的异常

先天萎缩或者发育不全
增生或者肥大
发育不良
胰管畸形
胰腺分裂症
环状胰腺
旋转畸形
异位胰腺
胰腺囊肿
动脉、血管和淋巴管畸形
胰腺肿瘤
囊性纤维化

1672 胰腺分裂症

成年人胰腺起源于腹侧和背侧的胰腺芽，其在妊娠第八周末发生融合。胰腺腺体的大部分起源于背侧芽，包括胰头的前上方部分、胰体和胰尾，通过 Santorini 导管或者副胰管引流到微小的乳突。腹侧芽变成胰头的后下方部分。腹侧胰腺芽的引流通过 Wirsung 导管进入主要的 Vater 乳头。随着腹侧和背侧胰腺及其导管系统的融合，Wirsung 导管变成主要的胰管，在接近90%的人群中 Santorini 导管通常都会随着微小乳突一起退化。这两个导管系统不能融合就会导致解剖异常，例如胰腺分裂症。在这种疾病中，Wirsung 导管非常细小，Santorini 导管成为主要的导管系统，通过微小的乳头与十二指肠保持交通。这种构型可见于4%~11%的尸体解剖中，在内镜逆行胰胆管造影术（ERCP）中占到3.25%。

先天性短胰腺

先天性胰腺短缩是一种罕见的畸形，报道称可发生于多脾综合征的个体中[75]，同时也可以是一种单独的畸形[162]。它也可见于共用一套十二指肠的联体婴儿中。这种情况下，胰腺显得较钝，在胰体和胰尾部缺乏胰腺组织，可能是由于背侧胰腺芽发育不全所致[75,162]。尽管胰腺实质部分缺乏，但是胰腺的功能总体上仍保持正常[84]。

手术解剖

胰腺由胰头、胰体和胰尾组成，但是这些区域没有明确的解剖学分界线。胰头位于 L2 的右侧，胰体处于 L1 前面，胰尾上升到 T12 的左侧。腹主动脉和下腔静脉在脊椎前方起到了一定的缓冲作用，然而某些外力（例如座位的安全带和驾驶方向盘损伤）会导致胰体部的钝性创伤。

事实上全部的胰腺都位于腹膜外。解剖学上的连续性是通过横结肠系膜、小肠系膜的腹膜反折，以及脾肾韧带和膈结肠韧带建立的。因此，肠系膜表面存在以直接扩散方式从胰管中溢出的胰酶[132]。这些解剖学上的关系对于理解急性胰腺炎患者的不同影像学改变所代表的病理生理学含义有重要意义。

脾动脉提供了胰腺大部分的血液供应，和脾静脉一起走行在胰腺上边。总体上脾动脉似乎是胰头血液供应中最多的一支。通过胰十二指肠动脉的上动脉和下动脉，胰头与十二指肠一起分享血液供应，其可使胰头部的手术操作变得更为复杂。胰腺的血液回流是向后经细小的分支血管进入肠系膜上静脉。

胆总管的胰腺部分（第三部分）有几个解剖变异值得注意：(1) 胆总管可能部分被胰腺舌部所覆盖（44%），(2) 胆总管可能完全被胰腺所覆盖（30%），(3) 胆总管的后表面可能是暴露的（16.5%），(4) 胆总管可能被胰腺的两个舌部所覆盖（9%）。在进行涉及胰头的手术时，外科医生必须警惕这些变异[166]。

胰腺炎

儿童时期胰腺炎是一种罕见的疾病，然而对于每一个有不明原因的急性或者反复发作性腹痛的儿童，都必须要考虑有胰腺炎的可能。除了在多器官衰竭中所发生的胰腺炎以外，总体上儿童胰腺炎的预后良好。无论胰腺炎有何病因，在所有类型的胰腺炎中都可见到某些普遍性的特征。然而，因为许多种疾病都会导致胰腺炎，所以患者的治疗必须是高度个体化的。

急性胰腺炎

临床上，急性胰腺炎定义为伴有血清胰酶水平升高的一次或者反复发作性腹痛。形态学上相关分类是急性局限性胰腺炎、弥漫肿胀性胰腺炎。急性期以后，症状开始缓解，血液生化指标检查和解剖学上的变化回归正常。急性和慢性胰腺炎之间存在连续性，反复发作性急性胰腺炎可能会进展成具有典型的临床和形态学特征的慢性胰腺炎。

病因学

虽然成年人中的胰腺炎通常与酒精滥用或者胆道疾病有关，但是儿童胰腺炎的病因更为多样化[150,175,191,207,214]。大多数儿童急性胰腺炎病例是由于全身性感染、创伤、胆总管结石病、胰胆管系统异常和药物（表 107-2）所致[153,175]。少见的病因还包括特发性疾病、代谢性疾病以及其他各种疾病，例如家族性胰腺炎和 Crohn 病[153,175]。

胰腺炎中有 6%～33% 的病例与胆道或者胰管疾病有关[23,40,180,191,207,214]，胆总管囊肿和胆石症是最为常见的原因。胆总管囊肿常与胰管和胆道的畸形融合（胰胆管融合畸形）有关，可能会形成一段较长的共同管道，使得胆汁反流到胰管中[126,17]。共同管道易见于 ERCP 中，这种管道通常是扩张性的，并包含有蛋白质栓或者结石，可导致梗阻性胰腺炎或者黄疸。

673 儿童胆石症经常与各种溶血性疾病有关，包括球形细胞增多症、β-珠蛋白生成障碍性贫血（地中海贫血）和镰状细胞贫血病。胆石症也可以由肥胖症和应用全胃肠外营养导致。胰管发育畸形在胆石症中的作用，例如胰管分离和 Vater 壶腹部狭窄，只是近来才被人们所认识[26,28,66,125,154,181,214]。不伴有胆总管囊肿的胰胆管融合畸形正在引起临床上的关注，因为它在超声检查中容易被忽略；大多数有这种疾病的患者有胰腺炎引起的反复发作性腹痛[107,125,181,202]。Tagge 等[181]发现 61 例胰腺炎患者中有 6 例（10%）有胰胆管融合畸形。他们注意到有胰胆管融合畸形的患者通常有反复发作的腹痛，复发性或慢性胰腺炎也与胰胆管的融合畸形有关。

表 107-2　儿童急性胰腺炎的病因

- 全身性感染
  - 腮腺炎
  - 风疹
  - 柯萨奇病毒 B
- 创伤
  - 钝性腹部创伤
  - 医源性创伤（例如手术、ERCP）
- 胰胆管系统畸形
  - 胰胆管融合畸形
  - 胰腺分裂症
  - Oddi 括约肌压力过高
  - 胆总管囊肿
  - 胆总管结石病
- 药物
  - 硫唑嘌呤
  - 四环素
  - L-门冬酰胺酶
  - 免疫抑制剂
  - 丙戊酸
- 代谢性疾病
  - 高甘油三酸酯血症
  - 高钙血症
  - 囊性纤维化
- 肝移植
- 混合性疾病
- 特发性疾病

（ERCP = 内镜逆行胰胆管造影术）

严重的腹部创伤可即刻造成急性症状[198]。然而，程度稍轻的创伤可导致迟发性发作和亚急性的临床表现。在所有曾有模糊不清病史的急性胰腺炎儿童中，都应该考虑到有儿童虐待的可能[214]。最后，在进行腹部手术或者 ERCP 的过程中，也可造成医源性损伤[163]。

药物可导致 8%～25% 的胰腺炎病例。使用某种免疫抑制药物可能与急性胰腺炎有关；然而，在我们的经验中，这种类型的急性胰腺炎对加贝酯反应良好，但是必须在早期大剂量应用。导致胰腺炎的大多数药物通常包括去羟肌苷、硫唑嘌呤、巯嘌呤、L-门冬酰胺酶和丙戊酸[62,118,180,190,206,207]。近来有报道称肝移植是导致急性胰腺炎的一个可能因素。在儿童中这种并发症的发生率和死亡率分别为 1.9% 和 43%[186]。肝移植术后发生的急性胰腺炎和一些高危因素，例如暴发性肝功能衰竭的诊断、再移植、肝移植时进行广泛的解剖、肾下动脉移植的使用，有很强的相关性[41]。

胰蛋白酶原基因和囊性纤维化跨膜转导调节因子（*CFTR*）基因的某些变异可导致急性复发性胰腺炎。许多特发性胰腺炎患者都有复合的杂合子基因型，其中 *CFTR* 基因的等位基因都是异常的，因此组成了不同程度的囊性纤维化。也有许多关于慢性胰腺炎和一些 *CFTR* 突变之间相关性的报道，这些相关性存在于有囊性纤维化的患者和携带有单基因突变的患者中[22,117,215]。

某种情况下，在出生以前就已经开始了胰腺的破坏。Shwachman-Diamond 综合征，一种常染色体隐性遗传病，近来被定位于 7 号染色体的着丝粒区域[58]，有这种综合征的婴幼儿在出生时就有胰腺功能不足，通常只有极低的血清胰蛋白酶原水平，提示到出生时几乎全部的胰腺外分泌功能都已经发生萎缩[38]。

诊断

急性胰腺炎的诊断基于临床病史、体格检查、实验室检查、诊断性影像学检查。通过淀粉酶分泌组织检测淀粉酶同工酶也已经用于增加诊断的精确性。血清脂肪酶水平也可以补充胰腺炎检测，增加诊断结果的阳性率[68]。目前已经提出了一套急性胰腺炎的新评分系统，与 Ranson 和 Glasgow 评分系统相比具有更好的敏感性[31]。参数包括年龄（<7 岁）、体重（<23 kg）、入院时白细胞计数（>18 500）、乳酸脱氢酶水平（>2000）、48 小时的低谷 Ca^{2+} 水平（<8.3 mg/dl）、48 小时的低谷白蛋白水平（<2.6 g/dl）、48 小时的液体潴留［>75 ml/(kg · 48 h)］和 48 小时的血液尿素氮水平升高（>5 mg/dl）。

拍摄胸部 X 光平片和腹部立位平片可以排除小肠穿孔[150,153]。偶尔，可以见到不透射线的胆结石、充气的右侧结肠，或者一段扩张的小肠肠袢（特征环）。左侧基底部胸膜的渗出相对比较常见，肺野的斑点状阴影是全身细胞因子释放的一种特征。通过应用水溶性造影剂来增强上消化道的影像学检查偶尔是有效的，尤其是在强烈怀疑有十二指肠或者小肠损伤的创伤病例中。

超声和 CT 扫描对检查胰腺病变是有效的[59,91]。创伤导致的腹部器官损伤，尤其是胰腺损伤，适合进行 CT 检查。

1674 ERCP 极少适合于急性胰腺炎患者；然而，在有不明原因的胰腺炎患儿中，ERCP 最终变成必需检查[28,66,125,181]。这种技术在伴有胰胆管融合畸形的复发性胰腺炎病例中非常实用[28,66,99,125,181]。

然而，ERCP 是一种可加重胰腺炎的损伤性技术，在胰腺炎的急性期通常不是首选方法。磁共振胰胆管成像（MRCP）是获得胰腺胆管影像的一种无创技术。MRCP 可在超过 96% 的患者中显示出胆总管，发现胆总管结石的敏感性为 71%～100%，超出了超声检查（20%～65%）和 CT 扫描（45%～85%）的敏感性。在超过 80% 的患者中可成功看到更为细小的胰管[83]。我们以前评价了 MRCP 在儿童急性胰腺炎患者中的作用[164]。患儿分为两组：第一组为 7 名超声诊断有胆总管囊肿的患儿，第二组为 9 名没有明显病因的急性胰腺炎的患儿。第一组的 7 名患儿中有 6 例发现存在胰胆管融合畸形，而在第二组的 9 名患儿中则只有 1 例出现此畸形。在第一组的患儿中发现 1 例有胰腺分裂症，但是在第二组的患儿中没有确定存在胰腺分裂症者。在第一组的患儿中有 1 例发现有主胰管扩张，在第二组中有 3 例。这些发现都提示 MRCP 在鉴别和排除儿童胰胆管结构异常中是一种潜在的有效方法。

治疗

急性胰腺炎的治疗有两个主要目的：（1）减少任何发病因素；（2）提供精确的支持治疗，包括大量应用镇痛药、应用胃肠外液体、维持营养需求、预防感染、抑制内分泌和外分泌的活性。

通常所需要的胃肠外镇痛药为麻醉药或者非甾体类消炎药，甚至可应用在轻度的胰腺炎患者中，因为胰腺炎的疼痛可以是非常剧烈的。传统上多应用哌替啶而不是吗啡，因为后者可导致 Vater 壶腹部的痉挛。

通常开始时给予鼻胃管吸引以减少呕吐和腹胀，然而除非患儿正在呕吐，鼻胃管减压的作用尚有疑问[48]。胃酸的吸引也可以通过限制胰泌素的释放来减少胰腺的外分泌。

必须停止口服喂养以减少对胰腺的刺激。早期给予全胃肠外营养以避免营养不良[165]。另外，在重症胰腺炎患儿中早期放置中央静脉导管可提供血管内液体支持和营养支持的通路。

应检测血细胞比容和血清中血糖及血钙的水平，仔细监测每小时的尿量。

虽然预防性应用抗生素的作用并没有得到证实，但是有坏死性胰腺炎的患儿可能会受益。其他治疗策略包括推荐使用生长抑素、高血糖素、抗胆碱能药、组胺阻滞剂和蛋白酶抑制剂，但是直到现在它们尚未显示出有明确作用。

在急性胰腺炎中，手术治疗以前试图控制疾病时都必须使用标准的内科治疗。儿童急性胰腺炎很少需要进行手术治疗，但是如果诊断不明确或者在急性期以后出现了并发症，例如假性囊肿或者是脓肿，偶尔也需要手术治疗。在有潜在的胰胆管融合畸形的急性胰腺炎患儿中，想要治愈通常需要进行手术，纠正潜在的胰胆管融合畸形[153]。

在重症急性胰腺炎的处理中，一个主要的决策就是胰腺坏死或者感染是否需要以及需要何时进行手术治疗。在重症急性胰腺炎中，坏死性胰腺组织的感染是死亡的主要危险因素，是手术治疗的指征之一。另一方面，非手术的保守治疗可处理无菌性胰腺坏死，包括抗生素治疗。有报道称无菌性胰腺坏死的死亡率为 1.8%，而感染性坏死的死亡率为 24%[20]。早期手术与死亡率增加有关，如果手术治疗不可避免，应该延迟手术的进行[146]。

慢性复发性胰腺炎

慢性复发性胰腺炎的特征是上腹部反复发作的疼痛，合并不同程度的胰腺外分泌和内分泌功能不良。在儿童时期相对很少有报道慢性复发性胰腺炎的存在，但是对于有反复发作性腹痛的儿童要考虑到这种疾病的可能[30,43,54,92,138]。这种疾病导致了进展程度不同的不可逆的胰腺结构改变[54]。目前，这种疾病治疗最有争议的一个方面是适当的手术方式选择。

病因和病理生理学

在儿童中，慢性复发性胰腺炎最为常见的病因是创伤[60,179]、遗传性疾病[13,161]、全身性疾病[50]、胰胆管的畸形，例如胰腺分裂症[2]、环状胰腺[34]、胆总管结石病[72]。另外，各种罕见的疾病，包括代谢性疾病、内分泌紊乱、炎症性肠病[13]，都可以导致慢性复发性胰腺炎。慢性复发性胰腺炎的病因列于表 107-3 中。

某些先天性畸形影响胰腺及其周围组织[2,26,28,34,66,72,125]，其中一些与慢性复发性胰腺炎有关。Vater 乳头狭窄和共同管道胆汁反流所导致的胰液流出道梗阻可造成炎症，如果梗阻得到解除，这种炎症可能是可逆的。复发性胰腺炎一个相对常见的病因是胰腺分裂症[2]，其中大多数胰液流经微小的 Santorini 导管，可能是解剖和流体动力学因素导致胰液
5 反应性梗阻。一些病例报道称，在特发性的慢性胰腺炎患者中，胰腺分裂症的发生率升高[2,28]。环状胰腺是由于胚胎性胰腺原基的异常旋转或固定所致，也已经证实与慢性胰腺炎有关（图 107-1）[34]。胰胆管融合畸形伴有或者不伴有胆总管结石病，同样可导致慢性复发性胰腺炎[107,125,181]。

最近几年，已经鉴定出数个基因与遗传性和特发性慢性胰腺炎有关：*PRSS1*、*GFTR* 和 *SPINK1*。*SPINK1* 突变主要发现于没有家族史的患者中。这些突变最常见于特发性慢性胰腺炎患者，然而有遗传性慢性胰腺

表 107-3　儿童慢性复发性胰腺炎的病因

胰管的先天性畸形
胰胆管融合畸形
胰腺分裂症
环状胰腺
胆道疾病
胆总管结石病
胆石症
创伤
全身性感染
遗传性胰腺炎
高脂蛋白血症
甲状旁腺功能亢进症和高钙血症
囊性纤维化
先天性代谢异常
慢性炎症状态
Crohn 病
溃疡性结肠炎
系统性红斑狼疮
慢性纤维性胰腺炎
青少年热带性胰腺炎
特发性慢性胰腺炎

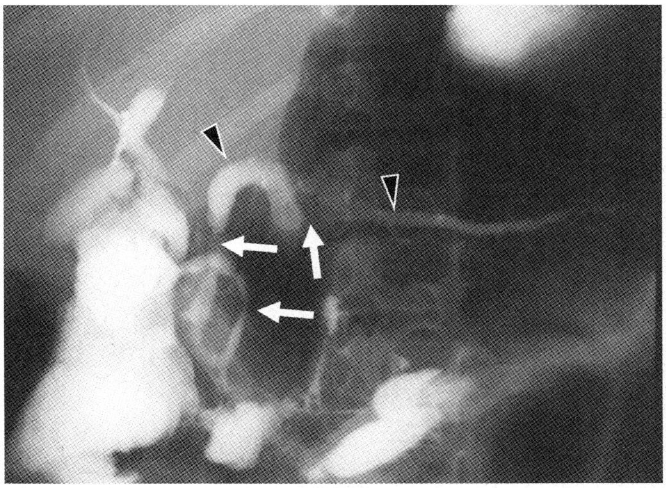

图 107-1　环状胰腺患儿的术前内镜逆行胰胆管造影术（ERCP）。显示出有复杂的胰管畸形伴有扩张（*箭头处*）和狭窄（*箭记号处*）。患儿进行了纵向胰空肠吻合术（Puestow 手术）。

炎的患者主要发生 *PRSS1* 的突变[211]。

诊断

血生化检测：对胰腺持久性损害的程度可以通过血液检测（胰酶检测）、粪便检测（胰酶检测、粪便中脂肪检测）和胰腺功能的无创检测例如胰腺的刺激试验（胰泌素）来评估。

影像学诊断：在30%~50%的慢性胰腺炎的青少年和成年人中，腹部立位平片可以显示胰腺有钙化斑。钙化斑是慢性胰腺炎的诊断特征，即使在临床上缺乏胰腺疾病的依据。然而，在有慢性复发性胰腺炎的儿童中，钙化斑的发生率较低，但是在遗传性胰腺炎的幼儿中，钙化斑的发生率较高[13]。

超声检查是儿童胰腺检查的理想手段。可能会发现胰管或者胆管扩张、钙化斑和并发症，例如假性囊肿、脓肿、结石和腹水。CT 扫描可观察到胰腺和胰管的大小（图 107-2），可有效发现在腹部平片和超声检查中可能遗漏的细小结石。在成年人和儿童中，ERCP 是诊断和处理慢性复发性胰腺炎的重要工具[26,28,30,66]。ERCP 可以发现胰胆管融合畸形伴有或者不伴有胆管的扩张[66,70,181]。在诊断胰胆管畸形中，ERCP 有接近 90% 的准确性。然而，如前所述，MRCP 技术在过去十年间得到了极大改进。MRCP 在许多胰腺和胆道疾病的诊断中与 ERCP 具有同样的价值，因为 MRCP 无创且更加安全，所以

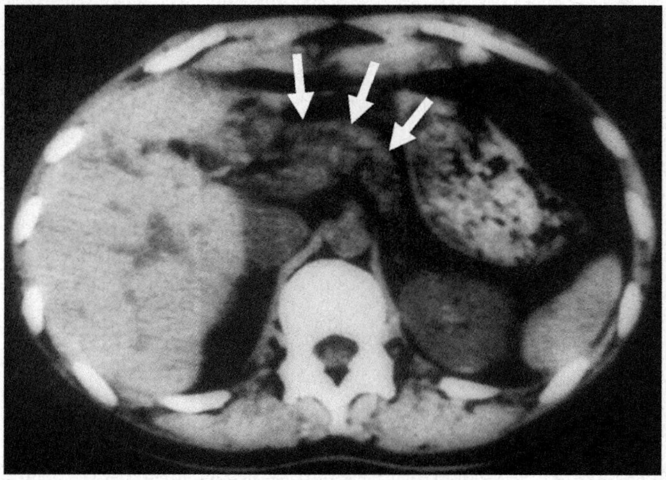

图 107-2　胰管不规则扩张（*箭记号处*）的患儿行 CT 扫描图像。患儿进行了纵向胰空肠吻合术（Puestow 手术）。

更为适合[83,164]。

手术治疗

慢性复发性胰腺炎手术治疗的目的是缓解疼痛、治疗并发症。关于胰腺的手术通常有三种类型：（1）括约肌成形术[89,133,154]，（2）经纵向胰空肠吻合术（Puestow）[148]或者端端胰空肠吻合术（Duval）来引流胰液[39]，（3）胰胃吻合术（Smith）[167]和胰切除术[49]。

数个研究小组已经证明，在谨慎选择的患者中括约肌成形术可成功控制慢性胰腺炎症状[52,133]。然而，正确使用这种手术方式需要通过胰管造影术来排除胰腺内胰管的梗阻。O'Neill 及其同事们[138]报道了在 7 例因慢性胰腺炎而进行括约肌成形术的儿童中有 6 例获得了良好的效果。

使用直接胰管减压手术通常的适应证是存在胰管扩张并有胰内胰管多发性狭窄的证据。引流手术重要的第二特征是通过避免切除大部分的胰腺组织来保留胰腺的内分泌功能。纵向胰空肠吻合术（Puestow 手术）应用于成年人中可在 70%~97% 的患者中成功消除或者缓解慢性胰腺炎的疼痛[147,167,204,208,209]。在儿童中，一些作者认为 Puestow 手术改善了胰腺的功能，缩短了住院时间，并使其朝着标准体重方向增加体重[35]。其他作者报道远端的胰切除术和胰空肠吻合术是有效的术式，而纵向胰空肠吻合术是无效的[205]。关于适当的手术方式，在儿童病例中值得进行进一步思考。

胰腺次全切除或者胰腺全切除术可伴发相当高的并发症发生率和死亡率，只适用于有难以处理的疼痛患者，这些患者都有弥漫性的胰腺实质损伤不伴有胰管扩张[67]。这种手术通常并不适用于儿童。

胰腺分裂症

在这个章节的第一部分已经描述了胰腺分裂症的胚胎学特征。当进行 ERCP 或者 MRCP 时，主乳头注射以后不能看到 Wirsung 管，或者 Wirsung 管较淡或不完全时，便要怀疑胰腺分裂症。MRCP 是一种有效而无创的诊断胰腺分裂症的工具（图 107-3）[164]，但是 ERCP 能够提供关于胰管的详细信息。如果 Vater

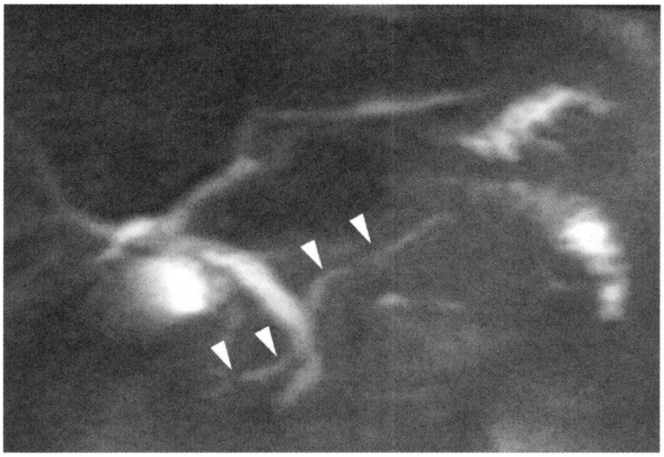

图 107-3　复发性胰腺炎患儿行磁共振胰胆管造影术（MRCP）的图像。Santorini 管是主要的胰管，它延伸至整个胰体和胰尾（*箭头处*）。

乳头注射造影剂以后怀疑有胰腺分裂症，就应该尝试寻找副乳头并将导管插入到副乳头中，但是因为乳头较小以及开口与十二指肠的角度关系，只有不到一半的病例可行副乳头导管插入。如果能够进入到副乳头中去，ERCP 就可显示 Santorini 管是主要的胰管，它延伸到整个胰体和胰尾。Santorini 管的成像偶尔显示有扩张、不规则或者狭窄，就提示存在慢性胰腺炎。

尸体解剖研究已经显示在 4%～11% 的患者中发现有胰腺分裂症，是胰腺最为常见的先天性畸形。当 Wirsung 管缺乏合并胰腺分裂症时，接近 10% 的受累患者有异常的解剖结构，其导致大多数甚至全部的胰腺分泌物引流都通过副乳头来完成[200]。

胰腺分裂症不应该被认为是一种疾病。然而，如果副乳头的流出道狭窄，就可导致胰腺炎。副乳头的狭窄可能是进行性的，因为流出道通常非常细小，而且没有炎症的证据。在不明原因的复发性胰腺炎患者中，胰腺分裂症的发生率可能会显著增高，在一组病例研究中发现有 25% 的患者具有胰腺分裂症[28]。Neblett 和 O' Neill 近来报道了胰腺分裂症在所有的胰腺炎儿童中检出率为 7.4%，在有复发性或者慢性胰腺炎的儿童中检出率为 19.2%。在 10 例胰腺分裂症患者中，8 例有完全性的胰腺分裂症，2 例则为不完全性的变异[134]。

胰腺分裂症合并胰腺炎时，治疗的主要目标是建立 Santorini 管的充分引流。当梗阻早期解除以后，这种疾病就不会进展为胰腺功能不全。纠治手术不仅可以保留胰腺功能，而且可以保证正常的生长和发育。

数个研究报告已经显示 Santorini 管的充分引流可以通过副乳头括约肌成形术来完成[2,115,167,196,201]。内镜下括约肌切开术已经得到临床应用，但是有报道称可出现副乳头再狭窄和症状的复发[93]。如果慢性胰腺炎已经发展到出现胰管扩张，就应该进行纵向胰空肠吻合术[138,148]。Neblett 和 O' Neill[134] 报道了 10 例胰腺分裂症患者中有 8 例进行了手术：7 例进行了经十二指肠的副乳头括约肌成形术，并有 2 例同时进行了主乳头的括约肌成形术（有 1 例同时行乳头中隔成形术）。3 名患者进行了纵向胰空肠吻合术，其中 1 名患者有中段胰管狭窄，另 2 例是因为括约肌成形术术后出现复发性胰腺炎不伴有内分泌和外分泌的胰腺 1677
功能不全。手术干预可直接缓解胰管梗阻，可能只涉及副胰管的括约肌成形术，或者连同主胰管的括约肌成形术及乳头中隔成形术一起进行。有更远端的胰管梗阻或者胰管扩张的患者，可能会从胰空肠吻合术中受益。在一个极其罕见的病例中，我们治疗了一名有胰腺分裂症、胆总管囊肿和胰胆管融合畸形等多种疾病共存的患者。图 107-4 显示术前 ERCP 和术中胆道造影的图像。这名患者进行了完全的胆总管囊肿切除和 Roux-en-Y 肝管空肠吻合术，随后进行经十二指肠乳头成形术，使得共同管道完全引流[106]。

胰腺囊肿和假性囊肿

胰腺囊肿在儿童中相对少见。囊肿的病因多样化，包括先天性和获得性的因素[199]。胰腺囊肿可以分为先天性的进行性囊肿、滞留性囊肿、肠道的重复畸形和假性囊肿。

先天性的进行性胰腺囊肿

先天性的进行性胰腺囊肿非常罕见，可能会在胎儿、婴幼儿、儿童或者成年人中遇到[3]。至今所有的儿科文献中只有 22 例相关报道[7,8,124,143]。这些囊肿在女性中多发。最常见于胰体和胰尾部，更多的是单腔性囊肿而非多腔性，内衬上皮细胞。囊肿内通常充填有混浊的黄色无菌液体，没有胰酶活性，不易发生粘连和感染。有报道称囊肿可同时发生在其他器官，

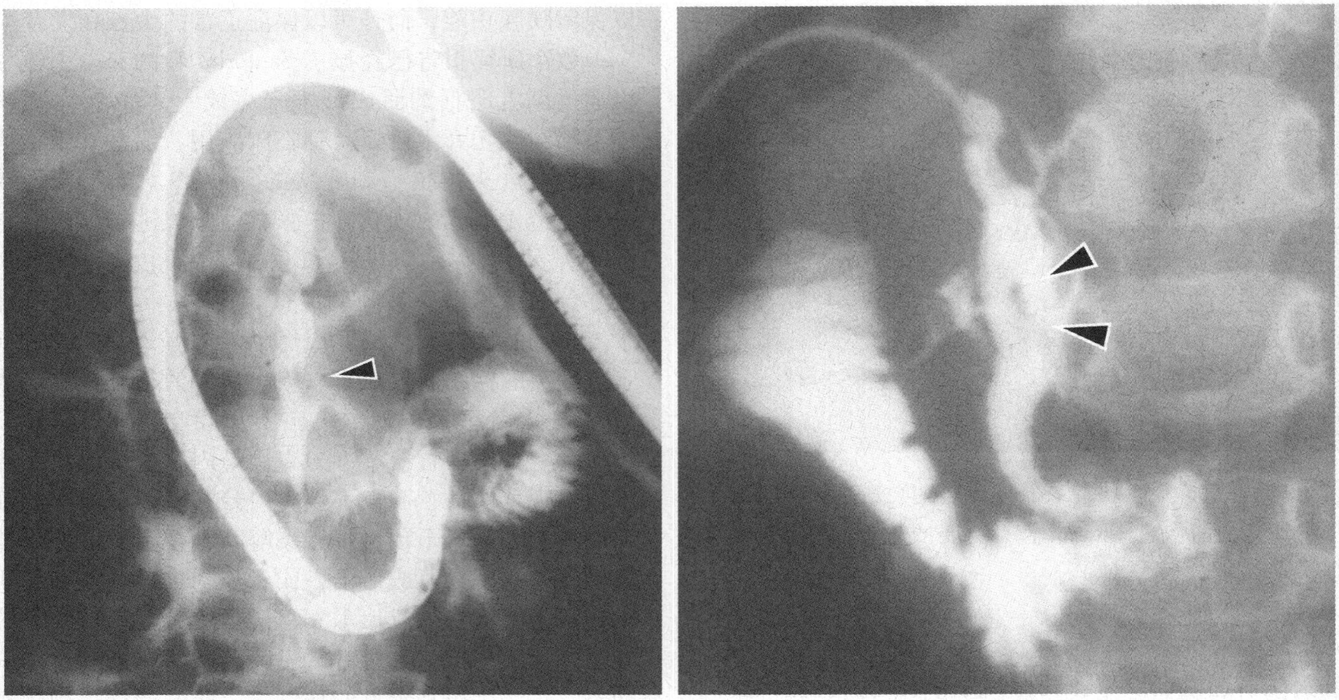

A　B

图 107-4　胆总管囊肿合并胰腺分裂症的患儿行（*A*）术前内镜逆行胰胆管造影术（ERCP）和（*B*）术中胆管造影术。也可以看到在胰内胆管中的隔膜（*箭头处*）。

例如 von Hippel-Lindau 病的特征是遗传性的小脑囊肿、视网膜的血管瘤、胰腺和其他器官的囊肿[79]。不认为与囊性纤维化同时发生的囊肿是胰腺假性囊肿，在这个章节中不进行讨论。

临床上，先天性的进行性胰腺囊肿是偶然发现的，或者是因为在产前时期出现羊水过多而被发现。出生以后，可能表现为没有症状的腹胀，或由于对临近器官外在的压迫而导致呕吐或者黄疸，或者是没有症状的腹部肿块。手术治疗包括胰体或胰尾囊肿的全部切除，以及胰头部囊肿的内引流术。

滞留性囊肿

胰腺的滞留性囊肿比较罕见，是由于腺体的慢性梗阻所导致[11]。这些囊肿内含有浑浊的液体，由胰腺外分泌的分泌物和高浓度的胰酶组成。这样的囊肿内衬胰管上皮细胞，除非是被慢性扩张或者是胰酶暴露引起的炎症所破坏[140]。

肠道的重复畸形

胰腺的肠道重复畸形比较罕见，通常伴有胃的重复畸形[136]。这种重复畸形最有可能的是由于由胰管形成的肠道憩室退化不全所导致[5]。所报道的许多涉及胰腺的肠道重复畸形病例囊肿与胰管相通，内衬胃型的上皮细胞，在其囊壁中含有异位的胰腺组织。

这些病例中最为常见的症状是反复发作性腹痛，常是饭后腹痛。伴有肠道重复畸形性囊肿的胰腺炎是由胰管梗阻所导致，囊肿内粘滞的分泌物或者血液以及囊肿内因消化性溃疡产生的碎片都可导致胰管梗阻[112,187]。在没有胰腺炎的病例中，腹部疼痛可以由于分泌物聚积以及肌肉收缩导致的囊壁张力所致[121]。

在胎儿 B 超检查中也可以发现胰腺的囊肿[101]。

到目前为止，文献中所有的肠道重复畸形性囊肿都可以通过完整切除治疗。有些囊肿需要进行胰管十二指肠切除术和内引流术[112]。

胰腺假性囊肿

临床特征

胰腺假性囊肿位于胰腺分泌物的集合部，囊肿内没有内衬上皮细胞，通常在胰腺损伤、炎症或者胰管梗阻以后发生[79]。在儿童中胰腺假性囊肿最为常见的原因是创伤和感染[123]。药物导致的急性胰腺炎，例如丙戊酸，也是胰腺假性囊肿的一种罕见原因[149]。

典型的囊肿位于胃后面的小网膜囊，由炎性结缔组织包裹的一个纤维素囊组成[15]。假性囊肿的囊壁也可以由临近组织组成，例如胃、十二指肠、结肠、小肠或者网膜。在大多数病例中囊液清澈或者呈麦秸色，可能包含有牙膏样的碎片。囊液淀粉酶的水平通常要高于 50 000 Somogyi U/ml[145]。

诊断

腹部钝性创伤史可提示存在胰腺假性囊肿，一种类似于胰腺炎的疾病，随后有数周到数月的无症状间歇期，在上腹部或者左上腹可扪及一个肿块。

腹痛是最为常见的症状，可伴有黄疸、胸痛、胃肠道梗阻的体征、呕吐、胃肠道出血、体重下降、发热和腹水。

B 超、CT 以及磁共振检查可有助于得出准确的诊断。这些检查对评估囊壁的厚度和在治疗期间观察囊肿内的变化有很大帮助（图 107-5）[14,48,59,97]。因为 ERCP 可以最终确定胰管的状态，指导外科干预，所以 ERCP 也是有效的检查手段[97,151,152,192]。

治疗

胰腺假性囊肿的最佳处理目前还存在争议。治疗选择包括从保守的药物治疗到手术引流[114,158,198]。常规处理包括持续 6 周的等待期的支持治疗，在此期间囊肿可自发消退，或者囊肿壁进行性的纤维化成熟，因此可以进行手术内引流到胃或者空肠[156,195]。这 6 周的等待期传统上已被人们接受，但是 CT 扫描中，早在 3～4 周时就可能显示出囊肿壁增厚，足以承受手术缝合。手术引流通常在成年人中进行，但是在儿童中存在争议，因为在这个年龄组中大多数的胰腺假性囊肿不通过手术引流就可自发消退，复发的风险较低[14,144]。

醋酸奥曲肽是一种长效的生长抑素类似物，已经显示可成功在胰腺术后降低胰腺的外分泌功能，最近在治疗胰腺假性囊肿中也获得成功[131]。

并发症的主要风险，例如感染、未经治疗的胰腺假性囊肿大出血或者严重症状持续，可能是更早进行手术治疗的指征。如果患者不能耐受大手术，则推荐进行外引流术[139]。有显著的证据提示内引流手术，尤其是经胃的囊肿胃造口术，在治疗胰腺假性囊肿中是有效的[90]。与此手术相比，其他学者[45,85,94]报道了经皮引流和内镜下透壁引流是安全有效的手术。然而通常认为，外引流术相比内引流术发生并发症的风险更高，例如瘘管形成和更高的复发率[25,42]。除非胰腺假性囊肿的囊壁已经成熟，足以耐受手术缝合，否则经胃的囊肿胃造口术不可能完成[96]。近来，研究显示，超过 6 周的假性囊肿患者以及囊肿直径大于 5 cm 的患者才能进行引流术，因为在确定诊断以后的最初 6 周内大多数胰腺假性囊肿会自发消退，并且 6 周后假性囊肿治疗的相关风险也会减少[96]。

虽然囊肿十二指肠造口术相对其他的手术操作较少应用，但囊肿紧密黏附于十二指肠是此手术的指征[71,157,212]。Roux-en-Y 囊肿空肠吻合术是最为广泛地应用于假性囊肿的内引流手术，此手术的并发症发生率和复发率最低[159]。

胰腺十二指肠吻合术或者远端胰腺切除术在理想条件下治疗假性囊肿患者都是有效的[145]。在假性囊肿位于胰体或胰尾部并有多发性小囊肿的患者中，可能需要进行远端的胰腺切除术[212]。

涉及胰头和胰腺钩状部分的囊肿并不适合于做内引流术，这种情况比较罕见，可能需要行近端的胰腺切除术，但是这样的切除手术应该只是作为一种最后的治疗手段[48,129,151,152]。

高胰岛素血症 1679

婴幼儿和儿童发生的低血糖有许多原因。在新生儿中，及时评估和治疗低血糖是必需的，因为持续的低血糖可能会导致永久性的脑损伤。1921 年，当 Banting 和 Best[9]分离出胰岛素作为有活性的激素时，就提出了胰腺在低血糖中的作用。在正常人群中，当

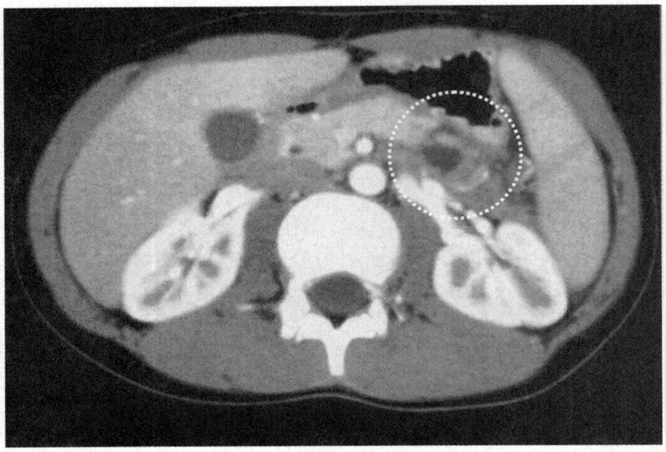

A

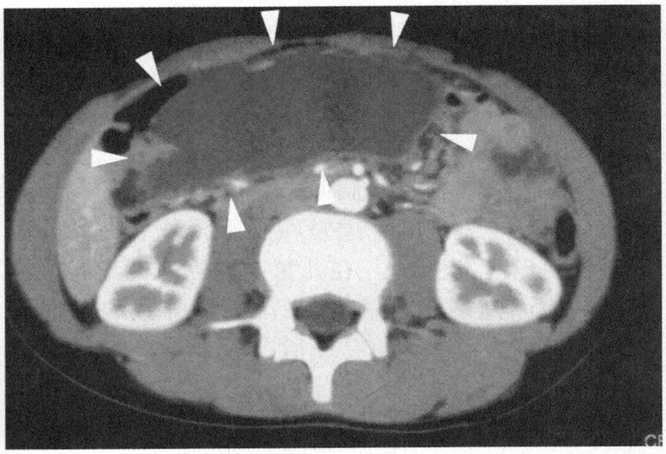

B

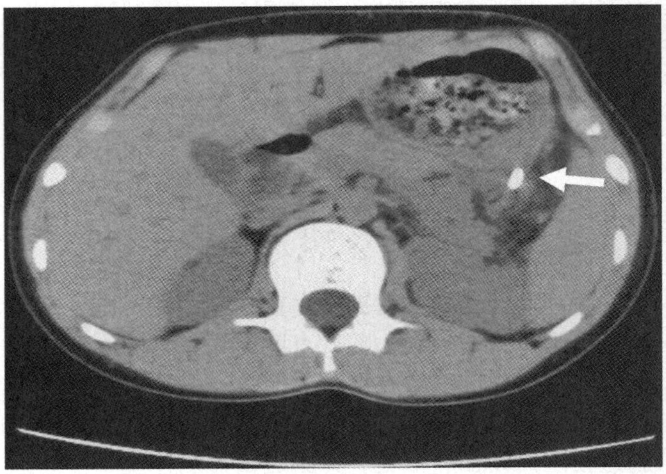

C

图 107-5　一名 12 岁男孩创伤后出现腹部胰腺假性囊肿的 CT 扫描图像。A. 胰体中断（*虚线环内*）。B. 外伤以后 2 周时发展成一个巨大的囊肿（*箭头处*）。C. 进行经皮穿刺外引流术（*箭记号处*）。

血糖下降到低血糖水平时，血清胰岛素水平较低；然而，在这些出现低血糖的高胰岛素血症人群中，胰岛素水平会不恰当地升高。在不到 5 年的时间里，以前被命名为胰岛母细胞增生症或者顽固性新生儿高胰岛素血症性低血糖（PHHI）的这种疾病，已经从分子、基因和临床水平进行了重新定义，从而可以合理地进行分类、诊断、治疗和预后（表 107-4）[168]。

病理生理学

胰腺的胰岛素分泌是一个复杂的、高度整合的过程，由营养物、激素和自主神经系统进行调节。这些信号作用于胰腺 β 细胞，其分泌胰岛素最终由三磷酸腺苷（ATP）敏感的钾离子通道（K_{ATP}）进行调节，

表 107-4　新生儿时期高胰岛素血症性低血糖的基因型分类

K_{ATP}通道缺陷
SUR1 突变
Kir6. 2 突变
杂合性缺失
葡萄糖激酶-激活突变
谷氨酸脱氢酶-激活突变
未定义的
常染色体显性遗传
常染色体隐性遗传
散发性
Beckwith-Wiedemann 综合征
β 细胞腺瘤-多发性内分泌肿瘤 Ⅰ 型

而 K_{ATP}可控制胰腺 β 细胞膜的极性。ATP/ADP（腺苷二磷酸）的摩尔比值保持了 K_{ATP}通道的通畅性，允许钾离子从正常的细胞内高浓度一侧流出细胞外，以保持细胞膜的极化。胰腺的 K_{ATP}通道由两种蛋白亚体组成——磺胺尿素受体 1（SUR1）和内向整流钾通道 Kir6.2，其独特的基因定位于 11 号染色体的临近位点（11p15.1）[4,141]。通过胰岛素非依赖性葡萄糖运输载体 GLUT2 转运到 β 细胞内的葡萄糖，通过葡萄糖激酶进行磷酸化，然后进行代谢，导致 ATP/ADP 比例的增加。ATP/ADP 比例增加会关闭 K_{ATP}通道，引发一系列事件，其特征是细胞内钾离子浓度升高、细胞膜去极化、钙离子内流以及胰岛素从储存的腺体中释放。这些基因的突变造成家族型的 PHHI。葡萄糖激酶和谷氨酸脱氢酶的活化性突变刺激了胰岛素在低血糖浓度时的异常分泌，因此产生了低血糖伴异常的高胰岛素血症[57,173]。葡萄糖激酶的基因定位于 7 号染色体上。

常染色体隐性遗传的 PHHI 大多数由 *SUR1/Kir6.2* 基因突变所致，而常染色体显性遗传的 PHHI 并不是由这类突变所致。目前，已经有两种已知病因引起常染色体显性遗传的 PHHI。其中一种是葡萄糖激酶基因中的功能获得性突变[57]，另外一种是在编码线粒体的谷氨酸脱氢酶基因中发生活化性突变[173]。

PHHI 病例中的大部分，也就是说大约有超过 95% 的病例是散发性的。局灶性的 PHHI 占所报道病例的 30%～40%，其余的 60%～70% 为弥散性[32,194]。局灶性 PHHI 的特征是胰岛样细胞的局灶性腺瘤增生，伴有小 β 细胞的细胞核紧密填充在一起。与此相反，在弥散性 PHHI 中，遍及胰腺的朗格汉斯细胞岛大小不规则，并伴含有巨大异常 β 细胞核的肥大的胰岛素分泌细胞。近来的研究显示，在 11 号染色体的 p15 区域出现母源等位基因的丢失和 K_{ATP}通道的突变，可导致高胰岛素血症[32]。另一方面，散发性 PHHI 伴有弥散表型的许多病例的病因学还不清楚。

Beckwith-Wiedemann 综合征是由染色体的 11p15.5 区域发生突变所致，在其发病机制中包括这个区域的重复序列。通常认为胰岛素样生长因子Ⅱ型（IGF-Ⅱ）的过度表达在躯体的过度生长和胚胎性肿瘤的发展中都起到了重要作用。到目前为止，还没有关于 K_{ATP}通道成分 SUR1/Kir6.2 的基因突变来解释高胰岛素血症和这种综合征伴有的低血糖的报道。

诊断

高胰岛素血症的诊断基于以下标准：（1）血浆胰岛素水平异常升高，与此有关的血糖水平在饭后和禁食期间的不同时间进行测量（例如胰岛素水平大于 10 μU/ml，同时伴有血糖水平小于 50 mg/dl）；（2）需要输注葡萄糖速率大于 10 mg/(kg · min) 以在没有尿糖的情况下保持血液中葡萄糖浓度大于 35 mg/dl；（3）在低血糖期间游离脂肪酸和血酮体的血浆浓度较低，因为胰岛素可抑制脂解作用和酮体产生；（4）尽管存在低血糖，还是对胰高血糖素有血糖反应。

在不具有 Beckwith-Wiedemann 综合征的特征和出生于非糖尿病母亲的巨大儿中，应该怀疑与 K_{ATP}通道中功能缺陷相关的高胰岛素血症。在这些婴幼儿中，可能会在出生后数小时或者数天内发生低血糖，因此诊断的可能性大。

另外一个试验是在低血糖时检测 IGF 结合蛋白 1（IGFBP1）的水平[104]。IGFBP1 的分泌实际上是由胰岛素所控制，血清中 IGFBP1 的浓度比血清胰岛素浓度更加稳定。在正常儿童和那些有不同程度内分泌或者代谢疾病而不是高胰岛素所致的低血糖儿童中，禁食期间 IGFBP1 的水平会上升，而 PHHI 的患者血清 IGFBP1 浓度接近对照组数值的 10%～20%。通常，这些数值小于 50 ng/ml，而对照组人群中数值接近 300 ng/ml。因此，在婴幼儿或者儿童发生低血糖的时候，异常的低 IGFBP1 浓度是诊断高胰岛素血症的另外一个指标。

经皮肝穿刺门静脉和胰腺静脉置入导管并连续检测胰岛素水平，这项技术已经应用于成年人中[82]，并且近来已经开始研究应用于儿童中。测量引流胰腺各部分的静脉中的葡萄糖、胰岛素、胰岛素-C 肽的比例以便定位病变部位。这些研究因为需要一定分析时间而有使用上的局限性。

鉴别诊断

对怀疑胰腺源性低血糖儿童的检查诊断是复杂的

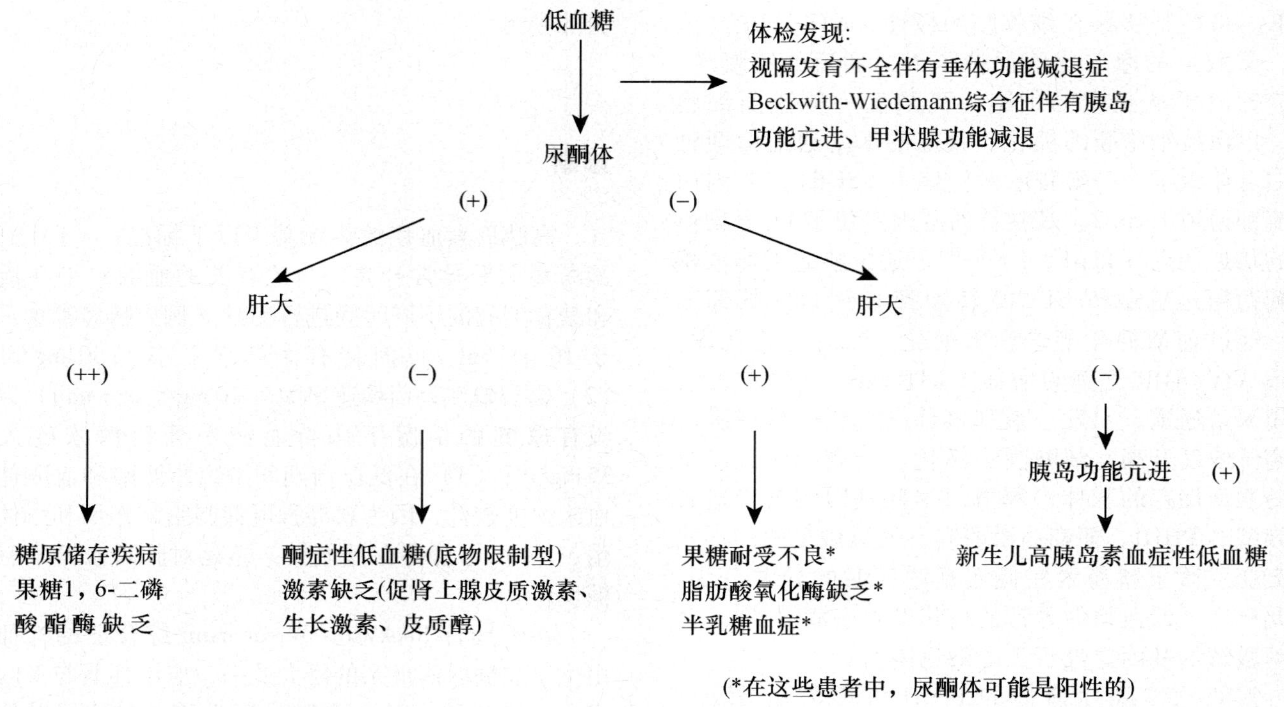

图 107-6 低血糖的鉴别诊断途径示意图。

(图 107-6)。低血糖的三个主要分类是高胰岛素血症、先天性代谢异常、内分泌功能障碍。内分泌疾病，例如肾上腺功能不足、全垂体功能减退症、单独的生长激素缺乏、甲状腺功能低下和先天性肾上腺增生，通常都可以通过体检和特异性的激素测定来鉴别。当存在肝大时，必须要考虑肝源性的疾病。

在小于 1 岁的儿童中，酮症性低血糖是最为常见的病因。通过低出生体重、经过整个夜间禁食后清早的症状和伴随的酮血症及酮尿症等病史，就可提示有
1681 酮症性低血糖。Stanley 和 Baker 具体描述了不同的先天性代谢异常的特异性生化检查诊断[172]。在这些儿童中，低血糖发作倾向于随年龄增长而自发消退。Beckwith-Wiedemann 综合征经常伴有低血糖，但会随着精心的内科治疗而自发消退。

治疗

内科处理

在 PHHI 中，分子缺陷和临床特征的相互关系呈现在表 107-5 中[168]。

内科治疗包括静脉提供 15%～20% 的葡萄糖以防止低血糖的发生。葡萄糖输液必须持续进行，调节至保持正常的血糖水平所需要的最小速率。通常需要放置中心静脉导管。

经常给予喂养以提供持续的葡萄糖摄入。多个药物试剂已经得到应用：二氮嗪、奥曲肽、胰高血糖素和丙酮二酰脲。

二氮嗪是主要的内科治疗药物。它作用于抑制 K_{ATP}通道的组分 SUR1，因此可防止钾离子通道的关闭，导致胰岛素分泌减少。通常初始剂量为 8～10 mg/(kg·d)，以后逐渐增加直到达到正常的血糖水平。最大剂量是 15～20 mg/(kg·d)[61,130]。治疗的成功率在 50%～75% 之间，但是在严重受累的新生儿中，成功率不到 50%。对二氮嗪缺乏反应可能反映出功能性的胰腺 K_{ATP} 通道的缺乏，如同在有 *SUR1/Kir6.2* 基因突变的患者中所见。钙离子通道阻滞剂，尤其是长效的生长抑素类似物奥曲肽，作为内科治疗药物可能会更加有效，有报道称在多达一半的受累婴幼儿中都获得了成功[56,102,108,185]。这些内科治疗方法的失败是进行胰腺切除术的明确指征，以避免出现长期的神经后遗症。

表 107-5 新生儿时期持久性高胰岛素血症性低血糖中分子缺陷与临床特征的关系

类型	巨大胎儿	低血糖/高胰岛素血症	家族史	分子缺陷	相关的临床、生化或者分子特征	对内科治疗的反应	推荐的手术方式	预后
散发型	出生时就存在	中度/重度，从出生第一天到数周	阴性	? SUR1/Kir6.2	在微腺瘤中存在杂合性缺失	总体上反应不佳，可能对生长抑素的反应要好过二氮嗪	如果冰冻切片显示β细胞团块伴有小核微腺瘤，则行部分胰腺切除术	极好
							如果冰冻切片显示β细胞中有巨核散播性增生，则行胰腺次全切除术（>95%）	密切随访；在 50% 的患者中会发生糖尿病，在 33% 的患者中出现持续性低血糖
常染色体隐性遗传	出生时就存在	重度，从出生第一天到数周	阳性	SUR1/Kir6.2	在某些人群中有血缘性特征	反应不良	胰腺次全切除术	密切随访
常染色体显性遗传	不常见	中度，通常在出生 6 个月以后才开始	阳性	葡萄糖激酶（激活）	无	非常好~极好	通常不需要手术/只有在内科治疗无效时才行部分胰腺切除术	极好
常染色体显性遗传	不常见	中度，通常在出生 6 个月以后才开始	阳性	谷氨酸脱氢酶（激活）	轻度的高氨血症	非常好~极好	通常不需要进行手术	极好
Beckwith-Wiedemann 综合征	出生时就存在	中度，约 6 个月以后会自发消退	阴性	倍增印记在染色体 11p15.1	巨舌，脐膨出，半侧身体肥大	良好	不推荐进行手术	低血糖预后极好，有相关的胚胎性肿瘤（Wilms 瘤、肝母细胞瘤）

手术治疗

对于已经给予最佳的内科治疗但还是不能维持正常禁食时血糖水平的患者，应该早期给予手术治疗，以避免未被发现的低血糖和脑损伤。手术目的是减少产生过量的胰岛素，但是这种手术是非生理性的和不精确的[29,172]。目前推荐的手术方案是做95%的切除，并只在十二指肠和胆道上留下胰腺组织的边缘[98,103,113,170]，而不是传统的做75%的胰腺切除（图107-7）。在整个手术过程中密切监测血糖水平。通过上腹部的横切口进行手术，进入小网膜囊内以暴露和搬动整个胰腺，再进行游离十二指肠的Kocher手法，然后沿着胰腺的行径密切检查红棕色的结节性腺瘤，摘除腺瘤并送冰冻切片分析。重要的是要知道腺
1683 瘤和弥漫性疾病合并存在，尤其是在婴幼儿中[169]。应该从胰头、胰体、胰尾部进行活检，做显微镜检查。如果没有发现局限性病变，将胰腺从左侧移动至右侧。胰尾从脾门处游离并保留。起源于脾血管的多个较短的胰腺血管给予结扎并切断。一旦胰体在肠系膜上动脉处得到游离，就可以看到门静脉。必须非常小心地游离胰腺的钩突，胰腺钩突部分包绕肠系膜上静脉。在95%～98%的包括胰腺钩突的胰腺切除术中，都必须鉴别出胆总管并进行保护。异位的胰腺组织应该切除。当发现是局灶性病变时，进行较少的胰腺组织切除比较适当，如同Cretolle等所展示的手术[29]。

手术以后要经常检测血糖水平。刚开始时可经常出现高血糖，但这是短暂的，总体上都需要增加葡萄糖供给以维持正常血糖水平，直到婴幼儿能够耐受口服喂养。偶尔也需要药物治疗，但是很少需要用到胰岛素。

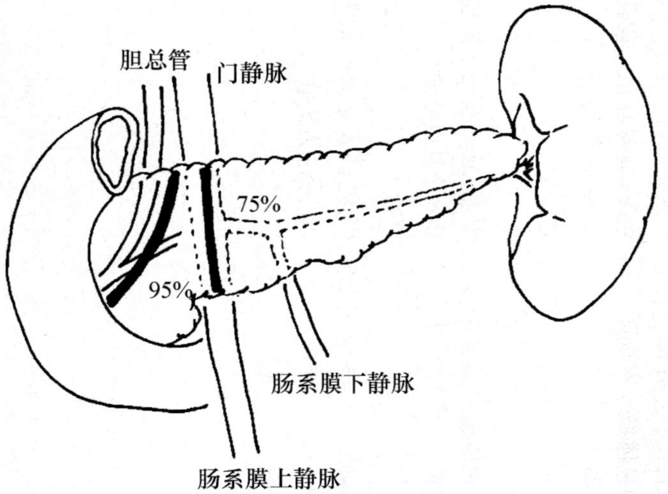

图107-7 胰腺的解剖范围。

结果

主要的术后并发症是持续性的低血糖和脑发育迟滞。然而，发生糖尿病的风险较低。Spitz等[170]报道了21例行95%胰腺切除术的患者中有4例发生了长时间的术后高血糖而需要胰岛素治疗，但是4例中只有1例需要长期的胰岛素治疗。脑发育迟滞可能在术前就已经存在了。

虽然手术的结果总体上与胰腺切除范围有关，但是并不是完全可以预测。Thomas等[182]发表的一篇综述显示，在165例患者中有125例进行了胰腺次全切除术（75%～90%）。125例患者中有35例（28%）需要进行第二次手术，有4名患者因为持续性低血糖而需要进行第三次手术。40名患者初次手术进行的是胰腺近全部切除术（95%～98%）。这些患者中有2例（5%）因为持续性低血糖而需要第二次手术。在进行胰腺近全部切除术的40名患者中，脑或者智力发育迟滞的发生率为12.5%。10%的患者需要二氮嗪治疗，7.5%的患者需要长期的胰岛素治疗。死亡率为2.5%。在1943年到1971年间进行的胰腺次全切除术的更早期经验中，死亡率为8.3%，而智力发育迟滞的发生率为52%。总体上术后的胰腺外分泌功能并没有受到损害[36,160]。Lovvorn等和其他的近期系列报道显示，没有出现患者死亡，并且并发症降低到最少[113]。

胰岛细胞性腺瘤

功能性的β细胞腺瘤（胰岛素瘤）可以导致高胰岛素血症，大多数的胰岛细胞性腺瘤经常出现在年长儿童中（也见于胰岛素瘤部分）。总体上，10%的胰岛细胞性腺瘤是恶性的，但是在儿童中恶性的β细胞腺瘤罕见。通常症状发生在4岁以后，但是有三分之一的胰岛细胞性腺瘤症状可发生在新生儿阶段[37]。

大多数胰岛细胞性腺瘤是实质性的，它们可能是

多发性的，或者与胰岛母细胞瘤有关。因为胰岛细胞性腺瘤体积较小，所以不能通过超声检查或者 CT 扫描来发现；相反，选择性的腹腔动脉造影术可以在 60% 的年长患者中确定诊断[75]。如果肿瘤位于胰头或者胰腺的中心部位，就可以进行肿瘤单纯切除。然而，大多数研究者推荐进行胰腺的 80%～90% 的远端切除术以控制不可触及的病变[192]。推荐进行术中胰岛素水平测定以避免遗漏病灶。

多发性内分泌肿瘤Ⅰ型（MEN-I）的特征是在肠道和胰腺中的内分泌组织，包括胰岛素分泌性肿瘤，但是通常会延迟到 10 岁以后才出现临床表现。多发性内分泌肿瘤Ⅰ型比较罕见，其发生率为每 10 000例中不超过 1 例。MEN-I 的基因已经被定位于 11 号染色体的长臂，是一种肿瘤抑制基因，与 11 号染色体短臂上的 K_{ATP}组分 SUR1/Kir6.2 中的功能性改变不相关[21]。

胰腺肿瘤

在婴幼儿和儿童中，胰腺肿瘤相对罕见。它们可以是囊性的或实质性的，可以是良性的或恶性的，可以有或没有激素活性。

1818 年，Todd[27]报道了第一例发生于一名 14 岁女孩的儿童单纯胰腺癌病例。1885 年，Bohn[12]报告了另外一例 7 个月大婴儿的单纯胰腺癌病例。1990 年，Grosfeld 等[65]报道了 13 例儿童胰腺肿瘤，包括 5 例胰岛素瘤，2 例黏液囊腺瘤，2 例胰腺横纹肌肉瘤，和 4 例胰腺癌。1992 年，Jaksic 等报道了 6 例儿童胰腺肿瘤[86]。直到现在英文文献中已经报道了超过 150 例的胰腺肿瘤[99,136,173,174,175,176]。

囊性肿瘤

胰腺的囊性肿瘤相对罕见。Howard 等[80]将这些病变分为：（1）囊腺瘤和囊腺癌，包括良性（微小囊性）囊腺瘤、良性和恶性的黏液性（巨大囊性）囊腺瘤和囊腺癌、乳头状-囊性上皮性肿瘤、腺泡细胞囊腺癌（在儿童中没有报道）；（2）畸胎瘤性囊肿。

囊腺瘤和囊腺癌

在儿童和成年人中，胰腺囊腺瘤比较罕见。直到目前，在儿童中只报道了 6 例，包括有 1 例为新生儿[17,65,69,87]。囊腺瘤和囊腺癌分为两组。因为巨大的黏液性囊性腺瘤有较大的潜在恶性，这些肿瘤应该与良性的浆液性囊腺瘤有所区别；浆液性囊腺瘤富含糖原，含有很少或者没有黏蛋白[23]。

浆液性囊腺瘤和囊腺癌

在儿童和成年人中，胰腺的浆液性囊腺瘤比较罕见，更常见于女性，主要见于胰体和胰尾部。这些肿瘤主要由小囊肿（微小囊性腺瘤）组成[77]。在超声检查和 CT 扫描中经常显示出有钙化。浆液性囊腺瘤不需要进行切除，除非它们造成了机械性梗阻，因为几乎所有的浆液性囊腺瘤都是良性的，没有潜在恶性。需要进行活检。浆液性囊腺癌事实上在儿童中并不存在，在成年人中也只有很少的病例报道[53,213]。

黏液性囊腺瘤和囊腺癌

胰腺的黏液性囊性肿瘤通常较大，经常是多囊性的肿瘤；它们形成乳头状，并内衬柱状的分泌黏液的上皮细胞，在女性中更为常见，主要见于胰体和胰尾部[116]。其他特征是囊内有巨大血管并出现黏膜上皮下出血。常见的鉴别诊断是胰腺炎伴有假性囊肿形成。胰腺的黏液性囊腺癌占胰腺所有恶性肿瘤的 1%，比通常的实质性胰腺肿瘤发生年龄更早，其发生率接近囊腺瘤的一半。胰腺的黏液性囊腺癌的临床和影像学表现类似于黏液性囊腺瘤的表现[10]。从病理上并不总是能够鉴别黏液性囊腺瘤和囊腺癌。在同一个肿瘤中通常也能明显地发现良性上皮细胞[23]，因此提示恶性的病灶可能发展于黏液性囊腺瘤中。一些文献记载更为保守的治疗能够导致在囊壁中发生致命的多形性腺癌[110]或者恶性肉瘤[64]。因此，黏液性囊腺瘤应该认为是一种癌前病变，在行不完全切除术或者袋形缝合术后，应该进行完整的切除[16,23]。然而，这种类型的胰腺恶性肿瘤的预后要显著好于常见的典型实质性胰管腺癌，因为它生长缓慢，并缺乏转移潜能[110]。

乳头状囊性上皮细胞肿瘤

最初的胰腺乳头状囊性内皮细胞肿瘤病例是由Franz在1959年报道的[47]。自从Kloppel及其同事们[95]描述了这些肿瘤为胰腺实质性和囊性腺泡细胞肿瘤以后，报道的儿童病例数不断增多。这些肿瘤主要发生于女孩和年轻女性，表现为巨大的包裹性肿块，通常伴有广泛性坏死和不同数量的囊性变。在组织学上，它们由小细胞以及形似内分泌肿瘤的假玫瑰花结构的实质性区域和呈乳头状结构的囊性区域组成[171]。在免疫组织化学上，实质性和囊性胰腺肿瘤的肿瘤细胞含有过碘酸希夫氏染色（PAS）阳性的颗粒，经常含有黄体酮受体。免疫学特点是与α-抗胰蛋白酶、α-抗糜蛋白酶、磷脂酶 A_2 和神经内分泌标志物如神经元特异性烯醇酶和突触体素呈免疫反应性。然而，总体上没有通常的胰腺癌标志物，例如癌胚抗原、CA19-9、组织多肽抗原[178]。这些肿瘤比常见类型的胰腺癌预后要好很多，但是仍有潜在恶性[100]。大多数病例中肿瘤切除以后呈现一种良性过程。我们经历过1例在初次临床评估时就已经转移到肝、脾和肺的病例。在日本有5%的病例会出现转移或者复发[77]。因此，需要完全切除肿瘤，因为与肿瘤的不良预后与转移有关。

儿童其他胰腺囊性肿瘤

1992年，Flaherty和Benjamin[46]报道了1例20个月大女孩的多囊性胰腺错构瘤。1990年，Mester等[122]回顾了10例胰腺囊性畸胎瘤病例，包括他们自己的1个病例。胰腺囊性畸胎瘤在年幼的患者中通常是良性的性腺外生殖细胞瘤，10名患者中有5例年龄小于11岁。

激素活性肿瘤

有内分泌活性的肿瘤通常是由其产生的症状而发现的，其中大多数起源于胰岛细胞。β细胞肿瘤分泌胰岛素；α细胞肿瘤分泌胰高血糖素；γ细胞肿瘤分泌胃泌激素；Δ细胞肿瘤分泌生长激素抑制素；Δ_1细胞肿瘤分泌血管活性肠肽（VIP），可能有P物质和分泌素。在儿童中，胰高血糖素瘤和生长激素抑制素瘤还没有被确定。

胰岛素瘤

胰岛素瘤是起源于胰岛细胞的最为常见的肿瘤，通常是良性的（90%）、实质性的（80%）病变，发生在大于4岁的儿童中[51,65,216]。血浆中胰岛素/葡萄糖比例大于1.0时具有诊断意义（正常是<0.4）[51]，这个比例随着禁食而增加。伴随的C肽水平测定可用于排除人为的低血糖。前胰岛素水平升高可提示为恶性肿瘤[64]。CT扫描、超声检查和动脉血管造影，以及经肝门静脉采血都可以用于胰岛素瘤的定位。肿瘤通常是散在的，包裹完整，大多数能够被摘除。术中超声检查的引入可确认不明显的病变灶。如果所有的肿瘤定位方法都没有成功，则建议行仔细切开腺体的远端胰腺切除术。大多数婴幼儿和儿童的胰岛素瘤都可以得到治愈。

胃泌素瘤

报道的第二常见的胰腺激素活性肿瘤是γ细胞肿瘤。与胃泌素瘤相关的临床综合征是指Zollinger-Ellison综合征[205]，其特征是高胃泌素血症并伴有重度消化性溃疡。这种综合征在儿童中非常罕见，只有44例病例报道[189]。胃泌素瘤是MEN-I综合征中的一部分，通常是一种恶性肿瘤，多中心生长，发现时已经远处转移[65]。通常在与胃泌素水平升高（>500 pg/ml）有关的消化性溃疡反复发作以后才得出诊断。静脉补钙和胰泌素刺激试验可用于诊断。CT扫描、经皮肝穿刺静脉采血和胃泌素分析可有效地进行定位。虽然全胃切除术是最为常见的治疗方法，但是随着胃酸分泌抑制剂的发展，例如 H_2 受体阻断药[33]和奥美拉唑（omeprazole）[120]，已经充分改变了胃泌素瘤的治疗方向。有胃泌素瘤的儿童通常需要终身进行药物治疗，需要服用生长抑素。虽然生长抑素有效，但由于它不仅降低了胃酸的分泌，也抑制了生长激素的分泌，所以不能长期服用。因此建议进行手术治疗，尤其是当剖腹手术时发现一个实质性的肿瘤而尚未发现远处转移证据的时候。然而，在那些内科治疗无效、有残留肿瘤或者有远处转移的患者中，还是需要进行全胃切除术[33,65]。

VIP 肿瘤（一种分泌肠血管活性肽的肿瘤）

在儿童中，VIP 肿瘤比其他胰腺起源的肿瘤更易涉及神经源性肿瘤，例如神经母细胞瘤或者神经节细胞瘤。只有 2 例儿童 VIP 肿瘤病例得到了报道[189]。由胰腺 VIP 肿瘤分泌的血管活性肠肽可能起源于胰岛中的神经细胞[51]。患者经常表现为伴有低钾血症和胃酸过少（WDHA 综合征）的大量水样腹泻、代谢性酸中毒和脱水继发的肾前性氮质血症。虽然内科治疗可包括链佐星和生长抑素的使用，但是不推荐长期使用生长抑素。只要可能都要手术根除产生肿瘤的腺体，因为 50% 的胰腺 VIP 肿瘤是恶性的[65]。

胰腺癌

胰腺癌在成年人中比较常见，但是在儿童中比较罕见。临床特征的不同点在于在成年人中梗阻性黄疸是初始发现的症状，而在儿童中腹部肿块为刚开始的临床特征[99]。儿童的胰腺癌可以分为 4 组：胰岛细胞癌、腺癌、胰母细胞瘤和其他种类胰腺癌。

胰岛细胞癌

在儿童中，胰岛细胞癌可能是或者不是功能性的。有功能的 β 细胞和非 β 细胞的胰岛细胞癌可发生于有低血糖联合 Zollinger-Ellison 综合征的婴幼儿和儿童中，但是并没有可触及的腹部肿块。β 细胞癌通常在胰岛素瘤开腹手术中发现[64]。四种功能性的儿童胰岛细胞癌都已经有所报道；所有的病例都通过手术根除来进行治疗，具有较高的长期存活率[81,177,188]。Wilson 报道了在 8 名有 Zollinger-Ellison 综合征的儿童中有 7 名存在非 β 细胞癌并有远处转移[210]。

儿童中非功能性胰岛细胞癌比成年人中更为常见。因为这些肿瘤通常是因触及腹部肿块而被发现，经常诊断时已经是晚期，许多受累婴幼儿和儿童在诊断时就有远处转移性病灶[64]。大多数非功能性肿瘤是巨大的实质性肿块，出现在胰腺腺体内的任何地方。总体上，虽然这些肿瘤大多数生长缓慢，但是可以进行积极的手术治疗，因为其具有潜在恶性[6]。

腺癌

胰腺的腺癌在儿童中非常罕见。1993 年，Vejcho[193] 回顾了 37 例胰腺腺癌病例。临床表现不同于成年人，发生腹痛并伴有黄疸的几率较低[188]。儿童中腹痛和可触及的上腹部肿块是最初的临床表现。分类仍然存在争议，分别基于肿瘤的活性、组织病理学以及免疫组织化学中的发现。Kloppe 等把腺癌分为三种类型：腺泡细胞性腺癌、实质性和囊性肿瘤（乳头状囊性肿瘤）及胰母细胞瘤[95]。腺泡细胞性腺癌在
儿童中更为常见[100,116]。腺泡细胞性腺癌儿童的预后 1686
比导管细胞类型的腺癌更好一些。导管细胞类型腺癌儿童的预后不理想，类似于成年人的预后[78]。CT 扫描和超声波检查是有效的诊断方法。对于局限性的病灶，胰腺十二指肠吻合术的预后良好。婴幼儿和儿童耐受胰腺切除根治术的能力好于成年人，死亡率较低，长期存活率较好[6]。

胰母细胞瘤

1977 年，Horie 等[78] 报道了 2 例胰腺癌病例，称之为胰母细胞瘤，是一种婴儿类型的胰腺癌。1984 年，Buchino 等[18] 回顾了 8 例胰母细胞瘤病例，其中 6 例手术根治以后得以存活。Grosfeld 等[65] 和 Jaksic 等[86] 各报道了 1 例病例。胰母细胞瘤有较好的预后，因为胰母细胞瘤有包膜完整的类器官结构，不会直接影响到主胰管系统。已经由 Buchio 等[18] 提出了胰母细胞瘤的诊断标准。虽然这些罕见病变的病理学尚未达成统一意见，但是可用于鉴别的命名似乎更为可取（例如胰岛细胞、胰管细胞、腺泡细胞、未分化的病变）[100]。

其他种类胰腺癌

文献中已经有以下儿童其他种类胰腺癌的病例报道：1 例单纯性胰腺癌[12]，1 例胰腺髓质癌[203]，6 例胰腺肉瘤（2 例淋巴肉瘤[203]、2 例囊腺瘤的肉瘤变[64,188]、2 例横纹肌肉瘤[65]），4 例未分化肉瘤[18,188] 和 2 例圆柱形细胞腺癌[12,27]。

（顾 松译 陈永卫校）

参考文献

1. Adams DJ, Harrison RG: The vascularization of the rat pancreas and the effect of ischemia on the islets of Langerhans. J Anat 1953;87:257.
2. Adzick NS, Shamberger RC, Winter HS, Hendren WH: Surgical treatment of pancreas divisum causing pancreatitis in children. J Pediatr Surg 1989;25:54.
3. Agha FP: Spontaneous resolution of pancreatic pseudocysts. Surg Gynecol Obstet 1984;158:22.
4. Aguilar-Bryan L, Nichols CG, Wechsler SW, et al: Cloning of the beta cell high-affinity sulfonylurea receptor: A regulator of insulin secretion. Science 1995;268:423.
5. Albu E, Buiumsohn A, Lopez R, Gerst PH: Gallstone pancreatitis in adolescents. J Pediatr Surg 1987;22:960.
6. Aszodi A, Leeming RA, Lash RH, et al: Giant nonfunctioning islet cell tumor requiring pancreaticoduodenectomy and complete liver revascularization. J Surg Oncol 1993; 53:273.
7. Auringer ST, Ulmer JL, Sumner TE, Turner CS: Congenital cyst of the pancreas. J Pediatr Surg 1993;28:1570.
8. Baker LL, Hartman GE, Northway WH: Sonographic detection of congenital pancreatic cysts in the newborn; report of a case and review of the literature. Pediatr Radiol 1990;20:488.
9. Banting FG, Best CH: The internal secretion of the pancreas. J Lab Clin Med 1922;7:251.
10. Becker WF, Welsh RA, Pratt HS: Cystadenoma and cystadenocarcinoma of the pancreas. Ann Surg 1965;261:845.
11. Bencosme SA: The histogenesis and cytology of the pancreatic islets in the rabbit. Am J Anat 1955;96:103.
12. Bohn A: [Cancer of the liver, the portal and retroperitoneal lymph glands and the pancreas in a 6 month old child.] Jahrb Kinderh 1885;23:143.
13. Bousvaros A: Acute and chronic pancreatitis. In International Seminars in Paediatric Gastroenterology and Nutrition, vol 4. Hamilton, Ontario, Canada, 1995, Decker Periodicals.
14. Bradley EL, Clements LJ: Spontaneous resolution of pancreatic pseudocysts. Implications for timing of operative intervention. Am J Surg 1975;129:23.
15. Brooks JR: Pseudocysts of the pancreas. In Brooks JR (ed): Surgery of the Pancreas. Philadelphia, WB Saunders, 1983.
16. Brugge WR, Lauwers GY, Sahani D, et al: Cystic neoplasms of the pancreas. N Engl J Med 2004;35:1218.
17. Brunschwig A: Surgery of Pancreatic Tumors, St Louis, CV Mosby, 1942.
18. Buchino JJ, Castello FM, Nagaraj HS: Pancreatoblastoma: A histochemical and ultrastructural analysis. Cancer 1984; 53:963.
19. Buchler M, Malfertheiner P, Uhl W, et al: Gabexate mesilate in human acute pancreatitis. German Pancreatitis Study Group. Gastroenterology 1993;104:1165.
20. Buchler MW, Gloor B, Muller CA, et al: Acute necrotizing pancreatitis: Treatment strategy according to the status of infection. Ann Surg 2000;232:619.
21. Chandrasekharappa SC, Guru SC, Manickam P, et al: Positional cloning of the gene for multiple endocrine neoplasia-type 1. Science 1997;276:404.
22. Cohn JA, Bornstein JD, Jowell PS: Cystic fibrosis mutations and genetic predisposition to idiopathic chronic pancreatitis. Med Clin North Am 2000;84:621.
23. Compagno J, Oertel JE: Mucinous cystic neoplasms of the pancreas with overt and latent malignancy (cystadenocarcinoma and cystadenoma): A clinicopathologic study of 41 cases. Am J Clin Pathol 1978;69:573.
24. Conklin JL: Cytogenesis of the human fetal pancreas. Am J Anat 1962;111:181.
25. Cooney DR, Grosfeld JL: Operative management of pancreatic pseudocysts in infants and children: A review of 75 cases. Ann Surg 1976;182:590.
26. Cooperman M, Ferrara JJ, Carey LC, et al: Idiopathic acute pancreatitis: The value of endoscopic retrograde cholangiopancreatography. Surgery 1981;90:666.
27. Corner BD: Primary carcinoma of the pancreas in an infant aged 7 months. Arch Dis Child 1943;18:106.
28. Cotton PB: Congenital anomaly of pancreas divisum as cause of obstructive pain and pancreatitis. Gut 1980;21:101.
29. Cretolle C, Fekete CN, Jan D, et al: Partial elective pancreatectomy is curative in focal form of permanent hyperinsulinemic hypoglycemia in infancy: A report of 45 cases from 1983-2000. J Pediatr Surg 2002;37:155.
30. Crombleholme TM, deLorimier AA, Wayu LW, et al: The modified Puestow procedure for chronic relapsing pancreatitis in children. J Pediatr Surg 1990;25:749.
31. DeBanto JR, Goday PS, Pedroso MR, et al: Acute pancreatitis in children. Am J Gastroenterol 2002;97:1726.
32. de Lonlay P, Fournet JC, Rahier J, et al: Somatic deletion of the imprinted 11015 region in sporadic persistent hyperinsulinemic hypoglycemia of infancy is specific of focal adenomatous hyperplasia and endorses partial pancreatectomy. J Clin Invest 1997;100:802.
33. Deveney CW, Deveney KE: Zollinger-Ellison syndrome (gastrinoma): Current diagnosis and treatment. Surg Clin North Am 1987;67:411.
34. Drey NW: Symptomatic annular pancreas in the adult. Ann Intern Med 1957;46:756.
35. Dubay D, Sandler A, Kimura K, et al: The modified Puestow procedure for complicated hereditary pancreatitis in children. J Pediatr Surg 2000;35:343.
36. Dunger DB, Burns C, Ghale GK, et al: Pancreatic exocrine and endocrine function after subtotal pancreatectomy for nesidioblastosis. J Pediatr Surg 1988;23:112.
37. Dunn JS, McLetchie NGB: Experimental alloxan diabetes in the rat. Lancet 1943;2:384.
38. Durie P: Pancreatic aspects of cystic fibrosis and other inherited causes of pancreatic dysfunction. Med Clin North Am 2000;84:609.
39. Duval MK Jr: Caudal pancreaticojejunostomy for chronic relapsing pancreatitis. Ann Surg 1954;140:775.
40. Eichelberger MR, Hoelzer DJ, Koop CE: Acute pancreatitis: The difficulties of diagnosis and therapy. J Pediatr Surg 1982;17:244.
41. Eghtesad B, Reyer JD, Ashrafi M, et al: Pancreatitis after liver transplantation in children: A single-center experience. Transplantation 2003;75:190.
42. Elechi EN, Callender CO, Leffall LD Jr, Kurtz LH: The treatment of pancreatic pseudocysts by external drainage. Surg Gynecol Obstet 1979;148:707.
43. Festen C, Severijnen R, vd Staak F, Rieu P: Chronic relapsing pancreatitis in childhood. J Pediatr Surg 1991; 26:182.
44. Finch WT, Sawyers JL, Schenker S: Prospective study to determine the efficacy of antibiotics in acute pancreatitis. Ann Surg 1976;183:667.
45. Firstenberg MS, Volsko TA, Sivit C, et al: Selective management of pediatric pancreatic injuries. J Pediatr Surg 1999; 34:1142.
46. Flaherty MJ, Benjamin DR: Multicystic pancreatic hamartoma: A distinctive lesion with immunohistochemical and ultrastructural study. Hum Pathol 1992;23:1309.
47. Frantz VK: Tumor of the pancreas. In Atlas of Tumor

Pathology, fascicles 27 and 28. Washington, DC, 1959, Armed Forces Institute of Pathology.
48. Frey CF: Pancreatic pseudocysts—operative strategy. Ann Surg 1978;188:652.
49. Frey CF: Role of subtotal pancreatectomy and pancreaticojejunostomy in chronic pancreatitis. J Surg Res 1981;31:36.
50. Frey C, Redo SF: Inflammatory lesions of the pancreas in infancy and childhood. Pediatrics 1978;32:143.
51. Friesen SR: An update on the diagnosis and treatment of rare neuroendocrine tumors. Surg Clin North Am 1987; 67:379.
52. Fuller RK, Loveland JP, Frankel MH: An evaluation of the efficacy of nasogastric suction treatment in alcoholic pancreatitis. Am J Gastroenterol 1981;75:349.
53. George DH, Murphy F, Michalski R, Ulmer BG: Serous cystadenocarcinoma of the pancreas: A new entity? Am J Surg Pathol 1989;13:61.
54. Ghishan FK, Greene HL, Avant G, et al: Chronic relapsing pancreatitis in childhood. J Pediatr 1983;102:514.
55. Gillette L, Lynch B: Annular pancreas. Ann Surg 1954; 139:374.
56. Glaser B, Hirch JH, Landau H: Persistent hyperinsulinism hypoglycemia of infancy: Long-term octreotide treatment without pancreatectomy. J Pediatr 1993;123:644.
57. Glaser B, Kesavan P, Heyman M, et al: Familial hyperinsulinism caused by an activating glucokinase mutation. N Engl J Med 1998;338:226.
58. Goobie S, Popovic M, Morrison J, et al: Shwachman-Diamond syndrome with exocrine pancreatic dysfunction and bone marrow failure maps to the centromeric region of chromosome 7. Am J Hum Genet 2001;68:1048.
59. Gorenstein A, O'Halpin D, Wesson DE, et al: Blunt injury to the pancreas in children: Selective management based on ultrasound. J Pediatr Surg 1987;22:1110.
60. Graham JM, Polorny WJ, Mattox KL, Jordan GL Jr: Surgical management of acute pancreatic injuries in children. J Pediatr Surg 1978;13:693.
61. Grant DB, Dunger DB, Burns EC: Long-term treatment with diazoxide in childhood hyperinsulinism, Acta Endocrinol (Copenhagen) 1986;279(Suppl):340.
62. Grauso-Eby NL, Goldfarb O, Feldman-Winter LB, McAhee GN: Acute pancreatitis in children from valproic acid: Case series and review. Pediatr Neurol 2002;28:145-148.
63. Gray SW, Skandalakis JE: The pancreas. In Embryology for Surgeons. Philadelphia, Williams & Wilkins, 1994.
64. Grosfeld JL, Clatworthy HW, Hamoudi AB: Pancreatic malignancy in children. Arch Surg 1970;101:370.
65. Grosfeld JL, Vane DW, Rescorla FJ, et al: Pancreatic tumors in childhood: Analysis of 13 cases. J Pediatr Surg 1990;25:1057.
66. Guelrud M, Mujica C, Jaen D, et al: The role of ERCP in the diagnosis and treatment of idiopathic recurrent pancreatitis in children and adolescents. Gastrointest Endosc 1994;40:428.
67. Guillemin G, Cuilleret J, Michel A, et al: Chronic relapsing pancreatitis; surgical management including 63 cases of pancreaticoduodenectomy. Am J Surg 1971;122:802.
68. Gumaste V, Dave P, Sereny G: Serum lipase: A better test to diagnose acute alcoholic pancreatitis. Am J Med 1992; 92:239.
69. Gundersen AE, Janis JF: Pancreatic cystadenoma in childhood. J Pediatr Surg 1969;4:478.
70. Gwozdz GP, Steinberg WM, Werner M, et al: Comparative evaluation of the diagnosis of acute pancreatitis based on serum and urine enzyme assays. Clin Chim Acta 1990; 187:243.
71. Hastings PR, Nance FC, Becker WF: Changing pattern in the management of pancreatic pseudocysts. Ann Surg 1975; 181:546.
72. Heikkinen ES, Salminer PM: Congenital choledochal cyst opening into the intraduodenal part of the common bile duct and complicated by cystolithiasis and acute pancreatitis. Acta Chir Scand 1954;150:183.
73. Heitz PU, Beglinger C, Gyr K: Anatomy and physiology of the exocrine pancreas. In Kloppel G, Heitz PU (eds): Pancreatic Pathology. London, Churchill Livingstone, 1984.
74. Hendricks SK, Sybert VP: Association of annular pancreas and duodenal obstruction, evidence for mendelian inheritance? Clin Genet 1991;39:383.
75. Herman TE, Siegel MJ: Polysplenia syndrome with congenital short pancreas. AJR Am J Roentgenol 1991;156:799.
76. Hermann RE: Common surgical problems. In Hermann RE (ed): Pancreatic Surgery. Chicago, Year Book, 1985.
77. Hirano T, Akoi Y, Ito T, et al: A case of solid and cystic tumor of the pancreas. J Jpn Soc Clin Surg 56:149, 1995.
78. Horie A, Yano Y, Kotoo Y, Miwa A: Morphogenesis of pancreatoblastoma, infantile carcinoma of the pancreas: Report of two cases. Cancer 1977;39:247.
79. Hough DM, Stephens DH, Johnson CD, Binkovitz LA, et al: Pancreatic lesions in von Hippel-Lindau disease: Prevalence, clinical significance, and CT findings. AJR Am J Roentgenol 1994;162:1091.
80. Howard JM, Jordan GJ Jr, Reber HA: Cysts of the pancreas. In Howard JM, Jordan GJ (eds): Surgical Diseases of the Pancreas, Philadelphia, Lea & Febiger, 1987.
81. Hurez A, Bedouelle J, Debray H, et al: Carcinoma of the islets of Langerhans with severe hypoglycemic manifestations in a nine year old child. Arch Franc Pediatr 1961;18:625.
82. Ingemansson S, Kuhl C, Larsson LI, et al: Localization of insulinomas and islet cell hyperplasias by pancreatic vein catheterization and insulin assay. Surg Gynecol Obstet 1978;146:725.
83. Jackson D: Pancreatitis: Etiology, diagnosis, and management. Curr Opin Pediatr 2001;13:447.
84. Jaffe R: The pancreas. In Stocker JT, Dehner LP (eds): Pediatric Pathology, 2nd ed. Philadelphia, Lippincott Williams & Wilkins, 2001, p 799.
85. Jaffe RB, Arata JA Jr, Matlak ME: Percutaneous drainage of traumatic pancreatic pseudocysts in children. AJR Am J Roentgenol 1989;152:591.
86. Jaksic T, Yaman M, Thorner P, et al: A 20-year-review of pediatric pancreatic tumors. J Pediatr Surg 1992;27:1315.
87. Jenkins JM, Othersen BH Jr: Cystadenoma of the pancreas in a newborn. J Pediatr Surg 1992;27:1569.
88. Johnson DD: Alloxan administration in the guinea pig: A study of the regenerative phase of the islands of Langerhans. Endocrinology 1950;47:393.
89. Jones SA, Steedman RA, Keller TB, Smith LL: Transduodenal sphincteroplasty (not sphincterotomy) for biliary and pancreatic disease. Am J Surg 1969;118:292.
90. Karaguzel G, Senocak ME, Buyukpamukcu N, Hicsonmez A: A surgical management of the pancreatic pseudocyst in children: A long-term evaluation. J Pediatr Surg 1995; 30:777.
91. Karp MP, Cooney DR, Berger PE, et al: The role of computed tomography in the evaluation of blunt abdominal trauma in children. J Pediatr Surg 1981;16:316.
92. Karp MP, Jewett TC, Cooney DR: Chronic relapsing pancreatitis in childhood caused by pancreaticobiliary ductal anomaly. J Pediatr Gastroenterol Nutr 1983;2:324.
93. Keith RG, Shapero TF, Saibil FG: Treatment of pancreatitis with pancreas divisum by dorsal duct sphincterotomy alone. Can J Surg 1982;25:622.

94. Kimble RM, Cohen R, Williams S: Successful endoscopic drainage of a posttraumatic pancreatic pseudocyst in a child. J Pediatr Surg 1999;34:1518.
95. Kloppel G, Morohoshi T, John HD, et al: Solid and cystic acinar cell tumour of the pancreas: A tumour in young women with favorable prognosis. Virchows Arch A Pathol Anat Histol 1981;392:171.
96. Kouchi K, Tenabe M, Yoshida H, et al: Nonoperative management of blunt pancreatic injury in childhood. J Pediatr Surg 1999;34:1736.
97. Kozarek RA, Christie D, Barclay G: Endoscopic therapy of pancreatitis in the pediatric population. Gastrointest Endosc 1993;39:665.
98. Kramer JL, Bell MJ, DeSchryver K, et al: Clinical and histologic indications for extensive pancreatic resection in nesidioblastosis. Am J Surg 1982;143:116.
99. Kuhn A: [Primary pancreatic carcinoma in infancy.] Klin Wochnschr 1887;24:494.
100. Lack EE, Cassady JR, Levey R, Vawter GF: Tumors of the exocrine pancreas in children and adolescents: A clinical and pathologic study of eight cases. Am J Surg Pathol 1983;7:319.
101. La Hei ER, Cohen RC: Antenatal detection of a pancreatic foregut duplication cyst. J Pediatr Surg 2001;36:501.
102. Lamberts SWJ, van der Lely AJ, de Herder WW, Holfland LJ: Octreotide. N Engl J Med 1996;334:246.
103. Langer JC, Filler RM, Wesson DE, et al: Surgical management of persistent neonatal hypoglycemia due to islet cell dysplasia. J Pediatr Surg 1984;19:786.
104. Levitt Katz LE, Satin-Smith MS, Collett-Solberg P, et al: Insulin-like growth factor binding protein-1 levels in the diagnosis of hypoglycemia caused by hyperinsulinism. J Pediatr 1997;131:193.
105. Lewis FP: The development of the liver. In Leibel F, Mall FP (eds): Human Embryology, vol 12. Philadelphia, JB Lippincott, 1912.
106. Li L, yamataka A Segawa O, Miyano T: Coexistence of pancreas divisum and septate common channel in a child with choledochal cyst. J Pediatr Gastroenterol Nutr 2001; 32:602.
107. Lilly JR, Stellin GP, Karrer FM: Forme fruste choledochal cyst. J Pediatr Surg 1985;20:449.
108. Lindley KJ, Dunne MJ, Kane C, et al: Ionic control of beta cell function in nesidioblastosis: A possible therapeutic role for calcium channel blockade. Arch Dis Child 1996; 74:373.
109. Liu HM, Potter EL: Development of the human pancreas. Arch Pathol 1962;74:439.
110. Logan SE, Voet RL, Tompkins RT: The malignant potential of mucinous cyst of the pancreas. West J Med 1982;136:157.
111. Loludice TA, Jarmolych J, Buhac I: A cause of obstructive jaundice. JAMA 1977;238:889.
112. Longmire WP 3rd, Rose AS: Hemoductal pancreatitis. Surg Gynecol Obstet 1973;136:246.
113. Lowvorn HN, Nance ML, Ferry RJ, et al: Congenital hyperinsulinism and the surgeon: Lessons learned over 35 years. J Pediatr Surg 1999;34:786.
114. Mabogunle OA: Pseudocysts of the pancreas in children: An African series. Ann Trop Paediatr 1988;8:241.
115. Madura JA: Pancreas divisum: Stenosis of the dorsally dominant pancreatic duct. Am J Surg 1986;151:742.
116. Mah PT, Loo DC, Tock EPC: Pancreatic acinar cell carcinoma in children. Am J Dis Child 1974;128:101.
117. Malats N, Casals T, Porta M, et al: Cystic fibrosis transmembrane regulator (CFTR) DeltaF508 mutation and 5T allele in patients with chronic pancreatitis and exocrine pancreatic cancer. PANKRAS II Study Group. Gut 2001;48:70.
118. Mallory A, Kern F Jr: Drug induced pancreatitis: A critical review. Gastroenterology 1980;78:813.
119. Mavridis G, Soutis M, Sakellaris D, Keramidas D: Annular pancreas, Acta Chir Hellen 1995;67:597.
120. McArthur KE, Collen MJ, Cherner JA: Omeprazole as a single dose is effective in Zollinger-Ellison syndrome. Gastroenterology 1984;86:1178.
121. Mellish RWP, Koop CE: Clinical manifestations of duplication of the bowel. Pediatrics 1961;27:397.
122. Mester M, Trajber HJ, Compton CC, et al: Cystic teratomas of the pancreas. Arch Surg 1990;125:1215.
123. Millar AJW, Rode H, Stunden RJ, Cywes S: Management of pancreatic pseudocysts in children. J Pediatr Surg 1988; 23:122.
124. Miles RM: Pancreatic cyst in the newborn. Ann Surg 1959; 149:576.
125. Miyano T, Ando KD, Yamataka A, et al: Pancreaticobiliary maljunction associated with nondilatation or minimal dilation of the common bile duct in children: Diagnosis and treatment. Eur J Pediatr Surg 1996;6:334.
126. Miyano T, Suruga K, Shimomura H, et al: Choledochopancreatic elongated common channel disorders. J Pediatr Surg 1984;19:165.
127. Miyano T, Yamataka A, Kato Y, et al: Choledochal cysts: Special emphasis on the usefulness of intraoperative endoscopy. J Pediatr Surg 1995;30:482.
128. Mizoguchi K: Anatomical studies on the opening of the ducts hepatopancreatica on the duodenal wall of Japanese. Showa Med J 1960;20:549.
129. Moor KL, Persaud TVN: Development of the pancreas. In Moor KL, Persaud TVN (eds): The Developing Human, 5th ed. Philadelphia, WB Saunders, 1993.
130. Moosa AR, Baker L, Lavelle-Jones M: Hypoglycemic syndrome in infancy and childhood. A surgeon's perspective. West J Med 1987;146:585.
131. Mulligan C, Howell C, Hatley R, et al: Conservative management of pediatric pancreatic pseudocyst using octreotide acetate. Am Surg 1995;61:206.
132. Myers MA: Intestinal effects of pancreatitis: Spread along mesenteric plan. In Dynamic Radiology of Abdomen; Normal and Pathologic Anatomy. Berlin, Springer-Verlag, 1976.
133. Nardi GL, Acosta JM: Papillitis as a cause of pancreatitis and abdominal pain: Role of evocative test, operative pancreatography and histologic evaluation. Ann Surg 1966; 164:611.
134. Neblett WW III, O'Neill JA Jr: Surgical management of recurrent pancreatitis in children with pancreas divisum. Ann Surg 2000;231:899.
135. Nestorowicz A, Glaser B, Wilson BA, et al: Genetic heterogeneity in familial hyperinsulinism. Hum Mol Genet 1998;7:1119.
136. Newman BM: Congenital abnormalities of the exocrine pancreas. In Lebenthal E (ed): Textbook of Gastroenterology and Nutrition in Infancy, 2nd ed. New York, Raven Press, 1989.
137. Odgers PNB: Some observations on the development of the ventral pancreas in man. J Anat 1930;65:1.
138. O'Neill JA Jr, Greene H, Grishan FK: Surgical implications of chronic pancreatitis. J Pediatr Surg 1982;17:920.
139. Othersen HB Jr, Moore FT, Boles ET: Traumatic pancreatitis and pseudocyst in childhood. J Trauma 1968;8:535.
140. Owor B: Chronic pancreatic disease in African children. Uganda Med J 1972;1:7.
141. Philipson LH, Steiner DF: Pas de deux or more: The sul-

fonylurea receptor and K+ channels. Science 1995; 268:327.
142. Philsalix C: Etude d'un embryon humain de 10 millimetres. Arch Zool Exp Gen Hist Nat Morph Hitol Evol Animaux Ser 2 1888;6:279.
143. Pilot LM Jr, Gooselaw JG, Isaacson PJ: Obstruction of the common bile duct in the newborn by a pancreatic cyst. Lancet 1964;84:204.
144. Pokorny WJ, Rafensperger JG, Harberg FJ: Pancreatic pseudocysts in children. Surg Gynecol Obstet 1980; 151:182.
145. Pollak EW, Michas CA, Wolfman EF: Pancreatic pseudocyst. Management in fifty-four patients. Am J Surg 1978; 135:199.
146. Poves I: Results of treatment in severe acute pancreatitis. Rev Esp Enfer Diag 2000;92:586.
147. Proctor HJ, Mendes OC, Thomas CG Jr, Herbst CA: Surgery for chronic pancreatitis: Drainage versus resection. Ann Surg 1979;189:664.
148. Puestow CB, Gillesby WJ: Retrograde surgical drainage of the pancreas for chronic relapsing pancreatitis. Arch Surg 1958;76:898.
149. Queizan A, Hernandez F, Rivas S: Pancreatic pseudocyst caused by valproic acid: Case report and review of the literature. Eur J Pediatr Surg 2003;13:60.
150. Ranson JHC: Acute pancreatitis. In Schwartz SI, Ellis H (eds): Maingot's Abdominal Operations, 8th ed. Norwalk, CT, Appleton-Century-Crofts, 1985.
151. Ravelo HR, Aldete JS: Analysis of forty-five patients with pseudocysts of the pancreas treated surgically. Surg Gynecol Obstet 1979;148:735.
152. Rescorla FJ, Cory D, Vane DW, et al: Failure of percutaneous drainage in children with traumatic pancreatic pseudocysts. J Pediatr Surg 1990;25:1038.
153. Rescorla F, Grosfeld JL: Pancreatitis. In Schiller M (ed): Pediatric Surgery of the Liver, Pancreas, and Spleen. Philadelphia, WB Saunders, 1991.
154. Richter JM, Schapiro RH, Mulley AG, Warshaw AL: Association of pancreas divisum and pancreatitis, and its treatment by sphincteroplasty of the accessory ampulla. Gastroenterology 1981;81:1104.
155. Rogers JC, Harris DJ, Holder T: Annular pancreas in a mother and daughter. Am J Med Genet 1993;45:116.
156. Sanfey H, Aguilar M, Jones RS: Pseudocysts of the pancreas, a review of 97 cases. Am Surg 1994;60:661.
157. Sankaran S, Walt AJ: The natural and unnatural history of pancreatic pseudocysts. Br J Surg 1975;62:37.
158. Sawyer SM, Davidson PM, McMullin N, et al: Pancreatic pseudocysts in children. Pediatr Surg Int 1989;4:300.
159. Scharplatz D, White TT: A review of 64 patients with pancreatic cysts. Ann Surg 1972;176:638.
160. Schonau E, Deeg KH, Huemmer HP, et al: Pancreatic growth and function following surgical treatment of nesidioblastosis in infancy. Eur J Pediatr 1991;50:550.
161. Scott HW Jr, Neblett WW, O'Neill JA Jr, et al: Longitudinal pancreaticojejunostomy in chronic pancreatitis with onset in childhood. Ann Surg 1984;199:610.
162. Shah KK, DeRidder PH, Schwab RE, Alexander TJ: CT diagnosis of dorsal pancreas agenesis. J Comput Assist Tomogr 1987;11:170.
163. Sherman S, Lehman GA: ERCP- and endoscopic sphincterotomy–induced pancreatitis. Pancreas 1991;6:350.
164. Shimizu T, Suzuki R, Yamashiro Y, et al: Magnetic resonance cholangiopancreatography in assessing the cause of acute pancreatitis in children. Pancreas 2001;22:196.
165. Sitzman JV, et al: Total parenteral nutrition and alternative energy substrates in treatment of severe acute pancreatitis. Surg Gynecol Obstet 1989;168:311.
166. Smanio T: Varying relation of the common bile duct with the posterior face of the pancreas in negro and white persons. J Int Coll Surg 1954;22:150.
167. Smith R: Progress in the surgical treatment of pancreatic disease. Am J Surg 1973;125:143.
168. Sperling MA, Menon RK: Hyperinsulinemic hypoglycemia of infancy. Pediatr Endocrinol 1999;28:695.
169. Spitz L, Bhargava RK, Grant DB, Leonard JV: Surgical treatment of hyperinsulinemic hypoglycemia in infancy and childhood. Arch Dis Child 1992;67:201.
170. Spitz L, Buick DG, Grant OB, et al: Surgical treatment of nesidioblastosis. Pediatr Surg Int 1986;1:26.
171. Stamm B, Burger H, Hollinger A: Acinar cell cystadenocarcinoma of the pancreas. Cancer 1987;60:2542.
172. Stanley CA, Baker L: Hyperinsulinism in infants and children: Diagnosis and therapy. Adv Pediatr 1976;23:315.
173. Stanley CA, Lieu YK, Hsu BY, et al: Hyperinsulinism and hyperammonemia in infants with regulatory mutations of the glutamate dehydrogenase gene. N Engl J Med 1998; 338:1352.
174. Stein ML, Rossi VC, Almeida AMC: [Carcinoma of the pancreas in the infant, presentation of a case.] Pediatr Pathol 1962;33:75.
175. Steinberg W, Tenner S: Acute pancreatitis. N Engl J Med 1994;330:1198.
176. Stewart SC, Stewart LF: A case of cancer of the pancreas in a 9 year old boy. Intern Clin 1915;2:118.
177. Stokes JM, Wohltmann HJ, Hartmann AF: Pancreatectomy in children. Arch Surg 1966;93:40.
178. Stommer P, Kraus J, Stolte M, Giede J: Solid and cystic pancreatic tumors. Clinical, histochemical, and electron microscopic features in ten cases. Cancer 1991;67:1635.
179. Stone HH: Pancreatic and duodenal trauma in children. J Pediatr Surg 1972;7:670.
180. Synn AY, Mulvihill SJ, Fonkalsrud EW: Surgical management of pancreatitis in childhood. J Pediatr 1987; 22:628.
181. Tagge EP, Smith SD, Raschbaum GR, et al: Pancreatic ductal abnormalities in children. Surgery 1991;110:709.
182. Thomas CG Jr, Cuenca RE, Azizkhan RG, et al: Changing concepts of islet cell dysplasia in neonatal and infantile hyperinsulinism. World J Surg 1988;12:598.
183. Thomas PM: Molecular basis for familial hyperinsulinemic hypoglycemia of infancy. Curr Opin Endocrinol Diabetes 1997;4:272.
184. Thomas PM, Cote GJ, Wohllk N, et al: Mutations in sulfonylurea receptor gene in familial persistent hyperinsulinemic hypoglycemia of infancy. Science 1995;268:426.
185. Thornton PS, Alter CA, Katz LE, et al: Short- and long-term use of octreotide in the treatment of congenital hyperinsulinism. J Pediatr 1993;123:637.
186. Tissieres P, Simon L, Debray D, et al: Acute pancreatitis after orthotopic liver transplantation in children: Incidence, contributing factors, and outcome. J Pediatr Gastroenterol Nutr 1998;26:315.
187. Traverso LW, Longmire WP Jr: Pancreatitis of unusual origin. Surg Gynecol Obstet 1975;141:383.
188. Tsukimoto I, Watanaber K, Lin JB, Nakajima T: Pancreatic carcinoma in children in Japan. Cancer 1973;31:1203.
189. Tudor RB: Childhood Disease Registry, Bismarck, ND, 1988.
190. Tudor RB: Pancreatitis and pancreatic pseudocysts. In Childhood Gastroenterology Registry, Report No. 3. Bismarck, ND, 1989.
191. Van Camp JM, Polley TZ, Coran AG: Pancreatitis in chil-

dren: Diagnosis and etiology in 57 patients. Pediatr Surg Int 1994;9:492.
192. Vane DW, Grosfeld JL, West KW, Rescorla FJ, et al: Pancreatic disorders in infancy and childhood: Experience with 92 cases. J Pediatr Surg 1989;24:771.
193. Vejcho S: Carcinoma of the pancreas in childhood: A case report of long term survival. J Med Assoc Thai 1993; 76:177.
194. Verkarre V, Fournet JC, de Lonlay P, et al: Paternal mutation of the sulfonylurea receptor (SUR1) gene and maternal loss of 11p15 imprinted genes lead to persistent hyperinsulinism in focal adenomatous hyperplasia. J Clin Invest 1998; 102:1286.
195. Wade JW: Twenty-five year experience with pancreatic pseudocysts. Are we making progress? Am J Surg 1985; 149:705.
196. Wagner CW, Golladay ES: Pancreas divisum and pancreatitis in children. Am Surg 1988;54:22.
197. Warkany J: Embryology as related to fibrocystic disease of the pancreas. 18th Report of the Ross Pediatric Research Conference. Columbus, OH, Ross Laboratories, 1956.
198. Warner RL, Othersen HB Jr, Smith CD: Traumatic pancreatitis and pseudocyst in children: Current management. J Trauma 1989;29:597.
199. Warren WD, Marsh WH, Sandusky WR: Pancreatic cysts: An appraisal of surgical procedures of pancreatic pseudocysts. Ann Surg 1958;147:903.
200. Warshaw AL: Pancreas divisum: A case for surgical treatment. Adv Surg 1987;21:93.
201. Warshaw AL, Richter J, Schapiro RH: The cause and treatment of pancreatitis associated with pancreas divisum. Ann Surg 1983;198:443.
202. Warshaw AL, Simeone J, Schapiro RH, et al: Objective evaluation of ampullary stenosis with ultrasonography and pancreatic stimulation. Am J Surg 1985;149:65.
203. Warthen RO, Sanford MD, Rice EC: Primary malignant tumor of the pancreas in a fifteen-month-old boy. Am J Dis Child 1952;83:663.
204. Way LW, Gadacz T, Goldman L: Surgical treatment of chronic pancreatitis. Am J Surg 1974;127:202.
205. Weber TR, Keller MS: Operative management of chronic pancreatitis in children. Arch Surg 2001;136:550-555.
206. Weetman RM, Baehner RL: Latent onset of clinical pancreatitis in children receiving L-asparaginase therapy. Cancer 1974;34:780.
207. Weizman Z, Durie PR: Acute pancreatitis in childhood. J Pediatr 1988;113:24.
208. White TT, Keith RG: Long term follow-up study of fifty patients with pancreaticojejunostomy. Surg Gynecol Obstet 1973;136:353.
209. White TT, Slavotinik AH: Results of surgical treatment of chronic pancreatitis. Report of 142 cases. Ann Surg 1979; 189:217.
210. Wilson SD: Zollinger-Ellison syndrome in children: A 25-year followup. Surgery 1991;110:696.
211. Witt H: Gene mutations in children with chronic pancreatitis. Pancreatology 2001;1:432.
212. Yellin AE, Vecchione TR, Donovan AJ: Distal pancreatectomy for pancreatic trauma. Am J Surg 1972;124:135.
213. Yoshimi N, Sugie S, Tanaka T, et al: A rare case of serous cystadenocarcinoma of the pancreas. Cancer 1992;69:2449.
214. Ziegler DW, Long JA, Philippart AI, Klein MD: Pancreatitis in childhood: Experience with 49 patients. Ann Surg 1988;207:257.
215. Zielenski J: Genotype and phenotype in caustic fibrosis. Respiration 2000;67:117-133.
216. Zollinger RM, Ellison EH: Primary peptic ulcerations of the jejunum associated with islet cell tumors of pancreas. Ann Surg 1955;142:709.

第 108 章

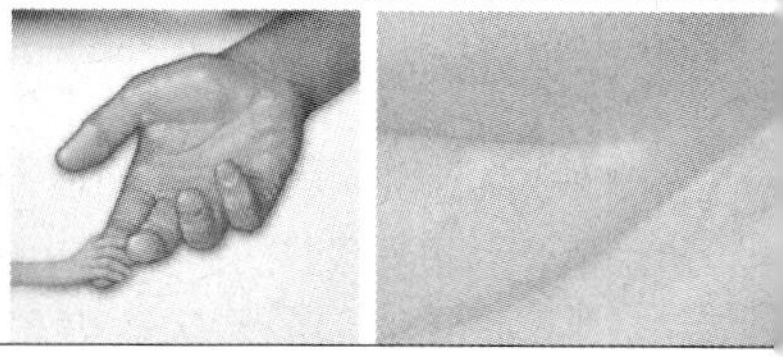

脾脏

Frederick J. Rescorla

691 脾脏的生理功能可以明确分为维持和储存红细胞以及免疫方面的功能。儿童因为发生红细胞变形性异常或者产生抗血小板抗体而导致脾脏红细胞或者血小板破坏过多，经常需要进行脾脏切除手术。脾脏作为一种免疫器官，其重要作用不仅可以导致脾脏外伤的非手术治疗，也会影响到选择性脾脏切除的时机，以及对特定疾病行脾脏部分切除术重新产生兴趣。脾脏切除技术随着先进的腹腔镜技术的出现而变化显著，然而，对于大多数的腹腔镜手术，腹腔镜脾脏切除术已经被认为是标准手术，但是缺乏随机对照研究的证据。腹腔镜脾脏切除技术及其与开腹脾脏切除术比较的结果，将在这个章节的后半部分进行讨论。

历史回顾

有关脾脏作用的争论已经有 300 多年的历史。Billroth 建立了脾脏微循环的开放循环理论，红髓的内皮束就取自他的名字。认识到脾脏作为健康和疾病状态下的功能性器官是在 20 世纪。一个更为重要的观察是在 1952 年由 King 和 Shumaker 进行的，他们注意到婴幼儿脾脏切除以后对感染的易感性[62]。脾脏在细菌性感染中的重要性促使小儿外科医生对脾脏外伤以后非手术治疗的作用进行研究[29]，并形成了一套完善的治疗儿童和成人脾脏外伤的方法。在手术治疗脾脏疾病中，另外一个显著的发展是 1991 年由 Delaitre 和 Maignien 首次报道的腹腔镜脾脏切除术[28]。腹腔镜脾脏切除技术很快成为儿童脾脏切除术的首选技术。

胚胎学和解剖学

脾脏的原基最初是在胚胎 8 ~ 10 mm 阶段胃和胰腺间见到的左背侧胃系膜的间质膨出。直到 10 ~ 12 mm阶段，见到真正的上皮组织，在与毛细血管的连接处出现了血窦。到胎儿生命的第四个月时，脾脏开始生成红细胞和白细胞，然而这种功能到怀孕晚期就停止了，临床上儿童时期脾脏极少作为显著的血细胞生成部位。脾脏解剖学上的排列与其各种不同的功能是一致的。血液通过脾动脉分支进入小梁动脉，经过进一步的分叉支，小动脉进入白髓。白髓由淋巴细胞和巨噬细胞组成，排列成围绕中央动脉的幼芽中心。远离中央动脉的分支血管递送悬浮的特殊物质进入白髓，这样可以促进针对特殊抗原的抗体形成[84,87,98,99]。脾脏中接近 20% 的体积是白髓，其余部分是红髓，由 Billroth 内皮束组成[108]。血液流经脾脏是通过一种“开放”或者“封闭”的方式。有 10%~20% 的血液通过“封闭系统”直接从毛细血管进入静脉窦。其余的血液直接流进红髓。这些细胞和其他的特殊物质必须以一种开放的方式在 Billroth 内皮束中经过，然后移行到血窦中，再进入小梁静脉。

功能

脾脏的功能与解剖学上的排列密切相关，可以分为维持红细胞稳定、免疫功能和储存红细胞。进入脾脏的底物紊乱时，可导致脾脏的某项功能亢进，以致需脾脏切除术。脾脏可以在红细胞寿命结束时破坏它，并且可以修复其他受损的红细胞。脾脏选择性地去除异常细胞例如球形红细胞，切除脾脏可增加这些

细胞的寿命。当血液流经脾脏时，Howell-Jolly 体
1692 （细胞核残余）、Heinz 体（变性的血红蛋白）和 Pappenheimer 体（铁颗粒体）被去除，而当脾脏切除以后，这些小体就可以在红细胞中见到。

脾脏免疫功能按特征可分为特异性和非特异性的免疫反应。脾脏特异性的免疫功能主要与抗原处理有关。在白髓的小动脉区域，抗原与巨噬细胞和 T 辅助细胞接触。作为细胞免疫反应的一部分，T 细胞对合成的细胞因子做出反应，然后活化 T 细胞经循环调整免疫反应。当抗原与巨噬细胞和 T 辅助细胞发生接触并运送至抗体合成细胞后，就可发生体液免疫反应[76]。

非特异性免疫反应功能涉及由巨噬细胞去除血液中的特殊物质。脾脏也是非特异性调理素的主要来源，其可以进一步活化补体系统，促进生物体的破坏。

免疫功能的另一方面仅仅是作为生物过滤器。如果只有少量的抗体来调理细菌，脾脏就在清除细菌方面承担了一个更重要的角色。这可能就是脾脏切除术后发生感染的年龄相关性差异的基础，因为年幼的儿童缺乏足够的抗体反应[87]。脾脏也作为一种储血器官，其在人类主要局限在血小板。在脾大的病例中，滞留在脾脏内的血小板比例就会增加，偶尔会导致血小板减少症。脾脏也是Ⅷ因子的储存器官。

解剖学上的异常

副脾

副脾是最常见的解剖异常，出现在 15%~30% 的儿童中。副脾最可能起源于没有与主要的脾脏组织发生融合的间质残留。副脾大部分（75%）位于脾门附近，胰尾紧跟其后；副脾沿着脾动脉、网膜、肠系膜和腹膜后腔出现，有时甚至会出现在阴囊中[32]。86% 为单个副脾，11% 有 2 个副脾，3% 出现 3 个或者 3 个以上的副脾[51,52]，而脾门为出现多个副脾的最常见部位。手术医生必须要认识到这些部位，常规检查有无副脾，因为遗漏一个副脾可能导致免疫性血小板减少性紫癜（ITP）或者遗传性球形细胞增多症复发。血小板减少性紫癜的复发经常在早期[45,116]，然而有报道称遗传性球形细胞增多症的复发可以延迟到术后 31 年[22]。

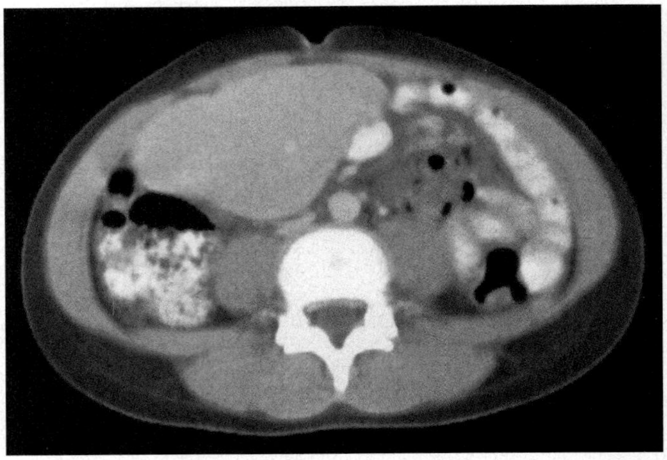

图 108-1 一个有间歇性腹痛和腹部肿块的 7 岁男孩行 CT 扫描图像见游走脾。腹腔镜脾固定术在左上腹区域固定。

游走脾

游走脾的特征是缺少与膈肌、结肠和后腹膜相连的韧带。游走脾的胚胎学基础可能与来自背侧肠系膜的脾韧带的发育不良有关[109]。有这种疾病的儿童经常表现为扭转和梗死，虽然他们也可以表现为间歇性的疼痛和腹部肿块（图 108-1）[50,72,82,103,104]，但是对于脾梗死需要进行脾切除术，在没有发生缺血和偶尔发现游走脾的病例中最好行脾固定术。脾固定术可以通过不同的技术完成，包括将脾放置到腹膜外腔的口袋中[104]、利用 Dexon 网眼篮固定[2]、缝合脾固定术[112]和结肠移位加胃固定术[16]。利用可吸收的网眼袋完成腹腔镜扭转复位和脾固定术，在脾门附近关闭网眼袋，然后将其固定在膈肌和后外侧的腹壁上。

脾囊肿

原发性的脾囊肿内层有一个上皮层，内部经常具有小梁。它们最可能起源于包括间皮表层到脾的实质。脾囊肿可没有症状，也可以表现为腹痛[121]、破裂[91]、脓肿[120]，或者是由于胃压迫而导致的症状。症状性囊肿通常大于 8 cm[121]。小的单纯性囊肿（<5 cm）可以观察，然而较大的、不断增大的囊肿或者出现症状的囊肿则需要进行最终的手术治疗。已经开始应用经皮穿刺吸引和硬化剂治疗，但是复发常

见，需要进行部分的脾切除术[78]。虽然先天性囊肿的乙醇硬化治疗已经有成功的报道，但是没有详细说明随访时间[1]。如果没有切除足够节段的囊肿，袋形缝合术可能与复发有关[80,114]。腹腔镜下囊肿部分切除术[64,100]和囊肿切除及部分脾切除术[13,47,123]已经有
693 非常成功的报道。利用超声谐波手术刀（Ethicon Endo-Surgery，Cincinnati，Ohio）[73,101,106]进行部分脾切除术及脾的边缘囊肿切除，或者在开腹手术[130]或腹腔镜手术[38,105]中利用缝合器设备来进行。利用烧灼术[105]、缝合术和网膜包裹缺损处也可以是有效的方法[106]。脾假性囊肿缺乏上皮衬里，最常见发生在外伤以后。较大的囊肿（>8.0 cm）、不断增大的囊肿和有症状的囊肿应该进行手术切除[117]。

无脾和多脾

无脾和多脾综合征有许多类似的特征。先天性无脾通常可合并复杂的先天性心脏病，以及双侧的“右面”，包括双侧的三叶肺、右侧胃和位于中部的肝脏[5]，也可以看到肠旋转不良[122]。在外周血涂片上可以看到 Howell-Jolly 小体，婴幼儿有发生无法抵抗性感染的风险。

多脾的病例中脾脏被分为多个脾肿块，经常与胆道闭锁有关。其他相关特征包括十二指肠前门静脉、器官反位、旋转不良、心脏缺陷[5]。这些儿童有足够的脾脏免疫功能。

脾脏性腺融合

脾脏性腺融合是指脾脏和左侧性腺之间发生早期融合[90]。残余物可以是连续的纤维素性束带，或者是不连续的脾脏组织黏附到性腺。其他异常特征是除了性腺融合外，在阴囊处发现异位的脾脏组织。

脾脏切除的指征

遗传性球形红细胞症

在北欧人的后裔中，遗传性球形红细胞贫血症是最常见的遗传性红细胞疾病。有接近 75% 的受累儿童为常染色体显性遗传方式，其余为新近发生的突变或者是常染色体隐性遗传疾病。锚蛋白或者血影蛋白中的膜缺陷导致变形能力差的球形红细胞形成。脾脏发生溶血的程度可从轻到重。大多数儿童有贫血、网织红细胞计数升高和轻度的胆红素水平升高。出现球形红细胞以及渗透脆性试验阳性，即可证实诊断。在受累的儿童中，再生障碍危象继发于细小病毒 B19 感染，导致红细胞生成抑制和由于红细胞进行性破坏而产生的血细胞比容下降[133]。对于中到重度的贫血，通常需要进行脾切除术。患儿常见有胆石症，随着患儿年龄的增长和溶血程度的加重，发生胆石症的概率会增加，因此在进行脾切除手术之前通常需要行胆囊超声检查。遗传性椭圆形红细胞增多症是一种与血影蛋白缺陷相关的类似疾病，但是大多数患儿没有症状，不会发生显著性溶血。

免疫性血小板减少性紫癜（ITP）

当抗血小板的自身抗体（通常是 IgG）结合到血小板时，就会发生免疫性血小板减少性紫癜（ITP），导致血小板在网织内皮系统中被破坏。治疗方法包括糖皮质激素（可以抑制网织内皮系统结合血小板-抗体复合物）、静脉注射免疫球蛋白（IVIG）（可以竞争性抑制巨噬细胞 Fc 受体结合血小板）、在 Rh 阳性的儿童中应用 Rho（D）免疫球蛋白（其结合到红细胞后使脾脏的能力饱和，并节约抗体包裹的血小板）和脾切除术。对糖皮质激素或 IVIG 有效，或者对两者都有效则提示脾切除术有效（97%），而对两者均无效则提示脾切除术有 70% 的可能性失败[25]。其他的学者发现，对 IVIG 有效的患儿与对糖皮质激素有效的患儿相比，脾切除术具有更好的疗效[57]。儿童时期的 ITP 通常是一种自限性的急性疾病，只有在慢性病例中才需要进行脾切除术。

镰状细胞病

镰状细胞病是由于正常血红蛋白 A 的 β 链中缬

氨酸替换了谷氨酸，导致血红蛋白A变成了血红蛋白S。当氧饱和度下降时，这些红细胞变硬，随后毛细血管发生阻塞，红细胞的寿命缩短。有纯合子镰状细胞性贫血和有血红蛋白镰状细胞病的儿童，有较高的发生疼痛危象和急性胸部综合征的频率。可以发生血红蛋白和血小板计数快速下降的脾脏血细胞破坏症。如果症状较重或者反复发作，进行脾切除术以减少进一步发作的机会。

珠蛋白生成障碍性贫血（地中海贫血）

地中海贫血是一组以α或β链血红蛋白异常产物为特征的疾病。地中海贫血的主要类型（Cooley贫血、β-地中海贫血）可导致在这组疾病中临床上最为严重的贫血。一些儿童会出现显著的脾大和脾脏血细胞破坏症。在重度贫血的儿童中，以及那些有显著的脾大和血小板或白细胞降低的病例中，应用脾切除术以减少输血的需求。

Gaucher病（戈谢病、家族性脾性贫血、葡萄糖脑苷脂酶缺乏症）

Gancher病是一种代谢性疾病，其特征为β-葡萄糖脑苷脂酶的缺陷，导致在脾脏、肝脏、骨髓和肺的巨噬细胞中产生过多的葡萄糖脑苷脂。这是一种常染色体隐性遗传性疾病，大多数发生于德国、波兰与苏联境内的犹太人。可以是重度的脾大，应用脾部分切除或者脾全部切除以缓解脾功能亢进和增加红细胞、白细胞和血小板计数[40]。然而，有脾部分切除术后复发的报道。

1694 脾脓肿

脾脓肿罕见，但是随着免疫受抑制儿童数量的增加而发病率不断增多。病原菌经常是真菌或者分枝杆菌[111]。患儿经常有发热、疼痛和血培养阳性。CT扫描经常可发现疾病扩散的特征，因此通常需要进行脾切除术。

脾切除术

开腹脾切除术

对于大多数的脾脏，甚至是脾大的病例，左上腹肋缘下切口可提供良好的术野暴露。向内侧牵拉脾脏，分离脾肾韧带、脾横隔韧带和脾结肠韧带。这种操作通常可以在一个相对较小的切口下完成，利用脾脏中部表面的凹陷，通过先游离脾下即可将脾脏搬移出腹腔。分离脾胃韧带和胃短血管，再分离脾门血管。如果胰腺非常靠近脾门，就可能需要切断韧带血管。仔细寻找副脾，如果有就应切除。另外一种开腹手术方法是利用侧面分离肌层的切口[43]，这种手术的平均住院时间为2.7天，与一些腹腔镜下手术类似[37,79,126]。脾切除术后的并发症相对罕见。报道脾切除术后可出现脾静脉、门静脉和肠系膜静脉的血栓形成，在评估脾切除术后的腹痛时应该考虑到这一点[110]。

腹腔镜下脾切除术

手术技术

应用于脾切除术的腹腔镜技术最初报道于1991年[28]，在随后的5年间这种技术已经成为大多数医院的首选方法。疼痛轻，因而应用止痛药少、住院时间短、切口美观，这些都是腹腔镜技术与开腹脾切除术相比的主要优势。对于那些不熟悉先进的腹腔镜技术的外科医生，腹腔镜手术有一个陡峭的学习曲线，并且对于脾大的病例手术可能是困难的，与开腹手术相比手术时间更长。在成人手术的研究中，腹腔镜技术发现副脾的效率一直存在疑问[45,116]，虽然在一系列的儿童开腹与腹腔镜脾切除术的比较中有相似的副脾发现概率[37,77,79,92,94,126]。

随着设备的小型化和先进技术如超声刀的应用，腹腔镜脾切除术已经得到了长足发展。虽然术前脾动脉栓塞在许多最初的成人病例中进行了报道[42]，但是并发症例如疼痛、脓肿、腹膜后的坏死也有发生[85,88]；一些医生发现在出血和需要输血的风险中两者没有差别。脾脏长度在20～30 cm之间的进行栓塞，脾脏大于30 cm的需要行开腹脾切除手术，但是大多数儿童时期脾大的病例中脾脏相对较小，所以这种技术似乎对于儿童来说没有必要[88]。对于成人巨大的脾脏，也曾经报道过采用手辅助的手术方法[48]，但是这额外的切口延长了住院时间，在儿童手术中似乎也没有必要。

虽然在一些最初的报道中利用了一种前路切口，但是目前大多数外科医生使用侧路切口，如图 108-2 中所描述。在笔者医院中，患者被置于接近 45 度的左侧抬高体位，轻度升高右侧胸腹以增加在左侧的通路。手术台旋转到患者的左侧以便于放置套针，然后再到右侧以获得右侧卧位便于手术操作。总的原则是助手使用两把抓钳通过上腹部中线的位置（见图 108-2中的 a 和 b）提起脾脏，提供周围组织的牵引。对于年幼的儿童和有较小脾脏的年长患者，在那些部位使用 3 mm 的手术器械，通过小的针刺切口直接放置到腹腔，而不需要使用套针。如果不使用套针，手术医生必须要清楚烧灼器传导损伤的风险。如果脾脏巨大，至少一个上腹部中线的套针必须适应 5 mm 的
95 手术器械。大多数的手术过程中，主刀医生左手（脐孔）握持镜头，右手持超声刀。脐孔最常见的是一个 15 mm 的入口以容纳直径 15 mm 的 Endocatch II（美国 Surgical 公司，Norwalk，CT）设备和血管内钉合器。使用 5 mm 的 30 度放大镜头，可以使它应用在左下腹，当应用血管内钉合器和通过脐孔放置回收设备时，镜头必须位于左下腹。

应用超音波谐波刀分离脾结肠韧带，使得结肠脾曲脱离脾脏（图 108-3A）。分离脾胃韧带，利用谐波超声刀切断胃短血管，因此外科医生很少需要更换器械（见图 108-3B）。由于脾脏和胃非常接近，大多数情况下游离脾脏上面是困难的，也必须小心以免损伤到膈肌。在脾门处找到的副脾通常和脾脏一起全部切除，其他较少的阴囊或者网膜的副脾则分别给予切除，通常从脐孔的切口进行切除。

然后从上极和下极将脾脏固定，处理脾门，通常或者使用谐波超声刀，或者使用血管夹和剪刀来游离脾脏下段的部分血管。外科医生必须作出决定，使用血管夹或血管内钉合器来处理其余的脾脏下极或者下
段的血管。如果血管逐一进行游离，外科医生必须有 1696
所准备，一旦发生出血，就应该利用抓钳控制近端的血管，夹闭血管或者钉合脾门剩余的血管。如果使用钉合器切断脾肾韧带，钉合器的后臂能够轻易地通过后侧到达脾门。操作时必须小心，以免损伤到胰尾部（见图 108-3C）。这时其他的辅助操作包括：使用吸盘抓钳以处置脾脏[44]，腹壁牵引装置[83]，绕脾门放置脐扎带以抬高并固定脾脏[102]。另外除了谐波超声刀和钉合器，可使用 LigaSure 血管闭合设备（美国 Surgical 公司，Norwalk，CT），其可利用双极电凝的能量和压力来达到封闭血管的效果[97]。也已经有报道称使用了达芬奇手术机器人[19]。

通过脐孔来放置 Endocatch II 回收袋。当回收袋张开时直径为 13 cm，袋深 23 cm，可容纳大多数儿童的脾脏。如果脾脏较小，对于一个 10 mm 或者 12 mm的脐戳孔，可以用一个 10 mm 的回收袋（Endopouch，Ethicon Surgery，Inc，Cincinnati，OH）来取脾脏。将脾脏放到回收袋中，将袋的颈部从脐孔拉出。通过回收袋外部的开口伸入手指或者环状钳，用以粉碎脾脏和取出脾脏的碎片（见图 108-3D）。已经有报道称可利用超声组织粉碎器（morcellator）和脂肪吸引器（liposucker）[66]来粉碎脾脏，还有一种技术是经阴道取出回收袋。在一些脾大的病例中，可能难以将脾脏放置到回收袋中[125]。Hebra 和其同事[54]利用一种去心设备在将脾脏放置到回收袋中以前减小脾脏的部分体积。对于遗传性球形红细胞贫血症的病例不推荐使用这种技术，因为脾组织

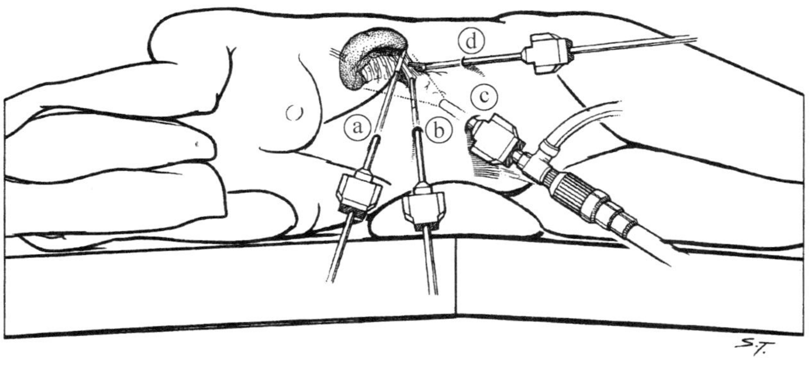

图 108-2　侧路切口时患儿的体位和腹腔镜套管大小以及部位：a 和 b，中线 3 或 5 毫米；c，脐部 12 或 15 毫米；d，左下腹 5 毫米。

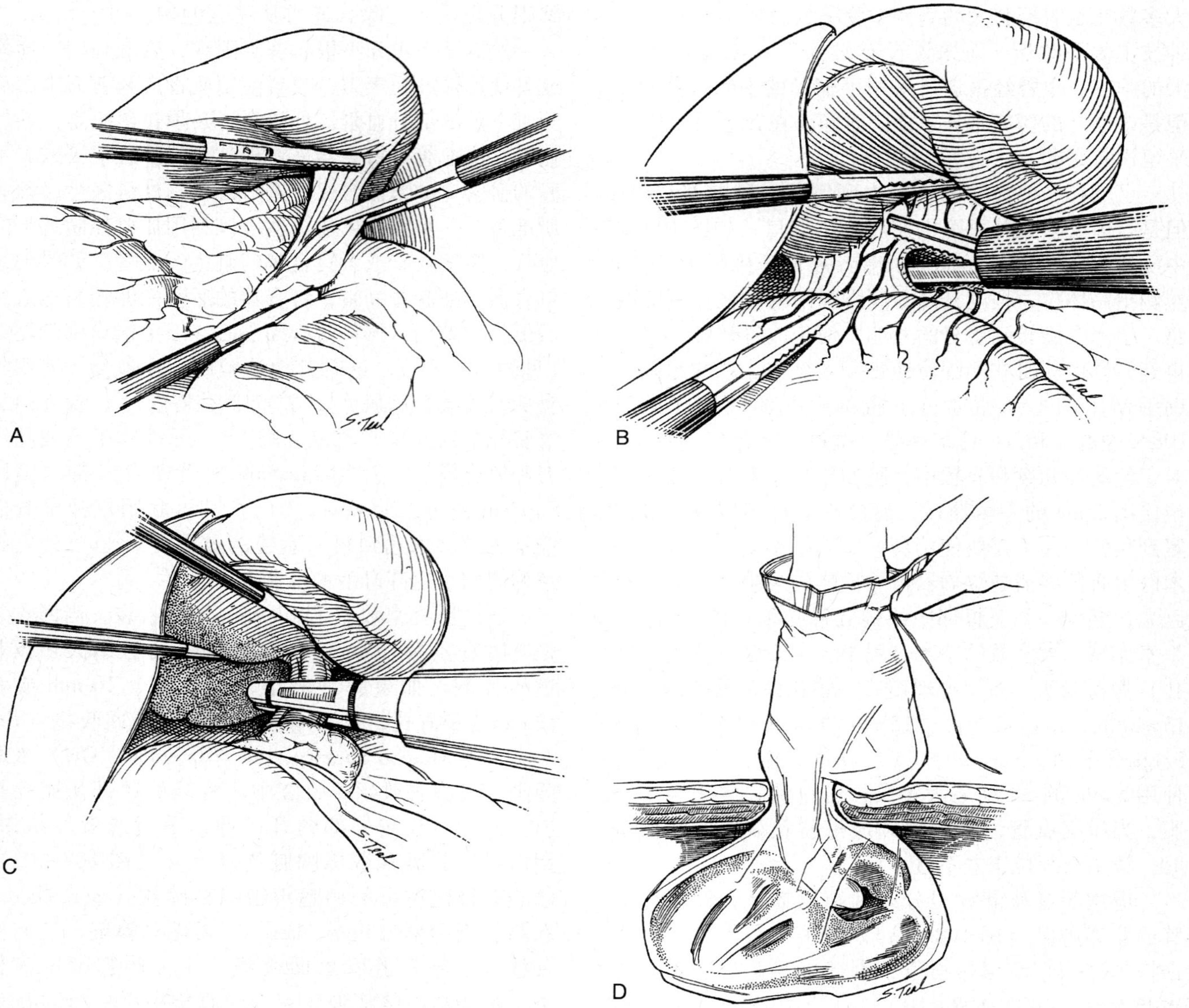

图 108–3　用谐波超声刀进行脾结肠韧带（A）和脾胃韧带（B）的分离。血管内钉合器用于分离脾门血管（C），放置入回收袋以后，从脐孔（D）中取出。用手指粉碎脾脏，用抓钳去除脾脏的碎片。

植入可能会导致复发性贫血。如果方便的话，5 mm 套管口的前筋膜层都应该关闭。在手术中应用的鼻胃管和 Foley 导尿管，在手术结束后去除。手术当天禁食后逐渐添加饮食，静脉应用吗啡和非甾体类消炎药以进行镇痛，当患儿能够进食液体时再给予口服镇痛药治疗。腹腔镜脾切除技术可应用到其他手术中，包括要行脾部分切除的疾病，如脾囊肿、游走脾行脾固定术以及创伤性脾脏外伤的治疗等[15,63]。

中转开腹手术

中转开腹脾切除手术最为常见的原因是由于脾脏巨大或者术中大出血，其在几个大宗病例数报道中发生率为 1.3%~2.8%[36,77,95,118,127]。恶性巨脾是一种更为困难的情况，作者发现，在成年人中恶性巨脾有 41% 行中转开腹手术，良性巨脾转为开腹手术的比例只有 3%[9]。在另外一些成年人病例研究中，Mahon 和 Rhodes 提出，对于脾脏重量小于 1 kg 的病例，中转开腹手术的比例是 0，而对于那些脾脏重量大于 1

kg 的病例，中转开腹手术的比例则为 60%[71]。在一些大宗的病例报道中已经发现，随着外科医生经验的增加，转为开腹手术的比例在下降[85,131]。一个对成年人 ITP 患者的多元分析确定了肥胖和外科医生经验为中转开腹手术的主要影响因素[27]。

副脾的探查

一些成年人的病例研究对腹腔镜是否能够充分探查副脾提出了质疑。尽管原发性副脾的发生率为 41%，但是有报道 18 例成年病例中有 9 例确定存在残留的脾脏功能[45]。在 3 个有症状的患者中就有 1 例在探查时发现存在副脾。实质性的破坏有 75% 的残留脾功能，而在那些没有实质性破坏的病例中只有 36% 的残留脾功能，因此强调需要避免脾脏破损。在另外一个研究中，9 例脾脏切除后失败的病例中就有 3 例有残留的脾功能[116]。虽然一些学者已经推荐术前进行 CT 扫描和（或）同位素闪烁扫描[36,81]，但是大多数医生放弃了这个做法，有些研究者提出腹腔镜手术有更高的副脾发现率[45,61]。一个研究报告利用术中同位素闪烁扫描来进行副脾的定位[21]。从 6 项儿科比较研究提供的数据中没有发现存在显著的差别[37,77,79,92,94,126]：在 128 例开腹脾切除术中发现副脾的比例为 20.3%，而 139 例腹腔镜脾切除术中发现副脾的比例则为 20.2%。在对 6 项成年人或者儿童的至少有 50 例腹腔镜脾切除术的大宗病例评价中，总共 585 例患者中发现副脾的比例是 14.7%[36,42,46,61,85,95]。也已经有报道腹腔镜切除遗漏副脾[4,115]，其中有 1 例是有症状的副脾，在因 ITP 而行开腹脾切除术后 30 年时才发现[14]。也已经有报道称在回收袋入口部位发生脾组织的植入[65]。

手术时间

大宗病例的比较研究都一致发现采用腹腔镜脾切除技术的手术时间相对更长[37,77,79,92,94,126]，一些研究报道随着手术医生经验的增加，手术时间在不断缩短[24,95]。在作者的医院中进行的一个 112 例腹腔镜脾切除的回顾分析中，发现最初的 50 例相对随后的 62 例手术时间更长（115 分钟 *vs* 98 分钟），但是两者之间的差别并不显著[95]。在后期相对较短的手术时间仍然要比由笔者及其同事报道的 83 分钟的开腹脾切除手术时间要长[94]。

疼痛

儿童的病例报道没有使用疼痛评分，而是依靠镇痛药物的使用来反映疼痛程度。所有现有的比较研究报道称，腹腔镜脾切除比开腹脾切除使用更少的相当吗啡剂量的镇痛药，但是两者之间的差别在 5 个研究中有 2 个没有达到统计学上的显著意义[8,23,79,92,94]。这个结果和成年人的研究结果是一致的，其指出在腹腔镜手术组有相同的生活质量和控制血液性疾病的效果，而疼痛较轻[124]。

住院时间

1697

住院时间的范围在 1.3～3.6 天，而最近的研究表明住院时间在 1.7～1.8 天[77,92,94]。所有的儿童比较研究都表明利用腹腔镜技术以后，住院时间变得更短（腹腔镜手术 1.3～3.6 天，开腹手术 2.5～4.9 天），缩短的程度在 18%～56%[37,77,79,92,94,126]。潜在的疾病可影响住院时间，镰状细胞病的婴幼儿和儿童比有 ITP 或遗传性球形红细胞贫血症的患儿需要更长的住院时间（2.5 天 *vs* 1.4 天）[94]。这是由于发生了术后急性胸部综合征的缘故。儿童单纯的脾大似乎对住院时间没有不利影响，因为遗传性球形红细胞贫血症的脾大是最为常见的脾切除手术指征，住院时间较短（1.4 天）。对从 1991 年到 2002 年间所有病例报道（主要是成年人病例）的 meta 分析（2940 例患者，2119 例行腹腔镜手术，821 例行开腹手术）表明，腹腔镜脾切除手术平均手术时间较长（腹腔镜手术 180 分钟，开腹手术 114 分钟；$P<0.0001$），但是住院时间较短（腹腔镜手术 3.6 天，开腹手术 7.2 天；$P<0.001$）[129]。腹腔镜手术未经证实的好处还包括可以促进儿童恢复全面的活动和回到学校读书，促使父母亲更早地恢复工作。已经发现进行腹腔镜脾切除的儿童恢复全面活动的时间比进行开腹手术的儿童提前 1～5 周[126]。另外，自身进行过脾切除手术的父母亲认为腹腔镜技术比开腹手术更好。

手术费用

大多数作者假定腹腔镜手术的住院时间较短，其抵消了手术时间长和应用一次性材料所造成的较高手术费用。来自比较研究的数据表明，有 3 个研究显示腹腔镜手术住院费用较高[23,59,126]，另有 3 个研究则显示腹腔镜手术住院费用较低[37,92,94]。各个医院各自决定其手术所需的费用或开销，以及使用手术室时间和住院天数，这种统计方法给比较研究造成了困难。现有的手术费用数据没有显示出任何一种手术具有手术费用上的优势。

并发症

对一个新手术最为重要的评价是术后并发症的评价。Clavien 分类系统[20]统计的手术并发症如下：

Ⅰ级：微小的、自发消退或者床边操作便可解决的问题（肺膨胀不全、胃扩张需要鼻胃管减压、体温 >38.5℃）。

Ⅱ级：有潜在的生命危险，通常需要干预的医源性的可导致住院时间加倍的并发症。

Ⅲ级：残留或者持久的残疾，医源性的器官切除。

Ⅳ级：由于并发症而导致的死亡。

这个评价系统应用于 1995 年到 2002 年间一组 344 例儿童腹腔镜脾切除术和 369 例儿童开腹脾切除手术的研究中。在这个评价中，Ⅰ级（腹腔镜手术 2.9% *vs* 开腹手术 4.9%；$P=0.18$）或者Ⅱ级（腹腔镜手术 6.7% *vs* 开腹手术 4.9%；$P=0.30$）并发症在两组之间没有统计学上显著性差异，在任何一组病例中都没有报道出现Ⅲ级或者Ⅳ级的并发症。

最大的成人单一机构比较研究（63 例腹腔镜手术，74 例开腹手术）表明，Ⅰ级和Ⅱ级手术并发症相当（5%～9%），但是Ⅲ级（41% *vs* 0）和Ⅳ级（3% *vs* 0）手术并发症在开腹手术中更高[42]。在 1991 年到 2002 年间所进行的 26 组比较研究（成人和儿童）的 meta 分析表明，总的并发症发生率腹腔镜脾切除手术为 15.5%，开腹脾切除手术为 26.6%（$P<0.0001$）[129]。腹腔镜手术组有更少的肺部、伤口和感染并发症（$P<0.0001$），但是当包括出血而转为开腹手术时，则有更多的出血并发症。

部分脾切除术

脾全切术并副脾切除术消除了脾源性溶血和先天性溶血性贫血的脾脏血液破坏。考虑到脾切除术后可发生无法抵抗的败血症，尤其是在年龄小于 5 岁的儿童中，这导致了部分脾切除术的出现。这种手术主要应用于溶血性贫血，例如遗传性球形红细胞贫血症，但也可以应用于 Gaucher 病[40]、Hodgkin 病[55]、外伤[89]、脾功能亢进伴囊性纤维化[119]以及脾囊肿切除术[105]、错构瘤[53]和血管瘤[7]。当这种技术应用于脾脏体积缩减术时，85%～95% 的疾病受累脾脏组织被切除，以留下接近 25% 的正常脾脏组织。脾脏血液供应的解剖学研究表明，86% 的脾脏有 2 支脾小叶动脉，12% 的脾脏组织有 3 支脾小叶动脉[69]。另外，77% 的脾脏组织有 4 支或者 5 支段血管，因此可以保留脾脏的上极或者下极段血管以供应 20%～25% 的脾脏组织。可以用缝合器缝合分离、烧灼切除或者谐波超声刀分离脾脏，可以用烧灼、氩气刀凝血或者局部使用止血剂的方法来止血。如果脾脏全部被游离，则残留的脾脏组织可以固定到后腹膜以防止扭转。这种手术可以在腹腔镜下用谐波超声刀进行，分离脾脏的同时又可提供止血（图 108-4）。

长期随访已经注意到红细胞半衰期延长，升高了血红蛋白水平，降低了网织红细胞计数和胆红素水平[6,96]，保存了脾脏的噬菌细胞功能，已经通过外周血涂片上消除 Howell-Jolly 小体和减少的去核红细胞数量得到证实[96]。其他参数包括肺炎链球菌特异性抗体的正常 IgM 和 IgG 滴度。脾脏的重新生长可发生在所有溶血性贫血的患儿中，但是重新生长的程度与溶血不相关。脾部分切除术后的并发症可包括进行性发生的胆石症（7%～22%），复发性贫血而需要进行输血，或者是随后行脾全切术[26,96]。在假设具有正 16

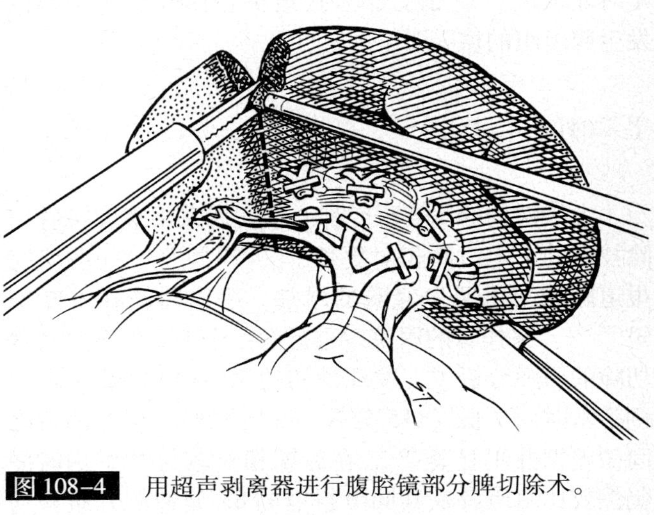

图 108-4　用超声剥离器进行腹腔镜部分脾切除术。

常的脾功能时必须要谨慎，因为有一例外伤患者在部分脾切除术后通过扫描发现有残留脾功能，但是13年后死于肺炎链球菌的感染[135]。该患儿没有接受过肺炎球菌的疫苗。推荐术前进行免疫接种，术后应用抗生素至少持续到发现脾脏免疫能力。

脾切除术后的败血症

发生脾切除术后暴发性感染（OPSI）是在1951年由King和Shumacker第一次报道的，他们报道了5例年龄小于6个月的婴幼儿因遗传性球形红细胞贫血症而进行脾切除[62]。所有5例患儿都发生了严重的感染，其中2例死亡。从此以后，许多报道都记录了这种风险，在儿童年龄小于5岁以及脾切除术后的最初数年内，这种风险的发生率成倍增加（60～100倍）。病因学上可能与有荚膜的细菌清除率下降[12]，以及免疫球蛋白水平的降低有关[17]。在幼年和童年时期脾脏显得尤其重要，因为在发生感染时噬菌细胞的功能几乎是脾脏所特有的[67]。

20世纪70年代所累积的报道资料[31]证实，脾切除术后OPSI的发生率为3.75%，死亡率为1.7%。在儿童病例中的发生率为4.1%，而在成年人中则为1.9%；在儿童中死亡率为1.8%，而在成年人中则为1.1%。其他研究显示在20世纪80年代和90年代，OPSI发生率的波动范围较大。在90年代中期，年龄小于15岁的儿童中总的OPSI的发生率波动在0.13%～8.1%之间，而成年人则为0.28%～1.9%[70]。在所有感染病例中，有50%～90%的病例为肺炎链球菌致病，全部的致死性感染中有60%与此有关[31,41,107,113]。流感嗜血杆菌感染占到了死亡病例的32%[56]，脑膜炎球菌和A组链球菌也是重要的病原菌。

迟发性感染导致死亡的风险也与不同的疾病状态有关，球形细胞增多症中死亡率为0.51%，ITP中死亡率为2.67%[33]。其他学者也发现，在年龄小于4岁的儿童中死亡率更高（死亡率：年龄小于4岁的儿童为8.1%，年长儿童为3.3%），大多数死亡病例发生于脾切除术后4年内[34,58]。由此可见，应提倡预防性应用青霉素。在儿童中相对成年人风险增加的是，致死性OPSI的发生率在儿童中为3.77%，而在成年人中则为0.39%。这些早期报道中有许多是发生在广泛应用疫苗接种和预防性使用抗生素以前，最近的研究显示OPSI的发生率降低到3.5%～3.8%[60,75]。疫苗接种可以降低细菌感染的风险[30]。

一项对比研究中，早期进行的脾切除没有进行免疫接种或预防性使用抗生素，而晚期进行的脾切除有70%进行了免疫接种并100%预防性使用抗生素，结果显示感染的发生率（6%～3.8%）和死亡率（3.9%～0.9%）都降低[60]。甚至在最近的研究中显示，感染的发生率与脾切除时的年龄有关（从出生到5岁：13.8%；大于5岁：0.5%）。历史上与OPSI有关的死亡率为50%～70%[10,49,70,113]，但是最近观察到的死亡率在10%左右[11,60]。

以前的研究显示，似乎可以用针对肺炎链球菌、脑膜炎球菌、流感嗜血杆菌的免疫接种和同时预防性使用抗生素来降低脾切除术后发生败血症的风险。随着疫苗的可得性增加，标准的推荐方案已包括术前免疫接种，并且许多儿童接受常规的儿童时期免疫接种来抵抗肺炎链球菌和流感嗜血杆菌。一些学者推荐终身预防性应用青霉素[74]，而其他学者推荐只需应用10年左右[134]。最高的OPSI发生率发生在儿童和脾切除术后2年之内，其长期的推荐方案还不清楚[128]。

在J. W. RILEY医院的儿童腹腔镜脾切除手术

在作者所在医院，腹腔镜脾切除是在1995年8月引进的，在4个月内这项技术便成为主要应用的技术。一共有190例儿童进行了腹腔镜脾手术，178例进行了脾切除，5例进行了部分脾切除，5例因上皮性或创伤性囊肿而进行了腹腔镜脾囊肿切除，2例进行了游走脾固定术。遗传性球形红细胞增多症是最为常见的脾切除手术指征，其次为ITP和镰状红细胞病伴脾脏血细胞破坏症。4例（2.2%）需要转为开腹手术：2例因为脾脏巨大，1例因为出血，1例是由于以前手术造成的粘连。平均住院时间是1.51天，遗传性球形红细胞增多症为1.23天，ITP为1.15天，镰状红细胞病伴脾脏血细胞破坏症为2.24天。一个 1699
溶血性贫血患儿因遗漏副脾而需要进行开腹副脾切除术，一个患儿因为没有预防性服用抗生素而死于脾切除术后的败血症。

（顾　松译　陈永卫校）

参考文献

1. Akhan O, Baykan Z, Oguzkurt L, et al: Percutaneous treatment of a congenital splenic cyst with alcohol: a new therapeutic approach. Eur Radiol 1997;7:1067.
2. Allen KB, Andrews G: Pediatric wandering spleen—the case for splenopexy: review of 35 reported cases in the literature. J Pediatr Surg 1989;24:432.
3. Al-Salem AH: Is splenectomy for massive splenomegaly safe in children? Am J Surg 1999;178:42.
4. Amaral JF, Meltzer RC, Crowley JP: Laparoscopic accessory splenectomy for recurrent idiopathic thrombocytopenic purpura. Surg Laparosc Endosc 1997;7:340.
5. Anderson C, Devine WA, Anderson RH, et al: Abnormalities of the spleen in relation to congenital malformations of the heart: A survey of necropsy findings in children. Br Heart J 1990;63:122.
6. Bader-Meunier B, Gauthier F, Archambaud F, et al: Long-term evaluation of the beneficial effect of subtotal splenectomy for management of hereditary spherocytosis. Blood 2001;97:399.
7. Bailez MM, Elmo G: Laparoscopic partial splenectomy for a hemangioma of the spleen. Pediatr Endosurg Innov Tech 2004;8:147.
8. Beanes S, Emil S, Kosi M, et al: A comparison of laparoscopic versus open splenectomy in children. Am Surg 1995;61:908.
9. Berman RS, Yahanda A, Mansfield PF, et al: Laparoscopic splenectomy in patients with hematologic malignancies. Am J Surg 1999;178:530.
10. Brigden ML: Overwhelming post-splenectomy infection—still a problem. West J Med 1992;157:440.
11. Brigden ML, Pattullo AL: Prevention and management of overwhelming postsplenectomy infection—an update. Crit Care Med 1999;27:836.
12. Brown EJ, Hosea SW, Frank MM: The role of the spleen in experimental pneumococcal bacteremia. J Clin Invest 1981;67:975.
13. Brown MF, Ross III, AJ, Bishop HC, et al: Partial splenectomy: The preferred alternative for the treatment of splenic cysts. J Pediatr Surg 1989;24:694.
14. Budzynski A, Bobrzynski A, Sacha T, et al: Laparoscopic removal of retroperitoneal accessory spleen in patient with relapsing idiopathic thrombocytopenic purpura 30 years after classical splenectomy. Surg Endosc 2002;16:1636.
15. Carbon RT, Baar S, Waldschmidt J, et al: Innovative minimally invasive pediatric surgery is of therapeutic value for splenic injury. J Pediatr Surg 2002;37:1146.
16. Caracicolo F, Bonatti PC, Castruci G, et al: Wandering spleen: Treatment with colonic displacement. J R Coll Surg Edinb 1986;31:242.
17. Chaimoff C, Douer D, Pick IA, et al: Serum immunoglobulin changes after accidental splenectomy in adults. Am J Surg 1978;136:332.
18. Chalkof EL, McCabe CJ: Fatal overwhelming postsplenectomy infection. Am J Surg 1985;49:534.
19. Chapman WH, Albrecht RJ, Kim VB, et al: Computer-assisted laparoscopic splenectomy with the da Vinci surgical robot. J Laparoendosc Adv Surg Tech A 2002;12:155.
20. Clavien PA, Sanabria JR, Strasberg SM: Proposed classification of complications of surgery with examples of utility in cholecystectomy. Surgery 1992;111:518.
21. Coventry BJ, Watson DI, Tucker K, et al: Intraoperative scintigraphic localization and laparoscopic excision of accessory splenic tissue. Surg Endosc 1998;12:159.
22. Crawford DL, Pickens PV, Moore JT: Hypertrophied splenic remnants in hereditary spherocytosis. Contemp Surg 1998;53:103.
23. Curran TJ, Foley MI, Swanstrom LL, et al: Laparoscopy improves outcomes for pediatric splenectomy. J Pediatr Surg 1998;33:1498.
24. Cusick RA, Waldhausen JH: The learning curve associated with pediatric laparoscopic splenectomy. Am J Surg 2201;181:393.
25. Davis PW, Williams DA, Shamberger RC: Immune thrombocytopenia: Surgical therapy and predictors of response. J Pediatr Surg 1991;26:407.
26. de Buys Roessingh AS, de Lagausie P, Rohrlich P, et al: Follow-up of partial splenectomy in children with hereditary spherocytosis. J Pediatr Surg 2002;37:1459.
27. Delaitre B, Blezel E, Samama G, et al: Laparoscopic splenectomy for idiopathic thrombocytopenic purpura. 2002;12:412.
28. Delaitre B, Maignien B: Splenectomy by the coelioscopic approach: Report of a case. Presse Med 1991;20:2263.
29. Douglas GJ, Simpson JS: The conservative management of splenic trauma. J Pediatr Surg 1971;6:565.
30. Ejstrud P, Kristensen B, Hansen JB, et al: Risk and patterns of bacteraemia after splenectomy: A population-based study. Scand J Infect Dis 2000;32:521.
31. Ellison EC, Fabri PJ: Complications of splenectomy. Surg Clin North Am 1983;63:1313.
32. Emmett JM, Dreyfuss ML: Accessory spleen in the scrotum: Review of literature on ectopic spleens and their associated surgical significance. Ann Surg 1943;117:754.
33. Eraklis AJ, Filler RM: Splenectomy in childhood: A review of 1413 cases. J Pediatr Surg 1972;7:382.
34. Eraklis AJ, Kewy SV, Diamond LK: Hazard of overwhelming infection after splenectomy in childhood. N Engl J Med 1967;276:1225.
35. Esposito C, Corcione F, Garipoli V, et al: Pediatric laparoscopic splenectomy: Are there real advantages in comparison with the traditional open approach? Pediatr Surg Int 1997;12:509.
36. Esposito C, Schaarschmidt K, Settimi A, et al: Experience with laparoscopic splenectomy. J Pediatr Surg 2001;36:309.
37. Farah RA, Rogers ZR, Thompson RW, et al: Comparison of laparoscopic and open splenectomy in children with hematologic disorders. J Pediatr 1997;131:41.
38. Feliciotti F, Sottili M, Guerrieri M, et al: Conservative ultrasound-guided laparoscopic treatment of posttraumatic splenic cysts: Report of two cases. Surg Laparosc Endosc 1996;6:322.
39. Fitzgerald PG, Langer JC, Cameron BH, et al: Pediatric laparoscopy splenectomy using the lateral approach. Surg Endosc 1996;10:859.
40. Fonkalsrud EW, Philippart M, Feig S: Ninety-five percent splenectomy for massive splenomegaly: A new surgical approach. J Pediatr Surg 1990;25:267.
41. Francke EL, Neu HA: Postsplenectomy infection. Surg Clin North Am 1981;61:135.
42. Friedman RL, Hiatt JR, Korman JL, et al: Laparoscopic or open splenectomy for hematologic disease: Which approach is superior? J Am Coll Surg 1997;185:49.
43. Geiger JD, Dinh VV, Teitelbaum DH, et al: The lateral approach for open splenectomy. J Pediatr Surg 1998;33:1153.

44. Gentilli S, Velardocchia M, Ferrero A, et al: Laparoscopic splenectomy. How to make it easier using an innovative atraumatic suction grasper. Surg Endosc 1998;12:1345.
45. Gigot JF, Jamar F, Ferrant A, et al: Inadequate detection of accessory spleens and splenosis with laparoscopic splenectomy: A shortcoming of the laparoscopic approach in hematologic diseases. Surg Endosc 1998;12:101.
46. Gigot JF, Legrand M, Cadiere GB, et al: Is laparoscopic splenectomy a justified approach in hematologic disorders? Primary results of a prospective multicenter study. Int Surg 1995;80:299.
47. Golinski D, Freud E, Steinberg R, et al: Vertical partial splenectomy for epidermoid cyst. J Pediatr Surg 1995; 30:1704.
48. Gossot D, Fritsch S, Celerier M: Laparoscopic splenectomy: Optimal vascular control using the lateral approach and ultrasonic dissection. Surg Endosc 1999;13:21.
49. Green JB, Shackford SR, Sise MJ, et al: Late septic complications in adults following from trauma: a prospective analysis in 144 patients. J Trauma 1986;26:999.
50. Greig JD, Sweet EM, Drainer IK: Splenic torsion in a wandering spleen, presenting as an acute abdominal mass. J Pediatr Surg 1994;29:571.
51. Halpert B, Alden ZA: Accessory spleens in or at the tail of the pancreas. Arch Pathol 1964;77:652.
52. Halpert B, Gyorkey F: Lesions observed in accessory spleens of 311 patients. Am J Clin Pathol 1959;32:165.
53. Havlik RJ, Touloukian RJ, Markowitz RI, et al: Partial splenectomy for symptomatic splenic hamartoma. J Pediatr Surg 1990;25:1273.
54. Hebra A, Walker JD, Tagge EP, et al: A new technique for laparoscopic splenectomy with massively enlarged spleens. Am Surg 1998;64:1161.
55. Hoekstra HJ, Tamminga RYJ, Timens W: Partial splenectomy in children: An alternative for splenectomy in the pathological stage of Hodgkin's disease. Ann Surg Oncol 1994;1:480.
56. Holdsworth RJ, Irving AD, Cuschieri A: Postsplenectomy sepsis and its mortality rate: Actual versus perceived risks. Br J Surg 1991;78:1031.
57. Holt D, Brown J, Terrill K, et al: Response to intravenous immunoglobulin predicts splenectomy response in children with immune thrombocytopenic purpura. Pediatrics 2003;111:87.
58. Horan M, Colebatch JH: Relation between splenectomy and subsequent infection. Arch Dis Child 1962;37:398.
59. Janu PG, Rogers DA, Lobe TE: A comparison of laparoscopic and traditional open splenectomy in childhood. J Pediatr Surg 1996;31:109.
60. Jugenburg M, Haddock G, Freedman MH, et al: The morbidity and mortality of pediatric splenectomy: Does prophylaxis make a difference? J Pediatr Surg 1999; 34:1064.
61. Katkhouda N, Hurwitz MB, Rivera RT, et al: Laparoscopic splenectomy: Outcome and efficacy in 103 consecutive patients. Ann Surg 1998;228:568.
62. King H, Shumaker HB Jr: Splenic studies: I. Susceptibility to infection after splenectomy performed in infancy. Ann Surg 1953;136:239.
63. Koehler RH, Smith S, Fry WR: Successful laparoscopic splenorrhaphy using absorbable mesh for grade III splenic injury: Report of a case. Surg Laparosc Endosc 1994;4:311.
64. Kum CK, Ngoi SS, Goh P, et al: A rare wandering splenic cyst removed with laparoscopic assistance. Singapore Med J 1993;34:179.
65. Kumar RJ, Borzi PA: Splenosis in a port site after laparoscopic splenectomy. Surg Endosc 2001;15:413.
66. Lai PB, Leung KL, Ho WS, et al: The use of liposucker for spleen retrieval after laparoscopic splenectomy. Surg Laparosc Endosc Percutan Tech 2000;10:39.
67. Lane PA: The spleen and children. Curr Opin Pediatr 1995;7:36.
68. Liu DC, Meyers MO, Hill CB, et al: Laparoscopic splenectomy in children with hematologic disorders: Preliminary experience at the Children's Hospital of New Orleans. Am Surg 2000;66:1168.
69. Liu DL, Xia S, Xu W, et al: Anatomy of vasculature of 850 spleen specimens and its applications in partial splenectomy. Surgery 1996;119;27.
70. Lynch AM, Kapila R: Overwhelming postsplenectomy infection. Infect Dis Clin North Am 1996;4:693.
71. Mahon D, Rhodes M: Laparoscopic splenectomy: Size matters. 2003;85:248.
72. Maxwell-Armstrong CA, Clarke EDV, Tsang TM, et al: The wandering spleen. Arch Dis Child 1996;74:247.
73. McLean AL, Broussard E, McCarter MD, et al: Laparoscopic marsupialization of nonparasitic splenic cysts. Contemp Surg 2000;56:541.
74. McMullen M, Johnston G: Long-term management of patients after splenectomy. BMJ 1993;307:1372.
75. Meekes I, van der Staak, van Oostrom C: Results of splenectomy performed on a group of 91 children. Eur J Pediatr Surg 1995;5:19.
76. Meyer AA: Spleen. In Greenfield LJ, Mulholland MW, Oldham KT, et al (eds): Surgery, 2nd ed. Philadelphia, Lippincott-Raven, 1997, p 262.
77. Minkes RK, Lagzdins M, Langer JC: Laparoscopic versus open splenectomy in children. J Pediatr Surg 2000;35:699.
78. Moir C, Guttman F, Jequier S, et al: Splenic cysts: Aspiration, sclerosis, or resection. J Pediatr Surg 1989; 24:646.
79. Moores, DC, McKee MA, Wang H, et al: Pediatric laparoscopic splenectomy. J Pediatr Surg 1995;30:1201.
80. Morgenstern L: Nonparasitic splenic cysts: Pathogenesis, classification, and treatment. J Am Coll Surg 2002;194:306.
81. Morris KT, Horvath KD, Jobe BA, et al: Laparoscopic management of accessory spleens in immune thrombocytopenic purpura. Surg Endosc 1999;13:520.
82. Muckmel E, Zer M, Dintsman M: Wandering spleen with torsion of pedicle in a child presenting as an intermittently-appearing abdominal mass. J Pediatr Surg 1978;13:127.
83. Nishizaki T, Takahashi I, Onohara T, et al: Laparoscopic splenectomy using wall-lifting procedure. Surg Endosc 1999; 13:1055.
84. Nossal GJV, Austin CM, Pye J, et al: Antigens in immunity: XII. Antigen trapping in the spleen. Int Arch Allergy 1966; 29:368.
85. Park AE, Birgisson G, Mastrangelo MJ, et al: Laparoscopic splenectomy: Outcomes and lessons learned from over 200 cases. Surgery 2000;128:660.
86. Park A, Heniford BT, Hebra A, et al: Pediatric laparoscopic splenectomy. Surg Endosc 2000;14:527.
87. Pearson HA: The spleen and disturbances of splenic function. In Nathan DG, Orkin SH (eds): Hematology of Infancy and Childhood, 5th ed. Philadelphia, WB Saunders, 1998, vol II, p 1051.
88. Poulin EC, Mamazza J, Schlachta CM: Splenic artery embolization before laparoscopic splenectomy. Surg Laparosc Endosc 1995;5:463.
89. Poulin EC, Thibault C, DesCoteaux JG, Cote G: Partial laparoscopic splenectomy for trauma: Technique and case report. Surg Laparosc Endosc 1995;5:306.
90. Putschar WGJ, Manion WC: Splenic-gonadal fusion. Am J Pathol 1986;32:15.

91. Rathaus V, Zissin R, Goldberg E: Spontaneous rupture of an epidermoid cyst of the spleen: Preoperative ultrasonographic diagnosis. J Clin Ultrasound 1991;19:235.
92. Reddy VS, Phan HH, O'Neill JA, et al: Laparoscopic versus open splenectomy in the pediatric population: A contemporary single-center experience. Am Surg 2001;67: 859.
93. Rescorla FJ: Laparoscopic splenectomy. In Langer JC, Albanese CT (eds): Pediatric Minimal Access Surgery: A Principle and Evidence Based Approach. New York, Marcel Dekker, in press.
94. Rescorla FJ, Breitfeld PP, West KW, et al: A case-controlled comparison of open and laparoscopic splenectomy in children. Surgery 1996;124:670.
95. Rescorla FJ, Engum SA, West KW, et al: Laparoscopic splenectomy has become the gold standard in children. Am Surg 2002;68:297.
96. Rice HE, Oldham KT, Hillery CA, et al: Clinical and hematologic benefits of partial splenectomy for congenital hemolytic anemias in children. Ann Surg 2003;237:281.
97. Romano F, Caprotti R, Franciosi C, et al: The use of LigaSure during pediatric laparoscopic splenectomy: A preliminary report. Pediatr Surg Int 2003;19:721.
98. Rowley DA: The effect of splenectomy on the formation of circulating antibody in the adult male albino rat. J Immunol 1950;64:289.
99. Rowley DA: The formation of circulating antibody in the splenectomized human being following intravenous injection of heterologous erythrocytes. J Immunol 1950; 65:515.
100. Salky B, Zimmerman M, Bauer J, et al: Splenic cyst—definitive treatment by laparoscopy. Gastrointest Endosc 1985;31:213.
101. Sardi A, Ojeda HF, King D: Laparoscopic resection of a benign true cyst of the spleen with the Harmonic scalpel producing high levels of CA 19-9 and carcinoembryonic antigen. Am Surg 1998;64:1149.
102. Schleef J, Morcate JJ, Steinau G, et al: Technical aspects of laparoscopic splenectomy in children. J Pediatr Surg 1997;32:615.
103. Schmidt SP, Andrews HG, White JJ: The splenic snood: An improved approach for the management of the wandering spleen. J Pediatr Surg 1992;27:1043.
104. Seashore JH, McIntosh S: Elective splenopexy for wandering spleen. J Pediatr Surg 1990;25:270.
105. Seshadri PA, Poenaru D, Park A: Laparoscopic splenic cystectomy: A case report. J Pediatr Surg 1998;33:1439.
106. Sierra R, Brunner WC, Murphy JT, et al: Laparoscopic marsupialization of a giant post-traumatic splenic cyst. JSLS 2004;8:384.
107. Singer DB: Postsplenectomy sepsis. In Rosenberg HS, Bolander RP (eds): Perspectives in Pediatric Pathology. Chicago, Year Book Medical Publishers, 1973, p 285.
108. Skandalakis PN, Colborn GL, Skandalakis LJ, et al: The surgical anatomy of the spleen. Surg Clin North Am 1993; 73:747.
109. Skandalakis LJ, Gray SW, Ricketts R, et al: The spleen. In Skandalakis JE, Gray SW (eds): Embryology for Surgeons, 2nd ed. Baltimore, Williams & Wilkins, 1994, p 334.
110. Skarsgard E, Doski J, Jaksic T, et al: Thrombosis of the portal venous system after splenectomy for pediatric hematologic disease. J Pediatr Surg 1993;28:1109.
111. Smith MD, Nio M, Carmel JE, et al: Management of splenic abscess in immunocompromised children. J Pediatr Surg 1993;28:823.
112. Stringel G, Soucy P, Mercer S: Torsion of the wandering spleen: Splenectomy or splenopexy? J Pediatr Surg 1982;17:373.
113. Styrt B: Infection associated with asplenia: risks, mechanisms, and prevention. Am J Med 1990;88:33.
114. Sullivan CA, Konefal SH: Epidermoid cyst of the spleen successfully treated by marsupialization. Clin Pediatr 1987;26:203.
115. Szold A, Schwartz J, Abu-Abeid S, et al: Laparoscopic splenectomies for idiopathic thrombocytopenic purpura: Experience of sixty cases. Am J Hematol 2000;63:7.
116. Targarona EM, Espert JJ, Balagué C, et al: Residual splenic function after laparoscopic splenectomy: A clinical concern. Arch Surg 1998;133:56.
117. Targarona EM, Martínez J, Ramos C, et al: Conservative laparoscopic treatment of posttraumatic splenic cyst. Surg Endosc 1995;9:71.
118. Terrosu G, Baccarani U, Bresadola V, et al: The impact of splenic weight on laparoscopic splenectomy for splenomegaly. Surg Endosc 2002;16:103.
119. Thalhammer GH, Eber E, Uranus S, et al: Partial splenectomy in cystic fibrosis patients with hypersplenism. Arch Dis Child 2003;88:143.
120. Thorne MT, Chwals WJ: Treatment of complicated congenital splenic cysts. J Pediatr Surg 1993;28:1635.
121. Tsakayannis DE, Mitchell K, Kozakewich HPW, et al: Splenic preservation in the management of splenic epidermoid cysts in children. J Pediatr Surg 1995;30:1468.
122. Tu ST, Wu JM, Yeh BH, et al: Intestinal obstruction in asplenia syndrome: Report of three cases. Acta Paediatr Sin 1994;35:70.
123. Uranüs S, Kronberger L, Kraft-Kine J: Partial splenic resection using the TA-stapler. Am J Surg 1194;168:49.
124. Velanovich V, Shurafa MS: Clinical and quality of life outcomes of laparoscopic and open splenectomy for haematological diseases. Eur J Surg 2001;167:23.
125. Vereczkei A, Illenyi L, Arany A, et al: Transvaginal extraction of the laparoscopically removed spleen. Surg Endosc 2003;17:157.
126. Waldhausen JHT, Tapper D: Is pediatric laparoscopic splenectomy safe and cost-effective? Arch Surg 1997;132:822.
127. Walsh RM, Heniford BT, Brody F, et al: The ascendance of laparoscopic splenectomy. Am Surg 2001;67:48.
128. West KW, Grosfeld JL: Postsplenectomy sepsis: Historical background and current concepts. World J Surg 1985;9:477.
129. Winslow ER, Brunt LM: Perioperative outcomes of laparoscopic versus open splenectomy: A meta-analysis with an emphasis on complications. Surgery 2003;134:647.
130. Yavorski CC, Greson KL, Egan MC: Splenic cysts: A new approach to partial splenectomy—case report and review of the literature. Am Surg 1998;64:795.
131. Yee LF, Carvajal SH, de Lorimier AA, et al: Laparoscopic splenectomy: The initial experience at University of California, San Francisco. Arch Surg 1995;130:874.
132. Yoshida K, Yamazaki Y, Mizuno R, et al: Laparoscopic splenectomy in children: Preliminary results and comparison with the open technique. Surg Endosc 1995;9:1279.
133. Young NS, Brown KE: Parvovirus B19. N Engl J Med 2004; 350:586.
134. Zarrabi MH, Rosner F: Serious infections in adults following splenectomy for trauma. Arch Intern Med 1984; 144:1421.
135. Ziske CG, Müller T: Partial splenectomy: Uses of error. Lancet 2002;359, 1144.

第八部分

泌尿生殖系统疾病

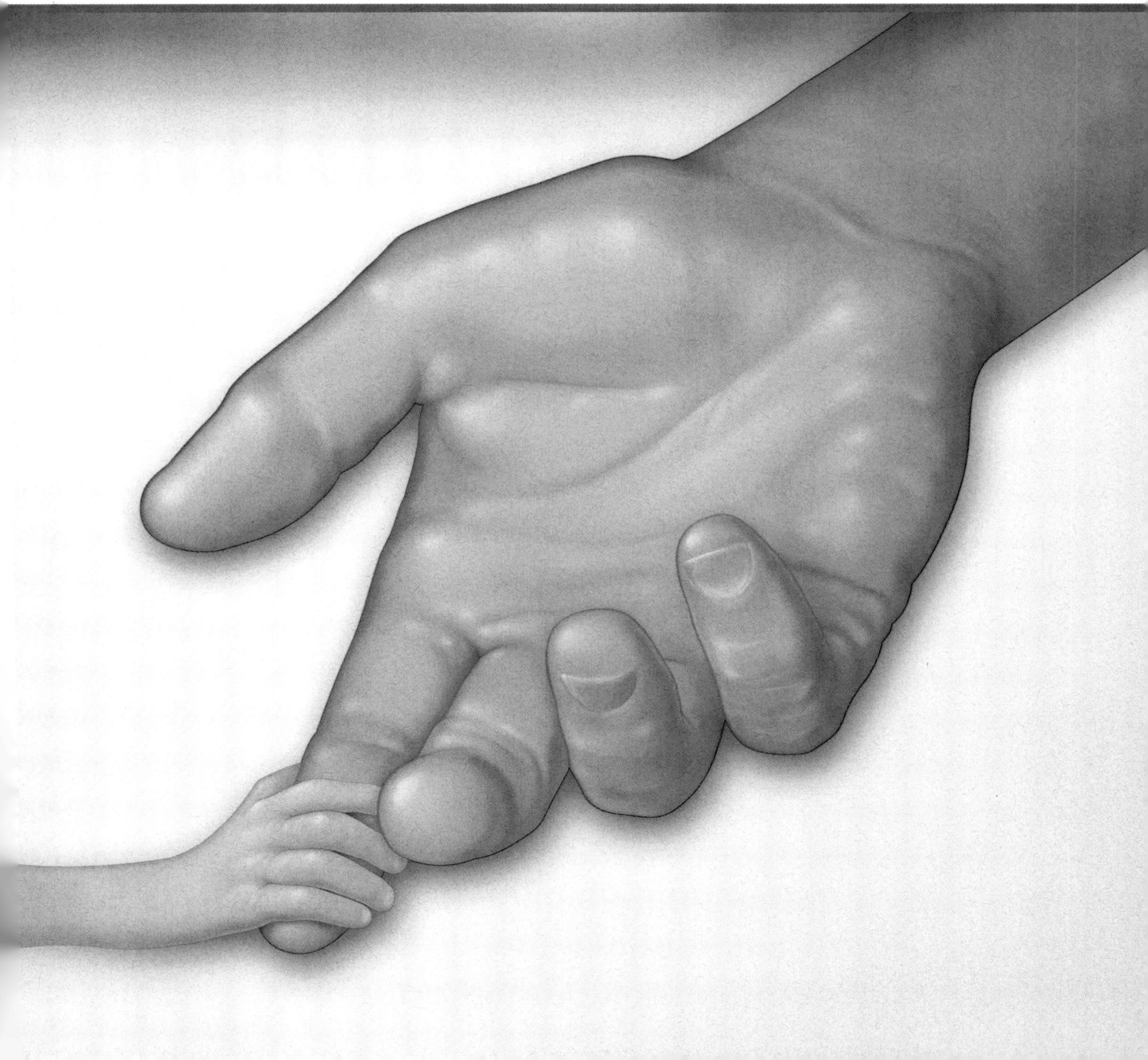

第 109 章

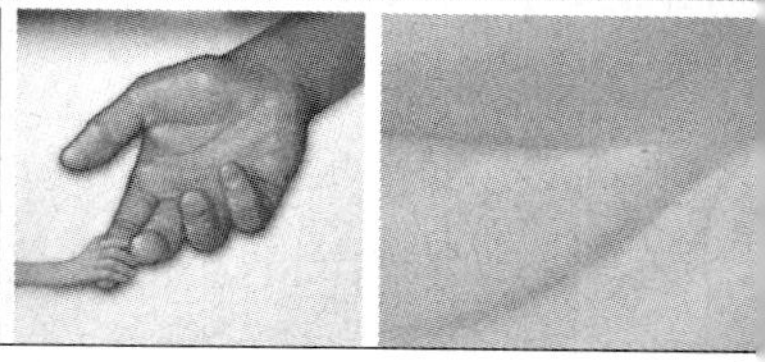

肾发育不全、发育不良以及囊性疾病

Kenneth I. Glassberg

肾的发育

705 现已证实，肾发育过程中有 400 多个基因参与调控。其中任何一个重要基因的缺陷均可导致特异性的肾发育异常，比如肾结构异常、肾发育不良或者肾囊性疾病。许多类型的肾囊性疾病都与基因的特异性突变有关。当这些基因正常时，它们在肾的发育过程中起到重要作用，一旦这些基因发生突变，将导致肾囊性疾病的发生。

肾发育是 wolffian 管（后期为输尿管芽）与后肾胚基相互作用的结果，两者相互传递信息，这些信息有的是主动发出的，而有的则是在收到对方信息后所作出的回应。肾发育的每一个阶段都要依赖于不同基因以及它们相应蛋白质产物的表达。例如，在胰岛素样生长因子 2（insulin-like growth factor-2，IGF-2）的作用下，后肾胚基的间充质细胞持续存在并且增殖，肾母细胞瘤 1 基因（Wilms tumor 1 gene，*WT1*）的表达会抑制 IGF-2，并产生一系列连锁反应，包括源自 wolffian 管的输尿管芽的发生和间充质细胞向上皮细胞的转变。后一种细胞的转变是由 *PAX2* 基因启动的。

由 wolffian 管形成输尿管芽的过程是一个由蛋白质介导的过程，这种蛋白质是由间充质细胞产生的，称为神经胶质细胞系来源的神经营养因子（glial cell line-derived neurotrophic factor，GDNF）。这种蛋白质在 wolffian 管尾端与酪蛋白激酶 c-ret 受体结合，可诱导输尿管芽的形成。输尿管芽不断延长，并且穿透其周围的间充质基质，在此处发生多级分叉。间充质（基质）细胞在每一个终末分叉的末端聚集成群，并分化为上皮、间质和内皮细胞以及后肾的区域性结构。上皮细胞首先形成球囊状的结构（肾小囊），并逐渐延长形成肾单位前的小管样结构，最终与未来会形成集合管的输尿管芽的终末分支相联系[16]。

输尿管芽分支减少，会同时伴有间充质细胞群数量的减少，并由此导致肾单位数量不足，形成诸如肾发育不全等疾病。输尿管芽分支末端与间充质细胞群之间相互作用太少，或者集合管与发育中的肾单位之间缺乏连续性，将会导致肾脏在结构上的发育始终处于幼稚状态，形成诸如肾发育不良等疾病。一些特异性生长因子的过度表达或不表达，会产生过度生长的肾脏疾病（如肾母细胞瘤）和肾囊性疾病。举例来说，前面提到过的 *IGF2* 基因在大多数散发性的肾母细胞瘤中为过度表达，而作为肿瘤抑制基因的 *WT1* 在许多有症状的肾母细胞瘤中发生突变。

肾发育异常

肾发育过程中的异常影响肾脏大小、形状或结构等情况称为肾发育异常。这类疾病主要由以下三种情况构成：发育不全、发育不良以及囊性发育不良（就像其他类型的肾囊性疾病一样）。肾发育不全指的是整个肾脏或某个肾段中的肾单位数量减少。有时在发育不良的肾脏或在发育不良的区域中有一些囊性改变，这些囊性改变可以是镜下改变或是肉眼改变，也可以是局灶性或弥漫性的。肾发育不良的特点为存在原始的小管，而这些小管一般被认为是在肾发育早期出现的结构，其特征性表现为小管周围包绕的平滑肌和胶原袖套，而缺乏弹性蛋白[10]。当发育不良和囊性改变这两种病变影响到整个肾脏时，这种情况就被认为是多囊性肾发育不良。多囊性肾发育不良可以随着时间而发生退化，最终演变成为小瘤样组织，有时也把这种情况称为肾不发育。这种病变一般表现为由细胞构成的小的组织团块，而没有明确的肾脏形态。肾脏严重发育不良时，集合系统发育极不成熟或缺乏。

肾不发育

Wolffian 管、输尿管芽或后肾胚基缺失会导致肾发育停止，亦称为肾不发育。出生时双侧肾不发育的发生率为 1/4000，多见于男性[31]。由于没有尿液生成，羊水过少，患儿出生时出现肺发育不成熟，气胸伴有 Potter 面容（眼距增宽，明显的内眦皮肤皱褶，
1706 下颏退化）。单侧肾不发育的患儿可以生存下来，其出生时的发病率为 1/450～1/1000[23]。准确判断单侧肾不发育的发生率十分困难，主要是因为在某些情况下（比如多囊肾），肾组织可以退化为组织小片，在影像学检查中不能被探及。

单侧肾不发育常常伴发其他泌尿系统异常，包括原发性膀胱输尿管反流（28%）、梗阻性巨输尿管（11%）以及肾盂输尿管连接部梗阻（3%）[6]。不论是单侧肾不发育还是肾脏异位，都可以伴随 müllerian 管缺陷和阴道不发育，这组伴发畸形被称为 Mayer-Rokitansky-Küster-Hauser 综合征。双侧肾不发育也可以是鳃弓-耳-肾综合征（branchio-oto-renal syndrome）的一个组成部分。

肾发育不全和发育不良性肾发育不全

肾发育不全是指整个肾脏或肾脏某一段的肾单位数量减少。发育不良性肾发育不全也有肾单位数量的减少，同时还可以存在一个肾形的发育不良区域。伴有异位输尿管开口的肾脏可以是一个完全性的肾发育不良、肾发育不全，也可以是发育不良性肾发育不全。异位输尿管开口可以继发于 wolffian 管处输尿管芽位点的异常，而且伴有肾脏发育的异常。

肾囊性疾病

肾囊肿（renal cyst）可以是先天性的、散在发作的，也可以是后天获得性的；单个或多个出现；可以是单侧或双侧。绝大部分来自肾单位和集合管。多囊性肾发育不良所包含的囊肿的形成源自肾单位发生前的一些肾小管结构。良性多房性囊肿实际上是一种瘤样结构，必须要与可能的恶性肿瘤区分开来。单房囊肿的起因不明，大多发生于正常的肾脏。

不同的肾囊肿从镜下到大体的大小各异。所有的囊肿内壁都覆盖有上皮细胞。有些囊肿外观呈现为扩张的小管样或集合管样结构，仍然保持与肾单位相延续。其他的则可能与肾单位分离，形成一个孤立结构。根据 Gardner 的建议[14]，任何管样结构，当其直径扩张超过正常状态下的四倍，就应当考虑为囊肿。

本章节所采用的分类方法是根据美国儿科学术委员会对泌尿外科方面的术语、命名以及分类上的建议，将各种情况分为遗传性与非遗传性疾病[18]。此外还加入了一些根据最近的发现而作出的改良（表 109-1）[16]。

从一开始，多囊性（*multicystic*）与多个囊性（*polycystic*）这两个词汇都具有“很多个囊”的意思，但所描述的情况是不同的。前者指一个发育不良的整体；而后者则指数个相互隔开的结构，绝大多数为遗传性的，而且绝大多数囊性病变在一生中的某个时候

表 109-1 肾脏囊性疾病的分类

表 109-1 肾脏囊性疾病的分类
遗传性
常染色体显性遗传性（成人型）多囊性肾脏疾病
常染色体隐性遗传性（婴儿型）多囊性肾脏疾病
青少年肾消耗性疾病-髓质囊性疾病复合疾病
青少年肾消耗性疾病（常染色体隐性遗传）
髓质囊性疾病（常染色体显性遗传）
先天性肾病（家族性肾病综合征，常染色体隐性遗传）
家族性发育不全性肾小球囊性疾病（常染色体显性遗传）
多发畸形综合征伴有肾囊肿（如结节性硬化、von Hippel-Lindau 病）
非遗传性
多囊肾（多囊性肾发育不良）
良性多房性肾囊肿（囊性肾瘤）
单纯性肾囊肿
髓质海绵肾
散发性肾小球囊性肾脏疾病
获得性肾囊性疾病
肾盏憩室（肾盂源性囊肿）

会与肾单位和集合管发生交通，但不是所有病变都伴随有发育不良。*多囊性肾脏疾病*的最常见情况是常染色体隐性遗传性多囊性肾脏疾病（autosomal recessive polycystic kidney disease，ARPKD）与常染色体显性遗传性多囊性肾脏疾病（autosomal dominant polycystic kidney disease，ADPKD）。这些情况可以进展为肾衰竭。

在外科方面具有较为重要意义的结构包括各种多房性囊肿结构以及伴随遗传性斑痣性错构瘤和结节性硬化的新生物。尽管多囊肾经常表现为一个腹部肿块，但很少需要进行手术切除。ADPKD 中比较大的囊肿可以通过腹腔镜手术进行去顶，但在儿童患者中，没有作者提到过进行去顶手术治疗。

常染色体显性遗传性（成人型）多囊性肾脏疾病

ADPKD 以往一般指的是成人多囊性肾脏疾病，这是因为这种疾病主要发生于成人；然而儿童甚至是胎儿也可以发生此病。ADPKD 是肾衰竭的最常见原因，在需要进行透析和移植的患者中约占 10%～15%[12]。这种疾病的发生率为 1/500～1/1000。双侧肾脏均可累及，一般是先出现于一侧，而后再出现于对侧。

遗传学：ADPKD 的发病涉及三种不同的基因突变：第 16 号染色体上的 *PKD1* 约占所有发病的 90%[30,32]，4 号染色体上的 *PKD2* 约占 5%～10%[13,29]，*PKD3* 目前还没有定性。外显率被认为是 100%，患者子代个体中有 50% 罹患此病。而根据 Gabow 的报道[13]，到 90 岁时 96% 的患者会出现 ADPKD 的表现。

1707

特征：由于 ADPDK 患者的后代中有 50% 的发病率，因此对其子女需要进行常规超声检查。到 25 岁时，至少有 85% 的个体会有囊肿表现，但绝大多数是无症状的[17]。ADPKD 患者的家庭成员由于存在较高的发病可能性，一般在 25 岁前都不能得到健康保险。

大多数患者在 30 岁至 70 岁之间出现症状，包括镜下和肉眼血尿、腰痛、高血压、由结石或血凝块引起的肾绞痛。在成人中，该疾病可伴发结肠憩室、肝囊肿、脑动脉瘤。其中肝囊肿在成人中的发生率远远高于儿童，而且主要出现在女性患者中。

ADPKD 有时也会发生于胎儿及婴儿；此年龄段约有 50% 的患儿肾脏较大，含有大的囊肿。有的患儿没有大的囊肿，而表现为肾脏的回声增强，这是由肾内扩张的小管和细管形成的多个界面造成的强超声反射引起的；后面这种表现是 ARPKD 的典型表现（图 109-1）。

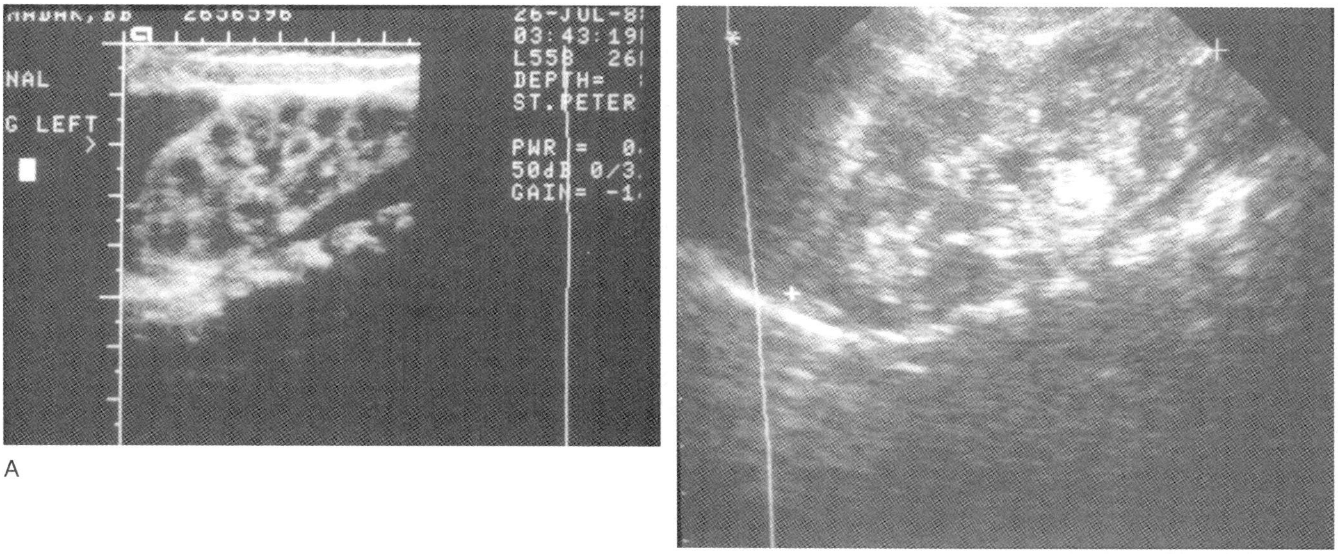

A　B

图 109-1　A. 一例新生儿常染色体显性遗传性多囊性肾脏疾病超声检查可见左肾多个囊肿。B. 新生儿常染色体隐性遗传性多囊性肾脏疾病，可见回声增强和多个小囊肿。（Courtesy of Walter Berdon，MD.）

以后这些囊肿会逐渐演变为肉眼可见的囊肿。当产前超声检查怀疑有 ADPKD 或 ARPKD 时，则需要对其父母进行基因学或超声检查。对这些儿童进行高血压监控十分重要，控制高血压能够推迟肾衰竭的发生。如果患者在年轻的时候出现血清肌酐水平增高、尿蛋白排泄增加以及高血压，那么这些患者的情况会迅速恶化，并且发展为肾衰竭。几乎所有的胎儿期和一岁内发病的患者最终都会进展为肾衰竭，不过在严密的监控下，肾衰竭的发生可以延迟。

常染色体隐性遗传性（婴儿型）多囊性肾脏疾病

目前已经明确，这种疾病也可以发生在青春期或 20 多岁，所以已经不再把这种疾病称为婴儿型多囊性肾脏疾病。ARPKD 是一种相对比较少见的疾病，大约每 40 000 个新生婴儿中发生一例[33]。所有的患者都会出现不同程度的先天性肝纤维化。一般情况下，年龄越小、肾脏病变越重的患者，其先天性肝纤维化的程度也越轻。

遗传学：这一疾病的遗传基因是位于第 6 号染色体上的 *PKHD1*[34]。ARPKD 不论轻重，均存在着这一基因的突变。由于本病具有常染色体隐性遗传的特点，所以仅有四分之一的子代个体发病，而父母双方均没有本病的表现。

临床特征：在宫内或出生时即被诊断为 ARPKD 的小儿，在出生后 2 个月内死于尿毒症或呼吸衰竭的并不少见。如果能够在出生后 1 个月后继续存活，那么在支持治疗下，其一年生存机会将有所提高。然而，所有的 ARPKD 患儿最终仍将进展为肾衰竭（图 109-2）。对于发病较晚的患儿，其高血压的出现也相对较晚，而且比较容易控制，同时肾衰竭的发展过程也比较慢。

1709 新生儿 ARPKD 可能会有巨肾表现。巨大的肾脏可以影响到呼吸，甚或导致胎儿娩出困难。病情严重者，可以表现为羊水过少、Potter 面容以及肢体畸形。一些少见的表现包括肾脏体积过大引起膈肌过度抬高，可以导致呼吸困难；在这种情况下，往往需要进行肾切除。

伴有严重的先天性肝纤维化的患者可以有门静脉高压、食管静脉曲张以及巨肝巨脾的表现。由门静脉高压引起的食管静脉曲张出血可能需要进行脾肾分流手术。产前超声检查的典型表现为肾脏明显增大，回声增强。这种增强回声是由肾内数量众多的小的镜下囊肿及扩张的管道和小管所产生的声波反射所致。随着时间的推移，可以进展为大的囊肿。患儿长大后，肾脏体积变小，这与 ADPKD 的情况相反。组织学检查可见集合管延长并明显扩张。本病无有效的治疗方法。治疗呼吸系统疾病可以有助于延长患儿的寿命。

具有肾囊肿表现的多发畸形综合征

有许多多发畸形综合征具有肾囊肿的特点。对外科医生来说比较有代表意义的是结节性硬化和遗传性斑痣性错构瘤。

结节性硬化

结节性硬化具有以下三联征表现：癫痫（80%）、皮脂腺腺瘤（75%）以及智力发育延缓（60%）[28]。皮脂腺腺瘤由纤维瘤样的肉色丘疹构成，位于面颊部。特征性病变为大脑的浅表皮层血肿，类似硬化的脑回，提示为结节性脑硬化的表现。血肿也会涉及身体的其他部位，尤其是肾脏及眼球。肾脏的其他病变还包括血管肌脂瘤和囊肿。

遗传学：25%～60% 的病例具有遗传特征，既可以散在发病，也可以表现出遗传特征的差异或不完全外显。到目前为止已经证实有两个基因与结节性硬化的常染色体显性遗传有关[5,21]，位于 9 号染色体上的 *TSC1* 与 16 号染色体上的 *TSC2*。后一基因缺陷发生的部位与 *PKD1* 相续，基因突变常与 ADPKD 的发生有关。两个 *TSC* 基因突变所产生的临床表现非常相似，这一事实说明这两个基因涉及同一进化路径。当其中任何一个基因不能合成正常的相应蛋白质时，所产生的结果是相似的。由于这两个基因中不论哪一个发生突变都可导致肿瘤的发生，因此这两个基因均被视为肿瘤抑制基因。

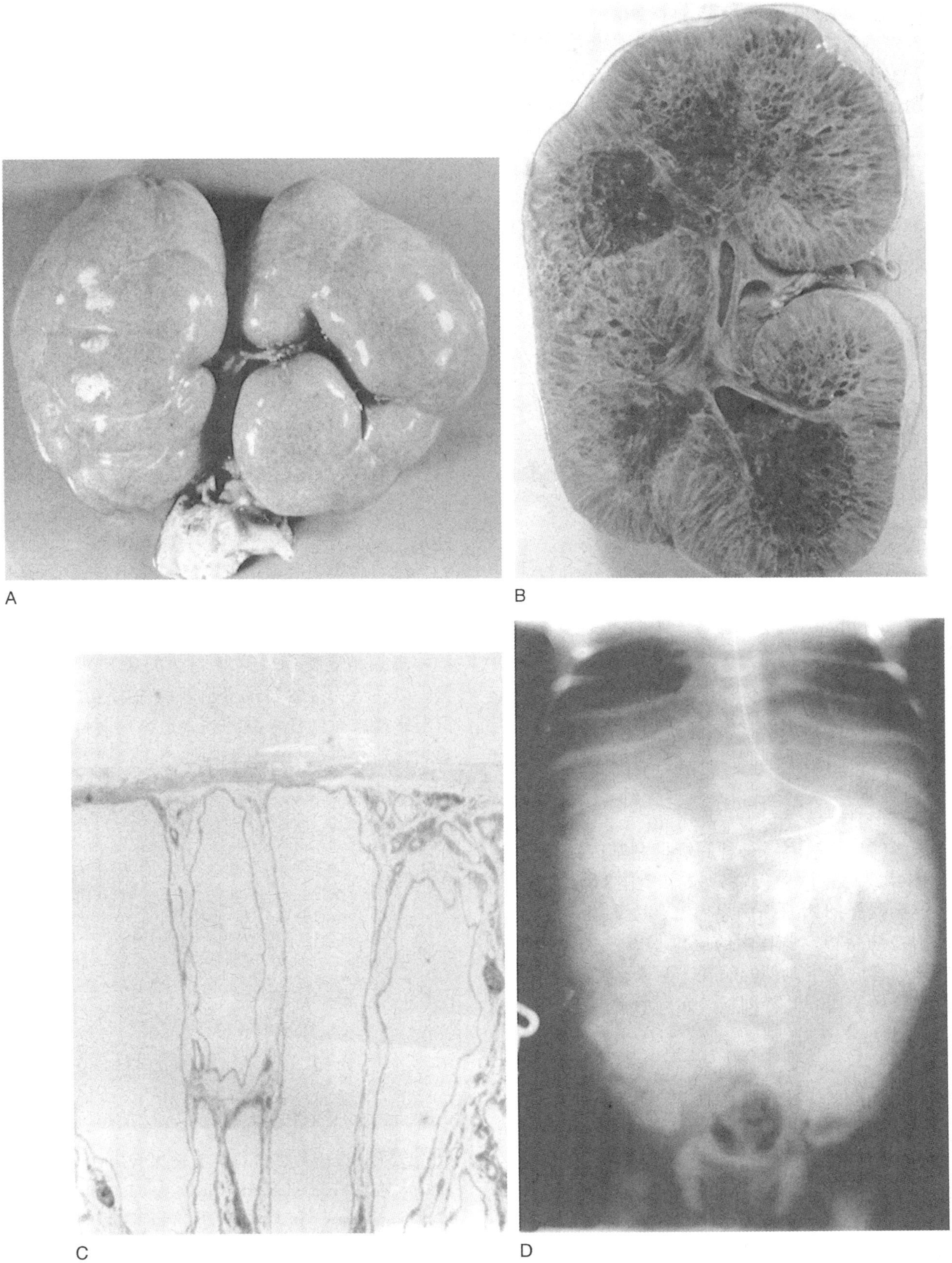

图 109-2　常染色体隐性遗传性多囊性肾脏疾病。A. 大体标本见互相融合的小的包膜下囊肿。B. 集合管呈放射状排列、变长、囊性扩张。C. 低倍光学显微镜下可见扩张的集合管。D. 静脉尿路造影可见特征性的“旭日征”，由造影剂浓集于扩张的集合管所引起。

临床特征：有 20% 的患者出现肾囊肿，而且大多在 3 岁以内发病，三分之一的肾囊肿患儿发病年龄小于 1 岁。由于有肾囊肿的存在，这一疾病可以在胎儿期通过超声检查进行产前诊断。如果产前诊断明确为本病，则此时认为继发于 16 号染色体的 *TSC2* 基因突变的可能性较大。在这些情况下，也可能出现相邻接的 *PKD1* 基因缺陷（对应于 ADPKD）。肾囊肿很少出现临床症状。过去很多患者在早期死于中枢神经系统病变，不过现在他们的生存时间已经延长，而且也许在将来会发现肾囊肿有影响肾脏功能的可能。

肾血管肌脂瘤发生于 40%～60% 的患者[7,19]。这种病变在 6 岁前很少见，而在 10 岁后则比较多见[4]。大的血管肌脂瘤有发生出血的可能。

在组织学检查上，囊肿有一致的表现，内衬肥大增生的嗜酸性细胞。理论上说，在结节性硬化患者中，这些增生的细胞有 2% 的机会发生肾细胞癌。最早报道有 7 岁的患儿发生肿瘤。

遗传性斑痣性错构瘤

这种常染色体显性遗传性疾病有以下表现：小脑成血管细胞瘤、视网膜血管瘤、胰腺囊肿、附睾和肾脏附睾囊腺瘤、嗜铬细胞瘤以及肾透明细胞癌。发病率约为 1/35 000[26]。

遗传学：*VHL* 基因（一种肿瘤抑制基因）位于 3 号染色体，具有显性遗传性；发病个体的子代中有 50% 可能会罹患此病。该病患者在出生时为杂合子，当该基因在某一特定器官内的等位基因发生突变时，即可在该器官内发生典型的病变。至今已经在不伴有遗传性斑痣性错构瘤的肾细胞癌病例中发现了不同的 *VHL* 基因突变。

临床特征：平均发病年龄在 35～40 岁，儿童期发病罕见。肾脏病变中最常见的是肾囊肿，在 76% 的患者中为首发表现[25]。有 10%～17% 的患者发生嗜铬细胞瘤[20,24]，而且这种情况似乎在家族发病中比较多见。有些患者由于中枢神经系统的毛细血管瘤而表现为癫痫发作。囊肿的内皮由增生细胞组成，这些患者发生肾细胞癌的机会明显增加。对于成年期患者，即使在刚发病时表现为单侧病变，也应当考虑到有发生双侧肾细胞癌的可能。30 岁以上的患者，尤其是当存在良性腺瘤样的小肿瘤时，应当每一至两年进行肾脏检查，通常为计算机断层扫描。

多囊性肾发育不良 171

这种病变属于涉及整个肾脏的完全性发育不良类型（图 109-3）。当发生于肾脏的某一极时，往往存在重复系统。如果患者患有双侧病变，则不可能存活，出现死产、羊水过少以及 Potter 面容。这种病变类型通常会伴有输尿管闭锁和无肾盂。如果肾盂存在，则作为肾盂积水型多囊肾对待（图 109-4）。当肾脏中实质性组织与少数囊泡混合存在时，则称为实质性囊性发育不良。不过，本病的典型表现是葡萄样外观，超声检查显示肾脏失去原有形态；囊肿形状不一，没有中央囊肿或内部囊肿，提示有一个肾盂存在（图 109-5）。这种类型的多囊肾需要与肾盂积水相鉴别，后者最大的囊肿为中央囊肿或内部囊肿，且与周围的囊肿相互交通，这些周围的囊肿即为扩张的肾盏。以往认为多囊肾的囊肿不存在相互之间的交通，但造影检查时向任一囊肿注入造影剂时都能够显示囊

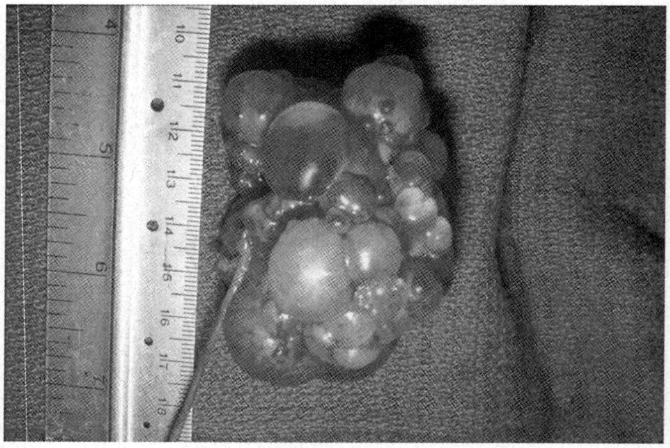

图 109-3 典型的多囊肾伴有输尿管闭锁。可见“葡萄串”外观。(From Shah SH, Glassberg KI: Multicystic dysplastic kidney disease. In Gearhart JP, Rink RC, Moriquand PDE [eds]: Pediatric Urology. Philadelphia, WB Saunders, 2001, p279.)（也见彩图）

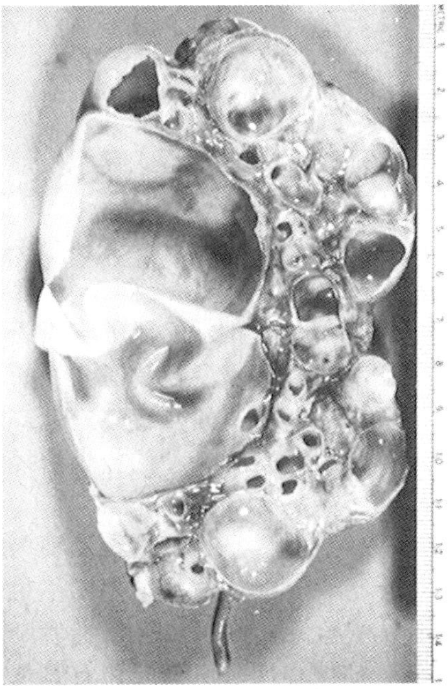

图 109-4　多囊性肾发育不良的肾盂积水结构。最大的囊肿位于中央内侧，较小的囊肿位于外周。

肿之间的交通（图 109-6）[17]。

临床特征：多囊性肾发育不良是肾囊性疾病中最为常见的类型，它与肾盂输尿管连接部梗阻是婴儿可触及腹部肿块的最主要原因。对侧检查很重要，因为 3%~12% 的多囊性肾脏疾病患儿同时患有对侧肾盂输尿管连接部梗阻，18%~43% 的患儿有对侧膀胱输尿管反流[1,2,11,32]。由于有输尿管反流发生的可能，应当对所有多囊性肾脏疾病患儿进行排尿性膀胱尿道造影检查。

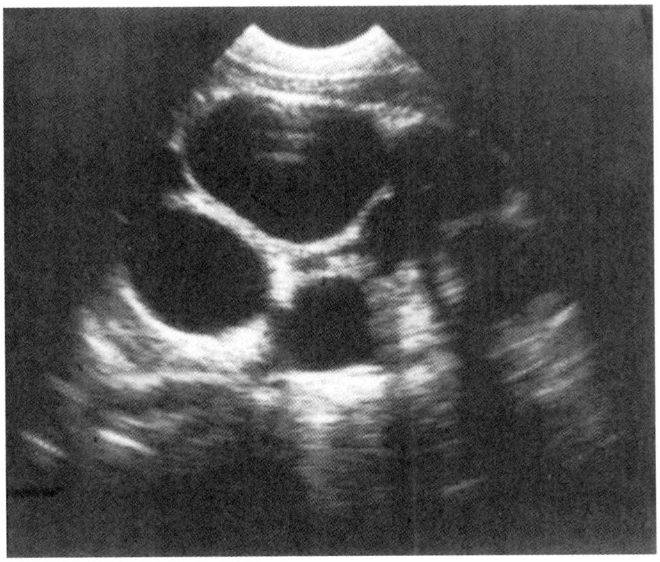

图 109-5　典型的多囊肾超声改变。可见三个大的囊肿，小的囊肿位于其间，肾实质很少。

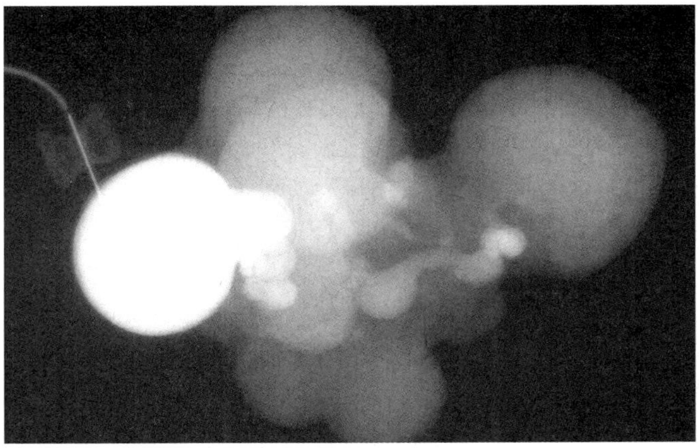

图 109-6　多囊性肾发育不良。向一个囊肿内注入造影剂后，所有的囊肿均可显影，表明囊肿之间存在管状的交通。尽管在超声影像中检查不出这些交通，但在切除后的标本中通过造影剂注入检查总是能够发现这些交通。

随着病情的进展，病变的肾脏一般可以通过触诊而在一岁以内发现。在使用超声以前，由于很难与肾脏肿瘤鉴别，同时也由于多囊肾中发现有肾母细胞瘤的少数病例报告，大多数的多囊肾都被切除。为了有助于鉴别多囊肾与肾盂积水，可以采用二巯基丁二酸（DMSA）扫描；多囊肾即使有功能，也十分低下，而肾盂积水肾功能很少丧失。对于多囊性发育不良
肾，必须作出决定是否行肾切除手术。超声影像学及 1711
其他影像学检查手段的应用提供了越来越精确的诊断，肾切除的概率也迅速下降。

大多数出现肾母细胞瘤的多囊性发育不良肾在病变检出前并不知道是否有多囊性病变。目前还不了解多囊性肾发育不良是否会导致肾母细胞瘤。有两篇文献报道了 120 例患者，其中 5 例发现有小结样肾肉瘤的肾源性残留[5,27]，1 例在肾门区发现有小的肾母细胞瘤，提示对这种类型病变的肾应当进行切除治疗。然而，有报告发现肾肉瘤也发生于正常的肾中，因此目前还不确定多囊肾中这些少见的瘤样小体是否意味着发生肾母细胞瘤的危险性增加。根据 Beckwith 的文献[3]，在肾母细胞瘤注册机构的 7500 个肾母细胞瘤

标本中，仅有5例发生于多囊肾中。Beckwith 统计得出多囊肾发生肾母细胞瘤的危险性比正常高出4倍，而这种低的发生率尚不足以提示可以进行预防性的肾切除手术。他指出即使发生了肾母细胞瘤，目前经过治疗以后的生存率也在90%以上。Zerres 等人[34]建议对多囊肾进行保守治疗，每三个月进行超声随访一次，直至8岁。他们通过计算得出，这种方案的花费为每人2000～5000美元，而相比之下，一个单纯肾切除手术的花费为5000～7000美元。

到现在为止，有一些个案报道指出多囊肾进展出现高血压表现，通过肾切除来治疗高血压。在美国儿科学会泌尿组的国立多囊肾注册机构的资料中，大多数患有囊性肾脏疾病的新生儿，其肾脏在5年内逐渐变小或保持原有大小，只有极少数人肾脏可以增大[33]。因而在超声检查中，变小的肾脏可以消失，这并不意味着肾脏本身消失，而是提示囊肿已经消失（图109-7）。内衬于囊壁的细胞依然存在，这一无定形的细胞群落构成了一个没有任何功能的肾脏残留（肾不发育）。

对多囊肾进行超声随访，习惯上在最初几年内每3～6个月一次，以后逐渐延长随访间歇直至8岁。尽管这样，目前还不清楚是否需要对影像学检查时肾脏已经消失或者肾脏始终保持稳定的患者继续进行随访。由于残留的细胞没有囊液，仅凭其本身形态不能够决定是否需要超声随访。

良性多房性囊肿（囊性肾瘤） 171

良性多房性囊肿是一种不伴有肾发育不良的肾脏新生物。这种病变体积较大，并且由一层厚的囊膜包裹。病变周围通常邻接有正常的肾脏实质。囊肿内的每一个病变囊腔大小从数毫米到数厘米不等，囊腔与囊腔之间无相互交通。囊肿内衬有立方上皮细胞或低的柱状上皮细胞。良性多房囊肿的分隔由纤维组织构成，无低分化组织或胚芽细胞。

当影像学检查，尤其是超声检查发现为多房性囊肿病变时，应当意识到仅凭这些条件尚不足以明确鉴别该病变是否为良性多房囊肿、多房性囊肿伴有部分分化的肾母细胞瘤、良性多房囊肿伴有肾母细胞瘤结节或者是囊性肾母细胞瘤。因此多房囊肿病变应当被 171
视为是一系列病变的集合，目前还没有报道从一种病变转化为另外一种病变（图109-8）。因为影像学无法区别这些病变，要明确诊断必须将病变部位切除（图109-9）。如果这些病变位于肾脏的一端，而且还保留有较多的正常肾脏实质，可以考虑进行部分肾切除手术。即使病变不是一个典型的良性多房囊肿，它也很少是一种侵袭性疾病。这些病变没有任何一个

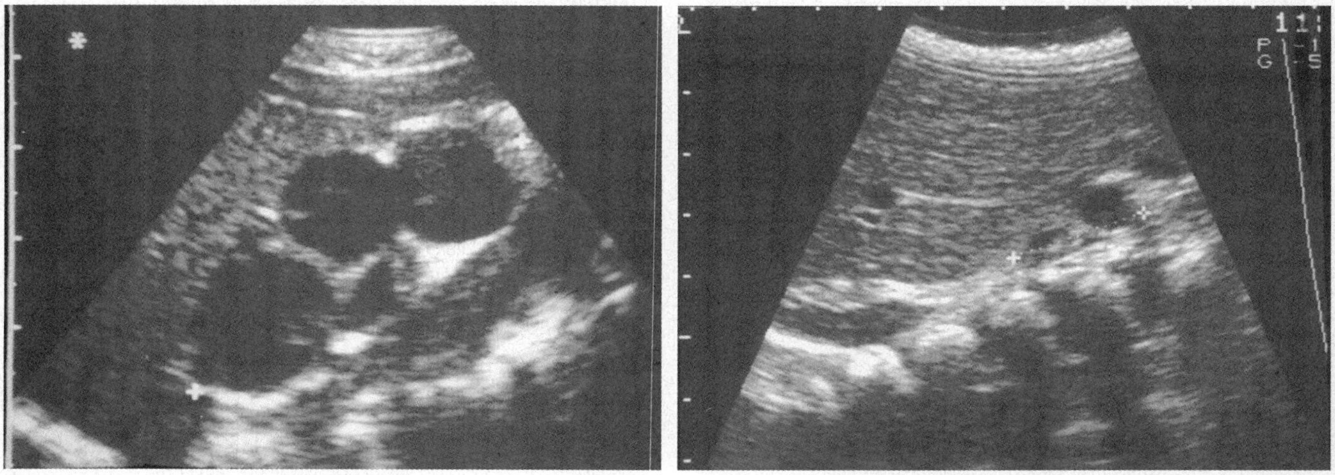

A　B

图109-7 A. 一例新生儿超声检查检出多囊肾。B. 在9个月时，囊肿缩小，肾脏很难探及。（From Shah SH，Glassberg KI：Multicystic dysplastic kidney disease. In Gearhart JP，Rink RC，Moriquand PDE［eds］：Pediatric Urology. Philadelphia，WB Saunders，2001，p284.）

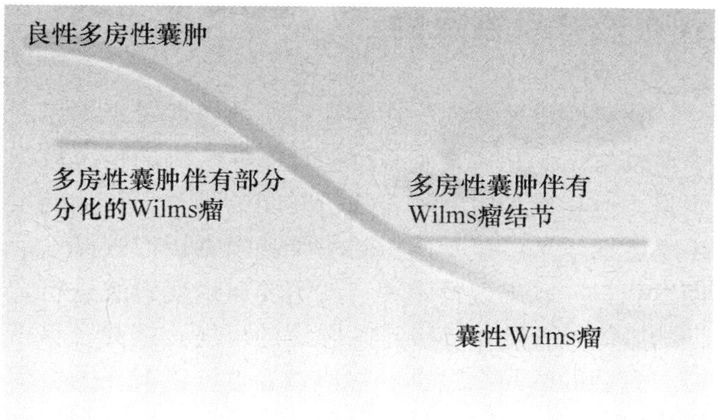

图 109-8　儿童期的几种多房性囊肿病变。由于影像学检查不能将这几种病变类型鉴别出来，所以必须依靠显微镜检查明确诊断。

涉及膨胀生长的结节，而且几乎根本不发生转移[9]。本病不应与肾母细胞瘤混淆，后者瘤体内含有坏死区域，在超声检查中的表现类似囊肿，这种表现往往代表着高侵袭性肿瘤。

单纯肾囊肿

单纯肾囊肿为肾内个别发生的病变，通常为卵圆形或圆形，边缘光滑。囊内一般为透明的或米色的液体，当产前超声发现该表现时，这种囊肿往往于出生后可以消失。当在儿童期发现该病变时，其处理方式

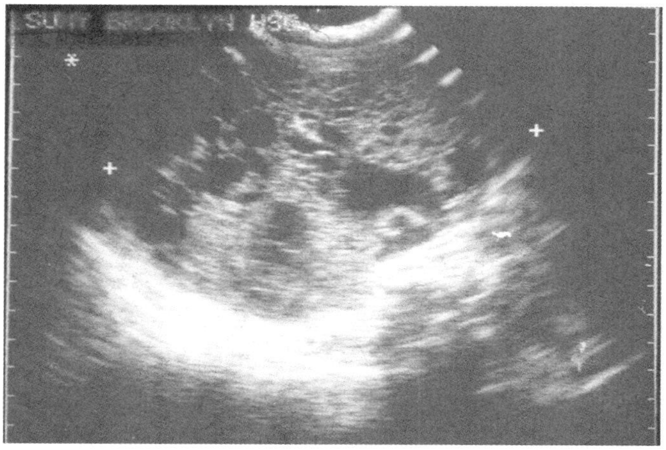

A

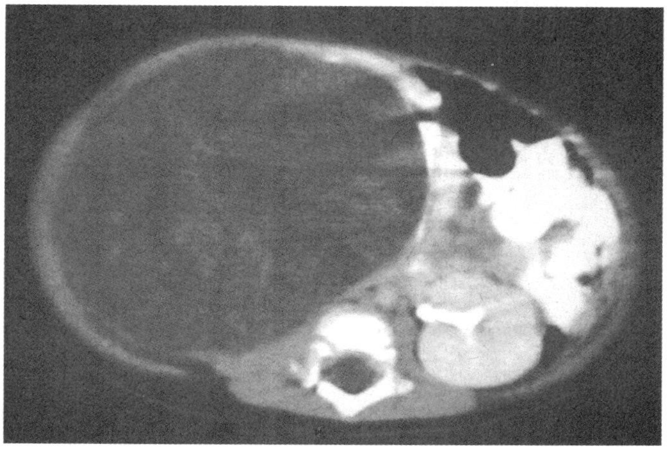

B

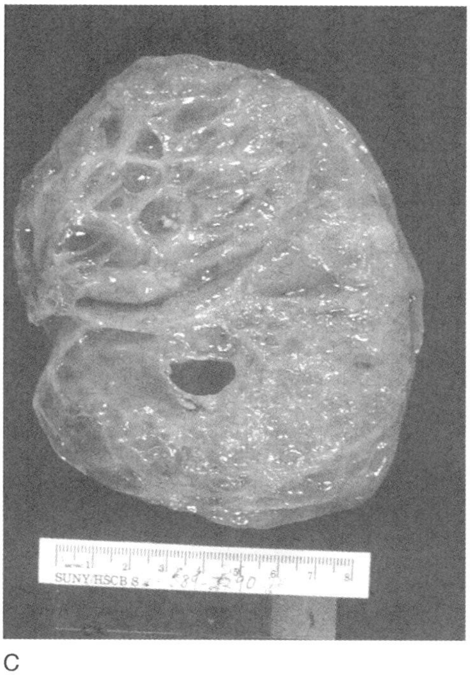

C

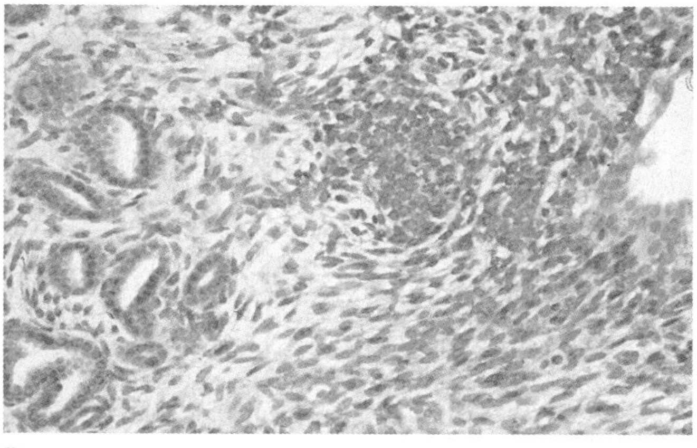

D

图 109-9　多房性囊肿伴有部分分化。A. 超声影像学检查发现肾脏肿块，其内为囊性结构。B. 在造影剂增强的 CT 扫描中，发现一个体积较大、边缘光滑的肾脏肿块，其内有细小的分隔，肾盏系统被推向一边。C. 肿块的大体标本可见有非交通性的小房。D. 显微镜下所见，可见胚芽细胞巢和小管系统，位于囊腔之间，为典型的多房性囊肿伴有部分分化的表现。（C 和 D 也见彩图）

与成人单纯性肾囊肿一样。由于以往认为儿童肾囊肿的发生较少，而且缺乏能够明确鉴定肾囊肿的方法，所以过去对肾囊肿的处理大多是采用手术治疗的方法。对儿童来说，肾囊肿罕有发生症状的。当在一个肾脏里发生的囊肿超过一个时，应当对患者进行随访观察，而且应当采用影像学方法对另一侧肾脏进行检查，以排除 ADPKD 中存在单侧多囊肾的原发不对称表现。

典型的良性单纯性囊肿的超声诊断标准如下：

1. 囊肿界限分明，囊壁薄而清晰，光滑，边缘清楚。

2. 囊肿内部无回声反射。

3. 囊肿的透声能力好。

4. 圆形或轻度卵圆形外观。

如果检查时均达到上述诊断标准，则不考虑有恶性病变的可能[19]。有时在肾脏的一极存在一簇肾囊肿，这时就需要鉴别是否有多房性囊肿的可能。如果所有的囊肿都是独立的，则应当考虑到单侧肾囊性疾病——一种单纯囊肿疾病的变异疾病[15]。虽然循证医学尚未对该病的随访作出任何推荐，但临床上最好还是建立连续的超声随访，随访间隔逐渐延长，以确保单纯肾囊肿的稳定，同时对 ADPKD 的不对称发病作出筛查。

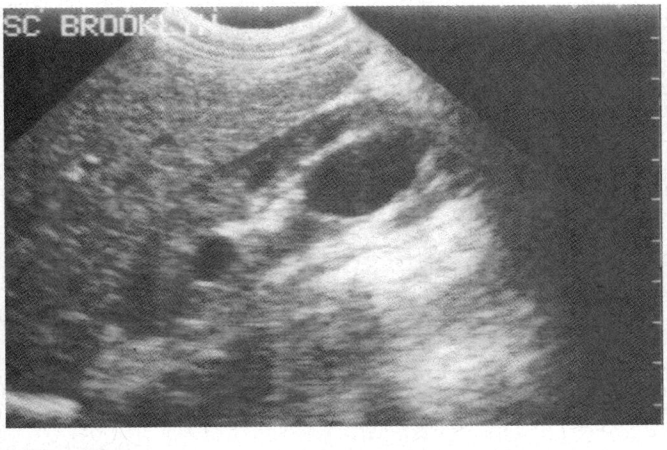

图 109-10 一例 7 岁儿童中的两个单纯性肾囊肿。可见超声检查时的肾外增强回声。这涉及声学放大效应，为单纯肾囊肿的典型表现，主要是由于声波通过囊肿与肾脏界面时反射增强。要特别注意的是，不要把这种表现与非典型的常染色体显性遗传性多囊性肾脏疾病的非对称性表现相混淆。

获得性肾囊性疾病

获得性肾囊性疾病在接受透析的慢性肾衰竭患者中比较常见。儿童发生获得性肾囊性疾病的情况较为少见，但在成人中，随着透析时间的延长，该病的发生率逐渐增加。接受透析的小年龄患者可以在儿童后期发病。一旦出现肾囊肿，就需要对病变肾脏进行定期的影像检查随访，以排除肿瘤的可能。接受肾移植后，囊肿的体积会缩小。移植患者也可以有新的肾囊肿形成，但一般体积都比较小。

肾盏憩室

肾盏憩室为一个卵圆形的、边缘光滑的囊，通常位于肾脏的一极，以上极多见。憩室通过一个狭窄的颈部与肾盂肾盏相交通。肾盏憩室也被称为肾盂源性囊肿，不过这一定义在憩室与肾盂交通时最为贴切。这些憩室内壁与肾盏一样，为平滑的移行上皮层。肾盏憩室为良性病变，但可以引发血尿或感染。由于憩室内的尿液淤滞，可以形成小的结石。

（赵海腾译 刘国华校）

参考文献

1. Al-Khaldi N, Watson AR, Zuccollo J, et al: Outcome of antenatally detected cystic dysplastic kidney disease. Arch Dis Child 1994;70:520.
2. Atiyeh B, Husmann D, Baum M: Contralateral renal abnormalities in multicystic-dysplastic kidney disease. J Pediatr 1992;121:65.
3. Beckwith JB: Editorial comment. J Urol 1997;158:2259.
4. Bernstein J, Gardner KD Jr: Cystic disease of the kidney and renal dysplasia. In Walsh PC, Gittes RF, Perlmutter AD, et al (eds): Campbell's Urology, 5th ed. Philadelphia, WB Saunders, 1986, p 1760.
5. Brook-Carter PT, Peral B, Ward CJ, et al: Deletion of the TSC2 and PKD1 genes associated with severe infantile polycystic kidney disease—a contiguous gene syndrome. Nat Genet 1994;8:328.
6. Cascio S, Paran S, Prori P: Associated urological anomalies in children with unilateral renal agenesis. J Urol 1999;162:1081.
7. Chonko AM, Weiss JM, Stein JH, et al: Renal involvement in tuberous sclerosis. Ann J Med 1974;56:124.
8. Dimmick J, Johnson HW, Coleman GU, et al: Wilms tumorlet, nodular renal blastema and multicystic renal dysplasia. J Urol 1998;142:484.
9. Eble JN, Bonsib SM: Extensively cystic renal neoplasms:

Cystic nephroma, cystic partially differentiated nephroblastoma, multilocular cystic renal cell carcinoma and cystic pelvis. Semin Diagn Pathol 1998;15:2.
10. Ericsson NO: Renal dysplasia. In Johnson JH, Goodwin WE (eds): Reviews in Pediatric Urology. Amsterdam, Excerpta Medica, 1974, p 25.
11. Flack CE, Bellinger MF: The multicystic dysplastic kidney and contralateral reflux: Protection of the solitary kidney. J Urol 1993;150:1873.
12. Gabow PA: Polycystic kidney disease: Clues to pathogenesis. Kidney Int 1991;40:989.
13. Gabow PA: Autosomal dominant polycystic kidney disease. N Engl J Med 1993;329:332.
14. Gardner KD Jr: Pathogenesis of human renal cystic disease. Annu Rev Med 1988;39:185.
15. Glassberg KI: Unilateral renal cystic disease [editorial]. Urology 1999;53:1227.
16. Glassberg KI: Normal and abnormal development of the kidney: A clinician's interpretation of current knowledge. J Urol 2002;167:2339.
17. Glassberg KI: Renal dysgenesis and cystic disease of the kidney. In Walsh PC, Retik AB, Vaughan ED Jr, Wein AJ (eds): Campbell's Urology, 8th ed. Philadelphia, WB Saunders, 2002, p 1950.
18. Glassberg KI, Stephens FD, Lebowitz RL, et al: Renal dysgenesis and cystic disease of the kidney: A report of the Committee on Terminology, Nomenclature and Classification, Section on Urology, American Academy of Pediatrics. J Urol 1987;138:1085.
19. Goldman SM., Hartman DS: The simple renal cysts. In Pollack HM (ed): Clinical Urography. Philadelphia, WB Saunders, 1990, p 1603.
20. Gomez MR: Tuberous Sclerosis. New York, Raven Press, 1979.
21. Horton WA, Wong V, Eldridge R: Von Hippel-Lindau disease: Clinical and pathological manifestations in nine families with 50 affected members. Arch Intern Med 1976; 136:769.
22. Kandt RS, Haines JL, Smith M, et al: Linkage of an important gene locus for tuberous sclerosis to a chromosome 16 member for polycystic kidney disease. Nat Genet 1992;2:37.
23. Kass EJ, Bloom D: Anomalies of the urinary tract. In Edelman CM (ed): Pediatric Kidney Disease. Boston, Little, Brown, 1992, p 2023.
24. Lagos JC, Gomez MR: Tuberous sclerosis: Reappraisal of a clinical entity. Mayo Clin Proc 1967;42:26 .
25. Levine E, Collins DL, Horton WA, et al: CT screening of the abdomen in von Hippel-Lindau disease. AJR Am J Roentgenol 1982;139:505.
26. Neuman HPH, Wiestler OD: Clustering of features of von Hippel-Lindau syndrome: Evidence for a complex genetic locus. Lancet 1991;337:1052.
27. Noe HN, Marshall JH, Edward OP: Nodular renal blastema in the multicystic kidney. J Urol 1989;127:486.
28. Pampigliana G, Moynahan EJ: The tuberous sclerosis syndrome: Clinical and EEG studies in 100 children. J Neurol Neurosurg Psychiatry 1976;39:666.
29. Peters DJM, Spiruit L, Sari JJ, et al: Chromosome 4 localization of a second gene for autosomal dominant polycystic kidney disease. Nat Genet 1993;5:359.
30. Pieke SA, Kimberling WJ, Kenyon KG, et al: Genetic heterogenicity of polycystic kidney disease: An estimate of the proportion of families unlinked to chromosome 16. Am J Hum Genet 1989;45:458.
31. Potter EL: Bilateral absence of ureters and kidneys: A report of 50 cases. Obstet Gynecol 1965;25:3.
32. Reeders ST, Bruening MH, Davies KE, et al: A highly polymorphic DNA marker linked to adult polycystic kidney disease on chromosome 16. Nature 1985;317:542.
33. Wacksman J: Multicystic dysplastic kidney. In Ball TP (ed): AUA Update Series, vol 17. Houston, American Urological Association, Office of Education, 1998, p 66.
34. Zerres K, Hansman M, Mallman R, et al: Autosomal recessive polycystic kidney disease: Problems of prenatal diagnosis. Prenat Diagn 1988;8:215.

第 110 章

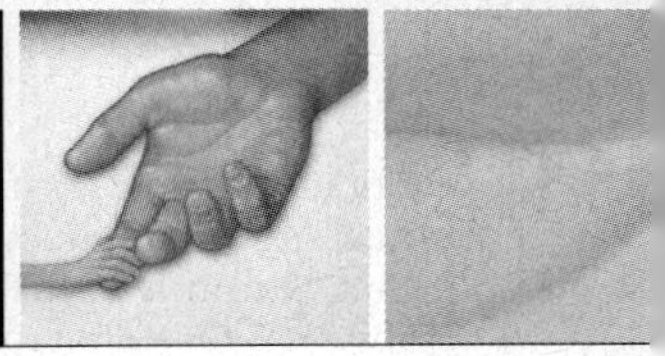

肾脏融合与异位

Pierre Mouriquand

胚胎学

1715 肾脏先天畸形的胚胎学方面涉及两个主要物质和三个过程。这两个主要物质是生肾物质（前肾、中肾和后肾）和输尿管芽（wolffian 结构）。三个过程是后肾组织的生发（肾脏构建）、肾脏的上升（头端迁移）以及肾脏的定位（分隔与旋转）。在这三个阶段发生异常（妊娠前 8 周）将会影响到肾脏的形态、数目和位置。

生肾索分为三个部分（图 110-1）[1]：最头端的节段构成前肾，中间的节段构成中肾，最尾端的节段构成后肾或肾脏。这一分类是完全按照解剖学来进行的，生肾物质从同一起源生发，并且按照从头端向尾端的方向表现出其特有的性质[26]。前肾（胚胎 8 体节阶段）完全退化，而其发出的管道形成中肾。在 23 体节的胚胎中，中肾形成中肾囊和排泄管，这些结构也将退化，仅剩一些胚胎残留，如男性的旁睾和女性的卵巢旁体[32]。后肾生成的位置位于生肾索中肾的尾端部分（后肾胚基）。

输尿管芽于妊娠 4~5 周时从中肾管靠近泄殖腔交界的部位发出。输尿管头端上升并与生肾索相遇，而后者开始发育成后肾并向头端迁移。输尿管头端开始发出一系列分支，形成肾盂、肾盏和一部分集合管[55]。肾脏向头端迁移的过程终止于妊娠第 8 周，其轴向 90 度旋转过程也于此时终止。在上升阶段，肾脏不断接受邻近的血管供应。最初的血管供应来自骶中动脉，然后是髂总动脉和肠系膜下动脉，最后是主动脉。肾脏的发育与输尿管芽来源的位置密切相关[44]。随后输尿管（在妊娠 35 天前的最初发育阶段是透水的）在胚胎 41 天前经历了一系列梗阻和腔化过程[2,60]。肌肉与神经的结构化以及尿液排泄系统的成熟是一个十分缓慢的过程（图 110-2），如果出现异常，会影响到整个尿路的解剖结构。在这一复杂的过程中发生任何延迟或位置异常，将有可能导致以下肾脏畸形[49]：肾不发育、多囊性肾发育不良和其他肾囊性疾病、先天性小肾、多肾以及巨肾（在第 109 章讨论）。在本章以下部分将讨论肾脏上升与融合过程发生异常所导致的畸形。

与肾脏上升过程异常相关的畸形（异位肾）

盆腔肾

在主动脉分叉以下的盆腔位置（骶骨或骨盆）是异位肾最常见的发生位置[71]。盆腔肾（图 110-3）通常为单侧，左侧略多见。约有 10% 的病例发生于双侧[58]。除了位置异常外，盆腔肾往往偏小，形状不规则，可伴有旋转不良和肾外型肾盏。

腰部或髂部异位肾

这些肾脏位于髂嵴以上和 L2 与 L3 水平以下的位置。这种肾脏很难与固定肾相鉴别，因为其输尿管长度正常，无旋转不良，可活动，而且一般能够被推到正常位置[58]。

胸腔肾

胸腔肾（图 110-4A 和 B）十分罕见（16 000 人

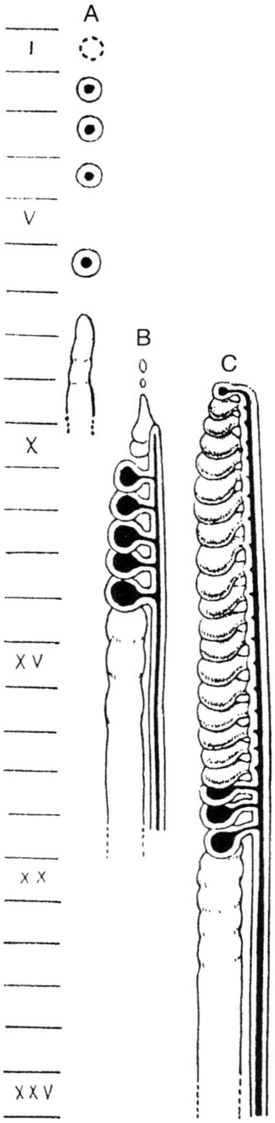

图 110-1　图中显示了人类肾脏的早期发育过程。A. 10 体节胚胎。B. 20 体节胚胎。C. 25 体节胚胎。罗马数字标注了体节的节段。圆圈标注了不参与肾脏构成的生肾节（基于 Torrey[72]）。（From Hamilton WJ, Boyd JD, Mossman HW [eds]: Human Embryology, 3rd ed. Cambridge, Heffer, 1962.）

发生 1 例）[5,6,13,19]，可能与中肾退化延迟有关（如生肾索持续存在）[34]。胸腔肾可以伴有心血管、肺以及脊椎畸形[45,51]。

伴发畸形

异位肾常伴有生殖系统和对侧泌尿系统畸形，如

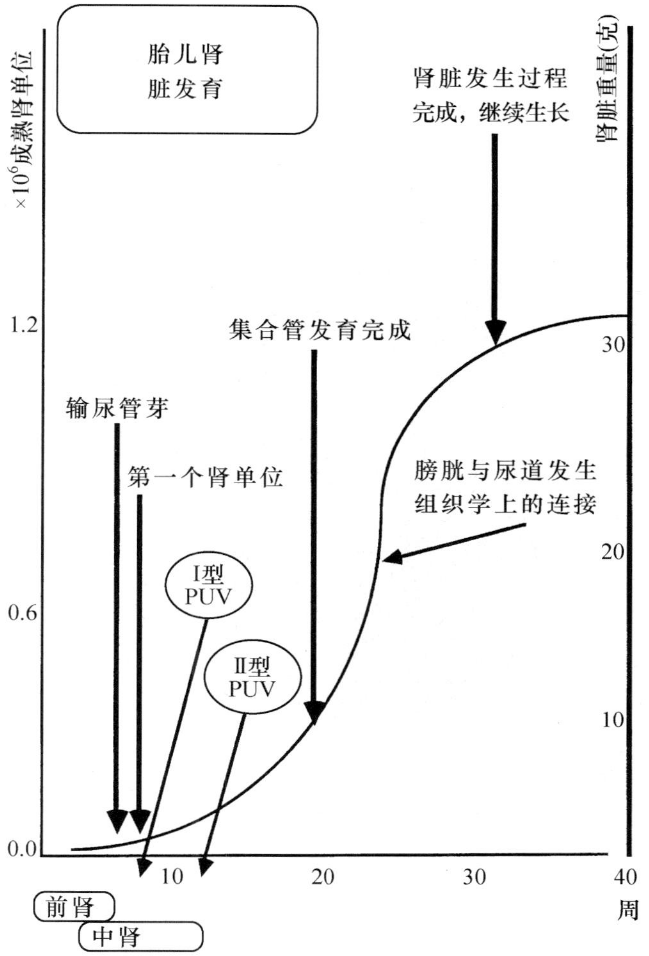

图 110-2　泌尿系统发生的时间表。PUV，后尿道瓣膜。

阴道缺失[35]、腔静脉后输尿管[37]、双角子宫、多肾[24]和对侧异位输尿管[11]。异位肾可以是某个复杂综合征中的一个表现，如 Mayer-Rokitansky-Küster-Hauser 综合征[7,69,70]、Fanconi 贫血[70]、联体畸形[68]。也有头端异位肾发生在脐膨出患者中的报道[3]。

异位肾的诊断

异位肾可以是偶然发现的，不需要手术治疗，也可以伴有尿液引流障碍或反流，需要进行外科手术治疗。同位素检查、超声影像学诊断、核磁共振显像（图 110-5）或静脉肾盂造影检查通常都能够确定异

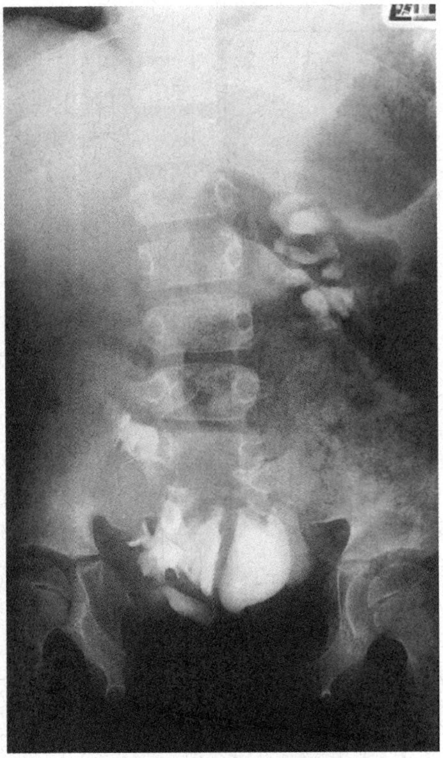

图 110-3 盆腔肾。(Courtesy of Professor Ⅰ. Gordon, Department of Radiology, Great Ormond Street Hospital, London.)

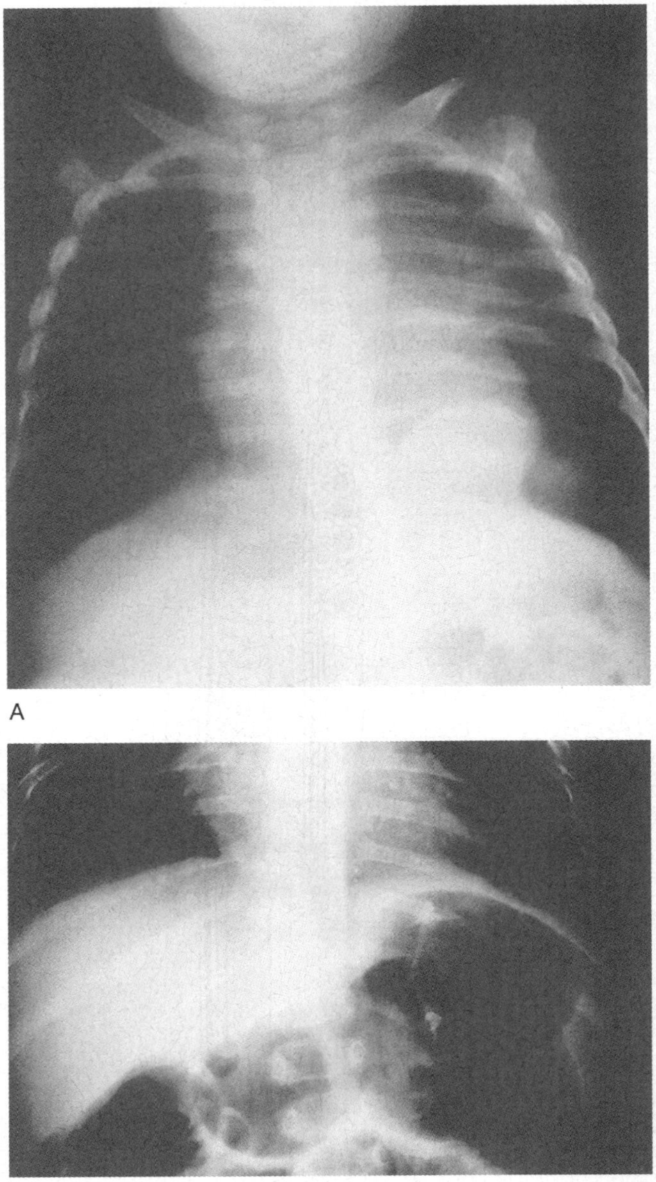

A

B

图 110-4 A 和 B. 胸腔肾(静脉尿路造影)。(Courtesy of Professor Ⅰ. Gordon, Department of Radiology, Great Ormond Street Hospital, London.)

位的肾实质。必要时，这些检查手段可能还要辅以逆行造影检查。CT 检查已经被认为是诊断异位肾的有效手段，对胸腔异位肾的诊断效果最佳[6]。产前检查可能会提示有异位肾存在，当合并有一定程度的扩张时，该诊断的准确性会大大提高。

与肾脏融合异常相关的畸形

马蹄肾

马蹄肾是肾脏融合异常中最为常见的畸形。马
蹄肾（图 110-6A 和 B，图 110-7A 和 B）的发生率
1717 为每 400～1800 例[28,14]尸检中出现 1 例。这种情况
在男性中较为多见。马蹄肾与其他肾融合畸形，如横过异位，在文献报道中被认为是家族多发的，包括双胞胎发病[17,30,40]。有 95% 的病例两肾下极有桥状的肾组织相互连接，连接的肾组织既可以是正常的肾组织，也可以是发育不良组织，甚至纤维组织。约 40% 的患者中，桥接的峡部组织位于第四腰椎水平，正好位于肠系膜下动脉起始部以下；在 20% 的病例中，该峡部位于盆腔；在其余的病例中，连接部位于肾正常位置的下极水平[35]。马蹄肾的峡部通常于大血管前方跨过，但有的从主动脉或下腔静脉后方绕过[16]。有的假设认为肠系膜下动脉卡在马蹄肾的峡部，从而阻止了肾脏的进一步上

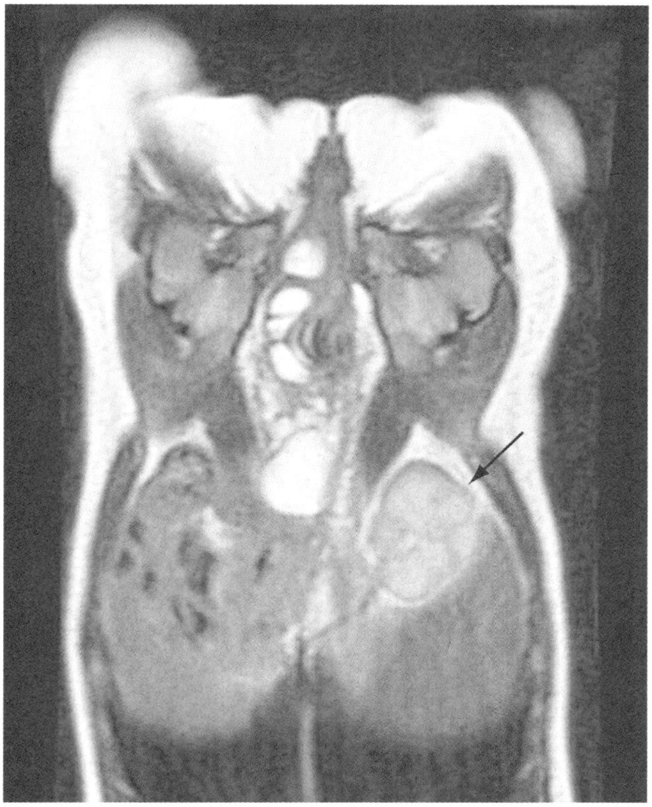

图 110-5　盆腔肾的核磁共振显像（*箭头处*）。（Courtesy of Professor J. P. Pracros, Department of Radiology, Debrousse Hospital, Lyon, France.）

升。有的马蹄肾融合部位发生在上极。输尿管从峡部前方弓形绕过。马蹄肾的血管供应差异较大[12]，在手术时必须牢记：30% 的患者只有一套肾血管，其内包括每个肾脏一根肾动脉。不过这些血管分支可能是不对称的，既可以是两支，也可以是三支。峡部的血供可以来自主动脉、肾动脉、肠系膜下动脉、髂总或髂外动脉或骶动脉。除此以外，也可以是所有的血管首先进入峡部，然后再供应其他部位[56]。以往的病例报告中曾经提到马蹄肾重复以及交通性肾重复的情况[62,75]。马蹄肾的一部分可以是发育不良的或是无功能的[10]。

伴发畸形比较多见，约占病例的 78%[77]。最常见的部位是中枢神经系统、胃肠道、骨骼以及心血管系统。在有 18 三体的儿童中，融合肾的发生率为 20%[8,74]。超过 60% 的 Turner 综合征患者存在肾脏畸形，包括马蹄肾[57]（7%）[36]。马蹄肾可以在较大年龄时因主动脉瘤而变得更为复杂[54]。

目前马蹄肾的诊断方法主要是利用以往提出的手段，同位素检查通常能够给出比较明确的诊断。在静脉尿路造影检查中，有造影剂充盈的肾盏向肾盂内侧移位，提示肾脏旋转不良，肾轴比较垂直并且向外侧 1718
移位，分泌性的囊腔位置较低，这些表现即可明确马蹄肾诊断。输尿管走向变异较大，但其上段也因峡部肾实质的存在而向外侧偏移。扩张的肾盂较为常见，主要是因为输尿管向前方成角（引起扭曲），也可能是由连接部异常或者迷行血管压迫连接部引起的肾盂输尿管交界处梗阻所造成。通常这些情况可以使马蹄肾伴有不同程度的尿液输送障碍，使得马蹄肾在产前即可获得诊断。膀胱输尿管反流也是马蹄肾的常见并发症（10%~80%）[15,57,62]。

马蹄肾患者的预后主要与其伴发的畸形有关。大多数马蹄肾患者终生可以不出现症状。不过，在伴有肾盂积水、反流、结石或组织发育不良的情况下，可能会出现反复尿路感染、疼痛、血尿，需要进行外科治疗。已有明确的证据表明马蹄肾患者发生肾母细胞瘤的风险较高，而且发生肾盂癌的风险也是正常人 3~4倍以上[47,67]。发生肿瘤（大多位于马蹄肾的桥接部位）后可以出现类似腹部疾病的表现。由肾脏迁移过程异常所产生的实质性肾峡部更易于发生肾细胞癌[36]。马蹄肾尤其容易发生原发性肾脏类癌瘤，而且可能来自肾脏中化生组织或畸胎瘤上皮的神经内分泌细胞[42]。有的病例被报道合并有神经节成神经细 1719
胞瘤[53]，也有的合并肾盏憩室伴发感染[64]。黄色肉芽肿性肾盂肾炎是马蹄肾的另一种并发症，是肾实质慢性炎症时的罕见并发症[33]。

对马蹄肾患者进行外科治疗的最常见指征是肾盂输尿管连接部梗阻。由于峡部可能不是造成梗阻的原因，所以大多数患者不再需要进行峡部切断手术[18]。如果肾脏的位置在正常情况所允许的范围内，而且病变为单侧，则推荐采用传统的前外侧后腹膜手术路径。如果肾脏的位置比较难于处理，或者病变为双侧，则最好采用经腹手术路径。输尿管肾盏造瘘术对于独立的尿路引流来说是一个不错的选择。肾盂内切开术是另外一个可以选择的方式，但比较适用于大年龄儿童[50]。

马蹄肾患者结石的发生率为 20%[58]，一般可以通过体外振波碎石或经皮手术进行治疗。腹腔镜半肾切除术治疗马蹄肾良性病变对于有经验的外科医生来说是一个很好的选择[76]。

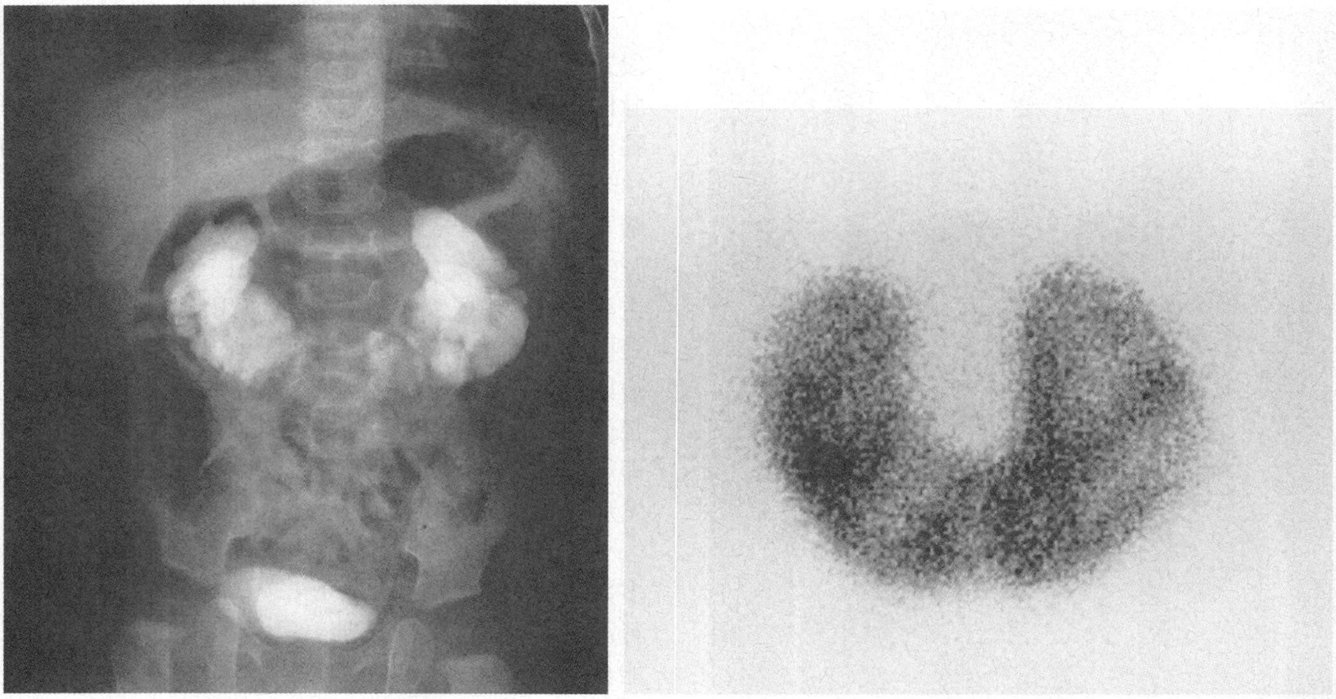

A　B

图 110-6　A 和 B. 马蹄肾［A. 静脉尿路造影；B. 二巯基丁二酸（DMSA）扫描］。(Courtesy of Professor Ⅰ. Gordon, Department of Radiology, Great Ormond Street Hospital, London.)

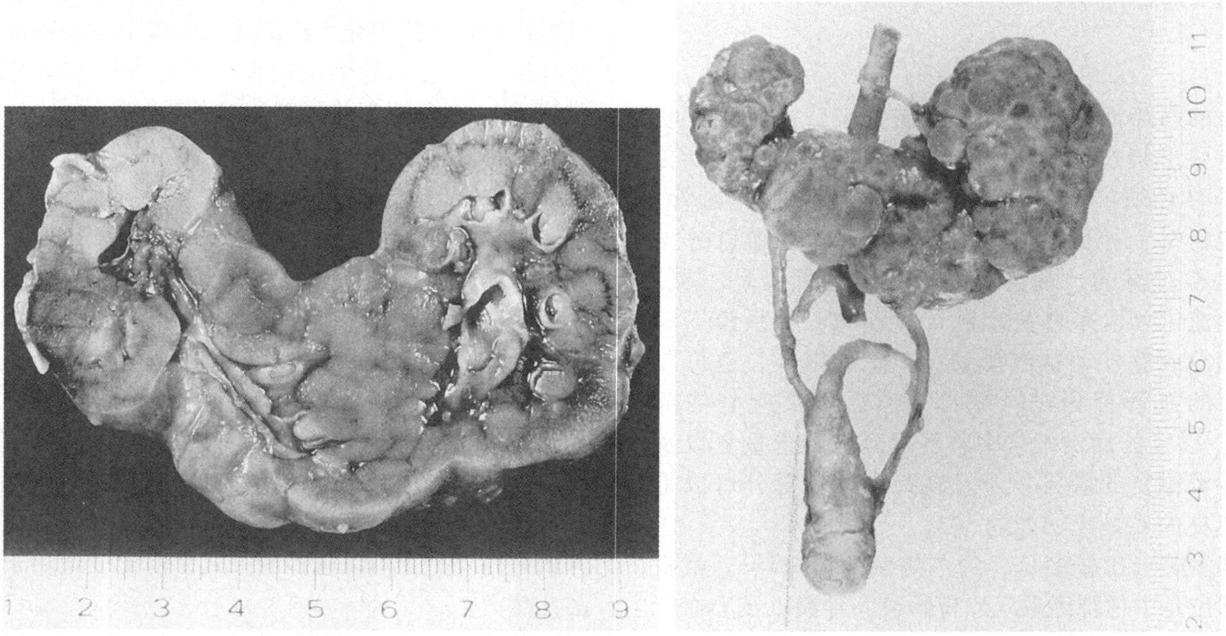

A　B

图 110-7　A 和 B. 马蹄肾病理标本。(Courtesy of Professor A. R. Risdon and Dr. G. Anderson, Department of Histopathology, Great Ormond Street Hospital, London.)

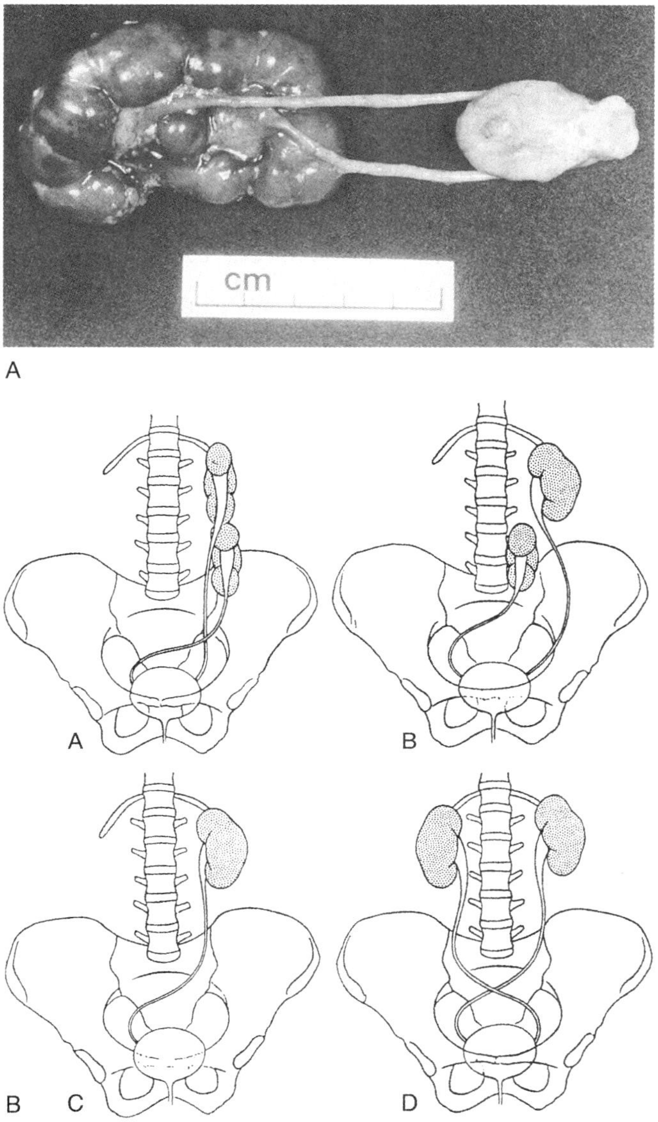

图 110-8　A. 肾脏横跨异位伴有肾融合。(From Professor A. R. Risdon and Dr. G. Anderson, Department of Histopathology, Great Ormond Street Hospital, London.) B. 四种不同类型的肾脏横跨异位：伴有融合（A），不伴有融合（B），孤立肾（C），双侧发生（D）。（From Ritchey M: Anomalies of the kidney. In Kelalis PP, King LR, Belman AB [eds]: Clinical Pediatric Urology, 3rd ed. Philadelphia, WB Saunders, 1992.）

肾脏横跨异位

肾脏横跨异位（图 110-8A 和 B）的发生率约为每 7000 个尸检中发现 1 例，在融合畸形中居第二位，仅次于马蹄肾[58]。肾脏横跨异位畸形有四种类型：(1) 伴有肾融合（85%），(2) 不伴有肾融合（<10%），(3) 孤立肾，(4) 双侧发生[1,39,46]。男性发病略多，左向右横跨的情况比右向左多见。融合的部位多发生于横跨肾的上极和正常位置肾的下极（单侧融合型）。肾盂位于肾脏的前方，旋转不完全。对于乙状肾或“S”形肾，融合的情况是一样的，只是肾脏旋转过程已经完成，此时两个肾盂的方向相反。有关肾脏不同程度融合的报道较少（如结节肾、“L”形肾和高位异位肾）[58]。继发于肾盂输尿管连接部梗阻的假性肾脏横跨异位也有报道[9]。静脉尿路造影、同位素检查、超声影像学、MRI 以及 CT 等检查可以明确异位的解剖类型。不过，有时这一诊断过程也会出现困难。肾脏的血管供应会有不同的变异[61]，有时也会出现血管跨越中线。大多数肾脏横跨异位是无症状的，在检查中偶然发现。如果需要手术治疗，对于横跨融合型的异位肾可以采用腹腔镜手术[4]。

肾脏横跨异位伴发畸形较为常见，包括骨骼畸形、肛门闭锁、心血管畸形[1,63]、生殖系统畸形[21,39]、脊柱裂[20]、膀胱输尿管反流、反流性肾病[73]、输尿管横跨异位、多囊性发育不良[52]、肾肿瘤[27,31]、输尿管嵌闭[59]以及睾丸肿瘤[41]。肾脏异位也可以是更为复杂的综合征中的一个表现，比如脊柱畸形、肛门闭锁、心脏畸形、食管气管瘘和（或）食管闭锁、肾不发育和发育不良、肢体缺陷综合征（VACTERL）[29]以及骈胝体发育不全[25,65]。这些不同 1720
畸形的组合可以解释文献中报道的一些并发症，如腹股沟疝患者合并横跨融合异位肾时，在疝修补手术时可能会误扎输尿管[38]。

（赵海腾译　刘国华校）

参考文献

1. Abeshouse BS, Bhisitkul I: Crossed renal ectopia with and without fusion. Urol Int 1959;9:63.
2. Alcaraz A, Vinaixa F, Tejedo-Mateu A, et al: Obstruction and recanalization of the ureter during embryonic development. J Urol 1991;145:410.
3. Aliotta PJ, Seidel FG, Karp M, Greenfeld SP: Renal malposition in patients with omphalocele. J Urol 1987;137:942.
4. Andersen RD, Van Savage JG: Laparoscopic nephrectomy of the lower kidney for crossed fused ectopia. J Urol 2000;163:1902.

5. Angulo JC, Lopex JI, Vilanova JR, Flores N: Intrathoracic kidney and vertebral fusion: A model of combined misdevelopment. J Urol 1992;147:1351.
6. Baillet AM, Escure MN: Apport de l'imagerie TDM au diagnostic de rein intrathoracique. J Radiol 1988;69:269.
7. Barakat AY, Seikaly MG, Der Kaloustian VM: Urogenital abnormalities in genetic disease. J Urol 1986;136:778.
8. Boatman DL, Kolln CP, Flocks RH: Congenital anomalies associated with horseshoe kidney. J Urol 1972;107:205.
9. Bolton DM, Stoller ML: Pseudo–crossed renal ectopia secondary to ureteric junction obstruction. J Urol 1995; 153:397.
10. Borer JG, Cargan FJ, Krantz R, et al: Unilateral single vaginal ectopic ureter with ipsilateral hypoplastic pelvic kidney and bicornuate uterus. J Urol 1993;149:1124.
11. Borer JG, Glassberg KI, Kassner EG, et al: Unilateral multicystic dysplasia in 1 component of a horseshoe kidney: Case reports and review of literature. J Urol 1994; 152:1568.
12. Boullier J, Chehval MJ, Purcell MH: Removal of a multicystic half of a horseshoe kidney: Significance of peroperative evaluation in identifying abnormal surgical anatomy. J Pediatr Surg 1992;27:1244.
13. Campbell MF: Renal ectopy. J Urol 1930;24:187.
14. Campbell MF: Anomalies of the kidney. In Campbell MF, Harrison JH (eds): Urology, vol 2, 3rd ed. Philadelphia, WB Saunders, 1970.
15. Cascio S, Sweeney B, Granata C, et al: Vesicoureteral reflux and ureteropelvic junction obstruction in children with horseshoe kidney: Treatment and outcome. J Urol 2002; 167:2566.
16. Dajani AM: Horseshoe kidney: A review of twenty-nine cases. Br J Urol 1966;38:388.
17. David RS: Horseshoe kidney: A report of one family. BMJ 1974;4:571.
18. Donahoe PK, Hendren WH: Pelvic kidney in infants and children: Experience of 16 children. J Pediatr Surg 1980; 15:486.
19. Donat SM, Donat PE: Intrathoracic kidney: A case report with a review of the world literature. J Urol 1988;140:131.
20. Dragun MJ, Flemming D, Knorr A, et al: Crossed fused renal ectopia in children with myelodysplasia. Urology 1994;44:562.
21. Eckford SD, Westgate J: Solitary crossed renal ectopia associated with unicornuate uterus, imperforate anus, and congenital scoliosis. J Urol 1996;156:221.
22. Evans DG, Rees HC, Spreadborough A, et al: Radial ray defects, renal ectopia, duodenal atresia and hydrocephalus: The extended spectrum for Fanconi anemia. Clin Dysmorphol 1994;3:200.
23. Fisher RM, Frank JD: Abnormal migration and fusion of the kidneys. In Gearhat JP, Rink RR, Mouriquand PDE (eds): Pediatric Urology. Philadelphia, WB Saunders, 2001, p 275.
24. Flyer MA, Haller JO, Fled M, Kantor A: Ectopic supernumerary kidney: Another cause of a pelvic mass. Abdom Imaging 1994;19:374.
25. Franco I, Rogan S, Fisher J, et al: Genitourinary malformations associated with agenesis of the corpus callosum. J Urol 1993;149:1119.
26. Fraser EA: The development of the vertebrate excretory system. Biol Rev 1950;25:159.
27. Gerber WL, Culp DA, Brown RC: Renal mass in crossed-fused ectopia. J Urol 1980;123:239.
28. Glenn JF: Analysis of 51 patients with horseshoe kidney. N Engl J Med 1959;261:684.
29. Golomb J, Ehrlich RM: Bilateral ureteral triplication with crossed ectopic fused kidneys associated with the VACTERL syndrome. J Urol 1989;141:1398.
30. Greenberg LW, Nelsen CE: Crossed fused ectopia of the kidneys in twins. Am J Dis Child 1971;122:175.
31. Gur U, Yossepowitch O, Baniel J: Transitional cell carcinoma in a fused crossed ectopic kidney. Urology 2003;62:748.
32. Hamilton WJ, Boyd JD, Mossman HW (eds): Human Embryology, 3rd ed. Cambridge, Heffer, 1962.
33. Hammadeh MY, Calder CJ, Corkery JJ: Pediatric xanthogranulomatous pyelonephritis in a horseshoe kidney. Br J Urol 1994;73:721.
34. Hawass ND, Kolawole TM, el Badawi MG, et al: Intrathoracic kidneys: Report of 6 cases and a review of the literature. Eur Urol 1988;14:83.
35. Hendren WH, Donahoe PK: Renal fusions and ectopia. In Welch KJ, Randolph JG, Ravitch MM, et al (eds): Pediatric Surgery, Chicago, Year Book, 1986.
36. Hohenfellner M, Schultz-Lampel D, Lampel A, et al: Tumor in the horseshoe kidney: Clinical implications and review of embryogenesis. J Urol 1992;147:1098.
37. Hubert J, Fournier G, Blum A, et al: Uretère rétrocave associé à une ectopie rénale pelvienne controlatérale: Apport du scanner tri-dimensionnel. Apropos d'un cas et revue de la littérature. Prog Urol 1994;4:262.
38. Hwang CM, Miller FH, Dalton DP, Hartz WH: Accidental ureteral ligation during an inguinal hernia repair of patient with crossed fused renal ectopia. Clin Imaging 2002;26:306.
39. Kakei H, Kondo H, Ogisu BI: Crossed ectopia of solitary kidney: A report of two cases and a review of literature. Urol Int 1976;31:470.
40. Kalra D, Broomhall J, Williams J: Horseshoe kidney in one of identical twin girls. J Urol 1985;134:113.
41. Key DW, Moyad R, Grossman HB: Seminoma associated with crossed fused renal ectopia. J Urol 1990;143:1015.
42. Krishnan B, Truong LD, Saleh G, et al: Horseshoe kidney is associated with an increased relative risk of primary renal carcinoid tumor. J Urol 1997;157:2059.
43. Lippe BL, Geffner ME, Dietrich RB: Renal malformation in patients with Turner's syndrome: Imaging in 141 patients. Pediatrics 1988;83:852.
44. Mackie GG, Stephens FD: Duplex kidneys: A correlation of renal dysplasia with position of the ureteral orifice. J Urol 1975;114:274.
45. Malek RS, Kelalis PP, Burke EC: Ectopic kidney in children and frequency of association with other malformations. Mayo Clin Proc 1971;46:461.
46. McDonald JH, McClellan DS: Crossed renal ectopia. Am J Surg 1957;93:995.
47. Mesrobian HGJ, Kelalis PP, Hrabovsky E, et al: Wilms tumor in horseshoe kidneys: A report from the national Wilms tumor study. J Urol 1985;133:1002.
48. Mollard P, Mouriquand P, Joubert P, Pouyau A: Urétéro-calicostomie pour hydronéphrose par maladie de la jonction de l'enfant et de l'dolescent: À propos de 35 cas. Chir Pediatr 1990;31:87.
49 Mouriquand PDE, Mollard P, Ransley PG: Dilemmes soulevés par le diagnostic antenatal des uropathies obstructives et leurs traitements. Pediatrie 1989;44:357.
50. Nakamura K, Baba S, Tazaki H: Endopyelotomy in horseshoe kidney. J Endourol 1994;8:203.
51. N'Guessen G, Stephens FD, Pick J: Congenital superior ectopic (thoracic) kidney. Urology 1984;24:219.
52. Nussbaum AR, Hartman DS, Whitley N: Multicystic

dysplasia and crossed renal ectopia. AJR Am J Roentgenol 1987;149:407.
53. Oguz A, Basaklar C, Gogus S, et al: Association of ganglioneuroblastoma with horseshoe kidney. Mater Med Pol 1994;26:35.
54. O'Hara PJ, Hakaim AG, Hertzer NR, et al: Surgical management of aortic aneurysm and coexistent horseshoe kidney: Review of a 31-year experience. J Vasc Surg 1993;17:940.
55. Osathanondh V, Potter EL: Development of human kidney as shown in microdissection—3 parts. Arch Pathol 1963; 76:271.
56. Perlmutter A, Retik A, Bauer S: Anomalies of the upper urinary tract. In Walsh P, Gittes PF, Perlmutter AD, et al (eds): Campbell's Urology. Philadelphia, WB Saunders, 1986.
57. Pitts WR, Muecke EC: Horseshoe kidneys: A 40 year experience. J Urol 1975;113:743.
58. Ritchey M: Anomalies of the kidney. In Kelalis PP, King LR, Belman AB (eds): Clinical Pediatric Urology, 3rd ed. Philadelphia, WB Saunders, 1992.
59. Rocklin MS, Apelgren KN, Slomski CA, Kandzari S: Scrotal incarceration of the ureter with crossed renal ectopia: Case report and literature review. J Urol 1989;142:366.
60. Ruano-Gil D, Coca-Payeras A, Tejedo-Mateu A: Obstruction and normal recanalization of the ureter in the human embryo. Its relation to congenital ureteric obstruction. Eur Urol 1975;1:287.
61. Rubinstein ZJ, Heitz M, Shanin N: Crossed renal ectopia: Angiographic findings in six cases. AJR Am J Roentgenol 1976;126:1035.
62. Segura JW, Kelalis PP, Burke EC: Horseshoe kidney in children. J Urol 1972;108:333.
63. Shaw MB, Cutress M, Papavassiliou V, et al: Duplicated inferior vena cava and crossed renal ectopia with abdominal aortic aneurysm: Preoperative anatomic studies facilitate surgery. Clin Anat 2003;16:355.
64. Shekarriz B, Upadhyay J, Bathold JS, Gonzales R: Infected caliceal diverticulum in a horseshoe kidney. J Urol 1998;160:842.
65. Shental J, Katz Z, Reich D: The persisting mesonephrotic duct syndrome in a neonate with agenesis of the corpus callosum. J Urol 1994;152:1590.
66. Smith DW: Recognizable patterns of human malformation: Genetic, embryologic and clinical aspects. In Smith DW (ed): Major Problems in Urology. Philadelphia, WB Saunders, 1970.
67. Smith-Behn J, Memo R: Malignancy associated with horseshoe kidney. South Med J 1988;81:1451.
68. Spitz L, Stringer MD, Kiely EM, et al: Separation of brachiothoraco-ischiopagus bipus conjoined twins. J Pediatr Surg 1994;29:477.
69. Strübbe EH, Willemsen WL, Lemmens JA, et al: Mayer-Rokitansky-Küster-Hauser syndrome: Distinction between two forms based on excretory urographic, sonographic, and laparoscopic findings. AJR Am J Roentgenol 1993; 160:331.
70. Tarry WF, Duckett JW, Stephens FD: The Mayer-Rokitansky syndrome: Pathogenesis, classification and management. J Urol 1986;136:648.
71. Thomson GJ, Pace JM: Ectopic kidney: A review of 97 cases. Mayo Clin Proc 1937;64:935.
72. Torrey TW: The early development of the human nephros. Contrib Embryol Carneg Instit 1954;35:175.
73. Wanatabe T: Reflux nephropathy in a patient with crossed renal ectopia with fusion. Pediatr Nephrol 2002;17:617.
74. Warkany J, Passarge E, Smith LB: Congenital malformations in autosomal trisomy syndromes. Am J Dis Child 1966; 112:502.
75. Wilson C, Azmy AF: Horseshoe kidney in children. Br J Urol 1986;58:361.
76. Yohannes P, Dinlec C, Liatsikos E, et al: Laparoscopic heminephrectomy for benign disease of the horseshoe kidney. JSLS 2002;6:381.
77. Zondek LH, Zondek T: Horseshoe kidney in associated congenital malformations. Urol Int 1964;18:347.

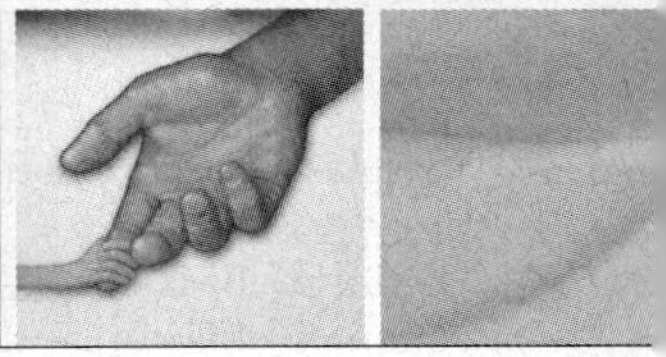

第 111 章

肾盂输尿管连接部梗阻

Byron D. Joyner 和 Michael E. Mitchell

肾盂积水的定义是：由于引流不充分或者由于尿液逆流，导致肾脏集合系统扩张。通常认为其原因主要是单纯性的机械性因素。更准确地说，肾盂积水是一个综合性的病征，是由肾小球的血流动力学与肾小管功能相互作用引起的[14]。肾盂积水一般都是通过产前超声检查发现的，约占新生儿所有尿路疾病的0.5%~0.6%。在出生以后新生儿中，有五分之一的产前肾盂积水会自行消退[24]。在出生后肾盂积水持续存在的新生儿中，有44%的肾盂积水由肾盂输尿管连接部（ureteropelvic junction，UPJ）梗阻引起[110]。因此，UPJ梗阻是产后肾盂积水的主要原因。

继发于UPJ梗阻的肾盂积水，其自然病程中的变化主要取决于肾盂内尿液阻力的大小。在高级别UPJ梗阻的肾脏中，不充分的引流导致静水压增高，肾盂扩张，同时尿液减少。肾盂内压的慢性增高会导致肾脏发生不可逆损害。而在低级别的UPJ梗阻中，肾脏处于一种自身稳定状态，经常会出现短时间的生长和改善。在这两种程度之间的病变，其可变范围很大，对于梗阻型的肾脏病变是否需要进行外科手术干预，目前还存在争议。

病因学/发病率

肾盂积水是通过产前超声检查出来的最为常见的异常，约占所有产前缺陷的50%[69,101]。所有妊娠中UPJ梗阻的发病率已经从0.02%上升到1%的筛查比例，而仅有1/500被认为是明显的肾盂积水[88,109]。UPJ梗阻在所有引起明显的先天性肾盂积水的病因中约占44%，由此可以换算出UPJ梗阻的发病率为每1250个出生婴儿中发生一例[10,74]。UPJ梗阻在男性中发病约为女性的两倍，特别是在新生儿阶段；有66%病例发生于左侧[52,105]，而成人则相反，发生于右侧的略多[16]。双侧发病的UPJ梗阻约占所有患者的10%~36%，在小年龄组的患者中所占的比例更高[7,105]。

Koff描述了在外科手术探查时发现的两种类型的UPJ畸形[59]（图111-1）。第一种类型是*外源性*异常，比较典型的是机械性因素所致，如横跨的血管、粘连束带、动静脉畸形、胎儿期遗留的皱襞[48,86]。外源性因素使得输尿管扭曲或压迫UPJ，造成输尿管成角，导致尿流受阻，肾盂积水进行性加重。与此类似，Östling也描述了出现在UPJ水平的输尿管皱褶（图111-2）[86]。从皱褶存在的意义上说，一般认为，这些皱褶的存在为小儿在出生两年内的轴向生长创造了条件，如果这些皱褶持续存在，就可能会造成外源性的梗阻。第二种类型，也是UPJ畸形最常见的类型，是*内源性*异常，传统上被认为是“无动力”节段。这种内源性异常会干扰输尿管向远端节段性输送尿液所需的蠕动波。在手术中可以看到，这些节段长

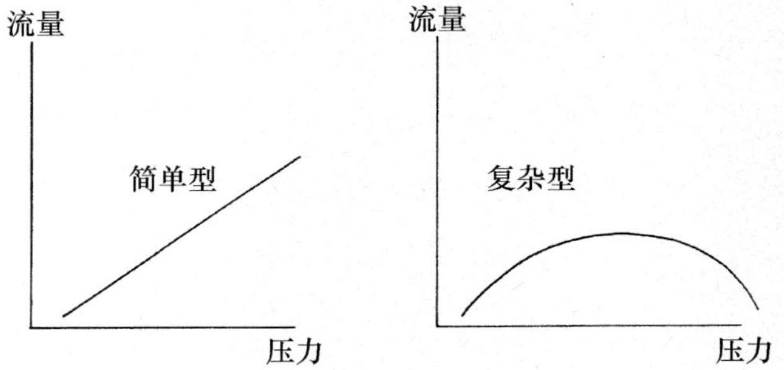

图 111-1 图中示意了人类肾盂积水中压力-流量关系中的简单和复杂两种类型。（From Koff SA：Pathophysiology of ureteropelvic junction obstruction：Clinical and experimental observations. Urol Clin North Am 1990；17：269.）

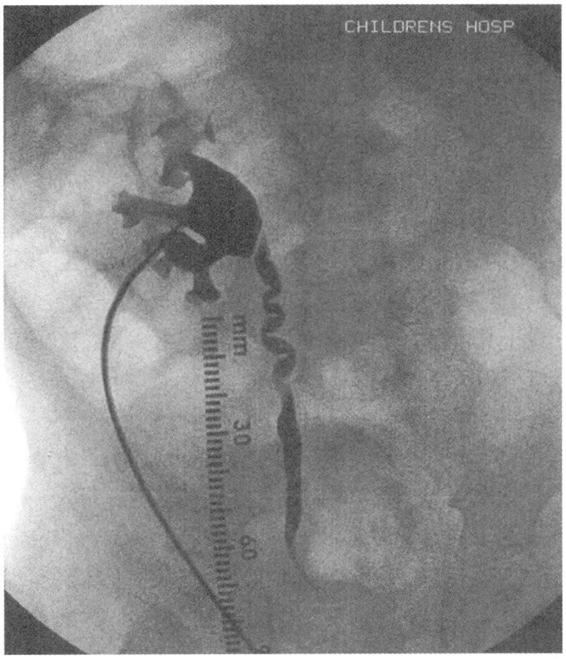

图 111-2　经皮肾造瘘造影检查显示胎儿 Östling 皱襞。（Courtesy of Children's Hospital & Regional Medical Center, Seattle.）

度不等，而且比其他部位的输尿管细。此外，这些节段虽然往往能够允许探针通过，但缺乏扩张的能力。在组织学表现上，病变节段的环肌纤维缺陷，排列紊
24 乱，形态上发育不良[32,80]。输尿管管径变小与肌肉缺陷两者结合在一起，被认为是造成内源性异常和阻碍尿液向输尿管远端输送的原因。其他用来描述这些 UPJ 梗阻类型的方法，是根据其容量依赖（外源性）和压力依赖（内源性）的特征来进行的[59,63]。Koff 通过实验和临床观察总结出：这些参数或者这些参数的组合可以解释 UPJ 梗阻的许多不同的临床表现[63]。

导致 UPJ 梗阻的第三种畸形是*腔内型*梗阻。腔内型梗阻病变的例子是输尿管瓣膜或良性纤维上皮性息肉[1,70]。这些异常可以导致部分性、间歇性梗阻，往往需要外科手术治疗（图 111-3）[35]。

胚胎学

在人类胚胎发生过程中，出现过三个独立而又相互依赖的肾脏系统：前肾、中肾和后肾——或真正的肾脏。最早出现并且持续时间最短的肾脏是前肾，许

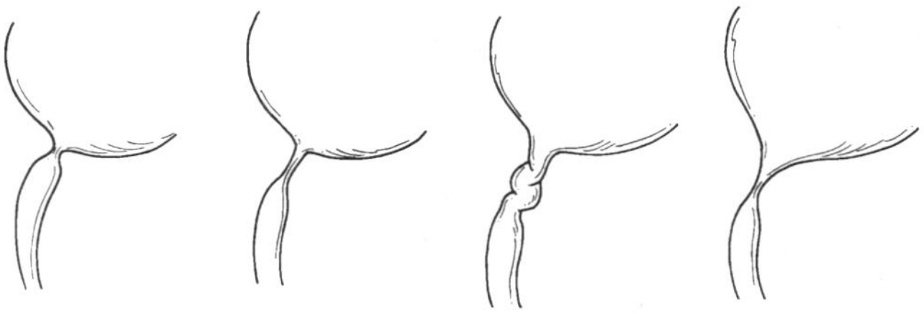

图 111-3　继发于狭窄的肾盂输尿管连接部梗阻：单纯型、节段型、匐行型和移行型。（Courtesy of Dr. F. Douglas Stephens.）（From Fung LCT, Lakshmanan Y: Anomalies of the renal collecting system: Ureteropelvic junction obstruction [pyelocalyectasis] and infundibular stenosis. In Belman AB, King LR, Kramer SA [eds]: Clinical Pediatric Urology, 4th ed. London, Martin Dunitz, 2002, p 561.）

多人认为是存在于发育中的胚胎颈部区域中一个退化结构。作者的观点是：前肾可能是肾脏双向发育中必不可少的构架。而根据现代理论的观点，前肾在妊娠第三周被中肾所取代。中肾不断延长形成一个管状结构，最终连接到尾端的中肾管或 wolffian 管。在妊娠第五周，管状系统的背侧中间壁向外侧呈憩室样生长，称为输尿管芽。就在中肾系统退化过程中，输尿管芽朝着原始后肾始基方向不断向上生长延长。两个结构相互接触后就会激发一系列过程，这一系列过程被称为肾脏发生。

在泌尿系统的发育过程中，有可能在四个不同的解剖部位发生机械性梗阻：输尿管肾盏、输尿管肾盂、输尿管膀胱以及膀胱尿道的连接处[3]。每一个部位都代表着两个或更多的胚胎结构的汇合处。目前还不能完全明确这些部位的具体情况，但它们在发育过程中容易出现异常。双向发育的特性启动了细胞复合体之间的信号交换和诱导过程。正常情况下，这一过程在每个解剖连接部位进行得极为精确。而在这些解剖部位上的偏差会导致小儿泌尿外科中最为常见的两个病理情况，即膀胱输尿管反流（VUR）和 UPJ 梗阻。

以往认为输尿管的双向腔化能够解释为什么最常见的梗阻部位位于腔化最后完成的末段：UPJ 和输尿管膀胱连接部（UVJ）[99]。然而最近发现这一双向腔化现象并不存在。腔化过程仅仅发生在输尿管的中间部分[6]。在现有的输尿管发生的实验模型和理论中，没有一个能够解释为什么 UPJ 是先天性输尿管梗阻最常见的发生部位。这方面的研究一直都是比较热门的领域。比如，一个使用了梗阻性肾病动物模型的新的

研究报告了一个可能的肾盂积水基因片断[12]。Chang等人描述了在小鼠模型内衬泌尿系统的间充基质中敲除编码钙调磷酸酶B1的基因（*Cnb1*），动物会因为输尿管丧失蠕动能力而发生肾盂积水。这一研究不仅指出肾盂是蠕动的调节部位，而且也解释了没有发现明显物理梗阻的先天性梗阻。

Ransley曾经提出发生在肾盂水平的另外一种尿路梗阻理论[95]。要了解这一理论，则需要明确在出生时肾脏所发生的改变。出生时，胎儿肾脏经历了一系列
1725 独立的生理过程。针对这一时期出现的过渡期肾脏学概念对于理解临床上发现的一过性肾积水来说是十分必要的。肾脏发生最终于妊娠36周时完成，而肾脏的生长发育还在持续进行。在最后三个月以及出生后的前10周内，肾小球滤过率（GFR）迅速增加[103]。在出生时，水和溶质排泄工作迅速从胎盘移交给新生儿肾脏。同时，肾血管的阻力也迅速增加，肾血液减少，GFR也降低。这一系列必不可少的事件建立了逐渐降低的排泄压力梯度和小管-肾盏梯度[95]。可能与这些相对应，肾内肾盂压力在新生儿UPJ梗阻的肾脏中实现了自主平衡的调节。而这种平衡一旦打破，就可能导致进行性的肾盂积水，肾功能迅速恶化。

临床特征

30年前，大多数UPJ梗阻的婴儿在初次就诊时表现为可以触及的腹部肿块[52]。而现在，表现为腹部肿块的UPJ梗阻在新生儿中不超过19%[103]。随着胎儿产前超声检查的不断深入应用，大多数UPJ梗阻患儿都可以在产前获得诊断。还有一些诊断为UPJ梗阻的患儿伴有一系列综合征。UPJ梗阻患儿的年龄分布似乎呈现双峰型：产后无症状的婴儿以及有症状的学龄期儿童。不过，偶尔会有一些婴儿因其他表现而被查出有UPJ梗阻，如生长缓慢、呕吐、喂养困难、继发于尿路感染的败血症，还有比较少见的与尿路结石相关的血尿症状。

出生前表现

在宫内发育第八周，中肾可以产生胎尿。一旦这一暂时性的肾脏结构退化以后，就由后肾产生尿液，并且一直持续整个宫内发育阶段。在妊娠12周内，肾功能足以完成钠的重吸收和尿素的浓缩工作。到妊娠12周时，胎儿肾脏产生尿液的速度达到50 ml/h[94]。羊水总数也由这些胎尿来维持，直至16周时，羊水总量能够保持在一个稳定的水平。因此，如果有足够的尿液分泌，就可以在妊娠第16～20周进行母体-胎儿超声检查[98]。大多数医疗中心在进行母体-胎儿超声检查过程中，可以在妊娠第17～19周探查到正常的肾脏，而对于集合系统明显扩张的肾脏，则可以早在第12～14周时检出[9]。

第一个产前检查发现尿路畸形的报告是在1970年发布的[38]。从那时起，美国医学生物疗效委员会超声协会认为胎儿超声筛查是安全的[2]。而这一结论的提出使得产科医生在这方面进行了大量的临床实践，也使得公众对此产生了极大的热情，从而开展了在妊娠中期三个月进行超声筛查的工作。尽管在美国现有的情况下，有关母体-胎儿超声检查的操作方案还在不断改进中，但还是在很大程度上依赖并沿用以往特定的惯例，并且根据各个机构的具体情况来进行检查[73]。

在产前超声检查广泛应用以前，大多数婴儿和学龄儿童都是在出现明显的尿路症状和体征以后才获得诊断；如今，绝大多数新生儿患儿都是通过产前检查获得诊断的。超声可以查出异常的解剖情况，但其对一些特殊的疾病过程没有特异性。超声检查中支持UPJ梗阻的特点包括：（1）单侧或有时有双侧的肾盂扩张；（2）羊水量正常；（3）没有明确的对侧输尿管扩张表现；（4）膀胱壁厚度正常，轮廓正常。在具有典型肾盂积水临床表现的病例中，UPJ的诊断会比较直观。而更多见的情况是，在新生儿早期的影像学诊断中，区分真性梗阻性尿路疾病和一过性肾盂积水是十分复杂的工作。此外，有时在产前区分UPJ梗阻和多囊性肾发育不良也会有困难，需要进行连续的肾脏超声检查和其他作为补充手段的放射影像学检查进行随访。

胎儿泌尿学协会（SFU）组织制定了对不同程度肾盂积水进行分级的指导纲要（表111-1）（图111-4A到D）[29,72]。一旦胎儿符合这些诊断标准，医生就应当考虑到UPJ梗阻引起肾盂积水的可能性，并且将相关情况告知患儿父母。对于男性胎儿来说，如果发现为双侧肾盂积水，那么就基本上不考虑UPJ梗阻，这是因为与双肾积水相对应的有可能是一个完全不同而且更为紧急的膀胱出口梗阻疾病，比如由后尿道瓣膜引起的双肾积水。

表 111-1　胎儿泌尿协会的肾盂积水分级

SFU 分级	描述
1	肾脏中部结构轻度分离，不涉及肾盏，肾实质正常
2	肾脏中部结构分离，累及未扩张的肾盏
3	肾盂明显分离扩张，超出肾脏边缘，肾盏不规则扩张，肾实质正常
4	肾盏变大、扩张（可向外突出）；肾实质变薄，小于或等于同侧（正常）肾脏厚度的 50%

产前咨询

应当告知患儿父母肾盂积水的假设诊断，并给予适当忠告。教育和沟通在整个产前咨询过程中极为必要。绝大多数产前检测到的泌尿生殖系统异常都不需要进行产后外科干预[11,107]。事实上，仅仅有 1%~25% 的患儿在 4 年的随访中需要外科治疗[71,96]。因此，要极力建议父母在产前与产后向小儿泌尿科医生咨询。继发于梗阻的单侧肾盂积水，其实际存活率为 100%。这种单侧肾盂积水的预后非常理想，为了达到这一效果，产后随访十分必要，以便跟踪肾盂积水的进程，同时与患儿家庭一起建立治疗守则。也正是因为这个原因，要向患儿父母极力推荐到小儿泌尿科医生处。 1726

产后表现

UPJ 梗阻的患儿症状各异，如发作性的腰痛或腹

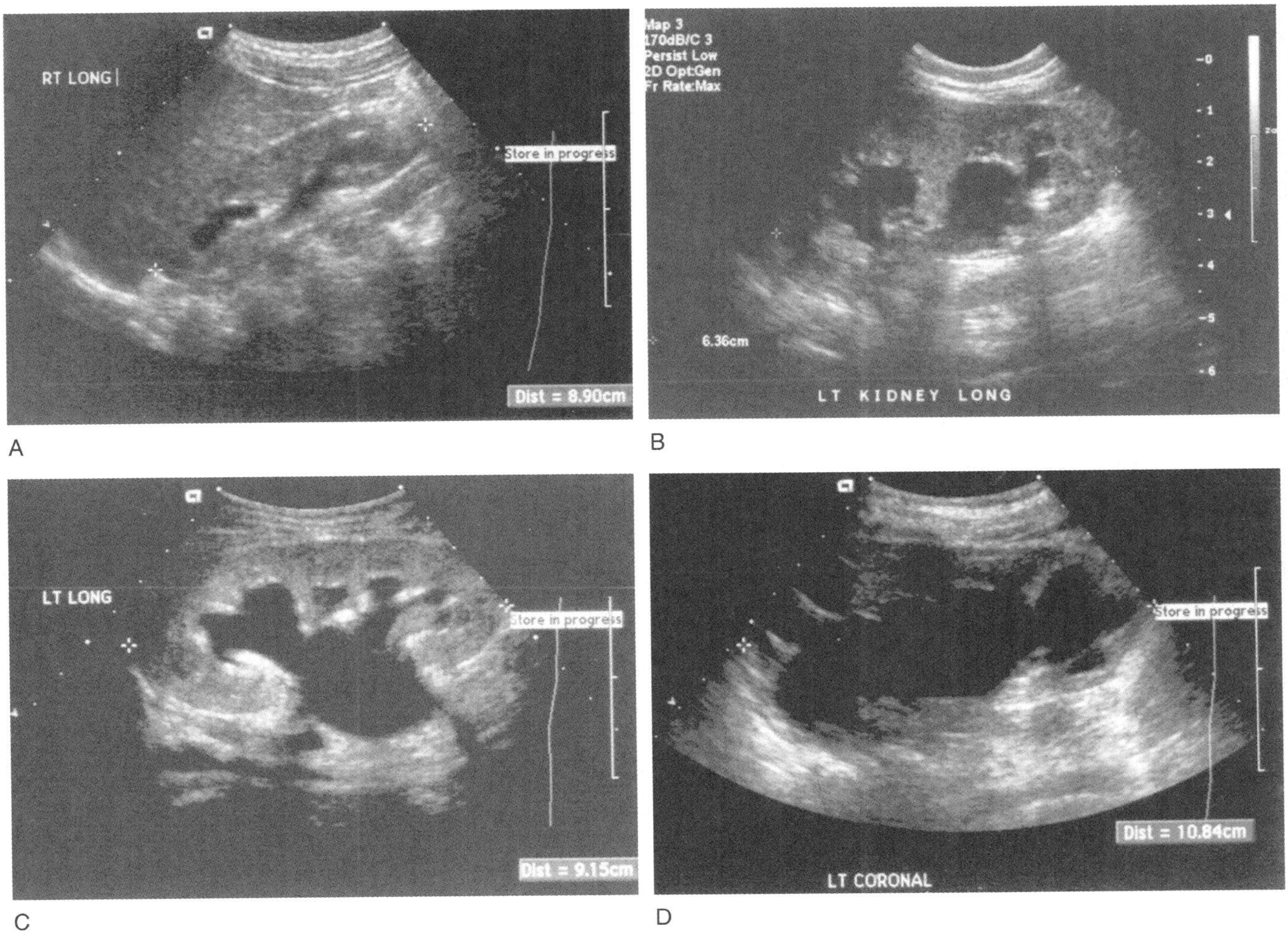

图 111-4　由胎儿泌尿协会提供的肾脏超声扫描分级方案。A. 肾盂积水 SFU 分级 1 级。B. 肾盂积水 SFU 分级 2 级。C. 肾盂积水 SFU 分级 3 级。D. 肾盂积水 SFU 分级 4 级。（Courtesy of Children's Hospital & Regional Medical Center，Seattle.）

痛以及尿路感染等。比较典型的表现是与 Dietl 危象相关联的周期性腹痛，常常伴有呕吐。在对性质不清的胃肠道疾病进行全面评估以后，就应当想到可能会有 UPJ 梗阻。结石可能会伴发于 UPJ 梗阻，事实上，UPJ 梗阻伴发肾结石的发生率是静脉尿路造影检查无症状人群的 17 倍[67]。血尿有可能是 UPJ 梗阻的最初表现。在轻微创伤后，扩张的集合系统中脆弱的黏膜血管会发生破裂出血。一些 UPJ 梗阻患儿有隐袭起病的表现，出现多年的食欲减退，生长缓慢。这些患儿一般多发现有左侧的 UPJ 梗阻。扩张的肾盂表现为肿块压迫胃部的特征，出现早期与过饱相关的食欲减退
1727 和呕吐。还有一些儿童表现为难以理解的尿脓毒症。Snyder 等曾经报道，UPJ 梗阻的患儿在度过新生儿时期后，有 30% 以尿路感染为首发症状[105]。

诊断

由于肾盂积水涉及范围很广，制定一系列鉴别诊断具有实际作用。其中一种方法是建立肾盂积水分型，比如梗阻型与非梗阻型。梗阻型肾盂积水的原因包括 UPJ 梗阻（发病率 44%）、UVJ 梗阻（发病率 21%）、多囊性肾发育不良、输尿管囊肿、集合系统重复畸形（发病率 12%）、后尿道瓣膜（发病率 9%）、异位输尿管、尿道闭锁、骶尾部畸胎瘤、子宫阴道积液。非梗阻型肾盂积水的原因包括 VUR（14%）、生理性扩张、梅干腹综合征（prune-belly syndrome）、肾囊性疾病、巨肾盏病（表 111-2）[77,92]。

表 111-2　肾盂积水的鉴别诊断

梗阻	非梗阻
肾盂输尿管连接部梗阻	膀胱输尿管反流
输尿管膀胱连接部梗阻	生理性扩张
多囊性肾发育不良	梅干腹综合征
输尿管囊肿	肾囊性疾病
集合系统重复	巨肾盏症
后尿道瓣膜	
异位输尿管	
尿道闭锁	
骶尾部畸胎瘤	
子宫阴道积液	

常规检查诊断 UPJ 梗阻并不困难，而诊断有明确意义的 UPJ 梗阻对于婴儿来说还有一定的难度。尽管有新的诊断方法对梗阻肾脏的特征进行定量评价，并且能够检查出异常的解剖结构，但是这些结果还不能同梗阻的程度以及肾脏进行性恶化的潜在进程有必然的相关性。在目前的影像学检查手段中，还没有任何一种能够准确评估有潜在梗阻可能的肾脏是不是有进行性的肾功能丧失。由于这些限制，在临床工作中可以采用几种相关的放射学检查方法，从生理学角度诊断那些可能需要进行外科干预的明显的 UPJ 梗阻。

静脉尿路造影

静脉尿路造影（IVU）是尿路疾病诊断中的一种非侵入性的放射学手段。作为一种影像学检查，对于肾功能和梗阻程度来说，它可以将解剖形态和功能信息结合起来。对超声检查中不明确的解剖情况比较有用，但在通常情况下，IVU 已经不太用于评价梗阻性尿路疾病的儿科患者。本文的叙述只是将这种方法作为补充手段。

尽管超声检查和同位素检查在很大程度上替代了 IVU，但是 IVU 在 UPJ 梗阻的诊断中还是有其特有的长处[97]。肾梗阻可以通过以下情况得到诊断上的提示：造影剂延迟显影或不显影、排出延迟、肾影轮廓变圆、造影剂稀释或者皮质系统变薄。在选择的患者中，如果病史上有矛盾或者检查结果不确切，可以进行大剂量的 IVU 检查来模拟一种满负荷的状态。在条件选择正确的情况下，可以获得优质的放射学图像，对一些患者可以明确诊断。

IVU 检查存在一些缺点。在新生儿病例中不作为首选，主要是因为这一阶段的肾功能还不成熟，即使是正常的肾脏，在出生后 4～6 周时，还不能完成尿液的酸化和浓缩功能。因此，IVU 检查时使用的静脉造影剂在新生儿肾脏中的显像能力很差。与其他类似的肾功能检查方法一样，IVU 很难鉴别患儿是处于脱水状态还是肾功能低下。

肾脏超声

肾脏超声的应用已经广泛普及，费用相对低廉，无创安全，无放射性，能够了解较多的解剖上的图像

信息。这些突出的优点使得超声检查能够广泛地应用于母体-胎儿和出生后的影像学诊断。也正因为超声的广泛应用，使得产前和产后尿路扩张的诊断率得到了提高。事实上，对于产前发现的肾盂积水来说，出生后最常用的首选检查手段就是肾脏超声。超声检查也是出生后发热性尿路感染的标准检查方法之一。肾脏超声在肾盂积水诊断中的准确率很高，能够提供 UPJ 梗阻的准确信息，包括肾盂扩张和肾盏扩张、对侧输尿管不扩张、正常充盈和排空的膀胱以及正常的膀胱壁厚度。在单侧肾盂积水病例中，超声检查可以看到患侧肾实质与对侧相比出现萎缩表现。

25 年前，小儿泌尿科医生之间达成共识，肾盂积水的量与梗阻的程度之间不存在相关性。Ransley 和同事最终确定了这一共识[96]。其研究发现，在肾盂最大前后径不超过 10 mm，并且没有肾盏和肾锥体扩张（SFU 分级为 1 级的肾盂积水）的新生儿和婴儿病例中，很少出现肾盂积水进行性加重和肾功能变差。在所有最初为非手术组但最终需要手术治疗的患者中，其产前肾盂前后径都超过了 12 mm。然而，他们也发现肾盂直径并不是一个用于预后的理想的阳性指
28 标，因为在研究中仅有 34% 的达标患者需要进行肾盂整形手术。在这些患者中，这种轻度的肾盂积水可能只是生理性的，由胎儿肾盂顺应性较高的自然特征所引起。对于肾外型肾盂的表现需要进行慎重考虑，有些病例可能会被误诊为病理性肾盂积水（图 111-5A 和 B）。有肾外型肾盂表现的患者一般都不伴有肾盏扩张，此时应当考虑为一种正常情况。

Koff 和其同事们建议采用序列化的超声检查来预测单侧 UPJ 梗阻是否进展[61]。除了能够监测 UPJ 梗阻的一过性发作，使用序列化的超声可以检测肾脏轴向生长的情况，作为 UPJ 梗阻是否进展的指标。在单侧 UPJ 梗阻的患者中，对侧正常肾脏的生长速度可以间接反映梗阻的情况[62]。应用肾脏生长-功能曲线时，对侧正常肾脏出现代偿性肥大，这种情况可能表明单侧的肾梗阻是进行性加重的。反过来说，如果对侧正常肾脏出现生长缓慢的表现（代偿性萎缩），则提示患侧梗阻肾脏的功能在迅速恢复，甚至超过正常，意味着不存在梗阻。然而由于操作者测量肾脏长度的方法并不统一，导致 Koff 的数据还没有得到验证。

无论哪一种 UPJ 梗阻的处理规范，序列化的超声检查都是一个十分重要的工具，但其中也存在问题，主要是因为检查间期需要等待一段时间，而在这段时间里肾脏的损伤可能会持续发生。比如肾皮质变薄，这一指标十分重要，但往往比较晚才发现。与比较少见的广泛的肾皮质变薄相比，局灶性的肾皮质丧失更加容易查出。受到 Koff 及其同事们研究的影响[61]，现在习惯上认为对单侧肾盂积水的患者来说，对侧肾脏代偿性的增生可能会是肾盂积水病变持续进展的危险指标[61]。不过，要对肾脏增生作出可行的超声诊断，需要对肾脏长度和容量进行连续的随访测定，这样就会限制超声对早期干预的指导作用[19]。

肾脏超声对肾盂积水的诊断十分准确，然而就像其他许多检查手段一样，也有其局限性。超声不能对梗阻作出诊断，主要是因为肾盂积水的程度既不能说

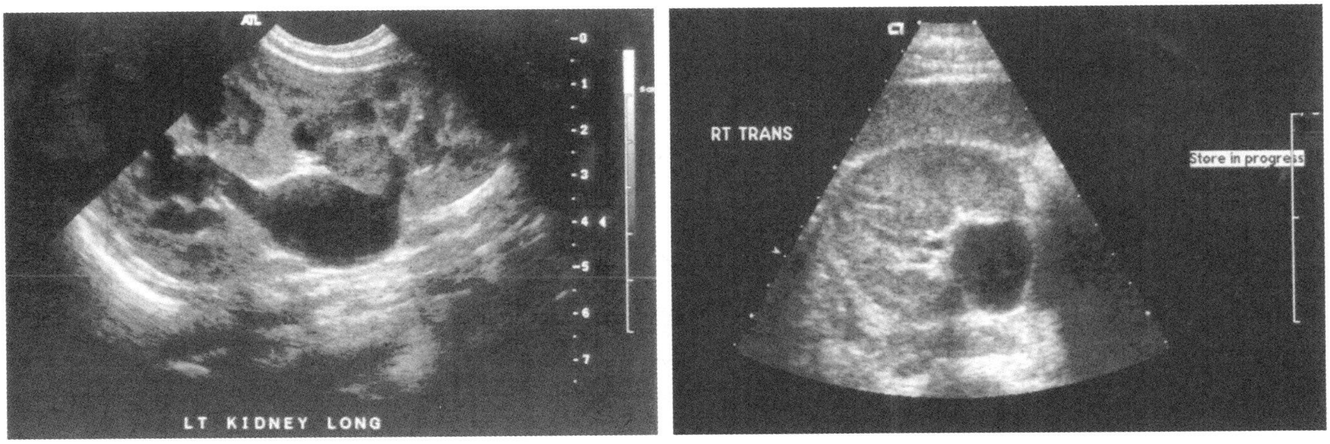

A B

图 111-5 A. 肾脏超声检查发现伴有肾内型肾盂的肾盂输尿管连接部梗阻。B. 肾脏超声检查所见非梗阻型肾外型肾盂。(Courtesy of Children's Hospital & Regional Medical Center, Seattle.)

明是否存在梗阻，也不能预测肾盂积水是否能够缓解[60]。这一特点在新生儿中尤其明显，因为此时肾盂积水可以是一过性的，同时也可能与小儿的水化状态和膀胱的充盈程度有关。进一步说，超声检查不能够提供与肾功能相关的任何信息。

锝 99m 肾脏核素扫描

分肾功能是对明显的梗阻进行功能性诊断的最为重要的检查参数，同时也是预测先天性 UPJ 梗阻外科治疗最佳时机的指标。肾脏核素扫描是评价总肾功能和分肾功能的检查手段之一。肾脏核素扫描主要使用三种放射性药物，其特性与其各自的生物学活性相关。锝 99-二乙基三胺五乙酸（^{99m}Tc-DTPA）和锝 99-巯基乙酰三甘油（^{99m}Tc-MAG-3）主要是在肾脏内浓聚，并可以从肾小球自由滤过[54]。DTPA 在肾小管内既不被分泌，也不被重吸收，而 MAG-3 是由肾小管分泌的。由于每一种试剂几乎都能被完全排泄，所以它们可用于检测分肾功能和尿液引流情况。第三种试剂是锝 99-二巯基丁二酸（^{99m}Tc-DMSA），可以与肾小管细胞紧密结合，因此可以用于检测分肾功能，以及检测临床上明显的肾皮质病变，如肾瘢痕。

目前至少已经发表了三份具有代表意义的方案， 172
以缩小临床使用的各种指导的分歧：核医学协会针对小儿利尿性肾图提出的核医学操作指南、缓和性利尿性肾图以及利尿性肾图委员会在第九届放射核素协会会议上关于肾脏泌尿学方面达成的共识[17,18,84]。所有这些在方法上都基本相同，在结果解释上也相似。从原则上说，一个没有明显梗阻存在的集合系统，在注射呋塞米（速尿）后的清除半衰期（也就是放射性药物制剂排出一半所需的时间）小于 10 分钟。如果超过 20 分钟就可以认为是异常的，存在有高级别的梗阻。清除半衰期介于 10 分钟和 20 分钟之间则认为是不明确的。半衰期不能被看做是判断梗阻的唯一标准。在大多数检查中，对结果的解释还需要结合其他可以得到的数据，如曲线分析和分肾功能，当然还要联系临床具体情况（图 111-6）。

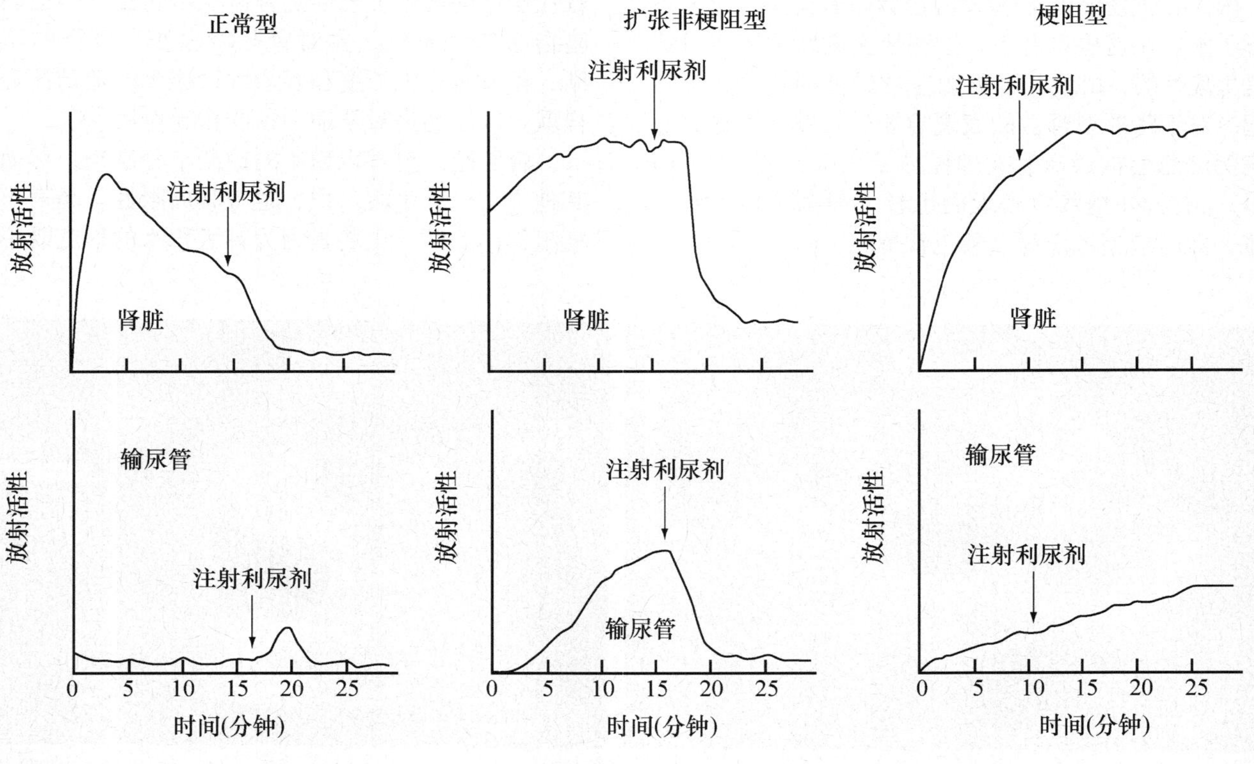

图 111-6　利尿性肾扫描的典型表现：正常、扩张非梗阻和梗阻[63]。（From Fung LCT, Lakshmanan Y: Anomalies of the renal collecting system: Ureteropelvic junction obstruction [pyelocalyectasis] and infundibular stenosis. In Belman AB, King LR, Kramer SA [eds]: Clinical Pediatric Urology, 4th ed. London, Martin Dunitz, 2002, p 594.）

肾图检查目前已经成为判断 UPJ 梗阻引起功能异常的最常用检查，主要是因为在其他检查中表现为严重肾盂积水（SFU 分级 3 或 4 级）的大多数病例，在利尿性肾图中可以反映出梗阻[72,111]。根据这些检查结果，由^{99m}Tc-DTPA 和^{99m}Tc-MAG-3 肾扫描测定的分肾功能可以作为决定是否需要进行外科手术干预的判断标准[23]。35% 的分肾功能对于决定是继续观察还是干预治疗非常重要。如果新生儿第一次检查时患侧的分肾功能大于 35%，那么该患儿可以继续保守观察，每三个月进行一次超声检查。相反，如果第一次检查时分肾功能小于 35%，或者同位素扫描复查时功能下降达到 10%[40]，那么就应当考虑进行外科干预治疗。

肾脏闪烁扫描法是评价总肾和分肾功能的检查手段之一，但不用于肾功能不全或肾功能不成熟以及集合系统非常扩张的患者。其他影响肾脏闪烁扫描法检查的因素包括地方习惯、检查时间、水合状态、膀胱充盈程度、蓄积效应、操作类型、肾脏对利尿剂的反应以及对肾功能超常概念的理解（图 111-7）[17,18,36,81,83,108]。肾功能超常指的是单侧肾盂积水患儿的积水肾脏分肾功能超过 55%。目前还不能够确定这种分肾功能超

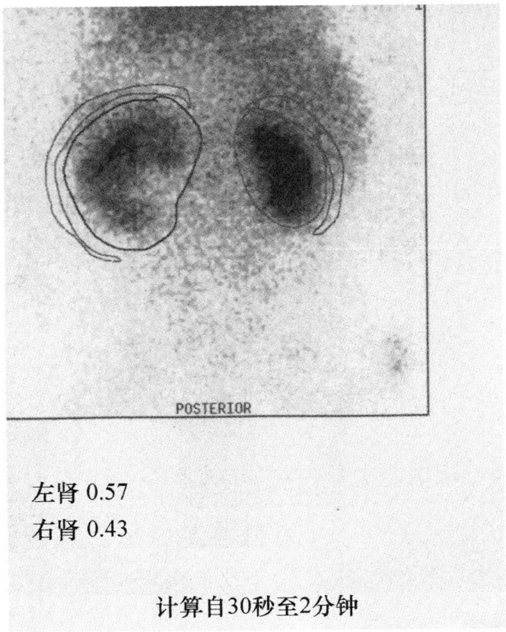

图 111-7　MAG-3 肾脏闪烁扫描：6 个月婴儿肾功能异常。该患儿产前超声检查发现有 SFU 分级 4 级肾盂积水，产后证实有高级别的左肾盂输尿管连接部梗阻。（Courtesy of Children's Hospital & Regional Medical Center, Seattle.）

常现象是真实的还是人为的，而且目前也没有对这种患者的治疗达成共识。Oh 及其同事对肾功能超常的受试者进行检查，认为这种患侧梗阻肾脏的功能超常现象可能不是真正意义上的高功能，而仅仅是对慢性梗阻的一种病理性代偿机制[83]。因为这一原因，Oh 告诫说，对分肾功能进行判断时应当警惕这种情况。Khan 及其同事认为肾功能超常是一种人为现象，可以通过应用 MAG-3 和使用合适的计算机软件进行多 1730
种算法计算等手段来避免[57]。

排尿性膀胱尿道造影

众所周知，VUR 是儿童最常见的下尿路疾病，可以与儿童最常见的上尿路疾病 UPJ 梗阻伴随出现[68]。这种伴发关系的确切原因目前还不了解[8]。不过现在已经知道大约有 9%～14% 的 UPJ 梗阻患者同时存在 VUR。反之，在 VUR 患者中，有 1% 发现同时存在 UPJ 梗阻。这些伴随关系发生的概率虽然很低，但是能够影响肾脏的功能，改变治疗方案。因此，不论年龄大小以及性别差异，排尿性膀胱尿道造影（VCUG）是临床上评价所有产前肾盂积水婴儿的标准方法[28,47]。

近来一些研究者对这一标准提出了质疑[119]。在一个回顾性调查中，有 106 个患者因 UPJ 梗阻而接受了肾盂整形手术，伴发于 UPJ 梗阻的低级别反流在肾盂整形术后自行消退。此外，伴发于 UPJ 梗阻的所有高级别反流都很容易通过肾脏超声检出。他们总结出 VCUG 这种检查应当仅仅限用于 UPJ 梗阻伴有超声检查显示输尿管扩张的患者。在评价这种处于两难境地的患儿时需要特别谨慎，对于这种情况的处理十分微妙，同时也很复杂。以前有报告提出产前肾盂积水和 VUR 有人种间的差别，Horowitz 与其他人证实了这一点[4,47,66]。黑人产前肾盂积水的婴儿没有 VUR 发生，而在非黑色人种中的发生率则为 17.6%，提示 VCUG 这种检查对于黑色人种不应当视为常规检查，而在非黑色人种中还是一项标准检查。

到目前为止，VUR 的主要检查手段还是标准的放射学 VCUG 检查。这是一项有痛苦并且有创的检查方法，对某些病例来说存在着生理上的不准确性。20 多年前，人们尝试了一些替代方法。Hofmann 提出一种实时的超声学检查方法，以替代检查 VUR 时所用

的 VCUG[44]。尽管这一方法在欧洲取得了成功，但在美洲还是没有得到推广。近来的一些报告提出采用其他方法来减少评估儿童 VUR 时所需要的辐射量，包括直接的核素放射学排尿性膀胱造影以及回波放大的排尿性超声造影检查[55]。这些方法都有其优点和缺点，彼此不能够完全互相替代，而且也没有一个具有与标准 VCUG 相同的效果。

核磁共振尿路造影

最近，动态钆增强核磁共振尿路造影技术（Gd-MRU）因其无电离辐射和无可比拟的三维影像而得到推崇。Wen 等人在大鼠中应用 Gd-DTPA 增强的 MR 成像，发现这种技术能够鉴别出梗阻和非梗阻的集合系统病变[117]。最近 Kirsch 应用类似技术，对 200 个接受过 Gd-MRU 系统评估的肾盂积水患儿进行了队列研究[58,87]。与超声和肾脏闪烁扫描相比，Gd-MRU 能够提供更为清晰的泌尿生殖系统解剖影像和极好的空间分辨率（图 111-8）。这种检查结果比较稳定，可重复性高，线性回归系数为 0.99。这一检查也有其局限性，通常需要在全麻或使用镇静剂的条件下进行，在图像的处理上也比较麻烦[45]。尽管这一技术目前还没有得到广泛应用，但 MRU 已经被认为是针对 UPJ 梗阻患者的较为可信的检查手段，包括解剖和功能上的诊断[58]。

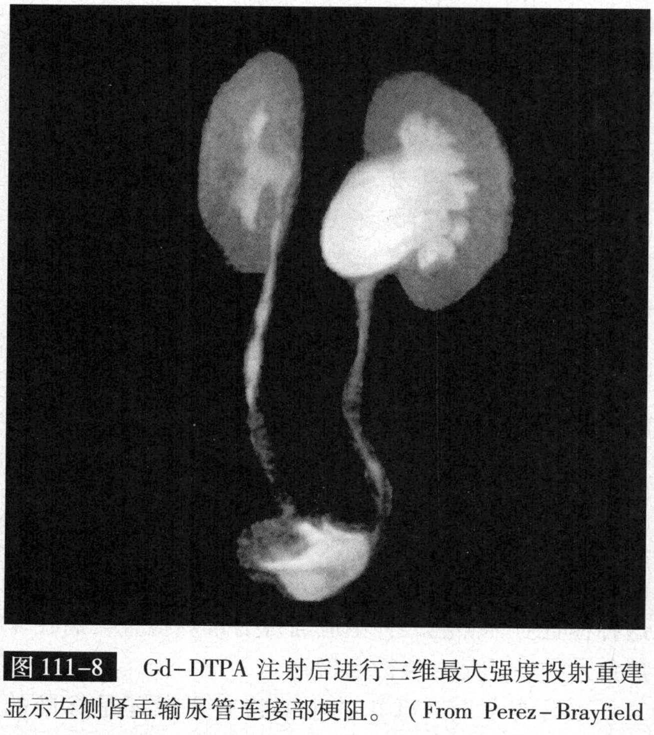

图 111-8 Gd-DTPA 注射后进行三维最大强度投射重建显示左侧肾盂输尿管连接部梗阻。（From Perez-Brayfield MR, Kirsch AJ, Jones RA, Grattan-Smith JD: A prospective study comparing ultrasound, nuclear scintigraphy and dynamic contrast-enhanced magnetic resonance imaging in the evaluation of hydronephrosis. J Urol 2003；170：1331.）

逆行肾盂造影

这种放射影像学检查手段目前已经很少应用于 UPJ 梗阻的临床诊断。在 108 例接受肾盂整形的患儿中，没有一个患儿因为逆行肾盂造影（RPG）检查而改变外科手术的方式或既定的手术方案[100]。然而在开放性肾盂整形手术前仍然经常进行逆行肾盂造影检查。在诊断过程中，往往很难得到有关 UPJ 与其他解剖结构之间的精确定位信息。因此，为了比较准确地定位

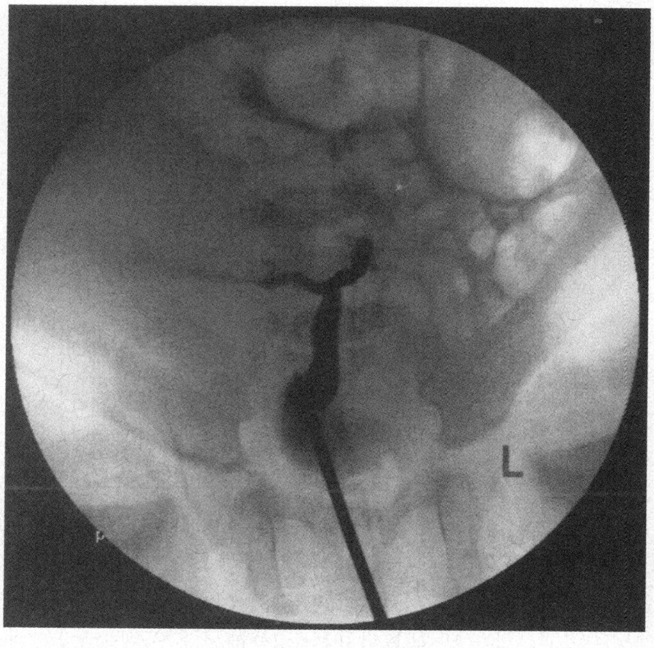

图 111-9 右侧逆行性肾盂输尿管造影显示右侧肾盂输尿管连接部梗阻，可见吹风样的造影剂进入扩张的肾盂。注意近端输尿管与扩张肾盂的偏差。（Courtesy of Byron Joyner, MD, Children's Hospital & Regional Medical Center, Seattle.）

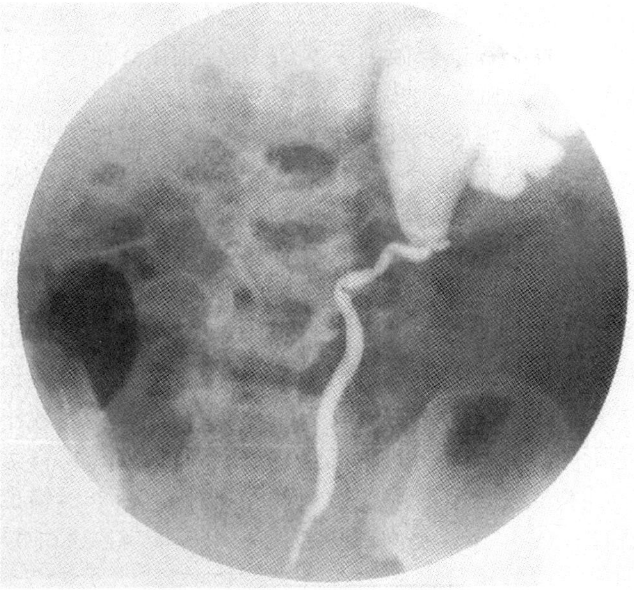

图 111-10　术前逆行性左侧肾盂输尿管造影显示匐行的肾盂输尿管连接部梗阻。左髂嵴与脊椎可作为定位切口的标志。(Courtesy of Richard Grady, MD, Children's Hospital & Regional Medical Center, Seattle.)

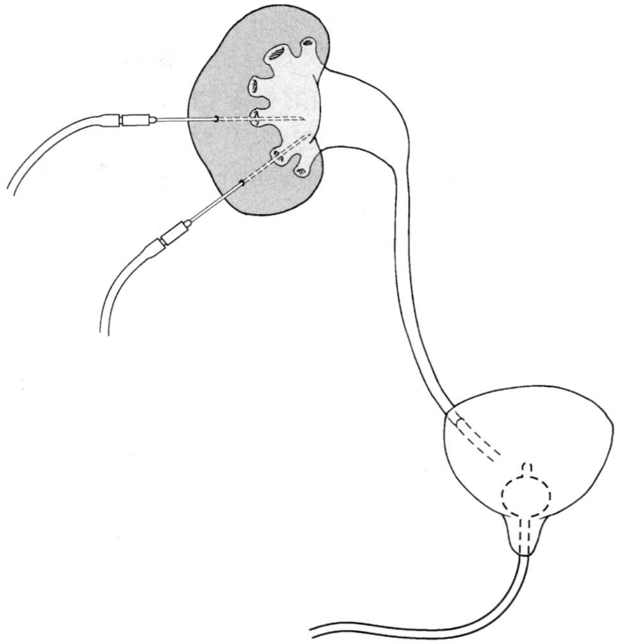

图 111-11　Whitaker 压力灌注试验。(From Fung LCT, Lakshmanan Y: Anomalies of the renal collecting system: Ureteropelvic junction obstruction [pyelocalyectasis] and infundibular stenosis. In Belman AB, King LR, Kramer SA [eds]: Clinical Pediatric Urology, 4th ed. London, Martin Dunitz, 2002, p 596.)

梗阻位置，以及排除潜在远端梗阻的可能性，可以进
31 行逆行肾盂造影检查（图 111-9 和图 111-10）[51]。

压力-流量测定

灌注激发试验最初由 Bäcklund 等人于 1965 年提出，后来由 Whitaker 于 1973 年推广。这是一项标准的压力流量研究，也简称为 Whitaker 试验（图 111-11）[5,118]。该试验可以检测输尿管在已知流率时的阻力，用肾盂和膀胱之间所自发产生的压力差来表示。试验结果不受肾脏 GRF 的影响，而且同期的顺行性肾盂造影能够较好地提供可疑梗阻段的解剖定位。当其他检查无法确定肾盂积水是否由梗阻引起时，则可利用这项检查提供帮助。这一试验的理论前提是梗阻限制了尿液的流动。因此当利尿出现时，肾盂压力就会增加。所以，不论在何种利尿速率下，相对膀胱压力明显增高的肾盂压力可以反映梗阻的存在。在 10 ml/min 流速的条件下，肾盂和膀胱的压力差小于 13 cmH_2O，则可以认为是正常。压力差在 14～20 cmH_2O 之间，则认为是轻度梗阻；压力差超过 35 cmH_2O 为明显梗阻。

进行 Whitaker 试验时，需要经皮肾盂穿刺，而且小儿患者往往需要全麻，因此在常规检查中不易被接受。这一试验一般仅在梗阻诊断不明确时才会应用，因而
很少应用于临床。此外，Whitaker 试验需要有严格的 1732
操作规范和精确的测量，以防止技术上的误差。近来，有人对 Whitaker 试验作了更接近生理的改进，用压力水平代替灌注速率并保持恒定，以更好地对 UPJ 梗阻进行分类[116]。从功能上讲，压力流量试验对于流速变量不敏感。正常肾盂压力小于 7 cmH_2O，在正常输尿管蠕动时，肾盂压力甚至可以小于 0。因此，如果在 7 cmH_2O 或以下的压力水平时没有产生尿流，则反映流出阻力增加，提示有梗阻存在。

生物化学标志物

输尿管梗阻在临床和实验研究中都可以导致细胞水平的肾脏损伤[39,89]。这样的研究结果使得研究人

员想到是否有可能存在着一类生物化学标志物，可以预测肾盂内压力增高者的产后肾功能情况，比如某些UPJ梗阻的病例[82]。预期的标志物包括尿钠、钙和β_2-微球蛋白。其他的一些生物化学标志物还在不断发现之中。近来，有研究表明集合系统压力持续上升能够诱发肾脏的异常改变，包括小管压力增加、肾血流减少、GFR降低以及肾小管功能紊乱[15,37]。Fung和Atala在非梗阻猪动物模型中做了相关研究，使其尿液流出需要克服预设的压力梯度，研究发现一种反映急性肾细胞损伤的标志物——N-乙酰-β-右旋氨基葡萄糖苷酶出现了进行性升高[34]。其他类似的研究发现，由压力诱导的肾功能紊乱和肾脏细胞损伤可能是相互依赖的过程[15,41]。其他很多在临床和实验研究中所涉及的生化标志物都与梗阻性尿路疾病的病理发生有关，而且可能作为预测肾脏疾病预后的标志物，包括尿液中的单核细胞趋化肽1（MCP-1）和表皮生长因子（EGF）、转化因子β（TGF-β）、尿液α_1-微球蛋白，以及p53和p21（WAF-1）表达[27,42,50,78]。梗阻性尿路疾病的生化标志物——尤其是针对UPJ梗阻——至今还没有完全明确，把它们作为肾功能的预测指标还不可信。由于缺乏测量肾梗阻的标准的生化和生理标志物，所以对于可疑的UPJ梗阻患者，还必须进行一系列放射学检查，以评估肾脏的功能和解剖形态。

术前血管造影

在病史采集和基本的放射学检查后，一旦确定了UPJ梗阻的诊断，通常需要考虑是否有下极迷行血管引起梗阻病变的可能性。这一特殊的解剖变异在年长儿童和成人UPJ梗阻中十分重要，因为这种情况可能影响外科手术方式的选择。

UPJ梗阻中迷行血管的发生率在文献报道中差别较大，从11%到79%，主要与描述UPJ梗阻的定义不同有关[52,112]。肾下极血管从邻近的UPJ处横跨称为“迷行血管”。一般认为，迷行血管主要是加重梗阻病变，而不是诱发梗阻[75]。如果在内镜手术前没有认识到这一情况，那么迷行血管的存在就会增加术后并发症的发生机会。有些影像学检查有助于判断迷行血管的存在，包括数字减影动脉血管造影、螺旋CT、增强彩色多普勒检查、腔内超声以及核磁共振血管造影。血管造影对检查下极迷行血管十分重要，尤其是对准备进行微创手术的UPJ梗阻患者[56]。已有针对迷行血管的回顾性综述发表[113]。

对小儿泌尿外科医生来说，有关术前血管造影检查判断迷行血管的问题还存在争议。对大多数UPJ梗阻的患儿来说，外科处理方法为开放手术、腹腔镜手术或机器人手术，而不是肾盂内切开，如果盲目使用这种方式，将不可避免地造成迷行血管损伤。到目前为止，小儿泌尿内腔镜手术的应用出于以下原因而受到限制：（1）现有的泌尿内腔镜设备大小还不适用于3岁以下的儿童；（2）大多数小儿外科医生所接受的训练是进行开放的离断式肾盂整形术，腹腔镜手术在合适的情况下是一个不错的选择；（3）开放手术和腹腔镜手术都能够在术中辨别出前位的迷行血管。

处理

尽管产前超声和众多的产后检查已经得到了广泛应用，但目前对UPJ梗阻的自然病程还不是很清楚。对单侧肾盂积水的治疗不能仅仅根据B超检查中肾盂扩张的程度，也不能基于利尿性肾图中有无梗阻[64,111]。一些调查者提出，在所有产前肾盂积水病例中，有近50%～80%可以在随访过程中自然缓解[21,43]。其余的在三年随访过程中出现进行性肾盂积水加重，同时有肾功能的降低[31]。目前还不清楚造成这些不同结局的原因是什么。由于缺乏对UPJ梗阻自然病程的了解，致使目前对这一疾病的治疗已经分为两个学派：观察等待和早期干预。

对于单侧疑似UPJ梗阻的轻度肾盂积水（肾盂扩张，但无肾盏扩张）患者来说，在处理上没有很大的分歧，这类患者的长期并发症发生率相对较低，一般不需要进行外科干预。同样，在对严重肾盂积水（肾盂肾盏扩张，并伴有肾皮质变薄）的处理上，目前的意见也比较一致，有肾功能降低、感染和有症状时，均提示需要进行外科治疗[98]。此外对双侧UPJ梗阻患者的处理也是统一的，本章不做具体描述。目前对UPJ梗阻治疗上的争议主要存在于三个方面，第一个就是中等程度的肾盂积水（肾盂肾盏扩张，不伴有肾皮质变薄），这种肾脏可能会在不出现相应肾功能损失的情况下自行好转，但也可能会出现另外一种不可预见的情况，也就是第二个方面，即不能预测在观察期间肾脏是否会逐渐变差。最后一个方面就是外科手术是否可以逆转 UPJ 梗阻导致的肾功能损伤。

密切观察

对于单侧 UPJ 梗阻的观察包括序列化的影像学检查，以及足够的细致和耐心。从目前已有的众多针对 UPJ 梗阻治疗的规范来看，已经能够说明没有任何一种方法是绝对的。不过，在一般情况下，对一个产前诊断肾盂积水的婴儿进行评估时，总的来说从直接体检和产后超声开始。体格检查能够了解小儿的生命体征、一般状况和总体情况。呼吸窘迫和呕吐在某些病例中可能是腹部肿块的伴发病症，而在多数情况下，此时的腹部肿块是没有获诊的。

产后超声应当在出生至少两天后进行，这是因为产后的相对脱水状态和生理性少尿可能会导致假阴性结果。这个规则也有例外，就是男性新生儿双侧肾盂积水伴有膀胱壁增厚，往往提示一种比较紧急的情况，如继发于后尿道瓣膜的膀胱出口梗阻。肾超声提示有 UPJ 梗阻时应当采取其他检查手段，以明确或排除梗阻的存在。进一步的影像学检查应当考虑到其他引起肾盂积水的原因，并以此为检查的选择依据，这是因为有很多情况可以出现类似肾盂积水的表现，或者在有或没有尿路梗阻的情况下出现集合系统扩张。这些情况包括生理性肾盂扩张、UPJ 梗阻、集合系统重复畸形伴有异位输尿管（或伴发输尿管囊肿）、巨输尿管、MCDK、UVJ 梗阻、后尿道瓣膜、梅干腹综合征、肾囊性疾病、肾盂旁肾囊肿以及巨肾盏病。此外，新生儿肾髓质和锥体常见的超声透过现象也可能被认为是肾盂积水，这种奇特的现象可以与肾盂积水的表现相混淆，但随着肾实质发育的成熟而逐渐消失，一般发生于出生后第三个月。超声随访没有明确的肾盂积水表现。

出生后的肾脏超声检查可以排除上述的一些诊断。对于 UPJ 梗阻来说，多个非交通性的肾盏在超声表现上并不常见，这种表现更多见于肾盂旁囊肿或 MCDK。肾盂旁囊肿在儿科患者中比较罕见，不要误认为是肾盂积水[20]。MCDK 能够通过同位素闪烁扫描法确诊，多用 DMSA 扫描，可以看到患侧肾功能丧失。

如果出生后的超声检查证实有明确的肾盂积水表现，则应当对患儿给予每天一次的预防性口服抗生素（阿莫西林，15 mg/kg）。这种疗法对有产前肾盂积水患儿来说，几乎能够完全控制尿脓毒症的发生[73]。在预防性治疗的基础上，还要通过 VCUG 检查来排除 VUR 的可能，即使出生后的超声检查没有任何异常发现，VUR 也可以发生[120]。在产前诊断为肾盂积水的患儿中，有 20% 的病例出生后超声检查呈阴性表现，这就是要对所有这些患儿进行 VCUG 检查的原因[21]。对于不伴有 VUR 的产后肾盂积水患儿是否使用预防性抗生素，目前还存在争议[33,46,115]。

外科手术

外科手术治疗 UPJ 梗阻的目的，是通过建立没有 1734
梗阻的肾盂引流来保留肾功能。对此有两种技术方案。第一种是*转移瓣技术*，利用肾盂组织来扩大狭窄的 UPJ 节段（图 111-12A 到 F）。第二种技术是*离断式肾盂整形术*，这是目前普遍应用的技术[16]，包括完全切除狭窄（功能异常）段，修剪肾盂（如果有必要的话），将肾盂和输尿管在相对应的位置进行重新吻合。这两种技术没有任何一个能够完全适用于所有可能的解剖变异。肾盂的解剖连同其他手术中的具体发现决定手术方式的选择。举例来说，当在手术
过程中证实有迷行血管时，与此对应的手术方式应当 1735
是离断式肾盂整形术，这样可以切除无动力节段，同时可以将血管放置于 UPJ 的后方。转移瓣技术在这种情况下不适用。通过制定合理的选择依据，任何一种手术方法都能够使 UPJ 梗阻的手术成功率达到或超过 90%~95%[48,76]。

在施行肾盂整形手术时，对患儿采用适当的全麻，并选择性使用局部阻滞麻醉。患儿体位摆放于俯卧切石位，以进行肾穿刺造影。尽管对此还存在争议[51]，但目前还是利用这一操作来判断病变的性质，同时帮助选择手术时的最佳暴露部位。在肾穿刺造影后放置 Foley 导尿管，重新将患儿放置于适合所选手术方式的体位。在进行开放式的肾盂整形手术时，有几种腹膜后路径可供选择，包括前肋下、腰部和腰背部。对于婴儿来说，作者选用的是前肋下肌层分开路径，这一路径可以通过较小的切口来获得良好的手术

暴露。（对大儿童来说，可以使用腰部切口来推移腹膜和较厚的肌束。）

患儿采用改良的俯卧位，患侧抬高 15～20 度角，对于年龄较小的患儿，可以将双上肢放置于一侧。手术操作台在患儿髂前上棘水平上凸弯曲，以暴露前腹壁和腰部区域。在肋下约两指宽水平，沿 Langer 线做

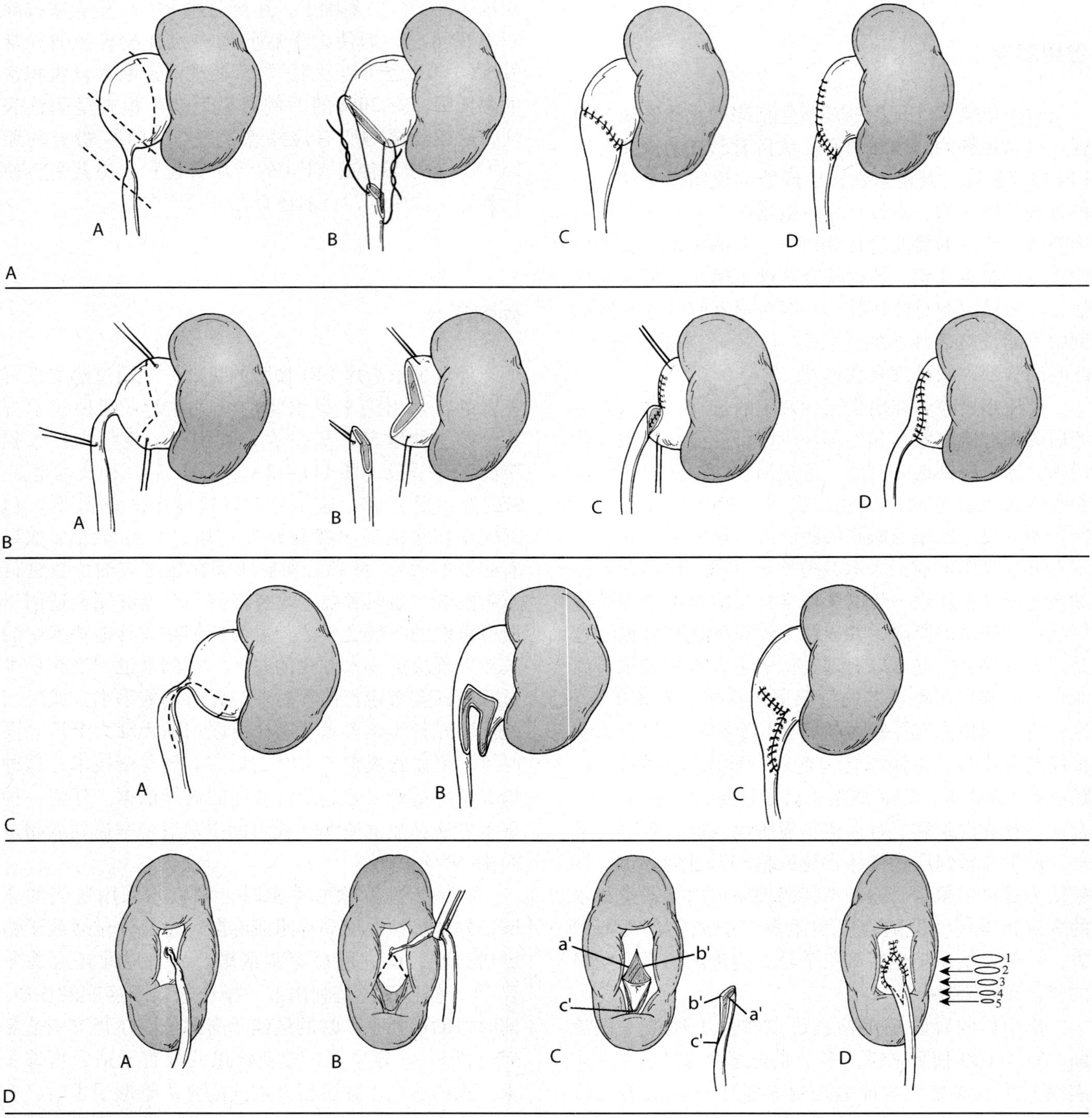

图 111-12 A. 离断式肾盂整形术。B. Anderson-Hynes 肾盂整形术。C. Foley Y-V 肾盂整形术。D. 用于治疗高位近端输尿管连接的 Foley Y-V 肾盂整形术的变化术式。

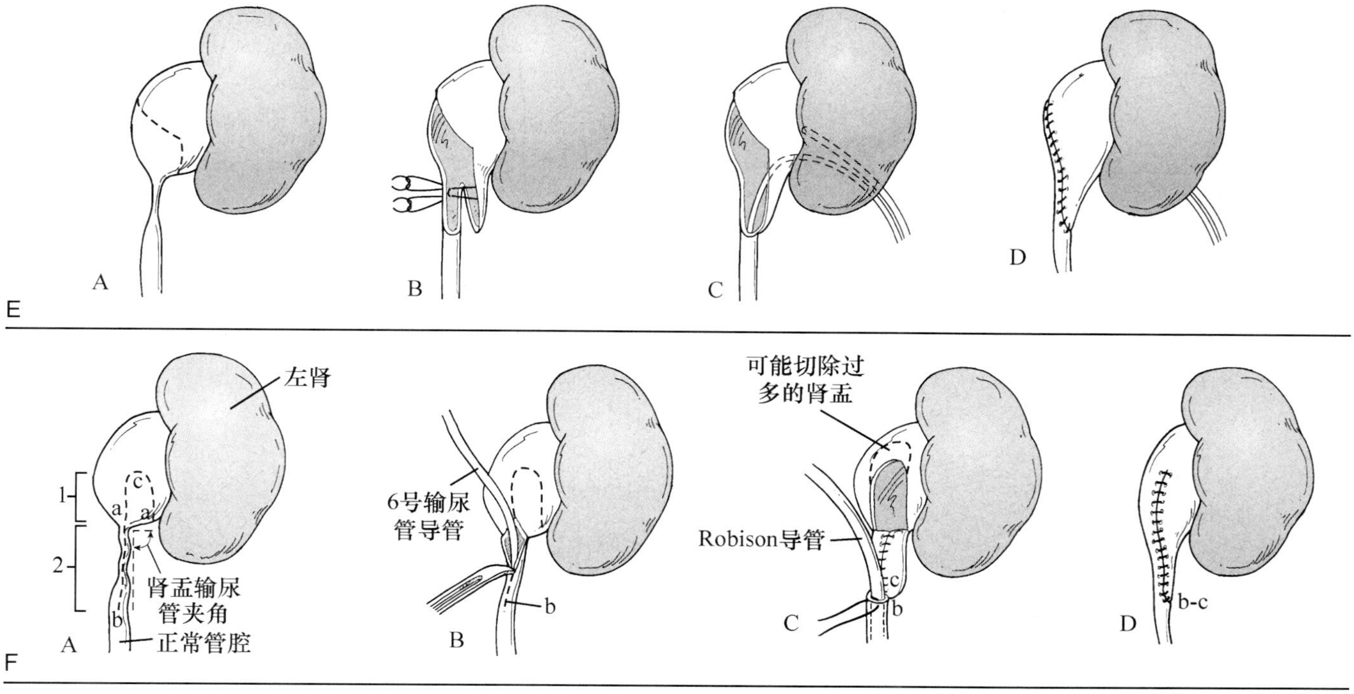

图 111-12　（续）E. 螺旋瓣。F. Scardino-Prince 垂直瓣肾盂输尿管整形术，用于长段型近端输尿管狭窄。（From Fung LCT，Lakshmanan Y：Anomalies of the renal collecting system：Ureteropelvic junction obstruction ［pyelocalyectasis］ and infundibular stenosis. In Belman AB，King LR，Kramer SA ［eds］：Clinical Pediatric Urology，4th ed. London，Martin Dunitz，2002，p 612.）

一 3～4 cm 切口。采用钝性分离方法将肌层分开，不需要切断肌肉。这种方法可以提供充分暴露，同时减少术后疼痛。将腹膜向内侧推开，垂直切开 Gerota 筋膜。使用环形自动牵开器可以很好地暴露肾脏和肾盂。

当肾脏和肾盂暴露以后，应当仔细检查组织的解剖关系，以便决定如何选择最佳的手术方式。*离断式肾盂整形术*适用于大多数 UPJ 梗阻病例。不过，有三种解剖上的异常需要采用相应的三种不同转移瓣技术：Foley Y-V 肾盂整形术、螺旋瓣技术或者是 Scardino-Prince 垂直瓣技术。第一种方法主要用于梗阻段长度超过 1.5～2 cm 者；第二种适用于肾盂较小，不需要进行肾盂修裁的患儿；最后一种方法在大多数情况下同样也可以用 Foley Y-V 方法来替代，主要用于当输尿管在较高的位置与肾盂交汇时。在这些病例中，将肾盂修裁成漏斗状，以构建成相应的引流系统。

在决定进行离断式肾盂整形术后，就应当对肾盂修裁的大小进行估计。原则上用牵引线做成“钻石”状定位，用肌腱剪刀沿牵引线边缘剪开肾盂。在剪开肾盂时，应当采用推剪的方式由上至下进行，这种方式能够使肾盂切缘轮廓平滑，有利于更好地与输尿管吻合。输尿管近端狭窄段需要向远端切除足够的长度，以达到正常健康的输尿管口径。1736
在进行输尿管与肾盂吻合之前，应当检查远端输尿管的长度，以保证吻合口处于无张力状态。肾盂输尿管的吻合从最低处开始，用 7-0 单丝可吸收缝线进行连续锁边缝合。在吻合时，要注意缝合相对较多的外膜层和较少的黏膜层，以实现不漏水吻合的目的。进行吻合时可以放置临时性的输尿管支撑管，以减少形成“靠背样”梗阻的危险。此外，也可以使用双“J”形输尿管支撑管，应用 Seldinger 方法将其植入到输尿管远端和膀胱，这种支撑管可以留置 4～6 周。

背侧腰部切开入路可以提供非常满意的暴露效果，尤其是对比较少见的双侧 UPJ 病变病例（图 111-13）。对于肋下入路，可以采用钝性分离肌肉的方法，在相对较短的距离内到达腹膜后。背侧腰部切开入路所能

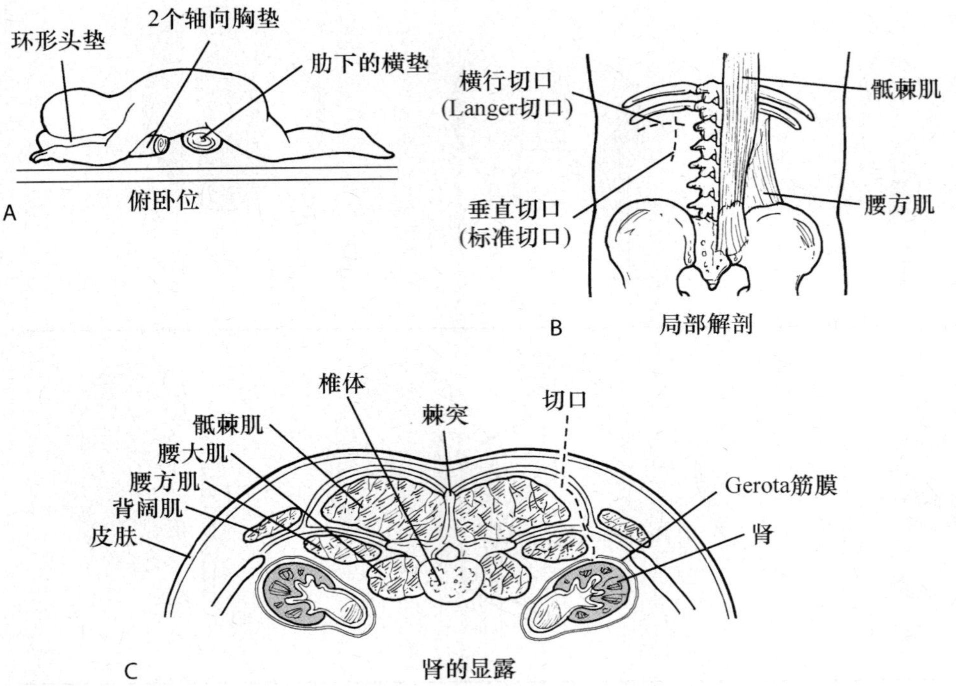

图 111-13 背侧腰部切开入路。(From Sheldon CA, Duckett JW: Infant pyeloplasty. AUA Update Series 1988; 7 [Lesson 37]: 293.)

提供的远端输尿管暴露范围有限，在实施前必须对输尿管的解剖进行准确定位。因此，在这种情况下可以采用肾盂穿刺造影。

儿童肾盂输尿管连接部梗阻的微创手术

在一些微创外科经验丰富的儿童医院，实施腹腔镜和机器人肾盂整形术是切实可行的，并且能够取得较好的效果[90]。

微创外科的指征和益处已经在成人中得到证实[79,106]。成人 UPJ 梗阻治疗的微创外科技术包括球囊扩张、经皮顺行肾盂内切开术、逆行切开线球囊法肾盂内切开术、输尿管镜逆行肾盂内切开术以及腹腔镜肾盂整形术。尽管技术上的发展使微创外科手段能够用于治疗 UPJ 梗阻患儿，但是开放式肾盂整形术依然是手术的金标准，其成功率一直都在 90% 以上[53]。

对儿童来说，微创手术选择的指征还不明确，所以泌尿内镜手术还不普遍[22]。最近一项研究比较了内镜肾盂整形术和开放式肾盂整形术治疗小儿 UPJ 梗阻，研究发现这两种方式的成功率分别为 88% 和 93%[102]。尽管在手术成功率的比较上两者差距很小，但在手术时间和住院花费上，内镜肾盂整形术要高出很多。考虑到目前的情况，利用微创外科手术治疗 UPJ 梗阻的优势不是很大。开放式肾盂整形术操作时间短，手术费用相对较少，并且具有长期效果。

小儿腹腔镜肾盂整形手术与其他儿童微创外科手术面临着同样的挑战[26]。多数小儿泌尿外科手术是重建性手术，而非破坏性手术，这使得很多操作者在提高基本的腹腔镜操作技能方面受到限制。大多数小儿外科医生都比较喜欢稳妥，同时相应的病例种类也比较少，使得微创手术时间较长，而且住院费用较高。这些实际情况限制了微创技术的应用。即使是在学术中心，很多小儿外科医生也既没有接受腹腔镜技术培训，也没有时间参加相关课程。这些情况连同其他问题限制了腹腔镜肾盂整形手术在儿科领域的普及。尽管腹腔镜肾盂整形手术在前十年间得到了较多关注，但面临的技术难题仍然较多，需要较长的学习曲线。成功率最高的腹腔镜肾盂整形手术都是在三级医疗中心，由经过高级腹腔镜培训的有经验的医生施行。对于比较小的肾内型肾盂或者是有过既往开放式肾盂整形手术史患者，腹腔镜肾盂整形术是相对禁忌的，即使对于有经验的操作者来说也是这样，因为这

17

些情况下可能会出现意想不到的技术困难和不必要的风险[65]。

在小儿微创外科中，机器人是另外一个令人振奋的不断发展的领域。这一新技术提供了完美的三维成像效果、前所未有的体内器械控制能力以及手术者位置上的改进。通过机器人技术，可以使腹腔镜经验较少的泌尿科医生迅速掌握治疗 UPJ 梗阻所需的体内器械操控技能，从而推动微创外科的发展[49,79]。

疗效

一个成功的肾盂整形手术始于术前尽可能早地发现肾功能损害的征象。根据一些调查者的研究，对于那些早期检出梗阻并且在肾损害发生前进行手术的患儿来说，肾功能有恢复的机会[13,14]。遵循外科原则可以提高手术成功率[30]。选择合适的小儿操作器械非常重要，对组织的无创操作也同样重要，包括仔细分离、减少外膜和外膜旁血管的损伤。输尿管肾盂吻合应当做到不漏水而且无张力。腹膜后间隙需要放置有效的引流。最后，肾盂整形手术后是否需要常规使用输尿管支撑和经皮肾造瘘还是一个有争议的话题[104]。肾盂整形术后放置输尿管支撑管最可能的原因是确保有效的尿液引流，维持输尿管口径，确保吻合对线对位。反对在肾盂整形术后放置输尿管支撑管最多见的原因是异物留置并可能会成为感染中心，并且对于小儿来说，取出内支撑管时需要基础麻醉。在作者所在医院，输尿管支撑管是有选择性地放置的，主要用于孤立肾患者、有 Östling 皱襞的新生儿或者经过一次失败的肾盂整形术的患者。如果留置了双 J 形输尿管支撑管，应当在手术 6~8 周后取出。

小儿肾盂整形手术的目的在于减轻肾盂积水，保存肾功能。手术以后，可通过多种放射学检查和临床观察来进行评价。肾脏超声判断肾盂整形手术成功，主要根据肾盂积水的 SFU 分级、患侧肾脏的一过性轴向生长和肾皮质逐渐增厚。成功的肾盂整形手术在利尿性肾扫描中的表现为尿液引流和分肾功能均得到改善。对于大年龄儿童，肾盂整形手术成功与否还表现为症状是否消失。

根据这些标准，肾盂整形手术治疗 UPJ 梗阻的成功率高达 98%[48,85,91]。由于成功率很高，有人提出如果术后 3 个月的利尿性肾扫描结果满意，就可以不再进行泌尿科随访。其他调查者认为，理想的随访应当持续 2 年[93]。作者的意见是在肾盂整形手术 3 个月后进行肾脏超声检查，6 个月后进行利尿性肾扫描，此后 2 年期间每年复查肾脏超声。当然，对于术前 DMSA 扫描发现有肾瘢痕的患者，应当在肾盂整形术后进行每年一次的血压检查。

肾盂整形术后并发症可以分为急性和迟发性。急性并发症在婴儿中发生机会相对较多[105]。对于术中尿培养阳性患儿来说，术后肾盂肾炎是最为常见的并发症，需要静脉应用抗生素治疗。迟发性的肾盂输尿管吻合口开放主要是由水肿引起的，可以导致吻合口周围长期漏尿。有趣的是，跨越吻合口的输尿管支撑并不能减少这一并发症的发生。对于肾盂整形术后肾盂积水或其症状持续存在的患者，通过放置经皮肾造瘘管可能会得以缓解。在这些患者中，有的可能需要进行第二次肾盂整形手术或者肾切除手术。迟发性的并发症可以有临床症状，也可以为放射学表现上的进行性加重。无论是哪一种情况，都需要明确采取什么手段，包括肾造瘘管或输尿管支撑管，来改善临床症状或肾功能。原则上，肾盂整形手术失败后的再次手术不宜在 2 个月内进行。治疗继发性的 UPJ 梗阻有 5 种基本的手术方式：改良的肾盂整形术、输尿管肾盏吻合术、肾盂内切开术、腹腔镜手术以及肾切除手术[25,114]。

小结

UPJ 梗阻是最为常见的先天性尿路梗阻，由于病变不同，临床表现不能预测，致使其治疗上也比较复杂。在许多患者中，由于梗阻是非进行性的，故仅仅靠观察即可。而在其他患者中，若放射学检查发现有肾功能恶化或进行性肾盂积水，则需要进行外科手术。遗憾的是，到目前为止还没有明确的指标决定什么样的肾脏需要手术治疗。不过，随着生物化学标志物方面的进展以及放射学手段的改进，以后对于可疑 UPJ 梗阻患儿可以在最早的时间内决定是否手术干预，以防止肾功能损害。

（赵海腾译　刘国华校）

参考文献

1. Adey GS, Vargas SO, Retik AB, et al: Fibroepithelial polyps causing ureteropelvic junction obstruction in children. J Urol 2003;169:1834.
2. American Institute for Ultrasound in Medicine, 1993.
3. Anderson JC, Weiss RM: Physiology and evaluation of ureteropelvic junction obstruction. J Endourol 1996;10:87.
4. Askari A, Belman B: Vesicoureteral reflux in black girls. J Urol 1982;127:747.
5. Bäcklund L, Grotte G, Reuterskiöld A: Functional stenosis as a cause of pelvi-ureteric obstruction. Arch Dis Child 1965;40:203.
6. Baker LA, Gomez RA: Embryonic development of the ureter: Acquisition of smooth muscle [abstract A1715]. J Am Soc Nephrol 1996;7:1593.
7. Bernstein GT, Mandell J, Lebowitz RL, et al: Ureteropelvic junction obstruction in the neonate. J Urol 1988;140:1216.
8. Bomalaski MD, Hirschl RB, Bloom DA: Versicoureteral reflux and ureteropelvic junction obstruction: Association, treatment options and outcome. J Urol 1997;157:969.
9. Bronstein M, Yotte JM, Brandes JM: First and early second-trimester diagnosis of fetal urinary tract abnormalities using transvaginal sonography. Prenat Diagn 1990;10:653.
10. Brown T, Mandell J, Lebowitz R: Neonatal hydronephrosis in the era of sonography. Am J Radiol 1987;148:959.
11. Callan NA, Balkemore K, Park J, et al: Fetal genitourinary tract anomalies: Evaluation, operative correction and follow-up. Obstet Gynecol 1990;75:67.
12. Chang CP, McDill BW, Neilson JR, et al: Calcineurin is required in urinary tract mesenchyme for the development of the pyeloureteral peristaltic machinery. J Clin Invest 2004;113:1051.
13. Chertin B, Fridmans A, Knizhnik M, et al: Does early detection of ureteropelvic junction obstruction improve surgical outcome in terms of renal function? J Urol 1999;162:1037.
14. Chiou YY, Chiu NT, Wang ST, et al: Factors associated with the outcomes of children with unilateral ureteropelvic junction obstruction. J Urol 2004;171:397.
15. Chisholm GD: Pathophysiology of obstructive uropathy. In Chisholm GD, Fair WR (eds): Scientific Foundations of Urology. Chicago, Year Book, 1990, p 59.
16. Clark WR, Malek RS: Ureteropelvic junction obstruction. Observations on the classic type in adults. J Urol 1987; 138:276.
17. Conway JJ: "Well-tempered" diuresis renography: Its historical development, physiological and technical pitfalls, and standardized technique protocol. Semin Nucl Med 1992;22:74.
18. Conway JJ, Maizels M: The "well-tempered" diuretic renogram: A standard method to examine the asymptomatic with hydronephrosis or hydroureteronephrosis. A report from combined meetings of The Society of Fetal Urology and members of the Pediatric Nuclear Medicine Council—The Society of Nuclear Medicine. J Nucl Med 1992;33:2047.
19. Cost GA, Merguerian PA, Cheerasarn SP, Shorliffe LMD: Sonographic renal parenchymal and pelvicaliceal areas: New quantitative parameters for renal sonographic followup. J Urol 1996;156(2S):725.
20. Cronon JJ, Amis ES, Yoder IC, et al: Peripelvic cysts: An impostor of sonographic hydronephrosis. J Ultrasound Med 1982;1:229.
21. Dejter SW, Gibbons MD: The fate of infant kidneys with fetal hydronephrosis but initially normal postnatal sonography. J Urol 1989;142:661.
22. Docimo SG: Pediatric endourology—coming into focus [editorial]. J Urol 1999;162;1731.
23. Duckett JW: When to operate on neonatal hydronephrosis. Urology 1993;42:617.
24. Ebel K: Uroradiology in the fetus and newborn: Diagnosis and follow-up of congenital obstruction of the urinary tract. Pediatr Radiol 1998;28:630.
25. Ellsworth PI, Walker RD, Elder JS: Management of the failed pyeloplasty. AUA Update Series 1997;16(Lesson 17):130.
26. Esposito C, Lima M, Mattioli G, et al: Complications of pediatric urological laparoscopy: Mistakes and risks. J Urol 2003;169:1490.
27. Everaert K, Delanghe J, Vande Wiele C, et al: Urinary alpha 1-microglobulin detects uropathy: A prospective study in 483 urological patients. Clin Chem Lab Med 1998;36:309.
28. Farhat W, McLorie G, Geary D, et al: The natural history of neonatal vesicoureteral reflux associated with antenatal hydronephrosis. J Urol 2000;164:1057.
29. Fernbach SK, Maizels M, Conway JJ: Ultrasound grading of hydronephrosis: Introduction to the system used by the Society for Fetal Urology. Pediatr Radiol 1993;23:478.
30. Flahsner SC, King LR: Ureteropelvic junction. In Kelalis PP, King LR, Belman BA (eds): Clinical Pediatric Urology, 3rd ed. Philadelphia, WB Saunders, 1992, p 693.
31. Flashner SC, Mesrobian HG, Flatt JA, et al: Non-obstructive dilation of the upper urinary tract may later convert to obstruction. Urology 1993;42:569.
32. Foote JW, Blennerhassett JB, Wiglesworth FW, MacKinnon KJ: Observations on the ureteropelvic junction. J Urol 1970;104:252.
33. Freedman ER, Rickwood AMK: Prenatally diagnosed pelviureteric junction obstruction: A benign condition? J Pediatric Surg 1994;29:769.
34. Fung LCT, Atala A: Constant elevation in renal pelvic pressure induces an increase in urinary *N*-acetyl-beta-D-glucosaminidase in a nonobstructive porcine model. J Urol 1998;159:212.
35. Fung LCT, Lakshmanan Y: Anomalies of the renal collecting system: Ureteropelvic junction obstruction (pyelocalyectasis) and infundibular stenosis. In Bellman AB, King LR, Kramer SA (eds): Clinical Pediatric Urology, 4th ed. London, Martin Dunitz, 2002, p 559.
36. Fung LC, McLorie GA, Khoury AE, et al: Contradictory supranormal nuclear renographic differential renal function: Fact or artifact? J Urol 1995;154:667.
37. Fung LCT, Stecker FE, Khoury AE, et al: Intrarenal resistive index correlates with renal pelvis pressure. J Urol 1994; 152:607.
38. Garrett WJ, Grunwald G, Robinson DE: Prenatal diagnosis of fetal polycystic kidney by ultrasound. Aust N Z J Obstet Gynaecol 1970;10:7.
39. Gillenwater JY: The pathophysiology of urinary tract obstruction. In Walsh PC, Retik AB, Stamey TA, Vaughn ED Jr (eds): Campbell's Urology, vol 1, 8th ed. Philadelphia, WB Saunders, 1992, p 499.
40. Gordon I: Antenatal diagnosis of pelvic hydronephrosis: Assessment of renal function and drainage as a guide to management. J Nucl Med 1991;32:1649.
41. Gottschalk CW, Mylle M: Micropuncture study of pressures in proximal tubules and peritubular capillaries of the rat kidney and their relation to ureteral and renal venous pressures. Am J Physiol 1956;185:430.
42. Granaliano G, Gesualdo L, Bartoli F, et al: MCP-1 and EGF renal expression and urine excretion in human congenital obstructive nephropathy. Kidney Int 2000;58:182.
43. Grignon A, Filion R, Filiatrault D, et al: Urinary tract obstruction in utero: Classification and clinical applications. Radiology 1986;160:645.

44. Hofmann V: Ultraschalldiagnostik beim vesico-ureteralen Reflux im Kindesalter. Z Urol Nephrol 1981;74:249.
45. Hollman GA, Elderbrook MK, VanDenLangenberg B: Results of a pediatric sedation program on head MRI scan success rates and procedure duration times. Clin Pediatr (Phila) 1995;34:300.
46. Holsy YL, Williot P, Danais S: Transitional neonatal hydronephrosis: Fact or fantasy? J Urol 1986;136:339.
47. Horowitz M, Gershbein AB, Glassberg KI: Vesicoureteral reflux in infants with prenatal hydronephrosis confirmed at birth: Racial differences. J Urol 1999;161:248.
48. Houben C, Wischermann A, Borner G, Slany E: Outcome analysis of pyeloplasty in infants. Pediatr Surg Int 2000;16:189.
49. Hubert J: Robotic pyeloplasty. Curr Urol Rep 2003;4:124.
50. Jabbour ME, Goldfischer ER, Anderson AE, et al: Failed endopyelotomy: Low expression of TGF beta regardless of the presence or absence of crossing vessels. J Endourol 1999;13:295.
51. Jayanthi VR, Churchill BM, Thorner PS, et al: Bilateral congenital midureteral adynamic segments. Urology 1995;45:520.
52. Johnston JH, Evans JP, Glassberg KI, Shapiro SR: Pelvic hydronephrosis in children: A review of 219 personal cases. J Urol 1977;117:97.
53. Karlin GS, Badlani GH, Smith AD: Endopyelotomy versus open pyeloplasty: Comparison in 88 patients. J Urol 1988;140:476.
54. Kass EJ, Fink-Bennett D: Contemporary techniques for the radioisotopic evaluation of the dilated urinary tract. Urol Clin North Am 1990;17:273.
55. Kenda RB: Imaging techniques for the detection of vesicoureteral reflux: What and when? Nephrol Dial Transplant 2001;16:4.
56. Khaira HS, Platt JF, Cohan RH, et al: Helical computed tomography for identification of crossing vessels in ureteropelvic junction obstruction—comparison with operative findings. Urology 2003;62:35.
57. Khan J, Charron M, Hickeson MP, et al: Supranormal renal function in unilateral hydronephrotic kidney can be avoided. Clin Nucl Med 2004;29:410.
58. Kirsch AJ: Magnetic resonance urography for the evaluation of pediatric hydronephrosis: The state of the art. Podium presentation at the 53rd Annual Meeting of the Society for Pediatric Urology, 2004, San Francisco.
59. Koff SA: Pathophysiology of ureteropelvic junction obstruction: Clinical and experimental observations. Urol Clin North Am 1990;17:263.
60. Koff SA: Neonatal management of unilateral hydronephrosis: Role for delayed intervention. Urol Clin North Am 1998;25:181.
61. Koff SA, Peller PA, Young DC, Pollifrone DL: The assessment of obstruction in the newborn with unilateral hydronephrosis by measuring the size of the opposite kidney. J Urol 1994;152:596.
62. Koff SA, Peller PA, Young DC, Pollifrone DL: Diagnostic criteria for assessing obstruction in the newborn with unilateral hydronephrosis using the renal growth–renal function chart. J Urol 1995;154:662.
63. Koff SA, Thrall JH: The diagnosis of obstruction in experimental hydroureteronephrosis: Mechanism for progressive urinary tract dilatation. Invest Urol 1981;19:85.
64. Konda R, Sakai K, Ota S, et al: Ultrasound grade of hydronephrosis and severity of renal cortical damage on ^{99m}Technetium dimercaptosuccinic acid renal scan in infants with unilateral hydronephrosis during followup and after pyeloplasty. J Urol 2002;167:2159.
65. Kumar U, Turk TM, Albala DM: The treatment of adult ureteropelvic junction obstruction: Issues and answers. AUA Update Series 2001;20(Lesson 36):282.
66. Kunin CM: A ten year study of bacteriuria in schoolgirls: Final report of bacteriologic, urologic and epidemiologic findings. J Infect Dis 1970;122:382.
67. Leary FJ, Myers RP, Greene LF: The value of excretory urography as a screening test in asymptomatic patients. J Urol 1972;107:850.
68. Lebowitz RL, Blickman JG: The coexistence of ureteropelvic junction obstruction and reflux. AJR Am J Roentgenol 1983;140:231.
69. Lettgen B, Meyer-Schwickerath M, Bedow W: [Prenatal ultrasound diagnosis of the kidneys and efferent urinary tract: Possibilities, applications and dangers.] Monatsschrift Kinderheilkunde 1993;141:462.
70. Macksood MJ, Roth DR, Chang CH, Pearlmutter AD: Benign fibro epithelial polyps as a cause of intermittent ureteropelvic junction obstruction in a child: A case report and review of the literature. J Urol 1985;134:951.
71. Madarikan BA, Hayward C, Roberts GM, Lari J: Clinical outcome of fetal uropathy. Arch Dis Child 1988;63:961.
72. Maizels M, Reisman ME, Flom LS, et al: Grading nephroureteral dilation detected in the first year of life: Correlation with obstruction. J Urol 1992;148:609.
73. Mandell J: Diagnosis and management of intrauterine urinary tract disorders. In O'Donnell B, Koff SA (eds): Pediatric Urology. Oxford, Butterworth-Heinemann, 1997, p 315.
74. Mandell J, Blyth B, Peters C, et al: Structural genitourinary defects detected in utero. Radiology 1991;178:193.
75. Martin X, Rouvière O: Radiologic evaluations affecting surgical technique in ureteropelvic junction obstruction. Curr Opin Urol 2001;11:193.
76. McAleer IM, Kaplan GW: Renal function before and after pyeloplasty: Does it improve? J Urol 1999;162:1041.
77. Merguerian P: The evaluation of prenatally detected hydronephrosis. Monogr Urol 1995;16(3):1.
78. Morrissey JJ, Ishidoya S, McCracken R, Klahr S: Control of p53 and p21 (WAF1) expression during unilateral ureteral obstruction. Kidney Int 1996;57:S84.
79. Munver R, Del Pizzo JJ, Sosa RE, Poppas DP: Minimally invasive surgical management of ureteropelvic junction obstruction: Laparoscopic and robot-assisted laparoscopic pyeloplasty. J Long-Term Effects Med Implants 2003;13:367.
80. Murnaghan G: The dynamics of the renal pelvis and ureter with reference to congenital hydronephrosis. J Urol 1958;30:321.
81. Nguyen HT, Gluckman GR, Kogan BA: Changing the technique of background subtraction alters calculated renal function on pediatric mercaptoacetyltriglycine renography. J Urol 1997;158:1252.
82. Nicolini U, Spelzini F: Invasive assessment of fetal renal abnormalities: Urinalysis, fetal blood sampling and biopsy. Prenatal Diagn 2001;21:964.
83. Oh SJ, Moon DH, Kang W, et al: Supranormal differential renal function is real but may be pathological: Assessment by 99m technetium mercaptoacetyltriglycine renal scan of congenital unilateral hydronephrosis. J Urol 2001;165:2300.
84. O'Reilly PH: Consensus Committee of the Society of Radionuclides in Nephrourology. Standardization of the renogram technique for investigating the dilated upper urinary tract and assessing the results of surgery. BJU Int 2003;91:239.
85. O'Reilly PH, Brooman PJ, Mak S, et al: The long-term results of Anderson-Hynes pyeloplasty. BJU Int 2001;87:287.
86. Östling K: The genesis of hydronephrosis particularly with regard to the changes at the ureteropelvic junction. Acta Chir Scand 1942;86(Suppl 72):1.

87. Perez-Brayfield MR, Kirsch AJ, Jones RA, Grattan-Smith JD: A prospective study comparing ultrasound, nuclear scintigraphy and dynamic contrast enhanced magnetic resonance imaging in the evaluation of hydronephrosis. J Urol 2003;170:1330.
88. Peters CA: Lower urinary tract obstruction: Clinical and experimental aspects. Br J Urol 1998;81(Suppl):22.
89. Peters CA, Carr MC, Lais A, et al: The response of the fetal kidney to obstruction. J Urol 1992;148:503.
90. Peters CA, Schlussel RN, Retik AB: Pediatric laparoscopic dismembered pyeloplasty. J Urol 1995;153:1962.
91. Pohl HG, Rushton HG, Park JS, et al: Early diuresis renogram findings predict success following pyeloplasty. J Urol 2001;165:2311.
92. Preston A, Lebowitz RL: What's new in pediatric uroradiology. Urol Radiol 1989;11:217.
93. Psooy K, Pike JG, Leonard MP: Long-term followup of pediatric dismembered pyeloplasty: How long is long enough? J Urol 2003;169:1809.
94. Rabinowitz R, Peters MT, Vyas S, et al: Measurement of fetal urine production in normal pregnancy by real-time ultrasonography. Am J Obstet Gynecol 1989;161:1264.
95. Ransley PG: Impaired renal function in the newborn: Nature of the injury (panel discussion). Society of Pediatric Urology, May 18, 1986, New York.
96. Ransley VM, Murphy JL, Mendoza SA: Postnatal management of UPJ obstruction detected antenatally. Dialogues Pediatr Urol 1985;8:6.
97. Rickard M, Whitaker RH: Pelviureteric junction obstruction in association with severe vesicoureteral reflux: A diagnostic dilemma. Urol Radiol 1984;6:1.
98. Roth JA, Diamond DA: Prenatal hydronephrosis. Currt Opin Pediatr 2001;13:138.
99. Ruano-Gil D, Coca-Payeras A, Tejedo-Maten A: Obstruction and normal recanalization of the ureter in the human embryo: Its relation to congenital ureteric obstruction. Eur Urol 1975;1:287.
100. Rushton HG, Salem Y, Belman AB, Majd M: Pediatric pyeloplasty: Is routine retrograde pyelogram necessary? J Urol 1994;152:604.
101. Saari-Keppainen A, Karjalainen O, Ylostalo P, Heinonen OP: Ultrasound screening and perinatal mortality: Controlled trial of systematic one-stage screening in pregnancy. The Helsinki Ultrasound Trial. Lancet 1990;336:387.
102. Schenkman EM, Tarry WF: Comparison of percutaneous endopyelotomy with open pyeloplasty for pediatric ureteropelvic junction obstruction. J Urol 1998;159:1013.
103. Sheldon CA, Duckett JW: Infant pyeloplasty. AUA Update Series 1988;7(Lesson 37):290.
104. Smith, KE, Holmes N, Lieb JI, et al: Stented versus nonstented pediatric pyeloplasty: A modern series and review of the literature. J Urol 2002;168:1127.
105. Snyder HM III, Lebowitz RL, Colodny AH, et al: UPJ obstruction in children. Urol Clin North Am 1980; 7:273.
106. Soper NJ, Barteau JA, Clayman RV, et al: Comparison of early postoperative results for laparoscopic versus standard open cholecystectomy. Surg Gynecol Obstet 1992;174:114.
107. Steele BT, DeMaria J, Toi A, et al: Neonatal outcome of fetuses with urinary tract abnormalities diagnosed by prenatal ultrasonography. CMAJ 1987;137:117.
108. Taylor A Jr, Thakore K, Folks R, et al: Background subtraction in technetium-99m-MAG3 renography. J Nucl Med 1997;38:74.
109. Thomas DFM: Fetal uropathy: Review. Br J Urol 1990;66:223.
110. Tripp BM, Homsy YL: Neonatal hydronephrosis—the controversy and the management. Pediatr Nephrol 1995;9:503.
111. Ulman I, Jayanthi VR, Koff SA: The long-term followup of newborns with severe unilateral hydronephrosis initially treated nonoperatively. J Urol 2000;164:1101.
112. Uson AC, Cox LA, Lattimer JK: Hydronephrosis in infants and children. II. Surgical management and results. JAMA 1968;205:327.
113. Van Cangh PJ, Nesa S, Galeon M: Vessels around the ureteropelvic junction: Significance and imaging by conventional radiology J Endourol 1996;10:111.
114. Varkorakis IM, Bhayani SB, Allaf ME, et al: Management of secondary ureteropelvic junction obstruction after failed primary laparoscopic pyeloplasty. J Urol 2004; 172:180.
115. Velicer CM, Heckbert SR, Lampe JW, et al: Antibiotic use in relation to the risk of breast cancer. JAMA 2004; 292:827.
116. Wåhlin N, Magnusson A, Persson AEG, et al: Pressure flow measurement of hydronephrosis in children: A new approach to definition and quantification of obstruction. J Urol 2001;166:1842.
117. Wen JG, Chen Y, Ringgaard S, et al: Evaluation of renal function in normal and hydronephrotic kidneys in rats using gadolinium diethylenetetramine-pentaacetic acid enhanced dynamic magnetic resonance imaging. J Urol 2000;163:1264.
118. Whitaker RH: Methods of assessing obstruction in dilated ureters. Br J Urol 1973;45:15.
119. Yerkes EB, Adams MC Pope JC IV, Brock JW III: Does every patient with prenatal hydronephrosis need voiding cystourethrography? J Urol 1999;162:1218.
120. Zerin JM, Ritchey ML, Chang AC: Incidental vesicoureteral reflux in neonates with antenatally detected hydronephrosis and other renal abnormalities. Radiology 1993;187:157.

第 112 章

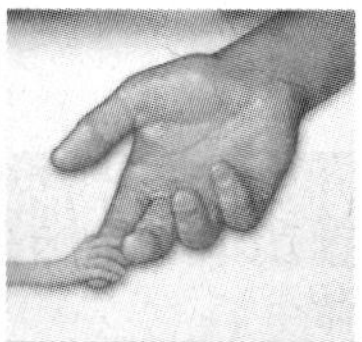

肾感染、脓肿、膀胱输尿管反流、尿路结石以及肾静脉血栓

Leslie T. McQuiston 和 Anthony A. Caldamone

尿路感染、肾脓肿以及膀胱输尿管反流

741 在婴儿与儿童中，泌尿道是除了呼吸道以外最多见感染的部位。由于儿童尿路感染（urinary tract infection，UTI）在诊断上有一些问题，所以其发病率很难确定。小年龄儿童可能仅仅表现为发热和发育迟缓，不伴有特异性的尿路症状或体征。UTI 的诊断和治疗对小儿来说十分重要，这主要考虑到其长期并发症问题，包括肾瘢痕、高血压以及肾功能下降。通过一些研究发现，在小年龄患儿发热性尿路感染中，肾瘢痕的发生率可以高达 40%～50%[92]。在 2 个月到 2 岁的发热患儿中，约有 5% 的患儿被诊断为尿路感染[2,55]。在儿科患者中，UTI 的发病具有明显的年龄和性别特点（表 112-1）。UTI 在女孩中的发病率高于男孩；据报道，在 1～5 岁的女孩中，UTI 的发病率为 1%～3%，而在此年龄段的男孩中却很少有 UTI 的发病报道[42]。一些研究表明，在未经过包皮环切手术的男孩，尤其是不超过 1 岁的男孩中，UTI 的发病率比包皮环切的男孩高出 5～20 倍[3,89]。在过去几年中，对 UTI 发病机制以及预测患者肾功能受损的影响因素有了更深的理解。

表 112-1 尿路感染发病的年龄和性别情况

年龄（岁）	女性（%）	男性（%）
<1	6.5	3.3
1～2	8.1	1.9

From American Academy of Pediatrics, Committee on Quality Improvement, Subcommittee on Urinary Tract Infection: Practice parameter: The diagnosis, treatment, and evaluation of the initial urinary tract infection in febrile infants and young children. Pediatrics 1999; 103: 843.

发病机制

细菌主要通过四个途径进入泌尿道：上行性、血源性、淋巴性以及直接侵入。血源性途径最多见于免疫力低下的儿童或新生儿，因为其免疫系统发育还不成熟。直接侵入可以发生于那些有瘘管的患儿，如阴道或胃肠道与泌尿生殖道交通的瘘管。在细菌通过尿道侵入的情况下，上行性渠道是最常见的途径。宿主因素包括抗感染能力，是 UTI 发病机制中的一个重要因素。UTI 在婴儿中的发生率较高，这可能与新生儿免疫系统发育不成熟有关，也可能与出生后第一年出现的尿道旁细菌过多迁移有关[17]。细菌从胃肠道迁移到尿道旁黏膜，然后可以上行到膀胱，继而再上行到肾脏（表 112-2）[35]。一些细菌的特征，如细菌菌毛的存在，可使细菌对尿道上皮细胞产生黏附作用，并且提高细菌的致病性。

鉴别肾盂肾炎与低位的 UTI 比较困难，其原因是细菌在尿路位置的高低与其引起的临床症状之间缺乏必然联系。不过在大年龄儿童中，肾盂肾炎的诊断可以参考有无发热、腰痛以及全身症状。在应用合适的抗生素后，仍持续发热超过 48 小时，提示可能有上尿路感染。婴儿出现发热性 UTI 时，应当考虑到肾盂肾炎的存在，并给予相应治疗。

表 112-2　感染的病原体

病原体	注释
大肠杆菌	占感染的 70%~90%
铜绿假单胞菌	最常见的非肠源性革兰阴性病原体 有时可见于免疫力低下的患者
肠球菌	最常见的革兰阳性病原体
B 组链球菌	新生儿少见
金黄色葡萄球菌	提示来源于另外的部位（脓肿、骨髓炎、细菌性心内膜炎）
变形杆菌	大于 1 岁的男孩
念珠菌，凝固酶阴性的葡萄球菌	见于接受过尿路操作的患者
克雷白杆菌	有时可见于免疫力低下的患者

Adapted from Handel LN, Caldamone AA: Urinary tract infections in the pediatric population. Lebanese Med J 2000; 52: 194.

表 112-3　尿路感染的危险因素

解剖畸形
膀胱输尿管反流
梗阻
其他：憩室、阴唇粘连
女性
未进行包皮环切的男性
排尿异常
便秘
器械操作
有 P 菌毛的细菌
排尿训练
性活动、妊娠

危险因素

尽管细菌的致病性在 UTI 的发生中扮演了重要角
1742 色，而宿主方面的一些因素也可以促进 UTI 的发生，包括年龄、性别、菌群因素、便秘、泌尿生殖系统畸形、性行为、遗传因素以及医源性因素（表 112-3）[93]。影响发病的最为重要的因素是年龄和性别。出生 3 个月以内，男婴的 UTI 发病风险是女婴的 5~8 倍[88]。超过这一年龄段后，女性的发病率又超过男性。在学龄前阶段，女孩发生的有症状感染是男孩的 10~20 倍[89]。

UTI 往往被认为是泌尿生殖道解剖畸形的一个标志。对这些畸形的早期诊断十分重要，如果延误诊断，可能会导致复发性感染和肾实质的丧失。梗阻性畸形如肾盂输尿管连接部梗阻、后尿道瓣膜、异位输尿管、输尿管囊肿和尿道憩室，有增加 UTI 发生的风险。肾脏畸形如肾乳头坏死、无功能肾以及单侧的髓质海绵肾，同样会增加患者对 UTI 的易感性。

膀胱输尿管反流（vesicoureteral reflux，VUR）指尿液从膀胱向肾脏的异常流动，这种情况同样可以提供机会使细菌从膀胱迁移到肾脏。VUR 本身并不会导致 UTI，对于 UTI 的产生，必须在 VUR 存在的基础上合并有菌尿。这一规则的例外情况是，小儿有明显的VUR且有明显的来自反流尿的残余尿。VUR在普通人群中的发生率大约为 1%，而在有菌尿的儿童中的发生率为 20%~35%[19,36]。在小于 1 岁的小儿中，有超过 60% 的患儿在初次 UTI 后被发现有 VUR[55]。这一数字在 2～3 岁时降到 30%，在成人时为 5% 以下[55]。随着小儿的生长，黏膜下隧道变长，黏膜下隧道长度与输尿管管径比值增加。此外，充盈与排尿压力也随着时间的变化而发生改变，这也有利于改善 VUR。所有这些因素，连同膀胱动力学和排尿方式的改变，均可以增加 VUR 自行缓解的机会。依照国际反流分级系统，VUR 被分成Ⅰ到Ⅴ级。Ⅰ级和Ⅱ级通常能够随着时间的延长而消失或改善，而Ⅳ级和Ⅴ级一般不能够自行缓解，需要进行干预治疗。

功能性异常如神经性膀胱，能够通过提高泌尿道压力、不完全排空膀胱以及经常进行器械导尿等使 UTI 的易感性增加。UTI 在排尿功能异常的患者中也很常见，可能与不完全排空膀胱、尿潴留以及尿路压力异常增加有关。有些情况如膀胱不稳定、排尿次数过少、Hinman 综合征、便秘等可伴有排尿功能异常。尿道旁与包皮处细菌菌群同样可以增加 UTI 的风险。包皮需氧菌群在出生后第一个月最多，6 个月后减少，而在 5 岁后比较少见[56,93]。

临床表现

患有 UTI 的儿童，尤其是 2 岁以下的小儿，并不都表现出典型的排尿困难、尿频、尿痛症状，体格检查的意义也不是很大。因此，对于婴儿和年幼的小儿，保持较高的警惕十分重要。对于 2 岁以下的儿童，父母所提供的可能是一些非特异性表现，如发热、紧张、呕吐或腹泻；父母也可能提供诸如发育迟
43 缓或喂养困难等情况。婴儿常常仅表现为发热症状。2～5 岁的儿童常常表现为与上呼吸道感染一致的发热和腹痛症状。在经过排尿训练后，患儿开始表现出相对比较特异性的症状，如发热、排尿困难、腰痛、尿急迫感。

诊断

确诊小儿 UTI 至关重要，而标本的采集方法能够影响到诊断的准确性（表 112-4）。这些采集方法包括中段尿、清洁尿、耻骨上抽吸、经尿道膀胱插管导尿以及会阴集尿袋。在经过排尿训练的小儿中，清洁尿方法收集的标本污染率为 30% 左右[58]。最无菌的方法也是尿液采集的金标准方法是耻骨上抽吸，不过这种方法常不能得到家长或初诊医生的接受。耻骨上抽吸方法的禁忌证是那些已经明确有泌尿生殖道解剖畸形的患者。

表 112-4　诊断尿路感染的标准

标本采集方法	菌落计数（纯培养物）	感染可能性（%）
耻骨上抽吸	革兰阴性细菌：任何数量	>99
	革兰阳性细菌：大于几千	
经尿道插管导尿	>100 000	95
	10 000～100 000	感染的可能性很大
	1000～10 000	可疑，复查
	<1000	感染的可能性小
清洁尿（男孩）	>10 000	可能感染
清洁尿（女孩）	3 次标本 >100 000	95
	2 次标本 >100 000	90
	1 次标本 >100 000	80
	50 000～100 000	可疑，复查
	10 000～50 000	如有症状，则为可疑，复查；如果无症状，感染可能性小
	<10 000	感染可能性小

Adapted from Handel LN, Caldamone AA: Urinary tract infections in the pediatric population. Lebanese Med J 2004; 52: 194.

经尿道膀胱插管导尿方法是值得推荐的方法，其假阳性率比会阴集尿袋方法低。阳性尿培养的敏感度为 95%，特异度也达到了 99%[2]。在未经过排尿训练的小儿中，采用会阴部集尿袋比较普遍，但这种方法的污染机会较高，其假阳性结果的发生率为 85%[2]。在 UTI 可疑程度较低的患儿中可以采用这种方法。目前推荐的方法是，在尿常规检查呈阳性表现或者通过集尿袋方法尿培养呈阳性结果后，再采用经尿道插管导尿或耻骨上抽吸的方法。

通过尿液分析，同时结合尿液镜检出现尿亚硝酸盐、中性粒细胞酯酶、细菌以及镜下白细胞等指标，可以使敏感度提高到 99.8%，特异度为 70%[2,58]。然而，即使在尿液分析或镜下分析中这些指标均呈阴性，也不能排除 UTI 诊断。只有尿液培养才是准确诊断 UTI 的方法。在最终的尿液培养结果出来前，要对患儿进行处理，这主要是因为 5 岁以下儿童发生肾瘢痕的风险较高。

影像学

对于 UTI 后影像学检查的作用还存在争议[39]。进行影像学检查最主要的目的是明确患儿后继 UTI 和肾损害的风险。影像学检查包括对肾脏和膀胱的解剖形态检查，以及鉴别有无 VUR 的功能性检查。现行的美国儿科协会指导推荐，对所有 2 岁以下的初发 UTI 患儿进行肾脏和膀胱超声检查[2]。对这些患儿进行超声检查的目的是明确是否存在先天性的尿路结构上的异常，如肾盂积水（图 112-1）。另外，超声检查可以发现任何可能的肾实质异常，如囊肿，也可以鉴别有无肾周积液。超声检查还可以明确鉴别输尿管扩张、膀胱壁增厚（图 112-2）、集合系统重复（图 112-3）、输尿管囊肿（图 112-4）、膀胱憩室和结石。如果有急性肾盂肾炎，超声检查可以显示肾脏局部或弥漫性变大，皮质回声异常。多项研究显示 UTI 后有 5%～10% 的患者有梗阻性病变，20%～50% 有 VUR[50]。因此，推荐对所有患 UTI 后的婴儿和儿

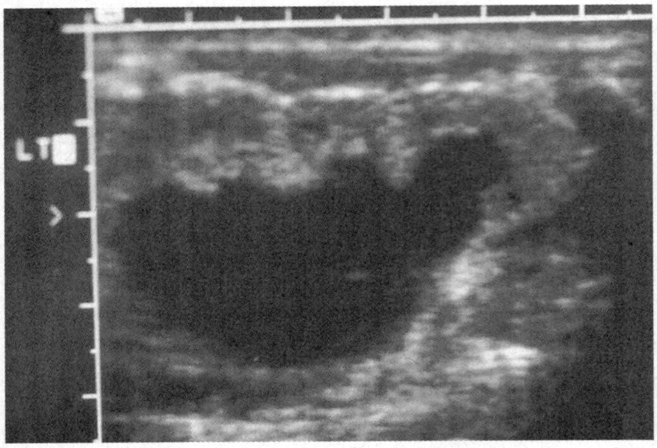

图 112-1　肾脏的矢状面超声显示肾盂和肾盏积水。

童进行上尿路和下尿路的影像学检查。这些检查一般包括肾脏和膀胱超声，以及排尿性膀胱尿道造影（VCUG）。按照性别，推荐对所有年龄的初发 UTI 男孩和 5 岁以下的初发 UTI 女孩进行超声和 VCUG 检查。
1744 此外，对于 5 岁以上的女孩来说，影像学检查的指征是患有肾盂肾炎者，或者复发 UTI 者（表 112-5）。

儿童 UTI 最常见的伴发疾病是 VUR，在 UTI 患儿中约占 20%～35%。VCUG 用于检查有无 VUR 的存在（图 112-5）。标准的 VCUG 检查是通过将含碘造影剂注入膀胱，然后在充盈期和排尿期进行摄片。美国儿科协会推荐将 VCUG 检查作为 VUR 诊断的首选检查，尤其对于男性患者，以排除后尿道瓣膜（图112-6）[2]。

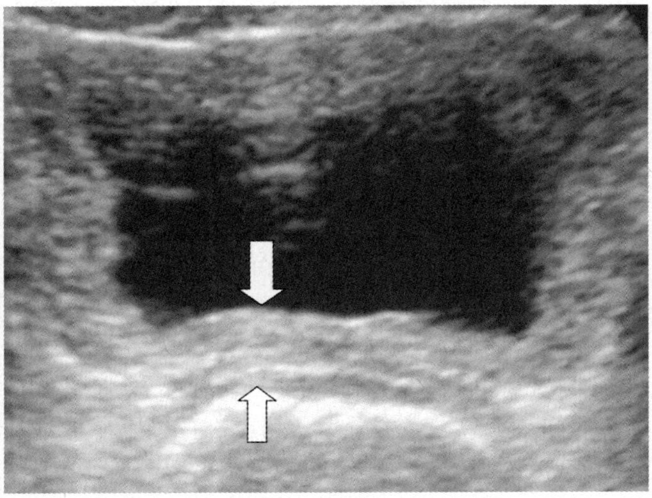

图 112-2　膀胱的横断面超声显示膀胱后壁增厚（*箭头*）。

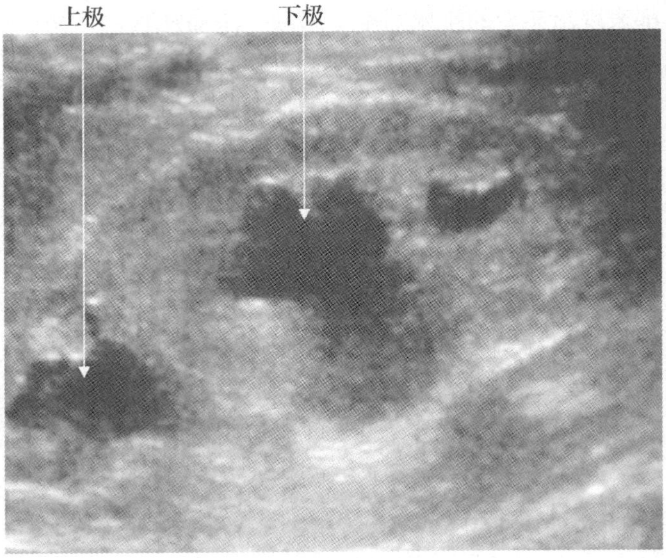

图 112-3　肾脏的矢状面超声显示重复的集合系统。

以往的推荐标准是在 UTI 后 4～6 周进行 VCUG 检查，这是因为膀胱壁炎症会造成反流，可能出现假阳性结果。最新的研究表明，早期（发生感染 7 天内）和晚期进行 VCUG 检查其结果没有区别[62]。只要患者无发热表现，并且培养结果呈阴性，VCUG 可以在任何时候进行，以防止在检查时感染的尿液被动逆行。

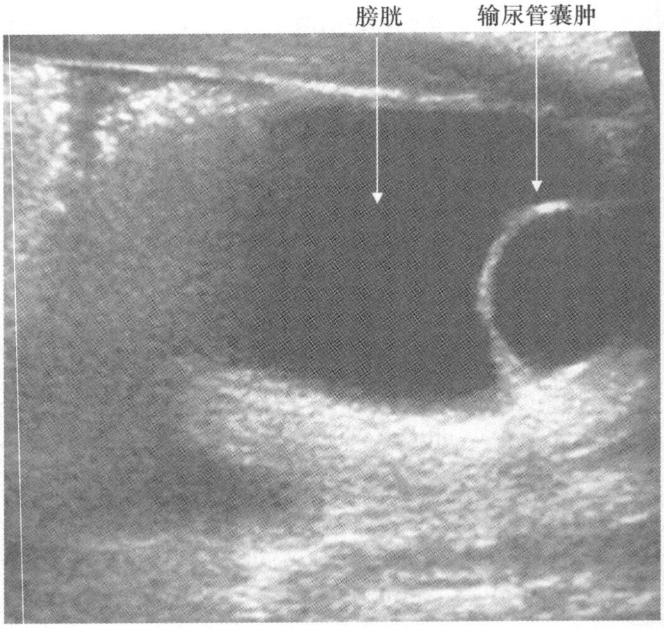

图 112-4　膀胱的横断面超声显示左侧输尿管囊肿。

表 112-5　小儿泌尿生殖系统影像检查

检查方法	检查所见	检查指征
肾脏/膀胱 US	脓肿 两个肾脏表现 肾脏大小 肾盂积水表现（见图 112-1） 膀胱壁增厚（见图 112-2） 排尿后残余尿 集合系统重复（见图 112-3） 输尿管囊肿（见图 112-4）	有过一次 UTI 的所有男孩
VCUG	膀胱输尿管反流（图 112-5） 后尿道瓣膜（见图 112-6）	有过一次 UTI 的所有男孩和超过 5 岁的女孩
MAG3 利尿性扫描	肾功能 肾梗阻	US 发现肾盂积水，VCUG 未见反流
DMSA 肾脏扫描	肾盂肾炎	诊断急性肾盂肾炎 评估肾瘢痕

DMSA：二巯基丁二酸；MAG3：巯基乙酰三甘油；US：超声检查；UTI：尿路感染；VCUG：排尿性膀胱尿道造影。

Adapted from Handel LN，Caldamone AA：Urinary tract infections in the pediatric population. Lebanese Med J 2004；52：194.

肾皮质的二巯基丁二酸（DMSA）显像对儿童肾
45 盂肾炎的检查既敏感又特异[50,87]。摄取稀疏区表示急性肾盂肾炎或肾瘢痕。在 DMSA 出现以前，其他的影像学检查发现有约 17% 的菌尿患儿有肾瘢痕；现在应用 DMSA 检查显示该比例为以前的两倍[92]。DMSA 的应用应当仅限于疑有急性 UTI，但诊断还不明确且高度怀疑为肾盂肾炎者。如果 DMSA 的检查结果影响患者的治疗方案，那么它也能用于评估这些患者 UTI 后肾瘢痕的情况。

巯基乙酰三甘油（MAG3）或二乙基三胺五乙酸（DTPA）结合利尿剂应用，可以用于评估不伴有 VUR 的肾盂积水患者的肾功能和排泄情况，判断梗阻是否存在。在检查中假阳性与假阴性结果均可出现，所以在解释检查结果时必须谨慎，必须与临床相联系。

肾脓肿是肾盂肾炎的潜在并发症，多发于免疫力

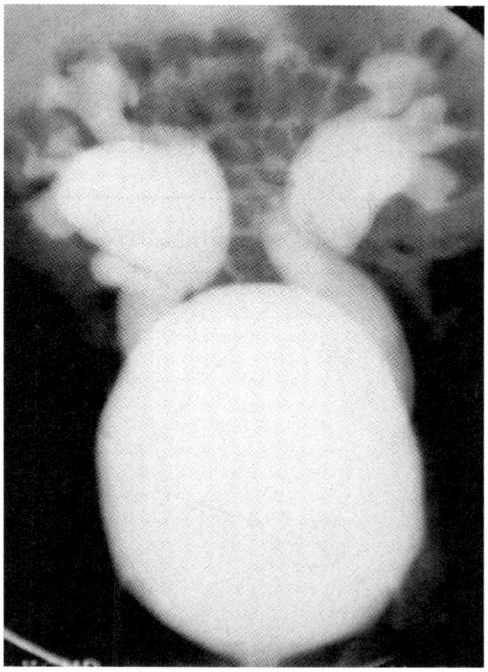

图 112-5　排尿性膀胱尿道造影显示膀胱输尿管反流。

低下的患者。革兰染色阳性病原体如金黄色葡萄球菌和链球菌可以是其致病菌。超声检查和计算机断层扫描（CT）是最好的诊断手段。治疗上有长期应用抗

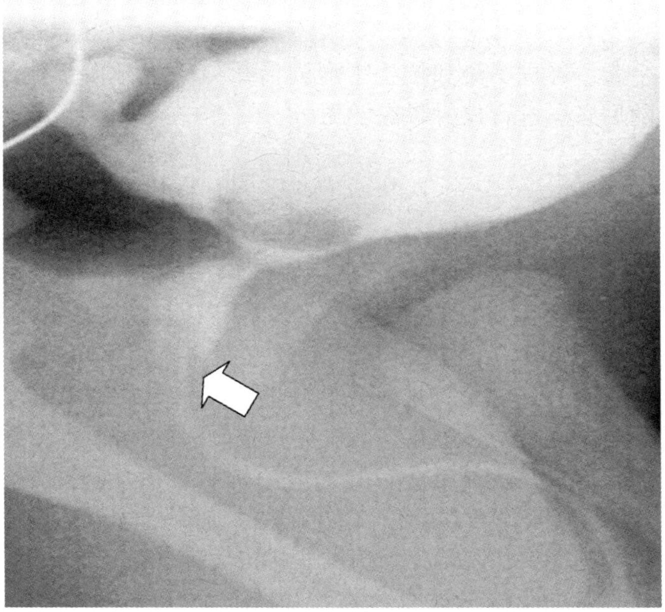

图 112-6　排尿性膀胱尿道造影显示后尿道瓣膜（*箭头*）。

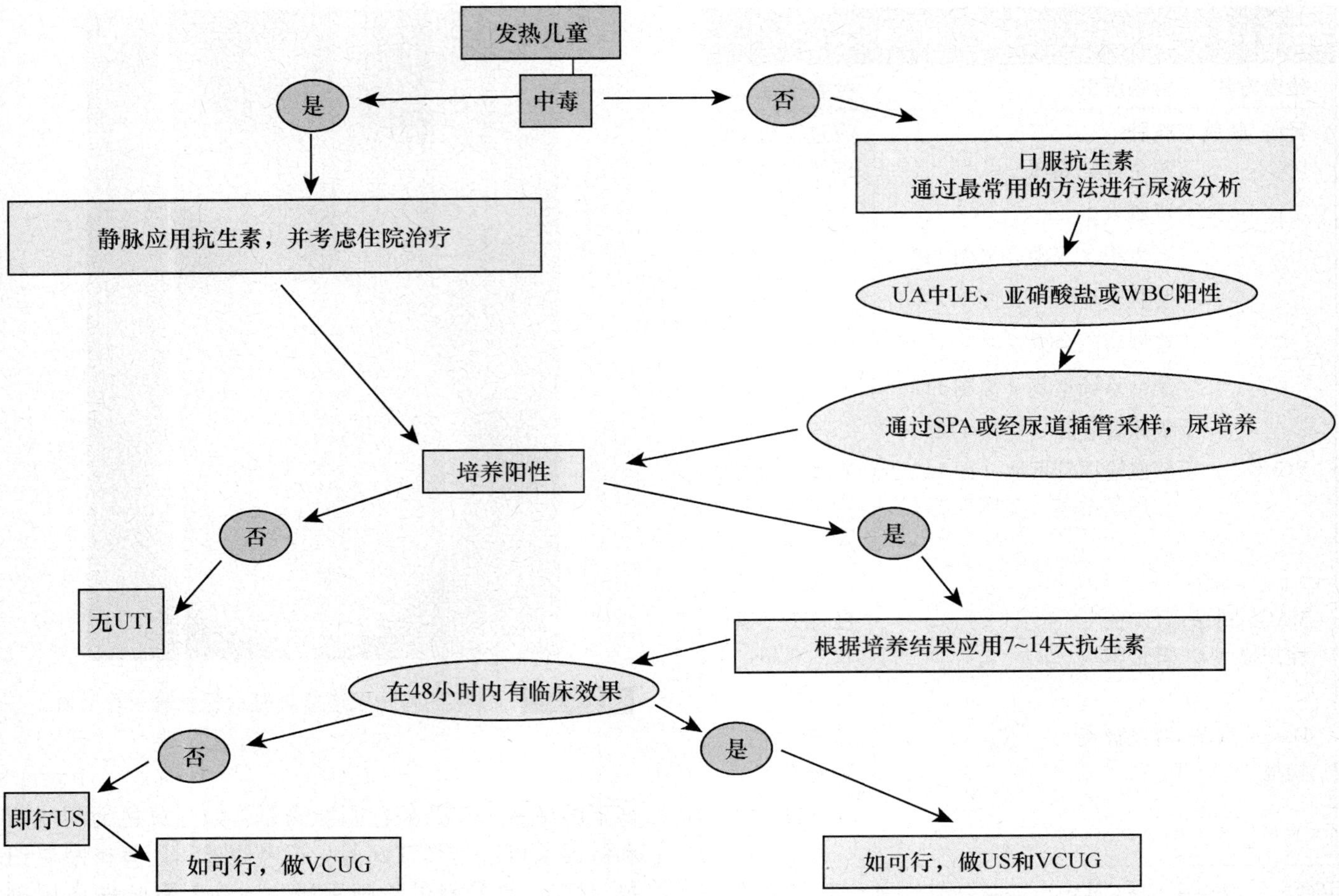

图 112-7 尿路感染（UTI）治疗的流程图。LE，白细胞酯酶；SPA，耻骨上吸引术；UA，尿液分析；US，超声检查；VCUG，排尿性膀胱尿道造影；WBC，白细胞。

生素、经皮引流和抗生素灌注治疗或手术开放引流。随后必须进行放射影像学随访。

治疗

由于有发生儿童肾瘢痕的风险，积极的诊断和治疗至关重要（图 112-7）。治疗方案需要根据不同的因素来制订，尤其是患儿的年龄和疾病的严重程度。小于 4 周的发热患儿其菌血症和脓血症的风险明显增加，需要住院并给予胃肠外应用抗生素治疗。同样，任何小于 5 岁的疑有 UTI 的患儿，如表现有全身症状，则需要住院治疗。美国儿科协会推荐对于有脱水表现、不能耐受口服药物治疗并且有中毒症状的患儿，应当给予静脉抗生素治疗[2]。此外，对于免疫力低下、疑有脓尿或菌血症或者口服给药治疗无效的儿童，应当考虑住院治疗。如果患儿能够耐受口服抗生素，而且父母能够保持随访并同医生进行交流，那么可以对患儿进行门诊治疗。

初步的抗生素治疗需要覆盖常见的病原体抗菌谱。一旦取得细菌培养和药物敏感试验结果，就应当调整抗生素以覆盖特定的病原体。对于以往曾患过 UTI 的患者，在选择初步抗生素时可以参考以前的细菌培养结果。对于住院治疗的儿童，应胃肠外给药如氨基糖苷类药物联合氨苄西林或头孢菌素，连续应用 48～72 小时，直到患儿发热停止，病情稳定，并且达到药敏效果。在患儿病情稳定后，可以根据药敏结果更换口服抗生素。大多数研究建议对于有发热症状的年幼儿童，疗程应当持续 7～10 天[47,108]。美国儿科协会建议非复杂性的 UTI 治疗疗程为 7～10 天，而对涉及肾脏或有中毒表现的患儿的治疗疗程为 14 天[2]。对于 6 周以下的婴儿，氨苄西林和庆大霉素或氨苄西林和头孢菌素是很好的首选治疗。头孢曲松是一个例外，因其可能增加年幼婴儿发生核黄疸的危险。对于那些可能有假单胞菌或肠球菌感染的儿童，氨苄西林和庆大霉素是给药首选，头孢菌素对肠球菌无效。使用庆大霉素时，尤其对于肾功能不全的患儿来说，应当密切监测药物水平。

如果患者临床情况比较稳定，建议使用广谱口服抗生素。对于临床表现较好的患儿，磺胺异噁唑或甲氧苄啶-磺胺甲基异噁唑（TMP-SMZ）、头孢菌素或呋喃妥因是比较常用的药物。由于有核黄疸和体液紊乱的风险，TMP-SMZ 不应用于 2 个月以下的小儿。呋喃妥因是通过尿液排泄的，在血液中不能达到有效的治疗浓度，所以不适用于有发热表现的 UTI 婴儿或者病变可能累及肾脏的小儿。近来氟喹诺酮类药物已经应用于儿科患者[30,88]。表 112-6 给出了常用的抗生素小结。

对于所有的 UTI 患儿应当考虑预防性使用小剂量抗生素，直到对肾脏进行全面的超声和 VCUG 评估。患有 VUR、复发性 UTI、不完全性梗阻或者免疫力低下的患儿，也要考虑使用预防性抗生素。理想的预防性用药可以使尿中排泌的抗生素水平增高，同时还能保持较低的血药浓度。阿莫西林、呋喃妥因和 TMP-SMZ 是这类药剂中最常用的药物。不过，由于大肠杆菌对阿莫西林表现出越来越高的耐药性，使得此药在有症状的儿科患者中的应用受到限制。一般情况下，用于预防性治疗的抗生素应当有别于治疗急性感染的抗生素。

表 112-6　用于治疗小儿尿路感染的抗生素

给药方法	抗生素	其他信息
胃肠外	氨苄西林和庆大霉素	检查庆大霉素水平
	氨苄西林和头孢菌素	不覆盖肠球菌或假单胞菌
	头孢曲松和头孢噻肟	不适用于 2 个月以下的婴儿
口服	TMP-SMZ	不适用于 2 个月以下的婴儿
	阿莫西林	增加大肠杆菌的耐药性
	呋喃妥因	如涉及肾脏，单用此药还不充分
	头孢菌素	不覆盖肠球菌或假单胞菌
	环丙沙星	最近已经允许应用于儿童

TMP-SMZ：甲氧苄啶和磺胺甲基异噁唑。

Adapted from Handel LN，Caldamone AA：Urinary tract infections in the pediatric population. Lebanese Med J 2004；52：194.

对于各项检查正常却有反复 UTI（定义为在 6 个月期间有三次或更多次的感染）的患者，有必要使用预防性抗生素。在这些患者中，还需要考虑到其他因素，如患者的年龄以及对 UTI 的生物学易感性。开始应用预防性抗生素的儿童，其感染的机会通常会减少，不过一旦停止使用预防性抗生素，其再次发生 1747
UTI 的风险程度又可回到原先的水平，对这些患者要进行细致的筛查以排除排尿功能紊乱和便秘。对于无症状菌尿，目前的建议是在严格随访的基础上不给予抗生素治疗。

VUR 的治疗需要考虑到以下一些因素：发病年龄、反流级别、有无排尿功能异常、伴发疾病以及对治疗方案的依从程度。将 VUR 分为原发性和继发性两种是有益处的。原发性反流是指膀胱输尿管连接部先天异常，导致输尿管隧道过短以及输尿管后的逼尿肌缺陷。缺乏输尿管后的逼尿肌支撑阻止了膀胱充盈期的输尿管闭合（图 112-8）。继发性反流是指其他解剖或功能上的异常所导致的反流，比如膀胱出口梗阻或膀胱输尿管连接部的异常（表 112-7）。

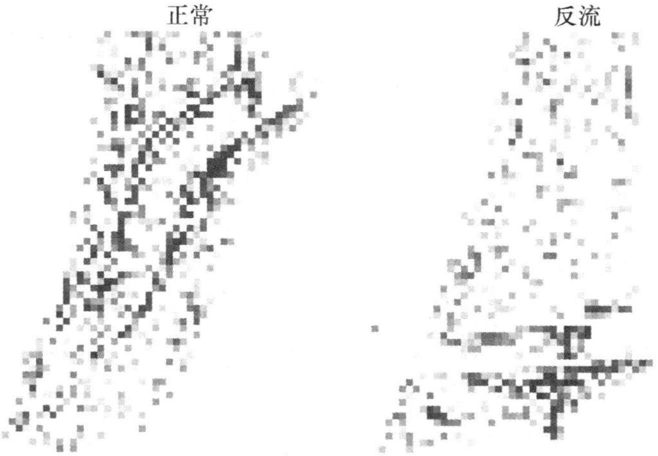

图 112-8　正常解剖和反流时输尿管膀胱连接部（UVJ）解剖。注意 UVJ 反流时缺乏逼尿肌支撑。

表 112-7　继发性反流的原因

解剖性
后尿道瓣膜
输尿管囊肿
憩室
异位输尿管
梅干腹综合征
膀胱外翻
功能性
排尿功能障碍
神经性膀胱
脊髓发育不良
骶骨发育不良

在大多数 VUR 患者中，预防性抗生素、UTI 的监控、规律性的排尿、便秘的治疗、定期超声和 VCUG 随访是治疗的主要环节[24]。对于外科治疗的指征问题还存在争议，不过大多数人对于以下情况的意见比较一致：严重的高位 UTI、在应用预防性抗生素的情况下依然有新生的肾瘢痕、肾脏生长缓慢、不能继续原有的治疗方案、高等级的 VUR（年幼婴儿除外）、膀胱输尿管连接部有明确的解剖缺陷和经过 2 年以上的随访 VUR 持续存在。

对于已经明确有排尿功能异常的 VUR 患儿，需要密切关注。现在已经明确，如果排尿功能异常（包括便秘）得到了很好的治疗，那么严重 UTI 和肾瘢痕的发生率以及手术治疗 VUR 的必要性都会明显降低[49,65,79]。排尿功能异常也是输尿管再植手术失败的主要原因[70]。

膀胱内和膀胱外入路的手术方式有很多种，所有这些手术都需要建立一段黏膜下的输尿管，有充分的后壁肌肉支撑，以提供必要的输尿管对膀胱充盈和收缩时的协调功能，防止尿液逆流（图 112-9 至图 112-11）。这种手术平均需要住院 48 小时，并发症发生率为 4%，其中 2%～2. 5% 是因为输尿管梗阻，另外 2%～2. 5% 是因为持续的 VUR。小儿膀胱输尿管反流指导小组指出，总的外科手术成功率为 95. 1%[24]。

Matouschek[64] 于 1981 年提出通过内镜注射聚四氟乙烯（Teflon）治疗尿失禁和 VUR 的概念。Puri 和 O'Donnel 对这一方法进行了改进和推广，1984 年用于小猪模型，然后应用于 VUR 患儿[16,74]。这种治疗方法的术后反应较小，可以作为门诊手术来施行（图 112-12 和 112-13）。由于有微粒迁移和诱发恶变的潜在危险[63]，现在已经不再使用 Teflon[70]。现在已经研究出很多其他的注射用药剂，并已用于动物模型和人类的 VUR 治疗。成功率接近 75%～80%，主要依赖于反流的程度和注射剂量的大小[48,53,82,98]。如今，国际中普遍使用的药物是聚糖苷巨球（Deflux）以及多聚二甲基硅氧烷和聚乙烯吡咯啉（Macroplastique）的混合物。

尿路结石

历史回顾和发病率

已有报道，早在公元前 4800 年的埃及木乃伊中，其膀胱和肾脏中就存在尿路结石[10]，并且对尿石症发病机制和治疗方法的研究由来已久。尽管小儿尿

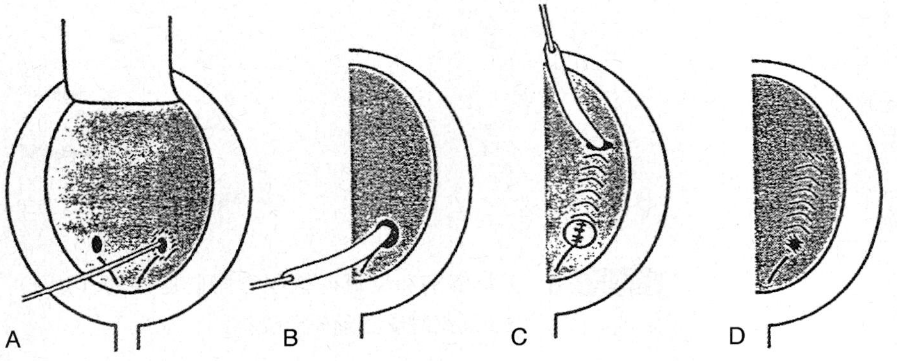

图 112-9　Leadbetter-Politano 输尿管再植术。A. 通过膀胱中线切口进行输尿管插管。B. 在输尿管周围解剖逼尿肌，直到输尿管完全游离。C. 用直角钳在膀胱内做出新的裂隙，建立黏膜下隧道，关闭逼尿肌缺损。D. 将输尿管穿过黏膜下隧道，制作输尿管出口。（From Rowe M, et al: Essentials of Pediatric Surgery. St Louis, Mosby-Year Book, 1995. ）

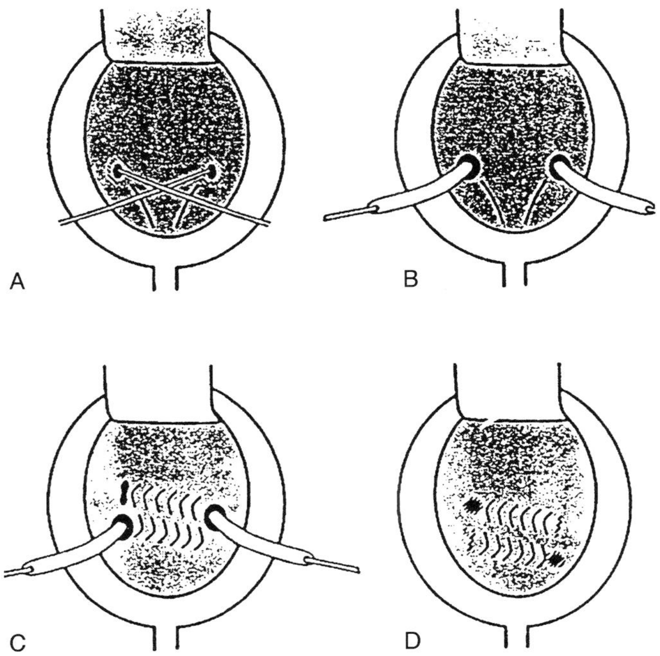

图 112-10　Cohen 横过三角区输尿管再植术。A. 双侧输尿管插管。B. 双侧输尿管游离，方法同 Leadbetter-Politano 手术。C. 关闭输尿管周围的逼尿肌，创建正常口径的裂隙，并且建立双侧跨三角区的隧道。D. 输尿管穿过相应的黏膜下隧道，并做输尿管开口成形。（From Rowe M, et al: Essentials of Pediatric Surgery. St Louis, Mosby-Year Book, 1995.）

石症已经发现了几个世纪，但是其临床表现、诊断和治疗方法仍在不断变化之中。

大约 7% 的结石发生于 16 岁以下的儿童[11]。传统上认为，尿石症分为膀胱结石和上尿路结石，分别多见于发展中国家和工业化发达地区。其中上尿路结石在儿童中的发病率远低于成人。同样，与成人结石相比较，小儿更多表现为代谢性因素以外的原因，如 UTI、解剖畸形和外科手术后的改变。现在，在没有上述易感因素的儿童中，上尿路结石的发病率也呈普遍上升趋势[1,85]，结石的类型也发生了改变。对尿石症患儿进行代谢评估的重要性已经得到体现，即使在地方性膀胱结石的好发区，其结石成因也与饮食有关。随着越来越精细的内镜设备和准确定位的体外冲击波碎石（ESWL）技术的出现，现在小儿结石病的治疗方法已经与成人十分接近。

结石病变谱

尽管有许多相关因素，但尿路结石形成最基本的概念是尿液浓缩。当一种溶质加入到溶剂中时，溶质会发生溶解，直到达到一定浓度，此时溶液呈饱和状态。超过这一浓度，溶质会在溶液中形成结晶，同时这些结晶会不断变大。超过饱和点后发生浓缩，结晶沉淀，形成晶核，这就是尿石形成的基础。结晶形成和聚合是结石形成的必要条件。这些过程同时受到抑

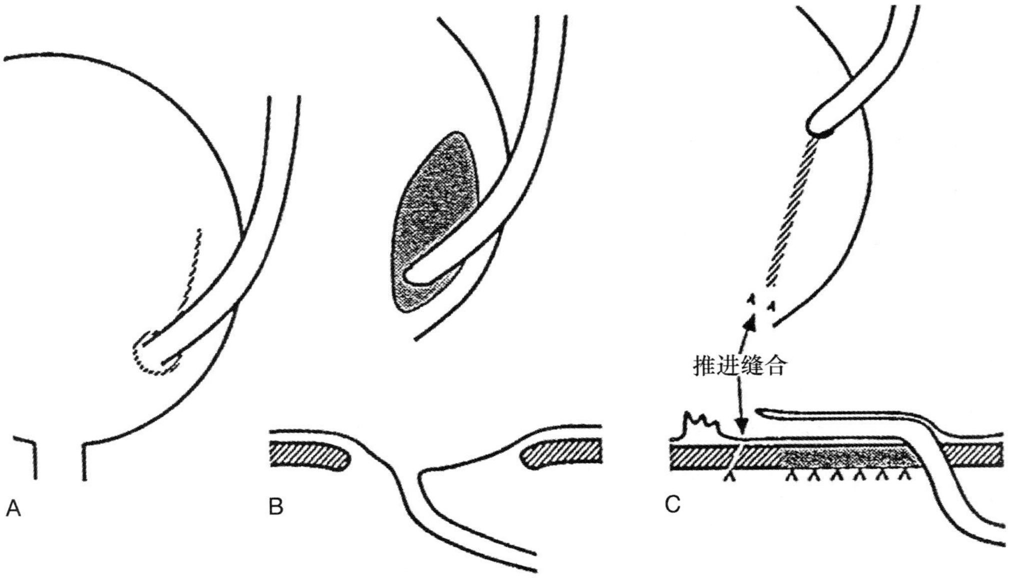

图 112-11　膀胱外逼尿肌修复术——改良的 Lich-Gregoir 手术。A. 膀胱外游离输尿管数公分，然后向尾端切开逼尿肌，并在输尿管插入处环形切开。B. 使输尿管仅与膀胱黏膜相连。C. 远端输尿管向前推移并缝合两针固定，然后缝合逼尿肌覆盖输尿管表面，重新建立一个更长的隧道。（From Rowe M, et al: Essentials of Pediatric Surgery. St Louis, Mosby-Year Book, 1995.）

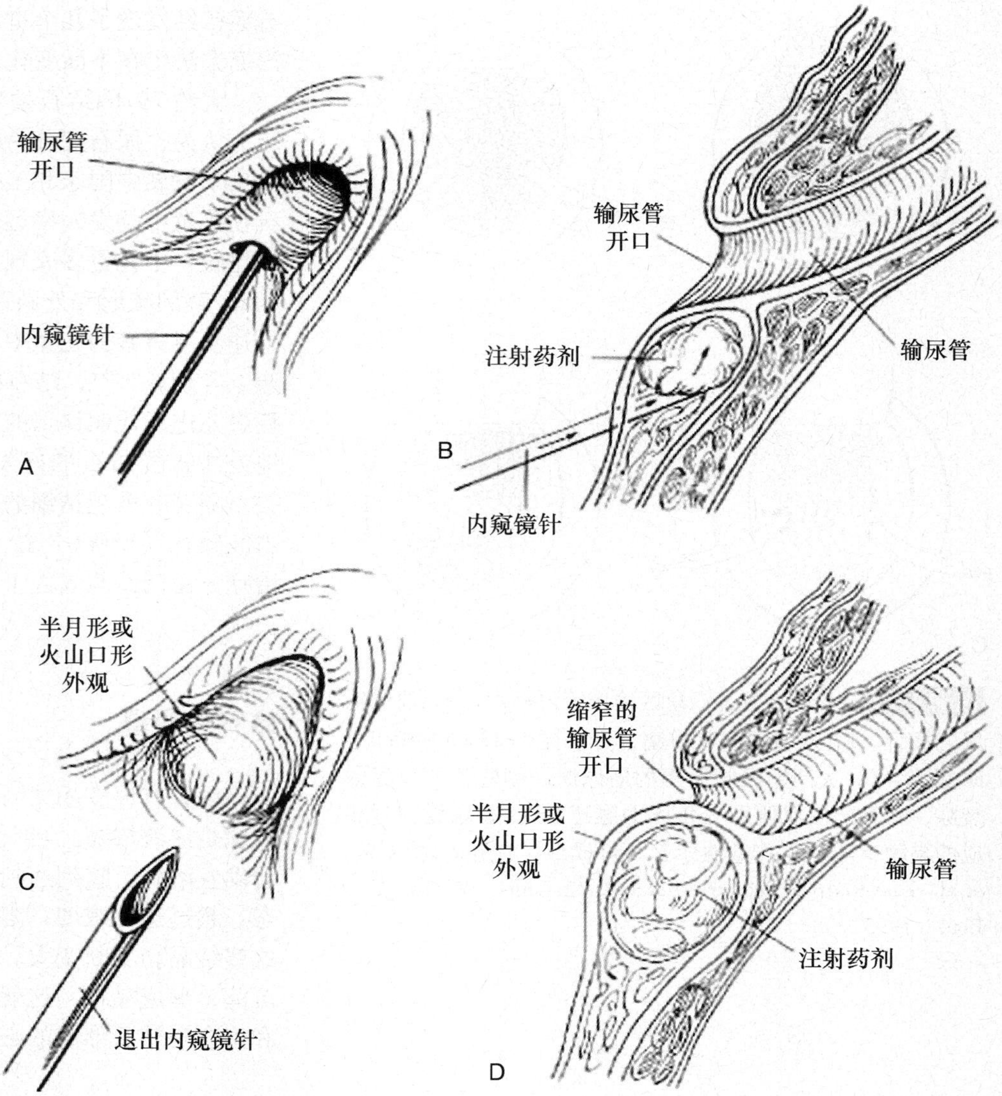

图 112-12　反流连接部的内镜治疗技术。A. 针刺入 6 点位置，针孔面向上。B. 在输尿管下缓慢注射。C. 注射后外观。D. 注射药物的正确位置。（From Russinko PJ, Tackett LD: Endoscopic correction of reflux. In Caldamone AA [ed]: Atlas Urol Clin North Am 2004; 12: 55.）

制因素和促进因素的影响。枸橼酸盐、镁、磷酸盐、肾钙素、黏蛋白（Tamm-Horsfall 蛋白）是结晶形成和聚合的抑制因素。细菌感染和解剖畸形如梗阻和尿流缓慢可以促进结晶聚合和滞留，增加临床上尿石症发生的风险[66,80]。许多关于儿童尿石症的研究表明
1750 代谢异常患者的比例可达 92%，高钙尿和低枸橼酸尿是最常见的[8,71,72,80,100-102]。值得注意的是，即使是在伴有尿石症和解剖梗阻的儿童中，尿液代谢异常的发生率也很高[66,72,81]。与感染相关的结石在 6 岁以下的小儿中发生率较高[21]。大约 12% 的结石患儿查不出明显的危险因素[96]。尿石症可以因其发病原因分为代谢性、解剖性、感染性或特发性。在有些病例中，这些发病因素可以互相重叠交错，其间的关系见表 112-8。

结石可以根据其位置分为上尿路（肾脏和输尿管）或下尿路（膀胱和尿道），也可以分为有症状和无症状。这些分类方法可能会对治疗方法的选择有一定影响。

临床表现

成人上尿路结石特征性的表现是出现肾绞痛症状。这种疼痛较剧烈、间歇出现、难以控制，常常伴有恶心和呕吐。不过这些表现在儿童中并不多见。尽管典型的肾绞痛也出现于儿童，但是更多见

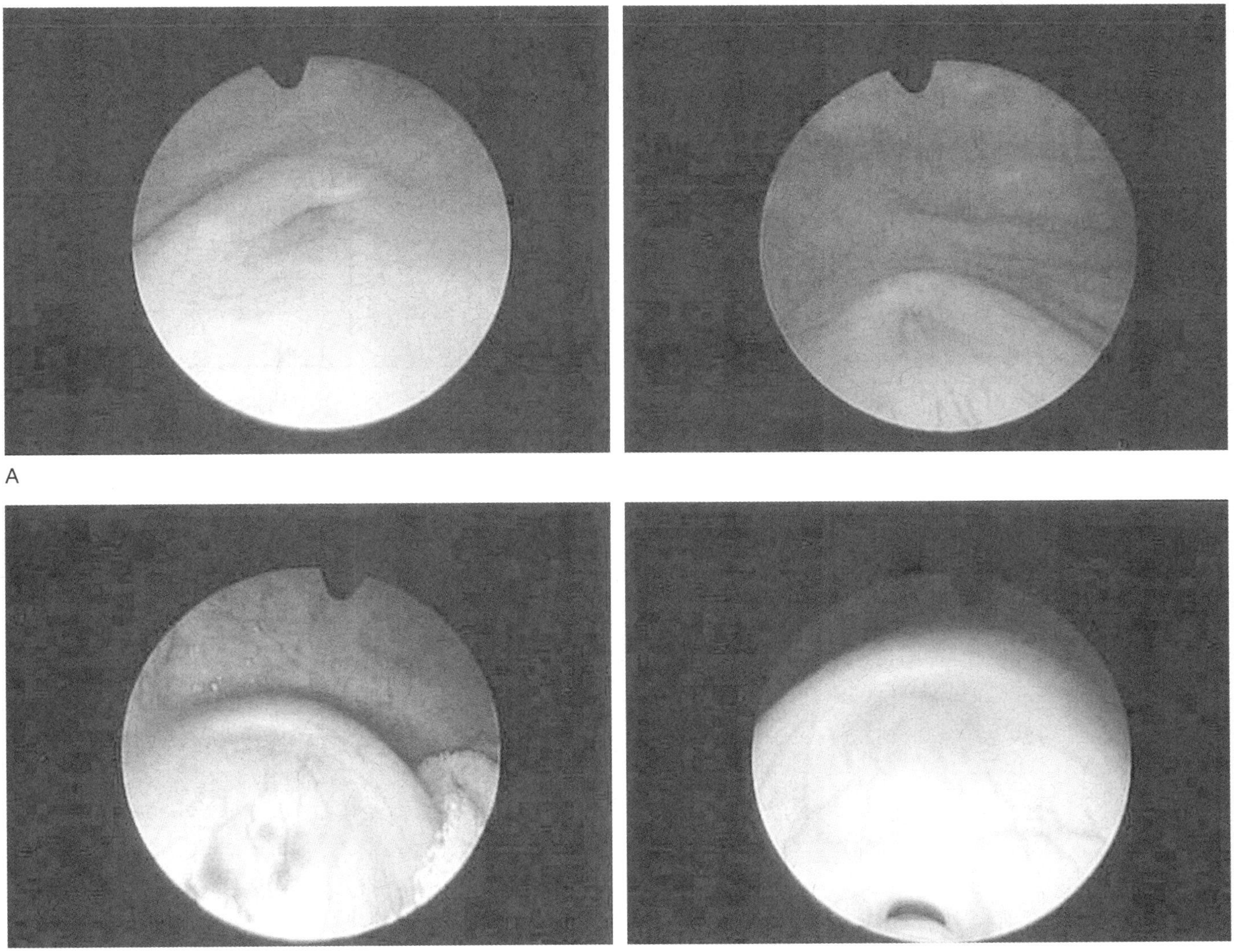

A

B

图 112-13　内镜注射。A. 注射前的左右输尿管开口。B. 注射后左右输尿管开口呈现半月形或火山口形外观（也见彩图）。

的是患儿因为 UTI 或血尿行影像学检查时发现上尿路和下尿路的结石。患儿也可以表现为非特异性的腹痛，伴有镜下血尿，有时可出现出口梗阻的表现（图 112-14）。

诊断

病史采集和体格检查对于排除其他原因引起的腹痛和背痛很有帮助。采集病史时应当包括饮食习惯和排尿情况。存在结石的证据之一是有肾结石的阳性家族史，这种情况出现于高达 37% 的尿石症患儿[69]。其他可以提示小儿患有结石的潜在情况包括：甲状旁腺功能亢进、肾小管酸中毒、炎性肠道疾病、癫痫病接受生酮膳食治疗[29]、囊性纤维化和 Dent 病[27]。常规进行尿液分析和尿培养，以明确有无镜下血尿、尿酸碱度、沉淀物结晶和 UTI。同时还要检查血清电解质、血尿素氮、肌酐、钙、尿酸、磷酸、镁。在对现有结石治疗后，应通过 24 小时尿液分析对患者进行结石风险评估。

影像学检查包括腹部平片、超声、静脉肾盂造影和 CT 平扫。对成人来说，标准的影像学检查是 CT 平扫，敏感度和特异度都很高。然而对儿童来说，尽管

表 112-8 儿童尿石症的临床诊断

诊断	Mayo 临床中心（N=221）患者数量（%）	北美（N=492）[#] 患者数量（%）	欧洲（N=481）[#] 患者数量（%）
代谢异常	115（52.0%）*	162（32.9）**	59（12.3）
特发性高钙尿	38	39	36
流动性降低	8	39	4
尿酸结石	8	22	2
地方性结石（尿酸盐）	0	10	0
胱氨酸尿	15	15	9
高草酸尿	25	12	5
肾小管酸中毒	4	10	2
其他	38**	25	1
泌尿生殖系统发育异常	66（29.9）*	160（32.5）	145（30.1）
感染			
原发性	41（18.6）*	21（4.3）	209（43.5）
所有原因	-	215（43.7）	358（74.4）
原因不明	55（24.9）	139（28.3）	68（14.1）

[#]Data from Polinsky MS, Kaiser BA, Bacuarte HJ: Urolithiasis in childhood. Pediatr Clin North Am 1987; 34: 683.

*代谢性异常经常会与泌尿生殖系统畸形和感染并存

**一个患者有不止一种异常

From Liebermann E: Importance of metabolic contributions to urolithiasis in pediatric patients [editorial]. Mayo Clin Proc 1993; 68: 313.

有些专家建议将 CT 作为第一线影像学检查手段，但所有这些检查的使用价值都有限[75,76]。其他专家推荐开始时使用腹部超声检查，主要是因为儿童尿路结石的表现差异大，而且也考虑到放射性辐射的因素[26,95]。腹部平片作为一线检查手段的帮助不大，但由于其对结石的成像作用，可以考虑用于辅助制订治疗方案。

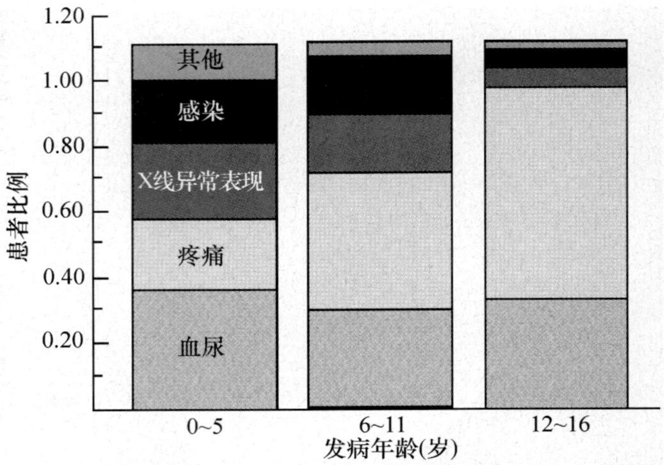

图 112-14 1965—1987 年间 Mayo 临床中心收治的 221 例儿童和青春期尿石症患者就诊时的临床表现。（From Milliner DS, Murphy ME: Urolithiasis in pediatric patients. Mayo Clin Proc 1993; 68: 241.）

治疗

初期治疗方案的确定要考虑到四个主要因素：临床情况、结石成分、结石大小和结石位置（表 112-9）。在有潜在的尿路梗阻合并发热或完全性梗阻的情况下，要确保立即解除梗阻，可以采用放置输尿管支撑管或经皮肾造瘘的方法。要在放置输尿管支撑管和经皮肾造瘘两者之间选择，需根据医生的情况、现有资源的情况以及患者的身材大小和解剖因素来选择。对儿童来说，肾造瘘引流可以不通过基础麻醉而实施，并可以作为首选。在梗阻解除并且给予抗感染治疗后，可进行针对取石的根治性治疗。

最常见的上尿路结石成分是草酸钙，这种结石辐射无法透过，溶解治疗无效。对一水草酸钙结石来说，ESWL 治疗可能无效，而 ESWL 对最常见的二水草酸钙的疗效较好。尿酸结石是透光结石，在尿 pH 低的环境下形成。一般可以在 CT 平扫中利用 Hounsfield 技术发现其特征性表现。尿酸结石可能通过溶石进行治疗，也可以利用碳酸氢钠和枸橼酸钾碱化尿液（pH >6.5）来预防。如果症状不消失，可以在溶石治疗的同时采用输尿管支撑或肾造瘘的方法暂时解除梗阻。鸟粪石结石一般都会伴发感染，所以在整个治疗过程中应当同时给予抗生素。由于鸟粪石（磷酸铵镁）结石通常比较大，或呈鹿角状外观，所

表 112-9 影响结石治疗的因素

因素	治疗要点
临床表现	
双侧梗阻	
孤立肾梗阻	对于所有这些表现，需要急诊通过支撑管或肾造瘘解除梗阻
发热/UTI 伴有潜在的梗阻	
难治性疼痛	
结石成分	
尿酸	考虑进行溶石治疗
鸟粪石（磷酸铵镁）	在整个治疗过程中持续应用抗生素治疗
胱氨酸	对 ESWL 治疗反应差
草酸钙	不透光结石，对 ESWL 治疗反应好
结石大小	
<4 mm	大约有 90% 的自行排出机会
4~6 mm	大约有 50% 的自行排出机会
>6 mm	大约有 10%~20% 的自行排出机会
结石位置	
肾脏	ESWL 或 PCNL
近端输尿管	输尿管镜取石（顺行）或 ESWL
远端输尿管	输尿管镜取石（逆行）或 ESWL
膀胱	膀胱切开取石或膀胱碎石取出

ESWL：体外冲击波碎石；PCNL：经皮肾穿刺取石；UTI：尿路感染。

以这种结石的一线治疗方法一般都是经皮肾穿刺取石
52 (percutaneous nephrostolithotomy，PCNL)。胱氨酸结石治疗往往比较困难且容易复发，小的肾脏胱氨酸结石可以通过 ESWL 治疗，而大的结石则很可能需要 PCNL或输尿管镜取石治疗[94]。

结石的大小指标可以用于判断该结石能否自行排出。成人中小于 4 mm 的结石排出机会是 90%，4~6 mm之间的结石自行排出的可能性约为 50%，对于超过 6 mm 的结石，其自行排出的可能性在 10%~20% 之间。有趣的是，儿童患者中通过 ESWL 治疗所产生的小结石或结石碎片也表现出与成人一样的排出机会，这在理论上可以通过输尿管的柔韧性和蠕动能力来解释[32,80,103]。因此，对于不伴发热或输尿管完全梗阻的患儿，在支持治疗中鼓励进水（口服或静脉）和止痛都是合理的初期治疗。研究表明，患者对短期的部分梗阻是可以耐受的，所以这种治疗可以在门诊进行 3~4 周，以促进结石自行排出。对于 4 mm 以上的梗阻性结石，自行排出的机会明显降低，提示需要尽早治疗。对于非梗阻性结石，可以选择性治疗。大于 2 cm 的结石 ESWL 治疗后排空效果较差。国立健康协会在 1998 年举办的研讨大会中推荐，对大于 2 cm 的结石可以采用 PCNL 作为一线治疗。“三明治疗法”是指将 PCNL 和 ESWL 结合在一起，是对大结石治疗的另一种医疗方法。

结石大多位于肾盂或肾盏、近端输尿管、远端输尿管或膀胱。部位不同意味着需要采用不同的处理措施。以肾结石来说，ESWL 和 PCNL 都可以采用。ESWL 或输尿管镜取石适用于治疗输尿管结石，而膀胱碎石取出和膀胱切开取石术则用于膀胱结石的治疗。

ESWL 最早于 19 世纪 80 年代早期提出[15]，是一种无创伤、耐受良好的治疗，但对许多年龄较小的儿童和需要特别照顾的婴儿来说，需要在基础麻醉下实施。现已经对体重仅 6.8 公斤的儿童进行了成功治疗。这一操作适用于近端输尿管结石，甚至包括一些远端输尿管结石。不过，女性输尿管中段以下的结石是这种治疗的禁忌证，主要是因为冲击波可能会对发育中的卵巢造成不可预知的影响。通过一到两次的治疗后，排石率为 70%～97%（平均 85%）[6,18,43,54,61]。ESWL 治疗的并发症包括不完全的结石碎片形成、碎片残留、石街、肾周血肿、发热、肾绞痛、冲击波出入部位的擦伤和淤斑[31]。尽管 ESWL 的远期和长期效果还不明确，但短期随访结果表明没有出现与肾功能和高血压相关的并发症[11,31,60,105]。

PCNL 需要放置肾造瘘管、基础麻醉，并进行住院治疗。一旦放置了肾造瘘管，就需要对通道进行扩张，以适应肾镜和电动液压或超声碎石钳[91]。这种方法的最佳适应证是大的伴有肾盂积水的肾结石或者是 ESWL 难治的结石（胱氨酸或一水草酸钙结石）。PCNL 和 ESWL 两者可以结合在一起，对于有些病例来说是最理想的治疗，称为三明治疗法。PCNL 还可能结合经肾造瘘管的 Renacidin 或 hemiacidrin 灌洗治
1753 疗，用于感染性结石，排石率接近 100%。然而对于儿童，取净结石可能需要多次手术。PCNL 的并发症包括集合系统穿孔、出血、灌洗液外渗、气胸、肠管损伤和碎片残留。

随着输尿管镜和设备向越来越小的方向不断发展，输尿管镜取石技术在小儿中的应用已经成为现实。输尿管结石可以通过顺行或逆行的方法进行输尿管镜取石，结石可以完整取出，或者结合激光、超声或液压碎石器（Swiss 碎石器）碎石。输尿管镜取石术治疗的成功率可能超过 95%[14,18,38,43,84,90]。术后留置输尿管支撑管 24～72 小时，以防止输尿管痉挛或水肿引起的狭窄。并发症包括输尿管穿孔、输尿管狭窄、反流、结石向近端移位以及结石通过输尿管穿孔部位脱落。

尽管小儿尿石症的微创治疗有较高的成功率，但是仍有 17% 的患者需要开放性的外科手术治疗[43]，这其中有约 45% 的患者可能会因此导致肾功能下降[34]。一些解剖畸形如肾盂输尿管连接部梗阻或梗阻性巨输尿管，需要对伴发的结石同时进行治疗，防止其复发，并且使肾功能保持在最佳状态[40,41]。

膀胱碎石术或经尿道膀胱结石碎石术适用于除很大结石外的所有结石。通过电动液压碎石器使结石变成碎片，然后通过灌洗方法使膀胱结石排出。膀胱结石已经越来越多地发生于接受过膀胱扩大术的患儿，尽管对这种患者进行开放手术完整取出结石还存在争议，但这是一种比较谨慎的选择，可以降低由于结石碎片残留引起结石复发的风险[13,20,86]。

结石复发

儿童尿石症有复发风险的时间比成人长，所以儿童结石总的复发率比较高。因此，对于患过一次尿石症的儿童，强烈推荐进行彻底的代谢性评估。要做 24 小时尿液的结石风险分析，至少包括尿量、pH、钙、肌酐、尿酸、枸橼酸、草酸和镁。在儿童期进入成人期的过程中，预防结石复发的基础是使患儿保持无石状态、检查和治疗代谢性异常、控制尿路感染、纠正解剖上的畸形。

肾静脉血栓

肾静脉血栓是指由于肾或肾内静脉急性广泛的闭锁而产生的一系列临床异常。Rayer 早在 150 多年前就对肾静脉血栓进行了首次描述[83]。在几十年的时间里，肾静脉血栓很少能够在临床上得到诊断，一般都是在手术或尸检中被发现。一旦在临床上发现这种疾病，首选治疗就是单纯肾切除，这种治疗指导一直持续到 19 世纪 60 年代早期[46,104]。在 1964 年，Stark 报道通过保守治疗可以取得很好的效果[97]，提示侵袭性的外科干预没有必要。抗凝剂和溶栓药物的应用还有争论，没有足够的儿童相关病例数目，同时也缺乏评价这些干预治疗利弊的对照试验。

病因

肾静脉血栓是一种婴儿期的疾病，大约有 80% 的病例在出生一个月内发病[4]。导致肾静脉血栓的原因有肾血流减少、血黏度增加和高凝状态。由于新生儿期肾脏灌注压低，有双重肾内毛细血管网，所以新生儿肾脏特别容易罹患此病。很多因素可以促成血液

浓缩，随着静脉血流缓慢，患者血栓形成的风险增加。此外，有近 50% 的患者在血栓发生前可能存在畸形[51,109]。血栓形成过程可以源于肾静脉主干，也可以是小的肾内静脉[37]。血栓可以是单侧或双侧的，但源于下腔静脉的血栓比较罕见[22]。

临床上新生儿肾静脉血栓的诱发因素包括早产[51]、围生期窒息、红细胞增多症、青紫型先天性心脏病[45]、母体患有糖尿病[7,77]、败血症、先天性肾病综合征[33,57]、巨细胞病毒感染[106]、休克、腹泻和脱水[5]、抗活化蛋白 C 现象[51]、V 因子 Leiden 基因杂合型[109]以及母体应用利尿剂和糖皮质激素[9]。已发现肾静脉血栓与肾上腺出血有关，并可通过产前超声检出[25,28,78]。

对于超过一个月的婴儿，肾静脉血栓通常会伴有低血容量，如胃肠道液体丢失或烧伤[5,23,33]，或与肾脏疾病有关，如肾病综合征[45,59]。肾静脉血栓可以继发于长时间的下腔静脉插管，由血栓扩展到肾静脉而引起[44]。

临床表现

临床表现不一，与年龄、血栓范围和血栓的急进情况有关。肾静脉血栓可以在产前即存在，或出现于没有易感疾病的健康儿童。新生儿的典型表现为可触及的肿块或肉眼血尿，不过这些表现仅仅出现于 13% 的获诊患儿[106]。在出现下肢肿胀、腹壁浅静脉扩张时，应当考虑到腔静脉血栓的可能。肾静脉血栓同样也可能出现于患有易感疾病的婴儿，也可以出现于既往有肾脏疾病（肾病综合征）的大年龄儿童。在大年龄儿童中的表现为急性腹痛、血尿和可触及的肿块。

54

诊断

肾静脉血栓往往伴有血小板减少（血小板计数 $<75\,000/mm^3$），这是由肾静脉血栓对血小板截流所造成的。还可出现特征性的消耗性凝血性疾病，表现为凝血酶原时间延长、纤维蛋白降解产物增加。白细胞增多的情况很常见，还有各种类型的贫血表现。血浆中的电解质变化很大，与易感疾病和肾功能有关。尿液检查经常发现血尿和蛋白尿，应当考虑进行凝血酶原异常的筛查。

影像学

腹部 X 线片检查可见增大的肾影，或者有类似肾血管的树状饰带影，但在通常情况下，这些表现都是正常的[12]。肾脏超声多普勒检查是一种较好的检查方法，用于评价肾脏肿块以及显示肾静脉和下腔静脉。具有诊断意义的影像包括静脉中的血栓和增大的肾脏。在疾病的初发期和恢复期可以通过肾脏核素扫描进行肾功能监测，如锝 99m－DMSA 或锝 99m－MAG3。CT、核磁共振以及下腔静脉造影用于明确血栓的范围（是否涉及下腔静脉），或者排除引起栓子或血栓的罕见原因（如肾脏外部压迫或来自于肾脏肿瘤的栓子）。

治疗

由于肾静脉血栓相对比较少见，而且目前还缺乏相关的临床对照研究，因此现在还没有一种普遍接受的理想治疗方法。尽管以前对急性期的患者进行过肾切除或血栓切除手术，但是这些治疗实际上并非一定要在急性期实施，现在这些方法仅限于累及下腔静脉的解剖学梗阻[97]。最初治疗应当包括纠正或治疗所有的易感性因素、积极补充液体和电解质、防止静脉血栓的脱落和传播。治疗中抗凝药物和溶栓药物的应用还存在争议，因为缺乏相关的对照试验。在最近的 16 例肾静脉血栓的回顾性研究中，9 例应用了肝素或依诺肝素或同时应用了这两种药物，其中有 6 例患儿肾功能保持正常，而另外 7 例没有应用抗凝药物治疗的患儿都不能维持正常的肾功能[99,109]。比较合理的方案包括对没有影响到腔静脉的单侧肾静脉血栓进行积极的支持治疗，尤其是对那些较易发生出血性并发症的患者。对于病变涉及腔静脉的单侧肾静脉血栓或者双侧肾静脉血栓，由于存在肺栓塞和肾衰竭的风险，可以考虑应用肝素治疗。对于双侧肾静脉血栓和肾衰竭的患者，可以考虑应用溶栓治疗。肝素治疗时间应当持续 7～14 天，如表 112－10 所示[4]。尽管肝素治疗已经成功应用于临床，但在新生儿中还

表 112-10 全身应用肝素的治疗和调整方案

1. 负荷量：肝素 75 U/kg IV 超过 10 分钟
2. 初始维持量：小于 1 岁婴儿 28 U/(kg·h)；大于 1 岁儿童 20 U/(kg·h)
3. 调整肝素用量以使 APTT 维持在 60~85 秒（假定这一指标反应 0.35~0.70 的抗 Xa 因子水平）

APTT（秒）	单次剂量（U/kg）	停用时间（分钟）	速率改变（%）	复测 APTT
<50	50	0	+10	4 小时
50~59	0	0	+10	4 小时
60~85	0	0	0	次日
86~95	0	0	-10	4 小时
96~120	0	30	-10	4 小时
>120	0	60	-15	4 小时

4. 在首剂肝素应用后及每次调整肝素输注速度后，每 4 小时测定血 APTT
5. 当 APTT 值达到治疗范围后，每天测定 CBC 和 APTT

APTT：活化部分凝血活酶时间；CBC：全血细胞计数

From Andrew M, Brooker LA: Hemostatic complications in renal disorders of the young. Pediatr Nephrol 1996; 10: 88.

有出血性并发症的报道[73,107]。小分子量肝素是比较安全的选择，在早产儿或足月新生儿中[68,109]，还要在用量选择上特别注意。已有报道全身或局部应用链激酶或尿激酶进行溶栓治疗[22,33,73]。全身应用链激酶的潜在并发症包括出血和过敏反应，选择性的局部应用并发症较少。由于在许多研究中对溶栓药物应用的方法、次数以及疗程都不一致，所以在这方面很难建立一个标准化的方案。

结果

随着对肾静脉血栓及其不同易患因素的认识和治疗水平的不断提高，患者的存活率已经上升到 80%~85%[4]。绝大多数死亡都是由于其原发疾病，而不是肾梗死。长期并发症包括高血压、肾萎缩和慢性 UTI，对这些疾病还没有进行系统的评估。在肾功能方面，其结果可以从完全恢复到无功能。利用放射性核素闪烁扫描进行阶段性监测，可以比较详细地随访评价肾功能的恢复情况。肾萎缩伴肾素性高血压以及萎缩肾单位的反复 UTI 都是进行肾切除的合理指征。

（赵海腾译 刘国华校）

参考文献

1. Al-Eisa AA, Al-Hunayyan A, Gupta R: Pediatric urolithiasis in Kuwait. Int Urol Nephrol 2002;33:3.
2. American Academy of Pediatrics, Committee on Quality Improvement, Subcommittee on Urinary Tract Infection: Practice parameter: The diagnosis, treatment, and evaluation of the initial urinary tract infection in febrile infants and young children. Pediatrics 1999;103:843.
3. American Academy of Pediatrics, Task Force on Circumcision: Circumcision policy statement. Pediatrics 1999; 103:686.
4. Andrew M, Brooker LA: Hemostatic complications in renal disorders of the young. Pediatr Nephrol 1996;10:88.
5. Arneil GC, MacDonald AM, Sweet EM: Renal vein thrombosis. Clin Nephrol 1973;1:119.
6. Ather MH, Noor MA: Does size and site matter for renal stones up to 30-mm in size in children treated by extracorporeal lithotripsy? Urology 2003;61:212.
7. Avery ME, Oppenheimer EH, Gordon HH: Renal vein thrombosis in newborn infants of diabetic mothers. N Engl J Med 1957;256:1134.
8. Battino BS, DeFoor W, Coe F, et al: Metabolic evaluation of children with urolithiasis: Are adult references for supersaturation appropriate? J Urol 2002;168:2568.
9. Belman AB: Renal vein thrombosis in infancy and childhood. Clin Pediatr 1976;15:1033.
10. Belman AB, Kaplan GW: Calculus disease. In Belman AB, Kaplan GW (eds): Genitourinary Problems in Pediatrics. Philadelphia, WB Saunders, 1981.
11. Borman V, Nagel R: Urolithiasis in childhood—a study of 181 cases. Urol Int 1982;37:178.
12. Brill PW, Mitty HA, Strauss L: Renal vein thrombosis: A cause of intrarenal calcification in the newborn. Pediatr Radiol 1977;6:172.
13. Cain MP, Casale AJ, Kaefer M, et al: Percutaneous cystolithotomy in the pediatric augmented bladder. J Urol 2002;168:1881.
14. Caione P, De Gennaro M, Capozza N, et al: Endoscopic manipulation of ureteral calculi in children by rigid operative ureteroscopy. J Urol 1990;144:484.
15. Chaussy C, Schmiedt E, Jocham D, et al: First clinical experience with extracorporeally induced destruction of kidney stones by shock waves. J Urol 1982;127:417.
16. Chertin B, Colhoun E, Velayudham M, et al: Endoscopic treatment of vesicoureteral reflux: 11 to 17 years of followup. J Urol 2002;167:1443.
17. Chon CH, Lai FC, Shortliffe LM: Pediatric urinary tract infections. Pediatr Clin North Am 2001;48:1441.
18. Choong S, Whitfield H, Duffy P, et al: The management of paediatric urolithiasis. BJU Int 2000;86:857.
19. Decter RM: Vesicoureteral reflux. Pediatr Rev 2001; 22:205.
20. DeFoor W, Minevich E, Reddy P, et al: Bladder calculi after augmentation cystoplasty: Risk factors and prevention strategies. J Urol 2004;172:1964.
21. Diamond DA, Rickwood AM, Lee PH, Johnston JH: Infection stones in children: A twenty-seven-year review. Urology 1994;43:525.
22. Duncan BW, Adzick NS, Longaker MT, et al: In utero arterial embolism from renal vein thrombosis with successful postnatal thrombolytic therapy. J Pediatr Surg 1991;26:741.
23. Duncan RE, Evans AT, Martin LW: Natural history and treatment of renal vein thrombosis in children. J Pediatr

Surg 1977;12:639.
24. Elder JS, Peters CA, Arant BS, et al: Pediatric Vesicoureteral Reflux Guidelines Panel summary report on the management of primary vesicoureteral reflux in children. J Urol 1997;157:1846.
25. Errington ML, Hendry GM: The rare association of right adrenal hemorrhage and renal vein thrombosis diagnosed with duplex ultrasound. Pediatr Radiol 1995;25:157.
26. Eshed I, Witzling M: The role of unenhanced helical CT in the evaluation of suspected renal colic and atypical abdominal pain in children. Pediatr Radiol 2002;32:205.
27. Faerber GJ: Pediatric urolithiasis. Curr Opin Urol 2001; 11:385.
28. Fishman JE, Joseph RC: Renal vein thrombosis in utero: Duplex sonography in diagnosis and follow-up. Pediatr Radiol 1994;24:135.
29. Furth SL, Casey JC, Pyzik PL, et al: Risk factors for urolithiasis in children on the ketogenic diet. Pediatr Nephrol 2000;15:125.
30. Gendrel D, Chalumeau M, Moulin F, Raymond J: Fluoroquinolones in paediatrics: A risk for the patient or for the community? Lancet Infect Dis 2003;3:537.
31. Goel MC, Baserge NS, Babu RV, et al: Pediatric kidney: Functional outcome after extracorporeal shock wave lithotripsy. J Urol 1996;155:2044..
32. Gofrit ON, Pode D, Meretyk S, et al: Is the pediatric ureter as efficient as the adult ureter in transporting fragments following extracorporeal shock wave lithotripsy for renal calculi larger than 10 mm? J Urol 2001;166:1862.
33. Gonzalez R, Schwartz S, Sheldon CA, Fraley EE: Bilateral renal vein thrombosis in infancy and childhood. Urol Clin North Am 1982;9:279.
34. Gough DCS, Baillie CT: Paediatric anatrophic nephrolithotomy: Stone clearance—at what price? BJU Int 2000;85:874.
35. Handel LN, Caldamone AA: Urinary tract infections in the pediatric population. Lebanese Med J (accepted for publication).
36. Hellerstein S: Recurrent urinary tract infections in children. Pediatr Infect Dis 1982;1:271.
37. Hepler AB: Thrombosis of renal veins. J Urol 1934;31:527.
38. Hill DE, Segura JW, Patterson DE: Ureteroscopy in children. J Urol 1990;144:481.
39. Hoberman A, Charron M, Hickey RW, et al: Imaging studies after a first febrile urinary tract infection in young children. N Engl J Med 2003;348:195.
40. Husmann DA, Milliner DS, Segura JW: Ureteropelvic junction obstruction with simultaneous renal calculi: Long-term follow-up. J Urol 1995;153:1399.
41. Husmann DA, Milliner DS, Segura JW: Ureteropelvic junction obstruction with concurrent renal pelvic calculi in the pediatric patient: Long-term follow-up. J Urol 1996; 156:741.
42. Jakobsson BJ, Esbjorner E, Hansson S: Minimum incidence and diagnostic rate of first urinary tract infection. Pediatrics 1999;104:222.
43. Jayanthi VR, Arnold PM, Koff SA: Strategies for managing upper tract calculi in young children. J Urol 1999;162:1234.
44. Kaplan BS, Chesney RW, Drummond KN: The nephrotic syndrome and renal vein thrombosis. Am J Dis Child 1978; 132:367.
45. Karafin L, Stearn TM: Renal vein thrombosis in children. J Urol 1964;92:91.
46. Kaufman JH: Renal vein thrombosis. Am J Dis Child 1958; 95:377.
47. Keren R, Chan E: A meta-analysis of randomized, controlled trials comparing short- and long-course antibiotic therapy for urinary tract infections in children. Pediatrics 2002;109:E70.
48. Kirsch AJ, Perez-Brayfield MR, Scherz AC: Minimally invasive treatment of vesicoureteral reflux with endoscopic injection of dextranomer/hyaluronic acid copolymer: The Children's Hospitals of Atlanta experience. J Urol 2003;170:21.
49. Koff SA, Wagner TT, Jayanthi VR: The relationship among dysfunctional elimination syndromes, primary vesicoureteral reflux and urinary tract infections in children. J Urol 1998;160:1019.
50. Kraus SJ: Genitourinary imaging in children. Pediatr Clin North Am 2001;48:1381.
51. Kuhle S, Massicotte P, Chan A, Mitchell L: A case series of 72 neonates with renal vein thrombosis: Data from the 1-800-No-Clots Registry. Thromb Haemost 2004;92:729.
52. Kurzock EA, Huffman JL, Hardy BE, Fugelso P: Endoscopic treatment of pediatric urolithiasis. J Pediatr Surg 1996; 31:1413.
53. Lackgren G, Wahlin N, Skoldenberg E, et al: Long term followup of children treated with dextranomer/hyaluronic acid copolymer for vesicoureteral reflux. J Urol 2001;166:1887.
54. Landau EH, Gofrit ON, Shapiro A, et al: Extracorporeal shock wave lithotripsy is highly effective for ureteral calculi in children. J Urol 2001;165:23.
55. Layton KL: Diagnosis and management of pediatric urinary tract infections. Clin Fam Pract 2003;5:367.
56. Lerman SE, Liao JC: Neonatal circumcision. Pediatr Clin North Am 2001;48:1539.
57. Levy PR, Tao W: Nephrotic syndrome in association with REV1 in infancy. J Pediatr 1974;85:359.
58. Liao JC, Churchill BM: Pediatric urine testing. Pediatr Clin North Am 2001;48:1425.
59. Llach F, Pepper S, Massry SG: The clinical spectrum of renal vein thrombosis: Acute and chronic. Am J Med 1980; 9:819.
60. Lottmann HB, Archambaud F, Hellal B, et al: 99m Technetium-dimercapto-succinic acid renal scan in the evaluation of potential long-term renal parenchymal damage associated with extracorporeal shock wave lithotripsy in children. J Urol 1998;159:521.
61. Lottmann HB, Archambaud F, Traxer O, et al: The efficacy and parenchymal consequences of extracorporeal shock wave lithotripsy in infants. BJU Int 2000;85:311.
62. Mahant S, To T, Friedman J: Timing of voiding cystourethrogram in the investigation of urinary tract infections in children. J Pediatr 2001;139:568.
63. Malizia AA, Reiman HM, Myers RP, et al: Migration and granulomatous reaction after periurethral injection of Polytef (Teflon). JAMA 1984;251:3277.
64. Matouschek E: Die Behandlung des vesikorenalen refluxes durch transurethrale einspritzung von teflonpaste. Urologe A 1981;20:263.
65. McKenna PH, Herndon CD: Voiding dysfunction associated with incontinence, vesicoureteral reflux and recurrent urinary tract infections. Curr Opin Urol 2000;10:599.
66. Menon M, Resnick MI: Urinary lithiasis: Etiology, diagnosis, and medical management. In Walsh PC, et al (eds): Campbell's Urology, 8th ed. Philadelphia, WB Saunders, 2002.
67. Metreweli C, Pearson R: Echographic diagnosis of neonatal renal vein thrombosis. Pediatr Radiol 1984;14:105.
68. Michaels LA, Gurian M, Hegyi T, Drachtman RA: Low molecular weight heparin in the treatment of venous and arterial thromboses in the premature infant. Pediatrics 2004;114:703.
69. Milliner DS, Murphy ME: Urolithiasis in pediatric patients.

Mayo Clin Proc 1993;68:241.
70. Noe HN: The role of dysfunctional voiding in failure or complication of ureteral reimplantation for primary reflux. J Urol 1985;134:1172.
71. Noe HN: Hypercalciuria and pediatric stone recurrences with and without structural abnormalities. J Urol 2000; 164:1094.
72. Noe HN, Stapleton FB, Jerkins GR, Roy S 3rd: Clinical experience with pediatric urolithiasis. J Urol 1983;129:1166.
73. Nuss R, Hays T, Manco-Johnson M: Efficacy and safety of heparin anticoagulation for neonatal renal vein thrombosis. Am J Pediatr Hematol Oncol 1994;16:127.
74. O'Donnell B, Puri P: Technical refinements in endoscopic correction of vesicoureteral reflux. J Urol 1998;140:1101.
75. Onen A, Jayanthi VR, Koff SA: Unenhanced spiral CT: The imaging method of choice in diagnosing renal ureteric calculi in children. BJU Int 2000;85:38.
76. Oner S, Oto A, Tekgul S, et al: Comparison of spiral CT and US in the evaluation of pediatric urolithiasis. JBR-BTR 2004;87:219.
77. Oppenheimer EH, Esterly JR: Thrombosis in the newborn: Comparison between infants of diabetic and nondiabetic mothers. J Pediatr 1965;67:549.
78. Orazi C, Fariello G, Malena S, et al: Renal vein thrombosis and adrenal hemorrhage in the newborn: Ultrasound evaluation of 4 cases. J Clin Ultrasound 1993;21:163.
79. Palmer LS, Franco I, Rotario P, et al: Biofeedback therapy expedites the resolution of reflux in older children. J Urol 2002;168:1699.
80. Pietrow PK, Pope JC 4th, Adams MC, et al: Clinical outcome of pediatric stone disease. J Urol 2002;167:670.
81. Polinsky MS, Kaiser BA, Bacuarte HJ: Urolithiasis in childhood. Pediatr Clin North Am 1987;34:683.
82. Puri P, Chertin B, Velaydham M, et al: Treatment of vesicoureteral reflux by endoscopic injection of dextranomer/ hyaluronic acid copolymer: Preliminary results. J Urol 2003; 170:1541.
83. Rayer PRO: Trate des Maladies des Reins. Paris, JB Bailliere, 1841.
84. Reddy PP, Barrieras DJ, Bagli DJ, et al: Initial experience with endoscopic holmium laser lithotripsy for pediatric urolithiasis. J Urol 1999;162:1714.
85. Rizvi SA, Naqvi SA, Hussain Z, et al: Pediatric urolithiasis: Developing nation perspectives. J Urol 2002;168:1522.
86. Roberts WW, Gearhart JP, Mathews RI: Time to recurrent stone formation in patients with bladder or continent reservoir reconstruction: Fragmentation versus intact extraction. J Urol 2004;172:1706.
87. Russinko PJ, Tackett LD: Endoscopic correction of reflux. In Caldamone AA (ed): Atlas Urol Clin North Am 2004;12:55.
88. Schaad UB: Fluoroquinolone antibiotics in infants and children. Infec Dis Clin N Amer 2005;19:617.
89. Schlager TA: Urinary tract infections in infants and children. Infect Dis Clin North Am 2003;17:353.
90. Schuster TG, Russell KY, Bloom DA, et al: Ureteroscopy for the treatment of urolithiasis in children. J Urol 2002;167:1813.
91. Segura JW: Role of percutaneous procedures in the management of renal calculi. Urol Clin 1990;17:207.
92. Shortliffe LD: Urinary tract infections in infants and children. In Walsh P, Retik A, Vaughan ED, Wein A (eds): Campbell's Urology, 8th ed. Philadelphia, WB Saunders, 2002.
93. Shortliffe LM, McCue JD: Urinary tract infections at the age extremes: Pediatrics and geriatrics. Am J Med 2002; 113(Suppl 1A):55S.
94. Slavkovic A, Radovanovic M, Siric Z, et al: Extracorporeal shock wave lithotripsy for cystine urolithiasis in children: Outcome and complications. Int Urol Nephrol 2002-2003; 34:457.
95. Smith SL, Somers JM, Broderick N, Halliday K: The role of the plain radiograph and renal tract ultrasound in the management of children with renal tract calculi. Clin Radiol 2000;55:708.
96. Stapleton FB: Clinical approach to children with urolithiasis. Semin Nephrol 1996;16:389.
97. Stark H: Renal vein thrombosis in infancy. Am J Dis Child 1964;108:430.
98. Stenberg A, Lackgren G: A new bioimplant for the endoscopic treatment of vesicoureteral reflux: Experimental and short-term clinical results. J Urol 1995;154:800.
99. Streif W, Goebel G, Chan AK, Massicotte MP: Use of low molecular mass heparin (enoxaparin) in newborn infants: A prospective cohort study of 62 patients. Arch Dis Child 2003;88:365.
100. Tefekli A, Esen T, Ziylan O, et al: Metabolic risk factors in pediatric and adult calcium oxalate urinary stone formers: Is there any difference? Urol Int 2003;70:273.
101. Tekin A, Tekgul S, Atsu N, et al: A study of the etiology of idiopathic calcium urolithiasis in children: Hypocitraturia is the most important risk factor. J Urol 2000;164:162.
102. Tekin A, Tekgul S, Atsu N, et al: Ureteropelvic junction obstruction and coexisting renal calculi in children: Role of metabolic abnormalities. Urology 2001;57:542.
103. Van Savage JG, Palanca LG, Andersen RD, et al: Treatment of distal ureteral stones in children: Similarities to the American Urological Association guidelines in adults. J Urol 2000;164:1089.
104. Verhagen AD, Hamilton JP, Genel M: Renal vein thrombosis in infants. Arch Dis Child 1965;40:214.
105. Vlajkovic M, Slavkovic A, Radovanovic M, et al: Long-term functional outcome of kidneys in children with urolithiasis after ESWL treatment. Eur J Pediatr Surg 2002;12:118.
106. Vorticky LH, Balfour HH Jr: Cytomegalovirus and renal vein thrombosis in a newborn infant. Am J Dis Child 1974;1276:742.
107. Weinschenk N, Pelidis M, Fiascone J: Combination thrombolytic and anticoagulant therapy for bilateral renal vein thrombosis in a premature infant. Am J Perinatol 2001; 18:293.
108. Williams G, Lee A, Craig J: Antibiotics for the prevention of urinary tract infection in children: A systematic review of randomized controlled trials. J Pediatr 2001;138:868.
109. Zigman A, Yazbeck S, Emil S, Nguyen L: Renal vein thrombosis: A 10 year review. J Pediatr Surg 2000;35:1540.

第 113 章

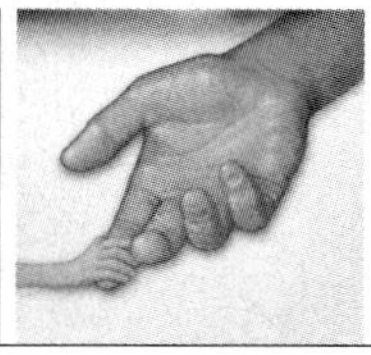

输尿管重复畸形和输尿管囊肿

Victor E. Boston

758 输尿管重复畸形和输尿管囊肿的解剖、临床表现和治疗十分复杂。明确了解肾脏、输尿管和膀胱的胚胎发育过程，对理解这些疾病的变异和重要性非常重要，是选择合理治疗方案的基础。

定义

以往对输尿管重复畸形和输尿管囊肿的定义还存在混淆。1984 年，美国儿童学会委员会泌尿学分会在定义、命名和分类方面做出了目前被广为接受的阐述[33]。

重复系统 指一个肾脏具有两个肾盂肾盏系统。*完全重复* 指一个肾脏拥有两条输尿管，并分别引流入膀胱或膀胱以下部位。*不完全重复* 指一个肾脏拥有两条输尿管，这两条输尿管最终融合成一条通道，并通过一个开口引流入膀胱。*分支系统* 是不完全重复的一种形式。

上极和下极输尿管 指分别引流肾脏上极和下极的输尿管。*上位输尿管开口和下位输尿管开口* 指分别与上极输尿管和下极输尿管相对应的输尿管开口。异位输尿管指引流到异常部位的输尿管。

输尿管囊肿 是输尿管下端与下尿路上皮交界处的囊性扩张。*膀胱内输尿管囊肿* 完全位于膀胱内，而 *异位输尿管囊肿* 则有一部分位于膀胱颈下方。输尿管囊肿在仅有单一输尿管的情况下称为 *单系统*，而在伴有双输尿管的情况下则称为 *双系统*。

胚胎学

在发育期胚胎后部的两侧，出现过三个排泄系统：前肾、中肾和后肾。这些结构在妊娠第三周开始出现，并按照时间和空间顺序从胚胎头端向尾端依次出现。肾脏发育源于后肾胚基。在发育过程中，前肾与中肾最终完全消失，留下中肾管结构作为仅存的原始排泄管道。中肾管远端与发育中的膀胱和泌尿生殖窦相交通，并且在胚胎第四周发育得比较明显[84]。正常的胚胎发育过程中，在接近妊娠第四周末时，中肾管在末端向内侧弯曲进入泄殖腔（图 113-1A），并在此处出现一个外生组织（输尿管芽）[84]。这一附属结构在一开始时是一个实体的细胞束，随后会发生腔化[17]。输尿管芽向外上方朝着发育中的肾脏方向生长，并与后肾胚接触，促使肾小球和肾脏的近端及远端小管的正常发育（图 113-1B）。输尿管芽自身演变成输尿管、肾盂、肾盏以及肾脏的乳头小管和集合管。这一相互作用过程发生在一个限定的时间窗内，否则就会出现肾发育不良[54,68]。

泄殖腔分成前方的泌尿生殖窦和后方的消化管。在妊娠第八周，中肾管远端末端加上输尿管芽延续段上方的小部分泄殖腔，通过不断地分化生长，合并成为发育中的膀胱下部后壁和泌尿生殖窦（图 113-1C）。 1759
在这一阶段，中肾管位于输尿管开口的下内方，称为 wolffian 管。经过这一迁移过程，使得正常输尿管开口位于膀胱三角区的上外侧角[75]。

男性中肾管发育成为附睾、输精管和精囊，并在尿道外括约肌上方精阜水平进入后尿道。与之伴行的输尿管芽同样也在外括约肌上方处连接发育中的膀胱和尿道。最初发生于发育中的肾脏内侧区域的睾丸开始与中肾管相接。在下降到内环深处过程中，输精管（中肾管）在输尿管前方跨过，并在精阜水平处呈弓形向下内侧进入的精囊[75]。

女性中肾管演变为 Gartner 管，紧靠阴道侧壁。

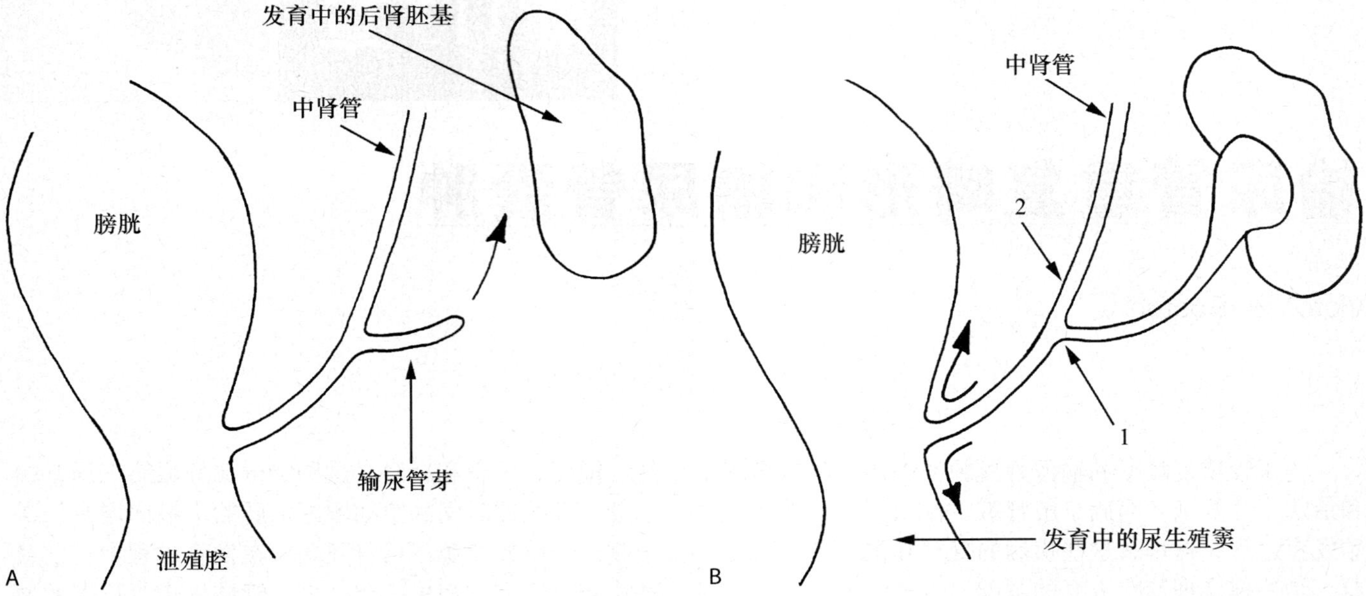

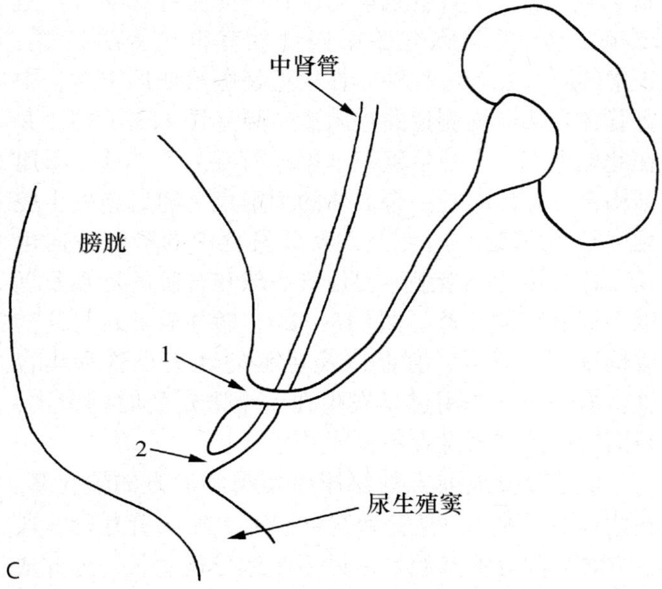

图 113-1　A. 在妊娠第四周末，中肾管远端出现芽状突起，朝向发育中的肾脏（后肾）胚基生长。B. 在妊娠第五周，输尿管芽与胚胎肾的胚基接触，诱导肾小球、近端和远端小管的发育。集合管、乳头管、肾盏、肾盂和输尿管发生自输尿管芽。这一相互作用的过程发生在一个适当的时间窗内，否则就会出现肾发育不良。中肾管的下端展开加入发育中的膀胱和尿生殖窦。输尿管芽开口（1）和伴行的中肾管（2）迁移并参与组成这些结构的一部分。C. 在妊娠第八周，中肾管的末端与其在输尿管芽上方的一小段展开分化生长，构成发育中的膀胱和尿生殖窦后壁的下部。在此阶段，中肾管（2）变成男性输精管，位于输尿管开口（1）的下内侧。

旁中肾管（müllerian 管）从中肾管内侧发出。在胚胎的尾端，这些结构与中肾管残迹的远端相结合，并在此处穿破中线处的泄殖腔。因此，由于性别分化生长的关系，输尿管芽及与其伴行的旁中肾管结构一起迁移到前庭、阴道、子宫颈、子宫或直肠等部位[75]。

如果单一的输尿管芽继续分支，可以导致不同程度的不完全性输尿管重复畸形。如果这一过程发生在妊娠第五周输尿管芽到达后肾胚基以后，会形成分支肾盂。如果输尿管分叉发生在妊娠第五周以前，会形成两条输尿管，可在输尿管全长任何地方发生分支，但在膀胱内仅有一个输尿管开口。

当在中肾管有两条输尿管芽同时发出时，会发生完全性输尿管重复畸形（图 113-2A）[16]。与单一系统一样，在妊娠第八周左右，中肾管远端末端加入输尿管芽延续段上方的小部分泄殖腔，通过不断地分化生长，合并成为发育中的膀胱下部后壁和尿生殖窦。最终形成的上极输尿管位于下极输尿管的下内侧（图 113-2B 和 C）。

两个输尿管芽的最上方最后发育。这样的结果是：越是上方的输尿管芽，与肾脏上极接触的时间越

17

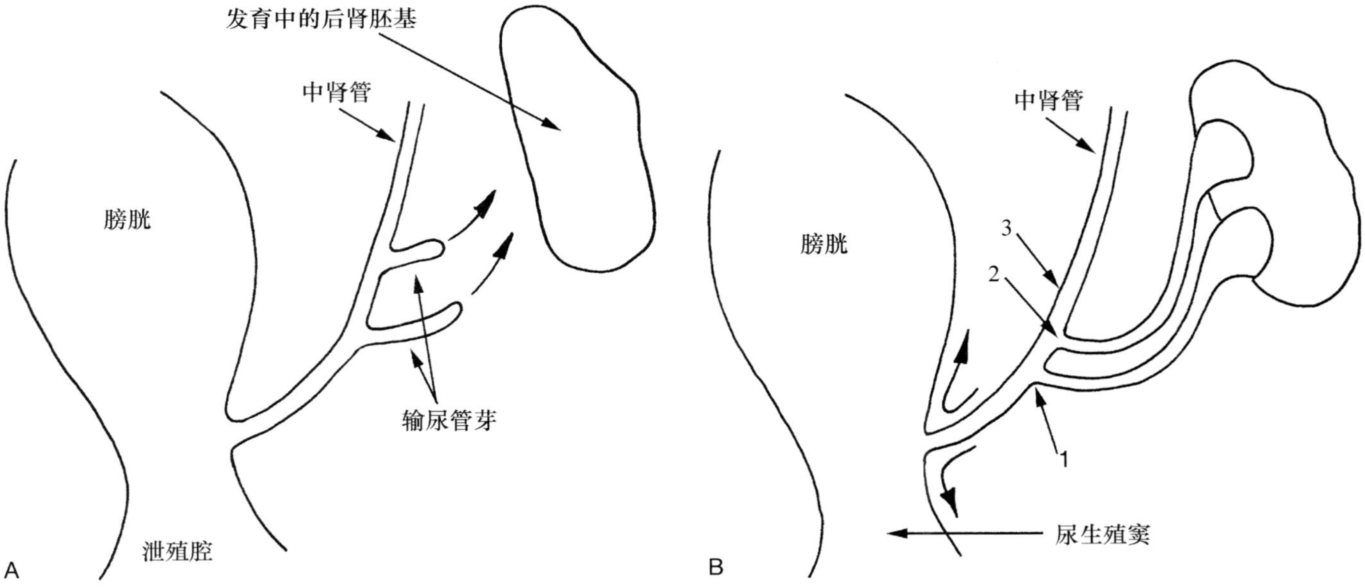

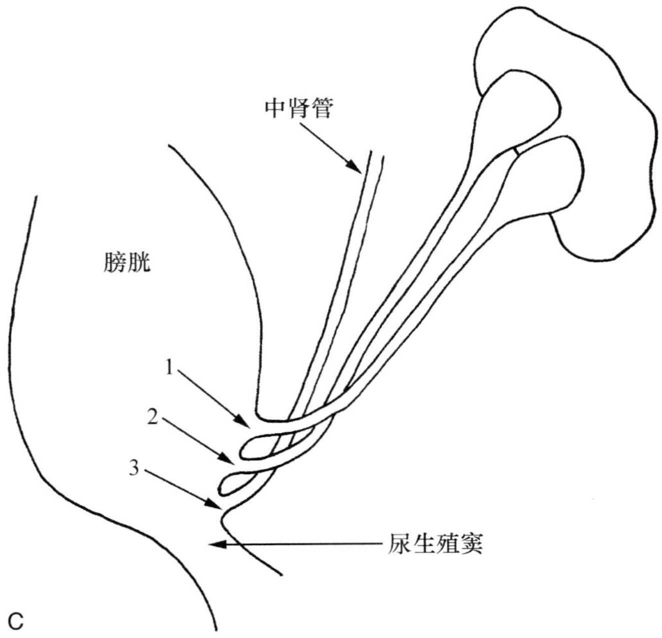

图 113-2　A. 妊娠第四周前后，两条输尿管芽从中肾管远端发出。B. 两条输尿管芽的头端最后发育。如果延时太久，上极输尿管芽就不会诱导发育中的肾脏胚基，可能导致肾脏上极的肾不发育。中肾管下端部分扩展，并加入发育中的膀胱和尿生殖窦。输尿管芽开口（1 和 2）和伴行的输尿管迁移，并参与组成这些结构的一部分。C. 在妊娠第八周左右，中肾管远端和其在输尿管芽上方的一小段（3）展开并分化生长，加入发育中的膀胱和尿生殖窦后壁的下部。注意下极输尿管芽（1）位于上极输尿管芽（2）和中肾管远端（3）的上方。

晚，越是不能诱导正常的肾脏发育。在重复畸形的临床实践中，肾发育不良往往发生在肾脏上极[68]。

中肾管上输尿管芽的发生部位也非常重要。如果这个部位太靠近远端，那么发育的输尿管就会与膀胱结合过早，其最终在膀胱壁迁移到达的位置也会过于偏向上外侧。在这个位置与逼尿肌相连会出现功能异常，导致膀胱输尿管反流（VUR）的发生[7,75,77]。在重复畸形的临床实践中，VUR 发生在下极输尿管的机会比发生在上极输尿管更多。如果输尿管芽的发生部位更靠近中肾管的近端，那么输尿管进入发育中的泌尿生殖窦和膀胱的时间会比较晚。在变异较小的病例中，上极输尿管可以出现在膀胱，但其在三角区开口的位置比正常情况更靠近下内方。在更为极端的病例中，输尿管根本不进入膀胱。此时，男性输尿管开口部位可能沿着位于膀胱颈下后尿道部的中肾管或其衍生结构的下端。应当注意到，在所有具有这些异常情况的男孩中，上极输尿管进入外括约肌上方的泌尿道，因此并不会出现尿失禁现象。而对于女孩来说，情况有所不同。在发育过程中，中肾管可以从发育中的膀胱尾侧任何地方发出，多见于阴道穹窿[75]。不论是完全性或不完全性的重复，有时其中的一根输尿管不能同发育中的后肾胚基相遇，此时会形成一条盲端输尿管，与肾脏没有任何连接[56]。

在罕见的情况下，会发现一种倒置的 Y 样畸形，对这种现象的解释是从中肾管尾端发出两条输尿管芽，在其上升进入后肾胚基前于头端相互融合[48]。至于输尿管开口的位置，与完全性输尿管重复畸形所见到的基本一致。

更为罕见的情况是输尿管三重畸形[61]。虽然在一些病例报告中提出由中肾管发出三条重复的输尿管芽，但大多数都通过一个单一的输尿管开口引流入膀胱。这提示为单一输尿管芽的三重畸形。输尿管的四重畸形也曾经有过报道，但这种情况非常罕见[11]。

输尿管芽在开始表现为实质性的组织束，随后会发生腔化。现在认为中肾管交界处的腔化过程障碍在输尿管囊肿的发生过程中起到一定作用[17]。然而，这个部位的胚胎学发生机制比较复杂，可能还存在其他重要的影响因素[76]。理论上说，输尿管囊肿既可以发生在正常的单一系统的输尿管，也可以发生在重复系统的输尿管。在实际情况中，大多数输尿管囊肿发生在重复系统，并且大多影响到上极半肾的输尿管[76]。当出现单一系统输尿管囊肿时，可以预计其在膀胱内的正常位置[85]。然而，在有上极输尿管的情况下，它可以位于膀胱三角区下内方以下的任何位置。此外，对女孩来说，这个位置还可以超出尿道，出现在中肾管开口的位置。在男孩和女孩的重复系统中，最常见的输尿管囊肿的位置是在膀胱颈部[33]。

不完全性输尿管重复畸形

分支的肾盂相对比较常见，但通常没有症状，出现在 10% 的人群中。当不完全性输尿管重复发生在肾盂水平以下时，有 50% 发生在中段输尿管，而各有 25% 分别发生在近端和远端输尿管[45]。在一些少见的情况下，输尿管一端呈盲端，可能是因为一个输尿管芽不能成功地诱导后肾胚基[63]。

有时这些畸形可因尿路感染（UTI）或腰部不适而出现症状[3]。可以发生 VUR，认为与重复畸形有关。发生从一条输尿管向另一条输尿管反流的情况很罕见，可能会导致尿潴留和感染。目前认为这种表现最可能发生在输尿管分支位于远端的情况下，而在输尿管膀胱壁段分支的时候极少出现[15,79]。偶尔可以发现有肾盂输尿管梗阻，通常发生在下极输尿管（图 113-3）[59]。

过去，不完全性输尿管重复畸形一般都是通过静脉肾盂造影检查进行诊断的（图 113-4），但是现在已经很少进行这种检查。目前对这种疾病的诊断在大多数情况下都是在检查 VUR 时同时发现的。两条输尿管显影既可以出现在排尿性膀胱尿道造影（MCUG）[45]，也可以出现在应用巯基乙酰三甘油（MAG3）或二乙基三胺五乙酸（DTPA）同位素扫描的排尿间接膀胱造影。

在有症状的病例中，治疗方法是使用预防性抗生素。当药物治疗无效时，需要进行外科干预。手术方式包括：如果重复的输尿管在膀胱附近[4]，则行两条输尿管的再植手术；如果重复输尿管位于较高水平，则在切除一条输尿管远端末端后，再行肾盂输尿管吻合术或输尿管输尿管吻合术[13]。

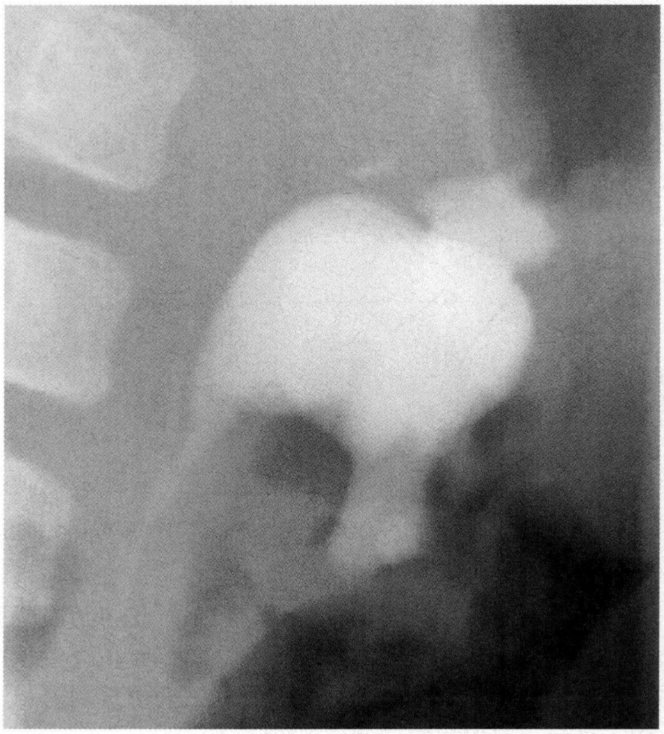

图 113-3 静脉尿路造影显示左肾的不完全性输尿管重复畸形，伴有典型的下极输尿管的肾盂输尿管连接部梗阻。

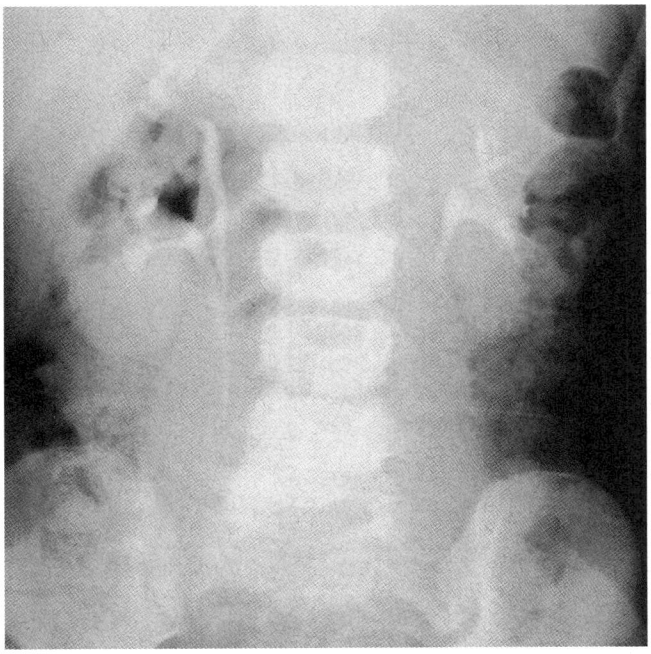

图 113-4　静脉尿路造影显示无症状、非梗阻、不完全的右侧输尿管重复畸形。

完全性输尿管重复畸形和输尿管囊肿

完全性输尿管重复畸形的发病率和表现

尸检显示完全性输尿管重复畸形的发病率大约为 0.8%[16,58]。左右输尿管重复的几率大致相等，大约有 40% 为双侧输尿管重复畸形[78]。女性发病的机会是男性的两倍[64]。在有尿路症状的患者中，如伴有 UTI 的患者，有大约 4% 的输尿管重复畸形的发病率[37]。有三分之二伴有 UTI 表现的重复畸形的患儿会出现 VUR[29]。该病有明显的家族发病倾向，有 12.5%~30% 的同胞亲属也有重复畸形[6,8,9]，提示该病的遗传特征为不完全外显的常染色体显性遗传[6,82]。

对于一些女孩来说（不包括男孩），如果输尿管开口位于尿道外括约肌以下的部位，那么在临床上就可以表现为滴尿性尿失禁。这种现象即使是在患儿有正常排尿行为时也可以出现。

此外，这种畸形既可以伴有 VUR，也可以伴有梗阻，这两种伴发异常均可以导致 UTI 和肾瘢痕。完全性输尿管重复畸形病例中，有 90% 的患儿其重复的上极肾有明显的原发性肾发育不良，这是由于上极输尿

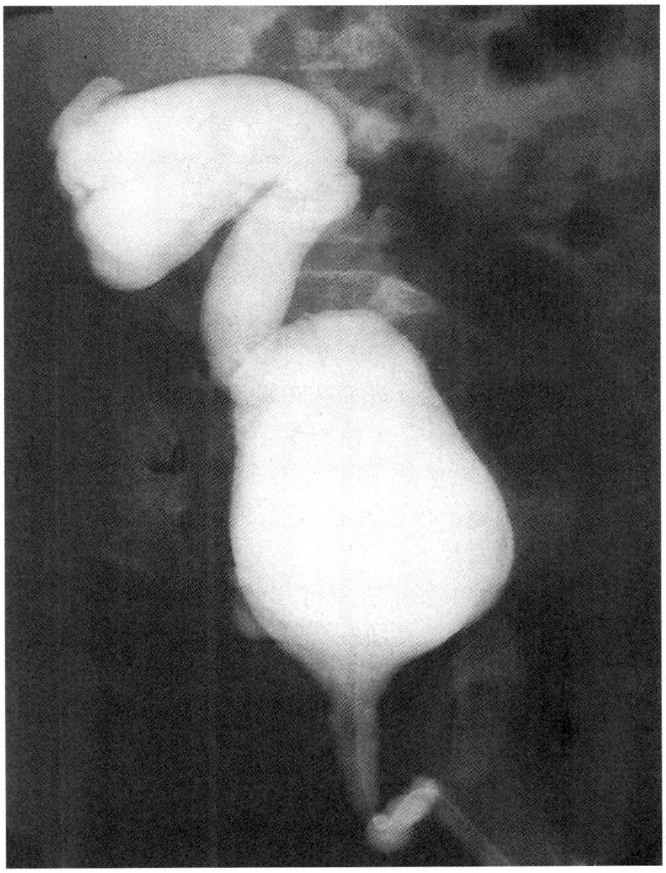

图 113-5　一个有尿路感染症状儿童的排尿性膀胱尿道造影显示，右侧完全性重复系统的下极输尿管的 5 级膀胱输尿管反流。

管芽对后肾胚基异常诱导所致[14]。这种异常与妊娠第五周到第六周输尿管芽与后肾胚基接触过晚有关。现已知这种发育不良在异位输尿管开口的病例中表现最多，尤其是在那些输尿管开口位置位于或低于尿道外括约肌水平的病例中[31,54,62,68]。无论是肾发育不良还是肾瘢痕，最终都可以导致高血压表现[37,49,53]。

VUR 一般发生在下极输尿管（图 113-5）；这种情况与输尿管膀胱连接有关，此时输尿管进入膀胱逼尿肌的位置高于正常输尿管开口，并且在膀胱三角区靠近外侧的顶部[23]。然而，有时反流也可以发生在上极输尿管，或出现更为矛盾的现象，即在 10% 的病例中，反流会发生在患有输尿管囊肿的输尿管中[19,69]。当上下两极都出现反流时，输尿管的开口往往相当靠近，并且位于外侧异位的位置。

同样，完全性输尿管重复畸形也可以发生典型的

肾盂输尿管交界处梗阻，这种情况大多发生在下极输尿管，其发病率要高于正常人群[30,80]。

输尿管囊肿的发病率和表现

尸检结果显示输尿管囊肿的发病率为每 4000 个儿童中有 1 例[16]。女性发病的可能性比男性高 4～7 倍[27]。左侧发病比右侧略为多见[67]。有 10% 的输尿管囊肿是双侧的[67]，60%～80% 是异位输尿管[55]，而且有 80% 的输尿管囊肿发生于重复畸形的上极输尿管[12]。单系统输尿管囊肿不多见，好发于男性，可伴有其他畸形，包括肾脏畸形如肾融合或异位[43]，以及多囊性肾发育不良[85]。

输尿管囊肿一般都在进行其他检查时被发现，如无症状的肾盂积水、可触及的腰部肿块、UTI，偶尔可因输尿管囊肿脱出尿道而出现于外阴时发现。

输尿管囊肿可以与其他畸形一起发生各种不同
1763 组合形式，从比较单纯的单系统到复杂的重复畸形的输尿管囊肿。由于大多数输尿管囊肿是异位的，所以与其相连的肾单位往往是无功能的[40]。大约有 10%～15% 与输尿管囊肿相连肾单位的位置相对正常，位于膀胱三角区，有一些残留的功能，此时有保留价值[32]。

输尿管囊肿通常都会使上极半肾的输尿管发生梗阻，一般会对相应肾单位造成明显的损害[24]。在极端情况下，当输尿管囊肿脱出尿道，造成尿道梗阻，会影响到所有的肾单位。输尿管囊肿是女孩尿道梗阻最常见的原因[51]。当发现有重复输尿管囊肿时，VUR 出现在患侧者（图 113-6）有 50%，而出现在对侧者有 25%[12,14,19]。

完全性输尿管重复畸形和输尿管囊肿的诊断

没有进行产前诊断的儿童大多表现为有症状的 UTI，这在新生儿期可能是非常严重的，有可能会危及生命[32,36]。很多患儿会伴有 VUR 或异位输尿管囊肿梗阻。前面已经提到，如果存在异位输尿管，当输尿管开口在尿道外括约肌以下时，女孩会表现为持续滴尿的尿失禁[69]。这种病史对于诊断至关重要。男孩异位输尿管连接在输精管或精囊时可以表现为附睾炎[34,44,73]。有时，一些没有明显 VUR 或梗阻的患儿要到成人时才能获诊[64]。

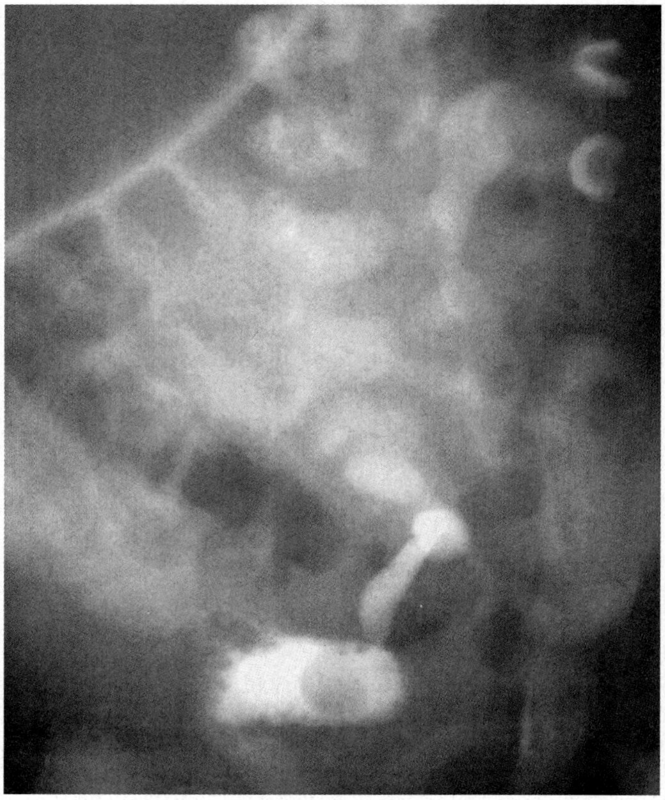

图 113-6 排尿性膀胱尿道造影显示左侧上极输尿管囊肿，伴有同侧完全重复系统下极输尿管的 4 级膀胱输尿管反流。

对肾脏的产前超声筛查可以发现不同程度的肾盂积水，能够预测输尿管囊肿[83]。尽管没有证据表明对有产前诊断的患儿进行治疗可以影响肾脏的预后，但是这样做可以减少有症状 UTI 的发作频率[70,81]。这些患儿需要进一步的超声评估和 MCUG 检查，而且必要时还可进行静脉肾盂造影和核磁共振（MRI）复查。肾盂造影对明确解剖畸形很有帮助，在肾单位有功能的情况下往往能够发现与其相应的输尿管囊肿（图 113-7）[26,40]。然而，当受累的半肾无功能时，影像学上的表现会非常隐蔽，因而在超声、二巯基丁二酸（DMSA）扫描、静脉尿路造影（IVU）检查时很容易漏掉[26,40,60]。在这些情况下进行 MRI 检查则很有帮助（图 113-8）[35]。在大多数病例中，有一定程度的肾盂积水，并很容易通过超声检查探测到（图 113-9）[22]。此外，膀胱的超声检查往往也会发现在 MCUG 上并不明显的输尿管囊肿（图 113-10）。有时

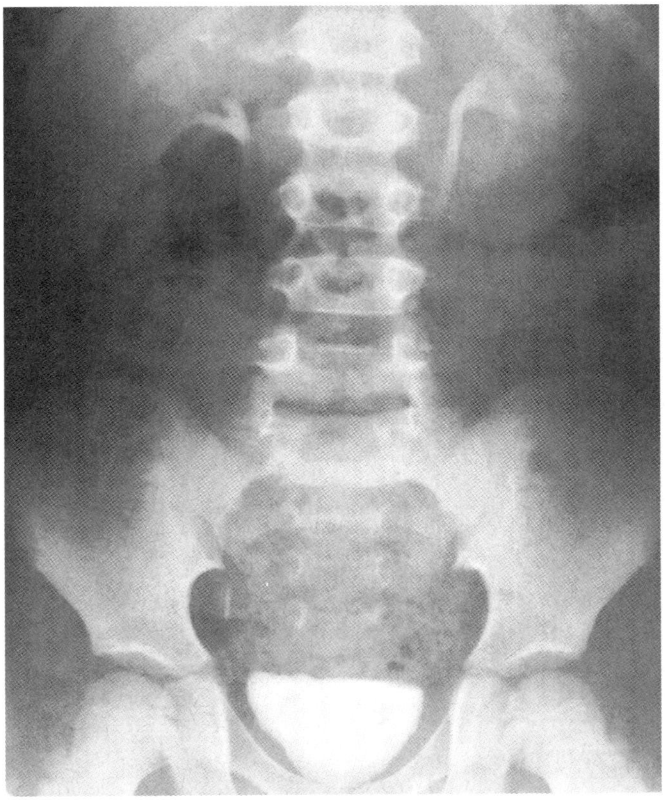

图 113-7　静脉尿路造影显示双侧膀胱内输尿管囊肿，合并有功能的单一系统肾单位。

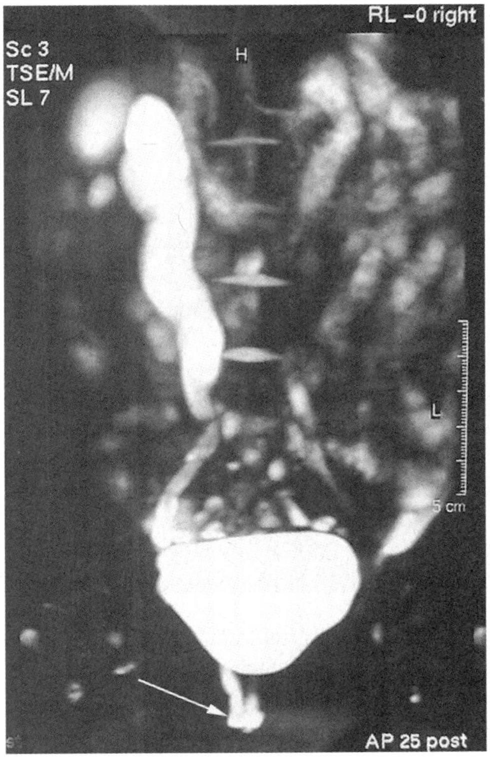

图 113-8　一个滴尿性尿失禁女孩的 T2 相核磁共振显像。注意右侧肾脏上极半肾的肾盂积水，这在肾盂造影检查时为无功能表现。箭头表示输尿管汇入阴道。

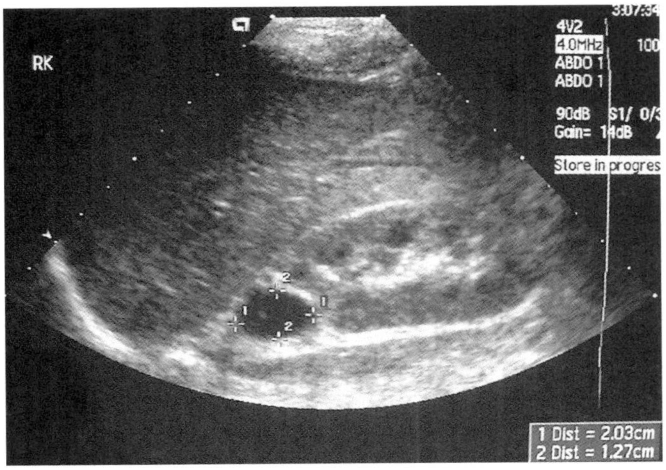

图 113-9　右肾超声扫描显示重复畸形的上极半肾肾盂积水。注意下极相对正常，在上下半肾之间存在明确分界。

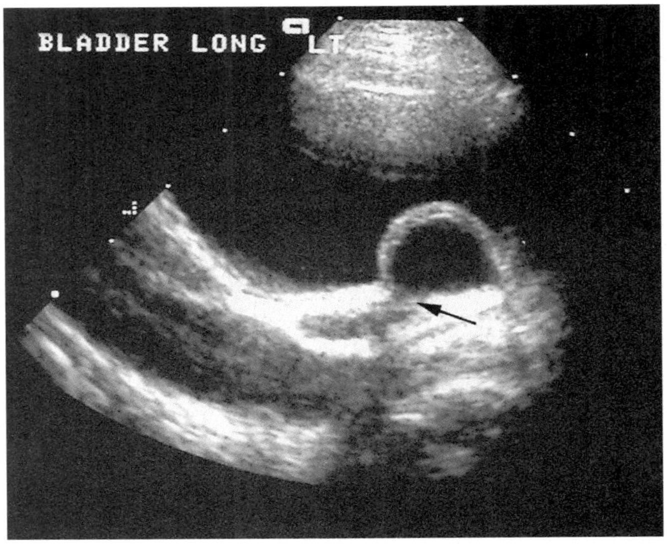

图 113-10　膀胱的矢状面超声扫描显示膀胱基底部的输尿管囊肿。注意输尿管（箭头）连接入输尿管囊肿的位置。

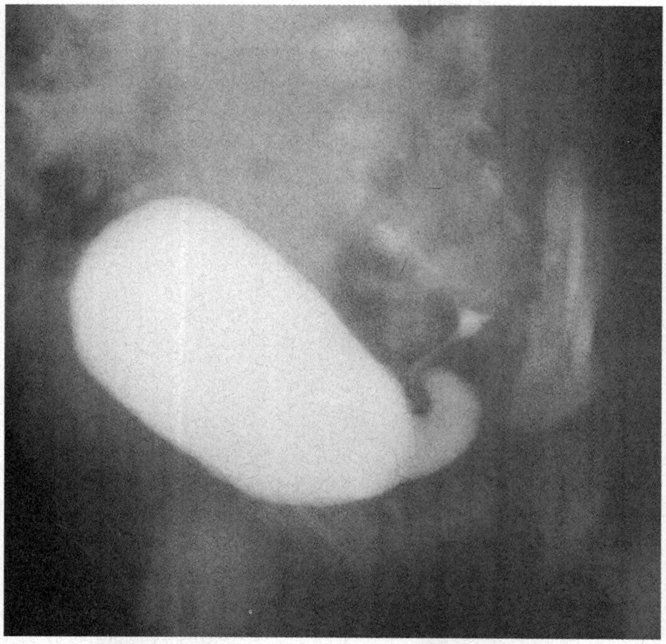

图 113-11 排尿性膀胱尿道造影显示输尿管囊肿向上极输尿管逆向脱垂，膀胱输尿管反流入左侧完全重复系统的下极输尿管。其表现可能会与膀胱憩室混淆。

1764 在排尿时，输尿管囊肿会沿着输尿管管腔向膀胱后膨出，从而与膀胱憩室相混淆（图 113-11）[21]。上极功能丧失发生在 90% 的异位输尿管病例中，在 DMSA 扫描中表现为放射稀疏缺损（图 113-12）；在 IVU 上表现为下极半肾移位所造成的典型“垂花”样表现。（图 113-13）[40,60]。在这些情况下，IVU 影像上所见的输尿管通常偏离其正常途径，从无功能上极半肾的输尿管外侧位置呈螺旋状下行（图 113-14）。

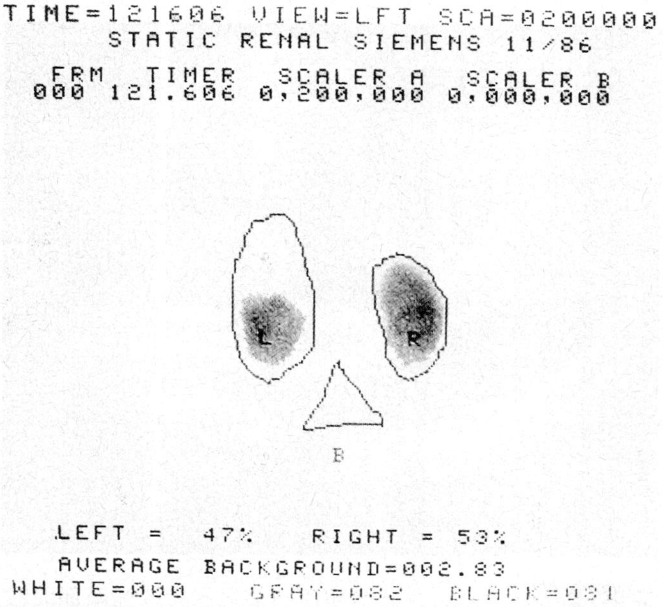

图 113-12 DMSA 同位素扫描显示左侧完全重复系统上极半肾功能差。上极输尿管伴有输尿管囊肿。

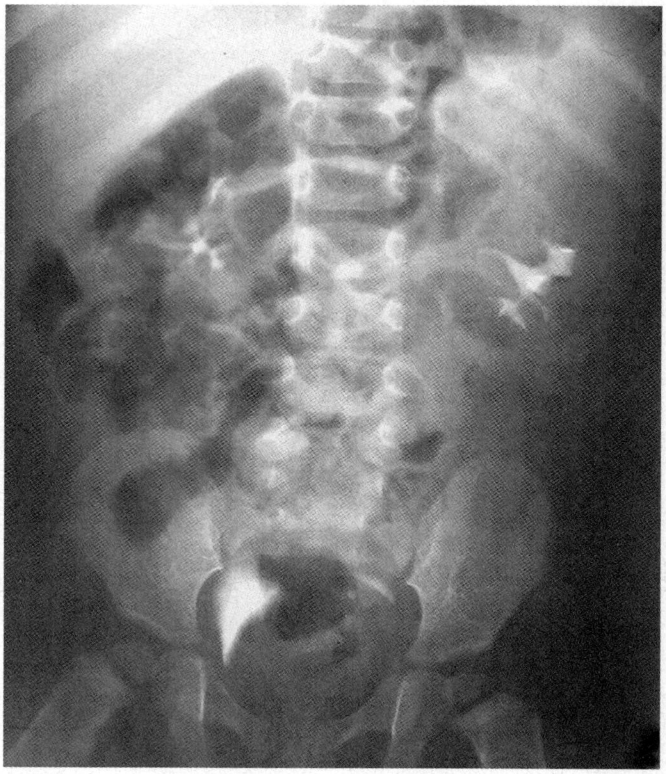

图 113-13 静脉尿路造影显示左侧“垂花”征。注意输尿管囊肿占据了左侧大部分膀胱基底部，下极半肾功能相对正常，被无功能的上极半肾肾盂积水压迫向下外方移位。

由于小婴儿的早期同位素数据指标不稳定，所以放射性同位素 DMSA 扫描评估肾功能、肾瘢痕或发育
不良，以及 MAG3 或 DTPA 肾扫描评估梗阻的检查应 176
当推迟至 6～8 周。MAG3 或 DTPA 的间接排尿性放射性核素扫描可以用来替代 MCUG 来评估 VUR。这对较大的儿童非常有用，这些患儿对 MCUG 检查从生理上和心理上都会感到不适应。

完全性输尿管重复畸形和输尿管囊肿的治疗

由于输尿管重复畸形和输尿管囊肿的病理变化很大，所以在治疗上应当做到个体化。治疗的主要目标

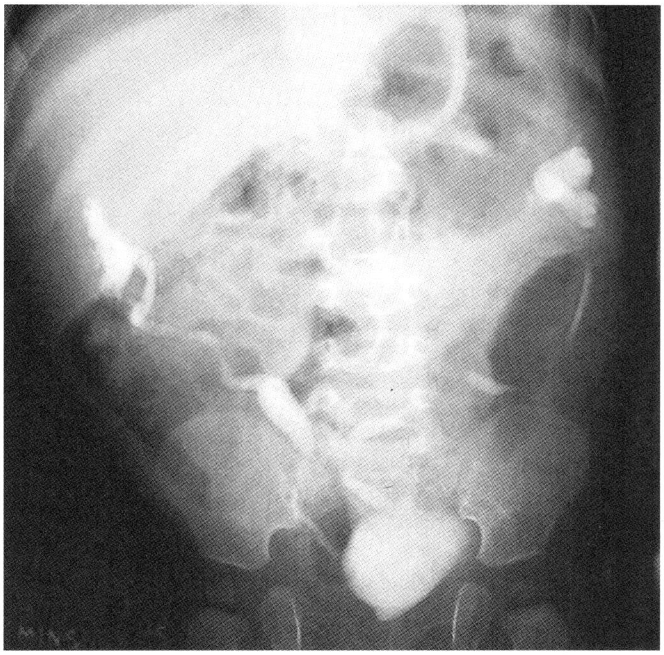

图 113-14　双侧完全重复系统的无功能梗阻性上极半肾输尿管静脉尿路造影。未见有功能的双侧上极半肾显影，仅见的异常表现为有功能的下极部分向外下方移位。注意下极输尿管呈螺旋形向膀胱走行，提示有未显影的上极输尿管肾盂积水存在。在这一病例中，存在一个膀胱内输尿管囊肿，但在造影中未显示。

是降低肾功能恶化的风险，控制症状，避免外科干预对膀胱功能造成的损害。在治疗上并不是所有的病例都需要进行手术，近来治疗的趋势不断向保守治疗发展。治疗主要针对 VUR、输尿管囊肿、肾盂输尿管梗阻以及继发于异位输尿管的尿失禁——输尿管重复畸形和输尿管囊肿的主要并发症，以下对这些分别进行讨论。

膀胱输尿管反流

与许多人的观念相反，有相当一部分发生于重复
66 畸形的反流可以随着时间推移而自行缓解。这种情况在 1 级或 2 级 VUR 中发生的机会（达 85%）比在高级别 VUR 中出现的机会更多[10,39,52,60]。为了使患儿保持在无症状的状态（就像原发性 VUR 一样），可以在开始就给予预防性抗生素。应当对这些患儿进行仔细随访，包括连续性的 DMSA 扫描，以检查有无肾瘢痕形成及其进展情况。VUR 既可以通过间接 MAG3 或 DTPA 膀胱造影，也可以通过 MCUG 检查来进行评估。如果发现有肾瘢痕进展伴肾功能下降，或者预防性抗生素不能控制有症状的上尿路 UTI，就需要进行外科手术干预[2,57]。

内镜治疗

目前内镜治疗重复畸形 VUR 的价值还存在争议。最近的数据表明，尽管这一技术用于治疗重复畸形 VUR 的成功率比用于原发性 VUR 的成功率要低，但仍然是一个有效手段，为疾病的治疗提供了一个选择[39,52,60]。开始，内镜手术采用 Teflon 胶，将其注入输尿管开口的下方[65]。由于考虑到含氟碳氢化合物的迁移和长期效果，近来引进 Deflux 作为一种成功率更高的制剂，取代 Teflon 植入物[46]。这种物质是聚糖苷-透明质酸聚合物[50,66]，从后方对输尿管开口起到压迫作用，这样可以通过两个机制防止膀胱输尿管反流的发生。第一，改变了输尿管开口轴向，使其从原来与输尿管平行的方向变为与输尿管垂直的方向，从而起到了“活瓣”的作用。第二，植入物本身可以形成一个黏附于下方膀胱逼尿肌的纤维囊。当膀胱三角区在排尿期发生收缩时，输尿管开口由于附着于其下的纤维囊而发生向内向下的移位，由此增加了膀胱壁段的长度。这一机制对于减少 VUR 的发生非常重要。在注射时将穿刺针通过内镜的操作鞘，使其斜面朝上于输尿管开口下方六点的位置注射药物（见第 112 章）。在重复畸形病例中，由于输尿管开口位置比较靠近，注射药物应当在上极半肾输尿管开口（位于内下方）的下方。穿刺于两个输尿管开口下方进针，在直视下注射药物，直至两个输尿管开口均受压。一般在注射时很少使用超过 0.3 ml 的药物。当输尿管开口分开的距离超过数毫米时，可以分别进行穿刺注射；不过，在下极输尿管开口下方进行注射时需要特别注意，因为上极输尿管有插入位置错误的可能。

开放式输尿管膀胱吻合术

输尿管再植手术是治疗 VUR 和输尿管梗阻的常规手术方法。由于有很多膀胱畸形是基于重复畸形的，所以在游离输尿管时很有可能损伤到膀胱出口[71]。也有很多病例存在原发性膀胱功能异常，这

与后尿道瓣膜病例中所见到的一样，可能与膀胱出口梗阻有关[1]。正因为如此，在手术前进行尿流动力学检查非常明智。当两个输尿管开口位于膀胱三角区相对正常的位置时，应当将两者都从膀胱底部进行游离，即使反流仅发生在下极输尿管。这一操作非常必要，因为这两条输尿管共用同一外膜，并拥有共同的血管供应[28]，仅仅游离病变的输尿管可能会导致一条或两条输尿管发生缺血性改变。除此以外，还可以在共鞘以上的部位游离两条输尿管。然后输尿管段可通过膀胱壁改变行程，可以采用膀胱内跨三角区技术或膀胱外的操作方法进行。这两种方法都是建立一个黏膜下隧道，其长度至少应当超过输尿管口径的 3 倍，从而形成一种“活瓣”机制。

当存在输尿管囊肿时，上述情况会比较复杂，治疗中还要考虑到输尿管囊肿的位置以及与之相对应的肾单位的功能（见后）。如果相应的肾单位已经无功能，而且患儿有临床症状，则应当考虑采用切除手术。为了不破坏膀胱颈部的解剖结构和功能，要采取比较保守的切除方法，一般需要在距膀胱 2～3 cm 处切除病变输尿管和受影响的肾脏部分。这些已经成功地通过开放手术或内镜手术完成。手术后输尿管残端一般很少影响预后，如果存在有症状的 VUR，可以通过内镜手术解决。

开放式输尿管输尿管吻合术

当一条输尿管有反流以及膀胱基底部的解剖结构比较复杂时，一种既简单效果又好的方法是将患侧输尿管吻合到对侧正常的输尿管上[2,51]，而患侧输尿管的远端向下方游离到膀胱外切除。

输尿管囊肿

治疗方法的选择要根据输尿管囊肿的大小和位置以及相应半肾的功能来决定。治疗方法很多，从简单的减压到切除。

切开减压

对于位于尿道的输尿管囊肿，不管是原发于尿道，还是从膀胱中脱垂到尿道，一般需要采取一些减压方法来避免由膀胱出口梗阻引起的长期并发症。单独切除无功能的肾脏和输尿管，而不切除输尿管囊肿往往不足以避免下段输尿管感染的发生。如果选择了这种方法，还应当结合囊肿减压或切除手术。对大多数病例来说，减压手术是比较好的选择，方法最简单，并发症最少[41]。

以前对输尿管囊肿进行大范围的切开去顶手术。这种做法存在一定问题，即如果输尿管囊肿来自于尿道，那么囊肿的表皮就不可能被完全切除，其皱褶会形成瓣膜样结构，可以导致尿道梗阻的发生[5]。此 176
外，术后的 VUR 几乎不可避免。因此，在去顶手术后通常都需要进行抗反流手术，这样就不如与一期手术同时实施。这种治疗方法损伤较大，困难也比较多，同时并发症发生的机会也比较高[71]。

内镜技术一般用于一些简单的输尿管囊肿切开病例，对囊肿既可以使用热切开，也可以进行单纯刺破[20,72,74]。在操作过程中有一点极为重要，即不能过度充盈膀胱，否则会使输尿管囊肿受压，难以发现。如果发生这种情况，可以在腰部按压患侧肾脏，这样有可能帮助输尿管囊肿重新充盈。选择输尿管囊肿表面的切开减压部位十分重要，如果可能，切开部位不应当选择在膀胱基底部的输尿管管腔表面。这可以通过术前超声定位来进行（见图 113-10）。这样可以减少术后的 VUR 并发症。单纯切开减压一般可以使输尿管变小，同时也使二期手术更容易进行。此外，伴发的下极输尿管 VUR 通常会自行消退。如果 VUR 持续存在，可以在实施根治性外科手术前，先尝试通过内镜注射 Teflon 或 Deflux 治疗[25]。

部分肾输尿管切除术

对于有症状的无功能肾单位伴有梗阻或发育不良的上半肾来说，通常需要进行部分肾输尿管切除手术。在具体实施时，应当首先从远端进行输尿管囊肿减压（前文已述）；否则其内残留的不流动液体会导致远端输尿管感染，进而会影响到后期膀胱基底部的重建手术（如果必须进行的话）。部分肾切除术包括区分正常的下半肾和无功能的上半肾，并切除相应肾单位下方的输尿管，切除输尿管时应尽可能靠近膀胱，又不能影响到下极输尿管。对于切除病变输尿管远端所引起的并发症已经在前文提到，并且在下文中会更详细描述。

手术操作既可以通过开放手术也可以通过内镜技

术来进行。后者可以更为有效地游离病变输尿管远端，但鉴别正常和异常半肾的准确性稍差[42]。内镜手术的时间也明显长于开放手术。目前还没有有关对比开放手术和内镜手术预后的资料。

在开放手术时，病变上半肾的输尿管和肾盂通常是扩张的，比较容易鉴别。在对上半肾的支配血管进行分离后，打开病变输尿管的近端，从此处将手指插入肾盂，这就能更好地鉴别病变半肾的界限，在不损伤下半肾肾盏的情况下判断正常和异常肾组织的相对无血管区断面[38]。此后一般不需要修补肾脏断面，以免对下半肾造成进一步损伤。在同一切口切除输尿管支至骨盆入口水平。

膀胱基底部重建

如前所述，一般不需要进行膀胱基底部重建手术。然而，有时在某些情况下需要进行输尿管囊肿和远端输尿管切除。这往往会造成比较明显的缺损，需要进行精确的解剖重建，否则膀胱颈部和后尿道的破坏会导致尿失禁[71]。幸运的是，输尿管直接开口到尿道的情况比较少见，大多开口于膀胱颈或以上水平。但输尿管囊肿常常会波及尿道，需要完全切除囊肿的上皮边缘，并进行细致修补，否则由于残留的囊肿边缘会形成“瓣膜样”结构，或者输尿管囊肿切缘形成瘢痕狭窄，会造成尿道梗阻[5]。由于上述原因，通常需要与输尿管囊肿一起同时游离无病变的下极输尿管。如果要切除上极输尿管，要将两条输尿管同时游离到共鞘上方。另外一种做法是在分离两条输尿管时先剥离病变输尿管的外膜，以保留“正常”输尿管的血管供应。在任何情况下，都要对膀胱基底部和出口的缺损进行修补，而不紧缩出口，然后对保留下来的下极输尿管进行再植手术，手术方法可以采用跨三角区或膀胱外的操作方法，以确保前文所提到的足够的黏膜下隧道长度。重建手术有比较明确的术后排尿异常的可能性，建议应当事先考虑到这些并发症，在术前进行尿流动力学检查，并在必要时术后复查[1,71]。

肾盂输尿管连接部梗阻

在重复畸形病例中，梗阻通常发生在下半肾，而且多见于男孩[30,80]。对于手术的选择还没有明确的循证依据。大多数外科医生都是根据受累肾单位的大小和功能来决定的。肾盂积水增大，或者同位素检查显示病变部分的肾功能下降，都提示需要进行外科干预。然而对于生长中的儿童来说，仅靠这些指标有时很难做出客观评价。出现于年长儿童中的腰痛，尤其是青春期前的儿童，同时在 MAG3 或 DTPA 同位素扫描中有明确的肾盂输尿管连接部梗阻的客观证据，都是外科治疗的指征。

手术方式是肾盂成形术，或者向无病变的上极输尿管进行肾盂输尿管吻合术，同时切除受累的下极输尿管远端[30,59,80]。在病变肾单位功能严重受损时进行部分肾输尿管切除手术。

异位输尿管伴尿失禁

对女性尿失禁伴有异位输尿管肾单位病例的手术
治疗相对比较简单。一般来说病变不会累及膀胱，而 1768
且输尿管无梗阻性病变。通过内镜或开放手术可进行部分肾输尿管切除术，输尿管切除到骨盆入口水平，不缝合输尿管残端。输尿管末端很少会出现异常，一般不需要切除。

小结

输尿管重复畸形和输尿管囊肿代表了一系列在解剖学和胚胎学上相互重叠的畸形病变。大多数非反流和非梗阻的重复畸形病例在临床上没有明显表现，一般不需要进行治疗；其他病例都会有明显的疾病表现。大多数不完全性重复畸形症状不明显。完全性的重复畸形通常也无症状，但可伴有 VUR 或输尿管囊肿。本病多见于女孩，两侧发病率相同，双侧发病者占 40%。

VUR 是重复畸形最常见的并发症，在有症状 UTI 病例中占 65%；反流通常发生在下极输尿管。对 VUR 可以进行密切观察，低级别的 VUR 很可能自行消退。

仔细询问病史对明确尿失禁的原因很有帮助。但对尿失禁患者还要进行选择性的影像学检查，以进一步明确解剖上的异常；这些检查包括超声影像、同位素扫描、MCUG、IVU 和 MRI。

基于这些检查资料，对每一个病例都要确定治疗方案，要特别强调防止肾功能恶化、控制症状、避免影响膀胱功能的手术治疗。对于肾功能受损或不能控制症状的 UTI 病例，可以采用内镜或开放手术治疗。输尿管囊肿可以采用内镜单纯穿刺或切开治疗。根治性重建手术引起继发性膀胱功能损害的风险较大，应当仅用于较为复杂的不能通过其他方法治疗的病例。

（赵海腾译 刘国华校）

参考文献

1. Abrahamsson K, Hansson E, Sillen U, et al: Bladder dysfunction: An integral part of the ectopic ureterocele complex. J Urol 1998;160:1468-1470.
2. Ahmed S, Boucaut HA: Vesicoureteral reflux in complete ureteral duplication: Surgical options. J Urol 1988;140:1092-1094.
3. Albers DD, Geyer JR, Barnes SD: Clinical significance of the blind-ending branch of a bifid ureter: Report of 3 additional cases. J Urol 1971;105:634-637.
4. Amar AD: Treatment of reflux in bifid ureters by conversion to complete duplication. J Urol 1972;108:77-78.
5. Ashcraft KW, Hendren WH: Bladder outlet obstruction after operation for ureterocele. J Pediatr Surg 1979;14:819-824.
6. Atwell JD, Cook PL, Howell CJ, et al: Familial incidence of bifid and double ureters. Arch Dis Child 1974;49:390-393.
7. Atwell JD, Cook PL, Strong L, Hyde I: The interrelationship between vesico-ureteric reflux, trigonal abnormalities and a bifid pelvicalyceal collecting system: A family study. Br J Urol 1977;49:97-107.
8. Aubert J, Irani J, Baumert H: Familial ureteral duplication and ureterocele: Two sisters and their father. Eur Urol 2000;37:714-717.
9. Babcock JR Jr, Belman AB, Shkolnik A, Ignatoff J: Familial ureteral duplication and ureterocele. Urology 1977;9:345-349.
10. Ben Ami T, Gayer G, Hertz M, et al: The natural history of reflux in the lower pole of duplicated collecting systems: A controlled study. Pediatr Radiol 1989;19:308-310.
11. Bhandarkar AD, Raju AM, Rao MS: Single unilateral ectopic bifid ureter with contralateral orthotopic quadrufid ureter—a rare combination. J Postgrad Med 1997;43:104-105.
12. Brock WA, Kaplan GW: Ectopic ureteroceles in children. J Urol 1978;119:800-803.
13. Busslinger MI, Kaiser G: Surgical significance of the duplex kidney with bifid ureter. Eur J Pediatr Surg 1992;2:150-151.
14. Caldamone AA, Snyder HM III, Duckett JW: Ureteroceles in children: Followup of management with upper tract approach. J Urol 1984;131:1130-1132.
15. Campbell JE: Ureteral peristalsis in duplex renal collecting systems. Am J Roentgenol Radium Ther Nucl Med 1967;99:577-584.
16. Campbell MF: Anomalies of the ureter. In Campbell MF, Harrison JH (eds): Urology, 3rd ed. Philadelphia, WB Saunders, 1970, pp 1487-1670.
17. Chwalla R: The process of formation of cystic dilatations of the vesical end of the ureter and of diverticula at the ureteral ostium. Urol Cutan Rev 1927;31:499.
18. Conway JJ, Maizels M: The "well tempered" diuretic renogram: A standard method to examine the asymptomatic neonate with hydronephrosis or hydroureteronephrosis. A report from combined meetings of the Society for Fetal Urology and Members of the Pediatric Nuclear Medicine Council–the Society of Nuclear Medicine. J Nucl Med 1992;33:2047-2051.
19. Cooper CS, Passerini-Glazel G, Hutcheson JC, et al: Long-term followup of endoscopic incision of ureteroceles: Intravesical versus extravesical. J Urol 2000;164:1097-1099.
20. Coplen DE, Duckett JW: The modern approach to ureteroceles. J Urol 1995;153:166-171.
21. Cremin BJ, Funston MR, Aaronson IA: "The intraureteric diverticulum," a manifestation of ureterocoele intussusception. Pediatr Radiol 1977;6:92-96.
22. Dalla Palma L, Bazzocchi M, Cressa C, Tommasini G: Radiological anatomy of the kidney revisited. Br J Radiol 1990;63:680-690.
23. de Caluwe D, Chertin B, Puri P: Long-term outcome of the retained ureteral stump after lower pole heminephrectomy in duplex kidneys. Eur Urol 2002;42:63-66.
24. DeFoor W, Minevich E, Tackett L, et al: Ectopic ureterocele: Clinical application of classification based on renal unit jeopardy. J Urol 2003;169:1092-1094.
25. Diamond T, Boston VE: Reflux following endoscopic treatment of ureteroceles: A new approach using endoscopic subureteric Teflon injection. Br J Urol 1987;60:279-280.
26. Diard F, Eklof O, Lebowitz R, Maurseth K: Urethral obstruction in boys caused by prolapse of simple ureterocele. Pediatr Radiol 1981;11:139-142.
27. Eklof O, Lohr G, Ringertz H, Thomasson B: Ectopic ureterocele in the male infant. Acta Radiol Diagn (Stockh) 1978;19:145-153.
28. Ellsworth PI, Lim DJ, Walker RD, et al: Common sheath reimplantation yields excellent results in the treatment of vesicoureteral reflux in duplicated collecting systems. J Urol 1996;155:1407-1409.
29. Fehrenbaker LG, Kelalis PP, Stickler GB: Vesicoureteral reflux and ureteral duplication in children. J Urol 1972;107:862-864.
30. Fernbach SK, Zawin JK, Lebowitz RL: Complete duplication of the ureter with ureteropelvic junction obstruction of the lower pole of the kidney: Imaging findings. AJR Am J Roentgenol 1995;164:701-704.
31. Gartell PC, MacIver AG, Atwell JD: Renal dysplasia and duplex kidneys. Eur Urol 1983;9:65-68.
32. Geringer AM, Berdon WE, Seldin DW, Hensle TW: The diagnostic approach to ectopic ureterocele and the renal duplication complex. J Urol 1983;129:539-542.
33. Glassberg KI, Braren V, Duckett JW, et al: Suggested terminology for duplex systems, ectopic ureters and ureteroceles. J Urol 1984;132:1153-1154.
34. Gravgaard E, Garsdal L, Moller SH: Double vas deferens and epididymis associated with ipsilateral renal agenesis simulating ectopic ureter opening into the seminal vesicle. Scand J Urol Nephrol 1978;12:85-87.
35. Gylys-Morin VM, Minevich E, Tackett LD, et al: Magnetic resonance imaging of the dysplastic renal moiety and ectopic ureter. J Urol 2000;164:2034-2039.
36. Hagg MJ, Mourachov PV, Snyder HM, et al: The modern endoscopic approach to ureterocele. J Urol 2000;163:940-943.
37. Hartman GW, Hodson CJ: The duplex kidney and related

abnormalities. Clin Radiol 1969;20:387-400.
38. Hurwitz RS: Easy method of upper-pole heminephroureterectomy in duplex systems in children. Urol Clin North Am 1990;17:115-119.
39. Husmann DA, Allen TD: Resolution of vesicoureteral reflux in completely duplicated systems: Fact or fiction? J Urol 1991;145:1022-1023.
40. Husmann DA, Ewalt DH, Glenski WJ, Bernier PA: Ureterocele associated with ureteral duplication and a nonfunctioning upper pole segment: Management by partial nephroureterectomy alone. J Urol 1995;154:723-726.
41. Husmann DA, Strand B, Ewalt D, et al: Management of ectopic ureterocele associated with renal duplication: A comparison of partial nephrectomy and endoscopic decompression. J Urol 1999;162:1406-1409.
42. Janetschek G, Seibold J, Radmayr C, Bartsch G: Laparoscopic heminephroureterectomy in pediatric patients. J Urol 1997; 158:1928-1930.
43. Johnson DK, Perlmutter AD: Single system ectopic ureteroceles with anomalies of the heart, testis and vas deferens. J Urol 1980;123:81-83.
44. Jonas P, Sidi A, Hertz M, Many M: A unique combination of congenital genitourinary anomalies in a child. J Urol 1977;118:349-350.
45. Kaplan N, Elkin M: Bifid renal pelves and ureters: Radiographic and cinefluorographic observations. Br J Urol 1968;40:235-244.
46. Kershen RT, Atala A: New advances in injectable therapies for the treatment of incontinence and vesicoureteral reflux. Urol Clin North Am 1999;26:81-94.
47. Klauber GT, Crawford DB: Prolapse of ectopic ureterocele and bladder trigone. Urology 1980;15:164-166.
48. Klauber GT, Reid EC: Inverted Y reduplication of the ureter. J Urol 1972;107:362-364.
49. Kumar R, Madan MS: Renal duplication with hypertension. J Pediatr Surg 1970;5:380-381.
50. Lackgren G, Wahlin N, Skoldenberg E, et al: Endoscopic treatment of vesicoureteral reflux with dextranomer/ hyaluronic acid copolymer is effective in either double ureters or a small kidney. J Urol 2003;170:1551-1555.
51. Lashley DB, McAleer IM, Kaplan GW: Ipsilateral ureteroureterostomy for the treatment of vesicoureteral reflux or obstruction associated with complete ureteral duplication. J Urol 2001;165:552-554.
52. Lee PH, Diamond DA, Duffy PG, Ransley PG: Duplex reflux: A study of 105 children. J Urol 1991;146:657-659.
53. Levy JB, Vandersteen DR, Morgenstern BZ, Husmann DA: Hypertension after surgical management of renal duplication associated with an upper pole ureterocele. J Urol 1997; 158:1241-1244.
54. Mackie GG, Stephens FD: Duplex kidneys: A correlation of renal dysplasia with position of the ureteric orifice. Birth Defects Orig Artic Ser 1977;13:313-321.
55. Mandell J, Colodny AH, Lebowitz R, et al: Ureteroceles in infants and children. J Urol 1980;123:921-926.
56. Marshall FF, McLoughlin MG: Long blind-ending ureteral duplications. J Urol 1978;120:626-628.
57. Miyakita H, Ninan GK, Puri P: Endoscopic correction of vesico-ureteric reflux in duplex systems. Eur Urol 1993; 24:111-115.
58. Nation EF: Duplication of the kidney and ureter: A statistical study of 230 new cases. J Urol 1944;51:456-465.
59. Ossandon F, Androulakakis P, Ransley PG: Surgical problems in pelviureteral junction obstruction of the lower moiety in incomplete duplex systems. J Urol 1981;125:871-872.
60. Pattaras JG, Rushton HG, Majd M: The role of 99m technetium dimercapto-succinic acid renal scans in the evaluation of occult ectopic ureters in girls with paradoxical incontinence. J Urol 1999;162:821-825.
61. Perkins PJ, Kroovand RL, Evans AT: Ureteral triplication. Radiology 1973;108:533-538.
62. Perrin EV, Persky L, Tucker A, Chrenka B: Renal duplication and dysplasia. Urology 1974;4:660-664.
63. Peterson LJ, Grimes JH, Weinerth JL, Glenn JF: Blind-ending branches of bifid ureters. Urology 1975;5:191-195.
64. Privett JT, Jeans WD, Roylance J: The incidence and importance of renal duplication. Clin Radiol 1976;27:521-530.
65. Puri P: Endoscopic correction of vesicoureteral reflux. Curr Opin Urol 2000;10:593-597.
66. Puri P, Chertin B, Velayudham M, et al: Treatment of vesicoureteral reflux by endoscopic injection of dextranomer/ hyaluronic acid copolymer: Preliminary results. J Urol 2003; 170:1541-1544.
67. Royle MG, Goodwin WE: The management of ureteroceles. J Urol 1971;106:42-47.
68. Schulman CC: [Ureter malformations and renal dysplasia—an embryological concept]. Urologe A 1978;17:273-277.
69. Sen S, Ahmed S, Borghol M: Surgical management of complete ureteric duplication abnormalities. Pediatr Surg Int 1998;13:61-64.
70. Shankar KR, Vishwanath N, Rickwood AM: Outcome of patients with prenatally detected duplex system ureterocele; natural history of those managed expectantly. J Urol 2001; 165:1226-1228.
71. Sherman ND, Stock JA, Hanna MK: Bladder dysfunction after bilateral ectopic ureterocele repair. J Urol 2003;170: 1975-1977.
72. Singh SJ, Smith G: Effectiveness of primary endoscopic incision of ureteroceles. Pediatr Surg Int 2001;17:528-531.
73. Slaughenhoupt BL, Mitcheson HD, Lee DL: Ureteral duplication with lower pole ectopia to the vas: A case report of an exception to the Weigert-Meyer law. Urology 1997;49:269-271.
74. Smith C, Gosalbez R, Parrott TS, et al: Transurethral puncture of ectopic ureteroceles in neonates and infants. J Urol 1994;152:2110-2112.
75. Tanagho EA: Embryologic basis for lower ureteral anomalies: A hypothesis. Urology 1976;7:451-464.
76. Tanagho EA: Ureteroceles: Embryogenesis, pathogenesis and management. J Contin Educ Urol 1979;7:451.
77. Tanagho EA, Hutch JA: Primary reflux. J Urol 1965;93: 158-164.
78. Timothy RP, Decter A, Perlmutter AD: Ureteral duplication: Clinical findings and therapy in 46 children. J Urol 1971;105:445-451.
79. Tresidder GC, Blandy JP, Murray RS: Pyelo-pelvic and uretero-ureteric reflux. Br J Urol 1970;42:728-735.
80. Ulchaker J, Ross J, Alexander F, Kay R: The spectrum of ureteropelvic junction obstructions occurring in duplicated collecting systems. J Pediatr Surg 1996;31:1221-1224.
81. Upadhyay J, Bolduc S, Braga L, et al: Impact of prenatal diagnosis on the morbidity associated with ureterocele management. J Urol 2002;167:2560-2565.
82. Whitaker J, Danks DM: A study of the inheritance of duplication of the kidneys and ureters. J Urol 1966;95: 176-178.
83. Whitten SM, McHoney M, Wilcox DT, et al: Accuracy of antenatal fetal ultrasound in the diagnosis of duplex kidneys. Ultrasound Obstet Gynecol 2003;21:342-346.
84. Williams PL: Embryology—urinary and reproductive systems.

In Gray's Anatomy: The Anatomical Basis of Medicine and Surgery, 38th ed. London, Churchill Livingstone, 1995, pp 199-204.

85. Zerin JM, Baker DR, Casale JA: Single-system ureteroceles in infants and children: Imaging features. Pediatr Radiol 2000;30:139-146.

第 114 章

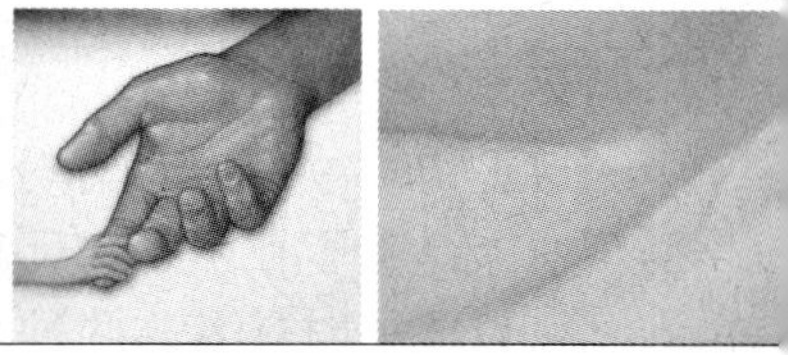

巨输尿管和梅干腹综合征 (Prune-Belly Syndrome)

Mark C. Adams 和 W. Hardy Hendren III

巨输尿管

771 输尿管异常扩大称为巨输尿管，此时输尿管可以过度延长屈曲。一般情况下，输尿管有两个主要的病理类型，分别是梗阻和明显的膀胱输尿管反流（图 114-1）。如果一条巨输尿管末端开口于膀胱颈部或尿道，那么该输尿管在膀胱充盈期可能表现为梗阻，而在膀胱颈部与尿道开放的排尿期可以表现为反流。一些病例的膀胱是正常的，其发生病变的部位是远端输尿管末端。而在其他病例中，巨输尿管可以继发于膀胱功能异常。例如在一些男性后尿道瓣膜所引起的严重尿道梗阻中，可以发现有明显的巨输尿管病变。切除后尿道瓣膜可以减轻排尿期膀胱内压，同时也减轻输尿管内的压力。与此类似，继发于脊髓脊膜膨出的神经性膀胱可以导致膀胱出口的生理性梗阻，同时也引起继发性巨输尿管。有时巨输尿管仅仅是一种形态上的异常表现，除了扩张以外并不伴有梗阻及反流。具有这种病理生理表现的巨输尿管可以根据

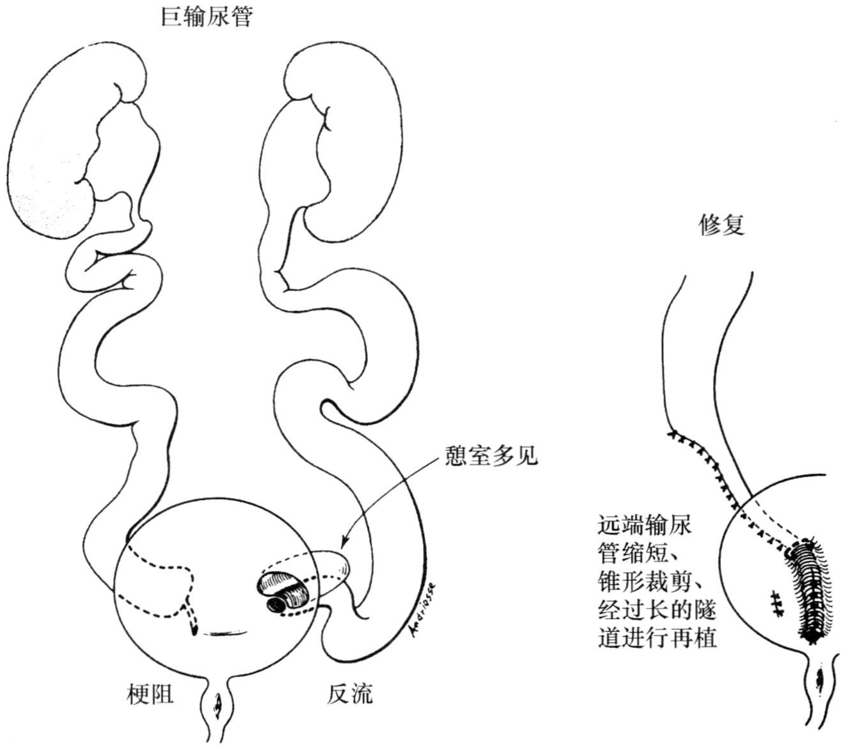

图 114-1 巨输尿管的类型和远端修复手术示意图。

1977 年提出的国际分类方法进行分类[69]。

除了梗阻型和反流型巨输尿管以外，一些输尿管可能同时具有这两种表现。在病理生理上表现为远端无动力节段和较短的黏膜下隧道。在这种情况下，可能会因为反流或向膀胱引流能力低下而使肾盂积水发生的可能性增加。

当病变为下段输尿管内部异常时，则巨输尿管可能是单侧性的，这种情况尤其多见于典型的梗阻型巨输尿管。这些病例通常都有输尿管末端纤维化，由各种组织学和超微结构的异常导致梗阻[35,39]。有人把这种异常称为无动力节段，然而这与先天性巨结肠的远端结肠和失弛缓症中下端食管的无动力节段是完全不同的概念。梗阻型巨输尿管的输尿管开口通常在外观上没有明显异常，很难看到真正的狭窄，在插入输尿管导管时一般也不会遇到困难。反流型巨输尿管的输尿管开口通常都会异常扩大，事实上，在一些病例中可以比较容易地将内镜插入巨输尿管。在原发性反流中，存在不完全的单向瓣膜机制，其发生原因与膀胱壁内黏膜下输尿管的长度和口径有关。

很多输尿管膨出和异位输尿管都伴有巨输尿管，尤其是患有集合系统重复畸形的女婴病例，这些病例一般都有患侧下极输尿管的反流（见第 113 章）。巨输尿管很少由于尿流过多引起，比如尿崩症。Prune-belly 综合征也有整个泌尿系统发育异常的表现，包括输尿管延长迂曲。显微镜切片检查可以发现输尿管管壁的肌肉组织减少，结缔组织增生，病变发生于下段输尿管的机会高于中上段输尿管。

巨输尿管主要发生于两类患者群。新生儿发病者主要出现于产前超声检查有肾盂积水的随访患者。相对于其他先天性上尿路畸形，在这类患者中巨输尿管的发生率高于年长的有症状儿童。在年长儿童中最常见的表现为尿路感染，还有一些儿童表现为由于梗阻而引起的间歇性疼痛或血尿。婴儿期的表现可以是发育迟缓。在泌尿系统检查时，一旦遇到巨输尿管表现，就必须对整个泌尿系统进行全面检查，以进一步明确巨输尿管的原发或继发类型。一般首先对肾脏与输尿管进行超声检查，可是静脉肾盂造影对诊断同样很有帮助。对于梗阻的诊断大多是通过利尿性放射性核素影像检查来确定，利尿后的排尿曲线是非常有意义的指标。在分析时应当注意到该曲线所反映的内容包括整个上尿路系统（同侧肾脏和输尿管），仅仅测
1772 量尿液从肾脏向输尿管引流而忽略向膀胱的引流，则会导致假阴性结果。尤其是对于有产前肾盂积水的新生儿，在描述放射性核素肾扫描结果时，必须考虑到肾脏的功能情况，如果分肾功能明显下降，则应当作为外科手术治疗的指征。在连续的肾扫描检查中发现有肾功能逐渐下降，则是明显的指征，需要尽快实施手术治疗。通过肾穿刺注入造影剂进行顺行性肾盂造影检查，对于一些有选择的病例可以更好地明确解剖情况，并测量和记录上尿路与膀胱之间的压力差。膀胱造影检查对于有反流的病例是必须进行的，可以了解输尿管的解剖异常。如果怀疑有膀胱异常，那么对这些患者进行尿流动力学检查评估很有意义。在进行连续的影像学检查时，暂时性放置导尿管引流也同样有助于区别原发性和继发性巨输尿管。膀胱镜检查可以了解下段输尿管的形态，但仅在实施重建手术时才进行。如前文所述，梗阻型巨输尿管开口的外观形态一般是正常的；反流型巨输尿管的输尿管开口通常会异常扩大，呈“高尔夫球洞”外观。如果原发病变是膀胱动力异常，则采用抗胆碱能药物治疗加或不加间歇性导尿，可以使输尿管扩张有所改善。如果患者患有尿道瓣膜病变，可以通过电切治疗。由于瓣膜病变所导致的疾病严重程度不同[22]，所以在治疗上应进行选择。对一些患者进行瓣膜电切，而其他患者在瓣膜电切后进行早期巨输尿管修复，或者个别情况下，在瓣膜电切后马上进行巨输尿管重建手术[21]。

由于宫内超声的广泛应用，使得许多巨输尿管患者在早期获诊。患病婴儿在出生后即需进行完整的泌尿系统评估。非梗阻非反流的巨输尿管可能在出生后自行缓解，所以对那些轻中度排泄梗阻型的婴儿，若肾功能尚可，可以在一个限定的时间段内进行连续性的观察随访，以了解是否出现自行缓解[3,37]。如果缓解不明确，应当考虑进行外科手术。在不存在反流的情况下，膀胱后输尿管管径是评价肾盂积水缓解可能性以及手术必要性的客观指标[40]。

总之，巨输尿管手术指征需要根据病因来确定。原发梗阻性巨输尿管、肾功能差（在肾扫描中总肾功能小于等于 35%～40%）、复发性感染、肾瘢痕、随访检查中肾功能下降或者有临床症状，这些都是手术治疗的明确指征。双侧巨输尿管或者孤立肾巨输尿管都会影响到全肾功能，应当考虑更为积极的治疗。最后，经过合理的观察期后仍不出现缓解，也是手术治疗的指征。发生于巨输尿管中的反流，除了肾功能正常的新生儿以外，一般都很难自行缓解，需要进行手术治疗。对于继发性反流，在治疗原发性膀胱出口梗阻或膀胱功能紊乱以后，也可能自行缓解。当需要进

行干预治疗时，已经明确采用修复的方法疗效较好，即使对新生儿的较大输尿管亦是如此。有时也需要进行经皮穿刺输尿管造瘘手术，应用于有感染的病例，
773 以及用于肾功能很差、且不确定是采用手术修复抑或手术切除肾脏的新生儿病例。这种情况下，暂时性的经皮肾穿刺造瘘引流有效而且并发症较少。因此，现在已经很少采用经皮输尿管造瘘手术。

手术方法

在需要进行手术修复的病例中，有超过 50% 的患者仅需要对输尿管下端进行重建手术[18,20,55,57,74]。尽管近端输尿管可能会有迂曲的表现，但在输尿管下端重建解除梗阻或反流后，近端的异常往往会改善。这种手术需要在抗反流的基础上耐心细致地操作。尽可能减少对输尿管的钳夹，以免损伤管壁。游离输尿管时要有足够的长度，以便修剪和再植于膀胱壁，避免成角，而且保持其处于无张力状态。操作时要保护输尿管的血供。输尿管进入膀胱的部位应当位于膀胱后壁的固定位置，以免其在膀胱充盈时发生梗阻或成角。黏膜下隧道的长度和输尿管管径要有足够的比例，以防止发生反流，这一比例一般为 4 或 5 比 1。

下端巨输尿管修复手术

图 114-2 显示下端巨输尿管修复的手术步骤。作者建议采用耻骨上水平皮肤切口，对筋膜层建议选择纵行的垂直切口，这样不仅可以很好地暴露膀胱，还可以很容易地显示输尿管的中下三分之一。使用 Denis Browne 通用牵开器可以提供满意的暴露。常规手术中很少会对中段三分之一的输尿管进行暴露和分离，如果有必要，可采用向内侧翻转结肠的方法完成。

如图 114-2A 所示，为便于操作，可以将一塑料导管插入并缝合于输尿管开口。在膀胱内环形分离输尿管开口后，开始从膀胱内向外侧游离输尿管，直至游离操作不能继续进行为止。在黏膜下隧道内附着于输尿管的肌肉和血管都需要进行分离，然后在膀胱侧进行电凝止血，注意不要在输尿管侧进行电凝操作。在膀胱外分离时，要沿着腹壁下静脉进行。遇到脐外侧韧带后结扎切断该韧带，以便向内上方牵开腹膜。对输尿管前方结构由下向上进行分离以后，可以将输尿管提出并暴露于切口外。如果紧贴膀胱进行分离，则有可能损伤膀胱的神经支配，应减少类似的操作。在向上方游离输尿管时，所有的输尿管旁组织都应当向输尿管侧保留，以保护输尿管的侧支血管供应（图 114-2B）。将输尿管从其内侧的腹膜上分离下来时，应当尽可能多地分离腹膜，而不是输尿管。在男性患者中，还应当分辨并保护腹膜表面的输精管。

对于输尿管过度迂曲以及再手术的病例，必须向内侧翻转结肠，以便更容易地向高处游离输尿管。对这种病例建议采用垂直的中线切口。向输尿管充注生理盐水可以更方便地游离输尿管。

仔细游离输尿管后，要在输尿管外侧壁表面潜行分离输尿管旁组织，然后将其切开并暴露将要进行裁剪的一侧输尿管壁（图 114-2C）。作者从 1959 年起，于开始的 20 年里进行巨输尿管修复手术时采用特制的输尿管钳，在裁剪输尿管时帮助切除过多的输尿管壁。一些外科医生仍然认为这种方法非常有效。不过在最近几年，作者已经不再使用这种方法，主要是因为在裁剪过程中不使用输尿管钳时，这些有血管供应的输尿管旁组织可以很容易地被分离并保留，然后再覆盖修裁好的输尿管。对于输尿管的修剪段可以事先用记号笔标记好，然后进行裁剪（图 114-2D）。切除多余的输尿管壁后，在放置于膀胱壁内时，应将切口侧朝向膀胱肌肉层面而不是黏膜面。有时在此处可以发现有输尿管外膜层的主要血管供应支，此时应当避开并保护该血管供应。操作时很重要的一点是不要把输尿管修剪得太狭窄，而且还要注意完成输尿管缝合需要保持 3～4 mm 的输尿管周径。缝合输尿管时可以使用 10 French 的导管作为支撑，但在婴儿中使用 8 French的导管可能会更合适。缝合时要注意不要将导管包绕过紧。

缝合输尿管时采用连续锁边缝合方式（图 114-2E），在最后几针时使用间断缝合更有益，可以方便再植时对末端的修剪。然后将保留下来的输尿管周围组织缝合，覆盖封闭第一层缝合好的切口。这两层缝合应当使用细的可吸收缝线。为方便操作，可以保留输尿管末端作为操作时的牵引，当再植时输尿管第一针固定缝合后切除末端，此时还应当同时切除梗阻巨输尿管的无动力节段。

选择输尿管进入膀胱的新入口（图 114-2F）非常重要。一种错误的做法是将该入口选择在过于靠近

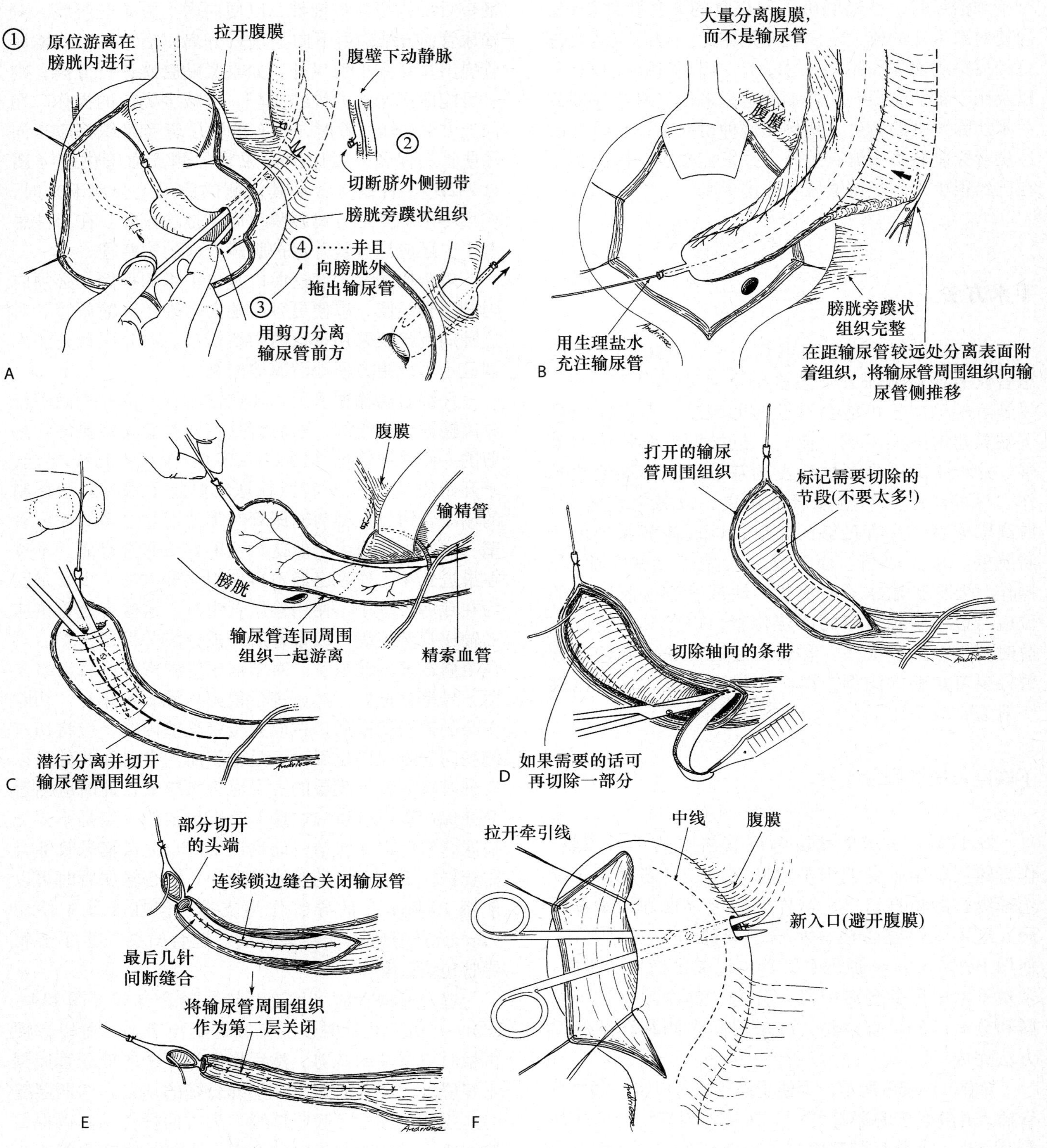

图114-2　远端输尿管修复手术。A. 原位膀胱内游离。B. 膀胱外游离。C. 打开输尿管周围组织。D. 修剪远端输尿管。E. 关闭远端输尿管。F. 建立新的入口。

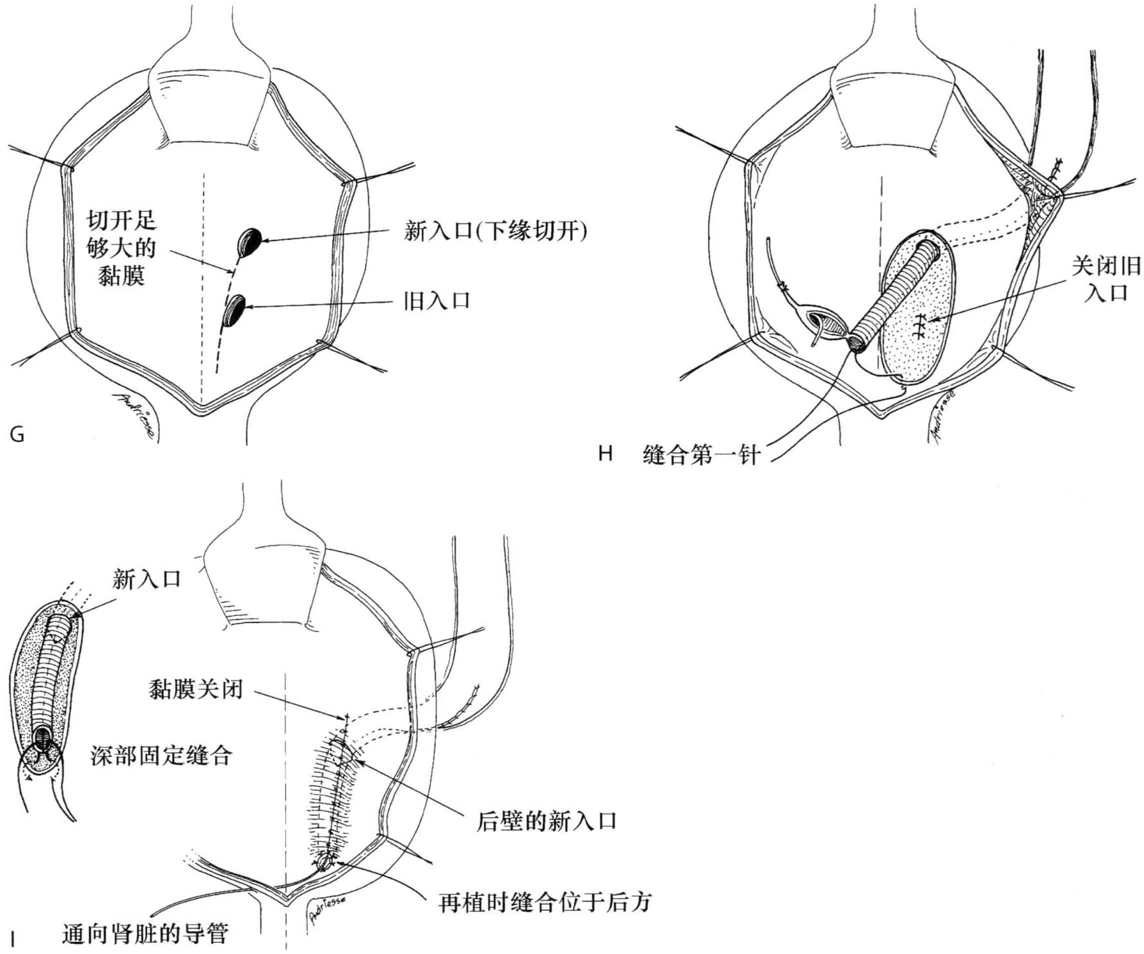

图 114-2　（续）G. 为锥形再植建立一个床。H. 在其隧道内缝合锥形的输尿管。I. 完成修复手术。

外侧处，这会导致输尿管成角，在膀胱充盈时造成梗阻。如果将入口选择于膀胱后壁，就不会出现这样的问题。新的入口要足够大，使其不能对输尿管造成压迫。在新的入口下缘处切开可以使输尿管更为平缓地进入膀胱，但此时要特别注意避免在此处损伤男性输精管。

输尿管入口建立后，在输尿管预置的出口处切开膀胱黏膜，切口的宽度要以容纳输尿管为宜（图 114-2G），这比建立黏膜下隧道的过程还要精确。在此处将输尿管与其背侧的膀胱肌肉缝合，这种做法是有益处的。对于一些膀胱（如 prune-belly 综合征和神经源性膀胱），要提起膀胱黏膜十分困难，需要进行烦琐的锐性分离。此后紧密缝合旧输尿管入口处的膀胱肌层。如果在术前存在输尿管旁憩室，那么在手术时还要切除原始输尿管入口处的膀胱黏膜，同时切除憩室。

然后要将输尿管缝合固定于输尿管床上（图 114-2H）。在出口处的远端固定缝合逼尿肌和黏膜以及输尿管全层，出口其余部分的缝合只需黏膜对黏膜缝合。裁剪过的输尿管后壁要朝向膀胱肌肉层面。裁剪 1775
过的输尿管从近端开始要有足够的长度，使其能够超出膀胱输尿管入口以外。修裁后的输尿管末端锥形管道应当平缓过渡，以避免向外突出形成类似憩室样的结构。

图 114-2I 显示了修复完成后的形态，黏膜层覆盖于裁剪后的输尿管表面。从对侧膀胱壁插入一 5 号鼻饲管，经输尿管进入肾脏，引流留置到术后 10～12 天。极少数情况下需要使用双“J”管支撑，也很少需要肾造瘘引流。以上所述及的巨输尿管修复手术是作者推荐应用的。有些外科医生倾向使用跨三角区输

尿管再植手术（cross－trigonal reimplantation technique），但这种做法仅适用于三角区宽度大于长度的情况，只有在这种情况下才能够提供足够长的黏膜下隧道。反流和非反流巨输尿管都可以在膀胱外进行修复[41,54]。对于双侧巨输尿管的患者，作者常规进行同期双侧下段输尿管的修复手术。

对于修复手术后的膀胱引流，最好使用直管引流，而不要使用经尿道的 Foley 导管，以避免球囊压迫或激惹对输尿管修复手术造成影响。极少数情况下可以使用耻骨上导管引流，如同期进行于膀胱出口的尿失禁手术。术后 10～12 天经输尿管引流管进行造影检查，以排除尿液渗漏，而这种情况很少发生，造影后拔除输尿管引流管。如果为双侧手术，则两侧同时进行造影检查。在拔除任何一侧输尿管导管后都要测定尿量，以明确同侧肾脏的引流情况。

输尿管折叠手术

经典的巨输尿管修复手术包括切除部分输尿管管壁，以缩减其周径，这也是作者建议的方法。输尿管折叠手术可以考虑用于中度扩张的输尿管，即便这种手术方法对于输尿管扩张明显或管壁增厚的患者来
1776 说，在再植手术时会造成输尿管壁过于臃肿。这种手术方法是由 Starr[71] 和 Kalicinski 等[30] 提出的，用于减少输尿管血管损伤的可能性。作者相信，如果采用如图 114-4 的手术方式，这种情况会罕有发生。在任意一种折叠方式中，可以先插入大小合适的支撑管，再放置无损伤钳，沿多余的输尿管作出标志线。另外，放置无损伤钳可以避开输尿管外膜中比较大的血管支。撤除无损伤钳后，可以应用两种方法中的任何一种来折叠输尿管壁。Starr[11] 所描述的方法是沿钳夹标志线采用内翻缝合方法，使过多的输尿管壁折叠起来，以减少输尿管管腔的大小（图 114-3）。Kalicinski 等人[30] 采用水平连续褥式缝合方法去除过多的输尿管管腔，然后再用连续缝合将这一分开的附属管腔折叠缝合到输尿管壁上（图 114-4）。组织学检查显示这一折叠的部分会在数月后发生闭锁，而另一部分管腔会持续开放[2]。

内镜注射

自从早期的输尿管下注射聚四氟乙烯（Teflon）

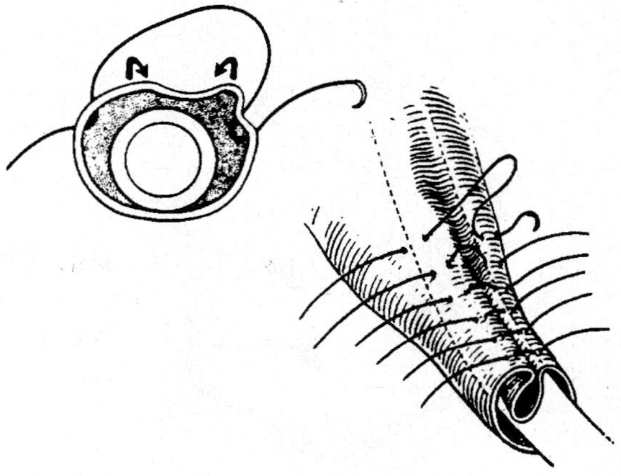

图 114-3 输尿管折叠时采用细的可吸收缝线间断内翻缝合。（From Keating MA，Retik AB：Management of failures of ureteroneocystostomy. In McDougal WS［ed］：Difficult Problems in Urologic Surgery. Chicago，Year Book，1989，p 131.）

治疗反流的报告出现后[45]，内镜治疗也开始应用于反流性巨输尿管。该治疗方法不适用于梗阻性巨输尿管。现已证实高级别的反流很难通过内镜根除，这与开放手术的结果一样。正常大小的输尿管一次注射治疗反流的成功率为 60%～80%。尽管经过第二次或第三次治疗后成功的可能性会增加，但在反流性巨输尿管治疗中的失败率还是超过 20%[8]。经过长期随访，

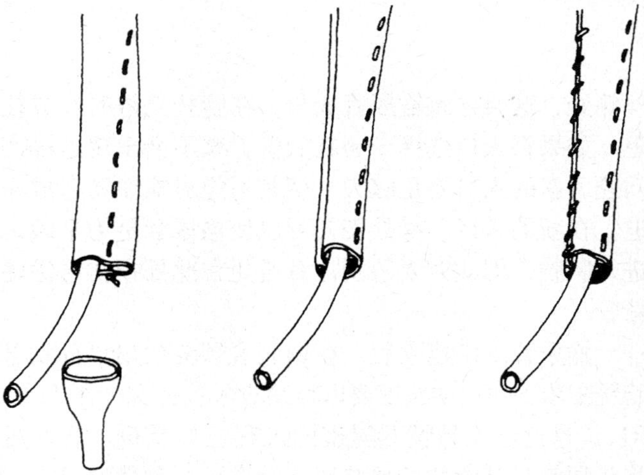

图 114-4 用连续水平褥式缝合分离出多余的管腔。然后将多余的部分折叠并缝合于主输尿管壁上。（From Kalicinski ZH，Kansy J，Kotabinsia B，et al：Surgery of megaureters：Modification of Hendren's operation. J Pediatr Surg 1977；12：183.）

复发率很低[7]。由于微粒迁移和自身免疫的原因，现在美国已经不赞成使用聚四氟乙烯。具有生物相容性和生物可降解的材料已经开始应用，而应用最广泛的材料是聚糖苷/透明质酸聚合物（Deflux，Q-Med Scandinavia，Uppsala，Sweden）[72]。这种材料比 Teflon 更容易使用，而且对所有级别的反流同样有效，也包括巨输尿管[6,32,59]。注射时输尿管水肿以及在黏膜下与输尿管间隙增加生物植入物注射的使用量，可以提高治疗效果，减少药物向近端迁移（图 114-5）[32]。内镜注射已经用于更为复杂的反流患者，包括继发性反流、重复畸形以及经尿道切开输尿管膨出后的反流[33]。治疗效果最不好的情况是对异位输尿管开口反流进行注射治疗。对于接受过生物植入物注射治疗的患者，再进行开放式输尿管再植手术的难度很大，然而文献中报道的成功率与那些直接进行再植手术的成功率相似。一般来说，开始时要将输尿管与生物植入物一同进行游离，并且把受影响的输尿管远端节段切除。

作者应用直接巨输尿管修复手术已经有 45 年的历史，取得了较好的效果，并一直推荐这种治疗方式。对少数巨输尿管患者也采用了注射治疗，主要是针对那些经历过手术并且采用较长的黏膜下隧道后仍然发生残余尿反流伴输尿管扩张的患者。

近端输尿管修复

如果原发的病理改变仅是膀胱输尿管梗阻或严重的反流，那么在远端输尿管修复术后大多不需要处理近端输尿管梗阻。然而对于近端输尿管的情况有以下几点需要强调。首先，以往有反流或梗阻的下段输尿管经过成功修复后，其迂曲的形态会有改善，成角会解除，扩张程度降低（图 114-6），如果患者的临床表现较好，最好再继续等待几个月或更长的时间再决定是否进行近端输尿管的修复手术。近端的输尿管可能会在远端输尿管修复后迅速发生更为明显的扩张表现，这是由再植部位周围组织水肿所引起的，需要进行反复的肾脏影像学检查以排除真性梗阻。如果远端输尿管修复好，近端输尿管仍然持续迂曲扩张，就应当依照图 114-7 的方式进行裁剪。这一裁剪过程有时仅需切除引起引流不畅的成角节段，尤其是位于肾盂

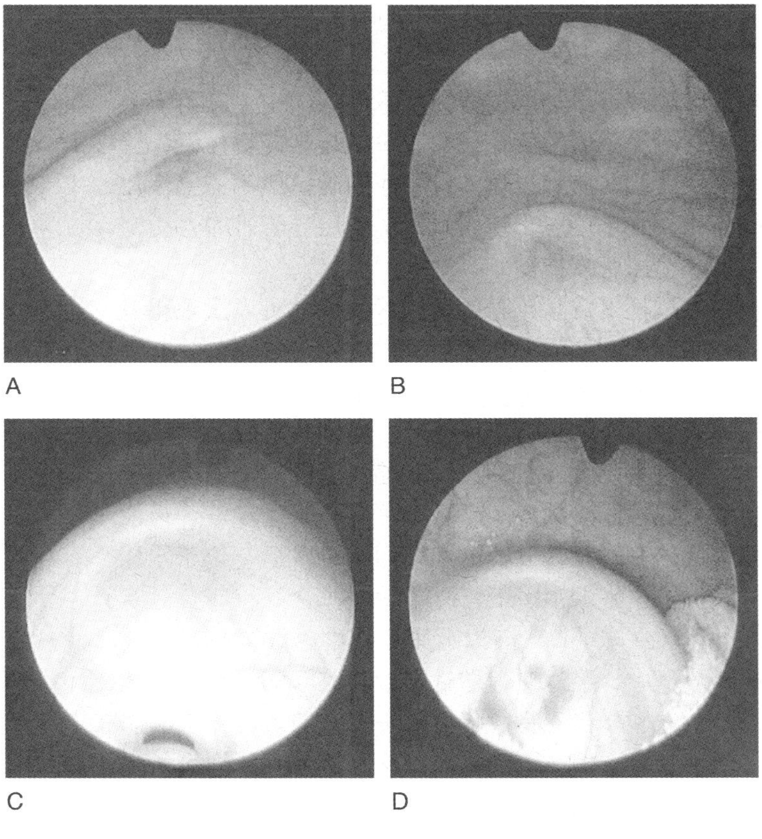

图 114-5　内镜下注射。A 和 B. 反流开口。C. 注射针插入输尿管下方的黏膜下间隙。D. 注射后的接合处。（Courtesy of Anthony Caldamone，MD）.

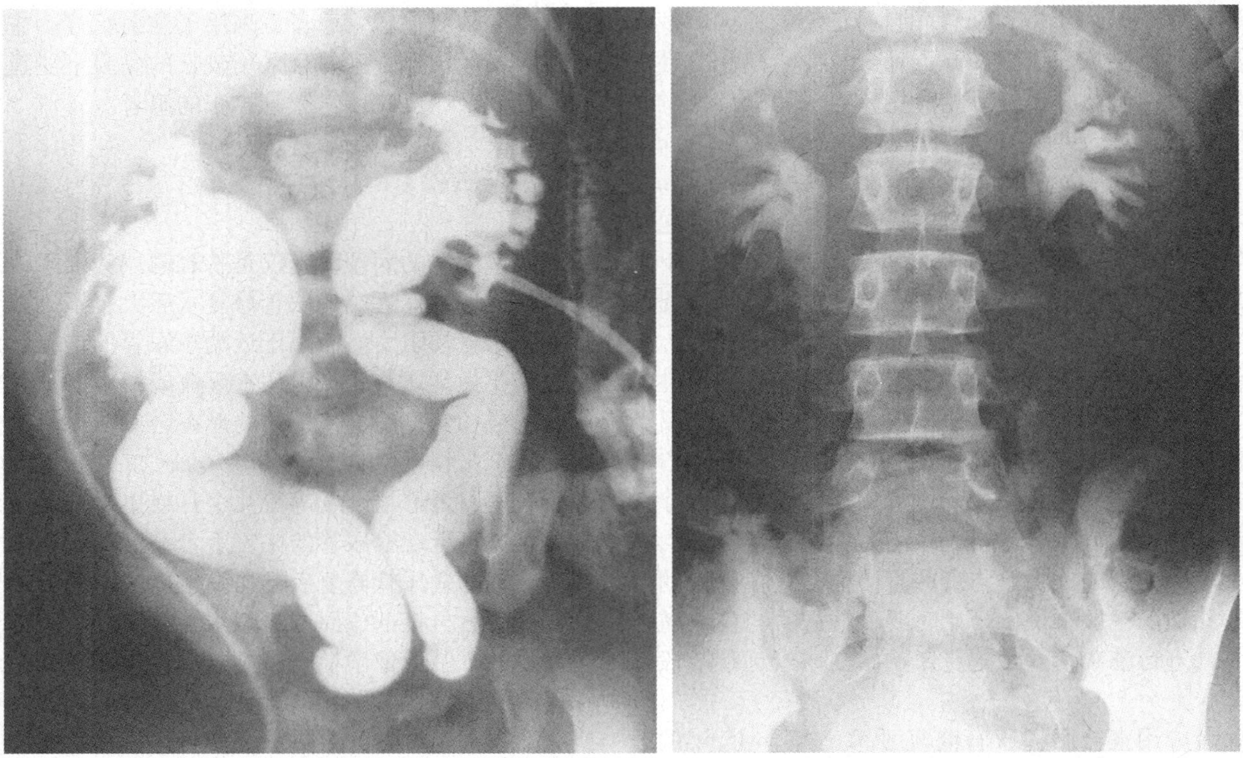

A B

图 114-6 反流型巨输尿管。A. 4 周患儿术前大量反流。预先放置肾造瘘管没有必要。B. 双侧巨输尿管修复术后 13 年的静脉肾盂造影检查。注意仅行远端输尿管修复手术后，近端有明显改善。

1778 输尿管连接部位的成角。在严重的病例中，裁剪还要缩减近端输尿管的管径。在原位纵行切开输尿管，修剪其宽度。在修剪近端节段输尿管时一般不需要使用操作钳。手术后应当使用肾造瘘术用导管暂时性引流或放置输尿管支撑管。

在透视下观察扩张的输尿管的活动可以发现很有意思的现象。如果输尿管的管壁不能够紧贴在一起，那么即使有输尿管的蠕动存在，也是无效的。尿液在输尿管中随着蠕动波来回搅动，而不是有效地排入膀胱。图 114-8 显示了一条扩张输尿管的蠕动研究。手术前，在输尿管的各个水平都可以看到蠕动波，但波幅都比较小，是无效的蠕动；而在手术后，位于输尿管裁剪部位下端 10 cm 处的蠕动波非常好，而且是有效的，但在末端 15 cm 以上则不存在这样的蠕动。在一些病例中，经过对近端输尿管长时间的观察，由于持续扩张和排空不良，仍需要进行裁剪。在作者的患者当中，有一例在下端输尿管修复手术 8 年后做了近端输尿管的修复手术，使其上尿路肾盂积水显著改善，肌酐清除率明显提高。

并发症

对于一个有经验的外科医生来说，将正常大小输尿管（不伴有反流或梗阻）再植入正常膀胱的手术成功率应当达到 98%，而巨输尿管修复手术的成功率则未达到这一水平。图 114-9 列出了巨输尿管修复手术的主要并发症[24]。当出口过于靠近外侧、隧道长度过短或者输尿管远端过于宽大时，则有可能导致反流。比较罕见的原因是在插入输尿管支撑管时，由于支撑管太硬，刺破输尿管隧道的起始部分，导致输尿管进入膀胱转折处穿孔，从而形成瘘管造成反流。使用柔软的 5 号婴儿塑料饲养管可以避免这一问题。导致术后梗阻的最常见原因是输尿管通过膀胱壁新入口时受压，这种情况多见于新入口的位置过于靠近外 17
侧，致使输尿管在膀胱充盈时发生成角。这就间接强

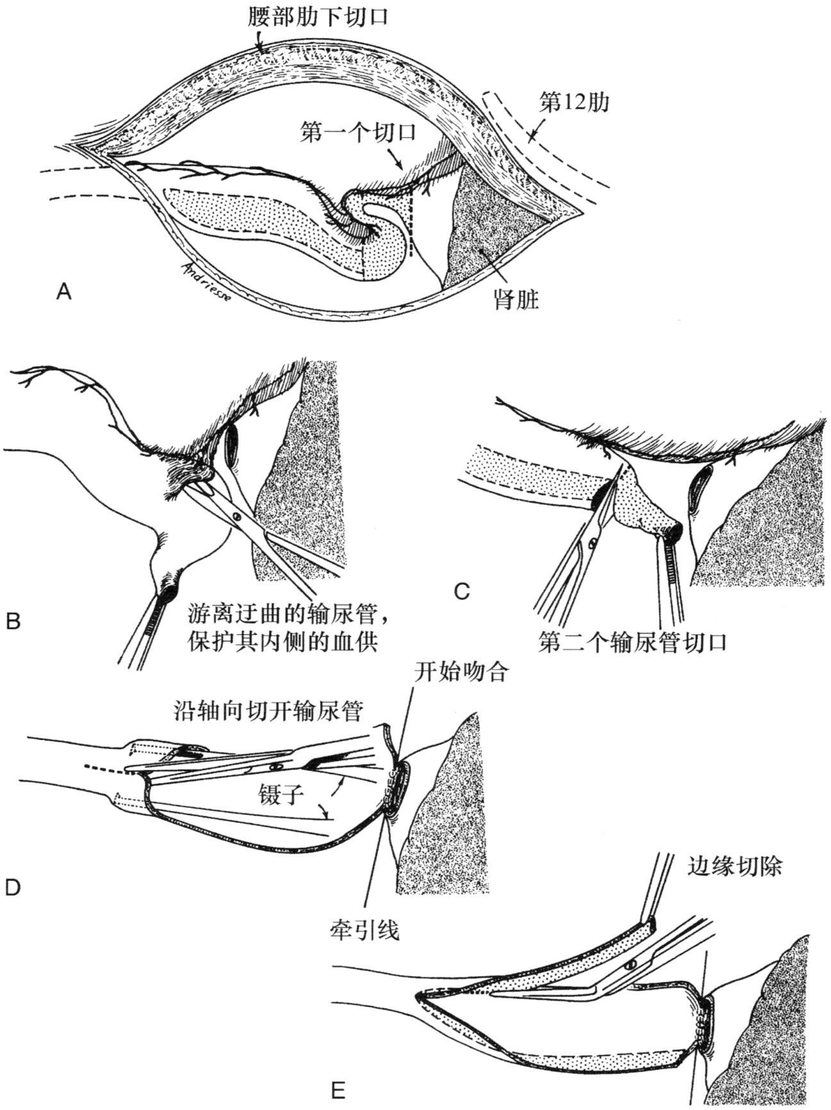

图 114-7 近端输尿管伸直加锥形裁剪，作者有四分之一的患者进行了这种手术，这些患者的输尿管迂曲并且有梗阻表现，尤其是在肾盂输尿管连接处最为明显。有些患者的输尿管近端扩张，不能有效排空。对近端输尿管进行修剪能够改善其排空活动。

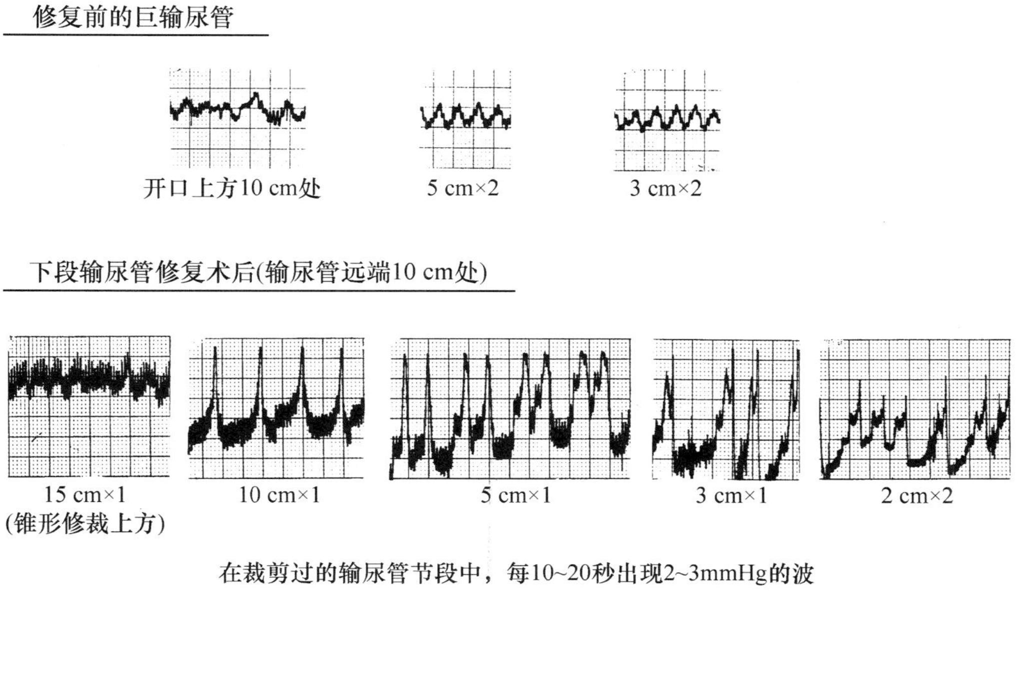

图 114-8 输尿管蠕动研究。在手术前输尿管下段的蠕动波是无效的，但在经过下段锥形裁剪后明显改善。在本研究中，修裁段以上的近端扩张输尿管蠕动波仍然处于无效状态。

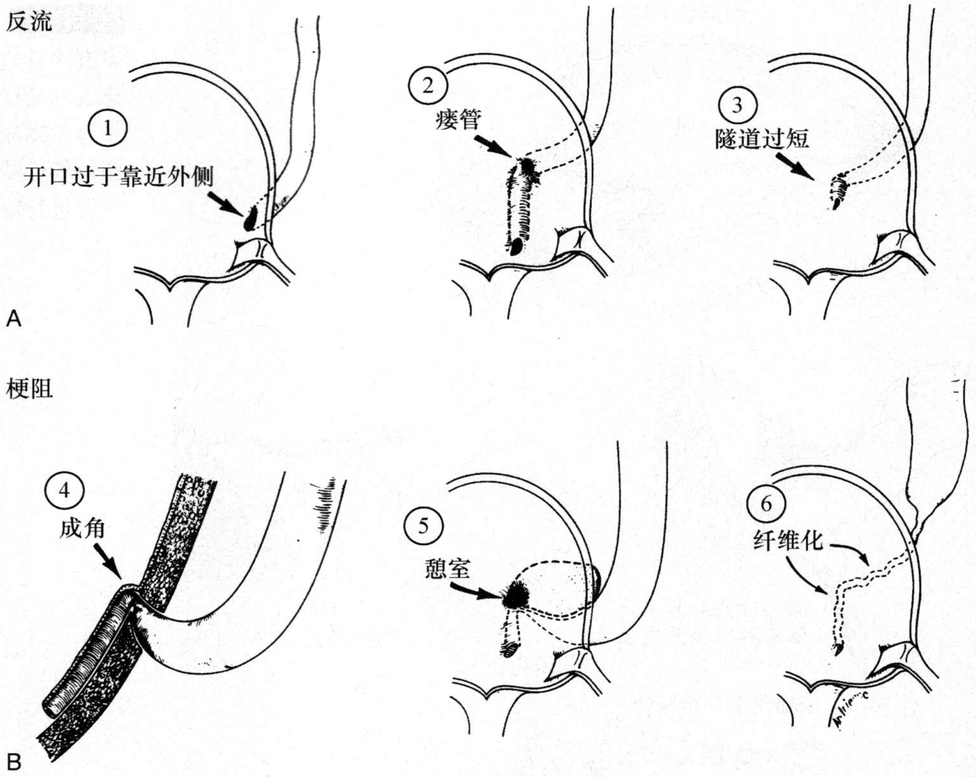

图 114-9　巨输尿管手术失败的最常见并发症。

调了将新入口建立在膀胱后壁的重要性，而不是位于膀胱侧壁。在某些病例中，将膀胱和入口固定于腰大肌上会有助于预防这种并发症。有时会在新建的入口部位发现有憩室形成，如果憩室过大，就会引起输尿管梗阻。输尿管远端纤维化也是可以避免的，这需要在游离输尿管时手法轻柔，保护输尿管的血液供应，在裁剪输尿管时不要使其过于狭窄，避免大范围修裁伤及远端输尿管的血供。

在作者对 294 例患者（男性 217 例，女性 77 例）404 条巨输尿管裁剪的经验中，包括 75 例 1 岁以下的婴儿，治疗梗阻型巨输尿管的成功率为 93%，高级别
1780 反流巨输尿管的成功率为 83%。在正常膀胱（130 例）中的操作成功率高于明显异常膀胱（164 例），后者包括后尿道瓣膜、神经性膀胱、输尿管膨出、梅干腹综合征以及膀胱外翻。大多数第二次进行的输尿管手术最终也获得了成功（图 114-10）。其他方法包括横跨输尿管输尿管吻合术、膀胱扩大术[28]、输尿管下注射聚糖苷微球以及在 2 例患者中进行的回肠裁剪代输尿管手术。其他作者也报告了类似结果[30,50,52,55]，而且不管是用切开裁剪还是折叠的方法，都会有问题发生。不管怎样，反流型巨输尿管修复手术后，发生继发性反流和梗阻并发症的情况多于梗阻型巨输尿管。胶原沉积增加以及异常的胶原-肌肉分布已经被发现存在于反流性巨输尿管，而在原发性梗阻型巨输尿管远端无动力节段以上却没有这种异常[36]。这种内在性的差异可能是两种类型巨输尿管产生不同结果的原因。

总结

输尿管的功能是在低压状态下将尿液从肾脏输送到膀胱。当输尿管发生明显扩张，蠕动时其管壁不能相互闭合，那么输尿管就不能有效地实现这一功能。当输尿管贮存的尿液超过其输送的尿液量时，其内静止的液体就会有利于细菌生长，这在合并由膀胱输尿管连接处功能不全引起反流的情况下更容易发生。巨输尿管可以通过修复手术治疗，其成功率较高。在操作时应当减少对扩张输尿管的钳夹，游离输尿管时要仔细，以保护输尿管的血供。发生梗阻时，要完全切除输尿管远端无动力节段，而后近端扩张的输尿管可裁剪到正常大小。作者认为通过锥形裁剪可以较好地

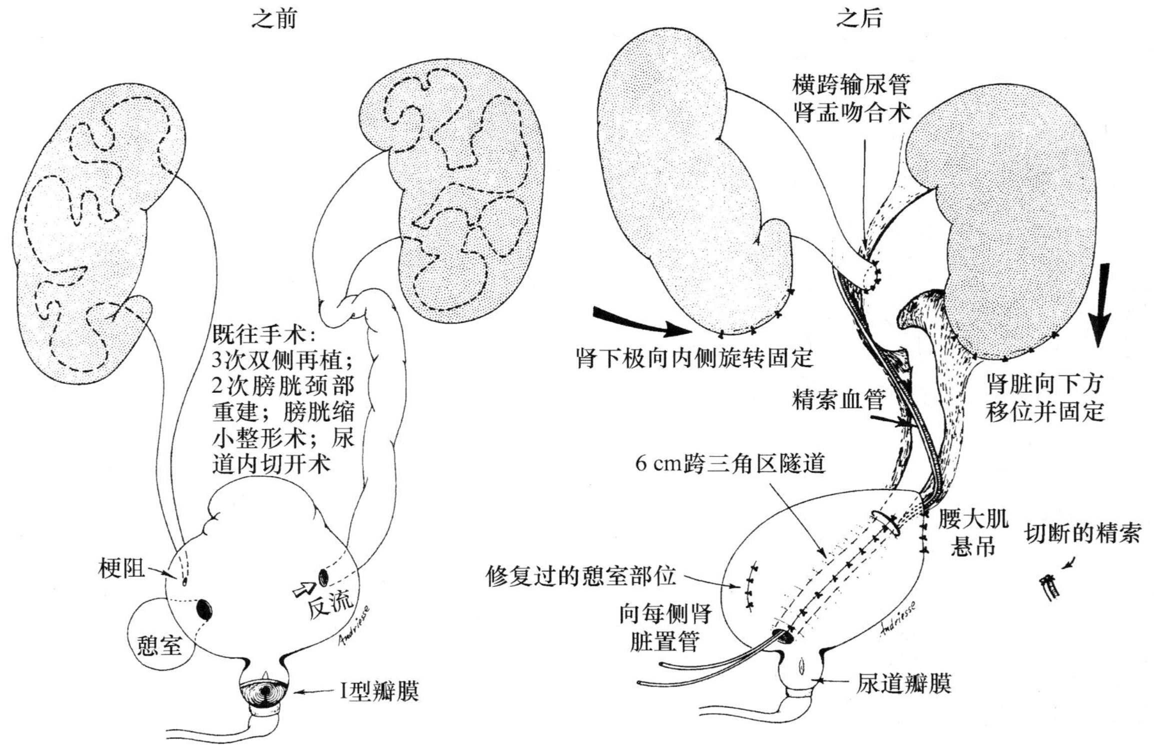

图 114-10　一个 14 岁的男孩在经过三次输尿管再植手术后，在右侧仅留下短的梗阻型巨输尿管，同时在左侧还有大量的反流。通过锥形裁剪和第四次再植手术，左侧输尿管恢复满意，手术同时将肾脏向下方牵移和膀胱向上方悬吊，相对延长了输尿管的长度[23]。术中采用精索血管来加强输尿管的血供。右肾则通过横跨输尿管肾盂吻合术引流。术中同时治疗了憩室和尿道瓣膜。

实现这一目的，而对于扩张程度不重、管壁不很厚的输尿管，也可以采用折叠方法进行操作。然后再根据抗反流手术的原则将重建好的输尿管再植入膀胱。这些修复手术发生梗阻并发症的机会稍高，而特别是持续反流的发生机会高于那些没有输尿管扩张的病例。这些并发症发生于反流型巨输尿管的机会大于梗阻型巨输尿管。而内镜注射治疗反流型巨输尿管的应用效果还需要更长期的随访和更多中心的经验总结来明确。

梅干腹综合征

一些罕见而怪异的巨输尿管是在梅干腹综合征患者中发现的，这一综合征的定义由 William Osler 于 1901 年描述，这些患者的腹壁肌肉先天发育缺陷，致使外观异常[46]。皮肤不规则皱起，外观类似梅干。这种病症也被称为 Eagle-Barrett 或三联综合征，这是因为它包含三个主要表现：腹壁肌肉缺陷、肾盂输尿管积水和隐睾[34,73]。本病病因不明，有人提出早期尿路梗阻[47]和尿性腹水[43]可能是其发病原因，或者是原始中胚层发育障碍导致产生腹壁和泌尿生殖系统改变[67]。几乎所有的患者都是男性，但也有女性发病的报道[60]。作者从 1968 年起治疗了 40 例梅干腹综合征患者，仅有 2 例是女性。文献报道有双胎都发病[56]、双胎之一发病以及染色体嵌合异常的同胞连续发病[19]。这些病例提示有基因致病的可能，但还不了解其确切的遗传学类型。与大多数病理学改变一样，梅干腹综合征的腹壁和泌尿系统异常的程度也轻重不等。

腹壁

图 114-11 显示了 4 例梅干腹综合征患者的腹壁

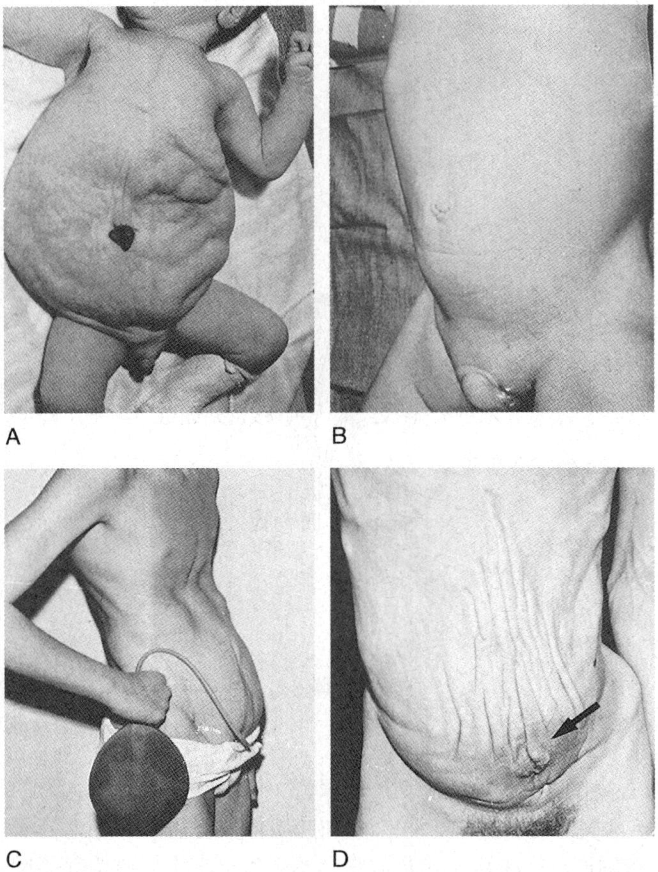

图 114-11 梅干腹综合征的不同腹壁外观。A. 新生儿严重梅干腹综合征的典型表现。可以看到腰部下垂，由于肌肉缺陷，腹壁菲薄，使得深部的肠袢清晰可见。B. 8 周的男孩患有轻度的梅干腹综合征。可以看到下腹部轻度皱褶以及深部扩大的膀胱。腹壁松弛，但比 A 中的患者发育好。C. 18 岁的患者具有梅干腹综合征典型的腹部隆起表现。可以看到胸骨下端内陷，这在此类患者中非常普遍。从婴儿期起就做了肾盂造瘘和膀胱造瘘。该患者接下来做了尿路重建手术。D. 16 岁的患者有明显的腹壁皱缩，有长期的输尿管造瘘（*箭头*）。该患者有脊柱后侧凸畸形。患者接下来做了尿流复道手术。

情况。在典型的病例中，腹壁松弛隆起，近看可以发现粗糙的皮肤皱褶。腹壁可以极为菲薄，甚至可以很容易看到扩张的输尿管袢和肠袢，观察到蠕动。在这种严重的病例中，腹壁的完整性很差，触诊时很容易扪及腹腔内容物。腹部隆起及肋缘明显凸出，这些都是很常见的表现，胸骨下端一般都是凹陷的。小儿长大以后皮肤通常都会变得光滑，然而其下腹部会明显隆起呈壶状外观。腹壁的组织学检查发现肌层缺如或发育不良，尤其是在下部和中央部分[1]。正常的肌群关系可能会保留下来，也可能融合成一纤维组织层。神经分布是完整的[44]。下胸壁支持结构缺陷在很多这类患儿中导致无效的咳嗽机制，使其更容易罹患呼吸系统感染。腹壁松弛也可以导致膀胱和肠功能低下。有趣的是患者伤口愈合机制不受影响，而且在手术修补后腹壁的外观和功能会有所改善。最早期也是最简单的治疗方法包括中线切开，在切除多余的皮肤以及双侧变薄的腹壁后关闭切口。Randolph 等人[62]提出采用近乎水平的切口，从双侧最低处的肋尖到耻骨联合，并切除其中间部分。Ehrlich[12,13] 和 Monfort[42,49] 及其同事报道的手术方法保留了中间部分的肌肉筋膜条带，在其表面用外侧比较好的肌肉、筋膜和皮肤覆盖（图 114-12）。这两种方法都能提供良好的暴露，以利于同期进行睾丸固定和泌尿生殖系统重建手术。

肾脏和输尿管

梅干腹综合征患者的肾脏结构和功能变异很大。在一些病例中，肾脏严重发育不良，小儿在出生后不久即死于继发于肾衰竭的肺发育不良（图 114-13）[65,66]。而病变的另一端是患者的肾脏相对正常。有超过半数的梅干腹综合征患者有肾发育不良的情况[66]，其严重程度是决定患者预后的重要因素。同一个患者两侧肾发育不良的程度也会有很大不同。在伴有膀胱出口梗阻和肛门闭锁的患者中，肾发育不良的程度比较严重[58]。

这种病变程度轻重不一的情况不仅可以见于肾实质的镜下表现，也出现于肾脏的集合系统，表现为扩张和少见的形态异常（图 114-14）。输尿管呈现特有的扩张、延长，严重扭曲，其严重程度远远超过男性高等级膀胱出口梗阻的相应表现，如尿道瓣膜中的表现。有些患者输尿管壁中缺乏肌肉成分，而其他患者中的肌肉发育则比较好。一般情况下，输尿管上端组织学结构的保留程度比远端输尿管好[48]。输尿管壁胶原成分增加，而肌肉成分减少，这些表现在严重反流的病例中尤其明显[16]。有些患者的肾盂输尿管连接部极度扭曲，但不发生梗阻，而其他患者则会出现肾盂输尿管连接部梗阻的表现。一些患者的输尿管蠕动能力很差，而其他患者的输尿管虽然有主动的蠕

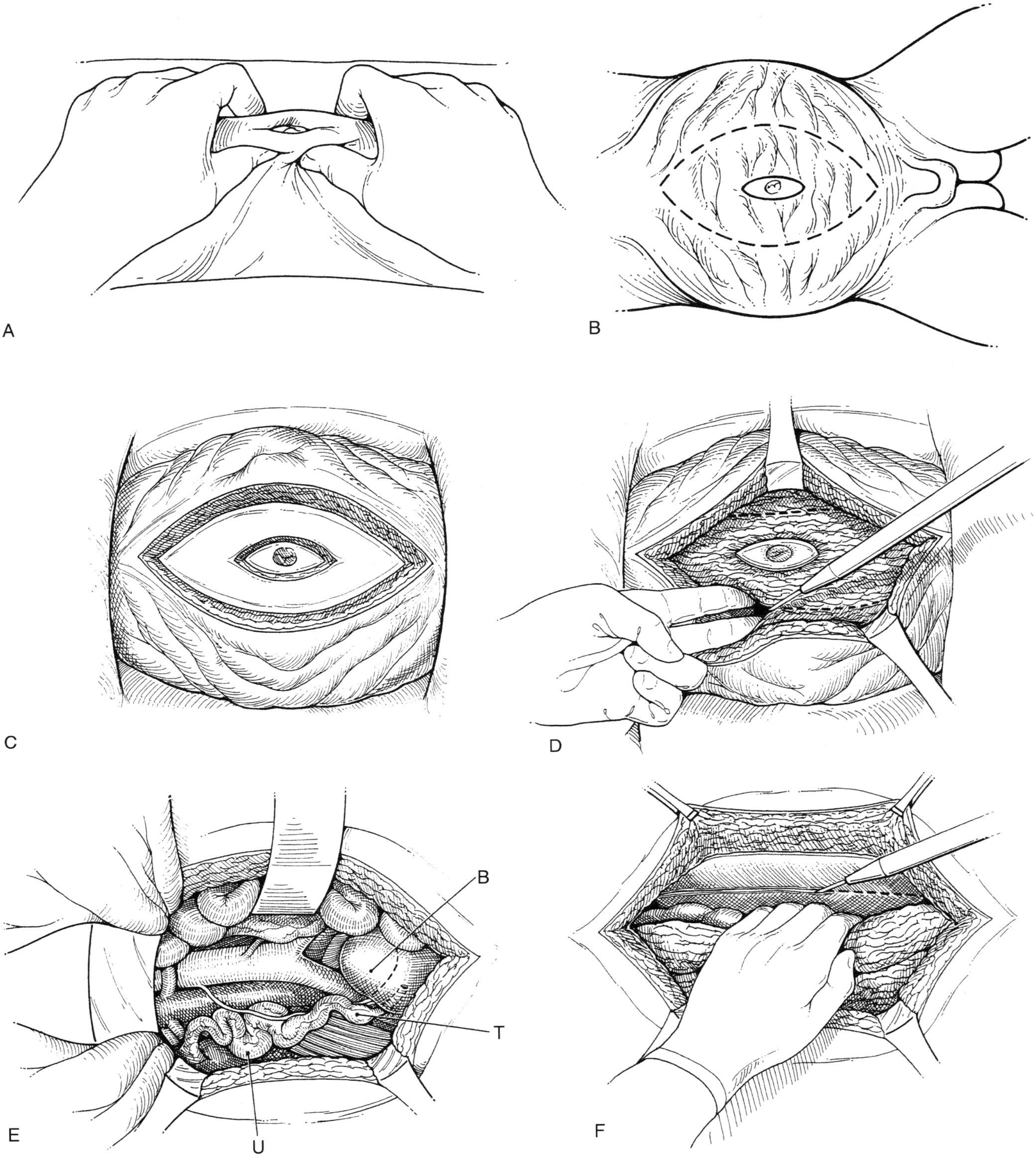

图 114–12　Monfort 腹壁整形术操作方法。A. 使腹壁呈帐篷样隆起，标记出多余的腹壁。B. 描画出腹壁切口外线，另外内部圆形切口保留脐部。C. 用电刀切除皮肤（仅表皮和真皮）。D. 在腹直肌外侧缘切开两侧腹壁，从腹壁上血管到腹壁下血管，以建立一个中部肌筋膜板。E. 向外侧牵开中部肌筋膜板，为同时进行的经腹膜泌尿生殖系统手术提供充分的暴露。B，膀胱；T，睾丸；U，输尿管。F. 用电刀在外侧腹壁肌肉的壁腹膜画线标记，准备完成腹壁整形手术。

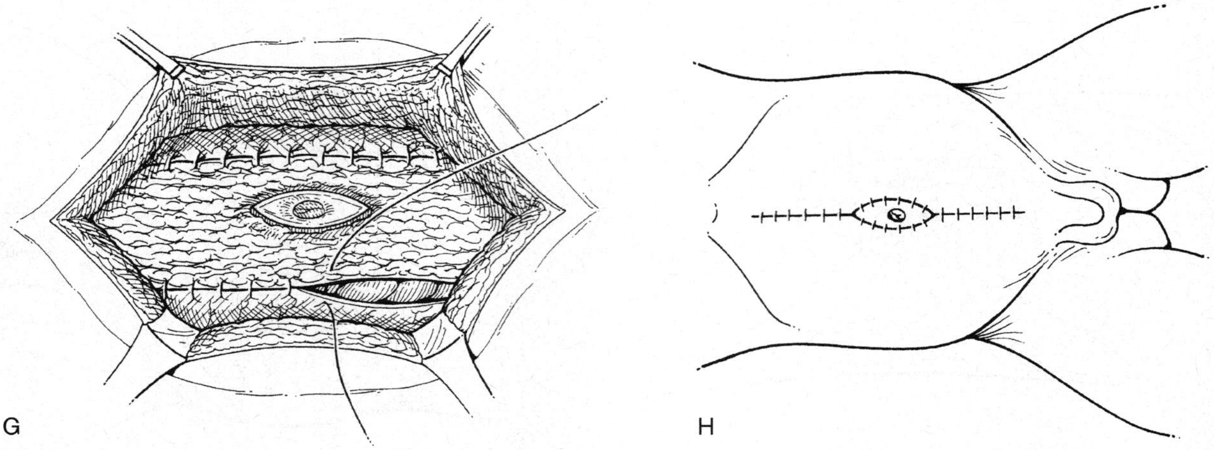

G　H

图 114-12　（续）G. 将中部肌筋膜板的边缘与标记线处的侧腹壁肌肉缝合。H. 将外侧皮瓣向中线处靠拢缝合，在外侧皮瓣与中部肌筋膜板之间放置立闭式引流。于中线处连同保留的脐部一起关闭皮肤切口。（H，From Woodard JR，Perez LM：Prune - belly syndrome. In Marshall FF［ed］：Operative Urology. Philadelphia，WB Saunders，1996.）

动，但这些蠕动同时也是无效的，其原因主要是输尿管壁在蠕动时不能够闭合。反复的尿路感染会导致输尿管壁炎症和纤维化，进而加重已有的病变。发生在肾脏病变水平的肾盂积水通常比输尿管和膀胱病变引起的肾盂积水要轻一些，而且保留下来的肾实质有时也会比远端扩张病变保留下来的肾实质要好。梅干腹综合征患者大多数（85%）都会发生反流[17]，但由于泌尿系统形态异常，使反流很难分级，不过由于反流量很大，干扰了膀胱的动力学活动，使患者容易罹患尿路感染。

膀胱

梅干腹综合征患者的膀胱容量往往很大。一些膀胱表现为大的憩室样穹顶，波及脐尿管区域（见图

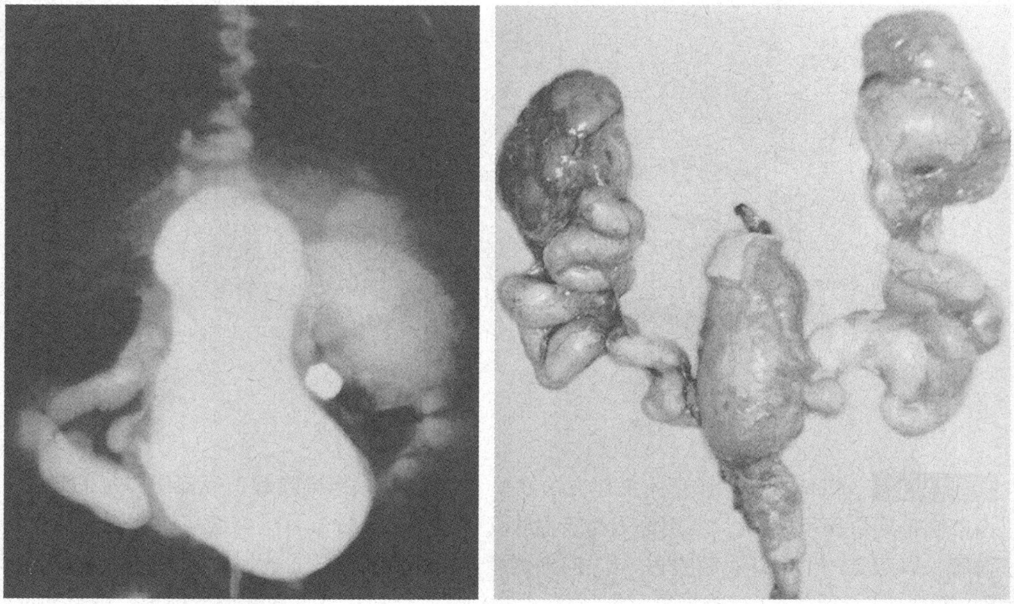

A　B

图 114-13　1 例新生儿梅干腹综合征，该患儿于出生后 1 周死于尿毒症。A. 膀胱造影显示膀胱扩大拉长，有憩室样的穹顶，这在梅干腹综合征中比较常见。可见大量反流进入扩张卷曲的输尿管。B. 尿路尸检标本。可见膀胱与脐部以及囊性发育不良的肾脏相连。

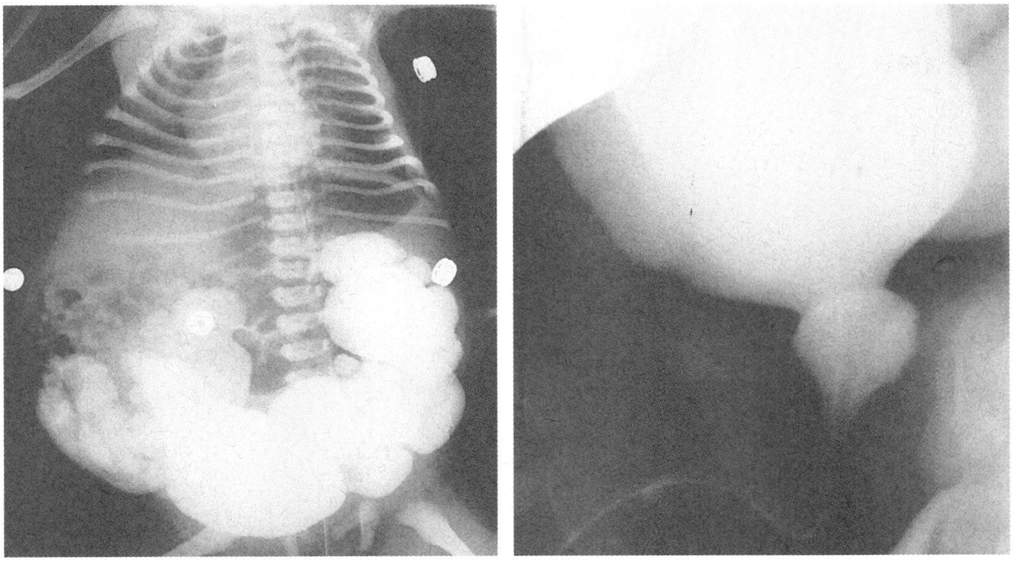

A　B

图 114-14　重症梅干腹综合征病例的典型表现。A. 膀胱造影。可见膀胱扩大伴有倒置的小泡样外观，以及大量反流进入卷曲的输尿管。如果将输尿管伸直，其长度可以超过患者的腿长。B. 膀胱尿道造影。可见膀胱壁光滑，膀胱颈开放，以及心形的尿道。

114-14）。对于尿道闭锁患者，膀胱穹顶部可以通过未闭的脐尿管向脐部引流。内镜检查可以发现膀胱壁通常比较光滑，无小梁形成。输尿管开口往往偏外侧，而且多少向正常位置偏头端的方向移位。输尿管开口常常极度扩大，这与大多数病例中所见的大量反流表现相一致。膀胱颈部异常增宽，并且呈漏斗状向心形扩张的前列腺尿道延续。在大体表现上，膀胱壁增厚，血管十分丰富。膀胱壁增厚并不是肌肉肥大的结果，组织学检查可以证实为肌肉和大量的胶原以及纤维组织。如果膀胱不发生扩张，那么它在功能上还是一个容量正常而且顺应性良好的贮袋。大量反流、逼尿肌收缩能力下降、充盈感降低、腹壁支持缺乏以及穹顶部的憩室样畸形，可以妨碍膀胱正常的排空活动。尽管有这些问题，大约还是有一半患者会出现自主排尿[31]，人们也注意到这种排尿质量也会出现自发性的改善和恶化。对于某些患者，需要考虑通过切除穹顶部来缩小膀胱[5,53]。穹顶部切除可以改善某些患者的膀胱排空，减少排尿后尿液残留。对于一些儿童梅干腹综合征患者，可以通过间歇导尿来帮助膀胱排空[31]。

尿道

后尿道扩张可能继发于先天缺陷或周围环绕的前列腺组织发育不良。男性梅干腹综合征患者排尿性膀胱造影中前列腺尿道呈心形外观，尿道外括约肌就位于前列腺尖部下方水平。尿道外括约肌水平的前列腺尿道变细并不一定造成尿道梗阻，但是有些男性患者合并有尿道闭锁[63]。有时一些患者合并有先天性尿道狭窄。在作者治疗的 38 个男性患者中，真性尿道瓣膜 5 例；19 例有瓣膜样狭窄，一般位于精阜根部水平。伴有膀胱排空障碍的患者可以通过切开这些皱襞来进行有效的治疗（图 114-15）。除了闭锁以外，前尿道也可以出现异常，表现为先天性巨尿道，这种梭形异常会使阴茎整体发育受到影响。一旦发现有前尿道畸形，一般需要对其进行手术修复。尿道发育不良需要通过开放式尿道成形术进行修复（图 114-16）。巨尿道可以通过修剪尿道黏膜纠正，再用数层尿道周围组织进行重叠覆盖。

睾丸 1785

大多数男性梅干腹综合征都伴有双侧腹腔型隐睾。睾丸的体积比正常要小，而且位于腹股沟内环深面，很像女性的卵巢。精索也比正常短，一般都伴有睾丸附睾分离。输精管可以发生扭曲，并且闭锁不少见。与输精管连接的盆腔腹膜通常都有大量的血管供应，这就提供了采用 Fowler-Stephens 手术进行睾丸

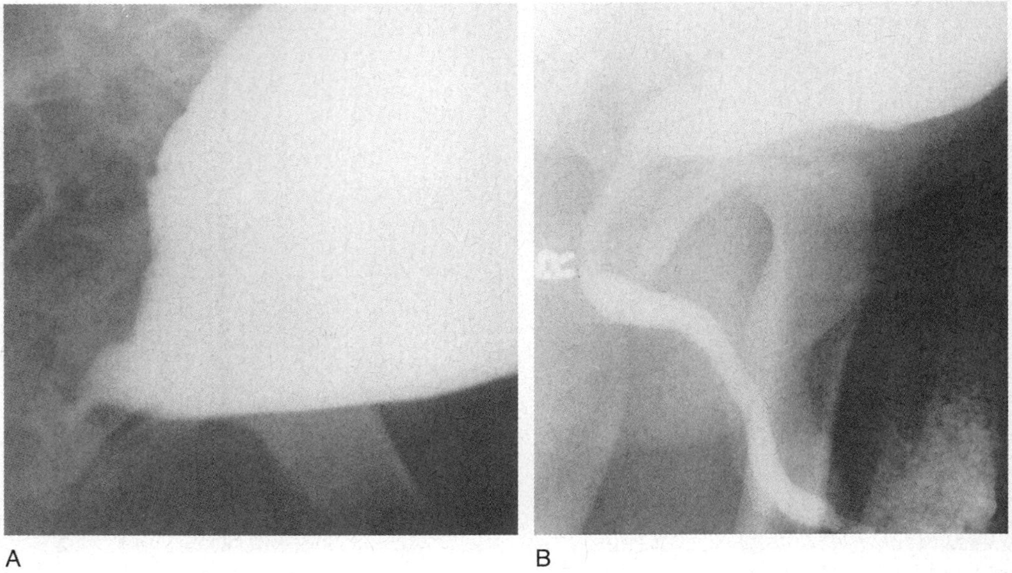

图 114-15 排尿性尿道造影。A. 术前检查发现典型的近端尿道扩张，膀胱颈增宽，并在精阜根部突然中断，此处为尿道瓣膜。B. 术后 7 个月检查显示原瓣膜梗阻处尿流通畅，整个尿道管径正常。

固定的可能性[15]。这种手术方法涉及在睾丸上方腹腔内分离精索，即游离睾丸的同时将输精管与其带侧支血管的宽条盆腔腹膜一同游离。睾丸固定手术的目的是将睾丸放入阴囊，在这个位置可以对睾丸的恶变情况进行监测，并且会对患儿的心理产生影响。尽管在 Leydig 细胞功能的作用下，第二性征发育出现阴茎生长并且性欲基本正常，但还没有见到有关本病患者可以生育的报道。大多数手术医生都发现将小婴儿的高位睾丸下降到阴囊内是一个很容易的过程，所需下降的距离相对较短。近来腹腔镜睾丸固定术也已经用于梅干腹综合征患者[10]，这一操作特别适用于分期的 Fowler-Stephens 手术。

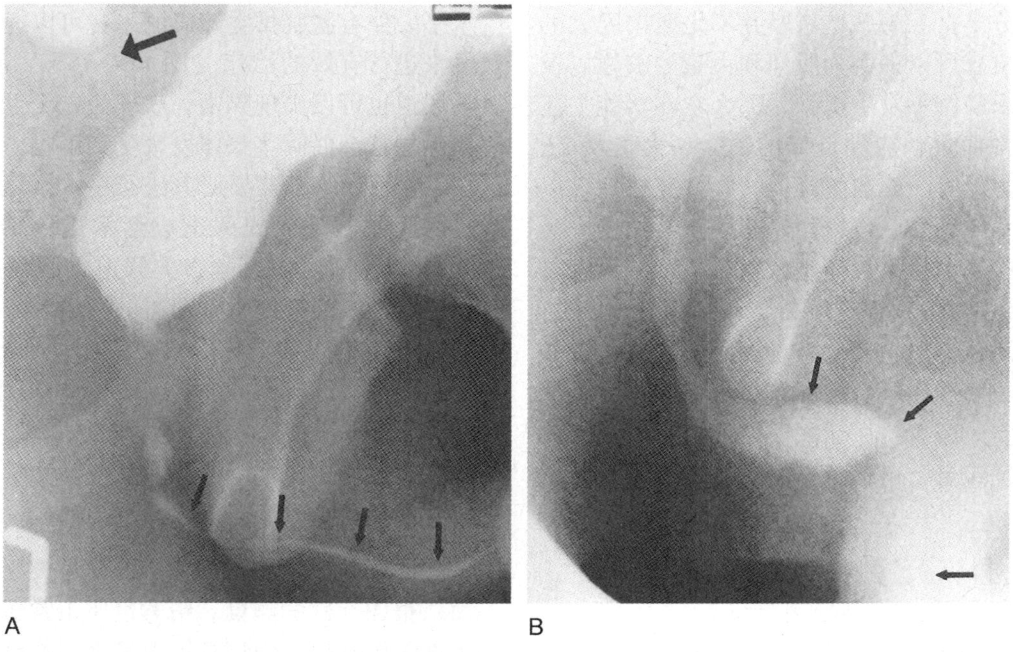

图 114-16 膀胱尿道造影。A. 术前。可见尿道发育不良（*小箭头*）以及由输尿管瓣膜引起的少见的巨输尿管梗阻（*大箭头*）。B. 将长段包皮补片植入尿道后的术后检查。

786 其他异常

许多梅干腹综合征患者都存在骨骼肌肉或矫形学上的异常，需要对这些异常进行治疗[4,38]。这些患者大多数合并结肠旋转不良和游离，但很少发生由中肠扭转引起的小肠梗阻。本病也可以合并肛门闭锁。由作者治疗过的所有女性梅干腹综合征患者都有泄殖腔畸形。在一些严重的病例中可以有肺发育不良，这些患者容易发生感染。漏斗胸是很常见的并发症，其腹壁肌肉也很薄弱。梅干腹综合征也可以伴有各种类型的先天性心脏病。

临床治疗

新生儿梅干腹综合征容易发生败血症，应当仔细对其进行评估。任何采用导管的检查都应当在使用抗生素和严格无菌技术的基础上进行。扩张的尿路可以容纳大量尿液而且引流很差，有细菌进入后很容易发生感染。有些肾发育不良的患儿肾功能极差，可能会早期死于肾衰竭。测定血清肌酐水平，特别是血清肌酐清除率可以合理地评价婴儿的肾功能水平。

婴儿梅干腹综合征是小儿泌尿外科领域里最具争议的话题。一方面有人建议对这些患者进行观察随访，尽可能少地采用外科干预[11,70,78]。另一方面的意见是建议在有适应证的情况下采用大的重建手术治疗[9,14,21,26,27,29,61,76,77]。应当强调的是，在对梅干腹综合征婴儿进行较大的重建手术时，需要专业麻醉医生在场，而且需要全程监护，同时还需要有相关手术经验的外科医生进行操作。更进一步说，比较大的重建手术一定要在患儿全身情况良好的情况下进行，包括肺功能良好，没有尿路感染。Woodard 和 Zucker 认为对于任何侵袭性操作都应当慎重考虑，因为这些手术操作难度较大，而且患者容易发生肺部并发症[77]。

目前有关治疗上的争议大部分是围绕尿路重建手术。在腹腔内睾丸的处理上已经基本一致，即早期就应当通过睾丸固定术使其下降。并且，很多患者及其家庭仅仅出于心理上的原因，要求对腹壁进行修复重建手术。作者认为，如果需要，可以在尿路重建的同时进行修复手术。只要患者肺功能能够承受，倾向于通过一次时间比较长的手术来解决所有的问题，而不是让患者接受多次手术。

当初期检查明确有梗阻存在时，不管梗阻部位是位于肾盂输尿管连接部，还是膀胱输尿管连接部，抑或是膀胱出口，都应当对其进行纠正（图 114-17）。大多数患者都有前面所提到的肾发育不良的病变基础，应当避免继发于梗阻的进一步病变。以作者的经验，大多数患有这种综合征的患者在存在膀胱输尿管反流的情况下，最终都需要进行手术修复。反流的常规分级方法并不适用于这类患者，而且梅干腹综合征患者的反流量也很大。对接受预防性抗生素治疗的患者进行早期观察，以此可以进一步评价膀胱的排空功能，同时也可以评估泌尿系统的其他功能。如果反流持续存在，最好采取措施纠正。如果反流患者发生尿路感染，或者肾功能变差，则应当尽早进行针对反流的修复手术。

在考虑梅干腹综合征患者的泌尿系统情况时，可以按照 Smith 和 Woodard 的描述将其分为三种类型[68]，这样做对治疗非常有利。这种分类方法大致与肾发育不良的程度相关。Ⅰ型患者同时存在严重的肾发育不良和肺发育不良，不能存活，针对泌尿系统的治疗不能挽救患者的生命。Ⅲ型患者一般是轻度或不完全类型的梅干腹综合征，肾功能相对较好。尽管与没有本综合征的患者相比，某些患者的尿路扩张可以比较严重，但在没有感染的情况下早期修复手术可以推迟进行。Ⅱ型患者的肾发育不全程度和肾功能情况介于前二者之间，这些患者通常具有梅干腹综合征的所有表现以及泌尿系统的滞留。毫无疑问，不论是否施行手术干预，其中的一些患者还是会进展到肾功能不全[64,78]。很多因素会影响梅干腹综合征患者，目前还很难对特定患者的自然病程作出预测，细致的随访观察至关重要。如果Ⅱ型患者发生感染、反流或肾功能恶化，作者建议采取手术治疗。观察和手术治疗常相互结合。作者相信，通过纠正梗阻和反流、改善膀胱排空以及预防感染这些手段，可以预防一些具有临界功能的患者进一步恶化，或者至少能够拖延肾功能不全发生的时间。

作者已经对 40 例梅干腹综合征患者进行了重建手术；12 例为初次治疗患者（图 114-18 和图 114-19），28 例为以往曾在其他地方接受过手术的再次治疗患者。后面这 28 例患者中，有 24 例接受了尿流改道手术[25,27]。这表明梅干腹综合征患者发生尿脓毒症的频率很高，需要采用不同的手术方法进行改道（图 114-20）。作者建议对这些患者应当在改道的基

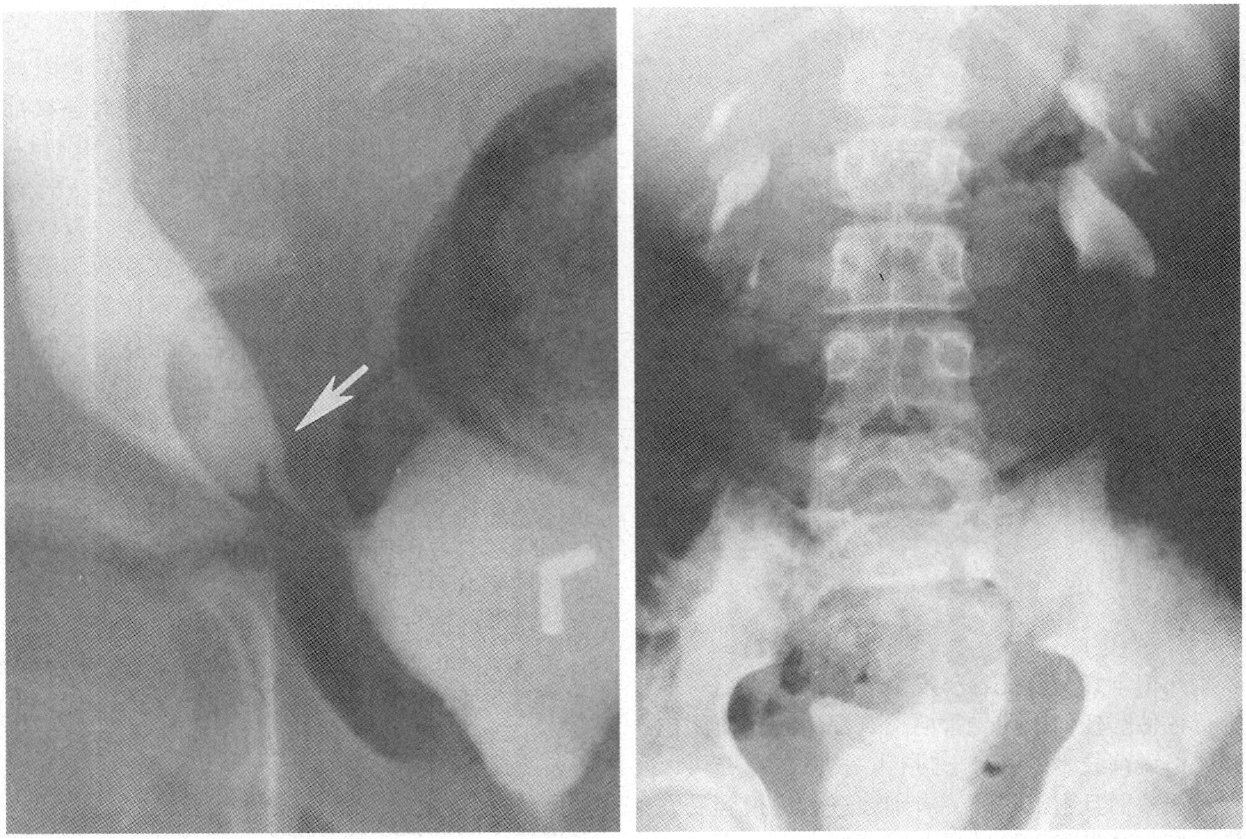

A B

图 114-17 图 114-16 和图 114-20 中同一患者的静脉肾盂造影检查。A. 右侧巨输尿管中的输尿管瓣膜（*箭头*）。B. 尿流复道手术 3 年后的静脉肾盂造影。

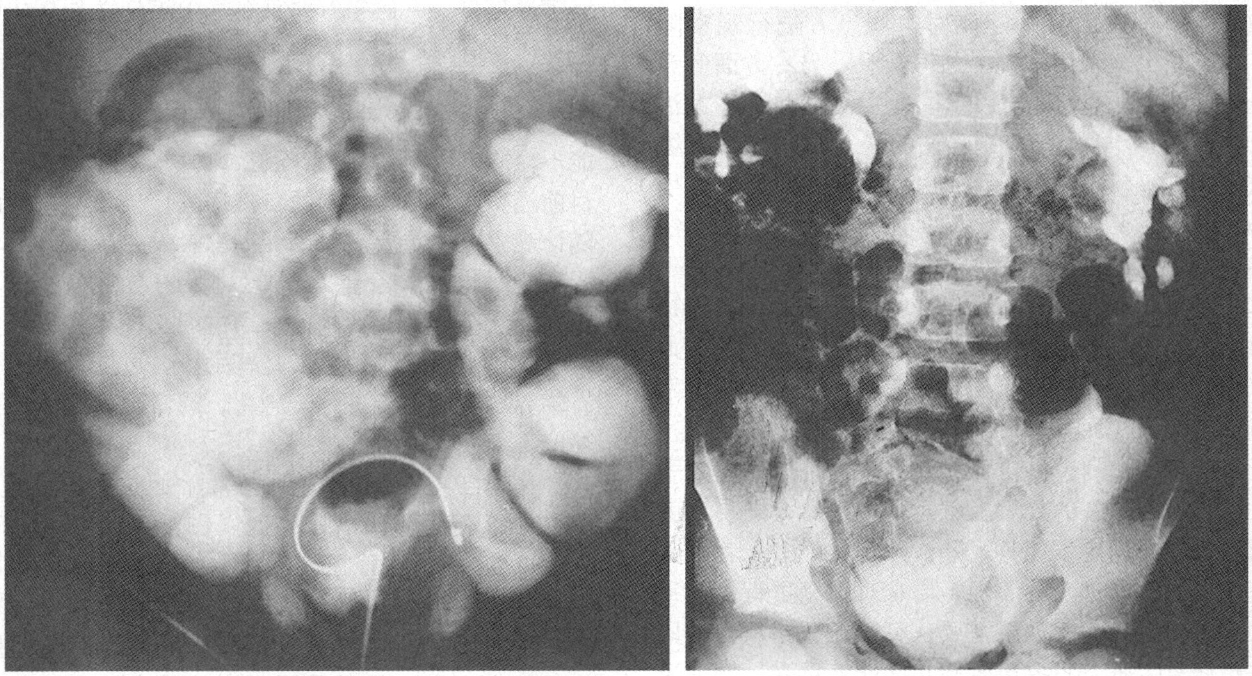

A B

图 114-18 婴儿梅干腹综合征。A. 术前膀胱造影。双侧大量的输尿管反流显示了迂曲延长的输尿管，右侧明显。可见左肾集合系统形态异常。该患儿接受了全尿路重建手术。B. 7 岁时的静脉肾盂造影。患者状态良好，无尿路症状。可见左输尿管显影，管径正常。很难将尿路外观的改善与患儿生存时间和健康状况联系在一起。解剖见图 114-19。

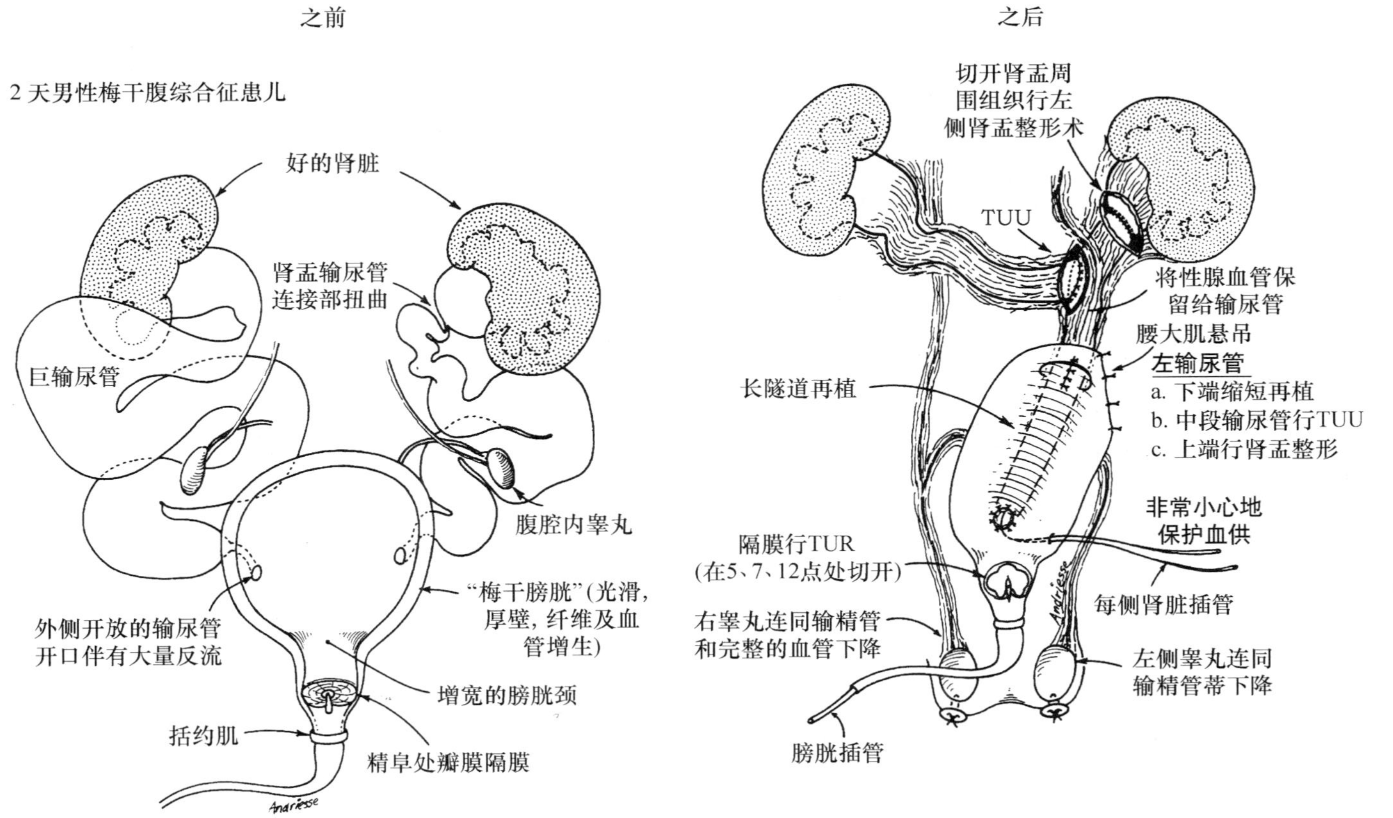

图 114-19　梅干腹综合征婴儿：术前和术后的解剖。TUR，经尿道切除；TUU，横跨输尿管输尿管吻合术。X 线表现见图 114-18。

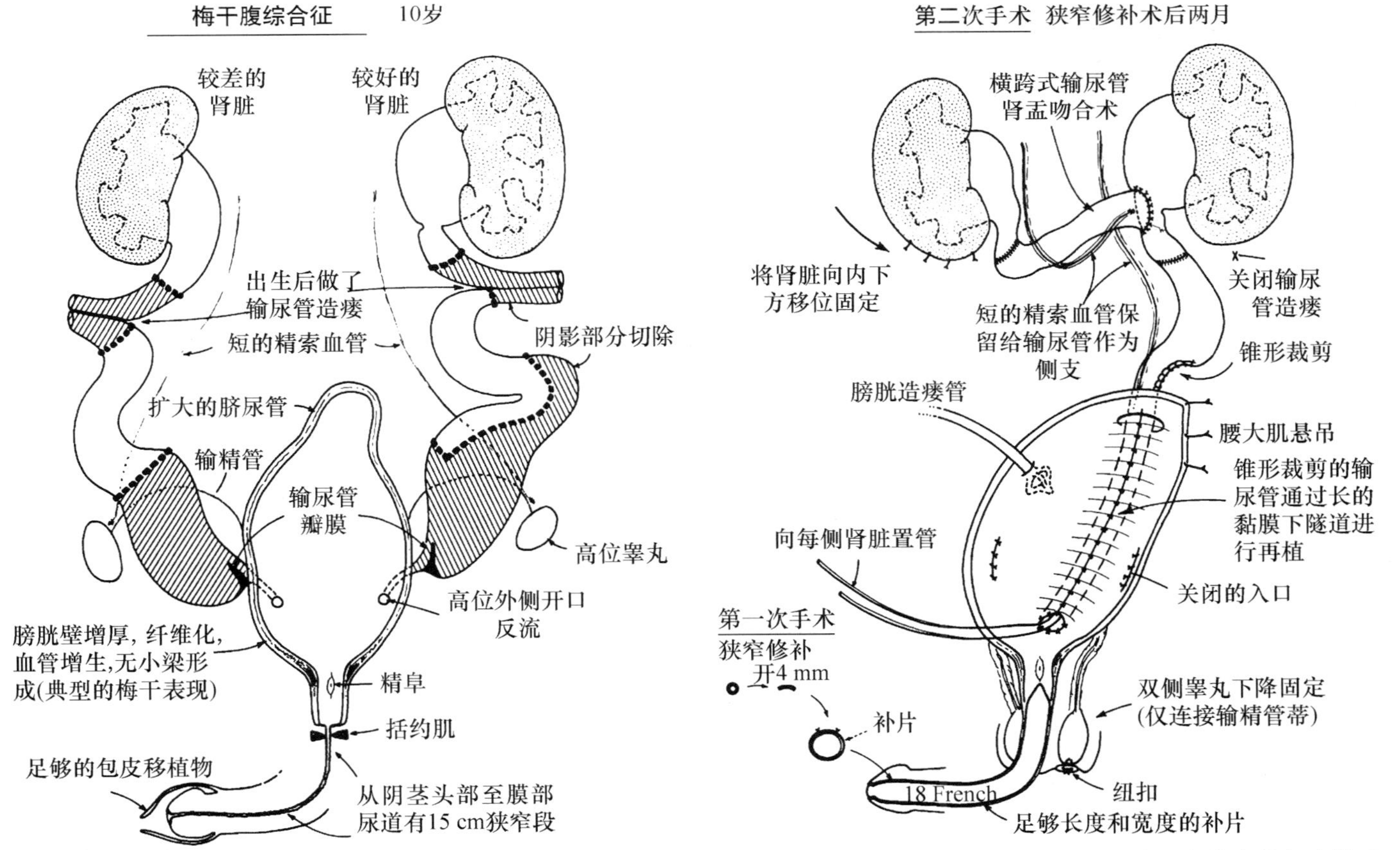

图 114-20　患有梅干腹综合征的 11 岁男孩，有异常的解剖表现，做过长期的输尿管造瘘。在手术 1 中，应用长的岛状包皮做了扩大的尿道成形术。两个月后，施行尿路重建手术，去除造瘘，同时做双侧睾丸下降固定手术。患者排尿正常，无尿失禁表现。肾功能正常［血清肌酐，0.9 mg/dl；肌酐清除率，106 L/(m^2 · d)］。肾盂造影见图 114-17。患者现在 35 岁，健康状况良好。

础上进行重建手术。12 例曾接受过肾切除手术，只
有一个肾脏留存。40 例患者中有 35 例存活（术后
4~30年）。8 例患者接受了肾移植手术。有 8 例以上
的患者因为其现有的肾功能情况，有可能需要肾移植
治疗。5 例患者死亡。1 例婴儿因为血友病失血和没
有给予足够的监护而在住院期间死亡，另 1 例婴儿在
1789 术后 2 个月因肺吸入死于家中。3 例为后期死亡：1
例发生在肾移植术后 3 年，另 1 例于移植成功后 10
年死于交通意外，还有 1 例于重建术后 11 年在透析
过程中发生败血症死亡。应当注意到这组患者是经过
选择的，并不能反映所有未经过选择的梅干腹综合征
患者肾功能不全的死亡率。

总结

一些严重的巨输尿管出现于梅干腹综合征患者，这些患者通常都会伴有其他的临床表现。在治疗上存在两种不同的观点：一是对经过选择的患者进行积极的手术重建，另一观点则支持“观察等待”。外科干预实际上也是一种保守措施，以减少尿液滞留和尿路感染，阻止肾功能不全的发生以及综合征病程的进展。重建手术非常需要，但在技术上比较困难，并且需要多方面的麻醉专业技术来维持接受手术患儿的代谢平衡。这种手术需要在专门的医疗中心进行，而且中心里需要集中专业的重建外科手术医生，以及配有所有必需的支持系统。

（赵海腾译 刘国华校）

参考文献

1. Afifi AK, Rebiez JM, Andonian SJ, et al: The myopathology of the prune belly syndrome. J Neurol Sci 1972; 15:153.
2. Bakker HHR, Scholtameijer RJ, Klopper PJ: Comparison of 2 different tapering techniques in megaureters. J Urol 1988; 140:1237.
3. Baskin LS, Zderic SA, Snyder HM, et al: Primary dilated megaureter: Long-term followup. J Urol 1994;152:618.
4. Brinker MR, Palutsis RS, Sarwark JF: The orthopaedic manifestations of prune-belly (Eagle-Barrett) syndrome. J Bone Joint Surg Am 1995;77:251.
5. Bukowski TP, Pearlmutter AD: Reduction cystoplasty in the prune belly syndrome: A long-term followup. J Urol 1994; 152:2113.
6. Capozza N, Caione P: Role of the endoscopic treatment of vesicoureteral reflux. A 16-years' experience. Minerva Pediatr 2003;55:607.
7. Chertin B, Colhoun E, Velayudham M, Puri P: Endoscopic treatment of vesicoureteral reflux: 11 to 17 years of followup. J Urol 2002;167:1443, discussion 1445.
8. Chertin B, De Caluwe D, Puri P: Endoscopic treatment of primary grades IV and V vesicoureteral reflux in children with subureteral injection of polytetrafluoroethylene. J Urol 2003;169:1847.
9. Cukier J: Resection of the urethra with the prune belly syndrome. Birth Defects 1977;5:95.
10. Docimo SG, Moore RG, Kavoussi LR: Laparoscopic orchidopexy in the prune belly syndrome: Case report and review of the literature. Urology 1994;45:679.
11. Duckett JW Jr: The prune-belly syndrome. In Kelalis PP, King LR, Belman AB (eds): Clinical Pediatric Urology. Philadelphia, WB Saunders, 1976.
12. Ehrlich RM, Lesavoy MA: Umbilicus preservation with total abdominal wall reconstruction in the prune-belly syndrome. Urology 1993;43:3.
13. Ehrlich RM, Lesavoy MA, Fine RN: Total abdominal wall reconstruction in the prune-belly syndrome. J Urol 1986; 136:282.
14. Fallat ME, Skoog SJ, Belman AB, et al: The prune belly syndrome: A comprehensive approach to management. J Urol 1989;142:802.
15. Fowler R, Stephens FD: The role of testicular vascular anatomy in the salvage of the high undescended testicle. Aust N Z J Surg 1959;29:92.
16. Gearhart JP, Lee BR, Partin AW, et al: A quantitative histological evaluation of the dilated ureter of childhood. II: Ectopia, posterior urethral valves and the prune belly syndrome. J Urol 1995;153:172.
17. Goulding FJ, Garrett RA: Twenty-five year experience with the prune belly syndrome. Urology 1978;7:329.
18. Hanna MK, Jeffs RD: Primary obstructive mega-ureter in children. Urology 1975;6:419.
19. Harley LM, Chen Y, Rattner WH: Prune belly syndrome. J Urol 1972;108:174.
20. Hendren WH: Operative repair of megaureter in children. J Urol 1969;101:491.
21. Hendren WH: A new approach to infants with severe obstructive uropathy: Early and complete reconstruction. J Pediatr Surg 1970;5:184.
22. Hendren WH: Posterior urethral valves in boys. A broad clinical spectrum. J Urol 1971;106:298.
23. Hendren WH: Reoperation for the failed ureteral reimplantation. J Urol 1974;111:403.
24. Hendren WH: Complications of megaureter repair. J Urol 1975;113:238.
25. Hendren WH: Complications of ureterostomy. J Urol 1978; 120:269.
26. Hendren WH: Prune-belly syndrome. In Devine CJ Jr, Stecker JF (eds): Urology in Practice. Boston, Little, Brown, 1978.
27. Hendren WH: Urinary tract refunctionalization after long-term diversion. A 20-year experience with 177 patients. Ann Surg 1990;212:478.
28. Hendren WH, Hendren RB: Bladder augmentation: Experience with 129 children and young adults. J Urol 1990;144:445.
29. Jeffs RD, Comisarow RH, Hanna MK: The early assessment for individualized treatment in the prune belly syndrome. Birth Defects 1977;13:97.
30. Kalicinski ZH, Kansy J, Kotarbinska B: Surgery of mega-

ureters—modification of Hendren's operation. J Pediatr Surg 1977;12:183.
31. Kinahan TJ, Churchill BM, McLorie GA, et al: The efficiency of bladder emptying in the prune belly syndrome. J Urol 1992;148:600.
32. Kirsch AJ, Perez-Brayfield MR, Scherz HC: Minimally invasive treatment of vesicoureteral reflux with endoscopic injection of dextranomer/hyaluronic acid copolymer: The Children's Hospitals of Atlanta experience. J Urol 2003;170:211.
33. Perez-Brayfield M, Kirsch AJ, Hensle TW, et al: Endoscopic treatment with dextranomer/hyaluronic acid for complex cases of vesico-ureteral reflux. J Urol 2004;172:1614.
34. Kroovand RL, Al-Ansari RM, Perlmutter AD: Urethral and genital malformations in prune belly syndrome. J Urol 1982;127:94.
35. Lee BR, Partin AW, Epstein JI, et al: A quantitative histological analysis of the dilated ureter of childhood. J Urol 1992; 148:1482.
36. Lee BR, Silver RI, Partin AW, et al: A quantitative histologic analysis of collagen subtypes: The primary obstructed and refluxing megaureter of childhood. Urology 1998; 51:820.
37. Liu HY, Dhillon HK, Yeung CK, et al: Clinical outcome and management of prenatally diagnosed primary megaureters. J Urol 1994;152:614.
38. Loder RT, Guiboux JP, Bloom DA, et al: Musculoskeletal aspects of prune-belly syndrome. Description and pathogenesis. Am J Dis Child 1992;146:1224.
39. McLaughlin AP, Pfister RC, Leadbetter WF, et al: The pathophysiology of primary megaloureter. J Urol 1973;109: 805.
40. McLellan DI, Retik AB, Bauer SB, et al: Rate and predictors of spontaneous resolution of prenatally diagnosed primary nonrefluxing megaureter. J Urol 2002;168:2177.
41. McLorie GA, Jayanthi VR, Kinahan TJ, et al: A modified extravesical technique for megaureter repair. Br J Urol 1994;74:715.
42. Monfort G, Guys JM, Bocciardi A, et al: A novel technique for reconstruction of the abdominal wall in the prune belly syndrome. J Urol 1991;146:639.
43. Monie IW, Monie BJ: Prune belly syndrome and fetal ascites. Teratology 1979;7:19.
44. Nunn IN, Stephens FD: The triad system: A composite anomaly of the abdominal wall, urinary system and testes. J Urol 1961;86:782.
45. O'Donnell B, Puri P: Treatment of vesicoureteric reflux by endoscopic injection of Teflon. BMJ 1984;289:7.
46. Osler W: Congenital absence of abdominal muscles, with distended and hypertrophied urinary bladder. Bull Johns Hopkins Hosp 1901;12:331.
47. Pagon RA, Smith DW, Shepard TH: Urethral obstruction malformation complex: A cause of abdominal muscle deficiency and the "prune belly." J Pediatr 1979;94:900.
48. Palmer JM, Teluk H: Ureteral pathology in the prune belly syndrome. J Urol 1974;111:701.
49. Parrott TS, Woodard JR: The Monfort operation for abdominal wall reconstruction in the prune belly syndrome, J Urol 1992;148:688.
50. Parrot TS, Woodard JR, Wolpert JJ: Ureteral tailoring: A comparison of wedge resection with infolding. J Urol 1990; 14:328.
51. Passerini-Glazel G, Araguna F, Chiozza L, et al: The P.A.D.U.A. (Progressive augmentation by dilating the urethra anterior). J Urol 1988;140:1247.
52. Perdzynski W, Kalicinski ZH: Long-term results after megaureter folding in children. J Pediatr Surg 1996;31:1211.
53. Perlmutter AD: Reduction cystoplasty in prune belly syndrome. J Urol 1976;116:356.
54. Perovic S: Surgical treatment of megaureters using detrusor tunneling extravesical ureteroneocystostomy. J Urol 1994; 152:622.
55. Peters CA, Mandell J, Lebowitz RL, et al: Congenital obstructed megaureters in early infancy: Diagnosis and treatment. J Urol 1989;142:641.
56. Peterson DS, Fish L, Cass AA: Twins with congenital deficiency of abdominal musculature. J Urol 1972;107:670.
57. Pfister RC, Hendren WH: Primary megaureter in children and adults. Urology 1978;12:160.
58. Potter EL: Abnormal development of the kidney. In Potter EL (ed): Normal and Abnormal Development of the Kidney. Chicago, Year Book, 1972, p 154.
59. Puri P, Chertin B, Velayudham M, et al: Treatment of vesicoureteral reflux by endoscopic injection of dextranomer/hyaluronic acid copolymer: Preliminary results. J Urol 2003; 170:1541, discussion 1544.
60. Rabinowtiz R, Schillinger JF: Prune belly syndrome in the female subject. J Urol 1977;118:454.
61. Randolph J, Cavett C, Eng G: Surgical correction and rehabilitation for children with "prune-belly" syndrome. Ann Surg 1981;193:757.
62. Randolph J, Cavett C, Eng G: Abdominal wall reconstruction in the prune belly syndrome. J Pediatr Surg 1981;16:960.
63. Reinberg Y, Chelimsky G, Gonzalez R: Urethral atresia and the prune belly syndrome—report of 6 cases. Br J Urol 1993;72:112.
64. Reinberg Y, Manivel JC, Fryd D, et al: The outcome of renal transplantation in children with the prune-belly syndrome. J Urol 1989;142:1541.
65. Reinberg Y, Manivel JC, Pettinato G, et al: Development of renal failure in children with the prune belly syndrome. J Urol 1991;145:1017.
66. Rogers LW, Ostrow PT: The prune belly syndrome. Report of 20 cases and description of a lethal variant. J Pediatr 1973;83:786.
67. Smith DW: Recognizable Patterns of Human Malformation. Philadelphia, WB Saunders, 1970, p 5.
68. Smith EA, Woodard JR: Prune-belly syndrome. In Retik AB, Vaughan ED, Wein AJ (eds): Campbell's Urology, vol 3, 8th ed. Philadelphia, WB Saunders, 2002, p 2117.
69. Smith ED: Report of working party to establish an international nomenclature for the large ureter. Birth Defects Original Articles Series 1977;13(5):3.
70. Snow BW, Duckett JW: Prune belly syndrome. In Gillenwater JY, Grayhack JT, Howards SS, et al (eds): Adult and Pediatric Urology. Chicago, Year Book, 1987.
71. Starr A: Ureteral plication: A new concept in ureteral tapering for megaureter. Invest Urol 1979;17:153.
72. Stenberg A, Lackgren G: A new bioimplant for the endoscopic treatment of vesicoureteral reflux: Experimental and short-term clinical results. J Urol 1995;154:800.
73. Williams DI, Burkholder GV: The prune belly syndrome. J Urol 1967;98:244.
74. Williams DI, Hulme-Moir I: Primary obstructive megaureter. Br J Urol 1970;42:140.
75. Woodard JR, Parrott TS: Orchiopexy in the prune belly syndrome. Br J Urol 1978;50:348.
76. Woodard JR, Parrott TS: Reconstruction of the urinary tract in prune belly uropathy. J Urol 1978;119:824.
77. Woodard JR, Zucker I: Current management of the dilated urinary tract in prune belly syndrome. Urol Clin North Am 1990;17:407.
78. Woodhouse RJ, Kellett MJ, Williams DI: Minimal surgical interference in the prune belly syndrome. Br J Urol 1979; 51:475.

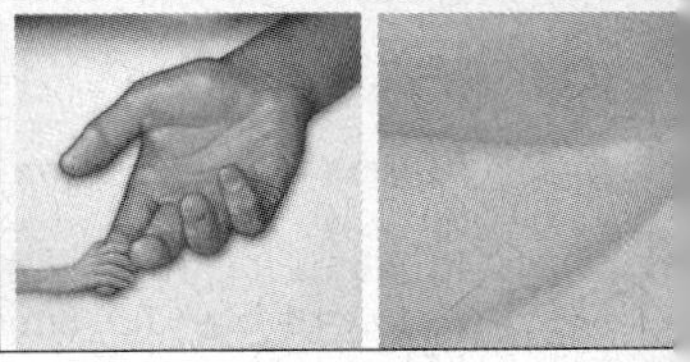

第 115 章

非可控性与可控性尿流改道

Elizabeth Yerkes、Peter Metcalfe 和 Richard C. Rink

1791 尿流改道有非可控性与可控性两种方式。非可控性改道的尿液贮袋是连接于体外的（造瘘袋或儿童尿布），在贮满时一般需要排空或丢弃。可控性尿流改道的尿液贮袋常规需要通过清洁间歇导尿（CIC）排空。一般情况下，由胃肠道节段而非膀胱做成的贮袋都是所谓的可控性尿液贮袋（CUR）。在儿童中，需要进行尿路重建的原发疾病是脊柱裂、膀胱外翻、后尿道瓣膜或者完全性的泄殖腔畸形。这些疾病中，病变的膀胱可以通过重建手术治疗，很少使用真正的 CUR 治疗。不过，大多数患者需要进行肠道膀胱成形术和建立用于插管的腹壁通道，因此，这也是可控的贮尿袋，这部分内容也将在本章讨论。本章节所使用的“尿液复道术”一词指将患儿以往所接受的非可控性尿流改道转变为可控性的改道。尽管尿液复道术在历史上具有重要意义，但由于已经很少在现代小儿泌尿外科重建中使用，所以这部分内容不在本章节中讨论。

历史上，永久性的非可控性尿流改道用于保护肾脏免受膀胱压力增高导致的破坏，或者是用于治疗尿失禁。现代临床实践中，通过 CIC 和抗胆碱能药物来对膀胱功能紊乱进行内科治疗，在很大程度上减少了外科手术干预的指征[84]。尿流动力学的专业知识能够对高危患者进行鉴别，提供更加积极的治疗[94]。手术技术的发展提供了安全压力下的贮尿能力，从而避免了永久性尿流改道的使用，但永久性尿流改道对部分患者来说还是适宜的选择。暂时性的尿流改道对某些患者来说是必要的，但很少作为第一线方案来治疗膀胱和上尿路疾病。

非可控性尿流改道

虽然对所有儿童来说，治疗的目的是获得排尿控制，但最主要的是保护上尿路的完整性。现在仍然使用一些暂时性或永久性的非可控性尿流改道，以保护上尿路功能，防止感染，或者是用于那些自我照料能力非常有限的患者，简化日常护理。

暂时性尿流改道应用最多的患者是婴儿和小年龄的儿童，可以简单地采用尿布来收集尿液。大多数永久性非可控性尿流改道需要造口术装置，以使尿液收集卫生。与使用 CIC 的可控性方式相比，非可控性造瘘有污秽的瘘口，体表外观不理想，这种造瘘最好不用于儿童。但对有选择的患者和家庭来说，这种改道方式仍然是一种比较理想的选择。

膀胱皮肤造口

膀胱皮肤造口是目前儿童最常使用的非可控性尿流改道方式，但这种方法极少作为第一线治疗，其应用指征也有限。对于患有神经性膀胱或不安全贮尿压力的婴儿，如果 CIC 和抗胆碱能药物治疗失败，或者患儿家庭不能或不愿意接受上述治疗，那么此时就需要进行膀胱皮肤造口术。一些未成熟婴儿由于尿道过细，不能够安全地进行后尿道瓣膜切除手术，这也是膀胱皮肤造口的适应证。这种患者生长到一定程度，可以进行瓣膜切除时，就应当关闭膀胱造口。如果年幼婴儿患有严重膀胱输尿管反流，并且在应用预防性抗生素的情况下仍然出现反复的尿路感染，那么通过膀胱造口治疗可能会有一定益处[80,110]。改善膀胱和上尿路的引流能力可以减少尿路感染的发生机会。在泄殖腔持续存在的情况下，尽管通过共同通道间歇导尿，但如果患者仍然出现难治性的肾盂积水、阴道积 179
液或尿路感染，也可以作为膀胱造口的一种少见指征。

理想的情况下，膀胱造口可以对膀胱内容物提供低压引流，同时维持最少的残余尿状态。很多临床应用已经证实了膀胱造口的这一优点[17,60,61,80,106,110]。它可以使上尿路扩张得以改善，肾功能保持稳定或提高。反流的消退或者输尿管扩张程度的改善使患者在再植手术中不需要进行输尿管修裁[80,110]。尽管开放造口中细菌迁移的情况很常见，但是有症状的感染和尿脓毒症的发生机会减少。有人担心对非神经性膀胱病变进行长期的膀胱造口引流，可能会因为缺乏周期性的膀胱充盈和排空而导致膀胱不能正常发育[32,109]，不过有些研究已经否定了这一论调[63,69,110]。

只要尿路能够维持稳定，膀胱可以长期保持清洁状态，膀胱造口就很容易关闭。膀胱造口既可以通过一期关闭，也可以结合可控性尿流改道来关闭。一些患者及其家庭不愿意关闭膀胱造口，或者发现膀胱造口和尿布引流是一种可以接受的永久性维持低压状态的方法。膀胱造口，不管是否使用造瘘连接装置，都可以在没有可控改道条件的成人中应用[60]。

多年来，膀胱皮肤造口手术采用两种方式。Lapides 提出将膀胱前壁肌瓣提出，并且向深部嵌插腹壁皮瓣以形成膀胱皮肤造口[83]。最常用到的手术方法由 Blocksom 于 1957 年提出[13]，并且 Duckett 加以改良[36]（图 115-1）。Blocksom 膀胱造口术通过脐与耻骨中点处一个小的横切口进行。切开筋膜，将腹膜向上方推离膀胱穹顶部。切断脐尿管残留，将膀胱顶部拖出皮肤。筋膜层与膀胱壁缝合，形成相当于 24 French 大小的缺损，然后缝合膀胱做成嵌入式造瘘口。

膀胱皮肤造口术的并发症包括造瘘口狭窄、脱垂、造瘘口周围皮肤炎症和膀胱结石。瘘口狭窄在膀胱壁僵硬肥厚的情况下比较多见，类似后尿道瓣膜。不将造瘘口做在膀胱顶部可能会导致膀胱后壁从造瘘口处脱垂，这也是 Blocksom 手术比 Lapides 膀胱造口术优越之处。脱垂可以通过手法回纳，应用暂时性的导管引流，并且对低位造口部位进行纠正。皮炎对某些患者来说是一个令人烦恼的并发症，可以应用氧化锌防护油脂，或治疗局部严重的真菌感染。如果膀胱造口处状态良好而且上尿路引流通畅，那么膀胱结石一般不太常见。

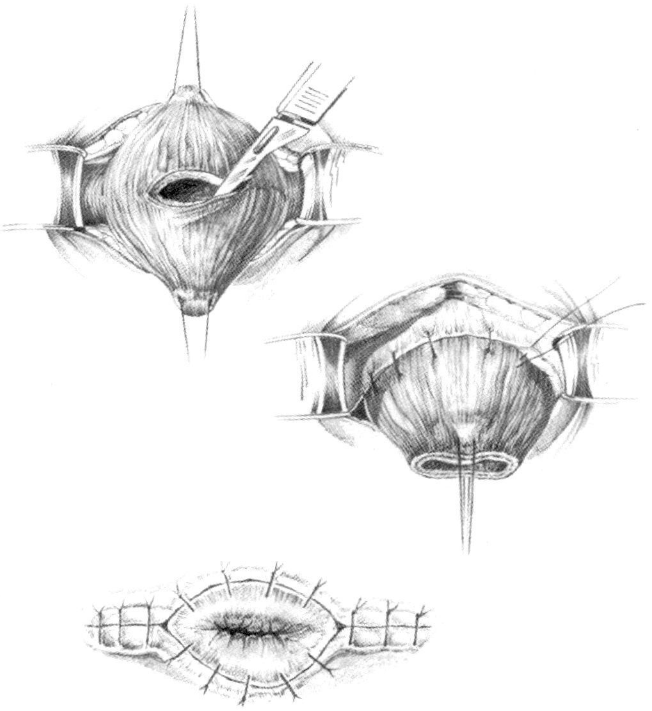

图 115-1 Blocksom 膀胱造口术，图中标示出了膀胱穹顶部的切口、表面筋膜的固定以及外翻的造瘘口。

输尿管皮肤造口术

用于膀胱上方临时尿流改道的输尿管造瘘术今天已经极少使用。以往这种方法主要用于引流伴有尿脓毒症的严重上尿路扩张患者[102]，或者有严重梗阻时加强肾脏的引流。目前对儿童可以通过经皮或内镜方法实现这些病变处的引流，但对于很小的婴儿，其输尿管的大小限制了该方法的使用[123]。通过袢式或末端输尿管皮肤造口术进行低位转流可暂时解决问题（图 115-2 和 115-3），其后期需要进行的手术包括输尿管膀胱吻合术。这种转流可以使输尿管口径变细，因而可以减少再植时手术的复杂程度。肾脏水平的改道手术能够通过腰部切口进行，可以做成袢式输尿管造口、Sober 输尿管造口或末端输尿管造口。袢式输尿管造口操作比较简单，对于暂时性的改道来说是比较理想的选择。在肾盂输尿管连接部位下方的输尿管末端造口会增加输尿管重建手术的难度，仅在严重的膀胱功能紊乱时作为比较少见的永久性改道[123]。Sober输尿管造口术是将输尿管近端作为引流口，远端与肾盂重新吻合，这种方法目前很少用，

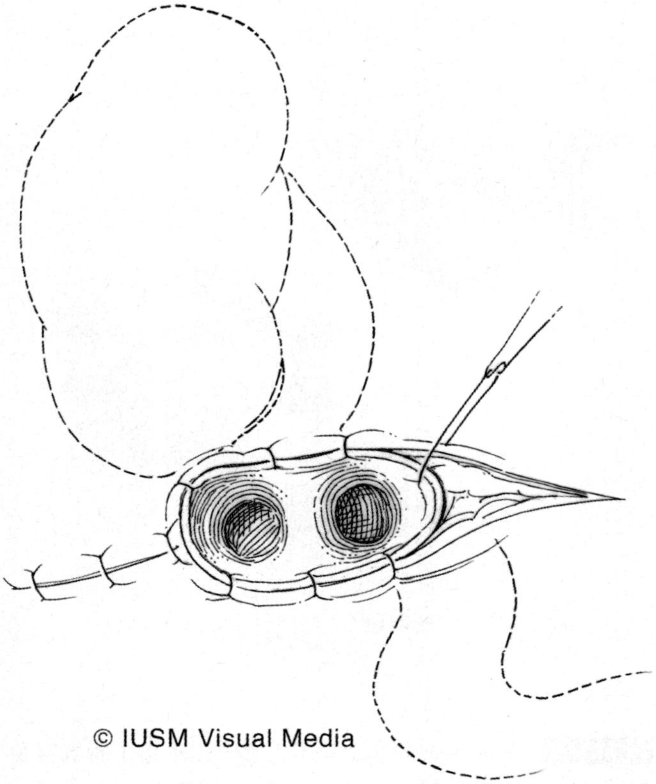

图 115-2 袢式输尿管造口术操作比较简单，因此可以很好地用于暂时性改道。

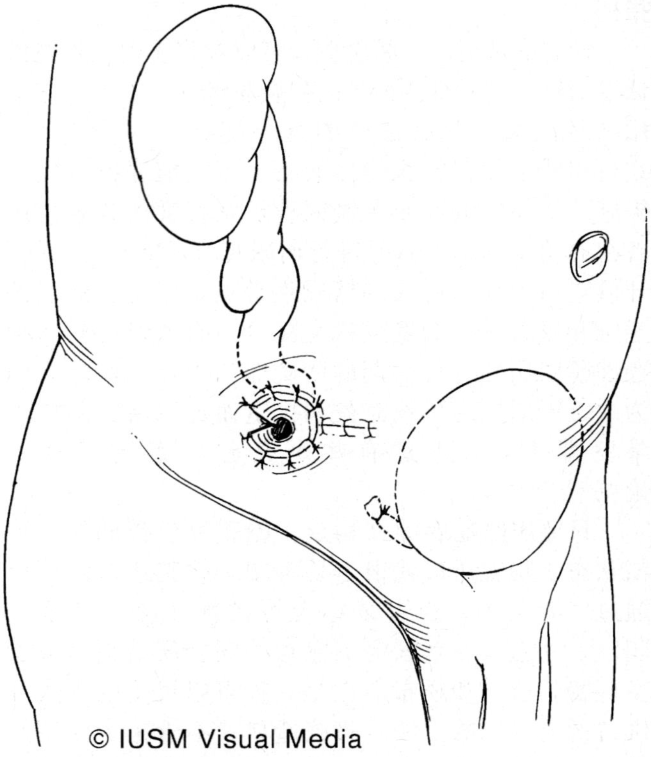

图 115-3 输尿管末端造口术，需要在后期去改道手术时进行再植。

其操作难度较大，不太适用于急性疾病期间的改道。但从另一方面来看，这种改道方式能够提供有效的转流，并且能够使尿流顺行流入膀胱[88]。不管采用何种方式，都应当仔细保护输尿管内侧的血供和外膜的血管，与皮肤做吻合时要保持无张力状态。由于大多数病例中的输尿管相对扩张，所以很少发生造瘘口狭窄。

对于某些后尿道瓣膜患者，如果采用膀胱改道后仍不能使肾功能得以改善，那么选择膀胱以上尿流改道可能会有所帮助[88]。持续的膀胱输尿管连接处梗
1793 阻就是这样一种情况。输尿管造口和肾盂造瘘能够提供上尿路最大限度的引流，而经皮肾穿刺造瘘对受影响的肾脏来说是一种创伤更小的暂时性方法[43]。由于引流的改善或者仅仅是由于肾脏不断发育成熟，一些患者在膀胱近端改道后会出现肾功能的改善[144]。对于膀胱皮肤造口，还要考虑在改道以后瓣膜膀胱可能会出现发育障碍。而对孤立肾患者采用袢式输尿管造口或输尿管末端造口，将会使膀胱失去功能。不过有些研究提示，膀胱功能障碍在很大程度上是由于膀胱以下的梗阻所致的膀胱壁异常，而不是由于膀胱以上的尿流改道[62,69]。

肾盂皮肤造口

与输尿管皮肤造口相比，现在通过肾盂造口进行近端改道的适应证更有限，这种转流方式的争论也都比较类似。作为从肾盂直接进行引流的方法，肾盂造口可以用于一些肾盂输尿管交界处梗阻的暂时性引流，也可以用于前文讨论过的后尿道瓣膜。肾盂造口需要利用非常扩张的肾外型肾盂在皮肤位置做无张力吻合。由于肾盂处的血供比较丰富，所以在后期根治性手术时，关闭肾盂造口是一个相对简单的过程。

回肠贮袋/结肠贮袋

永久性的膀胱以上尿流改道是比较可靠的治疗方

法，在过去几十年里非常流行，用于治疗神经性膀胱、膀胱出口梗阻和严重的尿失禁。大多数肠管都可以用于建立转流贮袋，而应用最多的还是回肠（图 115–4）和结肠。比较简单的反流性以及经隧道非反
794 流性输尿管肠管吻合都可以用于具体操作中。与回肠贮袋相比，结肠贮袋最大的优点是结肠可以提供更可靠的抗反流再植条件。

在一些病例中，回肠贮袋转流后发生上尿路功能下降的风险超过 50%[75,128,129]，尽管这一风险对于接受过膀胱癌膀胱切除的老年患者来说没有太大关系，但对儿童来说，由此所产生的对肾脏的长期影响则十分重要。由于在输尿管和结肠之间能够实现非反流吻合，这就使结肠贮袋在理论上优于回肠贮袋。不过在现实情况中，接受结肠贮袋的患者发生上尿路功能下降的占 26%～48%，而发生持续性输尿管反流的占 8%～58%[58]。回肠和结肠贮袋术后发生吻合口狭窄的机会大致相似（9%～22%）[58,75]。

Koch 及其同事对接受回肠贮袋转流治疗和接受 CIC 治疗的脊髓脊膜膨出患者进行了队列对比研究[75]，回肠贮袋组患者发生肾功能下降、肾结石以及肾盂肾炎的明显多于导尿组。两组患者均出现骨密度下降，而且骨折的发生率也相同，不过转流组患者生长曲线下降，脊柱弯曲发生相对较多，矫形术后发生并发症也较多。在非可控改道中，由于将肠管作为泌尿道使用，会并发代谢上的异常改变。

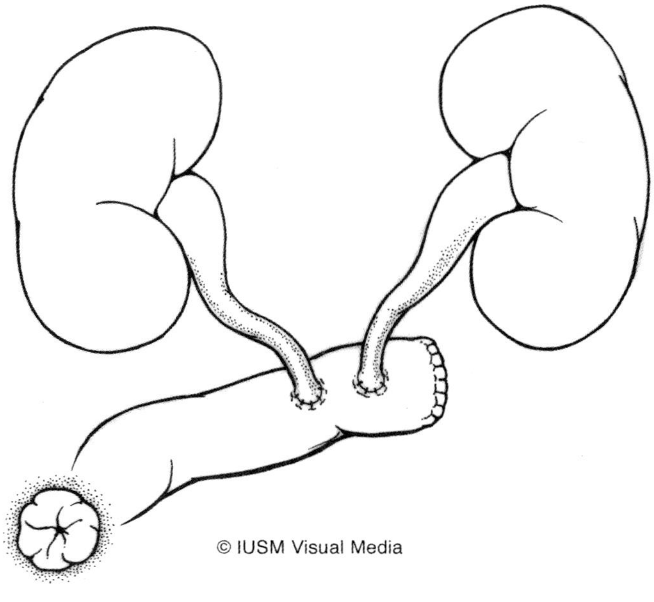

图 115–4 回肠贮尿袋是标准的永久性膀胱近端改道方法，适用于无膀胱的患者。

应用贮袋转流的其他并发症包括造瘘口狭窄、造瘘口脱垂、造瘘口旁疝以及造瘘口周围皮炎。造瘘口狭窄的发生率为 8%～61%，仔细的手术操作是避免造瘘口并发症的最好方法，包括保护肠管血供、建立一条直的而且口径足够大的筋膜层窗口、将贮袋与筋膜层充分固定。将瘘口做成乳头状凸起可以使其更好地与其功能相适应，而且还能避免狭窄的发生。

术后菌尿是很普遍的现象，在输尿管肠吻合以及贮袋自身状况良好的情况下，这种菌尿并不会对上尿路造成损伤[49,58]。转流尿液的静止状态会导致上尿路结石的发生，从而引起相关并发症。尿液和细菌混合可以产生亚硝胺，这种物质在游离的肠段内有诱发恶变的作用[44,58]。

Austen 和 Kalble 对世界上已经发表的文献作了回顾，在大量采用肠管的不可控性和可控性改道的患者中收集了 81 例肿瘤患者[8]。这一数字不包括很多在输尿管乙状结肠吻合术后发生恶变的病例。12 例回肠贮袋和 5 例结肠贮袋病例有肿瘤发生，平均潜伏期分别是 22 年和 10 年。发生于结肠贮袋的肿瘤主要是腺癌，在回肠贮袋中还可以发生移行细胞癌、鳞状细胞癌、类癌以及退行性肿瘤。肠段的慢性炎症可能在癌变中起到一定作用。建议对这些患者进行肿瘤的早期监测。

贮袋转流手术的术前准备包括彻底的机械灌肠和抗生素准备，术前一天胃肠外应用抗生素以保持尿液无菌。对于患有严重的肠神经源性疾病的患者，可能还需要一天以上的彻底清洁灌肠准备。另一重要的术前准备是肠造瘘治疗师对患者的多个体位进行检查，标示出两侧的造瘘口位置。脊髓脊膜膨出患者在坐位时，其腹壁轮廓可以发生很大的变化，造瘘口位置选择不当会增加患者术后的不适感。

非可控性回肠膀胱造口术

非可控性回肠膀胱造口术最早由 McGuire 及其同事们于 1994 年提出[127]，主要用于治疗成人继发于脊髓损伤和多发性硬化的膀胱与括约肌功能障碍。这些患者采用其他方法控制膀胱压力和尿失禁治疗失败，并且不愿或不能应用可控性改道治疗。许多患者由于

长期留置导尿管出现了严重的并发症。有一系列应用疗效极好的报道，通过这种方法保留了患者的肾功能，降低了患者尿路感染和结石的发生率，减少了造瘘口的并发症[7,41,86,104]。回肠膀胱造口术是以弹出式瓣膜的方式来维持安全的膀胱内压力，造瘘口的漏尿点压力低，并有中等量的残余尿[104]。

非可控性回肠膀胱造口适用于那些活动能力受限、社会支持度较低的患儿。尽管这种做法也需要一个永久性的造瘘口，但与标准的贮袋改道相比，更有利于保护肾功能。此外，这种手术也不会破坏膀胱输尿管连接部。即使患儿以后没有能力进行自我导尿，其家长一般也很难接受永久性的改道。而且，尽管患儿必须通过重建手术保留上尿路功能，一些家庭也不能够承担膀胱扩大术后或可控性尿液贮袋的护理措施。在这些情况下，就可以考虑应用带有非可控性输出袢和宽大开口的回肠补片扩大膀胱的非可控性回肠膀胱造口术。在手术初期可以考虑建立一个 Mitrofanoff 导尿通道。如果患者家庭最终愿意接受可控性改道和长期的膀胱扩大手术，就可以消除回肠瘘口，转为可控性改道[29]。

术前准备需要对肠道进行彻底清洁，并使尿液无菌。预先仔细选择造口位置，一般选择于右下腹，以保证与造口装置的连接。在冠状面将膀胱切为两片，准备与游离的回肠肠段缝合。于回肠系膜对侧缘打开肠管近端并与膀胱连续缝合。回肠段的长度要根据体型以及所需扩大的膀胱容量而定[86]。将乳头状的瘘口做在右下腹，无论膀胱是否减压，用 22 French 的
1795 导管支撑 3 周，以保证回肠膀胱缝合的口径。如果膀胱容量扩大很多，则应当放置耻骨上导管，以保证最充分的围术期引流。对于尿道功能丧失或严重的术前急迫性尿失禁的患者，还要进行膀胱颈或尿道手术，以增加出口阻力。

可控性尿流改道

可控性尿流改道有许多不同的手术方法，以改善或替换生理性的下尿路，其命名方式一般是根据手术方法或提出这种方法的外科医生的名字命名。手术方式的选择在很大程度上根据手术医生的经验和偏好，但主要依据是患者的原发病理改变。重建手术根据患者自身的解剖情况以及相关功能缺陷来设计。小儿的下尿路重建手术与成人手术有本质上的不同。在成人的重建手术中，由于其解剖形态比较固定，手术方式（如 Koch 贮袋、Indiana 贮袋、Mainz 贮袋）一般在术前就可以确定下来。而对患有诸如泄殖腔外翻疾病的小儿来说，其解剖形态千变万化，治疗中所要求的理想贮尿装置、低压贮袋、无漏尿和反流的导尿手段等都必须与重建手术中所能取得的组织材料相对应。无论什么情况，手术目的都是增加膀胱容量，改善流出道的状况，避免输尿管与 CUR 吻合时出现并发症。CUR 适用于患者生理膀胱丧失或不可用时。对患有膀胱发育不良综合征、泄殖腔外翻、继发于创伤或恶性肿瘤的盆腔器官破坏的患者，可以考虑使用 CUR。

可控性尿流改道现在已经十分普遍，但必须认识到做这种手术需要具有多方面的外科手术技能，同时也要掌握其所涵盖的各种疾病诊断。从定义上来看，这种治疗是创建一个贮袋，并必须能够通过间歇导尿来排空。这包括对完整但病变严重的膀胱进行扩张，或者完全利用其他替代组织建立一个贮袋。手术的目的和原则一样：建立一个理想的尿液贮袋，容易排空，并发症最少。因为胃肠道来源充足、容易取得，所以是最常用的组织材料。胃肠道生理上的可变性使得手术医生能够用于患者的手术重建。然而这些复杂的手术并不是没有并发症，对此要充分理解，并在具体应用中加以考虑。

膀胱扩大术

膀胱扩大术是小儿泌尿外科医生必不可少的治疗方法。在很多下尿路疾病的治疗上起到重要作用，包括神经性膀胱、后尿道瓣膜和膀胱外翻。在现代临床应用中通常还包括可控性的用于插管的腹壁造瘘口，造瘘材料可以使用阑尾（Mitrofanoff 通道）和裁剪的回肠（Monti 通道），还有可能需要进行其他手术来提高膀胱颈部的控尿能力。最好的排空方式是通过生理尿道间歇排空，但这在膀胱颈部重建以后往往不太可能实现。

就像前面讨论的一样，患有严重下尿路功能障碍的儿童需要通过尿液改道来进行治疗。由 Lapides[84,85] 提出的 CIC 操作保证了所有儿童都能够安全地排空膀胱，这也促进了下尿路重建手术的发展，维持了泌尿道的完整性，避免了使用体外集尿装置。尿

流动力学检查的发展也提高了我们的预测能力，可以预测什么类型的患者能够通过重建手术取得最好的效果，从而避免肾功能降低[94]。与之平行发展的内科学的进步也保证了这些复杂患者的生存时间，并且把治疗的重点转移到与生活质量密切相关的排尿控制上[51,143]。近来在导尿通道技术方面的发展更加简化了护理过程，使这一技术更加普及[57]。

下尿路重建的主要目的是在安全压力下贮存尿液而且不发生漏尿。足够的贮尿量需要有低压、高顺应性的大体积贮袋，而有限的收缩性和有效的括约肌机制也是实现可控的条件。

大多数扩大手术是通过胃肠道节段来实现的，这主要是因为肠管材料比较容易取得，而且比较容易成形。回肠是目前最常用的材料[46,115,116]，而使用乙状结肠的也比较多。以前也使用胃和回盲部肠管，但目前在儿科中使用得不多[3,19,130,132]。由于胃肠道管壁非常充裕，完全可以提供足够大的容量，通过去肠管化和其自身的弹性可满足低压贮器的需要[56,79]。然而，由于胃肠道同时还具有分泌[15,120]和吸收[72]的特性，也使其成为最常见并发症的发病原因。

膀胱扩大手术的成功需要合理地选择患者[30]、患者具有进行 CIC 的能力及意愿[82,120]、选择适当的用于扩大的材料以及对各种并发症的认识和治疗。

患者的评估和选择

患者、家庭以及整个治疗小组都要参与与大手术相关的决策工作。将胃肠道应用于泌尿道的最常见风险包括黏液分泌、尿路感染、膀胱和肾结石、代谢改变以及有生命危险的癌变和自发性穿孔，这些并发症都必须向患者及其家庭解释并取得理解[15,82,120]。护理患儿的每一个人都必须了解正确的护理方法，包括
96 强制性的 CIC 和定期膀胱冲洗[82,120,121]。

临床评价包括完整的病史和体检，尤其应当注意有无橡胶制品过敏，这有可能会成为致命的并发症。术前评估包括肾脏-膀胱超声检查（RBUS）和排尿性膀胱尿道造影（VCUG）。还需要进行血清化学分析，这是因为肾功能不全时可能不允许使用胃肠道进行手术[82]。最初有人提出将肌酐清除率小于 60 ml/min 作为使用回肠做可控贮袋的禁忌证[96,135]，然而扩大术后常使肾功能稳定下来，并且有机会在肾移植前接受重建手术。尿流动力学检查也是十分必要的，可以了解流出道阻力、膀胱容量和贮尿期压力。膀胱镜检查可以明确解剖形态，并且确保不存在不利于重建手术的情况[120]。

通过上述这些检查和评估，最终可以制定一个比较全面的外科治疗方案。最终的手术方案还要包括肠段的选择、是否要对患者进行同期的输尿管再植手术、膀胱颈部的手术方法以及如何建立导尿通道等等。神经性膀胱患者往往同时接受肠管顺行性排便控制手术，一般选择阑尾，以利其神经性病变肠管的排空[103]。在选择手术方式的时候，必须考虑到这一点，如果患者的阑尾已经用于排便控制手术，那么在手术时还需要选择额外的回肠段作为导尿用的通道。

术前准备通常包括肠道准备，这与前文所提到的通道转流手术一样。还需要围术期应用抗生素保持尿液无菌，这在接受脑室腹腔转流手术的患者中尤其重要[149]。

对所有患者都要进行长期随访。术后随访后，如果确定没有并发症出现，则要对患者进行年度检查，包括询问病史、体检，测定肌酐和电解质水平、超声检查以及术后每 5～10 年进行膀胱镜检查[82,120]。

胃肠道膀胱成形术

大多数因为膀胱动力异常而接受下尿路重建手术的患儿可以保留其原有的膀胱，但必须进行膀胱扩大手术以降低的膀胱内压力，限制其收缩，提高膀胱的顺应性。重建手术一般需要利用胃肠道节段，但手术中必须将其重新塑形和去肠管化，以克服其内在收缩特性所造成的影响[3,56,79,98]。最大的贮尿容量需要由球状的外形来提供[56]，将膀胱大范围地切成两片可以实现这一目的，还可以防止憩室样作用的产生。作者推荐采用膀胱旁正中切口，这样可以向瘘口提供更多的逼尿肌。这种做法的优点是能够得到更多逼尿肌的肌肉支持，有利于导尿通道的再植和控制（图 115-5）。将回肠进行 U 形或 S 形折叠能够增加其半径和容量[82]（图 115-6），从而最大限度地增加球体的容量。这种成形方式，连同沿肠管系膜对侧缘去管化，都起到了破坏肠管收缩能力的重要作用，否则完整的肠管可以产生 40～100 cmH_2O 的收缩压力[40,89,90]。一个重建手术医生在进行扩大手术时，应本着宁大勿小

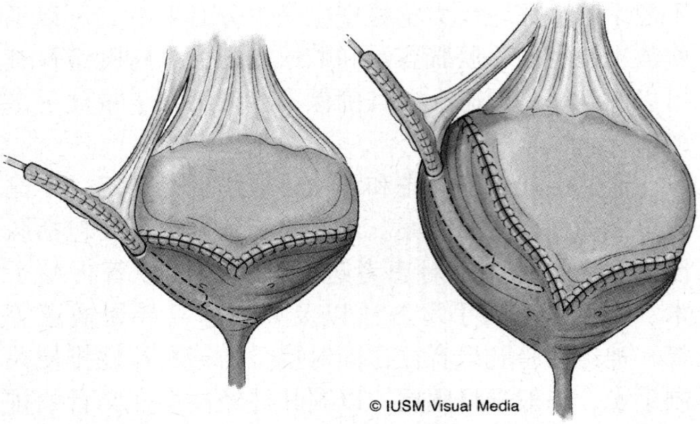

图 115-5　采用旁正中切口的膀胱成形术使逼尿肌运用更加灵活，能够获得更好的肌肉支撑，这在导尿通道再植操作中十分重要。

的原则[120]。不管在手术中选取了哪一段肠管，都必须用可吸收缝线进行紧密缝合。膀胱内放置耻骨上导管引流，并将导管固定在腹壁上，同时放置膀胱周围引流。

回肠膀胱成形术

回肠作为被选择肠段主要是因为其内在的低收缩特性、来源充分和容易进行操作[46,115,116]。在儿童病例中，切取 20～30 cm 肠管，远端边缘距回盲瓣 15～20 cm，以防维生素 B_{12} 和胆盐吸收障碍[79,114]。现已
1797 知道回肠的黏液分泌比结肠少，同时其穿孔率也比乙状结肠低[35]。应用回肠的一个内在的缺点是很难建

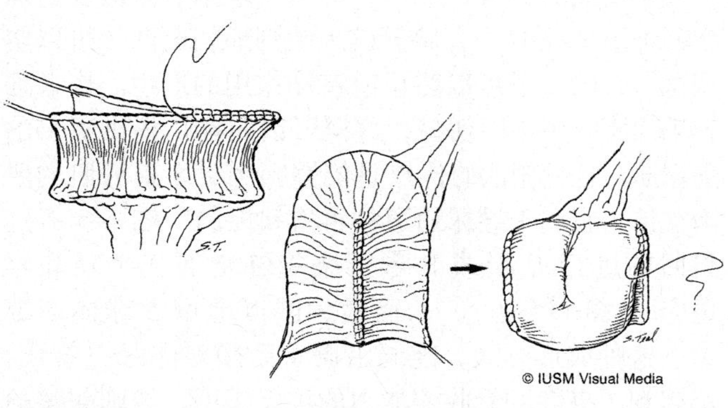

图 115-6　理想的膀胱扩大术能够同时增加容量和顺应性，这在控尿和肾脏保护中是必需的。

立一条用于输尿管再植的黏膜下隧道，或者用于插导尿管的通道。

乙状结肠膀胱成形术

应用乙状结肠的优点是肠管离膀胱较近，而且在神经性病变的患者中肠管扩张也很明显。术中游离 15～20 cm 肠管，并用抗生素冲洗。由于乙状结肠自身收缩能力较强，需要完全彻底地对其进行去管化处理[132]。与回肠扩大术相比，乙状结肠的自发穿孔发生机会较高[117]，可能与其自身收缩压力较高有关[111]。

回盲肠膀胱成形术

回盲部肠管的主要优点是其血供较好，应用回盲部肠管有两种手术方法，每一种都有很多变化。一种是将回肠和盲肠一同去管化成形[82]，另一种是仅将盲肠去管化，回肠用于建立可控性造瘘口[19]。这种手术仅在少数情况下用于神经性病变患者，主要是因为丧失回盲瓣后可能会导致难治性的腹泻[99]。

胃膀胱成形术

胃的吸收能力比其他肠段差，而其分泌氢离子的特征有利于慢性肾功能不全和代谢性酸中毒的患者[3,108]。在大弯侧沿胃网膜右血管游离一段 10～15 cm 宽的胃壁，穿过横结肠的大网膜到达膀胱。最初人们相信这种方法对所有需要膀胱扩大的患者来说都是最好的选择，但目前其应用已经受到限制，主要是因为血尿–排尿困难综合征，其发生率可以达到 70%。

可控性导尿通道

膀胱扩大手术和膀胱颈部手术明显降低了患者自发排空膀胱的能力，同时也增加了不完全排空的发生。如果不严格坚持定时 CIC，就有可能增加尿路感

染、尿石症[107]以及膀胱自发穿孔的风险[6,122]。1980 年，Mitrofanoff 提出可控性通道的原则，将阑尾通过黏膜下隧道再植入膀胱[100]。现在所说的“Mitrofanoff 原则”指使用任何合适的管道，将其通过有足够肌肉支持的黏膜下隧道植入，使其具有瓣膜功能，提供可靠的控尿机制（图 115-7）。

Mitrofanoff 原则得到了普遍支持，这种方法也可以使用其他各种组织，主要是因为阑尾（图 115-8）并不总是可用或可获得的，尤其是在同时进行 Malone
798 顺行性可控灌肠的情况下。也有应用胃、结肠、膀胱、输尿管和输卵管的成功报道*。Yang[148]和 Monti 及其同事[101]改进了回肠通道，提高了泌尿生殖道重建手术的可靠性，最大限度地减少了肠管损失，并能获得长达 15 cm 的肠管通道（图 115-9）[21,141]。

一条可控性的导尿通道需要柔软的管道、直的通道以及较短的腹内节段。阑尾膀胱造口需要完全游离右半结肠，以保证其足够的活动度。切除部分应当包含盲肠，因为这样做可以保证有足够大的皮肤瘘口，或者通过卷管来增加造瘘长度[16,33]。然后仔细游离阑尾，游离时应连同阑尾系膜一起，以保证其充足的血管供应。Monti-Yang 技术需要游离 2 cm 的回肠，沿系膜对侧缘打开，再将其包绕 12 French 导管重新卷管。然后将通道再植入膀胱，因其一定厚度的肌层对于可控性瓣膜机制是一个理想的条件；有文献报道还可以成功地使用胃和结肠带来实现这一目的。向回肠进行再植操作是一个非常具有挑战性的过程，需要做一个浆肌层沟槽或做 Ghoniem 再植。瘘口位置可以隐藏于脐部，或者放置于右下腹，主要是根据手术者的偏好而定。不管放在什么位置，都要保证能让 12 French 导管容易通过，通道走向要尽可能直和没有张力。达到要求后，要将通道和膀胱用永久性缝线固定于腹壁上。很多精巧的皮瓣技术可以用于减少瘘口狭窄的发生机会，所有技术都要求进行通道口的皮瓣嵌入操作。术后留置导管 2～3 周，第一次的导尿操作通常要在病房中进行。所有照料患儿的家庭成员都要学会正确的导尿技术。

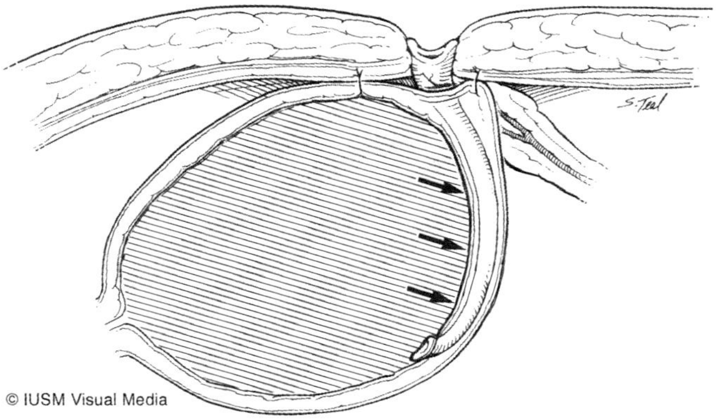

图 115-7　Mitrofanoff 原则指出一条可控性的导尿通道需要柔软的管道，在膀胱内压力升高的情况下会自行关闭，实现对尿液的控制。

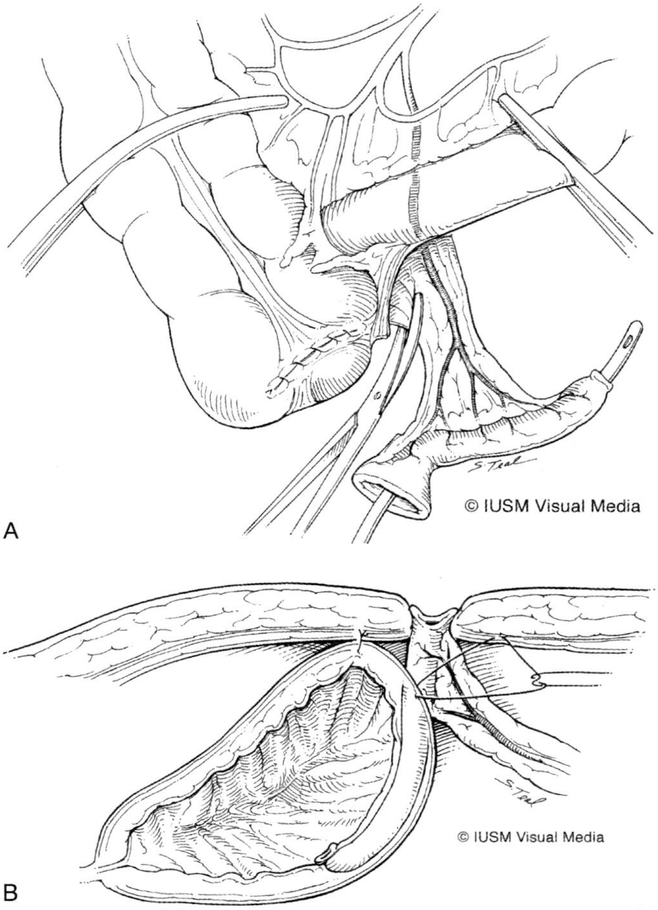

图 115-8　A. 阑尾是比较容易取得和游离的，要保证其血管供应。B. 阑尾很容易进行膀胱黏膜下植入，从而提供可靠的导尿通道。

有两篇已经发表的最大样本的文献报道，造瘘口控尿能力相当好，达到了 90%～99%[21,64]。并发症主

* 见参考文献 12，20，21，27，33，38，67，101，142，145，146 和 148。

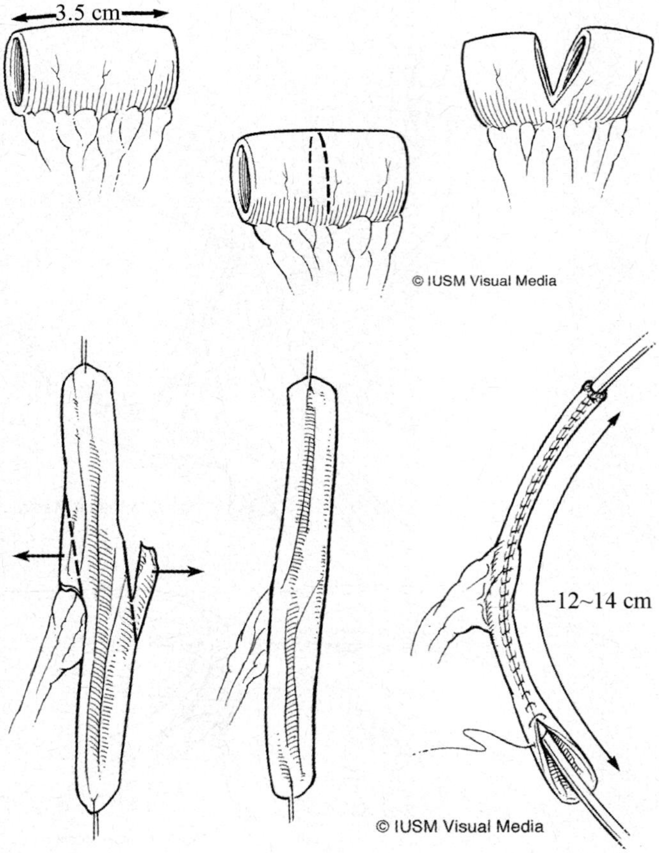

图 115-9　正常情况下，一条 2 cm 长的回肠段可以沿系膜对侧缘打开并重新卷管，做成一个有效的通道。一条更长一些的肠段（3.5 cm）部分切开，两端卷管，采用 Monti 方式螺旋再吻合，以适用于更长的通道。

要与导尿困难有关，绝大多数发生在皮肤水平，也可以发生在深部通道。所报道的瘘口狭窄的发生率为 5%~25%[45,64]，在回肠卷管中的发生率相对更低[21]。

一些作者提出应用膀胱自身组织的可控性导尿通道技术。最初由 Casale 提出的“膀胱内通道”由 Rink 进行了改良，尽管文献所报道的排尿控制率达到了 100%，但这一技术的造瘘口狭窄发生率也达到 45%。如果不经腹手术，则这一技术还比较有用，但它实际上已经被阑尾膀胱造口术和回肠再成形膀胱造口术所取代。

这些通道技术实现了较好的排尿控制效果，其导尿方式也比较容易被接受。对于那些尿道敏感以及肥胖和使用轮椅的女性患者来说，这种方式可以提供更多的方便。它同样也可以方便护理人员的工作，而更重要的是增加了患者的独立性。

可控性贮尿囊（袋）

如果整个膀胱都被非泌尿系统的组织（通常是胃肠道）所替代，并且需要通过其他方式而不是尿道排空，那么这种替代方式就称为可控性尿流贮袋。尽管这一名词在过去几十年里非常流行而且又进行了多次精简解释，但在今天的儿科领域却很少使用，主要是因为儿童的膀胱大多可以通过重建手术得以修复[120]。

一些疾病如膀胱发育不良或恶性病症导致膀胱切除，这些情况需要进行全膀胱替代。泄殖腔外翻的患者同样也需要膀胱替代。在有需要的情况下，可以通过替代手术使这些复杂疾病的患者获得对排尿的控制。不管手术操作如何完美，患者的不适应状态都会导致各种各样的并发症发生，所以针对患者选择手术过程与选择膀胱扩大手术一样重要。术前评估方法与膀胱扩大术前的评估非常相似，需要获取充分的临床信息、代谢、解剖以及功能上的数据，以确定具体的手术方案。

可控性尿流改道的目的包括建立大容量和高顺应 179
性的贮尿袋、抗反流输尿管再植、可控性的皮肤造瘘以及最少的并发症。

尽管胃肠道可以用于作为贮尿袋，但与膀胱扩大手术相比还存在关键性的区别。结肠和胃的应用十分重要，这是因为在输尿管的抗反流吻合和导尿通道的吻合中，结肠带和胃壁肌层的作用更加可靠。在儿童中有三种最常用的可控性贮尿袋类型，分别是单独由回肠做成的贮尿袋（Kock 贮尿袋）、胃与回肠的复合型贮尿袋以及回盲贮尿袋（Indiana 贮尿袋）[64]。其中每一种类型都有不同的变化，而所有这些都以减少并发症和有利于操作为目的。不过由于在文献报道中，这些手术在儿童中应用的数量比较少，而且每个贮尿袋在具体操作中都有不同，同时也没有关于这些方式的直接对比，所以现在还不能确定哪一种是最理想的贮尿袋[64,121,147]。因此重建外科的手术医生应当熟练掌握其中一些技术，每一种技术在临床应用中都有其各自的优点。

Kock 贮尿袋

Kock 最先于 1971 年提出了一种可控性的回肠造口技术[76,77]，并在此基础上于 1982 年发展形成了

Kock 贮尿袋[78]。这种可控性回肠贮尿袋是作为非原位膀胱替代物来应用的，直至今天还有一定程度的流行[1,2,31]。它需要构造一个可控性的输出道乳头以及一个抗反流作用的输入袢。这一手术通常需要应用机械式吻合器，而这有可能成为其最主要并发症的来源（结石形成），也是其应用后期失效的原因[11]。

在成人需要切取 80 cm 的回肠，利用近端 15～20 cm 肠管的顺蠕动特点形成抗反流机制，远端 12～15 cm 用于可控性皮肤造口。在儿童中，这些长度数字可以根据患儿的大小适当减少。肠管全层套叠，并用胃肠道吻合器固定三道，也有人提出应用可吸收缝线固定[134]。比较大的改动包括去除吻合器远端 6 个吻合钉[11]、剥除远端肠系膜[53]以及使用可吸收吻合钉[71]。

胃回肠贮尿袋

把胃和回肠结合在一起做成一个复合型贮尿袋，将其并发症相互抵消，而使这两个胃肠节段的优点都能得到充分发挥。其代谢紊乱能够互补，酸性的胃液分泌可以在回结肠内被中和成可吸收物质[9,91,95]。更进一步说，易患短肠综合征的高风险患者，如泄殖腔外翻患者，通过这种贮尿袋方式，可以最大限度地减少具有吸收作用的组织丧失[120]。然而，这种贮尿袋手术是一种非常复杂的重建操作，需要进行两个吻合，手术时间长，但对一些特殊患者来说，仍然是一个很有价值的选择。

Indiana 贮尿袋

由于回盲瓣具有潜在的控尿和抗反流能力，所以应用回盲节段肠管的贮尿袋技术已经得到普及。现在已经有很多相关的手术方法，都是为了提高经皮控尿能力、简化手术操作、减少术后并发症。Gilchrist 和 Merricks 所提出的套入技术目前还在应用，Indiana 小组[124]对这一贮尿袋技术进行了改良。Indiana 贮尿袋是利用盲肠去管化形成贮尿袋，将输尿管以抗反流方式植入结肠带，回肠向回盲瓣折叠套入，并采用 Lembert 缝合法固定（图 115-10）。文献报道的控尿率达到 95%～99%[113,124]，这在很大程度上与其大容量有关[25]。并发症的发生机会在可以接受的范围内，约为 0.6%[124]，但不是所有的手术医生都有这么高的成功率报告[23]。尽管 Indiana 贮尿袋在成人中应用非常广泛，但在儿童中的应用却很有限，这主要与切除回盲瓣后可能导致腹泻有关。

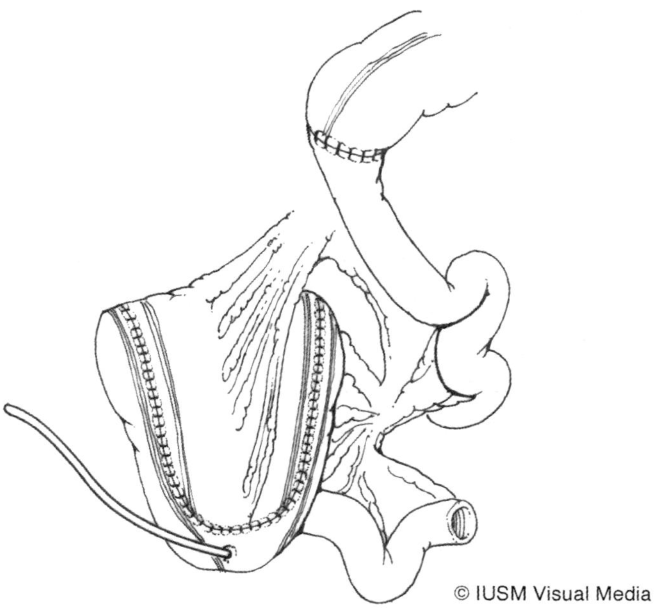

图 115-10　Indiana 贮尿袋利用回盲瓣实现对尿液的控制，并将盲肠作为尿液贮袋。

将肠管应用于泌尿道所发生的并发症

尽管将胃肠道应用为尿液贮尿袋的做法比较普遍，但这种做法有可能会导致很多并发症出现，而且有的并发症可能很严重。大致将并发症分为：（1）由结构缺陷所导致的并发症，（2）由肠管损失而导致的并发症，（3）由肠液分泌所导致的并发症，（4）由吸收所导致的并发症。

结构异常所导致的并发症 1800

这类并发症包括需要再次进行扩大手术、自发性穿孔和长期潜在恶变可能。有 6% 的患者需要再次进行扩大手术[111]，而且绝大多数是因为肠管持续性收缩而导致的高膀胱内压[52,92]。其临床特征性的表现为尿失禁或超声检查肾盂积水，这一并发症可以通过尿流动力学检查证实。

自发性穿孔是致命的并发症，临床上不能低估这一并发症。早期的尿漏可能是由于技术操作上的失误，而晚期的并发症则可能来源于肠管，一般在距离吻合线 1 cm 左右处发生[120]。患者的症状出现较迟，可能是由于其神经性病变推迟了症状的出现，从而极有可能导致败血症和死亡，所以需要非常警惕这种情况发生的可能性。通过膀胱 CT 增强检查明确诊断，治疗方法一般是开腹一期缝合穿孔[122]，也可以对某些患者通过导管引流进行保守治疗，现在也有这方面的成功报道[136]。

腺癌的发生也是一个值得关注的问题。据文献报道，大多发生于输尿管乙状结肠吻合术后[39,47,59,131,138]。病变来源于肠管和输尿管的连接处，其癌变的发生率是正常人群的7000 倍[59]。尽管有报告指出癌变可以早在扩大术后 3 年内发生[24,66]，但其平均潜伏期为 21.5～26 年[8,59]。在作者所在的医疗机构中，500 名接受扩大手术的患者有 3 例发生癌变，而这 3 例患者都死于代谢性疾病，其从疾病诊断到接受扩大手术的平均时间为 19 年[137]。虽然大多数外科医生都认识到这一危险，但直至目前为止，还没有针对术后监测而制定的明确指导策略。作者推荐在扩大手术后的前 5～10 年中每年进行一次膀胱镜检查[8,120]。

肠管损失

肠切除手术会使患者有肠梗阻的危险，其发生率大约在3%左右[42,98,117,120]。由于这些肠梗阻很多是由扩大的肠管系膜处的内疝所引起，所以 Leonard 及其同事建议对这些患者进行早期探查，以减少用于扩大手术的肠管发生缺血坏死的危险[87]。

由于 CUR 或扩大手术而切除部分胃肠道节段，这在一般情况下都是可以接受的；不过有报告提出在这些患者中有 10%～54% 出现肠功能紊乱[55,133]。切除回盲瓣可能会导致顽固性的腹泻和大便失禁，尤其是患有神经性病变的患者[48,70]。远端回肠的损失也可以导致腹泻，其发生机制是肝肠循环被中断[10]；不过如果远端 15～20 cm 肠管被完整保留下来，这一并发症一般不会发生。应用阴离子交换树脂通常可以成功地治疗轻症患者[82]。

接受 Kock 贮尿袋手术的患者在切除 80 cm 小肠后，有高达 35% 的人会出现维生素 B_{12} 缺乏[4]，而在接受回肠膀胱成形手术的患者中则不会出现这种并发症[125,140]，其原因可能是后一种手术在儿童患者中仅有 25 cm 以下的肠管被切除。

由肠管分泌引起的并发症

胃液分泌的酸性环境可能会导致血尿-排尿困难综合征，出现在 9%～70% 的患者中[28,87,97,120]。这是非常棘手的并发症，会导致膀胱痉挛、耻骨上疼痛、排尿困难、肉眼血尿以及生殖器表皮脱落。这在敏感体质的患者中表现得尤其严重，发生率接近 75%[82,105,119]。对于轻症患者可以采用抗组胺药物或质子泵抑制剂治疗[105]，但也可能需要采用碳酸氢钠溶液灌洗[37,112]。酸性物质的丢失可以导致严重的低钾血症、低氯血症、代谢性碱中毒，这些可以因伴发胃肠道炎症而进一步加重。

所有肠管都有持续性的黏液分泌，尽管在回肠中的分泌量相对较少[54,117,118]，但都会导致膀胱的排空不全，使患者容易罹患尿路感染和膀胱结石[120]。膀胱结石发生于 7%～25% 的扩大手术患者[14,65,107]，有两篇病例数量最多的文献报告其发生率为 10%～15%[34,65,81]。这样高的风险可能与黏液中钙磷水平增高有关[68]。鸟粪石成分提示最常见的病因为存在产尿素酶细菌。扩大手术中最常见的系统性酸中毒会降低抑制结石的作用，从而也促进结石的发生[107]。预防手段主要是定期进行 CIC 以及每天进行膀胱灌洗。治疗方法主要通过开放手段或内镜手段实施[14,35,81,107]，而开放手术一般仅用于处理较大的结石。

菌尿现象在进行 CIC 的患者中非常普遍，尤其是在接受过肠膀胱成形手术的患者中更加多见。尿路感染大多表现为尿液有恶臭味，其症状可以包括血尿、尿失禁加重、耻骨上疼痛或者黏液分泌增多[120]。Rink 及其同事报道在回肠膀胱扩大术的患者中，有症状的尿路感染的发生率为 22.7%，而在胃膀胱成形术患者中的发生率仅为 8%[117]。文献报告发热性尿路感染的总发生率为 14%。对于无症状菌尿一般不进行治疗，除非尿培养发现有产尿素酶细菌生长或者有毒力很强的细菌生长。然而治疗可降低结石形成的风险。

由于吸收引起的并发症

由于肠管有吸收功能，所以使用肠管作为尿液贮袋可能会出现明显的代谢性改变。结肠和回肠吸收铵盐、氢离子和氯离子，会导致高氯性代谢性酸中毒。对于肾功能正常的患者，这一并发症是可以承受的[74]，但对其他患者来说，就需要针对这一并发症进行内科治疗。离子吸收的程度主要与肠管接触面积的大小和接触时间的长短有关，所以，如果有明显的酸中毒表现，就要进一步检查有无不完全排空的情况[120]。尽管不是所有患者都会出现酸中毒表现，但绝大多数患者血氯水平都有增加，不过仍会维持在正常水平[98]。酸中毒动员体液缓冲系统，会导致骨骼
301 矿物质的丢失。虽然有人认为这会导致身体生长障碍，但有关这一观点还存有争议。在动物模型实验和膀胱外翻的患者中已经证实存在这种表现[18,73,93]，并且文献报道有 15%～20% 的膀胱外翻患者身高不足[50]。不过在发病率更高的脊髓发育不良患者中，很难证实有这种相关关系。酸中毒可以引起低枸橼酸尿症，增加肾脏和膀胱结石形成的风险[107]。

一些药物如苯妥英（大仑丁）与甲氨蝶呤比较容易从肠道吸收，应当密切监测其浓度水平[126]。葡萄糖同样可以从肠道吸收，所以对高血糖症患者进行尿液监测的结果并不可靠[139]。

小结

由 Lapides 提出的 CIC 使下尿路重建手术产生了变革，它打开了儿童一期重建手术的大门，能够保持尿路的完整性，淘汰了永久性的非可控性尿流改道，也极大限制了暂时性尿流改道的指征。Mitrofanoff 原则提供了更加积极的方式，使儿童获得完全控尿的能力。尽管受治患儿在独立性和社会行为方面得到了很大改善，但重建手术同时也带来了很多新的并发症，有些甚至是致命的。大家都清楚，决定手术方式的最主要因素是患者和家庭的意愿。患者及其家庭必须愿意而且能够每天进行 4 小时一次的间歇导尿，并且一直持续下去。这些重建手术需要得到一个团队的支持，包括家庭、手术者、护士，而且需要进行终身随访。

（赵海腾译　刘国华校）

参考文献

1. Abd-El-Gawad G, Abrahamsson K, Hanson E, et al: Early and late metabolic alterations in children and adolescents with a Kock urinary reservoir. BJU Int 1999;83:285-289.
2. Abd-el-Gawad G, Abrahamsson K, Hanson E, et al: Evaluation of Kock urinary reservoir function in children and adolescents at 3-10 years' follow-up. Scand J Urol Nephrol 1999;33:149-155.
3. Adams MC, Mitchell ME, Rink RC: Gastrocystoplasty: An alternative solution to the problem of urological reconstruction in the severely compromised patient. J Urol 1988;140:1152-1156.
4. Akerlund S: Urinary diversion via the continent ileal reservoir: Functional characteristics and long-term outcome. Scand J Urol Nephrol Suppl 1989;121:1-36.
5. Alexander F, Kay R: Cloacal anomalies: Role of vesicostomy. J Pediatr Surg 1994;29:74-76.
6. Anderson PA, Rickwood AM: Detrusor hyperreflexia as a factor in spontaneous perforation of augmentation cystoplasty for neuropathic bladder. Br J Urol 1991;67:210-212.
7. Atan A, Konety BR, Nangia A, et al: Advantages and risks of ileovesicostomy for the management of neuropathic bladder. Urology 1999;54:636-640.
8. Austen M, Kalble T: Secondary malignancies in different forms of urinary diversion using isolated gut. J Urol 2004;172:831-838.
9. Austin PF, DeLeary G, Homsy YL, et al: Long-term metabolic advantages of a gastrointestinal composite urinary reservoir. J Urol 1997;158:1704-1707; discussion 1707-1708.
10. Barrington JW, Fern-Davies H, Adams RJ, et al: Bile acid dysfunction after clam enterocystoplasty. Br J Urol 1995;76:169-171.
11. Benson M, Olsson C: Continent Cutaneous Urinary Diversion. Philadelphia, Elsevier Science, 2003.
12. Bihrle R, Klee LW, Adams MC, et al: Early clinical experience with the transverse colon-gastric tube continent urinary reservoir. J Urol 1991;146:751-753.
13. Blocksom BH Jr: Bladder pouch for prolonged tubeless cystostomy. J Urol 1957;78:398-401.
14. Blyth B, Ewalt DH, Duckett JW, et al: Lithogenic properties of enterocystoplasty. J Urol 1992;148:575-577; discussion 578-579.
15. Bruce AW, Reid G, Chan RC, et al: Bacterial adherence in the human ileal conduit: A morphological and bacteriological study. J Urol 1984;132:184-188.
16. Bruce RG, McRoberts JW: Cecoappendicovesicostomy: Conduit-lengthening technique for use in continent urinary reconstruction. Urology 1998;52:702-704.
17. Bruce RR, Gonzales ET Jr. Cutaneous vesicostomy: A useful form of temporary diversion in children. J Urol 1980;123:927-928.
18. Bushinsky DA, Kittaka MK, Weisinger JR, et al: Effects of chronic metabolic alkalosis on Ca^{2+}, PTH and 1,25(OH)2D3

in the rat. Am J Physiol 1989;257:E578-E582.

19. Cain M, Hussman D: Cecal bladder augmentation with a tapered catheterizable stoma: A modification of the Indiana pouch. Presented at the meeting of the American Academy of Pediatrics, Urology Section. 1994, Dallas.
20. Cain MP, Casale AJ, Rink RC: Initial experience using a catheterizable ileovesicostomy (Monti procedure) in children. Urology 1998;52:870-873.
21. Cain MP, Casale AJ, King SJ, et al: Appendicovesicostomy and newer alternatives for the Mitrofanoff procedure: Results in the last 100 patients at Riley Children's Hospital. J Urol 1999;162:1749-1752.
22. Cain MP, Rink RC, Yerkes EB, et al: Long-term followup and outcome of continent catheterizable vesicostomy using the Rink modification. J Urol 2002;168:2583-2585.
23. Canning D: Continent Urinary Diversion. Philadelphia, WB Saunders, 1998.
24. Carr LK, Herschorn S: Early development of adenocarcinoma in a young woman following augmentation cystoplasty for undiversion. J Urol 1997;157:2255-2256.
25. Carroll PR, Presti JC Jr, McAninch JW, et al: Functional characteristics of the continent ileocecal urinary reservoir: Mechanisms of urinary continence. J Urol 1989;142:1032-1036.
26. Casale AJ: Continent vesicostomy: A new method utilizing only bladder tissue. Presented before the 60th annual meeting of the American Association of Pediatrics, New Orleans, 1991.
27. Casale AJ: A long continent ileovesicostomy using a single piece of bowel. J Urol 1999;162:1743-1745.
28. Chadwick Plaire J, Snodgrass WT, Grady RW, et al: Long-term followup of the hematuria-dysuria syndrome. J Urol 2000;164:921-923.
29. Cheng E: Personal Communication, 2005.
30. Clark T, Pope JC 4th, Adams C, et al: Factors that influence outcomes of the Mitrofanoff and Malone antegrade continence enema reconstructive procedures in children. J Urol 2002;168:1537-1540; discussion 1540.
31. Clementson Kockum C, Helin I, Malmberg L, et al: Pediatric urinary tract reconstruction using intestine. Scand J Urol Nephrol 1999;33:53-56.
32. Close CE, Carr MC, Burns MW, et al: Lower urinary tract changes after early valve ablation in neonates and infants: Is early diversion warranted? J Urol 1997;157:984-988.
33. Cromie WJ, Barada JH, Weingarten JL: Cecal tubularization: Lengthening technique for creation of catheterizable conduit. Urology 1991;37:41-42.
34. DeFoor W, Minevich E, Reddy P, et al: Bladder calculi after augmentation cystoplasty: Risk factors and prevention strategies. J Urol 2004;172:1964-1966.
35. Docimo SG, Orth CR, Schulam PG: Percutaneous cystolithotomy after augmentation cystoplasty: Comparison with open procedures. Tech Urol 1998;4:43-45.
36. Duckett JW Jr: Cutaneous vesicostomy in childhood: The Blocksom technique. Urol Clin North Am 1974;1:485-95.
37. Dykes EH, Ransley PG: Gastrocystoplasty in children. Br J Urol 1992;69:91-95.
38. Figueroa TE, Sabogal L, Helal M, et al: The tapered and reimplanted small bowel as a variation of the Mitrofanoff procedure: Preliminary results. J Urol 1994;152:73-75.
39. Filmer RB, Spencer JR: Malignancies in bladder augmentations and intestinal conduits. J Urol 1990;143:671-678.
40. Fowler JE Jr: Continent urinary reservoirs. Surg Annu 1988;20:201-225.
41. Gauthier AR Jr, Winters JC: Incontinent ileovesicostomy in the management of neurogenic bladder dysfunction. Neurourol Urodyn 2003;22:142-146.
42. Gearhart JP, Albertsen PC, Marshall FF, et al: Pediatric applications of augmentation cystoplasty: The Johns Hopkins experience. J Urol 1986;136:430-432.
43. Ghali AM, El Malki T, Sheir KZ, et al: Posterior urethral valves with persistent high serum creatinine: The value of percutaneous nephrostomy. J Urol 2000;164:1340-1344.
44. Gittes RF: Carcinogenesis in ureterosigmoidostomy. Urol Clin North Am 1986;13:201-205.
45. Glassman DT, Docimo SG: Concealed umbilical stoma: Long-term evaluation of stomal stenosis. J Urol 2001;166:1028-1030.
46. Goldwasser B, Webster GD: Augmentation and substitution enterocystoplasty. J Urol 1986;135:215-224.
47. Golomb J, Klutke CG, Lewin KJ, et al: Bladder neoplasms associated with augmentation cystoplasty: Report of 2 cases and literature review. J Urol 1989;142:377-380.
48. Gonzalez R, Cabral B: Rectal continence after enterocystoplasty. Dial Pediatr Urol 1987;(10):3-4.
49. Gonzalez R, Reinberg Y: Localization of bacteriuria in patients with enterocystoplasty and nonrefluxing conduits. J Urol 1987;138:1104-1105.
50. Gros DA, Dodson JL, Lopatin UA, et al: Decreased linear growth associated with intestinal bladder augmentation in children with bladder exstrophy. J Urol 2000;164:917-920.
51. Hagglof B, Andren O, Bergstrom E, et al: Self-esteem before and after treatment in children with nocturnal enuresis and urinary incontinence. Scand J Urol Nephrol Suppl 1997;183:79-82.
52. Hedlund H, Lindstrom K, Mansson W: Dynamics of a continent caecal reservoir for urinary diversion. Br J Urol 1984; 56:366-372.
53. Hendren WH: Urinary diversion and undiversion in children. Surg Clin North Am 1976;56:425-449.
54. Hendren WH, Hendren RB: Bladder augmentation: Experience with 129 children and young adults. J Urol 1990;144:445-453; discussion 460.
55. Herschorn S, Hewitt RJ: Patient perspective of long-term outcome of augmentation cystoplasty for neurogenic bladder. Urology 1998;52:672-678.
56. Hinman F Jr: Selection of intestinal segments for bladder substitution: Physical and physiological characteristics. J Urol 1988;139:519-523.
57. Horowitz M, Kuhr CS, Mitchell ME: The Mitrofanoff catheterizable channel: Patient acceptance. J Urol 1995; 153:771-772.
58. Husmann DA, McLorie GA, Churchill BM: Nonrefluxing colonic conduits: A long-term life-table analysis. J Urol 1989; 142:1201-1203.
59. Husmann DA, Spence HM: Current status of tumor of the bowel following ureterosigmoidostomy: A review. J Urol 1990;144:607-610.
60. Hutcheson JC, Cooper CS, Canning DA, et al: The use of vesicostomy as permanent urinary diversion in the child with myelomeningocele. J Urol 2001;166:2351-2353.
61. Hutton KA, Thomas DF: Selective use of cutaneous vesicostomy in prenatally detected and clinically presenting uropathies. Eur Urol 1998;33:405-411.
62. Jaureguizar E, Lopez Pereira P, Martinez Urrutia MJ, et al: Does neonatal pyeloureterostomy worsen bladder function in children with posterior urethral valves? J Urol 2000; 164:1031-1033; discussion 1033-1034.
63. Jayanthi VR, McLorie GA, Khoury AE, et al: The effect of temporary cutaneous diversion on ultimate bladder function. J Urol 1995;154:889-892.
64. Kaefer M, Tobin MS, Hendren WH, et al: Continent

urinary diversion: the Children's Hospital experience. J Urol 1997;157:1394-1399.
65. Kaefer M, Hendren WH, Bauer SB, et al: Reservoir calculi: A comparison of reservoirs constructed from stomach and other enteric segments. J Urol 1998;160:2187-2190.
66. Kalble T, Tricker AR, Friedl P, et al: Ureterosigmoidostomy: Long-term results, risk of carcinoma and etiological factors for carcinogenesis. J Urol 1990;144:1110-1114.
67. Keating MA, Rink RC, Adams MC: Appendicovesicostomy: A useful adjunct to continent reconstruction of the bladder. J Urol 1993;149:1091-1094.
68. Khoury AE, Salomon M, Doche R, et al: Stone formation after augmentation cystoplasty: The role of intestinal mucus. J Urol 1997;158:1133-1137.
69. Kim YH, Horowitz M, Combs A, et al: Comparative urodynamic findings after primary valve ablation, vesicostomy or proximal diversion. J Urol 1996;156:673-676.
70. King L: Protection of the Upper Tracts in Children. Chicago, Year Book Medical, 1987.
71. Kirsch AJ, Olsson CA, Hensle TW: Pediatric continent reservoirs and colocystoplasty created with absorbable staples. J Urol 1996;156:614-617.
72. Koch MO, McDougal WS: The pathophysiology of hyperchloremic metabolic acidosis after urinary diversion through intestinal segments. Surgery 1985;98: 561-570.
73. Koch MO, McDougal WS: Bone demineralization following ureterosigmoid anastomosis: An experimental study in rats. J Urol 1988;140:856-859.
74. Koch MO, McDougal WS, Reddy PK, et al: Metabolic alterations following continent urinary diversion through colonic segments. J Urol 1991;145:270-273.
75. Koch MO, McDougal WS, Hall MC, et al: Long-term metabolic effects of urinary diversion: A comparison of myelomeningocele patients managed by clean intermittent catheterization and urinary diversion. J Urol 1992;147: 1343-1347.
76. Kock NG: Ileostomy without external appliances: A survey of 25 patients provided with intra-abdominal intestinal reservoir. Ann Surg 1971;173:545-550.
77. Kock NG: Construction of a continent ileostomy. Schweiz Med Wochenschr 1971;101:729-734.
78. Kock NG, Nilson AE, Nilsson LO, et al: Urinary diversion via a continent ileal reservoir: Clinical results in 12 patients. J Urol 1982;128:469-475.
79. Koff SA: Guidelines to determine the size and shape of intestinal segments used for reconstruction. J Urol 1988; 140:1150-1151.
80. Krahn CG, Johnson HW: Cutaneous vesicostomy in the young child: Indications and results. Urology 1993;41: 558-563.
81. Kronner KM, Casale AJ, Cain MP, et al: Bladder calculi in the pediatric augmented bladder. J Urol 1998;160: 1096-1098; discussion 1103.
82. Kropp B, Cheng E: Bladder Augmentation: Current and Future Techniques, 4th ed. London, Martin Dunitz, 2002.
83. Lapides J, Ajemian EP, Lichtwardt JR: Cutaneous vesicostomy. J Urol 1960;84:609-614.
84. Lapides J, Diokno AC, Silber SJ, et al: Clean, intermittent self-catheterization in the treatment of urinary tract disease. J Urol 1972;107:458-461.
85. Lapides J, Diokno AC, Gould FR, et al: Further observations on self-catheterization. J Urol 1976;116:169-171.
86. Leng WW, Faerber G, Del Terzo M, et al: Long-term outcome of incontinent ileovesicostomy management of severe lower urinary tract dysfunction. J Urol 1999;161:1803-1806.
87. Leonard MP, Dharamsi N, Williot PE: Outcome of gastrocystoplasty in tertiary pediatric urology practice. J Urol 2000;164:947-950.
88. Liard A, Seguier-Lipszyc E, Mitrofanoff P: Temporary high diversion for posterior urethral valves. J Urol 2000;164: 145-148.
89. Light JK: Enteroplasty to ablate bowel contractions in the reconstructed bladder: A case report. J Urol 1985;134: 958-959.
90. Light JK, Engelmann UH: Reconstruction of the lower urinary tract: Observations on bowel dynamics and the artificial urinary sphincter. J Urol 1985;133:594-597.
91. Lockhart JL, Davies R, Cox C, et al: The gastroileoileal pouch: An alternative continent urinary reservoir for patients with short bowel, acidosis and/or extensive pelvic radiation. J Urol 1993;150:46-50.
92. Lytton B, Green DF: Urodynamic studies in patients undergoing bladder replacement surgery. J Urol 1989; 141:1394-1397.
93. McDougal WS, Koch MO, Shands C 3rd, et al: Bony demineralization following urinary intestinal diversion. J Urol 1988;140:853-855.
94. McGuire EJ, Woodside JR, Borden TA, et al: Prognostic value of urodynamic testing in myelodysplastic patients. J Urol 1981;126:205-209.
95. McLaughlin KP, Rink RC, Adams MC, et al: Stomach in combination with other intestinal segments in pediatric lower urinary tract reconstruction. J Urol 1995;154:1162-1168.
96. Mills RD, Studer UE: Metabolic consequences of continent urinary diversion. J Urol 1999;161:1057-1066.
97. Mingin GC, Stock JA, Hanna MK: Gastrocystoplasty: Long-term complications in 22 patients. J Urol 1999; 162:1122-1125.
98. Mitchell ME, Piser JA: Intestinocystoplasty and total bladder replacement in children and young adults: Followup in 129 cases. J Urol 1987;138:579-584.
99. Mitchell ME, Rink RC: Pediatric urinary diversion and undiversion. Pediatr Clin North Am 1987;34:1319-1332.
100. Mitrofanoff P. [Trans-appendicular continent cystostomy in the management of the neurogenic bladder]. Chir Pediatr 1980;21:297-305.
101. Monti PR, Lara RC, Dutra MA, et al: New techniques for construction of efferent conduits based on the Mitrofanoff principle. Urology 1997;49:112-115.
102. Mor Y, Ramon J, Raviv G, et al: Low loop cutaneous ureterostomy and subsequent reconstruction: 20 years of experience. J Urol 1992;147:1595-1597; discussion 1597-1598.
103. Mor Y, Quinn FM, Carr B, et al: Combined Mitrofanoff and antegrade continence enema procedures for urinary and fecal incontinence. J Urol 1997;158:192-195.
104. Mutchnik SE, Hinson JL, Nickell KG, et al: Ileovesicostomy as an alternative form of bladder management in tetraplegic patients. Urology 1997;49:353-357.
105. Nguyen DH, Bain MA, Salmonson KL, et al: The syndrome of dysuria and hematuria in pediatric urinary reconstruction with stomach. J Urol 1993;150:707-709.
106. Noe HN, Jerkins GR: Cutaneous vesicostomy experience in infants and children. J Urol 1985;134:301-303.
107. Palmer LS, Franco I, Kogan SJ, et al: Urolithiasis in children following augmentation cystoplasty. J Urol 1993;150:726-729.
108. Piser JA, Mitchell ME, Kulb TB, et al: Gastrocystoplasty and colocystoplasty in canines: The metabolic consequences of acute saline and acid loading. J Urol 1987;138:1009-1013.
109. Podesta ML, Ruarte A, Gargiulo C, et al: Urodynamic findings in boys with posterior urethral valves after treat-

ment with primary valve ablation or vesicostomy and delayed ablation. J Urol 2000;164:139-144.

110. Podesta ML, Ruarte A, Herrera M, et al: Bladder functional outcome after delayed vesicostomy closure and antireflux surgery in young infants with 'primary' vesicoureteric reflux. BJU Int 2001;87:473-479.

111. Pope JC 4th, Keating MA, Casale AJ, et al. Augmenting the augmented bladder: Treatment of the contractile bowel segment. J Urol 1998;160:854-857.

112. Reinberg Y, Manivel JC, Froemming C, et al: Perforation of the gastric segment of an augmented bladder secondary to peptic ulcer disease. J Urol 1992;148:369-371.

113. Ring KS, Hensle TW: Urinary diversion. In Kelalis PP, King LR, Belman AB (eds): Clinical Pediatric Urology, 3rd ed. Martin Donitz, 1992, p 865-903.

114. Rink R, Mitchell M: Role of Enterocystoplasty in Reconstructing the Neurogenic Bladder. St. Louis, Mosby–Year Book, 1990.

115. Rink R, McLaughlin K: Indications for enterocystoplasty and choice of bowel segment. Prob Urol 1994:389-403.

116. Rink R: Choice of materials for bladder augmentation. Curr Opin Urol 1995:300-305.

117. Rink R, Hollensbe D, Adams M: Complications of augmentation in children and comparison of gastrointestinal segments. AUA Update Series 1995;14:122-128.

118. Rink R, Adams M: Augmentation Cystoplasty, 7th ed. Philadelphia, WB Saunders, 1998.

119. Rink R, Renschler T, Adams M, et al: Long term follow-up of the first gastrocystoplasty series. Presented before the annual meeting of the European Society of Pediatric Urology, Tours, France, 2000.

120. Rink R, Yerkes E, Adams M: Augmentation Cystoplasty. Philadelphia, WB Saunders, 2001.

121. Rink RC: Bladder augmentation: Options, outcomes, future. Urol Clin North Am 1999;26:111-23, viii-ix.

122. Rosen MA, Light JK: Spontaneous bladder rupture following augmentation enterocystoplasty. J Urol 1991;146:1232-1234.

123. Rosen MA, Roth DR, Gonzales ET Jr: Current indications for cutaneous ureterostomy. Urology 1994;43:92-96.

124. Rowland R: Present experience with the Indiana pouch. World J Urol 1995;(14):92-98.

125. Salomon L, Lugagne PM, Herve JM, et al: No evidence of metabolic disorders 10 to 22 years after Camey type I ileal enterocystoplasty. J Urol 1997;157:2104-2106.

126. Savarirayan F, Dixey GM: Syncope following ureterosigmoidostomy. J Urol 1969;101:844-845.

127. Schwartz SL, Kennelly MJ, McGuire EJ, et al: Incontinent ileo-vesicostomy urinary diversion in the treatment of lower urinary tract dysfunction. J Urol 1994;152:99-102.

128. Schwarz GR, Jeffs RD: Ileal conduit urinary diversion in children: Computer analysis of followup from 2 to 16 years. J Urol 1975;114:285-288.

129. Shapiro SR, Lebowitz R, Colodny AH: Fate of 90 children with ileal conduit urinary diversion a decade later: Analysis of complications, pyelography, renal function and bacteriology. J Urol 1975;114:289-295.

130. Sheldon CA, Gilbert A, Wacksman J, et al: Gastrocystoplasty: Technical and metabolic characteristics of the most versatile childhood bladder augmentation modality. J Pediatr Surg 1995;30:283-287; discussion 287-288.

131. Shokeir AA, Shamaa M, el-Mekresh MM, et al: Late malignancy in bowel segments exposed to urine without fecal stream. Urology 1995;46:657-661.

132. Sidi AA, Aliabadi H, Gonzalez R: Enterocystoplasty in the management and reconstruction of the pediatric neurogenic bladder. J Pediatr Surg 1987;22:153-157.

133. Singh G, Thomas DG: Bowel problems after enterocystoplasty. Br J Urol 1997;79:328-332.

134. Skinner DG, Lieskovsky G, Boyd S: Continent urinary diversion. J Urol 1989;141:1323-1327.

135. Skinner DG, Studer UE, Okada K, et al: Which patients are suitable for continent diversion or bladder substitution following cystectomy or other definitive local treatment? Int J Urol 1995;2:105-112.

136. Slaton JW, Kropp KA: Conservative management of suspected bladder rupture after augmentation enterocystoplasty. J Urol 1994;152:713-715.

137. Soergel TM, Cain MP, Misseri R, et al: Transitional cell carcinoma of the bladder following augmentation cystoplasty for the neuropathic bladder. J Urol 2004;172: 1649-1651; discussion 1651-1652.

138. Sohn M, Fuzesi L, Deutz F, et al: Signet ring cell carcinoma in adenomatous polyp at site of ureterosigmoidostomy 16 years after conversion to ileal conduit. J Urol 1990; 143:805-807.

139. Sridhar KN, Samuell CT, Woodhouse CR: Absorption of glucose from urinary conduits in diabetics and nondiabetics. BMJ (Clin Res Ed) 1983;287:1327-1329.

140. Stein R, Lotz J, Andreas J, et al: Long-term metabolic effects in patients with urinary diversion. World J Urol 1998;16:292-297.

141. Sugarman ID, Malone PS, Terry TR, et al: Transversely tubularized ileal segments for the Mitrofanoff or Malone antegrade colonic enema procedures: The Monti principle. Br J Urol 1998;81:253-256.

142. Suzer O, Vates TS, Freedman AL, et al: Results of the Mitrofanoff procedure in urinary tract reconstruction in children. Br J Urol 1997;79:279-282.

143. Thomas DF: Surgical treatment of urinary incontinence. Arch Dis Child 1997;76:377-380.

144. Tietjen DN, Gloor JM, Husmann DA: Proximal urinary diversion in the management of posterior urethral valves: Is it necessary? J Urol 1997;158:1008-1010.

145. Van Savage JG, Khoury AE, McLorie GA, et al: Outcome analysis of Mitrofanoff principle applications using appendix and ureter to umbilical and lower quadrant stomal sites. J Urol 1996;156:1794-1797.

146. Woodhouse CR, Malone PR, Cumming J, et al: The Mitrofanoff principle for continent urinary diversion. Br J Urol 1989;63:53-57.

147. Woodhouse CR, Pope AJ: Alternatives to urinary diversion with a bag: Results in 100 patients. Br J Urol 1993;72: 580-585.

148. Yang WH: Yang needle tunneling technique in creating antireflux and continent mechanisms. J Urol 1993; 150:830-834.

149. Yerkes EB, Rink RC, Cain MP, et al: Shunt infection and malfunction after augmentation cystoplasty. J Urol 2001; 165:2262-2264.

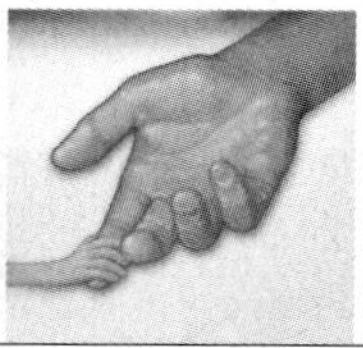

第 116 章

膀胱功能障碍

Martin Kaefer

805 膀胱功能障碍的范畴可以从简单的排尿异常到非常复杂的疾病，包括神经性膀胱功能障碍。膀胱功能障碍常见的症状是尿失禁（湿裤）。需要引起父母和孩子关注的是这种看似相对简单的临床表现可能反映了相当棘手和隐匿的疾病，包括下尿路和上尿路的损伤。本章从医生对有排尿症状孩子的最基本的评估开始，接着介绍与膀胱功能障碍相关的放射影像学及尿流动力学检查，最后对一些特殊疾病及其治疗进行讨论。

病史和体格检查

对膀胱功能障碍患儿的评估应该首先建立白天和夜晚的排尿症状记录。如表 116-1 所列，传统上将排尿症状分为刺激性表现和梗阻性表现。本章讨论的每个病例都存在这些症状。例如，患有梗阻性后尿道瓣膜男孩的父母可能不会谈及其孩子有尿潴留的表现，但是可以记录到尿频和尿急（继发于膀胱过度扩张后的激惹性增加）。这时需要确定孩子是否存在尿路感染，如果有则需要了解是否伴有发热。后一症状有助于将膀胱炎与明显的肾盂肾炎区别开来。医生还应该询问孩子是否有便秘，因为这可以反映出一种潴留情况（如排出障碍的病例）或神经性肠功能紊乱（如各种形式的脊髓神经管闭合不全）。如果考虑后一种诊断，应注意是否有下肢运动减弱或感觉改变。

表 116-1　排尿症状
刺激性
排尿困难
尿急
急迫性尿失禁
尿频
梗阻性
尿潴留
排尿延迟
排尿中断（开始和结束时）
排尿紧张
排尿不尽感

对有膀胱症状的患儿的体格检查应该包括腹部、背部、外阴部和下肢。腹部检查特别要注意是否能触及粪块和是否可以触诊或叩诊到膀胱，或是否两者皆有。

背部检查很重要。如发现腰脊椎处皮肤有毛发斑或有痣反映了神经外胚层的迁移异常，这往往是腰骶部脊髓束形成异常的征象。腰骶椎处皮肤凹陷同样也反映异常情况（图 116-1）。臀纹不对称进一步提示潜在的脊髓发育异常。两组臀部肌群神经支配的减弱程度不一可由臀纹不对称反映出来。比如，如果右侧臀部神经受损害的程度大于左侧，则右侧萎缩会严重一些，结果就是臀纹会向右侧倾斜。关于隐匿的脊髓神经管闭合不全的这种臂部不对称的临床表现，应该清楚也可能是一种继发于孩子生长发育过程的表现。因此，背部检查不仅在对患者初次评估时进行，而且在对持续性排尿疾患患者回访时也要进行。图 116-2 展示了脊髓栓系的概念。有以上任何一种皮肤表现的患者都应该进行腰骶部核磁共振（MRI）检查。

对男孩外阴部的检查应该包括沿着整个尿道的 1806
触诊。质地变硬可能是尿路感染或狭窄的表现。因为脊髓发育不良患儿中隐睾的发生率高，所以要注

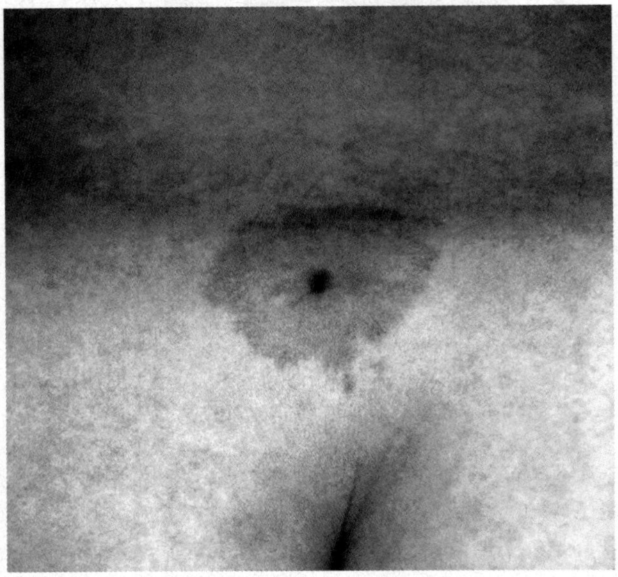

图 116-1　皮肤表现提示有潜在的脊髓栓系。一个 10 岁的患神经性膀胱的男孩，在体格检查中发现腰椎部有一胎痣、腰椎部凹陷和臀肌纹路的不对称。腰骶部核磁共振检查发现脊髓内脂肪瘤导致了脊髓栓系。

意检查睾丸的位置[19,49]。检查肛门并确认其在会阴部的位置和括约肌的张力是否正常。最后，应该记录任何下肢反射或运动力量的减弱，因为这些可能是神经肌源性疾病尤其是腰骶部脊髓栓系疾病的外部表现。

对每个有排尿症状的患儿都应该进行尿液分析。记录尿中红细胞、白细胞、糖和蛋白质的情况。尿比重低可能反映肾功能不全导致的尿液浓缩能力下降。

膀胱功能障碍的放射影像学检查和尿流动力学检查

膀胱超声

膀胱超声是最基本的影像学检查方法，能提供膀胱是否有明显病理变化的情况。如果排除了感染，膀胱壁增厚可能反映膀胱出口梗阻情况下膀胱的部分代偿增生。膀胱出口梗阻包括解剖上梗阻（如后尿道瓣膜）或是功能上梗阻（如逼尿肌-括约肌协同失调）(图 116-3)[39]。测定排尿后的残余尿量是评价患者是否能够完全排空膀胱的好方法。

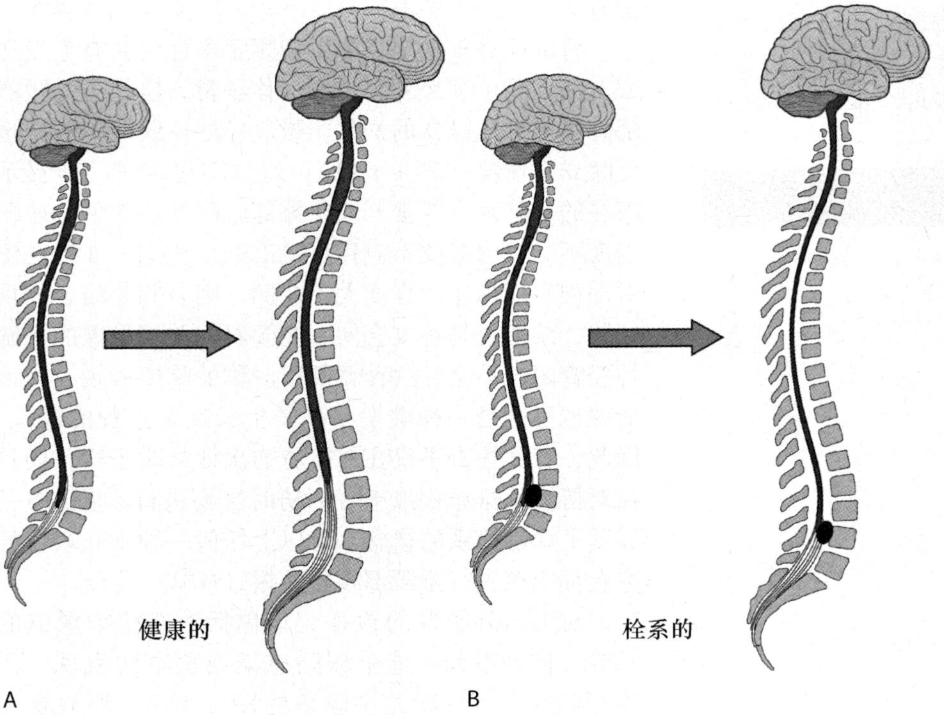

图 116-2　A. 正常的脊髓。脊柱骨生长快于脊髓。结果脊髓提升到较高的位置。B. 合并有脊髓脂肪瘤的异常脊髓解剖。当脊髓生长时，脊髓束不能向上浮起且被拉伸。这种拉伸导致了远端脊髓束的相对供氧不足，接着造成远段脊髓的神经损伤。

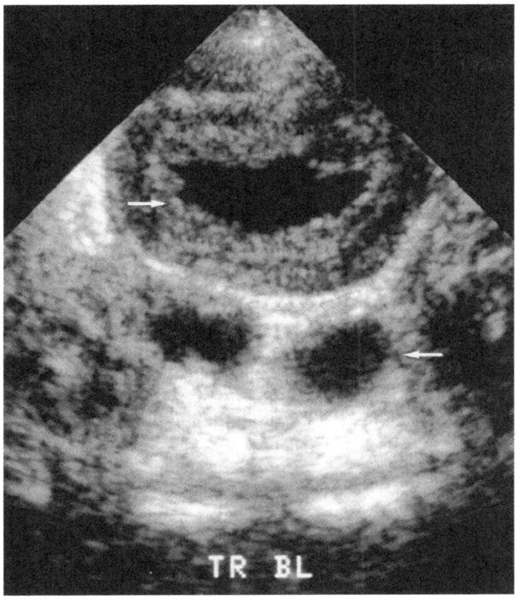

图 116-3　后尿道瓣膜患儿的膀胱超声。注意膀胱壁明显增厚（*左箭头*）和输尿管远端扩张（*右箭头*）。

排尿性膀胱尿路造影

将放射造影剂灌注入膀胱可以提供膀胱、膀胱颈和尿道的解剖学信息。图 116-4 提示了神经性膀胱功
07 能紊乱患者的典型放射学表现。由于慢性的高压性尿潴留，膀胱壁增厚且形成多发性憩室。在许多情况下排尿造影阶段提供了最有价值的信息，因为只有在这个时候膀胱颈部和尿道才能得到适当评估。这方面的典型例子是后尿道瓣膜的患者。膀胱颈部和梗阻近端的尿道明显扩张，膀胱本身出现小梁和形成憩室。不论是解剖上还是功能上的膀胱出口梗阻，患者膀胱输尿管反流都很常见。

尿流动力学评估

尿流动力学检查能够帮助深入了解膀胱功能信息。它能记录膀胱容量、膀胱充盈压、膀胱充盈时患者的感觉以及膀胱颈部有效开放的能力和逼尿肌是否能与外括约肌协同排尿。

在放置尿流动力学检查导管前，要求患儿排尿测定尿流率。然后将导管经尿道放入膀胱（或经耻骨上

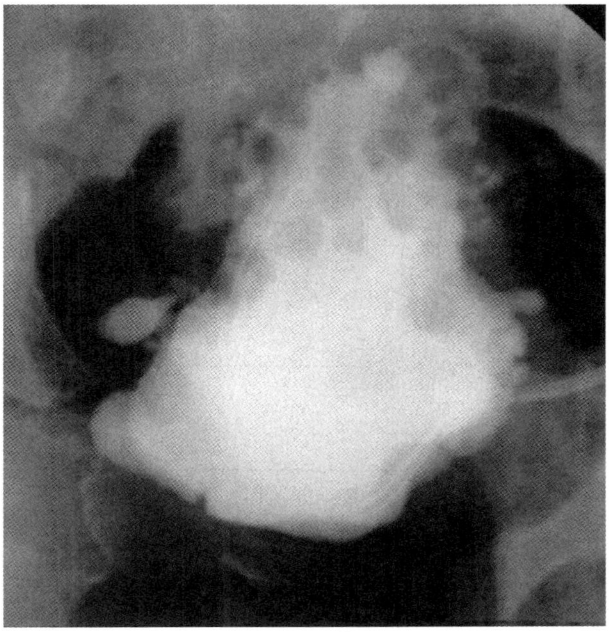

图 116-4　一例继发于脊髓脊膜膨出的神经性膀胱患儿的典型排尿性膀胱尿路造影图像。膀胱壁的顶部较基底部增厚，呈现“圣诞树”样的影像。

膀胱穿刺放置导尿管），测定膀胱内压力。膀胱压测定后，排空膀胱并测定残余尿和该残余量时膀胱的压力[43]。这项技术被证明能有效测定膀胱是否存在高静止压。接着将肌电图测定电极放置在会阴部，电极可以是表面电极，也可用针形电极直接刺入外括约肌复合体内。通过这些电极对肌肉电活动的记录来测定膀胱充盈和排空时外括约肌的功能。通常情况下，外括约肌在储尿阶段是活跃的。在要排尿前膀胱颈部放松时外括约肌变成静止状态（图 116-5A）。括约肌在排尿前不能放松称为逼尿肌-括约肌协同失调。这种现象通常在神经性膀胱功能障碍的患者身上可以记录到（图 116-5B）。

然后向膀胱内缓慢注入生理盐水来测量膀胱容量，而且测定压力-容量之间的关系来了解膀胱壁的顺应性。期望的膀胱容量百分比由患者实际容量除以根据年龄测算的正常容量后取得[44]。在充盈阶段注意记录膀胱有无非抑制性收缩，它反映了膀胱的敏感性。图 116-6 显示了顺应性膀胱和低顺应性、不稳定性膀胱的压力描记图的区别。充盈阶段注意记录漏尿点时压力。

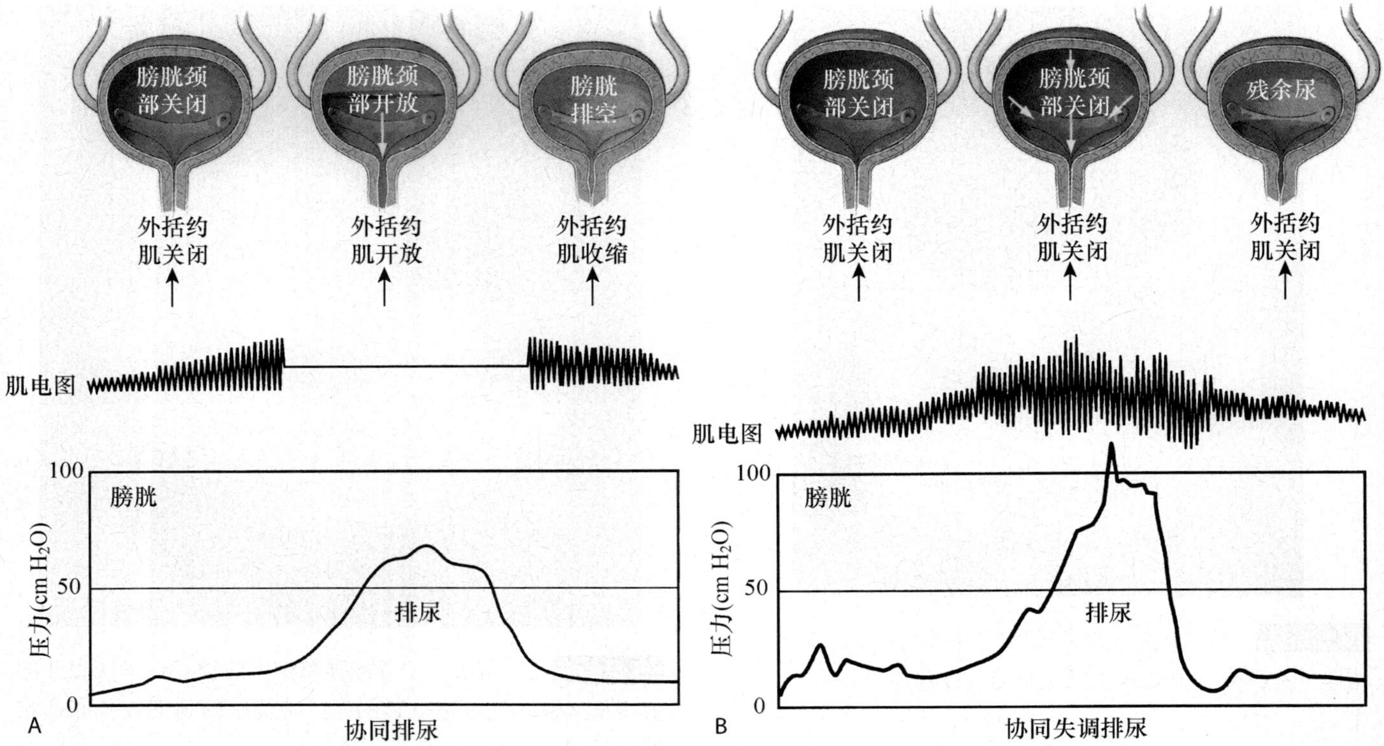

图 116-5 A. 协同排尿。尿道外括约肌的电活动持续活跃。在逼尿肌收缩前，外括约肌活动静止使得尿道阻力明显下降并易于以后的排空。*底部曲线*代表膀胱内压。B. 不协调排尿。在神经性膀胱功能紊乱的病例中，通常可以看到膀胱和括约肌活动的不协调。当膀胱开始收缩时，外括约肌活动增强，导致了出口压增高和有效排尿失败。*底部曲线*代表膀胱内压。

膀胱功能障碍的神经性因素

继发于脊髓发育不良的神经性膀胱

脊髓发育不良，定义为脊椎管和脊髓的发育异
1808 常，是造成神经性膀胱最常见的原因。遗传因素也起了部分作用。如果家庭中有一个脊髓发育不良的孩子，则每个弟妹可能有 2%~5% 的概率再次发生这种情况。早期研究报道发病率为 1/1000[69]。但是，在最近 20 年发病率有了稳定下降。这可能与普遍的围生期补充叶酸（一种脊髓正常形成的重要代谢物）以及终止妊娠有关[10,61]。日常饮食补充叶酸能够减少大约 50% 的脊髓发育不良发病率。

最常见的脊髓发育不良包括脑脊膜脱垂（脑脊膜膨出）以及在许多病例中出现的神经组织（脊髓脊膜突出）超出了椎管腔范围。对脊髓发育不良的孩子（图 116-7）首先应进行泌尿系评估，包括肾脏超声和排尿性膀胱尿路造影。另外，要经常进行间歇性

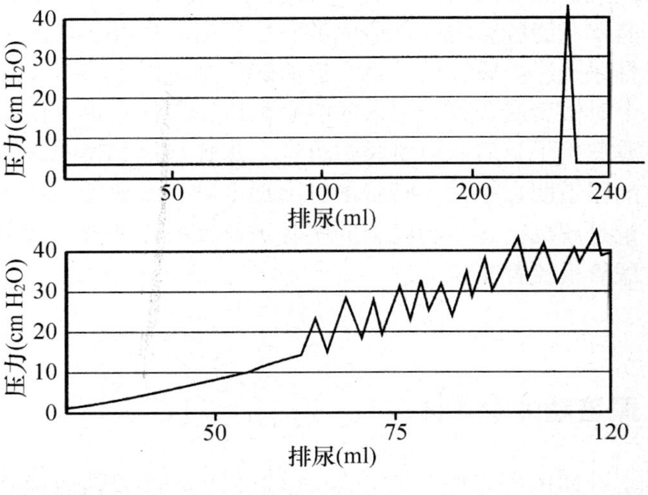

图 116-6 顺应性好的膀胱和低顺应性膀胱的典型尿流动力学描记。*上图*，顺应性好的膀胱。当膀胱充盈时，许多因素作用使得保持低膀胱内压直到开始排尿收缩。*下图*，逼尿肌反射亢进之低顺应性膀胱。当膀胱充盈时，膀胱内压力急剧上升。功能障碍的逼尿肌的激惹性通过许多小的压力曲线反映出来（比如无抑制收缩）。

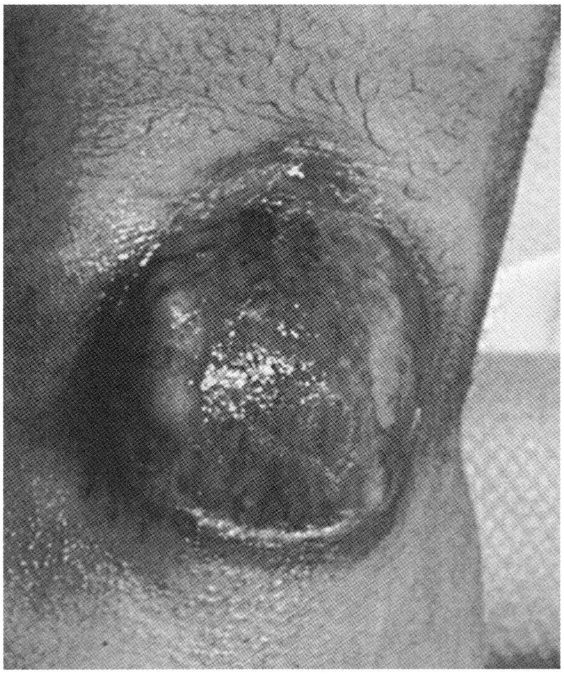

图 116-7 一例脊髓发育不良患儿的照片。脊髓束及合并的脂肪瘤脱出，有表皮覆盖。

清洁导尿（CIC）来测定孩子是否持续有残余尿增多。肾脏超声可以了解是否有肾积水。15% 的新生儿可能被检查出泌尿道异常，3% 显示因为脊髓椎管闭合障碍继发肾输尿管积水，10% 膀胱出口梗阻引
309 起下尿路功能异常（可能是高膀胱内压力的反映）继而发生子宫内畸形[2,7]。肾脏超声还可用以检查评估肾融合畸形，这在脊髓发育不良患者中较为常见[38]。

排尿性膀胱尿路造影检查的目的是发现膀胱输尿管反流，这种情况存在于 3%~5% 的脊髓发育不良新生儿[20]。反流常发生在那些逼尿肌张力高或逼尿肌-括约肌协同失调的孩子身上。如果没有恰当的措施来降低膀胱内压力，经常处于膀胱高压的孩子大约 30% 会产生新的反流。如前所述，做几次导尿可以决定膀胱是否能有效排空。如果随意导尿测定的膀胱容量超过了和年龄对应的预测容量，则应教会父母亲出院后进行一天 3 次的 CIC[44]。

泌尿系统随访内容包括在出生后 3 个月时进行尿流动力学检查。不鼓励更早地进行此检查，因为婴儿椎管闭合损伤将持续到 2 个月。尿流动力学检查有两个目的。第一，它作为基线以供将来动力学评估比较。尿流动力曲线的变化可能最早（通常在下肢功能变化前）提示在脊髓脊膜膨出关闭后发生了脊髓栓系，可能需要外科手术干预。

尿流动力学评估的第二个目的是测定膀胱总的储尿特点和括约肌的功能。可以进行膀胱收缩性和外括约肌活动的三种特殊结合情况的评定。Bauer 等人发现 19% 的患者表现出协同排尿，45% 的患者为协同失调排尿，余下 36% 的患者将表现为完全的失神经支配状况[3]。这种分类系统对于预测长期的肾脏和膀胱功能很重要，从而确定出哪些人可能得益于积极的治疗来减轻进展性的泌尿道损伤。Bauer 等人还指出在出生后 3 年内，排尿协同失调的患者发生泌尿道损伤的几率很高。他们发现 71% 的逼尿肌-括约肌失调的新生儿有泌尿道损伤，这可以在初查或以后的研究中发现；相反，相似的变化只发生于 17% 的协同排尿儿童以及 23% 的完全失神经支配的个体身上。值得注意的是，少数协同排尿或者失神经排尿并最终被证明发生上尿路损害的患儿会转变为高出口阻力。

对于继发于脊髓脊膜膨出的神经性膀胱功能障碍患者必须进行经常随访，因为他们的膀胱功能会随着时间变化（该变化可能影响上尿路和控尿）。有许多引起膀胱动力学变化的原因，最重要的是脊髓栓系[52]。

治疗神经性膀胱的基本目的是保护肾脏和膀胱的功能。一旦孩子到达控尿年龄，就要增加其他以控尿为目的的治疗。CIC 和抗胆碱能药物是治疗的基础，可以保证低压储尿。Edelstein 等证明如果积极有效地应用 CIC 和抗胆碱能药物治疗高风险患者——即那些具有高出口阻力、逼尿肌-括约肌协同失调或高收缩性膀胱（所谓对抗膀胱动力）者，上尿路损伤的概率明显减少[17]。Keaefer 等人接着用大量患者证明应用上述治疗后膀胱功能得到了长期保护（图 116-8）[44]。在他们的研究中发现因膀胱长期恶化而需要外科膀胱扩大术的患者比例减少了 2.5 倍。如果用这些药物治疗不足以降低膀胱内压，而且在出生后几年内出现进展性的肾盂积水，则需要进行外科皮肤膀胱造口手术。

同样对尿失禁最初也采取保守治疗（比如 CIC 和抗胆碱能药物）来降低膀胱内压。如果这些措施不能充分改善膀胱容量和顺应性，就可以应用肠膀胱成形术来扩大膀胱[27,65]。手术可以提供足够的膀胱出口

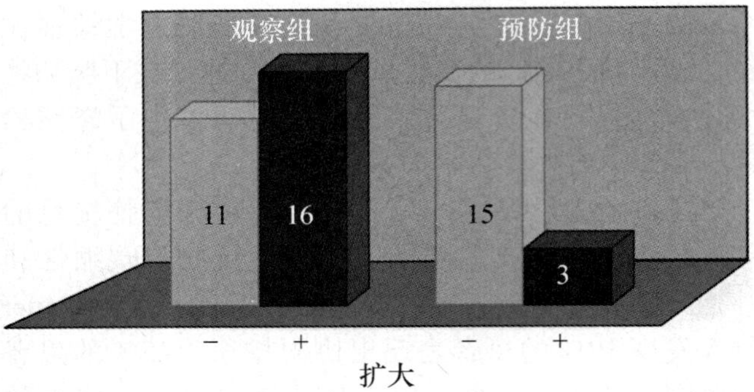

图 116-8 脊髓脊膜膨出患者相关治疗后膀胱恶化的发生率。观察组的患者是那些在出生时就被注意到有对抗膀胱动力存在，但只是在上尿路恶化或失禁更严重的情况下才进行间歇性导尿和抗胆碱能药物治疗来降低膀胱内压。这组患者平均治疗时间开始于 4.1 岁。预防组的患者也属于此类型，但在出生后 3 个月内便进行治疗来降低膀胱内压。观察组行膀胱扩大的几率是预防组的 2 倍多，差异具有统计学意义（42% 比 17%）。（From Kaefer M，Pabby A，Kelly M，et al：Improved bladder function after prophylactic treatment of the high risk neurogenic bladder in newborns with myelomeningocele. J Urol 1999；162：1068.）

阻力维持稳定的控尿状态[16]。

1810 隐匿性脊髓栓系症

一些先天性的缺陷可能会影响脊髓的发育，但是并没有导致椎管腔的开放。这样的缺陷发生率大约为 1/4000 活产儿[6]。这些损害可能不会引起明显的神经体征，但很多会在脊椎下段出现皮肤异常（见体格检查部分）。肛门直肠畸形患儿的脊髓栓系发生率高（大于 50%），有报道病变程度和直肠病变的程度成正比[24,68,70]。但是，一项近期研究提出直肠病变在提肌上和在提肌下患者之间没有明显的差别[24]。所有在脊柱下段有皮肤异常或有肛门直肠畸形的患者均应进行 MRI 检查以了解脊髓的病变情况[58]。出生后 6 个月内可用超声评估脊髓栓系[13]。

隐匿性脊髓栓系症的泌尿系统症状可出现如厕训练困难、获得尿控后又出现尿失禁（尤其在青春期当生长迅速引起脊髓束张力增加时）、复发性尿路感染或污裤（或以上症状同时发生）等。

虽然大多数发现有隐匿性脊髓栓系症的新生儿的体格检查可以极为正常，但 1/3 患者在 18 个月前的尿流动力学检查中可以显示下尿路的功能异常[45]。相反，实际上所有没有经历过手术的隐匿性神经管闭合不全的个体在 3 岁后都有异常的尿流动力学表现。

一旦 MRI 发现有脊髓栓系的征象（比如脊髓圆锥位于第二腰椎以下或有明显的椎管内脂肪瘤），应该做出判断是否需要神经外科干预。神经损伤的第一信号常常为尿流动力学表现异常。因而对所有 MRI 阳性表现的患者均应行尿流动力学检查。如果决定不纠正脊髓栓系，就应该每年随访尿流动力学检查，这样可以尽早察觉到将来的神经缺陷而及时采取适当的预防措施，防止发生不可逆的神经损伤。

骶骨发育不全

骶骨发育不全的患者通常会有神经性膀胱功能不全。骶骨发育不全的病因还不明确。然而现在发现胰岛素依赖的母亲有 1% 的机会产出该畸形的孩子，而且 16% 的骶骨发育不全患儿有患糖尿病的母亲[63,72]。因为这些患儿下肢感觉正常，只有极少或没有整形外科畸形，所以潜在的病变常常被忽略。约 20% 有这种情况的患儿直到 3～4 岁才被检查出来[25]。本病较为典型的表现是臀部扁平和低位短小的臀纹。脊椎下段侧位片显示骶椎缺失可以明确诊断。所有患者的腰骶椎 MRI 都显示 T12 椎体突然中断征象[62]。尿流动力学实验显示，几乎同等数量的患儿分别表现出上运动神经元（比如张力亢进、反射亢进）和下运动神经元（张力低下）的病变（30% *vs* 40%），但是 25% 的患者没有膀胱功能障碍的表现[5]。病变椎骨的数量与神经元病变类型没有关系。与脊髓发育不良或隐匿性脊髓束畸形病变相比，本病的损害较为稳定。很少看到随着这些患儿的长大出现进展性的去神经支配样的尿流动力学改变。用抗胆碱能药物来治疗无抑制收缩或放松高张逼尿肌，或两者兼用，但 CIC 只用来治疗膀胱排空能力差的患者。

脑瘫

脑瘫是指发生于围生期的一种大脑非进展性的

损伤（比如缺氧），往往会导致神经肌肉功能低下[50]，发病率为新生儿的 1/1000。很小的早产儿
811 在重症监护室存活率升高后，脑瘫的发病率也增高。虽然在尿流动力学检查中发现占较高百分比的患儿有无抑制性收缩，但大多数患儿有能力完全控制排尿[12]。尿失禁最常在身体不便而不能及时去卫生间的情况下发生的。因此，患儿获得控制排尿能力比预想的年龄晚，要到患儿适应以后。适当开设足够的残疾人便利通道将为许多具有这种情况的患儿提供很大帮助。

由于脑瘫患儿面临许多身体上的问题，因而尿流动力学检查只用于那些看上去是可以训练的、不会因为身体损害造成太大障碍的以及在儿童后期还没有实际控制能力的患儿。同样，只有在出现了泌尿道感染时才进行上下尿路的造影。

通常治疗以应用抗胆碱能药物去除无抑制性收缩为中心，但是必须严密监测残余尿量以确保每次排尿时完全排空。CIC 用于那些不能自行排空膀胱的患儿。这些患儿还有严重的便秘倾向，大多是因为摄水少和身体活动受到限制造成的。便秘可能破坏膀胱的稳定和排空，经证明对这些患儿采取通便治疗对尿失禁亦有益处。对保守治疗没有反应的小部分患儿经选择性背部神经切断术可以改善膀胱功能、减少无抑制性收缩和增加顺应性[35]。

膀胱功能障碍的解剖学因素

后尿道瓣膜

儿童群体中最多见的解剖性膀胱出口梗阻因素为男孩的后尿道瓣膜。其他造成膀胱出口梗阻的原因有尿道狭窄、前尿道憩室和位于膀胱出口部位的梗阻性输尿管囊肿[1,36,55]。

后尿道瓣膜的发生率为新生男婴的 1/5000 ~ 1/8000。儿童中临床表现多种多样，主要取决于梗阻的程度。因尿道瓣膜造成严重膀胱出口梗阻的新生男婴，其典型表现为腹部中线可能触诊到包块（扩张膀胱）、有腹水表现（肾脏的尿渗漏）或两者皆有。在大多数严重病例中，患儿由于在宫内肺发育期缺少羊水导致肺发育不全，出生后可出现呼吸窘迫的情况。如果儿童在较大年龄时才发现后尿道瓣膜，则梗阻常不严重。这些患儿典型首发表现为出现排尿功能障碍、泌尿道感染和极其偶然的肾衰竭征象（比如身材矮小）。今天，随着产前超声的广泛开展，大多数膀胱出口梗阻的男孩在出生前就可以得到诊断[8]。

尿道的解剖性梗阻导致了肾和膀胱的病理改变，如膀胱壁增厚、憩室形成以及后尿道不同程度扩张（图 116-9）。30% ~ 50% 的患者有膀胱输尿管反流。

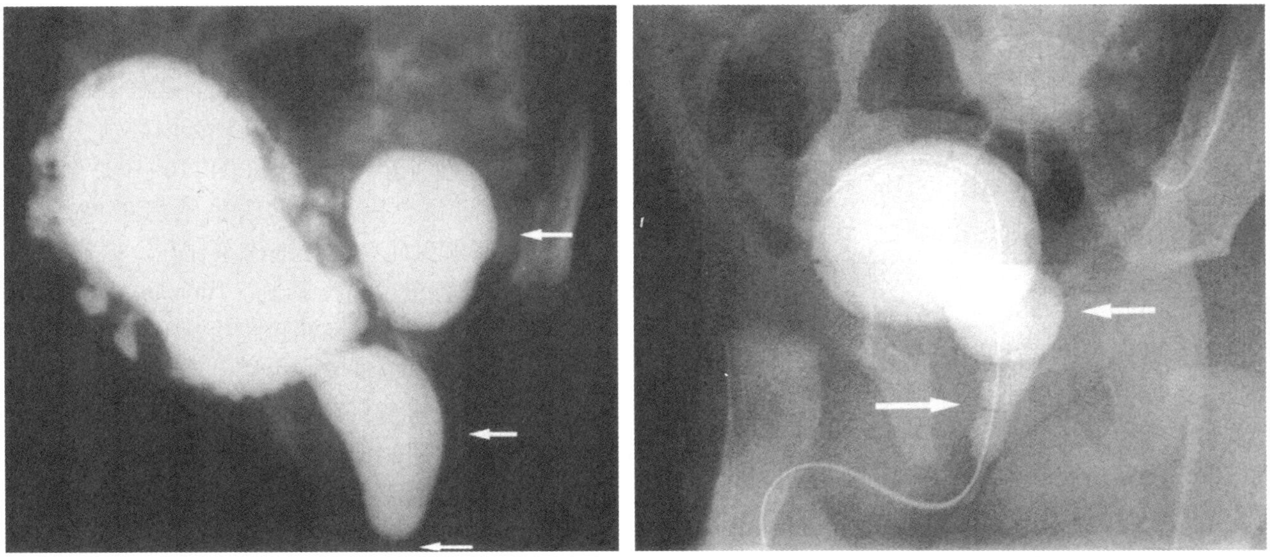

A　B

图 116-9　后尿道瓣膜患儿排尿性膀胱尿路造影。A. 严重病例表现出膀胱代偿功能不全，有多发性的大小憩室（*最上方箭头*）、扩张的后尿道（*中间箭头*）。*下面箭头* 显示瓣膜梗阻的位置。B. 膀胱轻度变化的病例。*上面箭头* 指扩张的后尿道。*下面箭头* 指后尿道瓣膜本身产生的阴影。

1812 这些患者中大约有 1/3 一旦梗阻解除后反流可以缓解。但是即使没有膀胱输尿管反流，上尿路仍然会有损伤，这是因为下尿路功能障碍导致了膀胱壁增厚。膀胱的组织学表现为细胞的肥大和细胞外基质的沉积，导致低膀胱容量和顺应性下降。

内镜下瓣膜叶的切除几乎可以安全地用于所有足月儿。当患儿尿道太小不能容纳膀胱镜时可以采用顺行瓣膜切开[73]。虽然电灼电极是最常用的切除瓣膜的设备，但电钩、钕: YAG 激光和顺行球囊导管治疗同样有效[11,18,48]。

当尿道梗阻解除后，膀胱功能障碍可能会继续存在。最多见的膀胱功能障碍表现为白天尿失禁并可持续到上学年龄以后。最初认为存在尿失禁是因为内镜下行瓣膜切除时损伤了尿道括约肌，或是因为最初的梗阻导致了膀胱括约肌的异常发育，或两者皆有。但是对这些患儿的尿流动力学检查却清楚显示，在瓣膜切除后仍看到膀胱功能障碍持续存在。许多研究者证明有三种原发性逼尿肌功能异常表现：膀胱张力亢进、逼尿肌反射亢进和逼尿肌瘫痪[4,22,40,64]。进一步研究显示，随着患儿长大，尿流动力学表现会有所改变。一项由 Holmdahl 等人进行的研究证明，许多新生儿期收缩亢进且低顺应性的患儿后来的尿流动力学显示出与逼尿肌瘫痪相关[33,34]。许多继发于后尿道瓣膜的膀胱功能障碍的患儿也表现出异常的膀胱感觉和不能感觉到膀胱胀满[47]。除了持续性膀胱功能障碍外，通常存在的问题是肾损伤和并发的尿液浓缩功能低下。大量的残余尿加重了下尿路功能障碍。

对后尿道瓣膜患儿功能障碍膀胱的治疗是依据其功能障碍的严重程度和性质以及膀胱排空能力。有高压排尿动力学表现的患儿往往可以得益于抗胆碱能药物治疗来改善顺应性。对于年幼的自然排空膀胱能力受损的患儿需要进行 CIC。如果大年龄患儿能够坚持严格按时间排尿，则可以不进行白天的导尿。近来 Koff 和助手提倡夜间留置导尿以提供有效的膀胱排空，通过改善夜间引流证明了肾积水和膀胱顺应性的明显改观[46,47]。虽然保守治疗通常对改进膀胱动力而取得效果（保持膀胱容量足够低来维持可接受的膀胱压），但一小部分患者仍需要行膀胱扩大来改善膀胱容量和顺应性[40]。后尿道瓣膜患儿的尿道感觉常没有变化，并且许多患儿通过阴茎导尿时感觉到疼痛。可以在前腹壁建立一个可控性导尿通道，这样可以改善生活质量，通过导尿改善膀胱的顺应性[42]。

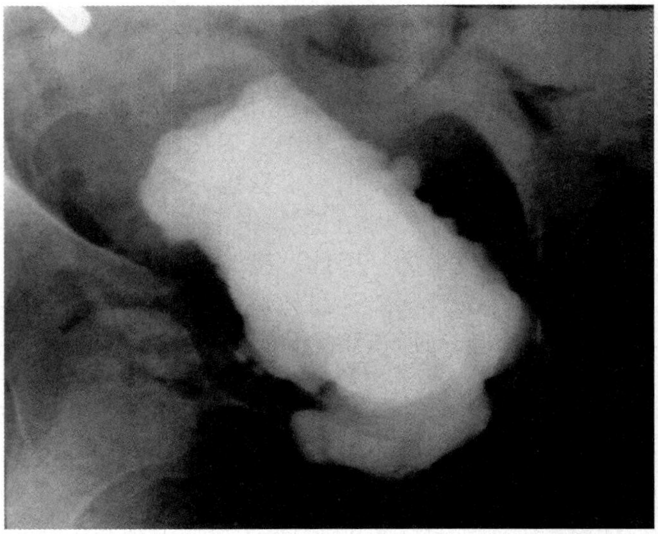

图 116-10　一例 Hinman 综合征患儿排尿性膀胱尿路造影。膀胱壁增厚后产生了明显的膀胱轮廓不规则表现。

非神经性、非解剖性膀胱功能障碍

排出功能障碍综合征

非解剖性膀胱出口梗阻或神经性疾病引起的膀胱功能障碍通常被称为排尿功能障碍。这个定义还包括与尿液潴留相关的各种症状。该综合征中最严重的情况指那些重度尿潴留的患儿表现出膀胱解剖上的变化，如上尿路的扩张和瘢痕形成。这些表现实际上与在神经性膀胱功能障碍中的表现难以区别（所以称之为非神经源性神经性膀胱）（图 116-10）[29,30]。如放射学发现问题严重则提示医生给患者做腰骶部的 MRI，以了解患儿有无脊髓栓系存在。尿流动力学检查表现为低容量、高压膀胱。Hinman 综合征的治疗方法类似于真正的神经性膀胱功能不全。结合抗胆碱能药物和 CIC 来降低膀胱内压。如果保守治疗不足以降低膀胱储尿压力，则进行膀胱扩大。与真正的神经 18
性病变患者不同的是，许多这种患儿有导尿疼痛感且可以从前腹壁的可控性尿流改道手术中受益。

另一方面，大多数有该综合征的患儿由于有相关的尿潴留表现而具有进展性排尿刺激症状和高度尿路感染的倾向。在过去十年里，逐步明确了许多患者有便秘。大量的粪便负荷可能对膀胱功能造成明显的损伤。因此，现在排出功能障碍综合征的概念越来越常

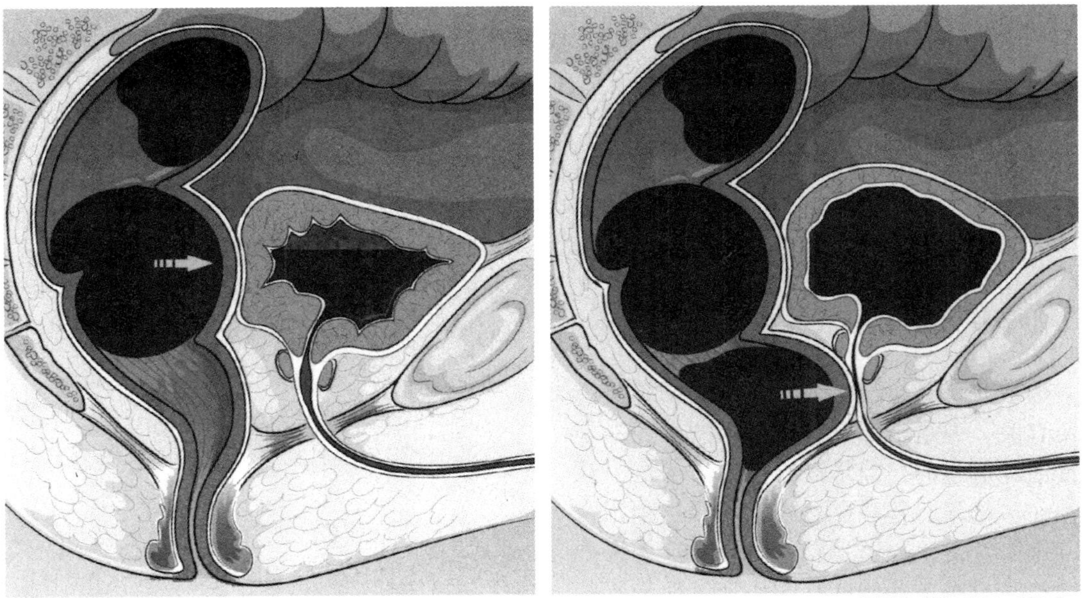

© IUSM, Office Of visual Media
C. M. Brown

图 116-11　便秘对膀胱功能的影响。*左图*，直肠内粪便可以提升膀胱后部，导致膀胱的不稳定。*右图*，严重的便秘可以造成对膀胱颈部外在的压迫，阻碍膀胱的排空。

见，很大程度上取代了排尿功能障碍。

有这种情况的患儿经常不能完全排空肠道或膀胱。结果膀胱排空差，导致膀胱持续性的扩张，使患儿有急迫性尿失禁的倾向。如果患儿不能完全排空膀胱，那么膀胱常达到充盈状态，可表现为尿频的症状。排尿后大量的残余尿导致患儿有尿路感染的倾向。便秘时由于粪块影响到膀胱的后部，可能引起膀胱刺激表现，而且对于严重的病例还可以阻碍膀胱的排空（图 116-11）。Dohil 等人证明在对便秘患儿进行肠道治疗后改善了膀胱排空功能，排尿后残余尿由治疗前的 66% 下降到治疗后的 21%[15]。慢性便秘与明显的肛门内括约肌肥大及异常的肛门括约肌肌电图表现是有关系的[54]。这可以使尿道括约肌和盆底活动增加，也就解释了与排尿失调以及不完全排空的相关关系。

放射影像学如有以下表现常高度提示该综合征的诊断，即腹部平片上看到大量粪块、膀胱超声发现大量残余尿以及在排尿性膀胱尿路造影中发现膀胱颈部的“陀螺状”影像（图 116-12）。

对排出障碍综合征患儿的治疗有：（1）定时排尿，即要求患儿每两小时排一次尿；（2）双排尿，即要求患儿在感觉排空膀胱后再次排尿（尽量减少大量残余尿量的几率）；（3）建立良好的排便习惯，可以通过食用纤维素、应用大便软化剂以及用足够的时

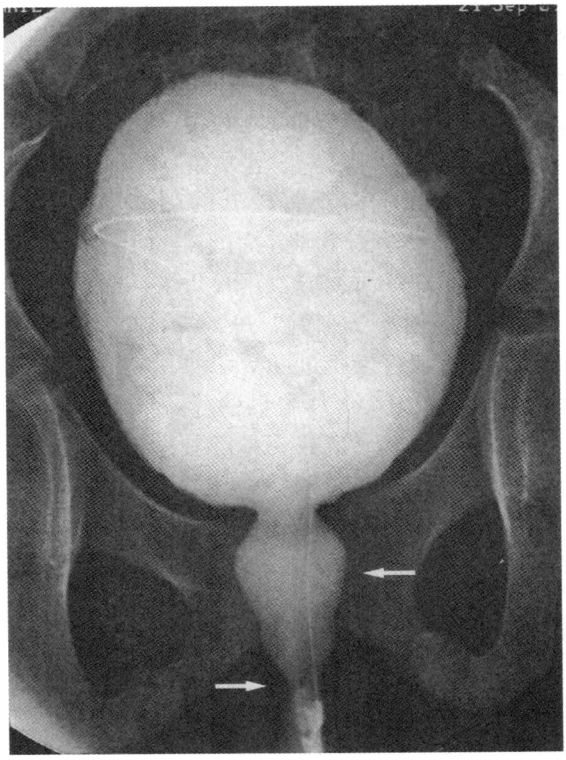

图 116-12　一例排出功能障碍综合征患儿的排尿性膀胱尿路造影，显示出膀胱充盈时有小憩室和远端尿道的扩张（*上面箭头*）。*下面箭头* 指的是外括约肌的位置，因为不能放松导致近端尿道成球囊状（称为陀螺状畸形）。

间去完成排空来养成。应用适当的足底部支托器可能对身体取得平衡状态十分有利，从而得到足够的放松。当这些保守方法不能使排尿/排便充分放松时，生物反馈法则是有效的方法。许多方法被用来进行生物反馈，包括视频游戏法[28]。

膀胱过度活动综合征

虽然大多数被儿科医生诊断为尿失禁和尿频的患儿多与尿潴留有关，但是小部分有该症状的患儿却是因为膀胱过度活动造成的，但是没有证据证明这些儿童存在神经损伤。结果，膀胱充盈或即便只达到正常
1814 膀胱容量的一半时常常也会诱发膀胱收缩。这类患儿既没有尿潴留也没有肠道功能紊乱的表现，而且膀胱超声测定显示残余尿不多。对于这种情况的有效治疗方法是抗胆碱能药物治疗。这些药物是乙酰胆碱竞争性抑制剂，能够阻断神经递质的毒蕈碱效应。抗胆碱能药物治疗效果明显。主要的副作用有口干、面红和便秘。最突出的问题是便秘，因为膀胱过度活动的患儿有便秘的倾向，而便秘又会加剧膀胱过度活动，因而抵消了药物的疗效。奥昔布宁（0.2 mg/kg，每天2～3次）是最常用的抗胆碱能药物。托特罗定是新的用于成人的抗胆碱能药物，显示了与奥昔布宁相似的较好的治疗效果，而具有较低的副作用发生率[56]。托特罗定还能安全有效地应用于儿童[32]。托特罗定的普通剂量是0.01 mg/kg，每天2次。对于那些已经耐受药物治疗的孩子来讲，每天1次的支持-松弛运动也是一种方法。膀胱过度活动症有自限性，即使是最顽固的病例在18个月内也会缓解[9]。如抗胆碱能药物治疗不能缓解，就需要对该患者进行彻底的尿流动力学检查。

夜间遗尿

不管是膀胱功能的问题，还是夜间没有足够的尿液浓缩功能，或与夜间难于觉醒有关，夜间尿床的问题通常在膀胱功能障碍章节中讨论[31]。各种研究显示在7岁以上的孩子中，单纯夜间遗尿的发生率为6%～10%。5～20岁患儿中自发痊愈率平均为15%[21]，许多遗尿的患儿最终可以正常控尿。

夜间遗尿是一种与遗传有关的多种起源的复杂疾病。从发病上来讲，遗传因素起了重要作用。50%的患儿具有阳性家族病史。在家族中，不同成员的湿裤方式可以相同，也可以不同。研究表明夜间遗尿的发生率在同卵双胞胎中为46%，在异卵双胞胎中为19%[37]。最常见的遗传方式为常染色体显性遗传。

各种病理生理学机制都在起作用，包括夜间多尿、夜间膀胱过度活动且膀胱容量小以及觉醒障碍[14]。而且，这些异常可以同时存在。人类尿液的产生有明显的生理周期，夜间尿量较白天减少50%以上。这种周期在儿童由夜间释放精氨酸抗利尿激素增多控制，就如血管紧张素Ⅱ和醛固酮一样[66,67]。长期以来，发现一些夜间遗尿的患儿其夜间产尿明显多于非遗尿的孩子。这些孩子对类似精氨酸抗利尿激素的去氨加压素（DDAVP）反应良好[59]。虽然发现一部分遗尿患儿的夜间功能膀胱容量较小，但是单纯夜间遗尿患儿膀胱功能异常的情况却相当少见。不论尿床是源于尿液浓缩能力、夜间功能性膀胱容量，还是其他一些还未发现的原因，尿床发生时不能觉醒的现象比较突出。这使许多人坚信睡眠障碍是遗尿症的根本原因，遗尿症患儿总是处于深睡眠状态。然而大量研究仍不能有力证明睡眠方式的异常。

夜间遗尿的治疗有许多方法。如果可能，白天的排尿异常症状应该给予纠正。应该要求患儿有规律排尿和避免在感到膀胱胀满后仍延迟排尿。与治疗便秘一样，尿急和尿频症状都应处理。有报道在便秘充分控制后，遗尿症的治愈达72%以上[53]。为了减少夜间多尿，上床前数小时就应限制进水。午后和晚饭的
低钙、低钠饮食可能也有帮助作用。应该教患儿在睡 18
前排尿，以减少夜间膀胱内尿量。

6岁以后仍有遗尿应该用药物、尿床警报仪器或两者皆用结合治疗。去氨加压素较易给药且对于控制尿量非常有效。睡前口服剂量为0.2和0.6 mg，或鼻内剂量为20和40 μg。在许多试验中报道，有60%～70%的患者对去氨加压素有反应（定义为可减少50%的夜间尿床量）[23]。其他意见包括应用三环抗抑郁药丙米嗪（盐酸丙米嗪），可以直接作用于膀胱平滑肌而且起到拟交感作用。与抗胆碱能药物相对较短的半衰期不同，血液中丙米嗪水平的增强需要数天，因而这种药物真正显效常需要2周时间。大约50%的遗尿患儿应用后有效，但是若不坚持治疗，有相当一部分患儿会复发。有报道只有17%的患儿在丙米嗪治疗期间能做到干燥，并且在停药6个月后还能继续

保持[60]。丙米嗪治疗的主要缺点是对心脏的毒副作用，即便是治疗剂量时仍然存在[71]。虽然并不期望抗胆碱能药物能有效治疗真正的单纯性夜间遗尿症，但这种药物偶尔还是有效的。

警铃治疗是夜间遗尿最有效的治疗方法。对全世界文献的 meta 分析显示有 68% 的平均成功率[31]。据报道在治疗时间达 6 个月时的效果可高达 90%[57]。虽然许多患儿不能觉醒，但是他们在警报响起时会停止排尿。因此，要求父母亲能帮助唤醒患儿并带去洗手间排尿。一旦内衣更换后应重新安置警报器。警报器治疗的实际机制还不明了，但是显然属于行为治疗的范畴。

（何 蓉译 文建国校）

参考文献

1. Austin PF, Cain MP, Casale AJ, et al: Prenatal bladder outlet obstruction secondary to ureterocele. Urology 1998;52:1132.
2. Bauer S: The management of spina bifida from birth onwards. In Whitaker RH, Woodard JR (eds): Paediatric Urology. London, Butterworths, 1985, p 87.
3. Bauer S, Hallet M, Khoshbin S: The predictive value of urodynamic evaluation in the newborn with myelodysplasia. JAMA 1984;152:650.
4. Bauer SB, Dieppa RA, Labib KK, et al: The bladder in boys with posterior urethral valves: A urodynamic assessment. J Urol 1979;121:769.
5. Boemers T, Van Gool J, deJong T, et al: Urodynamic evaluation of children with caudal regression syndrome (caudal dysplasia sequence). J Urol 1994;151:1038.
6. Bruce D, Schut L: Spinal lipomas in infancy and childhood. Brain 1979;5:92.
7. Chiaramonte R, Horowitz E, Kaplan G: Implications of hydronephrosis in newborns with myelodysplasia. J Urol 1986;136:427.
8. Cromie WJ, Lee K, Houde K, et al: Implications of prenatal ultrasound screening in the incidence of major genitourinary malformations. J Urol 2001;165:1677.
9. Curran MJ, Kaefer M, Peters C, et al: The overactive bladder in childhood: Long-term results with conservative management. J Urol 2000;163:574.
10. Czeizel A, Dudas I: Prevention of the first occurrence of neural-tube defects by preconceptual vitamin supplementation. N Engl J Med 1992;321:1832.
11. Deane AM, Whitaker RH, Sherwood T: Diathermy hook ablation of posterior urethral valves in neonates and infants. Br J Urol 1988;62:593.
12. Decter RM, Bauer SB, Khoshbin S, et al: Urodynamic assessment of children with cerebral palsy. J Urol 1987; 138:1110.
13. Dick EA, Patel K, Owens CM, et al: Spinal ultrasound in infants. Br J Radiol 2002;75:384.
14. Djurhuus JC, Rittig S: Current trends, diagnosis, and treatment of enuresis. Eur Urol 1998;33(Suppl 3):30.
15. Dohil R, Roberts E, Jones KV, et al: Constipation and reversible urinary tract abnormalities. Arch Dis Child 1994;70:56.
16. Donnahoo KK, Rink RC, Cain MP, et al: The Young-Dees-Leadbetter bladder neck repair for neurogenic incontinence. J Urol 1999;161:1946.
17. Edelstein RA, Bauer SB, Kelly MD, et al: The long-term urological response of neonates with myelodysplasia treated proactively with intermittent catheterization and anticholinergic therapy. J Urol 1995;154:1500.
18. Ehrlich RM, Shanberg A, Fine RN: Neodymium:YAG laser ablation of posterior urethral valves. J Urol 1987;138:959.
19. Ferrara P, Rossodivita A, Ruggiero A, et al: Cryptorchidism associated with meningomyelocele. J Pediatr Child Health 1998;34:44.
20. Flood H, Ritchey M, Bloom D: Outcome of reflux in children with myelodysplasia managed by bladder pressure monitoring. J Urol 1994;152:1574.
21. Forsythe WI, Redmond A: Enuresis and spontaneous cure rate. Study of 1129 enuretis. Arch Dis Child 1974;49:259.
22. Glassberg KI, Schneider M, Haller JO, et al: Observations on persistently dilated ureter after posterior urethral valve ablation. Urology 1982;20:20.
23. Glazener CMA, Evans JHC: Desmopressin for nocturnal enuresis in children (Cochrane review). Cochrane Database Syst Rev 2000;(2):CD002112.
24. Golonka NR, Haga LJ, Keating RP, et al: Routine MRI evaluation of low imperforate anus reveals unexpected high incidence of tethered spinal cord. J Pediatr Surg 2002;37:966.
25. Guzman L, Bauer S, Hallet M: The evaluation and management of children with sacral agenesis. Urology 1983; 23:506.
26. Hassan JM, Pope JCT, Brock JW 3rd, et al: Vesicoureteral reflux in patients with posterior urethral valves. J Urol 2003; 170:1677.
27. Hendren WH, Hendren RB: Bladder augmentation: Experience with 129 children and young adults. J Urol 1990;144:445.
28. Herndon CD, Decambre M, McKenna PH: Interactive computer games for treatment of pelvic floor dysfunction. J Urol 2001;166:1893.
29. Hinman F: Non-neurogenic neurogenic bladder (the Hinman syndrome): 15 years later. J Urol 1986;136:769.
30. Hinman F, Baumann F: Vesical and ureteral damage from voiding dysfunction in boys without neurologic or obstructive disease. J Urol 1973;109:727.
31. Hjalmas K, Arnold T, Bower W, et al: Nocturnal enuresis: An international evidence based management strategy. J Urol 2004;171:2545.
32. Hjalmas K, Hellstrom AL, Mogren K, et al: The overactive bladder in children: A potential future indication for tolterodine. BJU Int 2001;87:569.
33. Holmdahl G, Sillen U, Bachelard M, et al: The changing urodynamic pattern in valve bladders during infancy. J Urol 1995;153:463.
34. Holmdahl G, Sillen U, Hanson E, et al: Bladder dysfunction in boys with posterior urethral valves before and after puberty. J Urol 1996;155:694.
35. Houle A, Vernot O, RJ: Bladder function before and after sacral rhizotomy in children with cerebral palsy. J Urol 1998; 160:1088.
36. Hsiao KC, Baez-Trinidad L, Lendvay T, et al: Direct vision internal urethrotomy for the treatment of pediatric urethral strictures: Analysis of 50 patients. J Urol 2003;170:952.
37. Hublin C, Kaprio J, Partinen M, et al: Nocturnal enuresis in a nationwide twin cohort. Sleep 1998;21:579.
38. Hunt GM, Whitaker RH: The pattern of congenital renal

anomalies associated with neural-tube defects. Dev Med Child Neurol 1987;29:91.
39. Kaefer M, Barnewolt C, Retik AB, et al: The sonographic diagnosis of infravesical obstruction in children: Evaluation of bladder wall thickness indexed to bladder filling. J Urol 1997;157:989.
40. Kaefer M, Keating MA, Adams MC, et al: Posterior urethral valves, pressure pop-offs and bladder function. J Urol 1995; 154:708.
41. Kaefer M, Pabby A, Kelly M, et al: Improved bladder function after prophylactic treatment of the high risk neurogenic bladder in newborns with myelomeningocele. J Urol 1999; 162:1068.
42. Kaefer M, Retik AB: The Mitrofanoff principle in continent urinary reconstruction. Urol Clin North Am 1997; 24:795.
43. Kaefer M, Rosen A, Darbey M, et al: Pressure at residual volume: A useful adjunct to standard fill cystometry. J Urol 1997;158:1268.
44. Kaefer M, Zurakowski D, Bauer SB, et al: Estimating normal bladder capacity in children. J Urol 1997;158:2261.
45. Keating M, Rink R, Bauer S: Neuro-urologic implications of changing approach in management of occult spinal lesions. J Urol 1988;140:1299.
46. Koff SA, Gigax MR, Jayanthi VR: Nocturnal bladder emptying: A simple technique for reversing urinary tract deterioration in children with neurogenic bladder [abstract 60]. Presented at the 2004 Meeting of the American Academy of Pediatrics.
47. Koff SA, Mutabagani KH, Jayanthi VR: The valve bladder syndrome: Pathophysiology and treatment with nocturnal bladder emptying. J Urol 2002;167:291.
48. Kolicinski Z: Foley balloon procedure in posterior urethral valves. Dialogues Pediatr Urol 1988;11:7.
49. Kropp KA, Voeller KK: Cryptorchidism in meningomyelocele. J Pediatr 1981;99:110.
50. Kuban K, Leviton A: Cerebral palsy. N Engl J Med 1994; 330:188.
51. Lackgren G, Hjalmas K, van Gool J, et al: Nocturnal enuresis: A suggestion for a European treatment strategy. Acta Paediatr 1999;88:679.
52. Lais A, Kasabian N, Dyro F: Neurosurgical implications of continuous neuro-urological surveillance of children with myelodysplasia. J Urol 1993;150:1879.
53. Loening-Baucke V: Urinary incontinence and urinary tract infection and their resolution with treatment of chronic constipation of childhood. Pediatrics 1997;100:228.
54. Lofthouse C, Odeka EB: The problem of constipation in children: Understanding the issues. Gastroenterology 1998;8:68.
55. Merrot T, Chaumoitre K, Shojai R, et al: Fetal bladder rupture due to anterior urethral valves. Urology 2003;61:1259.
56. Millard R, Tuttle J, Moore K, et al: Clinical efficacy and safety of tolterodine compared to placebo in detrusor overactivity. J Urol 1999;161:1551.
57. Moffat MEK: Nocturnal enuresis: A review of the efficacy of treatments and practical advice for clinicians. J Dev Behav Pediatr 1997;18:49.
58. Mosiello G, Capitanucci ML, Gatti C, et al: How to investigate neurovesical dysfunction in children with anorectal malformations. J Urol 2003;170:1610.
59. Neveus T, Tuvemo T, Lackgren G, et al: Bladder capacity and renal concentrating ability in enuresis: Pathogenic implications. J Urol 2001;165:2022.
60. Nijman RJM, Butler R, van Gool J, et al: Conservative management of urinary incontinence in childhood. In Abrams P, Cardozo L, Khoury S, Wein A (eds): Incontinence, 2nd International Consultation on Incontinence, Paris, July 1-3, 2001. Plymouth, United Kingdom, Health Publication, 2002, p 515.
61. Palomaki G, Williams J, Haddow J: Prenatal screening for open neural-tube defects in Maine. N Engl J Med 1999; 340:1049.
62. Pang D: Sacral agenesis and caudal spinal cord malformations. Neurosurgery 1993;32:755.
63. Passarge E, Lenz K: Syndrome of caudal regression in infants of diabetic mothers: Observations of further cases. Pediatrics 1966;37:672.
64. Peters CA, Bolkier M, Bauer SB, et al: The urodynamic consequences of posterior urethral valves. J Urol 1990;144:122.
65. Rink RC: Bladder augmentation. Options, outcomes, future. Urol Clin North Am 1999;26:111.
66. Rittig S, Knudsen UB, Norgaard JP, et al: Abnormal diurnal rhythm of plasma vasopressin and urinary output in patients with enuresis. Am J Physiol 1989;256:F664.
67. Rittig S, Knudsen UB, Norgaard JP, et al: Diurnal variation of plasma atrial natriuretic peptide in normals and patients with enuresis nocturna. Scand J Clin Lab Invest 1991;51:209.
68. Shaul D, Harrison E: Classification of anorectal malformation: Initial approach, diagnostic test, and colostomy. Semin Pediatr Surg 1997;6:187.
69. Stein S, Feldman J, Freidlander M: Is myelomeningocele a disappearing disease? Pediatrics 1982;69:511.
70. Tsakayannis DE, Shamberger RC: Association of imperforate anus with occult spinal dysraphism. J Pediatr Surg 1995;30:1010.
71. von Gontard A, Lehmkuhl G: [Drug therapy of enuresis.] Zeitschrift Kinder Jugendpsychiatrie Psychotherapie 1996;24:18.
72. Wilmshurst J, Kelly R, Borzyskowski M: Presentation and outcome of sacral agenesis: 20 years' experience. Dev Med Child Neurol 1999;41:806.
73. Zaontz MR, Firlit CF: Percutaneous antegrade ablation of posterior urethral valves in premature or underweight term neonates: An alternative to primary vesicostomy. J Urol 1985;134:139.

第 117 章

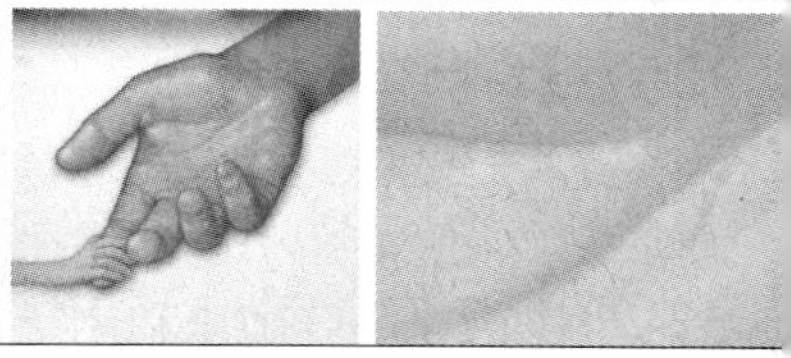

膀胱的结构性疾病，膀胱扩大

Eugene Minevich 和 Curtis A. Sheldon

817 要对一个异常膀胱进行有效的手术治疗，熟悉正常排尿和异常排尿的知识很重要（见第 116 章）。控尿的好坏取决于膀胱内压和膀胱出口阻力之间的复杂平衡。膀胱内压与许多参数有关，但只有顺应性既能反映肌张力又能反映间质弹性。这个指标不是恒定的，会随着膀胱容量而变化。因此，尿量、残余尿量以及膀胱排空频率决定了膀胱运动顺应性的大小。病理变化（如逼尿肌无抑制收缩或间质纤维化）可以明显改变顺应性和膀胱内压（见第 116 章）。

膀胱出口阻力的大小取决于多个参数的共同作用。腹内压突然增高时括约肌反射性收缩机制可以防止尿失禁；相反，逼尿肌收缩时膀胱出口括约肌反射性放松，此时出现自主排尿。另外，尿道括约肌中横纹肌的自主收缩可增强支持作用，防止尿失禁。但在某些情况下，膀胱括约肌反射性收缩和不适当的自主收缩机制（比如功能失调性排尿）可能会导致危险的膀胱高压。而且，在逼尿肌-括约肌协同失调的情况下，会出现有尿意时膀胱出口括约肌不能放松的情况。膀胱出口结构上的梗阻可能由先天性的解剖梗阻（如后尿道瓣膜）或后天获得性的病变（如狭窄）所引起。

不协调排尿对组织结构产生的影响变异较大。膀胱表现为逼尿肌肥大和小梁形成。小囊和憩室可能会继续发展，引起尿道感染和尿石症。可能还会发生间质纤维化，并导致进行性膀胱顺应性丧失。尤其应该关注的是膀胱高压对肾功能的影响。即使没有膀胱输尿管反流，肾盂内压力和膀胱内压力之间仍然存在紧密联系[56]。肾盂压力大于 40 cmH_2O 时肾乳头变形，这可能会改变肾小管向乳头引流的方向并导致肾内反流[124]。这会增加肾盂肾炎的发病几率。

膀胱内压对于最终肾功能的重要性在后尿道瓣膜中较为明显地体现出来（见第 120 章）[101]。膀胱输尿管反流和肾发育不良综合征是指那些先天性、单侧、严重肾发育不良合并瓣膜的患者。受累肾脏（通常左侧）通常功能很差或没有功能。但是对侧肾功能很好，显然是受到了胎儿期“瞬间消失”（pop-off）机制的保护，因膀胱与发育不良肾脏的扩张系统相通缓解了膀胱压力，使对侧肾脏得到了保护[42]。另外，出生时伴有尿腹的患儿（通常表明有肾穹窿的破裂）可以有很好的肾功能，推测可能是因为同样的机制。对合并有先天性憩室的后尿道瓣膜患儿也进行了类似的研究[101]。

神经性膀胱患儿（如脊髓发育不良患儿）的膀胱压力和肾脏预后紧密相关。膀胱漏尿点压力大于 40 cmH_2O时常提示上尿路病变的预后较差[80]。尿流动力学检查的最大尿道压力也被证实有类似的关联[22]。此外，膀胱内压的升高对移植肾会产生不利影响[23,99]。

另外，伴随膀胱内压升高的健康儿童其尿道感染和膀胱输尿管反流的发生风险会增高[64]。盐酸奥昔布宁通过降低膀胱内压可以明显减轻反流和尿道感 1818
染[65,107]。膀胱高压患者的抗反流手术失败风险要明显高于正常膀胱压的患者[93]。

外科医生必须认识到膀胱损伤的原因不能依赖终末期异常来确定，因为各种导致膀胱损伤的原发性疾病大部分重叠在一起。慢性潴留、感染、结石或手术导致的继发性病变也可以混淆结果。原发和继发病变都可以引起非特异性的肌肉、间质和膀胱上皮的变化。而且，没有人能以这些原发性疾病和情况比如脊髓发育不良、后尿道瓣膜、梅干腹综合征和肛门闭锁的基础知识来预测膀胱的功能状态。因此，在计划重大手术措施时应用正规的尿流动力学检查测定膀胱生理特性是必需的。

虽然膀胱功能不良会损害肾脏的概念已被接受，

但是很少有人知道肾脏疾病会导致膀胱损伤。原发性肾脏疾病引起的多尿实质上会改变膀胱功能。它可以引起膀胱高压和广泛性逼尿肌肥大，如果失代偿，膀胱就会高度扩张、松弛、低压以至不能完全排空。这些效应还会伴随继发性的肾疾病（如多尿伴后尿道瓣膜）。这些病变损害了肾髓质，引起浓缩能力的丧失，因此发生的多尿又会进一步损伤膀胱。

膀胱出口梗阻是膀胱和肾脏进行性损害的主要因素。结构性病变尤其重要，如尿道狭窄或后尿道瓣膜。逼尿肌-括约肌协同失调也是个重要问题，这种情况可以是自主性的或非自主性的。后者是指尿道周围括约肌在逼尿肌收缩时不恰当地收缩（而不是舒张）。患儿表现为在逼尿肌无抑制活动时为了防止尿失禁而关闭膀胱出口，或在膀胱胀满时以此来延迟排尿。这样的活动还可以用来防止疼痛性溢尿。这种活动体现在临床 Vincent 屈膝现象中，即孩子坐在脚上、蹲着或两腿挤压在一起来帮助增加膀胱出口阻力，阻止排尿。因为它能产生不良后果，所以外科医生应该去找寻具有这种综合征的患儿。

“瓣膜膀胱”是证明这些因素相互影响的最好例子（图 117-1）。由于膀胱壁肥大的效应，比如已改变的顺应性和无抑制性逼尿肌收缩，因此即使是在瓣膜切除后膀胱仍然在较高的压力下工作。膀胱可能不能完全排空，继而发生膀胱输尿管反流。排尿时，尿液流入尿道但也可以反流入肾脏。患者完成排尿后，肾内尿液又即刻回到膀胱内。这些尿量连同膀胱功能异常引起的排尿后的残余尿量，迫使膀胱连续在高储尿压力范围内工作，结果对肾脏产生不利影响。

最近，随着外科手术技术方面的进展，即通过重建的泌尿道进行间歇导尿的成功应用以及对早期改道手术的借鉴和学习[48]，使得大多数解剖结构已破坏的患儿能够通过进行重建手术达到控尿的目的，也保护了肾功能。实际上这些重建原则现在已被应用于所有泌尿道异常，并且成功的可能性很大。即使当患儿患有终末期肾疾病并最终需要肾移植时，重建方案也是可取的。重建手术要达到低压储尿和膀胱完全排空 181
等要求。通常，这样的重建手术用来治疗膀胱外翻、后尿道瓣膜以及与脊髓脊膜膨出、骶骨闭合不全或 VATER 复合畸形（脊椎缺陷、肛门闭锁、食管闭锁合并气管食管瘘，以及桡骨和肾发育不良）相关的神经性膀胱。其他需要重建的疾病包括泌尿生殖窦、泄殖腔畸形、泄殖腔外翻和双侧单一异位输尿管。所有这些情况通常涉及异常储尿压力和排空问题。

膀胱和尿道疾病

膀胱和尿道的解剖性疾病

原发性结构异常应引起重视，而后尿道瓣膜是最

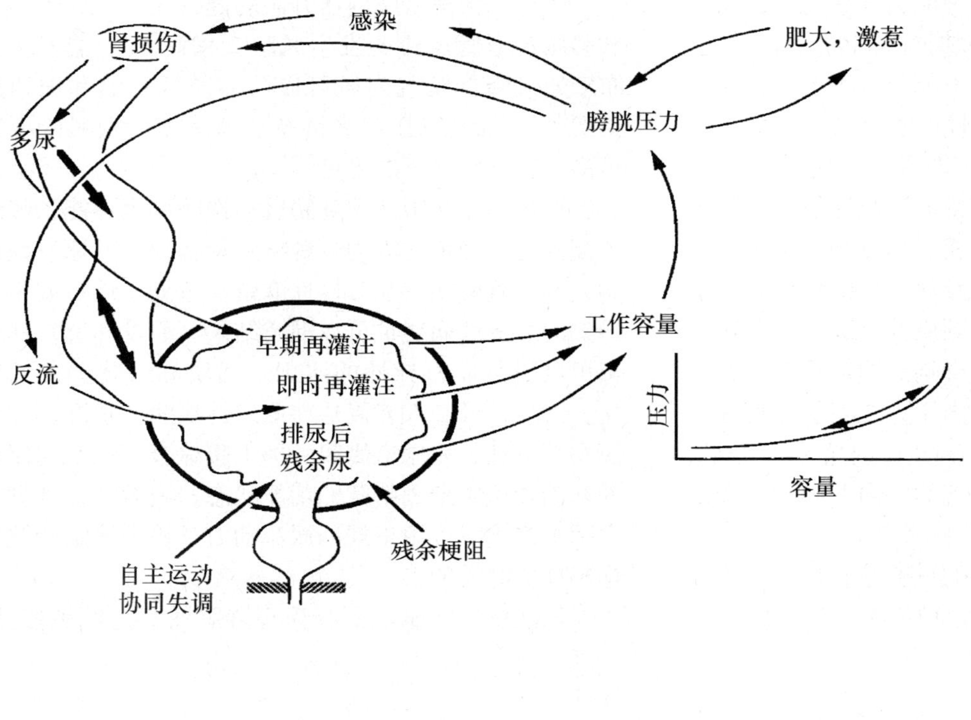

图 117-1　“瓣膜膀胱”的病理生理学。（From Sheldon CA，Snyder HM：Structural disorders of the bladder，augmentation. In Grosfeld JL，et al [eds]：Pediatric Surgery. St Louis，CV Mosby，p 114.）

好的例证（图 117-2），这是男婴中最常见的下尿路梗阻的原因。尽管这些畸形也会在第 120 章中讨论，但是本部分主要考虑与膀胱及上尿路相关的问题。后尿道瓣膜的三种类型已经被描述[134]。Ⅱ型可能并不存在。Ⅰ型和Ⅲ型都存在尿道腔内的瓣膜，可能厚也可能薄，但都覆盖了移行上皮（图 117-3）。在最常见的瓣膜类型（Ⅰ型）中，斜行的梗阻性瓣膜从精阜起源而远端终止于膜性尿道附近。Ⅲ型代表梗阻性瓣膜，起源于与尿道轴较为垂直的方向，并且比Ⅰ型病例更加远离尿道。

梗阻的结果是近端尿道拉长并扩张，逼尿肌肥大使膀胱颈变得相对狭窄。远端尿道口径正常，因此导致扩张的近端尿道和细的远端尿道之间有一个突然的过渡。膀胱显示出逼尿肌肥大，并且因为有小梁、小囊以及憩室的存在，膀胱变得不规则。上尿路的典型表现是严重的肾积水，伴有或不伴有膀胱输尿管反流。肾脏损害常见，而且从出生时就已经存在，即使去除瓣膜后也不会完全恢复。

大多数患者在婴儿期就被发现：25%～50% 的病例在新生儿期被发现，超过 2/3 的病例在出生后 1 年被检查出来。随着围生期超声检查的发展，宫内诊断变得普遍。宫内超声检查发现男婴有厚壁膀胱和肾积水则高度提示此诊断。肾积水的新生儿会表现为明显扩大的膀胱或扩张的肾脏。婴儿会出现尿路感染，或因为氮质血症而发育不良，但是在大一些的患儿中，其首发症状可能是尿失禁。用力排尿时尿流细，有时表现为滴尿，然而很多患儿和父母通常不会发现有问题，同样也不应忽视对这一类患儿的调查。

诊断性评估方法包括上尿路的超声检查和排尿性膀胱尿路造影检查（VCUG）。通过肾扫描评估肾功能。如果患儿的瓣膜成功切除后还有肾积水、反流、氮质血症或尿失禁存在，则具备尿流动力学检查的指征。

婴儿首先应该通过膀胱导尿、静脉复苏以及必要的呼吸支持来稳定病情。可以应用 5 或 8 French 婴儿胃管来引流尿液，因为大号的导管或球囊导管会引起剧烈的逼尿肌收缩而使得尿流不能通过输尿管膀胱交界处。大多数病例接下来要切除瓣膜（见图 117-3）。早产儿因尿道太细而不能经内镜施行电灼，可以顺行切除或膀胱造瘘；但是随着近年来膀胱镜的小型化，这些操作已很少采用。有严重反流尤其是伴有氮质血症的病例也可采用膀胱造瘘术。作者发现那些进行

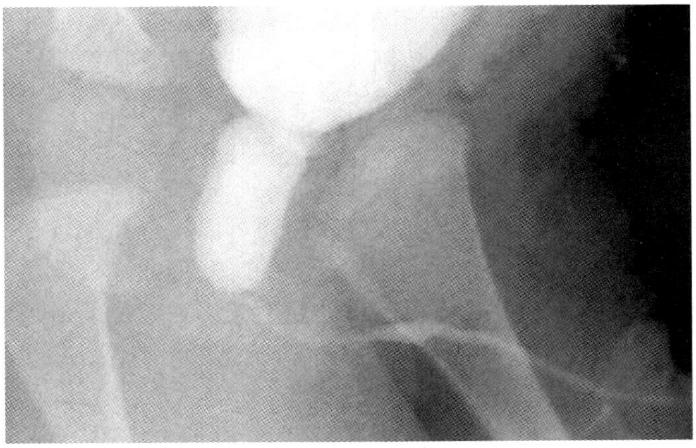

图 117-2 后尿道瓣膜的放射影像学表现。

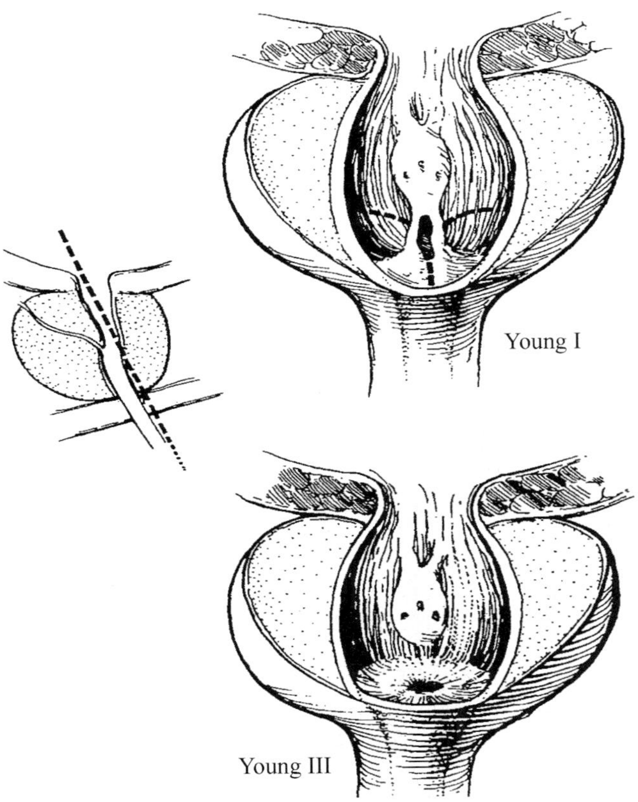

图 117-3 后尿道瓣膜的解剖结构。根据瓣膜结构，经尿道电灼通常选择在 5 点和 7 点的位置。（如提到过的Ⅰ型和Ⅲ型。）经筛选的病例可能在 12 点处电灼更好一些。（From Sheldon CA, Bukowski TP: Male external genitalia. In Rowe MI, O'Neill JA, Jr., Grosfeld JL, et al [eds]: Essentials of Pediatric Surgery. St Louis, Mosby-Year Book, 1995, p 775.）

了充分导管引流后仍情况不稳定、并持续氮质血症或败血症以及肾积水的病例，可能还需经皮肾造瘘直至达到足够稳定的状态后再进行手术。

少数患严重氮质血症并且对导尿没有反应的患儿可以通过经皮肾盂穿刺造瘘进行上尿路的引流。这种低压引流使肾功能得到恢复，因而可以将透析或肾移植延后至患儿稍大时进行。经皮膀胱造瘘或经皮肾盂造瘘都是可逆的。值得注意的是不应该在干燥的尿道中进行瓣膜电灼（如患儿行膀胱造瘘或肾盂造瘘后），因为这样会导致尿道狭窄。

在第 120 章中详细描述了前尿道瓣膜[106,126]、Cowper 管囊肿（图 117-4）[5,74]、尿道息肉、男性和女性重复尿道（图 117-5 和 117-6）以及尿道憩室的诊断和治疗。这些病变导致的膀胱结构改变多与梗阻
1820 相关。其他先天性尿道梗阻性病变包括椭圆囊肿和异位输尿管囊肿。获得性的梗阻病变有狭窄和尿道缩窄。膀胱外翻畸形、尿道上裂、尿道下裂和其他一些结构性病变在其他章节讨论（见第 118 和 119 章）。

膀胱憩室可能是膀胱出口梗阻的原因或结果。这种膀胱上皮褶皱袋通过逼尿肌缺陷处突出于膀胱，常常发生在输尿管裂隙处。感染和结石可能诱发引流较差的憩室出现症状。出现在输尿管裂隙处的憩室通常会使膀胱输尿管交界处变形，这足以引起输尿管反流或是梗阻。如果向远端突出于膀胱出口之下，则会导致膀胱出口梗阻（图 117-7）[111]。

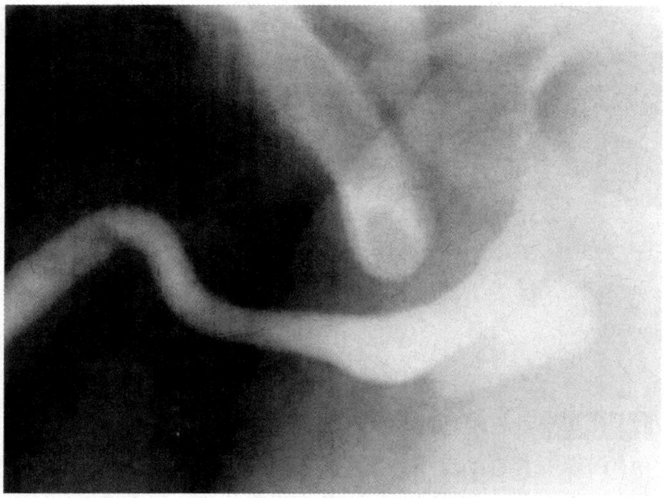

图 117-4 Cowper 管囊肿的放射影像学表现和引起的憩室。（From Sheldon CA, Snyder HM: Structural disorders of the bladder, augmentation. In Grosfeld JL, et al [eds]: Pediatric Surgery. St Louis, CV Mosby, p 114.）

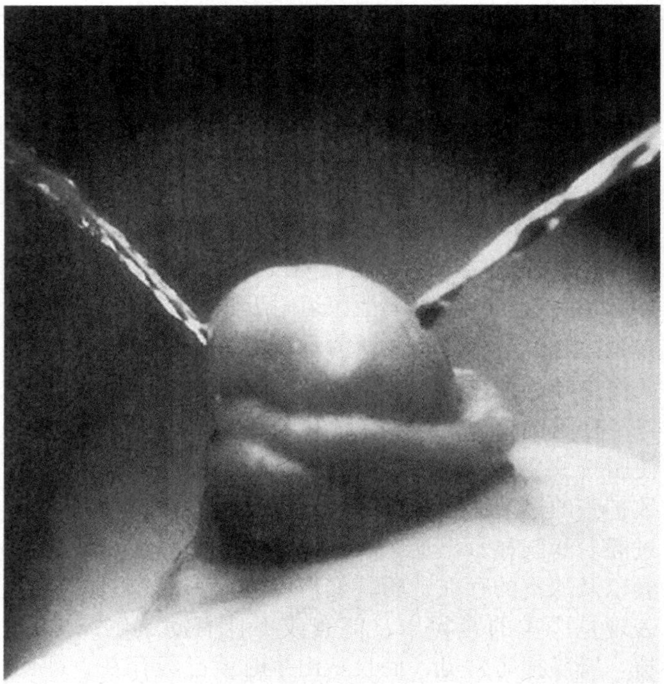

图 117-5 重复尿道。（From Sheldon CA, Bukowski TP: Male external genitalia. In Rowe MI, et al [eds]: Essentials of Pediatric Surgery. St Louis, Mosby-Year Book, 1995, p 779.）

小憩室若引流好不会引起膀胱输尿管反流，故不需要手术干预。多数有症状的患儿其憩室都需要行开放切除手术。远离三角区的憩室容易经膀胱外或膀胱内切除。但是三角区起源的憩室的处理就需要特别小心，因为距离输尿管和输精管很近。通常必须同时进行输尿管再植术。

膀胱和尿道功能的神经源性疾病

外科医生常常会遇到原发性的膀胱神经支配异常
问题（神经性膀胱）。脊髓发育不良是一种特别常见 182
的营养障碍疾病。脊髓脊膜膨出，即神经组织和脊膜突出于椎管腔外，是最常见的缺陷。脊膜膨出只包括脊膜的突出，而脂肪脊膜膨出则包括了突出的神经组织和脊膜及其周围的脂肪组织。这些病变引起的下尿路症状多种多样，但都不能通过观察神经损害平面来预测。因而，尿流动力学检查是最基本的检查手段。上尿路恶化的风险可以通过尿流动力学检查来进行预

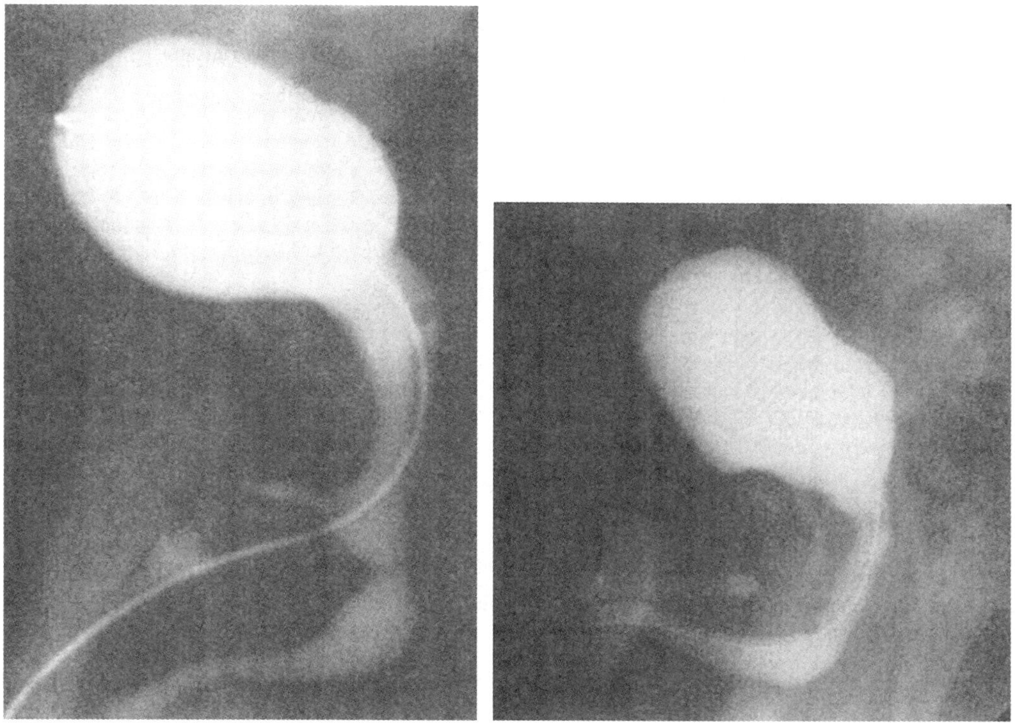

A　B

图 117-6　A. 完全尿道重复的放射影像学表现。B. 不完全尿道重复的放射影像学表现。（From Sheldon CA, Bukowski TP: Male external genitalia. In Rowe MI, O' Neill JA, Jr., Grosfeld JL, et al [eds]: Essentials of Pediatric Surgery. St Louis, Mosby-Year Book, 1995, p 779.）

测。现在已经公认漏尿压力超过 40 cmH_2O[80] 和排尿协同失调[3] 时，上尿路预后差（图 117-8 和 117-9）。协同失调时上尿路恶化的风险超过 70%；相对来讲，与括约肌协同和括约肌去神经化相关的上尿路恶化发生率为 15%～25%。遗憾的是，神经损害往往是动态变化的，如果开始时协同失调不存在，以后可能会发 1822

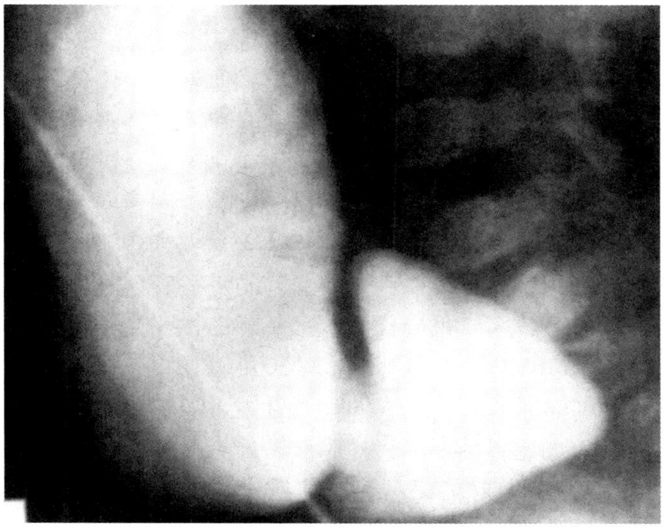

图 117-7　膀胱憩室挤切膀胱颈下方并导致膀胱出口梗阻。（From Sheldon CA, Essig KA: Congenital bladder diverticulum causing bladder outlet obstruction: Case report and review of literature. Pediatr Surg Int 1994; 9: 142.）

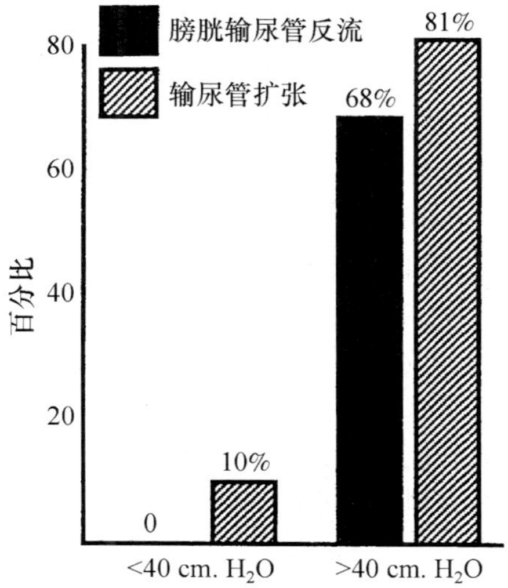

图 117-8　与尿道开放压力相关的上尿路损伤风险。（From McGuire EJ, Woodside JR, Borden TA, et al: Prognostic value of urodynamic testing in myelodysplastic patients. J Urol 1981; 126: 208.）

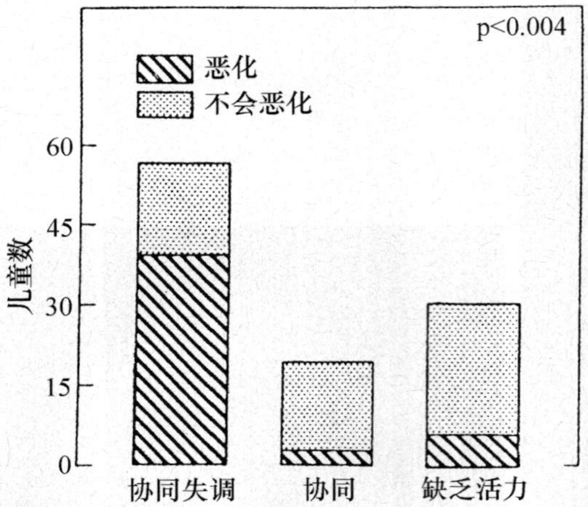

图 117-9 协同失调、能够协同、括约肌活力缺乏情况下尿路的恶化。（From Bauer SB：Early evaluation and management of children with spina bifida. In King LR［ed］：Urologic Surgery in Neonates and Young Infants. Philadelphia，WB Saunders，1988，p 256.）

生。协同失调的发展往往和脊髓栓系有关，随着患儿长大可以导致脊髓损伤或脊髓根部损伤。最大风险在出生后 2 年内，尤其是第一年，但是这种损伤可以在整个儿童时期都存在。

隐匿性（闭合性）脊髓神经管闭合不全包括脊髓栓系、椎管腔内脂肪瘤、皮样囊肿或窦道、脊髓纵裂和马尾肿瘤。这些患儿通常会有泌尿系异常，包括尿路感染和尿失禁。幸运的是许多患者的皮肤异常表现很明显。皮肤凹陷、皮肤标志、皮下脂肪瘤或骶骨突出处的毛发斑、皮肤血管畸形和色素沉着可能提示其下方有脊髓的病变。任何有尿失禁或其他膀胱功能失调症状的患儿如果存在上述表现，都需要排除隐匿性脊髓神经管闭合不全。这些诊断可以通过尿流动力学检查和脊髓核磁共振来证实，或者出生后 6 个月内通过脊髓超声检查证实。大约 45% 的患儿存在泌尿道功能异常。这些病变可能是上运动神经元或下运动神经元或混合性病变。因而，膀胱功能必须经过尿流动力学检查来测定而非推测。

另外造成神经性膀胱的重要因素是骶骨发育不全，通常见于肛门闭锁患儿或糖尿病母亲的孩子。这种情况的特征是先天性骶骨全部或部分缺如。体检中提示此病变的表现是异常臀纹或直接触诊到骶骨不完整。可以通过前后位和侧位的腰骶椎影像学检查证实其诊断。这类患儿中大约 75% 存在尿路功能异常[7]。半数患者有高反射性膀胱，通常为括约肌机制亢进和逼尿肌-括约肌协同失调。大约半数患儿为无反射性膀胱，其中括约肌结构通常已经部分或完全去神经化。

很多功能性的膀胱和尿道异常没有明显的神经性或结构性改变，这些异常情况包括无抑制性逼尿肌过度活动、膀胱张力低下和逼尿肌-括约肌协同失调。常能确定的原因是感染性或行为性因素，但是有时原因仍然难以确定。

解剖和神经源性联合疾病

第三类需要膀胱重建的婴儿是那些同时出现功能和结构性膀胱异常的患儿，如肛门闭锁和泄殖腔畸形。对于这些病例，在出生早期就应该进行解剖学评价，且要求完成一些最基本的检查，如肾脏超声、VCUG 和脊髓超声。解剖异常再加上功能异常造成了泌尿系统发病风险的增高。一项 McLorie 等人对 484 例患儿的连续研究发现晚期肾脏疾病的高风险率[81]。他们发现 6.4% 的高位肛门闭锁患儿以及 1.1% 的低位肛门闭锁患儿会死于肾衰竭。60% 的高位病变患儿和 20% 的低位病变患儿可伴有无瘘管性生殖泌尿系统畸形。实际上 1/3 以上的患儿会发生上尿路畸形，而双侧上尿路畸形发生率为 14%。

作者接连对 90 例肛门闭锁患儿进行了回顾性分析，发现 18% 有明显的神经性膀胱功能紊乱[110]。高位肛门闭锁患儿面临的风险最大。但是，一些低位病变的患儿也会出现神经性膀胱功能紊乱。许多患儿需要治疗处理脊髓栓系，因为有进行性的膀胱、尿道、直肠肛门和下肢神经支配损伤的风险。

研究回顾分析了 23 例为保存上尿路或正常控尿而接受重建手术的肛门闭锁患者，证明了发现这些异常的重要性[113]。如图 117-10 所示，9% 的患者有晚期肾脏疾患，65% 的患者有明显的肾脏畸形，57% 的患者有膀胱输尿管反流。30% 的患者会出现输尿管畸形，而 70% 的患者会有神经性膀胱功能紊乱问题。这些患者需要一个广泛的泌尿道重建操作（图 117-11）。特别需要注意的是，43% 的患者需要进行输尿管再植，43% 的患者需要膀胱扩大，35% 的患者需要 Mitrofanoff 新尿道，22% 的患者需要进行膀胱颈部重建。男性肛门闭锁患儿由于先天性的直肠尿道瘘导致尿道不规则而难以通过尿道导尿。尿道的感觉仍存在，这

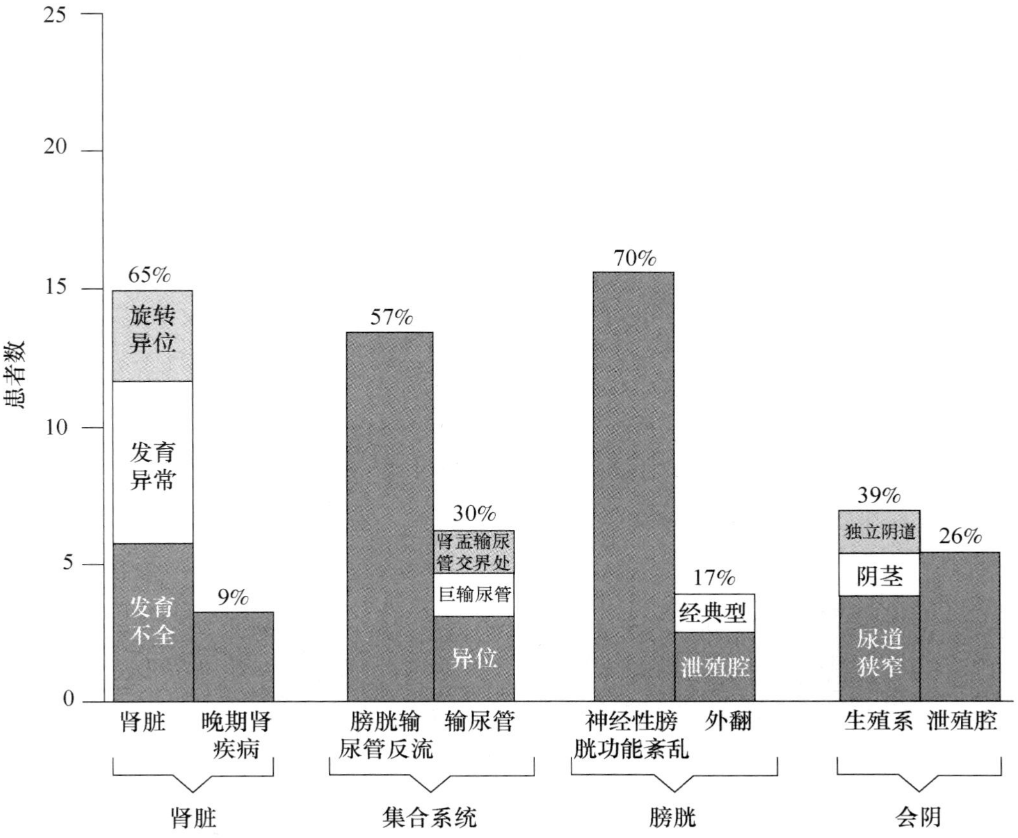

图 117-10 肛门闭锁合并的泌尿生殖系畸形。（From Sheldon CA，Gilbert A，Lewis AG，et al：Surgical implications of genitourinary tract anomalies in patients with imperforate anus. J Urol 1994；152：196.）

时可能需要做一个 Mitrofanoff 新尿道以便于进行间歇导尿。

本文描述的其他病变可能也需要膀胱重建。膀胱和阴道出口共用共同通道的泌尿生殖窦畸形的患儿可能合并有神经性膀胱功能紊乱。除了进行尿道和阴道重建外，有必要对薄弱的膀胱出口进行重建。由于其他一些和神经性膀胱功能紊乱相关的情况，可能需要膀胱扩大术。膀胱外翻和泄殖腔外翻是典型的需要行全尿路重建的病例。梅干腹综合征病例（第 114 章）通常行内科治疗，但有时需要外科干预。这些患者的典型特征为拥有一个内压低且不能完全排空的低张膀胱，膀胱不规则且有感染倾向。长时间后一些患者可失去膀胱容量和顺应性，因而通常需要进行尿流动力学检查以便于治疗。

重建手术原理

泌尿道重建的目的是为了保护上尿路、获得社会所能接受的控尿能力、最大限度地便于患儿护理以及增加其自理的可能性。对于有上尿路损伤风险的儿童，在其新生儿时期就应该进行评估而且开始进行保护上尿路的治疗。控尿能力的评估和治疗在入学前进行，以便于社会综合考虑。

一般而言，在外科干预前首先对泌尿道进行内科治疗。治疗方法包括间歇导尿以排空膀胱、抗胆碱治疗降低膀胱内压以及 α-肾上腺素治疗加强膀胱出口阻力。只有当内科治疗没有成效的情况下才采用外科手术。当准备进行泌尿道重建时，应仔细进行术前评估，这点很关键，而且要根据患者的个体需要制订重建方案。

尿路重建后必须使尿路功能平衡以保证长期效应，这包括四点[84]。第一是要有足够的膀胱（储备）容量和顺应性以做到低压储尿。理想的膀胱容量是指白天能有间隔 4 小时的导尿或间断性排尿，夜间 8 小时间隔而且不会超过最大压力或出现急迫性尿失禁。第二是指达到足够的膀胱出口阻力而保证控尿。第三是指必须有便利可靠的机制进行膀胱（储尿器）的排空。当然，理想的情况是能自然排

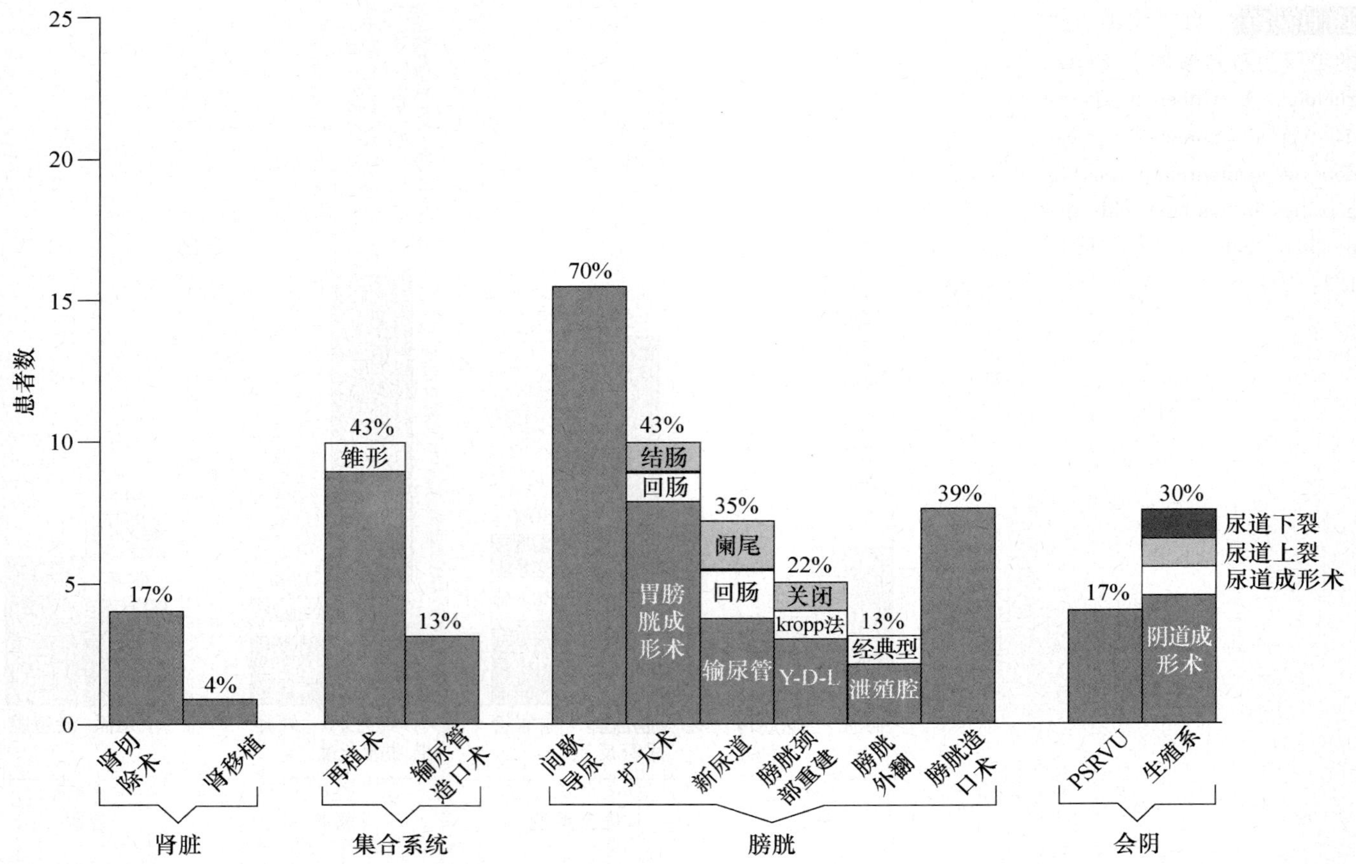

图 117-11 肛门闭锁患者的外科手术方式。Y-D-L., Young-Dees-Leadbetter 方法。(From Sheldon CA, Gilbert A, Lewis AG, et al: Surgical implications of genitourinary tract anomalies in patients with imperforateanus. J Urol 1994; 152: 197.)

尿，否则需间歇导尿。

天然的尿道排尿可能较易被接受，但已证明经此导尿很困难或不舒服（防止依赖性），所以有必要用一种替代的导尿管道。最终要没有梗阻和没有反流地将无菌性上尿路尿液引流入膀胱（储尿器），这样保护上尿路的效果才令人满意。

膀胱容量或顺应性不足的纠治方法

生理因素

可以通过膀胱扩大来提高膀胱容量和顺应性。行扩大术的指征必须包括以下临床症状，比如膀胱功能紊乱导致的尿失禁且内科治疗无效，以及由于不能获得足够的低压储尿容量而导致的上尿路恶化。另外，还包括测得的膀胱容量明显小于根据患儿年龄推算的容量。膀胱容量推算公式为：*容量（盎司）= 年龄（岁）+ 2* [61]。必须考虑到由于膀胱出口没有控制力而使膀胱呈低压引流状态，这时要想达到理想的功能膀胱容量较为困难。用 Foley 球囊导管堵住膀胱颈后得到的膀胱内压测量图可以提供可靠的功能膀胱容量数据。在获得最有效果的治疗期间，膀胱压力超过 35～40 cmH_2O，并伴随有等同于白天 4 小时内和夜晚 8 小时内产生的尿量时，建议考虑行膀胱扩大术。

关于膀胱扩大有一些重要的重建原则。首先注意膀胱容量的处理。如果行肠膀胱扩大，必须保留完整的逼尿肌以产生高压，通过尿流动力学检查发现结合部分就像一个大憩室[125]。如果肠道组织是加在完整的神经性膀胱上或是损伤的膀胱上，那么这种憩室的减压效应可能代替膀胱的扩大效应（即不能达到膀胱加强的效果）。从膀胱前面的膀胱颈水平到后面三角区呈矢状切开膀胱可以避免这种问题（“蛤式膀胱成形”）。必要时重建膀胱，即把膀胱从球状变成扁平片状，这样逼尿肌不可能再收缩产生明显的高压情况[9,10]。

正如膀胱扩大后膀胱高压的重要来源是膀胱逼尿肌一样，扩大膀胱使用的卷起的肠管部分本身也会产生压力。由于蠕动收缩，压力范围可在 60～100 cmH_2O 之间[72]。Kock 根据以上现象提出了理论，即通过一个“袋状”结构使肠段变成一个不能有效进行蠕动的储尿器[60]。将肠管沿长轴对称剖开后重新缝合，破坏环肌（“去管化”）抑制蠕动。一旦不能蠕动，储尿器就可以低压扩张和储备尿液（图117-12）[51,62]。另外肠管部分的几何容量也会明显扩大[51]。另一个
825 重要概念是适应（图 117-13）。众所周知，重建的膀胱以后会逐渐增大。恒压下，半径越大则提供的容量越大——再次强调去管化肠管进行膀胱扩大的优势。

在选择扩大物来源时要考虑到如下因素。解剖因素比如考虑到供应血管的游离度，则偏爱回肠、乙状结肠和回盲部，以及胃大弯部分。同时也要考虑到能否植入输尿管或做一个 Mitrofanoff 新尿道。另外重要的一点就是应避免腹膜腔的操作，所以对腹膜透析或脑室腹腔转流管的放置持保留意见。这样的情况下最好采用输尿管扩大或自体扩大术。

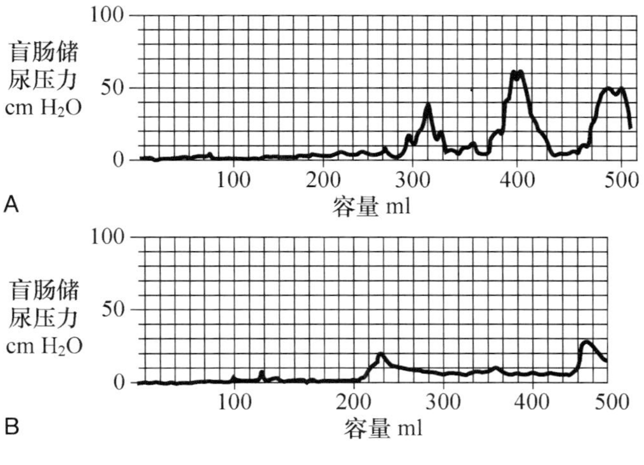

图 117-12　盲肠储尿器的尿流动力学表现。A. 肠管产生了高压蠕动波。B. 肠管杯片样操作后瓦解了蠕动，使得储尿容量增大但压力没有增高。（From Goldwasser HR, Webster GD：Augmentation and substitution enterocystoplasty. J Urol 1986；135：221.）

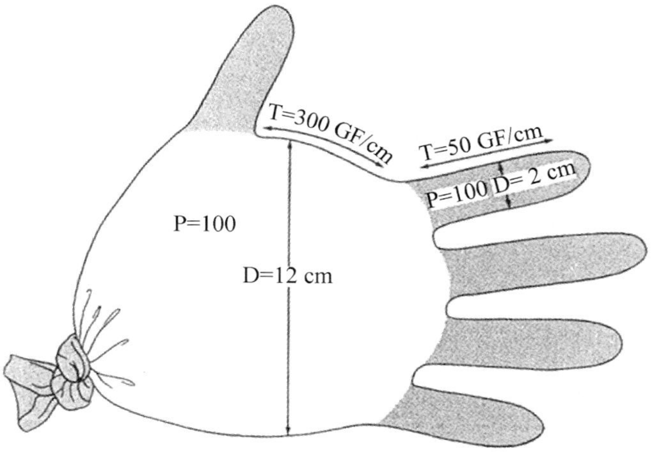

图 117-13　用膨胀的外科手套来说明拉普拉斯关系。虽然压力（P）均匀散开，但是直径（D）越大的部分其张力（T）就越大。（From Hinman F：Selection of intestinal segments for bladder substitution：Physical and physiological characteristics. J Urol 1988；139：522.）

扩大物来源的选择可能受到患者原发疾病的限制。短肠综合征的患者无法承受用回盲部或回肠肠段。处于临界排便控制的患者（比如肛门闭锁或脊髓发育不良）也不能承受回盲瓣或吸收水分的右半结肠的缺失。代谢结果可能是最重要的影响因素，如吸收性酸中毒和发育迟缓，这些可以因为慢性肾功能不全而恶化，这时可以采用自体扩大、输尿管扩大或胃膀胱成形技术。由于重建手术必须因人而异，即便是行胃膀胱扩大、自体扩大或输尿管扩大时，外科医生也必须熟悉各种重建替代物，并给患者做相应的准备，包括肠道准备。

小肠膀胱扩大手术

回肠膀胱成形术（图 117-14）是一种膀胱扩大最常用的技术[52,120]。膀胱呈“蛤”形切开。游离回肠 20～40 cm 并沿长轴对称切开，将其塑形为“杯片”状后用 3-0 Vicryl 缝线与膀胱片吻合（内翻锁边缝合）。肠道端端吻合恢复连续性。这种技术的优势在于操作简单，但是在回肠上进行抗反流输尿管再植或做 Mitrofanoff 新尿道不如在膀胱本身或其他扩充物上可靠。

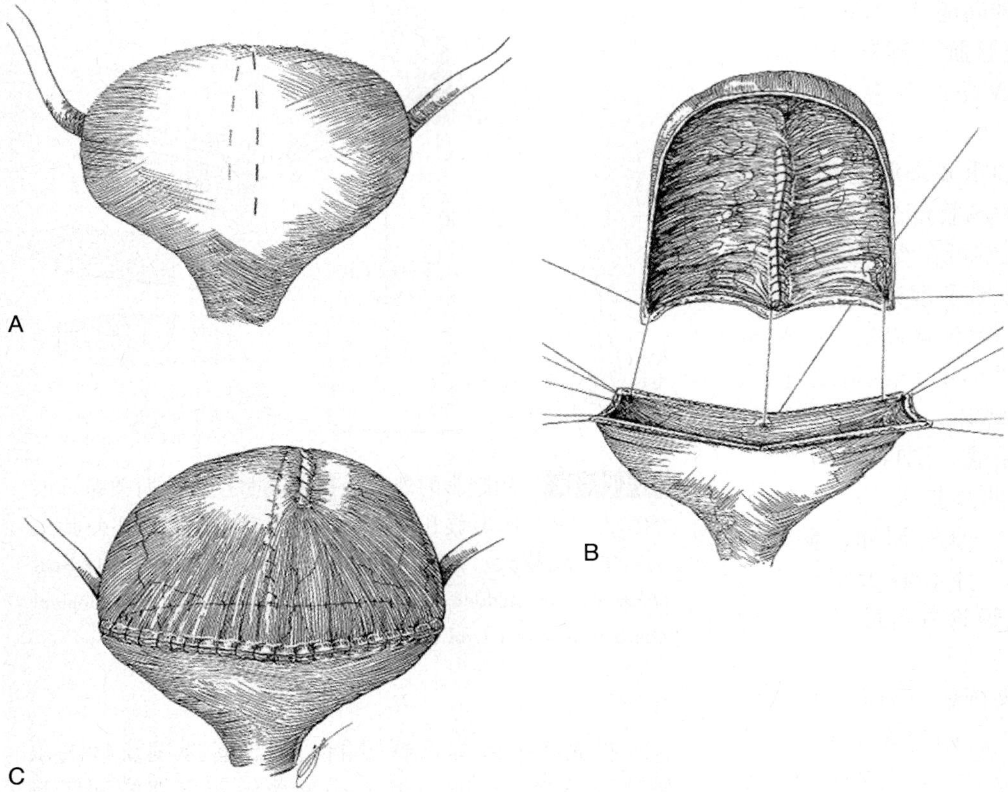

图 117-14　“蛤”式回肠膀胱成形技术。A. 小容量、高压膀胱。B. 膀胱被纵向切开备用，回肠去管腔化而做成杯片状。C. 将杯片状回肠吻合于膀胱。（From Minevich E, Sheldon CA：Urinary tract reconstruction for continence and renal preservation. In Ziegler MM, Azizkhan RG, Weber TR, et al［eds］：Operative Pediatric Surgery. Norwalk，CT，Appleton & Lange，2003，p 915.）

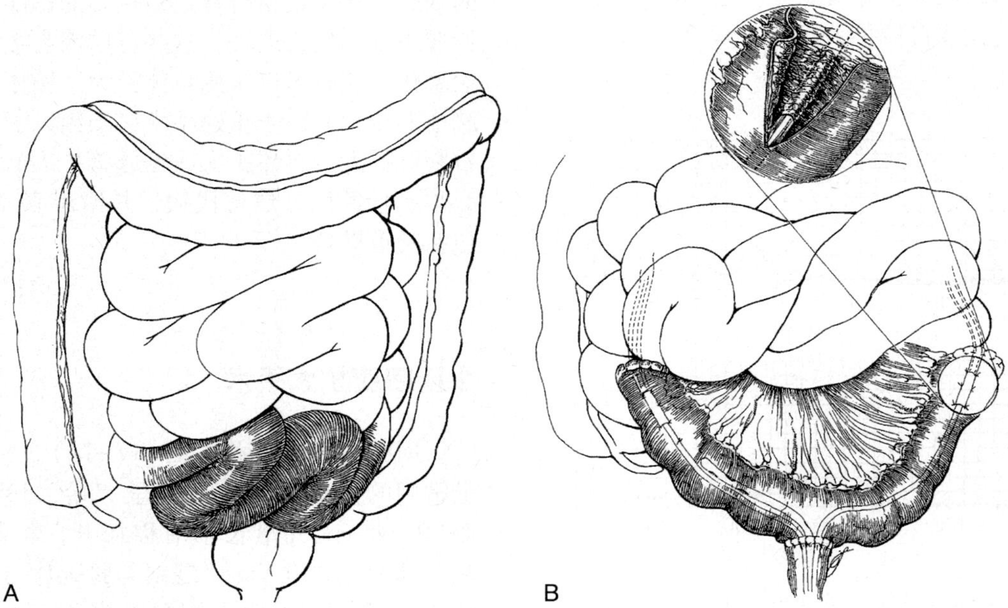

图 117-15　Camey 肠膀胱成形术。A. 将一段 35～40 cm 长的回肠原封不动地吻合于尿道残端，做成了可控性肠道储尿器。B. 在储尿器两侧将输尿管穿行于肠黏膜下 3～4 cm，可产生有效的抗反流结果。（From Minevich E，Sheldon CA：Urinary tract reconstruction for continence and renal preservation. In Ziegler MM，Azizkhan RG，Weber TR，et al［eds］：Operative Pediatric Surgery. Norwalk，CT，Appleton & Lange，2003，p 916.）

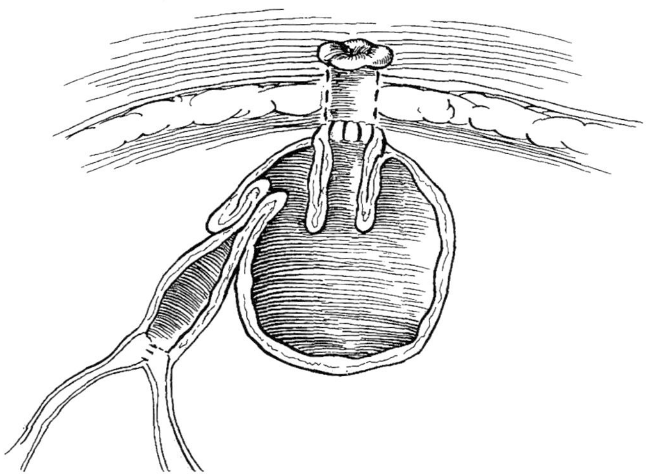

图 117-16　Kock 袋。一段 70 cm 的回肠重新改建成为一个蠕动袋，并且有两个乳头瓣结构。最近的改造方法包括将一个乳头瓣固定于储尿器壁，使之成为一个固定的翼状瓣膜。（From Minevich E，Sheldon CA：Urinary tract reconstruction for continence and renal preservation. In Ziegler MM，Azizkhan RG，Weber TR，et al［eds］：Operative Pediatric Surgery. Norwalk，CT，Appleton & Lange，2003，p 917.）

其他应用小肠进行膀胱扩大或替代的技术包括 Camey 法（图 117-15）[13]、Kock 袋（图 117-16）[60] 和回肠代新膀胱[59,94]。这些操作在获得控尿方面不太成功，而且许多医生发现其并发症和再次手术的发生率很高。

回盲部膀胱扩大手术

因为盲肠的自然构造看起来是理想的膀胱替代物，故泌尿科医生偏爱用回盲部肠段进行膀胱重建[38]。这种方法简单易行，而且在把扩张的输尿管再植于回肠方面有很大优势。回盲瓣犹如套叠瓣样可防止反流，但遗憾的是套叠瓣抗反流机制并不稳定。因此可引进各种对回盲瓣的外科改进方法，力求减少反流机会。对于那些处于排便控制边缘的患者（比如脊髓脊膜膨出或 VATER 复杂畸形），最大的影响便是丧失回盲瓣后出现的排便失控风险。

当盲肠或回盲部完整地用于进行膀胱扩大时，夜
326 间尿失禁成为许多研究发现的问题[130]。这个问题很可能是完整肠段的肠蠕动引起的，因为当应用杯状补片技术时，夜间尿失禁问题就很少见到了。其他应用回盲瓣的可控性分流方法有 Maintz 袋[128]、Penn 袋[31]、Indiana 袋[103] 以及 Florida 袋[97]。这些技术中，Indiana 袋在儿科中应用最为广泛，但也产生了不同的结果[6]。

大肠膀胱扩大手术

Mathisen 报道了用乙状结肠来扩大膀胱，其方式类似于先前介绍的回肠膀胱成形术[76]。这种方法也很简单，而且可以在结肠带上很好地进行输尿管抗反流再植或 Mitrofanoff 新尿道再植。这种方法看起来与其他肠段在膀胱排空能力、感染及外科并发症方面没
有区别[108]。如果患者先前曾因肛门闭锁进行过重建 1827
手术，那么此方法会影响直肠的血供，因为直肠肛门依靠的是递减式血供。尽管对超过 33% 的患者来讲尿失禁仍是个问题[98]，但是关于应用结肠再塑新膀胱的成功经验已有报道[95,98]。

胃膀胱扩大手术

Mitchell 等开创了应用胃壁组织进行尿路重建的新时代（图 117-17）[1]。他们证明了胃壁膀胱成形术的高成功率、通用性，以及在氮质血症的情况下也可耐受。这种方法可以减少感染、黏液产生和结石形成的风险，而且提供了很好的适应性。输尿管和 Mitrofanoff 新尿道再植也很容易。作者对胃壁膀胱成形术或胃代膀胱进行了长期随访，发现控尿率达 91%，所有患者的肾功能稳定[28,114]，只有 1 例患者出现上尿路的恶化，其问题是间歇导尿不适应。另外，胃膀胱成形术也被证明对那些终末期肾疾患并面临肾移植的患儿是很好的疗法[28,114]。自身尿道[15]、输尿管新尿道[86,114] 以及阑尾新尿道已被成功重建于胃代膀胱[112]。这种方法的缺点是会发生血尿-排尿困难综合征。

输尿管和自体膀胱扩大手术

输尿管膀胱扩大术[21]（图 117-18）和自体膀胱扩大术[16]（图 117-19）有较大的发展前途，因为这

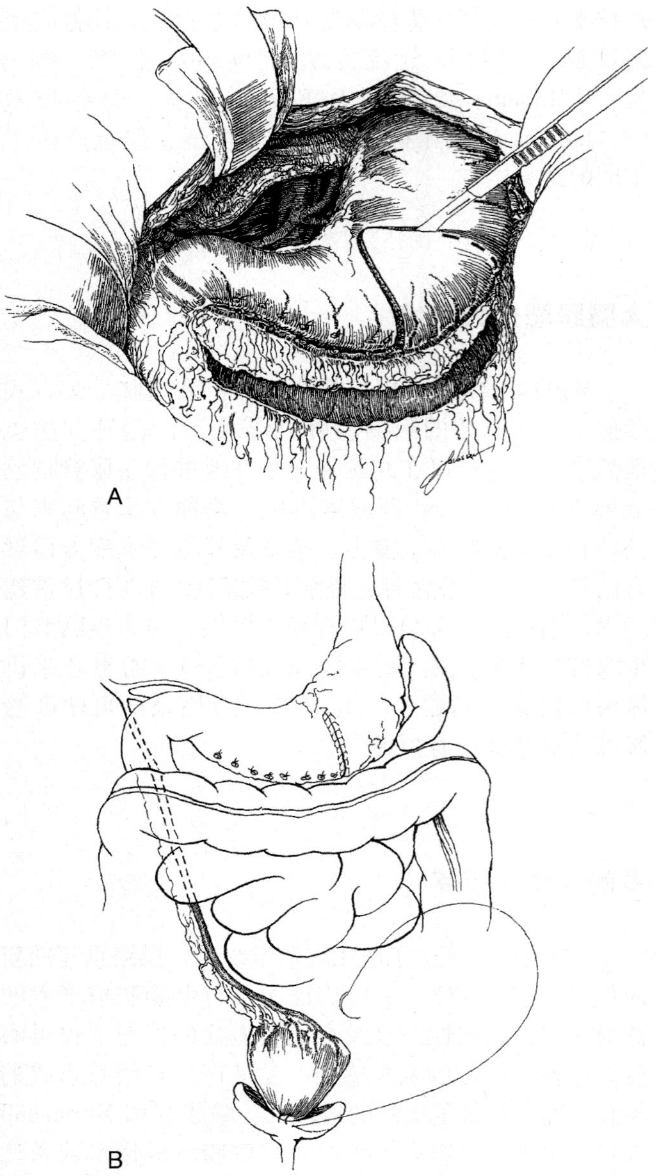

图 117-17 胃膀胱成形术。A. 保护胃网膜右侧血管和楔形游离出胃基底部。B. 将胃网膜右侧血管从腹膜后移至需扩大的手术部位。关闭胃切口。（From Minevich E，Sheldon CA：Urinary tract reconstruction for continence and renal preservation. In Ziegler MM，Azizkhan RG，Weber TR，et al [eds]：Operative Pediatric Surgery. Norwalk，CT，Appleton & Lange，2003，p 918.）

样可以防止吸收性代谢疾病，而且可以完全通过腹膜外途径完成手术。但是由于本身表面积的固有限制，这种方法难以获得足够的容量和顺应性[73]。在输尿管膀胱成形术中，所需输尿管是通过切除肾脏或输尿管输尿管吻合后得到的。但遗憾的是，用这种方法很难得到足够大的输尿管。另外，最近有报道说输尿管扩大术后能否获得长期的低储尿压和足够的容量还需要进一步观察[53]。 1828

纠治膀胱出口缺乏阻力的方法

保持控尿能力主要依靠膀胱出口阻力和膀胱压力之间的复杂平衡。要保持控尿，无论是在休息还是在体位改变、咳嗽、打喷嚏、用力时，膀胱出口阻力都要超过膀胱内压力。对那些在低压储尿情况下仍尿失禁的患儿需要行膀胱出口重建。很难评估那些高压或低容量患儿的膀胱出口情况，这些参数异常本身就可引起尿失禁。在这种情况下腹压漏尿点压大于 1829
100 cmH_2O以上提示有较好的控尿机制[129]。已证明尿道压力曲线和静止漏尿点压力并不是可靠的判断括约肌能力的参数。有许多控尿手术可供选择以增加控尿能力，包括增加尿道长度、膀胱颈悬吊、压迫尿道或完全关闭尿道。

Young 开展的早期工作试图通过后方逼尿肌的卷管化来延伸已有尿道[133]。这种方法后来被 Dees[26]和 Leadbetter[69]改进，即取一段（4～5 cm）膀胱后壁组织来进行卷管以延伸尿道。剥去两侧三角形状的膀胱上皮，剥离后残余面围绕一根小导管（8 或 10 French）[37]，靠拢形成新尿道[37]。临近的逼尿肌自行靠拢于黏膜管外以增加肌肉支持（图 117-20）。前尿道通常用缝合固定或应用压力悬吊带固定。各种各样的技术方法已有描述[63,70]。

这种技术的目的就是要使患儿具有控尿能力，以及在逼尿肌收缩情况下能够自然排尿。当逼尿肌不能有效收缩排空膀胱时，就需要间歇导尿。这项技术的优势是允许自行排尿、应用自体组织以及提供“突然排空”机制。但是这种方法减少了膀胱容量，导尿变得比较困难，而且导尿可能会损伤已经建立的控尿机制和导致重建失败。

对行 Young-Dees-Leadbetter 膀胱颈重建的患者给予附加 Mitrofanoff 新尿道，这样可以建立一个间歇导尿通道，对于所有重建患者，尤其是在术后早期是很有益处的。当患者学会应用重建尿道排尿后，通过简单的门诊手术即可关闭 Mitrofanoff 通道。由于其不会漏尿，因此也可以原位保留。

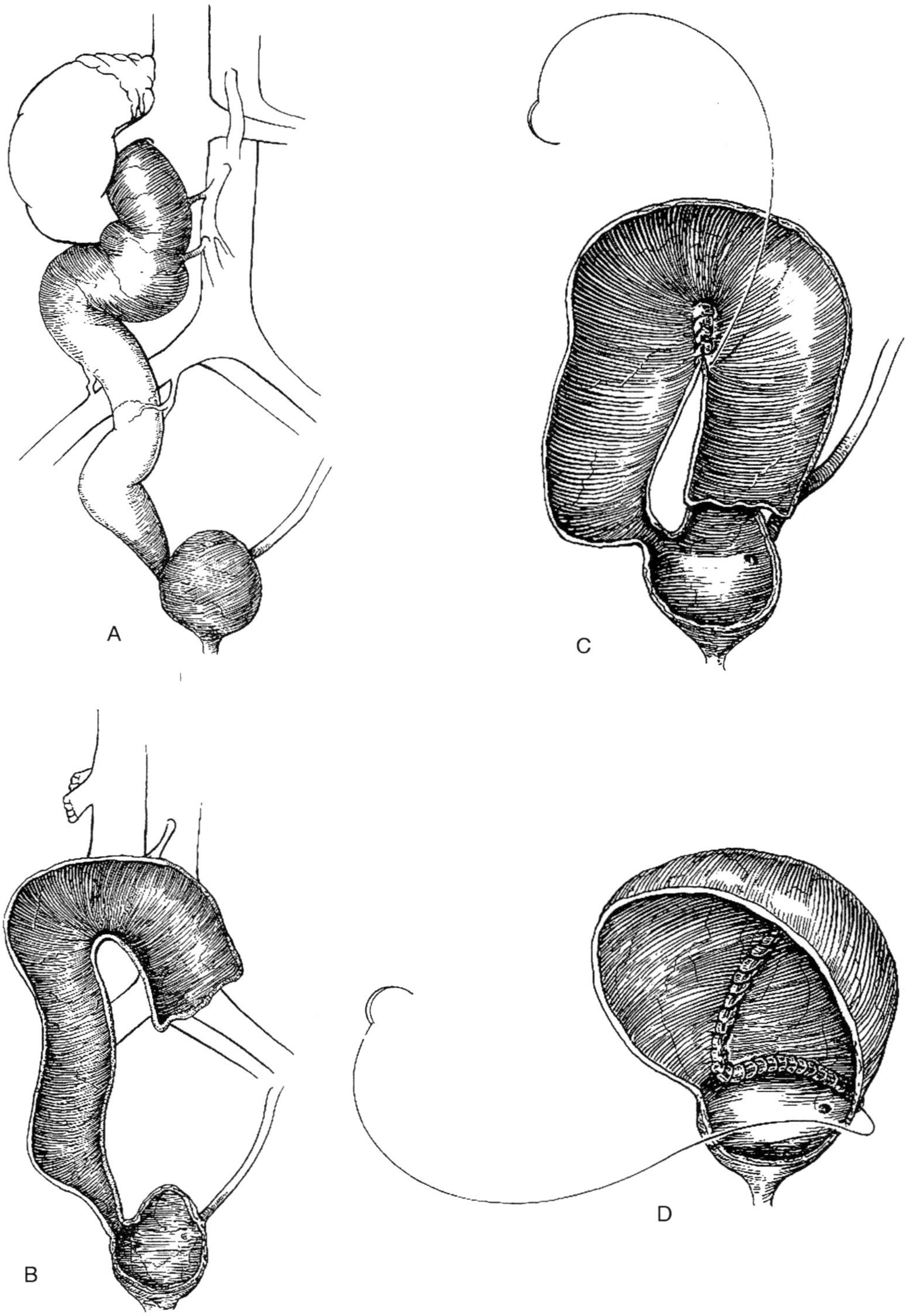

图 117-18　输尿管膀胱扩大术。A. 输尿管正常血供。B. 转移输尿管后去管腔化。C. 输尿管再塑成 U 形袋。D. 输尿管吻合于已呈“蛤”状的膀胱上。（From Minevich E，Sheldon CA：Urinary tract reconstruction for continence and renal preservation. In Ziegler MM，Azizkhan RG，Weber TR，et al［eds］：Operative Pediatric Surgery. Norwalk，CT，Appleton & Lange，2003，p 919.）

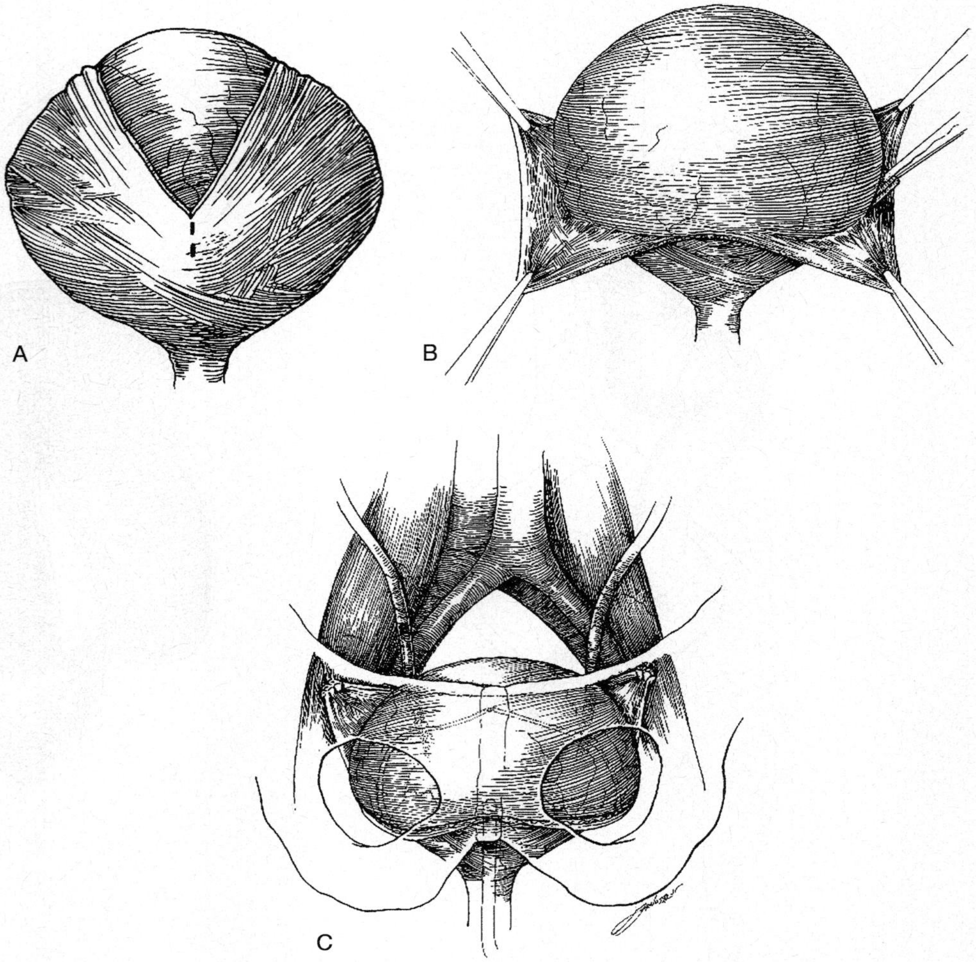

图 117-19　膀胱自体扩大术。A. 切开逼尿肌。B. 将逼尿肌从膀胱上皮剥离下来。C. 膀胱充盈时膀胱上皮膨出。（From Minevich E, Sheldon CA：Urinary tract reconstruction for continence and renal preservation. In Ziegler MM, Azizkhan RG, Weber TR, et al［eds］：Operative Pediatric Surgery. Norwalk, CT, Appleton & Lange, 2003, p 920.）

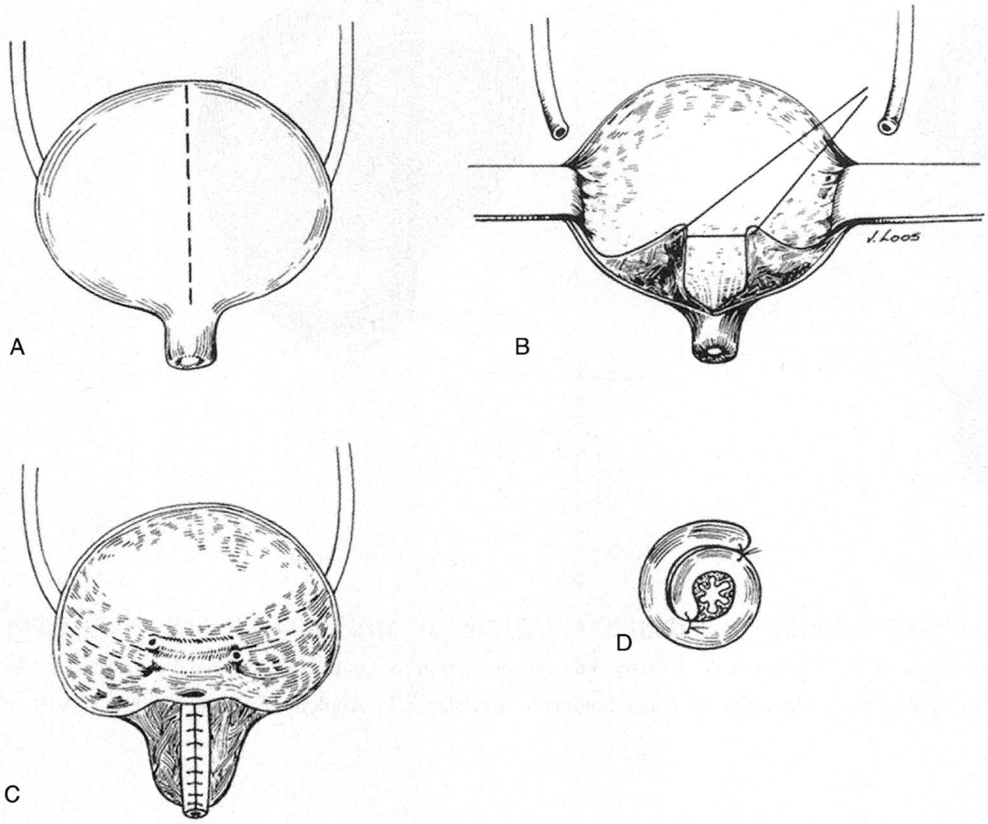

图 117-20　Young-Dees-Leadbetter 膀胱颈重建。A. 切开膀胱前壁。B. 切除膀胱三角区基底部黏膜。C. 黏膜带卷管化和输尿管再植。D. 逼尿肌交叉缝合。（From Sheldon CA, Bukowski TP：Bladder function. In Rowe MI, O'Neill JA, Jr., Grosfeld JL, et al［eds］：Essentials of Pediatric Surgery. St Louis, Mosby-Year Book, 1995, p 742.）

Kropp 方法（图 117-21）包括将与尿道相延续的膀胱前壁组织卷管化形成一段延伸的尿道，然后尿道管埋于膀胱上皮下[66]。这种方法应用自身组织来获
831 得控尿能力，但是导尿比较困难。Pippi Salle 改进方法[96]，即应用逼尿肌条高嵌体（保留后方膀胱组织），能使导尿容易一些。不论是 Kropp 管还是 Salle 高嵌体都没有提供“突然排空”机制，因此自然排尿的可能性减小，而且膀胱容量减少。

另外一个增加膀胱出口阻力的方法是筋膜吊带。通常应用一种活体的筋膜带，这种移植带可以通过内镜辅助横过阴道放置[79]，或者开放手术尿道后切开放置[32]。另一种替代方法是用筋膜条带在身体同侧锥形固定（图 117-22）[50]。后一种方法尤其适用于那些去神经控制但括约肌解剖机制未破坏而且需要行膀胱扩大的患儿。这些方法技术发展很快而且操作相对简单，包括应用自身组织，而且是可逆性操作。它们可以作为 Young-Dees-Leadbetter 方法的辅助操作。如果没有过度成角，自然排尿还是有可能的，而且还可以保持“突然排空”机制；但是过度成角可能会干扰自然排尿或导尿。

人工尿道括约肌（图 117-23）被证明在压迫尿道和提高膀胱出口阻力方面有效。应用最普遍的是现代 AS800 型，由环绕于膀胱颈部或球部尿道的袖带、一个腹内储水装置以及一个留置在阴囊或阴唇的活性压力球囊组成。袖带压力是恒定控制的，直到泵被挤压后液体从袖带流至储水球囊里，这时膀胱得以排空。控制系统中的延迟充盈阻力装置可以在袖带自动从储水球囊中取水再充盈前提供 1～2 分

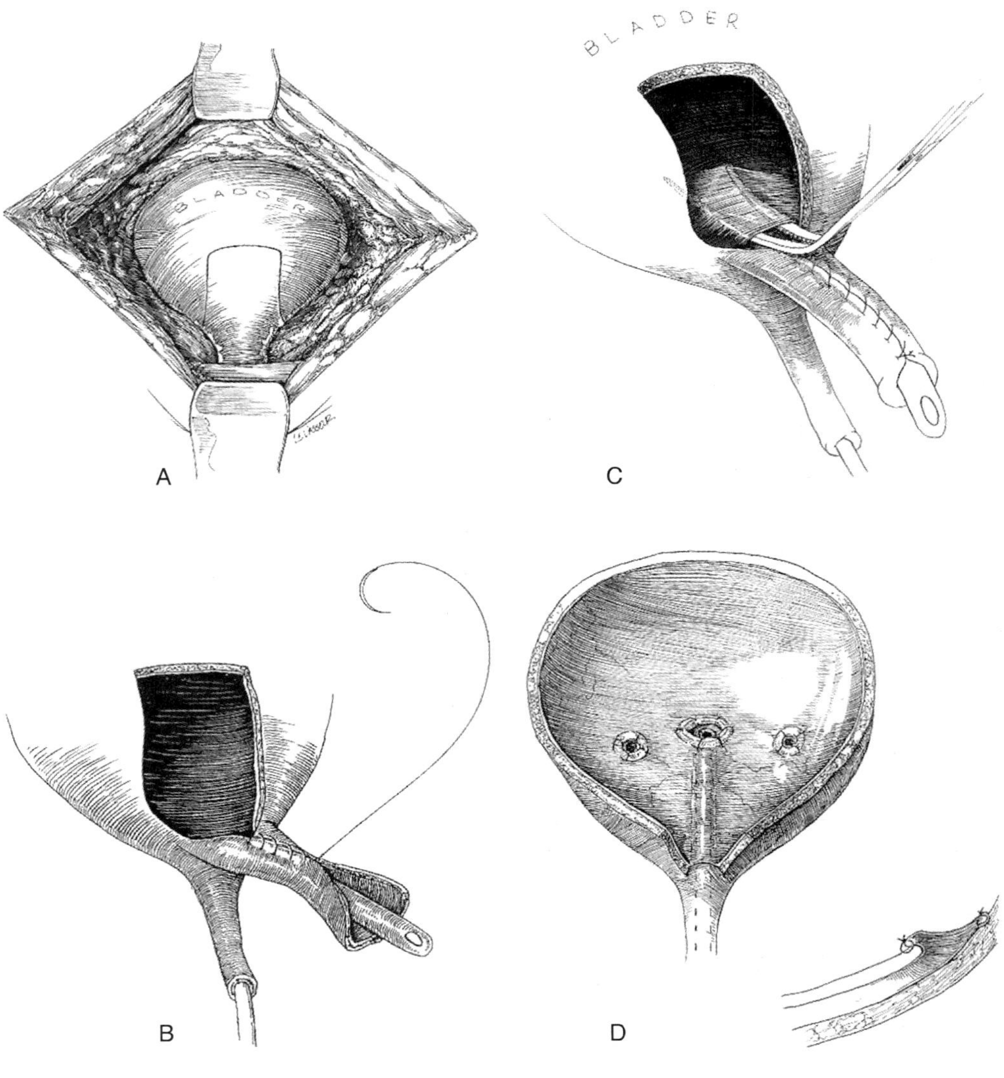

图 117-21 Kropp 方法。做一个逼尿肌管（前面，在后面制成管状也可以）并且从黏膜下隧道植入膀胱以形成一个有效的瓣膜。A. 前方膀胱瓣外观。B. 前方膀胱带卷管化。C. 自膀胱底部做出黏膜下隧道。D. 前方的膀胱管再植于黏膜下隧道。（From Minevich E, Sheldon CA：Urinary tract reconstruction for continence and renal preservation. In Ziegler MM, Azizkhan RG, Weber TR, et al［eds］：Operative Pediatric Surgery. Norwalk, CT, Appleton & Lange, 2003, p 925.）

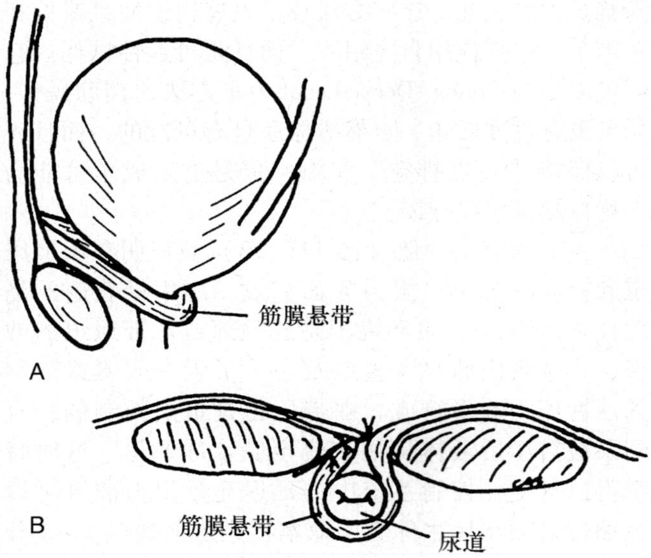

图 117-22 应用筋膜悬带来加强膀胱出口张力。A. 侧位矢状面外观。B. 冠状位外观。（From Sheldon CA：Urinary reconstruction［rather than diversion］for continence in difficult pediatric urologic disorders. Semin Pediatr Surg 1996；5：10.）

钟的尿道压力降低时间。压力控制球囊的压力范围多种多样，通常选择 60～70 cmH_2O 的球囊作为儿童重建压力[87]。高压力可能会因为压迫影响血供造成尿道腐蚀[2]。

有许多证明膀胱扩大后应用人工尿道括约肌治疗有效的报道[44,49,67,82]。这种技术的优势在于可以自然排尿，但也有不利之处。装有人工尿道括约肌装置的患者会遇到许多机械问题。最常见的问题就是袖带渗液或导管打结而需要手术纠正。最严重的并发症是袖带周围从括约肌到尿道的腐蚀和感染问题。后者往往需要去除装置。

最后，可能需要进行尿道关闭手术。这显然是一种确保控尿的极有效的方法，但往往是最后的选择[55,92]。单纯缝合膀胱颈部黏膜是没有效果的，因为可以发生再通的情况。尿流改道因为有肌肉加强（近端和远端），所以可以减少这种风险。这种方法往往需要建立一个导尿通道，这将在下一章节中讨论。这种方法的优势在于其成熟性和技术简单。但是该操作也将患儿置于形成膀胱结石的风险之中，且难以逆转。另外，由于缺乏“排空”机制，尿道关闭
1832 后，当患者不能规律地导尿排空膀胱时会增加膀胱破裂的风险。

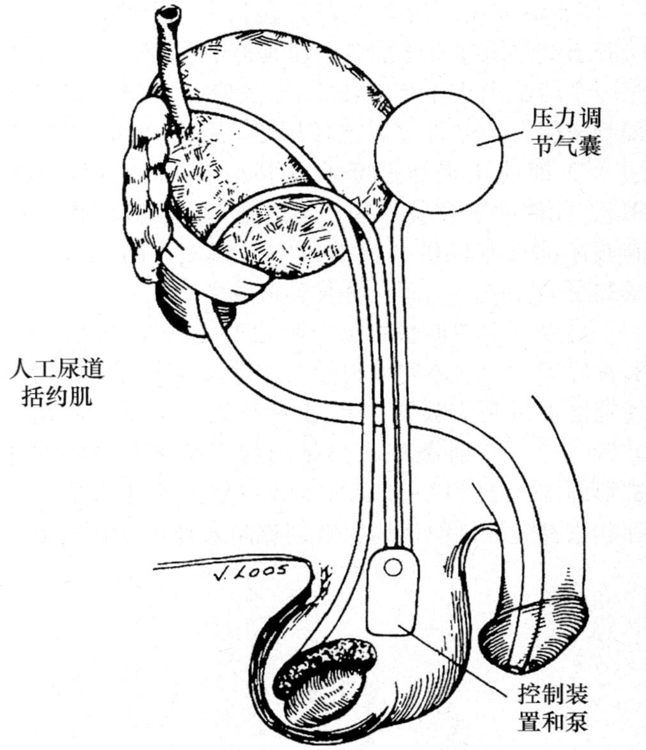

图 117-23 人工尿道括约肌。（From Sheldon CA，Bukowski TP：Bladder function. In Rowe MI，O' Neill JA，Jr.，Grosfeld JL，et al［eds］：Essentials of Pediatric Surgery. St Louis，Mosby-Year Book，1995，p 743.）

可控性尿液引流的替代方法

以上章节中描述的操作方法都需要建立一个从膀胱连接到腹壁或会阴部的可控性引流尿液的管道。如果是由于先前的手术操作或先天性的扭曲，或是患者生理上的限制而导致了导尿困难，就有指征建立导尿通道来代替自身尿道。这种方法是针对尿道的功能替代且基于以下原理，即管道有足够长度承受外力压迫，而且其出口阻力要超过膀胱（储尿器）内压。这种方法能成功获得控制能力是依赖于达到了可控性的储尿器-新尿道之间的平衡。新尿道产生的阻力必须超过膀胱的压力，不论是在静止期还是在膀胱内压突然升高时，如姿势的突然变化、腹内压突然增加（咳嗽、打喷嚏、紧张和体位突然变化）等，尿液均不会流出。新尿道的正常工作要求较低压力的膀胱（储尿器）。因此，可能需要进行肠膀胱扩大或替代，

以及包括去管化的重新塑形。膀胱有足够大容量很重要。在膀胱内尿液增加到压力容量曲线显示膀胱顺应性将要变低前进行间歇性导尿引流。

其他方法有乳头瓣（如回盲瓣或回回套叠瓣）以及翼状瓣（图 117-24）方法。乳头瓣本身不稳定，因为长时间后基底部的压力控制机制会分散，往往导致瓣膜失效和失禁。翼状瓣比较耐用，它的控尿机制由于储尿器壁的参与而较为稳定。

Mitrofanoff 新尿道是翼状瓣机制的例子，对儿童尤为适用[88]。这种方法是在膀胱和皮肤之间建立起一个可控性的导尿通道（新尿道）。它提供了单向翼状瓣膜机制，即允许导管顺行进入膀胱。翼状瓣还能可靠地防止尿失禁（图 117-25）。阑尾是最常用来进行 Mitrofanoff 管成形的组织。它连同阑尾系膜从盲肠上游离下来，通过逼尿肌切开或膀胱切开建立一个长长的黏膜下隧道。Mitrofanoff 新尿道的盲肠端经腹取出置于皮肤上，U 形瓣膜插入技术用来减少开口狭窄的风险。Mitrofanoff 新尿道的原理已被证明非常有用，可以再植于膀胱、结肠和胃，且具有同等效果[33,112]。多处可作为新成形尿道出口的选择，如下腹部、脐部和会阴部[112]。通过盲肠卷管化延长阑尾的方法可以扩大这种技术应用的范围[25,107,112,118]。Mitrofanoff 原理和这些技术的扩展成功地适用于各种情况下的下尿路可控性重建。

如果不能应用阑尾，可以用锥形裁剪的回肠段（超过 12～14 French），尽管近来回肠横行卷管肠段使用得较多[11,12,18]。回肠膀胱吻合的长度受到所用肠段圆周的限制，这使其在一些病例中的应用受到限制。Casale 介绍了一种可以使可控管道长度加倍的方 1833
法[17]。当已行或准备进行肾切除，或准备进行经输尿管输尿管吻合术时，输尿管可以作为 Mitrofanoff 管道的材料来源[90]。因为回肠管道重建较容易，所以除非有适应证时才采用经输尿管吻合术。如果输尿管存在反流，需要同时进行输尿管再植。其他可控性导尿方法包括 Benchekroun 方法[4]、Indiana 袋[103]、Koch 袋[119] 以及半 Koch 法[102]。虽然这些方法没有 Mitrofanoff 翼状瓣在儿童中应用广泛，但是在某些情况下也被证明是有用的。

Mitrofanoff 管道最常见的并发症是开口狭窄，而这是需要纠正的[11,71]。偶尔还可以看见息肉肉芽组织生长[100]。作者观察了一例在摩托车事故外伤后做了胃膀胱成形-Mitrofanoff 管手术的患者[83]。由于缺血坏死导致 Mitrofanoff 新尿道不通或者丧失功能的情况非常少见。

与排便失禁的协调问题

泌尿道重建时必须要考虑肛门直肠的功能。如果

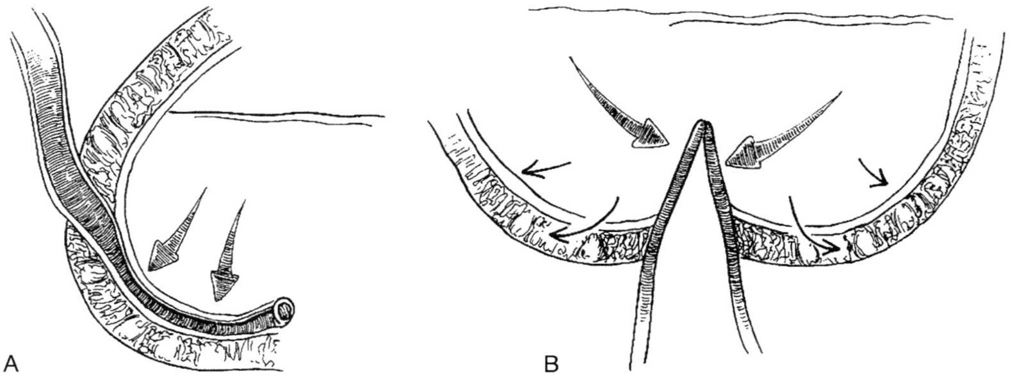

图 117-24　A. 翼状瓣。B. 乳头状瓣。乳头状瓣具有可控性，因为瓣膜周边受到储尿器压力的压迫。但遗憾的是，膀胱内压力也可以在瓣膜基底部向侧边分散，这样可能减弱或者完全抵消了瓣膜的控制机制。翼状瓣是可控的，因为黏膜下肠段被充盈的储尿器压住（就像膀胱输尿管反流时进行的输尿管再植一样）。与乳头状瓣不同，翼状瓣由于固定于储尿器壁内故较稳定。因此储尿器充盈不会导致控尿机制的丧失。（From Minevich E，Sheldon CA：Urinary tract reconstruction for continence and renal preservation. In Ziegler MM，Azizkhan RG，Weber TR，et al［eds］：Operative Pediatric Surgery. Norwalk，CT，Appleton & Lange，2003，p 928.）

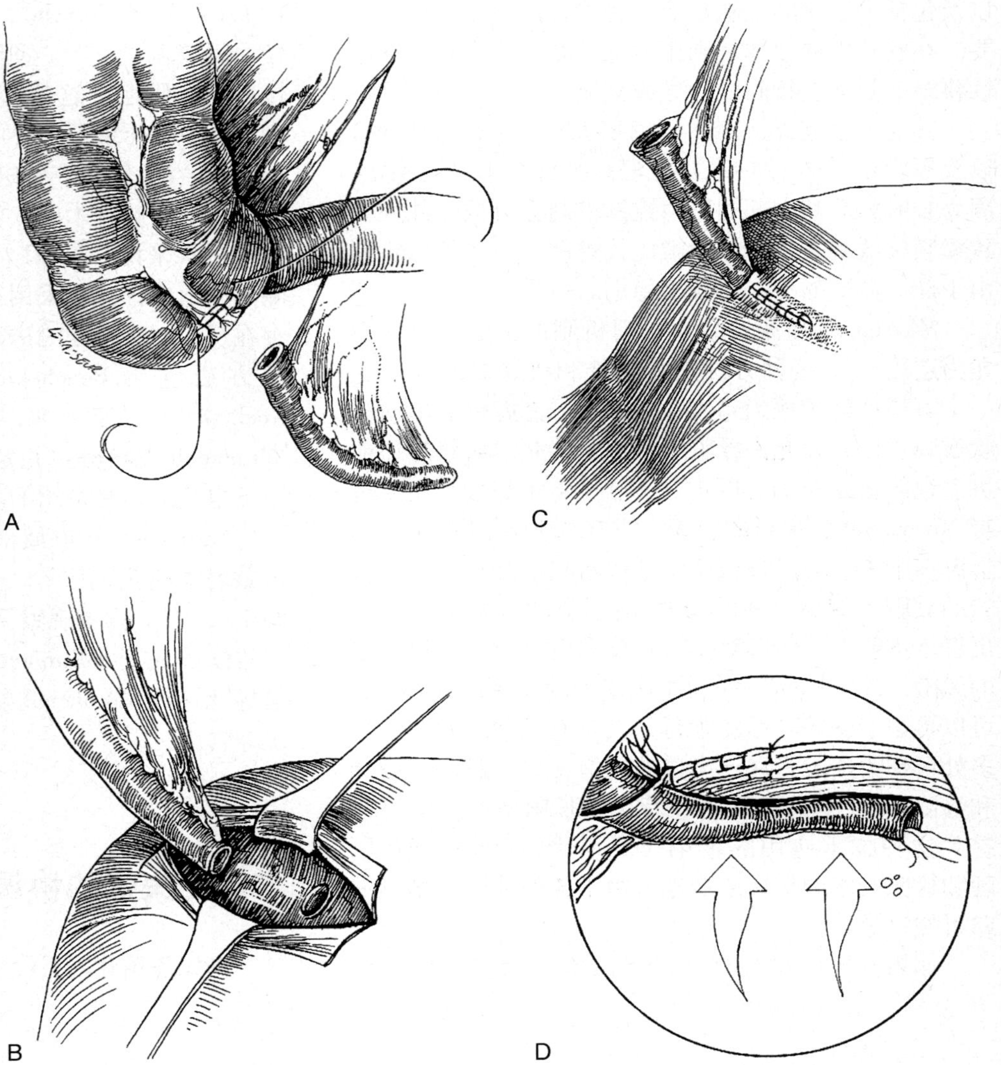

图 117-25 Mitrofanoff 方法。A. 阑尾连同系膜游离，盲肠段关闭。B. 膀胱外切开至黏膜开口，将阑尾远端黏膜开口种植于此。C. 逼尿肌缝合覆盖在阑尾外，阑尾近端开口植于皮肤作为导尿开口。D. 这张图示描绘了应用 Mitrofanoff 方法后的可控性翼状瓣机制；膀胱内压上升后对抗逼尿肌而压迫管腔，因此管腔被夹闭而产生控尿。（From Minevich E，Sheldon CA：Urinary tract reconstruction for continence and renal preservation. In Ziegler MM，Azizkhan RG，Weber TR，et al［eds］：Operative Pediatric Surgery. Norwalk，CT，Appleton & Lange，2003，p 929.）

患者能够控尿却还因为排便失禁而使用尿布，那么这种治疗很难被认为是成功的。而且，持续性的污便增加了泌尿道感染的风险，重建的膀胱和上尿道情况也进行性恶化。控尿治疗使胃肠道功能显著下降。比如抗副交感神经治疗可能导致严重的便秘，回盲部膀胱成形术可能会引发排便失禁。

进行尿路重建时要考虑到难治性排便失禁的问题，因此术前需评估。因为多数患者可以应用非手术方法进行治疗，如饮食控制、膨胀剂、行为纠治及灌肠，故手术重建以前必须详细履行这些干预措施。

1834 如果患者经过这些治疗症状仍难以控制，那么顺行可控性灌肠（图 117-26）则不失为一种很好的替代方法[75,117,123,131]。当非手术治疗无效或者灌肠有效但又无法被患者接受时，则有指征进行此操作。

顺行灌肠方法和 Mitrofanoff 新尿道的操作相似。阑尾或卷管后的回肠段[132]植于盲肠带上，另一端经腹壁开口于皮肤。阑尾或回肠段的准备与 Mitrofanoff 方法一样。沿盲肠前方的结肠带切开，将其与管道吻合，黏膜隧道的远端形成黏膜开口。管道被肌肉覆盖且远端经腹开口于皮肤。患者坐在便桶上，将一根导管伸入可控性盲肠造口处，每天 1 次（有时每天 2 次）。顺行灌肠液由自来水和食盐组成，在重力作用下进行灌洗。

尿路重建和终末期肾疾病

有报道在 20%~30% 的儿童病例中，先天性泌尿

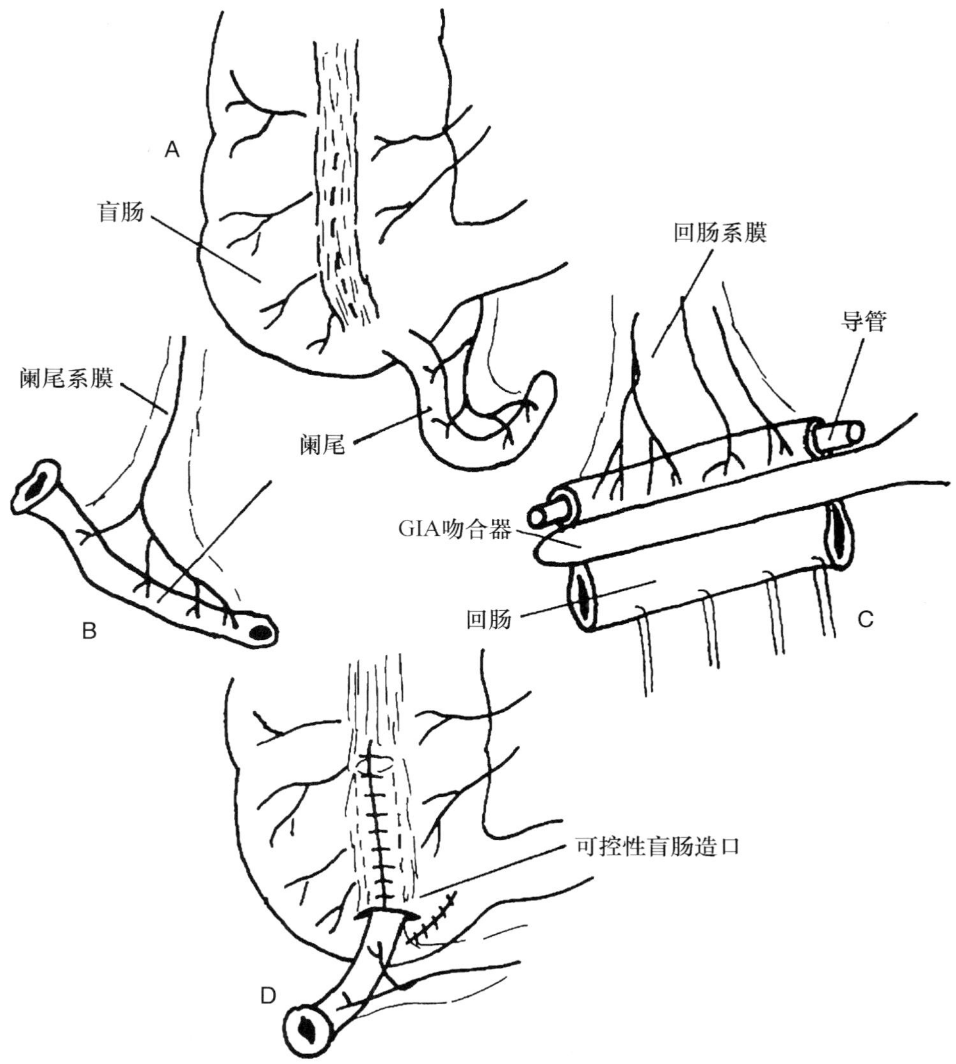

图 117-26 用来进行顺行可控灌肠的可控性盲肠造口术。A. 解剖出阑尾和盲肠前方的结肠带。B. 阑尾连同血管蒂游离。C. 另一种方法是取一段回肠并截短，带蒂游离。E. 可控性盲肠造口术后外观。（From Sheldon CA：Urinary reconstruction ［rather than diversion］ for continence in difficult pediatric urologic disorders. Semin Pediatr Surg 1996；5：14.）

系疾病是导致终末期肾疾病的原因[21,78]。尿路感染、同种异体移植物的功能不良、术后并发症、移植物的损伤证明先天性泌尿系疾病对成功进行肾脏移植有着不利影响。免疫抑制时，对移植物和受体而言，尿路感染是特别有害的。由后尿道瓣膜导致肾衰竭的移植受体，其尿路感染风险较高[43,89]。原发病为膀胱输尿管反流和移植时持续反流至自身肾脏的患者，会出现以上类似问题[8]。

这些数据说明有明显泌尿系疾病史的患者在移植前必须进行充分评估[109]。明显的膀胱输尿管反流应该通过输尿管再植或肾切除来解决。如果可能要避免肾切除，因为其产生的尿量可以保持膀胱功能，而且如果移植物失败，移植前后的透析治疗还是可供选择的。保持内生性（促）红细胞生成素的生成，可以避免频繁输血后的致敏作用。另外，保留输尿管对于以后的移植重建非常重要，也可能会发生一些输尿管的并发症。肾切除的指征包括存在复发性的尿路感染、具有尿路感染倾向的上尿路解剖特点、难治性高血压、严重的蛋白尿和严重多尿。

必要时，可以通过侧腹部切口或腰背部切口进行肾切除，以前常用的经腹手术现在很少采用。这些操作不会影响腹膜透析。腹腔镜方法也可用于肾切除。如果考虑需要行双侧肾切除且希望先做移植（以避免透析），应先切除功能最差的肾。如果第二个肾可以提供足够的肾功能，就可以避免透析。当进行肾移植时，可以从移植切口将剩余的肾取出。

通过药物或间歇导尿（或两者皆用）来降低膀胱内压，必要时行膀胱扩大术。进行移植前，手术切口的设计很重要。这样可以减少对正在或预期进行的腹膜透析的影响，也可减少对将进行的移植手术的影响。避免丧失透析用的腹膜腔入口的最好方法就是腹膜外路径对泌尿道进行手术，这样肾切除和输尿管再植会比较容易。

膀胱功能障碍的外科重建已成功实施，且已证明可以使移植手术结果更令人满意[27]。这样的方法有利于保护同种异体移植物和完全控尿，最好将移植物与肠段管道结合。移植适用于任何甚至是解剖结构最为复杂的终末期肾疾病的患儿[30,115]。移植物连接到重建膀胱有以下原则：（1）避免干性重建。如果移植的间歇时间长，重建膀胱的容量和顺应性将丧失。可以不切除自体肾脏（如果存在的话）或利用活的同种异体移植物，以便掌控时间。（2）再吸收性酸中毒的风险可以发生在移植前自体肾引流尿液至重建膀胱时，也可能发生在移植以后移植物随时间延长而衰竭时，可以通过避免应用小肠和结肠进行膀胱重建来减轻上述风险。胃膀胱成形术、应用输尿管和肾盂扩大术及自体扩大术都可以减少潜在的再吸收性酸中毒的可能。（3）自体扩大术和应用输尿管扩大术有腹膜后操作的潜力，因而可以避免对现有或将来的腹膜透析或脑室腹腔转流的干扰。（4）如果有可能，将输尿管再植于自体膀胱是最好的。如果不可能，则只有以结肠、回盲部或胃作为扩大术的材料时才能进行可靠的抗反流吻合。（5）进行移植时，必须仔细识别和保护扩大膀胱和相应的 Mitrofanoff 新尿道的血供。

并发症

急腹症

急腹症对于经历过泌尿道重建手术的患者，尤其是在膀胱扩大或肠代储尿器操作后，是需要特别关注的问题。这种操作下最常见的外科腹部急症是扩张膀胱或肠储尿器的穿孔，以及小肠梗阻。即便原因未明，大多数穿孔还是和神经性膀胱残余部分扩大术相关[29]。超过 2/3 的此类患者经历过间歇导尿，并且完全控尿是一个常见因素。虽然临床表现就是那些急腹症的情况，但是症状可以是非特异性；即使如此，也应高度怀疑急腹症。重要的是应该认识到重建手术多年后还可能发生破裂。神经管闭合不全或脊髓束受伤以及应用类固醇的肾移植患者由于感觉异常可能会混淆诊断。膀胱造影对确立诊断非常必要，但是会有一些假阴性的情况[34,105]。腹部 CT（膀胱或储尿器造影）是建立诊断最准确的方法。然而，当行膀胱扩大术后的患者在间歇导尿时出现腹痛、发热或呕吐时都应该怀疑有穿孔的可能，除非症状可以用其他原因解释。可能需要行剖腹探查来确定诊断。不常见但很重要的鉴别诊断有小肠梗阻、假膜性肠炎、中毒休克综合征以及脑室腹腔转流并发症[108]。

在尿路重建后进行剖腹探查术需要格外注意。当然，选择性的剖腹手术应按程序正规地对扩大或可控性改道的肠段进行准备。医生在膀胱内置入一根导管以利其排空和缩小而达到识别的目的，另一根导管则放入导尿管道，比如 Mitrofanoff 新尿道。应该努力识别和保护肠系膜用来供应重建用的胃或肠段的血管。如果可能，需要一位有经验的泌尿重建科医生在场。

代谢并发症

当胃肠组织结合到尿路后可能会发生代谢紊乱。这些代谢紊乱是由于溶质主动和被动地通过胃肠道壁进入血液造成的[46,77]。这些代谢紊乱的特征和严重度与每个患者所用胃肠组织的自然状态、吸收表面的范围、停留时间、代谢储备有关。代谢变化的代偿机制由肾、肝、肺承担。以上任一脏器的损害可能会使潜在的代谢缺陷恶化。症状包括酸-碱平衡状态改变、血清电解质成分异常、高氨血症和骨质脱矿质作用。

空肠、回肠或结肠段用于膀胱扩大可以导致酸中毒。在 20%~40% 的病例中发现酸中毒和空肠管道相关[24,58]。在空肠中，根据浓度梯度进行溶质的被动扩散。高渗尿进入空肠后会导致钠、氯和水分的丢失，引起低钠血症、低氯血症和容量浓缩后的浓缩性酸中毒[20]。另外，肾血流减少会导致继发性高醛固酮血症，从而使得高渗尿和高血钾的发生增多。后者会因为酸中毒引发的钾的移位而更加恶化。

将回肠和结肠段接于泌尿道产生的代谢问题是钠（与氢交换）和碳酸氢盐（与氯交换）的主动分泌，以及氨、氢和氯的重吸收。重要的是氨的吸收量，可以解释回肠或结肠段接触尿液后的许多异常情况。由氨产生的氢离子被血清中的碳酸氢盐缓冲，并生成了水和 CO_2。后者很容易通过肺排出，造成慢性代偿性呼吸性碱中毒。另外，通过骨质缓冲后引起不同程度的骨质去矿化和继发性的甲状旁腺功能亢进，这与高钙尿症、高磷酸尿症、高草酸尿症、低枸橼酸尿症、低钙血症和低镁血症时出现的情况一样。渗透性利尿和酸中毒联合可以导致全身性的钾消耗。

代谢性碱中毒是胃膀胱成形术的并发症。虽然不常见[28]，但是低钾-低氯性代谢性碱中毒也有报道[68,85]。盐皮质激素剩余和钾/氯的消耗结合后，可能会发生碳酸氢盐的过度吸收。

将肠段和泌尿道结合起来后发生低钾血症、低钙血症及低镁血症的潜在可能值得注意[77]。有报道称会发生足以使肌肉瘫痪的严重的低钾血症。虽然低钙血症很少严重到产生临床症状，但其还是和激惹、震颤、手足抽搐以及昏迷相关，甚至致命。低镁血症也很少能引起严重症状，但是可以表现出感觉异常、人格改变、谵妄、精神错乱、虚弱、震颤、手足抽搐以及癫痫发作，同样可以致命。

用肠段进行泌尿道重建而发生的高氨血症可以导致感觉改变和昏迷。如前所述，由肾小管产生、由尿素经过分解反应生成的铵离子从肠段中主动吸收并大量存在于尿液中。

也许对于结合肠段的最重要的关注点还是患儿的生长和发育问题。一些研究数据有力证明了这些患者的线性生长缺陷[35,127]。肾功能下降的患者尤其令人担忧。他们更可能发生代谢损害，并且损害更为严重，因为生长和发育通常早已受到严重影响。

也有有力证据显示肠段结合于泌尿道对于骨质矿化有着重要影响[45]。由于肾小管对钙重吸收的下降、肠道对钙磷吸收以及维生素 D 代谢的下降，代谢性酸中毒引起了骨质矿化缺陷和骨疾病以及线性生长障碍。碱化剂治疗在阻止和逆转这种去矿化疾病中取得了部分成功。

血尿-排尿困难综合征

尽管作者经验很少[28]，但是仍然发现血尿-排尿困难综合征是胃膀胱重建术的重要并发症[19]。这种并发症的特征是严重的疼痛和血尿。这是由于胃膀胱成形术后尿中酸液分泌造成了尿路上皮的腐蚀[91]。通过对血尿-排尿困难综合征患儿的内镜检查，发现尿道受累比膀胱本身还要多一些。主要有三种重要因素导致产生这种并发症：酸液的高度分泌、极度少尿[114]以及膀胱颈无力。真正的酸液高度分泌很少见，经推测造成这种情况的主要机制是高胃泌素血症，这在一些病案中有过报道[41]。H_2受体阻断药和质子泵抑制剂如奥美拉唑对这种综合征显示出了相当疗效。

胃肠道功能的改变

肠段和泌尿道的结合可能导致胃肠道功能的改变。有胃膀胱成形术后胃功能改变的报道[39]。功能变化包括体重减轻、饮食不耐受、倾倒综合征、胃排空延迟以及食管炎。作者通过回顾对胃膀胱成形术后的食管炎患者进行的长期随访（至少随访 5 年）发现，在研究了 44 例连续的患者后并没有发现胃功能或者是酸-碱状态的改变[28]。手术技术重点必须放在避开迷走神经、避免胃幽门部的切开以及避免 His 角的牵拉扭曲（比如胃造口管所致）上，这些可能导致胃食管交界处无张力。 1837

另一个从理论上应该关注的问题是切除了足够多的壁细胞组织后，由于内生因子的减少而干扰维生素 B_{12} 的吸收。需要长期随访后才能作出这样的结论。回肠也是维生素 B_{12} 的吸收部位，已证明回肠切除与维生素 B_{12} 的减少有关。这种情况表现为巨细胞贫血和脊髓小脑退行性疾病，但是由于机体对维生素 B_{12} 的储备，所以症状可能在许多年后才表现出来。

一些可能与肠切除相关的肠吸收不良的结果有腹泻、维生素缺乏以及排便失禁。腹泻最常见，这是由于细菌移位和胆汁酸重吸收能力下降（伴发或不伴发脂肪泻）所造成的[122]。回肠切除造成的吸收不良与切除的长度直接相关。切除回肠的长度超过 100 cm（成人同样）就会在一定程度上造成胆汁酸重吸收减少，而且不能通过增加肝脏的合成来代偿。结果是胆汁池缩小，出现脂肪泻。这类患者因为胆汁池缩小造成的主要后果还有胆石症，和尿石症一样，在回肠切除后发生概率明显增高。胆汁酸重吸收变化所造成的腹泻（伴有或不伴有脂肪泻）由于回肠内容物快速排空入结肠而变得更加严重，并可能造成渗透性腹泻。

虽然大多数数据来自成年患者，但是经历过回盲瓣切除的患儿有 10% 将会出现慢性腹泻。通过把回盲肠段回复到其在胃肠道的正常位置而恢复肠道的连续性，可以解决以上问题[40]。

尽管有资料报道，大多数患儿应用了肠道和胃后还是能够表现出相当好的耐受力，但是在进行尿路重建时应当谨慎注意避免大段肠段或回盲瓣的切除，尤其是在那些已经有损害的情况下。这类患者包括先前存在吸收不良或短肠综合征者，以及排便控制力处于边缘状态的病例，由于其丧失了粪便浓缩能力而会使污粪变得更加严重。后一种情况包括脊髓脊膜膨出和肛门闭锁患者，通常需要泌尿道重建。

恶变

作者对重建后发生尿路肠道恶变的认识多数来源于输尿管乙状结肠吻合术的经验[54,116]。新成形尿道和可控性改道发生恶变的概率都较低[36,104,121]。最近还有一项关于肠膀胱扩大后发生恶变的报道[121]。对于大多数病例，手术和发生癌症之间的一段时间非常重要。潜伏期中有一些重要表现清楚提示了癌变效应。而且，早期监测诊断是有可能的。显然，长期随访很重要。

（何　蓉译　文建国校）

参考文献

1. Adams MC, Mitchell ME, Rink RC: Gastrocystoplasty: An alternative solution to the problem of urologic reconstruction in the severely compromised patient. J Urol 1988; 140:1152.
2. Barrett DM, Furlowm WL: Incontinence, intermittent self-catheterization and the artificial genitourinary sphincter. J Urol 1984;132:268.
3. Bauer SB: Early evaluation and management of children with spina bifida. In King LR (ed): Urologic Surgery in Neonates and Young Infants. Philadelphia, WB Saunders, 1988.
4. Benchekroun A, Essakalli N, Faik M, et al: Continent urostomy with hydraulic ileal valve in 136 patients: 13 years of experience. J Urol 1989;142:46.
5. Bevers RF, Abbekerk EM, Boon TA: Cowper's syringocele: Symptoms, classification and treatment of an unappreciated problem. J Urol 2000;163:782.
6. Bihrle R: The Indiana pouch continent urinary reservoir. Urol Clin North Am 1997;24:773.
7. Boemers TM, van Gool JD, de Jong TP, et al: Urodynamic evaluation of children with the caudal regression syndrome (caudal dysplasia sequence). J Urol 1994;151:1038.
8. Bouchot O, Guillonneau B, Cantarovich D, et al: Vesicoureteral reflux in the renal transplantation candidate. Eur Urol 1991;20:26.
9. Bramble FJ: The treatment of adult enuresis and urge incontinence by enterocystoplasty. Br J Urol 1982;54:693.
10. Bramble FJ: The clam cystoplasty. Br J Urol 1990;66:337.
11. Cain MP, Casale AJ, King SJ, et al: Appendicovesicostomy and newer alternatives for the Mitrofanoff procedure: Results in the last 100 patients at Riley Children's Hospital. J Urol 1999;162:1749.
12. Cain MP, Casale AJ, Rink RC: Initial experience using a catheterizable ileovesicostomy (Monti procedure) in children. Urology 1998;52:870.
13. Camey M, Richard F, Botto H: Ileal replacement of bladder. In King L, Stone AR, Webster GD (eds): Bladder Reconstruction and Continent Urinary Diversion. Chicago, Year Book, 1991, p 389.
14. Capitanucci ML, Iacobelli BD, Silveri M, et al: Long-term urological follow-up of occult spinal dysraphism in children. Eur J Pediatr Surg 1996;6(Suppl 1):25.
15. Carr MC, Mitchell ME: Gastrocystoplasty and bladder replacement with stomach. In Marshall FF (ed): Textbook of Operative Urology. Philadelphia, WB Saunders, 1996, p 500.
16. Cartwright PC, Snow BW: Bladder autoaugmentation: Early clinical experience. J Urol 1989;142:505.
17. Casale AJ: A long continent ileovesicostomy using a single piece of bowel. J Urol 1999;162:1743.
18. Castellan MA, Gosalbez R Jr, Labbie A, et al: Clinical applications of the Monti procedure as a continent catheterizable stoma. Urology 1999;54:152.
19. Chadwick Plaire J, Snodgrass WT, Grady RW, et al: Long-term followup of the hematuria-dysuria syndrome. J Urol 2000;164:921.
20. Cher ML, Roehrborn CG: Incorporation of intestinal segments into the urinary tract. In Hohenfellner A, Wammack R (eds): Continent Urinary Diversion. Edinburgh, Churchill Livingstone, 1992.
21. Churchill BM, Aliabadi H, Landon EH, et al: Ureteral bladder augmentation. J Urol 1993;150:716.
22. Churchill BM, Gilmour RF, Williot P: Urodynamics. Pediatr Clin North Am 1987;34:1133.
23. Churchill BM, Sheldon CA, McLorie GA, et al: Factors influencing patient and graft survival in 300 cadaveric pediatric renal transplants. J Urol 1988;140:1129.
24. Clark SS: Electrolyte disturbance associated with jejunal conduit. J Urol 1989;142:1201.
25. Cromie WJ, Barada JH, Weingarten J: Cecal tubularization: Lengthening technique for creation of catheterizable conduit. Urology 1991;38:41.
26. Dees JE: Congenital epispadias with incontinence. J Urol 1949;62:513.
27. DeFoor W, Minevich E, McEnery P, et al: Lower urinary tract reconstruction is safe and effective in children with end stage renal disease. J Urol 2003;170:1497, discussion 1500.
28. DeFoor W, Minevich E, Reeves D, et al: Gastrocystoplasty: Long-term followup. J Urol 2003;170:1647, discussion 1649.
29. DeFoor W, Tackett L, Minevich E, et al: Risk factors for spontaneous bladder perforation after augmentation cystoplasty. Urology 2003;62:737.
30. DeFoor W, Tackett L, Minevich E, et al: Successful renal transplantation in children with posterior urethral valves. J Urol 2003;170:2402.
31. Duckett JW, Snyder HM, Use of the Mitrofanoff principle in urinary reconstruction. World J Urol 1985;3:191.
32. Elder JS: Periurethral and puboprostatic sling repair for

incontinence in patients with myelodysplasia. J Urol 1990; 144:434.

33. Elder JS: Continent appendicocolostomy: A variation of the Mitrofanoff principle in pediatric urinary tract reconstruction. J Urol 1992;148:117.
34. Elder JS, Snyder HM, Hulbert WC, et al: Perforation of the augmented bladder in patients undergoing clean intermittent catheterization. J Urol 1988;140:1159.
35. Feng AH, Kaar S, Elder JS: Influence of enterocystoplasty on linear growth in children with exstrophy. J Urol 2002; 167:2552, discussion 2555.
36. Filmer RB, Spencer JR, Malignancies in bladder augmentations and intestinal conduits. J Urol 1990;143:671.
37. Franco I, Kolligian M, Reda EF, et al: The importance of catheter size in the achievement of urinary continence in patients undergoing a Young-Dees-Leadbetter procedure. J Urol 1994;152:710.
38. Gil-Vernet JM Jr: The ileocolic segment in urologic surgery. J Urol 1965;94:418.
39. Gold BD, Bhoopalam PS, Reifen RM, et al: Gastrointestinal complications of gastrocystoplasty. Arch Dis Child 1992; 67:1272.
40. Gonzalez R, Sidi AA, Zhang G: Urinary undiversion: Indications, technique, and results in 50 cases. J Urol 1986; 136:13.
41. Gosalbez R, Woodard JR, Broecker BH, et al: Metabolic complications of the use of stomach for urinary reconstruction. J Urol 1993;150:710.
42. Greenfield SP, Hensle TW, Berdon WE, et al: Unilateral vesicoureteral reflux and unilateral nonfunctioning kidney associated with posterior urethral valves—a syndrome? J Urol 1983;130:733.
43. Groenewegen AAM, Sukhal RN, Nauta J, et al: Results of renal transplantation in boys treated for posterior urethral valves. J Urol 1993;149:1517.
44. Hafez AT, McLorie G, Bagli D, et al: A single-centre long-term outcome analysis of artificial urinary sphincter placement in children. BJU Int 2002;89:82.
45. Hafez AT, McLorie G, Gilday D, et al: Long-term evaluation of metabolic profile and bone mineral density after ileocystoplasty in children. J Urol 2003;170:1639, discussion 1641.
46. Hall MC, Koch MO, McDougal WS: Metabolic consequences of urinary diversion through intestinal segments. Urol Clin North Am 1991;18:725.
47. Harris CF, Cooper CS, Hutcheson JC, et al: Appendicovesicostomy: The Mitrofanoff procedure—a 15-year perspective. J Urol 2000;163:1922.
48. Hendren WH: Urinary tract re-functionalization after long-term diversion. A 20-year experience with 177 patients. Ann Surg 1990;212:478, discussion 494.
49. Herndon CD, Rink RC, Shaw MB, et al: The Indiana experience with artificial urinary sphincters in children and young adults. J Urol 2003;169:650, discussion 654.
50. Herschorn S, Radomski SB: Fascial slings and bladder neck tapering in the treatment of male neurogenic incontinence. J Urol 1992;147:1073.
51. Hinman F Jr: Selection of intestinal segments for bladder substitution: Physical and physiological characteristics. J Urol 1988;139:521.
52. Homsy YL, Reid EC: Ileocystoplasty. Urology 1974;4:135.
53. Husmann DA, Snodgrass WT, Koyle MA, et al: Ureterocystoplasty: Indications for a successful augmentation. J Urol 2004;171:1247.
54. Husmann DA, Spence HM: Current status of tumor of the bowel following ureterosigmoidostomy: A review. J Urol 1990;144:607.
55. Jayanthi VR, Churchill BM, McLorie GA, et al: Concomitant bladder neck closure and Mitrofanoff diversion for the management of intractable urinary incontinence. J Urol 1995;154:886.
56. Jones DA, Holden D, George NJ: Mechanism of upper tract dilatation in patients with thick walled bladders, chronic retention of urine and associated hydroureteronephrosis. J Urol 1988;140:326.
57. Kaefer M, Retik AB: The Mitrofanoff principle in continent urinary reconstruction. Urol Clin North Am 1997;24:795.
58. Klein EA, Montie JE, Montague D, et al: Jejunal conduit urinary diversion. J Urol 1986;135:244.
59. Kock NG, Ghoneim M, Lyche K: Replacement of the bladder by the urethral Kock pouch: Functional results, urodynamics, and radiological features. J Urol 1989;141:1111.
60. Kock NG, Norlen L, Philipson BM, et al: The continent ileal reservoir (Kock pouch) for urinary diversion. World J Urol 1985;3:146.
61. Koff SA: Estimating bladder capacity in children. Urology 1983;21:248.
62. Koff SA: Guidelines to determine the size and shape of intestinal segments used for reconstruction. Estimated influence of bowel length and radius on achievement of augmented bladder volume. J Urol 1988;140:1150.
63. Koff SA: A technique for bladder neck reconstruction in exstrophy: The cinch. J Urol 1990;144:549.
64. Koff SA, Lapides J, Piazza DH: Association of urinary tract infection and reflux with uninhibited bladder contractions and voluntary sphincteric obstruction. J Urol 1979;122:373.
65. Koff SA, Murtagh DS: The uninhibited bladder in children: Effect of treatment on recurrence of urinary infection and on vesicoureteral reflux resolution. J Urol 1983;130:1138.
66. Kropp KA, Angwafo FF: Urethral lengthening and reimplantation for neurogenic incontinence in children. J Urol 1986;135:533.
67. Kryger JV, Spencer Barthold J, Fleming P, et al: The outcome of artificial urinary sphincter placement after a mean 15-year follow-up in a paediatric population. BJU Int 1999;83:1026.
68. Kurzrock EA, Baskin LS, Kogan BA: Gastrocystoplasty: Long-term followup. J Urol 1998;160:2182.
69. Leadbetter GWJ: Surgical correction of total urinary incontinence. J Urol 1954;91:261.
70. Lepor H, Jeffs RD: Primary bladder closure and bladder neck reconstruction in classical bladder exstrophy. J Urol 1983;130:1142.
71. Liard A, Seguier-Lipszyc E, Mathiot A, et al: The Mitrofanoff procedure: 20 years later. J Urol 2001;165:2394.
72. Light JK, Engelmann UH: Reconstruction of the lower urinary tract: Observations on bowel dynamics and the artificial urinary sphincter. J Urol 1985;133:594.
73. MacNeily AE, Afshar K, Coleman GU, et al: Autoaugmentation by detrusor myotomy: Its lack of effectiveness in the management of congenital neuropathic bladder. J Urol 2003;170:1643, discussion 1646.
74. Maizels M, Stephens FD, King LR, et al: Cowper's syringocele: A classification of dilatations of Cowper's gland duct based upon clinical characteristics of 8 boys. J Urol 1983; 129:111.
75. Malone PS, Ransley PG, Kiely EM: Preliminary report: The antegrade continence enema. Lancet 1990;336:1217.
76. Mathisen W: Open-loop sigmoido-cystoplasty. Acta Chir Scand 1955;110:227.
77. McDougal WS: Metabolic complications of urinary intestinal diversion. J Urol 1992;147:1199.
78. McEnery PT, Stablein DM, Arbus G, et al: Renal transplanta-

tion in children. A report of the North American Pediatric Renal Transplant Cooperative Study. N Engl J Med 1992;326:1727.
79. McGuire EJ, Wang C, Usitalo H, et al: Modified pubovaginal sling in girls with myelodysplasia. J Urol 1986;135:94.
80. McGuire EJ, Woodside JR, Borden TA, et al: Prognostic value of urodynamic testing in myelodysplastic patients. J Urol 1981;126:205.
81. McLorie GA, Sheldon CA, Fleisher M, et al: The genitourinary system in patients with imperforate anus. J Pediatr Surg 1987;22:1100.
82. Miller EA, Mayo M, Kwan D, et al: Simultaneous augmentation cystoplasty and artificial urinary sphincter placement: Infection rates and voiding mechanisms. J Urol 1998;160: 750, discussion 752.
83. Minevich E, Sheldon CA: Gastrocystoplasty–ileal Mitrofanoff stoma fistula. J Urol 1999;161:271.
84. Minevich E, Sheldon CA: Urinary tract reconstruction for continence and renal preservation. In Ziegler MM, Azizkhan RG, Weber TR (eds): Operative Pediatric Surgery. Norwalk, CT, Appleton & Lange, 2003.
85. Mingin GC, Stock JA, Hanna MK: Gastrocystoplasty: Long-term complications in 22 patients. J Urol 1999;162:1122.
86. Mitchell ME, Adams MC, Rink RC: Urethral replacement with ureter. J Urol 1988;139:1282.
87. Mitchell ME, Rink RC: Experience with the artificial urinary sphincter in children and young adults. J Pediatr Surg 1983;18:700.
88. Mitrofanoff P: Cystostomie continente trans-appendiculaire dans le traitement des vessies neurologiques. Chir Pediatr 1980;21:297.
89. Mochon M, Kaiser BA, Dunn S, et al: Urinary tract infections in children with posterior urethral valves after kidney transplantation. J Urol 1992;148:1874.
90. Mor Y, Kajbafzadeh AM, German K, et al: The role of ureter in the creation of Mitrofanoff channels in children. J Urol 1997;157:635.
91. Nguyen DH, Bain M, Salmonson K, et al: The syndrome of dysuria and hematuria in pediatric urinary reconstruction with stomach. J Urol 1993;150:707.
92. Nguyen HT, Baskin LS: The outcome of bladder neck closure in children with severe urinary incontinence. J Urol 2003;169:1114, discussion 1116.
93. Noe HN: The role of dysfunctional voiding in failure or complication of ureteral reimplantation for primary reflux. J Urol 1985;134:1172.
94. Pagano F: The vesica ileale padovana. In Holenfellner P, Wammack R (eds): Continent Urinary Diversion. Edinburgh, Churchill Livingstone, 1992, p 122.
95. Parra R: A simplified technique for continent urinary diversion: An all-stapled colonic reservoir. J Urol 1991; 146:1496.
96. Pippi Salle JL, de Fraga JCS, Amarante A, et al: Urethral lengthening with anterior bladder wall flap for urinary incontinence: A new approach. J Urol 1994;152:803.
97. Pow-Sang JM, Helal M, Figueroa E, et al: Conversion from external appliance or internal urinary diversion to a continent urinary reservoir (Florida pouch I and II): Surgical technique, indications and complications. J Urol 1992; 147:356.
98. Reddy P, Lange P, Fraley E: Total bladder replacement using detubularized sigmoid colon: Technique and results. J Urol 1991;145:51.
99. Reinberg Y, Gonzalez R, Fryd D, et al: The outcome of renal transplantation in children with posterior urethral valves. J Urol 1988;140:1491.
100. Restrepo NC, Decter RM, Phillips PP, et al: Appendiceal granulation polyps: A complication of Mitrofanoff procedure. Urology 1994;43:219.
101. Rittenberg MH, Hulbert WC, Snyder HM 3rd, et al: Protective factors in posterior urethral valves. J Urol 1988; 140:993.
102. Robertson GN, King L: Bladder substitution in children. Urol Clin North Am 1986;13:333.
103. Rowland RG, Bihrle R, Mitchell ME: The Indiana continent urinary reservoir. J Urol 1987;137:1136.
104. Rowland R, Regan F: The risk of secondary malignancies in urinary reservoirs. In Hohenfellner A, Wammack R (eds): Continent Urinary Diversion. Edinburgh, Churchill Livingstone, 1992, p 299.
105. Rushton HG, Woodard JR, Parrott TS, et al: Delayed bladder rupture after augmentation enterocystoplasty. J Urol 1988;140:344.
106. Scherz HC, Kaplan GW, Packer MG: Anterior urethral valves in the fossa navicularis in children. J Urol 1987; 138:1211.
107. Scholtmeijer RJ, van Mastrigt R: The effect of oxyphenonium bromide and oxybutynin hydrochloride on detrusor contractility and reflux in children with vesicoureteral reflux and detrusor instability. J Urol 1991; 146:660.
108. Shekarriz B, Upadhyay J, Demirbilek S, et al: Surgical complications of bladder augmentation: Comparison between various enterocystoplasties in 133 patients. Urology 2000;55:123.
109. Sheldon CA, Churchill BM, McLorie GA, et al: Evaluation of factors contributing to mortality in pediatric renal transplant recipients. J Pediatr Surg 1992;27:629.
110. Sheldon C, Cormier M, Crone K, et al: Occult neurovesical dysfunction in children with imperforate anus and its variants. J Pediatr Surg 1991;26:49.
111. Sheldon CA, Essig KA: Congenital bladder diverticulum causing bladder outlet obstruction: Case report and review of literature. Pediatr Surg Int 1994;9:141.
112. Sheldon CA, Gilbert A: Use of the appendix for urethral reconstruction in children with congenital anomalies of the bladder. Surgery 1992;112:805.
113. Sheldon CA, Gilbert A, Lewis AG, et al: Surgical implications of genitourinary tract anomalies in patients with imperforate anus. J Urol 1994;152:196.
114. Sheldon CA, Gilbert A, Wacksman J, et al: Gastrocystoplasty: Technical and metabolic characteristics of the most versatile childhood bladder augmentation modality. J Pediatr Surg 1995;30:283.
115. Sheldon CA, Gonzaleas R, Burns MW, et al: Renal transplantation into dysfunctional bladder: The role of adjunctive bladder reconstruction. J Urol 1994;152:972.
116. Sheldon CA, McKinley RD, Hartig PR, et al: Carcinoma at the site of ureterosigmoidostomy. J Dis Colon Rectum 1983;26:55.
117. Sheldon CA, Minevich E, Wacksman J, et al: Role of the antegrade continence enema in the management of the most debilitating childhood recto-urogenital anomalies. J Urol 1997;158:1277, discussion 1279.
118. Sheldon CA, Minevich E, Wacksman J: Modified technique of antegrade continence enema using a stapling device. J Urol 2000;163:589.
119. Skinner DG, Lieskovsky G, Boyd SD, Continuing experience with the continent ileal reservoir (Kock pouch) as an alternative to cutaneous urinary diversion: An update after 250 cases. J Urol 1987;137:1140.
120. Smith RB, van Cangh P, Skinner DG, et al: Augmentation

enterocystoplasty: A critical review. J Urol 1977;118:35.
121. Soergel MT, Cain MP, Misseri R, et al: Transitional cell carcinoma following augmentation cystoplasty for neuropathic bladder. Paper presented at a meeting of the American Academy of Pediatrics, 2003, New Orleans.
122. Steiner MS, Morton RA: Nutritional and gastrointestinal complications of the use of bowel segments in the lower urinary tract. Urol Clin North Am 1991;18:743.
123. Tackett LD, Minevich E, Benedict JF, et al: Appendiceal versus ileal segment for antegrade continence enema. J Urol 2002;167:683.
124. Thomsen H: Pyelorenal backflow. Danish Med Bull 1984;31:348.
125. Turner-Warwick R, Ashken HM: The functional results of partial subtotal and total cystoplasty. Br J Urol 1967; 39:3.
126. Van Savage JG, Khoury AE, McLorie GA, et al: An algorithm for the management of anterior urethral valves. J Urol 1997;158:1030.
127. Wagstaff KE, Woodhouse CJ, Duffy PG, et al: Delayed linear growth in children with enterocystoplasties. Br J Urol 1992;69:314.
128. Wammack R, et al: The Maintz pouch. In Holenfellner P, Wammack R (eds): Continent Urinary Diversion. Churchill Livingstone, Edinburgh, 1992, p 131.
129. Wan J, McGuire EJ, Bloom DA, et al: Stress leak point pressure: A diagnostic tool for incontinent children. J Urol 1993;150:700.
130. Whitmore WF, Gittes RF: Reconstruction of the urinary tract by cecal and ileocecal cystoplasty: Review of a 15-year experience. J Urol 1983;129:494.
131. Yerkes EB, Cain MP, King S, et al: The Malone antegrade continence enema procedure: Quality of life and family perspective. J Urol 2003;169:320.
132. Yerkes EB, Rink RC, Cain MP, et al: Use of a Monti channel for administration of antegrade continence enemas. J Urol 2002;168:1883, discussion 1885.
133. Young HH: An operation for the cure of incontinence associated with epispadias. J Urol 1922;7:1.
134. Young HH, Frontz WA, Baldwin JC: Congenital obstruction of the posterior urethra. J Urol 1919;3:289-365; J Urol 2002;167:265, discussion 268.

第 118 章

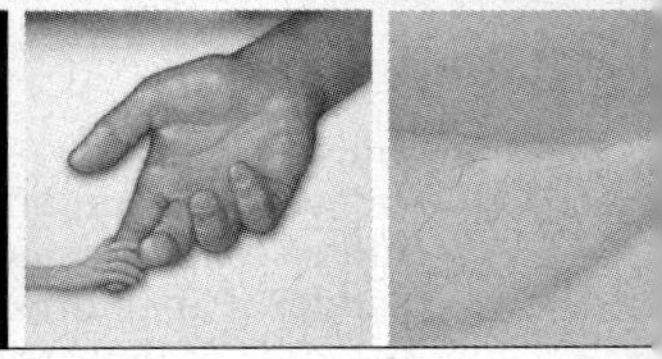

膀胱和泄殖腔外翻

John W. Brock III、Romano T. DeMarco 和 James A. O'Neill, Jr.

膀胱外翻

(John W. Brock Ⅲ和 Romano T. DeMarco)

1841 对膀胱外翻症的最先描述发现于大约公元前 2000 年亚述人的碑文上，此碑文现在存放在伦敦的大不列颠博物馆内。1597 年，Von Grafenberg 对膀胱外翻进行了描述，直到 1780 年 Chausseir 才确定了*膀胱外翻*这一术语。Mowat 在其 1748 年的工作中首先对膀胱外翻进行了完整地描述[96]。

正如 1849 年 MacKay 和 Syme[80] 的设想一样，膀胱外翻最初的治疗方法包括将一个外部的泌尿容器放在外翻膀胱的表面。后来 Syme[118] 还想出将输尿管乙状结肠吻合作为可控性尿流改道的方法。首次使用该方法的患者最后死于肾盂肾炎。1869 年，Thiersch[119] 描述应用外翻膀胱的两侧边缘来包裹可以达到 100 ml 的膀胱容量，但患者尿失禁及尿路败血症成为主要问题。

1894 年 Maydl[83] 应用了一种更为成功的尿流改道方法，主要包括将带有输尿管的膀胱三角区移植到直肠上。随后描述的输尿管乙状结肠吻合技术经过 Coffey[20]、Nesbitt[97] 以及 Leadbetter 和 Clarke[76] 等人的逐步改进提高后，避免了乙状结肠-输尿管反流问题。然而，这种技术常引起感染、电解质紊乱以及有可能诱发癌症[8]。尿流改道优先考虑提供控尿能力和控制感染，但是主要问题是解剖结构变化和性功能障碍。

成功发展的有效的尿流改道方法还包括膀胱闭合和重建。Trendelenburg[121] 报道了双侧骶骨截骨，应用骨盆环来保证前方膀胱及腹壁的闭合。1924 年 Burn[5,12] 和 1933 年 Janssen[58] 采纳了 Trendelenburg 的方法均成功进行了手术，但直到 1942 年 Young[130] 报道了第一例女性膀胱外翻关闭膀胱后能够控尿的病例。然后于 1948 年 Michon[88] 报道了 1 例成功进行了全部畸形重建手术的男性病例。

尽管如此，1970 年 Marshall 和 Muecke[82] 在对 329 例病例进行了回顾分析后得出结论，在那些完成了全部重建手术的患者中只有 19% 得到了令人满意的外观。其他作者也得出了相似的不理想的结论，指出还应该在尿流改道方法上更加努力精益求精[70,125]。以后，Lepor 和 Jeffs[77]、Mesrobian 等人[86] 以及 Hollowell 和 Ransley[52] 报道了经过分期重建手术，即尿道成形术、尿道上裂修补以及必要的膀胱扩大后，75%~80% 的患者能够控制排尿。1999 年，Grady 和 Mitchell[46] 在经过了成功手术实践后提倡在新生儿期进行完全初期膀胱外翻修补（CPER），与分期操作相比更令人满意。这种结论促使许多医院改变了对膀胱外翻新生儿的初期手术方法。

发病率

根据大量人群研究，膀胱外翻发病率估计为 1/10 000~1/50 000活产儿[73,75]。不同类型的男女比例在 2.3:1 到 4:1 之间[109]。这些数据说明膀胱外翻是一种罕见畸形，尤其是在女性中。

那些经过重建术后存活到成年的膀胱外翻患者，如果有机会成为父母亲，则需要考虑家族性再发病的风险。Ives 等人[56] 认为有 1/100 遗传的可能，但是 Shapiro 等人[109] 经过对 2500 例患者的调查发现遗传率只有 1/275。对同卵双生子的研究发现其 1 人或 2 人发生膀胱外翻的差异很大[56,109]。这就是膀胱外翻患者今后同胞的发病风险其实很小的原因，但遗传方式还未明确。尽管如此，这样的发病概率相对于普通人群仍明显增高——Shapiro 等人估计可达到 400 倍[109]。

胚胎学

经典的膀胱外翻的概念通过外观描述就可以推断
342 出来：如同用剪刀的一片刀刃将一个正常人的尿道剪开直至膀胱，而另一片刀刃则将腹壁皮肤剪开，膀胱和尿道在前，耻骨分开，而且切缘展开就像是打开了一本书。为了解释这种现象，胚胎学发生和重塑模型实验方面进行了许多努力[3,89,100]。解剖上的差异比如泄殖腔外翻将在本章节的附录中阐述，其中揭示了孕第四周至第十周期间这种组织结构的胚胎发生和起源，包括后肠的异常分化。

最初发育时，总泄殖腔通过泄殖腔膜与羊膜腔分隔开来，泄殖腔膜占据了腹壁脐部以下的位置[89]。泄殖腔膜内外胚层之间的间叶细胞向内生长可以形成下腹壁肌肉和耻骨。同时，泌尿直肠隔膜下降将泄殖腔分隔成前方的膀胱和后方的直肠，这层隔膜与后部残余的泄殖腔膜汇合，最终穿通形成肛门和泌尿生殖道的开口（图 118-1）。泄殖腔膜穿通前，两侧生殖结节移至泄殖腔膜前方中线上并融合。

近来的胚胎理论与 Muecke[95] 的实验研究有关，他在 1964 年指出在鸡胚胎 2～3 周时于泄殖腔膜上放置一塑料楔状物可阻止前部的泄殖腔膜的形成，导致膀胱外翻。Marshall 和 Muecke[81] 以及 Pohlman[103] 研究后强调由于泄殖腔膜的过度发育导致了基础缺陷，从而阻止了间叶组织的迁移和下腹壁及耻骨的正常发育。前部泄殖腔膜破裂的确切位置和时间决定了不同的发育异常，尽管经典的膀胱外翻占据了超过一半的病例数。

解剖异常

膀胱外翻可以被认为属于膀胱外翻复合畸形解剖异常的范畴[13]。这些异常包括耻骨分离、女性尿道上裂、男性尿道上裂、经典膀胱外翻、膀胱上瘘、重复膀胱外翻、膀胱外翻合并肛门闭锁和泄殖腔外翻（图 118-2）。与泄殖腔膜不同程度过度发育相关的是腹壁发育程度的多样性。在严重的经典膀胱外翻和泄殖腔外翻病例中，往往在外翻膀胱上方合并有脐部膨出。

在经典的膀胱外翻中，外翻的膀胱大小不一。外翻的膀胱板可以很大，同时有耻骨分离，一侧或两侧的膀胱板边缘可能很小并发育不全（图 118-3）。虽然出生时上尿路通常是正常的，但输尿管肾盂积水可能会发生。出生后随着时间流逝，膀胱黏膜由于慢性炎症、水肿和纤维化而发生化生。这样，随之会发生慢性输尿管梗阻和输尿管肾盂积水。这些因素需加以考虑，因为这关系到最终的重建方式和时间的选择。

临床表现

一般而言，具有各种膀胱外翻复合畸形的病例往往为足月产，没有相关的生理问题。严重的膀胱外翻

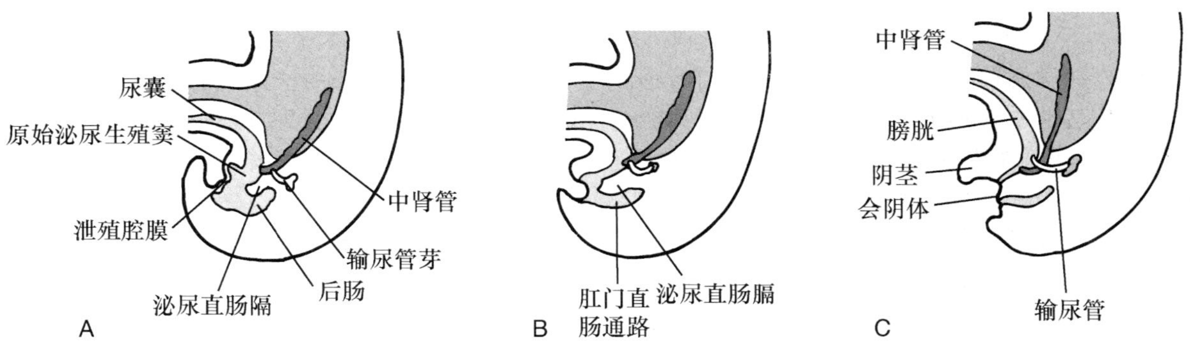

图 118-1　泄殖腔分裂成泌尿生殖窦和直肠。A. 孕第五周末期。B. 孕第七周。C. 孕第八周。（Adapted from Sadler TW：Langman's Medical Embryology，8th ed. Philadelphia，Lippincott Williams and Wilkins，2000，p 316.）

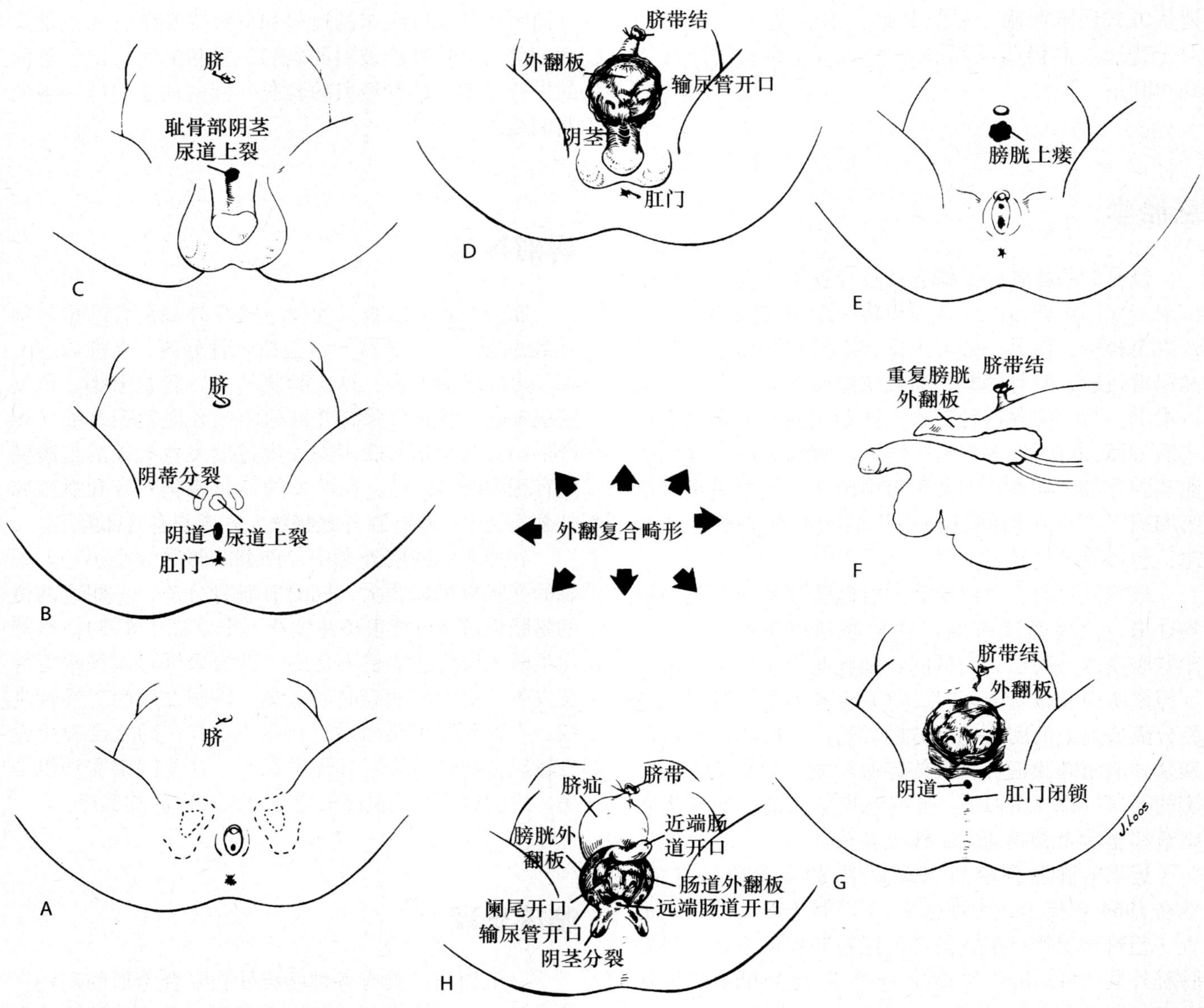

图 118-2 外翻复合畸形种类。A. 耻骨分离。B. 女性尿道上裂。C. 男性尿道上裂。D. 经典的膀胱外翻。E. 膀胱上瘘。F. 重复膀胱外翻。G. 膀胱外翻合并肛门闭锁。H. 泄殖腔外翻。

尤其是泄殖腔外翻病例早产发生率增高。经典的膀胱外翻病例很少有其他系统的异常情况。然而，在其他形式的膀胱外翻-尿道上裂复合畸形病例中往往合并多种异常。比如，膀胱上裂或泄殖腔外翻的病例常见有骨骼缺损、脊髓脊膜膨出和心血管畸形。

出生时，典型的外翻膀胱显而易见（图 118-4）；由于耻骨联合分离程度不同，膀胱壁背侧翻转程度也不同。尿液从翻转的膀胱壁下端边缘渗漏出来，但是输尿管开口可能不明显。脐部紧靠于膀胱板上缘，合并小的脐疝或脐膨出很常见。外翻的膀胱黏膜在出生时可能是正常的或者有一些数量不等的炎性息肉；接着，由于暴露和慢性炎症，黏膜表面增厚并呈水螅状（图 118-5）。虽然出生时膀胱壁肌肉有顺应性和适度的弹性，但随着时间推移，由于长时间暴露引发的慢性炎症，肌肉可能变得纤维化、坚硬和不能弯曲。

所有的膀胱外翻病例都存在一定程度的耻骨分离，这种分离导致耻骨支与坐骨及髂骨结合部的向外旋转和翻转。严重病例的髋骨和髋关节结合呈向下和向外分离。Sponseller 等人[114]运用计算机 X 线断层摄影术（CT）对骨盆进行三维重建显像，注意到膀胱

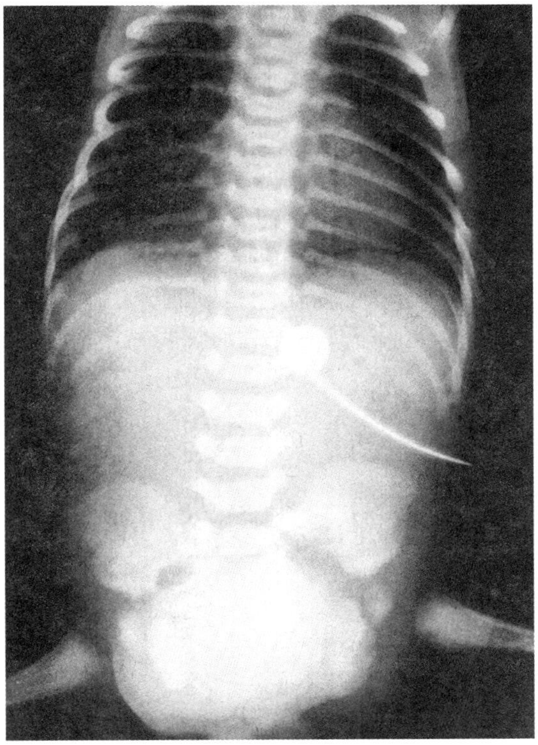

图 118-3　膀胱外翻新生儿平片显示了外翻膀胱呈软组织块影、耻骨分离以及髋关节后旋。

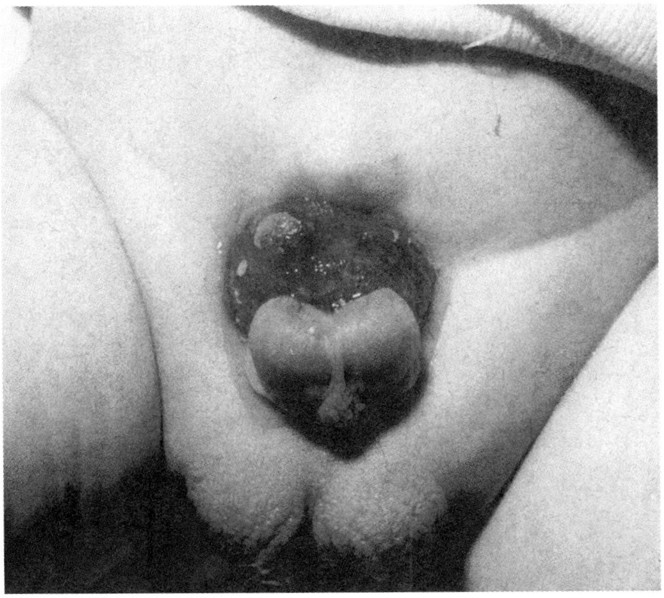

图 118-4　一例典型膀胱外翻男性新生儿的特征性表现。有小的膀胱板及在其上界还有一小的疝。阴茎缩短，阴茎体分得很开且伴随龟头分裂。特征性的表现是这些患者的尿道板短。

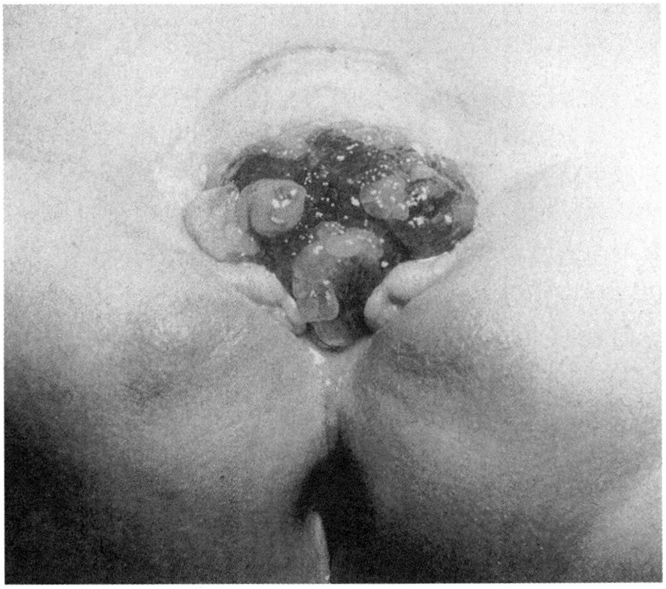

图 118-5　当出生后膀胱暴露超过 1 星期，黏膜会受影响而发生炎症，出现典型的水螅状赘生物，如同这例女性新生儿。避免这种并发症需出生后尽可能即行膀胱关闭术。

外翻儿童的骨盆骨骼有一些异常。这些包括髋臼 Y 形软骨组织之间的距离增大、髂骨前部的外旋和缩短（30%）、髂骨后部的外旋和髋臼的后倾。另外，Stec 等人[117]运用三维 CT 显像技术显示，膀胱外翻病例相对于年龄一致的对照组骶髂关节角增大了 10 度，骨盆向下过度旋转了 14.7 度，而骶骨体积增大了 42.6%。Stec 等人[116]通过三维 CT 显像也发现骨盆底 1844
肌肉组织的明显不同，尤其是肛提肌的定向。

有趣的是当患儿开始走路时，由于臀部关节的外旋会有一种特征性的蹒跚步态。然而下肢长骨的内旋不久便可以纠正这种问题。正如 Cracchiolo 和 Hall[23] 及 Kelly[66] 的报道，大多数患儿很少有甚至没有运动系统的问题或缺陷。

已经提及经典的膀胱外翻往往伴有一个小的脐疝，除非大的疝，一般不需要特殊治疗。膀胱外翻患儿也常常合并有腹股沟疝。由于筋膜有很大缺损，因此疝具有直疝和斜疝的特征。这种筋膜缺损向两侧延伸至腹直肌且超越腹直肌鞘，在分开的盆骨之间向下延伸到泌尿生殖膈。斜疝的形成归结于大的持续突起的鞘膜、大的腹股沟内外环和腹股沟管斜度的缺失。要修补这样的腹股沟疝应包括疝囊高位结扎和固定腹横筋膜，直疝修补则需用 Coop 筋膜通过各种方式建立内斜度。另外，睾丸可能没有下降。但是在大多数病例中，睾丸是回缩性的，最终将停留在阴囊内，并不需要行睾丸固定术。

在膀胱外翻患者中，因为脐部和肛门之间距离缩短使得会阴部显得短而宽。肛门通常前移而直接位于
1845 泌尿生殖膈的后方，对应于前腹壁大的三角筋膜缺损的后界。直肠通路和肛门通常是正常的，但也可出现狭窄而需要扩张。在极少数病例中肛门是异位的，可以存在直肠会阴瘘或直肠阴道瘘。显然，肛门括约肌也向前移位，并且肛提肌复合体分叉。后者导致10%~20%的患者出现会阴底部的薄弱和直肠脱垂。由于外翻膀胱的慢性炎症刺激，婴儿期可以引起异常负荷，导致直肠脱垂情况加重。未进行膀胱外翻纠治的婴儿可以出现一定程度的肛门失禁，尽管随着时间延长通常可以改善。直肠脱垂在膀胱关闭后进行处理。

男性生殖器缺陷

大多数膀胱外翻病例为男性，不论患者是否即将进行功能性关闭或尿流改道，对生殖器的评估都是重建计划中的重要组成部分。以往观点认为阴茎体直径正常，但是由于耻骨分离较宽使得其显得短，且阴茎体有明显的翘起，有缩短的尿道裂槽和阴茎海绵体脚附着异常（图 118-6）[27]。最近，Sliver 等人[111]发现男性膀胱外翻患者的阴茎体全长和前面部分明显缩短，提示阴茎体缩短与先天性阴茎体和骨盆异常相关[111]。事实上，其缩短程度，尤其当合并明显背屈时，可能非常严重，以致阴茎体和龟头接近于精阜。

大多数病例中，功能性的阴茎重建可以完成。但是对于一些阴茎严重短小的少见个案，性别转换较为合适。如果考虑进行性别转换，则患儿出生时需要一位有经验的医生和多学科团队一起完成详细的评估鉴定。

体检发现龟头呈特征性扁平状，阴茎体对半翻转，包皮堆积于阴茎体腹侧表面。阴茎体根部和阴囊分开很宽。正常时阴茎体和自主海绵体神经穿过前列腺的后外侧表面，但对于膀胱外翻患者则转移到了两边[107]。Hanna 和 Williams[49]在检查时发现射精管和输精管正常，并且在后尿道的开口明显（图 118-7）。另外，少见的变异还包括重复阴茎以及龟头和阴茎体的单侧发育不良。

女性生殖器缺陷

在女性病例中，阴蒂呈特征性分裂，同时伴有阴唇、阴阜、耻骨的对半分裂（图 118-8）。尿道和阴道短，阴道开口通常移至前方而且常常狭窄。除了偶见的重复阴道和子宫病外，患者子宫、输卵管和卵巢通常是正常的。因为膀胱外翻患者的骨盆底薄弱，常发生子宫脱垂的现象，直到前壁修补手术完成。

图 118-6　典型的男性膀胱外翻。正常男性会阴（A）和膀胱外翻（B）。注意会阴三角区的缺陷。1. 阴茎海绵体；2. 阴茎头；3. 尿道海绵体；4. 球海绵体肌；5. 坐骨；6. 坐骨耻骨支；7. 耻骨；8. 坐骨海绵体肌和阴茎脚；9. 泌尿生殖膈；10. 肛门和肛门外括约肌。

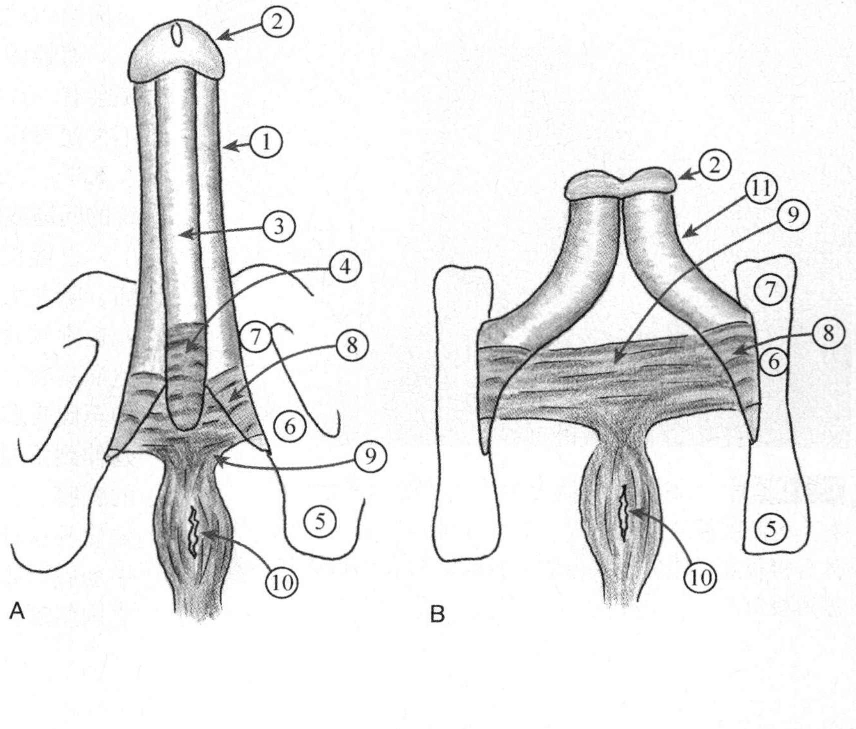

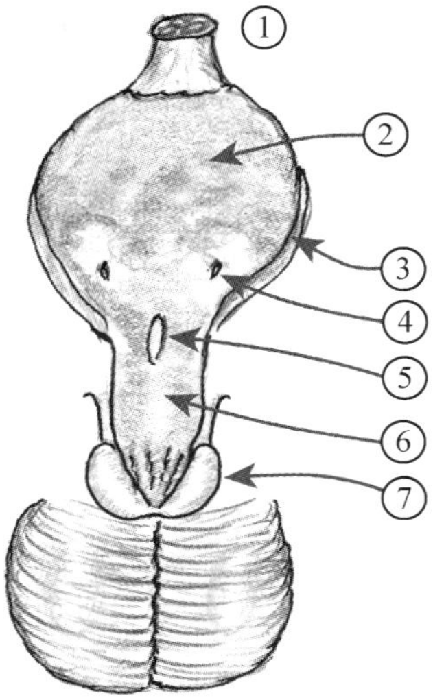

图 118-7 典型的男性膀胱外翻。阴茎被向下拉以暴露其背面。1. 脐带；2. 膀胱黏膜；3. 外翻周围组织；4. 左侧输尿管开口；5. 精阜；6. 尿道板；7. 阴茎头。

346 膀胱外翻的少见变异

隐匿性膀胱外翻

隐匿性膀胱外翻患者常常有特征性的耻骨联合分离和腹直肌异常。尿道呈卷管封闭状，但是膀胱可能

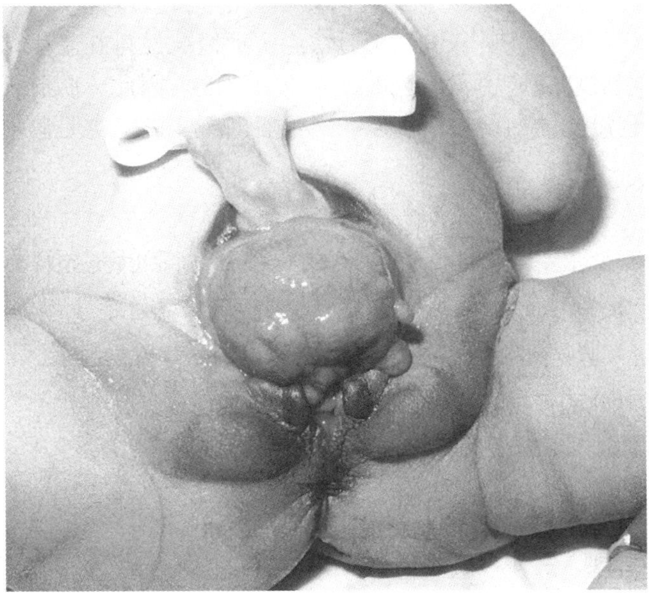

图 118-8 女性经典膀胱外翻的特征性表现。泌尿生殖膈后移导致肛门和泌尿生殖道之间的距离缩短。

只有一层皮肤覆盖[17]。可能有小的膀胱皮肤瘘或一小片不与泌尿系相通的异位膀胱黏膜。一些作者比如Turner 等人[122]和 Williams[124]描述了具有分裂变异的患者，包括耻骨分离、膀胱上瘘和重复膀胱外翻。这些变异常见于女性，且合并有先前描述的生殖器异常。

重复膀胱外翻

重复膀胱外翻患者存在耻骨分离，外翻膀胱片正好位于脐部下方，一个正常或较正常稍小的完整的膀胱在其下方（图 118-2F）。外翻的重复膀胱黏膜片是干燥的。在这些病例中，阴茎可能有不正常的短小，并可能有重复阴茎的尿道上裂。

膀胱上瘘

在膀胱上瘘患者中，耻骨和腹直肌通常是分裂的，不过膀胱突出仅表现在脐部以下水平（见图118-2E）。在前腹壁常有与膀胱相通的小通道，膀胱通过该通道表现出不同程度的脱垂。这种异常能够与脐尿管的开放区别，因为膀胱外翻复合畸形有特殊的耻骨联合与肌肉分离。

假性膀胱外翻

在假性膀胱外翻患者中，有些发现常与经典的膀胱外翻相关，包括脐部低位和附着于中度分离盆骨上的腹直肌有不同程度的分裂。膀胱充盈时可以突出于分裂的下腹壁，尿路却完全正常。

产前诊断

Barth[6]、Jaffe[57]和 Mirk[90]等已经描述了膀胱外翻产前超声的表现。膀胱在孕 15 周时可以有明显显像，每 1~3 小时排空 1 次。因此，如果膀胱影像缺失但是有正常的肾脏和羊水，且脐部位置是低位，则怀疑是膀胱外翻。孕后期，疑似耻骨分离可提示存在膀胱外翻。Gear-

hart 等人[35]回顾了产下膀胱外翻婴儿的 25 位妇女的产前超声，发现：(1) 膀胱缺失占 71%；(2) 下腹壁突出占 47%；(3) 男性胎儿阴囊前移且小阴茎占 57%；(4) 脐带低位占 29%；(5) 髂嵴的异常增宽占 18%。有了准确的产前诊断，父母可以接受劝告，制订早期进行产后
1847 处理的计划。产前诊断还可以使孕妇考虑在分娩前去往合适的三级医疗中心，使得孕妇和全家都能与对此病有经验的健康医疗人员近距离接触。

诊断检查

出生后，体格检查通常能提供早期修补手术计划的大多数所需信息。体格检查可以对膀胱板的尺寸和生殖器缺陷进行评估。应用肾脏超声（US）可以检测是否有肾盂积水或其他上尿路畸形。

另外，那些合并有其他器官系统畸形的患者或是疑似患者应该接受非常规的诊断评估（比如全血细胞计数、血清尿素氮和血糖水平、常规放射线检查）。对于早产的低体重儿，应该对未成熟肺进行评估。对于已经多年接受分阶段膀胱和下尿路重建的患者，或者是那些经过了初期修补的随访患者，需增加影像学和功能性检查，包括肾脏 US 、排尿性膀胱尿路造影（VCUG）和放射性核素以及尿流动力学检查。

治疗

膀胱外翻的治疗方法大体有两种（图 118–9）[5,9,18,40,45,46]。第一种方法是应用先进技术一次或分阶段进行功能性的下尿路重建。第二种方法包括外翻膀胱的切除和尿流改道替代法，这种方法只用于初期重建选择不合适或者是反复功能重建失败时。关于功能性重建，当男孩的阴茎组织不足而不利于男性倾向时应该考虑性别转换。随着尿道上裂修补技术的发展，男女之间的性别转换现在已不再普遍。要对患者进行性别转换必须经过多学科的讨论和广泛咨询，应该在其他所有选择都不能实施的情况下才加以考虑。

分阶段功能性重建

现代对膀胱外翻治疗的分阶段重建步骤最先由 Jeffs[60]在 20 世纪 70 年代提出，之前的患者经过各种单一阶段修复手术后效果较差，包括尿失禁和肾损伤[32,33,67,82,85]。图 118–9 提供了分期功能性重建的大体时间原则。第一阶段在出生时实施，可以保护上尿路和利于以后的控尿性重建。第二阶段男孩的典型选择是在出生 6 个月到 1 岁时进行，希望最大限度保证生殖器的结构和功能，以及增加出口阻力来促进膀胱的生长。最后，大约 4 岁时，对膀胱颈部进行修补，目的是获得社会生活所需的控制力和增强自尊。图 118–10描述的是女孩的初期膀胱关闭和尿道重建，图 118–11 展示了男孩第一阶段术后的完成效果。

近代儿科麻醉和术后重症监护情况使得在新生儿期成功完成主要的手术操作成为可能。因此，膀胱外翻患儿的初期重建可以在出生后即刻实施，这是骨盆

图 118–9　新生儿膀胱外翻患儿的远端生殖泌尿系重建手术方法。CPER，完全的初期外翻修补。

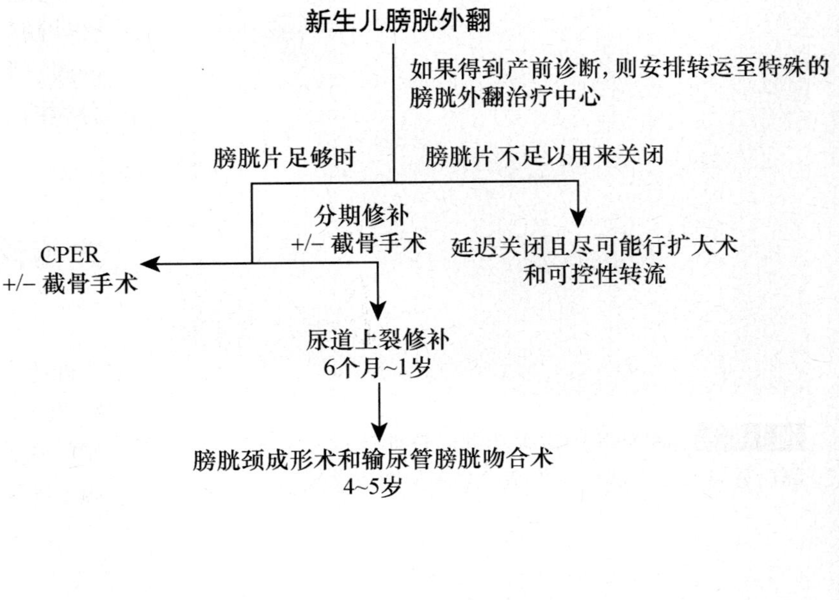

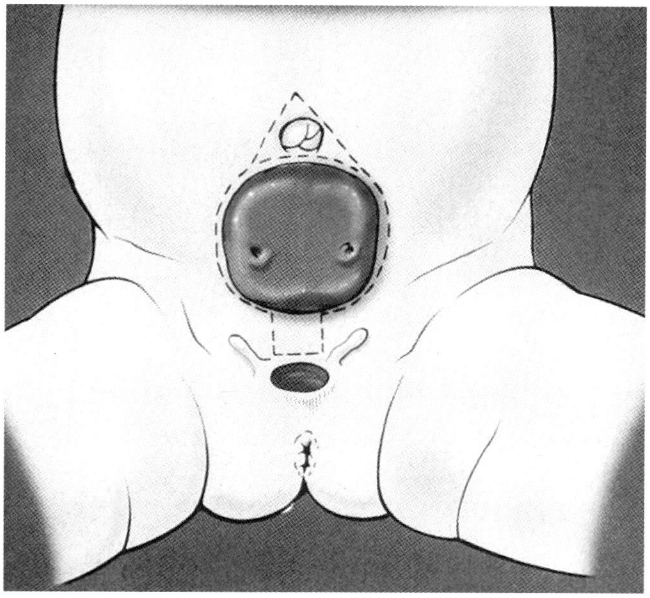

图 118-10　女性经典膀胱外翻的特征性表现和用于修补的切口。

环柔韧性最好的时期。而且，在新生儿期重建可以防止膀胱板暴露后不可避免的损伤和瘢痕化。另外，因
48 为刚出生时胃肠道和泌尿生殖道的细菌定居最少，所以很少发生手术后的严重感染。

手术前准备包括对所有内脏系统进行评估，保证没有生理上的严重畸形。如前所述，许多患有经典膀胱外翻的婴儿没有这些表现。要采取一些措施来避免对暴露的膀胱黏膜造成损伤，包括给膀胱板盖上柔软湿润的敷料（最好是聚四氟乙烯树脂或硅橡胶补片）以防损伤，以及去除脐带夹和脐带残端缝线以防止机械性损伤。在术前和术后应用抗生素。手术时患儿应有较宽泛的手术准备范围，包括乳头水平以下的躯体前部和后部使其可以翻转。因为手术时间长且应激强，全面监护和良好的静脉通路非常关键。

图 118-11 展示男孩初期膀胱关闭和尿路重建技术[78]。应用最广的技术基于 Jeffs 等人[38,40,59-61]和 Duckett 以及 Caldamone[29]的描述，包括将外翻的膀胱转换为不能控尿的尿道上裂。

用 5-0 Prolene 缝线牵引阴茎头，用输尿管导管保护两侧输尿管开口（见图 118-11A 和 G）。沿着膀胱板的外缘切开，仔细操作不要涉及任何的腹壁皮肤。切口向远端延伸至前列腺尿道的两侧以暴露精阜，保留较宽的膀胱颈部和前列腺尿道板。切除脐带以减少伤口感染的风险，脐部整形通常在初期重建手术时或以后进行。对于尿道长度有疑问的患儿，Duckett 建议利用外翻侧边制成翼状皮瓣[27]（见图 118-11E）。但是需要说明并非所有外科医生都会利用这样的翼状结构。Gearhart 等人[38,42]报道根据他们对于边翼的经验，约有 40% 的并发症发生率。尿道狭窄是最常见的并发症，与边翼组织的缺血有关。Duckett[27]尚未报道这些问题具有相同的发生率。这些边翼的益处之一就是通过延长尿道将膀胱板从阴茎上分离后，膀胱可以游离到骨盆的深部。

膀胱必须充分游离且保护好血供。阴茎海绵体尽量充分地从耻骨支下方解剖出来且要保留好神经血管束。阴茎体应仔细地靠拢于中线以利于阴茎的延长。外翻膀胱的周围边翼亦应游离延展于远端尿道板的周边，这样能够防止缺血。然后，边翼组织靠拢于中线并由可吸收缝线材料连于膀胱基底部。从腹腔引出输尿管支撑管，从耻骨上引出蘑菇头导尿管以及小硅橡胶尿道支撑管后将膀胱和新尿道进行卷管。现在存在一些争论，即是否将输尿管支撑管放置在那些有膀胱裂开倾向的患者身上。作者尚未发现这样的病例，且认为如果不放管输尿管阻塞的风险会加大。膀胱关闭后，耻骨接近于前方来防止膀胱关闭处和尿道重建处于高张力和发生破裂。大多数外科医生认为关闭耻骨环利于术后恢复以及之后获得控制力。可应用单股不吸收单纤丝缝线或是 Teflon 线关闭耻骨环，注意缝线材料的放置，使得线结缝合在耻骨前方，这样可以避免对耻骨下软组织的侵蚀。

在耻骨支关闭于中线后，使腹直肌筋膜和皮肤进一步覆盖新关闭的膀胱和尿道，或者由筋膜边翼覆盖[99]。耻骨的闭合可以不需要或最小限度使用到筋膜边翼来关闭腹壁。刚出生的患儿耻骨关闭一般不需要行截骨术，但是出生超过 3～4 天的患儿通常需要进行截骨手术，因为那时的耻骨环已经丧失弹性（图 118-12）。这种情况下，患儿将在术后进行 4～6 周的 Bryant 牵引或外固定。

女性患儿膀胱外翻的早期关闭手术相似。膀胱游离的方法和男孩相同，外翻膀胱边翼同样被伸展应用。膀胱和新尿道的闭合方式也与前面描述的一样。应用这种技术时，要将一牵引线固定在阴道上方，并且当新尿道成形时要充分游离阴道。把阴道向下放置使得开口处的远端有个角度。这是个重要的技术要点，因为如果阴道腹侧开放，将会使后来的重建操作很困难。耻骨关闭有保护作用，患儿将进行 Bryant 牵引。 1850

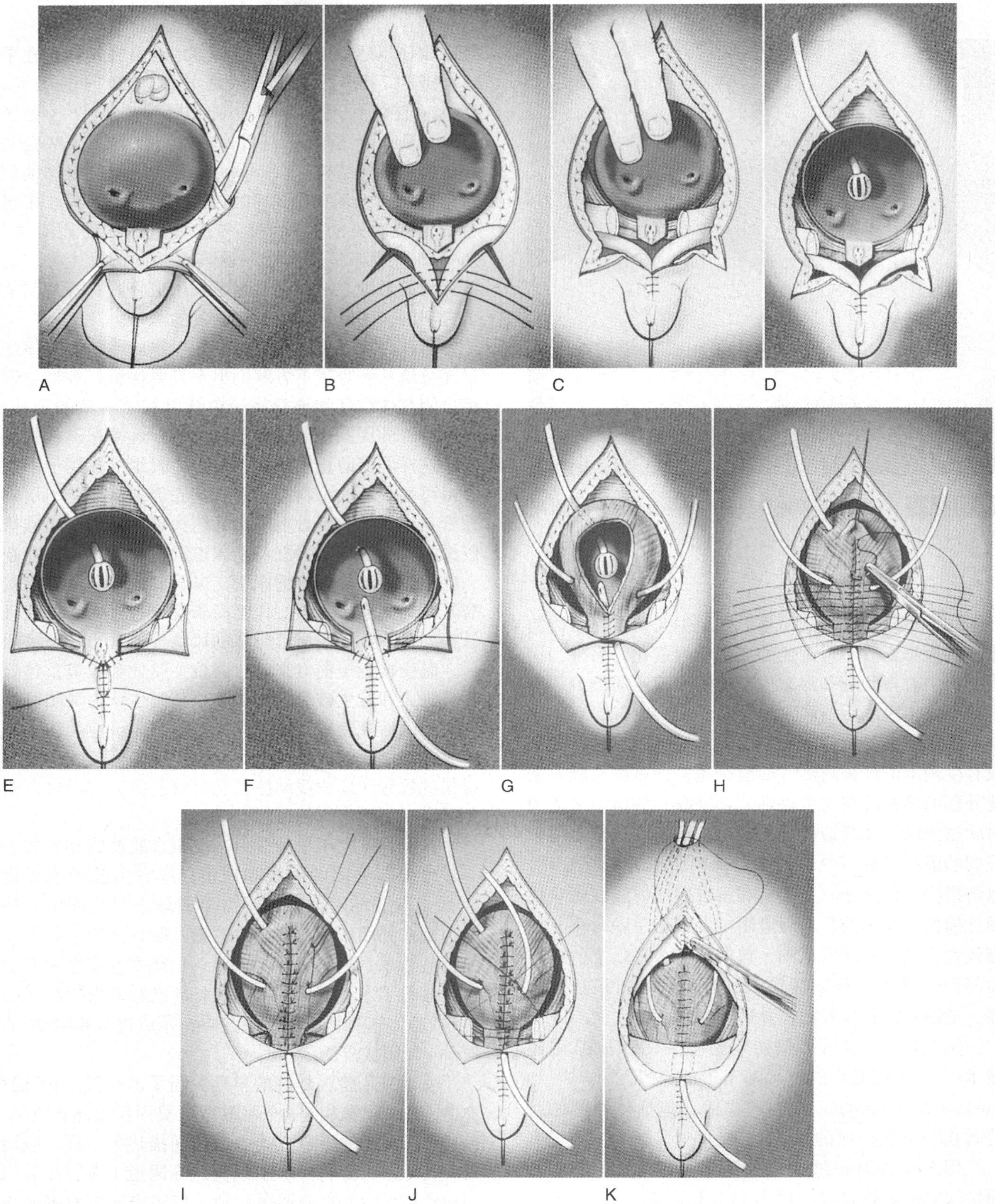

图 118-11 男性膀胱外翻修补系列图示。A. 完成沿着膀胱和尿道板周围的切开。B. 内翻膀胱板和靠拢阴茎体，这是尿道上裂修补的第一步。也要注意外翻膀胱下极周围的切开。C. 阴茎体上方皮肤关闭，且阴茎体部分从耻骨上游离。D. 放置耻骨上引流管。E. 进一步关闭下方的皮肤，接近于尿道板。现在外翻膀胱周围边翼就明显了。F. 尿道板准备以包绕导管行卷管缝合。G. 尿道板卷管缝合，输尿管导管分别放置于两条输尿管内并且各自从膀胱两侧引出。膀胱也即将行包裹缝合。H. 完成膀胱和尿道的包裹缝合，将各个引流管放置妥当。I. 膀胱和尿道板两层缝合关闭后，膀胱被放入盆腔并缝合固定。J. 尽量将耻骨支缝合靠拢。K. 引流管向上穿出，并关闭筋膜、皮下组织和皮肤。耻骨闭合对膀胱和腹壁的关闭起保护作用。

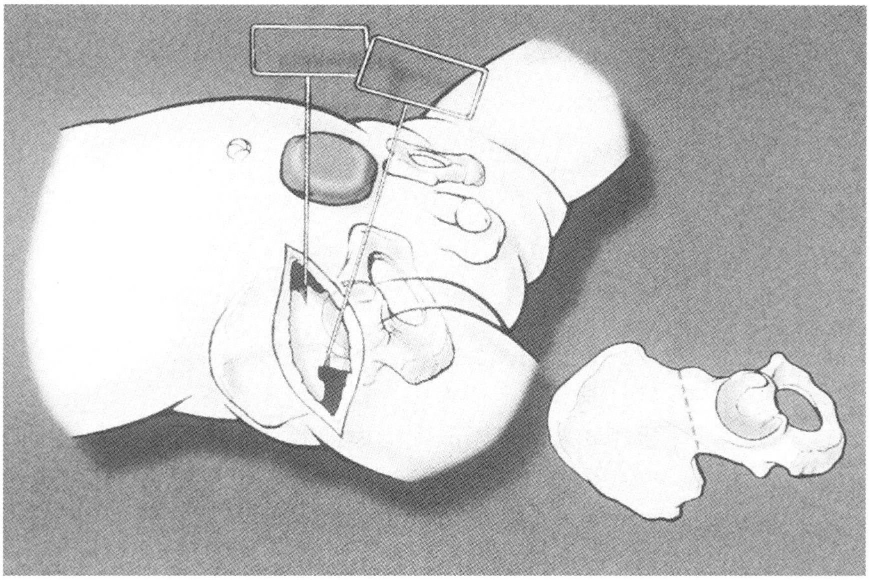

A

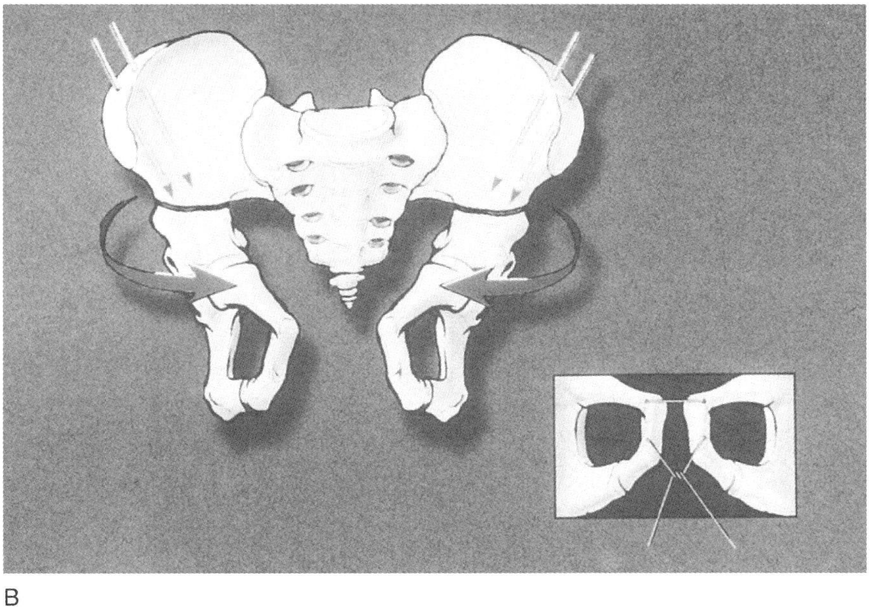

B

图 118-12 A. 通常在新生儿期闭合耻骨，因为那时耻骨有自然的弹性。如果没有在新生儿期或延迟进行手术，则耻骨缺乏弹性后就要进行前路或后路的截骨手术。这是前路髂骨截骨手术的位置。B. 外固定钉固定骨盆，耻骨支靠拢于中线。

第一阶段重建手术后的随访男女之间相似。观察研究包括残余尿的测定和肾脏超声检查。因为几乎所有的病例都存在膀胱输尿管反流，所以抗生素抑制治疗要继续。如果残余尿水平持续上升，应该检查排除尿道狭窄。

最后，大多数患者还需要进行抗反流手术，这种反流至少部分和输尿管的方向异常相关。如果过多的残余尿和上尿路扩张持续存在，那么在出生后一年内进行抗反流手术是必要的，但这种情况是较少见。大多数病例的膀胱尺寸逐步增长，并不需要进行抗反流手术直到行膀胱颈重建以获得控尿力。从技术上讲，大多数外科医生喜欢用横向三角（cross-trigonal）技术或头端三角输尿管再植（cephalotrigonal ureteral reimplantation）技术，这样可以最大可能地延长尿道[14,16]。

尽管大多数外科医生相信耻骨靠拢于中线有利于保护初步关闭的膀胱，促进将来的控尿能力，以及帮助膀胱、膀胱颈和尿道在骨盆内解剖复位，但是骨盆截骨术还是存在争议（见图 118-12）。一些学者，包括 Marshall 和 Muecke[82] 以及 Csontai 等人[24] 提倡靠 1851
拢耻骨而不进行截骨术。其他人采用耻骨支前路或上路截骨术，尤其是当以后的手术操作不需要翻转患者时。其他学者，比如 Mollard[93]，喜欢髂骨后路截骨术。Kelly[66]仅仅动用耻骨支的内层骨膜和肌肉组织。Gearhart[34]推荐对出生超过 72 小时的患儿、失去骨盆柔韧性的患儿以及骨盆分离等于或超过 4 cm 的患儿采取前路和垂直的髂骨截骨手术。

另外，耻骨靠拢于中线还利于延长再造阴茎的长度。现在都知道骨盆闭合时是否采用了截骨方式与活动没有长远关系。Kelly[66]，众多学者之一，发现若在儿童时期没有纠正骨盆分离，患者的步态也不会受影响，即儿童早期的蹒跚步态会自行纠正。唯一有影响的是髋关节内旋受到一定程度的限制，但是这不会影响活动，甚至可以奔跑。

男性病例第二阶段的修补包括阴茎重建[28]。手术在出生后 6～12 个月时进行。Gearhart 和 Jeffs[37]发现除了最大限度的生殖器重建外，尿道上裂的修补和尿道成形也有利于增大膀胱容量，这可能是尿液流出道阻力增加的结果。各种尿道延长手术的目的是能提供充足的空间而没有排尿狭窄感，促进控尿力并且能够轻松导尿[62,63,74,106]。尿道上裂第一期修补在初期膀胱关闭和近端尿道重建时进行，包括将阴茎体从耻骨支上分离。这种分离在一定程度上可以防止阴茎体的损伤和缺血。外翻膀胱边翼的构建可以促进尿道延长。至少在初期，阴茎背屈可以通过尿道板的分开得到部分松解。近端类型的单独尿道上裂通常和尿失禁有关。为膀胱外翻病例实施第一期重建手术时，将缺陷转变成单独的尿道上裂。在一定程度上将阴茎体从耻骨上分离下来是必要的；但是因为有损坏阴茎血供的风险，所以并不希望彻底分离。如果发生这种情况，会导致长期勃起功能障碍。

尿道上裂修补

关于尿道上裂修补，其目的是使阴茎有足够的长度且能够适度下垂以及松解阴茎背屈[30,50,51]。而且，重建尿道使得尿从阴茎头排出。这方面有很多技术，而且近来有了明显进步[1,4,7,10,94]。1989 年，Ransley 等人[105]描述了 Cantwell-Ransley 术式，即将阴茎尿道转移至腹侧且充分纠正背屈，尿瘘发生率较低（图 118-13）[65,70]。这种方法使阴茎体充分游离于耻骨，其背侧的尿道板经背侧和腹侧的两阴茎体游离后保留完整。如果游离后尿道板未束缚于阴茎，则保留其完整。如果这样会缩短阴茎和导致永久性背屈，则要将其分割开来，包皮内板或游离移植物可用以增加尿道[25,26,28,123]。然后尿道卷成管状，将阴茎体在中部横行切开，尿道从中间转移至腹侧。在尿道上方行海绵体吻合。这种阴茎体内部的旋转得以覆盖新建尿道。据 Gearhart 等人报道，相对于以前的手术，这种方法的并发症明显减少[39,41,43]。

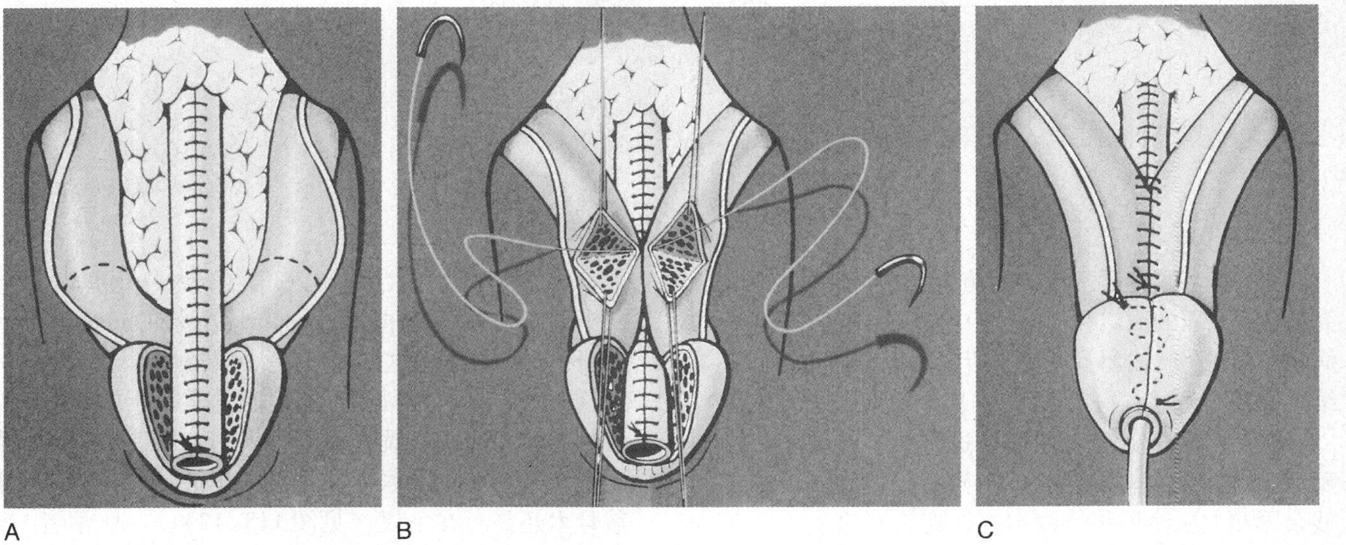

图 118-13 A-C. Cantwell-Ransley 尿道上裂修补术式的步骤。这种手术可使尿道得以延长，阴茎体合拢保证血供，并完全覆盖尿道。

852 Mitchell 和 Bagli[91] 报道，Cantwell-Ransley 术式又有了改进。改进方法是在阴茎体修补前先充分游离分解。依靠单独的阴茎海绵体和龟头血供，阴茎的三个部分（尿道板、右侧和左侧的阴茎海绵体）得以分离（图 118-14）。这使得龟头和尿道板独立，且可以使两侧的阴茎海绵体分离。最后，可以通过旋转松解来纠正背屈。

膀胱颈重建

膀胱外翻患儿最后阶段的重建手术包括控尿机制的建立，一般在 4 岁左右施行[101]。其间患者通过超声检查或阻抗体积描记法确保上尿路系统的引流通畅。这对于防止尿路感染和确保足够的尿路引流、避免肾盂积水非常重要。也要测定膀胱容量以利于决定合适的重建手术。Jeffs 等人[61] 报道，在进行膀胱颈重建后膀胱容量必须达到 60 ml 以上来保证能获得足够的功能容量。其他人则认为需要更大的膀胱容量，并依靠膀胱扩大手术以提供适合尿液储备的膀胱容量。

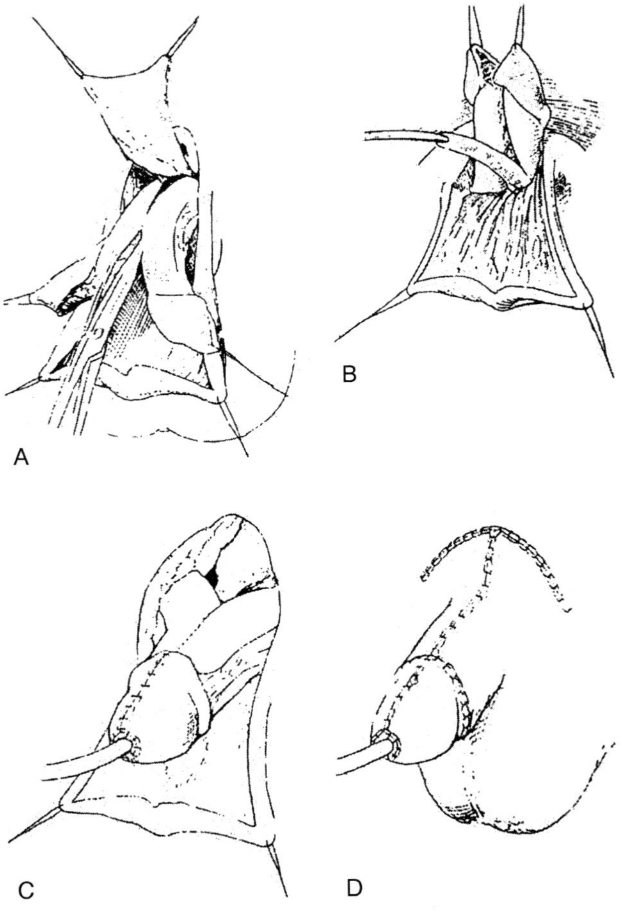

图 118-14　阴茎完全分解技术图示。A. 阴茎体分离和龟头对半分开。B. 尿道卷管缝合并转移至腹侧。C. 阴茎体在背侧重新靠拢缝合。D. 远端龟头关闭完成修补。（Adapted from Mitchell ME, Bagli DK: Complete penile disassembly for epispadias repair: The Mitchell technique. J Urol 1996; 155: 300.）

在许多用于重建膀胱颈部的操作中，Young-Dees-Leadbetter 技术的应用最为广泛（图 118-15）。在这种方法中，将输尿管移位并再植于膀胱内近头端位置，可以采用横向三角技术或是头端三角技术[15,21]。膀胱板的尾端标出 1.5～2 cm 宽、3.5 cm 长的区域。膀胱三角两侧朝向尾端的部分剥去黏膜，尾端组织卷成管状。这样三角区的膀胱肌转移到了新的膀胱颈的侧边，就像背心盖住短裤一样遮蔽了新尿道。这种肌肉覆盖黏膜管的操作完全在腹内进行。如果膀胱容量足够，则可以关闭膀胱，或应用肠膀胱扩大手术以提高膀胱容量[84]。最后，膀胱颈部重建通过将膀胱颈和尿道缝合于耻骨前方来加强。

手术以后，输尿管支撑管留置大约 1 周，Malecot 导管放置 3～4 周。不用放置尿道支撑管。患者在这段时间内持续接受抗生素治疗，还要应用抗痉挛药物防止膀胱痉挛。夹闭耻骨上导管开始排尿试验，如果残余尿少则可以去除耻骨上导管。手术时测定静水压来测试输出口阻力。作者认为阻力大于 50 cmH_2O 是控尿所必需的[13,44]。

对于那些膀胱颈重建术后仍旧尿失禁的患者，要确保膀胱的最大储尿容量[102]。最后，小容量的患者需要进行扩大手术将膀胱内压减少到能够控尿的水平。所有节段的小肠都可用来行膀胱扩大，但是对于经典膀胱外翻，回肠组织为首选。对于泄殖腔外翻患者，当肠管长度有问题时可以成功地应用胃壁组织手术。膀胱扩大成形术在第 117 章中讨论。

根据作者的经验，膀胱外翻患者可以在膀胱颈重建后获得社会生活需要的控尿能力。但是，经过膀胱外翻分期修补和膀胱颈重建后，在获得了社会生活需要的控尿能力和具有适当的排尿能力的患者中，有 75% 还存在与排空相关的临床问题，这可以通过尿流动力学检查进行客观评定[129]。排空差以及那些做过膀胱扩大的患者通常需要间歇性清洁导尿，但是那些具有膀胱外翻-尿道上裂复合畸形的

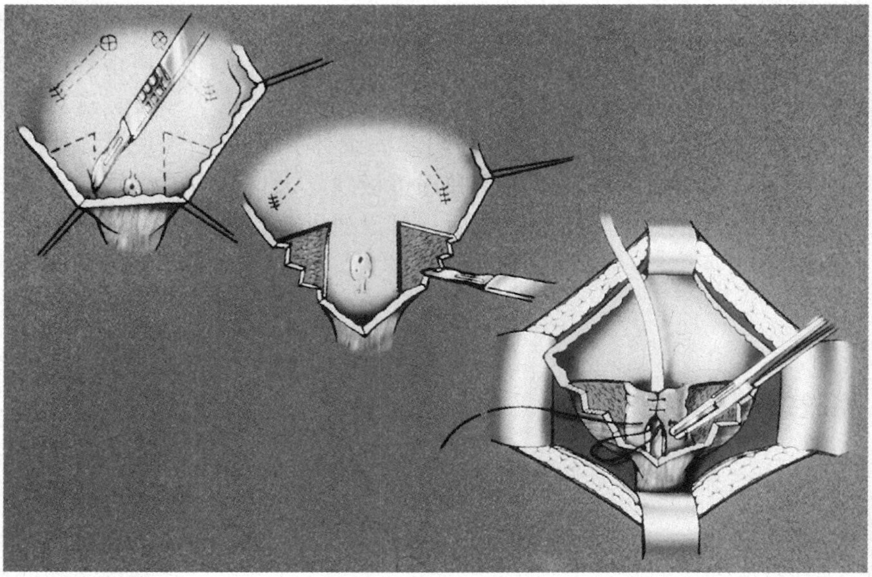

A

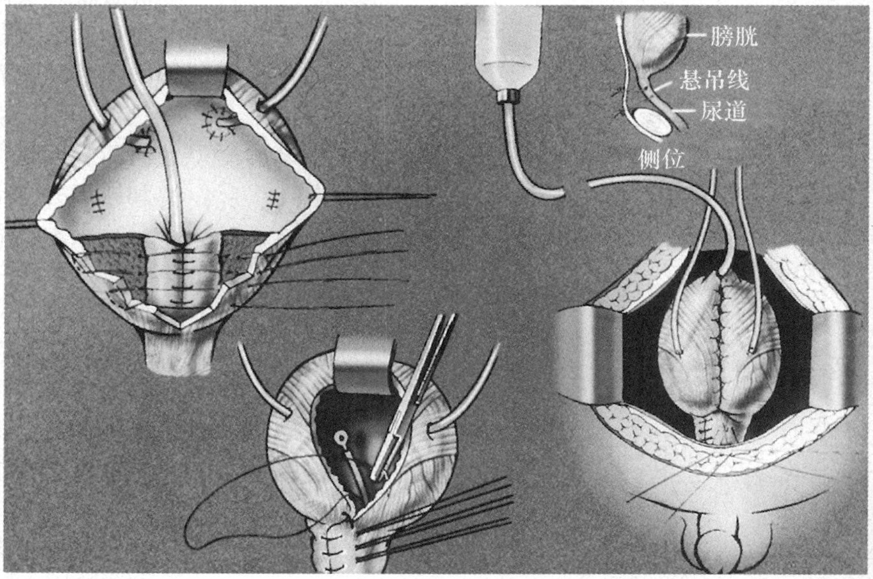

B

图 118-15　A 和 B. Young-Dees-Leadbetter 手术方法治疗膀胱外翻。用这种方法，输尿管适当再植以防止反流，修裁膀胱基底部以供以后延长尿道和加强膀胱颈部。这样可提供足够压力以促进膀胱容量扩大而不会产生尿道梗阻。

患儿由于尿道重建后呈弯折状而难以进行导尿。Mitrofanoff 方法的应用明显使上述治疗得到了改观[92]。这种方法是通过抗反流法将阑尾吻合于膀胱，另一端拖出腹壁成为可控性导尿开口。这种方
1853 法显著改善了患儿通过导管排空膀胱的能力。Mitrofanoff 方法在第 117 章中讨论。

是否有足够的控尿能力通常在修补术后 1 年内知道。对于术后仍有失禁的患者可有一些选择，包括用填充剂来加强出口的阻力[123]、重复 Young-Dees-Leadbetter 手术而可做或不做膀胱扩大、人工尿道括约肌、关闭膀胱颈而只保留一个可控性导尿开口以及尿流改道。

大多数女性患儿直到 4 岁左右才需要进行生殖系重建。到那时，如果没有做过初期重建手术，就要将分裂的阴蒂合拢，即把两半阴蒂靠中线部分的黏膜去除后缝合到中线。如果阴道开口并非合适地位于腹侧或有狭窄，就需要进行阴道成形术。但是许多女性患儿这方面的生殖系整形在第一阶段的重建中已成功完成，接下来要解决阴道狭窄或阴阜整形。

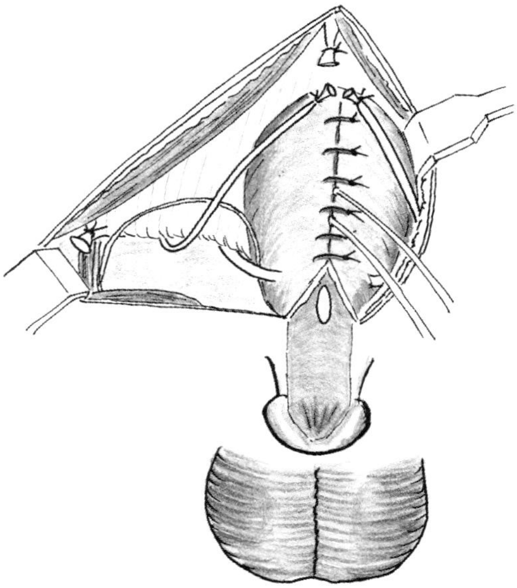

图 118-16　应用 Kelly 方法的第一阶段手术。皮肤切口要深至能够暴露腹直肌和会阴。关闭膀胱。先期进行右侧腹股沟疝修补手术。行输尿管置管。

Kelly 修补

1995 年，Kelly[66] 提出了分阶段修补膀胱外翻的另一种方法。这种方法包括彻底转移所有括约肌软组织和重塑阴茎，以达到控尿能力并且获得满意的生殖器功能。在男性患儿中，这种重建要分三步；女性患儿则只需两步。

354 在新生儿阶段，关闭膀胱顶和修补腹股沟疝（图 118-16）。膀胱关闭于中线，固定于直肠肌群的后面，并在膀胱颈水平的中线部位保留一个临时的尿流开口。固定输尿管支撑管并从尿流出口处引出作为术后数天的肾引流。直肌群靠近中线的部分在耻骨上尿流开口的下方靠拢。如果腹肌和耻骨分离较宽，可以用前面直肌的边翼来关闭腹部。垂直牵引腿部皮肤、在床上抬高臀部有利于术后数天的护理。

Kelly 法的第二阶段修补大约在患儿 3～6 个月时进行。最初的切口从尿道板开始至阴茎背部。阴茎脱套，最后被分解成独立的海绵体和尿道。再把切口向上延伸至腹壁。切除下腹壁的瘢痕，开放中线部分的筋膜和膀胱。然后，进行经三角区的或头端三角法的输尿管再植手术。

接下来对靠近骨盆壁中线部位的所有软组织结构进行根本游离（图 118-17）。游离骨盆前壁表面的骨膜，从耻骨前壁表面开始持续移向坐骨耻骨支和坐骨，将肛提肌从耻骨分离。这种侵袭性的切口可以使尿道周围括约肌、肛提肌群以及阴茎脚得以游离。这些肌群和阴茎脚以后将在没有张力和会阴部神经及血管牵拉的情况下合拢于中线。

因为膀胱外翻患儿的球海绵体肌、坐骨海绵体 1855
肌、会阴横肌和尿道括约肌群分布异常，它们呈一块连续的肌肉体与肛门外括约肌相延续。该肌群位于阴茎体后方，可以通过电刺激仪识别，将其从阴茎脚上分离并与尿道外括约肌一起覆盖在尿道周围（图 118-18）。

然后将尿道卷管放置于阴茎体的前部，在阴茎阴囊交界处暂时行一个尿道造口术。膀胱尾端关闭延续于卷管化后的尿道。尿道内外括约肌和肛提肌一起包绕在尿道周围。

阴茎体向中间靠拢缝合，注意保证缝合适当以防止产生阴茎的腹屈或背屈。然后在远端重建龟头。

在大约 3 岁时，获得控尿力以后可进行第三阶段手术。修补尿道下裂方法包括将多余的包皮转移制成新尿道。如果患儿只有很少量的转移包皮，则可以用会阴部阴茎阴囊开口处的皮瓣来覆盖。

女性患儿应用相似的方法进行两个阶段的手术纠治。第一阶段男女相似，但在第二阶段有些不同。女性尿道在阴道口尾端卷管化。切开尿道黏膜两边并卷成管形。将内外括约肌组织、肛提肌和骨膜从骨盆分离下来并覆盖在尿道阴道周围，使它们成为一体，然后放置在骨盆后部。这种安置使得尿道阴道正好位于短肌肉束之间。在阴道口后方行一 Y-V 切开，并向后中线延伸至少 1.5 cm。两半分裂的阴蒂体向中线靠拢并将各自的阴蒂头并拢。

应用这种技术于 19 例患者中取得了 73% 的控尿率[66]。7 例患者得到了正常的白天和夜间的控尿能力，可以有完全或接近完全的排空，这些评估基于直接询问、体格检查和 VCUG 而做出。7 例患者有社会生活所需的控尿力但是需要经常排尿而防止湿裤，而且他们偶尔会有漏尿。5 例患者经过上述阶段的修补仍有尿失禁。

一期重建

一期 CPER 在数十年前已有描述。然而，最初的

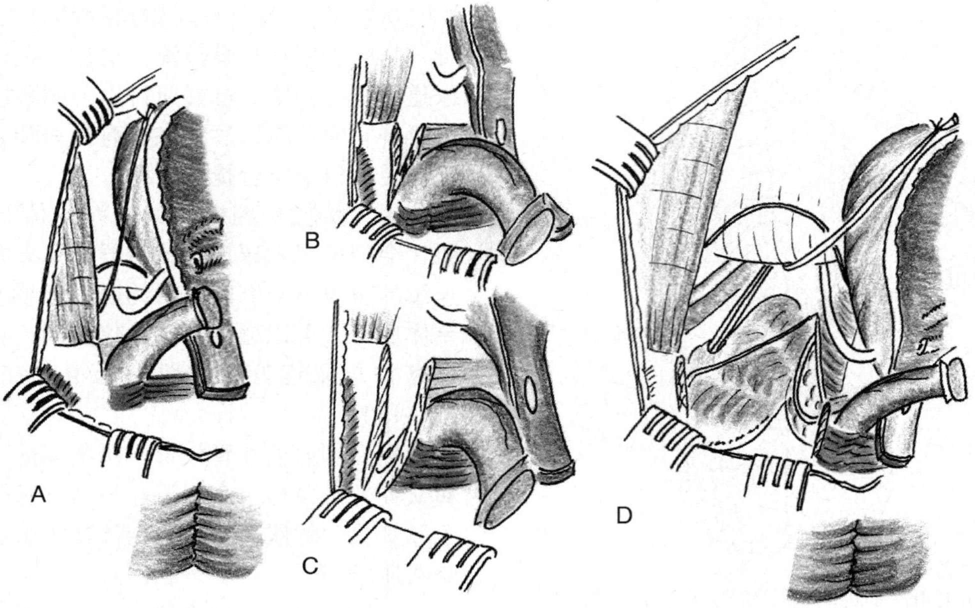

图 118-17　应用 Kelly 方法的第二阶段手术：软组织游离。A. 腹膜外切口延伸暴露肛提肌的上面，而皮下切口暴露耻骨、坐骨耻骨支和坐骨。B. 切开耻骨骨膜，显露出下面耻骨的一部分，这样可以暴露和扩大膀胱周围的空间，使得肛提肌从两侧骨盆壁上分离。C. 分离骨膜和下面的骨骼、软骨直至坐骨。通过向内侧牵拉肛提肌和坐骨直肠窝脂肪可以识别外阴部的神经血管束在骨盆壁两侧贴近坐骨棘的地方。外阴部的神经血管束行走于骨盆前壁，此处可能会受到不可逆的损伤。D. 开放骨盆侧壁和盆腔脏器之间的空间，将外阴部的神经血管束仔细地剥向坐骨棘。进行横向三角输尿管再植术，保留输尿管导管 1 周。

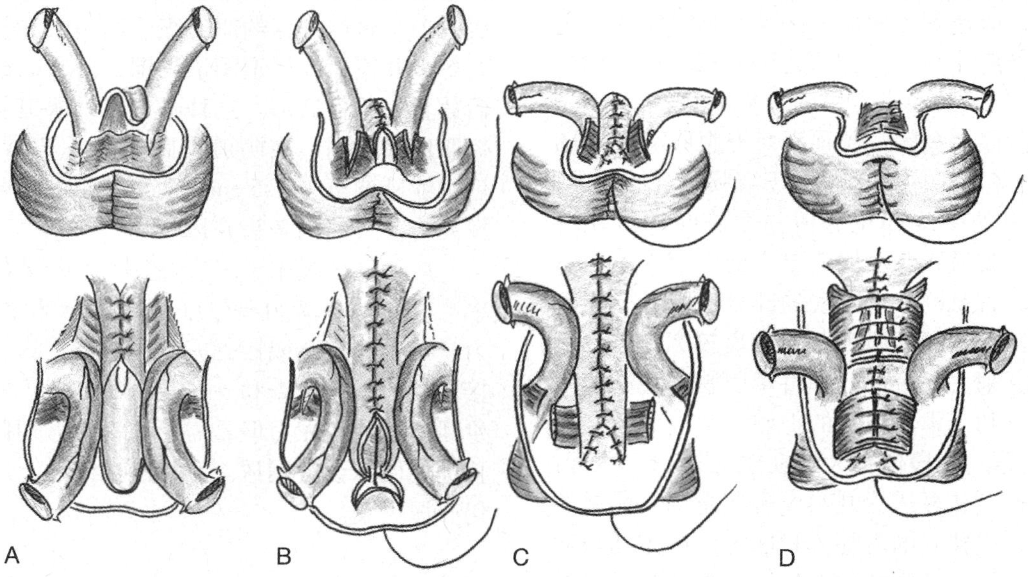

图 118-18　第二阶段 Kelly 手术：尿道管和括约肌的再造。A. 尿道板的卷管操作。B. 阴茎阴囊型尿道下裂尿道口的重建。一根粗线从尿道下裂尿道口穿入，穿过尿道管，从膀胱壁穿出。C. 尿道重建完成。区分出泌尿生殖膈并游离，此刻准备围绕远端尿道合并重建"外括约肌"。D. 泌尿生殖膈缝合成"外括约肌"。将膀胱颈部的纤维和肌肉组织游离，并围绕膀胱颈和近端后尿道进行缝合。

结果令人失望，肾功能恶化率高且控尿能力低[85]。最近，Grady 和 Mitchell[46] 做了一些工作，重新修改了这种方法。在新生儿期将整个阴茎分解并结合 CPER 在初期获得了令人振奋的 80% 的控尿率[46]。在新生儿期应用这种一期重建方法较大孩子容易，通过产生出口阻力使得新生儿建立起早期的膀胱功能，以后产生良好的控尿能力。新生儿的骨盆很柔韧并且可延展性强，也不存在膀胱纤维化，而膀胱纤维化从理论上讲是导致大孩子一期重建失败的原因[47]。Grady 和 Mitchell 假设 CPER 可能有一些其他理论上的优点，包括早期膀胱充盈排尿循环的建立以及出生后尽早正常发育的可能性。这些优点能保持正常的低压排尿，并且不需要今后的分期手术[104]。

CPER 方法在膀胱外翻儿童中可用来对膀胱、膀胱颈和尿道前面的缺陷部分进行修正。但是单纯进行膀胱缺损关闭而不把膀胱颈和尿道放置在骨盆下部，解
356 剖异常仍然存在。CPER 将下尿道放置于骨盆下部，将近端尿道放置于骨盆膈以内，这是较为正常的解剖结构，使得周围包绕的骨盆肌肉有利于控制尿道。

CPER 包括将男性患儿的整个阴茎分解，Grady 和 Mitchell 认为把尿道板从阴茎体上分离下来可以减轻尿道前部的张力[47]。这种附加的操作得以将尿道板向前拉伸，可以限制随后的近端尿道及膀胱颈部进入到盆腔内。将尿道上裂修补和初期膀胱关闭联合进行，这样可以向下深部分离联合腱使得膀胱、膀胱颈和尿道置于下方。

CPER 首先从双侧输尿管开口放置导管开始，分别在分裂的龟头每侧都缝上牵引线。这些牵引线先水平放置，当阴茎体从背侧尿道和海绵体上游离后，一齐在垂直方向旋转。

在上面，膀胱板从邻近皮肤上以类似重建手术第一阶段的方法进行分离。切口向前延伸至阴茎腹侧呈环形切开。切开平面位于 Buck 筋膜和其上组织结构之间，并延续到阴茎体上中线。在两侧切开以及将阴茎皮肤和肉膜从 Buck 筋膜上分离时要小心，以避免损伤神经血管束，这些神经血管束局限在阴茎两侧[127]。

尿道板从远端切开并延伸至近端的膀胱颈。接着，将阴茎分解为三个部分：右侧和左侧阴茎体、相互独立的半个龟头、尿道板及其附着的海绵体。从近端和腹侧开始切开并向远端分解这三个部分是最容易操作的[91]。尿道可以在这个时候进行卷管或者以后当尿道转移至阴茎体腹侧时再行卷管。

阴茎切开后，要进行骨盆底的切开，即取两侧深部平行切口切开，向后达后尿道的近端，就像 Grady 和 Mitchell[46] 所描述的（图 118-19）。还有一种就是 Vanderbilt 儿童医院采用的方法，即取一个简单的中

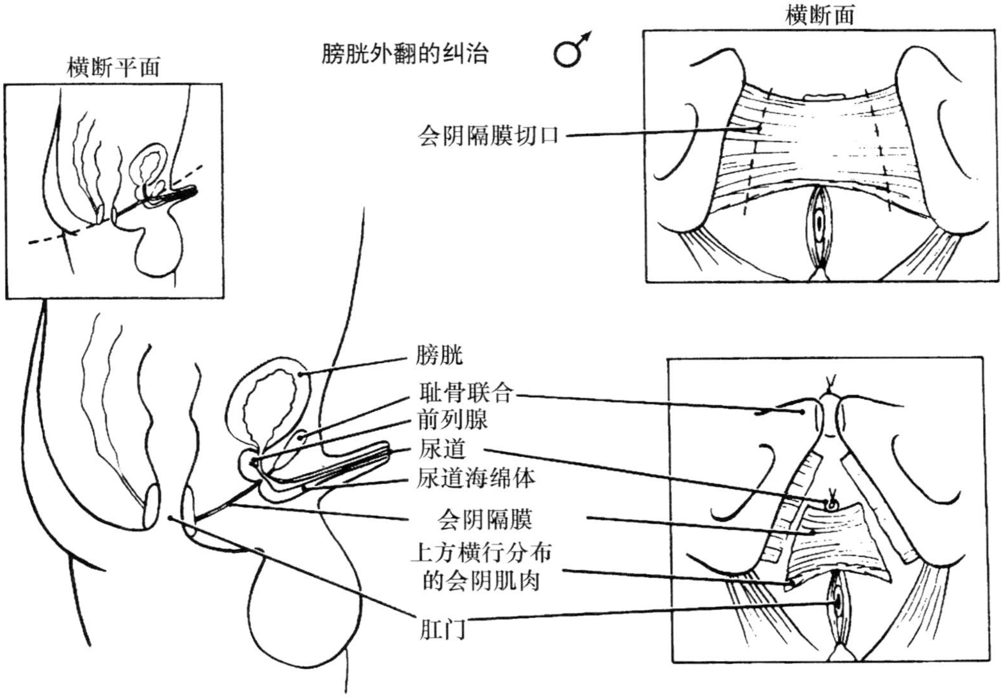

图 118-19　男性膀胱外翻修补的盆底示意图。沿尿道两边切开并分离联合腱束使得膀胱放置于盆腔后部。（Adapted from Grady RW, Mitchell ME：Complete primary repair of exstrophy. J Urol 1999；162：1416.）

线切口通过联合腱束，足够地切开联合腱束并与周围组织结构分离，使膀胱、膀胱颈和后尿道可以安置在骨盆的后部。

原则上膀胱和尿道的关闭通常在盆底游离切开后进行（图 118-20）。作者通常是在安全可靠地放置好耻骨上引流和输尿管导管后再两层关闭膀胱。如果先前未做好尿道，则用两层卷管做出尿道并且要稳妥放置好尿道支撑管。

接着将膀胱、膀胱颈和远端尿道放置于骨盆深部。在无不当张力的情况下，应用留置于联合腱束前方的 8 号 PDS 缝线缝合联合腱束。将膀胱放于后部并
1857 重新将耻骨联合靠拢后，评估阴茎体的发育状况。如果存在任何潜在的影响阴茎血供的问题，都有必要将关闭的耻骨联合再拆开，并且考虑进行截骨手术。

接着直肌筋膜靠拢，尿道转移至阴茎的腹侧。旋转左右侧阴茎体使其靠拢，然后间断缝合，最后牵引线保持向下。尿道此时可以稳妥地安置在阴茎体的腹侧。龟头成形方式类似于尿道下裂。偶尔会碰到尿道不够长而达不到龟头的情况，此时患儿先带着尿道下裂外观回家，今后再做整形手术。在行 CPER 时，男性患儿的尿道延长不适宜采用膀胱外翻周围的边翼组织，应用阴茎腹侧的转移皮瓣可以覆盖阴茎体。

手术之后应采取任何可以想到的方法对患者制动，这样可以减轻膀胱关闭后侧面的张力。作者一般采用 Bryant 牵引 2～3 周。另外，由于术后膀胱输尿管反流的高发生率，应采用小剂量的抑菌剂。

CRER 还成功应用于各种女性膀胱外翻-尿道上裂病例。作者近来报道了 6 例采用此技术的病例[2]。将膀胱颈部和尿道与阴道分离，这样可以将阴道置于远端而膀胱置于靠头侧。在各种膀胱外翻的女性患儿中可以发现尿道一分为二地位于阴道上方两边，按照传统的描述，外翻膀胱周围的边翼可以反过来用于延长尿道。尿道可以延长 30 mm，膀胱颈部用一条松软的耻骨阴道悬带固定。两个有尿道上裂的女孩采用相同的方法，在游离尿道后应用边翼延长尿道，而后获得重建。所有这一类患儿均具备干燥间歇期而没有持续性的滴尿，一个患儿在排尿训练期间偶尔湿裤，但也能保持 2 小时的干燥间歇。上述两个尿道上裂的患儿获得了白天以及夜晚的控尿能力。

尽管 CPER 的早期控尿率令人鼓舞，但近来的调查却不太乐观。Grady 等人[48]报道，在对 CPER 术后患者进行长期随访调查后发现，虽然 77% 的患者可以控制排尿，但是有超过 70% 的患者需要进行第二次膀胱颈修补来获得自控。现在该专家小组在初期关闭时就对膀胱颈和近端尿道进行裁剪，以希望能加强控制排尿的能力。随访中也有一些患者需要通过 Mitrofanoff 操作进行间歇性导尿来有效排空膀胱。而且，在最初接受手术的患者中有 50% 由于尿路感染而进行反流手术[46]。Grady 和 Mitchell[46]描述在他们的第一批患者中行 CPER 后遗留有尿道下裂的问题。最近以来，El-Sherbiny 等人[31]报道在接受 CPER 后的新生儿和闭合失败的儿童中尿道下裂的发生率为 59%。这些发现提示应对 CPER 技术进行改进，包括将近端尿道完全放置于后部和盆底以不同的方法切开，以希望获得更好的控尿率。

尿流改道

尿流改道适用于那些没有足够的膀胱板用于初期

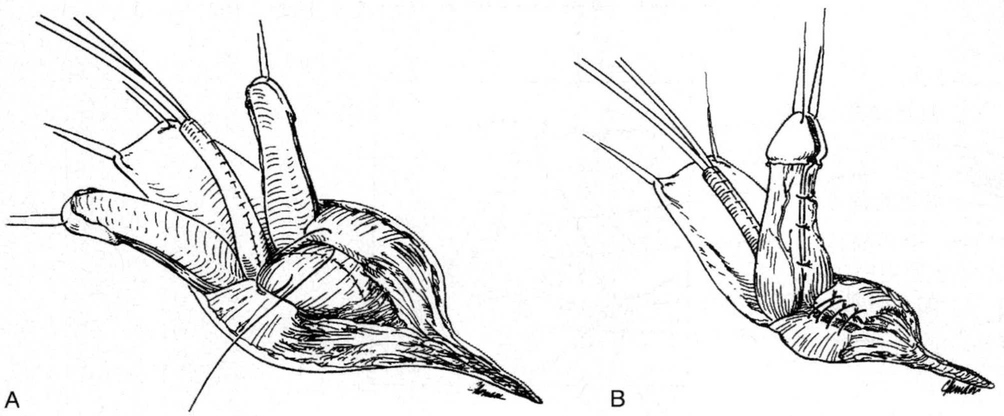

图 118-20　A. 将尿道板和膀胱作为一个连续单位进行关闭。B. 通过把膀胱、膀胱颈和尿道放置于骨盆后部将尿道移至阴茎体腹侧。（Adapted from Grady RW, Mitchell ME: Complete primary repair of exstrophy. J Urol 1999; 162: 1417.）

关闭或所有重建手术方法都失败的患者。尿流改道的倡导者坚持认为，低控尿率和膀胱的不完全排空导致关于膀胱重建可能性问题增多。虽然这些问题存在，但是在那些经过了分期重建手术后完全尿失禁的患者中，只有10%～20%需要进行尿流改道[108]。

从尿流改道的历史来看，第一种方法是输尿管乙状结肠吻合手术，这种手术因为没有腹壁造口已被普遍接受。但是据报道会发生间歇性的肾盂肾炎、高氯性酸中毒、输尿管梗阻、排便失禁和输尿管结肠吻合处的腺癌[28,112,113,131]，需要终生监测。尿流改道经设
358 计后有各种各样的方法，包括一期和分期手术以及可控性改道。其他的改道方式在第 115 章中描述。与接受分期重建术的患儿相比，尿流改道术后的患儿更易发生肾功能损害[54]。

并发症

膀胱关闭的最严重的早期并发症为膀胱裂开[22,98]。据报道在那些后来发生膀胱裂开的患者中伤口感染者达 42%[79]。其他和裂开有关的因素包括肠道病变未经处理而导致的腹胀、膀胱下垂和关闭术后 6 天内尿道及耻骨上引流管的滑出，可导致腹膜浸渍而引起以后的感染和膀胱裂开[14,55]。Jeffs 等人[61]发现关闭术后放置在尿道的引流管和裂开亦有关系。

膀胱裂开的处理依然是个难题。处理意见有：（1）尿流改道；（2）重新关闭膀胱成尿道样管状，并引流尿液直到以后行扩大术；（3）保持膀胱的外翻状态直至大约 4～6 个月后重新关闭。Sponseller 等人[115]描述的前路截骨手术及外固定对于成功进行膀胱再关闭是有帮助的。外固定可以在愈合期间（4～6 周）固定住骨盆环，这是成功所必需的。作者已经重新关闭了 4 例患者的裂开膀胱，没有 1 例患者再次出现裂开。

对于那些已进行了尿道上裂修补手术但仍没有获得足够的膀胱容量的患者，膀胱扩大整形仍是最可行的方法。这个手术可以在膀胱颈重建和尿道再植时进行，甚至可以在膀胱颈重建失败后进行以获得足够的储尿容量。作为获得排尿控制能力的方法，在功能性膀胱重建术后进行膀胱扩大术的必要性显而易见。印第安纳州的专家小组[110]近期报道在该地区的膀胱外翻病例中有 69% 需要进行膀胱扩大，再结合膀胱颈修补而获得控尿力。

膀胱颈重建失败会导致尿失禁。有控尿力被定义为有 3 个小时干燥间歇期，通常在重建术后 1 年内获得。治疗意见在本章节其他处进行讨论。

尿道上裂修补术后最常见的并发症是尿道皮肤瘘，发生率在 35%～50%。现代的手术方式，比如 Cantwell－Ransley 和 Mitchell 方法，尿瘘发生率较低[41,43]。另外，男性病例仍然存在阴茎长度减少和残余背屈的问题。大一些的患儿可以得益于阴茎体从耻骨支上的进一步游离。如 Kramer 和 Jackson[69]以及 Monfort 等人[94]描述的长斜方形和其他形状的皮瓣可以提供良好暴露下的进一步游离。

阴茎背屈的纠正还需要其他操作[53,71]。皮肤转移和尿道延长技术对于阴茎体和尿道板的延长是必要的[51,122]。Koff 和 Eakins[68]描述了采用阴茎体旋转技术来伸直阴茎使之处于稍朝下的方向。Ransley[104,105]和 Mitchell[91]的新技术在进行尿道上裂修补的初期就具备了应对这些解剖问题的潜力，减少了后续问题的产生。

对于经历了一期和分期膀胱重建的膀胱外翻患者，护理上的进步延长了他们的寿命，并且降低了成年时并发症的发生。特别是腺癌较为棘手[128]。在膀胱外翻患者中膀胱腺癌的发生率大约是普通人群的 250 倍[64]。这可能是慢性炎症、感染和膀胱暴露于腹壁后化生的结果。腺癌也可以在膀胱扩大术后发生，是因为胃肠道黏膜长时间接触尿液所致[36]。现在还不能肯定成功进行了膀胱关闭后是否可以减少这种癌症的风险，只有进行长期随访才能确定。膀胱外翻患者还可能发生的肿瘤类型有鳞状细胞癌和横纹肌肉瘤。

膀胱外翻患者无论男女其生殖器重建后的生育能力都是一个问题[72]。Shapiro 等人[109]调查了 2500 例膀胱外翻和尿道上裂的患者，统计出有 38 例男患者做了父亲而有 131 例女患者生育了孩子。这项研究表明男女患者都有可能生育后代，但是成功率远远低于正常人群。不容置疑，男患者生育能力低与初期关闭时损伤了精阜以及逆行射精有关。如 Woodhouse 等人[126]报道膀胱外翻患者的性欲很高，并且大多数尿道上裂修补后的患儿其阴茎勃起机制未受影响[127]。

许多膀胱外翻关闭后成功怀孕的病例被报道。Clemetson[19]在 1958 年回顾报道了 45 名膀胱外翻的妇女产下了 49 个孩子。在 1986 年 Burbige 等人[11]的一项研究中显示了 11 名妇女的 14 次怀孕史，其中 9 次正常

生产，3 次自然流产，2 次选择性流产。子宫下垂是最常见的并发症，11 例患者中有 7 人发生。先前进行过尿流改道的妇女应用自然阴道生产，而那些经历过功能性膀胱关闭的妇女则采用剖宫产，这样可以减轻对盆底的压力和避免对括约肌机制的创伤性损害[73]。

膀胱外翻：总结

对大多数膀胱外翻的患者来讲，重建手术是可行的。Hollowell 和 Ransley[52]、Ransley 等人[105]、Lepor 和 Jeffs[77]以及 Toguri 等人[120]报道有 80% 的控尿率，并且 Mesrobian 等人[86,87]报道有 74% 的长期控尿率。作者的患者在进行了下尿道重建后已经达到了 80%
1859 的控尿率。近来的趋势越来越倾向于对没有足够膀胱容量的患者，或控尿操作包括单纯关闭和膀胱颈重建失败的患者进行膀胱扩大。然而，要强调的是多数患者需要长期随访和多次手术干预来获得控尿能力。毋庸置疑，长期的控尿能力肯定会得到进一步改善。

无论哪种情况，都需要多年内进行多次重建手术，尤其是在一生中的塑形阶段；当生殖器定性成为一个重要因素时，社会和心理调节就成为主要问题。外科重建方法中应该考虑到这些问题。80% 的患者可以良好调节，希望这个结果在将来会有进步。

泄殖腔外翻

(James A. O'Neill, Jr.)

泄殖腔外翻的历史回顾

泄殖腔外翻在文献中是指泄殖腔的外翻、内脏外翻和膀胱肠道裂沟。1709 年 Littre 进行了首例报道，接着 1812 年 Meckel 、1900 年 von Recklinghausen 和 Schwalbe 报道了一系列病例[163,173]。1900 年，Steinbüchel[172]描述了第一例新生儿泄殖腔外翻的部分手术修补，但是这名患儿在出生后 5 天死亡。1960 年，Rickham[163]报道了第一个成功修补且存活的病例，全部的纠治分阶段完成。但是，多数泄殖腔外翻重建手术都是徒劳的，因为早产、短肠综合征、败血症和肾及中枢神经系统发育不良，这些并发因素使得死亡率高达 90%。由于对这种畸形的重建操作很原始，加上多次复杂手术的围术期护理的缺陷，导致了生存率较低，生存者的预后较差。1979 年，Welch[173]报道了波士顿儿童医院泄殖腔外翻患儿的死亡率为 50%。然而，由于护理方面的巨大改观和手术方法的革新，现在的生存率超过了 90%，努力方向转移到了改善这些患者的生活质量上。

发病率

泄殖腔外翻较为罕见，根据一些报道其发病率大约为 1/200 000～1/400 000 活产儿。虽然一些研究表明男女发生比例为 2∶1，但是其他研究（包括本文作者的研究）提出发生比例基本相似。如果考虑到产前明确诊断而以后胎内死亡的病例，则总的发病率要高于刚才引用的数据。在所有膀胱外翻畸形中，各种类型的泄殖腔外翻占 10%，包括合并耻骨联合分离的所有畸形[161]。

胚胎学

近来对膀胱外翻复合畸形的胚胎学解释在本章节中占了主要一节。关于膀胱外翻的各种研究，比如来自 Keppler-Noreuil[151]以及 Evans 和 Chudley[139]的研究，提供了现代形态发生方面的信息。这些研究，包括 Oostra 等人[160]的广泛回顾研究，表明将泄殖腔外翻定义为原始胚胎期中线的缺陷畸形较多中心胚胎期缺陷更为合理。各种膀胱外翻复合畸形的表现同间叶细胞向内生长以及泄殖腔膜破溃的时间和程度不同有关。这种发育过程中的胚胎缺陷提示了同源基因的病源作用，比如*HLXB 9*突变造成了直肠肛门和脊髓的畸形。Keppler-Noreuil[151]的研究分析了 OEIS 复合畸形（脐膨出-膀胱外翻-肛门闭锁-脊髓畸形）后发现环境因素和基因因素作用等同。同样，Evans 和 Chudley[139]假设疾病与一个或多个*HOX* 基因末端的错误表达相关，可能位于 10 号位或 11 号位，导致胚胎尾端的间叶细胞异常发生和增生扩散。

目前显示在胎儿发育的第四周到第八周，在某些部位会发生上述异常。现在认为若泌尿直肠隔下降到泄殖腔膜的水平而破溃，则会发生典型的膀胱外翻；如果泌尿直肠隔没有充分下降，那么肠管就会发生在膀胱两半的中间。然而，Lakshmanan 等人[152]对早期致病理论提出质疑，他们通过应用产前超声的数据，指出泄殖腔膜持续存在至少至孕 18 周。Bruch 等人[135]提出泄殖腔外翻不存在发育抑制的问题，但可能是异常胚胎发生的问题。Lakshmanan 和 Bruch 都报道了异卵双胞胎的泄殖腔外翻病例，但是在同卵双胞胎病例的报道中却提示两人都有泄殖腔外翻的只占一半。Smith 等人[167]报道了非双胞胎姊妹中的泄殖腔外翻病例。

泄殖腔外翻患者可以合并有许多畸形，这个事实可以支持本症在胚胎早期发生。以下这些畸形在泄殖腔外翻中的发生率要高于其在典型膀胱外翻中的发生率[136,149,156,167]。肠道畸形包括盲肠外翻、肛门闭锁、后肠闭锁和中肠短小而导致的吸收功能障碍倾向和生长障碍。脐膨出可以发生于许多病例。脊髓畸形很常见，包括骶骨和椎骨的异常、脊髓脊膜膨出、脊髓栓系和盆底肌肉组织薄弱。肾脏畸形，比如肾发育不全、融合畸形和异位肾都较常见。男性一般有较小、没有充分发育的阴茎结构；女性往往有阴道重复、较
860 宽的阴蒂对半分裂和偶尔发生的阴道发育不全或闭锁。

解剖学上的变异

正如先前提到的，如 Manzoni 等人[156]所述，泄殖腔外翻的表现和泌尿直肠隔的下降水平相关。各半膀胱通常以各自为中心分布于两侧，外翻的肠管一般是盲肠。但是，各半膀胱可能会在肠管的上方或下方汇合。膀胱可能完全被覆盖也可能只覆盖了一侧。作者曾经见过两例泄殖腔外翻的病例其膀胱完全被覆盖，其外观和隐匿性膀胱外翻很相似，但是在膀胱下方是回盲部组织结构。外阴部表现也各种各样。阴茎或阴蒂可以分裂得很宽、联生或甚至隐藏在外翻膀胱的下方[165]。重复子宫或阴道可能发生在 2/3 的女性患者身上，阴道发育不良可能发生在 1/3 的女性患者身上。一般都会同时存在腹股沟疝，男孩还会伴发有睾丸未降。

骨骼畸形，包括先天性髋关节脱位、马蹄内翻足和各种各样的下肢发育缺陷都较常见，发生于约 50% 的患者身上。Sponseller 等人[169]描述了膀胱外翻复合畸形的各种骨盆畸形的解剖学表现，但共同的特征是耻骨分离。

图 118-21 展示了外翻肠道组织的典型表现。可

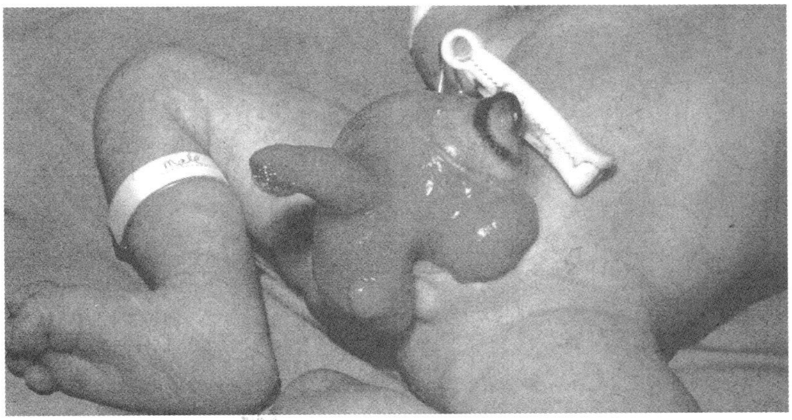

A

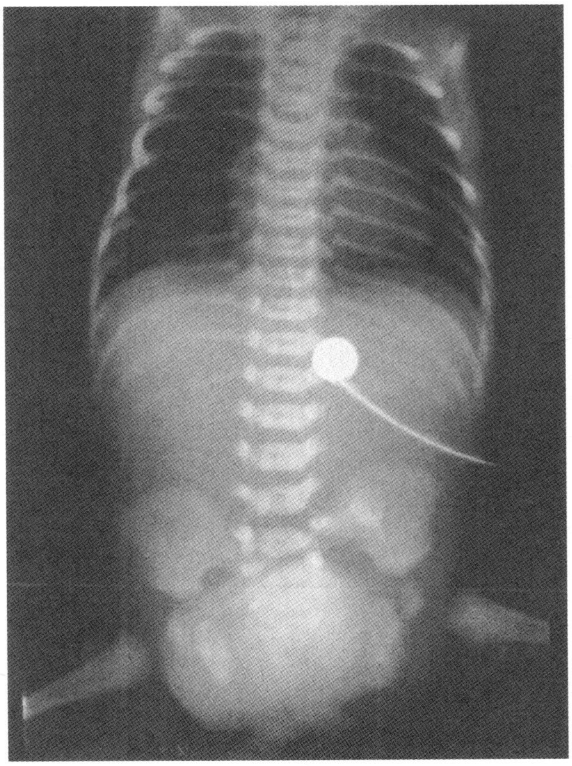

B

图 118-21　A. 一例女性新生儿泄殖腔外翻的典型外观表现。膀胱分裂成两半，盲肠外翻在中央如岛状，并有两个开口，一个通向阑尾，另一个通向末端回肠。中心的肠道卷管化并且放置在腹壁的左侧作为结肠造口，保留阑尾。两侧的膀胱合拢到中线上，内翻成管形放置于盆腔内，将耻骨支向中线靠拢，完整关闭腹壁。在第二阶段，尿道上裂修补时进行尿道重建，重复阴道重建为一。B. 相同患者的放射平片显示了外翻膀胱和肠道的软组织密度，以及耻骨支分离较宽。

能有复杂裂隙，但外观只有一个明显开口，也可能多个开口都很明显，比如上方有近端开口而远端肠道开口位于下方。一个或两个阑尾开口即重复阑尾的情况经常存在。虽然曾经提到过营养吸收障碍由小肠长度短导致，但是这个问题也会发生于小肠长度正常的患儿身上。并发的肠道畸形还包括旋转不良、肠道重复、肠闭锁和 Meckel 憩室。

各种各样的心血管和肺部畸形，包括先天性青紫型和非青紫型心脏病以及双主动脉弓，这些都曾有报道但发生率相对较少。在 Howell 等人[148]和 Davidoff 等人[138]对一系列病例的报道中，脊髓脊膜膨出发生于 50% 的患者身上。大多数病例局限于腰部，但是也遇到过一例骶部和一例胸部脊髓脊膜膨出。也有其他相似情况的报道。对于严重的脊椎神经管闭合不全病例，不建议进行治疗。

产前诊断

超声检查可以使泄殖腔外翻在产前得到明确诊断。在 Austin 等人[132]的回顾分析中，22 例病例中有 19 例仅通过超声获得了正确诊断。现在认为膀胱充
1861 盈缺损、前腹壁中线大部缺损和并发脊椎畸形都是特征性的表现。另外，下肢畸形、肾脏数量和位置的异常、肾积水、脑积水和耻骨分离也都有提到。近来产前孕母和胎儿核磁共振检查（MRI）提高了诊断的准确性。虽然胎儿镜在过去曾经应用于泄殖腔外翻的诊断，但是孕母和胎儿 MRI 可以避免这种侵入性检查的风险。另外一个产前正确诊断的优点在于明确性别。产前超声或 MRI 提供的资料以及通过羊水诊断获得的染色体组型，可以给父母亲提供更多机会考虑性别的问题。

泄殖腔外翻中对子宫的手术处理超出了此章节的讨论范围，这也正处在实验室研究阶段。迄今为止，只有膀胱外翻复合畸形中的脊髓分裂部分在产前被提到。

治疗

在产前确定有泄殖腔外翻的婴儿最好被送往一个特定治疗中心，这个中心集中了高危孕妇并具有处理新生婴儿畸形的丰富经验。出生时不需要许多诊断性检查，因为产前检查已经提供了准确的资料。所有病例在新生儿时期的生理状况都应保持稳定，这些婴儿最好经多学科团队诊治且由一名外科医生协调。最初的评估者应该包括新生儿学专家，因为许多这类婴儿可能是早产或是小于胎龄或两者皆有。考虑到呼吸窘迫综合征、新生儿败血症、坏死性小肠结肠炎和其他早产儿的并发症，对这些疾病的治疗也应该成为治疗计划的一部分。如果需要延迟初期手术，则脐膨出囊膜必须要保护好。应该预防性使用抗生素，因为经常会有尿路梗阻的情况。一期和分期重建手术的一般纲要列于图 118-22。

一般而言，泄殖腔外翻纠治有两种方法。Gearhart 和 Jeffs[141,143]已经透彻阐述了传统的分期手术方法。初期的全部修补方法已由 Howell 等人[148]、Zderic 等人[174]、Hendren[147]和 Mitchell 及 Plaire[159]描述。在过去的 20 年里，作者倾向于只要有可能就在出生后的 2～3 天由小儿普外科和泌尿外科医生联合进行初期的全部修补手术。但是，虽然想在出生时进行最大限度的重建，但对于早产且合并有肝脏外突的巨大脐膨出的病例仍然不可能进行。任何产前确定可能有尿路梗阻或其他肾脏畸形的婴儿都需要特殊关注。另外，性别确定能够在出生时完成，这是应该做的。本文将在后面部分讨论。

一份完整的泄殖腔外翻患者治疗计划应在出生后尽可能早地经多学科讨论并制定出来，而且要考虑到所有的问题，如生殖泌尿道、胃肠道、腹壁、性别确定和许多并发畸形的处理，包括脊椎神经管
闭合不全的治疗。畸形种类在表 118-1 中列出。利 186
用新生儿骨盆的柔韧性，理想的修补是在出生后 48 小时内进行。

泄殖腔外翻患儿在新生儿期的完整修补包括胃肠道的重建，即肠造口、膀胱和后部阴茎尿道的闭合、尿道上裂的修补和腹壁的关闭，不进行膀胱颈重建。偶尔需要进行双侧髋骨或垂直髂骨截骨手术[166,170]。

腹壁缺损

对于通常存在的脐膨出的较好处理方法是进行腹壁的全层修补。这一般可以完成的，尤其是在耻骨合拢后。对于早产婴儿，脐膨出和外翻组织占据了腹壁的大片面积，可以应用硅橡胶袋进行分期闭合或行不

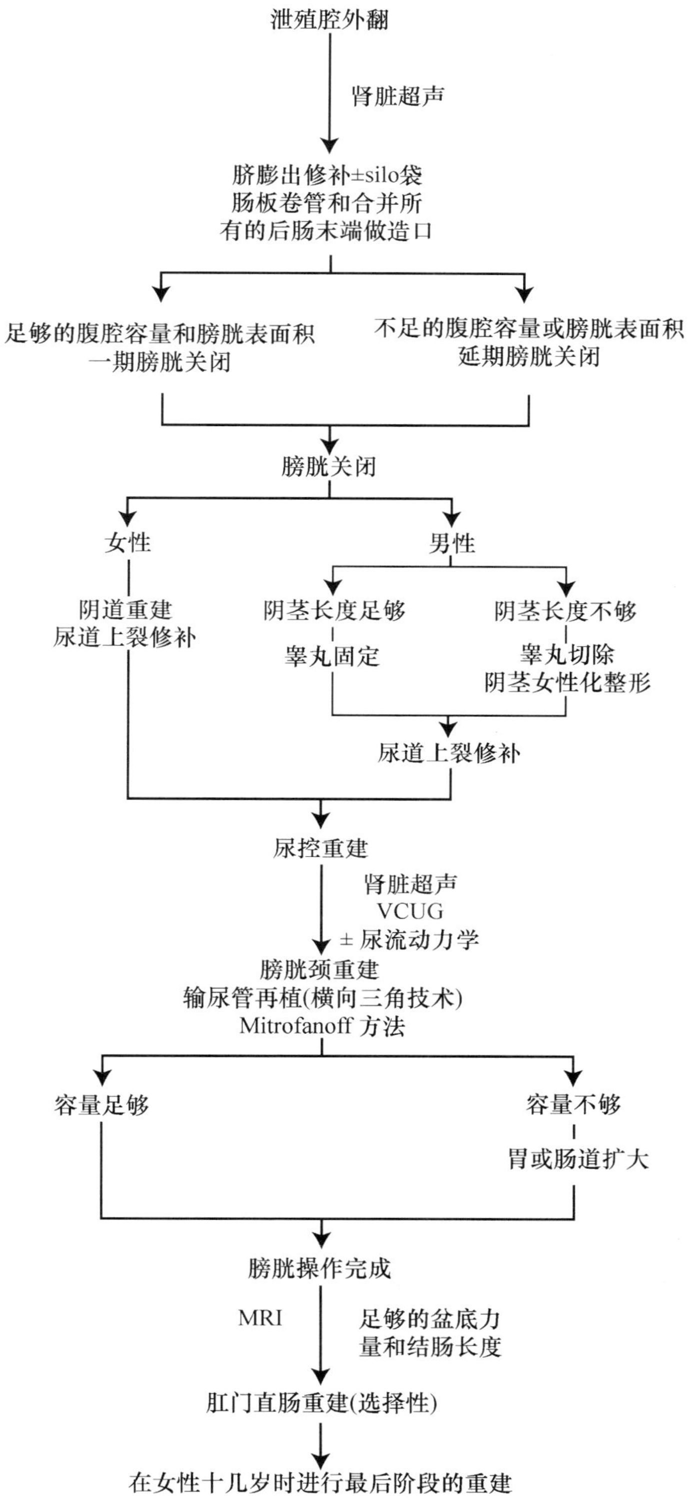

图 118-22　重建手术的概念。MRI，核磁共振显像；VCUG，排尿性膀胱尿路造影。

表 118-1　泄殖腔外翻患者的异常表现谱
脐膨出和腹壁缺陷
耻骨分裂
膀胱外翻中间介入了结肠组织
回盲部外翻
上面开口脱垂回肠
下面有一个或重复开口通向短小的后肠盲端
重复阑尾残端在中间位置
肛门闭锁
外生殖器分裂
小阴茎
隐睾
阴蒂和阴唇分裂
重复苗勒氏管结构
膀胱黏膜基础上的重复阴道外翻
阴道闭锁
脊髓脊膜膨出，脊髓囊状突出
其他缺陷
马蹄内翻畸形足
椎骨畸形（脊柱侧凸）
髋关节脱位
肾脏畸形
发育不良或多囊肾
巨输尿管
肾盂积水
融合畸形，异位

缝合筋膜的初期修补。这种初期修补能够在至少 80% 的病例中做到。

胃肠道重建

虽然确有短肠综合征的报道，但大多数泄殖腔外翻患者都能依靠足够长度的胃肠道正常地生长发育。不论小肠长度是否正常，都要尽一切努力来保存所有的肠道组织；第一是为了吸收功能，第二是因为可以用肠段组织来进行泌尿道重建。虽然 Rickham[163] 在 1960 年报道外翻的回盲部对于生存很重要，但是在

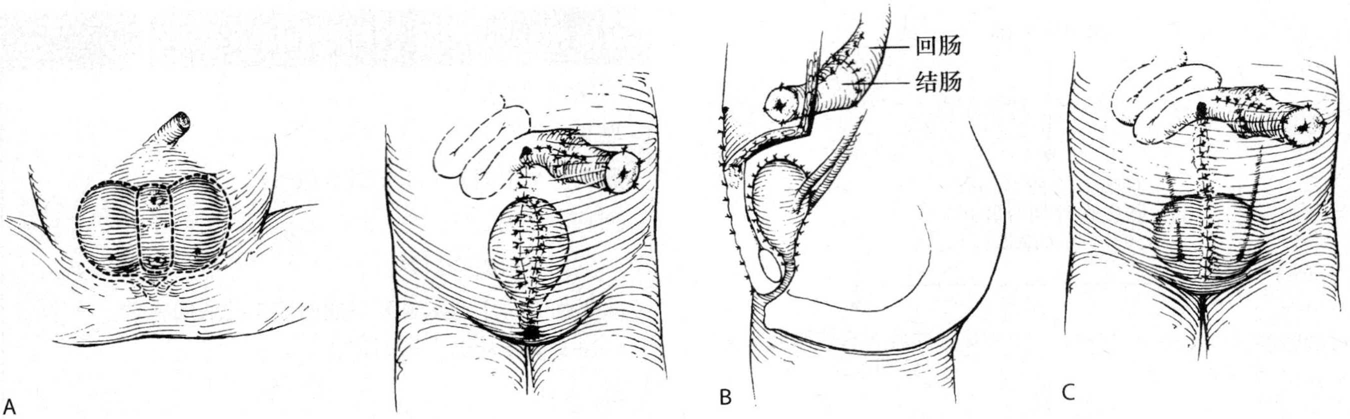

A　B　C

图 118-23　泄殖腔外翻的修补。A 和 B. 分开肠道黏膜和膀胱黏膜，回盲部卷成管状且拖出作为结肠造口的末端。如同完全的膀胱外翻修补术，膀胱各半被翻入，耻骨支靠拢。C. 其他方法是当不可能行卷管操作时，膀胱各半靠拢于中线并保持开放以等待分期手术。脐膨出关闭。

后来的 20 年里回肠造口术仍被普遍接受。1983 年，Howell 等人[148]重申了应最大限度保留肠道长度而不能摒弃结肠残段的原则。

修补手术时，膀胱侧边和外翻肠道之间的黏膜结合部分应该切开，要保留每块肠道黏膜和皮肤（图 118-23 和 118-24）。折叠回盲板成管状以重建回盲结合部。其边缘不要修裁以进行端端吻合术，因为黏膜表面组织将会缺失并且血供受损。当存在结肠重复时，每个肠段都要保留。后肠的末段通常存在且可能分开存在，与重建的回盲段邻近，或是可以用来延长结肠的长度。应该保留一个或重复阑尾时的两个阑
1863 尾，这是为了以后的胃肠道重建。将重建回盲段的末端作成肠造口从腹壁侧边脱出，以避免对腹壁闭合部的污染。如果需要，结肠段末端可以在今后的重建手术时重新定位。定位时应该考虑到合理有效地放置矫治器。偶尔会碰到患者有完整的结肠且前方还有肛门，这时可能需要行肛门成形术。外翻的盲肠板较小的患者，有时候其卷管化后的肠道会狭窄，但是因为狭窄处离造口的地方很靠近，所以可以用球囊扩张而避免重新再造。

作者尚未遇到过患者由于吸收障碍引发长期的营养问题，但是就像完全胃肠道外营养一样，适应期延长比较常见。所有的早期回肠末端造口患者都有营养问题。Davidoff 等人[138]报道通常患者需要 4 周的完全

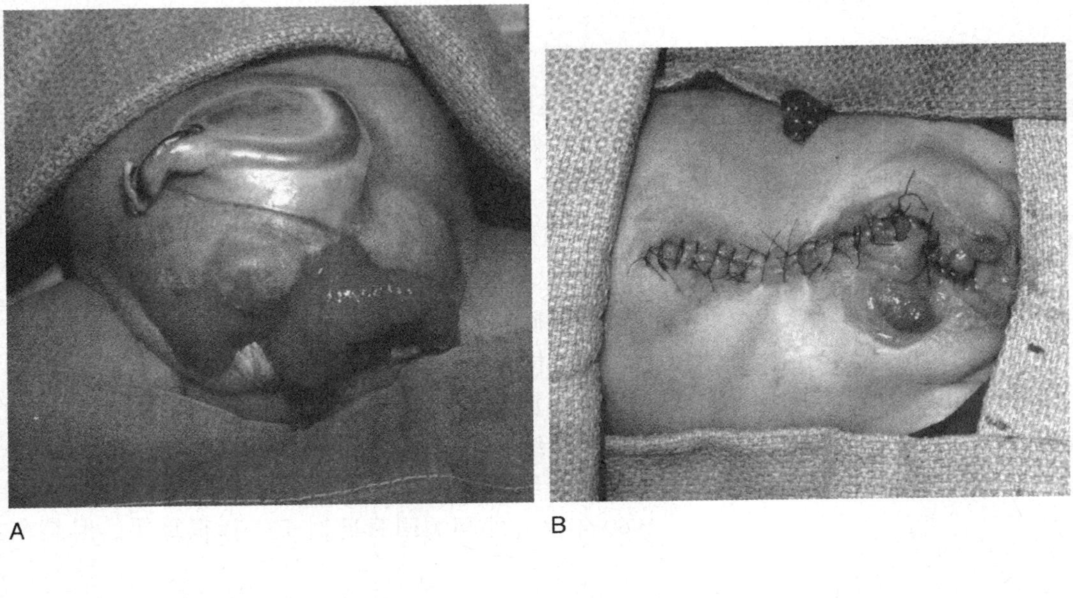

A　B

图 118-24　A. 一例女性泄殖腔外翻新生儿的典型表现，合并有脐膨出和两侧较小的膀胱板。从中央的盲肠可见有回肠脱垂。B. 对于这例患者，新生儿期的最初重建包括中央盲肠的卷管和腹壁左侧的结肠造口手术，由于膀胱板太小不能进行卷管所以留在体外。计划以后进行膀胱重建和泌尿生殖系重建。

胃肠道外营养，并且多数患者在 2 周内不能进行肠内喂养。

对于考虑在以后阶段要进行完全肛门直肠重建的患者，当经 CT 或 MRI 评估有脊髓神经管闭合不全或盆底肌发育缺陷时，将不再重建而保留永久的结肠造口。Lund 和 Hendren[155] 描述了 32 例患者中有 16 例经过根治（结肠连续）手术，但只有 3 例最终获得控制能力。在 Hendren 的报道中[147]，41 例泄殖腔外翻患者的结果得到了评估。41 例中有 7 例没有进行手术，15 例进行了结肠造口术，19 例行结肠根治术（连续性），其中有 3 例后来又回到了大便失禁的状态。大多数患者依靠灌肠排泄。Soffer 等人[168] 描述了 25 例泄殖腔外翻患者，最初都设法保留了结肠并且适应粪便排出。1 年后，对患者形成固态粪便并通过排泄口的能力进行评估。正常的结肠长度、形成固体粪便的能力以及肠道成功控制通过排泄口是进行根治手术的适应证。所有的 25 例患者经过了结肠根治手术。2 例结肠少于 10 cm 的患者进行了回肠造口术，1 例排便失禁，4 例有控制能力但偶尔污粪，11 例肠道处理控制得很干净，3 例完全得到控制，还有 4 例年龄太小无法评估。这些结果与多数完全肛门直肠重建手术相比更为乐观。从费城儿童医院的一系列患者调查来看，22 例泄殖腔外翻中有 20 例进行了永久性的结肠造口。3 例进行了根治手术，但其中 2 例又转回了结肠造口，还有 1 例进行灌肠治疗。针对根治手术后大便失禁患者的治疗还有 Malone 或左侧 Monti-Malone 法来进行顺行结肠冲洗[146,153]。

总的来讲，完全的肛门直肠重建还是一个未定的问题。大多数经过根治手术的患者大便失禁，而那些并发脊髓神经管闭合不全的患者得不到控便能力。因而，大部分患者，多数为短结肠，最好行末端结肠造口，但偶尔有些患者可备选进行结肠根治手术。此外，得到一致同意的是要保留这些患者的每一部分肠道组织。

泌尿道重建

泄殖腔外翻患者的泌尿道重建原则类似于对典型膀胱外翻患者的处理，这在本文前面已经阐述。手术处理的第一阶段是切除脐膨出以及仔细把肠道和膀胱分开。如图 118-23 中所示，尽可能先关闭膀胱。进行手术时，外科医生必须考虑到婴儿的大小和条件以及可利用膀胱黏膜组织的尺寸和容量。如果将合并有 1864
呼吸窘迫综合征的早产儿的膀胱和腹壁完全关闭有一定困难，或者膀胱组织不足，那么膀胱两半可以先简单靠拢并且留在腹壁外以等待以后的操作，但是膀胱有可能会发生纤维化（见图 118-24）。另一个替代方法就是进行膀胱的初期关闭，但是不要试图去关闭膀胱颈部。如果施行膀胱的初期关闭，则通过耻骨靠拢使膀胱在骨盆内是保证关闭完全的最佳方法，可进行或不进行髂骨截骨术。对于有足够膀胱组织的足月儿，除了初期膀胱关闭和耻骨靠拢外，作者更倾向于关闭膀胱颈，可以用或不用尿道侧边翼。如果开始时未施行膀胱颈部重建，那么可以和后来的控尿性重建手术、输尿管再植术和生殖器重建术一起进行。应用胃肠道部分行控尿性重建手术时，最好延后大约 4 年进行，到那时大多数患者有了稳定的胃肠功能且整个胃肠道长度和口径都有增加，尤其是阑尾。在本章节的主要部分对这些操作进行了详细阐述。Gearhart 等人[10-12,35] 倾向于分期操作，这样可以避免膀胱裂开后的严重并发症。其他人关于一期完全重建的经验都表明不会促进这种潜在并发症的发生[148,159,174]。

对于膀胱板组织不够的患者，将来可能会通过胎儿组织工程技术施行膀胱扩大[140]。但是如前所述，膀胱扩大和控尿重建的标准技术仍然是治疗的主要依据。

Grady 和 Mitchell[145] 证明一期全部外翻修补术较分期修补可以获得更好的控尿能力，并发症发生率也明显低于以前关于一期修补的报道。总的说来，多数患者可能会得到控尿力，但是多数只有在膀胱颈部重建后的其他操作中达到此效果[137,150,155]。许多证据表明在新生儿期接受了完全的尿道和膀胱修补的患者可以得到更好的储尿功能和最终的控尿能力，但是这还需要更多的数据来证明[159,174]。如前所述，重建的焦点问题转向了提高生存质量，这需要通过减少失禁出口的数量、提供保证正常活动的工具和改善外观来做到[157]。

Bolduc 等人[134] 观察到达 1/4 的膀胱外翻患者存在明显的上尿道病变，表现形式有肾瘢痕化或肾盂积水。控尿手术方法无法预测这些情况，膀胱颈关闭和其他形式的膀胱颈重建同样安全。换句话说，肾损害显然是一个原先就已经存在的问题。

Schober 等人[164] 近来关注高发的受神经源性畸形影响的长期尿控问题，强调了 Mitrofanoff 型重建手术的重要性，包括膀胱颈关闭和建立可控性导尿开口。他们指出阴茎短小或缺失占男性患者的1/3，而且这样的患者几乎没有生育能力。大多数女性患者拥有双角状子宫却有正常的输卵管和卵巢。有一些应用辅助技术成功妊娠的报道已经发表。

Baker Towell 和 Towell[133] 呈交了一份比较性分析研究，主题是关于泄殖腔外翻和一般患者在社会适应能力和生存质量方面的情况。泄殖腔外翻患者的评分与患有其他慢性疾病患者评分相当，提示儿童时期的性别评定或再选择未必会造成生理、情感或行为上的问题。他们认为需要进行长期的随访研究。因而，不论这种多系统畸形有多么复杂的本质，都有可能通过坚定积极的方法，使得大多数泄殖腔外翻婴儿得到接近于正常或至少是满意的社会生活和调控能力[155,157,159,164,174]。

生殖器重建

生殖器重建的总原则已经讲过。先前的报道提出，由于外生殖器短小，对泄殖腔外翻的患者进行男性化重建不太可能。由于这个原因，许多外科医生提出有此种畸形的男性患儿在新生儿初期手术时要转变为女性。近些年来，关于性别处理问题的争论更加激烈。显然，这个问题只是针对那些具有男性基因但解剖上却有功能缺陷的患者。

许多人认为新生儿的性别是中性的，孩子的性别确定根本上取决于性别培养。Zderic 等人[174] 描述了对早期性别转换的观察，而且报道了令人满意的长期随访结果。但是，对早期的性别转换进行修改还是必要的，因为至少一些泄殖腔外翻患者有足够的阴茎组织，可以通过现代技术得以重建，并且可以应用睾酮行补充治疗[159]。另外，越来越多的证据表明胎脑发育亦受到雄性激素的影响[162]。虽然泄殖腔外翻男性患者得到了性别的重新评定，结果令人满意，但长期的随访也证明一些患者希望重新转为男性。因而，只要阴茎成形术可行，就应该延迟性别的再评定。对于阴茎很小或没有阴茎残迹的患者，性别转换可能是唯一选择。

泄殖腔外翻的男性患儿具备组织学和结构均正
1865 常的睾丸，这与女性患儿有卵巢一样[158]。许多女性患儿有卵巢囊肿，但不是所有的病例都需要治疗[144]。男性患儿合并的先天性畸形如尿道下裂较难治疗，但卷管、切割尿道板行尿道成形修补还是有希望的[171]。

脊髓神经管闭合不全

泄殖腔外翻患者中近50%有各种各样的脊髓脊膜膨出。脂肪脊膜膨出患者的病变外覆皮肤，通常合并有脊髓栓系，以后需要进行修补。开放性的脊髓脊膜膨出通常需要关闭，脑积水时要进行转流手术，因此需要小儿神经外科医生加入治疗小组。通常采用两种方法。当有证据表明脑脊液渗漏或即将发生脊膜破裂时应该优先关闭脊髓脊膜膨出。另外，如果背部缺损可以延迟4～6周关闭，那么关闭前腹壁缺损就会比较容易。如果能够对脊髓脊膜膨出的包膜提供非常仔细的保护，则后一种方法可以安全实施。对于合并有脊髓脊膜膨出的泄殖腔外翻患者，当考虑通过骨盆截骨来靠拢耻骨时，必须选择背侧髂骨截骨的替代方法，比如前路髂骨截骨或前路耻骨截骨术。除非耻骨靠拢时张力极高，否则作者不主张进行截骨手术。

骨骼畸形

针对泄殖腔外翻婴儿各种骨骼畸形进行的小儿整形外科处理最好加入到整个治疗计划中。处理的一般原则和那些只患有骨骼畸形的患者的处理原则一样。比如，畸形足在出生后即刻被安置于矫正器中，有指征时行夹板固定和矫正手术。骨骼畸形患者如半椎体患者，若处于进展性的明显脊柱侧凸的危险中，则应该积极治疗。如果这些患者想尽可能早地得到良好的生存质量，那么理疗学家、临床医学家和社会工作者们都应该加入到这些患者的治疗中。

根据髋关节的功能和步态，应用或不用截骨方法进行耻骨分离初期闭合可以使这些患者有机会获得近乎正常的步态[166,170]。

泄殖腔外翻：结果

20世纪60年代泄殖腔外翻患者总生存率大约在20%左右，到20世纪70年代上升至50%[163,173]。到20世纪80年代，大多数报道的生存率达到了90%，并一直保持到今天[148,149,154,155,174,175]。现在，死亡与极度早产、肾发育不良或其他复杂致命畸形有关。有趣的是严重的心血管畸形在泄殖腔外翻患者中并不常见。

与泄殖腔外翻患者治疗相关的各种并发症和典型的膀胱外翻患者相似，这些在本章节的主体部分已经描述过。然而，膀胱裂开在泄殖腔外翻中发生的机会要高于典型的膀胱外翻。胃肠道疾病发病率特点和处理的方法在先前已经阐述，但是大多数患者最终可以获得满意的胃肠道功能。

（何 蓉译 文建国校）

参考文献

膀胱外翻

1. Abasiyanik A, Guvenc H, Koseoglu B: Penopubic flaps technique for the repair of epispadias with or without exstrophy: A preliminary report. J Pediatr Surg 1996;31:1225.
2. Adams MC, Pope JC IV, Brock JW III: Exstrophy/epispadias in the female: Complete primary repair [abstract]. Paper presented at the annual meeting of the AAP, 2002, Boston.
3. Ambrose SS, O'Brien DP III: Surgical embryology of the exstrophy-epispadias complex. Surg Clin North Am 1974; 54:1379.
4. Arap S, Giron AM, deGoes GM: Complete reconstruction of bladder exstrophy: Experimental program. Urology 1976; 7:413.
5. Arap S, Nahas WC, Giron AM, et al: Incontinent epispadias: Surgical treatment of 38 cases. J Urol 1988;140:577.
6. Barth RA, Filly RA, Sondheimer FK: Prenatal sonographic findings in bladder exstrophy. J Ultrasound Med 1990;9:359.
7. Ben-Chaim J, Peppas DS, Jeffs RD, et al: Complete male epispadias: Genital reconstruction and achieving continence. J Urol 1995;153:1665.
8. Bennett AH: Exstrophy of bladder treated by ureterosigmoidostomies: Long term evaluation. Urology 1973;2:165.
9. Boyce WH: A new concept concerning treatment of exstrophy of the bladder: 20 years later. J Urol 1972;107:476.
10. Brzezinski AE, Homsy YL, Laberge I: Orthoplasty in epispadias. J Urol 1986;136:259.
11. Burbige KA, Hensle TW, Chambers WJ, et al: Pregnancy and sexual function in women with bladder exstrophy. Urology 1986;28:12.
12. Burns JE: A new operation for exstrophy of the bladder. JAMA 1924;82:1587.
13. Caldamone AA: Anomalies of the bladder and cloaca. In Gillenwater JY, et al (eds): Adult and Pediatric Urology. St Louis, Mosby-Year Book, 1991.
14. Canning DA, et al: A computerized review of exstrophy patients managed during the past thirteen years [abstract]. Paper presented at the annual meeting of the AUA, 1989, Dallas.
15. Canning DA, Gearhart JP, Jeffs RD: Cephalotrigonal reimplant as an adjunct to bladder neck reconstruction [abstract]. Paper presented at the annual meeting of the AUA, 1990, New Orleans.
16. Cantwell FV: Operative technique of epispadias by transplantation of the urethra. Ann Surg 1895;22:689.
17. Cerniglia FR Jr, Roth DR, Gonzales ET Jr: Covered exstrophy and visceral sequestration in a male newborn: Case report. J Urol 1989;141:903.
18. Chisholm TC, McFarland FA: Exstrophy of the Urinary Bladder. Chicago, Year Book Medical Publishers, 1982.
19. Clemetson CA: Ectopia vesicae and split pelvis: An account of pregnancy in a woman with treated ectopia vesicae and split pelvis, including a review of the literature. J Obstet Gynaecol Br Emp 1958;65:973.
20. Coffey R: Transplantation of the ureter into the large intestine in the absence of a functioning bladder. Surg Gynecol Obstet 1921;32:383.
21. Cohen SJ: Ureterozystoneostomie, eine neue antirefluxtechnik. Akt Urol 1975;6:1.
22. Connor JP, Lattimer JK, Hensle TW, et al: Primary closure of bladder exstrophy: Long-term functional results in 137 patients. J Pediatr Surg 1988;23:1102.
23. Cracchiolo A 3rd, Hall CB: Bilateral iliac osteotomy: The first stage in repair of exstrophy of the bladder. Clin Orthop 1970;68:156.
24. Csontai A, Merksz M, Pirot L, et al: Results of surgical treatment in children with bladder exstrophy. Br J Urol 1992; 70:683.
25. Devine CJ, Horton CE: Hypospadias and epispadias. Clin Symp 1972;20:24.
26. Devine CJ Jr, Horton CE, Scarff JE Jr: Epispadias. Urol Clin North Am 1980;7:465.
27. Duckett JW: Use of paraexstrophy skin pedicle grafts for correction of exstrophy and epispadias repair. Birth Defects Orig Artic Ser 1977;13:175.
28. Duckett JW: The island flap technique for hypospadias repair. Urol Clin North Am 1981;8:503.
29. Duckett JW, Caldamone AA: Bladder exstrophy. AUA Update Series 1984;13:2.
30. Duckett JW Jr: Epispadias. Urol Clin North Am 1978;5:107.
31. El-Sherbiny MT, Hafez AT, Ghoneim MA: Complete repair of exstrophy: Further experience with neonates and children after failed initial closure. J Urol 2002;168:1692.
32. Engel RM: Bladder exstrophy: Vesicoplasty or urinary diversion? Urology 1973;2:20.
33. Ezell WW, Carlson HE: A realistic look at exstrophy of the bladder. Br J Urol 1970;42:197.
34. Gearhart JP: Exstrophy, Epispadias, and Other Bladder Anomalies. Philadelphia, WB Saunders, 2002, p 2136.
35. Gearhart JP, Ben-Chaim J, Jeffs RD, et al: Criteria for the prenatal diagnosis of classic bladder exstrophy. Obstet Gynecol 1995;85:961.
36. Gearhart JP, Jeffs RD: Augmentation cystoplasty in the failed exstrophy reconstruction. J Urol 1988;139:790.
37. Gearhart JP, Jeffs RD: Bladder exstrophy: Increase in capacity following epispadias repair. J Urol 1989;142:525.
38. Gearhart JP, Jeffs RD: State-of-the-art reconstructive surgery for bladder exstrophy at the Johns Hopkins Hospital. Am J Dis Child 1989;143:1475.
39. Gearhart JP, Jeffs RD: Complications of Exstrophy and Epispadias Repair, 2nd ed. Philadelphia, WB Saunders, 1990.
40. Gearhart JP, Jeffs RD: Management and Treatment of Classic Bladder Exstrophy. Philadelphia, WB Saunders, 1990.
41. Gearhart JP, Leonard MP, Burgers JK, et al: The Cantwell-Ransley technique for repair of epispadias. J Urol 1992; 148:851.
42. Gearhart JP, Peppas DS, Jeffs RD: Complications of paraexstrophy skin flaps in the reconstruction of classical bladder exstrophy. J Urol 1993;150:627.

43. Gearhart JP, Sciortino C, Ben-Chaim J, et al: The Cantwell-Ransley epispadias repair in exstrophy and epispadias: Lessons learned. Urology 1995;46:92.
44. Gearhart JP, Williams KA, Jeffs RD: Intraoperative urethral pressure profilometry as an adjunct to bladder neck reconstruction. J Urol 1986;136:1055.
45. Grady RW, Carr MC, Mitchell ME: Complete primary closure of bladder exstrophy: Epispadias and bladder exstrophy repair. Urol Clin North Am 1999;26:95.
46. Grady RW, Mitchell ME: Complete primary repair of exstrophy. J Urol 1999;162:1415.
47. Grady RW, Mitchell ME: Exstrophy and Epispadias Anomalies, 4th ed. Philadelphia, Lippincott Williams & Wilkins, 2002.
48. Grady RW, et al: The complete primary repair of exstrophy (CPRE) technique for repair of bladder exstrophy and epispadias: Long-term follow-up. Paper presented at the annual meeting of the AAP, 2003, New Orleans.
49. Hanna MK, Williams DI: Genital function in males with vesical exstrophy and epispadias. Br J Urol 1972; 44:169.
50. Hendren WH: Penile lengthening after previous repair of epispadias. J Urol 1979;121:527.
51. Hinman R: A method of lengthening and repairing the penis in exstrophy of the bladder. J Urol 1958;79:237.
52. Hollowell JG, Ransley PG: Surgical management of incontinence in bladder exstrophy. Br J Urol 1991;68:543.
53. Horton CE, Devine CJ Jr, Devine PC, et al: Aesthetic reconstructive genital surgery. Clin Plast Surg 1981;8:399.
54. Husmann DA, McLorie GA, Churchill BM: A comparison of renal function in the exstrophy patient treated with staged reconstruction versus urinary diversion. J Urol 1988; 140:1204.
55. Husmann DA, McLorie GA, Churchill BM: Closure of the exstrophic bladder: An evaluation of the factors leading to its success and its importance on urinary continence. J Urol 1989;142:522.
56. Ives E, Coffey R, Carter CO: A family study of bladder exstrophy. J Med Genet 1980;17:139.
57. Jaffe R, Schoenfeld A, Ovadia J: Sonographic findings in the prenatal diagnosis of bladder exstrophy. Am J Obstet Gynecol 1990;162:675.
58. Janssen P: Die Operation der blasenektopie ohne inanspruchnahme des Intestinums. Zentralbl Chir 1933;60:2657.
59. Jeffs RD: Exstrophy of the Urinary Bladder. Chicago, Year Book Medical Publishers, 1986.
60. Jeffs RD, Charrios R, Mnay M, et al: Primary Closure of the Exstrophied Bladder. Philadelphia, WB Saunders, 1972.
61. Jeffs RD, Guice SL, Oesch I: The factors in successful exstrophy closure. J Urol 1982;127:974.
62. Johnston JH: Lengthening of the congenital or acquired short penis. Br J Urol 1974;46:685.
63. Johnston JH: The genital aspects of exstrophy. J Urol 1975; 113:701.
64. Justrabo E, Poulard G, Arnould L, et al: [Invasive adenocarcinoma with epidermoid carcinoma on the site of bladder exstrophy: Histochemical and immunocytochemical study]. Arch Anat Cytol Pathol 1991;39:223.
65. Kajbafzadeh AM, Duffy PG, Ransley PG: The evolution of penile reconstruction in epispadias repair: A report of 180 cases. J Urol 1995;154:858.
66. Kelly JH: Vesical exstrophy: Repair using radical mobilisation of soft tissues. Pediatr Surg Int 1995;10:298.
67. King LR, Wendel EF: Primary cystectomy and permanent urinary diversion in the treatment of exstrophy of the urinary bladder. In Russell S, et al (eds): Current Controversies in Urologic Management. Philadelphia, WB Saunders, 1972.
68. Koff SA, Eakins M: The treatment of penile chordee using corporeal rotation. J Urol 1984;131:931.
69. Kramer SA, Jackson IT: Bilateral rhomboid flaps for reconstruction of the external genitalia in epispadias-exstrophy. Plast Reconstr Surg 1986;77:621.
70. Kramer SA, Kelalis PP: Assessment of urinary continence in epispadias: Review of 94 patients. J Urol 1982;128:290.
71. Kramer SA, Mesrobian HG, Kelalis PP: Long-term followup of cosmetic appearance and genital function in male epispadias: Review of 70 patients. J Urol 1986;135:543.
72. Krisiloff M, Puchner PJ, Tretter W, et al: Pregnancy in women with bladder exstrophy. J Urol 1978;119:478.
73. Lattimer JK, Beck L, Yeaw S, et al: Long-term followup after exstrophy closure: Late improvement and good quality of life. J Urol 1978;119:664.
74. Lattimer JK, Macfarlane MT: A urethral lengthening procedure for epispadias and exstrophy. J Urol 1980;123:544.
75. Lattimer JK, Smith MJ: Exstrophy closure: A followup on 70 cases. J Urol 1966;95:356.
76. Leadbetter WF, Clarke BG: Five years' experience with ureteroenterostomy by the "combined" technique. J Urol 1954;73:67.
77. Lepor H, Jeffs RD: Primary bladder closure and bladder neck reconstruction in classical bladder exstrophy. J Urol 1983;130:1142.
78. Lepor H, Shapiro E, Jeffs RD: Urethral reconstruction in boys with classical bladder exstrophy. J Urol 1984;131:512.
79. Lowe FC, Jeffs RD: Wound dehiscence in bladder exstrophy: An examination of the etiologies and factors for initial failure and subsequent success. J Urol 1983;130:312.
80. MacKay J, Syme J: Congenital exstrophy of the urinary bladder. Month J Med Sci 1849;9:934.
81. Marshall VF, Muecke EC: Variations in exstrophy of the bladder. J Urol 1962;88:766.
82. Marshall VF, Muecke EC: Functional closure of typical exstrophy of the bladder. J Urol 1970;104:205.
83. Maydl K: Uber die Radikaltherapie der Blasenectopie. Wien Med Wochenschr 1894;44:25.
84. McLaughlin KP, Rink RC, Adams MC, et al: Stomach in combination with other intestinal segments in pediatric lower urinary tract reconstruction. J Urol 1995;154:1162.
85. Megalli M, Lattimer JK: Review of the management of 140 cases of exstrophy of the bladder. J Urol 1973;109:246.
86. Mesrobian HG, Kelalis PP, Kramer SA: Long-term followup of cosmetic appearance and genital function in boys with exstrophy: Review of 53 patients. J Urol 1986;136:256.
87. Mesrobian HG, Kelalis PP, Kramer SA: Long-term followup of 103 patients with bladder exstrophy. J Urol 1988;139:719.
88. Michon L: Conservative operations for exstrophy of the bladder with particular reference to urinary incontinence. Br J Urol 1948;20:167.
89. Mildenberger H, Kluth D, Dziuba M: Embryology of bladder exstrophy. J Pediatr Surg 1988;23:166.
90. Mirk P, Calisti A, Fileni A: Prenatal sonographic diagnosis of bladder extrophy. J Ultrasound Med 1986;5:291.
91. Mitchell ME, Bagli DJ: Complete penile disassembly for epispadias repair: The Mitchell technique. J Urol 1996;155:300.
92. Mitrofanoff P: Cystomie continente trans-appendiculaire dans le traitement des vessies neurologues. Chir Ped 1980;21:297.
93. Mollard P: Bladder reconstruction in exstrophy. J Urol 1980;124:525.

94. Monfort G, Morisson-Lacombe G, Guys JM, et al: Transverse island flap and double flap procedure in the treatment of congenital epispadias in 32 patients. J Urol 1987;138:1069.
95. Muecke EC: The role of the cloacal membrane in exstrophy: The first successful experimental study. J Urol 1964;92:659.
96. Murphy LJT: The History of Urology. Springfield, Ill, Charles C Thomas, 1972.
97. Nesbitt RM: Ureterosigmoid anastomosis by direct elliptical connection: A preliminary report. J Urol 1949;61:728.
98. Oesterling JE, Jeffs RD: The importance of a successful initial bladder closure in the surgical management of classical bladder exstrophy: Analysis of 144 patients treated at the Johns Hopkins Hospital between 1975 and 1985. J Urol 1987;137:258.
99. Parkash S, Bhandari M: Rectus abdominis myocutaneous island flap for bridging defect after cystectomy for bladder exstrophy. Urology 1982;20:536.
100. Patton BM, Barry A: The genesis of exstrophy of the bladder and epispadias. Am J Anat 1952;90:35.
101. Perlmutter AD, Weinstein MD, Reitelman C: Vesical neck reconstruction in patients with epispadias-exstrophy complex. J Urol 1991;146:613.
102. Peters CA, Gearhart JP, Jeffs RD: Epispadias and incontinence: The challenge of the small bladder. J Urol 1988;140:1199.
103. Pohlman AG: The development of the cloaca in human embryos. Am J Anat 1911;21:1.
104. Ransley PG: Epispadias Repair. London, Butterworths, 1988.
105. Ransley PG, Duffy PG, Wollin M: Bladder Exstrophy Closure and Epispadias Repair, 4th ed. Edinburgh, Butterworths, 1989.
106. Schillinger JF, Wiley MJ: Bladder exstrophy: Penile lengthening procedure. Urology 1984;24:434.
107. Schlegel PN, Gearhart JP: Neuroanatomy of the pelvis in an infant with cloacal exstrophy: A detailed microdissection with histology. J Urol 1989;141:583.
108. Schwarz GR, Jeffs RD: Ileal conduit urinary diversion in children: Computer analysis of followup from 2 to 16 years. J Urol 1975;114:285.
109. Shapiro E, Lepor H, Jeffs RD: The inheritance of the exstrophy-epispadias complex. J Urol 1984;132:308.
110. Shaw MB, Rink RC, Kaefer M, et al: Continence in classic bladder exstrophy. Paper presented at the annual meeting of the AAP, 2002, Boston.
111. Silver RI, Yang A, Ben-Chaim J, et al: Penile length in adulthood after exstrophy reconstruction. J Urol 1997;157:999.
112. Spence HM, Hoffman WW, Fosmire GP: Tumour of the colon as a late complication of ureterosigmoidostomy for exstrophy of the bladder. Br J Urol 1979;51:466.
113. Spence HM, Hoffman WW, Pate VA: Exstrophy of the bladder. I. Long-term results in a series of 37 cases treated by ureterosigmoidostomy. J Urol 1975;114:133.
114. Sponseller PD, Bisson LJ, Gearhart JP, et al: The anatomy of the pelvis in the exstrophy complex. J Bone Joint Surg Am 1995;77:177.
115. Sponseller PD, Gearhart JP, Jeffs RD: Anterior innominate osteotomies for failure or late closure of bladder exstrophy. J Urol 1991;146:137.
116. Stec AA, Pannu HK, Tadros YE, et al: Pelvic floor anatomy in classic bladder exstrophy using 3-dimensional computerized tomography: Initial insights. J Urol 2001;166:1444.
117. Stec AA, Pannu HK, Tadros YE, et al: Evaluation of the bony pelvis in classic bladder exstrophy by using 3D-CT: Further insights. Urology 2001;58:1030.
118. Syme J: Ectopia vesicae. Lancet 1852;2:568.
119. Thiersch C: Ueber die entstchugsweise und operative behandlung der Epispadie. Arch Heilbundle 1869;10:20.
120. Toguri AG, Churchill BM, Schillinger JF, et al: Continence in cases of bladder exstrophy. J Urol 1978;119:538.
121. Trendelenburg F: De la cure operatoire de l'exstrophie vesicale et de l'epispadias. Arch Klin Chir 1892;43:394.
122. Turner WR Jr, Ransley PG, Bloom DA, et al: Variants of the exstrophic complex. Urol Clin North Am 1980;7:493.
123. Vyas PR, Roth DR, Perlmutter AD: Experience with free grafts in urethral reconstruction. J Urol 1987;137:471.
124. Williams DI: Split Symphysis Variants. New York, Springer-Verlag, 1947.
125. Williams DI, Keeton JE: Further progress with reconstruction of the exstrophied bladder. Br J Surg 1973;60:203.
126. Woodhouse CR, Ransley PG, Williams DI: The patient with exstrophy in adult life. Br J Urol 1983;55:632.
127. Woodhouse CR, Kellett MJ: Anatomy of the penis and its deformities in exstrophy and epispadias. J Urol 1984;132:1122.
128. Woodhouse CR, Strachan JR: Malignancy in exstrophy patients [abstract]. Scarborough, England, British Association of Urological Surgeons, July 11, 1990.
129. Yerkes EB, Adams MC, Rink RC, et al: How well do patients with exstrophy actually void? J Urol 2000;164:1044.
130. Young HH: Exstrophy of the bladder: The first case in which a normal bladder and urinary control have been obtained by plastic operation. Surg Gynecol Obstet 1942;74:729.
131. Zabbo A, Kay R: Ureterosigmoidostomy and bladder exstrophy: A long-term followup. J Urol 1986;136:396.

泄殖腔外翻

132. Austin PF, Homsey YL, Gearhart JP, et al: The prenatal diagnosis of cloacal exstrophy. J Urol 1998;160:1179-1181.
133. Baker Towell DM, Towell AD: A preliminary investigation into quality of life, psychological distress and social competence in children with cloacal exstrophy. J Urol 2003;169:1850-1853.
134. Bolduc S, Capolicchio G, Upadhyay J, et al: The fate of the upper urinary tract in exstrophy. J Urol 2002;168:2579-2582.
135. Bruch SW, Adzick NS, Goldstein RB, Harrison MR: Challenging the embyrogenesis of cloacal exstrophy. J Pediatr Surg 1996;31:768-770.
136. Caldamone AA: Anomalies of the bladder and cloaca. In Gillenwater JY, et al (eds): Adult and Pediatric Urology. St Louis, Mosby-Year Book, 1991.
137. Capolicchio G, McLorie GA, Farhad W, et al: A population based analysis of continence outcomes and bladder exstrophy. J Urol 2001;165:2418-2421.
138. Davidoff AM, Hebra A, Balmer D, et al: Management of the gastrointestinal tract and nutrition in patients with cloacal exstrophy. J Pediatr Surg 1996;31:771-773.
139. Evans JA, Chudley AE: Tibial agenesis, femoral duplication, and caudal midline anomalies. Am J Med Genet 1999;85:13-19.
140. Fauza DO, Fishman SJ, Mehegan K, Atala A: Videofetoscopically assisted fetal tissue engineering: Bladder augmentation. J Pediatr Surg 1998;33:7-12.
141. Gearhart JP: Bladder exstrophy: Staged reconstruction. Curr Opin Urol 1999;9:499-506.
142. Gearhart JP: Complete repair of bladder exstrophy in the newborn: Complications and management. J Urol 2001;165:2431-2433.

143. Gearhart JP, Jeffs RD: Techniques to create urinary continence in the cloacal exstrophy patient. J Urol 1991;146: 616-618.
144. Geiger JD, Coran AG: The association of large ovarian cysts with cloacal exstrophy. J Pediar Surg 1998;33:719-721.
145. Grady RW, Mitchell ME: Complete primary repair of exstrophy. J Urol 1999;162:1415-1420.
146. Griffiths DM, Malone PS: The Malone antegrade continence enema. J Pediatr Surg 1995;30:68-71.
147. Hendren WH: Cloaca, the most severe degree of imperforate anus: Experience with 195 cases. Ann Surg 1998;228:331-346.
148. Howell C, Caldamone AA, Snyder H, et al: Cloacal exstrophy—optimal management. J Pediatr Surg 1983;18: 365-369.
149. Hurwitz RS, Manzoni GA, Ransley PG, Stephens FD: Cloacal exstrophy: A report of 34 cases. J Urol 1987;138:1060-1064.
150. Husmann DA, Vandersteen DR, McLorie GA, Churchill BM: Urinary continence after staged bladder reconstruction for cloacal exstrophy: The effect of coexisting neurological abnormalities on urinary continence. J Urol 1999;161:1598-1602.
151. Keppler-Noreuil KM: OEIS complex (omphalocele-exstrophy-imperforate anus-spinal defects): A review of 14 cases. Am J Med Genet 2001;99:271-279.
152. Lakshmanan Y, Bellin PB, Gilroy AM, Fung LC: Antenatally diagnosed cloacal exstrophy variant with intravesical phallus in a twin pregnancy. Urology 2001;57:1178.
153. Liloku RB, Mure PY, Braga L, et al: The left Monti-Malone procedure: Preliminary results in seven cases. J Pediatr Surg 2002;37:228-231.
154. Lund DP, Hendren WH: Cloacal exstrophy: Experience with 20 cases. J Pediatr Surg 1993;28:1360-1368.
155. Lund DP, Hendren WH: Cloacal exstrophy: A 25-year experience with 50 cases. J Pediatr Surg 2001;36:68-75.
156. Manzoni GA, Ransley PG, Hurwitz RS: Cloacal exstrophy and cloacal exstrophy variants: A proposed system of classification. J Urol 1987;138:1065-1068.
157. Mathews R, Jeffs RD, Reiner WG, et al: Cloacal exstrophy—improving the quality of life: The Johns Hopkins experience. J Urol 1998;160:2452-2456.
158. Mathews RI, Perlman E, Marsh DW, Gearhart JP: Gonadal morphology in cloacal exstrophy: Implications in gender assignment. BJU Int 1999;84:99-100.
159. Mitchell ME, Plaire C: Management of cloacal exstrophy. In Zderic SA, et al (eds): Pediatric Gender Assignment: A Critical Reappraisal. New York, Kluwer Academic/Plenum Publishers, 2002.
160. Oostra RJ, Baljet B, Verbeeten BW, Hennekam RC: Congenital anomalies in the teratological collection of Museum Vrolik in Amsterdam, the Netherlands. III. Primary field defects, sequences, and other complex anomalies. Am J Med Genet 1998;80:46-59.
161. Parrott TS, Skandalakis JE, Gray SW: The bladder and urethra. In Skandalakis JE, Gray SW (eds): Embryology for Surgeons. Baltimore, Williams & Wilkins, 1994.
162. Reiner WG, Gearhart JP: Discordant sexual identity in some genetic males with cloacal exstrophy assigned to female sex at birth. N Engl J Med 2004;350:333-341.
163. Rickham PP: Vesicointestinal fissure. Arch Dis Child 1960; 35:97-100.
164. Schober JM, Carmichael PA, Hines M, Ransley PG: The ultimate challenge of cloacal exstrophy. J Urol 2002;167: 300-304.
165. Shaw MB, West K, Gitlin J, et al: Intravesical phallus in cloacal exstrophy. Urology 2003;61:644.
166. Silver RI, Sponseller PD, Gearhart JP: Staged closure of the pelvis in cloacal exstrophy: First description of a new approach. J Urol 1999;161:263-266.
167. Smith NM, Chambers HM, Furness ME, Haan EA: The OEIS complex (omphalocele-exstrophy-imperforate anus spinal defects) recurrence in sibs. J Med Genet 1992;29:730-732.
168. Soffer SZ, Rosen NG, Hong AR, et al: Cloacal exstrophy: A unified management plan. J Pediatr Surg 2000;35:932-937.
169. Sponseller PD, Bisson LJ, Gearhart JP, et al: The anatomy of the pelvis in the exstrophy complex. J Bone Joint Surg 1995;77:177-189.
170. Sponseller PD, Jani MM, Jeffs RD, Gearhart JP: Anterior innominate osteotomy in repair of bladder exstrophy. J Bone Joint Surg Am 2001;83:184-193.
171. Stein R, Thuroff JW: Hypospadias and bladder exstrophy. Curr Opin Urol 2002;12:195-200.
172. Steinbüchel W: Veter Nabelschurburch und blassen Bauchspalte mit codken Bildung von sciten des Dunndormers. Arch Gynaeckol 1900;60:465-469.
173. Welch KJ: Cloacal exstrophy. In Ravitch MM, et al (eds): Pediatric Surgery. Chicago, Yearbook Medical Publishers, 1979.
174. Zderic SA, Canning DA, Carr MC, et al: The CHOP experience with cloacal exstrophy and gender reassignment. In Zderic SA, et al (eds): Pediaric Gender Assignment: A Critical Reappraisal. New York, Kluwer Academic/Plenum Publishers, 2002.
175. Ziegler MM, Duckett JW, Howell CG: Cloacal exstrophy. In Welch KJ, et al (eds): Pediatric Surgery. Chicago, Yearbook Medical Publishers, 1986.

第 119 章

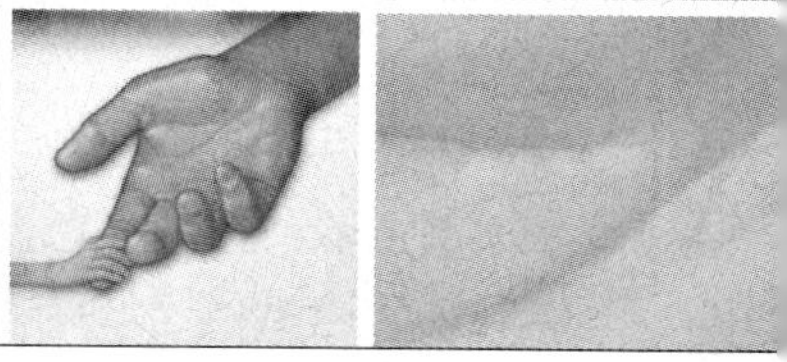

尿道下裂

Laurence S. Baskin

尿道下裂是一种最常见的先天性畸形，大约每 250 名新生儿中就有 1 人患病，或者粗略估计，每 125 名成活男婴中就有 1 人发病[118]。尿道下裂的定义是尿道、包皮和阴茎腹侧正常发育过程的终止。这将导致一系列的畸形发生，尿道可能在阴茎体的任何位置开口，或者在阴囊部，甚至是在会阴部（图 119-1）。尿道下裂常伴有阴茎下弯或痛性勃起。如果不予矫正，严重的尿道下裂患者需要采取坐姿排尿，并因对性生活的恐惧而避免与异性亲密接触。严重尿道下裂和阴茎弯曲的新生儿在出生时可能会出现“不典型外阴”，导致难以迅速、准确地确定其性别。

根据尿道口位置不同，对尿道下裂进行分类（图 119-2）。前位尿道下裂包括龟头型（尿道开口于龟头腹侧）、冠状沟型（尿道开口于冠状沟）或阴茎体远端型（尿道开口于阴茎体远端 1/3 处）。中间位的尿道下裂尿道开口于阴茎体中间的 1/3 处。后位尿道下裂尿道开口于阴茎体后 1/3 至会阴之间的任何位置，可以进一步分为近端阴茎体型（尿道开口于阴茎体后 1/3）、阴茎阴囊型（尿道开口于阴茎体与阴囊交界处）、阴囊型（尿道开口于阴囊表面或生殖膨大之间）以及会阴型（尿道开口于阴囊或生殖膨大后）。把尿道下裂细分为前位、中间位和后位对手术

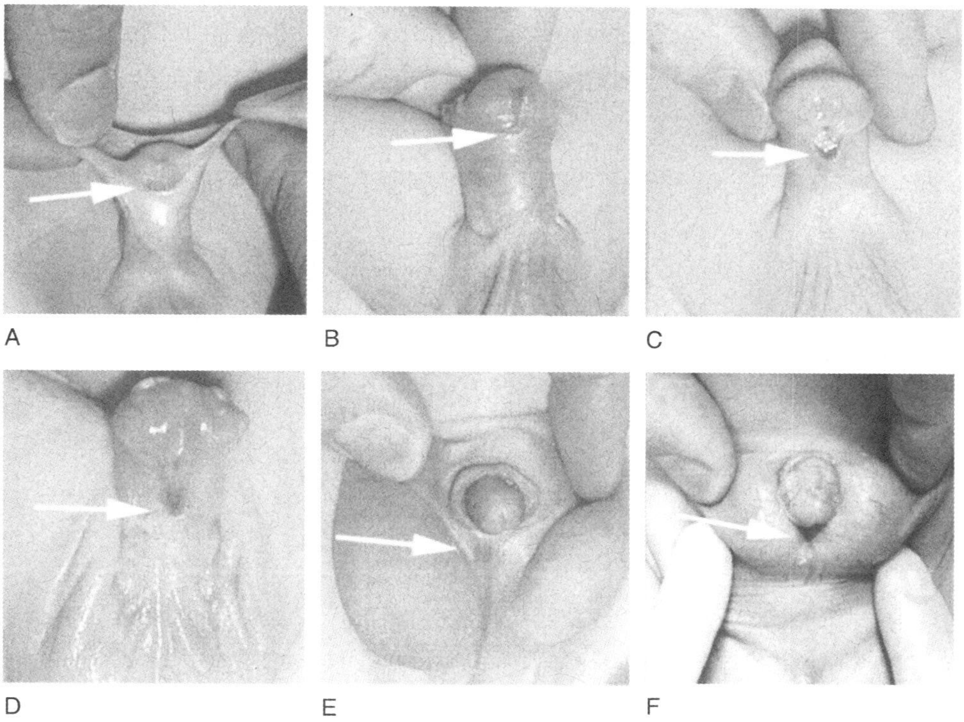

图 119-1 轻度至重度尿道下裂。A. 轻度尿道下裂，尿道开口于龟头。B. 轻度尿道下裂，尿道开口于冠状沟边缘。C. 中度尿道下裂，尿道开口于阴茎体远端。D. 中度尿道下裂，尿道开口于阴茎体中段。E. 重度尿道下裂，尿道开口于阴茎阴囊交界处。F. 重度尿道下裂，尿道开口于阴囊（*箭头* 指示尿道下裂患者的尿道开口位置）。注意阴茎腹侧包皮缺损，背侧包皮赘生。合伴阴茎下弯的尿道下裂，疾病程度更为严重。（From Baskin LS：Hypospadias and urethral development. J Urol 2000；163：951-956.）

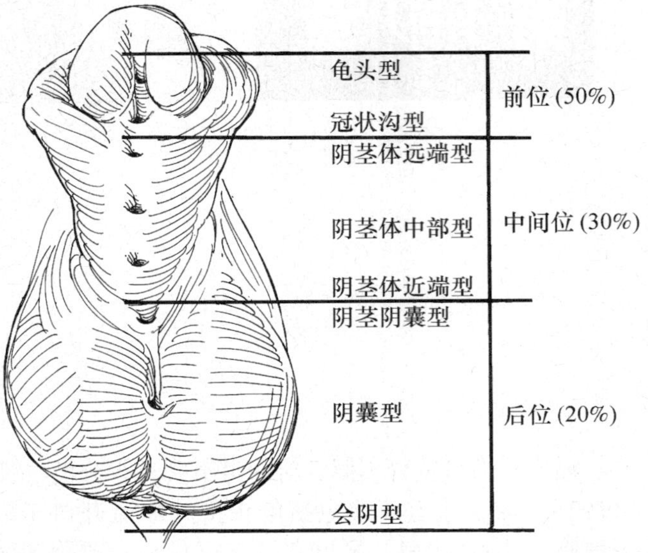

图 119-2　尿道下裂分型和发病率：前位、中间位和后位。

方式的选择并非一定有用，而且这些分类并没有兼顾阴茎下弯的程度（图 119-3）。前位尿道下裂合并严
1871 重阴茎下弯的患者也许需要进行更为广泛的手术来纠治联合畸形。

历史回顾

希腊文化里，人们对半男半女的阴阳神灵 Hermaphrodite 尤为崇敬。许多雕像也刻画了这种畸形的外生殖器，这也许象征了人们对雌雄同体的一种神往。因此，也就不难理解为什么直到公元一、二世纪以后，亚历山大港的外科医生 Heliodorus 和 Antyllus 才开始尝试通过切除阴茎远端下弯的部分来纠正这一畸形[132]。性生活方面，尿道的异位开口可引起*阳痿*。根据私人医生 Fernal 的记述，法国国王 Henry 二世同样患有尿道下裂。Henry 与 Catherine de Medici 成婚后多年未育，直到 Fernal "建议他的患者采取*动物交媾姿势*，才使其克服了这一困难[155]"。以后，Henry 二世生养了三个法国国王和其他七个孩子。

胚胎学

外生殖器的男性化是一个复杂的发育过程，涉及基因编码、细胞分化、激素信号转导、酶活性以及组织更新等[12]。在怀孕的第一个月末，胚胎后肠和将来的尿生殖系统发育，到达腹侧的泄殖腔膜[39]。泄殖腔膜把尿直肠分隔成两半，即后半部分的肛门和前半部分的尿生殖膜。后者周围出现三个隆突，最头端的一个是生殖结节，另两个紧靠尿生殖膜两侧的隆突是生殖膨大。此时，男女外生殖器并没有根本上的区别。垂体分泌的促黄体生成素在体内形成激素高峰，刺激睾酮反应性分泌，这种情况下，外生殖器将趋向男性化（图 119-4）。男性化的第一个标志就是肛门和生殖结构之间的距离增加，继而出现阴茎增

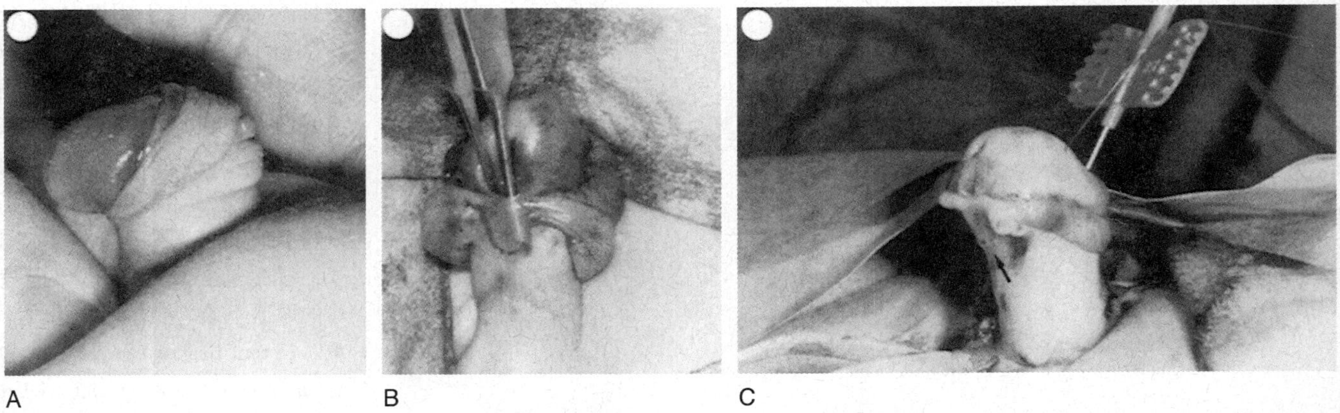

图 119-3　A. 冠状沟型尿道下裂，合并阴茎下弯。B. 阴茎腹侧包皮薄弱，术中不宜采用。C. 皮肤、肉膜松解（阴茎伸直）后，向后切开尿道口（*箭头位置*），为 onlay 岛状皮瓣手术做准备。（From Baskin LS, Duckett JW, et al: Changing concepts of hypospadias curvature lead to more onlay island flap procedures. J Urol 1994; 151: 191.）

长，由尿道沟延续而来的阴茎体尿道形成，以及包皮发育[77,87]。

在孕第八周以前，外生殖器停留在未分化阶段（见图 119–4）。位于阴茎腹侧面的尿道沟夹在一对尿道褶之间（图 119–5），阴茎体部的尿道由内胚层尿道褶边缘向中间融合而成，尿道沟的外胚层边缘融合形成尿道中缝。到孕第十二周时，冠状沟形成，龟头从阴茎体上凸显出来。此时，尿道褶在阴茎体的中线处完全融合。在孕第十六周期间，龟头部尿道开始发育。龟头尿道形成的机制尚存在争议（见图 119–5）。有证据提示有两种可能的解释：（1）内胚层细胞分化；（2）外胚层组织从龟头处主动向内侵袭（图 119–6）。

解剖和免疫组织化学的研究结果支持内胚层细 1872
胞分化理论，其依据是整个尿道的上皮属于尿生殖窦起源[101]。男性尿道的全长，包括龟头部，都是由进入生殖结节生长的背侧尿道板与腹侧的尿道褶融合而形成的。在相应的间质诱导下，尿道上皮能够分化为复层鳞状上皮，细胞具有特征性的角质染色颗粒，该现象支持龟头部尿道是由内胚层细胞分化的理论[100]。而对于第二种理论，即尿道上皮是由外胚层细胞内向性生长而来的解释，目前尚无证据证明[68]。

正常尿道发育形成的同时包皮也开始发育。在大约孕第八周时，在阴茎体两侧出现了幼稚的包皮褶

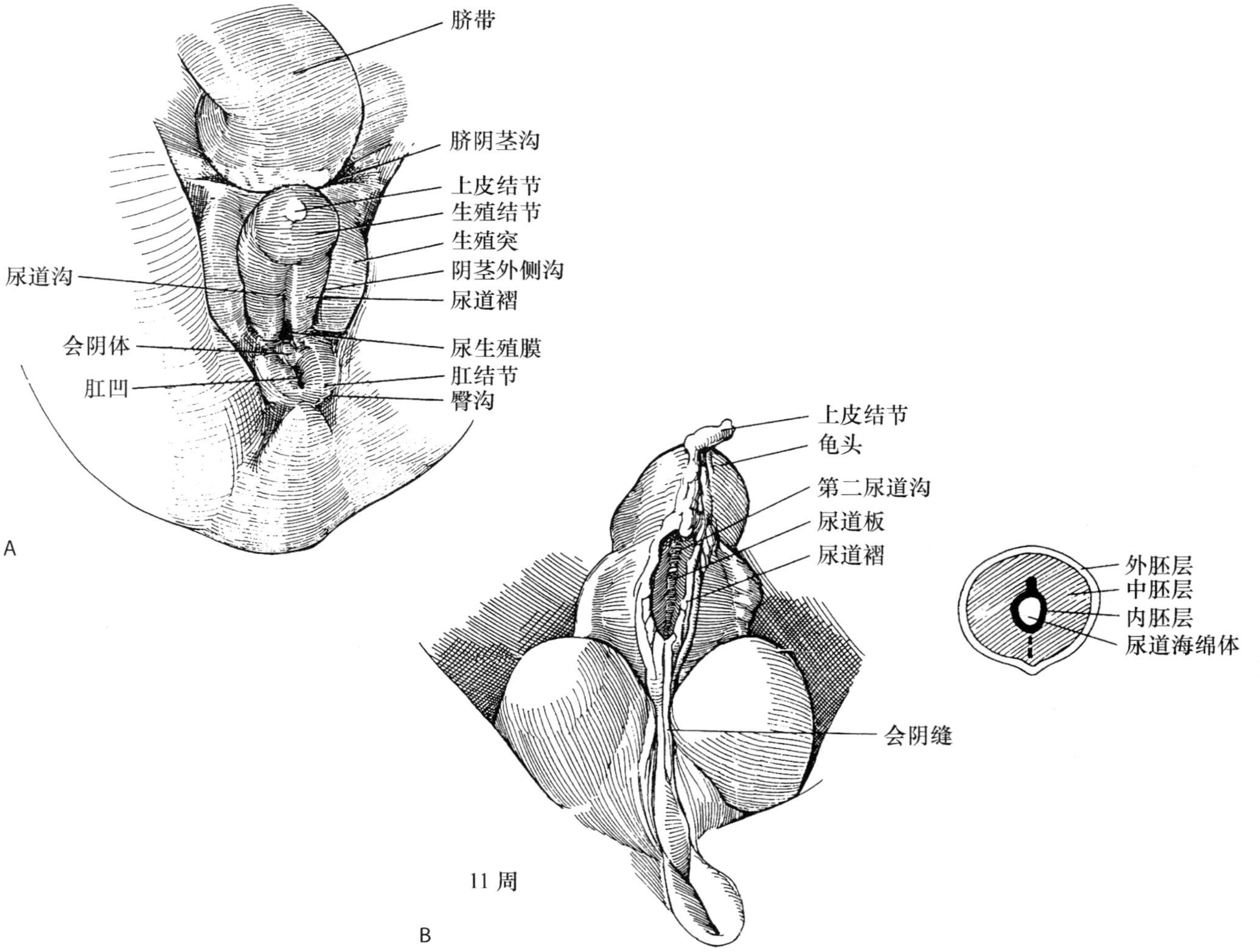

图 119–4 阴茎和尿道的发育。A. 怀孕大约 8 周时的未分化期，注意在生殖结节尾端斜面上形成的初级尿道沟。在肛凹和会阴体上方的尿生殖膜两侧，出现成对的生殖（阴唇阴囊）肿大。B. 第 11 孕周，尿道闭合。从肛门附近开始，邻近的外胚层尿道褶在尿道板上方融合，形成尿道的阴茎体部分，位于冠状沟的远端尿道最后闭合。

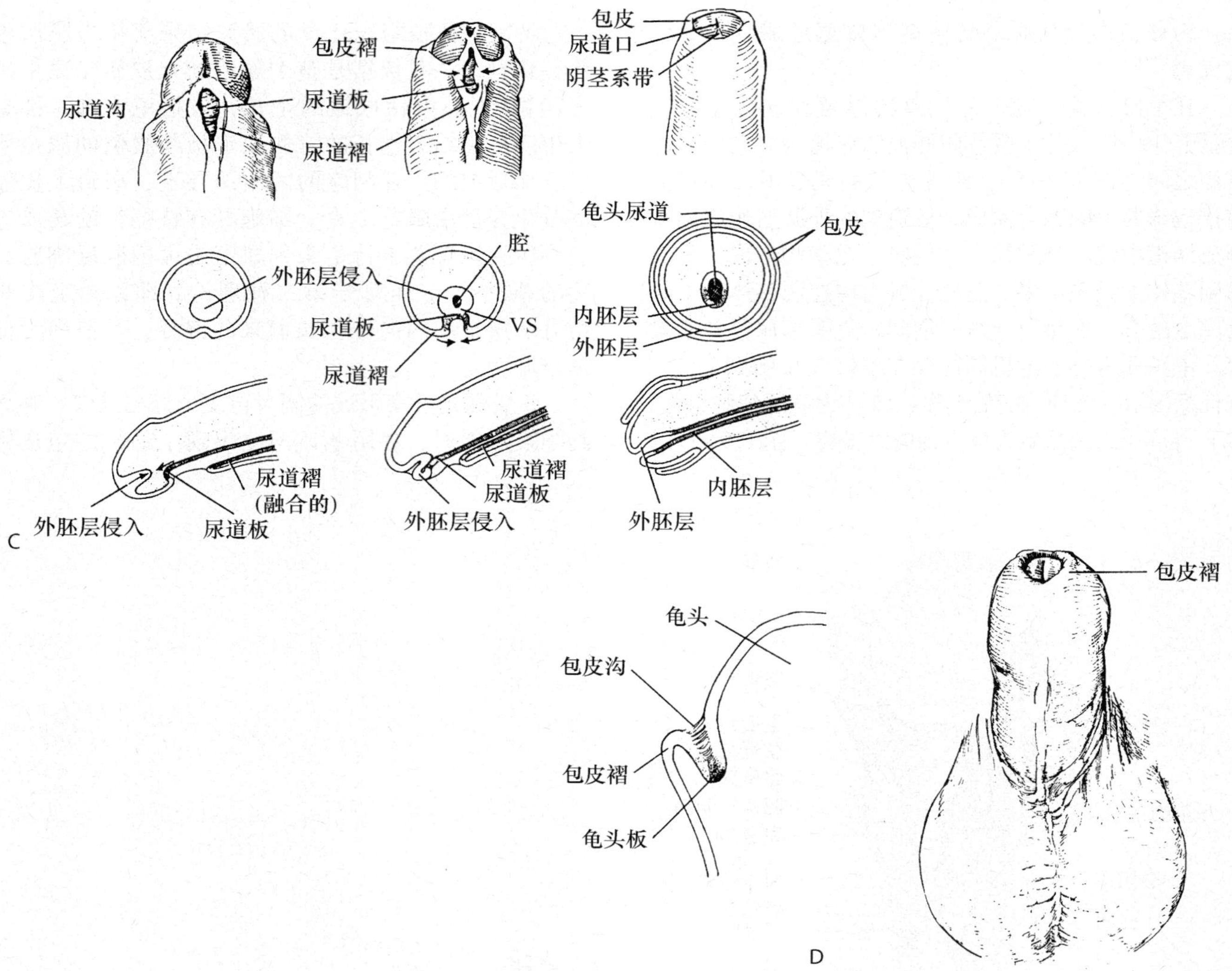

图 119-4 （续）C. 龟头尿道和舟状窝形成于怀孕晚期。外胚层组织由龟头顶端向间质侵袭性生长。侵入生长的外胚层底部与向前延伸的尿道板顶端接触，双侧壁结构崩溃，两者互相贯通。D. 龟头板的上皮细胞分化形成包皮，包皮褶和龟头之间形成冠状沟。（From Hinman F Jr：Surgical Anatomy of the Genitourinary Tract. Philadelphia，WB Saunders，1994，pp 418-470.）

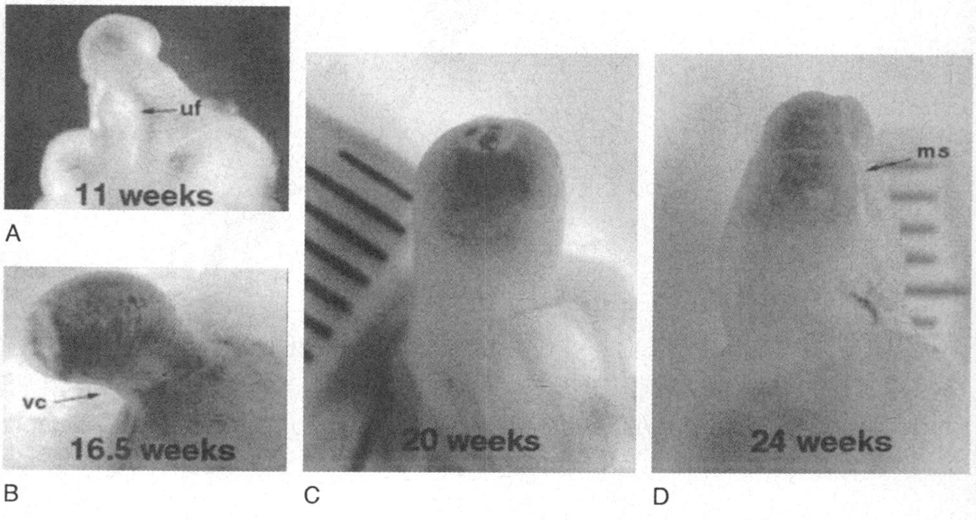

图 119-5 第 11、16.5、20 和 24 孕周时，正常男性外生殖器的发育。A. 注意开放的尿道和突起的尿道褶（uf）。B. 注意发育过程中出现的阴茎自然弯曲阶段。C. 包皮完整形成，阴茎弯曲已经纠正。D. 继续生长阶段，可见位于中线的皮肤缝隙（ms）。

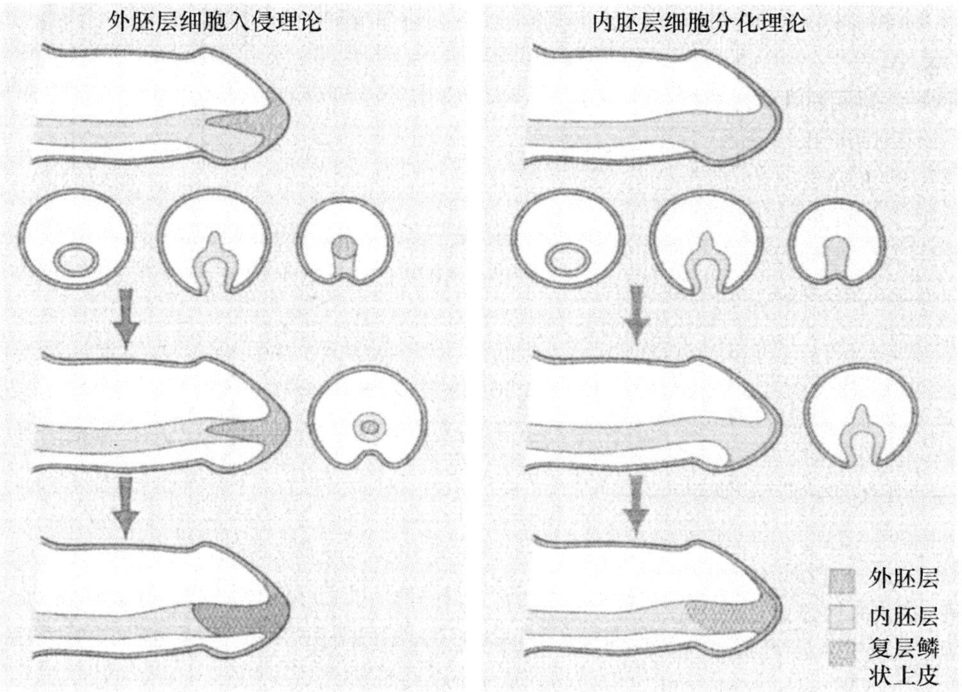

图 119-6 尿道发育的两种理论：旧学说认为尿道发育为外胚层侵入，新学说认为尿道发育为内胚层细胞分化所致。(From Kurzrock EL, Baskin LS, et al: Ontogeny of the male urethra: Theory of endodermal differentiation. Differentiation 1999; 64: 115-122.)

皱，褶皱向龟头背侧靠近，逐渐在冠状沟近端形成平脊。平脊并不完全围绕龟头，其在腹侧遭到龟头尿道的阻挡，否则可能出现龟头尿道发育不完全（见图 119-5A）。这样，随着间充质在包皮和龟头层次之间的生长，包皮褶皱逐渐向远端延伸。在包皮褶皱（包皮）遮盖整个龟头之前，上述过程会一直持续（见图 119-5C）。通常在出生时包皮已经融合，但继发性的蜕皮变化使包皮再次回缩。如果生殖褶没有融合，则不能形成腹侧包皮；于是尿道下裂患者就会发生阴茎腹侧包皮缺如，而背侧包皮过度赘生的现象（见图 119-1）。

由男性基因引起的雄激素的出现使"被动"或自发的女性化过程终止，阴茎开始分化发育[38]。在分子水平，睾酮必须在微粒体酶 2，5α-还原酶作用下转化为双氢睾酮（5α-dihydrotestosterone，DHT）才具有活性，从而诱导阴茎完全分化，使其具有典型的男性尿道与龟头[158]。血浆中睾酮与其蛋白质载体分离，通过被动扩散进入细胞[93]。一旦睾酮进入细胞，则立即与雄激素受体（AR）结合，继而诱导分子构象变化。AR 保护睾酮免受蛋白水解酶降解[93]。睾酮构象变化时需要 AR 二聚体参与、DNA 结合和转录激活，这些都是睾酮表达的必要条件。雄激素结合过程使热休克蛋白移位，这样或许能解除其对受体二聚体形成或 DNA 结合的限制。进入细胞核以后，AR 复合体与雄激素反应基因中的雄激素依赖 DNA 序列结合，并激活该基因。DHT 同样与 AR 结合，并能增加雄激素活性，产生这一效应的部分原因是 DHT 与 AR 的离解速度较慢[70]。

发病率

包括挪威、瑞典、英格兰、威尔士、匈牙利、丹麦、意大利和法国在内的一些欧洲国家以及美国都分别报道，在 20 世纪 60 年代、70 年代和 80 年代[117]，尿道下裂的发病率正不断上升。最近，国际情报交换所出生缺陷监测系统（International Clearinghouse for Birth Defects Monitoring Systems，ICBDMS）搜集数据加以分析，以明确疾病的增长趋势是否属于全球范围、发病率的上升是否还将持续以及发病是否存在地域特征等。ICBDMS 的数据表明尿道下裂的发病率不断上升并不是全球趋势，其在美国、挪威和丹麦的情况尤其值得注意[117]。另外，数据还显示，在物质生活不丰富或工业不发达（基于国民生产总值）的地区尿道下裂发病率并不上升，而在英格兰、加拿大及荷兰北部，发病率的增长势头从1985年以后也得到遏制[117]。

要从国际出生缺陷监测数据中得出确定性的结论比较困难。各地不同的报告制度、诊断标准和临床医生对报告的依从性都影响到统计结果的正确性。但是在美国，有两个独立的监测系统采用了相同的诊断标准对尿道下裂进行统计，结果仍然证明疾病的发病率有了明显上升。尽管这些监测程序并非完美无缺，但其提供的数据依然有保证[118]。

亚特兰大居民先天性缺陷项目（Metropolitan Atlanta Congenital Defects Program，MACDP）囊括了佐治亚州亚特兰大的22所医院，对登记在册的出生人口的患病情况做了统计，结果表明从1968年到1993年，尿道下裂的发病率几乎翻了一倍（$P < 10^{-6}$），年平均增长率为2.9%[118]。没有任何一所当地医院对此负有责任。严重的尿道下裂，即尿道开口于阴茎体、阴囊或会阴的患者数上升特别显著。在1968年至1990年间，严重病例的数量从每10 000名活产儿中的1.1人上升到2.7人。到1993年，这一年均数据达到了每10 000名活产儿中5.5人（$P < 10^{-6}$）[118]。

出生缺陷监测项目（Birth Defect Monitoring Program，BDMP）搜集了全国范围内的出院新生儿数据，同样显示尿道下裂的发病率在不断上升。具体发病率从1970年每10 000名活产儿（包括所有男婴和女婴）中的20.2上升到1993年每10 000名活产儿中的39.7（$P < 10^{-6}$）[118]。

两个独立的监测项目结果都报告尿道下裂的发病率增加了近一倍，而两个监测系统同时得出错误的发病率上升的结论似乎不太可能。换言之，如果结论是由于敏感度上升而造成的，那么就意味着监测项目初始少记录了近一半的先天性缺陷患者。这应该不太可能，因为无论是MACDP还是BDMP，在上述年代的疾病确证数据里都没有明显差异。医生对疾病的诊断报告习惯可能因时间不同而改变，尤其是在对轻度尿道下裂的报告方面。事实上，MACDP在关于轻重度尿道下裂所占比例上的报告却不一致，在1968年至1982年间是4.2，而1983年
1875 至1993年间是2.6，出现了下降。然而，另一个值得关注的问题是，随着轻重度尿道下裂的比例下降，未分类型的尿道下裂病例数也同样下降，这使得数据更难以解释。人们怀疑是否有轻度尿道下裂病例漏报的可能。尽管如此，这些纵向的研究报告仍然支持尿道下裂在美国的发病率逐渐增长。

伴发畸形

尿道下裂最常见的伴发畸形是隐睾和腹股沟斜疝。一项系列研究统计，9.3%的尿道下裂患者存在隐睾；隐睾在后位尿道下裂患者中的发病率高达32%，中间位中的发病率是6%，前位中的发病率是5%[95]。这些调查者们同时发现，所有尿道下裂患者中伴发斜疝者占总数的9%，在后位尿道下裂患者中此比例上升为17%。Ross等[136]报道尿道下裂患者伴发隐睾和腹股沟斜疝的比例基本相似，为16%左右。Cerasaro等[34]发现301名尿道下裂患者中18%伴发这些畸形。严重病例中，前列腺囊肿的发病率非常高。例如，Devine等[44]发现在44例后位尿道开口的患者中有6人（14%）存在前列腺囊肿，7例会阴型尿道下裂的患者中有4人（57%）存在前列腺囊肿，20例尿道开口于阴茎阴囊交界处的患者中有2人（10%）存在前列腺囊肿，17例尿道开口于阴茎体的患者没有一例存在前列腺囊肿。Shima等[142]统计发现29例龟头型尿道下裂患者中有1例伴发前列腺囊肿，74例阴茎体型尿道下裂患者中有3例伴发前列腺囊肿，122例阴茎阴囊型尿道下裂患者中有11例伴发前列腺囊肿，29例阴囊会阴型尿道下裂患者中有10例伴发前列腺囊肿；因此，在151例阴茎阴囊型或会阴型尿道下裂患者中，前列腺囊肿的发病率是14%。结合两组数据，严重尿道下裂患者伴发前列腺囊肿的发生率为11%。通常，前列腺囊肿的并发症只有感染和置放导管困难[130]。

由于外生殖器比膀胱水平以上的尿路部分形成较晚，所以尿路畸形的发病率低不足为奇。McArdle和Lebowitz[105]发现200例尿道下裂患者中只有6例（3%）发生生殖泌尿道畸形。Cerasaro等[34]发现1.7%（4/233）的尿道下裂患者有严重畸形。Aellan[9]统计瑞典患者发现，只有1%的尿道下裂患者存在肾脏畸形，而7%的患者存在其他系统畸形。通过回顾分析169例患者的临床资料，Shelton和Noe[141]认为无需常规对尿道下裂患者的尿路情况进行检查评价。Khuri等[95]在一项研究中回顾了1076例患者，发现尿道下裂伴发的尿路畸形主要包括肾盂输尿管交界处梗阻、严重的膀胱输尿管反流、肾发育不全、肾母细胞瘤、盆腔肾、

肾交叉异位以及马蹄肾等。他们认为尿道下裂合并腹股沟斜疝或隐睾的患者无需接受进一步的尿路检查，但对于尿道下裂伴发其他系统器官畸形的患者需要进行腹部超声对其上尿路系统进行筛查。

对服用己烯雌酚的妇女所生的 500 名男孩进行泌尿生殖畸形研究，发现 2% 患有尿道下裂，4.4% 的阴茎尿道存在畸形[69]。Gupta 和 Goldman[73] 指出，花生四烯酸级联代谢障碍能引起中线融合缺陷，如腭裂和尿道下裂。尿道下裂还常常和一些著名的综合征以及肾母细胞瘤等相关。

发病原因

尿道下裂发病率不断上升，使人们开始注意其病因、治疗和预防。到目前为止，对尿道下裂疾病还没有彻底了解，对疾病的预防与改善治疗尚无切实有效的方法。譬如，在最近的一项研究中，33 名患有严重尿道下裂（阴囊型或阴茎阴囊型）的患者接受了一系列的检查，包括临床体检、超声、核型、内分泌评价和 AR 基因及 5α-还原酶基因的分子遗传分析，检查的目的是为了对尿道下裂的发病原因进行分类和明确。12 名（36%）患者诊断明确，其余 64% 的患者归类为尿道下裂病因不明[3]。其他研究者曾试图将尿道下裂与雄激素代谢或 AR 异常联系起来。譬如，Gearhart 等[65] 在研究中证实，尿道下裂男孩包皮上的 AR 或 5α-还原酶水平不存在缺陷。Allera 等[5] 分析了 9 名严重尿道下裂患者，发现其中仅有 1 人存在 AR 基因开放读码框缺陷。Sutherland 等[150] 同样证明 AR 基因突变与尿道下裂之间很少有关联。应用单股构象多态型分析，发现 40 名远端尿道下裂患者中有 1 人 AR 基因的外显子发生了两处错义突变。分子生物学技术已经阐明，AR 基因缺陷确与单独的尿道下裂疾病之间存在关联。但是，这些缺陷只对相当小的一部分患者的发病原因进行了解释，由此提示，尿道下裂的发病因素还有许多未解之谜。

遗传缺陷

尿道下裂发病原因仍然未知，一定程度上反映了正常阴茎和尿道发育的复杂性，对其发生的分子和细胞基础依然无法明了[157]。已经知道，受精以后的 7～12周是阴茎尿道褶的融合阶段[12]。胎睾具有合成睾酮的能力，在激素刺激下尿道褶逐渐融合导致阴茎形成。胚胎期尿生殖窦和外生殖器充分男性化时，睾酮需要转化成 DHT，而这一过程必须依赖 5α-还原酶。

逐渐地，研究者对阴茎产生和尿道下裂病因的研究方向发生了转变，即从睾酮和 DHT 对细胞形态发育的作用机制转到其他一些细胞信号的作用上。正常泌尿生殖系的胚胎发育需要上皮-间质细胞之间的相互作用。有人提出假说，认为上皮和间质细胞之间信号传导缺失将会导致尿道下裂[100]。举例来说，前列腺的发育需要尿生殖窦上皮中睾酮依赖的 *Sonic hedgehog*（Shh）的表达[120]。Shh 缺失的小鼠中，阴茎发育受到抑制，同时存在泄殖腔缺陷[21,164]。缺失 1876
纤维母细胞生长因子 10 的小鼠，其尿道开口位置偏近、龟头扁平，同时存在尿道下裂畸形[164]。研究人员将有希望发现某种遗传信号分子，这种信号分子与阴茎上皮和间皮的相互作用有关，在阴茎的发育过程中起重要作用。

另一个关于尿道下裂病因的调查领域涉及同源异型盒（homeobox，Hox）基因的表达与调节。这些基因在转录水平发生调节，在控制胚胎发育方面起到重要作用。Hox A 和 Hox D 的基因簇在泌尿生殖道的长轴区域范围内表达。单一 *Hox A* 和 *Hox D* 基因功能丧失的转基因小鼠出现了同源性转换和泌尿生殖道的形态学缺陷[25,48,82,121]。患有手-足-生殖器综合征的男性存在常染色体异常，其特征性的常染色体区异常就是出现 *Hox A13* 突变，患者有严重程度不一的尿道下裂表现，这一现象说明或许 *Hox A13* 在正常阴茎的发育中具有重要意义[49,63,109]。进一步研究发现，胚胎期特定 Hox 基因的表达受激素调节[103]。譬如，雌激素与合成的雌激素 DES 对小鼠的 *Hox A9*，*Hox A10*，*Hox A11* 和 *Hox A13* 有抑制作用。因此，除了 Hox 基因缺陷以外，胚胎期异常的激素调节或表达可能会扰乱 Hox 基因的正常表达并导致生殖道畸形。

激素受体缺陷

如前所述，研究 AR 对解释尿道下裂的病因帮助甚微。事实上，一些研究已经证明尿道下裂患者中很少有 AR 的缺陷或编码序列的突变[78,106]。另外，Bentvelsen 等[26]比较了尿道下裂的男性患儿和同龄男性儿童包皮上的 AR 表达，发现两组间平均 AR 含量不存在显著差异。

酶的缺陷

尽管睾酮的作用非常重要，但是如果认为所有尿道下裂的形成都是由这一遗传缺陷造成的，似乎不可能。Holmes 等[79]认为睾酮的生化合成路径中有三个关键酶，这些酶的缺陷将造成尿道下裂的发生，其中包括羟类固醇脱氢酶、17α-羟化酶和 17，20-裂解酶。48 名睾丸完全下降合并不同程度尿道下裂的男性患儿与接受包皮环切手术的正常同龄男童进行配对比较，实验室检查项目包括孕烯醇酮、黄体酮、11-去氧皮质酮、17-羟孕烯醇酮、17-羟孕酮、11-脱氧皮质醇、皮质醇、脱氢表雄酮、雄烯二酮、雄烯二醇、睾酮、双氢睾酮等。观察焦点集中在雄激素合成的前几个步骤上，发现 12 名尿道下裂患者对促肾上腺皮质激素（ACTH）刺激应答正常。比较尿道下裂患者和正常对照组的雄激素前体和激素代谢过程，两者间不存在明显差异。个体对 ACTH 的反应不同，但各类型的尿道下裂患者和正常人群组间无显著差异。这些数据表明，从胆固醇到双氢睾酮的胆固醇代谢过程并不是造成尿道下裂的主要原因。

环境因素和内分泌破坏因素

过去，通常认为环境因素不是造成尿道下裂的主要原因[74,149]。而最近，在先天性畸形的研究中，多种分析病因的模型已经把环境污染作为影响因素之一加以考虑。譬如，家族中有人患有尿道下裂，如果其一级亲属再次患病，以前则常认为遗传因素是造成疾病的主要原因；但目前研究证明，除遗传因素以外，还有许多其他的原因。由于家族成员暴露于同一环境中，因此有学者提出应该把环境影响同样考虑进去。特别是有潜在的环境效应作用时，可加强遗传缺陷的表达，所以在分析尿道下裂病因时应该注意到环境暴露这一问题[13,62]。

对尿道下裂危险因素的研究引出了许多与疾病有关的患者父母的危险因素。在对先天性疾病的母系危险因素的传统研究中，母亲的年龄和初产年龄与尿道下裂有密切联系。但也有学者对母亲年龄与尿道下裂的关联存在置疑[74]。尿道下裂的父系危险因素主要包括阴囊与睾丸的畸形[152]、精母细胞活力低下以及精子形态异常[62]。有人提到，目前尿道下裂发病率上升也由于更多的不育症患者得到治疗，导致更多生育能力低下的男子繁衍后代。如 Fritz 和 Czeizel 提出，这一“放松选择的假说反映了由具备生育能力和不具备生育能力（生育能力低下）的夫妇所生养孩子的再分布状态，这可能是今天男性生殖器癌症和缺陷增加的原因，并导致精子数量下降”[62]。

除了双亲的危险因素以外，文献中普遍认为低出生体重与男孩尿道下裂有关[61]。Fredell 等[61]检查了发育不均一的单卵双生子的尿道下裂，发现双生子中尿道下裂男孩的出生体重仅仅是正常男孩的 78%。与正常单卵双生子比较，体重同样在统计学上存在显著差异。在另一项研究中发现，尿道下裂患儿胎盘的重量比对照组男孩低[149]。

1995 年的 meta 分析显示，在孕期的前三个月应用黄体酮和口服避孕药并不增加患尿道下裂的风险[125]。研究中没有包括 DES 的暴露因素。但是，其他一些项目中并没有把黄体酮列为孕期暴露因素来研究。最近，在另一项研究结果中提及，母亲在孕期一味进食素食会增加孩子患尿道下裂的可能。该研究观察了参与雅芳孕期与儿童期纵向研究项目（Avon Longitudinal study of pregnancy and Childhood）的母亲生育的 7928 名儿童，对其中 51 名尿道下裂患者进行了分析。作者假设素食者比杂食者更多地暴露于植物雌激素的影响下。植物雌激素可能来自于大豆，后者含有大量的异黄酮，或可能与杀虫剂和肥料中存在的内分泌阻断成分有关[123]。

虽然这些危险因素可能并不直接导致尿道下裂，但是却提供了一些额外的信息，这些信息也许能为将来的研究提供一个方向，为研究发展揭示一条出路。举例来说，现在越来越多的证据说明在低出生体重新生儿中，雄激素对女孩的影响比对男孩的影响更大[47]。同样，雄激素对男性生殖管道的发育也起到关键性作用。这样，在孕期暴露于某一抑制雄激素发挥作用的因素下可影响胎儿的体重增长，在尿道下裂和低体重出生儿的发育方面起到关键作用。

逐渐增长的尿道下裂的发病率与其他难愈的男性生殖健康的研究结果相平行，其中包括睾丸癌的逐年增加[29]、隐睾发病率增加、精液和精子质量下降[33]等。在一项调查研究中发现，有 8% 的隐睾患者存在泌尿生殖系的畸形，其中大于 50% 的患者有尿道下裂[36]。在过去的 50 年里，畸形发病率的不断上升恰伴随着工业生产和化学合成物使用的增加，这使得人们研究疾病发生过程中环境因素所起的重要作用的兴趣大大增加[13,153]。目前有报道阐述，野生动植物的研究结果结合实验室的数据已经说明，一些天然化学物质和人工化合物中所含有的成分能模仿激素拮抗作用，或者干扰内分泌系统和生殖系统的发育[37,133]。暴露于己烯雌酚和黄体酮作用下的胎鼠，出生时存在尿道下裂[96]。内分泌阻断物是否确实影响男性生殖健康，尤其是造成尿道下裂的产生，这一点还很难得到确证[143]。但无论如何，全球公众健康组织对内分泌阻断物的研究兴趣正逐渐增加，这将是疾病研究领域中的一个长期课题[59,71,86]。

正常阴茎与尿道下裂解剖

要开展尿道下裂修补手术，不仅需要对正常阴茎解剖有全面的认识，同时还要对尿道下裂阴茎的解剖有深入的了解。人类的阴茎由一对阴茎海绵体构成，外覆一层质厚、有弹性的白膜，海绵体之间有中线间隔（图 119-7）[18,20,77,162,163]。尿道海绵体位于阴茎腹 1878
侧，紧靠阴茎海绵体之间。Buck 筋膜位于阴茎海绵体之外，并分裂形成单独小室分别围绕海绵体。最近

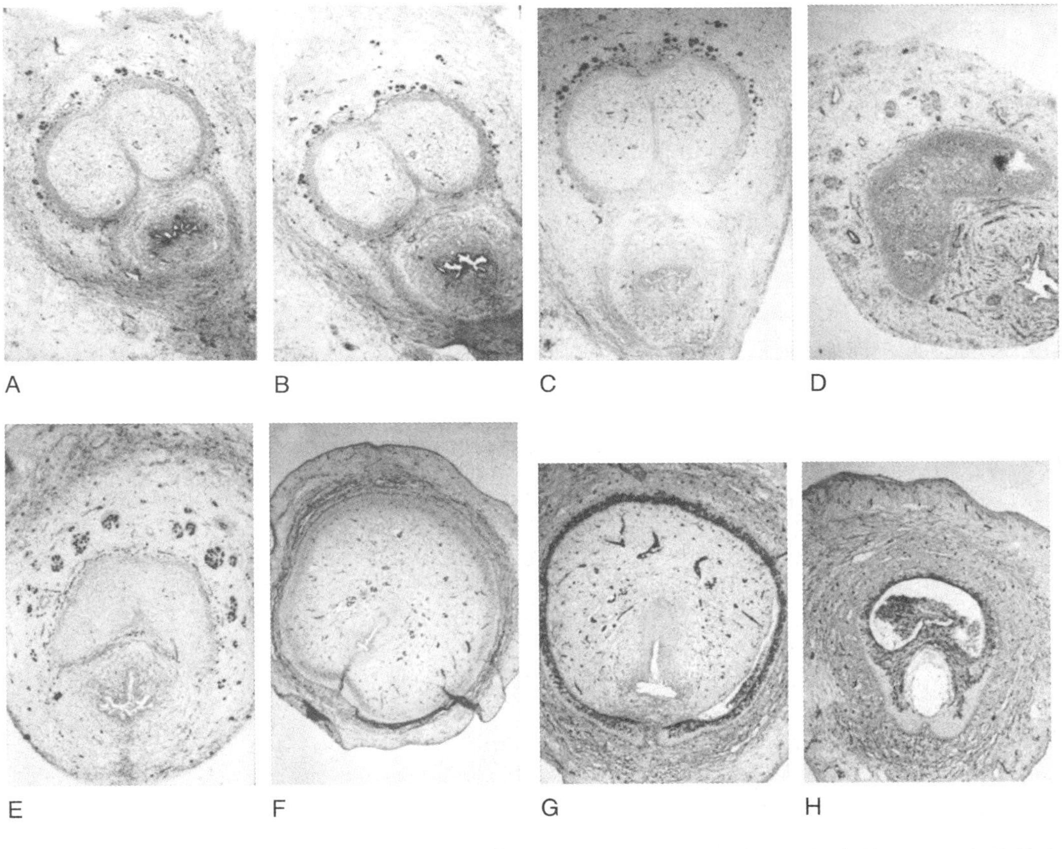

图 119-7　25 孕周时，正常人类胎儿的阴茎。A 至 H. 横切面，远端至近端，神经元标志物 S-100 免疫染色（25 ×）。注意被染成棕色的 S-100 神经元标志物的位置，完全围绕在海绵体周围，沿阴茎体向上延伸到尿道海绵体连接处，只在 12 点的位置出现缺如现象（A 至 D）。到近端阴茎海绵体分开的位置，神经侧向分布到耻骨支下缘，定位于 11 点和 1 点，形成假想的三角区。到此位置（E），神经已从海绵体（约为海绵体直径的一半）垂直延伸到最远距离，在 11 点和 1 点位置延续（F，G），形成更为紧密的结构，远离尿道。（From Baskin LS，Erol A，et al：Anatomical studies of hypospadias. J Urol 1998；160：1108–1115.）

的研究表明，神经血管束存在于 Buck 筋膜深层，并且在阴茎脚汇合形成阴茎体处，神经血管束围绕海绵体呈放射样生长，并分布于阴茎海绵体与尿道海绵体的所有连接处（见图 19-6 及图 119-7）[2,162]。这一概念完全否定了以前经典的教条学说，即认为神经血管束沿阴茎背侧 11 点和 1 点位置生长的说法。Buck 筋膜上是肉膜，肉膜紧靠皮肤。这一层次含有包皮的供应血管。包皮的血液供应包括两条阴部外下动脉和阴茎浅动脉的分支[76]，这些动脉分别形成前侧支与后侧支。在尿道下裂手术时，岛状皮瓣的经典血液供应途径来源于前外侧浅血管。术中游离 onlay 岛状皮瓣、管状皮瓣及去上皮化的带蒂皮瓣时必须仔细保留上述血管，这是手术成功的关键因素。外侧皮肤依赖皮下固有层血管而成活。

在解剖学上，与正常阴茎相比较，尿道下裂阴茎在神经分布、海绵体与白膜构造以及血管供应方面都没有明显异常，只是在尿道海绵体和龟头局部有畸形（图 119-8 和图 119-9）[18,19,162,163]。正常阴茎与尿道下裂阴茎的神经束都起自于尿道表面以上，略偏向侧面。由于两个阴茎脚聚合形成阴茎海绵体，神经束走行分为两条分支，各自围绕海绵体至阴茎腹侧尿道海绵体连接处，而并不局限于阴茎背侧的 11 点和 1 点位置（见图 119-7 和图 119-8）。与正常阴茎结构一样，尿道下裂的阴茎背侧 12 点处无神经分布。在阴茎海绵体开始分叉的位置，海绵体神经发出 nNOS 阳性神经，加入阴茎背侧神经，由此改变阴茎背侧神经远端的功能特性（见图 119-8）。相似地，位于阴茎腹侧的会阴神经起源于阴部神经，在阴茎海绵体和尿道海绵体连接处发生变化，即从 nNOS 阴性神经转变为具有 nNOS 活性。阴茎表面丰富的神经围绕或许是其维持勃起功能的重要保证[162]。

尿道下裂的阴茎与正常阴茎最大的不同在于血管分布（见图 119-9）。尿道下裂的阴茎具有巨大的内皮血管通道，通道内富含红细胞。与之相反，正常阴茎的尿道旁具有形态清晰的毛细血管围绕，呈放射状向龟头延伸。解剖尿道板，没有证据显示其发生纤维化或瘢痕[60]。尿道板上血管丰富，神经分布良好，具有与躯体广泛连接的肌肉和结缔组织（图 119-10）。这些特征或许能够解释在尿道下裂重建手术中出现的尿道板或海绵体愈合良好的现象[55,144]。

尿道下裂修复时需要注意三个主要畸形：（1）尿道开口异常；（2）阴茎下弯；（3）包皮缺陷和严重病况下出现的阴囊异常。

尿道异常

描述尿道下裂的基本特征主要根据尿道口的位置和构型。尿道口可能只是略偏向腹侧，位于龟头正常

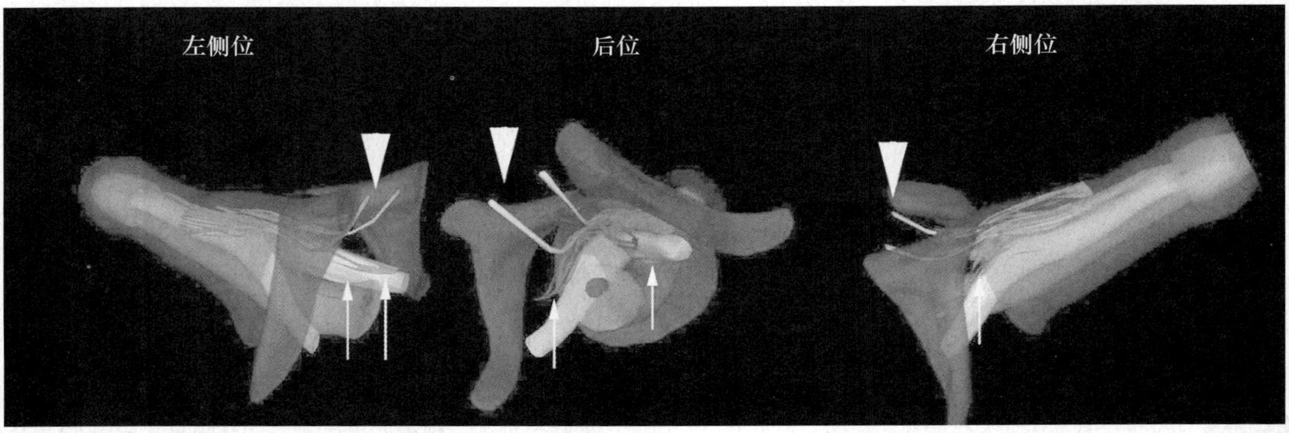

图 119-8 第 27 孕周时，人类胎儿阴茎正常结构的计算机三维重建。注意海绵体神经（白箭头）和背侧神经（楔形箭头）的路线远离沿坐骨结节行走的阴茎脚（白色）。海绵体神经到达阴茎起始端的路径更为直接，在耻骨弓下，神经进入海绵体深层。在靠近阴茎起始端的时候，海绵体神经发出分支与阴茎背侧神经联络，随后这些神经纤维呈 nNOS 免疫染色阳性。nNOS 染色阳性的背侧神经沿海绵体（灰色）延伸到龟头。随着阴茎背侧神经由 nNOS 染色阴性变为 nNOS 染色阳性，近端 nNOS 染色阴性的会阴神经也转变为 nNOS-免疫反应神经。

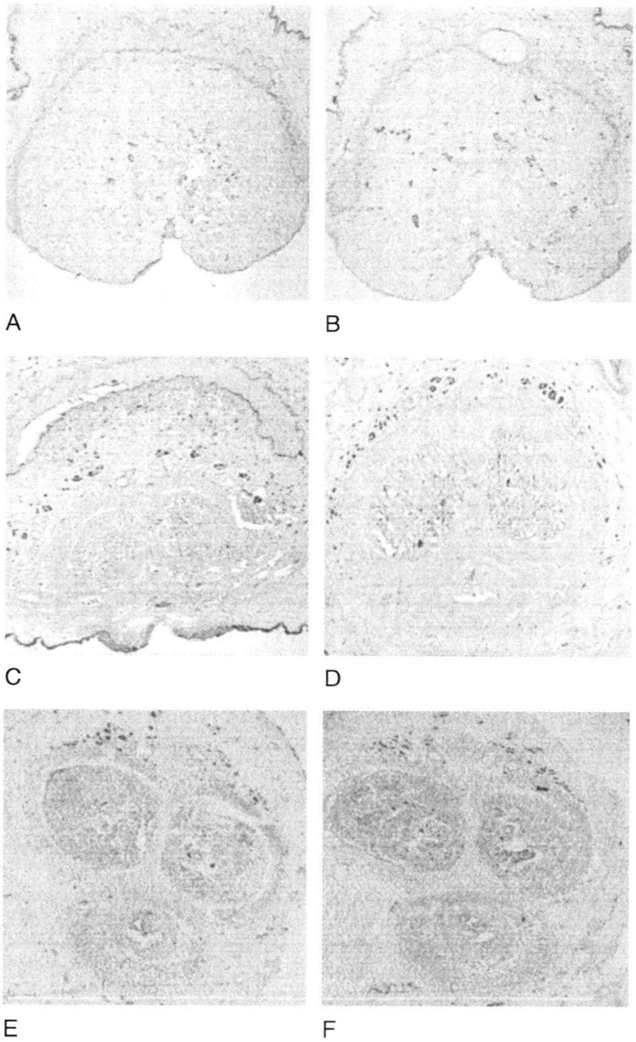

图 119-9　第 33 孕周时的尿道下裂阴茎。A 至 F. 横切面，由远端到近端，S-100 神经元标志物免疫染色（深染）（20×）。注意，除远端尿道和龟头形态异常以外（A 至 C），尿道下裂的阴茎的解剖结构与正常结构一致。（From Baskin LS, Erol A, et al: Anatomical studies of hypospadias. J Urol 1998; 160: 1108-1115.）

尿道开口处的盲端小凹下；也可以远在会阴处，形态似"阴道型尿道下裂"[161]。大多数患者的尿道口呈现一种过渡形态，其特征可通过形态、直径、弹性和强度来形容。尿道开口可以呈横向或纵向，或者在其表面上覆盖一层薄弱的皮肤。当包皮变异时可形成巨尿道口，此时远端尿道增大，而后在阴茎体部逐渐变细，形成正常口径的尿道[56]。尿道周围小管常有一小口，位于尿道口远端，经背侧进入尿道延伸一段距离。该结构一端为盲端，与排尿没有丝毫关系。尿道周围的小管与 Guérin 窦或 Morgagni 陷窝相对应[147]。除非它们无意间关闭而导致一个由上皮细胞构成的盲端贮袋，否则这些小管不会造成任何临床后果。

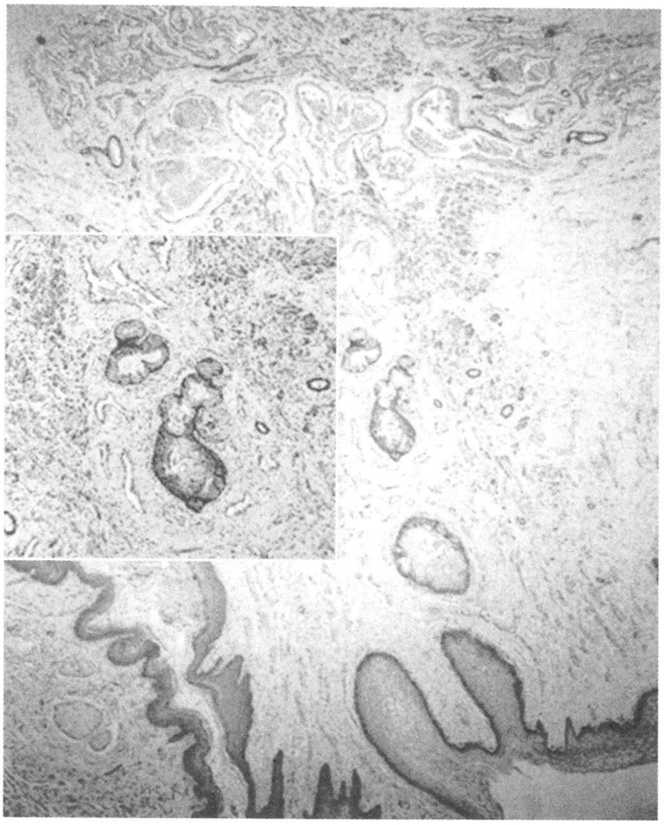

图 119-10　人类新生儿近端尿道下裂患者的尿道板（平滑肌纤维 α 肌动蛋白免疫染色，25×）。尿道板清晰可见，丝毫没有证据显示纤维化或瘢痕形成。尿道板内可见上皮网或尿道形成不良的迹象（*插图*）。

阴茎弯曲

阴茎弯曲的原因是阴茎腹侧正常结构的发育缺陷。阴茎弯曲又被称为阴茎痛性勃起，这一学术名称都表示在尿道口与龟头之间存在一条由结缔组织构成的索带，当阴茎勃起时，索带像绞索一样牵拉龟头，造成阴茎勃起障碍或疼痛。Mettauer[107] 认为这条索带由尿道海绵体退化形成。但是，尿道海绵体在孕期第四个月末时才形成尿道周围组织，这一点否定了上述假说。疾病表现为阴茎皮肤缺损、肉膜缺失、牵拉阴茎体腹侧时可触及引起勃起疼痛的真性纤维索带或阴茎海绵体腹侧发育不良等。

报道中偶尔提到阴茎的其他畸形，提示胚胎期造
1880 成尿道下裂的各种发育缺陷的变异。这些畸形可以表现为尿道发育过程中的缺陷（先天性尿道瘘）和一些不伴有尿道下裂的阴茎弯曲[40,131]。

皮肤与阴囊畸形

追根究源，阴茎皮肤缺损的本质是尿道形成过程出现紊乱的结果。尿道口远端的腹侧皮肤通常是缺如的，这可造成阴茎弯曲。尿道下裂患者常常没有阴茎系带。但有时，可以在舟状窝两侧发现系带插入的残迹。

尿道口近端的皮肤非常薄，甚至在插入导尿管或探针时，可以透过菲薄的皮肤看到操作器械。出现这种情况时，禁忌采取尿道口周围皮肤修补尿道（Mathieu 修补）。

一般来说，从尿道口到冠状沟的尿道板发育良好。即使在尿道开口非常接近阴茎体近端时，正常的尿道板也能保持弹性而没有纤维牵拉。这种情况下，人工勃起试验显示无阴茎下弯。尿道修补手术中可以选用正常的尿道板。但是，如果尿道板发育不良，在人工勃起时，尿道将像索带一样牵拉阴茎向腹侧弯曲。当这些引起痛性勃起的纤维组织离断以后，阴茎下弯能够得到充分矫正。

正常情况下，生殖结节在两个生殖膨大的头端发育。阴茎的位置可能向下移动，处于两个半阴囊之间发育，阴茎阴囊出现融合，阴茎陷入阴囊中间。近端尿道口与背侧阴茎之间形成斜向界线，进一步成为阴茎与阴囊之间的分界。

治疗

治疗的目标是重建一条无弯曲的阴茎，尿道口尽量靠近正常位置（龟头腹侧终点），以便正常地向前排尿和性交。为保证尿道下裂手术的成功应注意如下五个步骤：① 阴茎整形（阴茎伸直），② 尿道成形，③ 尿道口成形和龟头成形，④ 阴囊整形，⑤ 阴茎皮肤覆盖。上述步骤可以依次进行或按需整合，以获得手术成功（图 119-11）。本章将结合大量特殊的外科手术技巧来描述这些步骤。

前位尿道下裂

治疗前位尿道下裂取决于患儿家庭的文化背景。许多前位尿道下裂的患者无明显的功能障碍，阴茎下弯也不明显，能够直立排尿，尿线直。因此，手术中把尿道口前移到龟头正常位置的目的主要是为了美观。手术结果力求完美。目前，前位尿道下裂的手术属于门诊手术，经典的手术涉及尿道的步骤不多。手术方式的选择依靠尿道下裂阴茎的解剖特征。最常见的手术方式包括 MAGPI 术（meatal advancement glansplasty）、GAP 术（glans approximation procedure）、卷管尿道成形术（primary tubularization）、Mathieu 或称包皮翻转尿道成形术（flip-flap），以及 Snodgrass 或称为尿道板纵切卷管尿道成形术（tubularized incised plate urethroplasty）[51,55,104,144,145,165]。

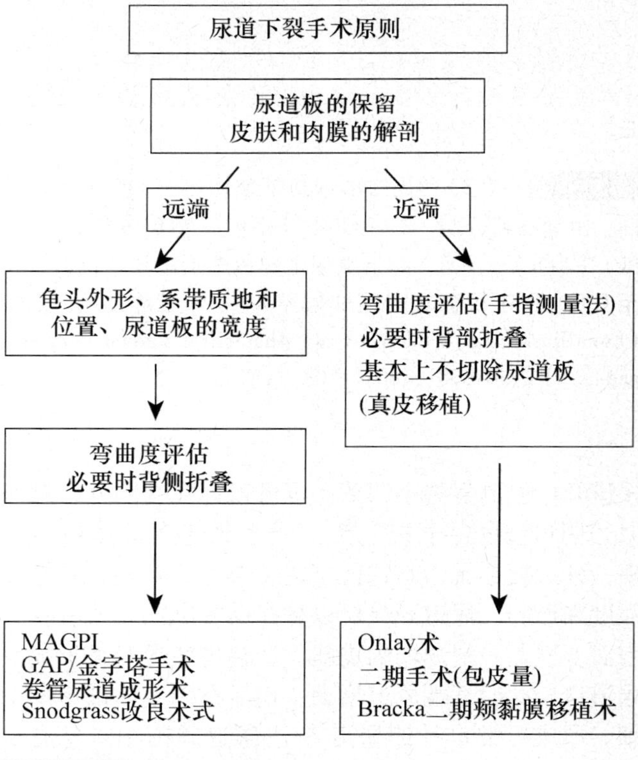

图 119-11 尿道下裂手术原则。

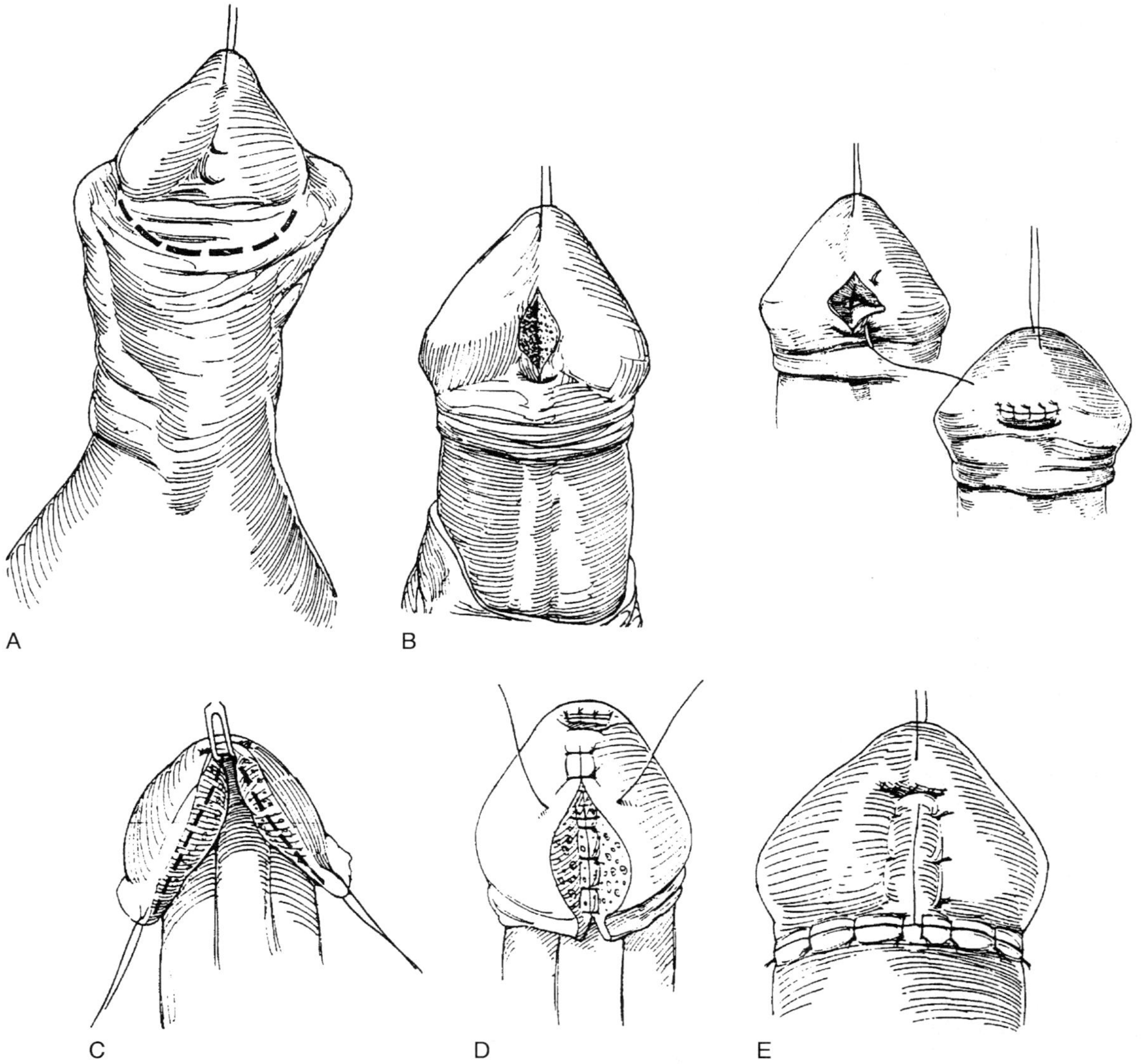

图 119-12 MAGPI 手术技巧。A. 首先于冠状沟下行包皮环切。B. 切除背侧皮桥后，Heineke-Mikulicz 法关闭尿道口背侧。C. 暴露龟头间质，关键步骤是将多余的皮肤修整切除（*虚线*），用 6-0 的铬线或皮肤拉钩将游离的尿道向前延伸。D. 尿道伤口表面两层缝合龟头间质，使尿道表面层次得以加强，龟头外观良好。E. 缝合包皮，使阴茎体皮肤如雪橇样。如果阴茎腹侧皮肤缺如，则可转移 Byar 皮瓣，在中线处缝合。（From Hinman F Jr：Atlas of Pediatric Urologic Surgery. Philadelphia，WB Saunders，1994，pp 575-578.）

MAGPI 手术

MAGPI 手术由 Duckett[51] 在 1981 年发明。该手术方法在选择合适的患者中疗效显著。能够以 MAGPI 方式进行手术的尿道下裂患者，其临床体征的特点是尿道开口于冠状沟或略偏于冠状沟之下，尿道口背侧龟头处有一层膜样组织，以至在排尿时引起尿流折射而偏向下方。尿道本身腹侧壁发育完好，海绵体厚实无闭锁。同时，尿道可以经游离向前移位（图 119-12）。

在尿道口近端、冠状沟下 5 mm 处环切包皮一圈，背侧包皮做成 Firlit 衣领样（见图 119-12A）。如脱袖套一样向阴茎阴囊交界处方向游离包皮，松解皮肤及肉膜下的所有纤维牵拉，尤其注意腹侧组织一定要充分松解，以此伸直阴茎。在这些病例中，腹侧纤维牵拉松解不充分是术后龟头下弯的最主要原因。包皮脱

1881 套样游离至阴茎根部时，阴茎扭转畸形能同时得到矫正。包皮游离之后，以人工勃起试验检查阴茎伸直程度。

背侧尿道板做一个 Heineke-Mikulicz 纵向切口，横行缝合，完成尿道口的前移（见图 119-12B）。更普遍的做法是把龟头组织连同龟头处的尿道壁楔行前移。横行缝合使得龟头皮桥平坦，背侧尿道得以前移到达龟头沟的龟头组织，用 7-0 的 Vicryl 可吸收线将前移的尿道口间断缝合、固定（见图 119-12C）。这样做可以缓解龟头下弯的幅度，使尿道口变得平坦，从而让尿流笔直向前。

龟头成形，重塑扁平的龟头为圆锥形外观（见图 119-12D）。旋转龟头两翼包绕尿道口近端，一个正常外观的圆锥形龟头得以成功重建。靠近龟头边缘的包皮需精确裁剪，与龟头两翼相称，于阴茎腹侧中线重新缝合。用 6-0 的 Vicryl 缝线间断缝合龟头深部组织，7-0 的铬线缝合表面上皮边缘（见图 119-12E）。这样，龟头系膜组织在龟头尿道上皮与龟头外层上皮之间愈合后，可以防止尿道口回缩。龟头两翼旋转后，成形的龟头外观与正常大致相同。尿道口的大小以探条测量确定，同时需要保证龟头成形时没有造成远端尿道管腔的狭窄。

1882 通常情况下，脱套以后的包皮足以再次缝合遮盖阴茎体（见图 119-12E）。如果腹侧包皮短缺，可以游离背侧包皮以 Byar 皮瓣的形式转移到腹侧进行替代。18 个月以下的患儿接受手术时不需要留置尿道支撑或导尿管。在阴茎下弯程度非常轻时，可以通过 MAGPI 手术保留包皮[46]。Polus 和 Lotte[122] 以及 Gilpin[66] 都曾在文献中提及在治疗不伴有阴茎下弯的前位尿道下裂时保留包皮的手术方式。

MAGPI 手术可以作为门诊手术加以应用，手术成功的关键在于选择合适的患者。为防止术后尿道退缩，术中必须做到充分前移尿道口并切实固定（图 119-13）。

GAP 手术

GAP 手术适用于一些冠状沟宽深的前位尿道下裂亚型的患者[165]。这些患者的龟头部没有遮挡尿流的横桥样组织隔膜而使尿流折向，这一表现也可见于更适合选用 MAGPI 术式的患者。在 GAP 手术中，口径宽大的尿道首先在支架管上卷成管状（图 119-14）。这种情况下，如果不适当地选择了 MAGPI 手术，术后就可能会产生龟头下弯、尿道回缩以及排尿时尿线呈散射状等情况。

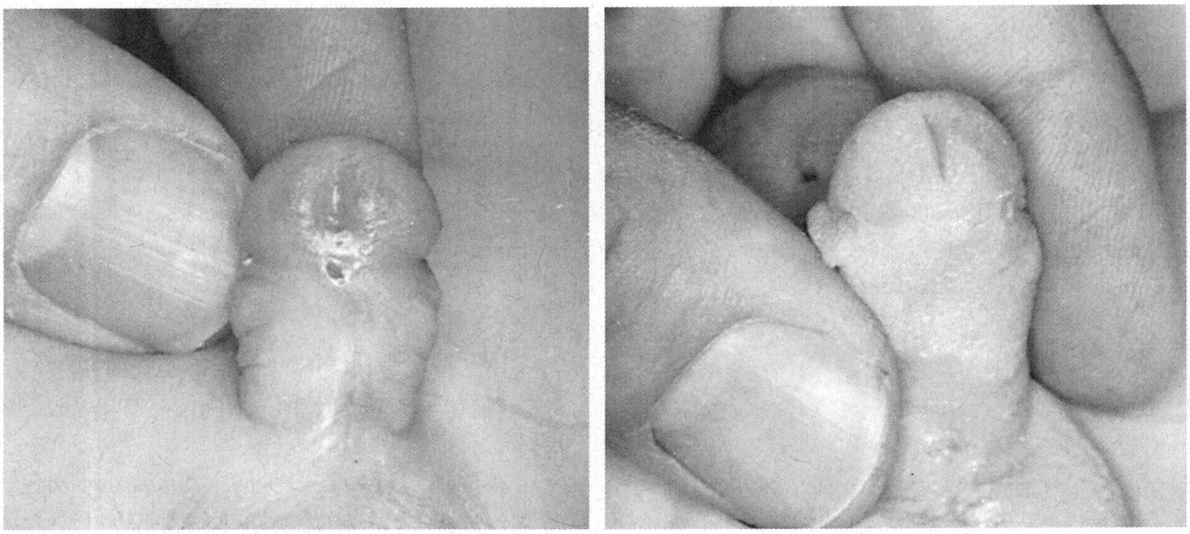

A B

图 119-13 A. 前位尿道下裂患者术前外观，可行 MAGPI 手术。注意尿道口背侧的蹼状组织。B. MAGPI 术后形态。（From Duckett JW, Baskin LA: Hypospadias. In Gillenwater J, et al [eds]: Adult and Pediatric Urology, 3rd ed. St Louis, Mosby-Year Book, 1996.）

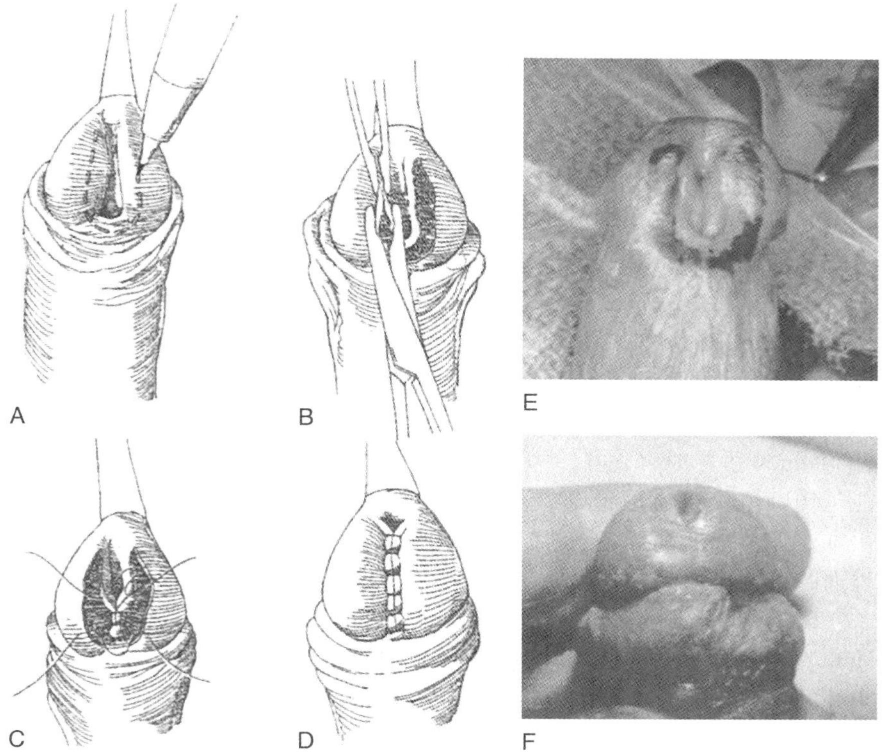

图 119-14　GAP 手术技巧。A. 初始切口。B. 去除上皮后暴露龟头间质。这是龟头两层缝合的关键保证，为尿道成形提供重要支持。C. 新尿道卷管，继而龟头闭合。D. 尿道修补完成。E. 前位尿道下裂患者外观形态，尿道口宽大，如裂开的鱼嘴，适用 GAP 手术。F. 术后观。

尿道松解术

另一个治疗冠状沟下尿道下裂的手术方式是尿道松解。Beck[22] 于 1917 年报道了这一方式，Koff[97]、Nasrallah 和 Minott[112] 以及 de Sy 和 Hoebeke[41] 使该手术得以重新应用。这一手术与 MAGPI 比较优点不多，而且需要更广泛地游离阴茎尿道。尿道口狭窄的发生率较高。

金字塔手术

另外一小部分患者只表现为前位尿道下裂。前位尿道下裂中有 6% 的患者包皮完整，包皮下尿道开口宽大，龟头扁平而无阴茎下弯（图 119-15）[54,56]。有时，这些只有在包皮环切术后才得以发现，从而使手术纠治更为复杂。Duckett 和 Keating[54] 为此创建了“金字塔”手术方式。沿龟头和阴茎远端仔细分离巨大的远端尿道，暴露尿道的四个象限（由此得名金字塔）。缝线收合尿道口以后将尿道包埋于龟头下，手术过程与尿道上裂修补术相似（见图 119-15C）。

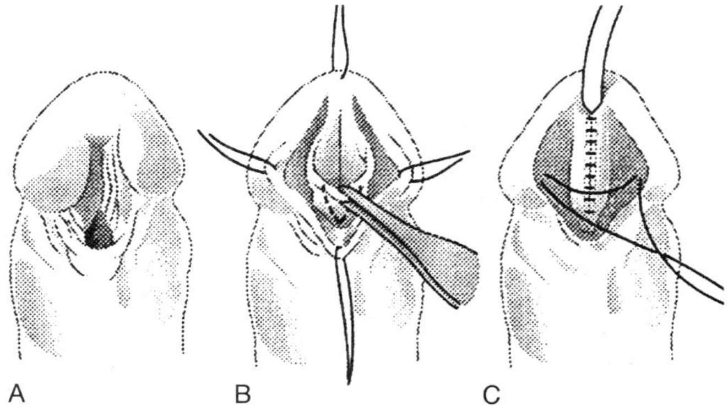

图 119-15　金字塔手术方式修补巨尿道口尿道下裂。A. 巨尿道口患者龟头缺损宽大，无阴茎下弯。正常新生儿尿道口为 12～14 French，患儿尿道口扩大到 22～24 French。通常情况下，该异常体征只在行包皮环切时才被发现，但是与包皮完整时的手术纠治过程相同。B. 手术过程涉及尿道周围游离、暴露尿道和龟头组织，然后移动异常扩大的楔形尿道。C. 在缝合的新尿道表面将暴露的龟头组织关闭。术中沿阴茎体和远端阴茎向近端仔细分离，充分暴露尿道的四象限是手术的关键技巧，金字塔手术设计的名称也源于此。尿道逐渐变细，将其包埋于龟头下的操作与修补尿道上裂相同。

Mathieu 或利用尿道口周围皮瓣的手术

当尿道口远离冠状沟而不能施行 MAGPI 手术时，或者当冠状沟太浅不适合采用 GAP 手术或原位卷管时（见后），可改用法国外科医生 Mathieu 于 1932 年介绍的将尿道口前移到龟头的手术方式[104]。该手术方式涉及尿道口周围皮瓣的运用，皮瓣依靠其原有的血管供应成活。为确保皮瓣成活，游离皮瓣的长宽之比不应大于 2∶1。如果不想保留任何皮下组织，皮瓣实际上也可以作为游离皮片来应用。皮瓣周围以带蒂包皮包绕作受体床，类似带血管蒂的皮瓣移植。在设
1883 计 Mathieu 手术时（图 119-16），必须保证腹侧皮肤能延伸到龟头正常尿道开口处。一些改良的 Mathieu 手术还涉及采用带蒂皮下组织两层缝合，加强尿道外表面的结构。

Radman[127] 进一步改良了 Barcat[11] 所改良的 Mathieu 手术，除尿道口周围皮瓣以外，还游离了龟头处的皮瓣，背向劈开龟头包埋尿道，将尿道向龟头顶端进一步延伸。Koff 等[98] 在 Mathieu 手术方面经验丰富，并报道手术效果极好。

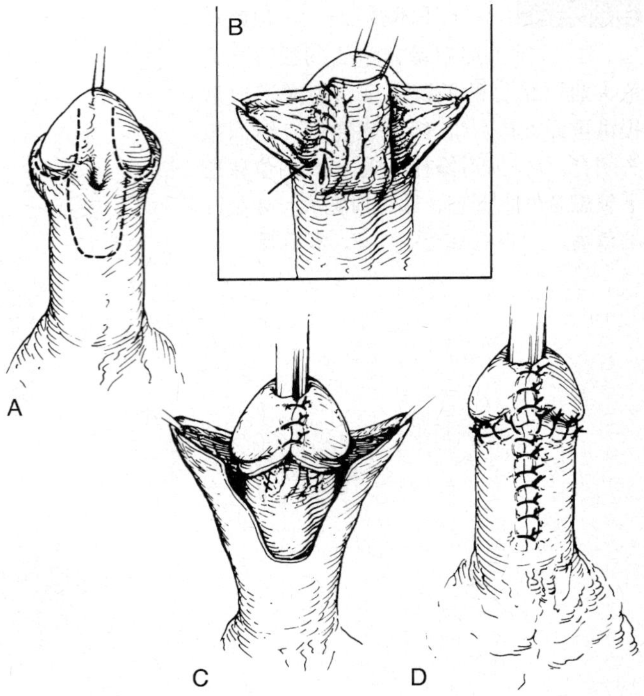

图 119-16 Mathieu 手术。A. 虚线勾出皮瓣轮廓。B. 旋转近端皮瓣，创建龟头侧面皮瓣。C. 龟头皮瓣遮盖新建尿道，按需移动包皮。D. 手术完成。（From Duckett JW：Hypospadias. In Walsh PC，Gittes RF，Perlmutter AD，et al ［eds］：Campbell's Urology，5th ed. Philadelphia，WB Saunders，1986，pp 1969–1999.）

Snodgrass 纵切尿道板尿道卷管成形术

历史上，当尿道沟不够宽大无法原位卷管时，手术路径需要改变，如选择 Mathieu 手术，或对于一些更严重的尿道下裂患者，需要行带蒂皮瓣移植。最近，Snodgrass 介绍了一种新的手术方式，即将尿道板切开，再行尿道卷管，尿道板随后二次愈合[144]（图 119-17）。手术的短期疗效显著，这一手术步骤得到广泛接受[145]。由于尿道板背侧切开，尿道口呈裂隙样，这是一个令人满意的术后外观。此种术式也已应用于更靠后的尿道下裂患者[146]。理论上讲，因瘢痕
1884 引起的尿道口狭窄是术后值得关心的一个问题，类似原发性尿道狭窄疾病。而对于后者，直视下行尿道切开手术会造成狭窄复发。但是，实际上，因手术导致的尿道口狭窄非常少见[35,84]。尿道下裂中，天然尿道板组织自身的血液供应丰富，连同海绵体血窦的充分营养，故似乎尿道板切开以后二次愈合不会造成局部瘢痕。尿道板切开卷管的尿道成形术有助于保留包皮（图 119-18）。为保留包皮，包皮切口只做于腹侧，因此有明显阴茎弯曲的患者不适用该手术方式。包皮三层缝合能防止皮肤瘘管的形成。包皮不能用作

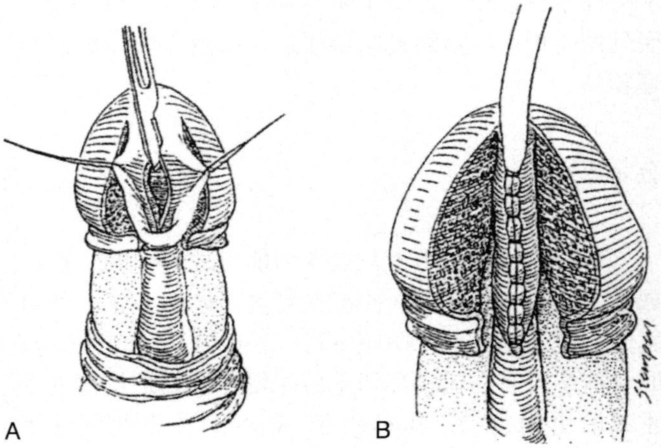

图 119-17 尿道板切开卷管尿道成形术。A. 深切尿道板背侧至海绵体组织。B. 新尿道卷管成形，继而龟头成形。

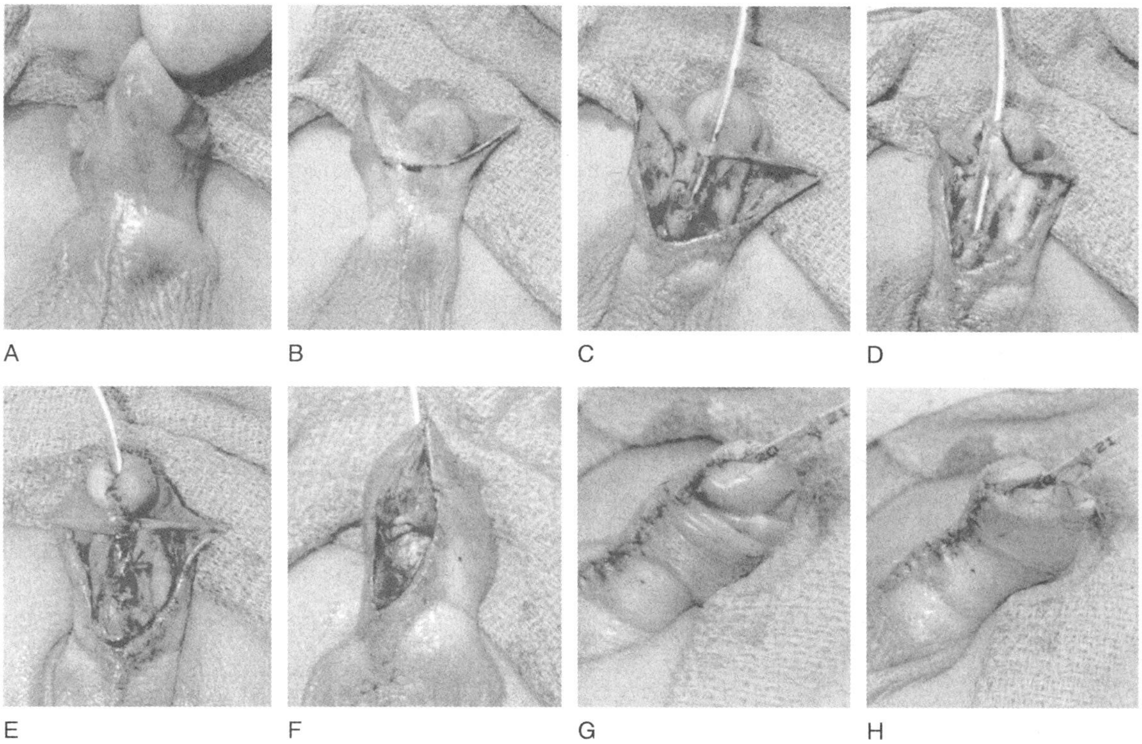

图 119-18 远端尿道下裂保留包皮的手术方式。A. 远端尿道下裂。B. 标记切口，为保留包皮做准备。C. 分离腹侧包皮。注意暴露的薄弱海绵体和远端尿道。D. 龟头两翼已被游离，依照 Snodgrass 手术方式完成远端尿道成形。E. 龟头成形，两层缝合组织。F. 重建包皮分成三层：（1）内侧包皮，（2）包皮下组织防止尿瘘，（3）外层包皮。G. 手术完成，包皮可退缩。H. 手术结束。

去上皮皮瓣，这在理论上增加了尿道瘘形成的可能性。

后位尿道下裂

尿道板保留手术

Duckett 普及了术中保留尿道板的概念，这是目前治疗后位尿道下裂和严重的前位尿道下裂的典型方式[16,52]。尿道板作为背侧尿道壁，腹侧尿道由包皮内板带血管蒂转移覆盖而形成。从广泛的临床经验得知，尿道板本身很少造成阴茎弯曲（图 119-19）。这一经验由大量的尿道板切除后行人工勃起试验验证，说明切除尿道板对改善阴茎下弯没有帮助（见图 119-19）[16]。进一步的实践经验证明，尿道板柔韧易弯曲，并且保留尿道板的辅助阴茎加强手术能够减少所引起的并发症，如近端吻合处的尿道瘘和狭窄等[14,16]。

为了松解勃起组织，采用保留尿道板但彻底剥离、暴露尿道海绵体的手术方式[108,110]的概念并没有获得成功。实际上，细致的解剖研究已经发现，在尿道下裂中，丰富的血管网络为尿道板提供了充足的血液供应。而提拉尿道板会侵犯这一血液供应网，对尿道板造成破坏[18]。因此，挪移尿道板的术式应该废止。

历史上，后位尿道下裂手术时都采用将异常尿道及周围组织全部切除直至暴露正常海绵体的方法。尿道由带血管蒂的包皮内板或外板卷管替代[8,50,148]。现在，在大多数尿道下裂（包括会阴型尿道下裂）的治疗中，尿道板均可保留，缺损的尿道由带血管蒂的游离皮瓣转移替代。在一些少见的尿道下裂病例中，尿道板需要切除，可以考虑二期手术修复（见后述）。

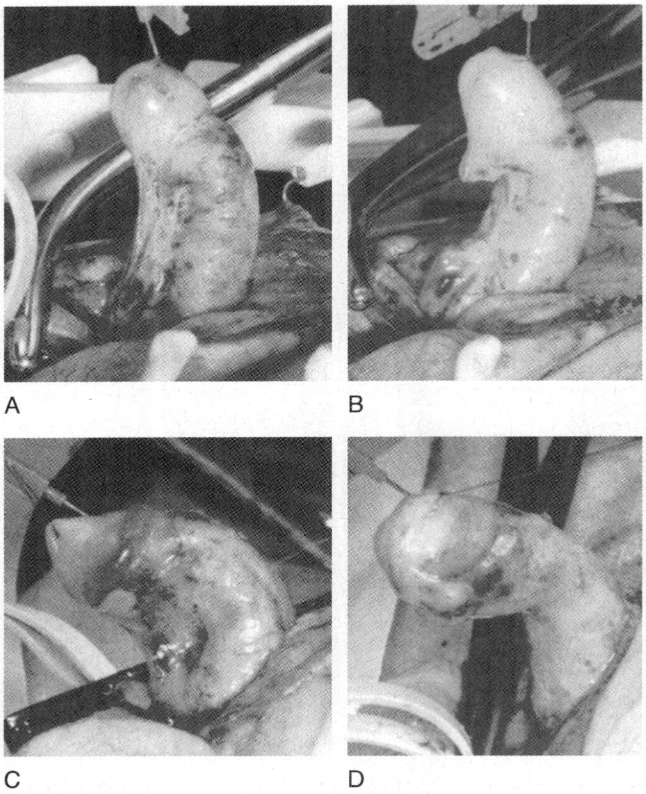

图 119-19 A. 尿道板保留的阴茎下弯。B. 切除尿道板后，阴茎仍然严重下弯。C. 尿道板保留的阴茎下弯。D. 切除尿道板后，阴茎仍然严重下弯。广泛的经验表明，尿道板很少是造成阴茎下弯的原因。

Onlay 包皮岛状皮瓣法

尿道下裂患者供应包皮组织的血液丰富，并且容易界定（见图 119-18）[76,88]。阴茎背侧绝大部分表皮组织血液供应充足，血管沿长轴纵向分布[124]。由阴茎皮肤上分离部分包皮内板，可以建立一岛状皮瓣。除背侧包皮的远端以外，背侧包皮和阴茎皮肤的血液供应均来自于其宽大的基底，而非依靠皮下组织。术中，可以切除阴茎皮瓣的边缘不予利用。

所有后位尿道下裂（包括伴有或不伴阴茎弯
1885 曲）的患者开始手术时都要保留尿道板的完整性。这一手术技巧同样可以运用于阴囊型和会阴型尿道下裂之中。对于防止近端尿道狭窄的发生，保留背侧尿道板的完整性是必要的。在 onlay 岛状皮瓣法治疗尿道下裂中，良好的血液供应使尿道瘘的发生率下降到约 5%~10%（图 119-20）[16]。Rushton 等[137]介绍，对于尿道缺损比较短的患者，可以选择包皮的一半做游离皮瓣替代尿道，而将留下的另一半包皮作为第二层遮盖物在皮瓣表面覆盖加强。onlay 岛状皮瓣法的长期效果很好[16,58,108]。在严重的尿道下裂中，可以把包皮设计成马蹄形，桥接于尿道缺损间（见图 119-20K）。

横裁包皮卷管岛状皮瓣法

在保留尿道板的概念普及以前，横裁包皮卷管岛状皮瓣法应用广泛（图 119-21）。目前，虽然长期随访显示尿道憩室的并发症导致了较高的再手术率，但该手术方式仍然成功用于必须切除尿道板的严重尿道下裂患者。在一些改良方法中，人们对近端吻合口采用斜形间断缝合，以减少术后尿道狭窄的发生。也有医生把新建的尿道固定到海绵体上，防止尿道憩室的形成，并有利于导尿操作。这些改进方法还包括在龟头下做宽大的隧道以弥补海绵体缺陷，可以避免术后尿道口狭窄[50]。如今，二期横裁包皮卷管岛状皮瓣法常规应用于尿道下裂修补术中。

二期尿道下裂修补术 188

在阴茎弯曲纠正后将背侧的包皮转移到腹侧，这是手术治疗严重尿道下裂时的另一种可选择的方法（图 119-22）。在严重的病例中，有时需要切除尿道板以纠正阴茎下弯。手术中可能需要皮瓣移植，但是不推荐在皮瓣成活以前行尿道成形手术。Byar 皮瓣能够从阴茎背侧转移到腹侧，建立的移植覆盖物可以在随后的尿道成形手术中加以利用[128]。有时阴茎下弯的纠正并不需要切除尿道板，这种情况下，可以把背侧的包皮缝合到保留下来的尿道板的每一侧（见图 119-22D）。二期手术的开展至少需要与一期手术间隔 6 个月以上。为方便二期手术对龟头的操作，常在一期手术时把背侧包皮卷入龟头的两翼下。新建的尿道用皮下组织覆盖加强，以避免发生尿道瘘。

Bracka 二期颊黏膜移植修补术

对有过手术史的严重尿道下裂患者，Bracka 提出了二期颊黏膜移植修补术[30]。在一期手术中，予阴

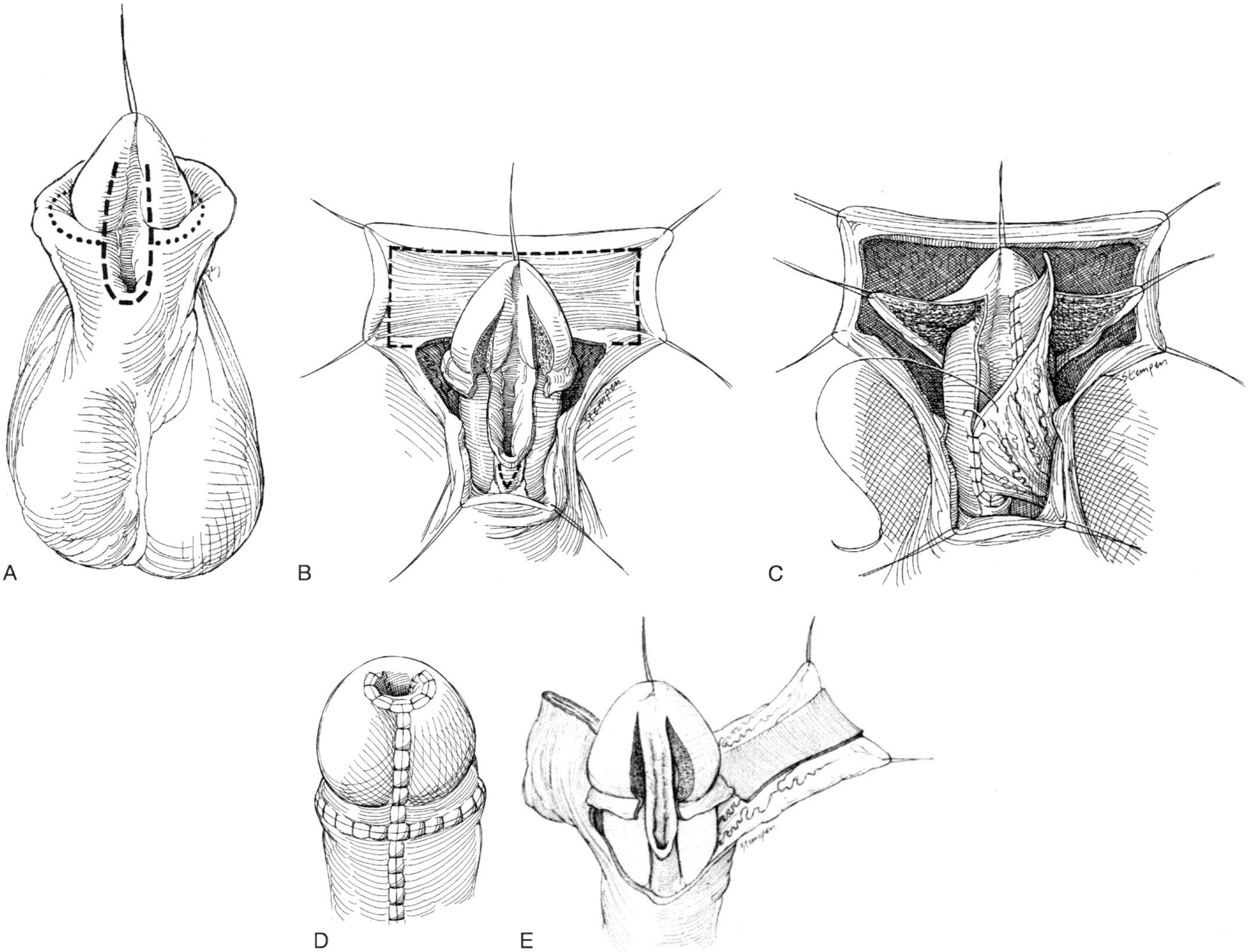

图 119-20　尿道下裂 onlay 岛状皮瓣手术。A. 围绕尿道板做 U 形切口，背侧尿道板保留约 8 mm 宽。B. 皮肤和皮下组织脱鞘，在包皮内板上设计 onlay 岛状皮瓣。沿海绵体平面和龟头间质分离龟头两翼。C. 阴茎阴囊型尿道下裂阴茎下弯时保留尿道板。D. 用 7-0 线，将 onlay 皮瓣连续缝合到尿道板上。对于 1 岁儿童，皮瓣修裁到 12 French 左右，以防组织过多导致尿道憩室形成。尿道口建立后，龟头两翼于新尿道表面合拢。按经典的 Byar 皮瓣重组法关闭阴茎皮肤。E. 包皮切开，原位游离短血管的 onlay 岛状皮瓣。该方法适用于小 onlay 手术，残存包皮可被用于第二层组织遮盖。

茎以手术伸直，切除瘢痕尿道（图 119-23 和 119-24）。从两颊或嘴唇处获得颊黏膜，移植到准备好的移植床上[15]。为防止移植区形成血肿将移植的颊黏
87 膜掀起，应严密缝合。在一期手术中，分离龟头两翼，为二期手术创建裂隙样的尿道口做准备。二期尿道成形术需要在一期手术以后至少 6 个月再予施行。二期手术中，需要对过多的颊黏膜进行修裁，龟头两层缝合（见图 119-23 和 119-24）。颊黏膜卷管成新尿道，用皮下组织进行第二层覆盖。

阴茎弯曲

随着尿道下裂手术向保留尿道板改进，阴茎弯曲的纠正方法也在不断改良。Gittes 和 McLaughlin[67] 在 1974 年提出人工勃起试验，为检查阴茎弯曲以及评价术中对此纠正的程度提供了检查标准。操作时，在阴茎根部扎上止血带，向海绵体注射生理盐水。两条阴茎海绵体充满生理盐水后就可以明确阴茎弯曲的程度，以及验证切除纤维组织后的治疗是否成功。在进

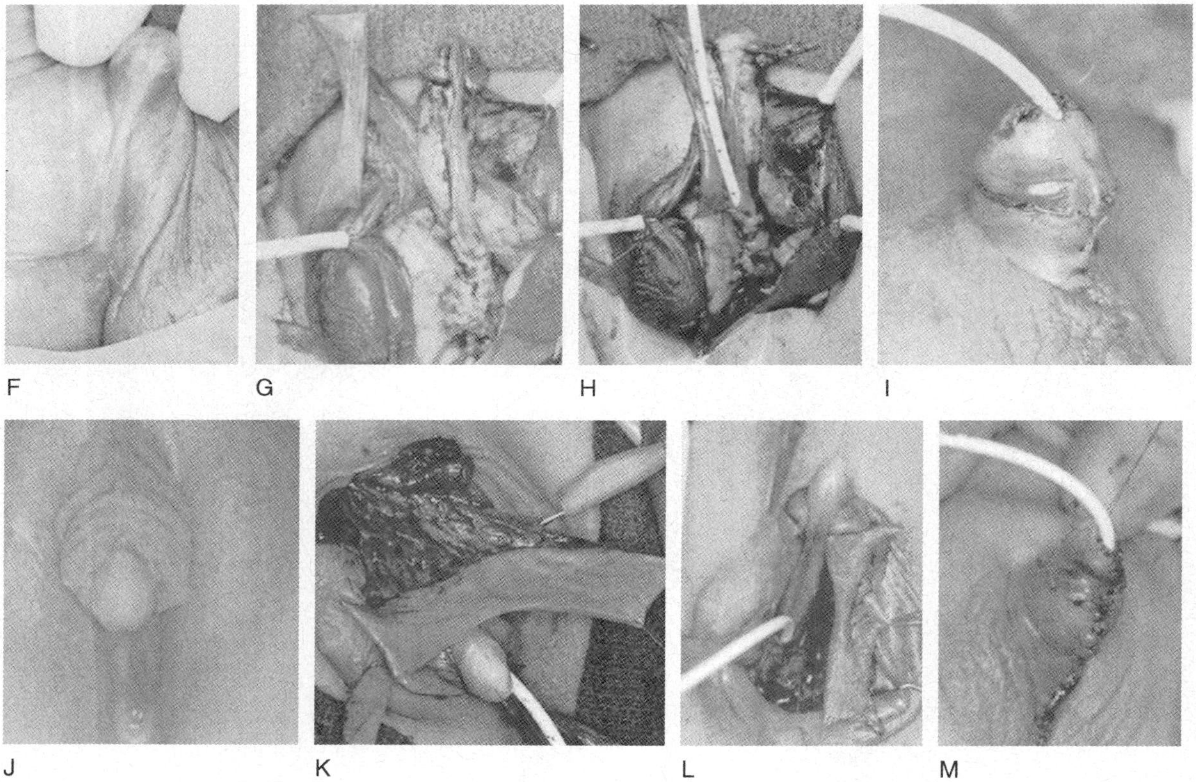

图 119-20　（续）F. 阴茎阴囊型尿道下裂，适用 onlay 岛状皮瓣手术。G. 保留尿道板，皮瓣游离。H. 将 onlay 皮瓣缝合到尿道板上。I. 手术完成。J. 会阴型尿道下裂。K. 马蹄形带血管蒂的 onlay 岛状皮瓣，桥接于长段尿道缺损上。L. 旋转 onlay皮瓣，桥接于缺损的尿道上。M. 手术完成。

行尿道成形和一期手术以前，必须完全纠正阴茎弯曲畸形。只要确保使用的是注射用生理盐水，至今还未见有关人工勃起试验造成阴茎海绵体损伤的报道。

尿道下裂患者中，25% 的阴茎弯曲是因为阴茎腹侧纤维成条索样或扇面样牵拉造成的。切除这些纤维以后，阴茎得以伸直。当然，这一简单的解释并不适用于所有类型的尿道下裂，单纯地切断腹侧牵拉索带就能纠正阴茎下弯的观点也不总是正确的。Kaplan 和 Lamm[89]认为，阴茎下弯可能是胚胎正常发育终止所造成的，类似于睾丸未降。事实上，在胚胎发育过程中，所有的阴茎都经历过弯曲阶段（图 119-25）。因此，在一些阴茎弯曲的临床病例中，腹侧纤维组织明显缺如并不奇怪。同样，阴茎下弯也可能是由于阴茎海绵体的背侧与腹侧发育不同步而造成的，手术时可以通过缩短背侧白膜来纠正。有人提出，在一些尿道下裂患者中，阴茎弯曲是因为畸形的尿道与包皮异常附着而引起的[23]，因此通过手术松解两者之间的粘连就可以加以纠治，这样的阴茎弯曲也称为皮肤型阴茎下弯。另外，阴茎弯曲也可能是因为腹侧皮肤明显匮乏而引起（见图 119-25）[4]。Devine 和 Horton[45] 对阴茎下弯进行了分类（Ⅰ型至Ⅲ型），并认为Ⅲ型阴茎下弯可能由肉膜发育不全而引起，与皮肤型阴茎下弯相似。

对于真性纤维性阴茎弯曲而言，阴茎的弯曲方向朝向腹侧，尿道口和龟头之间的距离很短。于冠状沟下绕龟头环行一圈切开包皮，切口位置处于龟头之
下、尿道开口远端，并深及尿道海绵体白膜。向阴茎 188
体近端分离，从白膜上游离纤维组织粘连。术中采用锐性分离的原则，从阴茎的一侧分离向另一侧，直至阴茎下弯被矫正为止。在此分离过程中，尿道随着阴茎的伸直而退缩升高。在大多数病例中，造成阴茎下弯的组织围绕在尿道口周围，并随近端尿道延伸一段
距离。组织游离通常需要一直游离到阴茎阴囊交界 189
处，甚至到阴囊和会阴区。一旦尿道获得充分游离，阴茎的纤维牵拉就应当充分剥离，直到阴茎的两侧。术中操作要仔细，以弯剪平行于阴茎体表面进行分离，并以人工勃起试验验证游离成功与否。

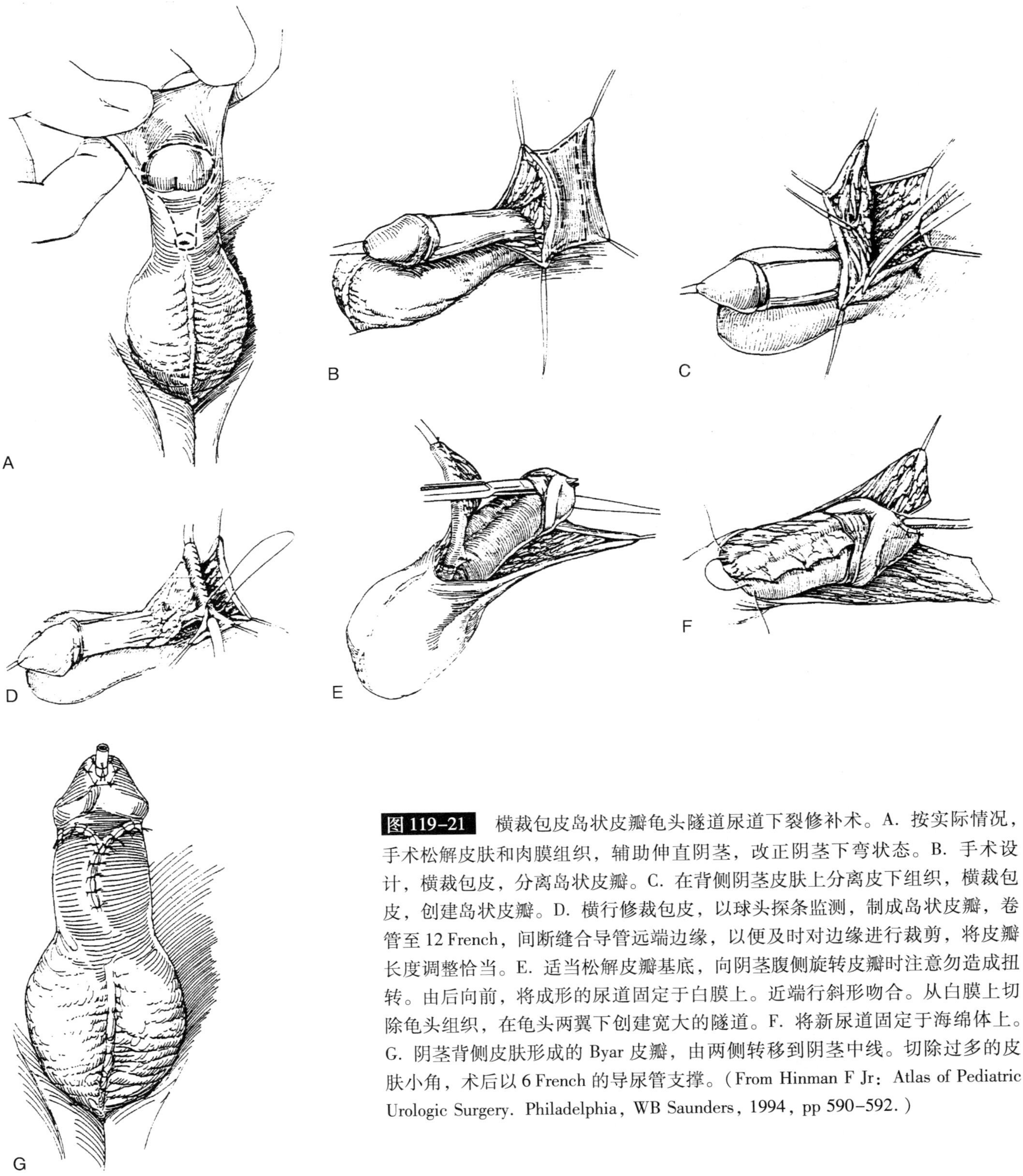

图 119-21　横裁包皮岛状皮瓣龟头隧道尿道下裂修补术。A. 按实际情况，手术松解皮肤和肉膜组织，辅助伸直阴茎，改正阴茎下弯状态。B. 手术设计，横裁包皮，分离岛状皮瓣。C. 在背侧阴茎皮肤上分离皮下组织，横裁包皮，创建岛状皮瓣。D. 横行修裁包皮，以球头探条监测，制成岛状皮瓣，卷管至 12 French，间断缝合导管远端边缘，以便及时对边缘进行裁剪，将皮瓣长度调整恰当。E. 适当松解皮瓣基底，向阴茎腹侧旋转皮瓣时注意勿造成扭转。由后向前，将成形的尿道固定于白膜上。近端行斜形吻合。从白膜上切除龟头组织，在龟头两翼下创建宽大的隧道。F. 将新尿道固定于海绵体上。G. 阴茎背侧皮肤形成的 Byar 皮瓣，由两侧转移到阴茎中线。切除过多的皮肤小角，术后以 6 French 的导尿管支撑。（From Hinman F Jr：Atlas of Pediatric Urologic Surgery. Philadelphia，WB Saunders，1994，pp 590-592.）

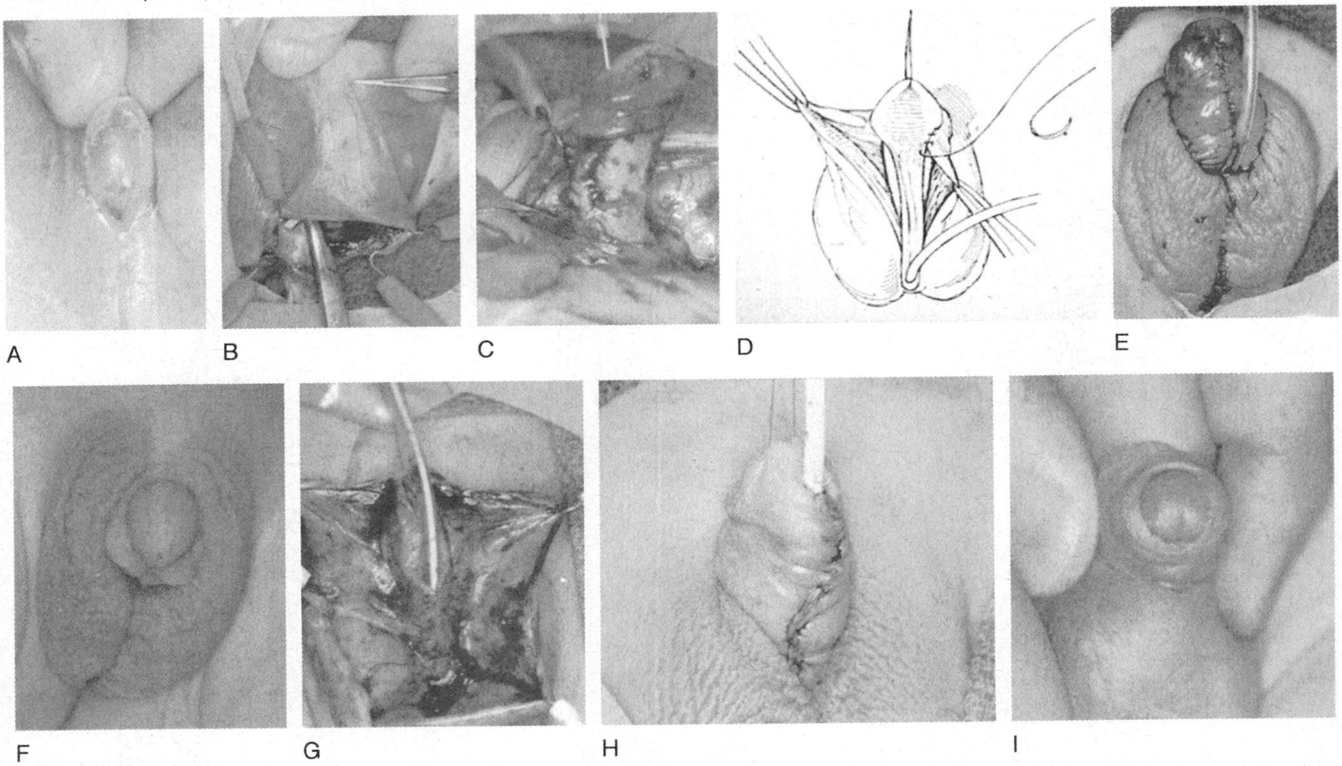

图 119-22 分期尿道成形手术。第一期手术包括纠正阴茎下弯，将背侧包皮转移到阴茎腹侧。A. 阴囊型尿道下裂，合并阴茎下弯和阴茎阴囊反位。B. 包皮附着至阴囊皮肤。C. 切除腹侧圈合的尿道板，伸直阴茎。D. 在一些经过筛选的患者中，尿道板可以保留，背侧包皮中线切开后向腹侧包绕阴茎体。E. 一期手术完成。F. 一期手术术后 6 个月，予二期尿道成形术。G. 尿道成形术。H. 手术完成。I. 术后 6 个月随访。

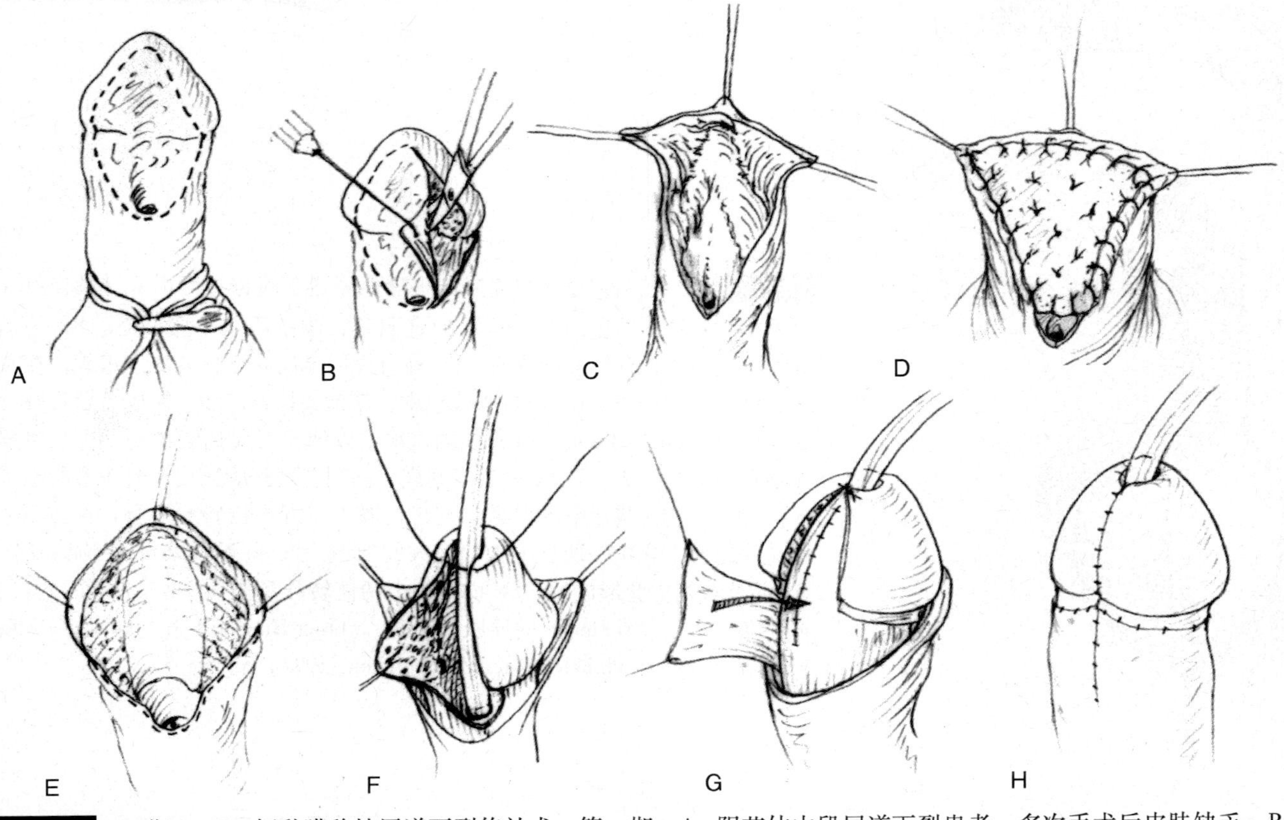

图 119-23 二期 Bracka 颊黏膜移植尿道下裂修补术。第一期：A. 阴茎体中段尿道下裂患者，多次手术后皮肤缺乏。B. 切除瘢痕组织。C. 分离龟头两翼。D. 游离颊黏膜遮盖在瘢痕上。一期手术以后 6 个月行二期手术：E. 暴露龟头间质，修剪颊黏膜，继而行尿道成形手术。F. 缝合尿道，开始尿道成形。G. 去上皮化的带血管蒂皮肤二次遮盖尿道伤口。H. 两层缝合，尿道成形，完成手术修补。

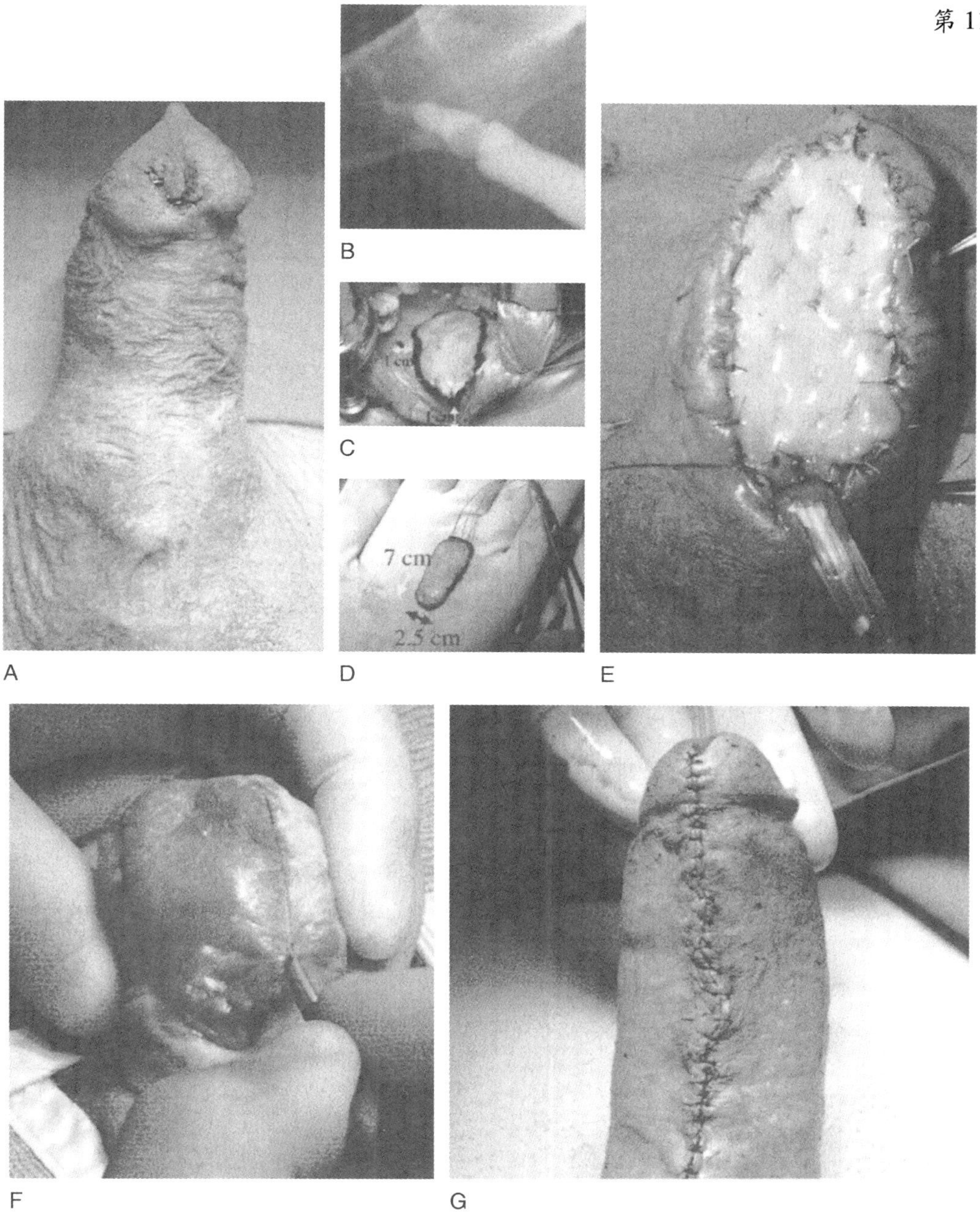

图 119-24　A. 多次手术患者，远端尿道狭窄。B. 尿道造影。C. 获得的颊黏膜大体观。D. 游离颊黏膜，准备移植。E. 切除瘢痕组织后，颊黏膜覆盖于阴茎腹侧。F. 术后 6 个月，颊黏膜伤口痊愈。G. 手术完成。

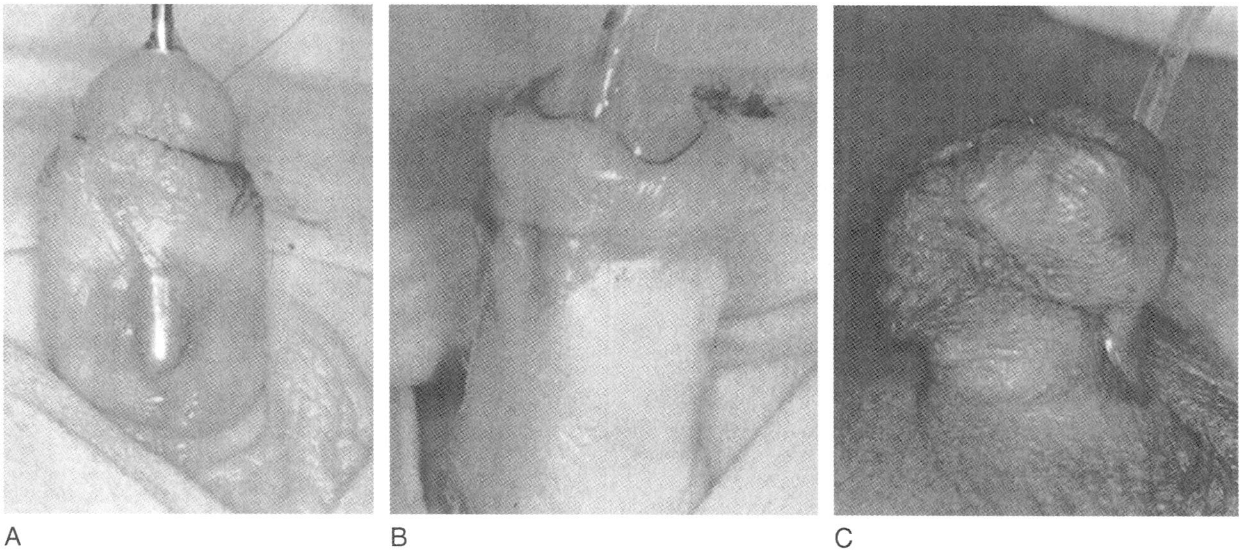

图 119-25　A. 先天性瘘管。B 和 C. 无尿道下裂的阴茎下弯。尿道海绵体异常发育引起阴茎下弯，需要尿道成形。

有几种方法已经用于纠正阴茎最后的弯曲。在背侧与腹侧海绵体之间沿冠状沟逐步小心侧切白膜外层是解除阴茎弯曲的有效方法。Koff 和 Eakins[99] 在治疗尿道上裂时的海绵体转位法也许可以同样应用于纠正尿道下裂的阴茎弯曲。理论上，在阴茎海绵体上缝线时可能会碰到神经血管束，而永久性地缝扎神经血管束可能造成组织淤血坏死或继发勃起功能障碍，所以人们在应用该手术方式时对此问题非常关注。尿道上裂中，神经血管束分布于阴茎两侧，远离手术损伤区域，但尿道下裂则不同，神经血管束直接分布于折叠缝合线下，容易被术者忽略。手术时，切口可以选择在两条阴茎海绵体的中隔处，实践证明这是一个不错的方法[43]。

如果充分切除所有的异常纤维组织后，人工勃起试验仍显示阴茎有下弯畸形，那么海绵体不对称可能是造成阴茎下弯的原因。历史上，阴茎弯曲的矫治采用改良的 Nesbit 背侧折叠术，即在一个椭圆形的范围内楔形切开白膜，再以不可吸收线将切口缝合[113]。在 19 世纪早期，这一手术方法就由美国外科之父 Syng Physick 首先提出，他采用背侧白膜折叠法来治疗阴茎下弯[116]。经过人工勃起试验，确定阴茎弯曲最严重的部位，于此部位渐次楔形切开白膜。然后，用不可吸收线横行缝合这些钻石样的切口，直至阴茎伸直。Nesbit 的手术方式被改良为阴茎背侧白膜折叠，来纠治海绵体不对称和尿道下裂中的阴茎下弯[14]。基于人类胚胎阴茎的解剖学研究，目前提倡的更为简单的手术径路选择在阴茎背侧中线的 12 点处，在此无神经区做切口，并将白膜折叠缝合[18]。缝合位置选择在背侧中线有效地避免了术中对神经血管的游离（图 119-26）[19]。中线折叠法可应用于所有从轻微至严重的阴茎下弯中（图 119-27）。但是，如果术中折叠部位需要超过两处，或必须超过四条缝线才能达到纠正阴茎弯曲的目的，就应该考虑其他手术方法，如完全切断尿道板、转移皮肤移植物进行替代等。人工勃起试验时，如果阴茎下弯不能被术者手指纠正，则不建议采用背侧白膜折叠法。该方法同样可用于矫治龟头下弯，但术中必须格外小心，不要损伤到供应龟头的神经血管束[18]。

在一些罕见病例中，腹侧的白膜组织非常缺乏，以至于需要将白膜切除而移植其他弹性组织。笔者首选真皮，手术方法如 Horton 和 Devine 所述[80]（图 119-28）。

硬性分离阴茎皮肤至阴茎阴囊交界处，可以松解

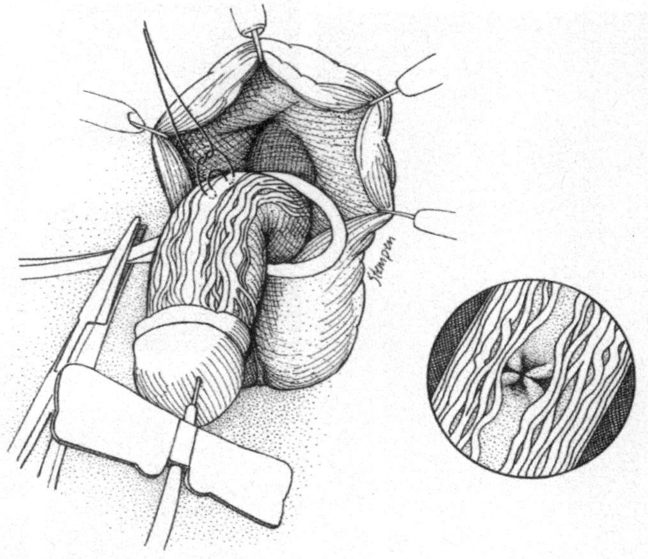

图 119-26 背侧中线折叠技术。操作中，在白膜无神经血管的 12 点位置平行、折叠缝合。该技术仅需要对阴茎进行很少的操作。术中无需切开海绵体或过分游离 Buck 筋膜。如果阴茎严重弯曲，最多可予两行并行折叠缝线纠正。

皮肤型阴茎下弯。在此过程之后，仍有大约 5% 的患者需要接受进一步的阴茎伸直操作[16,17]。在这些需要接受进一步操作才能伸直阴茎的患者中，超过 90% 可以通过白膜折叠的方法治疗，而无需切除尿道板。只有极少数的患者病症严重，需要采取尿道板切除和（或）皮肤移植才能完成阴茎伸直过程。

多次手术失败患者的治疗

一些尿道下裂患者经历了多次失败的手术，即使是那些经验丰富的外科医生，这样不幸的结果也同样可能发生。对于这些患者，先期创建的有问题的尿道常常需要废弃而进行重建。必要时阴茎还需要进一步伸直。在一些病例中，也许适合在尿道切除处先移植薄层筛网皮片，日后再将其卷成尿管[7,140]，或者移植游离的颊黏膜或皮肤[30-32]。过去，因为游离皮肤移植物的长期预后不如先前报道的那样好[75]，所以曾尝试移植膀胱黏膜替代尿道[92]。但可惜术后大约有 30% 的患者并发尿道口膀胱黏膜外翻[92]，每天常规行尿道扩张仍不能避免这一问题的出现。目前，口腔黏膜替代术已取而代之应用于这些复杂患者之

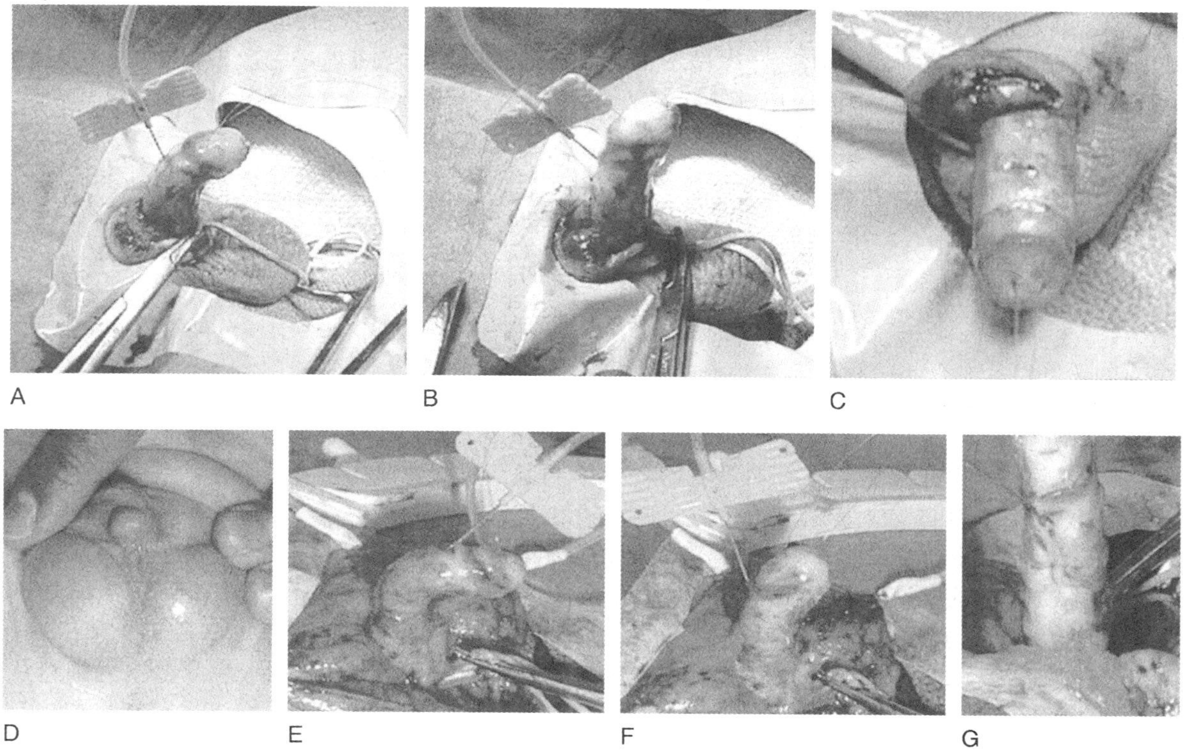

图 119-27　背侧中线折叠技术。A 至 C. 纠正轻度弯曲。D 至 G. 纠正中度至重度弯曲。注意阴茎背侧中线无神经区的两条 5-0 不可吸收的 Prolene 缝线。

中[15,53]。笔者推崇 Bracka 所介绍的二期手术方法(见图 119-23)[10,31,32]。

92 将来，在治疗难治性尿道下裂时也许可以用自身尿道上皮细胞培养出的自体物[134,135]。寻找适合泌尿道上皮细胞生长的基质可拓展该技术的应用范围。

手术技术问题

经过多年的发展，尿道下裂的治疗原则已经得到进一步改进，主要表现在由整形科医生培养精确、细致的手术操作手法，以及放大镜的使用。尖锐的虹膜

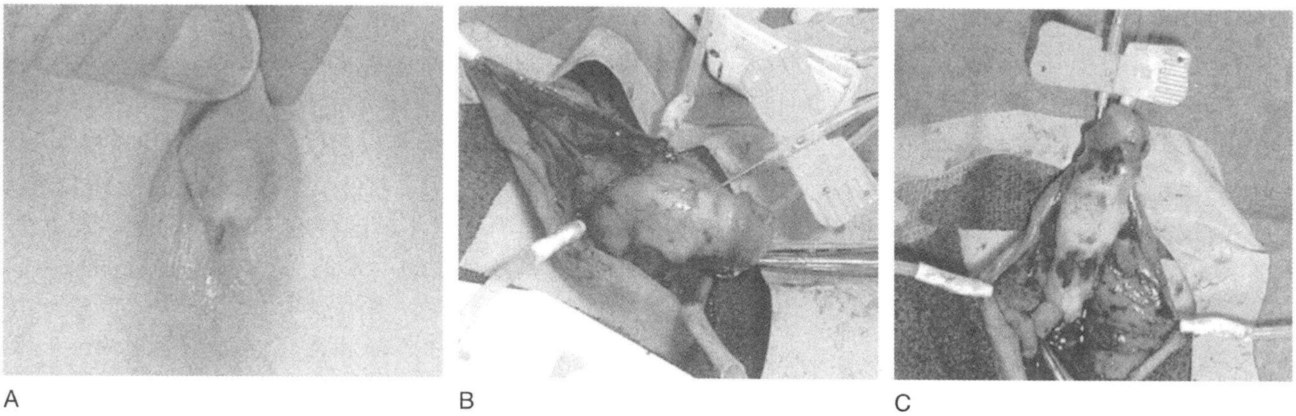

图 119-28　皮肤移植治疗严重阴茎腹侧弯曲。A. 阴囊型尿道下裂。B. 完全剥离皮肤和皮下组织后，阴茎弯曲成直角。C. 腹侧切开，准备移植皮肤。(From Hinman F Jr: Atlas of Urologic Surgery. Philadelphia, WB Saunders, 1989, pp 91-92.)

剪和精致的有齿镊是主要的手术器械。Castroviejo 持针器和 0.5 mm 镊子有助于术中用 7-0 的缝线做精细缝合。在测量尿道、吻合尺寸时需要使用球头探条，合适的探条也应用于探查尿道口。精细的泪小管探针适用于检查尿道瘘管和尿道周围管道。

止血方法

可以采取多种方法控制阴茎和龟头的出血。最简单的办法是在阴茎根部上止血带[115,126]，推荐的
1893 止血带持续应用时间从 20 分钟到 1 小时不等。笔者首选的方法是将 1∶100 000 的肾上腺素混合于 1% 的利多卡因（赛洛卡因）中，用 29 号细针注射入阴茎止血。使用时，药液经尿道周围渗透进入龟头，有助于龟头翼的操作。通常情况下，药液注射量为 1.0～1.5 ml。在吸入麻醉的条件下，避免肾上腺素引起心肌心律改变的安全范围比较大[91]。安全剂量是每公斤体重 1 ml 1∶100 000 肾上腺素溶液。笔者不支持肾上腺素引起血液淤滞的观点。止血的方法有许多种，笔者在使用 0.5 mm 精细镊时首选小电流的电刀（Bovie）。

止痛方法

考虑到术后出现的不适，可在术前进行骶尾神经阻滞麻醉[85]。如果尿道修补的时间超过 2 小时，手术结束时可以重复这一操作。有证据证明骶尾部阻滞麻醉还有利于减少手术出血量[72]。此外，可以选用 3 ml 0.5% 的布比卡因（丁哌卡因）在耻骨联合处注射，药液渗透入阴茎背侧神经束[160]。阴茎背侧阻滞麻醉有助于减少全身麻醉的药量，防止因阴茎勃起而造成的出血。

包扎方法

对于没有尿流改道的远端尿道下裂修补手术，笔者目前使用 Tegaderm 敷料完成术后包扎。术后 24～48 小时，患者父母亲在家中自行拆除敷料。对牵涉到尿流改道的尿道下裂修补，可以把阴茎压迫于腹壁上以更好地缓解张力，行“三明治”法包扎。一层 Telfa，阴茎腹侧覆盖经三次折叠的 4 ×4 英寸的纱布，再贴上中等大小的 Tegaderm 敷料固定。术后 48～72 小时在家中自行拆除敷料。笔者鼓励手术 48 小时以后每天带管洗澡两次，浸泡敷料以便其脱落。温水浴有助于清洁伤口，协助伤口愈合。

尿流改道

导尿管刺激膀胱三角区引起膀胱痉挛是一个严重问题，口服奥昔布宁能改善症状。另一个问题牵涉到引流管和集尿袋的连接。除非患者是成年人，否则笔者都避免使用 Foley 导尿管。对年龄为 6～18 个月的儿童，笔者首选“滴尿支撑管”。Kendall 制造了 6 French尿道下裂导尿管，而 5 French 和 8 French 的胃管同样有效。可以用圆针、5-0 的聚丙烯缝线将临时性支撑管缝合到龟头上。笔者采用这一方法后获得良好效果，使绝大多数尿道下裂的患者可以接受门诊手术。尿流改道要持续 3～10 天。如果改道时间少于 5 天，敷料脱落后建议患儿家长取出导尿管。术后患者接受随访 6 个月至 1 年，在排尿训练后及青春期后，都要求患者接受复诊。随访复诊时，对尿道不进行器械探查。在膀胱能控制小便的基础上，进行尿流率检查，以排除潜在的尿道狭窄。

手术年龄

尿道下裂修补手术的年龄在不断提前。Schultz 等[139]指出，疾病治疗的合适年龄应该是 6～18 个月之间，以尽量减少手术创伤对患者心理的影响。美国儿科学会对 18 个月以前进行生殖系手术的观点表示赞同[6]。18 个月以前，儿童尚不能完全辨认性别。目前笔者将手术年龄选择在 4～9 个月间，此时的阴茎已经具备足够的手术条件，与此前流行的 2～5 岁的手术年龄比较，手术成功率相似[42]。但是，由于条件（包括医疗方面和社会方面）的制约，手术时间往往会推迟。Kaplan 等[90]研究了 69 名婴儿期接受尿道修补手术的 6～10 岁患儿，发现与同龄正常儿童相比不存在更多病理心理方面的问题。

睾酮刺激

睾酮刺激可能诱发幼儿阴茎生长。药物使用的推荐方法是丙酸睾酮 25～50 mg（2 mg/kg），术前三次肌肉注射，间隔三周[38,64]。笔者认为，常规应用睾酮并无明显优点。而对于严重的病例，当阴茎短小如部分雄激素不敏感综合征，或出于疾病诊断的目的时，应用睾酮可能有所帮助。龟头发育不良的患者术前应用睾酮有利于手术开展。动物模型的研究结果提示，睾酮刺激可能对日后前列腺的成熟[111]和阴茎生长有害[83]。直到今天临床实践尚未对此有所证实。

并发症

尿道口狭窄

造成尿道口狭窄的原因是手术设计错误，或尿道成形、龟头成形时组织血液供应不良。术后扩张很少有治疗意义，而且给患者和家庭带来诸多痛苦。尿道内切开手术的长期效果亦不佳。如果尿道口狭窄临床表现明显（如并发瘘管、感染、憩室等），则需要行正式的手术修补，而其中的一些病例有必要接受二期手术（Bracka）[31,32]。如果尿道口狭窄持续存在，可以提起龟头两翼，切除下方瘢痕组织，交叉嵌入皮片。龟头尿道和尿道口的大量瘢痕可能是由尿道口周围皮片血液供应不良所引起的（如 Mathieu 或 Mustarde 手术）。

894 ### 尿道瘘

尿道瘘是尿道下裂手术中最常见的晚期并发症，其发生率已经成为评价手术效果的一个指标[129]。一期尿道下裂手术尿道瘘发生率的预计值在 10%～15% 之间。远端尿道梗阻常常与尿瘘持续有关。一旦瘘管成熟，关闭瘘管的手术可能失败，术后瘘管的高复发率令人失望。因此，一些医生主张在尿瘘手术时应贯彻以下原则，即皮瓣广泛游离、临近皮瓣转移、多层缝合及尿流改道[24,81,154,156]。笔者推荐术中使用放大镜和精细手术器械。以泪小管探针由瘘管外口伸入，明确瘘管上皮排列形态。手术切除范围自瘘口向下，深达尿道，以 7-0 的聚乙醇缝线内翻缝合瘘口周边。缝合结束后，挤压近端尿道，确保伤口密闭防水。两层缝合后，可应用“超级胶”作为伤口密闭剂。无需尿流改道。患者可由尿道自由排尿，术后当天可出院。

在施行尿瘘修补手术时需要明确是否同时伴有尿道狭窄或憩室，这一点非常重要。如果存在上述情况，那么只有在尿道狭窄或憩室改善后，才能保证尿瘘手术成功。有些时候，尿瘘修补同时需要行尿道口成形术。当瘘管靠近龟头时，最好打断尿道口与瘘口之间的皮桥，游离尿道内侧边缘，分两层向龟头方向渐进缝合（图 119-29）。

尿道狭窄

造成尿道狭窄的原因来自于初期手术时的一些技术问题。近端尿道狭窄可能是因为术中尿道内径计算错误引起新建尿道不够宽敞而造成，也可能是由于吻合口重叠而造成。为避免吻合口重叠，术中可以采用斜形吻合的方法，把尿道侧壁固定于白膜上。尿道口狭窄可能源于慢性干燥闭塞性龟头炎。该病变位于尿道口，甚至可向近端延伸进入成形的尿道。病变可能由尿道口周围血液供应不良所致，Mathieu 手术后发生概率较高。尿道口狭窄最可能的原因是靠近龟头顶端的尿道血液供应障碍。术中龟头隧道游离不充分，

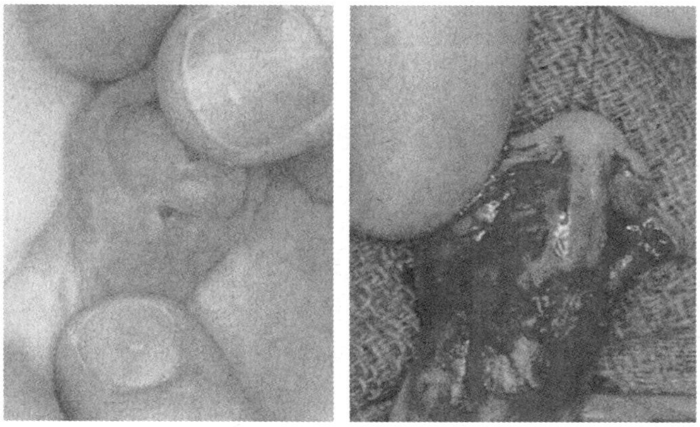

A　B

图 119-29　尿道下裂瘘。A. 冠状沟瘘，需要重新予以龟头成形手术。B. 保留尿道板，制备带一侧血管蒂的 onlay 皮瓣。

可能导致新建尿道受压，血液供应不良，继发尿道狭窄。一旦尿道狭窄形成，可以采取切除病变段尿道重新吻合的方法。重新吻合时，可选择带血管蒂的皮片转移，或是Bracka二期颊黏膜代尿道的方法[31,32,138]。笔者曾尝试采用直视下尿道内切开的方法治疗尿道下裂术后狭窄，但疗效欠佳[102]。

尿道憩室

梭形尿道憩室的形成可能与新建尿道过于宽敞而尿道口狭窄造成近端尿道气球样扩张有关。治疗时必须沿尿道纵轴切除扩张的憩室。更多见的手术操作是将阴茎包皮环行切开，包皮脱套样剥离到阴茎阴囊交界处，然后对尿道憩室进行裁剪缝合，这样做是为了避免在尿道伤口表面留置过多的重叠缝线。术中操作须谨慎，避免新建尿道与皮肤间瘘管形成。单独的尿道憩室可能由尿道下裂术后尿外渗进入邻近组织而引起，憩室表面常伴有尿道瘘管。Winslow等[159]曾报道利用憩室组织行二次尿道成形术。

结果

长期随访资料表明过去尿道下裂治疗主要针对年长儿，手术难度大[27,28,119,151]。尽管资料显示的疗效不甚理想，但这并不能反映现代水平[94]。Eberle等[57]在回顾性研究中报道，尿道下裂长期预后令人忧虑。42例后位尿道下裂患者成年以后，13例（13%）仍残存性别模糊、小阴茎、小睾丸、无法触及前列腺和男性乳腺发育等复杂问题。6例罹患Reifenstein综合征的患者具有严重的AR缺陷。为此，必须探寻更好的诊断方法，以便在婴儿期及早发现这一疾病。

目前，无论从外观上还是从功能上，尿道下裂的手术效果都明显好于过去。早期手术、一期尿道成形术的开展以及术后并发症的减少，都使我们对疾病治疗有了积极乐观的态度。借助人工勃起试验纠正阴茎下弯为理想的性生活提供了有力保障。通过手术，尿道口可以延伸至阴茎头端，除非患者伴发睾丸疾病，否则所有患者的生育能力都能得到显著提高。证据表明，新建的尿道可以随年龄而生长，很少有必要施行再次尿道改建手术。

尽早行尿道修复术最大限度减少了住院治疗，使患者与家长摆脱分离的焦虑和对去势的恐惧。我们完全可以自信地告诉家长，各型尿道下裂术后都能具备良好的外观与功能，患儿将不再背负心理上的创伤。 1895

总结

1. 尿道下裂应该在出生后1年以内手术，最佳手术年龄是4~6个月。在此年龄阶段，术后疼痛与导尿管不适症状轻微。同时，婴儿行动能力欠佳，使术后护理更加简便。
2. 应以形成裂隙样尿道口为目标，可以选择保留或不保留包皮，这一点取决于家长的态度。
3. 保留尿道板和发育不良的海绵体为再建尿道正常解剖结构提供了较大的可能性。
4. 中线折叠对治疗绝大多数阴茎下弯患者安全有效。（超过两处折叠可以选择另一种手术方式，如皮瓣移植。）
5. 少部分患者需要切除尿道板，二期手术得到普遍认同。
6. 带血管蒂的onlay岛状皮瓣移植法在尿道下裂的初次或再次手术时都有效。
7. 所有尿道成形术中，尿道伤口表面都应覆盖去上皮、带血管蒂的组织片。
8. 阴茎皮肤匮乏的患者最好采取Bracka二期颊黏膜代尿道手术。
9. 冠状沟瘘需要重做龟头成形术。

（孙 杰译 文建国校）

参考文献

1. Aigen AB, Khawand N, et al: Acquired megalourethra: An uncommon complication of the transverse preputial island flap urethroplasty. J Urol 1987;137:712-713.
2. Akman Y, Li YW, et al: Penile anatomy under the pubic arch: Reconstructive implications. J Urol 2001;166:225-230.
3. Albers N, Ulrichs C, et al: Etiologic classification of severe hypospadias: Implications for prognosis and management. J Pediatr 1997;131:386-392.
4. Allen TD, Spence HM: The surgical treatment of coronal hypospadias and related problems. J Urol 1968;100:504-508.
5. Allera A, Herbst MA, et al: Mutations of the androgen

receptor coding sequence are infrequent in patients with isolated hypospadias. J Clin Endocrinol Metab 1995;80: 2697-2699.
6. American Academy of Pediatrics: Timing of elective surgery on the genitalia of male children with particular reference to the risks, benefits, and psychological effects of surgery and anesthesia. Pediatrics 1996;97:590-594.
7. Angermeier KW, Jordan GH, et al: Complex urethral reconstruction. Urol Clin North Am 1994;21:567-581.
8. Asopa H, Elhence I, et al: One-stage correction of penile hypospadias using a foreskin tube: A preliminary report. Int Surg 1971;55:435-440.
9. Avellan L: The incidence of hypospadias in Sweden. Scand J Plast Reconstr Surg 1975;9:129-138.
10. Barbagli G, Palminteri E, et al: Penile urethral reconstruction: Concepts and concerns. Arch Esp Urol 2003;56: 549-556.
11. Barcat J: Plastic and Reconstructive Surgery of the Genital Area. Boston, Little, Brown, 1973.
12. Baskin LS: Hypospadias and urethral development. J Urol 2000;163:951-956.
13. Baskin LS, Colborn T, et al: Hypospadias and endocrine disruption: Is there a connection? Environ Health Perspect 2001;109:1175-1183.
14. Baskin LS, Duckett JW: Dorsal tunica albuginea plication for hypospadias curvature. J Urol 1994;151:1668-1671.
15. Baskin LS, Duckett JW: Buccal mucosa grafts in hypospadias surgery. Br J Urol 1995;76(Suppl 3):23-30.
16. Baskin LS, Duckett JW, et al: Changing concepts of hypospadias curvature lead to more onlay island flap procedures. J Urol 1994;151:191-196.
17. Baskin LS, Duckett JW, et al: Penile curvature. Urology 1996;48:347-356.
18. Baskin LS, Erol A, et al: Anatomical studies of hypospadias. J Urol 1998;160:1108-1115.
19. Baskin LS, Erol A, et al: Anatomy of the neurovascular bundle: Is safe mobilization possible? J Urol 2000;164:977-980.
20. Baskin LS, Lee YT, et al: Neuroanatomical ontogeny of the human fetal penis. Br J Urol 1997;79:628-640.
21. Baskin LS, Liu W, et al: Anatomical studies of the mouse genital tubercle. In Baskin LS (ed): Hypospadias and Genital Development. Philadelphia, Kluwer Academic/Plenum, 2004, pp 103-120.
22. Beck C: Hypospadias and its treatment. Surg Gynecol Obstet 1917;24:511-532.
23. Bellinger M: Embryology of the male external genitalia. Urol Clin North Am 1981;8:375-382.
24. Belman AB: De-epithelialized skin flap coverage in hypospadias repair. J Urol 1988;140:1273-1276.
25. Benson GV, Lim H, et al: Mechanisms of reduced fertility in Hoxa-10 mutant mice: Uterine homeosis and loss of maternal Hoxa-10 expression. Development 1996;122:2687-2696.
26. Bentvelsen FM, Brinkmann AO, et al: Decreased immunoreactive androgen receptor levels are not the cause of isolated hypospadias. Br J Urol 1995;76:384-388.
27. Berg R, Berg G: Penile malformation, gender identity and sexual orientation. Acta Psychiatr Scand 1983;68:154-166.
28. Berg R, Svensson J, et al: Social and sexual adjustment of men operated on for hypospadias during childhood: A controlled study. J Urol 1981;125:313-317.
29. Bergstrom R, Adami HO, et al: Increase in testicular cancer incidence in six European countries: A birth cohort phenomenon. J Natl Cancer Inst 1996;88:727-733.
30. Bracka A: A long-term view of hypospadias. Br J Plast Surg 1989;42:251-255.
31. Bracka A: Hypospadias repair: The two-stage alternative. Br J Urol 1995;76(Suppl 3):31-41.
32. Bracka A: A versatile two-stage hypospadias repair. Br J Plast Surg 1995;48:345-352.
33. Carlsen E, Giwercman A, et al: Declining semen quality and increasing incidence of testicular cancer: Is there a common cause? Environ Health Perspect 1995;103(Suppl 7):137-139.
34. Cerasaro TS, Brock WA, et al: Upper urinary tract anomalies associated with congenital hypospadias: Is screening necessary? J Urol 1986;135:537-538.
35. Cheng EY, Vemulapalli SN, et al: Snodgrass hypospadias repair with vascularized dartos flap: The perfect repair for virgin cases of hypospadias? J Urol 2002;168:1723-1726.
36. Cheng W, Mya GH, et al: Associated anomalies in patients with undescended testes. J Trop Pediatr 1996;42:204-206.
37. Colborn T, Short P, et al: Health effects of contemporary-use pesticides: The wildlife/human connection. Toxicol Ind Health 1999;15:61-67.
38. Conte F, Grumbach M: Pathogenesis, classification, diagnosis and treatment of anomalies of sex. In DeGroot (ed): Endocrinology. Philadelphia, WB Saunders, 1995.
39. Cunha G, Baskin L: Development of the penile urethra. In Baskin LS (ed): Hypospadias and Genital Development. Philadelphia, Kluwer Academic/Plenum, 2004, pp 87-100.
40. Daskalopoulos EI, Baskin L, et al: Congenital penile curvature (chordee without hypospadias). Urology 1993;42:708-712.
41. de Sy WA, Hoebeke P: Urethral advancement for distal hypospadias: 14 years' experience. Eur Urol 1994;26:90-92.
42. Devine CJ Jr: Chordee and hypospadias. In Glenn J, Boyce W (eds): Urologic Surgery. Philadelphia, JB Lippincott, 1983, pp 775-797.
43. Devine CJ Jr, Blackley SK, et al: The surgical treatment of chordee without hypospadias in men. J Urol 1991;146: 325-329.
44. Devine CJ Jr, Gonzales-Serva L, et al: Utricular configuration in hypospadias and intersex. J Urol 1980;123:407-411.
45. Devine CJ Jr, Horton C: Chordee without hypospadias. J Urol 1973;110:264-267.
46. Dewan PA: Distal hypospadias repair with preputial reconstruction. J Paediatr Child Health 1993;29:183-184.
47. de Zegher F, Francois I, et al: Androgens and fetal growth. Horm Res 1998;50:243-244.
48. Dolle P, Izpisua-Belmonte JC, et al: HOX-4 genes and the morphogenesis of mammalian genitalia. Genes Dev 1991; 5:1767.
49. Donnenfeld AE, Schrager DS, et al: Update on a family with hand-foot-genital syndrome: Hypospadias and urinary tract abnormalities in two boys from the fourth generation. Am J Med Genet 1992;44:482-484.
50. Duckett JW: Transverse preputial island flap technique for repair of severe hypospadias. Urol Clin North Am 1980; 7:423-431.
51. Duckett JW: MAGPI (meatal advancement and glanuloplasty): A procedure for subcoronal hypospadias. Urol Clin North Am 1981;8:513-520.
52. Duckett JW: The current hype in hypospadiology. Br J Urol 1995;76(Suppl 3):1-7.
53. Duckett JW, Coplen D, et al: Buccal mucosa in urethral reconstruction. J Urol 1995;153:1660-1663.
54. Duckett JW, Keating MA: Technical challenge of the megameatus intact prepuce hypospadias (MIP) variant: The pyramid procedure. J Urol 1989;141:1407-1409.
55. Duckett JW, Snyder HD: Meatal advancement and glanuloplasty hypospadias repair after 1000 cases: Avoidance of meatal stenosis and regression. J Urol 1992;147:665-669.
56. Duckett JW, Keating MA: Technical challenge of the megameatus intact prepuce hypospadias variant: the pyra-

mid procedure. J Urol 1989;141:1407-1409.
57. Eberle J, Uberreiter S, et al: Posterior hypospadias: Long-term followup after reconstructive surgery in the male direction. J Urol 1993;150:1474-1477.
58. Elder JS, Duckett JW, et al: Onlay island flap in the repair of mid and distal penile hypospadias without chordee. J Urol 1987;138:376-379.
59. Environmental Protection Agency, Endocrine Disruptor Screening and Testing Advisory Committee (EDSTAC): Final Report, 1998. Washington, DC, EPA.
60. Erol A, Baskin LS, et al: Anatomical studies of the urethral plate: Why preservation of the urethral plate is important in hypospadias repair. BJU Int 2000;85:728-734.
61. Fredell L, Lichtenstein P, et al: Hypospadias is related to birth weight in discordant monozygotic twins. J Urol 1998; 160:2197-2199.
62. Fritz G, Czeizel AE: Abnormal sperm morphology and function in the fathers of hypospadiacs. J Reprod Fertil 1996;106:63-66.
63. Fryns JP, Vogels A, et al: The hand-foot-genital syndrome: On the variable expression in affected males. Clin Genet 1993;43:232-234.
64. Gearhart JP, Jeffs RD: The use of parenteral testosterone therapy in genital reconstructive surgery. J Urol 1987;138: 1077-1078.
65. Gearhart JP, Linhard HR, et al: Androgen receptor levels and 5 alpha-reductase activities in preputial skin and chordee tissue of boys with isolated hypospadias. J Urol 1988;140: 1243-1246.
66. Gilpin D, Clements WD, et al: GRAP repair: Single-stage reconstruction of hypospadias as an out-patient procedure. Br J Urol 1993;71:226-229.
67. Gittes R, McLaughlin AI: Injection technique to induce penile erection. Urology 1974;4:473-475.
68. Glenister T: The origin and fate of the urethral plate in man. J Anat 1954;288:413-418.
69. Goldman A: Abnormal organogenesis in the reproductive system. In Wilson J, Fraser F (eds): Handbook of Teratology, vol 2. New York, Plenum Press, 1977, pp 391-419.
70. Griffin J, McPhau LM, et al: The androgen resistance syndromes: Steroid 5 alpha-reductase deficiency, testicular feminization and related disorders. In Scriver C (ed): The Metabolic and Molecular Bases of Inherited Disease, vol 3. Philadelphia, McGraw-Hill, 1995, pp 2967-2998.
71. Groshart C, Okkerman P, et al: Report to the European Commission: Identification of Endocrine Disruptors. First Draft Interim Report. Delft, the Netherlands, BKH Consulting Engineers, 1999.
72. Gunter JB, Forestner JE, et al: Caudal epidural anesthesia reduces blood loss during hypospadias repair. J Urol 1990; 144:517-519, 530.
73. Gupta C, Goldman A: Arachidonic acid cascade is involved in the masculinization of embryonic external genitalia in mice. Proc Natl Acad Sci U S A 1986;83: 4346-4349.
74. Harris EL: Genetic epidemiology of hypospadias. Epidemiol Rev 1990;12:29-40.
75. Hendren WH, Keating MA: Use of dermal graft and free urethral graft in penile reconstruction. J Urol 1988;140: 1265-1269.
76. Hinman F Jr: The blood supply to preputial island flaps. J Urol 1991;145:1232-1235.
77. Hinman F Jr: Penis and male urethra. In Hinman FJ (ed): UroSurgical Anatomy. Philadelphia, WB Saunders, 1993, pp 418-470.
78. Hiort O, Klauber G, et al: Molecular characterization of the androgen receptor gene in boys with hypospadias. Eur J Pediatr 1994;153:317-321.
79. Holmes NM, Miller WL, et al: Lack of defects in androgen production in children with hypospadias. J Clin Endocrinol Metab 2004;89:2811-2816.
80. Horton C, Devine C: Peyronie's disease. Plast Reconstr Surg 1973;52:503.
81. Horton C, Devine C, et al: Fistulas of the penile urethra. Plast Reconstr Surg 1980;66:407-418.
82. Hsieh-Li HM, Witte DP, et al: Hoxa 11 structure, extensive antisense transcription, and function in male and female fertility. Development 1995;121:1373-1385.
83. Hussman D, Cain M: Eventual phallic size is dependent on the timing of androgen administration. J Urol 1994;152: 734-739.
84. Jayanthi VR: The modified Snodgrass hypospadias repair: Reducing the risk of fistula and meatal stenosis. J Urol 2003;170:1603-1605.
85. Jensen B: Caudal block for postoperative pain relief in children after genital operations: A comparison between bupivacaine and morphine. Acta Anesthesiol Scand 1981; 25:373-375.
86. Jensen K: European Parliament's Committee on the Environment, Public Health and Consumer Protection. Report on Endocrine Disrupting Chemicals. Rapporteur, 1998.
87. Jirasek J, Raboch J, et al: The relationship between the development of gonads and external genitals in human fetuses. Am J Obstet Gynecol 1968;101:830.
88. Juskiewenski S, Vaysse P, et al: A study of the arterial blood supply to the penis. Anat Clin 1982;4:101-107.
89. Kaplan GW, Lamm DL: Embryogenesis of chordee. J Urol 1975;114:769-772.
90. Kaplan S, Hensle T, et al: Hypospadias: Associated behavior problems and male gender role development. J Urol 1989;141:45-A.
91. Karl H, Swedlow D, et al: Epinephrine-halothane interactions in children. Anesthesiology 1983;58:142-145.
92. Keating MA, Cartwright PC, et al: Bladder mucosa in urethral reconstructions. J Urol 1990;144:827-834.
93. Kelce WR, Wilson EM: Environmental antiandrogens: Developmental effects, molecular mechanisms, and clinical implications. J Mol Med 1997;75:198-207.
94. Kenawi M: Sexual function in hypospadias. Br J Urol 1975;47:883-890.
95. Khuri F, Hardy B, et al: Urologic anomalies associated with hypospadias. Urol Clin North Am 1981;8:565-571.
96. Kim KS, Torres CR, et al: Induction of hypospadias in a murine model by maternal exposure to synthetic estrogens. Environ Res 2004;94:267-275.
97. Koff S: Mobilization of the urethra in the surgical treatment of hypospadias. J Urol 1981;125:395-397.
98. Koff S, Brinkman J, et al: Extensive mobilization of the urethral plate and urethra for repair of hypospadias: The modified Barcat technique. J Urol 1994;151:466-469.
99. Koff S, Eakins M: The treatment of penile chordee using corporal rotation. J Urol 1984;131:931-934.
100. Kurzrock E, Baskin L, et al: Epithelial-mesenchymal interactions in development of the mouse fetal genital tubercle. Cells Tissues Organs 1999;164:1015-1020.
101. Kurzrock E, Baskin L, et al: Ontogeny of the male urethra: Theory of endodermal differentiation. Differentiation 1999;64:115-122.
102. Lofti A, Snyder H, et al: The treatment of urethral strictures: The contribution of clean intermittent catheterization to direct vision urethrotomy. J Urol 1991;145:810A.

103. Ma L, Benson GV, et al: Abdominal B (AbdB) Hoxa genes: Regulation in adult uterus by estrogen and progesterone and repression in mullerian duct by the synthetic estrogen diethylstilbestrol (DES). Dev Biol 1998;197:141-154.
104. Mathieu P: Traitement en un temps de l'hypospadias balanique et juxtabalanique. J Chir 1932;39:481.
105. McArdle F, Lebowitz R: Uncomplicated hypospadias and anomalies of upper urinary tract: Need for screening? Urology 1975;5:712-716.
106. McPhaul MJ, Marcelli M, et al: Genetic basis of endocrine disease. 4. The spectrum of mutations in the androgen receptor gene that causes androgen resistance. J Clin Endocrinol Metab 1993;76:17-23.
107. Mettauer JP: Practical observations on those malformations of the male urethra and penis, termed hypospadias and epispadias, with an anomalous case. Am J Med Sci 1842;4:43-47.
108. Mollard P, Mouriquand P, et al: Application of the onlay island flap urethroplasty to penile hypospadias with severe chordee. Br J Urol 1991;68:317-319.
109. Mortlock DP, Innis JW: Mutation of HOXA13 in hand-foot-genital syndrome. Nat Genet 1997;15:179-180.
110. Mouriquand PD, Persad R, et al: Hypospadias repair: current principles and procedures. Br J Urol 1995;76 Suppl 3:9-22.
111. Nasland M, Coffee D: The hormonal imprinting of the prostate and the regulation of stem cells in prostate growth. Proceedings of the 2nd NIADDK Symposium on the Study of Benign Prostatic Hyperplasia. Washington, DC, US Government Printing Office, 1985.
112. Nasrallah P, Minott H: Distal hypospadias repair. J Urol 1984;131:928-930.
113. Nesbit R: Plastic procedure for correction of hypospadias. J Urol 1941;45:699-702.
114. North K, Golding J: A maternal vegetarian diet in pregnancy is associated with hypospadias. The ALSPAC Study Team. Avon Longitudinal Study of Pregnancy and Childhood. BJU Int 2000;85:107-113.
115. Ossandon F, Ransley P: Lasso tourniquet for artificial erection in hypospadias. Urology 1982;19:656-657.
116. Pancoast J: Treatise on Operative Surgery. Philadelphia, Carrey & Hart, 1844.
117. Paulozzi L: International trends in rates of hypospadias and cryptorchidism. Environ Health Perspect 1999;107: 297-302.
118. Paulozzi L, Erickson D, et al: Hypospadias trends in two US surveillance systems. Pediatrics 1997;100:831-834.
119. Pegoraro V, Dal Poz R, et al: Controllo a lungo termine dell'pospadico operato. Estratto Urol 1979;46:1-9.
120. Podlasek CA, Barnett DH, et al: Prostate development requires Sonic hedgehog expressed by the urogenital sinus epithelium. Dev Biol 1999;209:28-39.
121. Podlasek CA, Duboule D, et al: Male accessory sex organ morphogenesis is altered by loss of function of Hoxd-13. Dev Dyn 1997;208:454-465.
122. Polus J, Lotte S: Chirurgie des hypospades: Une nouvelle technique esthetique et fonctionnelle. Ann Chir Plast 1965;10:3-9.
123. Price K, Fenwick G: Naturally occurring oestrogens in foods—a review. Food Addit Contam 1985;2:73-106.
124. Quartey J: One stage penile/preputial cutaneous island flap urethroplasty for urethral stricture: A preliminary report. J Urol 1983;129:284-287.
125. Raman-Wilms L, Tseng AL, et al: Fetal genital effects of first-trimester sex hormone exposure: A meta-analysis. Obstet Gynecol 1995;85:141-149.
126. Redman J: Tourniquet as hemostatic aid in repair of hypospadias. Urology 1986;28:241.
127. Redman J: The balanic groove technique of Barcat. J Urol 1987;137:83-85.
128. Retik AB, Bauer SB, et al: Management of severe hypospadias with a two-stage repair. J Urol 1994;152: 749-751.
129. Retik AB, Keating M, et al: Complications of hypospadias repair. Urol Clin North Am 1988;15:223-236.
130. Ritchey ML, Benson RJ, et al: Management of mullerian duct remnants in the male patient. J Urol 1988;140: 795-799.
131. Ritchey ML, Sinha A, et al: Congenital fistula of the penile urethra. J Urol 1993;151:1061-1062.
132. Rogers B: History of external genital surgery. In Horton C (ed): Plastic and Reconstructive Surgery of the Genital Area. Boston, Little, Brown, 1973, pp 3-47.
133. Rolland R, Gilbertson M, et al: Environmentally induced alterations in development: A focus on wildlife. Environ Health Perspect 1995;103(Suppl 4).
134. Romagnoli G, DeLuca M, et al: Treatment of posterior hypospadias by the autologous graft of cultured urethral epithelium. N Engl J Med 1990;323:527-530.
135. Romagnoli G, DeLuca M, et al: One-step treatment of proximal hypospadias by the autologous graft of cultured urethral epithelium. J Urol 1993;150:1204-1207.
136. Ross F, Farmer A, et al: Hypospadias—a review of 230 cases. Plast Reconstr Surg 1959;24:357-368.
137. Rushton H, Belman A: The split prepuce in situ onlay hypospadias repair. J Urol 1998;160:1134-1136.
138. Scherz HC, Kaplan GW, et al: Post-hypospadias repair urethral strictures: A review of 30 cases. J Urol 1988;140: 1253-1255.
139. Schultz J, Klykylo W, et al: Timing of elective hypospadias repair in children. Pediatrics 1983;71:342-351.
140. Secrest CL, Jordan GH, et al: Repair of the complications of hypospadias surgery. J Urol 1993;150:1415-1418.
141. Shelton TB, Noe HN: The role of excretory urography in patients with hypospadias. J Urol 1985;134:97-99.
142. Shima H, Ikoma F, et al: Developmental anomalies associated with hypospadias. J Urol 1979;122:619-621.
143. Skakkebaek NE, Rajpert-De Meyts E, et al: Germ cell cancer and disorders of spermatogenesis: An environmental connection? APMIS 1998;106:3-11.
144. Snodgrass W: Tubularized, incised plate urethroplasty for distal hypospadias. J Urol 1994;151:464-465.
145. Snodgrass W, Koyle M, et al: Tubularized incised plate hypospadias repair: Results of a multicenter experience. J Urol 1996;156:839-841.
146. Snodgrass W, Koyle M, et al: Tubularized incised plate hypospadias repair for proximal hypospadias. J Urol 1998; 159:2129-2131.
147. Sommer J, Stephens F: Dorsal ureteral diverticulum of the fossa navicularis: Symptoms, diagnosis and treatment. J Urol 1980;124:94-98.
148. Standoli L: Correzione Dell'ipospadias in tempo unico: Technica dell'ipospadias con tempo ad isola prepuziale. Rass Italia Chir Pediatr 1979;21:82-91.
149. Stoll C, Alembik Y, et al: Genetic and environmental factors in hypospadias. J Med Genet 1990;27:559-563.
150. Sutherland RW, Wiener JS, et al: Androgen receptor gene mutations are rarely associated with isolated penile hypospadias. J Urol 1996;156:828-831.
151. Svensson J, Berg R: Micturition studies and sexual function in operated hypospadiacs. Br J Urol 1983;55: 422-426.
152. Sweet R, Schrott H, et al: Study of the incidence of hypospa-

dias in Rochester, Minnesota 1940-1970, and a case-control comparison of possible etiologic factors. Mayo Clin Proc 1974;49:52-58.
153. Toppari J, Larsen JC, et al: Male reproductive health and environmental xenoestrogens. Environ Health Perspect 1996;104(Suppl 4):741-803.
154. Turner-Warwick R: The use of pedicle grafts in the repair of urinary tract fistulae. Br J Urol 1972;44:644-656.
155. Van der Meulen J: Hypospadias Monograph. Leiden, the Netherlands, AG Stenfert, Kroese, NV, 1964.
156. Walker R: Outpatient repair of urethral fistulae. Urol Clin North Am 1981;8:582-583.
157. Wilson JD, George FW, et al: The hormonal control of sexual development. Science 1981;211:1278-1284.
158. Wilson JD, Griffin JE, et al: Steroid 5 alpha-reductase 2 deficiency. Endocr Rev 1993;14:577-593.
159. Winslow BH, Vorstman B, et al: Urethroplasty using diverticular tissue. J Urol 1985;134:552-553.
160. Yeoman D, Cooke R, et al: Penile block for circumcision? A comparison with caudal block. Anesthesia 1983;38:862-866.
161. Young H: Genital Abnormalities, Hermaphroditism and Related Adrenal Diseases. Baltimore, Williams & Wilkins, 1937.
162. Yucel S, Baskin LS: Identification of communicating branches among the dorsal, perineal and cavernous nerves of the penis. J Urol 2003;170:153-158.
163. Yucel S, Baskin LS: Neuroanatomy of the male urethra and perineum. BJU Int 2003;92:624-630.
164. Yucel S, Liu W, et al: Anatomical studies of the fibroblast growth factor-10 mutant, Sonic Hedge Hog mutant, and androgen receptor mutant mouse genital tubercle. In Baskin L (ed): Hypospadias and Genital Development. Philadelphia, Kluwer Academic/Plenum, 2004, pp 123-145.
165. Zaontz MR: The GAP (glans approximation procedure) for glanular/coronal hypospadias. J Urol 1989;141:359-361.

第 120 章

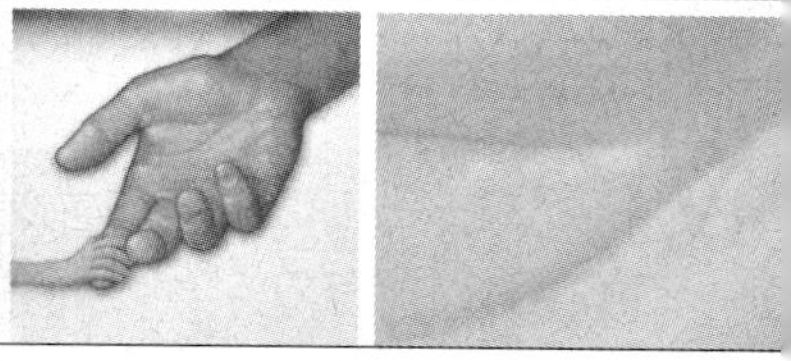

尿道、阴茎和阴囊畸形

J. Patrick Murphy 和 John M. Gatti

899 目前，产前就可以对尿道、阴茎和阴囊畸形进行评估。产前超声已成为产前诊断的重要工具，通过超声检查可以早期诊断出许多先天性泌尿生殖道畸形。实际上每例肾盂积水或者梗阻性的病变都可以在产前证实，但目前争论的焦点是产前治疗的有效性和适宜性。这点在后尿道瓣膜的治疗上尤为突出。对此采取的干预措施如膀胱羊膜腔转流和胎儿镜下尿道瓣膜切开均有过描述和应用，但是对预后是否有益还不是很确定[18,24,29]。

产前诊断令人喜忧参半。膀胱外翻的早期诊断可以给予胎儿家庭以忠告，也可以预先将新生儿转移至拥有治疗膀胱外翻专家的专业机构。但是，较为常见的肾盂积水却很少需要产前干预。除了这些，双亲的焦虑不安和医生的不确定往往诱发早产而将婴儿置于附加的危险中。家庭成员在患儿出生时常常处于困惑和失望中，并期望得到处理方法。父母亲会产生疑问，为什么产后匆忙转运却不立即给予干预治疗。产前干预和处理还在开展中，但这需要产科医生、围产科医生和产后处理这些畸形的外科医生之间进行培训和交流。

后尿道瓣膜

后尿道瓣膜（PUV）是尿道最常见的梗阻性畸形。新生儿男性发生率在 1/5000～1/8000 之间[33,42]。Hugh Hampton Young 是最先描述 PUV 并且对其进行分型的学者[125]。他将后尿道瓣膜分为 3 种类型：Ⅰ型、Ⅱ型和Ⅲ型。现在普遍认为Ⅱ型瓣膜为非梗阻性，而且仅涉及历史影响而已。95% 的 PUV 为Ⅰ型，表现为从精阜起源的膜状组织向远端延展插入邻近的膜性尿道前方，在精阜后方开放。病因可能是由于中肾管进入到泄殖腔时较正常偏前且在中线融合[114]。Ⅲ型瓣膜占 5%，表现为精阜远端有环形膜样组织，中央有开口，膜状组织偶尔会向远端移位而形成风向袋外观[27]。瓣膜的形成是因为泌尿生殖膜的不完全吸收所致。

目前，许多 PUV 病例是在产前通过超声检查提示有肾盂积水和（或）扩张、壁厚的膀胱而检测出来的。出生以后的超声可显示一个厚壁的膀胱和典型的扩张、延长的后尿道。肾盂积水的程度不同且可以是单侧或双侧的。体格检查可以发现扩张且张力高的膀胱、尿流无力、腹胀和可能具有的尿性腹水。如果胎儿受到羊水过少的影响，可能会产生呼吸窘迫和 Potter 综合征表现。大一点的患儿会发生尿路感染和排尿异常，尤其在白天会产生急迫性尿失禁。排尿性尿路造影通常的诊断标准是后尿道有扩张延长且突然过渡到远端的狭窄尿道，膀胱壁增厚伴有小梁小室形成，以及可能存在膀胱输尿管反流（图 120-1）。

PUV 的产前干预问题尚有争议。在过去的 10 年间产前超声诊断的准确性有了明显提高，但是非梗阻性疾病比如梅干腹综合征和严重的膀胱输尿管反流可能很难和 PUV 区别开来。产前干预包括早期分流、膀胱羊膜腔转流[29,30]、羊膜腔输注[57]、经皮胎儿膀胱镜[92,93,119]或是开放式胎儿手术[66]。所有这些操作对于胎儿和母亲都具有高风险性，包括早产、出血和感染。因此，只有那些拥有具备诊断和处理经验人员的治疗中心才可以考虑进行产前干预。在产前干预之 1900
前，即胎儿发育早期，可能已存在肾发育不良，解除梗阻的干预措施并不能使肾发育不良的情况逆转。因此大多数医生认为严重肾发育不良的胎儿并不是产前干预的理想人选。有许多参数来测定肾发育不良的严

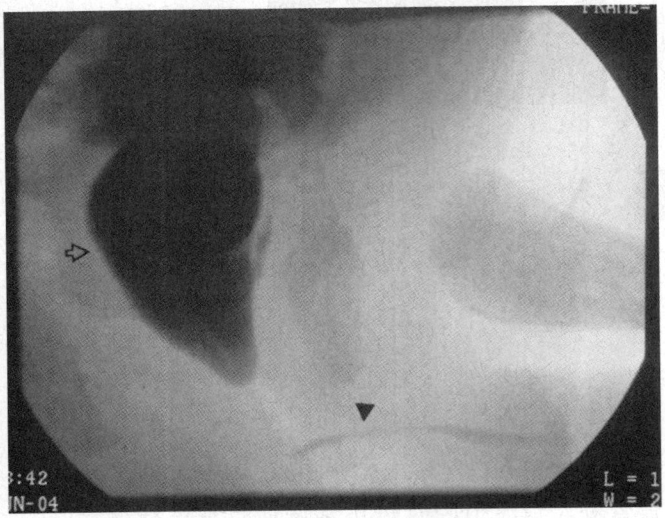

图 120-1　VCUG 显示了后尿道瓣膜影像表现，后尿道扩张（*空心箭头处*）和突然转变为狭窄的前尿道（*实心箭头处*）。有小梁形成的膀胱位于后尿道上方。

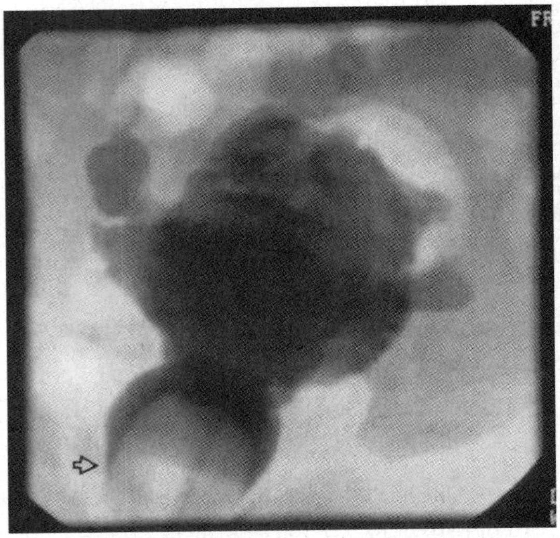

图 120-2　VCUG 显示了后尿道瓣膜和严重小梁形成的膀胱，Foley 球囊膨胀停留于扩张的后尿道内（*箭头处*）。

重程度。肾实质密度回声增高、肾实质囊性变和早期中度或重度的羊水过少都是严重肾发育不良的超声表现。经皮取出的胎儿尿样也可提示肾发育不良[18,24,39,112]。正常胎尿是低渗和低钠的，如果胎尿中钠超过100 mEq/L、渗透压超过 210 mOsm、尿蛋白超过20 mg/dl以及 β_2-微球蛋白超过 4 mg/L[71]，都提示存在严重的肾发育不良。具有这些影像学表现和尿检测指标的胎儿都不能获益于产前干预。与产后干预治疗相比，肾功能的总的长期预后并不能通过产前干预加以改善[29,30]。相反，那些做了产前治疗的患者似乎表现出了更加严重的梗阻，而且据说较那些产后处理的患者预后更差，当然这还存在争议。因此，产前治疗可能对这些高风险的患者有益。对 PUV 胎内干预最终作用的研究还在开展中，安全的新技术和早期治疗可能会改善预后[105]。

PUV 的产后治疗最初是进行膀胱引流。通常应用细而软的 5 或 8 French 鼻饲导管从尿道引流尿液。操作过程要小心以防止导管在扩张的后尿道中卷曲。膀胱超声可以确定其放置的合适位置。初期导尿时一般不用 Foley 导尿管，因为球囊在厚壁膀胱中会引起膀胱痉挛而影响尿液引流，或球囊可能会滑脱到扩张的后尿道中（图 120-2）。少数病例中，导尿管不能经尿道插入，只能进行经皮耻骨上穿刺。在开始的 24～48 小时内，液体和电解质治疗很重要。梗阻解除后多尿会使体液快速丧失，急需要水分和电解质的补充。酸碱平衡也同样重要，酸碱失衡可能会加重肾功能不全。要密切检测血清肌酐变化，其由肾脏排泄，应认识到在生命的最初几天里肌酐具有反映肾功能的价值。从以往处理看，当肌酐持续升高超过数天即要考虑进行耻骨上引流。然而，许多研究表明，相比标准的后尿道瓣膜切开或膀胱切开造口，耻骨上引流并不能对今后的肾功能起到改善作用[95,108,118]。没有必要进行预防性的抗生素应用，尤其是那些有肾盂积水或膀胱输尿管反流的患者。

当体液和电解质状况稳定后，大多数患者能够接受在内镜下行瓣膜切除术。随着纤维光学技术的进展，现在有了 7 French 标度的膀胱镜，可以进入到除了最小的早产婴儿以外的所有患儿的尿道。应用带有切割电流的 Bugbee 电极或小口径激光纤维[8]，放置在尿道中，在后退过程中对瓣膜的 5、7 和 12 点进行逐步切开。年长的儿童还可以用前列腺切除器进行操作，还有一些医生赞成经皮顺行电灼 PUV[126]。对于一些通过内镜不能进行瓣膜电灼的少见病例，可采用膀胱皮肤造口术。Blodksom 术式较受推崇，其方法是将膀胱顶提到皮肤处以减少膀胱塌陷的机会[9,22]。当患儿长大且医学上处于稳定期时，再通过内镜下行瓣膜切除和关闭膀胱造口。膀胱造口可能不会影响患儿远期的膀胱容量[42,81,91]。

近数十年来 PUV 患儿的远期预后有了改善，远期预后主要和三个因素紧密相关：（1）肾发育不良的程度，（2）伴或不伴有膀胱输尿管反流的尿路感染的发生率，（3）膀胱的功能状态。近 30 年来，患儿的总死亡率从 50% 降至 1%~3%[15,55]。新生儿护理水平的提高连同针对上述因素的治疗是预后改善的原因。肾发育不良是不可治愈的，但是对其他尿路感染和膀胱功能紊乱问题的关注能够减少和延缓肾进行性恶化的速度。在接受 PUV 治疗的患者中肾衰竭发生率高达 40%[95,108]。由于先进的医疗监护和免疫抑制治疗的应用，肾移植在这些患者的治疗中有所增加。移植成功者和那些没有明显尿路病变患儿的存活时间相当[53,82]。要注意对膀胱功能紊乱和急迫性尿失禁的高张膀胱的治疗，可以应用抗副交感神经疗法频繁排尿，对于延缓肾脏恶化或保护移植肾有重要意义。对于那些进行性膀胱肌源性失调和不能完全排空的膀胱，有必要进行间歇性清洁导尿和（或）整晚的膀胱引流。尿流动力学检查对于指导这类膀胱治疗很有帮助。在少数病例中行膀胱扩大术可能有必要[36,50,100,108]。膀胱输尿管反流（VUR）发生于大约一半的 PUV 患者[33,42,45]。这样高的发生率可能与膀胱高压有关，但是解剖发现与输尿管位置相关的原发性反流也很常见[47]。反流常常是双侧的，三分之一到二分之一的患者在瓣膜电灼后反流情况消失[33,45]。单侧输尿管反流有时与一侧扩张的发育不良并且功能较差的肾脏有关。这提示膀胱输尿管反流-肾发育不良（VURD）综合征对膀胱和对侧肾脏有一定的保护效应，即所谓的“popoff”机制，如继发于肾穹窿破裂后的大的膀胱憩室或尿性腹水[44,51,97]。

传统观点认为切除扩张且发育不良的肾和输尿管可以提高排泄率和减少感染几率[51]。最近更多的证据表明保留这些发育不良的肾单位并不会造成感染和影响肾功能，可以将其留在原位[58]。在那些应用常规方法治疗高压膀胱却不能奏效的少见病例，这些扩张的输尿管还可以在输尿管膀胱成形术时用做膀胱扩大的材料[14]。

在最初的 PUV 治疗时输尿管反流可以不处理[54]，只有那些尽管应用合适的药物预防和对膀胱功能失调进行适当治疗后还是反复尿路感染的患者，才需要进行输尿管再植术。VUR 的发生可能不会改变长期预后，除非有反复的尿路感染问题[45,52]。随着时间流逝，膀胱经过适当治疗后，扩张的输尿管可能回缩且膀胱壁会有改善。如果最后的确需要输尿管再植治疗，那么外科手术更容易改善效果。

男孩前尿道瓣膜

前尿道瓣膜发生几率远低于后尿道瓣膜，但是总的表现和对尿道的影响十分相似。它可以发生在前尿道的任何地方，在尿道球部略为多见[101]。它很有可能是由尿道腹侧的憩室发展而来。随着排尿时尿流向前，这种憩室样结构破坏了远端尿路，使得普通的尿道壁构成了一个梗阻性瓣膜[116]。其他的假设则认为由于原发性海绵体薄弱或尿道复制中断造成了这种病变[121]。放射影像学可以确定诊断，排尿性膀胱尿路造影显示出前尿道近端扩张而前尿道远端狭窄，常常还有一个微小的膜状组织。治疗方法可以通过内镜切除这些瓣膜，最好在直视下轻微灌洗尿道（防止强有力的灌注液将瓣膜展平）。肾盂积水和膀胱输尿管反流常常也和该病并存，治疗原则同后尿道瓣膜[41]。

有一种类似的病变为尿道舟状窝或称为 Guérin 瓣膜，是一种只发生在舟状窝处的尿道背侧憩室。这是一种少见的实性结构且需要切开，方式如前所述。由于病变靠近阴茎头端，所以可能很难诊断，但是龟头部的膀胱排尿造影可以显示远端病变[109]。

女孩尿道憩室

女性儿童尿道憩室很少见。这种病变可以表现为排尿困难、血尿或梗阻症状。由于女性尿道短，所以影像学诊断非常困难。但可以用膀胱镜来诊断，也可以用其来治疗，如果病变小可以采用内镜下憩室后唇切开[60]。

尿道狭窄

男孩的尿道狭窄情况多于女孩。尿道狭窄可以分为先天性、感染性、医源性或外伤性[56]。先天性狭窄极少见，但是可以存在尿道发育不全。感染性狭窄在儿童期不多见，而常常和性活跃青春期的淋菌性或滴虫性尿道炎有关系。长期留置导管而引发的感染在现代已经很少见。医源性狭窄发生在尿道手术或检查后。

前尿道外伤性狭窄可发生在骑跨伤后，即摔落在自行车横挡上时尿道被挤压在耻骨上。后尿道狭窄通

常发生于骨盆骨折导致的错位。在有尿道口出血、膀胱高跨和前列腺位于腹腔，以及行肛指检查或怀疑有
1902 骨盆骨折时，插管前都应进行逆行尿路造影，以防止因为插管使尿道从本来的部分断裂变成完全断裂。对于尿道部分断裂的情况，通常可采取内镜和荧光镜导管放入并留置导尿管的方法，这样要持续到伤口愈合而且行 RUG 检查时从导管周围注入的造影剂没有溢出。对于完全尿道断裂的初期治疗还有争议。先行耻骨上置管或膀胱造口，延迟大约 6 个月后再行重建手术的观点现在普遍被接受，但是一些学者提倡应用逆行尿道镜和顺行膀胱镜放置导管穿过缺损处，使得尿道先获得初步连接[87]。

狭窄的位置和长度决定治疗方案。大多数医生应用顺行膀胱镜结合逆行尿路造影来测定这些参数，但是有其他报道称采用术中超声显像测定更为准确[76]。短而薄弱的狭窄通常可以通过切开或扩张获得肯定的效果[85]。一些学者成功地应用渐进性尿道扩张来处理尿道发育不良[86]。对于球部尿道的长段狭窄或复发性狭窄的治疗，通常是切除狭窄部分，然后如同竹节样端端靠拢缝合。这需要耻骨下切开或阴茎体布局改变来覆盖长的间隔[75]。因为切除狭窄后再重新靠拢可能造成阴茎腹曲，舟状窝和下垂的尿道不够宽大。这些部位的长段狭窄治疗通常要用到皮瓣转移或是应用包皮边、阴茎体皮肤或颊黏膜[21]。这些患者需要长时期的随访，尽管大多数狭窄在一年内复发。

尿道闭锁

尿道闭锁和肾脏发育是矛盾的，除非膀胱和外界有替代通路来排出尿液，如开放的脐尿管。产前干预，即膀胱羊膜腔转流，可以帮助胎儿存活并分娩，但常常伴有明显的肾发育不良。这和梅干腹综合征有很强的联系[43]。围生期相关问题，即膀胱以下的尿路梗阻，必须最先解决，以后的重建将根据尿道发育程度的不同因人而异，不过大多数患儿最终还需要做某种可控性尿路转流手术解决问题。

女孩尿道狭窄

女孩尿道狭窄的概念尚未形成主流的说法。曾经认为女孩的尿路刺激、排尿梗阻或反复发作的尿路感染与尿路狭窄有关，而排尿性膀胱尿路造影能支持诊断，发现狭窄尿路位于泌尿生殖膈和括约肌水平。但现在认识到放射影像学和临床表现提示的只是排尿功能紊乱，与排尿时括约肌活动的不协调有关。尽管通过扩张后可以出现短期的外括约肌放松效应，但是并不主张尿道扩张，这是由于它不会产生长期效应，而且在过度扩张后有产生真正尿道狭窄的可能。

女孩尿道肿块

有多种病变可以以尿道肿块的形式存在于年轻女孩尿道中。该病变常常通过仔细检查就可获得诊断。尿道口病变包括尿道脱垂、输尿管囊肿脱垂、尿道囊肿或肉瘤。阴道病变可能会被误认为来源于尿道，包括 Gartner 管（卵巢冠纵管）囊肿、处女膜闭锁和肉瘤。

尿道脱垂最初发现于青春期前的非洲裔美国女孩，但是白种女孩也常常发病[26,98]。主要症状为污染内裤和排尿疼痛。体格检查可以发现在尿道口水平有一圈半透明的尿道组织突出，病变看似娇嫩的玫瑰，呈现出红色或紫色。可以试用坐浴法和雌激素乳膏治疗；当上法无效时，可以手术切除多余的尿道组织，再将尿道黏膜与邻近的尿道口上皮吻合。该手术并发症很少，但有出血、复发或尿道狭窄的可能。

输尿管囊肿脱垂也是水肿性质的肿块，但常较易区别，因其和周围的尿道口没有关系。症状包括有内裤污血、排尿疼痛或尿潴留。当超声检查发现有肾输尿管积水合并输尿管异位时可以确定诊断。如果输尿管囊肿不能自行消退，可以通过膀胱镜去顶减压，最后切除或再进行重建手术。

横纹肌肉瘤是最常见的原发性恶性肿瘤，可以累及婴儿和儿童的输尿管、阴道或膀胱，可能表现同以上症状。葡萄串样病变常呈外部生长并放射性生长于阴道或尿道阴道隔，一般在 2 岁前发病。尿道边缘至少部分不连续，这样可以将其和尿道脱垂区别开来。本病典型表现为葡萄状簇集团块从阴道口突出，会引起出血。放射影像检查可以充分评估肿块，并可以排除是否已向肺、肝或骨髓内转移。经组织学确诊后，可进行化学治疗、放射治疗和手术切除等多种治疗[83,103]。

处女膜闭锁表现为阴道口有肿块膨出，合并有阴道积液或子宫阴道积液，常常可在腹部触诊到扩张的子宫或阴道。尿道位于肿块的前方。治疗方法是进行切开和引流。

各种各样的囊肿都可发生在尿道口区域，包括上皮样囊肿、Skene 管囊肿、苗勒氏囊肿和午非氏管或 Gartner 管囊肿，可以行切除和引流，复发后再切除。
903 Gartner 管囊肿沿阴道壁分布并靠近膀胱，处理上要慎重，因为其胚胎来源于午非氏管或中肾管。因此，异位输尿管末端可能开口于囊肿，而囊肿破溃于阴道内会引起慢性滴尿失禁。尽管 Gartner 管囊肿在婴儿中不常见，但其是儿童期阴道膨胀增大的最常见的良性病变。一般可以没有症状，但一旦增大病变可能突出于阴道，并且和尿潴留或性活跃青春期的性交困难有关[80]。治疗方法通常采用袋形缝合术，但是当病变和异位输尿管相关时就需要近端重建，包括输尿管再植或肾切除。

尿道息肉少见，可引起间歇性出血或梗阻，可切除治疗[59]。

阴唇粘连

阴唇粘连，或称小阴唇融合，是由与外阴阴道炎有关的慢性炎症刺激或与尿失禁有关的慢性潮湿引起的。阴唇可以近乎完全靠拢融合，引起梗阻症状或不可控制的排尿障碍。最多见的症状是排尿后的不自主滴尿，这是因为坐位排尿时少量尿液积在这层隔膜上，当患儿处于站立位时滴尿于内裤上。慢性潮湿也可能引起瘙痒或尿痛等刺激症状，由于在这个粘连部位取样有一定障碍，所以留取无菌尿样较困难。

如果无尿路感染、尿痛、梗阻和尿失禁等情况，则不需要对阴唇粘连进行治疗，因为接近青春期时雌激素生理性释放，粘连通常可以缓解。如果对粘连进行治疗，可试用雌激素乳膏（0.01%）外用，每天 2 次，连续 2～4 周，但可能将近半数患者无效[79]。青春期前患儿长时间应用雌激素可能有外阴部色素沉着、乳芽发育或乳房压痛的风险。停止用药后以上症状可以逆转。有效的替代治疗是倍他米松乳膏（0.05%），一般一天 2 次，连续一个月[110]。

如果粘连持续存在或出现肥厚并继续进展，需要局部涂抹丙胺卡因 + 利多卡因（EMLA）乳膏后进行手术分离。用顶端带有棉花的涂药器或止血钳钝性向前后方向推开粘连部分。很重要的一点就是要在表皮损伤的小阴唇上涂抹润滑剂或抗生素油膏以防止再次粘连直至愈合。

Cowper 腺畸形

Cowper 腺（尿道球腺）成对位于尿道球部即泌尿生殖膈处，引流入球部尿道。当腺体引流出现梗阻时，可以形成一种表现如*空洞性脊髓突出*（syringoceles）的囊肿[70]。在尿道造影中可以表现为尿道球部有一充盈缺损或在破裂后呈现出充盈缺损的影像。作者认为大多数囊肿没有症状，一些囊肿可能会有终末血尿、尿道血迹、尿路感染或梗阻症状。一般治疗是内镜下去顶术，即把主要部分切除以防止梗阻，就像前面所讲的前尿道瓣膜的治疗一样。会阴开放手术只用于巨大囊肿[10]。

尿道息肉

尿道息肉一般发病于前列腺尿道，而且呈纤维肌性上皮结构并表面覆盖移行上皮[94]。偶尔也会发病于前尿道[16,88]，不论在哪个部位都会引起血尿、尿急或梗阻性症状。膀胱超声可以显示后尿道息肉（图 120-3），但是通常用排尿性膀胱尿路造影和膀胱镜检查诊断，膀胱镜下行切除治疗[38]。

前列腺囊肿 1904

前列腺囊肿是苗勒氏管的残余物，常见于具有两性特征的患者或有近端尿道下裂的患者。囊肿的增大可导致尿路症状，主要症状有尿路感染、排尿困难、尿急、血尿或附睾炎[120]。诊断通常依靠排尿性膀胱尿路造影或 RUG，超声可以检测到这些残余物，尤其是残余物较大时[61]。对那些有反复尿路症状的患者采用手术治疗。手术入路根据外科医生的经验可以选择经腹、经膀胱、经会阴、经后矢状（经直肠或直肠周围）或腹腔镜手术[7,63,73,106,120,124]。

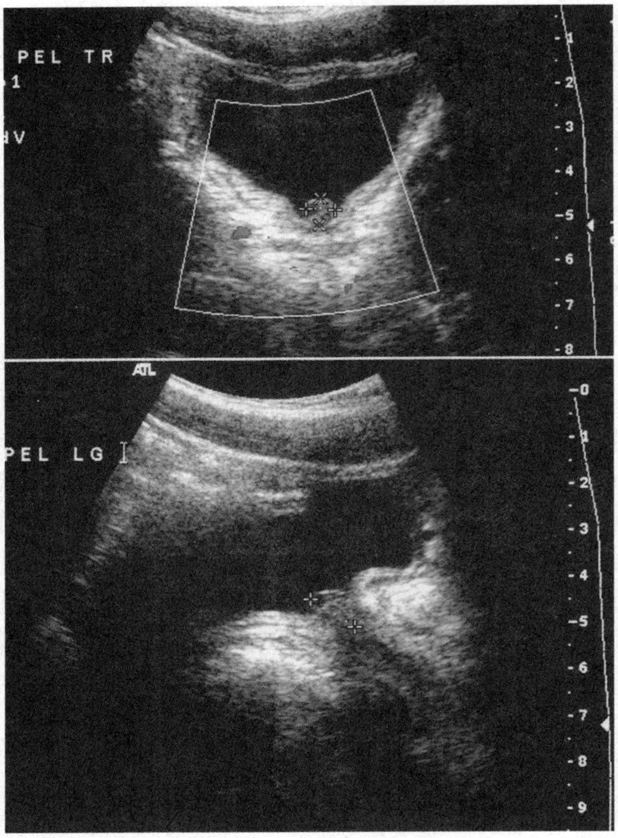

图 120-3　在膀胱内看到后尿道息肉的超声表现。上面影像显示膀胱的横断面，可见从后尿道升至膀胱内的息肉（*见指针*）。下面影像显示膀胱的纵切面，可以看到息肉从膀胱出口进入到后尿道（*见指针*）。

重复尿道

尿道重复较为罕见，常见于男性。尽管这种缺陷的胚胎学解释还有争议，但是多种多样的异常说明并没有共同的病因学可以解释所有表现。尿道重复可以连同膀胱重复直到龟头重复。在男性中，重复尿道呈矢状面排列于一个单一的阴茎体内[23]。较少见的病例表现为重复尿道并排分布在宽大或重复阴茎的龟头上（图 120-4）。矢状面排列的重复尿道中，位于腹侧的尿道一般较为正常，经过前列腺和括约肌。这条尿道可以开口在龟头顶端到肛门周围区域的任何地方。

背侧尿道可以开口在从尿道上裂到耻骨周周区域的阴茎体的任何部位。如果存在阴茎背屈和较宽的耻骨联合，提示可能合并有膀胱外翻复合畸形[4,90,99,104]。这条背侧尿道可以与膀胱或腹侧尿道相通（图 120-5），

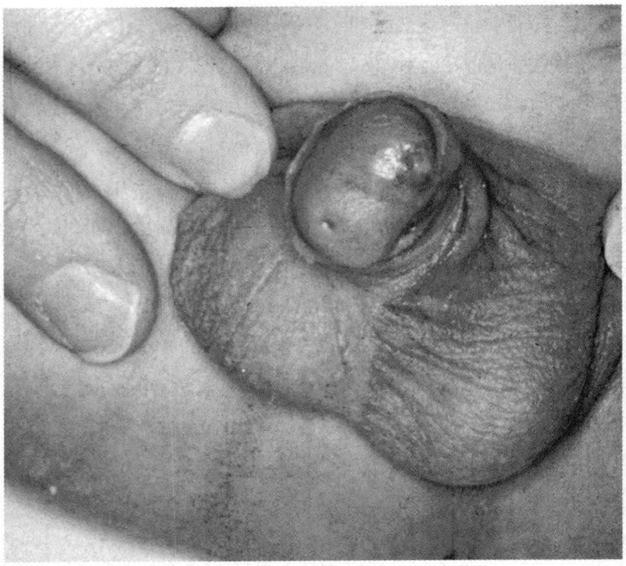

图 120-4　重复尿道在龟头两侧分别开口而且阴茎呈逆时针扭转。

但也可能在耻骨联合下方以盲端结束。如果与膀胱或腹侧尿道有交通，则由于背侧尿道不穿过括约肌而可能导致尿失禁。对于有症状的患者，处理包括切除背侧多余的尿道并通过尿道整形纠正阴茎弯曲，必要时还要把腹侧尿道转移至龟头。对于极少数背侧尿道占优势而腹侧尿道多余的病例，要切除腹侧尿道治疗尿失禁。对于那些更少见的并排尿道，需要根据不同的解剖情况行个体化处理。所有类型的尿道重复病例都要求进行全尿路放射影像学造影检查。

女性尿道重复可能合并有完全的膀胱和生殖器重复，也可能同时有结肠闭锁和（或）泄殖腔畸形[32]。背侧多余的尿道可以位于耻骨区域，还有报道称其与脐尿管残余相通[65]。治疗方面也要根据上述特别的解剖情况行个体化处理，尽量保护膀胱组织和保证控尿能力。

巨尿道

巨尿道是尿道扩张中少见的类型。巨尿道分两种类型：舟形和纺锤形。舟形巨尿道的形成和尿道海绵体的发育异常有关，排尿时可以看到尿道前面部分形成膨胀。在比较严重的纺锤形巨尿道（图 120-6）中，病变涉及整个阴茎的海绵体，由于长期的排尿冲

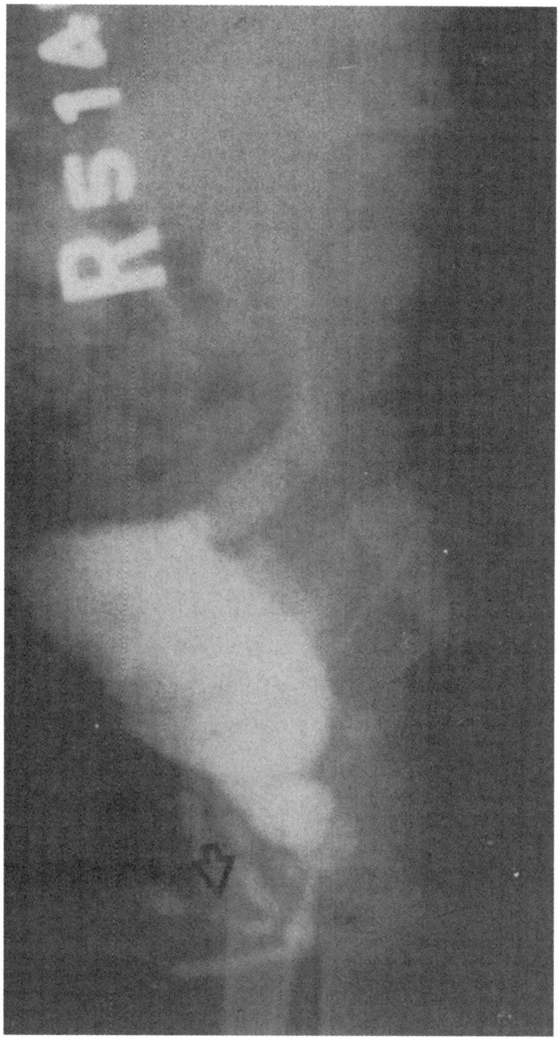

图 120-5 重复尿道位于背侧（箭头）且存在于耻骨上区域。

击造成尿道呈圆周状扩张[5]。这种病变一般在出生时可以发现，也可以在产前超声检查中得到诊断[102]。

该病的病因尚不清楚，可能与中胚叶发育缺陷有关，尤其和梅干腹综合征同时存在时[77]。肾脏-膀胱超声检测可排除其他的先天性畸形。因为扩张是非梗阻性的，为了美观，可行尿道成形手术，即切除多余的尿道组织和使尿道变细。

先天性尿瘘

先天性尿瘘较为罕见，通常发生于阴茎冠状沟下方的区域。因为合并有尿道下裂和阴茎下弯，提示其可能是尿道下裂畸形的组成部分。瘘口远端的尿道通常形态良好，但是如果龟头形态不佳，尿道可能较细。修补方法可以采用尿道下裂手术方式，也可以只是简单的多层瘘口关闭或是远端尿道和龟头进行复杂的重建[12,96]。

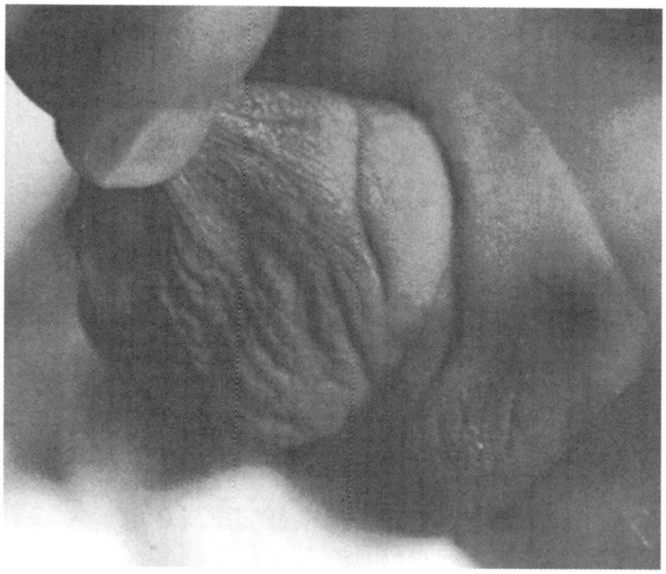

图 120-6 巨尿道，纺锤形。

包茎

*包茎*的定义是包皮不能上翻。出生时，生理性包茎是由于包皮和龟头的粘连使得包皮不能上翻。随着生长，因为上皮屑脱落或包皮垢在两层组织中堆积，使得两者分离。包皮垢通常被称为“包皮珠”，可能会被那些未受过相关教育的父母误认为是感染和化脓。随着自然勃起和本能的挤压，超过 90% 的孩子在 3～4 岁时可以上翻包皮[84]。

包皮不需要强行上翻，因为这样可能会造成包皮撕裂和瘢痕形成，如此恶性循环可造成病理性包茎。孩子超过 4 岁后还不能上翻包皮，或有包皮炎、龟头包皮炎发作时，可以试用倍他米松乳膏（0.05%）涂抹，一天 2 次，用药 1～2 个月后 90% 以上的患儿包皮可以上翻[67]。对糖皮质激素治疗耐受或有鼓包征提示有排尿梗阻的情况时，通常行阴茎包皮背侧姑息性切开或环切手术。

包皮环切术

包皮环切是泌尿学科最有争议的话题之一。美国儿科学会在1975年就制定了政策方针，即新生儿常规行包皮环切术而没有绝对的医疗适应证[117]。1999年，该学会又提出新的意见，即环切手术有一些医疗益处，但这不足以成为常规手术[2]。

包皮环切的提倡者认为环切后的男孩子有较低的尿路感染率、拉链伤害率或包茎发生率、性疾病传播率及成年后的阴茎癌发生率[17,64,69,123]。反对者则提出这种操作是非生理性的，可能没有必要，甚至是有害的。一些极端反对者们提出环切后男性的阴茎感觉下降、性交满意率下降，甚至可能出现高离婚率[40]。令人遗憾的是这种意见有情绪化的倾向，而且有大量的主观性“支持性研究”。Ganiats 和同事们分析后认为新生儿常规环切手术在经济方面及医疗方面的利弊可相互抵消，与费用及健康影响相比，个人的文化背景和宗教信仰是决定是否施行手术的关键[31]。

不管如何争论，包皮环切手术仍旧是美国最普遍的选择性手术之一，通常是由于美观和文化的原因。

包皮环切的风险在大范围人群中发生率很低（<1%），主要包括出血、感染、皮肤裂开、粘连、皮肤切除太多或太少和包皮狭窄等[1,122]。用于新生儿的环切方法主要有两种——Plastibell 法和 Gomco 夹法。两种方法并发症发生率相似，Plastibell 法感染发生率稍高，而 Gomco 夹法包皮裂开率较高[34]。Mogan 法还会引起龟头损伤，应该让有足够操作经验的人员执行这种方法。

技术方法

新生儿包皮环切可以在床边进行，或者当2～3个月龄时在手术室进行。作者提倡用局部麻醉，即在操作前施行表面或皮下麻醉。包皮处于无张力情况下在游离包皮上触摸冠状沟的界限给以标记，指示出合适的钳夹位置。用止血钳将龟头和粘连的包皮分离出间隙。用一把直的止血钳在包皮的背侧中线位置钳夹后剪开，以便放置器械进行操作。所有粘连处都要分离并取出包皮垢。手术要选择合适尺寸的止血钳，止血钳的圆锥部分应覆盖住龟头的大部分。一旦钳夹到位就把位于止血钳以上的多余包皮去除，先前标记的位置用止血钳进行咬合（Gomco）或用缝线结扎（Plastibell）。在止血钳上方牵拉包皮时应仔细操作，这样可以防止包皮在钳夹器上折叠以及包皮内板和近端阴茎皮肤在钳夹时对合不良。包皮内板和外板应等长切除，这样可以避免由于不适当的包皮内板过多或残留引起包皮过长复发，使得阴茎隐匿或埋藏。因为阴茎几乎完全不出血，所以包皮环切时不必应用电刀（图120-7）。

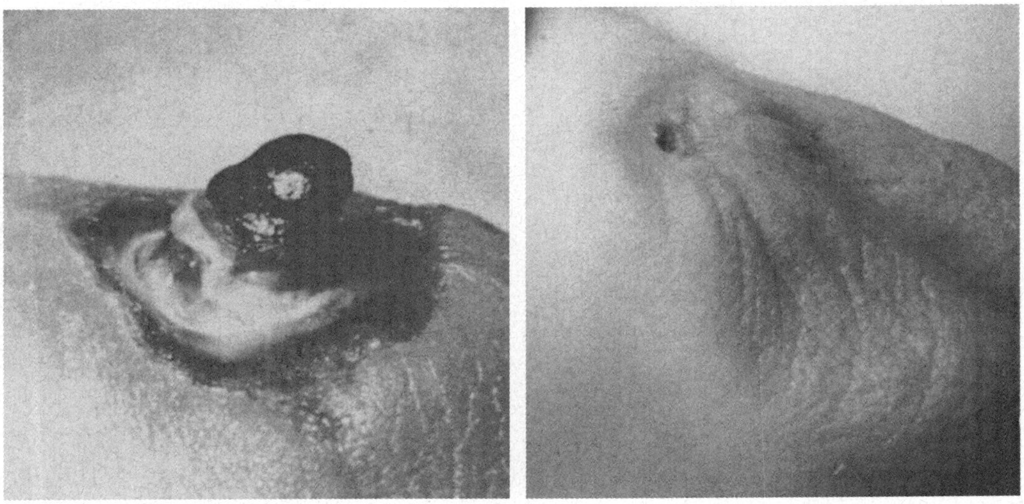
A B

图120-7 应用了金属夹基础上的电烙术造成新生儿包皮环切术的损伤。A. 术后即刻的表现。B. 手术后3个月的结果。

对于大一些的儿童，当麻醉风险减至最小时（6 个月以后），可在全身麻醉下进行操作。由于大孩子应用钳夹器械不可靠且尺寸不合适，所以作者所在的中心采用徒手器械操作。在切开前必须仔细标记近端和远端的切口，近端切口标记在冠状沟边缘上方，切除突出的包皮脂肪垫。多余的包皮沿阴茎标记线用电刀切除。应用电刀的好处是可以止血，但遇到大血管时需要结扎。切缘应用铬制缝线做皮下缝合，这样可以避免皮下缝线形成结节。手术部位可以涂抹少量的抗生素药膏，盖上纱布，纱布可以等待自然脱落或几天后取下。也鼓励术后 1 天就早期开始洗澡，在接下来的几个星期内，家长在手术部位涂抹药膏，至少一天 3 次。在手术结束时通常采取骶管阻滞或阴茎背部神经和环行阻滞麻醉，这样有助于术后镇痛。

尿道口狭窄

包皮环切术后大约有 10% 的男孩会出现尿道口狭窄[3]。若排除干燥性闭塞性龟头炎，则事实证明在未经过包皮环切术的男孩身上没有尿道口狭窄的发生。作者认为这是因为包皮环切后尿道口直接接触尿液（引起氨性皮炎）造成对尿道口的慢性刺激，或是因为在环切过程中处理包皮系带动脉时损伤了尿道口的脉管系统引起了出血。尿道口狭窄的典型病史是尿流细且向背侧偏斜，偏斜度往往大于 90 度。尿道口细小且通过 6 或 8 French
907 尿管时感到紧缩。尿道口狭窄可能与疼痛或出血污染内裤有关，也可能无关。这种疾病往往被过多诊断，那些有排尿疼痛而缺乏这些体征的患儿通常有排尿功能失调，伴有排尿时括约肌不协调。

尿道口狭窄的治疗方法是尿道外口切开术，即将腹侧尿道口周围组织用夹子或止血钳（作者采用无齿肠钳）夹住，然后大约切开至冠状沟边缘的一半。切开的边缘用抗生素药膏涂抹，家长也需积极配合进行药膏涂抹，每天 3 次至少一个星期以避免复发，当然复发并不常见。这个手术可以在诊室局麻下安全进行，也可在手术室进行[13]。

阴茎发育不全

先天性阴茎发育不全相当罕见，发病率为 1/1 000 000～1/3 000 000[46,107]。它是生殖结节部分或完全发育不良的结果。染色体型通常是 46，XY，而尿道常常开口于肛门周围或直肠[46,107]。本症往往合并一些畸形，包括隐睾症、肾脏畸形、膀胱输尿管反流、肛门畸形和心脏畸形[25,46,107]。越是近端尿道受累，合并畸形的发生率就越高，而且新生儿死亡率也越高[107]。对于女性性征明显的病例，按照惯例进行睾丸切除以及尿道、生殖器重建手术[46,115]。然而近年来有证据表明，尽管女性特征明显，但如果患者想要保留男性性征，则需经两性鉴定小组，包括泌尿学、内分泌和精神病学专家周密考虑，并得到家属的完全赞同后才能采取上述手术[20]。保留男性性征后待以后再重建新的阴茎，这种只是出于美观而限制功能的方法可能会得到赞同[20]。

阴茎重复畸形

新生儿阴茎重复发病率为 1/5 000 000[74,78]，重复程度不一，病因可能是中胚层联合异常或中胚叶遇到了两个尿道原基[49]。重复可表现为从仅有一个小的副阴茎到完全重复的尿道、龟头和阴茎体（图 120-8）。重复阴茎的大小尺寸不同，方向大多数是一边一个。合并的畸形有尿道下裂、阴囊异常、重复膀胱、肾脏异常、膀胱外

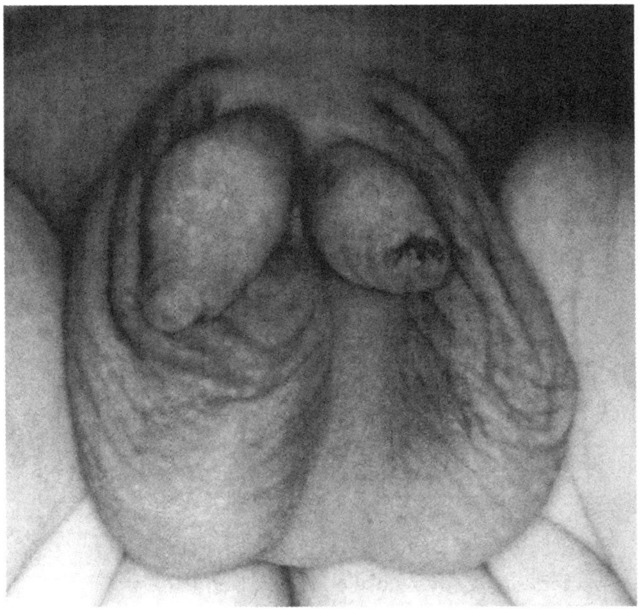

图 120-8　阴茎重复畸形，见两阴茎彼此相邻的结构。

翻和肛门及心脏畸形。进行全尿道造影、超声及核磁共振检查有助于评价阴茎的解剖发育情况[72]。外科手术方式必须根据缺陷程度的不同因人而异，可以是从简单的副阴茎切除到完全的重建手术[74]。

阴茎扭转

阴茎扭转是阴茎的一种旋转缺陷，常常呈逆时针方向且常合并有尿道下裂、阴茎下弯和包皮的背侧堆积。阴茎中轴线通常倾斜向左侧。小于90度的旋转一般没有症状且不需要纠正。外科手术治疗包括阴茎脱鞘、松解纤维组织和阴茎根部各个方向的非生理性束缚，使得阴茎适应于合适的位置[6]。在少见病例中，可能需要将阴茎根部固定于耻骨前方或应用肉膜瓣来旋转阴茎，这样可以使阴茎保持在合适的位置[28]。

阴茎阴囊反位和阴囊异位

阴囊是阴囊唇转移并向下中部的生殖结节折叠后形成的。可能是与引带缺陷相关的转移异常导致了阴囊畸形，包括阴茎阴囊转位、阴囊分裂或阴囊异位[111]。合并尿道下裂和阴茎下弯较多见。阴囊缺陷越是明显，其他畸形也越容易发生，包括骶尾部退化、VATER综合征、隐睾症和其他泌尿道畸形[48,68,111]。

明显的阴茎阴囊转位的修复需要应用各种各样的皮瓣技术。当合并有严重的尿道下裂需要包皮岛状皮
1908 瓣进行修补时，阴茎阴囊转位纠正往往在第二步进行，以避免引起岛状皮瓣的血供不良[35,89]。另外建议尿道下裂修补和阴囊转位纠治同步进行，但并发症趋于增加[19,37,62]。对于阴囊异位并发隐睾的病例，阴囊成形术和睾丸固定术常可同时完成。

（何 蓉译 文建国校）

参考文献

1. American Academy of Pediatrics: Report of the Task Force on Circumcision. Pediatrics 1989;84:388-391.
2. American Academy of Pediatrics, Task Force on Circumcision: Circumcision policy statement. Pediatrics 1999;103:686-693.
3. Allen JS, Summers JL, Wilkerson JE: Meatal calibration of newborn boys. J Urol 1972;107:498.
4. Al-Wattar KM: Congenital prepubic sinus: An epispadiac variant of urethral duplication: Case report and review of literature. J Pediatr Surg 2003;38:E10.
5. Appel RA, Kaplan GW, Brock WA, et al: Megalourethra. J Urol 1986;135:747-751.
6. Azmy A, Eckstein HB: Surgical correction of torsion of the penis. Br J Urol 1981;53:378-379.
7. Benedetto VD, Bagnara V, Guys JM, et al: A transvesical approach to mullerian duct remnants. Pediatr Surg Int 1997;12:151-154.
8. Biewald W, Schier F: Laser treatment of posterior urethral valves in neonates. Br J Urol 1992;69:425-427.
9. Blocksom BH Jr: Bladder pouch for prolonged tubeless cystostomy. J Urol 1957;78:398-401.
10. Brock WA, Kaplan GW: Lesions of Cowper's glands in children. J Urol 1979;122:121-123.
11. Brown MR, Cartwright PC, Snow BW: Common office problems in pediatric urology and gynecology. Pediatr Clin North Am 1997;44:1091-1115.
12. Caldamone AA, Chen SC, Elder JS, et al: Congenital anterior urethrocutaneous fistula. J Urol 1999;162:1430-1432.
13. Cartwright PC, Snow BW, McNees DC: Urethral meatotomy in the office using topical EMLA cream for anesthesia. J Urol 1996;156:857-858; discussion 858-859.
14. Churchill BM, Aliabadi H, Landau EH, et al: Ureteral bladder augmentation. J Urol 1993;150:716-720.
15. Churchill BM, McLorie GA, Khoury AE, et al: Emergency treatment and long-term follow-up of posterior urethral valves. Urol Clin North Am 1990;17:343-360.
16. Coleburn NH, Hensle TW: Anterior urethral polyp associated with hematuria in six-year-old child. Urology 1991;38:143-144.
17. Cook LS, Koutsky LA, Holmes KK: Circumcision and sexually transmitted diseases. Am J Public Health 1994;84:197-201.
18. Crombleholme TM, Harrison MR, Golbus MS, et al: Fetal intervention in obstructive uropathy: Prognostic indicators and efficacy of intervention. Am J Obstet Gynecol 1990;162:1239-1244.
19. DeFoor W, Wacksman J: Results of single staged hypospadias surgery to repair penoscrotal hypospadias with bifid scrotum or penoscrotal transposition. J Urol 2003;170:1585-1588; discussion 1588.
20. Diamond M: Pediatric management of ambiguous and traumatized genitalia. J Urol 1999;162:1021-1028.
21. Duckett JW, Coplen D, Ewalt D, et al: Buccal mucosal urethral replacement. J Urol 1995;153:1660-1663.
22. Duckett JW Jr: Cutaneous vesicostomy in childhood: The Blocksom technique. Urol Clin North Am 1974;1:485-495.
23. Effmann EL, Lebowitz RL, Colodny AH: Duplication of the urethra. Radiology 1976;119:179-185.
24. Elder JS, O'Grady JP, Ashmead G, et al: Evaluation of fetal renal function: Unreliability of fetal urinary electrolytes. J Urol 1990;144:574-578; discussion 593-594.
25. Evans JA, Erdile LB, Greenberg CR, et al: Agenesis of the penis: Patterns of associated malformations. Am J Med Genet 1999;84:47-55.
26. Fernandes ET, Dekermacher S, Sabadin MA, et al: Urethral prolapse in children. Urology 1993;41:240-242.
27. Field PL, Stephens FD: Congenital urethral membranes causing urethral obstruction. J Urol 1974;111:250-255.
28. Fisher C, Park M: Penile torsion repair using dorsal dartos flap rotation. J Urol 2004;171:1903-1904.

29. Freedman AL, Bukowski TP, Smith CA, et al: Fetal therapy for obstructive uropathy: Diagnosis specific outcomes [corrected]. J Urol 1996;156:720-723; discussion 723-724.
30. Freedman AL, Evans MI, Johnson MP: Complications of vesicoamniotic shunt placement for antenatal obstructive uropathy. J Urol 1997;157:3.
31. Ganiats TG, Humphrey JB, Taras HL, et al: Routine neonatal circumcision: A cost-utility analysis. Med Decis Making 1991;11:282-293.
32. Gastol P, Baka-Jakubiak M, Skobejko-Wlodarska L, et al: Complete duplication of the bladder, urethra, vagina, and uterus in girls. Urology 2000;55:578-581.
33. Gatti JM, Kirsch AJ: Posterior urethral valves: pre- and postnatal management. Curr Urol Rep 2001;2:138-145.
34. Gee WF, Ansell JS: Neonatal circumcision: A ten-year overview: with comparison of the Gomco clamp and the Plastibell device. Pediatrics 1976;58:824-827.
35. Germiyanoglu C, Ozkardes H, Altug U, et al: Reconstruction of penoscrotal transposition. Br J Urol 1994;73:200-203.
36. Ghanem MA, Wolffenbuttel KP, De Vylder A, et al: Long-term bladder dysfunction and renal function in boys with posterior urethral valves based on urodynamic findings. J Urol 2004;171:2409-2412.
37. Glassberg KI, Hansbrough F, Horowitz M: The Koyanagi-Nonomura 1-stage bucket repair of severe hypospadias with and without penoscrotal transposition. J Urol 1998;160:1104-1107; discussion 1137.
38. Gleason PE, Kramer SA: Genitourinary polyps in children. Urology 1994;44:106-109.
39. Glick PL, Harrison MR, Golbus MS, et al: Management of the fetus with congenital hydronephrosis II: Prognostic criteria and selection for treatment. J Pediatr Surg 1985;20:376-387.
40. Goldman R: The hidden trauma. In Circumcision. Boston, Vangard, 1997, pp 144-147.
41. Golimbu M, Orca M, Al-Askari S, et al: Anterior urethral valves. Urology 1978;12:343-346.
42. Gonzales ET: Posterior urethral valves and other urethral anomalies. In Walsh PC, et al (eds): Campbell's Urology. Philadelphia, WB Saunders, 2002, pp 2207-2330.
43. Gonzalez R, De Filippo R, Jednak R, et al: Urethral atresia: Long-term outcome in 6 children who survived the neonatal period. J Urol 2001;165:2241-2244.
44. Greenfield SP, Hensle TW, Berdon WE, et al: Unilateral vesicoureteral reflux and unilateral nonfunctioning kidney associated with posterior urethral valves—a syndrome? J Urol 1983;130:733-738.
45. Hassan JM, Pope JC 4th, Brock JW 3rd, et al: Vesicoureteral reflux in patients with posterior urethral valves. J Urol 2003;170:1677-1680; discussion 1680.
46. Hendren WH: The genetic male with absent penis and urethrorectal communication: Experience with 5 patients. J Urol 1997;157:1469-1474.
47. Henneberry MO, Stephens FD: Renal hypoplasia and dysplasia in infants with posterior urethral valves. J Urol 1980;123:912-915.
48. Hoar RM, Calvano CJ, Reddy PP, et al: Unilateral suprainguinal ectopic scrotum: The role of the gubernaculum in the formation of an ectopic scrotum. Teratology 1998;57:64-69.
49. Hollowell JG Jr, Witherington R, Ballagas AJ, et al: Embryologic considerations of diphallus and associated anomalies. J Urol 1977;117:728-732.
50. Holmdahl G, Sillen U, Hellstrom AL, et al: Does treatment with clean intermittent catheterization in boys with posterior urethral valves affect bladder and renal function? J Urol 2003;170:1681-1685; discussion 1685.
51. Hoover DL, Duckett JW Jr: Posterior urethral valves, unilateral reflux and renal dysplasia: A syndrome. J Urol 1982;128:994-997.
52. Hulbert WC, Duckett JW: Prognostic factors in infants with posterior urethral valves. J Urol 1986;135:121A.
53. Hyacinthe LM, Khoury AE, Churchill BM, et al: Improved outcome of renal transplant in children with posterior urethral valves. J Urol 1995;153:341A.
54. Johnston JH: Vesicoureteric reflux with urethral valves. Br J Urol 1979;51:100-104.
55. Johnston JH, Kulatilake AE: Posterior urethral valves: Results and sequelae. In Johnston JH, et al (eds): Problems in Pediatric Urology. Amsterdam, Excerpta Medica, 1972, p 161.
56. Kaplan GW, Brock WA: Urethral strictures in children. J Urol 1983;129:1200-1203.
57. Kilpatrick SJ: Therapeutic interventions for oligohydramnios: Amnioinfusion and maternal hydration. Clin Obstet Gynecol 1997;40:328-336.
58. Kim YH, Horowitz M, Combs AJ, et al: The management of unilateral poorly functioning kidneys in patients with posterior urethral valves. J Urol 1997;158:1001-1003.
59. Klee LW, Rink RC, Gleason PE, et al: Urethral polyp presenting as interlabial mass in young girls. Urology 1993;41:132-133.
60. Kohorn EI, Glickman MG: Technical aids in investigation and management of urethral diverticula in the female. Urology 1992;40:322-325.
61. Kojima Y, Hayashi Y, Maruyama T, et al: Comparison between ultrasonography and retrograde urethrography for detection of prostatic utricle associated with hypospadias. Urology 2001;57:1151-1155.
62. Koyanagi T, Nonomura K, Yamashita T, et al: One-stage repair of hypospadias: Is there no simple method universally applicable to all types of hypospadias? J Urol 1994;152:1232-1237.
63. Krstic ZD, Smoljanic Z, Micovic Z, et al: Surgical treatment of the Mullerian duct remnants. J Pediatr Surg 2001;36:870-876.
64. Lafferty PM, MacGregor FB, Scobie WG: Management of foreskin problems. Arch Dis Child 1991;66:696-697.
65. Liu KW, Fitzgerald RJ: An unusual case of complete urethral duplication in a female child. Aust N Z J Surg 1988;58:587-588.
66. Longaker MT, Golbus MS, Filly RA, et al: Maternal outcome after open fetal surgery: A review of the first 17 human cases. JAMA 1991;265:737-741.
67. Lund L, Wai KH, Mui LM, et al: Effect of topical steroid on non-retractile prepubertal foreskin by a prospective, randomized, double-blind study. Scand J Urol Nephrol 2000;34:267-269.
68. MacKenzie J, Chitayat D, McLorie G, et al: Penoscrotal transposition: A case report and review. Am J Med Genet 1994;49:103-107.
69. Maden C, Sherman KJ, Beckmann AM, et al: History of circumcision, medical conditions, and sexual activity and risk of penile cancer. J Natl Cancer Inst 1993;85:19-24.
70. Maizels M, Stephens FD, King LR, et al: Cowper's syringocele: A classification of dilatations of Cowper's gland duct based upon clinical characteristics of 8 boys. J Urol 1983;129:111-114.
71. Mandelbrot L, Dumez Y, Muller F, et al: Prenatal prediction of renal function in fetal obstructive uropathies. J Perinatol Med 1991;19(Suppl 1):283-287.

72. Marti-Bonmati L, Menor F, Gomez J, et al: Value of sonography in true complete diphallia. J Urol 1989;142:356-357.
73. Meisheri IV, Motiwale SS, Sawant VV: Surgical management of enlarged prostatic utricle. Pediatr Surg Int 2000;16: 199-203.
74. Merrot T, Anastasescu R, Keita M, et al: [An example of diphallia in children]. Prog Urol 2003;13:509-512.
75. Morey AF, Duckett CP, McAninch JW: Failed anterior urethroplasty: Guidelines for reconstruction. J Urol 1997;158: 1383-1387.
76. Morey AF, McAninch JW: Sonographic staging of anterior urethral strictures. J Urol 2000;163:1070-1075.
77. Mortensen PH, Johnson HW, Coleman GU, et al: Megalourethra. J Urol 1985;134:358-361.
78. Mughal SA, Soomro S, Shaikh JM: Double phallus. J Coll Physicians Surg Pak 2003;13:534-535.
79. Muram D: Treatment of prepubertal girls with labial adhesions. J Pediatr Adolesc Gynecol 1999;12:67-70.
80. Muram D, Jerkins GR: Urinary retention secondary to a Gartner's duct cyst. Obstet Gynecol 1988;72:510-511.
81. Narasimhan KL, Kaur B, Chowdhary SK, et al: Does mode of treatment affect the outcome of neonatal posterior urethral valves? J Urol 2004;171:2423-2426.
82. Nguyen HT, Peters CA: The long-term complications of posterior urethral valves. BJU Int 1999;83(Suppl 3):23-28.
83. Nussbaum AR, Lebowitz RL: Interlabial masses in little girls: Review and imaging recommendations. AJR Am J Roentgenol 1983;141:65-71.
84. Oster J: Further fate of the foreskin: Incidence of preputial adhesions, phimosis, and smegma among Danish schoolboys. Arch Dis Child 1968;43:200-203.
85. Pansadoro V, Emiliozzi P: Internal urethrotomy in the management of anterior urethral strictures: Long-term followup. J Urol 1996;156:73-75.
86. Passerini-Glazel G, Araguna F, Chiozza L, et al: The P.A.D.U.A. (progressive augmentation by dilating the urethra anterior) procedure for the treatment of severe urethral hypoplasia. J Urol 1988;140:1247-1249.
87. Patterson DE, Barrett DM, Myers RP, et al: Primary realignment of posterior urethral injuries. J Urol 1983;129: 513-516.
88. Perimenis P, Panagou A: Re: Acute urinary retention caused by anterior urethral polyp. Br J Urol 1992;70:695.
89. Pinke LA, Rathbun SR, Husmann DA, et al: Penoscrotal transposition: Review of 53 patients. J Urol 2001;166:1865-1868.
90. Pippi Salle JL, Sibai H, Jacobson AI, et al: Bladder exstrophy associated with complete urethral duplication: A rare malformation with excellent prognosis. J Urol 2001;165: 2434-2437.
91. Puri A, Grover VP, Agarwala S, et al: Initial surgical treatment as a determinant of bladder dysfunction in posterior urethral valves. Pediatr Surg Int 2002;18:438-443.
92. Quintero RA, Hume R, Smith C, et al: Percutaneous fetal cystoscopy and endoscopic fulguration of posterior urethral valves. Am J Obstet Gynecol 1995;172:206-209.
93. Quintero RA, Johnson MP, Romero R, et al: In-utero percutaneous cystoscopy in the management of fetal lower obstructive uropathy. Lancet 1995;346:537-540.
94. Raviv G, Leibovitch I, Hanani J, et al: Hematuria and voiding disorders in children caused by congenital urethral polyps: Principles of diagnosis and management. Eur Urol 1993;23:382-385.
95. Reinberg Y, de Castano I, Gonzalez R: Influence of initial therapy on progression of renal failure and body growth in children with posterior urethral valves. J Urol 1992;148: 532-533.
96. Ritchey ML, Sinha A, Argueso L: Congenital fistula of the penile urethra. J Urol 1994;151:1061-1062.
97. Rittenberg MH, Hulbert WC, Snyder HM 3rd, et al: Protective factors in posterior urethral valves. J Urol 1988; 140:993-996.
98. Rudin JE, Geldt VG, Alecseev EB: Prolapse of urethral mucosa in white female children: Experience with 58 cases. J Pediatr Surg 1997;32:423-425.
99. Salle JL, Sibai H, Rosenstein D, et al: Urethral duplication in the male: Review of 16 cases. J Urol 2000;163:1936-1940.
100. Salomon L, Fontaine E, Guest G, et al: Role of the bladder in delayed failure of kidney transplants in boys with posterior urethral valves. J Urol 2000;163:1282-1285.
101. Scherz HC, Kaplan GW, Packer MG: Anterior urethral valves in the fossa navicularis in children. J Urol 1987;138:1211-1213.
102. Sepulveda W, Berry SM, Romero R, et al: Prenatal diagnosis of congenital megalourethra. J Ultrasound Med 1993;12: 761-766.
103. Shapiro E, Strother D: Pediatric genitourinary rhabdomyosarcoma. J Urol 1992;148:1761-1768.
104. Sharma SK, Kapoor R, Kumar A, et al: Incomplete epispadiac urethral duplication with dorsal penile curvature. J Urol 1987;138:585-586.
105. Shimada K, Hosokawa S, Tohda A, et al: Follow-up of children after fetal treatment for obstructive uropathy. Int J Urol 1998;5:312-316.
106. Siegel JF, Brock WA, Pena A: Transrectal posterior sagittal approach to prostatic utricle (mullerian duct cyst). J Urol 1995;153:785-787.
107. Skoog SJ, Belman AB: Aphallia: Its classification and management. J Urol 1989;141:589-592.
108. Smith GH, Canning DA, Schulman SL, et al: The long-term outcome of posterior urethral valves treated with primary valve ablation and observation. J Urol 1996;155: 1730-1734.
109. Sommer JT, Stephens FD: Dorsal urethral diverticulum of the fossa navicularis: Symptoms, diagnosis and treatment. J Urol 1980;124:94-97.
110. Sorensen C, Furness P, Koyle MA: Betamethasone Cream for Treatment of Labial Adhesions. Boston, American Urological Association, South Central Section, 2003.
111. Spears T, Franco I, Reda EF, et al: Accessory and ectopic scrotum with VATER association. Urology 1992;40:343-345.
112. Spitzer A: The current approach to the assessment of fetal renal function: Fact or fiction? Pediatr Nephrol 1996;10:230-235.
113. Starr NB: Labial adhesions in childhood. J Pediatr Health Care 1996;10:26-27.
114. Stephens FD: Congenital Malformations of the Urinary Tract. New York, Praeger, 1983, p 577.
115. Stolar CJ, Wiener ES, Hensle TW, et al: Reconstruction of penile agenesis by a posterior sagittal approach. J Pediatr Surg 1987;22:1076-1080.
116. Tank ES: Anterior urethral valves resulting from congenital urethral diverticula. Urology 1987;30:467-469.
117. Thompson HC, King LR, Knox E, et al: Report of the ad hoc task force on circumcision. Pediatrics 1975;56:610-611.
118. Tietjen DN, Gloor JM, Husmann DA: Proximal urinary diversion in the management of posterior urethral valves: Is it necessary? J Urol 1997;158:1008-1010.
119. Welsh A, Agarwal S, Kumar S, et al: Fetal cystoscopy in the management of fetal obstructive uropathy: Experience in a single European centre. Prenat Diagn 2003;23:1033-1041.
120. Willetts IE, Roberts JP, MacKinnon AE: Laparoscopic excision of a prostatic utricle in a child. Pediatr Surg Int

2003;19:557-558.
121. Williams DI, Retik AB: Congenital valves and diverticula of the anterior urethra. Br J Urol 1969;41:228-234.
122. Wiswell TE, Geschke DW: Risks from circumcision during the first month of life compared with those for uncircumcised boys. Pediatrics 1989;83:1011-1015.
123. Wiswell TE, Hachey WE: Urinary tract infections and the uncircumcised state: An update. Clin Pediatr (Phila) 1993;32:130-134.
124. Yeung CK, Sihoe JD, Tam YH, et al: Laparoscopic excision of prostatic utricles in children. BJU Int 2001;87:505-508.
125. Young H, Frantz W, Baldwin J: Congenital obstruction of the posterior urethra. J Urol 1919;3:289.
126. Zaontz MR, Firlit CF: Percutaneous antegrade ablation of posterior urethral valves in premature or underweight term neonates: An alternative to primary vesicostomy. J Urol 1985;134:139-141.

第 121 章

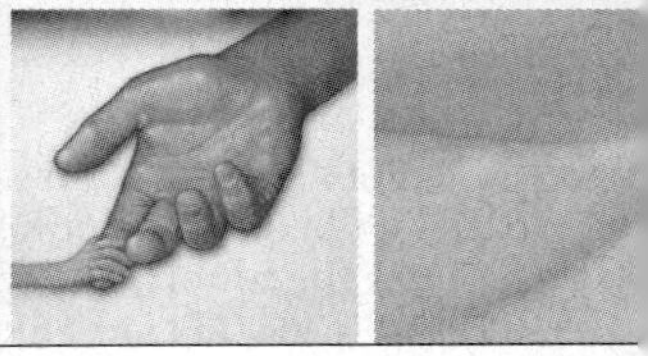

两性畸形

Patricia K. Donahoe、Jay J. Schnitzer 和 Rafael Pieretti

哺乳动物性别分化的发育生物学

1911 男性或女性外观的形成是一系列分子和形态学精确变化的结果。中胚叶位于内胚叶与外胚叶之间，是两者的媒介，早期胚胎的泌尿生殖嵴在此生成（图121-1）[48]。泌尿生殖嵴包含了未分化性腺和中肾组织，是产生生殖管道——午非氏管和苗勒氏管的场所。嵴的形成需要一些重要的基因，包括肾母细胞瘤因子（*WT1*）和类固醇生成因子（*SF-1*）。如果基因缺失，则不能形成性腺和邻近结构。*WT1* 基因突变的小鼠性腺和肾脏缺如[29]，而 *SF-1* 突变时体内性腺和肾上腺缺失[44]（见图 121-1）；人体中 *SF-1* 的同源基因缺失会造成类似表现[1]。表 121-1 中罗列了其他一些在发育早期起到重要作用的基因。同时，与午非氏管和苗勒氏管发育有关的重要基因也要表达。午非氏管的发育需要 *PAX2* 作用，可能还牵涉到 *PAX8*，上述两种基因配对存在，在果蝇的发育过程中起重要作用。苗勒氏管的形成需要一系列分泌因子的作用，这些因子的表达受 WNT 蛋白家族调控[64]。

在泌尿生殖嵴形成过程中，原始生殖细胞必须从胚胎外的外胚叶依次迁移，经过胚胎外胚层、原条、基底尿囊、后肠肠壁，最后进入泌尿生殖嵴并寄居于未分化性腺内。这一复杂的迁移过程受到一些基因[52]和蛋白的调控，其中包括 Fragilis、Stella、BMP4[71]，以及其他一些需要进一步阐述的基因和蛋白[48]。到达性腺后，具有有丝分裂活性的 XY 生殖细胞在减数分裂抑制因子的影响下停滞于 G_0 期。影响 XX 生殖细胞第一次减数分裂的因子至今未知。

性腺开始分化时，机体表达一些小分子转录因子，如位于 Y 染色体短臂上的基因 *SRY*，以及位于染色体 17q 上的与 SRY 相关的常染色体基因 *SOX 9*。事实上，在 1959 年认识到 45，X Turner 综合征的表现时[23]，就已经知道睾丸分化需要 Y 染色体信号[38]。然后细胞遗传学研究逐渐把男性分化区域定位于 Y 染色体的短臂上。后来，Page 等[60]比较了一系列因染色体缺失或移位而造成 XX 型男性和 XY 型女性的患者，把睾丸决定基因更精确地定位于 Y 染色体短臂的假常染色体区附近。之后，Sinclair 等[77]把一个编码 DNA 结合蛋白的单拷贝基因命名为 Y 染色体性别决定区（*SRY*），该基因存在于性腺嵴，在睾丸分化前表达[43]。*SRY* 表达的蛋白与核蛋白同源，属于高迁移率蛋白（HMG）。将 *SRY* 基因转染 XX 雌性小鼠胚胎后，部分比例的转基因鼠出现了睾丸发育，并且具备了雄性解剖与功能特征[42,43]。

除了 Y 染色体以外，常染色体与 X 因子在性别分化中也起了重要作用。譬如，在与性别反转相关的屈肢骨发育不良的病例中发现[24,80,82]，17 号染色体长臂上的突变导致了 SRY 相关基因产物 SOX9 的缺陷，而 SOX9 可促成性别分化。另外，分析 *SRY* 完整的 46，XY 的女性两性畸形，使人们在 X 染色体的短臂上找到了剂量敏感性性别基因（DSS）的倒错，而在女性性别分化时，这一基因的复制是必需的[5]。上述染色体区域中含有 *DAX-1* 基因，重复的性染色体 X 可能对睾丸分化存在负面影响，与抑制睾丸发育有关。9 号染色体短臂远端 9p[7]和 10 号染色体长臂远端 10q[86]的缺陷与性别反转有关。因此，尽管 *SRY* 是管理性别分化的主要开关基因，但是从 X 染色体和特定的常染色体上下传的分子信号同样决定了泌尿生殖嵴转化为性别特异性的性腺。这些负责卵巢分化的基因目前正在被研究，但是另一条 X 染色体也可能需 19
要研究。这一发现使人们对先前认为的卵巢发育是睾丸发育停滞以后的自发过程有了重新认识。

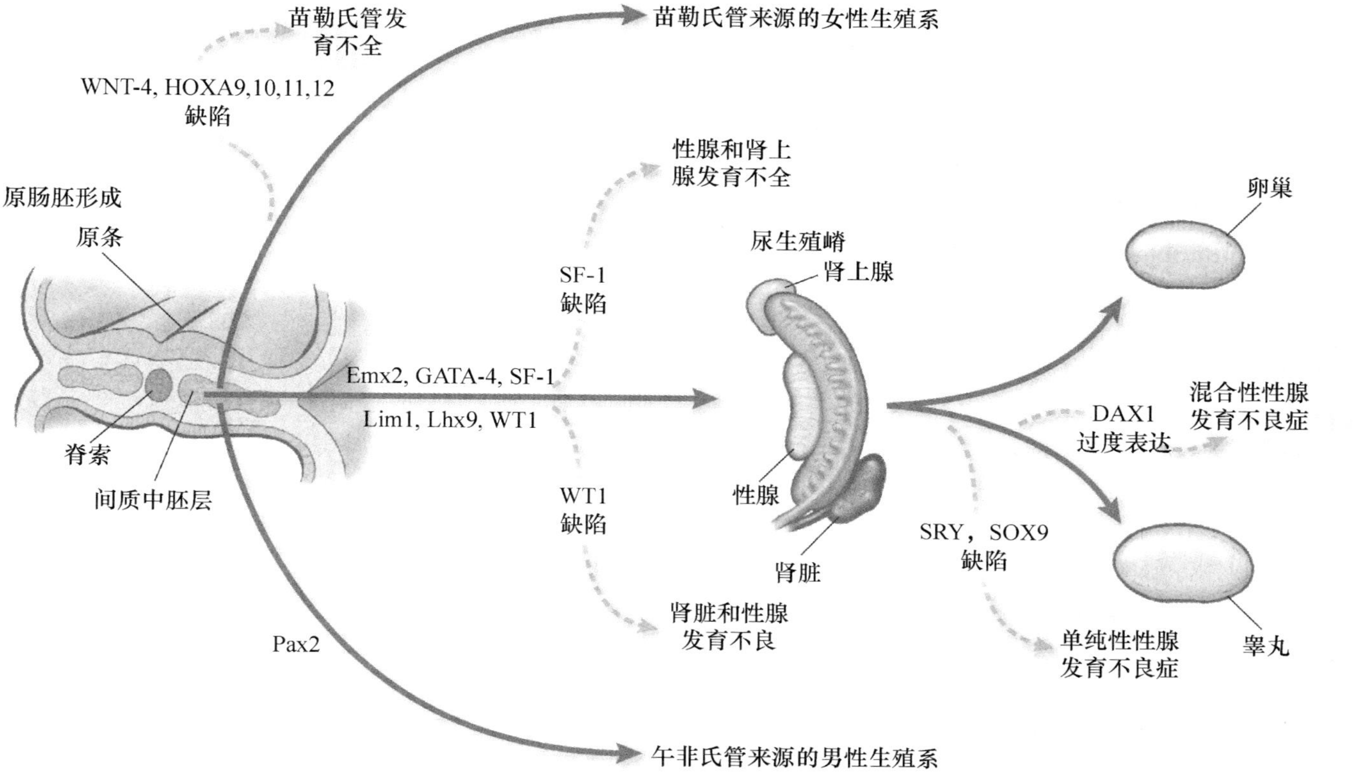

图 121-1 一些基因突变可能导致相关蛋白的缺失或过度表达，造成一系列涉及苗勒氏管或午非氏管、性腺、肾脏和肾上腺的发育不良疾病。*DAX1* 在 X 染色体上造成基因重复，引起先天性肾上腺发育不良；*Emx2*，空气门同源基因；*GATA-4*，编码的蛋白质连接到 GATA DNA 序列；*HOXA*，同源基因蛋白；*Lim1*，肢体发育涉及的重要同源基因；*Lhx9*，lim 同源基因家族；*Pax2*，配对的同源异形基因；*SF-1*，类固醇生成因子 1 基因；*SRY*，Y 染色体性别决定区；*SOX9*，SRY 同源基因 9；*WNT-4*，介导苗勒氏管间质发育的蛋白；*WT1*，Wilms 肿瘤抑制基因 1。（From MacLaughlin DT，Donahoe PK：Sex determination and differentiation. N Engl J Med 2004；350：367-378.）

同样，睾丸也能合成一种促成睾丸下降的蛋白质，称作类胰岛素生长因子 3（Insl3）[57,89]。因此，胚胎必须在发育之初就拥有合适的染色体核型（如女性 46, XX；男性 46, XY）才能保证正常的性别分化。生殖细胞必须准确地迁移到后肠，继而定居于腹膜后。在那里，细胞在泌尿生殖嵴聚集，向卵巢或睾丸转化。生殖细胞向泌尿生殖嵴迁移的同时可能介导形成特定性腺，继而产生性腺分泌激素。远侧受体在细胞外激素和蛋白的刺激下，激活细胞内信号传递途径和体细胞基因，引起细胞形态和生化发生变化，形成正常表现型的男性与女性[21]。

在所有哺乳动物的胚胎期，雄性和雌性的原始生殖管道会并存一小段时间。在睾丸缺如时，子宫、输卵管和上三分之一阴道的始基在女性体内自发发育。而附睾、输精管和精囊腺的始基，即午非氏管的发育需要睾酮刺激。胎儿睾丸由生精小管组成，周围围绕以支持细胞（Sertoli 细胞）和由间质分化形成的间质细胞（Leydig 细胞），能合成分泌男性分化所需的两种产物，即苗勒氏管抑制物质（MIS）和睾酮[40]。前者可抑制苗勒氏管的分化，后者能刺激午非氏管结构的形成。外生殖器原基自行发育产生阴蒂、小阴唇和大阴唇。在 5α-还原酶作用下，睾酮还原为双氢睾酮，这是外生殖器完全分化成阴茎和阴囊的必要条件[35]。随着阴茎生长，泌尿生殖褶融合形成尿道的阴茎部分，阴囊阴唇隆起在中线互相融合形成阴囊。睾酮在性别分化中的作用将在今后的章节里做进一步讨论。女性化发育是一个主动过程，能够不依靠卵巢独立存在。尽管雌激素在性别分化过程中的作用依然不明，但 X

染色体短臂上相关基因的重复似乎是抑制男性性征产生的必要因素，如已经明确定位的 *DAX-1* 基因转录后编码一种蛋白，可以阻止类固醇的生成[5,88]。

胚胎睾丸同样合成分泌 MIS。苗勒氏管抑制物是由 Jost[40]提出的，他发现将睾丸移植入雌兔体内后，除了可以刺激午非氏管形成以外，还能引起苗勒氏管退化。苗勒氏管的退化特征是细胞出现程序性死亡。由于这一重要发现，MIS 已经被分离提纯[9,67]用于克
1913 隆 *MIS* 基因[10]。MIS 的 C 端的生物活性与一组进化保留蛋白具有同源性，这些蛋白就是平时常常说到的转化生长因子 β（TGF-β）家族，包括 MIS、激活素（activin）、抑制素（inhibitin）、成骨生长因子（bone morphogenesis factor）、*果蝇* decapentaplagia、*非洲蟾蜍* Vg1 等[10]。MIS 配体与异源受体结合，该受体由至少两种丝氨酸-苏氨酸激酶跨膜单位组成，属于Ⅱ型受体[78]，可磷酸化或激活Ⅰ型受体[31]，使信号向下游传导，引起一系列分子水平变化，导致苗勒氏管退化。这些物质已经被研发成一种抗增殖剂，用来对抗苗勒氏管起源的肿瘤、卵巢癌[28,50]、子宫内膜癌[68]、宫颈癌[4]、乳腺癌[34,75,76]和前列腺癌[34]等。*MIS* 基因异常可导致苗勒氏管残留综合征。患有该综合征的男子与正常不同，体内苗勒氏管异常残留，终生存在不退化，通常伴发隐睾[6,33]。

两性畸形的病理生理

新生儿外生殖器畸形的形成大多与发育异常有关，可以将这些异常原因归为三大类（表 121-1）。在第一类中，基因型为女性的患者受到过量的雄激素刺激，表现出男性体征，引起生殖器异常，需要药物或外科干预（或两者都采用）。第二类两性畸形是因为雄激素产量不足或活力不够而引起，患者的基因型属于男性。第三类畸形因基因突变引起，造成性腺缺如、分化不完全或不对称[21]。了解这些畸形的病理生理变化是必要的，也是及时准确诊断疾病及制订治疗方案所不可或缺的条件。

女性基因型（46，XX）的雄激素过多

造成雄激素过多或女性男性化的最常见原因是负责将黄体酮转化为糖皮质激素和盐皮质激素的肾上腺酶类 P450 缺陷（细胞色素 P450 氧化酶，可使多种底物代谢），导致先天性肾上腺增生症（congenital adrenal hyperplasia，CAH）或肾上腺性征综合征，也称为女性假两性畸形[84]。该综合征在男性和女性中都能发病，但只有女性发病时才会引起生殖器外观异常。肾上腺分化始于孕 11 周时，晚于性腺和生殖道的分化。因此，雄激素过多主要影响外生殖器、生殖结节和泌尿生殖褶的发育，而这些结构的分化都开始于胚胎 11 周以后。生殖结节在过多雄激素的刺激下，能够演变为阴茎结构，而不再是阴蒂。泌尿生殖嵴融合形成阴囊外观，不同于阴唇。卵巢正常位于腹腔内。

CAH 病例中，90% 的病因是 *P450c21* 或 21-羟化酶基因即目前已知的 *CYP21*（表 121-2）突变。功能性基因 *CYP21B* 和无功能性假基因 *CYP21A* 的重新结合造成位于染色体 6p 的 HLA 位点的基因发生突变。功能性基因与假基因混合后将不能正常发挥作用[27,55,58,85]。其余 CAH 病例受种族影响，与 P450c11、3β-羟类固醇脱氢酶、CYP17 或 StAR 缺陷有关[17,54,61]。在一些罕见病例中，CAH 的发生由外源性雄激素刺激造成，譬如过去曾应用这些激素来预防流产。糖皮质激素和盐皮质激素的缺乏可负反馈影响垂体功能，引起促肾上腺皮质激素过多分泌，继而造成肾上腺束状带、球状带和网状带增生，网状带功能亢进的结果即出现雄激素分泌过多。17-羟孕酮堆积在 P450c21 附近，导致孕烯醇酮和孕酮及其 17-羟衍生物过量，继而又造成睾酮及其还原产物双氢睾酮产量过剩（图 121-2）。体内 17-羟孕酮的升高可以通过指尖采血获知[62]。目前，聚合酶链反应（PCR）、基因测序及原位杂交荧光技术（FISH）已经用于宫内诊断[17]。

这些患有肾上腺性征综合征的 46，XX 基因型女性卵巢正常，病变部位位于肾上腺。患者子宫和输卵管结构也正常。但是，由于向会阴迁移失败，阴道深度缩短。在严重男性化时，阴道与尿道连接于前列腺位置；当男性化程度轻微时，两者的连接部位将更靠近远端。外生殖器形态因阴蒂增大程度不同而各异，时而轻微，时而严重，一些患者的阴蒂形态甚至形同正常的阴茎。男性化时，阴唇部分融合形成阴唇阴囊褶；在一些更为严重的病例中，阴唇完全融合成阴囊外观。由于卵巢正常，性腺不会下降到阴唇阴囊褶或融合的阴囊内[16]。因此，患有双侧隐睾的婴儿需要

接受染色体核型检查，以明确其是否具有 Y 染色体。所有的酶缺陷疾病都会影响皮质醇的生物合成。负反馈的缺失会造成促皮质醇激素产量上升，进一步刺激肾上腺引起肾上腺增生，造成生化反应链上与缺陷酶邻近的产物合成增加，其中以雄激素类甾体物质更为明显。同时，促黑激素产量升高，造成外生殖器和乳晕色素沉着。

男性基因型（46，XY）的雄激素不足

造成46，XY 基因型男性化不足的原因可能是睾酮产量不足、雄激素受体缺陷或无法将睾酮转化为双
916 氢睾酮。所有这些类别的缺陷都能导致男性假两性畸形[13]。雄激素产量缺陷（见图 121-2）是遗传性酶缺陷的结果，包括类固醇急性调节蛋白（StAR）缺陷，可导致类脂性肾上腺增生（以前认为是胆固醇碳链裂解酶、P450scc 或 CYP11A$_1$ 的缺陷所致）。CYP11A$_1$（20，22-碳链裂解酶）、CYP17（17-羟化酶或裂解酶）、3β-羟化类固醇脱氢酶（3β-HSD）和17β-羟化类固醇脱氢酶（17β-HSD）以前被认为是17-酮类固醇还原酶，在胆固醇转化到睾酮的代谢中，这些酶同时或相继发挥作用[53]。对这些患者应用绒毛膜促性腺激素刺激试验，睾酮含量不上升或仅轻微上升。相反，MIS 水平却正常或高于正常。睾丸可能下降不全或/和发育弱小。在正常 MIS 的影响下，患者体内不存在苗勒氏管结构。由于睾酮缺乏，阴茎可能短小或存在尿道下裂[27]。

雄激素不敏感可以继发于受体缺陷之后。大多数异常是由雄激素受体点突变引起的[46,79]，目前能够通过 PCR 和 DNA 测序技术检测。很少见到大的基因缺失。临床表现由轻微到严重不等，完全的男性化不足通常被称为睾丸女性化综合征，患者几乎彻底呈现女性外观。血清睾酮水平可能上升，MIS 正常或在一些病例中明显升高，苗勒氏管退化正常。性腺对称，
917 睾丸可能下降，也可能位于腹腔内。但是，不是所有46，XY 的男性假两性畸形都能检测到雄激素受体基因编码区的缺陷。一些非编码启动子、3′非翻译区或其他转录因子及其协同因子的缺陷也可能是造成男性假两性畸形的原因，对于这些亚类患者病因的分子定位尚未明确。

3β-HSD 的作用是将 3β-羟类物质还原为 3-酮类，将 C5-6 之间的双键异构化到 C4-5 位置，从而把孕烯醇酮转化为孕酮，或者把 17-羟孕烯醇酮转化为 17-羟孕酮。这些步骤对产生糖皮质激素和盐皮质激素是必需的。同样，具有活性的 3β-HSD 也是脱氢表雄酮（DHEA）转化为雄烯二酮所必需的。构型不同的 3β-HSD 也存在于胎盘中，但功能尚未明确。另一个酶链反应中涉及的非 P450 酶是 17β-HSD，能将雄烯二酮转化为睾酮。

5α-还原酶 2 型基因的突变造成另一种男性假两性畸形。由于缺乏有效的酶，外周靶组织尤其是外生殖器内的睾酮不能转化为双氢睾酮[35,83]。这一非 P450 酶依赖于还原型 NADPH（烟酰胺腺嘌呤二核苷酸磷酸）。酶作用于生殖器引起阴茎嵴的延长和腹侧融合，阴茎嵴包绕尿道，使尿道口由会阴部移位到阴茎头端[13]。阴唇阴囊褶在其后方融合，形成阴囊结构。这一常染色体隐性遗传的严重尿道下裂可合并隐睾、阴茎阴囊反位和前列腺囊增大。5α-还原酶具有睾酮和 NADPH 辅因子结合位点，这些结合位点的点突变与有缺陷的表现型（疾病）相关。然而，目前已知 5α-还原酶有两个异构体形式[2]，位于第 19 号染色体的 2 型酶主要在外生殖器上表达。在这些基因型为男性的患者中，发生于青春期的一种矛盾的女子男性化及其导致的性别认知错误主要由 5α-还原酶 1 型异构体活性增强所致。

性腺发育和分化异常

性染色体异常通常表现为性腺不发育、发育不全或非对称性发育。这些异常患者性腺或者呈双侧条索状，如同完全不发育一样；或者两侧发育不对称，如同混合性腺发育不良或真两性畸形。性腺完全不发育的 46，XY 男性患者的 Y 染色体可能存在缺陷，或者是假常染色体 1A1 区的基因缺失[60]，或者是 *SRY* 基因的点突变[41]。基因突变可能与肢体畸形有关，这是一种严重的疾病，患者染色体 9p 的远端靠近 *SRY* 相关基因 *SOX 9* 的位置出现基因易位[24,82]。另一种由 *WT1* 基因突变造成的 Frasier 综合征[3]同样可能引起性腺完全不发育。条索状性腺无法双向发育，只能合成产生少量或根本不能生成睾酮及 MIS 此类的终产物；促性腺激素水平代偿性上升。苗勒氏管结构保存，患者表现型为女性。

表 121-1 两性畸形综合征:诊断和治疗

疾病	诊断特点	体格检查	性别选择	内科治疗	手术治疗
雄激素过量的女性(女性假两性畸形)					
先天性肾上腺皮质增生症(肾上腺性征综合征)	染色体核型 46,XX 电解质:高钾、低钠 雄激素水平高 17-羟孕酮水平高 MIS 0 *CYP21* 测序 染色体 FISH	性腺对称 阴蒂肥大 生殖窦造影:泌尿生殖窦缺损 阴唇阴囊增大	女性	氢化可的松或可的松 + 氟氢可的松 胚泡选择 从第 6 孕周开始,宫内类固醇替代	围术期应激类固醇 阴蒂退缩术 阴道外置术 阴唇阴囊切除术
雄激素水平低下的男性(男性假两性畸形)					
睾酮缺乏症	染色体核型 46,XY 睾酮水平低下 酶基因测序:*17-KS OH*, *P450scc*, *3β-HSD*, *CYP17* FISH	对称,睾丸下降不全,小睾丸 严重的尿道下裂	如果是男性	术前睾酮刺激 青春期应用睾酮	分期尿道下裂修补术 阴茎阴囊反位纠正术 睾丸固定术
		无苗勒氏管结构	如果是女性	青春期应用雌激素/黄体酮	性腺切除术
雄激素受体缺陷症睾丸女性化(完全雄激素不敏感症)	染色体核型 46,XY 睾酮水平高 MIS 水平高 雄激素受体基因测序 FISH	女性表现型 无苗勒氏管结构	女性	青春期应用雌激素/黄体酮	婴儿期:性腺切除术 青春期:阴道替代术
Reifenstein 综合征(不完全雄激素不敏感症)	染色体核型 46,XY 睾酮水平正常 MIS 轻微升高 PCR 检测雄激素受体基因 FISH CGH	如睾酮缺乏症	如果是女性 如果是男性	青春期应用雌激素/黄体酮 如睾酮缺乏症(如上所述)	婴儿期:性腺切除术,阴蒂退缩术,阴唇阴囊缩减术 青春期:阴道替代术 如睾酮缺乏症

5α-还原酶缺陷症	染色体核型 46,XY 睾酮水平高 DHT 水平低下 MIS 水平高 5α-还原酶 2 型基因测序 FISH	严重的阴茎阴囊型尿道下裂 睾丸对称，下降不全，睾丸结构正常 阴茎阴囊反位	男性	术前睾酮刺激 DHT 替代	尿道下裂修补术 阴茎阴囊反位纠正术
染色体异常					
单纯性腺发育不全症	染色体核型 46,XY 候补基因测序：*SRY*,*SOX 9*,*DAX-1* 睾酮缺乏 MIS 缺乏 FISH CGH	女性表现型 阴道存在 性腺缺如 对称	女性	青春期应用雌激素/黄体酮	性腺切除术
混合性腺发育不良症	染色体核型 45,X/46,XY 或 46,XY 睾酮水平低下 MIS 水平低下 *DAX-1* 基因测序 FISH CGH	非对称性腺：条索状性腺和睾丸 泌尿生殖窦缺陷 阴蒂肥大	如果是女性	青春期应用雌激素/黄体酮	阴蒂退缩术 阴道外置术 阴唇阴囊缩减术 性腺切除术
			如果是男性	术前睾酮刺激 青春期应用睾酮	
真两性畸形	染色体核型 46,XX 睾酮水平正常或低下 MIS 水平正常或低下 CGH	非对称睾丸、卵巢或卵睾 泌尿生殖窦缺陷 阴蒂肥大	如果是女性	青春期应用雌激素/黄体酮	阴蒂退缩术 阴道外置术 阴唇阴囊缩减术 保留正常卵巢或极化的卵巢组织
			如果是男性	术前睾酮刺激 青春期应用睾酮	分期尿道下裂修补术 阴茎阴囊反位纠正术 苗勒氏管切除术 保留输精管和正常睾丸或中间的睾丸组织 睾丸固定术？ 假体？

CGH,比较基因组杂交;DHT,双氢睾酮;FISH,荧光素原位杂交;MIS,苗勒氏抑制物;PCR,聚合酶链反应;UG,尿生殖系。

表 121-2 类固醇合成酶命名

旧名称	新名称——蛋白质	新名称——基因
睾丸		
20，22-碳链裂解酶	P450scc（侧链裂解）	*CYP11A*
17-羟化酶	P450c17	*CYP17*
17-裂解酶	P450c17	*CYP17*
3β-羟类固醇脱氢酶（3β-HSD）	相同	相同
17-酮类固醇还原酶	相同	相同
肾上腺		
21-羟化酶	P450c21	*CYP21*
11-羟化酶	P450c11	*CYP11B1*
18-羟化酶	P450c11	*CYP11B2*

混合性腺发育不良合并染色体核型45，X/46，XY是迄今为止最常见的畸形[20,70]。患者的性腺发育不对称，通常一侧是发育不良的小睾丸，另一侧是条索状性腺[15]。这些患者中，大多数保留了苗勒氏管。小睾丸可以产生足量的睾酮促成男性化发育和阴茎的形成。阴道向会阴迁移失败，并与尿道汇合成尿生殖窦，两者交汇点与膀胱颈之间的距离大于CAH患者。值得注意的是，40%混合性腺发育不良患者的染色体核型是46，XY，一些患者的两侧性腺均为睾丸或条索状卵巢。第二条X染色体的缺失可能与卵巢早期发育不良有一定关系。混合性腺发育不良疾病中至少存在两种生殖细胞，造成性腺嵌合。睾丸分化程度由XY基因型的细胞决定，细胞所占的百分比还同时影响性腺的对称程度。Y染色体缺失的原因可能是细胞有丝分裂时，复制配对的染色体向两极迁移过程中未

肾上腺和性腺类固醇激素的生物合成

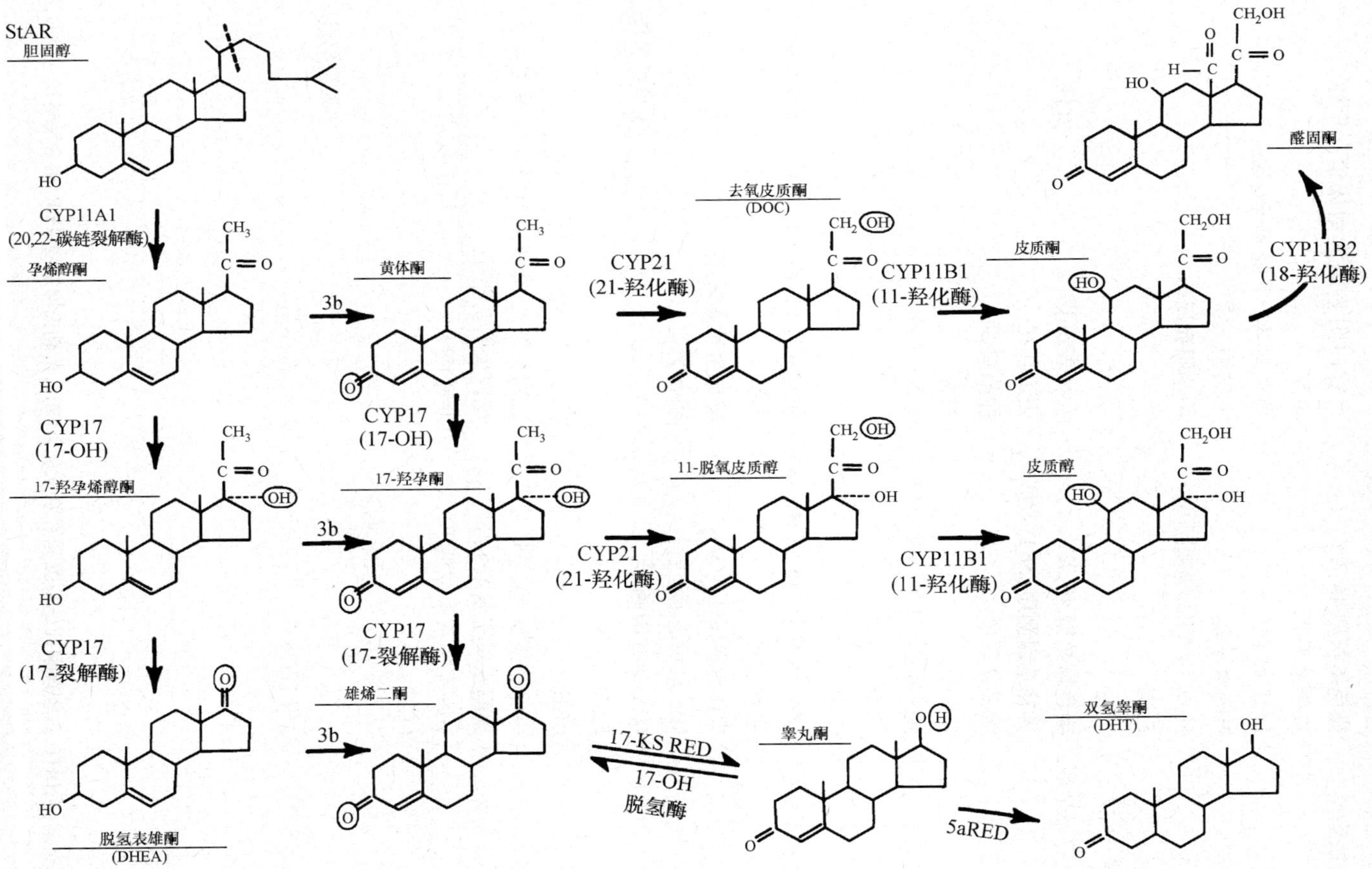

图 121-2 胆固醇到类固醇激素合成途径。粗体字母是酶的新名称，括号内是该酶的旧名称。CYP21、CYP11或3β-羟类固醇脱氢酶缺乏可导致先天性肾上腺增生症。CYP11A_1、CYP17、3β-羟类固醇脱氢酶和17-酮类固醇还原酶缺陷可造成睾酮合成减少，导致男性假两性畸形。

分离而造成的[18,23,48]。由于产前遗传检查愈发普遍，目前已经在外形正常的男性中发现少部分细胞存在 45, X/46, XY 嵌合核型。

除班图（Bantu）人以外，真两性畸形非常罕见，发病原因难以解释[14,81]。90% 以上的患者具有 46, XX 核型。这些患者中，许多以性腺不对称为特征，发育不良的睾丸和卵巢同时存在，分别位于腹部两侧，或出现性腺重合造成一侧或两侧卵睾的形成。当睾丸和卵巢同时出现于一个性腺的时候，睾丸通常位于性腺中央，卵巢出现在性腺两极[59]。尽管造成畸形的原因尚未在分子学上得到阐明，但可观察到包含有 *SRY* 基因的染色体碎片偶尔会易位到 X 染色体的某个隐蔽位置[8]。然而，这些患者中却没有检测出 *SRY* 基因。尽管早期睾丸存在分化现象，但却没有明显的精子发生[14]，这一点可能会反映由 Y 染色体介导的其他必要功能的缺失。苗勒氏管在睾丸组织一侧退化，而在中线和卵巢侧残存，同时阴道在更远的位置融入尿道，成为尿生殖窦缺损。性腺非对称发育的原因至今仍然是个谜。

诊断

对生殖器存在两性畸形的婴儿必须给予迅速、全面的评估，以明确其性腺种类。必须尽可能减少疾病对家庭和患儿将来造成的精神损害，这一点非常重要。因此，将患者介绍到一个对这些复杂疾病
918 有着丰富经验的、由内分泌专家和小儿外科医生组成的专家组通常会有所帮助。尽管许多综合征能影响后来的性发育，但只有四种情况会造成出生阶段的两性畸形，即女性假两性畸形（又称为肾上腺性征综合征和 CAH）、真两性畸形、男性假两性畸形和混合性腺发育不良等。患有完全性性腺发育不良征的儿童，纵然染色体核型是 46, XY，典型表现仍然是女性外观。性别的培养并不依赖于技巧娴熟的外科医生，对这一点一定要有清楚的认识。应该采用两种筛查标准以明确疾病类别，包括性腺是否对称及 Y 染色体是否存在（表 121-3）。两性畸形的诊断概要可参见表 121-1。

第一种标准是通过体检明确性腺是否对称，第二种标准是性染色体快速分析。目前通过 PCR 或 FISH 技术，*SRY* 探针可被用来探查 Y 染色体短臂末端。性腺对称与否由其彼此相对位置决定，或者位于腹股沟外环上方，或者位于腹股沟外环下方。性腺对称时，两侧性腺同时位于环口的上方或下方，此时各种生化缺陷是造成性腺畸形的主要原因。例如，在男性或女性假两性畸形时，生化缺陷对两侧性腺的影响效果相同。当一侧性腺位于腹股沟环上方，另一侧性腺位于腹股沟环下方时，性腺属于非对称性。非对称性腺出现于染色体畸形，如混合性腺发育不良或真两性畸形时，典型表现为优势睾丸下降，优势卵巢仍然位于外环上方。患有肾上腺性征综合征女性假两性畸形以及绝大多数真两性畸形患者的染色体核型是 46, XX。男性假两性畸形或混合性腺发育不良患者多携带 Y 染色体。

初期评估之后，需要对 46, XX 双侧对称性隐睾的患者进行 17-羟孕酮的快速分析，以及时发现 *CYP21* 异常。美国部分州对新生儿的 17-羟孕酮进行普遍筛查。详细的病史、体格检查，结合 PCR 或 FISH 技术，可以明确造成缺陷的突变基因或缺失基因（表 121-4），进而可以更进一步确诊这些疾病以及指导性别取向。然后，应用超声、磁共振、放射线增强显像及膀胱镜等多种检查手段，结合精确的实验室检查了解睾酮合成酶的异常，这些结果为诊断提供了更详尽的资料，为性别的决定提供高度精确的参考。

表 121-3　快速诊断方法

Y 染色体缺如或异常		Y 染色体存在	
对称	不对称	对称	不对称
女性假两性畸形（先天性肾上腺增生症）	真两性畸形	男性假两性畸形	混合性腺发育不良

这两种诊断标准——Y 染色体的存在或缺如以及性腺发育对称或不对称，使患儿能够迅速地被划分到其中一种两性畸形诊断中，准确率在 90% 左右。

表 121-4 涉及性别决定和发育的基因突变及其相关的两性畸形

基因（定位）	蛋白质及其功能	突变表现型
WT1（11p13）	转录因子	Frasier 综合征，Denys-Drash 综合征合并肾母细胞瘤
SF-1（9q33）	转录因子，细胞核受体	性腺和肾上腺发育不良
SOX 9（17q24）	高迁移率（HMG）蛋白转录因子	屈肢骨发育不良和男性性腺发育不良或 XY 性反转
DAX-1（Xp21.3）	转录调节因子，细胞核受体	性腺发育不良和先天性肾上腺发育不良
SRY（Yp11）	HMG 蛋白转录因子	性腺发育不良，XX 性反转
MIS（AMH）Ⅱ型受体（12q12-13）	丝氨酸苏氨酸激酶受体	持续苗勒氏管综合征
MIS（AMH）（19p13）	分泌蛋白，胎儿苗勒氏管退化因子，Leydig 细胞抑制因子	持续苗勒氏管综合征
AR（Xq11-12）	雄激素受体，配体转录因子	男性假两性畸形，雄激素不敏感综合征（完全性或部分性）
HSD17B3（9q22）	17-羟类固醇脱氢酶-17-酮类固醇还原酶 3	男性假两性畸形
SRD5A2（5p15）	5α-类固醇还原酶 2 型	男性假两性畸形（可能在青春期出现男性化）
CYP17（10q24q25.）	17-羟化酶，20，22-裂解酶	男性假两性畸形
CYP21（6q21.3）	21-羟化酶	先天性肾上腺增生症，女性假两性畸形
HSD3B2（1p13.1）	3β-羟类固醇脱氢酶 2 型	先天性肾上腺增生症
CYP11B1（8q24）	11β-羟化酶	先天性肾上腺增生症
StAR（8p11.2）	类固醇生成急性调节蛋白	先天性肾上腺类脂组织增生症

From MacLaughlin DT, Donahoe PK: Sex determination and differentiation. N Engl J Med 2004; 350: 367-378.

诊断时需要仔细观察阴茎的大小和阴茎阴囊的相对位置。尽管阴茎的尺寸存在很大差别，但仍然有一些数据值得借鉴[22,27]。足月时，阴茎的平均长度是 3.5 ±0.4 cm，胎龄 35 周时的长度是 3.0 ±0.4 cm，胎龄 30 周时的长度是 2.5 ±0.4 cm。足月儿阴茎的直径平均是 1 cm 左右。足月儿阴茎长度小于 1.5 ±0.7 cm 时，通过手术做成女性外观的可能性更大。但这种选择在 17-酮类固醇还原酶或 5α-还原酶缺陷时例外，这是因为这些病例体形较大（P. K. Donahoe 个人观察结果）或在青春期时存在性别倒错现象，所以笔者个人以为，还是倾向于选择男性性别。由于出生时子宫仍然受到胎盘人绒毛膜促性腺激素的影响而质地较硬，早期进行肛门指检可以发现其存在。检查男性患者时要注意尿道下裂是否存在和尿道口相对阴茎顶端的位置。检查女性患者时要注意阴道入口与膀胱颈、会阴的关系，以及阴道的长度。睾丸质地比卵巢致密，借此特点可以通过触诊性腺来区分睾丸和卵睾。附睾包绕睾丸周围，耐心检查可以和腹股沟卵巢区分开[21]。尿道下裂的阴茎位置靠后，阴囊常常处于阴茎前。

女性假两性畸形

如果患者是家族中的先证者，则很难诊断其是女性假两性畸形。如果亲属中已经有成员患病，则需要对这种常染色体缺陷疾病提高警惕，羊膜穿刺细胞核型分析有助于疾病的产前诊断。但是，临床上常见一些症状不典型的患者未被列入疑似病例。这些患者大多足月娩出，可能只有阴蒂肥大，腹腔性腺不对称，阴道未下降到会阴并在膀胱颈远端与尿道融合。很多亚型患者存在精阜结构，尿道与阴道的交汇点非常靠近膀胱颈[32]。受胎盘刺激，在患者精阜水平可能触诊到增大的前列腺。阴唇阴囊褶起皱、增大，一些患者甚至出现完全融合成阴囊的情况。除正常卵巢结构以外，患者子宫、输卵管形态正常。但是，由于没有很好地向会阴迁移，患者阴道短缩。膀胱镜检时测量

919 膀胱颈到阴道瘘的距离非常有必要，有助于为将来的手术重建制定精确的治疗计划。阴蒂作为外生殖器的特征，增生程度从轻微到严重，形态各异，一些患者的阴蒂外观如同男性阴茎。阴唇可能男性化形成阴唇阴囊褶，严重病例中可出现完全融合的阴囊形态。由于卵巢正常，性腺不会下降到阴唇阴囊褶或融合的阴囊内[16,20]。这些女性的染色体核型都是 46, XX，体内不能检测到 MIS，指血血清分析可发现 17-羟孕酮升高。患者体内睾酮含量同样上升，伴随血清促黑激素的升高，外生殖器和乳晕出现色素沉着。以 PCR 技术选择合适的探针可以发现 *P450c21* 基因发生点突变[85]。出生时，电解质水平通常正常，但是随着由母体带来的类固醇激素的下降，出生 5～7 天以后，血清钾水平将明显升高，而血清钠含量下降。结果造成心电图中 T 波倒置，如果不加注意，可出现心脏骤停。在更为罕见的 3β-HSD 缺陷患者中，17-羟孕烯醇酮、孕烯醇酮和 DHEA 含量升高。P450c11 缺陷的患者，血清 11-脱氧皮质醇、去氧皮质酮含量上升。如果不出现延误诊断的情况，这些患者的性别通常都会选择为女性，除非患儿已经长期被当作男孩抚养[11,17]。

男性假两性畸形

睾酮缺乏或不足

根据定义，男性假两性畸形的染色体核型是 46, XY，外生殖器男性化不足。睾酮-雄激素生物合成通路中的酶缺陷是造成本病的原因之一，患者血清基础睾酮水平低下，绒毛膜促性腺激素刺激效果不明显，只有少量甚至无睾酮生成。由于生化反应中涉及的酶的编码基因已经得到克隆，所以可以采用 PCR 技术检测 *StAR*、*3β-HSD*、*CYP17* 和 17-酮类固醇还原酶基因的缺陷。通常，患者睾丸小，双侧对称性下降不全；阴茎发育短小，多为严重尿道下裂。在正常 MIS 的影响下，患者体内无苗勒氏管结构。一些患者的外观表现完全如女性[25-27]。性别取向由阴茎大小所决定。一般而言，如果患者的阴茎发育很差，最好将其当作女孩抚养；如果阴茎发育比较理想，则首先选择做男性，因为患者对外源性雄激素敏感。17-酮类固醇还原酶缺陷少见，对此类患者的性别选择需予特别考虑，一般认为选择男性比较好（P. K. Donahoe，私人交流）。

雄激素受体缺陷

与睾丸女性化一样，雄激素受体严重缺陷的患者可造成雄激素受体完全缺乏[87]。由于患者表现为女性，所以应该按照女孩抚养。由于存在高浓度的有生物学活性的 MIS，患者体内无苗勒氏管结构。睾丸通常位于腹股沟区，触诊时睾丸的坚韧手感和附睾形态可区别于卵巢。患者染色体核型为 46, XY。尽管雄激素受体缺陷，睾酮水平和 MIS 含量却很高。以 PCR 或基因测序技术检测雄激素受体基因，能够定位疾病分子缺陷，明确诊断。 1920

雄激素受体不完全缺陷只造成 46, XY 患者部分男性化，畸形程度由轻微到严重不等。如同睾酮缺陷综合征一样，患儿阴茎发育短小，合并尿道下裂。睾丸小而对称，通常下降不全，无苗勒氏管结构。睾酮水平正常，MIS 含量上升。大多数畸形是由雄激素受体基因点突变造成的[46,79]，可通过 PCR 技术或 DNA 测序技术检测。仅罕见病例中存在大量基因缺失。性别取向由阴茎尺寸所决定。

5α-还原酶缺陷

5α-还原酶的作用是将睾酮转化为脱氢睾酮，该酶的缺陷也会造成男性假两性畸形。正常情况下，5α-还原酶作用于生殖器区，使阴茎嵴伸长和腹侧闭合，将尿道口从会阴处移到阴茎龟头中间[13]。但 5α-还原酶缺陷患者的这一过程表现异常，造成严重的阴茎阴囊型尿道下裂。睾丸结构正常，两侧对称，可完全下降到阴囊，也可发生隐睾。阴唇阴囊褶从后方开始融合，形成阴囊囊袋。这些患者的前列腺囊都比较大。再次强调，所有患者的染色体核型是 46, XY。血清睾酮水平比较高，但双氢睾酮含量低下。MIS 处于正常范围。应用 PCR 和全 DNA 测序技术可了解基因型，检测 5α-还原酶 2 型基因的点突变。由于青春期时患者将面临第二性征的出现，所以把这些孩子当作男孩抚养更为恰当。但是，需要注意的是，我们的社会只承认两种性别，没有人愿意接受这两种性别以外的第三种性别，所以在决定患儿性别时必须十分慎重，这是摆在所有人面前的一大障碍[2,35,36]。

染色体异常

单纯性腺发育不良

单纯性腺发育不良患者出生时，外观如同女性。通过羊膜腔穿刺分析染色体核型是46，XY的胎儿，产前B超发现其表现型却并非如预计而是属于女性时，可以对疾病进行早期诊断，这是一项新的诊断技术。疾病的躯体表现比较少，明显的异常包括足背水肿和Turner综合征的一些表现。苗勒氏管结构存在，但不能触摸到性腺。无法检测到睾酮和MIS，由此提示性腺发育不良。候补基因突变包括*SRY*、*SOX 9*、*WT 1*和*SF-1*等[48]。

混合性腺发育不良

患有混合性腺发育不良患者的两侧性腺不对称，一侧为条索状性腺，另一侧为发育不良的睾丸。通常，患者体内保留苗勒氏管结构[15,20,70]，阴蒂发育过于肥大。最常见的染色体核型是45，X／46，XY嵌合型，但有大约40%的患者染色体核型属于46，XY。由于睾丸发育不良，睾酮与MIS水平可能低下。性腺有恶变倾向，即使早在新生儿期间，也可出现性腺胚细胞瘤和（或）精原细胞瘤[49,56,74]。这些肿瘤可造成性腺扭转和明显缺失，罕见引起单侧睾丸发育不良或条索状卵巢。由于性腺胚细胞瘤可出现于任何年龄阶段，所以治疗通常有性腺切除、再造女性生殖道以及考虑将患儿当作女孩抚养等方法。目前对混合性腺发育不良疾病的认识已经达到了分子水平。研究发现，X染色体关联基因*DAX-1*可抑制睾丸分化（或本身是一种抑制分子），该基因可能在混合性腺发育不良疾病中起到一定作用[37]。但是，只有在找到有丝分裂中引起染色体配对和分离的决定基因以后，才有可能最终明确疾病的发生机制。

真两性畸形

造成真两性畸形的原因至今不明[14,81]。患有这种疾病的患者体内同时存在两种或两种以上性腺，两侧性腺表现为不对称性，可以是一侧睾丸，另一侧为卵睾，当然还存在其他各种不同的性腺组合方式。性腺混合时，睾丸组织总是位于中间位置，而卵巢组织位于两极[59]。瘤性转化不是这些性腺的特征表现。苗勒氏管结构在睾丸组织一侧发生退化，在卵巢一侧保留，同时子宫位于中线位置，阴道与尿道结合形成泌尿生殖窦缺陷，阴蒂增生肥大。90%的患者染色体核型是46，XX，睾酮和MIS含量低下或偶尔正常。尽管存在早期的睾丸分化[14]，但精子发生不明显，反映了必须由Y染色体介导的一些功能出现缺失。患者体内不能检测到*SRY*[51]，而造成疾病的分子生物学机制和引起两侧性腺不对称的原因至今仍是个谜。选择患儿性别需要参照其外观表现，这其实是由占主要地位的性腺所决定的。

内科处理

女性假两性畸形

男性化的女性假两性畸形是患者在新生儿期间发生致命并发症的危险因素。由于来自母体的皮质素能够透过胎盘进入胎儿体内，并逐渐从脂肪组织中释放出来，所以临床可见的肾上腺生殖危象直到出生以后5～7天才显示出来。加强临床监护措施、及时给予正确的代谢治疗可预防严重并发症的发生。糖皮质激素替代疗法，如口服氢化可的松8～10 mg/(m^2·d)，分2～3服下，或者使用醋酸可的松肌肉注射，25 mg/(m^2·d)，每3天一次[45]，可有效防止急性肾上腺功能不全引起的严重代谢异常。

对男性化症状严重的婴儿，或者男性化症状较轻但存在家族性失盐型女性假两性畸形史的患儿，可选择氟氢可的松（9α-氟皮质醇）0.05～0.2 mg/d治疗。尽管一些临床医生在开始治疗以前会参考患者的血清电解质水平和肾素活性，但最近有更多的证据表明，采用氟氢可的松治疗肾上腺功能障碍的自由度非常大，即使对男性化症状非常轻微的患儿，也同样可以应用该治疗方法。 192

出现肾上腺危象的婴儿需要等渗液水化治疗。第一个小时内，需要输注一半剂量的5%～10%葡萄糖生理盐水。这一用药方法能迅速纠正体内钠和氯离子的失平衡状态，但高钾和酸中毒状态改变缓慢。血清17-羟孕酮水平的显著提高是监测治疗有效性的指标。婴儿（平均体表面积 0.25 m^2）出现肾上腺危象时采用氢化可的松琥珀酸钠 25 mg（2 mg/kg）治疗，年长儿的用药剂量可达 50～100 mg。这些前体物质同时具备了糖皮质激素和盐皮质激素的活性，其中盐皮质激素的活性相当于 0.1 mg 氟氢可的松。接受手术治疗的婴儿也可采取类似的用药方案。告知患者那些可能促成肾上腺功能不良的因素，如高热、暴露于高温环境或手术之中。母乳和配方奶中钠含量低，因此需要额外添加食盐。必须仔细监测生长量表，以避免不充分及时的治疗或过度抑制肾上腺功能，以及慢性肾上腺功能不全。

目前，产前诊断和治疗是可行的[12,63]。可以在性别分化以前，即胎龄第 5 或 6 周时，选用地塞米松治疗抑制胎儿出现男性化。地塞米松穿透胎盘，抑制胎儿肾上腺功能，降低胚胎雄激素产量，并由此降低宫内男性化程度。胎儿性别由染色体分析结果所决定，标本取自羊膜穿刺或绒毛膜绒毛。采用 PCR 和 DNA 测序技术可以分析 *CYP21* 基因。对男性胎儿或未受影响的女性胎儿，可以中止治疗。对于受累女性胎儿，治疗将持续至足月分娩。目前，能够在早期胚泡阶段施行胚胎选择或遗传干预，可以事先选择 *CYP21* 基因正常的胚泡，继而将其导入先前有过 *CYP21* 基因突变胎儿怀孕史的母亲体内。

男性假两性畸形

阴茎发育不良的男性假两性畸形患者，如果存在睾酮生物合成障碍或雄激素抵抗的情况，则通常把他们选择为女性。但是，对于那些 5α-还原酶或 17β-羟化类固醇还原酶缺陷的患者，很难在刚出生时就为其确定性别。被指定为女性的患者需要在早期接受手术纠正外生殖器和切除性腺，但直到青春期时才给予激素，届时，患者将需要雌激素和孕酮治疗。青春期晚期时，可计划实施阴道替代手术。

如果将婴儿的性别选择为男性，则需要使用 10～25 mg 庚酸睾酮或环戊丙酸睾酮肌肉注射治疗，每月一次，连续 3 个月，以确认阴茎对雄激素敏感，并达到在术前增加阴茎长度的目的。如果阴茎条件许可，则应该在出生 1 年以内给予修补手术。这样做的优点是可以尽早提高激素的敏感度。每月肌肉注射睾酮连续 3 个月，经过 1～3 个疗程以后，在进行尿道下裂修补手术以前必须有至少 1 个月不应用睾酮的间歇期，以降低睾酮注射伴发的性机能亢进。这些患儿往往需要接受分期手术，而如果需要给予睾酮治疗，一般选择在二期手术以前。青春期开始以后，将重新予以睾酮替代治疗。如果可能，应给 5α-还原酶缺陷的患者以双氢睾酮替代治疗。否则，应该应用更高剂量的睾酮，从而克服酶阻断效应。

染色体异常

对于混合性腺发育不良或是真两性畸形的患者，如果选择成为女性，则不必在孩童期给予激素替代治疗。但是，如果选择成为男性，则在尿道下裂手术以前需要给予睾酮刺激。手术后治疗中止，直到青春期开始，重新应用激素。如果指派患者性别为女性，青春期开始时应采用雌激素和孕酮进行替代治疗。单纯性腺发育不良的患者既不需要手术治疗，也不需要药物治疗，雌激素和孕酮的替代疗法应始于青春期阶段。对各种 *WT1* 亚型缺陷的患者应随访其肾功能变化。*SF-1* 基因突变可造成先天性肾上腺功能低下综合征，激素替代治疗复杂。阴道再建计划应在青春期以后再做考虑。

手术修补

术前准备

在每次整形手术以前都应该对患者实施膀胱镜检查，推荐使用 Storz 或 Wolff 品牌的镜检设备。上述两种设备有较细的光源和较大的工作通道，提供了较好的光亮度和较大的操作空间，手术操作时能提供良好的照明，水流量大以便更好地扩张尿道，以及可能根据情况放置引导钢丝或导管。高速水流下行尿道球囊扩张，可使术者能很好地判断位于尿道后壁的阴道口形态（图 121-3）。在某些病例中，阴道开口可能只有针尖大小。

多年来，一直认为建立一些与年龄相称的标准值是非常必要的，其中包括尿道长度（从膀胱颈到尿道

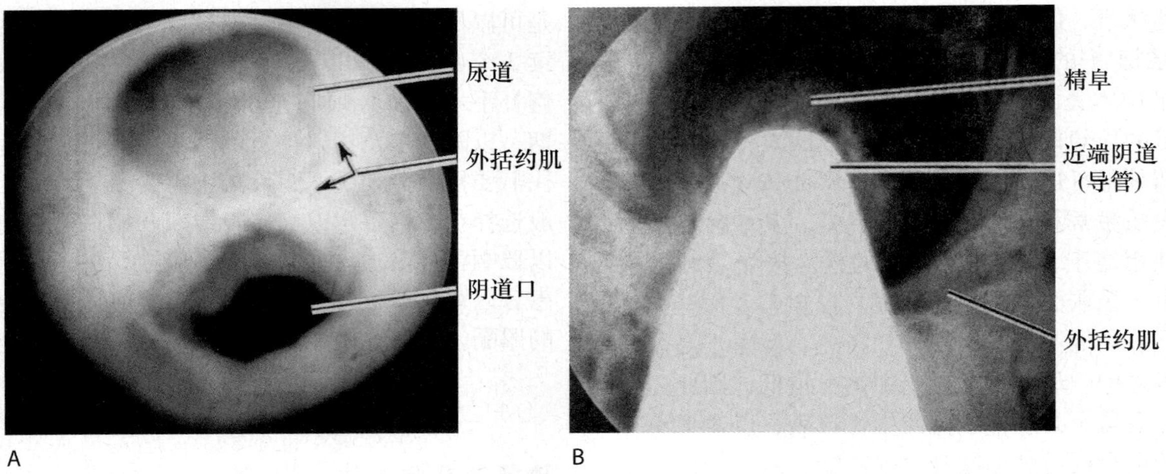

图 121-3 膀胱镜检查显示阴道进入近端尿道抑或远端尿道。A. 清楚显示阴道开口于远端尿道。B. 严重男性化的女性假两性畸形患者，导管显示阴道开口位于精阜。

阴道汇合处的距离）、泌尿生殖窦长度（尿道阴道汇合处到会阴的距离）以及阴道的长度（子宫颈到尿道阴道汇合处的距离）等。目前，作者根据阴道与尿道汇合点是位于精阜以上还是以下来建立一些简单的判断标准。所有汇合点位置平行或高于精阜的患者，认为处于高位，而汇合点位置低于精阜的患者则认定为低位。然而，还可以通过简单的测量为临床提供更精确的数据。例如，可以在 3 或 4 French 的尿道导管上间隔 1cm 标注刻度，将导管尖端放置于膀胱颈的位
1922 置，以刻注标度的导管为标尺进行测量。用同样的方法可以获得阴道长度。这些相关的测量数据应该予以记录，根据与年龄相对应的长度标准，选择制订相应的手术方案。

女性假两性畸形、混合性腺发育不良及真两性畸形患者的子宫颈位于阴道最上端。男性假两性畸形患者体内或者存在一个小的前列腺囊，或者有一个更深、更宽大的腔道，但近端无子宫颈结构。这种前列腺囊肿的特征是位于扁平精阜中央，周围无前列腺组织。阴道内留置 Fogarty 导管，膀胱内留置略小的 Foley 导尿管，将两者缚在一起。然后，将瘘管位置较远的患者置于截石位，行会阴重建术。而对近端泌尿生殖窦缺陷的患者，可以在全身准备完善后，改成俯卧位，将阴道和尿道分离。

充分的术前肠道准备非常重要。由于大多数患儿在早晨接受手术，所以这一准备工作应该在家完成。进行低位修补手术者，术前 2 天每天应该予以枸橼酸镁。而进行高位修补手术者，术前 3 天可连续 2 天口服一种聚乙二醇等张溶液 GoLYTELY，术前 1 天接着应用枸橼酸镁。对于一些患者，可以使用昂丹司琼以防止出现恶心症状，也可以通过细经鼻胃管给 GoLYTELY。GoLYTELY 必须在术前至少 24 小时停药，以防手术中发生泄漏。枸橼酸镁能使肠道收缩，术前最后一天使用，可防止出现肠瘘。口服新霉素和红霉素能减少细菌浓集。

如同先前所提到的，开始麻醉诱导时，可按照患儿体重给予应激剂量的类固醇。类固醇在术中持续应用，术后再持续应用 2～3 天，初始剂量为通常剂量的两倍，然后逐渐减量。应用地塞米松的儿童在手术当日可不必再应用药物，但服用泼尼松的患儿需要在手术当日早晨给予常规剂量的药物。术后服药方法由内分泌医生会诊决定。药物剂量由手术时间和范围以及住院时间而定。

女性再建手术

所有诊断为女性假两性畸形的新生儿，只要染色体核型属于 46, XX，就应该将其性别指定为女性，而不必顾忌患儿男性化的程度。一旦确定这些患者的性别为女性，就应该予以会阴重建手术。类似的手术同样可用于男性化不足的部分患者中，包括男性假两性畸形、混合性腺发育不良或真两性畸形等。修复手

术的主要依据是阴蒂退缩和阴道外置。前者的目的是缩短阴蒂，保留其感觉和勃起功能；后者是为了改善泌尿生殖窦未迁移到会阴的缺陷。患儿男性化程度越严重，阴道与尿道的汇合点位置就越高，手术的难度也越大。另外，需要通过手术将阴唇阴囊褶修裁变薄、伸长，以创建正常外观的大阴唇。无论怎样，只要条件允许，都应该同时完成阴蒂退缩、阴唇阴囊褶缩减及阴道外置手术，以便可以对周围组织进行充分利用[72,73]。

大多数患儿都可选择截石位进行手术。对畸形严重的患者，阴道在非常靠近膀胱颈的位置进入尿道时，可考虑后位手术径路。对于这些患者，也可以考虑游离整个泌尿生殖窦，手术操作可以在截石位完成。

行阴蒂整形手术时（图 121–4A），先在紧贴龟头基底部下环切包皮一圈，预留一小部分包皮以待以后缝合（见图 121–4A）。然后，如同手术修补尿道下裂一样，把阴蒂脱鞘，在中线位置切开阴蒂皮肤，创建 1923
Byar 皮瓣（见图 121–4B）。背侧切口足够长能包裹正常长度的阴蒂，使龟头无张力地骑坐于耻骨联合前女

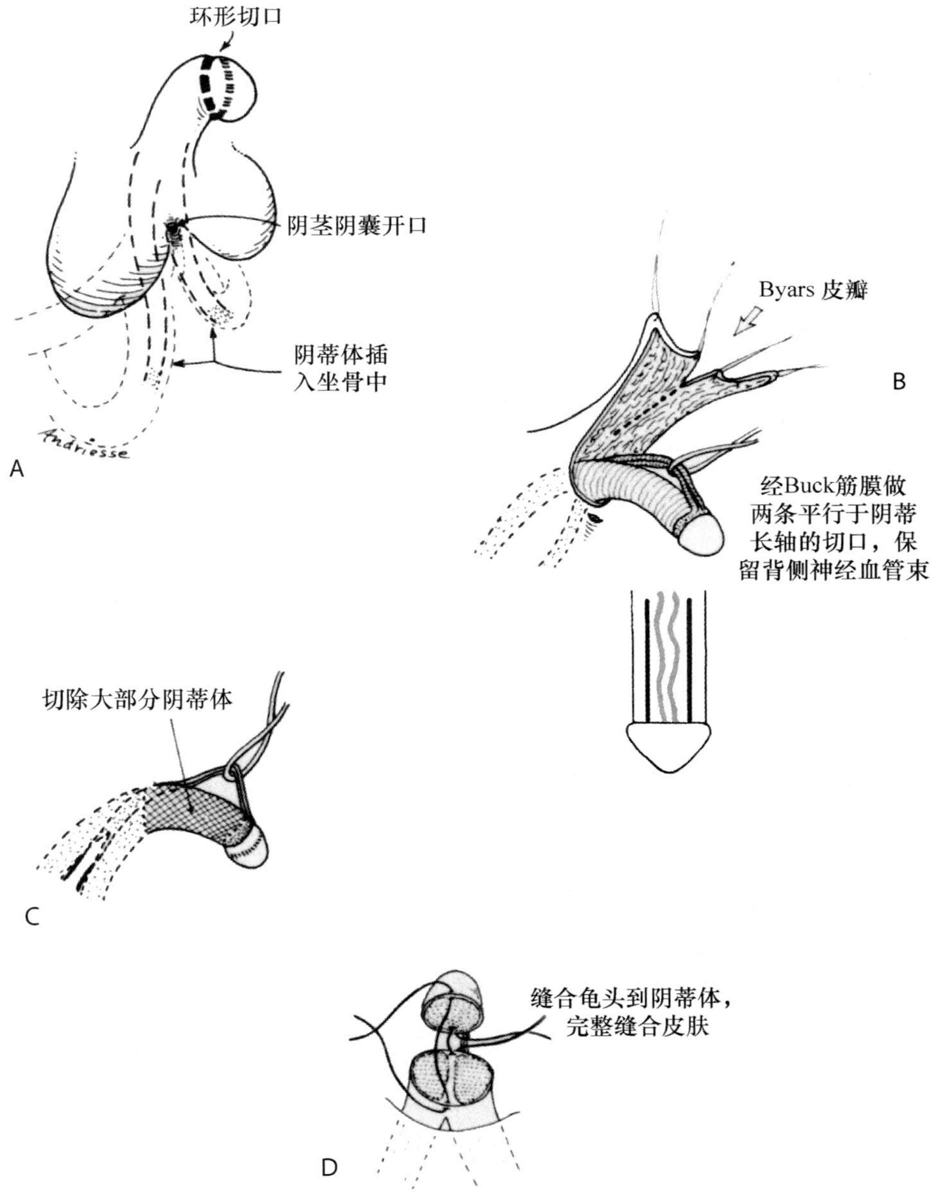

图 121–4　阴蒂退缩术。A. 于肥大的龟头下做环形切口。B. 背侧的阴蒂体皮肤明显，游离后在中线位置切开，以显微操作手段将背侧的神经血管束细致分离、保留。C. 于龟头基底和海绵体分叉之间切除阴蒂体。D. 用不可吸收的细线将龟头间断缝合到阴蒂体基底部。

性阴蒂的位置。经 Buck 筋膜做两条平行的纵切口，保留背侧神经血管束（见图 121–4B，*插图*）。阴茎的背侧动脉支源于阴部动脉，经坐骨粗隆穿 Alcock 管而来（图 121–5）。阴茎背侧动脉途经两侧海绵体中线，汇合于阴茎背侧正中。行走在每条阴茎海绵体中的动脉在中线位置与对侧血管交通，完成整个龟头的血管网分布。尚不清楚腹侧血管过渡到背侧的位置所在，但经验显示阴蒂具有良好的血液供应，由此设想动脉汇合点应该处于阴茎海绵体的近端。游离包皮的操作应选择在海绵体表面的筋膜层（见图 121–4C），手术时应用显微外科器械和放大镜。由阴蒂海绵体上提起神经血管束和 Buck 筋膜，向近端游离一直到阴蒂根部海绵体分叉处。然后，可以在龟头基底和海绵体分叉处之间切断阴蒂中间体，操作时注意要上提神经血管束避免其被误切。一些外科医生采用了不同的手术方法，沿阴蒂腹侧做两条平行纵切口，并由此切除海绵体组织。切除海绵体时需要仔细止血，但也要小心避免过度烧灼组织，以免造成局部纤维化及影响将来的勃起功能。多余的背侧神经血管束需要向上移位，海绵体残端与龟头吻合时可选用 4–0、5–0 或 6–0的不可吸收线间断缝合，具体缝线规格需参考患
1924 儿年龄和阴蒂尺寸（见图 121–4D）。肥大的龟头可以通过手术修裁，保留暴露的组织作为新的阴蒂。在大部分病例中，可以对阴蒂腹侧和两侧进行修剪，然后可以在冠状沟下缘把保留或残存的龟头缝合到近端游离的 Byar 皮瓣上（见图 121–4D）。

图 121–6A 描述了减少阴唇阴囊皱褶及阴道外置手术中的切口位置和皮瓣的选择。游离阴道，于中线位置切开阴道后壁，将直肠前的 U 形皮瓣向前插入阴道切口位置并与其吻合。这样，就在会阴部重建了阴道口。如果患儿的阴道尿道汇合位置很高，可以在龟头基底部游离一片向后延伸的岛状皮瓣，向内侧旋转，与游离后的阴道前壁吻合，重建阴道开口。吻合以后的阴道开口仍然可以在后壁中线上切开，经后方径路再次扩大阴道口。

图 121–6B 从矢状位展示了局部解剖结构，阴道进入尿道如泌尿生殖窦。在大多数男性化严重的 CAH 等女性假两性畸形病例中，阴道进入尿道的位置非常靠近膀胱颈。而对于一些男性化症状较轻的女性假两性畸形、混合性腺发育不良、真两性畸形的病例，阴道在尿道的远端与其汇合。高位泌尿生殖窦比较罕见，尽管其手术复杂，术后继发狭窄的可能性大，但所有畸形的手术原则相同。图 121–6C 中展现了一个插入直肠的手指，这样可以让术者明确尿道和直肠间的薄弱间隔。手术时将插入直肠的手指向后牵拉，可以避免损伤直肠。

如果尿道阴道瘘的位置偏高，或者接近膀胱颈，并且尿道和阴道共壁，则可以采取 Rink 等[69]介绍的

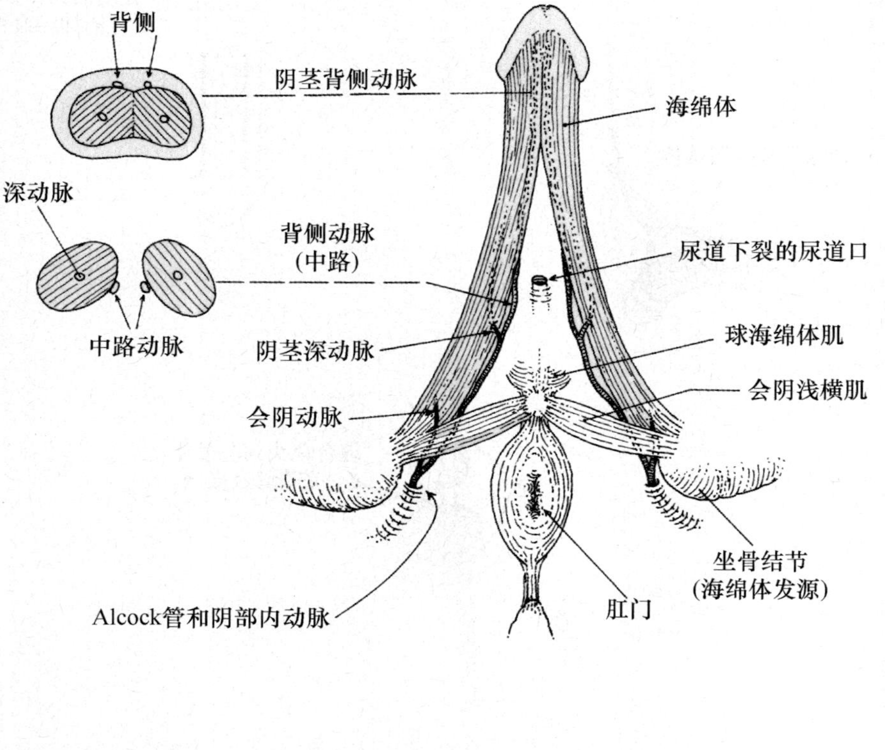

图 121–5　阴茎神经血管束解剖。阴部内动脉存在于坐骨结节处的 Alcock 管中，并在此分叉。会阴动脉经腹侧向阴囊延伸。阴茎背侧动脉行经于中间位置，其中的一个分支向深部走行演变为阴茎背深动脉。每条内侧血管围绕同侧的海绵体蜿蜒，行经海绵体内侧与背侧，在海绵体连接处，演变为阴茎背侧动脉。

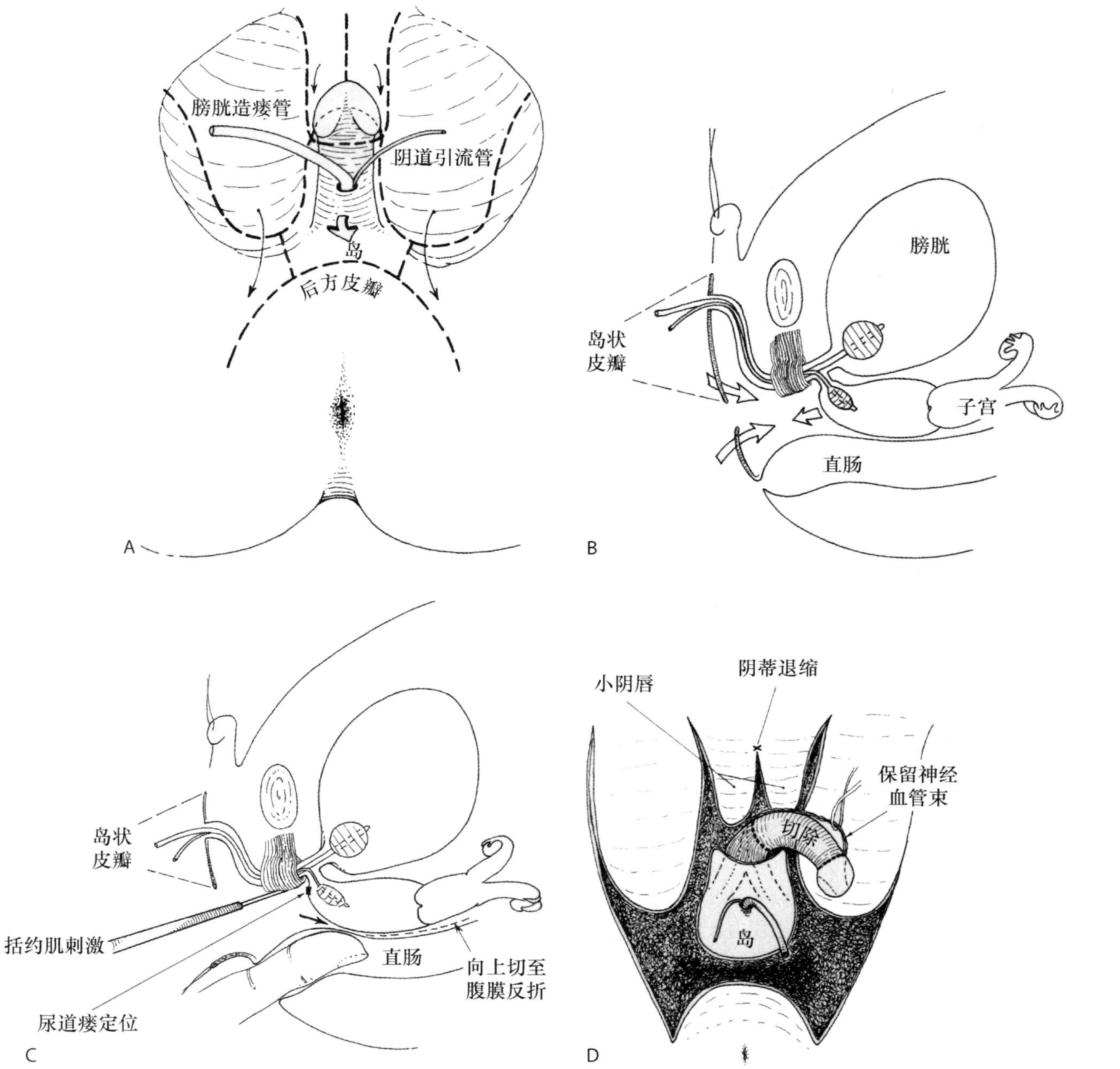

图 121-6　女性重建手术。A. 膀胱截石位时，从术者方向观察到的切口位置。B. 矢状位观，显示前方岛状皮瓣（*右箭头*）向下向内转移，以及内侧的后方皮瓣。小箭头显示从尿道上离断下来的阴道必须转位经过的距离。C. 向后分离阴道和直肠之间空隙，并开始向前从尿道上游离出阴道。D. 皮瓣分离结束。

后路手术方法而无需游离直肠，这样可以为局部分离提供必要的暴露条件。如同其他所描述的手术技巧一样，这一手术步骤可以应用于婴儿，而不必顾虑阴道位置。术前消毒范围包括整个下半身，从剑突一直到趾端，以便必要时患者体位可以不断地在俯卧位和仰卧位之间变化。

如果患者的瘘管位置较高，笔者推荐手术中首先游离阴道。内镜检查之后，将患者转到俯卧位，从后位做一倒 U 形皮瓣，皮瓣角位于两侧会阴体处。在中线位置切开，将泌尿生殖窦从后方的直肠上游离下来

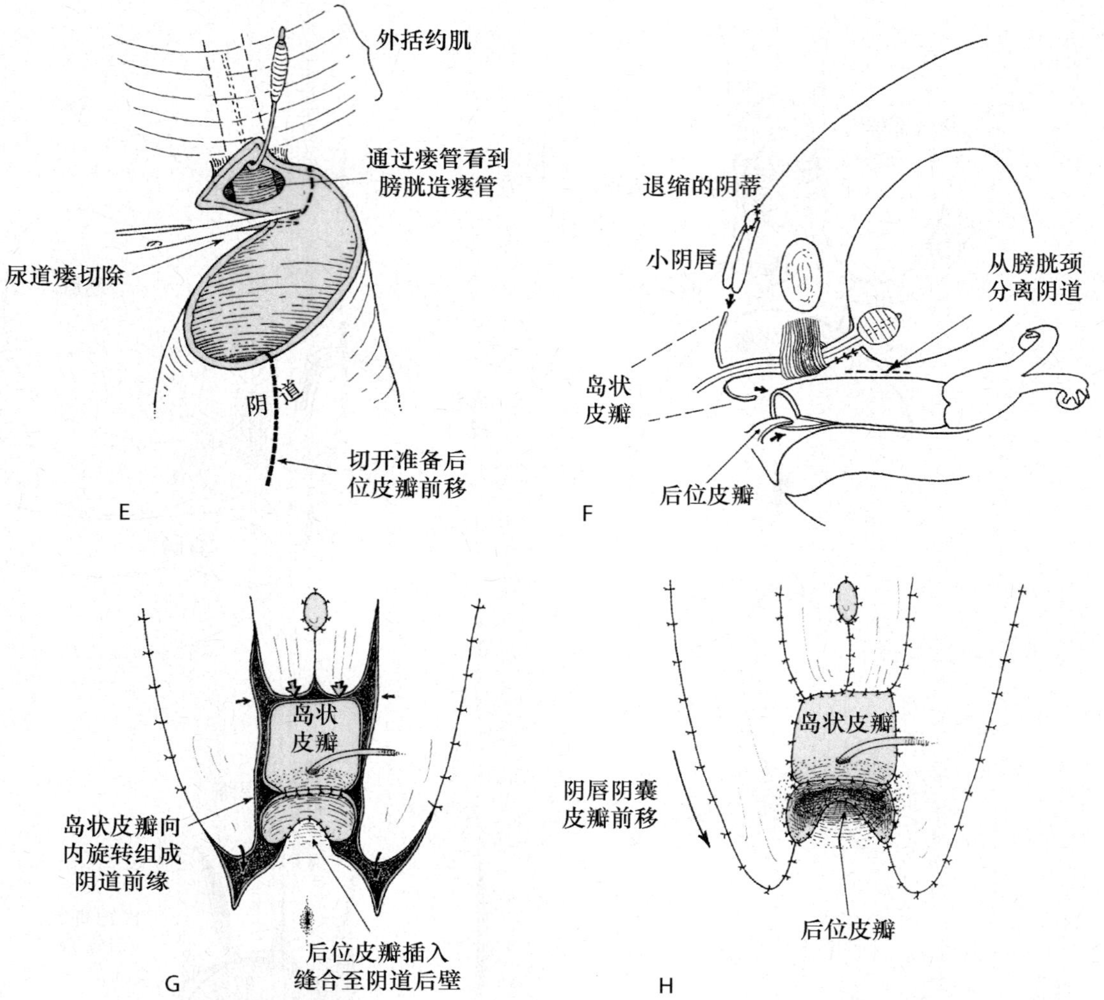

图 121-6　(续) E. 从尿道上分离阴道。F. 在尿道和直肠后分离前平面。G. 阴唇阴囊皮瓣前移遮盖缺损，前位岛状皮瓣向内旋转，后位 U 型皮瓣扩大阴道入口。H. 重建完成。

(图 121-7A)。然后，可以很容易地分离出直肠，在直肠内插入一个小的牵引器，将直肠向上牵拉，不必新做切口或离断直肠。由中线切开泌尿生殖窦后壁，从尿道口一直到尿道阴道交汇处（图 121-7B）。将远端阴道后壁一直切开到近端，暴露此处宽大的阴道腔。然后从阴道口置入牵引器，向上牵拉暴露前壁的阴道尿道瘘。局部注射 1∶200 000 的肾上腺素有助于从尿道处分离出阴道（见图 121-7B），非常靠近膀胱颈时可使用小巧的 Beaver 刀片，将有利于组织精确游离（图 121-7C）。由于尿道后壁和阴道前壁之间拥有非薄的共同的间充质组织，两者几乎共壁，所以这里手术操作最难。将倒 U 形皮瓣缝合到阴道后壁上（图 121-7D）。尿道管建立以后，在其表面再予以一层组织缝合加强，以避免尿道阴道瘘复发。如果可能，可以把阴唇阴囊的脂肪覆盖在尿道阴道之间，阻止瘘管复发。此时，在正中线位置重建的阴唇皮瓣或岛状皮瓣可以轻易地与阴道前壁吻合。广泛游离阴唇阴囊褶，去脂、修剪、向后移位，如 Y-V 成形术一样在阴道口两侧创建大阴唇（见图 121-6A）。如果阴蒂明显肥大，则在患者转为仰卧位时施行阴蒂成形术。该手术在游离阴道之后进行，但由于翻转体位时可能损伤到脆弱的吻合口，所以应该先于阴道外置手术。为扩大阴道入口，曾于阴道前壁分离过岛状皮瓣，之后遗留的皮肤缺损可以由阴蒂过

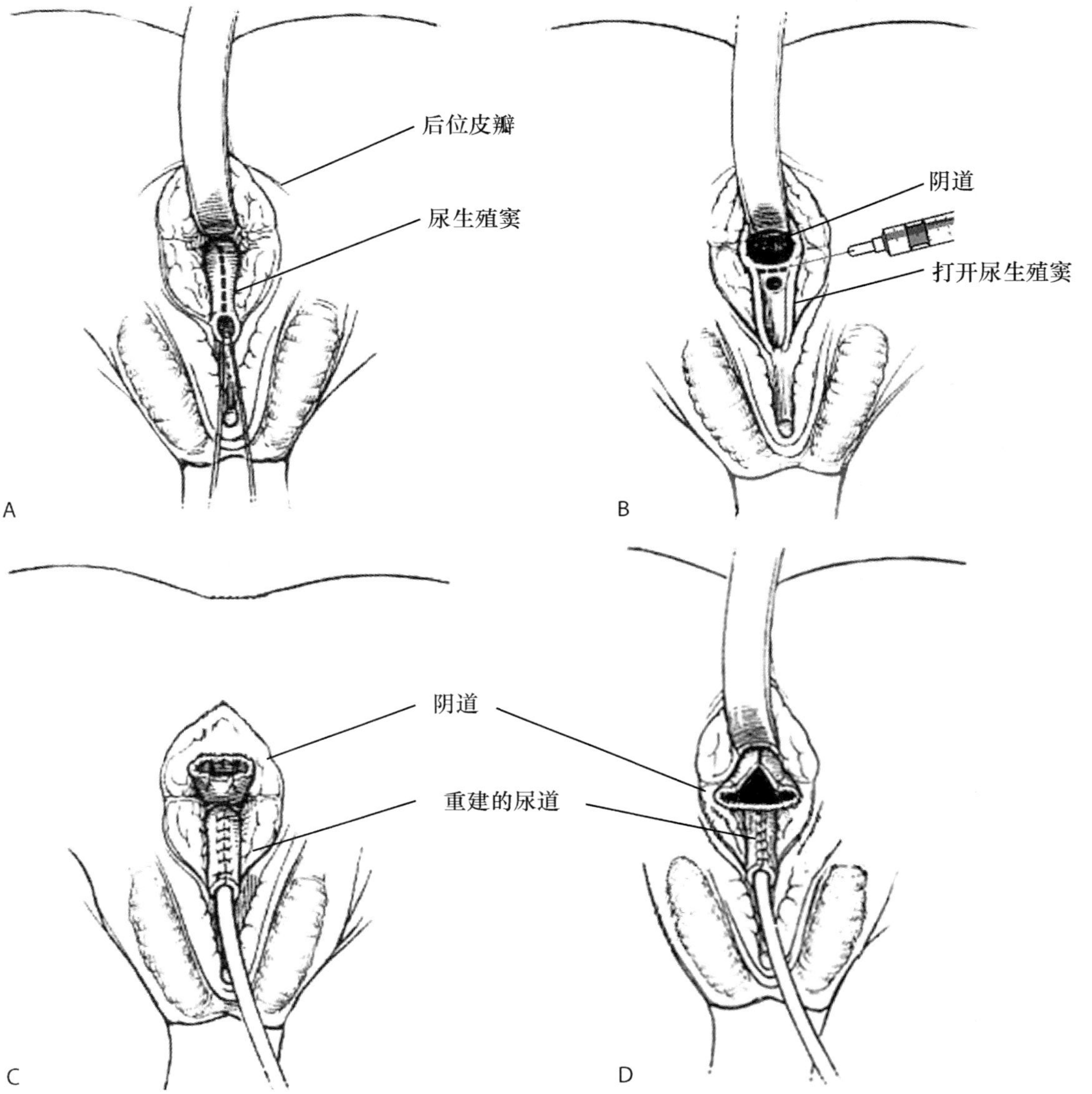

图 121-7　后路手术径路。A. 常用的从后位翻转的 U 型皮瓣。沿后壁或背侧表面长轴切开泌尿生殖窦，向上游离至阴道合流处。B. 阴道后壁打开，于扩大的阴道内置放窄的韧性牵拉器。向上提拉阴道，协助将阴道从尿道和膀胱颈上分离下来。局部注射稀释的肾上腺素（1∶200 000）有助于分离该处脆弱组织。该操作过程困难，应用小的 Beaver 刀片可能有帮助。C. 阴道分离后，尿道卷管。D. 开放阴道，U 型皮瓣插入扩大阴道入口。

多的皮肤来遮盖（见图 121-6G）。如果新建的尿道足够长，则可以把新尿道口设在会阴更靠近正常位置的地方，并打开远端泌尿生殖窦形成一个潮湿的入口。术后早期需要留置一根细的 Foley 导管。然而，如果可以经耻骨上皮肤留置导管将尿流改道，并结合尿道硅橡胶管支撑，则术后防止瘘管复发的效果会更好。

另一种治疗高位阴道的手术方法是全泌尿生殖窦松解术（TUM），由 Pena[66] 于 1997 年介绍用以修复泌尿生殖窦缺陷。环形游离泌尿生殖窦后，能够将其从耻骨上分离出来（图 121-8）。这样，那些向前牵拉尿道和阴道的无血管纤维韧带就得到松解，但操作可能增加损伤支配外括约肌的神经的危险，造成尿失禁。围绕泌尿生殖窦持续松解，直至可以无张力地将 1926

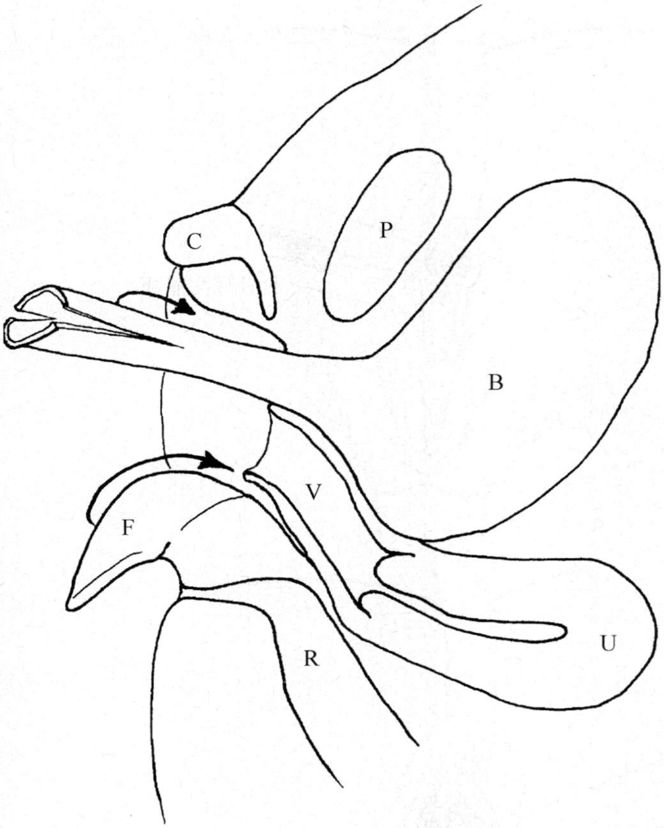

图 121-8　全泌尿生殖窦松解术（TUM）。环切泌尿生殖窦后可以向上一直松解到耻骨后，然后将其整体向下移位直至尿道阴道合流处降至会阴处。切开泌尿生殖窦，与上方的阴蒂缝合，以创建潮湿的阴道入口。后壁与 U 型翻转的皮瓣缝合。不必试图从尿道上分离出阴道。C. 阴蒂；F. 皮瓣；P. 耻骨；R. 直肠；U. 子宫；V. 阴道。（Adapted from Pena[66].）

尿道阴道瘘下降到会阴。也可以部分游离泌尿生殖窦到达耻骨膀胱韧带，这样可以减少外括约肌去神经损伤的可能。

作者认为，后矢状位径路是外科手术治疗 CAH 的一大进步。同样，经验表明，在截石位完成 TUM 手术也是一种安全的方法。但是，接受这一手术的患者必须进行长期随访，评估其控制小便的能力。一些研究小组报道其行 TUM 手术的经验，称术后没有患者继发尿失禁[19,30,39,47]。Jenak 等[39]建议把过多的泌尿生殖窦从腹侧打开，将其黏膜排列成行构建阴道前庭。Farkas 等[19]建议从背侧部分切开多余的泌尿生殖窦，留下足够长的尿道并且将开放的窦道黏膜瓣翻转形成外置阴道的前壁和侧壁。

高位泌尿生殖窦的另一种手术方法是 Passerini-Glazel 介绍的阴蒂阴道成形术[65]。在这一术式中，阴蒂退缩时保留了供应龟头的神经血管束。背侧和腹侧分离以后，沿长轴缝合阴蒂皮肤，完成阴道外置步骤。多余的皮肤向下向后转移，缝合到开口扩大的远端泌尿生殖窦上。然后，圆柱形的阴蒂和新建尿道得以成形，将其嵌入会阴，与游离以后的真实阴道相吻合。

男性再建手术

如果睾酮产量低下、受体对雄激素不敏感或者 5α-还原酶无力将睾酮转化为双氢睾酮，则会产生男性第一性征不足。这种情况可同样出现在混合性腺发育不良和真两性畸形中。对所有确认为男性的患者，治疗方案大体相似。在这些患者中，大多数表现为小阴茎合并严重的阴茎下弯，尿道开口于阴茎阴囊交界处，位于分裂的阴囊之间，有时还伴有阴茎前阴囊， 1927
可见皱褶的阴囊皮肤位于小阴茎之前（图 121-9A）。阴茎包皮不完整，背侧包皮堆积，术中注意保护这些包皮组织以便利用。术前睾酮治疗对小阴茎手术整形是有帮助的，同时可以明确阴茎对睾酮刺激是否敏感。由于小阴茎和严重的阴茎下弯合并存在，笔者推荐对这些患者采取分期手术的方法。

第一次修复手术主要目的是纠正阴茎弯曲、伸直阴茎，同时把背侧累赘的包皮转移到阴茎腹侧，一方面修补腹侧包皮缺损，另一方面为二期手术创建新尿道做准备。一旦包皮被环切并游离至阴茎阴囊交界处以后，就用人工勃起试验明确阴茎下弯的严重程度。然后，需要切除阴茎腹侧所有的瘢痕组织，这些瘢痕代表了闭锁的海绵体残留，必须从龟头下开始完全将其切除直至近端海绵体分叉处（图 121-9B）。这些属于尿道下裂亚型的患者，由于阴茎弯曲部位非常靠近阴茎海绵体的分叉，所以手术中出血较多，由此给新建的尿道带来许多失败的风险，因此作者建议对这些患者采取分期手术。图 121-9C 展示了如何分离背侧堆积的包皮组织，并将其转移覆盖到阴茎腹侧的操作步骤。与横行切口比较，纵向切口可以更好地保留血管，避免阴茎远端血液供应障碍，并有利于背侧包皮 192
遮盖腹侧缺损。如图所示，C 和 C’吻合，旋转远端打开的包皮至龟头顶。B 和 B’在阴茎腹侧吻合，皮

图 121-9　Ⅰ期男性重建手术。A. 严重阴茎弯曲的小阴茎外观，合并阴茎阴囊型尿道下裂和阴囊分裂。B. 阴茎弯曲纠正后，海绵体伸直。C. 展开背侧赘生的包皮。D. 沿长轴游离阴茎体，将背侧皮肤转移到阴茎腹侧，如帽子样遮盖腹侧阴茎体。E. Ⅰ期手术完成。

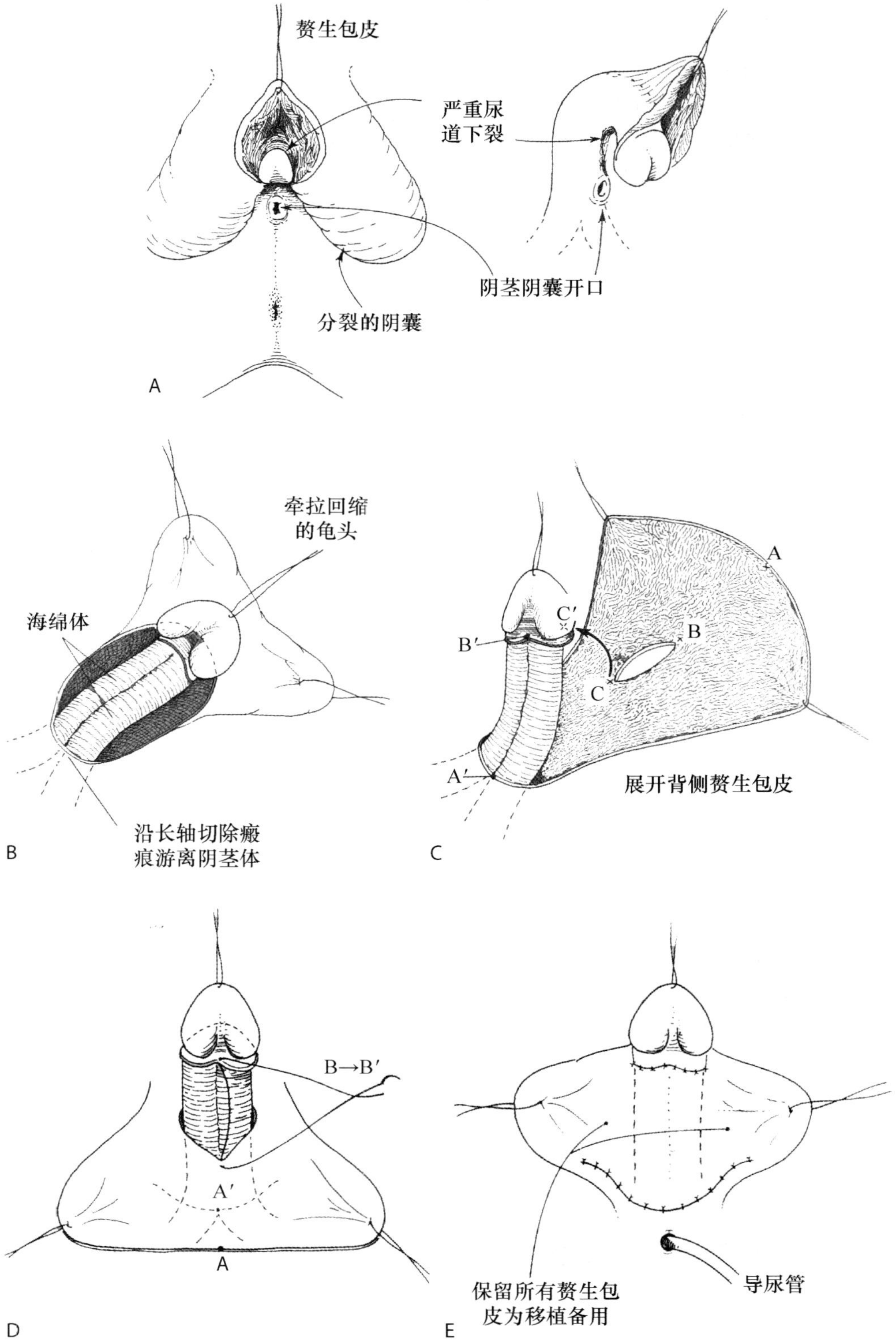

肤移位后 A 与近端会阴 A' 相吻合。这样就得到了足够覆盖阴茎体腹侧的皮肤，并为以后的尿道重建手术准备了丰富的尿道移植物。皮瓣合适并不再引起阴茎下弯，这一点非常重要（图 121-9D）。会阴尿道口留置 Foley 导管引流膀胱尿液。转移的包皮皮瓣裁剪后重新缝合，持续引流尿液 4～5 天，直至患者痊愈（图 121-9E）。

一期手术后 4～6 个月，当局部水肿消退、腹侧包皮变得柔软光滑以后，就可以计划行尿道下裂二期修补手术，即在阴茎阴囊交界处的尿道口和龟头顶点之间重建新的尿道。术前重要的一点是要考虑阴茎的大小，部分小阴茎需要行手术增大。如果阴茎持续不发育，则可每月给予睾酮，连续 2～3 次。为防止术后卧床休息期间阴茎频繁勃起，术前需要至少 4 周的激素停顿期。如图 121-10A 所示，将当时位于腹侧的丰富包皮卷管后可形成新的尿道。在近端，阴囊中线处的皮肤近乎没有毛发，可以卷管与近端尿道口吻合。可将多侧孔的 Jackson-Pratt 管支撑于近端阴囊中线皮瓣和远端背侧包皮构成的新尿道内（图 121-10B）。皮下组织以光滑的丙交酯乙交酯共聚物 910（Vicryl）可吸收缝线连续缝合，将阴囊中线皮瓣卷管。包皮重新定位后展平，按需

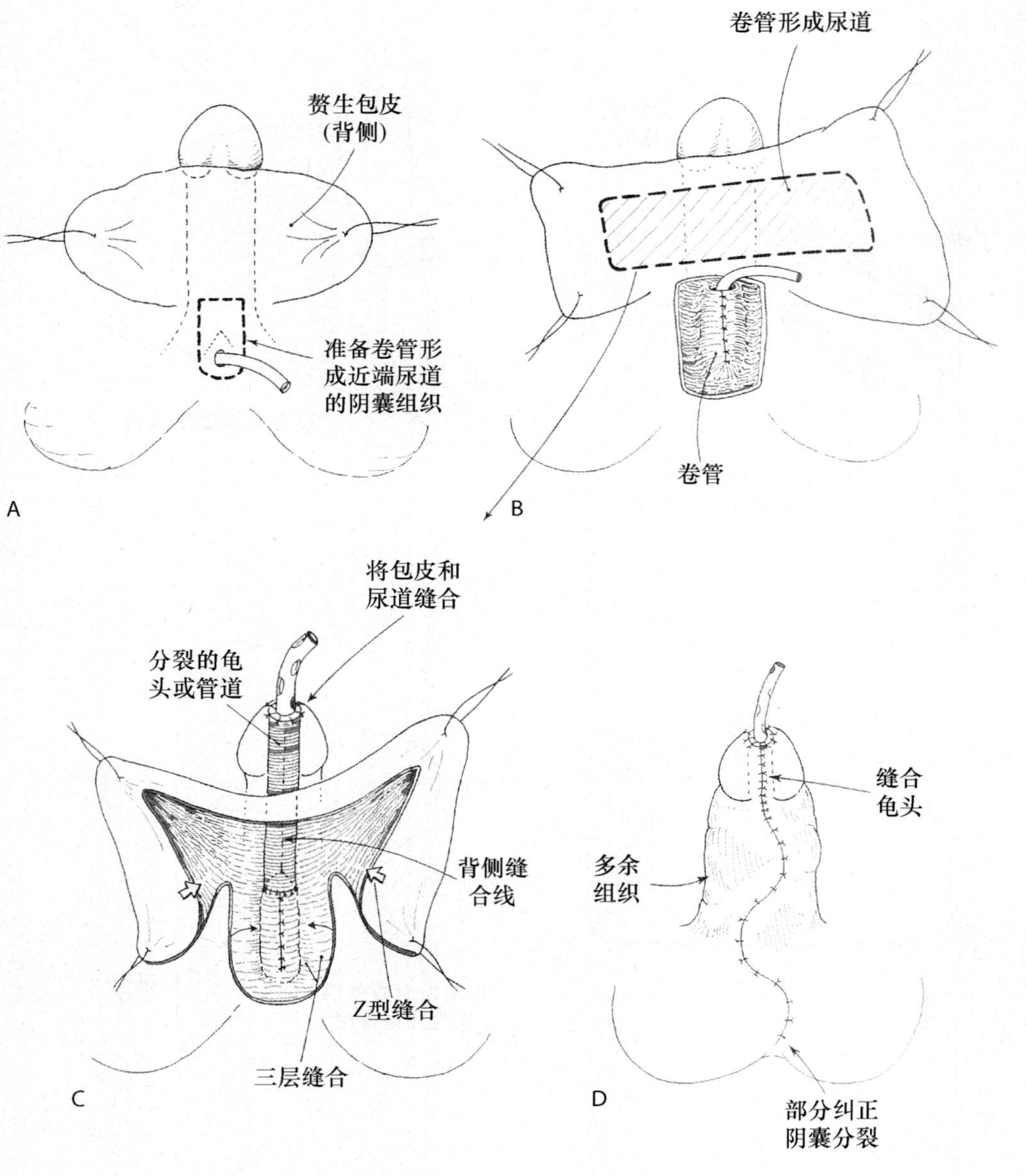

图 121-10 Ⅱ期男性重建手术。A. 设计复合尿道移植物。B. 阴囊组织卷管形成近端尿道，在多余的腹侧皮瓣上设计新尿道移植物的轮廓。C. 完成远端尿道移植，置放硅胶支撑管，创建通向尿道口的隧道。D. 最后缝合尿道，闭合外层伤口，利用背侧转移到腹侧后的过多的包皮组织分三层缝合。

要裁剪适当长度和宽度的游离移植物，准备将其一端与阴囊中线卷管后形成的尿道相连接，另一端向远端延伸，与龟头固定。1 岁以内的儿童，最合适的尿道宽度是 12mm。移植物切取以后，将包皮去脂，置于盛有生理盐水的硅胶容器内防止干燥萎缩。这一步骤在膀胱黏膜代尿道或口腔黏膜代尿道手术中更显重要。再次以 Vicryl 缝线连续缝合。斜切移植物以防与卷管后阴囊中线皮瓣吻合后出现狭窄，阴囊中线皮瓣也向反方向斜切。内翻缝合背侧包皮形成的新尿道，翻转面朝向海绵体。在完成近端尿道吻合以前，新形成的尿道管近端应超过原尿道口。因为即使是最细的 Foley 导管也易于在近端吻合口处成角，所以避免将其应用于阴茎短小的患者身上，而代之以外周尿道造瘘术，以及采用多侧孔的 Jackson-Pratt 支撑管并将其近端放过吻合部位。

根据龟头分离的程度不同，或者把新建的尿道埋藏于裂开的龟头深部，然后再将龟头聚拢缝合，或者在龟头顶点中线处打孔，尿道以皮下隧道的形式从龟头开口处引出（图 121-10C）。在隧道形成期间，千万不要扭转移植物。然后将远端龟头上皮与移植物间断缝合，注意尿道口必须宽敞以防术后狭窄。支撑管与龟头缝合，防止术后早期滑脱。新尿道表面需以组织遮盖加强，尤其在吻合口近端，需要向阴茎体方向游离组织，以 2～3 层额外层次遮盖于尿道表面，这样就在近端吻合口、阴囊中线移植物（尤其在缝合线朝外的地方）和更远端的新尿道移植物表面创建了大量间质层。根据不同的患者，残余的腹侧皮肤用不同的式样 Z 形缝合（图 121-10D）。注意不能把龟头对合得太紧，并应仔细选择硅橡胶支撑管，以使小阴茎不会明显外凸。如果需要，可以纵行劈开 7 号硅橡胶支撑管以适合较小的龟头。

膀胱引流可以在手术前于会阴部尿道造瘘，或耻骨上膀胱造瘘。阴囊中线卷管成新尿道以后，需要修剪近端阴茎体和阴囊的皮肤，这样也能部分纠治阴囊分裂。任何多余的组织都应留下，以便术后出现狭窄或瘘管而再行手术修补时加以利用。为达到引流的目
29 的，可以在局部留置一个小的独立的 Z 形开口。在度过出现瘘管和狭窄的风险期以后，可以对此进行修裁。如果龟头分裂且较小，可以保留远端腹侧阴茎体皮肤 5 mm，向远侧旋转，以缓解龟头下新尿道的压力。使用 Tegaderm 敷料直接覆盖于阴囊底和阴茎体上以适当加压，可以把术后血肿和水肿减少到最小。龟头缝合一针以固定支撑管。

在一些罕见的病例中，可利用的组织比较少，不能同时满足制作新尿道和覆盖阴茎腹侧的双重需要，此时可以考虑膀胱黏膜代尿道的手术方法。尽管这一方法常常是有效的，但黏膜伸缩和（或）干燥是该方法的明显缺点。在做吻合时需要持续灌注，并避免移植黏膜过于宽大，这些都很重要。术后导尿支撑管 1930
拔除以后，必须坚持每天扩张远端尿道以防膀胱黏膜暴露于空气中后发生尿道口粘合。扩张时，要求父母将 Hegar 扩张管置入尿道口下 1cm，从术后 10～14 天开始坚持每天 1～2 次。

一些性别选择为男性的真两性畸形或混合性腺发育不良的患者，体内残留的苗勒氏管可能扩张（图 121-11A）。这种情况通常见于二期手术以后的患者，由于远端尿道的建立，可能出现尿道阻力增加，排尿时尿流回流至苗勒氏管，造成管腔扩张。难治型的苗勒氏管异常引起反复发作的尿路感染和（或）附睾炎。对于这些患者，应该予以手术切除苗勒氏管。当输精管经过扩张的阴道外侧壁时，试图将其保留。在输精管进入精阜以前，必须充分估算其行经路线。预计每条输精管的行经路线，在其两侧分别做一切口（图 121-11B）。切除苗勒氏管的剩余结构，包括偶尔出现的显著扩张的阴道。然后，将包含输精管的阴道壁条卷管，从泌尿生殖窦到输精管入口处，黏膜内翻缝合（图 121-11C）。可以用可吸收线行连续缝合，通常一层缝合即可。对于混合性腺发育不良的患者，如果体内存在卵巢结构，可以切除这些与指定性别不符的器官。

阴茎体向远侧移位的患者，皱褶的阴囊出现在阴茎前（图 121-12A）。这种畸形常合并阴囊分裂，需要纠治。但是，重要的是，这类手术应该拖延至新尿道和阴茎腹侧伤口完全治愈以后进行。这是因为在手术纠治阴茎阴囊反位时需要游离并移除用于尿道下裂 1931
修补的皮瓣。阴茎阴囊反位手术与尿道成形手术之间应间隔至少 6 个月以上。将牵拉阴茎基底的皮肤松解，游离一块方形皮瓣，向尾端移位，以此伸长阴囊，进而纠正阴囊分裂畸形。然后，向前、向头端牵拉阴茎，转移腹壁皮瓣覆盖于阴茎腹侧基底（如图 121-12B 至 F 中，B 与 B’吻合）。在手术延伸阴茎的过程中，向上牵拉阴茎使其表现为勃起形态以后才能旋转腹壁皮瓣向后、向阴茎尾端，这一点非常重要。否则，很容易把阴茎移出阴阜顶端，造成无法接受的阴茎弯曲外观。由腹壁旋转而来的皮瓣必须有足够的长度以围绕阴茎基底半圈并与另一侧皮瓣吻合，

图 121–11　外科处理残留的苗勒氏管。A. 男性残留苗勒氏管结构时，所有的操作都必须遵循保护输精管的原则。如图所示，苗勒氏管常进入扩张的阴道侧壁，行经于黏膜和肌层之间，或穿行于肌层中。B. 保留含有输精管的阴道壁条带，将其卷管，切除残余的阴道和子宫。C. 从输精管进入阴道壁的入口开始关闭残留的阴道条带，直至狭窄的颈部，输精管在此位置进入尿道。

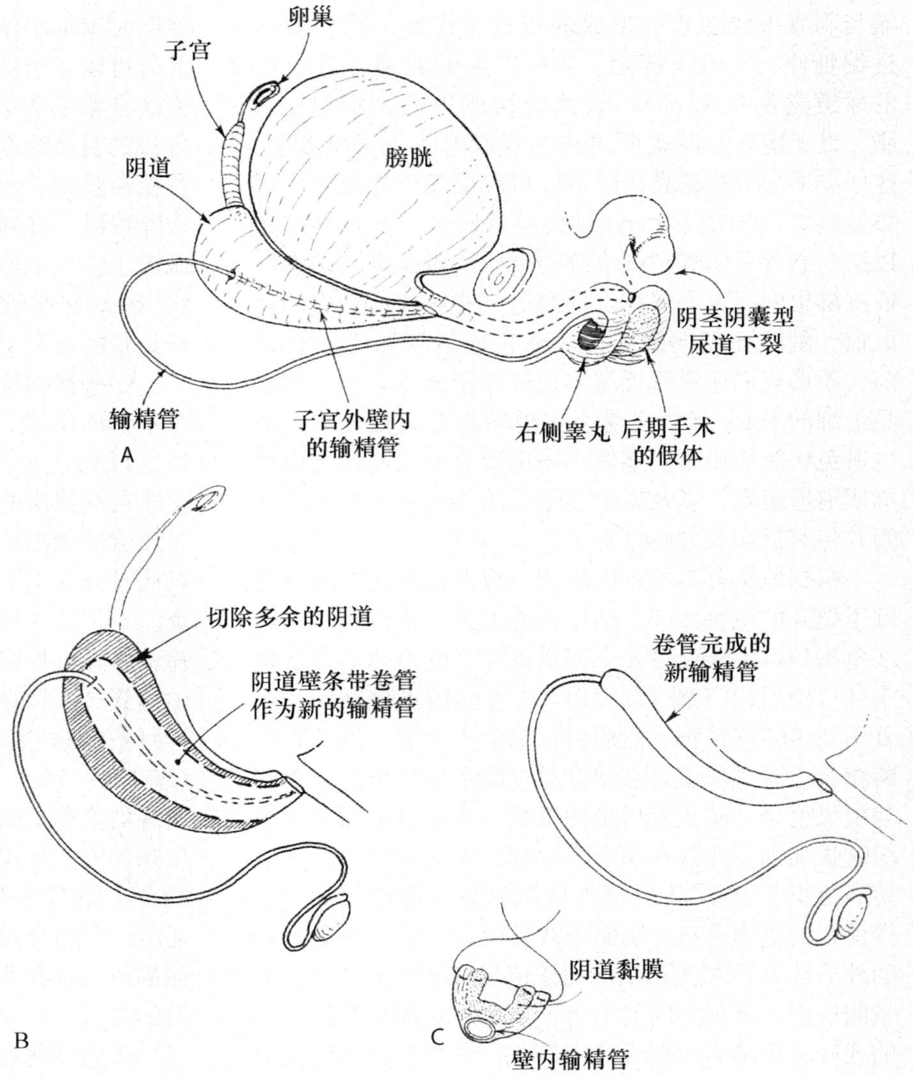

两侧皮瓣吻合时不能有张力。新建阴囊在两侧和中线位置缝合关闭，以完成修复和纠正阴囊分裂畸形。在阴茎腹侧伤口痊愈以前，患者需要卧床休息，并接受尿流改道。

小结

两性畸形的发病原因涉及众多病理生理异常，不同类型的疾病治疗必须加以系统全面的考虑，需要小儿外科医生和内分泌医生联手协作。家长必须参与决定，目的是为了尽可能地给患儿创造最高质量的生活。为达到最好的手术效果，需要医生考虑到方方面面的细致问题。所有这些努力的最终目的只有一个，那就是哪怕不能生育，也能给患者将来提供良好的、有功能的性生活。

（孙　杰译　文建国校）

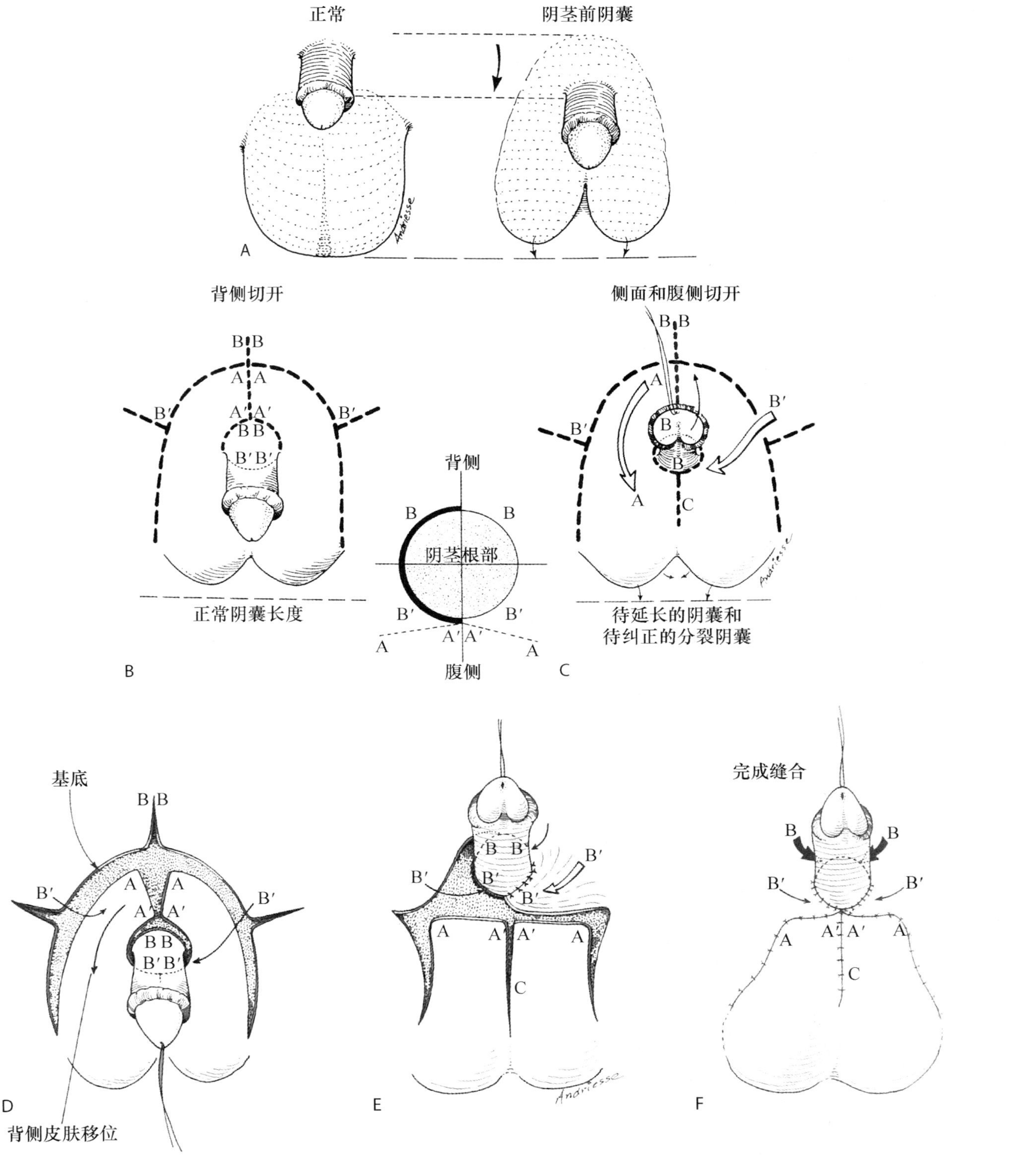

图 121-12　手术纠正阴茎阴囊反位和阴囊分裂。A. 纠正表现型错位的患者，其阴囊组织终止于阴茎背侧基底前，与阴囊分裂相关。B 和 C. 通过一系列背侧、侧面和腹侧的切口，完成阴囊后置和阴茎前移。D. 广泛提升基底宽大的腹部皮瓣，以保留足够的血液供应。E. 前位的腹壁皮肤需充分游离，以利其前移至阴茎腹侧皮肤时不存在张力。这一措施非常重要，不然可能造成阴茎前面或背侧皮瓣牵拉如蹼状。F. 用细的可吸收线缝合剩余的伤口。阴囊皮肤向尾端转位，阴囊得以延长，阴囊分裂的外观也得以改善。

致谢

We thank Rafael Pieretti Vanmarcke, MD, for his invaluable skills in updating the original diagrams done by Paul Andreissi, and for adapting the drawings that Richard Rink, MD, kindly gave us permission to use. We also thank David MacLaughlin, PhD, for his inestimable contributions to our understanding of the molecular mechanisms of sex differentiation. This chapter is dedicated to W. Hardy Hendren, MD, and John D. Crawford, MD, for all they taught us about the care of these children over the years.

参考文献

1. Achermann JC, Ito M, Hindmarsh PC, Jameson JL: A mutation in the gene encoding steroidogenic factor-1 causes XY sex reversal and adrenal failure in humans. Nat Genet 1999;22:125-126.
2. Andersson S, Berman DM, Jenkins EP, Russell DW: Deletion of steroid 5 alpha-reductase 2 gene in male pseudohermaphroditism. Nature 1991;354:159-161.
3. Barbaux S, Niaudet P, Gubler MC, et al: Donor splice-site mutations in WT1 are responsible for Frasier syndrome. Nat Genet 1997;17:467-470.
4. Barbie TU, Barbie DA, MacLaughlin DT, et al: Müllerian inhibiting substance inhibits cervical cancer cell growth via a pathway involving p130 and p107. Proc Natl Acad Sci U S A 2003;100:15601-15606.
5. Bardoni B, Zanaria E, Guioli S, et al: A dosage sensitive locus at chromosome Xp21 is involved in male to female sex reversal. Nat Genet 1994;7:497-501.
6. Belville C, Josso N, Picard JY: Persistence of müllerian derivatives in males. Am J Med Genet 1999;89:218-223.
7. Bennett CP, Docherty Z, Robb SA, et al: Deletion 9p and sex reversal. J Med Genet 1993;30:518-520.
8. Berkovitz GD, Fechner PY, Marcantonio SM, et al: The role of the sex-determining region of the Y chromosome (SRY) in the etiology of 46,XX true hermaphroditism. Hum Genet 1992;88:411-416.
9. Budzik GP, Powell SM, Kamagata S, Donahoe PK: Müllerian inhibiting substance fractionation by dye affinity chromatography. Cell 1983;34:307-314.
10. Cate RL, Donahoe PK, MacLaughlin DT: Müllerian inhibitory substance. In Sporn MB, Roberts AB (eds): Handbook of Experimental Pharmacology. Berlin, Springer-Verlag, 1990.
11. Dasgupta R, Schnitzer JJ, Hendren WH, Donahoe PK: Congenital adrenal hyperplasia: Surgical considerations required to repair a 46,XX patient raised as a male. J Pediatr Surg 2003;38:1269-1273.
12. David M, Forest MG: Prenatal treatment of congenital adrenal hyperplasia resulting from 21-hydroxylase deficiency. J Pediatr 1984;105:799-803.
13. Donahoe PK, Crawford JD, Hendren WH: Management of neonates and children with male pseudohermaphroditism. J Pediatr Surg 1977;12:1045-1057.
14. Donahoe PK, Crawford JD, Hendren WH: True hermaphroditism: A clinical description and a proposed function for the long arm of the Y chromosome. J Pediatr Surg 1978; 13:293-301.
15. Donahoe PK, Crawford JD, Hendren WH: Mixed gonadal dysgenesis, pathogenesis and management. J Pediatr Surg 1979;14:287-300.
16. Donahoe PK, Schnitzer JJ: Evaluation of the infant who has ambiguous genitalia, and principles of operative management. Semin Pediatr Surg 1996;5:1-12.
17. Donohoue PA, Parker K, Migeon CJ: Congenital adrenal hyperplasia. In Scriver CR, Beaudet AL, Sly WS, Valle D (eds): The Metabolic and Molecular Bases of Inherited Disease. New York, McGraw-Hill, 1995, pp 2929-2966.
18. Engle E, Forbes A: Cytogenetic and clinical findings in 48 patients with congenitally defective or absent ovaries. Medicine 1965;44:135-164.
19. Farkas A, Chertin B, Hadas-Halpren I: 1-Stage feminizing genitoplasty: 8 years of experience with 49 cases. J Urol 2001;165:2341-2346.
20. Federman DD: Abnormal Sexual Development: A Genetic and Endocrine Approach to Differential Diagnosis. Philadelphia, WB Saunders, 1967.
21. Federman DD, Donahoe PK: Ambiguous genitalia—etiology, diagnosis, and therapy. In Kreigsberg RA (ed): Advances in Endocrinology and Metabolism. Chicago, Mosby, 1995, pp 91-116.
22. Flatau E, Josefsberg Z, Reisner SH, et al: Penile size in the newborn. J Pediatr 1975;87:663-664.
23. Ford CE, Jones KW, Polani PE, et al: A sex-chromosome anomaly in a case of gonadal dysgenesis (Turner's syndrome). Lancet 1959;1:711-713.
24. Foster JW, Dominguez-Steglich MA, Guioli S, et al: Campomelic dysplasia and autosomal sex reversal caused by mutations in an SRY-related gene. Nature 1994;372:525-530.
25. Grumbach MM, Conte FA: Disorders of sexual differentiation. In Wilson JD, Foster DW (eds): Williams Textbook of Endocrinology. Philadelphia, WB Saunders, 1985, pp 312-401.
26. Grumbach MM, Conte FE: Disorders of sex differentiation. In Wilson JD, Foster DW, Kronenberg HM, Larsen PR (eds): Williams Textbook of Endocrinology, 9th ed. Philadelphia, WB Saunders, 1998, pp 1303-1425.
27. Grumbach M, Hughes I, Conte F: Disorders of sex differentiation. In Larsen PR, Kronenberg HM, Melmed S, Polonsky KS (eds): Williams Textbook of Endocrinology, 10th ed. Philadelphia, WB Saunders, 2003, pp 842-1002.
28. Ha TU, Segev DL, Barbie D, et al: Müllerian inhibiting substance inhibits ovarian cell growth through an Rb-independent mechanism. J Biol Chem 2000;275:37101-37109.
29. Hammes A, Guo JK, Lutsch G, et al: Two splice variants of the Wilms' tumor 1 gene have distinct functions during sex determination and nephron formation. Cell 2001;106:319-329.
30. Hamza AF, Soliman HA, Abdel Hay SA, et al: Total urogenital sinus mobilization in the repair of cloacal anomalies and congenital adrenal hyperplasia. J Pediatr Surg 2001; 36:1656-1658.
31. He WW, Gustafson ML, Hirobe S, Donahoe PK: The developmental expression of four novel serine/threonine kinase receptors homologous to the activin/TGF-beta receptor family. Dev Dyn 1993;196:133-142.
32. Hendren WH, Crawford JD: Adrenogenital syndrome: The anatomy of the anomaly and its repair. Some new concepts. J Pediatr Surg 1969;4:49-58.
33. Hoshiya M, Christian BP, Cromie WJ, et al: Persistent müllerian duct syndrome caused by both a 27-bp deletion and a novel splice mutation in the MIS type II receptor gene. Birth Defects Res Part A Clin Mol Teratol 2003;67:868-874.
34. Hoshiya Y, Gupta V, Segev DL, et al: Müllerian inhibiting substance induces NFκB signaling in breast and prostate cancer cells. Mol Cell Endocrinol 2003;211:43-49.
35. Imperato-McGinley J, Guerrero L, Gautier T, Peterson RE: Steroid 5alpha-reductase deficiency in man: An inherited form of male pseudohermaphroditism. Science 1974; 186:1213-1215.

36. Imperato-McGinley J, Zhu YS: Androgens and male physiology in the syndrome of 5alpha-reductase-2 deficiency. Mol Cell Endocrinol 2002;198:51-59.
37. Ito M, Yu R, Jameson JL: DAX-1 inhibits SF-1-mediated transactivation via a carboxy-terminal domain that is deleted in adrenal hypoplasia congenita. Mol Cell Biol 1997;17:1476-1483.
38. Jacobs PA, Ross A: Structural abnormalities of the Y chromosome in man. Nature 1966;210:352-354.
39. Jenak R, Ludwikowski B, Gonzalez R: Total urogenital sinus mobilization: A modified perineal approach for feminizing genitoplasty and urogenital sinus repair. J Urol 2001;165: 2347-2349.
40. Jost A: Recherches sur la differenciation sexuelle de l'embryon du lapin. Arch Anat Microsc Morphol Exp 1947;36:271-315.
41. Koopman P: SRY and SOX9: Mammalian testis-determining genes. Cell Mol Life Sci 1999;55:839-856.
42. Koopman P, Gubbay J, Vivian N, et al: Male development of chromosomally female mice transgenic for SRY. Nature 1991;351:117-121.
43. Koopman P, Munsterberg A, Capel B, et al: Expression of a candidate sex-determining gene during mouse testis differentiation. Nature 1990;348:450-452.
44. Lala DS, Rice DA, Parker KL: Steroidogenic factor I, a key regulator of steroidogenic enzyme expression, is the mouse homolog of fushi tarazu-factor I. Mol Endocrinol 1992;6:1249-1258.
45. Lee MM, Donahoe PK: Ambiguous genitalia. In Bardin W (ed): Current Therapy in Endocrinology and Metabolism. Toronto, BC Decker, 1992, pp 232-240.
46. Lubahn DB, Joseph DR, Sullivan PM, et al: Cloning of human androgen receptor complementary DNA and localization to the X chromosome. Science 1988;240:327-330.
47. Ludwikowski B, Oesch Hayward I, Gonzalez R: Total urogenital sinus mobilization. BJU Int 1999;83:820-822.
48. MacLaughlin DT, Donahoe PK: Sex determination and differentiation. N Engl J Med 2004;350:367-378.
49. Manuel M, Katayama KP, Jones HW: The age of occurrence of gonadal tumors in intersex patients with a Y chromosome. Am J Obstet Gynecol 1976;124:293-300.
50. Masiakos PT, MacLaughlin DT, Maheswaran S, et al: Human ovarian cancer, cell lines, and primary ascites cells express the human müllerian inhibiting substance (MIS) type II receptor, bind, and are responsive to MIS. Clin Cancer Res 1999;5:3488-3499.
51. McElreavey K, Vilain E, Abbas N, et al: XY sex reversal associated with a deletion 5′ to the SRY HMG box in the testis-determining region. Proc Natl Acad Sci U S A 1992; 89:11016-11020.
52. McLaren A: Mammalian germ cells: Birth, sex, and immortality. Cell Struct Funct 2001;26:119-122.
53. Miller WL: Molecular biology of steroid hormone synthesis. Endocr Rev 1988;9:295-318.
54. Miller WL: Steroid 17alpha-hydroxylase deficiency—not rare everywhere. J Clin Endocrinol Metab 2004;89:40-42.
55. Mornet E, Boue J, Raux-Demay M, et al: First trimester prenatal diagnosis of 21-hydroxylase deficiency by linkage analysis to HLA-DNA probes and by 17-hydroxyprogesterone determination. Hum Genet 1986;73:358-364.
56. Muller J, Skakkebaek NE, Nielsen OH, Graem N: Cryptorchidism and testis cancer: Atypical infantile germ cells followed by carcinoma in situ and invasive carcinoma in adulthood. Cancer 1984;54:629-634.
57. Nef S, Parada LF: Cryptorchidism in mice mutant for Insl3. Nat Genet 1999;22:295-299.
58. New MI, Wilson RC: Steroid disorders in children: Congenital adrenal hyperplasia and apparent mineralocorticoid excess. Proc Natl Acad Sci U S A 1999;96:12790-12797.
59. Nihoul-Fekete C, Lortat-Jacob S, Cachin O, Josso N: Preservation of gonadal function in true hermaphroditism. J Pediatr Surg 1984;19:50-55.
60. Page DC, Mosher R, Simpson E, et al: The sex-determining region of the human Y chromosome encodes a finger protein. Cell 1987;51:1091-1104.
61. Pang S: Congenital adrenal hyperplasia. Endocrinol Metab Clin North Am 1997;26:853-891.
62. Pang S, Pollack MS, Loo M, et al: Pitfalls of prenatal diagnosis of 21-hydroxylase deficiency congenital adrenal hyperplasia. J Clin Endocrinol Metab 1985;61:89-97.
63. Pang SY, Pollack MS, Marshall RN, Immken L: Prenatal treatment of congenital adrenal hyperplasia due to 21-hydroxylase deficiency. N Engl J Med 1990;322:111-115.
64. Parker KL, Schimmer BP, Schedl A: Genes essential for early events in gonadal development. Cell Mol Life Sci 1999;55:831-838.
65. Passerini-Glazel G: A new 1-stage procedure for clitorovaginoplasty in severely masculinized female pseudohermaphrodites. J Urol 1989;142:565-568.
66. Pena AJ: Total urogenital mobilization—an easier way to repair cloacas. J Pediatr Surg 1997;32:263-268.
67. Picard JY, Josso N: Purification of testicular anti-müllerian hormone allowing direct visualization of the pure glycoprotein and determination of yield and purification factor. Mol Endocrinol 1984;34:23-29.
68. Renaud EJ, MacLaughlin DT, Oliva E, et al: Endometrial cancer is a receptor-mediated target for müllerian inhibiting substance. Proc Natl Acad Sci U S A 2005;102:111-116.
69. Rink RC, Pope JC, Kropp BP, et al: Reconstruction of the high urogenital sinus: Early perineal prone approach without division of the rectum. J Urol 1997;158:1293-1297.
70. Robboy SJ, Miller T, Donahoe PK, et al: Dysgenesis of testicular and streak gonads in the syndrome of mixed gonadal dysgenesis: Perspective derived from a clinicopathologic analysis of twenty-one cases. Hum Pathol 1982;13:700-716.
71. Saitou M, Barton SC, Surani MA: A molecular programme for the specification of germ cell fate in mice. Nature 2002; 418:293-300.
72. Schnitzer JJ, Donahoe PK: Surgical treatment of congenital adrenal hyperplasia. Endocrinol Metab Clin North Am 2001;30:137-154.
73. Schnitzer JJ, Donahoe PK, Tash J, Poppas DP: Single stage reconstruction for infants with congenital adrenal hyperplasia. Endocrinologist 2003;13:190-194.
74. Scully RE: Gonadoblastoma: A review of 74 cases. Cancer 1970;25:1340-1356.
75. Segev DL, Ha TU, Tran TT, et al: Müllerian inhibiting substance inhibits breast cancer cell growth through an NFkappa B-mediated pathway. J Biol Chem 2000;275: 28371-28379.
76. Segev DL, Hoshiya Y, Stephen AE, et al: Müllerian inhibiting substance regulates NFkappaB signaling and growth of mammary epithelial cells in vivo. J Biol Chem 2001;276: 26799-26806.
77. Sinclair AH, Berta P, Palmer MS, et al: A gene from the human sex-determining region encodes a protein with homology to a conserved DNA-binding motif. Nature 1990; 346:240-244.
78. Teixeira J, Shah P, Donahoe PK: Developmental expression of a candidate müllerian inhibiting substance type II receptor. Endocrinology 1996;137:160.
79. Tilley WD, Marcelli M, Wilson JD, McPhaul MJ: Characterization and expression of a cDNA encoding the

human androgen receptor. Proc Natl Acad Sci U S A 1989; 86:327-331.

80. Tommerup N, Schempp W, Meinecke P, et al: Assignment of an autosomal sex reversal locus (SRA1) and campomelic dysplasia (CMPD1) to 17q24.3-q25.1. Nat Genet 1993;4:170-174.
81. van Niekerk W: True hermaphroditism. Am J Obstet Gynecol 1976;126:890-907.
82. Wagner T, Wirth J, Meyer J, et al: Autosomal sex reversal and campomelic dysplasia are caused by mutations in and around the SRY-related gene SOX9. Cell 1994;79:1111-1120.
83. Walsh PC, Madden JD, Harrod MJ, et al: Familial incomplete male pseudohermaphroditism, type 2: Decreased dihydrotestosterone formation in pseudovaginal perineoscrotal hypospadias. N Engl J Med 1974;291:944-949.
84. White PC, New MI: Molecular genetics of congenital adrenal hyperplasia. Baillieres Clin Endocrinol Metab 1988;2: 941-965.
85. White PC, New MI: Genetic basis of endocrine disease 2: Congenital adrenal hyperplasia due to 21-hydroxylase deficiency. J Clin Endocrinol Metab 1992;74:6-11.
86. Wilkie AOM, Campbell FM, Daubeney P, et al: Complete and partial XY sex reversal associated with terminal deletion of 10q: Report of 2 cases and literature review. Am J Med Genet 1993;46:597-600.
87. Wilson JD, Harrod MJ, Goldstein JL, et al: Familial incomplete male pseudohermaphroditism, type 1: Evidence for androgen resistance and variable clinical manifestations in a family with Reifenstein syndrome. N Engl J Med 1974;290:1098-1103.
88. Zazopoulos E, Lalli E, Stocco DM, Sassone-Corsi P: DNA binding and transcriptional repression by DAX-1 blocks steroidogenesis. Nature 1997;390:311-315.
89. Zimmermann S, Steding G, Emmen JM, et al: Targeted disruption of the Insl3 gene causes bilateral cryptorchidism. Mol Endocrinol 1999;13:681-691.

第 122 章

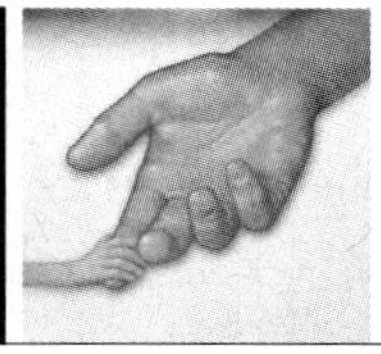

女性生殖道畸形

Jay L. Grosfeld 和 Arnold G. Coran

1935 绝大多数女性生殖道畸形是先天性的，出生时就有。在一些病例中，生殖道畸形是在检查泌尿系统疾患时发现的，或者作为一些与特定类型疾病有关的异常出现。少数患者到青春期时出现原发性闭经，还有些患者继发出现与感染、异物、外伤、肿瘤等有关的情况。最近 20 年，随着围产学、产科学、新生儿学和儿童放射学的发展，对女婴生殖道畸形的认识和护理研究也不断深入。目前，这类疾病中有些已经能够通过宫内 B 超明确诊断。要了解这些可能出现的复杂的先天性畸形，首先必须全面掌握女性泌尿生殖道的胚胎发育。

胚胎学

女性生殖道由苗勒氏管或中肾旁管发育而来。怀孕 3 周时，来自中肾管（午非氏管）的输尿管芽开始生长，与中肾胚基一起，最终形成肾脏和输尿管。在胎睾组织不存在的情况下，机体不产生雄激素和苗勒氏管抑制物质（MIS），输尿管芽远端的午非氏管结构被泌尿生殖窦吸收。怀孕 6 周时，配对的中肾旁管（苗勒氏管）沿午非氏管排列出现，相互接触。怀孕 6～8 周，成对出现的苗勒氏管越过午非氏管两侧，在中线融合。融合发生于头尾两端，形成腔室。然后，融合的苗勒氏管在苗勒氏结节处与泌尿生殖窦结合。怀孕 10 周时，苗勒氏管在中线位置形成一个管腔结构，称为子宫阴道管。两侧没有发生融合的部分苗勒氏管保持独立状态，最终形成输卵管结构。尾端融合的苗勒氏管增厚演变为子宫（子宫底和子宫体）和子宫颈。

阴道的确切胚胎学起源尚不明确。Koff 认为[72]，阴道上端三分之二到五分之四的部分可能来源于融合的苗勒氏管，下端三分之一到五分之一的部分来源于泌尿生殖窦。尽管有证据支持阴道形成的二元学说，但两者在阴道构成上的确切分布仍不明确。怀孕 9 周时，融合的苗勒氏管将泌尿生殖窦推向尾端，形成苗勒氏结节。阴道的形成由苗勒氏结节处开始，子宫阴道管在此与泌尿生殖窦结合。在怀孕 3～5 个月时，苗勒氏结节增厚伸长，两侧内胚层组织向内凹陷，称作窦阴道球。随着窦阴道球的生长，苗勒氏结节逐渐退化，子宫阴道腔和泌尿生殖窦之间的距离加长。怀孕 15～26 周时，窦阴道球完成生长，产生一条实质性的索带组织，称为原发性阴道板。索带从泌尿生殖窦开始空腔化，向头端延伸，形成阴道远端三分之一的部分。到怀孕 5 个月的时候，近端和远端阴道管腔贯通，阴道完全形成。生殖道畸形的产生可能出现于上述胚胎发育、管腔融合及空腔化的任何过程中。发育障碍可造成组织器官发育不全；管腔融合障碍可引起各种畸形，包括产生器官重复畸形；空腔化异常可导致阴道隔膜的形成。在胚胎发育过程中，苗勒氏管和午非氏管关系密切，因此临床上常见生殖系统和泌尿系统畸形同时存在。

女性外生殖器的分化出现在第 12～16 孕周。在缺乏胎儿雄激素（尤其是双氢睾酮）的条件下，生殖始基被动地发育形成女性外生殖器。生殖结节轻度
生长，形成阴蒂。尿道褶形成小阴唇而不发生融合，1936
未融合的生殖肿大形成大阴唇。泌尿生殖沟保持开放，形成阴道前庭[68]。

阴道发育不全

造成完全性阴道缺如或发育不全（也称作 Mayer

-Rokitansky 综合征）的原因可能是苗勒氏管没有能够到达泌尿生殖窦的位置，这涉及输尿管阴道腔或阴道板的异常发育。这一情况出现在怀孕第 4～12 周，属于散发的、多基因遗传、受多因素影响的异常现象[36]。至今没有发现与此相关的特发性遗传异常。Mayer[81]在 1829 年首先报道了一名伴有阴道发育不全的多发性畸形的死产儿。Rokitansky[112]（1838 年）和 Küster[74]（1910 年）曾进一步报道了类似的临床病例，并发现了伴随有正常卵巢和外生殖器的子宫发育不良病症（图 122-1A）。继而，Hauser 及其同事们[52]在 1961 年描述了这一疾病常伴发的肾脏和骨骼异常。于是，就以这些报道者名字的组合来命名这一畸形即 Mayer-Rokitansky-Küster-Hauser（MRKH）综合征。阴道发育不全的发病率是每 4000～5000 名活体女婴中出现 1 例[18]。这些患儿的染色体核型都是典型的 46，XX，具备正常发育的第二性征，通常在青春期阶段出现闭经[114]。这些患者的子宫形态变化不一，从正常到没有管腔的双角子宫。患者很少有月经现象，但会出现周期性腹部绞痛，可能与子宫内膜的功能有关。75% 的患者阴道缺如，25% 的患者阴道短小（通常短于 2.5 cm）（见图 122-1B）。大多数患者具备双侧输卵管和卵巢。但是，MRKH 综合征患者中偶尔出现单侧[70]或双侧性腺发育不全[100]。Plevraki 和同事们[100]注意到一名卵巢缺如患者体内出现睾丸特异蛋白 1-Y 连锁基因的表达。

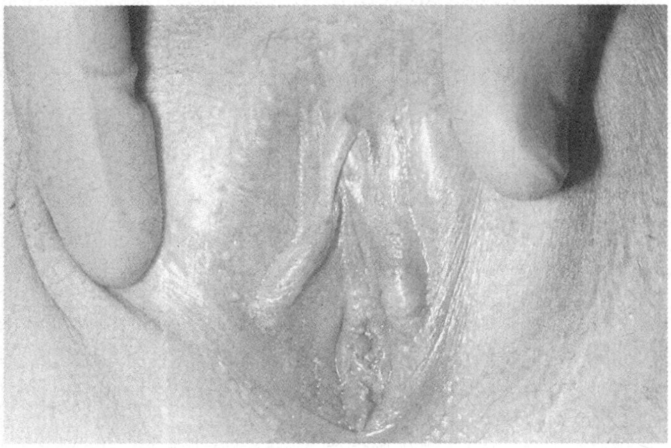

A

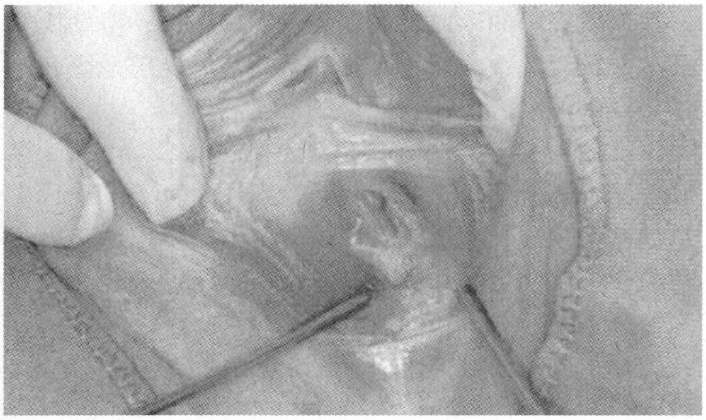

B

图 122-1 A. 13 岁阴道发育不全女孩的外阴。正常的外观形态表明疾病易被漏诊。B. 将小扩张器探入苗勒氏管凹。残留阴道深度 2.0 cm。

先天性阴道缺如伴尿路畸形的现象非常普遍，大约三分之一的此类患者存在肾脏畸形[37,47]。其中，最常见的肾脏畸形包括一侧肾发育不良、单侧或双侧异位肾。同样，肾融合畸形如马蹄肾或肾横过异位也很常见。

Griffin 和同事们[47]报道，大约有 12% 的 MRKH 患者存在骨骼畸形。其中三分之二的患者存在脊柱、四肢或肋骨异常。6% 的骨骼畸形患者属于 Klippel-Feil 类型，即存在颈胸体节的发育障碍[49]。1979 年，Duncan 和同事[30]报道了这些畸形的发生频率，并建议将其统称为 MURCS。这一简称是由苗勒氏管发育不全、肾发育不全和颈胸体节关联症的英语首字母缩写拼合而成的。MRKH 综合征可能会伴随 TAR 综合征（血小板减少合并桡骨缺如）[8,47]而出现，很少合并肛门直肠畸形[121]。有人观察到 MRKH 合并手部放射显像异常及听力丧失[129,130]。

1964 年，曾有报道在安曼人群中发现 McKusick-Kaufman 综合征（MKS），疾病包括因阴道闭锁或发育不全造成的子宫阴道积液、轴后多指症以及先天性心脏病等[83,117,123]。这是一种常染色体隐性遗传病，并发现其与 *MKKS* 基因突变有关。MKS 患者在症状上与 Bardet-Biedl 综合征（BBS）重叠[123]。BBS 患儿存在生殖器畸形和多指，另外还可能罹患色素沉着性视网膜炎、听力残疾、向心性肥胖及心脏畸形等。10%～15% 的 BBS 患者体内 *MKKS* 基因发生突变。染色体 20p12 上的 *BBS6* 基因异质性也可导致 BBS 疾病。

诊断

通常，阴道发育不全在青春期阶段就可诊断，伴

随有闭经。大约有 15% 的闭经女孩患有 MRKH 综合征。当闭经女孩同时伴发畸形（如骨骼、肾脏）时，
937 应考虑是否罹患 MRKH 综合征。近几年，产前超声已经能够发现阴道积液。同样，产前磁共振也能明确诊断。偶尔，腹部肿块的婴儿在新生儿期可以诊断出阴道闭锁。对于婴儿或者年长患者，完整的体格检查，包括借助阴道镜和膀胱镜、盆腔超声、计算机断层摄影（CT）、MRI[110] 以及腹腔镜等手段，可以明确疾病类型，并同时了解尿路畸形情况。超声、MRI 和内镜检查可以避免不必要的放射线损伤。

治疗

阴道发育不全的治疗需根据患者的不同解剖特点，因人而异。治疗时，需要评价和综合考虑器官的功能、患者的生育能力和心理问题，注意患者生理和心理的成熟性[31,32]。治疗的目的是给患者提供适当的性功能，治疗子宫和阴道缺如造成的心理创伤。这些患者是可以生儿育女的，通常情况下患者双侧卵巢功能正常，所以可以提供的一种治疗选择是体外受精、借腹生子[41,98]。心理学研究表明，与无法性交比较而言，生育障碍是 MRKH 综合征患者最需要克服的问题[31,101]。术前与患者本人和家庭沟通是必需的，治疗时间的选择也非常重要。如果患者子宫正常，而阴道短小没有到达会阴，那么在月经初潮来临以前，需要通过手术对阴道进行整形[22]。如果只是阴道远端缺如，可以游离后面和侧面的皮瓣并转入邻近的阴道以提供阴道入口。但是，这样的手术在大多数患者中难以完成，而且长期效果不够稳定。如果患者子宫缺如，则可以考虑在性活动开始以前行阴道重建手术。

尽管建立新子宫还不可行，但有很多方法可以重建阴道。正常女性的阴道由分层排列的非角质立方上皮构成，向后上方倾斜，后壁平均长度为 9.0 cm，前壁平均长度为 7.5 cm。阴道黏膜中无腺体，子宫颈分泌的黏液对阴道有润滑作用。理想状态下，新建的阴道应该定位准确（斜向后上方），有足够的空间容量，替代组织保持弹性（黏膜或皮肤），不会始终潮湿也不散发恶臭，没有毛发，并且至少在阴道入口处保留感觉功能[102]。阴道重建术应简单易行、一期完成、容易重复操作、病死率低并且预后良好（即性生活满意而无痛苦）。理想的手术步骤难以确定，并且各个专家对 MRKH 患者的阴道重建技巧有各自独特的见解[31,45,58,60,75]。

非手术治疗

1938 年，Frank 介绍了用 Pyrex 管对 6 位 MRKH 综合征患者进行每天扩张阴道凹 20 分钟的治疗[38]。1983 年，Rock 和同事报道，阴道强力（被动）扩张只对 43% 的患者有治疗作用[111]。患者不配合会影响治疗效果。Edmonds 注意到使用严谨的治疗程序和由经验丰富的护理专家参与，并通过循序渐进的扩张方法治疗能配合的患者，可改善疗效[31]。2002 年，美国妇产科学院制定的规则中建议将阴道扩张定为治疗的首选方法[1]。但是尚缺乏阴道扩张后对疗效的认真评价和在前瞻性随机研究中与其他治疗方法的对比。扩张治疗对阴道长度大于 2.5 cm 的患者是有利的（见图 122-1B）[108,111]。但性交过程中，阴道的长度、干涩及性交困难仍然是扩张后的遗留问题。

手术治疗

阴道重建的手术方法有许多种，包括皮瓣插入阴道成形（Abbe-McIndoe 术）[71,82]、各种筋膜皮肤[120]和肌层皮肤瓣膜转移［臀-大腿皮瓣、股薄肌、腹直肌[78]、Malaga 皮瓣[40]、Singapore 皮瓣[67,141]、Williams 外阴阴道成形术[144]、外阴阴道皮瓣（大阴唇莲花样皮瓣）[148]、小阴唇马蹄形皮瓣[103]、组织扩张后的阴唇皮瓣[9]］、真空辅助伤口闭合下的全层皮肤移植[50] 以及利用羊膜[3,87] 和腹膜[24] 等。Soong 和助手[125]、Rangaswamy 和同事[107] 以及 Templeman 及其同事们[132] 描述了腹腔镜下应用腹膜组织重建阴道的方法。Vecchietti[140] 手术过程包括经腹进行腹内牵引盆底引起会阴部的阴道区内陷。这一过程需要剖腹术或经腹腔镜径路完成，术后长期扩张。Wharton 手术[119,143] 只是简单地在阴道内留置一个以避孕套包裹的模型并维持数月。使用盲肠、小肠或乙状结肠进行肠代阴道手术已经作为替代同样类型手术的方式[45,58,60,89]。一些更流行的手术方式将在此详细论述。

过去 30 年里，最流行的阴道替代物是由 McIndoe 提出的分层厚皮移植片[82]。McIndoe手术中使用的是

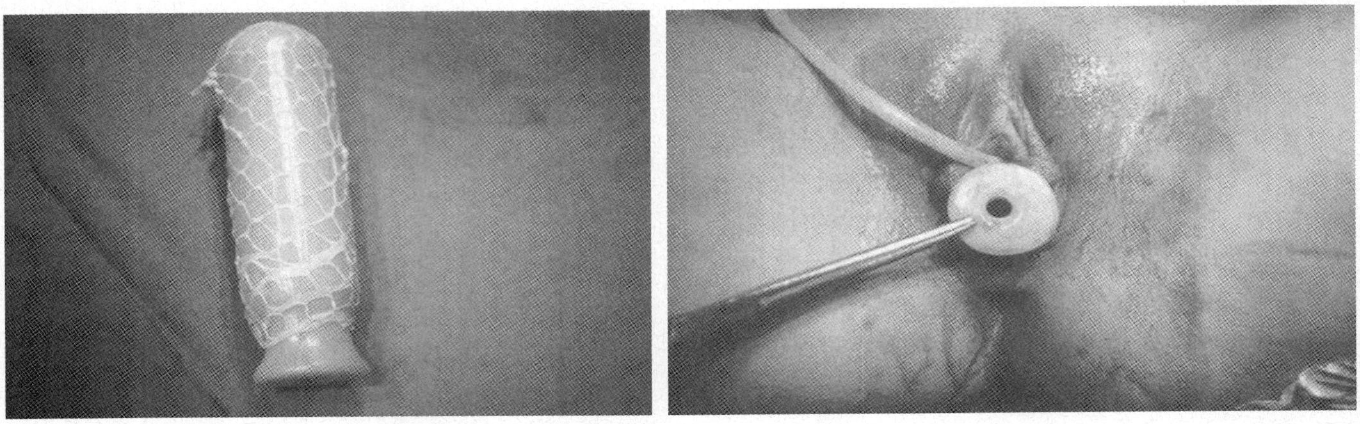

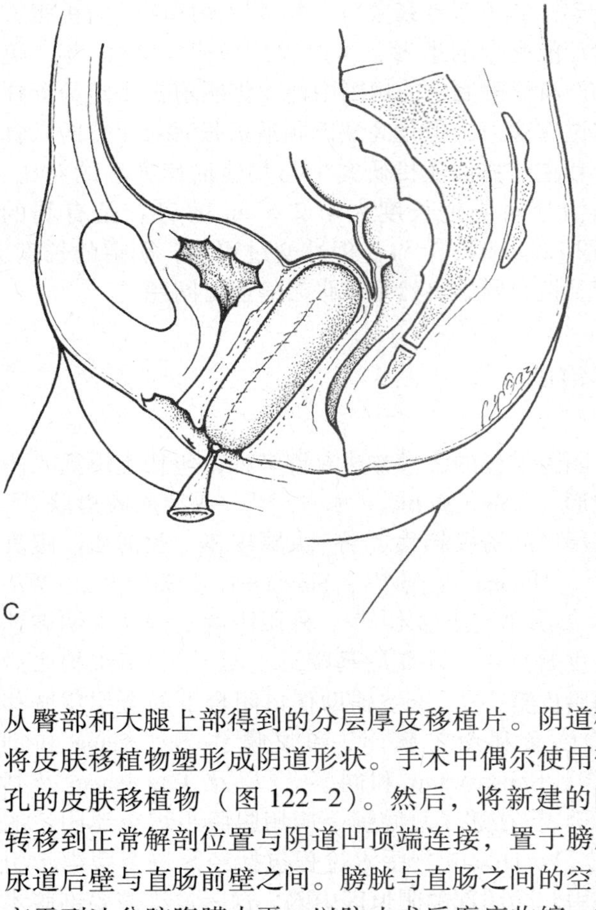

图 122-2　McIndoe 手术过程。A. 将带筛孔的分层厚皮移植片缝合到阴道模具上。B. 在膀胱和直肠之间游离出空间，将模具置放其中。C. 模具侧面观。

从臀部和大腿上部得到的分层厚皮移植片。阴道模具将皮肤移植物塑形成阴道形状。手术中偶尔使用带筛孔的皮肤移植物（图 122-2）。然后，将新建的阴道
1038 转移到正常解剖位置与阴道凹顶端连接，置于膀胱和尿道后壁与直肠前壁之间。膀胱与直肠之间的空间游离需到达盆腔腹膜水平，以防止术后瘢痕收缩。将阴道模具缝合在会阴皮肤边缘，防止移位。模具压迫性坏死导致的术后血肿和瘘管形成是早期的并发症，使用充气式的阴道模具可减少上述风险。据报道，术后并发症的发生率小于 10%。尽管有少数积极的报道[7,21]，但这一术式依然受到需要定期的长时间的家庭阴道扩张制约。该手术的缺点包括阴道干涩以及由于皮瓣挛缩引起的阴道狭窄、短浅和性交困难[25]。术后需要应用抗生素和止痛剂，定期在麻醉下更换新的、更大规格的阴道模具。对术后性生活的满意程度没有确切的调查结果[32]。在英国，羊膜是手术首选材料，可以避免裁剪自身移植物。但是，获取羊膜需要选择性地行剖宫产手术，建立组织材料库，并严格筛查供体以防 HIV 感染和 Creutzfeldt-Jakob 病[32]。俄罗斯和美国的医生多选择腹膜行阴道重建手术，但需要开腹或借助腹腔镜[24,115,132]。如前所述，为克服分层厚皮移植片转移后出现的收缩问题，人们选择了多种全层皮瓣移植的方法。使用带有毛发的全层皮瓣作为供体对阴道重建术造成的缺点是毛发生长问题，以及由此造成的性交困难。这一术式在供体部位也造成创口[32,144]。利用会阴组织重建阴道会损伤外生殖器 10

外观，而且 Williams 外阴阴道成形术后形成的异常转角将引起性交困难，并造成不理想的手术结果。使用组织扩张器扩张小阴唇治疗阴道短小被证明有效，但最新的结果还不能证明治疗后的阴道具有足够长度，并能适应性生活的需要[9,103]。经证实，自体颊黏膜移植可成功用于阴道成形术[92]。Lin 和其同事[76]报道了 8 例使用颊黏膜行阴道成形手术的病例。该技术需要阴道支撑物和术后扩张。术后并发症包括一例可能来源于肉芽组织的阴道出血和一例膀胱损伤。人工真皮和重组的基本纤维母细胞生长因子（bFGF）也被应用于阴道重建手术中，希望以此加速阴道黏膜上皮愈合，及减少因肉芽组织形成而造成的阴道血性分泌物[88]。由于研究对象较少，尚不能对此技术的有效性做出结论。

Vecchietti 手术需要开腹[140]（或腹腔镜[34]），缝线从上方穿过会阴膜，之后穿过一个塑料橄榄，并从腹部穿出固定。腹腔关闭后，缝线与固定于患者腹部的牵引器相连，牵引一周到 10 天。压力作用在塑料橄榄上，造成阴道内陷，产生阴道穹窿。早期阴道的长度是 10～12 cm，据报道阴道解剖和功能方面的成功率达到 100%[16]。并发症主要是少数患者出现膀胱和直肠瘘。这种牵引治疗的方法会引起患者不适，且治疗后需要长期扩张阴道，因此该方法在美国并没有得到广泛应用。Wharton 法[143]包括将一个避孕套包裹的模具插入新阴道内，促使阴道肉芽组织上皮化。该过程需要较长时间，因为阴道上皮生长需要 3～6 个月，而且常伴有阴道肉芽组织不断地排出血性分泌物。Schätz 和其同事[118]采用扩张疗法治疗了 3 例患者，以循序渐进的方式逐渐增加 Hegar 扩张器的尺寸，对原始苗勒氏管进行扩张。采用透热电疗将两个腔隙融合，平滑肌组织排列形成新的阴道腔。阴道顶由膀胱和直肠处的腹膜反折覆盖。Sheares 法是 Wharton 法[119]的改良，并在临床上得到应用。该手术方法是阴道内留置可调节的支撑管。连续 8 天应用抗生素和止痛剂，Foley 导尿管留置一周以防尿潴留。术后 1 周在麻醉下重新放置新的阴道模具。模具每天 24 小时留置阴道内，连续 3 个月，这之后只在晚间于阴道内留置模具，一直持续到开始规律的性生活。儿童置换新的阴道模具需要全身麻醉。新建的阴道长度应该为 7～10 cm，宽两指。部分患者在开始性生活初期有阴道润滑不够和性交困难的情况，可给予阴道润滑剂治疗。接受这一治疗的 2 名女性患者对性生活满意[118]。该疗法的主要缺点包括需要长期留置阴道模具、反复置换模具时需要全身麻醉、阴道润滑程度不够以及缺乏长期随访资料。

肠管代阴道成形术

由于先前手术方式的众多缺点，肠管代阴道手术得以流行。孤立小肠代阴道手术是 Baldwin 于 1904 年提出的[5]，最早在 1907 年施行[6]。Ruge 于 1914 年[116]最早施行乙状结肠代阴道手术。1940 年，Fall[33]介绍了该手术的临床经验，但由于缺乏有效的抗生素，手术死亡率很高，因此并没有得到推广。1972 年，经 Pratt[102]介绍，小肠和结肠代阴道手术再次引起人们的重视，之后文献对此进行了散在报道*。

目前，乙状结肠间段是替代阴道的首选部位。乙状结肠因先期手术而不能应用时，可考虑改用盲肠替代。尽管偶尔也会选择小肠进行阴道替代手术，但由于其黏膜形成过剩、组织脆弱，造成性交困难，因此效果并不令人满意。

术前 24 小时，需要以 GoLYTELY 对患者实行肠道准备。皮肤切开前 30～45 分钟，全身应用抗生素。手术在膀胱截石位下完成，患者双脚踩在脚镫上，这样可以同时对腹部和会阴进行消毒准备。膀胱留置 Foley 导尿管，盆腔和腹腔可以采用 Pfannenstiel 或更低的腹部中线切口进入。最近数年来，腹腔镜的应用使手术造成的创伤减小到最低程度[106,134,138]。术中可探查腹腔和生殖器官。如发现原始的双角子宫，则将其切除。少数情况下，可能发现发育正常的子宫，将其保留，并与阴道吻合。卵巢应保留在原位，以避免日后行激素替代，并利于将来患者需要时采取体外受精、借腹生子的医疗措施[31,41]。

借助左结肠动脉和痔上动脉的血液供应，可以游离 10～15 cm 的乙状结肠，此段容量足够新阴道所需。结肠过长会造成黏液分泌过剩，因此肠管长度应短。在两把 Bainbridge 肠钳之间离断乙状结肠，两断端之间肠管或者以吻合器钉合，或者用手工缝合（图 122-3）。对患有 Mayer-Rokitansky 综合征或阴道发育不全的患者，在阴道凹顶端做一切口，于膀胱后壁和直肠前壁之间分离一个空腔，一直向上到腹膜反折水平。通常可以将孤立肠管以同步顺蠕动的形式或者反 1940

* 见参考文献 20，27，39，45，59，60，89，104，106，134 和 142。

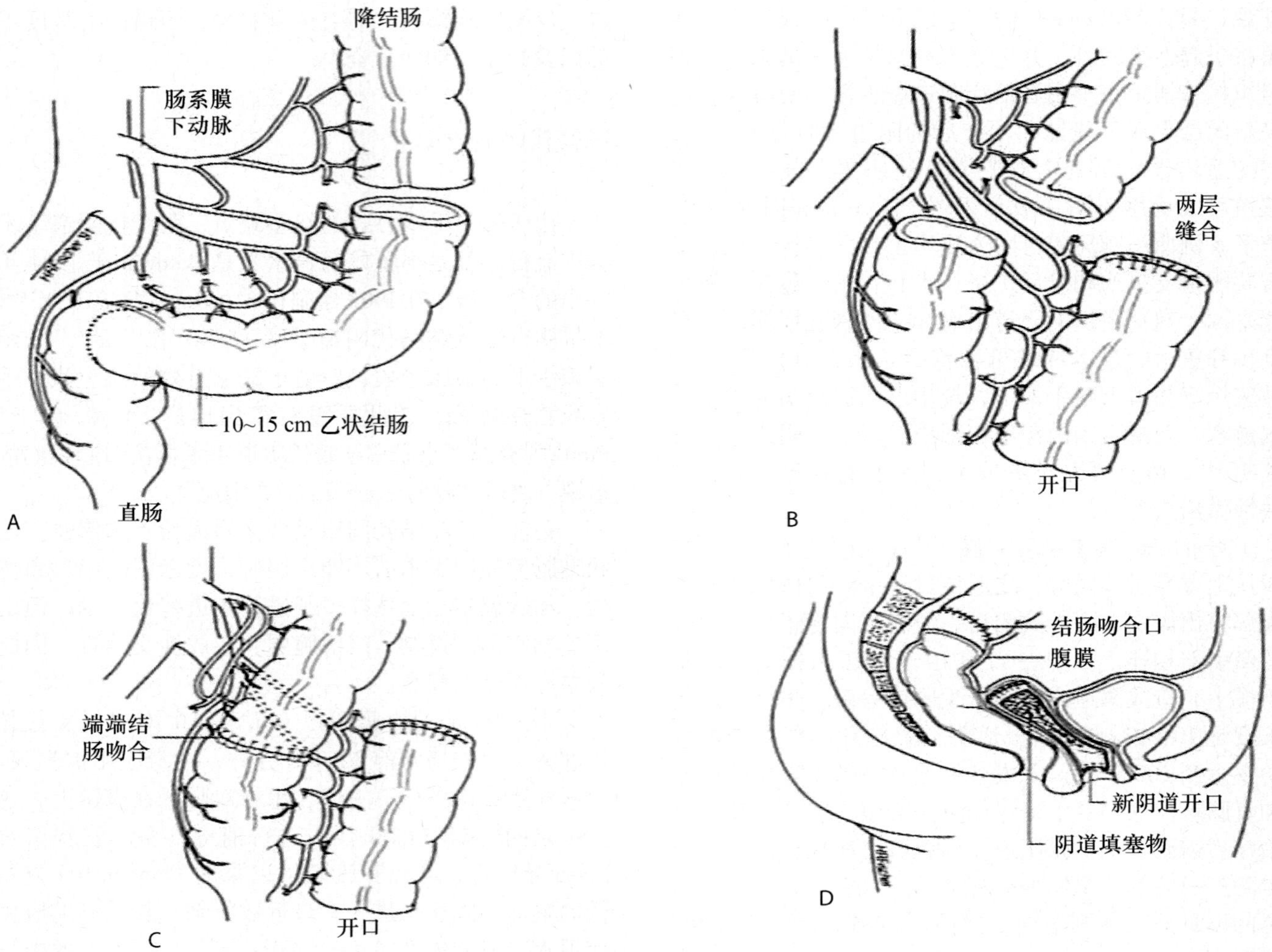

图 122-3 手术在膀胱截石位下完成，患者双脚踩在脚镫上。手术采用 Pfannenstiel 切口，或者采用腹腔镜进行。A. 游离 10～15 cm 的乙状结肠。B 和 C. 新阴道的近端做两层缝合封闭，乙状结肠远近端做端端吻合。D. 将游离的新阴道置入膀胱后壁和直肠前壁之间的空腔内，远端与残余的阴道或者小的会阴皮肤开口用可吸收缝线做单层间断缝合，将插入的结肠段和腹膜后腔做间断缝合防止脱垂。术后新阴道用凡士林纱布填塞。

转 180 度下降到会阴，具体方式根据系膜的长度而定。新阴道的近端用可吸收缝线两层缝合形成新的阴道顶，然后用可吸收缝线（3-0 Vicryl 或者 PDS）将插入的结肠段远端和会阴皮肤做间断单层缝合，最后用不可吸收缝线将插入的结肠段和腹膜后腔做三点间断缝合固定，防止新阴道的脱垂。

全身性抗生素可以用到术后 24 小时，镇痛药物可以用到术后 48 小时。如果有需要可以口服镇痛药物。术后新阴道用凡士林纱布填塞 5 天，期间用 Foley 导尿管排空膀胱。术后第五天，患者可以走动和进食，此时可以出院。一般术后 3 周和 3 个月各复查一次，如果出现阴道狭窄，需要进行麻醉下阴道扩张。一般不要求患者常规自行做阴道扩张。在术后 6 周之内应避免骑自行车，其他活动可以适当进行。

结果

我们对 36 名患者进行了乙状结肠代阴道重建术，包括 14 名 MRKH 综合征患者，还包括睾丸女性化综合征（10 例）、泄殖腔畸形（8 例）、阴道肿瘤（3

例）和混合性性腺发育不良（1 例）患者。术后均未发生阴道狭窄。所有性活跃期患者不需要润滑剂均能获得满意的性生活，没有出现性交困难或黏液分泌过多的问题。随访中阴道入口扩张良好，没有发现严重的并发症。

1941 Hensle 和 Reiley 介绍了他们对 30 名年龄在 1～20 岁之间的患者行小肠阴道替代手术的经验[26,60]。对达到生育年龄的 20 名患者进行信访，获得了 14 例手术的长期疗效资料。其中 10 名妇女（71%）获得了满意的性生活，4 人（29%）婚配，另有 3 人（21%）结婚后离异。只有 1 名患者主诉性交困难，该患者先前接受的是回肠代阴道手术，术后出现阴道狭窄而在家常规行阴道扩张，并需要再次予以手术整形。其余 13 名患者无日常阴道扩张的需要。研究者由此得出结论，回肠代阴道手术效果不佳，建议所有的病例予乙状结肠代替阴道。一名患者出现肠管脱垂，需要再次手术固定。Burger[20] 同样报道了 1 名回盲肠代阴道手术后出现狭窄的病例。Wesley 和 Coran[142] 报道了 6 名接受乙状结肠代阴道成形术的患者，其中 4 人在青春期手术，另 2 人于婴儿期手术。文献发表时有 3 人性生活良好，无需阴道润滑剂。Turner-Warwick 和 Kirby[137] 报道了 13 名接受结肠盲肠代阴道术的病例，其中 3 人需要再次予小手术改进阴道入口，另 1 人出现阴道肠管脱垂而需要环形切除多余的肠管。13 名患者中 7 人性生活活跃。Novak[89] 报道了 63 名乙状结肠代阴道手术后有 2 人出现间置肠管坏死，另有 2 人出现肠管脱垂。63 人中 59 人得到治愈。Syed 和同事们[131] 报道了 18 名年龄在 18 个月至 8 岁之间接受乙状结肠代阴道手术的患者资料，其中 3 人术后出现改道肠管的结肠炎。笔者没有对小年龄患者施行过类似手术，也没有见到上述并发症的出现。鉴于 Syed 和同事们[131] 的报道，Edmonds[32] 建议不要对低龄儿童施行该手术。在日本，Hiroi 和同事们[63] 报道了唯一一例乙状结肠代阴道手术后肠管出现恶变的病例。在术后 30 年，发现了一例黏液腺瘤。

根据作者和其他许多学者的经验，认为乙状结肠是替代阴道的最好组织材料。与其他许多方法不同，采用乙状结肠重建的阴道与正常相似，具有适当的容量，可以在性生活时分泌足够的润滑液，并且对于大多数患者而言，术后无需常规扩张。将新阴道的长度控制在 9.0～10.0 cm 之间可以避免黏液过多分泌的风险。那些已经认识到的并发症，如肠管阴道脱垂，可以通过在腹膜后固定乙状结肠来避免。使用乙状结肠而不是小肠进行手术可以消除一些其他的并发症，包括阴道狭窄和黏液产生过量等，详见前述。将来，通过腹腔镜技术可进一步降低伤口愈合不良和腹腔粘连等并发症，使手术更加完美[106,135,138]。

先天性阴道梗阻

先天性阴道梗阻可能是胎龄 5 个月时阴道空腔化不完全而造成的。处女膜出现在窦阴道球和泌尿生殖窦的连接处，通常在胎儿期穿孔。未发生穿孔的处女膜造成处女膜闭锁症[32]。处女膜闭锁导致整个阴道扩张，称为阴道积液；或者导致阴道和子宫同时扩张，称为子宫阴道积液。先天性阴道梗阻的最常见原因是处女膜闭锁（图 122-4A）[134]，相对少见的病因是阴道近端病损，如阴道高位横隔（见图122-4B）[15]。阴道高位横隔与阴道前壁部分发育不良和持续存在的泌尿生殖窦共同通道有关。

诊断

处女膜闭锁可以在胎儿期作出诊断[145]。胎儿阶段，闭锁的处女膜表现为一层薄膜，伴有阴道扩张（透超声肿块）和大阴唇伸展。处女膜闭锁和阴道积液可以早在怀孕第 4～6 个月时诊断出来[146]。阴道梗阻的新生儿通常表现为下腹部中线处肿块。这些患儿常伴有尿路梗阻。腹部的肿块实际上是扩张的阴道。

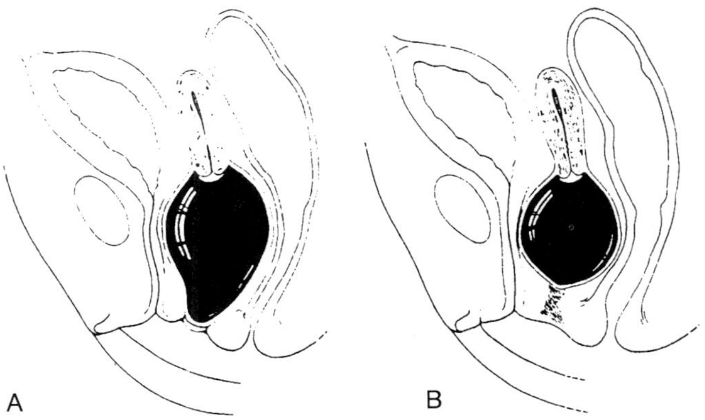

图 122-4　先天性阴道梗阻。A. 处女膜闭锁。B. 高位阴道横隔。

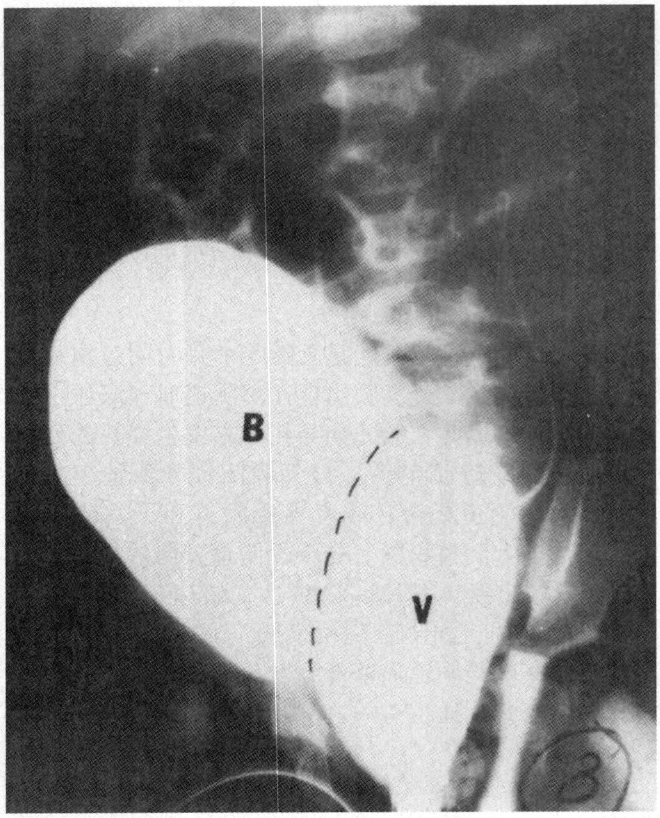

图 122-5　新生儿经皮阴道穿刺造影显示梗阻的阴道（V），同时膀胱（B）造影显像，以及左侧孤立肾和输尿管逆行造影。

子宫颈腺体在母体雌激素的刺激下不断分泌黏液，这些黏液堆积是造成阴道扩张的原因。腹部超声显示中线处巨大的透超声肿块。肿块引起膀胱向前移位，并向后顶推直肠。通过腹膜或前腹壁经皮细针穿刺吸引和注射造影剂有助于诊断（图 122-5）。如果出生时没有肿块，则通常需要到青春期时才能诊断出该疾病。青春期时处女膜闭锁的临床表现包括闭经、周期性腹痛和继发于阴道积血或子宫阴道积液的腹部肿块（图 122-6）。阴道口视诊可发现因阴道积血而凸出的
1942 蓝紫色膜性肿块。

婴儿和年幼儿常发现阴唇融合。融合的阴唇可表现为原发性皮桥结构，常因梗阻造成尿路感染。皮桥的分割可在全身麻醉条件下施行。阴道粘连更常见于 1～5 岁的幼女，因慢性刺激或缺乏足够的雌激素而造成疾病。分解阴道粘连的手术可在门诊施行，从而显示正常的阴道口。常规应用雌激素油膏（倍美力，Premarin）可有效防止阴唇再次粘连。

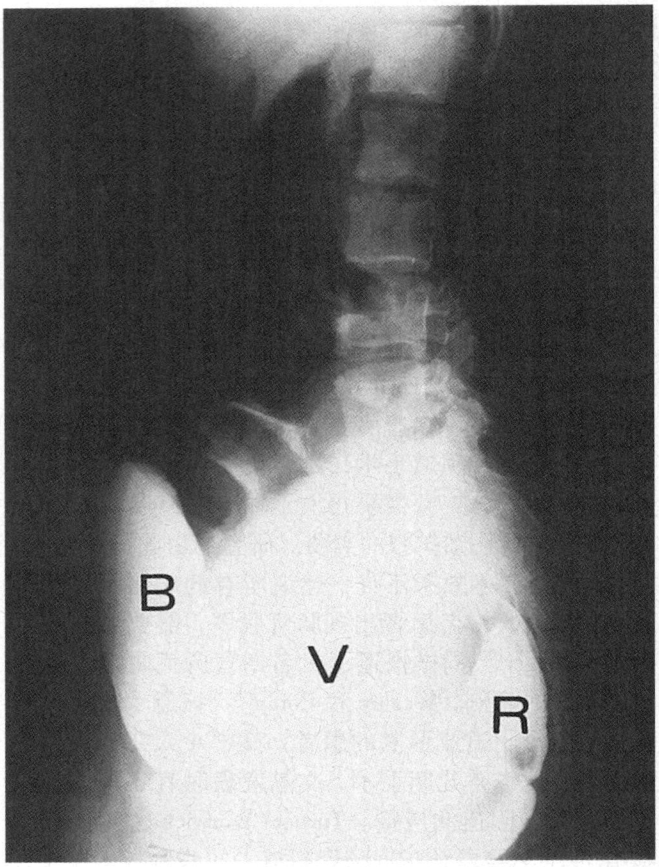

图 122-6　造影检查侧面观，患者腹部中线肿块推压，使膀胱（B）向前移位，直肠（R）向后移位。V 代表梗阻的阴道。

治疗

阴道梗阻的治疗需要结合患者解剖特点。新生儿期间治疗处女膜闭锁可以在无麻醉的条件下切开凸出的阴道入口。对于年长儿，可以在处女膜表面做一个十字形切口，从而起到充分引流的良好效果。引流手术前必须明确低位阴道隔没有伴发泌尿生殖窦共同通道或其他泌尿道畸形。

高位阴道隔膜和阴道前壁部分发育不良比较少见，但很难纠治。造成这种畸形的原因是构成阴道的苗勒氏管和泌尿生殖窦没有完全融合[32]。垂直融合不完全会导致不同部位和厚度的阴道隔膜形成。Rock 和同事们[111]将这些畸形分成高位（46%）、中间位（35%～40%）和低位（15%～20%）。阴道缺如越严重，隔膜的位置也越高。畸形可能同时伴随其他发育

异常，涉及尿路、子宫、肛管和直肠等。临床症状包括青春期无月经及周期性的腹痛[32]。疾病诊断通常是在出现外科急腹症症状时，腹部触诊发现肿块，以及因子宫阴道积液造成尿潴留时。偶尔，患者表现腹膜刺激症状，这是因为输卵管积血由输卵管伞部倒流入腹腔而造成的。治疗这些患儿前必须仔细体检。盆腔超声诊断阴道积血具有特异性。伴有或不伴有共同泌尿生殖窦的高位阴道横隔的最佳治疗手段是予阴道
943 前壁引流，切除阴道隔膜，同时经会阴将高位和低位阴道拖出，用可吸收缝线将其缝合固定于会阴。如果同时存在直肠、肛管向前移位，则很难施行精巧的阴道成形手术（尤其在婴儿期）。更合适的手术是先经泌尿生殖窦行初期引流，延期再予阴道重建。低位阴道隔膜的手术效果优于高位阴道隔膜[32]。为防止术后阴道狭窄行二次手术，术后常予阴道扩张。高位阴道隔膜术后常发生子宫内膜异位症，并且高位阴道隔膜患者的生育率只有 20%[111]。

融合异常

阴道重复

怀孕大约 9 周时胚胎发育异常可能造成两侧苗勒氏管完全或部分融合障碍，由此产生阴道和子宫重复畸形。这些畸形很常见[28]，可包括两个子宫和两个子宫颈伴有两个独立的阴道（双子宫）或一个单独的阴道（双角子宫）。畸形也可能表现为由两个子宫融合成一个子宫颈和阴道（单颈双子宫或双角子宫）（图 122-7）。

阴道完全重复时，其中的一个可能存在梗阻，另一个可能开放（图 122-8）[15,134]。当异位输尿管插入重复、闭锁的阴道时会出现腹部肿块，此时诊断易与尿路畸形混淆[73,85]。通常，外生殖器表现正常。通过超声检查发现新生儿腹部低回声肿块，应鉴别诊断双子宫和一侧阴道梗阻。肿块向前推挤膀胱，同时将正常的阴道顶向后方（图 122-9）。阴道镜有助于诊断，可在一侧阴道壁的较高位置发现向外凸出的肿块。简单地切开造成梗阻的隔膜就能获得充分的引流，但是为防止患侧细菌聚集和局部脓肿形成，常需要予以进一步的手术分割隔膜[19,32]。有些情况下，需要对患者施行正规的剖腹手术以提供充分引流和明

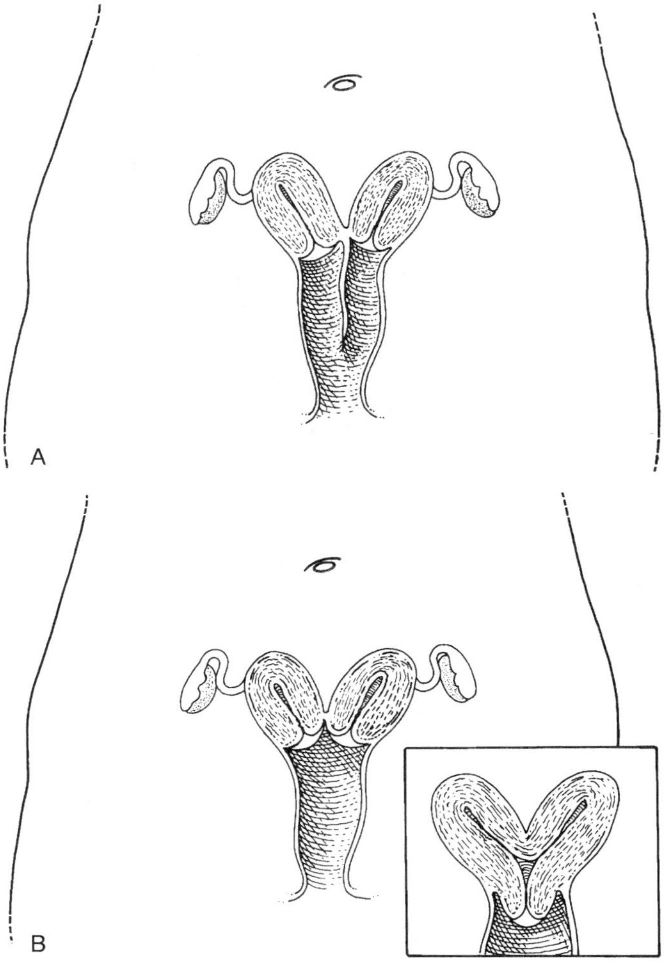

图 122-7 子宫（A）阴道（B）融合异常。

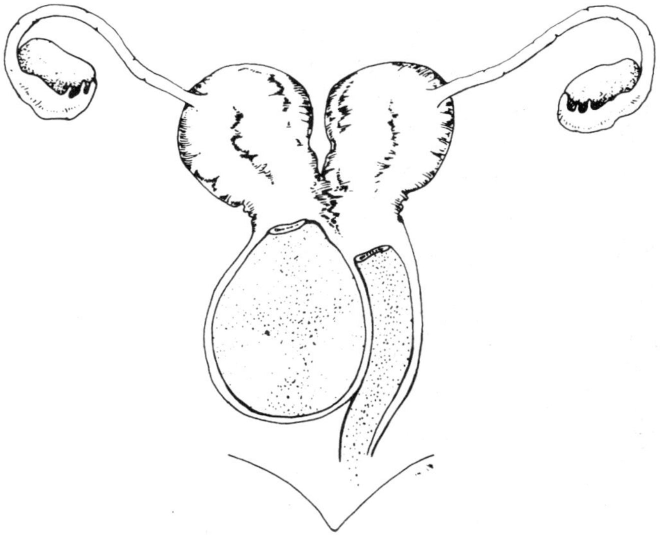

图 122-8 双子宫重复阴道患者单侧阴道梗阻。病变通常伴发闭锁阴道侧的肾发育不全。

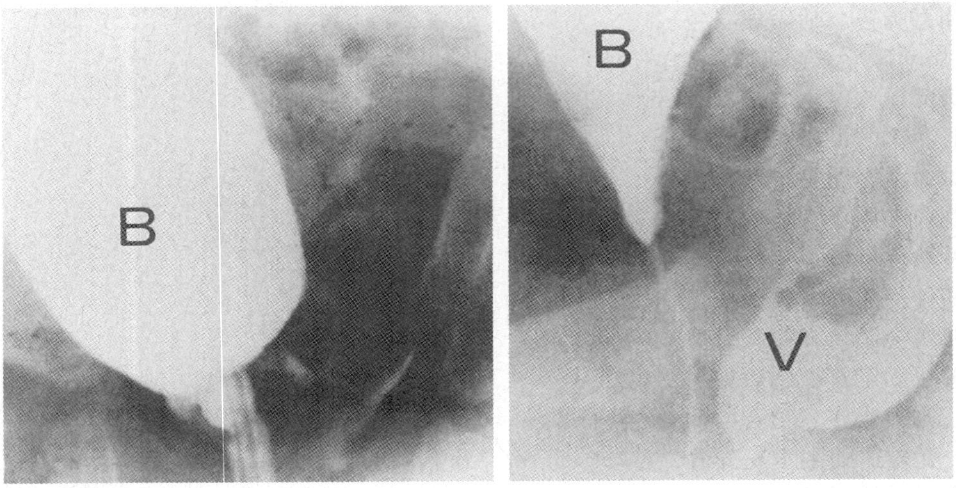

A B

图 122-9 双子宫重复阴道患者，膀胱造影（A）和阴道造影（B）显示单侧阴道梗阻。膀胱（B）和正常阴道（V）分离。

确诊断。对于大多数患者，分割阴道隔膜是治疗的全部内容，因为已有不少报道发现双角子宫的两侧角能分别孕育胎儿、足月顺产，由此说明梗阻侧阴道和子宫的生育能力并非一定遭受损伤。对于处于青春期的女孩，即使有月经现象，但仍发生周期性的盆腔不适和腹部肿块，同样应该考虑阴道重复畸形的可能。超声影像可发现低回声肿块，肿块内有散在的增强声影。阴道造影显示正常子宫和阴道被肿块推移。典型的盆腔 MRI 上可见正常喇叭形的子宫位于扩张、积血的阴道上方。T1 加权像上，阴道积血表现为高亮

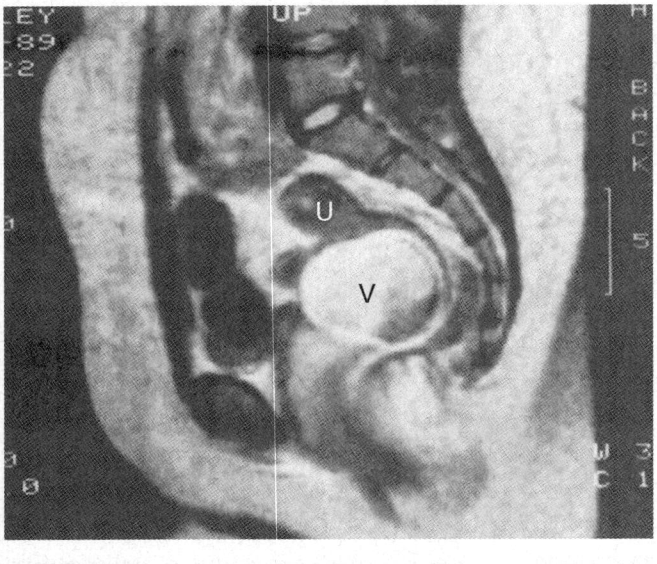

图 122-10 盆腔磁共振显示正常如喇叭形的子宫（U）和梗阻的阴道（V）。

信号（图 122-10）。青春期和幼儿期女性患儿的治疗方法大致相同，可通过阴道顺利完成。 194

泌尿生殖窦畸形

泌尿生殖窦是泌尿道和生殖道的共同开口。共同开口的泌尿生殖窦是两性胚胎发育期的正常阶段。正常女性胎儿在胎龄 9 周时，泌尿生殖窦已经融合，如果发生苗勒氏管发育停滞，则可出现尿道阴道合流或泌尿生殖窦共同开口[146]。阴道分化抑制可导致日后继发性地出现临床可见的泌尿生殖窦异常（图 122-11）。胚胎早期病变造成长段泌尿生殖窦的出现，合并短阴道和高位尿道开口。相反，胚胎晚期发生的病变可造成短小的泌尿生殖窦和基本正常的阴道，尿道开口位置较低[79]。早期缺陷，即阴道和尿道在高位进入泌尿生殖窦，常合并肛门前移，这一表现提示尿道直肠隔形成不良。

诊断

正确评价泌尿生殖窦畸形以前必须充分了解患者的解剖结构。逆行泌尿生殖窦造影（图 122-12）有助于了解泌尿生殖窦共同通道的长度，掌握阴道和尿道的解剖关系[56]。造影时，可以将一个钝性的连接管置放于会阴开口，通过它向泌尿生殖窦内滴注造影

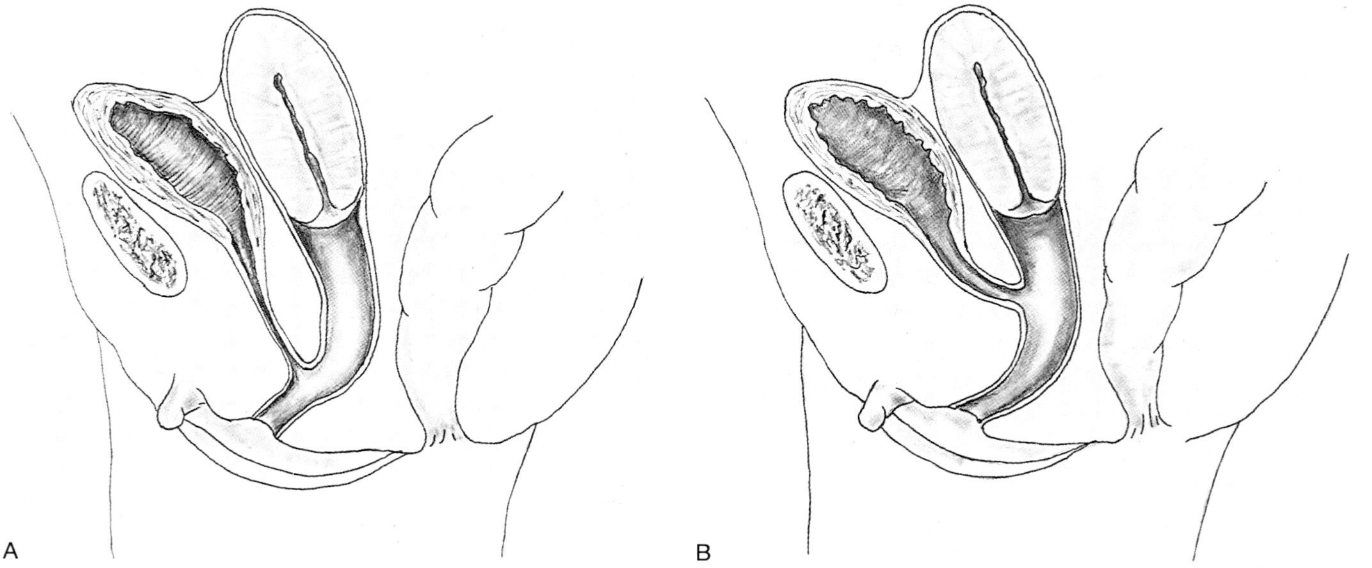

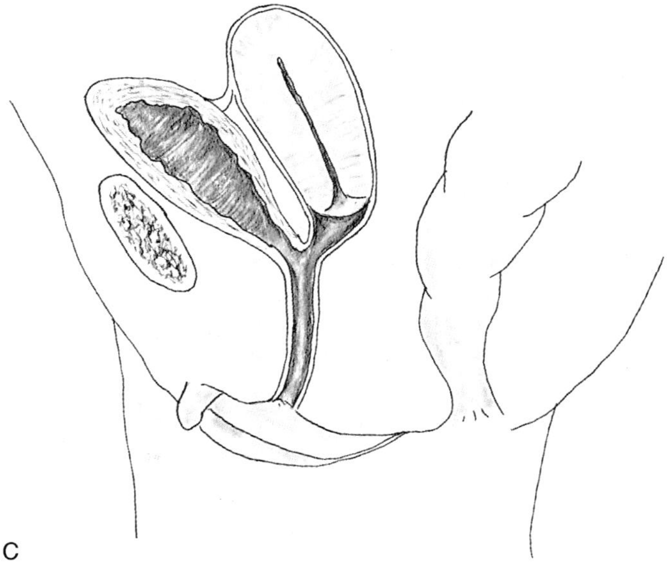

图 122-11　A. 低位合流的泌尿生殖窦。B. 阴道与尿道汇合于泌尿生殖窦中部。C. 高位合流，阴道与泌尿生殖窦汇合于尿道括约肌水平。

剂。每个患者都需要接受膀胱镜和阴道镜的检查。

治疗

一旦明确缺损的解剖情况，就可以针对性地选择各种不同的治疗方法。对低位的泌尿生殖窦畸形，其共同通道较短，可以简单地施行 U 形皮瓣阴道成形手术[53]。对高位膀胱和阴道合流的泌尿生殖窦畸形，Donahoe 和 Gustafson[29] 提倡采用会阴 U 形皮瓣倒置，结合双侧臀部皮瓣转移的方法来扩大阴道。但是，泌尿生殖窦常伴发肛门前移，在利用会阴皮瓣成形阴道以前需要手术将肛门向后迁移[57]。如果阴道进入泌尿生殖窦的位置过高，则需要从泌尿生殖窦游离出阴道
部分，并行拖出式阴道成形术。阴道和膀胱合流位置 1945
较高时，需要行拖出式阴道成形术，并在阴道前壁创建新的尿道[55]。一些患者泌尿生殖窦持续存在，阴道插入窦道的位置较高，对此 Passerini 生殖道阴道成形术或许具有治疗意义[93]。Peña 建议对所有共同通道长度大于 3 cm 的患者都予以泌尿生殖窦前移[97]。这样可以改善手术效果，减少术后发生阴道和尿道狭窄的可能性，降低尿道阴道瘘的发生率（图122-13）[97]。

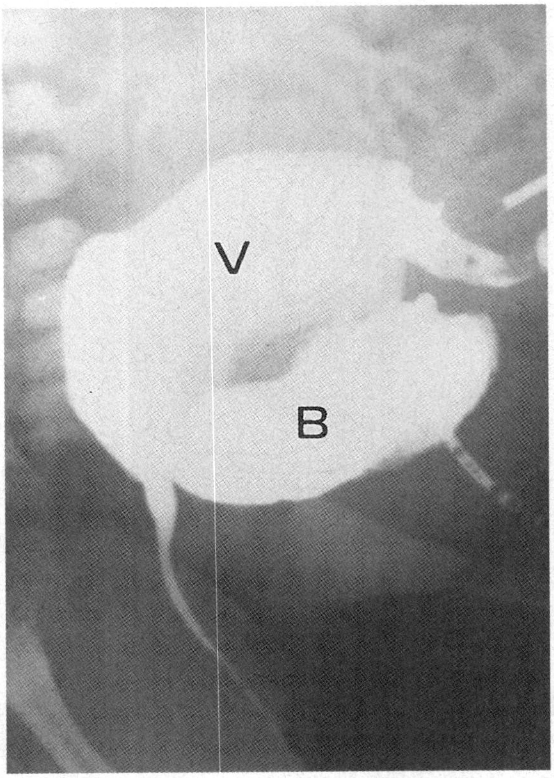

图 122-12　泌尿生殖窦逆行造影，显示膀胱（B）和阴道（V）高位合流，进入长段泌尿生殖窦。

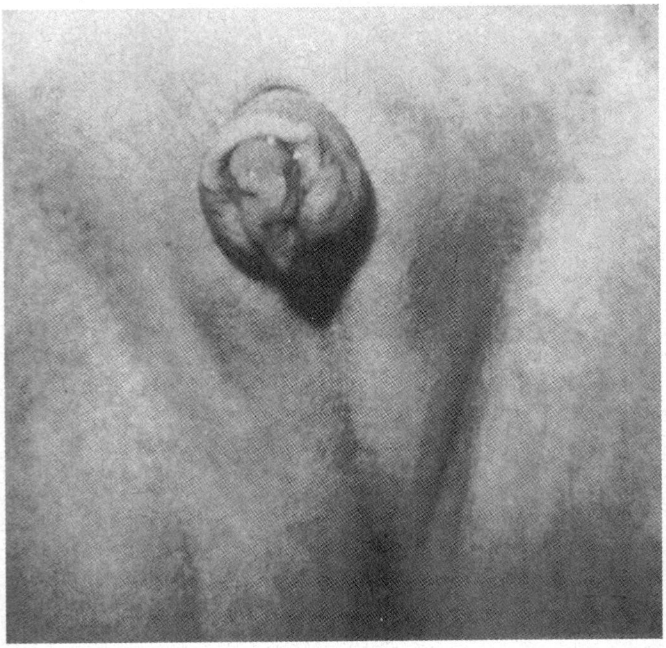

图 122-14　泄殖腔畸形患者的会阴外观。

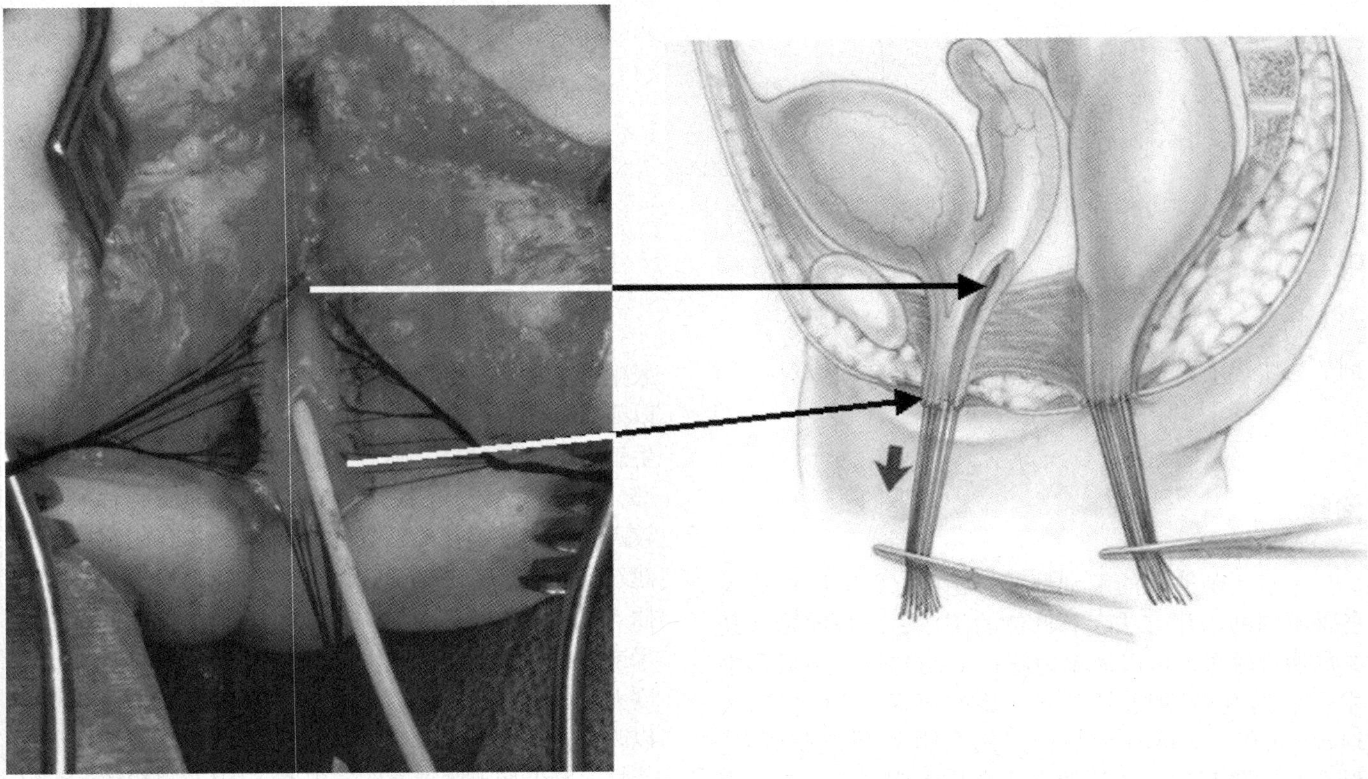

图 122-13　Peña 介绍的全泌尿生殖窦前移手术图解。上方箭头显示阴道水平。下方箭头显示泌尿生殖窦最远端部分。尿道内可见导管插入。（Courtesy of Dr. Alberto Peña）

泄殖腔畸形

泄殖腔畸形结合了泌尿生殖窦畸形和肛门直肠异常[44]。在胚胎早期发育过程中的泄殖腔期，尿囊和后肠互相融合[127]。怀孕 4 ~ 6 周时，尿直肠隔将尿囊与直肠分隔开。如果不出现分隔，将产生共同通道的泄殖腔。患有上述畸形的患者出生时表现为腹胀和会阴异常外观。通常，患者没有肛门或阴道，但会阴部存在一个单独的开口。生殖器外观像男性，类似阴茎的结构向腹侧弯曲（图 122-14）。膀胱可直接进入会阴开口，伴随相对正常长度的尿道。相反，膀胱也可以在非常高的位置进入泄殖腔，开口位置接近膀胱颈。直肠进入泄殖腔的位置同样可以在高位或者低位（图 122-15）[65]。泄殖腔畸形患者常伴发阴道异常，其中最多见的是阴道重复畸形。这些新生儿中也可出
1947 现明显的会阴梗阻，导致阴道积液和梗阻性泌尿道病理改变（图 122-16）。

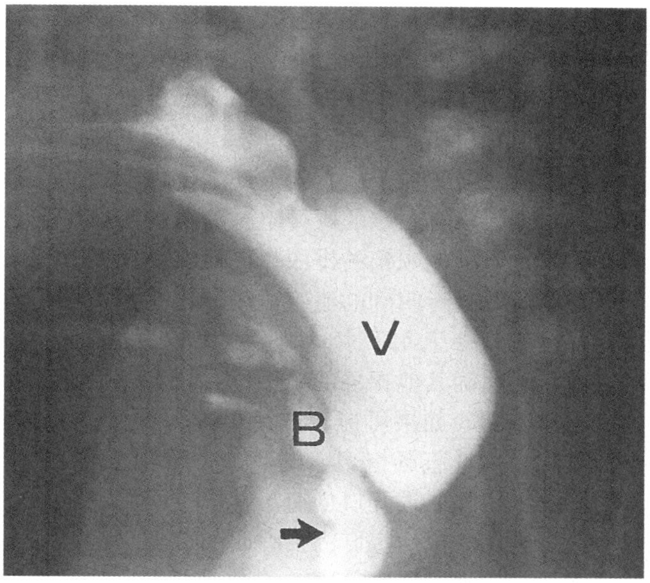

图 122-16 泄殖腔畸形患者膀胱（B）和阴道（V）顺行造影。图片上可见扩张的泌尿生殖窦（箭头）和会阴出口相对梗阻。

诊断

经会阴开口行逆行造影可确诊泄殖腔畸形。通过这一检查，一般可以同时显示泌尿生殖道和胃肠道系统。最近，Blask 和同事们[12]报道了超声检查对 9 名泌尿生殖窦梗阻或泄殖腔畸形患者的诊断意义。在腹部盆腔超声影像上，膀胱受到扩张的阴道挤压，通常很难辨别。在典型的声图上，明显扩张的阴道内充溢着尿液和阴道分泌的液体与组织碎片，使其很容易与扩张的膀胱相区别。但是，泄殖腔畸形的所有组分常难以通过简单的超声或逆行造影明确。因此，广视野膀胱镜检查或开腹手术是唯一能够明确畸形具体结构的手段。完全了解患者的解剖形态是治疗的首要原则[69]。有关泄殖腔外翻的叙述可参见第 116 章。

治疗

治疗任何一种类型的泄殖腔畸形都是一项复杂的

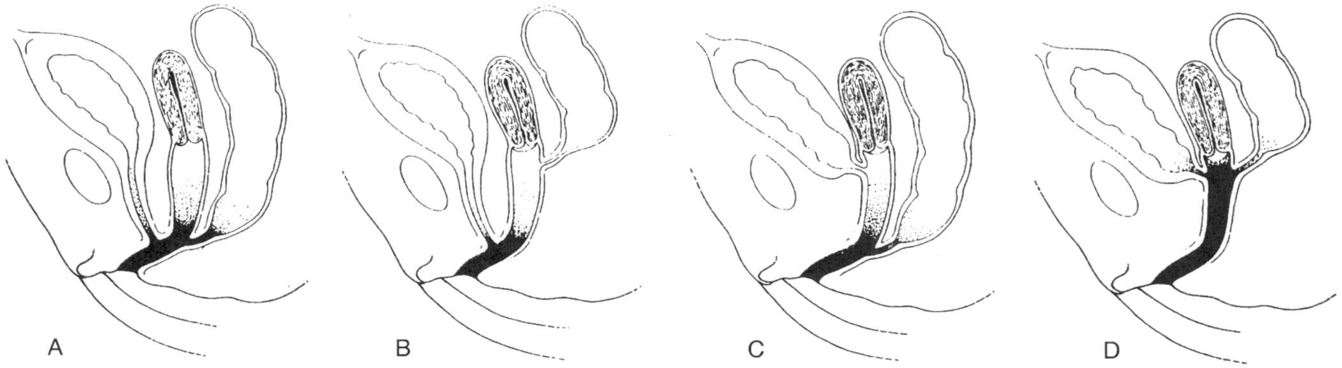

图 122-15 A 到 D，近端到远端不同类型的泄殖腔畸形。

工程，是对小儿外科和小儿泌尿科医生的巨大挑战。很明显，在开始治疗之前必须了解胃肠道的病理情况。如果直肠开口于泌尿生殖窦的较低位置，则可在会阴部予简单的肛门后切手术[54]。直肠开口位置较高更为常见，需要先予以结肠造瘘术，再予后期直肠拖出术。如果没有明显的尿梗阻，简单的泌尿生殖窦后切手术足以提供顺畅的排尿，使症状得到缓解。

对年长儿进行明确的泄殖腔畸形再建手术更为简单，并且应该将患儿手术时间定在 1 岁以后[105]。手术以前必须明确其他相关的畸形不会严重影响手术麻醉或术后苏醒。如果可能，尽量通过一次手术完成。在行肛门后切或直肠拖出术时，应使肛门充分靠后，以为阴道入口和尿道开口创造足够的空间。定位肛门时应使用电刺激仪确定肛门括约肌的位置。一旦直肠游离成功，处理泄殖腔前壁的剩余手术步骤与治疗泌尿生殖窦相似[53]。对于大多数高位的直肠畸形，最好的手术路径是后矢状路径（见第 101 章）。Peña 和其同事们指出，泌尿生殖窦共同通道的长度是决定手术路径的关键。共同通道长度大于 3.0 cm 的患者需
1948 要接受剖腹手术，而处于平均长度 2.3 cm 的患者则不需要[97]。共同通道长的患者合并尿路畸形的概率较高，因此需要接受更复杂的手术。

结果

Peña 和 de Vries[94,95] 报道了经后矢状路径同时有效治疗泄殖腔异常涉及的三种畸形（图122-17）。他们描述了采用这一手术方法对 54 名泄殖腔畸形患者进行治疗的早期结果[94]。术后随访表明，其中的 26 人能自主控制排便，21 人仅偶尔出现“污粪”现象。在 19 名骶骨发育正常的患者中，只有 5 人存在尿失禁现象，而 7 名骶骨发育不良的患者中有 5 人出现尿失禁。这些患者中 20 人术后接受了阴道镜检查，结果表明，14 人阴道入口和阴道腔完好，5 人阴道入口存在不同程度的狭窄。6 名患者因阴道尿道瘘需要接受二期手术纠治。在一篇近期的综述中，Peña 和同事回顾了 339 名泄殖腔畸形患者，其中 265 名患儿接受了一期手术修补，另外 74 名患者在外地手术失败[97]。高位缺损、共同通道长度超过 3.0 cm 的患者功能恢复不理想。总体而言，54% 的患者小便控制良
1949 好，24% 的患者通过尿道间歇性导尿可保持内裤不湿，22% 的患者在接受 Mitrofanoff 阑尾造瘘手术后不出现小便滴沥现象。这些患者中，泄殖腔共同通道长的患者有 78% 需要间歇性导尿。相对而言，那些共同通道小于 3.0 cm 的患者中，只有 28% 需要间歇导尿。所有患者中，60% 的患者有自主排便，其中 28% 没有“污粪”现象，72% 偶尔出现“污粪”。全部患者中 40% 有大便失禁，但对肠道训练反应良好[97]。

阴道口肿块

出现在阴道口、阴唇之间的肿块往往诊断困难。鉴别诊断包括尿道黏膜脱垂、异位输尿管囊肿脱垂、卵黄囊瘤脱垂、横纹肌肉瘤（葡萄状肉瘤）。掌握疾病临床本质、理解诊断和治疗的标准非常重要。

尿道黏膜脱垂

尿道黏膜脱垂（图 122-18）几乎仅发生在 3～9 岁的黑人女孩中[135]。受累儿童通常表现为内裤中血性斑点，以及阴道入口处坏死肿块。组织外观红肿、质地脆弱，尿道前壁脱垂、梗死。尽管病变组织源形态与成人尿道肉阜毛细血管瘤相似，但其发病原因仍不明确。正确诊断疾病依赖于对疾病本质的认识，无需特殊的检查手段。保守治疗包括坐浴、局部应用雌激素乳膏和抗生素等，总的治疗有效率仅有三分之一[139]。药物治疗易造成尿道黏膜脱垂复发。通常，手术只需要切除脱垂部分的黏膜，将正常尿道缝合至尿道口上[108]。术后并发症少，部分患者出现尿道口狭窄。Valerie 和同事们[139] 注意到，尿道黏膜脱垂切除以后的复发率在 1/20 左右。

异位输尿管囊肿脱垂

异位输尿管囊肿可以表现为阴唇之间阴道入口处的肿块（图 122-19）[77]。肿块通常光滑、色白或轻度水肿，从尿道口中脱出。肿块上方一般可见尿道开口。静脉尿路造影术可明确诊断，图像显示下极集合系统向下外侧推移（即垂花征，如百合花下垂）。患

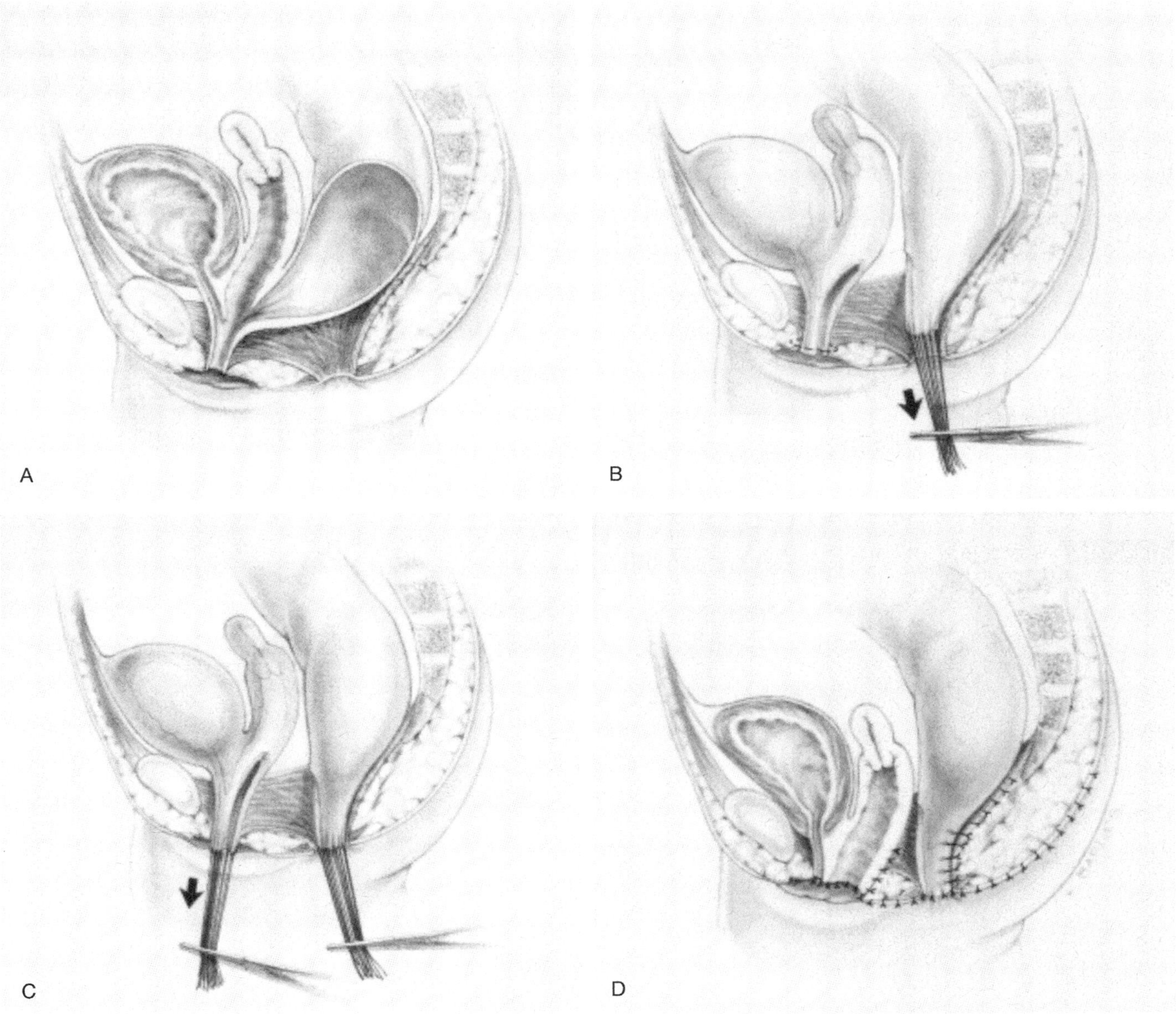

图 122-17　Peña 推荐的后矢状路径修补泄殖腔畸形。A. 图解表示膀胱泄殖腔瘘和直肠泄殖腔瘘进入泄殖腔内，会阴单一开口。B. 分离直肠瘘管，完成肛门成形手术。C. 游离泌尿生殖窦。D. 分离尿道，创建阴道开口。(Courtesy of Dr. Alberto Peña.)

侧输尿管由中线向外侧移位，膀胱表现为充盈缺损(见图 122-19)[90]。目前，新生儿期间的疾病处理是经尿道切开输尿管囊肿。1993 年，费城儿童医院报道了接受内镜下异位输尿管切开术的 24 名患者的系列随访结果[13]。该治疗方法使 75% 的患者摆脱了囊肿压迫症状，50% 的患者的上极肾功能得到了保存。47% 的患者术后出现膀胱输尿管反流，其中一半的儿童需要接受二期手术纠正反流。如果检查发现病变侧的上极肾功能很差，则传统的治疗方法是将上半肾切除，切除手术同时可合并切除输尿管，也可将其置于腹膜后。

葡萄状肉瘤

膀胱或阴道的葡萄状肉瘤或横纹肌肉瘤是最常见的下泌尿生殖系统恶性肿瘤，好发于婴儿期[62]。肿

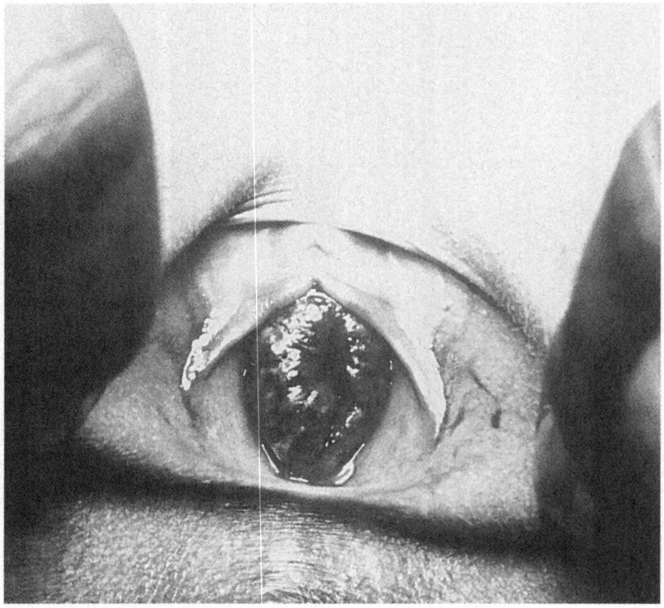

图 122-18 9 岁女孩尿道黏膜脱垂。注意脱垂组织外观充血坏死。

瘤可从阴道口脱垂。临床症状一般表现为内裤上的血性斑点，通过阴道镜和活检得以确诊[124]。如同疾病名称一样，病变外观为分叶状的葡萄样肿块。肿瘤范围需借助盆腔超声和 CT 确定。原发部位（外阴阴道处）的葡萄状肉瘤预后良好，超过 90% 的患者接受保留生育能力的手术（包括阴道镜下肿瘤切除）和多联化疗治疗后存活[2,10,80,124]。详细治疗方法参见第 32 章。

卵黄囊瘤

阴道是卵黄囊瘤的好发部位。肿块可脱垂于阴道口，或表现为阴道斑点状渗出或出血[14]。从病理角度分类，这类肿块属于内胚窦瘤（生殖细胞肿瘤），通常造成患者血清甲胎蛋白水平升高。生殖细胞肿瘤 195

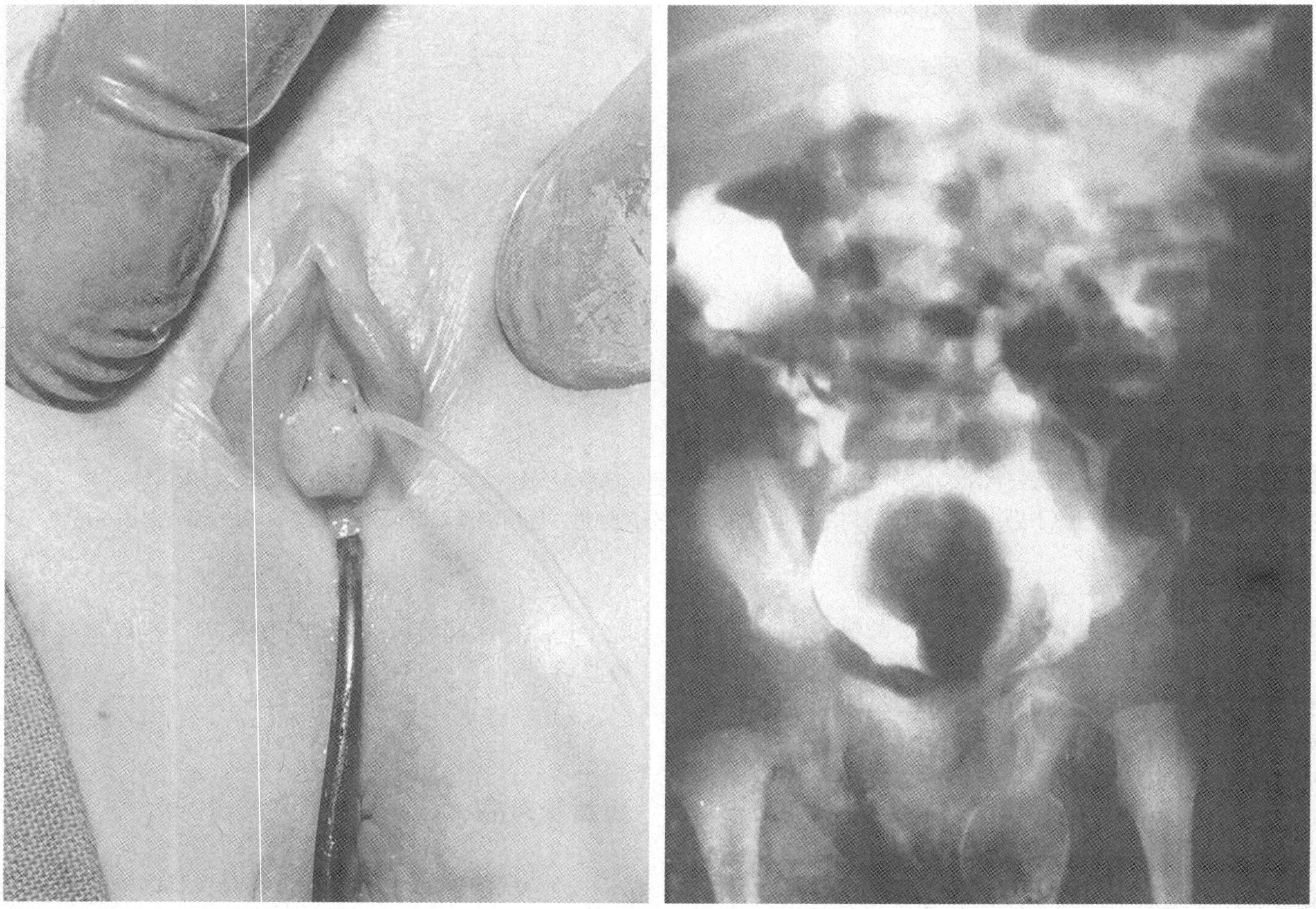

A B

图 122-19 A. 3 岁女孩输尿管囊肿脱垂。注意脱垂的囊肿呈白色、光滑外观。B. 异位输尿管囊肿患者静脉尿路造影显示右侧下极集合系统被推向侧面和后方（垂花征），伴随膀胱充盈缺损。

的化疗方案以铂为基础，一般预后良好（生存率达 85%）。保存生育力的手术结合佐剂化疗疗效显著[4,51]。事实上，一些病例显示，单纯予以化疗同样可以使肿瘤消退[86]。相关的深入讨论可参见第 34 章。

其他阴道入口病损

其他表现为阴唇之间肿块的病损包括低位、单纯的处女膜闭锁。这一病变在新生女婴中表现为阴唇之间突出的肿块（图 122-20）[109]。在母体雌激素的刺激下，女婴的处女膜闭锁常合并有不同程度的阴道积液。疾病诊断简单，如果及早发现，经处女膜切开引流后可获治愈。

女婴的尿道旁囊肿同样可表现为阴唇之间的肿块[11]。肿块压迫造成尿道口和阴道口偏向一侧。体检时，可辨认出正常的尿道和阴道开口（见图 122-20）。这些囊肿可能是 Skene 腺或 Gartner 管的胚胎残留。绝大多数囊肿可自行破裂，但仍有部分肿块需要经手术切开引流。Gartner 管囊肿是午非氏管的残留，可伴发单侧肾发育不良[64]和集合系统重复畸形，异位输尿管开口可与阴道相连，有些罕见病例输尿管可直接与囊肿本身连接[42,113]。1973 年，Goldstein 和同事[42]最先描述了 Gartner 管和一侧肾发育不良之间的关系。报道中的两例患者同时存在双角子宫。由于异位输尿管开口于阴道或 Gartner 管壁上，患者常表现为反复尿路感染和尿失禁[23,43]。一旦明
951 确尿路畸形，可予 Gartner 囊肿切除或造袋手术。

其他阴道肿瘤

血管瘤

如同在其他组织中一样，血管瘤同样可发生于阴道内。阴道血管瘤偶见广泛发展，影响到会阴、肛门和直肠壁周围的皮肤和皮下组织[17]。由于血管瘤的自身特性，即可在出生后的数月或数年内自行消退，故疾病治疗首推保守疗法。如并发溃疡或出血等情况，需要加以应用皮质激素和 α-干扰素[17]。保守治疗失败后可考虑手术切除。有关血管瘤的进一步信息

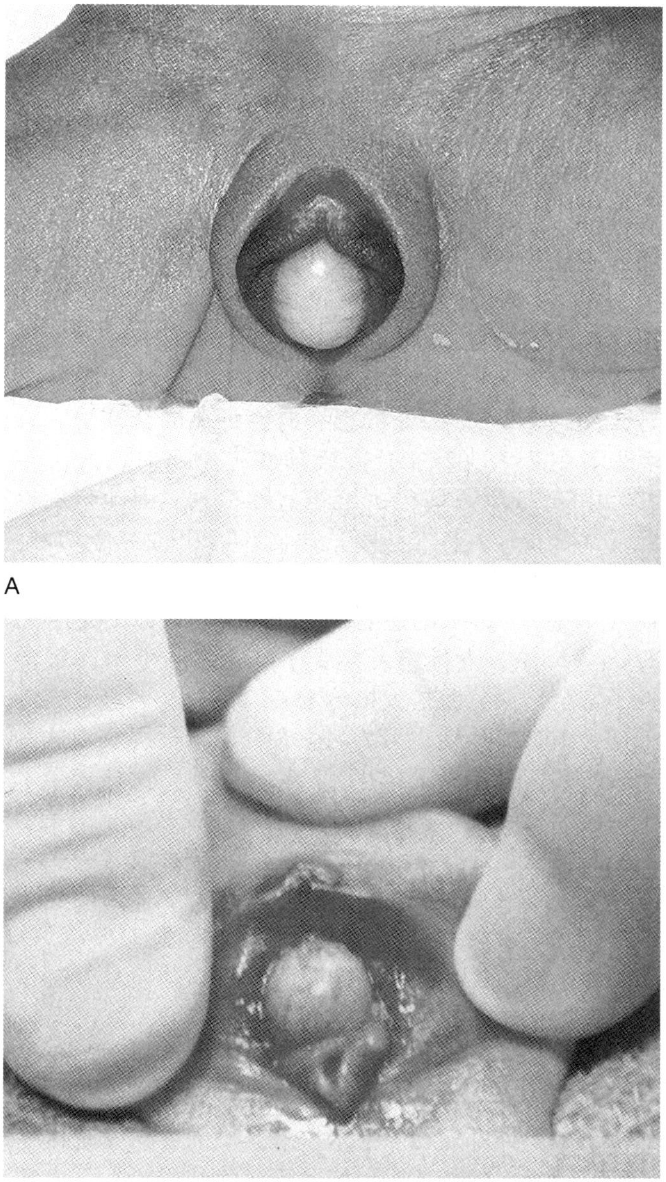

A

B

图 122-20 A. 新生儿膨出的处女膜。注意中线位置。B. 1 岁女孩尿道旁囊肿。在这些病例中，尿道和阴道开口向旁边移位，但仔细体检仍可将其辨认。

可参见第 130 章。

子宫颈和阴道腺癌

儿童发生子宫颈和阴道腺癌的机会很少。偶尔（<3%）在青春期性活跃期间可见子宫颈上皮内的

新生物，建议每年进行巴氏涂片检查。1971 年，Herbst 和同事们[61]报道了一名年轻的青春期怀孕女孩罹患阴道透明细胞腺癌的个案，该患者在怀孕期间服用了己烯雌酚。建议该患者的后代在年满 14 岁或月经来潮以后接受妇科检查，并在这之后每年接受常规体检。也曾报道发现一名阴道出血的婴儿患阴道透明细胞腺癌[147]。2004 年，McNall 及其同事们[84]回顾了 37 名 18 岁以前罹患阴道或子宫颈中肾管腺癌和透明细胞腺癌的患者，年龄从 7 个月到 18 岁不等。最常见的临床表现是阴道出血（89%）和（或）阴道渗液（16%）。62% 的患者有己烯雌酚暴露史。37 名患者中 8 人（21%）在确诊阴道肿瘤时已发生转移。由于 13 岁以前很少给予盆腔检查，因此疾病诊断常常延误。9 名（36%）患者没有出现月经初潮。肿瘤 FIGO 分期结果表明，76% 的患者属于Ⅰ期或Ⅱ期（早期），24% 的患者属于Ⅲ期或Ⅳ期（晚期）。22 名（58%）女性患者接受了肿瘤根治手术（根治性子宫全切或盆腔扩大根治术）：其中 19 名患者疾病分期为Ⅰ期或Ⅱ期，另 3 名患者分期未被提及。这些患者中的 7 人接受了放疗。7 名（18%）女孩接受了单纯肿瘤切除手术，其中 3 人术后接受放疗，另有 1 人同时接受了放疗和化疗。7 名晚期患者没有接受手术，其中 3 人接受化疗，3 人接受放疗，1 人接受了放疗化疗联合治疗。疾病的总体治愈率为 71%（27/38）。10 名患者死于疾病进展或复发。肿瘤复发是预后不良的标志。复发部位涉及肺（6 人）、淋巴结或软组织（2 人）和脑（1 人）。那些接受肿瘤切除手术的患者，3 年生存率估计在 85% 左右。尽管只有 7 人接受了单纯肿瘤切除手术，且其中的 4 名儿童接受了辅助治疗，但是比较单纯肿瘤切除和根治性手术的患者后发现，前者（保守手术）预后优于后者（3 年生存率 100% vs 78%）。研究中没有评价肿瘤尺寸。7 名单纯肿瘤切除的患者中有 2 人分期为Ⅲ期，而所有接受扩大根治术的患者都属于Ⅰ期或Ⅱ期。在统计学
1952 上能反映生存率的预测指标中，只有手术切除和诊断时是否发生转移这两项有意义。数据表明，保守手术联合辅助治疗能消除对根治手术的需要。确定这一观察结果尚需大样本前瞻性研究。由于肿瘤发生罕见，此项研究困难重重。由于已经有报道发现治疗后晚期复发的患者，因此肿瘤患者需要接受长期随访[35,66]。

（孙　杰译　文建国校）

参考文献

1. American College of Obstetrics and Gynecology: Committee Opinion: Nonsurgical diagnosis and management of vaginal agenesis. No. 274, July 2002. Int J Gynaecol Obstet 2002;79:167.
2. Andrassy RJ, Hays DM, Raney RB, et al: Conservative surgical management of vaginal and vulvar pediatric rhabdomyosarcoma: A report from the Intergroup Rhabdomyosarcoma Study Ⅲ. J Pediatr Surg 1995;30:1034.
3. Ashworth MF, Morton KE, Dewhurst J, et al: Vaginoplasty using amnion. Obstet Gynecol 1986;67:443.
4. Arora M, Shrivastav RK, Jaiprakash MP: A rare germ-cell tumor site: Vaginal endodermal sinus tumor. Pediatr Surg Int 2002;18:521.
5. Baldwin JF: The formation of an artificial vagina by intestinal transplantation. Ann Surg 1904;40:398.
6. Baldwin JF: Formation of an intestinal transplantation. Am J Obstet Dis Woman Child 1907;56:636.
7. Beemer W, Hopkins MP, Morley GW: Vaginal reconstruction in gynecologic oncology. Obstet Gynecol 1988;72:911.
8. Behera M, Couchman G, Walmer D, Prfice TM: Mullerian agenesis and thrombocytopenia absent radius syndrome: A case report and review of syndromes associated with Müllerian agenesis. Obstet Gynecol Surv 2005;60:453.
9. Belloli G, Campobasso P, Musi L: Labial skin-flap vaginoplasty using tissue expanders. Pediatr Surg Int 1997;12:168.
10. Bernal KL, Fahmy L, Remmenga S, et al: Embryonal rhabdomyosarcoma (sarcoma botryoides) of the cervix presenting as a cervical polyp treated with fertility-sparing surgery and adjuvant chemotherapy. Gynecol Oncol 2004;95:243.
11. Blaivas JG, Pais VM, Retik AB: Paraurethral cysts in female neonate. Urology 1976;7:504.
12. Blask AR, Sanders RC, Gearhart JP: Obstructed ureterovaginal anomalies: Demonstration with sonography. Radiology 1991;179:79.
13. Blyth B, Passerini-Glazel G, Camuffo C, et al: Endoscopic incision of ureteroceles: Intravesical versus ectopic. J Urol 1993;149:556.
14. Bochner BH, De Filippo RE, Hardy BE: Endodermal sinus tumor of the vagina. J Urol 2000;163:1293.
15. Bowman J, Scott R: Transverse vaginal septum. Obstet Gynecol 1954;3:441.
16. Borruto F: Mayer-Rokitansky-Küster syndrome: Vecchietti's personal series. Clin Exp Obstet Gyencol 1992;19:273.
17. Bouchard S, Yazbeck S, Lallier M: Perineal hemangioma, anorectal malformation, and genital anomaly: A new association? J Pediatr Surg 1999;34:1133.
18. Bryan AL, Nigro JA, Counseller VS: One hundred cases of congenital absence of the vagina. Surg Gynecol Obstet 1949;88:79.
19. Burbige KA, Hensle TW: Uterus didelphys and vaginal duplication with unilateral obstruction presenting as a newborn abdominal mass. J Urol 1984;132:1195.
20. Burger RA, Riedmiller H, Knapstein PG, et al: Ileocecal vaginal construction. Am J Obstet Gynecol 1989;161:162.
21. Buss JG, Lee RA: McIndoe procedure for vaginal agenesis: Results and complications. Mayo Clin Proc 1989;64:758.
22. Counseller VS, Flor FS: Congenital absence of the vagina: Further results of treatment and a new technique. Surg Clin North Am 1957;37:1107.
23. Currarino G: Single vaginal ectopic ureter and Gartner's duct cyst with ipsilateral renal hypoplasia and dysplasia (or agenesis). J Urol 1982;123:988.

24. Davydov SN, Zhvitiashvili OD: Formation of vagina (colpopoiesis) from peritoneum of Douglas pouch. Acta Chir Plast 1974;16:35.
25. de Souza AZ, Maluf M, Perin PM, et al: Surgical treatment of congenital uterovaginal agenesis: Mayer-Rokitansky-Küster-Hauser syndrome. Int Surg 1987;72:45.
26. Dean GE, Hensle TW: Intestinal vaginoplasty. Curr Surg Tech Urol 1994;7:1.
27. Del Rossi C, Attanasio A, Del Curto S, et al: Treatment of vaginal atresia at a missionary hospital in Bangladesh: Results and follow up of 20 cases. J Urol 2003;170:864.
28. Dewhurst CJ: Congenital malformations of the genital tract in childhood. Br J Obstet Gynaecol 1968;75:377.
29. Donahoe PK, Gustafson ML: Early one stage surgical reconstruction of the extremely high vagina in patients with congenital adrenal hyperplasia. J Pediatr Surg 1994;29:352.
30. Duncan PA, Shapiro LR, Stanzel JJ, et al: The MURCS association: Müllerian duct aplasia, renal aplasia, and cervicothoracic somite dysplasia. J Pediatr 1979;95:399.
31. Edmonds DK: Congenital malformations of the genital tract. Obstet Gynecol Clin North Am 2000;27:49.
32. Edmonds DK: Congenital malformations of the genital tract and their management. Best Pract Res Clin Obstet Gynaecol 2003;17:19.
33. Fall FH: A simple method for making an artificial vagina. Am J Obstet Gynecol 1940;40:906.
34. Fedele L, Bianchi S, Zanconato G, Raffaelli R: Laparoscopic creation of a neovagina in patients with Rokitansky syndrome: Analysis of 52 cases. Fertil Steril 2000;74:384.
35. Fishman DA, Williams S, Small W Jr, et al: Late recurrences of vaginal clear cell adenocarcinoma. Gynecol Oncol 1996; 62:128.
36. Folche M, Pigem I, Konje JC: Müllerian agenesis: Etiology, diagnosis, and management. Obstet Gynecol Surv 2000; 55:644.
37. Fore SR, Hammond CB, Parkes RT, Anderson EE: Urologic and genital anomalies in patients with congenital absence of the vagina. Obstet Gynecol 1975;46:410.
38. Frank RT: The formation of an artificial vagina without operation. Am J Obstet Gynecol 1938;35:1053.
39. Freundt I, Toolenaar TA, Huikeshoven FJ, et al: A modified technique to create a neovagina with an isolated segment of sigmoid colon. Surg Gynecol Obstet 1992;174:11.
40. Giraldo F, Solano MJ, Mora M, et al: The Malaga flap for vaginoplasty in the Mayer-Rokitansky-Küster-Hauser syndrome: Experience and early term results. Plast Reconstr Surg 1996;98:305.
41. Goldfarb JM, Austin C, Peskin B, et al: Fifteen years experience with an in-vitro fertilization surrogate gestational pregnancy programme. Hum Reprod 2000;15:1075.
42. Goldstein AI, Ackerman ES, Woodruff R, Poyas J: Vaginal and cervical communication with mesonephric duct remnants: Relationship to unilateral renal agenesis. Am J Obstet Gynecol 1973;116:101.
43. Gotoh T, Koyanagi T: Clinicopathological and embryological considerations of single ectopic ureters opening into Gartner's duct cyst: A unique subtype of single vaginal ectopia. J Urol 1987;137:969.
44. Gough MH: Anorectal agenesis with persistence of cloaca. Proc R Soc Med 1959;52:886.
45. Graziano K, Teitelbaum DH, Hirschl RB, Coran AG: Vaginal reconstruction for ambiguous genitalia and congenital absence of the vagina: A 27-year experience. J Pediatr Surg 2002;37:955.
46. Griesinger G, Dafopoulos K, Schultze-Mosgau A, et al: Mayer-Rokitansky-Küster-Hauser syndrome associated with thrombocytopenia–absent radius syndrome. Fertil Steril 2005;83:452.
47. Griffin JE, Edwards C, Madden JD, et al: Congenital absence of the vagina. Ann Intern Med 1976;85:224.
48. Grio R, Ambroggio GP, D'Addato F, et al: A new method of neovagina in Rokitansky's syndrome: A review of the literature and description of a series. Min Ginecol 2002;54:161.
49. Gunderson CH, Greenspan RH, Glaser GH, Lubs HA: The Klippel-Feil syndrome: Genetic and clinical reevaluation of cervical fusion. Medicine (Baltimore) 1967;46:491.
50. Hallberg H, Hollstrom H: Vaginal reconstruction with skin grafts and vacuum-assisted closure. Scand J Plast Reconstruct Surg Hand Surg 2003;37:97.
51. Handel LN, Scott SM, Giller RH: New perspectives on therapy for vaginal endodermal sinus tumors. J Urol 2002; 168:687.
52. Hauser GA, Keller M, Koller T, Wenner R: Das Rokitansky-Küster syndrome: Uterus bipartitus solidus rudimentarius cum Vagina solida. Gynaecologia 1961;151:11.
53. Hendren WH: Surgical management of urogenital sinus abnormalities. J Pediatr Surg 1977;12:339.
54. Hendren WH: Construction of female urethra from vaginal wall and a perineal flap. J Urol 1980;123:657.
55. Hendren WH: Urogenital sinus and anorectal malformation: Experience with 22 cases. J Pediatr Surg 1980;15:628.
56. Hendren WH, Crawford JD: Adrenogenital syndrome: The anatomy of the anomaly and its repair. Some new concepts. J Pediatr Surg 1969;4:49.
57. Hendren WH, Donahoe PK: Correction of congenital abnormalities of the vagina and perineum. J Pediatr Surg 1980;15:751.
58. Hendren WH, Atala A: Use of bowel for vaginal reconstruction. J Urol 1994;152:752.
59. Hensle TW, Dean GE: Vaginal replacement in children. J Urol 1992;148:677.
60. Hensle TW, Reiley EA: Vaginal replacement in children and young adults. J Urol 1998;159:1035.
61. Herbst AL, Ulfelder H, Poskanzer DC: Adenocarcinoma of the vagina. Association of maternal stilbestrol therapy with tumor appearance in young women. N Engl J Med 1971; 284:878.
62. Hilgers RD, Malkasian GD Jr, Soule EH: Embryonal rhabdomyosarcoma (botryoid type) of the vagina. Am J Obstet Gynecol 1970;107:484.
63. Hiroi H, Yasugi T, Matsumoto K, et al: Mucinous adenocarcinoma arising in a neovagina using the sigmoid colon 30 years after operation: A case report. J Surg Oncol 2001; 77:61.
64. Holmes M, Upadhyay V, Pease P: Gartner's duct cyst with unilateral renal dysplasia presenting as an introital mass in a new born. Pediatr Surg Int 1999;15:277.
65. Johnson RJ, Palken M, Derrick W, Bill AH: The embryology of high anorectal and associated genitourinary anomalies in the female. Surg Gynecol Obstet 1972;135:759.
66. Jones WB, Tan LK, Lewis JL Jr: Late recurrence of clear cell adenocarcinoma of the vagina and cervix: A report of three cases. Gynecol Oncol 1993;51:266.
67. Joseph VT: Pudendal-thigh flap vaginoplasty in the reconstruction of genital anomalies. J Pediatr Surg 1997; 32:62.
68. Jost A: Embryonic sexual differentiation. In Jones HW Jr, Scott WW (eds): Hermaphroditism, Genital Anomalies and Related Endocrine Disorders, 2nd ed. Baltimore, Williams & Wilkins, 1971.
69. Kay R, Tank ES: Principles of management of the persistent cloaca in the female newborn. J Urol 1977;117:102.

70. Kaya H, Sezik M, Ozkaya O, Kose SA: Mayer-Rokitansky-Küster-Hauser syndrome associated with unilateral gonadal agenesis: A case report. J Reprod Med 2003;48:902.
71. Keser A, Bozkurt N, Taner OF, Sensoz O: Treatment of vaginal agenesis with modified Abbe-McIndoe technique: Long-term follow up in 22 patients. Eur J Obstet Gynecol Reprod Biol 2005;121:110.
72. Koff AK: Development of the vagina in the human fetus. Contemp Embryol 1933;24:61.
73. Krishnan A, Baez L, Kirsh A: Single ectopic ureter inserting into a duplicated imperforate hemivagina: A rare cause of fetal abdominal mass. Urology 2003;62:144.
74. Küster H: Uterus bipartitus solidus rudimentarius cum Vagina solida. Z Geburtshife Perinatol 1910;67:692.
75. Laufer MR: Congenital absence of the vagina: In search of the perfect solution. When, and by what technique, should a vagina be created? Curr Opin Obstet Gynecol 2002; 14:441.
76. Lin WC, Chang CY, Shen YY, Tsai HD: Use of autologous buccal mucosa for vaginoplasty: A study of eight cases. Hum Reprod 2003;18:604.
77. Mandell J, Colodny AH, Lebowitz R, et al: Ureteroceles in infants and children. J Urol 1980;123:921.
78. Marcos R, Perez-Brayfield EA, Smith EA, et al: Vaginal reconstruction using a vertical rectus abdominis myocutaneous flap in a child: A case report. J Pediatr Surg 2001; 36:1070.
79. Marshall FF, Jeffs RD, Sarafyan WK: Urogenital sinus abnormalities in the female patient. J Urol 1979;122:568.
80. Martelli H, Oberlin O, et al: Conservative treatment for girls with nonmetastatic rhabdomyosarcoma of the genital tract: A report from the study committee of the International Society of Pediatric Oncology. Eur J Cancer 1999;34:1050.
81. Mayer CAJ: Uber Verdoppelungen des Uterus und ihre Arten, nebst Bemerkungen uber Hasenscharte und Wolfsrachen. J Chir Auger 1829;13:525.
82. McIndoe AH: Treatment of congenital absence and obliterative conditions of vagina. Br J Plast Surg 1950; 2:254.
83. McKusick VA, Bauer RL, Koop CE, Scott RB: Hydrometrocolpos as a simply inherited malformation. JAMA 1964;189:813.
84. McNall RY, Nowicki PD, Miller B, et al: Adenocarcinoma of the cervix and vagina in pediatric patients. Pediatr Blood Cancer 2004;43:289.
85. Mirza M, Moriquand P: Ectopic ureter entering a uterovaginal duplication. Br J Urol 1993;72:250.
86. Neels NJJ, Tissing WJE, Pieters R, et al: Treatment of an infant with a vaginal yolk sac tumor and distant metastases with chemotherapy only. Pediatr Blood Cancer 2004; 43:296.
87. Nisolle M, Donnez J: Vaginoplasty using amnionic membranes in cases of agenesis of the vagina. J Gynecol Surg 1992;8:25.
88. Noguchi S, Nakatsuka M, Sugiyama Y, et al: Use of artificial dermis and recombinant basic fibroblast growth factor for creating a neovagina in a patient with Mayer-Rokitansky-Küster-Hauser syndrome. Hum Reprod 2004;19:1629.
89. Novak F, Kos L, Plesko F: The advantages of the artificial vagina derived from sigmoid colon. Acta Obstet Gynecol Scand 1978;57:95.
90. Nussbaum AR, Lebowitz RL: Interlabial masses in little girls. Am J Res 1983;141:65.
91. Owens SB, Morse WH: Prolapse of the female urethra in children. J Urol 1968;100:171.
92. Ozgenel GY, Ozcan M: Neovaginal reconstruction with buccal mucosal grafts. Plast Reconstr Surg 2003;111:2250.
93. Passerini-Glazel G: A new one-stage procedure for clitorovaginoplasty in severely masculinized female pseudohermaphrodites. J Urol 1989;142:565.
94. Peña A: The surgical management of persistent cloaca: Results in 54 patients treated with a posterior sagittal approach. J Pediatr Surg 1989;24:590.
95. Peña A: Atlas of Surgical Management of Anorectal Malformation. New York, Springer-Verlag, 1990.
96. Peña A, deVries PA: Posterior sagittal anorectoplasty: Important technical considerations and new applications. J Pediatr Surg 1982;17:796.
97. Peña A, Levitt MA, Hong A, Midulla P: Surgical management of cloacal malformations: A review of 339 patients. J Pediatr Surg 2004;39:470.
98. Petrozza JC, Gary MR, Davis AJ, Reindollar RH: Congenital absence of the uterus and vagina is not commonly transmitted as a dominant genetic trait: Outcomes of surrogate pregnancies. Fertil Steril 1997;67:387.
99. Pittock ST, Babovic-Vuksanovic D, Lteif A: Mayer-Rokitansky-Küster-Hauser anomaly and its associated malformations. Am J Med Genet A 2005;135A:314.
100. Plevraki E, Kita M, Goulis DG, et al: Bilateral ovarian agenesis and the presence of the testis-specific protein 1-Y-linked gene: Two new features of Mayer-Rokitansky-Küster-Hauser syndrome. Fertil Steril 2004;81:689.
101. Poland ML, Evans TN: Psychologic aspects of vaginal agenesis. J Reprod Med 1985;30:340.
102. Pratt JH: Vaginal atresia corrected by the use of small and large bowel. Clin Obstet Gynecol 1972;96:639.
103. Purushothaman V: Horse shoe flap vaginoplasty—a new technique of vaginal reconstruction with labia minora flaps for primary vaginal agenesis. Br J Plast Surg 2005; Epub July 22.
104. Radhakrishnan J: Colon interposition vaginoplasty: A modification of the Wagner-Baldwin technique. J Pediatr Surg 1987;22:1175.
105. Raffensperger JG, Ramenofsky ML: The management of a cloaca. J Pediatr Surg 1973;8:647.
106. Rajimwale A, Furness PD III, Brant WO, Koyle MA: Vaginal reconstruction using sigmoid colon in children and young adults. BJU Int 2004;94:1143.
107. Rangaswamy M, Macado NO, Kaur S, Machado L: Laparoscopic vaginoplasty using a sliding peritoneal flap for correction of complete vaginal agenesis. Eur J Obstet Gynecol Reprod Biol 2001;98:244.
108. Redman JF: Conservative management of urethral prolapse in female children. Urology 1982;19:509.
109. Reed MH, Griscom WT: Hydrometrocolpos in infancy. Am J Res 1973;118:1.
110. Reinhold C, Hricak H, Forstner R, et al: Primary amenorrhea evaluation with MR imaging. Radiology 1997;203:383.
111. Rock JA, Reeves LA, Retto H, et al: Success following vaginal creation for müllerian agenesis. Fertil Steril 1983;39:809.
112. Rokitansky K: Uber die sogenannten Verdoppelungen des Uterus. Med Jb Ost Staat 1938;26:39.
113. Rosenfeld DL, Barone JG, Lis E, et al: A "flipped" kidney in utero in an infant with a double collecting system and a Gartner's duct cyst with a vaginal ectopic ureter. Pediatr Radiol 1995;25:466.
114. Ross GT, Vande Weile RL: The ovaries. In Williams RH (ed): Textbook of Endocrinology, 5th ed. Philadelphia, WB Saunders, 1974.
115. Rothman D: The use of peritoneum in the construction

of a vagina. Obstet Gynecol 1972;40:835.
116. Ruge E: Ersatz der Vagina durch die flexur mittels Laparotomie. Dtsch Med Wochenschr 1914;40:120.
117. Schaap C, de Die-Smulders CE, Kuijten RH, Fryns JP: McKusick-Kaufman syndrome: The diagnostic challenge of abdominal distension in the neonatal period. Eur J Pediatr 1992;151:583.
118. Schätz T, Huber J, Wenzl R: Creation of a neovagina according to Wharton-Sheares-George in patients with Mayer-Rokitansky-Küster-Hauser syndrome. Fertil Steril 2005;83:437.
119. Sheares BH: Congenital atresia of the vagina—a technique for tunneling the space between the bladder and rectum and construction of a new vagina by a modified Wharton technique. J Obstet Gynecol Br Emp 1960;67:24.
120. Selvaggi G, Monstrey S, Depypere H, et al: Creation of a neovagina with use of a pudendal thigh fasciocutaneous flap and restoration of uterovaginal continuity. Fertil Steril 2003;80:607.
121. Shreeprasad P, Kalrao V, Patankar SS: Mayer-Rokitansky syndrome and anorectal malformation. Indian J Pediatr 2004;71:1133.
122. Slavotinek AM, Biesecker LG: Phenotypic overlap of McKusick-Kaufman syndrome with Bardet-Biedl syndrome: A literature review. Am J Med Genet 2000;95:208.
123. Slavotinek AM, Dutra A, Kpodzo D, et al: A female with complete lack of mullerian fusion, postaxial polydactyly and tetralogy of Fallot: Genetic heterogeneity of McKusick-Kaufman syndrome or a unique syndrome? Am J Med Genet 2004;129:69.
124. Solomon LA, Zurawin RK, Edwards CL: Vaginoscopic resection for rhabdomyosarcoma of the vagina: A case report and review of the literature. Pediatr Adolesc Gynecol 2003;16:139.
125. Soong YK, Chang FH, Lai YM, et al: Results of modified laparoscopically assisted neovaginoplasty in 18 patients with congenital absence of vagina. Hum Reprod 1996;11:200.
126. Stenchever MA, et al: Comprehensive Gynecology, 4th ed. St. Louis, CV Mosby, 2001.
127. Stephens FD, Smith ED: Anorectal Malformations in Children. Chicago, Year Book Medical, 1971.
128. Stone DL, Slavotinek A, Bouffard GG, et al: Mutation of a gene encoding a putative chaperonin causes McKusick-Kaufman syndrome. Nat Genet 2000;25:79.
129. Strubbe EH, Thijn CJ, Willemsen WN, Lappohn R: Evaluation of radiographic abnormalities of the hand in patients with Mayer-Rokitansky-Küster-Hauser syndrome. Skel Radiol 1987;16:227.
130. Strubbe EH, Cremers CW, Dikkers FG, Willemsen WN: Mayer-Rokitansky-Küster-Hauser syndrome. Am J Otol 1994;15:431.
131. Syed HA, Malone PS, Hitchcock RJ: Diversion colitis in children with colovaginoplasty. BJU Int 2001;87:857.
132. Templeman C, Hertweck P, Levine R, Reich H: A new technique for the creation of a neovagina. J Pediatr Adolesc Gynecol 2000;13:99.
133. Therrell BL, et al: Results of screening 1.9 million Texas newborns for 21-hydroxylase deficient congenital adrenal hyperplasia. Pediatrics 1998;101:583.
134. Tompkins P: Imperforate hymen and hematocolpos. JAMA 1939;113:913.
135. Thoury A, Detchev R, Darai E: Sigmoid neovagina by combined laparoscopic-perineal route for Rokitansky syndrome. Gynecol Obstet Fertil 2002;30:938.
136. Trotman M, Brewster E: Prolapse of the urethral mucosa in prepubertal West Indian girls. Br J Urol 1993;73:503.
137. Turner-Warwick R, Kirby RS: The construction and reconstruction of the vagina with the colocecum. Surg Gynecol Obstet 1990;170:132.
138. Urbanowicz W, Starzyk J, Sulislawski J: Laparoscopic vaginal reconstruction using a sigmoid colon segment: A preliminary report. J Urol 2004;171:2632.
139. Valerie E, Gilchrist HF, Frischer J, et al: Diagnosis and treatment of urethral prolapse in children. Urology 1999;54:1082.
140. Vecchietti G: Neovagina nella syndrome di Rokitansky-Küster-Hauser. Attuat Ostet Ginecol 1965;11:131.
141. Wee JT, Joseph VT: A new technique of vaginal reconstruction using neurovascular pudendal-thigh flaps: A preliminary report. Plast Reconstr Surg 1989;83:701.
142. Wesley JR, Coran AG: Intestinal vaginoplasty for congenital absence of the vagina. J Pediatr Surg 1992;27:885.
143. Wharton LR: A simple method of constructing a vagina: Report of four cases. Ann Surg 1938;107:842.
144. Williams EA: Congenital absence of the vagina—a simple operation for its relief. J Obstet Gynaecol Br Emp 1964;71:511.
145. Winderl LM, Silverman RK: Prenatal diagnosis of congenital imperforate hymen. Obstet Gynecol 1995;85:857.
146. Witschi F: Development and differentiation of the uterus. In Mack HC (ed): Prenatal Life. Detroit, Wayne State University Press, 1970.
147. Yavuz H, Arslan A, Avsaz AF: Vaginal clear cell adenocarcinoma in an infant. Pediatr Hematol Oncol 1996;13:577.
148. Yii NW, Niranjan NS: Lotus petal flaps in vulvo-vaginal reconstruction. Br J Plast Surg 1996;49:547.

第九部分

特殊的小儿外科疾病

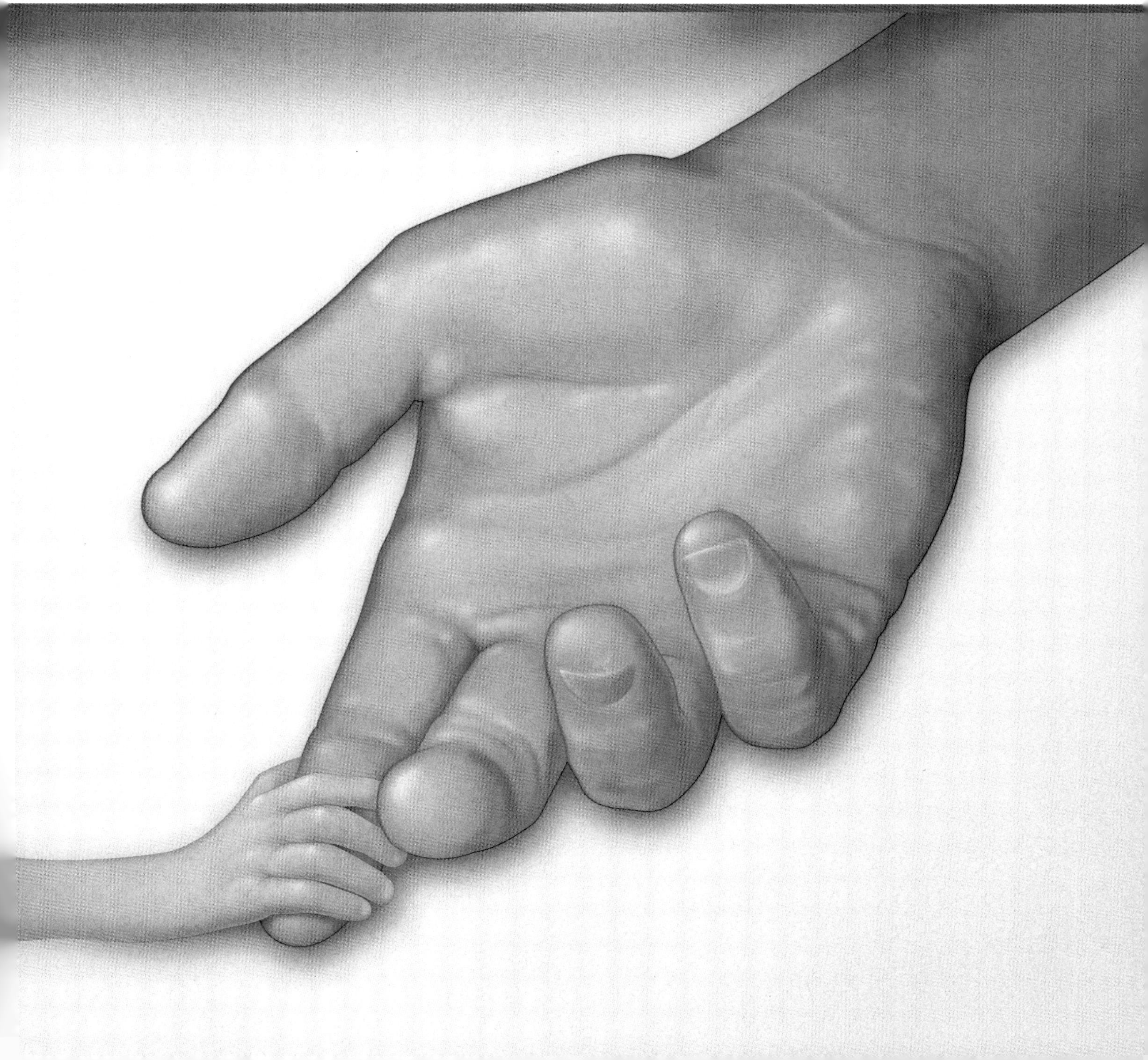

第 123 章

先天性心脏病和大血管畸形

Eric Devaney、Richard Ohye 和 Edward L. Bove

动脉导管未闭

959 动脉导管是一种正常的胎儿结构，是肺动脉干或近端左肺动脉（PA）和近端降主动脉之间的交通（图 123-1）。在胎儿发育过程中，这个血管为离开右心室的血流绕开高阻力的肺血管床，并直接跨越体循环提供了通路。从组织学来说，主动脉和肺动脉的中层由环形排列的弹性纤维构成，而动脉导管的中层主要由平滑肌细胞组成。正常出生后，肺通气引起的氧张力上升预示着动脉导管的关闭。一个足月婴儿，其动脉导管通常在出生后 12～24 小时内完全关闭。闭合的动脉导管留下一个纤维条索，称之为动脉韧带。导管关闭失败就导致所谓的动脉导管未闭（PDA）。孤立性 PDA 的发生率约为 1 人/1200 例活产婴儿，约占全部先天性心脏病的 7%[39]。早产儿的 PDA 发病率更高（高于 20%）[68]，这种缺陷可能是孤立性的，或者合并许多其他畸形。在一些肺血流不足（例如肺动脉闭锁）或体循环血流不足（例如重症主动脉缩窄）的心脏缺损中，需要持续的动脉导管未闭。前列腺素维持动脉导管开放这一发现，在改善这类患者的存活率方面发挥了重要作用[28]。

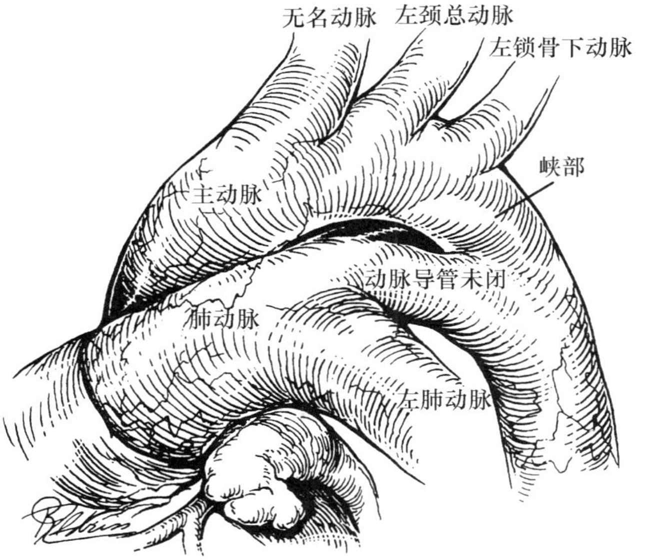

图 123-1 左侧胸廓切开时的动脉导管未闭（PDA）解剖。导管从肺总动脉（PA）延伸，并进入在左锁骨下动脉（LSA）远端的近端降主动脉。(From Hillman ND, Mavroudis C, Backer CL: Patent ductus arteriosus. In Mavroudis C, Backer CL [eds]: Pediatric Cardiac Surgery, 3rd ed. Philadelphia. Mosby, 2003.)

自然病史和诊断

PDA 的病理生理学涉及跨导管的血液分流。导管的大小和肺循环及体循环血管阻力的比值决定了分流血量。出生时，肺血管阻力大幅度降低，并在出生后第一个星期持续降低。这导致跨导管的左向右血流。过量的肺血流可引起充血性心力衰竭，且在极端病例中，可能会发生低血压和体循环灌注不良。对于活过婴儿期的大型 PDA 患者，有发展成肺血管梗阻性病变的风险。在这些病例中，当肺血管阻力超过体循环血管阻力时，可能会引起 Eisenmenger 生理学状态，引起跨动脉导管的反向分流（从左向右分流变成右向左分流），导致发绀和最终的右心室（RV）衰竭。一些小型 PDA 的患者可能直到成人期前都无症状。也有报道在长期合并 PDA 时存在心内膜炎（和动脉内膜炎）[16]。

1960 PDA 的临床表现取决于分流量和并发的心脏缺损。左向右分流引起心脏左侧部分的容量超负荷。婴儿充血性心力衰竭的体征通常包括呼吸急促、心动过速和喂养不良。年长儿可能会有反复呼吸道感染、疲劳和发育障碍。体格检查包括脉压增宽和心前区搏动。听诊显示一个连续的“机器样”杂音，沿胸骨左上缘听诊最佳。放射影像所见包括肺血管纹理增多和心脏左侧增大，通常与分流程度成正比。心电图可证实左心室（LV）肥大和左心房（LA）扩大。超声心动图是目前选用的诊断方法，并且能排除其他合并的缺损。心导管的主要适应证有两个。第一，怀疑有肺动脉高压的年长患者可用心导管来评估肺血管梗阻性病变。第二，由于经心导管技术的发展，可以对一些选择性病例进行导管封堵。

治疗

有三种关闭动脉导管的治疗方案：药物治疗、手术关闭和血管内器械封堵。吲哚美辛是一种前列腺素抑制剂，有助于刺激早产儿 PDA 的关闭[36]。对足月儿却罕有奏效。用法是每剂 0.1～0.2 mg/kg，静脉用药，间隔 12 或 24 小时，共用 3 剂。这种方法在近 80% 的早产儿中取得成功。已知吲哚美辛有很多可能的副作用，包括高血压、减少胃肠道血流、减少肾血流和干扰血小板功能。吲哚美辛治疗的禁忌证包括败血症、肾功能不全和出血性疾病。在两次完整的吲哚美辛治疗失败后，应谋求手术关闭导管。

PDA 的手术径路通常是经左后外侧第三和第四肋间隙的胸廓切口开胸术（图 123-2）。纵行分开覆盖在近端胸部降主动脉上的胸膜。因此迷走神经被向内侧吊起。然后开始游离，以明确远端的主动脉弓横部和动脉导管。在一些病例中，动脉导管可能是最大的血管结构，因此关键的是不要将之与主动脉相混淆。一旦解剖明确，轻柔地游离导管。导管组织极脆且易碎，特别是早产儿，因此不推荐直接对其进行操作。喉返神经在后方绕过动脉导管，在游离时必须加以保护。可用手术夹或丝线结扎来关闭动脉导管，或者在两道结扎间加以切断（图 123-3）。在大多数病例中都选用后者；但是对于早产儿，最安全的方法是用手术夹夹闭。通常在新生儿重症监护病房内进行此手术操作，这可避免患者搬运引起的问题[18,72]。

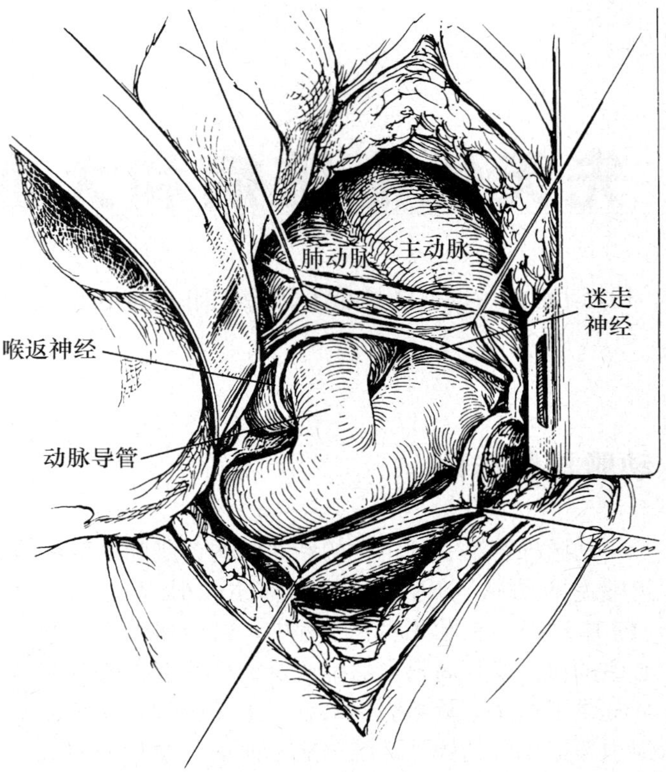

图 123-2 通过左侧胸廓切口暴露未闭的动脉导管（PDA）。打开并翻起纵隔胸膜，保护迷走神经和喉返神经。（From Hillman ND, Mavroudis C, Backer CL: Patent ductus arteriosus. In Mavroudis C, Backer CL [eds]: Pediatric Cardiac Surgery, 3rd ed. Philadelphia. Mosby, 2003.）

最近，采用电视辅助胸腔镜进行 PDA 结扎[15]。这个方法有减少疼痛和缩短住院时间的潜在好处。缺点包括一个较长的学习曲线和增加手术时间。

已发展出一些血管内器械以经心导管封堵 PDA[19,31,58]。已证明这些器械是很成功的，以至于在大多数中心，经心导管封堵成了封堵小型或中型年长婴儿和儿童 PDA 的治疗选择。大型动脉导管的患者采用手术治疗。

结果

采用手术或经心导管方法关闭 PDA 的死亡率接近零。手术治疗的潜在并发症包括气胸、喉返神经损伤和乳糜胸。大多数患者在 PDA 结扎术后的预期寿

图 123-3　控制未闭的动脉导管（PDA）的不同技术。A. 单纯结扎。B. 结扎和使用血管夹。C 和 D. 结扎及外膜荷包缝线缝合。（From Hillman ND, Mavroudis C, Backer CL: Patent ductus arteriosus. In Mavroudis C, Backer CL [eds]: Pediatric Cardiac Surgery, 3rd ed. Philadelphia. Mosby, 2003.）

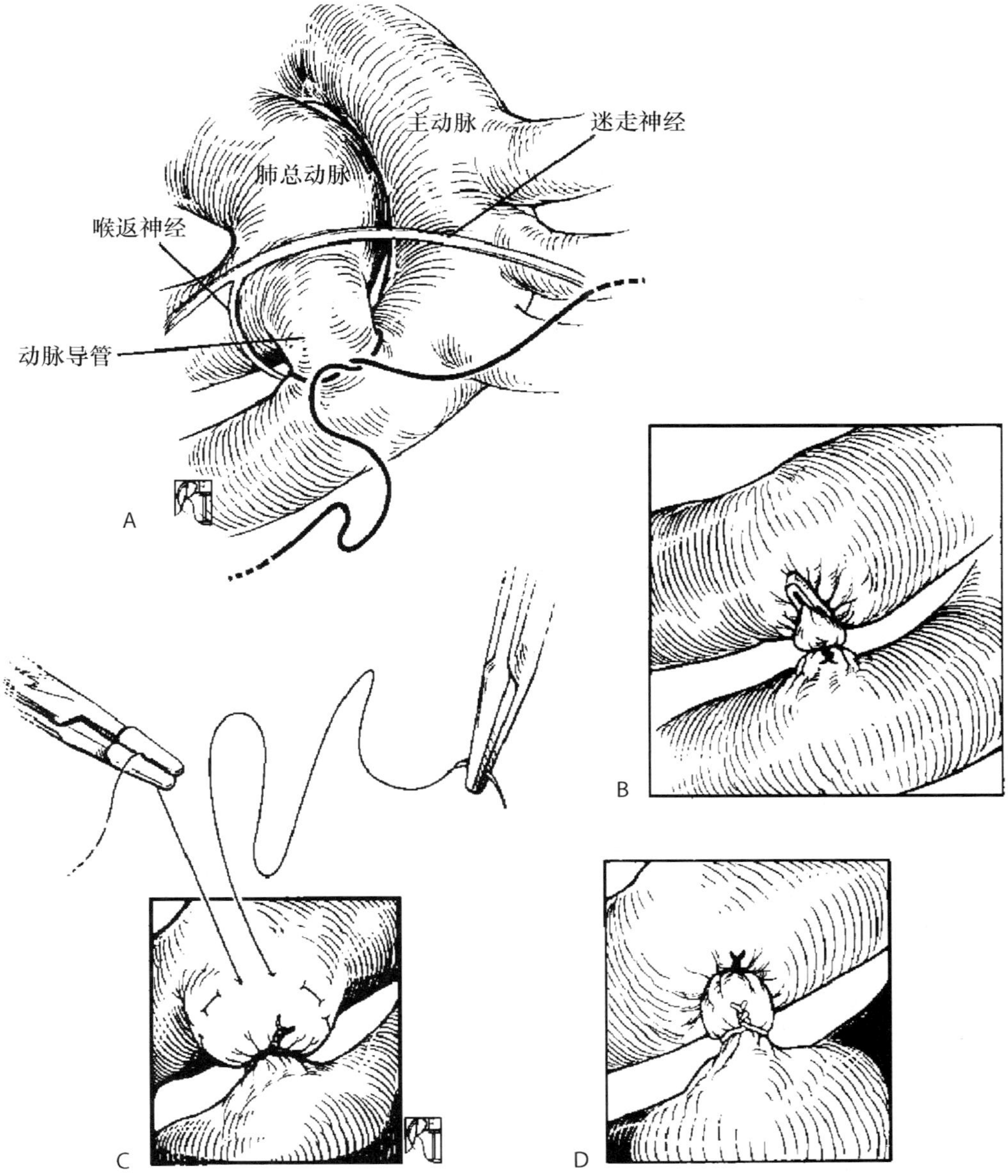

61 命应该是正常的。早产儿的长期存活主要取决于早产的程度和合并存在的畸形。

主动脉缩窄

主动脉缩窄是一种胸部降主动脉近端，靠近动脉导管（或动脉韧带）连接处的先天性狭窄。这会造成血流梗阻，并引起左心室（LV）的压力负荷。主动脉缩窄的发病率约 0.5 例/1000 个活产婴儿，占先天性心脏病的 5%[39]。主动脉缩窄通常合并其他心脏缺损，包括主动脉双叶瓣（超过 50% 的病例）、PDA 和室间隔缺损（VSD）。可能会有其他左侧梗阻性病变，包括主动脉弓发育不良、主动脉狭窄、二尖瓣狭窄和左心室发育不良。

自然病史和诊断

根据解剖、年龄和症状分为两种表现形式（图 123-4）。婴儿型缩窄患者症状在出生后第一周内出现。这些婴儿存在严重主动脉梗阻，因此其下半身血

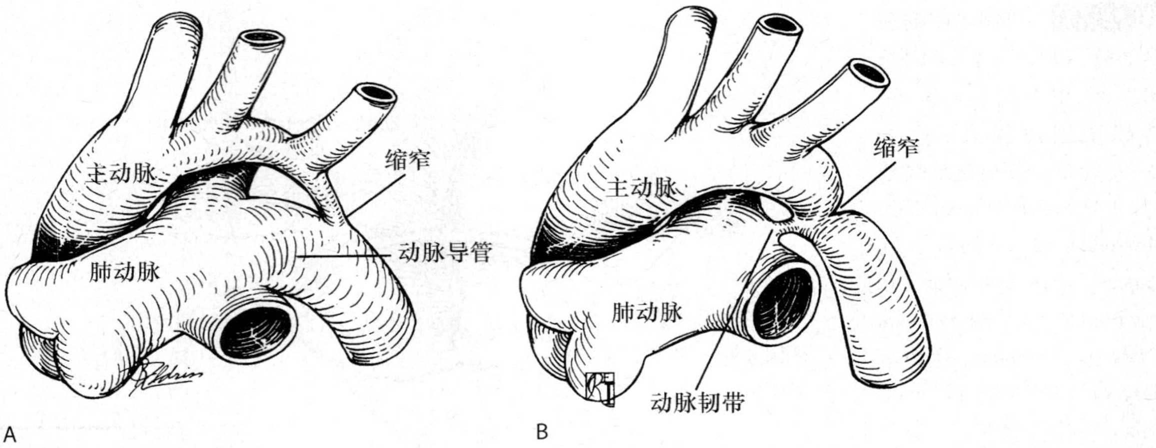

图 123-4　A. 婴儿型主动脉（Ao）缩窄。峡部（在左锁骨下动脉到动脉导管连接处之间的主动脉）发育不良，且降主动脉的大部分血流来自动脉导管。B. 成人型缩窄，可见动脉导管旁的主动脉狭窄和一个明显的后侧扩大。动脉导管收缩形成动脉韧带。（From Backer CL，Mavroudis C：Coarctation of the aorta. In Mavroudis C，Backer CL [eds]：Pediatric Cardiac Surgery，3rd ed. Philadelphia. Mosby，2003.）

液灌注依赖于动脉导管的血流。随后，动脉导管的自发关闭（这也可能加重了主动脉梗阻）致使缩窄处远端的组织缺血。因此造成的左心室压力负荷可能导致充血性心力衰竭。患者会表现出休克，且有严重的酸中毒、少尿和远端脉搏消失。如果不进行治疗，这些患者可能无法存活。

第二种表现形式有时被称作成人型缩窄。成人型缩窄的患者通常在婴儿期无症状，而在以后的人生中出现高血压。这些患者普遍产生广泛的侧支以作为梗
1962 阻部分的旁路。这些患者的预期寿命有限，因为在生命晚期会出现心力衰竭，且存在心内膜炎（通常涉及主动脉双叶瓣）或血管内膜炎（在狭窄后的主动脉部位有喷射性湍流）、主动脉破裂以及颅内出血（浆果动脉瘤，即颅内小动脉瘤，在主动脉缩窄患者中更常见）的累加风险[65]。

主动脉缩窄通常可临床诊断。有显著缩窄的新生儿可能在出生时表现正常，但是在导管闭合后将出现心力衰竭的体征，诸如易激惹、呼吸急促和喂养困难。下肢没有脉搏，且上肢脉搏也可能微弱。胸部放射影像可能显示有心脏肥大和肺静脉充血。心电图显示左心室劳损的状态。超声心动图通常是诊断性的，证实在缩窄位置的解剖狭窄和降主动脉中血液脉动消失；也可以证实其他心脏缺损。

年长儿童和成人通常在手臂和腿之间存在压力阶差，这可以通过测量所有肢体的袖带血压加以鉴别。放射影像可证实有肋骨凹迹，这是由产生大型的肋间侧支血管引起的，侧支血管侵蚀肋骨的下缘。年长患者的超声心动图通常足以证实诊断，但是计算机断层扫描（CT）和磁共振影像（MRI）提供了优良的解剖细节，有助于治疗决策。通常无需心导管。

治疗

主动脉缩窄通常需要手术治疗，但是对于患病新生儿的紧急药物治疗需要注意。在出生后 7～10 天给予前列腺素 E_1，通常对于保持导管再开放是有效的；当出生后 2 周以后，其有效性减弱。对于主动脉缩窄患者的复苏，静脉内补液、变力性药物和纠正贫血可能也是重要的。

通过左侧第三或第四肋间的左后外侧胸廓切口，对缩窄进行外科暴露。切开覆盖在左锁骨下动脉和近端胸部降主动脉上的纵隔胸膜，游离松解降主动脉、主动脉弓横部、头臂血管和动脉导管（或韧带）。需要仔细操作以防损伤迷走神经及其喉返分支。通常从外观上的狭窄和后方的凹陷可明确缩窄段，但是内部的狭窄通常是更加严重的。对于年龄小于 2 岁的患者，可在静脉内给予一剂肝素（100 单位/千克）。通过使用夹钳来控制主动脉的近端和远端。通常，近端夹钳放置在主动脉弓横部的无名动脉和左颈动脉之

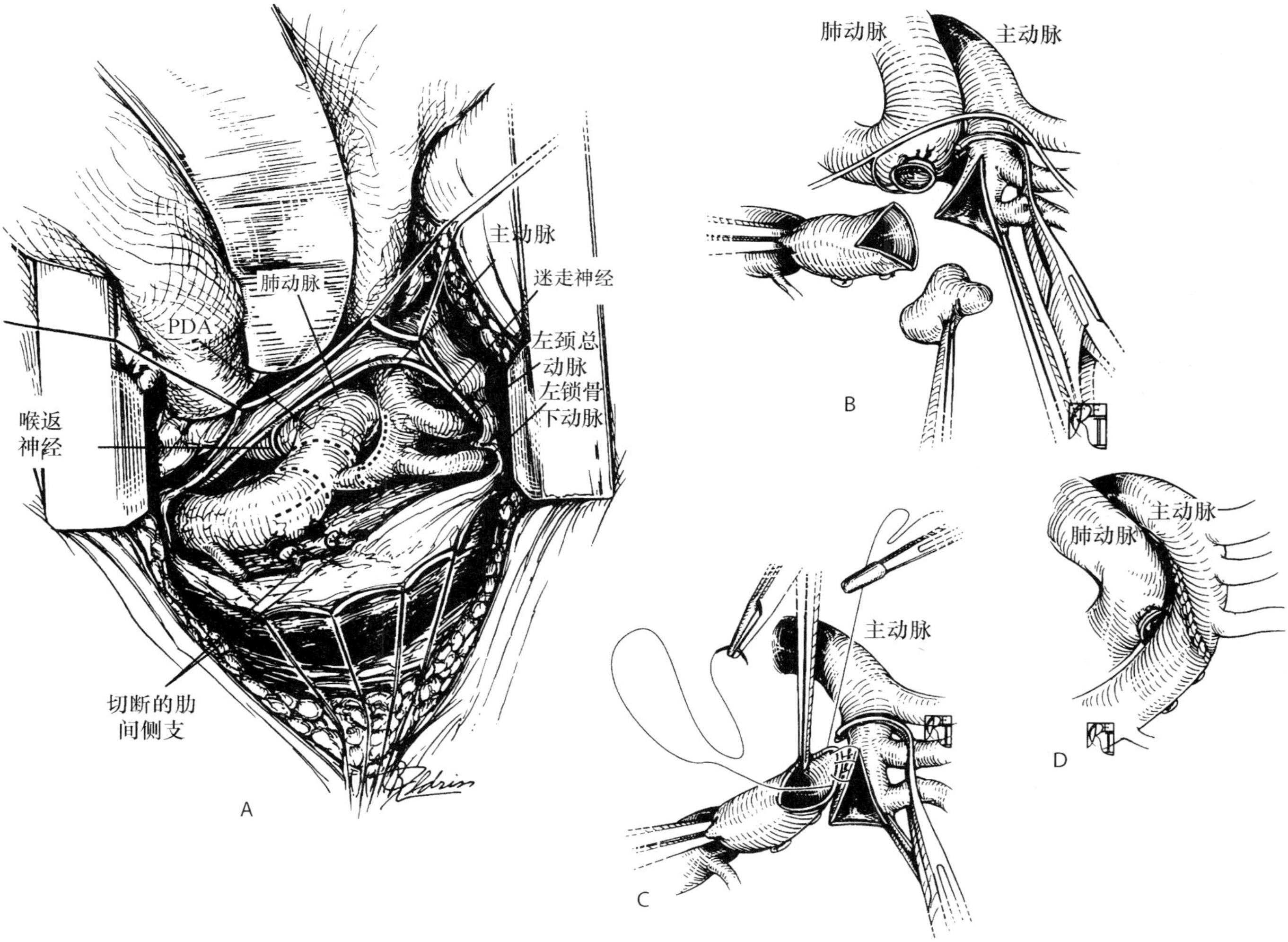

图 123-5　切除和扩大端端吻合。A. 通过左后外侧胸廓切口进行暴露。游离松解血管，且在必要时切断肋间血管。B. 结扎并切断动脉导管。建立近端和远端的控制，切除缩窄段。分别沿小弧和大弧剪开近端和远端的主动脉。C. 采用连续缝合技术进行吻合。D. 修复完成。（From Backer CL, Mavroudis C: Coarctation of the aorta. In Mavroudis C, Backer CL [eds]: Pediatric Cardiac Surgery, 3rd ed. Philadelphia. Mosby, 2003.）

间，同时夹住左颈动脉和左锁骨下动脉。对于婴儿和儿童，优先选用的缩窄手术方法是切除后行扩大端端吻合修复（图 123-5）[7]。对缩窄段进行大范围切除，然后沿内弧剪开近端主动脉，远端主动脉沿外弧剪开，最后进行扩大端端吻合。

年长儿童和成人可能无法进行解除及一期修复而不造成吻合口张力过大，这可能导致出血或瘢痕形成而使缩窄复发。在这些病例中，有采用另一种方法的适应证。对于儿童，希望其能进一步生长，可通过补片主动脉成形术对缩窄进行修复[6,24]。所需的初步游离较少。对近端和远端加以控制后，在跨狭窄区域做一个纵行的主动脉切口，然后缝一块聚四氟乙烯
（PTFE）补片来扩大缩窄。通过避免使用环形人造材 1963
料，保留了自体主动脉组织的生长潜能。成人不再考虑生长，切除缩窄段后可使用相应的植入假体建立连接（PTFE 或 Dacron 涤纶）。

在手术修复缩窄时，脊髓损伤是一个主要问题。无良好侧支形成的患者，主动脉阻断可能会引起脊髓缺血，从而可能导致截瘫。标准的预防措施包括建立浅低温（35℃），保持近端主动脉较高的血压和最短的主动脉阻断时间。侧支血流不够的年长儿童和成人，可采用左心转流技术（左心房插管，引流氧合血

液，使用离心泵将血液输送入股动脉或远端主动脉）来维持远端主动脉的灌注[78]。总的来说，主动脉缩窄术后的截瘫发生率低于1%[12]。

修复以后，患者可能会出现严重的高血压。可静脉内使用β受体阻断药（例如艾司洛尔）或血管扩张剂（例如硝普钠）加以治疗。高血压不加以控制的话，会导致肠系膜动脉炎。高血压通常会在术后数日到数周内消退，但是年长儿童和成人可能需要持久的抗高血压治疗。认为在婴儿期修复缩窄引起后期高血压的风险最小[67]。

尝试使用经导管治疗作为缩窄的最初治疗，但是这种方法是有争议的[17,57,73]。这一方法的局限性包括缩窄复发，可能需要多次介入治疗，以及股脉管系统损伤（为了获取入口）和动脉瘤形成。通常推荐使用球囊血管成形术来治疗术后缩窄复发，其有效率在90%[35,37,80]。

1964 结果

新生儿缩窄修复的早期死亡率为2%～10%，而年长儿童和成人约为1%[7,74]。切除并端端吻合后的缩窄复发率为4%～8%[7,61]。缩窄修复后的长期生存取决于合并的缺损和高血压的持续情况。

房间隔缺损

房间隔缺损（ASD）是排在第三位的最常见的先天性心脏缺损，每1000名活产婴儿中发生1例，占先天性心脏缺损的10%[39]。为了理解ASD的命名，对正常的房间隔解剖进行回顾是有必要的。在胚胎发育过程中，原发隔最初将共同心房分隔开。在原发隔下方存在原发孔，在原发隔与心内膜垫融合时关闭。在原发隔的中部形成继发孔，然后继发隔将之覆盖，继发隔沿原发隔右侧，从心房的顶部向下延伸。这一过程形成了一个活瓣，使来自下腔静脉的血流可在继发隔下方优先流动，并通过继发孔进入左心房。出生后，继发隔与原发隔融合，因此将心房之间的交通封闭（图123-6）。

ASD可根据胚胎学进行分类。最常见的缺损是继发孔ASD（80%），当继发孔太大，继发隔无法将之完全覆盖时产生（图123-7）。出生后继发隔和原发隔融合失败导致一个持续的缝隙样交通，这就

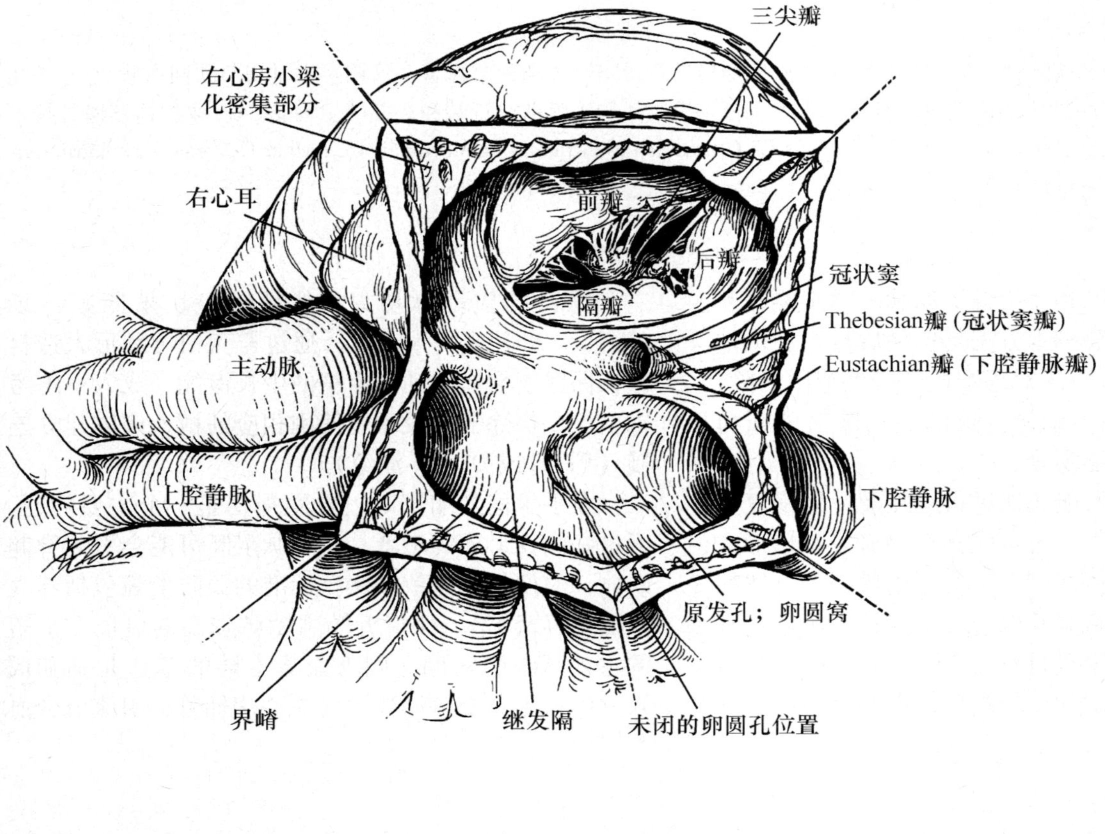

图123-6 外科医生从右心房切口观察到的正常心房内解剖。（From Backer CL, Mavroudis C: Atrial septal defect, partial anomalous pulmonary venous connection, and scimitar syndrome. In Mavroudis C, Backer CL [eds]: Pediatric Cardiac Surgery, 3rd ed. Philadelphia. Mosby, 2003.）

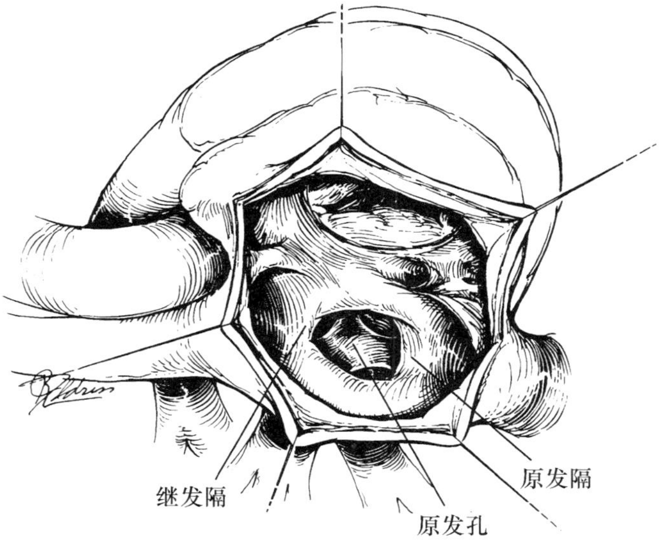

图 123-7　原发孔房间隔缺损。注意在正常卵圆窝位置的原发隔缺损。(From Backer CL, Mavroudis C: Atrial septal defect, partial anomalous pulmonary venous connection, and scimitar syndrome. In Mavroudis C, Backer CL [eds]: Pediatric Cardiac Surgery, 3rd ed. Philadelphia. Mosby, 2003.)

是已知的卵圆孔未闭（PFO）。原发孔 ASD（10%）表现为持续存在的原发孔，是因为原发隔与心内膜垫融合失败引起的。这一缺损在房室间隔缺损（AVSD）的章节中加以讨论。静脉窦型 ASD（10%）是由于静脉通路与心房的融合异常引起的；这些缺损可位于房间隔的高位，邻近上腔静脉开口处，或较少见地位于房间隔的低位，下腔静脉的开口处（图 123-8）。静脉窦型 ASD 通常并发部分肺静脉异位引流，经常是右上肺静脉在上腔静脉与心房连接处引流入上腔静脉。一种罕见类型的 ASD 是无顶冠状窦隔缺损。当在冠状窦和邻近房间隔的左心房之间缺少共同壁时，会发生这种畸形。这种无顶的冠状窦导致右心房和左心房在冠状窦位置存在交通。

自然病史和诊断

心房水平的分流主要发生在舒张期，并取决于心房缺损的大小，且更重要的是心室相对顺应性。换言 1965
之，血流优先流入顺应性更好的心腔。出生时，两个心腔的顺应性相等，但是当肺血管阻力降低时，右心室重构，并变得更赋顺应性。结果，出生后的跨 ASD 分流为左向右。这造成了心脏右侧的容量负荷。这种容量负荷是一种在舒张期由于额外的静脉血回流进入心腔引起的负担。

ASD 引起的容量超负荷通常可以良好地耐受。因此，患者多数是无症状的。婴儿的充血性心力衰竭是罕见的。儿童可能会产生劳累性呼吸困难，无法耐受运动或出现反复呼吸道感染的症状。ASD 未加治疗的年长患者可能会发展成房性心律失常，且成人可能会发展成充血性心力衰竭和右心室功能障碍。肺血管梗阻性病变可能会成为 ASD 未加治疗时的晚期并发症；

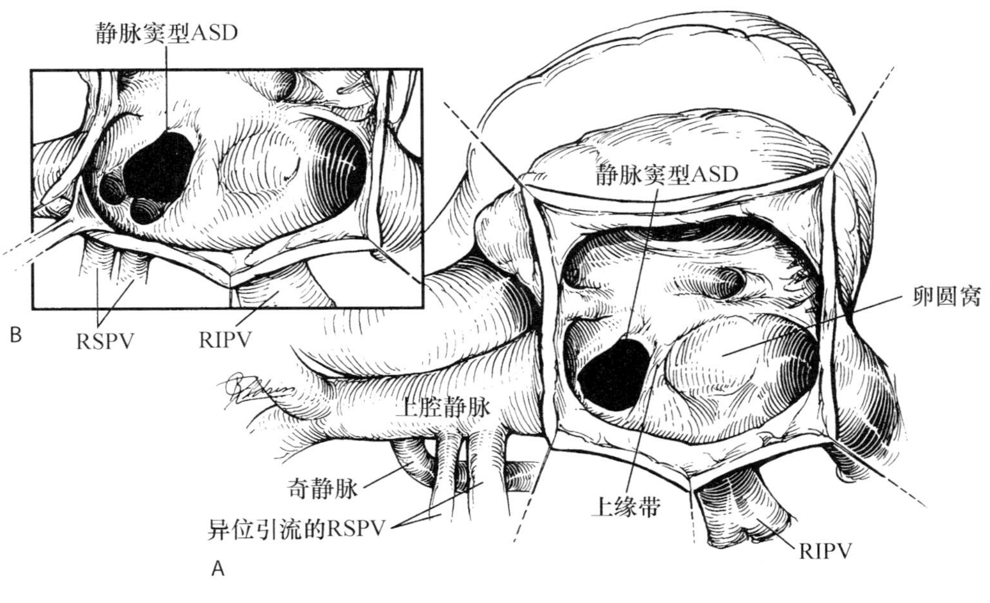

图 123-8　静脉窦型房间隔缺损。A. 缺损在上缘带头端的上腔静脉与心房连接处附近。注意异位引流到上腔静脉（SVC）的右上肺静脉（RSPV）和正常引流的右下肺静脉（RIPV）。B. 其他类型静脉窦型 ASD 合并的邻近缺损的异位引流 RSPV。(From Backer CL, Mavroudis C: Atrial septal defect, partial anomalous pulmonary venous connection, and scimitar syndrome. In Mavroudis C, Backer CL [eds]: Pediatric Cardiac Surgery, 3rd ed. Philadelphia. Mosby, 2003.)

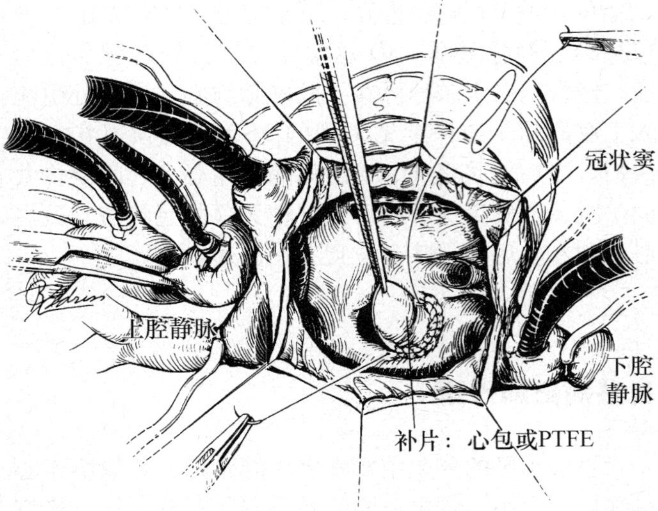

图 123-9 补片关闭继发孔房间隔缺损。采用双腔静脉插管，在主动脉阻断后，通过主动脉根部灌注停搏液，使心脏停搏。PTFE：聚四氟乙烯。（From Backer CL, Mavroudis C: Atrial septal defect, partial anomalous pulmonary venous connection, and scimitar syndrome. In Mavroudis C, Backer CL [eds]: Pediatric Cardiac Surgery, 3rd ed. Philadelphia. Mosby, 2003.）

年龄在 20～40 岁之间的大型 ASD 未经治疗的成人，14% 产生重度肺动脉高压。反常栓塞也是一个重要的 ASD 潜在并发症。

在体格检查中，ASD 患者有第二心音固定分裂和胸骨左上部的收缩期喷射性杂音，这是因为肺动脉相对狭窄引起的（跨过正常肺动脉瓣的血流增多）。胸部放射影像显示心脏肥大，且心电图大多证实有不完全性右束支传导阻滞。超声心动图证实 ASD 的临床诊断，并对解剖进行分类。很少需要用于诊断目的心导管（评估年长患者的肺血管阻力），但是取而代之的是广泛使用的介入治疗（器械封堵）。

治疗

由于 ASD 的远期并发症，因此推荐对所有有症状的缺损患者和肺循环与体循环血流比值（Qp/Qs）大于 1.5 的无症状患者进行修补。通常在学龄期前对儿童进行手术。可使用手术方法或在心导管室内采用器械的方法关闭 ASD。

手术修补 ASD 是相对简单的（图 123-9）。推荐对于大型继发孔缺损和大多数其他类型的 ASD 进行手术关闭。通过正中切口暴露心脏。需要采用双 1966
腔静脉插管和浅低温心肺转流进行手术。主动脉阻断，采用停搏液使心脏停搏，通过右心房切口暴露房间隔，然后使用补片关闭缺损（PTFE 或自体心包），并采用聚丙烯线连续缝合。如果有肺静脉异位回流，可建立板障将血流通过房间隔缺损重新定向。小型缺损或 PFO 无需补片，可直接缝合。所有病例都要仔细进行左心房排气，以避免空气栓塞的并发症。

小型到中型的继发孔 ASD 或 PFO 现在可用经心导管技术关闭[63]。在大多数中心，器械封堵这些缺损现在变成了标准治疗。

结果

两种方法关闭 ASD 都非常成功[20]。死亡率低于 1%。很少发生并发症。儿童期接受房间隔修补的患者的长期生存是正常的[49]。

室间隔缺损

室间隔缺损（VSD）是最常见的先天性心脏畸形（除主动脉双叶瓣以外），每 1000 名活产婴儿中有 4 例，占先天性心脏病的 40%[39]。在位置、大小和存在的缺损数量上的报道各家不同。常有合并的心脏缺损。VSD 是心室分隔失败造成的。最常见的分类是根据其位置划分的：膜周（80%）、流入道（5%）、流出道（10%）或小梁部（5%）（图 123-10）。膜周型最常见，位于三尖瓣、二尖瓣和主动脉瓣环接触位置的膜部区域。流入道缺损位于三尖瓣隔瓣下方。流出道缺损也称作室上嵴或双动脉下型。这些缺损的上缘是双侧半月瓣。流出道缺损在亚洲人群中常见。小梁部（或肌部）VSD 的边缘全部由肌肉构成，它们通常是多发性的，可能合并膜周或流出道缺损。VSD 的大小不同。当 VSD 的大小（或多个缺损的大小总和）接近主动脉瓣环的大小时，定义为非限制性 VSD。

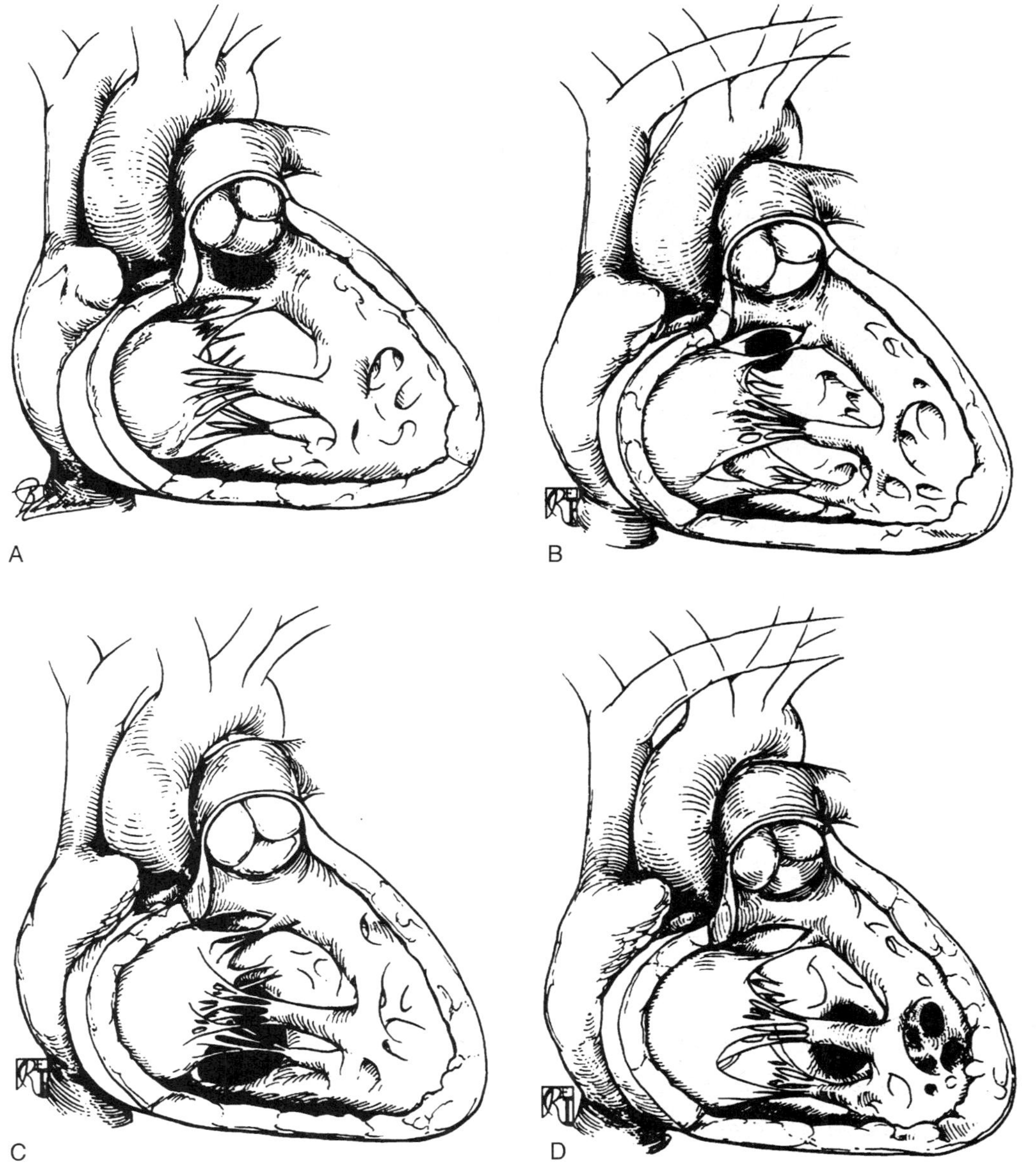

图 123-10 根据位置划分的室间隔缺损（VSD）类型。A. 流出道（室上嵴，双动脉）。B. 膜周。C. 流入道。D. 小梁部（肌部）。（From Mavroudis C, Backer CL, Jacobs JP: Ventricular septal defect. In Mavroudis C, Backer CL [eds]: Pediatric Cardiac Surgery, 3rd ed. Philadelphia. Mosby, 2003.）

自然病史和诊断

VSD 的生理学主要涉及收缩期的左向右分流。这引起了心脏左侧的容量负荷（左心房和左心室在舒张期接受的静脉回流增多）。右心室容量负荷不增加（血流直接从左心室通过 VSD 射入肺循环），但这却是一个压力负荷。跨 VSD 的分流量取决于缺损的大小和肺循环与体循环血管阻力的比值。因为出生后头几个星期的肺血管阻力降低，跨 VSD 的分流可能增大。因此，出生时无症状的 VSD 可能最终引起严重的充血性心力衰竭。

VSD 患者的自然病史存在差异。大部分的 VSD 是限制性的，在出生后第一年可能自发关闭[52]。大型 VSD 的患者因充血性心力衰竭而产生症状。如果 VSD 不加以治疗，过量的肺血流在 1～2 岁时就引起肺血管梗阻性病变。较小的 VSD 可能仍无症状。流出道 VSD 的患者，邻近的主动脉瓣可能会发生瓣叶脱垂和主动脉关闭不全[53]。

大型 VSD 婴儿的心力衰竭体征包括呼吸急促、肝大、喂养不良和发育障碍。体格检查时，胸骨左缘有全收缩期杂音。心前区有搏动。通常，较小的缺损杂音较响。肺血管梗阻性病变的患者可能没有杂音，

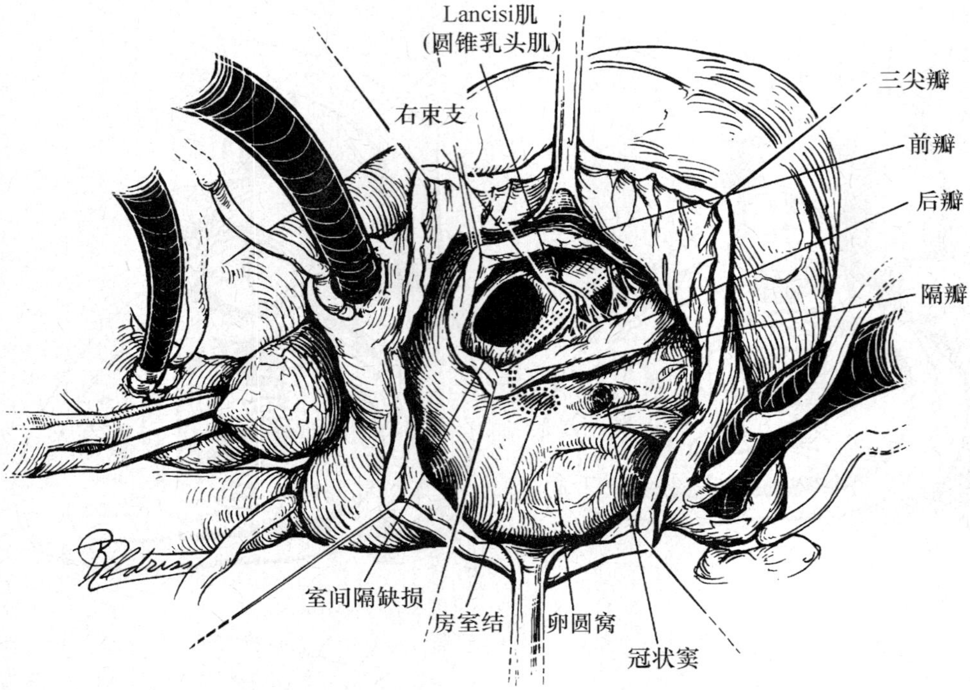

图 123-11 外科医生所见的经右心房暴露膜周室间隔缺损（VSD）。三尖瓣隔瓣和前瓣拉开，以暴露 VSD。传导组织用从房室（AV）结沿 VSD 后下缘画出的虚线标明。在关闭这些缺损时，缝线在室间隔的右心室面要离开缺损边缘几个毫米，以防传导损伤。（From Mavroudis C, Backer CL, Jacobs JP: Ventricular septal defect. In Mavroudis C, Backer CL [eds]: Pediatric Cardiac Surgery, 3rd ed. Philadelphia. Mosby, 2003.）

但是第二心音的肺动脉部分明显。胸部放射影像显示肺血管纹理增多和心脏肥大。心电图有明显的右心室肥大。

小型 VSD 患者的分流小，且通常无症状，仅有全收缩期杂音。中型 VSD 患者会根据分流程度表现出症状和体征。

1967 超声心动图可诊断大多数病例。可精确鉴别解剖，并排除存在的合并畸形。对有 VSD 的年长儿童和成人选择性地进行心导管检查，以判定肺血管阻力，并评估对肺血管扩张药物的反应。

治疗

VSD 患者的治疗取决于缺损的大小、缺损的类型、分流量和肺血管阻力。总的来说，表现出难治性充血性心力衰竭或发育障碍的大型缺损患者应接受早期手术修补。如果充血症状可通过药物治疗加以调整，手术可推迟到 6 个月大时进行。中型缺损的患者可安全地进行随访。如果在学龄期前未自发关闭，再考虑手术。对于很小的 VSD，且 Qp/Qs 小于 1.5，则无需关闭。这些患者有较小的远期心内膜炎的风险，但是通过合适的抗生素预防治疗可以将此风险降低到最小[22]。如同以前所注意到的，流出道 VSD 的患者有发生瓣叶脱垂引起主动脉关闭不全的显著风险；因此，所有流出道缺损应进行关闭。晚期发现的大型 VSD 的年长儿童和成人必须接受心导管检查，以评估肺血管系统。肺血管阻力固定高于 8～10 Wood 单位·平方米是手术关闭 VSD 的禁忌证。

经正中切口进行手术关闭（图 123-11）。这需要心肺转流，采用双腔静脉插管。输注心脏停搏液后，行右心房切口，经三尖瓣暴露室间隔。这可提供对膜周、流入道和大多数流出道缺损的评估。大多数小梁部缺损也可通过此方法加以暴露。一些流出道 VSD 可通过肺动脉切口获得最佳暴露，因为缺损就在瓣膜下方。众所周知，位于心室尖端的小梁部缺损难以暴露，可能需要进行心尖部的心室切口（左心室或右心室）。一旦缺损暴露，通常采用 PTFE 补片和聚丙烯
线连续缝合关闭，但是其他中心可能偏爱使用其他材 196
料或者间断缝合技术。当关闭 VSD 时，传导组织的解剖知识非常重要。房室结是一个位于 Koch 三角（由冠状窦、Todaro 腱和三尖瓣隔瓣的瓣环附着处构成）顶端的心房结构。此结随后发出 His 束，在膜部室间隔下方穿过房室连接处。此束然后分叉形成沿肌部室间隔两面下行的右束支和左束支。当存在膜周 VSD 时，His 束穿过缺损的后下缘，通常在左心室

面。在此危险区域内，缝线必须在缺损的右心室面进行浅缝，并距离缺损边缘几个毫米。His 束也沿流入道 VSD 的后下缘走行，而在流出道和小梁部缺损时，传导组织距离较远。

肺动脉（PA）环扎术是一种姑息手术，目的是在患者因合并疾病或复杂解剖（例如多发性小梁部 VSD）而无法进行手术关闭缺损时，保护肺循环免于过量血流的损害。可通过胸骨切口或胸廓切口放置肺动脉环扎带。收紧环扎带，并测定近端和远端的压力，以使远端肺血管压力接近体循环的二分之一。然后应该将环扎带缝合在肺总动脉的外膜上，以防移位。向远端移位可能会导致一侧或双侧肺动脉分支狭窄（和发育不良），而向近端异位可能会导致肺动脉瓣畸形。最后，当患者可进行 VSD 关闭时，必须拆除环扎带。在大多数的病例中，也将需要对肺总动脉进行修补（切除瘢痕并一期关闭或者补片修补）。

最近，经心导管技术得以发展，可在心导管室内完成一些 VSD 的封堵。

结果

VSD 修复手术的死亡率在 1% 左右[48]。主要的并发症包括传导结构的损伤以及三尖瓣或主动脉瓣的损伤。组织水肿可能会引起短暂的心脏传导阻滞，但是永久的心脏传导阻滞只发生于 1%～2% 的病例[48]。术后的传导阻滞一般在术后 7～10 天出现。如果正常传导无法建立，则需要安装起搏器。VSD 补片或缝线引起的三尖瓣环变形或牵扯可能会造成三尖瓣关闭不全。缝合不当也能造成主动脉瓣的损伤（特别是在膜周部和流出道的 VSD）。5% 的病例可能出现 VSD 残留，当分流明显时（Qp/Qs > 1.5）需要行再次修补手术。术中常规行超声心动图显像评估瓣膜功能和残余分流量。

房室间隔缺损

房室间隔缺损（AVSD）为一组先天性疾病，表现为各种位于房室瓣上下的各种房室间隔缺损。其他常用的 AVSD 的名称包括房室通道缺损、心内膜垫缺损和共同房室。这类相应的间隔缺损常常合并房室瓣畸形。AVSD 包括不完全性 AVSD，也称为原发孔 ASD，其仅有一个直接位于房室瓣上方的房间隔缺损，并有两个分隔的房室瓣口。严重病例包括完全性 AVSD，即同时有 ASD 和 VSD 以及一个共同的房室瓣。AVSD 约占先天性心脏畸形的 4%，并时常合并其他心脏畸形。有心脏畸形的 Down 综合征患者中，30%～40% 的人有 AVSD[69]。

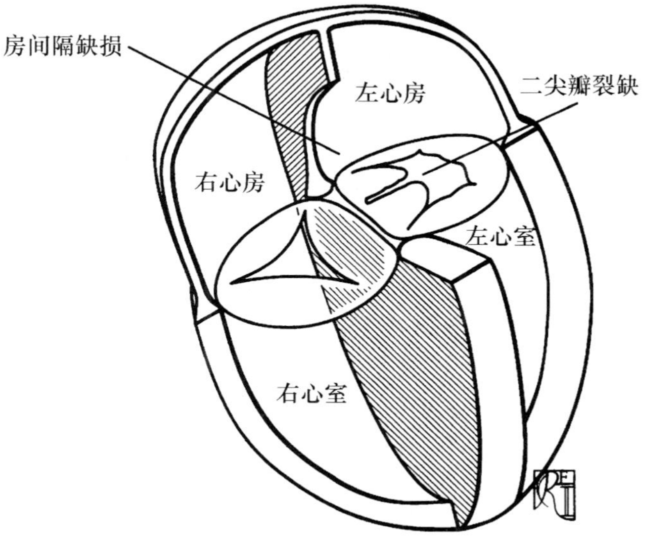

图 123-12　不完全性房室间隔缺损。（From Backer CL, Mavroudis C：Atrioventricular septal defect. In Mavroudis C, Backer CL［eds］：Pediatric Cardiac Surgery, 3rd ed. Philadelphia. Mosby, 2003.）

AVSD 的胚胎学畸形是正常的心内膜垫发育失败，导致了不同程度的房间隔和室间隔缺损以及房室瓣畸形。AVSD 通常根据房室瓣形态分为不完全性和完全性。不完全性或部分性缺损有两个分离的房室瓣口（图 123-12）。不完全性 AVSD 的二尖瓣常常合并前瓣叶裂缺。虽然大多数不完全性 AVSD 患者没有心室水平的分流，但是 AVSD 的不完全性和完全性的分类仅取决于瓣膜解剖，而不是有没有 VSD。无心室水平分流的不完全性缺损也指原发孔 ASD，而那些有 VSD 的被描述为中间性或过渡性 AVSD。完全性 AVSD 有一个共同房室瓣口，使得一个单独的五叶瓣覆盖在右心室和左心室上方（图 123-13）。

Rastelli 及其同事[64]对 AVSD 进行了进一步分类，根据共同瓣上桥瓣的形态学将其分为 A、B 和 C 三型

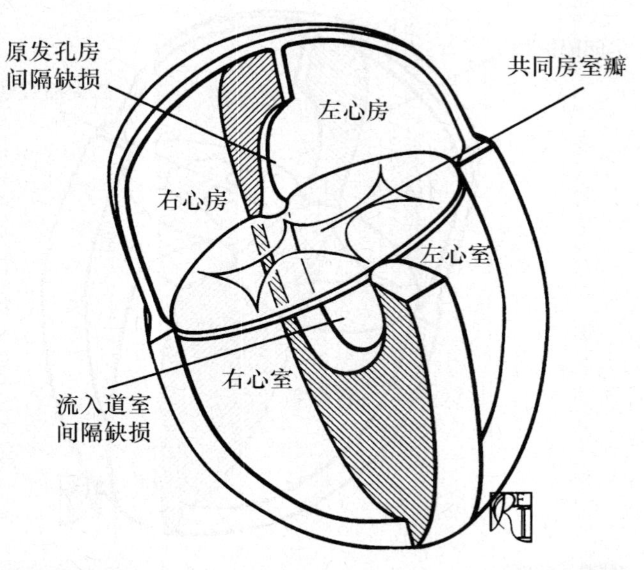

图 123-13　完全性房室间隔缺损。(From Backer CL, Mavroudis C: Atrioventricular septal defect. In Mavroudis C, Backer CL [eds]: Pediatric Cardiac Surgery, 3rd ed. Philadelphia. Mosby, 2003.)

(图 123-14)。Rastelli A 型缺损的瓣叶在室间隔水平有分割，并通过许多腱索附着在室间隔嵴上。B 型完全性 AVSD 罕见，其特征为来自左侧房室瓣的腱索附着在右心室的乳头肌上。Rastelli C 型缺损的上桥瓣是“自由漂浮”的，因为其未分隔，且不附着在室隔嵴上。

如果左右两侧房室瓣对等享有共同房室瓣开口，这种 AVSD 称为平衡型缺损。偶尔有瓣膜开口不平衡，其中一侧占优势。在显著的右侧优势时，左侧房室瓣和左心室发育不良，且时常合并其他左侧畸形，包括主动脉狭窄、主动脉发育不良和缩窄。相反，显著的左侧优势时，合并有右心室发育不良、肺动脉狭窄或闭锁，以及 Fallot 四联症（TOF）。

在 AVSD 手术治疗中，传导组织的位置很重要，因为在修补时，这些组织有被损伤的风险。房室结对着冠状窦向后下方移位。His 束沿室隔嵴的左侧面，向前上方走行，在延续为右束支前发出左束支。

AVSD 合并的心脏畸形包括 PDA（10%）和 TOF（10%）[10]。左侧房室瓣的重要畸形包括单一乳头肌（降落伞样二尖瓣）（2%~6%）和双开孔二尖瓣（8%~14%）[27]。3% 的 AVSD 患者有左上腔静脉残存合并或不合并无顶冠状窦。右心室双出口（2%）的解剖非常复杂，或可能甚至无法进行手术根治[10]。如同以前提到的，主动脉下狭窄或房室瓣冗余组织引起的左心室流出道梗阻占 4%~7%[59,71]。合并大动脉错位和左心室流入道梗阻罕有报道[10,59]。

自然病史和诊断

AVSD 显著的血流动力学特征是房室水平的左向右分流。没有心室水平的分流时，血流动力学和临床表现类似典型的继发孔 ASD 合并右心房（RA）和右心室容量超负荷。体格检查时有心前区搏动、

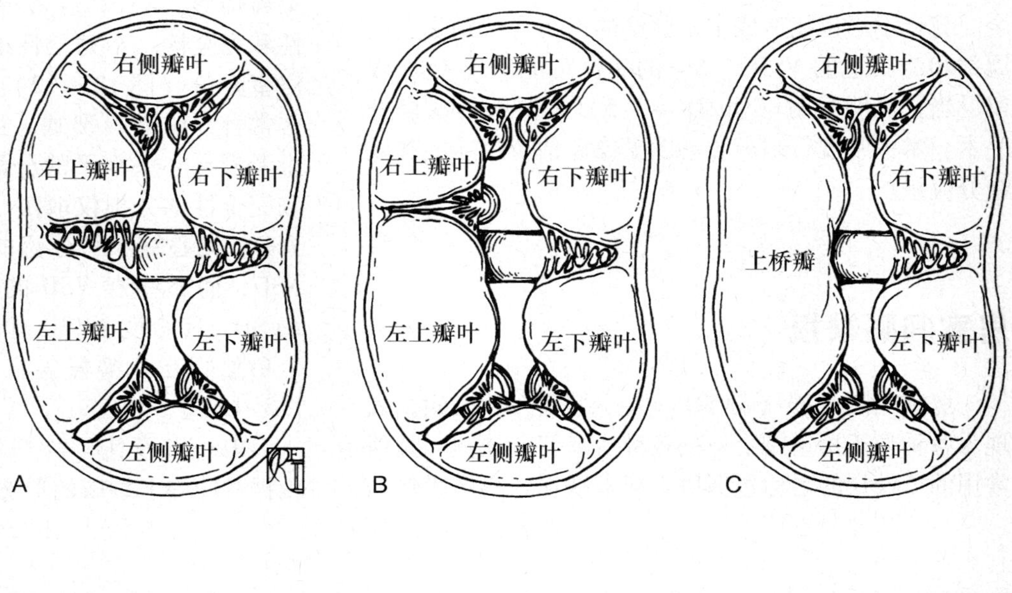

图 123-14　Rastelli 分类。(From Backer CL, Mavroudis C: Atrioventricular septal defect. In Mavroudis C, Backer CL [eds]: Pediatric Cardiac Surgery, 3rd ed. Philadelphia. Mosby, 2003.)

肺动脉流出道杂音和固定增宽的第二心音分裂。心电图显示电轴左偏、心房扩大导致的 P 波高大和 PR 间期延长。胸部放射影像通常显示轻度心脏肥大和肺血管纹理增多。多普勒超声心动图对于房间隔缺损、无心室水平分流和存在的任何房室瓣畸形有诊断作用。仅在成年期诊断的患者或者体检或放射影像学检查有肺血流减少的患者有心导管检查的适应证。肺血流减少可能是肺血管病变或合并右侧梗阻性病变引起的。肺血管阻力固定高于 10 单位 · 平方米是手术关闭的禁忌证。

如果仅有一个非复杂性的 ASD，则数十年的慢性容量超负荷的自然史会导致心房扩大和心律失常、心室功能障碍以及潜在的肺血管病变。因此，有手术修补的适应证，且通常在 2～4 岁时进行手术。

完全性 AVSD 患者有心房和心室水平的分流。这些患者通常在婴儿早期即有充血性心力衰竭的症状和体征。完全性 AVSD 可发生中度或更重的左侧房室瓣反流，使临床症状恶化。体格检查时，心前区搏动强烈，听诊在胸骨左缘有收缩期杂音，左侧房室瓣反流引起心尖部的高调杂音和共同房室瓣的舒张中期血流杂音。胸部放射影像证实明显的心脏肥大和肺循环容量超负荷。心电图显示双心室肥大、心房扩大、PR 间期延长、电轴左偏和逆时针转位的额面电轴。多普勒超声心动图具有诊断价值，可判定心房和心室水平的分流、瓣膜结构和任何合并的畸形。对于年龄大于 1 岁的患者、有肺血管阻力增高的患者或一些需要进一步评估合并其他重大心脏畸形的患者，应该进行心导管检查。

因为存在大型左向右分流，并且合并的房室瓣反流有恶化的可能，所以高达 90% 的未经治疗的完全性 AVSD 患者在 1 岁前出现肺血管病变。由于小气道病变、慢性通气不足和 P_{CO_2} 升高，21 三体患者比染色体正常的患者更早出现肺血管梗阻性病变。最初进行积极的药物治疗，以缓解充血性心力衰竭的症状。应在 3～6 个月时进行选择性手术纠治。如果药物治疗失败，则有早期手术干预的适应证。

治疗

对不完全性或完全性 AVSD 的治疗是手术完全修复。目前，肺动脉环扎的姑息手术在这种病变的治疗中发挥的作用非常有限。肺动脉环扎的适应证可能包括那些合并复杂心脏畸形、功能性单心室需要最终进行 Fontan 手术和临床条件差而无法经受重大心脏手术的患者。

大多数患者取正中胸骨切口路径，常规建立心肺 1971
转流。很少使用深低温停循环技术，但可能在极低出生体重的新生儿进行手术时需要。仅有心房水平分流的不完全性 AVSD 的手术类似继发孔 ASD 采取的方法。

修补完全性 AVSD 有两种广泛使用的方法：单片法技术和双片法技术。无论采取哪种方法，目的都是要关闭 ASD 和 VSD，并将共同房室瓣分割为两个无狭窄的有功能的瓣膜。二尖瓣前瓣裂缺通常加以关闭，以减少远期二尖瓣反流的风险。

对于双片法技术，ASD 和 VSD 分别使用补片关闭（图 123-15B）。对于单片法技术，将上桥瓣和下桥瓣沿界限分割成左右两部分，使用单一补片关闭室间隔缺损和房间隔缺损，然后将瓣叶的分割边缘重新悬吊在补片上（见图 123-15A）。对于小型 VSD，可

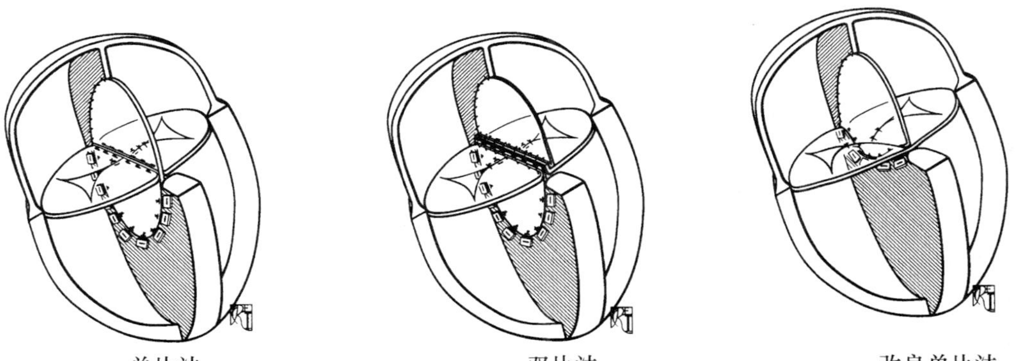

单片法　A　双片法　B　改良单片法　C

图 123-15　使用单片法（A）、双片法（B）和改良单片法（C）技术进行房室间隔缺损的手术修补。（From Backer CL, Mavroudis C: Atrioventricular septal defect. In Mavroudis C, Backer CL [eds]: Pediatric Cardiac Surgery, 3rd ed. Philadelphia. Mosby, 2003.）

采用改良单片法。这种方法采用单一补片直接缝合在VSD边缘，将桥瓣瓣叶夹缝在补片和VSD的室隔嵴之间（见图123-15C）。

结果

手术死亡率主要与任何合并的心脏畸形和左侧房室瓣反流有关。非复杂性不完全性AVSD的手术死亡率为0～0.6%。合并左侧房室瓣反流使死亡率升高到4%～6%[70,71]。对于完全性AVSD，无左侧房室瓣反流的死亡率约为5%，相比有明显反流的死亡率为13%[71]。

有或无反流的患者其手术死亡率的差异强调了仔细处理左侧房室瓣的重要性。此外，AVSD术后大部分再次手术是因为左侧房室瓣反流。10%～15%的患者术后有显著的房室瓣反流，7%～12%的患者需要再次手术进行修补或者换瓣[34,50,62]。

持续永久性完全性心脏阻滞的发生率为1%[40,71]。由于房室结或His束水肿或损伤，术后即刻的心脏阻滞可能是一过性的。但是，右束支阻滞常见（22%）[40]。

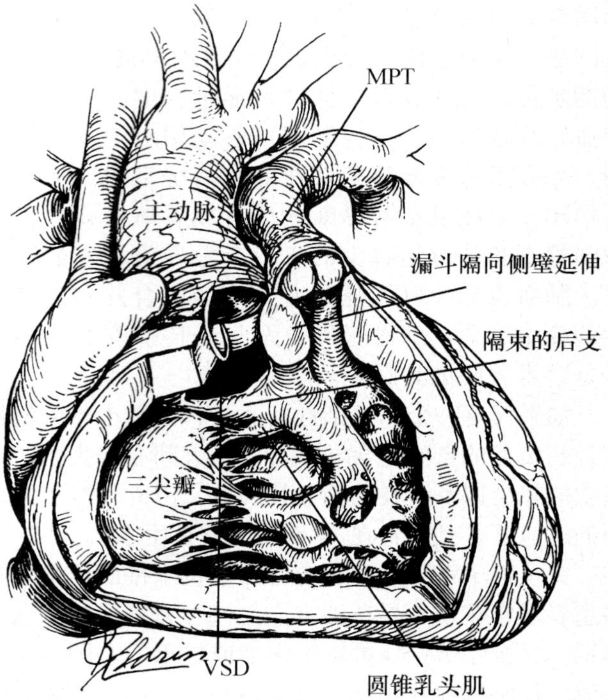

图123-16 Fallot四联症的病理解剖。室间隔缺损（VSD）为非限制性。漏斗隔对位不良，引起主动脉骑跨和挤入右心室流出道。注意发育不良的肺动脉干（MPT）。（From Hirsch JC，Bove EL：Tetralogy of Fallot. In Mavroudis C，Backer CL［eds］：Pediatric Cardiac Surgery，3rd ed. Philadelphia. Mosby，2003.）

Fallot 四联症

Etienne Fallot在1888年首次描述了Fallot四联症（TOF）。其病理解剖包括四个部分：VSD、主动脉骑跨、肺动脉狭窄和右心室肥厚（图123-16）。TOF的解剖也可能与一个单独的胚胎学缺损有关：漏斗隔的前向对位不良[75]。正常的漏斗隔将原始的流出道分开，并与室间隔融合。漏斗隔前向对位不良使之与室间隔融合失败而造成了VSD，也使主动脉移位到VSD和右心室上方。对位不良的漏斗隔挤入了右心室流出道，造成了肺动脉狭窄和继发的右心室肥厚。粗大的肌束从漏斗隔与室间隔连接部位向右心室游离壁延伸，并造成了右心室流出道的梗阻。肺动脉瓣常有狭窄，且瓣叶增厚，大多数病例呈双叶瓣。可能有冠状动脉的畸形，5%的病例为左前降支起源于右冠状动脉。25%的病例为主动脉右弓。合并畸形包括ASD、完全性AVSD、PDA或多发VSD。

TOF是最常见的发绀型先天性心脏病。每1000名活产婴儿中有0.6例，占所有先天性心脏病患者数量的5%[39]。

自然病史和诊断

1972

TOF患者出现发绀是因为跨室间隔缺损的右向左分流。发绀的程度与右心室流出道梗阻的程度呈正比。严重程度各不相同，有些患者在新生儿期就出现症状，而其他的则无症状。间歇性发生的缺氧是一种众所周知的TOF临床表现。缺氧发作的病因学尚有争议，但是很明显与一过性的肺循环和体循环血流不平衡有关。血容量不足、外周血管扩张（例如洗澡后）或漏斗部痉挛可能会诱发缺氧发作。有新生儿缺氧发作的报道，但可能在3～18个月之间的发生率更高。可能会观察到年长儿童以自发性蹲踞来消除缺氧发作。认为这种蹲踞体位可增加体循环血管阻力，从

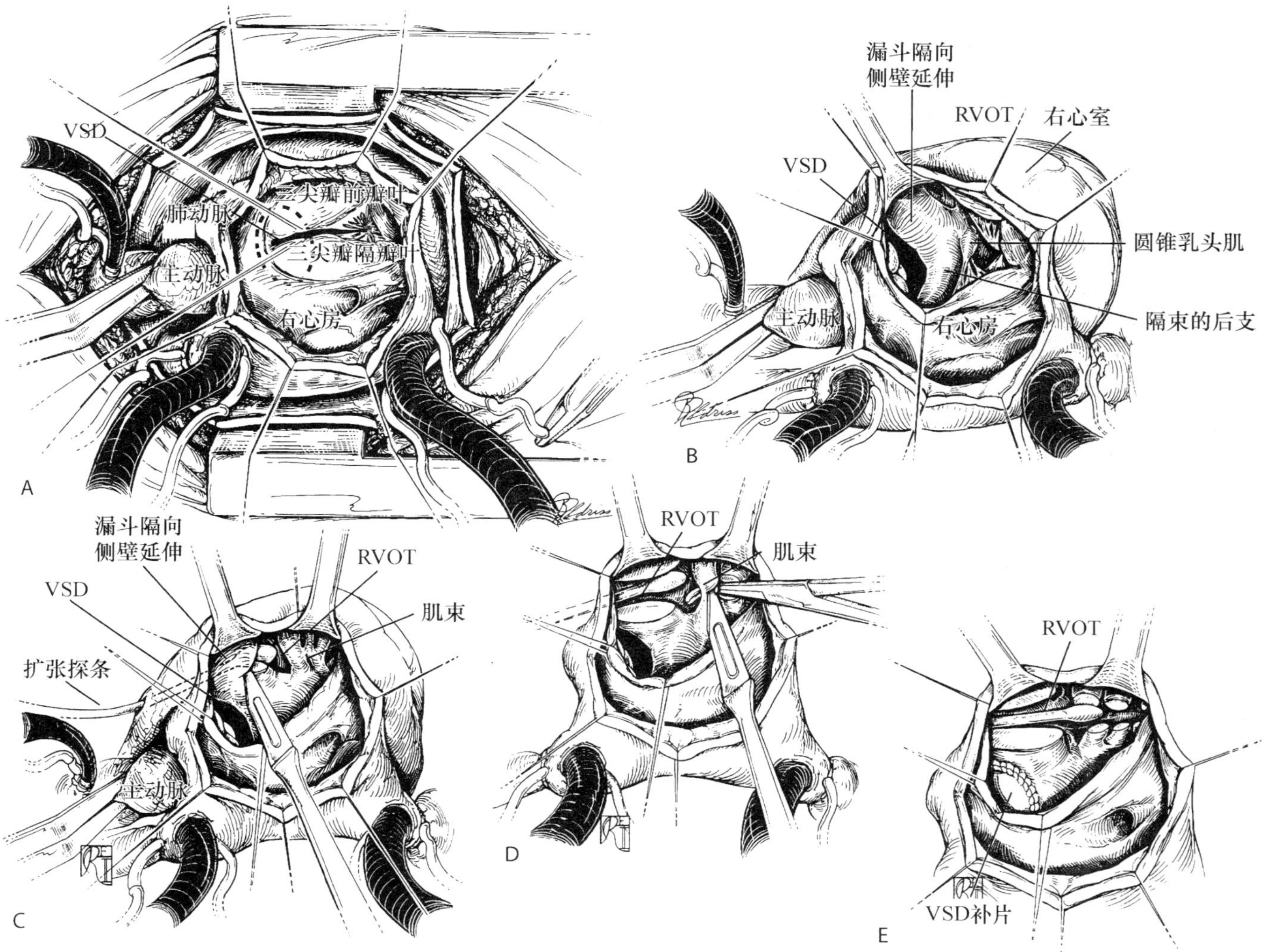

图 123-17　经心房路径治疗 Fallot 四联症。A. 虚线标出了室间隔缺损（VSD）的位置。B. 三尖瓣隔瓣和前瓣悬吊缝线，以便暴露 VSD。C 和 D. 使用扩张探条证实右心室流出道（RVOT）的路径，可切断或切除肥厚的肌束。E. 采用补片关闭 VSD。（From Hirsch JC, Bove EL: Tetralogy of Fallot. In Mavroudis C, Backer CL [eds]: Pediatric Cardiac Surgery, 3rd ed. Philadelphia. Mosby, 2003.）

而增加肺循环血流。

未经治疗的 TOF 的远期并发症包括杵状指和杵状趾、劳累后严重呼吸困难、脑脓肿（继发于右向左分流）、反常栓塞以及红细胞增多（可引起脑血栓形成）。大多数未经治疗的 TOF 患者不可能长期生存。

体格检查发现最多的是发绀。通常第一心音正常而第二心音单一。胸骨左缘有收缩期肺动脉喷射性杂音。年长儿童和成人会出现杵状指（趾）。胸部放射影像的特征显示为靴形心，这是由于右心室肥厚引起心尖上翘造成的。可能会有右位主动脉弓。心电图显示右心室肥厚。超声心动图可明确诊断，且大多数病例无需心导管检查。

治疗

TOF 药物治疗的目的是在于治疗和预防缺氧发作。有缺氧发作的患者应给予氧气和镇静，如果有酸中毒也应给予纠正。贫血婴儿可能需要输血。可使用 α 激动剂来提高体循环阻力，以增加肺血流。一些中

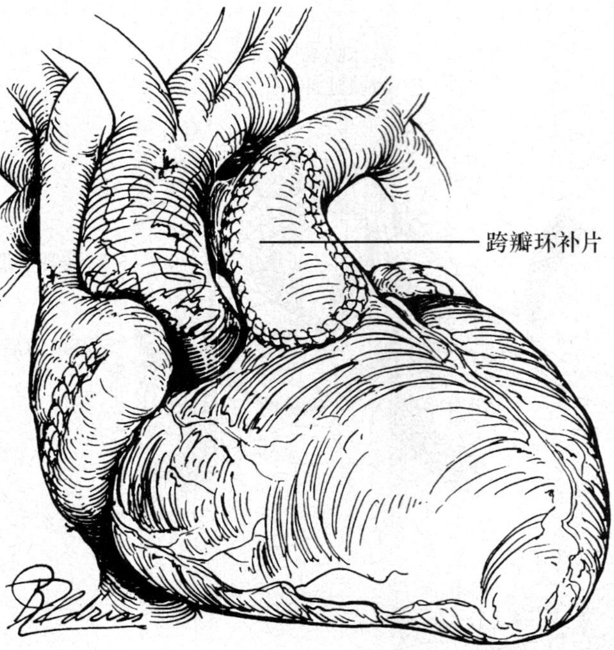

图 123-18 采用跨瓣环补片来扩大发育不良的肺动脉瓣环和肺动脉总干。（From Hirsch JC，Bove EL：Tetralogy of Fallot. In Mavroudis C，Backer CL［eds］：Pediatric Cardiac Surgery，3rd ed. Philadelphia. Mosby，2003.）

心采用 β 阻断剂进行长期治疗，以降低缺氧发作的发生率。

所有的 TOF 患者应该接受手术治疗。总的来说，无症状的患者应该在 4～6 个月之间进行择期手术。严重发绀新生儿和有缺氧发作的婴儿有早期手术的适应证。

经典的 TOF 纠治手术分为两期。第一期手术是建立体肺分流来缓解发绀。第二期手术是根治手术。目前，大多数的中心优先采用一期手术根治。一些患者（例如合并多发先天性畸形、严重并发疾病或异常的冠状动脉跨过发育不良的漏斗部的患者）仍然有进行初期姑息手术建立分流的适应证。改良 Blalock-Taussig 分流是今日最常用的分流类型，在无名或锁骨下动脉和同侧肺动脉之间置入管道（PTFE）。可在或不在心肺转流下建立分流。

采用正中胸骨切口和双腔静脉插管的心肺转流进行 TOF 的根治手术（图 123-17）。经心房途径，将阻塞右心室流出道的肌束切除或分开，使用补片关闭 VSD。根据肺动脉瓣的状态，可能要进行肺动脉瓣膜切开。对一些肺动脉瓣环或漏斗部严重发育不良的病例，可能需要右心室流出道跨瓣环补片来解除梗阻（图 123-18）。我们的基本观点是采用最小的右心室切口，以保护右心室功能。当有异常的冠状动脉跨过右心室漏斗部时，可能无跨瓣补片的适应证；这种病例需要在右心室（经单独的心室切口）和肺总动脉 1973
之间架设管道（冷冻保存的同种带瓣管道或生物学异种移植物）。需跨瓣补片的患者可能将会发生肺动脉关闭不全。只要三尖瓣功能完好，大多数患者可很好耐受。一些成人患者由于慢性肺动脉瓣关闭不全而发生右心室衰竭，且可能需要植入肺动脉瓣[23,25]。

结果

TOF 术后的早期死亡率为 1%～5%[38,41]。远期并发症包括右心室流出道梗阻复发、管道失去功能和由于慢性肺动脉瓣关闭不全引起的右心室功能障碍。20 年的实际生存率是 86%，功能状态良好。

大动脉错位

大动脉错位（TGA）是一种常见的先天性心血管畸形，其心室动脉连接不一致。这种不一致的解剖是由主动脉发自形态学右心室和肺动脉发自形态学左心室引起的。TGA 分为右位或 d-TGA 和左位或 l-TGA。l-TGA 合并双侧心房心室连接不一致（右心房与左心室连接，左心房与右心室连接）和心室动脉连接不一致，也称为先天性纠正性 TGA。l-TGA 是 TGA 的罕见变异，其超出本章节的讨论范围。

d-TGA 是引起婴儿发绀的最常见因素，约占全部
先天性心血管畸形的 10%[29]。缺损可进一步分为室间 197
隔完整（IVS）的 d-TGA（55%～60%）和 d-TGA 合并 VSD（40%～45%）；肺动脉狭窄会引起明显的左心室流出道梗阻，这在室间隔完整的 d-TGA 中罕见，在d-TGA/VSD病例中约占 10%[42]。

自然病史和诊断

如不加干预，d-TGA 基本是致命的：未经治疗，30% 的新生儿将在出生后第一周内死亡，50% 在出生

后第一个月内死亡，70% 在 6 个月内死亡，90% 在 1 岁前死亡[45]。

临床特征取决于血流混合程度和肺血流量。这些因素与 d-TGA 特殊的解剖亚型有关。

室间隔完整（或小型 VSD）的 d-TGA 婴儿在心房和 PDA 水平的血液混合有限。ASD 可能是限制性的，且 PDA 大多在出生后第一周关闭。随着混合程度降低，患者发绀更明显，并将最终出现心血管功能衰竭。幸运的是，大部分这类婴儿在生命早期出现症状，有 56% 在出生后 1 小时内被护士或医生发现，在第一天内被发现者占 92%[44]。

合并大型 VSD 的 d-TGA 有额外的血液混合机会，并可增加肺血流。d-TGA/VSD 的新生儿可能仅有轻度发绀，可能最初会被忽视。但是通常在 2～6 周内将出现充血性心力衰竭的症状与体征。呼吸急促和心动过速变得明显，而发绀可能仍为轻度。听诊特征与充血性心力衰竭合并肺血流增多相一致，包括全收缩期杂音、第三心音、舒张中期隆隆音、奔马律和第二心音窄分裂及其肺动脉部分增强。有 d-TGA 和明显肺动脉狭窄的新生儿在出生时表现出严重发绀。程度较轻的肺动脉狭窄将引起不同程度的发绀。

根据临床表现常怀疑是否为 d-TGA。胸部放射影像显示蛋型心和上纵隔影较窄，轻度心脏肥大和肺血管纹理增多。超声心动图具有诊断性。目前很少需要进行心导管检查。

治疗

对于所有类型的 d-TGA，有必要保持心脏右侧和左侧之间的氧合血和脱氧血有足够混合。d-TGA 的血液循环是两个分离的回路，肺循环和体循环是并联的（图 123-19）。在心脏两侧之间无交通的话，脱氧血无法到达肺，氧合血无法到达体循环。大多数患者在手术之前需要有两个水平的分流。d-TGA/IVS 病例通过输注前列腺素 E_1 保持 PDA 开放和确保合适大小的 ASD 来获得足够分流，包括在必要时进行房间隔球囊切开术。偶尔，d-TGA/VSD 合并轻度肺动脉狭窄或没有肺动脉狭窄的患者，在心房和心室水平有足够的分流，可停用前列腺素 E_1。存在明显的肺动脉狭窄时，将需要前列腺素 E_1 来提供足够的肺血流。采用这些治疗策略来减轻患者的症状，直到可以

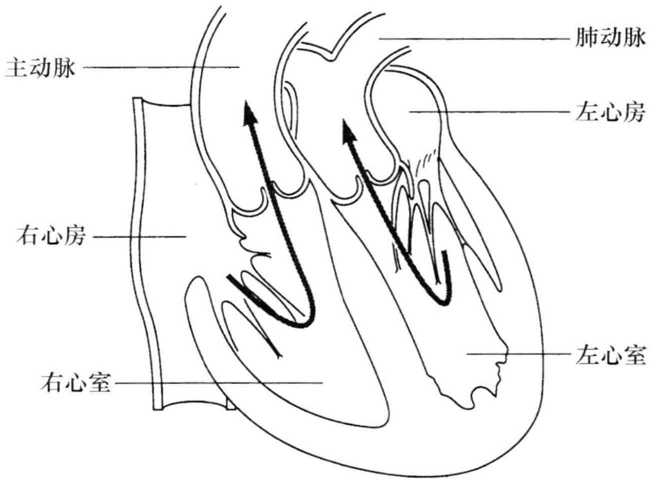

图 123-19　室间隔完整的 d-TGA 的解剖。（From Bove EL，Lupinetti FM：Congenital heart disease and cardiac tumors. In Greenfield LJ，Mulholland MW，Oldham KT，Zelenock GB［eds］：Surgery Scientific Principle and Practice. Philadelphia，JB Lippincott. 1993.）

实施根治手术。当没有诸如临床状况恶化等不利因素 1975
的情况下，目前对于所有 d-TGA 的治疗都是新生儿期根治。

无肺动脉狭窄的 d-TGA

目前对 d-TGA 的治疗是动脉调转手术（ASO）。经胸骨正中切口和标准的心肺转流技术实施手术。断开主动脉和肺总动脉（图 123-20A）。使用 Lecompte 法将肺动脉换位到主动脉前方，将远端的主动脉吻合到近端的肺动脉上（见图 123-20B）。从主动脉上取下冠状动脉，并带有冠状动脉开口处的主动脉壁组织，形成一个纽扣状的结构，并转移到近端的肺动脉上去（见图 123-20C）。采用裤状的自体心包补片重建近端主动脉（见图 123-20D），并与远端的肺动脉吻合。ASD 或如果有 VSD 也一并关闭。

有室间隔缺损和肺动脉狭窄的 d-TGA

如果有显著的肺动脉狭窄，可实施 Rastelli 手术，因为 ASO 会引起体循环的左心室流出道梗阻。Rastelli 手术将 VSD 用作左心室到主动脉的出口。在肺动脉

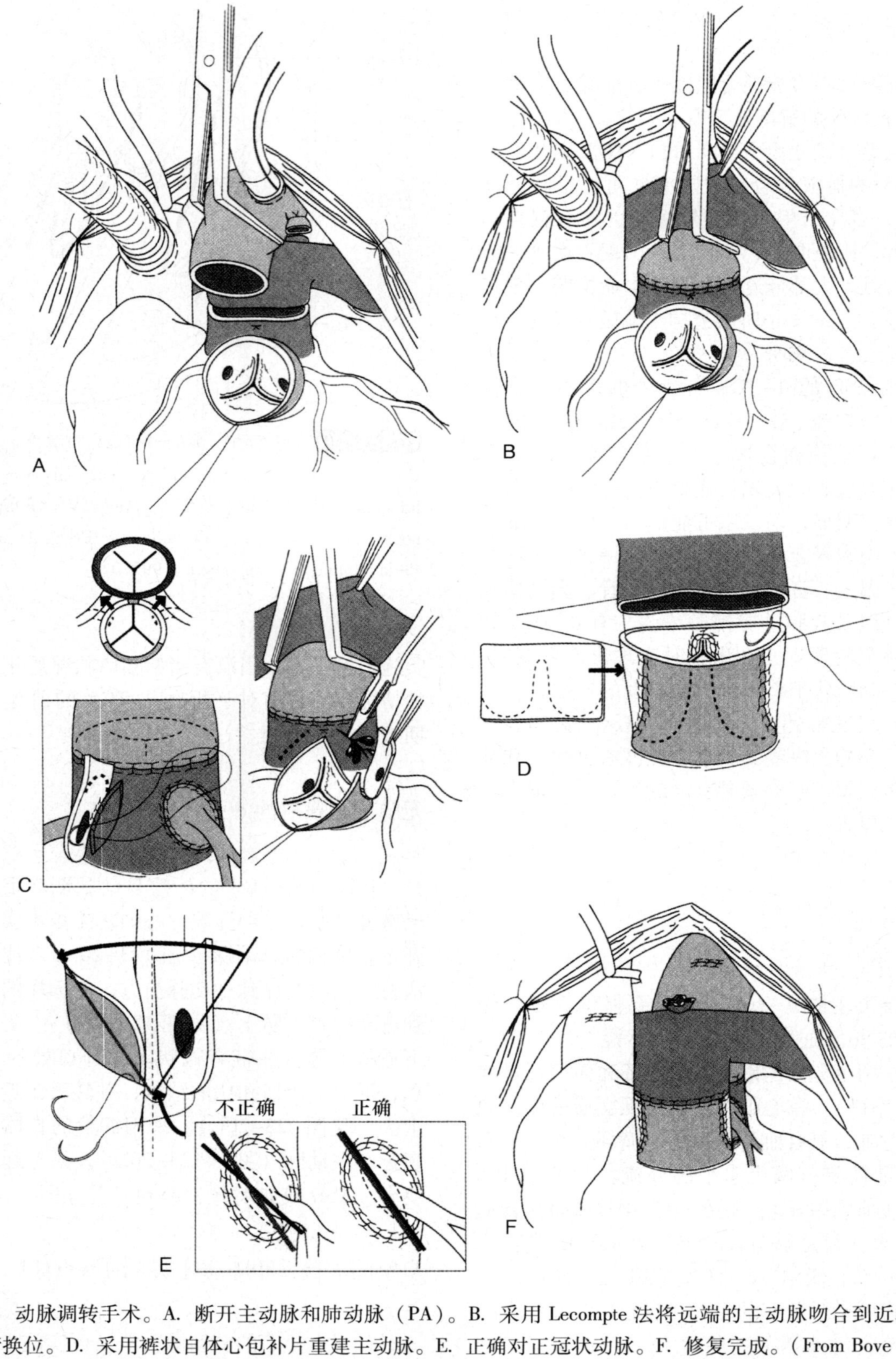

图 123-20 动脉调转手术。A. 断开主动脉和肺动脉（PA）。B. 采用 Lecompte 法将远端的主动脉吻合到近端的肺动脉。C. 冠状血管换位。D. 采用裤状自体心包补片重建主动脉。E. 正确对正冠状动脉。F. 修复完成。（From Bove EL，Lupinetti FM：Congenital heart disease and cardiac tumors. In Greenfield LJ，Mulholland MW，Oldham KT，Zelenock GB［eds］：Surgery Scientific Principle and Practice. Philadelphia，JB Lippincott. 1993.）

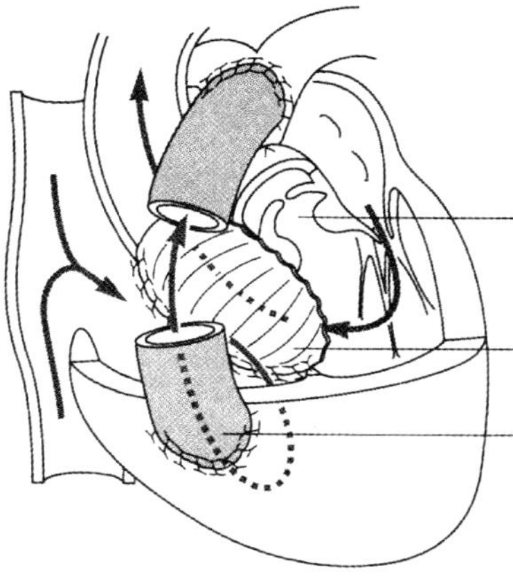

图 123-21　Rastelli 手术。（From Bove EL, Lupinetti FM: Congenital heart disease and cardiac tumors. In Greenfield LJ, Mulholland MW, Oldham KT, Zelenock GB [eds]: Surgery Scientific Principle and Practice. Philadelphia, JB Lippincott. 1993.）

瓣环处结扎并断开肺动脉。VSD 补片将 VSD 和主动脉瓣一起包住，形成一个从左心室到主动脉的隧道（图 123-21）。采用管道连接右心室漏斗部和远端肺动脉来重建右心室-肺动脉的连接。

结果

目前 ASO 的医院存活率为 90%～95%[13,33,42,46]。d-TGA/IVS 的死亡率通常低于 d-TGA/VSD 或 d-TGA/VSD/肺动脉狭窄。d-TGA/IVS 的医院死亡率为 3.5%～7.6%，相比 d-TGA/VSD 为 9.4%～13.1%[13,33]。5 年到 10 年和 15 年的生存率分别为 87.9%～93% 和 86%～88%[13,33,46]。再次手术的最常见原因是肺动脉瓣上狭窄，发生率为 3.9%～16%[33,46]。

最近关于 101 例接受 Rastelli 手术后 25 年患者的研究显示，医院死亡率为 7%，在此研究的后 7 年中没有死亡[43]。5 年、10 年、15 年和 20 年的实际生存率分别为 82%、80%、68% 和 52%。

单心室和左心发育不良综合征

很多先天性心血管畸形都导致功能性单心室的解剖结构，最常见的是三尖瓣闭锁、肺动脉闭锁、非平衡性 AVSD 和左心发育不良综合征（HLHS）。最常见的是 HLHS。在美国，每年约有 1000 例 HLHS 婴儿出生。这是最常见的重症先天性心脏病，占所有在出生后第一年中诊断畸形的 7%～9%[29]。所有单心室病变共同的生理学表现是仅有一个可以支持心排出量的心室。它们也共同需要进行二期或三期手术来进行重建，最终进行 Fontan 手术。初期手术的目的是维持足够的心排出量和氧饱和度，为最终的 Fontan 手术做准备。适合行 Fontan 手术的患者应包括这些特征：良好的心室功能、肺血管阻力低、无流出道梗阻和没有明显的房室瓣或半月瓣反流。其他治疗方法是心脏移植。

自然病史和诊断

这些病变的自然病史取决于肺血流量和体循环流出道梗阻的程度。肺血流严重受限或有明显体循环流出道梗阻的患者将在动脉导管关闭后迅速死亡。肺血流过多且无体循环流出道梗阻的患者将在数十个月大时死于肺血管梗阻性病变，这取决于肺循环超负荷的程度。偶尔，患者可能在合适的体循环与肺循环血流比值上取得“平衡”，罕有病例可以活到成年期。但是，这些患者的治疗选择仍是分期重建直至 Fontan 手术，因为即使一个完美平衡的循环，也会使心脏容量超负荷，最终会造成心力衰竭。一般的，这一情况仅可使患者无需在新生儿期进行控制肺血流的初期手术。

治疗

由于合适的供体数量有限，长期使用免疫抑制剂的不确定影响和植入心脏的寿命有限，所以大多数中心制定了一个分期重建的策略，作为单心室病变的主要治疗。分期重建包括一系列的两次或三次手术。新生儿期的初期手术可能需要，也可能不需要。在 4～6 个月大时进行双向 Glenn 手术或半 Fontan 手术，然后在 18～24 个月时进行 Fontan 手术。

初期姑息手术

体循环和肺循环血流比率不平衡的患者需要在新

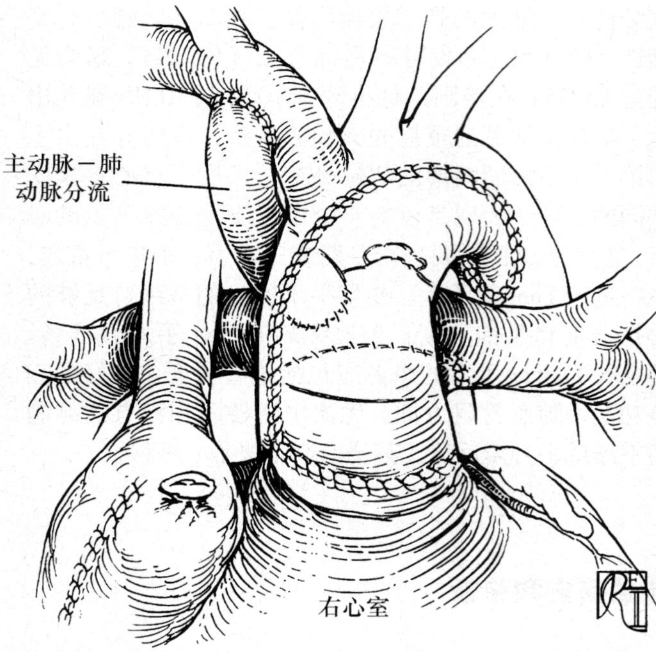

图 123-22 Norwood 手术完成图。（From Ohye RG，Mosca RM，Bove EL et al：hypoplastic left heart syndrome. In Mavroudis C，Backer CL［eds］：Pediatric Cardiac Surgery，3rd ed. Philadelphia. Mosby，2003.）

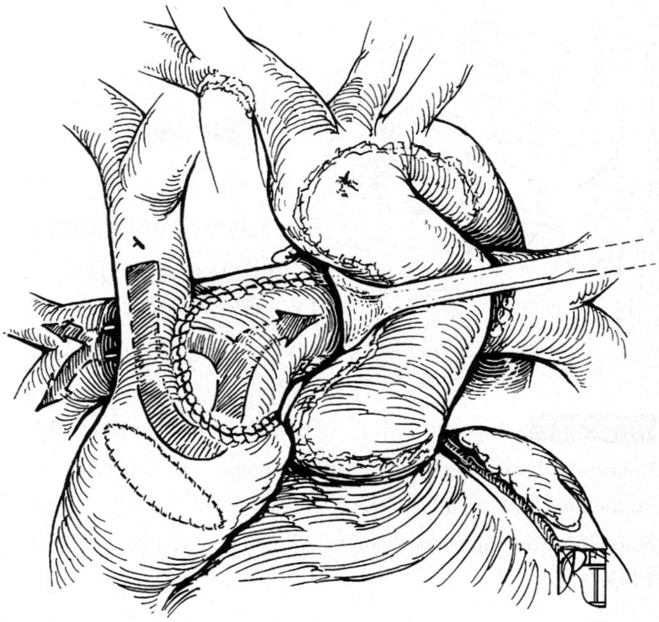

图 123-23 半 Fontan 手术完成图。（From Ohye RG，Mosca RM，Bove EL et al：hypoplastic left heart syndrome. In Mavroudis C，Backer CL［eds］：Pediatric Cardiac Surgery，3rd ed. Philadelphia. Mosby，2003.）

生儿期进行初期手术。此第一期重建手术的目的在于提供无梗阻的体循环和冠状循环血流、非限制性的肺
1977 静脉回流和流量受控的肺血流。对于体循环血流无梗阻且肺血流过多的患者，可进行肺动脉环扎或离断后建立体肺分流来控制肺循环超负荷。对于体循环血流无梗阻，但肺血流不够的患者，建立体肺分流。最常见的单心室（HLHS）患者有体循环梗阻和肺血流过多，需要实施初期的 Norwood 手术。在 Norwood 手术时，在近端的肺动脉上重建主动脉，以便使单一右心室能射血入主动脉。然后建立体肺分流来提供肺动脉血流（图 123-22）。此分流可来自无名动脉（改良 Blalock-Taussig 分流）或来自右心室。

双向 Glenn 分流或半 Fontan 手术

为了将右心室承担压力负荷的时间缩减到最短，通常在 4～6 个月实施半 Fontan 手术或双向 Glenn（BDG）吻合。BDG 吻合时要拆除体肺分流，并将上腔静脉通过端侧吻合直接连接到右肺动脉上。在此第二期手术之后，肺动脉血流全部由上腔静脉提供。半 Fontan 术是一种改良的 BDG 手术。半 Fontan 术包括在上腔静脉/右心房连接部位和肺动脉的侧侧吻合，常规扩大肺动脉分支，并用临时性补片将肺动脉和右心房隔开（图 123-23）。

Fontan 手术

通常在 18～24 个月之间实施最终的 Fontan 手术。我们对 HLHS 解剖采用的 Fontan 技术是侧隧道全腔肺连接（图 123-24）。在 Fontan 手术时，下腔静脉的静脉血直接回流到肺动脉。其他中心使用心外管道连接下腔静脉和右肺动脉。

结果 197

最近，在单心室患者的手术效果上取得了巨大的飞跃。最令人瞩目的变化是那些在 20 年前都要死亡的 HLHS 患者，现在的生存率得到极大改善。风险最高的分期手术依然是 Norwood 手术。在 20 世纪 90 年

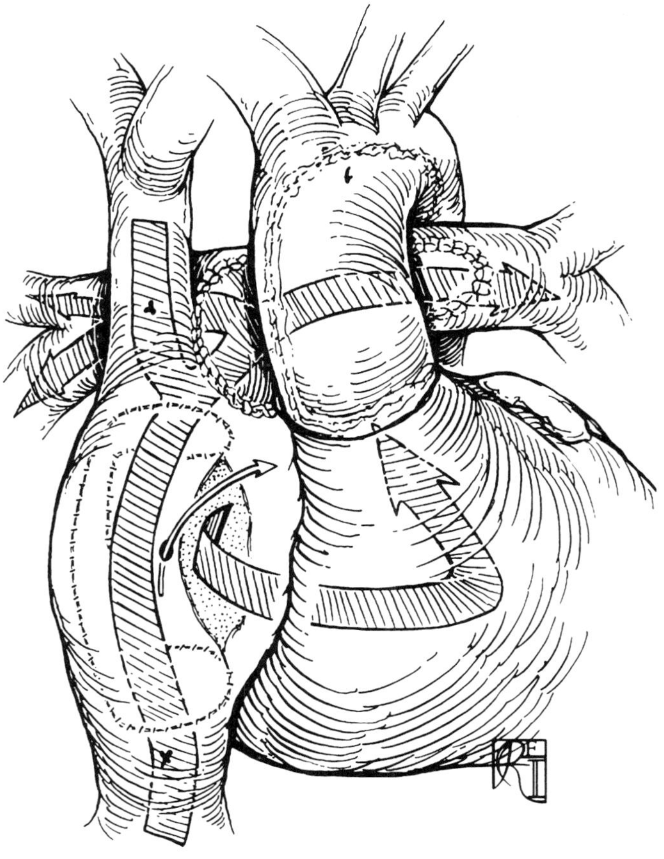

图 123-24 Fontan 手术完成图。（From Ohye RG，Mosca RM，Bove EL et al：hypoplastic left heart syndrome. In Mavroudis C，Backer CL［eds］：Pediatric Cardiac Surgery，3rd ed. Philadelphia. Mosby，2003.

代，美国的 Norwood 手术死亡率约 40%[32]。近来，一些高级中心报道的医院存活率约 90% 或更高[1,47,60,66]。报道的半 Fontan 和 Fontan 手术的效果非常优秀，两种手术存活率为 98%[11,26]。

血管环和吊带

血管环由一系列主动脉弓、肺动脉和头臂血管的畸形组成。这些病变的显著临床症状是不同程度的气管食管压迫。这些血管畸形可分为完全性血管环和部分性血管环。完全性血管环可分为双主动脉弓和右位主动脉弓合并左侧动脉韧带。这两种又可以进一步根据特殊的解剖进行细分（表 123-1）。不完全性血管环包括锁骨下动脉异位、无名动脉压迫

表 123-1 血管畸形的解剖分类和分型

畸形发生率[70,71,74,79,80]	%
完全性血管环	65～82
双主动脉弓	38～55
右侧优势	73～81
左侧优势	15～20
双侧均衡	3～11
右位主动脉弓，左侧动脉韧带/导管	24～55
迷走左锁骨下动脉	65～92
镜像分支	8～35
右侧动脉韧带	0～3
不完全性血管环	14～29
无名动脉压迫	80～87
右锁骨下动脉异位	13～20
肺动脉吊带	2～9

From Ohye RG，Wild LC，Mutabagani K，Bove EL：Vascular rings and slings. In Franco KL，Putman JB（eds）：Advanced Therapy in Thoracic Surgery. Hamilton. Ontario，BC Decker，2004.

和肺动脉吊带。其他罕见的变异包括左位主动脉弓合并右位降主动脉和右动脉韧带，以及左位主动脉弓合并右锁骨下动脉异位和右动脉韧带。在所有先天性心脏病患者中，临床上症状显著的血管环的发生率为 1%～2%。

有报道血管环和肺动脉吊带会合并其他心脏缺损，包括 TOF、ASD、肺动脉分支狭窄、主动脉缩窄、AVSD、VSD、主动脉弓中断和主肺动脉窗。11%～20% 的血管环患者合并显著的心脏畸形[4,76,79]。基本上右位主动脉弓合并的其他畸形的发生率更高。

在胚胎发育的第四周末，在背主动脉和腹侧根之间形成第六对主动脉弓或鳃弓。随后动脉弓退化并移行，形成解剖学上正常发育或异常发育的主动脉及其分支。大多数的第一、第二和第五弓退化。第三弓形成颈总动脉和近端的颈内静脉。右侧第四弓形成近端的右锁骨下动脉。左侧第四弓形成了从左颈动脉到左锁骨下动脉之间的主动脉弓。右侧第六弓的近端部分变成了右肺动脉的近端部分，而远端部分退化。同样，近端的左侧第六弓形成了近端左肺动脉，且远端第六弓变成动脉导管（图 123-25）。

两个肺动脉血管前体通过血管发生过程的联合、新生血管的重新发育和血管发生、已有血管的出芽及移行形成了肺动脉。如同先前所提到的，近端肺动脉基于第六弓，而原始肺芽最初的血液供应来自内脏神

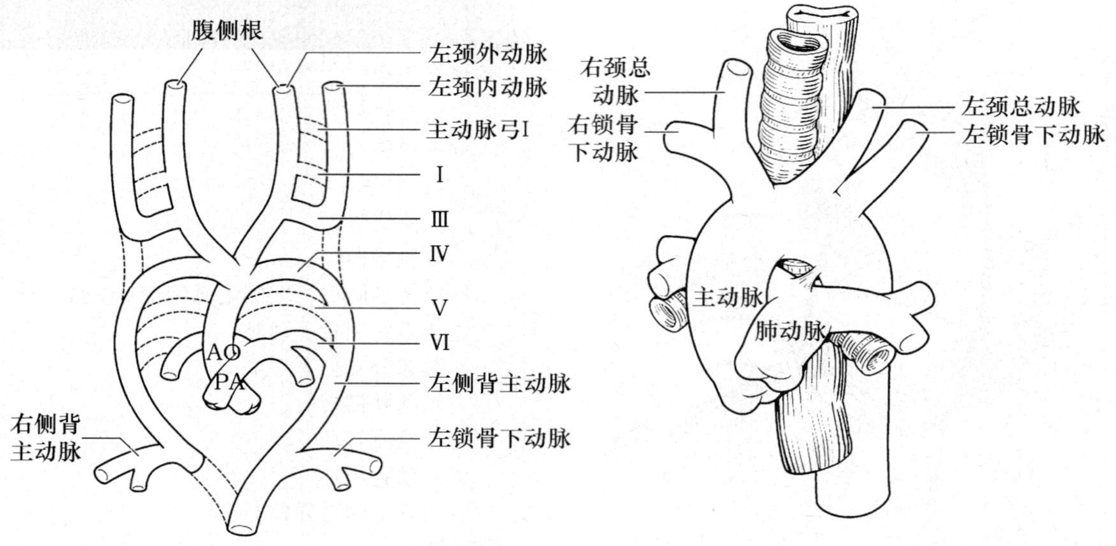

图 123-25　正常主动脉弓的发育。AO：主动脉；PA：肺动脉。（From Ohye RG，Wild LC，Mutabagani K，Bove EL：Vascular rings and slings. In Franco KL，Putman JB［eds］：Advanced Therapy in Thoracic Surgery. Hamilton. Ontario，BC Decker，2004.）

1979 经丛。最后，这两个肺动脉节段联合在一起，并形成了肺实质的血管网（图 123-26）。

自然病史和诊断

完全性血管环的儿童都在出生后第一周到第一个月内出现症状。一般双主动脉弓儿童的症状比那些右位主动脉弓合并左侧动脉韧带的患者出现得更早。在年龄更小的组中，主要是呼吸道症状明显，饮水都可以良好耐受。呼吸道症状可能包括喘鸣、非排痰性干咳、呼吸暂停或频繁呼吸道感染。典型的咳嗽似“海豹吼叫”或是“刺耳”的。这些症状可能类似哮喘、呼吸道感染或反流，且血管环儿童通常最初都被误诊。如果吞咽固体实物，则吞咽困难会变得明显。

不完全血管环患者的表现不同。无名动脉压迫的儿童通常会在出生后 1～2 年内出现呼吸道症状。虽

图 123-26　正常的肺动脉发育。（From Ohye RG，Wild LC，Mutabagani K，Bove EL：Vascular rings and slings. In Franco KL，Putman JB［eds］：Advanced Therapy in Thoracic Surgery. Hamilton. Ontario，BC Decker，2004.）

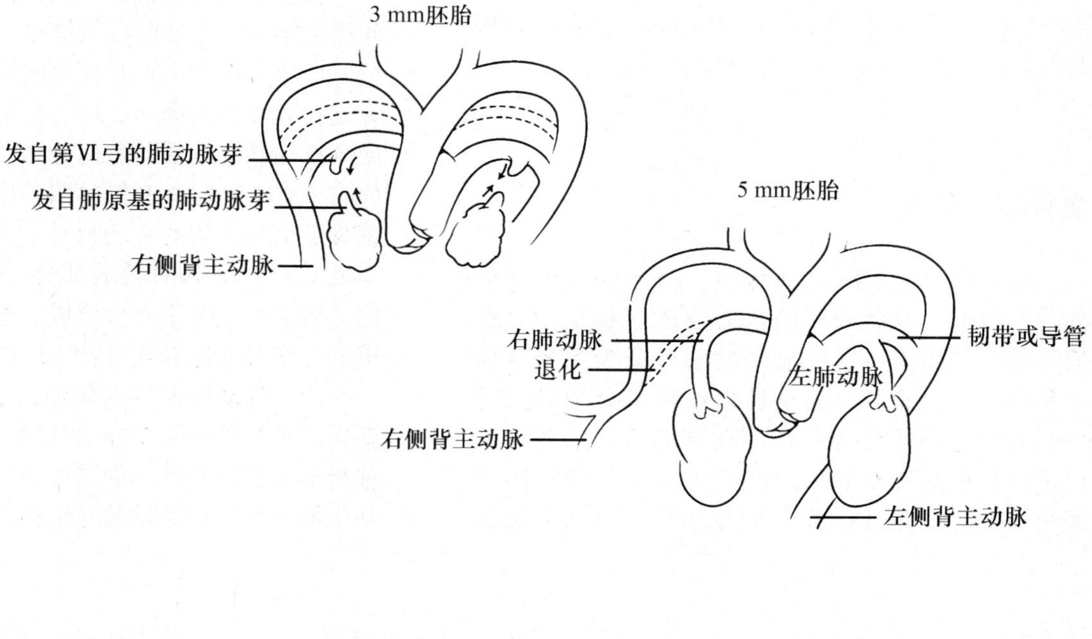

然在弓畸形中最常见的是右锁骨下动脉异位，占人群的 0.5%~1%，但是其罕有引起症状。通常，当发生症状时，患者常七八十岁了，因为迷走血管扩张和钙化，动脉压迫后方的食管，引起食管压迫性咽下困难。右锁骨下动脉异位很少引起儿童症状，除非其管腔异常巨大或合并气管软化。

肺动脉吊带儿童一般在出生后第一周或第一月内出现呼吸道症状。如果有完全性血管环，则呼吸道症状包括喘鸣、非排痰性干咳、呼吸暂停或频繁呼吸道感染，可能类似其他病症而引起误诊。30%~40% 的
1980 肺动脉吊带患者合并完全性气管环，导致气管局部狭窄或弥漫性狭窄。

因为症状表现不同且有许多可用的诊断测试方法，所以血管环的诊断方法各异。怀疑有哮喘或气管软化的儿童可能应到胸腔科医生处就诊，并通过胸部影像和支气管镜来进行诊断。在一些情况下，在评估合并的心脏畸形时，可以通过超声心动图得以诊断。通常是从胸部放射影像开始进行诊断的。辅助检查可包括食管钡餐造影、CT、MRI 和支气管镜。CT、MRI 和支气管镜是判断肺动脉吊带患者气管解剖的重要方法。超声心动图也具有诊断作用，且可用于排除其他心脏畸形。在过去广泛使用的气管图和心导管现在已经很少应用了。

治疗

完全性血管环

双主动脉弓

当右侧背主动脉退化失败的时候会发生双主动脉弓（图 123-27）。两个主动脉弓形成了完整的环，包绕气管和食管。大部分病例的右侧主动脉弓占优势，其次是左侧优势，双侧均衡最少见（见表 123-1）。左右颈动脉和锁骨下动脉通常发自其相应的主动脉弓。通常动脉韧带和降主动脉保留在左侧。

双主动脉弓的手术路径是经左后外侧胸廓切口。通过在第三或第四肋间的保留肌肉的小切口可方便地完成手术。向前下牵开肺，暴露后纵隔。在辨明迷走神经和膈神经后，切开胸膜。然后在非优势主动脉弓上能保留头臂血流的部位上放置两个血管夹，并在这两个夹子中间断开。如果对断开部位不确定的话，先在不同部位临时阻断主动脉弓，并监测各肢体的脉搏和血压。如果有闭锁节段，就在闭锁点断开。在韧带/导管和非优势主动脉弓区域的食管和气管周围进行游离，以便让血管结构回缩，并松解任何残余的梗阻性粘连。

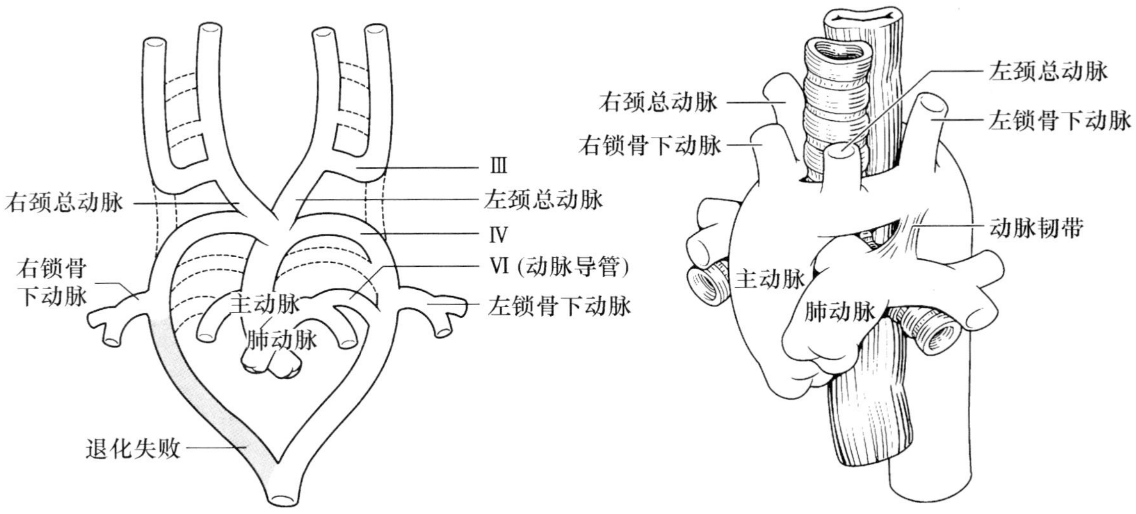

图 123-27　双主动脉弓的形成。(From Ohye RG, Wild LC, Mutabagani K, Bove EL: Vascular rings and slings. In Franco KL, Putman JB [eds]: Advanced Therapy in Thoracic Surgery. Hamilton. Ontario, BC Decker, 2004.)

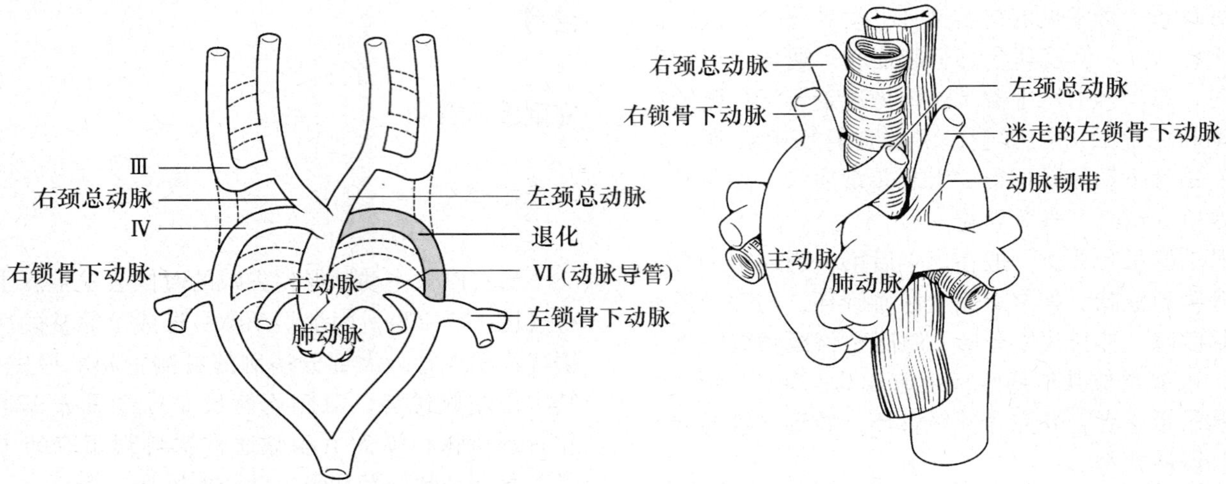

图 123-28 右位主动脉弓合并迷走左锁骨下动脉和食管后左侧动脉韧带的形成。(From Ohye RG, Wild LC, Mutabagani K, Bove EL: Vascular rings and slings. In Franco KL, Putman JB [eds]: Advanced Therapy in Thoracic Surgery. Hamilton. Ontario, BC Decker, 2004.)

右位主动脉弓合并左侧动脉韧带

右位主动脉弓合并左侧动脉韧带有三种解剖变异。如果左侧第四弓在主动脉和左锁骨下动脉间退化，会造成右位主动脉弓合并左锁骨下动脉异位。动脉韧带位于食管后，在左肺动脉和迷走左锁骨下动脉间形成间桥，形成一个完全性血管环（图 123-28）。如果左侧第四弓在左锁骨下动脉起始部以后，但在主动脉弓到达背主动脉与第六弓（变成动脉导管）交通之前的部位退化，就会形成镜像分支。食管后动脉韧带直接起源于降主动脉，或起源于发自降主动脉的 Kommerell 憩室，就形成了完全性血管环（图 123-29）。如果在左侧第四和第六弓之间仍有交通，就有镜像分支及发自前方镜像左锁骨下动脉的动脉韧带，血管环就不会形成（图 123-30）。

右位主动脉弓合并食管后左侧动脉韧带的手术径路和双主动脉弓一样。断开动脉韧带，并松解任何在

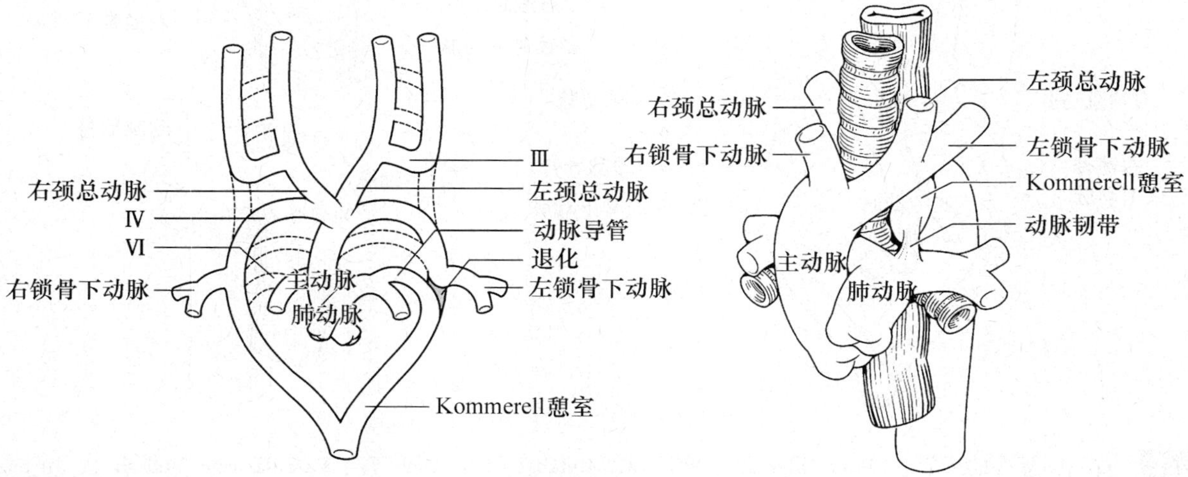

图 123-29 右位主动脉弓合并镜像分支和食管后动脉韧带。(From Ohye RG, Wild LC, Mutabagani K, Bove EL: Vascular rings and slings. In Franco KL, Putman JB [eds]: Advanced Therapy in Thoracic Surgery. Hamilton. Ontario, BC Decker, 2004.)

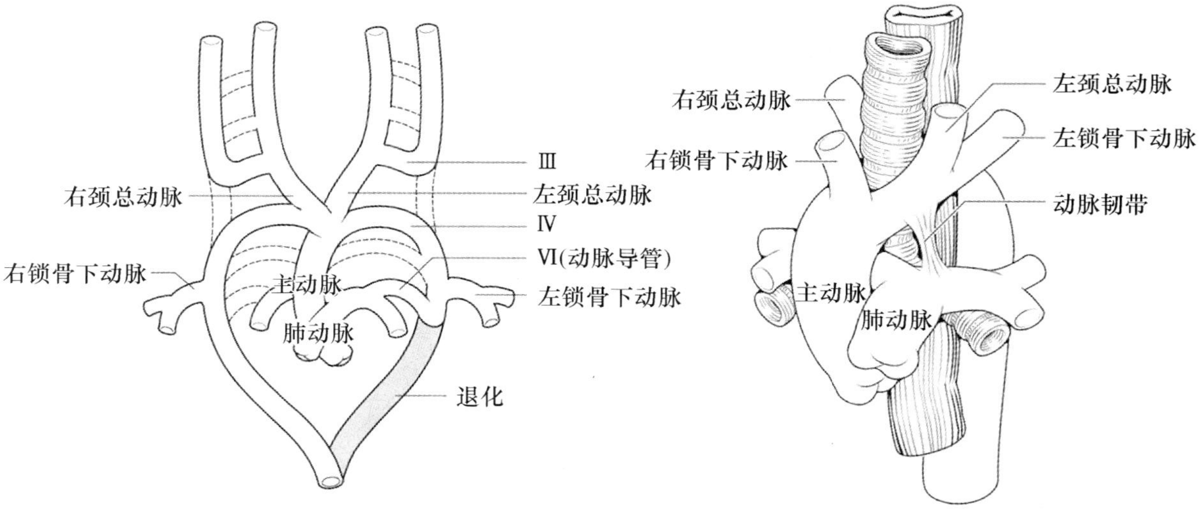

图 123-30 右位主动脉弓合并镜像分支和左侧动脉韧带，不形成血管环。（From Ohye RG，Wild LC，Mutabagani K，Bove EL：Vascular rings and slings. In Franco KL，Putman JB［eds］：Advanced Therapy in Thoracic Surgery. Hamilton. Ontario，BC Decker，2004.）

食管和气管周围的粘连。偶尔有 Kommerell 憩室引起
982 压迫，甚至在断开动脉韧带后仍引起压迫的报道。这样，如果憩室特别明显，就可能要切除或将憩室向后悬吊在椎前筋膜上。

不完全性血管环

无名动脉压迫

在无名动脉压迫综合征中，主动脉弓和动脉韧带位于其正常位置的左侧。但是，无名动脉部分或完全自中线左侧发出（图 123-31）。如果动脉在气管前方自左向右走行，会引起气管压迫。无名动脉压迫综合征症状可能很轻，也可能很严重。如果是症状轻的儿童，且气管镜下发现气管压迫很轻，可以进行观察，因为症状可能随着生长而消除。手术适应证包括呼吸暂停、严重呼吸窘迫、明显的喘鸣或反复呼吸道感染。

已经阐述了一些纠治无名动脉压迫综合征的方法。这包括单纯切断、切断后重新种植到升主动脉右

图 123-31 无名动脉压迫综合征的胚胎起源。（From Ohye RG，Wild LC，Mutabagani K，Bove EL：Vascular rings and slings. In Franco KL，Putman JB［eds］：Advanced Therapy in Thoracic Surgery. Hamilton. Ontario，BC Decker，2004.）

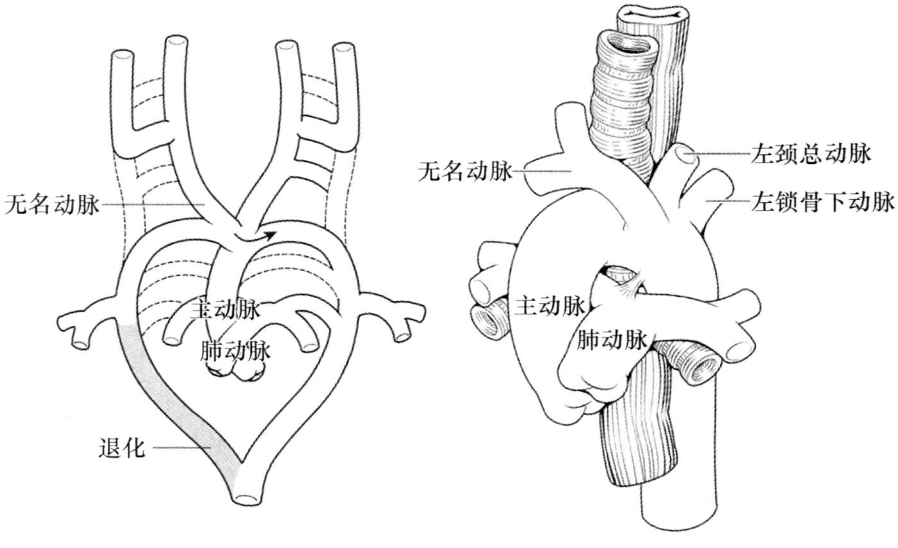

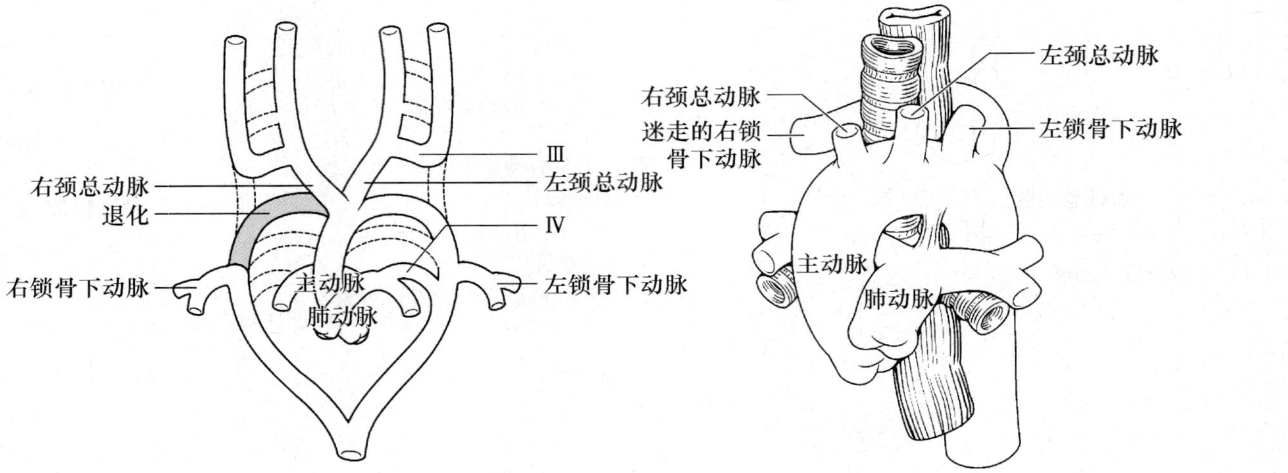

图 123-32 左位主动脉弓合并右锁骨下动脉异位。（From Ohye RG，Wild LC，Mutabagani K，Bove EL：Vascular rings and slings. In Franco KL，Putman JB［eds］：Advanced Therapy in Thoracic Surgery. Hamilton. Ontario，BC Decker，2004.）

侧和胸骨后悬吊。悬吊是目前使用最多的技术。通过左前、右前或右侧乳下前外侧胸廓切口进行暴露。一旦暴露了无名动脉，不要对动脉进行游离。通过不对无名动脉进行周围游离，将血管吊起时也可将气管向前拉起。带垫聚丙烯缝线穿过部分无名动脉和无名动脉起始部的主动脉壁。在支气管镜引导下，临时性地松开缝线，有助于合理地在血管和胸骨后安置缝线。一旦支气管镜证实气管得到了满意的重新开放，就将缝线穿过胸骨并固定。

左位主动脉弓合并右锁骨下动脉异位

当第四弓在右颈总动脉和右锁骨下动脉之间退化时，就会发生右锁骨下动脉异位（图 123-32）。此时右锁骨下动脉起源于左位的升主动脉，在食管后方从左向右走行。虽然动脉会在后方压迫食管，但罕见引起儿童症状。手术治疗为经左后外侧切口单纯切断。很少需要在右颈动脉或主动脉弓上重新种植。

肺动脉吊带

正常情况下，右侧和左侧第六主动脉弓构成了其相应的肺动脉的近端部分。如果近端的左侧第六弓退化，且左肺芽向右侧移行与右肺动脉相遇，就会形成肺动脉吊带（图 123-33）。30%～40% 的肺动脉吊带患者会合并完全性气管环和气管狭窄[9]。有报道肺动脉韧带多合并右上叶支气管起源于气管[3]。

起初对肺动脉吊带的修复包括在非心肺转流下切断左肺动脉并换位到气管前。在这些早期报道中，左肺动脉血栓形成的发生率高。因此一些作者建议断开气管，并换位到左肺动脉后。如果在气管重建的过程中气管可进行断开，那么这些方法是合理的。但是，目前大多数作者建议重新种植左肺动脉，且效果优良。经胸骨正中切口，在心肺转流下进行手术，以确保手术时良好的视野。无需主动脉阻断。将左肺动脉从右肺动脉上离断下来，换位到气管前方，并重新种植到肺总动脉上。 198

任何气管重建都要在支气管镜的支持下进行。已报道的气管重建技术很多，最常用的是切除后一期吻合，对短段狭窄采用滑动气管成形术（slide tracheoplasty），长段狭窄采用肋软骨或心包补片修补。

需右侧胸廓切口治疗的血管环

超过 95% 的无并发心脏缺损的血管环可通过左侧胸廓切口进行手术。对于存在右侧动脉韧带的罕见病例需要进行右侧胸廓切口。在左位主动脉弓合并右位降主动脉的情况下，会发生右侧动脉韧带，韧带在降主动脉和右肺动脉之间形成间桥，成为一个完整的环。报道在左位主动脉弓合并右锁骨下动脉异位时也有右侧动脉韧带。在这种病例中，动脉韧带可能发自

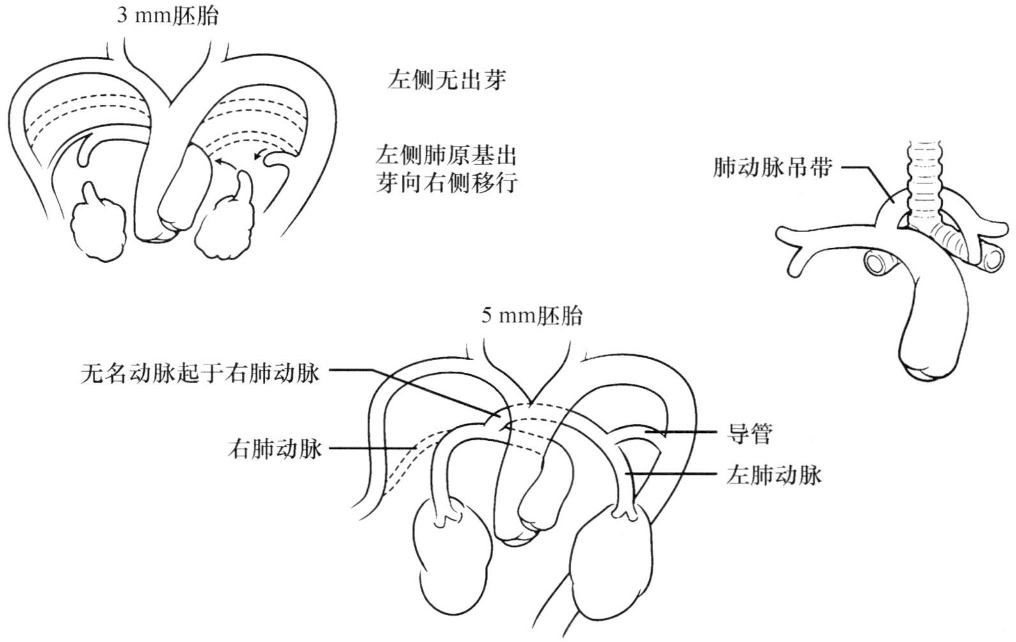

图 123-33 肺动脉吊带的形成。（From Ohye RG, Wild LC, Mutabagani K, Bove EL: Vascular rings and slings. In Franco KL, Putman JB [eds]: Advanced Therapy in Thoracic Surgery. Hamilton. Ontario, BC Decker, 2004.）

异位的锁骨下动脉、主动脉弓的憩室或直接从左位主
1984 动脉弓到右肺动脉。此外，在右颈动脉近端有闭锁段的双主动脉弓更容易经右胸切口加以离断。这些畸形的治疗方法和左侧血管环离断的方法相同，注意右侧喉返神经也绕过右侧动脉韧带。

视频辅助胸腔镜手术

Burke 及其同事和我们中心报道了使用机器人技术[55]或不使用机器人技术[14]的视频辅助胸腔镜手术（VATS）治疗血管环。两种方法所进行的胸腔镜下的离断手术，仅限于那些需要离断非连通性血管结构的患者。无手术死亡，且所有手术都是通过胸腔镜完成的。

结果

血管环手术的死亡率为 0.5%～7.6%，在最新的系列报道中存活率进一步提高[3,51,76,79]。大多数的死亡与其他心脏缺陷或呼吸道感染和呼吸衰竭有关。Backer 及其同事[8]报道了一组 16 例采用左肺动脉离断并重新种植治疗肺动脉吊带的患者，全部需要进行气管重建。没有手术死亡率，且一例晚期死亡是呼吸道并发症引起的。在这一报道和其他报道中，主要并发症的发生率和死亡率都与气管重建有关[8,77]。

（孙彦隽译　刘锦纷校）

参考文献

1. Azakie A, Martinez D, Sapru A, et al: Impact of right ventricle to pulmonary artery conduit on outcome of the modified Norwood procedure. Ann Thorac Surg 2004;77:1727-1733.
2. Bacha EA, Scheule AM, Zurakowski D, et al: Long-term results after early primary repair of tetralogy of Fallot. J Thorac Cardiovasc Surg 2001;122:154-161.
3. Backer C: Vascular rings and pulmonary artery sling. In Mavroudis C (ed): Pediatric Cardiac Surgery, 2nd ed. St. Louis, Mosby, 1994.
4. Backer CL, Ilbawi MN, Idriss FS, DeLeon SY: Vascular anomalies causing tracheoesophageal compression: Review of experience in children. J Thorac Cardiovasc Surg 1989; 97:725-731.
5. Backer CL, Idriss FS, Zales VR, et al: Surgical management of the conal (supracristal) ventricular septal defect. J Thorac Cardiovasc Surg 1991;102:288-295; discussion 295-296.
6. Backer CL, Paape K, Zales VR, et al: Coarctation of the aorta: Repair with polytetrafluoroethylene patch aortoplasty. Circulation 1995;92(9 Suppl):II132-II136.
7. Backer CL, Mavroudis C, Zias EA, et al: Repair of coarctation with resection and extended end-to-end anastomosis. Ann Thorac Surg 1998;66:1365-1370; discussion 1370-1371.
8. Backer CL, Mavroudis C, Dunham ME, Holinger LD: Pulmonary artery sling: Results with median sternotomy,

cardiopulmonary bypass, and reimplantation. Ann Thorac Surg 1999;67:1738-1744; discussion 1744-1745.
9. Berdon WE, Baker DH, Wung JT, et al: Complete cartilage-ring tracheal stenosis associated with anomalous left pulmonary artery: The ring-sling complex. Radiology 1984; 152:57-64.
10. Bharati S, Kirklin JW, McAllister HA Jr, Lev M: The surgical anatomy of common atrioventricular orifice associated with tetralogy of Fallot, double outlet right ventricle and complete regular transposition. Circulation 1980;61:1142-1149.
11. Bove EL: Current status of staged reconstruction for hypoplastic left heart syndrome. Pediatr Cardiol 1998;19: 308-315.
12. Brewer LA 3rd, Fosburg RG, Mulder GA, Verska JJ: Spinal cord complications following surgery for coarctation of the aorta: A study of 66 cases. J Thorac Cardiovasc Surg 1972;64: 368-381.
13. Brown JW, Park HJ, Turrentine MW: Arterial switch operation: Factors impacting survival in the current era. Ann Thorac Surg 2001;71:1978-1984.
14. Burke RP, Wernovsky G, van der Velde M, et al: Video-assisted thoracoscopic surgery for congenital heart disease. J Thorac Cardiovasc Surg 1995;109:499-507; discussion 508.
15. Burke RP, Jacobs JP, Cheng W, et al: Video-assisted thoracoscopic surgery for patent ductus arteriosus in low birth weight neonates and infants. Pediatrics 1999;104:227-230.
16. Campbell M: Natural history of persistent ductus arteriosus. Br Heart J 1968;30:4-13.
17. Cooper RS, Ritter SB, Rothe WB, et al: Angioplasty for coarctation of the aorta: Long-term results. Circulation 1987;75:600-604.
18. Coster DD, Gorton ME, Grooters RK, et al: Surgical closure of the patent ductus arteriosus in the neonatal intensive care unit. Ann Thorac Surg 1989;48:386-389.
19. Cowley CG, Lloyd TR: Interventional cardiac catheterization advances in nonsurgical approaches to congenital heart disease. Curr Opin Pediatr 1999;11:425-432.
20. Cowley CG, Lloyd TR, Bove EL, et al: Comparison of results of closure of secundum atrial septal defect by surgery versus Amplatzer septal occluder. Am J Cardiol 2001;88:589-591.
21. Craig RJ, Selzer A: Natural history and prognosis of atrial septal defect. Circulation 1968;37:805-815.
22. Dajani AS, Taubert KA, Wilson W, et al: Prevention of bacterial endocarditis. Recommendations by the American Heart Association. Circulation 1997;96:358-366.
23. de Ruijter FT, Weenink I, Hitchcock FJ, et al: Right ventricular dysfunction and pulmonary valve replacement after correction of tetralogy of Fallot. Ann Thorac Surg 2002;73:1794-1800; discussion 1800.
24. del Nido PJ, Williams WG, Wilson GJ, et al: Synthetic patch angioplasty for repair of coarctation of the aorta: Experience with aneurysm formation. Circulation 1986;74:I32-I36.
25. Discigil B, Dearani JA, Puga FJ, et al: Late pulmonary valve replacement after repair of tetralogy of Fallot. J Thorac Cardiovasc Surg 2001;121:344-351.
26. Douglas WI, Goldberg CS, Mosca RS, et al: Hemi-Fontan procedure for hypoplastic left heart syndrome: Outcome and suitability for Fontan. Ann Thorac Surg 1999;68: 1361-1367; discussion 1368.
27. Draulans-Noe HA, Wenink AC, Quaegebeur J: Single papillary muscle ("parachute valve") and double-orifice left ventricle in atrioventricular septal defect convergence of chordal attachment: Surgical anatomy and results of surgery. Pediatr Cardiol 1990;11:29-35.
28. Elliott RB, Starling MB, Neutze JM: Medical manipulation of the ductus arteriosus. Lancet 1975;1:140-142.
29. Fyler D: Report of the New England Regional Infant Cardiac Program. Pediatrics 1980;65:375-461.
30. Gersony WM, Peckham GJ, Ellison RC, et al: Effects of indomethacin in premature infants with patent ductus arteriosus: Results of a national collaborative study. J Pediatr 1983;102:895-906.
31. Goyal VS, Fulwani MC, Ramakantan R, et al: Follow-up after coil closure of patent ductus arteriosus. Am J Cardiol 1999;83:463-466.
32. Gutgesell HP, Gibson J: Management of hypoplastic left heart syndrome in the 1990s. Am J Cardiol 2002;89: 842-846.
33. Haas F, Wottke M, Poppert H, Meisner H: Long-term survival and functional follow-up in patients after the arterial switch operation. Ann Thorac Surg 1999;68:1692-1697.
34. Hanley FL, Fenton KN, Jonas RA, et al: Surgical repair of complete atrioventricular canal defects in infancy: Twenty-year trends. J Thorac Cardiovasc Surg 1993;106:387-394; discussion 394-397.
35. Hellenbrand WE, Allen HD, Golinko RJ, et al: Balloon angioplasty for aortic recoarctation: Results of Valvuloplasty and Angioplasty of Congenital Anomalies Registry. Am J Cardiol 1990;65:793-797.
36. Heymann MA, Rudolph AM, Silverman NH: Closure of the ductus arteriosus in premature infants by inhibition of prostaglandin synthesis. N Engl J Med 1976;295: 530-533.
37. Hijazi ZM, Fahey JT, Kleinman CS, Hellenbrand WE: Balloon angioplasty for recurrent coarctation of aorta: Immediate and long-term results. Circulation 1991;84:1150-1156.
38. Hirsch JC, Bove EL: Tetralogy of Fallot. In Mavroudis C, Backer CL (eds): Pediatric Cardiac Surgery, 3rd ed. Philadelphia, Mosby, 2003.
39. Hoffman JI, Kaplan S: The incidence of congenital heart disease. J Am Coll Cardiol 2002;39:1890-1900.
40. Kadoba K, Jonas RA, Mayer JE, Castaneda AR: Mitral valve replacement in the first year of life. J Thorac Cardiovasc Surg 1990;100:762-768.
41. Karl TR, Sano S, Pornviliwan S, Mee RB: Tetralogy of Fallot: Favorable outcome of nonneonatal transatrial, transpulmonary repair. Ann Thorac Surg 1992;54:903-907.
42. Kirklin J: Complete transposition of the great arteries. In Kirklin J (ed): Cardiac Surgery. New York, Churchill Livingstone, 1993, pp 1383-1467.
43. Kreutzer C, De Vive J, Oppido G, et al: Twenty-five-year experience with Rastelli repair for transposition of the great arteries. J Thorac Cardiovasc Surg 2000;120: 211-223.
44. Levin DL, Paul MH, Muster AJ, et al: d-Transposition of the great vessels in the neonate: A clinical diagnosis. Arch Intern Med 1977;137:1421-1425.
45. Liebman J: Natural history of transposition of the great arteries: Anatomy and birth and death characteristics. Circulation 1969;40:237-262.
46. Losay J, Touchot A, Serraf A, et al: Late outcome after arterial switch operation for transposition of the great arteries. Circulation 2001;104(12 Suppl 1):I121-I126.
47. Mair R, Tulzer G, Sames E, et al: Right ventricular to pulmonary artery conduit instead of modified Blalock-Taussig shunt improves postoperative hemodynamics in newborns after the Norwood operation. J Thorac Cardiovasc Surg 2003;126:1378-1384.
48. Mavroudis C, Backer CL, Jacobs JP: Ventricular septal defect. In Mavroudis C, Backer CL (eds): Pediatric Cardiac Surgery, 3rd ed. Philadelphia, Mosby, 2003.
49. Meijboom F, Hess J, Szatmari A, et al: Long-term follow-up

(9 to 20 years) after surgical closure of atrial septal defect at a young age. Am J Cardiol 1993;72:1431-1434.
50. Minich LL, Tani LY, Pagotto LT, et al: Size of ventricular structures influences surgical outcome in Down syndrome infants with atrioventricular septal defect. Am J Cardiol 1998;81:1062-1065.
51. Mitchell J: Vascular rings, slings and other arch anomalies. In Kaiser L (ed): Mastery of Cardiothoracic Surgery. Philadelphia, Lippincott-Raven, 1998.
52. Moe DG, Guntheroth WG: Spontaneous closure of uncomplicated ventricular septal defect. Am J Cardiol 1987;60: 674-678.
53. Momma K, Toyama K, Takao A, et al: Natural history of subarterial infundibular ventricular septal defect. Am Heart J 1984;108:1312-1317.
54. Newfeld EA, Sher M, Paul MH, Nikaidoh H: Pulmonary vascular disease in complete atrioventricular canal defect. Am J Cardiol 1977;39:721-726.
55. Ohye R: Robotics in pediatric cardiac surgery. Presented before the 40th annual meeting of the Society of Thoracic Surgeons, San Antonio, Texas, 2004.
56. Ohye R: Vascular rings and slings. In Franco KL, Putman JB (eds): Advanced Therapy in Thoracic Surgery. Hamilton, Ontario, BC Decker, 2004.
57. Ovaert C, McCrindle BW, Nykanen D, et al: Balloon angioplasty of native coarctation: Clinical outcomes and predictors of success. J Am Coll Cardiol 2000;35: 988-996.
58. Patel HT, Cao QL, Rhodes J, Hijazi ZM: Long-term outcome of transcatheter coil closure of small to large patent ductus arteriosus. Cathet Cardiovasc Interv 1999;47:457-461.
59. Piccoli GP, Ho SY, Wilkinson JL, et al: Left-sided obstructive lesions in atrioventricular septal defects: An anatomic study. J Thorac Cardiovasc Surg 1982;83:453-460.
60. Pizarro C, Malec E, Maher KO, et al: Right ventricle to pulmonary artery conduit improves outcome after stage I Norwood for hypoplastic left heart syndrome. Circulation 2003;108(Suppl 1):II155-II160.
61. Presbitero P, Demarie D, Villani M, et al: Long term results (15–30 years) of surgical repair of aortic coarctation. Br Heart J 1987;57:462-467.
62. Puga FJ: Reoperation after repair of atrioventricular canal defects. Semin Thorac Cardiovasc Surg Pediatr Card Surg Annu 1998;1:123-128.
63. Purcell IF, Brecker SJ, Ward DE: Closure of defects of the atrial septum in adults using the Amplatzer device: 100 consecutive patients in a single center. Clin Cardiol 2004;27: 509-513.
64. Rastelli G, Kirklin JW, Titus JL: Anatomic observations on complete form of persistent common atrioventricular canal with special reference to atrioventricular valves. Mayo Clin Proc 1966;41:296-308.
65. Reifenstein GH, Levine SA, Gross RE: Coarctation of the aorta: A review of 104 autopsied cases of the "adult type," 2 years of age or older. Am Heart J 1947;33:146-168.
66. Sano S, Ishino K, Kawada M, et al: Right ventricle-pulmonary artery shunt in first-stage palliation of hypoplastic left heart syndrome. J Thorac Cardiovasc Surg 2003;126:504-509; discussion 509-510.
67. Seirafi PA, Warner KG, Geggel RL, et al: Repair of coarctation of the aorta during infancy minimizes the risk of late hypertension. Ann Thorac Surg 1998;66:1378-1382.
68. Siassi B, Blanco C, Cabal LA, Coran AG: Incidence and clinical features of patent ductus arteriosus in low-birth-weight infants: A prospective analysis of 150 consecutively born infants. Pediatrics 1976;57:347-351.
69. Spicer RL: Cardiovascular disease in Down syndrome. Pediatr Clin North Am 1984;31:1331-1343.
70. Stewart S, Alexson C, Manning J: Partial atrioventricular canal defect: The early and late results of operation. Ann Thorac Surg 1987;43:527-529.
71. Studer M, Blackstone EH, Kirklin JW, et al: Determinants of early and late results of repair of atrioventricular septal (canal) defects. J Thorac Cardiovasc Surg 1982;84:523-542.
72. Taylor RL, Grover FL, Harman PK, et al: Operative closure of patent ductus arteriosus in premature infants in the neonatal intensive care unit. Am J Surg 1986;152: 704-708.
73. Tynan M, Finley JP, Fontes V, et al: Balloon angioplasty for the treatment of native coarctation: Results of Valvuloplasty and Angioplasty of Congenital Anomalies Registry. Am J Cardiol 1990;65:790-792.
74. van Heurn LW, Wong CM, Spiegelhalter DJ, et al: Surgical treatment of aortic coarctation in infants younger than three months: 1985 to 1990. Success of extended end-to-end arch aortoplasty. J Thorac Cardiovasc Surg 1994;107:74-85; discussion 85-86.
75. Van Praagh R, Van Praagh S, Nebesar RA, et al: Tetralogy of Fallot: Underdevelopment of the pulmonary infundibulum and its sequelae. Am J Cardiol 1970;26:25-33.
76. van Son JA, Julsrud PR, Hagler DJ, et al: Surgical treatment of vascular rings: The Mayo Clinic experience. Mayo Clin Proc 1993;68:1056-1063.
77. van Son JA, Hambsch J, Haas GS, et al: Pulmonary artery sling: Reimplantation versus antetracheal translocation. Ann Thorac Surg 1999;68:989-994.
78. Wong CH, Watson B, Smith J, et al: The use of left heart bypass in adult and recurrent coarctation repair. Eur J Cardiothorac Surg 2001;20:1199-1201.
79. Woods RK, Sharp RJ, Holcomb GW 3rd, et al: Vascular anomalies and tracheoesophageal compression: A single institution's 25-year experience. Ann Thorac Surg 2001;72:434-438; discussion 438-439.
80. Yetman AT, Nykanen D, McCrindle BW, et al: Balloon angioplasty of recurrent coarctation: A 12-year review. J Am Coll Cardiol 1997;30:811-816.

第 124 章

神经管缺陷、脑积水、难治性癫痫和中枢神经系统感染的处理

Jodi L. Smith

神经管缺陷

1987 人类胚胎发育最早、最关键的时期是神经胚形成的时期，此时产生神经管（NT），它是成人整个中枢神经系统即脑和脊髓（SC）的基础。神经管在神经胚形成的第一和第二期形成。神经胚形成第一阶段包括神经板（NP）的形成以及随后经形态学改变而形成神经管。神经胚形成的第二阶段涉及上皮索（即髓索）的形成以及随后腔化形成神经管。人类大脑和 S2 以上的脊髓是由第一阶段神经胚演变而来的，而 S2 以下的脊髓及终丝由第二阶段的神经胚演变而来。一个世纪以来，研究者已经通过很多不同的动物模型和实验去探究一期和二期神经胚形成的机制。当人类神经管形成出错时，就会产生神经管缺陷（neural tube defects，NTD）。

神经管缺陷在人类先天性畸形中最为常见。这一类复杂的先天性畸形的发生是由于形成脑和脊髓的神经管在胚胎发育的最初几个星期内未能闭合。根据有无神经组织的外露，神经管闭合不全常分为开放性和闭合性两种类型。开放性神经管闭合不全是由于原始神经胚形成障碍所致，表现为神经管及其表面的膜异常，并且表面覆盖的皮肤缺损。闭合性神经管闭合不全是由于神经胚形成的第二阶段出错，表现为神经管及其表面的膜异常，但其表面有完整的皮肤覆盖。开放性神经管闭合不全包括无脑畸形、囊性脊柱裂（即脊髓裂、脊髓脊膜膨出和脊膜膨出）、枕骨裂脑露畸形和脑膨出。闭合性神经管闭合不全包括隐性脊柱裂、脂肪瘤畸形（如脂肪瘤和脂肪脊髓脊膜膨出）、脊髓裂畸形（脊髓纵裂、双脊髓畸形）、神经管原肠囊肿、皮肤窦和骶骨发育不良（尾骨退化）。

无脑畸形或脑组织缺如是由于神经管头端部分未能闭合而导致，患儿通常在出生时或出生后数天内死亡。囊性脊柱裂（即脊髓裂、脊髓脊膜膨出和脊膜膨出）是由于尾端神经管发育不全所致，畸形发育的神经组织和（或）脊膜通过裂开的椎管、肌肉和皮肤
突出到皮肤外（图 124-1）。开放性神经管闭合不全 1988
可以是严重的颅脊柱裂畸形，即整个神经管闭合不全，也可以是局限性、单一椎体水平的神经管闭合不全。近期的研究显示围孕期补充叶酸能够减少 50%~70% 神经管闭合不全的发生和复发[34,98]，然而发生这一类畸形的患儿仍占新生活产儿的 1/1000。换言

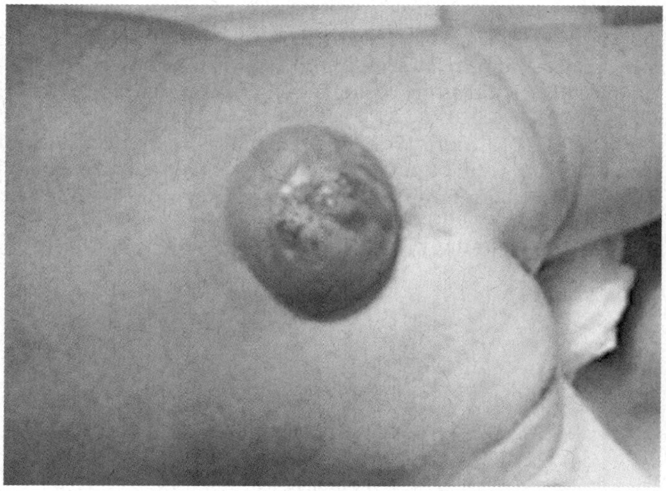

图 124-1 出生 3 小时的由超声产前诊断为 L5 ~ S1 脊髓脊膜膨出的男婴。

之，在美国，包括选择性终止妊娠在内，每年约有 4000 名或每天有 11～12 名怀孕妇女怀有神经管闭合不全胎儿，这类严重的畸形可导致胎儿夭折、婴儿死亡、终身残疾和花费大量医疗费用。为了根除神经管闭合不全，我们必须花大量精力从细胞学、分子学等方面研究神经管形成的机制。

胚胎学

通过对大量的人类胚胎和动物胚胎如鸡、鼠等的研究，我们已经弄清楚人类正常神经管发育的大部分机制。原始神经胚形成有 4 个空间和时间上相互重叠的阶段：(1) 神经板的产生，(2) 神经板的成形，(3) 神经板的弯曲，(4) 神经皱襞的融合（图 124-2A 至 E）[126,132]。

神经板形成出现在胚胎发生的早期，此时脊索中胚层/嘴侧内胚层诱导表面的外胚层增厚，局部增厚的外胚层形成由假柱状上皮细胞组成的扁平状神经板。随后，扁平状神经板开始变形，头尾侧伸长，中间二侧变窄，尖底进一步增厚（图 124-3A 至 E），这一变化使得扁平神经板随后弯曲成长管形而非球囊形结构。

神经板弯曲开始于神经板成形期间并涉及 3 个形态发生期的关键阶段：(1) 绞合点的形成，(2) 神经皱襞的形成，(3) 神经板的折叠（图 124-4）[132]。神经板的弯曲以 1 个中间绞合点（MHP）和 2 个背外侧绞合点（DLHP）的形成而开始[127]。每个绞合点组成了神经板的局部，并连接、固定于相邻组织（即前脑下方的脊索前板中胚层和脊索尾侧形成中间绞合点，表皮外胚层向两侧形成背侧绞合点），同时形成了一条纵形的沟（图 124-2C，2E）。在绞合点内的神经板沟的产生是神经上皮细胞形状改变的结果。在中间绞合点或未来的神经管顶板，神经中央板固定到前脑底层的脊索前板中胚层和更尾侧的脊索。这些组织相互诱导、交互，导致中央神经上皮细胞变短，形成楔状[131]。脊索诱导的中央神经上皮细胞又导致了中央纵沟的形成。同样地，在成对的背外侧绞合点，背外侧神经板固定到双侧神经皱襞的表皮样外胚层上，背
外侧神经上皮细胞呈楔形样改变，导致背外侧纵沟的 1989
形成。接着当每侧神经板侧缘的基底膜开始附着在相邻的表皮外胚层中间的基底膜时，最后与绞合点形成有时间和空间关联的神经板折叠包括神经皱襞的上升和汇合。

中间绞合点形成后，其每侧的神经板侧面无沟部分向背侧提升，并沿神经沟纵轴旋转，集中于中央沟，形成了初始的神经皱襞和外圈神经沟（即在神经皱襞的上升过程中，神经板呈 V 型延长）。在未来的脑水平，神经皱襞（即神经板侧缘的双薄层外胚层结

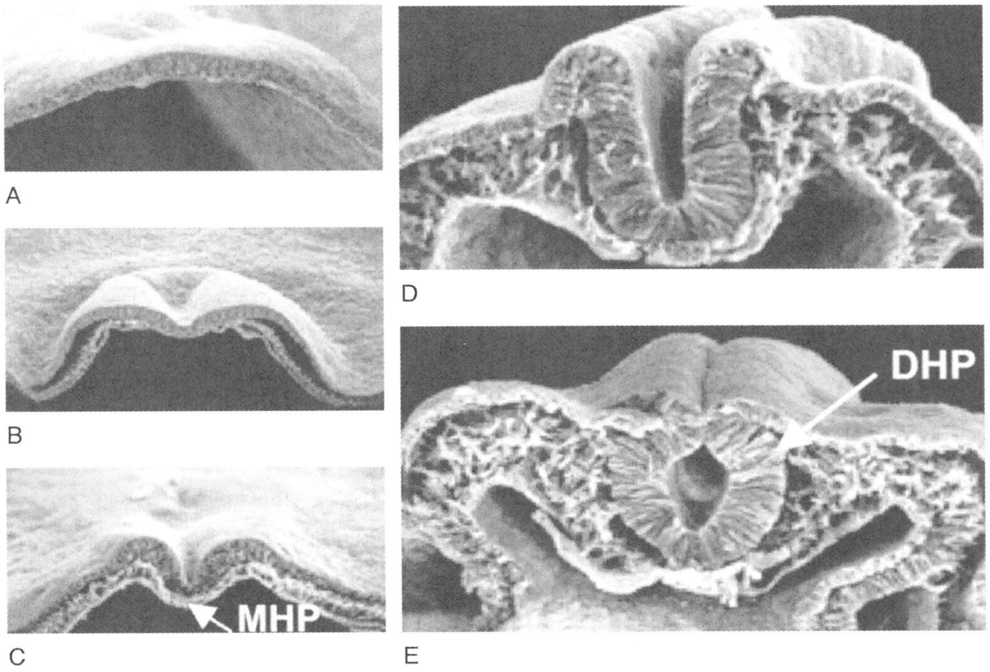

图 124-2　A 至 E. 鸡胚胎横断面电子显微镜扫描显示第一阶段神经胚形成的四期—神经板的产生、成形和弯曲以及神经皱襞的融合。在神经胚形成的第一阶段，神经管即中枢神经系统的前体是由外胚层扁平神经板发展而来。MHP，中间绞合点；DHP，背侧绞合点。（Adapted from Smith JL, Schoenwolf GC: Neurulation: Coming to closure. Trends Neurosci 1997; 20:510.）

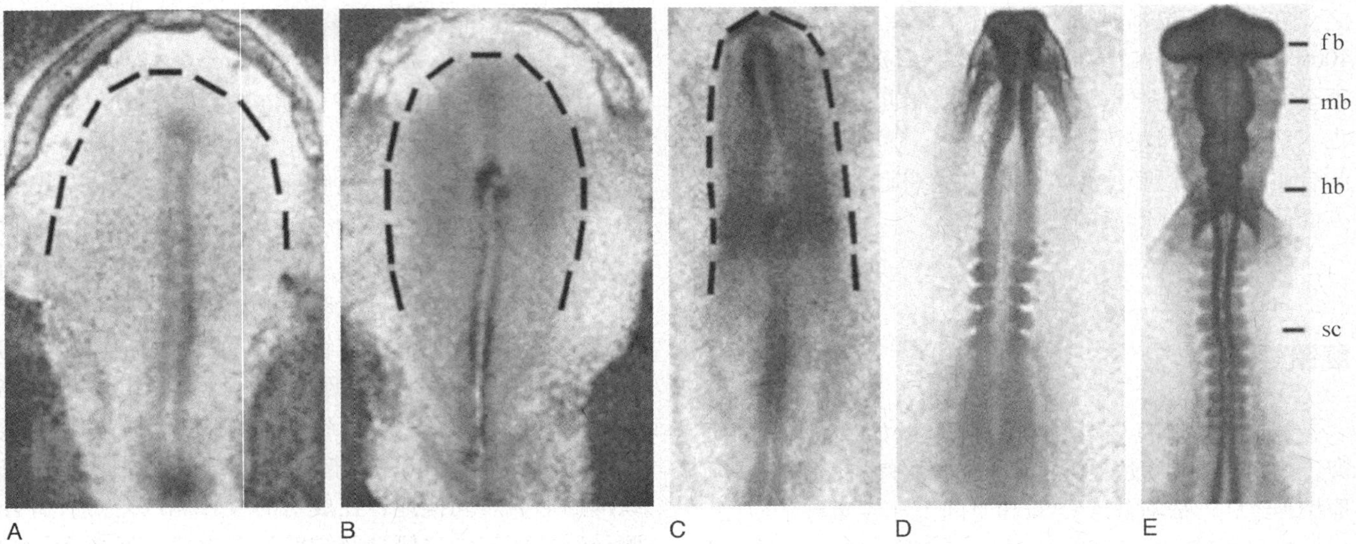

图 124-3 在 Hamburger 和 Hamilton 4 到 10 + 期[54]，光镜显示的鸡胚胎背侧观。A. 扁平神经板（4 期）形成的初期。B. 有脊索的扁平神经管（头期，5 期）。C. 神经袖套期（6 期）显示头尾侧伸长和中外侧变窄这一神经板成形的特征。A 到 C 的虚线显示神经板头侧的近端边界。D. 初始的神经管（8 + 期）。E. 神经管的定形（10 + 期）。fb，前脑；hb，后脑；mb，中脑；sc，脊髓。（Adapted from Smith JL，Schoenwolf GC：Neurulation：Coming to closure. Trends Neurosci 1997；20:510.）

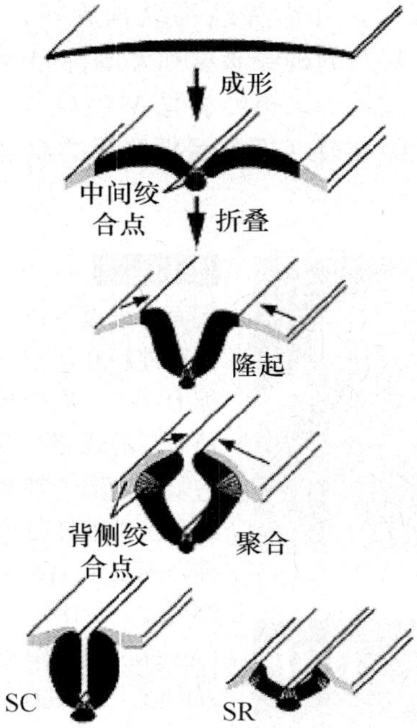

图 124-4 示意图显示第一阶段在未来的中脑/后脑水平神经管形成的主要形态学发生情况，以及脊髓（SC）及其长菱形窦道（SR）水平的不同形态学改变。（Adapted from Smith JL，Schoenwolf GC：Neurulation：Coming to closure. Trends Neurosci 1997；20:510.）

构，每侧都由神经上皮的内层及表皮外胚层的外层组成）朝背侧中线会合，各自沿纵轴旋转集中于对应的背外侧沟。神经皱襞在背侧近中线处因互相会合而完成靠近。相反，在未来的脊髓上，当神经皱襞形成时神经板背侧附着在相邻的表皮外胚层上，但背外侧神经上皮细胞没有变成楔形，从而使得背外侧沟无法形成。结果，当神经皱襞上升时，每侧神经板的一半对合，导致神经管内腔暂时性闭塞。最后，在尾侧神经孔闭合区域的菱形窦水平，神经板皱襞折叠，就像在未来的脑水平一样，这一过程包括中间绞合点和成对的背侧绞合点的形成，在绞合点周围神经皱襞分别上升会合。当神经皱襞在背侧中线融合时，神经沟及头端、尾端的神经孔闭合。当神经管顶板、相关的神经嵴和上面的表皮外胚层（或表皮）形成时，这一过程结束。

人类的神经板在排卵后 16 天就可以看见，此时假柱状上皮在中线处连接到其下方的脊索上。在侧面，神经上皮靠近表皮外胚层的鳞状上皮。排卵后 17～19 天，可以看到中线处的神经沟；排卵后 19～21 天，可以看到侧侧相连的神经皱襞。此时神经皱襞上升，在背侧中线处会合，神经沟也闭合，形成神经管。起初神经皱襞在尾侧后脑或颅脊髓处融合。整个神经沟和头、尾侧神经孔的闭合在 4～6 天内完成，尾侧神经孔在排卵后 25～27 天闭合。

多年以来，神经胚形成被视为简单的、由内在力量控制的、全或无的过程，其中神经板或者向上卷曲成管状或者不向上卷曲。此外，通过顶微丝的收缩，神经上皮细胞从柱状变成楔形，这被认为是神经板变化的内在力量。然而最新的研究进展告诉我们这种传统的神经胚形成观点是错误的。神经胚形成是一个高度复杂的、多因素过程，不仅需要来自神经上皮细胞的内在力量，也需要由表皮外胚层细胞产生的外在力量，内外力量结合起作用[126,132]。

“神经胚形成多因素模型”已被用来解释由基础细胞行为产生的引起形态改变的内在和外在力量，例如神经胚形成使扁平的假复层外胚层细胞即神经板转变为成人中枢神经系统的前体即长形神经管[132]，这一过程中存在细胞形状、位置、数量的改变以及相互影响。根据这一模型，由拉长的、重新排列的和非随机头尾侧分割的神经上皮细胞产生的内在力量控制着神经胚的形状，由神经上皮细胞楔入产生的内在力量控制着神经板皱起。外在力量是由表皮外胚层细胞形状改变而产生的，即由低的立方形变成鳞状，也可由表皮外胚层细胞由尾侧向中间会合延伸的重新排列产生，以及由从头侧到尾侧、从中间向两侧的细胞非随机导向性分裂而产生。这种表皮外胚层细胞行为的变化控制着表皮外胚层头尾侧的伸长以及中间表皮外胚层的扩张，最终控制着神经皱襞上升、会合和融合。

流行病学

脊柱裂的发病率为 1‰～2‰，由于遗传的因素，在某些人群中发病率更高。其在全球的发病率存在明显差异。例如在英国，发病率最高的地方主要在爱尔兰和威尔士，包括活产和死产儿在内，脊髓脊膜突出的发病率为 3‰～4‰，而无脑畸形发病率更可高达 6‰。在美国，发病率明显下降，非洲裔美国人活产儿的发病率为 0.1‰～0.4‰，而白种人群中该发病率为 1‰。

病因学

神经管缺陷如脊髓脊膜膨出的确切病因学及特定的基因仍未阐明，可能受遗传及环境多因素的影响。除了在神经胚形成阶段出现问题阻碍神经管闭合外，在神经胚形成后出现问题（如未受保护的神经系统暴露在羊水中）也能对神经管的发育及随后的神经功能产生有害作用。另外，各种致畸剂也被证明是产生神经管缺陷的原因，卡马西平、丙戊酸和叶酸缺乏是神经管缺陷的主要原因。另一方面，围孕期补充叶酸被证明能减少神经管缺陷的发生及复发[34,98]，这也证明叶酸的缺乏至少部分上是神经管缺陷的原因之一。然而，叶酸预防神经管缺陷的确切机制仍不清楚。尽管如此，1992 年 9 月美国公共卫生组织强烈推荐美国育龄期妇女在怀孕前口服叶酸每天 0.4mg，以降低胎儿产生神经管缺陷的危险。另外，若怀孕期服用丙戊酸（已知的叶酸拮抗剂），则胎儿患神经管缺陷的风险为 1%～2%。

病理

开放性神经管缺陷最常见的两种类型为囊性脊柱裂中的脊髓脊膜膨出和脊膜膨出。脊髓脊膜膨出是活产儿中最常见的 NTD，由开放的神经基板组成，并由薄层上皮细胞中间带所包绕，再依次由正常皮肤围绕（见图 124-1）。神经基板的背侧（即暴露部分）组成了外翻神经管的内侧，并与脊髓头侧的中央管相连。相反，神经板的腹侧组成了外翻神经管的外侧，这里原本应该是神经管关闭的地方。腹侧或运动神经根由基板腹侧面发出，在两侧分别由侧面向中央走行。背侧或感觉神经根在运动神经根的旁边进入基板的外围。蛛网膜囊和蛛网膜
下腔位于神经基板的下方。皮肤和硬膜之间的连接 1991
位于皮下，距皮肤边缘只有几毫米。紧贴硬膜的是硬膜外间隙，内含有脂肪。棘突是缺如的，并且棘突周围的肌肉、发育不良的椎板以及椎弓根均外翻。在多数病例中，神经基板到脊髓头侧这一段是正常的；然而，有时会伴有脊髓裂畸形（即脊髓纵裂）、动静脉畸形、表皮样囊肿或脂肪瘤。另外，多数脊髓脊膜膨出患儿伴有相关的神经系统畸形如脑积水、Chiari Ⅱ畸形以及因为骶神经根病变而引起的下肢畸形和泌尿生殖系统畸形。脊膜膨出是有皮肤覆盖的畸形，其特点为仅有硬膜从背侧骨缺损处（脊柱裂）膨出，与脊髓脊膜膨出不同的是脊髓和

神经根没有疝出到被皮肤覆盖的硬脊膜囊内，患儿通常也不合并相关的神经系统畸形。

神经管缺陷的诊断

开放性神经管缺陷如无脑畸形、脊髓脊膜膨出可在产前通过测定羊水或母亲血清的 α-甲胎蛋白（AFP）而诊断。胚胎早期的主要血清蛋白 AFP 可以从开放的神经管内漏到羊水中。产前诊断开放性神经管缺陷的第一步是在怀孕 15 和 20 周时抽取孕妇血液检测 AFP。通过孕期和 AFP 水平，可以估算开放性神经管缺陷的风险。例如怀孕 20 周的妇女，若血清 AFP 浓度超过 1000 ng/ml 就应该考虑胎儿患神经管缺陷的可能性。孕期超过 15 周时通过测定血清 AFP 水平检出开放性神经管缺陷的准确率大于 75%。若母亲血清 AFP 还不能确诊，则可检测羊水内的 AFP，其准确率可达 98%。另外，胎儿超声也可以诊断开放性神经管缺陷。有时候，有经验的超声医生甚至可以查出胎儿闭合性神经管缺陷。如果脊髓脊膜膨出的产前诊断成立，则父母会进行广泛的产前咨询并计划剖宫产分娩。

评价和治疗

新生儿脊髓脊膜膨出表现为囊性的突出物，内含神经基板及脑脊液（CSF）（见图 124-1）。出生时囊的大小取决于腹侧积聚于神经板内的脑脊液量。这些患儿可能合并有其他相关的中枢神经系统畸形，如 Chiari Ⅱ 畸形、脑积水、脊髓积水、脑干畸形、胼胝体发育不良和多小脑回畸形。出生后这些患儿需要立即进行全身体检，包括测量头围，以及评价生命力（特别是哭声和吸吮力），肛门括约肌功能，上下肢运动和感觉功能以及脊膜膨出缺损的部位、水平及大小。另外，还需评估脑积水、Chiari Ⅱ 畸形的症状和体征，以及相关的矫形方面的畸形如畸形足和脊柱后侧凸。

手术前，要求新生儿俯卧位以防囊肿破裂及外力损伤神经基板。另外，囊肿表面需用无菌生理盐水纱布覆盖，以防外露的神经组织干燥。放置静脉导管并应用抗生素。给予头颅超声或 CT 检查用以评价脑室的大小，从而决定是否需要分流手术。最初，脑室大小可以正常或轻度增大，一旦囊肿修补后，脑室常常明显增大。与脊髓脊膜膨出相关的脑积水的发生率为 80%～90%。

脊髓脊膜膨出通常都是在出生 24～48 小时内手术，除非患儿身体条件无法耐受手术或麻醉[52]。手术的目的是把神经基板关闭到椎管腔内，重建有益于神经元功能的内环境[93]。手术涉及：（1）将神经基板从中间带分离下来，重建基板并使其进入椎管，同时保护好所有神经组织；（2）在缺损边缘从硬膜外隙分离硬膜，并密闭缝合，但需给新建的神经管留下足够的硬膜下空间；（3）手术纠正明显的后凸畸形；（4）游离脊柱旁肌肉和筋膜并向中线缝合；（5）皮肤及皮下组织通常需要筋膜下四周游离减张，然后在中线处无张力缝合。

常见的术后并发症为脑脊液漏、伤口愈合不良或脊髓栓系。通过严密缝合硬膜及放置引流管治疗脑积水，脑脊液漏的发生率大为减少。可能发生伤口愈合不良，特别是对于大的脊髓脊膜膨出，可以通过患儿保持俯卧和从湿到干的敷料改变进行预防。但是，目前还没有减少脊髓脊膜膨出修补术后脊髓栓系发生的方法。

胎儿外科治疗神经管缺陷

胎内修补脊髓脊膜膨出被认为是改善神经功能的一种手段，因为有一种学说认为神经组织暴露于羊水可能会导致二次损伤和残疾，因此尽早在宫内修补脊髓脊膜膨出可以减轻甚至完全消除这种损害。另外，通过宫内关闭神经基板，阻止脑脊液渗漏，还有可能纠正一些神经管缺陷的潜在后遗症如需做分流手术的 199
脑积水和 Chiari Ⅱ 畸形。

1990—1999 年间，一家专门机构开展了一项非随机观察性研究，比较了 29 例在孕 24～30 周进行宫内脊髓脊膜膨出修补手术的胎儿和 23 例病情相当但在出生后行标准修复手术的患儿的结果，包括是否需要行腹腔分流手术、产科并发症、分娩时胎龄和出生时体重[24]。研究结果提示宫内修补术能减少后脑疝及需要行分流手术的脑积水的发病率，然而该研究还显示宫内手术增加了羊水过少的风险，并可因子宫提前收缩而需住院治疗，出现分娩提前（33.2 周比 37.0 周）以及新生儿体重较轻（2172 g 比3075 g）。

这项研究的其他问题包括样本量较小，随访期较短。

虽然已有初步证据表明宫内手术能减轻后脑疝的严重程度以及降低脑积水的发生率，但这些结论仍有待进一步证实。最近的一项研究显示与产后脊髓脊膜膨出修补术相比，在孕 20～28 周期间手术并不能显著改善下肢的功能[142]，并且还会带来因宫内手术而产生的其他风险。目前为了进一步了解宫内手术的利弊，一项关于宫内修补术与传统出生后修补术的随机调查研究正在进行[138,145]。在宫内手术的利与弊未完全阐明之前，我们不应该将宫内修补术治疗脊髓脊膜膨出视为一种优先考虑的方法并加以提倡。

相关畸形

脊髓脊膜膨出常常伴有其他中枢神经系统畸形。例如 90% 以上的脊髓脊膜膨出患儿患有 Chiari Ⅱ 畸形和脑积水。Chiari Ⅱ 畸形是一个涉及颅骨、硬膜和后脑的复杂畸形，包括颅骨凹陷、后颅窝狭小、横窦及窦汇低位、大脑镰破孔、心形天幕切迹伴小脑向上疝出、延髓纽结、嘴形顶盖、中间团块状突出、上隐窝扩大、第四脑室拉长、脊髓积水，以及小脑蚓部、第四脑室、延髓和脑桥通过枕骨大孔下移（图 124－5A～B）。
Chiari Ⅱ 畸形在新生儿期常表现为呼吸声尖锐、呼吸 1993
暂停、吞咽困难或鼻反流、哭声微弱或无、上肢或下肢（或四肢）无力或痉挛。儿童或青少年表现更为隐匿，可以是晕厥发作、眼球震颤、低位颅神经麻痹、反射亢进和四肢肌张力增高。脑核磁共振检查是最好的影像学诊断方法。

对于有症状（即脑干受压症状和体征）的 Chiari Ⅱ 畸形患儿，治疗方法采用后颅窝和（或）颈髓减压手术。这是一个有挑战性的手术，因为窦汇及横窦位置很低（即靠近枕骨大孔），小脑通常紧贴延髓并且第四脑室上下移位。在做减压手术以前，脑积水的患者必须确保分流管通畅，因为脑积水同样可以产生与 Chiari Ⅱ 畸形相似的脑干压迫症状及体征。即便分流管重度阻塞，脑室也可能没有明显扩大，CT 检查可能难以发现，因此检查分流是否通畅应当在脊髓脊膜膨出的 Chiari Ⅱ 畸形患者进行减压手术之前，通过

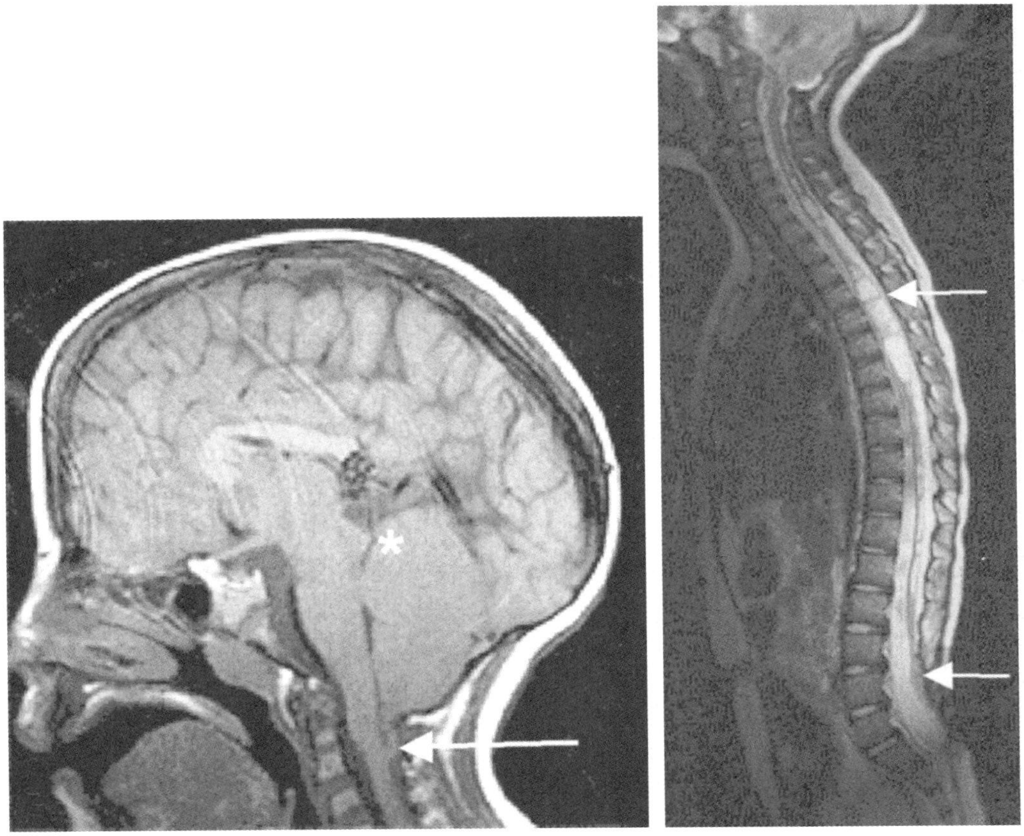

A　B

图 124－5　曾行脊髓脊膜膨出宫内修补术的 5 岁女孩。A. 矢状面脑核磁共振影像（MRI）显示 Chiari Ⅱ 畸形伴有小脑和顶盖板孔向上疝入（星头），以及小脑扁桃体向下疝入到枕骨大孔（箭头）。B. 脊柱矢状面 MRI 显示脊髓空洞从 C5 到 L2（上面的箭头）。脊髓和圆锥末端在 L4（下面的箭头）伴有脊髓栓系。

分流装置穿刺、分流装置内注射放射性核素以及分流管探查确定。

80%~95%的脊髓脊膜膨出可以合并脑积水。此类患者中脑积水的诱因可以是 Chiari Ⅱ畸形、导水管狭窄、第四脑室出口梗阻、后颅窝硬膜静脉窦受压而导致的静脉引流异常、开放性脊髓脊膜膨出伴脑脊液漏以及其他中枢神经系统畸形。治疗脑积水通常采用脑室腹膜分流手术，即将脑脊液分流到腹膜腔内再吸收。对于严重的症状性脑积水，分流手术可以与脊髓脊膜膨出修补术同时进行，也可以在修补术后几天内再次麻醉后进行，以减少感染的风险。

隐性脊柱裂——闭合性神经管缺陷

在神经胚形成的第二阶段，神经管的尾侧从尾芽开始发育，后者是由颅内原始条纹的残端分化出来的。此阶段又分为三期：（1）脊髓的形成；（2）脊髓内形成许多小的管腔；（3）这些管腔互相融合成一整条长的中央管，并由周围层呈放射状的脊髓细胞包绕[125]。当神经胚形成的第二阶段出错时，会产生闭合性神经管缺陷，即覆盖的皮肤是完好的，但尾侧的神经管及其覆盖的膜发育异常。尾侧脊髓发育异常包括隐性脊柱裂、终丝牵拉或增厚、脂肪瘤畸形（如腰骶脂肪瘤、脂肪脊髓脊膜膨出和终丝脂肪浸润）、脊髓裂畸形（即脊髓纵裂、双脊髓）、神经管原肠囊肿、皮肤窦道和骶骨发育不全/尾骨退化，这些病变都会引起脊髓栓系[153]。脊髓栓系因脊髓圆锥被牵拉，引起缺血缺氧，而导致神经功能进行性受损。

隐性脊柱裂常伴有皮肤特异性改变，这可作为判断有无脊髓栓系的标志，特别是当这些改变发生在臀沟以上区域时。这些皮肤特异性改变有腰骶多毛症（即毛发丛）、皮肤窦道、骶部皮肤小凹陷、毛细血管瘤、尾部皮赘和皮下脂肪瘤。有这些病变的患者需要做进一步检查，包括全脊柱的 MRI，寻找脊髓栓系。相反，如果皮肤特征性改变如小凹陷等在臀沟下面，多表明是一个良性病变如潜毛窦，无神经损害，不需要进一步治疗。

除了皮肤特征性改变外，脊髓栓系综合征和隐性脊柱裂的患儿常有：（1）脊髓和椎体发育畸形；（2）骨科畸形，如脊柱侧弯、下肢萎缩或不对称以及足畸形；（3）进行性神经功能减退，如下肢无力、感觉丧失、神经根病变、下肢痉挛、反射亢进以及步态异常；（4）泌尿系统功能障碍，如神经性膀胱和尿失禁；（5）排便功能障碍。另外，肛门直肠、泌尿系畸形患者的尾侧脊髓畸形及相关的脊髓栓系发生率较高，如泄殖腔外翻、残留性泄殖腔、阴茎阴囊转位、肛门闭锁以及 VATER（椎管缺损、肛门闭锁、气管食管瘘伴食管闭锁以及桡骨和肾发育不良）[154]。虽然对同时存在的泄殖腔发育及尾端脊髓畸形的解释还不清楚，但泌尿生殖系统、肛门直肠系统及末端神经管至少部分存在密切的时空上的联系。由于合并畸形及脊髓栓系的发生率很高，所以肛门直肠畸形及泌尿生殖系畸形的患者需要常规行 MRI 扫描，以评价无症状的脊髓栓系。

脊髓脂肪瘤畸形如终丝脂肪变性、脂肪脊髓脊膜膨出和脊髓脂肪瘤能引起脊髓栓系，也是需要手术治疗的闭合性神经管缺陷的最常见类型。终丝脂肪变性表现为短的、增粗的终丝部分或完全被脂肪浸润[55,72,153]。脂肪脊髓膨出表现为一个由皮肤覆盖的皮下脂肪瘤向内部延伸，通过腰骶筋膜、椎板、硬膜及软膜的缺损进入到低位的脊髓内。脊髓脂肪瘤是脂肪脊髓脊膜膨出的一种类型，包括圆锥脂肪瘤。大多 199
数脂肪瘤畸形患儿，出生时神经功能并未受损，多因为皮下脂肪瘤或者前面描述的皮肤特征性变化而前来就诊。

脊髓栓系的自然病程是神经系统进行性恶化，表现为在体重及身高的快速增长期，出现感觉、运动、直肠及膀胱功能病变[55]。因而，早期预防性脊髓栓系松解手术适用于所有患者，用以稳定神经功能，预防不可恢复的神经损伤。手术采用显微外科技术，术中运用肛门括约肌肌电图及体表感觉诱发电位监测神经功能，通过术中刺激神经根以鉴别功能性和非功能性神经根。对于终丝脂肪变性，手术采用后路正中切口，L4~L5 或 L5~S1 部分椎体切除，于中线剪开硬脊膜，暴露终丝。电刺激终丝，确认无神经功能后切下一小段终丝并送病理检查。对于脂肪脊髓脊膜膨出或脊髓脂肪瘤，手术方法包括从腰骶部筋膜缺损处将皮下脂肪瘤与脊髓或终丝脂肪瘤分离，没有必要完全切除皮下脂肪瘤，因为这会使表面的皮肤缺血，影响伤口愈合[72]。接着，在椎管缺损的头端切开椎板，以暴露正常解剖结构，然后小心地逐步从头向尾分离至切除脂肪瘤并进入椎管腔处，接下来的步骤如下：（1）将圆锥从其附着的脂肪瘤、软脊膜及硬脊膜上分离下来；（2）用激光刀或超声吸引器缩减髓内脂肪团块，以减轻脊髓和圆锥的压力；（3）切断终丝；

（4）扩大、密闭缝合硬膜；（5）严密缝合脊柱旁肌肉、腰骶筋膜及皮肤。手术相关的并发症包括麻醉风险、神经功能和（或）泌尿系统功能恶化、脑脊液漏和感染。

其他类型的隐性脊柱裂包括脊髓裂畸形（即脊髓纵裂）、皮肤窦道和神经管原肠囊肿。在脊髓裂畸形中，脊髓在矢状面一分为二，每半个脊髓拥有各自分开的硬脊膜囊（Ⅱ型）或共同拥有同一个硬脊膜囊（Ⅰ型）[107]。脊髓裂畸形的表面皮肤具有典型的毛发丛样特征。在Ⅱ型，增粗的终丝或（和）中线处的骨嵴形成了脊髓栓系；在Ⅰ型，硬脊膜和半脊髓之间的纤维隔膜或束带造成脊髓栓系。为了预防神经和泌尿功能损伤，需要行脊髓栓系松解手术，即切除中线处的骨嵴或切除硬脊膜和半脊髓之间的纤维束带及隔膜，以及切断终丝。

儿童的皮肤窦道通常表现为皮肤特征性变化、神经功能受损、感染或化学性脊膜炎或合并有上述各种表现[1,45]。皮肤窦道为神经管未完全闭合的残留物，表层外胚层和皮肤附属器与神经外胚层完全分离断开失败，使得从皮肤的开口到筋膜、硬膜或脊髓之间留有一个衬有上皮细胞的管道[107]。皮肤窦道在神经轴中线处的任何地方均可发生，可伴有脑脊液流出、硬膜内皮样囊肿或表皮样囊肿、脊髓裂畸形和脊髓栓系。相关的皮肤病变可发生在臀沟以上神经中轴上，包括皮肤小凹、毛细血管瘤、毛发丛、皮赘和皮下脂肪瘤。在皮肤小凹处，可能有囊内容物或脑脊液流出或局部感染的征象，如红斑或硬结。MRI 是可供选择的神经影像学诊断工具，因为它能显示皮肤窦道以及相关的病理表现，如脊髓栓系、肿瘤、瘘管或脊髓裂畸形。然而，对于某些小的或不在扫描切面上的皮肤窦道，则 MRI 难以发现[1]。所以，对于臀沟上方神经中轴处的皮肤特征性病变，即使 MRI 未发现异常，也需要手术探查。手术包括完全切除皮肤小凹和窦道、硬膜内探查、完全切除任何连接到硬膜内的连接物或肿块、解除脊髓栓系。及时的诊断和适当的硬膜内探查手术是预防感染（包括脊膜炎）、保护或改善神经功能的保证。

椎管内神经管原肠囊肿是少见的先天性畸形，内附有消化道黏膜[153]。此病变的发生是由于原始外胚层和内胚层持续的异常连接，常伴有椎体畸形和其他形式的隐性脊柱裂如脊髓裂畸形、脂肪瘤、皮肤窦道和脊髓栓系。椎管内神经管原肠囊肿的患者可有皮肤特征性改变或脊髓压迫症状，如疼痛和神经功能障碍。治疗方法为囊肿完全切除以及其他相关畸形的手术，包括脊髓栓系松解手术。要求做到肉眼完全切除，因为次全切除的复发率很高[115]。

做过脊髓栓系松解手术的隐性脊柱裂和脊髓栓系患者，若出现神经功能或泌尿功能进行性恶化，则预示着脊髓栓系的复发，其复发率可达 15%[73]。所以，长期的神经和泌尿功能随访能保证脊髓再栓系的患者得到及时手术。

结果和预后 1995

对神经管缺陷的治疗已有 50 年的历史。以前，新生儿患有神经管缺陷时或者暂时不予治疗，或者给予选择性手术，结果大多数患儿死于脑膜炎、脑积水、脓毒血症或这三种疾病的任意组合。然而，在近 30 年内，几乎在所有的美国儿童医疗中心都能对有神经管缺陷的新生儿给予及时积极的治疗，包括开放性神经管缺陷的早期手术关闭和早期分流手术治疗脑积水，这些措施使得绝大多数的患儿智力基本正常。

开放性神经管缺陷的初期闭合手术只是治疗的第一步。一般说来，这些患儿还需要长期、定期地到医疗机构接受随访，在那里，需要有一个由儿童保健科、神经外科、泌尿科、矫形外科的儿科医生以及理疗师、康复师、职业治疗师、护士和营养师组成的团队为患儿诊治。这个团队是患儿得到长期治疗并最终取得良好结果的保证。经过适当的治疗，这些患儿能够像正常人一样生活以及繁衍后代。例如，近期有一篇 20～25 年的随访研究报道，神经管缺陷患儿经过及时手术和长期治疗，都已进入大学读书，很多患者已经有了合适的工作[21]。经过积极的治疗和多学科协作，患儿长期存活至成年和老年的现象已非常普遍。

神经外科医生必须时刻警惕脊髓脊膜膨出的患儿及成人神经功能恶化。神经变性的最常见原因除分流功能障碍外，还有产生症状的脊髓栓系。几乎所有脊髓脊膜膨出的脊髓都是低位的，末端位于腰部或骶部区域。患者可以没有任何新的神经方面的不适主诉。然而，尽管经受了精细手术，关闭了闭合不全的神经管，但仍有至少 20% 的脊髓脊膜膨出患者会出现有症状的脊髓栓系。这些患者在随访中通常出现一个或多个症状或体征：步履艰难、背部疼痛、下肢无力、感觉丧失、新的足畸形出现、尿流动力学指标的改变或尿失禁。当出现一个或多个这些症状或体征时，对于同时伴有脑积水的患者，必须先评价分流功能。当确定分流管功能正常后，考虑行脊髓栓系松解手术，将神经板和神经根从背侧硬膜上游离下来，解除脊髓栓系。但是，对于常规术后 MRI 检查显示有脊髓栓系而没有症状的患者，暂不考虑再次手术。

脑积水

脑积水是儿科常见疾病，因脑脊液容量过多导致脑室扩大、皮层变薄（图 124-6A 和 B）和颅内压升高（ICP）。先天性脑积水的发病率为 0.9‰～1.8‰[81]，每年死亡率约为 1%。治疗方法为脑脊液分流手术，包括有阀门调节的置管脑脊液分流手术以及内镜第三脑室造瘘术，目的是预防因颅内压升高而造成的神经损害。脑积水的及时治疗能改善患儿智力，有效延长生命。

脑积水是由于脑脊液的产生与吸收失平衡而造成的，多数情况下是由于脑脊液吸收功能障碍所引起。只有脉络丛乳头状瘤例外，这种患者的脑积水至少部分是由于脑脊液分泌过多而引起。脑脊液容量增加继发于脑脊液吸收功能损伤和（或）脑脊液产生过多，
1996 进而导致脑室进行性扩张。在部分儿童中，脑脊液可通过旁路吸收，从而使得脑室不再进行性扩大，形成静止性或代偿性脑积水。一份详细的有关未手术的脑积水自然病程的分析资料显示，45% 以上脑积水患儿的脑室不进行性扩大[79]。儿童代偿性脑积水不需要行脑脊液分流手术，然而在某些情况下，如发热和感染，能打破平衡，引起失代偿，使得颅内压增高。因而，对于不需要分流手术的代偿性脑积水，必须密切监测可能发生的失代偿的症状和体征，如头痛、呕吐、共济失调和视觉症状。

脑脊液的形成是一个能量依赖性的、颅内压力非依赖性的过程，每天约产生 450ml，或每分钟产生 0.3ml。侧脑室、第三脑室和第四脑室里的脉络丛产生 50%～80% 的脑脊液，其余 20%～50% 的脑脊液由脑室的室管膜和脑实质作为脑的代谢产物而产生。脑脊液的流向是从头端向尾端，流经脑室系统，从 Luschka 孔和 Magendie 孔流出，进入脑皮层和脊髓的蛛网膜下腔。之后脑脊液再穿过天幕切迹，通过大脑半球凸面，最后被蛛网膜颗粒吸收入静脉系统。

与脑脊液的形成相反，脑脊液的吸收是能量非依赖性的过程，以大流量的方式进入位于蛛网膜下腔和硬膜内静脉窦之间的蛛网膜颗粒内。脑脊液的吸收依赖于从蛛网膜下腔通过蛛网膜颗粒到硬膜静脉窦之间的压力梯度。当颅内压力正常时（即 $<7\ cmH_2O$ 或 5 mmHg），脑脊液以 0.3ml/min 的速率产生，此时脑脊液还没有开始吸收。当颅内压增高时，脑脊液开始吸收，其吸收率与颅内压成正比。此外，还有其他一

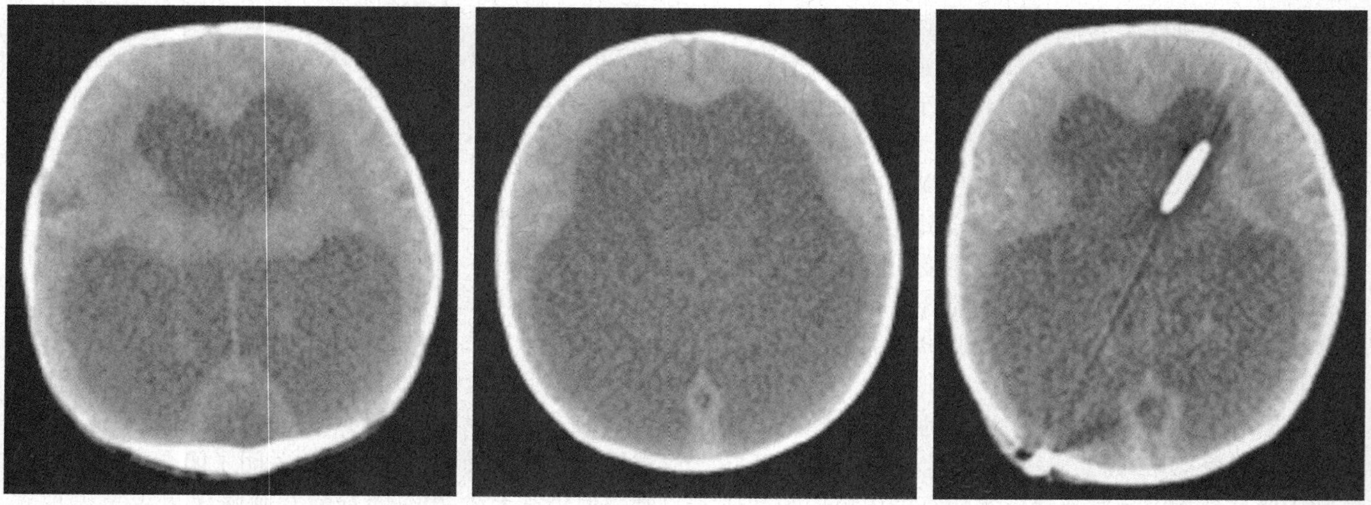

A B C

图 124-6 出生 5 天的女婴患有先天性导水管狭窄引起的重度阻塞性脑积水。A 和 B. 头部 CT 显示脑室重度扩张。C. 头部 CT 显示分流管放置术后 1 天。

些可能存在的脑脊液吸收途径，如淋巴系统、鼻黏膜、鼻旁窦以及颅内和脊神经的神经根鞘，当颅内压升高时，它们也可能参与脑脊液的吸收，但是目前尚缺乏这些吸收途径的确切证据。

脑室通路的阻塞或者吸收障碍使得脑室内压增高，梗阻近端以上的脑室进行性扩张。其病理表现为脑室扩张，通常以枕角最先扩张，皮层变薄，室管膜破裂，脑脊液渗入到脑室旁的白质内，白质受损以及瘢痕增生，颅内压升高，脑疝，昏迷，最终死亡。

病因学

脑积水的病因学是根据阻塞的部位而定的。如果阻塞部位在蛛网膜颗粒以上，则阻塞部位以上的脑室选择性扩大，此时称阻塞性脑积水或非交通性脑积水。例如，导水管阻塞引起侧脑室和第三脑室扩大，并与第四脑室不成比例。相反，如果是蛛网膜颗粒水平阻塞，引起脑脊液吸收障碍，则侧脑室、第三脑室和第四脑室均扩张，蛛网膜下腔脑脊液容量增多，此时的脑积水称为非阻塞性脑积水或交通性脑积水。脑积水不包括脑萎缩引起的脑室扩大，此时的脑积水不是真正的脑积水。

脑积水的阻塞部位可以在室间孔，常见原因有先天性的狭窄或闭锁，颅内囊肿如蛛网膜下腔或脑室内的蛛网膜囊肿、邻近脑室的脑穿通性囊肿和胶样囊肿，肿瘤如下丘脑胶质瘤、颅咽管瘤和室管膜下巨细胞性星形细胞瘤，以及血管畸形。阻塞部位在导水管水平是另外一种常见的阻塞性脑积水（见图 124-6A 和 B）。导水管阻塞的原因包括脊髓脊膜膨出和相关 Chiari Ⅱ畸形患者的小脑向上通过小脑幕切迹疝出、Galen 静脉血管畸形、炎症或出血引起的导水管处神经胶质增生、松果体区肿瘤和顶盖胶质瘤。另外，阻塞性脑积水还可以由以下原因引起：由第四脑室和后颅窝肿瘤导致的脑室流出道梗阻，如髓母细胞瘤、室管膜瘤和毛细胞性星形细胞瘤；Dandy-Walker 综合征，即后颅窝有一个大的与扩大的第四脑室相通的囊肿造成了流出道梗阻（即 Luschka 侧孔和 Magendie 正中孔的梗阻）；以及 Chiari Ⅱ畸形，即由于后颅窝狭小，第四脑室疝入到枕骨大孔引起梗阻。

对于交通性或非阻塞性脑积水，梗阻部位可以发生在基底池水平。此时，脑脊液在椎管和脑皮层的蛛网膜下腔之间受阻，无法到达蛛网膜颗粒从而被吸收。结果，侧脑室、第三脑室和第四脑室均扩大。常见原因有先天性感染，化脓性、结核性和真菌性感染引起的脑膜炎，动脉瘤破裂、血管畸形或外伤引起的蛛网膜下腔出血，早产儿脑室内出血伴胚层出血，基底蛛网膜炎，软脑脊膜癌病，神经类肉瘤病和使脑脊液蛋白水平升高的肿瘤。梗阻部位还可以发生在蛛网膜颗粒水平，原因是蛛网膜颗粒的阻塞或闭锁，导致
蛛网膜下腔和脑室扩大。另外，梗阻部位还可以发生 1997
在硬膜静脉窦水平，其原因为静脉流出梗阻。这种梗阻可见于存在颈静脉孔狭窄的软骨发育不全或多骨缝闭合的狭颅症患者、先天性心脏病右心房压力增高患者，以及硬膜静脉窦或上腔静脉血栓的患者。静脉流出道梗阻能引起静脉压升高，最终导致脑皮层静脉引流减少、脑血流量增加、颅内压升高、脑僵硬度增加、脑脊液吸收减少。在婴儿，由于前囟和颅缝未闭，静脉压升高和脑脊液吸收减少导致婴儿头围增大，伴有颅缝分裂以及脑室增大。相反，若颅缝和前囟已闭，升高的静脉压使静脉怒张，导致颅内压升高，此时，患者尽管存在脑脊液吸收减少，仍有脑室系统受压，产生假性脑瘤的临床表现。

严重脑积水表现为脑室极度扩张而脑皮层菲薄，脑电图出现背景皮层活动贯穿全脑，在脑脊液分流术后受压的大脑皮层至少有部分可以得到恢复（见图 124-6A 和 B）。相反，积水性无脑畸形是由于受两侧大脑前动脉和大脑中动脉供血的脑组织全部或几乎全部缺失，从而使颅腔内充满了脑脊液，而非脑组织（图 124-7A 和 B）。颅腔的形态和硬膜仍旧完好，内含有丘脑、脑干和少量的由大脑后动脉供血的枕叶。双侧的颈内动脉阻塞和感染是积水性无脑畸形的最常见原因。脑电图表现为皮层活动消失。这类患儿过于易激惹，停留在原始反射，哭吵、吸吮力弱，语音及微笑落后。脑脊液分流手术有可能控制进行性扩大的头围，但对于神经功能的改善没有帮助。

临床表现

婴儿脑积水表现为易激惹、昏睡、生长发育落后、呼吸暂停、心动过缓、反射亢进、肌张力增高、头围进行性增大、前囟饱满、骨缝裂开、头皮薄、头皮静脉曲张、前额隆起、上眼睑不下垂及眼球向上运动障

图 124-7 患有脑积水的出生 2 天的女婴。A. 显示上矢状窦（箭头）和少量的右颞下极及枕部皮层（三角箭头）。B. 刚出生后的头部 CT 扫描见少量的右后侧脑皮层（箭头）。整个大脑半球几乎被脑脊液取代。

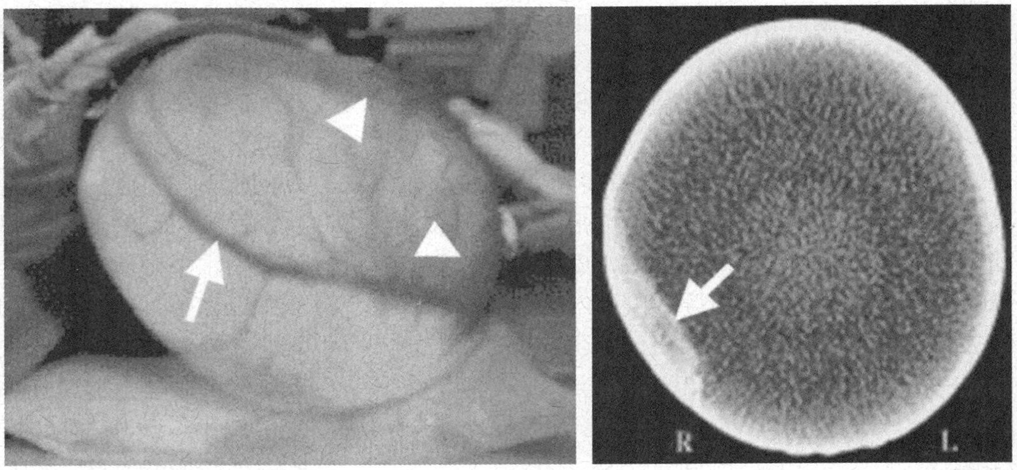

A B

碍（即顶盖受压导致的两眼“落日征”）、意识减退、视盘水肿以及第三、第四、第六对颅神经麻痹。在儿童，由于颅缝已经闭合，脑积水可以表现为头痛（尤其在早晨）、恶心、呕吐、昏睡、视盘水肿、视力下降、认知功能和行为能力下降、记忆障碍、注意力减退、学习成绩下降、步态改变、双眼不能上视、复视（特别是第六对颅神经麻痹）和抽搐。

脑积水的影像学特征

脑积水的颅骨平片常常显示破壶样外观和冠状缝裂开。CT 和 MRI 常可见颞角扩张，脑沟、基底池和大脑半球间裂消失，额角和第三脑室球形扩张，胼胝体上拱和（或）萎缩以及与脑脊液经室管膜吸收有关的脑室周围水肿。

良性脑外积水（也称婴儿良性轴外积液）是一个很少需要手术的疾病，其特征为双侧前方蛛网膜下腔（如脑沟和脑池）扩大，脑室正常或轻度扩大，前囟搏动明显，头围进行性扩大，超过正常儿头围的
1998 百分线。良性脑外积水的婴儿由于头围大，运动发育可能轻度落后。其发病机制尚未清楚，可能与脑脊液吸收不良有关。通常有明显的大头家族史。大约在 12~18 个月龄，扩大的头围趋于稳定，从而使得身体的生长能够赶上头围的生长。大约到 2 岁，脑积水自然缓解，不需要分流手术。虽然这一疾病通常不需要手术，但是有必要密切监测患儿的头围、头部 CT 或超声以评价异常扩大的脑室。

处理

治疗的目的是获得理想的神经功能，预防或恢复因脑室扩大压迫脑组织引起的神经损伤。最好的结果是手术后大脑皮质厚度恢复至少在 2.8 cm 以上[166]。患有脑积水的婴儿在出生后 5 个月内做分流手术，则达到这一理想结果的可能性较大。

脑积水的治疗方法是手术，手术方式的选择依赖于脑积水的原因。例如，对于阻塞性脑积水的患儿，手术方法是去除阻塞（如肿瘤）；对于交通性脑积水的患儿或阻塞性脑积水而阻塞部位无法手术去除的患儿，需要做脑脊液分流手术，分流管的一端放置在脑室内分泌脑脊液且接近梗阻处的部位，另一端放置在远处可以再吸收脑脊液的地方。最常用的远端部位是腹腔、右心房、胸膜腔、胆囊、膀胱/输尿管和基底池（即第三脑室造瘘），而腹腔是目前选择最多的部位（即脑室腹腔分流术），除非存在腹腔脓肿或吸收障碍。当腹腔有病变时，如手术后广泛的腹腔粘连、腹膜炎、病理性肥胖和早产儿坏死性小肠结肠炎，脑室心房分流术是另外一种可以选择的方法。如果腹腔和心房都不能利用，那么对于 7 岁以上的患儿，还可以选择脑室胸腔分流术。

脑脊液分流系统至少包括三个组成部分：脑室端管，通常放置在侧脑室的枕角或额角（见图 124-6C）；远端管，用来将脑脊液引流到远端可以被吸收的地方；以及阀门。传统的调压管通过打开一个固定的调压装置来调节脑脊液单向流动。这种压力调节取决于阀门的性质，一般分为低压、中压和高压（典型的分别为

5、10 和 15 cmH_2O）。一旦阀门打开，对脑脊液流动产生一个很小的阻力，结果，当直立位时，由于地心引力的作用，可以产生一个很高的脑脊液流出率，造成很大的颅内负压，此过程称为“虹吸现象”。

由于虹吸可以造成脑室裂隙现象，极大地增加了脑室端分流管阻塞的可能性，因此，某些分流管被设计成能限制脑脊液过度流出的结构，尤其是当直立位时[152]。例如，Delta 阀（Medtronic PS Medical，Goleta，CA）就是一种标准的振动膜型的压力调节阀，内有抗虹吸装置，用来减少直立位时脑脊液的过度分流。Orbis-Sigma 阀（Cordis，Miami）包含一个可变阻力的流量控制元件，当压力进行性升高时，通过不断缩小流出孔达到控制脑脊液过度分流的目的。虽然这些新的阀门被誉为预防过度分流、增进治疗效果的有效装置，然而，最近的随机调查在比较了 3 种分流装置（即普通的可调压阀、Delta 阀和 Orbis-Sigma 阀）治疗儿童脑积水的效果后发现，这 3 种分流装置在分流手术的失败率方面并没有显著性差异。最近又出现两种可编程的调压管，当此种分流管被埋入体内后，仍可在体外重新设置压力，此种分流管被广泛地应用在小儿脑积水上。虽然有大量的各种类型的分流管用于治疗脑积水，但是至今还没有前瞻性的随机双盲多中心的试验证明哪一种分流管比其他分流管更有效。

脑室腹腔分流术是儿童脑积水脑脊液分流的首选方法。手术在气管插管全身麻醉下进行，手术前静脉预防性应用抗生素。抗生素预防性应用的效果已经被证实，并给出了推荐的抗生素种类[41,78]。将患者放置在手术床头端边缘，靠近手术者，头部放在凝胶垫圈上，偏向置管侧的对侧，用凝胶卷垫在肩膀下，使头颈和躯干拉直，以利于建立皮下隧道置管。皮肤准备前，先用记号笔根据脑室端钻骨孔置管的位置（如额部或枕部）描出头皮切口，在仔细的皮肤准备后，再用笔将皮肤切口重新涂描一遍。腹部切口通常在右上腹或腹中线剑突下 2～3 横指距离。铺无菌巾后贴含碘贴膜，在骨孔周边切开一弧形切口，掀开皮瓣，切开骨膜，颅骨钻孔，电凝并打开硬脑膜、蛛网膜和软脑膜。

接着，切开腹部切口，打开进入腹腔的通道，轻柔地探查证实已进入腹腔。用皮下通条在头部与腹部切口之间打一皮下通道。在即将放置分流装置之前才将其从消毒盒中取出，并浸泡在抗生素溶液中，准备安装入人体内。分流管远端装置包括阀门穿过皮下隧道并放置在隧道内，隧道外管道用浸泡过抗生素的纱布包裹，避免与皮肤接触。接着，脑室段分流管通过探针置入脑室，也可在超声和（或）脑室镜的引导下，将分流管精确地插入到脑室内理想的位置。脑室镜还能穿破脑室内的隔膜，使脑脊液互相流通。

一旦分流管插入脑室并有脑脊液流出，就根据术前头部 CT 测得的数据，将分流管剪成需要的长度，与分流系统的远端装置连接，再用 2-0 或 3-0 线打结，固定接口。然后，提起远端分流管，证实有脑脊液流出后，将管毫无阻力地放入到腹腔内。抗生素溶液冲洗伤口后，两层缝合伤口。伤口要求仔细对合，严密缝合，最后用无菌纱布覆盖。

大多数安置了分流管的患儿将长期依赖于分流管，因此，这些患儿需要长期随访以确定分流管工作正常，因为分流障碍的发生率还是相当高的。例如，一项关于 1719 例儿童脑积水分流手术的回顾性调查发现[122]，手术后 10 年分流障碍发生的可能性为 70%，远远高于术后近期分率障碍的发生率（即术后第一年的发生率为 30%，以后每年 2%～5% 递增）。另外，术后 10 年感染的发生率为 9%，并且分流障碍发生的时间因原因不同而各不相同。其他研究报道小儿脑积水分流术后第一年分流障碍发生率为 40%[16,111]。另外一项有关分流阀门设计的随机调查报道[40]，在一所每年有很多脑积水分流手术的医疗中心，由富有经验的小儿神经外科医生操作，第一年分流障碍的发生率为 40%，第二年为 60%，感染的发生率为 8%。

脑脊液分流障碍主要有以下三方面原因：（1）机械故障，（2）感染，（3）过度分流或分流不足（即功能障碍）。近端阻塞（即脑室端管道阻塞）是分流管机械故障的最常见原因[122]。其他原因包括分流管远端的阻塞或分流装置其他部位的阻塞（如抗虹吸装置的阻塞）；由腹腔炎症引起腹腔假性囊肿的形成，导致腹腔端管道阻塞；腹腔内脑脊液重吸收障碍引起的腹水；分流管折断；分流管接口脱落；分流管移位；远端分流管长度不够；近端或远端管道位置放置不妥当；感染；过度分流，可导致硬膜下积液、脑室裂隙、颅缝早闭或脑压过低。Sainte-Rose 及其同事的研究发现[122]，2/3 的分流障碍起因于分流管阻塞或折断，阻塞导致的分流障碍占 56.1%，而折断部位几乎总是发生在连接器部位。另外，他们还发现，由分流管近端阻塞引起的分流障碍在脑室裂隙患者中的发生率明显高于具有正常或扩大脑室患者的发生率，并且腹腔段末端为裂隙状的管道阻塞的发生率也明显高于末端为开口状的管道。

再次分流失败在儿童中很常见，可引起很多并发症，少数还可能引起死亡。一项关于儿童反复分流障碍危险因素的前瞻性单机构观察性研究显示，第一次分流手术的时间很关键，如果第二次分流修复术距离第一次分流管安置术的时间不到 6 个月，则分流障碍发生的危险性很高。患儿第一次接受脑积水分流手术时的年龄也是分流障碍的主要危险因素，小于 40 周以及 40 周和 1 岁之间做脑积水分流手术的患儿分流障碍的发生率要高于大于 1 岁时手术的患儿。脑室内出血、脑膜炎和肿瘤引起的脑积水也容易引起分流障碍反复发作。患儿在做分流手术同时再接受其他手术，也会增加分流障碍的机会。

大多数分流障碍的诊断是很容易的，因为患儿有急性颅内压升高的明显症状和体征，如烦躁、头痛、呕吐和昏睡，如果不及时手术，会很快发展成昏迷和死亡。Sainte-Rose 及其同事报道[122]，1.05% 的死亡直接与分流障碍有关。也有些分流障碍的儿童会出现一些更为微妙的变化，如学习成绩退步、注意力不集中或行为改变。这些微妙的变化说明患儿脑室正随着时间延长而逐渐扩大，并且可能在发作时明显扩大。相反，急性恶化常常仅有脑室的轻度扩大。当怀疑有分流障碍时，需做头部 CT 扫描，并与以前正常时的头部 CT 扫描相比较，以判断脑室是否扩大。同时还需对管道系统进行检查以判断分流管接口是否脱落、脑室内以及整个分流管的位置、远端分流管的长度。

一旦怀疑有分流障碍，必须确定出现障碍的部
2000 位，最常见的原因是脑室端导管被脉络丛、胶质、结缔组织、软脑膜、室管膜或脑组织（或上述组织的任意组合）阻塞，特别在裂隙样脑室中更易发生[122]。近端分流管阻塞会出现颅内压急剧升高，需要急诊行分流管更换手术。为了减少近端分流管阻塞的发生率，外科医生利用头颅解剖标志，将分流管放入室间孔前方的侧脑室前角或枕角以避免被脉络丛包绕[122]。自从 20 世纪 90 年代早期纤维内镜开始应用以来，外科医生为了避开脉络丛的包绕，开始在脑室镜的引导下，通过直视手术将分流管放入脑室内。虽然有许多非对照性研究报道此种手术可以减少脑室端分流管的阻塞[140]，但是一项多中心的随机试验研究显示，脑室镜直视下分流管放置手术与非脑室镜辅助下分流管放置术相比，二者产生的分流障碍发生率无显著差异[75]。同时该研究通过术后影像学检查发现，无论是否在脑室镜直视下放置分流管，只有 2/3 的分流管放置于远离脉络丛区域。这一结果提示脑室镜直视下手术对分流管的精确放置并没有帮助。但是，这项研究还发现，术后影像学证实分流管远离脉络丛的患者，分流障碍的发生率确实很低。

远端分流障碍的原因可以是分流管折断、远端分流管长度不够、分流管感染和远端脑脊液吸收障碍。由于分流管材料是硅胶组织，所以会随时间延长而钙化裂开。裂开常发生，在锁骨上方，因为这里活动度大，接口处也是容易裂开的地方。所以需要探查整个分流管，确定是否存在连续中断的地方，特别是接口处。如果发现断裂，就必须更换分流管。另外，如果远端分流管太短，需要做分流管延长手术。

分流管感染也能引起远端分流障碍，是继机械梗阻后引起分流障碍的第二大原因。对于每次分流手术，分流管感染的发生率为 2%~8%[40]，而对于一套分流系统，感染的可能性为 5%~15%。分流管感染引起的后果非常严重，包括智力和局部神经功能损伤、大量的医疗花费甚至死亡。大多数感染发生在分流管埋置术后的头 6 个月[41]，约占 90%，其中术后第一个月感染的发生率为 70%。最常见的病原菌为葡萄球菌（表皮葡萄球菌占 20%，金黄色葡萄球菌占 20%），其他为棒状杆菌、链球菌、肠球菌、需氧的革兰阴性杆菌和真菌。6 个月以后的感染非常少见，且多为正常皮肤的惰性细菌如表皮葡萄球菌和痤疮丙酸杆菌。由于大多数感染是因为分流管与患者自身皮肤接触污染引起的，所以手术中严格操作非常重要。

分流术后感染包括伤口感染并累及分流管、脑室感染、腹腔感染和感染性假性囊肿。感染的危险因素包括小年龄、皮肤条件差、手术时间长、伴有开放性神经管缺陷、术后伤口脑脊液漏或伤口裂开、多次的分流管修复手术以及合并有其他感染。感染的患者常有低热（在 100℉ 到 102℉ 之间）或有分流障碍的征象，还可以有脑膜炎、脑室内炎症、腹膜炎或蜂窝织炎的表现，或者合并有上述各种表现。临床表现为易激惹、头痛、恶心和呕吐、昏睡、食欲减退、腹痛、分流管处皮肤红肿、畏光和颈强直。头部 CT 显示脑室大小改变或无变化。

一旦怀疑分流感染，患者必须进行分流管摄片（即头颅前后位、侧位的摄片，胸部和腹部的摄片）以及头部 CT 扫描。分流管摄片可以了解管道的连续性、可供穿刺的分流储器位置、分流相关问题的可能来源以及其他可能的感染源如肺炎。头部 CT 能显示脑室端管道的位置、脑室的大小和内容物，包括在严重的革兰阴性菌脑室炎症时出现的脑室和局限性化脓性积液。

如果患者主诉腹痛或有腹胀表现，需要给予腹部 CT 或超声检查，以确定有无腹腔内脑脊液假性囊肿。另外，还有必要行外周血白细胞计数和血培养，因为分流感染的患者常有血白细胞升高和血培养阳性。最后，还需要行多脏器检查，以确定有无合并感染。

如果怀疑有分流感染，应抽取分流管内的脑脊液化验。穿刺前先刮去穿刺部位的毛发，并用聚乙烯酮碘消毒皮肤。采用无菌技术用 25 号蝶形针穿过皮肤下向储液囊穿刺，测定分流管近端和远端的流量，同时留取脑脊液做细胞计数和分类，蛋白、糖测定，革兰染色和培养以及药物敏感试验。脑脊液送化验后，开始静脉应用广谱抗生素。

如果脑脊液检查证实感染（即脑脊液培养分离出细菌、脑脊液中性粒细胞和蛋白增多或脑脊液糖减少），需手术拔除分流管，脑室外引流并留置中心静脉
2001 管道。全身合理应用抗生素（即敏感的能穿透血脑屏障的抗生素），直到感染得到控制，此时新的分流管可重新安置。治疗期间必须监测脑脊液。目前，由于存在不同情况，抗生素的疗程从 2 天到 3 周不等[155]。目前正在研究在不牺牲疗效的前提下，努力缩短住院日、减少并发症，并最大限度地提高抗生素疗效。作者所在研究所的抗生素治疗至少持续至连续 2 次间隔 48 小时以上的脑脊液培养阴性，并且炎性物质吸收。除了抗生素治疗方面的一些问题外，分流感染还会引起脑室内脑脊液腔隙性分隔、智力受损（IQ 下降高达 8～10 分）、癫痫风险增加及死亡率增加[41]。

分流管过度引流即分流过度，也归类为分流失败。多数分流管无论是高压还是低压都会产生过度分流[152]。过度分流能引起硬膜下血肿、低颅内压综合征或脑室裂隙综合征。硬膜下血肿是由于脑室塌陷，致使脑皮层从硬膜上被牵拉下来，桥静脉撕裂出血。虽然硬膜下血肿多能自行吸收而无需治疗，但是对于有症状或进行性增多的硬膜下血肿仍需手术，以利于脑室再膨胀，消除硬膜下间隙。手术方法为钻孔外引流或埋置低压分流管于硬膜下内引流。除了并发硬膜下血肿外，过度分流还能引起低颅压综合征，产生头痛、恶心、呕吐、心动过快和昏睡，这些症状在体位改变时尤其容易发生。当低颅压综合征的患者呈现直立位时，会引起过度分流，造成颅内负压，出现剧烈的体位性头痛，必须躺下才能缓解[48,112]。如果症状持续存在或经常发作并影响正常生活、学习，就需要行分流管修复术，重新埋置一根压力较高的分流管或加装抗虹吸装置，或者埋置压力较高的抗虹吸分流管。

过度分流还能引起裂隙样脑室，即在放置了分流管后，脑室变得非常小或呈裂隙样。在以前的回顾性研究中，裂隙脑室的发生率占 80%[152]，有趣的是 88.5% 的裂隙脑室患者可以完全没有症状，而在 11.5% 有症状的患者中，仅 6.5% 的患者需要手术干预。脑室裂隙综合征的症状偶尔发生，表现为间断性的呕吐、头痛和昏睡。影像学表现为脑室非常小，脑室外脑脊液间隙减少，颅骨增厚，没有颅内脑脊液积聚的空间[152]。此时，脑室壁塌陷，包绕并阻塞脑室内分流管，使之无法引流[152]。最后，脑室内压力升高，脑室略微扩大，分流管恢复工作。由于分流管间断性的阻塞、工作，引起升高的颅内压波动，造成神经功能急性损伤。而且，由于颅内空间的限制，已经没有额外的空间允许颅内容量增加，包括脑血容量的增加。结果，任何可以引起脑血管扩张（如偏头痛）或脑血流增加（如夏天在户外烈日下运动或游戏）的因素，都会引起颅内压升高，产生症状[152]。脑室裂隙综合征的患儿在分流管阻塞的早期就会出现症状，头部 CT 扫描常常显示与其平常的裂隙脑室状态相比脑室大小无变化。

对于分流功能正常的急性神经功能减退的患儿，药物治疗可能起到作用，如用脱水剂呋塞米或乙酰唑胺降低颅内压，直到升高的压力消退。某些患者用抗偏头痛的药物如赛庚啶、普萘洛尔等也可能有效。如果药物治疗无效，则需手术干预。手术方法包括脑室端分流管的更换、分流阀压力上调以增加阻力、加装抗虹吸或流量控制装置、分流管同侧的颞下去骨瓣减压以及上述几种方法的联合应用。颅内压监护仪是有用的，可以辨别高颅压波动引起的颅高压头痛与真正的过度分流造成颅内负压引起的低颅压头痛。颅内压监护仪还对辨别其他原因引起的与分流手术无关的颅内压正常的头痛有帮助。

侧脑室放置脑积水分流管后，有时会出现孤立性第四脑室扩张，这在有出血后脑积水病史的患儿中尤其容易发生，出血后脑积水可由与早产有关的脑室内出血、感染后脑积水或反复分流感染/室管膜炎所引起。在这种情况下，脑脊液的过度分流可以引起裂隙样脑室或导水管狭窄或两者同时存在。一旦发生导水管狭窄，则由于导水管解剖或功能上的梗阻，使得第四脑室无法与第三脑室相交通。同样，由于第四脑室出口（即 Luschka 孔和 Magendie 孔）的梗阻，使得第四脑室和基底池不能交通。闭塞的第四脑室产生的脑

脊液使得脑室进行性扩大，出现头痛、吞咽困难、低位颅神经麻痹、共济失调、昏睡、痉挛性四肢轻瘫和恶心/呕吐。婴儿可有屏气发作和心动过缓。对于有症状的患儿，可以另外行第四脑室腹腔分流术，也可以放置一根分流管于第四脑室内，再通过 Y 型接口将其与相邻的幕上分流管在阀门上方相连通。然而，当脑室随着脑脊液的引流而缩小时，脑干向后方正常位
2002 置后移，导致第四脑室内的分流管可能会碰伤脑干[33]。另外，大约 40% 的患儿术后 1 年内需要再次更换分流管[80]。还有一种治疗方法是枕下开颅开放性手术，将第四脑室与蛛网膜下腔和基底池打通，必要时还可以同时再放置一根分流管连通第四脑室与脊髓的蛛网膜下腔[31,148]。近来，内镜手术又备受推崇，即采用内镜下导水管成形术和放置支撑管的脑室间造瘘术，以建立孤立的第四脑室与幕上脑室系统之间的通路[49]。

内镜第三脑室造瘘术（ETV）能被用来治疗某些类型的阻塞性脑积水，如导水管狭窄和松果体区肿瘤引起的阻塞性脑积水。如果该手术成功，则不需要行分流手术，避免了分流所带来的各种并发症。但是，该手术却不适合治疗交通性脑积水，对于小于 1 岁的婴幼儿成功率也很低。用于治疗大儿童和成年人的获得性阻塞性脑积水的成功率最高，使约 70% 的该类患者脱离了分流管[30,121]。在小于 3 岁的儿童中，成功率在 40%～50% 之间。对于存在病理改变的患者，成功率也很低，如肿瘤、已经做过分流手术、曾有过蛛网膜下腔出血、曾做过全脑放疗以及第三脑室底瘢痕显著增生者，其成功率仅为 20%[53]。

第三脑室造瘘术是在冠状缝前中线旁 2.5～3cm 额骨上钻一骨孔[121]，将镜鞘插过室间孔以保护周围组织，防止内镜反复进出时损伤脑组织。硬性或软性内镜插入镜鞘，通过室间孔进入第三脑室，在第三脑室底中线处的乳头小体开裂处前方造瘘，瘘口包括第三脑室底后缘，再用 2 号球囊扩张管通过反复充气和放气将造瘘口扩大。造瘘完成后，再将内镜伸入脚间池，观察蛛网膜，确定没有多余的蛛网膜阻碍脑脊液流入蛛网膜下腔。

有关第三脑室造瘘术的并发症的发生率现在越来越明确。因技术原因而不能完成手术的超过 26%[23]，而主要并发症为血管损伤继发出血[143]。其他报道的并发症有心跳暂停、尿崩症、抗利尿激素分泌过多综合征、硬膜下血肿、脑膜炎、脑梗死、暂时性第三和第六对颅神经麻痹、短期记忆障碍[23,143]。第三脑室造瘘术的风险还包括感染、周围相邻脑结构损伤（如下丘脑、腺垂体、视交叉），以及动脉损伤引起的术中破裂出血或外伤后动脉瘤形成造成的迟发性出血。少部分患者还有远期的手术失败，表现为颅高压症状的复发，动态 MRI 可以通过评价脑脊液在第三脑室造瘘口处的流通情况而判断造瘘口是否通畅。如果造瘘口不够通畅，有必要行内镜探查，尝试再次行造瘘口穿通术，若原造瘘口处瘢痕增生无法再次手术穿通，只得行脑室腹腔分流术。

结果和预后

未经治疗的脑积水预后差，50% 的患儿在 3 岁前死去[165]，仅 20%～23% 能活到成年。活到成年的脑积水患儿中，仅有 38% 有正常智力[79]。脑积水分流术技术的发展使得儿童脑积水的预后有了很大改善。许多做了分流手术的脑积水患儿可以有正常的智力，参加正常的社会活动。认知发育和寿命主要取决于潜在疾病的自然病程。约 50%～55% 脑积水分流术后的儿童智商超过 80，语言认知能力优于非语言认知能力[27,38,63]。然而，癫痫常预示脑积水分流术后的儿童有较差的智力，无癫痫者中约 66% 的智商高于 90，而有癫痫者中这一比例仅为 24%[20]。不幸的是，分流并发症反复出现的脑积水患儿预后差。

儿童癫痫外科

癫痫是儿童时期常见的疾病[57]。在美国和加拿大，癫痫的发病率为 0.5%～1.0%[9,57,58]，而且大约超过 50% 的癫痫病例在 5 岁以前就发病[32,57]。通常，儿童癫痫一开始使用抗癫痫药物治疗。然而，20%～25% 的儿童癫痫不能通过药物治疗来控制发作[22,101]，而且现在认识到开始于儿童时期的癫痫发作是由已知的结构性病灶导致的，并不能通过药物来控制，而且很少随儿童发育自发缓解[2]。反复发作的抽搐以及药物的副作用对大脑发育有负面影响，并能导致神经认知功能的严重障碍[2,3,25,59,61,147,150]。而且，慢性癫痫发作可影响儿童教育，导致学习困难和相关的社会心理影响，如学前教育的儿科检查评估得分低下、行为困难、学校表现较差、抑郁、兴奋和自我尊重感

2003 差[61,62,67]。因为儿童时期难治性癫痫是进行性发展的，可导致患儿身体虚弱以及智力和行为功能的退化，所以应给予积极治疗。癫痫外科为难治性癫痫儿童提供了有效的治疗方法。外科治疗的目的是尽可能切除癫痫病灶而不产生新的神经缺陷，或不比已有的情况更差。

癫痫手术的指征是：（1）儿童癫痫发作持续，而且至少经过 2～3 个合适的抗癫痫药物单独或联合足量用药的试验性治疗，每种药物都使用至最大耐受剂量；（2）癫痫发作明显降低了儿童的生活质量；（3）单侧局限性的癫痫病灶，这个病灶能可靠的重复确认；（4）切除癫痫病灶不会导致不可接受的神经缺陷[2,15,97,105]。一旦儿童癫痫药物治疗失败，应立即进行术前准备，因为早期手术治疗对功能恢复至关重要[2,6,105]。

术前评估

术前评估的主要目的是确定癫痫发作的区域（即癫痫病灶）及其与重要皮质功能区的关系[2,147]。对难治性且能致残的儿童癫痫进行的初始评估包括非侵入性的癫痫综合征鉴定和药物治疗的优化。对患儿进行全面的神经系统病史询问和体格检查、基线脑电图检查和高分辨率脑 MRI 行全颞叶薄层冠状扫描［如三维扰相梯度回波序列（3D-SPGR）扫描］、液体衰减反转恢复（FLAIR）序列和磁共振波谱技术。基线脑电图能确定癫痫病灶，以及鉴定抽搐和癫痫综合征，从而为疾病诊断提供重要信息[103]。基线脑电图上有意义的局灶性表现包括：局部慢波、快活动的局部衰减和局部癫痫样的放电（如棘波和尖波）。成功局部切除手术的良好预后因素包括癫痫样活动的单一病灶表现[103]。MRI 可用来评估局部结构异常（例如细胞结构）或异常病灶（例如肿瘤），这些异常可导致儿童癫痫。当 MRI 局部异常的表现和基线脑电图上癫痫发作的位置相符合时，可增加致癫痫区域认定的可靠性，增加手术后控制癫痫发作的可能性[17,103,105]。MRI 检查可看到与药物难治性癫痫有关的结构性异常，包括低分化肿瘤，如神经节神经胶质瘤（图 124-8A 到 C）、胚胎发育不良性神经上皮肿瘤（DNET）、星形细胞瘤、少突神经胶质细胞瘤和多形性黄色星形细胞瘤；发育性异常，如皮质发育不

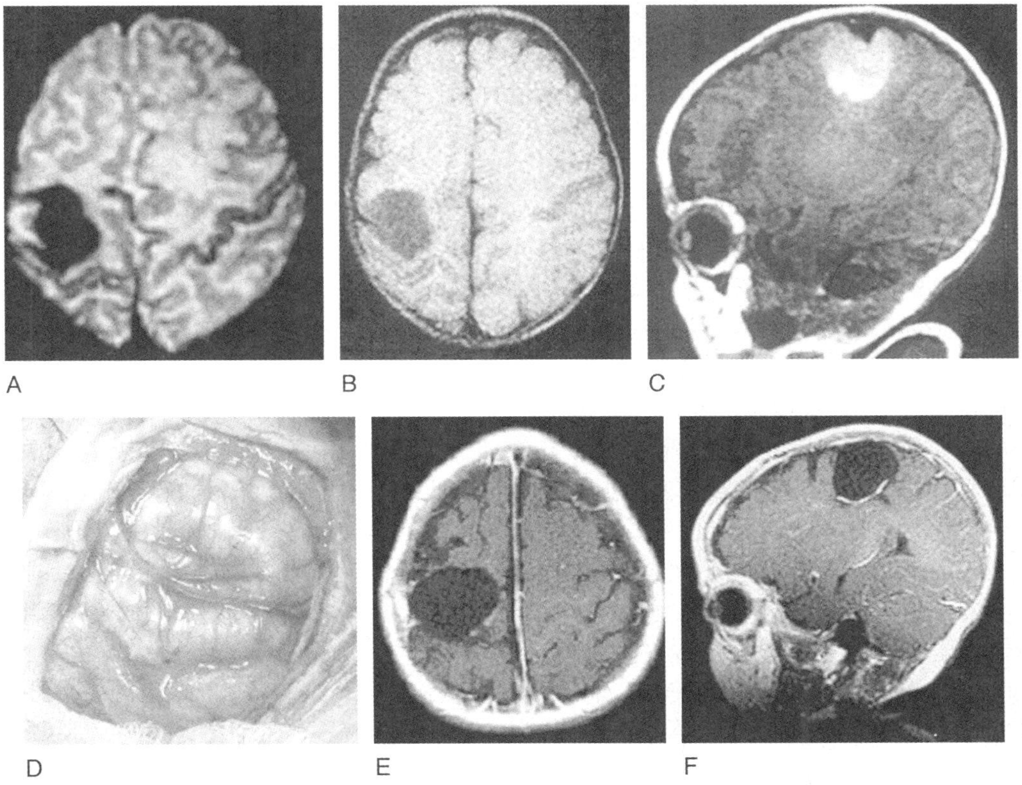

图 124-8　3 个月女婴每天 30～60 次癫痫发作，使用三种抗惊厥药。A 到 C. 脑 MRI 显示右后前方一个 2.5×2.5×2 cm 肿块。术前视频脑电图定位在 MRI 显示的非正常区域。患儿接受了肿块完全切除及切除术中脑电图定位的邻近致癫痫区。最终病理诊断为神经节神经胶质瘤。患儿现在 33 个月，无肿瘤复发，有轻微残余的痉挛性左侧偏瘫，已完全没有癫痫发作，不再使用任何抗惊厥药物。

2004 良和局部神经元异常移位（例如灰质异位）；血管异常，如海绵状血管瘤和动静脉畸形；继发性创伤后或局部缺血后脑软化病灶；以及颞叶中央硬化[103]。

如果初始评估提示可能存在一个癫痫灶，则需要进行另外的检查以进一步确定癫痫灶，包括采用表面电极（即头皮电极）的延时视频基线脑电图监测、功能神经影像学检查［正电子发射扫描（PET）或单光子计算机发射扫描（SPECT），或二者同时进行检测］，以及神经心理测试，可以向颈动脉内注射或不注射异戊巴比妥钠（即 Wada 试验）。延长的视频基线脑电图监测包括脑活动和临床行为的同步记录，这是术前评估的基础[60,103]。它结合了经头皮电极同步基线脑电图记录和同步持续实时声音/视频记录儿童典型癫痫发作的技术，因此能够确定儿童癫痫灶位于哪一侧及其具体部位。当怀疑为颞部病灶时，可以放置蝶骨电极来记录中央颞叶的活动。另外，当对癫痫持续监测时，抗癫痫药物可逐渐撤出直到记录到一些典型癫痫发作。在大部分病例中，视频基线脑电图使我们能够确定患者是否患有癫痫，是全身还是部分性发作，以及部分性发作从哪里开始[15,105]。当对一个儿童考虑进行癫痫手术时，理想的情况是发现癫痫在基线脑电图上是高度刻板的，所有癫痫从相同区域发生[105]。偶尔，视频基线脑电图会提示存在独立的双侧癫痫灶，尤其是在继发于多病灶异常的癫痫儿童中，例如结节性硬化中所见[14]。在这类病例中，如果癫痫主要从一侧发生，则患儿仍然有进行癫痫手术的指征；然而，必须认识到这样做不可能彻底控制癫痫[105]。

用 PET[28,29,33] 和 SPECT[102] 做的神经功能影像同样能通过检测整体和局部的脑的功能性异常来提供有价值的定位信息。然后这个信息可以和基线脑电图上观察到的电生理异常以及 MRI 上的解剖异常相比较。PET 是非侵袭性的功能影像学检查，它通过判断放射性核素[18F]脱氧葡萄糖（FDG）摄取的范围来测量局部脑葡萄糖的利用或代谢。在癫痫发作间期，从 PET 上看癫痫灶是一个葡萄糖代谢减退区域。这个检查对定位皮质发育异常的局灶区域、中间颞叶硬化和其他与表面基线脑电图定位的致癫痫区域相符合的结构性异常尤其有帮助。SPECT 是另一种非侵袭性的功能性影像学检查，它通过灌注放射性示踪剂如 ^{99m}Tc 六甲基丙二基胺肟（^{99m}Tc-HMPAO）来测量区域脑血流。它可在特殊的时间点及时提供局部脑血流的快照[3]。在癫痫发作间期，癫痫灶是低代谢的和血流较低的区域。结果，在 SPECT 扫描上可发现这些区域相对血流灌注不足[99]。相反，在发作期的 SPECT 研究中，如果在癫痫发作时注射示踪剂，可发现癫痫灶区域过度灌注，因为作为代谢需求增加的结果，在癫痫发作时到癫痫灶的血流明显增加。发作时的 SPECT 比发作间期的 SPECT 在定位致癫区域方面更加可靠[56,86,135]，而且发作时 SPECT 比发作间期 PET 更具可行性，因为不像发作间期 PET 那样必须在给予示踪物后短期进行，发作时 SPECT 可以在给予示踪物后合适的时期进行[105]。功能影像学检查，如 PET 和 SPECT，已经减少了近 90% 的儿童颅内监测的需要[28,56,86]。

术前评估的另一个重要因素是确定脑功能区和癫痫灶位置之间的关系。这可帮助预测切除癫痫灶后的风险。神经心理学测试在术前评估中有重要作用[103]。这些测试能通过确定与患者潜在病灶有关的神经系统功能异常区域来定侧和定位[71]。例如，从优势半球颞叶开始发作的癫痫患者可能有言语记忆或语言采集的缺失，而视觉空间的记忆缺失提示癫痫发作在非优势半球颞叶。言语和视觉空间记忆均明显缺失提示双侧颞叶损伤和可能为双侧癫痫灶。另外，术前神经心理测试能帮助预测术后认知功能的预后，并可作为基线来监测疾病的进展、成功治疗和治疗的副作用[3,103]。而且，术后神经心理测试能用来辨别残留或导致的认知缺陷，还能帮助计划心理教育干预措施以处理任何神经心理损伤。

颈内动脉注射异戊巴比妥（即 Wada 试验）同样可以使用于儿童癫痫的诊断中，尤其在年长儿中，可以确定哪一侧大脑半球是语言优势半球，查明每侧大脑半球对记忆功能的相对作用[3,15,83,139]。在这些研究中，进行脑血管造影和分别注射异戊巴比妥到每侧颈内动脉中。颈内动脉注射异戊巴比妥导致同侧脑功能的阻滞，这可模仿外科切除同侧大脑半球的作用。一次成功的注射可通过对侧轻偏瘫和同侧基线脑电图减慢来证明。随后进行语言和记忆测试来确定计划切除半球的对侧半球是否能支持足够的语言和记忆功能。Wada 试验是查明语言优势半球和评价颞叶切除后残留记忆能力的最理想的方法。然而，在年幼儿童中进行 Wada 试验通常比较困难，因为必须让他们保持清醒和配合。

术前检查的结果可决定患者是否有进行癫痫手术的指征，或是否需要额外的检查来更加精确地指出癫痫灶的位置和语言皮质区域。在由癫痫学家、神经外

2005 科医生、神经系统放射学家和其他癫痫外科组成员参加的多学科临床会议中，对前面提到的结果进行综述以后决定患者有无手术指征。儿童神经外科医生讨论手术的风险和好处，决定手术路径，以及最终决定是否实施手术[103]。通常从视频基线脑电图、MRI、PET中获得的结果提供最有力的指征[15]，当明显有确定的局部癫痫发作区域，并与基线脑电图、放射影像、神经心理学及临床证据一致时，建议采取手术治疗[97]。癫痫手术成功的可能性随独立因素集中在单一部位的数量增加而增加[15,46,84,135]。

在一些患儿中，手术或许是良好的选择，但数据资料却不确定或不一致。这些患儿包括那些有正常或非定位的影像学检查和视频基线脑电图确定癫痫发作而没有足够定位的患儿、癫痫灶比影像学检查观察到的结构性病灶更广泛的患儿，以及癫痫灶邻近语言皮质的患儿。对于这些患儿，可能需要延长的、侵入性的颅内基线脑电图监测以获得更精确的定位信息[4,5,15,68,69,97]。颅内基线脑电图监测有以下优点：(1) 它可帮助确定病灶周围致癫痫区域的范围，以及依次引导切除的范围；(2) 它可通过查明这些癫痫是否从单一的可手术的致癫痫带发出，帮助确定儿童多发性结构性病灶和多病灶发作间波释放是否是手术指征；(3) 它能显示邻近癫痫灶的语言皮质区域，以决定能否安全地切除癫痫灶而不产生新的神经缺陷或比现有的症状更加严重。

这个技术包括植入表面电极，如将网格或带状电极植入一个薄而柔软的塑料片中，直接放置在皮质表面，可通过开颅术和打开硬脑膜放置网格电极，或通过骨孔在硬膜下放置带状电极[146]。在关闭硬脑膜前，可给硬膜下放有网格电极的患者配置一个颅内压监测仪，以方便手术后监测和处理由放置网格电极引起的颅内压升高。颅内压监测在延长的发作后期病例中尤其有帮助，因为它能帮助鉴别出血或水肿造成的神经功能恶化和发作后的昏睡[97]。另外，将带状电极和网格电极缝合到硬脑膜上可使手术后发生位置移动的风险降至最小，电极头经隧道到达远处出口部位可使感染的风险降至最小。必须扩大硬脑膜下间隙以放置电极的病例可进行硬脑膜成形术，进行骨瓣松弛复位，两层关闭头皮切口，紧密关闭电极出口周围皮肤以防止脑脊液漏，电极用4-0尼龙线固定在头皮上可防止电极位置移动。如果有必要，可以用框架基础系统引导放置多接触深部电极来获取准确的皮质表面下深部结构的基线脑电图记录。深部电极检测皮质的有限区域，对描绘大的致癫痫区域没有帮助。然而深部电极检测对从中间颞叶结构如海马和杏仁核发出癫痫的儿童有帮助，但并不能确定癫痫起源于哪一侧[5]。

植入表面电极后，应摄术后头颅X光片来证实电极的位置，预防性静脉应用抗生素和小剂量皮质激素，并进行持续视频基线脑电图监测。该患儿一直监测到记录到一些典型癫痫发作为止。一旦记录到数量合适的儿童典型癫痫发作，则开始进行皮质刺激研究以标记出功能皮质和诱发先兆或癫痫发作，这可进一步帮助定位癫痫灶[3,15,97]。然后按照电刺激、结构和功能方面的资料做出手术计划，接着该患儿被送回手术室，在那里重新进行开颅手术和按计划进行癫痫灶切除手术。在第二次手术前重复拍摄头颅X光片，并和前面的头颅X光片进行比较以证明电极的位置和评估电极的移动。很少出现不能发现致癫痫灶或切除致癫痫灶导致不能接受的神经功能缺陷的情况。在这些病例中，去除硬膜下电极，不进行切除致癫痫灶的手术而直接进行关颅[97]。

尽管颅内基线脑电图监测能帮助决定癫痫手术的可行性和安全性，但这是个侵入性的操作，并有一些可能的风险，包括出血、感染、脑脊液漏、电极移位、颅内压升高，甚至导致死亡[69,164]。放置带状电极的并发症发生率是1%～3%[161]，而放置深部电极的并发症发生率是3%～10%[136]。放置网格电极的并发症发生率比放置带状电极更为多见。感染的风险随侵入性监测的持续时间延长而增加，并可通过预防性给予抗生素而降低。在许多病例中，放置网格电极的额外手术不是必需的[5,68,106]。取而代之的是在手术同时进行术中脑皮层电图记法，通过发作间棘波释放部位、背景基线脑电图模式的差异，以及采用术中躯体感觉诱发电位鉴定临界功能皮质（例如主要感觉运动皮质），从而做出皮质切除的精确范围[5,123]。

癫痫手术的类型

在儿童癫痫手术中，有三种类型的手术用来治疗难治性癫痫：(1) 切除术，把致癫痫皮质切除；(2) 切断术，把癫痫样放电的关键路径中断；(3) 植入术，使用电刺激[103,104,147]。所进行手术的类型根据术前得到的检查结果来决定。

2006 切除手术

致癫痫皮质切除手术的特定类型包括：对难治性复杂性部分癫痫行前颞叶切除，同时行扁桃体海马切开术；对无病损癫痫行扩大颞叶切除术[97]；对由结构性病灶如皮质异常、脑内错构瘤、肿瘤（见图127-8A到F）和血管异常引起的癫痫行多叶、单叶和局部皮质切除[147]；以及大脑半球切除术，即切除手术的极限，包括彻底切除（解剖性）或离断（功能性）异常的大脑半球，并被报道是所有缓解癫痫的手术中最为成功的方法之一[104,110,114]。大脑半球切除术适合于一侧大脑半球严重损伤和对侧半球相对完整的患者，它在严重单侧运动性癫痫已经有对侧轻偏瘫和偏盲症的儿童中特别有效。大脑半球切除术的指征包括：Rasmussen 综合征[149]、Sturge-Weber 综合征[47]、半侧巨脑[151]、弥漫性半球皮质发育异常、婴儿偏瘫和大脑梗死。当术前的检查显示儿童癫痫是从整个大脑半球发起时，切除该侧大脑半球但保留同侧的基底节（解剖性大脑半球切除）或通过切除少量皮质组织而离断该侧大脑半球（功能性大脑半球切除术或大脑半球径路切开术），可以使75%～80%的患者癫痫发作明显减少（80%或更多）并且认知功能得到改善[36,147,149,159]。

颞叶癫痫是成人和青少年手术指征中最常见的定位相关癫痫，但在婴儿和儿童中少于颞叶外癫痫[43,82]。在颞叶癫痫中，患者通常经历复杂部分性发作以及口和手的自动症，这些症状发作前可能有先兆。尽管在成人和青少年中导致颞叶癫痫的最常见原因是中间颞叶硬化症，但在婴儿和儿童中则没有这种情况[42,162]。取而代之的是，颞叶癫痫在这个年龄组的最常见原因是先天性脑发育异常，如皮质发育异常、低分化肿瘤和血管异常[6,44]。在病灶相关颞叶癫痫的患儿中，作为颞叶肿块导致的症状，癫痫的来源通常不是病灶自身而是病灶周围的边缘[39]，这些患者良好的预后取决于恰当地确定病灶周围致癫痫带的范围和沿着病灶切除这个癫痫带区域。

当诊断检查的结果显示癫痫起源于单个颞叶时，建议进行手术治疗。颞叶的侧面新皮质和中间基底段都可以导致儿童癫痫[2,3]。颞叶的中间基底段由梭状回和海马回以及杏仁核海马复合体组成。已经有一些报道描述了在难治性单侧起源的颞叶中间基底段儿童癫痫中切除颞叶来源癫痫灶的手术方法[147]。例如，可以行前颞叶切除术加杏仁核海马切开术[3,104,134]。这两步手术涉及在颞上回下首先切除大约3.5 cm前颞叶（从颞顶沿着颞中回用尺测量）和软膜下分离技术。这样可暴露颞角和中间颞叶结构，包括海马、杏仁核和海马回。随后通过显微镜下软膜下分离切除中间结构，分离后部界限到达盖板水平。在难治性单侧起源的中间基底段儿童癫痫中，切除受累的中间颞叶和彻底切除中间的颞部结构，有超过75%的机会可以使儿童癫痫发作明显减少或使癫痫儿童免于药物治疗[2,3,6,94,147]。

在儿童癫痫手术指征中，颞叶外癫痫比颞叶中间基底段癫痫更多见[43]。癫痫样异常可以位于额部、顶部或枕部，经常不能准确定位[156-158]。而且，在儿童难治性癫痫中，通常并不少见累及超过一叶的病例[97]。当癫痫灶位于颞叶外并且影像学检查中无病损相关性（非病灶性，颞叶外癫痫）时，患者经常需要侵入性的颅内监测和电刺激研究以限定和准确定位癫痫灶，并画出与致癫痫皮质相关的语言脑功能区[15,97]。这些癫痫可能是临床静息的，提示是顶部或侧面额部病灶；复杂部分性发作提示额叶病灶；如合并黑矇症，提示为枕叶病灶。确定切除边缘是基于手术前植入硬膜下电极做颅内监测和电刺激研究后确定的致癫痫脑回，或手术中脑皮层电图和功能皮质地图。随后在手术显微镜下行皮质切除术，彻底切除致癫痫灶是联合软膜下分割技术的切除手术。大约2/3的颞叶外癫痫儿童（病灶性或非病灶性）手术后获得明显改善[7,129]。

切除手术合并的风险通常和脑切除的区域或多个区域有关，包括视野缺损（例如对侧上象限盲或由于损伤 Meyer 环/后颞叶切除时视觉放射而导致的“天空馅饼”缺损）、人为偏瘫、语言和记忆缺失、损伤邻近血管导致的中风（例如在颞叶切除时损伤大脑中动脉的 sylvian 分支），以及颅神经麻痹（例如在切除海马时损伤到第三颅神经）。主要并发症例如中风和轻瘫的发生率为2%～5%[128,129]。

切断手术

切除致癫痫灶是癫痫外科的主要方法。然而，在一些儿童中，致癫痫区域在功能关键的皮质区域（例如感觉运动、语言或视觉的皮质，或具有一种以上功能的区域），且不能被安全地切除。这些儿童可能有

2007 做切断手术的指征——将癫痫灶和其他脑部进行隔离的手术[104]。例如，如果手术前评估显示一个儿童的癫痫灶在脑的语言区，如同运动皮质那样，切除病灶可能导致不能接受的神经功能缺陷，例如对侧瘫痪或无力。为防止上述情况发生，癫痫起源于语言皮质的儿童可以进行“切断”类型的手术，即多处软膜下横切[95,97,104]。这种类型手术的可行性是基于观察到正常皮质功能是垂直路径投射，而癫痫是通过水平路径投射。用一个细的头端小球状的探针来切断语言皮质区的水平纤维，因而阻止突发释放的水平传播且不损伤功能皮质的垂直柱。切断手术在手术显微镜直视下于皮质凸面浅表下进行，每个切割和脑回长轴成直角并相互平行，间距 5 mm，直到覆盖整个致癫痫区域。通过这项技术，手术患者癫痫发作频率明显减少，而没有出现任何持久的神经系统缺陷。在颞叶外癫痫中，通过多处软膜下横切而获得的癫痫控制效果可以与通过切除手术获得的效果类似[133]。

胼胝体切开术是另一种类型的切断手术，其可以在不能确定癫痫灶或有多处癫痫灶时采用。在这个手术中，通过双侧额部颅骨切开路径，胼胝体的前 2/3 或整个胼胝体被切开[88,107,147]。这个手术适合于经典的有症状性全身性癫痫伴多种发作类型和多个致癫痫区的患者，这些患者有某种程度的发育延迟和智力落后[15,103]。切开胼胝体会引起大脑半球的分离和防止癫痫放电的快速两侧泛化。手术治疗的指征包括：无张力性癫痫发作（落下发作）的易于猛然摔倒和使头部受伤的一类患者，和有 Lennox-Gastaut 综合征的患者。在合适的患者中，这种手术非常有效。例如，在无张力性癫痫发作的患者中，近 80% 可能完全或几乎完全停止发作。然而，癫痫很少能完全免于发作，没有肌阵挛性发作的患者在胼胝体切开术后没有效果或出现不一致的反应。另外，胼胝体切开术合并许多可能的副作用，其中一些可能是有相当破坏性的，包括语言障碍（例如全哑到开始说话迟钝）、无力、部分发作频率和程度增加，以及优势半球在左侧的患者出现分离综合征，包括左侧触觉命名不能、左侧动用障碍、假血红蛋白、右侧味觉命名不能、损害右手的空间综合障碍，导致难以临摹复杂图形、自发语言减少和不能自制[147]。

预后

癫痫手术的成功预后因素取决于：（1）通过彻底术前评估指导选择合适和适时的患者；（2）临床、电生理学和神经放射学资料具有良好相关性；（3）彻底或接近彻底地切除癫痫灶；（4）没有手术相关的损伤。患者手术后进行常规基线脑电图、MRI 和神经心理测试，并按照癫痫减少的百分比和手术后的时间长短分级。术前神经心理学测试的结果也可以和术后的测试结果进行比较，查明手术对儿童行为和认知的影响。通过这种方式，术后神经心理测试能帮助确定残留或导致的认知缺陷，辅助计划心理教育干预来处理这些缺陷。患者手术后继续服用抗惊厥药物 1～2 年。那些术后不再发作癫痫，并且基线脑电图表现相对良好的患者可以逐级停止服用抗癫痫药物。

一些研究显示了癫痫术后的预后（尤其在对结构性病灶引起的难治性癫痫行多叶、单叶和局部皮质切除时）与病理及病灶部位的相关性[103,147]。与儿童难治性癫痫相关的结构性病灶包括：发育性病灶，如局部皮质发育异常和错构瘤；血管性病灶，如海绵状血管瘤和动静脉畸形；低度恶性的肿瘤，如 DNET、神经节神经胶质瘤、神经节瘤、星形细胞瘤、多形性黄色星形细胞瘤和少突神经胶质瘤；缺血性或缺氧性损伤；创伤性损伤；以及中间颞叶硬化[103,147]。在一个重要的导致儿童难治性癫痫的原因——局部皮质发育不良中，手术治疗的效果在手术后前 2 年内非常好；然而，始终没有癫痫发作的患者的百分比随时间延长而减少。例如，在一项病例研究中[90]，尽管有 65% 的皮质发育不良患者在 2 年里没有发作癫痫，但是只有 40% 的患者在 5 年里仍然没有癫痫发作，而 10 年里没有发作癫痫的患者只占 33%。在其他的病例研究中平均随访时间为 3.6 年，皮质发育不良儿童不再发作癫痫的比例是 52%[163]。中颞叶硬化在儿童中相对少见，与在成人中的观察结果类似[90,163]，绝大多数患此类疾病的儿童和青少年在外科手术后癫痫不再发作的比例很高。DNET 是一种良性皮质病灶，具有囊性或微小囊性成分且常合并皮质发育不良[103]。与皮质发育不良不同，DNET 相关的致癫痫区域存在于皮质内邻近病灶的部位而不存在于 DNET 本身[50]。因此，全部切除这些病灶并在切除前辅以脑皮层电图记法来确定毗邻处致癫痫皮质，能使大约 75% 的患者彻底告别癫痫[116]。在有神经节神经胶质瘤的癫痫患者中（见图 124-8A 到 F），彻底手术切除是首选的治疗方法，并且是预测不再发作癫痫的最重要因素[76]，大约 78% 的患者逐渐脱离抗癫痫药物治疗而没有癫痫发作[70]。

2008 手术治疗的目标是彻底去除癫痫发作或能采用癫痫药物治疗完全控制癫痫，以及使儿童在长期认知、行为和社会发展上获得改善。在儿童中，手术治疗癫痫能减少发作频率和程度，并可限制常由慢性未控制性癫痫所导致的认知和心理损害。然而，外科治疗必须在合适的时机进行以使儿童发挥出他们最大的潜能和达到教育、职业和社会目标[103]。

与任何手术操作一样，癫痫手术操作同样具有风险，产生新的永久性神经缺陷或加重已有缺陷的风险必须与彻底去除癫痫或明显减少发作频率的潜在好处相比较。癫痫手术的风险包括切除或损伤语言皮质，损伤投射纤维、联系纤维或切除皮质下的连合纤维，损伤 Meyer 环导致对侧“天空馅饼”（pie-in-the-sky）视野缺损，损伤切除区域血管导致缺血损伤或血管分布区域中风，损伤邻近颅神经。尽管手术操作有风险，但是对合适病例早期手术治疗能阻止正在发育中大脑的进行性损伤改变，包括进展性心理和智力损害，允许合适的脑发育，减少不希望出现的药物治疗副作用，并使许多癫痫儿童有正常的、有价值的生活。当前，手术是唯一可彻底治愈癫痫的治疗方法，早期通过广泛的术前评估来确定合适的手术指征是获得成功预后的首要因素[108]。

迷走神经刺激

迷走神经刺激，即放入可植入的神经控制假体（NCP；Cyberonics，Houston），是儿童癫痫外科治疗最近的发展，并在多种药物治疗失败且没有指征进行切除或切断术的药物难治性癫痫儿童中，作为一种有效的治疗选择而受到越来越多的欢迎。这些儿童大多每天有多次广泛或局灶的癫痫发作（或两种都有），这些发作起源于两侧大脑的多个部位，没有皮质切除指征或已经在先前的皮质切除中失败。放置迷走神经刺激仪包括将包扎好的螺旋状铂金分叉电极环绕在颈部区域的左侧迷走神经上，然后将分叉的螺旋状前端连接到一个脉冲发生器上，这个脉冲发生器依次插入左胸区域的皮下或肌肉下的间隙[10,104]。它们一起释放间歇电刺激左颈迷走神经——通常每 5 分钟释放 30 秒。电脉冲通过上升感觉细胞核（例如孤束核）传导到脑皮质，对整个中枢神经系统的神经元兴奋性产生影响[11]。尽管已经有假说认为这些喙侧脉冲通过破坏由异常神经元组以不受控制的同步形式发放的异常电活动来阻止癫痫活动，但是调节癫痫的确切机制仍不清楚[9,8,120]。

脉冲发生器有八个设计参数，这些参数可以由膝上或手提计算机控制遥感程序杆通过皮肤进行非侵袭性的调节。刺激参数根据患者的耐受程度和癫痫发作频率来进行调整，在耐受时停止服用抗癫痫药物。迷走神经刺激另外的好处是能使用手提磁铁控制癫痫发作活动。例如，在癫痫先兆或发作开始时，患者或其家庭成员可以简短地将手提磁铁经过放置发生器的胸口袋。这会触发重叠在基线输出上的刺激链，可减弱甚至停止即将发生的癫痫发作[11]。迷走神经刺激的其他好处包括：保证治疗的顺应性、长期持续的有效性[96]和总体生活质量及认知功能的改善[11]。迷走神经刺激会产生副作用，包括声嘶、咽喉疼痛、咳嗽、呼吸困难和感觉异常。这些反应多间歇发生，伴随刺激释放时出现，然后有特征性的迅速消失[96,124]。迷走神经刺激的手术并发症很少，包括左侧声带损伤、低度面部轻瘫、心动过缓和有 1.1% 的感染比例需要取出迷走神经刺激仪[11]。尽管迷走神经是副交感神经系统的主要传出神经，但通过 NCP 系统的迷走神经刺激并没有显示出对心脏节律、肺功能、胃肠道运动或分泌的不利影响[124]。

先前的研究显示药物和手术难治性癫痫的儿童和青少年从迷走神经刺激中获得了实在的好处，许多患者癫痫发作明显减少，并且一些患者能减少使用抗惊厥药物的数量[100,109]。特发性的癫痫患者和那些起源于结构性病因的癫痫患者具有适当的迷走神经刺激指征[11]。特别是迷走神经刺激已经显示出在 Lennox-Gastaut 综合征患者中具有较高的有效性，一项病例研究显示 6 个儿童中的 5 个发作频率减少 90%[64]。而且，已经显示使用磁铁使一些患者发作持续时间减少，并且在其他一些患者中可减少发作后昏睡[109]。在一项针对药物难治性癫痫患儿发作频率和生活质量的回顾性分析中，29% 的患儿使用迷走神经刺激后癫痫发作频率减少 90% 以上，39% 的患儿癫痫发作减少了 50%~90%，13% 的患儿癫痫发作频率减少低于 50%。尽管使用迷走神经刺激控制癫痫发作是有可能的，但彻底控制癫痫发作的可能性非常低[11]。

中枢神经系统化脓性感染

中枢神经系统化脓性感染包括颅内感染，如脑

2009 脓肿、硬膜下积脓、硬膜外脓肿、颅骨骨髓炎、Pott瘤（结核球）、急性化脓性脑膜炎[14]；以及椎管内感染，如脊髓脓肿、硬脊膜外脓肿、椎间盘炎症及椎体骨髓炎。颅内感染可危及生命，在有高热、头痛并存在颅内伤口和窦道的患儿中，鉴别诊断时必须考虑到颅内感染。同样，椎管内感染可引起神经损伤，尤其是在诊断延误时后果更为严重。在患儿出现背痛、脊髓紧张和发热时必须考虑椎管内感染。下面我们讨论与小儿神经外科相关的中枢神经系统化脓性感染的治疗。

颅内感染

典型的硬膜外、硬膜内和脑实质内化脓性感染是耳鼻系统、中耳和外伤后感染以及免疫抑制引起的神经外科并发症，常表现为神经系统急症[31]。硬膜外脓肿的部位在硬膜外和颅盖骨或颅底骨之间，硬膜下脓肿发生在硬膜和蛛网膜之间的硬膜下间隙，脑脓肿是指在脑实质内的局限性的化脓性坏死灶。

发病率

有报道的儿童颅内感染的发病率仍很低。在患者很多的小儿神经外科中心，硬膜外的孤立脓肿发生率为每年1例，硬膜下脓肿为每年1～2例[108,130]，脑脓肿每年不到1～3例[31]。虽然儿童颅内感染相对不多见，但是如果不及时诊断和处理，感染会迅速致死。及早的诊断［CT和（或）MRI］、积极的抗生素治疗以及适时、充分地手术治疗大的脓肿是成功治疗的保证。治疗过程中需要靠神经影像学检查监测，以判断感染是否吸收。

病因学

颅内感染的原因包括：（1）临近组织感染的直接延伸，如鼻房窦炎、中耳炎、乳突炎或静脉传播；（2）穿透性颅脑外伤或神经外科手术的直接接种；（3）远处感染通过血源传播。鼻房窦、乳突气室、眼眶或颅骨等附近组织感染是引起硬膜外脓肿的最常见原因。硬膜外脓肿的原因还可以是先天性皮肤窦道、外伤（特别是穿通伤）、开颅手术、应用颅钳以及鼻房窦和颅底手术等的并发症[51]。硬膜下脓肿最常见的原因是额窦、筛窦、中耳和乳突气室炎症[8,92]。其他原因有附近头皮、帽状腱膜下间隙、颅盖骨或硬膜外间隙的感染（或上述几个地方的联合感染），脑膜炎或已有的硬膜下渗出或血肿引起的继发感染[13]，脑实质内脓肿破裂到硬膜下腔以及硬膜下穿刺或硬膜下放置分流管。

在儿童中，脑脓肿的最常见原因是鼻房窦、中耳和牙齿感染的直接或间接传播[160]。在青少年中，额叶脑脓肿常由急性额窦炎引起[31]。在患有先天性心脏病或肺内右向左分流疾病的儿童中，从远处感染源的血运性传播如肺部感染、皮肤感染、骨髓炎和细菌性心内膜炎仍旧是脑脓肿形成的重要发病机制[118]。在新生儿中，细菌性脑膜炎由柠檬酸杆菌、变形杆菌、沙雷氏菌或肠杆菌引起，在大多数患儿中可并发脑脓肿形成[118]。而且，直接的脑内播种如穿透性颅脑外伤、眼眶穿通伤、颅骨复合骨折、头皮伤、面部感染、脑脊液漏和外伤后脑膜炎都能导致儿童脑脓肿的产生。脑脓肿发生的部位取决于细菌入侵的路径，例如，耳或乳突气室炎症常引起同侧的大脑半球或颞叶脓肿，鼻房窦炎常引起额叶脓肿的形成，血运性传播的脓肿常发生在大脑中动脉分布区域。

脑脓肿培养出的常见需氧菌有葡萄球菌、链球菌、肠杆菌和嗜血杆菌，常见厌氧菌有类杆菌、胨链球菌、梭形杆菌、韦永球菌、丙酸杆菌和放线菌属。在许多病例中，脓液培养出的细菌是多样的，既含有厌氧菌又含有需氧菌[31]。然而，有些病例尽管已及时留取标本，却仍无法分离出细菌。根据培养出的细菌，细菌学诊断常可推断颅内感染的来源。例如，鼻房窦感染引起的颅内感染经常培养出厌氧和（或）需氧链球菌，革兰阴性菌感染如类杆菌和嗜血杆菌常提示有耳源性感染，金黄色葡萄球菌感染常提示由颅骨复合骨折和神经外科操作引起。真菌感染如念珠菌、霉曲菌、诺卡菌和隐球菌，常导致器官移植或恶性肿瘤化疗后免疫抑制以及宿主防御机制损伤的患儿发生脑脓肿[137]。

病理表现 2010

从鼻房窦、乳突气室或中耳到硬膜外和硬膜下间隙或到脑实质的感染传播途径，是板障血管或供给硬膜外层的滋养层血管发生感染性血栓性静脉炎的结果[31]。一旦感染进入板障层，细菌便会在该层内迅速扩散，并波及颅骨的广泛区域。偶尔，骨髓炎症可引起骨膜下脓肿，导致表面头皮肿胀（图 124-9A 和 B）。一旦炎症进入硬膜下间隙，可在硬膜下腔内快速扩散，因为这一间隙在脑表面、大脑镰和天幕的两侧、枕大孔以及脊髓硬膜下腔互相连通。硬膜下感染灶直接作用在暴露的脑组织上，导致脑皮层静脉阻塞和感染性血栓性静脉炎，最终引起脑梗死和水肿。脑水肿还能产生显著的占位效应，引起相应的脑组织受压和脑疝。

细菌种植到已有的坏死灶或直接的颅脑外伤、血肿，或感染性血栓性静脉炎引起的脑梗死，造成脑脓肿的形成。一旦细菌在脑实质内形成病灶，便会产生急性炎症反应，导致多形核白细胞浸润和水肿。病灶中心最后坏死和液化，周围由炎性细胞、新生血管和成纤维细胞包绕[31]，成纤维细胞再产生致密的胶原胶囊，并且周围可见水肿以及神经胶质增生。伴有周围水肿带的脑脓肿可引起颅内压显著增高，导致脑疝和死亡。而且脓肿一旦破入脑室系统或通过皮层进入蛛网膜下腔，可造成病情突然恶化甚至死亡。

临床表现

颅内感染的儿童常有脑外伤、鼻或耳流脓性分泌物、发热或头痛的病史。如果是硬膜外脓肿，典型病例常是急性起病，伴有发热、头痛或耳原发病灶处疼痛。如果是骨膜下脓肿引起的硬膜外脓肿，通常在额窦、乳突气室或板障区域可触及患者的头皮压痛、肿胀、有波动感（见图 124-9A 和 B）。当感染播散至硬膜下腔时，对相邻的硬膜和脑的占位效应逐步增加，使头痛逐渐加剧。最后，当脓肿增大、脑疝出现时，患者出现局灶性神经系统症状，伴有意识障碍[130]。

当脓肿播散到硬膜下间隙时，随着脑水肿、梗死及脑疝的出现，患者出现急速的神经功能减退，并有典型的颅内压升高及全身系统感染征象，如身体不适、发热、寒战、假性脑膜炎、呕吐、头痛、局灶性神经系统病变和精神症状[51]。另外，硬膜下脓肿的患儿还可以在继发于骨膜下脓肿（Pott 瘤）的受累乳突或鼻窦处有头皮压痛和水肿（见图 124-9A 和 B），25%～50% 的患者可伴有局灶性癫痫[31]。硬膜下脓肿可以在幕上也可以在幕下，或者两处同时存在（见图 124-10A 到 C）。典型的后颅窝硬膜下脓肿可有全身发热、头痛和颈强直，但是一般没有局灶性的神经系统症状及癫痫[19]。

脑脓肿的临床表现各不相同，主要是根据脓肿的 2011
位置、大小、数量、细菌的毒力以及患者的年龄和抵抗力而定[31]。儿童和青少年脑脓肿的症状和体征是：（1）全身感染，包括身体不适、发热、寒战和颈强直；（2）脓肿的占位效应以及周围脑水肿引起的颅

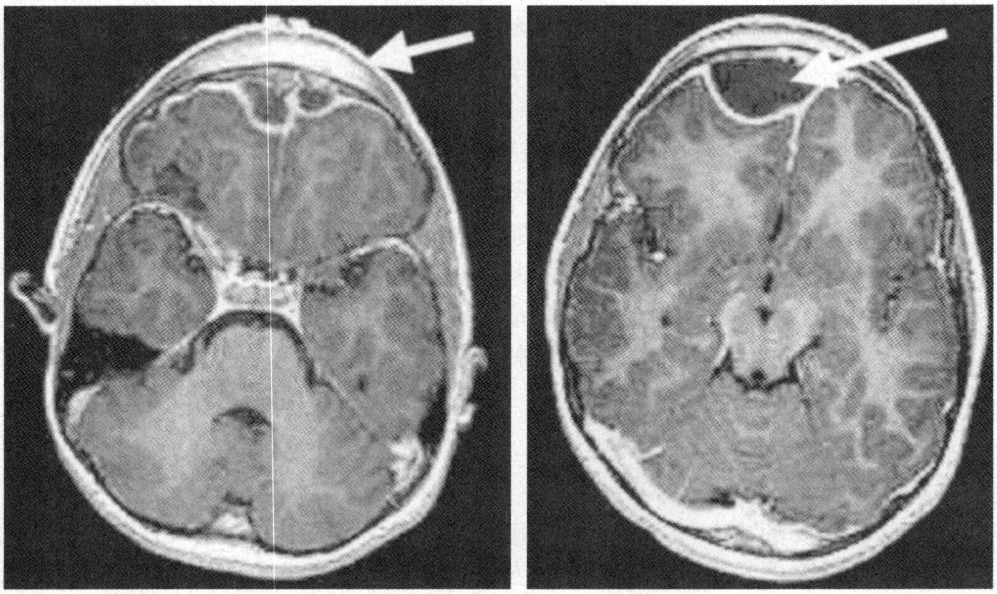

A　　B

图 124-9　A 和 B，为一个 5 岁男孩的轴向磁共振影像，有喉链球菌感染病史，口服抗生素 2 周，随后出现发热、寒战、头痛、前额中部进行性肿胀、呕吐和昏睡。A. 额部骨膜下脓肿（即 Pott 瘤；A. 箭头）和硬膜外脓肿（B. 箭头）很明显。通过保留骨瓣的脓肿引流、积极的抗生素治疗，感染完全吸收，没有留下神经系统后遗症。

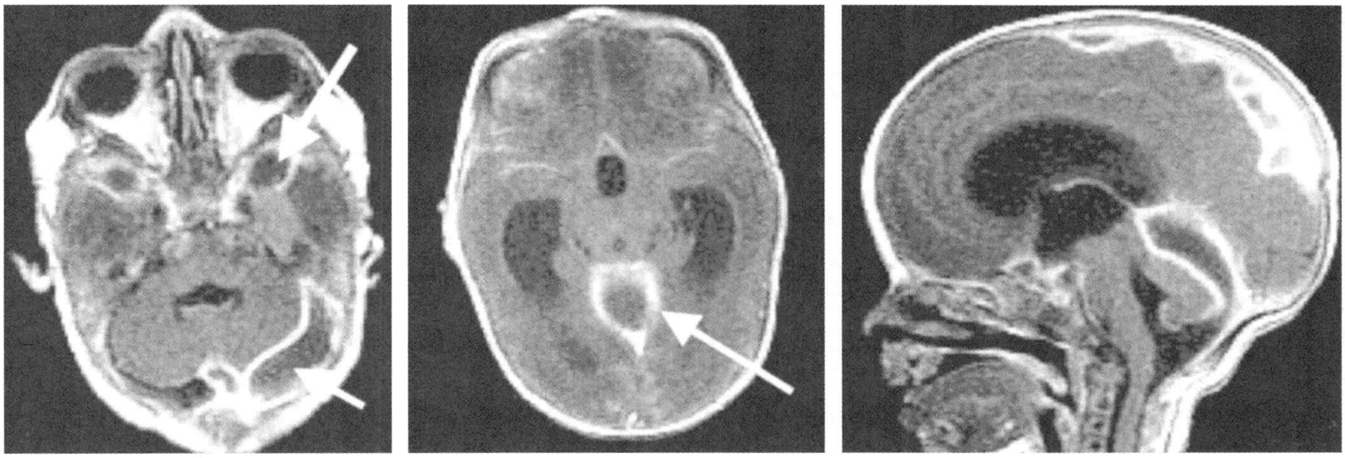

A　B　C

图 124-10　轴向（A 和 B）和矢状位（C）脑核磁共振影像（MRI）。一个 35 周的早产男婴，患有脑膜炎，病原体不明，给予大量抗生素，其中不包括甲硝唑。他开始出现抽搐、呼吸困难，需要气管插管。MRI 显示广泛的硬膜下积脓，向两侧延伸，幕上幕下均有（箭头）。脓肿引流时的培养结果为脆弱类杆菌。通过继续应用抗生素并加用甲硝唑，感染最终得以消除。孩子现在已快 4 岁，不再服用抗癫痫药，没有留下神经系统后遗症。

内压升高表现，如头痛、呕吐和意识减退；（3）反映脓肿所在位置的神经损伤症状，如脓肿压迫额叶后部或颞叶沟回疝引起的轻偏瘫，脓肿在颞叶功能部位引起的语言障碍，颞后部或枕叶脓肿引起的视野障碍，小脑脓肿引起的眼球震颤、眼球运动障碍、共济失调和肌张力减退。婴儿脑脓肿的表现有颅内压升高的症状和体征，包括易激惹、昏睡、呕吐、前囟饱满、前额饱满以及头围增加。至少 25%～50% 的幕上脑脓肿患儿在其病程中表现有局灶性或全身性的癫痫[65]。

诊断

怀疑脑脓肿的患者应该进行头颅增强 CT 或 MRI 检查（或二者都做）。头颅增强 CT 扫描能够快速诊断，而 MRI 能够提供精确的术前脓肿定位以及有利于监测脓肿吸收情况。根据颅内感染的类型、程度和阶段，这些检查能够显示硬膜增强、脓肿壁、脑水肿低密度区、静脉梗死灶以及早期的脑炎。矢状位和冠状位扫描有助于发现感染的窦腔以及颅顶骨和颅底骨脓液的积聚。脑脓肿的增强 CT 和 MRI 扫描特征为病灶周围环形强化伴周围水肿。尤其是在 MRI 图像上可表现为 T1 像的病灶中央低信号区、病灶周围环形强化，T2 像病灶中央高信号影伴周围低信号的脓肿壁以及最外层的水肿带[113]。

有帮助的实验室检查为周围血细胞计数、血沉和 C-反应蛋白，这些指标在脑脓肿时都会轻度升高[65]。血培养也有可能找到致病菌，尤其是在硬膜外和硬膜下脓肿时[65]。由于脑脊液检查诊断率低，并且有脑疝的风险，所以在影像学诊断前不要做脑脊液检查，特别是在怀疑有占位性病变时。手术引流时留取脓液做细菌学检查[31]。这些培养有助于确定细菌的抗生素敏感性，从而指导用药。标本的采集以及需氧菌和厌氧菌培养技术的掌握有助于获得阳性的培养结果。

治疗

高度怀疑是保证及时诊断的基础。成功的治疗需要手术引流、合适的抗生素治疗以及小儿神经外科医生和感染科医生的密切合作。一旦确诊，立即全身应用抗生素[31]。尽管术前应用抗生素可能产生某些骨浸润，但不太可能影响培养结果。2012

初次选择的抗生素很难针对致病菌。不同的原发感染灶其致病细菌也不相同[31]。因此，对原发病灶的认识有助于抗生素的选择。例如，原发感染灶在额窦，最可能的致病菌是链球菌，抗生素选择甲硝唑和青霉素或第三代头孢菌素。如果原发病灶未知，抗生素应当包括耐酶青霉素、第三代头孢菌素和甲硝唑，用以覆盖需氧及厌氧的链球菌、其他厌氧菌和葡萄球菌。虽然理想的治疗时间一直无法确定，但是静脉抗生素必须一直用到全身的感染征象消失，颅内的感染灶缩到最小[18,130]。有学者推荐再口服抗生素 2~3 个月，以预防复发[91]。

除了全身应用抗生素，颅内感染的儿童还需要皮质激素及抗癫痫药物治疗。皮质激素如地塞米松对减轻感染引起的脑水肿是有效的，并且尚未发现会使炎症反应加重。所以，在发病的急性期应用激素能减轻颅内压，预防脑疝。由于25%~50%的患儿颅内感染时可伴有抽搐，所以一旦诊断成立，应该给予预防性抗癫痫药物。

脑脓肿外科手术除了有助于细菌学诊断、指导抗生素应用外，还能引流脓液，减小脑脓肿体积，降低颅内压。如果找到原发灶，并且患儿条件允许，还应对原发灶行手术干预[31]。脓肿引流手术可通过开颅手术进行，也可通过小骨窗手术或骨孔手术进行。移除的骨瓣要正好够大以达到脓肿或脓液。如果硬膜外脓肿发生的部位曾经做过骨瓣手术，那么在做脓肿手术时常常需要去除骨瓣，以后再行颅骨修补手术。如果硬膜外脓肿在颅面部，且面积广泛，去除骨瓣后需要做大范围颅面重建手术，并且可能造成不可弥补的缺陷，那么骨瓣可以在术中回纳，但必须用抗生素溶液做广泛的硬膜外冲洗和清创，并且全身抗生素要用到感染完全消失[31]。所有患者必须行神经影像学随访以监测评价治疗效果。

对于硬膜下脓肿，采用开颅手术、颅骨穿通术或骨孔手术，在立体 CT 或 MRI 导向下，精确定位脓肿位置使得最小限度地切开骨瓣和打开硬膜。硬膜剪开后，留取脓液做需氧和厌氧菌培养，抽出脓液，用抗生素溶液彻底冲洗硬膜下腔。颅骨切开后如果没有骨髓炎和硬膜外脓肿，骨瓣可以回纳。由于骨瓣可能难以愈合，造成骨瓣吸收或死骨形成，所以必须密切监测骨瓣的愈合情况。如果硬膜下脓肿复发，有必要再次行脓肿引流。由流感嗜血杆菌脑膜炎引起的婴幼儿硬膜下积液，一般不需要手术干预，除非积液产生占位效应，患者由于颅内压升高出现症状，才考虑手术。手术方式为前囟侧方的穿刺引流或骨孔手术去除硬膜下积液，这种积液一般是无菌的[31]。

对于脑脓肿的治疗，有报道采用静脉抗生素治疗，结合神经外科手术，甚至可以不用手术，仅采用药物保守治疗。然而单独的抗生素治疗需要经常靠神经影像学检查随访，以确定治疗效果。同时，有必要密切监测患者的神经系统变化以及意识改变。发生如下情况时必须立即手术：（1）患者神经系统症状加重；（2）CT 或 MRI 表现有明显的占位效应；（3）抗生素治疗 2 周，脓肿缩小不明显。

脑脓肿治疗有两种手术方法：针刺穿刺引流，同时放置或不放置引流管；以及脓肿摘除术。超声引导或立体定向可以精确确定脓肿的位置，有利于穿刺及引流管放置入脓腔。在脓肿穿刺时，通过超声还可以了解到脓肿缩小的情况。用注射器缓慢抽取脓液，生理盐水冲洗后，将引流管留置在脓腔内几天，直至脓液引流停止。如果脓肿是多房性的，引流常常难以奏效，此时需要手术切除。小骨瓣切口，掀开骨瓣，打开硬膜，选择无功能区进入脑实质，保护好周围的白质不受损伤，完整切除脓肿，术后给予较长时间的抗生素治疗。

预后

预后是否良好取决于是否快速诊断和治疗。而且，神经系统的恢复和存活还取决于得到确诊时患者的情况及治疗方案。所以，早期的诊断和及时积极的治疗，合理应用抗生素以及手术摘除脓肿，是减少颅内化脓性感染引起的并发症及降低其死亡率的关键。2013
由于及时的诊断以及合理的抗生素治疗，脑脓肿的死亡率已经由过去的 32% 下降到现在的 10%。然而，脑脓肿破入脑室引起的死亡率很高，为 23.8%~80%[141,167]。脑脓肿经治疗后，远期的神经系统后遗症仍占约 44%[26]。另外，治疗后存活的儿童仍常留有学习障碍[118]和癫痫后遗症[91]。

椎管内感染

脊髓硬膜外脓肿在儿童中很少见[66]，因而常常漏诊，直到典型的神经损害症状出现时才发现[119]。由于病程进展很快，因此需要急诊手术减压，以预防不可恢复的截瘫。皮肤和黏膜的感染如疖疮、咽炎和牙齿的脓肿是引起椎管硬膜外脓肿最常见的血行传播的感染源[12,60,87]。其他原因有椎体炎症、脊柱旁脓肿，以及盆腔、后腹膜及后纵隔化脓性病灶的直接扩散。这种直接扩散可通过穿过椎间孔的静脉传播，或者细菌直接种植在由于钝性外伤引起的硬膜外血肿上[66]。儿童最常见的硬膜外脓肿的病原菌为金黄色葡萄球菌，有时也可能分离出厌氧菌和革兰阴性杆菌。

硬膜外脓肿 80% 发生在脊髓的背侧。在 C1 到 S2 范围之间，硬膜与后方的后纵韧带粘连。结果积聚在硬膜外后方或后侧方的脓肿上下广泛扩散，但被椎板和黄韧带局限于背侧。虽然硬膜外感染可以发生在椎管纵轴的任何节段，但是文献报道最常见的部位还是在胸部下段及腰部[87]。硬膜外一旦发生感染，脓液积聚在椎体和黄韧带的深部，外面包绕一圈已经形成血栓的静脉和肉芽组织。由于硬脊膜强大的屏障阻挡着感染，所以脑脊膜炎很少发生，除非做腰穿使得感染扩散。但是脓肿压迫以及脊髓动静脉血栓形成均导致脊髓损伤[87]。

临床上，患有硬膜外脓肿的儿童可能会发热和身体不适，典型的表现可有背部疼痛、脊柱压痛或放射痛。背痛常发生在胸部中段向胸壁四周放射。疼痛经常持续存在，可因咳嗽或运动而加剧。患者常表现颈项强直以及脓肿部位剧烈的叩击痛。感染的原发灶有可能很明显。脊髓受压的症状常表现为急性的进行性腿部肌力减退和感觉丧失，膀胱和肠道功能障碍。

如果儿童怀疑有脊柱硬膜外脓肿，需要进行外周血细胞计数、血沉及 C-反应蛋白检查，这些指标常会升高。另外，还需做血培养以明确病原体。可选择的确诊方法为全脊柱 MRI 平扫或平扫加增强，可以显示脓肿的部位、程度。不建议做腰穿检查。如果不具备 MRI 检查条件，而必须以脊髓造影作为确诊的手段时，腰穿部位必须尽可能地远离怀疑脓肿的部位。

一旦硬膜外脓肿确诊，必须立即治疗，以预防神经系统后遗症的产生。首先需要静脉应用抗生素治疗，选择的抗生素必须能有效对付葡萄球菌、厌氧菌和革兰阴性杆菌。注射用抗生素至少需要持续 4～8 周。虽然有一些文献报道单独用抗生素治疗也能成功治愈那些尚未出现神经症状的脓肿患者[12]，但是在大多数病例中，成功的治疗需要靠药物和手术的联合治疗。急诊手术的目的是引流脓液，给脊髓和神经根减压，尤其是脓肿范围很广的时候。手术方法是后入路椎板切开减压，引流脓性物质。切开一个或两个椎体平面，暴露脓肿的一端或两端，用引流管冲洗，并且引流足以解决问题。如果手术减压需要切开多个椎板，则术后需要密切关注脊柱后凸及脊柱不稳定的情况，因为这可能是多椎板切除儿童的远期并发症[12]。

预后与患者术前神经功能状况有关[89]。如果能够早期诊断、及时治疗，预后是非常好的。如果患者有轻度的运动功能障碍，并且在 36 小时内得到及时治疗，也有可能获得好的结局[35]。然而，一旦孩子出现截瘫，想要康复几乎是不可能的。因此，早期诊断和及时正确的治疗是硬脊膜外脓肿儿童获得康复的最重要的保证。在过去几十年，由于没有及时建立合适的治疗方法，导致硬脊膜外脓肿的死亡率一直保持在 14% 左右[35]。

（鲍　南译　金惠明校）

参考文献

1. Ackerman LL, Menezes AH: Spinal congenital dermal sinuses: A 30-year experience. Pediatrics 2003;112:641.
2. Adelson PD: The surgical treatment of temporal lobe epilepsy in children. In Albright AL, Pollack IF, Adelson PD (eds): Principles and Practice of Pediatric Neurosurgery. New York, Thieme, 1999, p 1111.
3. Adelson PD: Temporal lobectomy in children with intractable seizures. Pediatr Neurosurg 2001;34:268.
4. Adelson PD, Black PM, Madsen JR, et al: Use of subdural grids and strip electrodes to identify a seizure focus in children. Pediatr Neurosurg 1995;22:174.
5. Adelson PD, O'Rourke DK, Albright AL: Chronic invasive monitoring for identifying seizure foci in children. Neurosurg Clin N Am 1995;6:491.
6. Adelson PD, Peacock WJ, Chugani HT, et al: Temporal and extended temporal resections for the treatment of intractable seizures in early childhood. Pediatr Neurosurg 1992;18:169.
7. Adler J, Guisseppe E, Winston K, et al: Results of surgery for extratemporal partial epilepsy that began in childhood. Arch Neurol 1991;48:133.
8. Amar AP, Heck CN, DeGiorgio CM, et al: Experience with vagus nerve stimulation for intractable epilepsy: Some questions and answers. Neurologia Med Chir 1999;39:489.
9. Amar AP, Heck CN, Levy ML, et al: An institutional experience with cervical vagus nerve trunk stimulation for medically refractory epilepsy: Rationale, technique, and outcome. Neurosurgery 1998;43:1265.
10. Amar AP, Levy ML, Apuzzo MLJ: Vagus nerve stimulation for intractable epilepsy. In Rengachary SS (ed): Neurosurgical Operative Atlas, vol 9. Chicago, American Association of Neurological Surgeons, 2000, p 179.
11. Amar AP, Levy ML, McComb JG, et al: Vagus nerve stimulation for control of intractable seizures in childhood. Pediatr Neurosurg 2001;34:218.
12. Bair-Merritt MH, Chung C, Collier A: Spinal epidural abscess in a young child. Pediatrics 2000;106:1.
13. Bakker S, Kluytmans J, den Hollander JC, et al: Subdural empyema caused by *Escherichia coli*: Hematogenous dissemination to a preexisting chronic subdural hematoma. Clin Infect Dis 1995;21:458.
14. Bebin EM, Kelly PJ, Gomez MR: Surgical treatment for

epilepsy in cerebral tuberous sclerosis. Epilepsia 1993; 34:651.
15. Benbadis SR, Wyllie E: Evaluation of intractable seizures in children. In Albright AL, Pollack IF, Adelson PD (eds): Principles and Practice of Pediatric Neurosurgery. New York, Thieme, 1999, p 1095.
16. Bierbauer KS, Storrs BB, McLone DG, et al: A prospective, randomized study of shunt function and infection as a function of shunt placement. Pediatr Neurosurg 1990;16:287.
17. Blume WT, Girvin JP, McLachlan RS, et al: Effective temporal lobectomy in childhood without invasive EEG. Epilepsia 1997;38:164.
18. Bok A, Peter J: Subdural empyema: Burr holes or craniotomy? A retrospective computerized tomography–era analysis of treatment in 90 cases. J Neurosurg 1993;78:574.
19. Borovich B, Johnston E, Spagnuoloa E: Infratentorial subdural empyema: Clinical and computerized tomography findings. Report of three cases. J Neurosurg 1990;72:299.
20. Bourgeois M, Sainte-Rose C, Cinalli G, et al: Epilepsy in children with shunted hydrocephalus. J Neurosurg 1999;90:274.
21. Bowman RM, McLone DG, Grant JA, et al: Spina bifida outcome: A 25-year prospective. Pediatr Neurosurg 2001;34:114.
22. Braathen G, Theorell K: A general hospital population of childhood epilepsy. Acta Paediatr 1995;84:1143.
23. Brockmeyer D, Abtin K, Carey L, et al: Endoscopic third ventriculostomy: An outcome analysis. Pediatr Neurosurg 1998;28:236.
24. Bruner JP, Tulipan N, Paschall RL, et al: Fetal surgery for myelomeningocele and the incidence of shunt-dependent hydrocephalus, JAMA 1999;282:1819.
25. Camfield CS, Chaplin S, Doyle A-B, et al: Side effects of phenobarbital in toddlers; behavioral and cognitive aspects. J Pediatr 1979;95:361.
26. Carey ME, Chou SN, French LA: Long-term neurological residua in patients surviving brain abscess with surgery. J Neurosurg 1971;34:652.
27. Casey AT, Kimmings EJ, Kleinlugtebeld AD, et al: The long-term outlook for hydrocephalus in childhood. Pediatr Neurosurg 1997;27:63.
28. Chugani HT: PET in preoperative evaluation of intractable epilepsy. Pediatr Neurol 1994;9:411.
29. Chugani HT, Chugani DC: Basic mechanisms of childhood epilepsies: Studies with positron emission tomography. Adv Neurol 1999;79:883.
30. Cinalli G, Sainte-Rose C, Chumas PD, et al: Failure of third ventriculostomy in the treatment of aqueductal stenosis in children. J Neurosurg 1999;90:448.
31. Cochrane DD, Dobson SR, Steinbok P: Intracranial suppuration: Epidural abscess, subdural empyema, and brain abscess. In McLone DG (editor-in-chief): Pediatric Neurosurgery: Surgery of the Developing Nervous System, 4th ed. Philadelphia, WB Saunders, 2001, p 973.
32. Cowan LD, Bodensteiner JB, Leviton A, et al: Prevalence of the epilepsies in children and adolsescents. Epilepsia 1989; 30:94.
33. Cummings TJ, Chugani DC, Chugani HT: Positron emission tomography in pediatric epilepsy. Neurosurg Clin N Am 1995;6:465.
34. Czeizel AE, Dudas I: Prevention of the first occurrence of neural-tube defects by periconceptional vitamin supplementation, N Engl J Med 1992;327:1832.
35. Danner RL, Hartman BJ: Update of spinal epidural abscess: 35 cases and review of the literature. Rev Infect Dis 1987;9:265.
36. Davies KG, Maxwell RE, French LA, et al: Hemispherectomy for intractable seizures: Long-term results in 17 patients followed for up to 38 years. J Neurosurg 1993;78:733.
37. Dollo C, Kanner A, Siomin V, et al: Outlet fenestration for isolated fourth ventricle with and without an internal shunt. Childs Nerv Syst 2001;17:483.
38. Donders J, Canady AI, Rourke BP: Psychometric intelligence after infantile hydrocephalus. Childs Nerv Syst 1990;6:148.
39. Drake JM, Hoffman HJ, Kobiashi J, et al: Surgical management of children with temporal lobe epilepsy and mass lesions. Neurosurgery 1987;2:92.
40. Drake JM, Kestle JRW, Milner R, et al: Randomized trial of cerebrospinal fluid shunt valve design in pediatric hydrocephalus. Neurosurgery 1998;43:294.
41. Drake JM, Sainte-Rose C: The Shunt Book. New York, Blackwell Scientific, 1995.
42. Duchowny M: The syndrome of partial seizures in infancy. J Child Neurol 1992;7:66.
43. Duchowny M: Epilepsy surgery in children. Curr Opin Neurol 1995;8:112.
44. Duchowny M, Lewin B, Jayakar P, et al: Temporal lobectomy in early childhood. Epilepsia 1992;33:298.
45. Elton S, Oakes WJ: Dermal sinus tracts of the spine. Neurosurgical Focus [serial online], January 10(1), Article 4, 2001. Available at http://www.aans.org/education/journal/neurosurgical/jan01/10-1-4.pdf.
46. Engel J Jr, Rausch R, Lieb JP, et al: Correlation of criteria used for localizing epileptic foci in patients considered for surgical therapy of epilepsy. Ann Neurol 1981;9:215.
47. Erba G, Cavazutti V: Sturge-Weber syndrome: Natural history and indications for surgery. J Epilepsy 1990;3(Suppl 1):287.
48. Foltz EL, Blanks JP: Symptomatic low intracranial pressure in shunted hydrocephalus. J Neurosurg 1988;68:401.
49. Fritsch MJ, Kienke S, Manwaring KH, et al: Endoscopic aqueductoplasty and interventriculostomy for the treatment of isolated fourth ventricle in children. Neurosurgery 2004; 55:372.
50. Fukuda M, Kameyama S, Tomikawa M, et al: Epilepsy surgery for focal cortical dysplasia and dysplasia and dysembryoplastic neuroepithelial tumor. No Shinkei Geka 2000;28:135.
51. Galbraith J, Barr V: Epidural abscess and subdural empyema. Adv Neurol 1974;6:257.
52. Gaskill SJ: Primary closure of open myelomeningocele. Neurosurgical Focus [serial online], February 16(2), Article 3, 2004. Available at http://www.aans.org/education/journal/neurosurgical/feb04/16-2-3.pdf.
53. Greenberg, MS: Handbook of Neurosurgery, 5th ed. New York, Thieme, 2001, p 175.
54. Hamburger V, Hamilton HL: A series of normal stages in the development of the chick embryo. J Morphol 1951;88:49.
55. Harrison MJ, Mitnick RJ, Rosenblum BR, et al: Leptomyelolipoma: Analysis of 20 cases. J Neurosurg 1990; 73:360.
56. Harvey AS, Bowe JM, Hopkins IJ, et al: Ictal ^{99m}Tc-HMPAO single photon emission computed tomography in children with temporal lobe epilepsy. Epilepsia 1993;34:869.
57. Hauser W: Seizure disorders: The changes with age. Epilepsia 1992;4:S6.
58. Hauser WA: Epidemiology of epilepsy in children. Neurosurg Clin N Am 1995;6:419.
59. Herranz JL, Armijo JA, Artega R: Clinical side effects of phenobarbital, primidone, phenytoin, carbamazepine, and valproate during monotherapy in children. Epilepsia 1988;29:794.
60. Holmes GL: Partial complex seizures in children: An analysis of 69 seizures in 24 patients using EEG FM radiotelemetry and videotape recording, Electroencephalogram Clin

Neurophysiol 1984;57:13.
61. Holmes G: The long-term effects of seizures on the developing brain: Clinical and laboratory issues. Brain Dev 1991;13:393.
62. Holmes G: Epilepsy in the developing brain: Lessons from the laboratory and clinic. Epilepsia 1997;38:12.
63. Hoppe-Hirsch E, Laroussinie F, Brunet L, et al: Late outcome of the surgical treatment of hydrocephalus. Childs Nerv Syst 1998;14:97.
64. Hornig G, Murphy JV, Schallert G, et al: Left vagus nerve stimulation in children with refractory epilepsy: An update. South Med J 1997;90:484.
65. Idriss ZH, Gutman LT, Kronfol NM: Brain abscesses in infants and children: Current status of clinical findings, management and prognosis. Clin Pediatr (Phila) 1978;17:738.
66. Jacobsen FS, Sullivan B: Spinal epidural abscess in children. Orthopedics 1994;17:1131.
67. Jalava M, Sillanpaa M, Camfield C, et al: Social adjustment and competence 35 years after onset of childhood epilepsy: A prospective controlled study. Epilepsia 1997;38:708.
68. Jayakar P: Invasive EEG monitoring in children: When, where, and what? J Clin Neurophysiol 1999;16:408.
69. Jayakar P, Duchowny M, Resnick TJ: Subdural monitoring in the evaluation of children for epilepsy surgery. J Child Neurol 1994;9(Suppl 2):S61.
70. Johnson JH Jr, Hariharan S, Berman J, et al: Clinical outcome of pediatric gangliogliomas: Ninety-nine cases over 20 years. Pediatr Neurosurg 1997;27:203.
71. Jones-Gotman M, Smith ML, Zatorre RJ: Neuropsychological testing for localizing and lateralizing the epileptogenic region. In Engel J Jr (ed): Surgical Treatment of the Epilepsies, 2nd ed. New York, Raven Press, 1993, p 245.
72. Kanev PM, Lemire RJ, Loeser JD, et al: Management and long-term follow-up review of children with lipomyelomeningocele, 1952-1987. J Neurosurg 1990;73:48.
73. Kanev PM, Nierbrauer KS: Reflections on the natural history of lipomyelomeningocele. Pediatr Neurosurg 1995;22:137.
74. Katz BZ, Yogev R: Bacterial and viral meningitis and encephalitis. In McLone DG (editor-in-chief): Pediatric Neurosurgery: Surgery of the Developing Nervous System, 4th ed. Philadelphia, WB Saunders, 2001, p 991.
75. Kestle JRW, Drake JM, Cochrane DD, et al: Lack of benefit of endoscopic ventriculoperitoneal shunt insertion: A multicenter randomized trial. J Neurosurg 2003; 98:284.
76. Khajavi K, Comair YG, Prayson RA, et al: Childhood ganglioglioma and medically intractable epilepsy. A clinicopathological study of 15 patients and a review of the literature. Pediatr Neurosurg 1995;22:181.
77. Krauss WE, McCormick PC: Infections of the dural spaces. Neurosurg Clin N Am 1992;3:421.
78. Langley JM, LeBlanc JC, Drake JM, et al: Efficacy of antimicrobial prophylaxis in placement of cerebrospinal fluid shunts: Meta-analysis. Clin Infect Dis 1993;17:98.
79. Laurence KM, Coates S: The natural history of hydrocephalus. Detailed analysis of 182 unoperated cases. Arch Dis Child 1962;37:345.
80. Lee M, Leahu D, Weiner HL, et al: Complications of fourth ventricular shunts. Pediatr Neurosurg 1995;22:309.
81. Lemire RJ: Neural tube defects. JAMA 1988;259:558.
82. Lobel DA, Park YD, Lee MR: Surgical treatment of epilepsy in children. Contemp Neurosurg 2004;26:1.
83. Loring DW, Meador KJ, Lee GP, et al: Amobarbital Effects and Lateralized Brain Function: The Wada Test. New York, Springer-Verlag, 1992.
84. Luders H, Dinner DS, Morris HH, et al: EEG evaluation for epilepsy surgery in children. Clev Clin J Med 1989;56 (Suppl 1):S53.
85. Luken MG, Whelan MA: Recent diagnostic experience with subdural empyema. J Neurosurg 1980;52:764.
86. Lynch BJ, O'Tuama L, Holmes GL, et al: Correlation of Tc99-m HMPAO SPECT with EEG monitoring: Prognostic value for outcome of epilepsy surgery in children. Ann Neurol 1992;32:433.
87. Mackenzie AR, Laing RBS, Smith CC, et al.: Spinal epidural abscess: The importance of early diagnosis and treatment. J Neurol Neurosurg Psychiatry 1998;65:209.
88. Madsen JR, Black PM: Corpus callosotomy. In Albright AL, Pollack IF, Adelson PD (eds): Principles and Practice of Pediatric Neurosurgery. New York, Thieme, 1999, p 1147.
89. Maslen DR, Jones SR, Crisplin MA, et al: Spinal epidural abscess: Optimizing patient care. Arch Intern Med 1993;153:1713.
90. Mathern GW, Giza CC, Yudovin S, et al: Postoperative seizure control and antiepileptic drug use in pediatric epilepsy surgery patients: The UCLA experience, 1986-1997. Epilepsia 1999;40:1740.
91. Mathisen GE, Johnson JP: Brain abscess. Clin Infect Dis 1997;25:763.
92. Mauser HW, Van Houwelingen H, Tulleken CA: Factors affecting the outcome in subdural empyema. J Neurol Neurosurg Psychiatry 1987;50:1136.
93. McLone DG: Repair of the myelomeningocele. In Rengachary SS, Wilkins RH (eds): Neurosurgical Operative Atlas, vol 3. Chicago, American Association of Neurological Surgeons, 1993, p 38.
94. Meyer FB, Marsh WR, Laws ER, et al: Temporal lobectomy in children with epilepsy. J Neurosurg 1986;64:371.
95. Morrell F, Whisler WW, Bleck TP: Multiple subpial transection: A new approach to the surgical treatment of focal epilepsy. J Neurosurg 1989;70:231.
96. Morris GL, Mueller WM: Vagus nerve stimulation study group E01-E05: Long-term treatment with vagus nerve stimulation in patients with refractory epilepsy. Neurology 1999;53:1731.
97. Morrison G: Extratemporal epilepsy surgery in children. In Albright AL, Pollack IF, Adelson PD (eds): Principles and Practice of Pediatric Neurosurgery. New York, Thieme, 1999, p 1127.
98. MRC Vitamin Study Research Group: Prevention of neural tube defects: Results of the Medical Research Council Vitamin Study. Lancet 1991;338:131.
99. Mullan BP, O'Connor MK, Hung JC: Single photon emission computed tomography. Neuroimaging Clin N Am 1995; 5:647.
100. Murphy JV, Hornig G, Schallert G: Left vagal nerve stimulation in children with refractory epilepsy: Preliminary observations. Arch Neurol 1995;52:886.
101. National Institutes of Health: Surgery for epilepsy. Consensus Statement 1990;8:1.
102. Newton MR, Berkovic SF, Austin MC, et al: SPECT in the localization of extratemporal and temporal seizure foci. J Neurol Neurosurg Psychiatry 1995;59:26.
103. Nordli DR Jr, Kelley KR: Selection and evaluation of children for epilepsy surgery. Pediatr Neurosurg 2001; 34:1.
104. Ojemann SG, Peacock WJ: Surgical treatment of epilepsy. In McLone DG (editor-in-chief): Pediatric Neurosurgery: Surgery of the Developing Nervous System, 4th ed. Philadelphia, WB Saunders, 2001, p 1025.
105. Olson DM: Evaluation of children for epilepsy surgery.

Pediatr Neurosurg 2001;34:159.
106. Olson DM, Chugani HT, Shewmon DA, et al: Electrocorticographic confirmation of focal positron emission tomographic abnormalities in children with intractable epilepsy. Epilepsia 1990;31:731.
107. Pang D, Dias MS, Ahab-Barmada M: Split cord malformation. Part I: A unified theory of embryogenesis for double SC malformations. Neurosurgery 1992;31:451.
108. Pattisapu J, Parent A: Subdural empyemas in children. Pediatr Neurosci 1987;13:251.
109. Patwardhan RV, Stong V, Bebin EM, et al: Efficacy of vagal nerve stimulation in children with medically refractory epilepsy. Neurosurgery 2000;47:1353.
110. Peacock WJ: Hemispherectomy. In McLone DG (editor-in-chief): Pediatric Neurosurgery: Surgery of the Developing Nervous System, 4th ed. Philadelphia, WB Saunders, 2001, p 1035.
111. Piatt JH Jr, Carlson CV: A search for determinants of cerebrospinal fluid shunt survival: Retrospective analysis of a 14-year institutional experience. Pediatr Neurosurg 1993;19:233.
112. Pudenz RH, Foltz EL: Hydrocephalus: Overdrainage by ventricular shunts. Surg Neurol 1991;35:200.
113. Pyhtinen J, Paakko E, Jartti P: Cerebral abscess with multiple rims of MRI. Neuroradiology 1997;39:857.
114. Rasmussen T: Hemispherectomy for seizures revisited. Can J Neurol Sci 1983;10:71.
115. Rauzzino MJ, Tubbs RS, Alexander E, et al: Spinal neurenteric cysts and their relation to more common aspects of occult spinal dysraphism. Neurosurgical Focus [serial online], January 10(1), Article 2, 2001. Available at http://www.aans.org/education/journal/neurosurgical/jan01/10-1-2.pdf.
116. Raymond AA, Halpin SF, Alsanjari N, et al: Dysembryoplastic neuroepithelial tumor. Features in 16 patients. Brain 1994;117:461.
117. Rekate HL: Classification of slit-ventricle syndromes using intracranial pressure monitoring. Pediatr Neurosurg 1993;19:15.
118. Renier D, Flandin C, Hirsch E, et al: Brain abscesses in neonates: A study of 30 cases. J Neurosurg 1988;69:877.
119. Rubin G, Michowiz SD, Ashkenasi A, et al: Spinal epidural abscess in the pediatric age group: Case report and review of the literature. Pediatr Infect Dis J 1993;12:1007.
120. Rutecki P: Anatomical, physiological, and theoretical basis for the antiepileptic effect of vagus nerve stimulation. Epilepsia 1990;31(Suppl 2):S1.
121. Sainte-Rose C, Chumas PD: Endoscopic third ventriculostomy. Tech Neurosurg 1995;1:176.
122. Sainte-Rose C, Piatt JH, Renier D, et al: Mechanical complications in shunts. Pediatr Neurosurg 1991;17:2.
123. Salanova V, Morris HHD, Van Ness PC, et al: Comparison of scalp electroencephalogram with subdural electrocorticogram recordings and functional mapping in frontal lobe epilepsy. Arch Neurol 1993;50:294.
124. Schachter SC, Saper CB: Progress in epilepsy research: Vagus nerve stimulation. Epilepsia 1998;39:677.
125. Schoenwolf GC, DeLongo J: Ultrastructure of secondary neurulation in the chick embryo. Am J Anat 1980;158:43.
126. Schoenwolf GC, Smith JL: Mechanisms of neurulation: Traditional viewpoint and recent advances. Development 1990;109:243.
127. Schoenwolf GC, Smith JL: Epithelial cell wedging: A fundamental cell behavior contributing to hinge point formation during epithelial morphogenesis. In Keller RE, Fristrom D (eds): Control of Morphogenesis by Specific Cell Behaviors, vol 1, Seminars in Developmental Biology. London, WB Saunders, 1990, p 325.
128. Sinclair DB, Aronyk K, Snyder T, et al: Pediatric epilepsy surgery at the University of Alberta: 1988-2000. Pediatr Neurol 2003;29:302.
129. Sinclair DB, Aronyk K, Snyder T, et al: Extratemporal resection for childhood epilepsy. Pediatr Neurol 2004;30:177.
130. Smith H, Hendrick E: Subdural empyema and epidural abscess in children. J Neurosurg 1983;58:392.
131. Smith JL, Schoenwolf GC: Notochordal induction of cell wedging in the chick neural plate and its role in neural tube formation. J Exp Zool 1989;250:49.
132. Smith JL, Schoenwolf GC: Neurulation: Coming to closure. Trends Neurosci 1997;20:510.
133. Smith MC: Multiple subpial transection in patients with extratemporal epilepsy. Epilepsia 1998;39(Suppl 4):S81.
134. Spencer DD, Spencer SS, Mattson RH, et al: Access to the posterior medial temporal lobe structures in the surgical treatment of temporal lobe epilepsy. Neurosurgery 1984;15:667.
135. Spencer S: The relative contributions of MRI, SPECT, PET imaging in epilepsy. Epilepsia 1994;35(Suppl 6):S72.
136. Sperling MR, O'Connor MJ: Comparison of depth and subdural electrodes in recording temporal lobe seizures. Neurology 1989;39:1497.
137. Storrs BB: Intracranial tuberculous, fungal, and parasitic infections of the central nervous system. In McLone DG (editor-in-chief): Pediatric Neurosurgery: Surgery of the Developing Nervous System, 4th ed. Philadelphia, WB Saunders, 2001, p 1009.
138. Sutton LN: Fetal neurosurgery for myelomeningocele. Contemp Neurosurg 2003;25.
139. Szabo CA, Wyllie E: Intracarotid amobarbital testing for language and memory dominance in children. Epilepsy Res 1993;15:239.
140. Taha JM, Crone KR: Endoscopically guided shunt placement. Tech Neurosurg 1996;1:159.
141. Takeshita M, Kagawa M, Yato S, et al: Current treatment of brain abscess in patients with congenital heart disease. Neurosurgery 1997;41:1270.
142. Tubbs RS, Chambers MR, Smyth MD, et al: Late gestational intrauterine myelomeningocele repair does not improve lower extremity function. Pediatr Neurosurg 2003;38:128.
143. Tuli S, Alshail E, Drake JM: Third ventriculostomy versus cerebrospinal fluid shunt as a first procedure in pediatric hydrocephalus. Pediatr Neurosurg 1999;30:11.
144. Tuli S, Drake JM, Lawless J, et al: Risk factors for repeated cerebrospinal shunt failures in pediatric patients with hydrocephalus. J Neurosurg 2000;92:31.
145. Tulipan N: Intrauterine closure of myelomeningocele: an update. Neurosurgical Focus [serial online], February 16(2), Article 2, 2004. Available at http://www.aans.org/education/journal/neurosurgical/feb04/16-2-2.pdf.
146. Uematsu S: Detection of an epileptic focus and cortical mapping using a subdural grid. In Rengachary SS, Wilkins RH (eds): Neurosurgical Operative Atlas, vol 2. Chicago, American Association of Neurological Surgeons, 1992, p 67.
147. Villarejo F, Comair YG: Surgical treatment of pediatric epilepsy. In Choux M, Di Rocco C, Hockley AD, Walker ML (eds): Pediatric Neurosurgery. London, Churchill Livingstone, 1999, p 1717.
148. Villavicencio AT, Wellons JC, George TM: Avoiding complicated shunt systems by open fenestration of symptomatic fourth ventricular cysts associated with

hydrocephalus. Pediatr Neurosurg 1998;29:314.
149. Vining EPG, Freeman JM, Brandt J, et al: Progressive unilateral encephalopathy of childhood (Rasmussen's syndrome): A reappraisal. Epilepsia 1993;34:639.
150. Vining EPG, Mellits D, Dorsen M, et al: Psychological and behavioral effects of antiepileptic drugs in children: A double blind comparison between phenobarbital and valproic acid. Pediatrics 1987;80:165.
151. Vivegano F, Bertini E, Boldrini C, et al: Hemimegalencephaly and intractable epilepsy: Benefits of hemispherectomy. Epilepsia 1989;30:833.
152. Walker ML, Fried A, Petronio J: Diagnosis and treatment of the slit ventricle syndrome. Neurosurg Clin N Am 1993;4:707.
153. Warder DE: Tethered cord syndrome and occult spinal dysraphism, Neurosurgical Focus [serial online], January 10(1), Article 1, 2001. Available at http://www.aans.org/education/journal/neurosurgical/jan01/10-1-1.pdf.
154. Warf BC, Scott RM, Barnes PD, et al: Tethered SC in patients with anorectal and urogenital malformations. Pediatr Neurosurg 1993;19:25.
155. Whitehead WE, Kestle JR: The treatment of cerebrospinal fluid shunt infections. Results from a practice survey of the American Society of Pediatric Neurosurgeons. Pediatr Neurosurg 2001;35:205.
156. Williamson PD, Boon PA, Thadani VM, et al: Parietal lobe epilepsy: Diagnostic consideration and results of surgery. Ann Neurol 1992;31:193.
157. Williamson PD, Spencer DD, Spencer SS, et al: Complex partial seizures of frontal lobe origin. Ann Neurol 1985;18:497.
158. Williamson PD, Spencer SS: Clinical and EEG features of complex partial seizures of extratemporal origin. Epilepsia 1986;27(Suppl 2):S46.
159. Winston KR, Welch K, Adler JR, et al: Cerebral hemicorticectomy for epilepsy. J Neurosurg 1992;77:889.
160. Wong TT, Lee LS, Wang HS, et al: Brain abscesses in children—a cooperative study of 83 cases. Childs Nerv Syst 1989;5:19.
161. Wyler AR, Walker G, Richey ET, et al: Chronic subdural strip electrodes recordings for difficult epileptic problems. J Epilepsy 1988;1:171.
162. Wyllie E, Chee M, Granstrom ML, et al: Temporal lobe epilepsy in early childhood. Epilepsia 1993;34:859.
163. Wyllie E, Comair YG, Kotagal P, et al: Seizure outcome after epilepsy surgery in children and adolescents. Ann Neurol 1998;44:740.
164. Wyllie E, Luders H, Morris HH III, et al: Subdural electrodes in the evaluation for epilepsy surgery in children and adults. Neuropediatrics 1988;19:80.
165. Yashon D, Jane JA, Sugar O: The course of severe untreated infantile hydrocephalus. Prognostic significance of cerebral mantle. J Neurosurg 1965;23:509.
166. Young HF, Nulsen FB, Weiss MH, et al: The relationship of intelligence and cerebral mantle in treated infantile hydrocephalus (IQ potential in hydrocephalic children). Pediatrics 1973;52:38.
167. Zeidman SM, Geisler FH, Olivi A: Intraventricular rupture of a purulent brain abscess: Case report. Neurosurgery 1995;36:189.

第 125 章

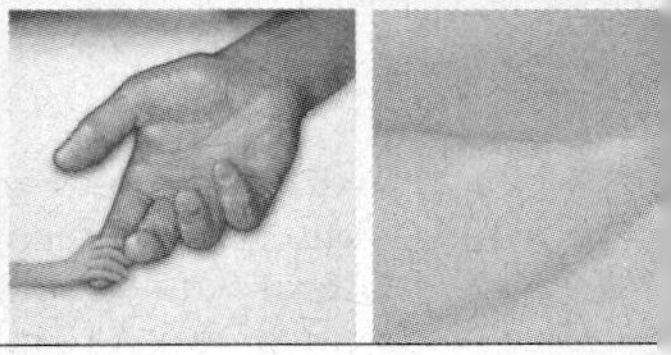

主要先天性骨科疾病

Kosmas Kayes 和 William Didelot

发育性髋关节发育异常（Developmental Dysplasia of the Hip，DDH）

命名/发病率/病因

2018 儿童的髋关节发育异常包括一个很宽的疾病谱，但所有病例都表现为一定程度的股骨头和髋臼的不适应。它可以是很轻的髋臼发育不良，髋臼没有完全发育好（股骨头可以在正常位置或处于轻度半脱位状态），也可以是股骨头完全脱位，完全和髋臼分开。在这两者之间的情况称为不稳定的髋关节，股骨头位于髋臼内，但可以通过轻柔的手法将其从髋臼内脱出或令其处于半脱位状态，或者股骨头处于部分的半脱位状态，有些可以完全脱出但有些则不能[1,6]。另一种类型的髋关节脱位被称为畸形性髋关节脱位，通常与某些神经肌肉疾病有关，例如脊髓脊膜膨出、多关节挛缩或者某种综合征。这种髋关节脱位是僵硬的、固定的脱位，在出生前就存在，对于一般使用在普通髋关节脱位病例上的非手术治疗方法没有反应。绝大多数的髋关节脱位可以在出生时通过体检或 B 超检查发现，但髋关节不稳定的病例直到 1 岁以内才会有所发现。仍然有一些类型的髋关节发育异常直到青少年阶段还没有被查出，通常会表现为髋部疼痛但体检没有什么发现。这种疾病的命名在最近 15 年已经从“先天性髋关节脱位”转变为“发育性髋关节发育异常”（DDH）。这种变化反映了许多明确的信息，即在出生时髋关节的畸形并不明显，并且很少有完全脱位的情况，更多的畸形是在发育过程中出现的[7,31]。

髋关节发育异常是儿童髋关节最多见的疾病。平均每 1000 个新生儿中有 1 名为髋关节脱位，有 10 个存在髋关节半脱位或发育不良。在出生后 2 周内，大多数髋关节会自身夹紧。在这种情况下，10 000 个孩子中大约有 4 个将最终出现髋关节脱位、半脱位或发育不良。女性的发病率明显高于男性，比例为 4∶1，造成这种情况的原因被认为与胎儿对母亲怀孕期间分泌的松弛激素的敏感性有关；女孩会由于松弛激素的作用产生全身关节韧带的一过性松弛，而男孩却不会（因为他们对松弛激素不敏感）。左侧的髋关节异常占 60%，可能与宫内母亲的骶骨压迫髋关节有关，因为大多数胎位是左枕前位。这种疾病的发病率在本土美洲人以及那些有用襁褓包裹孩子习惯的民族中比较高[6]。

髋关节发育异常的发生原因是多方面的。基因、生理学方面的因素以及机械性因素，如出生前和出生后体位，都对其发生有一定的影响。基因是一方面的原因，因为有阳性家族史的孩子发生 DDH 的概率很高，在同胞或双胞胎中同样很高。机械体位因素也是一方面的原因，包括子宫内压迫或异常体位，如第一胎、臀位、羊水过少以及多胞胎都是高危因素。产后体位同样重要，因为有用襁褓包裹孩子传统的民族以及本土美洲人的孩子 DDH 的发病率明显高于其他民族[33,46,53,54]。

诊断

病史和筛查

早期发现 DDH 是非常重要的，越早实施治疗，预后越好。与新生儿相关的病史包括是否是第一胎、宫内体位情况、是否有 DDH 的家族史、是否有相关的骨科或泌尿生殖系统先天性异常、是否是多胞胎以及是否有羊水过少。最大的高危因素是臀位产，第二位的是阳性家族史。

绝大多数的病例通过美国儿科协会制定的筛查计划被早期发现。这一计划包括一系列的体格检查，分
2019 别在孩子出生时及出生后 2 周进行，随后正常的孩子，在 1、2、4、6、9 及 12 个月时复诊随访。对于存在高危因素的孩子，这一计划要严格执行。在这些孩子中，影像学的检查是可以选择的。对于臀位产的女孩，推荐使用影像学检查。对于存在高危因素的孩子，在 4 个月以内要用 B 超检查，4 个月以后摄片检查。尽管可能有个别晚期脱位和发育不良的病例直到出生后很久才被发现，但为此而用影像学检查全部新生儿是没有必要的[3,4,15,20]。不是所有的髋关节发育异常都在出生时表现出症状，一些病例在出生后的几个月内都不表现出体检时的异常。一些病例直到很晚都没有表现出症状，除非用影像学的检查方法；这些病例可能随后在十几岁时出现髋部的疼痛症状。

体格检查

随着孩子年龄的增长，体检的发现也有所不同。对于出生后 3 个月内的孩子，最可靠的体检发现是 Barlow 试验或 Ortolani 试验阳性。在做 Barlow 试验时，髋关节处于屈曲 90 度自然内收体位，膝关节屈曲 90 度，检查者用虎口和手掌抓住患儿的膝关节，拇指在大腿的内侧，4 个手指在大腿的外侧，在内收髋关节的同时，轻轻地将大腿向后外侧推挤，试图将位于髋臼内的股骨头向后方推出。Ortolani 试验的做法与前者相似，所不同的是，用力的方向是将患儿的大腿推向前上方，外展髋关节，试图将已经脱位的股骨头复入髋臼内。在评估时，外展程度的平衡也是很重要的，任何程度的外展不对称都需要进一步检查。皮纹的不对称已经被证明可靠性较低。

超过 3 岁的髋关节发育异常，往往髋关节已经完全脱位，并且无法复位。或许偶尔还可以复位，但只能达到半脱位的程度。在这种情况下，Barlow 试验和 Ortolani 试验已经不再有意义。外展不对称往往是最有提示性的表现，同样的体征还有双腿不等长或 Galeazzi 征阳性，即屈髋屈膝 90 度时一侧的膝盖高于另一侧，也是肢体长度不等的表现。实际上，由于脱位的髋关节向后方移位，因此看上去患侧的腿显得短一些。在能够行走的年龄段，最明显的表现是双腿不等长及骨盆倾斜。患儿可以由于外展肌缩短（无力）产生 Trendelenburg 步态和屈髋挛缩。如果髋关节脱位是双侧的，患儿会出现腰椎前凸加剧。

影像学检查

B 超和 X 光骨盆平片是评估髋关节发育异常的有力工具，但它们的应用时间有所不同。对于 3 周到 4 个月的孩子，B 超是诊断髋关节异常的可靠手段。诊断的可靠性在很大程度上取决于检查者的技术以及读片者的经验。在美国不推荐对所有的新生儿进行 B 超检查。B 超可以通过确定股骨头软骨的位置来评估半脱位的程度，还可以通过测量从髂翼到髋臼后壁的 α 角来评估髋臼的发育程度（图 125-1）。它还可以显示盂唇、关节囊、髂腰肌和股骨头骨化中心。α 角是 2020
在冠状面上测量的，它指的是髂翼垂直线与髋臼骨顶平行线之间的夹角。α 角大于 60 度被认为是正常的。β 角被用来测量盂唇，以及间接测量股骨头的覆盖程度，但不常用来评估髋关节发育异常的程度。还有一种动态的检查方法是通过横断面的扫描来完成的，在做 Barlow 试验时测量半脱位的程度或股骨头的稳定性。

在小于 3～4 个月的孩子中，由于髋臼的骨化中心刚开始形成，骨盆平片的可靠性较低。超过这个年龄段后，摄片检查是监测髋关节发育异常的最具诊断意义和最有效的方法[18]。在预约骨盆摄片时，前后位片和蛙式位片是常规要求完成的（称为正位片和蛙式位骨盆片）。在正位片上要测量一些重要的参数（图 125-2）。Shenton 线指的是从闭孔上缘画半圆形的线，一般该线和股骨颈位于同一水平。如果该线中断，则表明股骨头相对髋臼的位置偏高。Hilgenreiner 线指双侧三角软骨位置连线的水平线。从髋臼外侧缘向 Hilgenreiner 线做垂线，可以将一侧的髋关节划分为 4 个象限。股骨近端干骺端的内侧尖端应该位于内下象限，否则说明髋关节没有复位。髋臼指数指的是从三角软骨到髋臼外侧缘的连线与 Hilgenreiner 线的夹角。正常儿童 1 岁时该角度应小于 25 度。髋臼指数越高说明髋臼的发育越差。

观察评估髋关节发育不良的最好方法是在麻醉下向髋关节注入一些造影剂，然后进行透视检查（关节造影）。造影剂可以显示股骨头软骨的轮廓，显示其与髋臼确切的关系。还可以显示盂唇和股骨头圆韧带

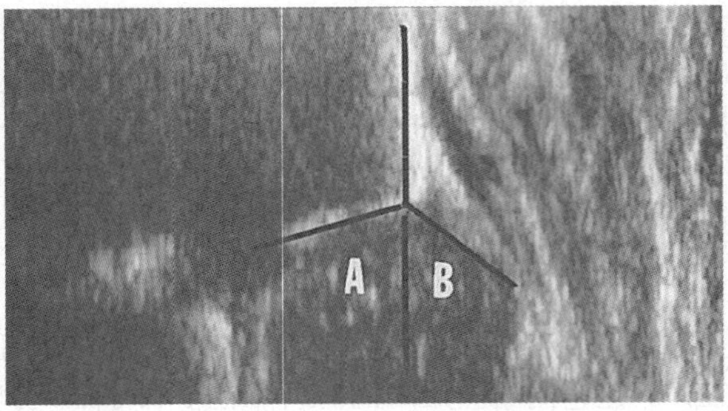

A

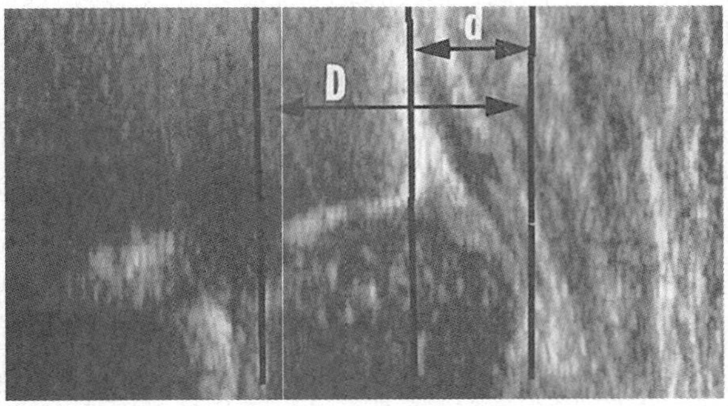

B

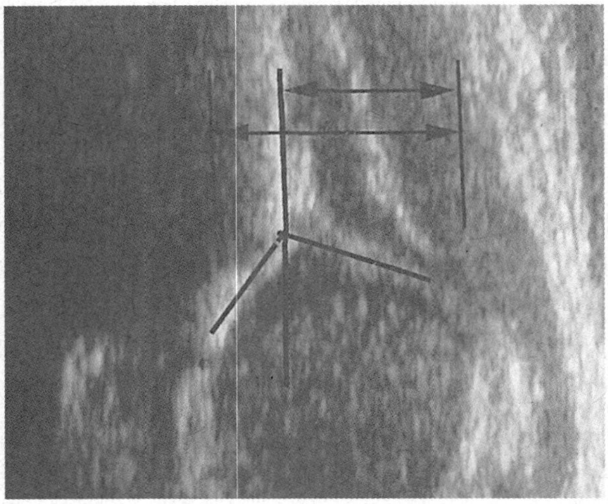
C

图 125-1　A. 标准的正常婴儿髋关节 B 超冠状面图像。α 角（A）相对应的是髋臼的骨顶（正常大于 60 度）。β 角（B）对应的是髋臼的软骨骨顶（正常小于 50 度）。B. 测量股骨头覆盖的百分率：d/D × 100（正常 50%）。C. 一个发育不良的髋关节的 B 超冠状面图像。α 角为 40 度；股骨头处于半脱位状态，只有 25% 的覆盖率。

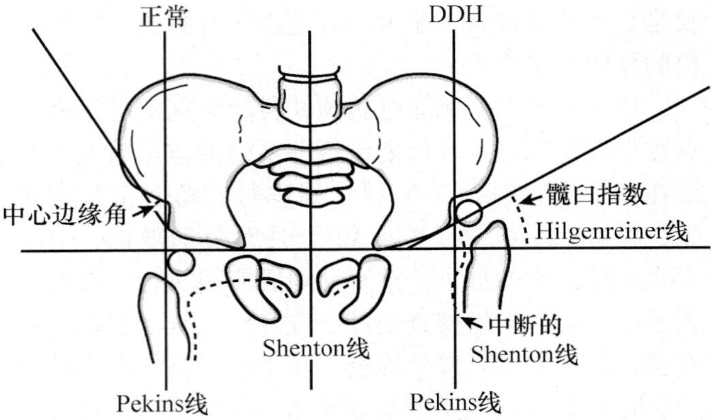

图 125-2　骨盆平片的测量图解。DDH，髋关节发育异常。

的位置以及是否在关节内侧间隙有造影剂的集中显影，如果有则说明关节很松弛或者复位不理想。尽管超声对于评价髋关节的位置很有帮助，但如果对于髋关节的位置和稳定性有疑问，可以选择做关节造影检查。它对于评价闭合复位的髋关节以及在重建矫形手术前制订手术计划非常有帮助。CT 可以用于评价闭合或切开复位后石膏固定的髋关节位置情况。MRI 在 DDH 疾病方面应用较少，但最近有研究显示在术后髋关节评估方面，它与 CT 同样有效，并且可使患者免受 X 线辐射。

解剖/病理解剖

髋关节的发育起始于构成股骨头和髋臼的软骨细胞。在胚胎 7 ~ 8 周时在股骨头和髋臼之间形成一个裂口，形成关节。所以最初的髋关节是处于复位状态的，先前讨论的那些因素导致的是后期的髋关节不稳定。在孕 11 周，髋关节完全形成。在出生后 4 个月之前，股骨头仍然是软骨性的，4 个月时骨化中心开始出现。在生长发育停止之前髋臼和股骨头相互影响共同发育，保持着髋关节的同心圆复位状态。一个缺乏股骨头刺激的髋臼无法正常发育。如果髋关节在早期是稳定的，那么关节会自行对一些发育不良进行塑形，最终形成一个正常的关节。股骨头脱位的时间越久，最终产生正常髋关节解剖形态的可能性就越小。在出生后的第一年，髋臼的塑形能力最强，在 4 ~ 5 岁前仍然存在一定的塑形能力，在此之后塑形的潜力极小。

与髋关节发育异常相关的解剖结构（表 125-1）在不同病例中作用各不相同。内收肌逐渐挛缩。对于

表 125-1 阻挡复位的因素
内收肌
髂腰肌
内侧关节囊
内翻的盂唇
股骨头圆韧带
脂肪垫
髋臼横韧带

全脱位的髋关节，髂腰肌可能是复位的一个很大的阻碍因素。它会在关节囊的前外侧产生一个沙漏形的压迫切迹，阻挡股骨头的复位。股骨头圆韧带连接股骨
2021 头中心小凹和髋臼深部，它可以增生肥大，阻挡股骨头同心圆复位。脂肪垫是指堆积在髋臼内侧壁的一些脂肪和纤维组织，它可以在尝试复位髋关节时使股骨头向外侧移位。盂唇和髋臼的软骨边缘可以内翻折叠或变钝阻挡股骨头复位。髋关节的前内侧关节囊可以挛缩。髋横韧带在髋臼内壁和后壁之间下方跨过髋关节也会阻挡股骨头向内复位。随着孩子年龄的增大，这些因素会变得越来越明显，给完成复位造成很大困难。

治疗

治疗有两个目的：第一个目的是将股骨头复位，并且使其稳定在髋臼内；第二个目的是确保各种髋臼发育不良的塑形。如果达到了第一个目的，并且完成了同心圆复位，那么随着孩子的进一步生长，髋臼还会进一步得到塑形。由于在出生后第一年塑形潜力最大，所以尽可能早地进行治疗相当重要。治疗的计划流程取决于孩子的年龄和髋关节发育异常的程度。以下是可以帮助完成复位和稳定髋关节的各种方法：

Pavlik 吊带
闭合复位加石膏固定
切开复位加关节囊缝合术
股骨短缩截骨
髋臼手术

治疗将根据患儿的年龄被分段讨论。前面提到的治疗方法有些只在某个年龄段使用有效，而另一些则可以跨越整个年龄段应用。

0～6 个月

如果在出生时体检就发现阳性体征（Barlow 或 Ortolani 试验阳性），建议立即请骨科医生会诊。有证据表明，在出生后的两周内绝大多数髋关节会逐渐稳定，所以在两周内的早期治疗目前有争议，但大多数学者仍然建议早期立即治疗。不论是哪种情况，必须进行密切地随访。Pavlik 吊带是治疗这一年龄段患儿的理想选择，它可以应用于小于 6 个月及轻于 20 磅的患儿（图 125-3）。如果髋关节处于脱位状态，或者是可以复位的，那么 Pavlik 吊带是最好的选择。它是一种主动的治疗，在保持髋关节稳定位置的基础上允许髋关节部分活动。吊带使髋关节保持在屈曲 90～100 度并外展的体位上以达到稳定髋关节的目的。每天需佩戴吊带 24 小时，及时地调整和纠正吊带所保持的体位对于降低并发症的发生率非常重要。吊带治疗可能导致股骨头无菌坏死（AVN，在以后的章节内

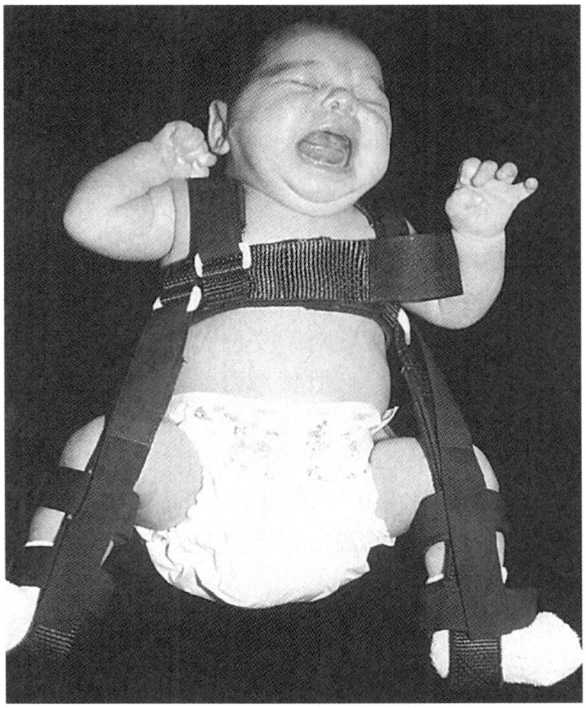

图 125-3 接受 Pavlik 吊带治疗的婴儿。通过前方吊带维持髋关节屈曲大约 100 度，通过后方吊带（未显示）限制髋关节的内收。

讨论），这一并发症的产生被认为与过度屈曲髋关节后外展带过紧有关。一旦实施治疗，吊带需要在一周内检查一次以明确吊带是否合适以及是否能够被患儿家庭所接受。治疗的时间长度大约是患儿被诊断时年龄的两倍，也有一些学者推荐不论诊断时的年龄有多大，至少要佩戴吊带治疗 3 个月。当临床检查和影像学检查都显示正常后，可以去除吊带。这种治疗对于 90% 以上的 Barlow 试验阳性（髋关节在位，但是可以被脱出）患儿有效[28,35,36]。如果髋关节是 Ortolani 试验阳性（髋关节是脱位的，但可以被复位），这种吊带治疗也会有效，但必须连续应用 3 周以上。

吊带佩戴的方式首先是将患儿的双上臂穿过上方吊带，确保胸部吊带位于患儿乳头水平。然后将足部穿入马镫形吊带，将尼龙搭扣扣住。前方的吊带从胸带一直延伸至足带，应将其放松至股骨与身体纵轴呈 90 度角的位置。为了防止股骨头无菌坏死以及股神经一过性麻痹，髋关节不应屈曲超过 90 度。后方的外展带不应过紧，只要髋关节内收不超过中线即可。

在这个时间段内，如果髋关节不能通过轻柔的手法得到复位或者对于 Pavlik 吊带治疗两周没有反应，
2022 可以应用闭合复位来治疗。关节造影检查通常在全身麻醉下进行，检查髋关节的稳定性。如果在关节造影中达到了复位标准，可以进行髋关节人字石膏固定，髋关节被固定在屈曲 90 度、外展 30～60 度的安全角度内。如果需要通过极度外展来保持复位的稳定性，则需要切开复位。如果需要通过极度的外展髋关节来保持石膏内髋关节的稳定，则有股骨头无菌坏死的危险。关节内侧的间隙应该很小（小于 3～5 毫米），否则闭合复位的成功率很低。那些阻挡髋关节复位的障碍物可以通过逐渐挤压来使其收缩，否则需要仔细考虑切开复位的必要性。对于复位前的牵引目前仍存在争议，即对于其能降低股骨头无菌坏死的发生率这一观点，有的研究支持，有些则不支持[34,36,48]。通常采用 Bryant 牵引方式对患儿进行牵引（即髋关节屈曲 90 度，膝关节屈曲 10～20 度），牵引 1～2 周后进行闭合复位。在牵引的最后几天内，逐步外展髋关节以便为复位创造条件。

在闭合复位后，患儿被固定在人形位石膏内 6～8 周。通常在术后进行一次 CT（或 MRI）检查，以确保复位成功。一般在 6～8 周时再进行一次关节造影检查，以评估髋关节发育进展情况。石膏可以延续到 6～12 周，然后全天或夜间使用外展支具来刺激髋臼的发育。一些学者推荐应用某些类型的外展支具直到摄片检查髋关节发育正常为止[41]。

6～12 个月

随着患儿年龄增大，如果髋关节仍然没有复位（图 125-4），一些代偿性的改变会逐渐加剧，常常需要一些更积极的方法来克服阻挡复位的障碍。在这个年龄段，没有使用 Pavlik 吊带的指征。如果能够实现轻柔的同心圆式的稳定复位，那么闭合复位的方法还是可以使用的。如果在早期需要通过过度的外展来维持髋关节的稳定，那么发生并发症的危险将会增加，主要是股骨头无菌坏死。在这种情况下可以考虑手术切开复位。一些学者认为除非闭合复位可以立即得到一个非常完美的同心圆复位，而且非常稳定，否则都应该考虑手术切开复位，他们认为切开复位比被动的、头臼不适应的闭合复位安全。切开复位的目的与闭合复位相同，都是为了达到股骨头和髋臼的同心圆稳定复位。在切开复位时，目前有两种进路最常用来达到以上目的，这两种进路各有各的优点。

Smith-Peterson 前侧切开应用的是阔筋膜张肌和缝匠肌之间的间隙。它是最常用的进路，并且通过这一进路，所有阻挡股骨头复位的结构都能被暴露出来。内收肌和髂腰肌可以被延长，盂唇可以被切开或松解，圆韧带和脂肪垫被切除。虽然髋横韧带位于髋臼的深层，但需要的时候也可以将其切除。紧缩前方的关节囊（关节囊成形）有助于提高复位的稳定性。

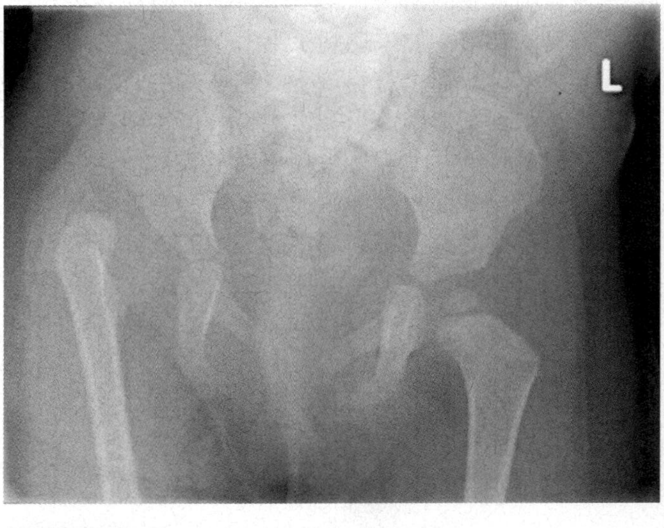

图 125-4 右侧髋关节脱位，左侧是正常的。

一些学者认为这是切开复位操作中最重要的部分，但有证据表明它在稳定关节方面并没有像以往认为的那样发挥非常重要的作用。术后患儿仍然要石膏固定 6～8 周。这一进路对于较大患儿来说是一个较好的选择，髋臼的矫形手术也可以通过这一切口进行。

Ludloff 内侧进路对于技术的要求更高。它常被用于小年龄患儿，由于患儿较小，使得操作的难度更大。这一切口位于腹股沟处内收肌之间，从内收短肌浅层到深层。它可以提供好的进路并能暴露阻挡复位的内侧结构。由于盂唇和前外侧关节囊不能被暴露，因此，关节囊成形术不能通过这一切口来进行。有研究显示，通过这一切口复位时股骨头无菌坏死的发生率较高，因为存在损伤内侧旋支血管的危险。如果股骨头已经移位到髋臼的上方，那么通过这一切口来进行复位是非常困难的。

如果在 X 线片上看到股骨头已经高于髋臼水平，并且软组织严重挛缩，那么股骨短缩截骨有助于获得更加稳定的复位以及减小对股骨头的压力。它有助于降低股骨头无菌坏死的发生率以及增加髋关节的稳定性。如果存在严重的髋外翻或股骨头前倾角明显增大，截骨可以通过一些调整来纠正这些畸形。切口位于大粗隆下方水平，在骨愈合完成之前通过钢板和螺钉来固定截骨端。股骨短缩截骨对于行走期的大年龄患儿来说，基本上都是需要的。

行走期年龄，大于 12 个月

一旦患儿的髋关节开始负重，则适应性的变化开始发生，并且闭合复位成功的概率变得更小。大多数的髋关节需要切开复位，其中许多需要股骨短缩截骨（图 125-5）[14,43]。随着患儿年龄的增大，髋臼塑形的潜力逐渐减小，一些孩子可能需要骨盆截骨来更好地覆盖股骨头并提供更为稳定的复位（图 125-5）。骨盆截骨手术可以采用好几种方式进行，其主要的目的
023 是通过改变髋臼的方向来更多地覆盖股骨头外侧和前方。如果能够获得更多的覆盖及良好的头臼适应度，那么随着时间的推移，髋关节通过塑形达到正常解剖结构的潜力将增大[10,17]。

一些髋关节发育异常的病例到年龄很大时仍然没有被发现。对于超过 4 岁的患儿，手术切开复位髋关节的风险将增加。一些学者建议对 8 岁以内的孩子尝试复位。如果大年龄的孩子双侧髋关节都是脱位的，则医生应该考虑保持这种脱位状态，因为脱位的关节在产生退行性关节炎之前，可以保持很长一段时间而没有大碍。另一种髋关节发育异常的表现为在青春期早期至晚期出现髋关节疼痛，在 X 线片上可以发现这些病例存在髋关节发育不良。这些髋关节没有脱位，但髋臼对于股骨头的覆盖程度有缺陷，股骨头处于不同程度的半脱位状态。在这样的病例中可以采用某种类型的手术改变髋臼的方向来获得更好的头臼相容性和更好的股骨头覆盖率。这样做的目的是希望借此来推迟进一步的退行性关节改变。很多证据表明在 DDH 的自然史中残留髋关节发育不良会导致髋关节退行性关节炎产生，并最终导致需要进行髋关节置换。所有针对 DDH 的直接治疗目的都是要尽量延迟这一过程的进展*。

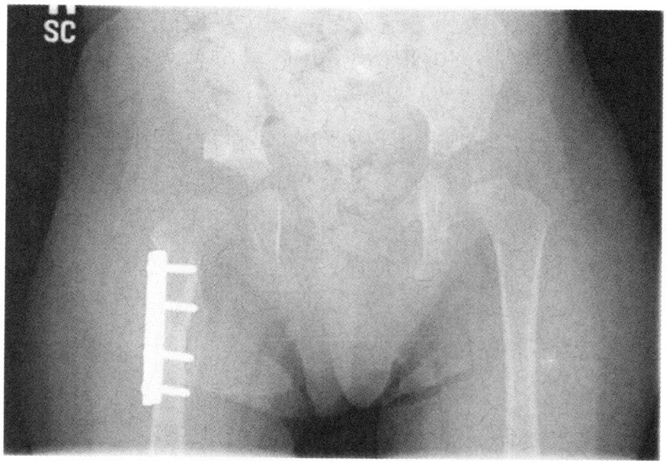

图 125-5　股骨截骨应用钢板和螺钉固定，合并骨盆截骨（箭头）。

并发症

股骨头无菌坏死

如果用苛刻的眼光看长期随访的 DDH 治疗后的 X 线片，60% 的病例存在股骨头无菌坏死。所有形式的治疗都会使股骨头的血供处于危险状态。股骨头无菌坏死的具体病因目前还不清楚，但被认为与闭合复

* 见参考文献 4，8，11-13，16，26-28，32，35，38-40，45，47。

位时对于股骨头压力过高或者在手术时损伤了内旋分支血管有关。在年幼的患儿中，他们的软骨性股骨头被认为具有保护性，小年龄的股骨头无菌坏死患儿有很大的机会痊愈。股骨头无菌坏死可能导致骨骺板生长阻滞，产生股骨颈变短或在骨骼成熟时产生髋内翻或外翻畸形。但是，最终的结果在任何年龄中都是无法预料的[13]。

髋关节再次脱位

有一些髋关节无法通过常规的治疗方式达到稳定，无论是应用 Pavlik 吊带或者是手术治疗。即使经过切开复位骨性手术后，随着时间的推移髋关节还会出现半脱位，甚至全脱位。这种情况往往需要另一次手术治疗，这将增加股骨头无菌坏死的发生率，同时也是长期疗效差的一个预示因素[13,29]。

先天性足部畸形

跖骨内收

命名/发病率/病因

跖骨内收畸形的表现是前半足内收，使得足的内侧缘凹陷，外侧缘凸出（图 125-6）。后足正常，活动自如。发病率约为千分之一，没有性别差异[59]。最可能的病因是宫内体位的压迫。它和髋关节发育异常有时合并发生。

诊断/影像学检查

这种畸形在患儿俯卧位时最易被检查出来，检查
2024 患足的外侧缘可以发现其向内侧偏离，外观突出。畸形的严重程度可以通过测量足跟等分线来明确。足跟等分线是指沿足跟方向向足趾划的垂线。正常情况下该线应通过第二和第三趾之间。轻度的跖骨内收时，该线通过第三趾；畸形加重时，该线会通过第四甚至第五趾。除了前足的内收，足其他部分是正常的。后足正常，踝关节背屈正常。踇外展肌可能会过度活动使得第一趾内收（踇趾返祖现象）。X 光摄片可以评估足部的骨性结构，但除非有其他方面的考虑，否则一般在对这种畸形的诊断中不需要使用。

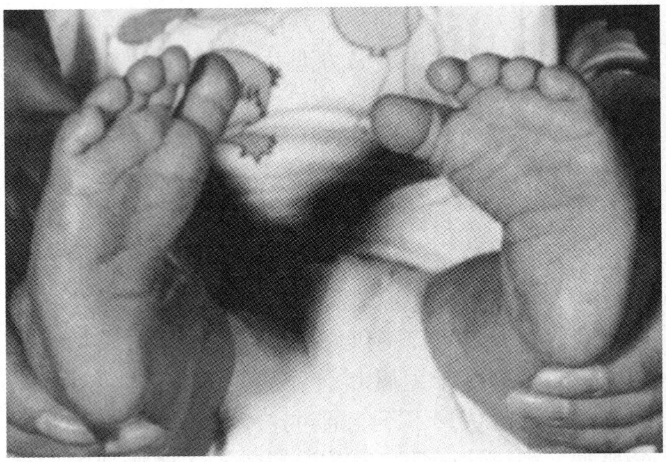

图 125-6 跖骨内收。

治疗

这种畸形的自然史是，如果畸形是柔软的，可以被动纠正到超过中立位，那么大部分跖骨内收能够自发地得到纠正[57]。如果畸形非常严重并且没有得到治疗，那么以后可能会由于第五跖骨基底部的凸出和足内侧缘的凹陷而产生穿鞋不适。它也可能是儿童内八字行走步态产生的原因之一。绝大部分这种畸形不需要治疗或者可以通过家长的手法按摩得到恢复。如果畸形持续存在或者足部僵硬不能被动纠正，可以通过牵引石膏固定加以解决。如果 5 岁以后仍然存在这种畸形，可以考虑手术治疗。对年龄过小的患儿做软组织关节松解手术会导致足部的僵硬。过去实施的跖骨截骨术目前仍在应用。在 5 岁以前等待畸形自行恢复，5 岁以后应用舟状骨撑开楔形截骨加骰骨闭合楔形截骨术是比较可靠的方法[55,56,88]。

柔软型扁平足

命名/发病率/病因

扁平足畸形指的是足内侧纵弓消失。这种表现在

小年龄的儿童中较多见，尤其是当他们刚开始走路时。这些孩子中许多都有关节松弛，当足部负重时，支持足弓的韧带松弛，不能支持体重导致足弓塌陷。胫后肌可能会力量不足，从而导致扁平足产生。

诊断/影像学检查

诊断需要通过临床体检得出。在负重时足的内侧纵弓消失，表现为扁平足的外观。足非常柔软，当足部不负重或足尖负重时，足弓再次出现。当患儿用足趾行走时，足跟像正常一样向内翻位置旋转，同时足弓出现。影像学检查方面，在侧位 X 光片上可以看到距骨呈跖屈位，与第一跖骨不排成一列；然而，如果没有怀疑患儿有其他足部的疾病，一般不需要进行摄片检查。

治疗

如果足是柔软的，那么这种畸形不需要任何治疗。需要告知家长并向其保证这种畸形无需治疗，并且应用支具不会对足弓的形成有任何帮助。许多孩子随着年龄的增长，关节松弛好转，畸形会逐渐得到纠正，足弓会重新出现。如果患儿出现症状，可以考虑通过不同类型的植入物（通常是硅胶、金属螺钉或者 U 型钉）来制动或稳定距下关节。同时可以考虑跟骨或者骰骨的撑开楔形截骨[66-68]。距下关节融合术应用于那些最严重的病例，即出现持续的足部疼痛并且应用其他方法治疗无效的病例。

如果足部不是柔软的，当患儿用足尖站立时，足弓没有出现，则这种畸形属于僵硬型扁平足。这种畸形会对患儿以后的生活造成影响，对于患有这种严重畸形并伴有疼痛的病例可以考虑手术治疗。治疗的结果并不确定，一些患者可能最终还需要通过距下关节融合手术来解除疼痛。

先天性马蹄内翻足

命名/发病率/病因

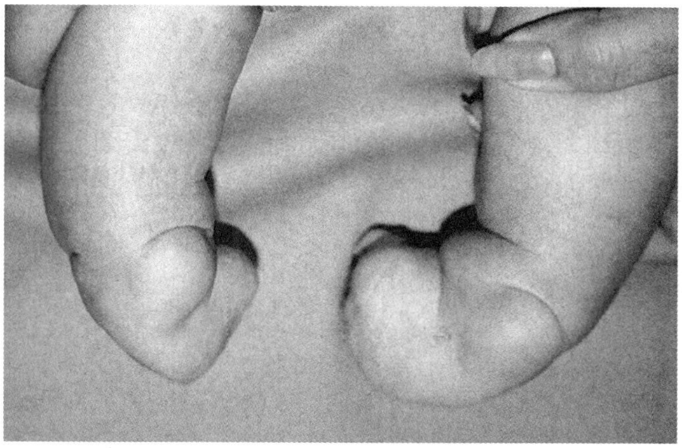

图 125-7　双侧先天性马蹄内翻足患儿显示部分畸形表现。患儿俯卧位，可以明显地显示出后足的内翻。双足内旋，并有马蹄畸形。

先天性马蹄内翻足指的是足部存在以下几种不同程度的畸形：跖骨内收、前足旋后、跟骨或后足内翻以及踝关节马蹄畸形（图 125-7）。因此这种畸形也被称为足部马蹄内翻畸形。畸形的严重程度变化范围很大，从可以通过轻度的牵引治疗得到解决的姿势性马蹄足到通过石膏矫形都无法矫正而必须手术的僵硬型马蹄足。确切的发病原因现在还不清楚，但发病的原因包括体位和遗传等多方面的因素。体位因素可以
是任何缩小胎儿在宫内环境的因素，如羊水过少、第 2025
一胎以及多胞胎等。许多僵硬、持续存在的马蹄内翻足与一些神经肌肉性疾病或者一些综合征有关，如脊柱裂、骨畸形性发育不良、骶骨发育不良以及多关节挛缩等。那些与这些情况中的一种或几种无关的畸形足被认为是发育缺陷的结果。由于表现形式多样，分类非常困难[71,73,80]。

诊断/影像学检查

诊断通常可以通过前面提到的体格检查来完成。由于跖骨内收和旋后的原因，前足向内偏移，导致前足几乎和胫骨相接触，跟骨内翻并且上移，在后跟脂肪垫部位无法触及跟骨结节。在足内侧弓可以出现不同深度的皮肤褶皱凹陷。最后，跟腱非常紧张，导致跟骨上移。偶尔由于畸形程度非常轻，诊断可能会难于做出，但这样的情况非常少见。如果足没有背屈不足，以及跟骨没有内翻，那么这种畸形不是真正的先天性马蹄内翻足。

在新生儿期进行摄片检查是没有必要的，因为那时绝大多数跗骨之间都没有骨化。距骨跟骨指数或跟骨轴线和距骨轴线之间的角度可以在正位片和侧位片上测量。在任何位置上该角度都要大于30度，小于30度则提示这两块骨趋向于平行。在正常足的正侧位片上，它们应该是处于分叉位置上的。随着患儿年龄的增长，摄片检查有助于监测治疗的进程。

解剖/病理解剖

在正常情况下，跟骨和距骨在轴线平面和矢状平面上是处于分叉位置的。在马蹄内翻足畸形中，由于跟骨内翻，导致这两块骨趋向平行。这一畸形和跖骨内收畸形是先天性马蹄内翻足最主要的骨性畸形。足的第一轴线跖屈畸形，舟状骨相对距骨头向内侧背侧半脱位。距骨通常较小，距骨颈短，形态异常。软组织畸形方面包括严重的跟腱挛缩，胫后肌、趾长屈肌、踇长屈肌挛缩。这些肌腱通过足的内侧部分，偶尔它们还会和其他肌腱的一些条索相融合。这些肌腱经常被包裹在一些瘢痕组织内，形成所谓的Henry结节。跖腱膜同样也非常紧张。[70]

治疗

对先天性马蹄内翻足的治疗常需要某些手法矫正和石膏矫正，并且许多畸形足需要手术治疗。被Ponseti所推崇的手法加石膏矫形的治疗方法已经有30年的历史，但直到最近5~10年，这一方法才在小儿骨科界被广泛采纳。这一方法已经取得了很好的近期疗效，最近对一些大孩子的随访显示畸形的纠正得到了维持[72,74,77,78]。治疗的过程包括6~8次经过手法矫正后的长腿石膏筒固定。第一步是纠正足部第一轴线的跖屈畸形，使其和其他跖骨的轴线方向一致。在这个阶段，石膏不能提供很大的矫正作用，但可以改善第一跖骨的跖屈畸形，并且逐步消除足弓内侧的皮肤褶皱凹陷。接下来的几次石膏固定逐步纠正足的旋后和内收畸形，使足的方向和胫骨方向一致，最终达到轻度的过度矫正，即轻度外翻的体位。最后一次石膏矫正通过缓慢地使足部背屈来尝试纠正马蹄畸形。值得注意的是，在没有完全纠正内翻畸形时不要迅速纠正马蹄畸形，否则会出现摇椅足畸形。在大部分的畸形足矫正过程中，需要进行跟腱切断术来达到松解跟腱的目的，使得跟骨下降至足跟脂肪垫部位，使足能够进行背屈。这个操作可以在医生的诊室里进行，可不需要镇静，随后可以进行最后一次石膏固定，使足处于轻度背屈及外旋的体位。石膏固定3周，然后患儿佩戴最后的Denis Browne外展矫形鞋，防止畸形复发。矫形鞋在患儿9个月以前需要全天佩戴，然后夜间佩戴和部分时间佩戴直至4岁。畸形复发主要是由于没有按照要求佩戴矫形鞋或无法佩戴矫形鞋导致的。

如果跟腱挛缩和足旋后畸形复发，则患者需要接受后路松解，即切开跟腱延长术以及全部或一半的胫后肌转移至足的外侧部分。这一手术通常可以成功地将足纠正到功能体位。

一些骨科医生仍然坚持手术治疗，他们认为手法矫正和石膏固定不能提供足够的矫正。为了提供足够的矫正，需要进行彻底的距下关节松解术。跟腱、胫后肌、踇长屈肌和趾长屈肌需要被延长，跟舟足底韧带和骨间韧带需要被切除。距舟关节需要被松解，舟状骨需要向外侧复位至距骨头前方。在外侧，腓骨肌腱膜需要被松解。对于严重关节间瘢痕导致的僵硬足，需要松解关节囊。当矫形完成时，过度纠正或矫正不足都可能存在，并且随着时间的推移，畸形复发和足的过度矫形都可能发生[79,81,82]。Ponseti方法似乎可以使畸形得到更好的临床矫正，无论是足的外观还是功能。

在法国，由Dimeglio发展推出的一种技术取得了良好效果。这一技术是每天由专职的理疗师对畸形足进行手法矫正，以及在特殊的机器上对畸形足进行被动运动锻炼。这一技术过分依赖操作者的经验和技术，在美国还没有得到推广。虽然到5岁时畸形的复发率极低，但无论采用什么治疗计划，最终没有一个畸形足能够达到临床和放射影像上的完全正常。

先天性膝关节脱位

先天性膝关节脱位包括一系列的疾病谱，从能够自行纠正的轻度体位性脱位到必须通过手术治疗的僵硬型脱位（图125-8）。这种畸形经常发生在患有脊髓脊膜膨出、多关节挛缩及其他一些综合征如Larson综合征的患儿身上。这种畸形经常和DDH、马蹄内翻足及跖骨内收伴随发生。当发现有膝关节脱位时，非常重要的是检查髋关节有无发育异常。出生时膝关节脱位表现为膝关节过伸，由于髋关节屈曲，导致患

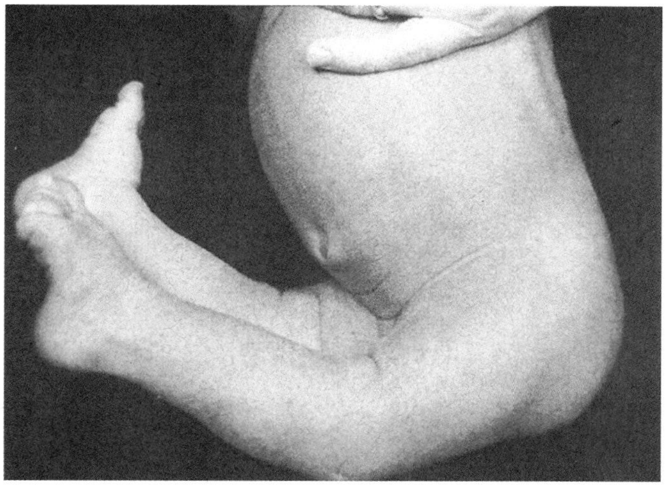

图 125-8　先天性膝关节脱位。

足紧贴患儿头部表面。畸形的病理表现为以下的一种或全部：股四头肌挛缩、髌上囊消失、侧副韧带紧张以及腘绳肌向前方半脱位。

如果畸形是由于宫内体位压迫导致的，那么畸形相对较轻，膝关节仍然能适当屈曲。在几周内膝关节能够自行恢复，或者可以通过轻柔的手法活动帮助促进这种畸形的恢复。系列矫形石膏或许对于畸形的恢复有帮助，如果并发髋关节发育异常，则一旦膝关节的活动度能够适合佩戴吊带，就必须佩戴 Pavlik 吊带治疗。

严重的挛缩畸形和真正的脱位在治疗的早期就会表现出来，因为它们对牵引治疗和系列矫形石膏治疗的反应很小。在治疗后的 3 个月这种表现就能被证明。如果在这段时间内膝关节不能恢复 30 度的屈曲，可以考虑进行手术治疗。手术包括以下的一种或几种，根据畸形的严重程度而定。手术的第一步是 V-Y 股四头肌成形术或 Z 形肌腱延长术，然后如果需要的话可以松解前方的关节囊，腘绳肌肌腱后移，固定侧副韧带。应使膝关节达到 90 度屈曲的程度，然后用石膏固定膝关节于屈曲 45～60 度的位置上 3～4 周。

先天性髌骨脱位

真正的先天性髌骨脱位非常少见。这种情况必须与那些后天性的习惯性髌骨脱位相鉴别。在先天性髌骨脱位的病例中，髌骨发育很差甚至缺如，股骨滑车非常平坦。外侧支持带非常紧张，髌骨向外侧完全脱位。髌骨经常和髂胫束粘连，不能越过股骨外侧髁复位。经常出现膝外翻畸形，同时有膝关节屈曲畸形。在这种情况下，通常需要手术治疗，包括广泛的外侧支持带松解，一直要松解到大粗隆水平，内侧折叠，以及腘绳肌转移固定术或半侧髌韧带转移术。

先天性脊柱畸形

先天性脊柱侧凸非常少见。它是一种脊柱的发育异常，典型的情况是生成障碍和分节异常[101]。先天性意味着畸形在出生时即存在。椎体的畸形在出生时即存在，然而，临床发现的外观畸形通常要在出生后几年才被发现，这取决于发生生长不平衡的程度。单发的椎体异常可能是散发的，但是多发性椎体异常可能是遗传的[103]。真正的发病率目前还不清楚，因为有些椎体异常造成的畸形很小，容易被忽略。

胚胎期脊柱的发育发生在孕 4～6 周。在第六周之前，脊柱间充质机质细胞形成完毕。椎体的形成缺陷就发生在这一时期。这种形成缺陷包括形成障碍、分节障碍以及节段融合。最终的临床畸形的产生取决于椎体畸形的类型、部位以及它对脊柱生长平衡性的影响。

脊柱的分节障碍最易发生在胸椎或胸腰椎部位。它可以是单侧的或是双侧的。单侧的分节障碍也称为“棒状骨桥”，会导致脊柱生长不平衡（图 125-9）。

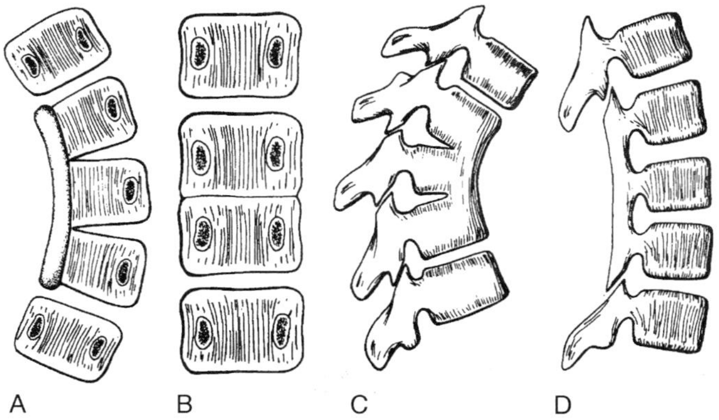

图 125-9　分节障碍。A. 单侧未分节棒状骨桥导致脊柱侧凸，通常进行性加重。B. 双侧分节障碍导致的融合椎体。C. 前方分节缺陷导致的后凸畸形。D. 后方分节障碍导致的前凸畸形。（Adapted with permission from Winter RB: Congenital Deformities of the Spine. New York, Thieme-Stratton, 1983.）

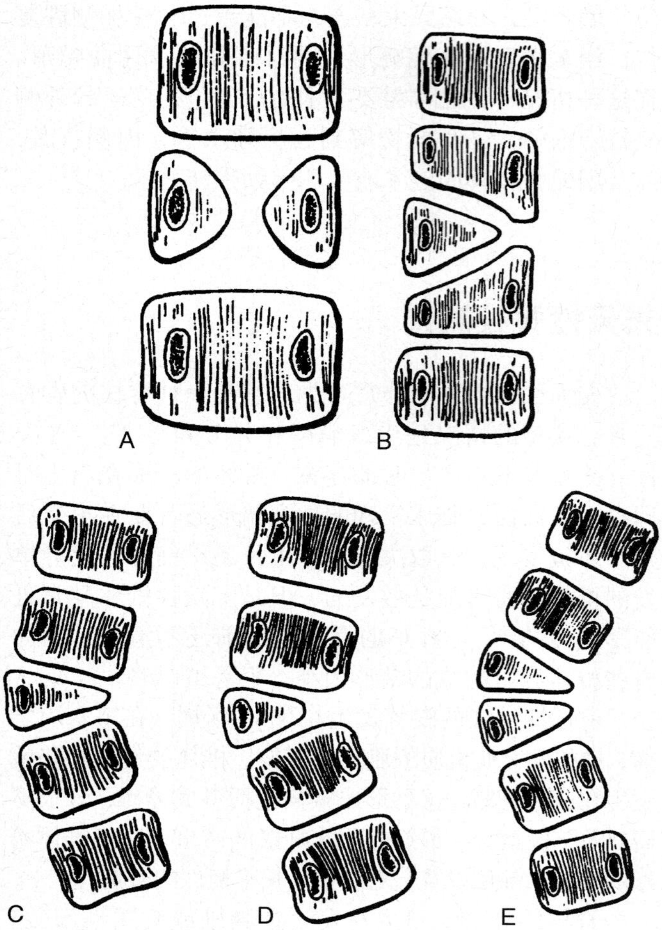

图 125-10 形成障碍。A. 前方中心形成障碍（“蝴蝶椎体”），通常是非进行性的。B. 嵌入型半椎体，注意存在相适应的邻近椎体，造成的畸形很小。C 到 E. 分别为楔形、游离型、多发型半椎体，显示不同的椎体楔形程度，以及逐渐增加的进展趋势。（Adapted with permission from Bradford DS, Hensinger RM: The Pediatric Spine. New York, Thieme, 1985.）

2027 在最初摄片时这种畸形可能并没有表现出来，但如果在 X 线片上发现相应的肋骨融合，则需要高度怀疑存在椎体分节障碍。畸形通常进展很快。最终的畸形程度取决于骨性融合的部位。侧方的棒状骨桥会导致脊柱侧凸，前方的棒状骨桥会导致脊柱后凸，而后方的棒状骨桥则导致脊柱前凸。病变的部位也可组合而导致脊柱后侧凸或前侧凸。到目前为止，最常见的是脊柱侧凸，然后是脊柱后凸，脊柱前凸非常少见。双侧受累的椎体导致一块融合椎体，造成的畸形很小。

椎体形成障碍可以表现为轻度的椎体楔形变到严

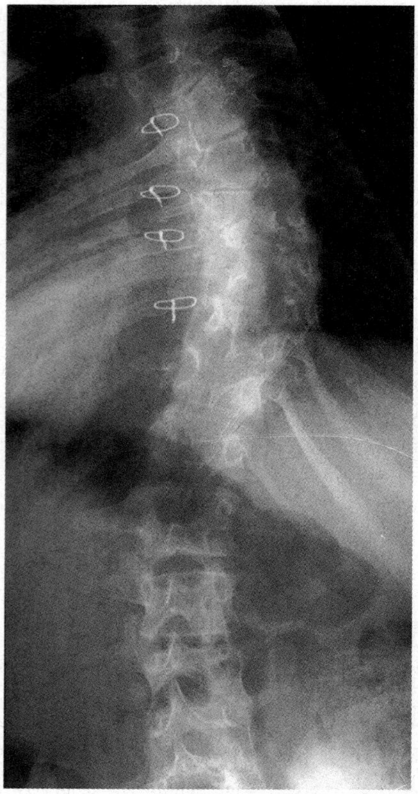

图 125-11 包括分节障碍和形成障碍的多发性畸形。注意在凸侧有肋骨融合，提示存在棒状骨桥。

重的半侧椎体完全缺失（半椎体畸形）（图 125-10）。它可以发生在脊柱的任何部位。半椎体畸形非常常见。如果发生在胸椎，会出现相应的多余肋骨。临床上表现出的畸形程度取决于半椎体的部位以及半椎体的生长潜力。侧方的半椎体会导致脊柱侧凸，而后方的半椎体会导致脊柱后凸。

剩下的畸形是混合型的或者由于其病理变化复杂而很难被分型（图 125-11）。临床上，畸形的数量变化不等，取决于缺陷的程度。但是，进展最快的畸形是一侧半椎体畸形合并对侧的未分化棒状骨桥[98]。这种畸形迅速进展，需要手术介入治疗，并且通常在诊断后就要进行手术。

神经轴的形成和骨性椎管相结合，据报道椎管内畸形的发生率高达 40%[90,100]。70% 的病例存在皮肤表面的异常，包括皮肤凹陷、脂肪瘤、片状毛发增生及痣。脊髓纵裂是最多见的发育畸形[94]。脊髓纵裂是指脊髓或马尾在矢状位上被分裂开，将其劈裂开的是从后方椎体发出的骨性或纤维软骨性结构。如果出

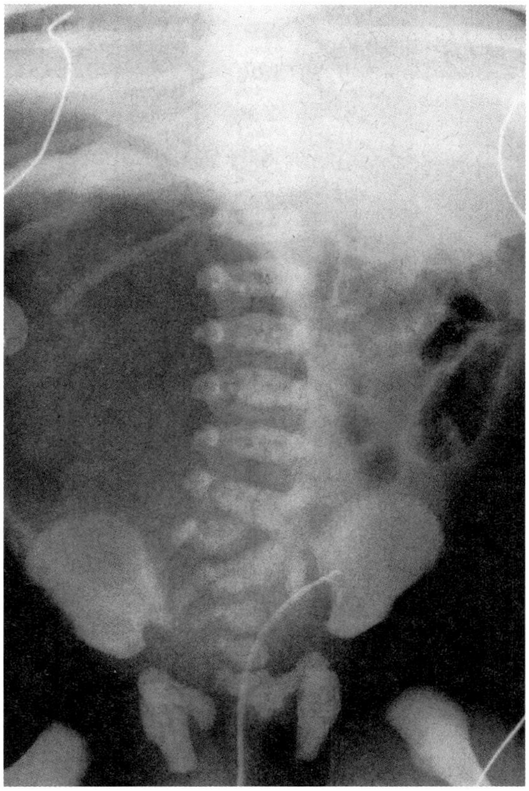

图 125-12　在肛门闭锁患儿肾-输尿管-膀胱 X 光片上的偶然发现，注意 S1 半椎体畸形。

现症状或在进行脊柱的矫形手术之前，需要将其切除。其他的椎管内畸形包括脊髓栓系、脊髓空洞症、表皮囊肿、脂肪瘤和畸胎瘤。对于这类病例必须进行详细的神经学检查，一旦怀疑有异常，需要进行 MRI 检查。

此时伴发其他系统畸形的概率是 60%[87]。包括生殖泌尿系统，25%；Klippel-Feil 综合征（颈椎棘突融合），25%；和心血管系统，10%。消化系统的
028 畸形也可能出现，以及与 VATER 综合征（并发椎体形成缺陷，桡骨发育异常及肾发育异常）相关的气管食管瘘和肛门闭锁。其他骨骼肌肉系统畸形包括 Sprengel 畸形（先天性高肩胛症）、胸廓畸形，四肢发育缺陷相对较少见。所有的病例都需要进行肾 B 超检查以明确是否有潜在的畸形，因为泌尿生殖系统的畸形很难通过单一的体格检查发现。

先天性脊柱侧凸畸形的患儿在出生时可能存在或不存在脊柱畸形。如果存在脊柱畸形，那么典型的畸形是脊柱向侧方偏移。这种情况容易与先天性肌性斜颈（见第 57 章）或婴儿型特发性脊柱侧凸（胸段的脊柱弯曲）相混淆。这两种情况下都会造成出生时出现临床畸形表现，但 X 线片却没有显示椎体发育异常。极常见的情况是，椎体的畸形是在检查其他系统的问题时被发现的（图 125-12），最初发现可以在任何年龄。可以通过 X 线片表现作出诊断，但 MRI 和 CT 检查有助于进一步了解畸形的病理变化。

除了观察之外没有什么更好的非手术治疗方法。与其他对支架治疗有反应的脊柱侧凸不同，先天性脊柱侧凸一般不应用支架治疗。理想的治疗模式是在脊柱病变加剧之前进行手术支撑固定。

先天性脊柱侧凸的手术方法的选择取决于畸形的类型、畸形的部位以及遗留的生长能力。治疗的目标是使病变进展停止，在骨骼成熟时达到脊柱的平衡。椎体生长最迅速的时期是在 2 岁之前和青春期。因此，在这些时期内临床畸形会迅速变化，需要密切监测。这类患者的手术并发症较高。当手术尝试纠正侧凸畸形时，患者极易出现神经系统并发症。理想状态是，当患者的畸形具有很大的进展可能性时，在侧凸角度较小时进行支持固定[95]。其他进展可能性小和进展情况不明确的患儿需要密切随访，摄片检查。在侧凸弧度不再进展或脊柱仍然处于平衡状态时，手术治疗应被推迟。总的来说，50% 的侧凸是稳定的，25% 的侧凸进展缓慢，25% 的侧凸进展迅速。

手术是先天性脊柱侧凸的最终治疗方法。其应用指征是迅速进展的侧凸畸形，以及引起脊柱失平衡的畸形。根据畸形的类型和发生部位，有一系列的手术方法可以选择。尝试纠正侧凸畸形有很高的神经损伤风险。原位融合被认为是金标准[102]，在进展性畸形或有进展趋势但脊柱仍处于平衡状态的畸形中有应用指征。对于年龄小的患儿，必须应用前后路融合以平衡残留的生长能力。对于脊柱残留的生长能力很小的大年龄患儿，单纯的后路融合固定就足够了。半侧骨骺阻滞固定术是原位融合的一种变化方式。它包括仅融合凸侧的椎体部分，而允许凹侧的骨骺继续生长，使得畸形得到纠正。由于是逐渐地纠正畸形，故降低了神经损伤的风险。半椎体切除术在腰椎病变中应用较多，因为腰椎的脊柱失平衡非常明显，并且该部分相应节段的神经马尾在牵拉等损伤方面相对较为安全（图 125-13）。少数情况下，半椎体切除也可在胸椎或胸腰椎节段中应用[91]。但要取得良好的疗效，通常需要前路和后路都暴露。脊柱截骨术和椎体切除术在最严重的病例中应用，包括那些具有极其严重的侧凸失

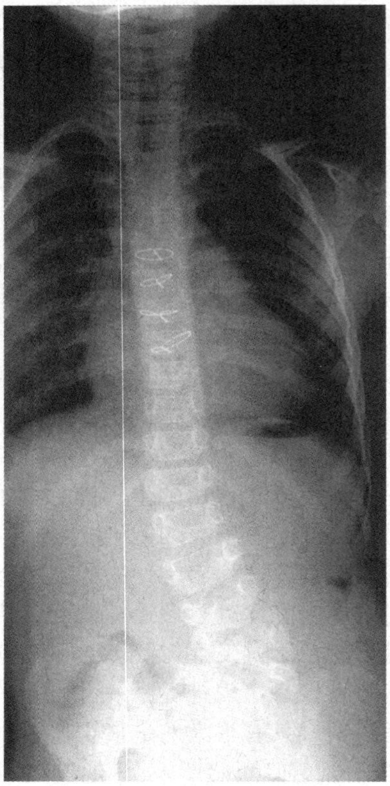

图 125-13 左侧 L5 半椎体畸形导致脊柱失平衡。这是进行半椎体切除术的理想位置。

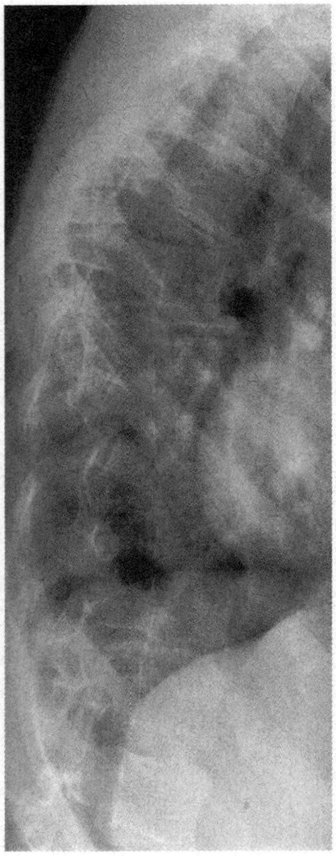

图 125-14 后方半椎体畸形合并前方形成障碍导致后凸畸形。

平衡并且无法通过其他标准术式解决的畸形。由于是对畸形的迅速矫正，所以这类手术有很大的神经损伤风险，绝大多数医生将这类手术作为补救性的手术。

脊柱的前路进路包括传统的经胸入路或者是胸腹联合入路。在这些患者中，由于有其他伴随畸形的存在，以及经胸手术后肺功能有进一步损伤，因此术后发病率很高。在一些情况下，视频辅助的胸腔镜手术非常有用[99]。在应用这种技术时，对于脊柱的显露是足够的，但一些设备仍需要改进，以便能够更完整的切除椎间盘以及进行前路融合固定。应用这一技术后，术后的肺部病变将减轻。

先天性脊柱后凸畸形是先天性脊柱侧凸畸形的变异形式，通常继发于前方椎体发育障碍（图 125-14）[96]。它也可以是由于前方或更常见的前侧方棒状
2029 骨桥导致分节异常而引起。由于存在进展性以及涉及神经组织，这类畸形预后很差。如果没有及时发现，会造成截瘫。先天性脊柱后凸畸形需要在诊断后就进行手术支撑固定，以防止病情进一步恶化。支架没有应用价值。由于畸形的变异性很大，故单一的手术方式不能适用于所有情况。总的来说，如果患儿小于 5 岁，后凸畸形小于 50 度，那么单纯的后路融合就足够了；如果超过 5 岁，畸形更为严重，那么需要前后路的融合术[97]。

骶骨发育不全或者部分或完全骶骨缺失是另一种类型的先天性脊柱畸形。它的发生与母亲的胰岛素依赖型糖尿病有关[89]，尽管最近这二者之间的联系被质疑。它经常与消化系统和泌尿生殖系统的畸形伴发。神经系统受累的情况多变，经常导致髋关节、膝关节和足部的畸形。该病的预后和治疗方式取决于畸形的程度、脊柱的稳定性、神经系统受累的平面以及相关其他畸形的情况。总的来说，只有那些脊柱和骨盆之间有稳定接触的患儿能够行走[92]。他们可能需要手术来矫正下肢的畸形。大部分脊柱和骨盆之间没有稳定关系的患儿将无法行走，其治疗目的是改善坐姿的平衡。

（葛翼华译　赵　黎校）

参考文献

发育性髋关节发育异常

1. Bennett JT, MacEwen GD: Congenital dislocation of the hip. Recent advances and current problems. Clin Orthop 1989; 247:15.
2. Bialik V, Fishman J, Katzir J, Zeltzer M: Clinical assessment of hip instability in the newborn by an orthopaedic surgeon and a pediatrician. J Pediatr Orthop 1986;6:703.
3. Boeree NR, Clarke NMP: Ultrasound imaging and secondary screening for congenital dislocation of the hip. J Bone Joint Surg Br 1994;76:525.
4. Castelein RM, Sauter AJ, de Vlieger M, van Linge B: Natural history of ultrasound hip abnormalities in clinically normal newborns. J Pediatr Orthop 1992;12:423.
5. Cheng JC, Chan YL, Hui PW, et al: Ultrasonographic hip morphometry in infants. J Pediatr Orthop 1994; 14:24.
6. Coleman SS: Congenital dysplasia of the hip in the Navajo Indian. Clin Orthop 1968;56:179.
7. Coleman SS: Developmental dislocation of the hip: Evolutionary changes in diagnosis and treatment. J Pediatr Orthop 1994;14:1.
8. Drummond DS, O'Donnell J, Breed A, et al: Arthrography in the evaluation of congenital dislocation of the hip. Clin Orthop 1989;243:148.
9. Eggli KD, King SH, Boal DK, Quiogue T: Low-dose CT of developmental dysplasia of the hip after reduction: Diagnostic accuracy and dosimetry. AJR Am J Roentgenol 1994; 163:1441.
10. Faciszewski T, Kiefer GN, Coleman SS: Pemberton osteotomy for residual acetabular dysplasia in children who have congenital dislocation of the hip. J Bone Joint Surg Am 1993;75:643.
11. Fish DN, Herzenberg JE, Hensinger RN: Current practice in use of pre-reduction traction for congenital dislocation of the hip. J Pediatr Orthop 1991;11:149.
12. Fleissner PR Jr, Ciccarelli CJ, Eilert RE, et al: The success of closed reduction in the treatment of complex developmental dislocation of the hip. J Pediatr Orthop 1994; 14:631.
13. Gabuzda GM, Renshaw TS: Reduction of congenital dislocation of the hip. J Bone Joint Surg Am 1992;74:624.
14. Galpin RD, Roach JW, Wenger DR, et al: One-stage treatment of congenital dislocation of the joint in older children, including femoral shortening. J Bone Joint Surg Am 1989; 71:734.
15. Garvey M, Donoghue VB, Gorman WA, et al: Radiographic screening at four months of infants at risk for congenital hip dislocation. J Bone Joint Surg Br 1992;74:704.
16. Grill F, Benshael H, Canadell J, et al: The Pavlik harness in the treatment of congenital dislocating hip: Report of a multicenter study of the European Paediatric Orthopaedic Society. J Pediatr Orthop 1988;8:1.
17. Gulman B, Tuncay IC, Dabak N, Karaismailoglu N: Salter's innominate osteotomy in the treatment of congenital hip dislocation: A long-term review. J Pediatr Orthop 1994; 14:662.
18. Harcke HT: Imaging in congenital dislocation and dysplasia of the hip. Clin Orthop 1992;281:2.
19. Hensinger RN: Congenital dislocation of the hip. CIBA Clin Symp 1979;31:1.
20. Hernandez RJ, Cornell RG, Hensinger RN, et al: Ultrasound diagnosis of neonatal congenital dislocation of the hip. J Bone Joint Surg Br 1994;76:539.
21. Herring JA, Cummings DR: The limb-deficient child. In Morrissy RT, Weinstein SL (eds): Lovell and Winter's Pediatric Orthopaedics, 4th ed. Philadelphia, Lippincott-Raven, 1996.
22. Hinderaker T, Daltveit AK, Irgens LM, et al: The impact of intra-uterine factors on neonatal hip instability: An analysis of 1,059,479 children in Norway. Acta Orthop Scand 1994; 65:239.
23. Hummer CD, MacEwen GD: The coexistence of torticollis and congenital dysplasia of the hip. J Bone Joint Surg Am 1972;54:1255.
24. Ilfeld FW, Westin GW, Makin M: Missed or developmental dislocation of the hip. Clin Orthop 1986;203:276.
25. Ishii Y, Weinstein SL, Ponsetti IV: Correlation between arthrograms and operative findings in congenital dislocation of the hip. Clin Orthop 1980;153:138.
26. Jones GT, Schoenecker PL, Dias LS: Developmental hip dysplasia potentiated by inappropriate use of the Pavlik harness. J Pediatr Orthop 1992;12:722.
27. Kahle WK, Anderson MB, Alpert J, et al: The value of preliminary traction in the treatment of congenital dislocation of the hip. J Bone Joint Surg Am 1990;72:1043.
28. Kalamchi A, MacFarlane R 3rd: The Pavlik harness: Results in patients over three months of age. J Pediatric Orthop 1982;2:3.
29. Kasser JR, Bowen JR, MacEwen GD: Varus derotation osteotomy in the treatment of persistent dysplasia in congenital dislocation of the hip. J Bone Joint Surg Am 1985; 67:195.
30. Kershaw CJ, Ware HE, Pattison R, Fixsen JA: Revision of failed open reduction of congenital dislocation of the hip. J Bone Joint Surg Br 1993;75:744.
31. Klisic PJ: Congenital dislocation of the hip: A misleading term. J Bone Joint Surg Br 1989;71:136.
32. Malvitz TA, Weinstein SL: Closed reduction for congenital dysplasia of the hip. J Bone Joint Surg Am 1994;76:1777.
33. McKinnon B, Bosse MJ, Browning WH: Congenital dysplasia of the hip: The lax (subluxatable) newborn hip. J Pediatr Orthop 1984;4:422.
34. Mubarak SJ, Beck LR, Sutherland D: Home traction in the management of congenital dislocation of the hips. J Pediatr Orthop 1986;6:721.
35. Mubarak S, Garfin S, Vance R, et al: Pitfalls in the use of the Pavlik harness for treatment of congenital dysplasia, subluxation, and dislocation of the hip. J Bone Joint Surg Am 1981;63:1239.
36. Mubarak SJ, Leach J, Wenger DR: Management of congenital dislocation of the hip in the infant. Contemp Orthop 1987;15:29.
37. Pavlik A: Stirrups as an aid in the treatment of congenital dysplasias of the hip in children. J Pediatr Orthop 1989; 9:157.
38. Quinn RH, Renshaw TS, DeLuca PA: Preliminary traction in the treatment of developmental dislocation of the hip. J Pediatr Orthop 1994;14:636.
39. Race C, Herring JA: Congenital dislocation of the hip: An evaluation of closed reduction. J Pediatr Orthop 1983; 3:166.
40. Ramsey PL, Lasser S, MacEwen GD: Congenital dislocation of the hip: Use of the Pavlik harness in the child during the first six months of life. J Bone Joint Surg Am 1976;58:1000.
41. Rachbauer F, Sterzinger W, Klestil T, et al: Acetabular development following early treatment of hip dysplasia by Pavlik harness. Acta Orthop Trauma Surg 1994;113:281.
42. Rosendahl K, Markestad T, Lie RT: Ultrasound screening

for developmental dysplasia of the hip in the neonate: The effect on treatment rate and prevalence of late cases. Pediatrics 1995;96:982.
43. Schoenecker PL, Strecker WB: Congenital dislocation of the hip in children. Comparison of the effects of femoral shortening and of skeletal traction in treatment. J Bone Joint Surg Am 1984;66:21.
44. Stanton RP, Capecci R: Computed tomography for early evaluation of developmental dysplasia of the hip. J Pediatr Orthop 1992;12:727.
45. Tavares JO, Gottwald DH, Rochelle JR: Guided abduction traction in the treatment of congenital hip dislocation. J Pediatr Orthop 1994;14:643.
46. Tredwell SJ: Neonatal screening for hip joint instability: Its clinical and economical relevance. Clin Orthop 1992; 281:63.
47. Viere RG, Birch JG, Herring JA, et al: Use of the Pavlik harness in congenital dislocation of the hip. J Bone Joint Surg Am 1990;72:238.
48. Weinstein SL: Traction in developmental dislocation of the hip. Is its use justified? Clin Orthop 1997;338:79.
49. Weinstein SL: Developmental hip dysplasia and dislocation. In Morissy RT, Weinstein SL (eds): Lovell and Winter's Pediatric Orthopedics, vol 2, 5th ed. Philadelphia, Lippincott Williams and Wilkins, 2001, p 905.
50. Weinstein SL, Mubarak SJ, Wenger DR: Developmental hip dysplasia and dislocation: Part 1. J Bone Joint Surg Am 2003;85:1824.
51. Weinstein SL, Mubarak SJ, Wenger DR: Developmental hip dysplasia and dislocation: Part 2. J Bone Joint Surg Am 2003;85:2024.
52. Weintroub S, Grill F: Ultrasonography in developmental dysplasia of the hip. J Bone Joint Surg Am 2000;82:1004.
53. Wilkinson JA: Etiologic factors in congenital displacement of the hip and myelodysplasia. Clin Orthop 1992; 281:75.
54. Yngve D, Gross R: Late diagnosis of hip dislocation in infants. J Pediatr Orthop 1990;10:777.

跖骨内收

55. Bleck EE: Metatarsus adductus: Classification and relationship to outcome of treatment. J Pediatr Orthop 1983;3:2.
56. Brink DS, Levitsky DR: Cuneiform and cuboid wedge osteotomies for correction of residual metatarsus adductus: A surgical review. J Foot Ankle Surg 1995;34:371.
57. Farsetti P, Weinstein SL, Ponseti IV: The long-term functional and radiographic outcomes of untreated and nonoperatively treated metatarsus adductus. J Bone Joint Surg Am 1994;76:257.
58. Ghali NN, Abberton MJ, Silk FF: The management of metatarsus adductus et supinatus. J Bone Joint Surg Br 1984;66:376.
59. Harley BD, Fritzhand AJ, Little JM, et al: Abductory midfoot osteotomy procedure for metatarsus adductus. J Foot Ankle Surg 1995;34:153.
60. Heyman CH, Herndon CH, Strong JM: Mobilization of the tarsometatarsal and intermetatarsal joints for the correction of resistant adduction of the fore part of the foot in congenital clubfoot or congenital metatarsus varus. J Bone Joint Surg Am 1958;40:299.
61. Jacobs JE: Metatarsus varus and hip dysplasia. Clin Orthop 1960;16:203.
62. Katz K, David R, Soudry M: Below-knee plaster cast for the treatment of metatarsus adductus. J Pediatr Orthop 1999; 19:49.
63. Kite JH: Congenital metatarsus varus. J Bone Joint Surg Am 1967;49:388.
64. Ponseti IV, Becker JR: Congenital metatarsus adductus: The results of treatment. J Bone Joint Surg Am 1966; 48:702.
65. Smith JT, Bleck EE, Gamble JG, et al: Simple method of documenting metatarsus adductus. J Pediatr Orthop 1991; 11:679.

柔软型扁平足

66. Bruyn JM, Cerniglia MW, Chaney DM: Combination of Evans calcaneal osteotomy and STA-peg arthrodesis for correction of the severe pes valgus planus deformity. J Foot Ankle Surg 1999;38:339.
67. Giannini BS, Caccarelli F, Benedetti MG, et al: Surgical treatment of flexible flatfoot in children, a four-year follow up study. J Bone Joint Surg Am 2001;83(Suppl 2):73.
68. Roye DP Jr, Raimondo RA: Surgical treatment of the child's and adolescent's flexible flatfoot. Clin Podiatr Med Surg 2000;17:515.
69. Wenger DR, Maudlin D, Speck G, et al: Corrective shoes and inserts as treatment for flexible flatfoot in infants and children. J Bone Joint Surg Am 1989;71:800.

先天性马蹄内翻足

70. Carroll NC: Pathoanatomy and surgical treatment of the resistant clubfoot. Instr Course Lect 1988;37:93.
71. Cowell HR, Wein BK: Current concepts review: Genetic aspects of clubfoot. J Bone Joint Surg Am 1980;62:1381.
72. Dobbs MB, Rudzki JR, Purcell DB, et al: Factors predictive of outcome after use of Ponseti method for the treatment of idiopathic clubfeet. J Bone Joint Surg Am 2004;86:22.
73. Goldner JL: Congenital talipes equinovarus—fifteen years of surgical treatment. Curr Pract Orthop Surg 1969; 4:61.
74. Ippolito E, Farsetti P, Caterini R, Tudisco C: Long-term comparative results in patients with congenital clubfoot treated with two different protocols. J Bone Joint Surg Am 2003;85:1286.
75. McKay DW: New concept of and approach to clubfoot treatment, I: Principles and morbid anatomy. J Pediatr Orthop 1982;2:347.
76. McKay DW: New concept of and approach to clubfoot treatment, Section III: Evaluation and results. Correction of the clubfoot. J Pediatr Orthop 1983;3:141.
77. Morcuende JA, Dolan LA, Dietz FR, Ponseti IV: Radical reduction in the rate of extensive corrective surgery for clubfoot using the Ponseti method. Pediatrics 2004;113:376.
78. Noonan KJ, Richards BS: Nonsurgical management of idiopathic clubfoot. J Am Acad Orthop Surg 2003;11:392.
79. Ryoppy S, Sairanen H: Neonatal operative treatment of clubfoot. J Bone Joint Surg Br 1983;65:320.
80. Simons GW: A standardized method for the radiographic evaluation of clubfeet. Clin Orthop 1978;135:107.
81. Thompson GH, Richardson AB, Westin GW: Surgical management of resistant congenital talipes equinovarus deformities. J Bone Joint Surg Am 1982;64:652.
82. Turco VJ: Resistant congenital clubfoot—one stage posteromedial releases with internal fixation. J Bone Joint Surg Am 1979;61:805.

先天性膝关节脱位

83. Curtis BH, Fisher RL: Congenital hyperextension with anterior subluxation of the knee. J Bone Joint Surg Am 1969;51:255.
84. Ferris B, Aichroth P: The treatment of congenital knee dislocation. Clin Orthop 1987;216:135.
85. Nogi J, MacEwen GD: Congenital dislocation of the knee. J Pediatr Orthop 1982;2:509.
86. Ooishi T, Sugioka Y, Matsumoto S, Fujii T: Congenital dislocation of the knee. Clin Orthop 1993;287:189.
87. Beals RK, Robbins JR, Rolfe B: Anomalies associated with vertebral malformations. Clin Orthop 1993;1:99.
88. Beals RK, Rolfe B: VATER association: A unifying concept of multiple anomalies. J Bone Joint Surg Am 1989; 71:948.
89. Blumel J, Evans EB, Eggers GWN: Partial and complete agenesis or malformation of the sacrum with associated anomalies; etiologic and clinical study with special reference to heredity; a preliminary report. J Bone Joint Surg Am 1959;41:497.
90. Bradford DS, Heithoff KB, Cohen M: Intraspinal abnormalities and congenital spine deformities: A radiographic and MRI study. J Pediatr Orthop 1991;11:36.
91. Deviren V, Berven S, Smith JA, et al: Excision of hemivertebrae in the management of congenital scoliosis involving the thoracic and thoracolumbar spine. J Bone Joint Surg Br 2001;83:496.
92. Guille JT, Benevides R, DeAlba LCC, et al: Lumbosacral agenesis: A new classification correlating spinal deformity and ambulatory potential. J Bone Joint Surg Am 2002;84:32.
93. Kalter H: Case reports of malformations associated with maternal diabetes: History and critique. Clin Genet 1993; 43:174.
94. McMaster MJ: Occult intraspinal anomalies and congenital scoliosis. J Bone Joint Surg Am 1984;66:588.
95. McMaster MJ, Ohtsuka K: The natural history of congenital scoliosis: A study of 251 patients. J Bone Joint Surg Am 1982;64:1128.
96. McMaster MJ, Singh H: Natural history of congenital kyphosis and kyphoscoliosis. A study of one hundred and twelve patients. J Bone Joint Surg Am 1999;81:1367.
97. McMaster MJ, Singh H: The surgical management of congenital kyphosis and kyphoscoliosis. Spine 2001;26:2146.
98. Nasca RJ, Stelling FH, Steel HH: Progression of congenital scoliosis due to hemivertebrae and hemevertebrae with bars. J Bone Joint Surg Am 1975;57:456.
99. Regan JJ, Mack MJ, Picetti GD: A technical report on video-assisted thoracoscopy in thoracic spinal surgery. Spine 1995;20:831.
100. Winter RB, Lonstein JE, Denis F, et al: Prevalence of spinal canal or cord anomalies in idiopathic, congenital, and neuromuscular scoliosis. Orthop Trans 1992;16:135.
101. Winter RB, Moe JH, Eilers VE: Congenital scoliosis: A study of 234 patients treated and untreated. J Bone Joint Surg Am 1968;50:1.
102. Winter RB, Moe J, Lonstein J: Posterior spinal arthrodesis for congenital scoliosis: An analysis of the cases of 290 patients 5-19 years old. J Bone Joint Surg Am 1984; 66:1187.
103. Wynne-Davies R: Congenital vertebral anomalies: Aetiology and relationship to spina bifida cystica. J Med Genet 1975;12:280.

第 126 章

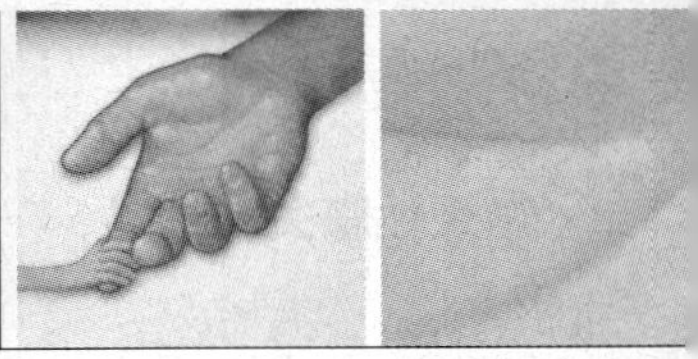

骨与关节感染

Robert M. Kay 和 William L. Oppenheim

2033 在抗生素出现前，骨、肌肉感染常会导致慢性窦道、反复感染甚至死亡[121]。尽管现代医学及外科手术有了长足的发展，但骨与关节感染仍是威胁儿童健康的常见疾病。治疗的目的在于早期清除感染，尽可能减少其对正常组织的破坏，控制远期后遗症的发生。每一位患儿应根据其症状出现时间、累及部位、病原体、对感染的反应以及固有的免疫应答能力来制订个性化的治疗方案。

急性血源性骨髓炎（AHO）

病理生理学

急性血源性骨髓炎是最常见的儿童骨骼肌肉系统感染[23,35,100,147,162]。在抗生素出现前，常导致患儿死亡[121]。在未发育成熟的骨骼中，人们认为感染是由菌血症以及局部创伤共同作用所致。任何因素单一作用不会引起典型的骨髓炎表现[102,119,130,158]。儿童长骨骺板具有独特的解剖结构和血液循环特点，所以易于受到局部感染。而成年人其感染可发生于骨的任何部位，常与创伤有关。

菌血症一般源自患儿近期的感染或其身体其他部位的感染，如上呼吸道感染、尿路感染、中耳炎、皮肤感染（如脓疱病）[38,61]。尽管一般来讲菌血症源自远处转移，但是邻近组织感染播散也可造成 AHO。也有闭合骨折后骨髓炎的报道，但较罕见[18]。因此，许多儿童时期的感染在播散到骨骼之前，及时、有效的治疗可以控制急性骨髓炎的发生[26]。

感染更易发生于长骨干骺端，尤其是下肢长骨。这可能是由于生长期儿童干骺端小动脉终末吻合支的血液流动缓慢，以及此处网状内皮组织系统功能不完善（图 126-1）[35,38,102]。创伤后脓毒性血栓在血肿部位聚集，部分是因为此处细菌的黏附性增加[58]。婴幼儿的危险性更大，因其免疫系统发育不完善，同时留置导管的应用也会增加潜在感染的发生率[46]。12～18个月前的小儿，感染可迅速扩散累及骨骺；在较年长儿童中，则由于其骨骺远、近端独立循环的形成而不会发生此种扩散[22,107]。

一旦细菌定居于干骺端，宿主的防御系统会试图将其清除，可能造成感染的完全消散、部分感染或者慢性感染。若感染局限于骨内，则形成 Brodie 脓肿，放射线片上表现为邻近骨骺形成骨膜下脓肿。如局部感染没有被控制，则会沿 Volkmann 管道扩散，穿过干骺端形成骨膜下脓肿。若骺板位于关节内，细菌可以透过骺板进入关节腔导致关节炎。骨膜下脓肿形成，压力增高，进一步影响血供，导致缺血、骨破坏及感染持续扩散的恶性循环。

尽管金黄色葡萄球菌是儿童时期最常见的致病菌，但病原菌根据患儿的年龄而不同*。据报道，在不同研究中，44%～88%细菌培养阳性者为金黄色葡萄球菌感染[26,35,100,132,162]。B 族链球菌和革兰阴性菌在新生儿中多见。4～5 岁未接受 B 型流感嗜血杆菌（HIB）疫苗患儿多为流感嗜血杆菌感染。在上述人群中，流感嗜血杆菌引起的 AHO 在小于 2 岁的患儿中约占 10%，在
5 岁以内患儿中占 5%[35,105]。若治疗不彻底，可能引 2034
起继发性脑脊髓膜炎。接受过 HIB 免疫的儿童，Kingella kingae（KK）为常见的病原菌[48,90,166]。

罕见的机会性感染则见于特异性高危人群，如重

---

* 见参考文献 26，30，35，37，38，61，66，100，105，132，138 和 162。

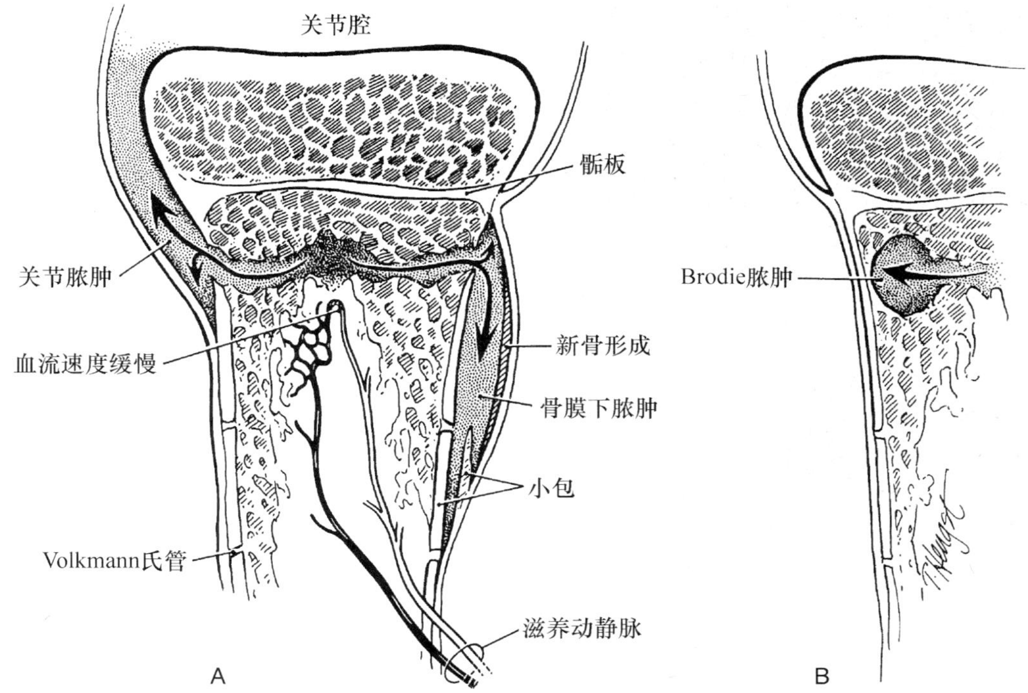

图 126-1　A. 儿童骨与关节感染的发病机制：一般血源性播散的感染导致感染停留于长骨干骺端，这部分是由于此处血流缓慢。感染可以随 Volkmann 管播散形成脓肿。陈旧性的坏死骨可不完全吸收（小包）。也可见到骨膜下新骨形成。如果干骺端位于关节囊内（如儿童的髋关节和膝关节），感染可以播散至关节，导致化脓性关节炎。B. 如果感染位于干骺端而没有及时清除，则形成 Brodie 脓肿。

症监护室患儿院内感染[61,66]，镰状红细胞病患儿对沙门杆菌属易感（除金黄色葡萄球菌外）[36,41,52,61,95]。运动时脚部刺伤与假单胞杆菌感染有关[15,41,77]。结核分枝杆菌感染多见于人口密集城市、发展中国家和 HIV 感染流行区域。美国西南部有球孢子菌感染流行，而 Lyme 病在美国东北部和中部流行。

临床表现

发热、局部疼痛、拒动为 AHO 患儿的常见表现。10 岁以内患儿 60%～85% 有此症状[23,35,100,105,162]。男女比例为 2∶1，大于 10 岁患儿中此比例可达 4∶1[37,38,61,100,105,132]。新生儿中仅有体征，或者仅有嗜睡、食欲缺乏或不能吮吸等急性血源性骨髓炎的症状。患者拒动（假瘫）也是新生儿和小婴儿的一个常见表现（图 126-2）。

50%～70% 的儿科骨髓炎发生于股骨和胫骨（图 126－3）[23,26,35,131,162]。一般为单发，2%～7% 为多发[23,26,35,132,162]。

完整病史和体格检查非常重要，医生应详细询问有无潜在的感染源如近期出现的皮肤破损、中耳炎、上呼吸道感染、尿路感染等。感染可能发生的高危因素包括医疗条件、免疫状况、近来所患疾病以及症状持续时间。

体检时，局部的肿、痛、热明显。虽然患儿在体检过程中的情绪改变如哭闹程度对症状的判断有帮助，但是这些在年幼以及精神紧张患儿中可能难于鉴别。

影像学表现

除病史以及体检外，非常重要的是平片检查，尤其是对于病变部位明确的患儿[55,86,129]。在 AHO 早期，深部软组织肿胀的 X 线片仅表现为软组织层次不清；2035
1～2周后，会出现骨质溶解、骨膜抬高、骨膜下新骨形成以及 Brodie 脓肿的典型表现（见图 126-4）。

超声表现与平片的改变是平行的[1,67,68,85,92,93,109,117]，

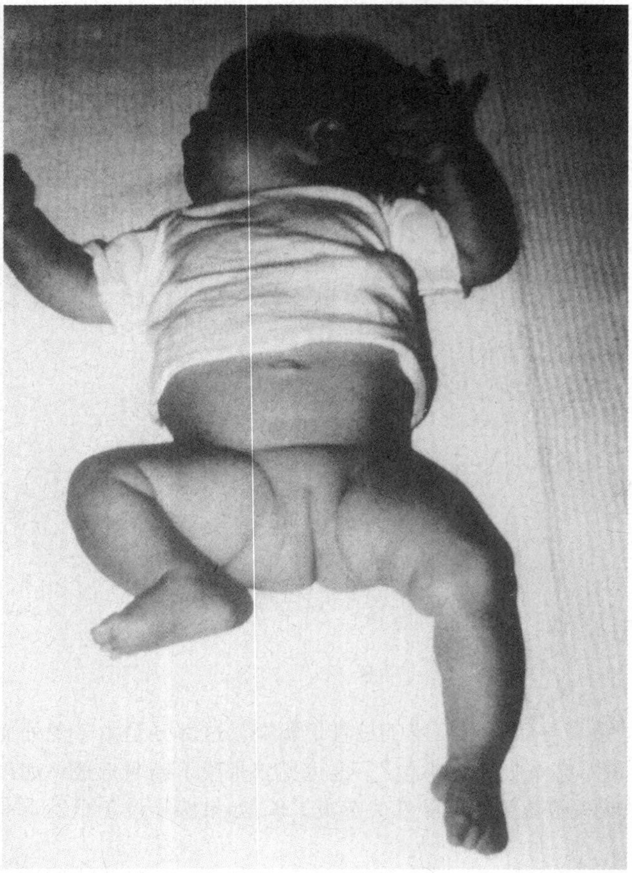

图 126-2 新生儿假性瘫痪，可见不对称性下肢活动，这是由于儿童拒绝活动患肢。

超声对于皮质下脓肿的诊断有重要价值[1,68]。

对于定位新生儿、幼儿的病变部位，以及评价任何年龄患儿脊柱、骨盆等深部感染，三相骨扫描有重要价值。骨扫描的灵敏度为 84%~100% 不等，而特异度为 70%~96%[14,24,25]。骨扫描对新生儿骨骼肌肉感染的评价非常重要，因为此类患儿约有一半表现为多处累及（"转移性"骨髓炎）[37,105]。如果感染进一步发展，可以引起骨坏死，出现冷点而不是典型的热点。扫描表现为冷点的骨髓炎患儿，其感染程度通常重于那些表现为热点的患儿[112]。针抽吸试验 24 小时内不会影响骨扫描的结果[17]。因此，抽吸试验不必等到骨扫描完成后再进行。

血白细胞计数在成人中具有一定的应用价值，但对于怀疑有骨骼肌肉感染的儿童价值不大[83]。

断层扫描对于 AHO 患儿意义不大，尽管其对于确诊和判断感染累及程度有一定价值。CT 可以清楚显示晚期死骨以及骨破坏，但是在平片上同样可以看到[55]。因此，对于疑诊 AHO 的患儿，CT 检查作用不大。其对于疾病晚期判断平片上不显影的死骨以及骨脓肿引流时的手术设计有一定的帮助。

MRI 在诊断骨髓炎方面具有高度的敏感性和特异性，并可以用来确诊和评价骨和软组织受累及的程度[33,55,80,84,86]。MRI 优于 CT 之处在于软组织显影，包括窦道和软组织脓肿，并对 AHO 患儿的评估有重要意义。MRI 常用于骨盆骨髓炎，尤其是当感染波及骨盆后部时。儿童骨盆骨髓炎与软组织感染包括脓肿形成密切相关，因此推荐使用 MRI[64,156]。另外，MRI 可以区别骨髓炎与蜂窝织炎。

实验室检查

应进行白细胞分类计数。虽然白细胞增多和（或）核左移常见，但正常时也不能排除骨髓炎[37,38,132]。C 反应蛋白（CRP）水平和血沉（ESR）在 AHO 中常升高。急性期 CRP 升高及治疗后降低均较 ESR 敏感[111,123,138,154]。若 CRP 在抗生素治疗后不能迅速降低，则提示该患儿高危。

血培养可明确致病菌从而行抗生素治疗。骨膜下穿刺抽吸可以在脓液形成时进行。若骨膜下穿刺未能抽出脓液，可在患儿镇静和全身麻醉下进行骨穿刺。

穿刺抽液应做革兰染色、培养，以及需氧菌、厌氧菌、分枝杆菌和真菌药敏试验。也应做血培养及其他体液培养（唾液、血清、尿液等），因为这些检查在 AHO 患儿中常呈阳性，即使穿刺抽液结果为阴性[35,61,138]。血培养阳性常是唯一阳性表现，在指导抗生素应用方面意义重大[35,61,138]。

微生物学

2037

金黄色葡萄球菌是所有年龄患儿中最常见的病原菌。除此外，新生儿常见病原菌包括 B 族链球菌和革兰阴性棒状菌。

1 个月至 5 岁正常发育的小儿，最常见的病原菌为金黄色葡萄球菌、肺炎双球菌和链球菌[61,101,138]，KK 也有渐增加的趋势（一组调查中小于 3 岁的骨关节感染患儿 KK 感染达 17%），而流感嗜血杆菌降低；

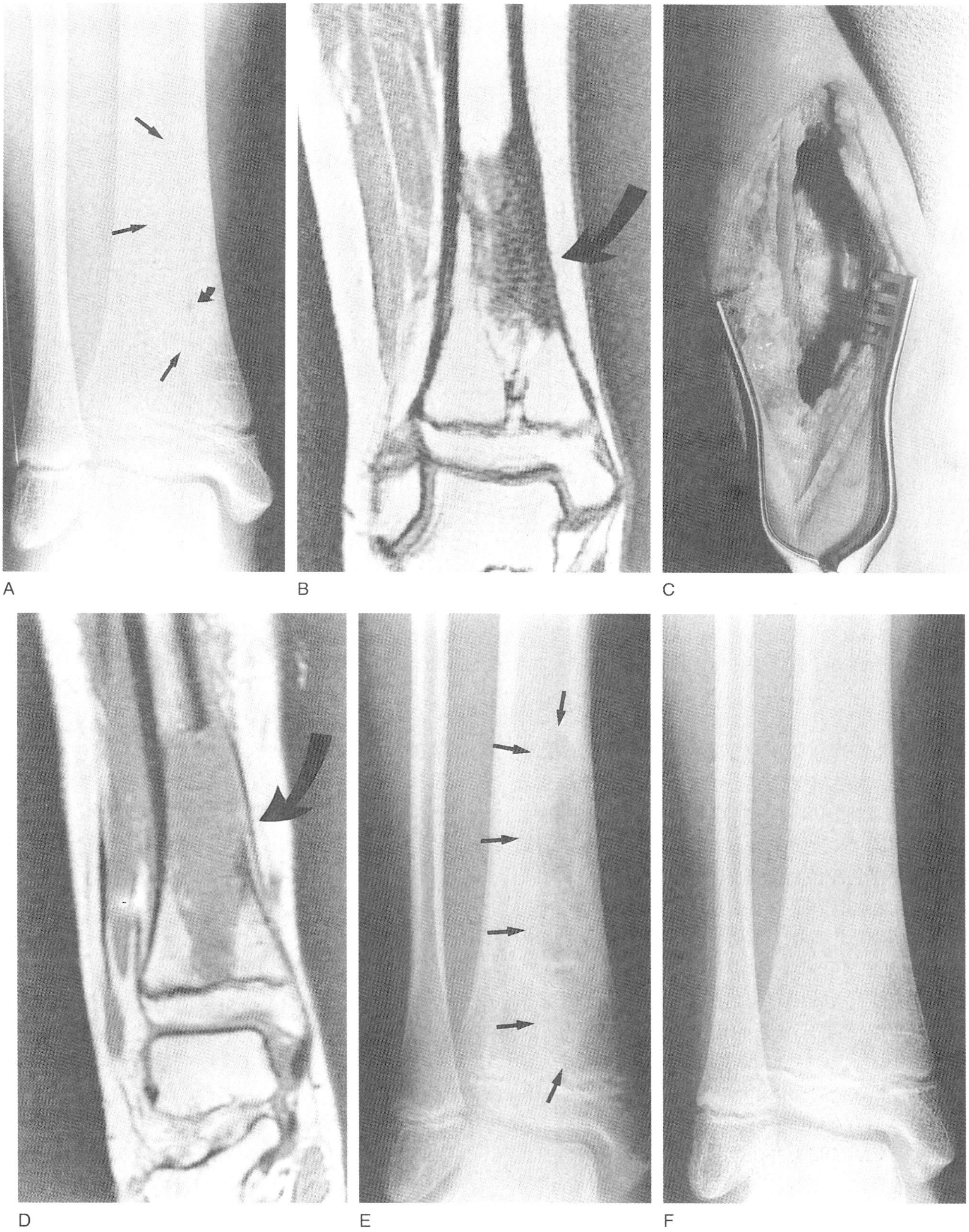

图 126-3 11 岁男孩，10 岁曾患骨髓炎，1 年后疼痛复发。A. 胫骨远端 X 线显示骨硬化性骨髓炎（直箭头所指），伴有透明区（弯箭头所指），与骨样骨瘤的表现相似。B. MRI 的 T1 加权图像显示累及区域（箭头所指）。C. 术中摄片显示彻底清除胫骨远端病灶。D. 术后 MRI 证实。E. 二次清除手术后 1 个月，胫骨缺损处行骨移植（箭头所指）。F. 骨移植后 9 个月，胫骨表现基本正常。

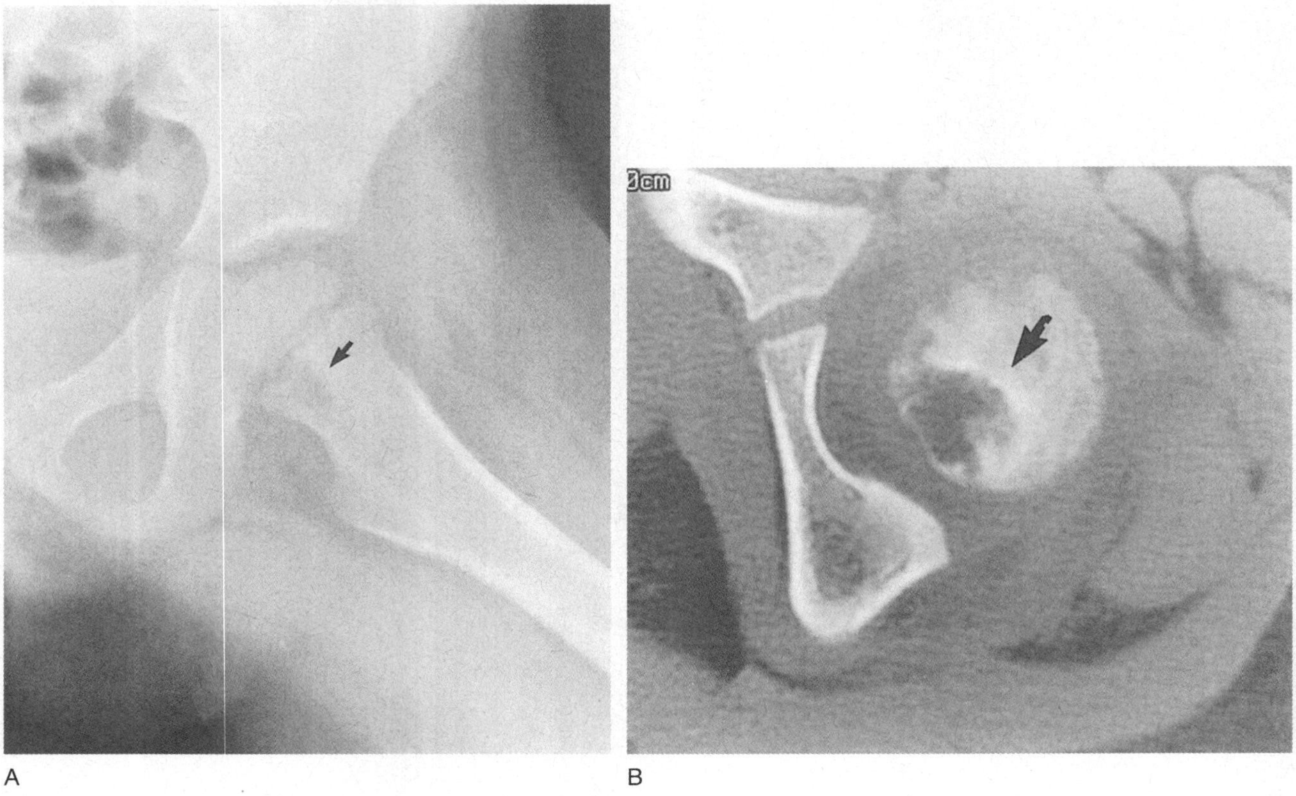

图 126-4 3 岁女孩左股骨近端 Brodie 脓肿，跛行几周。平片（A）和 CT 扫描（B）对 Brodie 脓肿的显示一致。切开活检为骨髓炎；清除病灶，行脂肪植入（由于累及骨骺）。患儿术后应用抗生素 6 周。

幸运的是在儿科骨骼肌肉感染患儿的治疗中，KK 对于大多数抗生素敏感[48,90,166]。HIB 疫苗出现前，3 岁以内 AHO 患儿约 10%～15% 为 HIB 感染。流感嗜血杆菌是 4 岁以内未接受完整 HIB 免疫儿童的主要病原菌。在流感嗜血杆菌所致的儿童细菌性关节炎病例中，30% 有发生脑脊髓膜炎的危险[125,133]。

在 5 岁以上儿童中，金黄色葡萄球菌多为 AHO 的致病菌。

社区获得性耐甲氧苯青霉素金黄色葡萄球菌（CA-MRSA）感染有增高的趋势[62,70,71,97,104,128]，最近两项研究表明，CA-MRSA 存在于 0.6%～0.8% 的正常健康儿童中[71,104]。Sattler 等报告 144 例 CA-MRSA 感染儿童中有 63 例（44%）为抗甲氧苯青霉素菌株感染[128]。CA-MRSA 占社区获得性骨骼肌肉金黄色葡萄球菌感染的 15%～20%[62,128]。目前，CA-MRSA 感染者较院内感染者对抗生素敏感[62,70,71,99,104,128]。70%～100% 的 CA-MRSA 感染者对克林霉素敏感，90%～100% 对庆大霉素敏感，90%～100% 对甲氧苄氨嘧啶-磺胺甲基异噁唑敏感[62,70,128]。多数菌株对红霉素抵抗，并且即使其对克林霉素敏感[62,97]，也可能在抗生素治疗过程中出现耐药性[97]。

治疗

治疗的目的在于快速去除感染，降低死亡率和减少长期后遗症的发生。抗生素仍是达到上述目的的主要途径*。患肢固定制动数日可能减轻症状。

早期抗生素应用以革兰染色结果为参照，若无法检测到细菌则需参考患儿年龄、免疫状况以及可疑病原体，选择一种强效的抗生素（表 126-1）。在MRSA 感染高危地区，需要咨询当地的传染病专家来选择合适的抗生素。

* 见参考文献 49，61，101，105，106，126，136，138，149 和 150。

表 126-1　急性骨髓炎常见病原体及常用抗生素

患儿年龄	常见病原体	抗生素和剂量
<1 个月	B 族链球菌 金黄色葡萄球菌† 肠道革兰阴性棒状菌	苯唑西林* [150~200 mg/(kg·d)] 和庆大霉素 [6.0~7.5 mg/(kg·d)] 或 苯唑西林* [150~200 mg/(kg·d)] 和头孢噻肟 [150 mg/(kg·d)]
1 个月~5 岁	金黄色葡萄球菌† B 型流感嗜血杆菌 (HIB)‡ 肺炎双球菌 链球菌 *Kingella kingae*	非 HIB 免疫 苯唑西林* [150~200 mg/(kg·d)] 和头孢噻肟 [100~150 mg/(kg·d)] 或 头孢呋辛 [100~150 mg/(kg·d)] HIB 免疫 头孢唑林 [100 mg/(kg·d)] 或 苯唑西林* [150~200 mg/(kg·d)] 或 克林霉素 [30~40 mg/(kg·d)]
>5 岁	金黄色葡萄球菌†	头孢唑林 [100 mg/(kg·d)] 或 苯唑西林* [150~200 mg/(kg·d)] 或 克林霉素 [30~40 mg/(kg·d)]

* 可以用萘夫西林代替苯唑西林。
† 考虑到金黄色葡萄球菌的耐药性，可以加用万古霉素或者克林霉素。
‡ HIB 感染在完全免疫儿童中罕见。

新生儿的早期抗生素治疗需要选择一种能够覆盖金黄色葡萄球菌、B 组链球菌和革兰阴性大肠杆菌的抗生素。合理的抗生素包括半合成青霉素（苯唑西林或萘夫西林）和庆大霉素的联合应用。另外，也可以选用半合成青霉素和头孢噻肟的联合治疗。

在 1 个月至 4 岁幼儿中，其免疫状况在抗生素选择上起到重要作用。未接受 HIB 免疫的儿童需应用抗生素清除金黄色葡萄球菌、肺炎双球菌和链球菌，此外还包括流感嗜血杆菌。可选择半合成青霉素（苯唑西林或萘夫西林）与头孢噻肟合用或单用头孢呋辛[61,101,138]。对于 HIB 免疫过的患儿，头孢唑林可以作为首选。在 MRSA 感染高发地区，可在前面用药的基础上加用万古霉素或克林霉素。

在大于 4 岁的儿童中，金黄色葡萄球菌为常见的病原菌。单一药物治疗可选用半合成青霉素（苯唑西林或萘夫西林）或加用头孢唑林[61,101,138]。对于 MRSA感染高发地区，则需在前面用药的基础上加用万古霉素或克林霉素。

患儿首次出现 AHO 时，很少考虑手术治疗。若在强效抗生素应用的第一个 24~48 小时内，临床症状无明显改善，则考虑行前述放射学检查。手术指征包括骨膜下脓肿或累及大量正常骨组织。手术包括冲洗和病灶清除，去除坏死组织。术中需采集病灶培养物。Swiontkowski 推荐使用激光多普勒血流仪以更准确地定位必须清除的病灶范围，尽管多数医生认为价值不大[146]。

首选静脉内给药，过渡到肠道内给药的时间存在争论。只有患儿和家长很想采用口服抗生素方式，才会选择这种治疗方法。Peltola 等研究一组急性葡萄球菌骨髓炎患儿后，认为在 4 天内可以转为口服给药，并且无长期后遗症[111]。

抗生素治疗推荐总疗程 4~6 周*。抗生素疗程小

* 见参考文献 49，61，101，105，106，126，136，138，149 和 150。

于3周者复发率远高于大于3周者[35]。

用于治疗骨骼肌肉感染的口服给药剂量远大于常规治疗软组织感染的剂量（见表126-1）。对于门诊患儿，全血细胞计数、血沉、C反应蛋白需每周检
2039 测。血清细菌滴度目前不需要常规检测。

并发症

AHO的并发症与患儿年龄、对感染的抵抗力、感染的器官，以及确诊和开始治疗的时间有关[121]。如前所述，小于12～18个月的患儿，骨骺和骺板由于骨骺血供的因素而处于高危状态[22,107]。骨骺损伤可导致肢体不等长和（或）成角畸形。

Perlman等报道骨髓炎患儿中的1/3会有邻近关节的感染[113]。若不能及时发现，关节感染可导致关节的破坏。软骨损伤后不能再生的特性使得细菌性关节炎较骨髓炎更需要及时处理。

脑脊髓膜炎也是一种严重的并发症，尤其是流感嗜血杆菌感染，因此静脉大剂量应用抗生素至少3～5天。不能根治的急性感染可发展为慢性骨髓炎，常年疼痛，间歇引流，甚至截肢[105]。长期引流的伤口可并发鳞状细胞癌。

Maraqa等报道了门诊患儿肠外给药治疗儿科骨骼肌肉感染后的并发症[96]。172例中4例（2.2%）发展为慢性或复发感染。并发症与静脉留置导管有关者占30%，非导管相关者占32%，无明确原因的并发症占5%。在门诊患者抗生素治疗过程中，药物不良反应发生率为32%，26%需再次入院治疗。64%的门诊患儿顺利完成肠外抗生素治疗。

化脓性关节炎

病理生理学

化脓性关节炎的病因可能为血源性、直接感染或者邻近长骨骨骺感染通过皮质播散至关节所致*。对多项研究的系统回顾显示，41%的化脓性关节炎发生于膝关节，25%发生于髋关节，13%发生于踝关节，10%发生于肘关节[60]。

临床表现

化脓性关节炎的临床表现与急性骨髓炎类似，但是发病年龄较小。小于2岁的幼儿在化脓性关节炎患儿中占40%～50%[11,75,91]。男性与女性之比为2:1。幼儿可表现为拒动、疼痛、发热，而新生儿仅表现为精神差、苍白等症状，白细胞计数正常，无发热[46]。

在较大儿童中，体检发现类似于急性骨髓炎，但是关节激惹与拒动更典型。通常患膝或患髋呈屈曲位，拒绝检查者活动。髋关节和膝关节发病约占所有病例的70%[11,60,75,133,147]，踝关节占10%。

CRP有时可以高于急性骨髓炎，尽管这两类疾病可能同时存在[154]。急性骨髓炎患儿若CRP在24小时内接近正常的2倍，则表明可能同时存在化脓性关节炎。白细胞分类计数和血沉应常规检查，但是在疾病早期多为正常。CRP在起病早期即可升高，其升高程度高于血沉，并且在感染得到充分治疗后迅速恢复正常。

化脓性关节炎与中毒性滑膜炎难于鉴别，后者是一种髋关节非感染性渗出。化脓性关节炎一般可以有白细胞计数升高，CRP、ESR升高，高热，并且中毒性表现较中毒性滑膜炎重[34]。但是，在一些临床以及实验室检查上，二者有相同之处。中毒性滑膜炎患儿也表现为患肢不愿负重，但较化脓性关节炎的程度轻[88]。Kocher等报道，与滑膜炎相比，化脓性关节炎的高危因素包括拒绝负重、ESR≥40 mm/h、白细胞计数>12 000/ml、发热。若这些危险因素同时存在，则可以区分这两种疾病[88]。

中毒性滑膜炎常表现为一个平台期或在就诊后12～24小时症状减轻。若患儿有滑膜炎症状，但无此过程，那么更需要进行进一步检查，怀疑为化脓性关节炎。

髋关节超声能够检查出髋关节内渗出，但是仅从渗出的多少或者产生回声的能力难于将其与无菌性渗出相鉴别[168]。尽管彩色多普勒可以从股骨头的血运来发现一些异常，但是从实验室检查或临床上并不能区别无菌性渗出与化脓性渗出[143,144]。

---

*见参考文献2，11，30，46，60，75，91，99，113和147。

表 126-2　中毒性滑膜炎和化脓性关节炎的典型生化表现

指标	中毒性滑膜炎	化脓性关节炎
白细胞计数（个/毫升）	<15 000	>50 000
多核细胞（%）	<25	>90
糖含量（血糖百分比 %）	>65	~30

若诊断不确定或者疑为化脓性关节炎，则可以抽吸关节液行革兰染色、细胞计数以及糖定量检查。中毒性滑膜炎的关节液表现为细胞计数低、中性粒细胞减少和糖含量增加（表 126-2）。若革兰染色发现细菌，则可证实化脓性关节炎，同时做药敏试验。

在儿童中，髋关节穿刺需要在麻醉或者持续镇静
2040 下进行，膝关节穿刺可以在门诊进行。若髋关节内无液体抽出，那么可以做关节造影以确定针头位于关节囊内。推荐使用肝素化注射器以防血液凝固，因为凝血可能对细胞计数产生干扰。若细胞学检查后尚余部分样品，可将一滴关节液置于两指指间。由于聚合透明质酸的存在，当两手指分离时，指尖会有少许粘着感。若无粘着感，则可能存在感染。

滑膜液培养的阳性率在化脓性关节炎中为 50%~80%[145]。在急性骨髓炎中，血培养和其他一些相关分泌物的培养可以更准确地检测出病原体。临床和实验室检查证实为化脓性关节炎的患儿，血培养也为阳性，而关节穿刺的阴性率为 30%[147]。

葡萄球菌和链球菌的感染占化脓性关节炎的 50%~70%；在未接受 HIB 免疫的儿童中，流感嗜血杆菌占 25%[60,75,147]。淋病奈瑟球菌感染多见于新生儿、发育期青少年和滥交者[44,60,73,74,110,118,122,159,163]。

化脓性关节炎可与腰大肌脓肿相混淆[137,138]。患有腰大肌脓肿的儿童，髋关节屈曲可以减轻伸髋旋转所致的疼痛（腰大肌征）。有时，还可以有脊柱、腹部或者泌尿生殖系统的疼痛，超声、CT、MRI 可以将腰大肌脓肿与化脓性关节炎相区别。

微生物学

化脓性关节炎中，金黄色葡萄球菌是各年龄组最常见的病原菌。除此之外，新生儿多见 B 族溶血性链球菌和肠道革兰阴性短棒状细菌的感染。

对于 1 个月至 5 岁完整免疫的儿童，最常见的致病菌为金黄色葡萄球菌、KK、肺炎双球菌和化脓性链球菌[60,145]。HIB 对于免疫系统尚未发育完善的儿童来说是一个巨大的威胁，但目前随着疫苗的普及，它的感染已经非常稀少了。

在大于 5 岁的儿童中，金黄色葡萄球菌和 A 组链球菌是多数急性血源性骨髓炎的致病菌，如前所述，性活跃期青少年和性滥交者易发生淋球菌性关系炎。

越来越多的骨髓炎和化脓性关节炎由 CA-MRSA 感染而引起，在近来的两项研究中，由 CA-MRSA 引起的感染占到了金黄色葡萄球菌性骨骼肌肉感染的 15%~20%。具体的感染情况已在前文中述及。再强调一次，在 MRSA 感染高危地区，需要咨询当地传染病专家来选择不同的抗生素。

治疗

治疗的目的在于尽可能快地控制感染，减少关节损伤。在化脓性关节炎发生后几小时内，即可在实验室或临床上观察到关节软骨的破坏*。感染部位的冲洗对预后有重要作用。与骨髓炎发生骨损伤后可以再生不同，关节软骨在化脓性关节炎中受到的破坏是无法修复的。

冲洗包括手术引流（切开或关节镜），或者反复的关节穿刺。手术可对患病关节进行彻底的冲洗，破坏多囊腔隙间的隔膜。术后早期应放置引流管。一些学者提倡反复抽吸关节（膝关节或者踝关节），尽管这种方法较放置引流管有一定缺陷，如初始引流不够彻底，以及反复穿刺使患儿遭受痛苦和多次镇静、麻醉等。

无论哪种方法，抗生素都需要与引流同时应用[60,87]。再一次强调，革兰染色用来指导每次用药，但是若革兰染色未发现细菌或者随后的培养无阳性结果，则需应用与急性骨髓炎类似的强效抗生素治疗。在新生儿中，抗生素治疗包括半合成青霉素（苯唑西

* 见参考文献 2，7，11，27-29，46，56，75，76，114，133 和 136。

表 126-3　化脓性关节炎的常见病原体和常用抗生素

年龄	常见病原体	抗生素和剂量
<1 个月	B 族链球菌	苯唑西林* [150～200 mg/(kg·d)] 和庆大霉素 [6.0～7.5 mg/(kg·d)]
	金黄色葡萄球菌†	或
	肠道革兰阴性棒状菌	苯唑西林* [150～200 mg/(kg·d)] 和头孢噻肟 [150 mg/(kg·d)]
1 个月～5 岁	金黄色葡萄球菌†	非 HIB 免疫
	流感嗜血杆菌 B 型 (HIB)‡	苯唑西林* [150～200 mg/(kg·d)] 和头孢噻肟 [100～150 mg/(kg·d)]
	Kingella kingae	或
	A 族链球菌	头孢呋辛 [100～150 mg/(kg·d)]
	肺炎双球菌	HIB 免疫
		头孢唑林 [100 mg/(kg·d)]
		或
		苯唑西林* [150～200 mg/(kg·d)]
		或
		克林霉素 [30～40 mg/(kg·d)]
>5 岁	金黄色葡萄球菌†	头孢唑林 [100 mg/(kg·d)]
		或
		苯唑西林* [150～200 mg/(kg·d)]

*可以用萘夫西林代替苯唑西林。

†考虑到金黄色葡萄球菌的抗药性，可以加用万古霉素或者克林霉素。

‡HIB 感染在完全免疫儿童中罕见。

林或萘夫西林）和氨基糖苷类抗生素（表 126-3）。5 岁以下儿童治疗可以选用苯唑西林或萘夫西林加用头孢噻肟，或者仅用头孢呋辛。大于 5 岁儿童可选用苯唑西林或萘夫西林。

在 MRSA 感染高发区，对疑有骨骼肌肉感染的儿童，应在前述用药的基础上加用万古霉素或者克林霉素。

并发症

因为化脓性关节炎可以造成关节软骨的破坏，所以并发症常见[7,27-29,142]。最终的诊断依赖于治疗前症状持续的时间、患儿的年龄和致病菌[114,142,145,147]。小
2041 于 1 岁者预后可能更差，因为此类患儿诊断较晚，治疗前症状持续时间长。由于诊断和治疗的延误，常会使小患儿的预后差[22,107]。葡萄球菌和大肠杆菌感染的预后较流感嗜血杆菌差[147]。尽管影像学表现比临床症状重，但是关节面的破坏常见[7]。脑膜炎（尤其是流感嗜血杆菌感染引起的脑膜炎）可能会十分严重。肢体不等长、旋转或者成角畸形也见于骨骺损伤的长期后遗症[7,108,114,142,145]。KK 与其他致病菌相比，其感染不会产生严重的并发症，预后较好[48,90,166]。

其他感染

亚急性骨髓炎

亚急性骨髓炎隐性起病[3,38,54,65,120]，由低毒性致病菌或者残余致病菌所致。可波及骨骺板、骨骺和长骨干骺端，甚至可以穿过骨骺。病程由几周至数月不等，起病至就诊时，放射线平片已有改变。这些骨性改变可能与原发性骨肿瘤相混淆，包括小圆细胞肿

瘤；因此，可能需要取活检明确诊断。金黄色葡萄球菌是最常见的致病菌，尽管培养多为阴性。

髂骨骨髓炎

髂骨骨髓炎占儿童骨髓炎的 1%～2%[6,10]。患儿有孤立性髋关节疼痛，可被误认为化脓性髋关节炎。Beaupre 和 Carroll 描述了三种临床表现：腰椎间盘综合征、臀肌综合征和腹部综合征[6]。表现为腰椎间盘综合征的患儿症状与腰椎间盘突出相似，背部疼痛经常放射到臀部和/或大腿。腹部综合征类似于急腹症，甚至有报道在这些患儿就诊时误认为阑尾炎并行切除术者[6,10]。不论其临床表现如何，体格检查在髋骨有压痛，FABER 试验（髋关节屈曲、外展、外旋）时有疼痛，骨盆外侧有压迹。放射线表现为正常，或者可能在骶髂关节有硬化带和（或）溶解性变化。骨扫描和（或）MRI 在明确诊断时有一定价值[24,63]。骨扫描通过针孔核准技术可以清楚显示病变。Haliloglu 等提出 MRI 对于骶髂关节感染敏感，但是不能将其与骶髂关节炎相区分[63]。多数病例培养后有金黄色葡萄球菌感染。尽管对于顽固性病例可以采用关节冲洗，但是多数仅使用抗生素即可。

慢性复发性多发性骨髓炎

慢性复发性多发性骨髓炎（CRMO）是骨髓炎的
2042 少见类型，仅在近几十年方认识到[8,13,40,47,103,141]。早期与急性骨髓炎难于鉴别。多累及 2～10 处（许多部位可能为无症状），并且女性多于男性。可以表现为皮肤缺损，包括掌跖脓疱病[40,81]。平均发病年龄 10～15岁。常见部位有肢体末端、干骺端、长骨、颈椎和脊柱[40]。

早期放射线检查表现为干骺端溶解性变化，而后渐硬化[81]；但是，此时不排除肿瘤可能。骨扫描可以帮助显示受累程度，并且显示在无症状位点的摄取量增加[81,103]。随着急性骨髓炎进展，CT 表现为骨破坏，并且 MRI 显示累及骨髓[81]。切开组织活检进行微生物及病理学检查，对早期诊断有一定帮助。培养常表现为阴性，病理学改变与骨髓炎一致。在数月至数年的病程中，可反复改善和恶化，恶化时不需重复手术或者培养。抗生素不会改变疾病进程。可以用非固醇类抗炎药物治疗以减轻症状。

椎体骨髓炎

椎体骨髓炎占儿童骨髓炎的 0～3%，典型病例发生于 10 岁以内[37,43,105,132,148,152]。患儿表现为腰痛、局部压痛、发热和拒绝行走[53]。这些患儿拒行任何脊柱运动，脊柱生理弧度消失。骨扫描、MRI 可以明确诊断，尽管 MRI 对早期感染更为敏感，并且能更准确地反映骨和软组织受累及的程度[94,152]。常见病原菌为金黄色葡萄球菌。应进行血培养，虽然多数结果为阴性。静脉应用抗生素 4～6 周，支具保护。一般不需要椎间盘针吸活检。

椎间盘炎

对于椎间盘炎和椎体骨髓炎是否是不同的疾病，或者是一种疾病的不同表现，仍存在一定争论[53]。椎间盘炎的临床表现与椎体炎类似，有腰部疼痛、局部压痛、发热和拒绝行走[12,39,43,53,59]。拒绝负重和脊柱活动这点是一致的。椎间盘炎多见于 2～3 岁的幼儿[43,152]。椎间盘炎是否为感染所致尚无定论。放射线表现为椎间隙狭窄，严重病例显示终板的破坏。金黄色葡萄球菌为常见病原菌。虽然许多病例可通过制动而好转，但是严重病例常应用抗生素治疗。

镰状细胞性贫血患儿的感染

患有镰状细胞性贫血的患儿，其罹患骨髓炎的危险性增高[36,41,52,135]。这可能与血流缓慢、贫血、缺氧和局部缺血有关。镰状细胞危象与骨骼肌肉感染难于区分。这两种情况的患儿均可表现为骨痛和发热，实验室检查可见白细胞增多、炎症标志物（ESR、CRP）升高。在一些病例中，骨骼肌肉感染可以使镰状细胞性贫血患儿贫血加重[82]。

镰状细胞性贫血患儿 247 例主诉骨骼肌肉症状入院，Dalton 等报道其骨骼肌肉感染发病率为 1.6%[32]。骨和骨髓扫描在区别危象和感染时非常有效[134]。超声、骨扫描、MRI也可以协助诊断[127,155,164]。沙门杆菌为镰状细胞性贫血患儿常见病菌，金黄色葡萄球菌也常见[21,36,41,52,95]。治疗与其他的急性骨髓炎相同，但是在选择抗生素时应当考虑沙门杆菌感染。病理性骨折也有报道，在急性病例中多于慢性病例[21,36,41,52,95]。

足部穿刺伤

在足部穿刺伤中，感染发生率近15%，其中有1%～2%深部骨或（和）关节感染（图126-5）[45]。深部感染常与跟骨骨突骨软骨炎相混淆，并且大于90%的病例由假单胞杆菌所致[61,72,77,115,147]。在无感染存在时，可以在运动员的鞋子中发现致病菌。在受伤后几天至几周，由于局部红、肿、痛，行走困难而就诊。确诊后需要静脉应用抗生素和外科手术治疗。抗生素包括氨基糖苷类，治疗至少1～3周[61,72,77]。

骨与关节结核

骨结核仍是全世界的一个重要健康问题。全世界每年有八百多人新感染，并且有二百多人死于结核病。多数病例发生于发展中国家[160]。2002年，有15 000多例在美国，其中近1000例是小于15岁的儿童。2%～5%的结核病累及骨或关节[19]。骨骼肌肉结核感染50%累及脊柱[116,157]。Rasool报道，42例中5
2044 例（12%）为多发，50例中6例（12%）出现生长紊乱[116]。涂片和培养明确诊断，同时进行药敏实验[157]。X线片上可以看到破坏和变形，但是为非病理性[42,116,157]。MRI对于诊断有意义，并且可以与其他疾病相区别[4,57]。治疗主要是采用抗结核药物。肢体末端有囊性变时，可以行病灶刮除；多个椎体累及、有神经性症状或者有渐进性变形时，需要行脊柱手术治疗[78,79,157]。

Lyme关节炎

Lyme病由伯氏疏螺旋体所致，由硬蜱传播。美国大于90%的病例发生于康涅狄格州、罗德岛州、纽约州、新泽西州、宾夕法尼亚州、威斯康星州、马里兰州和马塞诸塞州[140]。近90%仅表现为游走性红斑[50]。Lyme关节炎发生频率各异，但是早诊早治者少见。大样本儿童Lyme病患者，6%发生关节炎，许多并无皮肤破损[50]。也有心脏和神经系统受累及的报道[50,51,140]。

累及关节者包括1～4个关节的周期性或持续性（4周内）发作[124]。Rose等也发现这种病有累及少关节、多关节和迁移的形式[124]。膝关节累及达到90%[5,139,140,161]。Lyme关节炎可能与化脓性关节炎混淆。对于非典型Lyme病，免疫学检查可证实诊断。滑液中红白细胞计数经常大于40 000～50 000/ml，中性粒细胞大于75%[51,161]。在一项研究中，4%（84例中3例）有眼部感染；所有3例患儿均出现与炎症有关的眼部症状。

阿莫西林或多西环素可提供适当的抗生素作用范围。及时应用抗生素可使慢性关节炎症状的发生率低于5%[51]。

淋球菌性关节炎

此病在性发育期青少年和受虐儿童中多见[44,60,73,74,110,118,122,159,163]。约有1%的淋球菌感染者有系统感染症状，表现为发热、皮疹、关节痛和腱鞘炎[60]。尽管可以影响到多个关节，但是多累及膝关节和手[163]。受累关节常采用冲洗和清创术，尽管也可以采用多次穿刺。滑膜液培养常无阳性表现。颈椎、阴道、肛门、口腔、皮肤和（或）血培养可能会有阳性表现[60]。需要特殊培养基（如巧克力琼脂和Thayer-Martin琼脂）。推荐采用三代头孢菌素进行肠外抗生素治疗1～2周。

放线菌骨髓炎

伊氏放线菌多在口咽部，是一种共生菌[167]。软组织创伤后可以变为病原菌。50%以上的骨髓炎发生于面颈部，尤其是局部感染后易发于颚部[9,98,147,151,167]。40%的放线菌骨髓炎可以波及椎体，几乎均伴有其他病变。较少累及四肢，多由开放性骨折直接蔓延、直接创伤或者人咬伤所致；仅有3%的四肢病变被认为与血源性传播有关[9,98,147,151]。

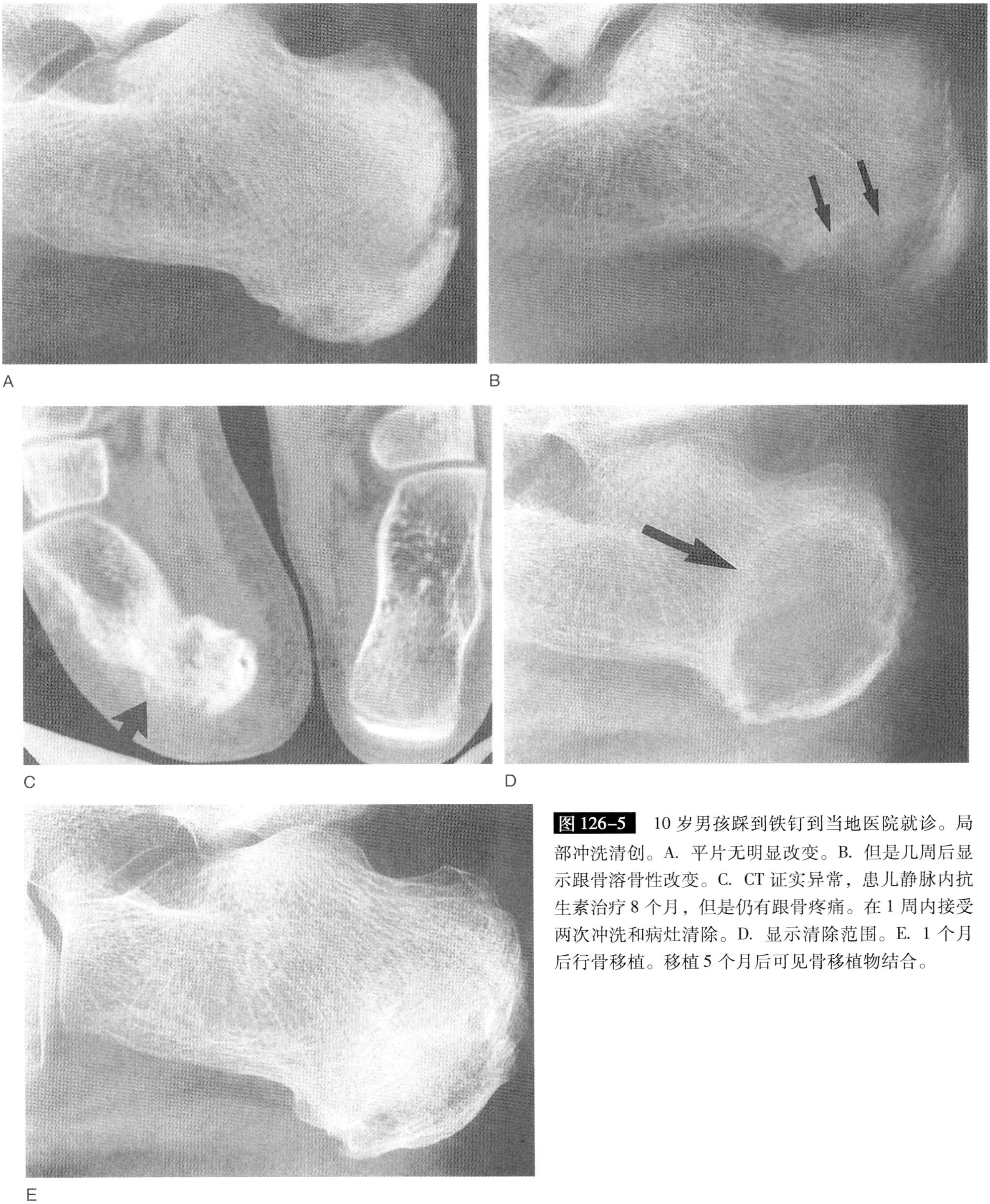

图 126–5　10 岁男孩踩到铁钉到当地医院就诊。局部冲洗清创。A. 平片无明显改变。B. 但是几周后显示跟骨溶骨性改变。C. CT 证实异常，患儿静脉内抗生素治疗 8 个月，但是仍有跟骨疼痛。在 1 周内接受两次冲洗和病灶清除。D. 显示清除范围。E. 1 个月后行骨移植。移植 5 个月后可见骨移植物结合。

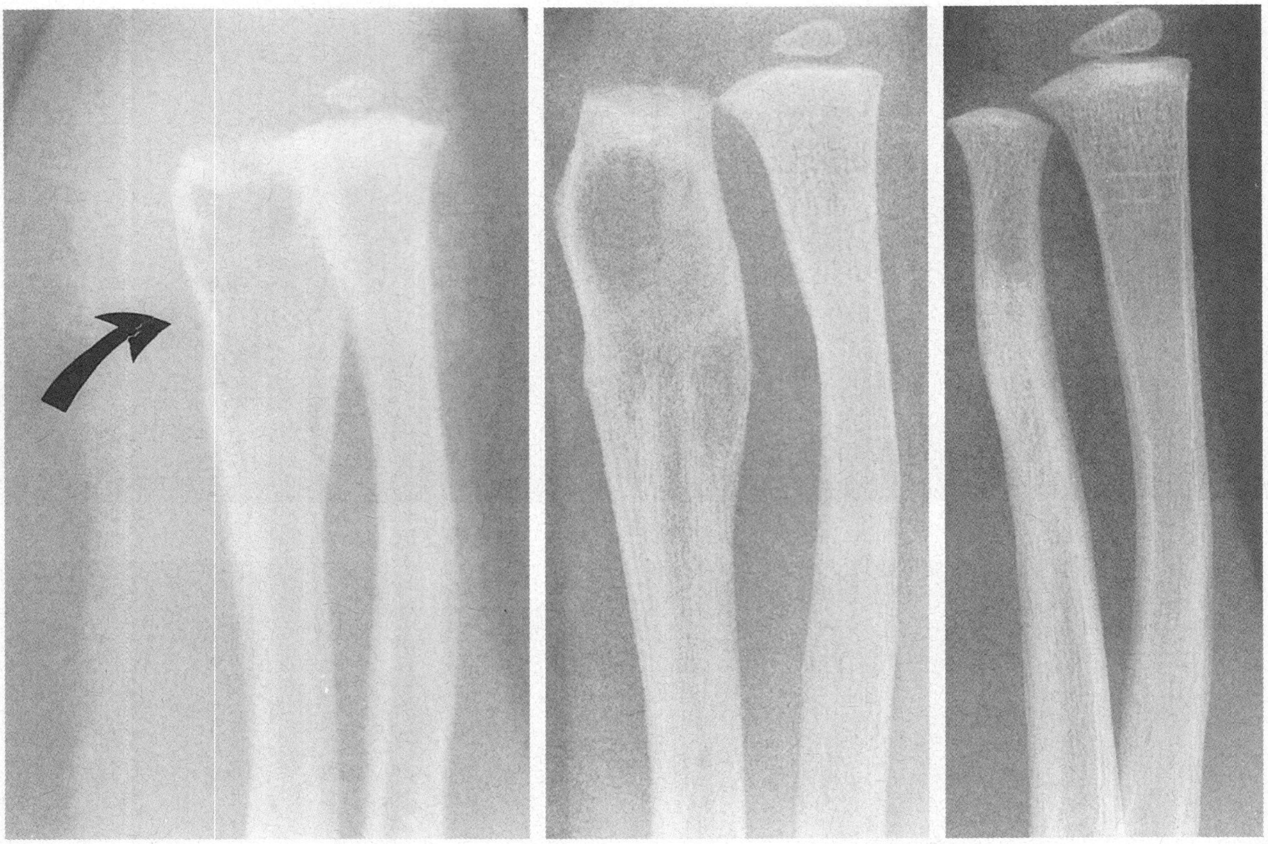

A　B　C

图 126-6　14 个月男孩右前臂远端肿胀 1 个月，ESR 为 41 mm/h。A. 平片可见尺骨远端有溶骨性改变。诊断可以是感染和肿瘤。患儿行切开活检和病灶清除。病理学检查显示为球孢子菌病。患儿口服两性霉素 B 6 个月后口服氟康唑。B. 术后 2 个月 X 线。C. 术后 12 个月 X 线显示尺骨已愈合并再塑形。

球孢子菌骨髓炎

粗球孢子菌属南美土壤中的真菌。具有免疫能力的宿主一般有中度上呼吸道感染，数周或数月内感染消失[155]。5%~10% 的感染人群表现为慢性肺炎或者呈播散性[155]。播散性疾病可以影响骨、肌肉、皮肤或者脑脊膜。在一组研究中，14 例中有 9 例（64%）为多处发病[31]。肌肉骨骼系统的球孢子菌骨髓炎因不能被精确诊断而延误。白细胞计数和血沉正常。皮肤试验可证实曾经暴露于粗球孢子菌，并且免疫学检查（尤其是 IgG）在评价临床表现和系统疾病严重性方面有重要意义。但是，穿刺或组织活检培养的进一步证实也是有必要的。

多数病例需要手术清除病灶，同时静脉应用两性霉素 B（图 126-6）。有作者报道联合手术及药物治疗的效果优于单纯采用药物治疗[16]。尽管治疗得当，但肌肉骨骼系统球孢子菌骨髓炎的死亡率在最近的研究中仍然高达 12%~17%。

总结

骨关节感染仍是儿童保健的重要问题。在应用抗生素以前，多种感染性疾病导致了较高的死亡率。今天，人们已通过早诊早治限制了其慢性并发症。尽管在早期使用广谱性抗生素，但是仍然应当根据具体的致病菌选用特异性的药物。（常用药物以及剂量见表 126-4。）发现晚的患儿常需要清创。即使做到早诊早 2046
治，长期并发症如关节炎、慢性骨髓炎、骺板阻滞、肢体不等长以及成角畸形等长期后遗症仍时有发生。

（葛翼华译　赵　黎校）

表 126-4 儿童骨骼肌肉感染常用抗生素

药物	给药方式	剂量	给药间隔	最大剂量
阿米卡星	静脉/肌注	15~20 mg/(kg·d)	q8~12 h	1.5 g/d
阿莫西林	口服	80~100 mg/(kg·d)	q6~8 h	
氨苄西林	口服	100~200 mg/(kg·d)	q6 h	12 g/d
头孢唑林	静脉	100 mg/(kg·d)	q8 h	6.0 g/d
头孢噻肟	静脉	100~200 mg/(kg·d)	q6~8 h	12 g/d
头孢他啶	静脉/肌注	150 mg/(kg·d)	q6~8 h	6.0 g/d
头孢曲松	静脉/肌注	50~100 mg/(kg·d)	q12~24 h	4.0 g/d
头孢呋辛	静脉/肌注	75~150 mg/(kg·d)	q6~8 h	6.0 g/d
头孢氨苄	口服	100~150 mg/(kg·d)	q6	4.0 g/d
环丙沙星*	静脉	30 mg/(kg·d)	q12 h	800 mg/d
	口服	30 mg/(kg·d)	q12 h	1.5 g/d
克林霉素*	静脉	30~40 mg/(kg·d)	q6~8 h	4.8 g/d
	口服	20~40 mg/(kg·d)	q6~8 h	1.8 g/d
双氯西林	口服	75~100 mg/(kg·d)	q6	
庆大霉素	静脉/肌注	5.0~7.5 mg/(kg·d)	q8 h	
甲氧西林	静脉/肌注	200 mg/(kg·d)	q6	
萘夫西林	静脉	100~150 mg/(kg·d)	q6	
苯唑西林	静脉	150 mg/(kg·d)	q6	12 g/d
青霉素*	静脉	150 000 U/(kg·d)	q6	24×10^6 U/d
	口服	125 mg/(kg·d)	q4~6 h	3.0 g/d
磺胺甲噁唑/甲氧苄啶	静脉/口服	10 mg/(kg·d) (甲氧苄啶)	q12 h	
万古霉素	静脉	40 mg/(kg·d)	q6 h	4.0 g/d

* 指出不同用药途径的每日剂量和最大剂量。

数据见参考文献 60，61，101，138 和 145。

参考文献

1. Abernethy LJ, Lee YC, Cole WG: Ultrasound localization of subperiosteal abscesses in children with late-acute osteomyelitis. J Pediatr Orthop 1993;13:766-768.
2. Almquist EE: The changing epidemiology of septic arthritis in children. Clin Orthop 1970;68:96-99.
3. Andrew TA, Porter K: Primary subacute epiphyseal osteomyelitis: A report of three cases. J Pediatr Orthop 1985;5:155-157.
4. Andronikou S, Jadwat S, Douis H: Patterns of disease on MRI in 53 children with tuberculous spondylitis and the role of gadolinium. Pediatr Radiol 2002;32:798-805.
5. Bachman DT, Srivastava G: Emergency department presentations of Lyme disease in children. Pediatr Emerg Care 1998;14:356-361.
6. Beaupre A, Carroll N: The three syndromes of iliac osteomyelitis in children. J Bone Joint Surg Am 1979;61:1087-1092.
7. Betz RR, Cooperman DR, Wopperer JM, et al: Late sequelae of septic arthritis of the hip in infancy and childhood. J Pediatr Orthop 1990;10:365-372.
8. Bjorksten B, Gustavson KH, Eriksson B, et al: Chronic recurrent multifocal osteomyelitis and pustulosis palmoplantaris. J Pediatr 1978;93:227-231.
9. Blinkhorn RJ Jr, Strimbu V, Effron D, et al: "Punch" actinomycosis causing osteomyelitis of the hand. Arch Intern Med 1988;148:2668-2670.
10. Bohay DR, Gray JM: Sacroiliac joint pyarthrosis. Orthop Rev 1993;22:817-823.
11. Borella L, Goobar JE, Summitt RL, et al: Septic arthritis in childhood. J Pediatr 1963;62:742-747.
12. Boston HC Jr, Bianco AJ Jr, Rhodes KH: Disk space infections in children. Orthop Clin North Am 1975;6:953-964.
13. Bousvaros A, Marcon M, Treem W, et al: Chronic recurrent multifocal osteomyelitis associated with chronic inflammatory bowel disease in children. Dig Dis Sci 1999;44:2500-2507.
14. Boutin RD, Brossmann J, Sartoris DJ, et al: Update on imaging of orthopedic infections. Orthop Clin North Am 1998;29:41-66.
15. Brand RA, Black H: *Pseudomonas* osteomyelitis following puncture wounds in children. J Bone Joint Surg Am 1974;56:1637-1642.
16. Bried JM, Galgiani JN: *Coccidioides immitis* infections in bones and joints. Clin Orthop 1986;235-243.
17. Canale ST, Harkness RM, Thomas PA, et al: Does aspiration

of bones and joints affect results of later bone scanning? J Pediatr Orthop 1985;5:23-26.
18. Canale ST, Puhl J, Watson FM, et al: Acute osteomyelitis following closed fractures: Report of three cases. J Bone Joint Surg Am 1975;57:415-418.
19. Centers for Disease Control and Prevention: Reported tuberculosis in the United States, 2002. Atlanta, U.S. Department of Health and Human Services, CDC, September 2003.
20. Centers for Disease Control and Prevention: Trends in tuberculosis morbidity—United States, 1992-2002. MMWR Morb Mortal Wkly Rep 2003;52:217-220, 222.
21. Chambers JB, Forsythe DA, Bertrand SL, et al: Retrospective review of osteoarticular infections in a pediatric sickle cell age group. J Pediatr Orthop 2000;20:682-685.
22. Chung SM: The arterial supply of the developing proximal end of the human femur. J Bone Joint Surg Am 1976;58: 961-970.
23. Cole WG, Dalziel RE, Leitl S: Treatment of acute osteomyelitis in childhood. J Bone Joint Surg Br 1982;64:218-223.
24. Connolly LP, Connolly SA, Drubach LA, et al: Acute hematogenous osteomyelitis of children: Assessment of skeletal scintigraphy-based diagnosis in the era of MRI. J Nucl Med 2002;43:1310-1316.
25. Connolly LP, Treves ST, Connolly SA, et al: Pediatric skeletal scintigraphy: Applications of pinhole magnification. Radiographics 1998;18:341-351.
26. Craigen MA, Watters J, Hackett JS: The changing epidemiology of osteomyelitis in children. J Bone Joint Surg Br 1992;74:541-545.
27. Curtiss PH Jr: Cartilage damage in septic arthritis. Clin Orthop 1969;64:87-90.
28. Curtiss PH Jr, Klein L: Destruction of articular cartilage in septic arthritis: I. In vitro studies. Am J Orthop 1963;45A: 797-806.
29. Curtiss PH Jr, Klein L: Destruction of articular cartilage in septic arthritis: II. In vivo studies. J Bone Joint Surg Am 1965;47:1595-1604.
30. Dagan R: Management of acute hematogenous osteomyelitis and septic arthritis in the pediatric patient. Pediatr Infect Dis J 1993;12:88-92.
31. Dalinka MK, Dinnenberg S, Greendyk WH, et al: Roentgenographic features of osseous coccidioidomycosis and differential diagnosis. J Bone Joint Surg Am 1971;53:1157-1164.
32. Dalton GP, Drummond DS, Davidson RS, et al: Bone infarction versus infection in sickle cell disease in children. J Pediatr Orthop 1996;16:540-544.
33. Dangman BC, Hoffer FA, Rand FF, et al: Osteomyelitis in children: Gadolinium-enhanced MR imaging. Radiology 1992;182:743-747.
34. Del Beccaro MA, Champoux AN, Bockers T, et al: Septic arthritis versus transient synovitis of the hip: The value of screening laboratory tests. Ann Emerg Med 1992;21: 1418-1422.
35. Dich VQ, Nelson JD, Haltalin KC: Osteomyelitis in infants and children: A review of 163 cases. Am J Dis Child 1975; 129:1273-1278.
36. Diggs LW: Bone and joint lesions in sickle-cell disease. Clin Orthop 1967;52:119-143.
37. Dirschl DR: Acute pyogenic osteomyelitis in children. Orthop Rev 1994;23:305-312.
38. Dormans JP, Drummond DS: Pediatric hematogenous osteomyelitis: new trends in presentation, diagnosis, and treatment. J Am Acad Orthop Surg 1994;2:333-341.
39. Early SD, Kay RM, Tolo VT: Childhood diskitis. J Am Acad Orthop Surg 2003;11:413-420.
40. Earwaker JW, Cotten A: SAPHO: Syndrome or concept? Imaging findings. Skeletal Radiol 2003;32:311-327.
41. Ebong WW: Pathological fracture complicating long bone osteomyelitis in patients with sickle cell disease. J Pediatr Orthop 1986;6:177-181.
42. Eren A, Atay EF, Omeroglu H, et al: Solitary cystic tuberculosis of long tubular bones in children. J Pediatr Orthop B 2003;12:72-75.
43. Fernandez M, Carrol CL, Baker CJ: Discitis and vertebral osteomyelitis in children: An 18-year review. Pediatrics 2000;105:1299-1304.
44. Feroli KL, Burstein GR: Adolescent sexually transmitted diseases: New recommendations for diagnosis, treatment, and prevention. MCN Am J Matern Child Nurs 2003;28: 113-118.
45. Fitzgerald RH Jr, Cowan JD: Puncture wounds of the foot. Orthop Clin North Am 1975;6:965-972.
46. Frederiksen B, Christiansen P, Knudsen FU: Acute osteomyelitis and septic arthritis in the neonate, risk factors and outcome. Eur J Pediatr 1993;152:577-580.
47. Gamble JG, Rinsky LA: Chronic recurrent multifocal osteomyelitis: A distinct clinical entity. J Pediatr Orthop 1986;6:579-584.
48. Gamble JG, Rinsky LA: *Kingella kingae* infection in healthy children. J Pediatr Orthop 1988;8:445-449.
49. Gentry LO: Antibiotic therapy for osteomyelitis. Infect Dis Clin North Am 1990;4:485-499.
50. Gerber MA, Shapiro ED, Burke GS, et al: Lyme disease in children in southeastern Connecticut. Pediatric Lyme Disease Study Group. N Engl J Med 1996;335:1270-1274.
51. Gerber MA, Zemel LS, Shapiro ED: Lyme arthritis in children: Clinical epidemiology and long-term outcomes. Pediatrics 1998;102:905-908.
52. Givner LB, Luddy RE, Schwartz AD: Etiology of osteomyelitis in patients with major sickle hemoglobinopathies. J Pediatr 1981;99:411-413.
53. Glazer PA, Hu SS: Pediatric spinal infections. Orthop Clin North Am 1996;27:111-123.
54. Gledhill RB: Subacute osteomyelitis in children. Clin Orthop 1973;96:57-69.
55. Gold RH, Hawkins RA, Katz RD: Bacterial osteomyelitis: Findings on plain radiography, CT, MR, and scintigraphy. AJR Am J Roentgenol 1991;157:365-370.
56. Goldstein WM, Gleason TF, Barmada R: A comparison between arthrotomy and irrigation and débridement and multiple aspirations in the treatment of pyogenic arthritis: A histological study in a rabbit model. Orthopedics 1983; 6:1309.
57. Griffith JF, Kumta SM, Leung PC, et al: Imaging of musculoskeletal tuberculosis: A new look at an old disease. Clin Orthop 2002:32-39.
58. Gristina AG, Naylor PT, Myrvik QN: Musculoskeletal infection, microbial adhesion, and antibiotic resistance. Infect Dis Clin North Am 1990;4:391-408.
59. Gutierrez KM: Diskitis. In Long SS, Pickering LK, Prober CG (eds): Principles and Practice of Pediatric Infectious Diseases. New York, Churchill Livingstone, 2003, pp 481-484.
60. Gutierrez KM: Infectious and inflammatory arthritis. In Long SS, Pickering LK, Prober CG (eds): Principles and Practice of Pediatric Infectious Diseases. New York, Churchill Livingstone, 2003, pp 475-481.
61. Gutierrez KM: Osteomyelitis. In Long SS, Pickering LK, Prober CG (eds): Principles and Practice of Pediatric Infectious Diseases. New York, Churchill Livingstone, 2003, pp 467-474.
62. Gwynne-Jones DP, Stott NS: Community-acquired methicillin-resistant *Staphylococcus aureus:* A cause of musculoskeletal

sepsis in children. J Pediatr Orthop 1999;19:413-416.

63. Haliloglu M, Kleiman MB, Siddiqui AR, et al: Osteomyelitis and pyogenic infection of the sacroiliac joint: MRI findings and review. Pediatr Radiol 1994;24:333-335.
64. Hammond PJ, Macnicol MF: Osteomyelitis of the pelvis and proximal femur: Diagnostic difficulties. J Pediatr Orthop B 2001;10:113-119.
65. Hoffman EB, de Beer JD, Keys G, et al: Diaphyseal primary subacute osteomyelitis in children. J Pediatr Orthop 1990; 10:250-254.
66. Holzel H, de Saxe M: Septicaemia in paediatric intensive-care patients at the Hospital for Sick Children, Great Ormond Street. J Hosp Infect 1992;22:185-195.
67. Howard CB, Einhorn M, Dagan R, et al: Ultrasound in diagnosis and management of acute haematogenous osteomyelitis in children. J Bone Joint Surg Br 1993;75:79-82.
68. Howard CB, Einhorun MS: Ultrasound in the detection of subperiosteal abscesses. J Bone Joint Surg Br 1991;73: 175-176.
69. Huppertz HI, Munchmeier D, Lieb W: Ocular manifestations in children and adolescents with Lyme arthritis. Br J Ophthalmol 1999;83:1149-1152.
70. Hussain FM, Boyle-Vavra S, Bethel CD, et al: Current trends in community-acquired methicillin-resistant *Staphylococcus aureus* at a tertiary care pediatric facility. Pediatr Infect Dis J 2000;19:1163-1166.
71. Hussain FM, Boyle-Vavra S, Daum RS: Community-acquired methicillin-resistant *Staphylococcus aureus* colonization in healthy children attending an outpatient pediatric clinic. Pediatr Infect Dis J 2001;20:763-767.
72. Inaba AS, Zukin DD, Perro M: An update on the evaluation and management of plantar puncture wounds and *Pseudomonas* osteomyelitis. Pediatr Emerg Care 1992;8:38-44.
73. Ingram DL: *Neisseria gonorrhoeae* in children. Pediatr Ann 1994;23:341-345.
74. Ingram DM, Miller WC, Schoenbach VJ, et al: Risk assessment for gonococcal and chlamydial infections in young children undergoing evaluation for sexual abuse. Pediatrics 2001;107:E73.
75. Jackson MA, Burry VF, Olson LC: Pyogenic arthritis associated with adjacent osteomyelitis: Identification of the sequela-prone child. Pediatr Infect Dis J 1992;11:9-13.
76. Jackson MA, Nelson JD: Etiology and medical management of acute suppurative bone and joint infections in pediatric patients. J Pediatr Orthop 1982;2:313-323.
77. Jacobs RF, McCarthy RE, Elser JM: *Pseudomonas* osteochondritis complicating puncture wounds of the foot in children: A 10-year evaluation. J Infect Dis 1989;160:657-661.
78. Jain AK: Treatment of tuberculosis of the spine with neurologic complications. Clin Orthop 2002;75-84.
79. Jain AK, Sinha S: Tuberculosis of the thoracic spine. J Bone Joint Surg Br 2003;85:150; author reply 150.
80. Jaramillo D, Treves ST, Kasser JR, et al: Osteomyelitis and septic arthritis in children: Appropriate use of imaging to guide treatment. AJR Am J Roentgenol 1995;165:399-403.
81. Jurriaans E, Singh NP, Finlay K, et al: Imaging of chronic recurrent multifocal osteomyelitis. Radiol Clin North Am 2001;39:305-327.
82. Juwah AI, Nlemadim A, Kaine W: Clinical presentation of severe anemia in pediatric patients with sickle cell anemia seen in Enugu, Nigeria. Am J Hematol 2003;72:185-191.
83. Kaiser S, Jacobsson H, Hirsch G: Specific or superfluous? Doubtful clinical value of granulocyte scintigraphy in osteomyelitis in children. J Pediatr Orthop B 2001;10: 109-112.
84. Kaiser S, Jorulf H, Hirsch G: Clinical value of imaging techniques in childhood osteomyelitis. Acta Radiol 1998;39: 523-531.
85. Kaiser S, Rosenborg M: Early detection of subperiosteal abscesses by ultrasonography: A means for further successful treatment in pediatric osteomyelitis. Pediatr Radiol 1994;24:336-339.
86. Kleinman PK: A regional approach to osteomyelitis of the lower extremities in children. Radiol Clin North Am 2002;40:1033-1059.
87. Kocher MS, Mandiga R, Murphy JM, et al: A clinical practice guideline for treatment of septic arthritis in children: Efficacy in improving process of care and effect on outcome of septic arthritis of the hip. J Bone Joint Surg Am 2003; 85:994-999.
88. Kocher MS, Zurakowski D, Kasser JR: Differentiating between septic arthritis and transient synovitis of the hip in children: An evidence-based clinical prediction algorithm. J Bone Joint Surg Am 1999;81:1662-1670.
89. Kushwaha VP, Shaw BA, Gerardi JA, et al: Musculoskeletal coccidioidomycosis: A review of 25 cases. Clin Orthop 1996:190-199.
90. Lundy DW, Kehl DK: Increasing prevalence of *Kingella kingae* in osteoarticular infections in young children. J Pediatr Orthop 1998;18:262-267.
91. Lunseth PA, Heiple KG: Prognosis in septic arthritis of the hip in children. Clin Orthop 1979:81-85.
92. Mah ET, LeQuesne GW, Gent RJ, et al: Ultrasonic features of acute osteomyelitis in children. J Bone Joint Surg Br 1994;76:969-974.
93. Mah ET, LeQuesne GW, Gent RJ, et al: Ultrasonic signs of pelvic osteomyelitis in children. Pediatr Radiol 1994;24: 484-487.
94. Mahboubi S, Morris MC: Imaging of spinal infections in children. Radiol Clin North Am 2001;39:215-222.
95. Mallouh A, Talab Y: Bone and joint infection in patients with sickle cell disease. J Pediatr Orthop 1985;5:158-162.
96. Maraqa NF, Gomez MM, Rathore MH: Outpatient parenteral antimicrobial therapy in osteoarticular infections in children. J Pediatr Orthop 2002;22:506-510.
97. Marcinak JF, Frank AL: Treatment of community-acquired methicillin-resistant *Staphylococcus aureus* in children. Curr Opin Infect Dis 2003;16:265-269.
98. Mesgarzadeh M, Bonakdarpour A, Redecki PD: Case report 395: Hematogenous *Actinomyces* osteomyelitis (calcaneus). Skeletal Radiol 1986;15:584-588.
99. Morrey BF, Bianco AJ Jr, Rhodes KH: Septic arthritis in children. Orthop Clin North Am 1975;6:923-934.
100. Morrey BF, Peterson HA: Hematogenous pyogenic osteomyelitis in children. Orthop Clin North Am 1975; 6:935-951.
101. Morrissy RT: Bone and joint sepsis. In Morrissy RT, Weinstein SL (eds): Lovell and Winter's Pediatric Orthopaedics. Philadelphia, Lippincott Williams & Wilkins, 2001, pp 459-505.
102. Morrissy RT, Haynes DW: Acute hematogenous osteomyelitis: A model with trauma as an etiology. J Pediatr Orthop 1989;9:447-456.
103. Mortensson W, Edeburn G, Fries M, et al: Chronic recurrent multifocal osteomyelitis in children: A roentgenologic and scintigraphic investigation. Acta Radiol 1988;29:565-570.
104. Nakamura MM, Rohling KL, Shashaty M, et al: Prevalence of methicillin-resistant *Staphylococcus aureus* nasal carriage in the community pediatric population. Pediatr Infect Dis J 2002;21:917-922.
105. Nelson JD: Acute osteomyelitis in children. Infect Dis Clin North Am 1990;4:513-522.

106. Nelson JD, Bucholz RW, Kusmiesz H, et al: Benefits and risks of sequential parenteral-oral cephalosporin therapy for suppurative bone and joint infections. J Pediatr Orthop 1982;2:255-262.
107. Ogden JA, Lister G: The pathology of neonatal osteomyelitis. Pediatrics 1975;55:474-478.
108. Ono CM, Albertson KS, Reinker KA, et al: Acquired radial clubhand deformity due to osteomyelitis. J Pediatr Orthop 1995;15:161-168.
109. Oudjhane K, Azouz EM: Imaging of osteomyelitis in children. Radiol Clin North Am 2001;39:251-266.
110. Palusci VJ, Reeves MJ: Testing for genital gonorrhea infections in prepubertal girls with suspected sexual abuse. Pediatr Infect Dis J 2003;22:618-623.
111. Peltola H, Unkila-Kallio L, Kallio MJ: Simplified treatment of acute staphylococcal osteomyelitis of childhood. The Finnish Study Group. Pediatrics 1997;99:846-850.
112. Pennington WT, Mott MP, Thometz JG, et al: Photopenic bone scan osteomyelitis: A clinical perspective. J Pediatr Orthop 1999;19:695-698.
113. Perlman MH, Patzakis MJ, Kumar PJ, et al: The incidence of joint involvement with adjacent osteomyelitis in pediatric patients. J Pediatr Orthop 2000;20:40-43.
114. Peters W, Irving J, Letts M: Long-term effects of neonatal bone and joint infection on adjacent growth plates. J Pediatr Orthop 1992;12:806-810.
115. Puffinbarger WR, Gruel CR, Herndon WA, et al: Osteomyelitis of the calcaneus in children. J Pediatr Orthop 1996;16:224-230.
116. Rasool MN: Osseous manifestations of tuberculosis in children. J Pediatr Orthop 2001;21:749-755.
117. Riebel TW, Nasir R, Nazarenko O: The value of sonography in the detection of osteomyelitis. Pediatr Radiol 1996; 26:291-297.
118. Rimsza ME, Niggemann EH: Medical evaluation of sexually abused children: A review of 311 cases. Pediatrics 1982;69: 8-14.
119. Rissing JP: Animal models of osteomyelitis: Knowledge, hypothesis, and speculation. Infect Dis Clin North Am 1990;4:377-390.
120. Roberts JM, Drummond DS, Breed AL, et al: Subacute hematogenous osteomyelitis in children: A retrospective study. J Pediatr Orthop 1982;2:249-254.
121. Robertson DE: Acute hematogenous osteomyelitis. J Bone Joint Surg 1938;20:35.
122. Robinson AJ, Watkeys JE, Ridgway GL: Sexually transmitted organisms in sexually abused children. Arch Dis Child 1998;79:356-358.
123. Roine I, Arguedas A, Faingezicht I, et al: Early detection of sequela-prone osteomyelitis in children with use of simple clinical and laboratory criteria. Clin Infect Dis 1997; 24:849-853.
124. Rose CD, Fawcett PT, Eppes SC, et al: Pediatric Lyme arthritis: Clinical spectrum and outcome. J Pediatr Orthop 1994;14:238-241.
125. Rotbart HA, Glode MP: *Haemophilus influenzae* type b septic arthritis in children: Report of 23 cases. Pediatrics 1985;75:254-259.
126. Sabath LD, Garner C, Wilcox C, et al: Effect of inoculum and of beta-lactamase on the anti-staphylococcal activity of thirteen penicillins and cephalosporins. Antimicrob Agents Chemother 1975;8:344-349.
127. Sadat-Ali M, al-Umran K, al-Habdan I, et al: Ultrasonography: Can it differentiate between vaso-occlusive crisis and acute osteomyelitis in sickle cell disease? J Pediatr Orthop 1998; 18:552-554.
128. Sattler CA, Mason EO Jr, Kaplan SL: Prospective comparison of risk factors and demographic and clinical characteristics of community-acquired, methicillin-resistant versus methicillin-susceptible *Staphylococcus aureus* infection in children. Pediatr Infect Dis J 2002;21:910-917.
129. Schauwecker DS, Braunstein EM, Wheat LJ: Diagnostic imaging of osteomyelitis. Infect Dis Clin North Am 1990; 4:441-463.
130. Scheman RJ, Janota M, Lewin P: The production of experimental osteomyelitis. JAMA 1941;117:1525.
131. Schutzman SA, Teach S: Upper-extremity impairment in young children. Ann Emerg Med 1995;26:474-479.
132. Scott RJ, Christofersen MR, Robertson WW Jr, et al: Acute osteomyelitis in children: A review of 116 cases. J Pediatr Orthop 1990;10:649-652.
133. Shaw BA, Kasser JR: Acute septic arthritis in infancy and childhood. Clin Orthop 1990;212-225.
134. Skaggs DL, Kim SK, Greene NW, et al: Differentiation between bone infarction and acute osteomyelitis in children with sickle-cell disease with use of sequential radionuclide bone-marrow and bone scans. J Bone Joint Surg Am 2001;83:1810-1813.
135. Smith JA: Bone disorders in sickle cell disease. Hematol Oncol Clin North Am 1996;10:1345-1356.
136. Smith JW: Infectious arthritis. Infect Dis Clin North Am 1990;4:523-538.
137. Song J, Letts M, Monson R: Differentiation of psoas muscle abscess from septic arthritis of the hip in children. Clin Orthop 2001;258-265.
138. Song KM, Sloboda JF: Acute hematogenous osteomyelitis in children. J Am Acad Orthop Surg 2001;9:166-175.
139. Sood SK: Lyme disease. Pediatr Infect Dis J 1999;18: 913-925.
140. Sood SK, Ilowite NT: Lyme arthritis in children: Is chronic arthritis a common complication? J Rheumatol 2000;27: 1836-1838.
141. Stanton RP, Lopez-Sosa FH, Doidge R: Chronic recurrent multifocal osteomyelitis. Orthop Rev 1993;22:229-233.
142. Strong M, Lejman T, Michno P, et al: Sequelae from septic arthritis of the knee during the first two years of life. J Pediatr Orthop 1994;14:745-751.
143. Strouse PJ, DiPietro MA, Adler RS: Pediatric hip effusions: Evaluation with power Doppler sonography. Radiology 1998;206:731-735.
144. Strouse PJ, DiPietro MA, Teo EL, et al: Power Doppler evaluation of joint effusions: Investigation in a rabbit model. Pediatr Radiol 1999;29:617-623.
145. Sucato DJ, Schwend RM, Gillespie R: Septic arthritis of the hip in children. J Am Acad Orthop Surg 1997;5: 249-260.
146. Swiontkowski MF: Surgical approaches in osteomyelitis: Use of laser Doppler flowmetry to determine nonviable bone. Infect Dis Clin North Am 1990;4:501-512.
147. Syriopoulou VP, Smith AL: Osteomyelitis and septic arthritis. In Feigen RD, Cherry JD (eds): Textbook of Pediatric Infectious Diseases. Philadelphia, WB Saunders, 1992.
148. Tay BK, Deckey J, Hu SS: Spinal infections. J Am Acad Orthop Surg 2002;10:188-197.
149. Tetzlaff TR, Howard JB, McCraken GH, et al: Antibiotic concentrations in pus and bone of children with osteomyelitis. J Pediatr 1978;92:135-140.
150. Tetzlaff TR, McCracken GH Jr, Nelson JD: Oral antibiotic therapy for skeletal infections of children: II. Therapy of osteomyelitis and suppurative arthritis. J Pediatr 1978;92: 485-490.

151. Thisted E, Poulsen P, Christensen PO: Actinomycotic osteomyelitis in a child. J Laryngol Otol 1987;101:746-748.
152. Turpin S, Lambert R: Role of scintigraphy in musculoskeletal and spinal infections. Radiol Clin North Am 2001;39:169-189.
153. Umans H, Haramati N, Flusser G: The diagnostic role of gadolinium enhanced MRI in distinguishing between acute medullary bone infarct and osteomyelitis. Magn Reson Imaging 2000;18:255-262.
154. Unkila-Kallio L, Kallio MJ, Peltola H: The usefulness of C-reactive protein levels in the identification of concurrent septic arthritis in children who have acute hematogenous osteomyelitis: A comparison with the usefulness of the erythrocyte sedimentation rate and the white blood-cell count. J Bone Joint Surg Am 1994;76:848-853.
155. Vaz A, Pineda-Roman M, Thomas AR, et al: Coccidioidomycosis: An update. Hosp Pract (Off Ed) 1998;33: 105-108, 113-115, 119-120.
156. Viani RM, Bromberg K, Bradley JS: Obturator internus muscle abscess in children: Report of seven cases and review. Clin Infect Dis 1999;28:117-122.
157. Watts HG, Lifeso RM: Tuberculosis of bones and joints. J Bone Joint Surg Am 1996;78:288-298.
158. Whalen JL, Fitzgerald RH Jr, Morrissy RT: A histological study of acute hematogenous osteomyelitis following physeal injuries in rabbits. J Bone Joint Surg Am 1988;70: 1383-1392.
159. White BD: Red eyes and red rash with fever: An uncommon initial presentation for staphylococcal obturator abscess with adjacent ischial osteomyelitis. J Am Osteopath Assoc 1991;91:807-812.
160. WHO: Tuberculosis: Fact Sheet No. 104. Geneva, World Health Organization, 2002.
161. Willis AA, Widmann RF, Flynn JM, et al: Lyme arthritis presenting as acute septic arthritis in children. J Pediatr Orthop 2003;23:114-118.
162. Winters JL, Cahen I: Acute hematogenous osteomyelitis: A review of sixty-six cases. J Bone Joint Surg Am 1960; 42:691.
163. Wise CM, Morris CR, Wasilauskas BL, et al: Gonococcal arthritis in an era of increasing penicillin resistance: Presentations and outcomes in 41 recent cases (1985-1991). Arch Intern Med 1994;154:2690-2695.
164. Wong AL, Sakamoto KM, Johnson EE: Differentiating osteomyelitis from bone infarction in sickle cell disease. Pediatr Emerg Care 2001;17:60-63; quiz 64.
165. Wrobel CJ, Chappell ET, Taylor W: Clinical presentation, radiological findings, and treatment results of coccidioidomycosis involving the spine: Report on 23 cases. J Neurosurg 2001;95:33-39.
166. Yagupsky P, Dagan R: *Kingella kingae:* An emerging cause of invasive infections in young children. Clin Infect Dis 1997;24:860-866.
167. Yung BC, Cheng JC, Chan TT, et al: Aggressive thoracic actinomycosis complicated by vertebral osteomyelitis and epidural abscess leading to spinal cord compression. Spine 2000;25:745-748.
168. Zawin JK, Hoffer FA, Rand FF, et al: Joint effusion in children with an irritable hip: US diagnosis and aspiration. Radiology 1993;187:459-463.

第 127 章

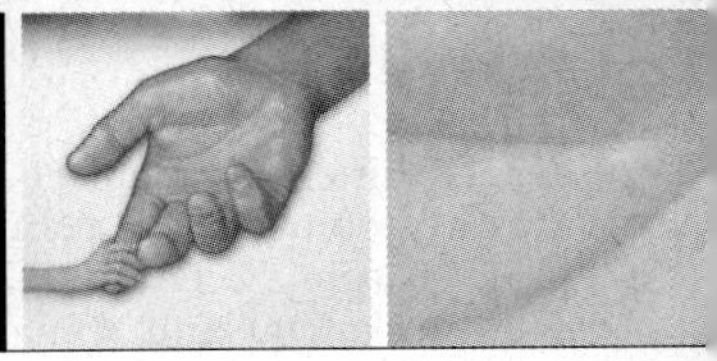

儿童截肢手术

Randall T. Loder

对于一个儿童截肢患者的治疗涉及小儿外科学的各个方面，包括对于儿童生理和心理的康复治疗。儿童截肢患者在发病原因、手术原则和康复治疗方面与成人截肢患者截然不同。不仅在生理康复方面不同，而且在心理康复方面的不同与生理方面同样重要。和许多儿童骨科方面的问题一样，在照料一名儿童截肢患者时，必须时刻牢记儿童的生长潜力，这种生长能力是除了空间方面的需要考虑的三维因素之外的第四维因素。

儿童截肢手术包括两大类型：先天性的和获得性的。先天性截肢包括那些发生在宫内的在出生时即存在的肢体残缺，或者更常见的是一些先天性肢体缺陷最终治疗的结果。获得性截肢通常是由于创伤或后天疾病（肿瘤、感染）导致的。

儿童截肢在许多方面和成人不同[43]。在儿童中，截肢的最主要原因是先天性疾病、创伤感染以及肿瘤；而在成人，截肢最主要的原因是由于肢体的缺血病变（如糖尿病引起的小血管病变）。多发性肢体缺陷在儿童中更为多见，这是由于病因的不同造成的（如儿童的病因是先天性缺陷、暴发性紫癜、创伤等，而成人的病因是血管疾病）。由于儿童会持续生长，截肢后的残留肢体也会继续生长。就像儿童长大过程中不断需要更大的衣服一样，儿童截肢患者由于残留肢体逐渐长大，需要不断更换新的假肢。因此，在仔细考虑手术方案时必须考虑清楚是否要破坏骨骺板。在儿童截肢患者中有一种独特的现象——残肢过度生长，这是由于在一个横断骨骼的截肢残端，骨骼代偿性的生长造成的。由于这种原因，在儿童中相比横断骨骼的截肢术，关节离断术更为常用。儿童截肢患者的活动水平要明显高于那些由于血管疾病造成截肢的成人。因此，对于残留肢体的结构功能的要求及假肢合适程度的要求是不同的。对于心理社会方面的挑战，儿童要比成人更为严峻。但幻觉现象在儿童中没有成人那么常见。

儿童截肢术的指导性原则是尽量多地保存肢体长度，保存生长板，尽量进行关节离断术而不进行经骨离断术，以及尽量多地保留关节。

先天性肢体缺陷所致的截肢

目前，许多先天性肢体发育缺陷可以在产前诊断出来[16,28]。满怀期待的家长经常在孩子出生前就来向骨科医生咨询肢体发育缺陷以及它的预后和治疗方案。经典的肢体发育缺陷分类方法是 Frantz 和 O'Rahilly[24] 提出的（图 127-1）[34]。肢体发育缺陷可以是末端型的，也可以是中间型的。末梢发育缺陷指的是缺损水平远端的部分完全受累。中间型的发育缺陷指的是发育缺陷位于肢体的中部，近端和远端的肢体完好。这两种类型均可被分为横断型和轴旁型。横断型发育缺陷指全部的肢体发育缺陷，而轴旁缺陷指的是肢体的内侧或外侧的发育缺陷。轴旁肢体发育缺陷（先天性纵向肢体结构缺失）又可被细分为轴前（如桡侧或胫侧发育缺陷）或轴后（如尺侧或腓侧发育缺陷）。

股骨发育缺陷（近侧股骨灶性缺损）

以往认为的近侧股骨灶性缺损（PFFD），目前被命名为先天性股骨发育缺陷。这一术语更好地反映了疾病发生的范围，从轻度的股骨短缩到完全的股骨缺失。有两种分类方法被应用：传统的 Aitken 分类

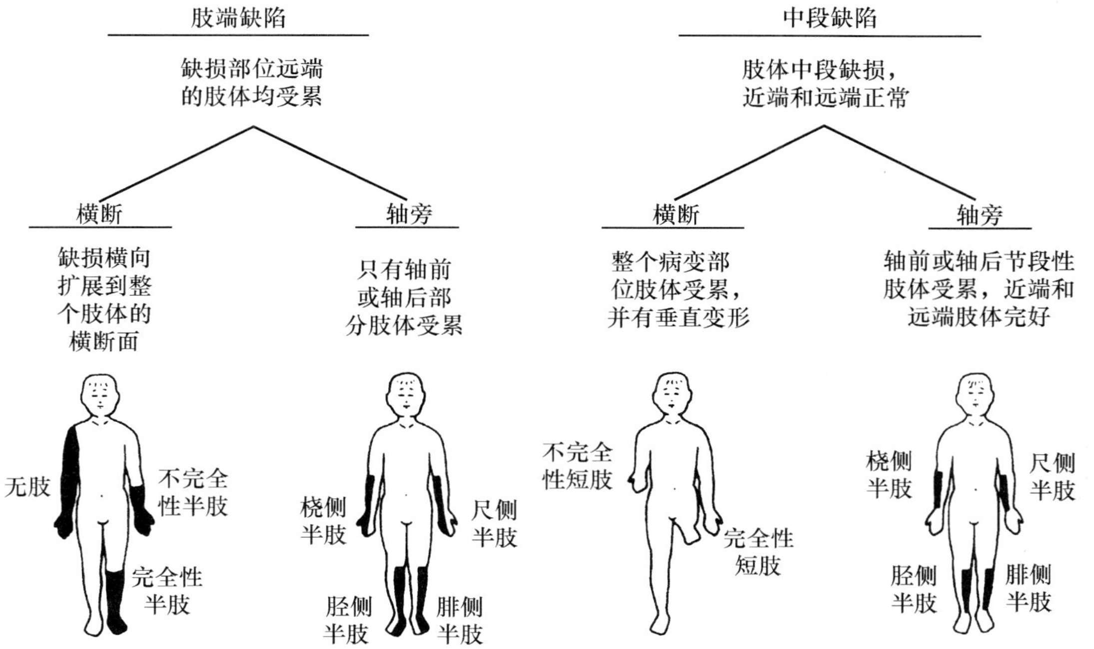

图 127-1　Frantz 和 O'Rahilly 对于先天性肢体缺陷的分类。[From Herring JA, Cummings DR: The limb-deficient child. In Morrissy RT, Weinstein SL (eds): Lovell and Winter's Pediatric Orthopaedics. Philadelphia, Lippincott-Raven, 1996, with permission.]

法[3]和最近的 Gillespite 和 Torode[26,27]分类法（图 127-2A 和 B）[72]。存在典型 PFFD 的孩子，表现为大
2051 腿短缩、外展、外旋、屈曲体位（图 127-3）。常合并腓侧发育缺陷。如果伴有腓侧发育缺陷则患儿的足是跖屈畸形的。

决定治疗方案的因素包括和对侧相比患侧肢体的长度、髋关节的稳定性，以及是单侧还是双侧受累。对于儿童的 Gillespie A 型肢体发育缺陷，肢体延长/肢体等长手术是通常选择的治疗方法[61]。对于儿童的 Gillespie B 型肢体发育缺陷，可以选择应用假肢。对于患儿存在足部跖屈畸形的情况可以佩戴非标准的假肢；如果是足部畸形，可以做足部切除（Syme 截肢术）以便于佩戴标准的假肢。然而，对于患儿来说令其满意并可获得较好的功能通常是不进行截肢而佩戴非常规的假肢[41]。如果患肢的长度低于对侧的膝关节水平而且足部的运动功能良好，Van Nes 旋转矫形术是一种可选的方案[42,74]。在这种手术中，足部被旋转 180 度，肢体在膝关节或胫骨水平（或两者同时）缩短，使得反向旋转的足部位于对侧的膝关节水平。缩短肢体可以使旋转肢体时不牵拉神经血管结构并且使足部正好位于对侧的膝关节水平。这时的患"足"变成了功能上的膝关节并且患肢可以通过佩戴一个膝关节以下的假肢来代替一个非常规的膝关节以上的假肢。这个手术的优点是减少能量消耗以及能够获得比进行足部切除加佩戴膝关节以上假肢更好的功能[23]。缺点是不美观，通常不能被家属和患儿接受。对于那些 Gillespie C 型肢体发育缺陷的患儿建议佩戴假肢，可以进行或者不进行髂股之间的融合[70]。患有 PFFD 的患儿通常不需要手术或佩戴假肢，除非有明显的肢体不等长。

腓骨缺损

腓骨缺损是下肢最常见的先天性发育缺陷。这种发育缺陷[2,71]通常伴随外侧足趾及跖骨等结构的缺失、跗骨桥，以及僵硬的马蹄外翻足畸形[29]；踝关节为球窝关节；脊柱后突伴随皮肤凹陷；以及膝关节交叉韧带缺失（图 127-4）[65]。同时还伴有不同程度的股骨发育不良，从轻度的股骨外踝发育不良到先天性的股骨短缩和 PFFD。这些患儿可以有上肢的畸形，典型的是尺侧发育缺陷综合征。

类型		股骨头	髋臼	股骨干	股骨和髋臼成份骨骼成熟度的关系
A	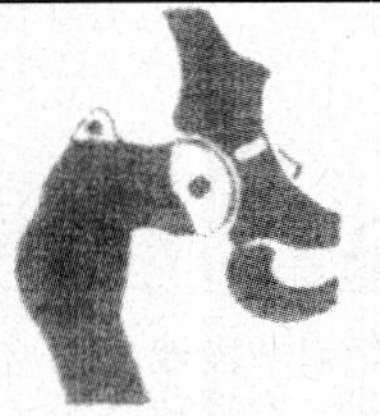	存在	正常	短	股骨内的骨连接 股骨头位于髋臼内 转子下成角内翻，多形成假关节
B	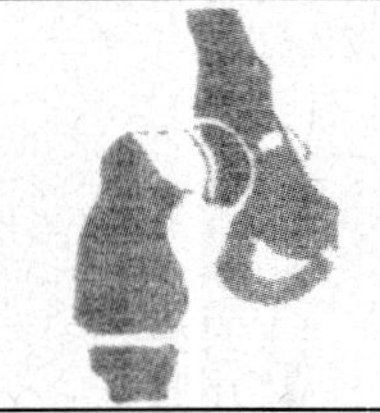	存在	正常或轻度发育异常	短，近端变形	股骨头和股骨干无骨性连接 股骨头位于髋臼内
C	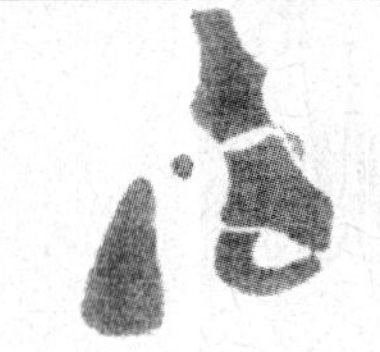	缺损或为小骨	严重发育异常	短，近端变细	股骨干和近端小骨的有骨性连接 股骨与髋臼不形成关节
D	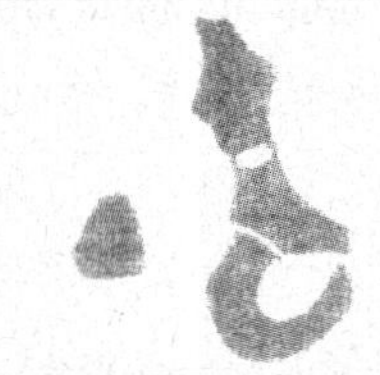	缺损	缺损 闭孔扩大 双侧骨盆呈方形	短，畸形	（无）

A

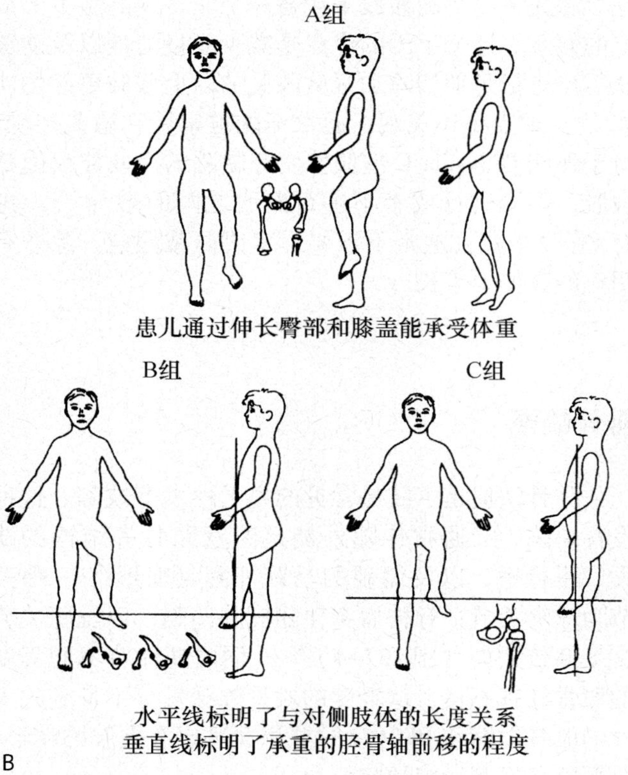

B

图 127-2　先天性股骨缺损的分类。A. Aitken 近侧股骨灶性缺损分类，有 4 种类型，从 A 到 D。B. Gillespie 和 Torode 的股骨缺损分类。A 组包括单纯股骨短缩的病例，B 组包括 Aitken A、B 和 C 型的病例，C 组包括 Aitken D 型的病例（股骨大部分缺失）。［A, From Tachdjian MO: Pediatric Orthopedics. Philadelphia, WB Saunders, 1990; B, from Gillespie R: Classification of congenital abnormalities of the femur. In Herring JA, Birch JG (eds): The Child with a Limb Deficiency. Rosemont, IL, American Academy of Orthopaedic Surgeons, 1998, p 63, with permission.］

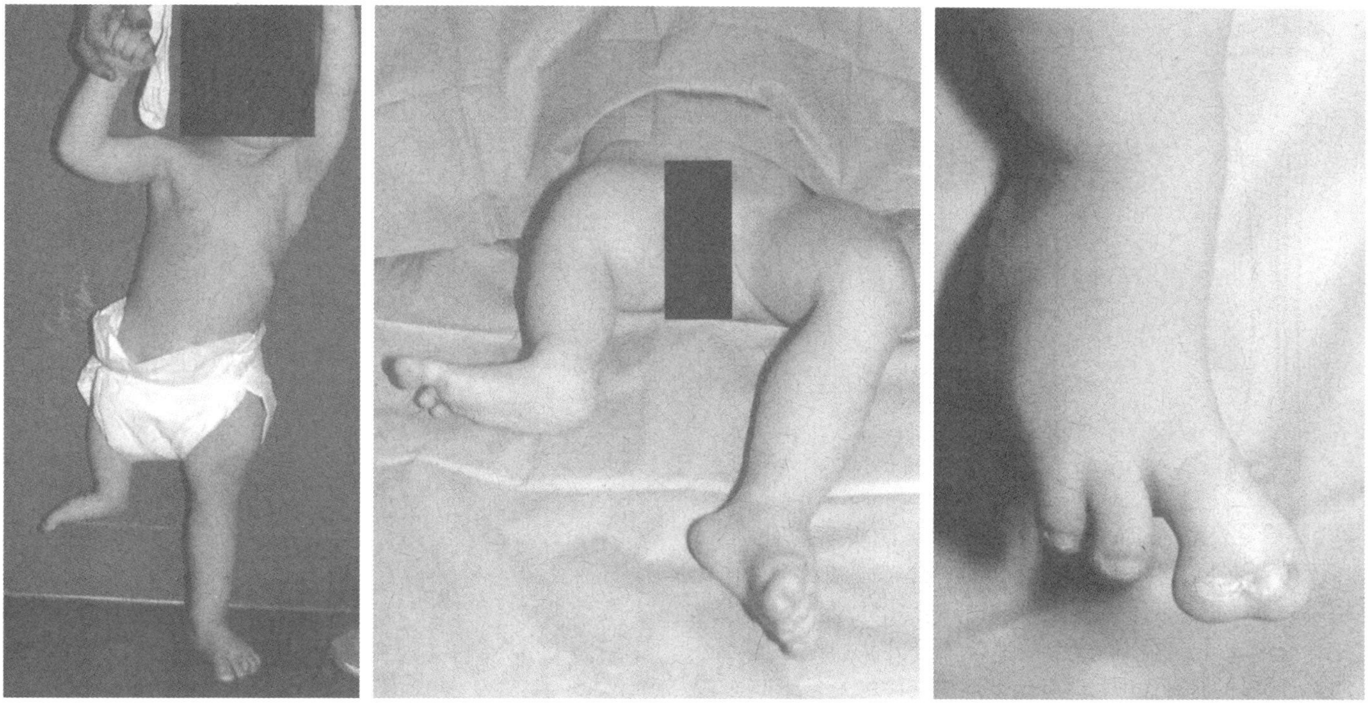

A　B　C

图 127-3　近侧股骨灶性缺损的临床照片。A. 当患儿站立时，注意大腿明显短缩并且外旋，踝关节大约接近对侧膝关节的水平。如果患儿存在这种畸形，并且踝关节的活动功能很好，那么这个孩子是进行 Van Nes 旋转矫形术的理想病例。B. 仰卧时，可以发现髋关节明显的屈曲外展。C. 可以注意到足部短小，并且只有 4 条发育线，最大的足趾存在复杂多趾畸形。

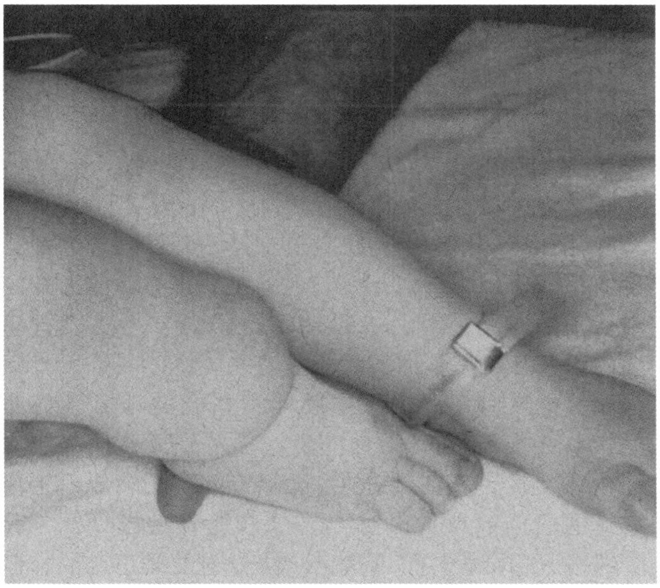

图 127-4　一个腓侧半肢畸形的患儿。腿部短缩，脊柱后凸，足部仅有 3 条发育线，并为马蹄外翻足。

最常用的分类是 Achterman 和 Kalamchi[2] 的分类方法（图 127-5），这是一种将双侧足部功能和肢体不等长包括在内的新的分类系统（表 127-1）[6]。治疗方法取决于足部的功能及其再塑形的潜力以及肢体不等长的程度。随着肢体延长新技术的开展，目前保存足部和延长肢体的可能性增大，而在以往通常是进行足部切除和佩戴假肢[13,18,32,50,53,56]。然而，对于严重的畸形，肢体延长加足部重建手术并不能修复踝关节的稳定性和距下关节的运动功能。在许多组病例中，大部分力图达到跖屈足部外观，恢复肢体等长的手术操作的效果都不令人满意。早期的结果良好，但长期随访就会有各种问题出现[12]。因此，足部切除（Syme 或 Boyd 截肢术）加佩戴假肢仍然是治疗严重腓侧发育缺陷的常用方法。肢体延长术适合于那些一侧足部跖屈，但具有稳定的髋关节、膝关节和踝关节的患儿[13]。存在轻度腓侧发育缺陷的患儿可以通过
肢体延长术达到很好的功能效果[39]。 2054

传统的足部切除术的指征是踝关节不稳定、超过短缩肢体的 30%、僵硬的马蹄外翻足畸形，以及异

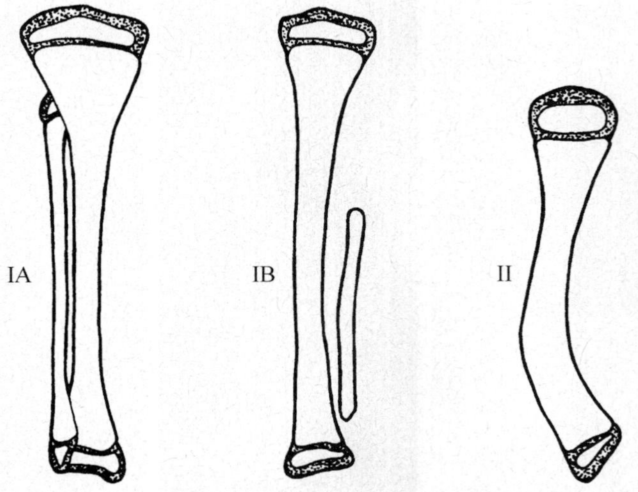

图 127-5　Acterman 和 Kalamchi 的腓骨缺损的分类。Ⅰ型包括部分腓骨仍存在的病例。IA 型，腓骨近端的骨骺位于胫骨骨骺板以远的水平，而腓骨远端生长板位于接近距骨顶的水平。在 IB 型中，腓骨部分缺失，缺失至少 30%～50% 的腓骨长度，腓骨远端不能支持踝关节。Ⅱ型，腓骨完全缺失。[From Herring JA, Cummings DR: The limb-deficient child. In Morrissy RT, Weinstein SL (eds): Lovell and Winter's Pediatric Orthopaedics. Philadelphia, Lippincott-Raven, 1996, with permission.]

表 127-1　腓骨缺损功能分类和治疗原则

分类	治疗
Ⅰ型：有功能的足	
IA：0～5% 的不等长	矫形支具/骺骨干固定术
IB：6%～10% 的不等长	骺骨干固定术 ± 骨延长术
IC：11%～30% 的不等长	1～2 次骨延长手术（或截肢）
ID：>30% 的不等长	>2 次骨延长手术或者直接截肢
Ⅱ型：无功能的足	
ⅡA：上肢有功能	早期截肢
ⅡB：上肢无功能	考虑保肢手术

From Birch JG, Lincoln TL, Mack PW: Functional classification of fibular deficiency. In Herring JA, Birch JG (eds): The Child with a Limb Deficiency. Rosemont, IL, American Academy of Orthopaedic Surgeons, 1998, p161, adapted with permission.

常的踝关节或距下关节活动（或两种皆有）。对于大部分严重畸形的病例，截肢手术的效果要优于做肢体延长和足部矫形手术[50]。截肢后，患儿的活动能力强、足部疼痛少、并发症少。早期截肢手术加假肢佩戴的优点是很少需要二次手术，患儿长大后不会有痛苦的记忆，且功能良好[18,33]。总的来说，对于腓侧发育缺损的治疗方案的选择无论是对家长还是对医生来说都是非常困难的，它取决于许多因素：足部的情况、相关的畸形、家属的要求及其传统文化对于截肢的看法和接受程度。

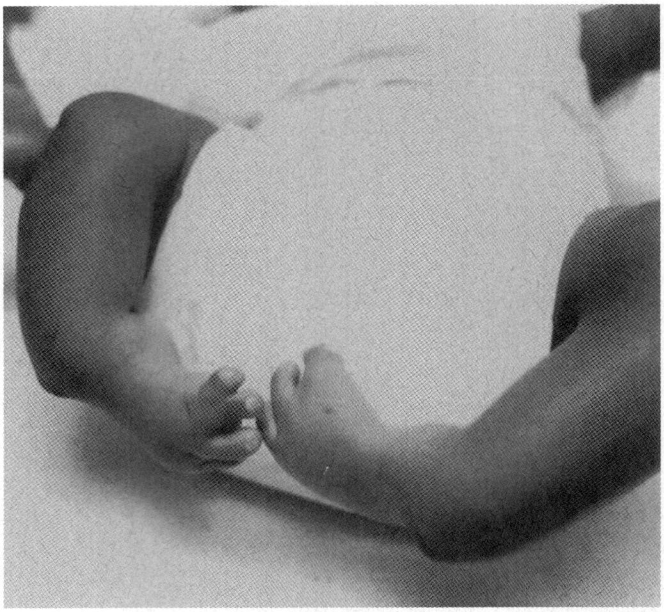

图 127-6　双侧胫侧半肢畸形病例。腿部短缩，马蹄内翻足畸形。

胫骨缺损

胫骨缺损相对腓骨缺损较少见。其发病率大约是每一百万个活体新生儿中有 1 例发病，是目前已知的唯一一种通过基因遗传的骨骼发育缺陷[14]。腓骨缺损的患儿常伴有其他的骨骼肌肉系统畸形（如股骨缺损和尺骨缺损）而没有主要器官系统的畸形（如心血管系统），而胫骨缺损的患儿除了先天性手部或脊柱畸形，通常合并有其他主要器官系统的畸形而不伴有骨骼肌肉系统的畸形[67,69]。和股骨缺损相同，胫骨缺损也包括很广的疾病谱。腓骨通常是正常的，但胫骨和足部有不同程度的发育缺陷。一般来说，患侧的腿较短，膝关节屈曲，马蹄内翻足畸形（图 127-6）[18,22,67]。足部的足趾少于或多于 5 个，可以出现跗

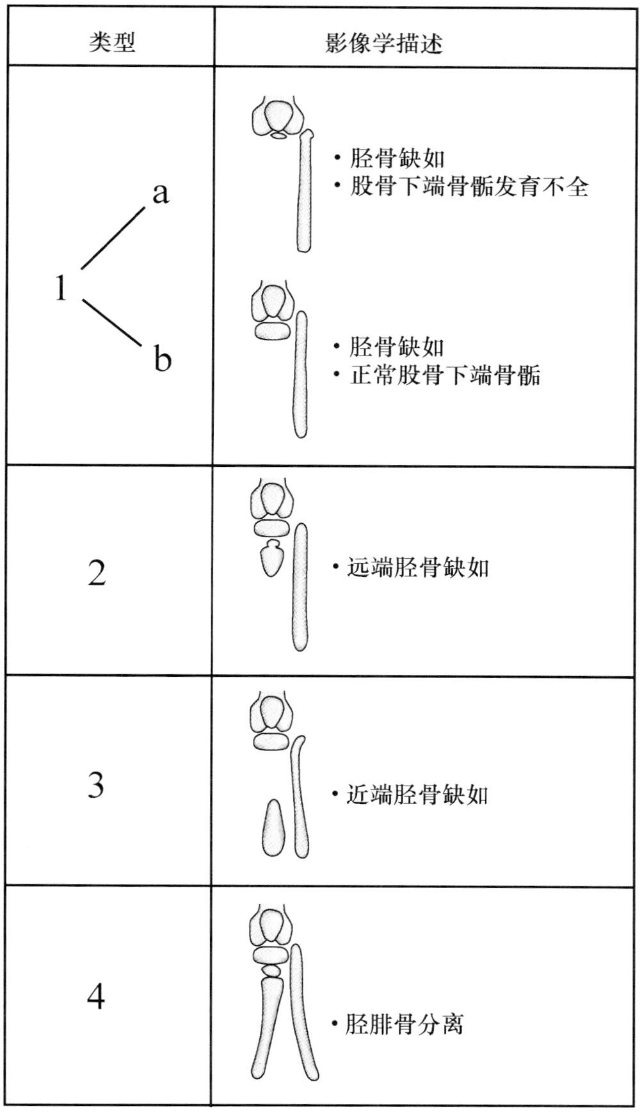

图 127-7 Jones 的胫侧半肢畸形分类。[From Herring JA, Cummings DR: The limb-deficient child. In Morrissy RT, Weinstein SL (eds): Lovell and Winter's Pediatric Orthopaedics. Philadelphia, Lippincott-Raven, 1996, with permission.]

骨桥[16]。

最常用的分类方法是 Jones 等的分类方法[40]（图 127-7）[34]。治疗方案取决于是否存在膝关节屈曲性挛缩，股四头肌的主动功能和足部的功能/畸形。对于那些胫骨完全缺失的病例（Jones Ⅰ型），以往尝试的治疗方法是腓骨中置，重建胫骨切除足部，佩戴假肢。然而，在大部分病例组中这种方法完全失败。因此目前推荐早期膝关节离断手术加佩戴假肢来治疗 Jones Ⅰ型胫骨缺损[19,47,67]。对于其他类型，不同的重建方案有一定的成功率[69]。

创伤导致的截肢

创伤是导致儿童截肢的主要原因。在最近的一个病例回顾报告中，来自 2 座姐妹城市的 2 所 Shriners 儿童医院的 235 名患儿由于创伤导致进行截肢手术 256 例[46]，其平均年龄为（7.9 ± 5.0）岁。92% 的病例是单一肢体截肢，8% 的病例需要对 2～4 个肢体进行截肢手术。下肢占 63%，上肢占 37%。截肢的原因中，割草机损伤占 30%，农场机械损伤占 24%，交通事故占 16%，火车轧伤占 9%，其他机器损伤占 6%，爆炸物损伤（爆竹或炸弹）占 4%，烧伤占 3%，枪伤占 3%，各种复杂创伤占 5%。在另一个相似的病例回顾报告中，Harborview 医学中心报道了 74 例儿童创伤截肢病例，其中 22% 是割草机损伤，16% 是交通事故损伤，14% 是农场机械损伤，8% 为枪伤[75]。

尽管爆炸损伤导致的截肢仅占美国总的创伤截肢
的 4%[46]。但这种原因可能是世界范围内儿童创伤截 2055
肢的最主要原因，因为存在大量以往战争残留下来的地雷未被挖出。目前全世界大约有一亿一千万颗残留的地雷，分布在 60 个国家，每年致残致死大约 26 000 人[45,59]，其中一半是儿童[5,77]。这些大量的地雷损伤对于那些原本经济就很困难的国家的医疗保健系统造成了额外严重的负担[57,77]，并且产生了大量的康复方面的问题[15,37]。由于地雷造成的损伤如此普遍，以至于有“地雷足”这样的说法[15,37]。

一个肢体要损伤到什么程度才能被认为是无法挽救的而要采取截肢手术呢？决定因素是进行保肢手术技术上的能力，以及在保肢手术成功的前提下所能达到的远期肢体功能和应用假肢的功能对比。主要要考虑的问题是主动的肌肉/运动功能、感觉、关节活动度/稳定性，以及在生长期儿童中还要考虑的肢体长度问题。保存肢体失败会造成大量的花费、多次的手术、住院时间延迟，以及心理方面的创伤（包括对于家长和孩子）[8]。为了帮助外科医生预测哪些肢体无法通过保肢手术加以挽救，下肢损伤严重程度评分已被采用。目前最常用的评分标准是毁损肢体严重程度评分系统［Mangled Extremity Severity Score（MESS）］

表 127-2　毁损肢体严重评分系统（MESS）变量表

变量	描述	分数
骨骼/软组织损伤	低能量损伤（稳定、单纯骨折、民间的枪伤）	1
	中等能量损伤（开放性骨折或多发骨折、脱位）	2
	高能量损伤（近距离枪伤或军队的枪伤、碾压伤）	3
	极高能量损伤（以上的损伤＋严重的污染、软组织撕脱）	4
肢体缺血*	脉搏减弱或消失但末梢灌注良好	1*
	无脉；感觉异常，毛细血管再充盈减弱	2*
	肢体冷、麻痹、感觉丧失、麻木	3*
休克	收缩压始终高于 90 mmHg	0
	一过性的低血压	1
	持续的低血压	2
年龄	<30	0
	30～50	1
	>50	2

MESS 评分结果是将 4 个变量参数的得分相加所得。

*如果缺血时间超过 6 小时，则相应的得分翻倍。

From Johansen K, Daines M, Howey T, et al: Objective criteria accurately predict amputation following lower extremity trauma. J Trauma 1990; 30: 568, adapted with permission.

（表 127-2）[31,35,38]。MESS 提出了 4 项损伤特征：组织的损伤程度、肢体缺血严重程度、是否存在休克，以及患儿的年龄。如果 MESS 评分大于 7 分，那么有截肢的阳性指征。然而，大部分的这些评分系统适用于成人，目前还没有根据患儿年龄不同的一系列评分标准。MESS 对于儿童创伤仍有一定的预测能力[20]，但这一领域仍需进一步的研究。

处理儿童毁损肢体或接近截肢手术的治疗方式包括基本的外科常规。立即进行冲洗清创，切除坏死组织，然后进行合适的骨骼固定是首要的。骨折的固定非常重要，包括应用外固定（如外固定支架）、内固定，或二者兼用，这取决于骨折的特点。固定可以降低感染的风险，并且可以改善软组织损伤，包括血管神经损伤的治疗效果。多次、反复的冲洗清创，及分期地切除坏死组织在最初的 2～3 天是必要的，直至伤口清洁为止。当发生软组织覆盖缺损时，需要进行整形手术，如果单纯分层皮肤植皮不够的话，需要应用局部游离皮瓣或带血管的游离皮瓣移植手术治疗。

当严重的创伤造成截肢或者肢体明显不能被保存时，清创冲洗、切除坏死组织、延迟关闭伤口是必要的。在儿童中应尽量保存肢体，在靠近远端处截肢。在评估了患儿佩带假肢的功能后，如果在最初的截肢水平上有问题，还可以进行翻修手术，将截肢平面向近端靠近。

儿童的肢体再植/血运重建

随着显微外科技术的不断发展，肢体的再植和血运重建已成为可能。然而，成功实施肢体再植/血运重建手术并不能代表能够达到完全的功能恢复。当面对一个创伤性截肢的患儿时，外科医生常常被问及，这个肢体还能被再植吗。最多见的是上肢截肢术。在儿童上肢的创伤性截断损伤或血供损伤中，截断肢体的存活率在那些仅需要重建血供的肢体中要高于那些需要再植的肢体（88%对 63%），因为前者有残留的完整的桥状连接组织以及重建血供后比再植后有更多潜在的静脉回流。同样的撕裂伤造成的截肢经过再植手术后相比碾压伤来说要有较高的存活率（72%对 53%）。肢体经过血运重建后的成活率和年龄无关，再植手术后的成功率却与年龄有关。小于 9 岁的孩子再植手术后的成活率要高于大于 9 岁的孩子（77%对 52%）[66]。对于年龄非常小的患儿，成活率反而要有

2056

所降低，原因是对于细小血管吻合的技术要求增高，以及碾压和撕脱损伤的比率增加[9]。对于手指的截肢，如果截肢水平位于指浅屈肌腱止点的远端，即中节指骨的基底部以远，那么手指的主动运动功能要好很多。

在儿童中，普遍认为截肢损伤部分应该尽量进行再植手术[4,62,66]。尤其是当上肢的损伤包括拇指和多个手指，或截肢平面较高（腕关节和前臂）时，应尽一切努力进行再植手术。如果肢体缺损的细菌培养是阴性的，即使将来的功能预后很差，也要尽量进行肢体再植手术[10]。再植手术的相对禁忌证是热缺血时间过长（没有肌肉的手指缺血超过 12 小时，存在肌肉组织的更近端的截肢端缺血超过 6 小时）、只有一侧边缘的手指残端、碾压伤或撕脱伤、多节段损伤伴有威胁生命的损伤、无法依从术后的康复锻炼，以及截肢残端无意中被冷冻破坏。直接放置截肢残端于冰块上会导致冷冻破坏，这样会妨碍手术的成功。正确处理残肢的方法是，用湿的生理盐水或林格液纱布包裹然后放置在无菌的塑料袋中，再将这个塑料袋放入一个盛有冰的大的容器内，这样可以避免残肢直接和冰接触。干冰已经不再使用了[9]。

疾病导致的截肢

肿瘤

当外科医生面对一个可能有恶性肢体肿瘤的患儿时，要考虑做活检。尽管活检看似是一个简单的操作，但必须仔细安排，以便和以后的手术相配合，无论以后是做保肢手术还是截肢手术[48,49]。如果操作失败，有可能由于肿瘤污染导致无法完成保肢手术，在有些病例中甚至会降低患儿的生存率。因此，做活检手术的外科医生应是进行最终手术的同一位医生。

和所有的肿瘤一样，肢体的恶性肿瘤也是分期的。肿瘤的分期对于活检是非常重要的。最常用的分期分类是 Enneking 等提出的分期标准[17]。组织学的分级分为低度恶性（G1）或高度恶性（G2），部位上的分类被分为区域内肿瘤（T1），区域外肿瘤
057 （T2），或转移肿瘤（M）（表 127-3）。“区域”这一句词指的是一些能够阻碍肿瘤扩散的天然屏障所分割出的肢体的解剖区域空间。这样的分界线是骨皮质和

表 127-3　肢体恶性肿瘤的九级分级系统

分期	恶性程度	部位
ⅠA	低度恶性（G1）	区域内（T1）
ⅠB	低度恶性（G1）	区域外（T2）
ⅡA	高度恶性（G2）	区域内（T1）
ⅡB	高度恶性（G2）	区域内（T2）
Ⅲ	任何程度局部病灶加远端转移	任何部位

From Mirra JM：Bone Tumors. Philadelphia，Lea & Febiger，1989，adapted with permission.

筋膜。例如，如果一个骨肉瘤完全局限在其原发的骨皮质内，则其分级为 IA（高度恶性，区域内肿瘤）。同样，一个原发于股四头肌的滑膜肉瘤从四头肌筋膜扩散到皮下组织内则为ⅡB（高度恶性及区域外肿瘤）。

区分肿瘤的分期对于决定手术切除的范围和边界是非常重要的。4 个主要的切除边界是肿瘤内切除、肿瘤边界切除、肿瘤广泛切除，以及放射扩大切除（图 127-8）[11]。肿瘤内切除仅仅切除病灶的一部分，留下其余的病灶、反应区域、卫星病灶及跳跃病灶在正常组织内。肿瘤边界切除指的是在关节囊外的平面切除炎症反应区域的全部肿瘤，卫星肿瘤灶和跳跃病灶被留置在体内。广泛切除指的是切除肿瘤的范围扩大到反应区域外的正常组织。放射性扩大切除需要切除肿瘤扩散的整个区域范围。在做任何肌肉骨科肿瘤的切除手术时，肿瘤不需要被完全暴露出来，最终是将肿瘤连同周围正常组织一并切除，在最小的范围内达到最大边界的切除。

在过去，截肢是治疗儿童肢体恶性肿瘤最常用的方法。随着技术的不断进步如影像学检查（核磁共振、CT）、化疗方案的完善，包括辅助化疗的应用，外科手术技术无论是活检技术还是以后的重建手术（大范围的同种异体骨移植、内固定的新技术，以及人工关节的发展），这些技术的进步使得保肢手术成为可能。同样的，儿童肢体肉瘤的总体生存率和预期寿命也随着技术的进步得到了较大的提高。正是由于这些原因，目前大部分患有肢体恶性肿瘤疾病的患儿可以接受保肢治疗而不是截肢手术。

当选择进行截肢手术而不是保肢手术或旋转矫形手术时，总的生存率是相似的[60]。尽管并发症产生的几率较大，但接受保肢手术的患儿其生存质量和总

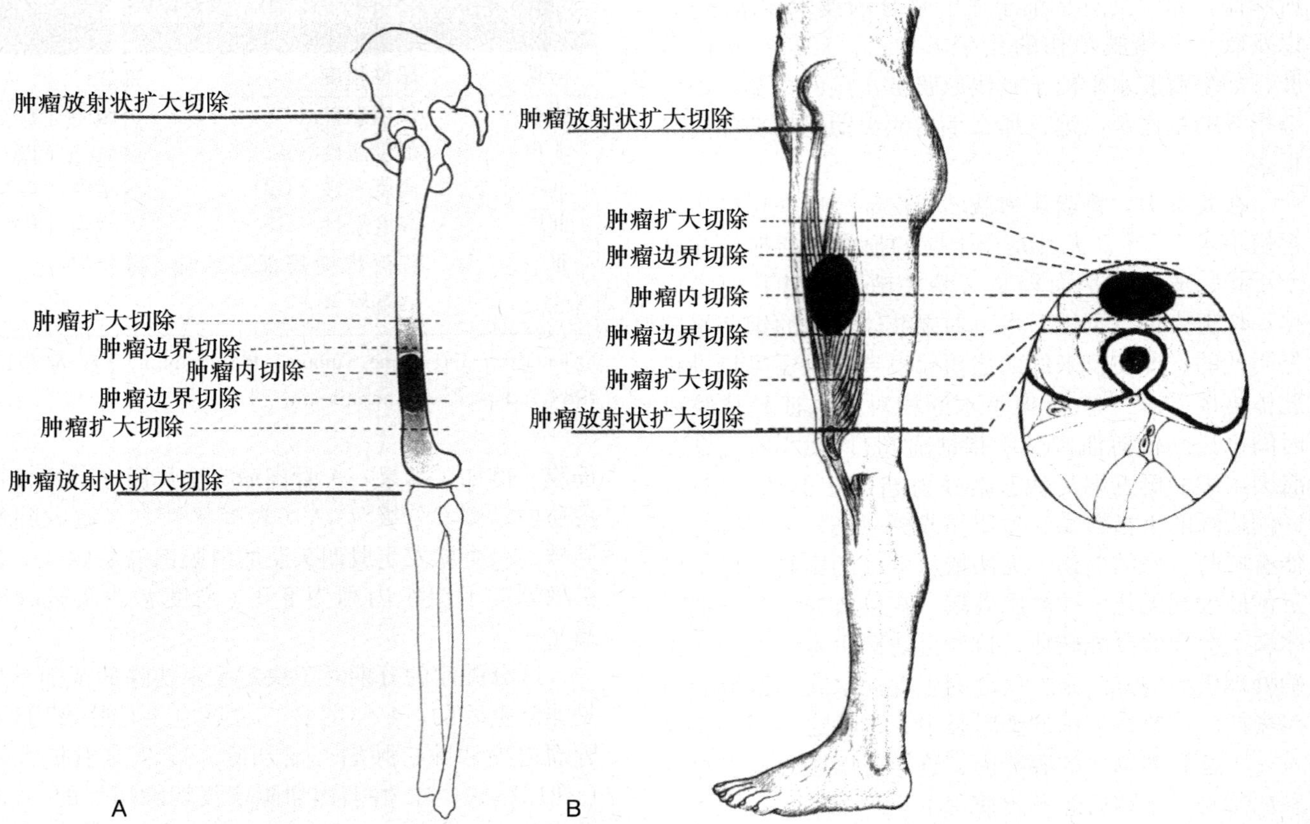

图 127-8 根据九级法分级而制定的切除肢体恶性肿瘤的 4 个手术边界平面。A. 针对骨肿瘤。B. 针对软组织肿瘤。(From Campanacci M: Bone and Soft Tissue Tumors. New York, Springer-Verlag, 1990, with permission.)

的功能水平明显提高[25,30,55,63,64]。旋转矫形手术的功
能结果特别好[51]，如果肿瘤的解剖位置合适，家长/
患儿能够接受旋转矫形后的外观，那么还是强烈建议
做这种手术。总而言之，是选择做截肢手术还是保肢
2058 手术取决于肿瘤的分级、分期、游离切除肿瘤的能
力，以及肿瘤对于辅助化疗的反应[44]。

败血症/暴发性紫癜

暴发性紫癜非常少见，但会导致严重的感染性休克和 DIC，造成皮肤皮下组织出血坏死。最初的表现为扩散性的斑疹，迅速进展为全层皮肤坏死并伴有大量脓液产生。伴有广泛的软组织坏死可导致截肢。大多数病例是由于脑膜炎双球菌感染导致的，也可以是链球菌等其他病原体导致的[36,78]。对于儿童暴发性紫癜的急性期治疗包括静脉应用抗生素（抗菌谱应包括脑膜炎双球菌和链球菌）、扩容、加强通气和应用血管活性药物。筋膜切开术要在早期积极应用，这可以减少深层的软组织受累，缩小截肢的范围。暴发性紫癜经常造成干性坏疽，在这种情况下，截肢要等到坏疽的边界完全清晰时再进行，这样有助于尽量多地保存肢体[36,79]。远期的并发症包括对于横断骨骼的截肢残端的软组织覆盖，以及随着患儿的生长由于部分骨骺存在或骨骺阻滞导致的肢体成角畸形和长骨畸形。

血管疾病

除了创伤和暴发性紫癜导致的微血管病变，其他的血管疾病同样会造成肢体截肢。新生儿的肢体缺血有多种原因，潜在的病理变化是动脉闭塞[7,21]。早产儿是动脉闭塞的高危人群。动脉闭塞可能是由

于血液高凝状态或血栓栓塞性疾病造成的。新生儿的纤溶系统较弱，导致他们相对成人更容易发生血栓。经动脉进行的导管介入治疗同样可以引起血栓形成及动脉栓塞闭塞。由于血液高凝状态导致的新生儿动脉闭塞通常发生在生后 1 周内，而动脉导管插入术引起的动脉闭塞常发生在生后 8 周[1]。无论是什么原因、什么年龄、肢体缺血及随后发生的坏疽都将导致截肢。和暴发性紫癜一样，对于损伤/缺血的肢体，建议等待界限清晰和发展到干性坏疽阶段再进行截肢。通过这一阶段的观察能够尽量多地保存肢体。只有在出现感染扩散的情况下要进行早期截肢和清创。长期后遗症并不明显，患儿可以通过佩戴假肢达到较好的功能。

残端过度生长现象和幻觉现象

残端肢体的过度生长现象是儿童截肢患者特有的一种现象。造成残端过度生长的原因是在生理条件下局部的成骨作用。经过干骺端的截肢手术最易出现残端过度生长。干骺端是成骨最活跃的部位，软骨成骨和骨膜成骨形成都非常活跃。这种联合的成骨作用可能在截肢或损伤后造成局部很好的成骨环境。无论是经骨干的或是经干骺端的截肢残端的过度生长，都和成骨的骨膜及可能过度活跃的骨髓前体细胞有关。而在进行关节离断术后的局部组织内不存在活跃的成骨组织。

如果残端的过度生长造成一定的问题，需要再次进行残端修整术以便能够继续佩戴假肢。最明显的原因是骨骼生长穿透了皮肤。其他需要进行残肢修整的指征包括：囊肿形成、骨骼过度生长导致疼痛等[1]。在一个包括 1015 名骨骼未成熟的截肢患者的统计中，约 6% 的病例由于过度生长需要进行残肢修整手术[1]。最近的一组病例报告残肢修整手术的比率高达 27%[58]。决定是否需要行残肢修整手术包括以下 3 个主要因素：最初截肢时的年龄、截肢的类型（先天性或获得性）、截肢的水平（横断骨骼的或关节离断术）。截肢时年龄大于 12 岁的患儿需要再次行残端修整手术的可能性较小[17]。获得性截肢手术可能需要再次行残端修整手术，其中最常见的是获得性的膝关节下截肢术（50%），先天性截肢的患儿很少需要再次修整残端（4%）[1]。截肢的水平也很重要，横断骨骼的截肢容易产生残端过度生长，需要进行残端修整，发生率排列如下：胫骨、肱骨、腓骨、股骨。关节离断术需要进行残端修整术的概率是 0%[158]。残端修整手术需要切除周围的滑囊/囊肿，然后扩大切除过度生长的骨骼，通常要切除 2～3 cm，以利于周围软组织覆盖。

幻觉现象（患肢存在幻觉及患肢疼痛）在成人截肢患者中是一种常见现象。在儿童中，传统上认为发生的概率明显低于成人。然而，最近对于儿童和青少年的研究表明这种现象并不少见。一项儿童截肢患者的统计报道显示，42% 患肢存在幻觉，29% 存在患肢疼痛[80]。幻觉现象在接受截肢手术的儿童中要比在先天性截肢的患儿中更常见[80]。儿童烫伤和电击伤导致的截肢发生患肢疼痛的概率明显高于烧伤[73]。多达 20% 的先天性截肢患儿患肢存在幻觉[52]。患肢疼痛在恶性肿瘤导致的截肢患者（48%）中的发生率要高于创伤导致的截肢患者（12%）[68]；对于恶性肿瘤进行的化疗也可能是导致这些儿童产生患肢疼痛的危险因素。

（葛翼华译　赵　黎校）

参考文献

1. Abraham E, Pellicore RJ, Hamilton RC, et al: Stump overgrowth in juvenile amputees. J Pediatr Orthop 1986;6:66.
2. Achterman C, Kalamchi A: Congenital deficiency of the fibula. J Bone Joint Surg Br 1979;61:133.
3. Aitken GT: Proximal femoral focal deficiency: Definition, classification and management. In Aitken GT (ed): Proximal Femoral Focal Deficiency: A Congenital Anomaly. Washington, DC, National Academy of Sciences, 1969, p 1.
4. Beris AE, Soucacos PN, Malizos KN: Microsurgery in children. Clin Orthop 1995;314:112.
5. Bilukha OO, Brennan M, Woodruff BA: Death and injury from landmines and unexploded ordnance in Afghanistan. JAMA 2003;290:650.
6. Birch JG, Lincoln TL, Mack PW: Functional classification of fibular deficiency. In Herring JA, Birch JG (eds): The Child with a Limb Deficiency. Rosemont, IL, American Academy of Orthopaedic Surgeons, 1998, p 161.
7. Blank JE, Dormans JP, Davidson RS: Perinatal limb ischemia: Orthopaedic implications. J Pediatr Orthop 1996;16:90.
8. Bosse MJ, MacKenzie EJ, Kellam JF, et al: A prospective evaluation of the clinical utility of the lower-extremity injury-severity scores. J Bone Joint Surg Am 2001;83:3.
9. Boulas HJ: Amputations of the fingers and hands: Indications for replantation. J Am Acad Orthop Surg 1998;6:100.
10. Buncke GM, Buntic RF, Romeo O: Pediatric mutilating hand injuries. Hand Clin 2003;19:121.

11. Campanacci M: Bone and Soft Tissue Tumors. New York, Springer-Verlag, 1990.
12. Cheng JCY, Cheung KW, Ng BKW: Severe progressive deformities after limb lengthening in type-II fibular hemimelia. J Bone Joint Surg Br 1998;80:772.
13. Choi IH, Kumar SJ, Bowen JR: Amputation or limb-lengthening for partial or total absence of the fibula. J Bone Joint Surg Am 1990;72:1391.
14. Clark MW: Autosomal dominant inheritance of tibial meromelia. J Bone Joint Surg Am 1975;57:262.
15. Coupland RM, Korver A: Injuries from antipersonnel mines: The experience of the International Committee of the Red Cross. BMJ 1991;303:1509.
16. Dreyfus M, Baldauf J-J, Rigaut E, et al: Prenatal diagnosis of unilateral tibial hemimelia. Ultrasound Obstet Gynecol 1996; 7:205.
17. Enneking WF, Spanier SS, Goodman MA: A system for surgical staging of musculoskeletal sarcoma. Clin Orthop 1980;153:106.
18. Epps CH Jr, Schneider PL: Treatment of the hemimelias of the lower extremity. J Bone Joint Surg Am 1989; 71:273.
19. Epps CH Jr, Tooms RE, Edholm CD, et al: Failure of centralization of the fibula for congenital longitudinal deficiency of the tibia. J Bone Joint Surg Am 1991; 73:858.
20. Fagelman MF, Epps HR, Rang M: Mangled extremity severity score in children. J Pediatr Orthop 2002;22:182.
21. Farrar MJ, Bennet GC, Wilson NIL, et al: The orthopaedic implications of peripheral limb ischaemia in infants and children. J Bone Joint Surg Br 1996;78:6.
22. Fernandez-Palazzi F, Bendaham J, Rivas S: Congenital deficiency of the tibia: A report on 22 cases. J Pediatr Orthop B 1998;7:298.
23. Fowler E, Zernicke R, Setoguchi Y, et al: Energy expenditure during walking by children who have proximal femoral focal deficiency. J Bone Joint Surg Am 1996;78:1857.
24. Frantz CH, O'Rahilly R: Congenital skeletal limb deficiencies. J Bone Joint Surg Am 1961;43:1022.
25. Fuchs B, Kotajarvi BR, Kaufman KR, et al: Functional outcome of patients with rotationplasty about the knee. Clin Orthop 2003;415:52.
26. Gillespie R: Classification of congenital abnormalities of the femur. In Herring JA, Birch JG (eds): The Child with a Limb Deficiency. Rosemont, IL, American Academy of Orthopaedic Surgeons, 1998, p 63.
27. Gillespie R, Torode IP: Classification and management of congenital abnormalities of the femur. J Bone Joint Surg Br 1983;65:557.
28. Goncalves LF, De Luca GR, Vitorello DA, et al: Prenatal diagnosis of bilateral proximal femoral hypoplasia. Ultrasound Obstet Gynecol 1996;8:127.
29. Grogan DP, Holt GR, Ogden JA: Talocalcaneal coalition in patients who have fibular hemimelia or proximal femoral focal deficiency. J Bone Joint Surg Am 1994;76:1363.
30. Ham SJ, Koops HS, Veth RPH, et al: Limb salvage surgery for primary bone sarcoma of the lower extremities: Long-term consequences of endoprosthetic reconstructions. Ann Surg Oncol 1998;5:423.
31. Helfet DL, Howey T, Sanders R, et al: Limb salvage versus amputation: Preliminary results of the Mangled Extremity Severity Score. Clin Orthop 1990;256:80.
32. Herring JA: Symes amputation for fibular hemimelia: A second look in the Ilizarov era. Instr Course Lect 1992: 41:435.
33. Herring JA, Barnhill B, Gaffney C: Syme amputation: An evaluation of the physical and psychological function in young patients. J Bone Joint Surg Am 1986;68:573.
34. Herring JA, Cummings DR: The limb-deficient child. In Morrissy RT, Weinstein SL (eds): Lovell and Winter's Pediatric Orthopaedics. Philadelphia, Lippincott-Raven, 1996.
35. Howe HR Jr, Poole GV, Hansen KJ, et al: Salvage of lower extremities following combined orthopaedic and vascular trauma. A predictive salvage index. Am Surg 1987;53:205.
36. Huang DB, Price M, Pokorny J, et al: Reconstructive surgery in children after meningococcal purpura fulminans. J Pediatr Surg 1999;34:595.
37. Jacobs LGH: The landmine foot: Its description and management. Injury 1991;22:463.
38. Johansen K, Daines M, Howey T, et al: Objective criteria accurately predict amputation following lower extremity trauma. J Trauma 1990;30:568.
39. Johnston CE II, Haideri NF: Comparison of functional outcome in fibular deficiency treated by limb salvage versus Syme's amputation. In Herring JA, Birch JG (eds): The Child with a Limb Deficiency. Rosemont, IL, American Academy of Orthopaedic Surgeons, 1998, p 173.
40. Jones D, Barnes J, Lloyd-Roberts GC: Congenital aplasia and dysplasia of the tibia with intact fibula. J Bone Joint Surg Br 1978;60:31.
41. Kant P, Koh SH-Y, Neumann V, et al: Treatment of longitudinal deficiency affecting the femur: Comparing patient mobility and satisfaction outcomes of Syme amputation against extension prosthesis. J Pediatr Orthop 2003; 23:236.
42. Kostuik JP, Gillespie R, Hall JE, et al: Van Nes rotational osteotomy for treatment of proximal femoral focal deficiency and congenital short femur. J Bone Joint Surg Am 1975;57:1039.
43. Krajbich JI: Lower-limb deficiencies and amputations in children. J Am Acad Orthop Surg 1998;6:358.
44. Kumta SM, Cheng JCY, Li CK, et al: Scope and limitations of limb-sparing surgery in childhood sarcoma. J Pediatr Orthop 2002;22:244.
45. Letts M, Davidson D: Epidemiology and prevention of traumatic amputations in children. In Herring JA, Birch JG (eds): The Child with a Limb Deficiency. Rosemont, IL, American Academy of Orthopaedic Surgeons, 1998.
46. Loder RT: Demographics of traumatic amputations in children. Implications for prevention strategies. J Bone Joint Surg Am 2004;86:923.
47. Loder RT, Herring JA: Fibular transfer for congenital absence of the tibia: A reassessment. J Pediatr Orthop 1987;7:8.
48. Mankin HJ, Lange TA, Spanier SS: The hazards of biopsy in patients with malignant primary bone and soft tissue tumors. J Bone Joint Surg Am 1982;64:1121.
49. Mankin HJ, Mankin CJ, Simon MA: The hazards of the biopsy, revisited. J Bone Joint Surg Am 1996;78:656.
50. McCarthy JJ, Clancy GL, Chang FM, et al: Fibular hemimelia: Comparison of outcome measurements after amputation and lengthening. J Bone Joint Surg Am 2000;82:1732.
51. McClenaghan BA, Krajbich JI, Pirone AM, et al: Comparative assessment of gait after limb salvage procedures. J Bone Joint Surg Am 1989;71:1178.
52. Melzack R, Israel R, Lacroix R, et al: Phantom limbs in people with congenital limb deficiency or amputation in early childhood. Brain 1997;120:1603.
53. Miller LS, Bell DF: Management of congenital fibular deficiency by Ilizarov technique. J Pediatr Orthop 1992;12:651.
54. Mirra JM: Bone Tumors. Philadelphia, Lea & Febiger, 1989.
55. Nagarajan R, Neglia JP, Clohisy DR, et al: Limb salvage and

amputation in survivors of pediatric lower-extremity bone tumors: What are the long-term implications? J Clin Oncol 2002;20:4493.
56. Naudie D, Hamdy RC, Fassier F, et al: Management of fibular hemimelia. Amputation or limb lengthening. J Bone Joint Surg Br 1997;79:58.
57. O'Connell C: The aftermath of war: In the minefields of Mozambique. Can Med Assoc J 2000;163:1590.
58. O'Neal ML, Bahner R, Ganey TM, et al: Osseous overgrowth after amputation in adolescents and children. J Pediatr Orthop 1996;16:78.
59. Pearn J: Children and war. J Paediatr Child Health 2003; 39:166.
60. Postma A, Kingma A, de Ruiter JH, et al: Quality of life in bone tumor patients comparing limb salvage and amputation of the lower extremity. J Surg Oncol 1992;51:47.
61. Price CT, Noonan KJ: Femoral lengthening with monolateral half-pin devices. In Herring JA, Birch JG (eds): The Child with a Limb Deficiency. Rosemont, IL, American Academy of Orthopaedic Surgeons, 1998, p 133.
62. Raimondi PL, Petrolati M, Delaria G: Replantation of large segments in children. Hand Clin 2000;16:547.
63. Renard AJ, Veth RP, Schreuder HWB, et al: Function and complications after ablative and limb-salvage therapy in lower extremity sarcoma of bone. J Surg Oncol 2000; 73:198.
64. Rödl RW, Pohlmann U, Gosheger G, et al: Rotationplasty—quality of life after 10 years in 22 patients. Acta Orthop Scand 2002;73:85.
65. Roux MO, Carlioz H: Clinical examination and investigation of the cruciate ligaments in children with fibular hemimelia. J Pediatr Orthop 1999;19:247.
66. Saies AD, Urbaniak JD, Nunley JA, et al: Results after replantation and revascularization in the upper extremity in children. J Bone Joint Surg Am 1994;76:1766.
67. Schoenecker PL, Capelli AM, Millar EA, et al: Congenital longitudinal deficiency of the tibia. J Bone Joint Surg Am 1989;71:278.
68. Smith J, Thompson JM: Phantom limb pain and chemotherapy in pediatric amputees. Mayo Clin Proc 1995;70:357.
69. Spiegel DA, Loder RT, Crandall RC: Congenital longitudinal deficiency of the tibia. Int Orthop 2003;27:338.
70. Steel HH, Lin PS, Betz RR, et al: Iliofemoral fusion for proximal femoral focal deficiency. J Bone Joint Surg Am 1987;69:837.
71. Stevens PM, Arms D: Postaxial hypoplasia of the lower extremity. J Pediatr Orthop 2000;20:166.
72. Tachdjian MO: Pediatric Orthopedics. Philadelphia, WB Saunders, 1990.
73. Thomas CR, Brazeal BA, Rosenberg L, et al: Phantom limb pain in pediatric burn survivors. Burns 2003;29:139.
74. Torode IP, Gillespie R: Rotationplasty of the lower limb for congenital defects of the femur. J Bone Joint Surg Br 1983; 65:569.
75. Trautwein LC, Smith DG, Rivara FP: Pediatric amputation injuries: Etiology, cost, and outcome. J Trauma 1996;41:831.
76. Turker R, Mendelson S, Ackman J, et al: Anatomic considerations of the foot and leg in tibial hemimelia. J Pediatr Orthop 1996;16:445.
77. Walsh NE, Walsh WS: Rehabilitation of landmine victims—the ultimate challenge. Bull World Health Org 2003;81:665.
78. Warner PM, Kagan RJ, Yakuboff KP, et al: Current management of purpura fulminans: A multicenter study. J Burn Care Rehabil 2003;24:119.
79. Wheeler JS, Anderson BJ, De Chalain TMB: Surgical intervention in children with meningococcal purpura fulminans—a review of 117 procedures in 21 children. J Pediatr Surg 2003; 38:597.
80. Wilkins KL, McGrath PJ, Finley GA, et al: Phantom limb sensations and phantom limb pain in child and adolescent amputees. Pain 1998;78:7.

第 128 章

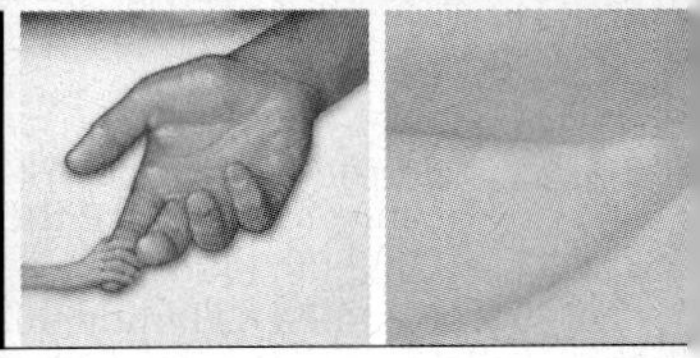

皮肤、结缔组织、肌肉、肌腱和手的先天性缺损

Edward P. Miranda 和 Stephen J. Mathes

2061 细胞增殖、分化和退化是人胚胎发生的特征，随后的发育过程是复杂的并具有潜在的畸变可能。但是，在怀孕期间发生畸变和损伤十分频繁，有证据显示孕期自发的流产高达 33%[49,86,87]，此时通过人绒毛膜促性腺激素测定可检测到受精卵植入。这种流产有时反而是好事情，如较大的染色体畸形患儿即使生下来可能也无法存活[30]。这种对于畸变的选择并不是非常精确，因为仍然会有一些不致死亡的畸形儿出生。

发生率和发病风险

较大的畸形表现为结构上的异常，从而导致医学和社会学的后果。较大的畸形发生率在新生儿为 2%~3%[14,31,38,83]。较小的畸形主要是结构上的变化，并不会带来明显的医学或者社会负担。15% 的新生儿至少有一种可辨认的畸形。较大的和微小的异常之间的区别非常明显，因为所有人类的畸形都是以一种连续的状态存在。但是，即使是最微小的生理畸变也可能使患儿处于心理社会的孤立状态，因此需要适当的手术治疗。

皮肤和软组织

胚胎学

皮肤、肌肉、结缔组织和肌腱的发生是在胚胎的第 3 周开始的。在此期间，出现原始的条纹并促进了三胚层胚胎（外胚层、中胚层和内胚层）、脊索和体节的形成[53]。

表皮的发生

皮肤是人体最大的器官，由两层组成：真皮和表皮。皮肤有许多功能而不仅仅是人体和外界环境之间的屏障[53]。皮肤可以调节体温、感知觉，并起到屏障的作用，防止水分丢失和微生物入侵，同时也是一种主要的神经调节免疫器官[50]。表皮系统也是非言语交往的中介，皮肤的出现有助于人与人之间的识别和本体感觉。

表皮本身来源于外胚层细胞的单细胞层，在怀孕 4 周时形成周皮[62]。早期的表皮是单层的，暴露于羊水中，通过表皮可以参与重要的盐水交换。随时间的推移，在胚胎第 3 个月，表皮扩展至 3 个细胞层（基底层、中间层和表层）。表皮继续生长，在第 6 个月分化已达到有效的屏障功能。显微镜下，皮肤与新生儿表皮相似，可以见到：基底层（最内层）、棘层、颗粒层和角质层（最外层）。角质化细胞在存活期间从基底层逐渐向角质层发展并最终脱落。这样的迁移是以渐进性的分化和角质颗粒在基底颗粒层的聚集形式为特征。中间层对外界环境维持一种屏障作用。基底层内残留有角质细胞的干细胞，可以再生成为皮肤的其他层[53]。

其他几种细胞迁移至表皮以辅助其功能。黑素细 206
胞是神经嵴源性细胞，首先迁移至真皮，而后迁移至表皮。这些细胞可以产生黑色素以防止紫外线的损伤。大约在胚胎第 3 周，表皮内可见 Langerhans 细胞。Langerhans 细胞是骨髓源性，在表皮层中排列有特异的抗原递呈细胞，形成免疫性的网络，以向 T 细胞察觉和递呈外源性抗原[53]。

表皮和其他中胚层组织的发生

在胚胎发育第 3 周，在原线头端出现原结。间充质细胞从结的地方开始迁移，并形成中线细胞索，称为脊索。这一过程持续发展，直至形成口咽膜。由于内胚层和外胚层的紧密联结，而不能继续伸展。脊索产生脊柱并且诱导外胚层形成神经板，即神经系统的始基[53]。

随着脊索的形成，胚胎内的中胚页在两侧增厚，形成一对轴旁中胚层的纵柱。在第 3 周末，这些轴旁中胚层条索分成成对的立方体称为体节。最终，42～44对体节以头尾向的顺序发育。体节是大多数中轴骨骼、肌肉组织和相关真皮的部分前体[53,59,78]。

胚胎第 3 周间充质的出现对于器官发生是必要的。在第 8 周，面部和手已成人形。在胚胎第 12 周，腭已形成并可以通过外生殖器辨别性别。在中胚层分化和发育过程发生中断（间充质细胞迁移、脊索、体节），准确地反映了在皮肤、结缔组织、肌肉和肌腱发生的先天性畸形的多样性。对于此类广泛的畸形，对缺陷的解剖学认识和系统的分析对于形成有效的治疗方案是非常必要的[53]。

缺陷的分析和治疗技术

任何一种缺陷的结构异常，可细分为正常组织异位、局部正常组织缺乏以及组织构成的畸变。

正常组织异位

正常组织先天性异位来源于胚线的融合，由于临近组织的异常生长导致解剖标记移位，或者旋转不良。内脏异位可对患者无任何影响。右位心可以无任何临床症状。但是，在多数病例，异位有较大的影响。异位的程度取决于正常发育的异常造成的串联事体。脊柱裂是躯干尾端背侧的缺陷，在胚胎发育的第 4 周，由于多种软组织和脊椎骨骼缺损所致。当椎管闭合异常时，脊髓可以通过躯干的缺损处疝出，并发生脊髓脊膜膨出。随后可以发生一系列的异常[47,81]。异位的脊髓可以发生退行性改变，并且下肢无神经支配，因此可以导致纤维脂肪替代肌肉组织，结果形成畸形的、不可逆转的下肢瘫痪。

及时的手术介入将异位的正常组织还纳入其原始解剖部位，可以打断异常的顺序并且可能恢复正常的功能和形态。实验动物中，在宫内修复脊椎管缺损，可以中止神经系统异常的继续发展[48]。这种方法目前在人类还处于研究阶段，并且有潜力校正大多数畸形。

生理上的畸形不十分明显，例如面裂，更多的是受到社会的压力[35,66,80]。这些压力不应当被低估。甚至是功能损害并不明显，怪异的外形仍然会受到影响和社会的排斥。历史上，面裂的新生儿死亡的危险较高。尽管这样的危险在现代治疗手段下几乎已被消除，但是社会对于这些患者的接纳则取决于他们恢复正常面部结构的能力及其能够展示一些技能如演讲的能力[20,26]。对缺陷的分析经常会发现在先天性唇裂中有较小的软组织缺损。可见畸形的大小与面部标记异位的程度是成比例的。手术将异位的结构复位至正常的解剖位置是纠正畸形的最理想的情况。除了修复的技术方面，时机的选择非常重要，因为要考虑到社会的接纳和语言的发展。在 18 个月以前进行腭裂的修补可以使患儿获得较好的语言能力。

局部正常组织缺乏

由于组织缺乏或者缺陷所致的结构畸形对整形外科医生提出了很高的要求。异源性或者自体材料在先天性缺损的重建过程中得到了应用，用于治疗组织缺乏或者缺陷所致的先天性畸形。异体组织重建具有不受供体量的限制、无供体部位缺损以及易于应用等优点。但是，自体组织重建对于先天性畸形更有优势，因为这样的组织能够与活的自体结构完全结合，维持了生长的潜能和创伤的修复，并且在愈合后能够抵抗 2062
感染。然而，异体物手术植入在青少年时期最为明智，在特殊的临床环境下，维持了良好的重建标准，例如先天发育不全的乳房畸形[37]。

有多种外科手术方式，可达到自体组织的最佳化应用。非血管组织移植方法较简单，并且是替代皮肤、肌肉、结缔组织和肌腱的有效途径。这项技术在供体部位能够完全自我修复的情况下，是首选的方法。此外，移植床血管形成良好，对于营养移植物直到新生血管形成也是非常有必要的。当血管床不适合移植物或者在重建过程中要求有专门的组织时，应用专门组织自身的血供进行整块皮瓣转移[15,44]。组织移植的方法取决于供体和受体部位的距离。游离微血管皮瓣移植是供体部位与受体部位的距离太远时的一种非常好的移植方法。

组织扩展是一种非常有效的方法，适用于那些供体部位少，同时又能够产生结构完整的软组织。带头皮的头发移植治疗表皮发育不全就是非常好的例子，阐明了组织扩增后的潜能[67]。牵拉骨生长技术是另一个相似的例子。该项使骨延长的技术首先是由 Ilizarov 提出的，用于长骨的延长，现在也可用于面部骨骼。逐步的面部骨骼延长，不伴有供区的畸形，对于治疗半面矮小患者的下颌骨发育不全是非常有效的[52]。

组织结构的畸变

组织中相关细胞成分的不平衡可能会导致明显的畸形而不伴有组织的缺失。皮肤缺损，如先天性巨大色素痣和葡萄酒斑，都是由于过多地表达了某种特殊细胞或组织的畸形。在先天性巨大色素痣中，黑素细胞相关痣细胞在真皮层过度增殖。在出生后，这些细胞蜕变成为黑素瘤的危险性增加，因此需要进行手术切除。表皮葡萄酒斑是由于真皮中异常的微血管组织积聚后过度发育所致。这些病变不具有分裂活性并且也没有形成新生物的潜能。但是，它们可毁损面容并且会受到社会歧视。由于继发的瘢痕和畸形，一般并不采用直接的切除。选择性的激光切除部分血管组织对于治疗这种畸形是一种有效的方法。

许多局部的先天性畸形并不会造成很大的影响，通常认为是正常组织的变异。例如，先天性掌长肌腱缺如有 15%~20% 的发生率。这样的畸形是不需要治疗的。但是，当功能或者形态受到影响时，在重建前认真地分析正常结构异位的程度、组织缺损的程度以及迷行组织的构成是非常必要的。合适的手术时机通常可阻止一系列可预知的继发性畸形。

特殊的解剖部位

皮肤

先天性皮肤发育不全

先天性皮肤发育不全（ACC）是一种罕见的先天性异常，以全层皮肤缺失和部分皮下组织缺失为特征。头皮累及比率约为 85%，偶尔会累及全部头盖组织，包括颅顶和硬脊膜的缺失。确切的发生率并不清楚，在文献报道中少于 300 例。ACC 的诊断靠临床诊断，并且一般在出生时即能发现，尽管出生前超声诊断也有报道。病变一般表现为一层薄的、透明的膜或者是干燥的瘢痕代替正常的皮肤，无毛囊。头顶部是最常波及的部位。对于小的缺损，自然病程表现为来自侧缘的上皮形成，但是巨大的缺损通常不能关闭并且需要进行治疗。广泛的头皮缺损的死亡率为 20%~30%[36,85]。

ACC 的流行病学并不十分清楚。已有报道 ACC 与其他的缺陷有关，包括肢体畸形、脐膨出和裂。治疗经常是针对那些巨大的缺损以及那些伴有骨缺损的患者。颅顶部累及骨的患者可能由于矢状窦的出血而使患者处于危险状态，故需要早期的手术治疗[36]。一般采用皮瓣或者皮肤移植来修复缺损，或者两者同时使用。骨性的颅骨重建通常需要延迟到患儿 2 岁后进行；偶尔，骨性的硬脑膜可以自发的产生新骨来填补缺损。正常毛发的重建需要通过头皮的组织扩展和在患儿 5~7岁时用局部皮瓣覆盖感染处来完成[69,79,85]。

先天性黑素细胞痣和巨大色素痣

先天性痣由巨大的、成簇的、产生色素的黑素细胞在真皮聚集而成，在出生时即产生大量的色素。与普通的后天性痣相比，先天性痣体积巨大，有更多的细胞质，位于真皮的深层。小的先天性痣的发生率为每 100 个新生儿中有 1 名，巨大的先天性痣为每 20000 个新生儿中有 1 名[7]。出生后，区别是先天性还是获得性非常困难，即使是从组织学上也难于鉴别。先天性黑素细胞痣根据 206

大小可以分为：小型，直径小于1.5 cm；中型，直径 1.5 ~19.9 cm；大型（巨大），大于 20 cm[10,11]。

先天性痣具有转变成为黑素瘤的可能性，也是这些病变需要进行手术治疗的主要原因。但是，对于其恶变的真正危险性并不确定。巨大的先天性痣（GCN），其恶变率约为 1%~31% 不等，但是 GCN 患者总的数目并不清楚，因为这些数据由于其范围太大而不十分可靠。近来一项数据表明 GCN 患者黑素瘤的总体发生率为 8.2%，需要进行手术切除。恶性黑色素瘤发生的危险也是非常大的，60% 的 GCN 相关性黑色素瘤在头十年内发生，但有几项研究显示许多恶性变在 3 岁左右发生。小的先天性痣恶变为黑色素瘤也有报道，其恶变率约为 2.6%~4.9%[88]。

巨大色素痣（GHN）是先天性痣的一种特殊亚型。这些由黑色素细胞组成的表皮缺损非常广泛，并且包绕了整个解剖部位，可超过体表面积的 20%（见图 128-1）。这些痣通常表现为多毛伴良性表面结节，是由局部的神经外胚层组织分化而来[34]。当头部或者躯干上部被累及时，20% 的患者可以观察到神经方面的异常。伴有 GHN 的软脑膜黑皮病、脑积水、癫痫发作以及脊髓病的神经学表现与神经外胚层的发育是一致的[34]。

GHN 可毁损面容并在出生时即可以诊断[74]。GHN 患儿的父母通常在早期即开始寻求治疗。一些患有 GHN 的新生儿在出生后不久即发现患有恶性黑色素瘤，因此需要早期进行手术切除。GHN 病变连续的切除同时应用皮下组织扩张器，可以美化患病部位，减少恶变的危险[39]。在出生 6 个月内，婴儿皮肤逐渐增加的顺应性和弹性为发现巨大的痣提供了很多机会[43]。在这一时间，结节或增加的色素区域将被切除。随后切除的时机是建立在痣的外观变化的基础上，以及父母决定进行完整切除的时间。反复切除可以在儿童早期完整去除病变。完整切除痣同时进行皮肤移植可能会产生瘢痕以及收缩变形，不只在痣切除的区域，在皮肤供体部位也是如此。应用序贯切除同时扩展邻近正常部位的皮肤来覆盖痣切除的部位，这样不会产生额外的瘢痕。

皮脂腺痣

皮脂腺痣（SN）是一种实性的、边界清楚、斑状的突起于皮肤表面的病变。SN 多发生于头皮、两鬓或者耳前区，有时在出生时即可诊断。儿童组织学分析显示表皮异常增生伴有毛囊和皮脂腺发育不全。在青春期，皮脂腺成熟，上皮细胞增生。在成人，有 6%~50% 可以发展为基底细胞癌（BCC）[71]。

在儿童期对 SN 的治疗存在一定争议。早期报道 BCC 在青少年的发病率约 10%~15%，现已被大量的回顾性研究驳斥。研究显示良性上皮样细胞病变的发生率低，并且在 16 岁之前切除的病变无一例发生 BCC。但是，在成人中，仍然有相当多的文献报道了 SN 相关性 BCC 的发生。其治疗方法为切除，但是延迟至青少年时期才进行切除是不明智的[71,82]。

先天性蹼

先天性蹼（翼状胬肉）最多见于颈部（翼状颈皮）。在颈部，皮肤呈厚襞状，皮下组织从乳突向侧方延伸至肩峰。病变一般为双侧，并可以使局部结构扭曲变形，包括后发际线，其边界通常向外侧移位至颈部从而表现为短颈畸形。蹼的表现与在腋襞和脚的表现类似。

先天性蹼可以单独发生，或者与其他先天性畸形同时发生，但是病因尚不清楚[27]。某些局部畸形例如 Klippel-Feil 综合征即表现为这种发育性缺损。颈蹼通常为 Turner 综合征的表现之一。蹼可以导致功能性或者外观性残疾（或二者皆有）。可通过多个 Z 形成形术加延长术完成矫正，一般在 1~6 岁进行[70]。

先天性乳房畸形

胚胎学

乳房在胚胎的第 5 周由外胚层发育而来。双侧乳腺嵴从腋窝延伸至腹股沟。在胚胎第 7~8 周，乳腺嵴逐渐退化，仅留下胸壁前方和腋窝。在胚胎 10~14 周以后，原始的乳房组织侵入胸部间充质组织并开始形成腺体。间充质包围乳腺并形成层状与 Camper 筋膜（最外层）相连续并且第 2 层将乳房从胸壁下肌肉组织中分离。Camper 筋膜环绕在乳房前方所有的部分，除了小巢深部。结缔组织网通过乳腺形成 Cooper 韧带，起到悬吊乳房的作用。输乳管约在胚胎 20 周时形成，腺体组织逐渐发育至青春期末[51,54,61]。

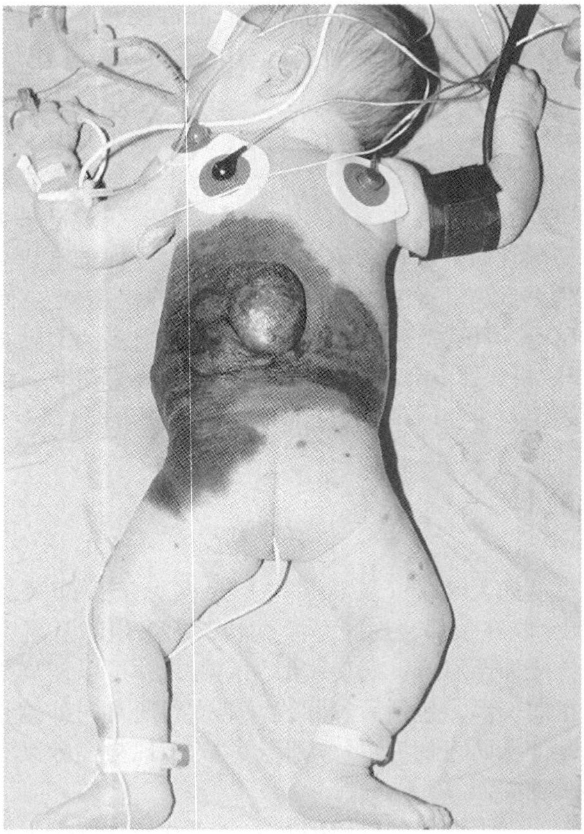
A

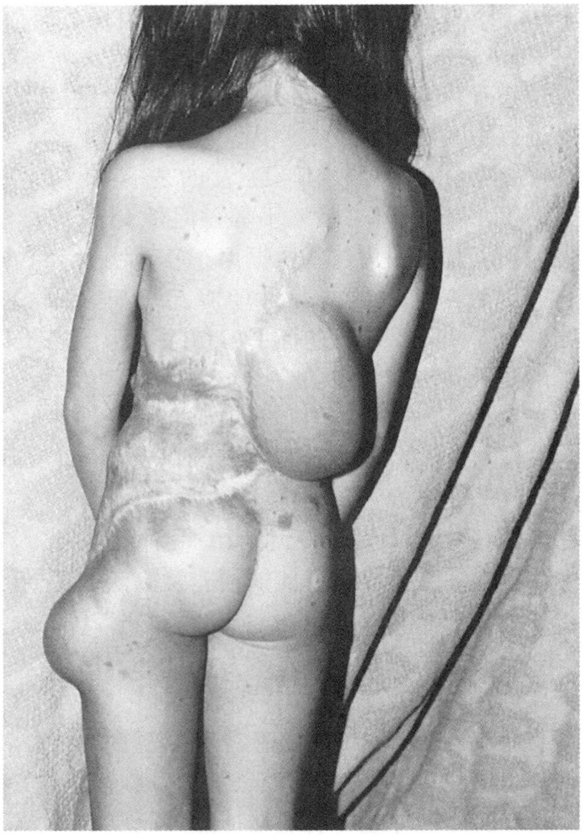
B

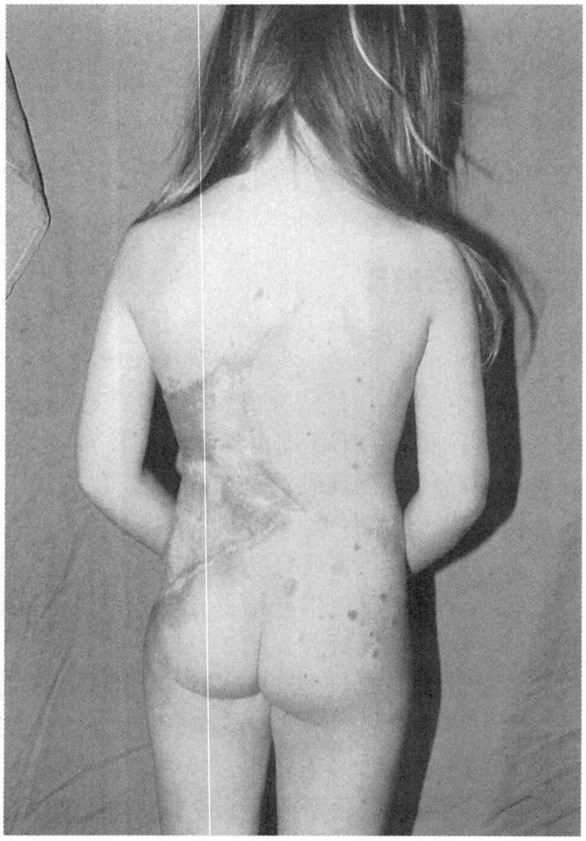
C

图 128-1　A. 先天性巨大色素痣。该婴儿巨大的中线部肿块证实是恶性神经嵴细胞瘤，出生时已经存在。B. 恶性肿瘤被完全切除。切除后植入多个组织扩张器有利于创面覆盖。C. 切除了大部分痣。

2066 多乳头和多乳房

多乳头（多乳头畸形）和多乳房（多乳房畸形）是相对多见的先天性畸形，多乳头的发生率大约为 0.2%～2.5%，多乳房的发生率为 0.1%～1.0%。可见这些畸形沿着乳腺嵴从腋窝至腹股沟。多乳头和多乳房是由于孕期乳腺嵴正常凋亡退化异常所致。多乳头在出生时即可做出诊断。常见的多乳头部位是正常乳房的下方，最常见的副乳部位是腋窝[1,51]。

多乳头和多乳房就诊的主要原因是美观问题，但是也可以对激素变化有正常的反应，从而与正常的乳房相似，包括在青春期增大和哺乳期分泌乳汁。这些病变的治疗一般是采用简单的切除，但是应慎重考虑，因为影响正常乳房的疾病也可以影响到多余的乳房，应排除乳房肿块。此外，有几种其他疾病与多乳头和多乳房相关，包括在男性患者，睾丸肿瘤的发病率较高。其他有争论性的疾病包括泌尿生殖道畸形和肾细胞癌[13,25,84]。

先天性乳房缺失

完全的一侧或双侧乳房缺失非常少见，可以独立发生或与其他的多种发育性综合征同时发生，包括 Poland 综合征，Ullrich-Turner 综合征和 AREDYLD 综合征（肾小管缺乏、外胚层发育不良、脂肪缺乏性糖尿病）（图 128-2A～E）。先天性双侧乳房缺失非常少见，在文献中几乎没有报道。孟德尔氏遗传有可能，但是病因并不明确，致畸原可能也起到一定作用。由于该病少见，最佳治疗方法的研究并不充分。有成功应用自体组织，包括横向的腹直肌 TRAM 皮瓣移植重建新生乳房的报道。也可以选择组织扩展和移植[51]。

结节状乳房疾病

结节性乳房疾病最早由 Rees 和 Aston 在 1976 年首次报道，因为其表现与结节状根类似而得名（图 128-3A～D）[65]。尽管在文献报道中，对于这一术语和结节状乳房的描述还存在混淆，但是一般表现为乳房的不对称，并且有公认的下列表现：88% 行乳房增大成形术的女性有乳房不对称，29% 有乳房基底部收缩[68]。真正的结节状乳房非常少见，且不是仅依靠不对称或者是收缩，而是依靠乳房组织通过收缩的筋膜环向深部疝出至乳晕来确诊的。确切的发生率尚不确定，并且似乎没有可遗传的基因学因素[51]。

致密的筋膜环可以导致乳房在青春期发育不对称，并且最终腺体组织通过其疝出，引起乳晕的扩大。这可能与 1/4 或者超过 1/4 的发育不良有关，并且下方的缺损最常见。下方乳腺褶通常会抬高[63]。

结节状乳房通常在十几岁时由于外观的异常而被发现。这种异常由常见的不对称变异而来，因此治疗方法一般不同。接近 90% 为双侧发病，其中大概有 1/4 患者表现为乳腺组织严重的发育不良[51]。

对于结节状乳房的治疗存在一定争议，但是通常有几项基本原则。患者在乳房发育停止之前不适宜采用手术治疗。几乎在所有的病例中，疝出的乳房组织会引起乳晕的扩大，因此需要进行乳晕环切使其缩小。这一切口还可以到达筋膜环，其收缩的条带必须进行松解。建立了正常的乳房下褶和自然的下方轮廓后，建议同时进行局部组织的重组，但这两步之后的手术计划并不十分明确[28]。对于发育不良或者是不对称的乳房，组织扩张、植入移植物或者二者同时使用可有助于组织重组，但是仅使用植入物的效果不甚理想，乳房下褶皱畸形较常见[42,51]。

男子女性型乳房（婴幼儿和青少年）

男子女性型乳房，或者男子乳房异常表现比较常见，但是复杂的畸形包括先天性和获得性（图 128-4A～D）[9,51,56]。总的发生率为 32%～40%，在青少年男性中发生率为 65%[56]。男子女性型乳房多为双侧（报道为 25%～75%）[18,55]。

尽管许多男子女性型乳房的个别原因已被阐明，但是男性乳房的发育多继发于雌激素相对于睾酮的过量分泌——可以来源于绝对的雌激素分泌增多、睾酮的缺乏或者受体抵抗[24]。有关男子女性乳房的病因将在其他章节详细讨论[24]。男子女性型乳房可以分为先天性和获得性，或者称为生理性或病理性。在男孩，多数病例为先天性和生理性，在新生儿或者青少年时期发现。在宫内高母体雌激素水平可以导致乳房组织发育（新生儿男子女性型乳房），出生后几周内会复原。在青少年，雌二醇-睾酮比例的升高可以导致 65% 的男孩出现可以察觉的男子女性型乳房；但是，大多数如果不进行认真体检是不易发现的。

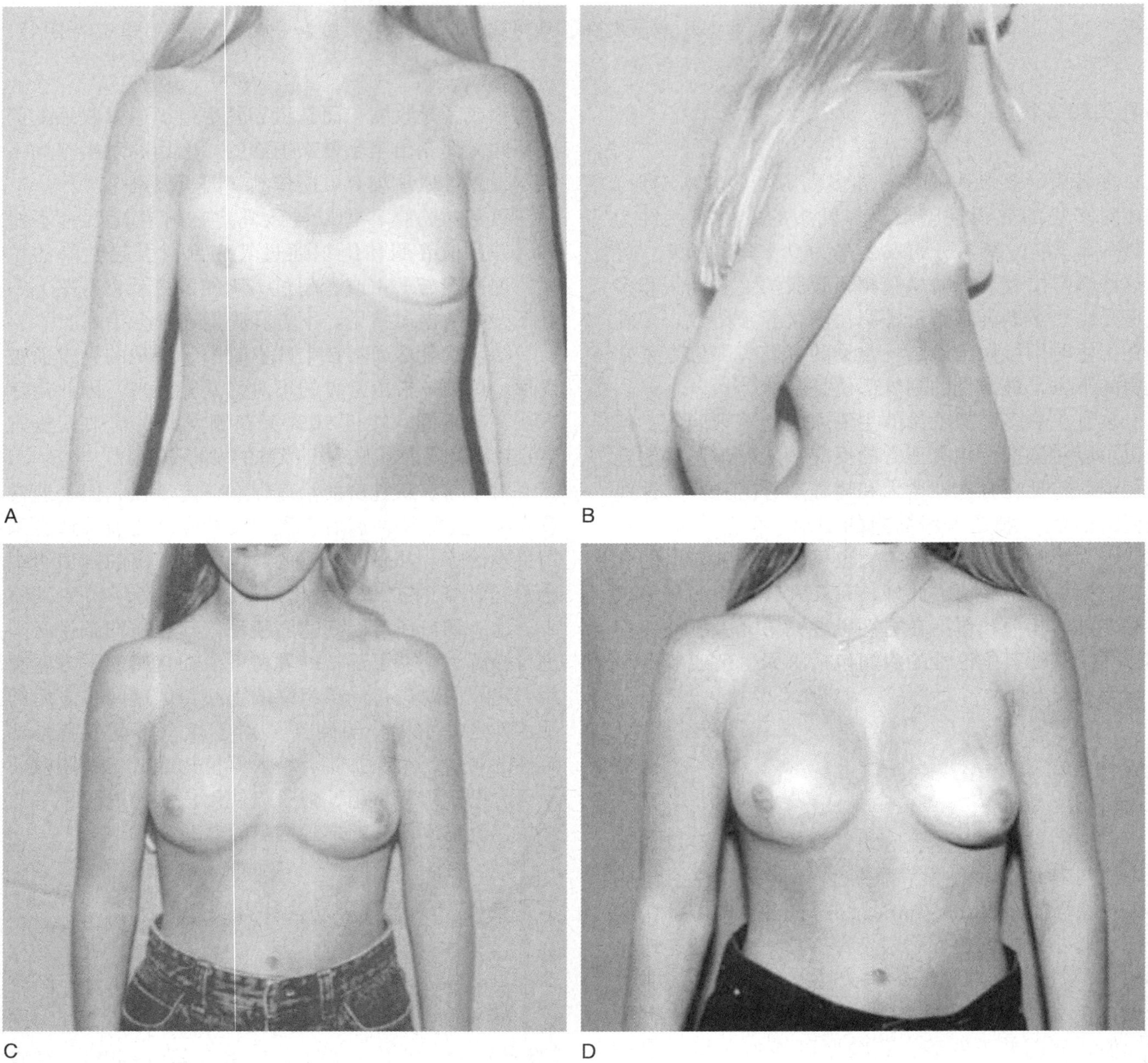

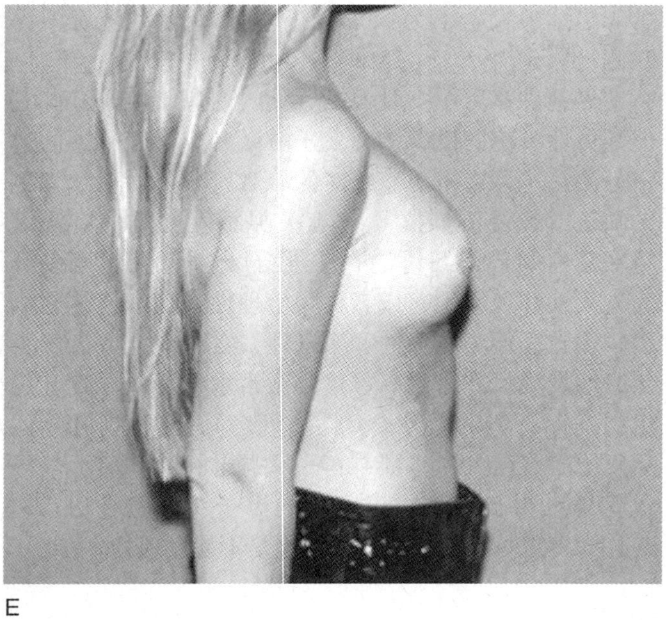

图 128-2 先天性乳房缺如。A. 术前正位，可见右半胸乳房缺如。B. 侧位观。C. 扩张器置入，以准备充足的皮肤覆盖重建乳房。D. 术后正位观，患者在右侧乳房的位置植入永久盐水假体。E. 侧位观，可以看到预扩展的皮肤可以植入足够的永久假体和保持良好的外形。

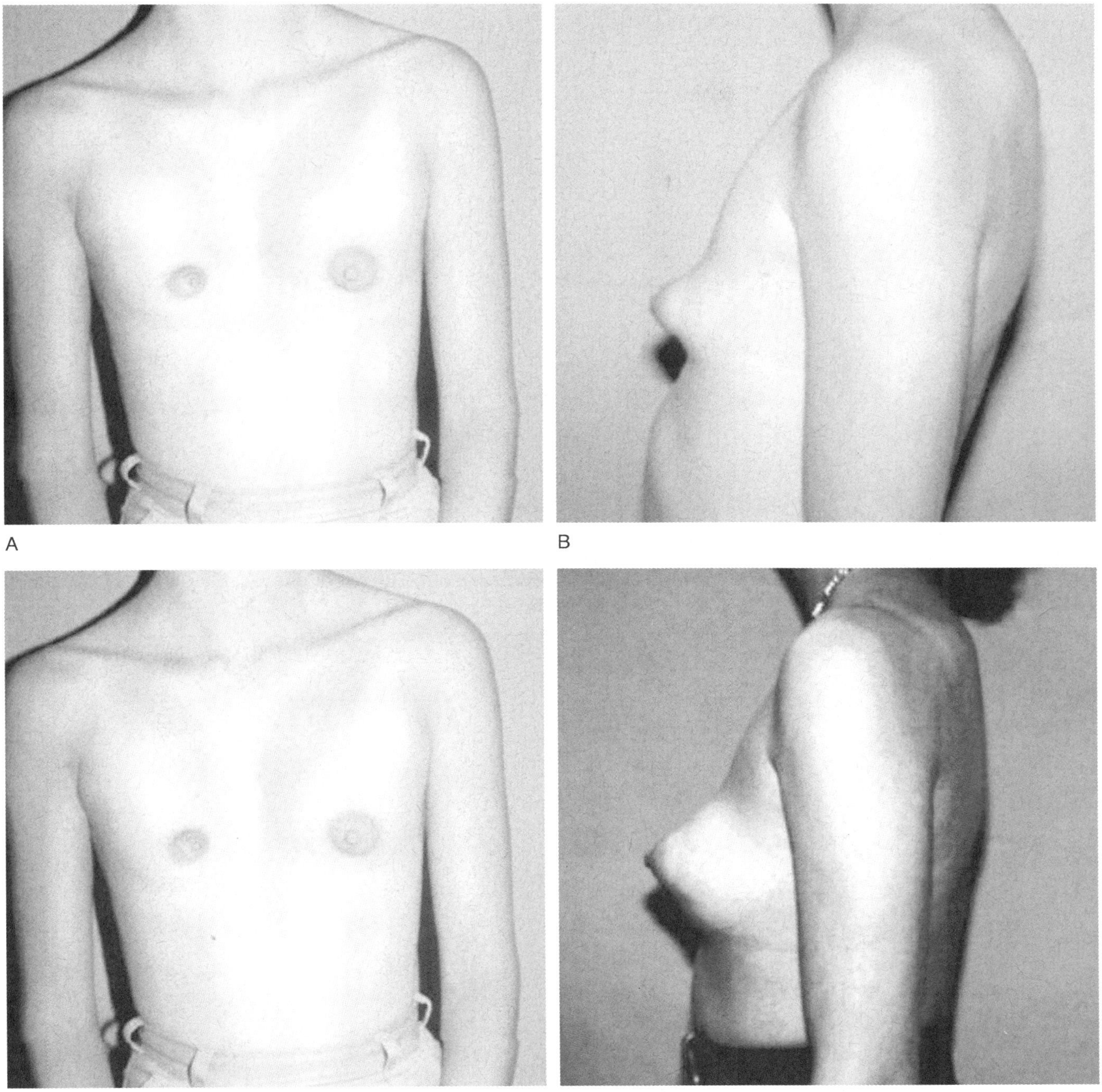

图 128-3　结节状左乳，伴有轻度漏斗胸。A. 术前正位，先天性乳房和中胸部畸形。B. 侧位观，结节状乳房畸形。C. 术后松解先天性束带，应用植入物重建乳房外形。D. 术后侧位观。

2068 儿乎所有的病例在青春期末会复原[8,51]。病理性男子女性型乳房在儿童和青少年相对较少，但是需要引起特别注意，尤其是在 Klinefelter 综合征中，其乳腺癌发病率增加了 60 倍（单纯的男子女性型乳房，其发生乳腺癌的危险性并不增加）[33]。

尽管青少年男子女性型乳房一般是自限性的，在青春期末可复原，但持续存在的男子女性型乳房（出现超过一年，青春期结束后不能自行消失）如果不行

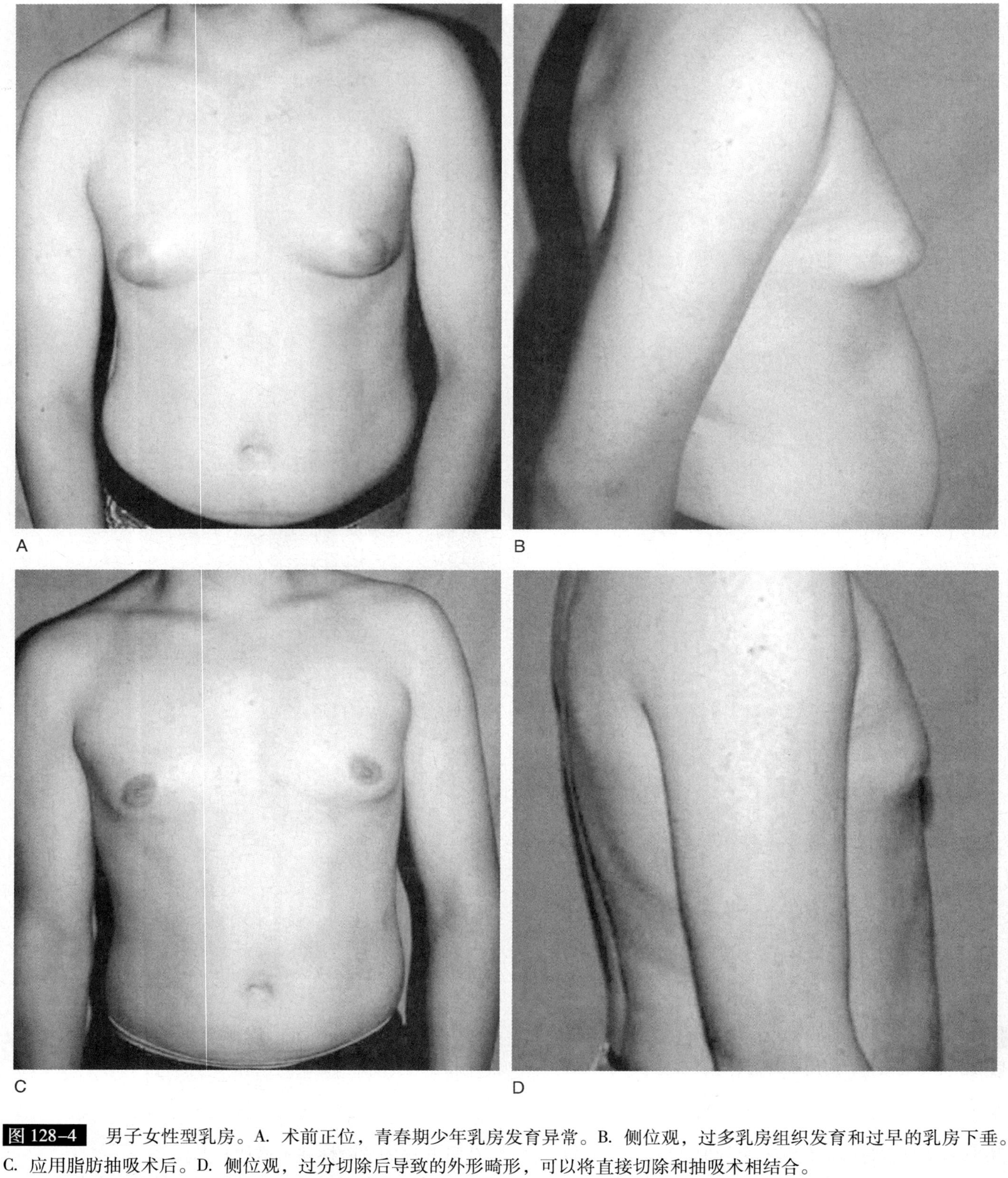

图 128–4　男子女性型乳房。A. 术前正位，青春期少年乳房发育异常。B. 侧位观，过多乳房组织发育和过早的乳房下垂。C. 应用脂肪抽吸术后。D. 侧位观，过分切除后导致的外形畸形，可以将直接切除和抽吸术相结合。

手术治疗一般不会复原，因为异常的乳房必然会发生纤维化[6]。对于整形外科医生来讲，男子女性型乳房
2069 最初就诊是由于外观的不美观，但是，仍然需要进行细致的病史询问和体格检查。尽管男子女性型乳房在一般人群中或者经过儿科医生体检发现的病例一般都是不复杂的，并且是良性的，但有证据表明需手术治疗的男子女性型乳房是更复杂的亚型。尤其是几项大型研究发现在患有女性型乳房且需手术治疗的男性患
2070 者中，其患双侧睾丸和非黑色素皮肤癌的危险性增加。睾丸癌的风险在年轻男性明显增高，其标准化发病率据统计高达 6.7[19,60]，故必须加强对睾丸和皮肤的检查以及预防皮肤癌的教育。

对于青少年男子女性型乳房患者，原则上采用非手术治疗，因为几乎所有的病例在 2 年内都能复原[45]。对于持续存在的病例，治疗取决于乳房的大小和下垂的程度。治疗方法多样，包括经乳晕切口乳房切除术、抽吸辅助脂肪切除术（SAL）、超声辅助脂肪切除术（UAL）。药物为基础的治疗成功率低。对于乳房较小的病例、通过乳腺内切口简单的切除即可，另外 SAL 和 UAL 均可以应用。对于乳房较大的病例、基底广泛的乳房伴有轻微的或无下垂者，最好采用经乳晕切除和 SAL/UAL 联合使用。所有的乳房组织均可通过切口去除，但是额外的抽吸技术可以有利于胸部更好的塑形，从而避免内凹畸形。巨大的乳房伴有严重下垂者的治疗方法是有争论的，通常需要切除额外多余的皮肤同时进行乳房切除和游离乳头移植，但是，仍然很难达到满意的外观[51]。

血管畸形

包括血管瘤、毛细血管畸形（葡萄酒色痣）、毛细血管扩张、淋巴管畸形（水囊状淋巴管瘤）和静脉以及复合畸形将在第 130～133 章中论述。

肌肉、肌腱和结缔组织

关于 Ehlers-Danlos 和 Marfan 综合征在第 59，74 和 123 章有论述。

裂

裂的畸形，包括单侧唇裂、腭裂和复杂的颅面裂，在第 50 和 51 章中讨论。

先天性睑下垂

上睑提肌先天性发育异常在出生时即与一侧或双侧上睑下垂不同（图 128-5A，5B）。这种缺陷是由于动眼神经上支发育异常所致，尽管这种理论存在一

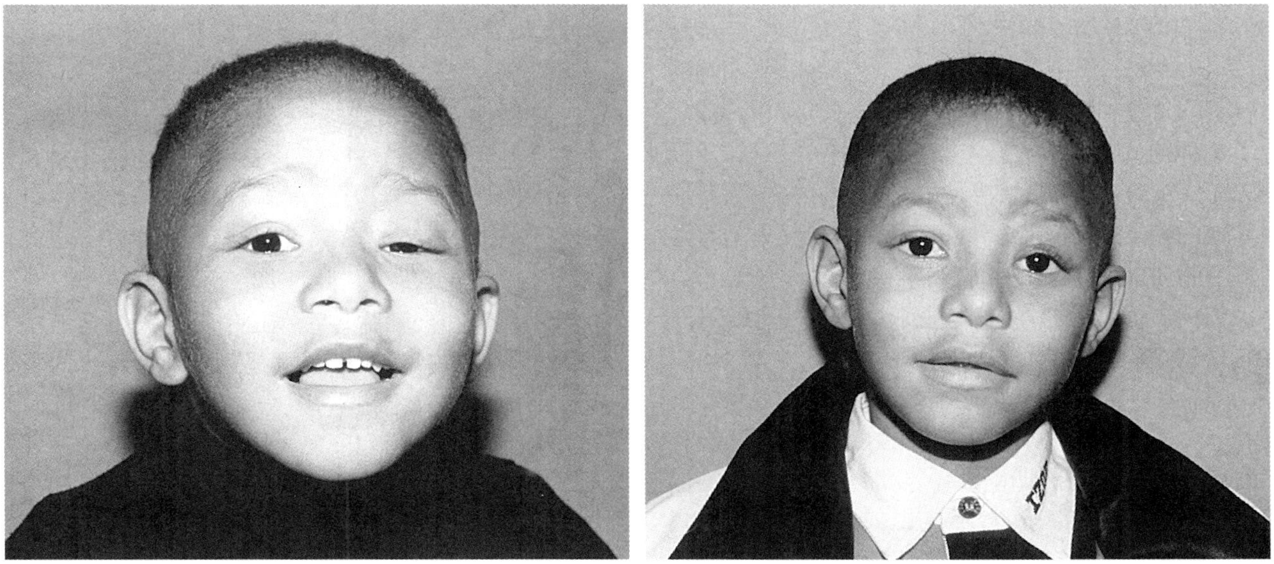

A　　B

图 128-5　A. 先天性左眼睑下垂。B. 睑板至额肌筋膜吊带术加上眼睑下垂矫形术后。

定争议，但是一些证据显示这种发育缺陷在于肌肉本身。尽管正常的乳头和调节反射显示动眼神经核本身并未受影响。但因其有上直肌无力，故提示第三对颅神经发育异常，有证据显示，这种缺陷为常染色体显性遗传，且外显率多样。

严重的睑下垂有弱视的危险，需要进行早期的矫正。通过眉弓的悬吊，应用额肌替代提肌在严重的病
2071 例可以选用。轻度的病例应当延迟至患儿 3～4 岁时再进行治疗，此时容易看到精细的睑结构并且便于操作。如果有足够的提肌，将其腱膜切除后短缩也可以起到矫正的作用[29,64]。

Poland 综合征

在 1841 年，一位名叫 Alfred Poland 的医学生，报道了一些罕见的尸体解剖学发现：单侧的胸肌、上肢和手发育不全。其表现多样，发生率约为1∶30 000，女性易发，与男性比例为 2∶1 至 3∶1[22,32]。

Poland 综合征的病因学理论上是由于在胚胎 6～7 周时，锁骨下血供受阻所致。在这一时间，肋骨向前、向内侧发育，压迫锁骨下动脉呈 U 型。动脉壁的张力可能导致血管的扭结和阻断。血流量减少的位置，可能决定了缺损处组织的位置，可以包括胸壁、胸肌、乳房，以及上肢和手。血管方面的研究显示患侧锁骨下动脉血流量减少，多数累及到锁骨下或椎体的近端动脉，并显示可以引起骨颈畸形，在 Klippel-Feil 综合征和或者 Mobius 综合征的第 6 对、第 7 对脑神经先天性麻痹中可以见到。Poland 综合征、Klippel-Feil 综合征和 Mobius 综合征具有共同的表现，支持了这种疾病的胚胎发生相同[16,17,23,46]。

Poland 综合征的基本特征是胸大肌的胸骨头缺失，其他的特点是乳房或乳头的发育不全或者不发育、皮下脂肪缺乏、胸部和腋窝毛发增多、同侧肢体畸形，包括短缩和并指等。其他肌肉也可以受到不同程度的累积，包括胸肌的缺如（图 128-6A～F）和前锯肌、冈上肌、背阔肌、外斜肌的发育不良。胸廓本身也可以由于前外侧肋骨的缺如而受到波及，可能有肺脏的疝出或者胸壁的凹陷。手部的畸形更多见，包括指关节粘连、并指、发育不良，或者中指骨缺如。发生并指的患儿应当很大程度上怀疑是 Poland 综合征，因为并指病例中有 10% 报道患有该综合征[2,22]。

尽管手部的畸形对功能方面的影响较轻，并且与并指的表现有关。在轻度的 Poland 综合征中，其治疗最初是因为美观的原因。对于更严重的病例，尤其是那些累及胸廓的患儿，稳定胸壁是首要的，因为所有胸腔内结构的重建都建立在此基础之上。小的胸壁畸形一般可以用同侧的背阔肌皮瓣重建。主要的胸壁畸形需要用骨性或者网格状假体进行更好的稳定。分裂肋骨自体移植和 Marlex 网片可以用于中重度缺损，并可以用背阔肌皮瓣转移覆盖。转移的背阔肌皮瓣可以复制缺失的胸大肌前方的腋窝褶皱，并且可以增加软组织的覆盖度。余下的形态异常可以通过异体移植治疗[4,22,58]。

重建 Poland 综合征的女性患儿乳房通常是具有挑战性的。在严重的病例，一般乳房的重建是作为二期手术在青春期晚期、胸壁稳定数年以后进行。在背阔肌后方植入移植物非常有效。成功的应用游离组织移植也有报道。在那些皮肤外膜发育不良者，青春期早期进行组织扩张可以增加软组织，以备后期修复之用，并且可以减轻由于乳房缺失所导致的心理上的压力[3,40,72]。

斜颈

在第 57 章中有论述。

手

胚胎学

手臂肢芽在第 31 天出现，在胚胎发育的第 14 阶段与外胚层下方的缘脉的形成相吻合。鳍状手在大约第 33 天时形成。指放线在第 41 天最为明显，但是直到第 47 天才开始分离。指间区域自发凋亡从而使手指分离。正中动脉为胚胎期手部供血，在第 5 和第 6 周被尺动脉和桡动脉替代。正中动脉仅维持正中神经和骨间的血供。背侧和腹侧芽基分别分化成为背侧和掌侧的前臂肌肉，从第 5～8 周，在表面和深部形成。手的内部肌肉来源于第 5 胚层；深部的小鱼际和鱼际肌肉在第 7 周最后分离；在第 5 周，间充质聚集和软骨化；第 6 周，指节软骨化结束；第 7 周籽骨形成；第 8 周以胚胎发生结束为标记，大多数最终形态形成。而后主要进行胚胎的生长发育，其间，主要是指甲的发育和软骨的骨化[53]。

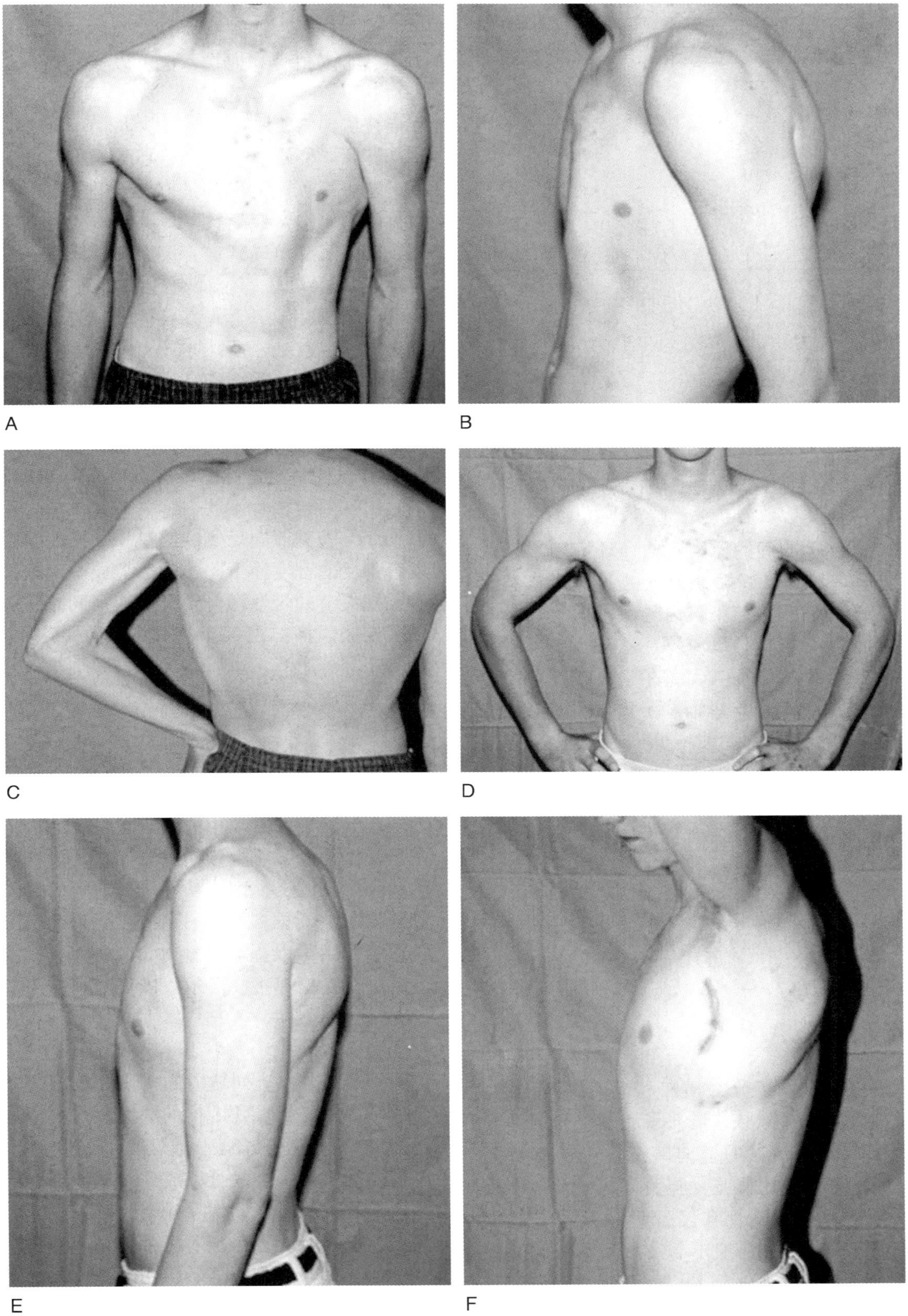

图 128-6 Poland 综合征左侧胸部不对称性鸡胸。A. 术前正位，左侧胸肌缺如。B. 侧位观。C. 胸部后位观，检测是否有左边背阔肌，等张收缩可见肌肉外侧缘。D. 术后正位观，背阔肌功能性转移至前半侧胸廓，矫正了外形并且维持了背阔肌的功能。E. 术后侧位观，切口被上肢所遮盖。胸廓前方背阔肌的外形与胸大肌类似，无后方供体部位胸廓畸形。F. 术后侧位观，上肢外展可见采集肌肉的切口。

表 128-1 先天性手部畸形国际手外科协会分类系统

1. 形成异常
2. 分化异常
3. 重复畸形
4. 过度生长
5. 发育不良
6. 先天性束带综合征
7. 全身骨骼畸形

发生率

上肢畸形的发生率估计为每 10 000 人中有 18 人
2073 发生至每 626 名活产儿中有 1 例发生[8,37]。疾控中心数据显示在每 1000 例活产儿中，横向的缺陷为 0.8，并指为 0.9，白种人多指为 0.2，黑人为 0.12[12]。病例中有 40%~50% 无明确的原因。估计环境因素导致的肢体畸形占 10%[75]。妊娠期前 3 个月，风疹、巨细胞病毒、弓形体、水痘感染可以导致轴向缺陷。影响肢体发育的化学污染包括反应停、乙醇、苯妥因和华法林。一些遗传性综合征（孟德尔遗传或其他遗传模式）也会伴有骨骼畸形。短指、手指弯曲变形、并指、多指可见于 21 三体；屈曲指见于 18 三体；多指见于 13 三体。

先天性手部异常：分类和治疗

国际手外科协会建立了一项 7 级的分类系统对于手部畸形进行分类，如表 128-1 所示[76]。

形成障碍

形成障碍可以进一步分为横向和纵向发育停滞。横向缺损又称为先天性截肢，最严重者发生于肩部导致无肢。肘下缺损是常见的横向畸形，止于前臂上方。在婴儿时期开始使用假肢，腕关节缺失女孩多于男孩。在这种情况下，桡骨和尺骨骨骺远端骨骼缺如，但是旋前和旋后功能一般不受影响。在双侧缺失中，优势臂实行 Krukenberg 手术，在非优势臂佩戴假肢。Krukenberg 手术将前臂骨分为相对捕握的两肢。渐进性的长度的恢复限制了纵向的缺损，可以是桡侧、尺侧、中心型或者完全性（海豹肢）。

侧缺损：桡侧缺损可以影响桡骨、舟状骨、斜方肌、小多角骨和拇指，也可以伴有肌肉肌腱、神经和血管结构异常。在典型的桡侧畸形手中，前臂短，手向桡侧偏斜，拇指缺失或浮动。这种缺损在胚胎第 1 周即开始。桡侧干的发育与心脏隔膜的发育为同一时间，这可以解释桡侧列的缺损同时伴有房间隔缺损，可见于 Holt-Oram 综合征中。桡侧缺损也伴有椎体的缺损、肛门闭锁、气管食管瘘和食管闭锁、桡骨和肾发育不良（VATER 综合征），同时有血液方面的疾病如 Fanconi 贫血和血小板减少症同时桡骨缺失（TAR 综合征）。治疗应在出生后尽快开始，传统的方法包括连续石膏牵拉尺侧，延长并游离腓骨移植也在研究中。

尺侧缺损：尺侧列缺损少见并且能够与环指或小指缺损、肘部、肱骨或者肩部束带（Poland 综合征）同时出现。与桡骨不同，腕关节呈拱形，尺骨缺失可以不伴有腕关节向尺侧的偏移。缺损的严重程度根据发育不良的程度而不同，从部分或全部缺损伴或不伴有肱桡关节的骨性融合到尺侧缺损同时腕关节呈截肢样改变。假体如肘关节内置装置可以提高肢体的功能。在部分患者，可以将尺侧骨残端与桡骨融合以提高肘关节的稳定性。

拇指缺损：对于拇指缺损的处理取决于其严重性。对于拇指不发育，第 1 指的拇指成形术是最成功的恢复功能性对掌作用的方法。足部的踇指代拇指术由于受体神经和肌腱结构的缺如以及大脑缺乏对拇指活动和感觉的支配而成功率较低。短的拇指可以通过骨延长术被延长。加宽第 1 指蹼距离和肌腱移植以建立对掌作用可以提高功能。浮动拇指一般将其切除，同时进行食指拇指成形术以恢复对掌作用。

裂手：裂手、螯状指和分裂手都是描述中间型（第 2、3 或 4）排列缺损的术语。典型的缺损包括部分或全部中心指或几个指的缺失。非典型的缺损是并指（中心指残端与第二或第四指融合）或者多指。多指类型包括多余的骨性成分。功能决定治疗，外观是次要的考虑因素。切除残余的第三掌骨可以帮助较深的裂隙闭合。骨切开术可矫正邻近指的旋转畸形。

分化障碍

分化障碍包括软组织和骨骼的分离障碍以及先天

性肿瘤。指骨融合（指关节粘连）并不常见，通常
2074 与并指同时发生。并指本身常见，多见于中指和无名指。真正的分化障碍要与 Poland 综合征的枝状并指（短的蹼指）以及与继发于束带的远端指节融合的有隙并指相区别。综合征表现有并指症状的有 Apert 综合征、Pfeiffer 和 Goltz 综合征、Chotzen 综合征（尖头并指畸形）、眼齿生殖器综合征以及 13 三体。

如果并指长度不同并且指骨有骨性融合，有隙并指应当在 1 岁之前进行分离。如无这些症状，分离手术可以在 2～3 岁进行。Apert 综合征的并指畸形非常复杂，对整形外科医生提出了一个挑战，即要恢复手的功能包括捕握和指间的感觉（图 128-7）。在这一点上，三指手优于四指手和一个拇指[21]。拇指和小指在 1 岁之前进行分离。余下的指在 6～9 个月内进行分离。Apter 综合征的另一个特征是拇指向桡侧弯曲。拇指截骨和植骨术在 4～7 岁时进行，在拇指和食指间的虎口部位行 Z 字成形术。

先天性屈曲畸形： 软组织分化失败可以导致先天性屈曲畸形。拇指呈钩状或者拇-掌面挛缩。拇长伸肌、拇短伸肌、拇长展肌肌力缺如或者减弱。在婴儿时期可以用夹板固定或者手法矫正，手术矫形应延迟直到患儿 3 岁。钩状的拇指必须要与扳机指相区别，扳机指是在第一指间关节滑车处长屈肌形成一个结节，使指节关节和掌指关节伸直受限。由于 30% 的扳机指可以自愈，手术治疗应在患儿 3 岁以后进行。

手指弯曲变形最常影响小指的中间指节，在许多综合征中可以见到（如 Treacher Collins 和 Silver-Russell 综合征，口面指和眼齿指发育不良）。屈曲指是指先天性近指节间关节屈曲挛缩，通常发生在小指，可与一些综合征同时发生，如 Marfan 腘窝翼状赘蹼以及口面指和眼齿指发育不良。如果残疾或畸形，挛缩可以通过分离跖表浅屈肌腱和延长掌侧皮肤同时进行全层皮瓣移植进行松解。在较严重的病例，可以施行关节成形术或者关节固定术。先天性多关节挛缩表现为多个部位的关节非进行性挛缩，影响到四肢和脊柱。在上肢，肩关节屈曲和内旋，肘关节屈曲或者伸
2075 展，腕关节屈曲并向尺侧偏移或者伸展，以及向桡侧偏移，拇指和余指屈曲，向尺侧偏移。

发生于手部的孤立的多关节挛缩称为“风吹手”，表现为掌指关节屈曲并向尺侧偏移，是由于掌筋膜和韧带的畸形所致，伴或不伴腱和韧带的畸形。增厚的皮下纤维束带和挛缩的掌指侧皮肤导致了畸形

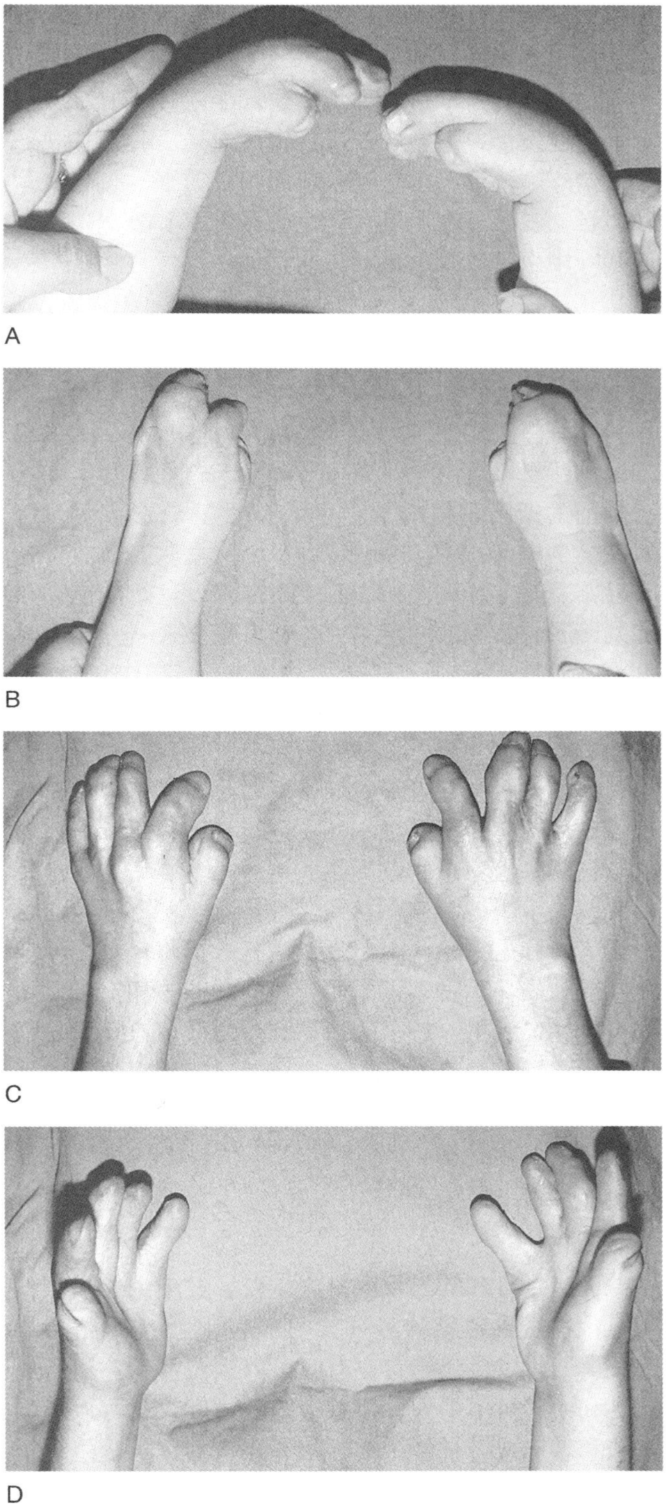

图 128-7　A. 婴儿 Apert 综合征，有典型的并指畸形。B. 复杂的双侧有隙并指。C 和 D. 并指分离术后外观。

的形成。还可继发掌骨头畸形。由于掌侧韧带和皮肤挛缩，拇指屈曲，外展受限。

应在婴儿时期进行夹板固定和手法矫正。如果畸形进行性发展，通常在青春期发展迅速，提示应进行手术治疗。矫形手术包括松解掌指关节囊、韧带和内在肌腱，复位外在肌腱，行掌骨截骨术和分离掌部皮肤和纤维束带，随后进行皮肤移植。

部分重复畸形

部分重复畸形多在胚胎发育早期出现。多指是常见的手部畸形，轴背的小指重复畸形的发生率多于轴前的拇指重复畸形。中心型重复畸形少见。附属肢体的畸形应尽早手术治疗。手术矫正轴前多指有时需延迟至12个月以后，此时可以进行功能评价和判断及保存优势拇指（一般为尺侧拇指）。侧副韧带甚至肌腱和骨，可被切除用来重建余指，或者行Bilhaut-Cloquet手术，从邻近两拇指的中间作切口，切除中心楔形物后，将两拇指剩余外侧部分融合。如果拇指类似食指并且不能处于对掌位时，可以行旋转截骨术，转移肌腱（如Huber通过腱膜将指短展肌移位）同时加宽第1指蹼距离。

镜像手表现为7或8个手指，1或2个示指，2个无名指和中指，两个尺骨，桡骨、拇指缺如，伸肌薄弱或缺失。手丧失了抓握或捏的功能。相对指需要进行重建，并去除过多的指；圆角皮肤可以用来做成宽的指蹼。腕关节固定术在青春期早期即可进行。通过切除一个尺骨鹰嘴后可以改善肘关节活动性。

过度生长

巨指指骨和软组织的过度生长。典型的Ⅰ型巨指与正中神经或者尺神经（少见）的脂肪纤维错构瘤有关。通常发生于指骨，有时可以累及掌骨。尽管屈肌腱和血管可不受累，但软组织的过度生长可以影响皮肤和淋巴或者神经结构。相邻几指的巨指较之单个手指的巨指多见。正中神经错构瘤可压迫腕管内的结构。Ⅱ型巨指是von Recklinghausen病（神经纤维瘤）的一部分。沿着主要的外周神经分布，多见于正中神经。与Ⅰ和Ⅱ型相反，Ⅲ型巨指（骨肥厚型）不伴有神经的扩大但是可以沿着正中神经的感觉支分布。治疗包括骺骨干固定术、骨骺阻滞、骺板切除、多重脱指技术、纵向指截骨术、软组织减量、末梢神经切除和部分或全部指切除术。皮瓣坏死是巨指修复后的常见并发症。

发育不良

发育不良畸形依据其发育不良的程度和受累的组织表现多样。枝形并指（短指）多在一些综合征中见到，为常染色体显性遗传；先天性缺指是指骨或掌骨的完全缺失；短掌骨少见，通常直到青春期快速生长时才能发现，伴发的综合征包括假性甲状旁腺机能亢进症、Turner综合征和猫叫样哭泣。通常不必治疗，但是延长受累的尺侧掌骨可以增加手掌的大小有利于抓握。延长术的操作包括骨移植或者牵拉成骨作用[41,57,73]。短的指骨是造成枝形指骨的主要原因。小指的中节指骨是手部骨骼中长度变化最大的，尤其在女孩。除了截骨术矫正偏移之外，手术干预没有太大意义。指骨延长对于功能没有明显改善。

束带畸形

手部束带畸形发生于胚胎发育期。主流学说认为是羊膜带包裹在肢体周围导致局部的缺血和坏死。另一种解释是内在的缺陷引起的出血或者局部肢体的缺陷导致了浅表组织的坏死。坏死区域愈合后形成环形瘢痕，在肢体损伤后继发出现羊膜带[77]。肢体远端较之近端易于受到影响。束带瘢痕对于远端肢体形成神经病理性压迫。在指骨，有隙并指是由于组织坏死和融合所致，表现为融合处指骨近节和远节的横断沟槽或者截肢。对于多数的缩窄环，可单纯或者分期手术切除同时进行Z字成形术。宽大的束带环需要进行局部皮瓣的转移覆盖缺损处。融合指的治疗因人而异，分离包括交叉皮瓣、完全截肢、延长或者游离指移植。

小结 2076

严重程度不同的多种畸形可由先天性皮肤、肌肉、结缔组织和肌腱的缺失所致。肢体的任何一处解剖部位都可能受到影响。在决定手术的治疗指征和时机时，功能受损的严重性以及畸形的程度、与畸形相关的社会压力都必须考虑在内。正确的治疗计划取决于精确的诊断和对于缺损部位的分析。几乎所有的缺损都能够通过正常结构异位的程度、组织的缺失、组织构成的畸变进行系统评价。然后针对每一处具体的畸形制定手术矫形方案。甚至对于最复杂的畸形，可应用系统的方法简化和优选安全的治疗方案。

（葛翼华译　赵　黎校）

参考文献

1. Abramson DJ: Bilateral intra-areolar polythelia. Arch Surg 1975;110:1255.
2. Al-Qattan MM: Classification of hand anomalies in Poland's syndrome. Br J Plast Surg 2001;54:132.
3. Argenta LC, VanderKolk C, Friedman RJ, Marks M: Refinements in reconstruction of congenital breast deformities. Plast Reconstr Surg 1985;76:73.
4. Avci G, Misirlioglu A, Eker G, Akoz T: Mild degree of Poland's syndrome reconstruction with customized silicone prosthesis. Aesthetic Plast Surg 2003;27:112.
5. Baldwin HC, Manners RM: Congenital blepharoptosis: A literature review of the histology of levator palpebrae superioris muscle. Ophthalm Plast Reconstr Surg 2002;18:301.
6. Bannayan GA, Hajdu SI: Gynecomastia: Clinicopathologic study of 351 cases. Am J Clin Pathol 1972;57:431.
7. Bauer BS, Corcoran J: Treatment of large and giant nevi. Clin Plast Surg 2005;32:11.
8. Bowe J, Conway H: Congenital deformities of the hands. Plast Reconstr Surg 1956;18:286.
9. Carlson HE: Gynecomastia. N Engl J Med 1980;303:795.
10. Castilla EE, da Graca Dutra M, Orioli-Parreiras IM: Epidemiology of congenital pigmented naevi: I. Incidence rates and relative frequencies. Br J Dermatol 1981;104:307.
11. Castilla EE, da Graca Dutra M, Orioli-Parreiras IM: Epidemiology of congenital pigmented naevi: II. Risk factors. Br J Dermatol 1981;104:421.
12. Centers for Disease Control and Prevention: Congenital Malformation Surveillance Report. Atlanta, US Public Health Service, US Department of Health and Human Services, 1984.
13. Cheong JH, Lee BC, Lee KS: Carcinoma of the axillary breast. Yonsei Med J 1999;40:290.
14. Chung CS, Myrianthopoulos NC: Congenital anomalies: Mortality and morbidity, burden and classification. Am J Med Genet 1987;27:505.
15. Ciresi KF, Mathes SJ: The classification of flaps. Orthop Clin North Am 1993;24:383.
16. Cobben JM, Robinson PH, van Essen AJ, et al: Poland anomaly in mother and daughter. Am J Med Genet 1989;33:519.
17. Cobben JM, van Essen AJ, McParland PC, et al: A boy with Poland anomaly and facio-auriculo-vertebral dysplasia. Clin Genet 1992;41:105.
18. Cohen IK, Pozez AL, McKeown JE: Gynecomastia. In Courtiss EH (ed): Male Aesthetic Surgery. St Louis, CV Mosby, 1991.
19. Daniels IR, Layer GT: Testicular tumours presenting as gynaecomastia. Eur J Surg Oncol 2003;29:437.
20. Elmendorf EN 3rd, D'Antonio LL, Hardesty RA: Assessment of the patient with cleft lip and palate. A developmental approach. Clin Plast Surg 1993;20:607.
21. Flatt A: The Care of Congenital Hand Anomalies. St Louis, CV Mosby, 1977.
22. Fokin AA, Robicsek F: Poland's syndrome revisited. Ann Thorac Surg 2002;74:2218.
23. Fraser FC, Ronen GM, O'Leary E: Pectoralis major defect and Poland sequence in second cousins: Extension of the Poland sequence spectrum. Am J Med Genet 1989;33:468.
24. Glass AR: Gynecomastia. Endocrinol Metab Clin North Am 1994;23:825.
25. Goedert JJ, McKeen EA, Javadpour N, et al: Polythelia and testicular cancer. Ann Intern Med 1984;101:646.
26. Goldberg R, Motzkin B, Marion R, et al: Velo-cardio-facial syndrome: A review of 120 patients. Am J Med Genet 1993;45:313.
27. Graham JM Jr, Smith DW: Dominantly inherited pterygium colli. J Pediatr 1981;98:664.
28. Grolleau JL, Lanfrey E, Lavigne B, et al: Breast base anomalies: Treatment strategy for tuberous breasts, minor deformities, and asymmetry. Plast Reconstr Surg 1999;104:2040.
29. Han K, Kang J: Tripartite frontalis muscle flap transposition for blepharoptosis. Ann Plast Surg 1993;30:224.
30. Hassold T, Chen N, Funkhouser J, et al: A cytogenetic study of 1000 spontaneous abortions. Ann Hum Genet 1980;44:151.
31. Holmes LB, Kleiner BC, Leppig KA, et al: Predictive value of minor anomalies: II. Use in cohort studies to identify teratogens. Teratology 1987;36:291.
32. Hurwitz DJ, Stofman G, Curtin H: Three-dimensional imaging of Poland's syndrome. Plast Reconstr Surg 1994;94:719.
33. Jackson AW, Muldal S, Ockey CH, O'Connor PJ: Carcinoma of male breast in association with the Klinefelter syndrome. BMJ 1965;5429:223.
34. Jerdan MS, Cohen BA, Smith RR, Hood AF: Neuroectodermal neoplasms arising in congenital nevi. Am J Dermatopathol 1985;7(Suppl):41.
35. Kapp-Simon KA: Psychological interventions for the adolescent with cleft lip and palate. Cleft Palate Craniofac J 1995;32:104.
36. Kim CS, Tatum SA, Rodziewicz G: Scalp aplasia cutis congenita presenting with sagittal sinus hemorrhage. Arch Otolaryngol Head Neck Surg 2001;127:71.
37. Lamb DW, Wynne-Davies R, Soto L: An estimate of the population frequency of congenital malformations of the upper limb. J Hand Surg [Am] 1982;7:557.
38. Leppig KA, Werler MM, Cann CI, et al: Predictive value of minor anomalies. I. Association with major malformations. J Pediatr 1987;110:531.
39. Llaneras MR, Morgan RF, Pham ST, et al: Congenital giant hairy nevus: Implications for treatment. J Emerg Med 1989;7:25.
40. Longaker MT, Glat PM, Colen LB, Siebert JW: Reconstruction of breast asymmetry in Poland's chest-wall deformity using microvascular free flaps. Plast Reconstr Surg 1997;99:429.
41. Magnan B, Bragantini A, Regis D, Bartolozzi P: Metatarsal lengthening by callotasis during the growth phase. J Bone Joint Surg Br 1995;77:602.

42. Mandrekas AD, Zambacos GJ, Anastasopoulos A, et al: Aesthetic reconstruction of the tuberous breast deformity. Plast Reconstr Surg 2003;112:1099, discussion 1109.
43. Marchac D, Weston J: Abdominoplasty in infants for removal of giant congenital nevi: A report of three cases. Plast Reconstr Surg 1985;75:155.
44. Mathes SJ, Nahai F: Reconstructive Surgery: Principles, Anatomy and Technique. St Louis, Quality Medical, 1997.
45. McGrath MH: Gynecomastia. In Jurkiewicz MJ, Mathes SJ, Krizek TJ, Ariyan S (eds): Plastic Surgery: Principles and Practice. St Louis, CV Mosby, 1990.
46. Mentzel HJ, Seidel J, Sauner D, et al: Radiological aspects of the Poland syndrome and implications for treatment: A case study and review. Eur J Pediatr 2002; 161:455.
47. Meuli M, Meuli-Simmen C, Yingling CD, et al: Creation of myelomeningocele in utero: A model of functional damage from spinal cord exposure in fetal sheep. J Pediatr Surg 1995;30:1028, discussion 1032.
48. Meuli-Simmen C, Meuli M, Hutchins GM, et al: Fetal reconstructive surgery: Experimental use of the latissimus dorsi flap to correct myelomeningocele in utero. Plast Reconstr Surg 1995;96:1007.
49. Miller JF, Williamson E, Glue J, et al: Fetal loss after implantation. A prospective study. Lancet 1980;2:554.
50. Miranda E, Granstein RD: Neuropeptide and cytokine mediated regulation of Langerhans cell function. Excerpta Medica International Congress Series 1998;1159:101.
51. Mathes SJ, Seyfer AE, Miranda EP: Congenital anomalies of the chest wall. In Mathes SJ (ed): Plastic Surgery. Vol. 6. Philadelphia, Saunders/Elsevier, 2006; p. 457.
52. Mofid MM, Manson PN, Robertson BC, et al: Craniofacial distraction osteogenesis: A review of 3278 cases. Plast Reconstr Surg 2001;108:1103, discussion 1115.
53. Moore K: The Developing Human: Clinically Oriented Embryology, 4th ed. Philadelphia, Saunders, 1988.
54. Nelson MM, Cooper CK: Congenital defects of the breast—an autosomal dominant trait. S Afr Med J 1982; 61:434.
55. Neuman JF: Evaluation and treatment of gynecomastia. Am Fam Physician 1997;55:1835.
56. Nuttall FQ: Gynecomastia as a physical finding in normal men. J Clin Endocrinol Metab 1979;48:338.
57. Ogino T, Kato H, Ishii S, Usui M: Digital lengthening in congenital hand deformities. J Hand Surg [Br] 1994; 19:120.
58. Ohmori K, Takada H: Correction of Poland's pectoralis major muscle anomaly with latissimus dorsi musculocutaneous flaps. Plast Reconstr Surg 1980;65:400.
59. Olivera-Martinez I, Thelu J, Dhouailly D: Molecular mechanisms controlling dorsal dermis generation from the somitic dermomyotome. Int J Dev Biol 2004;48:93.
60. Olsson H, Bladstrom A, Alm P: Male gynecomastia and risk for malignant tumours—a cohort study. BMC Cancer 2002;2(1):26.
61. Osbourne M: Breast development and anatomy. In Harris J (ed): Breast Diseases, 2nd ed. Philadelphia, Lippincott, 1991, p 1.
62. O'Shaughnessy RF, Christiano AM: Inherited disorders of the skin in human and mouse: From development to differentiation. Int J Dev Biol 2004;48:171.
63. Panettiere P, Del Gaudio GA, Marchetti L, et al: The tuberous breast syndrome. Aesthetic Plast Surg 2000; 24:445.
64. Pearl RM: Improved technique for fascial sling reconstruction of severe congenital ptosis. Plast Reconstr Surg 1995; 95:920.
65. Rees TD, Aston SJ: The tuberous breast. Clin Plast Surg 1976;3:339.
66. Richman LC: Neuropsychological development in adolescents: Cognitive and emotional model for considering risk factors for adolescents with cleft. Cleft Palate Craniofac J 1995;32:99.
67. Rivera R, LoGiudice J, Gosain AK: Tissue expansion in pediatric patients. Clin Plast Surg 2005;32:35.
68. Rohrich RJ, Hartley W, Brown S: Incidence of breast and chest wall asymmetry in breast augmentation: A retrospective analysis of 100 patients. Plast Reconstr Surg 2003; 111:1513, discussion 1520.
69. Ross DA, Laurie SW, Coombs CJ, Mutimer KL: Aplasia cutis congenita: Failed conservative treatment. Plast Reconstr Surg 1995;95:124.
70. Rossillon D, De Mey A, Lejour M: Pterygium colli: Surgical treatment. Br J Plast Surg 1989;42:178.
71. Santibanez-Gallerani A, Marshall D, Duarte AM, et al: Should nevus sebaceus of Jadassohn in children be excised? A study of 757 cases, and literature review. J Craniofac Surg 2003;14:658.
72. Shamberger RC, Welch KJ, Upton J 3rd: Surgical treatment of thoracic deformity in Poland's syndrome. J Pediatr Surg 1989;24:760, discussion 766.
73. Smith RJ, Gumley GJ: Metacarpal distraction lengthening. Hand Clin 1985;1:417.
74. Straker H: Giant pigmented hairy nevi. Arch Dermatol 1968; 98:93.
75. Swanson AB, Swanson GD: Flynn's hand surgery. In Jupiter JJ (ed): Congenital Limb Malformations: Classification and Treatment, 4th ed. Baltimore, Williams & Wilkins, 1983.
76. Swanson AB, Swanson GD, Tada K: A classification for congenital limb malformation. J Hand Surg [Am] 1983; 8:693.
77. Tada K, Yonenobu K, Swanson AB: Congenital constriction band syndrome. J Pediatr Orthop 1984;4:726.
78. Tajbakhsh S, Sporle R: Somite development: Constructing the vertebrate body. Cell 1998;92:9.
79. Theile RJ, Lanigan MW, McDermant GR: Reconstruction of aplasia cutis congenita of the scalp by split rib cranioplasty and a free latissimus dorsi muscle flap in a nine month old infant. Br J Plast Surg 1995; 48:507.
80. Tobiasen JM, Hiebert JM: Clefting and psychosocial adjustment. Influence of facial aesthetics. Clin Plast Surg 1993; 20:623.
81. Urui S, Oi S: Experimental study of the embryogenesis of open spinal dysraphism. Neurosurg Clin North Am 1995;6:195.
82. van der Putte SC: Apoeccrine glands in nevus sebaceus. Am J Dermatopathol 1994;16:23.
83. Van Regemorter N, Dodion J, Druart C, et al: Congenital malformations in 10,000 consecutive births in a university hospital: Need for genetic counseling and prenatal diagnosis. J Pediatr 1984;104:386.
84. Velanovich V: Ectopic breast tissue, supernumerary breasts, and supernumerary nipples. South Med J 1995; 88:903.
85. Verhelle NA, Heymans O, Deleuze JP, et al: Abdominal aplasia cutis congenita: Case report and review of the literature. J Pediatr Surg 2004;39:237.

86. Whittaker PG, Taylor A, Lind T: Unsuspected pregnancy loss in healthy women. Lancet 1983;1:1126.
87. Wilcox AJ, Weinberg CR, O'Connor JF, et al: Incidence of early loss of pregnancy. N Engl J Med 1988; 319:189.
88. Zaal LH, Mooi WJ, Sillevis Smitt JH, van der Horst CM: Classification of congenital melanocytic naevi and malignant transformation: A review of the literature. Br J Plast Surg 2004;57:707.

第 129 章

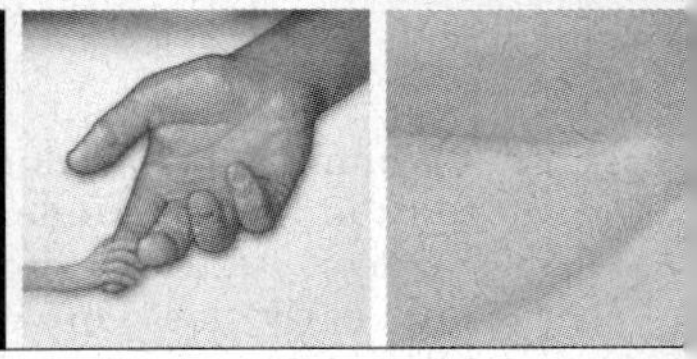

联体双胎

James A. O'Neill, Jr.

2079 几个世纪以来，社会对待联体双胎的态度逐渐发生了变化，由宗教背景下对他们的排斥到迄今被认为是更具人性化的一种形式。联体双胎是最少见、最复杂、最富挑战的先天畸形之一。它需要所有外科专家中最富有创造力的医生来治疗。历史资料显示，Spitz 和 Kiely 指出最早有关联体双胎的是艺术人工制品，如一尊双身体雕塑，描绘的是公元前 6000 年的寄生式联体双胎[68]。一座女性双胎雕像被安放在土耳其安卡拉的博物馆内，而其他公元前 80 年石制的臀联双胎雕塑，在意大利佛罗伦萨的圣马可博物馆内可以看到。第一个历史性的有关联体双胎的文献在 Pliny 的著作中可以看到。但最早完整的例子是在 1100 年由英国的 Biddendeu 夫人作的描述，这些使人难以忘记的联体双胎出现在每年一次的宗教仪式上。在这些宗教仪式上，表现人体解剖的蛋糕被出售，蛋糕上表现的为肩部和臀部相连，大多数畸形学家不接受这种相连，但臀联双胎被认可，他们的历史与几个其他的历史性的案例也被 Bonderson 详细记录下来[6]。最早分离联体双胎的记载是在公元 970 年[66]，美国试图分离一例 30 岁男性的坐骨联体双胎。分离后其中一个死亡。在 1678 年，Pare 出版了第一篇有关联体双胎解剖和病因分析的科学报告[49]。在 1670 年，Durston 描绘了在联体双胎中的一个患有孤立性食管闭锁[17]。

Seller 认为这种发育不同时性的类型揭示了联体双胎本身是一种畸形，并且每一例双胎个体至少有一半的几率发生畸形[56]。1869 年，Koeing 报道通过结扎脐部水平的组织桥首次成功分离一例脐部联体双胎，但实际上手术是由瑞士巴塞尔的 Johannes Fatio 做的，并且 Koeing 只是一个旁观者[35,52]。

Sills 等人、Anderson、Spencer 和其他人也发表了一些有趣的历史性回顾，这些回顾提供了有关那些未做分离手术而存活的联体双胎的有趣信息，并且在当时他们是如何适应社会的[2,25,58,62]。

1811 年，著名的 Bunker 双胎出生在暹罗，“联体婴”这个术语由此产生[25]，这对双胎生活在 P. T. Barnum 马戏团许多年了，给人们留下了非常奇特的印象。他们是正常的个体，并且本质上有可纠治的畸形，即使在那个时代成功分离只是一个简单的操作，但 Bunker 双胎从没被分开。到目前为止，有报道超过 1200 例联体双胎中，约 250 例成功分离，在这些分离者中，其中一个或两个已经存活很长一段时间。大多数后期的病例是从 1960 年开始报道的。

发病率与胚胎学

典型的单合子双胎发生率为每 1000 名活产婴儿中有 4 例，当母亲服用生育药物时，其发生率似乎更高。双合子、异卵双胎的发生率约每 1000 名活产儿中有 10～15 例，双胎出生率约为每 90 名活产婴儿中有 1 对，联体双胎发生率约为每 50 000 名活产婴儿中有 1 例，所报道的发生率范围从美国的 1/10 000 到南非的 1/50 000[13,47]，有多组更高比率的联体双胎的报道[18,46]。寄生胎或非对称性联体双胎更少并且其发生率约每 1 000 000 名活产儿中有 1 例或 2 例，这种双胎形式亦是单合子的[24]。

Spencer 报道 1% 的联体双胎是死产的，40%～60% 只存活 1 天，剩下的是有可能分离的[62]。在死产的联体双胎中，男性为主，这是因为单合子双胎多为男性。近来报道产前诊断的联体双胎有超过 1/4 死于子宫内，超过一半生后立即死亡，仅有 20% 的存活者[39]，这将表现出一个更真实的数据，存活主要基

2081 于联体的类型和范围，然而，联体双胎存活较长时间能成为分离候选者的多为女性，其与男性的比例约为 3∶1。

在 1948 年，Rock 和 Hertig 证实受精后第 6 天，细胞簇构成了人类的受精卵，变成了所谓的胚泡[53]。胚胎、羊膜、卵黄囊的内细胞团发育形成了在胚泡一极的细胞聚集。在怀孕的第 1 周，内细胞团内的细胞是全能的，可分裂成两个胚盘，这些胚盘可发育成两个同样的人。在怀孕前 7 天，受精卵分裂形成单合子双胎，它有相同的性别和核型，同享一个羊膜和卵黄囊。双合子或异卵双胎由两个分开的卵细胞受精而成，每个胚胎有它自己的羊膜、卵黄囊和脐带，这样的双胎有相同或相反的性别，并有不同的核型。

虽然联体双胎在胚胎发育早期就有明显的变化，但确切的原因尚未明确。Zimmerman 描述了有关联体双胎的胚胎学经典理论[77]。他的研究认为联体双胎是由于怀孕前 7 天内细胞团不完全分裂所致；在受精后第 13 至 16 天，这一时期被认为可发生单合子双胎。有关后期分裂引起的复杂融合的确切原因仍不清楚，复杂融合的范围广泛，胚胎的不完全分裂似乎与多种器官系统完全分化受限有关。一个双受精胚胎的不完全分裂的后期理论被大多数研究者所接受。另一方面，Spencer 提出另一个理论，该理论认为联体双胎是由于开始两个独立的单合子胚盘，继发性融合所导致的[60]。然而，在邻近外胚层的区域不会发生融合，Spencer 还认为寄生胎、胎中胎、畸胎瘤以及无心畸胎都是由一个胚胎的死亡或退化所导致的[61]。尽管 Spencer 的 Meta 分析有很大意义，但是融合和分裂的理论仍未被证实。

分类

最常见的临床分类是由 Potter 和 Craig 提出的（图 129-1），列举了联体双胎最常见的形式[50]。表 129-1 的分类法在文献中被普遍应用。在所有的描绘中，术语“双胎”，希腊单词意思是“合在一起”。按出现频率排序，最常用的术语是胸联双胎、脐部联胎、臀联双胎、坐骨联胎、头联双胎和附头联胎以及常常同时发生的一些联体，如胸腹联体。另外，Spencer 描述了一种有用的分类，该分类来自于研究的观点，它基于胚胎的数据分析和综合 1200 多例病例进行的畸胎学的仔细分析[59,62]，将联体双胎分成腹和背连接形式，连接部位只有 8 个解剖位点中的一个，它的分类中包括许多少见的联体形式，但在文献中没有被广泛应用。

产前诊断和产科处理

许多作者已经对联体双胎的超声检查结果做过描述[7,30,337]。一些报道指出，在怀孕第 10 周运用该技术能够早期诊断[4]，随着技术的进步，包括三维重建，许多病例被发现[1]。超声发现联体双胎的表现包括在系列检查中双胎的体位固定，在双胎之间缺乏分开的膜结构，并且不能证明有两个膀胱，尤其在中期伴随有水肿或羊水过多（图 129-2）。尽管具有三维重建的 CT 扫描已经开始使用，但它有辐射并且不比超声显示得更清晰[33,37]。另一方面，具有三维重建的 CT 证实是一种有用的补充方法，尤其对心脏的评估[11,22,41,65]，产前超声心动图（ECHO）相当有用，通常比生后的 ECHO 更精确。产前超声、ECHO 和三维成像的 MRI 常能提供足够的信息来帮助家庭决定是否继续妊娠[73]。在我们对产前研究的经验中，早在怀孕 20 周就可获得联体心脏解剖的精确轮廓，但该检查在妊娠晚期进行最可靠。产前超声不仅能证实联体双胎的存在，同时亦能发现发生多胎的特有并发症，如双生胎儿血液交换综合征、无心双胎、双胎内的一胎死亡以及继发性羊水过少或羊水过多[31,40]，妊娠早期三维彩色多普勒超声显像对研究血管解剖非常有用[41]，通常在孕早期行腹部二维超声和经阴道超声，接下来运用彩色多普勒、MRI 以及三维超声[73]。产前 MRI 对诊断不对称性联胎也有帮助[12]。

Sills 等人和许多其他学者[48,158]回顾了大量联体双胎的产科处理，联体双胎是高危妊娠，臀先露多见。因此，产前超声对制定产科治疗计划很重要。尽管文献报道许多联体双胎可经阴道生产，但是最安全且适当的方法是剖宫产，由于双胎中的一个心脏不成熟或是单个心脏以及逆向动脉灌流的发生，双胎将会出现迅速的心功能恶化（衰竭），剖宫产为宫外分娩期的治疗提供了机会[8,45]。因为宫内窘迫在联体儿中常见，所以应阻止早产的发生，在羊膜穿刺的引导下，使胎 2081
儿肺发育成熟。在生产时，胎儿情况决定了如何采取进一步的支持疗法以及进行必要的系列诊断性评估。

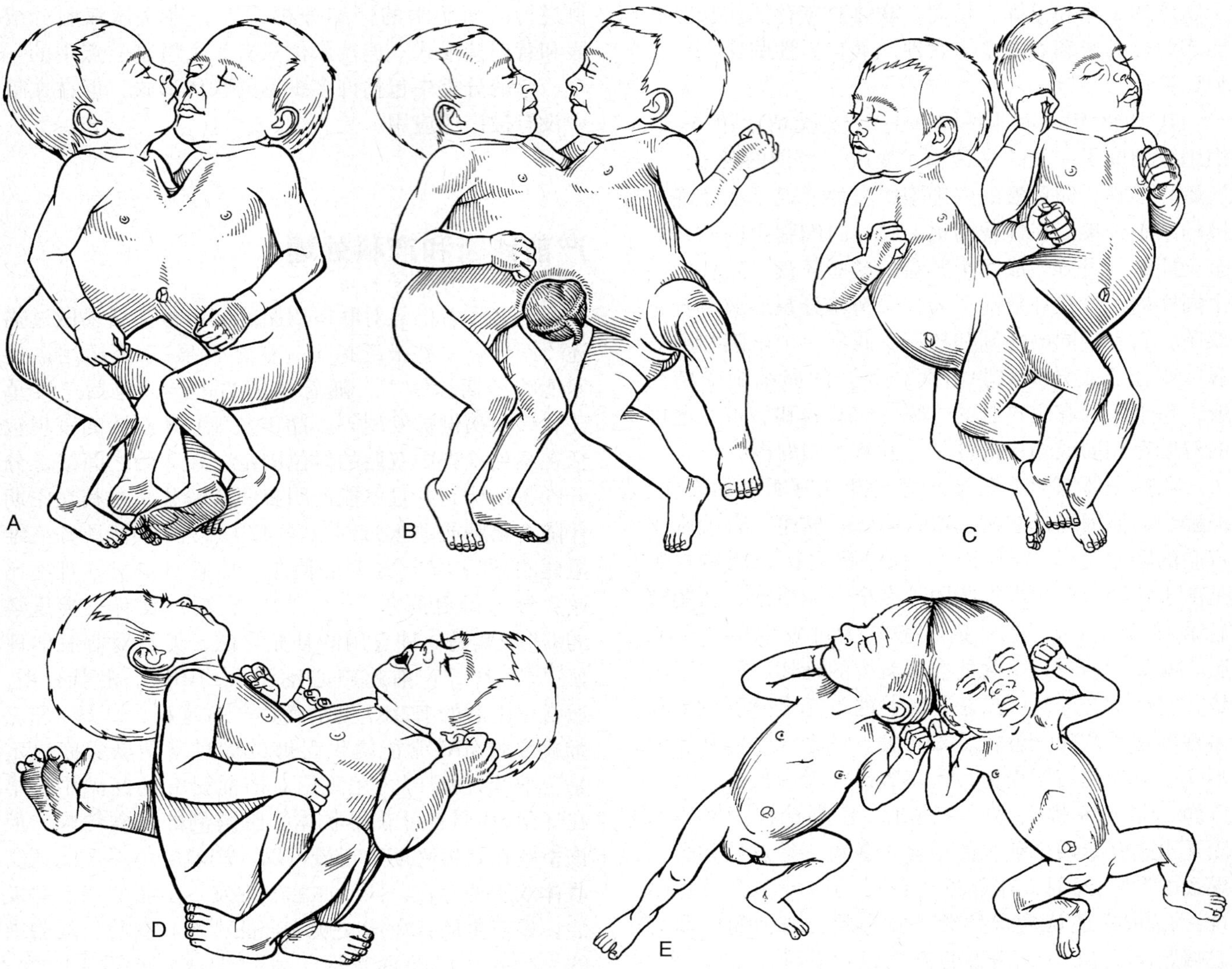

图 129-1 联体双胎的各种类型。A. 胸联双胎。B. 脐部联胎，有时亦称为胸脐联胎。C. 臀联双胎，亦有一种三足畸胎。D. 坐骨三腿联体，亦有一种四足畸胎。E. 头联双胎。

表 129-1 联体双胎的分类

类型	发生率（%）	受累器官
胸联双胎	74	心脏、肝、肠管
脐部联胎	1	肝、胆道、肠管
臀联双胎	17	脊柱、直肠、泌尿生殖道
坐骨联胎	6	骨盆、肝、肠道、泌尿生殖道
头联双胎	2	大脑、矢状窦

术前诊断性检查

表 129-1 列举了各种形式的联体双胎常累及的器 2082
官。产前评估对受累的各个器官系统是最直接的，因为总体上，器官重建对多种畸形器官是标准的方法，减轻了器官共用和发育不良的程度，除了标准的放射影像外，根据患儿的状况及耐受应激的能力来同时进行侵入性的操作。此外，诊断性检查进行的时机与预期分离的时间有关，如果将这些检查放在围生期后期进行，与生后立即进行相比可能更加精确且造成的生理影响更小。

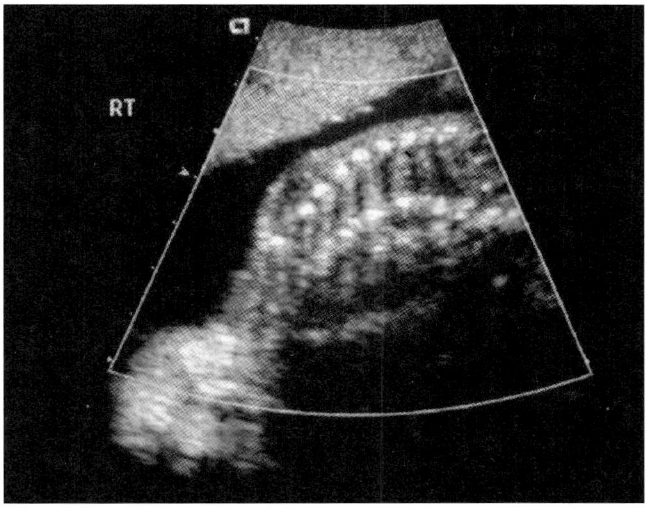

图 129-2　这个产前超声显示有 2 个脊柱，通过另外的影像检查发现是胸联双胎的腹部相连，并共用 1 个心脏。

表 129-2 列举了我们和其他人发现的各种检查方法，对各种形式的联体双胎的评估有帮助，其目的是获得尽可能多的有关精确解剖和功能的信息以指导治疗方案的制定。对每一个没有了解清楚的器官系统，亦必须进行彻底研究。在所有的联体双胎中，其中一个胎儿要小于另一个，而且在一半的病例中，其中一个胎儿有更多的畸形[40,48,62,68]，必须了解这些不同之处，因为总的来说，在进行分离时，尤其当组织结构不能均匀分配时，要尽可能保留较正常的胎儿的正常组织，这对涉及中枢神经系统的状况尤其重要，因为一个胎儿可能未发育完全或者可能已有脑室内出血。

表 129-2　联体双胎中有用的诊断检查

联体类型	诊断方法
胸联双胎	胸片、ECG、超声心动图、三维 MRA、选择性心导管检查、血气分析
脐部联胎	胸和腹部平片、上消化道造影、DISIDA 肝扫描、三维 MRI
臀联双胎	胸、腹和下肢平片；上、下消化道造影
坐骨联胎	膀胱镜、膀胱造影、静脉肾盂造影、肾扫描、阴道造影、螺旋 CT 和三维重建、脊柱 MRI，如需要可做主动脉造影
头联双胎	CT 和三维重建、MRA
非对称性联体	胸和腹部平片，有些病例中可行胃肠道造影

头颅超声、CT 和 MRI 对评估大脑和畸形都有帮助[11,33,37]。MRI 尤其适用于头联双胎和臀联双胎，可对大脑和脊髓进行彻底评估[19,41]，尽管在头联双胎中，脑血管造影被认为很有必要，但是核磁共振血管造影（MRA）和快速螺旋 CT 的出现使得许多病例不必再做传统的血管造影。

在术前，不管心脏是否相连，对所有联体双胎做血管系统评估是很有必要的，如前面所提到的，产前 ECHO 和心电图（ECG）比产后检查能提供更多更精确的有关心脏的信息。这是因为超声探头放在常见的脐突出部位较困难。但是，这些产后进行的检查可发现心脏分开的病例存在的畸形和心脏相连的面积和部位，以及发现心脏相连病例的心内和心外畸形。在过去，心导管检查是唯一能发现心内畸形和连接部的确切性质、血流方向和所有进出心脏血管的特点。但是，Fogel 等人进一步改良了心脏三维 MRA 技术，可提供精确的解剖信息，并可作为是否做心脏分离手术的基础[22]。Fogel 和同事的研究得到了 Spielman、Norwitz 和 Kingston 及其同事的证实[33,45,65]。目前，Fogel 等人分析了 139 例复杂心脏缺损和重建患者，认为三维重建 MRI 伴或不伴 MRA 是评价联体心脏最有用和损伤最小的方法[22]。到目前为止，心电图上出现单个 QRS 波不能作为心脏成功分离的指征。令人遗憾的是，与其他人研究相同，我们的研究认为出现两个独立的波亦不作为联体心脏能成功分离的指征。

尽管过去使用的放射性核素心血管造影可证实血流方向和交叉循环的程度，但是这项技术已被三维 MRA 取代。因为对于大多数拟行外科分离的双胎患儿，其共享的肝必须被分开，所以确定是否存在 1 条或 2 条下腔静脉是至关重要的。在许多联体双胎中，1 条下腔静脉引流至 2 个肝，这成为在制定分离方案时的关键因素。

由于联体双胎早产的高发率，所以肺功能受损较常见。如果胸腔相连，并且一个胎儿的胸廓小于另一个，在有心内或心外分流的病例中，则会出现氧合不足。胸部 X 线检查、动脉血气分析以及彻底的体格检查，对肺功能的评估是很重要的，后来的检查必须与对心脏评估所获得的信息相结合。

大多数联体双胎共享一个肝，并且可共享一套胰
2083 胆管系统，尤其存在十二指肠连接部时[43,47,68]，这是术前评估的一个关键点。因为我们有过这样的病例，脐坐骨联体双胎分享一个单独的胆管系统及胰腺，超声和放射性核素胆管显影并分别同时注入两个胎儿体内，是最有用的检查。三维 MRI/MRA 可提供额外的信息，所以目前运用血管造影对肝脏评估就没有必要了。

除了头联双胎外，其他所有联体双胎有可能共用部分胃肠道。最好的评估方法是采用上下消化道造影检查，常常需要使用各种造影剂来确定哪些结构是相连的。在这些病例中，记住常见的肠道共用形式是有帮助的。在胸联双胎和脐部联胎中，胃肠连接处常在十二指肠水平，当交汇在十二指肠第二段时，有可能只有一个胰腺及一套肝外胆道系统。在坐骨联胎和臀联双胎中，肠道交汇处通常在 Meckel 憩室发生部位的末端回肠。在另外一些病例中，有共用单个结肠或偶尔除了共用的乙状结肠外，其余肠道是分开的情况。

内镜下的影像学检查是评估泌尿生殖器的最好方法（见图 129-7），这些评估方法包括 B 超、肾盂造影、膀胱造影、增强 CT 以及放射性功能核素检查[46,75]，其目的是测定肾功能状况，肾、输尿管、膀胱的数目和部位。因为大多数联体双胎是女性，确切的阴道或泌尿生殖窦的检查很重要，超声、阴道镜和阴道 X 线摄片有助于发现是否为单个或双阴道，子宫颈、尿生殖窦的存在和缺失或者是否有阴道积液。在这些复杂的尾部连接的病例中，测定这些空腔脏器的数目、大小和位置，对制定分期重建方法很重要。在男性联体双胎分离前，决定是否需要做性别改变，对外生殖器和性腺的评估很重要。

坐骨联胎和臀联双胎的尾部连接，其脊柱、骨盆、下肢共用的程度不同[46]，常规 X 线摄片、CT 和 MRI 检查是必须做的，CT、三维 MRI 重建和 CT 扫描对决定外科手术方案是最有帮助的诊断方法（图 129-3）。当下肢共用时，在坐骨联体三腿双胎中，有时需要做主动脉造影，以发现共用肢体血供的确切特点，除非彩色多普勒检查能明确显示血管的解剖，对双胎来说，下肢能否被分离还是共用至关重要。

自从皮肤扩张器运用于分离前的联体双胎，精确估计联体双胎共用皮肤的范围就显得不那么必要了（图 129-4）。我们开发了一种准确的方法，使用间断分开注射和进行灌注定位法来评估共用皮肤的程度，但这种技术现在只适用于皮肤扩张器无效或者认为有必要做的急诊病例中。

早期报道强调术前评估联体双胎的甲状腺和肾上腺功能很重要，但是除了在相当少的病例中，我们发现这些检查是不必要的。

伦理思考

随着技术的不断提高，有更多的联体双胎被分离，有关伦理讨论和分析的文献明显增多，公众争论的重点是 Lakeberg 双胎，他们是心脏相连，只有一个胎儿可能存活[15,72]。类似的争论还有英国曼彻斯特
的 Maltese 联体双胎，他们共用 1 个心脏，直到法院 2084
作出决定，才允许进行分离手术[5,14,34,38,43]。对于对外科医生和其他有关人员而言，关于这个话题伦理方面的讨论是非常熟悉的。

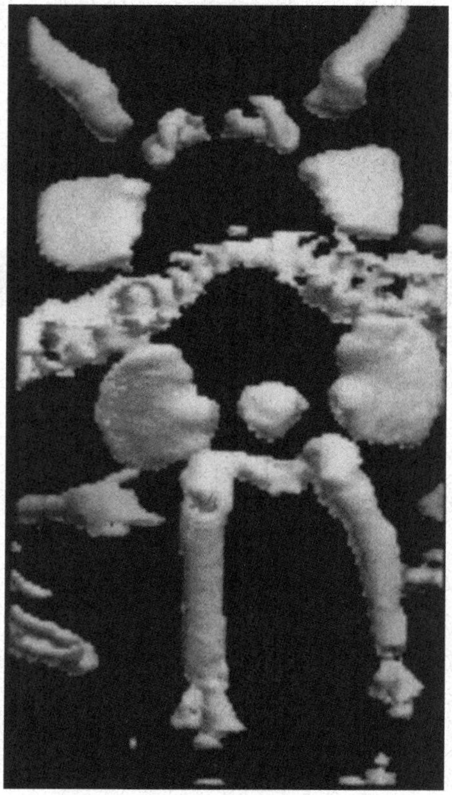

图 129-3 通过计算机三维重建的坐骨三腿联体的成像，清晰地显示了共用的肢体和骨盆的解剖，当制定分离和重建计划时，可通过各个角度进行影像观察。

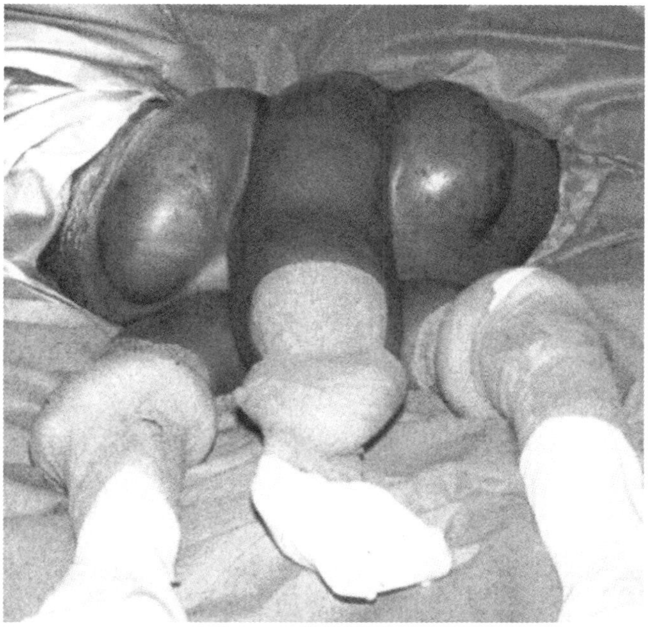

图 129-4 注意如何放置皮下皮肤扩张器，并为坐骨三腿联体双胎的患儿提供腹部和骨盆关闭所需的足够多的皮肤。

基于产前检查做出的产前诊断和影像学的准确描述是非常可靠的。有丰富联体儿分离经验的小儿外科医生，去劝告患儿父母了解有关成功分离的可能性及在外科技术、术后护理、重建和康复上取得的进展是最有说服力的[67]，这种信息使父母处于一个最佳的角度来决定是否希望继续妊娠。在患儿出生前后，家庭的隐私权应受到尊敬和保护，因为必须要作出决定及达成一致观点，所以小儿外科团队必须与家人建立紧密且相互信任的关系，有必要进行详细和反复讨论。尤其是术前评估显示仅一个患儿能存活或双胎中的一个可能遗留严重功能障碍时。此外，对于极少数分离后的双胎，期待治愈某种程度的畸形是现实的。在心脏相连以及只有 1 条下腔静脉引流至共用的肝和只有 1 套肝外胆管系统的联体双胎中，只有一个能存活，对外科医生和父母来说，做出选择牺牲其中一个患儿以换取另一个生存下来的决定是困难和令人伤心的。Annas、Thomasma 等人以及 Dougherty 和其他人已详细分析了这种可怕的选择[3,15,71,72]，如果在这种情况下不做分离，那么两个患儿都会死亡，了解了这一点有助于做出决定的。要了解手术本身不能决定哪一个患儿能生存，而是由其解剖学特点来决定的。Thomasma 等人分析认为不仅要进行后期的伦理考虑，而且要进行社会、费用因素以及其他同时期的问题的考虑[50,72]。

如果能达到一定程度的生存质量，我们倾向于做联体分离，即便只能一个生存，总比两个都死亡要好，这种判断是基于丰富经验的基础上作出的，器官和共用结构的最佳分配是基于解剖和获得的资料的基础上。分离时器官处理需要个别考虑，当两个联体双胎之间没有明显区别时，要最大限度维持两个患儿器官的完整性。然而，如其中一个智力和生理方面受损，我们认为分配应倾向于更加健康的患儿。尽管我们有这样的观点认为如果有可能挽救一个患儿的，决不能让 2 个患儿都死亡。需要强调的是，父母有最终权力来决定接受或拒绝外科分离。在曼彻斯特的病例中，英国法院认为作为社会的代表，法院有权力作出决定。每一个病例都是不同的，必须最大限度照顾到父母和他们的孩子的情感和权力。

分离时机

在不成熟的器官系统中，由于严重的器官功能不全和生理功能减弱，急诊分离往往伴随有较高的死亡率，我们发现生后 6 个月之内进行的急诊分离手术比生后 6 个月以后分离的有较高的死亡率[48]。回顾我们的经验以及从文献上获得的信息，建议尽可能在可选择的基础上，在生后 9~12 个月进行分离，但 Spitz 和 Kiely 指出在生后 2~4 个月选择性分离手术是安全的，这可能是正确的[68,69]，为什么年长儿的麻醉处理较容易且对血液丢失和生理影响的耐受比新生儿要好，这是可以理解的。如果外科分离延迟至 1 岁以后，那么对联体双胎独立的个性发展不利，但我们发现在几个月内分离是可以采纳的。急诊条件下可进行强行分离，即便是在新生儿中。这包括在出现一胎死产、肠梗阻、脐膨出破裂、心力衰竭、尿路梗阻或呼吸衰竭时。

可在联体双胎 4 个月或更大时进行分离，这时可提供足够的时间进行详细的术前评估以及召集所有的专家商议一个成功的分离手术方案。 2085

术前计划和麻醉管理

联体双胎的成功分离是有经验的小儿外科专家和

麻醉师组成的团队共同完成的。对所有收集到的信息和术前及术后监护人员，所有外科、麻醉及诊断技师和护士以及其他术中相关人员和监护人员开一个小组讨论会是必要的。我们发现，根据诊断检查了解共用器官的特点有助于构建模型和描绘各种器官系统，且有利于预期的分离手术的成功实施。但近来我们发现，三维 MRI 和 MRA 可以从各种不同的视角进行观察甚至更为有用，所有成员在术前进行模拟操练已成常规，并使每个成员了解下一步该如何做，尽管有些决定必须在术中做出，但是成员所面临的许多问题大多在术前要做出计划。

必须配备有两组完整的外科专家团队，同时必须有两组有经验的麻醉医生团队，并知道如何共同努力工作。因为大量出血、低血容量、低温是主要的危险因素，麻醉医生必须能够处理。我们常规放置桡动脉和中心静脉导管，并且在联体双胎中留置其他静脉通路。两个患儿分别监测，包括动静脉压、ECG、氧饱和度、二氧化碳浓度、食管温度、尿量和血气分析，只有一个例外，那就是联体双胎中预计只有一个存活，那么就只监测预期存活的那一个。根据共用循环的程度，慎重地调整静脉使用镇静剂的剂量，加大肌松药的运用，主要是因为在一定时间内，只有一个患儿在行气管插管。一般药物和静脉补液量根据双胎的总体重计算，每个患儿给予一半量。只有非常有经验的医生可参与麻醉管理，包括气管插管。我们发现短效吸入性麻醉剂加上高浓度氧易于管理。在许多病例，分离过程时间很长，需要特殊的管理技术，例如 Wong 等人所描述的一个历时 5 天的头联双胎的分离[76]。

一旦所有的监护、静脉通路和气管插管被仔细确认后，两组麻醉医生将双胎抬起，以便进行彻底的全身消毒和铺巾。在大多数病例，我们认为将患儿放在垫子上，并抬高 30 度是有好处的，便于外科和麻醉医生手术操作。尽管开始分离时只需一组术中护理人员，但一旦分离后，就需要两组护理人员了。在外科医生使用仪器以及准备前，要提前了解联体双胎中每个患儿的重建特点，在分离手术时，每个外科专业组应协同工作。主刀医生必须指导整个手术的全过程。因为他要负责发挥每个人的作用，并且要在手术过程中出现任何变化时作出决策。手术途径一方面基于相关的解剖及既定的手术步骤，另一方面是为了达到最大程度的暴露。

器官系统重建的方法

一般来说，一旦对各结构的分配已作出决定，器官重建的标准方法是有序进行的，有时需要新的技术或特殊裁剪重建技术，特别是对于皮肤和胃肠道的处理。

皮肤

在胸联双胎、坐骨联胎、臀联和头联双胎中，存在广泛的共用皮肤，并且在分离后，面临关闭创面的皮肤不足，使用皮肤扩张器是有用的，可增加覆盖创面的皮肤量。头部、胸腹部、四肢和会阴部的覆盖和体腔的关闭通常面临皮肤缺损的问题。Filler 报道通过使用扩张器扩大腹膜腔，使坐骨联胎增加腹壁面积[28]。然而，我们和其他人更倾向于使用皮下扩张器，尽可能多地在身体的背侧和腹侧面上以及下肢的上半部分放置扩张器（见图129-4）[47,48]，腹膜腔放置皮肤扩张器有感染的风险并且限制了胃肠功能。

即使可通过几个皮肤小切口将扩张器放在皮下，但在新生儿时期，放置皮下皮肤扩张器常引起皮肤糜烂。我们倾向等待至少 4 周，甚至更长时间。因为这个时期的婴儿对放置皮肤扩张器更易耐受，能多次进行注射使其扩张。一般需要 6～8 周或更长时间，才能达到皮肤扩张的最大效果，放置的最佳时间根据分离的时间来决定。

中枢神经系统 2086

中枢神经系统共用有两种形式：头联双胎形式，它有不同程度的大脑共用；另一种形式为部分脊髓共用。

臀联双胎和一些坐骨联胎可共用椎体和脊髓的各个部分，我们和 Fieggen 等人报道的双胎有共用的骶部和分开的脊髓，但有部分细丝共用需要仔细分离[19,48]。在这些病例中，我们倾向于分期进行分离，首先分离骶后部，仔细分离共用的细丝，留下骶部前半部分作固定，在二期手术时进行分离。在这种情况中，应预计会出现各种程度的膀胱和肛门括约肌功能不良。

头联双胎占联体双胎的 2%，并可分成部分和完全联体两种形式，受累结构取决于相连处是否在头顶部、枕部或者部分颅骨。Buchelz 等人建立了一种更切合实际的分型方法，取决于脑组织融合的位置和程度以及术中阻断的静脉结构[9]。超过 30 对分离手术的报道，包括最近的一些报道显示，大多数手术失败，除了少数脑组织共用的联体双胎之外，少数存活者的远期效果并不令人满意[36]。最近做的头联双胎是脑组织分开的，但上矢状窦共用，有一些获得成功，如 Campbeu 等人、Drummond 等人的报道和来自洛杉矶、达拉斯和纽约的报道[10,16]。在所有的病例中，存在许多问题，远期结果仍不清楚。尽管有限的头联双胎分离获得成功，但是本质上讲，大脑完全共用的联体分离仍未获得成功。精确的影像检查在区别完全与部分头联双胎是必须的。

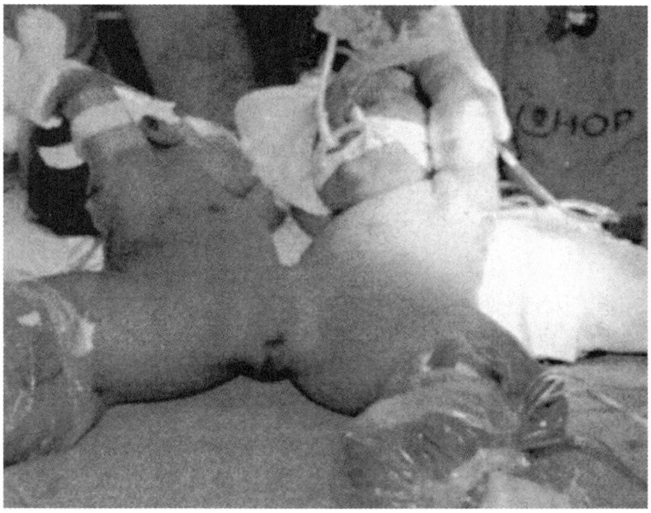

图 129-5 这对脐部联胎只共用肝一个相当大的部分，然而，一些脐部联胎亦共用十二指肠和部分胆道。

肝和胰胆系统

除了头联双胎外，所有前面或腹侧联体双胎几乎都有肝共用（图 129-5），对于肝，最关键的术前检查是了解是否每个肝都有各自的通向心脏的排出通路，或者是否只有 1 条下腔静脉引流至 2 个肝。如果没有肝静脉引流，则无法存活。一旦确定每个患儿有它自己的肝静脉系统，分离肝就容易了。选择肝的中心区域作为分离点。首先要分离出一圈有足够的距离，以放置大的夹子或吸引管，用可吸收缝线做二道交叉褥式缝合，以便在两者之间进行分离。然而，在分离时，个别出血的血管及胆管应用丝线结扎，以便能控制出血过多。如果患儿因处理心脏畸形而进行体外循环时，冷缺血状态下的肝分离必须迅速完成。

在肝分离时，应考虑到 2 个关键点，第一个是虽然大多数共用肝只有 1 个或 2 个大的横位门静脉连接，但静脉连接有时以较难控制的多静脉管道网状相连的形式出现。如果术前检查没有明确共用肝之间门静脉连接的特点，那么术中多普勒超声检查可能是有帮助的；第二个关键点，如果只有单个肝外胆道系统，在事先应决定肝的什么部位作为分离点，且术中必须做胆管造影。这样一个患儿有肝外胆道系统，而另一个患儿只有肝管，可做外引流或空肠 Roux-en-Y 吻合术。如果双胎只有一套胆道系统并共用一个胰腺，胰腺最好与肝外胆管系统一起保留。如果有两个小的胰腺牙基，每个患儿可获得一个，接下来考虑如何重建共用的十二指肠。在少数只有一套肝外胆道系统的双胎中，双胎中的另一个并不能得到什么。

胃肠道系统

肠道共用一般分为两种形式，尽管每一种有多种形式。第一种形式为十二指肠共用，位于第 2 或第 3 段，第 4 段和其余的肠道是分开的。当十二指肠近端
共用时，通常只出现一套胆道系统。当发生在十二指 2087
肠第 3 段时，可出现一些程度的胰胆管相连。如果胆道结构与十二指肠相连处是分开的，那么重建的方法是建立在确认并保留每个患儿的 Vater 壶腹的基础上，我们发现如果仅有一个壶腹，那么一个患儿有时需要做胆管再植。

胃肠道共用的第二种形式是回结肠或偶尔仅有结肠共用，在回结肠形式中，主要的相连点位于 Meckel 憩室的位置，其共用末端回肠和整个结肠，这些共用的肠管有来源于两个患儿的双重血供，在这种形式中，我们倾向于其中一个患儿保留回盲瓣，另一个保留肛门，且通常只有 1 个肛门，两个患儿得到一半共用的结肠，并至少有 1 个有括约肌[29,32]。尽管在过去，肛门闭锁的患儿通常要做结肠造瘘，但自从

1983 年起，我们采取立即行肛直肠重建，因为在这些患儿中，骨盆是开放的，并且在术中可广泛暴露。这种方法总体功能效果良好，引起的皮肤关闭问题要比做结肠造瘘少。在其他类型中，整个小肠和结肠大部是分开的，直肠、乙状结肠共用并通常只有 1 个肛门。因此，一个患儿拥有肛门和共用的直肠、乙状结肠，另一个患儿肠管末端终止于较短的结肠，并立即在肛门闭锁处做括约肌重建，通过该方法大多数病例可获得较好的排便功能。

心脏

因为大多数活产联体双胎主要是胸联双胎，心脏相连是一个常见的问题。另外，了解心内以及心外畸形很重要[23]。1979 年 Synhorst 等人报道成功分离一例心房水平相连的心脏联体双胎[70]，其中的一个术后 7 天死于严重右心发育不良综合征，另一个存活了几年。不幸的是，只有房桥相连的病例相当少见。另一方面，心室相连较常见，但心室分离几乎不可能[60]。我们尝试做过心室分离，但未获成功。其他的方法是牺牲其中一个，对选择存活的患儿采取断开大的血管并重建整个心脏。第三种修补方法是，在解剖基础上，进行联体心脏切开，体外重建以及自体移植。我们还未对联体双胎做过心脏异体移植，并且不认为对父母来说是一种合理的方法。正如作者所了解的，把全部的心脏组织给心室水平相连的双胎中的一个是唯一可行的方法，即使成功率很低。至于后一种方法，目前也只有两位患儿短期存活和一位患儿长期存活。

泌尿生殖系统

在坐骨联胎和臀联双胎中存在许多解剖变异，对泌尿生殖系统进行分期重建被认为是最满意的途径，而胃肠道倾向于立即做重建，与阴道和生殖器重建一样，许多患儿有泌尿生殖道共用，需要进行膀胱扩大并分期重建以促进正常排尿。我们对坐骨联胎的泌尿生殖道重建的经验是由 Hsu 等人总结的[28]。在文章中，我们将计划好的双重构建分成 I 期和 II 期重建过程。患者的分离是根据是否有 1 个或 2 个膀胱（图

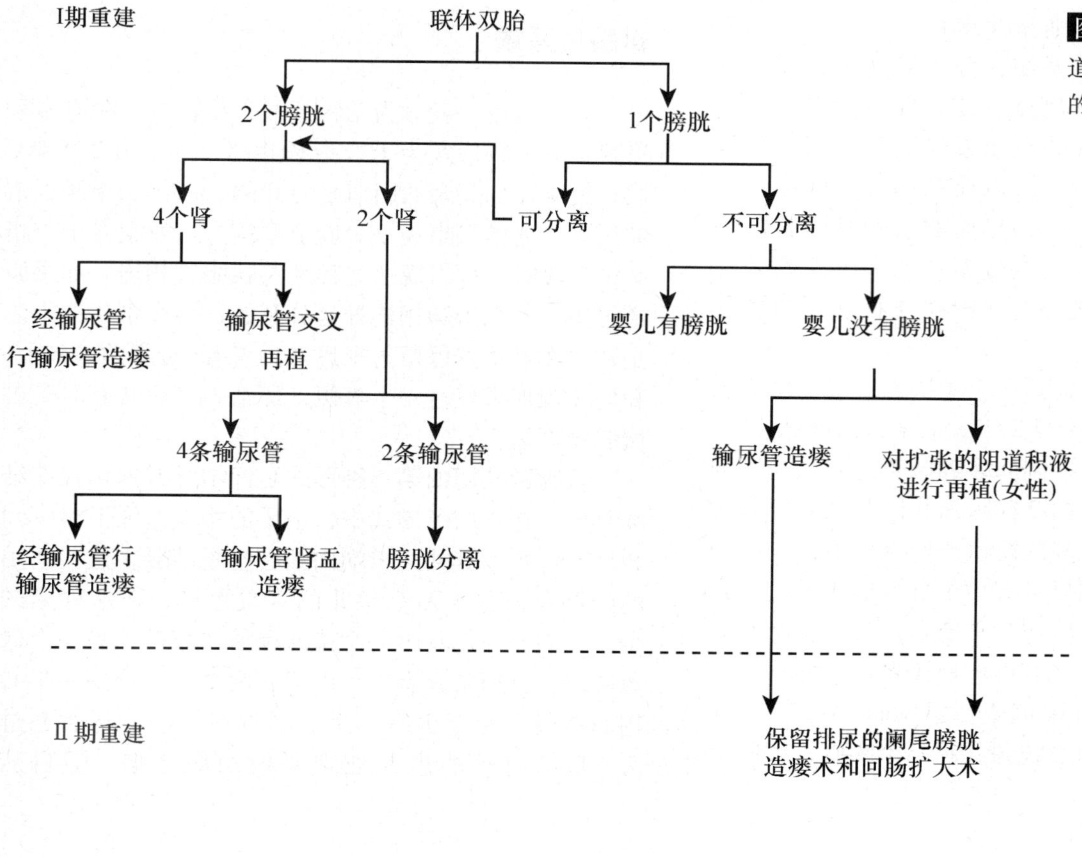

图 129-6　共用泌尿生殖道的坐骨联胎和臀联双胎的泌尿生殖道重建计划。

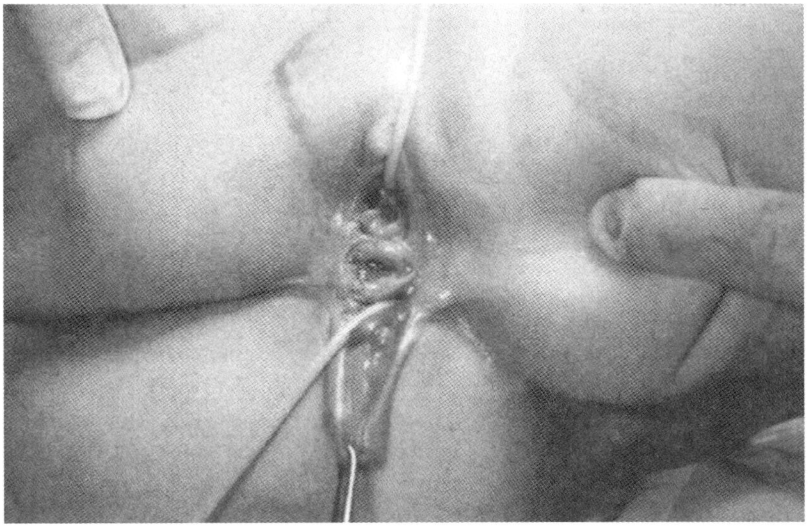

A

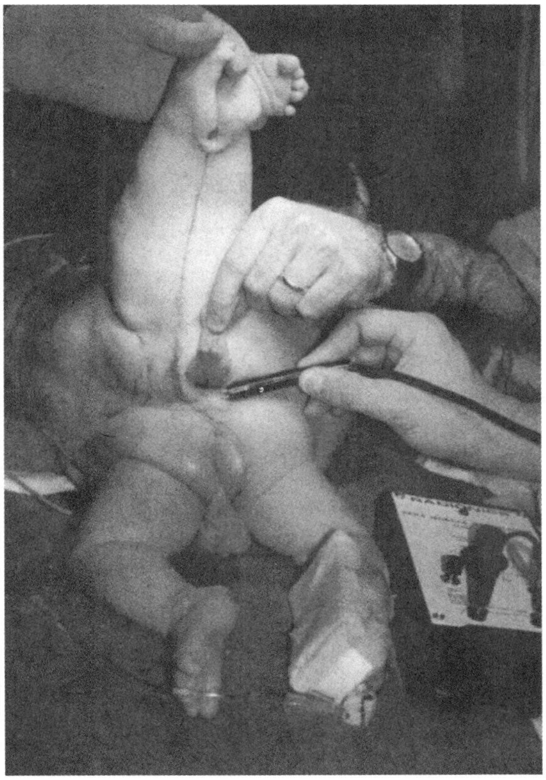

B

图 129-7 除了影像学造影检查结果，坐骨联胎的器官系统评价的具体细节。A. 女性。看清每一个孔是很重要的，在每一个尿道放置导管。向上，可以看见正常的尿道、2 个阴道和 1 个肛门。向下，只有 1 个泌尿生殖窦，用一根导管置入尿道内，导管放入泌尿生殖窦。B. 男性。一条线画在共用的腿和肛门周围，提示这是计划好的分离线。向下，可看到左边有 1 个正常外生殖器和 1 个肛门，双胎的右边为闭锁的肛门，但在电刺激下证实有外括约肌存在。注意双胎的右边有移位的外生殖器，需要适当再定位。

129-6）。以我们的经验，这种方法一直被认为是很有用的。如果只有 1 个膀胱，但有 1 个泌尿生殖窦，后者的结构可被用作膀胱的替代物，并且由 Holcomb 和我们小组报道可重建 1 个新的阴道[26]。在两个患儿共用 1 个膀胱的病例中，做出给每个患儿部分膀胱的决定是以膀胱基底的神经和血供为基础的。如果膀胱镜发现膀胱三角较小，那么共用的膀胱不能分成两个相同的部分，一个患儿给予大部分膀胱，且有满意的容量，另外一个患儿给予小部分膀胱，并做暂时性膀胱造瘘，接下来再做扩大整形以及做可控性导管样造瘘。

大多数女性坐骨联胎或臀联双胎中有单个外生殖器以及两个阴道（图 129-7），在两个女性患儿中，可保留生育能力。如果双胎共享 1 个正常的外生殖器，其中一个患儿需要做二次生殖器成形术。如果存在泌尿生殖窦或共同的泄殖腔，阴道和泄殖腔或泌尿生殖窦的连接处应做修补。男性双胎有 1 套或 2 套外生殖器，必须进行合适的分离，我们治疗过的双胎中 1 个患儿有阴茎移位需复位（见图 129-7）。尿道下裂较常见并且能进行常规修补。在只有 1 个阴茎的病例中，一个患儿要进行男性重建，而另一个要进行女性重建，在这个过程中，大阴唇可通过阴囊组织构建。

需要强调的是坐骨联胎的尿道尤其需要进行多期重建，如果没有出现并发症，要进行密切长期随访[28,57,75]。通过仔细观察和判断且进一步干预[28,57,75]，一般可维持正常的肾功能和较好地排尿，已进行阴道重建的女性患儿要一直监测到生长发育成熟，有正常的性能力和生育能力。这些患者的生活质量较高并对社会有较好的适应能力[27]。需要指出的是成功的生 2089
殖重建经常需要安全的骨盆修补，并且有时要做两侧髂骨切开术[32]。

腹壁

使用皮肤扩张器不仅延伸了表面覆盖的皮肤，

而且扩大了底下的腹壁，但是腹壁筋膜的关闭仍可能有困难。在这些病例中，我们在正中筋膜上使用可吸收网片，亦可用来覆盖坐骨三腿联体分离后骨盆侧面大的缺损，随访中显示可吸收网片可起到纤维素框架的作用。因为还没有发生过有腹腔内容物通过网片疝出的情况，我们亦用这些网片来进行胸壁的重建。

骨骼系统

涉及骨骼系统的骨盆相连双胎最大的问题是长期的病变和功能障碍。因此，矫形外科医生对联体双胎要考虑长期的功能和机能恢复是很重要的，Albent 等人报道了联体双胎矫形科处理的经验，提示这些患儿通常需要多次手术，并随访整个儿童和青少年时期[1,64]，以观察是否存在腹侧、侧面或背侧联体以及脊柱侧凸[19,42]。这些患儿中，脊椎畸形的发生率较高，并可导致脊柱畸形[64]，此外，双胎中的一个或另一个有缩小或不对称的胸壁，可能会发生潜在性脊柱侧凸。如果步态失衡与肢体缺失或骨盆畸形有关，则脊柱侧凸常见。由于发生脊柱侧凸的风险可能贯穿于整个儿童期，故有必要每年进行随访。无论胸廓相连的程度如何，我们的经验是要早期进行胸壁的矫形[21,47,48,55]。

坐骨联胎的处理对矫形外科医生最具挑战性，但一些臀联双胎需要矫形外科和神经外科医生共同来处理，因为存在骶部共用的问题。坐骨联胎根据两腿、三腿、四腿的数量进行划分，后者最常见。这些联体双胎通常能被成功分离。我们对联体双胎三腿畸形的主要经验是，每个患儿有 1 条正常的腿，并共用 1 条畸形的相互融合的腿。Albent 等人[1]已经总结了我们关于后者的部分经验[1]。第一个挑战是对骨盆和第 3 条共用腿的仔细评估。在早期报道中，第 3 条共用的腿通常要截肢并且皮肤用作骨盆和腹壁的关闭。然而，目前随着皮肤扩张器的运用，可尽可能多地保留肢体以维持其功能。自从 1980 年起，我们已开始运用后一种方法。只有在仔细评估骨盆的三维 CT 重建影像后，才能决定骨盆分离的合适位置。这种方法亦为决定是否将共用的第 3 条腿髋臼给予双胎中的一个或两者给予一部分提供了方便。这种决定取决于共用的肢体能否被分开，或者必须给予双胎中的一个。从前路分离骨盆通常是分离过程早期阶段最早的步骤之一，它涉及骨盆器官和会阴的分离和切割，后路分离通常最后进行。正如前面所提到的，目前利用可行的几个影像技术中的一个来评估共用肢体的血供，是评价和分离过程的一个非常重要的部分，这个评价决定是否能提供给一个或两个患儿主要的血液供应，并指导骨盆分离的位点。

在这种情况下，完成了分离过程后骨盆被广泛打开，我们认为要尽可能关闭骨盆，所以我们倾向于早期分离进行后路髋骨切开术，而不是后期处理。髋骨切开术不仅能提供关闭骨盆环的机会，而且能进行较好的皮肤关闭和会阴部的固定。因为坐骨联胎中的一个患儿通常只有一个下肢，较好的骨盆关闭可提高其最终适应一个合适的 bucket 类型的假体的能力。

仔细和频繁的矫形外科随访对了解长期机能恢复和功能很重要，必须记录术后的情况，包括畸形共用腿与正常腿的情况。髋脱位和足部畸形亦是常见的问题，髋脱位可反复发生，通常需要进行分期修复。我们已遇到的问题有马蹄状畸形、髋部的旋转畸形、反复髋脱位、髋的屈曲和外展挛缩和髋臼畸形。标准的矫形手术已被使用，并且大部分获得成功，但通常需要不断校正。在随诊这组患儿 20 多年后，我们发现精致的合适假体是提供长期的良好功能的关键，且在整个生长期需要校正。通过持续和密切的观察，这些患者可长期获得良好的功能，但在成人常有某些程度的功能障碍。但现代康复技术和矫形仪器已使其有了很大改观。随着术前影像、外科经验的提高以及康复技术的改善，使得有功能的膝盖的共用腿保留更长，功能更好成为可能，皮肤扩张器是实现这种可能的关键所在。

临床经验 2090

从 1957 年起已经治疗了 24 对完全的和 3 对不完全的联体双胎，除了 3 对外其余都是在近 20 年中进行的。在 27 对双胎中有 18 对接受了手术，有 24 位患儿活了下来。不幸的是，7 位患儿死于分离后的 1 个月至 10 年，主要是因为先天性心脏病，这在现在是可以纠治的。这个经验建议我们应通过早期手术来纠治明显的心脏畸形。

头联双胎

我们继续来关注一对头颅侧面相连的女性双胎，双胎中的一个患儿的左前额与另一个患儿的右侧颞枕部相连。她们已经 35 岁了，在过去的几年中，通过几次评估，因为脑组织和血管共用的程度以及少见的上矢状窦相连，医生认为是不可能分离的。这两个女人完全独立生存，令人惊奇的是她们是如何适应生存的环境，即便当她们在儿童期时，她们的状况是相当困难的。其中一个基本上是正常的，另一个稍小并因为复杂的泌尿生殖道畸形和小肠梗阻而经历了几次手术。她们一直没有计划进行分离手术，除非其中一个发生晚期疾病。我们曾会诊过一对头联双胎，该双胎具有复杂的大脑相连，其中一个有明显的畸形，故未做分离手术，最后患儿死亡。

胸联双胎

目前，已有 13 对胸联双胎被评估，有 7 对未分离，并被证实有非常复杂的心脏相连和有限的心室容积，由于患有先天性心脏病，他们最终在生后短时间内死亡。从 1971 年开始，在剩下的 6 对胸联双胎中进行了心脏分离[48]。在一对女性胸联双胎中，心脏在心室水平相连，双胎仅有少量的心室容积，后通过切除退化的心脏来进行心室分离，患儿维持心脏活力约 12 小时，但最终死于心力衰竭；另一对男性联体双胎，心脏相连于心房和心室两个水平，共用的肝脏只有一条肝静脉回流至下腔静脉，不幸的是下腔静脉引流入双胎中一个功能较差的心脏，另一个患儿的正常心脏与其相连，因为有难治性充血性心力衰竭，分离手术在生后 3.5 周进行，并且只有一个患儿能存活。在分离时，保留双胎的肝静脉引流并进行心脏自体移植，尽管这个心脏一开始功能是好的，但是该患儿还是在 10 小时后死于心衰。建议进行后一种手术，因为它能为重建一个植入的心脏提供机会，而这个心脏通常是异常的。

在 4 对女性胸联双胎中，大血管被分开并且有一对双胎死亡，对供体的心脏进行了不种程度的切除和重建，在所有病例中，主要的心脏结构被留下来给存活的患儿。第一例手术是在 1977 年进行的，患儿为 1 个月大并患有严重的先天性心脏病。除血管分离外无需重建，患儿存活了 4 个月但死于肝衰竭。值得注意的是，其心脏功能较好，如果无胆道梗阻可有长期存活的可能。从 1992 年起，这种类型的手术已进行了 3 例，2 例女性胸联双胎进行了血管分离并对选择存活的患儿进行了整个心脏置换，所以选择活下来的每个患儿心脏较正常并且有一定程度的可纠治性。对这些病例进行了详细观察后，有证据显示，在术后 8 ~ 10 小时死亡的患儿，由于供体心脏的冠脉血流量不足，以致不能维持其功能；换句话说，心脏出现了大面积的心肌梗死。在此经验基础上，用不同的方法对第 6 对女性胸联双胎进行了分离。在这些双胎中，进行血管分离估计无法存活。从主动脉的侧面到供体主动脉的末端构建主动脉 - 主动脉旁路，以确保在残余的供体心脏中有较好的冠脉血流。异常的肺静脉引流亦要被纠正。在其他病例中，双胎中一个患儿的心脏组织被完全保留，胸腔进行部分重建，以便完成纵隔关闭和膈肌重建。这个患儿存活了 10.5 个月，后因合并肺炎呼衰而死亡。有趣的是，在开普勒的红十字医院，亦尝试进行主动脉 - 主动脉旁路分流手术，并有一个患儿长期存活。

毫无疑问，大多数心室水平心脏相连的胸联双胎，因为伴有复杂的心脏畸形[23]，不能分离而存活下来[23]；另一方面，偶尔儿对胸联双胎至少有一个胎儿有正常的或容易被纠治的伴有正常流入和流出道的心脏。在这种病例中，尝试分离是合理的。获得成功的程度很有限，表明只有在某些有经验的医疗中心
内在该问题上继续努力可能是合适的，大多数使用的 2091
重建技术是非常标准的心内修补方法。

脐部联胎

目前已有两对女性脐部联胎接受治疗。一些胸部联胎同时伴有脐部相连。在第一对中，其解剖与 Bucker双胎相似，简单地行肝脏分离并作I期腹壁关闭（见图 129-5），这两个患儿目前已 12 岁了，发育良好；第二对双胎有巨大的脐部相连，在 6 个月大时进行分离，因为双胎中较小的患儿有严重的呼吸困难故有生命危险。由于患儿是早产并有呼吸窘迫综合征，故我们使用机械通气。这些患儿只有一套肝外胆道系统，该系统和十二指肠和空肠将给双胎中的一个，另一个患儿在肝脏的切缘放置引流管，以刺激胆道皮肤瘘的

形成，该瘘管是可以形成的。不幸的是，接受整个胆道系统的患儿，在分离后1个月死于梭状芽孢杆菌性腹膜炎和支气管肺发育不良，另一个患儿因持续的呼吸衰竭和主动脉下狭窄，在6个月大时死亡。

臀联双胎

在1957年，一对女性臀联双胎在2周大时进行了分离手术，每个患儿有她自己的直肠、膀胱和肾脏，但是她们共用一个阴道将不得不分开[48]。双胎中较大的患儿现已长大成人，有较好的直肠和膀胱功能，并已结婚；双胎中较小的一个因为Fallot四联症相关的并发症在10岁时死亡，她在今天是可以治疗的。

另外，我们有一些争论，是否坐骨联胎中的一个是真正的臀部相连，因为他们共用一个骶尾部，但其他观点支持我们将它归类为坐骨三腿联体双胎。

坐骨联胎

我们遇到过6对坐骨联胎，1对为四足畸胎，5对为三足畸胎，四足畸胎在1岁时分离，两个患儿较好，一个患儿现在已22岁了，基本上是正常的，另一个患儿在3岁时因误吞豌豆而死亡；5对三足畸胎中的3对之前已有描述[47]。所有5对三足畸胎都成功分离，但一个患儿在1978年死于胸壁关闭过紧。从那以后，皮肤扩张器和其他措施的运用已减少了这种情况的发生，这些患儿的胃肠道、泌尿和生殖道重建的具体细节已有讨论，这些三足畸胎患儿的治疗结果大多数是令人满意的，其随访时间为6～24年。

不完全或非对称性联体双胎

我们见过3对部分联体双胎，均为下肢和骨盆外部相连、外生殖器和肠道部分重复畸形。所有患儿在胸壁下部和上腹部相连。对比早期的对称类型的描述，他们亦被认为是一种不对称的联体双胎。在3对中2对有脐膨出，2对有先天性心脏病。所有患儿在生后短期内分离，所有患儿早期都存活。在手术时有一个共同的特征为血管连接处位于镰状韧带的附近。在一个病例中血流通过镰状韧带的大血管直接进入肝实质内；另两个病例，大血管通路进入肝静脉附近的肝上下腔静脉内。在3对双胎中的1对，有证据显示不完全双胎是单合子的正常双胎，3对非对称性双胎存活者中的一个患儿，在4个月时死于当时被认为是不可纠治的复杂先心病。

其他方面

联体双胎的分离是具有挑战性的，需要仔细和详细的计划，并需要许多专家，尤其是外科专家的参与。现代影像学是关键性的，许多技术具有相当的专业性，仅在少数医疗中心可进行。值得注意的是，没有哪一个学科在每次可能的重建手术中都拥有如此多的专家和及时的信息。尽管所有外科医生必须熟悉手术处理的每个方面，但是没有一个人能够或应该全部承担，尤其是承担复杂联体的处理如心脏相连，以及只有少数有类似经验的专门医疗中心能处理的联体，如独立胆道系统的处理。另外，对这些患儿应进行长期随访，因为只有通过这个方法才能获得分离后重建技术的有效性和了解患儿的生活质量，也可获得心理治疗和进行伦理分析的根源，以便为这些特殊患儿提供最佳的治疗。

（严志龙译　叶祖萍校）

参考文献

1. Albert MJ, Drummond DS, O'Neill JA, Watts H: The orthopedic management of conjoined twins: A review of 13 cases and report of four cases. J Pediatr Orthop 1992;2:300.
2. Anderson T: Documentary and artistic evidence for conjoined twins from sixteenth century England. Am J Med Genet 2002;109:155.
3. Annas GJ: Siamese twins: Killing one to save the other. Hastings Cent Rep 1987;17:27.
4. Bega G, Wapner R, Lev-Toaff A, Kulhman K: Diagnosis of conjoined twins at 10 weeks using three-dimensional ultrasound: A case report. Ultrasound Obstet Gynecol 2000; 16:388.
5. Bennett J: Siamese twins: Both lives must be equally respected. Br J Nurs 2000;9:1122.
6. Bondeson J: The Biddenden Maids: A curious chapter in the history of conjoined twins. J R Soc Med 1992;85:217.
7. Bonilla-Musoles F, Machado LE, Osborne NG, et al: Two-dimensional and three-dimensional sonography of conjoined twins. J Clin Ultrasound 2002;30:68.

8. Bouchard S, Johnson MP, Flake AW, et al: The EXIT procedure: Experience and outcome in 31 cases. J Pediatr Surg 2002;37:418.
9. Bucholz RD, Yoon KW, Shively RE: Temporoparietal craniopagus: Case report and review of the literature. J Neurosurg 1987;66:72.
10. Campbell S, Theile R, Stuart G, et al: Separation of craniopagus joined at the occiput. Case report. J Neurosurg 2002;97:983.
11. Casele HL, Meyer JR: Ultrafast magnetic resonance imaging of cephalopagus conjoined twins. Obstet Gynecol 2000; 95:1015.
12. Chen PL, Choe KA: Prenatal MRI of heteropagus twins. AJR Am J Roentgenol 2003;181:1676.
13. Cywes S, Millar AJW, Rode H, Brown RA: Conjoined twins: The Cape Town experience. Pediatr Surg Int 1997;12:234.
14. Dominic C: Separating the twins Jodie and Mary. Ethics Medics 2001;26:2.
15. Dougherty CJ: Joining in life and death: On separating the Lakeberg twins. Bioethics Forum 1995;11:9.
16. Drummond G, Scott T, Mackay D, Lipschitz R: Separation of the Baragwanath craniopagus twins. Br J Plast Surg 1991; 44:49.
17. Durston W: A narrative of monstrous birth in Plymouth, October 22, 1670: Together with the anatomical observations thereupon by William Durston, Doctor of Physics, and communication to Dr. Tim Clerk. Philos Trans R Soc 1670;5:2096.
18. El-Gohary MD: Siamese twins in the United Arab Emirates. Pediatr Surg Int 1998;13:154.
19. Fieggen G, Millar A, Rode H, et al: Spinal cord involvement in pygopagus conjoined twins: Case report and review of the literature. Childs Nerv Syst 2003;19:183.
20. Filler RM: Conjoined twins and their separation. Semin Perinatol 1986;10:82.
21. Fishman SJ, Puder M, Geva T, et al: Cardiac relocation and chest wall reconstruction after separation of thoracopagus conjoined twins with a single heart. J Pediatr Surg 2002; 37:515.
22. Fogel MA, Hubbard A, Weinberg PM: A simplified approach for assessment of intracardiac baffles and extracardiac conduits in congenital heart surgery with two- and three-dimensional magnetic resonance imaging. Am Heart J 2001;142:1028.
23. Gerlis LM, Seo JW, Ho SY, Chi JG: Morphology of the cardiovascular system in conjoined twins: Spatial and sequential arrangements in 36 cases. Teratology 1993; 47:91.
24. Gupta DK, Lal A, Bajpai M: Epigastric heteropagus twins—a report of four cases. Pediatr Surg Int 2001;17:481.
25. Guttmacher AF: Biographical notes on some famous conjoined twins. Birth Defects (OAS) 1967;3:10.
26. Holcomb GW, Keating MA, Hollowell JG, et al: Continent urinary reconstruction in ischiopagus tripus conjoined twins. J Urol 1989;141:100.
27. Hoyle RM, Thomas CG: Twenty-three-year follow-up of separated ischiopagus tetrapus conjoined twins. Ann Surg 1989;210:673.
28. Hsu H-S, Duckett JW, Templeton JM, O'Neill JA: Experience with urogenital reconstruction of ischiopagus conjoined twins. J Urol 1995;154:563.
29. Janik JS, Hendrickson RJ, Janik JP, et al: Spectrum of anorectal anomalies in pygopagus twins. J Pediatr Surg 2003;38:608.
30. Johnson DD, Pretorius DH, Budorick N: Three-dimensional ultrasound of conjoined twins. Obstet Gynecol 1997;90:701.
31. Kim JA, Cho JY, Lee YH, et al: Complications arising in twin pregnancy: Findings of prenatal ultrasonography. Korean J Radiol 2003;4:54.
32. Kim SS, Waldhausen JH, Weidener BC, et al: Perineal reconstruction of female conjoined twins. J Pediatr Surg 2002;37:1740.
33. Kingston CA, McHugh K, Kumaradevan J, et al: Imaging in the preoperative assessment of conjoined twins. Radiographics 2001;21:1187.
34. Knowles LP: The Maltese conjoined twins. Hubris in the court. Hastings Cent Rep 2001;31:47.
35. Koenig E: Sibi invicem adnati feliciter separate. Ephemerid Natur Curios 1689;2:145.
36. Lansdell H: Intelligence test scores from infancy to adulthood for a craniopagus twin pair neurosurgically separated at 4 months of age. Psychol Rep 1999;84:209.
37. Loller LP, Spevak T, Fishman EK: Conjoined twins: Multiorgan system evaluation by multidector CT and 3D volume rendering. J Comput Assist Tomogr 2001;25:870.
38. London AJ: The Maltese conjoined twins. Two views of their separation. Hastings Cent Rep 2001;31:49.
39. MacKenzie TC, Crombleholme TM, Johnson MP, et al: The natural history of prenatally diagnosed conjoined twins. J Pediatr Surg 2002;37:303.
40. Malone FD, D'Alton ME: Anomalies peculiar to multiple gestations. Clin Perinatol 2000;37:1033.
41. Martinez L, Fernandez J, Pastor I, et al: The contribution of modern imaging to planning separation strategies in conjoined twins. Eur J Pediatr Surg 2003;13:120.
42. McDowell BC, Morton BE, Janik JS, et al: Separation of conjoined pygopagus twins. Plast Reconstr Surg 2003; 111:1998.
43. Meyers RL, Matlak ME: Biliary tract anomalies in thoracoomphalopagus conjoined twins. J Pediatr Surg 2002;37:1716.
44. Moraczewkis AS: Against the separation of Jodie and Mary. Ethics Medics 2001;26:1.
45. Norwitz ER, Hoyle LP, Jenkins KJ, et al: Separation of conjoined twins with the twin reversed-arterial-perfusion sequence after prenatal planning with three-dimensional modeling. N Engl J Med 2000;343:399.
46. Omokhodion SI, Ladipo JK, Odebode TO, et al: The Ibadan coinjoined twins: A report of omphalopagus twins and a review of cases reported in Nigeria over 60 years. Ann Trop Paediatr 2001;21:263.
47. O'Neill JA: Conjoined twins. In O'Neill JA, Rowe MI, Grosfeld JG, et al (eds): Pediatric Surgery, 5th ed. St Louis, Mosby–Year Book, 1998, p 1925.
48. O'Neill JA, Holcomb GW, Schnaufer L, et al: Surgical experience with thirteen conjoined twins. Ann Surg 1988;208:299.
49. Paré A: The collected works of Ambroise Paré, London, 1634, Translated by Johnson T. Poundridge. New York, Milford House, 1968.
50. Potter EL, Craig JM: Pathology of the Fetus and Infant, 3rd ed. Chicago, Year Book, 1975.
51. Ratiu P, Singer P: The ethics and economics of heroic surgery. Hastings Cent Rep 2001;31:47.
52. Rickham PP: The dawn of paediatric surgery: Johannes Fatio (1649-1691): His life, his work and his horrible end. Prog Pediatr Surg 1986;20:94.
53. Rock J, Hertig A: The human conceptus during the first two weeks of gestation. Am J Obstet Gynecol 1948;55:6.
54. Ross AJ, O'Neill JA, Silverman DG, et al: A new technique for evaluating cutaneous vascularity in complicated conjoined twins. J Pediatr Surg 1985;20:743.
55. Saing H, Mok C-K, Lau JTK, Tam PKH: A method of repair of thoracic cage defects after separation of thoraco-

omphalopagus twins. Pediatr Surg Int 1987;2:113.
56. Seller MJ: Conjoined twins discordant for cleft lip and palate. Am J Med Genet 1990;37:530.
57. Shapiro E, Fair WR, Ternberg JL, et al: Ischiopagus tetrapus twins: Urological aspects of separation and 10-year follow up. J Urol 1991;145:120.
58. Sills ES, Vrbikova J, Kastratovic-Kotlica B: Conjoined twins, conception, pregnancy, and delivery: A reproductive history of the pygopagus Blazek sisters (1878-1922). Am J Obstet Gynecol 2001;185:1396.
59. Spencer R: Anatomic description of conjoined twins: A plea for standardized terminology. J Pediatr Surg 1996; 31:941.
60. Spencer R: Theoretical and analytical embryology of conjoined twins, parts I and II. Clin Anat 2000;13:36.
61. Spencer R: Parasitic conjoined twins: External, internal (fetuses in fetu and teratomas) and detached (acardiacs). Clin Anat 2001;14:428.
62. Spencer R: Conjoined Twins: Developmental Malformations and Clinical Implications. Baltimore, Johns Hopkins University Press, 2003.
63. Spencer R, Robichaux WH, Superneau DW, Lucas VW: Unusual cardiac malformations in conjoined twins: Thoracopagus twins with conjoined pentalogy of Cantrell and an omphalopagus twin with atretic ventricles. Pediatr Cardiol 2002;23:631.
64. Spiegel DA, Ganley TJ, Akbarnia H, Drummond DS: Congenital vertebral anomalies in ischiopagus and pygopagus conjoined twins. Clin Orthop 2000;381:137.
65. Spielmann AL, Freed KS, Spritzer CE: MRI of conjoined twins illustrating advances in fetal imaging. J Comput Assist Tomogr 2001;25:88.
66. Spitz L: Surgery for conjoined twins. Ann R Coll Surg Engl 2003;85:230.
67. Spitz L, Kiely E: Success rate for surgery of conjoined twins. Lancet 2000;356:1765.
68. Spitz L, Kiely EM: Experience in the management of conjoined twins. Br J Surg 2002;89:1188.
69. Spitz L, Kiely EM: Conjoined twins. JAMA 2003;289:1307.
70. Synhorst D, Matlak M, Roan Y, et al: Separation of conjoined thoracopagus twins joined at the right atrium. Am J Cardiol 1979;43:662.
71. Tendler MD: Siamese twins—the surgery: So one may live. Assia Jew Med Ethics 2001;4:22.
72. Thomasma DC, Muraskas J, Marshall PA, et al: The ethics of caring for conjoined twins. The Lakeberg twins. Hastings Cent Rep 1996;26:4.
73. Turner RJ, Hankins JDW, Weintraub JC, et al: Magnetic resonance imaging and ultrasonography in the antenatal evaluation of conjoined twins. Am J Obstet Gynecol 1986;155:645.
74. Watanatittan S, Niramis R, Suwatanaviroj A, Havanonda S: Conjoined twins: Surgical separation in eleven cases. J Med Assoc Thai 2003;3(Suppl):S633.
75. Wilcox DT, Quin PM, Spitz L, et al: Urological problems in conjoined twins. Br J Urol 1998;81:905.
76. Wong TG, Ong BC, Ang C, Chee HL: Anesthetic management for a five-day separation of craniopagus twins. Anesth Analg 2003;97:999.
77. Zimmerman AA: Embryologic and anatomic considerations of conjoined twins. National Foundation 1967;3:18.

第 130 章

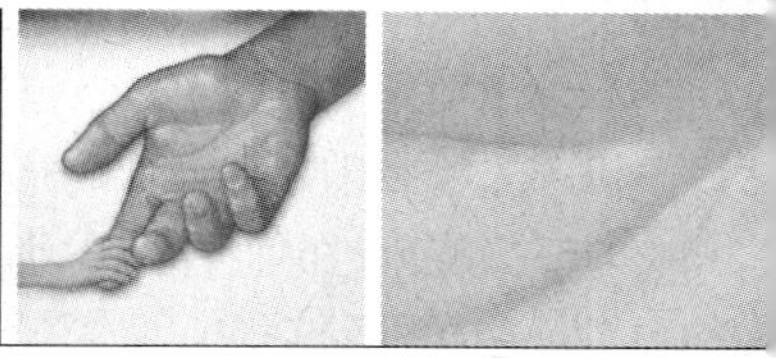

血管异常：血管瘤与血管畸形

Giannoula Klement 和 Steven J. Fishman

分类

2094 血管异常是一大组临床表现各不相同的疾病，范围从小的皮肤色素缺失到大的严重病变，可累及一个肢体或一个脏器从而危及生命[64,67]。长期以来，由于不同专业的临床医生对血管异常疾病的诊治不同，并且极少临床医生对此给予关注，因此妨碍了统一的血管异常病变分类系统的产生。这种命名杂乱的情况大部分是由于对血管异常疾病认识不足，以及不恰当的诊断和不恰当的治疗。尽管医生们喜欢拉丁术语，但这类疾病仍长期由本国术语描述。当母亲由于她婴儿的血管胎记受到责难时，这类病变被称为“母亲痣”（naevus maternus）[63]。细胞（和外科）病理学之父 Virchow 根据显微镜下的管腔结构将所有血管异常疾病命名为“血管瘤”（angiomas）并将其分类：单纯血管瘤、海绵状血管瘤和蔓状血管瘤[85]。Virchow 以前的学生 Wegener 提出了一种具有相似的组织学形态的分支“淋巴血管瘤”[86]。这一 19 世纪混合有普及的描述性术语的组织病理学命名系统，一直保存到本世纪的医学教科书中。Virchow 的“单纯血管瘤”变为同义词“毛细血管瘤”，也被称为“草莓状血管瘤”，他的“海绵状血管瘤”常常用于消退和从不消退的不同血管异常病变。严格的病理学分类没有与临床联系，对儿童血管异常疾病的诊断和治疗没有用处。陈旧、矛盾、不准确的疾病分类系统应该被摒弃。

最早根据血管异常病变的细胞学特征、结合临床表现和自然病程的生物学分类系统在 1982 年由 Mulliken 和 Glowacki 提出[65]，并被许多临床和基础研究确证[29,40]。1996 年，Mulliken 分类被国际血管异常研究协会（ISSVA，International Society for the Study of Vascular Anomalies）所采纳。根据血管异常病变的细胞学特征和临床行为将其分为肿瘤和畸形（表 130-1）。可根据临床表现、影像学、组织病理学、血流动力学等方面的不同而将这两类病变区分开来[58,59]。准确的命名是必需的，因为这两类病变的预后和治疗都不相同。

血管性肿瘤包括婴儿型血管瘤、迅速消退的先天性血管瘤、不消退的先天性血管瘤、簇状血管瘤和卡波西血管内皮瘤，以及其他少见类型。所有血管性肿瘤都远比常见的婴儿型血管瘤少见。血管瘤存在细胞的增殖。这类良性肿瘤在婴儿期生长迅速，儿童期逐渐消退，而在青春期和成人中几乎不出现。其他血管性肿瘤也存在动态的生命周期。

表 130-1 血管异常病变的生物学分类

血管肿瘤：
- 血管瘤（常见婴儿型）
- 迅速消退的先天性血管瘤（RICH）
- 不消退的先天性血管瘤（NICH）
- Kaposi 血管内皮瘤（KHE）
- 簇状血管瘤
- 其他少见类型

血管畸形：
- 毛细血管型（CM）
- 静脉型（VM）
- 淋巴管型（LM）
- 动静脉型（AVM）
- Klippel-Trenaunay 综合征（CLVM）
- 其他结合型（CVM、LVM、CAVM 等）

相反，血管畸形是一种发育异常，由异常的管道
2095 和静止的血管内皮细胞组成，几乎从不消退，有的甚至逐渐扩张。血管畸形可根据管道结构和血流动力学的不同再分类。慢流病变存在于毛细血管、淋巴管或静脉结构中，而快流病变包括动脉或动静脉异常。复杂血管畸形常伴有软组织及骨骼的过度生长，许多这类病变具有以人名命名的专有名称。

各种类型的血管异常病变可生长于身体任何器官系统。除常见于头面部外，亦可侵及胸腹壁或腔、实质器官、空腔脏器、脑等。可呈多发性。初始表现多为外表异常，亦可产生危险的临床症状，如疼痛、出血、肿块效应，甚至充血性心力衰竭。

由于分类混乱以及缺乏转诊中心，直到最近对血管异常病变的准确诊断仍然使普通儿科医生感到困难。根据病变的部位，患儿可能被转到皮肤科、整形外科、普外科、耳鼻喉科、矫形外科、神经外科、介入放射科或肿瘤科就诊。结果导致多种矛盾的诊断和不同的命名。这样，由于不确定的诊断，致使大部分病例得到不恰当或不正确的治疗。一些三级医学中心现在都建立了多学科的血管异常诊治中心，在诊断的准确性和治疗的标准化上都取得很大进步。90%以上的小儿血管异常病例可根据病史及体检作出正确的诊断[29]。对深部皮下、肌内或脏器内的病变诊断有困难，影像学和内镜检查对这些病例来说是需要的，可建立诊断，明确病变解剖范围。

发病机制

血管瘤

一个迅速生长的血管瘤由丰富的、分化迅速的血管内皮细胞组成（增殖期）。随着自发消退，血管内皮细胞活性逐渐降低（退化期）[65]。肿瘤“血管生成依赖”的概念最早由 Folkman 和 Klagsbrun 提出[35]，提示应深入研究血管瘤的生长周期。已知血管生成因子作用于血管内皮细胞和周围细胞，启动毛细血管网络的形成[35,61]。这一过程受血管内皮细胞生长抑制因子的紧密调节，以保持正常的微血管处于静止期。血管瘤是一种最纯粹的血管生成模型。它可能是由于局部正常的血管抑制因子减少或血管刺激因子产物增加所致。血管瘤自发的消退可能是由于血管抑制因子增加或促血管生成因子的下调。

常见的免疫组化标志物包括 glut-1、Fcγ RⅡ、Lewis Y 抗原、分层蛋白、3 型碘化甲腺氨酸脱碘酶等，它们表达水平的升高提示血管瘤可能来源于或部分为胎盘的正常前体[47,69]。

细胞免疫组化标志物可说明血管瘤临床分期[82]。迅速生长的血管瘤的生化特征是表达增殖细胞核抗原，它部分由血管生成肽血管内皮细胞生长因子（VEGF）和碱性纤维母细胞生长因子（bFGF）调节[56]。Ⅳ型胶原酶也在增殖期血管瘤表达，这说明胶原沉积是必需的，可为增生的毛细血管提供空间。血管生成多肽能促使增殖细胞的分化，以及组织型金属蛋白酶抑制剂（TIMP-Ⅰ）——一种新生血管形成的抑制剂的自分泌诱导剂。已知肥大细胞在增殖后期和退化早期表达，能分泌调节因子下调血管瘤生成[39,72]。总之无论哪种因素促使血管瘤由增殖期向退化期转化，都会出现肿瘤分化、内皮细胞老化以及实质被纤维和脂肪替代[22,46,82]。

血管畸形

血管畸形的四种主要分类都各有其特殊的组织病理学表现。复杂结合型在光镜下常难以鉴别。不同的血管异常其主要的细胞学特征是静止的内皮细胞层。然而，如果血栓产生，这在淋巴型、静脉型或结合的淋巴海绵样血管异常中常常见到，那么在栓子内常见到异常增生的新生毛细血管管道。

毛细血管病变由规则的、扩张的、薄壁毛细血管到静脉大小的管道组成，位于乳突层或网状真皮层上方。

淋巴型和静脉型的异常病变存在不同厚度的壁。骨骼和平滑肌都可能形成壁，淋巴细胞结节状聚合常常在结缔组织的间质见到。静脉畸形常常是薄壁的，带有稀疏的不规则的平滑肌岛。苍白的嗜酸性液体常常在淋巴异常以及有血液、栓子、静脉石形成的静脉畸形中见到。这些错误形成的静脉网络引流到邻近肿胀的缺乏静脉瓣的静脉。从临床和组织学表现两方面，结合的淋巴海绵样畸形都可能发生。

动静脉畸形（AVM）中的动脉形态是异常的，由基质内异常增生的平滑肌纤维组成厚壁。AVM 中不成熟的静脉表现为“动脉化”（反应性肌肉增生）。

尽管大部分的血管畸形是散发的，但不常见的家族病例和多样性，导致最近特异性基因突变的发现，甚至可能提供散发病例病因学的线索[13]。与遗传性
2096 出血性毛细血管扩张症（Rendu-Osler-Weber 综合征）相关的一个基因位于染色体 9q。一种常染色体显性遗传的皮肤肌肉血管畸形，三代家系基因图谱研究表明其基因异常位于染色体 9p，而与家族性颅内静脉异常有关的基因位于染色体 7p[24]。家族性的 *RASA1* 基因突变在多发的小毛细血管畸形、AVM、动静脉瘘或 Parkes Weber 综合征中被发现[24]。

血管瘤和血管畸形的鉴别

临床表现

血管瘤

血管瘤是婴幼儿时期最常见的良性肿瘤，它们不常在出生时出现，而常出现在新生儿期，多在出生后 2 周内出现。大约 30%～40% 在出生时见到的是皮肤病变的先兆：仅仅可见的“贫血痔”、毛细血管扩张或红色斑点，或一种淤斑样青肿（图 130-1A）。深部（皮下）或脏器的血管瘤可能直到 2～3 个月才表现出来。深部血管瘤表面的皮肤仅仅有轻微淡蓝色的突起。局部引流的静脉常见扩张。过去称深部血管瘤为“海绵样”，称浅表病变为“毛细血管样”，这种命名易混淆，不应再应用。事实上，没有完全的“海绵样”血管瘤。这类病变要么是深部的血管瘤，要么是被错误标记的静脉畸形。

大约 80% 血管瘤是单个生长的瘤体，20% 是多发病变[54]。这类肿瘤在女性中远比在男性中多发（比例 3∶1～5∶1）。这种女性占优势的情况甚至在面部血管瘤合伴胸腔畸形时更为明显[40]。发病率在白人婴儿中为 10%～12%[27]，在黑人婴儿中较低。在出生体重小于 1000g 的早产儿中发病率为 22%[2,45]。

血管瘤的特征是出生后 6～8 个月内生长迅速（增殖期）。随着肿瘤在表皮生长，皮肤变为鲜红色，突出皮肤或呈凸起状（图 130-1B）。

血管瘤至 1 岁末时生长达到高峰，肿瘤生长似乎与孩子生长成比例。这时，退化期表现开始出现。鲜

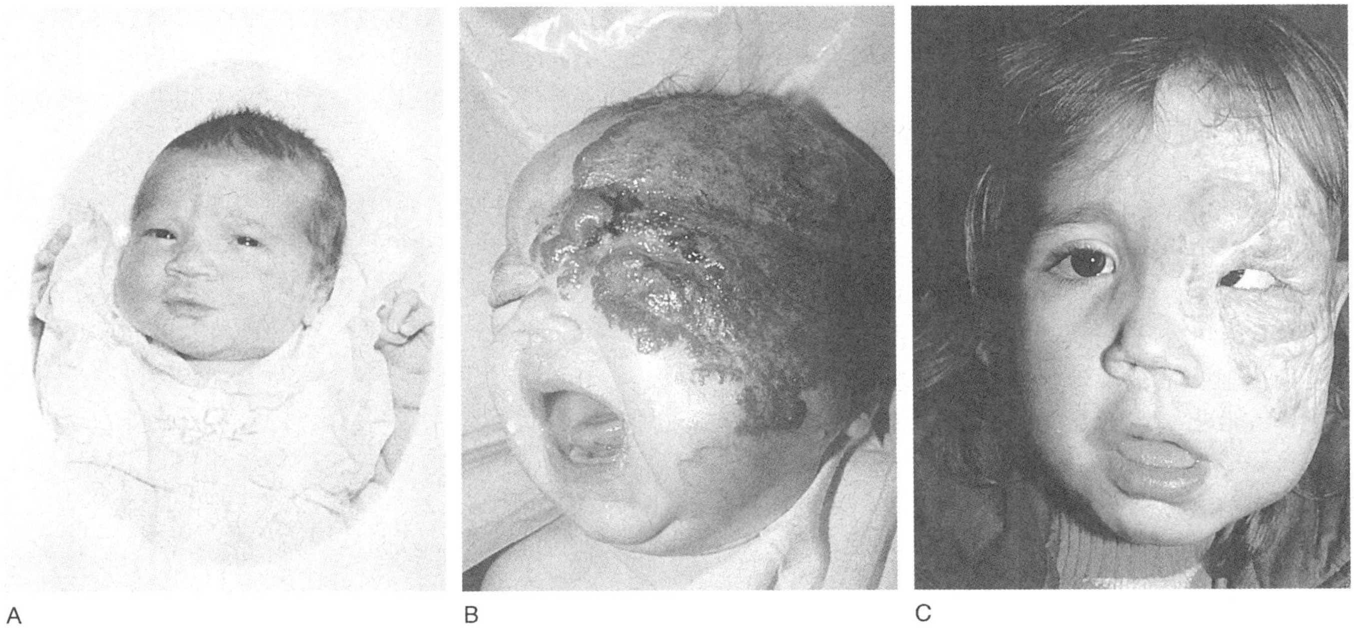

图 130-1　血管瘤自然病程。A. 新生儿期照片显示在左侧前额、头、面颊部浅的点状斑。B. 4 个月时，进展性的面部血管瘤（增殖期）伴有自发性溃疡，完全的眼眶阻塞，对糖皮质激素无反应。C. 4 岁时，退化期，可见残留眶周的瘢痕，斜视，左眼视力减退。

红色转为暗紫红色，皮肤逐渐苍白，呈不均匀灰色，无光泽，肿瘤触感缺乏张力。典型的血管瘤退化期持续到5～10岁（图130-1C）。

血管瘤消退与其大小、部位、外观等无关。大多数血管瘤是小而无害的，约50%的患儿可遗留正常皮肤[15]。分布广泛或突出体表的血管瘤亦可完全消退。大的血管瘤消退时，皮肤可能遗留血管扩张、绉样松弛皱襞、淡黄色斑、瘢痕（如增殖期有溃疡）、纤维脂肪残留物等。

与血管畸形不同，血管瘤很少产生骨骼畸形或肢
2097 体肥大。然而，大的面部血管瘤常引起软骨和骨的过度生长，导致面部骨骼继发性的血流增加或局部肿块效应。即使肢体有广泛的血管瘤，也几乎从未见到肢体骨骼的轴向过度生长[16]。

重要的一点是并非所有的血管瘤都为草莓样[58,67]。深部（皮下）的血管瘤部分位于颈部或躯干部，可能与淋巴型畸形混淆，但可以用超声或核磁共振（MRI）检查予以鉴别。血管瘤也可能与葡萄酒斑（毛细血管型畸形）相仿。血管瘤真正的特性是明显的引流静脉而且随后发生退化[31]。

另外必须注意的一点是，并非所有的草莓样病变都是血管瘤。最常与之混淆的病变是化脓性肉芽肿。这类相当常见的病变很少发生于6个月龄前（发病的平均年龄是6.7岁）[73]，而血管瘤在婴儿早期就出现并发展。化脓性肉芽肿的患儿常常没有病史或不存在先前的皮肤状况（尽管这种病变可能产生于葡萄酒斑上）。典型的化脓性肉芽肿是单个小的病变（平均直径6.5 mm）。它们生长迅速，从皮肤发出，形成一个蒂。表皮的破坏和结痂常见，并常因反复出血（常常大量出血）开始就医或去急诊。静脉畸形也常与血管瘤混淆。尽管皮肤是光滑的，但颜色可能相近。淋巴管畸形或淋巴静脉畸形，特别是出生时或婴儿期伴有病变内出血，常被误诊为血管瘤。体检对诊断有帮助，B超能进一步确定。婴儿的纤维肉瘤、横纹肌肉瘤或突起的神经胶质瘤也常被误诊为先天性或新生儿血管瘤[11]。MRI有诊断价值。任何血管病变如怀疑为恶性时都应行活检。

其他肿瘤

一种迅速消退的先天性血管瘤（RICH）在出生时即出现并生长充分[10]。这类少见的血管瘤在出生后不再生长并在8～14个月内消退。典型的RICH是突起的，呈圆顶型，红色到紫罗兰色，周围常有苍白晕（图130-2）。与典型的血管瘤不同，它们可能在产前检查中被发现。相反，更少见的不消退的先天性血管瘤（NICH）[27]从不消退并需要手术切除。高血流的先天性血管瘤病变可能导致高输出性心力衰竭。然而，这种需要治疗的情况在RICH中不常见。事实上，家庭和临床医生常常惊奇于RICH快速的自发消退。直到最近RICH被重新作为一个特殊的疾病而认识，被纳入到典型血管瘤临床记录中，由此可以解释以前被不合理地推论为“奇迹般消退”的情况。

Kaposi血管内皮瘤（KHE）常被认为是有“侵略性”的血管瘤。然而，已很清楚其在组织病理学和临床上与婴儿常见血管瘤有区别。KHE在出生时即表现或在出生后早期即发展，侵袭性很强。男女发病率相等。肿块常常呈紫红色，边界不清，有光泽，有张力，高于皮肤（图130-3）。常常发生于躯干、肩或大腿或腹膜后腔，更常见于外周。KHE常侵犯多个组织，包括皮肤、皮下和肌肉。与血管瘤不同，KHE可导致邻近骨骼的破坏性改变。组织学上，纺锤样内皮细胞占优势，带有细胞内裂隙样空间[87]。更重要的是，KHE常伴有Kasabach-Merritt现象（KMP，血管瘤血小板减少综合征），由于血小板陷阱导致消耗性血小板减少。血小板减少是很严重的（血小板计数 < 10 000/mm^3），由此导致胃肠道、胸膜肺、腹腔或颅内的出血。这种病变的患儿死亡率高达

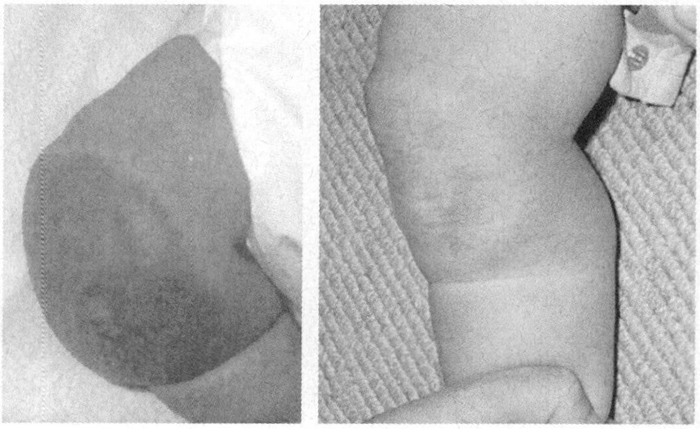

A　　B

图130-2　迅速消退的先天性血管瘤。A. 出生时生长完全。注意为圆形和有苍白晕。B. 1岁前未治疗，几乎完全消退。

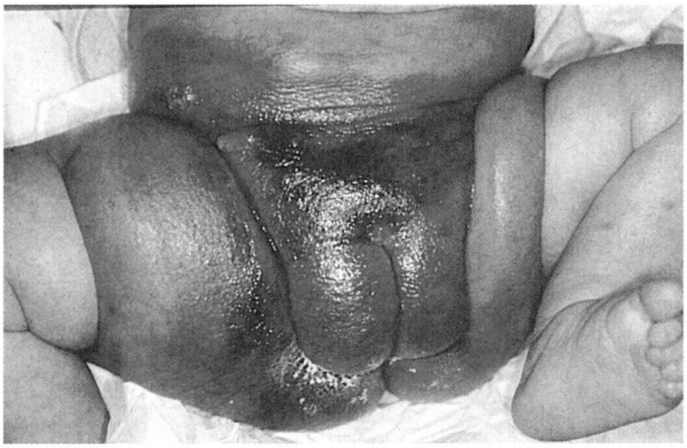

图 130-3　伴有 Kasabach-Merritt 现象（血小板计数为 6000/mm³）的 Kaposi 血管内皮瘤。注意下腹部和会阴部淤斑和水肿。

2098 20%～30%，必须早期治疗[23]。回顾性分析血管瘤伴有 KMP 的报道反映了在过去困难的是分类这些病变，而不是将两种病变重叠[76]。实际上，典型的婴儿型血管瘤从来不发生 KMP。尽管 KHE 可自发发展，但它仍然在整个儿童早期占优势，可能在儿童中期静止，存在于终生[6]。在成人后期，它的分布部位可能会产生肌肉骨骼疼痛综合征。

丛状血管瘤（也指“Nagakawa 血管母细胞瘤”）可以是先天性或获得性的。分布的部位与 KHE 类似，尽管丛状血管瘤倾向于更小。它们边界不清，有压痛，呈暗红色/紫红色，有丘疹或小半鞘翅。组织学检查最明显的是广泛分布在真皮层中间和下三分之一的带蓝色结节，或被称为“cannonballs”的丛状的毛细血管[49]。这种结节比血管瘤的结节更宽。这种病变细胞更丰富，而且大量的内皮细胞是纺锤形的。

毛细血管畸形

毛细血管畸形（从 19 世纪以来被称为“葡萄酒斑”）是一种有斑点的红色血管斑，出生时出现，并持续终生。毛细血管畸形可局限或广泛存在于面部、躯干、四肢。这种病变必须与常见的可消退的有斑点的红斑相区别。这种斑发生于 50% 的新生儿中，多位于眉间、眼睑、鼻、上唇或颈项部。这种斑又被称为新生儿斑、白鹳咬痕或天使之吻。

Sturge-Weber 综合征指面部毛细血管畸形合并同

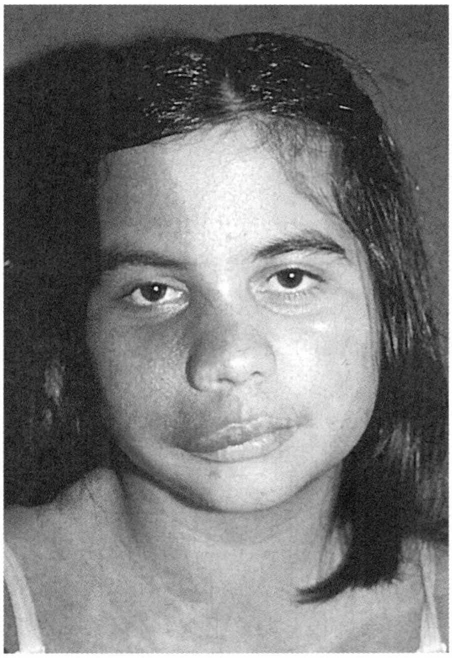

图 130-4　十几岁的女孩，右侧面部和胸部毛细血管畸形（葡萄酒斑）。有脑膜血管异常病变（Sturge-Weber 综合征）的患者必须行眶周检查和核磁共振检查。

侧颞叶和枕叶软脑膜血管异常。颅内血管异常可导致反复抽搐和对侧偏瘫，以及运动或认知功能的不同程度发育迟缓。三叉神经第一支（V1）眼神经感觉区及皮肤最常受累，上颌支（V2）或下颌支（V3）有毛细血管畸形时很少累及颅内。当病变累及 V1 区和 V2 区时，患者有很高的风险患青光眼（图 130-4）。

面部毛细血管畸形常导致肤色加深，皮肤出现增生性变化；增厚的紫色结节在青春期开始发展。这种皮肤改变很少发生于肢体畸形。面部毛细血管畸形有时伴有局部软组织及骨骼的过度增生。广泛的肢体毛细血管畸形可产生轴向和横向的肢体肥大，常在出生时表现。静脉曲张在儿童期不会发展，并且当儿童成长时肢体肥大不会恶化。肢体毛细血管畸形可为复杂血管畸形的一部分，如 Klippel-Trenaunay 综合征和 Parkes-Weber 综合征。在背侧中线的毛细血管畸形可作为一种信号，提示可能潜在枕部的脑膨出和颈部或腰部椎管闭合不全。

淋巴管畸形

淋巴管畸形在儿童早期表现，常常出生时即出现。这类病变与其他血管异常一样，通过影像学检查，产前检出率逐渐提高[55]。它们可以是局部小的病变，也可以是弥漫性的病变，侵及整个肢体、躯干或区域。它们可以是微囊的、大囊的或混合型的。术语“囊性水囊肿”指颈部大囊的淋巴管畸形，而“淋巴管瘤”实际上是一种微囊的淋巴管畸形，不应再在现代医学命名中应用。后缀“-oma”意味着肿瘤，因此常引起这一范围命名的混淆。临床上，典型的大囊病变是球形、肉色、比重依赖性的病变，而微囊病变几乎不能压缩。与所有畸形病变相同，淋巴管畸形的内皮细胞和平滑肌组成是静止的。然而，结缔组织包含淋巴细胞结节状集合，并包括滤泡的生殖中心。

淋巴管畸形依据淋巴液的流入和流出、炎症的情况和是否发生病变内出血而扩张或收缩。多数在出生时表现或在 2 岁前发生，然而有时突然在大儿童中表
2099 现（很少发生在青春期）。在怀孕前 3 个月末，产前 B 超即可能尽早发现大囊的淋巴管畸形[53]。这类病变可能发生在任何部位，但常见于面颈部、腋下和后背部（图 130-5A）。表皮受累皮肤可能表现为皱褶或小凹形成。婴儿纤维肉瘤可类似颈躯干部的淋巴管畸形[44]。

大囊性淋巴管畸形常见于颈部和腋下。在前额、口周、面颊部的畸形常常是大囊和微囊的混合，可导致面部不对称和变形。软组织和骨骼的过度生长是淋巴管畸形的特征。这种畸形是巨唇、巨舌、巨耳、巨颧最常见的基础[67]。面颈部的淋巴管畸形常伴有下颌骨的过度生长和咬合不正[71]。一个典型的伴有小囊泡的巨大舌头会导致说话困难，并伴有反复感染、肿胀、出血、牙齿卫生不佳和龋齿。在面颈部，微囊和大囊的畸形可导致气道梗阻，有时必须行气管切开。颈部和腋下的淋巴管畸形常常影响胸腔和纵隔，可能导致致命的反复胸膜和心包渗液（图130-5B）。肺的淋巴管异常可能导致肺水肿。肢体广泛的畸形与淋巴水肿（甚至象皮病）有关。骨骼的变形和增生也是肢体畸形的常见特征。少见的病种“骨消失病”（Gorham-Stout 综合征）可能是淋巴管畸形累及骨骼，进而导致进行性骨溶解所致。盆腔的淋巴管畸形可能表现为外阴淋巴管扩张、尿道出口梗阻、便秘或反复的感染。胃肠道的畸形（以前称为“淋巴管瘤病”）可导致低蛋白血症，继发于蛋白丢失肠病。

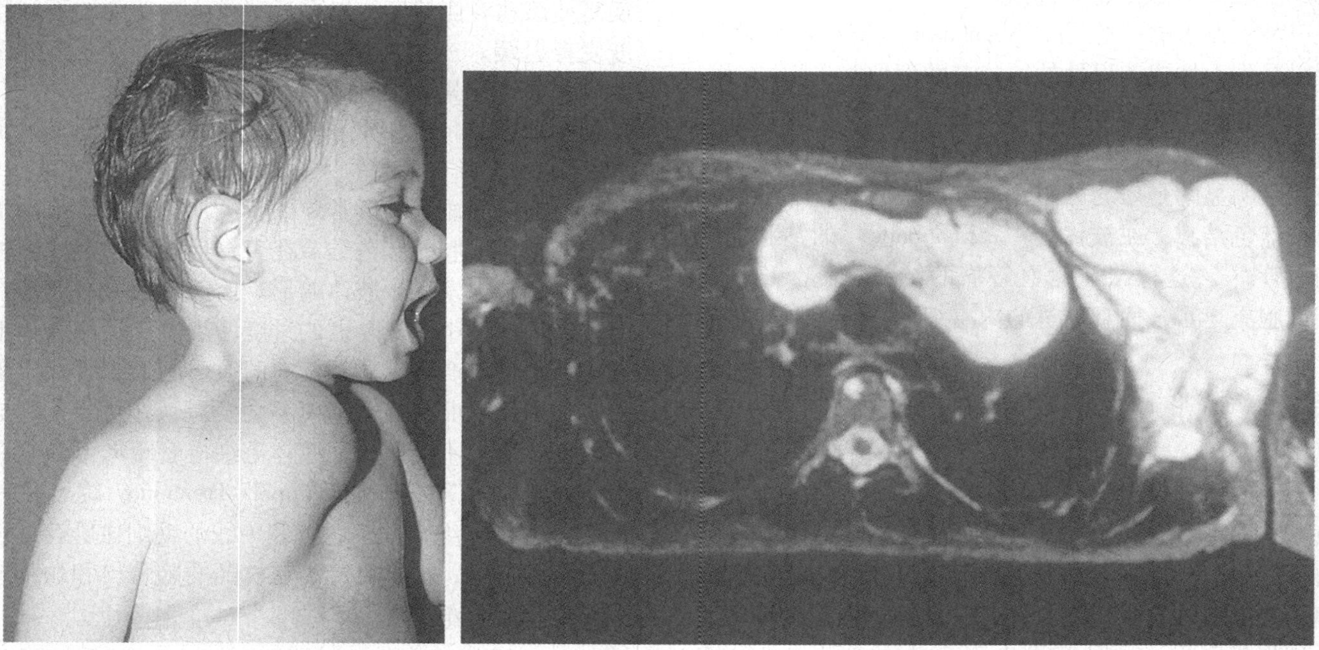

A　B

图 130-5　A. 胸部和腋下的大囊性淋巴管畸形累及臂丛，可能有纵隔扩张。B. 33 岁女性纵隔淋巴管畸形，从儿童时开始颈部手术超过 30 次。

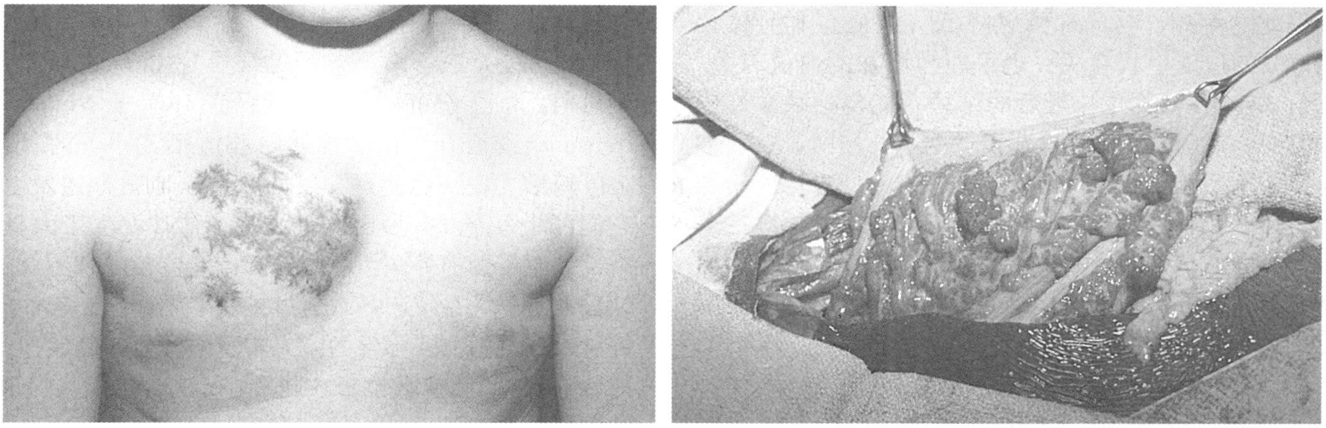

A B

图 130-6 A. 胸壁静脉畸形。B. 结肠的广泛静脉畸形伴有胃肠道出血。

静脉畸形

静脉畸形在出生时即存在，但并不总是非常明显。在以往的医学用语或文献中常错误地将其称为“海绵状血管瘤”。这种慢流的血管异常可表现为淡蓝色斑或软的蓝色肿块。静脉畸形可局限或广泛。可发生于任何部位：脸、四肢、躯干、口鼻部、生殖器、膀胱、脑、脊髓、肝、脾、空腔脏器、肺、骨骼肌和骨（图 130-6）。对美观的影响可能不重要，也可能是悲剧性的变形。这类病变容易压缩，当依靠时可出现加剧的肿胀。可产生血栓，并且早到 2 岁即可产生静脉石。静脉畸形随小儿生长成比例增大，缓慢
2100 恶化，并常在青春期增大。静脉畸形是最常见的有症状的血管畸形。充血肿胀或病变内血栓或两者同时存在均会引起不适。累及关节时导致关节积血或含铁血黄素关节病。

大多数静脉畸形为单发，亦有多发的皮肤病变产生。后一种血管畸形可能是遗传的[12]。家族性血管球静脉畸形（血管球病）是一种不常见的常染色体显性综合征，有较高的外显率，由多发的结节样皮肤静脉异常组成，可见于皮肤任何部位[14]。组织学上，这类病变与典型的静脉畸形不同，有大量的血管球细胞排列于扩张的静脉管道。触诊常常有压痛。

动静脉畸形

大多数小儿期快流血管异常为动静脉畸形（AVM）。单纯的动脉畸形（例如动脉瘤、狭窄或扩张）或动静脉瘘作为有症状的病变很少单独产生，它们常常与动静脉畸形伴发。这类畸形由滋养动脉、小或大的动静脉瘘以及增大的静脉所组成。AVM 在出生时即出现，在婴儿或儿童期逐渐明显。它们被认为由胚胎期畸形发生和异常动脉决定所导致。最后形成于高流量动脉床和不活跃的静脉网络之间的多种异常连接导致额外的血流射入静脉，由此形成脆弱的高度扩张的病变。

这类病变在儿童期常常表现不明显，被误认为血管瘤或葡萄酒斑。青春期或创伤可能促发其扩张，这促使 AVM 表现出快流性质的皮肤表现。皮肤变成红色或青紫色，在血管斑之下显示有肿块，局部温暖，有震颤和杂音（图 130-7）。临床表现特点常常是不

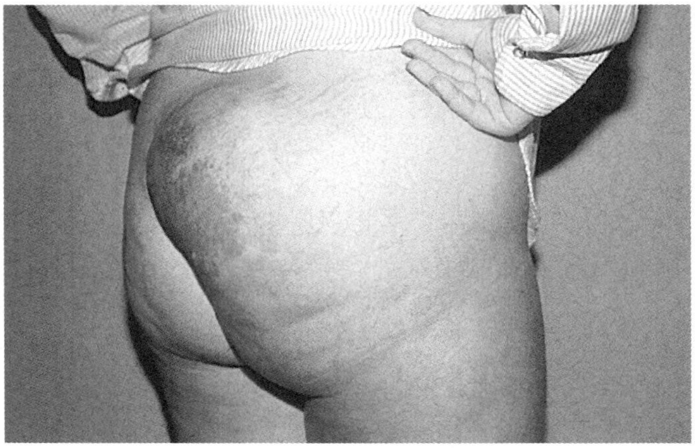

图 130-7 十几岁的女孩，出生时右臀发红，青春期扩张，显示为动静脉畸形。

同程度的疼痛，与局部给氧降低（缺血）和身体相关部分的过度生长有关，也可能与增加的血流有关。无论AVM在何部位，最后的结果可能包括缺血性皮肤改变、溃疡、顽固性疼痛以及间歇性出血，并且甚至在儿童期就可能出现。

超声和彩色多普勒检查可明确临床诊断。脉冲多普勒可确定动脉的输出（与正常一侧对照），从而用来监测AVM的进展。MRI可很好地记录畸形的解剖范围。Schobinger阶梯系统常常用于描述AVM的状态：

1. 第一级——一个粉蓝色且温暖的斑。多普勒超声显示动静脉分流。

2. 第二级——搏动，震颤，有杂音。

3. 第三级——营养不良性皮肤改变，溃疡，出血，疼痛。

4. 第四级——高输出量心力衰竭。

2101 复杂血管畸形

大多数复杂血管畸形都有命名，常常伴随软组织与骨骼的过度增生（见表130-1）。这些命名常常错误应用并令人误解，而与发病机制无关。根据血流动力学和畸形管腔结构的不同，可将其分为两类：慢流与快流。

慢流复杂血管畸形包括毛细血管-静脉畸形和毛细血管-淋巴管-静脉畸形。后者对应于Klippel-Trenaunay综合征，用于描述与肢体肥大有关的复杂血管畸形。皮肤病变是多发的，常以地图方式发生；它们可能有或没有淋巴血管滤泡，常常发生于大腿、臀部和躯干的前外侧。静脉异常可能包括发育不全或缺失的深静脉系统，导致通过扩张、无瓣膜、表浅的静脉来促进引流。异常的、无瓣膜的、位于胚胎边缘的Servelle静脉常常位于大腿和小腿的侧面，与不同的深静脉系统连接[78]。淋巴管发育不良也是原发缺陷，淋巴囊常见。肢体的扩张由小到奇形怪状（图130-8）。结合慢流异常常累及同侧臀部、会阴和后腹膜。扩张到盆腔导致血尿、便血、便秘、膀胱出口梗阻[5]。可能产生血栓性静脉炎和肺栓塞，在Klippel-Trenaunay综合征患者中有高发生率[68]。与其他半侧肥大综合征不同，Klippel-Trenaunay综合征患者患肾母细胞瘤的风险并不增加，B超扫描不是必需的[41]。

快流复杂血管畸形（例如毛细血管-动静脉畸形或毛细血管-动脉-淋巴管-静脉畸形）较少见。Parkes-Weber综合征属于此类病变。皮肤温度升高，杂音、震颤存在。动静脉瘘为多发，位于受累肢体

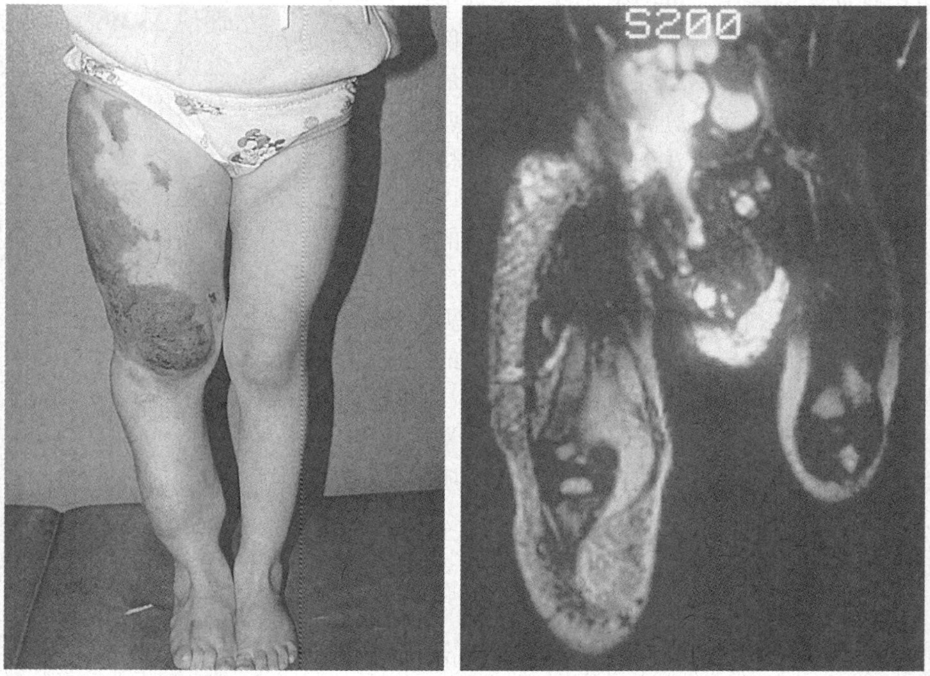

图130-8 A. 伴有下肢肥大的复合毛细血管-淋巴管-静脉畸形（Klippel-Trenaunay综合征）。B. MRI显示这一畸形的大囊性的淋巴管异常扩展到盆腔。

处，部分靠近关节。小儿童 MRI 及血管造影可能仅显示肢体弥散的血管过度形成，动静脉瘘随后才明显。

遗传性出血性毛细血管扩张症（HHT）也称为 Rendu-Osler-Weber 病，是一种基因问题，开始是毛细血管扩张病变，逐渐发展至皮肤、黏膜、肝、肺、脑的毛细血管-静脉分流，常见于 30 或 40 岁左右[42]。脑和肺的 AVM 和肝的血管异常会发展。两个影响转移生长因子-β 信号的基因被发现。HHT1 是由于 endoglin 的突变，它编码一种内皮细胞糖蛋白。HHT2 是由 activin 受体样激酶突变所引起。

变形杆菌综合征是一种相当少见的疾病，以不同的皮肤和皮下组织病变为特征，包括血管畸形、脂肪瘤、色素沉着和不同类型的痣，以及大头畸形、肢体不对称伴手足部分巨大发育和脑回状跖肌增厚。它是典型的肢体或指趾过度生长的局部巨大发育。半身肥大症和软组织过度生长导致骨骼畸形，如脊柱侧弯或脊柱后侧弯，可能导致呼吸危害。Joseph Merrick（也
2102 就是“象人”）曾被认为是神经纤维瘤病，现在回顾起来，其实应该是患了变形杆菌综合征。栓塞性事件增加的风险，例如深静脉血栓或肺栓塞，特别在男性中，促成了所有的发病率和病死率，甚至在幼儿中。诊断是复杂的，并以多种特殊的诊断标准为依据。变形杆菌综合征可能过分诊断，因为这个名字常常被给予其他难以确定的处于过度生长状态的患者。

Bannayan-Riley-Ruvalcaba 综合征是常染色体显性疾病，定位于 *PTEN* 基因，以大头、多发脂肪瘤、错构瘤性回肠和结肠息肉、Hashimoto 甲状腺炎、阴茎龟头的斑点和血管畸形为特征[57]。血管异常，包括毛细血管、静脉和动静脉畸形，有时是这个综合征的组成部分。

伴发异常

尽管教科书常常把血管瘤列为与有不同异常表现的综合征伴发的疾病，但这类名称常常是不正确的。常见的消退的婴儿斑或真正的血管畸形（毛细血管、淋巴管、静脉或动脉）与异形的综合征并不相关[19]。

然而，有很好的文献记载了真正的血管瘤伴畸形。术语 PHACES 综合征是最近提出的描述一种与后颅窝畸形、血管瘤、动脉异常、主动脉缩窄、心脏缺陷和眼异常相关的综合征的名词。中线的缺陷例如胸骨不联合和脐上脊也能被发现。一种广泛的异常曾被描述，受累婴儿仅仅有部分表现[36,74]。腰骶部血管瘤是几种皮肤病变之一［例如葡萄酒斑、achordoma（鹿尾）、毛发片］，被认为是隐性脊柱裂的信号（例如脂肪脑膜膨出、脊髓栓系和脊髓纵裂）[67]。

内脏表现

婴儿皮肤多发性血管瘤伴发潜伏内脏（特别是肝内）血管瘤的风险可能很高[18,81]。这种皮肤血管瘤的典型表现较小（直径小于 3～5 mm），暗红色，穹窿形。肝病变可能不伴有皮肤病变。有症状时，内脏血管瘤常常在出生后 1～16 周的小婴儿中进行评估。传统的三联征是充血性心力衰竭、肝大以及很少表现的贫血。肝血管肿瘤有不同的表现和临床过程[50]。许多婴儿由于皮肤多发病变而进行 B 超检查，发现无症状的单个或多个病变。病变导致高输出量心力衰竭证明病变内存在大血管动静脉、动脉门脉或门体循环的分流。不常见但很可怕的是，多发病变几乎完全替代肝脏致使肝巨大。这类病变不会导致高输出量心力衰竭，但是取而代之的是继发于腹腔间隙综合征的器官衰竭。另外，有巨大的肝血管瘤的婴儿可能有继发性甲状腺功能低下[47]，任何有明显临床病变的婴儿，即使新生儿期甲状腺刺激激素检测正常，也要重复检查。甲状腺功能低下是由于血管瘤表达的脱碘酶使甲状腺激素失活而导致。只有当血管瘤足够大使激素失活快于甲状腺分泌产生时，才导致临床甲状腺功能低下。理论上任何部位的血管瘤均可导致甲状腺功能低下，但所有的报道均与肝病变相关。大的单个的肝血管病变可在产前或出生后马上被发现，常常伴以一过性的血小板轻度减少，可能不是典型的婴儿型血管瘤，但是 RICH。它们通常迅速消退，不伴有其他严重的临床表现。早期报道的肝血管瘤病死率为 30%～80% 可能被过度夸大，因为没有包括先前无症状的未检测到的病变，并且缺乏对这类肿瘤临床变异的评价[8,20]。

肝 AVM 可能相当少见。诊断混淆可能是由于有些肝血管瘤通过快流大血管分流到实质[9,50]。少见通过活检或手术切除来区分肝内血管瘤与肝母细胞瘤、血管肉瘤、转移性神经母细胞瘤或间质错构瘤。

空腔脏器血管瘤与慢性发作性出血相关。与肝病变相似，它们亦常伴有皮肤多发性血管瘤。

血管畸形也常累及内脏，尤其是胃肠道（见图130-6）[32,34]。静脉病变更占优势。它们可能为局灶性、多发或弥散。用可弯曲的纤维光学食管十二指肠镜和结肠镜能可靠地评估胃肠道病变。最近介绍的无线胶囊肠镜可革命性地减小可视小肠检查的创伤。内镜检查较胃肠道造影更能证实和鉴定血管异常的特征。

皮肤血管畸形与胃肠道相似病变相关最早被Gascoyen在1860年描述[38]，但术语“蓝色橡皮疱痣综合征”（Blue rubber bleb nevus syndrome）在1958年由Bean提出[7]。这一综合征是少见疾病，多为散发，有报道是常染色体显性遗传。胃肠道静脉畸形是无蒂的或为息肉样，位于食管、胃、小肠和结肠，以及肠系膜，内镜很易见到。这类患者也可伴有血管畸形，
2103 累及腮腺、脑、肝、脾或其他器官。反复的消化道出血可较为严重，并且一旦出血明显，常常持续一生。有些患者需要每周输血。尽管有些患者接受上百次输血，但是突然的血流动力学不稳的严重出血并不常见[30]。一个静脉畸形可成为肠套迭的起始点。有些病例病变累及骨和关节，不适和功能丧失可能非常严重，甚至需要截肢。

胃肠道血管畸形也可能发生于Turner综合征中，也可以是独立的血管异常[17]。

静脉畸形常发生于肝脏。实际上，成人常见的肝内血管病变常常被称为血管瘤，而其实不是血管瘤，而是静脉畸形。婴儿的血管瘤不会持续存在或发生于成人期。

影像学特点

影像学检查用来描述血管异常的类型、流变学性质以及解剖范围。彩色多普勒超声检查可区分慢流或快流病变。增生期血管瘤产生明显的往返信号，即使有经验的超声医生也难以通过信号将其与AVM鉴别。超声最大的障碍是高度依赖于操作者，并且显示异常病变大小及其与邻近组织关系的能力受限。

MRI常常是最能提供信息的检查，因为它可提供血流动力学的信息和病变累及的范围。这种检测显示血管瘤由实质（固体）组成，在T1加权时为中等密度，T2加权为中等高密度[48,59]。周围和瘤体内有流空，证明快流通过滋养动脉进入扩张的引流静脉。在退化后期，退化的血管瘤变成慢流团块，脂肪组织占优势。

MRI可描述除皮肤毛细血管斑以外的所有血管畸形类型。静脉畸形在T2加权中有高信号密度，比脂肪组织亮。静脉石在T1和T2加权显示为分散的圆形空信号，是证实静脉畸形的依据。在T1加权序列，采用钆显示静脉畸形增强不均匀，淋巴管畸形则没有增强或只环型增强[59]。

为避免放射暴露，增强CT不常应用，尽管它能准确区分淋巴管、静脉和淋巴管静脉畸形。静脉石在CT上显示比在MRI上清晰。CT对评估骨内的血管畸形以及继发的骨改变更有价值。

血管造影是侵袭性的检查方法，很少应用于血管异常的诊断。它常常用于治疗性超选择性栓塞。血管造影（静脉造影）在评估和治疗某些静脉异常方面仍然有空间。

血管瘤治疗

观察

大多数血管瘤不需要治疗，但并不表明无事可做。首先，需要向家长全面细致地解释血管瘤的病程。照片记录对证实消退非常有用。通过定期的随访来评价肿瘤。经常观察是必要的，只要血管瘤巨大、溃疡、多发或位于解剖重要部位。

局部并发症：溃疡和出血

自发溃疡发生于5%的皮肤血管瘤，多位于口周或会阴部的血管瘤。经常更换尿布和大量使用隔离霜有助于预防溃疡。治疗主要为清洁换药，每日应用表面抗生素。如果焦痂形成，则需要更换敷料。溃疡的血管瘤常常在2周内再上皮化。曾报道脉冲染料激光治疗可减轻疼痛，促进创面愈合[1,62]。

血管瘤小点出血不常见，但常常吓坏父母亲。他们应该用干净的纱布压迫出血部位，维持压力10分钟。很少需要褥式缝合。

危险并发症的药物治疗

严重或危及生命的并发症是血管瘤药物治疗的指征。尽管约 20% 的血管瘤发生损伤、梗阻或危险的并发症，但只有不到 1% 是真正危及生命的。潜在的致命并发症包括充血性心力衰竭、气道梗阻、消化道出血等。

颈面部血管瘤能导致环状的上气道梗阻或吞咽困难。声门下的血管瘤在 6～8 周常常表现为隐匿的双相喘鸣，并可见颈面部的血管瘤。大的面部肿瘤生长扩张皮肤，并破坏正常的解剖结构。甚至很小的上眼睑血管瘤也能破坏角膜，导致散光以及继发弱视。病变累及边缘结构例如眼睑、唇、鼻孔、耳骨和耳廓时，可能遗留后
2104 遗症而难以手术纠治，此时也可以考虑药物治疗。

激素治疗

糖皮质激素仍然是治疗危重血管瘤的主要药物，阻止增殖，促进退化。糖皮质激素通过促进分化和抑制血管生成以加速血管瘤退化。它们主要的抗血管生成效应是抑制巨噬细胞分泌的血管生成前蛋白 VEGF 和 bFGF。而且，糖皮质激素抑制磷脂酶 A_2，该酶能释放花生四烯酸，是血管生成前因子前列腺素的前体[21]。最后，糖皮质激素抑制金属蛋白酶，金属蛋白酶通过分解细胞外基质促进血管生成[49]。

开始阶段选用泼尼松或泼尼松龙，2～3 mg/(kg·d)。对激素敏感的血管瘤 1 周内即有效果。通常，30% 的血管瘤消退加快，40% 处于稳定状态，30% 无反应。如果无反应，例如无色泽转淡、变软、生长消失，则甚至可考虑短期给予更高的治疗剂量至5 mg/(kg·d)，或更改药物。如果血管瘤有反应，疗程和剂量应根据瘤体部位和成熟度来调节。治疗 4～6 周后，剂量可减少。治疗后期，隔日口服能使疗效维持，并可减少药物并发症如生长迟缓和 Cushing 综合征样面容等。如剂量太小或药物撤退太快，可能出现反弹。激素治疗应持续至消退完全，平均治疗至 8～10 个月龄（图 130-9）。应密切监测患者副反应，如身体生长暂时减慢、Cushing 综合征样面容、行为变化（如易激惹、哭吵）、胃肠道溃疡、体重增加、感染、高血压或肥厚性心肌病。

瘤体内糖皮质激素注射适用于局限的面部血管瘤，尤其是位于上睑、鼻、颊、唇部的血管瘤。曾有

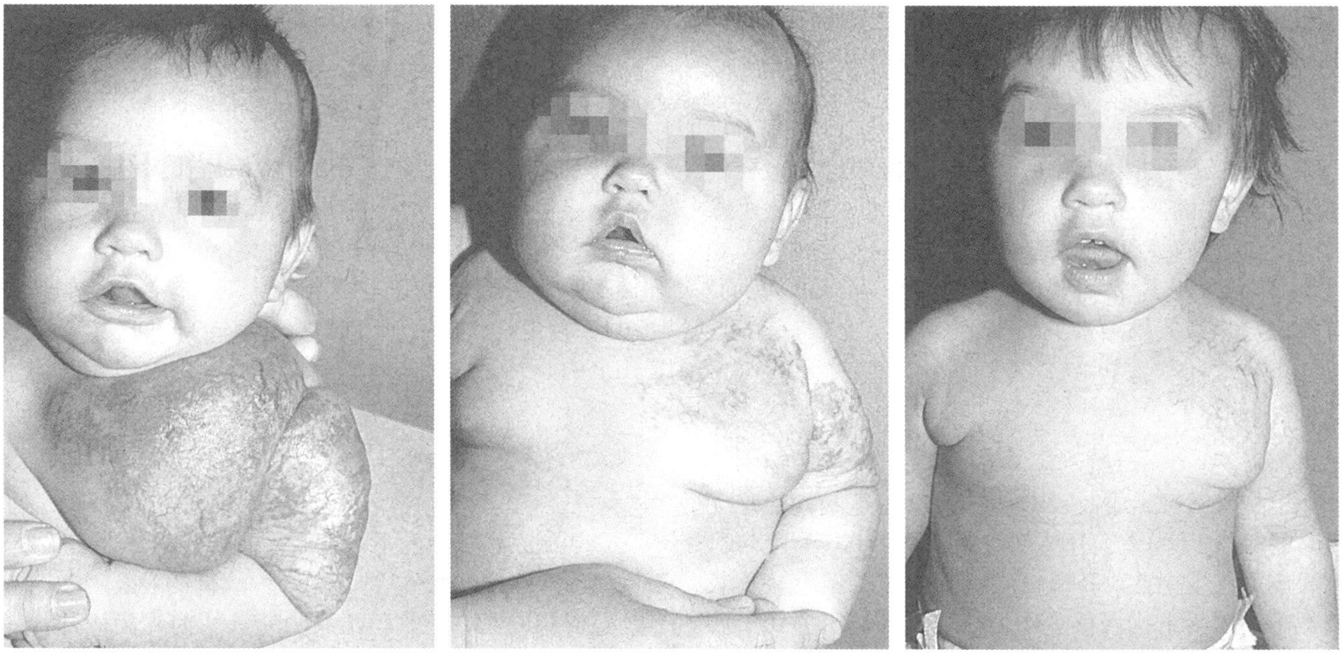

A　B　C

图 130-9　A. 3 个月女婴在胸部和上臂有一大的增殖期血管瘤。B. 口服糖皮质激素治疗 1 个月后（持续治疗 5 个月）。注意加速的消退和 Cushing 综合征面容。C. 1.5 岁时，持续自然消退。

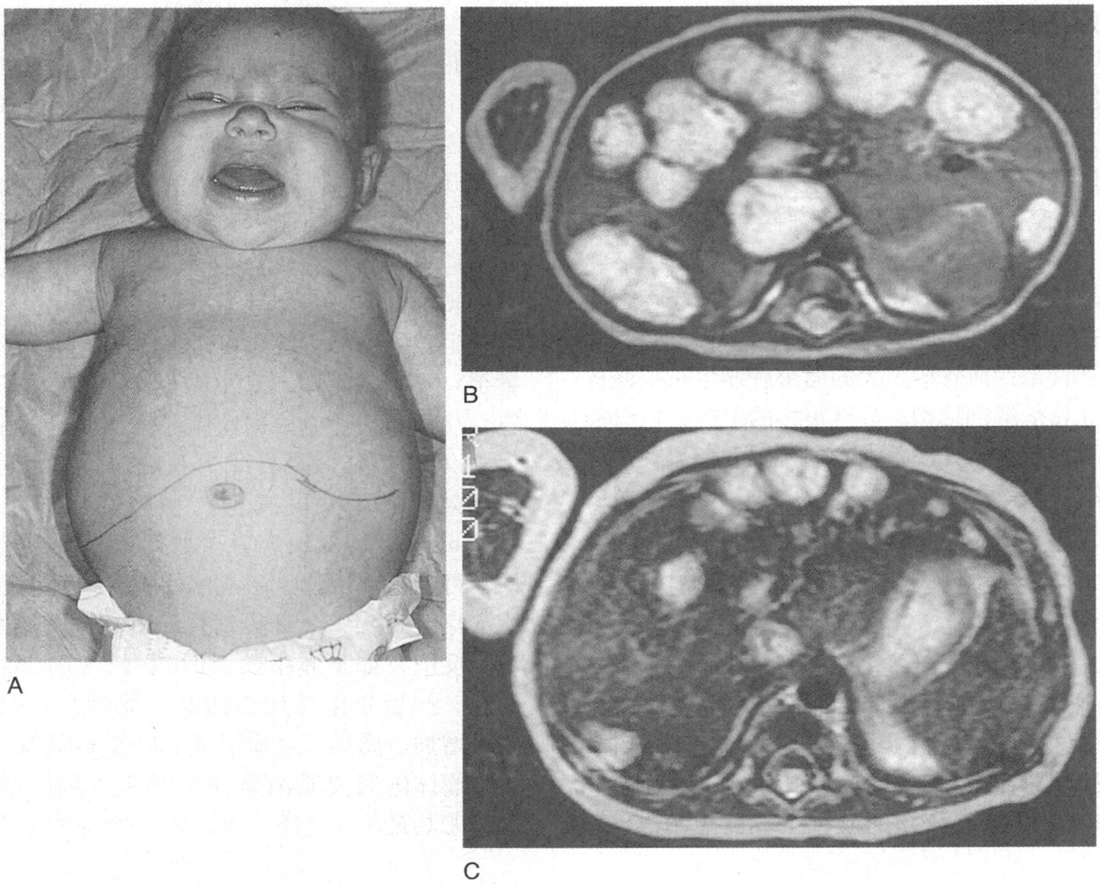

图 130-10　A. 婴儿多发肝内血管瘤导致充血性心力衰竭。B. 另一个孩子药物治疗前 MRI 显示多发肝内血管瘤（4 个月）。C. 第二个孩子接受 8 个月药物治疗后 MRI 影像。

2 例眶周血管瘤注射治疗后，由于视网膜动脉血栓性梗阻而致盲的报道，所以要保证小心、缓慢地注射[75]。曲安西龙注射应缓慢、低压，每次剂量不超过 3～5 mg/kg。常常需要 3～5 次注射，间隔 6～8 周。有效率与全身应用激素类似[52,80]。

其他药物

干扰素 α-2a 或 α-2b（IFN-α2）是激素治疗无效时的替换药物[28]。IFN 剂量为 200～300 万 IU/m^2，每天皮下注射一次。IFN 较激素起效慢，但直接比较较困难，因为干扰素很少作为一线用药，可能用于顽固性病变。IFN-α2 几乎促进所有的血管瘤以及大部分伴有血小板消耗的 KHE 的退化[8,28]。IFN-α2 治疗常常需要 6～12 个月（图 130-10）。因为 IFN-α2 治疗有显著的痉挛性双瘫的风险，尤其是小于 1 岁的婴儿[4,84]，所以它仅在经过慎重考虑后作为替代药物应 2105
用。接受 IFN-α2 治疗的儿童应该仔细评估神经系统和发育情况。作为治疗激素不敏感病变的干扰素的替代药物，每周低剂量静脉给予长春新碱（体重小于 20 kg 的儿童 0.5 mg/m^2 或 0.025 mg/kg）已于最近在几个中心开始应用[43]。

激光治疗

当激素治疗声门下血管瘤需要长时间才能有效时，激光治疗能抑制肿瘤[79]。有一种流行的观念：激光治疗对皮肤血管瘤有效。有些研究者认为光凝固法作用于早期的新生血管瘤，可以阻止肿瘤的扩张以及继发的并发症。脉冲染料激光治疗仅能渗透入真皮层 0.75～1.0 mm，能使血管瘤表面变淡[37]。尽管激光治疗对部分表浅血管瘤有效，但这部分血管瘤是可以自然消

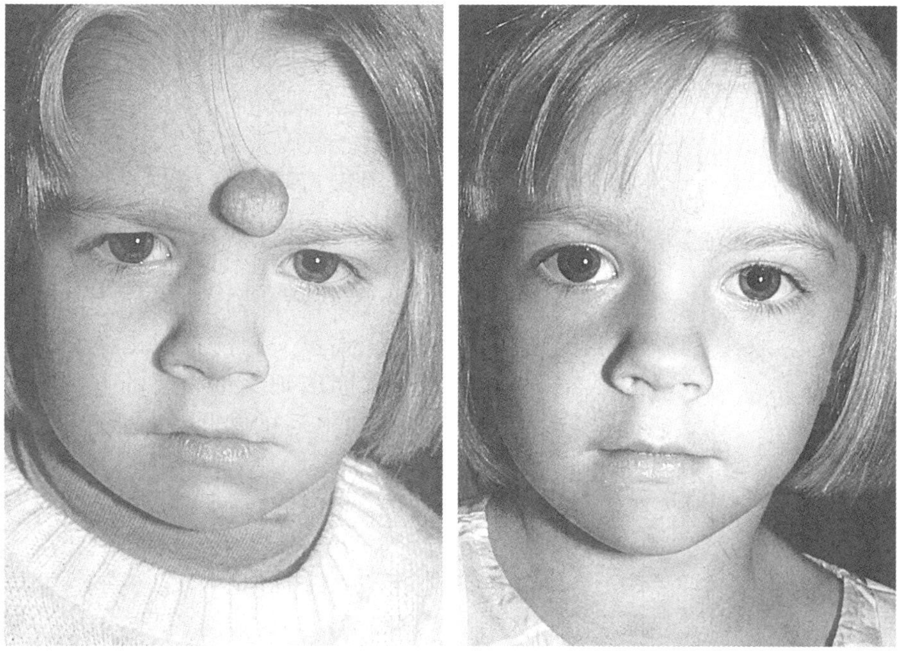

A　　B

图 130-11　A. 5 岁女孩前额带蒂的退化期血管瘤。B. 手术切除 2 个月后。

退的，而且消退后皮肤基本正常。对于深部或皮下血管瘤，没有证据表明反复的激光治疗能抑制其生长，促进其消退[77]。过度的激光治疗可能会导致皮肤丢失及永久的瘢痕，而且费用及时间的消耗亦是血管瘤反复激光治疗存在争议的问题。激光治疗对加速溃疡血管瘤的恢复是有用的[62]。对皮肤血管瘤消退后遗留的毛细血管扩张，激光治疗无疑是有效的。

外科手术

对局限的带蒂病变，尤其是部分瘤体反复出血、深部溃疡的病变，即使在增殖期也可考虑彻底手术切除（图 130-11）。眼睑血管瘤导致弱视，药物治疗无
2106 效，可手术切除以减轻对角膜的压力。

退化期血管瘤的切除，无论是分期手术还是完全手术，有时都是基于心理学的考虑。例如，一个大的唇部肿瘤或鼻尖部球状的血管瘤会使学龄前儿童感到不安。瘢痕的范围应该与儿童潜在的情感应激权衡。如果切除不可避免，瘢痕与血管瘤去除后效果相同，或瘢痕很易隐藏，这些都是可以手术的指征。

理想的是，退化相对完全（退化完全期）时经过很好计划后去除纤维脂肪组织和瘢痕或松弛的皮肤。凸出的血管瘤常常导致皮肤扩张，所以尽可能切除皮肤而不破坏正常解剖轮廓。瘢痕和实际组织缺失不常发生，这类副反应需要更复杂的重建步骤。

对于接近环形的病变，无论何时切除肿瘤，都能很好地标记，通过环形切除可立即到病变附近，用荷包缝合关闭，这种方法较传统的扁梭形切除和线形缝合要好。尽管 6～12 个月后需要二期手术，但最后的瘢痕远比较长的线状瘢痕好[66]。

肝血管瘤实质上从不需要切除。无症状的病变需要仔细观察，通过系列的体检和超声评估。大的单个的 RICH 型病变会迅速消退。对于高输出量心力衰竭，如果激素治疗无效，则可以由对婴儿治疗有经验的介入放射科医生进行高选择性的分流大血管栓塞，使之得到改善。除肝移植外，对肝脏被巨大弥漫性肿瘤占据导致腹腔间隙综合征的病例来说没有别的手术选择，这对于药物治疗无效而且不存在长期的重度甲状腺功能低下的病例是合理的考虑。

血管畸形的治疗

毛细血管畸形

脉冲染料激光治疗是婴儿和儿童毛细血管畸形的

标准治疗方法[3,83]。明显的淡化占病例的70%~80%，幼儿效果更好。脸部病变较肢体病变更有效。

淋巴管畸形

淋巴管畸形突然增大的两个原因是感染和瘤体内出血。淋巴管畸形的蜂窝织炎要求立即采用抗生素治疗。非激素类抗炎药物在这一疾病的加剧期也有益处。镇痛药、休息、时间对淋巴管畸形出血来说都是需要的。

手术切除是治愈这类畸形的唯一方法。需要分期手术时，每一次手术都要尽可能彻底地切除单一解剖
2107 区域的病变。广泛的病变即使经过多次手术也常常不能完整切除。不幸的是，脆弱的正常结构常常横跨畸形，而且深部的囊有大量的显微结构连接。术后即刻的并发症包括长期的引流、血肿和蜂窝织炎。疣状淋巴囊可在手术瘢痕内或附近产生。在手术后长期甚至数年，持续扩张的淋巴管畸形非常常见。

大囊性病变有时能用抽吸淋巴液再注入硬化剂如100%乙醇、十四烷基硫酸钠、博来霉素、OK-432（一种灭活的A型溶血性链球菌）等基本除去或至少减小[60,70]。不幸的是，硬化剂治疗后常见畸形持续或反复的肿胀。

淋巴管畸形累及纵隔结构或肺时令人苦恼。有些纵隔团块样病变多年无症状。大的病变可以手术切除或硬化剂治疗。更大的挑战是胸膜或心包积液或腹水发展，特别是当它们是乳糜液时。胸导管或中央淋巴导管的增强淋巴管造影可能有益，因为在某些情况下可能可以进行创新的个体化治疗[33]。

静脉畸形

弹力绷带支持袜治疗对肢体静脉畸形是必需的。低剂量阿司匹林对减轻栓塞发作的疼痛可能有效。静脉畸形可能通过手术切除或硬化剂治疗减轻。

直接对静脉畸形行注射治疗是有风险的，必须由训练有素的有经验的介入治疗医生进行。全身麻醉和实时荧光造影监测常常是需要的。局部压迫和其他操作防止高浓度的硬化剂进入体循环。局部并发症（如皮肤或黏膜起泡、全层坏死或神经损伤）和全身并发症（如肾毒性、一过性肺高压，甚至心搏停止）曾被报道。常常需要多次硬化剂治疗，可间隔几个月实施。静脉异常有再通或再发的倾向。

庞大的或广泛的软组织病变常常考虑手术切除。手足的静脉畸形切除对维持轮廓是有益的。失血可能是明显和快速的。有些病例术前硬化剂治疗对减少术中出血有用。肢体切除手术时止血带是有用的。多个大号的静脉内导管，以及准备好的血库和麻醉队伍是必需的。在伤口关闭前止住出血不太可能，然而皮肤关闭通常能达到少量止血的目的。患者和家属应预先被告知术后的血肿和伤口裂开常见，但是可处理的。

弥散的结肠静脉畸形导致严重出血，可通过部分结肠切除、肛门直肠黏膜剥离、结肠经肛门拖出等方法治疗[31]。注意避免损伤任何盆腔周围的静脉畸形，因为止血可能是不可能的。

蓝色橡皮疱痣综合征多发静脉畸形导致的出血可以通过单独根除每个病变来处理，可通过术中经口至肛门的全胃肠道内镜来鉴别[30]。尽管消耗时间长，但这一方法已成功地应用于初始10个患者中的9个，止住出血，并随访9年。在术前，这些患者需要上百次输血，术后则不再需要输血。

动静脉畸形（AVM）

AVM在婴儿和幼儿中常是静止的。虽然对无症状早期AVM进行栓塞或手术是有争议的，但是如果切除病变较容易而且没有严重的损伤，则上述方法可能是可行的。一般在儿童后期或青春期，当危险症状和体征增加时进行治疗（例如缺血性疼痛、顽固的皮肤溃疡、出血或高输出量心力衰竭）。

对一个AVM病灶采用高度选择性的动脉栓塞能减轻疼痛、出血或心力衰竭，尤其是那些外科手术可能导致肢体损毁或毁容的病例。栓塞仅能偶尔永久治愈AVM。单一的直接的动静脉连接提供了最乐观的可能。不能结扎动脉滋养血管或做近端栓塞。邻近动脉的迅速再通会供血给病灶，而且动脉结扎限制了以后对病灶进行合适的亚选择性动脉栓塞治疗。

外科手术用于彻底切除或暴露AVM。外科手术术前24~72小时行动脉栓塞能暂时性阻塞病灶。栓塞能减少术中出血，但不能改变切除的范围。畸形的

病灶必须广泛切除，常常包括覆盖的皮肤。手术切除原则与静脉畸形相似。栓塞与手术切除结合，之后必须监测患者，每年进行临床检查、超声或 MRI 检查。完全治愈不常见，但有可能。

复合血管畸形

对复杂病变基本上采取保守治疗。患有这种病变的儿童需要每年检查。对于病变累及肢体的病例，在 2 岁前要进行临床评估，通过放射学检查测量腿的长
2108 度。如果偏差大于 1.5 cm，就需要采用有跟鞋来防止跛行和背部的病变。骺骨干固定术能阻断较长肢体的生长，来匹配对侧肢体的生长，从而达到成人后最终的长度。MRI 和核磁共振血管造影能用来检测滋养动脉，鉴别异常静脉，判定深静脉系统是否有功能。弹力压迫袜被推荐应用于肢体静脉缺陷和深静脉有功能的病例。显著功能不全的曲张静脉有时可在儿童期手术治疗。已有报道在某些病例中重建深静脉系统[78]，但疗效可疑。在奇形怪状的肥大病例中，如果不能适合鞋或妨碍行走活动，则需要分期轮廓切除手术并可能需要选择截肢。躯干和会阴部复合血管畸形可以分期手术治疗。

（洪　莉译　夏慧敏校）

参考文献

1. Achauer BM, Vander Kam VM: Ulcerated anogenital hemangioma of infancy. Plast Reconstr Surg 1991; 87:861.
2. Amir J, Metzker A, Krikler R, et al: Strawberry hemangioma in preterm infants. Pediatr Dermatol 1986;3:331.
3. Ashinoff R, Geronemus RG: Flashlamp-pumped pulsed dye laser for port-wine stains in infancy: Earlier versus later treatment. J Am Acad Dermatol 1991;24:467.
4. Barlow CF, Priebe CJ, Mulliken JB, et al: Spastic diplegia as a complication of interferon alfa-2a treatment of hemangiomas of infancy. J Pediatr 1998;132:527.
5. Baskerville PA, Ackroyd JS, Lea Thomas M, et al: The Klippel-Trenaunay syndrome: Clinical, radiological and haemodynamic features and management. Br J Surg 1985; 72:232.
6. Bean WB: Blue Rubber-Bleb Nevi of the Skin and Gastrointestinal Tract. Springfield, IL, Charles C Thomas, 1958.
7. Beaubien ER, Ball NJ, Storwick GS: Kaposiform hemangioendothelioma: A locally aggressive vascular tumor. J Am Acad Dermatol 1998;38:799.
8. Berman B, Lim H: Concurrent cutaneous and hepatic hemangiomata in infancy: Report of a case and a review of the literature. J Dermatol Surg Oncol 1978;4:869.
9. Boon LM, Burrows PE, Paltiel HJ, et al: Hepatic vascular anomalies in infancy: A twenty-seven-year experience. J Pediatr 1996;129:346.
10. Boon LM, Enjolras O, Mulliken JB: Congenital hemangioma: Evidence of accelerated involution. J Pediatr 1996;128:329.
11. Boon LM, Fishman SJ, Lund DP, et al: Congenital fibrosarcoma masquerading as congenital hemangioma: Report of two cases. J Pediatr Surg 1995;30:1378.
12. Boon LM, Mulliken JB, Vikkula M, et al: Assignment of a locus for dominantly inherited venous malformations to chromosome 9p. Hum Mol Genet 1994;3:1583.
13. Bowers R, Graham, EA, Tomlinson KM: The natural history of strawberry nevus. Arch Dermatol 1960;82:667.
14. Boyd JB, Mulliken JB, Kaban LB, et al: Skeletal changes associated with vascular malformations. Plast Reconstr Surg 1984;74:789.
15. Brouillard P, Boon LM, Mulliken JB, et al: Mutations in a novel factor, glomulin, are responsible for glomuvenous malformations (“glomangiomas”). Am J Hum Genet 2002; 70:866.
16. Brouillard P, Vikkula M: Vascular malformations: Localized defects in vascular morphogenesis. Clin Genet 2003; 63:340.
17. Burge DM, Middleton AW, Kamath R, et al: Intestinal haemorrhage in Turner’s syndrome. Arch Dis Child 1981; 56:557.
18. Burman D, Mansell PW, Warin RP: Miliary haemangiomata in the newborn. Arch Dis Child 1967;42:193.
19. Burns AJ, Kaplan LC, Mulliken JB: Is there an association between hemangioma and syndromes with dysmorphic features? Pediatrics 1991;88:1257.
20. Cohen RC, Myers NA: Diagnosis and management of massive hepatic hemangiomas in childhood. J Pediatr Surg 1986;21:6.
21. Crum R, Szabo S, Folkman J: A new class of steroids inhibits angiogenesis in the presence of heparin or a heparin fragment. Science 1985;230:1375.
22. Dethlefsen SM, Mulliken JB, Glowacki J: An ultrastructural study of mast cell interactions in hemangiomas. Ultrastruct Pathol 1986;10:175.
23. Eerola I, Boon LM, Mulliken JB, et al: Capillary malformation–arteriovenous malformation, a new clinical and genetic disorder caused by *RASA1* mutations. Am J Hum Genet 2003;73:1240.
24. el-Dessouky M, Azmy AF, Raine PA, et al: Kasabach-Merritt syndrome. J Pediatr Surg 1988;23:109.
25. Enjolras O, Mulliken JB, Boon LM, et al: Noninvoluting congenital hemangioma: A rare cutaneous vascular anomaly. Plast Reconstr Surg 2001;107:1647.
26. Enjolras O, Riche MC, Merland JJ: Facial port-wine stains and Sturge-Weber syndrome. Pediatrics 1985;76:48.
27. Enjolras O, Riche MC, Merland JJ, et al: Management of alarming hemangiomas in infancy: A review of 25 cases. Pediatrics 1990;85:491.
28. Ezekowitz RA, Mulliken JB, Folkman J: Interferon alfa-2a therapy for life-threatening hemangiomas of infancy. N Engl J Med 1992;326:1456.
29. Finn MC, Glowacki J, Mulliken JB: Congenital vascular lesions: Clinical application of a new classification. J Pediatr Surg 1983;18:894.
30. Fishman SJ, Burrows PE, Leichtner AM, et al: Gastrointestinal

manifestations of vascular anomalies in childhood: Varied etiologies require multiple therapeutic modalities. J Pediatr Surg 1998;33:1163.
31. Fishman SJ, Burrows PE, Upton J, et al: Life-threatening anomalies of the thoracic duct: Anatomic delineation dictates management. J Pediatr Surg 2001;36:1269.
32. Fishman SJ, Fox VL: Visceral vascular anomalies. Gastrointest Endosc Clin N Am 2001;11:813.
33. Fishman SJ, Shamberger RC, Fox VL, et al: Endorectal pull-through abates gastrointestinal hemorrhage from colorectal venous malformations. J Pediatr Surg 2000; 35:982.
34. Fishman SJ, Smithers CJ, Folkman J, et al: Blue rubber bleb nevus syndrome: Surgical eradication of gastrointestinal bleeding. Ann Surg 2005;241:528.
35. Folkman J, Klagsbrun M: Angiogenic factors. Science 1987; 235:442.
36. Frieden IJ, Reese V, Cohen D: PHACE syndrome. The association of posterior fossa brain malformations, hemangiomas, arterial anomalies, coarctation of the aorta and cardiac defects, and eye abnormalities. Arch Dermatol 1996; 132:307.
37. Garden JM, Bakus AD, Paller AS: Treatment of cutaneous hemangiomas by the flashlamp-pumped pulsed dye laser: Prospective analysis. J Pediatr 1992;120:555.
38. Gascoyen M: Case of naevus involving the parotid gland, and causing death from suffocation. Trans Pathol Soc 1860;11:267.
39. Glowacki J, Mulliken JB: Mast cells in hemangiomas and vascular malformations. Pediatrics 1982;70:48.
40. Gorlin RJ, Kantaputra P, Aughton DJ, et al: Marked female predilection in some syndromes associated with facial hemangiomas. Am J Med Genet 1994;52:130.
41. Greene AK, Kieran M, Burrows PE, et al: Wilms tumor screening is unnecessary in Klippel-Trenaunay syndrome. Pediatrics 2004;113:e326.
42. Guttmacher AE, Marchuk DA, White RI Jr: Hereditary hemorrhagic telangiectasia. N Engl J Med 1995;333:918.
43. Haisley-Royster C, Enjolras O, Frieden LT, et al: Kasabach-Merritt phenomenon: A retrospective study of treatment with vincristine. J Pediatr Hematol Oncol 2002; 24:459.
44. Hayward PG, Orgill DP, Mulliken JB, et al: Congenital fibrosarcoma masquerading as lymphatic malformation: Report of two cases. J Pediatr Surg 1995;30:84.
45. Holmdahl K: Cutaneous hemangiomas in premature and mature infants. Acta Paediatr 1955;44:370.
46. Hopfel-Kreiner I: Histogenesis of hemangiomas—an ultrastructural study on capillary and cavernous hemangiomas of the skin. Pathol Res Pract 1980;170:70.
47. Huang SA, Tu HM, Harney JW, et al: Severe hypothyroidism caused by type 3 iodothyronine deiodinase in infantile hemangiomas. N Engl J Med 2000;343:185.
48. Huston J III, Forbes GS, Ruefenacht DA, et al: Magnetic resonance imaging of facial vascular anomalies. Mayo Clin Proc 1992;67:739.
49. Jones EW, Orkin M: Tufted angioma (angioblastoma). A benign progressive angioma, not to be confused with Kaposi's sarcoma or low-grade angiosarcoma. J Am Acad Dermatol 1989;20:214.
50. Kassarjian A, Zurakowski D, Dubois J, et al: Infantile hepatic hemangiomas: Clinical and imaging findings and their correlation with therapy. AJR Am J Roentgenol 2004;182:785.
51. Kisu T, Yamaoka K, Uchida Y, et al: A case of blue rubber bleb nevus syndrome with familial onset. Gastroenterol Jpn 1986;21:262.
52. Kushner BJ: The treatment of periorbital infantile hemangioma with intralesional corticosteroid. Plast Reconstr Surg 1985;76:517.
53. Langer JC, Fitzgerald PG, Desa D, et al: Cervical cystic hygroma in the fetus: Clinical spectrum and outcome. J Pediatr Surg 1990;25:58.
54. Margileth AM, Museles M: Cutaneous hemangiomas in children. Diagnosis and conservative management. JAMA 1965;194:523.
55. Marler JJ, Fishman SJ, Kilroy SM, et al: Increased expression of urinary matrix metalloproteinases parallels the extent and progression of vascular anomalies. Pediatrics 2005;116:35.
56. Marler JJ, Fishman SJ, Upton J, et al: Prenatal diagnosis of vascular anomalies. J Pediatr Surg 2002;37:318.
57. Marsh DJ, Kum JB, Lunetta KL, et al: PTEN mutation spectrum and genotype-phenotype correlations in Bannayan-Riley-Ruvalcaba syndrome suggest a single entity with Cowden syndrome. Hum Mol Genet 1999;8:1461.
58. Martinez-Perez D, Fein NA, Boon LM, et al: Not all hemangiomas look like strawberries: Uncommon presentations of the most common tumor of infancy. Pediatr Dermatol 1995;12:1.
59. Meyer JS, Hoffer FA, Barnes PD, et al: Biological classification of soft-tissue vascular anomalies: MR correlation. AJR Am J Roentgenol 1991;157:559.
60. Molitch HI, Unger EC, Witte CL, et al: Percutaneous sclerotherapy of lymphangiomas. Radiology 1995; 194:343.
61. Montesano R, Vassalli JD, Baird A, et al: Basic fibroblast growth factor induces angiogenesis in vitro. Proc Natl Acad Sci U S A 1986;83:7297.
62. Morelli JG, Tan OT, Weston WL: Treatment of ulcerated hemangiomas with the pulsed tunable dye laser. Am J Dis Child 1991;145:1062.
63. Mulliken JB: Cutaneous vascular anomalies. Semin Vasc Surg 1993;6:204.
64. Mulliken JB, Fishman SJ, Burrows PE: Vascular anomalies. Curr Probl Surg 2000;37:517.
65. Mulliken JB, Glowacki J: Hemangiomas and vascular malformations in infants and children: A classification based on endothelial characteristics. Plast Reconstr Surg 1982;69:412.
66. Mulliken JB, Rogers GF, Marler JJ: Circular excision of hemangioma and purse-string closure: The smallest possible scar. Plast Reconstr Surg 2002;109:1544.
67. Mulliken JB, Young AE: Vascular Birthmarks: Hemangiomas and Malformations. Philadelphia, WB Saunders; 1988.
68. Noel AA, Gloviczki P, Cherry KJ Jr, et al: Surgical treatment of venous malformations in Klippel-Trenaunay syndrome. J Vasc Surg 2000;32:840.
69. North PE, Waner M, Mizeracki A, et al: A unique microvascular phenotype shared by juvenile hemangiomas and human placenta. Arch Dermatol 2001;137:559.
70. Ogita S, Tsuto T, Deguchi E, et al: OK-432 therapy for unresectable lymphangiomas in children. J Pediatr Surg 1991; 26:263.
71. Padwa BL, Hayward PG, Ferraro NF, et al: Cervicofacial lymphatic malformation: Clinical course, surgical intervention, and pathogenesis of skeletal hypertrophy. Plast Reconstr Surg 1995;95:951.
72. Pasyk KA, Cherry GW, Grabb WC, et al: Quantitative evaluation of mast cells in cellularly dynamic and adynamic vascular malformations. Plast Reconstr Surg 1984; 73:69.

73. Patrice SJ, Wiss K, Mulliken JB: Pyogenic granuloma (lobular capillary hemangioma): A clinicopathologic study of 178 cases. Pediatr Dermatol 1991;8:267.
74. Reese V, Frieden LT, Paller AS, et al: Association of facial hemangiomas with Dandy-Walker and other posterior fossa malformations. J Pediatr 1993;122:379.
75. Ruttum MS, Abrams GW, Harris GJ, et al: Bilateral retinal embolization associated with intralesional corticosteroid injection for capillary hemangioma of infancy. J Pediatr Ophthalmol Strabismus 1993;30:4.
76. Sarkar M, Mulliken JB, Kozakewich HP, et al: Thrombocytopenic coagulopathy (Kasabach-Merritt phenomenon) is associated with kaposiform hemangioendothelioma and not with common infantile hemangioma. Plast Reconstr Surg 1997;100:1377.
77. Scheepers JH, Quaba AA: Does the pulsed tunable dye laser have a role in the management of infantile hemangiomas? Observations based on 3 years' experience. Plast Reconstr Surg 1995;95:305.
78. Servelle M: Klippel and Trenaunay's syndrome. 768 operated cases. Ann Surg 1985;201:365.
79. Sie KC, McGill T, Healy GB: Subglottic hemangioma: Ten years' experience with the carbon dioxide laser. Ann Otol Rhinol Laryngol 1994;103:167.
80. Sloan GM, Reinisch JF, Nichter LS, et al: Intralesional corticosteroid therapy for infantile hemangiomas. Plast Reconstr Surg 1989;83:459.
81. Stenninger E, Schollin J: Diffuse neonatal haemangiomatosis in a newborn child. Acta Paediatr 1993;82:102.
82. Takahashi K, Mulliken JB, Kozakewich HP, et al: Cellular markers that distinguish the phases of hemangioma during infancy and childhood. J Clin Invest 1994;93:2357.
83. Tan OT, Sherwood K, Gilchrest BA: Treatment of children with port-wine stains using the flashlamp-pulsed tunable dye laser. N Engl J Med 1989;320:416.
84. Vesikari T, Nuutila A, Cantell K: Neurologic sequelae following interferon therapy of juvenile laryngeal papilloma. Acta Paediatr Scand 1988;77:619.
85. Virchow R: Angiome. In Die Krankhaften Geshwulste. Berlin, Hirschwald, 1863.
86. Wegner G: Ueber Lymphangiome. Arch Klin Chir 1877;20:641.
87. Zukerberg LR, Nickoloff BJ, Weiss SW: Kaposiform hemangioendothelioma of infancy and childhood. An aggressive neoplasm associated with Kasabach-Merritt syndrome and lymphangiomatosis. Am J Surg Pathol 1993;17:321.

第 131 章

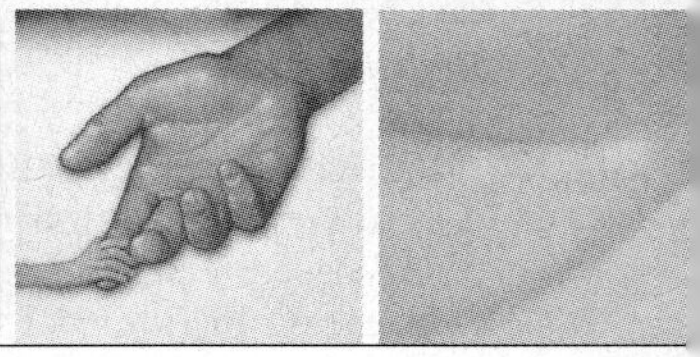

动脉疾病

James A. O'Neill, Jr.

2111 许多疾病可能会影响动脉系统。虽然单发的病种很稀少，但当累积在一起时，动脉疾病就相当多见了。表 131-1 列举了最常见的影响到动脉树的疾病，应用了一个有用的分类，包括先天性畸形、结缔组织疾病和获得性疾病。

先天性畸形

先天性动脉瘤

先天性动脉瘤很少见，常偶然发现，可能会影响任何动脉，但内脏动脉最常受影响[58]。先天性动脉瘤的破裂更不常见，尽管当血流紊乱或邻近的肾动脉分支受压而使肾动脉分支受影响时，其导致的高血压较常见。Kim 和同事曾报道一个 3 周大的婴儿患有先天性腹主动脉瘤伴有肾血管性高血压[33]。Latter 和同事描述了产前 B 超发现一个孕 34 周的胎儿患腹主动脉瘤[36]。目前这类病变的产前诊断较常见[41]。这些病例证明了某些动脉瘤的先天性特性，与获得性的病变相区分。Sarkar 及其同事指出大部分先天性动脉瘤的儿童在 5 岁前显现症状，并且这类病变常见于腹主动脉或其初始的分支，而不在四肢[66]。然而，我们和其他人偶尔见到婴儿和小龄儿童在肢体近端的动脉分支或在颅内动脉有先天性动脉瘤。这类病变是囊形或梭形的（图 131-1）。这类动脉瘤的病理学检查常常显示中层不发育所致的扩张，但不能说明深入的病因。Senzaki 和同事发表了他们观察到的儿童中与年龄相关的动脉弹性特征性改变[69]。这些研究证实外周和近端动脉壁的扩张性在出生后逐渐下降，于是问题出现了：为什么有些婴儿在某些动脉部位早熟而丧失弹性组织？尽管先天性动脉瘤在儿童中是单发的，但偶尔有报道描述了多发脏器的动脉瘤[67]。我们的经验与 Guzzetta 一样，在发病顺序上，先天性脏器动脉瘤最常发生于脾、肝及肾动脉，居于腹主动脉瘤之后[27]。我们曾见到一例 8 岁儿童患肾动脉瘤。

先天性动脉瘤在许多状态下显示为静止的，除非与临床症状相关，例如高血压、头痛或可触及的搏动的肿块。核磁共振血管造影（MRA）、CT 血管造影（CTA）或标准血管造影可确诊[46]。

因为先天性脏器动脉瘤如此不常见，而且很少见到破裂的报道，所以手术指征不确定。然而，根据我们见到的破裂动脉瘤的大小以及文献报道，我们认为如果脏器动脉瘤直径大于 2 cm 或者正在扩大，则需要修补。适当的治疗有手术切除，以及用自体或假体材料行动脉重建。尽管偶尔有动脉结扎的报道，但从生长和发育的观点来看，重建是最好的。无论是否可能，因为生长的需要我们喜欢应用自体材料重建。然而，Latter 和同事[36]以及 Saad 和 May[62]报道了应用假体材料成功地进行了主动脉重建。我们曾经应用栓塞的方法成功治愈了一例下极脾动脉动脉瘤，依靠胃短血管给予双侧血供。我们应用自体静脉治疗肾外的肾动脉瘤，予以切除和重建。Konan 和同事描述了经动脉的伴有脊髓动静脉畸形（AVMS）的动脉瘤栓塞[35]。Redekop 和同事描述了采用不同方法治疗伴有脑动静脉畸形的动脉瘤[59]。

动静脉畸形（AVM） 2112

大部分 AVM 是外周的和局限的（见第 130 章）。Szilagyi 和同事描述了根据胚胎分化程度进行的 AVM

表 131-1　动脉系统疾病分类

先天性畸形
动脉瘤
先天性缺失
畸形
动静脉畸形

结缔组织疾病
Marfan 综合征
Ehlers-Danlos 综合征
家族性囊性中层坏死
Turner 综合征
胱氨酸贮积症
肢骨纹状肥大

获得性疾病
与 Ehlers-Danlos 综合征相关的动脉瘤
Kawasaki 病
发育不良
创伤
感染
血栓形成
栓塞
炎症和免疫闭塞综合征
Williams 综合征
亚急性细菌性心内膜炎
中主动脉综合征
肾血管性高血压
小动脉疾病

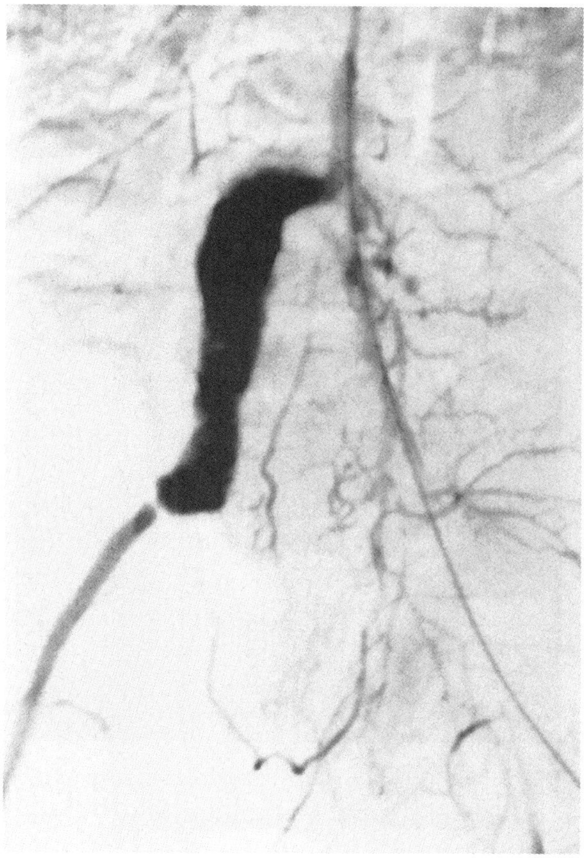

图 131-1　这个血管造影显示一个 4 岁男孩的髂总动脉先天性梭状动脉瘤，最终需要切除和通过插入移植重建。

分类，从微瘘型到大瘘型（图 131-2）[78]。Upton 和同事指出这类畸形根据动脉组分的尺寸和性质分为慢流和快流[85]。快流或微瘘型很难通过血管造影证实，症状和体征是轻微的；然而大瘘型临床表现明显，容易通过血管造影证实（见图 131-2）。尽管先天性 AVM 较常见，但幸运的是广泛的危及生命的类型十分少见。Tice 和同伴[81]以及 Upton 和同事[85]发现一半 AVM 发生在四肢，尤其是下肢。尽管许多报道证明上肢和颈部的 AVM 更可能产生生理后果，但是我们曾治疗过两个儿童，分别为 8 岁和 12 岁，盆腔和大腿患有广泛的 AVM，伴有严重的充血性心力衰竭。临床上浅表 AVM 可能表现为不同的血管瘤、血管痣，甚至为动静脉瘤性静脉曲张，常见于腿部。后者最早由 Parkes Weber 于 1907 年描述，当时他报道了这样的畸形伴有肢体的半身肥大[54]。在后一种情况中，肢体的过度生长不依赖于与这种病变相关的微瘘型 AVM。然而，对于一个肢体上的独立的大瘘型 AVM，受累肢体的迟发过度生长是由于血流增强和核心温度增高导致骨骺加速生长。Knudsen 和 Alden 报道了一个大范围的对小于 6 个月的小婴儿 AVM 的综述；AVM 见于头、颈、肠道、肝、肺和中央静脉系统，常常伴有严重的局部和全身的生理效应[34]。

症状和体征

AVM 最常见的症状和体征有疼痛、皮肤毁容、肢体或面部的肿胀。伴有搏动的静脉曲张、皮肤溃疡、出血以及邻近受累骨骼和软组织的过度生长常见于四肢的病变。AVM 相关的症状和体征在躯体的其他部位是不同的。例如在肠道，出血是最常见的表现，病变常常是多发的[10]；在肝脏，病变常常分类

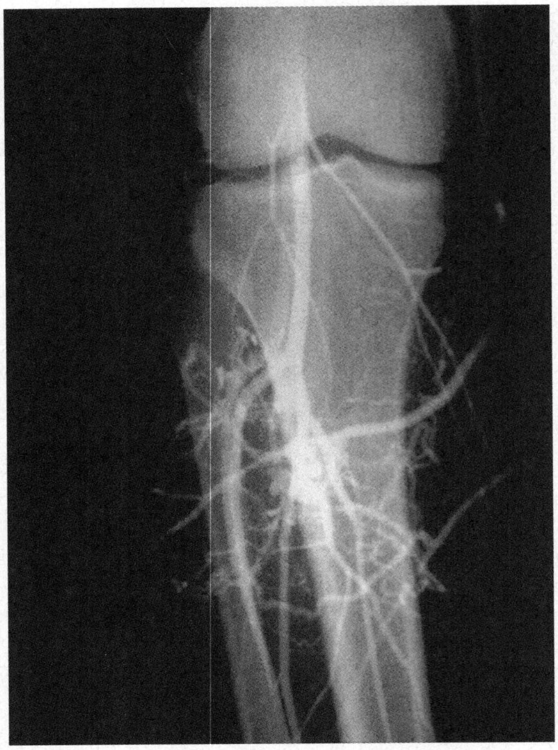

图 131-2　患儿表现为腿痛、肿胀和少许浅表静脉扩张。此处动脉造影显示一个大瘘型动静脉畸形伴有早期的静脉充盈。这种类型的病变大多不能完全切除。

为血管内皮瘤，由大的分流导致的顽固性充血性心力衰竭较常见，尤其在新生儿；肺 AVM 可能无症状，
2113 或伴有脑的栓塞性感染并发症。中枢神经系统的畸形产生抽搐，或由于颅内出血或压迫重要生命结构导致相应的症状。Knudsen 和 Alden 报道在小于 6 个月的小婴儿中，身体不同部位的有症状的 AVM 常常伴发难治性高输出量充血性心力衰竭[34]。

诊断

皮内或皮下有搏动的静脉曲张所伴有的多汗症和局部皮温升高是明显的体检发现，并且曲张静脉听诊和触诊可能表现为震颤和杂音。有趣的是，大而深的 AVM 可能伴有相关皮肤表面不明显的小血管瘤。多普勒检查常常显示大瘘连接的连续信号特征。先天性 AVM 典型的血管造影特点是：动脉扩张和扭曲、相关扩张血管的早期充盈、动静脉间连接的表现以及在动静脉管道间染料搞成泥浆样。然而后几种典型表现并非出现在所有病例中，仅在 60% 的 Szilagyi 病例中出现。血管造影可能不能证明广泛扩散的微瘘畸形，在这些病例中，可能需要皮肤和肌肉血流测定和对照的静脉血氧饱和度来建立诊断。Tanaka 和同事评估了脑 AVM 的血管结构，用血管造影将它们区分为动静脉瘘（AVF）型和丛型[80]。之后他们研究了这两种颅内 AVM 血管造影类型的组织学切片，发现二者是相似的。有趣的是，他们发现在病变的一侧有许多单个的血管与深部血管连接，而在另一侧与引流血管吻合。动静脉瘘和丛状类型的唯一区别是丛状类型基本上是 AVF 成球形。与创伤性 AVF 比较，先天性 AVM 通常有滋养动脉和引流静脉的复杂网络，限制了栓塞和结扎的价值。头颈部 AVM 中，有超过三分之一的病变累及深部的骨骼。我们曾遇到过患者在拔牙后大出血，是一个先前未被怀疑的 AVM 的最先表现。

尽管多普勒检查是一个非常好的扫描检查，但 MRA 或 CTA 可以提供更多的信息，尤其是对于广泛的畸形。在试图外科手术切除之前获得血管造影仍很重要，因为可以显示准确的解剖细节，但有可能最终被 MRA 或 CTA 取代。另外，术前栓塞是有用的技术，可用来控制手术中的出血。

治疗

第 130 章描述了治疗 AVM 的不同方法。非手术治疗对大多数 AVM 可以是有效的，尤其是症状限制在扩张的静脉或病变太广泛使切除不那么有效时。在这种情况下，外部弹力袜支持常常是最好的办法。使用弹力袜可使病变改善或至少保持稳定。

至于广泛 AVM 的手术治疗，单纯结扎或栓塞大的滋养血管是无效的，并常伴有并发症，例如组织广泛坏死。结扎后，这种 AVM 迅速发展侧支血流。另外，结扎可能阻碍应用术前栓塞来控制出血。对于颈内动脉受累病例，如果施行结扎并且大量侧支出现，那么在这之后应用栓塞是禁忌的，因为有颅内梗死的风险。我们保留先应用栓塞作为术前的治疗，尽管如果他们不幸成为手术候选者或拒绝广泛的根除手术，而可能进行一系列的长时间栓塞治疗。我们在切除术前 24 小时进行栓塞，因为栓塞之后侧支保持不变。限制性的手术切除常常导致症状复发和侧支循环形

成，所以目标应是尽可能完全切除畸形。

2114 对微瘘型 AVM，如伴有 Klippel-Trenaunay 综合征的病例，Gloviczki 和同事推荐用弹力袜压迫治疗，这常常是成功的[24]。有时部分切除皮肤病变可能对使用可压缩衣服支持有益。McCullough 和 Kenwright 的长期研究显示外科手术对处理下肢肥大常常有效[42]。不幸的是，尚没有理想可靠的方法治疗头颈部广泛的 AVM。尽管部分切除或血管造影栓塞能暂时减轻症状，如 Iglesia 和 Fellows 显示的那样[30]，但复发是常见的，尽管并不总是像开始时的表现那样严重。我们观察到盆腔或内脏的局部病变在栓塞治疗后明显改善。先天性 AVM 的患者大多都需要长期的多种形式的治疗，根据维护适当功能的原则明智地选择。最后，许多躯体广泛 AVM 的患者都不幸地需要截肢。

结缔组织疾病

最常见的结缔组织疾病可能是 Marfan 综合征。1896 年，Marfan 描述了一种常染色体显性遗传性疾病的特征性体形：高个、瘦弱、蜘蛛样指趾伴有关节的过度伸展性、眼晶状体脱位、下胸部隆起[40]。后来认识到随着患 Marfan 综合征个体的长大，他们也出现自发性气胸、腹股沟疝以及升主动脉动脉瘤，累及主动脉弓和冠状血管。Marfan 综合征的特征是进行性的退行性变，倾向于减少这些个体的寿命。这些患者血管疾病的特征是由于异常的弹力组织，致使中层囊性坏死伴有内层破裂。有可能根据皮肤活检诊断 Marfan 综合征。Wilson 及同伴研究证明，Marfan 综合征的心血管并发症是由于微纤维蛋白（一种主要的血管结缔组织组分）结构和功能的改变所致[90]。含微纤维蛋白的微纤维与内皮细胞相关，随后的研究表明在这些患者中血流调节的内皮细胞依赖的血管扩张受损。

其他胶原生成的疾病也可导致大动脉中层变性的发展，伴有动脉瘤形成和破裂。其中一种是 Ehlers-Danlos 综合征，一种遗传性疾病，以皮肤弹性过度和易损伤为特点。虽然后一种综合征动脉瘤常常在髂部和四肢发展，但腹主动脉常常受累（图 131-3）。Ehlers-Danlos 综合征的血管形式很可能与动脉瘤Ⅳ型相关，在Ⅲ型中胶原或缺失或数量异常[57]。后一种类型是由于Ⅲ型胶原基因（*COL3A1*）突变。除了动脉瘤形成和破裂外，肠道和尿道的破裂也是这种综合征的并发症。有趣的是这种Ⅲ型胶原的异常类型在典型的症状严重的综合征患者和轻度表现的患者中均可见到。因此，与基因（*COL3A1*）相关的Ⅲ型胶原异常可显示表型谱，但不能预示疾病的严重程度。尽管大部分有严重综合征的患者可在一种或两种主要并发症下存活，但Ⅳ型患者倾向于在青春期死亡。

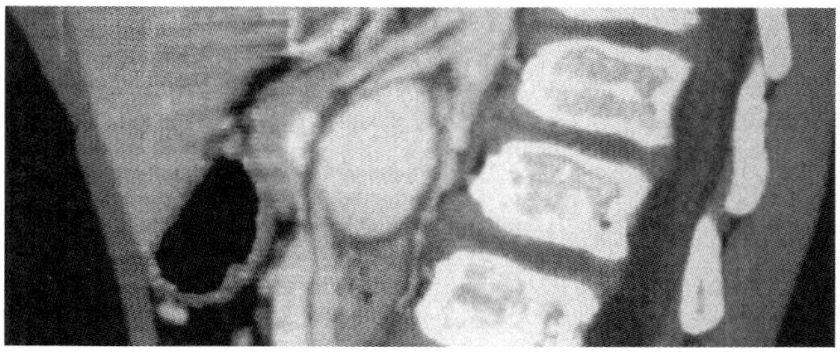

图 131-3　CT 血管造影显示一个 Ehlers-Danlos 综合征患儿体内的与腹部疼痛相关的肠系膜上动脉动脉瘤。这类患儿最好避免侵入性诊断步骤。

其他导致囊性中层退化变性和动脉瘤形成的疾病包括结核性硬化症、家族性囊性中层坏死、Turner 综合征、胱氨酸贮积症和肢骨纹状肥大[56]。最后一种情况包括一个或多个骨骨质增生伴有动脉瘤，尤其在锁骨下或腋动脉部位[2]。

如果怀疑有动脉瘤，常常应用多普勒影像检查和血管造影，除非是 Ehlers-Danlos 综合征Ⅳ型，但非侵入性方法如 MRA 或 CTA 则更好。一旦动脉瘤被确诊，应予切除，用假体移植物替代。这种方法常常成功应用于大多数此类结缔组织疾病的患者，除了 Ehlers-Danlos 综合征。因为这种疾病的血管胶原基质缺乏，缝合和钳夹受累血管可能导致血管壁破裂，使手术处理困难或不能手术。Cikrit 和同事提醒因为血管的易脆性应注意动脉修补[9]。如果手术不可避免，有时利用聚四氟乙烯树脂（Teflon）补片包裹动脉瘤或可能时仔细结扎近端和外周动脉瘤的远端。另外，Ehlers-Danlos 综合征患者处理较困难，有额外的出血和其他并发症[22]。

获得性疾病

动脉瘤

获得性动脉瘤常常由于外伤而导致（见第 22

章)。创伤性动脉瘤大多是假性动脉瘤，倾向于进行
2115 性增大。它们与钝性创伤或医源性动脉穿刺或透析损伤有关。假性动脉瘤的初期治疗可用压迫或栓塞，偶尔行切除和重建。栓塞引起的细菌性心内膜炎可能导致受累血管壁退化变性，常常自发性破裂，这已被 Nakayama 和同事证实[49]。急诊处理时常常要另外处理心脏病变。

Kawasaki 病可能产生单个或多个动脉瘤，可发生在身体任何部位。最常见和最常考虑到的是冠状动脉动脉瘤。该病的特征是手掌或足底疹、红斑和水肿，咽炎，结膜炎，颈部腺病及关节炎。大约 15% 的患者发展成冠状动脉动脉瘤，但近四分之一的患者超声心动图异常。除了患病儿童胆囊积水的发生率较高外，儿童冠状动脉动脉瘤表现与年轻成人可相似。小的、无症状的冠状动脉动脉瘤偶尔可以治愈，但大的动脉瘤发生栓子和心肌梗死的风险很高[1]。冠状动脉瘤要求冠状动脉搭桥，因为根本的问题是心肌缺血。与 Kawasaki 病相关的外周动脉动脉瘤常常是多发的、小的、梭状的，并且有自限性，常常不需要治疗，除非它们正在扩张并有症状。腋动脉是最常受累的血管[61]。

其他导致获得性动脉瘤的原因是巨细胞动脉炎、结节性多动脉炎及其他类型动脉炎。

表 131-2 动脉血栓和栓塞的原因

直接血管损伤
动脉和静脉置管
不慎外科损伤
注射刺激性和血管活性药物、麻醉药
医源性诊断损伤
肢体创伤
压迫
绷带、管形石膏和骨骼牵引
农场损伤
骨折

围生期原因
早产
败血症
难产或分娩
弥散性血管内凝血

其他
败血症
先天性心脏病
糖尿病
血管炎和胶原病
热损伤、电损伤
血管异常
肿瘤
放射
镰状红细胞病

血栓和栓塞

表 131-2 列出了导致动脉栓塞和栓子的多种原因。偶见患者，主要是婴儿，发生自发性动脉血栓。髂外动脉最易发生动脉血栓，不同脏器动脉及上肢近端血管也较易累及。婴儿血管容积相对较小，当败血症或其他原因导致慢流状态发生时尤其有风险。新生儿红细胞相对增多并且血液具有高黏度。Colburn 和同事研究显示有的婴儿，尤其是糖尿病母亲的后代，有严重的与高黏度综合征有关的发生在外周和脏器动脉内的栓子，或偶尔有大动脉分支的栓子[10]。与此相关的最早报道可能是 1914 年由 Von Khautz 列出的直到 15 岁的儿童个案报道[87]。从那时起有许多报道描述了自发性动脉血栓形成的病例，尤其在新生儿，大多与肢体坏疽和红细胞增多症或生理上不稳定有关。然而，在很多情况下原因不明。但有一点是明确的，即某些病例血栓形成开始于子宫。

我们发现栓子事件通常为一种模式。婴儿最常见的与红细胞增多症相关的脏器栓子表现为节段性肠坏死。与慢流状态和败血症相关的栓子倾向于导致肢体远端部位的皮肤坏死，以小血管栓子的模式出现。与栓塞和栓子有关的凝固性疾病包括镰状红细胞病、白血病、细菌性心内膜炎等[14,82]。与后面的疾病相关的栓塞和栓子程度有限，常常不需要手术干预。对婴儿高黏度综合征和红细胞增多症的处理可能需要血浆置换或换血，另外也可能需要溶栓、血栓切除或血管修补。如果有额外的凝血缺陷使这些婴儿具有颅内出血的相关风险，则不能采用动脉内灌注溶栓药物，例如组织纤维蛋白溶酶原激活剂（tPA）或尿激酶[77]。我们已成功地将这些技术用于某些没有并发症的患者。

由金黄色葡萄球菌及其他微生物导致的细菌性

心内膜炎患者常有栓塞并发症的风险。栓塞最初导致外周或脏器的梗阻，偶尔伴有真菌性动脉瘤形成。我们曾报道过治疗 8 例在主动脉瓣或二尖瓣有金黄色葡萄球菌心内膜炎的患者，他们产生主动脉或髂血管动脉瘤破裂，都需要分期修补[49]。然而，
2116 由其他微生物所致的细菌性心内膜炎导致的外周栓子常常只需要切除。根据我们的经验，发生大的外周血管栓子的最常见部位是股动脉，但发生在所有大的分支病变的梗阻均有报道。所以对细菌性心内膜炎患者必须仔细监测超声心动图，如果观察到瓣膜赘生物脱落，必须仔细寻找外周栓塞的临床证据。如果要避免血管变性和和真菌性动脉瘤，必须彻底取出感染性栓子。一旦发现感染性动脉瘤，必须治疗，在小年龄患儿中可行栓子切除或分期修复，但在大儿童和青春期患者中最好是切除和如果可能行另外的解剖旁路（图 131-4）。

我们也碰到过由于脐动脉插管引起血栓性或栓塞性并发症的患者。在一些病例中，这类并发症可能与葡萄球菌感染有关，继而导致真菌性动脉瘤形成。早先我们曾报道过一个包括 41 例患者的研究，病例的血栓或栓塞表现不同，与脐动脉插管有关，

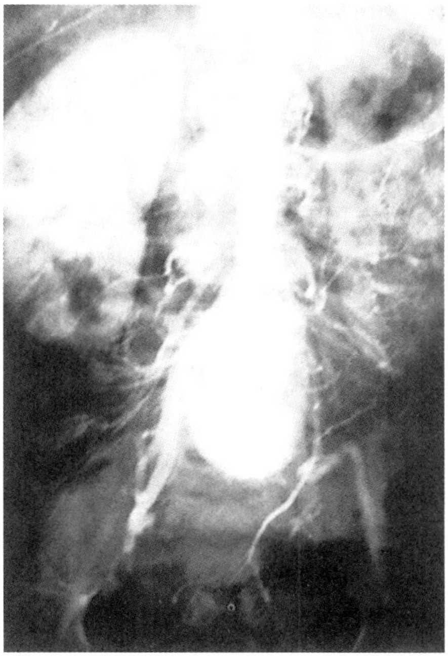

图 131-4　主动脉造影显示一个有细菌性心内膜炎二尖瓣疾病的 5 岁男孩有主髂动脉真菌性动脉瘤。动脉瘤因为渗漏被切除，之后的分期假体修复成功进行。

他们中大部分通过手术治疗[43]。Mendeloff 和同事最近报道了一个包括 46 例病例的综述，其中包括他们自己的 1 例与脐动脉插管有关的真菌性主动脉动脉瘤[44]。他们提出一种处理这类患者的规则，与我们的方法一致。从我们先前的报道开始，我们用动脉内灌注尿激酶或组织纤维蛋白溶酶原激活剂（tPA）的方法处理了几例这样的婴儿，80% 的病例取得成功。在主动脉或大分支梗阻的情况下，部分机体的存活遭受威胁，如果溶栓治疗不能立即解决问题，应行血栓切除。

除了上面提到的血栓和栓塞的病因外，Nehler 和同事报道的医源性血管损伤也是血栓和栓塞的常见原因[50]。他们指出这种损伤频率增加是因为腔内血管成形术和支架应用增加，这些都要求大号的动脉穿刺。他们进一步指出不同的内在血管装置是医源性血管损伤的来源，损伤范围从动脉破裂到血栓形成和栓塞。因为儿童血管尺寸更小、发生血液低流状态的频率更高，故如 Flanagan 和同事指出的，血栓和栓塞常发生于儿童[21]。脐、桡、肱、股和腋动脉是最常见的动脉通路，侵入过程常常与动脉痉挛和血栓形成有关。已经认识到最好不要通过动脉径路输注大量的液体和给予药物，因为有坏疽的高危风险。下列药物如碳酸氢钠、戊巴比妥、各种抗生素或收缩性药物可能导致痉挛、血栓和外周坏疽。尽管心脏插管偶尔必须通过腋动脉进行，但这一通路明显与上肢坏疽的发生率有关。应尽可能应用股动脉通路。在这些病例中如果临床有明显的外周缺血，并且可能发生明显的坏疽，则应考虑溶栓药物输注、血栓切除或动脉损伤修复，并且必须迅速进行。应用肝素抗凝也可能有效。

不管血管闭塞的部位在何处，以及是否由于血栓、栓塞或其他原因导致，症状和体征都伴随可预知的类型。重要的是根据基本的临床体征迅速诊断。动脉闭塞的表现包括脉搏缺失、冷、苍白、运动功能下降、反射消失及疼痛。运动功能下降和感觉降低是缺血的晚期征象。在动脉危害的早期（少于 4～6 小时），症状和体征可能不明显，鉴别动脉闭塞和痉挛有困难。外周血管多普勒检查常常用搏动波缺失证实真的闭塞，减弱波存在于痉挛病例。随着发病时间延长，根据连续的多普勒和临床检查得知，如果缺血超过 4～6 小时则不应考虑为痉挛所致。如果在 6～12 小时之内确诊，血管修复或溶栓治疗结果最好。因为有侧支循环，皮肤颜色可能保留，甚至在肢体先兆缺

血影响到深部组织时也可如此，虽然在这种情况下毛细血管充盈常常延迟。一般来说，先前的观察划界方
2117 法已不再采用，因为消除动脉梗阻的侵袭性方法使成功率达到75%~90%[21,53]。

闭塞综合征

颅内动脉

中风在儿童中少见，但如果发生则是破坏性的。一些疾病例如镰状红细胞病、神经纤维瘤病、青紫型先天性心脏病或特发性动脉炎是最常见的原因。在包含212例患者的综述中，Ganesan和同事采用详细的大脑显像和其他研究方法来观察动脉缺血性中风的危险因素[23]。在这些患者中，115例先前是健康的：在这组中，创伤和先前的水痘-带状疱疹病毒感染伴有颅内动脉异常是最常见的情况。其余患者都具有与个体疾病状态有关的已知危险因素。Strater和同伴进行了一项前瞻性的5年随访研究，对儿童期复发中风的危险因素进行评估，并鉴别先天性心脏畸形、血管病变、感染疾病、胶原组织疾病和代谢性疾病[76]。先前的复发中风病例对照研究显示其与遗传性高凝状态的危险因子相关。这种情况下复发中风的风险高达10%。Chabrier和同事研究了复发中风的风险机制[8]。动脉病性中风最常见。那些非进展性的患者一般结果较好，复发的风险降低；而那些有进展性动脉病的患者，例如烟雾病，结果较差，复发风险较高。Carvalho和Garg综述了儿童动脉中风的治疗，指出在大多情况下治疗是支持性的，但有时抗凝和溶栓对处理儿童急性中风是有用的[7]。在这类疾病中，大部分颅内动脉疾病的表现是轻度中风、一过性缺血和抽搐。据估计，儿童中风发病率大约是2.5/100 000[7]。烟雾病（Moyamoya disease）在日本文献中被描述，可能包括许多导致颅内动脉多发狭窄的疾病。术语“moyamoya”是日本语，描述了这类患者大脑动脉造影的模式；这个词翻译过来的意思是“烟雾弥漫的事物”，像吸烟时朝空气中喷出的烟雾。这种疾病可导致中风，但在少见的病变侵犯大脑中动脉近端或颅内颈内动脉的病例中，可能通过浅表的临时到大脑中动脉的吻合而减轻。Caldarelli和同事描述了利用肌瓣和脑-肌-血管联合术的技术[6]。在短期随访中，作者描述了大脑循环的改善，但与临床改善无关。这可能是因为在多数情况下外科治疗应用于大的中风发生后。

颅外动脉

1908年，Takayasu描述了一例升主动脉分支血管闭塞合并视网膜中央血管病变的病例[79]。Dean综述了儿童动脉病变，并指出Takayasu病除了累及弓状分支血管的起点外，颅外颈内动脉和椎动脉更远端部位的狭窄病变在儿童中很少见[17]。与烟雾病相同，Takayasu动脉炎是进展性的，可能累及降主动脉。Weyand和Goronzy发表了对大血管和中血管血管炎的病因分析[89]。他们指出大动脉的炎症，例如主动脉和它的主要分支，可由许多疾病导致，包括Kawasaki病、Behcet综合征、风湿性关节炎、梅毒和结核。主动脉炎和大血管动脉炎通常有两种类型：巨细胞动脉炎和Takayasu动脉炎。事实上，很难区分Takayasu动脉炎与纤维肌性发育不良，以及纤维肌性增生（FMH）。后者被认为是一种自身免疫性疾病，而巨细胞动脉炎和Takayasu动脉炎在病理生理学方面不同，涉及抗原递呈细胞、T细胞和巨噬细胞细胞免疫反应[32]。有证据显示Takayasu动脉炎可能发生于亚洲人，以进展的方式累及到整个动脉分支[31,71]。另一方面，在北美，腹腔脏器血管被首先累及。后者是FMH还是Takayasu动脉炎还不清楚。然而，北美形式似乎是非进展的，倾向于筋疲力尽，提供了手术干预的机会。阿司匹林和皮质激素可能会减轻巨细胞动脉炎和Takayasu动脉炎的进展，但尚无充分证据显示它们对FMH有效[15]。

其他可能引起颅外血管闭塞的疾病是Williams综合征。它是一种遗传性疾病，表现为先天性心脏病，尤其是肺动脉狭窄；在各类动脉狭窄中，锁骨下动脉和肾动脉最常受累；并有特殊面容[18]。Williams综合征患者与Takayasu病和FMH患者一样，通常存在肾血管性高血压。他们不仅有临床表型，也有广泛的弹力蛋白半合子状态，表现为狭窄性动脉病和相关的血管僵硬。锁骨下动脉和肾动脉与主动脉一样特别易受累[60]。我们发现气囊血管成形术对锁骨下动脉和其他上肢血管狭窄有效，但在我们的患者中肾动脉病变通常需要动脉重建，因为硬化位于开口部位。

表 131-3　肾血管性高血压的原因

先天性
动脉发育不良
神经纤维瘤病
Williams 综合征
主动脉缩窄
获得性
纤维肌性增生、肾动脉狭窄
中主动脉综合征
Takayasu 病
肾动脉创伤、吻合口狭窄
血栓或栓塞后肾动脉闭塞
肾炎、肾盂肾炎、肿瘤、溶血性尿毒症综合征
尿路梗阻

肾血管性高血压

纤维肌性增生（FMH）

如前面提到的，根据我们的经验，儿童肾血管性高血压的根本原因是 FMH[51]。导致肾血管性高血压
2118 的不同原因列于表 131-3。儿童高血压发病率估计在 1%~5%，后者是在青春期儿童中的比例，发病率接近先天性心脏病。然而，儿童高血压较先天性心脏病不易诊断，这是因为在这个年龄组中血压不是常规测量的指标。潜在的外科可纠治的高血压发生率大约是：出生到 5 岁年龄组为 80%，6～10 岁年龄组为 44%，11～20 岁年龄组为 20%[51]。最常见的外科可纠治的病因是肾血管疾病。肾动脉狭窄导致肾缺血，依次产生收缩血压的持续升高，这与 Goldblatt 和同事在 1934 年所指出的一样[25]。随后，发现肾缺血与肾素-血管紧张素轴的联系是疾病的原因。从那时起，我们和其他人报道了儿童中大宗的不同类型的肾动脉狭窄和中主动脉综合征病例的血管重建[51,52]。

病因

如表 131-3 所示，肾血管性高血压的特殊原因常常是显而易见的[72]。先天性或获得性疾病包括内分泌性、神经性、代谢性、肾脏感染和血管疾病等最常见的疾病。Wilson 和同事[90]以及 Dean[17]报道了先天性肾动脉狭窄和闭塞。虽然闭塞的原因不明，但有些病例明显发生于宫内并伴有肾发育不良。另外，导致肾动脉狭窄的先天性疾病还包括神经纤维瘤病和 Williams 综合征（图 131-5 和 131-6）[12,18,19]。最常见的获得性肾血管性高血压是 FMH。如前面提到的，FMH 可能是一种自身免疫性血管炎，病因不止一个，但受累动脉段的组织学表现证明肌层有不同程度的纤维增生和内膜有纤维发育不良。肾动脉狭窄常位于主动脉壁内的开口，虽然有时也碰到分支的病变。有时，FMH 合并主动脉和大脏器动脉狭窄，这种状况被认为是中主动脉综合征[52]。在神经纤维瘤病患者中，我们发现肾动脉开口闭塞的原因是肥厚的神经组织形成紧密的套囊，环绕肾血管的开口并累及肾动脉和邻近的主动脉血管壁。

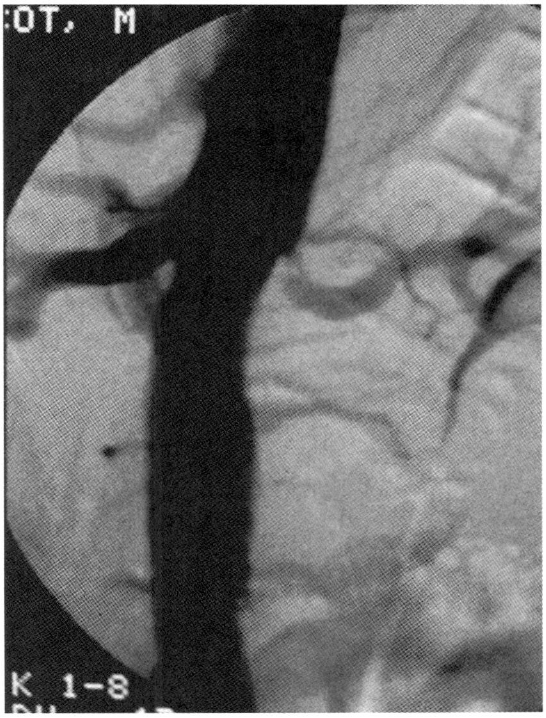

图 131-5　6 岁男孩有神经纤维瘤病和高血压，主动脉造影显示典型的由于动脉壁的神经受累而导致的左肾动脉开口狭窄。

临床表现

症状显现时，如出现头痛、易激惹、充血性心力

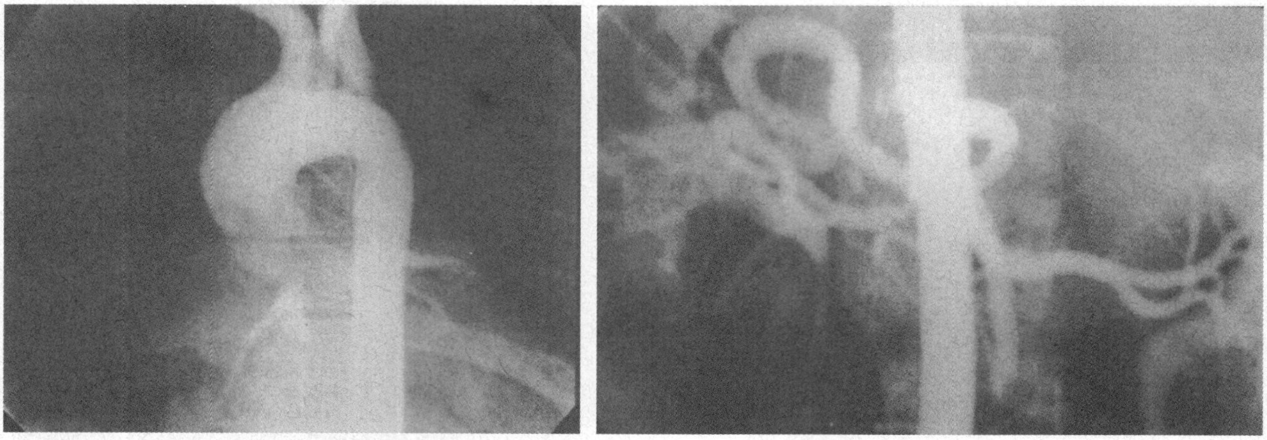

A　　B

图 131-6　A. 10 岁女孩有 Williams 综合征，主动脉弓造影显示左锁骨下动脉起始部狭窄。球囊扩张持久减轻病变，但不改善肾动脉狭窄。B. 此处显示的右肾动脉开口狭窄需要重建。由于狭窄长度短，有可能成功移植远端的血管进入动脉一侧，减轻高血压。

衰竭和脑病等即可诊断高血压。然而，在许多情况下，高血压首先在一个选择性手术麻醉前的评估中被发现。例如双侧肾动脉狭窄的患者出现恶性高血压表现，如充血性心力衰竭、视网膜病，甚至少尿性肾衰竭时，才使问题显现。在我们 70 多例不同病因导致的肾血管性高血压中，约一半患者有症状[51]。参照年龄血压的正常值，我们的患者均有高血压。大龄儿童血压常在 220～250/120～100 mmHg，小龄儿童患者血压相对低但仍然升高。在诊断和手术以前，应尽力
2119 控制血压，但经过最初的强化治疗后，仍发现血压常升高，尤其当患者激动或焦虑时。有一半时间可听到腹部杂音。但有时中主动脉狭窄的患者下肢脉搏消失，上下肢脉压差为 40～60 mmHg。

诊断研究

实验室研究在评估和处理肾血管性高血压方面的价值有限，尽管有些 FMH 的患者有血沉和 C 反应蛋白升高。一般来说，血沉在 6 个月内降到正常，因此我们以此指导修复的时机，因为在动脉炎活动期进行血管重建往往失败。

心电图和胸片可用来证实左心室衰竭的存在和程度。我们发现测量外周血浆肾素水平没有什么特殊价值，也没有通过不同的激发试验决定治疗方法。常规的儿茶酚胺检测可排除嗜铬细胞瘤，但在肾血管性高血压患者中正常。

影像学检查是诊断和治疗的关键。快速序列静脉尿路造影和放射性核素流体扫描是有用的，它们能显示病变侧造影剂排泄延迟，用以筛选单侧肾动脉狭窄。然而，它们对双侧肾动脉狭窄的病例没有用，所以这些研究的准确性是 60%。另外我们发现 MRA，尤其是 CTA 非常准确[86]。尽管 CTA 最终可能替代主动脉造影，但在目前我们仍然推荐主动脉造影及选择性肾动脉造影，因为它的准确性为 100%，并且有时，当有指征时，可同时进行腔内的球囊扩张（图 131-7）。我们的患者已使用限制体积的造影剂，尤其是肾功能损伤的患者。在分支血管病变的患者中，局部滴注硝酸甘油可用于明显显示这些狭窄病变，通过扩张正常血管和加亮由狭窄分支血管供血的缺血区域实现上述用途。

在大部分病例中，FMH 累及一侧或双侧肾动 2120
脉[63]。通常仅开口狭窄，然而有时动脉完全闭塞或血管长段狭窄。狭窄后扩张是规律。尽管 FMH 在年轻成人血管造影中有波纹样的表现，但在儿童中单一狭窄常见。

中主动脉综合征

中主动脉综合征是 FMH 的一个变异类型，但血管广泛受累，而不仅局限于肾动脉。有些作者认为中

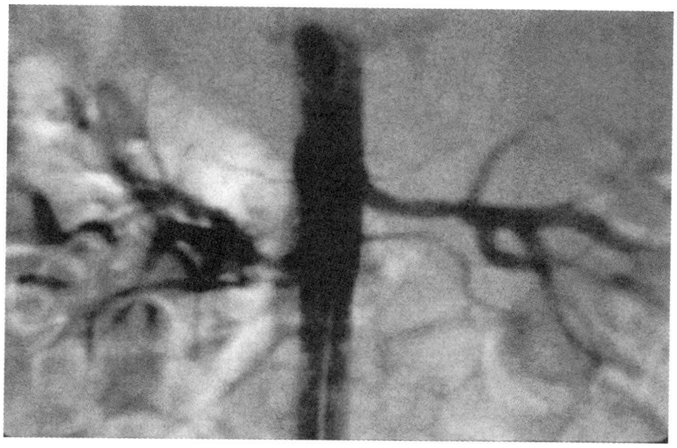

图 131-7　6 岁男孩的血管造影显示广泛的纤维肌性增生伴有双侧肾动脉狭窄。左肾动脉远端的轻度狭窄对手术扩张有反应。右肾动脉狭窄通过建立肾动脉旁路治疗，包括两个远端吻合。高血压缓解超过 8 年。

主动脉综合征是 Takayasu 动脉炎的一种形式，但某些特征可以区分这两种状况[11,65]。另一个描述中主动脉综合征的术语是主动脉峡下缩窄。我们描述了 17 例患者的中主动脉综合征，记录他们的诊断、病理发现、治疗和效果[52]。

大部分患者大于 5 岁，提示病变是获得性的。主动脉狭窄常位于肾上、肾下，或位于受累的肾动脉。病变局限于肾下主动脉很少见。尽管文献记载的 Takayasu 动脉炎倾向于具有进展性，尤其是在亚洲人群，但白种人的中主动脉综合征采用血管重建成功治疗，倾向于无复发。

大部分中主动脉综合征患者合并肾动脉狭窄，常常是双侧性的，症状严重，包括恶性高血压、充血性心力衰竭和偶尔的少尿性肾衰竭以及腿跛行。尽管我们的患者大部分有不同程度的腹腔动脉和肠系膜上动脉狭窄，但没有肠道缺血的体征。恶性高血压的体征包括严重的头痛、高血压性视网膜病和脑病。

实验室和其他检查证实我们的患者有肾功能减弱和充血性心力衰竭，但没有心肌缺血。所有中主动脉综合征的患者在血管造影上显示不同范围和部位的主动脉狭窄，并且在大多情况下，主动脉狭窄的中央段从主动脉裂孔到肠系膜下动脉水平。病变仅偶尔累及胸主动脉。常常累及双侧肾动脉，一侧或双侧肾动脉可能完全闭塞，血流依赖侧支循环。内脏肠系膜血管的狭窄程度特征性地刺激侧支的广泛形成，从肠系膜下动脉通过 Riolan 拱廊。

治疗

诊断和治疗前血压应予以控制，除非要进行肾切除或患者有少尿性肾衰竭。即便是后一种情况，也至少用硝普盐部分控制血压。儿童期降低血压的较好方法是联合应用 α-和 β-肾上腺素能阻滞剂和噻嗪类利尿剂。最有效的药物是米诺地尔、短效或长效的普萘洛尔及氢氯噻嗪。血管紧张素转化酶抑制剂的应用是有争议的，因为对有肾血管缺血的患者有直接的肾毒性，我们避免应用这类药物。对恶性高血压的短期治疗，我们发现应用硝普盐和酚苄明效果最好。术后应用这样的药物同样对肾再血管化的患者很有效。如果可能，外科修复应该推迟到恶性高血压缓解。

在过去几年，我们和其他许多作者报道将球囊扩张应用于 FMH 和放支架患者[19,83]。我们和几个作者也报道球囊血管成形术对许多侧支血管病变有持续的效果，但对肾开口病变的效果为一过性的[5,29,51,83]。因此，球囊血管成形术可避免肾动脉开口处狭窄患者发生肾功能损伤和充血性心力衰竭，但也常常需要手术修复。应用切开球囊置管也有短期成功的报道[28]。对儿童肾动脉开口狭窄的病例应用球囊扩张后静脉内支架尚没有足够的经验，但显示对血管狭窄合并先天性心脏病有短期或长期效果[5,70]。对小年龄患儿我们避免应用支架，尽管在未来不影响生长的不溶解支架可能成为一种方法。目前，外科手术修复仍然是最好的方法。

在过去，肾切除术是用于治疗肾血管性高血压唯一的方法。小婴儿的肾切除指征有血管修复困难、肾动脉广泛累及及手术失败者。对于不能耐受血管重建或扩张的节段性肾内病变者，或有分支肾动脉血管动脉瘤合并节段肾缺血的患者，部分肾切除可能有效。然而，一般来说，肾切除和部分肾切除应该是处理肾血管性高血压最后的手段。

外科医生必须熟悉根据血管病变的特点而选取的不同手术方法。肾动脉狭窄最理想的治疗方法是直接肾移植，但这种技术不适用于长段型肾动脉狭窄或中主动脉综合征。大多数肾动脉狭窄患者需要某种形式的搭桥。通常，大多数外科医生喜欢应用插入移植，端侧吻合到主动脉，端端吻合到肾动脉。Stoney 和同伴喜欢应用自体腹下动脉，但这种方法不总是可行，因为移植动脉可能没有充足的长度来插入[75]。另外，

FMH有时也可累及腹下动脉，对双侧肾动脉狭窄的
2121 病例移植双侧腹下动脉可能不是好方法，因为可能导致性功能障碍。我们和其他作者用由涤纶鞘保护的自体隐静脉来避免血管移植物产生动脉瘤[4,73]。这种方法成功率很高，长期随访没有发现术后内膜增生。其他可应用的方法包括补片血管成形和应用假体移植物。后两种方法较前面讨论的标准方法术后闭塞的发生率较高。

对于中主动脉综合征病例，已描述了许多治疗方法。Stanley和Fry报道应用补片血管成形和搭桥移植，但他们喜欢用假体补片对主动脉和肾动脉行广泛的补片血管成形[74]。Messina和同事、我们组及其他研究者倾向于应用主动脉-主动脉旁路，从胸降主动脉或从腹主动脉上段到分叉水平，而单侧或双侧肾动脉旁路从正常上主动脉或主动脉-主动脉旁路移植物发出[45,52]。针织涤纶用于5岁以下的主动脉-主动脉旁路移植，尽管绝大部分患儿年龄较大。另一方面，我们不喜欢用假体材料作为肾旁路[55]。Messina和同事[45]以及Stoney和同伴[75]喜欢进行内脏动脉重建，即使患者无症状，但我们在随访中没有发现这种方法是必要的[84]。尽管Lillehei和Shamberger报道了对中主动脉综合征的分期重建，但大多外科医生喜欢直接一期重建，并显示有良好的效果[38,43,45,47,74,75]。

对肾动脉狭窄和中主动脉综合征进行外科重建的成功率较高，死亡率较低。尽管偶尔有外科修复术后死亡的报道，但我们和其他人没有死亡病例，并且移植失败率在5%～10%之间。不幸的是，失败有时导致肾切除。95%以上的患者获得治愈或症状明显改善，但许多研究显示FMH有复发。我们碰到一例患者，在对侧肾动脉狭窄治疗14年后，由于肾动脉狭窄而致复发性高血压，所以必须对这些患者进行长期监测。

小动脉疾病和血管痉挛疾病

Athreya曾很好地总结了儿童期发生的许多小动脉非动脉粥样硬化性闭塞病变[3]。风湿性疾病最多，包括硬皮病、红斑狼疮、皮肌炎、幼年性风湿性关节炎、多动脉炎性结节及暴发性紫癜。据报道这些疾病合并小动脉进行性闭塞，尤其在手指和脚趾。当疾病进展到远端小动脉闭塞时，I型糖尿病的患者可能有类似的临床表现；不幸的是，这常常导致截肢。在以上提到的这些自身免疫性疾病中，许多有血管痉挛表现。

两个主要的综合征，Raynaud综合征和交感反射性营养不良，是儿童期发生的两类血管痉挛疾病。其他合并血管痉挛的疾病包括冻疮、冷球蛋白血症、抗磷脂抗体综合征和类似血管炎疾病。抗磷脂抗体包括抗心肌磷脂抗体和狼疮抗凝剂，它们与动脉和静脉血栓有关。

Raynaud综合征

Raynaud综合征指肢端动脉暂时性痉挛，由于寒冷和情绪应激引起。典型的临床表现是苍白，接着有青紫、麻木、疼痛，指端发红伴有温暖和麻刺感。当Raynaud综合征长期存在时，指尖丛萎缩和再吸收，有时合并溃疡。Raynaud综合征程度不同，由很轻及一过性到严重，常常合并先前提到的风湿性疾病和结缔组织疾病。在Raynaud综合征诊断前，重要的是排除胸腔出口综合征、摄取了拟交感神经药物和不同病毒的感染。

治疗方法包括治疗任何潜在的风湿性疾病，避免暴露于寒冷，口服硝苯地平或其他钙通道阻滞剂，对迫切的坏疽输注前列腺素E_1和前列环素，对有严重的顽固症状患者动脉内应用利舍平或行交感切除术。不幸的是，外科交感切除的长期结果并不乐观。

交感反射性营养不良

Mitchell和同事在1864年最先描述了交感反射性营养不良，它是一种神经损伤的并发症[48]。这个疾病的特点是严重、持续疼痛，并可被任何形式的皮肤刺激所加重。在运动时疼痛加重。尽管交感反射性营养不良常常有创伤病史，但有时没有。这个疾病不包括指端萎缩，儿童复原的前景通常较好。应激和心身障碍是常见的并发症。根本治疗是解决潜在的心身和应激问题。儿童需要物理治疗和主动运动，尽管有可能需要镇痛药。没有发现已知的药物或手术对治疗这种疾病有效。

抗磷脂抗体综合征

抗磷脂或抗心肌磷脂抗体的产生可以是自发的，或更常见的是作为系统性红斑狼疮的一部分[37]。血

管血栓形成和血小板减少与这些抗体存在相关关
2122 系[26]。主要自体抗原是β_2-糖蛋白Ⅰ，也涉及载脂蛋白H，一种结合心肌磷脂和其他磷脂的蛋白[88]。已知这些自身抗体干扰凝血级联瀑布。

仅有的完全有效的治疗是如果可能，针对这些疾病的主要表现直接治疗。凝血问题的最好治疗方法是采用华法林[13,39]。

（洪　莉译　夏慧敏校）

参考文献

1. Akagi T, Rose V, Benson LN, et al: Outcome of coronary artery aneurysms after Kawasaki disease. J Pediatr 1992; 121:689-694.
2. Applebaum RE, Caniano DA, Sun CC, et al: Synchronous left subclavian and axillary artery aneurysms associated with melorheostosis. Surgery 1986;99:249-253.
3. Athreya BH: Vasospastic disorders in children. Semin Pediatr Surg 1994;3:70-78.
4. Berkowitz HD, O'Neill JA. Renovascular hypertension in children. J Vasc Surg 1989;9:46-55.
5. Blum U, Krumme B, Fleugel P, et al: Treatment of ostial renal artery stenoses with vascular endoprostheses after unsuccessful balloon angioplasty. N Engl J Med 1997;336:459-465.
6. Caldarelli M, DiRocco C, Gagglini T: Surgical treatment of moyamoya disease in the pediatric age. J Neuro Surg Sci 2001;45:83-91.
7. Carvalho KS, Garg BP: Arterial strokes in children. Neurol Clin 2002;20:1079-1100.
8. Chabrier S, Husson B, Lasjaunias P, et al: Stroke in childhood: Outcome and recurrence risk by mechanism in 59 patients. J Child Neurol 2000;15:290-294.
9. Cikrit DF, Glover JR, Dalsing MC, Silver D: The Ehlers-Danlos specter revisited. Vasc Endovasc Surg 2002;36:213-217.
10. Colburn MD, Galibert HA, Quinones-Baldrich W: Neonatal aortic thrombosis. Surgery 1992;111:21-28.
11. Connolly JE, Wilson SE, Lawrence PL, Fugitani RM: Middle aortic syndrome: Distal thoracic and abdominal coarctation, a disorder with multiple etiologies. J Am Col Surg 2002; 194:774-781.
12. Criado E, Izquierdo L, Lujan S, et al: Abdominal aortic coarctation, renovascular hypertension and neurofibromatosis. Ann Vasc Surg 2002;16:363-367.
13. Crowther MA, Ginsberg JS, Julian J, et al: A comparison of two intensities of warfarin for the prevention of recurrent thrombosis in patients with the antiphospholipid antibody syndrome. N Engl J Med 2003;349:1133-1138.
14. de Chadarevine JP, Balarezo FS, Heggere M, Dampier C: Splenic artery and veins in pediatric sickle cell disease. Pediatr Dev Pathol 2001;4:538-544.
15. D'Souza SJ, Tsai Ws, Silver MM, et al: Diagnosis and management of stenotic aorto-arteriopathy in childhood. J Pediatr 1998;132:1016-1022.
16. De la Torre L, Carrasco D, More MA, et al: Vascular malformations of the colon in children. J Pediatr Surg 2002; 37:1754-1757.
17. Dean RH, Robaczewski D: Arteriopathies of childhood. Semin Pediatr Surg 1994;3:103-113.
18. Eronen M, Peippo M, Hiippala A, et al: Cardiovascular manifestations in 75 patients with Williams syndrome. J Med Genet 2002;39:554-558.
19. Estepa R, Gallego N, Orte L, et al: Renovascular hypertension in children. Scand J Urol Nephrol 2001;35:388-392.
20. Fink C, Peuster M, Hausdorf G: Endovascular stenting as an emergency treatment for neonatal coarctation. Cardiol Young 2000;10:644-646.
21. Flanagan DP, Keifer TJ, Schuler JJ, et al: Experience with iatrogenic pediatric vascular injuries: Incidence, etiology, management and results. Ann Surg 1983;198:430-442.
22. Freeman RK, Swegle J, Size MJ: The surgical complications of Ehlers-Danlos syndrome. Am Surg 1996;62:869-873.
23. Ganesan V, Prengler M, McShane MA, et al: Investigation of risk factors in children with arterial ischemic stroke. Ann Neurol 2003;53:149-150.
24. Gloviczki P, Hollier LH, Telander RL, et al: Surgical implications of Klippel-Trenaunay syndrome. Ann Surg 1983;196: 353-362.
25. Goldblatt H, Lynch J, Hanzell RF, et al: Studies on experimental hypertension: Production of persistent elevation of systolic blood pressure by means of renal ischemia. J Exp Med 1934;59:347-349.
26. Guvenc VG, Sarper N, Tuzlaci A, Gunaltay N: Transient antiphospholipid syndrome in an infant with segmental small bowel infarction. J Pediatr Surg 2004;39:124-127.
27. Guzzetta PC: Congenital and acquired aneurysmal disease. Semin Pediatr Surg 1994;3:97-102.
28. Haas NA, Ocker V, Knirsch W, et al: Successful management of a resistant renal artery stenosis in a child using a 4 mm cutting balloon catheter. Cathet Cardiovasc Interv 2002;56:227-231.
29. Hofbeck M, Singer H, Rupprecht T, et al: Successful percutaneous transluminal angioplasty for treatment of renovascular hypertension in a 15-month old child. Eur J Pediatr 1998;157:512-514.
30. Iglesia KA, Fellows KE: Contemporary interventional procedures for vascular disorders in children. Semin Pediatr Surg 1994;3:87-96.
31. Ishikawa K: Natural history and classification of occlusive thromboaortopathy (Takayasu's disease). Circulation 1978;57:27-35.
32. Johnston SL, Lock RJ, Gompels MM: Takayasu arteritis: A review. J Clin Pathol 2002;55:481-486.
33. Kim TS, Chung JW, Park JH, et al: Renal artery evaluation: Comparison of spiral CT angiography to intra-arterial DSA. J Vasc Interv Radiol 1998;9:553-559.
34. Knudson RP, Alden ER: Symptomatic arteriovenous malformation in infants less than 6 months of age. Pediatrics 1979;64:238-241.
35. Konan AV, Raymond J, Roy D: Transarterial embolization of aneurysms associated with spinal cord arteriovenous malformations: Report of four cases. J Neuro Surg 1999;90:148-154.
36. Latter D, Beland MJ, Batten A, et al: Congenital abdominal aortic aneurism. Can J Surg 1989;32:135-138.
37. Levine JS, Branch DW, Rauch J: The antiphospholipid syndrome. N Engl J Med 2002;346:752-763.
38. Lillehei CW, Shamberger RC: Staged reconstruction for middle aortic syndrome. J Pediatr Surg 2001;36:1252-1254.
39. Lockshin MD, Erkin D: Treatment of the antiphospholipid syndrome. N Engl J Med 2003;349:1177-1179.
40. Marfan BAJ: Un cas de déformation congénitale des quatre membres, bleus prononcée aux extremités, characterisée par l'allongement des os avec un certain degré d'amincisse-

ment. Bull Mem Soc Med Hop Paris 1896;13:220-221.
41. Marler JJ, Fishman SJ, Upton J, et al: Prenatal diagnosis of vascular anomalies. J Pediatr Surg 2002;37:318-326.
42. McCullough CJ, Kenwright J: The prognosis in congenital lower limb hypertrophy. Acta Orthop Scand 1979;50:307-312.
43. McTaggart SJ, Gulity S, Walker RG, et al: Evaluation and long-term outcome of pediatric renovascular hypertension. Pediatr Nephrol 2000;14:1022-1029.
44. Mendeloff J, Stallion A, Hutton M, et al: Aortic aneurysm resulting from umbilical artery catheterization: Case report, literature review, and management algorithm. J Vasc Surg 2001;33:419-424.
45. Messina LM, Riley LM, Goldstone J, et al: Middle aortic syndrome: Effectiveness and durability of complex arterial revascularization techniques. Ann Surg 1986;204:331-339.
46. Meyer JS, Fellows KE: Vascular imaging in children. Semin Pediatr Surg 1994;3:79-86.
47. Mickley V, Fleiter T: Coarctations of descending and abdominal aorta: Long-term results of surgical therapy. J Vasc Surg 1998;28;206-214.
48. Mitchell SW, Morehouse GR, Keen WW: Gunshot Wounds and Other Injuries of Nerves. Philadelphia, JB Lippincott, 1864.
49. Nakayama DK, O'Neill JA, Wagner H, et al: Management of vascular complications of bacterial endocarditis. J Pediatr Surg 1986;21:636-639.
50. Nehler MR, Taylor LM, Porter JM: Iatrogenic vascular trauma. Semin Vasc 1998;11:283-293.
51. O'Neill JA: Long-term outcome with surgical treatment of renovascular hypertension. J Pediatr Surg 1998;33:106-111.
52. O'Neill JA, Berkowitz H, Fellows KJ, Harmon CM: Midaortic syndrome and hypertension in childhood. J Pediatr Surg 1995;30:164-172.
53. O'Neill JA, Neblett WW, Born ML: Management of major thromboembolic complications of umbilical artery catheters. J Pediatr Surg 1981;16:972-978.
54. Parkes-Weber F: Angiomalformation in connection with hypertrophy of limbs or hemihypertrophy. Br J Dermatol 1907;19:231-233.
55. Paty PS, Darling RC, Lee D, et al: Is prosthetic renal artery reconstruction a durable procedure? An analysis of 489 bypass grafts. J Vasc Surg 2001;34:127-132.
56. Patzer L, Basche S, Misselwitz J: Renal artery stenosis and aneurysmatic dilatation of arteria sclerotis interna in tuberous sclerosis complex. Pediatr Nephrol 2002;17:193-196.
57. Pepin M, Schwarze U, Superti-Furga A, Byers PH: Clinical and genetic features of Ehlers-Danlos syndrome type IV, the vascular type. N Engl J Med 2000;342:673-680.
58. Rainio P, Biancar F, Leinonen S, Juvonen T: Aneurysm of the profunda femoris artery manifested as acute groin pain in a child. J Pediatr Surg 2003;38:1699-1700.
59. Redekop G, TerBurgge K, Montanera W, Willinisky R: Arterial aneurysms associated with cerebral arterial venous malformations: Classification, incidence, and risk of hemorrhage. J Neuro Surg 1998;89:539-546.
60. Rose C, Wessel A, Panku R, et al: Anomalies of the abdominal aorta in Williams-Beuren syndrome—another cause of arterial hypertension. Eur J Pediatr 2001;160:655-658.
61. Rowley AH, Gonzalez-Crussi F, Shulman ST: Kawasaki syndrome. Curr Probl Pediatr 1991;21:387-405.
62. Saad SA, May A: Abdominal aortic aneurysm in a neonate. J Pediatr Surg 1991;36:1423-1424.
63. Safian RD, Textor SC: Renal artery stenosis. N Engl J Med 2001;344:431-442.
64. Salaymeh KJ, Banerjee A: Evaluation of arterial stiffness in children with Williams syndrome: Does it play a role in evolving hypertension? Am Heart J 2001;142:549-555.
65. Sandman W, Sculte KM: Multivisceral fibromuscular dysplasia in childhood: Case report and review of the literature. Ann Vasc Surg 2000;14:496-502.
66. Sarkar R, Coran AG, Cilley RE, et al: Arterial aneurysms in children: Clinicopathologic classification. J Vasc Surg 1991;13:47-57.
67. Schiller M, Gordon R, Shifrin E, Abu-Dalu K: Mulitple arterial aneurysms. J Pediatr Surg 1983;18:27-29.
68. Schmidt B, Andrew M: Neonatal thrombosis: Report of a prospective Canadian and international registry. Pediatrics 1995;96:939-943.
69. Senzaki H, Akagi M, Hishi T, et al: Age-associated changes in arterial elastic properties in children. Eur J Pediatr 2002;161:547-551.
70. Shaffer KM, Mullens CE, Grifka RG, et al: Intravascular stents in congenital heart disease: Short- and long-term results from a large single-center experience. J Am Coll Cardiol 1998;31:661-667.
71. Sharma S, Rajani M, Talwar KK: Angiographic morphology in nonspecific aortoarteritis (Takayasu's arteritis): A study of 126 patients from North India. Cardio Vasc Intervent Radiol 1992;15:160-165.
72. Shinohara M, Shitara T, Hatakeyama S-I, et al: An infant with systemic hypertension, renal artery stenosis, and neuroblastoma. J Pediatr Surg 2004;39:103-106.
73. Stanley JC, Ernst CB, Fry WJ: Fate of 100 aortorenal vein grafts: Characteristics of late graft expansion, aneurysmal dilatation and stenosis. Surgery 1973;74:931-944.
74. Stanley JC, Fry WJ: Pediatric renal artery occlusive disease and renovascular hypertension. Surgery 1981;116: 669-675.
75. Stoney RJ, DeLuccia N, Ehrenfeld WK, Wylie EF: Aortorenal autografts: long-term assessment. Arch Surg 1981;116: 1416-1422.
76. Strater R, Becker S, von Eckardstein A, et al: Prospective assessment of risk factors for recurrent stroke during childhood—a 5-year follow-up study. Lancet 2002;360: 1540-1545.
77. Strife JL, Ball WS, Tobin RB, et al: Arterial occlusions in neonates: Use of fibrinolytic therapy. Radiology 1989;166:395-400.
78. Szilagyi DE, Smith RF, Elliott JP, Hageman JH: Congenital arteriovenous anomalies of the limbs. Arch Surg 1976; 111:422-429.
79. Takayasu M: A case with unusual changes of the central vessels in the retina. Nippon Ganka Gakkai Zasshi 1908; 12:554-556.
80. Tanaka R, Miyasaka Y, Fujii K, et al: Vascular structure of arterial venous malformations. J Clin Neurosci, 2000;7: 24-28.
81. Tice DA, Clauss RH, Keirle AM, Reed GE: Congenital arterial venous fistulae of the extremities: Observations concerning treatment. Arch Surg 1963;86:460-465.
82. Tsomi K, Karagiorga-Lagana M, Karabatsos F, et al: Arterial elastorrhexis in beta-thalassaemia intermedia, sickle cell thalassemia and hereditary spherocytosis. Eur J Haematol 2001;67:135-141.
83. Tyagi S, Kaul UA, Satsangi DK, Arora R: Percutaneous transluminal angioplasty for renovascular hypertension in children: Initial and long-term results. Pediatrics 1997;99:44-49.
84. Upchurch GR, Hanke PK, Eagleton MJ, et al: Pediatric splanchnic arterial occlusive disease: Clinical relevance and operative treatment. J Vasc Surg 2002;35:860-867.
85. Upton J, Coombs CJ, Mulliken JB, et al: Vascular malformations of the upper limb: A review of 270 patients. J Hand

Surg 1999;24:1019-1035.
86. Vade A, Agarwal R, Lim-Dunham J, Hartoin D: Utility of computed tomographic renal angiogram in the management of childhood hypertension. Pediatr Nephrol 2002; 17:741-747.
87. Von Khautz A: Spontane extremitatengangran im kindersalter. Z Kinderhelkd 1914;11:35-38.
88. Von Scheven E, Athreya BH, Rose CD, et al: Clinical characteristics of antiphospholipid syndrome in children. J Pediatr 1996;129:339-345.
89. Weyand CM, Goronzy JJ: Medium- and large-vessel vasculitis. N Engl J Med 2003;349:160-169.
90. Wilson DI, Appleton RE, Coulthard MG, et al: Fetal and infantile hypertension caused by unilateral renal arterial disease. Arch Dis Child 1990;65:881-884.

第 132 章

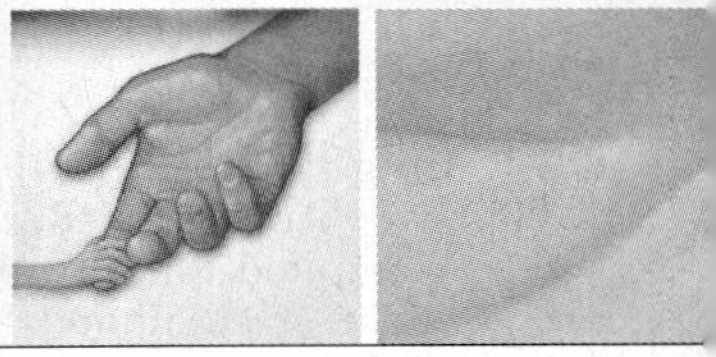

儿童静脉疾病

Michael C. Dalsing 和 Keshav Pandurangi

儿童静脉疾病的发生由炎性、免疫性、感染性或先天性原因导致。通常认为这些疾病并不少见。在一个系列研究中，有 516 例见于儿童期的急性血管问题，其中静脉疾病比例超过三分之一[125]。静脉疾病可分为先天性中央静脉异常、先天性外周静脉异常和静脉血栓。

这一章反映了这三类疾病及其主要分支，每一类都引起关注儿童静脉疾病的外科医生的特别关注。

先天性中央静脉异常

上腔静脉和下腔静脉异常

三对胚胎亚系统促成了完整的静脉系统循环回路：主要静脉前支（前主静脉）形成上腔静脉（SVC）和它的属支，主要静脉后支（下主静脉和上主静脉）形成下腔静脉（IVC）和它的属支，卵黄静脉形成门静脉和它的属支（图 132-1）。

大静脉干的异常常发生于上腔静脉和下腔静脉系统，很少发生于门静脉系统。上腔静脉重复伴有引流到冠状窦常无症状，没有临床意义，除非在心脏手术和心肺搭桥时被发现[31,73,129]。左侧上腔静脉常常无临床表现，但在行心肺搭桥时很重要。另一方面，异常的静脉系统回流到心脏产生不同程度的氧合不全，并伴发需要处理的其他心内异常[56]。预后常常依赖于并发心脏异常的严重程度而不是静脉自身的异常。

下腔静脉异常在人群中占 4%[133]。下腔静脉重复或左位的发生率为 0.2%～0.3%，常常在腹部影像检查，腔静脉造影或主动脉、肾、肾上腺手术中偶然发现[22,26,39]。下腔静脉发育不全较少见，可能是一种孤立的畸形[17]，或合并复杂心脏异常，例如多脾-无脾综合征。先天性下腔静脉梗阻可能继发于右心房的持续性下腔静脉瓣[103,127]，或来源于肝上网。尽管患者可能在不同的时期维持无症状，但最终发展为门脉高压而需要手术治疗[87,103]。腹部 CT 或超声检查用来确立诊断[39]。一旦作出诊断，应该行下腔静脉造影来准确显示静脉异常。腔静脉腔静脉搭桥和经颈静脉膜切除术曾成功进行[32,58]。血管内血管成形术和血管支架是可考虑的选择。中期结果显示对症状性中央静脉梗阻采用血管支架有暂时的作用，但要求定期随访和再干预以维持 2 年 79% 的开放程度[86]。

肾静脉发育异常与下腔静脉异常伴发，可导致主动脉后或环主动脉的左肾静脉。主动脉后静脉的产生伴有持久存在的左后肾静脉和左前肾静脉的退化。在左前、左后肾静脉持久存在的病例中，环主动脉的左肾静脉形成[38]。主动脉后左肾静脉发生率为 1.2%～2.4%，环主动脉左肾静脉发生率报道为 1.5%～8.7%[39]。这些异常常因为其他原因进行腹部影像检查时被偶然发现，只有在腹膜后手术或晚些时候进行腹主动脉重建时才有临床意义。

门静脉异常

门静脉异常包括分支模式变异、缺失、位置异常（十二指肠前位置）和重复。肝内门静脉正常分支变异从 1957 年开始被报道，人群中大约占 20%，临床表现常常不明显[36]。

先天性门静脉缺如（CAPV）是少见的先天性

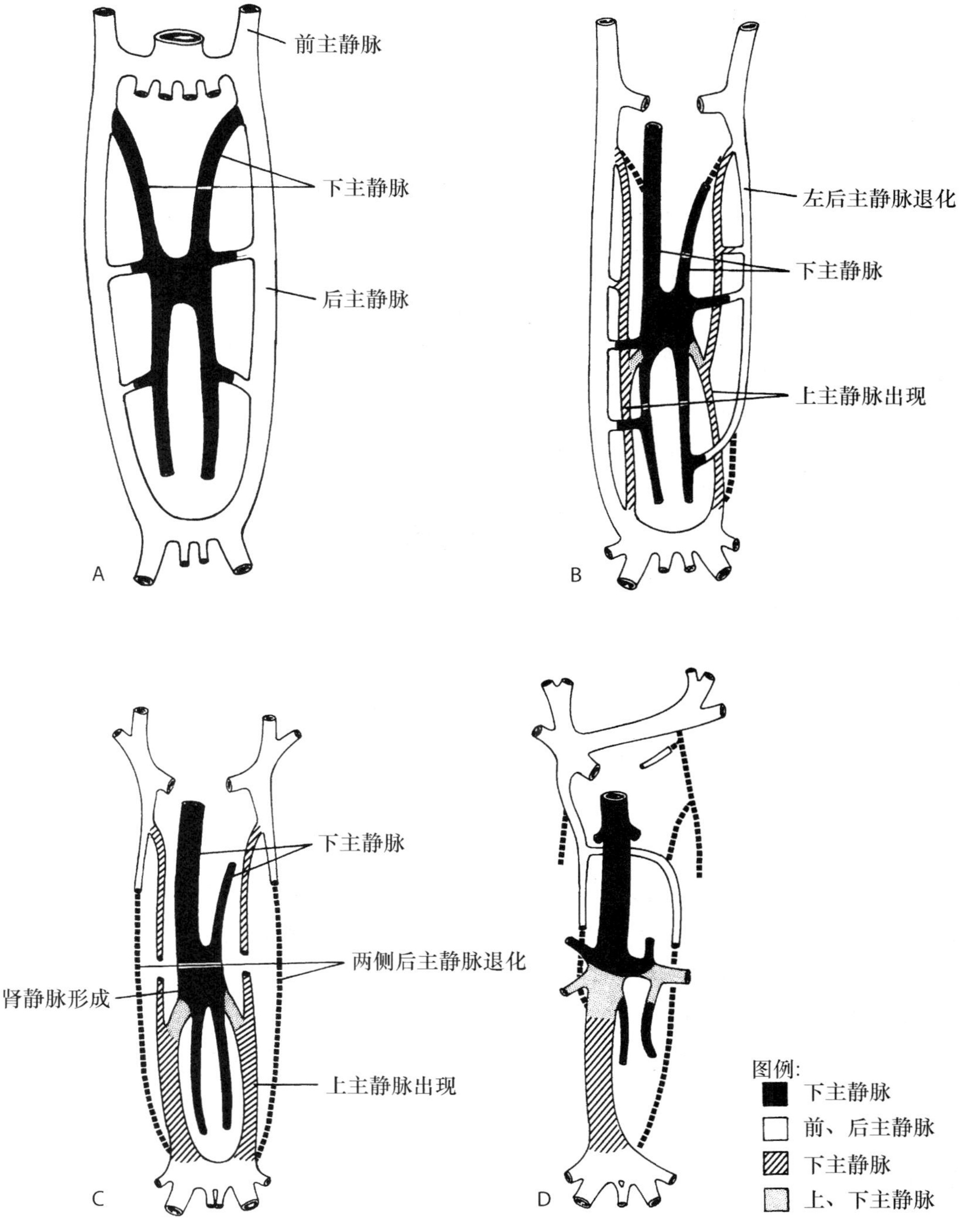

图 132-1 下腔静脉的发育。A. 在胚胎 6 周时，后主静脉占优势。B. 在胚胎 7 周，下主静脉占优势而后主静脉开始退化。C. 在胚胎 8 周，下主静脉形成肾上下腔静脉。上主静脉形成肾下下腔静脉。D. 成人下腔静脉。

畸形，由胚胎第 4～10 周发育异常所致。由于门静脉和肝静脉产生于卵黄静脉和脐静脉，故 CAPV 合并内脏和体循环交通。最早在 1793 年报道门静脉缺如和先天性肠系膜腔静脉分流的是 John Abernathy。从那以后，只有少数病例在文献中被描述。异常肠系膜腔静脉或肠系膜肾静脉连接也有描述[12,71]。这类异常大部分见于女孩[93]。CAPV 常常伴发其他先天性异常，例如心脏缺陷、胆道闭锁和多脾。心脏畸形常常见于 CAPV 患者，因为这种相关异常来源于相似的胚胎损伤和对门静脉缺失和分流的充血效应的补偿[118]。先天性门体循环分流被认识到是儿童期的一种重要疾病，必须与代谢性缺陷包括高血氨或半乳糖血症相区分。对有高水平血半乳糖的新生儿进行筛查有助于检测先天性门体循环分流[81]。

2126 多普勒超声常常被用来作为诊断门静脉异常的首选方法。尽管这种方法不能完全显示门静脉或它主要的分支，但它确实能显示门腔分流的异常类型。CT 和 MRI 能确证门静脉的缺失，它们都能显现门体分流。MRI 能描述多种平面的血管，比常规 CT 更容易鉴别门体分流[81]。也可应用经动脉门静脉造影、直接门静脉造影和脾门静脉造影，但这些有创技术正在被 MR 静脉造影（MRV）所取代[36]。尽管 Shinkai 和同事报道他们从新生儿到成人范围的患者没有经历有症状的门体性脑病[112]，但有小部分儿童和更多的成人存在门体性脑病和肝衰竭的症状。CAPV 常常在肝脏疾病，如胆道闭锁或肝肿瘤的手术或放射学检查中被偶然发现。对常规治疗无反应的症状性 CAPV 则有指征进行肝移植[112]。

十二指肠前门静脉是少见疾病，自从 1921 年由 Knight 首先描述以来文献报道有 82 例。大约一半病例临床表现为高位小肠梗阻，但仅有少部分梗阻被清楚地显示是由于异常门静脉导致。在大部分这类病例中，梗阻由合并畸形造成，如十二指肠隔膜、肠旋转不良和环状胰腺。剩下的一半十二指肠前门静脉病例无症状，在其他原因的手术中被偶然发现，不需要治疗。十二指肠前门静脉常常伴有心脏和胃肠道异常。对于由十二指肠前门静脉引起的十二指肠梗阻，最好的治疗方法是通过十二指肠十二指肠吻合或胃十二指肠吻合解除梗阻，由此门静脉可以置于十二指肠第二段和吻合口之间[77]。在无症状的患者中，门静脉重复或位于十二指肠前对因其他原因进行的胆道、十二指肠或肝脏手术造成危险，如果存在必须要给予确认。

静脉瘤

静脉瘤可以被很好地描述为一个单独的静脉扩张区域，以单个的管道与主要静脉结构连接，除外动静脉连接、假性动脉瘤或曲张的静脉节段[37]。在成人和儿童人群中这是少见病例。上腔静脉、下腔静脉、内脏血管的静脉瘤都曾被描述。在中央静脉中，上腔静脉静脉瘤最常见。上腔静脉静脉瘤大多在常规胸片检查中偶然被发现。上腔静脉静脉瘤自发破裂很少见。因为与外科手术修补有关的发病率和死亡率较高，在这一部位，对无症状和无增大的静脉瘤常规采取非手术治疗[16]。

另一方面，腹部静脉瘤大多是有症状的。这包括下腔静脉、肠系膜上静脉、脾静脉、门静脉和髂静脉静脉瘤。症状包括腹部疼痛、继发于瘘形成的肠道出血或血栓栓塞。诊断由静脉造影或动脉造影静脉期证实，后者在观察导致儿童症状的其他潜在原因时进行。CT 和 MRI 也可应用，特别是在腔内病变。在有关静脉瘤的文献综述中，Calligaro 和同事报道在腹部静脉瘤患者中，非手术治疗后大约有 41% 的患者有危及生命的并发症，并推荐在低风险患者中行预防性手术干预，完全或部分切除静脉瘤[16]。

门静脉瘤常常位于肠系膜上静脉和脾静脉的结合处，或在肝门左右门静脉分叉处。门静脉瘤少见，大约占患者的 0.07%。无创诊断手段，例如多普勒超声、CT、MRI 能作出门静脉瘤的诊断。然而，多普勒超声是单个最有用的诊断工具，进一步的检查可能不需要，除非计划进行外科手术。在大部分患者中，门静脉瘤是偶然发现的[131]。大的门静脉瘤可能造成十二指肠压迫、胆道梗阻、慢性门脉高压、破裂，和由于反复形成栓子导致门静脉完全堵塞。这些并发症均需要手术治疗。过去应用门腔分流，最近静脉瘤部分预防性切除或静脉瘤缝合术成为治疗选择，尤其是当静脉瘤生长或出现并发症时[36]。然而，小的静脉瘤常常无症状，倾向于长时间维持无变化，对这些患者而言，超声监测是可接受的治疗方法。

先天性外周静脉异常

独立静脉畸形

血管畸形在人群中大约占 1.5%，由动脉、毛细血管、静脉或淋巴管结构发育不良引起[98,132]。在 1988 年，"Hamburg 分类"重点聚焦于重要的病理解剖学特征和导致的治疗选择[8]。依据主要受累的血管系统，先天性血管畸形分为下列五组：动脉、静脉（即主要的静脉畸形，无论局限或弥散）、动静脉（即慢流或快流）、淋巴管（明显的囊性水囊肿和淋巴管瘤）和混合或结合畸形。而且，这些畸形可能发生在躯干和内脏或外周血管[9]。

单纯动脉病变在所有畸形中不到 1%。最常见的

2127 病变，大约占一半，缘于静脉。混合动脉和静脉的缺陷在畸形中占 15%～30%[98]。本章重点在于原发的静脉畸形。

尽管大部分这类畸形局限于静脉系统，而且散发于健康的个体，但已有报道其合并区域性解剖结构异常，例如见于 Klippel–Trenaunay 综合征。异常范围从无症状的新生儿斑到危及生命的状况。并非所有的血管畸形出生时即明显，许多在出生后数年或数十年出现。临床表现很大程度上依赖占优势血管的特征：动脉、毛细血管、静脉或淋巴管。症状包括可触及的肿块、水肿、静脉曲张、慢性静脉不全导致的溃疡、机械性杂音、肢体长度差异或其他不能解释的疼痛。增强 CT、血管造影、静脉造影、多普勒超声和 MRI 是当今用于评估畸形的技术。动脉造影是一种有创诊断技术，但能治疗选择性的患者。这一技术包括超选择性插管和螺圈栓塞治疗。多普勒超声是可携带的，无创伤性，能提供病变功能信息和解剖信息。MRI 也是血管畸形患者可选择的诊断方式，因为它能鉴别病变扩张到周围软组织和骨的范围[91]。它也能很好地作为怀疑畸形的初始诊断试验，尤其是对于婴儿和儿童，在这些患者中竞争性试验可能引发额外风险。静脉畸形的处理依据病变的类型、部位、范围和患者的症状。局限的病变可被观察到，特别是在有症状时。皮肤血管瘤表现为局部畸形，在别处讨论。

无瓣膜

在一项研究中，无瓣膜或静脉瓣缺如在先天性血管异常合并深静脉异常中占 4%～7%[33]。这种异常并不在出生时表现。它是一种常染色体显性异常，导致明显的静脉反流，当儿童直立姿势和开始行走时静脉高血压而最终导致慢性静脉功能不全。这些重力效应和流体静力的负荷可能在以后导致症状出现[23]。不明原因的严重肿胀和疼痛可能是最先的表现。若出现有症状的静脉功能不全而先前无深静脉栓子[35]或在青春期前出现静脉曲张，则应疑有瓣膜异常[133]。平滑和均匀的静脉 X 线照片对无瓣膜具有诊断价值，这与深静脉正常静脉 X 线照片的表现截然相反，后者由于瓣膜窦的扩张而具有不规则的轮廓[14,124]。多普勒超声是一开始可用于选择的筛查技术。升高或降低的静脉造影可证实瓣膜缺如，并提供解剖细节，有利于手术干预[99]。对无瓣膜后遗症的治疗常常是非手术的，包括肢体的抬高和逐步的压迫袜。早期曾报道将腋静脉瓣移植到下肢深静脉，75% 的患者症状改善，94% 的患者静脉淤滞溃疡得到治愈[116]。Raju 和同事曾报道 60% 的患者 5 年症状改善，60% 的患者 5 年无静脉溃疡复发[99]。这样的治疗是那些对保守治疗无效的无瓣膜患者的选择。

深静脉发育不全

真正的深静脉发育不全很少见。然而，纵向隔膜或“静脉马刺”，或左髂总静脉起始处的单纯狭窄在人群中占 20%（图 132–2）[133]。这些变异的假名包括 May–Thurner 综合征、Cockett 综合征[24]和髂压迫综合征。左髂总静脉压迫发生在右髂总动脉和第五腰椎之间。髂压迫综合征很少见，真正的发病率不清楚。尸体解剖发现人群中髂静脉压迫的发生率为 22%[80]。出现症状的大部分是女性，发生在生命的第二到第四个十年。症状范围从轻度单侧下肢肿胀、疼痛到深静脉血栓形成，可导致肺栓塞或慢性静脉功能不全。多普勒超声提供可疑诊断，但能由 MRV 确诊。症状治疗开始给予压迫袜和对 DVT（深部静脉血栓形成）者行抗凝治疗，但大部分患者需要手术干预[1]。在成人中，血管内支架提供了一种微创的选择，据报道 79%～89% 的患者 1 年开放[54,85]。对于年轻患者，长期的成功是最佳的，可能提供手术干预。外科手术包括隐静脉股–股静脉旁路移植或右髂动脉移位后行左髂总静脉补片血管成形术；报道有 67%～97% 的患者 3 年临床开放[117]。

发育不全存在时，常常合并淋巴管异常。对淋巴管疾病的讨论超出了这一章的范畴。深静脉主干发育不全或发育不良导致流出梗阻，伴有大的双侧浅表静脉的发育，据报道在静脉异常患者中占 8%[33]。有时胚胎静脉维持通畅并可为受累肢体提供流出。这类患者倾向于有肿胀、疼痛、静脉跛行、双侧静脉栓子和溃疡。静脉造影可用于诊断，但 MRI 更能确定异常的解剖结构和范围[124]。一旦解剖结构确定，治疗应该直接结扎连接浅表静脉系统的胚胎静脉的穿孔分支（在深静脉发育不全患者中），或终止错误形成的静脉相互连接（此处主要通过深静脉引流并被证实）[69]。注意到手术阻断大的侧支可能导致严重的并发症，但在代偿失调的患者中仍然需要考虑[44]。

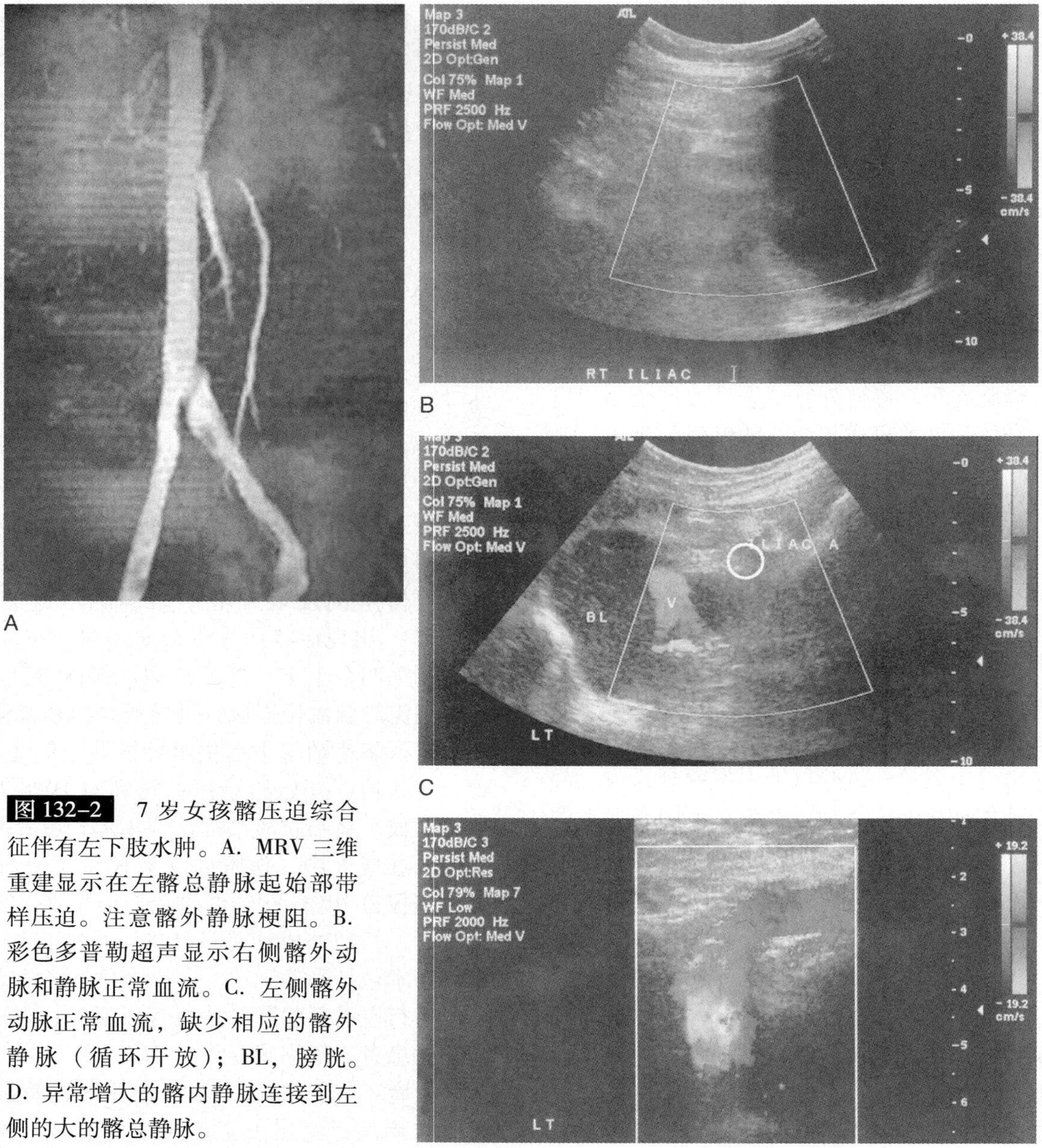

图 132-2 7 岁女孩髂压迫综合征伴有左下肢水肿。A. MRV 三维重建显示在左髂总静脉起始部带样压迫。注意髂外静脉梗阻。B. 彩色多普勒超声显示右侧髂外动脉和静脉正常血流。C. 左侧髂外动脉正常血流，缺少相应的髂外静脉（循环开放）；BL，膀胱。D. 异常增大的髂内静脉连接到左侧的大的髂总静脉。

2128 复杂静脉畸形

严重的先天性血管畸形的临床表现结合了动脉、静脉和淋巴管的发育异常。尽管复杂血管畸形发生少见，但临床表现的严重程度（即组织增生和骨骼过度生长）和问题的大小给人以深刻的印象，常常需要多学科的方法治疗。最常见的血管畸形是 Klippel-Trenaunay 综合征（KTS）、Parkes Weber 综合征和 Maffucci 综合征。治疗依据患者的年龄、病变的组织学特点和症状的严重程度。

KTS 合并毛细血管、静脉、淋巴管的畸形，无动静脉分流。临床症状与病变的范围和部位相关，从轻度静脉曲张到大的增大的肢体或累及躯干[55,106,133]。95% 的患者累及下肢，85% 的患者是单侧的（图132-3）。尽管综合征在出生时即存在，但受累儿童无症状。然而，KTS 患者中 75% 在 10 岁前出现症状[134]。KTS 患者中大约 20% 发现有髂股静脉畸形[42]。尽管持续坐骨静脉是少见异常，但

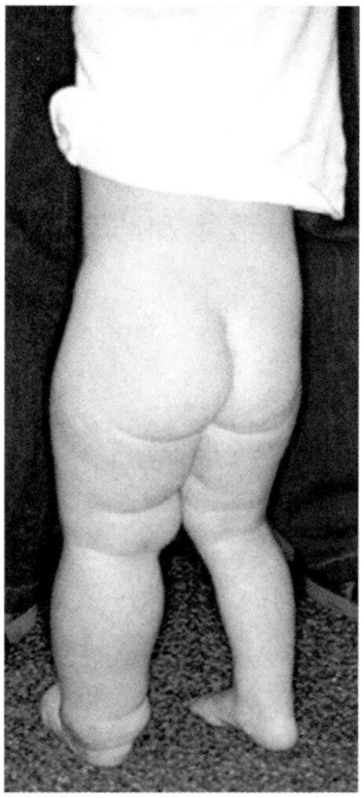

图 132-3　Klippel-Trenaunay 综合征。注意单侧下肢肥大、水肿，下肢长度有差异（也见彩图）。

常常合并存在。轻度症状患者应该用压力服治疗。突起的疣状毛细血管畸形常常是综合征的一部分，
2129 常表现反复的出血。硬化剂治疗对这种局部的皮肤病变特别有效[78,126]。最常见的异常是侧面的静脉异常，表现为静脉曲张[134]。有症状（疼痛和水肿最常见）时应该用静脉造影术和 MRI 广泛记录静脉异常。单独静脉造影术诊断持续坐骨静脉的敏感性为 70%[21]。MRI 强化了对深静脉闭锁的诊断，并在显示软组织畸形分布方面尤其出色[124]。诊断研究的主要目标在于手术切除浅静脉前证实深静脉系统的开放。非手术治疗包括压迫治疗和腿抬高，应该推荐给所有患者。Mayo 诊所注意到在有症状的患者中，浅表静脉手术可明显改善临床症状，虽然 50% 的患者静脉曲张复发[82]。尽管大部分 KTS 患者采用非手术治疗，但约 10% 的患者需要手术[49,82]。有些作者提倡对深静脉开放的患者行侵袭性曲张静脉切除，短期随访结果令人鼓舞[6]。

Parkes Weber 综合征的临床表现与 KTS 类似。临床鉴别是 Parkes Weber 综合征中存在动静脉瘘，而在 KTS 中不存在。由于存在具有快流特点的大动静脉瘘，因此有许多血流动力学的并发症，这是 Parkes Weber 综合征治疗的焦点[124]。少数情况是，这些瘘发生于中央部位，由主动脉或髂动脉的主要分支产生，表现为高输出量充血性心力衰竭[68,124]。大部分病变是手术无法治疗的，若手术干预，则并发症发病率显著。因此，栓塞硬化剂治疗，一种结合栓塞和硬化剂的治疗，成为大的症状性畸形的首选方法，并用于选择性病例中手术的辅助治疗。近年来报道用乙醇和 N-丁基氰基丙烯酸酯作为硬化剂，显示有良好的结果，能显著减少手术切除的并发症[66,67]。

Maffucci 综合征同时存在血管畸形和软骨发育异常。最常见的并发病变是大的皮下复杂静脉畸形。深静脉异常也可见到。约 20% 的患者遭遇恶性变化，常常是软骨肉瘤。在软骨发育不良病例中，新生物的风险达到 50%，要求对这些患者密切随访。系列放射学检查和可疑病变的活检可以建立诊断。外科手术切除是需要的，放疗没有治疗价值[134]。

静脉瘤和静脉曲张

颈部和肢体浅表的静脉瘤常常无症状，但常使父母或儿童感到忧虑和苦恼。颈内静脉瘤的鉴别诊断包括海绵状血管瘤、分支和肠源性囊肿，以及囊状淋巴管瘤。大部分颈内静脉瘤表现为无症状肿块，有良性的自然病史[16]。Valsalva 检查使颈内静脉瘤明显增大，有助于诊断[52]。彩色多普勒超声常常足以作出诊断。颈内静脉瘤唯一的手术指征是美容[64]。

肢体的静脉瘤分为深部和表浅病变。症状和推荐的治疗方法根据解剖部位而不同。深静脉瘤常常发生于腘静脉，表现为肢体疼痛并发肿块，或有时肿胀，以及具有明显的栓子栓塞的风险[98]。有的研究者尝试单独的抗凝治疗，但效果不良[37]。外科手术方法包括结扎、切线切除伴侧面的静脉缝合术或自体静脉补片，以及完整切除和移植物间置，通畅率高达 76%[16]。获得最好的长期通畅率应采用切线切除伴侧面的静脉缝合术。浅表系统的静脉瘤常常产生中等程度的下肢肿胀，伴或不伴有疼痛。这种扩张很少破裂，曲张静脉毁损面容常常是唯一的手术指征。

先天性外周静脉曲张更可能由静脉壁缺陷所致而不是瓣叶缺乏[47,70,97,101,121]。有报道原发性静脉曲张也见于上肢，用以支持这个疾病的遗传病因[128]。治疗范围从压力袜到切除扩张的曲张静脉，及除去反

流点。

2130 外周静脉路径和连接处的异常通常没有临床意义，尽管大隐和小隐静脉重复可能在成人表现为在成功的静脉剥脱术后复发表浅静脉曲张。

静脉血栓

遗传性凝血疾病

凝血系统基因的异常使婴儿和儿童易患血栓和血栓栓塞疾病。在静脉和动脉血栓并发症中，凝血异常包括活性蛋白 C（APC）抵抗（Leiden Ⅴ因子），以及抗纤维蛋白酶Ⅲ、蛋白 C 和蛋白 S 缺乏。少见的是原发抗磷脂综合征，表现为抗凝血狼疮、高半胱氨酸血症和家族性高脂血症[115]。这些高凝风险因子在婴儿肾脏和腹部脏器静脉血栓形成中起重要作用[51]。APC 抵抗在先天性高凝疾病中最常见，在一个系列研究中，APC 抵抗占血栓形成的儿童的 23%～30%[5]。Ⅴ因子失活、减少导致高凝状态，与正常人群相比，杂合子血栓形成的风险增加 7～10 倍，纯合子风险增加 79 倍[60,62,102]。在有高凝状态危险因子的患者中，也有研究证明先天性抗凝血酶Ⅲ缺乏者患静脉血栓的风险是先天性蛋白 C 缺乏和蛋白 S 缺乏患者的 4 倍（分别为 12% 比 2.8% 比 3.3%）[34]。

腔静脉血栓

儿童上腔静脉梗阻常由内在插管和起搏器导致的血栓引起。在需要中央静脉插管的新生儿中，16% 发生上腔静脉血栓[92]。也可见到恶性肿瘤和炎性结节的侵入和压迫。头部抬高和抗凝血治疗能减轻肿胀和青紫症状。

下腔静脉血栓可由髂股、肾或肝静脉血栓传播而来。常伴有严重的伴发疾病或脱水，这种状态可能表现为具有戏剧性的症状，包括水肿、青紫、溃疡或仅有下肢静脉曲张和下腹部侧支。中央静脉插管频率增加导致下腔静脉完全梗阻的发生率在需要这种治疗的婴儿中达 14.5%[92]。诊断根据腔静脉造影、CT 或 MRI 作出。急性暴发病例应该用溶栓或栓子切除和抗凝治疗。腔静脉梗阻导致的下肢慢性静脉功能不全采用升高和压迫袜治疗。长期研究显示下腔静脉血栓的预后可能主要依赖于血栓的范围。静脉曲张年轻时即存在，并随时间而恶化。30% 的患者在 10 年随访中可见血栓后综合征[50]。已知慎重应用中央静脉插管是减少下腔静脉血栓发生和防止长期并发症的最好方法。

肾、肠系膜和门静脉血栓

肾静脉血栓常常是原发过程，几乎总是伴有严重的伴发疾病或脱水。治疗和预后依赖肾脏受累及的严重程度和潜在的疾病过程。尽管有的病例肾功能不全有改善，但后期的高血压或感染仍要求肾切除[30]。肝素抗凝治疗可缩小血栓的传播范围，减少肺栓塞的风险。与儿童和青春期少年相比，新生儿肾静脉血栓很少好转。新生儿血栓中肾静脉血栓最常见，40% 的患儿有症状。血尿和血小板减少是最常见的症状，50% 的新生儿有此表现。与对照患儿相比，肾静脉血栓的新生儿中 67%～85% 至少有一种遗传性高凝风险[51,61,108]。多普勒超声是最常用的确诊方法。增强 CT 和 MRI 取代常规静脉造影。血栓常常起始于肾内小静脉，因此主要治疗包括支持和抗凝治疗[7,30,45]。已有在孤立双侧肾静脉血栓的病例中全身应用溶栓治疗的描述，其结果相互矛盾。预后仍然是严重的，新生儿肾静脉血栓的死亡率为 5%～13%[15,108]。

肠系膜上静脉血栓伴有肠道缺血同样有较高的死亡率。然而，不到 5% 的病例可能导致肠坏死[20]。系膜静脉血栓常常是亚急性的，没有特异性的表现，为痉挛性腹部疼痛、腹胀、厌食、不适。易患因素包括门脉高压、充血性心力衰竭导致的静脉淤滞、腹腔内败血症或静脉炎、恶性梗阻和高凝血状态[51]（恶性疾病，抗凝血酶Ⅲ、蛋白 C、蛋白 S 缺乏，抗心肌磷脂抗体，或深静脉血栓）。有些病例症状存在超过一个月。多普勒超声是可靠的非创伤性检查方法，但增强 CT 或 MRI 可提供更多解剖细节。如果出现腹膜炎体征或怀疑肠穿孔，需要进行剖腹探查和切除所有坏死肠段。如果肠管活力不能确定，则 24 小时内第二次行探腹手术是必要的。迅速的肝素抗凝治疗可减少坏死进一步传播的风险，从 30%～40% 降到 3%～5%[20]。如果潜在的疾病易导致静脉血栓，则长期的抗凝治疗可能是必需的。

2131 门静脉血栓少见，表现不一。急性门静脉栓塞可能没有特异性腹部症状。儿童慢性门静脉栓塞常表现为有门脉高压的趋势，例如胃肠道出血。先天性畸形、恶性疾病、血栓形成倾向、脐静脉插管、腹部手术、新生儿败血症和脐炎，以及创伤是门静脉血栓的易患因素。然而，多达 40% 的病例原因不明[89]。遗传性蛋白 C、蛋白 S、抗凝血酶Ⅲ缺乏的患者比正常人群血栓形成的风险高[51]。有趣的是，尽管激活蛋白 C 抵抗是最常见的静脉血栓的原因，但报道认为这不是门静脉血栓的促进因素[111]。多普勒超声可早期诊断门静脉血栓，甚至是在腹部疼痛作为唯一症状时，据报道其特异性为 90%[46]。与肾静脉和肠系膜静脉血栓相同，增强 CT 或 MRI 可提供更好的解剖细节。治疗包括直接针对门静脉血栓自身、导致的门脉高压以及其他并发症进行治疗。已证明抗凝可有效地治疗急性门静脉血栓。推荐门体分流以减少门脉高压，成功率达 90%[88]。

下肢血栓

在行中央静脉插管的患者中深静脉血栓（DVT）很常见，使发病率和病死率明显升高。加拿大静脉血栓前瞻性研究显示，正常人群中儿童 DVT 发生率是 0.07/10 000，成人人群是 2.5%～5%。这类静脉血栓的 58% 是下肢静脉血栓[3]。91%～96% 的儿童 DVT 中有并发症（如遗传性高凝血状态、严重脱水、败血症），并且在中央静脉插管患者中其发生率高达 77%[3,100]。对照成人的 DVT，儿童 DVT 仅有 4% 有特发性病因[3]。抗凝血酶Ⅲ、蛋白 C、蛋白 S 缺乏和激活的蛋白 C 抵抗是公认的儿童静脉血栓的危险因素[120]。遗传性高凝血疾病所致的血栓更严重，多发生在纯合子个体[110]。诊断常常根据多普勒超声作出，但因为小静脉和不同的血栓部位，儿童患者仍然选择性地应用静脉造影。治疗包括肢体抬高、抗凝（肝素，然后华法林）和压迫袜。对于中央静脉置管所致 DVT，溶栓治疗在新生儿中曾有尝试，但结果不一[130]。急性并发症包括静脉炎和炎症，需要手术干预。未治疗的 DVT 或残留血栓导致慢性静脉功能不全的症状。甚至应用适当的抗凝药物后，DVT 在儿童中仍有 8.1%～18.5% 的复发[3,74]。

上肢血栓

上肢静脉血栓的病因分为原发性和继发性。继发性静脉血栓常常是医源性的（中央静脉置管、起搏器）或由一种潜在的高凝状态引起。发现中央静脉置管直接与 36% 的上肢 DVT 相关[3]，中央静脉置管频率增加，上肢血栓发生增加。多普勒评估常用于有症状患者的诊断。抗凝治疗需要 3～6 个月，手臂症状保守治疗包括抬高、休息和弹力袜支持。对于有静脉通路的患者应该评估更有效的导管相关的血栓溶解。

原发性静脉血栓没有明显的原因可鉴别，有时是错误名称，因为自发“努力性”血栓（Paget－von Schroetter 综合征）以及胸腔出口的病理性压迫也包括在这一组中。症状可由胸腔出口的骨异常和锁骨下静脉压迫，或由于异常的腋胸肌压迫腋静脉，或正常位置肌肉群肌肉肥大引起[105,119]。努力性血栓常常产生于男性运动员占优势的手臂，在儿童和青春期不常见。常见表现是受累手臂的疼痛和肿胀，伴有水肿、青紫和明显的静脉侧支。在普通人群中，急性锁骨下－腋静脉血栓表现在生命的第三到第四个十年，有 10%～15% 的患者有肺栓塞的风险[53,75]，所以要求抗凝治疗。虽然进行了充分的抗凝，70%～80% 的患者仍然有症状[28,53]。一个更强大的治疗方法在过去 10 年曾得到提倡。尽管静脉多普勒超声能证明 DVT，但静脉造影可确定解剖结构，并且如果有指征允许溶栓治疗。因为有些解剖变异在一定部位压迫血管结构，因此推荐行受累上臂的延展和外展的动态静脉造影。推荐治疗是直接置管溶栓和接下来的抗凝治疗[25]。另外，在青春期和年轻成人患者中曾尝试经皮的腔内球囊血管成形术伴有或没有支架放置[63]。无胸腔出口减压时，这种血管内技术在 2 年有 6% 的成功率，可见破裂和支架变形[41,72]。有许多胸腔出口减压的外科方法，包括腋下、锁骨上以及锁骨上结合锁骨下的切口。我们喜欢结合锁骨上和锁骨下切口来完全减 2132
压胸腔出口，去除第一肋、前斜角肌和锁骨下肌，由此去除主要的潜在的外在静脉压迫。残留的静脉疾病要求另外的静脉成形术或旁路步骤。儿科患者表现同样的症状并具有出现相同并发症的风险。近来报道对儿童采用相似的治疗策略显示了良好的短期效果[123]。

静脉血栓并发症

血栓性静脉炎

血栓性静脉炎表现为疾病过程的广谱表现，包括：（1）非特异性、非化脓性血栓性静脉炎表现为疼痛、压痛和顺着静脉通路的发红；（2）化脓性血栓性静脉炎伴有腔内脓性渗出、静脉坏死和外周静脉脓肿。诊断由体检、血液研究和多普勒超声建立。无菌性静脉炎常常对局部治疗有反应，包括热浸泡和镇痛，其他方面健康的儿童不要求静脉切除。对于有发展的浅表脓毒性血栓性静脉炎，两个必要的条件是静脉血栓和血栓感染，常常伴有皮肤菌丛。最主要的临床特征是局部肿胀、红斑、硬结和可触及的索带。发热和压痛在大儿童中发生，更多见于新生儿[57]。大约 90% 的患者在静脉穿刺点发展为血栓性静脉炎[109]。革兰阳性病菌是最常见的病原菌，培养葡萄球菌菌属最常见。治疗开始去除导管，经验性应用抗生素。浅表脓毒性血栓性静脉炎的彻底治疗是根治性切除受影响的静脉段[4,57,84,96,109]。

深静脉的脓毒性血栓性静脉炎在儿童中少见。对于大多数病例，血栓感染发生于危重患者经皮穿刺的中央静脉置管。诊断需要高度怀疑，因为对重症患者和不能运动患者的体检受限。尽管多普勒超声能鉴别腘静脉和股静脉血栓，但增强 CT 应该用于怀疑髂股 DVT 的患者。CT 不仅揭示管腔内血栓和范围，而且可观察静脉周围的液体、软组织脓肿，其他受累器官也可以看到。治疗包括迅速去除存在的导管、使用抗生素、抗凝治疗和培养来鉴别微生物[59]。并发症包括脓毒性肺栓塞、骨髓炎和脓毒性关节炎[43]。对于保守治疗难以治愈的脓毒性病例，确定的静脉周围或皮下脓肿引流和静脉血栓切除结合动静脉瘘可能会挽救生命[59]。

颈内静脉血栓性静脉炎少见，但有咽部间隙感染的严重并发症。Lemierre 曾描述，这种综合征在青春期和年轻成人中可见，表现常常与咽炎或扁桃体炎相似。咽侧间隙的感染导致炎症和继发对颈内静脉内皮细胞的损伤。由于少见和症状不典型，诊断常被延误[2,122]。诊断由多普勒超声、增强 CT 或 MRI 确定。CT 和 MRI 较超声更敏感，报告的准确性接近静脉造影[11,79]。最常见的病原菌是坏死梭形杆菌。治疗主要采用抗生素，常常是青霉素，同时给予肝素抗凝治疗。脓毒性栓塞是常见的[76]。当抗生素治疗没有改善时，原发脓肿的手术引流（扁桃体周围，咽旁间隙脓肿）可能是必要的。很少需要颈内静脉结扎或切除。尽管采用全身性抗生素治疗，但仍有高达 18% 的患者可能死亡[48]。

肺栓塞

肺栓塞（PE）促使重症患儿发病率和死亡率明显增加。肺栓塞真正的发病率不清楚，但似乎比文献报告的要高。Andrew 和同事通过通气灌注肺扫描发现 DVT 患者中 70% 有肺栓塞。真正的肺栓塞发生率可能更高，因为仅对 23% 的高危患者评估了肺栓塞，这可能是由于在重症患儿中怀疑指数很低。14% 的肺栓塞发生是由于下肢 DVT，6% 由于上肢 DVT[3]。在 DVT 中全部的肺栓塞发生率是 17%（上肢或下肢）；当伴有 CVL 时，发生率为 56%。儿童肺栓塞的死亡率为 1.7%[74]。

通气灌注肺扫描常用于肺栓塞诊断，但正被螺旋 CT 所取代。肺血管造影仍然在选择性病例中使用[29]。治疗肺栓塞的可靠选择是抗凝、溶栓或手术。在儿童中治疗 DVT 和 PE 的临床试验尚未完善，成人指南不能外推至儿童。对于大于 2 个月的儿童，部分激活凝血酶原时间的目标为 60～85 秒，标准肝素治疗应该开始 5～10 天，重叠华法林 4～5 天。低分子量肝素是一种可接受的选择[113]。长期的抗凝常常是必需的以防止复发，并按照国际标准化比例（INR）提供华法林给药，该比例为 2～3[29,114]。通常，对于有栓子而没有潜在遗传性或持续获得性缺陷的患者，在血栓发作后华法林治疗 6 个月。其他患者应该终生 2133
接受抗凝治疗[110]。在更多的 DVT 患者和任何对抗凝有禁忌证的患者中应考虑手术放置一个下腔静脉过滤装置。对于有血流动力学危害和严重的有症状的大静脉近端血栓的肺栓塞患者，应该适当考虑溶栓治疗。尽管在一个系列研究中全身性溶栓治疗使 81% 的患者完全解决血栓，14% 的患者部分解决血栓[65]，但导管直接溶栓治疗的效果更好。长期的抗凝常常是必需的，以防止复发，并且提供国际正常比例（INR）的华法林给药，该比例为 2～3。最近，重组的活化蛋白 C 已被证明在成人败血症中对控制和治疗凝血和感染都有效，并在儿科急诊中应用[40]。必须根据个体基础考虑是否选择栓子切除。

遗传性前血栓形成障碍的存在影响了 DVT 和 PE

的处理效果，它使得一期自发性静脉血栓形成后复发性栓子出现的危险性大大增加。另外，儿童的凝血系统不同于成人，更容易影响血栓的形成和增殖以及对抗凝系统的反应。最初诊断为股静脉血栓并得到规范治疗的患者中 12.5% 出现 PE 复发。

血栓后综合征

深静脉和外周静脉异常能导致慢性静脉疾病症状。在先天性外周静脉异常的患者中，并发症见于较正常人群更小的年龄。历史上，根据体检发现（如静脉曲张、皮肤褪色、溃疡）诊断慢性静脉疾病是充分的，治疗局限于外周支持和溃疡给药。随着新的发展，静脉疾病可通过手术修复[10,27,107]。慢性静脉疾病的准确分类对患者的评估和治疗更为关键。在 1994 年，一个特别的美国静脉论坛发展了一个新的分类系统[94]。CEAP 分类代表一个临床（clinical，C）、病因（etiologic，E）、解剖（anatomic，A）和病理生理（pathophysiologic，P）的分类，并被广泛接受。C 构成分为6 类（表 132-1），E 根据静脉功能不全分为原发性、继发性或先天性，A 根据分布分为浅表的、穿孔的或深部分支，P 根据发展机制分为反流、梗阻或在下肢静脉定义的 18 节段中都有发生。这个分类系统最大的价值是标准化了关键要素，有静脉疾病的患者用这种方式不仅能与其他患者区分，而且可以分组，并且可以在不同机构的报道中用标准方式进行对照。在对慢性静脉疾病的治疗反应进行评估后，有几种改良被提出[104]。

由急性 DVT 的残留血栓或纤维性改变导致的慢性静脉功能不全及其后遗症称为*血栓后综合征*，它只是慢性静脉疾病的一个原因。尽管不如在成人中普遍（20%~67%），但血栓后综合征在先前有 DVT 的儿童中的比例最高达到 12%~18%[3,74]。症状包括疼痛、肿胀、棕褐色变色和受累肢体的溃疡（CEAP 分类：C_{2-6}）。这种表现在最初发作 DVT 时接受适当抗凝药物和弹力袜压迫治疗的患者中少见[95]。

表 132-1　慢性下肢静脉疾病临床分类

0 级	无可见或可触及的静脉疾病
1 级	毛细血管扩张，网状静脉，踝张开
2 级	静脉曲张
3 级	水肿没有皮肤改变
4 级	归因于静脉疾病的皮肤改变（如色素沉着、静脉性湿疹、脂性硬皮病）
5 级	确定的超过已治愈溃疡的皮肤改变
6 级	确定的超过活动性溃疡的皮肤改变

总结

与成人相比，儿童静脉疾病更多受到先天性畸形的影响，但许多症状等到成年期才表现出来。先天性畸形的潜在并发症决定了干预的水平，从观察到手术不等。

儿童静脉血栓形成有其独有的特点，比如肾静脉血栓形成。治疗的目的仍然是阻止血栓的进展，减少对器官的破坏和防止肺栓塞。要治疗这一类患儿必须掌握处理高凝状态的知识。

（洪　莉译　夏慧敏校）

参考文献

1. Akers DL Jr, Creado B, Hewitt RL: Iliac vein compression syndrome: Case report and review of the literature. J Vasc Surg 1996;24:477-481.
2. Alvarez A, Schreiber JR: Lemierre's syndrome in adolescent children—anaerobic sepsis with internal jugular vein thrombophlebitis following pharyngitis. Pediatrics 1995;96:354-359.
3. Andrew M, David M, Adams M, et al: Venous thromboembolic complications (VTE) in children: First analyses of the Canadian Registry of VTE. Blood 1994;83:1251-1257.
4. Arisoy ES, Correa-Calderon A, Kaplan SL: Primary deep venous septic thrombophlebitis in a child. J Pediatr 1994;124:439-441.
5. Aschka I, Aumann V, Bergmann F, et al: Prevalence of factor V Leiden in children with thrombo-embolism. Eur J Pediatr 1996;155:1009-1014.
6. Baraldini V, Coletti M, Cipolat L, et al: Early surgical management of Klippel-Trenaunay syndrome in childhood can prevent long-term haemodynamic effects of distal venous hypertension. J Pediatr Surg 2002;37:232-235.
7. Baum NH, Moriel E, Carlton CE Jr: Renal vein thrombosis. J Urol 1978;119:443-448.
8. Belov S: Classification of congenital vascular defects. Int Angiol 1990;9:141-146.
9. Belov S: Anatomopathological classification of congenital vascular defects. Semin Vasc Surg 1993;6:219-224.
10. Bhuller AS, Nachreiner RD, Dalsing MC: Pathophysiology of chronic venous insufficiency and new horizons in surgical management. Semin Intervent Radiol 2001;18:155-170.

11. Blomquist IK, Bayer AS: Life-threatening deep fascial space infections of the head and neck. Infect Dis Clin North Am 1988;2:237-264.
12. Braun P, Collin PP, Ducharme JC: Preduodenal portal vein: A significant entity? Report of two cases and review of the literature. Can J Surg 1974;17:316-319, 322.
13. Brock PA, Jordan PH Jr, Barth MH, et al: Portal vein aneurysm: A rare but important vascular condition. Surgery 1997;121:105-108.
14. Browse NL, Burnand KG, Thomas LM: The Klippel-Trenaunay syndrome. In Browse NL, Burnand KG, Thomas LM (eds): Diseases of the Veins: Pathology, Diagnosis and Treatment. New York, Edward Arnold, 1988, pp 609-625.
15. Brun P, Beaufils F, Pillion G, et al: Thrombosis of the renal veins in the newborn: Treatment and long-term prognosis. Ann Pediatr (Paris) 1993;40:75-80.
16. Calligaro KD, Ahmad S, Dandora R, et al: Venous aneurysms: Surgical indications and review of the literature. Surgery 1995;117:1-6.
17. Campbell M, Deuchar DC: Absent inferior vena cava, symmetrical liver, splenic agenesis, and situs inversus, and their embryology. Br Heart J 1967;29:268-275.
18. Chalmers EA, Gibson BE: Thrombolytic therapy in the management of paediatric thromboembolic disease. Br J Haematol 1999;104:14-21.
19. Chang TN, Tang L, Keller K, et al: Pylephlebitis, portal-mesenteric thrombosis, and multiple liver abscesses owing to perforated appendicitis. J Pediatr Surg 2001;36:E19.
20. Chen MC, Brown MC, Willson RA, et al: Mesenteric vein thrombosis: Four cases and review of the literature. Dig Dis 1996;14:382-389.
21. Cherry KJ, Gloviczki P, Stanson AW: Persistent sciatic vein: diagnosis and treatment of a rare condition. J Vasc Surg 1996;23:490-497.
22. Chuang VP, Mena CE, Hoskins PA: Congenital anomalies of the inferior vena cava: Review of embryogenesis and presentation of a simplified classification. Br J Radiol 1974; 47:206-213.
23. Cockett FB: The significance of absence of valves in the deep veins. J Cardiovasc Surg (Torino) 1964;15:722-727.
24. Cockett FB, Thomas ML: The iliac compression syndrome. Br J Surg 1965;52:816-821.
25. Comerota AJ: Catheter-directed thrombolysis for treatment of axillary-subclavian venous thrombosis. Perspect Vasc Surg Endovasc Ther 2001;14:51-56.
26. Crawford FA Jr, Wolfe WG: Interposition mesocaval H shunt associated with a left inferior vena cava. Surgery 1976;79: 678-681.
27. Dalsing MC: Chronic venous disease. In Greenfield LJ, Mulholland MW, Oldham KT, et al (eds): Surgery: Scientific Principles and Practice, 3rd ed. Philadelphia, Lippincott Williams & Wilkins, 2001, pp 1888-1897.
28. Donayre CE, White GH, Mehringer SM, et al: Pathogenesis determines late morbidity of axillosubclavian vein thrombosis. Am J Surg 1986;152:179-184.
29. Donnelly KM: Venous thromboembolic disease in the pediatric intensive care unit. Curr Opin Pediatr 1999;11:213-217.
30. Duncan RE, Evans AT, Martin LW: Natural history and treatment of renal vein thrombosis in children. J Pediatr Surg 1977;12:639-645.
31. Edwards JE, Du SJ, Alcott DL, et al: Thoracic venous anomalies: III. Atresia of the common pulmonary vein, the pulmonary veins draining wholly into the superior vena cava. AMA Arch Pathol 1951;51:446-460.
32. Eguchi S, Endo S, Yamaguchi A, et al: Inferior caval occlusion associated with the Budd-Chiari-syndrome: Treatment with bypass operation. J Cardiovasc Surg (Torino) 1966;7: 490-494.
33. Eifert S, Villavicencio JL, Kao TC, et al: Prevalence of deep venous anomalies in congenital vascular malformations of venous predominance. J Vasc Surg 2000;31:462-471.
34. Finazzi G, Barbui T: Different incidence of venous thrombosis in patients with inherited deficiencies of antithrombin III, protein C and protein S. Thromb Haemost 1994;71:15-18.
35. Friedman EI, Taylor LM Jr, Porter JM: Congenital venous valvular aplasia of the lower extremities. Surgery 1988;103: 24-26.
36. Gallego C, Velasco M, Marcuello P, et al: Congenital and acquired anomalies of the portal venous system. Radiographics 2002;22:141-159.
37. Gillespie DL, Villavicencio JL, Gallagher C, et al: Presentation and management of venous aneurysms. J Vasc Surg 1997;26:845-852.
38. Giordano JM: Embryology of the vascular system. In Rutherford RB (ed): Vascular Surgery, 5th ed. Philadelphia, WB Saunders, 2000, pp 46-47.
39. Giordano JM, Trout HH 3rd: Anomalies of the inferior vena cava. J Vasc Surg 1986;3:924-928.
40. Giroir BP: Recombinant human activated protein C for the treatment of severe sepsis: Is there a role in pediatrics? Curr Opin Pediatr 2003;15:92-96.
41. Glanz S, Gordon DH, Lipkowitz GS, et al: Axillary and subclavian vein stenosis: Percutaneous angioplasty. Radiology 1988;168:371-373.
42. Gloviczki P, Hollier LH, Telander RL, et al: Surgical implications of Klippel-Trenaunay syndrome. Ann Surg 1983;197: 353-362.
43. Gorenstein A, Gross E, Houri S, et al: The pivotal role of deep vein thrombophlebitis in the development of acute disseminated staphylococcal disease in children. Pediatrics 2000;106:E87.
44. Gorenstein A, Shifrin E, Gordon RL, et al: Congenital aplasia of the deep veins of lower extremities in children: The role of ascending functional phlebography. Surgery 1986; 99:414-420.
45. Gupta N, Gewertz BL: Acute occlusive events involving the renal vessels. In Rutherford RB (ed): Vascular Surgery, 5th ed. Philadelphia, WB Saunders, 2000, pp 1706-1712.
46. Gurakan F, Eren M, Kocak N, et al: Extrahepatic portal vein thrombosis in children: Etiology and long-term follow-up. J Clin Gastroenterol 2004;38:368-372.
47. Haardt B: Histochemical comparison of the enzyme profiles of healthy veins and varicose veins. Phlebologie 1986; 39:921-931.
48. Hagelskjaer Kristensen L, Prag J: Human necrobacillosis, with emphasis on Lemierre's syndrome. Clin Infect Dis 2000; 31:524-532.
49. Harris EJ Jr: Chronic venous and lymphatic diseases. In Porter JM (ed): Year Book of Vascular Surgery. St. Louis, Mosby, 2002, pp 518-520.
50. Hausler M, Hubner D, Delhaas T, et al: Long term complications of inferior vena cava thrombosis. Arch Dis Child 2001;85:228-233.
51. Heller C, Schobess R, Kurnik K, et al: Abdominal venous thrombosis in neonates and infants: Role of prothrombotic risk factors—a multicentre case-control study. For the Childhood Thrombophilia Study Group. Br J Haematol 2000;111:534-539.
52. Hughes PL, Qureshi SA, Galloway RW: Jugular venous aneurysm in children. Br J Radiol 1988;61:1082-1084.
53. Hurlbert SN, Rutherford RB: Primary subclavian-axillary vein thrombosis. Ann Vasc Surg 1995;9:217-223.

54. Hurst DR, Forauer AR, Bloom JR, et al: Diagnosis and endovascular treatment of iliocaval compression syndrome. J Vasc Surg 2001;34:106-113.
55. Jacob AG, Driscoll DJ, Shaughnessy WJ, et al: Klippel-Trenaunay syndrome: Spectrum and management. Mayo Clin Proc 1998;73:28-36.
56. Kabbani SS, Feldman M, Angelini P, et al: Single (left) superior vena cava draining into the left atrium: Surgical repair. Ann Thorac Surg 1973;16:518-525.
57. Khan EA, Correa AG, Baker CJ: Suppurative thrombophlebitis in children: A ten-year experience. Pediatr Infect Dis J 1997;16:63-67.
58. Kimura C, Shirotani H, Hirooka M, et al: Membranous obliteration of the inferior vena cava in the hepatic portion. (Review of 6 cases with 3 autopsies). J Cardiovasc Surg (Torino) 1963;4:87-98.
59. Kniemeyer HW, Grabitz K, Buhl R, et al: Surgical treatment of septic deep venous thrombosis. Surgery 1995;118:49-53.
60. Koeleman BP, Reitsma PH, Allaart CF, et al: Activated protein C resistance as an additional risk factor for thrombosis in protein C–deficient families. Blood 1994;84:1031-1035.
61. Kosch A, Kuwertz-Broking E, Heller C, et al: Renal venous thrombosis in neonates: Prothrombotic risk factors and long-term follow-up. Blood 2004;104:1356-1360.
62. Koster T, Rosendaal FR, de Ronde H, et al: Venous thrombosis due to poor anticoagulant response to activated protein C: Leiden Thrombophilia Study. Lancet 1993;342:1503-1506.
63. Kreienberg PB, Chang BB, Darling RC 3rd, et al: Long-term results in patients treated with thrombolysis, thoracic inlet decompression, and subclavian vein stenting for Paget-Schroetter syndrome. J Vasc Surg 2001;33:S100-S105.
64. LaMonte SJ, Walker EA, Moran WB: Internal jugular phlebectasia: A clinicoroentgenographic diagnosis. Arch Otolaryngol 1976;102:706-708.
65. Leaker M, Massicotte MP, Brooker LA, et al: Thrombolytic therapy in pediatric patients: A comprehensive review of the literature. Thromb Haemost 1996;76:132-134.
66. Lee BB: Critical issues in management of congenital vascular malformation. Ann Vasc Surg 2004;18:380-392.
67. Lee BB, Bergan JJ: Advanced management of congenital vascular malformations: A multidisciplinary approach. Cardiovasc Surg 2002;10:523-533.
68. Lindenauer SM: The Klippel-Trenaunay syndrome: Varicosity, hypertrophy and hemangioma with no arteriovenous fistula. Ann Surg 1965;162:303-314.
69. Loose DA: Surgical treatment of predominantly venous defects. Semin Vasc Surg 1993;6:252-259.
70. Ludbrook J: Valvular defect in primary varicose veins: Cause or effect? Lancet 1963;41:1289-1292.
71. Marois D, van Heerden JA, Carpenter HA, et al: Congenital absence of the portal vein. Mayo Clin Proc 1979;54: 55-59.
72. Meier GH, Pollak JS, Rosenblatt M, et al: Initial experience with venous stents in exertional axillary-subclavian vein thrombosis. J Vasc Surg 1996;24:974-981; discussion 981-973.
73. Miller G, Inmon TW, Pollock BE: Persistent left superior vena cava. Am Heart J 1955;49:267-274.
74. Monagle P, Adams M, Mahoney M, et al: Outcome of pediatric thromboembolic disease: A report from the Canadian Childhood Thrombophilia Registry. Pediatr Res 2000;47: 763-766.
75. Monreal M, Lafoz E, Ruiz J, et al: Upper-extremity deep venous thrombosis and pulmonary embolism: A prospective study. Chest 1991;99:280-283.
76. Moore BA, Dekle C, Werkhaven J: Bilateral Lemierre's syndrome: A case report and literature review. Ear Nose Throat J 2002;81:234-236, 238-240, 242 passim.
77. Mordehai J, Cohen Z, Kurzbart E, et al: Preduodenal portal vein causing duodenal obstruction associated with situs inversus, intestinal malrotation, and polysplenia: A case report. J Pediatr Surg 2002;37:E5.
78. Mulliken JB: Cutaneous vascular anomalies. Semin Vasc Surg 1993;6:204-218.
79. Nakamura S, Sadoshima S, Doi Y, et al: Internal jugular vein thrombosis, Lemierre's syndrome; oropharyngeal infection with antibiotic and anticoagulation therapy—a case report. Angiology 2000;51:173-177.
80. Negus D, Fletcher EW, Cockett FB, et al: Compression and band formation at the mouth of the left common iliac vein. Br J Surg 1968;55:369-374.
81. Niwa T, Aida N, Tachibana K, et al: Congenital absence of the portal vein: Clinical and radiologic findings. J Comput Assist Tomogr 2002;26:681-686.
82. Noel AA, Gloviczki P, Cherry KJ Jr, et al: Surgical treatment of venous malformations in Klippel-Trenaunay syndrome. J Vasc Surg 2000;32:840-847.
83. Nowak-Gottl U, Junker R, Kreuz W, et al: Risk of recurrent venous thrombosis in children with combined prothrombotic risk factors. Blood 2001;97:858-862.
84. O'Neill JA Jr, Pruitt BA Jr, Foley FD, et al: Suppurative thrombophlebitis—a lethal complication of intravenous therapy. J Trauma 1968;8:256-267.
85. O'Sullivan GJ, Semba CP, Bittner CA, et al: Endovascular management of iliac vein compression (May-Thurner) syndrome. J Vasc Interv Radiol 2000;11:823-836.
86. Oderich GS, Treiman GS, Schneider P, et al: Stent placement for treatment of central and peripheral venous obstruction: A long-term multi-institutional experience. J Vasc Surg 2000; 32:760-769.
87. Ohara I, Ouchi H, Takahashi K: A bypass operation for occlusion of the hepatic inferior vena cava. Surg Gynecol Obstet 1963;117:151-155.
88. Orloff MJ, Orloff MS, Girard B, et al: Bleeding esophagogastric varices from extrahepatic portal hypertension: 40 years' experience with portal-systemic shunt. J Am Coll Surg 2002;194:717-728; discussion 728-730.
89. Orloff MJ, Orloff MS, Rambotti M: Treatment of bleeding esophagogastric varices due to extrahepatic portal hypertension: Results of portal-systemic shunts during 35 years. J Pediatr Surg 1994;29:142-151; discussion 151-144.
90. Patel P, Weitz J, Brooker LA, et al: Decreased thrombin activity of fibrin clots prepared in cord plasma compared with adult plasma. Pediatr Res 1996;39:826-830.
91. Pearce WH, Rutherford RB, Whitehill TA, et al: Nuclear magnetic resonance imaging: Its diagnostic value in patients with congenital vascular malformations of the limbs. J Vasc Surg 1988;8:64-70.
92. Pippus KG, Giacomantonio JM, Gillis DA, et al: Thrombotic complications of saphenous central venous lines. J Pediatr Surg 1994;29:1218-1219.
93. Pohl A, Jung A, Vielhaber H, et al: Congenital atresia of the portal vein and extrahepatic portocaval shunt associated with benign neonatal hemangiomatosis, congenital adrenal hyperplasia, and atrial septal defect. J Pediatr Surg 2003; 38:633-634.
94. Porter JM, Moneta GL: Reporting standards in venous disease: An update. International Consensus Committee on Chronic Venous Disease. J Vasc Surg 1995;21:635-645.
95. Prandoni P, Lensing AW, Prins MR: The natural history of deep-vein thrombosis. Semin Thromb Hemost 1997;23: 185-188.

96. Pruitt BA Jr, Stein JM, Foley FD, et al: Intravenous therapy in burn patients: Suppurative thrombophlebitis and other life-threatening complications. Arch Surg 1970;100: 399-404.
97. Psaila JV, Melhuish J: Viscoelastic properties and collagen content of the long saphenous vein in normal and varicose veins. Br J Surg 1989;76:37-40.
98. Rachel E, Pearce WH: Venous malformations and aneurysms: Evaluation and treatment. In Gloviczki P, Yao JST (eds): Handbook of Venous Disorders—Guidelines of the American Venous Forum, 2nd ed. New York, Arnold, 2001, pp 439-449.
99. Raju S: Venous valve reconstruction. In Raju S, Villavicencio JL (eds): Surgical Management of Venous Disease. Baltimore, Williams & Wilkins, 1997, pp 338-356.
100. Revel-Vilk S, Chan A, Bauman M, et al: Prothrombotic conditions in an unselected cohort of children with venous thromboembolic disease. J Thromb Haemost 2003;1:915-921.
101. Rose SS, Ahmed A: Some thoughts on the aetiology of varicose veins. J Cardiovasc Surg (Torino) 1986;27:534-543.
102. Rosendaal FR, Koster T, Vandenbroucke JP, et al: High risk of thrombosis in patients homozygous for factor V Leiden (activated protein C resistance). Blood 1995;85: 1504-1508.
103. Rossall RE, Caldwell RA: Obstruction of inferior vena cava by a persistent eustachian valve in a young adult. J Clin Pathol 1957;10:40-45.
104. Rutherford RB, Padberg FT Jr, Comerota AJ, et al: Venous outcomes assessment. In Gloviczki P, Yao JST (eds): Handbook of Venous Disorders—Guidelines of the American Venous Forum, 2nd ed. New York, Arnold, 2001, pp 497-508.
105. Sachatello CR: The axillopectoral muscle (Langer's axillary arch): A cause of axillary vein obstruction. Surgery 1977;81:610-612.
106. Samuel M, Spitz L: Klippel-Trenaunay syndrome: Clinical features, complications and management in children. Br J Surg 1995;82:757-761.
107. Sanders BM, Dalsing MC: Deep vein valvular incompetence: Options for reconstruction. Perspect Vasc Surg Endovasc Ther 2001;14:89-106.
108. Schmidt B, Andrew M: Neonatal thrombosis: Report of a prospective Canadian and international registry. Pediatrics 1995;96:939-943.
109. Sears N, Grosfeld JL, Weber TR, et al: Suppurative thrombophlebitis in childhood. Pediatrics 1981;68:630-632.
110. Segel GB, Francis CA: Anticoagulant proteins in childhood venous and arterial thrombosis: A review. Blood Cells Mol Dis 2000;26:540-560.
111. Seixas CA, Hessel G, Ribeiro CC, et al: Factor V Leiden is not common in children with portal vein thrombosis. Thromb Haemost 1997;77:258-261.
112. Shinkai M, Ohhama Y, Nishi T, et al: Congenital absence of the portal vein and role of liver transplantation in children. J Pediatr Surg 2001;36:1026-1031.
113. Streif W, Goebel G, Chan AK, et al: Use of low molecular mass heparin (enoxaparin) in newborn infants: A prospective cohort study of 62 patients. Arch Dis Child Fetal Neonatal Ed 2003;88:F365-F370.
114. Streif W, Mitchell LG, Andrew M: Antithrombotic therapy in children. Curr Opin Pediatr 1999;11:56-64.
115. Sutor AH, Uhl M: Diagnosis of thromboembolic disease during infancy and childhood, Semin Thromb Hemost 1997;23:237-246.
116. Taheri SA, Heffner R, Meenaghan MA, et al: Technique and results of venous valve transplantation. In Bergan JJ, Yao JST (eds): Surgery of the Veins. New York, Grune & Stratton, 1985, pp 219-231.
117. Taheri SA, Williams J, Powell S, et al: Iliocaval compression syndrome. Am J Surg 1987;154:169-172.
118. Tanaka Y, Takayanagi M, Shiratori Y, et al: Congenital absence of portal vein with multiple hyperplastic nodular lesions in the liver. J Gastroenterol 2003;38:288-294.
119. Tilney ML, Griffiths HJ, Edwards EA: Natural history of major venous thrombosis of the upper extremity. Arch Surg 1970;101:792-796.
120. Tormene D, Simioni P, Prandoni P, et al: The incidence of venous thromboembolism in thrombophilic children: A prospective cohort study. Blood 2002;100:2403-2405.
121. Travers JP, Brookes CE, Evans J, et al: Assessment of wall structure and composition of varicose veins with reference to collagen, elastin and smooth muscle content. Eur J Vasc Endovasc Surg 1996;11:230-237.
122. Venglarcik J: Lemierre's syndrome. Pediatr Infect Dis J 2003;22:921-923.
123. Vercellio G, Baraldini V, Gatti C, et al: Thoracic outlet syndrome in paediatrics: Clinical presentation, surgical treatment, and outcome in a series of eight children. J Pediatr Surg 2003;38:58-61.
124. Villavicencio JL: Congenital vascular malformations of venous predominance: Klippel-Tranaunay syndrome. In Raju S, Villavicencio JL (eds): Surgical Management of Venous Disease. Baltimore, Williams & Wilkins, 1997, pp 445-461.
125. Villavicencio JL, Gonzalez-Cerna JL: Acute vascular problems of children. Curr Probl Surg 1985;22:1-85.
126. Villavicencio JL, Scultetus A, Lee BB: Congenital vascular malformations: When and how to treat them. Semin Vasc Surg 2002;15:65-71.
127. Watkins E Jr, Fortin CL: Surgical correction of a congenital coarctation of the inferior vena cava. Ann Surg 1964;159: 536-541.
128. Welch HJ, Villavicencio JL: Primary varicose veins of the upper extremity: A report of three cases. J Vasc Surg 1994; 20:839-843.
129. Wennerstrand JR: A case with a vena cava superior on both sides. Anat Anz 1963;112:338-343.
130. Wever ML, Liem KD, Geven WB, et al: Urokinase therapy in neonates with catheter related central venous thrombosis. Thromb Haemost 1995;73:180-185.
131. Yang DM, Yoon MH, Kim HS, et al: Portal vein aneurysm of the umbilical portion: Imaging features and the relationship with portal vein anomalies. Abdom Imaging 2003; 28:62-67.
132. Young AE: Pathogenesis of vascular malformations. In Mulliken JB, Young AE (eds): Vascular Birthmarks—Hemangiomas and Malformations. Philadelphia, WB Saunders, 1988, pp 107-113.
133. Young AE: Venous and arterial malformations. In Mulliken JB, Young AE (eds): Vascular Birthmarks—Hemangiomas and Malformations. Philadelphia, WB Saunders, 1988, pp 196-214.
134. Young AE, Ackroyd J, Baskerville P: Combined vascular malformations. In Mulliken JB, Young AE (eds): Vascular Birthmarks—Hemangiomas and Malformations. Philadelphia, WB Saunders, 1988, pp 246-274.

第 133 章

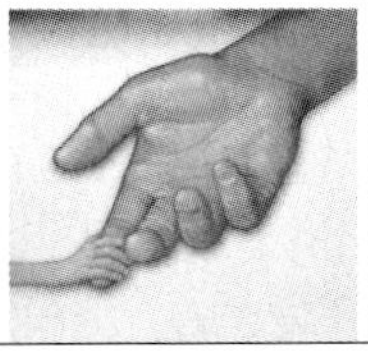

淋巴系统疾病

Eric W. Fonkalsrud

胚胎学和解剖

2137 Sabin[47]、Skandalakis[53]和其他一些学者详细地描述了淋巴系统的发现、分类和胚胎学的简史。淋巴系统的发育与静脉结构紧密相关，有一个内皮细胞层。孕 6 周时，颈部能分辨出成对的颈淋巴管囊，腰区能看到髂囊[43~46]。孕 8 周时，肠系膜根的底部可见腹膜后淋巴囊。乳糜池在腹主动脉背侧发育。成对的胸导管穿过胸腔向头侧发育，连接腹部的淋巴系统和颈部的静脉系统（图 133-1）。最后胸导管向头侧发出一支管道到达右胸，然后跨越到左侧，在颈锁关节左侧汇入静脉系统。头、颈、上臂接受从成对的颈淋巴囊来的淋巴管丛。围绕坐骨和股静脉的后囊接受来自后背、臀部及下肢的淋巴管。孕 9 周左右，结缔组织侵入淋巴囊形成淋巴结[29]。淋巴细胞进入淋巴结，形成淋巴管和滤泡。浅表淋巴管有瓣膜，由复杂的类似毛细血管样结构的皮肤网络组成，引流到有瓣膜的大的皮下管道。这些管道引流到第三级，更深层的位于筋膜上方的皮下脂肪层，此处的淋巴管有更多的瓣膜，并有薄的肌层，单向输送[40]。淋巴管造影显示皮下淋巴系统和与深部动脉平行的肌内淋巴系统的交通部分邻近局部淋巴结[28]。除非是病态[50]，浅表和深部的系统被认为在功能上是独立的。

淋巴系统分布于全身，可清除渗出液以及组织间液中的小分子和大分子物质。与血管相比，毛细淋巴管缺乏完整的基底膜，可以漏过大分子和细胞。这使无法通过静脉系统吸收的大分子的血浆蛋白和脂质可在细胞间扩散[7,38]。通常情况下，淋巴系统的压力为 0 mmH_2O 或负值[33]。

尽管有学者认为淋巴系统畸形是胚胎发育时淋巴系统梗阻、发育不全、发育异常或不发育的结果，但其病理生理学仍不清楚[60]。体液过多或引流系统缺陷可导致淋巴引流障碍。有学者认为淋巴系统畸形由原始淋巴囊退化产生[46]。淋巴管梗阻导致内皮层间隙扩张，形成范围小到显微管道的小囊肿，大到单房的囊肿。不同的是，损伤的或异常的原始淋巴囊可能不会以有序的或完整的方式来播散，由此导致淋巴液生成减少或形成异常的淋巴系统，进而导致淋巴水肿的临床表现。一个公认的观点认为淋巴管造影摄片显示的淋巴水肿、淋巴管瘤、淋巴管扩张和淋巴血管肉瘤与淋巴管发育不良、异常增生或肿瘤形成有关[21,27]。病理变异包括：（1）淋巴管瘤，由淋巴管畸形导致淋巴管扩张而形成连续的肿块；（2）淋巴管扩张，是由于淋巴管发育过程中淋巴管梗阻，实质或固态结构发育不良而形成扩张；（3）淋巴水肿，与原始皮下淋巴系统管缺失或发育不良有关。

淋巴管瘤

淋巴管瘤是良性的、错构瘤性质的淋巴系统肿瘤，其特征是有多发交通的淋巴管和囊性空间。直径大多小于 5 mm，几乎人体任何部位均可产生。超过 2/3 的淋巴管瘤在出生时即可出现，其余多在 2 岁前出现。产前 B 超偶尔在胎儿体内发现淋巴管瘤[34]。与血管瘤不同，淋巴管瘤很少会自发消退，有可能增大，偶尔会延伸到邻近组织。许多淋巴管瘤累及皮肤 2138
和皮下组织，并常常伴有其他类型的血管病变，尤其是静脉畸形[33]。在有些患儿，扩张的毛细血管和静脉管腔分散或邻近淋巴管瘤，称为血管淋巴管瘤。这类肿瘤可以是局限性的也可以是广泛性的，并可侵犯几乎所有的组织。

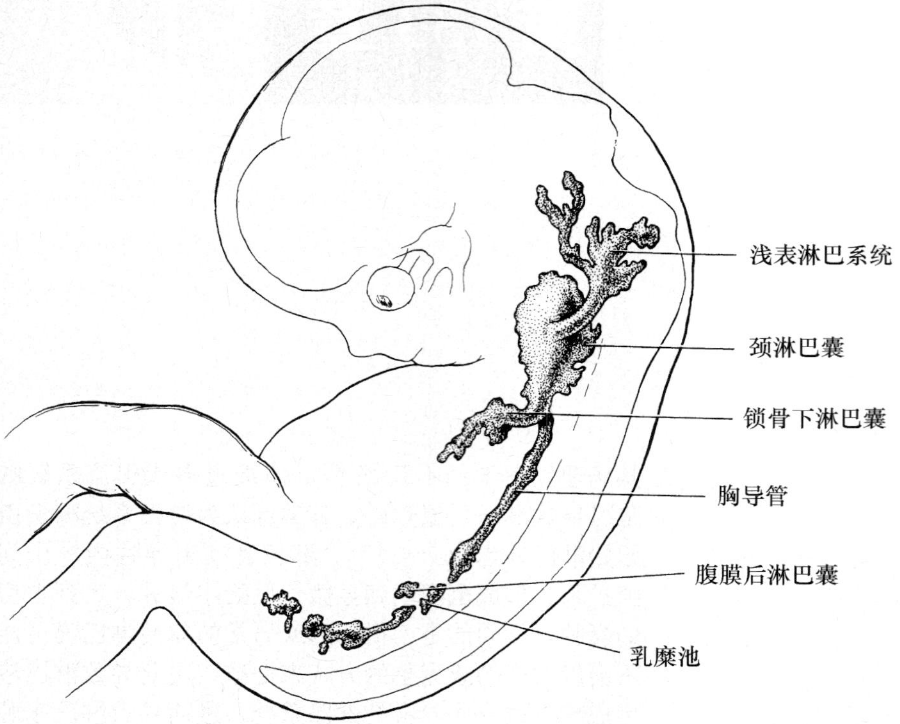

图 133-1 胎儿淋巴系统发育从颈、胸、髂区的原始静脉淋巴囊开始。

淋巴管瘤可分为：（1）单纯淋巴管瘤，由小的毛细血管大小的淋巴管组成；（2）海绵状淋巴管瘤，有扩张的淋巴管，常有纤维外膜覆盖；（3）囊性淋巴管瘤，通常指囊性水囊瘤[1]。

淋巴管瘤最常见的并发症是反复发作的蜂窝织炎和淋巴管炎，偶尔会引起败血症。淋巴管炎常伴有周围组织压迫引起明显的肿胀和疼痛。由于反复感染，这类病变可以发展为纤维化。淋巴管瘤皮肤囊肿的破裂伴随淋巴液和血液的渗漏，常常是蜂窝织炎的前奏。淋巴管炎，通常由链球菌或葡萄球菌引起，常发展迅速，需要迅速的抗感染治疗和适当制动。应该静脉给予抗生素，直到产生疗效，再逐渐改为口服。

淋巴管瘤浸润到周围组织使局部扩展，常难以完整切除。这类浸润型的淋巴管瘤常见于舌、颊、胸腔、腹膜后和四肢[37]（图 133-2），较囊性淋巴管瘤触诊更坚硬，由致密的结缔组织间质和淋巴管道内的微小淋巴管间隙（微囊肿）组成。新生儿呼吸窘迫可能由颈部淋巴管瘤压迫气道引起。舌的病变多位于中线，浸润口腔底部可导致双侧颌下肿胀。由于反复的损伤或感染，舌头可经常发生肿大，由于舌从口腔突出，可出现渗出，流涎过多，偶尔发生出血。

2139 囊性淋巴管瘤通常柔软、可压缩，照射可透光。这类病变可发生于全身，常见于颈部（图 133-3）、腋下、纵隔及腹股沟[13]。有些患儿，肿块可侵犯颈部和纵隔或腋下（图 133-4）。偶尔，囊性淋巴管瘤可见于肝、脾，肾较罕见。这些病变通常称为水囊状

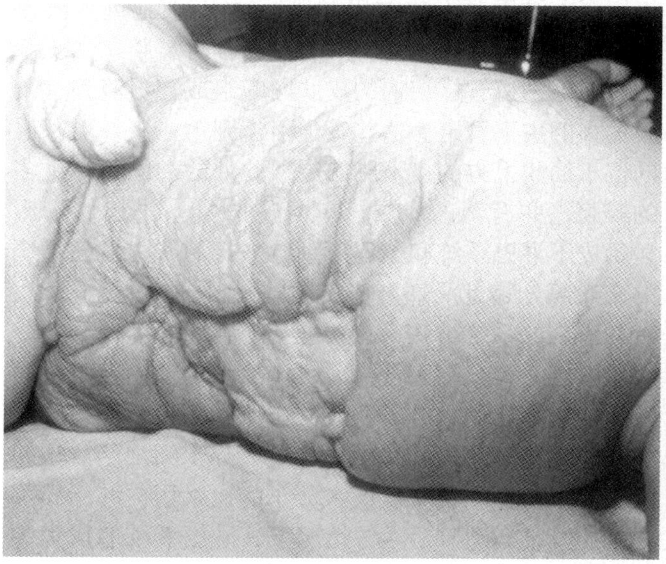

图 133-2 该 3 岁男孩淋巴管瘤累及左腿和外生殖器，行分期切除手术，包括病变的皮肤和皮下组织。

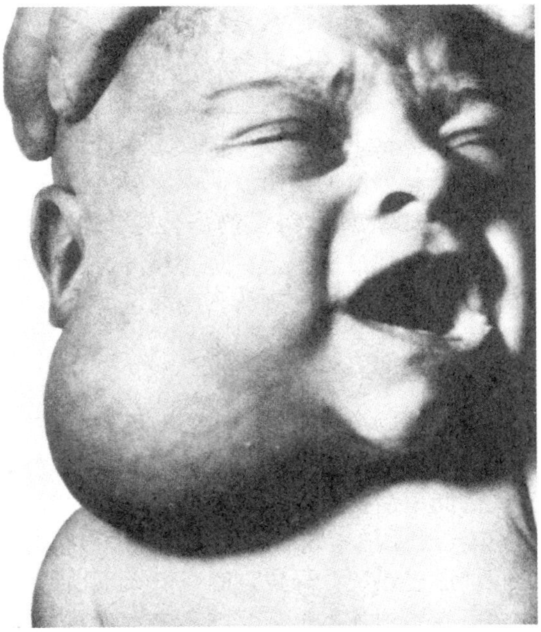

图 133–3　该 3 周大婴儿，颈部右前三角区可见水囊状淋巴管瘤。

淋巴管瘤。胚胎学上，这类病变被认为是由于发育中的淋巴海绵囊挤压断离，引起淋巴组织退化，与淋巴系统其余部分交通失败所致。囊性水囊瘤可能是单个

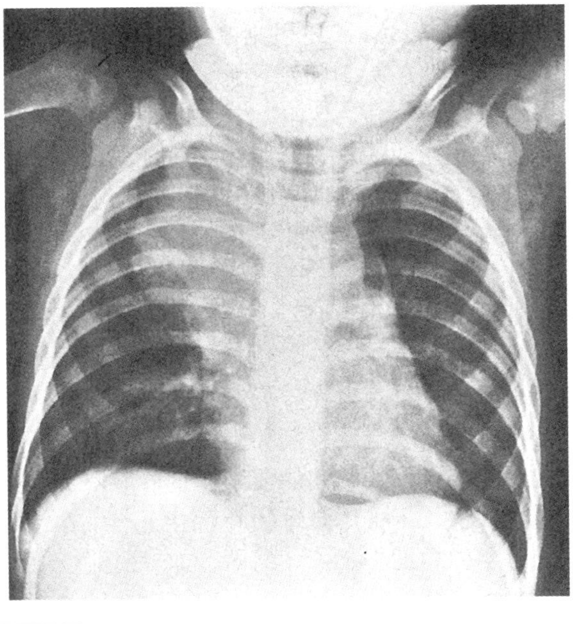

图 133–4　右颈部水囊状淋巴管瘤患儿的胸片，有大的纵隔扩张。

的，但多数在病变处有多发的非交通性小腔形成[1]。

不论皮肤的还是囊性的或皮下的淋巴管瘤的诊断，常以特异的临床表现为依据。如有疑问，超声可以确诊；然而，当病变浸润到机体深层结构而无法确定时，增强 CT 可准确显示病变的范围[1]。另一可选择的方法是 MRI。以上这些方法对侵犯颈、胸腔、后腹膜的淋巴管样病变尤其有用。MRI 对判断侵犯四肢淋巴系统的复杂血管病变更有价值。

淋巴管瘤治疗的指征包括毁形、体积巨大、慢性淋巴液渗出，以及经常发作的感染[18]。淋巴管瘤的治疗是尽可能切除[13]。这类病变是良性的，故切除过程中不要损伤重要的结构。完整切除的患儿中 5%~15% 复发，需要再次手术。即便淋巴管瘤囊性成分已被成功完整切除，切除区域的永久的皮肤侵犯并不少见。当病变较大，皮肤有渗出时，局部激光治疗可能有效。对不能切除的或复发的病变采用放疗、激素和硬化剂治疗一般无效。对难以手术切除的病例，瘤体内注射 OK–432，为一种冻干的低病毒链球菌和青霉素的孵育和相互作用下的单克隆抗体，有效率约 60%[14,17,35]。瘤体内注射博来霉素 A_5 曾作为首选治疗，报道有 55% 的患儿有效[36,56]；但偶尔可出现包括感染、胃肠道紊乱、肺纤维化等并发症。对头颈部巨大的、有明显微小囊性成分的淋巴管瘤，注射治疗无明显效果。纤维蛋白黏合剂注射曾有应用，偶有成功。

浸润型淋巴管瘤包绕正常结构，常向外生长，包绕神经丛，常切除困难。手术时间较长且技术难度大。必须熟悉复杂区域的解剖结构，例如头颈部、腋窝、纵隔、盆腔等。当手术切除淋巴管瘤时，一定要考虑到这是良性病变，尽量避免损伤重要的附属结 2140
构。当必需手术治疗危及生命的气道梗阻时，更是如此。当病变扩散到深部或重要结构时，应该切除淋巴管瘤主要部分，如有可能，应该尽可能完整切除，而 1/3 以上的病例需要分期手术[18]。淋巴管瘤很少能完整切除，除非是颈部局限的淋巴水囊瘤。完整切除不能以牺牲重要脏器为代价。

淋巴管扩张

淋巴管扩张可影响多个器官和组织，包括小肠、肺和骨。肠道的淋巴管扩张常见于 3 岁以下的儿童，

表现为腹泻、呕吐及生长发育迟缓，是蛋白丢失性肠病的病因之一[19]。小肠黏膜活检可确诊。病理显示小肠绒毛内淋巴管扩张，伴有小肠固有层的梗阻；较常见的可延伸到固有层、黏膜下层、浆膜甚至肠系膜，偶尔仅累及肠系膜。蛋白丢失的程度轻重不同。因为长链脂肪不能被扩张或梗阻的肠道淋巴系统吸收，故存在脂肪吸收不良。常见淋巴细胞减少和低蛋白血症。低丙种球蛋白血症也可见到。偶尔可见下肢凹陷性水肿。肠道淋巴管扩张的治疗包括添加中链三酰甘油和维生素的高蛋白、低脂饮食[42]。该饮食计划可以减少腹泻和低蛋白血症。肠道淋巴管扩张常因为范围太大而不能手术，偶尔随时间延长症状有所改善。干扰素-α 已用于治疗少数复杂患儿，偶有疗效。

肺淋巴管扩张在新生儿及婴儿早期由于肺实质淋巴系统梗阻可导致呼吸窘迫。肺淋巴管梗阻可导致肺水肿和胸膜渗出。常是双侧的，并向两肺扩散。该病常合并先天性心脏病，也有家族遗传的报道。有的病例可自行缓解，但大多数病例常迅速发展为呼吸衰竭，最终致死。年长患儿可表现为杵状指、呼吸困难、咯血。胸片显示间质液体，有或无胸膜渗出。肺活检可确诊。治疗为支持治疗，必要时采用胸腔穿刺或置胸管引流。用四环素或其他硬化剂行化学性胸膜固定术可防止反复的胸腔积液[13]。

骨淋巴管扩张可导致疼痛、畸形、病理性骨折，在 X 线片上可显示为溶解性改变。病变可累及除颅骨、指（趾）骨以外几乎所有的骨骼。骨淋巴管扩张可与其他部位的淋巴管瘤同时存在，尤其在躯干部和乳糜胸。病变会逐渐增大，直到开始破坏骨骼。颈椎淋巴管扩张如果椎体塌陷可能致死。放射学特征性表现可确诊。骨弥漫性淋巴管扩张没有特殊治疗方法，病变刮除并在缺损处充填自体骨片可
2140 能有效。

乳糜性腹水

乳糜性腹水可在生后早期出现，通常是由于肠系膜淋巴系统与胸导管的连接发育不全或缺失引起的。乳糜腹有可能是全身淋巴系统发育不良的表现，并有乳糜返流入肠道淋巴系统。增大的肠道淋巴系统可破裂到肠腔，肠道继发性丢失蛋白质和脂肪。乳糜尿病理生理与其相似，为淋巴系统破裂到肾盂[24,39]。

乳糜性腹水很顽固，可致死。死因可能为营养不良、低蛋白血症、脱水或败血症。治疗包括低脂或中链三酰甘油、高蛋白饮食，反复穿刺、全胃肠外营养。经腹腔静脉分流的内引流偶尔有效，然而，常发生引流阻塞。如疑有可纠正的病变是剖腹探查的指征。这时，放射性淋巴管造影是有用的方法，可以显示腹腔漏出的大致位置。有的乳糜漏可能会在手术中发现并结扎；如伴有乳糜胸，术前食用黄油或奶油可证实。

少数病例，肠道短段的局限的淋巴系统梗阻也会导致腹泻、呕吐和蛋白丢失。病变段肠切除可治愈。可疑病变的肠道活检有助于确定切除的范围。

CT 和放射性核素淋巴管造影可用于鉴别大的、梗阻的腹部淋巴系统，导致乳糜反流入下肢。这些淋巴管偶尔可以被结扎，可以改善淋巴水肿，纠正向阴囊的乳糜漏管。

先天性乳糜胸

先天性乳糜胸表现为乳糜向一侧或双侧胸腔渗出。原因可能是乳糜产生过度、淋巴管连接失败、淋巴结重吸收过少、肺淋巴系统异常或新生儿难产时损伤。婴儿可能合并纵隔移位、肺发育不良、充血性心力衰竭或积水。另外，还包括 21 三体综合征、先天性肺淋巴管扩张、食管闭锁、肺叶外型肺隔离症、羊
水过多。 2141

产前或出生时表现为胸膜渗出可能为乳糜胸。液体为浆液性，液体细胞计数淋巴细胞超过 60% 可诊断为乳糜胸[4,59]。如果患儿进食脂肪食物或牛奶，乳糜为牛奶样；显微镜检查显示乳糜微粒染色为脂肪。乳糜包括磷脂类型的脂肪、胆固醇、长链三酰甘油。蛋白质平均含量为 40 g/L，电解质和葡萄糖水平接近血浆水平。约一半患者在生后第 1 周出现症状。

治疗包括反复胸腔穿刺和引流以扩张肺。开始时患儿接受含中链三酰甘油的要素饮食口服喂养。如果液体集聚太快，可采用全胃肠外营养。非手术治疗持续多长时间的意见不统一；然而，如果引流持续 3～4 周，需要手术结扎胸导管[2]。术前进食黄油和奶油可帮助鉴别漏出部位。在大部分病例漏出点以上或以下结扎都是有效的。

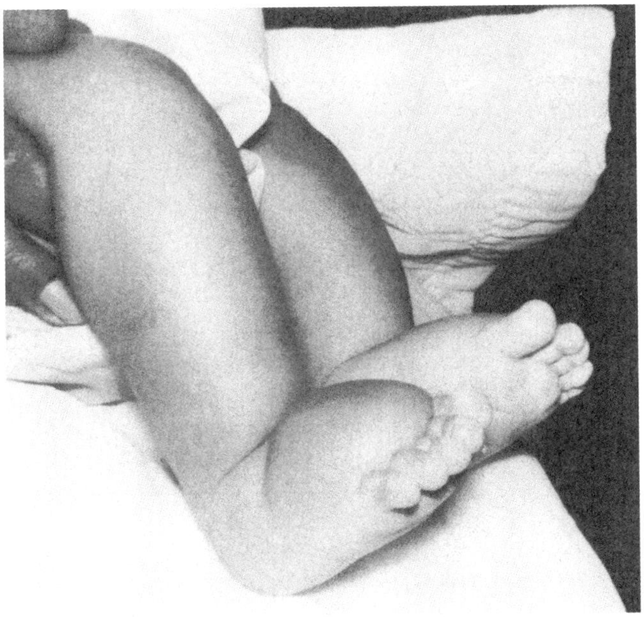

图 133-5　该 2 月大的婴儿，先天性淋巴水肿累及双侧下肢（腓骨和足背）。

淋巴水肿

淋巴水肿的确切病因不明，但一般在术语上是指由先天性淋巴系统发育异常或继发性淋巴管梗阻引起的组织间隙淋巴液异常积聚[48]。幼儿淋巴水肿的最常见病因是下肢原发性先天性淋巴系统畸形[26]。下肢淋巴水肿其他病因包括慢性感染（淋巴管炎）、丝虫病、昆虫叮咬、肿瘤、腹股沟或腋下的手术或辐射以及外伤[7]。单侧的下肢水肿可能是（少见）腹膜后的肿瘤或淋巴瘤压迫髂血管引起。双侧下肢水肿应该注意排除其他病因，例如低白蛋白血症、肾病综合征，以及腔静脉内肾母细胞瘤引起的两侧静脉梗阻。儿童上肢的淋巴水肿少见[12]。

根据发病年龄，原发性淋巴水肿可分为三类：(1) 先天性淋巴水肿，出生即有（图 133-5）；(2) 早发的淋巴水肿，在青春期早期出现，可能由于激素因素影响所致；(3) 迟发的淋巴水肿，在中年自发产生（大于 30 岁）[7,16,26]。Milroy 先天性家族性淋巴水肿占所有淋巴水肿的比例不到 2%，为常染色体单基因遗传。与常见于女孩（65%）的原发性淋巴水肿不同[32,48]，Milroy 病男女孩发病相等。受累家系在染色体 5q35.3 位置有单核苷酸替换。血管内皮生长因子受体 3（VEGFR3）基因图是关注的焦点[23]，因为只有淋巴管内皮表达 VEGFR3，且进一步的研究证明基因与家族性淋巴水肿有关。淋巴水肿也可伴有 Turner 综合征和 Noonan 综合征。下肢水肿也可在肠道淋巴管扩张和脑血管畸形的儿童中见到。

大多淋巴水肿的发病机制是下肢皮下淋巴管道的缺失、不发育或发育不良[25,41]。发育不良时，淋巴结和管道较小，且数量少。激素可能影响青春期女孩的早发的淋巴水肿的发展[7,25]。“黄甲”综合征是由甲床淋巴引流异常引起，导致趾甲脱色和营养不良改变。这些淋巴水肿综合征的儿童可伴有肺部疾病，包括慢性支气管炎和支气管扩张。

临床通常能确诊淋巴水肿[7,48]。多普勒超声及体积描记法可排除动静脉疾病[33]。放射性核素显像应用 Tc99m 硫黄胶体皮下注射 3 小时后可显示淋巴管道和梗阻部位[55]。90% 浅表淋巴系统发育不良的儿童病变侵犯远端而不是近端。MRI 也可以鉴别淋巴管瘤和淋巴水肿。淋巴管造影可提供有益的信息但偶尔可能导致淋巴管炎。淋巴水肿并发症包括持续性肿胀、肌性水肿伴有皮肤增厚、脱色、蜂窝织炎、淋巴管炎。反复发作的淋巴管炎需要长期预防性地应用抗革兰阳性菌的抗生素。

有许多研究者[41]，但不是全部[51]，认为淋巴系 2141
统分为浅表无瓣膜系统和深部有瓣膜系统。在淋巴水肿的病例，液体来自皮下组织的浅表系统池，液体产生超过引流能力[6]。富含蛋白的液体增加了血液渗透压，使水肿持续存在。如果肢体表面的皮肤长期受到牵拉，弹性纤维会失去张力。没有外来支撑，这些纤维不再能限制小的水肿回复正常。深部淋巴系统在筋膜以下，在肌肉内的部分是独立的，相互不影响[48]。普遍的观察发现在所有淋巴水肿病例中肌肉及其淋巴系统是有活性的，在可能的设计步骤中，尽量将淋巴输送到深部有瓣膜的系统，使液体能向上移动。

下肢淋巴水肿最初的保守治疗包括足部护理和卫生。慎重应用抗生素治疗和预防蜂窝织炎和局部应用抗真菌剂对治疗淋巴水肿是重要的[57,58]。控制体重被认为是有益的；然而，利尿剂作用不大。其他药物（例如泛酸、透明质酸酶）是实验性的未获得广泛使用[48]。华法林（香豆素）对治疗淋巴水肿可能有效，大约使水肿体积平均减轻 50%。华法林对淋巴水肿的治疗作用可能在于刺激皮肤巨噬细胞，促进局部蛋白水解和蛋白吸收。有些学者认为增加饮食中黄酮类摄入、限制长链三酰甘油，对保护血管内皮细胞、改善微循环有效[41]。

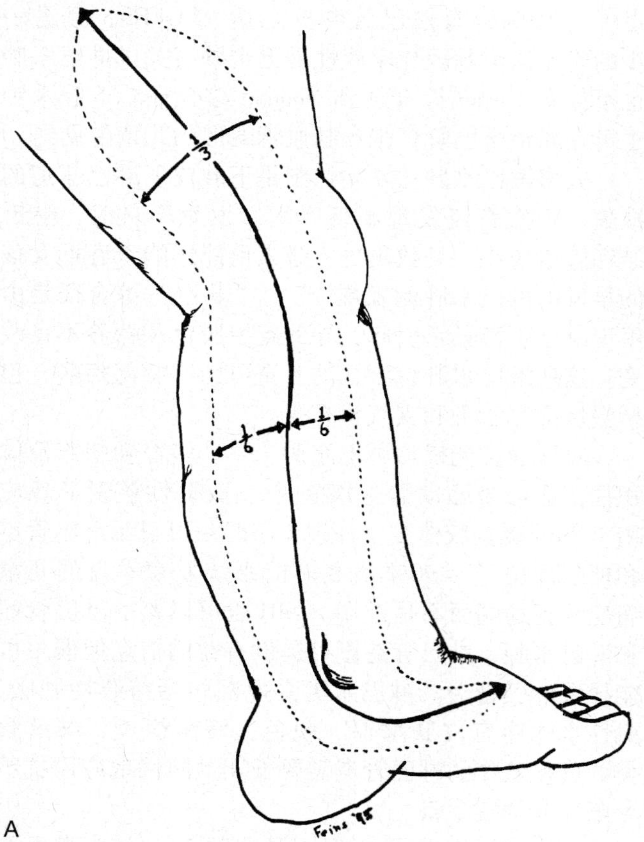

A

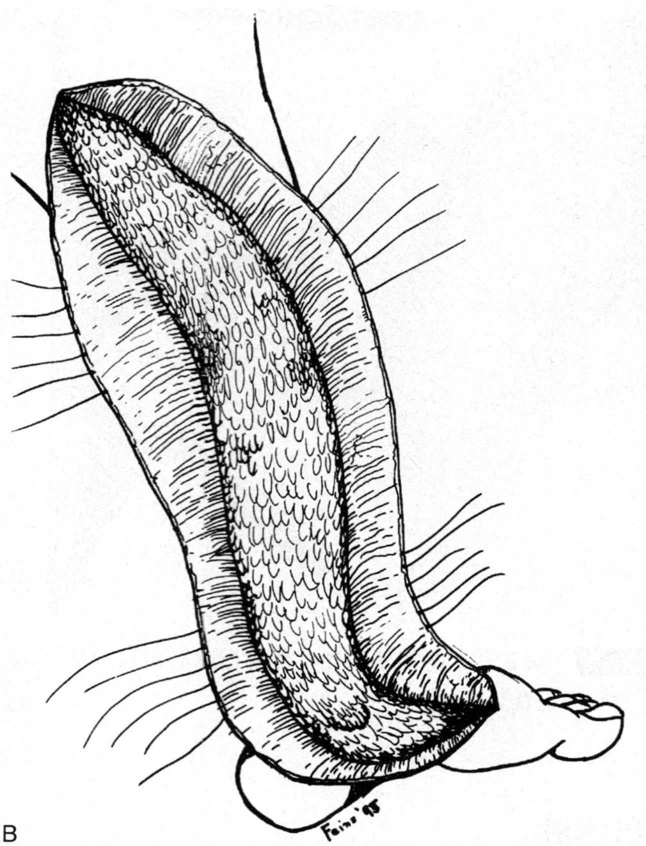

B

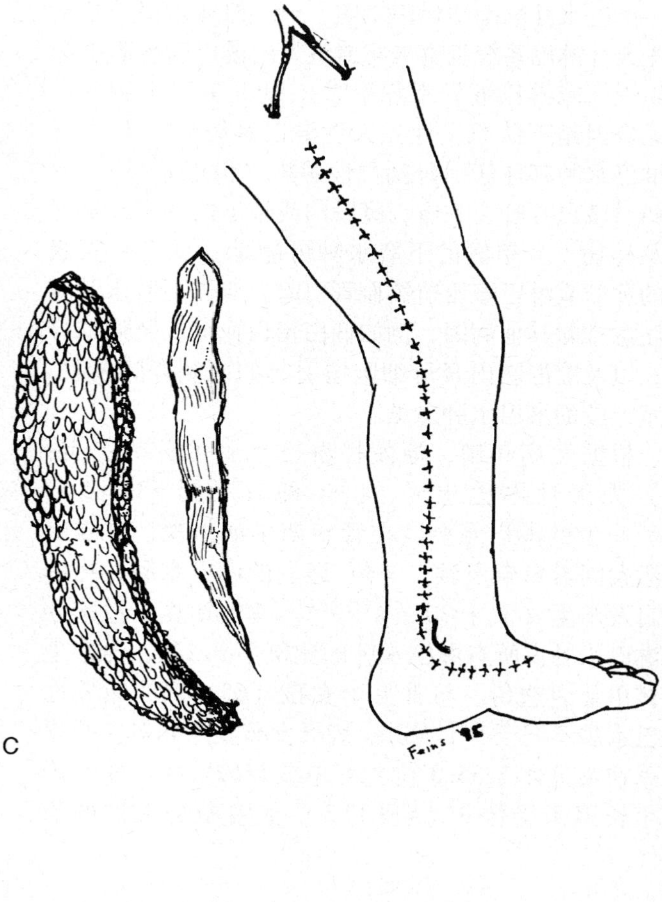

C

图 133-6　A. 对下肢早发或晚发的淋巴水肿，切口选择在腿的内面。垂直箭头显示切口的长度。水平箭头显示皮瓣的宽度。每一皮瓣占腿周径的 1/4 或 1/6，总暴露面积占肢体的 1/2～1/3。B. 皮瓣是薄层或全厚皮瓣。张力线置于表皮下层用以牵引，避免额外的皮肤操作。完全切除暴露的皮下组织和下层筋膜。C. 单片切除了皮下组织。单独切除了深筋膜。切口用 U 形钉关闭，皮瓣下置入 2 个大的 Hemovac 引流管。

长时间无压力站立可加剧淋巴液积聚；而行走或跑步可能会减缓这一过程。日间使用加压弹力袜，以及夜间抬高下肢可减轻肿胀，并减轻由于难看的腿部水肿引起的负性心理影响。在成长中的儿童支持袜应该每 4～6 个月更换一次。枕垫对夜间抬高下肢不适合，床脚垫高 10～12 英寸更有效。肺次序泵系统能减少淋巴水肿的程度以及在小儿站立和行走时液体再积聚。这种泵在夜间间歇性由脚趾到腹股沟压迫下肢。大约 85% 的淋巴水肿病例能用非手术方法成功治疗。远端肢体淋巴系统发育不良，但有正常盆腔和髂部淋巴管的病例很少出现严重问题。有近端梗阻性发育不良的病例，会产生更严重的淋巴水肿（15%），常要求手术干预。

儿童和年轻成人淋巴水肿的手术治疗是一个挑战，因为这种情况不常见，且有丰富经验的医生很少[26,51,57]。近来，没有形成一个治愈淋巴水肿的外科治疗方法。外科治疗指征为保守治疗失败，由于下肢体积和重量增加限制了日常活动。反复发作的蜂窝织炎和淋巴管炎，常导致疼痛，也是手术指征。大多数原发性淋巴水肿病例是女性，在青春期时外观和心理上的考虑也很重要。淋巴血管肉瘤少见，但长期直立性淋巴水肿常常是致命的并发症[20]。

尝试手术矫治淋巴水肿可追溯到 1841 年[53]，包括生理的和切除的方法。生理性手术基于重新连接[15,57]、重建[3,9]，或刺激淋巴系统途径生长的目标。这些方法包括应用大网膜桥或无功能带蒂的小肠，去除黏膜，置于受累肢体，作为潜在的淋巴引流来源[15,54]。这些方法对原发性淋巴水肿很少成功，除非在手术时切除大量的皮下组织，或除非病变是由于局部梗阻引起的继发性淋巴水肿。也尝试过运用显微外科技术吻合淋巴管静脉，但能否保持长期的通畅和这一技术的有效性目前尚不得而知，例如在乳腺切除术后的淋巴水肿[9]。

2142 因为淋巴在皮下组织产生和聚集，目前的治疗方法是切除这些肿胀组织，前提是筋膜下的淋巴管正常。1912 年，Charles[5] 报道成功切除水肿的皮肤和皮下组织直到肌层，再用其他部位移植的分层厚皮瓣覆盖裸露的表面。Charles 方法有缺点，包括术后外观较差、移植物脱失、慢性感染、外植角化、持续淋巴液渗出和皮肤感觉缺失，现在已很少应用。1936 年，Homans[22] 改良了这一手术方法，切除皮下组织到深筋膜，用薄层转移皮瓣来覆盖切除区域。最近，脂肪吸引去除皮下组织再加压包扎偶有应用，并取得了一些成功。

分期皮下淋巴管切除术，加充气止血带来减少失血，能明显减少早发和迟发淋巴水肿患儿肢体的肿胀，也可用于先天性淋巴水肿的病例[13,52]。术前行放射性核素淋巴管造影来证实筋膜下的淋巴管正常[16,55]。切除手术常分期进行，首先切除腿中间从踝到膝上的部分，至少 9 个月后侧面的部分再进行第二次手术[31,58]。薄层皮瓣与肌肉筋膜之下的皮下组织全部切除，剥离切除切口边缘的皮肤（图133-6）。如果可能，要识别腓总神经并避免损伤。彻底止血，伤口负压引流持续 1 周。镫形皮肤保留 2 周因为皮瓣
关闭愈合较慢。因为手术中切除了隐静脉系统，深部 2144
静脉系统功能必须良好，由术前静脉造影来确定。蓬松的有轻微压力的引流条应用 1 周左右。术后应用几周弹力支持裤，继而应用弹力袜数月。伤口引流可能每天约 100 ml；而在术后 7 天，引流量常小于 10 ml。每日应用皮肤保湿霜有助于减轻患肢的干燥。尽管分期淋巴管切除术不能完全治愈而且常有局部的复发，但多数作者认为这是目前最可靠而有效的手术方法[30,49]（图 133-7）。大约 80% 分期淋巴管切除术的患儿可获得长期满意的效果，虽然不确定支持袜能否对复发的肿胀起到最佳的控制。

组织结构继续改善常需 1 年多，同一部位的二次手术最好在这一间期后进行[31,58]。罕见的巨大肢体的患儿需要行三期手术。对淋巴水肿累及大腿的患儿，这一部位的手术要推迟到小腿手术完成以后进行。处理双侧病变时，一次尽量处理一侧肢体。如果第一次没有明显的并发症，对侧肢体的手术可以在几周后进行[11]。

尽管手术技巧类似，但上肢的原发性先天性淋巴水肿外科处理较下肢更加复杂，因为每一个手指及手的背侧和前臂常需要多次分期手术[12]。另外，术后患儿穿戴压力手套和弹力绷带很麻烦。某些上肢原发性淋巴水肿的患儿伴有会阴部淋巴水肿，但也可能会产生单独的会阴肿胀。阴唇下淋巴管切除术对大部分女性患儿是有效的。对阴茎和阴囊淋巴水肿，可通过在阴茎根部以下的阴囊横切口切除所有的皮下组织[8,10]。切除延伸到阴茎的 Buck 筋膜和睾丸被膜，注意避免损伤精索。切除多余的阴茎和阴囊皮肤。引流伤口，支持敷料，应用 Foley 导尿管 4～7 天，应用抗生素 7～10 天。

（洪 莉译 夏慧敏校）

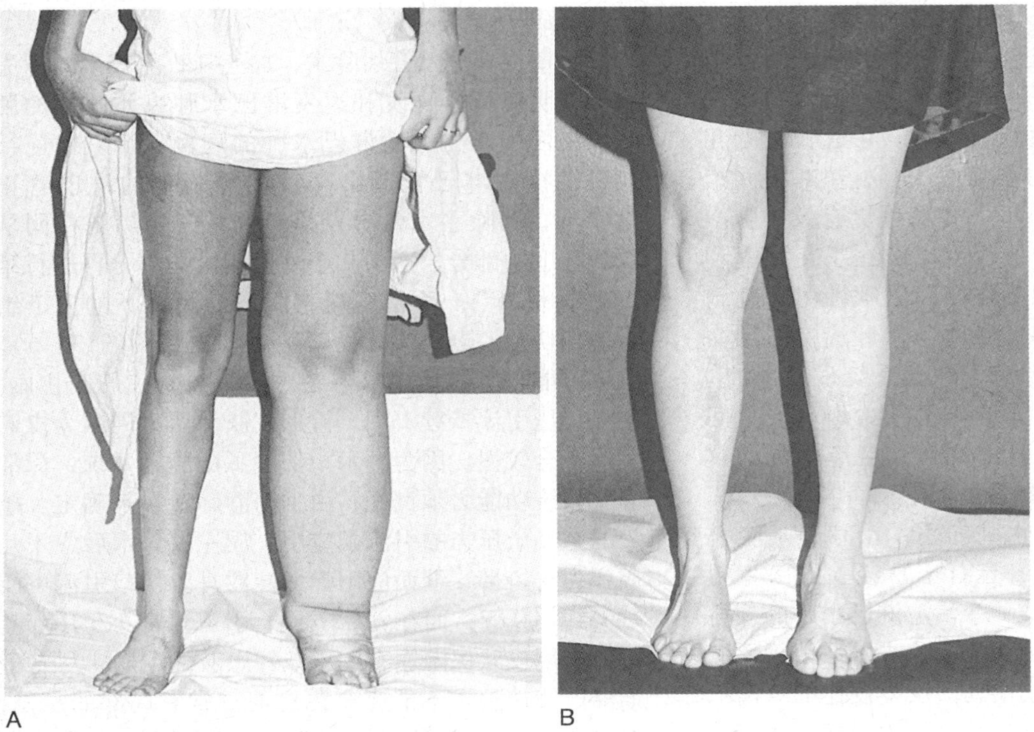

图 133-7 A. 该14岁女孩，左下肢早发性淋巴水肿。B. 同一个患者17岁时3次切除术后6个月。

参考文献

1. Alguahtani A, Nguyen LT, Flageole H, et al: Twenty-five years experience with lymphangiomas in children. J Pediatr Surg 1999;34:1164.
2. Anderson EA, Hertel J, Pedersen SA, Sorensen HR: Congenital chylothorax: Management by ligature of the thoracic duct. Scand J Thorac Cardiovasc Surg 1984;18:193.
3. Baumeister RG, Seifert J, Wiebecke B: Homologous and autologous experimental lymph vessel transplantation initial experience. Int J Microsurg 1981;3:19.
4. Benacerraf BR, Frigoletto FD: Mid-trimester fetal thoracentesis. J Clin Ultrasound 1985;13:202.
5. Charles RH: Lymphedema. In Latham A, English TC (eds): A System of Treatment, vol 3. London, Churchill, 1912.
6. Crockett DJ: Lymphatic anatomy and lymphedema. Br J Plast Surg 1965;28:12.
7. Dale WA: The swollen leg. Curr Probl Surg 1973;Sep:1.
8. Dandapat MC, Mohapatro SN, Sushanta KP: Elephantiasis of the penis and scrotum: A review of 350 cases. Am J Surg 1985;149:686.
9. Degni M: New techniques of lymphatic venous anastomosis for the treatment of lymphedema. J Cardiovasc Surg 1978; 19:577.
10. Feins NR: A new surgical technique for lymphedema of the penis and scrotum. J Pediatr Surg 1980;15:787.
11. Feins NR: Lymphatic disorders. In O'Neill JA Jr, Rowe MI, Grosfeld JL, et al (eds): Pediatric Surgery, 5th ed. St Louis, Mosby, 1998.
12. Fonkalsrud EW: A syndrome of congenital lymphedema of the upper extremity and associated systemic lymphatic malformations. Surg Gynecol Obstet 1977;145:228.
13. Fonkalsrud EW: Disorders of the lymphatic system. In Ravitch MM, Randolph JG, Welch K, et al (eds): Pediatric Surgery, 4th ed. Chicago, Mosby–Year Book, 1986.
14. Fujino A, Moriya Y, Morikawa Y, et al: A role of cytokines in OK-432 injection therapy for cystic lymphangioma: An approach to the mechanism. J Pediatr Surg 2003; 38:1806.
15. Goldsmith HS, Los Santos R, Beattie EJ Jr: Relief of chronic lymphedema by omental transposition. Ann Surg 1967; 166:572.
16. Gough MH: Primary lymphedema clinical and lymphangiographic studies. Br J Surg 1966;53:917.
17. Greinwald JH Jr, Burke DK, Sato Y, et al: Treatment of lymphangiomas in children: An update of Picibanil (OK-432) sclerotherapy. Otolaryngol Head Neck Surg 1999; 121:381.
18. Hancock BJ, St-Vil D, Luks FI, et al: Complications of lymphangiomas in children. J Pediatr Surg 1992;27:220.
19. Henzel JH, Pories WJ, Burget DE, et al: Intra-abdominal lymphangiomata. Arch Surg 1966;93:304.
20. Hermann JB, Gruhm JG: Lymphangiosarcoma of the chronically edematous extremity. Surg Gynecol Obstet 1957; 105:665.
21. Hilliard RI, McKendry JBS, Phillips MJ: Congenital abnormalities of the lymphatic system: A new clinical classification. Pediatrics 1990;86:988.
22. Homans J: The treatment of elephantiasis of the legs: Preliminary report. N Engl J Med 1936;215:1099.
23. Irrthum A, Karkkainen MJ, Devriendt K, et al: Congenital hereditary lymphedema caused by a mutation that inactivates VEGFR3 tyrosine kinase. Am J Hum Genet 2000;67:295.
24. Kelly ML Jr, Batt HR: Chylous ascites: An analysis of its etiology. Gastroenterology 1960;39:161.
25. Kinmonth JB, Taylor GW, Jantet GH: Chylous complica-

tions of primary lymphedema. J Cardiovasc Surg (Torino) 1964;5:327.
26. Kinmonth JB, Taylor GW, Tracy GD, Marsh JD: Primary lymphedema, clinical and lymphangiographic studies of a series of 107 patients in which the lower limbs were affected. Br J Surg 1957;45:1.
27. Levine C: Primary disorders of the lymphatic vessels: A unified concept. J Pediatr Surg 1989;24:233.
28. Malek P, Belan A, Kocandrle VL: The superficial and deep lymphatic system of the lower extremities and their mutual relationship under physiological and pathologic conditions. J Cardiovasc Surg 1964;5:686.
29. McClure CFW, Silvester CF: A comparative study of the lymphaticovenous communications in adult mammals. Nat Rec 1909;3:534.
30. Miller TA: A surgical approach to lymphedema. Am J Surg 1977;134:191.
31. Miller TA, Harper J, Longmire WP Jr: The management of lymphedema by staged subcutaneous excision. Surg Gynecol Obstet 1973;136:586.
32. Milroy WF: An undescribed variety of hereditary oedema. N Y Med J 1892;56:505.
33. Mulliken JB, Fishman SJ, Burrows PE: Vascular anomalies. Curr Probl Surg 2000;37:517.
34. Ogita K, Suita S, Taguchi T, et al: Outcome of fetal cystic hygromas and experience of intrauterine treatment. Fetal Diagn Ther 2001;16:105.
35. Ogita S, Tsuto T, Wakamura K, et al: OK-432 therapy in 64 patients with lymphangioma. J Pediatr Surg 1994; 29:784.
36. Okada A, Kubota, Fukuzawa M, et al: Injection of bleomycin as primary therapy of cystic hygromas. J Pediatr Surg 1992; 27:440.
37. Padwa BL, Hayward PG, Ferraro NF, et al: Cervicofacial lymphatic malformations: Clinical course, surgical intervention, and pathogenesis of skeletal hypertrophy. Plast Recontr Surg 1995;95:951.
38. Patterson RM, Ballard CL, Wasserman K, Mayerson HS: Lymphatic permeability to albumin. Am J Physiol 1958; 194:120.
39. Pomerantz M, Waldman TA: Systemic lymphatic abnormalities associated with gastrointestinal protein loss secondary to intestinal lymphangiectasia. Gastroenterology 1963; 45:703.
40. Puckett CL: Microlymphatic surgery for lymphedema. Clin Plast Surg 1983;10:133.
41. Rockson SG: Lymphedema [review]. Am J Med 2001;110:288.
42. Roisman S, Manny J, Shiloni E: Intra-abdominal lymphangioma. Br J Surg 1989;76:485.
43. Sabin FR: On the origin of the lymphatic system from the veins and the development of the lymph heart and thoracic duct in the pig. Am J Anat 1901;1:367.
44. Sabin FR: On the development of the superficial lymphatics in the skin of the pig. Am J Anat 1904;3:183.
45. Sabin FR: The development of the lymphatic nodes in the pig and their relation to the lymph hearts. Am J Anat 1905; 4:355.
46. Sabin FR: The lymphatic system in human embryos with a consideration of the morphology of the system as a whole. Am J Anat 1909;9:43.
47. Sabin FR: The development of the lymphatic system. In Keibel G, Mall FP (eds): Manual of Human Embryology, vol 2. Philadelphia, JB Lippincott, 1912, p 709.
48. Savage RC: The surgical management of lymphedema. Surg Gynecol Obstet 1985;160:283.
49. Sawhney CP: Lymphedema of the extremities; a new approach to its management. Br J Plast Surg 1980;33:445.
50. Schnur PL: Surgical treatment of lymphedema: A reappraisal. Vasc Surg 1977;11:182.
51. Serville N: Surgical treatment of lymphedema: A report of 652 cases. Surgery 1987;101:485.
52. Sistrunk WE: Further experiences with Kondolean operation for elephantiasis. JAMA 1918;71:800.
53. Skandalakis JE: I wish I had been there: Highlights in the history of lymphatics. Am Surg 1995;61:799.
54. Smith JW, Conway H: Selection of appropriate surgical procedures in lymphedema; introduction of hinged pedicle. Plast Reconstr Surg 1962;30:10.
55. Stewart G, Gaunt JI, Croft DN, et al: Isotope lymphangiography: A new method of investigating the role of the lymphatics in chronic limb edema. Br J Surg 1985;72:906.
56. Tanigawa N, Shimomatsuya T, Takahashi K, et al: Treatment of cystic hygroma and lymphangioma with the use of bleomycin fat emulsion. Cancer 1987;60:741.
57. Thompson N: Surgical treatment of chronic lymphedema of the lower limb. BMJ 1962;5319:1567.
58. Thompson N: The surgical treatment of chronic lymphedema of the extremities. Surg Clin North Am 1967; 47:445.
59. Van Aerde J, Campbell AN, Smith JA: Spontaneous chylothorax in newborns. Am J Dis Child 1984;138:961.
60. Witte MH, Witte CL: Lymphangiogenesis and lymphologic syndromes. Lymphology 1986;19:21.

索 引

注：索引中的页码与正文页面中两侧的原版页码相对应。
页码后跟的字母 f 指图；页码后跟的字母 t 指表；页码后跟的字母 b 指加框的信息资料。

A

B

C

D

E

F

G

H

I

J

K

L

M

N

O

P

Q

R

S

T

U

V

W

X

Y

Z